AIIMS-MAMC-PGI's
Comprehensive Textbook of

Diagnostic Radiology

AIIMS-MAMC-PGI's Comprehensive Textbook of

Diagnostic Radiology

SECOND EDITION

VOLUME 1

- Neuroradiology including Head and Neck Imaging
- Recent Advances and Applied Physics in Imaging

Editors

Manavjit Singh Sandhu MD FICR
Professor and Head
Department of Radiodiagnosis
Postgraduate Institute of Medical Education and Research, Chandigarh, India

Anju Garg MD
Director Professor and Head
Department of Radiodiagnosis
Maulana Azad Medical College
New Delhi, India

Arun Kumar Gupta MD FAMS
Professor and Head
Department of Radiodiagnosis
All India Institute of Medical Sciences
New Delhi, India

JAYPEE

JAYPEE BROTHERS MEDICAL PUBLISHERS
The Health Sciences Publisher
New Delhi | London | Panama

Jaypee Brothers Medical Publishers (P) Ltd.

Headquarters
Jaypee Brothers Medical Publishers (P) Ltd.
4838/24, Ansari Road, Daryaganj
New Delhi 110 002, India
Phone: +91-11-43574357
Fax: +91-11-43574314
Email: jaypee@jaypeebrothers.com

Overseas Offices
JP Medical Ltd.
83, Victoria Street, London
SW1H 0HW (UK)
Phone: +44 20 3170 8910
Fax: +44 (0)20 3008 6180
E-mail: info@jpmedpub.com

Jaypee-Highlights Medical Publishers Inc.
City of Knowledge, Bld. 235, 2nd Floor, Clayton
Panama City, Panama
Phone: +1 507-301-0496
Fax: +1 507-301-0499
E-mail: cservice@jphmedical.com

Jaypee Brothers Medical Publishers (P) Ltd.
Bhotahity, Kathmandu, Nepal
Phone: +977-9741283608
E-mail: kathmandu@jaypeebrothers.com

Website: www.jaypeebrothers.com
Website: www.jaypeedigital.com

Inquiries for bulk sales may be solicited at: jaypee@jaypeebrothers.com

AIIMS-MAMC-PGI's Comprehensive Textbook of Diagnostic Radiology (Volumes 1 to 3)

First Edition: 2016
Second Edition: **2019**

ISBN: 978-93-5270-704-1

Printed at: Replika Press Pvt. Ltd.

Dedicated to

THE SUPREME BEING

Who so mercifully helps us to accomplish gigantic tasks

so smoothly, effortlessly and so beautifully

Associate Editors

VOLUME 1

SECTION 1: Neuroradiology including Head and Neck Imaging

Paramjeet Singh MD
Professor
Department of Radiodiagnosis
Postgraduate Institute of Medical Education and Research
Chandigarh, India

Vivek Gupta MD DM
Professor
Department of Radiodiagnosis
Postgraduate Institute of Medical Education and Research
Chandigarh, India

Shailesh B Gaikwad MD
Professor and Head
Department of Neuroimaging and Interventional Neuroradiology
(CN Centre)
All India Institute of Medical Sciences
New Delhi, India

Ajay Garg MD
Professor
Department of Neuroimaging and Interventional Neuroradiology
(CN Centre)
All India Institute of Medical Sciences
New Delhi, India

SECTION 2: Recent Advances and Applied Physics in Imaging

Sanjay Sharma MD DNB MNAMS FRCR FICR
Professor
Department of Radiodiagnosis
Dr Rajendra Prasad Centre for
Ophthalmic Sciences
All India Institute of Medical Sciences
New Delhi, India

Ashu Seith Bhalla MD MAMS FICR
Professor
Department of Radiodiagnosis
All India Institute of Medical Sciences
New Delhi, India

Smriti Hari MD MAMS
Professor
Department of Radiodiagnosis
All India Institute of Medical Sciences
New Delhi, India

VOLUME 2

SECTION 3: Gastrointestinal and Hepatobiliary Imaging

Deep Narayan Srivastava MD MBA FAMS FICR
Professor
Department of Radiodiagnosis
All India Institute of Medical Sciences
New Delhi, India

Raju Sharma MD MAMS FICR
Professor
Department of Radiodiagnosis
All India Institute of Medical Sciences
New Delhi, India

SECTION 4: Genitourinary Imaging

Anupam Lal MD
Professor
Department of Radiodiagnosis
Postgraduate Institute of Medical Education and Research
Chandigarh, India

SECTION 5: Pediatric Imaging

Ashu Seith Bhalla MD MAMS FICR
Professor
Department of Radiodiagnosis
All India Institute of Medical Sciences
New Delhi, India

Sanjay Thulkar MD
Professor
Department of Radiodiagnosis
Dr BRA Institute—Rotary Cancer Hospital
All India Institute of Medical Sciences
New Delhi, India

VOLUME 3

SECTION 6: Chest and Cardiovascular Imaging

Sanjiv Sharma MD
Professor and Head
Department of Cardiac Radiology
Cardio-Thoracic Sciences Centre
All India Institute of Medical Sciences
New Delhi, India

Rashmi Dixit MD
Director Professor
Department of Radiodiagnosis
Maulana Azad Medical College
New Delhi, India

SECTION 7: Musculoskeletal and Breast Imaging

Anjali Prakash DMRD DNB MNAMS
Director Professor
Department of Radiodiagnosis
Maulana Azad Medical College
New Delhi, India

Contributors

Ajay Garg MD
Professor
Department of Neuroimaging and Interventional Neuroradiology (CN Centre)
All India Institute of Medical Sciences
New Delhi, India

Ajay Gulati MD MAMS
Additional Professor
Department of Radiodiagnosis
Postgraduate Institute of Medical Education and Research, Chandigarh, India

Ajay Kumar MD
Professor
Department of Radiodiagnosis and Imaging
Postgraduate Institute of Medical Education and Research, Chandigarh, India

Akshay Kumar Saxena MD Dip NBE
Professor
Department of Radiodiagnosis
Postgraduate Institute of Medical Education and Research, Chandigarh, India

Alpana Manchanda MD
Director Professor
Department of Radiodiagnosis
Maulana Azad Medical College
New Delhi, India

Amar Mukund MD
Associate Professor
Department of Radiodiagnosis
Institute of Liver and Biliary Sciences (ILBS)
New Delhi, India

Anil Chauhan
MBBS Board Certified in Radiology, USA
Fellow, Body Imaging
Department of Radiology
University of Texas MD Anderson Cancer Center, Houston, USA

Anil K Pandey PhD
Assistant Professor (Medical Physics)
Department of Nuclear Medicine
All India Institute of Medical Sciences
New Delhi, India

Anindita Sinha MD
Additional Professor
Department of Radiodiagnosis
Postgraduate Institute of Medical Education and Research, Chandigarh, India

Anish Bhattacharya DNB DRM MNAMS
Professor
Department of Nuclear Medicine
Postgraduate Institute of Medical Education and Research, Chandigarh, India

Anjali Prakash DMRD DNB MNAMS
Director Professor
Department of Radiodiagnosis
Maulana Azad Medical College
New Delhi, India

Anju Garg MD
Director Professor and Head
Department of Radiodiagnosis
Maulana Azad Medical College
New Delhi, India

Ankur Gadodia MD DNB FRCR
Consultant
Goyal MRI and Diagnostic Centre
New Delhi, India

Ankur Goyal MD DNB MNAMS
Assistant Professor
Department of Radiodiagnosis
All India Institute of Medical Sciences
New Delhi, India

Anmol Bhatia MD
Assistant Professor
Department of Radiodiagnosis and Imaging
Postgraduate Institute of Medical Education and Research, Chandigarh, India

Anuj Prabhakar DNB DM
Assistant Professor
Department of Neuroimaging and Interventional Neuroradiology (CN Centre)
All India Institute of Medical Sciences
New Delhi, India

Anupam Lal MD
Professor
Department of Radiodiagnosis
Postgraduate Institute of Medical Education and Research, Chandigarh, India

Arun Deep Arora MD
Former Senior Research Associate
Department of Radiodiagnosis
All India Institute of Medical Sciences
New Delhi, India

Arun Kumar Gupta MD FAMS
Professor and Head
Department of Radiodiagnosis
All India Institute of Medical Sciences
New Delhi, India

Arun Malhotra DRM PhD
Former Professor and Head
Department of Nuclear Medicine
All India Institute of Medical Sciences
New Delhi, India

Ashu Seith Bhalla MD MAMS FICR
Professor
Department of Radiodiagnosis
All India Institute of Medical Sciences
New Delhi, India

Atin Kumar MD DNB MNAMS
Professor
Department of Radiodiagnosis
Jai Prakash Narayan Apex Trauma Center
All India Institute of Medical Sciences
New Delhi, India

BR Mittal MD DRM DNB FICNM FAMS
Professor and Head
Department of Nuclear Medicine
Postgraduate Institute of Medical Education and Research, Chandigarh, India

Chandan Jyoti Das MD DNB MNAMS
Associate Professor
Department of Radiodiagnosis
All India Institute of Medical Sciences
New Delhi, India

Chandrashekhara SH MD DNB MNAMS
Associate Professor
Department of Radiodiagnosis
Dr BRA Institute—Rotary Cancer Hospital
All India Institute of Medical Sciences
New Delhi, India

Chirag Kamal Ahuja MD DM
Assistant Professor
Department of Radiodiagnosis and Imaging
Postgraduate Institute of Medical Education
and Research, Chandigarh, India

Deep Narayan Srivastava MD MBA FAMS FICR
Professor
Department of Radiodiagnosis
All India Institute of Medical Sciences
New Delhi, India

Devasenathipathy Kandasamy MD DNB FRCR
Associate Professor
Department of Radiodiagnosis
All India Institute of Medical Sciences
New Delhi, India

Ekta Dhamija MD
Assistant Professor
Department of Radiodiagnosis
Dr BRA Institute—Rotary Cancer Hospital
All India Institute of Medical Sciences
New Delhi, India

Gaurav S Pradhan MBBS DMRD DNB
Director Professor
Department of Radiodiagnosis
Maulana Azad Medical College
New Delhi, India

Gurpreet Singh Gulati MD
Professor
Department of Cardiac Radiology
Cardio-Thoracic Sciences Centre
All India Institute of Medical Sciences
New Delhi, India

Hina Arif Mumtaz MD DNB
Former Senior Research Associate
Department of Radiodiagnosis
Postgraduate Institute of Medical Education
and Research, Chandigarh, India

Jyoti Kumar MD DNB MNAMS
Professor
Department of Radiodiagnosis
Maulana Azad Medical College
New Delhi, India

Kartik Ganga MD
Fellow
Department of Cardiovascular Radiology
and Endovascular Interventions
All India Institute of Medical Sciences
New Delhi, India

Kirti Gupta
MD Neuropathology Fellowship (St Jude, USA)
Professor
Department of Histopathology
Postgraduate Institute of Medical Education
and Research, Chandigarh, India

Kumble S Madhusudhan MD FRCR MAMS
Associate Professor
Department of Radiodiagnosis
All India Institute of Medical Sciences
New Delhi, India

Kushaljit Singh Sodhi MD MNAMS FICR
Professor
Department of Radiodiagnosis
Postgraduate Institute of Medical Education
and Research, Chandigarh, India

Kusum Joshi MD PhD
Professor and Former Head
Department of Histopathology
Postgraduate Institute of Medical Education
and Research, Chandigarh, India

Mahesh Prakash MD MAMS FICR
Professor
Department of Radiodiagnosis
Postgraduate Institute of Medical Education
and Research, Chandigarh, India

Manavjit Singh Sandhu MD FICR
Professor and Head
Department of Radiodiagnosis
Postgraduate Institute of Medical Education
and Research, Chandigarh, India

Mandeep Garg MD FRCR
Professor
Department of Radiodiagnosis
Postgraduate Institute of Medical Education
and Research, Chandigarh, India

Mandeep Kang MD DNB MAMS FICR
Professor
Department of Radiodiagnosis
Postgraduate Institute of Medical Education
and Research, Chandigarh, India

Manisha Jana MD DNB FRCR
Associate Professor
Department of Radiodiagnosis
All India Institute of Medical Sciences
New Delhi, India

Manish Modi MD DM
Professor
Department of Neurology
Postgraduate Institute of Medical Education
and Research, Chandigarh, India

Manphool Singhal MD DNB MNAMS
Additional Professor
Department of Radiodiagnosis
Postgraduate Institute of Medical Education
and Research, Chandigarh, India

Mukesh Kumar Yadav MD
Assistant Professor
Department of Radiodiagnosis
Dr BRA Institute—Rotary Cancer Hospital
All India Institute of Medical Sciences
New Delhi, India

Naveen Kalra MD MAMS FICR
Professor
Department of Radiodiagnosis
Postgraduate Institute of Medical Education
and Research, Chandigarh, India

Nidhi Prabhakar MD DNB
Assistant Professor
Department of Radiodiagnosis
Postgraduate Institute of Medical Education
and Research, Chandigarh, India

Niranjan Khandelwal MD Dip NBE FICR FAMS
Former Head
Department of Radiodiagnosis
Postgraduate Institute of Medical Education
and Research, Chandigarh, India

Pankaj Gupta MD DNB
Assistant Professor
Department of Radiodiagnosis and Imaging
Postgraduate Institute of Medical Education
and Research, Chandigarh, India

Paramjeet Singh MD
Professor
Department of Radiodiagnosis
Postgraduate Institute of Medical Education
and Research, Chandigarh, India

Pratik Kumar PhD Dip RP
Professor
Medical Physics Unit
Dr BRA Institute—Rotary Cancer Hospital
All India Institute of Medical Sciences
New Delhi, India

Priya Jagia MD DNB
Professor
Department of Cardiovascular Radiology and Endovascular Interventions
All India Institute of Medical Sciences
New Delhi, India

Priyanka Naranje MD DNB MNAMS
Assistant Professor
Department of Radiodiagnosis
All India Institute of Medical Sciences
New Delhi, India

Punit Sharma MD
Former Senior Resident
Department of Nuclear Medicine
All India Institute of Medical Sciences
New Delhi, India

Radhika Batra MD DNB
Assistant Professor
Department of Radiodiagnosis
Maulana Azad Medical College
New Delhi, India

Radhika Srinivasan MD PhD
Professor
Department of Cytology and Gynec-pathology
Postgraduate Institute of Medical Education and Research, Chandigarh, India

Rajat Jain MD
Former Senior Resident
Department of Radiodiagnosis
Maulana Azad Medical College
New Delhi, India

Raju Sharma MD MAMS FICR
Professor
Department of Radiodiagnosis
All India Institute of Medical Sciences
New Delhi, India

Rakesh Kumar MD PhD
Professor
Department of Nuclear Medicine
All India Institute of Medical Sciences
New Delhi, India

Rakesh Kumar Vasishta MD FRCPath
Professor and Head
Department of Histopathology
Postgraduate Institute of Medical Education and Research, Chandigarh, India

Rama Mohan Reddy MD (Nuclear Medicine)
Former Senior Resident
Department of Nuclear Medicine
All India Institute of Medical Sciences
New Delhi, India

Rashmi Dixit MD
Director Professor
Department of Radiodiagnosis
Maulana Azad Medical College
New Delhi, India

Sameer Vyas MD DM MAMS
Additional Professor
Department of Radiodiagnosis and Imaging
Postgraduate Institute of Medical Education and Research, Chandigarh, India

Sanjay Sharma MD DNB MNAMS FRCR FICR
Professor
Department of Radiodiagnosis
Dr Rajendra Prasad Centre for Ophthalmic Sciences
All India Institute of Medical Sciences
New Delhi, India

Sanjay Thulkar MD
Professor
Department of Radiodiagnosis
Dr BRA Institute—Rotary Cancer Hospital
All India Institute of Medical Sciences
New Delhi, India

Sanjeev Kumar MD
Assistant Professor
Department of Cardiovascular Radiology and Endovascular Interventions
All India Institute of Medical Sciences
New Delhi, India

Sanjiv Sharma MD
Professor and Head
Department of Cardiac Radiology
Cardio-Thoracic Sciences Centre
All India Institute of Medical Sciences
New Delhi, India

Sapna Singh MD DNB MNAMS
Professor
Department of Radiodiagnosis
Maulana Azad Medical College
New Delhi, India

Satyam DNB MNAMS
Specialist
Department of Radiodiagnosis
Lok Nayak Hospital
New Delhi, India

SC Bansal MA MSc PhD
Former Lecturer
Department of Radiodiagnosis
Postgraduate Institute of Medical Education and Research, Chandigarh, India

Shailesh B Gaikwad MD
Professor and Head
Department of Neuroimaging and Interventional Neuroradiology (CN Centre)
All India Institute of Medical Sciences
New Delhi, India

Shamim Ahmed Shamim MD (Nuclear Medicine)
Assistant Professor
Department of Nuclear Medicine
All India Institute of Medical Sciences
New Delhi, India

Shashi Bala Paul PhD MAMS
Senior Scientist
Department of Radiodiagnosis
All India Institute of Medical Sciences
New Delhi, India

Shivanand Gamanagatti MD MAMS
Professor
Department of Radiodiagnosis
(Trauma Center Division)
All India Institute of Medical Sciences
New Delhi, India

Smita Manchanda MD DNB MNAMS
Assistant Professor
Department of Radiodiagnosis
All India Institute of Medical Sciences
New Delhi, India

Smriti Hari MD MAMS
Professor
Department of Radiodiagnosis
All India Institute of Medical Sciences
New Delhi, India

Subrat Kumar Acharya
DM FNASc FASc FNA JC Bose Fellow
Former Professor and Head
Department of Gastroenterology
All India Institute of Medical Sciences
New Delhi, India

Sudesh Prabhakar MD DM
Former Professor and Head
Department of Neurology
Postgraduate Institute of Medical Education and Research, Chandigarh, India

Sudha Suri MD
Former Emeritus Professor
Department of Radiodiagnosis
Postgraduate Institute of Medical Education and Research, Chandigarh, India

(Late) Sumedha Pawa MBBS MD
Director Professor
Department of Radiodiagnosis
Maulana Azad Medical College
New Delhi, India

Surabhi Vyas MD DNB MNAMS
Associate Professor
Department of Radiodiagnosis
All India Institute of Medical Sciences
New Delhi, India

Swati Gupta MD DNB FRCR
Assistant Professor
Department of Radiodiagnosis
Maulana Azad Medical College
New Delhi, India

Tulika Singh MD
Additional Professor
Department of Radiodiagnosis
Postgraduate Institute of Medical Education and Research, Chandigarh, India

Ujjwal Gorsi MD
Assistant Professor
Department of Radiodiagnosis
Postgraduate Institute of Medical Education and Research, Chandigarh, India

Uma Debi MD
Assistant Professor
Department of Radiodiagnosis
Postgraduate Institute of Medical Education and Research, Chandigarh, India

Veena Chowdhury MBBS MD
Former Professor of Excellence
Department of Radiodiagnosis
Maulana Azad Medical College
New Delhi, India

Veenu Singla MD
Professor
Department of Radiodiagnosis
Postgraduate Institute of Medical Education and Research, Chandigarh, India

Vikas Bhatia MD DM
Assistant Professor
Department of Radiodiagnosis
Postgraduate Institute of Medical Education and Research, Chandigarh, India

Virendra Jain MD FRCR
Former Senior Resident
Department of Radiodiagnosis
Maulana Azad Medical College
New Delhi, India

Vivek Gupta MD DM
Professor
Department of Radiodiagnosis
Postgraduate Institute of Medical Education and Research, Chandigarh, India

Preface

In 1996, a unique venture was jointly initiated by the faculty of Radiodiagnosis, All India Institute of Medical Sciences (AIIMS), New Delhi; Maulana Azad Medical College (MAMC), New Delhi; and Postgraduate Institute of Medical Education and Research (PGIMER), Chandigarh, India, to organize continuing medical education (CME) programs based on a series of imaging courses. An integral part of this endeavour was publishing books covering all organ systems. The aim was to provide state-of-the-art knowledge for postgraduate students as well as the practicing radiologists along with establishing a uniform pattern of teaching in radiology across the country.

The first series of seven imaging courses was successfully completed in the year 2000. A second series of these courses was then initiated in the year 2002 and was completed in 2004. This was also highly successful. The third series of seven extremely popular and successful courses covering all the organ systems and advances in physics was started in 2008 and was completed in 2013. Currently, the fourth series is underway.

Every course in each of the series has resulted in publication of a book. These books have been very popular amongst residents as well as among practicing radiologists.

Considering the popularity of these books, the editors, along with publishers, M/s Jaypee Brothers Medical Publishers (P) Ltd, New Delhi, India, decided to combine the individual books into three volumes—*AIIMS-MAMC-PGI's Comprehensive Textbook of Diagnostic Radiology*.

In keeping pace with newer developments in the field of diagnostic radiology and in order to cater to the contemporary needs of users, the second edition of *AIIMS-MAMC-PGI's Comprehensive Textbook of Diagnostic Radiology* is now being presented after a gap of three years since the previous edition of this book. It is anticipated that with such a complete coverage of all the subjects, the users will not have to refer to any other book during their routine learning of diagnostic radiology.

We are sure that residents and radiologists will find these comprehensive three volumes easy to handle and very useful in day-to-day practice.

We are once again grateful to all the contributors from the three apex academic institutions of India, i.e. AIIMS, New Delhi; MAMC, New Delhi; and PGIMER, Chandigarh, India.

We are thankful to M/s Jaypee Brothers Medical Publishers (P) Ltd, for helping us to make our dream come true.

Manavjit Singh Sandhu
Anju Garg
Arun Kumar Gupta

Acknowledgments

We would like to put on record our deep appreciation and gratitude:

To Professors Manorama Berry, Sudha Suri and Veena Chowdhury (Past Editors) the three pioneers who in 1996 took a bold initiative and started a unique teaching course now popularly known as AIIMS-MAMC-PGI's imaging course. Up to 2013, three series of these courses have been completed and the fourth series was started at the end of 2016. This course series has become extremely popular and every course is followed by the publication of a book which too is highly appreciated and popular.

To Professors Sima Mukhopadhyay, Sushma Vashisht and Niranjan Khandelwal who have been the Editors of past series and who contributed to organizing the earlier courses in their capacity as Heads of Departments.

To all the Associate Editors of the different course books who put in immense effort to bring the books out on time.

To all the Authors who contributed chapters without whom we could not have collected such an outstanding content of teaching and academic material.

To our respective hospitals for giving us the privilege and unique opportunity to work, which enabled us to amass data from patients and document images of diverse diseases that provide the reader with a wide spectrum of knowledge.

Our sincere and grateful thanks to Shri Jitendar P Vij (Group Chairman), Mr Ankit Vij (Managing Director), Mr MS Mani (Group President), Ms Chetna Malhotra Vohra (Associate Director–Content Strategy), Ms Pooja Bhandari (Production Head), Ms Kritika Dua (Senior Development Editor) and other members of M/s Jaypee Brothers Medical Publishers (P) Ltd, New Delhi, India, for their untiring coordination efforts in the production of this book.

We are very proud indeed at the culmination of two decades of these course series, to compile and present them together in the form of these three volumes of *AIIMS-MAMC-PGI's Comprehensive Textbook of Diagnostic Radiology*.

Contents

VOLUME 1

NEUROradiology INCLUDING HEAD AND NECK IMAGING, RECENT ADVANCES AND APPLIED PHYSICS IN IMAGING

SECTION 1: Neuroradiology including Head and Neck Imaging

SECTION 2: Recent Advances and Applied Physics in Imaging

VOLUME 2
GASTROINTESTINAL AND HEPATOBILIARY IMAGING, GENITOURINARY AND PEDIATRIC IMAGING

SECTION 3: Gastrointestinal and Hepatobiliary Imaging

SECTION 4: Genitourinary Imaging

VOLUME 3

CHEST AND CARDIOVASCULAR IMAGING, MUSCULOSKELETAL AND BREAST IMAGING

SECTION 6: Chest and Cardiovascular Imaging

Section 1

Neuroradiology including Head and Neck Imaging

CHAPTER 1

Evaluation of Plain X-ray Skull: A Systematic Approach

Niranjan Khandelwal, Sudha Suri, Vikas Bhatia

INTRODUCTION

In the past, skull radiograph was considered an essential step in the investigative protocol of a patient suspected to have a neurological disease. With the introduction of computed tomography (CT) and magnetic resonance imaging (MRI), there has been a tremendous decline in the usage of plain films and the indications for skull radiographs have been redefined.[1,2] The major indication for skull radiographs is in the evaluation of skeletal dysplasia, diagnostic survey in abuse, abnormal head shapes, infections and tumors affecting the skull bones, metabolic bone disease, leukemia and multiple myeloma. Abnormalities in skull radiographs may be seen in the form of change in the size, density and shape of the skull, as well as the other defects of the skull. In patients presenting with stroke, epilepsy, dementia or in postoperative cases, skull X-rays generally provide no useful information and MRI or CT is the investigation of choice.[3] In patients of trauma, CT should be the first line of investigation except in patients who suffer from facial and orbital fractures where plain films are helpful in orientation and in medicolegal cases.[4-6] Occasionally, skull X-rays may reveal linear fractures with more certainty than a CT scan.[4] In patients suspected to have intracerebral tumors, posteroanterior (PA) and lateral view of skull may provide additional information like detection of hyperostosis in case of meningiomas, presence of lytic and sclerotic metastasis in neuroblastomas and tram-track calcification in Sturge-Weber syndrome which may compliment the diagnosis on CT. The present chapter will describe the normal roentgen anatomy as seen in the basic views of skull followed by systematic approach to the analysis of the abnormal skull X-rays.[7-9]

An overview of the basic X-rays of skull is shown in **Table 1**.

LATERAL VIEW OF SKULL

A single lateral view of the skull **(Fig. 1A)** is the most common radiographic X-ray examination to be performed. A systematic approach to the examination consists of evaluation of the size and shape of the cranium, the thickness and density of the bones, the sutures, the vascular markings, the base of skull and the cranial cavity.

Size and shape of the skull is determined by examining the relative size of face and cranium. When the skull is longer and has a relatively shorter vertical diameter, it is referred to as *dolichocephalic*. On the other hand, when the vertical diameter is greater, it is termed as *brachycephalic*. The outer table, the inner table and the diploic space of the bones should be carefully examined for presence of any erosion, sclerosis or widening.

The normal sutures in adults are surrounded by a narrow area of increased density, a fact that helps in distinguishing fracture lines from sutures. Sutures are difficult to visualize in newborns but in children older than 3 years, the width of the suture should not be more than 2 mm. Width of the sutures can be best assessed at the top of the coronal suture in the lateral view. To see the sagittal and the lambdoid sutures, PA and Towne's views are performed. Vascular markings are seen along the

Table 1: Overview of the skull X-ray views.

View	*Patient positioning*	*Acquisition*	*Optimum view*	*Indications/information provided*
Lateral view	• Patient seated or standing • Affected side next to the bucky • Interpupillary line perpendicular to film and tube • Mid sagittal plane parallel to film	• Horizontal CR (central ray) : ¾" superior to EAM • Vertical CR : ¾"anterior to EAM	• Entire skull should be on the film • No rotation • Overlapping of ramus of mandible and orbits	• Most common radiographic X-ray of skull • Overview of the entire skull • Sella, clivus, anterior cranial fossa • Calcifications, suture, vascular markings, fractures
Towne view	• Position patients chin bringing the OML (orbitomeatal line) perpendicular to IR (image receptor) • Align midsagittal plane to CR	• Angle the CR 30 Degrees, • Center at two and a half inches above glabella. To pass through foramen magnum	• Ensure that the skull is straight with no rotation, include the entire skull in the field of view.	• Occipital bone, foramen magnum, dorsum sellae, the internal acoustic canals, mastoids and the condyles of mandible.
Caldwell view	• Place the patient's nose and forehead against the IR. • Flex the neck as needed to align the OML perpendicular to IR. • Align the midsagittal plane to the midline of the grid in order to avoid rotation or tilt.	• Angle 15 Degrees caudal and center as to exit the nasion.	• No rotation	• Frontal and ethmoid sinuses • Supraorbital rim fractures
Frontal view	• Place the patient's nose and forehead against the IR. • Flex the neck as needed to align the OML perpendicular to IR. • Align the midsagittal plane to the midline of the grid in order to avoid rotation or tilt.	• Center the CR as to exit the Nasion.	• No rotation	• Skull fractures • Superior orbital fissure • Greater and lesser wings of the sphenoid
Submentovertex view	• Tilt the patient's head back bringing the chin up until the inferior OML is parallel to the IR. • Be aware of any suspected cervical spine injury before performing this view. • Align the midsagittal plane perpendicular to the IR.	• CR is perpendicular to the inferior OML, center 1 and a half inch inferior to the mandibular symphysis.	• No rotation	• Foramen ovale • Foramen spinosum • Foramen lacerum • Specific situations such as looking for the skull base lesions, middle ear or inner ear lesions, nasopharyngeal masses or oropharyngeal lesions and sinus pathologies
Waters' view	• Patient seated close to bucky • Mentomeatal line perpendicular to film (closed mouth) • Mouth can be opened for sphenoid sinus (cantho-meatal line 35-40 degree to bucky)	• Horizontal CR exit through base of nose • Vertical CR mid sagittal	• Facial bones and sinus on the film • No rotation • Petrous ridges below floor of maxilla.	• Sinus diseases • Injury to maxilla and orbit

coronal suture due to middle meningeal vessels. Arterial grooves become narrower as they go distally. They may be confused with fracture lines but the latter are more radiolucent whereas vascular markings have a halo of increased density around them. Posterior branch of middle meningeal artery as it ascends upward and posteriorly sometimes causes a shadow over the temporal bone that should not be mistaken for a fracture. Enlargement

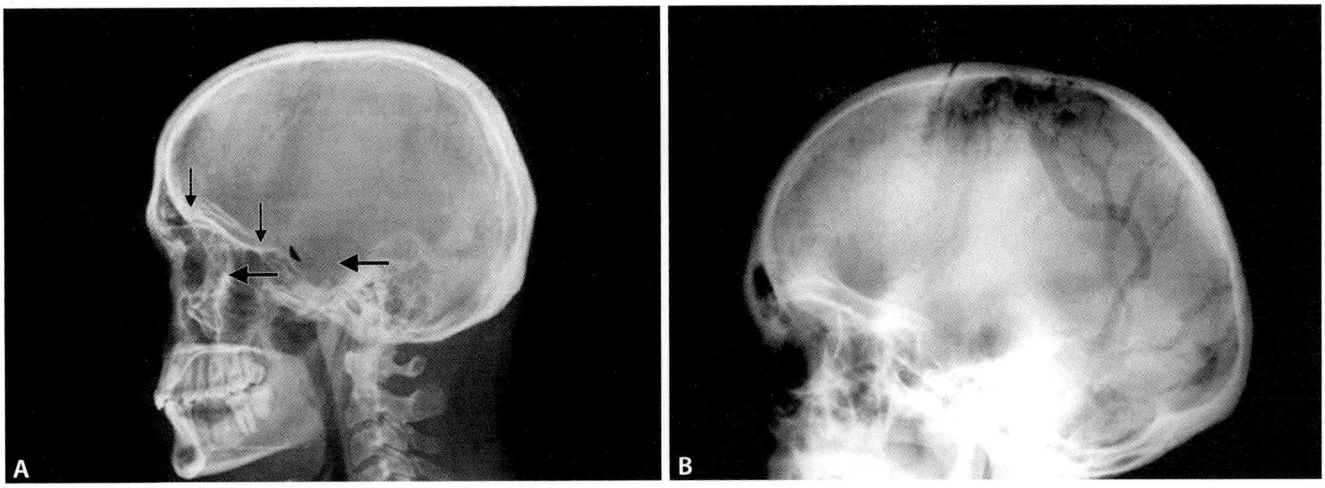

Figs. 1A and B: (A) Normal lateral view of skull demonstrates the normal coronal sutures, lambdoid sutures and the vascular grooves due to middle meningeal vessels posterior to coronal sutures. Note the two lines formed by the roof of the orbits ending posteriorly at the anterior clinoid processes. Arrow head marks the tuberculum sellae. Vertical arrows (anterior) show the cribriform plate and the (posterior) planum sphenoidale. Anterior horizontal arrow shows the greater wing of sphenoid bone forming anterior borders of middle cranial fossa. The dorsum sellae (horizontal arrows) with posterior clinoid processes above and the clivus posteriorly are well seen; (B) Lateral view of skull shows multiple dilated vascular markings in the parieto-occipital region in a case of parasagittal meningioma.

of the arterial grooves may occur in meningioma and arteriovenous malformations **(Fig. 1B)**.

Diploic venous channels are extremely variable in position but are generally seen in the frontal and parietal bones. Venous lakes may be seen as round or oval radiolucent areas and should not be confused with destructive lesions of the bone. Besides the arterial and diploic venous channels, the dural sinuses also produce grooves on the inner table of the skull.

The structures along the base of the skull should be carefully examined, in particular the three lines which represent the floor of the anterior cranial fossa. The upper two lines are formed by the roofs of the orbits, which end posteriorly at the anterior clinoid processes. The lower line is formed anteriorly by the cribriform plate of the ethmoid bone and posteriorly by planum sphenoidale ending at the tuberculum sellae, which marks the superior limit of the anterior wall of the sella turcica. A depression just anterior to the tuberculum sellae is called sulcus chiasmaticus. The roof of the sella posteriorly is formed by the dorsum sellae, which ends in the posterior clinoid processes. Sphenoid sinus is seen below the floor of the sella turcica. The pneumatization of this sinus shows considerable variation. Floor of the middle cranial fossa is formed by the greater wings of the sphenoid on each side, which appear as curvilinear shadows concave outward. These lines serve as a point of reference for locating the temporal lobe of the brain. The dorsum sellae continues as the clivus, which is followed by the occipital bone ending at the anterior margin of the foramen magnum. Clivus is seen to terminate just above the top of the odontoid process of the axis. The normal calcification may be seen in the falx cerebri, petroclinoid ligaments, tentorium, pineal body, habenular commissure and choroid plexus.

FRONTAL VIEW (FIG. 2)

Posteroanterior projection with 15-20° craniocaudal angulation is preferred to straight PA projection as the petrous pyramids are projected below the orbits and the superior orbital fissure as well as greater and lesser wings of the sphenoid are clearly visualized. PA view is also examined for shape of the skull, with special attention to the symmetry of the two sides. The bony landmarks, which require to be carefully examined for any erosions, sclerosis or lack of continuity include crista galli in the midline, planum sphenoidale, floor of the sella, lesser and greater wings of the sphenoid and the three lines of the orbit formed by the palpable superior border of orbit, highest point of roof of the orbit and the sphenoid ridge which represents the floor of the anterior cranial fossa. The floor of the posterior cranial fossa can also be seen inferiorly. Pacchionian depressions due to arachnoid granulations can be seen in both PA and lateral views as tiny radiolucent areas usually within 2.5-3 cm from the midline. Their margins are well defined superiorly, whereas inferiorly the margins fade away—a feature helpful in distinguishing these from destructive lesions.

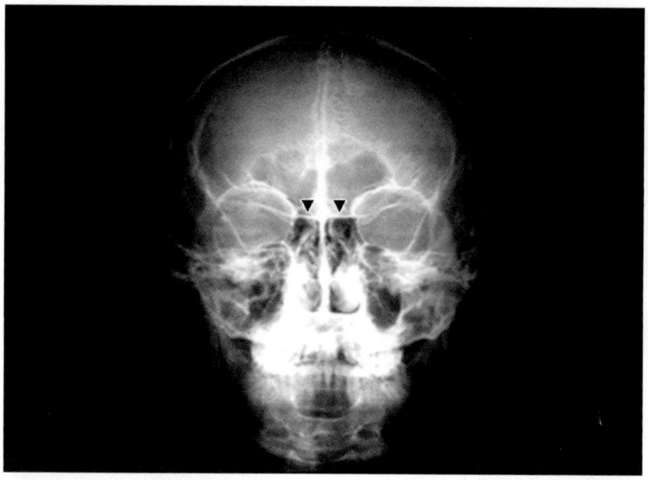

Fig. 2: Posteroanterior (PA) view with 15° caudal angulation demonstrates the dense vertical bony projection in the midline due to crista galli, lesser wings of the sphenoid on both sides joining to form the planum sphenoidale (arrow heads). Floor of sella is faintly visualized in the midline. Oblique line of the orbit is formed by the greater wing of sphenoid in its lower two-thirds and by the frontal bone in its upper one-third.

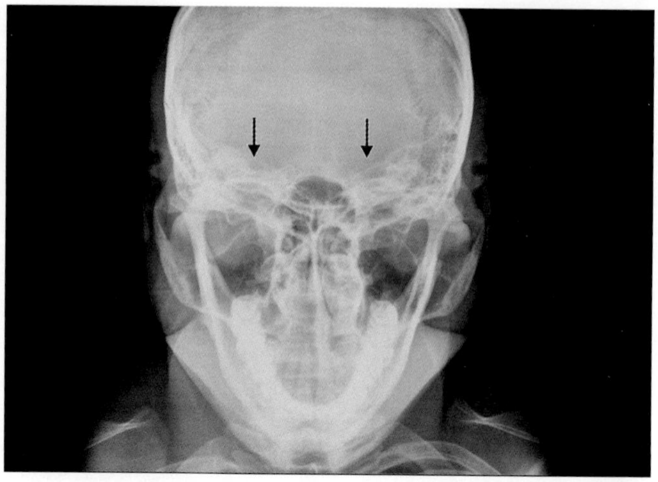

Fig. 3: Towne's view shows foramen magnum in the center with dorsum sellae projecting through it. The parallel lucencies (arrows) on either side represent the internal auditory canals. Further, laterally pneumatized mastoids air cells can also be seen.

TOWNE'S VIEW

Towne's view **(Fig. 3)** is performed by angling the tube 35° caudally from the orbitomeatal line. It is generally performed when pathology is suspected in the petrous pyramids. This projection also shows the occipital bone, foramen magnum, dorsum sellae, the internal acoustic canals, mastoids and the condyles of mandible.

BASAL VIEW

Basal view **(Fig. 4)** of the skull or the submentovertical view is an infrequent examination and is generally performed in specific situations such as looking for the skull base lesions, middle ear or inner ear lesions, nasopharyngeal masses or oropharyngeal lesions and sinus pathologies. The bony landmarks that should always be identified and carefully examined include three lines, constituted by the lateral wall of the maxillary antrum (S-shaped), the posterolateral wall of the orbit, and the anterior wall of the middle cranial fossa which is arched with concavity pointing posteriorly. The lesser wing of the sphenoid is seen just behind the anterior wall of middle cranial fossa. A transverse dense line in the center represents the anterior margin of sella. The medial and lateral pterygoid processes are projected over the sphenoid ridge. Sphenoid sinuses should be carefully seen as early bone destruction in patients of nasopharyngeal carcinoma or sphenoid sinus carcinoma is well demonstrated in this view.

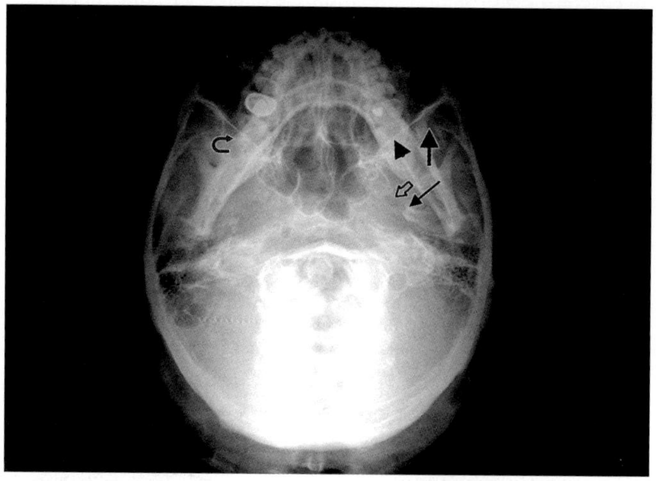

Fig. 4: Basal view of skull shows the nasopharynx, sphenoid sinus and ethmoid sinuses in the midline. Posteriorly odontoid process is seen to project into the foramen magnum posterior to the arch of atlas. Laterally, the foramen ovale (open arrow), foramen spinosum, (long arrow), Eustachian tube posterior to foramen spinosum and the carotid canal are well visualized. Anterolaterally, the three lines formed by the posterior wall of orbit (arrow head), maxillary sinus (S-shaped) (curved arrow) and the anterior wall of middle cranial fossa (thick arrow) (arched shadow with concavity posteriorly) should be looked for in each case. Medial and lateral pterygoid plates are well seen.

There are three important foramina seen in the basal view. Foramen ovale lying behind the pterygoid processes gives passage to the third division of the trigeminal nerve, accessory meningeal artery and superficial petrosal nerve. Foramen spinosum lying behind and lateral to foramen ovale transmits the middle meningeal artery.

Foramen lacerum is seen anterolateral to the petrous apex and has a well-defined medial margin produced by the internal carotid artery. The Eustachian canal is seen behind the foramen spinosum. The external auditory canal is seen behind the condyle of the mandible. Internal auditory canals and inner ear structures including semicircular canals should be carefully looked for. The clivus and foramen magnum are well seen through which the anterior arch of atlas and odontoid process of axis are seen to project. Jugular fossa and jugular foramen are seen laterally on each side of the junction of petrous portion of the temporal bone and occipital bone.

WATERS' VIEW

It is one of the standard views to study the maxillary and anterior ethmoidal sinuses. Waters' view **(Fig. 5)** is generally performed with the patient in sitting position to facilitate demonstration of any fluid level in the sinuses. Patient is instructed to keep the mouth open with nose and chin touching the cassette in order to visualize the sphenoid sinuses. It is performed by placing the orbitomeatal line at an angle of 35° with the plane of film by either raising the chin or by tilting the tube. It also gives clear picture of the roof of the orbits, destruction of which may be seen in mucocele of frontal sinus and in carcinoma of lacrimal gland.

CALDWELL'S VIEW

Caldwell's view is the best projection for examining the frontal and ethmoid sinuses. Patient is positioned directly facing the cassette in either sitting or prone position with midsagittal plane and orbitomeatal line perpendicular to the film with nose and forehead touching the cassette. Central ray is directed 15° caudally to the nasion.

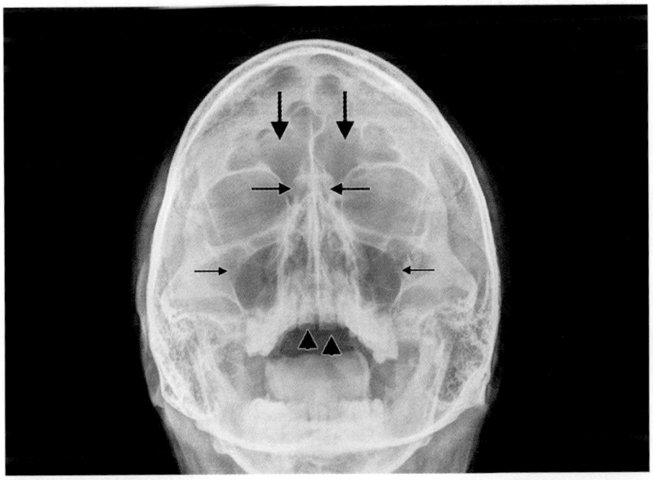

Fig. 5: Waters' view of skull shows bilateral maxillary antrum (lower horizontal arrows), frontal sinuses (vertical arrows), ethmoid sinuses (upper horizontal arrows) and lower margin of sphenoid sinuses (arrowheads).

The various abnormalities that can be detected on the plain skull X-rays can be categorized in the following groups:

- Abnormal density
- Abnormal contour of the skull
- Abnormal intracranial volume
- Intracranial calcification
- Increased thickness of the skull
- Single lucent defect
- Multiple lucent defects
- Sclerotic areas.

Abnormal Density

Generalized reduced density: Thinning of the skull bones with decreased bone density is seen in osteogenesis imperfecta, hypophosphatasia and achondrogenesis. In hypophosphatasia, there is decreased ossification of the skull and vertebrae or as isolated areas of unusually thin calvarial bone. Osteogenesis imperfecta shows increased osseous fragility leading to multiple fractures in addition to decreased density.

Focal reduced density: Focal areas of defective ossification can occur in the lacunar skull where in well-defined lucent areas are seen corresponding to nonossified fibrous bone and the lacunae are bounded by normally ossified bone.

Generalized increased density: It is seen in sclerosing bone dysplasias such as osteopetrosis, and pyknodysostosis. In osteopetrosis increased density is seen in the basal bones initially and later the calvaria becomes dense and thick. The density of facial bones is relatively less dense.

Localized increased density: It may be seen in fibrous dysplasia, osteoma, craniometaphyseal dysplasia, etc.

Abnormal Contour of the Skull

Normal contour of the skull is maintained by sutures, the intracranial contents and normal bone formation. Abnormality in any of these may result in abnormal contour of the skull.

Premature fusion of the sutures, craniosynostosis, is the most common cause of abnormal contour in children. If the suture closes early, the calvarium expands to accommodate the growing brain in the axis of the fused suture. Sagittal synostosis (scaphocephaly) is the most common form of isolated synostosis with M:F = 4:1.[10]

It leads to an elongated narrow boat-shaped skull. The closure of both coronal sutures and lambdoid sutures (*turricephaly)* produces a short wide skull with towering head, with bulging temporal areas and shallow orbits **(Fig. 6)**. The recessed supraorbital rims and hypoplasia of the basal frontal bone, gives cloverleaf-like skull appearance.

Plagiocephaly means skewed or oblique head. It results when there is unilateral such as coronal or lambdoid synostosis. Unicoronal synostosis is the second most common form of craniosynostosis, after sagittal synostosis. Two-thirds cases occur in female patients and 10% are familial in nature. In this condition, there is elongation of the orbit, elevation of the lateral portion of ipsilateral orbital rim (the harlequin eye appearance) and tilting of the nasal septum and crista galli toward the affected side. Margins of the affected sutures develop sclerosis. Any decrease or increase in the cerebral volume may result in abnormal contour.

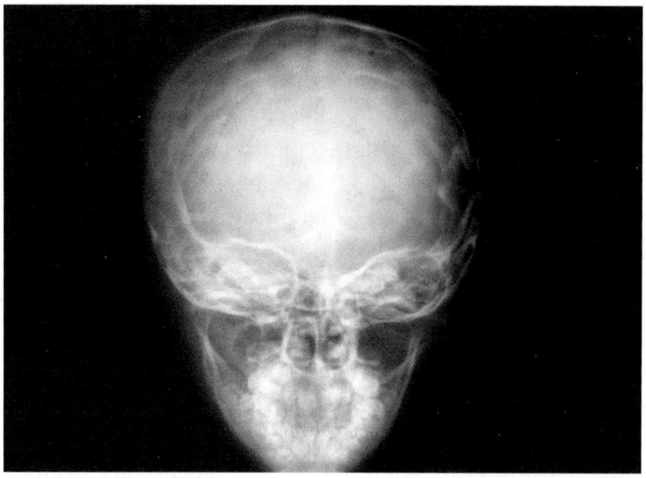

Fig. 6: Craniosynostosis. Anteroposterior (AP) view of skull shows silver beaten appearance due to exaggerated convolutional markings all over the skull vault. None of the sutures is seen.

Premature fusion of multiple sutures on one side is associated with signs of raised intracranial tension in the form of increased convolutional markings. The hemicalvarium on the ipsilateral side is smaller than the opposite side. The tables of bones of the skull are thickened and there may be elevation of the petrous pyramid on the same side.

Expansion of the bony calvarium due to the presence of slow growing intracerebral or subarachnoid space occupying lesions such as arachnoid cysts may also result in abnormal contour **(Figs. 7A and B)**. The bony vault bulges outward with thinning of the inner table. Chronic subdural hematomas may also cause expansion of the adjacent calvarium and may even erode the inner table. Calcifications when present facilitate the diagnosis.

Abnormal bone formation such as that occurs in achondroplasia characterized by defective endochondral ossification, results in shortening of the bones of the skull base as these bones develop from cartilage. Since the bones of the vault develop from membranous bones, these remain unaffected. The result is a small foramen magnum and enlarged cranium with frontal bossing and large jaws.

Abnormal Intracranial Volume

Size of the calvarium is dependent on the size of the intracranial contents. The most accurate way to determine abnormal cranial volume is to measure the skull directly

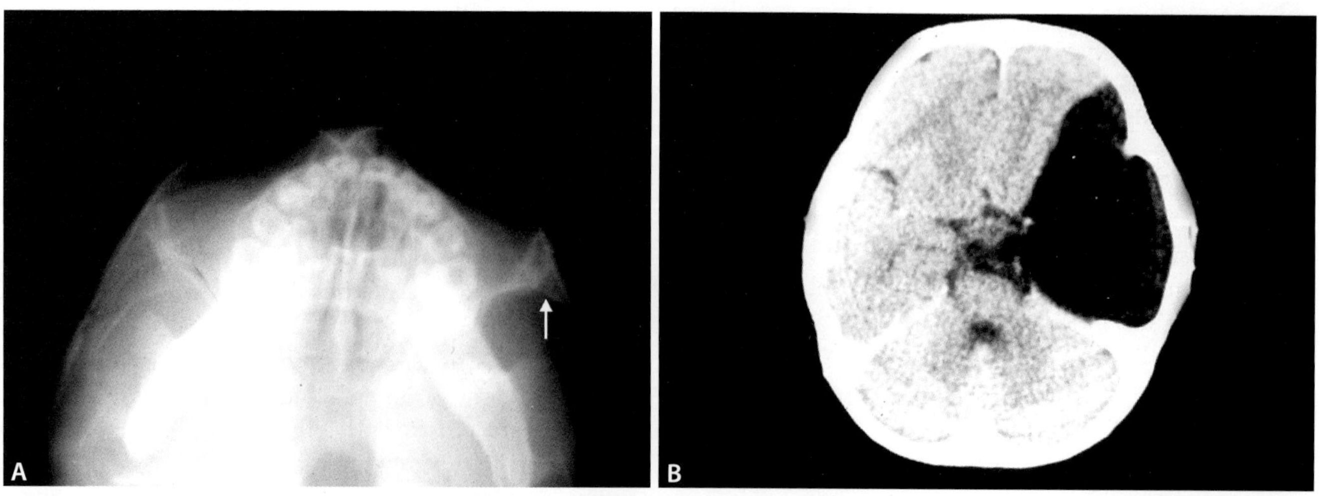

Figs. 7A and B: Arachnoid cyst. (A) Basal view of skull shows thinning and ballooning of anterior and lateral walls of the left middle cranial fossa (arrow); (B) Axial CT scan of the same patient shows a large left temporoparietal arachnoid cyst.

and compare the measurements to standard for age and body size. A simple method of assessing the size of the skull is to compare the skull vault to the size of the face. At birth, the volume of skull is approximately four times that of face. This ratio decreases to 3:1 by age 2 and 1.5:1 by adulthood.[8]

Enlarged head size may result from hydrocephalus, macrocephaly, hydranencephaly and in pituitary dwarfism. The most common cause of hydrocephalus in children is congenital obstruction of the ventricular system and is associated with raised intracranial tension. Sutures become wide due to expansion of the intracranial contents.

Small skull but otherwise normal contour is characteristically seen in microcephaly associated with mental retardation. Cranial sutures fuse early but this is a result of microcephaly and not the cause. The sinuses are large and the digital or convolutional markings are absent or decreased. It is important to differentiate premature closure of all the sutures from microcephaly with fused sutures. When multiple sutures fuse prematurely, the fusion does not occur simultaneously and the result is an irregular skull due to expansion of the skull in unusual directions to accommodate the brain. Clinically, signs of raised intracranial tension are present. Convolutional markings are exaggerated.

Increased thickness of the skull may result due to early cessation of brain growth or due to cerebral atrophy. Increased width of diploic space due to increased hematopoiesis is seen in hemolytic anemia. Progressive hydrocephalus leads to large bony calvarium and a decreased diploic space. However, if a ventricular shunt is performed and abnormal expansion ceases resulting in arrested hydrocephalus, the cranial sutures close and the inner table of bones of the skull become thicker and the diploic space becomes larger. A history of hydrocephalus and the presence of a ventricular shunt facilitate the diagnosis.

Among the hemolytic anemia producing hyperplasia of the bone marrow, thalassemia causes most marked changes. The diploic space is widened with striking radial striations, the "hair-on-end" appearance **(Fig. 8)**. The paranasal sinuses may also be completely obliterated due to widening of the diploic space of facial bones. Such changes may also be seen in other forms of anemia, such as sickle cell disease, hereditary spherocytosis, but the changes are much less marked.

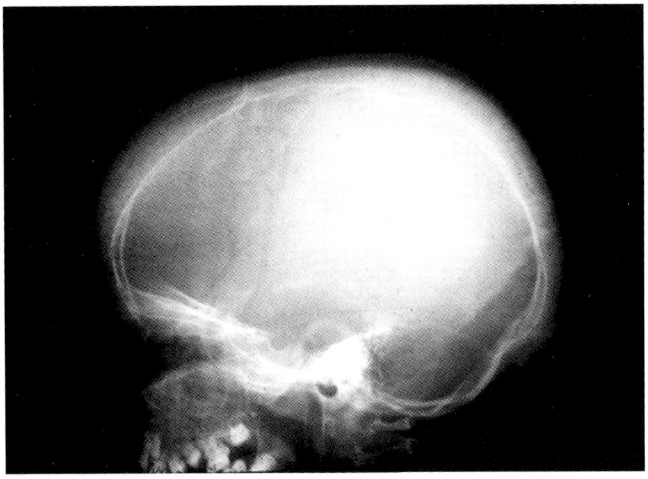

Fig. 8: Thalassemia. Lateral skull radiograph shows widened diploic space with coarsened trabeculae giving "hair-on-end" appearance typical of hemolytic anemia.

Table 2: Skull vault lucent areas.

Normal: Parietal foramina, vascular channels, pacchionian granulations, fontanelles
Neoplastic: • Myeloma • Metastasis • LCH (acute phase)
Inflammatory/infective diseases: • Osteomyelitis • TB • Hydatid • Syphilis
Vascular causes: • Hemangioma • Sinus pericranii
Metabolic: • Osteoporosis • Hyperparathyroidism
Miscellaneous: • Leptomeningeal cyst • Burr hole • Intradiploic arachnoid cyst • Neurofibroma • Paget's disease

Radiolucent Areas in Skull

When there is a single lucent lesion, the important considerations that help in deciding its nature are its location, associated soft tissue swelling, table of the bone involved and margins of the lytic lesion, whether sharp, ill-defined or sclerotic. Radiolucent defects in the skull bone may be due to variety of causes, which may be congenital or acquired **(Table 2)**. A sclerotic margin of the lesion sometimes also helps in narrowing down the differential diagnosis **(Table 3)**. Congenital causes may be parietal foramina, anomalous apertures, meningoencephalocele or dermal sinus. The acquired causes include trauma, infections, tumors and histiocytosis.

Table 3: Skull vault lucent areas with marginal sclerosis.

• Epidermoid
• Encephalocele/meningocele
• LCH (healing phase)
• Posttreatment metastasis
• Chronic osteomyelitis
• Fibrous dysplasia

Bilaterally symmetrical rounded lytic defects located in the posterior parietal bone are characteristic of parietal foramina and are of no clinical significance. Lytic defects due to meningoencephalocele are located in the midline in the frontal or occipital regions and have sharp margins. Associated soft tissue mass clinches the diagnosis. In the first 3 months of life, meningoencephalocele is generally associated with lacunar skull (craniolacunia) **(Fig. 9)**. A *dermal sinus* also occurs in the midline of the skull and may present as a radiolucent defect with a sharp slightly sclerotic border. It is generally associated with a lipoma or a nevus in the overlying soft tissues. These lesions may have an intracranial components which may require a CT scan for demonstration.

Fractures generally occur at the site of injury and may be associated with soft tissue swelling. *Linear nondepressed fractures* may be seen as radiolucent lines and should not be confused with sutures or vascular grooves. Fracture lines are nontapering, nonbranching and have sharp borders whereas vascular grooves have ill-defined borders and an undulating course. Sutures are seen in known anatomical positions and have saw tooth edges. *Depressed fractures* generally occur after severe trauma and are considered more serious than linear fractures. Radiologically, the depressed fragment presents as area of increased radiodensity surrounded by a radiolucent zone **(Fig. 10)**. In children, when the dura beneath the suture is torn, the arachnoid membrane herniates through the dura into the bony defect. The pulsations of the brain lead to progressive enlargement of the arachnoid collection resulting in expansion of the fracture line termed as growing skull fracture. The bulging membranes result in the formation of leptomeningeal cyst **(Fig. 11)**.

Infections of the skull are uncommon and generally follow trauma or arise secondary to infection elsewhere in the body. The radiographic appearance consists of mottled irregular lucencies, which have ill-defined borders and are associated with soft tissue swelling of the scalp.

Epidermoid tumors develop from a congenital inclusion of epithelial cells within the calvarium. Radiologically, these lesions present as well-defined lytic lesions, which have sclerotic border and are not necessarily located

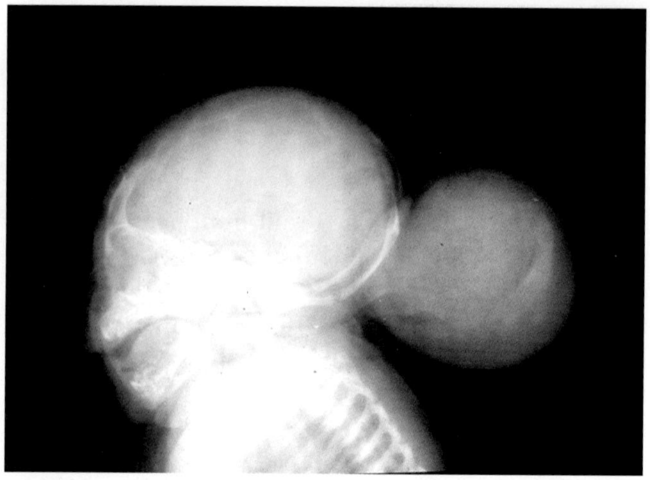

Fig. 9: Craniolacunia. Lateral skull radiograph in an infant shows multiple lucencies with intervening dense areas typical of craniolacunia. Note the associated occipital encephalocele and absence of sutural widening.

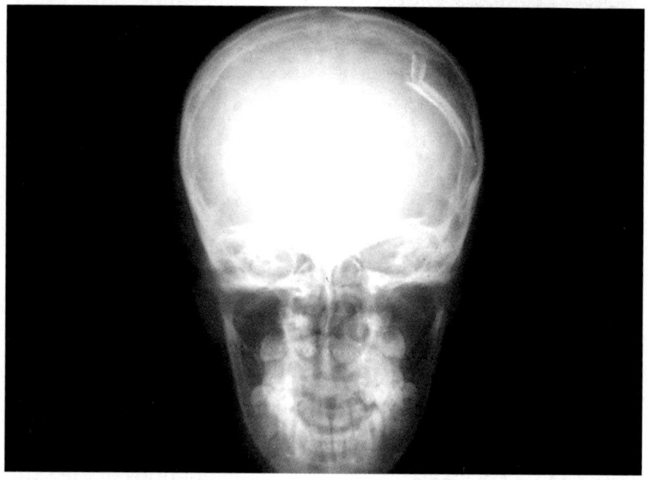

Fig. 10: Depressed fracture. Frontal radiograph shows the parallel dense lines due to depressed bone fragments and associated lucency due to absence of bone.

in the midline such as dermoid **(Fig. 12)**. Intracranial epidermoids may also produce a radiolucent shadow, which may mimick a lytic lesion **(Figs. 13A and B)**.

Malignant lesions such as primary osteosarcoma or metastasis can also produce lytic defects. Osteosarcoma causes gross destruction of the bone with ill-defined margins and soft tissue swelling **(Figs. 14A and B)**. Neuro-fibromatosis is a rare cause of a lytic defect seen along the suture. This defect is not due to the presence of neurofibroma but is a manifestation of mesenchymal defect. Intracranial mass lesions can also rarely present as lytic areas of the skull.

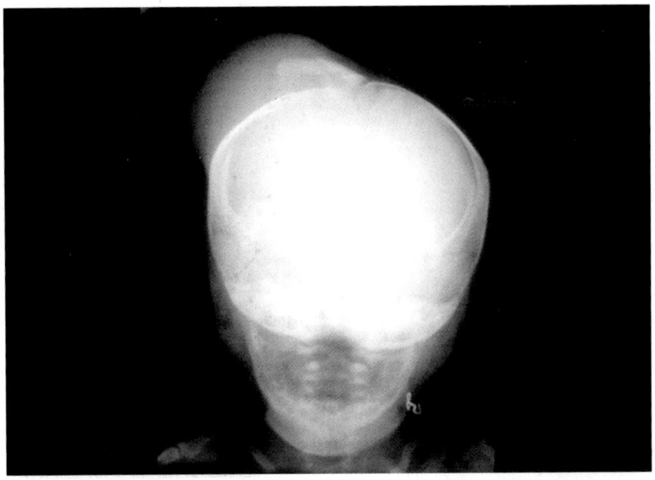

Fig. 11: Growing fracture. Posteroanterior (PA) skull radiographs in a child demonstrate fracture of the right frontal bone with thickening, sclerosis and wide separation of the fracture ends. Note the soft tissue swelling overlying this area.

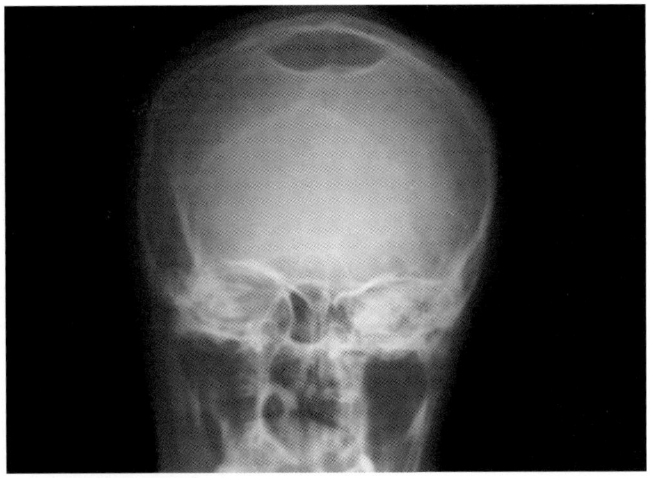

Fig. 12: Dermoid scalp. Skull radiograph shows a well-circumscribed lucency overlying the coronal suture.

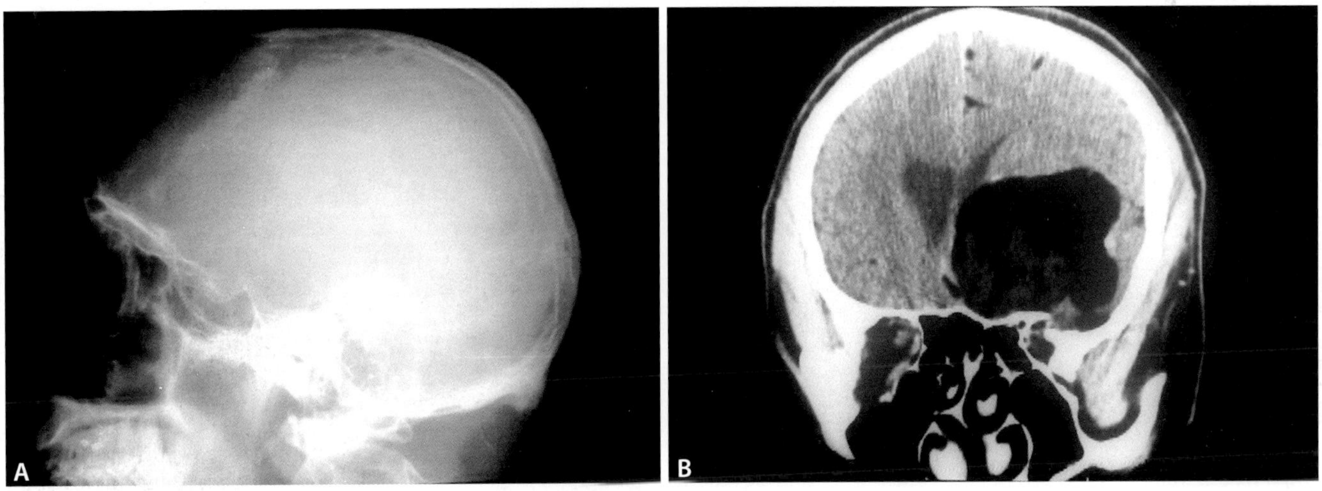

Figs. 13A and B: Single lucent lesion. (A) Skull radiograph shows a well-circumscribed lucency overlying the coronal suture mimicking a lytic lesion; (B) Coronal computed tomography (CT) scan in the same patient shows a large hypodense lesion due to epidermoid in the temporoparietal region. No lytic lesion of skull vault is seen.

Eosinophilic granulomas, Hand-Schüller-Christian disease and *Letterer-Siwe disease* all form part of a complex comprising histiocytosis. The severity ranges from mild in eosinophilic granuloma to very malignant course in Letterer- Siwe disease. A single lytic lesion having sharp nonsclerotic border and bevelled edges is characteristic of eosinophilic granulomas **(Fig. 15)**. Occasionally, a small bone is seen in the center representing button sequestrum. Lytic lesions in the other two variants are larger, multiple and punched out **(Fig. 16)**.

Multiple radiolucent defects in the skull in children may be due to craniolacunia, presence of wormian bones, increased convolutional makings due to raised intracranial tension, histiocytosis and metastasis from neuroblastoma **(Figs. 17A and B)**, leukemia or Ewing's sarcoma. In adults, multiple myeloma **(Fig. 18)**, metastasis and hyperparathyroidism **(Fig. 19)** are the usual causes.

Craniolacunia is due to a defect in ossification of the bones, which develop from membranous tissue. There are multiple radiolucent defects seen all over the cranial vault interspersed with strips of normal bone, which appear dense. Craniolacunia (lacunar skull) by itself is not of much significance, but it is generally associated with myelomeningocele or encephalocele

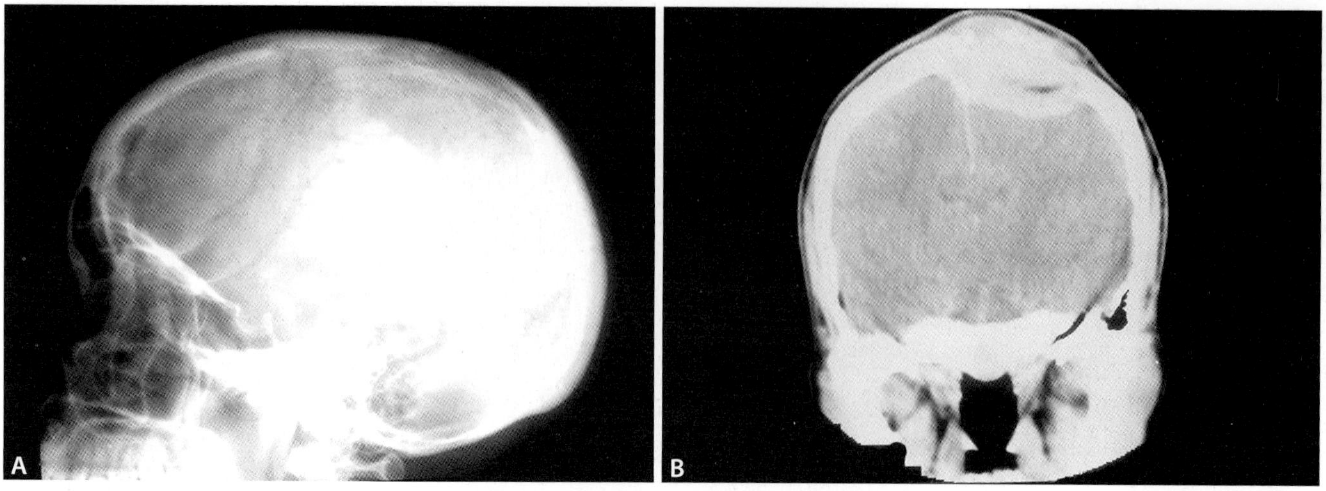

Figs. 14A and B: Osteosarcoma. (A) Large lytic area with irregular margin is seen affecting the left parietal bone; (B) Computed tomography (CT) scan of the same patient shows the soft tissue swelling, destruction of the bone and extradural extension of the tumor.

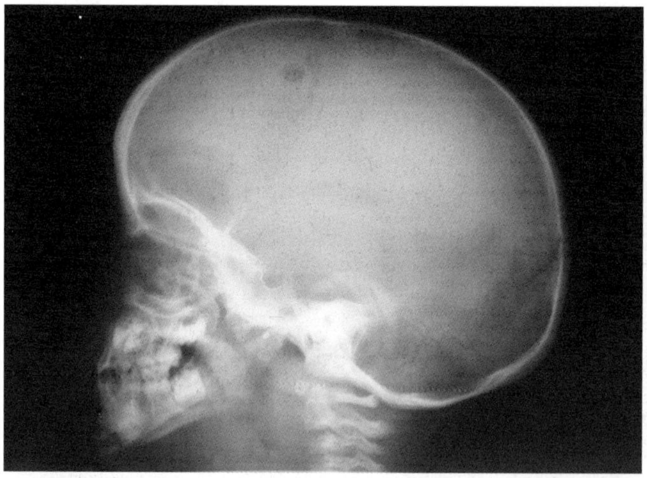

Fig. 15: Eosinophilic granuloma. Lateral skull radiograph shows a single lytic lesion having sharp nonsclerotic border and bevelled edges.

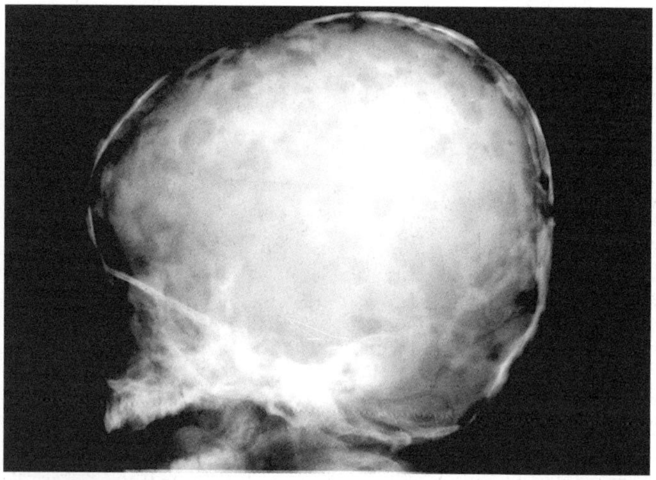

Fig. 16: Histiocytosis (Hand-Schüller-Christian disease). Lateral radiograph of skull shows multiple well-defined lytic lesions of the vault with bevelled edges characteristic of histiocytosis.

(***see* Fig. 9**). Appearance must not be confused with *increased convolutional markings* that result from raised intracranial tension and are seen as multiple radiolucent areas not exceeding the diameter of a finger. Convolutional marking may also be seen in normal children in the frontal and occipital region. Presence of increased convolutional markings in the parietal region should generally be considered abnormal. Wormian bones are seen along the sutures and results due to defective mineralization. Multiple wormian bones are seen in cleidocranial dysostosis, osteogenesis imperfecta, hypothyroidism and pyknodysostosis.

Lytic lesions seen in *multiple myeloma* are punched out, usually associated with osteoporosis and involve the mandible more frequently compared to *metastasis.* However, many times differentiation from metastasis may not be possible on radiological appearance alone. The sclerosis or sclerotic rim is very rare seen in 3% of cases in multiple myeloma and usually occur after therapy.[11] *Hyperparathyroidism* generally results in mottled demineralization **(Fig. 19)** but may sometimes cause multiple well-defined lytic areas **(Fig. 20)**.

Sclerotic Areas of the Skull

Areas of increased density in the skull may be seen in both normal as well as pathological conditions. Differential diagnosis depends on the localized vs generalized sclerosis **(Table 4)**. Osteopetrosis is a rare condition, which is characterized by diffuse thickening of the skull

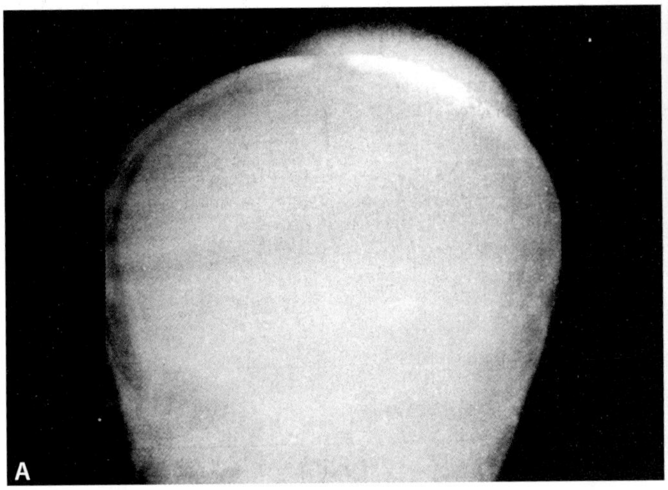

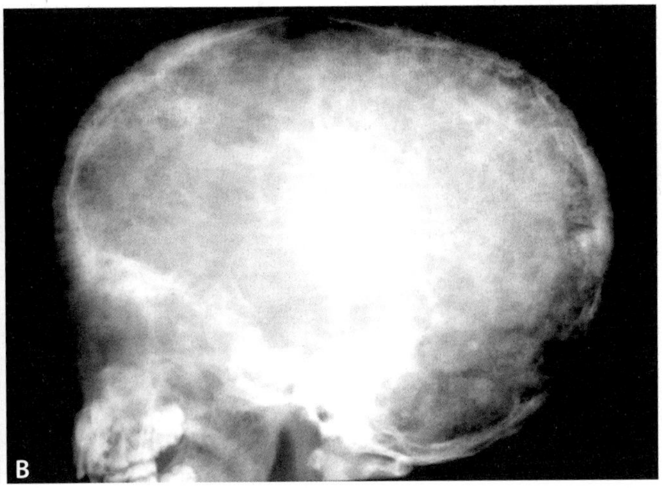

Figs. 17A and B: Metastatic lesions of the skull in a child with abdominal neuroblastoma. (A) Sutural metastasis: Frontal skull radiograph shows widening of the sagittal suture with an overlying soft tissue swelling; (B) Diffuse metastasis of skull vault: Lateral skull radiograph shows multiple lytic areas involving both tables of skull and diploic space. Note widening of coronal suture also.

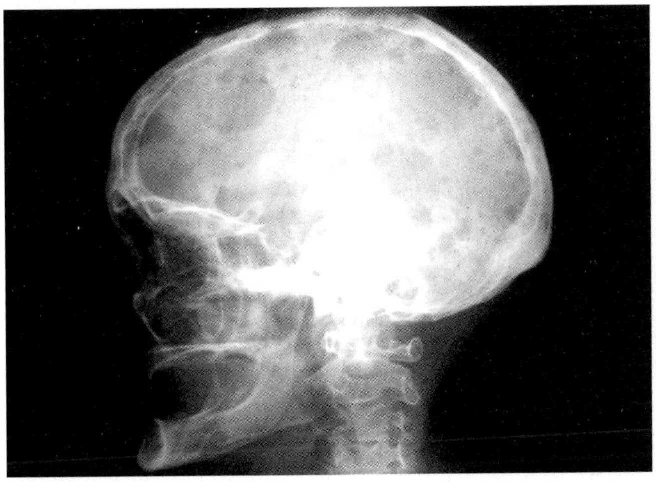

Fig. 18: Multiple myeloma. Lateral skull radiographs shows multiple well-defined punched out lytic lesions affecting the skull vault as well as mandible typical of myeloma.

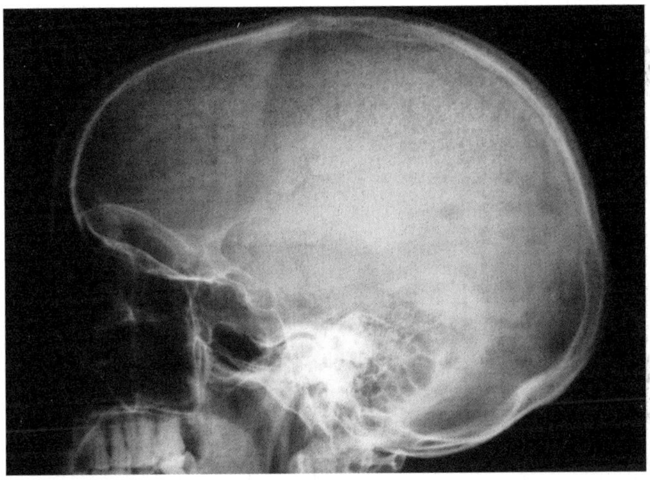

Fig. 19: Hyperparathyroidism. Lateral skull radiograph shows multiple lytic lesions with mottled appearance.

and face **(Fig. 21)**. Fibrous dysplasia may involve the vault or base of skull. There may be a single lesion or it may be part of syndrome *(McCune-Albright syndrome)* seen in females when it affects multiple bones and is associated with precocious puberty. The lesions are sclerotic with loss of normal trabecular pattern. Mixed types of lesions with sclerotic and lytic areas are also known to occur **(Figs. 22A to C)**. Paget disease in the mixed phase shows marked thickening of the diploic space, particularly the inner calvarial table, causing marked enlargement. The areas of sclerosis may be circular and occur in previous areas of osteoporosis. This pattern often creates focal areas of opacity giving "cotton wool" appearance at radiography **(Fig. 23)**. Multiple hyperostotic lesions affecting the calvarium measuring 5–10 mm in size may be seen in tuberous sclerosis in association with calcified lesion in periventricular region. Thickening of the frontal and parietal bones may occur in rickets due to presence of poorly mineralized bone, which on healing becomes dense. An *osteoma* affecting the skull bones is a benign tumor, which appears as a dense lesion projecting extracranially from the outer table of skull. Osteoma is also the most common benign tumor affecting the sinuses **(Fig. 24)**. Focal areas of hyperostosis are characteristic of *meningioma* **(Figs. 25A and B)**. When the hyperostosis affects the frontal bone, in a case of convexity meningioma, it must be differentiated from *hyperostosis frontalis interna* **(Fig. 26)**, the latter is generally seen in elderly females and

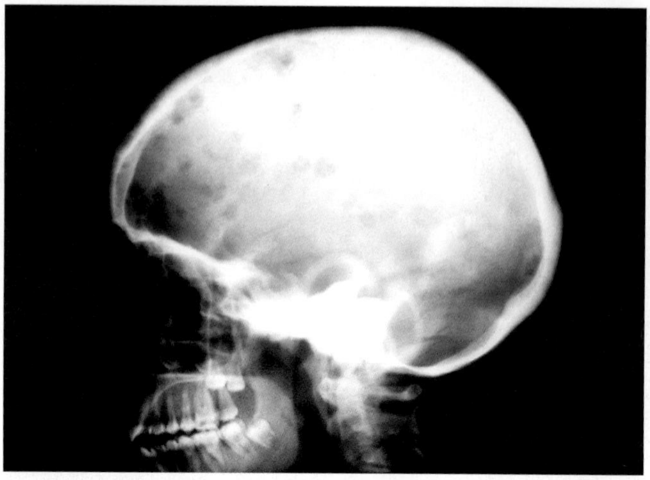

Fig. 20: Hyperparathyroidism. Lateral skull radiograph shows multiple well-circumscribed rounded lytic lesions involving skull vault with bone within bone appearance—an unusual feature of hyperparathyroidism.

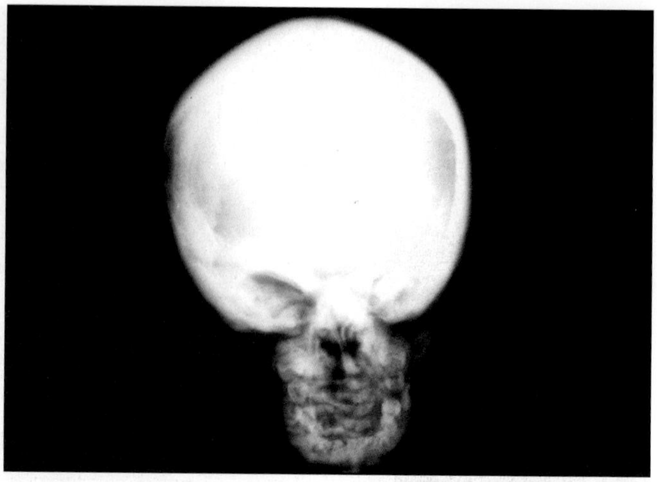

Fig. 21: Osteopetrosis. Frontal radiograph shows diffuse increased density affecting all bones of the skull vault as well as base.

affects the inner table with sparing of diploic space and does not cross the midline.

Intracranial Calcification

Presence of calcification can provide important clue to the diagnosis in several conditions intracranial calcification can be physiological or pathological **(Table 5)**. Although causes are numerous, some of these conditions have specific appearance, which can be diagnostic.

The most common physiological calcification occurs in the pineal gland. It is seen in the midline approximately 3 cm above and behind the posterior clinoids in the lateral view **(Fig. 27)**. Size of the pineal calcification is most important as any increase in size more than 10 mm is abnormal and raises the possibility of pinealoma.

Habenular commissure calcification has a characteristic appearance and is seen as a C-shaped structure open posteriorly. It lies above and anterior to pineal gland. Choroid plexus calcification is generally bilateral and may be unequal on the two sides. Other normal sites of calcification are the falx and anterior petroclinoid ligaments above the sella.

Tuberous sclerosis is a syndrome comprised of epilepsy, mental retardation and adenoma sebaceum. Multiple hamartomas occur in the brain as well as at other sites such as kidneys. Tumors consist of glial tissue and ganglion cells. In the brain they are usually multiple and are seen in the subcortical, subependymal and basal ganglia regions. Calcification is seen in 50% of the lesions **(Fig. 28)**.

Sturge-Weber syndrome is another important cause of intracranial calcification. Patients present with epilepsy and mental retardation and often have cutaneous hemangioma in the distribution of trigeminal nerve on the same side as calcification. Calcification has a typical tram-track appearance and is seen in the cerebral cortex **(Figs. 29A and B)**.

Basal ganglia calcification is an important feature of hypoparathyroidism and pseudohypoparathyroidism. Widespread irregular and punctate areas of calcification, which are diffusely scattered, are characteristic of Fahr's disease. In this condition, patients present with severe growth and mental retardation. The disease is hereditary and is characterized by microscopic deposits of iron and calcium in the basal ganglia, cerebellum and subcortical region. Infections due to toxoplasma and cytomegalovirus are important causes of intracranial calcification in the newborn. Calcifications are multiple and diffusely

Table 4: Skull vault sclerotic areas.

Generalized sclerosis	*Localized sclerosis*
• Paget's disease	• Metastasis
• Sclerotic metastasis	• Paget's disease
• Fibrous dysplasia	• Fibrous dysplasia
• Renal osteodystrophy	• Hyperostosis frontalis interna
• Myelofibrosis	• Meningioma
• Chronic hemolytic anemia	• Calcified hematoma
• Bone dysplasias e.g. osteopetrosis, pyknodystosis	
• Prolonged phenytoin treatment	
• Acromegaly	
• Fluorosis	

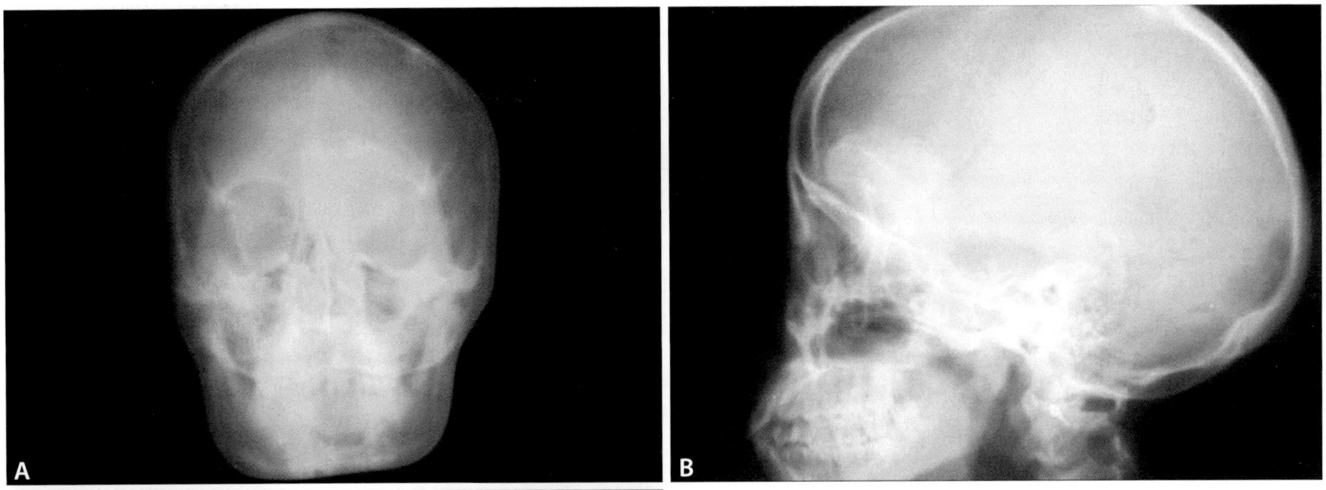

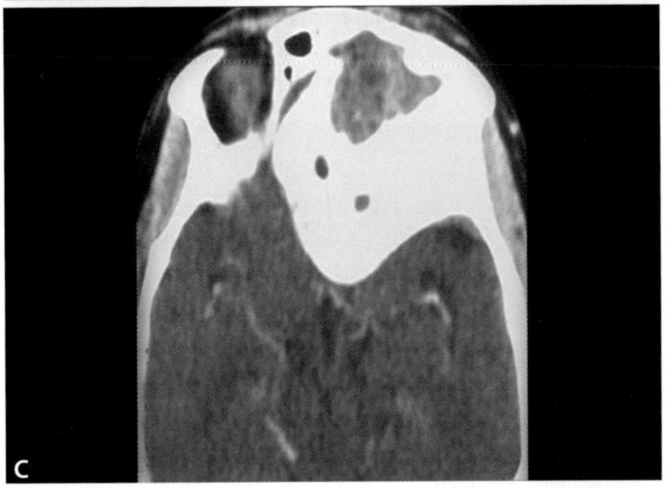

Figs. 22A to C: Fibrous dysplasia. (A) Frontal and (B) lateral views of skull reveal sclerotic lesion involving the frontal bone. The frontal sinus is opaque; (C) Axial computed tomography (CT) scan in the same patient shows expanded sclerotic frontal bone.

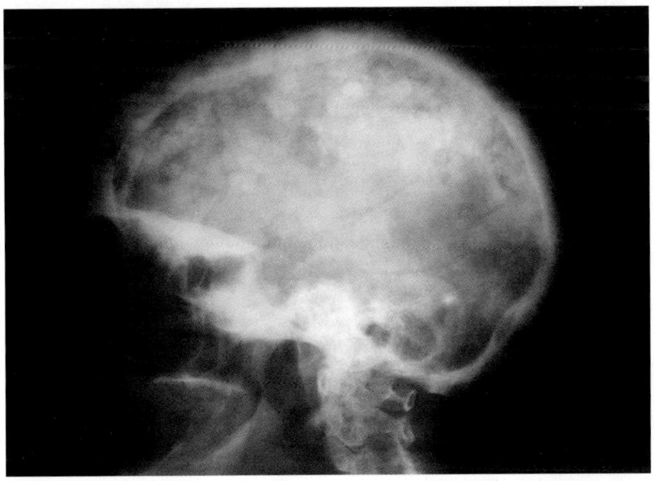

Fig. 23: Paget's disease. Lateral view of skull reveals focal areas of opacities in previous areas of osteoporosis giving "cotton-wool" appearance.

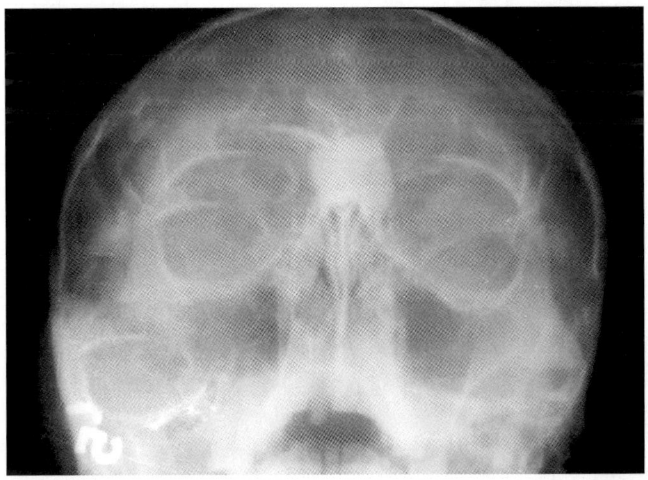

Fig. 24: Osteoma. Waters' view of skull shows osteoma of the frontal sinus.

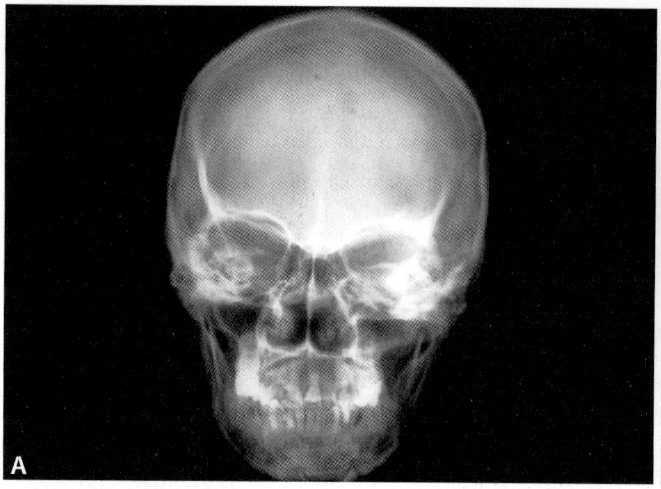

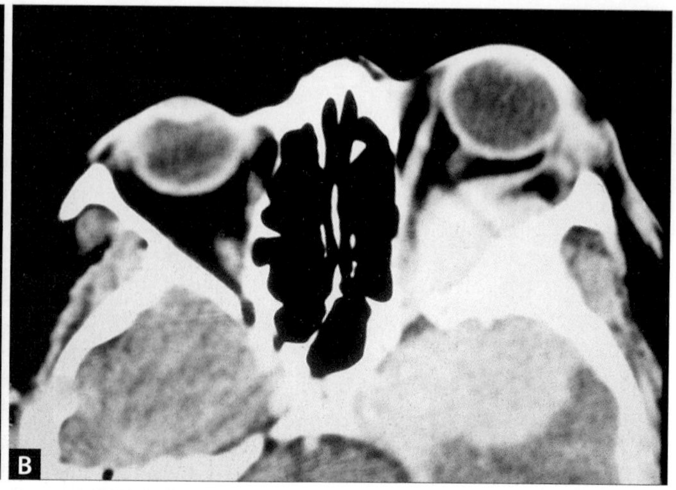

Figs. 25A and B: Sphenoid wing meningioma. (A) Posteroanterior (PA) view of skull shows hyperostosis of the left lesser and greater wings of the sphenoid bone typical of meningioma; (B) Contrast enhanced computed tomography (CT) scan in the same patient shows proptosis and hyperostosis of sphenoid wings with enhancing extradural mass due to meningioma on the left side.

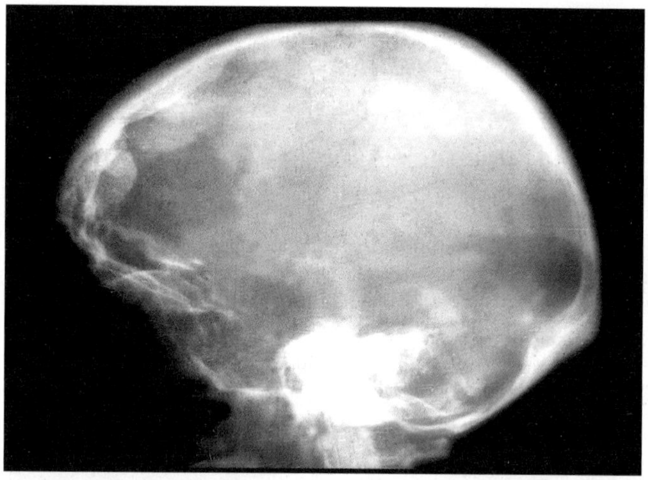

Fig. 26: Hyperostosis frontalis interna. Lateral skull radiograph shows irregular thickening of the frontal bone in an elderly female. The inner table is involved more than the outer table with sparing of diploic spaces.

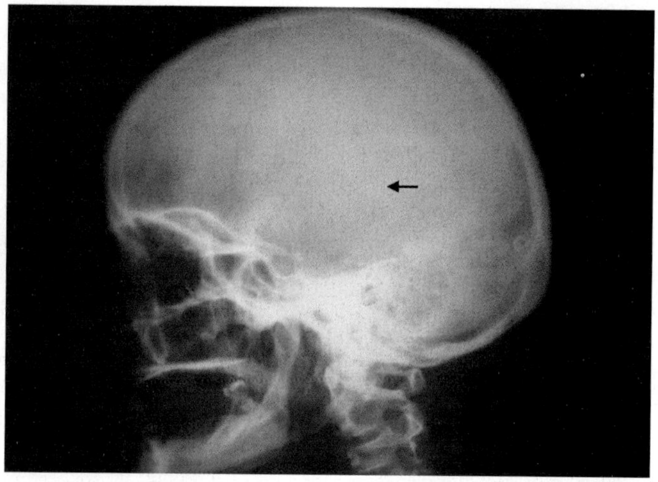

Fig. 27: Lateral view skull shows pineal gland calcification (arrow).

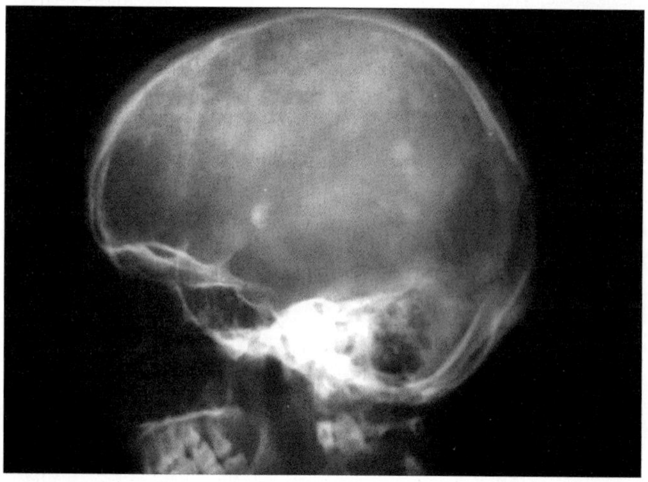

Fig. 28: Tuberous sclerosis. X-ray skull lateral view showing multiple calcified lesions.

Table 5: Causes of intracranial calcification.

Normal intracranial calcification/variants	***Abnormal intracranial calcification***
• Pineal • Habenular commissure • Basal ganglia • Dentate • Parasellar ligament • Arachnoid granulations • Choroid plexus • Dura	*Familial conditions:* • Tuberous sclerosis • Sturge-Weber syndrome • Idiopathic familial cerebrovascular calcinosis (Fahr's disease)
	Metabolic causes: • Hypoparathyroidism • Pseudohypoparathyroidism
	Inflammatory diseases: • Cytomegalic inclusion disease • Toxoplasmosis • Rubella • Abscess
	Vascular causes: • Arteriovenous malformation • Intracerebral hematoma • Subdural hematoma
	Neoplasms: • Craniopharyngioma • Astrocytomas • Oligodendrogliomas • Pinealoma

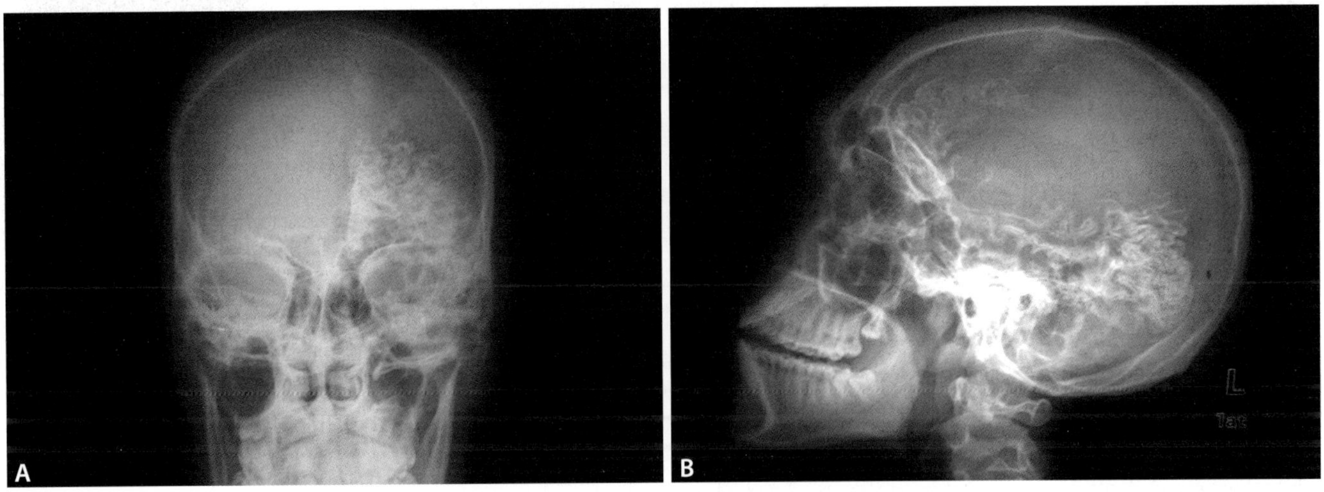

Figs. 29A and B: Sturge-Weber syndrome. (A) Posteroanterior (PA) and (B) lateral view of the skull shows gyriform calcification on the left side.

scattered in the brain parenchyma or paraventricular region. Bacterial infections may progress to cerebral abscess, which may get calcified.

Arteriovenous malformations calcify in 2–25% of all affected patients. Typically, calcification is in the form of an incomplete ring but may be nodular or amorphous. A large arc like calcification seen in the region of pineal gland in a newborn presenting with congestive heart failure and hydrocephalus is characteristic of vein of Galen aneurysm. Intracerebral or chronic subdural hematomas may reveal curvilinear calcification. A variety of tumors may show calcification. In children, suprasellar craniopharyngioma is the most common tumor, which reveals calcification whereas in adults oligodendrogliomas and meningiomas are the common tumors to calcify.

REFERENCES

1. Tress BM. The need for skull radiography in patients presenting for CT. Radiology. 1983;146(1):87-9.
2. Moseley I. Long-term effects of the introduction of noninvasive investigations in neuroradiology. Neuroradiology. 1988;30(3):193-200.

3. Rastogi SC, Barraclough BM. Skull radiography in patients with psychiatric illness. Br Med J. 1983;287(6401):1259.
4. Taveras JM. Anatomy and examination of skull. In: Interactive Review of Radiology. Lippincotts Williams and Wilkins, 1999.
5. Sanders R, MacEwen CJ, McCulloch AS. The value of skull radiography in ophthalmology. ActaRadiol. 1994;35(5): 429-33.
6. Baker HL Jr. The impact of computed tomography on neuroradiologic practice. Radiology. 1975;116(3):637-40.
7. Taveras JM. The skull. In: Taveras JM, Wood EH (Eds). Diagnostic Neuroradiology, 2nd edition. The Williams and Wilkins Company. 1986.pp.1-65.
8. Gerald B. Systematic radiographic evaluation of the abnormal skull. In: Rabinowitz JG (Ed). Pediatric Radiology. Philadelphia: JB Lippincott Company. 1978.pp.285-313.
9. Butler P, Jeffiree MA. The skull and brain. In: Butler P, Mitchell AWM, Ellis H (Eds). Applied Radiological Anatomy, 1st edition. Cambridge University Press. 2001.pp.17-60.
10. Kirmi O, J Lo S, Johnson D, et al. Craniosynostosis: aradiological and surgical perspective. Seminars in ULTRASOUND CT and MRI. 2009;30(6):492-512.
11. Baur-Melnyk A, Reiser M. Oncohaematologic disorders affecting the skeleton in the elderly. RadiolClin North Am. 2008;46(4):785-98.

CHAPTER 2

Normal Anatomy of Brain on CT and MRI

Paramjeet Singh

INTRODUCTION

An understanding of basic anatomy of the brain is vital to the planning and interpretation of neuroradiologic studies. Modern imaging techniques provide cross-sections of the brain similar to the dissected brain. Computerized tomography (CT) and magnetic resonance imaging (MRI) provides cross-sectional anatomy of the brain. Current MRI scanners and multidetector computerized tomography (MDCT) have expanded the scope of three-dimensional conceptualization of complex brain structures through multiplanar imaging and reconstructions from true volumetric data sets. Better tissue differentiation on MRI allows not only morphological, but also histological information to some extent. Recent advances in functional imaging and diffusion tensor imaging makes understanding of brain anatomy even more important. This chapter reviews the essentials of surface and cross-sectional anatomy of the brain as seen on CT and MRI.

TECHNIQUES AND NORMAL APPEARANCE

General Considerations

Noncontiguous axial CT sections are usually obtained at 15–20° angulation to the orbitomeatal line, while axial MRI sections are generally obtained parallel to it (along bicommissural plane or AC-PC line). MRI, owing to its multiplanar capability allows direct coronal and sagittal sections. However, MDCT scanners and newer MR techniques allow volumetric data acquisitions with reconstructions in desirable planes. T1- and T2-weighted (T1W and T2W) images are routinely obtained on MRI. The T1WI are excellent for showing anatomy while T2WI are highly sensitive in detecting brain pathology (details of MR sequences is beyond the scope of this chapter).

The white matter is hypodense to gray matter on CT. The cerebral white matter appears bright while the gray matter is relatively dark on T1WI. The relationship reverses as white matter becomes progressively darker on increasing the T2-weighting; the crossover occurring in the proton density images. The basal ganglia, red nucleus and putamen appear hypointense on T2WI due to their mineral contents.

The cerebrospinal fluid (CSF) shows low density on CT (0–15 HU) depending on its protein content. The CSF is hypointense on T1WI and extremely bright on T2WI due to its long T1 and T2 relaxation times. The CSF is in constant motion which may occasionally result in flow-related artifacts and loss of signal (flow void), classically seen in the region of cerebral aqueduct. The glomera of the choroid plexus within the lateral ventricles are seen as soft tissue density on CT and show homogeneous enhancement on contrast enhanced CT (CECT). On T2WI the choroid plexus appears heterogeneous due to the presence of calcification and cysts.

Visualization of blood vessels needs administration of iodinated contrast in CT. On MRI, major blood vessels are visualized without contrast administration and appear as flow voids on spin echo imaging or show flow-related enhancement on gradient echo imaging. Flow-related artifacts are often seen in phase encoding direction especially in long TR sequences and should not be mistaken for pathology. Familiarity with normal variations like dilated perivascular spaces is important. Modern MR imaging also provides a good understanding of white matter tracts through diffusion tensor imaging and functional areas of the brain through BOLD imaging.

Except for the intraorbital segment of the optic nerves, the remaining cranial nerves are usually not visualized on CT. On MR, using thin sections and fluid sensitive techniques like SPACE and CISS, the cisternal segments of most of the cranial nerves can be identified.

The inner meningeal layers are not normally visualized on noncontrast MRI and may show no or fine linear enhancement following contrast administration. Major dural folds like falx and tentorium appear hypointense on MRI and enhance after contrast administration along with the venous sinuses within them. Contrast-enhanced MR angiograms are increasingly used for demonstrating vascular anatomy.

The diploic space appears bright on T1WI due to its fat content and is outlined by the low signal intensity compact bones of the inner and outer tables of skull. CT better demonstrates the bony outlines. Similarly, it is superior to MR for visualization of intracranial calcification.

Normal Anatomy of Brain

Figure 1 shows the major subdivisions of brain. Brain consists of three major components.

1. The forebrain (prosencephalon) comprised of two cerebral hemispheres (telencephalon) and thalamus and surrounding gray matter, epithalamus, hypothalamus and subthalamus (diencephalon).
2. The basal ganglia
3. The midbrain (mesencephalon)
4. The hindbrain (rhombencephalon) comprised of cerebellum and pons (metencephalon), and medulla oblongata (myelencephalon).

CEREBRAL HEMISPHERES

Cerebrum consists of two hemispheres which are partially connected with each other through corpus callosum. Each cerebral hemisphere has three borders superomedial, inferomedial and inferolateral. The superomedial border separates the superolateral and medial surfaces, the inferolateral border separates the superolateral and inferior surfaces, and the inferomedial border separates medial surface and inferior surface.

Lateral Surface of the Cerebral Hemisphere (Fig. 2A)

The two cerebral hemispheres are incompletely divided by the interhemispheric fissure. The sylvian fissure (lateral fissure) separates the temporal lobe from the frontal and parietal lobes. Its anterior horizontal and anterior ascending rami extend into the inferior frontal gyrus. The posterior ramus passes backward and upward terminating into ascending and descending rami. The central sulcus separates the frontal from the parietal lobe **(Fig. 3E)**. It originates slightly behind the midpoint between the frontal and occipital poles on the superomedial

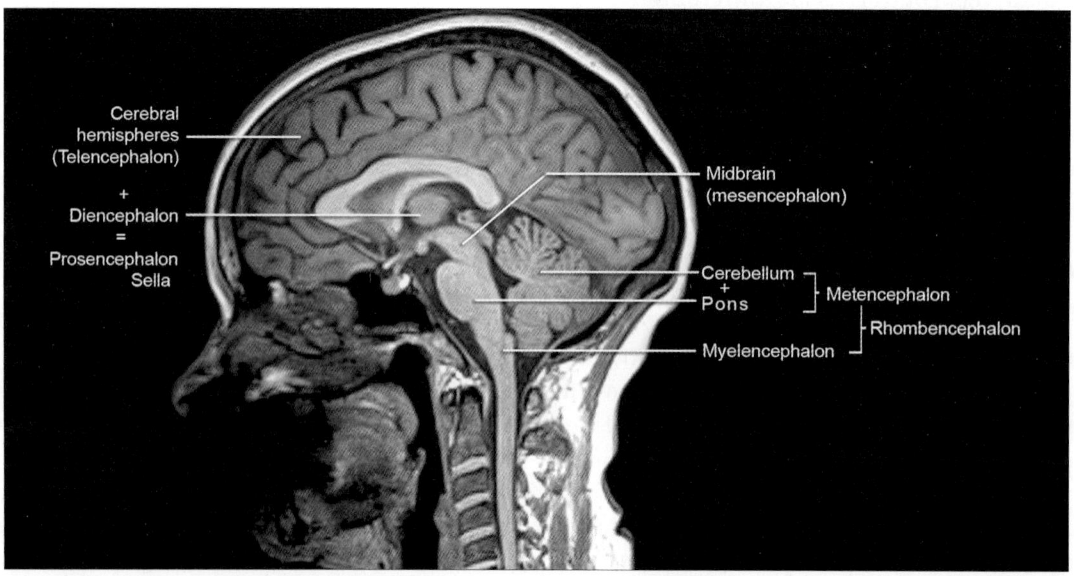

Fig. 1: Midline sagittal image of brain showing embryonal divisions.

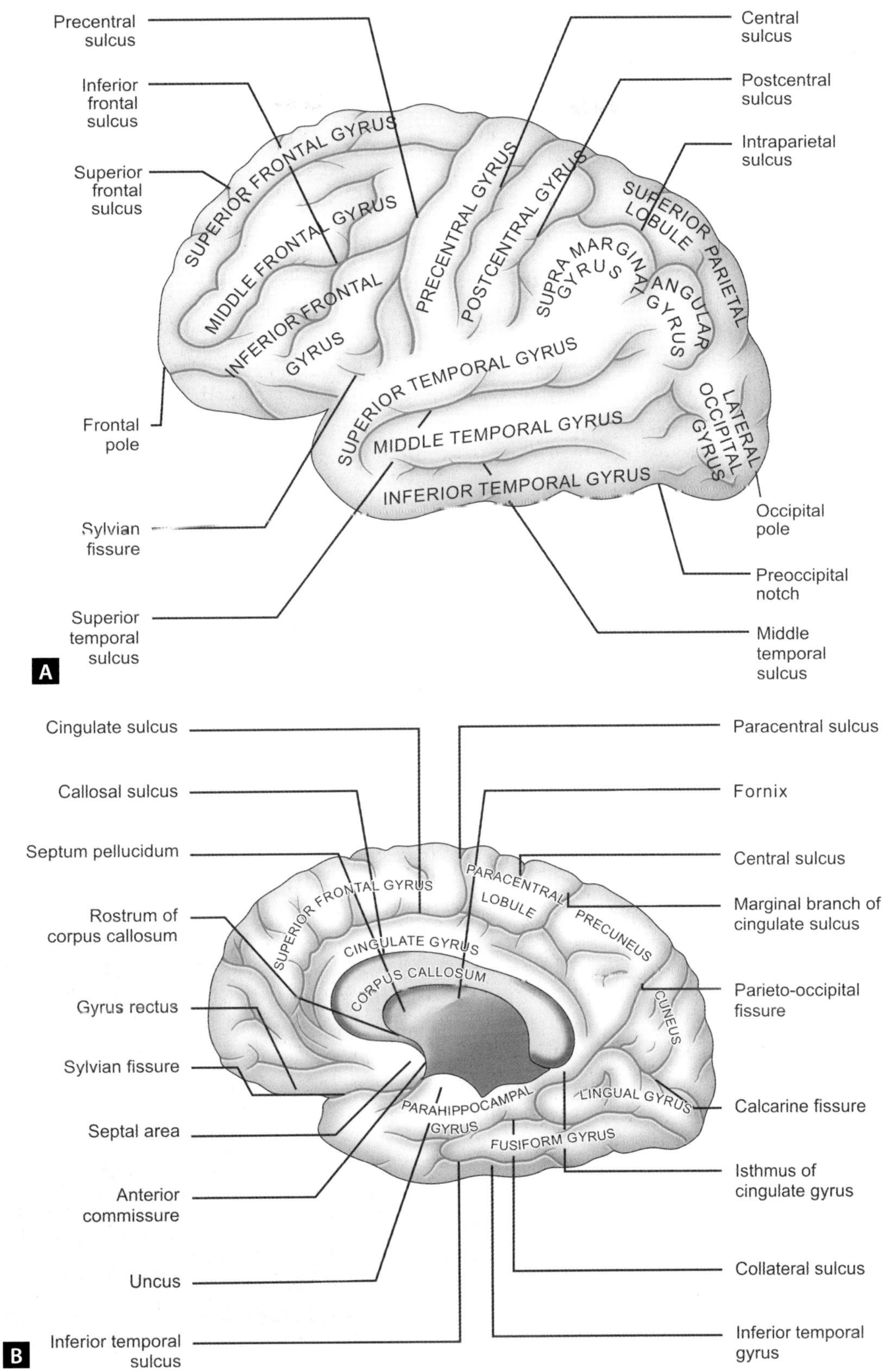
Precentral sulcus
Inferior frontal sulcus
Superior frontal sulcus
Frontal pole
Sylvian fissure
Superior temporal sulcus
A
Central sulcus
Postcentral sulcus
Intraparietal sulcus
Occipital pole
Preoccipital notch
Middle temporal sulcus
SUPERIOR FRONTAL GYRUS
MIDDLE FRONTAL GYRUS
INFERIOR FRONTAL GYRUS
PRECENTRAL GYRUS
POSTCENTRAL GYRUS
SUPRA MARGINAL GYRUS
SUPERIOR PARIETAL LOBULE
ANGULAR GYRUS
SUPERIOR TEMPORAL GYRUS
MIDDLE TEMPORAL GYRUS
INFERIOR TEMPORAL GYRUS
LATERAL OCCIPITAL GYRUS
Cingulate sulcus
Callosal sulcus
Septum pellucidum
Rostrum of corpus callosum
Gyrus rectus
Sylvian fissure
Septal area
Anterior commissure
Uncus
Inferior temporal sulcus
B
Paracentral sulcus
Fornix
Central sulcus
Marginal branch of cingulate sulcus
Parieto-occipital fissure
Calcarine fissure
Isthmus of cingulate gyrus
Collateral sulcus
Inferior temporal gyrus
SUPERIOR FRONTAL GYRUS
PARACENTRAL LOBULE
PRECUNEUS
CINGULATE GYRUS
CORPUS CALLOSUM
CUNEUS
LINGUAL GYRUS
PARAHIPPOCAMPAL GYRUS
FUSIFORM GYRUS

Figs. 2A and B

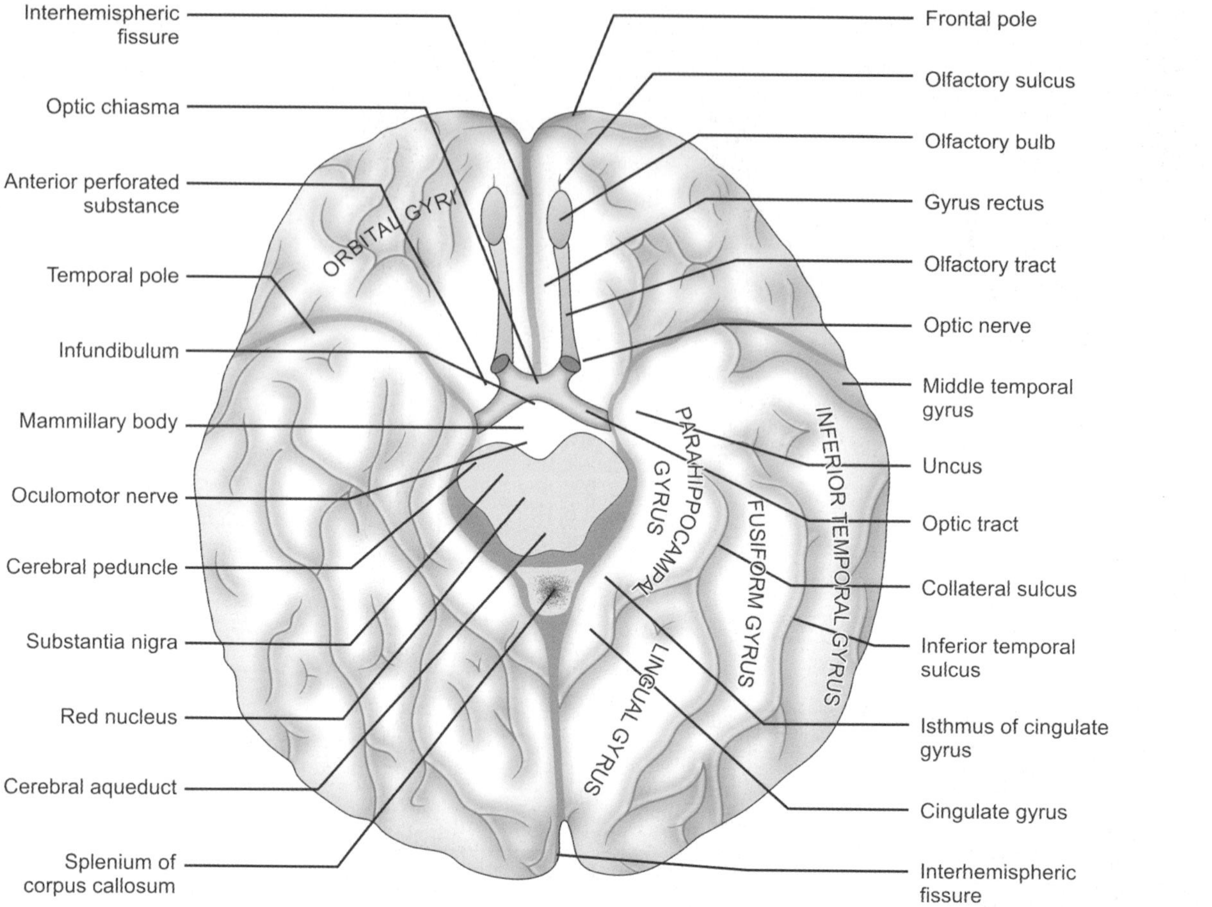

Fig. 2C

Figs. 2A to C: Diagrammatic representation showing anatomy of cerebral hemispheres on the (A) Lateral; (B) Medial; and (C) Inferior surface.

border and continues obliquely inferolaterally on the lateral surface. Various features on cross-sectional imaging identifying it are upper T or L sign (junction of superior frontal and precentral sulci), lower T sign (identifying inferior frontal sulcus and gyrus), Omega, Epsilon, and Sigmoidal hook signs (shapes of hand motor area or knob), U sign (subcentral gyrus bordering central sulcus inferolaterally), bracket sign (junction of marginal sulcus with interhemispheric fissure), etc. **(Fig. 6N)**.

The frontal lobe is bounded posteriorly by the precentral gyrus, which lies between the central and precentral sulci **(Fig. 3E)**. The precentral gyrus contains the primary motor area with inverse topographic representation of contralateral body parts. The superior frontal sulcus and inferior frontal sulcus divide the frontal lobe anterior to precentral gyrus into superior, middle and inferior gyri **(Figs. 3E, 3F, 5A, 5B, 6H and 5J)**. In front of the precentral gyrus is the premotor area, consisting of posterior part of the superior, middle and inferior frontal gyri. The Broca's

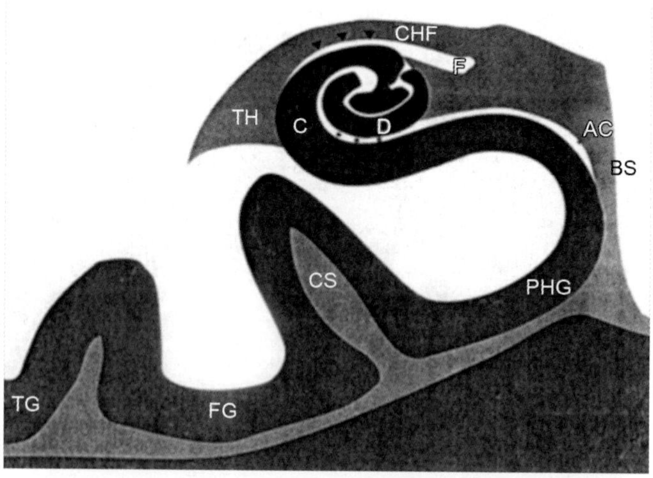

Fig. 2D: Line diagram and corresponding coronal T2 and inversion recovery images of right hippocampus.
Abbreviations: AC: Ambient cistern; BS: Brainstem; C: Cornu ammonis; CHF: Choroid fissure; CS: Collateral sulcus; D: Dentate gyrus; FG: Fusiform gyrus; F: Fimbria; TH: Temporal horn; TG: Inferior temporal gyrus; PHG: Parahippocampal gyrus.

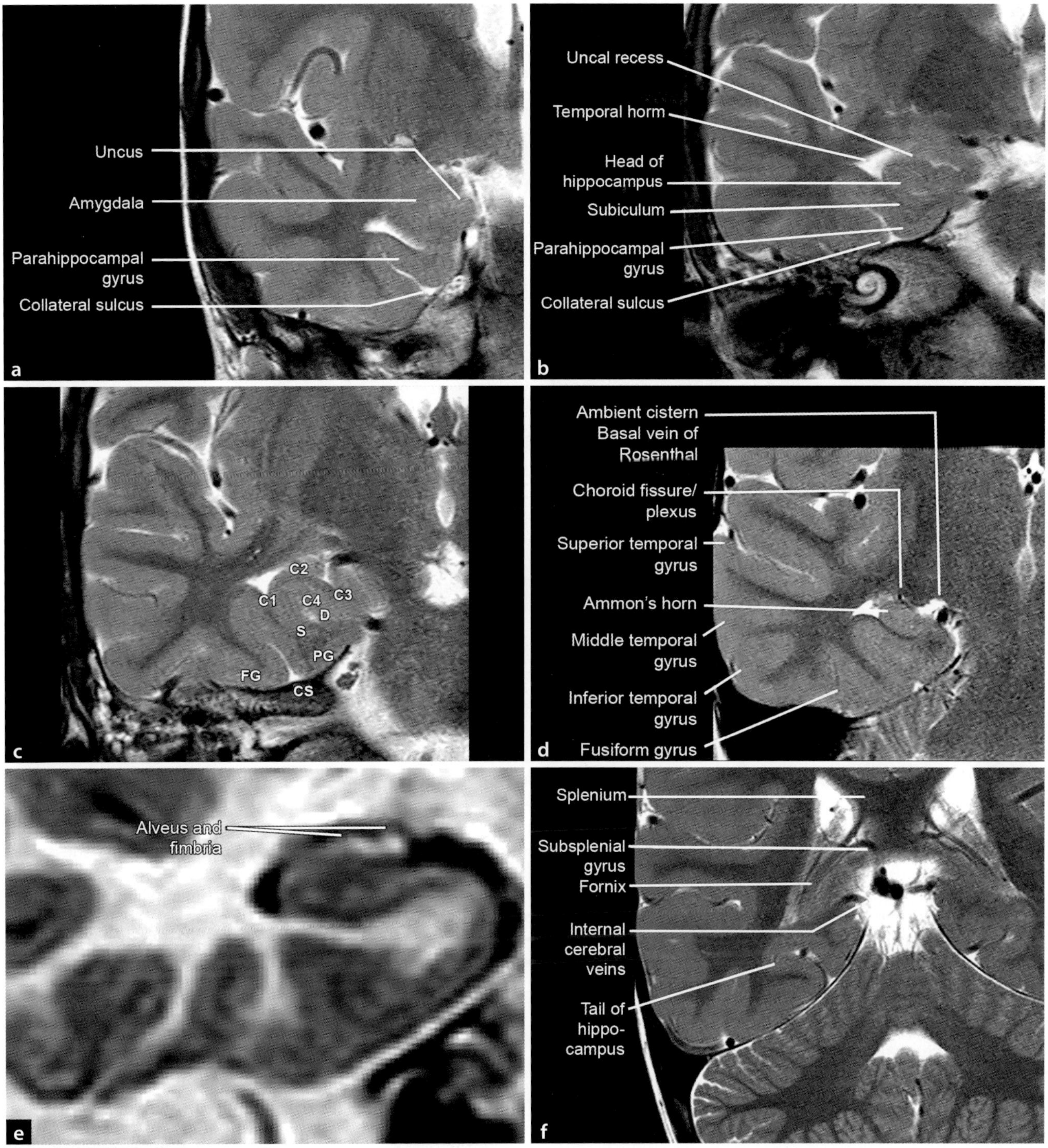

Fig. 2E (a to f): (a) At the level of amygdala; (b) At the level of head of hippocampus; (c) Internal anatomy of hippocampus. Sectors of Sommer C1 to C4; (d) At the level of body of hippocampus; (e) T1 image at the level of body of hippocampus; (f) Section at tail of hippocampus.
Abbreviations: G: Dentate gyrus; PG: Parahippocampal gyrus; CS: Collateral sulcus; FG: Fusiform gyrus.

area which is concerned with the motor mechanisms of speech also lies at the posterior part of the inferior frontal gyrus in the dominant lobe usually seen at the level of frontal horns on axial sections.

The convexity of the parietal lobe consists of the postcentral gyrus and the superior and inferior parietal lobules separated by the horizontally running intraparietal sulcus **(Figs. 3E and F)**. The postcentral gyrus is located

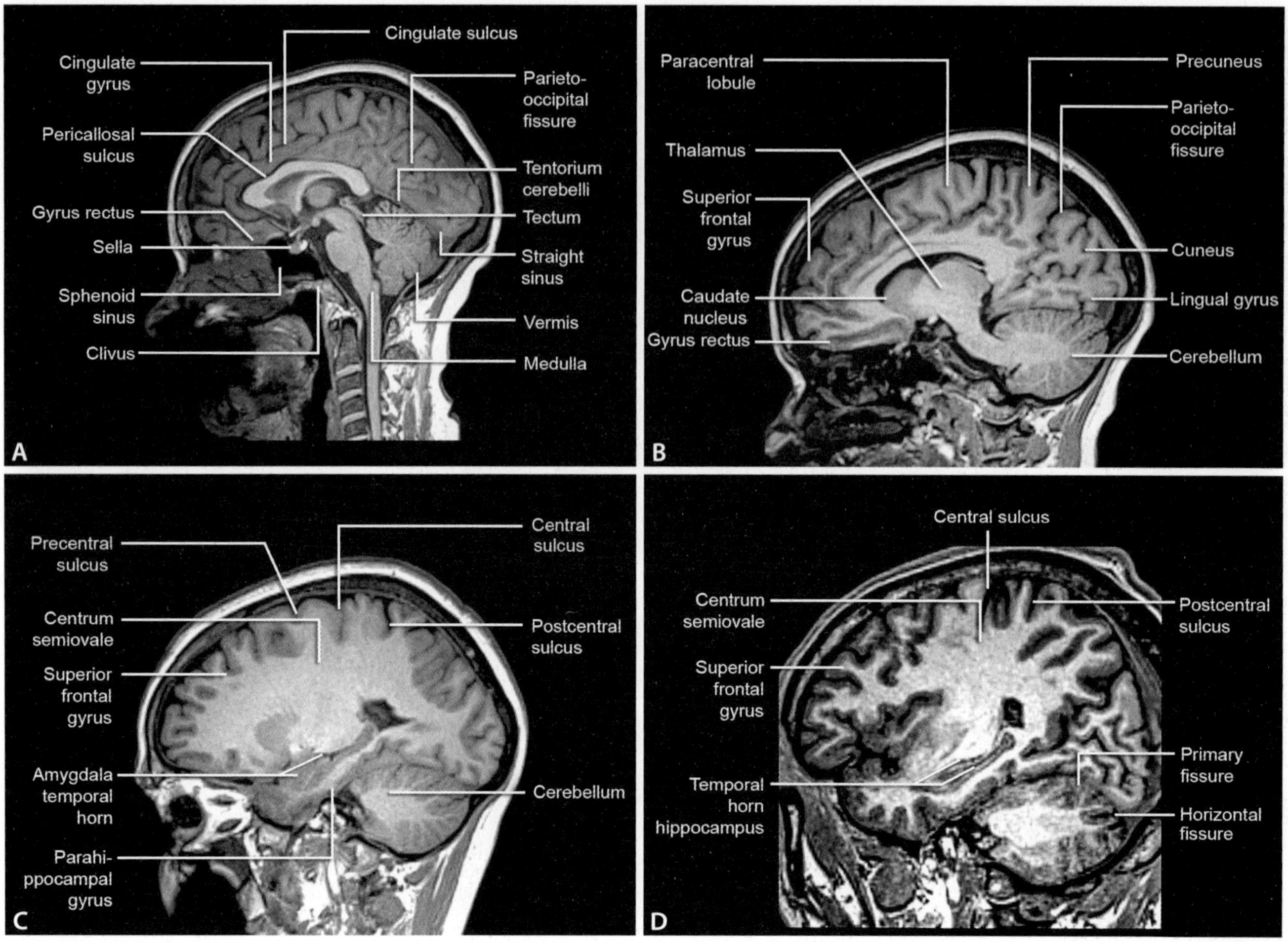

Figs. 3A to D: (A) Mid-sagittal MR section shows the entire length of the corpus callosum bordered above by the pericallosal sulcus. Cingulate gyrus and sulcus lie above it. The brainstem divisions, cerebellar vermis and the sellar/suprasellar anatomy are exquisitely shown on this section. The vein of Galen and straight sinus are seen behind the splenium leading to the torcula. A large rounded mass of gray matter within the 3rd ventricle represents interthalamic adhesion. The fornix is seen beneath the corpus callosum. The 3rd and 4th ventricles with the interconnecting aqueduct are well shown in this section. The tectal plate lies posterior to the aqueduct. The suprasellar cistern interpeduncular fossa, quadrigeminal plate cistern and cisterna magna are important cerebrospinal fluid (CSF) spaces identified in this section; (B to D) Parasagittal MR sections. The parieto-occipital fissure marks the boundary between parietal (precuneus) and occipital (cuneus) lobes. The calcarine fissure separates lingual gyrus from cuneus. The central, pre- and postcentral sulci and the related gyri can be followed. The parahippocampal gyrus can be seen following the temporal horn closely. The frontal lobe consists of superior and middle frontal gyri on these sections.

between the central and postcentral sulcus and contains the primary (somesthetic, tactile, thermal and kinesthetic) areas, with body representation corresponding to that in precentral gyrus. The inferior parietal lobule is further subdivided into the supramarginal and angular gyri, which are located around the terminal ascending ramus of the sylvian fissure and the superior temporal sulcus, respectively **(Fig. 3E)**. The temporal lobe is divided into superior, middle and inferior temporal gyri by two horizontally running sulci—the superior and middle temporal sulcus **(Fig. 3F)**. In the dominant cerebral hemisphere at the posterior portion of the superior temporal gyrus lies the Wernicke's area, linked with comprehension of language. A lesion of this area causes sensory aphasia. Another important area is the area for hearing—acoustic area, which is also located in the temporal lobe. It lies in that part of the superior temporal gyrus which forms the inferior wall of posterior ramus of lateral sulcus and is defined as the transverse temporal gyrus (Heschl's gyrus). This is best seen in the coronal sections.

The lateral surface of the occipital lobe consists of the lateral occipital gyri **(Fig. 5I)** (visual associative functions). The preoccipital notch indents the inferolateral border of

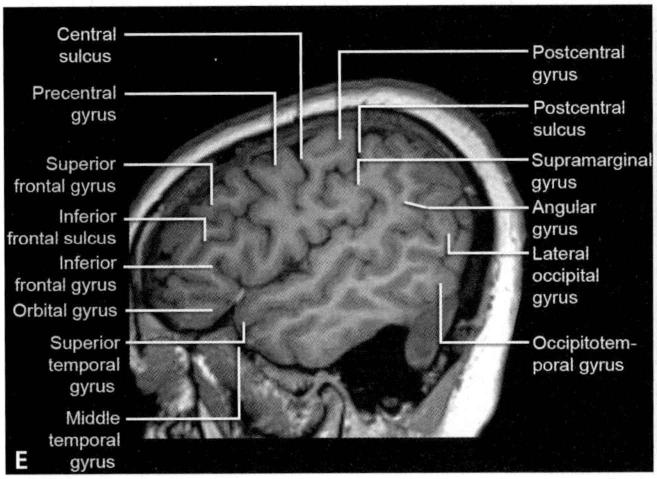

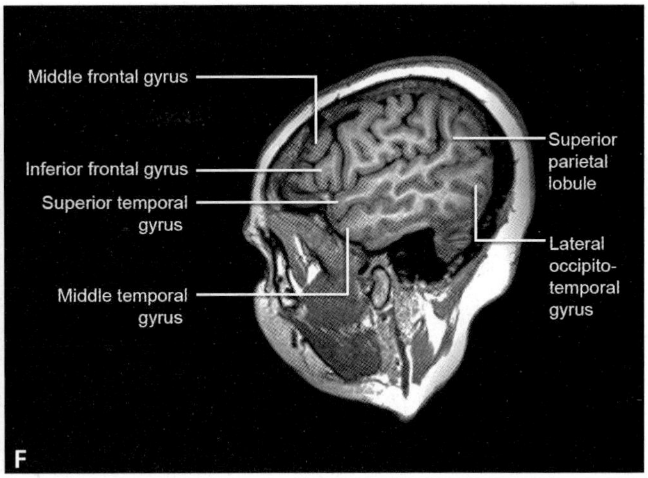

Figs. 3E and F: Sagittal MR sections at and lateral to Sylvian fissure. The Sylvian fissure can be traced anteriorly where its anterior ascending and horizontal rami form a V or Y configuration. These divide the inferior frontal gyrus into pars orbitalis, pars triangularis and pars opercularis giving it a characteristic M shape. Posteriorly the fissure ends in ascending and descending rami. The horse-shoe shaped supramarginal gyrus sits atop the ascending ramus. The middle frontal gyrus extends posteriorly to meet the precentral gyrus and the inferior frontal sulcus meets the obliquely coursing precentral sulcus. The central sulcus can be traced inferiorly to the subcentral gyrus. The superior and inferior temporal gyri are identified in the extreme lateral sections.

the hemisphere about 4 cm from the occipital pole. An imaginary line drawn from the superior end of the parieto-occipital fissure to the preoccipital notch marks the boundary between the occipital lobe and the parietal and temporal lobes. Insula (central lobe) is the part of cerebral cortex which lies in the depth of the lateral sulcus. It is formed by portions of the frontal, parietal and temporal lobes **(Figs. 5C and 6H)**.

Medial Surface of the Cerebral Hemisphere (Fig. 2B)

The corpus callosum is a large mass of nerve fibers which connect the cerebral hemispheres and forms most of the roof of the lateral ventricles. It is arbitrarily divided from front to back into rostrum, genu, body, and splenium **(Fig. 3A)**. The small anterior commissure ventral to the rostrum of the corpus callosum connects portions of the middle and inferior temporal gyri. The two lateral ventricles are separated by septum pellucidum **(Fig. 4C)** which extends from the inferior aspect of the body and genu of the corpus callosum to the superior aspect of the columns of the fornix **(Figs. 5C and D)**.

The callosal sulcus separates the corpus callosum from the cingulate gyrus. The cingulate sulcus separates the cingulate gyrus from the superior frontal gyrus anteriorly and the paracentral lobule posteriorly **(Figs. 3A and B)**. The central sulcus is deficient on medial surface and continuations of the precentral and postcentral gyri form the paracentral lobule on medial surface which is limited posteriorly by the marginal branch of the cingulate sulcus and anteriorly by the paracentral sulcus, a direct continuation of the precentral sulcus from the lateral surface. On the medial surface the parietal lobe (precuneus) is separated from the occipital lobe by parieto-occipital fissure **(Figs. 3B and C, 6J and K)**.

The calcarine fissure divides the medial surface of occipital lobe into the cuneus above and the lingual gyrus below **(Figs. 6H and I)**. The calcarine (primary visual) cortex, consisting of portions of the cuneate and lingual gyri lies along the banks of the calcarine fissure deep within the occipital lobe. At the inferolateral aspect of the occipital and temporal lobes lies the fusiform (lateral occipitotemporal) gyrus.

The limbic system is considered a separate lobe by some anatomists. Cingulate gyrus, parahippocampal gyrus, proper hippocampus, paraterminal gyrus and subcallosal area constitute the limbic system. Amygdala, although anatomically distinct, is functionally a part of limbic system. The cingulate gyrus lies above the corpus callosum and continues posteriorly behind the corpus callosum through the isthmus into the parahippocampal gyrus which is separated from the fusiform gyrus by the collateral sulcus. The uncus is the most anterior part of the parahippocampal gyrus which points medially and covers the amygdala which lies superior and anterior to head of hippocampus **[(Figs. 2E (a to f)]**.

Understanding of anatomy of hippocampus is important to interpret the MR findings in hippocampal

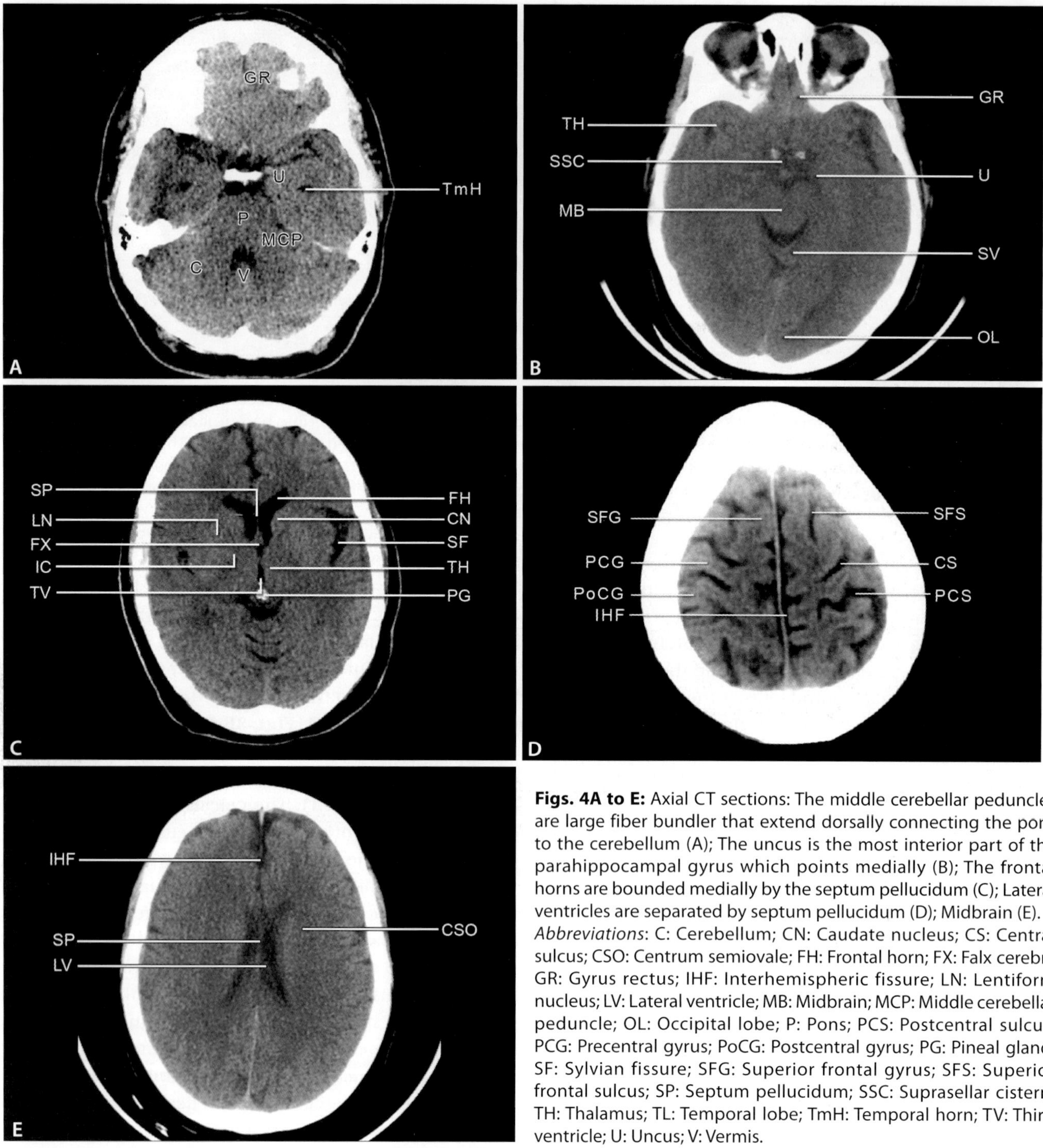

Figs. 4A to E: Axial CT sections: The middle cerebellar peduncles are large fiber bundler that extend dorsally connecting the pons to the cerebellum (A); The uncus is the most interior part of the parahippocampal gyrus which points medially (B); The frontal horns are bounded medially by the septum pellucidum (C); Lateral ventricles are separated by septum pellucidum (D); Midbrain (E).
Abbreviations: C: Cerebellum; CN: Caudate nucleus; CS: Central sulcus; CSO: Centrum semiovale; FH: Frontal horn; FX: Falx cerebri; GR: Gyrus rectus; IHF: Interhemispheric fissure; LN: Lentiform nucleus; LV: Lateral ventricle; MB: Midbrain; MCP: Middle cerebellar peduncle; OL: Occipital lobe; P: Pons; PCS: Postcentral sulcus; PCG: Precentral gyrus; PoCG: Postcentral gyrus; PG: Pineal gland; SF: Sylvian fissure; SFG: Superior frontal gyrus; SFS: Superior frontal sulcus; SP: Septum pellucidum; SSC: Suprasellar cistern; TH: Thalamus; TL: Temporal lobe; TmH: Temporal horn; TV: Third ventricle; U: Uncus; V: Vermis.

sclerosis in epilepsy. Hippocampus is located on the medial aspect of temporal lobe, superior to the parahippocampal gyrus, bounded superolaterally by the floor of the temporal horn of lateral ventricle. Anteroposteriorly hippocampus is divided into head, body and tail. It is composed of two interlocking U-shaped lamina of gray matter called cornu ammonis and dentate gyrus. The hippocampal fissure separates the subiculum (the superior flat part of parahippocampal gyrus) from the dentate gyrus. Cornu ammonis is connected with gray matter of parahippocampal gyrus through subiculum. The cornu ammonis (Ammon's horn) consists of C1, C2,

C3 and C4 sectors of Sommer. White matter tracts extend from cornu ammonis to alveus which lie on the superior surface of hippocampus and converge medially to form fimbria, which in turn is continuous with crus of fornix. Choroid fissure lies superomedial to hippocampus and the ambient cistern lies medially **(Fig. 2D)**.

Inferior Surface of the Cerebral Hemisphere (Fig. 2C)

The lingual and fusiform gyri course through this areas separated by collateral sulcus. The inferior temporal sulcus separates the inferior temporal gyrus from the fusiform gyrus **(Figs. 5I and J)**.

The inferior aspects of the occipital lobe and the temporal lobe sit over the tentorium of the cerebellum.

Olfactory nerve (CN I) originates from nasal mucosa and pierces cribriform plate to enter the cranium. On the inferior (orbital) surface of frontal lobe the olfactory bulb and the olfactory tract over lie the olfactory sulcus which runs in the anteroposterior direction. Area medial to this is called gyrus rectus. Area lateral to olfactory sulcus is divided into four parts by a H-shaped sulcus into anterior, posterior, medial and lateral orbital gyri **(Figs. 5A and B)**.

Optic nerves (CN II) extend from optic disc to optic chiasma and continues posteriorly as optic tracts leading to lateral geniculate body, pretectal nucleus and superior colliculus.

DIENCEPHALON

The diencephalon connects the cerebral hemispheres to the mid brain and is made of thalamus, hypothalamus, subthalamus and epithalamus. The hypothalamus lies within the floor and lateral walls of the third ventricle. It extends from the lamina terminalis anteriorly to the caudal aspect of the mammillary bodies and includes the tuber cinereum which gives rise to the pituitary stalk **(Fig. 6F)**.

Each thalamus is a large mass of gray matter in the lateral wall of the 3rd ventricle. It is bounded laterally by the posterior limb of the internal capsule and ventrally by the hypothalamic sulcus **(Fig. 6G)**. The interthalamic adhesion projecting through the 3rd ventricle forms a medial connection with the opposite thalamus. The dorsolateral margin of the thalamus forms part of the floor of the lateral ventricle. The posterior bulging portion of the thalamus is called the pulvinar **(Fig. 5F)**. It overhangs medial and lateral geniculate bodies.

Ventral to the pulvinar lie the medial and lateral geniculate bodies on each side of midbrain, together called the metathalamus. They relay auditory and visual information to their respective receptor areas of cortex. The subthalamus is bounded by the hypothalamus anteriorly, the internal capsule laterally, and the thalamus above. The subthalamic nucleus integrates and relays connections from the globus pallidus and the thalamus.

The most dorsal division of the diencephalon, the epithalamus, includes the habenular nuclei, posterior commissure and pineal body. The structure is a part of limbic system.

MIDBRAIN AND BRAINSTEM (PONS AND MEDULLA (FIG. 3A)

The midbrain consists of a smaller dorsal portion the tectum and larger ventral portion, the cerebral peduncles **(Fig. 6F)**. Aqueduct connecting the 3rd and 4th ventricles runs in the center of the junction of the tectum and cerebral peduncles **(Fig. 3A)**. Each cerebral peduncle has a ventral part—the crus and a dorsal part—the tegmentum, separated by substantia nigra. The red nucleus, another pigmented nucleus is located posterior and medial to the substantia nigra on each side. Pars compacta separates the substantia nigra and red nucleus **(Fig. 6L)**. The tectum consists of four rounded prominences—the two superior colliculi and two inferior colliculi or corpora quadrigemina. Each superior colliculus is connected to the *ipsilateral lateral* geniculate body through the superior brachium, where the optic tract ends. Similarly, the inferior colliculi are connected to the medial geniculate bodies through the inferior brachium thereby connecting it to the auditory cortex **(Fig. 6F)**.

The oculomotor nerves (CN III) exit from the caudal aspect of the interpeduncular fossa **(Fig. 7A)**. The paired trochlear nerves (CN IV) emerge from the dorsal surface of the brainstem caudal to the inferior colliculi, and wrap around the lateral aspects of the midbrain. The ventral and dorsal aspects of the cerebral peduncles are separated by semilunar substantia nigra with red nuclei on its dorsomedial aspect **(Fig. 6L)**.

The pons has a bulging ventral surface with a shallow midline basal sulcus. The middle cerebellar peduncles are large fiber bundles that extend dorsally connecting the pons to the cerebellum **(Fig. 4A)**. Emerging from the lateral aspect of the pons are the trigeminal nerves (CN V) **(Figs. 6D, 7B)**, while the paired paramedian abducens nerves (CN VI) exit ventrally from the pontomedullary junction. The facial nerves (CN VII) and the vestibulocochlear nerves (V III) emerge from the lateral aspect of the pontomedullary junction and pass through the cerebellopontine angle cistern **(Fig. 7C)**.

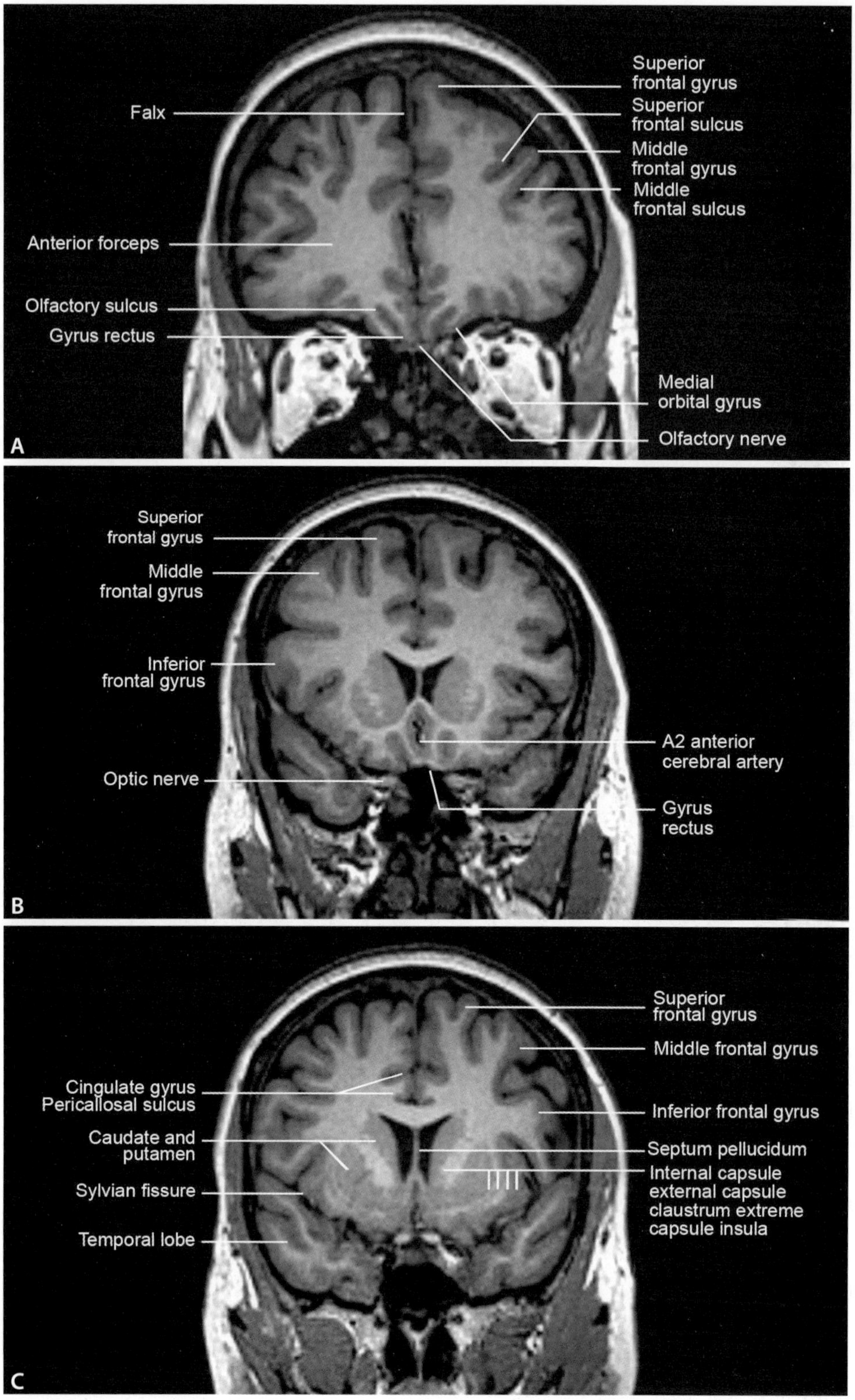
Falx
Superior frontal gyrus
Superior frontal sulcus
Middle frontal gyrus
Middle frontal sulcus
Anterior forceps
Olfactory sulcus
Gyrus rectus
Medial orbital gyrus
Olfactory nerve
A
Superior frontal gyrus
Middle frontal gyrus
Inferior frontal gyrus
A2 anterior cerebral artery
Optic nerve
Gyrus rectus
B
Superior frontal gyrus
Middle frontal gyrus
Cingulate gyrus
Pericallosal sulcus
Inferior frontal gyrus
Caudate and putamen
Septum pellucidum
Internal capsule external capsule claustrum extreme capsule insula
Sylvian fissure
Temporal lobe
C

Figs. 5A to C

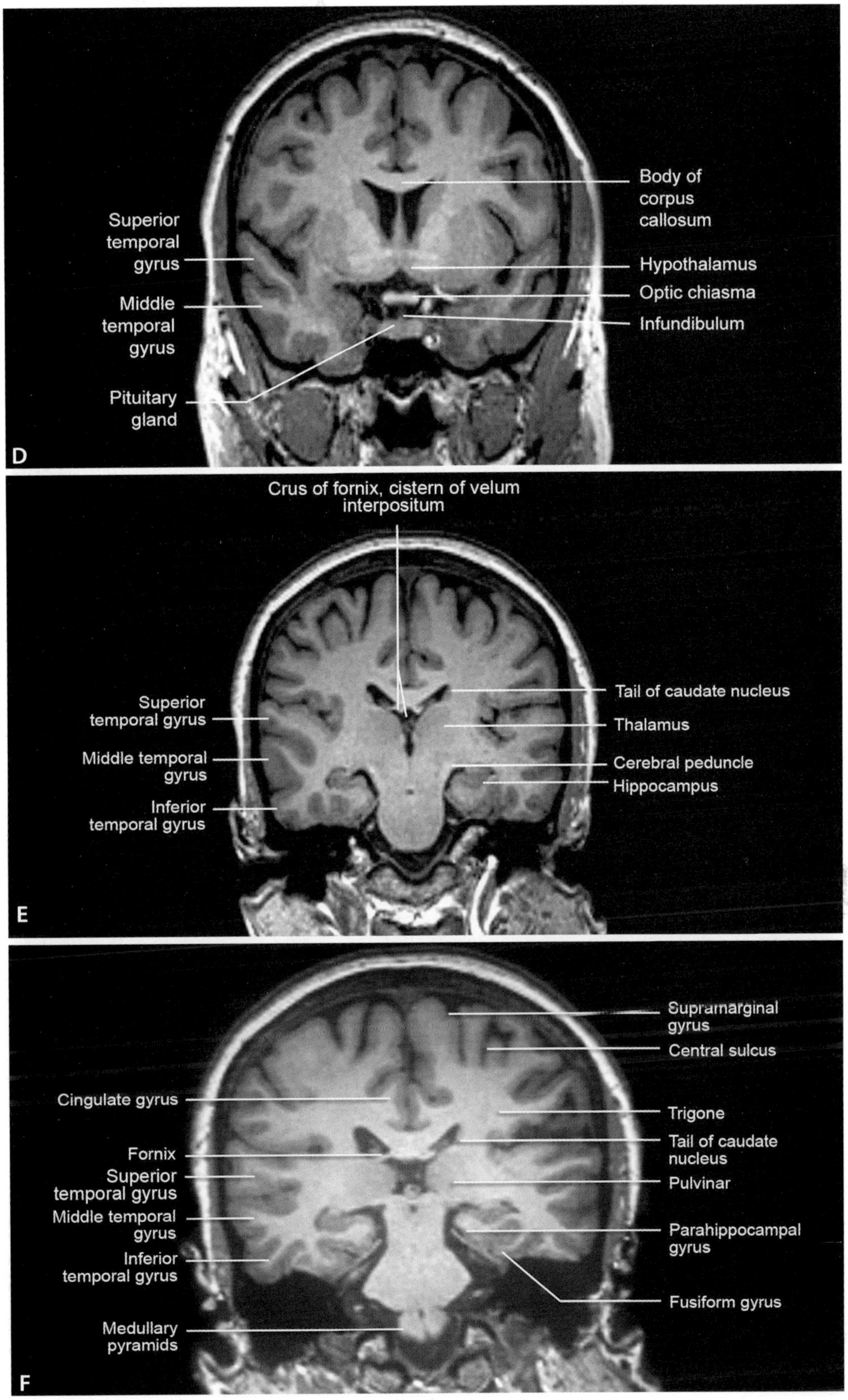
Superior temporal gyrus
Middle temporal gyrus
Pituitary gland
Body of corpus callosum
Hypothalamus
Optic chiasma
Infundibulum
D
Crus of fornix, cistern of velum interpositum
Superior temporal gyrus
Middle temporal gyrus
Inferior temporal gyrus
Tail of caudate nucleus
Thalamus
Cerebral peduncle
Hippocampus
E
Cingulate gyrus
Fornix
Superior temporal gyrus
Middle temporal gyrus
Inferior temporal gyrus
Medullary pyramids
Supramarginal gyrus
Central sulcus
Trigone
Tail of caudate nucleus
Pulvinar
Parahippocampal gyrus
Fusiform gyrus
F

Figs. 5D to F

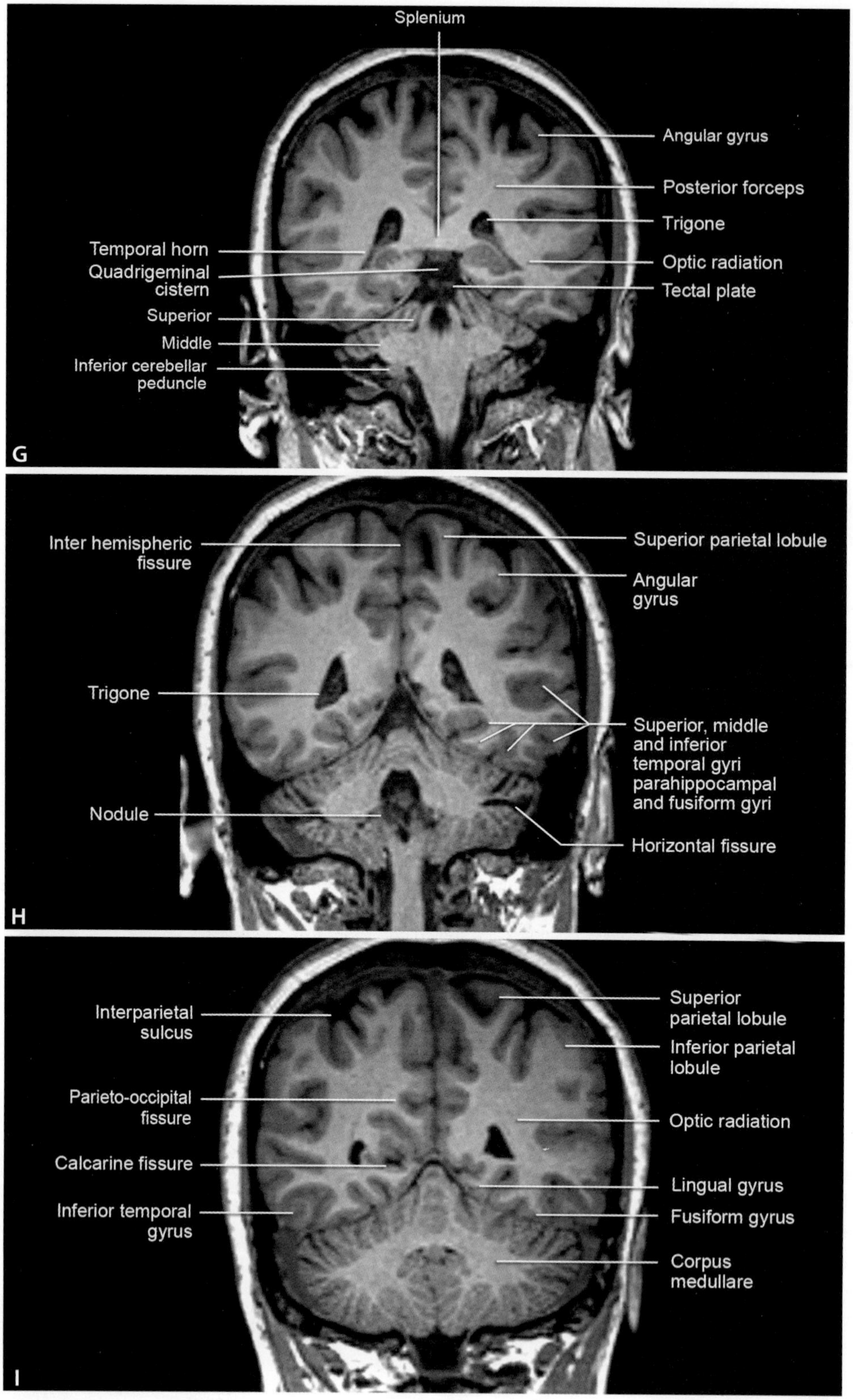
Splenium
Angular gyrus
Posterior forceps
Trigone
Optic radiation
Tectal plate
Temporal horn
Quadrigeminal cistern
Superior
Middle
Inferior cerebellar peduncle
G
Inter hemispheric fissure
Superior parietal lobule
Angular gyrus
Trigone
Superior, middle and inferior temporal gyri parahippocampal and fusiform gyri
Nodule
Horizontal fissure
H
Interparietal sulcus
Superior parietal lobule
Inferior parietal lobule
Parieto-occipital fissure
Optic radiation
Calcarine fissure
Lingual gyrus
Inferior temporal gyrus
Fusiform gyrus
Corpus medullare
I

Figs. 5G to I

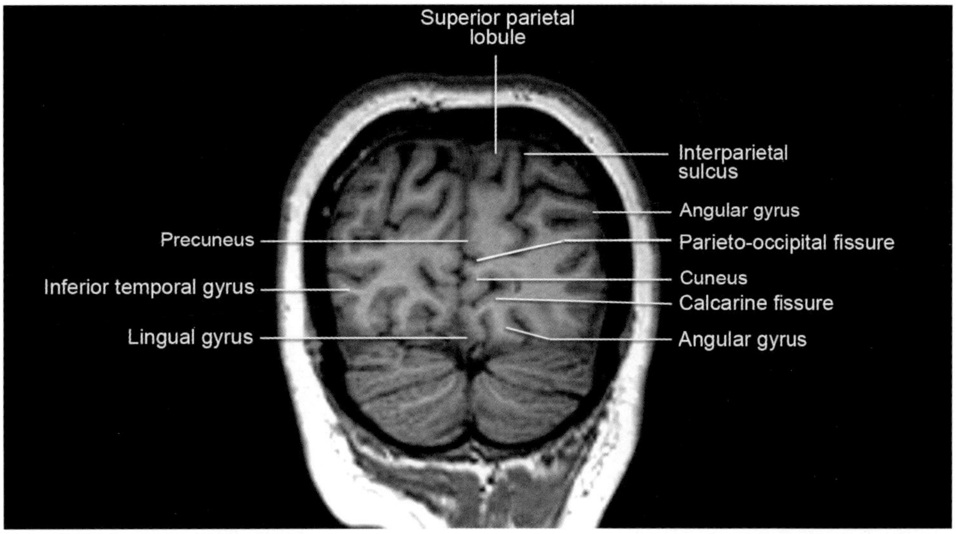

Fig. 5J

Figs. 5A to J: (A and B) Coronal MR sections anterior to the frontal horn. The entire slice contains frontal lobe. The olfactory nerve nestles between the gyrus rectus and medial orbital gyrus on the cribriform plate. (A) The more anterior section shows a continuous interhemispheric fissure which is interrupted by corpus callosum on the more posterior section. (B) The optic strut separates the optic nerve from superior orbital fissure; (C and D) Coronal MR sections through the frontal horn. The frontal horns are outlined by corpus callosum and caudate nucleus. The internal capsule, putamen, external capsule, claustrum and insula can be seen from medial to lateral. The two columns of fornix outline the foramen of Monro with septum pellucidum above it separating the two frontal horns. Optic chiasma can be identified above the pituitary gland and its infundibulum. In the parasellar area, the cavernous sinuses containing third, fourth, fifth and sixth nerves are outlined by low intensity dura; (E) Coronal MR sections at the third ventricle level. Mid third of the lateral convexity is parietal lobe and lower third is temporal lobe. Corpus callosum lies at the bottom of the interhemispheric fissure. The lateral ventricles (with crus fornix on its superior medial part) and third ventricle are seen more inferiorly. The interpeduncular fossa is seen as a CSF space below third ventricle. The tail of caudate nucleus lies on the lateral aspect of lateral ventricle. The medial temporal lobe consists of hippocampus with overlying choroid fissure; (F) Coronal MR sections through the body of lateral ventricle. This section cut through the splenium of corpus callosum with the cingulate gyrus lying just above it. Below it lie the quadrigeminal plate (tectum) and its cistern. The sections pass through the mid brain, pons and medulla. The lateral convexity consists entirely of parietal and temporal lobes; (G and H) Coronal MR sections through the trigone and occipital horns. Superior two-thirds of the lateral convexity of brain at this level consists of superior and inferior parietal lobules. The lower third belongs to the temporal lobe. The inferior surface of temporal lobe consists of parahippocampal, fusiform and inferior temporal gyri; (G) The section through trigones cuts the cerebellar peduncles while; (H) A more posterior section shows the cerebellar hemispheres, vermis and the tonsils; (I and J) Coronal MR sections posterior to the occipital horn. The interhemispheric fissure completely divides the two cerebral hemispheres. The lingual, fusiform and inferior temporal gyri are clearly identified. The precuneus and cuneus are separated by parieto-occipital fissure and between the cuneus and lingual gyrus lies the calcarine fissure.

The medulla oblongata connects the midbrain and the spinal cord. It measures 3 cm in length and 2 cm in width. On the ventral aspect of the medulla the paramedian pyramids form longitudinal protrusions on each side of the ventral median fissure. The paired ventrolateral sulci separate the medullary pyramids and the inferior olives **(Fig. 6A)**. The hypoglossal nerves (CN XII) emerge from the ventrolateral sulci. The rootlets of the glossopharyngeal (CN IX), vagus (CN X) and spinal accessory (CN XI) nerves exit from the dorsolateral sulcus which is located further laterally **(Fig. 7D)**. The paired cuneate and gracilis tubercles form longitudinal ridges on the dorsal aspect of the medulla oblongata just caudal to the fourth ventricles separated by posterior median sulcus.

CEREBELLUM

The cerebellum lies posterior to the pons and medulla. The superior, middle, and inferior cerebellar peduncles connect the cerebellum to midbrain, pons and medulla respectively. The narrowest leaf-like subdivisions of the cerebellar cortex are termed folia. The cerebellum consists of the midline cerebellar vermis connecting the paired lateral hemispheres. The hemisphere is divided into anterior lobe, middle lobe and flocculonodular lobe by deep fissures named primary fissure and posterolateral fissure **(Figs. 3D and 5H)**. A deep horizontal fissure divides it into superior and inferior halves. Caudal to the inferior vermis and between the cerebellar tonsils is the vallecula **(Fig. 6A)** which communicates with the fourth ventricle

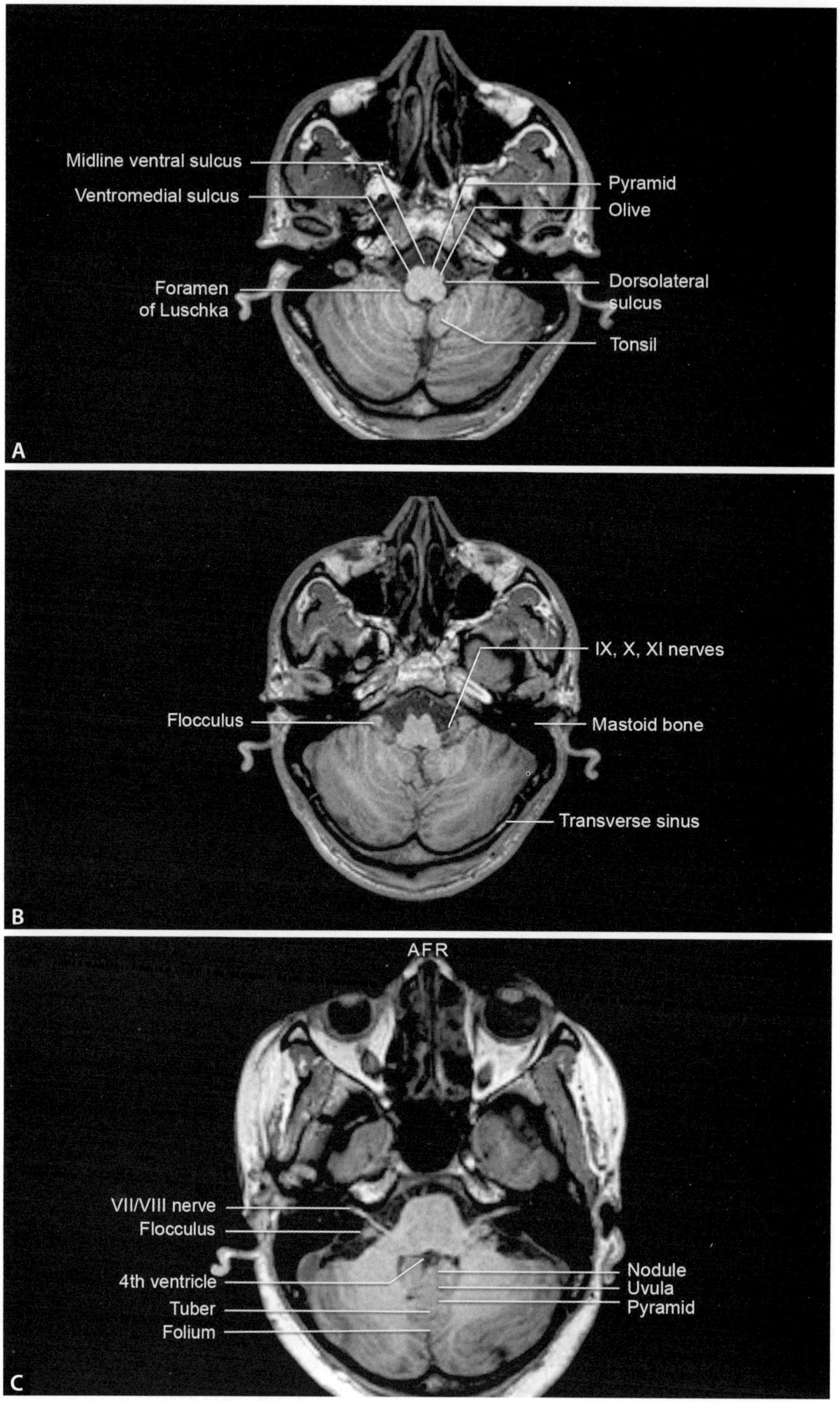
Midline ventral sulcus
Ventromedial sulcus
Foramen of Luschka
Pyramid
Olive
Dorsolateral sulcus
Tonsil
A
Flocculus
IX, X, XI nerves
Mastoid bone
Transverse sinus
B
AFR
VII/VIII nerve
Flocculus
4th ventricle
Tuber
Folium
Nodule
Uvula
Pyramid
C

Figs. 6A to C

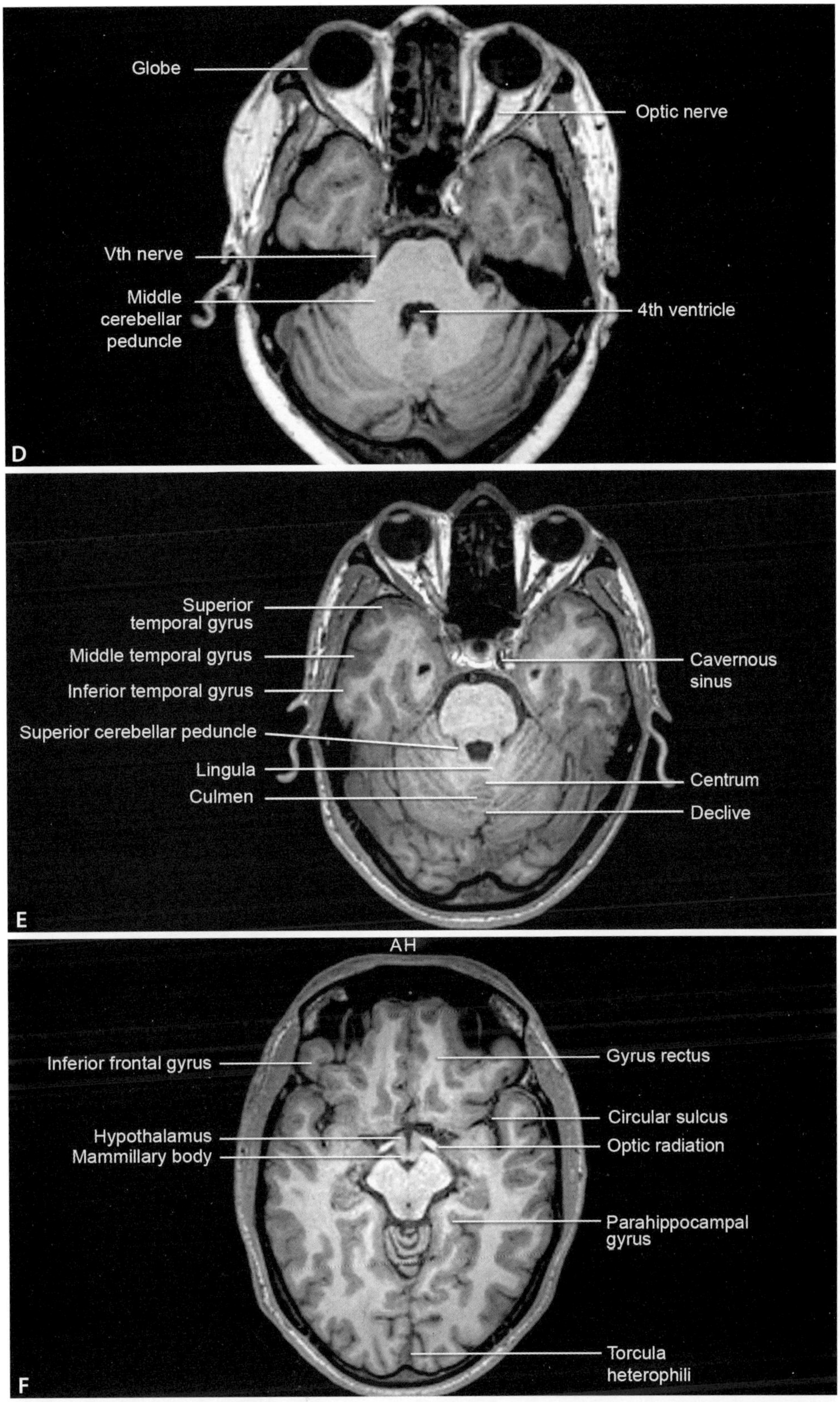
Globe
Optic nerve
Vth nerve
Middle cerebellar peduncle
4th ventricle
D
Superior temporal gyrus
Middle temporal gyrus
Inferior temporal gyrus
Superior cerebellar peduncle
Lingula
Culmen
Cavernous sinus
Centrum
Declive
E
AH
Inferior frontal gyrus
Gyrus rectus
Circular sulcus
Hypothalamus
Mammillary body
Optic radiation
Parahippocampal gyrus
Torcula heterophili
F

Figs. 6D to F

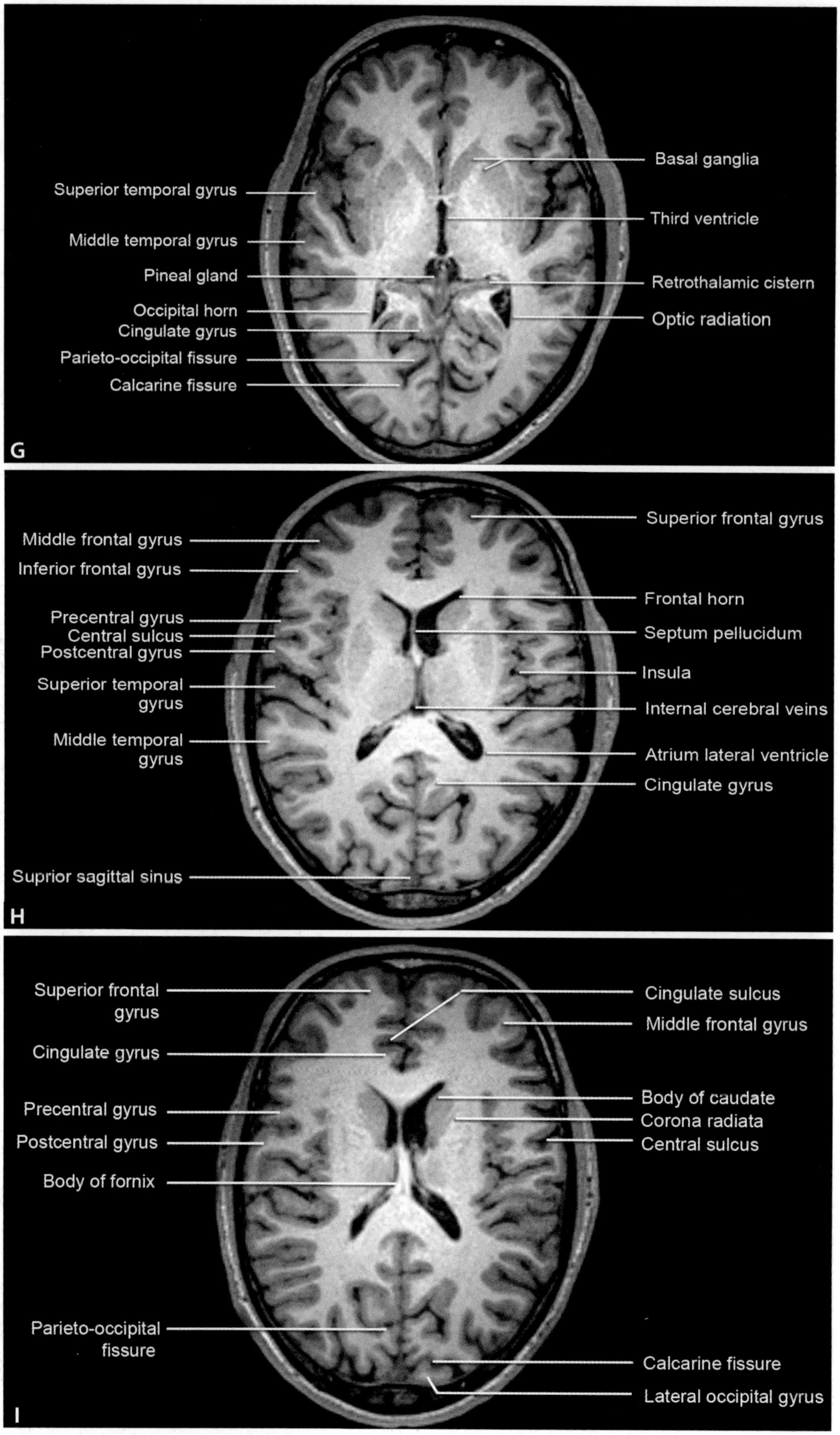
Superior temporal gyrus
Middle temporal gyrus
Pineal gland
Occipital horn
Cingulate gyrus
Parieto-occipital fissure
Calcarine fissure
Basal ganglia
Third ventricle
Retrothalamic cistern
Optic radiation
G
Middle frontal gyrus
Inferior frontal gyrus
Precentral gyrus
Central sulcus
Postcentral gyrus
Superior temporal gyrus
Middle temporal gyrus
Suprior sagittal sinus
Superior frontal gyrus
Frontal horn
Septum pellucidum
Insula
Internal cerebral veins
Atrium lateral ventricle
Cingulate gyrus
H
Superior frontal gyrus
Cingulate gyrus
Precentral gyrus
Postcentral gyrus
Body of fornix
Parieto-occipital fissure
Cingulate sulcus
Middle frontal gyrus
Body of caudate
Corona radiata
Central sulcus
Calcarine fissure
Lateral occipital gyrus
I

Figs. 6G to I

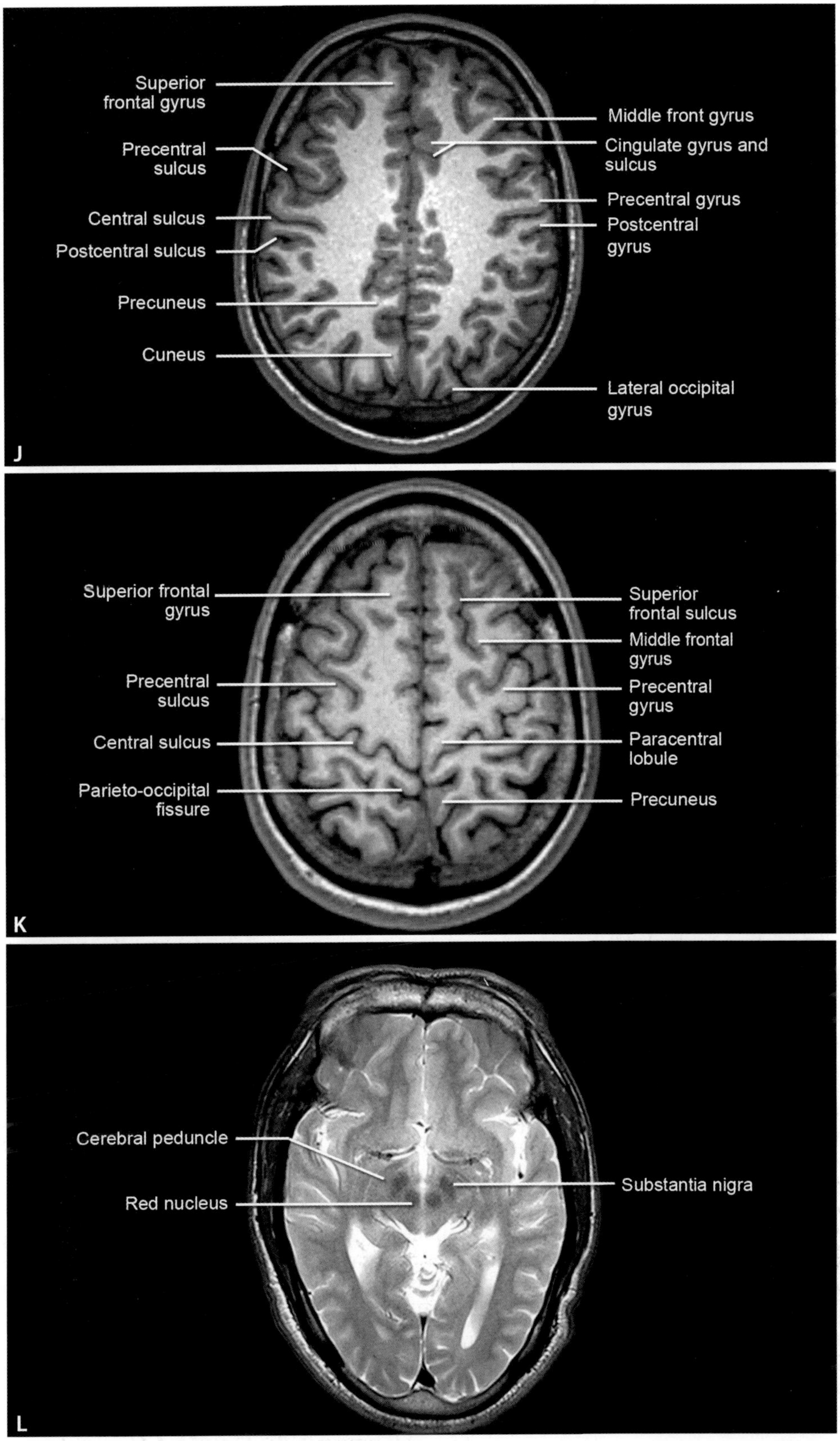

Superior frontal gyrus
Precentral sulcus
Central sulcus
Postcentral sulcus
Precuneus
Cuneus
Middle front gyrus
Cingulate gyrus and sulcus
Precentral gyrus
Postcentral gyrus
Lateral occipital gyrus
J
Superior frontal gyrus
Precentral sulcus
Central sulcus
Parieto-occipital fissure
Superior frontal sulcus
Middle frontal gyrus
Precentral gyrus
Paracentral lobule
Precuneus
K
Cerebral peduncle
Red nucleus
Substantia nigra
L

Figs. 6J to L

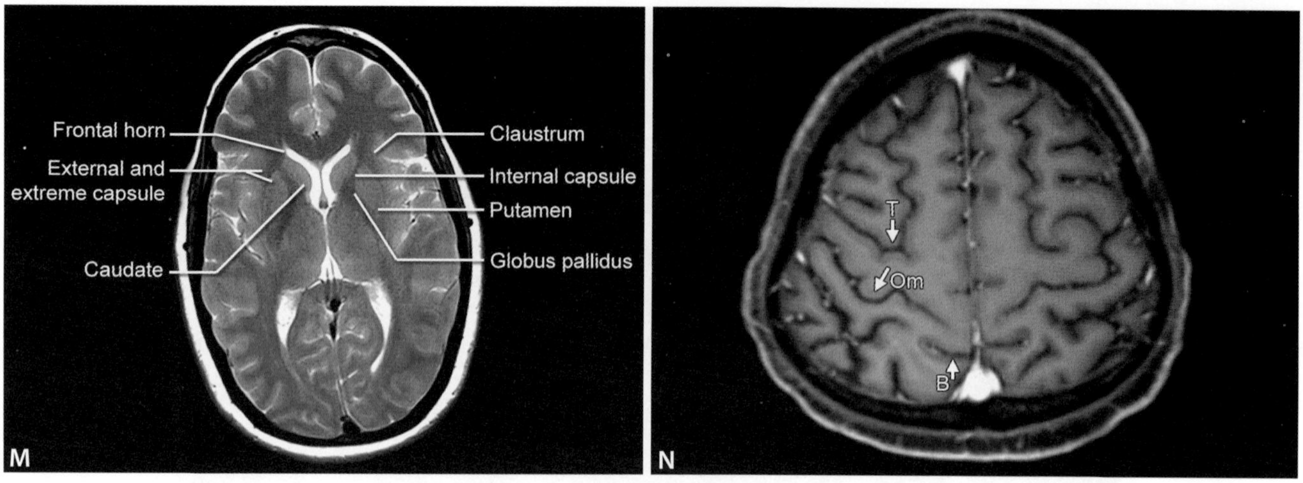

Figs. 6M and N

Figs. 6A to N: (A) T1-weighted axial MR section at the level of medulla shows the midline ventral sulcus, pyramids and olives separated by ventromedial sulcus. Dorsolateral sulcus is seen posterior to olives. Cerebellar tonsils are seen posterolateral to the medulla. Vallecula is seen posteriorly. Fourth ventricle with foramen of Luschka is seen posterior to medulla; (B) T1-weighted axial MR section at slightly higher level than Figure 2.6A shows the IX, X and XI cranial nerves seen as a common bundle exiting from the dorsolateral sulcus; (C) T1-weighted axial MR section through the pons. Pons is seen in front of the fourth ventricles. The CP angle cisterns lie lateral to the pons. Seventh and eight cranial nerves course through the cistern anterior to flocculus toward internal auditory canals. The inferior vermis and its various divisions are well seen; (D) T1-weighted axial MR section through middle part of fourth ventricle. Middle cerebellar peduncles connecting the pons with cerebellar hemispheres are well seen. Fifth nerves are seen emerging from the lateral surface of pons on both sides. Also seen are globes with optic nerve and lower part of temporal lobes; (E) T1-weighted axial MR section through the midbrain shows the superior cerebellar peduncles, and the parts of superior vermis. Anteriorly the olfactory nerve and gyrus rectus on each side of interhemispheric fissure are seen clearly. The structures of the middle cranial fossa-cavernous sinus, both temporal lobes with superior, middle and inferior temporal gyri, are also seen; (F) T1-weighted axial MR section at the level of midbrain. Inferiorly frontal and temporal lobes are seen separated by sylvian fissure. V-shaped tentorium outlining the superior vermis is seen with quadrigeminal plate and cistern located anterior to it. Parahippocampal gyrus and fusiform gyrus course forward from occipital pole to midbrain. Anterior to midbrain, mammillary bodies, optic radiations and hypothalamus are seen; (G) T1-weighted axial MR section at the level of lower third ventricle shows the basal ganglia, internal capsule, thalami and retrothalamic cistern. Peripherally superior temporal and middle temporal gyri are seen posterior to sylvian fissure. Frontal horns of lateral ventricles are seen anteriorly and occipital horns posteriorly. Pineal gland is seen posterior to the third ventricle. Optic radiations are seen ending in the occipital cortex. Also seen is the Y-shaped parieto-occipital fissure and calcarine fissure, the later forming the lateral boundary of lingual gyrus; (H) T1-weighted axial MR section at the level of mid-3rd ventricle showing various parts of frontal lobe, anteriorly and occipital lobes posteriorly. In the midline genu of the corpus callosum is seen anteriorly connecting the frontal lobes. Septum pellucidum is seen separating the frontal horns of lateral ventricles. Posteriorly in the midline splenium of the corpus callosum is seen forming posterior wall of 3rd ventricle and medial wall of atria of lateral ventricle. Peripherally the central sulcus is seen separating the frontal (precentral) and parietal (postcentral) lobes. The sylvian fissure separates the parietal lobe (post central gyrus) from the temporal lobe (superior temporal gyrus). In the depth of the sylvian fissure, portions of frontal, parietal and temporal lobe form the insula; (I) T1-weighted axial MR section at the superior part of 3rd ventricle shows the superior frontal gyrus and middle frontal gyrus separated by superior frontal sulcus. Body of fornix is seen anterior to 3rd ventricles which separate the lateral ventricles. The other structures seen in Figure 2.6H are also seen; (J and K) T1-weighted axial MR section at supraventricular level show the deep white matter of cerebral hemispheres, the centrum semiovale. The central sulcus characteristically dips posteriorly and leads to paracentral lobule. Posterior to it the precuneus and cuneus are separately seen. Only superior and middle frontal gyri are seen at this level; (L) T2-weighted axial MR section at midbrain level. Semilunar band of pigmented gray matter anteriorly—the substantia nigra, appears hypointense. Another area of hypointensity is seen dorsomedial to substantia nigra called the red nucleus. The substantia nigra and red nuclei are separated by pars compacta; (M) T2-weighted axial MR section at the level of basal ganglia. Slit like third ventricle in midline is flanked by thalamus on each side. The interhemispheric fissure anteriorly separates the two frontal lobes. Medial to the sylvian fissure, lie the insular cortex and external capsule. The caudate and lentiform nuclei with intervening internal capsule lie medially. Globus pallidus appears hypointense in comparison to putamen on T2-weighted images. Claustrum—a strip of gray matter lies between the external and extreme capsule; (N) Localization of central sulcus on axial section. Arrows and corresponding notations indicate upper T or L sign (junction of superior frontal and precentral sulci), Omega sign (shape of hand motor area) and bracket sign (junction of marginal sulcus with inter hemispheric fissure).

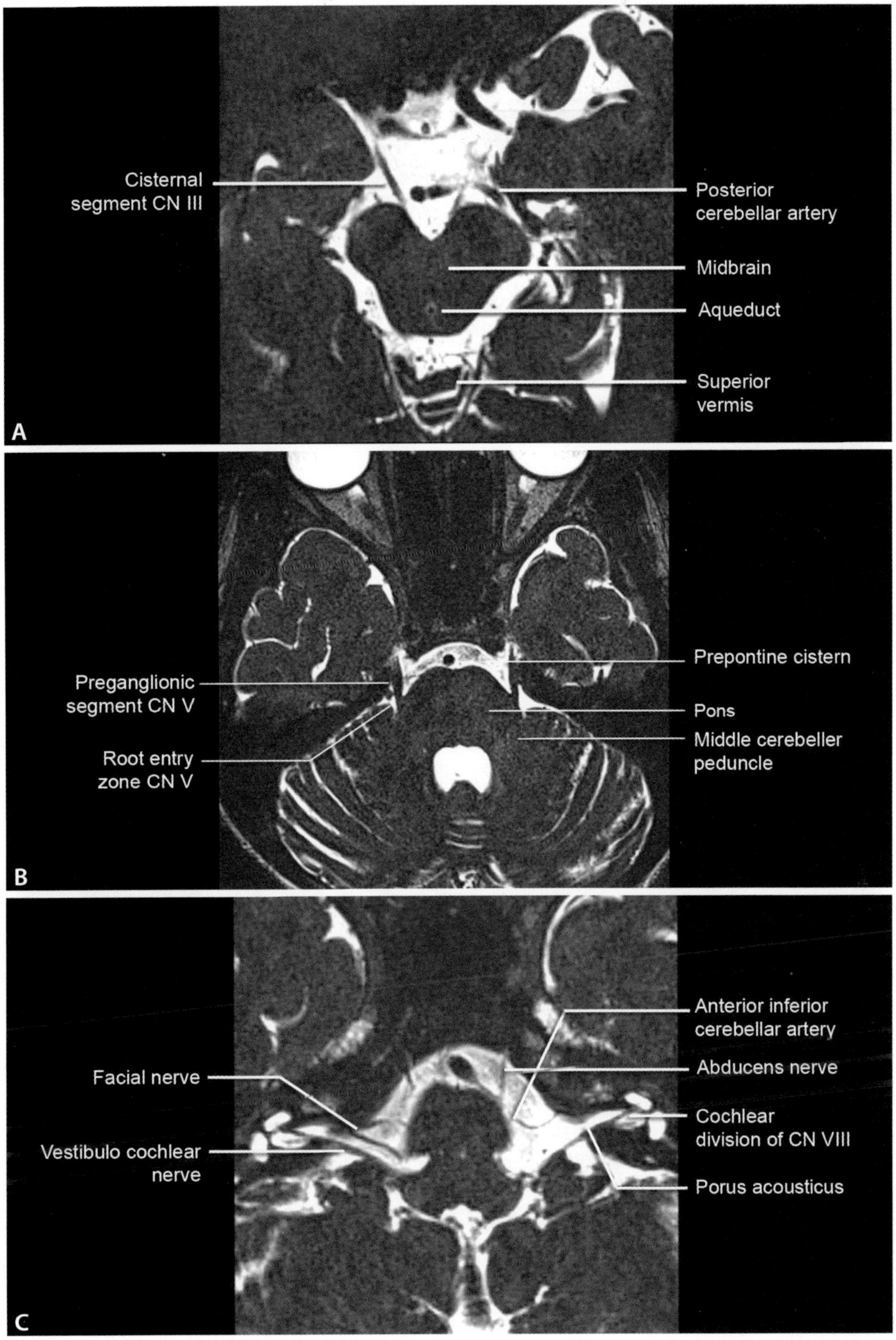
Cisternal segment CN III
Posterior cerebellar artery
Midbrain
Aqueduct
Superior vermis
A
Preganglionic segment CN V
Root entry zone CN V
Prepontine cistern
Pons
Middle cerebeller peduncle
B
Facial nerve
Vestibulo cochlear nerve
Anterior inferior cerebellar artery
Abducens nerve
Cochlear division of CN VIII
Porus acousticus
C

Figs. 7A to C

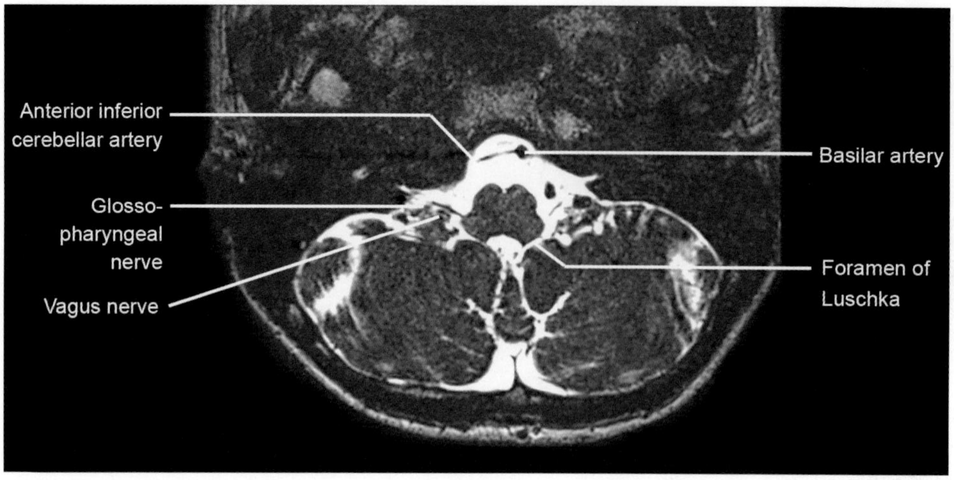

Fig. 7D

Figs. 7A to D: Axial MR cisternography sections using SPACE technique through (A) Midbrain; (B and C) Pons; and (D) Medulla show III, V, VI, VII, VIII, IX and X cranial nerves in relation to brainstem as labeled.

through the foramen of Magendie. The superior divisions of the vermis are lingula, centrum, culmen, declive and folium **(Fig. 6E)**. The inferior divisions are tuber, pyramid, uvula and nodule **(Fig. 6C)**. Immediately caudal to the inferior medullary velum is the nodulus of the vermis. The flocculus projects into the cerebellopontine angle cistern ventral to the inferior cerebellar peduncle **(Fig. 6B)**. The deep cerebral nuclei are laterally placed dentate and medially placed paired emboliform, globose and fastigial nuclei.

WHITE MATTER OF BRAIN (FIGS. 8A TO J)

The fiber connections of the cerebral cortex are divisible into three major groups **(Figs. 8A to H)**. Projection fibers are corticospinal, corticobulbar, corticopontine and cortico- thalamic tracts. Association fibers consist of subcortical U fibers, long projection fibers of cingulum, superior/inferior longitudinal fasciculi, uncinate fasciculus and superior/ inferior occipitofrontal fasciculi. The commissural fibers interconnecting the two hemispheres are corpus callosum, anterior and posterior commissure, hippocampal/habenular commissures and the hypothalamic commissure. The common central mass of white matter is known as the centrum semiovale **(Fig. 4D)**. Projection fibers passing through the corona radiata converge to form the internal capsule consisting of anterior and posterior limbs and the genu **(Figs. 4C and 6M)**. The brainstem tracts are also well shown **(Figs. 8I to J)**.

The columns of fornix which lie on either side of the foramen of Monro continue posteriorly as body of fornix. It is a C-shaped bundle of white matter forming the roof of III ventricle. Posteriorly it divides into the two crura which continue into the fimbria and alveus of hippocampal formation **(Fig. 2B)**. This is part of limbic system concerned with emotional and sexual behavior and recent memory.

VENTRICLES AND CISTERNS

The ventricular system consists of lateral, third, fourth ventricles and the cerebral aqueduct. The lateral ventricles communicate with the third ventricle by the foramen of Monro while the third ventricle communicates with the fourth ventricle via the aqueduct of Sylvius.

The lateral ventricles consist of frontal horns, body, trigone, occipital and temporal horns. Foramen of Monro defines the junction between frontal horns and body of lateral ventricles and the splenium of corpus callosum arbitrarily separates the body from the trigone. The frontal horns are bounded medially by the septum pellucidum **(Fig. 4C)**, inferiorly and laterally by the head of the caudate nucleus, and superiorly and anteriorly by the corpus callosum. The body is bounded superiorly by the corpus callosum, inferiorly by caudate nucleus and the thalamus, medially by the fornix and laterally by the body of the caudate nucleus **(Fig. 5E)**. The trigone contains large tuft of choroid plexus called glomus **(Fig. 5H)**.

The third ventricle is bounded laterally by the thalami, inferiorly by the hypothalamus **(Figs. 5D and E)**, anteriorly by the anterior commissure and lamina terminalis, posteriorly by the epithalamus and posterior commissure, and superiorly by the cistern of the velum interpositum and body of the fornix. The inferior aspect of third ventricle has downward invaginations called optic, infundibular

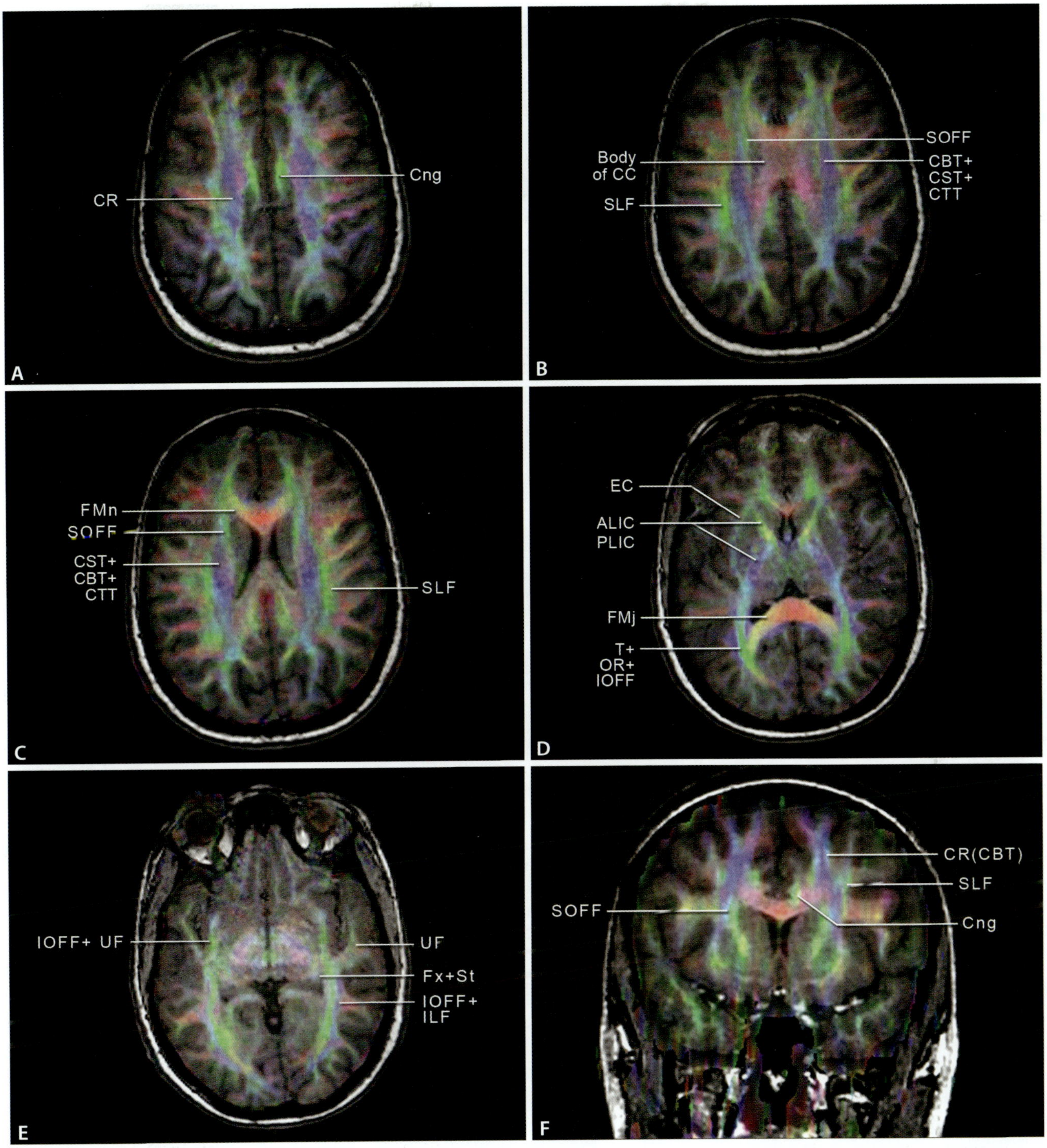

CR
Cng
A
Body of CC
SLF
SOFF
CBT+ CST+ CTT
B
FMn
SOFF
CST+ CBT+ CTT
SLF
C
EC
ALIC
PLIC
FMj
T+ OR+ IOFF
D
IOFF+ UF
UF
Fx+St
IOFF+ ILF
E
SOFF
CR(CBT)
SLF
Cng
F

Figs. 8A to F

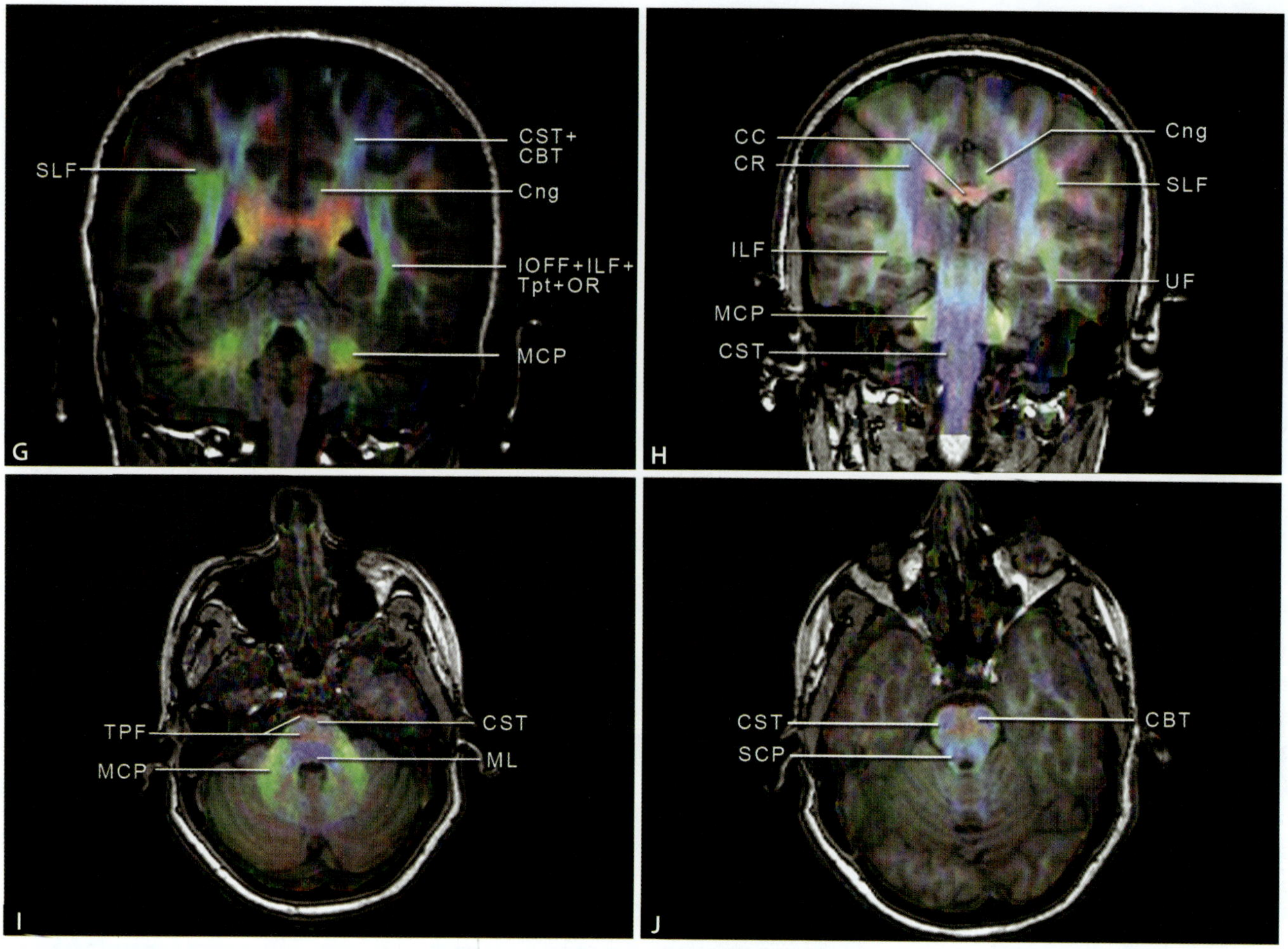

Figs. 8G to J

Figs. 8A to J: Fractional anisotropy maps superimposed on T1 weighted images of brain showing the white matter tracts. *Abbreviations*: ALIC: Anterior limb of internal capsule; CBT: Corticobulbar tract; Cng: Cingulum; CR: Corona radiata; CST: Corticospinal tract; CTT: Corticothalamic tract; FMj: Forceps major; FMn: Forceps minor; Fx: Fornix; ILF: Inferior longitudinal fasciculus; IOFF: Inferior occipitofrontal fasciculus; MCP: Middle cerebellar peduncles; ML: Medial lemniscus; OR: Optic radiation; PLIC: Posterior limb of internal capsule; SCP: Superior cerebellar peduncle; SLF: Superior longitudinal (arcuate) fasciculus; SOFF: Superior occipitofrontal fasciculus; St: Stria terminalis; TPF: Transverse pontine fibers; Tpt: Tapetum; UF: Uncinate fasciculus.

recesses anteriorly and, suprapineal and pineal recesses posteriorly.

The fourth ventricle is rhomboid in shape and lies between the pons and cerebellum. It communicates above with the third ventricle via the aqueduct and with subarachnoid space through posterior midline foramen of Magendie and posterolateral foramina of Luschka **(Fig. 6A)**.

The major cisterns at the base of the brain are suprasellar cistern, perimesencephalic cistern, prepontine and perimedullary cisterns and the cerebellopontine angle cistern. The suprasellar cistern is a five pointed CSF space, communicating anteriorly with interhemispheric fissure, laterally with Sylvian fissure and posteriorly with perimesencephalic cistern. It contains optic chiasma, internal carotid artery and circle of Willis and pituitary stalk **(Fig. 4B)**. The perimesencephalic cistern consists of interpeduncular, crural, ambient and quadrigeminal plate cisterns lying along the anterior, anterolateral, posterolateral and posterior aspects of the midbrain respectively. The upper end of basilar artery and the III cranial nerve lie within the interpeduncular cistern. Intimately related to the quadrigeminal plate cistern **(Fig. 5G)** are the pineal gland and the vein of Galen. The fourth cranial nerves course in the ambient cisterns around the midbrain.

The cerebellopontine angle cistern **(Figs. 5C, 7B and C)** is bounded medially by the middle cerebellar peduncle and the anteroinferior surface of the cerebellum and laterally by the temporal bone. It contains VII/VIII cranial nerves and anterior inferior cerebellar arteries. Prepontine cistern **(Figs. 7B and C)** lies anterior to the pons and contains basilar artery. The perimedullary cisterns surround the medulla and contain lower cranial nerves (CN IX, X and XI) and vertebral arteries **(Fig. 7D)**. Superior cerebellar cistern lies superior to the cerebellum and contains vein of Galen. The cisterna magna is a CSF space at the posteroinferior aspect of cerebellum and may be sometimes very large in normal people.

BASAL GANGLIA AND ADJACENT STRUCTURES

Basal ganglia represent central gray matter consisting of corpus striatum (caudate nucleus and lentiform nucleus) and claustrum a strip of gray matter lateral to the lentiform nucleus and amygdala at the roof of temporal horn. The caudate nucleus has a larger head anteriorly and a narrow posterior part, the tail, which follows the superolateral border of thalamus and the temporal horn into the amygdala. The lentiform nucleus is wedge shaped and comprised of globus pallidus medially and putamen laterally. External capsule, claustrum, extreme capsule and insular cortex lie lateral to the putamen in that order **(Fig. 5C)**. The internal capsule is bounded anteromedially by caudate head, laterally by lentiform nucleus and posteromedially by thalamus **(Figs. 6G and M)**.

SUGGESTED READING

1. Atlas S (Ed). Magnetic Resonance Imaging of the Brain and Spine, 5th edition. Philadelphia: Lippincott Williams & Wilkins; 2016.
2. Berry M, Standring SM, Bannister LH. Nervous system. In: Susan Standring (Ed). Gray's Anatomy, 41st edition—The Anatomical Basis of Clinical Practice, New York: Elsevier, Churchill Livingstone; 2016.
3. Butler P, Jeffiree MA. The skull and brain. In: Butler P, Mitchell AWM, Ellis H (Eds). Applied Radiological Anatomy, 1st edition. Cambridge University Press. 2001; pp. 17-60.
4. Lee SH, Rao KCVG, Zimmerman RA (Eds). Normal Anatomy in Cranial MRI and CT, 4th edition. New York: McGraw Hill Inc.; 1999. pp.105-37.
5. Patel VH, Friedman L. MRI of the Brain: Normal Anatomy and Normal Variants, 1st edition, Philadelphia: WB Saunders Company; 1997.
6. Scott WR, Hanaway J. Correlative anatomy of the brain. In: Radiology-Diagnosis-Imaging-Intervention, Vol. 3. Philadelphia: JB Lippincott Co.; 1986.
7. Snell RS (Ed). Snell's Textbook of Clinical Anatomy, 7th edition. Boston: Little Brown and Company; 2004. pp. 790-830.

CHAPTER 3

Normal Cerebral Angiography

Shailesh B Gaikwad, Ajay Kumar, Anuj Prabhakar

CEREBRAL ANGIOGRAPHY TECHNIQUE

INTRODUCTION

This is an important albeit invasive procedure wherein most cases of suspected vascular pathologies baring few exceptions are diagnosed. It is a direct examination of the blood vessels that provide not only the information of the vascular anatomy but also the flow dynamics.

Historical Background

Cerebral angiography was first introduced by Moniz. Moniz and Almeida Lima, performed the first cerebral angiography on living human patients in 1927.[1]

Definition

It is the demonstration of the cerebral vascular anatomy by direct injection of the iodinated contrast medium into the vessel.

Six Vessel Angiography

It includes the study of the following vessels:

1. Right internal carotid artery
2. Left internal carotid artery
3. Right external carotid artery
4. Left external carotid artery
5. Right vertebral artery
6. Left vertebral artery.

Indications[2]

- Evaluate intracranial circulation when CT or MR angiography is inconclusive either due to failure to visualize the pathology or patient factors like clips, coils or patient motion.
- Define presence/extent of atherosclerotic vessel disease, especially when information on the presence and nature of collateral supply is needed.
- Define etiology of hemorrhage.
- Define presence, location, and anatomy of intracranial aneurysms and arteriovenous malformations.
- Evaluate vasospasm related to subarachnoid hemorrhage.
- Investigate reversible cerebral vasoconstriction syndrome.
- Define presence/extent of trauma to cervicocerebral vessels.
- Define vascular supply to tumors.
- Define presence/extent of vasculitis.
- Evaluate pulsatile tinnitus or cranial bruit.
- Define presence of venous occlusive disease.
- Perform physiologic testing of brain function and balloon test occlusion.
- Determine presence of intracranial flow for the purpose of documenting angiographic brain death, especially when nuclear medicine blood flow study is inconclusive.
- Evaluate cerebral circulation before or after planned intervention.

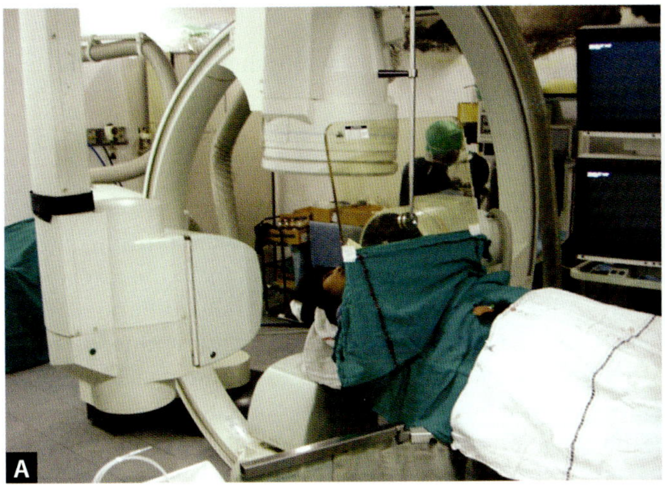

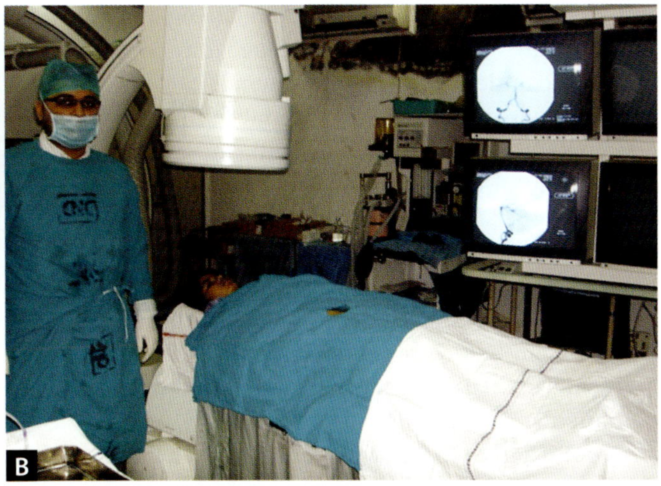

Figs. 1A and B: DSA biplane machine with monitors.

Contraindications

There are no absolute contraindications to cerebral angiography.[3] Relative contraindications include:

- Allergy to iodinated contrast agents
- Abnormal renal function
- Coagulopathy
- Local site infection
- Pregnancy.

Patient Preparation

Careful history taking is very important before the procedure. It is advisable to take informed consent from the patient in case of elective procedure and from relatives in case of emergency. Patient should be well hydrated before the procedure. Patient must have passed urine before the procedure. A detailed informed consent should be obtained including specific risks of the procedure. Laboratory parameters that should be evaluated include complete blood cell count, serum creatinine or glomerular filtration rate, prothrombin time and international normalized ratio, as dictated by the patients' clinical situation. Anticoagulants should be withheld when possible. Patients should eat nothing by mouth 6 hours before the procedure. The morning insulin dose should be reduced in half. Inguinal region should be shaved and prepared prior to the procedure.[3]

Requirements

- Digital subtraction angiography (DSA) machine **(Figs. 1A and B)**
- Catheterization equipment **(Fig. 2)**
- Disposables.

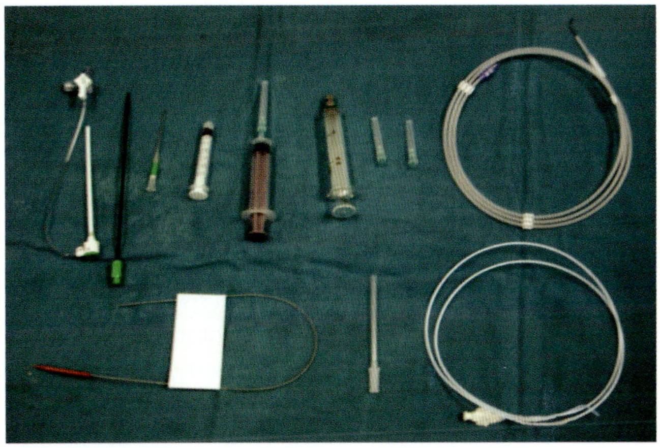

Fig. 2: Instruments required: (left to right) Sheath, dilator, puncture needle, syringes, terumo wire, short guidewire, single puncture needle, catheter.

Catheterization Equipment

Cleaning agents, blade no. 11, puncture needle, vascular sheath, mini-guidewire, various catheters, Terumo guidewire, and syringes.

Site of the Puncture

The common femoral artery (CFA) crosses the pelvic brim at the level of the inguinal ligament, which extends from the spine of the anterior superior iliac crest to the pubic tubercle. It then enters the femoral sheath which is made up of 3 compartments containing the femoral artery laterally and the vein medially. The medial and smallest compartment is called the femoral canal which contains lymphatic vessels and lymph nodes. Lateral to the femoral artery and outside the femoral sheath is the femoral nerve. The CFA represents an ideal site for arterial access and sheath insertion because it is relatively large, is less involved with atherosclerosis, and is readily compressible against the underlying head of the femur.

The ideal site of femoral arterial puncture (not skin puncture) is a point 1 cm lateral to the most medial aspect of the femoral head, midway between its superior and inferior border. Various landmarks have been utilized for identification of the femoral artery:

1. The skin crease may be used as a marker for the underlying inguinal ligament, and an arterial puncture 2 to 3 cm below the midpoint of the skin crease has been used. This technique may be inaccurate in obese patients.
2. A point 2 to 3 cm below the midpoint of a line between the anterior superior iliac spine and pubic tubercle (mid inguinal point) may be used as a site for femoral arterial cannulation **(Figs. 3 and 4)**.
3. Fluoroscopic landmark: The femoral head is identified. skin puncture done at the lower border of the femoral head, with the needle entering the skin at a 30° to 45° angle. Artery puncture is performed at the mid portion of the head of femur in its medial third.
4. Ultrasound-guided femoral arterial cannulation may be performed in obese patients or in those with a weak pulse.

Caudal punctures have an increased risk of hematoma, and pseudoaneurysms as there is lack of underlying bony structure and scaffolding by femoral sheath. High puncture above the inguinal ligament is associated with an increased risk of retroperitoneal hemorrhage due to lack of effective compression and tamponade. Infrainguinal puncture and bleeding may also cause retroperitoneal hemorrhage due to tracking of the blood upward underneath the ligament and into the retroperitoneal space.[4]

Preparation

Sterilize the site first with savlon, then with betadine and with spirit in the last.

Wipe with sterilized gauze piece.

Local Anesthesia

For local anesthesia (LA), give subcutaneous injection of 2% xylocaine without adrenaline. Palpate the artery with index, mid and ring finger of the left hand. Infiltrate 2–3 mL each on the either side of the artery. Care must be taken to not to inject LA into the vessel, before giving injection always check by withdrawing to rule out arterial puncture. Give injection slowly for the patient comfort **(Fig. 5)**.

Artery Puncture

- Give 3 mm wide and 3 mm deep, superficial skin incision at the puncture site by using 11 no. blade. It is

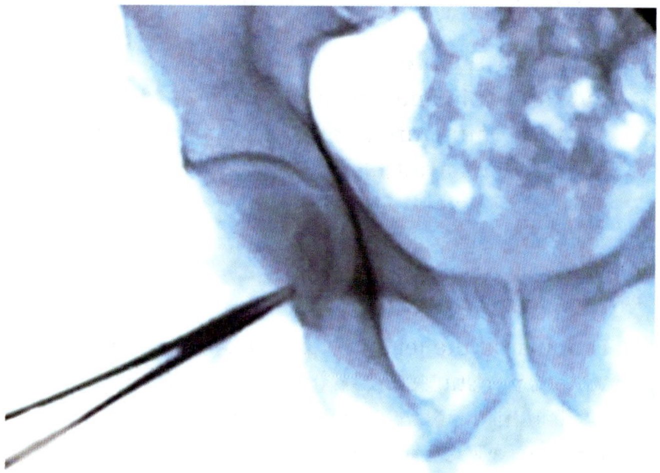

Fig. 3: Marking the site of puncture on fluoroscopy.

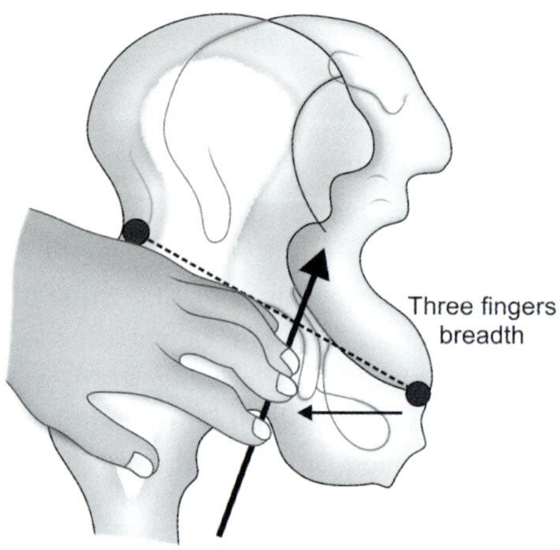

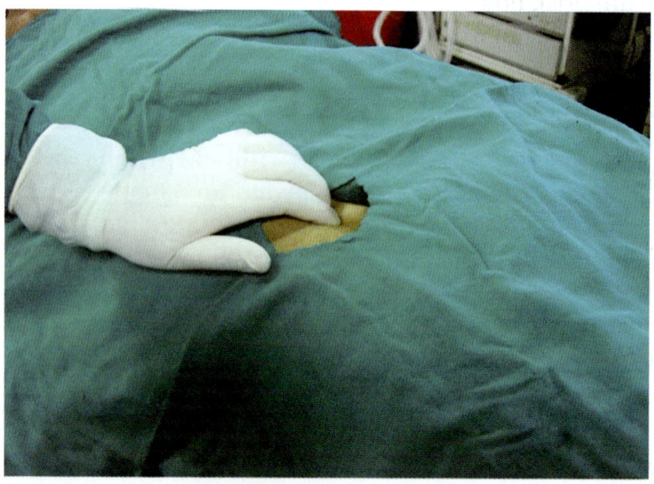

Fig. 4: Localization and palpation of femoral artery.

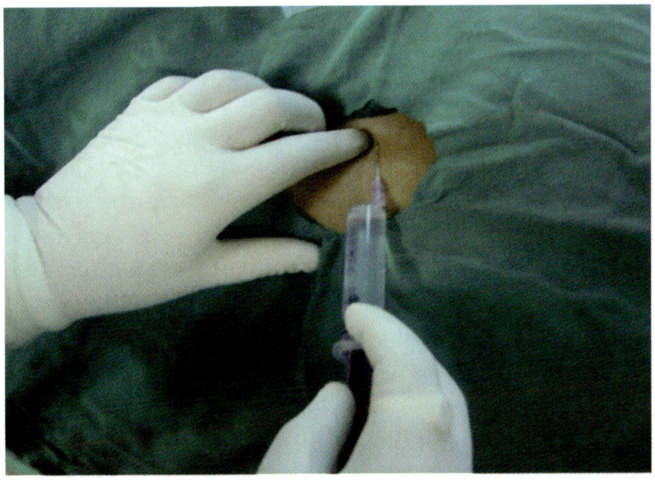

Fig. 5: Infiltrating local anesthetic at the site of puncture.

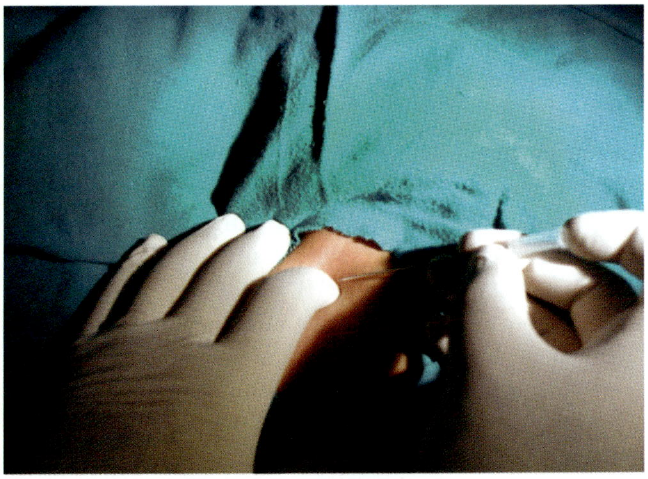

Fig. 6: Arterial puncture.

ideal to check the site under fluoroscopy before arterial puncture.

- **Seldinger technique:** Palpate femoral artery by the index, middle and ring finger, of the left hand. Take Medicut (puncture needle with needle inside and plastic cannula outside) in the right hand and advance toward the artery at about 45° angle. Feel the pulse of the artery through the needle in the right hand and as one feels it over femoral artery, enter artery with a jab **(Fig. 6)**. Remove the needle and slowly withdraw the cannula till the jet of the blood is obtained. Rule out venous puncture (blood will not come out in jets). After confirming arterial access introduce a 0.035-inch short J-tip guidewire, and remove the cannula. If resistance is encountered as the guidewire leaves the needle tip, the guidewire should be removed and the needle adjusted to ensure brisk flow. Lowering the hub of the needle before guidewire insertion or slight repositioning either laterally or medially will aid in smooth guidewire advancement. The guidewire must enter smoothly without resistance. Is case excess resistance is felt, the needle and guidewire complex must be removed and a fresh attempt should be made. Finally, introduce arterial sheath over the short guidewire.[4]
- Again check the position of the sheath by withdrawing blood using syringe. Arterial blood will come into syringe in pulsatile manner and with thrust.
- Inject 2500 unit of heparin (0.5 mL) and flush sheath with saline to flush in remaining part of heparin in the sheath lumen.

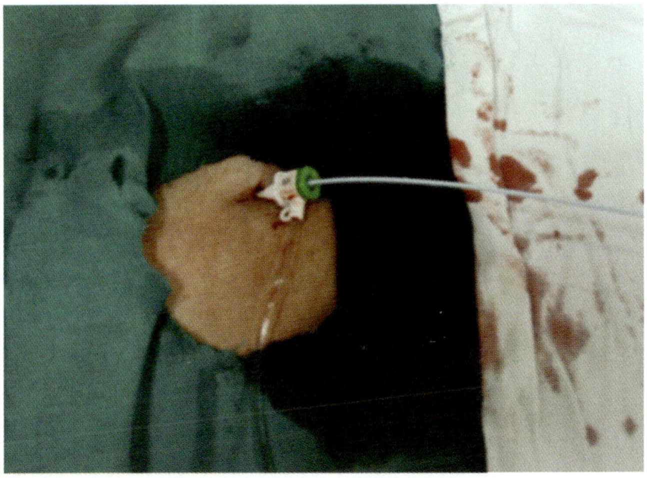

Fig. 7: Placement of arterial sheath.

- Take the desired catheter and start angiography **(Fig. 7)**.

Puncture Technique

It is of two types:

1. Single wall puncture
2. Double wall puncture.

In single wall puncture technique, only the anterior wall of artery is punctured and in double wall both anterior as well as posterior wall get punctured. Single wall is safe in experienced hands while double wall is safer in inexperienced hand as chances of dissection of artery are higher in single wall technique. In double wall technique the chance of posterior wall hematoma is high. Improper technique can lead to trauma of the vessel regardless of the type of needle used.

Procedure

The aortic arch anatomy will help determine the selection of the catheter. Types I and II arch configurations can be routinely catheterized with an angled catheter, while a reverse curve catheter is generally necessary to select vessels arising from Type III arches. In patients with atherosclerotic vessel disease a hydrophilic 0.035-inch wire with a curved tip such as the terumo wire (Terumo Interventional Systems, Somerset, NJ) is used. The guidewire is advanced into the artery followed by the catheter. As the wire is removed, an inadvertent vacuum effect may occur if the catheter is in a small artery or if the end hole is wedged against the wall of the artery. To prevent inadvertent air embolus, the guidewire should be removed slowly, keeping the catheter hub filled with heparinized saline by dripping or injecting it into the hub while the wire is withdrawn.[3] For Internal carotid artery (ICA) injection, an angled tip catheter and hydrophilic guidewire are needed. If a reverse curve catheter is used for common carotid artery (CCA) catheterization, an exchange of catheters is required over an exchange length guidewire placed in the external carotid artery.

While performing diagnostic angiography for vertebral arteries (VA), the left VA is preferred as it is mostly larger than the right in diameter. The right VA is catheterized only if the left VA is not accessible, right VA pathology is suspected, or when contrast does not reflux into the right posterior inferior cerebellar artery (PICA) on left VA injection. Extra care should be taken when VA injection is performed, as the VA is prone to vasospasm and dissection.[2]

For anterior intracranial cerebral angiography, standard AP Towne's view and lateral projections are used. Oblique images at 45 degrees may separate overlapping arteries. Special views like Stenvers view for middle cerebral artery (MCA) and submental vertex view for anterior communicating artery may be acquired if necessary. For vertebral arteriograms, the standard projections are AP (Towne's view) and lateral projections centered caudally and dorsally to cover the posterior circulation.[3]

Important Points to Remember

Check for free backflow of the blood in the catheter. Inject test amount 2–3 mL of contrast before taking run to check the exact position of the catheter and to check vascular spasm. Instruct the patient before every injection and inform the effect of the contrast like flushing and warm sensation or alteration in the taste, etc.

Postprocedural Management

Before removing the sheath, aspirate few milliliter of the blood to aspirate out any thrombus that could have formed during the procedure. If there is free backflow and if no clots are visible in the aspirate, the sheath can be safely removed. Compress the arterial puncture site which is about 0.5 cm above the skin puncture site (for about 20-min). Compress the actual puncture site with middle finger, compress above it with index finger and below it with ring finger. Puncture site should be clearly visible during compression so that hematoma formation can be avoided. Do not obliterate the pulse, distal pulse should be faintly palpable. Apply steady moderate pressure for 15 minutes, reduce the pressure in next 5-min. Never remove compression abruptly. After compression feel all distal pulses. If the patient has both an arterial and a venous sheath, the arterial sheath should be removed first and the venous sheath removed 5 minutes later. This technique avoids the risk of arteriovenous fistula formation and also preserves a venous access for medication administration in case of a vasovagal reaction.[4]

Bed rest is recommended for 8 hours after the procedure. The patient is instructed to avoid bending his/her leg. Check groin for hematoma formation. Monitor BP, pulse and neurological status of the patient. If patient is unable to pass urine then catheterize the patient until the patient is able to ambulate.

Complications

Complications may be neurological and non-neurological. Stroke is the main neurological complication. Non-neurological complications are renal failure, arterial occlusions requiring intervention, arteriovenous fistula, and hematoma requiring transfusions or surgical intervention. In a study by Kaufmann et al. 19826 consecutive patients undergoing DSA were retrospectively reviewed. Neurologic complications occurred in 2.63%, with 0.14% of these causing permanent disability. Deaths occurred in 0.06%. Access-site hematoma was the most common complication overall (4.2%). Patients suffering from atherosclerotic vascular disease, subarachnoid hemorrhage and frequent transient ischemic attack were more likely to have complications.[5]

CEREBRAL ANGIOGRAPHIC ANATOMY

ARTERIAL ANATOMY

The brain is supplied by the two internal cerebral arteries, and two vertebral arteries which join to form the basilar artery. The basilar artery divides into two posterior cerebral arteries which along with posterior communicating arteries form the posterior part of circle of Willis. The anterior part of circle of Willis is constituted by both anterior cerebral arteries, anterior communicating artery and internal cerebral arteries.

The internal carotid artery (ICA) is divided into the following segments as per the Bouthillier classification system:[6]

- C1 cervical—CCA bifurcation to entrance of carotid canal
- C2 petrous—extends up to posterior edge of formaen lacerum
- C3 lacerum—extends up to superior margin of petrolingual ligament
- C4 cavernous—extends up to proximal dural ring (anterior clinoid process)
- C5 clinoid—extends up to distal dural ring
- C6 ophthalmic—extends up to just proximal to the origin of Posterior communicating artery (PCom)
- C7 communicating—extends up to ICA bifurcation

ICA on each side enters the cranium by passing through the carotid canal in the petrous temporal bone (petrous segment). Petrous ICA give rise to Vidian artery (artery of pterygoid canal) and caroticotympanic artery which supplies middle and internal ear and occasionally the persistent stapedial artery. At times, the ICA courses posterolaterally than anteromedial (normal course) and presents as pulsatile retrotympanic mass called. Knowledge of this variant is necessary to differentiate it from glomus tympanicum so that hazardous biopsy can be avoided.

The ICA runs within the cavernous sinus to pierce the dura to enter the subarachnoid space adjacent to the anterior clinoid process. The cavernous ICA can be subdivided into ascending cavernous (C5), first posterior genu (C4), horizontal part (C3), second anterior genu (C2) and the rest of cavernous segment (C1). Meningohypophyseal artery arises near junction of C5 and C4. Meningohypophyseal artery branches supply the posterior pituitary, cavernous sinus, clival dura and sometimes III to VI cranial nerves. The horizontal part (C3) extends between first posterior (C4) and second anterior genu (C2). After second genu (C2), rest of the cavernous ICA is called as C1 segment **(Fig. 8)**. The inferolateral trunk arises from C4 segment and supplies the dura of the cavernous sinus and cranial nerves III, IV, V and VI. The superior hypophyseal trunk arises from supraclinoid ICA and supplies anterior pituitary. The ophthalmic artery arises from ophthalmic ICA **(Fig. 9)**. The anterior

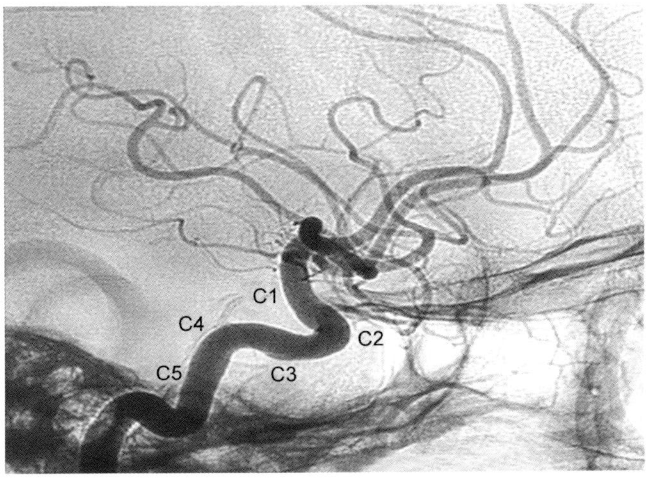

Fig. 8: ICA cavernous segments: Image showing cavernous ICA segments. C5 segment extends from carotid canal opening to first posterior genu (C4), horizontal segment (C3) extends between first posterior genu (C4) and second anterior genu (C2). Rest of cavernous ICA is called (C1).

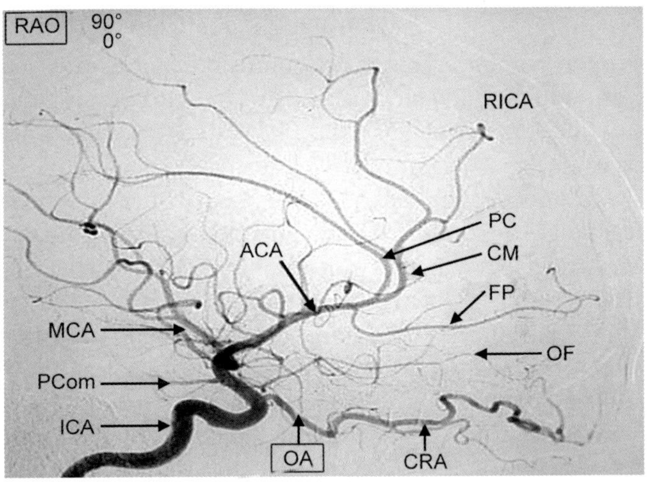

Fig. 9: Anterior circulation lateral view: Selective ICA angiogram lateral view showing different important branches (as annotated). *Abbreviations*: ICA: Internal carotid artery; OA: Ophthalmic a rtery; CRA: Central retinal artery, PCom: Posterior communicating artery; MCA: Middle cerebral artery; ACA: Anterior cerebral artery; OF: Orbitofrontal artery; FP: Frontopolar artery; CM: Callosomarginal artery; PC: Pericallosal artery.

choroidal artery arises from ICA just above PCom origin which arises posteromedially from communicating segment of ICA. The anterior choroidal artery supplies the choroid plexus of the lateral ventricles, medial temporal lobe and some striate branches to deep ganglionic structures **(Fig. 10)**. The PCom runs posteriorly to join the posterior cerebral arteries (branches of basilar artery) to complete the circle of Willis. PCom supplies the deep ganglionic structures including the thalamus.

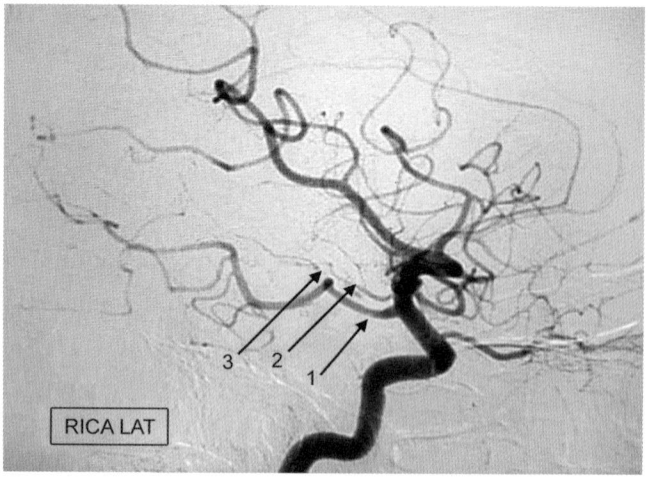

Fig. 10: Lateral ICA angiogram showing fetal PCA (1), anterior choroidal artery (2) and the plexal point (3), the point where artery enters the choroidal fissure.

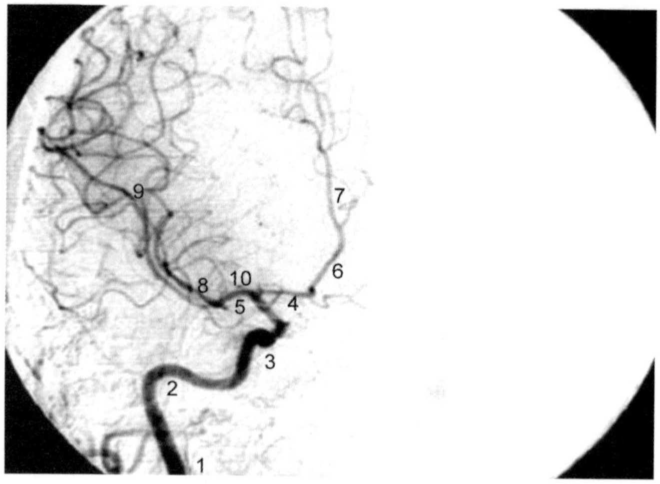

Fig. 11: Right internal carotid artery angiogram PA view. *Abbreviations*: 1: Cervical segment of ICA; 2: Petrous segment of ICA; 3: Cavernous segment of ICA; 4: Anterior cerebral artery (A1); 5: Middle cerebral artery (M1); 6: Anterior cerebral artery (A2); 7: Anterior cerebral artery (A3); 8: Middle cerebral artery (M2); 9: Middle cerebral artery (M3); 10: Lenticulostriate arteries.

The anterior cerebral arteries proceed medially within the interhemispheric fissure separated by the falx. Both anterior cerebral arteries are connected by the anterior communicating artery in the midline completing the anterior part of circle of Willis (located in the suprasellar cistern).

Anterior cerebral artery (ACA) is thus divided into three segments. Horizontal (A1) segment which extends from the ACA origin to its junction with the anterior communicating artery (ACom). The medial lenticulostriate arteries arise from A1 segment. A2 segment which extends from the junction of ACom to its bifurcation into pericallosal and callosomarginal arteries. The orbitofrontal and frontopolar arteries arise from A2 segment. The recurrent artery of Heubner which is a lenticulostriate branch may arise from proximal A2 segment and less commonly from A1 segment. A3 segment refers to the cortical branches that supply the anterior two-thirds of medial hemispheric surface and a small superior area over the convexities.

Middle cerebral artery (MCA) is also divided into three major segments. Horizontal (M1) segment: Extends from the origin of MCA to its bifurcation or trifurcation at Sylvian fissure. The lateral lenticulostriate arteries arise from M1 segment and supply the lentiform nucleus, parts of internal capsule and caudate nucleus. Insular (M2) segment: At its genu, the MCA divides into its insular (M2) branches, which loop over the insula and pass laterally to exit from sylvian fissure. Opercular (M3) segment: This gives off branches that emerge from the Sylvian fissure and ramify over the hemispheric surface. The insular and the opercular branches supply the temporal, parietal and variable parts of frontal and occipital lobes **(Figs. 11 and 12)**.

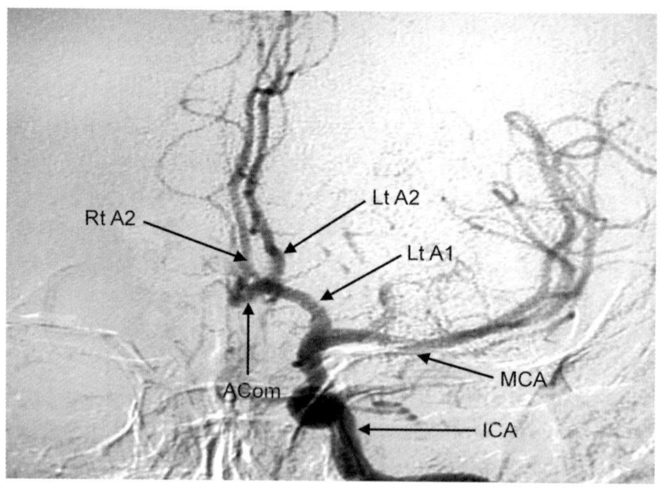

Fig. 12: Left ICA angiogram frontal view revealing ICA bifurcation, MCA, ACA segments and ACom (as annotated).

The two vertebral arteries (VA) arise from the respective subclavian arteries, course cephalad and enter the cranium through the foramen magnum. These unite in the posterior fossa, usually anterior to the medulla to form the basilar artery. Most of the time vertebral arteries are asymmetrical. In about 60% left vertebral artery is dominant, in 25% right can be dominant and in about 25% both vertebral artery can be symmetrical in size. Left vertebral artery can arise directly from aorta in small percentage.

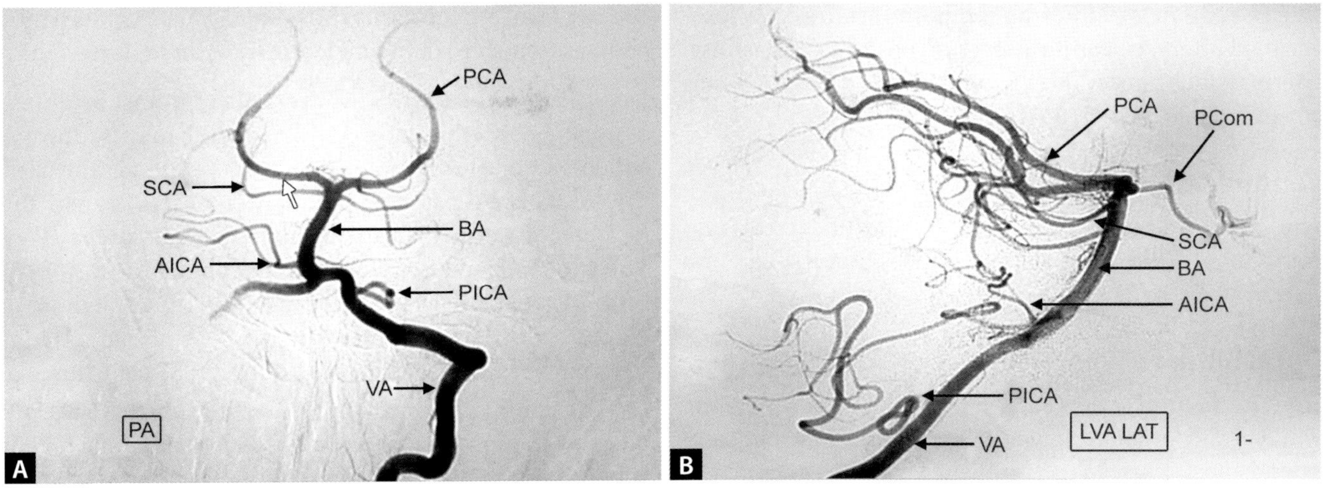

Figs. 13A and B: Posterior circulation frontal and lateral view showing the major arteries and their branches.
Abbreviations: VA: Vertebral artery; BA: Basilar artery; PICA: Posterior inferior cerebellar artery; AICA: Anterior inferior cerebellar artery; SCA: Superior cerebellar artery; PCA: Posterior cerebral artery; PCom: Posterior communicating artery).

The intracranial VA gives two major branches: Anterior spinal artery supplying the spinal cord and PICA on each side which supplies choroid plexus of fourth ventricle, medulla, cerebellar tonsils, inferior vermis and parts of cerebellar hemispheres.

Basilar artery (BA) runs anterior to pons in the prepontine cistern and terminates in the interpeduncular cistern by dividing into posterior cerebral arteries (PCAs). In prepontine cistern, it lies within the space marginated by lateral margin of clivus. Any further deviation from these boundaries is considered as dolichoectasia. In addition, the basilar artery gives off anterior inferior cerebellar artery (AICA) and superior cerebellar artery (SCA) on each side, just before bifurcation into posterior cerebral arteries. The anterior inferior cerebellar artery is the first major branch of basilar artery and most of the time (about 70%) arises as single vessel.

AICA courses posterolaterally within the CP angle cistern, whereas SCA curves around the pons and the midbrain just below the tentorial hiatus **(Figs. 13 and 14)**. The AICA supplies the VII, VIII CN, inferolateral pons, middle cerebellar peduncle and anterolateral surface of cerebellum. The SCA supplies the entire superior surface of cerebellum, vermis, deep cerebellar white matter and dentate nuclei. In addition, BA also gives off multiple short and long segment circumflex perforating branches which supply the ventral pons and rostral brainstem.

The PCAs are usually terminal branches of basilar artery but they can arise directly from supraclinoid ICA with hypertrophy of PCom and hypoplasia of ipsilateral P1 segment of PCA called as fetal PCA **(*see* Fig. 10)**. PCA on each side is divided into three major segments.

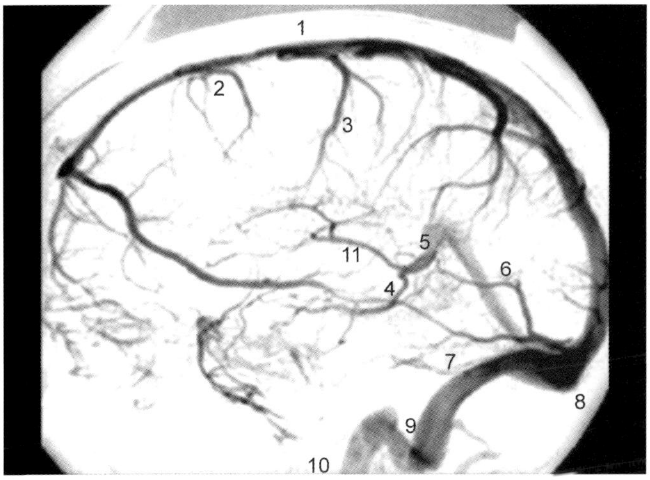

Fig. 14: Right internal carotid angiogram venous phase (lateral view).
Abbreviations: 1: Superior sagittal sinus; 2: Superior cerebral veins; 3: Vein of Trolard; 4: Basal vein of Rosenthal; 5: Vein of Galen; 6: Straight sinus; 7: Transverse sinus; 8: Torcular herophili; 9: Sigmoid sinus; 10: Internal jugular vein; 11: Internal cerebral vein).

Precommunicating (P1 or peduncular) segment: It extends from the origin of PCA to its junction with the PCom. The posterior thalamoperforating arteries and medial posterior choroidal artery usually arise from P1 segment. Ambient (P2) segment: It courses around the midbrain above the trochlear nerve and tentorial incisura. The lateral posterior choroidal artery and thalamogeniculate arteries arise from the P2 segment.

Quadrigeminal (P3) segment: It runs behind the midbrain in the quadrigeminal plate cistern. The major branches of P3 segment are inferior temporal arteries, parieto-occipital artery, calcarine artery and posterior pericallosal arteries which supply the occipital lobe and posterior part of parietal lobe **(Figs. 13A and B)**.

Venous Anatomy (Fig. 14)

The cerebral venous system is composed of two components, the dural venous sinuses and the cerebral veins.

Dural Sinuses

Superior sagittal sinus (SSS): It is situated in the midline and typically originates near the crista galli anteriorly and extends posteriorly to its confluence with the straight and lateral sinuses at the torcula.

Inferior sagittal sinus is situated in the inferior free margin of the falx cerebri and joins the vein of Galen to form the straight sinus.

Straight sinus courses backwards to unite with the SSS at the torcular herophili.

Transverse and occipital sinuses: The torcular herophili divides into the transverse (lateral) and occipital sinuses. The transverse sinuses course laterally around the tentorial attachment to form the sigmoid sinuses and drain into the internal jugular veins on either side. The occipital sinus is rudimentary.

Cavernous sinuses: The cavernous sinuses are the largest venous sinuses located in the parasellar region. Its major tributaries are superior and inferior ophthalmic veins. The ICA and 3rd, 4th, 6th, ophthalmic and maxillary divisions of 5th cranial nerves course within each sinus. Both cavernous sinuses communicate with each other, preclival venous plexus, sigmoid sinuses, and jugular bulb (through superior and inferior petrosal sinuses).

Cerebral Veins

These are divided into superficial (cortical) veins and deep veins.

Superficial cortical veins: These are variable in number and enter the SSS near the vertex. The larger veins which may be identified are superficial middle cerebral vein which runs along the sylvian fissure, vein of Trolard which courses from sylvian fissure to SSS and vein of Labbe which courses from sylvian fissure to the transverse sinus.

Deep cerebral veins: The medullary veins originate 1–2 cm below the cortex and course centrally toward subependymal veins which surround the lateral ventricles. The thalamostriate vein and septal vein join near the foramen of Monro to form the internal cerebral vein (ICV). The two ICVs and basal veins of Rosenthal (BVR) join to form the vein of Galen which runs under the splenium of corpus callosum and unites with the inferior sagittal sinus to form the straight sinus which joins the SSS at the torcula.

The major veins draining the posterior fossa are anterior pontomesencephalic vein, precentral cerebellar vein, superior and inferior vermian veins and hemispheric veins.

CONCLUSION

The above chapter was a brief review of the basic anatomy and techniques for cerebral angiography. DSA is the gold standard for detection of vascular pathologies in the brain. Despite its invasive nature and the recent advances in CT, MR technology its importance has not diminished in the current clinical scenario.

REFERENCES

1. Doby T. Cerebral angiography and Egas Moniz. Am J Roentgenol. 1992;159(2):364-4.
2. Wojak JC, Abruzzo TA, Bello JA, et al. Quality Improvement Guidelines for Adult Diagnostic Cervicocerebral Angiography: Update Cooperative Study between the Society of Interventional Radiology (SIR), American Society of Neuroradiology (ASNR), and Society of NeuroInterventional Surgery (SNIS). J Vasc Interv Radiol. 2015;26(11):1596-608.
3. Ahn SH, Prince EA, Dubel GJ. Basic neuroangiography: review of technique and perioperative patient care. Semin Interv Radiol. 2013;30(3):225-33.
4. Bangalore S, Bhatt DL. Femoral arterial access and closure. Circulation. 2011;124(5):e147-56.
5. Kaufmann TJ, Huston J, Mandrekar JN, et al. Complications of diagnostic cerebral angiography: evaluation of 19826 consecutive patients. Radiology. 2007;243(3):812-9.
6. Bouthillier A, van Loveren HR, Keller JT. Segments of the internal carotid artery: a new classification. Neurosurgery. 1996;38(3):425-32; discussion 432-3.

CHAPTER 4

Advances in Neuroimaging Techniques: Computed Tomography

Sameer Vyas, Paramjeet Singh, Niranjan Khandelwal

INTRODUCTION

Computed tomography (CT) technology has significantly evolved over the recent years with technical advancements to increase speed, improve image quality and reduce dose.[1,2] Introduction of spiral (helical) CT scans in 1990 which use slip ring technology allows continuous data acquisition of a volume by 360° gantry rotation during continuous table movement during the scan. The technique reduced slice thickness to submillimeter levels, allowed faster scanning and acquisition of a large volumetric data which can be used to generate thin slices and high resolution reformations of images in any desired plane from very thin isotropic voxels. Nowadays, CT has become valuable diagnostic tool and plays a very pivotal role in current clinical neuro-imaging. Main advantages of the CT include widespread availability, ease of clinical application, and noninvasive nature. There has been several advancement in CT technology, which include multidetector computed tomography (MDCT), dual-energy CT, portable CT, cone beam CT, phase contrast CT and iteractive reconstruction algorithms. Better collimation of the X-ray beams, higher heat capacity of the newer X-ray tubes and increased sensitivity of detector assembly have significantly upgraded the technology.[1]

In this chapter, we will first discuss the recent advances in the CT technology and then will elaborate the neuroimaging applications of CT.

RECENT ADVANCES IN CT TECHNOLOGY

Multidetector Computed Tomography

The introduction of multidetector computed tomography (MDCT) system into clinical radiology has brought a revolution in the field of medical imaging. MDCT are the latest techniques where multiple rows of detectors are used to acquire multiple slices per rotation through interweaving helices (2, 4, 16 up to 320 slices). 1 mm × 20 mm detectors are replaced with arrays of 1 mm × 1.25 mm channels in MDCT which can be arranged in a symmetrical, adaptive or hybrid fashion. MDCT uses high gantry speed (0.5–0.8 seconds) allowing faster imaging and larger volume coverage particularly for CT angiography.[3]

This technology allowed the maturing of traditional CT from plain axial cross-section imaging to a modern real- like three-dimensional (3D) tool with identical spatial resolution along all directions allowing excellent multiplanar reformations and high quality 3D reconstructions. The scan parameters can be manipulated by changing the collimation, detector configuration and reconstruction algorithm.[3] Retrospective data analysis allows flexibility of examination. Simultaneous development of efficient computer systems made possible postprocessing and analysis of enormous data sets.

The two chief benefits of helical or multislice CT are an increase in the speed and defined ability of performance of volume acquisitions.

1. *Increased speed:* Multidetector CT allows high-speed scanning, thinner sections or longer scan ranges. Increased scanning speed leads to less motion artifacts, especially in the cases of children and patients who are critically ill or are in trauma. Since scanning is rapid, more volume can be covered and more data of higher resolution can be acquired for better 3D reconstructions. The contrast requirement is also less compared with standard CT or better images can be obtained with the same amounts of contrast material.
2. *Volume acquisition:* A continuous volume acquisition in a helical CT makes sure that none of the lesions go as miss when a patient respirates or makes a movement. These improved 3D capabilities of multiplanar reformations and exhaustive 3D representations are the prime benefits for volume acquisition. This technology provides best result if the thickness of the chosen section is reduced to the minimum. The utility of volume rendering techniques has risen so much that interpretation of images has progressed from observation of aerial sections to evaluation of real 3D data sets.

Flat-panel volume computed tomography: Flat-panel volume computed tomography is recent development in the CT technology that allows coverage of a large volume per rotation. Fluoroscopic and dynamic imaging is possible with high spatial resolution.[6] It represents combining of different modalities like radiography, fluoroscopy, X-ray angiography, and volumetric CT into one system. Area detectors have replaced the detector rows in this new technology. The flat-panel detector with its wide Z-axis coverage makes the imaging of entire organs possible in a single axial acquisition. Intra-operative and vascular imaging is possible due to its fluoroscopic and angiographic modalities. The flat-panel volume CT is advantageous in comparison to multidetector CT as it allows ultra-high spatial resolution, real-time fluoroscopy, dynamic imaging capabilities, and whole-organ coverage in one rotation.[4] The main limitations of flat-panel volume CT is that it requires a higher radiation dose [needed to achieve a comparable signal-to-noise ratio], lower contrast resolution, and a slower scintillator that slows down the scanning process.

Dynamic computed tomography angiography: Inability to provide any dynamic (i.e. temporal resolved) information was a major limitation of MDCT compared to the gold standard of angiographic, digital subtraction angiography. But this limitation seems to be resolved with the recent introduction of a 320-detector row CT scanner that provides the possibility of dynamic volume scanning (four-dimensional scanning with the fourth dimension being the time).[5,6] Volumetric CT using 320 detector rows enables full brain coverage in a single rotation that allows for combined time-resolved whole-brain perfusion and four-dimensional computed tomography angiography (CTA). Its potential applications in neuroradiology are in stroke, steno-occlusive disease, arteriovenous malformations and dural shunts. The broad coverage enabled by it offers Z-axis c overage allowing for whole-brain perfusion and subtracted dynamic angiography of the entire intracranial circulation. It has the potential of scanning entire organs such as the heart and brain in a single rotation as it provides large maximum detector area that can be used for this scanner, therefore allowing the visualization of dynamic flow and perfusion, as well as motion of an entire volume at very short time interval.

Dual Energy Computed Tomography

Conventional CT demonstrate exquisite anatomic detail with high contrast and spatial resolution whereas Dual Energy Computed Tomography (DECT) provides insights into the material properties of the tissues.[7-9] With DECT, differentiation between tissues that have similar attenuation on conventional CT imaging is possible. The basic principle of DECT is based on that different material show different attenuation (absorption) of energy at varying energy of the incident X-rays (various kVp settings), and this difference in attenuation can be used for tissue characterization. DECT scanners can be performed by sequential acquisition of two separate scans (dual-source CT scanners, one at each energy level, Siemens Healthcare) or fast kV-switching systems (GE Healthcare), or dual-layer detection technology (simultaneous detection of multiple energies by multilayer detectors, Phillips Healthcare).[9] DECT analyzes the changes in attenuation of different materials at 2 disparate energy levels, and subsequently uses a process termed material decomposition to generate monochromatic DECT images. The methodology of image reconstruction varies based on the acquisition method, with single-source fast-kilovoltage switching images constructed from projection space data, whereas dual-source CT (where high-energy and lower-energy acquisitions are not coincident with each other in a helical acquisition) uses image domain material decomposition. DECT minimize the beam-hardening and photon-starvation artifacts, including implanted metal, dense intravenous contrast within central venous structures at the thoracic inlet level, and inherently dense bony structures.

DECT has several useful clinical applications in head and neck imaging for better clinical care, which include atherosclerotic plaque, metal artifact reduction and tumor characterization. Several studies had demonstrated that with DECT, there had been dose reduction or similar dose when compared to single-energy CT. It provides high temporal resolution and enables bone removed CT neuroangiographic images of diagnostic quality. In addition, calcified plaques and surgical clips can be removed by processing the data. Recent studies have reported contrast-enhanced dual-energy CT angiography had high diagnostic accuracy for the detection of intracranial aneurysm as compared with 3D digital subtraction angiography (DSA) at a lower radiation dose.

Cone Beam CT

Standard CT scanners uses the fan-beam geometry of the X-ray, whereas cone beam CT (CBCT) uses X-ray beam which is conical in configuration and enables a volume of tissue to be imaged in a single rotation.[1] By increasing the anode angle in the X-ray tube, there is increase in the cone angle of the X-ray beam. The data of the entire region of interest can captured in a single rotation by rectangular or round two-dimensional (2D) detector. The reconstruction algorithm most frequently used in CBCT is a modified Feldkamp algorithm, which is essentially a 3D adaptation of the filtered back-projection method used in fan-beam 2D reconstructions.

Recent advances in imaging technology have significantly improved the CBCT scanners. These include development of flat-panel detector arrays which are compact, relatively low-cost, high-quality and large-area; better X-ray tubes which are capable of multiple exposures necessary for cone-beam scanning and low-cost computers with processing power sufficient for cone beam image reconstruction in near real time. CBCT is typically implemented as a seat scanner such that the imaging chain is rotated around a vertical axis with the patient seated at the isocenter. The high resolution of flat-panel CBCT is advantageous for many clinical applications in dental imaging, temporal bone imaging, sinonasal imaging, and imaging of implanted devices (e.g., prostheses, endovascular coils, and stents).

Portable CT

Standard CT scanners are stationary and located in the radiology imaging department. The patients are required to travel to a CT suite for imaging, where there is a high-voltage power source with radiation shielding of wall and ceiling. These scanners are not suitable for the patients who are critically ill patients in intensive care units (ICUs) as well as patients undergoing surgery. There is significant higher morbidity (13–71%) in transporting the critically ill patient to the imaging area. The portable CT are used for imaging patients at bedside in ICUs (to minimize movement of critically ill patients) and for perioperative cross-sectional image in operation theatres (to provide fast check on surgical outcome).[10]

Though portable and mobile CT terms are used interchangeably, there is difference between portable CT and mobile CT. Portable CT represents CT system within the hospital that can be moved from place to place whereas mobile CT represents CT system that function as standalone unit, typically in a trailer. There are concerns of scattered radiations for staff and public from ionization radiation arising from the portable scanners in the scanning area (ICUs or operation theaters), as portable system cannot be shielded. Scatter shields on the front and back of the scanner can be used to reduce the scatter dose.

CereTom, produced by NeuroLogica is portable scanner designed specifically for head imaging. It attaches directly to a patient's bed and used for scanning of the head and neck. Though the cost of portable CT is higher than a standard CT scanner, portable head CT are considered to be economically and clinically beneficial in ICUs and operating rooms as the cost of staff personnel and equipment needed for the transport of a patient to and from the conventional scanner exceed in value. Many studies have shown that the portable CT images are of good diagnostic quality and the radiation dose is also near similar to that of standard CT.

Phase Contrast CT

Conventional CT technologies are based on absorption property of the X-ray only; but there are other physical properties of the X-rays penetrating through matter that could potentially contribute to other complementary information. Phase-contrast computed tomography (CT) is non-conventional CT imaging and an X-ray–based experimental imaging modality in which the phase shifts of X-rays passing through matter rather is used to generate tissue contrast.[11] It is based on refraction and interference effects of X-ray imaging, with higher contrast than conventional absorption-based X-ray attenuation. Experiments had shown that suggest that phase contrast CT yields higher contrast in biologic soft tissue than conventional X-ray imaging. The phase-shift information can be gathered with a variety of techniques, including propagation-based, analyzer-based, or crystal interferometer–based methods.

Most of these methods are based on monochromatic, parallel X-ray beams. It requires synchrotron X-ray sources or low-power microfocus X-ray tubes, which have limited availability and hence limits PCCT use in a potential clinical setting. With recent advances in technology, the phase-shift information can also be derived from grating-based phase-contrast CT when conventional X-ray tubes are used, which has lead to potential chances of phase-contrast CT to clinical applications. However, there are still many limitation of PCCT into medical imaging. Clinical applications of the PCCT include atherosclerotic carotid plaque characterization by its capability to differentiate various components of soft plaque, and *ex vivo* breast imaging by demonstrating excellent soft-tissue contrast. Without use of any contrast media, PCCT had shown ductal structures, collagen architecture and the three-dimensional outline of ductal carcinoma.

Advances in Image Reconstruction Algorithms

With the phenomenal advances in CT hardware, there has been significant improvement in the data processing methods, such as reconstruction techniques especially the iterative reconstruction (IR) CT algorithms.[1,12] Analytical approach of filtered back projection (FBP) was standard reconstruction method for diagnostic CT earlier. It was much faster and less perfect method, but has limitations like high image noise, streak artifacts, or low-contrast. These problems have been overcome by development of statistical and model based IR algorithms. By noise reductions in CT image processing, iterative reconstruction (IR) techniques allows substantial reduction in the radiation dose and improve image quality. IR techniques had shown enhanced diagnostic accuracy and artefact suppression. Image reconstruction in iterative reconstruction starts with an image assumption and then compares it to real time measured values while making constant adjustments until the two are in agreement. These algorithms essentially consist of a trial-and-error correction loop that is introduced in the image reconstruction process. Several iterative reconstruction software packages for CT are now commercially available, which includes iDose (Philips Healthcare, Best, Netherlands), ASiR (GE Healthcare, Milwaukee, WI), Adaptive Iterative Dose Reduction (Toshiba, Tochigi, Japan), and IRIS (Siemens, Erlangen, Germany).[1]

COMPUTED TOMOGRAPHY IN NEUROIMAGING

Computed tomography scan has been the workhorse of neuroimaging. It is a cost-effective and quick screening test with established role in cross-sectional imaging of craniospinal trauma, subarachnoid hemorrhage, stroke and evaluation of postoperative patients. In addition, it has a role in those patients in which MRI is contraindicated. The concept of CT imaging was challenged with the advent of MRI; however, with recent technology advancement like multidetector CT, the modality has seen a new resurgence. Many of these CT applications are current standards in clinical practice.

Computed tomography angiography now plays an expanded role in evaluation of subarachnoid hemorrhage by detecting vascular lesions like aneurysms and arteriovenous malformations. These patients are already on the CT table and it only requires and additional few minutes to obtain detailed information about possible causes of the hemorrhage. Most of the surgeons nowadays operate solely on the basis of a CTA exam. With MDCT, spatial resolution is excellent and the results are similar or even superior to angiography. There is an increasing use of the modality in imaging of stroke through CTA of intracranial and neck vessels, venography and CT perfusion imaging. The excellent reconstructions of CT data have also enhanced the utility of CT in neuroimaging, i.e. in spinal trauma and evaluation of craniovertebral junction.

NONCONTRAST CT OF HEAD

Helical CT has not caught on for routine imaging of the neurocranium and axial mode is still used for routine imaging; however, thin-sections obtained on multichannel scans have distinct advantage. Thin sections of the middle cranial and posterior fossa reduce the beam hardening artifacts and improve delineation of the brainstem and temporal lobe. A usual spiral protocol is 5 mm acquisition with thin sections (i.e. 1.5 mm) can be merged into thicker (2.5 mm or more) thus reducing noise and radiation dose. The data may be split back for high resolution reconstructions. Thus, there is now the option of not only axial but also coronal or sagittal images of the brain. The clinical usefulness of this technique, however, has not yet been tested. The technology has affected pediatric neuro applications in many ways. Increased speed has eliminated the need for sedation and a reconstruction of data obtained in least provocative position allows multiplanar depiction of anatomy.

Windowing in the CT is important concept in neuroimaging as changing this will cause significant difference in the appearance of the picture to bring the particular pathology to show particular structures.[13] Windowing helps in changing the grayscale component of a CT by changing the CT numbers. This is also known as gray-level mapping or contrast stretching. Windowing in CT has two components, window level and window width. The window level helps in adjusting the brightness of the image whereas the window width helps in adjusting the contrast. The window width is the measure of the range of CT numbers that an image contains as compared to window level or centre is the midpoint of the range of the CT numbers displayed. Typical window width or level in neuroimaging varies from institution to institution and vendor to vendor. Typical values in neuroimaging consists of for brain parenchyma (WW: 80 WL: 40), for subdural lesions (WW. 150-300 WL: 50-100) and for stroke (WW: 40 WL:40).

CT ANGIOGRAPHY

Catheter angiography; the gold standard for diagnostic neuroangiography, is an expensive and invasive procedure with a morbidity and mortality of 1.5–2%. High spatial resolution for visualization of small and tortuous vessels is required for imaging of vascular anatomy of head and neck region. In addition, to avoid venous enhancement fast acquisition is required. CTA of the craniocervical vessels thus has strikingly benefits from the technology of MDCT. At submillimeter collimation (0.5–0.75), the entire length of the carotids or the cerebral arteries is scanned in a few seconds in pure arterial phase. Finest anatomic detail can be achieved by this isotropic data set providing high quality 2D and 3D renderings of vascular anatomy through different reconstruction techniques.[14,15]

Magnetic resonance angiography (MRA) and color Doppler ultrasound (DUS) are some noninvasive alternatives. The limitations of MRA include motion artifacts, long examination times, loss of signal due to turbulence and in plane saturation leading to exaggeration of stenosis, poor demonstration of calcium and bony landmarks and limitations in evaluating postoperative patients with metallic clips and stents. Color Doppler (CD) is operator-dependent and limited in evaluating the intracranial vasculature.

Computed tomography angiography the current noninvasive modality of choice for neuroangiography, overcomes many of the disadvantages of MRA. It is faster, available in smaller centers, cheaper, sensitive to presence of calcium, displays bony landmarks and can be used in patients with aneurysm clips and other MR incompatible metallic hardware. CTA depends on volume expansion and opacification of blood in the vessel and hence more accurate. Drawbacks of CTA are the use of intravenous contrast and radiation exposure.

Technique: CT angiography evaluates the area from arch of aorta to vertex for cervicocerebral study in one sitting or from C1 to vertex for cerebral angiogram in 15–20 seconds. Typical parameters can be as follows: 120–140 kVp, 200–350 mAs, 1.25 mm cuts with 1 mm overlap, a pitch of 3 for head (1.25 mm/3.75 mm/rev) and 6 (1.25 mm/7.5 mm/rev) for neck and 0.5 second rotation time. 100 mL of contrast is injected at a rate of 4 mL/s by a power injector which can be chased by bolus tracking. When a threshold attenuation of 100 HU is reached as detected by the ROI placed in one of the common carotids, the scan starts automatically. Alternatively, a test bolus method (20 mL), using a single axial section dynamic study at C5 level can be used. An arbitrary delay of 15–20 seconds is also adequate for CTA of brain. A rapid intravenous injection of nonionic contrast, preferably from right hand, via pressure injector with flow rate of at least 3 mL/s achieves a luminal density of 150 HU which is considered to give best results. Higher rates do not offer any significant advantage.[15] The images are reformatted with section thickness of 1.25 mm and overlap of 1 mm at a narrow field of view (120 mm).

Image processing: There are various display technique for image processing in CT angiography, which include multiplanar reconstructions (MPR), maximum intensity projection (MIP), shaded-surface display (SSD) and volume-rendering technique (VRT).[15,16] MPR allows for viewing of the raw data in any desired plane along the course of the vessel and is good for relatively straight vessels such as the carotid arteries but is not very effective for vascular anatomies which are complex like circle of Willis. MIP images are obtained by projection of imaginary rays through the image data and mapping the maximum attenuation values. The attenuation value, i.e. vessel lumen, calcium and thrombus are well delineated but depth information is totally lost. The degree of stenosis is calculated accurately but there may be overlapping of vessels with bone. Surface shaded display computes all surface connecting neighboring pixels above a particular threshold. Unlike MIP it preserves depth information (displays complex anatomic relationship in region of vessel overlap) but loses attenuation information. It does not show interiors of the vessels, thrombus and wall calcification and as underestimates stenosis. VRT allows integration of all available information through most advanced 3D rendering algorithm. An opacity as well as color is assigned to all the voxels available and VR incorporates all the relevant data into the final resulting image. It overcomes many of the problems seen with MIP and SSD. Since some data loss is inherent with all postprocessing techniques, raw images should be analyzed in all cases.

Applications of CT Angiography

Extracranial Vasculature

Carotid artery stenosis: The detection and accurate quantification of carotid artery stenosis is important for appropriate treatment since carotid endarterectomy has a clear benefit in symptomatic patients with high grade stenosis (70–99%) [North American Symptomatic Carotid Endarterectomy Trial (NASCET)]. The gold standard of carotid evaluation has been conventional angiography but the risks associated with it, interobserver variability in interpreting stenosis (up to 7%), a tendency to overestimate stenosis (6%) and limited number of views are some of the limitations. CTA can provide infinite views for accurate estimation of eccentric or irregular stenosis, delineates mural calcium from luminal contrast and prevents inaccuracy in grading stenosis. Magnified axial images with a window setting half way between luminal contrast and wall are considered best to evaluate stenosis followed by MIP and SSD.[17] Length of thickness, thickness of slices presence of calcification and direction of vessel in the imaged volume also affect measurements.[17-19]

It is difficult to assess exact accuracy of CTA in carotid stenosis due to different criteria and parameters used on different machines; however, reported sensitivity for severe stenosis and occlusion has ranged from 88–100%, which correlates well with conventional angiography **(Figs. 1A to D)**. Lee et al. reported 100% accuracy for occlusion, 90% for critical stenosis (90–99%), greater than 95% for severe stenosis (70–89%), greater than 85% for moderate stenosis (50–69%) and 95% for minimal stenosis.[17-19] CTA also has a good correlation of plaque morphology (calcified, soft or ulcerated).

Computed tomography angiography has a higher accuracy compared to duplex ultrasound (DUS) and is comparable or slightly better than CE MRA (100% vs 93%) for assessing high-grade stenosis and distinguishing it from complete occlusion. This is crucial, as high-grade stenosis is an indication for carotid endarterectomy whereas complete occlusion is a contraindication to surgery. CTA also provides assessment of the brain parenchyma at the same time.

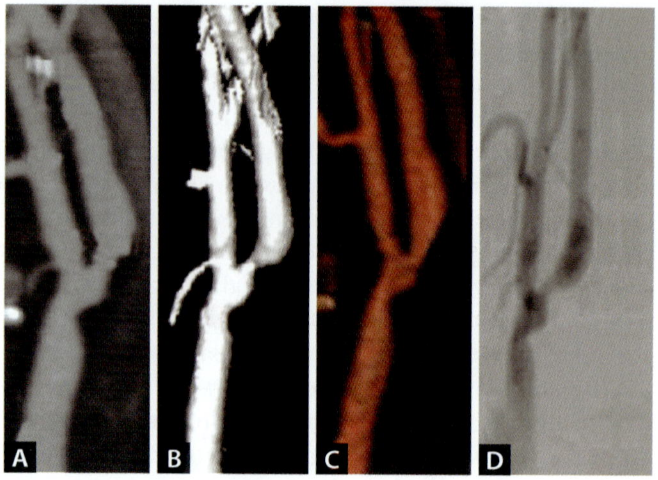

Figs. 1A to D: Left common and internal carotid artery stenosis: (A) MIP; (B) SSD; (C) VR and (D) DSA images showing moderate stenosis of distal common carotid and proximal internal carotid artery. The stenosis is not complete.

Dissections: Dissection of carotid or vertebral artery is an increasingly recognized cause of stroke in young is adequately evaluated with CTA and results are comparable to other noninvasive techniques like MRA and CD.[20] Subadventitial dissections, presence of intramural hematoma, stenosis, occlusions and pseudoaneurysms can be picked up.

Computed tomography angiography is not successful for hemodynamic of blood flow. MDCT can simultaneously evaluate the intracranial vasculature for tandem stenosis in same sitting. Polytrauma patients with a high index of vascular injury can also be evaluated by CTA. MDCT provides simultaneous assessment of vascular, soft tissue and vertebral injury in this setting.

Intracranial Vasculature

Aneurysms: Digital subtraction angiography is the gold standard for the evaluation of patients with subarachnoid hemorrhage secondary to suspected aneurysmal rupture, but it is time consuming, invasive and carries a less than 0.1% complication rate of permanent neurological deficit.[15] There is an associated increased risk of rebleed. As shown by some clinical studies, CTA seems suitable in the acute stage after subarachnoid hemorrhage (SAH) as it does not require intra-arterial catheterization, uses short scan times and can immediately follow the initial unenhanced CT examination.[21,22] Yang et al. had evaluated the diagnostic accuracy of CT Angiography for the small intracranial aneurysms by a large cohort study.[23] They demonstrated that CT angiography had high accuracy for detection of small cerebral aneurysms, including those smaller than

3 mm. However the sensitivities of CT angiography were lower for detection of aneurysms smaller than 3 mm and unruptured compared with aneurysms that were 3–5 mm and ruptured.

For diagnosed aneurysms, CTA provides a more detailed analysis of the sac morphology, neck, parent vessel caliber and its spatial relationship with aneurysm, additional vascular relationships and surrounding anatomy (bony and soft tissue landmarks) which helps in finding the appropriate options for treatment (surgical or minimally invasive endovascular) **(Figs. 2 to 4)**.

Computed tomography angiography is also a problem-solving modality in poorly defined aneurysms on DSA and particularly useful for evaluation of paraclinoid aneurysms for their anatomically complex relationships with bony and vascular structures **(Figs. 2A to D)**. CTA is significant in the characterization of giant aneurysms preceeding surgical or endovascular treatment and helps in the detection of pseudoaneurysms. CTA is also indicated in the assessment of postoperative/postintervention status of aneurysm.

Though conventional angiography is more sensitive for small aneurysms, CTA may show small thrombosed aneurysms not shown on DSA.[24] CTA can be very efficient for screening of vasospasm following SAH. It can be a screening technique to detect aneurysms in high-risk group patients such as those with strong family histories, though MRA is currently the modality of choice.

Computed tomography angiography and MRA have been found to be generally equivalent in their ability to detect and characterize aneurysms (>5 mm).[25] CTA however, is superior to MRA, as turbulent flow or slow flow may cause artifactual loss of signal in MRA.

Some drawbacks of CT angiography include bleak visibility of small arteries, difficulty in distinguishing the infundibular dilatation at the origin of an artery from an aneurysm, the kissing vessel artifact, display of venous

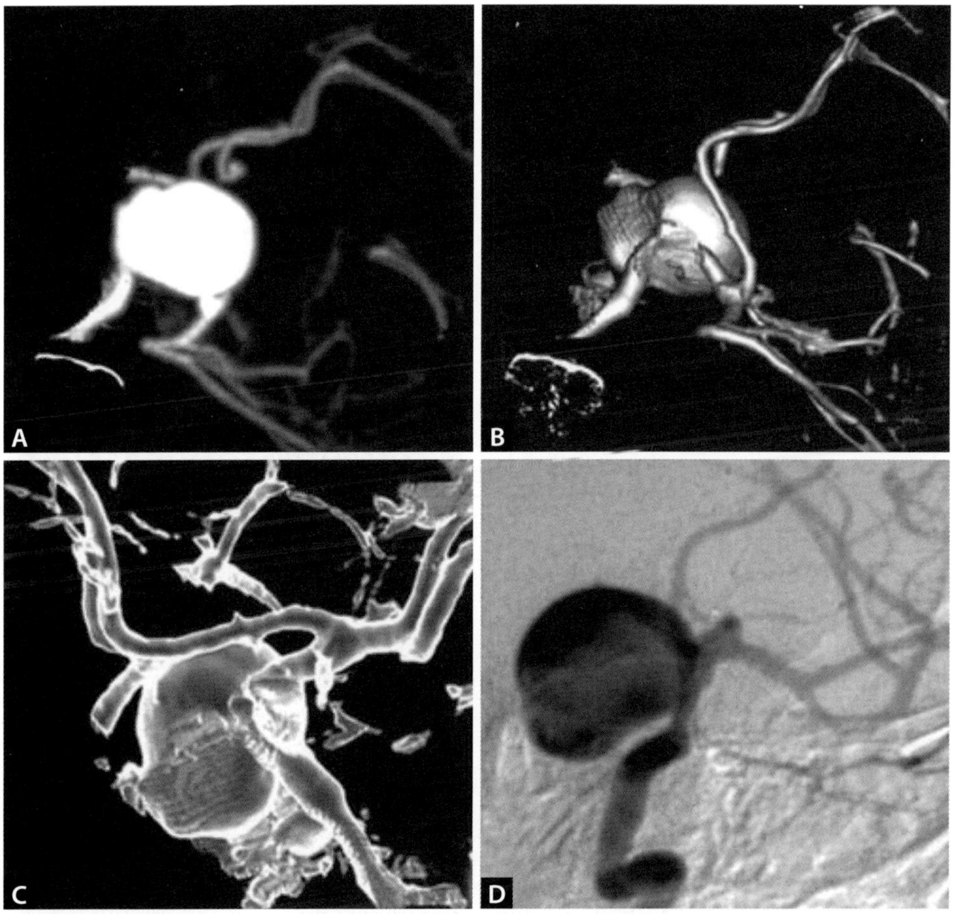

Figs. 2A to D: A giant carotico-ophthalmic aneurysm: Maximum intensity projection (A), volume-rendering (B and C) images; and digital subtraction angiography (D). The carotid artery is incorporated into the aneurysm. Postprocessing shows vascular relationship better than DSA.

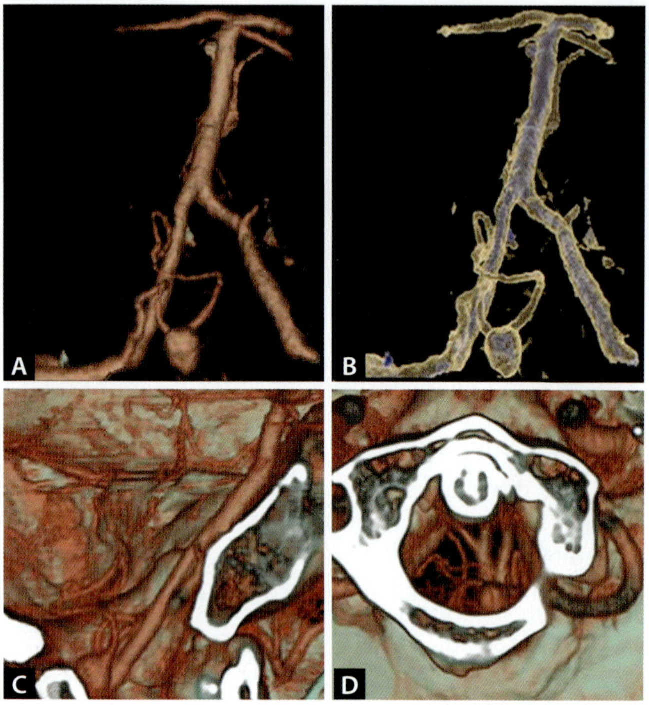

Figs. 3A to D: Posterior inferior cerebellar artery (PICA) aneurysm: volume-rendering images (A and B) posterior view showing the aneurysm arising from the left PICA. The relationship with C1 posterior arch was clearly shown (C and D) helping the decision for surgical approach.

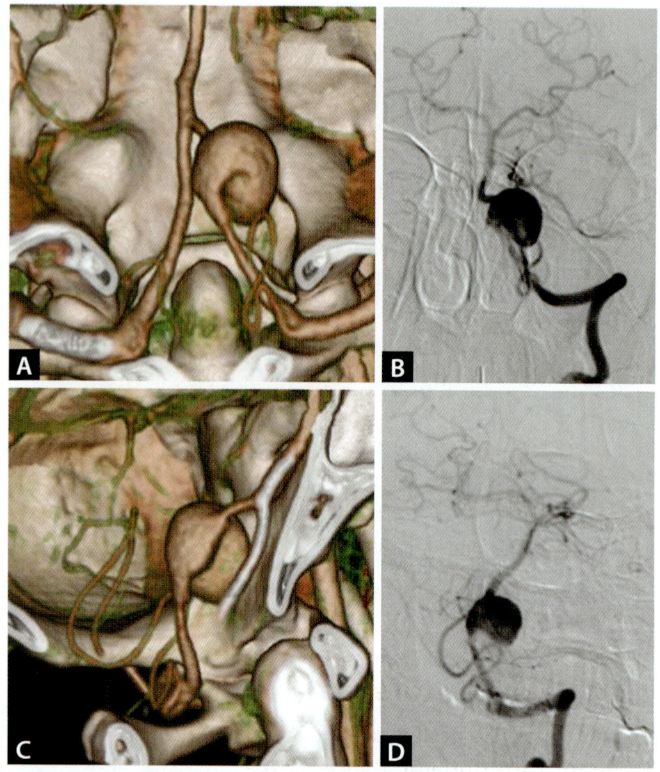

Figs. 4A to D: Left vertebral artery aneurysm: Volume-rendering (A and C) and digital subtraction angiography (B and D) showing left vertebral artery aneurysm with complex configuration better shown on computed tomography volume-rendering images.

structures that can simulate aneurysms, inability to identify thrombosis and calcification on three-dimensional images, and beam-hardening artifacts produced by aneurysm clips.

Arteriovenous malformations: CT angiography though has limited role in intracranial arteriovenous malformations (AVMs), it can visualize the feeding arteries, nidus and draining veins but optimal temporal information regarding arterial and venous phases may not be adequate as compared to DSA.[26] CTA does not possess a high spatial resolution which is required for detecting associated aneurysm, stenosis and small feeding vessels provided by conventional angiography. The major use of CTA today is in the evaluation of the AVM nidus during radiosurgery planning and post-treatment follow-up.[27]

Though any study has not yet compared the roles of CTA and MRA in AVMs yet each modality appears to have its own advantages and disadvantages but flow encoded MR may provide more information in AVM. Embolization material can interfere with delineation of vasculature on MRA but usually is not a problem with CTA.

Tumors: CT angiography can demonstrate vascular encasement by skull-base tumors. It also provides preoperative assessment of the 3D bony and vascular anatomy prior to tumor excision.

COMPUTED TOMOGRAPHY PERFUSION

It has been shown that cerebral blood volume when falls below 20 mL/100 g/min synaptic transmission in neurons fails and below 10 mL irreversible cell death occurs. Therefore tissue salvage is possible in areas with lesser degrees of compromise of blood flow. Computed tomography perfusion (CTP) is a rapid means to evaluate cerebral perfusion as there is a linear relationship between the contrast agent concentration and attenuation.[28-34] CTP is based on the central volume principle as per the equation: CBF = CBV/MTT [cerebral blood flow (CBF), cerebral blood volume (CBV), mean transit time (MTT)]. During the first pass of a bolus of contrast, there is a transient increase in attenuation proportional to the concentration of the agent in a given region. Contrast agent-time concentration curves are generated in an arterial and venous region of interest (ROI) (i.e. middle cerebral artery and superior sagittal sinus) and in the area of perfusion abnormality. Deconvolution of this data gives the MTT. Cerebral blood volume (CBV) is calculated as the area under the curve of parenchymal pixel and the arterial ROI. From this CBF can be calculated.[28]

Technique: Usually for anterior circulation stroke, four adjacent 5 mm slices are selected starting at the level of basal ganglia. About 50 mL of a nonionic contrast is injected at a rate of 3 mL/s. Five seconds later a continuous scan is initiated using 80 kVp, 190–200 mA at one second rotation for 50 seconds. The perfusion data is analyzed at a work station to generate color coded CBF, CBV and MTT maps. With the advent of 256 and 320 MDCT, whole brain perfusion CT can be performed which provides access to the entire brain with the administration of one contrast medium bolus so that ischemic region can be identified.[33-34]

Clinical Applications

Acute stroke: The goal is to identify potentially salvageable tissue for thrombolytic therapy. In a retrospective study, Eastwood et al. found significant difference in CBV, CBF and MTT in symptomatic hemisphere of which MTT was the best indicator for stroke.[30] A 35% decrease in CBF had a good correlation with ischemic penumbra in another study.[30] Early studies do indicate that CTP may enable predication of patients who would benefit from therapy and determine final infarct size.

Cerebrovascular reserve: In patients with chronic ischemia related to underlying stenotic lesions, the involved territory is maximally vasodilated due to autoregulation and cannot respond to acetazolamide challenge. An increase of 5% in CBF indicates insufficiency and a decrease in CBF indicates higher risk of stroke. CTP has been used to show low CBV and CBF in patients of SAH with moderate-to-severe vasospasm.[31,32]

Tumors: Many studies has shown that modified CTP technique has high permeability surface product (a measure of microvascular permeability) in tumors and may prove advantageous over MR in tumor perfusion studies. CTP can be used for preoperative grading of gliomas and can provide additional information about tumor hemodynamics.[33,34] In addition, perfusion computed tomography (PCT) maps are also useful for surgical biopsy and/or radiosurgery guidance to target the areas of increased CBV which can yield better histology and better response to treatment.

COMPUTED TOMOGRAPHY IMAGING OF ACUTE ISCHEMIC STROKE

Several studies have shown better neurological outcome in patients with acute stroke with thrombolytic therapy which were based on the imaging criteria. Multimodal CT (noncontrast CT, CT Angiography and perfusion CT) allows the assessment of the four Ps (parenchyma, pipes perfusion, and penumbra).[35-40] MDCT provides a 'one-stop-shop' approach for comprehensive noninvasive assessment of acute stroke patients by demonstrating the site of arterial occlusion and hemodynamic status of the brain parenchyma. A noncontrast scan is done to diagnose infarct, determine its extension and rule out hemorrhage. A CTA is an accurate technique for evaluation of vascular patency in acute stroke by allowing comprehensive evaluation of the intra- and extracranial vasculature. A CTA from the aortic arch to the intracerebral vessels helps to detect carotid plaques as possible causes of the event, distinguishes between proximal and distal occlusions of an intracranial artery, differentiates arterial from venous infarct and provides information about hypoperfusion and collateralization of blood flow. Finally, a CT perfusion scan distinguishes between penumbra of hypoperfused and umbra of nonperfused tissue in order to select patients who would benefit from thrombolytic therapy. The above information provides a rational basis on which to choose the optimal treatment for patients with acute stroke **(Figs. 5A to C)**. Due to limited availability of PET, SPECT and Xenon CT, CT and MR perfusion are the two practical choices. MRI imaging with DWI and PWI is equally powerful alternative and both CT and MR techniques are comparable in evaluating the tissue at risk in acute stroke according to a recent study.[40] However, widespread availability of CT in smaller centers is a big advantage.

COMPUTED TOMOGRAPHY VENOGRAPHY

Computed tomography venography allows visualization of the cerebral venous structures and has high sensitivity for depicting the cerebral veins and sinus compared to DSA.[41-43] MDCT venography is a fast, widely accessible, and cost-effective method for evaluating cerebral sinuses in emergency setting. MR venography (MRV) is currently the technique of choice for diagnostic evaluation and follow-up for patient with cerebral sinovenous thrombosis. Studies have shown CTV as comparable to accuracy of MRV in the diagnosis of dural sinovenous thrombosis.[41-43] CT venography overcomes flow-related artifacts (differentiates slow flow from thrombosis) seen

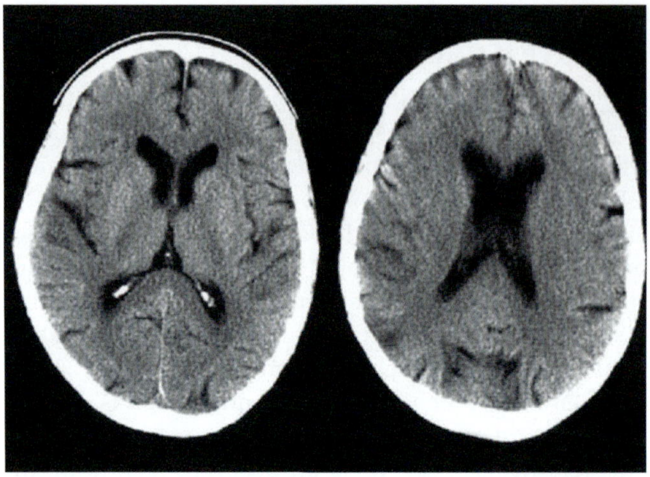

Fig. 5A: Noncontrast CT within 2 hours of stroke showing ill-defined hypodensity in the right parietotemporal region.

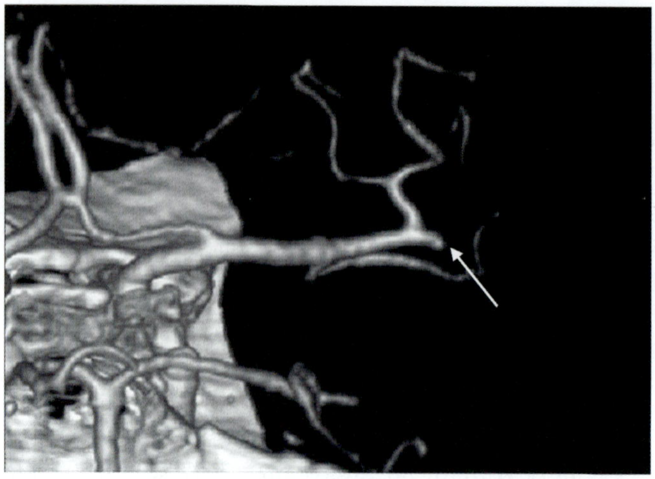

Fig. 5B: Computed tomography angiography in posterosuperior view showing complete occlusion of the inferior division of the right middle cerebral artery (MCA) (arrow).

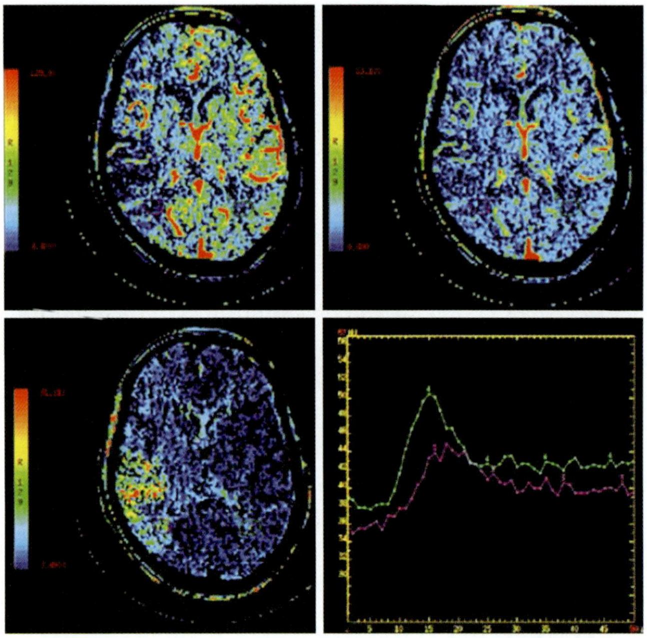

Fig. 5C: Cerebral blood flow, cerebral blood volume and mean transit time maps showing perfusion defect and a large ischemic penumbra. MTT maps shows delayed transit of contrast. Time attenuation curve of penumbra region showing less attenuation compared to normal side.

on time-of-flight (TOF) MR, takes less time and also helps in distinction of tumors that compress dural sinuses, from those which occlude them. However, CT needs contrast administration and lacks sensitivity of MR in showing venous infarction of brain. Overall, CTV is a reliable alternative to MRV in case MR is contraindicated in such patients or is not diagnostic.

Technique: Computed tomography venography is performed using 100 mL of intravenous contrast injected at the rate of 3 mL/s with power injector. After a scan delay of 40 seconds, 1 mm collimated sections with a pitch of 2:1 are done covering the skull.

Clinical Applications of CT Venography

Cerebral sinovenous thrombosis: Dural sinus thrombosis is difficult to diagnose clinically due to varied clinical presentation. The most commonly affected sinuses are the superior sagittal sinus, the transverse sinus and the sigmoid sinus. On CTV, a thrombosed dural sinus is seen as a filling defect and is often associated with contrast enhancement of the walls of the dural sinus as well as abnormal collateral venous drainage and tentorial enhancement **(Figs. 6A to E)**.

Tumors: CTV is also useful for showing venous invasion by meningioma.

MULTIDETECTOR COMPUTED TOMOGRAPHY OF SPINE

Multidetector CT has been a major advancement in imaging of trauma patients to facilitate rapid diagnosis before the patient can be shifted to operation theater. Bony abnormalities are depicted better with MDCT when compared to single slice CT. Current scanners with 16 or more detectors are used to scan from head to below hips using whole body single pass technique. Imaging metallic hardware, which was impossible due to streak artifacts in the single slice helical CT scanning can now be assessed

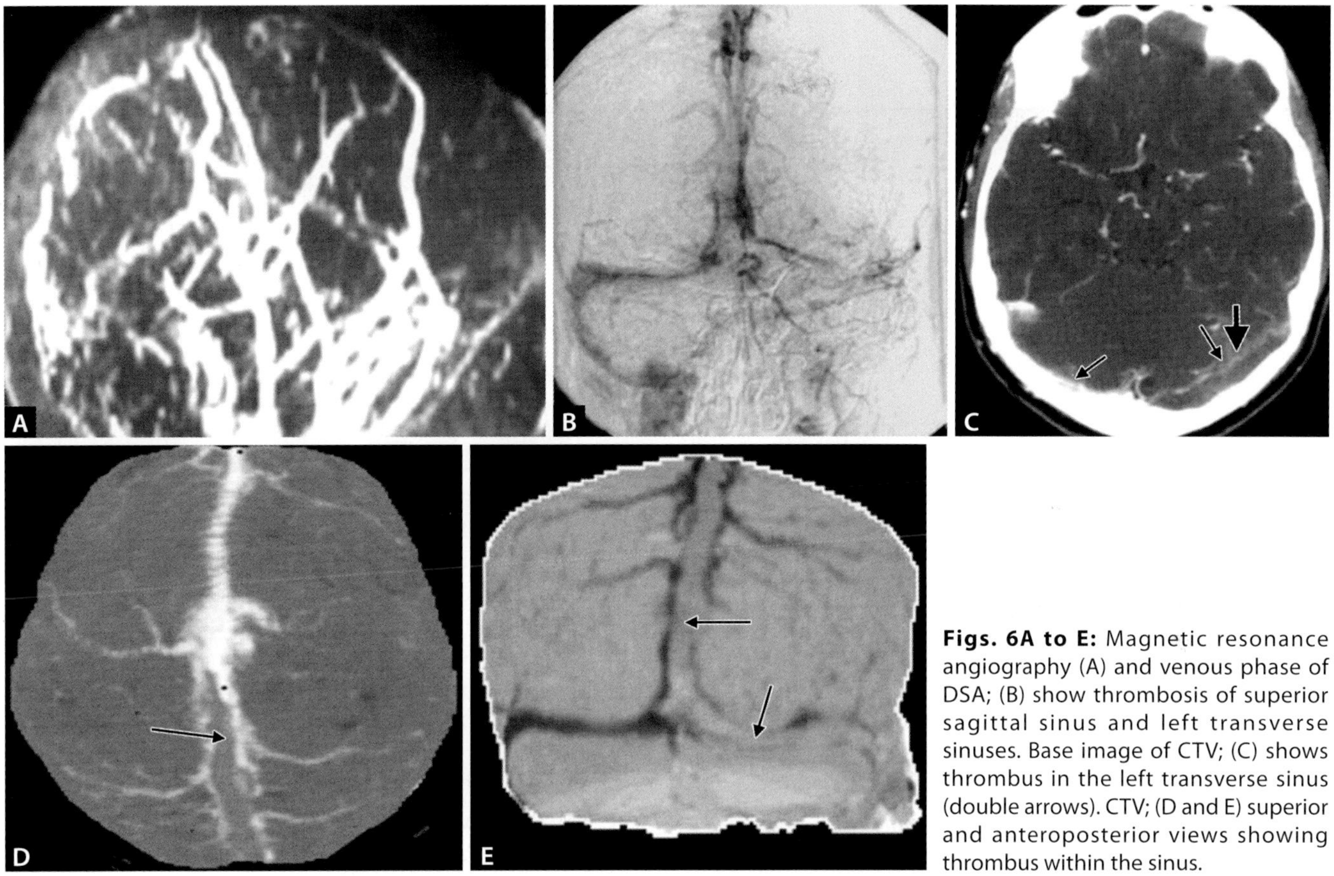

Figs. 6A to E: Magnetic resonance angiography (A) and venous phase of DSA; (B) show thrombosis of superior sagittal sinus and left transverse sinuses. Base image of CTV; (C) shows thrombus in the left transverse sinus (double arrows). CTV; (D and E) superior and anteroposterior views showing thrombus within the sinus.

easily with MDCT due to increase in the of detector rows.[44] With improvement of isotropic resolutions, multiplaner reformations now enable diagnosis that are not so apparent on axial images, i.e. transverse fractures and fusions. Understanding of complex spatial relationships of bone becomes easier which translates into increased confidence level of the radiologist. While 3D-CT may not add to diagnostic information achieved by use of 2D reformatted image but it does aid the surgeons to plan reconstructive surgery.

Clinical Applications

- *Trauma*
  - *Cervical trauma:* CT is cost effective in patients with closed head injury with high risk of associated cervical spine injury, i.e. in confirming and better depicting the extent of the injuries. MDCT gives excellent reformatted images to identify fractures in horizontal plane that may not be apparent otherwise **(Figs. 7A to C)**. Craniovertebral junction is one area well suited for reformatted images. Any associated vascular injury can also be simultaneously evaluated with CTA.
  - *Thoracolumbar trauma:* Combination of 5–10 mm routine abdominal sections for visceral injuries and plain radiography for lumbar spine fracture is inadequate. In such situations, MDCT due to thinner sections and better reformations is 97% sensitive for detection of unstable fractures as compared to 33% sensitivity of plain radiography.[45]
- *In degenerative diseases of spine:* CT is inferior to MRI for evaluating soft tissue detail. Main advantage of MDCT is to show bony canal, i.e. oblique reformations for foraminal stenosis. MDCT depicts trabecular anatomy in the bone marrow with remarkable clarity and early trabecular destruction by tumors is readily apparent. MDCT complements MR and plain radiographic assessment for marrow infiltrative disorders like multiple myeloma, detects vertebrae at risk for fracture and differentiate benign from neoplastic fractures.[46,47]
- Multidetector CT is also useful in evaluation of postoperative patients for hardware and in assessing progression of healing. The artifacts due to metallic hardware implants can be reduced by various advanced CT techniques. Maximizing the peak voltage and tube current, minimizing the detector collimation and pitch

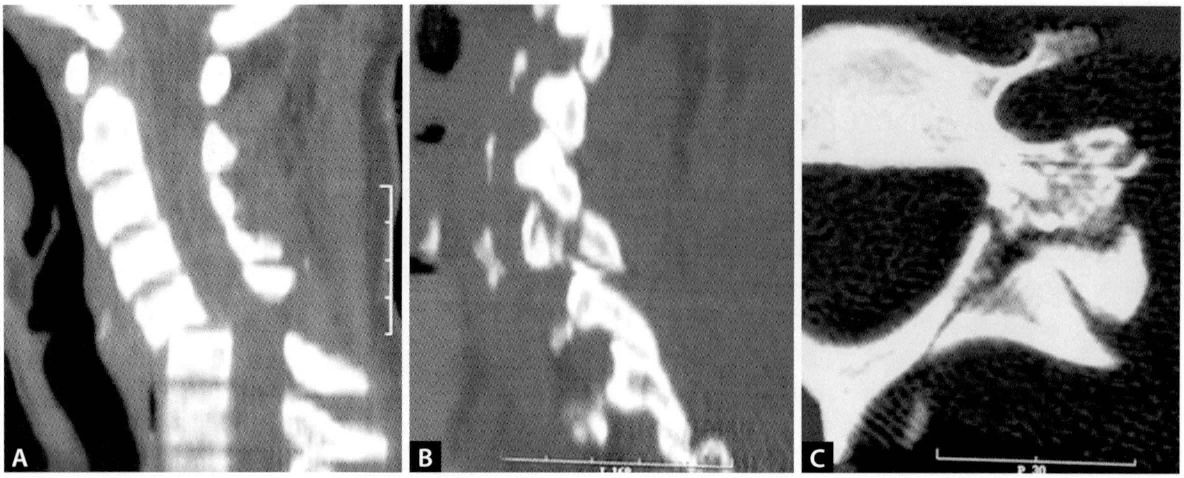

Figs. 7A to C: Sagittal reconstructed (A) helical CT images of cervical spine showing malalignment on CT. Parasagittal reconstructed image of CT (B) better shows the fracture and the locked facet. Axial image (C) shows fracture of lateral mass on left side.

during acquisition can help in reducing the artifacts. Using thin slice reconstruction, thicker slice reformats and 3D-VR techniques are also helpful in reducing the artifacts.[47]

- Numerous vascular conditions like aortic dissection, aortic aneurysm and aneurysm of artery of Adamkiewicz and post-intervention procedures like aortic stent graft placement can endanger the vascular integrity of artery of Adamkiewicz. In these conditions, MDCT angiography of spinal vasculature with adapted brain reconstruction algorithm may provide the details of perfusion and anatomy of artery of Adamkiewicz.[48]
- With multiplanar and 3D reformations, spinal deformities can be assessed in all planes allowing identification of previously unrecognized malformations and better characterization of previously identified deformities. MDCT has a role in depiction of postoperative bony fusions and in patients with indwelling hardware. However, MR still remains the modality of choice to evaluate disc abnormalities and post disc surgery scanning.[46]

RADIATION CONCERNS

Radiation hazard is a major issue as there is a manifold increase in the number of CT examinations performed currently. Helical CT provides a reduction in patient dose over "step and shoot" scans due to short scan times (higher pitch). However, it is known that increasing the pitch does not necessarily decrease the dose as there is an automatic increase in the tube current.[49,50] Further advancement in X-ray tube technology can accomplish decreased dose by modulating the X-ray tube current. The penumbra of the CT beam is a source of wasted radiation. Efforts are on to harvest these for diagnostic information. The organ-specific and shape-specific beam profiles are also being developed like tilted gantries which may reduce radiation to lens.

3D PRINTING

3D Printing is a technique which helps to generate anatomical models or 3D printed physical models from the volumetric medical imaging data (CT or MRI) with the help of computers.[51,52] This technique primarily consists of three steps, initially image segmentation is done, followed mesh refinement and then 3D printing. These have become more popular and cost effective in medicine due to segmentation algorithms advancement and more accessibility of three-dimensional (3D) printers. The 3D printing can be divided into three groups: extrusion printing, photopolymerization and powder-based printing. Extrusion printing is most common form of the 3D printing and is also known as Fused Deposition Modeling (FDM).[51] In this technique, material is melted and the desired shape is made layer by layer fashion, by depositing via a nozzle.

With the 3D printing, the patient-specific models can be made of various organs in the body (like liver and lungs) and anatomical regions of interest. Now there are open-source post-processing tools for the end-users, which help in segmentation of the anatomical structure or spatial model and then desired final product can be printed with the help of special 3D printers.[52] Physical models or prototypes can be made rapidly from the various virtual datasets of CT or MRI.

CONCLUSION

Extensive technical advances in CT have led to significant improvement in the image quality, speed and reduction in radiation dose. Several CT advancement, like multidetector computed tomography (MDCT), dual-energy CT, cone beam CT, portable CT, phase contrast CT and iteractive reconstruction algorithms have revolutionized the neuroimaging with extensive anatomic coverage and thinner sections. Entire cranial and extra-cranial vasculature can be noninvasively demonstrating with high spatial and temporal resolution. With the recent MDCT scanners, visualization of dynamic flow and perfusion as well as motion of an entire volume at a very short time interval is possible.

REFERENCES

1. Ginat DT, Gupta R. Advances in computed tomography imaging technology. Annu Rev Biomed Eng. 2014;16: 431-53.
2. Pelc NJ. Recent and future directions in CT imaging. Ann Biomed Eng. 2014;42(2):260-8.
3. Hu H. Multi-slice helical CT: Scan and reconstruction. Med Phys. 1999;26:5-18.
4. Gupta R, Cheung AC, Bartling SH, et al. Flat-Panel Volume CT: Fundamental Principles, Technology, and Applications. Radiographics. 2008;28:2009-22.
5. Salomon EJ, Barfett J, Willems PW, et al. Dynamic CT Angiography and CT Perfusion Employing a 320-detector Row CT. Klin Neuroradiol. 2009;19:187-96.
6. Brouwer PA, Bosman T, van Walderveen MA, et al. Dynamic 320-section CT angiography in cranial arteriovenous shunting lesions. Am J Neuroradiol. 2010; 31(4):767-70.
7. Hegde A, Chan LL, Tan L, et al. Dual Energy CT and its Use in Neuroangiography. Ann Acad Med Singapore. 2009; 38:817-20.
8. Zhang LJ, Wu SY, Niu JB, et al. Dual energy CT angiography in the evaluation of intracranial aneurysms: Image quality, radiation dose, and comparison with 3D rotational digital subtraction angiography. Am J Roentgenol. 2010; 194:23-30.
9. Ginat DT, Mayich M, Daftari-Besheli L, et al. Clinical applications of dual-energy CT in head and neck imaging. Eur Arch Otorhinolaryngol. 2016; 273(3):547-53.
10. Rumboldt Z, Huda W, All JW. Review of portable CT with assessment of a dedicated head CT scanner. Am J Neuroradiol. 2009; 30(9):1630-6.
11. Hetterich H, Willner M, Fill S, et al. Phase-contrast CT:qualitative and quantitative evaluation of atherosclerotic carotid artery plaque. Radiology. 2014; 271(3):870-8.
12. Geyer LL, Schoepf UJ, Meinel FG, et al. State of the Art: Iterative CT Reconstruction Techniques. Radiology. 2015; 276(2):339-57.
13. Mainali S, Wahba M, Elijovich L. Detection of Early Ischemic Changes in Noncontrast CT Head Improved with "Stroke Windows". ISRN Neurosci. 2014;2014:654980.
14. Westerlaan HE. Gravendeel J, Fiore D, et al. Multislice CT angiography in the selection of patients with ruptured intracranial aneurysms suitable for clipping or coiling. Neuroradiology. 2007;49:997-1007.
15. Kuszyk BS, Beauchamp NJ Jr, Fishman EK. Neurovascular applications of CT angiography. Semin Ultrasound CT MR. 1998;19(5):394-404.
16. Snyder KV, Mokin M, Bates VE. Neurologic applications of whole-brain volumetric multidetector computed tomography. Neurol Clin. 2014;32(1):237-51.
17. Anderson GB, Ashforth R, Steinke DE, et al. CT angiography for the detection and characterization carotid artery bifurcation disease. Stroke. 2000;31:2168-74.
18. Dillon EH, Van Leeuwen MS, Fernandes MA, et al. CT angiography: Application to the evaluation of carotid artery stenosis. Radiology. 1993;189:211-9.
19. Lee A, Boss J, Ngyuyen T, et al. Application of helical computed tomographic angiography in evaluation of carotid artery stenosis. Applied Radiology. 1998;26-30.
20. Link J, Brossman J, Penslcen V, et al. Common carotid artery bifurcation: Preliminary results of CT angiography and color coded duplex sonography compared with digital subtraction angiography. Am J Roentgenol. 1997; 168:361-5.
21. Leclerc X, Godefroy O, Salhi A, et al. Helical CT for the diagnosis of extracranial carotid artery dissection. Stroke. 1996;27:461-6.
22. Zouaori A, Sahil M, Mairo B, et al. Three-dimensional computed tomographic angiography in detection of cerebral aneurysms in acute subarachnoid hemorrhage. Neurosurgery. 1997; 41:125-30.
23. Yang ZL, Ni QQ, Schoepf UJ, et al. Small Intracranial Aneurysms: Diagnostic Accuracy of CT Angiography. Radiology. 2017; 285(3):941-52.
24. Hope JK, Wilson JL, Thomson FJ. Three-dimensional angiography in the dectection and characterization of intracranial berry aneurysms. Am J Neuroradiol. 1996;17:439-45.
25. Brown JH, Lustrin ES, Lev MH, et al. Characterization of intracranial aneurysms using CT angiography. Am J Roentgenol. 1997;169: 889-93.
26. Barboriak DP, Provenzale JM. MR arteriography of intracranial circulation. Am J Roentgenol. 1998; 171:1469-78.
27. Reiger J, Hoston N, Neuman, K et al. Initial clinical experience with spiral CT and 3D arterial reconstruction in intracranial aneurysm and arteriovenous malformations. Neuroradiology. 1996; 36:245-51.
28. Wintermark M, Reichhart M, Cuisenaire O, et al. Comparison of admission perfusion computed tomography and qualitative diffusion and perfusion weighted magnetic resonance imaging in acute stroke patients. Stroke. 2002; 33:2025-31.
29. Nabavi DG, Cenic A, Craen RA, et al. Assessment of cerebral perfusion: Experimental validation and the initial clinical experience. Radiology. 1999; 213:141-9.
30. Eastwood JD, Lev MH, Azhari T, et al. Perfusion scanning with deconvolution analysis: Pilot study in patients with

acute middle cerebral artery stroke. Radiology. 2002; 222:227-36.

31. Wintermark M, Reichhart M, Thiran JP, et al. Prognostic accuracy of cerebral blood flow measurement by perfusion computed tomography, at the time of emergency room admission, in acute stroke patients. Ann Neurol. 2002; 51:417-32.
32. Nabavi DG, LeBlanc LM, Baxter B, et al. Monitoring cerebral perfusion after subarachnoid hemorrhage using CT. Neuroradiology. 2001;43:7-16.
33. Murayama K, Katada K, Nakane M, et al. Whole-Brain Perfusion CT Performed with a Prototype 256-Detector Row CT System: Initial Experience. Radiology. 2009;250:202-11.
34. Ellika SK, Jain R, Patel SC, et al. Role of Perfusion CT in Glioma Grading and Comparison with Conventional MR Imaging Features. Am J Neuroradiol. 2007; 28:1981-7.
35. Srinivasan A, Goyal M, Azri FA, et al. State-of-the-Art Imaging of Acute Stroke. Radiographics. 2006; 26:75-95.
36. Ledezma CJ, Wintermark M. Multi-modal CT in Stroke Imaging: New Concepts. Radiol Clin North Am. 2009; 47(1):109-16.
37. Tomandl BF, Klotz E, Handschu R, et al. Comprehensive Imaging of Ischemic Stroke with Multisection CT. Radiographics. 2003; 23:565-92.
38. Zerna C, Assis Z, d'Esterre CD, et al. Imaging, Intervention, and Workflow in Acute Ischemic Stroke: The Calgary Approach. Am J Neuroradiol. 2016;37(6):978-84.
39. Wardlaw JM. Overview of Cochrane thrombolysis meta-analysis. Neurology. 2001; 57:S69-76.
40. Sunshine J. CT, MR and MR angiography in evaluation of patients with acute stroke. J Vasc Interv Radiol. 2004;15:S47-55.
41. Khandelwal N, Agarwal A, Kochhar R, et al. Comparison of CT Venography with MR Venography in cerebral sinovenous thrombosis. Am J Roentgenol. 2006; 187:1637-43.
42. Linn J, Erlt-Wagner B, Seelos KC, et al. Diagnostic value of multidetector-row CT angiography in the evaluation of thrombosis of the cerebral venous thrombosis. Am J Neuroradiol. 2007; 28: 946-52.
43. Ozsvath RR, Casey SO, Lustrin ES, et al. Cerebral venography: Comparison of CT and MR projection venography. Am J Roentgenol. 1997; 169:1699-707.
44. Buchwalter KA, Rydberg J, Kopecky KK, et al. Musculoskeletal imaging with multislice CT. Am J Roentgenol. 2001; 176:979-86.
45. Rhee PM, Bridgeman A, Acosta JA, et al. Lumbar fractures in adult blunt trauma: Axial and single slice helical abdominal and pelvic computed tomographic scans versus portable plain X ray. J Trauma. 2002; 53:663-7.
46. Crim JR, Tripp D. Multidetector CT of the spine. Semin in US, CT and MRI. 2004; 25:55-66.
47. Ohashi K, El-Khoury GY. Musculoskeletal CT: Recent advances and current clinical applications. Radiol Clinc N Am. 2009; 47: 387-409.
48. Boll DT, Bulow H, Blackam KA, et al. MDCT Angiography of the spinal vasculature and the artery of the Adamkiewicz. Am J Roentgenol. 2006; 187:1054-60.
49. Mahesh M, Scatarige JC, Cooper J, et al. Dose and pitch relationship for a particular multislice CT scanner. Am J Roentgenol. 2001; 177:1273-75.
50. Costello JE, Cecava ND, Tucker JE, et al. CT radiation dose: current controversies and dose reduction strategies. Am J Roentgenol. 2013; 201(6):1283-90.
51. Bücking TM, Hill ER, Robertson JL, Maneas E, Plumb AA, Nikitichev DI. From medical imaging data to 3D printed anatomical models. PLoS One. 2017;12(5):e0178540.
52. Bortolotto C, Eshja E, Peroni C, et al. 3D Printing of CT Dataset: Validation of an Open Source and Consumer-Available Workflow. J Digit Imaging. 2016;29(1):14-21.

CHAPTER 5

Advances in Neuroimaging Techniques: Magnetic Resonance Imaging

Paramjeet Singh, Niranjan Khandelwal, Sameer Vyas

Magnetic resonance imaging (MRI) is probably the most powerful tool in the radiologist's arsenal in diagnosing the brain and spinal pathologies. It has got tremendous role in providing into both the anatomical, pathological and functional aspects of a disease entity. Improvements have been directed toward reducing scan times and improving image quality through developing new pulse sequences, improved receiver coil technology, enhanced gradient performance, use of higher field strength magnets and application of more efficient data processing. Modern ultrafast sub-second sequences virtually freeze the physiological motion. On the other hand, with the advent of diffusion weighted imaging, perfusion imaging, spectroscopy it is now possible to provide an insight into the functional aspect of the disease. With advancement in MRI technology, it has emerged as a powerful tool not only for fast routine scanning, but also establishing its multiparametric applications into studying organ function, metabolism and physiology leading to an integrative approach.

In this chapter, we are going to discuss the hardware improvement in MRI including higher field strength MRI followed by faster scanning techniques and the different sequences exploring functional aspect of disease and finally briefly about the latest exciting developments on artificial intelligence. MR spectroscopy, functional MRI and 3D printing have been discussed in the other chapters in this book.

IMPROVEMENTS IN MR HARDWARE

During last few decades, tremendous improvement has been observed in the MR hardware particularly in the form of evolution of high field MRI. The technical design of magnets operating at 1.5 T has been the subject of an enormous engineering effort and area of research over the last 30 years and evolution of designs over years have led to a high level of performance and efficiency. In the last 15 years we observed similar evolution with 3T units. Currently further upgradation of magnetic strength is an area of major research.

High field strength MRI: A large number of MR systems operating at a field strength of 3 Tesla (and higher) have been installed worldwide and are gaining acceptance for clinical and research purpose particularly in neuroimaging. The US Food and Drug Administration cleared the first seven tesla (7T) magnetic resonance imaging device in October 2017 for clinical use. MR scanners with 9.4 T, 10.5 T and 11.75 T are also being used for research purposes in few institutions.

It is an established and well-recognized fact that increasing the static field strength increases the signal detected in MRI.[1-3] It primarily happens through two mechanisms: increasing magnetization and increasing detection efficiency. Spin polarization is produced by most MRI scanners by applying the static field to a spin system that is in thermal equilibrium with its surroundings a phenomenon known as Boltzmann polarization. In this setting, the equilibrium magnetization bears a linear relationship with field strength. The detected signal is proportional to the rate of spin precession, and this leads to a detection efficiency that increases linearly with field strength.[4] The combination of increased magnetization and increased spin detection efficiency leads to an increase in signal strength that is proportional to the square of the applied field. However, to determine the overall advantage of increasing the field strength and, therefore, the operating frequency, it is necessary to consider the frequency dependence of the noise voltages that are inevitably present. The noise voltages are superimposed on the signal voltage and will impair the ability to construct an image from the signal voltage unless the signal to noise ratio (SNR) of the system is sufficiently large. Without going into the complexity of physics it can be commented that the noise voltage is linearly proportional to the Larmor frequency and proportional to the square root of the tissue conductivity. In most tissues, the conductivity increases weakly with frequency, and, as a result, the thermal noise level generally increases slightly faster than linearly with increasing field strength.[5] The advantage of improved SNR can be exploited to increase speed and resolution judiciously, i.e. imaging time can be reduced for a similar SNR as 1.5 T or spatial resolution increased for an equal imaging time on both.[6]

SNR changes linearly with B0. However, in presence of inhomogeneity and changing tissue relaxation, linear increase in SNR may not be possible.[7] Besides the increase in SNR, the other tissue properties or imaging parameters which are also affected at higher field strength include resolution, T1 (in sec), T2* (in sec), apparent T2, sensitivity to susceptibility and spectral resolution in MRSI.[8] Two main advantages of higher field strength are increase in SNR and susceptibility induced contrast. These are especially helpful in functional imaging techniques [fMRI, blood oxygen level dependent (BOLD) contrast], MR spectroscopy and high resolution anatomical imaging (volumetric 3-dimensional imaging) within acceptable acquisition time. High field MRI is clinically very useful for imaging of epilepsy, brain tumors, multiple sclerosis, Alzheimer's disease and psychiatric illness. However, there are many technical challenges and limitations of higher field strength. Technical challenges include increased susceptibility artifacts and specific absorption rate (SAR), and inhomogeneous field (main and radiofrequency). Other limitations include very high cost, and imaging artifacts.

RAPID IMAGE ACQUISITION TECHNIQUES

Ever since the role of MRI has been established in clinical settings, researches are going on to reduce the MR acquisition time and at the same time maintaining high-image spatial resolution, contrast, and quality. The MR imaging techniques that can be employed for rapid image acquisition are discussed below in brief.

Echo-planar Imaging (EPI)

Echo-planar (or Echo volume) imaging is based on acquisition of all of the k-space following a single excitation pulse, and is the most direct approach for rapid image acquisition as well as reduce motion artifacts. EPI may be performed with a series of spin echoes (in which a series of 180-degree refocusing pulses are applied) or with a series of gradient echoes (created by alternating the polarity or direction of the readout gradient). Conventionally, EPI is associated with gradient echo acquisitions, while the spin echo variant is termed fast spin echo (FSE), turbo spin echo (TSE), or rapid acquisition with relaxation enhancement (RARE). Although sampling a different echo for each line in k-space is done in both gradient echo and spin echo approaches, the weighing of the acquired signal is differently. In gradient echo EPI, the different k-space lines have different T2* weightings as the signal is decaying as a function of T2*, while in spin echo EPI, each k-space line has a different T2 weighting as the signal is decaying by the longer T2 time constant. This difference is important with respect to image quality as chemical shift and local magnetic susceptibility artifacts (also known as off resonance effects) can modulate the gradient echo signals. However, these effects can be reduced with spin echo EPI. Other artifact concerns with EPI include ghosting, due to a mismatch in location of the echo center between k-space lines acquired with a positive readout gradient, and those acquired with a negative readout gradient; geometric off-resonance distortions; and fat signal ghosting.

EPI is an excellent tool for many neuroimaging sequences despite its limitations. It has got tremendous utility for functional imaging and diffusion tensor imaging, where the physiologic process under evaluation takes place rapidly (e.g. neuronal activity or blood perfusion) or the method is sensitive to subject motion. On present day MRI scanners, the individual gradient echoes that make up the EPI readout train is separated by temporal gap of less than 2 milliseconds. Thus, 64 to 128 echoes can be acquired following a single excitation pulse in time periods of 100 to 300 milliseconds. Although it is long relative to T2*, this is still short enough making sure there is still a measurable signal at the end of the echo train. Continuing advancements in gradient technology, specifically the rate at which gradients can be turned on and reach their maximum value (slew rate), have been critical to the success of EPI in many neuroimaging applications where precise morphologic information is not strictly necessary.

A simple way to decrease the effects of off-resonance distortions in EPI is to reduce the number of lines acquired following each RF excitation pulse. Multishot EPI divides the number of k-space lines into pieces (e.g. in a four-shot sequence, 128 k-space lines are broken down to 4 sets of 32). The reduced number of gradient echoes significantly reduces the sampling period and, therefore, the T2* weighting across the echo train. This reduces the spatial displacements caused by off-resonance effects by a factor equal to the number of shots used to acquire the k-c plane. Of course, multishot EPI sequences reduce the advantages of EPI, specifically the ability to "freeze" motion.

Fast Spin Echo Imaging

Hennig et al.[9] in the mid-1980s first introduced the spin echo EPI with the publication of the RARE method.[9] It uses RF-generated spin echoes as opposed to gradient echoes and is based on the RF pulse train known as the Carr-Purcell-Meiboom-Gill (CPMG) sequence,[10-12] in which a string of 180-degree pulses separated by intervals of 2τ follow an initial 90-degree excitation pulse. The basic RARE sequence had been modified in the early 1990s to allow for flexible T2 contrast manipulation.[13-17] After these initial modifications, gradually conventional spin echo sequences became replaced with newer versions of the RARE sequence, also referred to as FSE or TSE sequences. Currently, all MR vendors provide both single-shot and multiple shot versions of FSE sequences, under multiple trade names. Generally speaking, the multiple-shot versions of the FSE sequence has completely replaced conventional spin echo sequences which were used as the gold standard for brain lesion detection during the first decade of MR as the FSE sequences can produce comparable T2-weighted tissue contrast and image quality, provided by conventional spin echo imaging in much shorter scan time.[15,18-22] However, FSE has got lesser sensitivity to hemorrhage compared to conventional spin echo sequences[21] while the signal from fat (bright fat phenomenon) is higher in FSE imaging[23,24] as well as MT effects are also higher in FSE compared to conventional spin echo imaging.[25] Despite these limitations, FSE has almost completely replaced conventional spine echo imaging by virtue of reduced scan time.

Gradient and Spin Echo Imaging (GRASE)

The gradient and spin echo imaging can be combined to produce a novel imaging technique that allows rapid image acquisition as well as a unique image contrast. High spatial resolution 3D imaging in a much shorter time is possible with this technique[26] and has been incorporated into perfusion and diffusion imaging sequences.

Steady State Imaging Methods

Simply shortening TR, thereby allowing more data to be acquired in same acquisition time, can lead to acquisition of higher spatial resolution images or higher volumetric coverage. It can also be used to acquire same amount of data in reduced scan time. The technique involves repeated application of identical and, typically low-angle RF pulses with a time separation much less than T1 and T2; thereby not allowing the magnetization to fully relax back to equilibrium prior to each subsequent RF excitation pulse. The process of repeated excitation results in a steady state of magnetization so that the transverse and/or longitudinal magnetization before each RF pulse is constant. Although very rapid imaging is possible with this technique, the signal measured in steady state imaging is significantly less, as the magnetization is not allowed to fully recover and the RF pulses are often less than 30 degrees. Hence it is obvious that while the steady state sequences have very high signal efficiency (signal per unit time), the overall absolute SNR is less compared to conventional methods.

Steady state methods can either be spoiled or nonspoiled. If the transverse magnetization is spoiled before each RF pulse, only the longitudinal magnetization is in equilibrium. Hence, the images acquired in this spoiled situation (termed spoiled gradient, SPGR, or spoiled fast low angle shot, FLASH), show a strong T1 contrast. On the other hand, if the sequence is left unspoiled allowing the transverse magnetization to evolve or to be balanced so that the transverse magnetization is completely refocused prior to each RF pulse and both the longitudinal and transverse magnetizations will be brought into dynamic equilibrium. Images acquired under this condition [termed gradient recalled acquisition in the steady-state (GRASS); fast imaging with steady-state precession (FISP); fast field echo (FFE); reversed FISP (PSIF), or true FISP] have contrast that is a function of T1, T2, and/or T2*. The clinical applications of the gradient echo imaging are predominantly in the characterization of tissue susceptibility characteristics and can be used for demonstration of intracranial calcification and hemorrhages.

Partial Fourier Acquisitions

Echo-planar imaging, FSE and steady state imaging methods although offer rapid image acquisitions, these are frequently associated with a multitude of artifacts and image distortion which makes them incapable of high resolution, high-quality, and motion-free imaging. Hence, alternate approaches based on properties of Fourier transform have been proposed. Zero-padding and partial or half-Fourier acquisition are the main techniques for partial Fourier acquisitions. Zero-padding is the most basic approach and it involves "padding" the original lower-resolution k-space with zeros so as to increase the apparent extent of "acquired" k-space. Zero-padding is commonly associated with Gibbs ringing artifact, which occur due to the sharp boundary in k-space introduced along the border of the acquired k-space data, and the zero-filled portion. Half-Fourier acquisition is based on the fact that conjugate symmetry exists between pairs of points that lie equidistant from the origin of k-space, and on a diagonal line passing through the origin. Hence, only one-half of k-space need be acquired, with the other half synthesized from the acquired data—commonly known as partial or half-Fourier acquisition.[27]

Parallel Imaging

The term parallel imaging encompasses a group of methods which are generally designed to decrease scan time by sub/undersampling k-space data. In order to save scanning time in parallel imaging, some phase encoding lines are not collected. As a result, the field-of-view (FoV) of the image is reduced, which is likely to result into aliasing, or fold-over, artifacts. The term acceleration/reduction factor refers to the amount/factor by which the data is undersampled. For example, the acceleration factor, R = 2 if only half of the normally required data is collected. Parallel imaging reconstruction can be applied in order to remove the aliasing artifacts resulting from the smaller FoV. Parallel imaging can work in either the image domain or in k-space, but the common theme of all of these methods is that they employ the varying spatial sensitivities of a receiver coil array to reconstruct the aliased image.

The salient features of parallel imaging-based sequences are:

- The undersampled data is reconstructed by these the techniques and these are not new imaging sequences.
- Data needs to be acquired simultaneously and independently with multiple receiver channels having different sensitivity profiles.
- Contrast behavior of the underlying imaging sequence generally does not change by the parallel imaging.
- These techniques work either by decreasing the amount of time needed to perform an imaging sequence or increasing the resolution in a given specific measurement time, or combination of the two can be used.
- Main limitation is the reduction in the SNR in the reconstructed image by a factor greater than or equal to the square root of the reduction factor, as R-times fewer data points are acquired.

Currently, parallel MRI methods can be broadly classed based on whether the reconstruction and alias removal is performed in the image domain (e.g. sensitivity encoding, SENSE) or in the k-space domain [e.g. simultaneous acquisition of spatial harmonics (SMASH), generalized autocalibrating partially parallel acquisition (GRAPPA)]. No consensus exists as to which technique is universally superior. The choice may be both vendor- and case-specific. The major applications of parallel imaging are in MR angiography and dynamic postcontrast imaging.

These parallel MRI methods are summarized in **Flowchart 1**.

Compressed SENSE (CSENSE)

Another technique of reducing the acquisition time came into fray within the last decade known as compressed sensing. The basis of compressed sensing MRI (CS MRI) is image reconstruction from a k-space which is incompletely filled or under sampled.[28-30]

Originally, it was proposed as a general concept to accurately reconstruct a small number of random measurements.[29,30] The concept of CS-MRI was inspired from a similar imaging problem related to transmission and storage of huge volume of imaging dataset generated by modern-day scanners. The solution to this problem was permanently discarding certain data elements and thereby reducing file size—a process known as lossy image compression. Successful compression of medical images can be achieved even at compression ratios from 9:1 to 25:1 using a variety of algorithms, while preserving diagnostic efficacy at the same time. This led Lustig et al.[28] to raise the question that if the images are indeed compressible whether it is necessary to acquire the full dataset at all. Further they proposed that reconstruction of the same image generated from a fully sampled set could be possible from the simple measurement of the

Flowchart 1: Various parallel imaging methods.

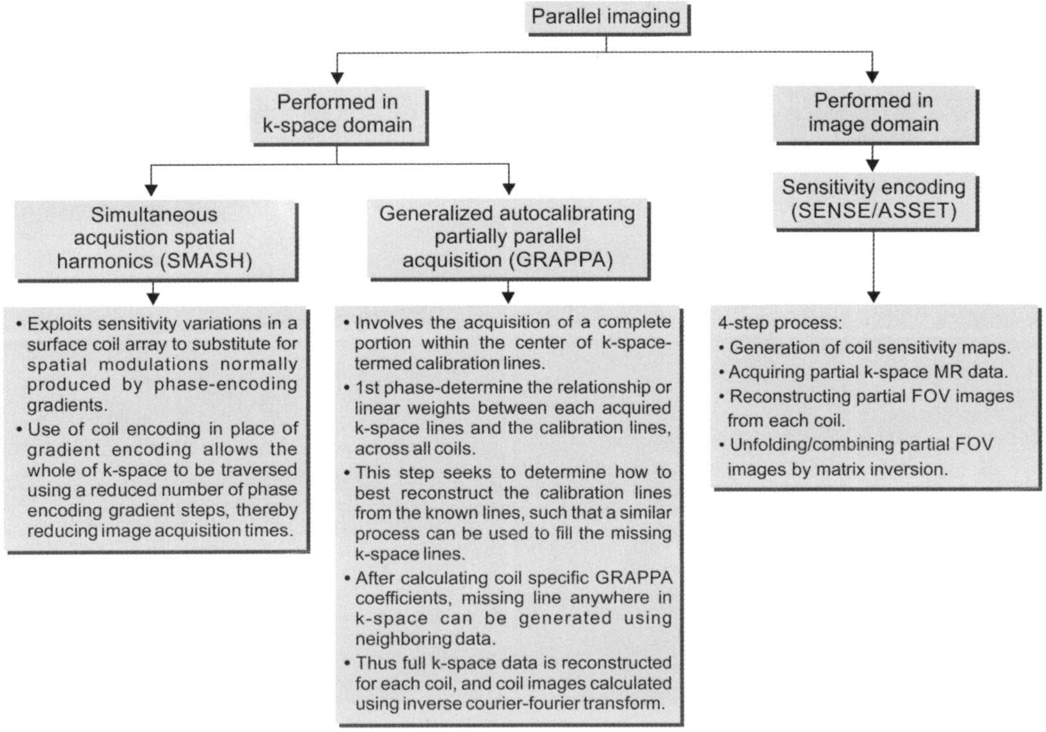

compressed information directly from the small number of measurements and it can be achieved by k-space undersampling as MRI measures Fourier coefficients only.

The successful utilization of compressed sensing is team play of data acquisition and image reconstruction. Lustig et al.[28] identified three criteria as being essential to ensure successful image recovery from subsampled data:

- Firstly, once the conversion with a mathematical transformation has been done, the object that is acquired should have a sparse representation.
- Secondly, subsampling of k-space should be done in such a way that incoherent, i.e. noise like artifacts are produced in the image as a result of aliasing.
- Finally, a nonlinear, iterative optimization, that simultaneously enforces a sparse representation of the resulting image, is used for reconstruction of the images, leading to removal of the noise like artifacts, while preserving its consistency to the acquired data.

The role of compressed SENSE in neuroimaging is still an area of research. Major application is in pediatric neuroimaging as it can significantly (~40–50%) reduce the acquisition time thereby reducing the sedation and anesthesia time and at the same time producing images of significant diagnostic quality **(Figs. 1A to H)**. Other potential application is acquisition of high resolution MR angiography images and in vessel wall imaging where images with lesser slice thickness can be acquired at similar time of acquisition using compressed SENSE algorithm.

Multiband or Multiplexed Imaging

Multiband is the latest addition to the suite of rapid MR acquisition methodologies. It aims to excite and acquire data from multiple imaging slices simultaneously.[31,32] Multiband RF pulses, which comprise two or more single-band pulses that each excites specific slices in a conventional 2D multislice acquisition, are used in this technique. To separate the received signal from each slice, parallel imaging methods such as SENSE can be used, provided there are sufficient coil sensitivity variations along the slice direction. Thus, the technique as originally proposed was limited to relatively largely spaced slices. To eliminate this issue, a phase shift can be introduced between excited slices, which can then be readily reconstructed using a phase constrained parallel MRI reconstruction method even in the absence of coil sensitivity differences. Though only developed in 2010, this technique has gained rapid acceptance in neuroimaging research applications particularly in functional MRI and arterial spin labeling (ASL) perfusion. Further, the ability to combine multi-band imaging with in plane SENSE acceleration offers the

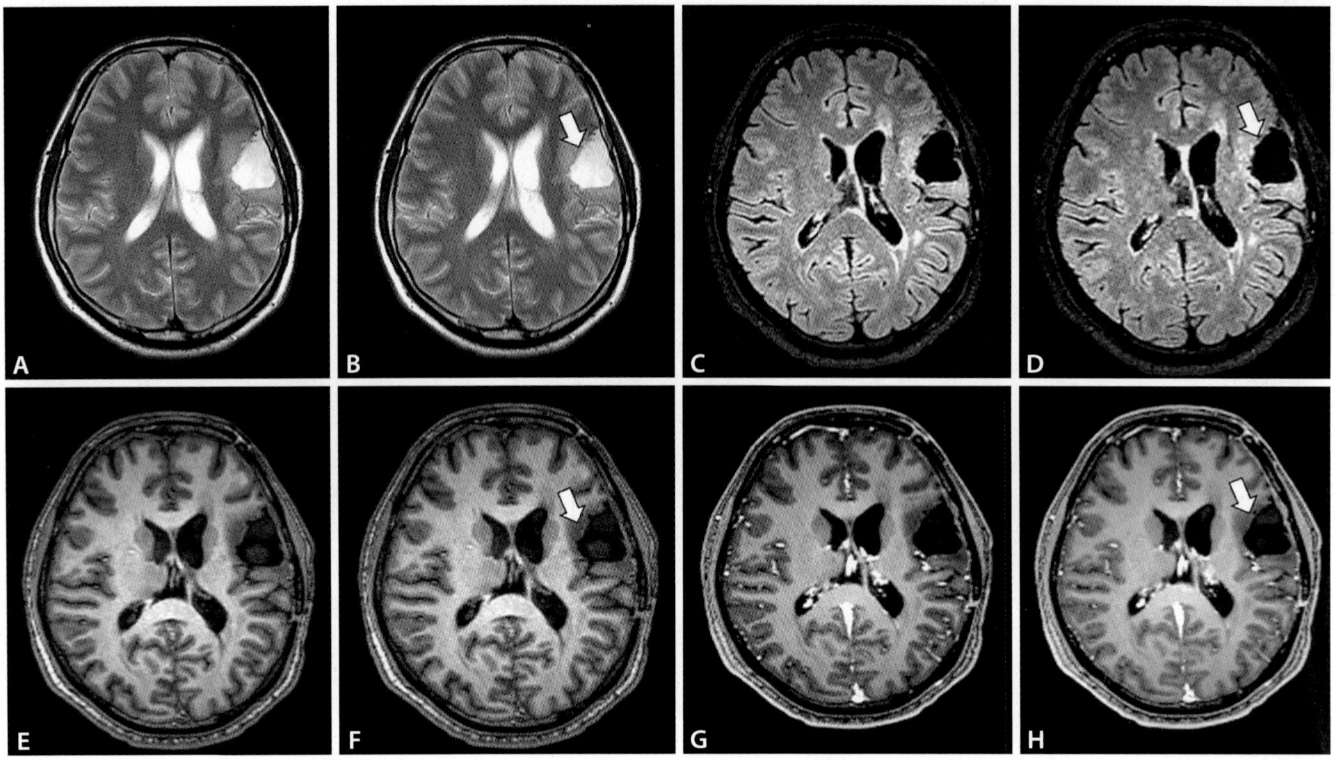

Figs. 1A to H: Contrast-enhanced MRI of a 13-year-old male child status postoperative for low grade glial tumor. (A and B) T2 axial sequences of brain acquired with conventional MRI and CSENSE MRI technique with acceleration factor of 2.4 respectively. (C and D) Axial reformatted image of 3D FLAIR sequences acquired with conventional MRI and CSENSE MRI technique with acceleration factor of 8. (E and F) Axial reformatted image of T1-GRE precontrast sequences acquired with conventional MRI and CSENSE MRI technique acquired with acceleration factor of 3.4. (G and H) Axial reformatted image of T1-GRE postcontrast sequences acquired with conventional MRI and CSENSE MRI technique acquired with acceleration factor of 4. Mild blurring of margin of postoperative cavity noted in T2, FLAIR, T1 pre- and postcontrast sequences acquired with C-SENSE (B, D, F and H) shown by arrow.

potential for significant reductions in overall acquisition time in multislice imaging techniques.

ADVANCED MR IMAGING TECHNIQUES

SUSCEPTIBILITY WEIGHTED IMAGING (SWI)

Susceptibility weighted imaging exploits the magnetic inhomogeneity where tissues of higher susceptibility distort the magnetic field and become out of phase from their neighbors at long echo times.[33] Thus, there is signal loss on magnitude images. It is fully velocity compensated high resolution 3D gradient echo sequence that uses magnitude and filtered phase information, separately and in combination to create a new source of contrast. Unlike initial experience with spoiled GRE, with advent of 3T and parallel imaging, it is now possible to image the entire brain with SWI in a short time. Delineation of small vessels particularly veins is exquisite on SWI, due to high T2* of deoxygenated blood. The technique provides additional clinical information in evaluation of traumatic brain injuries, coagulopathic and other hemorrhagic disorders, vascular malformations, cerebral infarctions, neoplasms, and neurodegenerative disorders associated with calcifications or iron depositions.[34]

Interpretation of SWI is dependent on the MR system. The appearance of hemorrhage and calcification in right and left-handed system are opposite to each other and the phase image should be evaluated very carefully for it. **Figure 2** summaries the appearance of hemorrhage and calcification in right and left handed systems.

Quantitative Susceptibility Mapping (QSM)

Quantitative susceptibility mapping is a relatively newer MRI technique that aim to extract the spatial susceptibility distribution of objects or tissues from the measured MRI phase or local field data by solving a known inverse problem.[35] With the advent of ultra-high field MRI resulting into increased sensitivity to magnetic susceptibility differences, it is now possible to achieve excellent anatomical contrast on T2*-weighted magnitude

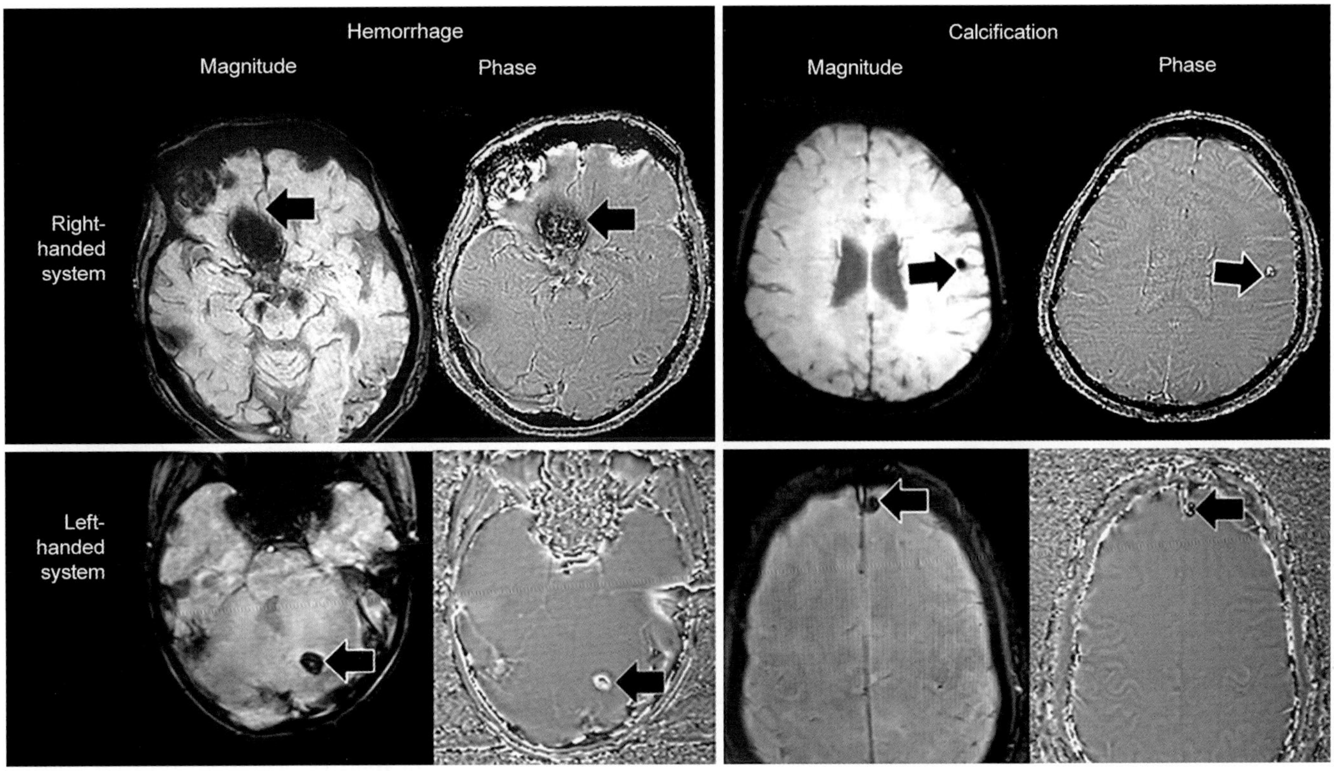

Fig. 2: Appearance of hemorrhage and calcifications (arrows) on magnitude and phase images on SWI in right and left-handed systems.

and phase images. Path-breaking work has been done in last decade for noninvasive quantification magnetic susceptibility in vivo.[35]

Following are the major sources of phase contrast in biological tissue—the heme and non-heme iron content, myelin, calcium and lipid.[36] The phase contrast for deep gray matter structures is dependent chiefly on the amount of iron.[36] The amount of iron deposition is related to aging as well as many neurodegenerative disorders.[36] MR signal magnitude and phase are determined by the level of deoxyhemoglobin, in case of veins in the brain. As deoxyhemoglobin level is directly related to oxygen saturation, it can be used as a surrogate marker of change in blood flow.[36] The cellular composition as well as arrangement may affect the magnetic properties of tissues in cases of white matter structures.[36] Bulk magnetic susceptibility is produced by the integration of the microscopic effects. On the contrary, depending on the geometry and orientation of the object, non-local phase effects are produced by bulk susceptibility. Therefore, although the phase information at any location is directly related to the local magnetic field of the source, it can be spatially distant to the source of susceptibility changes. Such non-local effects can make it difficult to quantify susceptibility changes using phase images.[36] The clinical applications of QSM include anatomical imaging of the human brain, traumatic brain injury, brain tumor, neurodegenerative disease, neurosurgical planning.[35,36]

Susceptibility Tensor Imaging (STI)

The dependence of gradient echo signal phase on the orientation of biological tissues with respect to the main magnetic field can be used to quantitatively determine orientation-independent magnetic susceptibility parameters by a newly developed MR technique known as susceptibility tensor imaging, which bears a conceptual similarity to diffusion tensor imaging (DTI).[37] The principal eigenvectors of the susceptibility tensor can be used for mapping of brain white matter fiber orientations and reconstruction of 3D white matter pathways. Myelin is the main determinant factor of the susceptibility anisotropy, contrary to diffusion anisotropy. Sensitivity of the susceptibility anisotropy of white matter to gadolinium-based contrast agents is another unique feature of STI.

STI has been shown to reproduce anatomical structures comparable to those with DTI while mapping major white matter fiber bundles in mouse brain.[37] In addition, STI, because of its unique sensitivity to oriented lipid molecules, can be a potentially new tool to assess the white matter integrity. In the setting of diseases like fetal alcohol spectrum disorder or multiple sclerosis, myelin formation during development and myelin breakdown in different neural diseases can potentially be studied using STI.[37]

DIFFUSION IMAGING

Diffusion Weighted Imaging (DWI)

Diffusion contrast depends on molecular motion of water. As initially described by Stejskal and Tanner in 1965, spin echo T2 EPI sequences can be sensitized to random diffusion of water molecules using bipolar gradients of equal magnitude and opposite polarity. The directional nature of net water movement of water in the white matter tracts (anisotropy) is depicted as signal loss on images by application of gradients in three orthogonal directions. This signal loss or diffusion weighting is determined by sequence specific parameter named "b value" (depending on strength, duration and interval of DW gradient) and tissue specific diffusivity factor called "ADC coefficient". Usually a "b value" 1000 sec/mm^2 allows good diffusion weighting in brain but it is used in tandem with a non-zero (20 sec/mm^2) value for calculations. Anisotropic images can be combined to yield isotropic mean diffusivity TRACE images (DWI) which are used for evaluating stroke and other routine purposes. Alternately ADC maps can be calculated to yield true magnitude images. These remove the inherent T2 contrast in these images which cause interpretative problems.[38,39]

The primary use of DWI has been in brain imaging due to its exquisitely unique sensitivity for ischemic stroke. This noninvasive test for cerebral tissue viability came at a vital time when thrombolytic and neuroprotective agents were entering clinical practice. It is a FDI-approved sequence for routine stroke protocol in neuroimaging now. Diffusion changes are detectable within minutes of cerebral ischemia (as early as 20 minutes in humans). This is due to cytotoxic edema (Na^+/K^+/ATPase pump failure) and squeezed extracellular compartment. DWI picks up infarcts with a sensitivity and specificity of 88–100% within 6 hours compared to conventional CT and MRI images which are abnormal only in less than 50% of cases **(Figs. 3A to G)**. Diagnosis of hyperacute infarction within this window period is vital for initiation of therapy. Infarcts appear bright on DWI (dark on ADC maps). The reduced ADC persists variably (usually ten days), returns to baseline and then remains elevated subsequently due to ensuing brain softening and gliosis. However, DWI changes may pseudonormalize after natural reperfusion or neuroprotective therapy within 1–2 days. DWI when assessed along with perfusion imaging is a better guide to treatment decisions and clinical outcome. DWI also has a role in the setting of acute on chronic ischemia, neonatal hypoxic injuries and venous thrombosis. More importantly DWI helps excluding stroke in an equivocal clinical setting, i.e. differentiating stroke from multiple sclerosis plaques and from other stroke mimics like vasogenic edema syndromes (hypertensive encephalopathy, eclampsia, meningioma cyclosporine toxicity, etc.) which are not associated with restriction of diffusion.[38]

The other uses of DWI are in diagnosing abscesses **(Figs. 4A and B)**, encephalitides and diffuse axonal injuries. All these conditions show high signal on DWI. It also help in characterizing tumors, i.e. differentiating epidermoids from cysts, by showing restricted diffusion in hypercellular tumors, i.e. lymphoma, malignant meningioma, differentiating necrotic from solid enhancing components, radiation necrosis from recurrent tumor (higher diffusion in necrosis) and postoperative cavity/cystic neoplasms from abscess in operated tumors.[38,39]

Diffusion Tensor Imaging

Dependency of molecular diffusion on the orientation of white matter fiber tracts (anisotropy) can be mapped spatially by acquiring relatively high-resolution DWI.[40] Computer algorithms allow the generation of white matter fiber tract maps from the tensor data. Tensor is a map of directional vectors in 3D space and it is a mathematic construct that describes the properties of an ellipsoid. The data for tensor must be measured along six or more collinear directions by gradients [multidirectional diffusion weighting (MDDW)- 6–256 directions]. From this data, diffusion coefficients or eigenvalues along the three principle directions, eigenvectors defining the orientation of fibers and fractional anisotropy (FA) can be calculated **(Fig. 5A)**. Thus, TRACE image (isotropic diffusion), ADC image (pure diffusion contrast from diffusion coefficients), FA maps with and without color codes (directional diffusion) and tensor image (calculated diffusion data with direction and velocity) are the data sets available for analysis from which fiber tracks can be constructed **(Fig. 5B)**.

Quantitative brain maps can be generated coregistering the 3D white matter fiber tracts on the anatomic images using Automated Image Registration Software. 3T due to its high SNR and reduced scan times allows sampling of high number of directions for DTI within an acceptable time. Higher b-values enhance anisotropy effects helping more complex evaluations like fiber tracking and tensor imaging more so for trajectory of crossing fiber. Susceptibility effects can be overcome using PAT, radial imaging or PROPELLER.

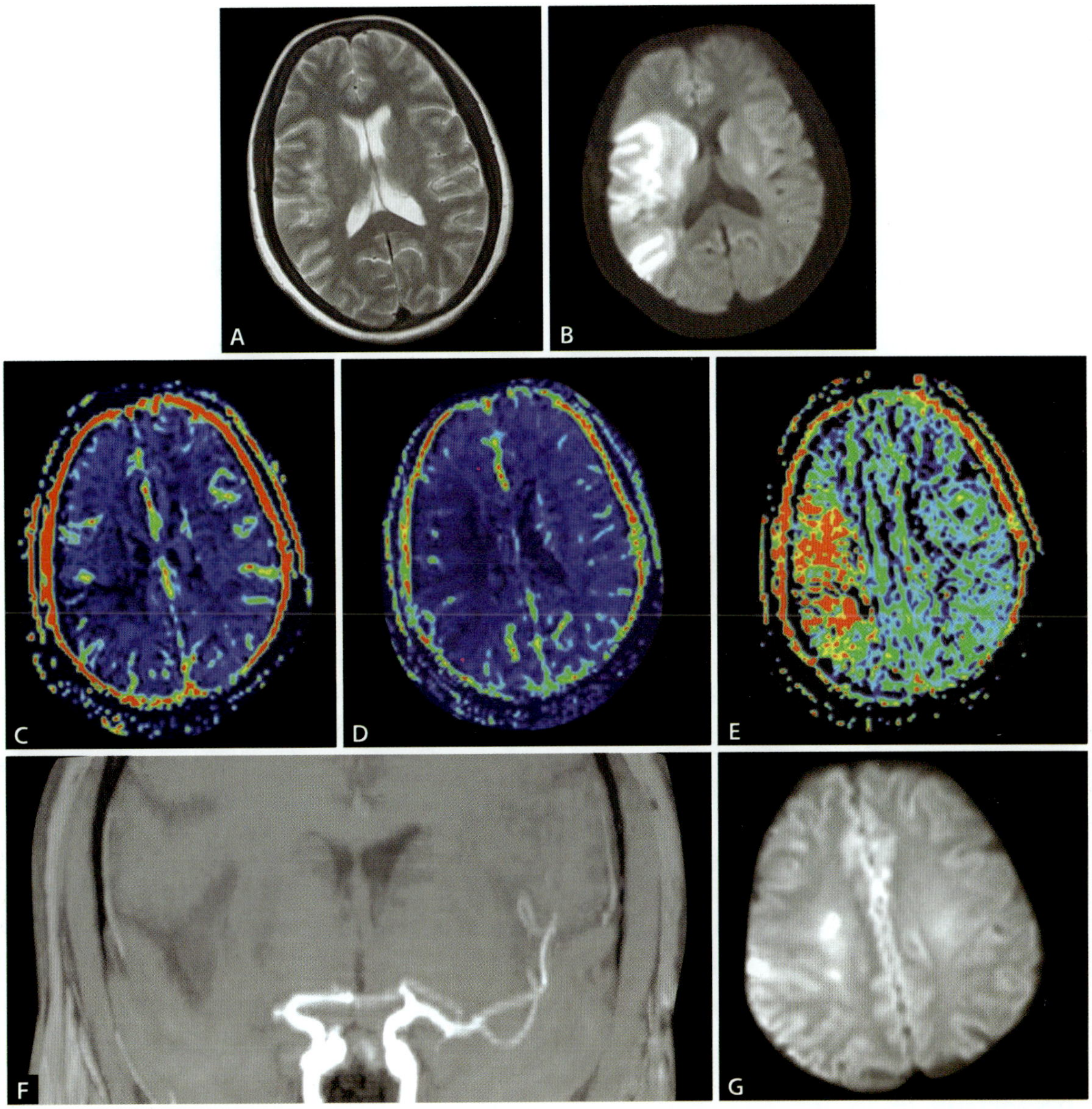

Figs. 3A to G: A 42-year-female with acute onset left hemiparesis. (A) T2W image-subtle signal changes along the right insula; (B) DWI–restriction in right MCA territory at the level of basal ganglia. Perfusion maps above the level of basal ganglia show normal color maps of CBV; (C) decreased CBF; (D) and raised MTT; (E) in the right MCA territory; (F) DWI showed no concordant extent of restriction at the corresponding level; (G) suggestive of DWI-PWI mismatch—evolving ischemic penumbra.

Clinical Applications

Diffusion tensor imaging is valuable in assessment of white matter structural integrity and connectivity. Use of DTI has been incorporated by various groups into imaging protocols of stroke, trauma (to study DAI and its long-term effects) and multiple sclerosis (loss of anisotropy in damaged white matter) **(Fig. 6)**. The disruption of fibers can be shown in all the above conditions.[40] It has been used to study brain development and included in a number of psychiatric protocols. The most advanced application is that of fiber tracking along with functional MRI to trace the connectivity of various areas of brain. Studies in schizophrenia have revealed disturbances of anisotropy which reflects possible functional disconnectivity. It can help surgical planning of tumors and when used along with cortical mapping technique, the entire functional unit can be shown. Some studies have also suggested that DTI can differentiate white matter tracts infiltrated with tumors (e.g. in high grade glioma) from those merely displaced (low grade tumor) **(Figs. 7A and B)**.[40,41]

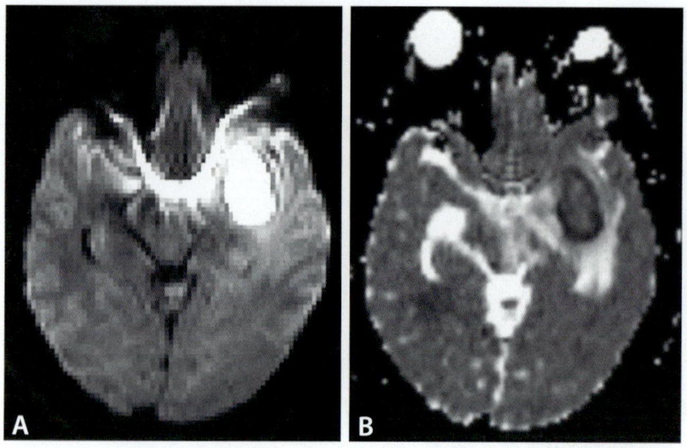

Figs. 4A and B: DW (A) and ADC; (B) images show diffusion restriction in the abscess cavity in left temporal lobe (bright on DWI and dark on ADC).

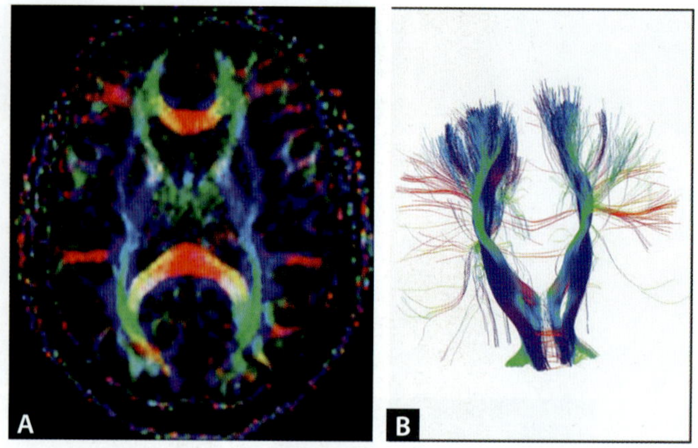

Figs. 5A and B: Directionally color coded FA map (A) and fiber tracking; (B) showing corticospinal tracts.

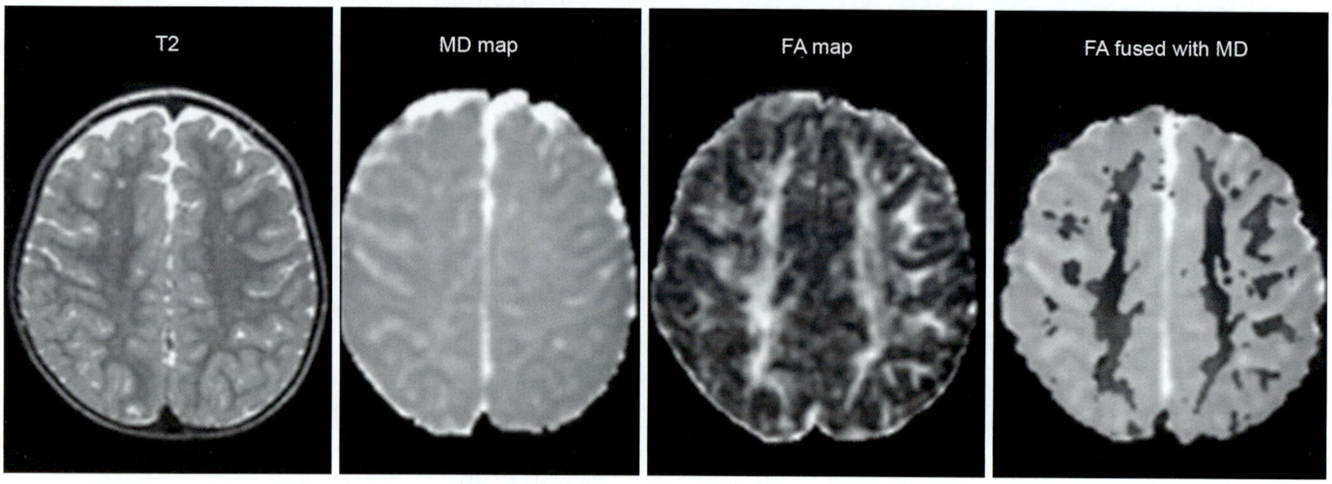

Fig. 6: Patient of multiple sclerosis with white matter subtle lesions on T2. FA data shows severe disruption of white matter anisotropy due to destruction of myelin.

Diffusion Spectrum Imaging

Diffusion spectrum imaging (DSI), first described by Wedeen et al.[42] can be considered as reference standard of diffusion imaging and is quiet suitable for in vivo application as it is capable of providing sufficiently dense q-space signal sample from which it is possible to derive a displacement distribution with the use of the Fourier transform.[39] A 6-dimensional image of both position and displacement can be obtained with the application of the Fourier transform over q-space in every brain position. Displacement distribution or the probability density function, which describe diffusion at each position, can provide a detailed description of diffusion and excellent resolution of the highly complex fiber organization, including fiber crossings. Diffusion spectrum imaging is generally used for fiber tractography, where only directional information is needed. Hence, by summing the probabilities of diffusion in each direction, probability density function (PDF) is normally reduced to an orientation distribution function.[39]

In DSI, strong diffusion weighting (b-value ~3000–8000 s/mm^2) with large number of diffusion encoding directions. It helps in delineating crossing fibers, which are not resolved by DTI model. The main limitation is long acquisition time.

q-Ball Imaging

q-ball imaging is most common algorithm used for extracting information from high angular resolution diffusion imaging (HARDI). HARDI is based on modeling a 3-dimensional orientation distribution function.[43] The general principle for all these techniques is dense sampling

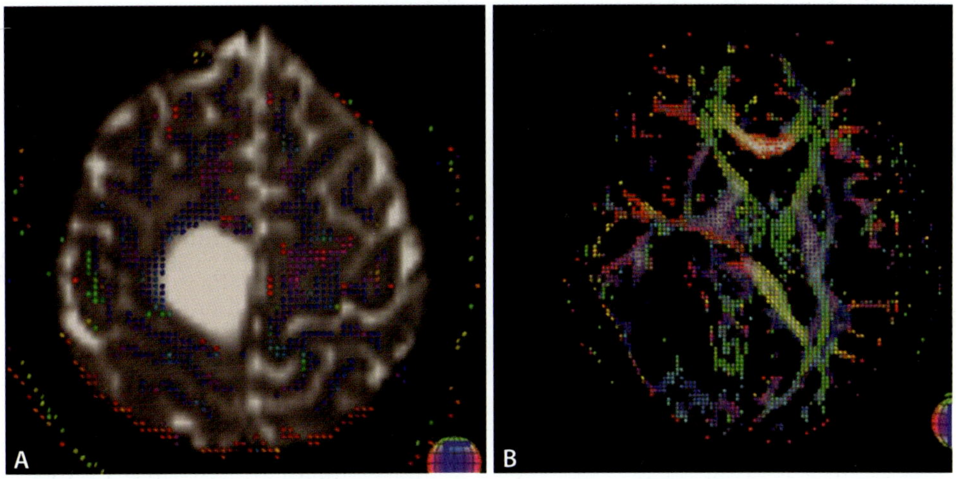

Figs. 7A and B: (A) The tensor and anatomy fusion image showing displacement of intact white matter in perirolandic area by the lesion in right high frontal cortex—DNET; (B) Tensor+ anatomy fusion image—white matter infiltration by glioblastoma multiforme leading to loss of anisotropy.

of the signal within a sphere with a constant high b value (>4000 s/mm^2) in q-space.[39] Various algorithms are used to calculate the orientation distribution function is from the resultant data. It helps in depiction of the crossing fibers, and is more clinically applicable. The images acquired with q-ball imaging closely resembles those acquired with DSI.[39] Further validation studies have to be done to determine the image quality for all brain regions and accuracy of fiber tracking with q-ball imaging. Besides q- ball imaging other heuristic methods based on persistent angular structure[44] and spherical deconvolution[45] can also achieve the same purpose.

Diffusion Kurtosis Imaging (DKI)

Diffusion kurtosis imaging is a new imaging technique as extension of the DTI technique which allows the estimation of diffusion as well as kurtosis parameters.[46,47] The DTI model is based on that diffusion occurs in a random unrestricted way and follows a Gaussian diffusion probability distribution function. However, water diffusion in human deviates from that strict Gaussian behavior due to the complexity of tissue and occurs in a restricted way. By incorporating and quantifying non-Gaussianity of water diffusion in tissues in its model, the diffusional kurtosis is a more accurate representation of restricted diffusion than DTI and may give additional biomarkers in various disease states (tissue structure and pathophysiology). DKI uses higher b-values than conventional DWI and gives dimensionless metric of the departure from a Gaussian form called kurtosis. The resulting kurtosis maps are reproducible. The three-dimensional kurtosis angular plots describe tissue-specific geometry for various brain regions and may show the potential of showing multiple fiber structures in a single voxel. Recent studies have shown that diffusion kurtosis imaging can provide information that is complementary of DTI.[46] It has been studied for various pathologies such as brain tumors, degenerative diseases, demyelinating diseases, and cerebrovascular diseases.

Main advantage of DKI is that it allows assessment of the cerebral cortex and basal ganglia which are isotropic structures and is main limitation of DTI. DKI can also improve estimation of the orientation distribution function (ODF) for optimizing white matter fiber tracking and the resolution of crossing fibers.[46]

Readout Segmented EPI-based Diffusion (RESOLVE Diffusion)

While DWI based on single shot echo-planar imaging (ss-EPI) requires less acquisition time, the diffusion weighted image quality in the head and neck regions like orbit, skull bases, temporal bone as well as in spine is often compromised due to the presence of magnetic susceptibility artifacts that can arise due to the presence of air, bone or fat in the vicinity of these structures. In addition two other problems have been encountered with DWI based on ss-EPI namely T2 blurring and long TE.[48] T2 blurring occurs as a result of long data sampling interval during the readout, which leads to broadening of point spread function and blurring of reconstructed image.[48] On the other hand long TE, which results from a combination of the diffusion-encoding gradients and the long data sampling interval, causes low signal to noise ratio (SNR).[48]

In order to address these problems, Porter and Heidemann[48] described a new method of acquiring diffusion-weighted images. This technique involves coupling of readout segmented EPI (rs-EPI), GRAPPA and 2D navigator reacquisition to obtain high resolution diffusion-weighted images. This technique has been popularized by the term RESOLVE (readout segmentation of long variable echo trains) sequence for DWI. This technique offers the advantages of high-quality, high-resolution DWI and DTI with reduced susceptibility and blurring artifacts making it applicable to challenging body regions including brain, skull-base, orbit, spine, breast, pelvis and prostate.[48] Besides that the technique is insensitive to motion-induced phase errors and there is reduced specific absorption rate (SAR) in comparison to turbo spin echo (TSE) based methods.[48]

Contiguous-Slice Zonally Oblique Multislice (CO-ZOOM) Diffusion

CO-ZOOM diffusion is another relatively newer technique for high resolution DWI and DTI. Dowell et al.[49] described its application in acquisition of optic nerve and spinal cord DTI. In this sequence, a modified ss-EPI sequence containing a refocusing RF pulse is used in presence of the phase-encoding (rather than slice-select) gradient to acquire the images. Hence it is possible to achieve excitation and refocusing of only a narrow volume; thereby eliminating the problem of signal aliasing associated with narrow FOVs. Two methods for the sequence have been described—for spinal cord cardiac gating is included to reduce the pulsation artifact, whereas inversion recovery (IR) cerebrospinal (CSF) suppression is used in the study the optic nerve in order to eliminate partial volume effects.[49] This technique is considered to be highly useful for diffusion imaging of small structures like spinal cord and optic nerve and achieves high resolution and less distortion due to susceptibility artifacts. Further nerve tracking analyses are also possible with this technique as continuous slices are acquired.

PERFUSION WEIGHTED IMAGING

Perfusion indicates the delivery of blood at the level of the capillaries. It is measured in units of mL/100 gm/minute. Delivery of oxygen and other nutrients to the tissue is closely related to perfusion. Hence measurement of perfusion, an essential physiologic parameter is crucial. The MR perfusion techniques are broadly classified into two groups—those using an exogenous contrast and those not using it.[50] The former includes two methods namely dynamic susceptibility contrast (DSC)—MRI and dynamic contrast enhanced (DCE)—MRI while the latter includes arterial spin labeling perfusion.

DSC perfusion: It measures signal reduction induced in the brain during passage of injected paramagnetic contrast agents which induce magnetic susceptibility effects (T2*).[51] Intravascular compartmentalized contrast produces large magnetic field gradients across the vascular boundaries leading to reduction in T2* and loss of signal which relates to proportion of vascularity. Best results are achieved with gradient based EPI with 2-second sampling rate over a minute. This can be plotted as a time intensity curve or concentration time curve. Integration of area under this curve yields regional cerebral blood volume (rCBV). Similarly mean transit time (MTT), total blood flow (rCBF), time to arrival (TTA) or time to peak (TPP) can also be calculated. High field MR provides better results due to higher SNR, longer T2*, faster scans, parallel imaging and requirement of lower optimal contrast volumes.

DCE perfusion: It depends on the injection of a gadolinium-based contrast agent. Dynamic acquisition of T1-weighted MR images are done before, during, and after bolus injection of a contrast agent. By applying the physical principles of tracer-kinetic modeling, the generated data can be interpreted in terms of physiological tissue characteristics.[50]

ASL perfusion: Brain perfusion can also be measured by spin labeling of arterial water by EPI signal tagging with alternating frequency (EPISTAR, ASL) or other techniques.[52] Two methods of ASL perfusion are described-pulsed ASL (PASL) and pseudocontinuous ASL (PCASL).[53] Pseudocontinuous ASL is method of choice for clinical application as it has high SNR. In this technique, train of short pulses in form of long labeling period (1–2 seconds) is designed to invert the inflowing blood magnetization in an adiabatic or pseudo steady-state manner. Hence it can be considered that blood is being continuously inverted as it flows through a "labeling plane" in the inferior-superior direction. In pulsed ASL, arterial blood is tagged by a short adiabatic inversion pulse (approximately in the order of 10 msec) to invert the blood water instantaneously in a particular region, typically located inferior to the brain. The main limitation of pulsed ASL is that it has low SNR.

Clinical Applications of MRP

PWI in Stroke: Ischemic brain after acute vascular occlusion shows reduced rCBV and elevated MTT and TTP as lack of signal drop after contrast arrival. The ischemic penumbra, i.e. "functionally impaired but not irreversibly damaged" area around an established infarction is identified when areas of PWI and DWI defect are compared. A mismatch; perfusion defect being larger than diffusion abnormality as seen in large arterial occlusion, denotes viable tissue at risk. The neurological deficit will likely to increase in such a situation and needs aggressive treatment. When there is a match between the two (PWI = DWI or PWI < DWI) infarct is presumed stable or already reperfused (***See* Figs. 3A to G**). Thus, an MRI stroke protocol should include T2 FSE and FLAIR sections of brain followed by MRA, DWI, PWI and a GRE sequence for hemorrhage. This comprehensive protocol should take less than 15 minutes on a modern state of the art MR scans.[51]

PWI of cerebral tumors: Tumor angiogenesis and vascularity determines biological aggressiveness of the cerebral neoplasms. These can be predicted by MR perfusion imaging. The technique is particularly useful for differentiating tumor necrosis from recurrent tumors (the former being avascular) and assesses response to treatment by antiangiogenetic chemotherapeutic agents (in terms of reduced rCBV post treatment). The rCBV correlates well with histological neovascularity and grades of gliomas. It progresses from lower values in low grade gliomas to high values in glioblastoma multiforme. PWI also acts as a guide in heterogeneous tumors for biopsy from more aggressive areas for appropriate staging. These areas may not necessarily show maximum enhancement on contrast enhanced MR or CT sections. Lymphomas show low vascularity and solitary metastases reduced perilesional contrast activity as compared to gliomas. Another possible role can be in atypical infections and demyelinating lesions mimicking neoplasms. Thus, PWI helps in diagnosing, characterizing and follow-up of brain neoplasms.[51]

***ASL perfusion*:** Clinical applications include early diagnosis of dementia and other neurodegenerative diseases, epileptogenic foci may be identified using ASL in seizure disorder patients and subtle functional changes in psychiatric disorders such as posttraumatic stress disorder or mild traumatic brain injury.[53]

MAGNETIC RESONANCE NEUROGRAPHY (MRN)

With the improvement of MR hardware and newer imaging technique, MR imaging of peripheral nerves is now quite feasible and has become an important adjunct to clinical examination and electrodiagnostic testing in the diagnosis of peripheral neuropathy. With MRN it is now possible to demonstrate the anatomy and pathology of the peripheral nerves in great details.

Role of MRN in Diagnosis of Peripheral Neuropathy[54]

1. Confirmation of clinical suspicion of peripheral neuropathy:
   a. Either by directly demonstrating the nerve abnormality or
   b. By showing the regional muscle denervation changes
2. Assessment of extent of the abnormality in nerve injuries.
3. Evaluation of the disease load in diffuse peripheral nerve lesions, such as hereditary neuropathies and neurofibromatosis.
4. Depiction of the lesions causing nerve entrapment or impingement.
5. Exclusion of the diagnosis of neuropathy by showing normal nerves and regional muscles.
6. To find out incidental lesions in the region of interest mimicking neuropathy symptoms.
7. Providing the image guidance for perineural medication injections.

Interpretation of MRN[54]

The mainstays of MRN are axial T1-weighted and fluid-sensitive fat suppressed T2-weighted images. The following parameters are generally evaluated in MRN-course, caliber and signal intensity (SI) of the nerve, fascicular pattern, size, and perineural fibrosis or mass lesions. The SI of normal nerves is intermediate (similar to muscle) on T1-weighted and intermediate to minimally increased SI on T2-weighted images. In cases of neuropathy, the nerve SI increases tremendously and the nerve may show fluid like SI of the adjacent vessels, on T2-weighted imaging. Various contributory factors are recognized for this signal change, e.g. vascular congestion; blockade of axoplasmic flow, leading to abnormal proximal accumulation of endoneurial fluid; and distal Wallerian degeneration changes. In addition to the nerve injuries, demonstration of denervation related changes in muscle bulk and SI acts as an indirect feature of peripheral neuropathy.

Classification of Nerve Injuries

Seddon et al.[55] classified the nerve injuries in 3 types:

1. *Neurapraxia—mildest type of injury*: Involve only the myelin sheath around the axon. MRN may show mild T2 hyperintensity with increased bulk of the nerve.
2. *Axonotmesis*: Complete rupture of axon leading to distal Wallerian degeneration with intact epineurium and perineurium. In addition to findings of neurapraxia,

MRN may show effacement, enlargement, or disruption of individual fascicles.

3. *Neurotmesis*: It refers to complete disruption of the nerve with complete loss of function. MRN can demonstrate the discontinuity of the nerve directly or fluid in the gap or granulation tissue between the torn nerve endings.

Sunderland[56] further classified nerve injuries into 5 types. While the first and second degree injuries correspond to neurapraxia and axonotmesis, the third-, fourth- and fifth-degree injuries reflect injuries to endoneurium, perineurium and epineurium, respectively. Neuroma, which appears as focal nerve enlargement with a partially or completely effaced fascicular pattern, is commonly found in fourth-degree nerve injuries.

MRN Protocol

The recommended protocol for MRN includes following sequences and can be completed within approximately 45 minutes.

- Axial 2D T1-weighted (3 mm isotropic reconstructions)
- Axial T2 SPAIR (3 mm)
- Coronal 3D STIR SPACE
- T2 SPACE (1 mm)
- 3D DW PSIF [reversed FISP (fast imaging with steady-state free precession)] imaging
- Postcontrast sequences to be used in case of suspected tumor, diffuse peripheral nerve lesions, inflammation, infections.

Future Directions

- DTI has been found to have promising results in demonstration of peripheral nerve imaging in animal models and healthy volunteers. It is possible to calculate ADC, FA and mean diffusivity from DTI besides tractography which is likely to provide more insight into the disease process.
- Whole body MRN though technically challenging to perform can be useful in diseases like neurofibromatosis.
- Gadofluoride M, a newer MR contrast, accumulates in nerves undergoing Wallerian degeneration and disappears with remyelination. By virtue of this property, it has been shown to be useful in demonstrating demyelination and remyelination in animal models.[54]

MAGNETIC RESONANCE ANGIOGRAPHY

Magnetic resonance angiography (MRA) uses inflow effects of blood in 2D and 3D TOF angiography or phase contrast technique in PC MRA. TOF MRA provides satisfactory images of extra and intracranial vasculature and is recommended for screening of aneurysms in asymptomatic patients. TOF MRA suffers from limitations like saturation effects and turbulence-related signal loss. An ultrafast 3D gradient echo version is used for CE MRA which overcomes many of these drawbacks.[57] The short TR nulls fat signal. Being fast, the sequence freezes motion and provides temporal (arterial and venous phases) and spatial resolution. This leads to better visualization of vascular bifurcations, distal vessels and quantification of stenosis and correlates better with other diagnostic modalities. CE MRA needs timing of the sequence with contrast bolus arrival so that data acquisition is in the center of the k-space. This is achieved by rapid contrast infusion with power injector and sequence triggering with test bolus. PAT enabled neurovascular MR coils allow imaging of neck and intracranial vessels at one sitting **(Figs. 8A and B)** and can be used in stroke protocols along with diffusion and perfusion imaging. CE MRA also better evaluates intracranial aneurysms (particularly giant aneurysms) and post coiling follow-up of aneurysms. Improved vessel to background signal, higher visibility of gadolinium, higher resolution, larger FOV, k-space reordering and keyhole techniques on 3T produces superior quality diagnostic angiograms with improved visualization of smaller vessels **(Fig. 9)**. TOF-MRA using C-SENSE can be an alternative technique to acquire MRA in a shorter time as well **(Figs. 10A to F)**.

Time resolved CE MRA with sub-second temporal resolution and digital substraction has become feasible and initial results are exciting (time resolved imaging of contrast kinetics, or TRICKS).[58] Using parallel imaging, key hole acquisition and CENTRA k-space sampling yields nearly isotropic volume acquisition. This allows direct observation of the fast hemodynamic changes associated with abnormal vasculature of AVM's and directionality of flow in unilateral carotid occlusion syndromes.[59] Generated MIP's show the angio-architecture of AVM in any spatial orientation with enough temporal resolution to differentiate between early arterial, arterial, parenchymal and venous phases **(Figs. 11A to G)**. When the technique fails to show smaller vessels, it can be combined with high spatial resolution MRA.

Degree of stenosis and plaque morphology is important predictors of stroke. High resolution MR imaging is a developing technique. It can characterize atherosclerotic plaques for instability (irregularity and ulceration) with 81% sensitivity and 90% specificity thus facilitating prognosis and decision making of plaque stabilizing therapy.[60]

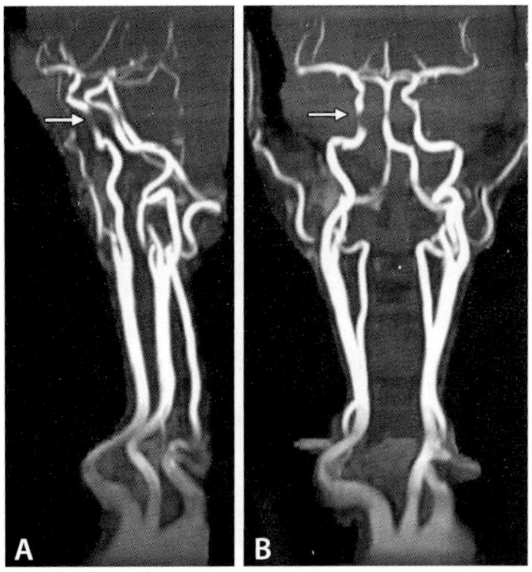

Figs. 8A and B: Oblique (A) and AP; (B) views of contrast-enhanced MR angiography of cervicocranial arteries showing a stenotic lesion of the right carotid artery (arrow).

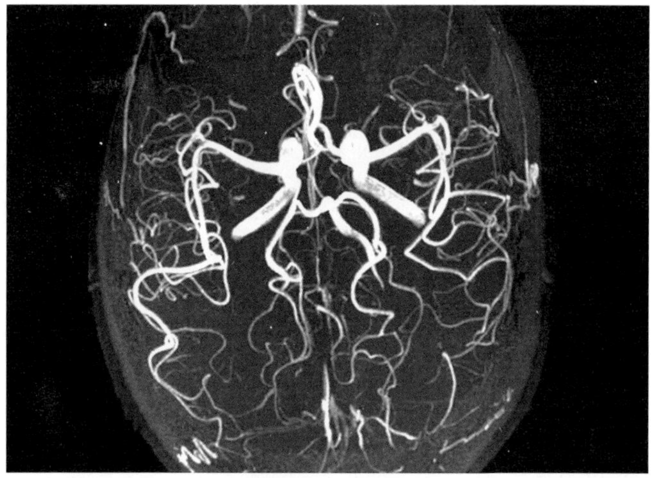

Fig. 9: Time of flight MRA; excellent angiogram due to background suppression and better flow-related signal leading to better distal smaller vessel visibility.

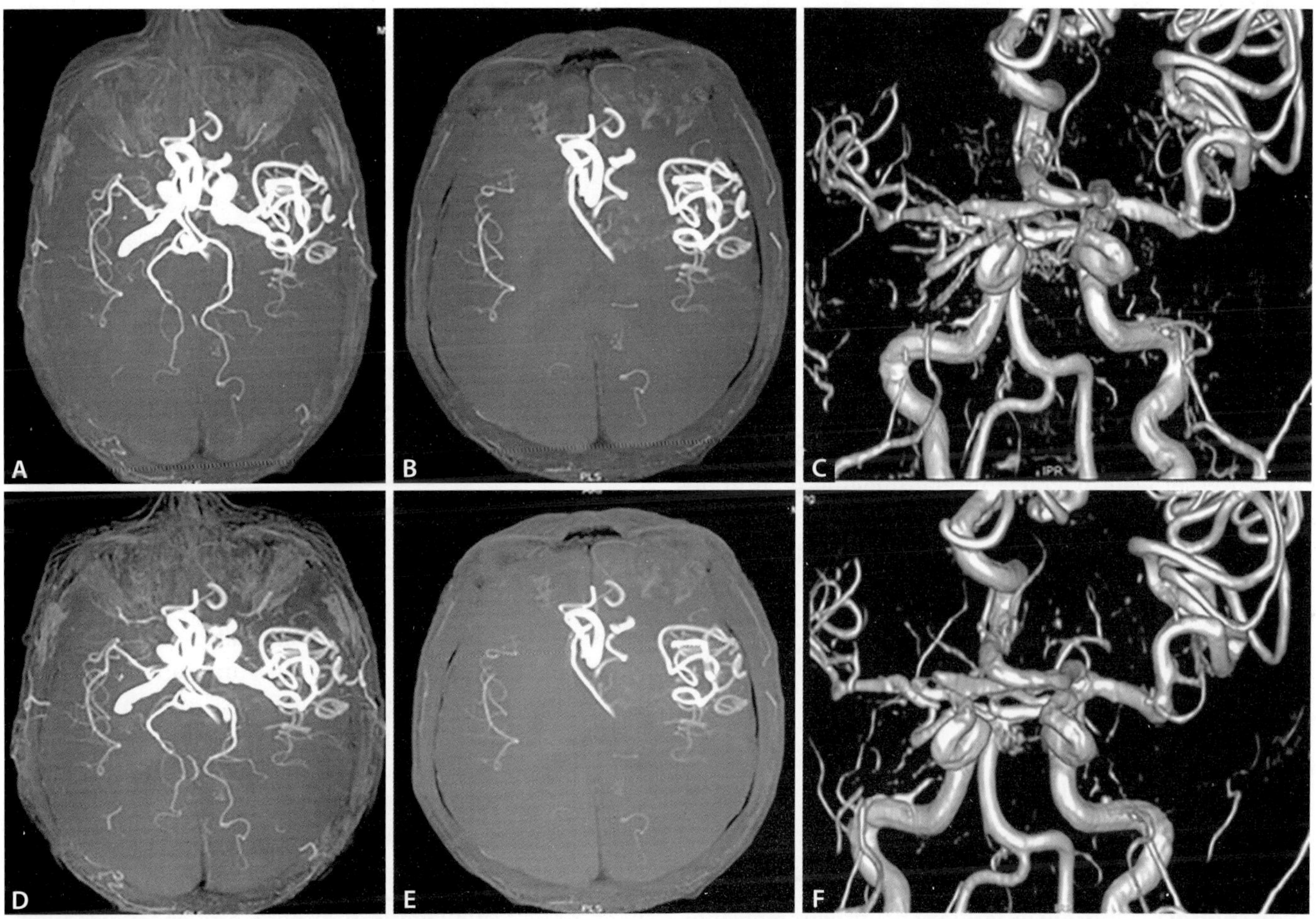

Figs. 10A to F: MRA of a 22-year-male patient presenting with headache: (A to C) MRA acquired with conventional technique and (D to F) MRA acquired with C-SENSE with acceleration factor of 3. (A and B) and (D and E) axial maximum intensity projection images and (C and F) volume rendered images. The images showed an arteriovenous malformation in left temporal region with multiple dilated feeding arteries with intervening nidus.

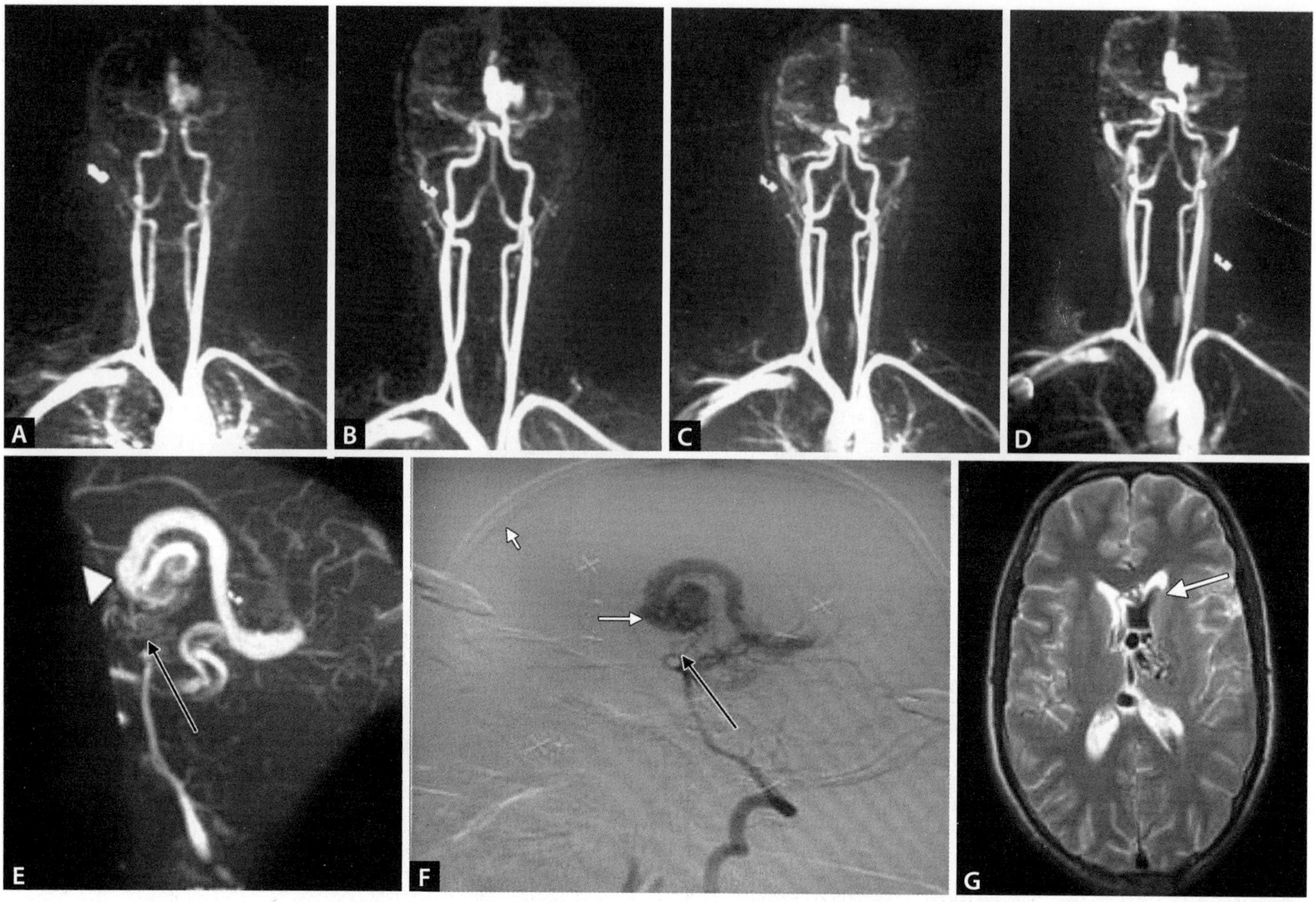

Figs. 11A to G: An 18-year-male with left thalamic AVM: (A to D) Sequential arterial, *nidus* and venous enhancement (white arrows) on time resolved MRA. (E) High spatial resolution MRA—lateral MIP projection with corresponding DSA (F). On DSA left VA run showing feeders (black arrow), *nidus* and draining veins [white arrowhead in MRA (E) similar to white arrow in DSA (F)]. (G) T2 TSE axial section.

VESSEL WALL MR IMAGING (VW-MR IMAGING)

It is not possible to adequately image the pathology hidden in the vessel wall by conventional imaging techniques like CTA, MRA or DSA which image the vessel lumen. High resolution vessel wall imaging using MRI has been developed over the past decade in order to overcome this pitfall of conventional angiographic modalities. Currently, vessel wall imaging for both intracranial and extracranial vessels has been developed and they are discussed here briefly.

Intracranial Vessel Wall Imaging

Essential technical requirements for intracranial vessel imaging are:[61]

High spatial resolution: By virtue of being extremely thin, the wall of the intracranial vessel is extremely difficult. Normal thickness of wall of the middle cerebral artery or basilar trunk is 0.2-0.3 mm, which is approximately 1/10th of the luminal diameter of these arteries and is smaller than the voxel dimensions currently available. However, as most of the disease condition is associated with wall thickening, the conspicuity of vessel wall increases in disease state. Besides it is possible to suppress the blood or CSF signal in the voxel. 3T is preferred over 1.5 T for VW-MR because of its intrinsically higher SNR. At 3T for a 2D sequence following parameters are considered standard-voxel size: 2.0 mm × 0.4 mm × 0.4 mm, scan duration-approximately 5–7 min for a 2–4 cm thick section of tissue. For 3D sequence, a 0.5 mm isotropic voxel (range 0.4–0.7 mm) can be used and the coverage time for circle of Willis and 2nd and 3rd order branches typically varies between 7 and 10 minutes.

Multiplanar 2D or 3D acquisitions: The vessel wall need to be visualized in both long and short axis plane for accurate interpretation of VW-MR imaging. One of the approaches for achieving this could be acquisition of the 2D sequence multiple times in orthogonal planes. However, as most intracranial vessels have a curved course rather than straight course. Hence, partial volume averaging can result from the vessel obliquity and curvature, confounding the appearance of the arterial wall. The other approach is to use a 3D (volumetric) sequence and viewing the images in different orthogonal 2D planes. It reduces scan time and provides the option of viewing the arterial wall in any plane of choice. Variable flip angle refocusing pulse, fast spin-echo sequences are generally used for 3D VW-MR acquisitions. The sequence is known by different names from different vendors, e.g. VISTA (volume isotropic turbo spin-echo acquisition; Philips Healthcare, Best, the Netherlands), SPACE (sampling perfection with application-optimized contrasts by using different flip angle evolutions; Siemens, Erlangen, Germany), and Cube (GE Healthcare, Milwaukee, Wisconsin). Despite the advantages of 3D sequences, some groups have found 2D images to have better quality for a particular vessel of interest. Hence, it may be prudent to include both 2D and 3D sequences.

Multiple tissue weightings: Baseline TOF MRA is used for localizing the abnormality. In cases with severe luminal narrowing or dilation, a contrast enhanced MRA may be required because of slow flow leading to signal drop on TOF MRA. T1-weighted vessel wall sequence, before and after gadolinium-based contrast agent administration, is the primary sequence used. Proton density sequence can be used because of its higher SNR compared to T1-weighted sequence; but as vessel wall signal approaches that of CSF on PD images, the vessel wall becomes less conspicuous on PD. The contrast enhancement on PD can also be less prominent compared to T1. A T2-weighted VW-MR sequence is also incorporated in the typical imaging sequence. Fat suppression is generally not required, unless imaging of external carotid branches in scalp needs to image in some specific situation like giant cell arteritis.

Suppression of MR imaging signal in blood and CSF: Suppression of MR signal from blood, CSF or brain parenchyma (if vessel is embedded in the brain parenchyma) is a mandatory prerequisite for good quality VW-MR. Use of spin echo sequences, presaturation bands and double inversion recovery are some of the techniques used to suppress the blood MR signal.

***Clinical applications*:** Intracranial VW-MR imaging is a useful adjunct to conventional imaging in many clinical conditions **(Figs. 12A to D)**. It is especially helpful in characterizing and differentiating between intracranial atherosclerotic plaque, vasculitis, reversible cerebral vasoconstriction syndrome, moyamoya disease, radiation induced arteriopathy and arterial dissection. In addition, it is also helpful to identify symptomatic, nonstenotic disease of the intracranial arteries. Recent studies have shown that is useful for prediction of future behavior of unruptured intracranial saccular aneurysms.[61]

Extracranial Vessel Wall Imaging

High resolution vessel wall MRI for cervical vessels is an important adjunct to ultrasonography and Doppler and CT angiography and has developed significantly over the last decade. Following information can be obtained from cervical VW-MR: (a) the degree of stenosis, (b) total volume of the plaque, (c) component of the plaques, and (d) surface morphology of the plaque, including ulceration and fibrous cap rupture.[62] A number of MR sequences including T1, T2 and PD-weighted sequences, and time-of-flight (TOF) imaging and black- and bright-blood sequences. The characteristics of carotid plaque on MR is summarized in **Table 1**.[62]

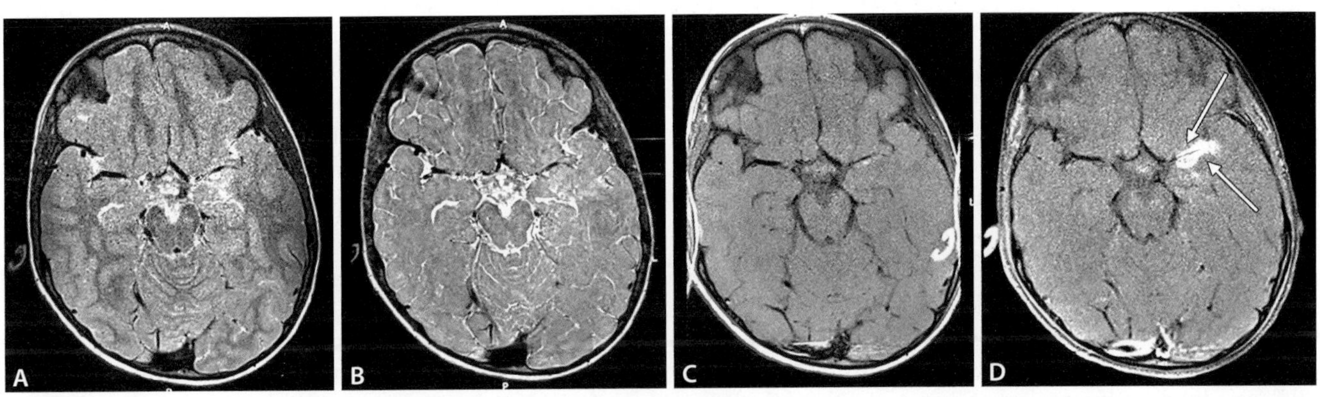

Figs. 12A to D: A 7-year-old girl with left middle cerebral artery (MCA) arteriopathy: T2 (A), PD (B) and T1 (C) MR images showing marked narrowing of left MCA with contrast-enhanced T1 MR images showing florid enhancement of the MCA wall (arrows in D).

Table 1: Carotid plaque morphology on MRI.

Sequence	Plaque Component					
	Lipid core	Fibrous tissue	Hemorrhage			Calcification
			Fresh (<1 week)	Recent (1–6 weeks)	Chronic (>6 weeks)	
3D TOF	Iso	Iso	Hyper	Hyper	Hypo	Marked hypo
T1-w	Iso/hyper	Iso/hyper	Hyper	Hyper	Hypo	Marked hypo
T2-w	Hypo	Iso/hyper	Iso/hypo	Hyper	Hypo	Marked hypo
PD-w	Iso/hyper	Iso/hyper	Iso/hypo	Hyper	Hypo	Marked hypo
Postcontrast T1-w	Nonenhancing	Enhancing	Nonenhancing	Nonenhancing	Nonenhancing	Nonenhancing

The following reading scheme can be followed for deciding carotid plaque morphology:[62]

1. Calcification: hypointense on all sequences
2. Recent/fresh hemorrhage: hyperintense on T1 and TOF MRA
3. Lipid core: focal decrease in signal intensity from PD weighted images to T2-weighted images.
4. Fibrous component: the remaining areas should be considered as fibrous component.

The plaque inflammation is a risk factor for plaque vulnerability and it is indicated by postgadolinium enhancement. Tissue specific agents like ultra-small superparamagnetic iron oxide particles can be issued for demonstration of plaque inflammation and uptake of these particles is found to be more commonly observed in the carotid plaques of symptomatic patients than asymptomatic patients.[62]

MAGNETIC RESONANCE ELASTOGRAPHY (MRE)

Elastography is radiologist's tool for virtual palpation. It can be used to assess the stiffness of tissues which cannot be palpated clinically, e.g. brain. It is a three step process and includes the following:

- *Firstly*, introduction of shear waves into the tissue under study by an external mechanical driver.
- *Secondly*, a phase contrast MR sequence with motion encoding gradient is used to study the motions.
- *Thirdly*, stiffness maps called elastograms are generated from the measure of displacements.

The role of MRE is well established for different organs of the body particularly liver. The applications of MRE in neuroimaging are relatively new and are discussed briefly. It has been found to be a highly accurate method for measuring brain stiffness. The test-retest repeatability has errors of 1%, 2% and 3–7% for measurement of global stiffness, lobar stiffness and stiffness of subcortical gray matter.[63] It is found that stiffness decreases with age in healthy volunteers and a strong relationship between viscoelasticity and behavioral performance exists. Furthermore, stiffness is found to decrease in diseases like multiple sclerosis and several neurodegenerative diseases including those related to dementia with a variable spatial pattern of stiffness changes observed in different types of dementia. Last but not the least, it is a promising tool for the preoperative assessment of consistency and adherence of intracranial tumors to neighboring tissues and thereby predicts surgical difficulty. Thus, MRE has a potential role in multitude of neurological diseases. However, further studies are required for its validation in the field of neuroimaging.

MAGNETIC RESONANCE FINGERPRINTING

Magnetic resonance fingerprinting (MRF) is a novel approach that does the data acquisition, post-processing and visualization in a completely different fashion.[64] Rather than doing a repeated, serial data acquisition for characterization of individual parameters of interest, MRF uses a pseudo randomized acquisition. In this method, the signals from different tissues have a unique signal evolution or "fingerprint" that is simultaneously a function of the multiple material properties under investigation. A pattern recognition algorithm is used for post processing so as to match the fingerprints to a predefined dictionary of predicted signal evolutions, which can then be translated into quantitative maps of the magnetic parameters of interest. Conceptually MRF is related to compressed sensing[28] and shares some of its benefits. For example, MRF does not suffer from the high sensitivity to measurement errors found in other faster acquisition methods and fully quantitative results can be obtained by MRF within a scanning time which is comparable to that of a conventional qualitative MR scan. Most importantly, while a limited set of parameters can be evaluated at a time using conventional MR techniques, it is possible many MR parameters can be concurrently examined quantitatively using

MRF given enough scan time. Thus, MRF opens the door to computer-assisted multi-parametric MR analyses, similar to genomic or proteomic analyses that could detect important but complex changes across a large number of MR parameters simultaneously. When an appropriate pattern recognition algorithm is used, MRF also provides a new and more robust behaviour in the presence of noise or other acquisition errors that may lead to the near complete suppression of deleterious effects stemming from these factors.

CHEMICAL EXCHANGE SATURATION TRANSFER (CEST) MRI

Chemical exchange saturation transfer magnetic resonance imaging is an emerging MR application that has the potential to provide molecular information of different pathologies as well as response to treatment. It is a novel MR technique by virtue of which it is possible to detect certain compounds which are too low to affect the MR contrast in standard sequences or to be detected by MR spectroscopic imaging at typical water imaging resolution.[65,66] For these compounds to be detected, they should be capable of exchanging protons with surrounding water molecules. Water in biological system exists in dynamic equilibrium between free and bound water. By saturating or irradiation of bond water, there is transfer of magnetization between them. Greatly enhanced sensitivity can be achieved as continuous build-up of magnetic saturation of water is possible, by virtue of this property. Thus, CEST MRI has immense potential in providing spectacular image contrast based on specific molecular compositions at relevant millimolar physiological concentrations.[65,66]

On MR imaging perspective, cellular proteins can be divided into two main types; bound proteins, and mobile proteins and peptides. Bound proteins are solid-like macromolecules whose protons have short T2 (~ μs) and are detected by conventional magnetization transfer (MT) contrast. On the other hand mobile protons and peptides have protons having long T2 (~ tens of ms) and can be detected by CEST MRI techniques like amide proton transfer.

Magnetization Transfer

The contrast depending on exchange of magnetization between different tissues (i.e. water pool and macromolecular pool) is called magnetization transfer (MT) contrast. The macromolecules transfer magnetization to water protons leading to a decrease in their relaxation time and loss of signal. Off resonance pulses are added to the routine MR pulse sequences to suppress the macromolecular pool (around 1000–2000 Hz) with subsequent reduction in signal intensity of background tissue in brain.[67]

The effect can be used qualitatively in clinical imaging, i.e. suppression of the background tissue in cerebral MRA for better contrast and small vessel detection, achieve better conspicuity of contrast enhancing lesions and to increase the cord CSF contrast on T2* images of spine. The MT effect can be quantitatively measured from images acquired with and without MT pulse saturation and expressed in form of MT ratio (MTR): Mo – Ms/Mo × 100% where Mo and Ms are signal intensities without and with MT pulse. MTR can be measured at the region of interest or for the entire brain with pixel to pixel coregistration.

Disorders of neural tissue often manifest as reduced MT ratios due to destruction of macromolecules (i.e. myelin). MT has been applied in multiple sclerosis to characterize plaques, determining total lesion load/ response to treatment and predict clinical course.[68] It has also been applied for studying myelination in developing brain, SLE, multisystem atrophy, amyotrophic lateral sclerosis, schizophrenia, Alzheimer's disease, etc. It is reliable in differentiating tuberculoma (low MTR) from pyogenic abscess and tumors.[69]

Amide Proton Transfer

Amide proton transfer (APT) is a variant of CEST MRI, and is also known as amide CEST. It is the most popular CEST MRI till date. Proteins and peptides of the tissue are the major known contributors to APT. The main neurological applications reported for APT are the detection of cancer and ischemic stroke.

Clinical Application of APT MRI

Cerebrovascular stroke: It is possible to identify ischemic regions of brain parenchyma in patients of ischemic stroke.[66] Increase in ATP hydrolysis takes place in setting of decreased cerebral blood flow leading to reduced bicarbonate buffering and local acidosis. This in turn leads to decreased exchange rate of amide protons as the chemical exchange of amide proton is catalyzed in an alkaline environment. This decrease in amide proton exchange leads to a decrease in APT MRI contrast in the ischemic tissue and this can be detected even with a relatively low 0.5 μT saturation power. Compared to the hypoperfused salvageable penumbra, the ischemic core shows much decreased APT. In animal models it has been found that hemorrhagic vs ischemic stroke can also be distinguished by hyperintense vs hypointense APT

MRI contrast. Thus, APT can be an important adjunct to anatomical MR imaging, diffusion and perfusion studies in the setting of stroke.

Multiple sclerosis: Accumulation of mobile proteins in the normal appearing white matter is the neuropathological and biochemical basis of the biochemical neuropathology of multiple sclerosis (MS). APT contrast increases as a result of this protein accumulation and can be detected at 7T and a moderate 2–3.5 μT saturation power.[66] Furthermore, spectral analysis of the CEST showed increased asymmetry around the amide CEST peak in lesions and normal-appearing white matter in the spine of MS patients compared to healthy white matter in healthy subjects.

Alzheimer's disease: Reduced mobile protein content related to Alzheimer's disease, can be detected by APT MRI, but it is yet to be translated to clinical studies.[66]

Brain tumor: APT at 3T and 7T magnetic field strengths has been found to have promising role in brain tumor imaging. The histopathological tumor grade bears a positive correlation with APT MRI contrast. APT MRI contrast has been shown to reduce with treatment. Correspondingly, lower APT MRI contrast is generated in pseudoprogression from post-treatment inflammation compared to recurrent glioma. High APT MRI contrast has been more correlated with high-grade gliomas than strongly enhancing imaging regions with gadolinium-based MRI contrast agents.[66]

Intracranial hemorrhage: High MTR is seen in acute hemorrhages compared to subacute hemorrhages regardless of the underlying pathology and thus can be useful in evaluation of hemorrhagic brain lesions.[70]

gluCEST MRI

It is an extremely difficult task to selectively detect only a single metabolite amidst multitude of metabolites within tissues as the MR frequencies of these metabolites overlap. Fortunately, Glutamate (glu) is an exception showing CEST peak at 3.0 ppm. For glutamate, the chemical exchange occurs for amine group, CEST detection of glutamate is further facilitated by its higher concentration in brain compared to other metabolites.[66]

gluCEST MRI, i.e. the imaging of glutamate with CEST MRI, has been done successfully in healthy brain tissue and the spinal cord. Strong CEST contrast is generated by a 3.6 μT saturation power. The relatively high saturation power is necessary for separation of the MR frequencies of glutamate and water, and the fast exchange rate of the labile protons on glutamate. However, as 7T MRI provides more selective saturation of glutamate than 3T, clinical gluCEST MRI studies have only been performed at 7T scanners.[66]

Strong correlation exists between the gluCEST ratio from gray and white matter to the ratio of glutamate concentration measured with 1H MR spectroscopy. Lateralization of temporal lobe seizure is possible with gluCEST MRI brain study correctly and the findings corroborated with MR spectroscopy. Relative glutamate concentrations in the spinal cord may serve as an additional biomarker for multiple sclerosis, which may complement the mobile protein content measurements made with APT MRI.[66]

POSITRON EMISSION TOMOGRAPHY AND MRI (PET/MRI)

Inability to perform simultaneous data acquisition producing artifacts and exposing the patient to significant radiation are major limitations of PET/CT.[71,72] Moreover, PET/CT has poor contrast in soft tissue as well as in complex anatomical regions like head and neck. An integrated PET/MR scanner (Siemens) which enables simultaneous acquisition of PET and MR imaging was launched in 2010, Munich, Germany.[73] There were many technical and practical hurdles before PET/MR was available for clinical imaging. Firstly, the photomultiplier (PMT)-based PET scanners do not work within or near the magnetic environment of an MR scanner. To overcome this, the developers used avalanche photo diode or silicon PMT-based PET detector systems.[74] Secondly, metallic objects such as surface coils used to get best MR image quality interfere with the gamma rays from PET, causing unwanted attenuation. This can be achieved by modification of surface coils to reduce their metal content. Thirdly, MR data are not readily usable for attenuation correction like PET/CT.[75] Therefore, quantification of PET data was not possible. Various approaches to overcome this problem are currently under investigation.[76]

Applications in neuroimaging: Besides oncological applications, PET/MRI has got few neurological applications.

- In patients with Alzheimer's disease, PET/MR can be used for the early diagnosis, evaluation of disease progression and therapy response. In addition, morphologic images are essential to exclude other causes of dementia like multi-infarct dementia or normal-pressure hydrocephalus.[77,78]
- Patients with refractory epilepsy despite medical treatment require surgery to resect the epileptogenic

focus.[79] For success of surgical procedure structural and functional imaging data is of outmost importance. Therefore, these patients needs to undergo a battery of imaging and non-imaging tests like morphologic MRI, functional MRI, PET, and EEG for correct localization of epileptic focus. The PET/MR will be useful in such patients and data can be obtained using single imaging test in one day rather than multiple imaging tests on different days.

ARTIFICIAL INTELLIGENCE IN NEURORADIOLOGY

Mimicking human cognitive function is the ultimate goal of artificial intelligence (AI). With the advent of AI, the healthcare system is observing a paradigm shift which is enforced by rapid progress of analytics techniques and increasing availability of healthcare data. The AI devices and techniques are broadly classified into two types, machine learning (ML) techniques and natural language processing (NLP) methods.[80] The machine learning techniques analyze structured data such as imaging, genetic and EP data. In the medical applications, the ML procedures attempt to cluster patients' traits, or infer the probability of the disease outcomes. On the other hand, NLP methods natural extract information from unstructured data such as clinical notes/medical journals to supplement and enrich structured medical data. The NLP procedures target at turning texts to machine-readable structured data, which can then be analyzed by ML techniques. The most common types of ML algorithms include neural network, support vector machine (SVM).[80]

Deep Learning

Deep learning has ushered a new era in the ML algorithms. Deep learning is a subset of supervised machine learning method. These techniques use some form of neural network based on their ability to automatically extract relevant features. Deep learning allows constructing an image-classification in shorter time as compared to experts. Rapid development of modern computing enables deep learning to build-up neural networks with a large number of layers, which is infeasible for classical neural networks. As such, deep learning can explore more complex nonlinear patterns in the data. Deep learning is gaining popularity as the data is becoming more complex and the volume of data increases. In the medical applications, the commonly used deep learning algorithms include convolution neural network (CNN), recurrent neural network, deep belief network and deep neural network.[80]

Major Applications of AI in Neuroimaging

Few of the major applications of AI in neuroimaging includes—brain tumor segmentation with MRI, early detection of Alzheimer's disease with fMRI, detection of stroke and possible reduction of gadolinium dose in clinical MR imaging. In fact, US Food and Drug administration (FDA) has granted a de Novo request for the first-ever computer-aided triage and notification platform to identify large vessel occlusion (LVO) strokes in CTA imaging in February 2018. Although the AI technologies are attracting substantial attentions in medical research, the real-life implementation is still unclear due to lack of standards of the safety and efficacy of AI systems.

ACKNOWLEDGMENTS

The authors acknowledge and thank Dr Nirmalya Ray, DM resident in Neuroradiology section of Department of Radiodiagnosis and Imaging, PGIMER, Chandigarh for active involvement and helping in writing the chapter.

REFERENCES

1. Chen CN, Sank VJ, Cohen SM, et al. The field dependence of NMR imaging. I. Laboratory assessment of signal-to-noise ratio and power deposition. Magn Reson Med. 1986;3:722-9.
2. Hoult DI, Chen CN, Sank VJ. The field dependence of NMR imaging. II. Arguments concerning an optimal field strength. Magn Reson Med. 1986;3:730-46.
3. Edelstein WA, Glover GH, Hardy CJ, et al. The intrinsic signal-to-noise ratio in NMR imaging. Magn Reson Med. 1986;3:604-18.
4. Middleton H, Black RD, Saam B, et al. MR imaging with hyperpolarized 3He gas. Magn Reson Med. 1995; 33:271-5.
5. Foster TH. Tissue conductivity modifies the magnetic resonance intrinsic signal-to-noise ratio at high frequencies. Magn Reson Med. 1992;23:383-5.
6. Scarabino T, Nemore F, Giannatempo GM, et al. 3.0 T magnetic resonance in neuroradiology. Eur J Radiol. 2003;48:154-64.
7. Duyn JH. The future of ultra-high field MRI and fMRI for study of the human brain. Neuroimage. 2012;62:1241-8.
8. Balchandani P, Naidich TP. Ultra-high-field MR neuroimaging. Am J Neuroradiol. 2015;36:1204-15.
9. Hennig J, Nauerth A, Friedburg H. RARE imaging: a fast imaging method for clinical MR. Magn Reson Med. 1986;3(6):823-33.
10. Carr H, Purcell E. Effects of diffusion on free precession in nuclear magnetic resonance experiments. Phys Rev. 1954;94(3):630-8.

11. Meiboom S, Gill D. Modified spin-echo method for measuring nuclear relaxation times. Rev Sci Instrum. 1958;29:688-91.
12. Maudsley AA. Modified Carr-Purcell-Meiboom-Gill sequence for NMR Fourier imaging applications. J Magn Reson (1969). 1986;69:488-91.
13. Mulkern RV, Wong ST, Winalski C, et al. Contrast manipulation and artifact assessment of 2D and 3D RARE sequences. Magn Reson Imaging. 1990;8:557-66.
14. Mulkern RV, Melki PS, Jakab P, et al. Phase encode order and its effect on contrast and artifact in single-shot RARE sequences. Med Phys. 1991;18:1032-7.
15. Melki PS, Mulkern RV, Panych LP, et al. Comparing the FAISE method with conventional dual-echo sequences. J Magn Reson Imaging. 1991;1:319-26.
16. Melki PS, Jolesz FA, Mulkern RV. Partial RF echo planar imaging with the FAISE method. I. Experimental and theoretical assessment of artifact. Magn Reson Med. 1992;26:328-41.
17. Melki PS, Jolesz FA, Mulkern RV. Partial RF echo planar imaging with the FAISE method. II. Contrast equivalence with spin echo sequences. Magn Reson Med. 1992;26:342-54.
18. Ahn SS, Mantello MT, Jones KM, et al. Rapid MR imaging of the pediatric brain using the fast spin-echo technique. Am J Neuroradiol. 1992;13(4):1169-77.
19. Constable RT, Smith RC, Gore JC. Signal-to-noise and contrast in fast spin echo (FSE) and inversion recovery FSE imaging. J Comput Assist Tomogr. 1992;16(1):41-7.
20. Jones KM, Mulkern RV, Mantello MT, et al. Brain hemorrhage: evaluation with fast spin-echo and conventional dual spin-echo images. Radiology. 1992;182(1):53-8.
21. Jones KM, Mulkern RV, Schwartz RB. Fast spin-echo MR imaging of the brain and spine: current concepts. Am J Roentgenol. 1992;158:1313-20.
22. Tice HM, Jones KM, Mulkern RV. Fast spin-echo imaging of intracranial neoplasms. J Comput Assist Tomogr. 1993;17:425-31.
23. Hardy PA, Henkelman RM, Bishop JE. Why fat is bright in rare and fast spin-echo imaging. J Magn Reson Imaging. 1992;2(5):533-40.
24. Hiramatsu K, Mulkern RV. A novel method for fat suppression in RARE sequences. Magn Reson Med. 1992;27(1):107-17.
25. Melki PS, Mulkern RV. Magnetization transfer effects in multislice RARE sequences. Magn Reson Med. 1992;24(1):189-95.
26. Feinberg DA, Kiefer B, Litt AW. High resolution GRASE MRI of the brain and spine: 512 and 1024 matrix imaging. J Comput Assist Tomogr. 1995;19(1):1-7.
27. McGibney G, Smith MR, Nichols ST. Quantitative evaluation of several partial Fourier reconstruction algorithms used in MRI. Magn Reson Med. 1993;30(1):51-9.
28. Lustig M, Donoho D, Pauly JM. Sparse MRI: the application of compressed sensing for rapid MR imaging. Magn Reson Med. 2007;58:1182-95.
29. Donoho DL. Compressed sensing. IEEE Transactions on Information Theory. 2006;52(4):1289-306.
30. Candes EJ, Romberg J, Tao T. Robust uncertainty principles: exact signal reconstruction from highly incomplete frequency information. IEEE Transactions on Information Theory. 2006;52(2):489-509.
31. Moeller S, Yacoub E, Olman CA. Multiband multislice GE-EPI at 7 Tesla, with 16-fold acceleration using partial parallel imaging with application to high spatial and temporal whole-brain fMRI. Magnetic Reson Med. 2010;63(5):1144-53.
32. Feinberg DA, Setsompop K. Ultra-fast MRI of the human brain with simultaneous multi-slice imaging. J Magn Reson. 2013;229:90-100.
33. Haacke EM, Mittal S, Wu Z, et al. Susceptibility-weighted-imaging: technical aspects and clinical applications, Part I. Am J Neuroradiol. 2009;30:19-30.
34. Mittal S, Wu J, Neelavalli EM, et al. Susceptibility-weighted-imaging: technical aspects and clinical applications, Part II. Am J Neuroradiol. 2009;30:232-52.
35. Deistung A, Schweser F, Reichenbach JR. Overview of quantitative susceptibility mapping. NMR Biomed. 2017;30(4). doi: 10.1002/nbm.3569.
36. Haacke EM, Liu S, Buch S, et al. Quantitative susceptibility mapping: current status and future directions. Magn Reson Imaging. 2015;33(1):1-25.
37. Li W, Liu C3, Duong TQ, et al. Susceptibility tensor imaging (STI) of the brain. NMR Biomed. 2017;30(4):e3540.
38. Schaefer PW, Grant PE, Gonzalez RG. Diffusion-weighted imaging of the brain. Radiology. 2000;217:331-45.
39. Hagmann P, Jonasson L, Maeder P, et al. Understanding diffusion MR imaging techniques: from scalar diffusion-weighted imaging to diffusion tensor imaging and beyond. Radiographics. 2006;26(Suppl 1):S205-23.
40. Sundgren PC, Dong Q, Go'mez-Hassan D, et al. Diffusion tensor imaging of the brain: review of clinical applications. Neuroradiology. 2004;46:339-50.
41. Bammer R, Acar B, Moseley ME. In vivo MR tractography using diffusion imaging. Eur J Radiol. 2003;45:223-34.
42. Wedeen VJ, Hagmann P, Tseng WY, et al. Mapping complex tissue architecture with diffusion spectrum magnetic resonance imaging. Magn Reson Med. 2005;54:1377-86.
43. Tuch DS, Reese TG, Wiegell MR, et al. Diffusion MRI of complex neural architecture. Neuron. 2003;40:885-95.
44. Jansons KM, Alexander DC. Persistent angular structure: new insights from diffusion MRI data. [Dummy version]. Inf Process Med Imaging. 2003;18:672-83.
45. Tournier JD, Calamante F, Gadian DG, et al. Direct estimation of the fiber orientation density function from diffusion-weighted MRI data using spherical deconvolution. Neuroimage. 2004;23:1176-85.
46. Steven AJ, Zhuo J, Melhem ER. Diffusion kurtosis imaging: an emerging technique for evaluating the microstructural environment of the brain. Am J Roentgenol. 2014;202:W26-33.

47. Fieremans E, Jensen JH, Helpern JA. White matter characterization with diffusional kurtosis imaging. Neuroimage. 2011;58:177-88.
48. Porter DA, Heidemann RM. High resolution diffusion-weighted imaging using readout-segmented echo-planar imaging, parallel imaging and a two-dimensional navigator-based reacquisition. Magn Reson Med. 2009;62: 468-75.
49. Dowell NG, Jenkins TM, Ciccarelli O, et al. Contiguous-slice zonally oblique multislice (CO-ZOOM) diffusion tensor imaging: examples of in vivo spinal cord and optic nerve applications. J Magn Reson Imaging. 2009;29(2):454-60.
50. Jahng GH, Li KL, Ostergaard L, et al. Perfusion magnetic resonance imaging: a comprehensive update on principles and techniques. Korean J Radiol. 2014;15:554-77.
51. Cha S. Perfusion MR imaging: basic principles and clinical applications. Magn Reson Imaging Clin N Am. 2003;11:403-13.
52. Wang J, Alsop DC, Li L, et al. Comparison of quantitative perfusion imaging using arterial spin labeling at 1.5 and 4.0 Tesla. Magn Reson Med. 2002;48:242-54.
53. Haller S, Zaharchuk G, Thomas DL, et al. Arterial spin labeling perfusion of the brain: emerging clinical applications. Radiology. 2016;281:337-56.
54. Chhabra A, Andreisek G, Soldatos T, et al. MR neurography: past, present, and future. Am J Roentgenol. 2011;197: 583-91.
55. Seddon HJ, Medawar PB, Smith H. Rate of regeneration of peripheral nerves in man. J Physiol. 1943;102:191-215.
56. Sunderland S. A classification of peripheral nerve injuries producing loss of function. Brain. 1951;74:491-516.
57. Sohn CH, Sevick RJ, Frayne R. Contrast-enhanced MR angiography of the intracranial circulation. Neuroimag Clin N Am. 2003;11:599-614.
58. Korosec FR, Frayne R, Grist TM, et al. Time-resolved contrast-enhanced 3D MR angiography. Magn Reson Med. 1996;36:345-51.
59. Taschner CA, Gieseke J, Thuc VL, et al. Intracranial arterio-venous malformation: time-resolved contrast-enhanced MR angiography with combination of parallel imaging, keyhole acquisition and k-space sampling techniques at 1.5 T. Radiology. 2008;246:871-9.
60. Hatsukami TS, Ross R, Polissar NL, et al. Visualization of fibrous cap thickness and rupture in human atherosclerotic plaques in vivo with high resolution magnetic resonance imaging. Circulation. 2000;102:959-64.
61. Mandell DM, Mossa-Basha M, Qiao Y, et al. Intracranial vessel wall MRI: principles and expert consensus recommendations of the American Society of Neuroradiology. AJNR Am J Neuroradiol. 2017;38:218-29.
62. Choi YJ, Jung SC, Lee DH. Vessel wall imaging of the intracranial and cervical carotid arteries. J Stroke. 2015;17:238-55.
63. Murphy MC, Huston J 3rd, Ehman RL. MR elastography of the brain and its application in neurological diseases. Neuroimage. 2017;S1053-8119(17)30821-2.
64. Ma D, Gulani V, Seiberlich N, et al. Magnetic resonance fingerprinting. Nature. 2013;495:187-92.
65. Wu B,Warnock G, Zaiss M, et al. An overview of CEST MRI for non-MR physicists. EJNMMI Phys. 2016;3:19.
66. Jones KM, Pollard AC, Pagel MD. Clinical applications of chemical exchange saturation transfer (CEST) MRI. J Magn Reson Imaging. 2018;47:11-27.
67. McGowan JC. The physical basis of magnetization transfer imaging. Neurology. 1999;53(5 Suppl 3):S3-7.
68. Santos AC, Narayanan S, de Stefano N, et al. Magnetization transfer can predict clinical evolution in patients with multiple sclerosis. J Neurol. 2002;249:662-8.
69. Gupta RK, Hussain M, Vatsal DK, et al. Comparative evaluation of magnetization transfer imaging and in vivo proton MR spectroscopy in brain tuberculomas. Magn Reson Imaging. 2002;20:375-81
70. Jeong HK, Han K, Zhou J, et al. Characterizing amide proton transfer imaging in haemorrhage brain lesions using 3T MRI. Eur Radiol. 2017;27:1577-84.
71. Chawla SC, Federman N, Zhang D, et al. Estimated cumulative radiation dose from PET/CT in children with malignancies: a 5-year retrospective review. Pediatr Radiol. 2010;40:681-6.
72. Mattsson S, Söderberg M. Radiation dose management in CT, SPECT/CT and PET/CT techniques. Radiat Prot Dosimetry. 2011;147(1-2):13-21.
73. Delso G, Fürst S, Jakoby B, et al. Performance measurements of the Siemens mMR integrated whole-body PET/MR scanner. J Nucl Med. 2011;52:1914-22.
74. Pichler BJ, Judenhofer MS, Catana C, et al. Performance test of an LSO-APD detector in a 7-T MRI scanner for simultaneous PET/MRI. J Nucl Med. 2006;47:639-47.
75. Hofmann M, Pichler B, Schölkopf B, et al. Towards quantitative PET/MRI: a review of MR-based attenuation correction techniques. Eur J Nucl Med Mol Imaging. 2009;36(Suppl 1):S93-104.
76. Zaidi H, Ojha N, Morich M, et al. Design and performance evaluation of a whole-body Ingenuity TF. PET-MRI system. Phys Med Biol. 2011;56:3091-106.
77. Ossenkoppele R, Tolboom N, Foster-Dingley JC, et al. Longitudinal imaging of Alzheimer pathology using [11C] PIB, [18F]FDDNP and [18F]FDG PET. Eur J Nucl Med Mol Imaging. 2012;39:990-1000.
78. Kenny ER, Blamire AM, Firbank MJ, et al. Functional connectivity in cortical regions in dementia with Lewy bodies and Alzheimer's disease. Brain. 2012;135:569-81.
79. Duncan J. The current status of neuroimaging for epilepsy. Curr Opin Neurol. 2009;22:179-84.
80. Jiang F, Jiang Y, Zhi H, et al Artificial intelligence in healthcare: past, present and future. Stroke Vasc Neurol. 2017;2(4):230-43.

CHAPTER 6

Magnetic Resonance Spectroscopy

Vikas Bhatia, Paramjeet Singh, Niranjan Khandelwal

INTRODUCTION

Nuclear magnetic resonance (NMR) and spectroscopy were introduced as experimental techniques as a method of delineating structure and composition of various physical and chemical materials. Subsequently, it was found to have many applications in medicine and *in vivo* magnetic resonance spectroscopy (MRS) evolved as a new molecular imaging technique to noninvasively determine the metabolites in any given living tissue which are measured as a result of their different chemical shifts or frequencies.[1] Most of the pathologic processes are characterized by metabolic changes earlier than anatomic changes during disease process and after treatment. Thus, MRS imaging provides information which can lead to early diagnosis, treatment plan and response assesment.[2]

MRS is a spectrum which tells us about the chemical and physical properties of a tissue based on the intensity and distribution of energy measured after a certain wavelength or frequency is allowed to interact with the tissue sample.

MR spectra is shown by those nuclei that contain an odd number of protons and neutrons, such as hydrogen-1, carbon-13, fluorine-19, phosphorus-31 as they exhibit a magnetic momentum to interact with the external magnetic field.[3] A major limitation of MRS is that only those metabolites with a concentration of more than 0.1 mM can be detected. However, with the recent development of hardware and localizing techniques, MRS offers a promising future to detect many different metabolites and their role in physiological and pathological conditions.

PRINCIPLE

Basic fundamental principles of magnetic resonance imaging (MRI) and MRS are same.[4] While MRI provides information on anatomy and pathology displayed as visual images, MRS basically obtains chemical information of the region of interest as a spectra which is displayed as numerical values. The simple MRI sequence block contains slice excitation by radio frequency pulse followed by application of slice encoding, phase encoding, and frequency-encoding gradients in mutually orthogonal planes. Whereas, in a classical spectroscopic imaging sequence, the MRS signal is acquired without a frequency-encoding gradient. Thus, acquired MRS signal contains different frequencies that correspond to the chemical shift with no spatial information. The amplitude of chemical shifts of various metabolites depends on the gyromagnetic ratio of the nuclei and intensity of external magnetic field **(Table 1)**. So, at a given external magnetic field, every chemically distinct nucleus shows slightly different resonating frequency—the *chemical shift*—giving rise to separate peaks in the MR spectrum. By the same principle, in a given standard chemical environment increasing the external magnetic field strength transforms into better separation of signal frequencies of various metabolites in MR spectrum. J coupling or spin-spin coupling is due to interactions with a neighboring nuclear spin and provides additional information.

Table 1: MRS: Properties of nuclei.

Nucleus	Spin quantum number	Natural abundance (%)	Gyromagnetic ratio (MHz/T)	Resonance frequency (MHz) at 1.5T	Resonance frequency (MHz) at 3T
^{1}H	1/2	100	42.6	63.9	127.7
^{31}P	1/2	100	17.2	25.9	51.7
^{19}F	1/2	100	40.1	60.1	120.2
^{23}Na	3/4	100	11.3	16.9	33.8
^{17}O	5/2	0.04	2.0	8.7	17.3
^{7}Li	3/2	92.6	16.5	24.8	49.7
^{13}C	1/2	1.1	10.7	16.1	32.1

Spectrum

An MRS provides *in vivo* biochemical information represented spectrum with the peaks in the spectra obtained correspond with various metabolites. The horizontal axis shows resonance frequency as ppm to the total resonance frequency. The vertical axis plots the concentrations or relative signal amplitude of metabolites.

Factors affecting the peak sharpness and line width are:

a. External magnetic field homogeneity
b. Inhomogeneity of the magnetic field due to susceptibility gradient
c. T2 time of the sample.

The spectra obtained are interpretated for the following **(Fig. 1)**:

- Center of the resonance frequency in ppm
- Height of peak
- Line width at half-height
- Area and shape of peak
- Characteristic of the peaks, e.g. single, doublet, triplet.

The display of the MR spectra as per convention include:

- *Up-field* is to the right represents lower frequencies and are shielded.
- *Down-field* is to the left represents higher frequencies and are deshielded.
- *Chemical shifts (in ppm)* is positive going to the left and is negative towards the right.

Zero setting is done by RF of a particular compound, e.g. phosphocreatine for ^{31}P-MRS and tetramethylsilane (TMS) for ^{1}H and ^{13}C MRS (at 4.8 ppm). Since TMS is not seen *in viva* known chemical like NAA at 2.0 ppm is used as chemical shift reference. The ppm scale describes the shifts in hertz from a reference peak divided by frequency of excitation. For example, ^{31}P-MRS acquired at 1.5 T shows resonance frequency at 25.86 MHz and 25.86 Hz is 1 ppm. The ppm scales provides easy comparison of data obtained in different fields.

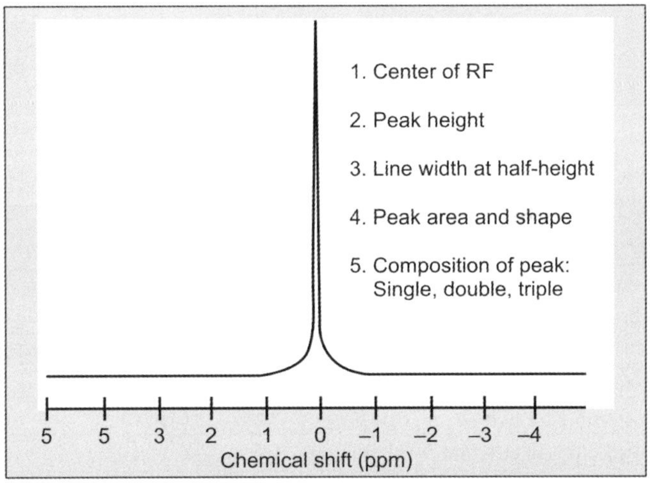

Fig. 1: Parameters for analysis of MR spectrum.

Spectrum and Echo Time

The metabolites and their spectral pattern on proton MRS depend on the time to echo (TE).[5] Various metabolites which are seen on long and short TE are summarized **(Tables 2 and 3)**.

The phenomenon of spin-spin coupling (J coupling) influences the appearance of spectra due to various metabolites obtained at different TE. It is emphasized that the frequency of resonating protons is affected by adjacent electrons and hence various chemical groups within the same molecule resonate at different frequencies. For instance, lactic acid, COOH-CHOH-CH3, the principle signal is due to CH 3 group at 1.33 ppm. As this group is connected to the CH group, coupling of proton signals is seen: resulting in splitting of CH 3

Table 2: Various metabolites with molecular concentrations.[7]

ppm	Spectral assignment	Approximate concentration mM/kg net wt
0.9–1.3	Macromolecules, amino acids, lipids	<0.5
1.35	Lactate	0.5
1.47	Alanine	<0.3
1.9	Acetate	0.2
2.02, 2.6	N-acetyl aspartate	7–10
2.1/2.5	Glutamate + Glutamine	6–10
2.4	Pyruvate succinate	0.3
3.02, 3.9	Creatine	5–7
3.2	Choline	5–7
3.36	Scylloinositol and taurine	1
3.56, 4.06	Myoinositol, glycine	5–7

Table 3: Visualization of metabolites based on TE values.[7]

	Large signals at long TE	Large signals at short TE	Small signals (short or long TE)
Normally present	NAA	Glutamate	N-acetyl-aspartyl-glutamate (NAAG
	Cr	Glutamine	Taurine, ethanolamine
	Cho	Myo-inositol	Glucose
Pathological	Lactate	Lipids	
	Succinate	Macromolecules	
	Pyruvate	Phenylalanine	
	Alanine		
	Glycine		

peak into a doublet with intensity ratio 1:1. Metabolites with doublet peaks (lactate, alanine) are usually seen as positive peaks around TE 280 ms with inversion at TE 140 ms. Triplets (e.g. glutamate/glutamine, aspartate), which have two neighboring protons, are seen at short TE or t intermediate TE). Quartets (e.g. myoinositol) tend to be seen at shortest TE.[6]

Observable Biochemicals on MRS

The *in vivo* MR spectroscopy before any postprocessing contains four types of compounds in its spectrum.[8]

1. Water with a concentration of about 40 M between 4.3 and 6 ppm.
   This water signal is required to be suppressed because its signal intensity is about four orders more than other visible metabolites.
2. Lipids, macromolecules, the macromolecules produce a broad signal on the background or are invisible in the MR spectra.
3. Metabolites having concentration >1 mM and molecular weight less than 2000 Da between 0.5 and 4 ppm.
   This is the most important group in clinical MR spectroscopy which comprises of approximately twenty compounds found in ^{1}H MR spectra of humans.
4. Metabolites having concentration <1 mM with molecular weight 2000 Da between 6 and 10 ppm. These are usually not evaluated in clinical MR spectroscopy due to limitation of time and SNR.

Hydrogen 1 (^{1}H-MRS)

Proton is abundantly present in the body and hence most suited for MRS. **Figures 2A and B** shows major spectral peaks from human brain using a 3T MRI system at TE = 135 ms (2A) and TE = 30 ms (2B). **Table 4** shows the major compounds as seen on ^{1}H-MRS with approximate concentration and chemical shift in ppm.

N-acetylaspartate (NAA) peak is seen as major upfield peak on ^{1}H-MRS. It is specifically present in CNS predominantly in mature neurons and axons. It is considered to be a sensitive marker density and viability of neurons.[9] This metabolite is seen in cortex and white matter of fetuses as early as 16 weeks of gestation. During the early years of life, rapid increase in levels of NAA and Cr is seen. After this, levels increase less than 1% a year until reaching adult values by age 16 years. Reduced levels of NAA are seen in pathologics such as degenerative disorders and stroke due to neuronal loss or injury. NAA–glutamate is present only in white matter (not in gray matter) and constitutes a resonance of around 20% near to 2.0 ppm overlapping with the NAA peak.

Choline (Cho) peak is seen at 3.22 ppm and is due to glycerophosphocholine (GPC) and glycerophospho-ethanolamine (GPE) constituting the phospholipid layer of the cell membrane. Raised levels of choline are seen in acute demyelinating lesions due to release of membrane phospholipids during active myelin breakdown. Raised choline is seen in brain tumors due to associated increased cellular density. Infants with active myelination stage also have increased levels of choline as compared to adults.

Creatine (Cr) peak at 3.02 ppm is due to sum of creatine and phosphocreatine and it does not indicate energy state of the cell. Concentration of total creatinine is relative constant throughout the brain with relative resistance to change. These properties make Cr to be used as an internal standard to normalize resonance intensities of other metabolites.

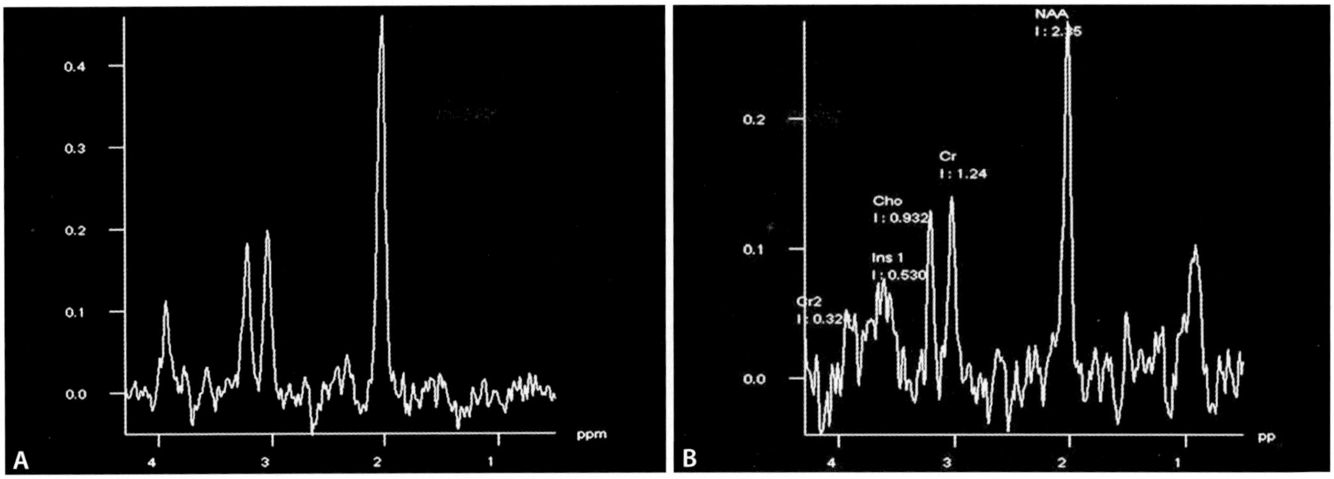

Figs. 2A and B: (A) Normal proton ^{1}H-MRS in brain (TE = 135 ms); (B) Normal proton ^{1}H-MRS in brain (TE = 30 ms).

Table 4: Differential diagnostic uses of metabolites in MRS.[7]

Metabolite (Normal cerebral concentration)	*Major resonance peak*	*Characteristics*	*Decreased*	*Increased*
1. Creatine (Cr) and phosphocreatine (PCr) (8 mM)	3.0 and 3.9 Singlet	Marker of brain metabolism	• Hypoxic injury • Ischemic injury • Neoplasms • Traumatic insult	Hyperosmolar increasing with age
2. Lactate (Lac) (1 mM: Not visible because of its low concentration)	1.3 Doublet Inverted at TE 144 ms	• Product of anaerobic metabolic activity • Indicates ischemia • Interrupted Krebs' cycle • Inhibition of PDH	Unknown	• Hypoxic/ischemic insult • Hemorrhage • Infections • Neoplasms
3. Myoinositol (mL) (5 mM)	3.5 Multiplet Short TE	• Marker of astrocytes • Regulation of cell volume • Indicates osmotic stress	• Stroke • Tumor • Hypoxia • Hyponatremia • SIADH	• Neonate • Renal dysfunction • DM • Recovery from hypoxic insult
4. N-acetyl aspartate (NAA) (8–9 mM)	2.0 Singlet	• Most prominent upright signal in normal brain tissue • Indicative of normal neuronal function	• Hypoxia • Infants • Ischemic injury • Seizure disorder • Demyelination • Neoplasms • Traumatic insult • Neurodegenerative disorders	• Canavan's disease • Recovery after axonal injury • PMD • Normal developing infant brain
5. Choline (Cho) (1.5 mM)	3.2 Singlet	• Required for Membrane synthesis • Increased levels seen after membrane degradation	• Hepatic encephalopathy • Stroke • SIADH • Cryptococcoma	• Traumatic injury • Neoplastic • Ischemic injury • Demyelination • Certain infections • Neonates
6. Lipid	0.9–1.3 Broad peak Short TE	• Indicates pathological process due to liberation of membrane lipids	Not detectable	• Voxel contamination, e.g. scalp • Necrotic neoplasm • Lymphoma • Tuberculoma • Brain abscess • Toxoplasmosis • Traumatic/ischemic insult

Contd...

Contd...

Metabolite (Normal cerebral concentration)	*Major resonance peak*	*Characteristics*	*Decreased*	*Increased*
7. Glutamine (Gln) and glutamate Glu) (Gln approx 5 mm, Glu approx 10 mm)	2.1–2.6 3.75 Multiplet Short TE	• Marker of astrocytes and increased levels may indicate replacement of neurons by astrocytes	• Traumatic injury • Hyponatremia • SIADH	• Hepatic encephalopathy • Hypoxic injury
8. Succinate	2.4 Singlet	Abscesses with anaerobic metabolism		Succinate >acetate indicative of parasitic abscesses
9. Acetate	1.9 Singlet	Abscesses with anaerobic metabolism		Acetate >succinate indicative of pyogenic
10. Amino acids	0.9 Doublet /triplet Inverted at TE 144 ms	Necessary for protein synthesis		Hypervalinemia Branched-chain ketonuria MSUD Brain abscess
11. Glycine	3.5 Singlet Long TE	Inhibitory neurotransmitter and antioxidant		Pyogenic abscess Hyperglycinemia tumor
12. Alanine	1.5 Doublet/triplet Inverted at TE 144 ms	Produced by transamination of pyruvate in hypoxic tissues		Pyogenic abscess Meningioma Central neurocytoma PNET
13. Trehalose	3.6–3.8	Disaccharide		Fungal infections

Lactate (lac) peak is formed due to anaerobic glycolysis and seen as doublet at 1.33 ppm.[10] Lactate accumulates when oxidative metabolism is unable to meet energy requirements leading to accelerated anaerobic glycolysis. Certain brain tumors, such as gliomas show elevated concentrations of lactate, because they show increased glycolysis independent of the adequacy of oxidative metabolic pathways. Elevated lactate is also seen in the extracellular environment of necrotic tissue and cysts as well as in areas of ischemic infarction.

Other metabolites such as myoinositol, glutamate/glutamine and glucose, may also be observed. Broad peaks at 0.9–1.3 ppm of lipid may obscure some of the metabolites, contaminate the spectra and need to be separated from lactate peak.[11] The differential diagnostic uses of metabolites of ^{1}H-MRS have been summarized in **Table 4.**[12]

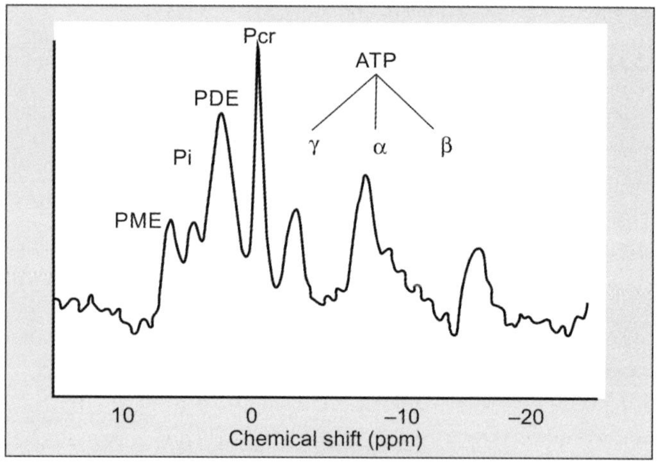

Fig. 3: Normal ^{3}1P-MRS of brain.

Phosphorus 31 (^{31}P-MRS)

It demonstrates the metabolites involved in the energy metabolism. **Figure 3** shows a typical ^{31}P-MRS spectrum of human brain. The first down-field peak is due to phosphomonoesters (PME) composed of phosphocholine, phosphoethanolamine and sugar phosphates. It is dependent on metabolic state of the cell. The next peak is due to inorganic phosphate (Pi) composed of monobasic and dibasic inorganic phosphate. In acidosis, there is chemical shifts of Pi towards up-field in contrast to shift of Pi to the down-field in alkalosis and can be used to estimate intracellular pH. The next phosphodiesters (PDE) peak is composed of glycerophosphocholine and phosphoethanolamine followed by phosphocreatine (PCr) peak. Then follows three peaks of ATP – γ, α, β. The β ATP is frequently used to assess ATP concentration.

The other nuclei like 13_{C}, 23_{Na}, 39_{K}, 19_{F}, 7_{Li}, 14_{N}, 15_{N} also exhibit MRS activity and are of research utility at present rather than of clinical significance.[13]

LOCALIZATION TECHNIQUES

The volume of interest when localized precisely leads to a clean spectra that are essential for accurate interpretation of MRS data. There are two types of localization techniques, i.e.(a) by using main magnetic field gradient (B0 field) and (b) by using RF field gradient (B1 field).

B_1 Field Gradient Methods

Surface Coils

Surface coil provides adequate localization of the metabolites insurface tissues close to the coil with good sensitivity. There is inherent inhomogeneity of surface coils. For studies requiring more precise localization or to quantitate metabolites, other localization methods are warranted. Surface spoiling by the use of grid of wires helps alpine eliminating signals from the surface of the tissue with preservation of signal originating from deep layer of the tissue.[14] Inhomogeneity of the surface coils can be used to advantage in localization methods by "rotating frame imaging". By this way, 2D Fourier transformation of the data, sets produces 1D metabolic map where sequential spectra represent greater distance from the surface coil.[15]

B_0 Field Gradient Methods

Static Field Gradient

By using static homogeneous magnetic field over a small volume, ^{31}P-MRS is possible in brain and liver. But this technique is difficult and has limited use.

Slice-selective B_0-gradient Techniques

DRESS

Depth-resolved surface spectroscopy (DRESS) is the simplest gradient localization method. A single plane-selective radiofrequency (RF) pulse is applied to the volume of tissue and data acquisition is done. This method is crude and suffers from lack of information at the center of RF pulse producing baseline artifacts. The sequence can also be used in slice-interleaved multislice mode (SLIT-DRESS). The water suppression is achieved by using a long, low amplitude Gaussian pulse.

3D Localization Methods

Two major localization techniques of the MRS signal are: Single voxel spectroscopy (SVS) and spectroscopic imaging (MRSI) or chemical shift imaging (CSI).

The pulse sequences used in single-voxel spectroscopy are as follows:

a. **STEAM:** The stimulated-echo acquisition mode (STEAM) of localization for ^{1}H-MRS is constituted by three 90° selective pulses, each applied with an orthogonal gradient for slice excitation. This sequence is simple and robust but there is approximately 50% signal loss. It is not suitable for observation of nuclei having short T2 values.[16]
b. **PRESS:** The point-resolved spectroscopy (PRESS) localization consists of a sequence of 90-180-180° pulses which are applied with orthogonal gradient. Unlike STEAM, no signal loss is seen. The PRESS sequence has the disadvantage that it cannot be applied in short TE values (<40 ms). Water suppression is done by using a gaussian pulse preceding the localization pulses. A variant of this sequence is MESA by using binomial (1331) pulse to achieve water suppression followed by a train of three 180-180-180° pulses.
c. **ISIS:** Image selected *in vivo* spectroscopy (ISIS) consists of three inversion pulses and a fourth nonselective pulse. It requires a minimum eight phase cycles to localize the signal. There is minimum loss from T2 relaxation and especially useful for nuclei having short T2 values like ^{31}P.

Chemical shift imaging (CSI): Using phase encoding strategies, it is possible to encode information from multiple voxels simultaneously. Phase encoding can be applied in multiple dimensions. Data are translated to extract chemical shift information from multiple positions using up to 4D Fourier transformations. MRSI has the advantage of obtaining multiple spectra in one data acquisition. The technique requires a larger volume homogeneous magnetic field as compared to than SVS.[4] The vast quantity of data generated with CSI make management, analysis and interpretation of CSI spectra a daunting challenge in the clinical setting.

Figures 4A to F show the various localization pulse sequence methods.

Single Voxel Versus Multivoxel Spectroscopy

Comparative description between the SVS and MRSI is shown in **Table 5**.

As the RF pulses have a nonrectangular profile, the spatial origin of signal in a voxel does not coincide with the rectangular shape of the voxel in MRSI and signal from one voxel is contaminated by signal in others leading to phenomenon known as voxel bleeding. This is more pertinent when interpreting the lipid signals in MRSI, because the lipid signal from the subcutaneous regions such as scalp is about a thousand times in magnitude than the signal of metabolites and can lead to significant voxel bleeding and interference with spectroscopy findings. For the same reason, SVS is usually the method of choice when

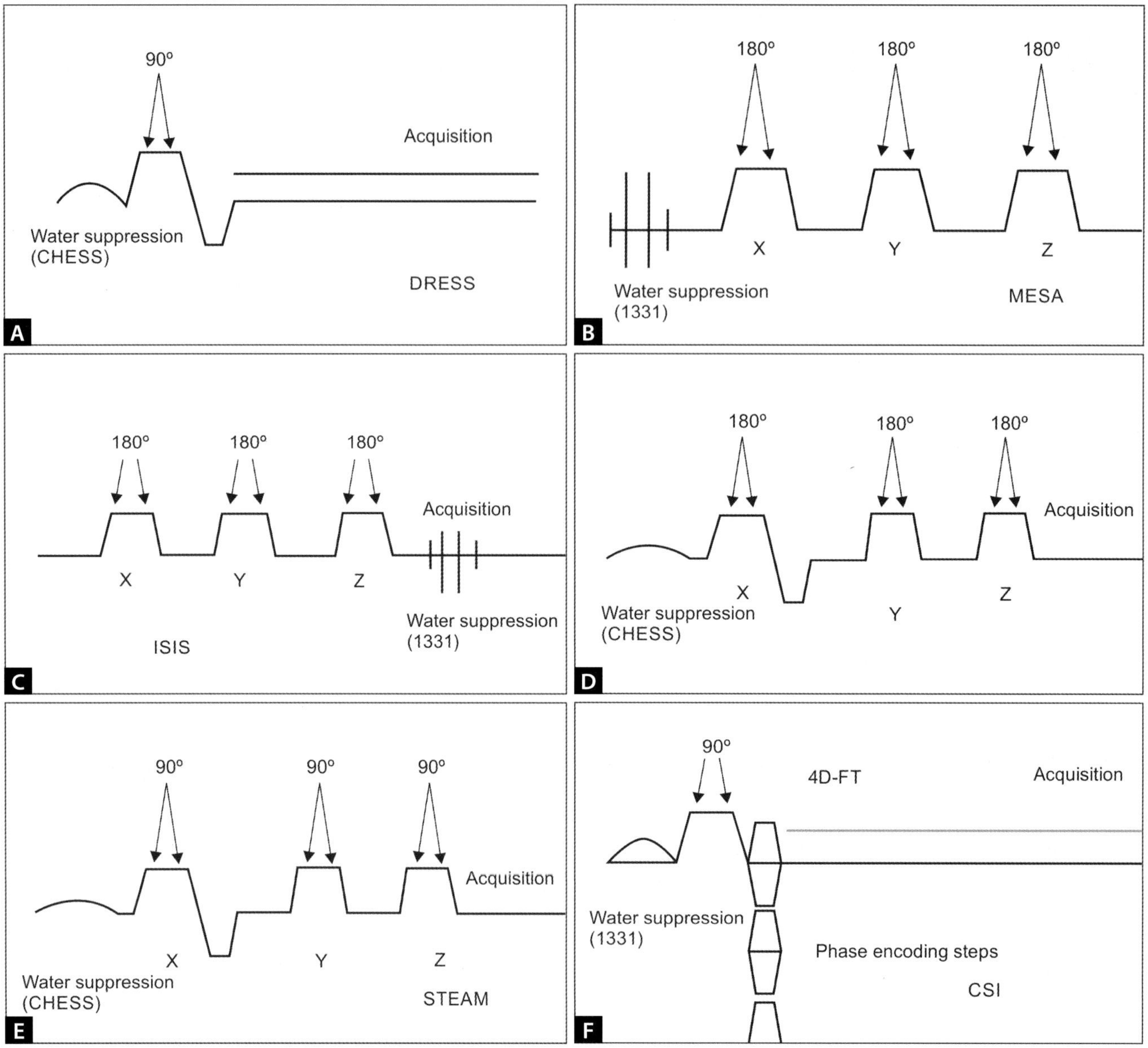

Figs. 4A to F: Different techniques of localization in MRS.

accurate quantification of metabolites is required where voxel bleeding phenomenon is not significant.[4]

Quantitative Spectroscopy

Measurement of the concentration of metabolites (quantification) is essential to facilitate distinction between normal and diseased tissue and for comparison of results from different laboratories. Quantification relies on calibration of resonance signals with internal or external standard or phantom. The area under a resonance signal is proportional to the number of nuclei, one can find out concentration of an unknown peak. Peak width relates to T2 relaxation. Peak width and height can also be used for quantification.

Data Acquisition and Analysis

The following steps are roughly the guidelines for proper spectral acquisition and analysis:

Voxel positioning: Accurate and proper or pure voxel positioning is essential to acquire good spectra (avoid scalp and CSF). Thin-slice high resolution image acquisition and the best positioning of the voxel within the image is the correct way to achieve best spectral information.

Table 5: Comparison between SVS and MRSI.[17]

Technique	*SVS*	*MRSI*
TE Voxel size (cm^3) Scan times (min) Shimming Lipid and water suppression Processing	Short or long 4–20 5–10 Local Good Simple processing	Usually long 1–4 5–30 Globalized Worse Processing time consuming
When to use	Single focal lesion or diffuse disease Single query, e.g. abscess vs tumor Complementary to MRSI (e.g. different TE in SVS) Areas close to skull	Multiple or heterogeneous lesions Diffuse disease Comparative assessment of brain regions required
Advantage	High data quality Fast Voxel boundaries better defined Automatic water reference acquisition Limited dataset can be used even if aborted early	Information about heterogeneity of the tissue Retrospective selection of the ROI can be done in the investigated volume Smaller voxel volumes used to assess metabolite distribution
Disadvantage	Selected volume is accurate placement of ROI required at time of investigation No information on spatial heterogeneity of lesion No information of normal brain	More processing required to minimize spectral loss due to insufficient lipid and water suppression Longer acquisition times Experienced needed to plan

Shimming: Adjustment of the magnetic field homogeneity over the voxel is time consuming. The largest source of variation is due to field inhomogeneity.

Water suppression: The large water signal must be suppressed completely to obtain weaker signal of tissue metabolites. There are three techniques to achieve water suppression:

1. Gaussian chemical shift selective (CHESS) pulses.
2. A narrow band pulse (<50 Hz) is applied prior to localization pulse.
3. Binomial pulse sequence (1331 pulse).

This sequence of RF pulses excite the metabolites of interest and not the water and can be used prior or later to localization pulses.

- Inversion recovery and long echo-times.
- *RF calibration*: The signal strength is optimized by adjusting the amplitude of the pulses.

Averaging: To improve SNR, multiple signals are acquired and average values are recorded.

- Fourier transformation (FT) and phase encoding.
- Baseline correction, curve fitting, relaxation time corrections and normal values in control subjects.
- These steps help in proper quantification and to produce uniformity of spectral studies.

CLINICAL APPLICATIONS OF MRS OF BRAIN

In the last few decades there is phenomenal growth of MRS both *in vitro* and *in vivo* applications. This chapter will focus mainly on the utility of ^{1}H-MRS in neurological disorders; although ^{31}P-MRS is useful in the investigation of mitochondrial diseases. Most centers studying the brain with spectroscopy heavily rely upon ^{1}H-MRS. There are several reasons for this: first, the hardware required for ^{1}H-MRS is the same as that used for conventional brain MRI and ^{1}H-MRS can be implemented on most standard commercial scanners operating at 1.5 tesla without the need for hardware modification that would be required to operate at a frequency other than that used for hydrogen. Second, because the MR is much more sensitive to protons as compared to phosphorus, ^{1}H-MRS provides spatial resolution that is best suitable for examining brain pathology. Third, the information available from changes in the level of NAA as measured by ^{1}H-MRS, provides specific chemical pathologic evidence of neuronal injury, information that cannot be obtained with any other MRS. The goal of clinical spectroscopy is to provide biochemical information to assist in the differential diagnosis when standard clinical images fail. There is a rapid growth of clinical MRS in brain as immobilization of head is relatively easy, close proximity of brain to surface and lack of lipid signals that may contaminate spectra. It is of diagnostic value for evaluating and monitoring the progression of stroke, ischemic injury, brain tumors, epilepsy, white matter disorders, Alzheimer's disease, HIV infection, etc.

Brain Tumors

Both proton and phosphorus spectroscopy provide diverse metabolic patterns in brain tumors. Proton MRS generally shows increased Cho/Cr ratio and lactate level, decreased NAA (or complete absence) and Cr. Cho is generally increased in solid portion of the tumor and decreased in the central necrotic portion. ^{31}P-MRS studies show decreased concentration of all metabolites relative to normal brain reflecting loss of viable tissue. Alkaline pH, increased PME, decreased PDE and P Cr are the typical findings in tumors.[18-22]

The following are the major clinical applications of MRS in patients with brain tumors:

Noninvasive diagnosis and grading of cerebral space occupying lesions.

Grading of glial tumors: Spectroscopy findings of astrocytomas reveal elevated choline, reduced Cr and NAA in comparison to the normal brain **(Figs. 5 and 6)**. A higher grade of malignancy is indicated by presence of lactate and lipid peaks reflecting tumor necrosis and hypoxia. Elevated choline peak reflects increased cellularity and membrane synthesis. Localized astrocytomas particularly pilocystic astrocytoma shows raised Cho, low NAA, and presence of a lactate peak—paradoxical findings that are more characteristic of malignant neoplasms than this clinically benign-behaving tumor.[23]

Differentiation between IDH mutant and wild type astrocytomas: IDH-mutant astrocytoma shows a 2-hydroxyglutarate (2-HG) peak resonating at 2.25 ppm which is not seen in wild type.[24]

Medulloblastoma: Medulloblastomas are characterized by high choline peak, absent or low lipid and taurine peak at 3.4 ppm (relatively specific).[25]

Meningiomas vs GBM: The distinction between an intra-axial GBM and an extra-axial lesion, such as meningiomas is not difficult in the majority of cases, occasionally such distinctions are problematic and in such cases ^{1}H-MRS helps in differentiating them. The spectra from the

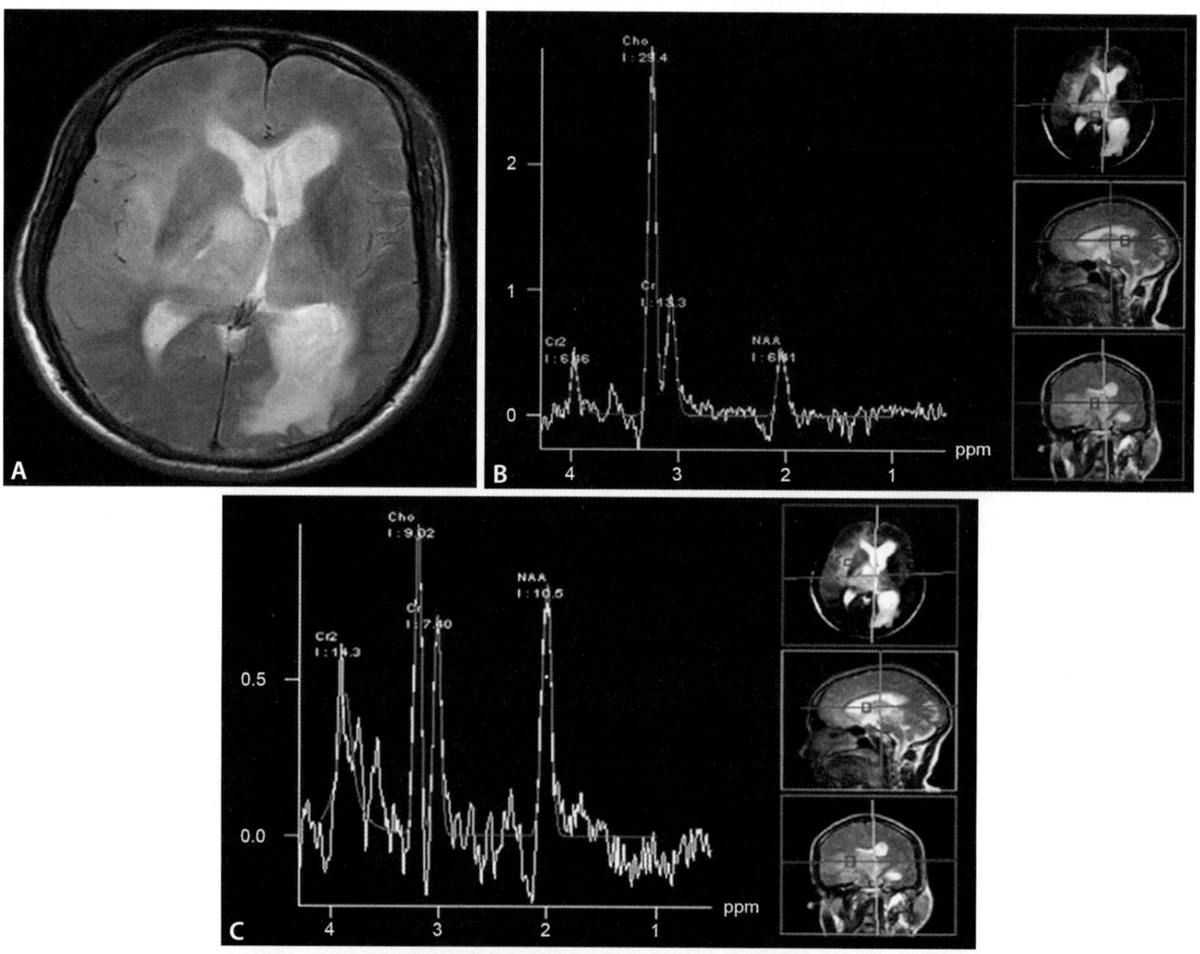

Figs. 5A to C: (A) T2W MR image shows infiltrating astrocytoma involving right thalamic region; (B) CSI ^{1}H-MRS (TE =135 ms) from the thalamic location shows increased choline and Cho/Cr ratio with decreased NAA; (C) The voxel placed in right insular region also shows increased choline/Cr, choline/NAA ratios suggestive of tumor infiltration.

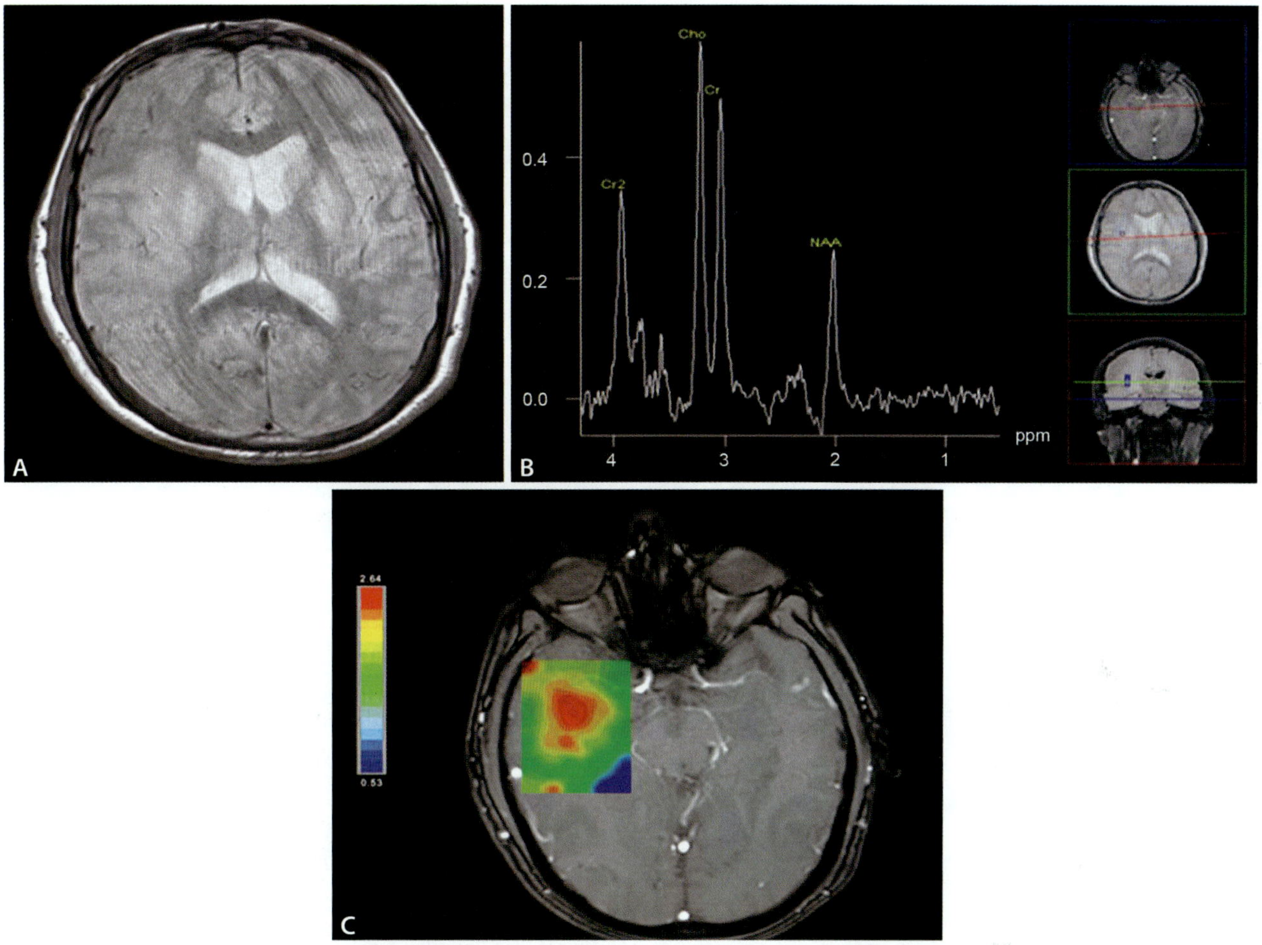

Figs. 6A to C: (A) T2W MR image shows ill-defined hyperintense lesion in right insular region; (B) CSI ^{1}H-MRS (TE = 135 ms) from the lesions shows increased choline and Cho/Cr ratio with decreased NAA; (C) Metabolic map shows mapping of choline/NAA ratios with the red-colored areas predicting the yield areas for pathologically higher grade foci of tumor.

meningioma show low NAA as well as a alanine peak[26] (Ala) **(Figs. 7A to C)**. Spectra from GBM on the other hand show a different metabolite profile as discussed earlier.

Metastases: Spectroscopy findings in metastases show reduction of NAA and Cr with high choline values similar to those of gliomas. They may also contain lipid/lactate peak depending on presence of necrosis. One characteristic that differentiates them from glioma is the defined margins of metastatis, with usually no abnormal spectroscopic findings in surrounding edema. Gliomas on the other hand usually show abnormal spectroscopic findings which can extend beyond the enhancing borders. **(Figs. 8A to C)**.

Lymphoma: These lesions show reduced NAA and high choline with infiltration of adjacent brain. MRS findings may be indistinguishable from gliomas.

Table 6 summarizes the commonly found metabolites in the evaluation of brain tumors.[20]

Tumor Extent (Edema vs Infiltration)

Spectroscopy can differentiate vasogenic edema from infiltration as in cases of vasogenic edema no abnormal metabolic ratios are seen whereas in cases of infiltration there is demonstrable raised choline and reduced NAA peaks **(Fig. 5C)**. Thus, MRS can aid in depiction of tumor margins for adequate resection and appropriate planning of radiation therapy.[7]

Therapeutic planning for gliomas: Utility of MRS for identifying tumor and predicting response to therapy: Metabolite maps from ^{1}H-MRS can be used to suggest regions of higher grade in tumors and to plan stereotactic biopsies and selective tumor resection **(Figs. 6A to C)**. Metabolic changes on chemical profile have also been used to predict chemotherapeutic sensitivity prior to intervention as well as to monitor the response to drug and radiation therapy.

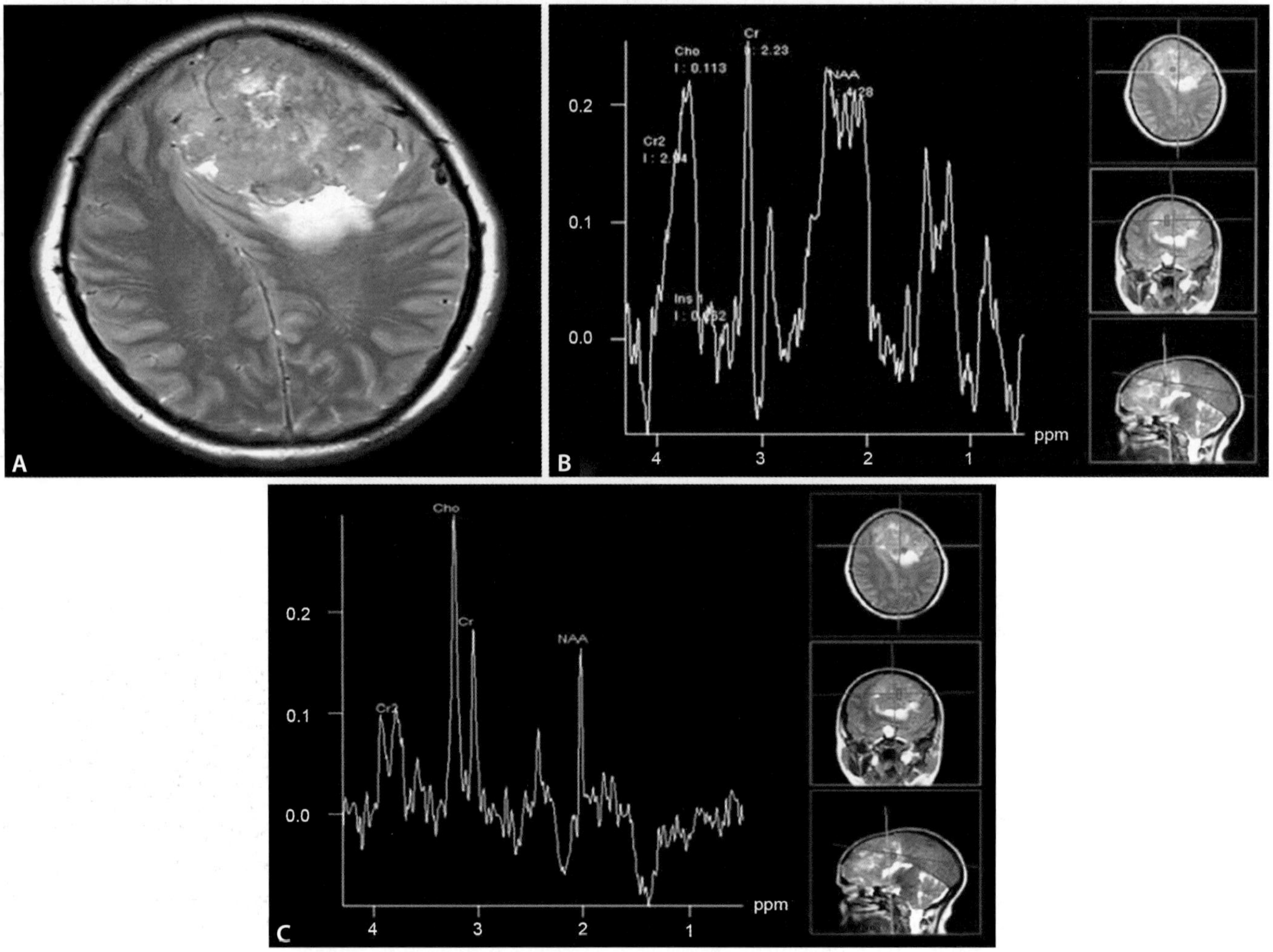

Figs. 7A to C: (A) T2W MR image irregular heterogeneous hyperintense lesion with central necrosis in left frontal location; (B and C) CSI 1H-MRS showing alanine peaks (1.4 ppm) at TE = 30 ms (everted) and TE = 135 ms (inverted) suggestive of meningioma.

Distinction between radiation necrosis and recurrent tumor in postoperative patients: This is the most common scenario for which MRS is utilized in clinical neuroimaging. This diagnostic dilemma has not been solved by any of the numerous advances in MRI because both of these pathologies are seen as heterogeneous mass lesions with enhancement and edema. MRS has been used to diagnose recurrent tumor, mainly based on relative increases in choline, as opposed to MRS in radiation necrosis, which generally shows low levels **(Figs. 9 and 10)**.[23-25]

Differentiation of Intracranial Ring Enhancing Lesions (Table 7)

Necrotic brain tumor vs abscess: Pyogenic brain abscesses shows resonance from amino acids, succinate, acetate and lactate peaks on MR spectroscopy. In contrast, spectra from the necrotic areas of tumors show only lactate peak. The tubercular abscesses and the necrotic tumors both may show lactate levels. But the necrotic high grade tumors significantly elevated Cho/NAA ratios whereas tubercular abscesses show high lipid peaks **(Figs. 11 and 12)**.[26-32]

Pyogenic abscess vs tubercular abscess: Pyogenic brain abscesses show presence of lipid/lactate and amino acid peaks with presence of other metabolites such as succinate and acetate **(Figs. 13 and 14)**, while tuberculous abscesses show only lipid and lactate levels **(Figs. 15A to C)**. Further etiological categorization of pyogenic abscess can also be done by MRS. Aerobic or anaerobic brain abscesses may be differentiated on MRS based on presence of acetate and succinate peaks which are seen only in anaerobic brain abscesses.[29]

Neurocysticercosis (NCC) vs intracranial tuberculoma: It is not always easy to distinguish NCC from tuberculomas

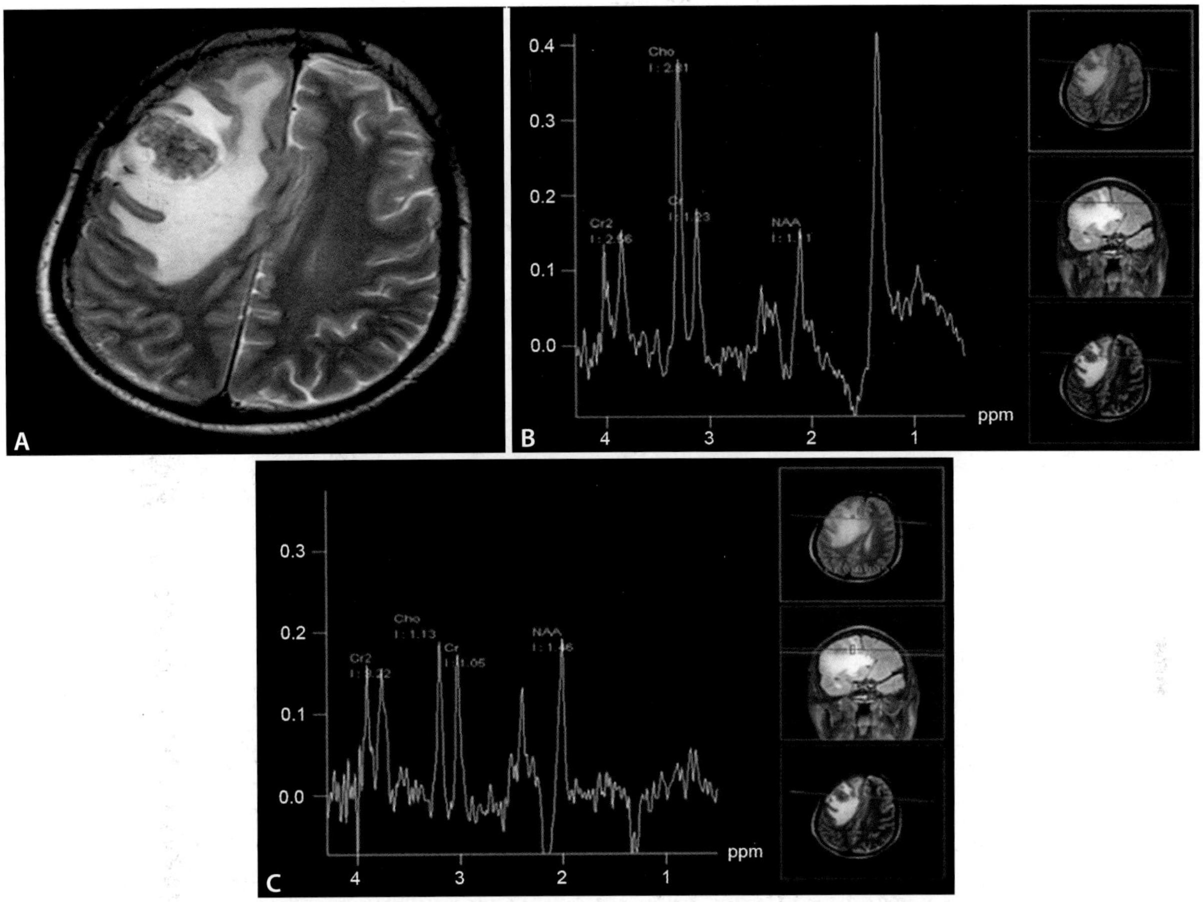

Figs. 8A to C: (A) T2W MR image showing heterogeneous lesion with intense perilesional edema in right frontal location; (B) CSI ^{1}H-MRS of the lesion shows marked increase in the Choline/NAA ratios with significant lipid lactate peaks suggestive of metastasis; (C) Voxel placed in perilesional edema shows no Cho/NAA ratio reversal.

Table 6: Metabolite patterns in brain tumors

	Major metabolic changes				
Major tumor types	***NAA***	***Cho***	***Cr***	***mI***	***Lip***
Grade II glioma	↓	↑	↓	↑↑/=	-
Grade III glioma	↓↓	↑↑	↓	↑/=	+/-
GBM	↓↓↓	↑↑↑	↓↓	=/↓	++
Lymphoma	↓↓	↑↑↑	↓↓	↓↓	++
Metastasis	↓↓	↑↑	↓↓	↓↓	++
Meningioma	↓↓↓	↑	↓↓	↓↓	+/-

based on the CT and MRI findings and MRS may act as a problem solving tool.[33] Evaluation of inflammatory granulomas with ^{1}H-MRS reveals very low level of normal metabolites in NCC with succinate peak **(Figs. 16A and B)** whereas tuberculomas are characterized by prominent lipid resonances due to large lipid fraction present in tubercular bacilli. Lipids are seen in more than 80% of tuberculomas while other nonspecific granulomas and NCC showed lipid in 20% of cases.[33,34] Studies have shown that tuberculomas had prominent lipids, higher choline and reduced NAA and Cr with a Cho/Cr ratio greater than 1 in all tuberculomas as compared to NCC.[35]

MRS IN PEDIATRICS

The metabolic spectra in developing brain are different from those of adult brain, a fact that is important to know before describing the pathological changes in the children.

Low NAA is seen at birth and shows rapid increase during first year with attainment of final values at the age of 3–5 years which is correlated with the ongoing neuronal maturation. Choline compounds show a high peak in neonatal age with decrease as cerebral maturation progresses. Myoinositol is the highest peak at 3.5 ppm on spectroscopy of newborn and it rapidly decreases with age.[36]

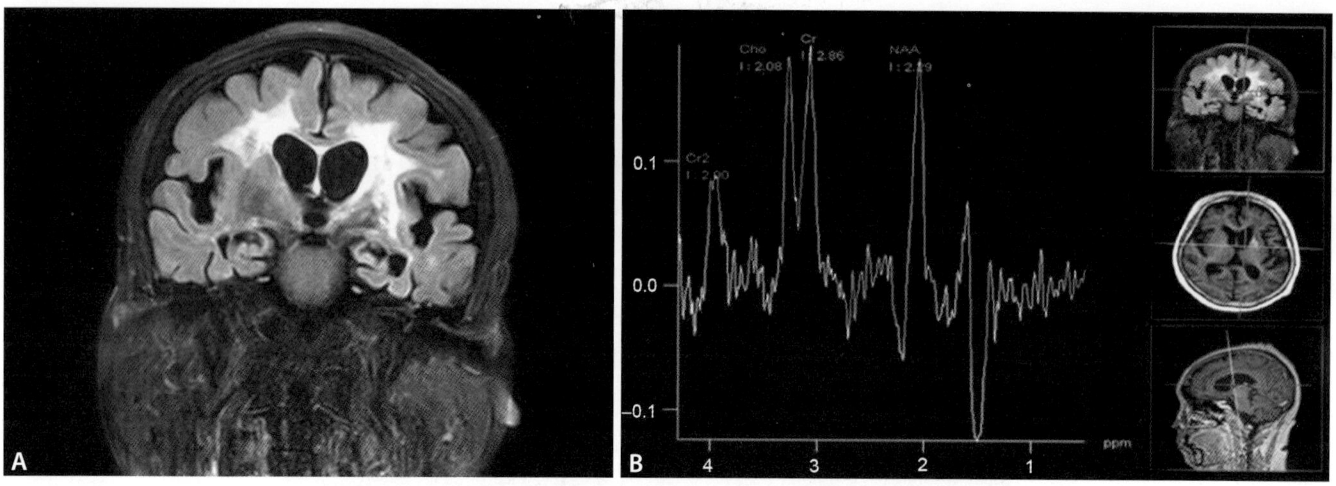

Figs. 9A and B: (A) Postcontrast T1W MR image of a postoperative and postradiotherapy of infiltrating astrocytoma showing irregular ring enhancing lesion in the postoperative location; (B) CSI ^{1}H-MRS TE = 135 ms) of the lesion shows marked increase in the Choline/NAA ratios with no significant lactate peaks suggestive of recurrent tumor.

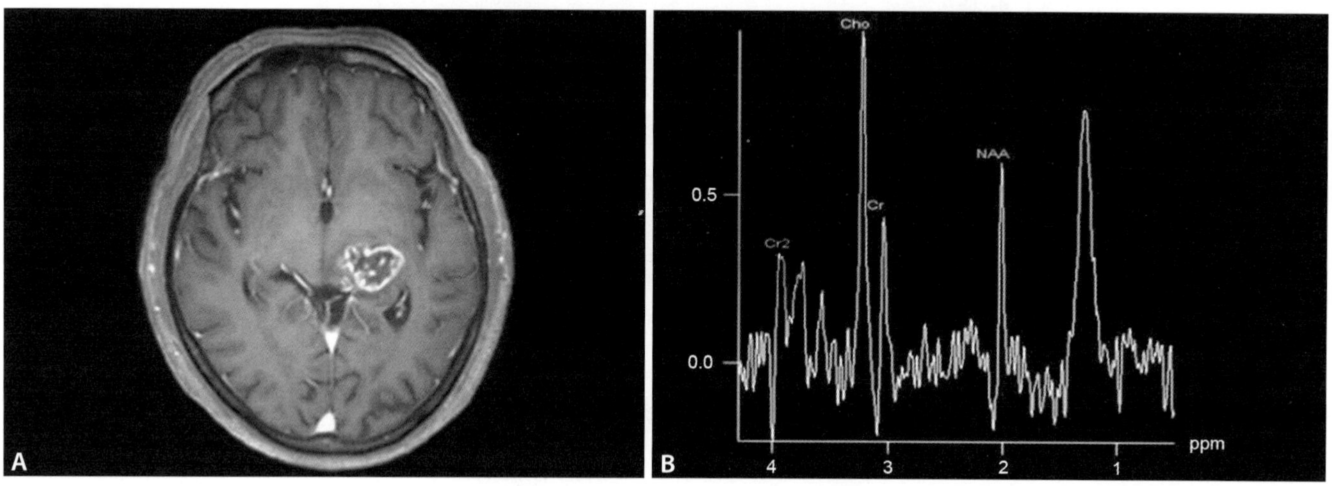

Figs. 10A and B: (A) FLAIR image of postradiotherapy of lymphoma showing hyperintense lesions in bilateral periventricular locations; (B) CSI ^{1}H-MRS of the periventricular lesion shows no significant increase in the Choline/NAA ratios with presence of inverted lactate peak.

Prematurity and Birth Asphyxia

In birth asphyxia, there is decrease in PCr/Pi ratio compared to control subjects.[37] Ratio of PCr/Pi below 0.8 is associated with poor prognosis.[38] There is also decrease in Pi/ATP ratio. Increase in lactate/NAA ratio and decrease in NAA level may convey poor prognosis.

Metabolic Disorders and Leukodystrophies

Hepatic encephalopathy is one acquired metabolic disorder that is currently diagnostic with ^{1}H-MRS. In this condition, ^{1}H-MRS shows an elevation of glutamine levels and a reduction in choline and myoinositol levels **(Figs. 17A and B)**.

Currently, the MR spectroscopy is not very sensitive *in vivo* to measure the specific metabolite or other markers e.g enzymes, proteins responsible for specific metabolic disorder. However, it can detect the secondary changes that results from these disorder and can help in diagnosis **(Table 8)**.

Examples of such situations include:

- Prominent NAA in Canavan's disease **(Figs. 18A and B)**
- Lactate peak in mitochondrial disorders[12]

Patients with PKAN (pantothenate kinase associated neurodegeneration) show spectral broadening due to magnetic inhomogeneity caused by iron deposition in the globus pallidus. Rare metabolic disorders like defective NAA synthesis due to N-acetylaspertase deficiency and

Table 7: MRS findings in various ring enhancing lesions.

Primary neoplasm/ glioma	Decreased NAA Raised choline Lactate peak 2 hydroxyglutarate at 2.25 ppm in mutant type astrocytoma
Metastasis	Decreased NAA Raised choline Lactate peak Normal spectra in edema
Pyogenic abscess	Lactate lipid peak Amino acid peak Acetate and succinate peak
Tubercular abscess	Prominent lipid peak Lactate peak
Fungal abscess	Variable NAA and choline Lipid lactate peak Amino acids Trehalose peak
Demyelination	Variable findings Increased choline NAA/cr higher than tumors Lactate Glutamate peak
Lymphoma	Raised choline Mild increase lipid/lactate Variably decreased NAA/Cr
Toxoplasma	Lipid lactate peak Suppressed normal metabolites

defective creatinine synthesis due to arginine: glycine amidinotransferase (AGAT) and guanidino acetate methyl transferase (GAMT) deficiency may not show any signal changes on conventional MR imaging. The spectroscopy in these disorders shows absence of NAA and creatine peaks respectively.[36]

MAGNETIC RESONANCE SPECTROSCOPY IN EPILEPSY

Lateralization in Temporal Lobe Epilepsy

Magnetic resonance spectroscopy can depict the metabolic changes that may precede any definitive imaging changes in the hippocampus in mesial temporal lobe epilepsy which can be seen as normal findings on conventional MRI.[37-40] Such findings are typical for bitemporal lesions or for extratemporal epilepsies. It is also very helpful for lateralization of epileptic focus.[41] There is reduction of NAA and NAA/(Cr + Cho) ratio in the ipsilateral hippocampus. NAA/Cr is also reduced in the ipsilateral frontal lobe in patients with frontal lobe epilepsy. Similarly, ^{31}P MRS shows increase in pH and decrease in Pi in the involved hippocampus or frontal lobe.[22] Alterations of metabolic activity and neuronal integrity persist inter-ictally and make it possible to lateralize the epileptic focus. Therefore, MRSI provides useful information in preoperative planning of epilepsy surgery.[42]

MRS in Neurodegenerative Diseases

Alzheimer's Disease

Alzheimer's disease (AD) is slowly progressive disease with loss of cognitive function and is one of the most common causes of dementia. The diagnosis is usually achieved in autopsy. There is decreased NAA and NAA/Cr in frontoparietal, temporal lobes and hippocampus. Myoinositol is found to be increased in AD but this is nonspecific. The ratio of NAA/Cr is not changed in NPH and therefore can be differentiate from AD. ^{31}P-MRS shows increased PME and decreased PCr in the initial stages of AD. As dementia worsens, the level of PME decreases and the level of PCr increases. ^{31}P-MRS can also distinguish AD from multiinfarct dementia (MID).[43] In MID, there is elevation of P Cr/Pi ratio in both the temporoparietal and frontal regions. Whereas PME and the ratio of PME/PDE are elevated in AD in the temporoparietal lobe. Pi is also elevated in the frontal and temporoparietal regions of AD. These spectral profiles are accurate in distinguish MID from AD in more than 100% cases.

Amyotrophic Lateral Sclerosis (ALS)

^{1}H-MRS in ALS has demonstrated decreased cortical NAA which was maximal in the motor cortex. The level of NAA has been found to decrease overtime as the disease progresses. Glutamate excitotoxicity has been proposed to be cause of neuronal loss in ALS. ^{1}H-MRS has shown increased signals from glutamate and glutamine in these patients. ^{1}H-MRS findings in patients after treatment with Riluzole (a drug that inhibits glutamate release from presynaptic terminals), the level of NAA increases in these patients which may reflect the reversal of injury.

Idiopathic Parkinson's Disease (IPD) versus Other Parkinsonian Syndromes

In IPD, the primary pathology is thought to be in the substantia nigra and the volume of nigral axonal terminals lost in the basal ganglia are too small to be measured by current MRS techniques and so in IPD, the metabolic resonances do not appear to be changed in the basal ganglia or in the cortex. In contrast, various other parkinsonian syndromes such as progressive supranuclear palsy and multisystem atrophy (MSA) demonstrate significant decreases of NAA/Cho and NAA/Cr in the lentiform nucleus and striatum.

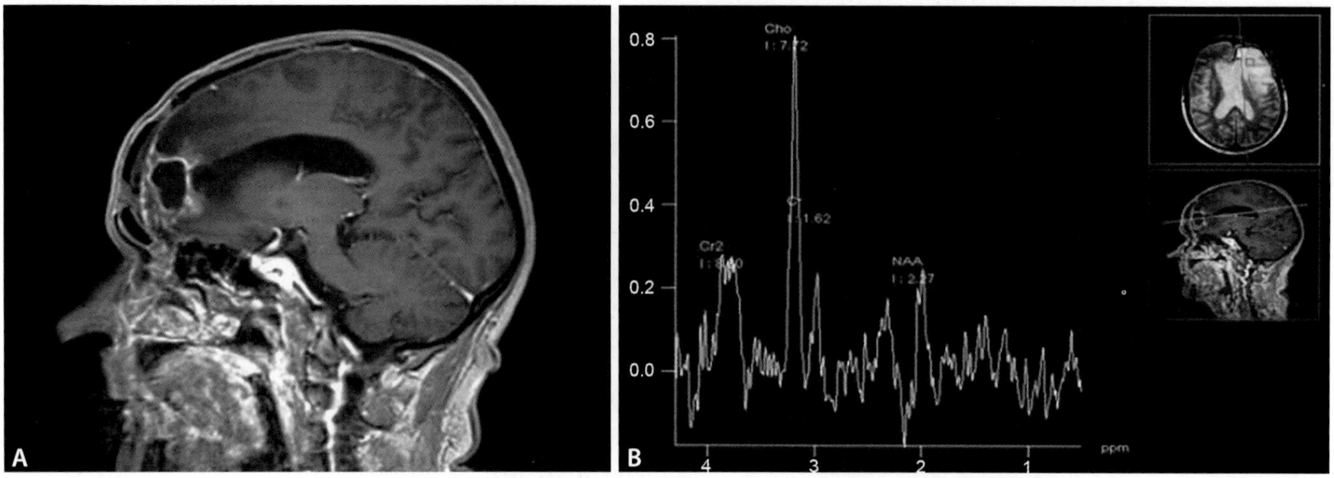

Figs. 11A and B: (A) Postcontrast MR image shows ring enhancing lesion in left thalamic location with mass effect—biopsy proven glioma WHO- grade IV; (B) CSI ^{1}H-MRS from the lesion at TE 135 ms shows Cho/NAA. Note the prominent lipid peak that may also be seen in gliomas.

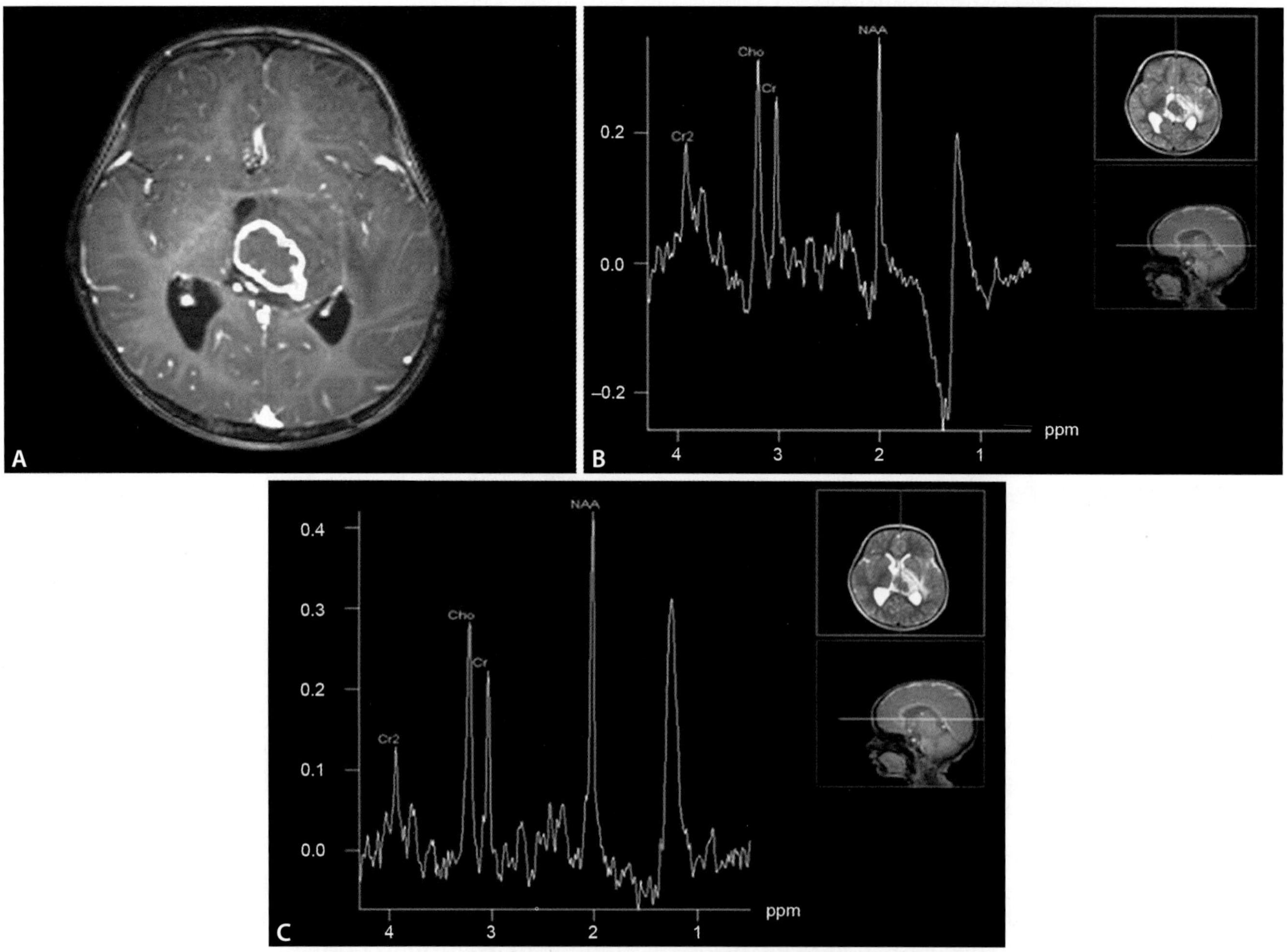

Figs. 12A to C: (A) Postcontrast MR image shows ring enhancing lesion in left thalamic location with mass effect; (B and C) CSI ^{1}H-MRS from the lesion at TE 135 ms and 30 ms shows lipid peak that is more prominent at low TE and the lactate doublet.

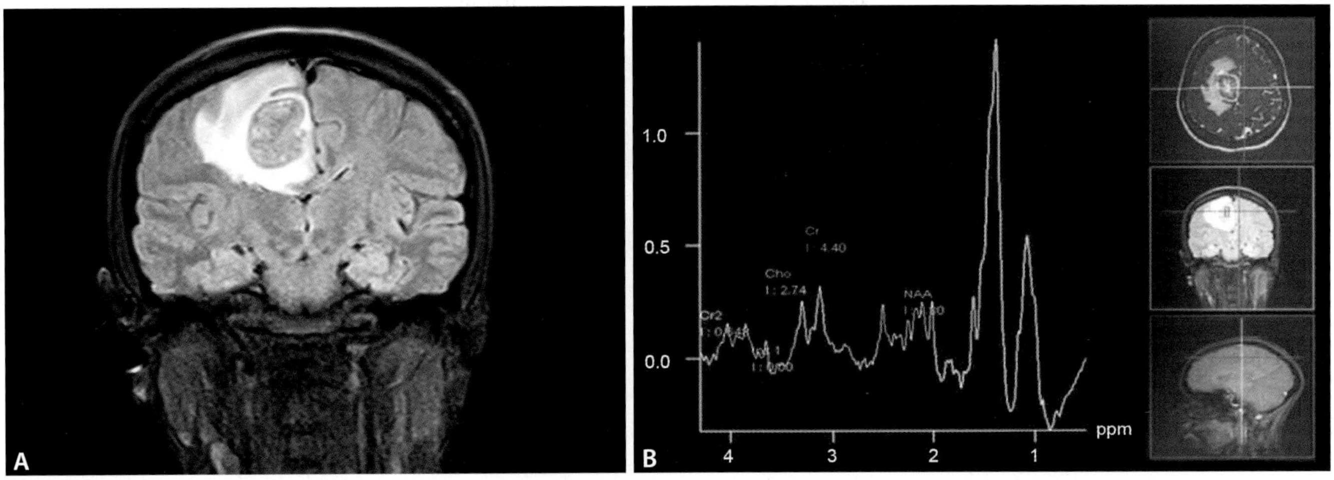

Figs. 13A and B: (A) FLAIR image shows heterogeneous ring lesion (pyogenic abscess); (B) CSI ^{1}H-MRS (TE = 30) shows decreased normal metabolites (NAA, Choline, Creatine) and increased amino acids (0.9 ppm), succinate (2.4 ppm) and lipid lactate peaks.

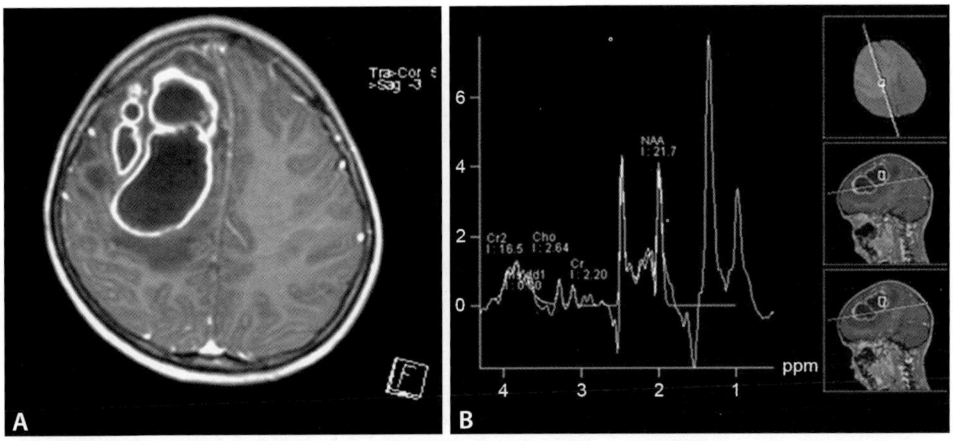

Figs. 14A and B: (A) Postcontrast axial images in a 10-year-old male patient show multiple ring enhancing lesions in right frontal lobe; (B) CSI ^{1}H-MRS (TE = 30) shows presence of increased amino acids (0.9 ppm), succinate (2.4 ppm) and lipid lactate peaks (1.3 ppm) s/o pyogenic abscess.

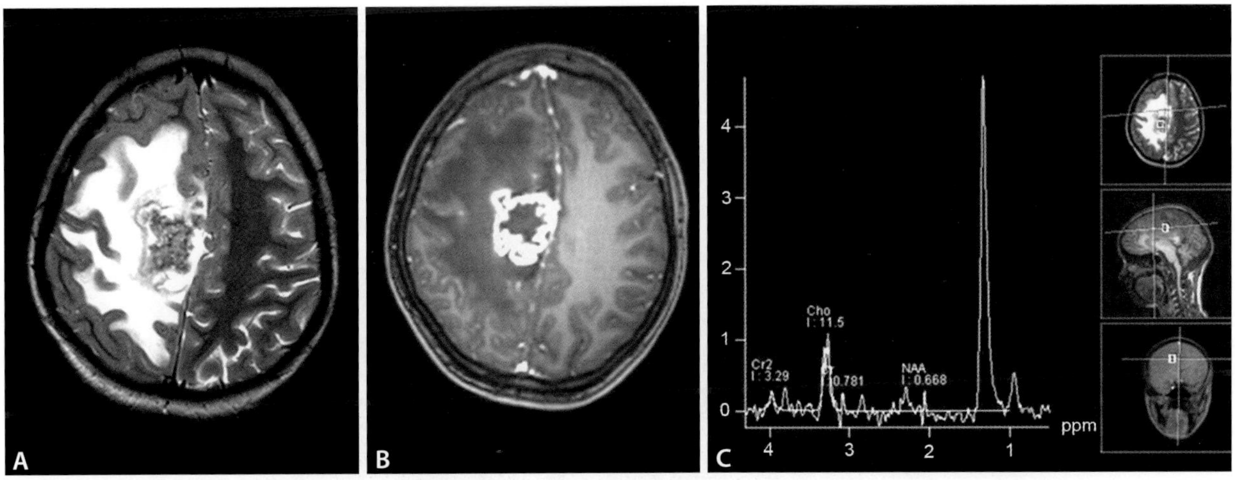

Figs. 15A to C: (A) Axial T2w images show heterogeneous hypointense lesion in right frontal lobe with surrounding marked edema. (B) Postcontrast MR image shows ring enhancement; (B and C) CSI ^{1}H-MRS from the lesion at TE 30 ms shows prominent lipid peak. Biopsy came out tuberculosis.

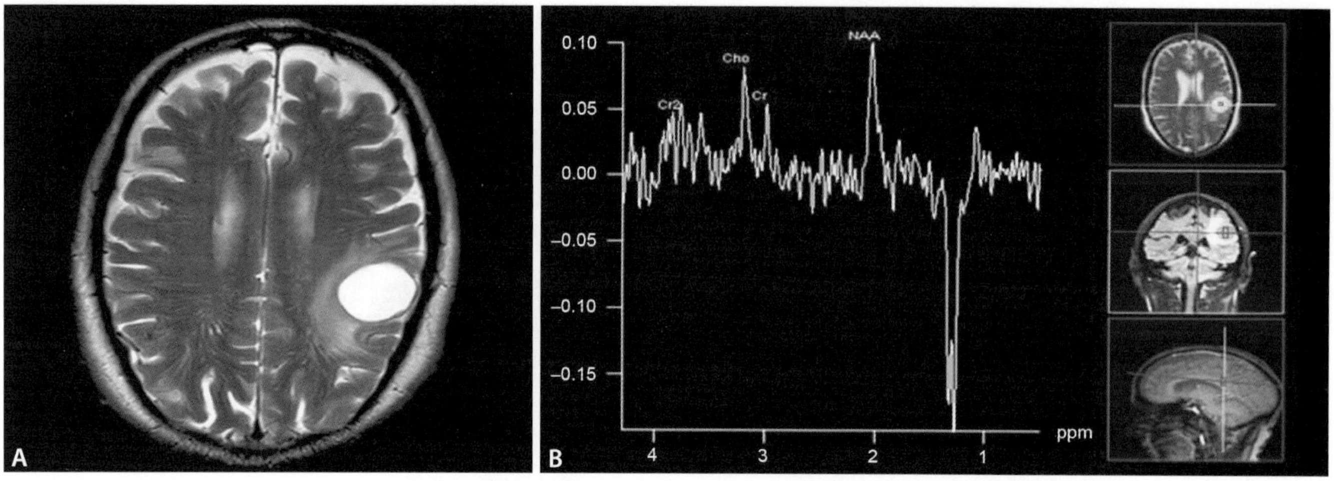

Figs. 16A and B: (A) 55-year-old patient with neurocysticercosis. (A) T2 axial MR image shows cystic lesion in left parietal cortex; (B) CSI ^{1}H-MRS (TE = 135 ms) shows lactate peak at 1.3 ppm with decreased normal metabolites.

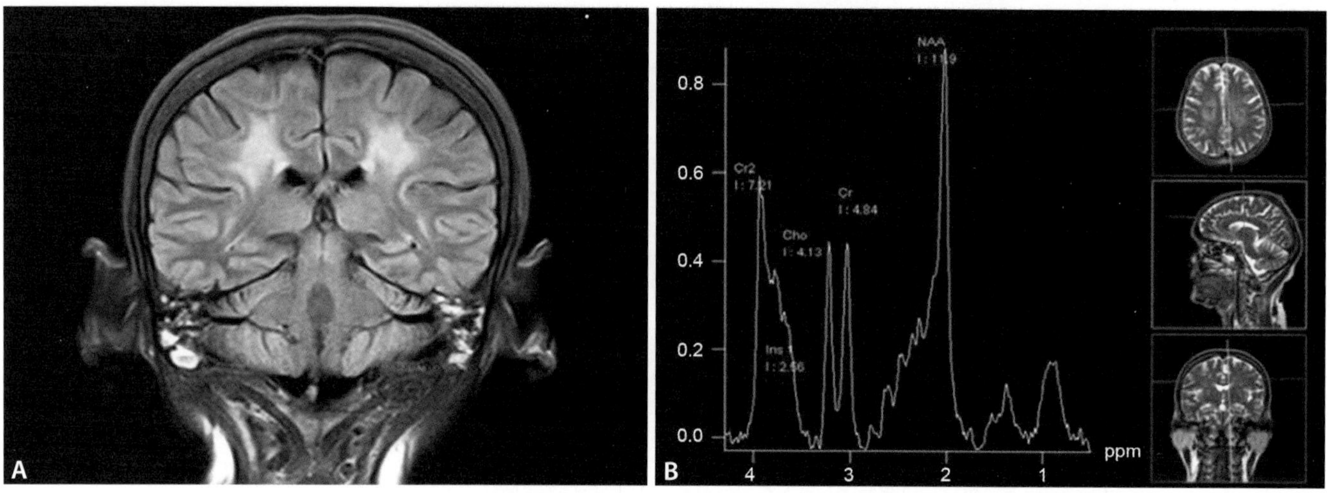

Figs. 17A and B: (A) 45-year-old patient with cirrhosis and encephalopathy. (A) FLAIR MR image shows hyperintensities in bilateral centrum semiovale; (B) CSI ^{1}H-MRS (TE = 30 ms) shows glutamate and glutamine peak at 2.5 ppm.

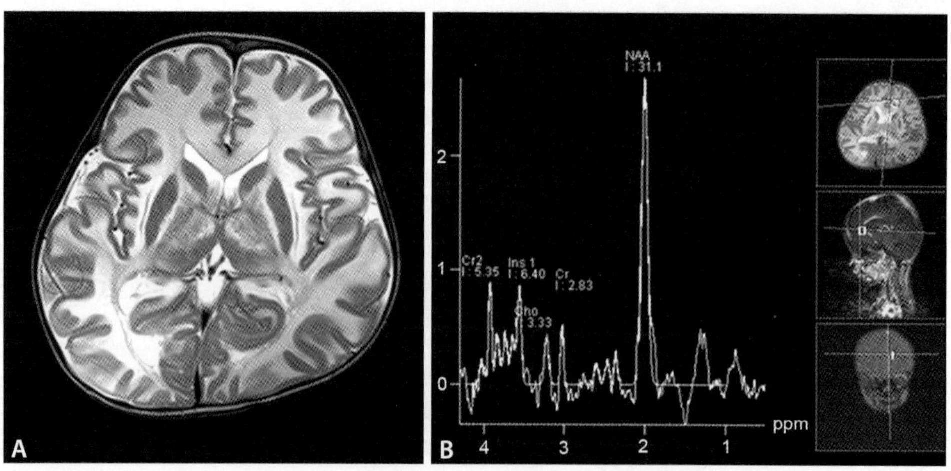

Figs. 18A and B: A 2-year-old child with developmental delay. (A) Axial T2-W MR images show extensive high-signal intensity areas throughout the white matter reaching up to the subcortical region, internal and external capsules, and corpus callosum; (B) MR spectroscopy shows raised NAA peak (arrow).

Table 8: Spectroscopic findings in hereditary metabolic disorders.

	Cho	*Cr*	*NAA*	*Lac*	*Others*
(A) Mitochondrial encephalomyopathies					
MELAS	↓	↓	↓	↑↑	
Leigh syndrome	↓	↓	↓	↑↑	
Menkes disease	n	↓	↓↓	↑↑	
SDH complex deficiency	↓	↓↓	↓↓↓	↑↑	suc
(B) Amino acid and organic acidurias					
Phenylketonuria	n	n	n		phe
Nonketotic hyperglycinemia	n	n	n		glycine
Maple syrup urine disease	n	n	↓↓	↑	BCA
Canavan disease	↓	↑	↑↑↑		
Glutaric aciduria type I	n	n	↓↓	↑	
Propionic academia	n	n	↓↓	↑	Glx
Urea cycle defects	↓	↓	↓	↑	Gln
(C) Lysosomal storage disease					
Metachromatic leukodystrophy	↑↑	↓	↓↓↓	↑	
Fucosidosis	n	n	↓	↑	
(D) Peroxisomal disorders					
X-linked adrenoleukodystrophy	↑↑↑	↓↓	↓↓↓	↑	
Adrenomyeloneuropathy	n	n	n		
(E) Leukoencephalopathies					
Alexander disease	↑↑↑	↓↓	↓↓↓	↑↑	
Megalencephalic leukoencephalopathy with subcortical cysts	↓↓	↓↓	↓↓	↑	
Leukoencephalopathy with vanishing white matter	↓↓	↓↓	↓↓	↑	
Leukoencephalopathy with involvement of brain stem and spinal cord and elevated white matter lactate	↑	n	↓↓	↑↑	
Cerebral autosomal dominant arteriopathy with subcortical infarcts and leukoencephalopathy (CADASIL)	n	n	↓↓	↑	
(F) Miscellaneous					
Creatine deficiency	n	↓↓↓	n		
Pelizaeus–Merzbacher disease	n	n/↑	n		

Huntington's Disease (HD)

This condition may affect neurons throughout the brain, but targets initially the cells in the basal ganglia. Studies have shown that in humans NAA/Cho is reduced both in the basal ganglia as well as in the cortex in patients with symptomatic HD. Although not always found, increase of LA have been observed in the occipital lobes, basal ganglia and frontal lobes of HD patients.

MAGNETIC RESONANCE SPECTROSCOPY IN DEMYELINATING DISEASES

Multiple Sclerosis

^{1}H-MRS shows normal spectrum in hyperacute plaques of MS. In demyelinating plaques, there is elevation of Cho/Cr ratio **(Figs. 19 and 20)**. In subacute to chronic plaques, there is decreased NAA/Cr ratio.[44] Acute active MS plaques (that enhances following Gd DTPA) often show increased lactate, mobile lipids and so called 'marker peaks' in the 2.1–2.6 ppm in region and this help in the differentiation from chronic (irreversible) MS plaques.[45] However, a MRS study in children with acute MS, did not show elevated lipid or lactate level. Inositol which is a marker for astrocyte becomes increased in chronic lesions.[46]

Normal appearing white matter (NAWM) in MS: The NAA/Cr ratio in normal appearing white matter drops one month after the occurrence of an acute lesion in areas distinct from the lesion, it is normalized after 6 months, and drops again, when relapses occur. It correlates well with total lesion load and disability.[47,48] Therefore, NAA

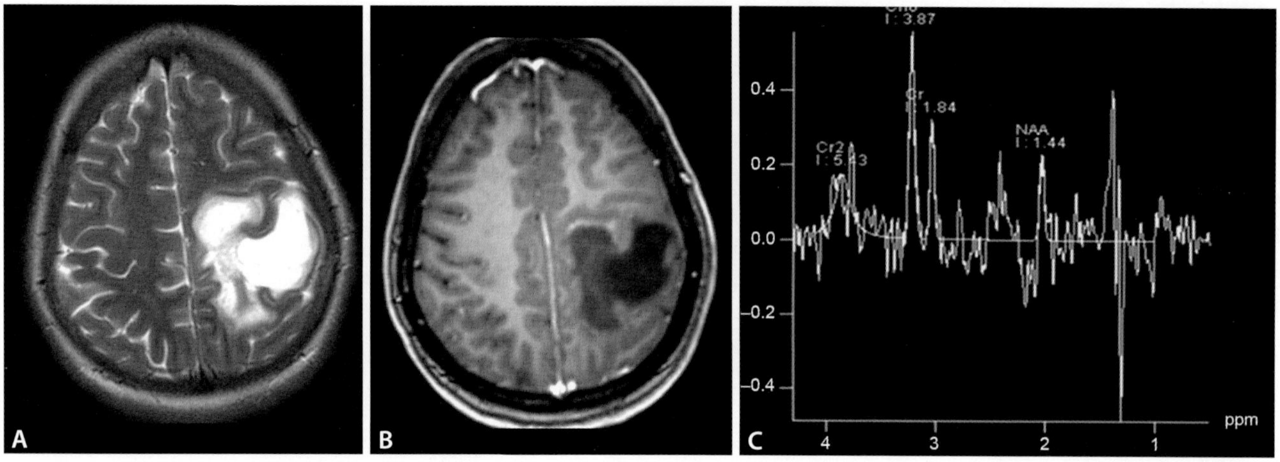

Figs. 19A to C: A 35-year-old patient with biopsy proven tumefactive demyelination. (A) T2W MR image shows a large hyperintense areas involving left frontal lobe; (B) T1 postcontrast image—lesion shows peripheral incomplete ring type enhancement; (C) CSI ^{1}H-MRS (TE = 135 ms) from the lesion shows increased choline, decreased NAA, lipid/ lactate peaks at 1.3 ppm and glutamate/glutamine peak at 2.4 ppm.

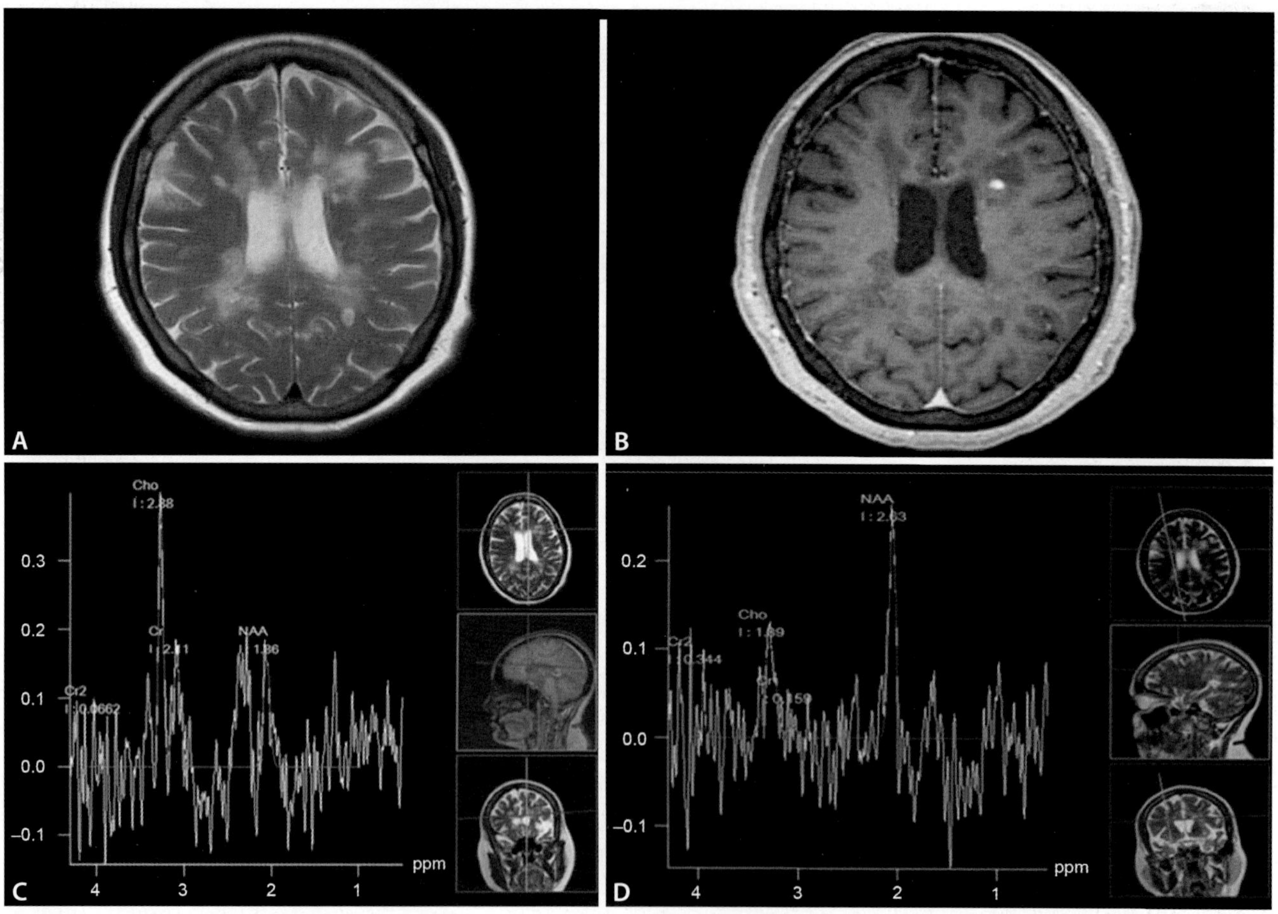

Figs. 20A to D: (A) A 30-year-old patient with primary progressive multiple sclerosis. (A) T2W MR image shows multiple hyperintense areas in periventricular location; (B) T1 postcontrast image—lesion in left periventricular location shows enhancement suggestive of acute lesion; (C) CSI ^{1}H-MRS (TE = 135 ms) from the left periventricular lesion shows increased choline and decreased NAA suggestive of acute lesion; (D) CSI ^{1}H-MRS (TE = 135 ms) from the lesion in right periventricular location shows normalized choline and NAA levels suggestive of chronic lesion.

or the NAA/Cr ratio is a good surrogate marker for the monitoring of neuroprotection in preclinical therapeutic studies.[49]

Tumefactive demyelination: MRS findings are characterized by reduced NAA, raised choline, lipid/lactate peaks and glutamate/glutamine peaks.

MAGNETIC RESONANCE SPECTROSCOPY IN HEAD TRAUMA

MRS provides a way to evaluate tissue viability following trauma and the results of MRS may provide insight as to how patients should be treated and whether treatment is effective, thus helping neurosurgeons make clinical decision. Studies have shown that the injured region had highly increased lactate signal and decreased NAA, Cr and Cho. Increase in lactate is related to ischemia after trauma and decrease of NAA, Cr and Cho is related to edema, which has a dilution effect.[7] A study conducted in the institute to evaluate the role of MR spectroscopy in diffuse axonal injury in patients with head injury who had a grossly normal CT by comparing the metabolic ratios in different regions of the brain in these patients with a control group. The author found that there was a highly significant decrease in both the NAA/Cr and NAA/Cho ratios in the splenium in patients with head injury as compared to the control group **(Figs. 21A to D)**. When the study group was further subdivided according to severity of head injury, there was a highly significant decrease in both the NAA/Cr and NAA/Cho ratios in the splenium in the severely injured groups to whereas the decrease in the metabolite ratios was not significant in the mild on moderately head injured group.

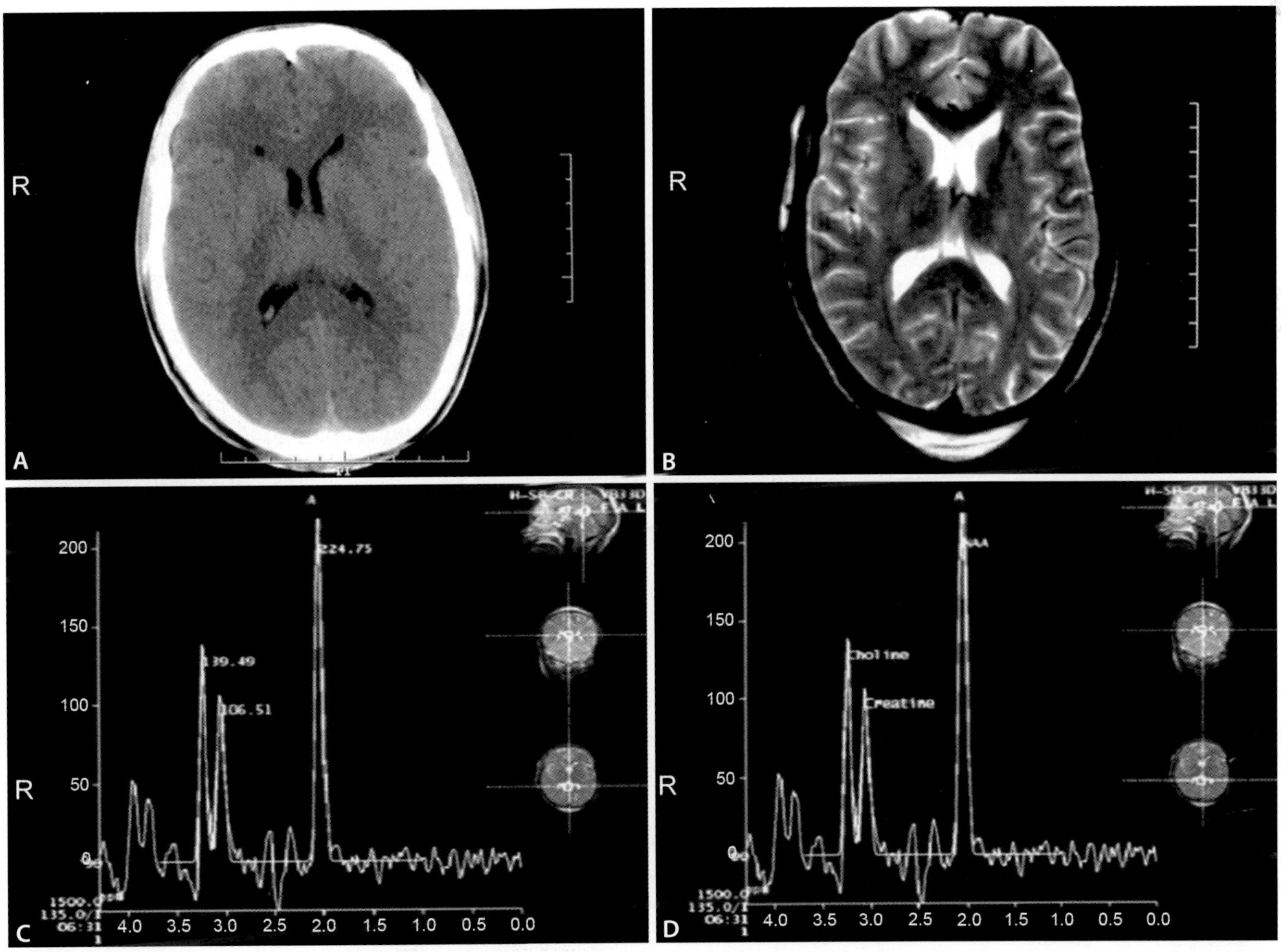

Figs. 21A to D: 23-year-old male patient with head injury with (A) Normal NCCT head; (B) Normal MR scan and (C and D) MRS shows decrease in NAA/Cho and NAA/Cr ratios in the splenium.

MAGNETIC RESONANCE SPECTROSCOPY IN STROKE

There is loss of NAA and increase in lactate level in the area of infarction and these finding correlate clinically with functional outcome and disability. In ischemic penumbra, there is increase in the lactate level without decrease in NAA. Chronic infarcts often show increased lactate.[50-52]

MAGNETIC RESONANCE SPECTROSCOPY IN PSYCHIATRIC DISEASES

In schizophrenia, there is increase in PCr/ATP and PCr/Pi ratios in the right temporal lobe with decrease in PME in left frontal lobe and elevated PDE and low PCr in both frontal lobes. MRS can also assess lithium levels during treatment. ^{1}H-MRS findings in schizophrenia have been inconsistent with some studies finding reduced NAA in various regions of the brain including frontal cortex, dorsolateral prefrontal cortex and temporal cortex. However, low NAA levels in the hippocampus is a more consistent finding.

MAGNETIC RESONANCE SPECTROSCOPY IN HIV/AIDS

It is generally agreed that conventional MRI is not sensitive to the detection of early stages of HIV infection of brain. Neurological disease is found in 30–40% of all AIDS patients and this frequency is increasing as treatment for other complications such as *Pneumocystis carinii* pneumonia have improved.

There is marked reduction of NAA/Cho and NAA/Cr ratios in the regions that appear normal on MRI study in HIV encephalopathy (direct HIV infection). Similar, findings may be seen with gross atrophy of brain in late stage of the disease.

It is observed that Cr resonance is stable overtime on an absolute scale. MRS can also help in the monitoring of drugs that helps in the management of AIDS patients. An important clinical problem in the AIDS patients is differentiating toxoplasmosis from lymphoma. In toxoplasmosis there is a large lipid peak whereas in lymphoma there is increase in Cho/Cr ratio. However, these results are not consistent and atypical spectra are observed in many cases. In PML, there is increase in lactate level. MRS, therefore, provides insights in the neurological problems in AIDS and can help in monitoring the new neuroprotective agents.[53]

CLINICAL SUCCESS

The initial widespread enthusiasm on MRS and MRSI as research methodology useful for clinical applications waned subsequently with many workers terming it as a largely an investigational tool.[1] But MRS does have particular clinical value for the lateralization of seizure focus in temporal lobe epilepsy for preoperative planning.[23] MRS can differentiate radiation necrosis from tumor recurrence, infarct from tumor, lymphoma from PML in HIV patient, monitor treatment response, etc.[20]

Artefacts in MR Spectroscopy

As with other MR sequences, MRS is a very sensitive technique and it is commonly affected by artifacts thereby reducing its diagnostic utility.

Field Inhomogeneity

Field inhomogeneity results in overlapping resonances, reduces the SNR and can result in inadequate water suppression. Broad line widths can result in serious degradation of the quality and interpretation of spectral data. These can result from variety of causes such as improper shimming and the presence of paramagnetic materials (e.g. metallic devices, hemorrhage, or calcifications) and air-tissue interfaces such as mesial anterior temporal and inferior frontal lobes. Iron containing structures such as striatum and substantia nigra also show broader line width.[53, 54]

Remedy: Reshimming or use of high-order shims with repetition of the procedure, or by slightly changing the region of interest slightly may overcome these artefacts.

Inadequate Water and Lipid Suppression

These may occur due to field inhomogeneity or the result of a failed optimization of water suppression pulse flip angles. Spurious water signals can come from outside the voxel in areas of poor field homogeneity degrading the MR spectra. Lipid signals in the scalp are of greater magnitude than metabolites and inadequate suppression can lead to inability to detect lactate and may interfere with NAA signal. Various lipid suppression methods have been described in literature. Adequately placed outer-volume suppression saturation bands may overcome this problem.

Remedy: Repeating the calibration or slightly altering the voxel position can overcome this problem. Spurious water signals can be suppressed using outer-volume suppression saturation bands .[54,55]

Head motion: Head motion may have a disastrous effect on MRS, with loss of resolution and SNR, lipid and water suppression problems, and erroneous voxel location.

Incorrect Voxel Placement

It is of paramount importance to correctly place the voxel at the region of interest for optimum results. Particularly in follow-up studies it is important that the sectra are recorded from the same location utilizing same technical parameters.

Remedy: Careful radiologist/technician supervision and use of institutional standardized MRS protocols can overcome this problem. Use of automated voxel placement and real time registration of localizer images to standard anatomical templates) may become increasingly used for such studies in future.

Incorrect Protocol

Adequate training and expertise of radiologists/technologists in using a particular choice of protocol for a particular study (e.g. short or long echo time, single- or multi-voxel) has to be encouraged. In general short echo time spectra should be used when compounds such as mI or Glx are required, while multivoxel methods are important for pathologies such as brain tumors. Very small lesions less than 1.0–1.5 cm in diameter may not be evaluated by MRS. Similarly lesions near areas of marked susceptibility may also result in poor spectra.

Out-of-voxel Magnetization

Slice profiles are not usually perfect and there will always be a small amount of residual magnetization originating from outside the voxel particularly from unsuppressed water or lipid signals.

Remedy: These can be minimized by using outer-volume suppression saturation bands and when proper crushing is used in conjunction with an optimum ordering of slice select gradients.[54, 55]

Chemical Shift Displacement Effects

When a slice-selective pulse is applied, the position of the slice depends on the frequency offset and the gradient strength. The voxel position of each metabolite will be slightly different, depending on the chemical shift and the strength of the gradient used. This is more of a problem at higher fields than lower.

Remedy: Use of the highest possible bandwidth RF pulses and high bandwidth saturation pulses to sharpen the edges of the excitation box.[55]

Fast MR Spectroscopy Techniques including Whole Brain MR Spectroscopy

A major limitation of standard MR spectroscopy techniques is long acquisition times, especially with 3D data acquisition. Fast CSI techniques have been shown to significantly reduce data acquisition times. These fast techniques were introduced to reduce the limitations associated with conventional spectroscopy techniques.

Parallel imaging: These include sensitivity encoding (SENSE), simultaneous acquisition of spatial harmonics (SMASH) and generalized autocalibrating partial parallel acquisition (GRAPPA). In these techniques, multiple receiver coils are used which increases signal sensitivity and spatial encoding by reducing the number of k-space lines and hence accelerating the image acquisition. These can have low SNR for which number of coil elements can be increased. [56-58]

Fast multivoxel techniques: A whole brain MRSI can be done by reducing the scanning time and motion sensitivity. Using the time-varying gradients during the readout MRSI can be accelerated. K-space trajectories mostly used in spectroscopic imaging are echo-planar and spiral trajectories reducing the acquisition time.[59]

Spiral MRSI: It is a fast spectroscopic imaging technique that traverses k-space by using spiral trajectories. Oscillating readout gradients are applied in a spectroscopic imaging sequence in two spatial dimensions during the data acquisition resulting in marked reduction in acquisition times. Data is then reconstructed onto a Cartesian k-space and Fourier transformation is applied Spiral MRSI thus leads to shorter imaging time, higher spatial resolution and increased SNR.[60]

Turbo spectroscopic imaging (turbo-MRSI): Acceleration of acquisition can be done by use of multiple-echo refocusing. It can be combined with parallel imaging techniques such as SENSE to improve SNR these can help in reduction of acquisition times by about eight folds compared to conventional MRSI techniques. Major drawbacks include reduced spectral resolution and SNR.[61, 62]

Echo-planar spectroscopic imaging (EPSI): These techniques have shown improved spatial and temporal resolution compared to typical conventional MRSI. These are particularly useful in whole brain MRSI as these can provide improved spatial and spectral encoding. Modification have been proposed to enhance the acceleration of data collection with use of SENSE-EPSI. These techniques have limitation in the form of contraction of spectral bandwidth and reduced SNR.

Whole Brain MRSI

The whole brain MRSI requires a volumetric echo planar spectroscopy imaging and lipid nulling through an inversion recovery preparation that enables acquisition of spectra from cortical surface and high-speed spectroscopy methods with reduced k-space acquisition and parallel techniques. Major applications have come up in neurodegenerative and psychiatric diseases. It can demonstrate metabolic changes in a larger brain area simultaneously in patients suffering from diseases causing diffuse metabolic changes.[63,64]

FUTURE DEVELOPMENTS

There is tremendous need to improve ease-in-operation, reliability, reproducibility and sensitivity of MRS. MR signals are week and SNR of spectra acquired at 1.5–2.0 T is barely adequate.

One touch MRS protocols where one can choose the position of voxel from the locator images and the system automatically performs all operation including data analysis and baseline correction will be the ideal goal. The plethora of localization technique causes more confusion. There is a need to standardize MRS protocol so as to have a uniform database and reproducibility. Improved instrumentation (3.0T or more) with autoshimming, reduced eddy currents, high SNR may further develop with increase in the use of phased array coils. Further improvements and developments will take place in absolute quantification of metabolites and to produce metabolic images from CSI data. Development of spectroscopic intracellular contrast agents and targeted labels may further improve clinical utility of MRS.

Despite its problems, MRS has a unique ability to noninvasively measure various metabolites in human body. It is a useful addition in basic biochemical research and clinical investigations.[8]

REFERENCES

1. Cousins JP. Clinical MR spectroscopy fundamentals, current applications and future potential. AJR. 1995;164:1337-47.
2. Bolinger L, Insko EK. Spectroscopy: Basic principles and techniques. In: Edelman RR, Hesselink JR, Zlatkin MB. (Eds): Body MRI. Philadelphia: WB Saunders. 1996.pp. 353-79.
3. Matson GB, Weiner MW. Spectroscopy in Magnetic Resonance Imaging. In: Stark DD, Bradley WG (Ed). St Louis: Mosby. 1999;181-211.
4. Skoch A, Jiru F, Bunke J. Spectroscopic imaging: basic principles. Eur J Radio. 2008;67:230-39.
5. Soares DP, Law M. Magnetic resonance spectroscopy of the brain: review of metabolites and clinical applications. Clin Radiol. 2009;64:12-21.
6. McLean MA, Cross JJ. Magnetic resonance spectroscopy: principles and applications in neurosurgery. Br J Neurosurg. 2009;23:5-13.
7. Callot V, Galanaud D, Le Fur Y, Confort-Gouny S, Ranjeva JP, Cozzone PJ. (1)H MR spectroscopy of human brain tumours: a practical approach. Eur J Radiol. 2008;67:268-74.
8. Hajek M, Dezortova M. Introduction to clinical in vivo MR spectroscopy. Eur J Radial. 2008;67:185-93.
9. Birken DL, Oldendorf WH. NAA: A literature review of compound prominent of proton spectroscopy of brain. Neurosci Biobehv Rev. 1989;13:23-31.
10. Rothman DL, Arias MF, Shulman GI. A pulse sequence for simplifying hydrogen NMR spectra of biological tissues. J Magn Reson. 1984;60:430-4.
11. Behar KL, Rothman DL, Spencer DD. Analysis of macromolecule resonances in 1H-MRS spectra of human brain. Mag Reson Med. 1994;32:294-8.
12. Gulati S, Shah T, Menon S, et al. Magnetic resonance spectroscopy in pediatric neurology. Ind J Paediatr. 2003;70:317.
13. Trabesinger AH, Meier D, Boesiger P. In vivo H NMR spectroscopy of individual human brain metabolites at moderate field strengths. J Magn Reson Imag. 2003;21:1295.
14. Chen W, Ackerman JJH. Surface coil spin echo localization in vivo via in homogenous surface spoiling magnetic gradient. J Magn Reson. 1989;82:655.
15. Garwood M, Schleich T, Ross BD, et al. A modified rotating frame experiment based on a Fourier series window function: Application to in vivo spatially localized NMR spectroscopy. J Magn Reson. 1985;65:239.
16. Frahm J, Merboldt KD, Hanicke W. Localised proton spectroscopy using stimulated echoes. J Magn Reson. 1987;72:502.
17. Bertoldo D, Watcharakorn A, Castillo M. Brain proton magnetic resonance spectroscopy. Introduction and overview. Neuroimag Clin N Am 2013; 23:359-80.
18. Usenius JP, Kauppinen RA, Vainio PA, et al. Quantitative metabolite patterns of human brain tumors: Detection by1H-NMR spectroscopy in vivo and in vitro. J Comput Assist Tomogr. 1994;18:705.
19. Negendank W. Studies of human tumors by MRS: A review. NMR Biomed. 1992;5:303.
20. Oberhaensli RD, Hilton-Jones D, Bore PJ, et al. Biochemical investigation of human tumors in vivo with phosphorus-31 magnetic resonance spectroscopy. Lancet. 1986;5:8.
21. Fulham MJ, Bizzi A, Dietz MJ, et al. Mapping of brain tumor metabolites with proton MR spectroscopic imaging: Clinical relevance. Radiology. 1992;185:675.
22. Kuesel AC, Sutherland GR, Halliday W, et al. 1H-MRS of high-grade astrocytomas: Mobile lipid accumulation in necrotic tissue. NMR Biomed. 1994;7:149.
23. Smith JK, Castillo M, Kwock L. MR spectroscopy of brain tumors. Magn Reson Imaging Clin N Am. 2003;11:415.
24. Choi C, Raisanen JM, Ganji SK, et al. Prospective longitudinal analysis of 2-hydroxyglutarate magnetic resonance spectroscopy identifies broad clinical utility for the management of patients with IDH-mutant glioma. J Clin Oncol. 2016 20; 34(33):4030-9.
25. Davies NP, Wilson M, Harris LM, Natarajan K, Lateef S, Macpherson L, et al. Identification and characterisation of

childhood cerebellar tumours by in vivo proton MRS. NMR Biomed. 2008;21:908–18.
26. Harting I, Hartmann M, Bonsanto MM, et al. Characterization of necrotic meningioma using diffusion MRI, perfusion MRI and MR spectroscopy: Case report and review of the literature. Neuroradiology.2004.46:189.
27. Garg M, Gupta RK, Husain M, Chawla S, Chawla J, Kumar R, et al. Brain abscess: etiological categorization with in vivo proton MR spectroscopy. Radiology. 2004;230: 519-27.
28. Gupta RK, Vatsal DK, Husain N, Chawla S, Prasad KN, Roy R, et al. Differentiation of tuberculous from pyogenic brain abscesses with in vivo proton MR spectroscopy and magnetization transfer MR imaging. AJNR J. 2001;22: 1503-9.
29. Castillo M, Kwock L, Mukherji S. Clinical applications of MR spectroscopy. AJNR. 1996;17:1-15.
30. Kimura T, Sako K, Gotoh T, Tanaka K, Tanaka T. In vivo single-voxel proton MR spectroscopy with ring like enhancement. NMR Biomed. 2001;14:339-49.
31. Lai PH, Ho JT, Chen WL, Hsu SS, Wang JS, Pan HB, et al. Brain abscess and necrotic brain tumors: discrimination with proton MR spectroscopy and diffusion-weighted imaging. AJNR. 2002;23:1369-77.
32. Jayasunder R, Singh VP, Raghunathan P, et al. Inflammatory granulomas: evaluation with proton MRS. NMR Biomed. 1999;12:139.
33. Cecil KM, Lenkinski RE. Proton MR spectroscopy in inflammatory and infectious brain disorders. Neuroimaging Clinics of North America. 1998;8:863.
34. Pretell EJ, Martinot C, Garcia HH, et al. Differential diagnosis between cerebral tuberculosis and Neurocysticercosis by magnetic resonance spectroscopy. J Comput Assist Tomogr. 2005;29:112.
35. Dezortova M, Hajek M Eur J Radiol. (1)H MR spectroscopy in pediatrics. 2008;67(2):240-921.
36. Cady EB, Costello AM, Dawson MJ, et al. Non-invasive investigation of cerebral metabolism in newborn infants by phosphorus nuclear magnetic resonance spectroscopy. Lancet. 1983;1:1059.
37. Bruhn H, Frahm J, Merboldt KD, et al. Multiple sclerosis in children: Cerebral metabolic alteration monitored by localized proton magnetic resonance spectroscopy in vivo. Ann Neurol. 1992;32:140.
38. Hajek M, Dezortova M, Krsek P. (1)H MR spectroscopy in epilepsy. Eur J Radiol. 2008;67:258.
39. Hugg JW, Laxer KD, Matson GB, et al. Lateralization of human focal epilepsy by 31P magnetic resonance spectroscopic imaging. Neurology. 1993;43:2011.
40. Garcia PA, Laxer KD, van der Grond J, et al. 31P magnetic resonance spectroscopic imaging in patients with frontal lobe epilepsy. Ann Neurol. 1994;35:217.
41. Stefan TH, Ederhart KE, W-Huk BE, et al. Clinical applications of 1H-MR spectroscopy the evaluation of epilepsies. What do pathological spectra stand for with regard to current results and what answers do they give to common clinical questions concerning the treatment of epilepsies. Acta Neurol Scand. 2003;108:223.
42. Pettegrew JW, Moossy J, Withers G, et al. 31P nuclear magnetic resonance study of the brain in Alzheimer's disease. J Neuropathol Exp Neurol. 1988;47:235.
43. Matthews PM, Francis G, Antel J, et al. Proton magnetic resonance spectroscopy for metabolic characterization of plaques in multiple sclerosis, Neurology. 1991;41:1251.
44. Grossman RI, Lenkinski RE, Ramer KN, et al. MR proton spectroscopy in multiple sclerosis. Am J Neuroradiol. 1992;13:1535.
45. Mader I, Rauer S, Gall P, Klose U. (1)H MR spectroscopy of inflammation, infection and ischemia of the brain. Eur J Radiol. 2008;67:250.
46. De Stefano N, Narayanan S, Francis SJ, et al. Diffuse axonal and tissue injury in patients with multiple sclerosis with low cerebral lesion load and no disability. Arch Neurol. 2002;59:1565-71.
47. De Stefano N, Narayanan S, Matthews PM, et al. In vivo evidence for axonal dysfunction remote from focal cerebral demyelination of the type seen in multiple sclerosis. Brain. 1999;122:1933-9.
48. Arnold DL. Evidence for neuroprotection and remyelination using imaging techniques. Neurology. 2007;68:S83-90, discussion S91-6.
49. Graham GD, Kalvach P, Blamire AM, et al. Clinical correlates of proton magnetic resonance spectroscopy findings after acute cerebral infarction. Stroke. 1995;26:225.
50. Barker PB, Gillard JH, van Zijl PC, et al. Acute stroke; evaluation with serial proton MR spectroscopic imaging. Radiology. 1994;192:723.
51. Hugg JW, Duijn JH, Matson GB, et al. Elevated lactate and alkalosis in chronic human brain infarction observed by 1H and 31P spectroscopic imaging (MRSI). J Cereb Blood Flow Metab. 1992;12:734.
52. Paley M. Proton spectroscopy of the human brain. In: Bradley WG, Bydder GM, (Eds). MartynDunitz, London. 1997;309-23.
53. Horská A, Calhoun VD, Bradshaw DH, Barker PB. Rapid method for correction of CSF partial volume in quantitative proton MR spectroscopic imaging. Magn Reson Med 2002; 48: 555–8
54. Ernst T, Chang L. Elimination of artifacts in short echo time H MR spectroscopy of the frontal lobe. Magn Reson Med 1996; 36: 462–8.
55. Hurd R, Sailasuta N. Elimination of artifacts in short echo proton spectroscopy. 5th Annual Meeting of the International Society of Magnetic Resonance in Medicine; Vancouver, BC, Canada; 1997. p. 1453
56. Pruessmann KP, Weiger M, Scheidegger MB, Boesiger P. SENSE: sensitivity encoding for fast MRI. Magn Reson Med. 1999;42(5):952–62.
57. Sodickson DK, Manning WJ. Simultaneous acquisition of spatial harmonics (SMASH): fast imaging with radiofrequency coil arrays. Magn Reson Med. 1997;38(4):591–603.

58. Griswold MA, Jakob PM, Heidemann RM, Nittka M, Jellus V, Wang J, Kiefer B, et al. Generalized autocalibrating partially parallel acquisitions (GRAPPA). Magn Reson Med. 2002;47(6):1202–10.
59. Posse S, Tedeschi G, Risinger R, Ogg R, Le Bihan D. High speed 1H spectroscopic imaging in human brain by echo planar spatial-spectral encoding. Magn Reson Med. 1995;33(1):34–40.
60. Block KT, Frahm J. Spiral imaging: a critical appraisal. J Magn Reson Imaging. 2005;21(6):657–68.
61. Martin AJ, Liu H, Hall WA, Truwit CL. Preliminary assessment of turbo spectroscopic imaging for targeting in brain biopsy. AJNR. 2001;22(5):959–68.
62. Stengel A, Neumann-Haefelin T, Singer OC, Neumann-Haefelin C, Zanella FE, Lanfermann H, Pilatus U. Multiple spin-echo spectroscopic imaging for rapid quantitative assessment of N-acetylaspartate and lactate in acute stroke. Magn Reson Med. 2004;52(2): 228–38.
63. Maudsley AA, Domenig C, Sheriff S. Reproducibility of serial whole-brain MR spectroscopic imaging. NMR Biomed. 2010;23:251–6.
64. Stagg CJ, Knight S, Talbot K, Jenkinson M, Maudsley AA, Turner MR. Whole-brain magnetic resonance spectroscopic imaging measures are related to disability in ALS. Neurology. 2013;80:610–5.

CHAPTER 7

Functional MRI

Anuj Prabhakar

INTRODUCTION

Functional magnetic resonance imaging (fMRI) is an MRI-based tool that is utilized for analysis and localization of brain function.[1] This technique has enabled neuroscientists to gain valuable insight into the changes that occur while our brain functions. It helps in advancing our knowledge of structural organization in the brain. fMRI is also useful in evaluation of brain function in a wide variety of pathologies and in assessment of the risk of functional compromise after surgery. This chapter provides a brief introduction to the fundamental principles of functional MRI and its applications.

PRINCIPLE OF fMRI AND BOLD CONTRAST

fMRI is useful in evaluation of the eloquent areas of the brain. fMRI technique is usually based upon blood-oxygenation-level dependent (BOLD) contrast. BOLD effect was initially described by Seiji Ogawa. Turner et al. first obtained an echo-planar imaging time series of oxygenation changes occurring in blood with a cat brain during a global oxygenation stress.[2] The BOLD contrast effect was subsequently demonstrated in human subjects in 1992.[3,4] BOLD-fMRI differentiates between active and inactive areas by exploiting the difference in magnetic properties of deoxygenated and oxygenated hemoglobin. This allows the investigator to recognize changes in the local blood flow in the brain. Oxy hemoglobin is diamagnetic in nature while deoxyhemoglobin is paramagnetic and aligns with the magnetic field in the MRI gantry.[1] This paramagnetic nature leads to an increase in field inhomogeneity. This causes a swift dephasing of the local transverse magnetization that reduces the transverse relaxation time (T2*) in the adjacent brain parenchyma.

There is coupling of the local blood flow and neuronal activity in the brain.[5,6] Whenever an external stimulus is provided to the brain there is an increase in the local neuronal activity of the area in the brain associated with that particular task. This leads to an increase in the energy consumption and oxygen utilization within the stimulated area. In order to supply the increased oxygen demand, there is an increase in the regional blood flow and volume. However, the relationship between oxygen demand and blood flow is not linear and paradoxically, the degree of oxygen delivery, outstrips the elevated oxygen requirement. This leads to an increase in the local concentration of oxygenated hemoglobin. There is a commensurate reduction in the amount of deoxygenated hemoglobin in the draining veins, venules and local capillaries. Therefore, the net result of this increase in the neural activity is a reduction in the paramagnetic effect induced dephasing due to deoxyhemoglobin. The T2* signal increases and these changes can be observed using MRI. BOLD fMRI signal changes are small in magnitude and vary between 2% and 5%.[7]

The change in MRI signal secondary to neuronal activation is known as the hemodynamic response function (HRF) **(Fig. 1)**. The BOLD response is delayed by 1–2 s after any stimulus, irrespective of its length. The response has a temporal width of 4–6 s. If the stimulus is

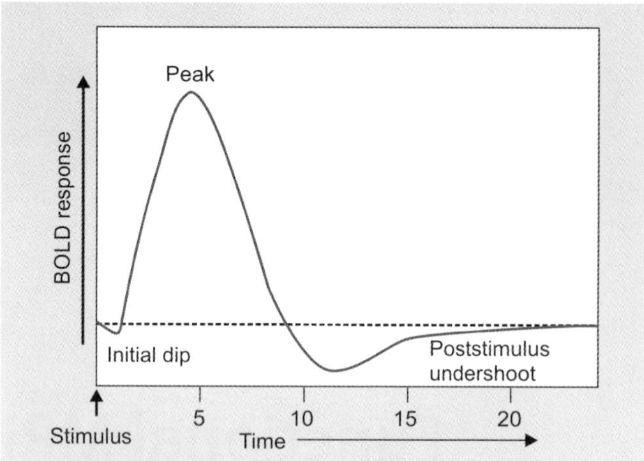

Fig. 1: Hemodymanic response function curve.

sustained for 20 s or longer, it usually reaches a plateau. Some investigators have described an initial fall in the BOLD signal that may last for 1–2 s before the usual increase. A matching transitory boost in deoxyhemoglobin concentration has been seen on optical imaging. There is a poststimulus undershoot that may last for approximately 30 s. Longer stimuli have longer poststimulus undershoot. BOLD response to multiple stimuli is not linear. This means that the response to two stimuli together is less than twice the integrated response of a single activation. Baseline cerebral blood flow (CBF) can also affect the extent of the BOLD effect after a stimulus. For example, if the CBF at baseline is increased by breathing carbon dioxide, the BOLD reaction for a particular task is reduced significantly.[8,9]

ADVANTAGES OF BOLD fMRI

There are many advantages in using fMRI over other conventional imaging methods while studying brain functions:[10]

- fMRI has better spatial resolution (1–4 mm in-plane resolution)
- The temporal resolution (0.1–1 sec) is also higher
- There is no need for radioactive isotopes
- fMRI is a non-invasive technique that can be easily replicated without any significant patient preparation
- The radiologist can acquire both anatomical and functional images in the same session
- There are no significant added costs.

Thus fMRI has become the most commonly used functional brain mapping modality.

LIMITATIONS OF BOLD TECHNIQUE

Susceptibility effects

T2* Gradient recalled echo echoplanar imaging (EPI) sequences are commonly used for BOLD imaging as they allow rapid scanning of the whole brain in a short time frame. However, these sequences are extremely sensitive to intravoxel dephasing. This occurs due to the changes in local magnetic field secondary to the variation in the magnetic susceptibility of different tissues contained within the voxel. Magnetic field gradients are generated which make the protons spin at different frequencies. Dephasing occurs with signal loss. This effect is maximized at areas of air tissue interface like orbitofrontal cortex or the medial and inferior temporal lobes. Activations related to visual and cognitive processing are seen in these areas. Susceptibility effects cause reduction in the sensitivity for this brain activation. Vascular clips, craniotomy hardware or stent grafts also cause significant artifacts during imaging. Another potential source of susceptibility artefacts is the presence of tumor-related hemorrhage in patients undergoing pre operative functional imaging for language or motor function.

Geometric Distortions

EPI sequences are prone to mislocalization of the BOLD signal in the phase encoding direction due to inhomogeneities in the magnetic field, especially if the bandwidth in the phase encoding direction is low. As previously discussed, regions in the brain that are adjacent to the air–soft tissue interface are more susceptible to distortions due to strong local variations in the magnetic field secondary to the susceptibility artefacts. Another source of distortion is the imperfection in linearity of the gradient waveforms. Few strategies may be utilized to correct and reduce image distortions. A field map may be acquired by applying a GRE sequence with 2 echoes at different TE. The field map is calculated by the difference in phase between the images acquired at different TE. This map can be used to map and correct the local field variations. The other technique used in correction of geometric distortion is the point spread function (PSF). Acquisitions using an additional phase encoding gradients are performed to calculate the PSF of each voxel. These PSFs encode the spatial information about the distortion and the overall distribution of intensities from a single voxel. Measuring the PSF allows the distortion in geometry and intensity to be corrected.

Venous Effects

The bold signal is dependent on local vasculature. At 1.5T and 3T BOLD activation may be localized to the adjacent draining vein and venules. This effect increases the likelihood of a false positive activation. It is seen more commonly in areas that are close to large draining veins like the superior sagittal sinus or it's draining cortical veins.

Physiologic Noise and Motion

Normal physiological functions like cardiac activity, respiration or had motion may contribute toward artefacts during acquisition of bold signal especially in resting state fMRI. Various techniques have been developed to mitigate the contribution by these effects to the BOLD signal.

Neurovascular Uncoupling

In a normal individual the activation of neurons and the subsequent hemodynamic changes are coupled in a predictable manner. There are many steps including initial neuronal firing followed by neurotransmitter release at synapses. This is followed by chemical mediator release from interneurons and astrocytes, resulting in vasoconstriction or vasodilatation. In patients who have structural lesions like tumors or arteriovenous malformations, alterations in the hemodynamic response lead to neurovascular uncoupling. This may lead to abnormally decreased or absent BOLD activation. Inadvertent resection of eloquent areas in such cases may cause permanent deficits.[4,7,10]

IMAGING ACQUISITION

BOLD fMRI is acquired using fast imaging read out. T2* weighted imaging is used. EPI sequences allow rapid whole brain coverage. A single-shot EPI technique is able to acquire multiple images at high speed (<100 ms/image). For example, the entire brain can be covered with 28 slices (slice thickness 5 mm) in less than 3 seconds. The TE ranges between 20–40 ms, and TR is between 1000 and 4000 ms. Using shorter TR (<1000 ms) reduces the temporal resolution; however the BOLD signal and the number of slices that can be acquired are also reduced. For this reason it is not generally used in clinical fMRI, which is performed on individual patients and therefore requires the greatest MR signal for both sensitivity and reliability. Single shot EPI is favored over multishot EPI, as it reduces motion artefacts in functionally impaired patients. At our institute the following parameters are used for fMRI in the routine clinical setting: EPI single shot; TR - 2000 ms; TE - 30 ms; Flip angle - 90; FOV - 230*230*140 mm; Voxel size- 3*3*4; Slice thickness - 4 mm; Slice gap - 0 mm; Number of slices- 35; Total scan duration- 5 min 14 sec; 150 dynamics.

fMRI EXAMINATION DESIGN

fMRI experiments are able to identify task evoked signal alteration in a sequence of MR images, and extract areas of activity using statistical analysis.[11] Those areas that show signal changes and correlate with the stimulus that has been applied can be recognized. Subsequently these are compared with the high-resolution T1-weighted anatomical images. Overall, there are two categories of task paradigms: block ('boxcar') designs and event-related designs **(Fig. 2)**. Block design paradigms are the most frequently used because of their simplicity, ease of implementation, and sensitivity. This design consists of repeated presentation of a task for at least 20 seconds followed by an alternate rest condition of similar duration.[3,6,12] The "rest" task must be chosen with care, as it should activate the various neural processes of the stimulus task except for the cognitive process that is being evaluated. The data collected from a block design experiment allow each task condition to be averaged to improve the signal-to-noise ratio (SNR) and then a simple "contrast" can be performed to compare the two conditions. Also, the averaging of BOLD signal over multiple repetitions compensates for any stimuli that may have been missed by the patient. The contrast can be obtained by performing a voxel-wise comparison between the BOLD signals recorded in the active and rest phases using parametric statistical analysis. Currently, most clinical fMRI procedures use block design. Block designs are very useful in clinical fMRI studies because the chief purpose in most clinical settings is to localize

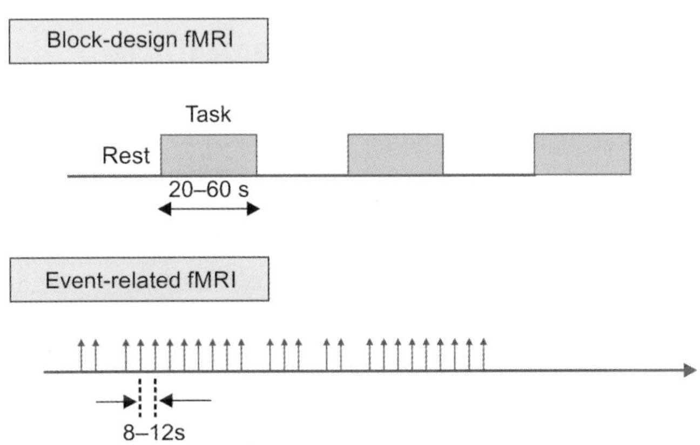

Fig. 2: Illustration showing difference in the technique used for block designs versus event-related paradigms.

and evaluate a focal activated region in the brain rather than define connectivity patterns in the whole brain. The prolonged duration required for each condition in a block design experiment, however, has many inherent design limits. For example, the long duration required for each condition limits the ability to study multiple conditions within the time constraints of a standard scanning session. The ability to extract temporal information about the brain responses is also limited because of the prolonged BOLD response. Excessive repetition of the active and rest phases may cause habituation.

Event-related fMRI paradigms utilize very brief stimuli that are presented at random of specific time points **(Fig. 2)**. They can be used to follow the course of neural processing in the brain.[13,14] The differences in the onset of activity produced by different stimuli can also be studied. Furthermore, as the stimuli appear at random time points, they are more statistically robust as compared to blocked designs. Therefore, event-related fMRI paradigms are useful to access questions that center upon the temporal performance of hemodynamic response, any changes that might occur with modification of the experimental context, and differences between various subjects. Event-related approach also avoids the habituation and fatigue that tends to arise in the box car design. Event-related experimental designs are used in most fMRI research on cognition, but their application in the clinical scenario is challenging. Firstly, complicated statistical methods are required to obtain the functional maps, however with increasing processing speed this technique has becoming feasible. Secondly, event-related designs require substantial validation and development prior to clinical use. Nevertheless, event-related designs offer more flexibility and are likely to achieve wider acceptance in the future.

fMRI EXAMINATION TASK PARADIGM

fMRI involves creating a paradigm which is presented to the patient, who is then required to is perform according to the provided instruction. A paradigm is a temporal allocation of stimuli that are used to elicit neuronal activation in a subject. Paradigms include active language, motor or memory tasks and passive auditory, tactile, or visual stimuli **(Figs. 3A and B)**.[15] Finger tapping is a dependable paradigm for localization of the hand activity in the primary motor cortex. A variety of language paradigms like verbal fluency with word generation, sentence comprehension, verb generation and picture naming. The use of multiple language paradigms increases the sensitivity and specificity of presurgical fMRI.[3,16] Verb generation is the

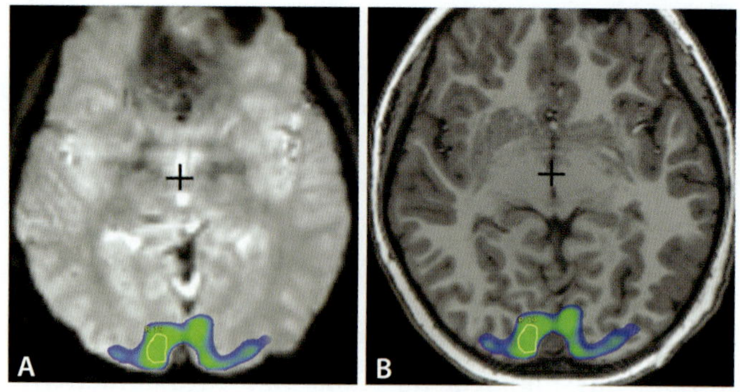

Figs. 3A and B: Visual checkerboard paradigm in fMRI: areas of activation (green blue color) are seen in bilateral occipital cortices superimposed on axial BOLD (A) and T1-weighted (B) images.

most commonly used and probably the most reliable test in the clinical arena. Instructions are simple: given a word think of the associated verb. Most patients understand it well and are compliant once inside the magnet. Various stimulus delivery packages are available in the market, e.g. Cogent (Laboratory of Neurobiology, Wellcome Trust, London, UK;), E-Prime (Psychology Software Tools, Inc.; Pennsylvania, USA), and Presentation (Neurobehavioral Systems, Inc.; California, USA). While presenting the paradigm it is essential to synchronize the stimulus delivery with the MRI sequence trigger. The task may be presented to the subject via an MRI compatible screen in the MRI scanner room, headphones or specially designed goggles.

POST-PROCESSING AND DATA ANALYSIS

Post-processing of clinical fMRI data generally adopts the approach used in conventional fMRI studies, which includes the following steps:

1. *Realignment*: All BOLD images acquired in a given time series are aligned to each other to correct for motion artifacts. The transformation information utilized in this process may be plotted as a graph. If the plot reveals motion larger than the size of the smallest voxel in any direction at a particular point of time the affected volume/dataset must be removed from the final analysis **(Fig. 4)**.
2. *Slice timing correction*: EPI sequences are acquired slice by slice in two dimensions. Therefore each slice is obtained at a different repetition time. If the statistical calculation is performed using the onset time relative to the first slice only, the delay in acquisition of the last slice will degrade the result of the fMRI scan. Slice timing correction must be performed to prevent this anomalous result.

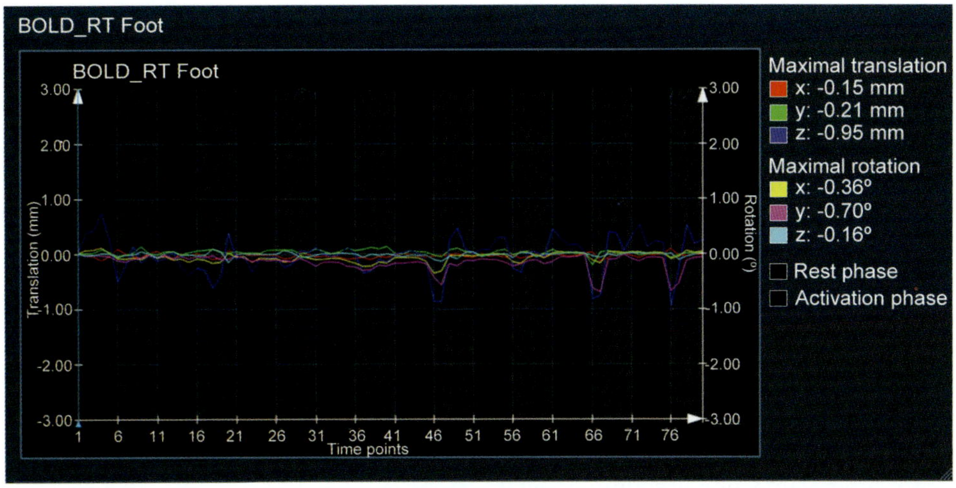

Fig. 4: Motion correction: Graph showing the patients head translation and rotation along all axis during rest and activation phases. If there is excessive motion at any time point, the corresponding EPI volume must be discarded from the final analysis.

3. *Coregistration*: In this step the EPI slices are coregistered with a high resolution anatomic scan in a voxel-wise manner. Segmentation of the anatomical image into gray matter, white matter, and cerebrospinal fluid is performed using tissue probability maps. Lastly the segmented images can be co-registered with the functional data.
4. *Normalization*: In clinical research the BOLD signal must be averaged across different subjects. The brain images of each patient are wrapped over the same stereotactic. This enables the researcher to evaluate the functional data from all subjects in a standard space. The most commonly used templates for normalization are the Montreal Neurological Institute (MNI) template, Talairach and Tournoux atlas, ICBM template.[17]
5. *Smoothing*: Smoothing of the fMRI images needs to be done prior to group-level statistical analysis, to superimpose corresponding areas of activity from the different subjects. Smoothening reduces noise and increases SNR. This step also suppresses the effect of anatomical and functional variability among individual subjects during group analysis.[18]
6. Statistical analysis is executed using a general linear model to compare the functional images obtained after performing the above steps to the design paradigm.
7. *Inference and interpretation of results*: Areas of functional activation are obtained after statistical processing. These can be superimposed on structural images or on 3D brain renders.

Clinical fMRI is mostly used for individual subjects and not group analysis. It is not essential to normalize the images. However, motion correction is extremely important in clinical setting. This is performed with rigid body transformation algorithms. Newer techniques for accurate motion correction and reduction of variation due to physiological causes are being developed.[16,19] A flow diagram of the various steps involved in fMRI is given in **Figure 5**.[20]

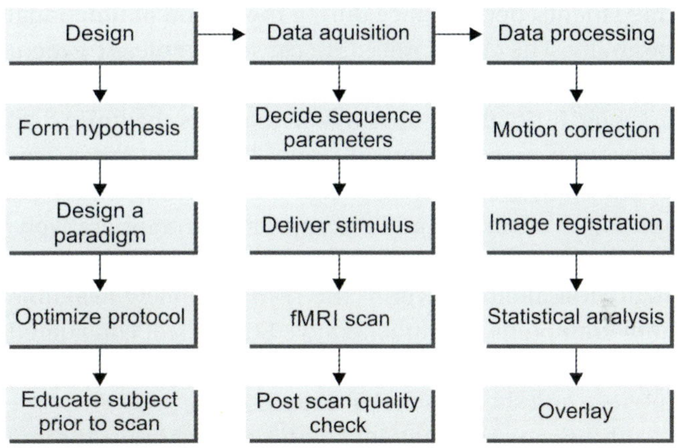

Fig. 5: Flow diagram depicting the various steps necessary for fMRI acquisition and analysis.[20]

CURRENT CLINICAL APPLICATIONS OF fMRI

Neurosurgical Planning

The capability to localize functional areas in patients makes fMRI very important in preoperative planning. Presurgical mapping is essential to: (a) to determine hemispheric dominance; (b) to select candidates for awake craniotomy;

(c) to guide the intraoperative surgical procedure; and (d) to assess the risk of postoperative neurologic deficits by measuring the distance between the margin of the lesion resection and critical functional structures.[16]

The "gold standard" for localizing foci of activation in the brain is electrical cortical mapping (ECM). ECM has several drawbacks. It is invasive in nature and the procedure takes a lot of time. Only a limited area of the brain is mapped. Another limitation is that the data from ECM is often accessible only during surgery after conclusions as regards to feasibility and surgical approach have already been drawn. The Wada test is another technique that is routinely used prior to epilepsy surgery. The dominant hemisphere for memory and language is recognized by the intra-arterial injection of sodium amytal into bilateral internal carotid arteries.[21] The drug causes temporary anesthetization of the brain tissue. Cerebral dominance for language and memory is determined on the patient's performance during the period of functional disability. The Wada procedure causes significant patient discomfort, and morbidity as compared to functional imaging. fMRI allows the surgeon to assess the functional areas prior to the surgery in a non-invasive manner. This information may be used to make choices regarding the suitability of surgery and the approach. Intraoperatively, it helps to familiarize the surgeon with the functional and structural anatomy within the restricted view available after craniotomy. If intraoperative ECM is still considered essential, fMRI directs the surgeon toward the regions of interest, and shortens the procedure.

The majority of patients with primary brain tumors can perform the various fMRI paradigms. Both motor and language paradigms can be performed. fMRI is highly sensitive in the detection of sensorimotor activation in healthy subjects and is also feasible in patients with lesions around the central sulcus **(Figs. 6A to F)**. Either volitional or passive paradigms may be used. Functional imaging is also useful in identifying functional areas in patients who have significantly distorted anatomy.[22] There is a good quality spatial correlation between motor fMRI and intraoperative ECM results. A distance of 10 mm or more between the functional cortex, as defined with fMRI, and the tumor has been found to be associated with significantly less risk of loss of function postoperatively.[23] The diagnostic performance of fMRI may change according to the grade of the glioma. Bizzi et al. reported higher sensitivity and lower specificity WHO grade II and III gliomas than in glioblastoma multiforme (GBM), particularly for fMRI of language.[24] This was postulated to be due to the neurovascular uncoupling or greater mass-effect seen in GBM. fMRI can also be used to predict deficits and study cortical reorganization.[22]

Epilepsy

Mapping of language and memory functions is possible using fMRI in temporal lobe epilepsy (TLE). This has both preoperative and prognostic significance. Various language paradigms are available to evaluate the Broca's area, Wernicke's area and the anterior temporal lobe language areas. Commonly used tasks include Verbal fluency, semantic decision, and verb generation. Evaluation of hemispheric dominance for language function can also be performed with fMRI using the lateralization index. Language mapping with fMRI has been seen to be more accurate as compared to Wada test in predicting naming ability post-surgery. The likelihood of postoperative preservation of naming function is higher if activation is noted in the left hippocampus during the pre-surgical fluency task, in right TLE patients. On the other hand, left TLE patients, who are more proficient in naming, show more activation in the left frontal lobe during various naming tasks. This suggests that the brain has a compensatory response to epileptic activity. Auditory and visual naming tasks may also help in predicting difficulties during naming after anterior temporal lobe resection.

Verbal or visual memory may be affected in approximately one-third of patients undergoing left or right anterior temporal lobe resection, respectively. Autobiographical, episodic and working memory related networks can be evaluated using fMRI in epilepsy patients. fMRI helps in prognosticating such patients.[25]

Dementia

Functional imaging offers substantial potential to recognize patients with prodromal dementia. The prefrontal cortex and the medial temporal lobe are implicated in working and secondary memory in healthy subjects. An increase in activation has been seen in the prefrontal cortex with increasing memory usage.[26] This is more evident during the initial, learning attempts.[27] Successful recall has been seen to be associated with increased activation.[27] The medial temporal lobe, the hippocampus and the parahippocampal cortex show activation during learning and recall. fMRI studies have revealed that modified patterns of activation in these memory-specific brain regions may be an indicator of brain dysfunction in early-stage dementia and mild cognitive impairment. Such markers may be used in clinical trials

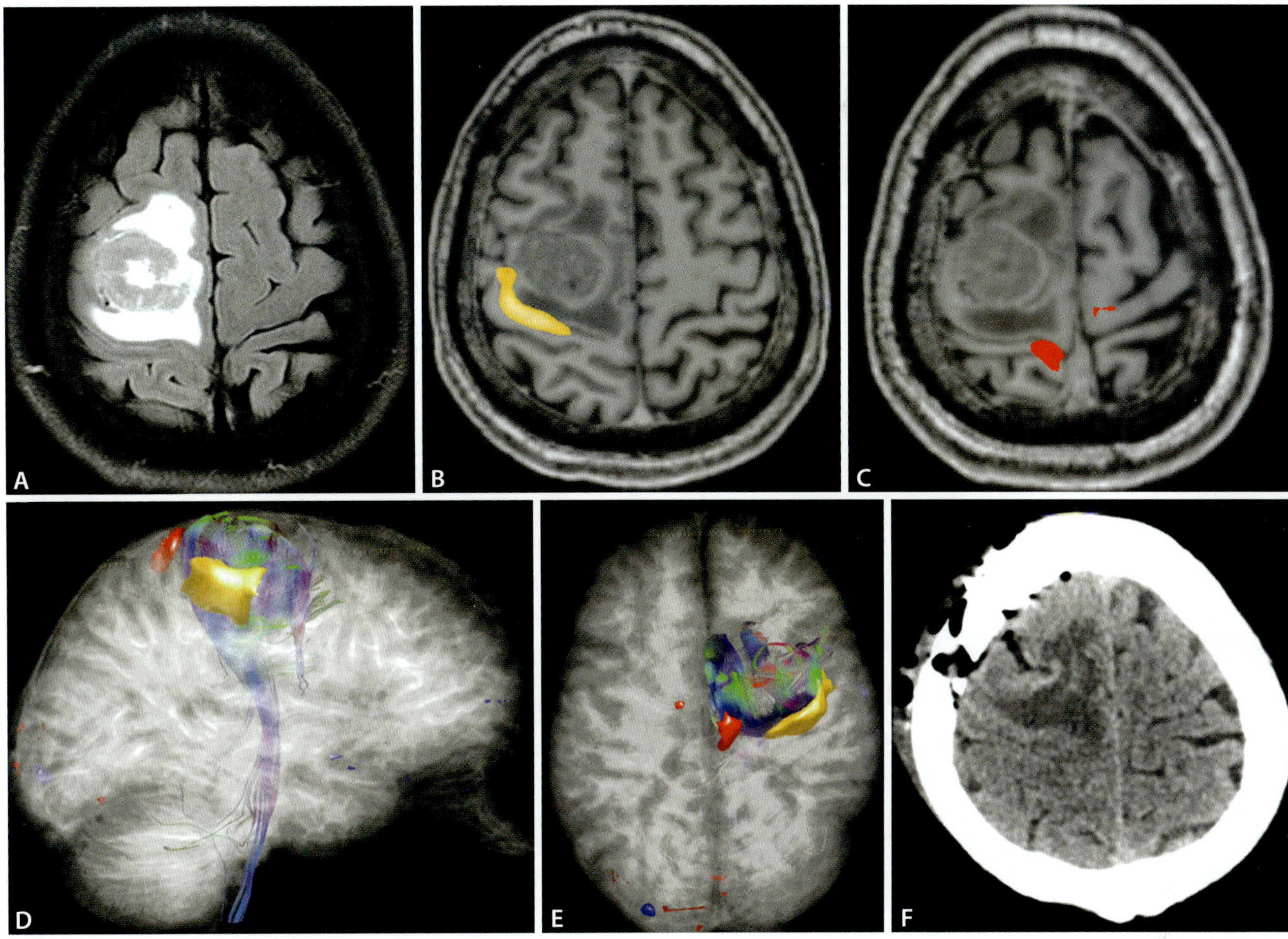

Figs. 6A to F: Pre-surgical fMRI: Axial FLAIR image (A) shows a well-defined lesion in the right high frontal region with surrounding edema. The right central sulcus is effaced and displaced posteriorly. Preoperative evaluation of motor area was performed using finger tapping; (B) and foot movement; (C) paradigms. The results were superimposed on axial T1-weighted images. The motor area corresponding to hand motion (orange area in B) has been displaced posteriorly and laterally. The foot motor cortex is also seen along the posterosuperior aspect of the edema. Composite glass brain images; (D and E) with functional and tractography data superimposed give an overview of both with matter tracts (purple, green) and activated areas (orange: hand motor, red: foot motor) surrounding the lesion. Such images allow the surgeons to decide their approach. Postoperative CT; (F) shows the anterolateral approach used in this patient that has spared the motor cortex and white matter tracts.

of cognition enhancing drugs, as the currently utilized measures may be weighed down by measurement error and variability of change with time.

Diminished intensity of activation has been shown in the frontal and temporal regions of patients with Alzheimer's disease. "At-risk" subjects have also shown mixed results in various studies. Both increased and decreased activation have been seen in this group as compared to the control group.[28,29] Increased activation in Alzheimer's or at-risk patients may be explained by compensatory-recruitment of a larger area of the brain as compared to the normal population for the same task. If significant neuronal loss has already occurred, decrease in BOLD activation may be seen, especially in tasks that exceed the patient's compensatory reserve.[28]

Defining Disease Based on Patterns of Brain Function

fMRI could be used to define different "phenotypes" in a particular disease state. This may be especially pertinent in diseases like dyslexia, in which clinical classification is. fMRI studies may also provide an insights into the pathophysiology of the disease process. For example, Eden et al. have demonstrated that there is no activation in the motion sensitive visual cortex when dyslexic patients are presented with a moving stimulus.[30] Subsequent studies have suggested that such insufficiency in the integrity of the cortical magnocellular pathway may serve as a clinical marker in the disorder.[31]

Psychiatric Disorders

Most of the major psychiatric illnesses are characterised by widely distributed disordered neural systems. There is no single brain region associated with a particular mental illness. However, there are a few exceptions. Anterior cingulate cortex hyperactivity has been shown to be associated with major depression. Normalization of activity has been seen after treatment in such patients.[32] In schizophrenia a reduction of activity has been seen in the same area.[33] However, fMRI is not used for individual diagnosis of mental illness in the clinical setting. Resting state fMRI and connectivity analysis are more appropriate for research in psychiatric disorders.

ADVANCES IN fMRI TECHNIQUE

Real-Time fMRI Neurofeedback

Real-time fMRI was developed by Cox et al.[34] The main difference between this technique and routine fMRI is in the speed of computation. The post-processing steps in real-time fMRI images are same as those in offline fMRI studies. However, with the advent of faster computer processing, better imaging sequences and algorithms, this process can be performed in a very small time frame. As the data is rapidly analyzed while the subject is in the MRI gantry, the results can be utilized to modulate his/her mental processes. The participants can learn to control multiple areas in the brain. Few studies have been performed which show that various brain areas including cingulate cortex, cingulate cortex, insular cortex, amygdala, motor, premotor and somatosensory cortices, visual and auditory cortex etc. may be controlled in this manner. Real-time fMRI neurofeedback has shown benefit in treatment of diseases like schizophrenia, depression, Parkinson's, tinnitus, and nicotine addiction.[34,35]

Resting State fMRI

Resting state fMRI (RSfMRI) scrutinizes synchronous activations between different areas in the brain that are at distinct locations physically. No external stimulus or task is given to the subject during RS fMRI. The patient lies awake, quietly in the MRI gantry throughout the sequence. The main aim of this technique is to identify the resting state networks. These networks are spatially distinct areas of the brain that are functionally connected with each other. A range of statistical techniques have been developed to identify resting state networks (RSNs) like seed-based analysis, independent component analysis, graph methods, clustering algorithms and multivariate pattern classification.

Various RSNs have been described. The most commonly studied network is the DMN. This network includes precuneus/posterior cingulate, lateral parietal cortex and the mesial prefrontal cortex. Other RSNs include the somatosensory network (primary and higher order motor and sensory areas), visual network (the occipital cortex), auditory network (Heschl gyrus, the superior temporal gyrus, and the posterior insula), language network (Broca and Wernicke areas with prefrontal, temporal, parietal, and subcortical regions), dorsal attention network (intraparietal sulcus and the frontal eye field), ventral attention network (temporoparietal junction and ventral frontal cortex), frontoparietal control network (lateral prefrontal cortex and the inferior parietal lobule) and the cingulo-opercular network (medial superior frontal cortex, anterior insula, and anterior prefrontal cortex). Each of these networks is thought to serve a distinct function.

RSNs have been studied in a variety of disorders such as epilepsy, Alzheimer's, major depressive disorder and schizophrenia.[36] However, RS fMRI is still an experimental tool at present. More research is necessary before it can be used in mainstream clinical practice.

CONCLUSION

Functional MRI is the new frontier for brain research. It gives an insight into brain connectivity, function and complexity. Significant research has been done on fMRI with newer techniques being developed rapidly. Presurgical evaluation of language, motor areas has become an essential tool for ensuring best possible patient outcome.

REFERENCES

1. Khanna N, Altmeyer W, Zhuo J, et al. Functional neuroimaging: fundamental principles and clinical applications. Neuroradiol J. 2015;28(2):87-96.
2. Bandettini PA. Twenty years of functional MRI: the science and the stories. NeuroImage. 2012;62(2):575-88.
3. Bandettini PA, Wong EC, Hinks RS, et al. Time course EPI of human brain function during task activation. Magn Reson Med. 1992;25:390-7.
4. Menon RS, Ogawa S, Kim SG, et al. Functional brain mapping using magnetic resonance imaging. Signal changes accompanying visual stimulation. Invest Radiol. 1992;27(Suppl 2):S47-53.

5. Thulborn KR. MRI in the management of cerebrovascular disease to prevent stroke. Neurol Clin. 2008;26(4):897-921, vii-viii.
6. Kwong KK. Functional Magnetic Resonance Imaging with Echo Planar Imaging. Milano: Springer Milan; 1996. pp. 73-90.
7. Zacà D, Agarwal S, Gujar SK, et al. Special considerations/ technical limitations of blood-oxygen-level-dependent functional magnetic resonance imaging. Neuroimaging Clin N Am. 2014;24(4):705-15.
8. Buxton RB, Uludağ K, Dubowitz DJ, et al. Modeling the hemodynamic response to brain activation. NeuroImage. 2004;23:S220-33.
9. Tootell RBH, Reppas JB, Dale AM, et al. Visual motion aftereffect in human cortical area MT revealed by functional magnetic resonance imaging. Nature. 1995;375:139-41.
10. Detre JA, Floyd TF. Functional MRI and its applications to the clinical neurosciences. The Neuroscientist. 2001;7:64-79.
11. Bandettini PA, Jesmanowicz A, Wong EC, et al. Processing strategies for time-course data sets in functional MRI of the human brain. Magn Reson Med. 1993;30:161-73.
12. Ogawa S, Tank DW, Menon R, et al. Intrinsic signal changes accompanying sensory stimulation: functional brain mapping with magnetic resonance imaging. Proc Natl Acad Sci. 1992;89:5951-5.
13. Dale AM. Optimal experimental design for event-related fMRI. Hum Brain Mapp. 1999;8:109-14.
14. Rosen BR, Buckner RL, Dale AM. Event-related functional MRI: Past, present, and future. Proc Natl Acad Sci. 1998;95:773-80.
15. Moritz C, Haughton V. Functional MR imaging: paradigms for clinical preoperative mapping. Magn Reson Imaging Clin N Am. 2003;11:529-42.
16. Baciu M, Kahane P, David D, et al. Hemispheric language dominance testing by fMRI in epileptic patients, using a rhyme detection task. NeuroImage. 2000;11:S268.
17. Mandal PK, Mahajan R, Dinov ID. Structural brain atlases: design, rationale, and applications in normal and pathological cohorts. J Alzheimers Dis JAD. 2012;31(03):S169-8.
18. Mikl M, Mareček R, Hluštík P, et al. Effects of spatial smoothing on fMRI group inferences. Magn Reson Imaging. 2008;26(4):490-503.
19. Bullmore ET, Brammer MJ, Rabe-Hesketh S, et al. Methods for diagnosis and treatment of stimulus-correlated motion in generic brain activation studies using fMRI. Hum Brain Mapp. 1999;7:38-48.
20. Conklin CJ, Faro SH, Mohamed FB. Technical considerations for functional magnetic resonance imaging analysis. Neuroimaging Clin N Am. 2014;24(4):695-704.
21. Sabbah P, Chassoux F, Leveque C, et al. Functional MR imaging in assessment of language dominance in epileptic patients. NeuroImage. 2003;18:460-7.
22. Gabriel M, Brennan NP, Peck KK, et al. Blood oxygen level dependent functional magnetic resonance imaging for presurgical planning. Neuroimaging Clin N Am. 2014;24(4):557-71.
23. Håberg A, Kvistad KA, Unsgård G, et al. Preoperative blood oxygen level-dependent functional magnetic resonance imaging in patients with primary brain tumors: clinical application and outcome. Neurosurgery. 2004;54:902-15.
24. Bizzi A, Blasi V, Falini A, et al. Presurgical functional MR imaging of language and motor functions: validation with intraoperative electrocortical mapping. Radiology. 2008;248:579-89.
25. Chaudhary UJ, Duncan JS. Applications of blood-oxygen-level-dependent functional magnetic resonance imaging and diffusion tensor imaging in epilepsy. Neuroimaging Clin N Am. 2014;24(4):671-94.
26. Courtney SM, Ungerleider LG, Keil K, et al. Transient and sustained activity in a distributed neural system for human working memory. Nature. 1997;386:608-11.
27. Gabrieli JDE, Poldrack RA, Desmond JE. The role of left prefrontal cortex in language and memory. Proc Natl Acad Sci. 1998;95:906-13.
28. Bookheimer SY, Strojwas MH, Cohen MS, et al. Patterns of brain activation in people at risk for Alzheimer's disease. N Engl J Med. 2000;343:450-6.
29. Small GW, Ercoli LM, Silverman DHS, et al. Cerebral metabolic and cognitive decline in persons at genetic risk for Alzheimer's disease. Proc Natl Acad Sci. 2000;97:6037-42.
30. Eden GF, VanMeter JW, Rumsey JM, et al. Abnormal processing of visual motion in dyslexia revealed by functional brain imaging. Nature. 1996;382:66-9.
31. Demb JB, Boynton GM, Heeger DJ. Brain activity in visual cortex predicts individual differences in reading performance. Proc Natl Acad Sci. 1997;94:13363-6.
32. Temple E, Poldrack RA, Protopapas A, et al. Disruption of the neural response to rapid acoustic stimuli in dyslexia: evidence from functional MRI. Proc Natl Acad Sci. 2000;97:13907-12.
33. Mayberg HS, Brannan SK, Tekell JL, et al. Regional metabolic effects of fluoxetine in major depression: serial changes and relationship to clinical response. Biol Psychiatry. 2000;48:830-43.
34. deCharms RC. Applications of real-time fMRI. Nat Rev Neurosci. 2008;9:20-9.
35. Emmert K, Kopel R, Sulzer J, et al. Meta-analysis of real-time fMRI neurofeedback studies using individual participant data: how is brain regulation mediated? NeuroImage. 2016;124:806-12.
36. Lee MH, Smyser CD, Shimony JS. Resting-state fMRI: a review of methods and clinical applications. Am J Neuroradiol. 2013;34(10):1866-72.

CHAPTER 8

Imaging and Interventions in Cerebral Ischemia

Shailesh B Gaikwad, Anuj Prabhakar

INTRODUCTION

Stroke is characterized as an acute, abrupt onset, central nervous system injury of vascular origin. The term "stroke" encompasses cerebral ischemia/infarcts, intracerebral hemorrhage and subarachnoid hemorrhage. The age adjusted prevalence rate for stroke in our country is 84–262/100,000 for rural areas and between 334–424/100,000 for urban areas.[1] 50–80% of strokes are ischemic in origin. Subarachnoid hemorrhage accounts for 1–7% of stroke cases and intracerebral hemorrhage is found in 7–27% of strokes, thus cerebral infarction is the major contributor towards morbidity and mortality in stroke. There is higher incidence of stroke amongst the younger age group and also among poorer population in India.[1] Imaging plays an important role in not only diagnosis and etiological classification of stroke, but also in its management, especially in the acute setting. A number of modalities may be utilized in imaging of cerebral ischemia and its effects on the brain parenchyma. The management of acute stroke has under gone rapid evolution and an interventional neuroradiologist has become an indispensible in management of acute ischemic stroke. In this chapter we shall discuss the pathophysiology, imaging and the various endovascular techniques that are utilized in these patients.

Pathophysiological Considerations

The cerebral blood flow is maintained by cerebral auto-regulation at a stable level. Under normal circumstances the rate of blood flow in the brain is directed by the cerebral vascular resistance which in turn is decided by the vessel diameter.[2] Auto regulation functions between 60–150 mm Hg mean arterial pressure. The brain is unable to compensate for changes in pressure either below or above this, leading to cerebral injury. When a major cerebral vessel undergoes acute occlusion, there is reduction of cerebral blood flow in the distribution of that particular vascular territory. This leads to a complex sequence of biochemical events that end with death of the involved neural tissue. Normal blood flow to the brain is approximately 50 mL/100 g brain tissue/minute. If the blood flow is reduced below 18 mL, the spontaneous and evoked electrical activity ceases, leading to neurological deficit. Failure of membrane ion homeostasis occurs at 10–12 mL/10 g/minute. Beyond this infarcts develop in the involved parenchyma **(Table 1)**. If the duration of ischemia lasts for more than 30 minutes, cytotoxic edema sets in.[1,3] At the cellular level, local depletion of oxygen or glucose causes a reduction in the production of high energy compounds. 5–10 minutes of complete occlusion may lead to an infarct.[4] Release of excitatory neurotransmitters,

Table 1: Cerebral blood flow (CBF) in the pathophysiology of acute ischemic stroke.

• Normal	CBF - 50–60 mL/100 g/min
• Oligemic State	CBF - 35 mL/100 g/min
• Ischemic State	CBF - 20 mL/100 g/min
• Infarction	CBF - <10 mL/100 g/min

oxygen free radicles and apoptosis occur. The ion gradient across cell membranes is lost leading to cytotoxic edema. Cytotoxic edema manifests as focal swelling of the brain parenchyma with effacement of sulci and loss of gray white matter differentiation. Vasogenic edema, that occurs due to extravasation of water through damaged endothelial cells, develops in 3–6 hours and may extend into the white matter.[5] Within 24–48 hours of infarction, in-growth of phagocytic microglial cells occurs with proliferation of new capillaries. These capillaries lack tight junctions, and are permeable to both large molecules and water. This process begins at the periphery of the infarct and proceeds centrally.[6,7] Slowly, the necrotic tissue is removed by the macrophages and the remnant cavities and cysts occupy the infarcted area with glial scar tissue. Over subsequent weeks, complete resorption of necrotic tissue takes place with resultant encephalomalacia and loss of volume.[8]

Significance of a Penumbra

Brain tissue is extremely sensitive to ischemia. In presence of complete occlusion of a major artery, the neuron can remain viable for approximately 2–3 minutes. It is estimated that about 1.9 million neurons die every minute. When the ischemia is incomplete, the injured brain continues blood supply from patent arteries and leptomeningeal collaterals. Therefore, acute cerebral ischemia may result in a central irreversibly infarcted tissue core surrounded by a peripheral zone of potentially salvageable (reversible ischemia) called a "Penumbra" **(Fig. 1)**. The transition from ischemia to irreversible infarction depends on the severity and the duration of reduction of blood supply.[9,10] The penumbra is a dynamic entity and its size is inversely related to the duration of the delay in recanalization. Imaging is currently directed to evaluate the size of the penumbra with the help of multidetector CT and MR imaging.

Etiology

Various systems have been proposed to classify arterial stroke subtypes. The simplest classification system is the ASCO phenotype system. This divides stroke into four subtypes: atherosclerotic, small vessel disease, cardioembolic and others.

Atherosclerotic strokes are the most common subtype of acute arterial stroke. They form approximately 40–45% of cases. Atherosclerotic disease may be intracranial, extracranial, or coronary. The prevalence of these subtypes varies with race and ethnicity. Intracranial atherosclerosis causes upto 30-50% of strokes in Asians.

Large artery infarcts are usually embolic in nature. Emboli arise from thrombi that develop at the site of an "at risk" ASVD plaque. Atherosclerotic plaques are most commonly found at the level of the carotid bifurcation. The cavernous internal carotid artery is the next most common site. The middle cerebral artery is the most frequently occluded intracranial vessel. A gene locus has been identified near TSPAN2 in patient who are susceptible to large artery atherosclerosis.

Small vessel disease represents 15–30% of all strokes. Small artery occlusions, (lacunar infarcts) are defined as lesions measuring less than 15 mm in diameter. They occur when the small penetrating vessels supplying the basal ganglia, thalami, pons, internal capsule and deep white matter are involved. These lesions may be clinically silent or may manifest with severe neurological impairment depending upon the site of infarct. Lacunar infarcts can

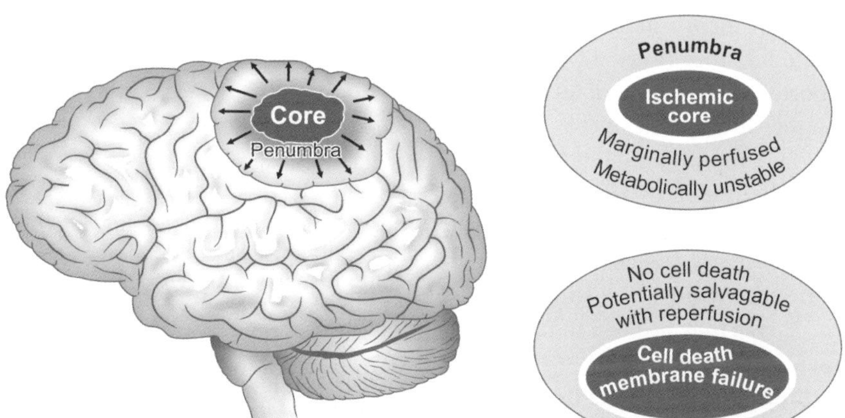

Fig. 1: Schematic diagram of brain involvement in acute ischemic stroke of MCA territory shows central core "representing the irreversible infarcted zone" and surrounded by the penumbra representing reversible ischemic zone if timely thrombolytic therapy is administered.

be embolic, atheromatous, or thrombotic in nature. Most involve penetrating arteries in the basal ganglia/thalami, pons, internal capsule and deep cerebral white matter.

Cardioembolic disease is a cause of 15–25% of major strokes. Myocardial infarction, arrhythmia (most often atrial fibrillation), and valvular heart disease may lead to release of emboli from the heart.

Other is a heterogeneous group that combines strokes with miscellaneous but known etiologies together with strokes of undetermined etiology (cryptogenic stroke).[11]

IMAGING IN ISCHEMIC STROKE

Rowley[12] has emphasized on the assessment of the four Ps—parenchyma, pipes, perfusion and penumbra as summarized in **Table 2**.

Table 2: Goals of imaging in the evaluation of acute stroke.

• Parenchyma	To evaluate for early imaging features of acute stroke and rule out hemorrhage
• Pipes	To identify an intravascular thrombus in either intracranial or extracranial circulation
• Perfusion	Evaluation of CBF, CBV, MTT
• Penumbra	Assess tissue at risk of infarct if ischemic insult continues without recanalization

Computed Tomography

The three main CT techniques used routinely for acute stroke evaluation are: 1. Noncontrast CT; 2. CT Angiography (CTA); 3. CT Perfusion.

Computed tomography is the initial imaging modality used in a patient presenting with ischemic stroke. Earlier, the main role of CT was to identify intracranial hemorrhage and to rule out other pathologies like neoplasms, that may mimic stroke. However, recent studies have pointed out that CT, in the context of use of thrombolytic therapy, has significant prognostic value in the evaluation of acute stroke patients.[13]

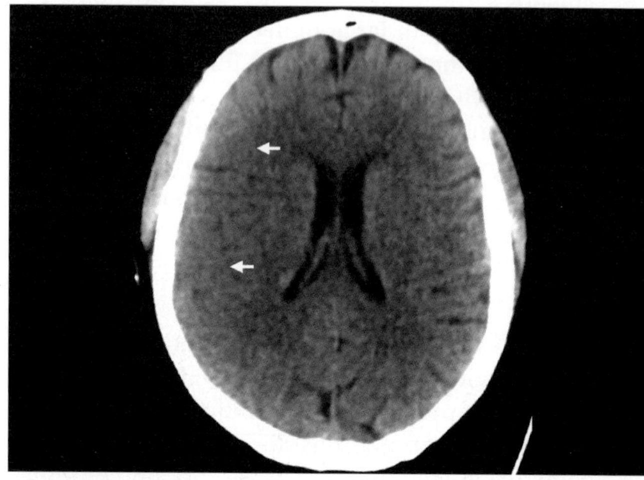

Fig. 2: NCCT head showing effacement of sulci with loss of gray white matter differentiation in the right MCA territory (arrows).

In the hyperacute stage of infarction, changes noticed on CT occur as a result of cytotoxic edema. The latter is seen as reduction in the density of gray matter in the ischemic tissue and obliteration of sulci and gray-white matter differentiation **(Fig. 2)**. In MCA territory infarction, these changes lead to the well-described insular ribbon sign and obscuration of lentiform nuclei due to acute ischemia of lenticulostriate territory **(Figs. 3A and B)**.[14,15] Various studies have reported a sensitivity of 56 to 90% in detection of such changes during initial 3–6 hours of ictus.[9] The extent of these CT identifiable changes at the time of presentation can help in identifying the subgroup of patients who will have a better outcome following thrombolytic therapy.[9] In the early stages, a hyperdense thrombus may be identified within MCA (dense MCA sign) **(Figs. 4A and B)**. [15,16] This may be seen in up to 50% of all cases.[16,17] Narrower window width (~8HU) and center level (~32 HU) settings improve lesion detection as compared to the default CT window. Increased clarity of early CT signs of infarct is associated with increased risk of haemorrhage. Also, involvement of more than 1/3rd MCA territory on NCCT increases the risk of hemorrhage after IV rTPa administration. However, various studies that utilized one-third rule showed that there was poor interobserver correlation.[18] Thus, the Alberta Stroke Program Early CT Score (ASPECTS) was proposed in 2001

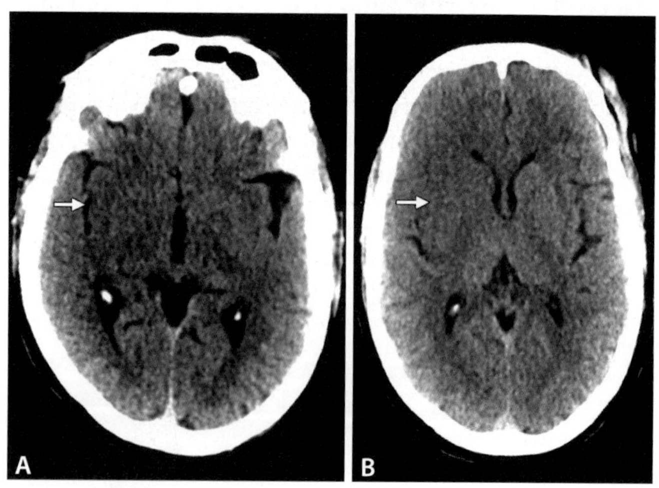

Figs. 3A and B: NCCT head showing (A) hypodensity involving the insular ribbon "Insular ribbon sign" (arrow); (B) Obscuration of right lentiform nucleus (arrow).

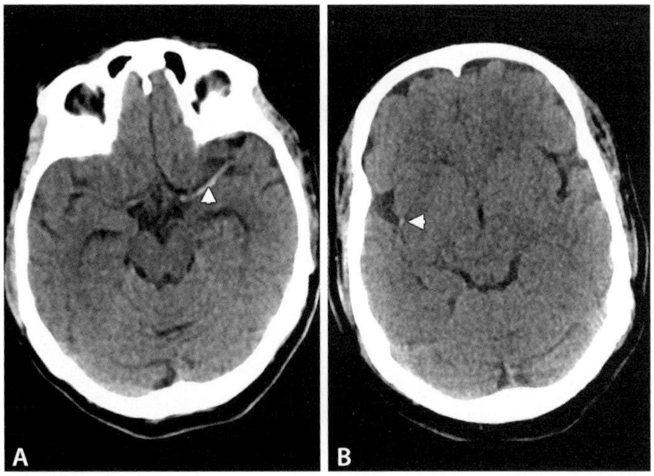

Figs. 4A and B: NCCT Head showing the hyperdense MCA sign secondary to an embolus lodged in the MCA (arrow head in A). If the embolus lodges in one of the M2 segmental arteries MCA dot sign is seen (arrowhead in B).

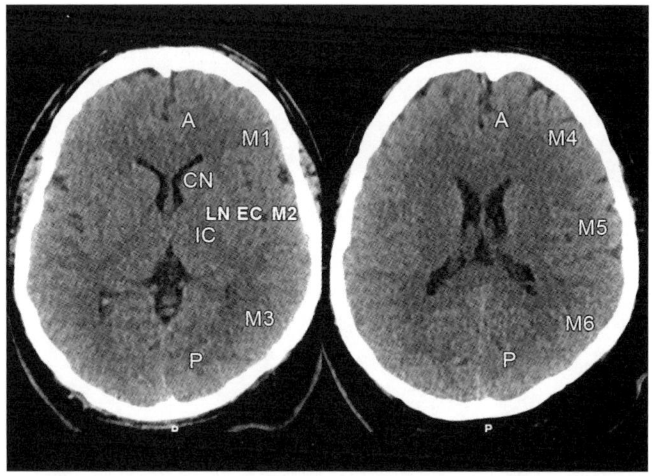

Fig. 5: The ASPECTS is determined from two standardized axial CT cuts, one at the level of the thalamus and basal ganglion and one adjacent to the most superior margin of the ganglionic structures, such that they are not seen. A single point is subtracted for an area of early ischemic change for each of the defined regions. A normal CT scan receives an ASPECTS of 10 points.

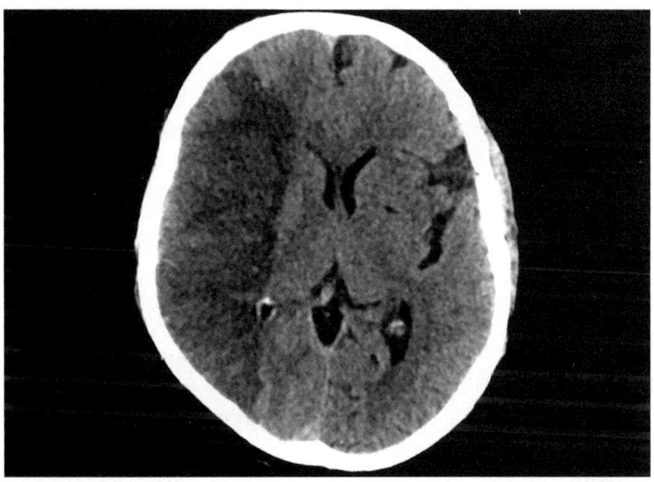

Fig. 6: Acute infarct 2 days after onset of symptoms. A wedge-shaped low density area involving both gray and white matter in the right MCA territory.

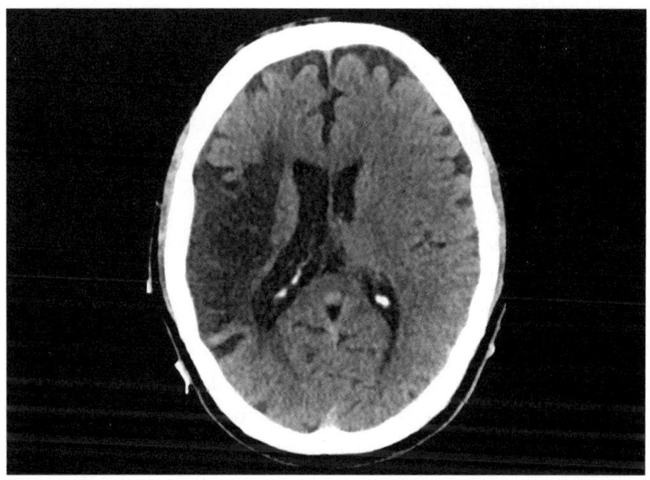

Fig. 7: Chronic infarct—Months to years after a strokeencephalomalacic changes result in volume loss of the affected brain. Calcification is rarely seen in chronic infarction.

to quantitatively assess acute ischemia on CT images by using a 10-point topographic scoring system[19] **(Fig. 5)**.

During the next few days, the density of the infarcted tissue decreases further, associated mass effect increases, and change can be seen in both grey and white matter **(Fig. 6)**. The infarct in acute and subacute stages can usually be easily identified. Sometimes, it may be possible to see a "fogging effect" in the subacute stage. This occurs due to increase in the attenuation of the infarcted tissue to a level approaching that of surrounding normal brain, thereby masking the infarct. This phenomenon is attributed to reopening of capillaries in the region with resultant hyperemia.[5] In the chronic stage; encephalomalacia is seen as area of low density with accompanying loss of volume in the form of dilated sulci and adjacent ventricular system **(Fig. 7)**.

CT Angiography

CT angiography is a recently introduced technique which aims at studying the vasculature by performing rapid sequence computed tomography through the area of interest at the time of maximum opacification

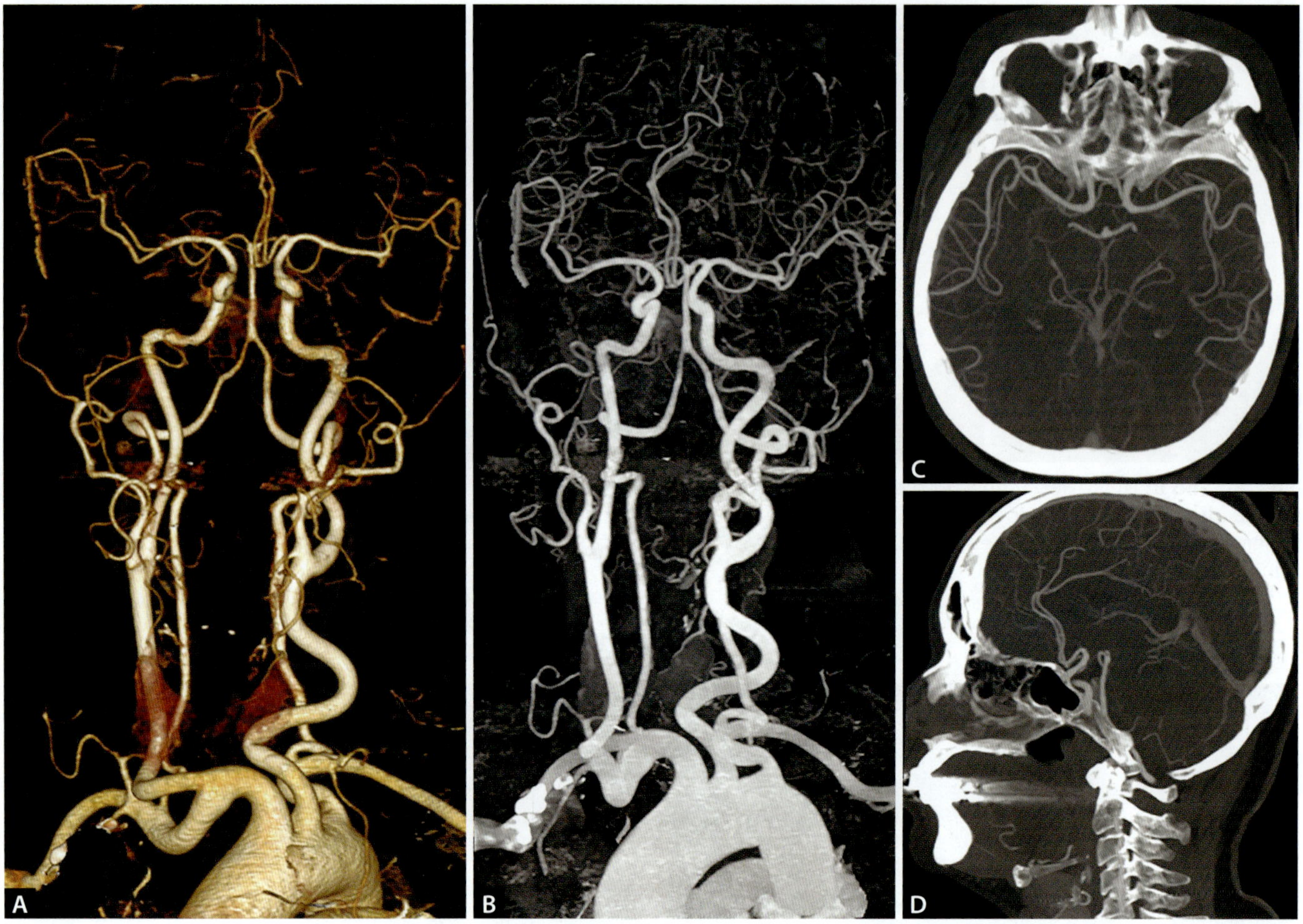

Figs. 8A to D: VRT (A), 3D MIP (B) and 2D MIP (C and D) CT angiography images. CTA is able to show the intra- and extracranial circulation in detail.

of the vessels with an intravenous bolus of contrast **(Figs. 8A to D)**. The data thus acquired can be processed to generate images similar to conventional angiograms.[20] CTA for patients of acute stroke must include both head and neck. The acquisition begins from the arch of aorta and should extend beyond the circle of Willis.[18] An acute thrombus is seen as an abrupt cutoff of the involved vessel without distal contrast opacification **(Figs. 9A and B)**. The thrombus location and extent is associated with subsequent recanalization rates in patients treated with IV TPa. Clot burden score can also be calculated on CTA images. When the CTA does not show occlusion, clot burden score is considered as 10. The intracranial circulation is divided into the infraclinoid ICA, supraclinoid ICA, proximal M1 segment, distal M1 segment, each M2 branch and the A1 segment. Two points each are deducted if the thrombus involves the supraclinoid ICA, proximal M1 segment or distal M1 segments. One point is deducted if the thrombus involves the either M2 branch, the infraclinoid ICA, or the A1 segment.[21] The distal branches may be reformed through pial collaterals. Multiphasic imaging is essential to evaluate the presence of collaterals.[22] Various collateral scoring systems have been described. The ASTIN/ SIR scoring system is given in **Table 3**.[23] The sensitivity and specificity of CTA for detection of intracranial occlusion is high and varies between 92 and 100 and between 82 and 100% respectively.[24]

ASITN/SIR, American Society of Interventional and Therapeutic Neuroradiology/Society of Interventional Radiology; CTA, CT angiography.[23]

CTA source images (CTASI) can also be utilized to detect ischemic regions. The sensitivity of CTASI and DWI for detection of ischemic regions is similar. DWI is superior at demonstrating smaller abnormalities. In strokes of less than 3 hour duration CTA SI has higher sensitivity to ischemia as compared to NCCT. CTSI also identifies the area that will ultimately undergo infarction as it provides an estimate of cerebral blood volume.

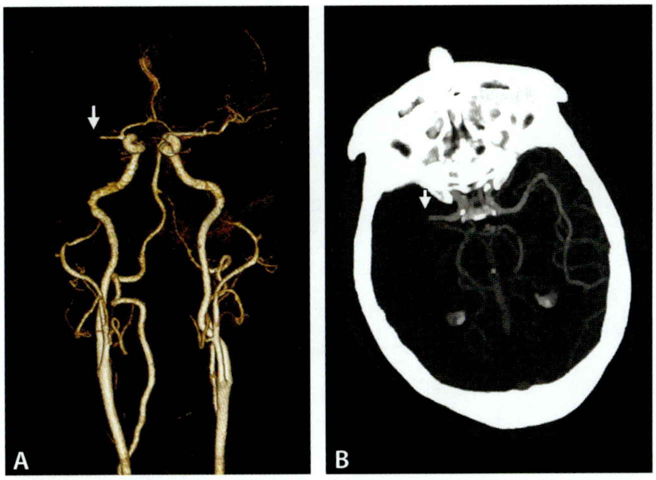

Figs. 9A and B: Acute thrombus in right MCA: VRT (A) and MIP(B) images showing abrupt cut off of the M1 segment of right MCA is seen without distal opacification (arrow).

Table 3: Modified version of the ASITN/SIR collateral score for dynamic CTA.

• 0—Non-existent or barely visible pial collaterals on the ischemic site during any point of time
• 1—Partial collateralization of the ischemic site until the late venous phase
• 2—Partial collateralization of the ischemic site before the venous phase
• 3—Complete collateralization of the ischemic site by the late venous phase
• 4—Complete collateralization of the ischemic site before the venous phase

In the extra-cranial circulation CTA is better than ultrasound for differentiating between complete and near complete occlusion. CTA also has 100% negative predictive value for excluding more than 70% stenosis when compared to DSA and functions well as a screening test. A large meta-analysis found CTA to have a sensitivity >90% and specificity >95% for detecting significant lesions compared with DSA.[24]

CT Perfusion Imaging

CT perfusion helps in identifying the tissue at risk. Various parameters are evaluated on CT perfusion. Cerebral blood volume (CBV) is defined as the volume of blood per unit of brain tissue (normal range 4-5 mL/100 g). Cerebral blood flow (CBF) is the volume of blood flow per unit of brain tissue per minute (normal range in gray matter = 50-60 mL/100 g/min). Mean transit time (MTT) refers to the difference between the time at arterial inflow and at venous outflow and time to peak enhancement, depicts the time required from the beginning of contrast injection to reach the maximum concentration within a region of interest.[9] In acute ischemic stroke, the penumbra will show an increase in the MTT with moderately or markedly decreased CBF and normal or increased CBV (80–100% or higher) **(Fig. 10)**, whereas infarcted tissue shows severely decreased CBF (<30%) and CBV (<40%) with increased MTT.[25]

Magnetic Resonance Imaging

Magnetic resonance imaging is more sensitive for detecting acute infarct as compared to CT.[26] During the initial few hours of ischemia, the findings on MRI are related to vascular occlusion and cytotoxic edema. The sensitivity of apparent diffusion coefficient (ADC) maps and diffusion-weighted imaging (DWI) are very sensitive for the diagnosis of acute stroke. An acute infarct is hypointense on ADC and hyperintense on DWI **(Figs. 11A to F)**. ADC maps may show hypointensity within minutes of stroke onset; however ADC and DWI maps may not be 100 % positive within the first 2-4 hours after stroke onset. Various studies have found a sensitivity of 90-95 % of DWI for diagnosis of hyper acute stroke. Addition of perfusion-weighted imaging improves the sensitivity in such cases.[27] "T2 shine-through," may occur at a later stage after infarction and is seen as a bright signal on both DWI and ADC maps **(Figs. 12A and B)**. Hypointensity on ADC is maximum at 2–3 days and persists for 7–10 days. Signal intensity is lowest on DWI 3–4 days after infarction, however hyperintense signal usually persists for about 10–14 days. Pseudonormalization, characterized by normal signal on ADC may be seen on ADC maps approximately 1–2 weeks after stroke onset. The signal intensity, however remains high on T2-weighted images.[28] Restriction on DWI, is secondary to cytotoxic edema and is usually considered irreversible, however partially reversibility has been documented, if early and effective reperfusion is achieved, especially in less than 3 h after arterial occlusion.[29]

Hyperintense signal may be seen on FLAIR imaging after 6–12 hours of symptom onset. A DWI - FLAIR mismatch indicates that the infarct may be less than 6 hours old.[28] Other changes in the brain parenchyma include hyperintensity on T2-weighted images accompanied by subtle mass effect and loss of gray-white matter differentiation on T1-weighted images. These changes are limited to grey matter during the initial few hours. In some cases, hypointensity may be observed on

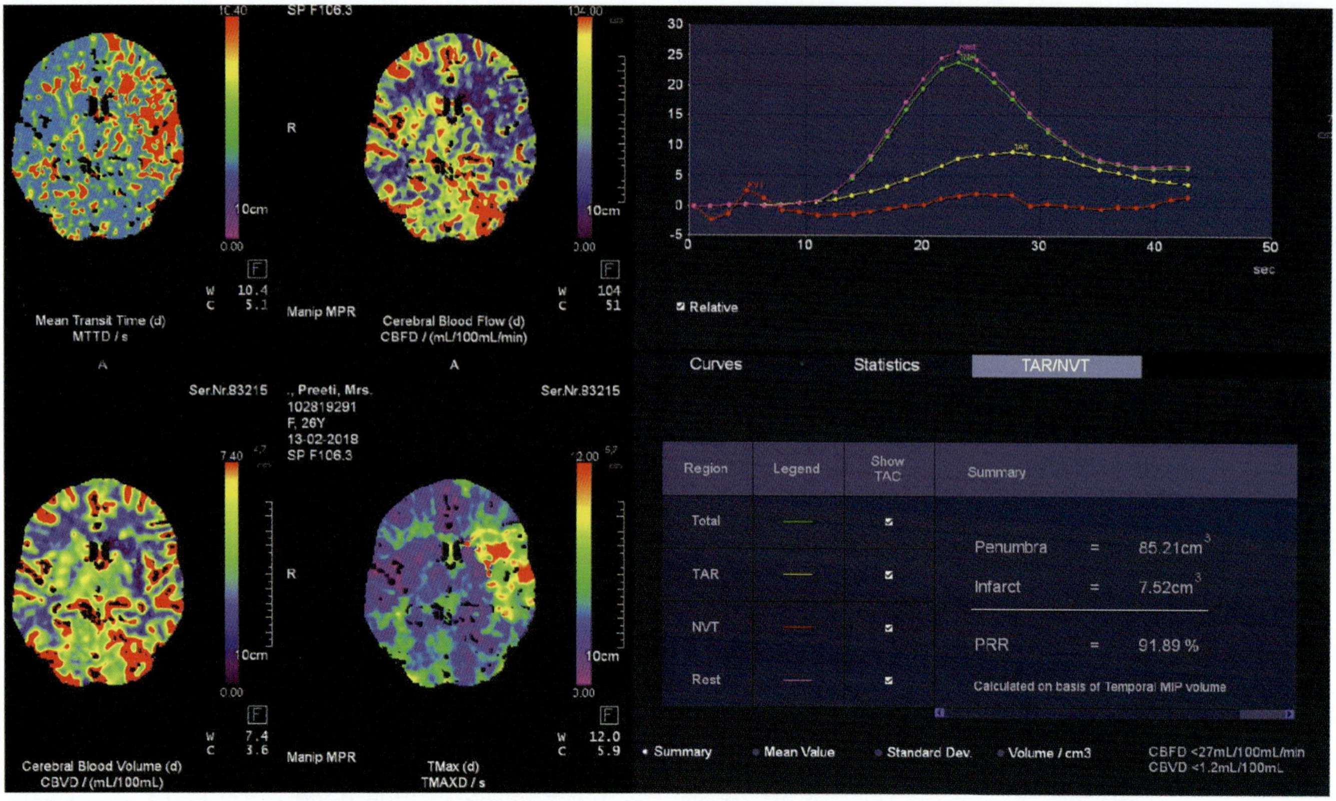

Fig. 10: CT perfusion: Penumbra shows an increased mean transit time with moderately decreased cerebral blood flow and normal cerebral blood volume. The percentage of penumbra can also be calculated.

T2-weighted images in the subcortical white matter. The cause for this hypointensity is not clear, but it may be related to presence of iron or free radicals. During next few days, intravascular and overlying meningeal enhancement can be seen in contrast-enhanced studies. The signal alteration and the mass effect become more conspicuous. During the subacute phase, sometimes T2 shortening may be observed in the infarct resulting in almost complete disappearance of the signal alteration observed initially on T2-weighted images. This is the "fogging effect" **(Figs. 13A to C)**. Contrast administration also shows prominent parenchymal enhancement in the infarcted tissue in the subacte phase **(Figs. 14A to D)**.[30] This is followed by resolution of meningeal/intravascular enhancement, reduction in mass effect.

Areas of T1 shortening, indicative of hemorrhage, may be seen in up to 20% of all infarcts.[25,30] T2*-weighted gradient-echo images and susceptibility-weighted images (SWI) may demonstrate areas of abnormal "blooming" in acute intracranial hemorrhage. The "artery susceptibility sign" is also seen on gradient imaging as blooming within the involved vessel. It is considered as MRI correlate of the hyperdense MCA seen on NECT **(Fig. 11D)**. The risk of hemorrhage after IV thrombolysis in patients with microhemorrhages depicted on SWI is unclear; Routine use of MRI to exclude cerebral microbleeds before administration of IV alteplase is not recommended.[31] In the chronic stage, encephalomalacia develops and is seen as focal area of altered signal associated with loss of volume.

As compared to CT MRI offers the capability to differentiate acute from chronic infarcts. Sub-clinical ischemic lesions and infarcts involving the posterior fossa are also better visualized on MRI. There is no radiation exposure and the spatial resolution is better. However MRI is more expensive with limited availability. The test is of longer duration as compared to CT and is more vulnerable to motion artifacts. Claustrophobia, metal implants, patient confusion, or cardiac pacemakers are also contraindication for MRI.[24]

Magnetic Resonance Angiography

Magnetic resonance angiography has come up as an effective, noninvasive tool to evaluate the vasculature. There are several different techniques that are available for evaluating intracranial vessels including 2-D time of flight

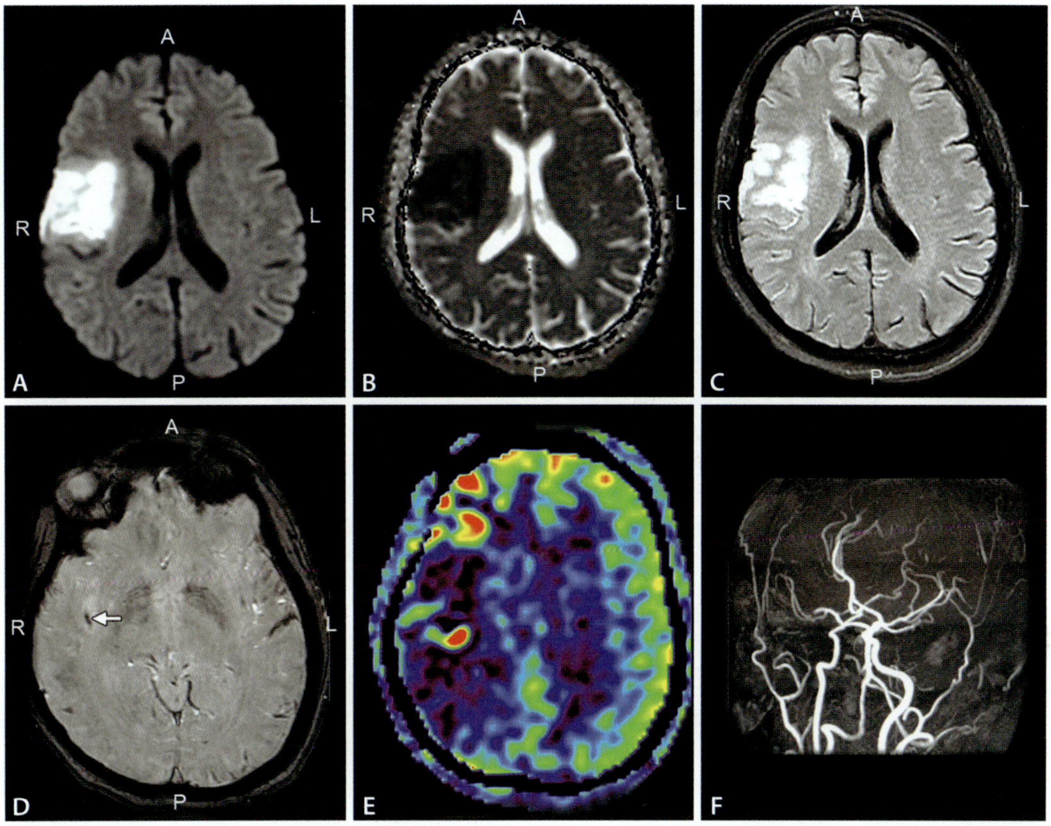

Figs. 11A to F: Axial DWI (A), ADC (B), FLAIR (C), SWI (D), ASL (E) and MIP TOF images (F) in a patient presenting with acute right MCA infarct. The lesion is bright on DWI, FLAIR and hypointense on ADC. SWI image is showing the hypointense thrombus within the MCA (arrow). ASL shows hypoperfusion of the involved area. MRA shows loss of normal flow-related signal in the right MCA distal M1 segment.

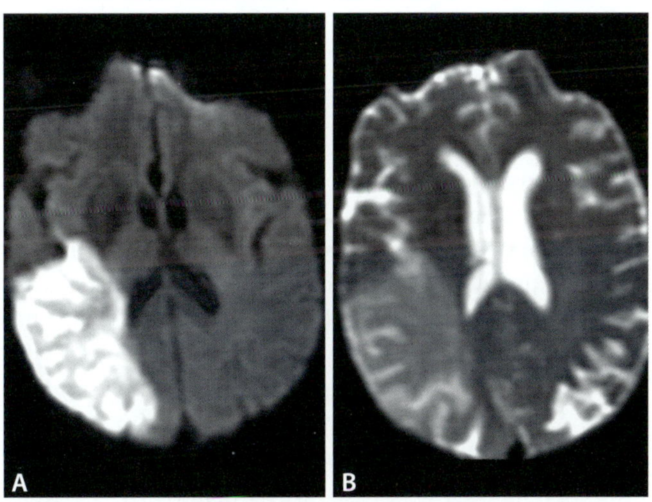

Figs. 12A and B: DWI and ADC images showing hyperintense signal - T2 shine-through.

(TOF), 3-D TOF, multiple overlapping thin-slab acquisition, and contrast-enhanced MRA. TOF angiography exploits the fact that the flowing blood continuously replaces the protons present within the vessel at a given point with fresh protons. The sequence is tailored such that the signal can be generated only from the protons in the flowing blood. Due to its simplicity and elegance, TOF technique is most frequently used in assessment of vessels. MRA allows noninvasive assessment of neck vessels as well as large intracranial vasculature.

Intracranial nonenhanced TOF MRA has a sensitivity of 80% to 90% for occlusions and 60% to 85% for stenosis, when compared with DSA or CTA. Although, TOF MRA is useful for identifying proximal large-vessel occlusions, it is not able to reliably identify branch or distal occlusions.[32] MRA has been shown to be better than Doppler US for distinguishing near total stenosis from occlusion of ICA.[33-35] In extracranial carotid disease 2D and 3D TOF MRA has a mean specificity of 88% and a mean sensitivity of 93% in diagnosing 70% stenosis. Contrast-enhanced MRA is more accurate as compared to nonenhanced techniques. It has specificity of 86% to 97% and sensitivitiy of 62% to 91%, when compared with DSA **(Figs. 15A to C)**.[24]

The spatial resolution is still not adequate enough to assess small intracranial vessels on 1.5T systems. However, with 3T MR system, it is now possible to image small

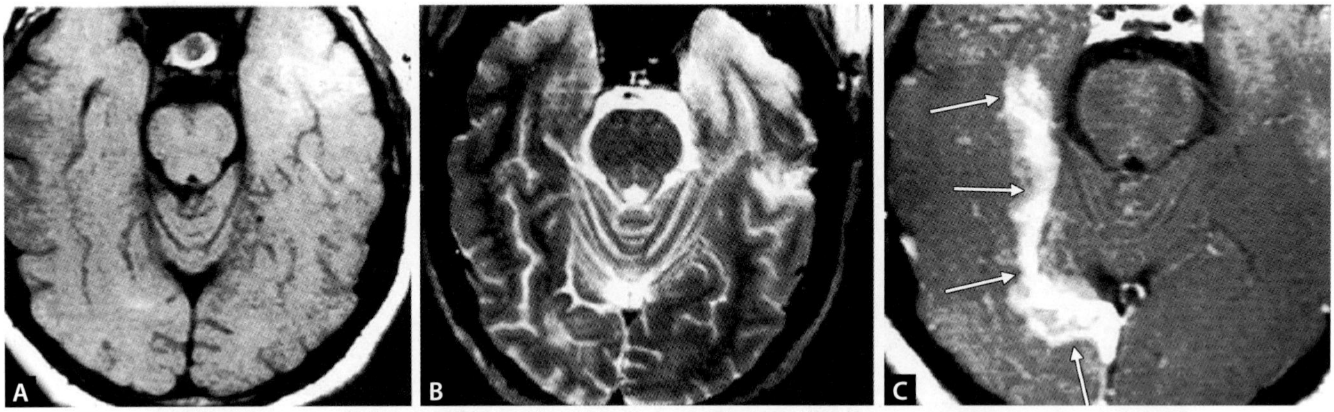

Figs. 13A to C: T1-weighted axial section (A) and T2-weighted section; (B) do not show presence of infarct which is seen as an enhanced area; (C) after contrast administration (arrows).

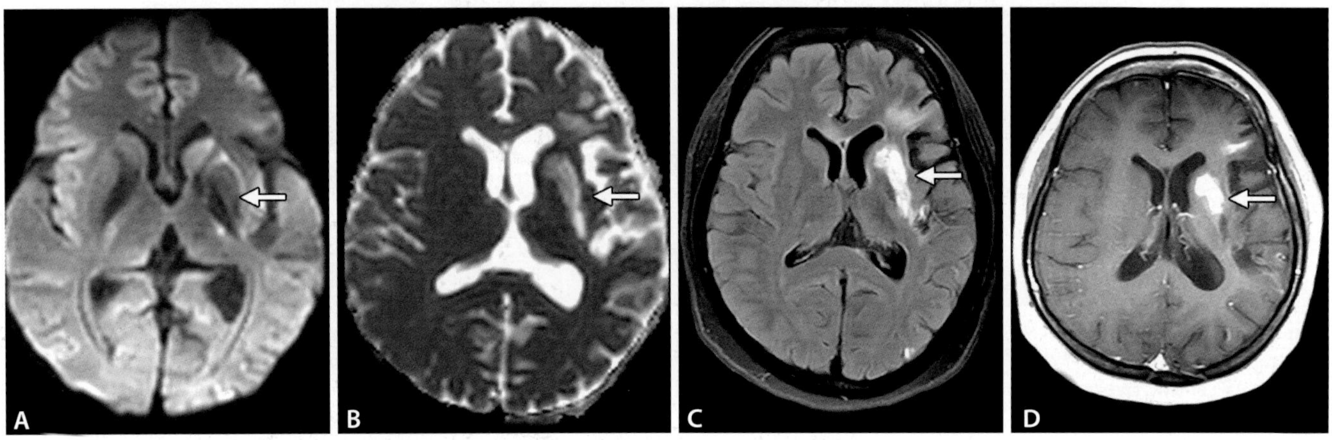

Figs. 14A to D: DWI (A), ADC (B), FLAIR (C) and post-contrast T1 (D) images in a subacute left basal ganglia infarct (arrows). The lesion is hypointense on DWI, hyperintense on ADC, FLAIR and is showing post-contrast enhancement.

intracranial vessels also. Disadvantages of MRA include its high cost, restricted availability, inability to evaluate small intracranial vessels and susceptibility to complex flow patterns. Additionally, some patients (e.g. claustrophobic, patients with metallic implants) may be unsuitable for MR evaluation and vessels at the root of neck and aortic arch are not so easy to image.

Combination of DWI and Perfusion in Evaluation of Acute Stroke

Perfusion MR is a technique that uses a rapid echo planar MR imaging sequence following the injection of contrast material. PW imaging demonstrates the alteration in physiologic state of the intracranial vasculature immediately after acute vascular occlusion. These changes may be characterized by a variety of qualitative flow-related maps including relative cerebral blood flow (rCBF), relative cerebral blood volume (rCBV) and mean transit time (MTT). Differences in perfusion and diffusion images may indicate the penumbra or the salvagable brain tissue **(Figs. 16 and 17)**. MTT maps show the largest area of abnormality and overestimate the final infarct size. Relative cerebral blood volume maps tend toward underestimation of the final infarct size. However, it has been seen that rCBV maps are closely correlated with changes in infarct size between initial and follow-up DWI maps. A mismatch between initial rCBV map and DWI more often predicts that there will be further extension of the infarct as compared to a mismatch between rCBV map and DWI.[18]

In acute stroke areas that show both diffusion and perfusion abnormalities represent infarcted tissue, while an area that shows only perfusion abnormalities with normal diffusion is likely to represent penumbra. Mismatch may also be seen in patients with symptomatic chronic cerebrovascular disease during challenge testing. In

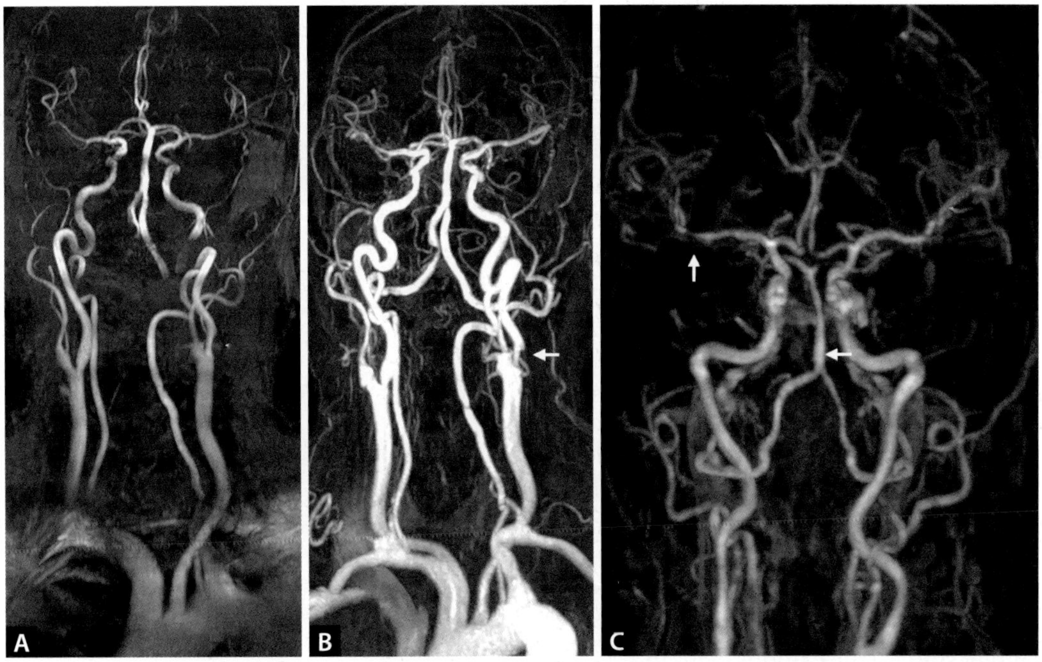

Figs. 15A to C: 3D TOF MRA (A), 3D Contrast-enhanced MRA (B) MIP images showing narrowing in left proximal ICA at the carotid bifurcation (arrows). CEMRA is not affected by vessel tortuosity or flow-related phenomena and shows the neck vessels with more clarity. 3D CEMRA MIP projection (C) shows intracranial atherosclerotic narrowing involving the right MCA M1 segment (arrow).

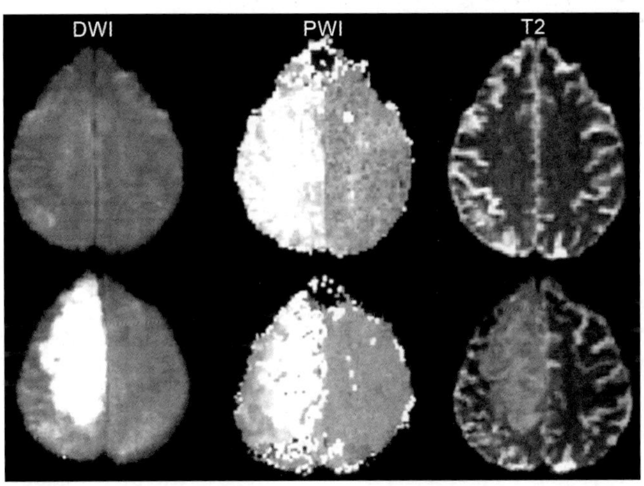

Fig. 16: Diffusion-weighted images and perfusion weighted images showing mismatch in the infarcted areas of the brain.

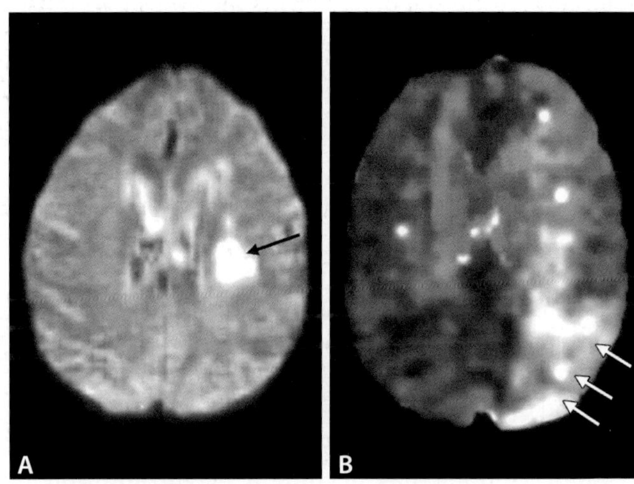

Figs. 17A and B: (A) Diffusion-weighted (black arrow) and (B) perfusion-weighted section showing mismatch (white arrows).

general, complete occlusion involving the proximal artery is more likely to cause a diffusion-perfusion mismatch as compared to distal or lacunar infarctions. In small vessel infarctions, diffusion-perfusion match is less, and the diffusion volume increases only slightly with time. In early reperfusion the diffusion volume may be larger than the perfusion abnormality. The perfusion abnormality may also be absent in early reperfusion.[18]

Carotid Ultrasound

Ultrasound (US) is an inexpensive, noninvasive, widely available tool, which can provide a reliable assessment of extracranial carotid arteries. A complete carotid US study includes a visual assessment of B-mode US image as well as evaluation of flow through the arteries using duplex and color Doppler. Normal carotid artery is visualized on US as two parallel echoic lines separated by an anechoic region.[36] The echogenic wall represents combined thickness of intima and media, and should not exceed 0.8 mm in width.[36] A plaque is seen as a hypoechoic to mildly echogenic eccentric area within the vessel lumen causing variable degree of stenosis. Presence of heterogeneity within the plaque may suggest possibility of hemorrhage, thrombosis, calcification or ulceration of the plaque.[37] US is reported to identify intraplaque hemorrhage with sensitivity and specificity of 90–94% and 75–88% respectively.[38,39] Heterogeneous and irregular plaques are known to be associated with a higher risk of stroke.[40]An ulceration within the plaque appears as a focal defect with sharp or overhanging margins.[41] Addition of color Doppler improves the detection of plaque ulcerations.[36] In addition to its role in atherosclerosis, US is also useful in documenting thickening of carotid arterial wall caused by various vasculitides, e.g. aortoarteritis and to monitor response to medical management in these cases.

Duplex Doppler study of the carotids helps in assessing the velocity of blood flow through the vessel. Normal end diastolic ICA velocity is less than 40 cm/s.[36] In presence of any narrowing of the vessel lumen, velocity of the blood flow at the site of narrowing increases. A number of studies have shown that the increase in the velocity can be used to assess the degree of luminal narrowing.[42-44] The velocity should be measured at or just distal to the site of stenosis as shown on B-mode US or color Doppler study. A number of studies have shown that carotid Doppler can diagnose critical carotid bifurcation stenosis with a sensitivity of 81–94% and a specificity of 78–91%.[33,34,43-45] It is advisable that each center must establish its own criteria for diagnosing critical stenosis.[46] Some of the criteria which have been used in the literature for diagnosing >70% stenosis include peak ICA systolic velocity of >230 cm/s, end diastolic ICA velocity of >100 cm/s and a ratio of peak systolic ICA to CCA velocity of >4.[47]

Color Doppler has become a useful addition to the sonographic evaluation of carotid arteries. Severe stenosis (>70%) with abnormal flow velocities can be easily identified as areas of aliasing with post stenotic turbulence.[41] Color Doppler has high sensitivity for detecting a thin streak of blood flow.[36] The distinction between near total stenosis and vessel occlusion is more accurately made. Another important usefulness of color Doppler is its ability to detect narrowing produced by anechoic plaques, which would otherwise be missed on B-mode US.

The shortcomings of US include its inability to evaluate the intracranial vasculature, chances of missing tandem lesions in ICA higher up in the neck, and inability to assess densely calcified plaques.

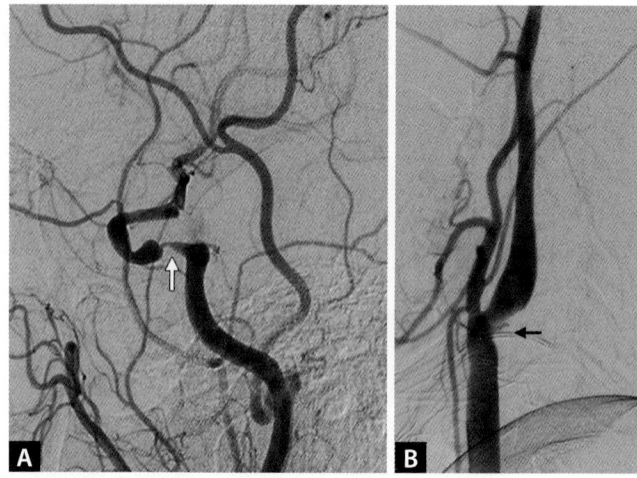

Figs. 18A and B: DSA is the gold standard for evaluation of both intra and extracranial circulation. Lateral view of ICA (A) shows narrowing in the petrous segment with reduced distal flow (white arrow). Lateral view of CCA; (B) in another patient shows narrowing with ulceration in the carotid bulb (black arrow).

Catheter Angiography

It is considered to be the gold standard for vascular studies. The technique allows assessment of vascular lumen of both intra and extracranial **(Figs. 18A and B)** vasculature with unmatched spatial resolution. Unlike MRA and Doppler, artifacts produced by complex flow patterns due to vascular loops or tortuosities do not degrade the technique. However, the procedure is invasive. Even with improvements in catheters, guidewires and contrast media, significant neurological complications may occur in 1–2% of all patients.[48] In spite of these potential risks, catheter angiography remains the investigation of choice in experienced hands for assessment of intracranial vasculature and is used as a problem-solving technique for the larger neck vessels. One limitation of the investigation is its inability to directly visualize the wall of the vessels. The latter information may be useful in certain situations like assessment of calcification in the wall, vasculitis and occult arterial dissections.

RECANALIZATION STRATEGIES IN ACUTE STROKE

New therapies are being developed to manage acute ischemic infarction. It is important to distinguish between tissue that has undergone infarction and tissue that is ischemic but will survive despite the reduced perfusion to use these therapies appropriately. Although ischemic tissue may be salvaged successfully, these strategies are associated with risks such as an increased chance of intracranial hemorrhage. Some of the recanalization strategies are discussed in brief:

Intravenous TPA

National Institute of Neurological Disorders and Stroke Study (NINDS trial): NINDS study showed that there was a benefit of intravenous (IV) tissue plasminogen activator, if it was administered within 3 hours of acute ischemic stroke onset.[49] In this study there was a trend towards an improvement in outcome despite the presence of hypodensity on early CT. The beneficial effects were noted in all stroke subtypes including suspected lacunar infarction. The benefits were sustained at 1 year. There were 12% absolutc (30% relative) differences in 2 groups in patients having minimal or no disability at 3 months (32% vs. 44%). Mortality rate of 17% vs. 25% was insignificant and symptomatic intracerebral hemorrhage within 36 hours was reported as 6.4% vs. 0.6%. In both the PROACT II and NINDS trial, clinical outcomes were significantly better in those patients receiving fibrinolytic therapy despite an increase in the rate of intracerebral hemorrhage in the drug group as compared to the placebo group.[50]

The study concluded that despite an increased incidence of symptomatic ICH, treatment within 3 hours improved clinical outcome at 3 months.

ECASS—European Cooperative Acute Stroke Study Trials

In ECASS 1 trial, TPA dose of 1.1 mg/kg (maximum 100 mg) was used, of which 10% of the entire dose was used as bolus. This study showed that there was an increased risk of fatal parenchymal haemorrhage (30% vs. 6.5%) after IV thrombolysis administered within 6 hours (median time of 4 hours) of stroke onset. This unacceptably high risk of ICH may be attributed to various reasons such as: i. increased dose, ii. Increased therapeutic window, iii. Inclusion of large number (17%) of patients who already had unrecognized abnormality on pretreatment CT. This, however, did not statistically affect significant outcome.[51]

The ECASS 2 trial also did not confirm a statistical benefit for IV Alteplase. A dose of 0.95 mg/kg, administered within 6 hours of stroke onset was found to be as safe as that administered within 3 hours. No statistical benefit could be confirmed when compared with a placebo. The extent of hypodensity was found to be a major risk factor for severe hemorrhagic transformation. The ECASS 3 trial demonstrated benefit of IV Alteplase beyond the three hour window that was established in the NINDS trialand extended it upto 4.5 hours.[51]

The 2018 AHA guidelines for the early management of patients with acute ischemic stroke recommend that IV Alteplase (0.9 mg/kg, maximum dose 90 mg over 60 minutes with initial 10% of dose given as bolus over 1 minute) may be given to selected patients who can be treated within 4.5 hours of ischemic stroke symptom onset. Intravenous therapy should be started as soon as possible. Patients who are eligible for IV Alteplase should receive the drug even if endovascular treatment is being considered.[52]

Intra-arterial Therapy

Endovascular treatment for acute stroke includes mechanical thrombectomy or fibrinolysis. The intra arterial route allows the neuro interventionist to extend the time window available for treatment of acute stroke and to target the large thrombi in the affected vessel directly.

The initial PROACT 1 and 2 trials evaluated the role if intra-arterial recombinant pro-urokinase in patients with acute ischemic stroke of less than 6 hours duration caused by middle cerebral artery occlusion. In the PROACT 1 trial patients with TIMI grade 0 or 1 with occlusion of M1/M2 were included. Recanalization efficacy was assessed at the end of 2 hours infusion and ICH causing neurological deterioration was assessed at 24 hours. Recanalization rates were 58% (partial or complete) vs. 14% for placebo and this difference was significant. Hemorrhagic transformation causing neurological deterioration within 24 hours of treatment was seen in 15.4% in r-proUK group and 7.1% of the placebo arm. Both recanalization and hemorrhage frequencies were influenced by heparin dose. However, neurological outcome was not significant.[53] Similarly, the results of the PROACT 2 trial also showed that arterial recanalization was achieved in 66% of patients who received recombinant prourokinase. Despite an increased risk of early intracerebral hemorrhage in the patients who received recombinant prourokinase (27.8% vs. 5.5% within 24 hours), 90 days mortality rates were not significantly different between the two groups (24% r-proUK vs. 27% control). This was the first randomised acute stroke trial to show a benefit of therapy as long as 6 hours after the onset of stroke.[54] Subsequently, first generation mechanical thrombectomy devices like the Merci retriever and the Penumbra aspiration system were introduced for mechanical thrombectomy. The initial multicenter prospective randomized controlled trials, including IMS 3, MR RESCUE and SYNTHESIS expansion evaluated intra-arterial fibrinolysis with or without first generation embolectomy devices. These failed to demonstrate benefit from endovascular intervention over IV Alteplase. However, there were various drawback and reservations regarding these trials. The imaging of patients enrolled in these trials was not adequate. Also, these studies suffered from a lack of proper selection of patients in the interventional arm. The newer thrombectomy devices were used in only a minority of patients.[55]

MR CLEAN was first randomized trial to demonstrate the benefit of current endovascular therapy combined with medical management over medical management alone for patients suffering from acute anterior circulation ischemic stroke with proximal arterial occlusion that could be treated within a time window of 6 h after stroke onset. A total of 500 patients were included (intervention arm, n = 233; Standard care -IV alteplase, n = 267). Retrievable stents were utilized for 81.5% of the patients in the endovascular group. There was a difference of 13.5% in the rate of functional independence in favor of the intervention (32.6% vs. 19.1%). There were no significant differences in the occurrence of symptomatic intracerebral hemorrhage or mortality.[56]

The DAWN trial was a multicenter prospective open label blinded end point RCT that evaluated 206 patients. It evaluated patients treated between 6–24 hours after stroke. Clinical imaging mismatch was used as the eligibility criteria in selection of patients for mechanical thrombectomy. This trial was stopped early at the first interim analysis. It demonstrated a benefit in functional outcome in the treatment group (mRS score 0–2, 49% versus 13%; adjusted difference, 33%; 95% CI, 21–44; posterior probability of superiority >0.999). This was the first RCT that gave evidence supporting mechanical thrombectomy after 6 hours in selected patients.[52]

The DIFFUSE 3 trial was randomized, multicenter and open-label. The outcome assessment was blinded. All those patients presenting 6–16 hours after symptom onset with remaining ischemic brain tissue that was not yet infarcted were included in the study. The inclusion criteria were proximal ICA or MCA occlusion, initial infarct size at presentation < 70 ml, and ratio of the penumbra volume to infarct volume on perfusion imaging of 1.8 or more. These patients were randomly assigned to thrombectomy with standard medical therapy or standard medical therapy alone. The trial was terminated early for efficacy after 182 patients had undergone randomization (92 to the endovascular-therapy group and 90 to the medical-therapy group). It was seen that the functional outcomes in patients who underwent endovascular management, as evaluated on the modified Rankin scale at 90 days, was better as compared to the medical therapy group. The mortality rate at 90 days was 14% in the endovascular-therapy group while the medical-therapy group had 26% mortality rate. There was no significant difference in the frequency of symptomatic intracranial hemorrhage between the two groups (7% and 4%, respectively). The frequency of serious adverse events (43% and 53%, respectively) was also similar. This trial underlined the importance of evaluating the penumbra/core mismatch using CT/MR perfusion imaging in patients who reach the hospital after 6 hours of stroke onset. It also expanded the criteria to identify patients who benefit from mechanical thrombectomy after 6 hours.[57]

As per the 2018 AHA guidelines for acute stroke Patients should receive mechanical thrombectomy if they meet all the following criteria: (1) prestroke mRS score should be between 0 to 1; (2) The occluding thrombus causing symptoms should involve the internal carotid artery or MCA (M1 segment); (3) age ≥18 years; (4) NIHSS score greater than or equal to 6; (5) ASPECTS greater than or equal to 6; and (6) Groin puncture for endovascular thrombectomy can be performed within 6 hours of stroke onset.[52]

There are no clear guidelines for endovascular management in posterior circulation stroke. Mechanical thrombectomy may be performed for basilar artery occlusion up to 12–24 hours after symptom onset, however a recent analysis of the Basilar Artery International Cooperation Study registry found that severe strokes at presentation treated beyond 9 hours after onset had poor clinical outcome.[58]

Technique

Access is made through a 6-F/8-F sheath. An initial angiogram is performed to assess exact location of occlusion and to assess hemodynamics of cerebral perfusion. Heparin is given in a bolus dose of 5,000 U followed by 1,000 U/hr for 2 hours or until the end of the procedure. A guide catheter is introduced into the affected internal carotid artery. Subsequently, a microcather is advanced into the occluded middle cerebral artery over a 0.14 microguide wire. Both microcatheter and microwire must be navigated across the site of occlusion. A stent retriever is then deployed at the site of the thrombus. This is a cylindrical self-expanding non-detachable stent that is mounted on a wire and deployed via the microcatheter. Once the stent is delivered into the vessel it self-expands within the thrombus pushing the clot against the wall of the artery, reestablishing blood flow to the brain. The stent is kept deployed for a few minutes, thus allowing it to ensnare the thrombus within its tines. The stent, microcatheter and the ensnared thrombus are then pulled out of the vessel while simultaneously aspirating with a 50-cc syringe through the guide catheter **(Figs. 19A to D)**.

Aspiration of the clot may also be performed using the penumbra device. This is a trackable reperfusion catheter with a large inner lumen that is deployed at the surface of the thrombus. A suction pump is used to generate negative pressure that allows the thrombus to be digested.

Various complications like sICH, SAH, IVH, vessel dissection, non-target emboli, vasospasm and stent dislocation may occur during mechanical thrombectomy.[59]

Acute Stroke Imaging Protocol (Flowchart 1)

Based on the experience at our institution and several others in the world, we recommend that whenever acute stroke patients arrive to the hospital within the first 6 hours after onset of symptoms, they undergo an unenhanced CT. If NCCT depicts hemorrhage, no thrombolytic therapy is offered. If the CT shows signs of hyperacute infarct or is normal, a CT angiography of the head and neck to identify the site arterial occlusion. Those patients who present within 4.5 hours after the onset of acute stroke are given IV TPA if there are no contraindications for the same. If a large vessel occlusion is seen (ICA, M1 MCA, A1 ACA) on CT angiography the patient is taken up for mechanical thrombectomy. CT/MR perfusion may be performed in patients who are outside the 6-hour time window or in patients presenting with wake up stroke. Such patients may be offered mechanical thrombectomy if significant penumbra is seen on perfusion imaging.

VASCULOPATHIES

Atherosclerotic Vascular Disease (ASVD)

In presence of identifiable risk factors, ischemic stroke in a large number of patients is assumed to be secondary to ASVD. The role of imaging in this group of patients is to identify those patients who can be expected to benefit

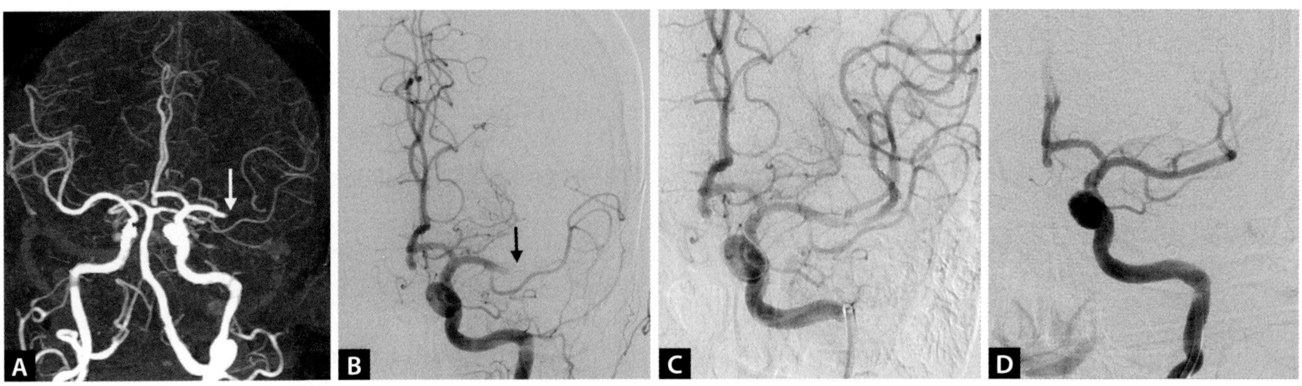

Figs. 19A to D: (A) A 55-year-old patient presented with right hemiparesis of 3 hours duration. CTA (A) and DSA; (B) revealed acute thrombus in left MCA M1 segment (arrows). Stent retriever was deployed; (C) and a single pass was taken. Post-procedure DSA; (D) revealed removal of the thrombus with good forward flow.

Flowchart 1: Acute stroke management protocol.

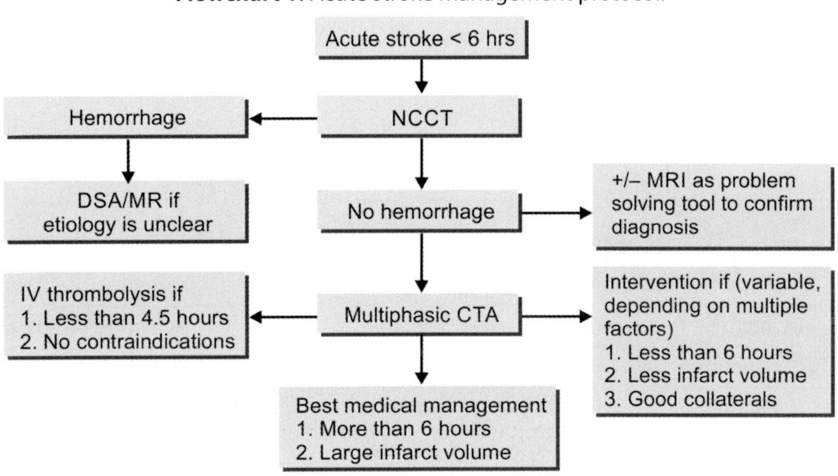

from intervention by reduction of future risk of stroke. On the basis of trials done so far, this group includes patients with nondisabling stroke in the anterior circulation with >70% stenosis and asymptomatic patients with >80% stenosis according to NASCET technique of stenosis measurement.[43-45] The initial screening is done by a noninvasive techniques, i.e. ultrasound, CTA or MRA. In view of its operator dependence of US, we feel that CTA/MRA should be the initial imaging modalities. Mural calcification, luminal irregularity, vessel stenosis, occlusion and thrombosis may be seen on CTA. Smooth plaques on CTA with extensive coalescent calcification are associated with decreased risk of rupture. A lipid rich core may be seen in larger plaques as subintimal hypodensity. High density subintimal foci are indicative of intra plaque haemorrhage. Both these findings represent an increased risk of plaque rupture. CTA may also reveal ulcerations in the form of contrast filled outpouchings. High resolution MRI can also be used to characterize plaque morphology. Hyperintense signal within the plaque on T1-weighted fat suppressed images represents hemorrhage. Marginal enhancement may occur around the plaque due to neo vascularity and is suggestive of an "at risk"plaque.[41] The MRI imaging appearance of plaque components is given in **Table 4**. Catheter angiography is a useful problem solving tool for confirmation of stenosis, evaluation of intracranial stenocclusive disease, ruling out any tandem lesions and to evaluate the hemodynamics in a patient.[41] Carotid artery stenting/carotid end arterectomy may be performed in selected patients who have significant stenosis at the carotid bifurcation.

Arterial Dissection

Dissection of the internal carotid artery is an important cause of stroke in young patients, responsible for up to 20% of all cases of stroke in young.[61] As a whole, arterial dissection is the cause of stroke in about 3% of all cases. It may be spontaneous or may occur secondary to blunt or penetrating trauma to the vessel. Catheter angiography has been traditionally used for the diagnosis of carotid dissection. Typical findings on angiogram include long segment tapering/narrowing of the cervical ICA extending from just beyond the carotid bulb up to the base of skull.[41] With the development of CTA, MRI and MRA, it is now possible to diagnose arterial dissection noninvasively **(Figs. 20A to C)**.[41,62] Apart from demonstrating luminal changes; wall hematoma can also be directly visualized. Associated pseudoaneurysms, if present, can also be visualized. Catheter angiography is needed only if any additional information is required **(Figs. 20A to F)**.

Aortoarteritis

Aortoarteritis is an important cause of stroke in young and middle-aged female patients in India. Clue to the diagnosis is usually evident in the form of differential limb pulses/blood pressures or hypertension due to renal artery involvement. Catheter angiography is invariably required for complete assessment in these patients as multiple vascular systems are usually involved. By virtue of its ability to visualize arterial wall, ultrasound serves as an excellent modality to document carotid arterial wall thickness and monitor response to medical therapy.

Fibromuscular Dysplasia

This is a non atherosclerotic, non inflammatory arteriopathy affecting medium and large size vessels. It is more common in females and occurs between 20–40 years of age. String of beads appearance, smooth long segment tubular narrowing or asymmetrical diverticulum like outpouchings may be seen.[41] Earlier catheter angiography **(Fig. 21)** was the investigation of choice for diagnosis of FMD for two reasons. One is that due to irregular areas of stenosis and dilatation seen in most cases of FMD, the flow pattern in the vessels is complex.[61] Secondly, FMD is known to be associated with intracranial aneurysms in up to 21-51% of cases. However, current generation

Table 4: MR classification of plaque components.[60]

		T1-weighted	*T2-weighted*	*Proton density–weighted*	*STIR*	*Contrast-enhanced T1-weighted*
Lipid-rich necrotic core		Iso/hyperintense	Iso/hypointense	Iso/hyperintense	Hypointense	Hypointense
Fibrous tissue		Isointense	Isointense	Isointense	Hyperintense	Hyperintense
Hemorrhage	Fresh	Hyperintense	Hypointense	Hypointense	Hypointense	Isointense
	Recent	Hyperintense	Hyperintense	Hyperintense	Hyperintense	Isointense
Calcification		Hypointense	Hypointense	Hypointense	Hypointense	Hypointense

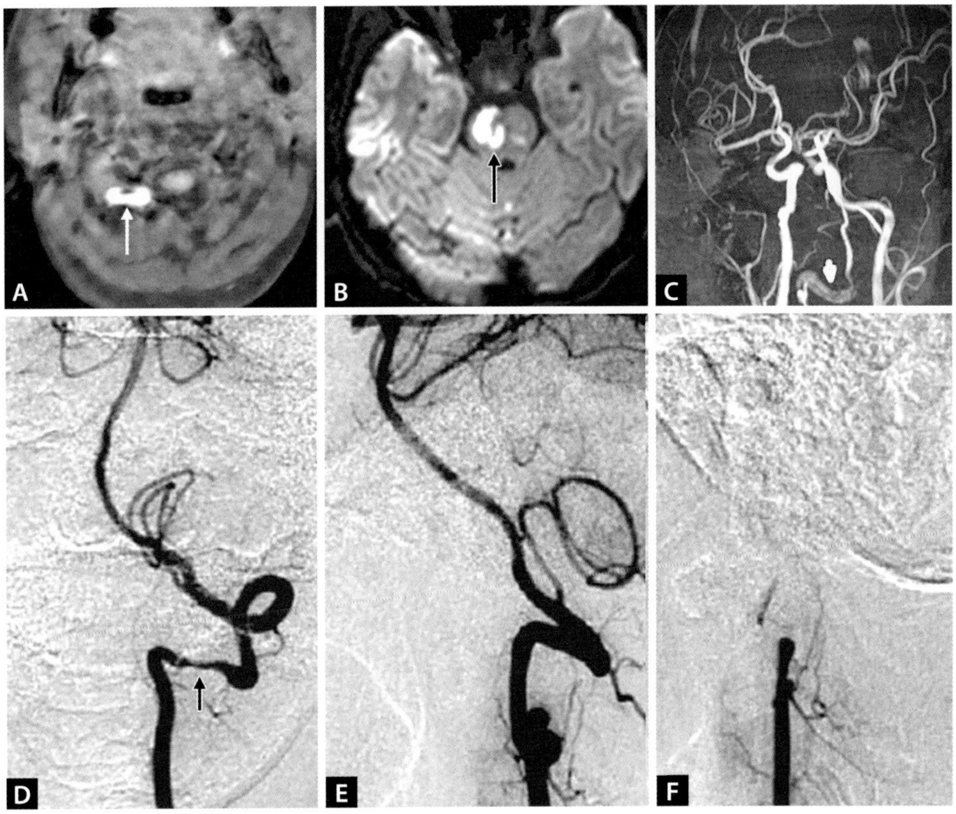

Figs. 20A to F: Axial T1 (A), Diffusion (B) and 3D MIP TOF (C) images in a case of right vertebral artery dissection show an eccentric hyperntense hematoma within the vessel wall (arrow, A) with pontine infarct (arrow, B). The right V3 segment shows loss of normal flow related signal (small arrow, C). The hyperintensity seen on TOF images in the right V3 segment is due to hematoma in the dissected segment. Left vertebral artery injection in AP (D), lateral flexion (E) and extension (F) in another patient show left vertebral irregularity and narrowing that is suggestive of dissection (arrow, D). The vessel is patent on flexion however, complete occlusion is noted on extension of neck.

CTA enables the radiologist to accurately diagnose FMD in cervicocephalic arteries and can also evaluate the intracranial circulation for aneurysms.[41]

Other Vasculopathies

This is an important, though uncommon, heterogeneous group of conditions, which can present with ischemic or hemorrhagic stroke. The diagnosis may be suggested by the related clinical features, e.g. stroke in young, stroke in the setting of disorders known to cause vasculitis or features suggestive of involvement of other organ systems, e.g. skin, kidneys, etc. Vascular imaging in these patients is needed to reach the diagnosis, to suggest areas suitable for biopsy, and to monitor response to treatment. Catheter angiography is most invariably required to assess the intracranial circulation. Sometimes, however, MRI and MRA may provide sufficient information needed for diagnosis, e.g. in Moya Moya disease particularly in the very young.

RECANALIZATION STRATEGIES IN ATHEROSCLEROTIC VESSEL DISEASE

Carotid Artery Stenting

Carotid artery stenting (CAS) is a minimally invasive procedure for management of carotid artery stenosis. The technique utilized in the North American Symptomatic Carotid Endarterectomy Trial is recommended for the analysis of stenosis. In this, the diameter at narrowest site in the stenotic segment is referenced to the most normal diameter immediately cephalad to the stenosis and not below.[63] The Stenting and Angioplasty with Protection in Patients at High Risk for Endarterectomy trial conducted in North America, favored CAS over CEA in a non-inferiority analysis. There was no difference between the long-term results at the end of 3 years between the CAS and CEA groups. However, this study has been criticized as it was terminated prematurely and most of the patients were asymptomatic. Later, 3 large randomized trials reported results favoring CEA over CAS. These were Stent-Protected

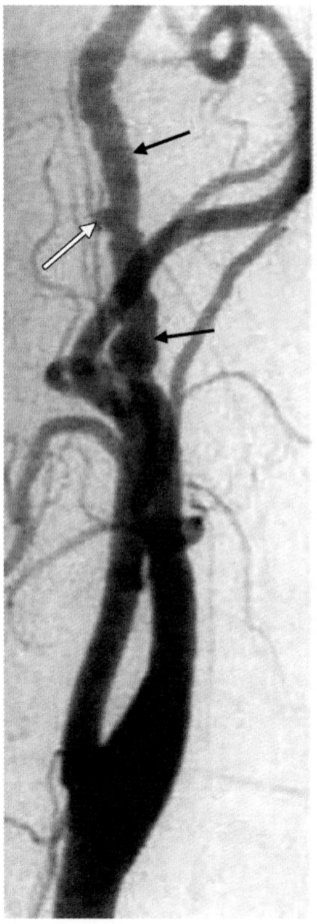

Fig. 21: Case of fibromuscular dysplasia (FMD) showing the string of beads appearance (arrows).

Angioplasty versus Carotid Endarterectomy (SPACE), Endarterectomy versus Angioplasty in Patients with Symptomatic Severe Carotid Stenosis (ECASS) and the International Carotid Stenting Study (ICSS). The SPACE trial was terminated prematurely as evidence of a significantly higher rate of death or stroke was seen in CAS patients as compared to CEA at 30 days. In the ICSS the rate of stroke, MI or death at 4 months was notably higher in CAS. However, these results showing inferior efficacy of stenting as compared with CEA are considered inconclusive due to certain pitfalls for e.g. EPDs were not required; there was variation in the sort of stent used. Also, dual antiplatelet therapy for CAS was not mandatory in these trials. The Carotid Revascularization Endarterectomy versus Stenting Trial (CREST), a multicenter, randomized trial included 2,502 patients. Both symptomatic and asymptomatic patients were enrolled in this study and assigned to either CAS or CEA. Only one stent type was used in all patients; embolus protection device was compulsory whenever technically feasible and antiplatelet therapy was given in all patients. The treating physicians were strictly evaluated and trained during in the lead-in phase. While evaluating the results significant difference was found between CAS and CEA in the rates of primary end point (p = 0.51). It was noticed that rate of stroke during the procedure was higher in the CAS (p = 0.01). On the other hand MI was more common during CEA (p = 0.03). Women, symptomatic patients and age more than 65 years were found to be associated with higher stroke and death rates in the stenting.[63,64]

Table 5: Indications for CAS over CEA.

• Recent history of acute coronary syndrome, cardiac failure or severe left ventricular systolic dysfunction, Myocardial infarction or history of myocardial infarction within the last 6 weeks, severe coronary artery stenotic lesions requiring revascularization
• Severe pulmonary dysfunction
• Recurrent lesions following carotid endarterectomy
• Complete occlusion of the contralateral carotid artery
• History of previous radiation therapy, radical neck surgery, tracheostomy
• Thick, short neck due to obesity or Inability to tilt the head backward
• Paralysis of the laryngeal nerve
• Common carotid bifurcation located in the upper part of the neck (at the level of cervical vertebrae 2–3)
• Lesion is located at the origin or proximal part of the common carotid artery
• Distal internal carotid artery stenosis
• Separated tandem lesions
• Carotid dissection

Best medical management is an essential for treatment for all patients suffering from carotid stenosis. The 2011 American College of Cardiology and American Heart Association (AHA) guideline recommended CAS as an alternative to CEA in average-surgical-risk symptomatic patients when the anticipated risk of periprocedural stroke or mortality is <6% (Class I, B). They preferred CAS to CEA when carotid lesions were anatomically unfavorable (Class IIa, B). They also recommended that CAS may be considered in highly selected asymptomatic patients with ≥60% angiographic stenosis (Class IIb,B). Indications for CAS over CEA are given in **Table 5**.

Contraindications for CAS include unfavorable aortic arch anatomy or a heavily calcified aortic arch or a type 3 aortic arch. Other relative contraindications for which carotid end arterectomy may be preferred include lipid-rich soft plaque, Intraplaque hemorrhage, extensive plaque (>15 mm in length), heavily calcified plaque, thin fibrous cap, a lesion located at a curve or history of severe allergic reaction to iodinated contrast.

Preparation

CAS is generally performed under local anesthesia via trans-femoral route. Sedation is avoided. If general anesthesia is employed, use of intraoperative EEG/brain mapping should be considered. CAS can cause dramatic changes in the patient's hemodynamics, leading to hypotension or bradycardia. Vasoactive medications must be available to treat any hemodynamically significant changes. An arterial line should be placed for invasive hemodynamic monitoring during the procedure. Patients should be on aspirin 150 mg and clopidogrel 150 mg OD for a period of at least 3 to 4 days preoperatively, and these should be continued in the postoperative period. If adequate pretreatment time is not available 300 mg Aspirin + 300 mg Clopidogrel may be administered 2 h prior to CAS. Full sterile precautions should be maintained throughout the procedure as with any invasive procedure.

Technique

The common femoral artery is punctured via the percutaneous route using the Seldinger technique. A short sheath (8F) is then placed over a 0.035 in the wire. Intravenous heparin (70–100 U/kg) is instilled. The Activated clotting time is kept between 250 and 300 seconds. Using an angled catheter with 0.35" guidewire, the common carotid artery is selectively cannulated and mapped. The guidewire is then advanced into the external carotid artery followed by advancement of the catheter into the external carotid artery. Over an exchange length guidewire, a 90 cm shuttle is advanced into the common carotid artery. Dedicated carotid arteriograms are performed in multiple views to identify the lesion. A 0.014 in wire should be used to traverse the lesion. An embolic protection device may be deployed at this point in the straight terminal segment of the ICA . This is followed by pre-dilation using a small profile balloon if the stenosis is severe **(Figs. 22A to C)**. Careful attention must be paid to the patient's hemodynamics during this maneuver. Subsequently an appropriately sized stent is deployed. A self-expanding stainless-steel or nitinol stent is preferred for the carotid artery. Nitinol stents do not undergo foreshortening. They are more flexible and they match the target vessel curvature better as compared to other stents. The length of stent to be utilised depends on the length of the lesion. Usually 20–40 mm length is used. The stent should cover 5 to 10 mm distal and proximal to the area of narrowing. As most carotid stenosis involve the carotid bulb and the proximal ICA, the stent has to be deployed from the ICA into the distal CCA. While sizing the stent a stent-to-artery ratio of 1.1:1 to 1.4:1 for the ICA is considered. For patients with a large size-mismatch between the ICA and CCA, tapered stents can be used. If there is significant residual stenosis after deployment of the stent (> 30%), balloon angioplasty may be performed **(Figs. 23A to C)**. The carotid sinus reflex may get activated during post-dilatation, occasionally requiring intravenous atropine or dopamine, depending on the patient's hemodynamic status. Finally, the EPD, if deployed, is removed followed by carotid and a cerebral angiography and removal of catheters and sheaths if the result is satisfactory.

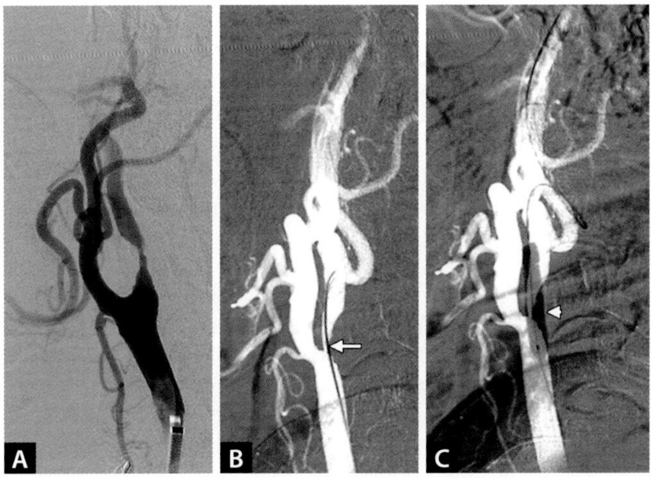

Figs. 22A to C: DSA image (A) showing severe ICA stenosis. The stenotic site was crossed by an 0.014 micro guidewire (B, arrow)) and predilatation was performed (C, arrowhead).

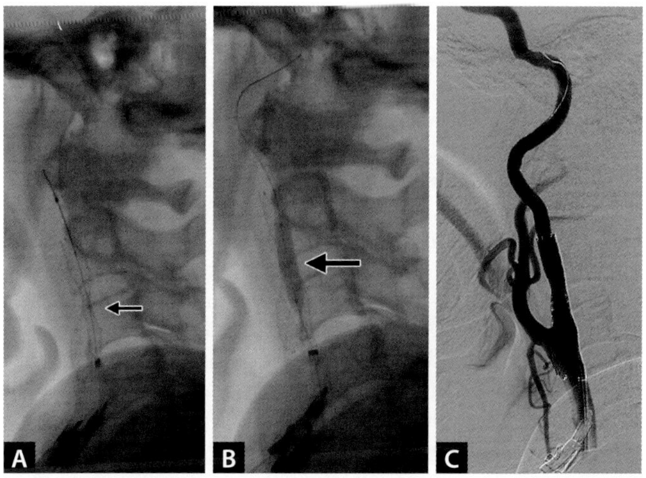

Figs. 23A to C: Fluoroscopy images. (A and B) showing stent deployment (thin arrow) and post-stent balloon dilatation (thick arrow). Check DSA (C) reveals normal opening of the stent with good forward flow.

Complications

Complications related to femoral artery access including bleeding, perforation, dissection, thrombosis, and distal embolization may occur. The stent may not deploy properly and can be associated with fracture.

CONCLUSION

CAS has evolved significantly over the past 2 decades. Large studies have shown that CAS, is a safe option for management of carotid artery stenosis in experienced hands. In certain high-risk patients, CAS is already recommended above CEA. Further improvement in technique and hardware, will lead to reduction of perioperative stroke rate. This will enable the CAS to become the standard of care for all patients.

REFERENCES

1. Bell BA, Symon L, Branston NM. CBF and time thresholds for the formation of ischemic cerebral edema, and effect of reperfusion in baboons. J Neurosurg. 1985 ;62(1):31-41.
2. Markus H. Cerebral perfusion and stroke. J Neurol Neurosurg Psychiatry. 2004;75(3):353-61.
3. Ter Panning B. Pathophysiology of stroke. Neuroimag Clin North Am. 1992;2:389-408.
4. Deb P, Sharma S, Hassan KM. Pathophysiologic mechanisms of acute ischemic stroke: An overview with emphasis on therapeutic significance beyond thrombolysis. Pathophysiology. 2010;17(3):197-218.
5. Taveras JM. Brain vascular disorders. Neuroradiology, 3rd edn. Taveras JM, editor. Maryland: William and Wilkins; 1996.
6. Sage MR. Blood brain barrier: Phenomenon of increasing importance to the imaging clinician. AJR. 1982;138:887-98.
7. DiChiro G, Timins EL, Jones AE. Radionuclide scanning and microangiography of evolving and complete brain infarctions. Neurology. 1974;24:418-23.
8. Einsiedel-Lechtape H, Kleihues P. Pathology of cerebral vascular insufficiency. In: Newton TH, Potts DG, (Eds). Radiology of the skull and brain: Anatomy and pathology. St. Louis: The CV Mosby Co; 1977.
9. Astrup J, Siesjo BK, Symon L. Thresholds in cerebral ischemia:The ischaemic penumbra. Stroke. 1981;12:723–5.
10. Hossmann KA. Viability thresholds and the penumbra of focal ischemia. Ann Neurol. 1994;36:557-65.
11. Osborn A, hedlund G. Arterial anatomy and strokes. In: Brain imaging, pathology and anatomy, 2nd edn. Philadelphia: Elsevier; 2018. pp. 197-252.
12. Rowley HA. The four Ps of acute stroke imaging; parenchyma, pipes, perfusion, and penumbra. AJNR. 2001;22:500-601.
13. Tomandi BF, Klotz E, Handschu R. Comprehensive imaging of ischemic stroke with multisection CT. Radiographics. 2003;23:565-92.
14. Tomura N, Uemura K, Inugami A. CT findings in cerebral ischemia: Obscuration of the lentiform nucleus. Radiology. 1988;168:463-7.
15. Truwit CL, Barkovich AJ, Gean A. Loss of insular ribbon: Another CT sign of acute middle cerebral artery infarction. Radiology. 1990;178:801-6.
16. Leys D, Pruvo JP, Godefroy O. Prevalence and significance of hyperdense middle cerebral artery in acute stroke. Stroke. 1992. 317-24 p.
17. Tomsick T, Brott T, Barsan W. Thrombus localization with emergency cerebral CT. AJNR. 1992;13(1);257-63.
18. Srinivasan A, Goyal M, Azri FA, Lum C. State-of-the-Art Imaging of Acute Stroke. RadioGraphics. 2006; 26(suppl_1):S75-95.
19. Pexman JH, Barber PA, Hill MD, et al. Use of the Alberta Stroke Program Early CT Score (ASPECTS) for assessing CT scans in patients with acute stroke. Am J Neuroradiol. 2001;22(8):1534-42.
20. Leclerc X, Godefroy O, Provo JP. Computed tomography angiography for the evaluation of carotid artery stenosis. Stroke. 1995;26:1577.
21. Treurniet KM, Yoo AJ, Berkhemer OA, et al. Clot Burden Score on Baseline Computerized Tomographic Angiography and Intra-Arterial Treatment Effect in Acute Ischemic Stroke. Stroke. 2016;47(12):2972-8.
22. Bouchez L, Sztajzel R, Vargas MI, et al. CT imaging selection in acute stroke. Eur J Radiol. 2017;96:153-61.
23. Seker F, Potreck A, Möhlenbruch M, et al. Comparison of four different collateral scores in acute ischemic stroke by CT angiography. J NeuroInterventional Surg. 2016;8(11):1116-8.
24. Jauch EC, Saver JL, Adams HP, et al. Guidelines for the Early Management of Patients With Acute Ischemic Stroke: A Guideline for Healthcare Professionals From the American Heart Association/American Stroke Association. Stroke. 2013;44(3):870-947.
25. Hoeffner EG, Case I, Jain R. Cerebral perfusion CT: Technique and clinical applications. Radiology. 2004;231:632-44.
26. Bryan RN, Levy LM, Whitlow WD. Diagnosis of acute cerebral infarction: Comparison of CT and MR imaging. AJNR. 1991;12(4);611-20.
27. Simonsen CZ, Madsen MH, Schmitz ML, et al. Sensitivity of diffusion-and perfusion-weighted imaging for diagnosing acute ischemic stroke is 97.5%. Stroke. 2015;46(1):98-101.
28. Allen LM, Hasso AN, Handwerker J, et al. Sequence-specific MR Imaging Findings That Are Useful in Dating Ischemic Stroke. RadioGraphics. 2012;32(5):1285-97.
29. Vilela P, Rowley HA. Brain ischemia: CT and MRI techniques in acute ischemic stroke. Eur J Radiol. 2017;96:162-72.
30. Mathews VP, Whitlow WE, Bryan RN. Cerebral ischemia and infarction. In: Atlas SW, editor. 2nd edn. Philadelphia: Lippincott-Raven Publishers; 1996.
31. Powers WJ, Derdeyn CP, Biller J, et al. 2015 American Heart Association/American Stroke Association Focused Update of the 2013 Guidelines for the Early Management of Patients With Acute Ischemic Stroke Regarding Endovascular

Treatment: A Guideline for Healthcare Professionals From the American Heart Association/American Stroke Association. Stroke. 2015;46(10):3020-35.
32. Bash S, Villablanca JP, Jahan R, et al. Intracranial vascular stenosis and occlusive disease: evaluation with CT angiography, MR angiography, and digital subtraction angiography. Am J Neuroradiol. 2005;26(5):1012-21.
33. Mittl RL, Broderick M, Carpenter J P, et al. Blinded reader comparison of MRA and duplex sonography for carotid artery bifurcation stenosis. Stroke. 1994;25:4-10.
34. North American Symptomatic Carotid Endarterectomy Trial: methods, patient characteristics, and progress. Stroke 1991;22:711-20.
35. Pryor JC, Setton A, Nelson PK, et al. Complications of diagnostic cerebral angiography and tips on avoidance. Neuroimaging Clin N Am. 1996. 6(3):751-8.
36. Polak JF, O'Leary DH, Kronmal RA. Sonographic evaluation of carotid artery atherosclerosis in the elderly. Relationship of disease severity to stroke and transient ischemic attack. Radiology. 1973;188:363-70.
37. Provenzale JM, Jahan R, Naidich TP, et al. Assessment of the patient with hyperacute stroke: Imaging and therapy. Radiology. 2003;229:347-59.
38. Merritt CRB, El B. The future of carotid sonography. AJR. 1992;158:37-9.
39. Steinke W, Hennerice M, Rautenberg W. Symptomatic and asymptomatic high grade carotid stenosis in Doppler color flow imaging. Neurology. 1992;42(1):131-8.
40. Moneta GL, Edwards JM, Chitwood RW. Correlation of NASCET angiographic definition of 70 to 99 percent ICA stenosis with duplex scanning. J Vasc Surg. 1993; 17(1):152-7.
41. Osborn A. Vasculopathy. In: Brain imaging, pathology and anatomy. 2nd ed. Philadelphia: Elsevier; 2018. pp. 277-326.
42. Frught WE, Mattes MA, Van Bemmelen PS. Color flow duplex scanning of carotid arteries. New velocity criteria based on ROC analysis for threshold stenosis used in the symptomatic and asymptomatic carotid trials. J Vasc Surg. 1994;19(5):818-27.
43. Neale ML, Chambers JL, Kelly AJ. Reappraisal of duplex criteria to assess significant carotid stenosis with special reference to reports from NASCET and ESCT. J Vasc Surg. 1994;20:642.
44. Patel MR, Kuntz KM, Klufas RA. Pre-operative assessment of the carotid bifurcation. Can MRA and duplex ultrasonography replace contrast angiography. Stroke. 1995;26(10):1753-8.
45. Kent KC, Kuntz KM, Patel MR. Operative imaging strategies for carotid endarterectomy. An analysis of morbidity and cost effectivenss in symptomatic patients. JAMA. 1995;274:888.
46. Rosovsky MA, Litt AW, Krinsky G. Magnetic resonance carotid angiography of the neck: Clinical implication. Neuroimaging Clin N Am. 1996;6(4):863-74.
47. Tahmasebpour HR, Buckley AR, Cooperberg PL, Fix CH. Sonographic Examination of the Carotid Arteries. RadioGraphics. 2005;25(6):1561-75.
48. Cumming MJ, Marrow IM. Carotid artery stenosis: A prospective comparison of CT angiography and conventional angiography. AJR. 1994;163-517.
49. National Institute of Neurological Disorders and Stroke rt-PA Stroke Study Group. Tissue plasminogen activator for acute ischemic stroke. N Engl J Med. 1995;333(24):1581-7.
50. Del Zoppo GJ, Higashida RT, Furlan AJ. PROACT: A phase II randomized trial of recombinant pro-urokinase by direct arterial delivery in acute middle cerebral artery stroke. Stroke. 1998;29:4-11.
51. Hacke W, Kaste M, Fieschi C, et al. Randomised double-blind placebo-controlled trial of thrombolytic therapy with intravenous alteplase in acute ischaemic stroke (ECASS II). The Lancet. 1998;352(9136):1245-51.
52. Powers WJ, Rabinstein AA, Ackerson T, et al. 2018 Guidelines for the Early Management of Patients With Acute Ischemic Stroke: A Guideline for Healthcare Professionals From the American Heart Association/American Stroke Association. Stroke. 2018 Jan 1;STR.0000000000000158.
53. Zeumer H, Freitag H-J, Zanella F, et al. Local intraarterial fibrinolytic therapy in patients with stroke: Urokinase versus recombinant tissue plasminogen activator (r-TPA). Neuroradiology. 1993;35:159-62.
54. Furlan A, Higashida R, Wechsler L, et al. Intra-arterial Prourokinase for acute ischemic stroke. JAMA. 1999; 282(21):2003-11.
55. Ding D. Endovascular Mechanical Thrombectomy for Acute Ischemic Stroke: A New Standard of Care. J Stroke. 2015;17(2):123.
56. Berkhemer OA, Fransen PSS, Beumer D, et al. A randomized trial of intraarterial treatment for acute ischemic stroke. N Engl J Med. 2015;372(1):11-20.
57. Albers GW, Marks MP, Kemp S, et al. Thrombectomy for Stroke at 6 to 16 Hours with Selection by Perfusion Imaging. N Engl J Med. 2018;0(0):null.
58. Lindsberg PJ, Pekkola J, Strbian D, et al. Time window for recanalization in basilar artery occlusion: Speculative synthesis. Neurology. 2015;85(20):1806-15.
59. Behme D, Gondecki L, Fiethen S, et al. Complications of mechanical thrombectomy for acute ischemic stroke—a retrospective single-center study of 176 consecutive cases. Neuroradiology. 2014;56(6):467-76.
60. Young VEL, Sadat U, Gillard JH. Noninvasive carotid artery imaging with a focus on the vulnerable plaque. Neuroimaging Clin N Am. 2011;21(2):391-405, xi–xii.
61. Provenzale JM. Dissection of the internal carotid and vertebral arteries: Imaging features. AJR. 1995;165:1099.
62. Willinsky R, TerBrugge K, Montanero W, et al. Micro-arteriovenous malformations of the brain: Superselective angiography in diagnosis and treatment. AJNR 1992;13(1):325-30.
63. Ahn SH, Prince EA, Dubel GJ. Carotid Artery Stenting: Review of Technique and Update of Recent Literature. Semin Interv Radiol. 2013;30(3):288-96.
64. Noiphithak R, Liengudom A. Recent Update on Carotid Endarterectomy versus Carotid Artery Stenting. Cerebrovasc Dis. 2017;43(1–2):68-75.

CHAPTER 9

Imaging of Subarachnoid Hemorrhage

Niranjan Khandelwal, Vivek Gupta

INTRODUCTION

Bleeding into the subarachnoid space is termed subarachnoid hemorrhage (SAH). It may be spontaneous or traumatic in onset, and may be trivial or massive in volume. Subarachnoid space can be the primary site of bleed or may be secondarily involved by extension of intracerebral hemorrhage (ICH). The causes of spontaneous SAH are:

- Ruptured intracranial aneurysms (75–80%)
- Arteriovenous malformations (AVMs) (5%)
- Cryptic vascular malformations (5–10%)
- Vasculitis
- Blood dyscrasias
- Primary and metastatic brain tumors (<2%)
- Spinal cord AVMs or tumors (<2%)
- Eclampsia (<2%)
- Anticoagulant therapy
- Unknown etiology (7–10%).

INCIDENCE

The incidence of SAH has been estimated to be about 10–28 per 100,000 person-years. However, some recent studies have found it to be much lower in the range of 6–8 per 100,000 person-years.[1] It carries a very high morbidity and mortality.[2,3] Ten percent of patients die before reaching the hospital. About 8% die from deterioration after the initial hemorrhage. Amongst the patients surviving the initial hemorrhage and treated without surgery, re-bleeding is the major cause of death in about 30–38% of cases. Vasospasm kills another 7% and causes severe deficit in another 7%.[2] The 30 days mortality rate for SAH is 46%.[4,5] It is further complicated by intracerebral hemorrhage (ICH) (20–40%), intraventricular hemorrhage (IVH) (15–35%) and subdural hemorrhage (SDH) (2–5%).

CLINICAL FEATURES

Sudden, severe "explosive" headache, vomiting, altered sensorium are common presentations. Usually the headache is described as "worst headache of the life". The usual age of presentation is 55–60 years; 20% of cases during sleep and 50% of patients have warning symptoms.[3] The risk factors are modifiable and non-modifiable. Among the latter group familial predisposition, presence of heritable connective tissue disorders like Ehler-Danlos disease, Autosomal dominant polycystic kidney disease (ADPKD) and Neurofibromatosis-I. Modifiable risk factors are hypertension, cigarette smoking, cocaine abuse, oral contraceptives, alcohol consumption, pregnancy, etc.[2-5]

GRADING SYSTEM OF SUBARACHNOID HEMORRHAGE

The clinical grading is important for estimating prognosis of SAH as well as to assess the operative risk. There are several grading systems and are listed in the Appendix.

DIAGNOSIS

- Lumbar puncture
- Computed tomography (CT)

- Magnetic resonance imaging (MRI)
- Conventional cerebral angiography
- CT angiography (CTA)
- Magnetic resonance angiography (MRA)
- Transcranial Doppler ultrasound.

Lumbar Puncture (LP)

Before the advent of CT, it was the only method to confirm the diagnosis of SAH. Presently, it is indicated only when CT is normal in patients with sudden, severe headache. There is risk of re-bleeding or neurological deterioration after LP and in two studies involving 165 patients with SAH, 17 (10%) patients experienced deterioration in their conditions within 24 hours of LP.[6,7] Opening pressure is usually elevated. Cerebrospinal fluid (CSF) is bloody not clearing with sequential tubes; Xanthochromia is present after 1–2 days of SAH. Presently with the availability of NCCT and MRI it is rare that a LP is required to establish the diagnosis of SAH.

Computed Tomography

Nonenhanced CT is the first step in the investigation of patients with suspected SAH. The probability of detecting hemorrhage is proportional to the clinical grade of the patient and the time after the hemorrhage. Three percent of 1553 patients had normal CT within 24 hours of confirmed SAH.[6] In a prospective series of 100 patients, SAH was detected in all patients within 48 hours of ictus, 85% after 5 days, 50% after one week, 30% after 2 weeks and almost nil after 3 weeks[8] **(Fig. 1A and B)**. Contrast enhanced CT helps in detecting the etiology of SAH, e.g. aneurysms (30–76%), AVMs (98–100%), tumors, etc. The volume and location of SAH on CT gives important prognostic information about vasospasm and outcome after the hemorrhage. In a prospective study, Fisher et al. reported a good correlation between the location and volume of blood and subsequent development of vasospasm. Increasing SAH on CT is associated with worsening clinical grade and poor outcome **(Table 1)**.[9]

CT is also helpful in detecting complications of SAH and surgery including ICH hydrocephalus and infarcts. CT can also predict aneurysm location and the side in more than 70% of cases.

- Bleed in interhemispheric fissure, frontal lobe or septum pellucidum indicates anterior communicating artery (ACoM) aneurysm **(Figs. 2A to C)**.
- Bleed in sylvian fissure or temporal lobe or interpeduncular cistern indicates posterior communicating artery (PCoM) aneurysm.
- Comma shaped bleed in sylvian fissure indicates MCA aneurysm.
- Bleed in interpeduncular cistern and/or brainstem suggests basilar top aneurysm **(Figs. 3A and B)**.

Magnetic Resonance Imaging

Conventional MRI (T1WI and T2WI) is not very sensitive in detecting SAH in acute stage (first 24–48 hours) in which situation CT is the preferred modality. FLAIR sequence has been found to be quite sensitive in detecting acute SAH. Since the application of inversion recovery pulse nulls the

Table 1: Modified Fisher grading scale and vasospasm (on CT).

Grade	*Features*	*Risk of vasospasm*
1.	Focal/diffuse thin SAH (<1mm)	24%
2.	Focal/diffuse thin SAH (<1mm) with IVH	33%
3.	Thick SAH (>1 mm)	33%
4.	Thick SAH (>1 mm) with IVH	40%

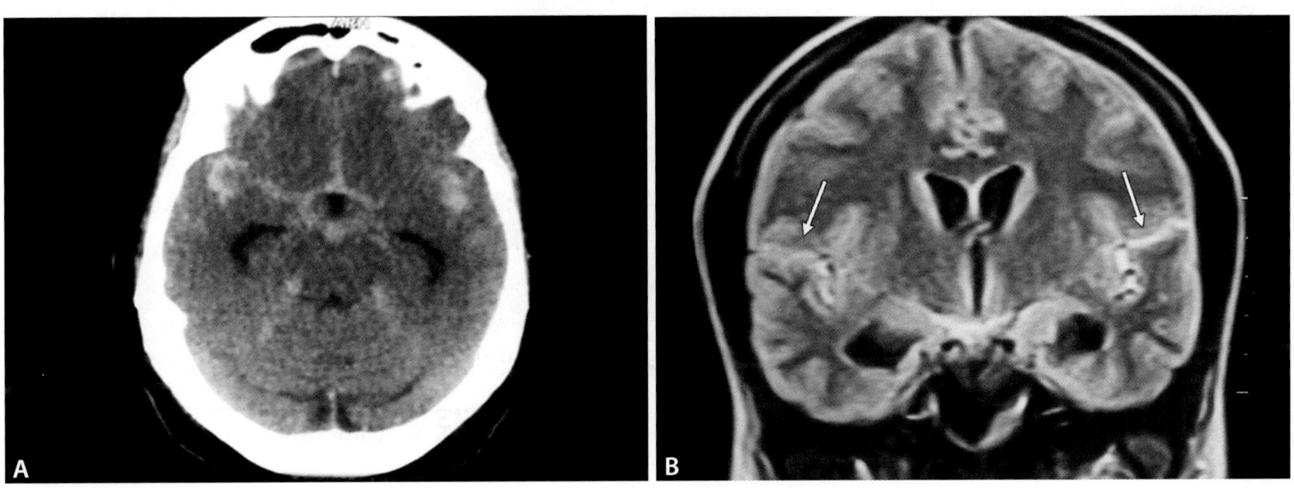

Figs. 1A and B: NCCT (A), and MRI–FLAIR (B), (different patients) showing acute subarachnoid hemorrhage (white arrows in B).

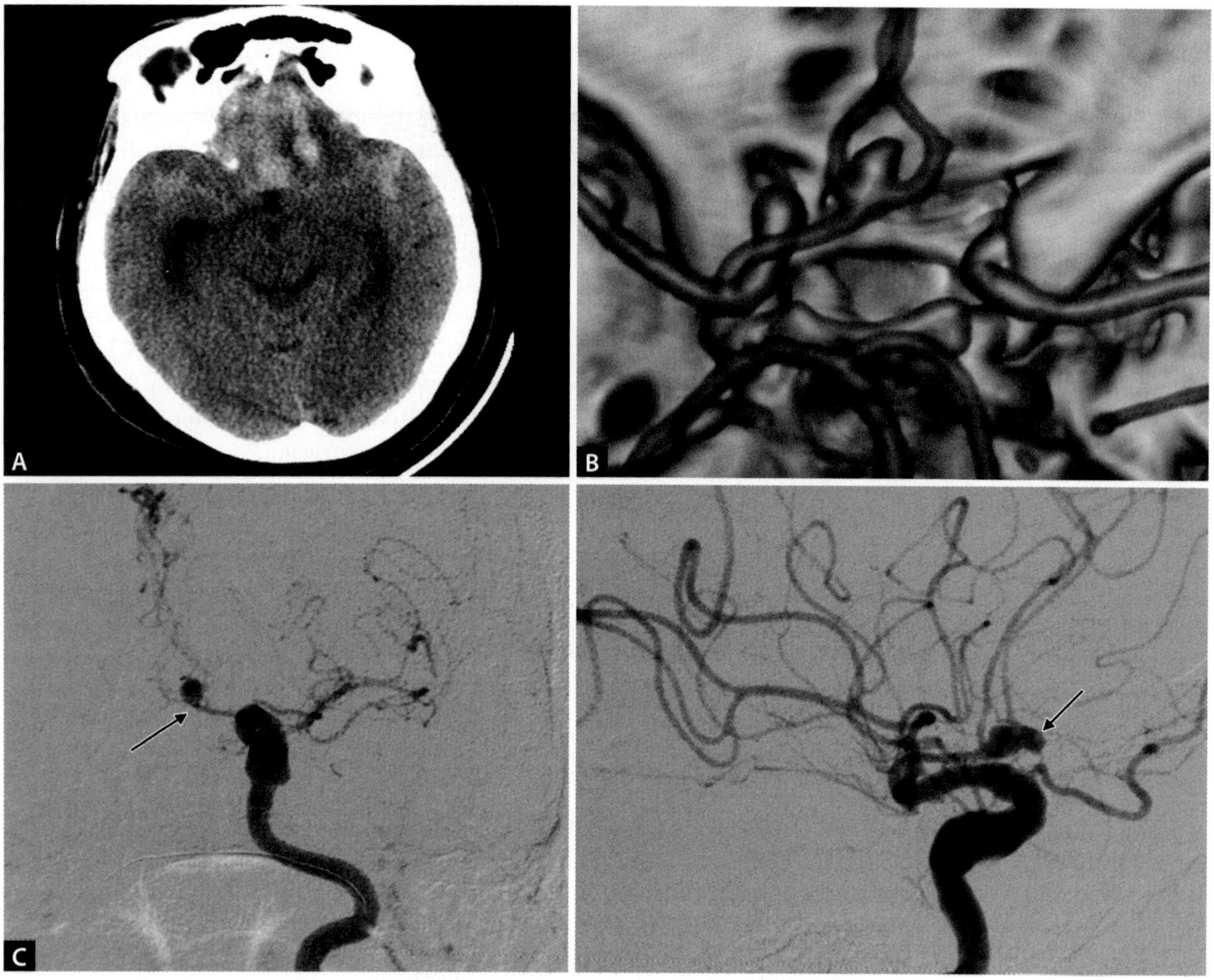

Figs. 2A to C: NCCT axial image shows hemorrhage in the anterior interhemispheric fissure (A) CT angiography VR image (B) and DSA AP and lateral views demonstrated anterior communicating aneurysm (arrows) (C).

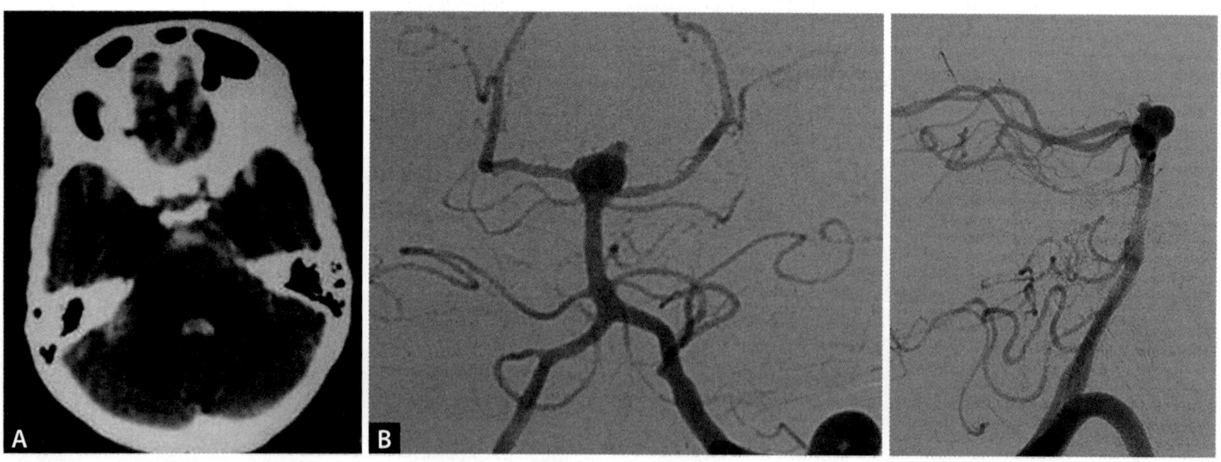

Figs. 3A and B: Acute hemorrhage in the prepontine and fourth ventricle (A) on NCCT due rupture of vertebrobasilar aneurysm (B).

signal of CSF on T2 weighted sequence the blood in the subarachnoid space can be seen with a high sensitivity **(Figs. 4A and B)**.[10]

However, with elapsing time in subacute and chronic SAH, MRI is the best modality (>after 48 hours to over 1 month) and can detect hemorrhage even when CSF

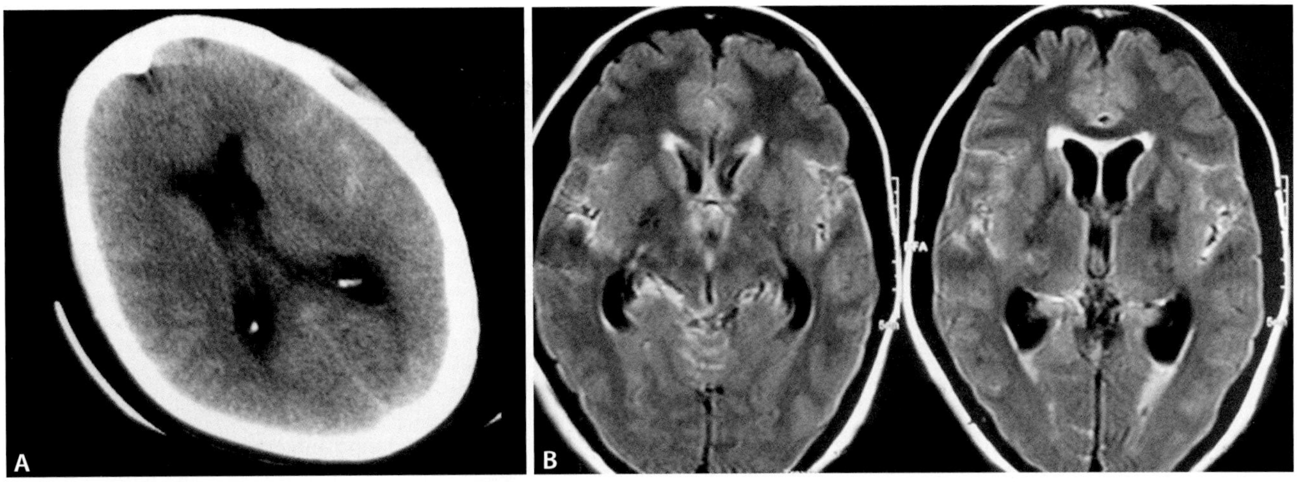

Figs. 4A and B: NCCT (A) and FLAIR (B) images to show subarachnoid bleed in bilateral Sylvian fissures (the acute hemorrhage appears hyperintense on FLAIR imaging).

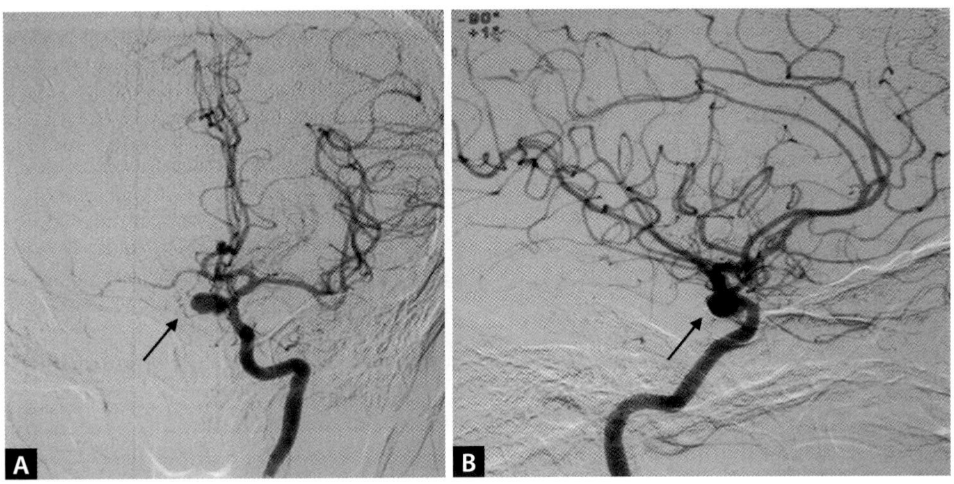

Figs. 5A and B: (A) AP and (B) Lateral. Angiographic views of left internal carotid artery showing an ICA aneurysm (arrows).

examination and CT become normal.[8] Standard spin echo (SE: T1, PD, T2) and gradient echo (GE) and susceptibility sequences are used. Contrast enhanced MRI helps in detecting the cause of SAH. MRI had a sensitivity of 95% and in no case CT was positive where MRI had failed.[9] This is because of formation of methemoglobin (usually after 4–5 days) which has paramagnetic properties and hence causes T_1 shortening. With mild SAH, the RBCs may be absorbed before methemoglobin is formed and it may be missed on MRI. GE sequences are especially helpful to observe the products of hemorrhage because of increased sensitivity to magnetic susceptibility. MRI also depicts complications of SAH, i.e. hydrocephalus, mass effect, infarcts, etc. It also helps in determining the etiology of SAH, e.g. aneurysms, AVMs, venous angiomas, tumors, etc. In cases of multiple aneurysms, it may help in determining which aneurysm has ruptured.

Cerebral Angiography

It is considered the gold standard and 4 vessel angiography should generally be performed in all cases of SAH. The role of angiography is to identify the cause of bleed, relationship of the cause to the parent vessel, define collateral circulation and assess vasospasm. Technically adequate angiography is essential. Magnification, subtraction and stereoscopic techniques delineate the cause of bleeding in most cases. Transfemoral catheterization of both internal carotid **(Figs. 5A and B)** and one vertebral artery is generally done. Contralateral vertebral artery catheterization is required if the visualization of the PICA is not seen through reflux. Selective injection of ECA may be required to rule out Dural AVMs. Cross compression study should routinely be done in all case of anterior or posterior communicating artery aneurysms and ICA aneurysm to delineate cross circulation.

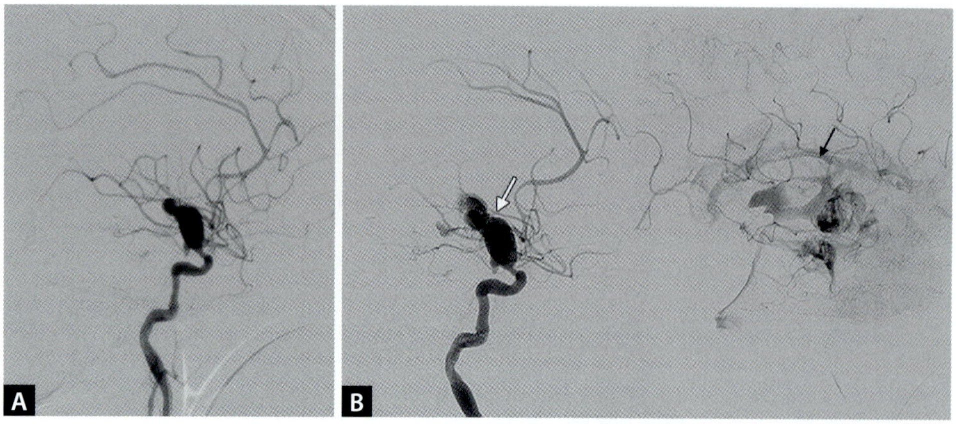

Figs. 6A and B: Lateral carotid angiogram shows a complex aneurysm with teat which bleed during angiography. Note the site of bleed (white arrow showing extravasation of contrast) and accumulation of blood in the ventricular system (black arrow).

The angiography should be done as early as possible after ictus. It can be deferred in patients showing rapidly deteriorating neurological status. The risks of angiography are well established. Ischemic events occur in 1.3% of patients in the first 24 hours after angiography. Neurological deterioration occurs in 1.8% of patients between 18 and 72 hours of angiography. Complications are directly related to the volume of contrast, serum creatinine level, number of catheters used, duration of the procedure and the patient's age. Rupture of aneurysm during angiography is rare (0.13%) but carries high mortality **(Figs. 6A and B)**.[11,12] 3D Rotational angiography is a technique in cerebral angiography which gives 3D model of the relevant artery without any bony or venous overlap. Since it can be rotated in any direction and orientation it can give very detailed anatomical information of the involved artery and the aneurysms. To establish the usefulness in detecting arteries less than 3 mm in size (which can be commonly missed on conventional DSA) a review of 350 datasets was done in a recent study. In addition to detecting all the large aneurysms, 94 additional small (<3 mm) aneurysms were detected on 3DRA.[13] This technique can also delineate the aneurysm volume, size, its relations to smaller branches close to neck and incorporation of the vessels **(Fig. 7)**.

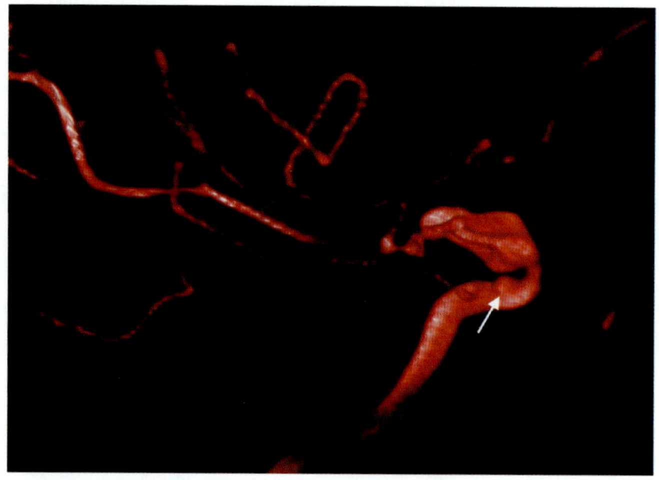

Fig. 7: 3DRA image of right ICA showing a paraclinoid aneurysm. Note a smaller sessile about 3 mm sized aneurysm proximal to it (arrow) which was not seen on DSA.

CT Angiography (CTA)

With the advent of multislice CT (MDCT), CT angiography has emerged as the alternative to the invasive cerebral digital subtraction angiography (DSA). An increasing number of centers are now treating aneurysms on the basis of findings of CTA with DSA being reserved for the negative cases or cases with diagnostic uncertainty.[14,15]

In a cohort of 223 patients, CTA was safely, effectively and reliably used as a sole modality for planning both operative clipping and endovascular coiling, with an apparent detection rate of 100%.[15] However, it is still to be universally accepted as a standard first line diagnostic test for evaluation for the SAH.

The advantages of three-dimensional representations of the arteries and their relationship to the surrounding structures are well documented. Additionally the ability to rotate the 3 D images into the identical projection encountered by the surgeon has tremendous advantages. Also, CTA has the ability to characterize the relevant preoperative surgical anatomy such as aneurysmal neck morphology, apical teats, calcification, thrombosis, parent and feeding vessels, diagnosing additional small aneurysms and collateral circulation at the circle of Willis **(Figs. 8 to 10)**.[16] Pitfalls of CT angiography include lack of visibility of small arteries, difficulty differentiating the infundibular dilatation at the origin of an artery from

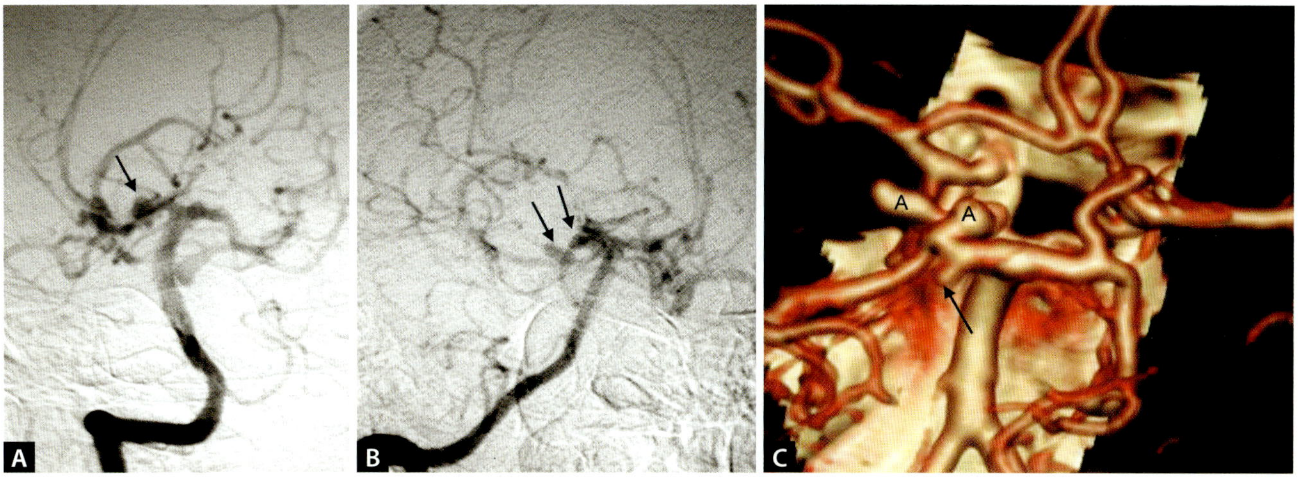

Figs. 8A to C: DSA-PA view of posterior circulation showing one right P1-segment aneurysm (A), oblique view showing another PCom. artery aneurysm (B). CTA reconstruction (C), showing an additional third aneurysm (arrow) in the proximal P1 segment not seen on DSA.

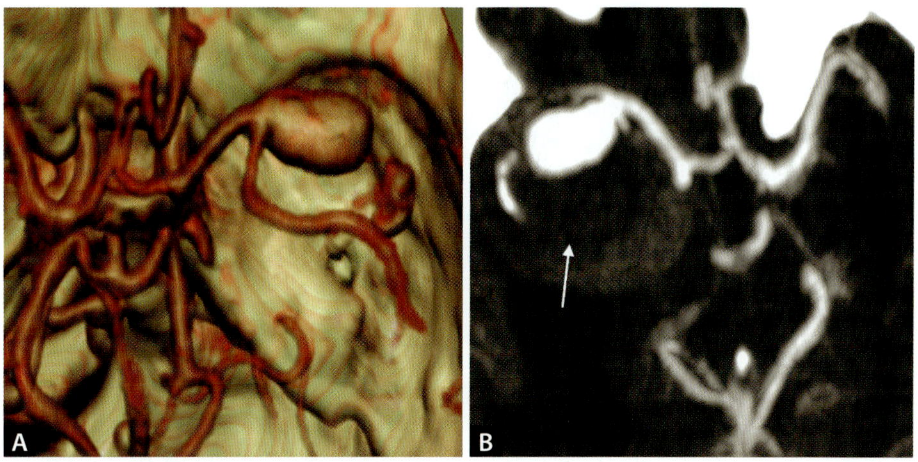

Figs. 9A and B: CTA-VR image (A) showing a large MCA aneurysm. However MIP image (B) showing a larger thrombosed portion (arrow) of the aneurysm surrounding the patent central aneurysm.

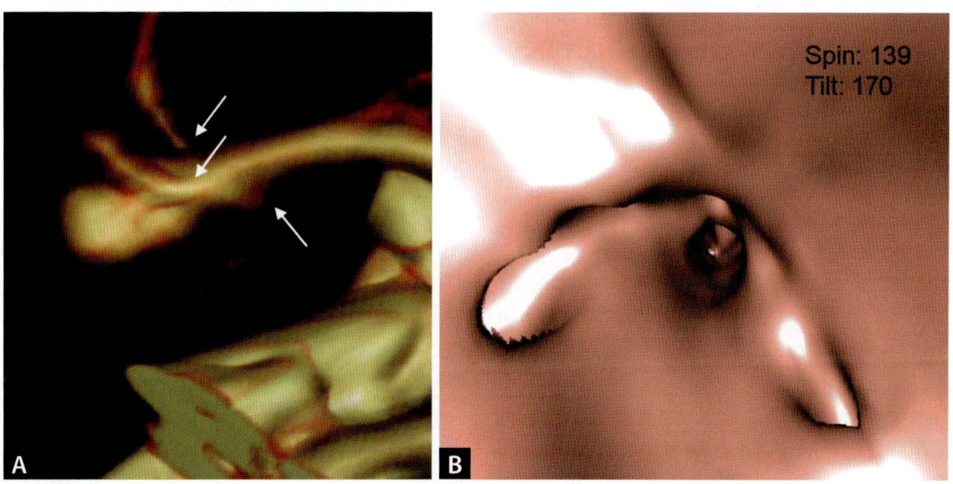

Figs. 10A and B: CTA VR image (A) showing multiple vessels arising in close relation to the neck (arrows) whose origins can be seen better on virtual angioscopy (B).

an aneurysm, the kissing vessel artifact, demonstration of venous structures that can simulate aneurysms, inability to identify thrombosis and calcification on three-dimensional images, and beam hardening artifacts produced by aneurysm clips.[17] Now with higher (128/320) slice spiral scanners it is feasible to obtain pure arterial phase images without any venous contamination. Also, it is possible to have high quality images with reconstruction interval of up to 0.24 mm which is close to the spatial resolution of the DSA which is about 0.32 × 0.32.

Standard parameters for the CT angiographic acquisition are 1.00 mm section thickness, 0.5 mm section interval, pitch of 3, and 120 kVp, 240 mAs, and 14.0 cm field of view. Scanning time is approximately 6 seconds for a 64-slice scanner which further reduces in a higher-slice CT. The scanning volume includes from the first cervical vertebra to the vertex. Approximately 80 mL of non-ionic low-osmolar iodinated contrast material is administered intravenously with a power injector at a rate of 4 mL/sec via an 18-gauge catheter positioned in a peripheral vein followed by 20 ml of saline flush (if dual head pressure injector is available). Contrast material is injected and scan initiated at a fixed delay of 16 seconds or a bolus chase technique is used which is more precise in capturing peak arterial phase.

The source images are reconstructed directly into 3 dimensional formats and recorded in maximum intensity projection (MIP), shaded surface display (SSD), volume rendering (VR) or in ray sum projection (projection of the sum of pixel values which is analogous to conventional angiography). The reported sensitivity and specificity of CTA in aneurysms over 3 mm in size are 90.4–95 and 100% respectively in recent studies.[18-20]

In a recent study comparing 64 slice CTA with DSA and 3DRA found sensitivity of 64 slice CTA for aneurysms >4 mm was 100% and for less than 4 mm was 92.3%.[21] In comparison to this, other studies have reported sensitivity of 4/16 slice CTs to diagnose aneurysms 3–4 mm to be in the range of 74–84%.[22-24]

Dual Energy CT

This new technology has made possible tissue differentiation and characterization on CT which was not possible before. This can be used as an added advantage in the work-up of SAH. Dual energy CT can help in removal of aneurysmal clip from the images with much lesser artifacts as compared to conventional CT angiography. Also, bone subtraction while post-processing CTA images is more reliable and comprehensive as compared to manual or automated/semi-automated algorithms.[25]

Magnetic Resonance Angiography

It is possibly the best noninvasive modality to evaluate the etiology of SAH. The various methods of imaging vascular flow and displaying it in multiple projections with MR are termed magnetic resonance angiography (MRA). The two principle techniques of data acquisition are time of flight (TOF) and phase contrast (PC) in both 2D and 3D planes. Multiple overlapping thin slab acquisition (MOTSA) with or without magnetization transfer has special value in the evaluation of circle of Willis.

A major limitation of time of flight technique is flow artifacts due to turbulent flow and in-plane saturation effects due to slow flow which hinders in the detection of small aneurysms.

The advent of 3D first pass gadolinium-enhanced gradient echo techniques with short repetition times have been shown to be technically superior with lesser artifacts related to flow alterations.[26] Also, MRA is useful as noninvasive tool for the follow-up imaging of coiled aneurysms.[27] Compared with DSA, 3D TOF MRA has sensitivity of 72–97% and specificity of 91–100% in detection of residual flow in aneurysms treated by platinum coils.[28,29] However, this sensitivity goes down significantly for aneurysms size <3 mm **(Figs. 11A to D)**.

Dynamic CEMR may help in detecting small aneurysms or AVMs. Blood oxygen level dependent (BOLD) contrast is a noninvasive functional MRI technique to localize a definable cortical function in relation to the site of AVM nidus as an aid to operative planning. The reported sensitivity and specificity of MRA in detecting aneurysms over 3 mm in size are 90.6 to 96 and 100% respectively in recent studies and are comparable to CTA.[18-20] It is the best screening modality for unruptured aneurysms or AVMs. It is of value in patients with angiographically negative SAH or in renal failure or where contrast injection is contraindicated.

Transcranial Doppler Ultrasound

It is used to study changes in cerebral artery flow velocity after SAH to correlate the onset of clinical vasospasm. Doppler flow velocity is proportional to the blood flow through the artery and inversely proportional to the cross-sectional diameter of the artery. There is rough correlation between angiographic vessels diameter and Doppler flow velocity.[30] Proximal middle cerebral artery (MCA) is normally studied. Mean MCA flow velocity (Normal value 60 cm/sec) of over 120 cm/sec is 100% specific and 59% sensitive, whereas velocity of over 200 cm/sec is 100% sensitive for detection of vasospasm on angiography.[30]

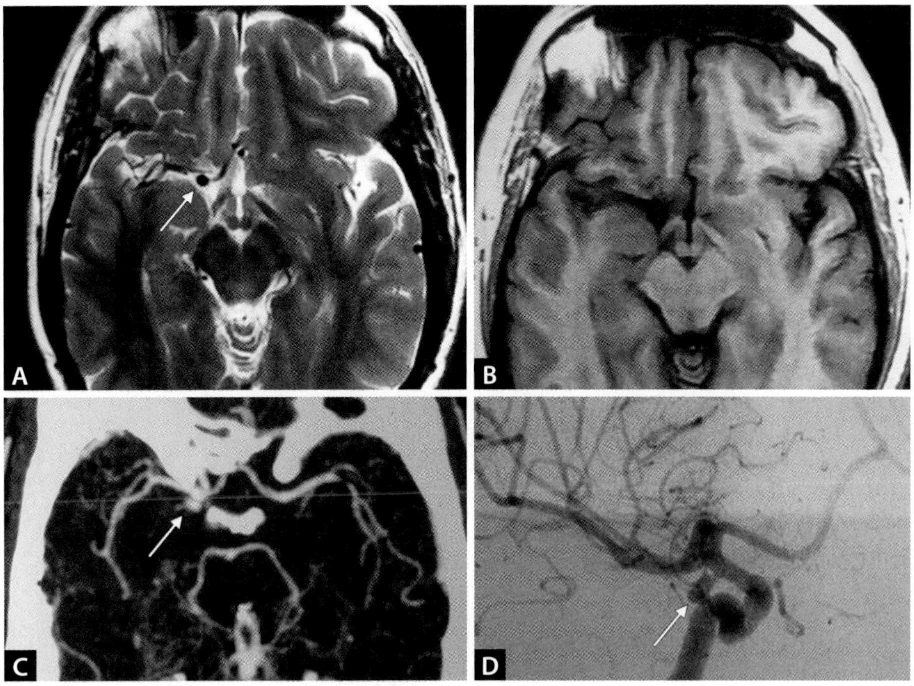

Figs. 11A to D: MR T2WI, T1WI (A and B) images showing a small RICA aneurysm (arrow) which was confirmed on CTA and DSA (C and D) to be a PCom. aneurysm.

ANEURYSMS

They result from focal degeneration of the arterial wall because of congenital factors which are aggravated by conditions like hypertension and smoking. These are the most common cause of SAH and occur in 1–14% of population. Only <2% occur during childhood.[31] They are of three types: Saccular (out pouching from arterial bifurcation), Fusiform (arterial dilatation) or Dissecting (pseudo-aneurysm) **(Figs. 12A to C)**. The ratio between ruptured versus unruptured aneurysm is 5:3 to 5:6.

The etiology of aneurysm may be:

- Congenital
- Infection (mycotic aneurysm)
- Trauma
- High flow state (AVM/AVF)
- Neoplasm (primary or metastasis)
- Miscellaneous, e.g. Arteritis, Moya Moya disease, SLE, drug abuse.

Increased incidence of aneurysm is seen in:

- Anomalous vessels (arterial) fenestration persistent trigeminal artery
- Aortic coarctation (8–10%)
- Polycystic kidney disease (10–30%)
- Fibromuscular dysplasia (7–10%)
- Connective tissue disorders (Marfan-Ehler-Danlos)
- High flow status, e.g. AVMs/AVFs
- Familial.

Clinical Presentation

The most common presentation is SAH followed by ICH (20–40%), IVH (15–35%) subdural bleed (2–5%) **(Figs. 13A to C)**. It may present with mass effect and cranial nerve palsy, infarcts, seizures or may be found incidentally on imaging.

Location

About 90–95% of aneurysm are found in carotid circulation, 5–15% in vertebrobasilar circulation and 15–20% aneurysms are multiple. Common locations are anterior communicating artery (30–35%), posterior communicating artery (30–35%) the middle cerebral artery bifurcation (20%), basilar top (5%) and PICA (5%) **(Figs. 14A and B)**.

Multiple Aneurysms

In 15–20% of cases, there may be multiple aneurysm of which 75% have two aneurysms, 15% have three aneurysms and 10% have more than three aneurysms. There is strong female predominance. Aneurysms can be bilaterally symmetrical (mirror aneurysm) or asymmetrical located on different vessels **(Fig. 15)**. In cases of multiple aneurysms, it is important to determine which aneurysm has actually ruptured. Clinical signs alone localize a ruptured aneurysm in only one-third of patients. The

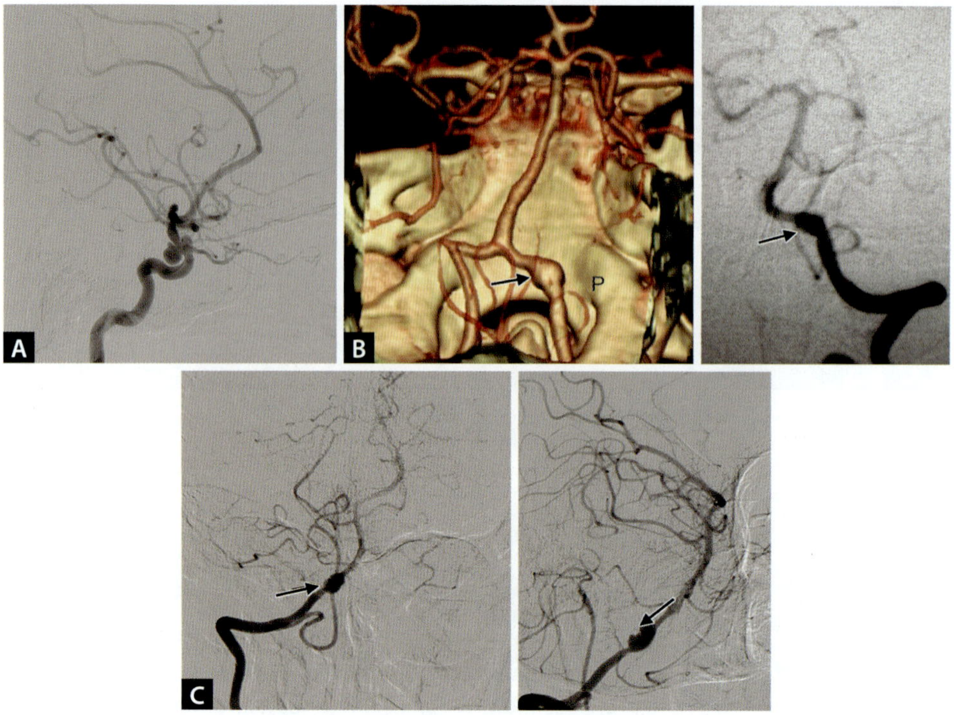

Figs. 12A to C: DSA image showing a ICA saccular aneurysm (A), a fusiform left vertebral aneurysm (arrow in B) and a dissecting right vertebral artery aneurysm (arrows in C).

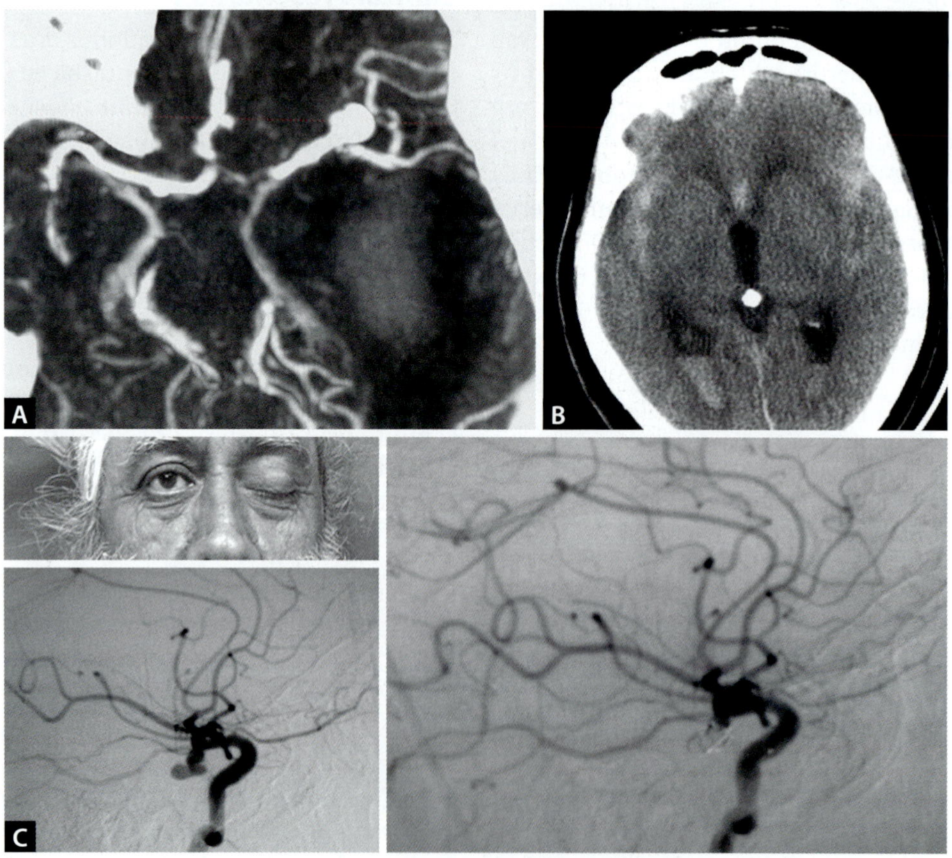

Figs. 13A to C: Aneurysm rupture presenting as parenchymal hemorrhage (A) and SAH with intraventricular hemorrhage (B). A nonruptured left PCom. aneurysm presenting with left ptosis (C).

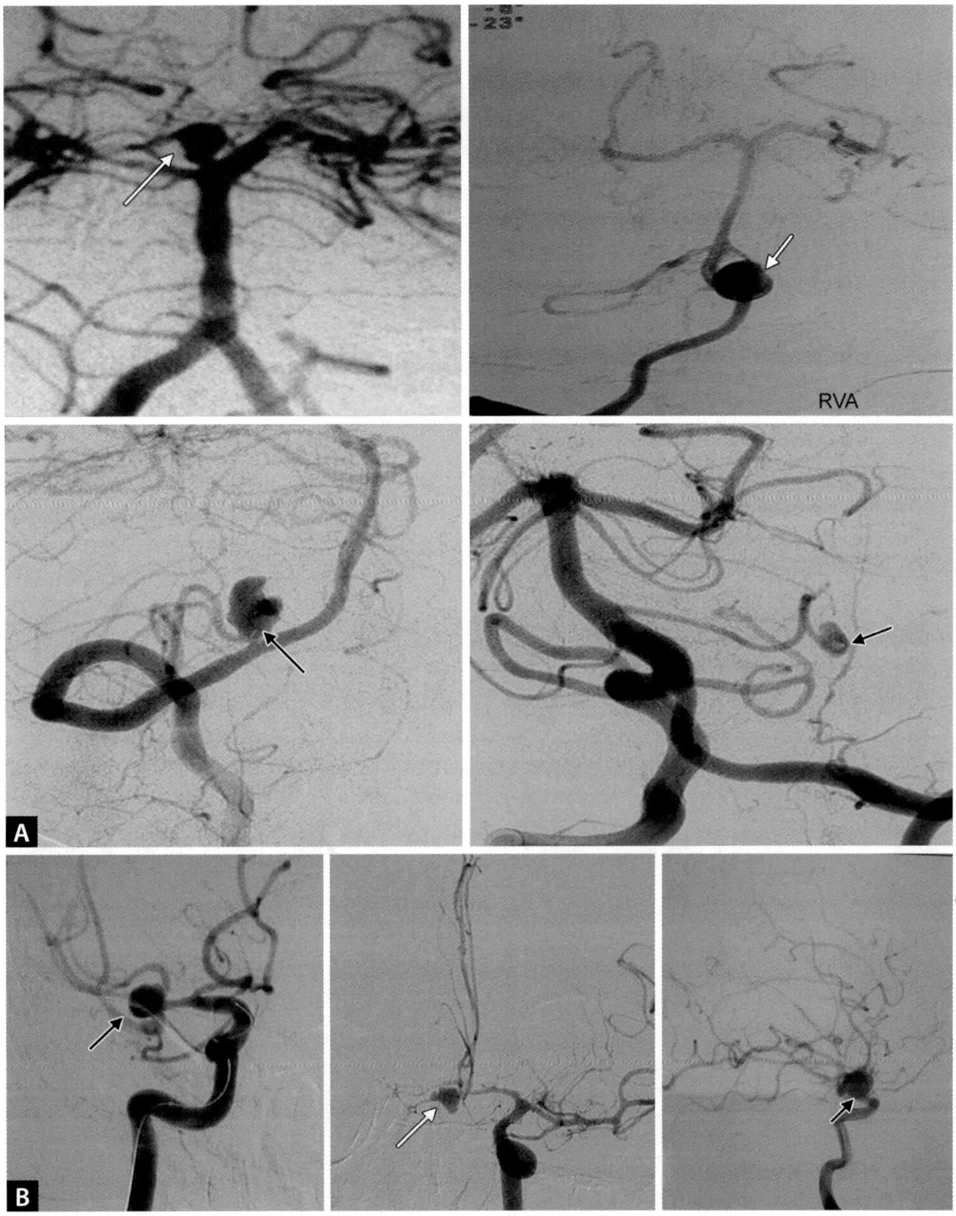

Figs. 14A and B: (A) Posterior circulation aneurysms—basilar top (long white arrow), vertebrobasilar junction (short white arrow), PICA aneurysm (long black arrow) and left AICA aneurysm; (B) Anterior circulation aneurysms. A MCA aneurysm (long black arrow), ACom. aneurysm (white arrow) and an ICA aneurysm (short black arrow).

imaging findings that are useful to determine the ruptured aneurysms are contrast extravasation (pathognomonic) presence of clot or mass effect on CT/MR and presence of SAH/vasospasm. The size location and configuration of the aneurysm are also helpful: proximally located aneurysm, largest aneurysm and the one having irregular configuration is the most likely the cause of bleed.

Unruptured Aneurysms

The risk of bleeding from unruptured aneurysm is not known and depends primarily on the size of the aneurysm.[32] Since aneurysms are not static and show increase in size on serial angiograms, surgery or interventional occlusion is needed. The critical size above which an unruptured aneurysms should be considered for treatment is debatable and varies from 3 mm–9 mm in various studies.[33] MR is the best modality to follow these patients under observation. In a recent study of follow-up of 181 unruptured aneurysms for a median period of 20 years (range- 1–39 years) the cumulative rates of rupture among 142 patients were 10.55% at 10 years and 30.3% at 30 years.[34]

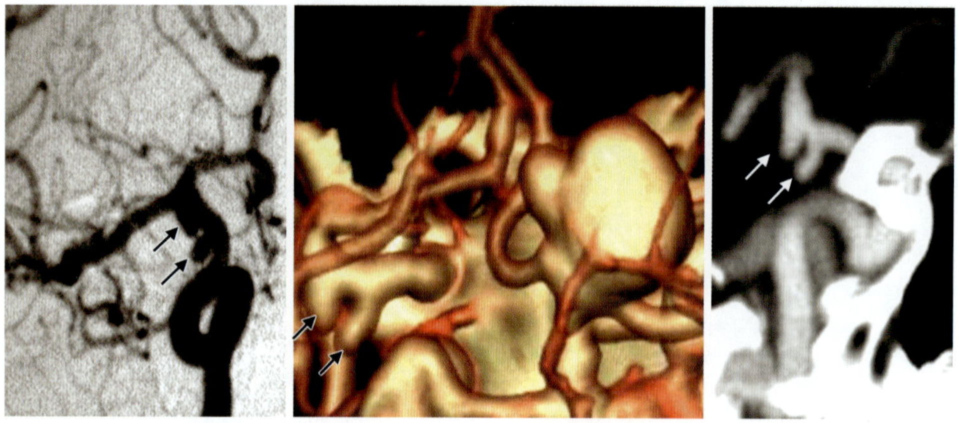

Fig. 15: DSA and CTA images showing two RICA aneurysms (arrows) and a large LICA bifurcation aneurysm.

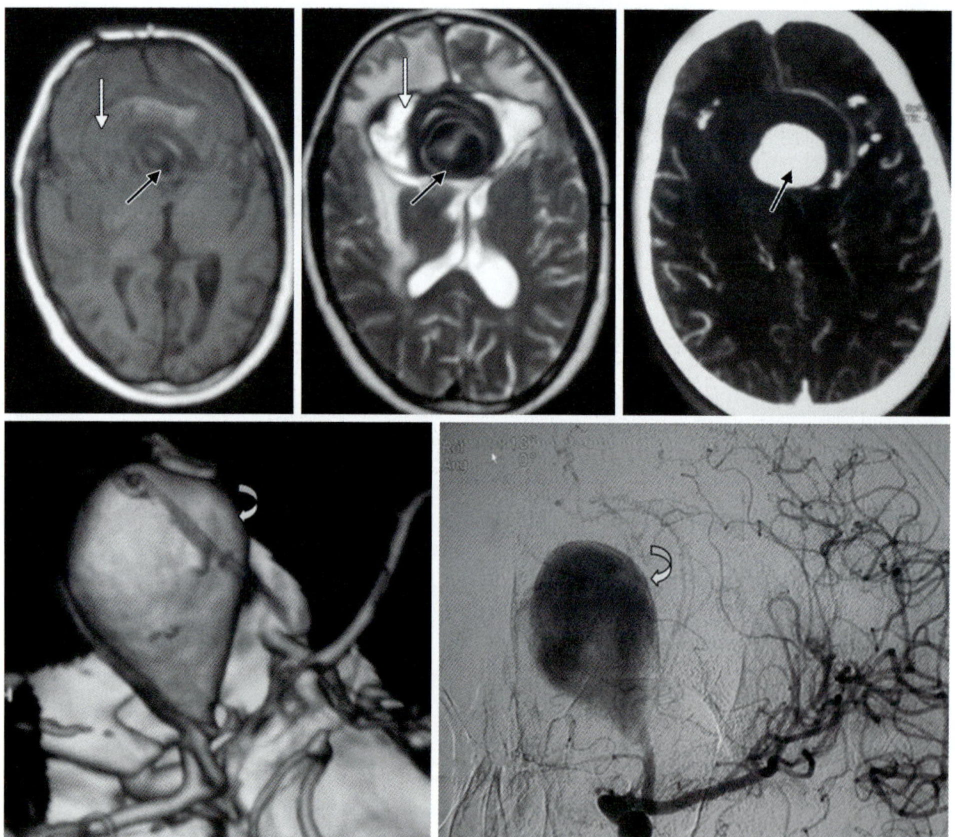

Fig. 16: Partially thrombosed aneurysm seen as a central area of flow void seen on T1WI, T2WI and CTA (black arrows) surrounded by variable signal intensity area seen as isointense on T1WI and hyperintense on T2WI (white arrows). CTA VR and DSA (below curved arrow) images showing it to be a large ACom. artery aneurysm.

Thrombosed Aneurysms

Partially thrombosed aneurysms have a patent lumen inside a thickened, often partially calcified wall that is lined with laminated clot. The residual lumen and outer rim may enhance strongly on CECT/CEMR. Completely thrombosed aneurysms show variable hyper density on NCCT with no contrast enhancement. On MR, partially thrombosed aneurysms show variable single intensity: an area of flow void surrounded by variable signal intensity, concentric layers with signal void outer rim is a common finding **(Fig. 16)**. Completely thrombosed aneurysm may be hyperintense on T1 and T2WI. It may be missed completely without the use of contrast MRI. Conventional angiography underestimates the size of thrombosed aneurysms and may show only mass effect.

Giant Aneurysms

Aneurysms less than 1 cm in diameter are called small aneurysms, large aneurysms are the ones between 1.0 cm and 2.5 cm. Aneurysms whose diameter exceeds 2.5 cm are termed giant aneurysms **(Figs. 17A and B)**. These usually present in middle aged women with mass effect; SAH does occur but is rare. They are commonly located in the extradural internal carotid artery, proximal MCA or apex of basilar artery. Conventional angiography fails to define the total extent of giant aneurysms because of associated thrombosis and associated extra-aneurysmal parenchymal changes. MRI is best imaging modality to evaluate these lesions.

Mycotic Aneurysms

These are defined an aneurysms that are the result of an infectious process involving the arterial wall and constitute 2–4% of all intracranial aneurysms. These occur in 3–15% of patients of subacute bacterial endocarditis **(Figs. 18A and B)**. The most common location is distal MCA branches (75–80%). They may be multiple (20%).[31,32]

Flow-related Aneurysms

The frequency of aneurysms with AVM has been reported from 2.7%–30%. They can occur in the proximal or distal feeding artery, inside the nidus (8–12%) or in the draining vein of the AVMs **(Fig. 19)**. There is increase in incidence of hemorrhage when AVM is associated with intranidal or venous aneurysm.[31,32]

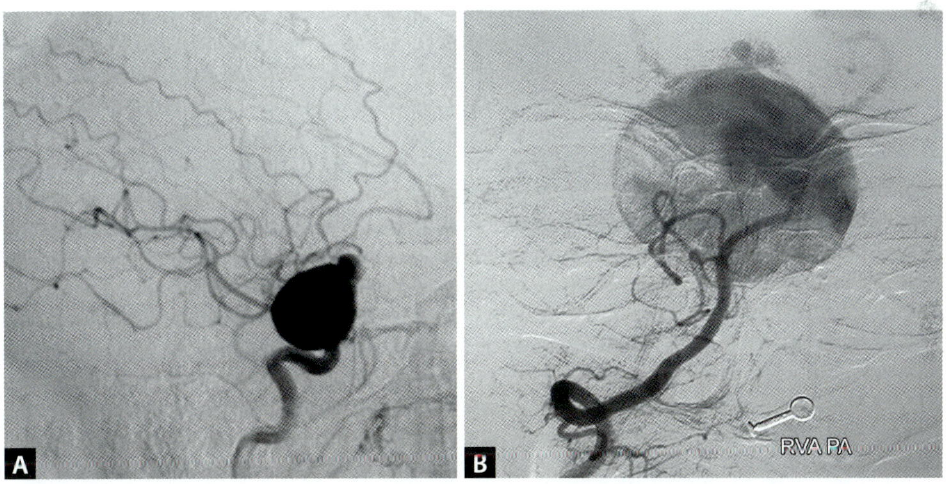

Figs. 17A and B: DSA projections showing giant ICA (A) and a giant left PCA (B) aneurysm.

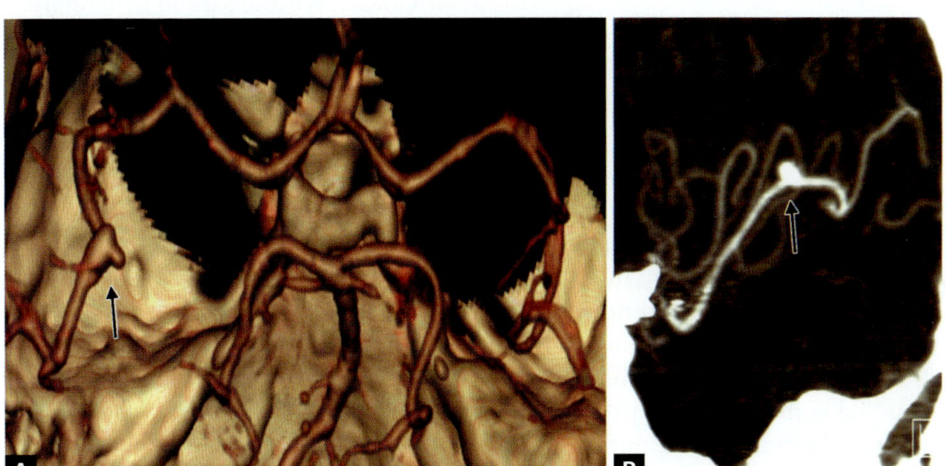

Figs. 18A and B: (A) CTA VR and (B) MIP images show an irregular aneurysm (mycotic) in the distal left MCA in a patient of subacute bacterial endocarditis.

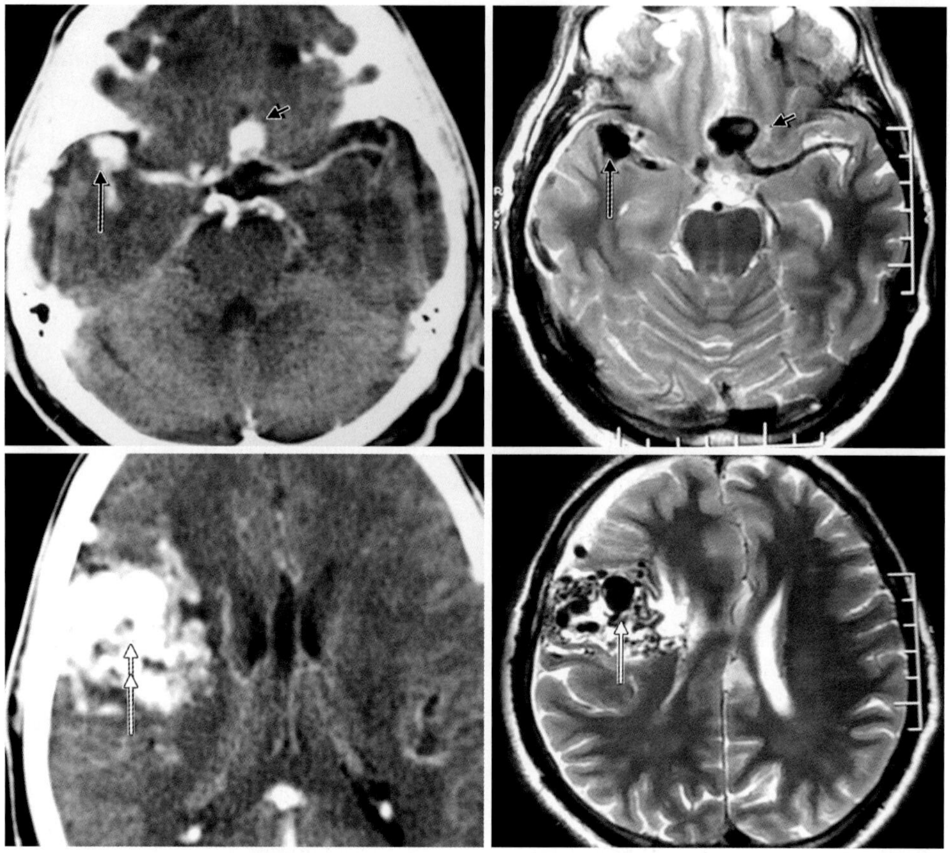

Fig. 19: CT and MR images showing flow-related aneurysms in right MCA (black arrows) and ACom. artery (small black arrow). Also seen is right parietal AVM with intranidal aneurysm (white arrows).

VASCULAR MALFORMATIONS

Vascular malformations are classified into 4 major pathologic types: (A) arteriovenous malformations (AVMs) (B) Capillary telangiectasias, (C) Cavernous angiomas, and (D) Venous angiomas.[35] The overall incidence is from 0.1%–4%.

AVMs can be (A) parenchymal (pial) (B) dural or (C) mixed (pial-dural) type.

Parenchymal AVMs

These are comprised of a complex network of abnormal vascular channels consisting of arterial feeders, the nidus and enlarged veins without an intervening capillary bed and normal brain parenchyma.[35,36] They are usually solitary (98%), but can be multiple (2%), especially in Rendu-Osler-Weber and Wyburn-Mason's syndromes. The common age at presentation is 20–40 years. The presenting clinical features include intracranial hemorrhage (55%), seizures (36%), headache and progressive neurologic deficit (9%). The risk of hemorrhage is 2–4% per year and rebleeding after initial hemorrhage is about 6% in the first year and slowly decreases thereafter.[37] Hemorrhagic complications with AVMs are common when these are peri or intraventricular in location, or have central (deep) venous drainage, or show intranidal aneurysm.

On CT, AVMs are iso to hyperdense and show intense serpiginous enhancement **(Figs. 20A to C)**. Calcification is present in 25–30% of cases. Secondary changes such as acute hemorrhage, edema, mass effect and ischemia are readily identified on CT. On MRI, they are usually seen as tightly packed honeycomb of "flow voids" on both T1 and T2 spin echo sequences. The feeding arteries, the nidus or the draining veins may be clearly seen on standard SE or time of flight (TOF) or phase contrast (PC) MRA techniques **(Fig. 21)**. Areas of increased signal may be seen in thrombosed vessels or in vessels with slow or turbulent flow. Hemorrhage in all stages, hypoperfusion because of steal phenomenon atrophy gliosis, mass effect, etc. are better seen on MRI than CT.

Recently with the use of 3T MR systems ultra fast acquisitions have become a possibility. Time resolved contrast enhanced MRA is one such technique which

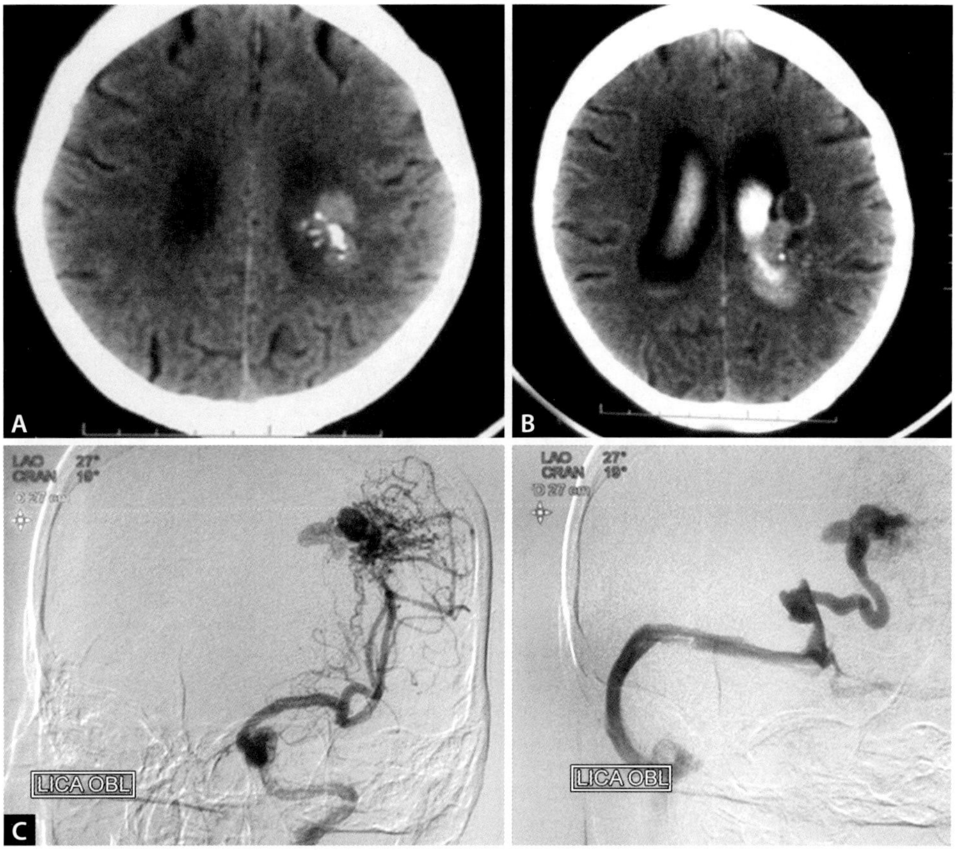

Figs. 20A to C: (A and B) Serpiginous hyperdense areas in the left periventricular region with IVH. Carotid angiogram; (C) Oblique projections show the arterial feeder, the nidus and venous drainage into deep venous system.

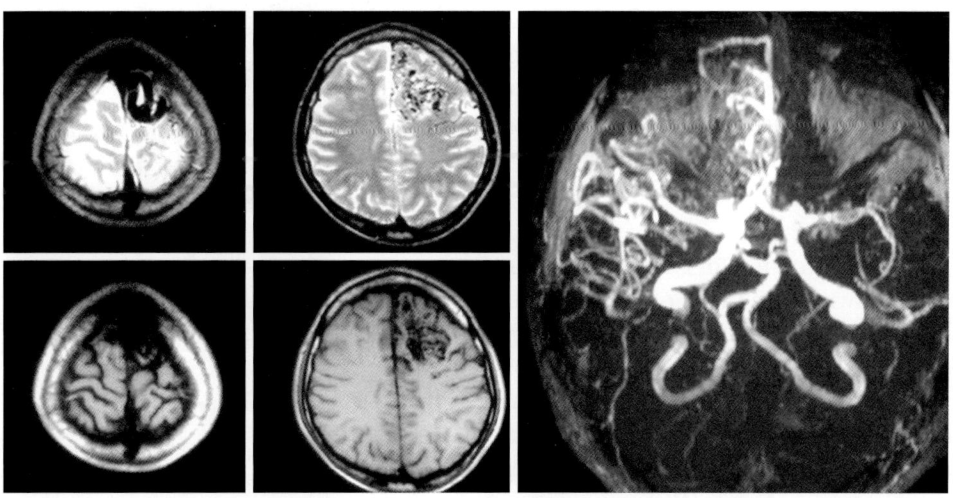

Fig. 21: MR (T2WI, T1WI and MRA) images showing multiple, tortuous flow voids in the left frontal region suggestive of AVM which is seen as bunch of vessels on MRA.

aims at capturing the dynamic information of the AVMs in addition to the diagnosis thereby offering an alternative to DSA. By combining parallel imaging, keyhole acquisition and k-space sampling now it is possible to image cerebral AVMs in early arterial phase, late arterial phase, parenchymal and venous phase. Studies have demonstrated a good co-relation of time resolved MRA and DSA in imaging location and number of arterial feeders, size of the nidus and number and type of venous drainage **(Figs. 22A to H)**.[38,39]

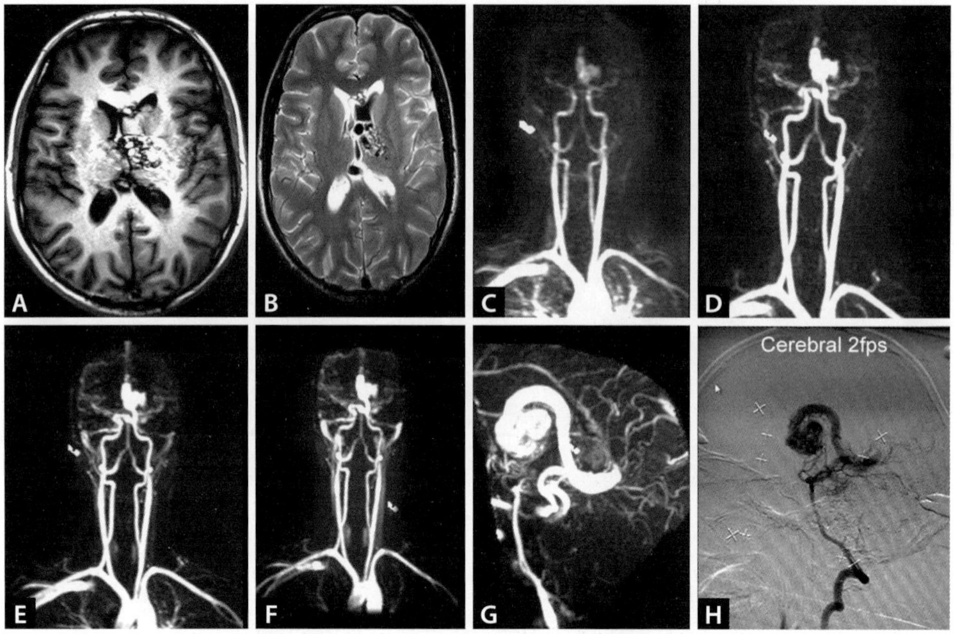

Figs. 22A to H: An 18-year-old male with left thalamic AVM T1W and T2WI showing AVM in left basal ganglia and thalamic region (A and B). Sequential arterial (C and D), nidus (E) and venous (F) enhancement on time resolved MRA Coronal projection. High spatial resolution MRA—lateral MIP projection (G) with corresponding DSA (H) –Lt. PCA run image showing feeders, nidus and draining veins.

Cerebral angiography is the gold standard in the evaluation of AVMs. It demonstrates tightly packed masses of enlarged feeding arteries, the nidus and tortuous draining veins. A flow related aneurysm (arterial, nidal or venous) may be seen in 8–12% of cases. Occasionally, AVM may involve entire lobe with no demonstrable nidus. Thrombosed AVMs may have normal angiogram (cryptic AVM). Occasionally arteries with slow blood flow may be seen till late in capillary phase and rare termed "stagnating arteries."[30]

Dural AVMs

These are abnormal vascular network with thickened dural arteries and veins within the wall of venous sinus without any discrete nidus. Unlike pial AVMs, dural AVMs are acquired secondary to the segmental thrombosis of the dural venous sinus. They usually present with pulsatile tinnitus, bruit, headache, visual impairment or papilledema. CT scan is usually normal except in situations like carotid cavernous fistula (CCF) where there can be enlarged cavernous sinus and dilated superior ophthalmic vein. MRI may also be normal. PC MRA can show the flow direction in the fistula. On angiography, most dural AVMs have multiple feeders from dural branches except in case of fistulae where there is a single dural artery. The dural sinus is usually occluded **(Fig. 23)**.

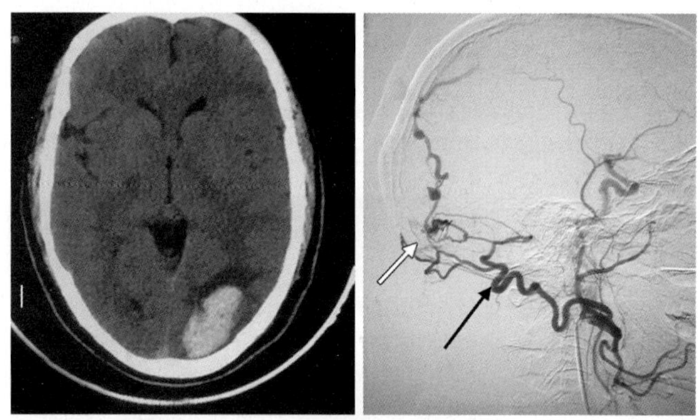

Fig. 23: NCCT image showing acute bleed in left occipital bleed secondary to the dural AV fistula being supplied by the posterior meningeal branch of the left vertebral artery (arrow). Site of the fistula is left sigmoid sinus, marked with white arrow.

Mixed Pial and Dural AVMs

When parenchymal AVM is of large size, it may recruit vascular supply from dural branches. Meningeal artery contributes in 15–50% of cases. On imaging, these AVMs show characteristics of both pial and dural AVMs.

CAPILLARY TELANGIECTASIAS

These are nets of dilated capillaries whose walls lack smooth muscle and elastic fibers and have intervening normal brain parenchyma. They are usually multiple and located in the pons, cerebellum or spinal cord. Most lesions are small and clinically silent, discovered incidentally on imaging. CT and MRI are usually normal except for faint increased density on contrast examination. MRI shows the product of hemorrhage as multiple hyperintense foci on T2WI and GE images.

Angiographically also, they are occult; rarely, a faint vascular stain may be seen.

CAVERNOUS ANGIOMAS

Cavernous angiomas are endothelial lined sinusoidal spaces not separated by neural tissues and are discrete multilobulated lesions that contain products of hemorrhage in various stages. They account for 8–16% of all intracranial vascular malformations.[36] The clinical features include seizures (60%), progressive neurological deficit (50%), hemorrhage (20%), hydrocephalus or they may present as incidental findings on routine imaging (50%). They can occur anywhere in the brain; 80% are supratentorial and 20% are infratentorial. On CT, they appear as iso or hyperdense lesions with minimal or no enhancement and show variable calcification. Mass effect or edema is conspicuously absent. On angiography they are "occult". MR shows the most characteristic and diagnostic findings in the form of "popcorn" like lesion with well delineated complex core of mixed signal intensity **(Figs. 24A to C)**. A low signal hemosiderin rim surrounds the lesion which becomes prominent or "blooms" on T2WI or gradient echo images.[31]

VENOUS ANGIOMAS

These are radially arranged dilated anomalous veins that coverage in an enlarged transcortical vein. There is no arterial component or intervening normal brain tissue or evidence of gliosis or hemosiderin. They are the most common vascular malformations found at autopsy and are located in deep cerebral or cerebellar white matter close to ventricle. They are usually solitary but can be multiple. Hemorrhagic complications occur but are rare. Computed tomography is usually normal or may show enhanced tuft of rounded or linear vessels (medullary veins). Magnetic resonance findings are often diagnostic: a stellate tangle of venous tributaries draining into a large dilated anomalous veins. "Flow void" vein is the characteristic findings, especially well seen on CEMR. Cerebral angiography shows normal arterial and capillary phase. Multiple enlarged medullary veins coverage into dilated transcortical vein giving rise to "medusa head" appearance seen in the venous phase **(Fig. 25)**.

Angiographically occult vascular malformations (AOVMs) are 10% of all vascular malformation and are due to:

- Thrombosed AVMs (44%)
- Cavernous angiomas (31%)
- Venous angiomas (10%)
- Capillary telangiectasia (4%)
- Unclassified or mixed angiomas (11%).

TRAUMATIC SUBARACHNOID HEMORRHAGE

Moderate to severe head trauma may produce SAH and a small percentage show associated aneurysms. "Pseudo SAH" may be seen with severe diffuse cerebral edema where brain becomes very low in attenuation and the circulating blood appears very hyperdense.[31] "Pseudodelta" sign on plain CT may be seen in posterior

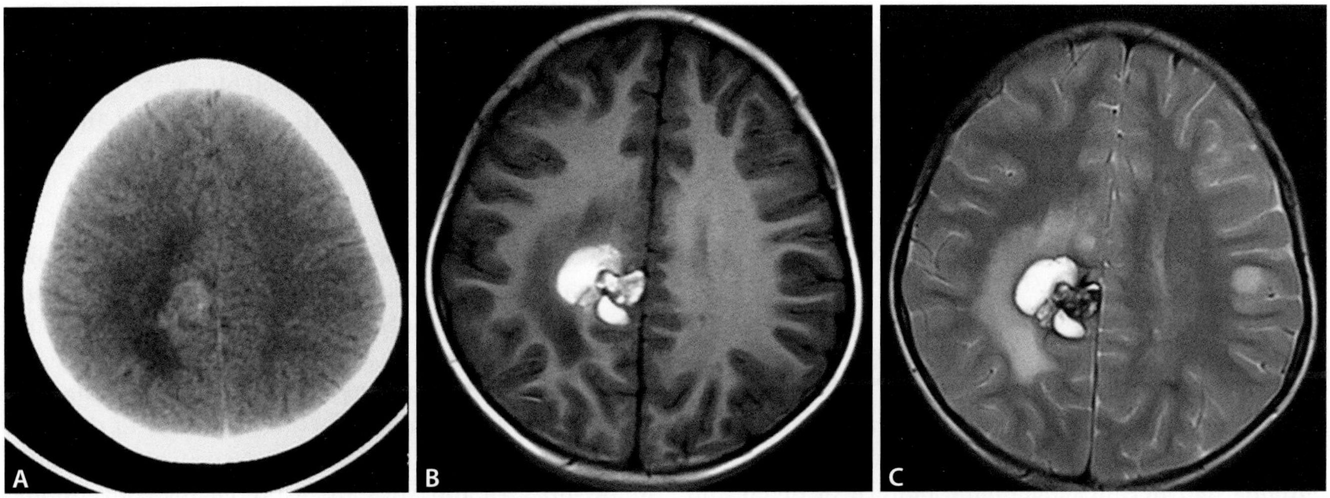

Figs. 24 A to C: NCCT, T1- and T2-weighted MR images shows hemorrhagic lesion (with both acute and chronic bleed) with typical "popcorn" appearance with surrounding hypointense rim on T2WI suggestive of cavernous angioma.

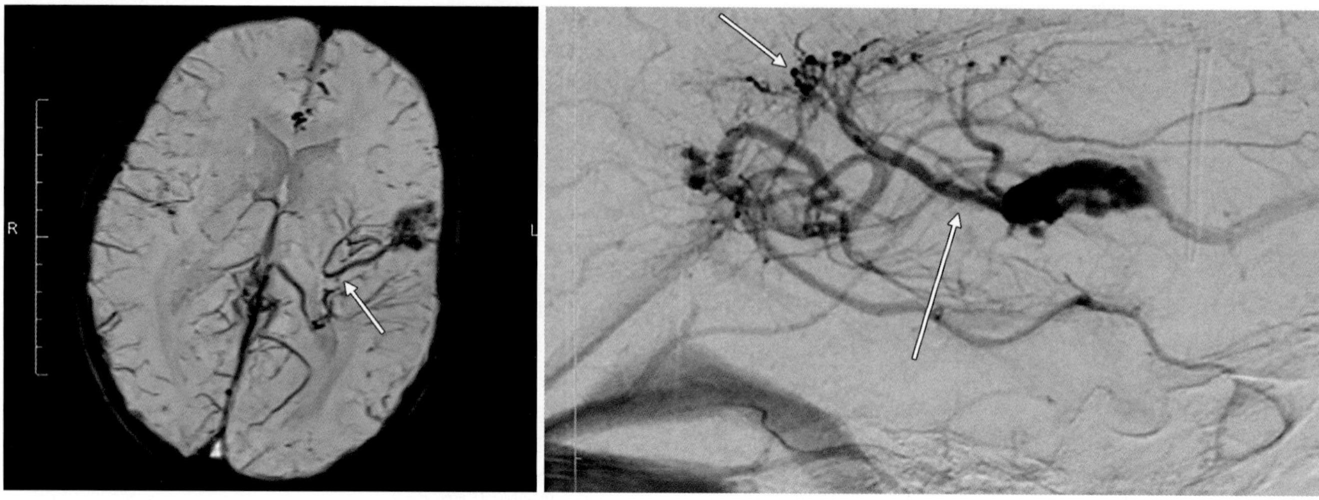

Fig. 25: MRI SWI image showing a prominent transcortical vein (left image). Venous phase of left ICA angiogram showing multiple medullary veins (small arrow) draining into a large vein (large arrow) a typical angiographic picture of venous angioma.

parafalcine or interhemispheric SAH and should not be mistaken for dural sinus thrombosis.[40]

Subarachnoid Hemorrhage of Unknown Etiology

The incidence of SAH of unknown etiology is about 7–10% of all SAH. The possible causes are:

- *Incomplete angiogram*: 1–2% of aneurysms occur at PICA origin and can be missed, if complete 4 vessels angiogram is not done.
- Obliteration of lesion by the hemorrhage.
- Aneurysm or AVM too small to be visualized.
- Cervical or upper thoracic AVM.
- SAH of nonaneurysmal etiology.

There is risk of rebleed (up to 0.5% per year) and delayed cerebral ischemia. In such cases a repeat angiography is required and is usually done after 6 weeks (may be after 3rd weeks) or till vascular spasm disappears. In a series of 92 cases of negative angiogram in SAH, an aneurysm was demonstrated on a second angiogram in 4 cases and on a third angiogram in 1 case only.[41] In a recent study conducted in the institute in 30 patients of negative DSA, the CTA showed aneurysms in 5 patients where DSA was negative. In one patient repeat DSA at 4 weeks showed small aneurysm (unpublished).

In another review of 61 patients of angiographically negative spontaneous SAH patients was done. In it 18 patients had perimesencephalic pattern of bleed and 34 patients had SAH without any demonstrable cause. Prognosis of both groups was found to be good.[42]

Non-aneurysmal SAH

Perimesencephalic SAH, vasculitis coagulation disorders and trauma are common causes for non-aneurysmal SAH. Perimesencephalic SAH is a distinct benign entity with good outcome and less risk of rebleed or vasospasm than other patients of SAH.

It is possibility due to rupture of small perimesencepalic vein. Cerebral angiography is normal. The criteria that establish the diagnosis on CT or MRI are:[43]

- Epicenter of hemorrhage is immediately anterior to the midbrain with extension into anterior part of ambient cistern or basal part of sylvian fissure.
- Absence of complete filling of anterior interhemispheric fissure.
- No more than minute amount of blood in lateral portion of sylvian fissure.
- Absence of frank intraventricular bleed.
- Repeat panangiography is not indicated in these patients.[31,32]

SUMMARY

The diagnosis of acute SAH can be made on CT but MRI is required in subacute and chronic SAH. There are various etiologies for SAH, the common being rupture of aneurysms and AVMs. Conventional four vessel angiography still remains the modality of choice for defining the location and detailed anatomy of the AVM for surgery, endovascular therapy as well for post-surgical follow-up. CTA and MRA are fast replacing conventional angiography for diagnostic purposes and have comparable specificity and sensitivity.

REFERENCES

1. Menghini VV, Brown RD Jr, Sicks JD, et al. Incidence and prevalence of intracranial aneurysms and hemorrhage in Olmsted Couty, Minnessota, 1965 to 1995. Neurology. 1998; 51:405-11.
2. Salis AL, Nibbelink DW, Torner JC (Eds). Aneurysmal subarachnoid haemorrhage : Report of cooperative study: Urban and Schwazzenberg Baltimore - Munich. 1981;370-85.
3. Parkarinen S. Incidence, etiology and prognosis of primary SAH. Acta Neurol Scandina. 1967;48:1-128.
4. Locksley H. Report on the cooperative study of SAH. J Neuosurg. 1966;25:219-39.
5. ICMR, Epidemiological study on SAH in INDIA (1972-75) ICMR Bull, New Delhi, 1987.
6. Patel MK, Clarke MA. Lumbar puncture and subarachnoid haemorrhage. Postgrad Med J. 1986;62:1021.
7. Kasell NF, Toner JC, Haley EC Jr. The international co-operative study on the timing of aneurysm surgery. I overall management results. J Neurosurg. 1990;73: 307-25.
8. Van Gijn J, Van Dongen KL. The time course of aneurysmal haemorrhage on computed tomograms. Neuroradiology. 1985;23:153-55.
9. Ogawa T, Inugamia A, Fujita H, et al. MR diagnosis of subacute and chronic subarachnoid haemorrhage. Comparison with CT. AJR. 1995; 165:1257-62.
10. Singer M, Atlas S, Drayer B. Subarachnoid space disease: diagnosis with fluid attenuated inversion recovery MR imaging and comparison with contrast-enhanced T1 weighted images: blinded reader study. Radiology. 1998;208:417-22.
11. Dion JE, Gates FC, Fox AJ, et al. Clinical events following neuroangiography. A prospective study. Stroke. 1987;18: 997-1009.
12. Khandelwal N, Kaur Baljeet, Malik N, et al. Rupture of intracranial aneurysms during angiography. JAPI. 1994;42:76-77.
13. Van Rooji WJ, Sprengers ME, de Gast AN, et al. 3D rotational angiography: the new gold standard in the detection of additional intracranial aneurysms. AJNR. 2008;29: 976-79.
14. Vekthuis BK, Van Leeuwen MS, Witkamp TD, et al. Computerized tomography angiography in patients with subarachnoid hemorrhage: From aneurysm detection to treatment without conventional angiography. J Neurosurg. 1999;91:761-7.
15. Hoh BL, Cheung AC, Rabinov JD, et al. Results of a prospective protocol of computed tomographic angiography in place of catheter angiography as the only diagnostic and pretreatment planning study for cerebral aneurysms by a combined neurovascular team. Neurosurgery. 2004;54:1329-42.
16. Wintermark M, Uske A, Chalaron M, et al. Multislice computerized tomography angiography in the evaluation of intracranial aneurysms: A comparison with intra-arterial digital subtraction angiography. J Neurosurg. 2003;98:828-36.
17. Takhtani D. CT Neuroangiography: A Glance at the Common Pitfalls and Their Prevention. AJR. 2005;185:772-83.
18. Harrison MJ, Johnson BA, Gardner GM, et al. Preliminary results on the management of Unruptured aneurysms with magnetic imaging angiography and computed tomography angio-graphs. Neurosurg. 1997;40:947-55.
19. Schwartz RB, Tice HM, Hooten SM, et al. Evaluation of cerebral aneurysms with helical CT: Correlation with conventional angiography and MR angiographs. Radiology. 1994;192:717-22.
20. Zouaou A, Sahel M, Marro B, et al. Three dimensional computed tomographic angiography in detection of haemorrhage. Neuro Surg. 1997;41:125-30.
21. McKinney AM, Palmer CS, Truwit CL, et al. Detection of aneurysms by 64-section multidetector CT angiography in patients acutely suspected of having an intracranial aneurysm and comparison with digital subtraction and 3D rotational angiography. AJNR. 2008;29:594-602.
22. Dammert S, Krings T, Moller-Hartmann W, et al. Detection of intracranial aneurysms with multislice CT: comparison with conventional angiography. Neuroradiology. 2004;46:427-34.
23. Tipper G, U King-Im JM, Price SJ, et al. Detection and evaluation of intracranial aneurysms with 16-row multislice CT angiography. Clin Radiol. 2005;60:565-72.
24. Yoon DY, Lim KJ, Choi CS, et al. Detection and characterization of intracranial aneurysms with 16-channel multidetector row CT angiography: a prospective comparison of volume rendered images and digital substraction angiography. AJNR. 2007;28:60-67.
25. Postma AA, Das M, Stadler AA, et al. Dual-Energy CT: What the Neuroradiologist Should Know. Curr Radiol Rep. 2015;3(5):16.
26. Parker DL, Goodrich KC, Alexander AL, et al. Optimized visualization of vessels in contrast enhanced intracranial MR angiography. Magn Reson Med. 1998;40:873-82.
27. Leclerc X, Navez JF, Gauvrit JY, et al. Aneurysms of the anterior communicating artery treated with Guglielmi detachable coils: Follow-up with contrast enhanced MR angiography. Am J Neuro Radiol. 2002;23:1121-27.
28. Okahara M, Kiyosue H, Hori Y et al. Three-dimensional time- of-flight MR angiography for the evaluation of intracranial aneurysms after endovascular packing with Guglielmi detachable coils: Comparison with 3D digital subtraction angiography. Eur Radiol. 2004;14:1162-8.
29. Yamada N, Hayashi K, Murao K, et al. Time-of-flight MR angiography targeted to coiled intracranial aneurysms is more sensitive to residual flow than is digital subtraction angiography. AJNR. 2004;25:1154-7.
30. Harders AG, Gillsbach JM. Time course of blood velocity changes related to vasospam in the circle of Willis measured by Transcranial Doppler Ultrasound. J Neurosurgery. 1987;66:718-24.
31. Osborn AG. Intracranial aneurysms. In: Diagnostic neuroradiology. Ed Mosby. 1994;248-329.

32. Atlas SW. Magnetic Resonance Imaging of Brain and Spine. (2nd Edn) Lipincott Raven. 1994;489-556.
33. Wiebers Do, Whiswant JP, Sundt TM. The significance of unruptured saccular aneurysms. J Neurosurg. 1987;66:23-29.
34. Juvela S, Porras M, Poussa K. Natural history of unruptured intracranial aneurysms: probability of and risk factors for aneurysm rupture. J Neurosurg. 2008;108:1052-60.
35. Russell DS, Rubinstein LJ. Pathology of Tumours of the Nervous System, (5th edn) Williams and Wilkins, Baltimore 1989.
36. Graves VB, Duff TA. Intracranial arteriovenous malformations: Current imaging and treatment. Invest Radiol. 1990;25:952-60.
37. Brown RDJ, Wiebers DO, Forbes G, et al. The natural history of Unruptured intracranial arteriovenous malformations. J Neurosurg. 1988;68:352-57.
38. Taschner CA, Gieseke J, Le Thuc V, et al. intracranial arteriovenous malformation: time resolved contrast enhanced MR Angiography with combination of parallel imaging, keyhole acquisition, and k-space sampling techniques at 1.5 T. Radiology. 2008;246(3): 871-79.
39. Saleh RS, Lohan DG, Villablanca JP, et al. Assessment of craniospinal arteriovenous malformations at 3T with highly temporally and highly spatially resolved contrast enhanced MR angiography. AJNR. 2008;29:1024-31.
40. Khandelwal N, Malik N, Pathak A, et al. Head Injury: Pseudodelta sign on CT. Australasian Radiology. 1992;36: 303-04.
41. Duong H, Meancon D, Tampieri D, et al. The negative angiograms in subarachnoid haemorrhage. Neuroradiology. 1996;38:15-19.
42. Gupta SK, Gupta R, Khosla VK et al. Nonaneurysmal non perimesencephalic subarachnoid hemorrhage: is it a benign entity? Surg Neurol. 2009;71:566-71.
43. Rienkel GJE, Wijdicks EFM, Vermeulen M, et al. Nonaneurysmal perimesencephalic subarachnoid haemorrhage. CT and MR patterns that differ from aneurysmal rupture. AJNR. 1991;12:829-34.

CHAPTER 10

Endovascular Management of Intracranial Aneurysms

Shailesh B Gaikwad

Intracranial aneurysms are localized pathological dilatations of cerebral arteries. They are the most common of the cranial vascular lesion encountered. Rupture of aneurysms is a neurologic event with grave consequences. Rapid advancements in neurointerventional techniques, equipments, and critical care have led to significant reduction in morbidity and mortality particularly in patients with ruptured aneurysm. We attempt to present scenario regarding endovascular treatment of intracranial aneurysms.

The exact prevalence of cerebral aneurysms is not accurately documented and varies widely in the published literature. It is accepted that about 3% to 5% of the population should harbor an intracranial aneurysm. In various adult autopsy studies[1] frequency ranges from 1% to 6%, where as in angiographic series;[2] the incidence of intracranial aneurysms varies from 0.65% to 7%. Berry aneurysms are multiple in about 20% to 30% of cases. Females more commonly harbor intracranial aneurysm with peak prevalence in the fourth and sixth decades. Aneurysms in the pediatric population are rare, accounting for 2% to 4% of all aneurysms. These are generally are found in males and tend to be of larger dissecting variety.[3,4]

Different types of intracranial aneurysms exist. They are classified on their shape, size, location, and cause. Majority of intracranial aneurysms are saccular ones whereas fusiform, dissecting, mycotic and traumatic aneurysms are relatively rare.

PATHOGENESIS

Pathogenesis of intracranial aneurysms remains incompletely understood. For instance, the exact origin of the defect in the parent vessel wall is not established clearly, but it does not seem to be congenital.[5,6] It is believed that intracranial aneurysms result from a combination of hemodynamic stresses and acquired arterial wall degenerative changes, even if inherited diseases may predispose aneurysmal formation by weakening the vessel wall. This idea also is reinforced by the relative rarity of cerebral aneurysms in children.[7]

Hemodynamic Factors

Hemodynamic stress plays the most important role in the development of intracranial aneurysms fact supported by their preferential sites of occurrence at arterial bifurcations and increased frequency in the presence of circle of Willis asymmetry and vascular anomalies such as fenestrations and in cases of high-flow arteriovenous malformations.[8] This hemodynamic stress mainly results in two distinct physical forces.

The impacting force, perpendicular to the vessel wall, corresponds to the inertial force of the bloodstream and can be considered as the local elevation of the pressure at the area where the blood flow impacts.[9] The "wall shear stress", parallel to the vessel wall, caused by the viscous friction of the bloodstream.[10]

Even though impacting forces are important for aneurysm formation, various flow models reveal that their contribution to the rupture of the aneurysms may be less than previously thought. More than hypertension itself, it is the resultant amplification of blood blow and subsequent change of wall shear stress that appears to be main determinant in arterial wall degeneration and subsequent aneurysmal rupture.[11]

Acquired/Degenerative Changes

Several medical conditions are associated with the development of intracranial aneurysms such as systemic lupus erythematosus, Takayasu disease, giant cell arteritis, ADPCKD, Ehlers-Danlos syndrome, Marfan syndrome, fibromuscular dysplasia, neurofibromatosis, pseudoxanthoma elasticum, hereditary hemorrhagic telangiectasia, coarctation of the aorta, and alpha1-antitrypsin deficency.[12-14]

Genetics also plays a role in the formation of intracranial aneurysms. If 2 first-degree relatives in the same family have an intracranial aneurysm with no heritable connective tissue disorder, immediate family members have up to a 17% incidence of harboring an unruptured aneurysm.[15] Furthermore, first-degree and second-degree relatives of a patient with aneurysmal subarachnoid hemorrhage (SAH) are at 4.1- to 6.6-fold increased risk for aneurysmal SAH.[16,17] Thereforc, screening is suggested in patients who have 2 or more family members with intracranial aneurysms.

Exogenous risk factors for the development of an intracranial aneurysm formation include cigarette smoking, cocaine use and heavy consumption of alcohol.[17,18] Infections, head trauma and intracranial neoplasms can rarely become primary causes of intracranial aneurysms.

TYPES OF ANEURYSMS

Saccular aneurysm: True aneurysm with all the layers of arterial wall as its covering. Majority of these aneurysm occur in the anterior circulation (90%), most commonly arising from the circle of Willis. Most common location is anterior communicating artery (35%) followed by the internal carotid artery (30%), including the carotid bifurcation, posterior communicating artery, and ophthalmic artery. The next most common location is the middle cerebral artery bifurcation (20%), followed by the basilar apex (5%). Vertebrobasilar junction, superior cerebellar artery and posterior inferior cerebellar artery account for less than ten percent of intracranial aneurysm.[19,20]

Dissecting aneurysm: Dissecting intracranial aneurysms are rare, originate from a dissection, which corresponds to a tear through the intima and internal elastic lamina with subsequent intramural hemorrhage.[21] The involved segment can become ectatic in response. Sometimes the tear may extend through the media and the adventitia resulting in pseudoaneurysm formation with or without SAH. Dissecting aneurysms can be acute or chronic. Acute dissecting aneurysms usually present with hemorrhage. Chronic dissecting aneurysms will more often induce compression of the adjacent structures.[22]

Atherosclerotic aneurysm: Atherosclerotic aneurysms are segmental arterial ectasia caused by atherosclerotic and degenerative changes. They are characterized by an enlarged and elongated course with a circumferential involvement of the parent vessel and lack of a well-defined neck. This gives them a fusiform morphology. Vertebrobasilar circulation is reported to be the most frequent site of occurrence.[23,24]

Mycotic aneurysm: Infectious (so-called mycotic) aneurysms are rare and account for 2% to 4% of all aneurysms. Most of infectious aneurysms occur in patients with infective endocarditis, the most common causative bacterium being *Streptococcus viridans*, while Aspergillus fumigatus is the most common agent causing fungal aneurysms.[25,26] These are often multiple and located distal to the circle of Willis, because they result from septic emboli in small cerebral arterial branches with resultant inflammation and necrosis.[27] Being fragile in nature, they usually rupture within the first weeks, with high morbidity and mortality.

Traumatic aneurysm: Account for less than 1% of all intracranial aneurysms, but they represent 5–15% of aneurysms in children. They are pseudoaneurysms, which develop after direct injury or shear of the arterial wall. Injury leads to formation of hematoma that first organizes and then recanalizes. Closed head injuries result in shearing or impaction of the arterial wall against a dural fold and are responsible for distal aneurysms of the pericallosal artery (most common) and the posterior cerebral or the superior cerebellar arteries.[28-30]

CLINICAL PRESENTATION

Subarachnoid hemorhage: Subarachnoid hemorrhage (SAH) resulting from ruptured cerebral aneurysms with consequent accumulation of blood in subarachnoid spaces. It is the most devastating presentation of cerebral aneurysm.

The patient will present with sever headache, often described as "worst headache of life" associated with varying neurological deficits. Patient with acute SAH may also have varying degree of neurological deficits.

Non-hemorrhagic neurological deficits: Aneurysm either due their mass effect or arterial pulsations can produce various neurological deficits. For example, giant cavernous ICA aneurysm can present with ipsilateral third, fourth or sixth cranial nerve palsies. Similarly large supraclinoid or Acom aneurysm may present with vision disturbances due to compression of optic apparatus. Large post fossa dissecting aneurysm may present with symptoms of brain stem compression or hydrocephalus. There is substantial clot burden associated with dissecting aneurysms, which has potential to cause ischemic stroke. Such a scenario is seen with dissecting MCA aneurysm.

Unruptured incidental aneurysm: Widespread use of CT and MR imaging has led to significant increase in numbers of intracranial aneurysms discovered incidentally, making the management of patients with unruptured intracranial aneurysms (UIAs) an increasingly relevant. We provide here a brief review of International Study of Unruptured Intracranial Aneurysms (ISUIA) to bring some perspective on this subject **(Table 1)**. The study analyzed 727 patients who had UIAs and no history of SAH (group 1 patients) and 722 patients who had UIAs and a history of SAH from another aneurysm (group 2 patients). Mean follow-up was about 7.5 years.[31]

The rupture rate for patients who had UIAs 7 mm or less in diameter was approximately less 1% per year. Aneurysmal location was important for predicting future UIA rupture, Posterior circulation and the posterior communicating artery aneurysm had greater risk of rupture as compared to anterior counterparts whereas carotid cavernous artery UIAs were associated with least risk.

Even though the above data suggests aneurysm with size less than 7 mm have < 1% annual risk of rupture, majority of ruptured aneurysm that present in our clinical practice are less than 7 mm. This observation compels us to understand the need for providing the patient with extensive preprocedural counseling given procedural risk and risk of future rupture.

DIAGNOSTIC EVAUATION

Whenever SAH is suspected, noncontrast head CT is cornerstone of the diagnosis with very high diagnostic yield. NCCT head not only conforms the diagnosis of SAH, but also provides valuable information regarding ventricular size, status of cerebral parenchyma and suspected location of the aneurysm **(Figs.1A to G)**. NCCT also remains a powerful tool for comparison and follow up.

MR imaging has limited role in evaluation of patient with SAH in emergency. However it is not infrequent for patient to get MRI for headache due to SAH. MRI revels altered signal intensity in sulcal spaces, most apparent on FLAIR images. T2 shortening (blooming) can be noted on gradient images, particularly well on SWI images. Careful attention must be paid so as not confuse cortical vein with surface SAH. MR imaging become important once we are concerned with large or giant aneurysm, where interest lies in assessing parenchymal status. MR vessel wall imaging is sometime done to delineate wall of the aneurysm. This becomes useful in understanding point of rupture and assessing fragility of the wall.

Imaging techniques for intracranial aneurysms include digital subtraction angiography (DSA) both 2D and 3D rotational angiography, multislice computed tomographic (MSCT) angiography, MR angiography, and transcranial Doppler ultrasonography.

Intra-arterial DSA is still the gold standard for evaluation of a patient with a suspected aneurysm, given its high spatial resolution; however with new generation MSCTA has a similar specificity and sensitivity for detecting an intracranial aneurysm, except for aneurysm smaller than 3 mm. The spatial resolution for DSA is 0.2 mm, and about 0.15 mm for 3D-DSA.[32] DSA is an invasive test with about 0.5–1% risk of permanent neurologic complications, whereas there is no risk of neurologic complications with MSCTA or MR angiography.[33,34]

The current spatial resolution of CT angiography is 0.4 to 0.7 mm.[32,35] When compared with DSA as the reference standard, CT angiography has an average reported specificity rate of 96% to 98% (90% to 94% for aneurysms smaller than 3 mm and up to 100% for aneurysms larger

Table 1: International Study of Unruptured Intracranial Aneurysms (ISUIA) study.

Aneurysm location	*< 7 mm group 1*	*< 7 mm group II*	*7–12 mm*	*13–24 mm*	*25+ mm*
Cav. ICA	0%	0%	0%	3%	6.4%
ACom/MCA/ICA	0%	1.5%	2.6%	14.5%	40%
Post circ. /Pcom	2.5%	3.4%	14.5%	18.4%	50%

Group 1 had no subarachnoid hemorrhage. Group 2 had subarachnoid hemorrhage from a separate aneurysm.

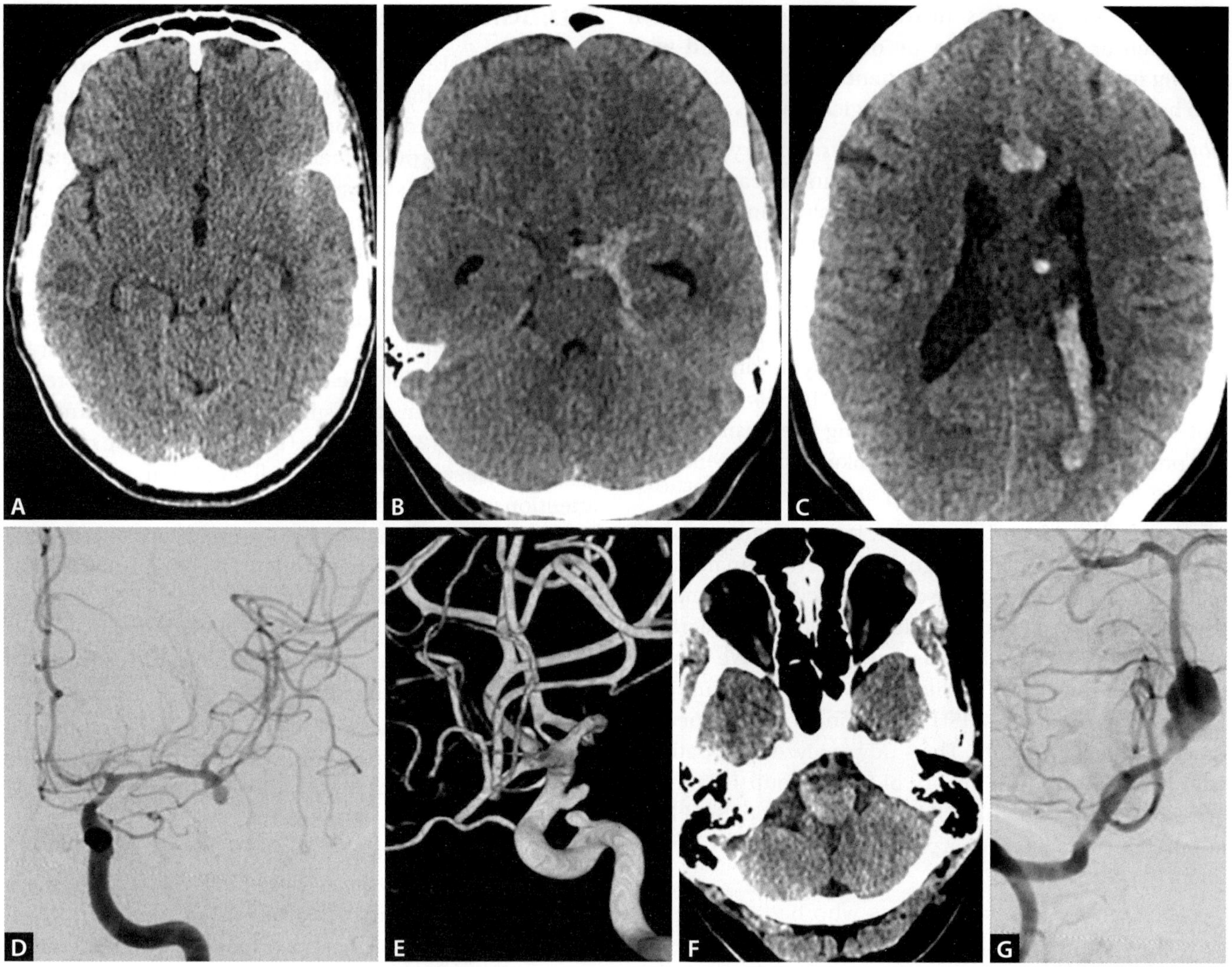

Figs. 1A to G: NCCT head in aneurysm. (A to C) show Fischer grade 2 (thin SAH), 3 (thick SAH) and 4 (thick SAH with IVH), respectively. Sentinel hematoma: Angiograms (D and E) of patient in A and B revealed left MCA bifurcation aneurysm and left Pcom aneurysm, respectively. Aneurysm presenting as mass effect: Dissecting vertebra-basilar junction aneurysm (G) compressing the brainstem (F).

than 4 mm) and sensitivity rates of 96% to 98%.[36] The spatial resolution of MR angiography at 1.5 T is on the order of 1 mm. With 3-T scanners, spatial resolution may reach 0.6 mm.[37] When compared with DSA, MR angiography reported specificity rates for detection of intracranial aneurysms ranging from 69% to 100%, with a sensitivity rate of 75% to 100%.[38,39]

As a matter of institute protocol all patient with suspected aneurysm undergo complete cerebral diagnostic angiography. This demonstrate size of the aneurysm and its orientation, length of neck, relationship between the aneurysm and parent artery and the status of rest of intracranial vessels. Some giant and complex aneurysms may require additional physiologic evaluation, including test occlusion and cross compression studies to determine the adequacy of collaterals, there by identifying if a patient can tolerate parent vessel occlusion.

If the first angiogram following SAH is negative, angiography should be repeated 1–2 weeks later. The recent use of 3D DSA has improved the pretreatment delineation of the aneurysm anatomy and of the surrounding vessels, however it could be misleading in presence of close approximation of vessels to the aneurysms.

PREPROCEDURE MANAGEMENT

Patient with acute SAH is an emergency[40] demanding immediate stabilization and management. The initial management is directed at ensuring basic life support. This includes ensuring adequate airway, ventilator, and circulatory support. History and physical examination are obtained to assess possible cause of SAH. Chest radiographs, electrocardiograms, blood work, serum electrolytes, cardiac and liver enzymes, coagulation profile and cross matching of blood is performed.

The clinical picture is classified according to the given algorithms[41] (WFNS: World Federation of Neurological Surgeons[42] and Hunt and Hess grade[43] respectively) **(Tables 2 and 3)**.

Patients are then managed in an intensive care setting, where close observation and frequent neurologic examinations can be done. Patients are kept nil orally until a final therapeutic decision on how to treat the aneurysm is taken. Majority of patients with SAH are hypovolemic, problem compounded by coexisting cerebral salt wasting or SIADH. Large bore IV access, and an arterial line if required is placed. Adequate normal saline with electrolyte supplementation is given with the goal of attaining/maintaining euvolemia. Role of IV dextrose in acute setting is controversial.

Extension of blood into cisterns and/or ventricles incites an inflammatory response and consequent adhesion formation. This hampers normal cerebrospinal fluid (CSF) circulation and results in hydrocephalus, documented in approximately 20–30 % of the cases. Treatment requires augmentation of CSF flow either through placement of external ventricular drain or lumbar drain. Excessive CSF drainage can result in sudden drop of the ICP, which may precipitate rebleeding. Hence drainage bag usually is placed at 18 to 20 cm above the head level. Improvement in CSF circulation not only improves ventricular status but also helps in counteracting development of cerebral vasospasm.[44] Persistent hydrocephalus may require VP shunt.

At authors' institute prophylactic anticonvulsants are currently administered to all patients with acute SAH. Rationale for this stems from the concern that a post SAH seizure could promote rebleeding of the aneurysm.[45]

Management of blood pressure in cases of acute SAH is complex and still slightly controversial. There is strong opinion to treat significantly elevated blood pressure because of increased incidence of rerupture in patients with continuous hypertension following SAH.[22] However moderated increase in blood pressure is a normal physiological response to SAH for maintaining cerebral perfusion. Hence care must be given to fact that sudden or exaggerated drop in blood pressure might precipitate cerebral ischemia due to underlying cerebral vasospasm.

Given high rates of rerupture in ruptured aneurysm, it is imperative that once the patient has been stabilized, next immediate goal should be occlusion of the aneurysm. This can be achieved either through endovascular route or via surgery (clipping). We will now summarize various endovascular methods to treat aneurysm.

Table 2: World Federation of Neurological Surgeons (WFNS) grade.

WFNS grade	*GCS score*	*Focal deficit*
I	15	Absent
II	14–13	Absent
III	14–13	Present
IV	12–7	Present or absent
V	6–3	Present or absent

Table 3: Hunt and Hess grade.

Hunt and Hess Category	*Criteria*
Grade I	Asymptomatic or minimal headache and slight nuchal rigidity
Grade II	Moderate-to-severe headache, nuchal rigidity, no neurological deficit
Grade III	Drowsiness, confusion or mild neurological deficit
Grade IV	Stupor, moderate-to-severe hemiparesis, early decerebrate rigidity and vegetative disturbances
Grade V	Deep coma, decerebrate rigidity—moribund appearance

ENDOVASCULAR TREATMENT

- *Endosaccular (treatment from within the aneurysm)*
  - Simple coiling without assistance
  - Balloon-assisted coiling
  - Stent-assisted coiling
  - Newer Devices
    - P-conus
    - Pulse Rider
    - WEB
    - Medina coils
- *Endoluminal (treatment from within the parent artery)*
  - Constructive: Parent vessel preserved
    - Flow Diverters
    - Covered Stents
  - Deconstructive: Parent vessel occlusion

SIMPLE COILING

How coiling of a simple aneurysm is done without any adjunctive device **(Figs. 2A to D)**.

Anesthesia

At the authors' institution, each endovascular aneurysm treatment is done under general anesthesia with complete

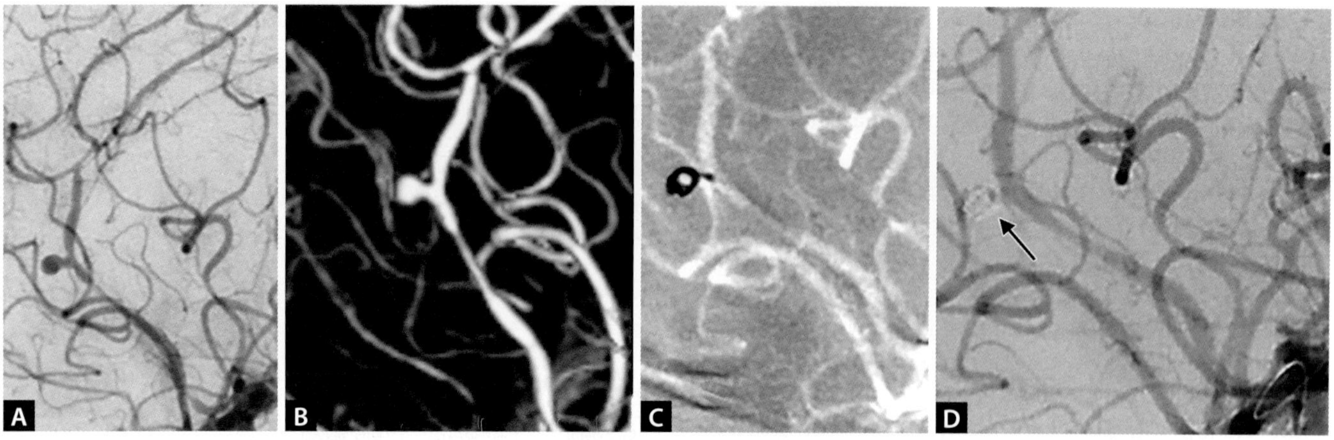

Figs. 2A to D: Conventional coiling: LICA angiogram (A) and 3D DSA; (B) reveal DACA aneurysm. Under roadmap; (C) aneurysm is coiled without use of adjunctive device. Control angiogram; (D) showing complete occlusion of the aneurysm (arrow).

hemodynamic and neurophysiological monitoring. The neuroanesthesiologist takes all necessary steps to avoid exaggerated blood pressure changes (spikes), especially while inducing or extubating the patient. Anesthesia is necessary to not only to maintain immobility but may also herald any intraoperative complication for example, intraprocedure aneurysmal rupture is manifested by immediate hypertension and bradycardia.

Access

Arterial sheath, generally 6F in caliber is introduced via femoral artery. If adjunctive devices are needed larger bore femoral puncture or simultaneous contralateral femoral puncture may be taken. After the sheath is inserted in the groin, 50 international units (IU) of heparin per kilogram is given intra-arterially as a bolus with intent to keep the ACT between 250 and 300 seconds.[43] Protamine sulfate for heparin reversal kept ready in neurointervention suite to be injected in unlikely case of aneurysmal rupture. The usual dose is 10 mg of protamine per 1000 IU of circulating heparin. Anti platelet regimen will be discussed under section on stent-assisted coiling.

Angiogram

A complete cerebral angiogram is performed before treatment with 5F catheter, including injections of the bilateral internal carotid and vertebral arteries. Additional 3D rotational images and cross compression studies are obtained to accurately define the morphology of the aneurysm and status of crossflow/collaterals.

After completion of diagnostic study, for therapeutic procedure a 6F guide catheter is introduced in target artery and positioned in close proximity to the aneurysm. It is necessary for the guide catheter to have a stable position for safe and smooth microcatheter navigation. Guide catheter should always be visible on working road map projection even during advancement of the coil through microcatheter into the aneurysm. Routinely used Guide catheters are the Neuron (Penumbra), Envoy (codman), or Chaperon (microvention). In case of tortuous aortic or neck anatomy Additionally a triple coaxial system consisting of a long sheath (Shuttle: cook) followed by guide catheter can be placed to straighten out the system and provide enhanced stability.[46-48]

Microcatheterization of Aneurysm

Catheterisation of an aneurysm is done via microcatheter-microwire combination under a constant visualization on roadmap. There is hydrophilic coating on outer wall of all microcatheters, which helps in minimizing friction and thus permit distal catheterization into the intracranial circulation. The various microcatheters used are Echelon (eV3), SL-10 (Stryker), Headway-17 (Microvention), etc. Microcatheters are shaped by steam heating of the tip to conform according to anatomy of artery and aneurysm. The ideal microcatheter position is governed by morphology of the aneurysm (shape, size, neck and relation to curve of parent artery). A well-positioned microcatheter should allow stable coil extrusion while maintaining its relation with parent artery and aneurysm.

Coiling

The choice of the coil is governed again by size, shape and neck of the aneurysm. The aim of the first coil or the framing coil is to create a frame or basket for the placement of subsequent coils. The framing coil also acts as bridge across the aneurysmal neck to prevent migrating of additional into the parent vessel. Size of the first coil is determined by largest dimension of the aneurysm. For proper approximation along the aneurysmal sac, the first coil should have largest and longest dimension possible. Well-apposed coil provides sound basket and stability to the subsequent coil mass.

First coil also called as framing coil is usually a 3D coil (complex shaped coil) and subsequent coils (filling coils) are generally helical coils. Under live roadmap keeping good profile of aneurysmal neck, successive coils are introduced into the aneurysm. Additional coils are introduced till they form dense coil mass and aneurysm is no longer opacifying on angiogram.

Once the aneurysm is obliterated, microcatheter is withdrawn slowly. Check angiogram is performed to assess the degree of aneurysm occlusion, patency of parent artery and status of the distal vasculature.

Once the procedure has been completed, femoral artery sheath is removed. Manual compression or closure device can be used to obtain hemostasis. Pressure with fingertips is maintained on the puncture site for usually 30 to 40 minutes if manual compression is used. The patient is then shifted to neuro ICU. Leg is kept immobilized for atleast 6 hours to prevent puncture site complications.[49]

BALLOON-ASSISTED COILING

An aneurysm is considered wide necked when the ratio between the maximum diameters of dome and neck is less than two. The aneurysms then become anatomically unfavorable for conventional coiling as chances of prolapsing of coils in parent artery increases. Moret et al. first described utility of balloon remodeling technique for such aneurysms.[50,51]

The technique consists of inflating a balloon (non detachable) in front of aneurysmal neck during coil placement. The balloon acts as a temporary bridge, allowing coils to be packed into the aneurysm sac without prolapsing into the artery. The coils remain molded within the aneurysm after deflation of the balloon, essentially "remodeling the arterial wall". It is routinely used today to treat wide-necked aneurysms particularly in patients with SAH, thus eliminating stent placement and the use of antiplatelet agents.

To treat wide-necked side-wall aneurysms, the neurointerventionist routinely uses compliant balloons, e.g. HyperGlide (Ev3, Irvine, CA), Ascent (Codman Neurovascular, Raynham, MA) and Scepter C (Microvention- Terumo, Inc, Tustin, CA).

Technique for balloon-assisted coiling **(Figs. 3A to H)** is essentially same as described previously. Under roadmap, first the deflated balloon first is navigated across the neck of the aneurysm. This is followed by catheterization of the aneurysm. The balloon is inflated across the neck of the aneurysm, causing temporary occlusion of the neck and parent vessel. Thus the balloon bridges the neck and allows formation of coil basket. Before the coil is detached, balloon is deflated to test the stability of the coil within sac. If no displacement of the coil loop is observed, the coil is detached. This procedure is repeated multiple times until the aneurysm no longer fills with contrast or has a dense coil mass within the confines of its lumen.

To treat an aneurysm located at arterial bifurcations or aneurysm with arteries arising from its neck, neurointerventionist use extra-compliant low-pressure balloon which conform to the irregularities of any vasculature space. When the balloon is inflated, ity partially herniates into the aneurysm neck or the origin of the arterial branches emerging from the neck of the aneurysm. This configuration secures the parent artery and arterial branches emerging from the neck of the aneurysm during coil placement. Example of extra compliant balloon are hyperform (eV3) and Septor -XC (Microvention).

STENT-ASSISTED COILING

Stent-assisted coiling is done for wide-necked and dysplastic aneurysms that are not amendable with simple or balloon assisted coiling. The stent acts as a scaffold that prevents the coils placed into the aneurysm sac from herniation into the parent vessel. The stent may also reduce the inflow into the aneurysm, promoting stasis and thrombosis of the aneurysm. In addition, the struts of the stent may provide a matrix for the growth of endothelial cells across the neck of the aneurysm.

Initially, balloon-expandable coronary stents were used; however being relatively stiff stents they were difficult to navigate into tortuous intracranial circulation and carried risk of possible rupture of the parent vessel. They were gradually replaced with self-expanding stents.

Self-expanding stents are broadly divided into two types either laser cut or braided. Laser cut stents are Neuroform (Stryker), Enterprise (Codman) and Solitaire (eV3). Braided stents are Leo (Balt Extrusion), and LVIS (Microvention).

Technique of Coiling with Stent Assistance (Figs. 4A to H)

The aneurysm may be coiled by different techniques using stent assistance. We briefly describe four different

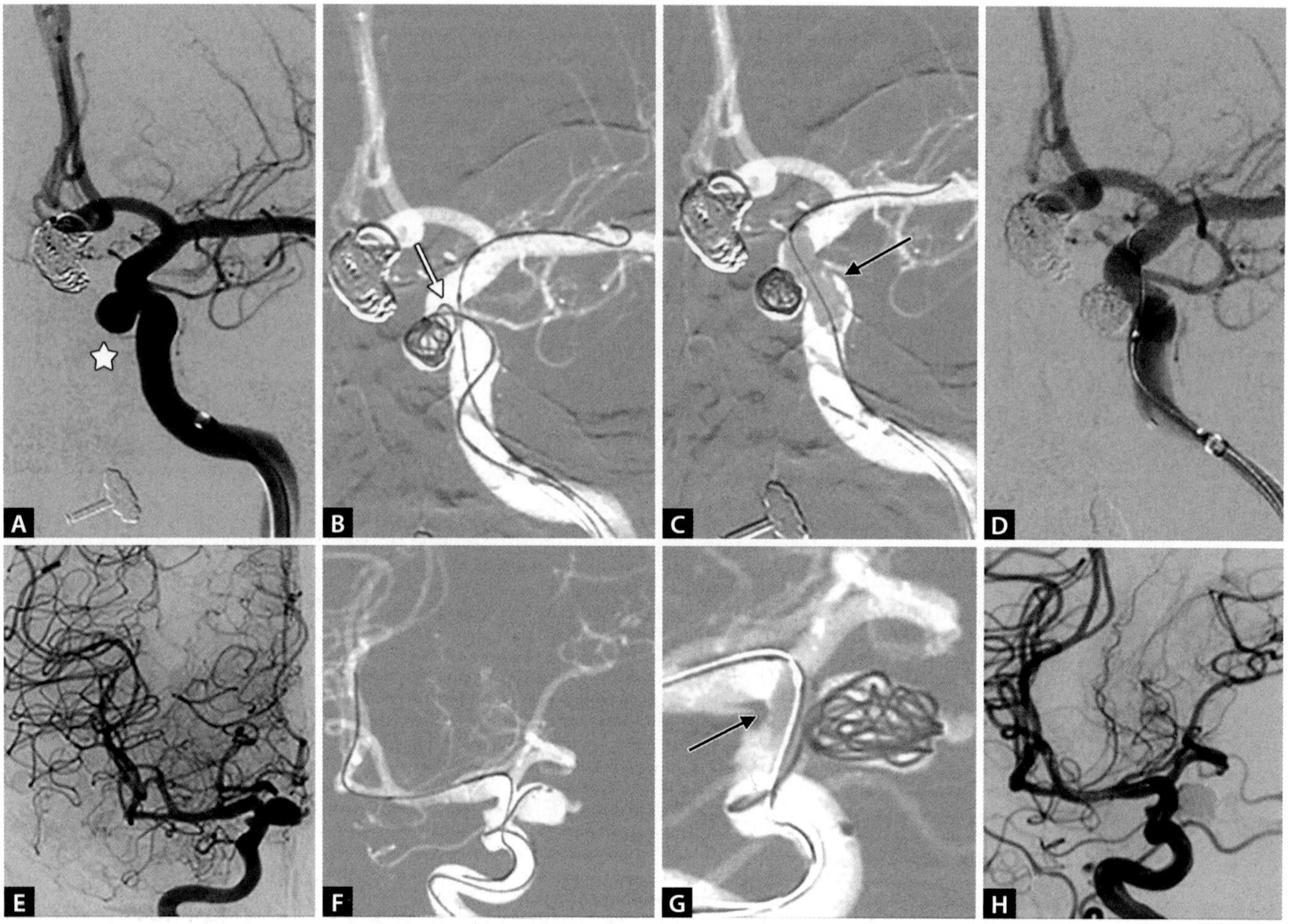

Figs. 3A to H: Balloon-assisted coiling: LICA angiogram (A) reveals left carotid cave aneurysm (*). Unassisted coiling; (B) resulted in herniation of coil loops in parent artery (white arrow). After balloon inflation; (C) (black arrow) the aneurysm is remodeled and completely coiled; (D). Another case with wide neck ruptured superior hypophyseal aneurysm; (E) is treated with balloon-assisted (black arrow) coiling; (F and G). Control angiogram; (H) showing complete obliteration of the aneurysm.

approaches for stent assisted coiling. "Jailing the microcatheter", in this technique aneurysm is first catheterized followed by deployment of stent across the aneurysm. This effectively jails the coiling catheter between parent artery and the stent, providing increased stability while coiling. In the second technique stent is first delivered across neck of the aneurysm, followed by placement of coiling catheter into the aneurysm sac through stent struts. Third technique involves coiling of aneurysm by routine balloon assisted manner, then the stent is placed across the neck of the aneurysm with an intention to decrease recanalization by promoting endothelial growth along the stent surface. Final technique also called as stent jack technique, involves partial deployment of a first coil before placement of stent across the aneurysm neck. After complete deployment of the stent, the first coil is detached. This in contrast to jailing technique, which involves only catheterization of aneurysm, not coil placement before stent deployment.

It becomes very important for an interventional neuroradiologist to understand anatomy of both aneurysm and parent artery on 3D rotational angiogram. Points to be considered when contemplating size of the stent are length of the neck, dimensions of parent artery at level of aneurysm as well as proximal and distal to the aneurysm. The diameter of the stent is then sized to be about 0.5–1 mm more than diameter of parent artery. Length of the stent is determined by the fact that middle of the stent should be across the aneurysmal neck with at least 5 mm coverage along both proximal and distal aspects of aneurysm neck.

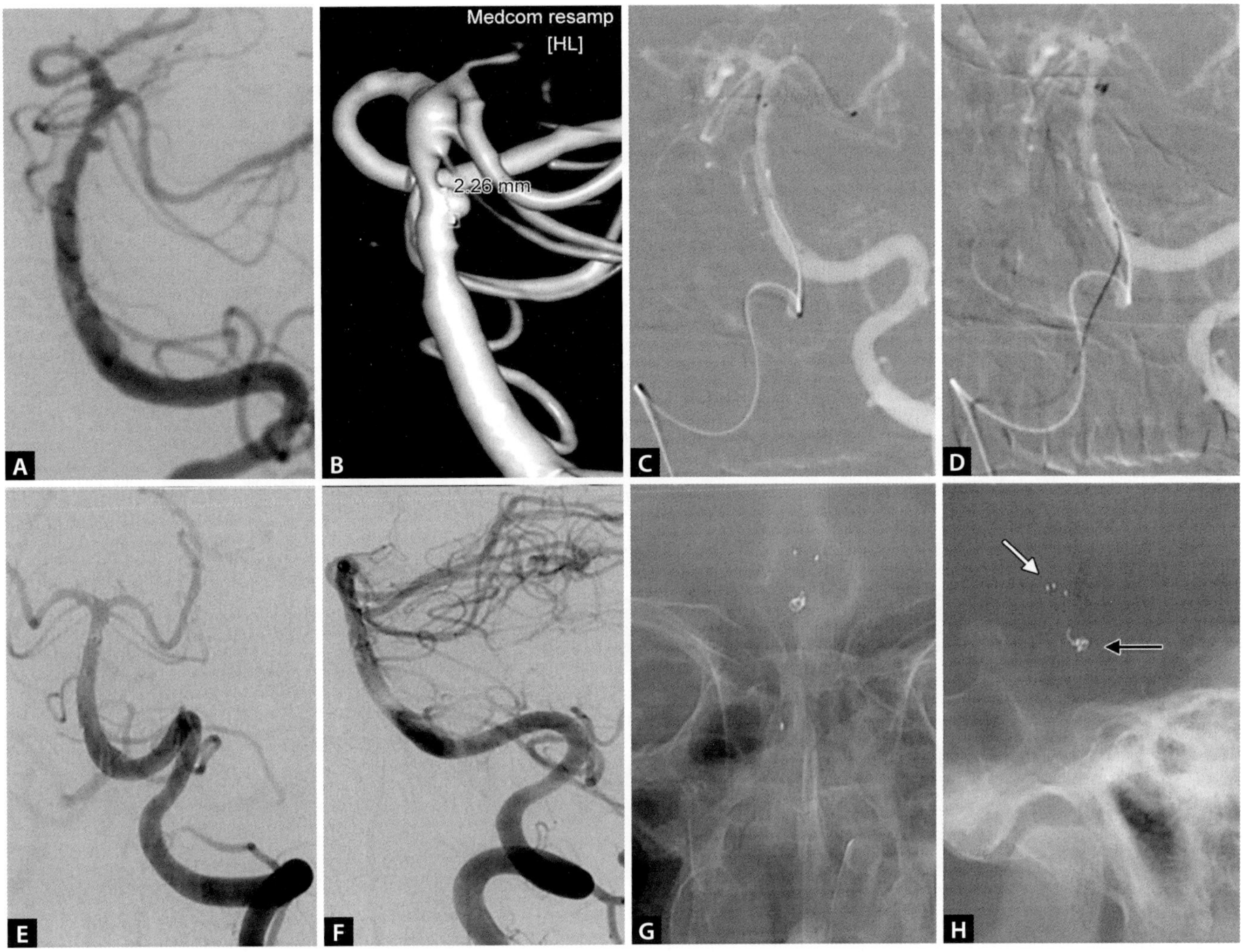

Figs. 4A to H: Stent Jack Technique (Stent-assisted coiling). LVA angiogram (A) and VRT image (B) show small dysplastic blister aneurysm in distal basilar artery. Under roadmap (C and D), first coil was partially placed with few loops were seen to be prolapsing into the parent artery, at this point stent was deployed to push the coil loops inside the aneurysm. Control angiogram (E and F) reveals occlusion of aneurysm with patent basilar artery. Native images (G and H) show stent markers (white arrow) and coil loops (black arrow), respectively.

PROTOCOL FOR ANTIPLATELET ADMINISTRATION IN CASES OF INTRACRANIAL STENTING

Stent is a foreign body, thus its placement into the cerebral vessel will incite inflammatory response with consequent platelet activation and clot formation. To prevent this, it is of utmost important to administer optimal antiplatelet agents before placement of an intracranial stent. The optimal dose and treatment regimen, however, has not been determined.

At authors institution dual antiplatelets are administered for at least 3 days prior to the procedure. Aspirin (150 mg/day orally) and clopidogrel (150 mg/day orally) are the drugs used. If a stent needs to be placed on an emergent basis the authors will administer dual antiplatelet 3 to 4 hours prior to the procedure. Dose of drugs is clopidogrel (300 mg orally) and aspirin (300 mg orally). If an emergency stent graft **(Figs. 5A to H)** needs to be placed during the procedure in a patient who has not been treated preoperatively with antiplatelet medications, the patient is loaded with abciximab (glycoprotein IIa/IIIb inhibitor) at the dose of 0.25 mg/kg the and subsequently dual antiplatelets are started. Few institutions may keep patient on continuous infusion of abciximab for 12 to 24 hours before shifting to dual antiplatelets.[52]

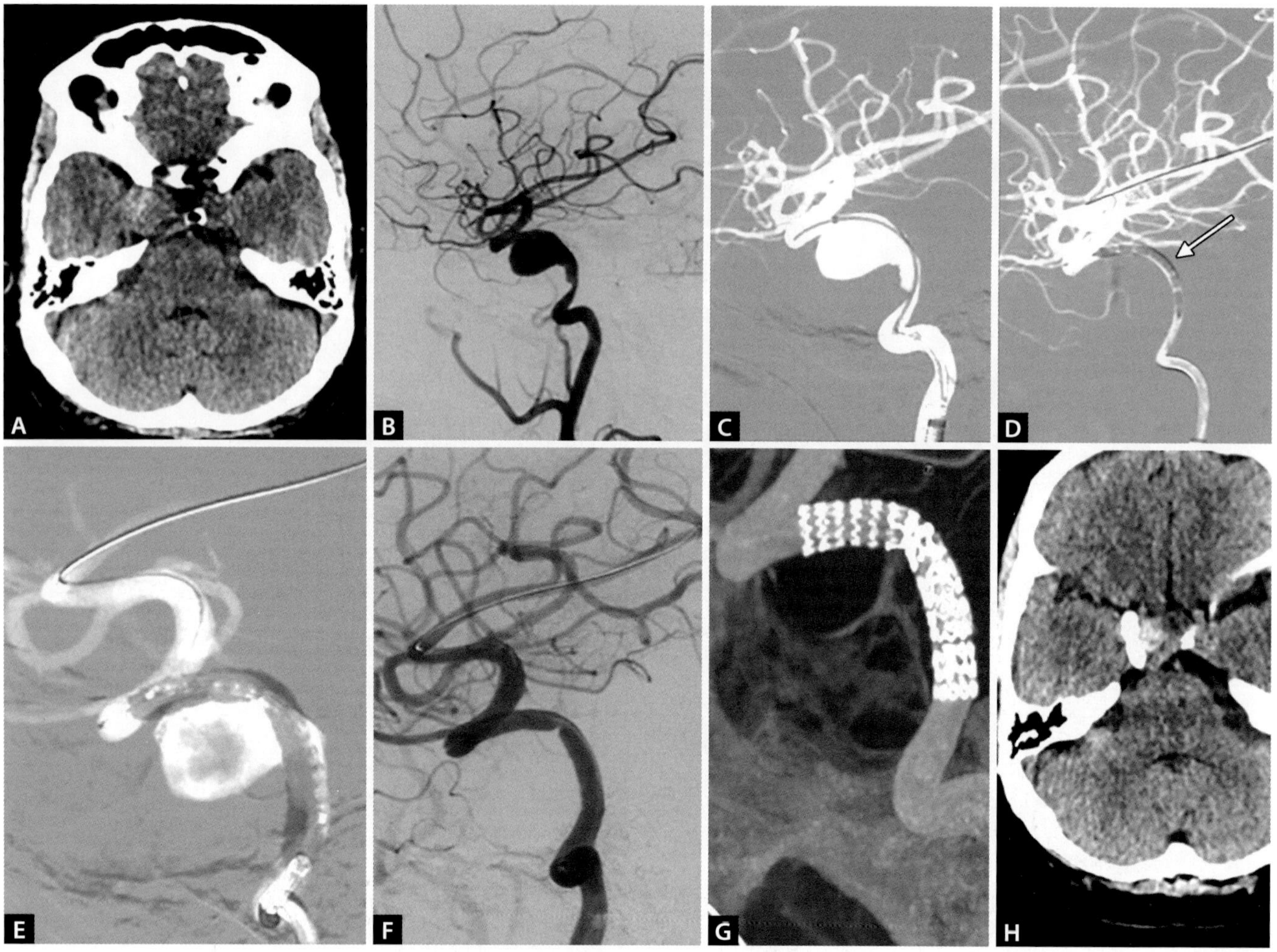

Figs. 5A to H: Covered stent placement: NCCT head (A) and RICA angiogram; (B) show partially thrombosed right cavernous ICA aneurysm. Subsequent balloon mounted stent graft (white arrow) (covered stent) is navigated; (C and D) and inflated; (E) across the aneurysm. Control angiogram; (F) shows occlusion of aneurysm with patent ICA. Follow-up CT; (G and H) documents shrinkage of aneurysm with resolution of its mass effect.

FLOW DIVERTERS

Over last decade revolutionary devices for treatment of complex aneurysm have appeared in markets called flow diverters.[53] Novelty of these devices lies in the fact that they treat aneurysms from endoluminal rather than conventional endosaccular approach **(Figs. 6A to F)**. Such stent-like devices are designed to reconstruct the parent vessel and to divert flow away from the aneurysm lumen without the use of coils.

Flow diverters are stent like devices has tighter scaffolding, providing a means over which endothelial cells can grow to seal off the neck of the aneurysm. The device promotes thrombus formation within the aneurysm by decreasing the hemodynamic effects within the aneurysm sac, spare side branches and perforators (fill via pressure gradient) promote neointimal remodeling (maintaining outflow in the side branches and perforators) and change the configuration of the parent vessel in relation to aneurysm.[54,55]

Flow diverters are braided stents with high metal coverage and low porosity. They are made of either chromium cobalt or nitinol wires. Number of wires range from 48 to 96. The various flow diverters available in market are Pipeline (Ev3), Silk (Balt), FRED (microvention), SURPASS (Stryker) and p64 (Phenox).

Current indication of flow diverters is wide necked large/giant intracranial aneurysm (>10 mm) not amenable to other endovascular treatment options. However with advancement in their design flow diverters are now also used for blister aneurysms, distal anterior

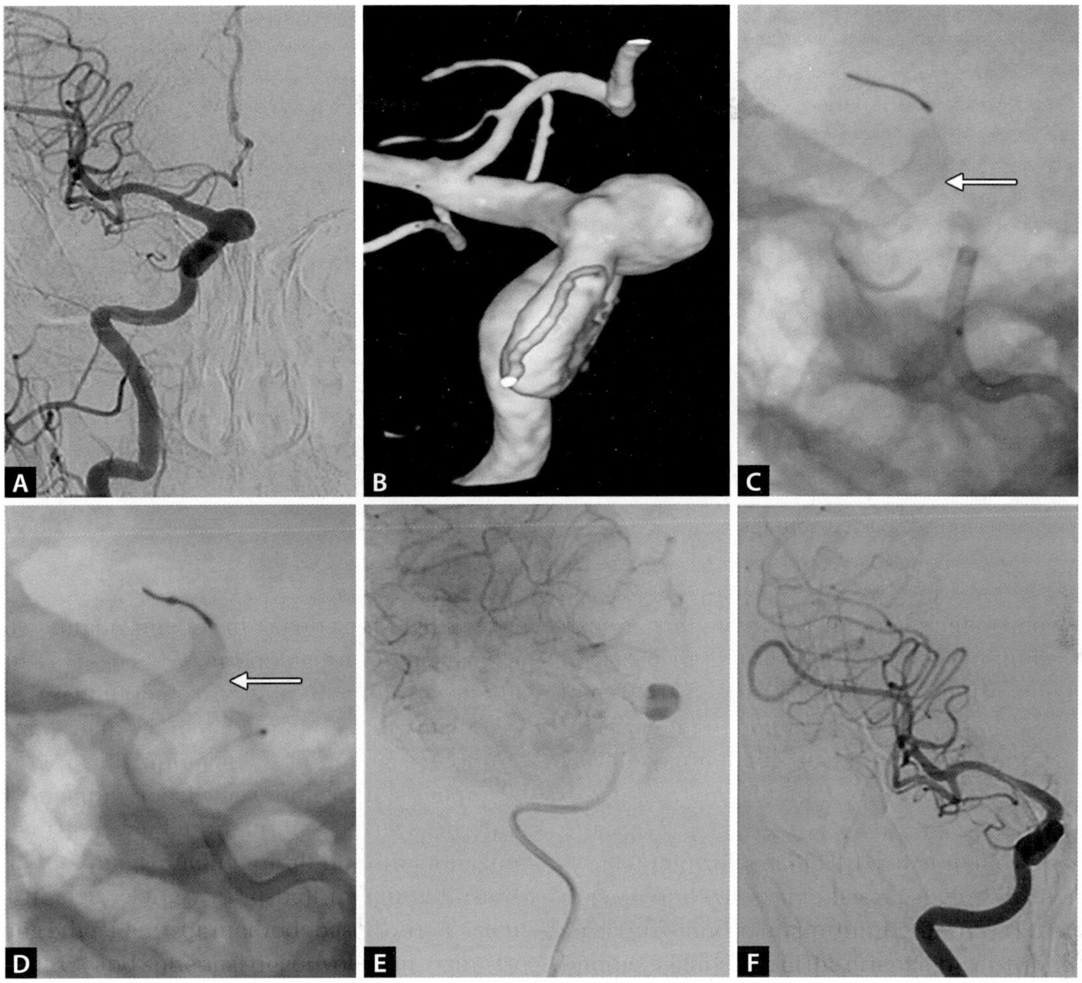

Figs. 6A to F: Flow diverter placement. RICA angiogram (A) and VRT image; (B) show wide neck superior hypophyseal aneurysm. Fluoroscopy-spots; (C and D) show deployment of FD (white arrows) across neck of the aneurysm. Control angiogram; (E) showing marked stasis in aneurysm. Follow-up angiogram after 1 year; (F) shows complete obliteration of aneurysm with remodeling of the parent artery.

circulation aneurysm and large posterior fossa dissecting aneurysms.[56,57]

Flow diverters are bulky devices with relative difficulty in their deployment across the aneurysm. Hence they are associated with higher incidence of both ischemic and hemorrhagic complications.

PARENT ARTERY OCCLUSION

Sometimes in very complex large dissecting aneurysms, preservation of parent artery may not be possible. In such situations it becomes imperative that parent artery be occluded. This can be done either with concomitant aneurysm occlusion **(Figs. 7A to E)** or as a stand-alone procedure **(Figs. 7F to J)**. The basic idea behind this technique lies in the fact that progression of these aneurysms is directly dependent on direction of the blood flow across them. If we are able to abolish/reverse this flow, the progression of the aneurysm may be arrested and with due passage of time the involved arterial segment will heal. The anatomy of arterial collaterals, competence of COW and possibility of development of new collaterals must be understood when contemplating parent artery occlusion (PAO). In majority of cases prior to arterial sacrifice, a temporary balloon test occlusion (BTO) is done to assess whether the patient can tolerate permanent occlusion of the artery. Once the patient tolerates BTO, parent artery is then occluded either with coils **(Figs. 7A to E)** or detachable balloons **(Figs. 7F to K)**. Possible complications include stroke, non-shrinkage of aneurysm on follow-up and closure of direct anatomical pathway for future intervention. However PAO is a time proven therapeutic option. Elegance of this technique is highlighted by the excellent long-term angiographic and

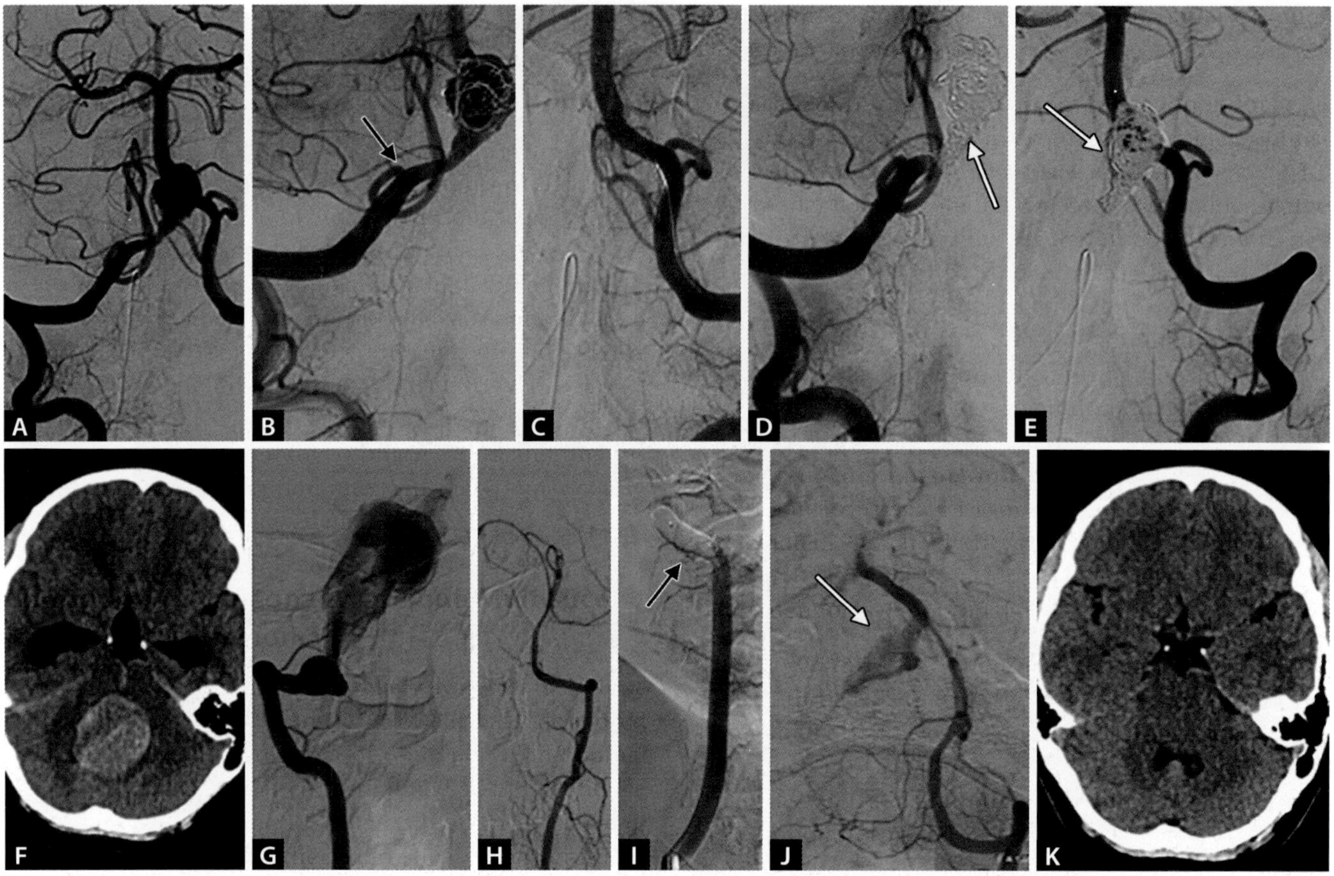

Figs. 7A to K: Parent artery occlusion: RVA angiogram (A) reveals vertebrobasilar dissecting aneurysm. It was treated by occlusion of aneurysm and V4 segment of RVA distal to origin of right PICA (black arrow in B) with stent placement from LVA to basilar artery (C). Control angiogram (D and E) revealed occlusion of both aneurysm and parent artery (coil mass marked by white arrows).
Parent artery occlusion with flow reversal: NCCT head (F) and RVA angiogram (G) reveals large dissecting right V4 segment aneurysm with hydrocephalus. LVA (H) is hypoplastic. After successful balloon test occlusion, RVA (I) was occluded with detachable balloon (black arrow). Postprocedure LVA angiogram (J) reveals reversal of flow in aneurysm (white arrow). Follow-up CT (K) after a year shows resolution of both aneurysm and hydrocephalus.

clinical results that are achieved with minimal intervention in complex aneurysms, which are otherwise a challenge to treat.

COMPLICATIONS OF ENDOVASCULAR COILING AND THEIR MANAGEMENT

Alongside the risks, the advantages and disadvantages of endovascular coiling should be weighed against the risk of surgical treatment or a conservative approach before treatment, to determine the best option for the optimal clinical outcome. Patients should be given their full options along with extensive information before treatment. In the case of a ruptured aneurysm this information should be given to the patient's relatives. The information provided must inform patient party in a comprehensive manner about therapeutic options, relative merits and demerits, cost of procedure, goals of treatment and estimated duration of ICU/hospital stay.

Every periprocedural or postprocedural complication needs to be examined thoroughly before corrective actions are taken.

Coil Migration/Malposition

Coil malposition refers to placement of coil outsides the confines of aneurysmal sac. Malposition of a coil usually results from poor coil choice, improper catheter position, or choice of technique not suitable for aneurysm. Most commonly it is a single loop of coil that protrudes into the parent vessel. Single loop plastered along the arterial wall will seldom causes a thromboembolic complication and thus we should refrain from overzealous treatment.

If thrombus forms around the loop of coil, a glycoprotein IIa/IIIb inhibitor can be given at the site of thrombus formation to dissolve the clot. If the coil gas to be removed, one of the retrieval devices like microsnare or retrievable stent must be used **(Figs. 8F to J)**. If coil

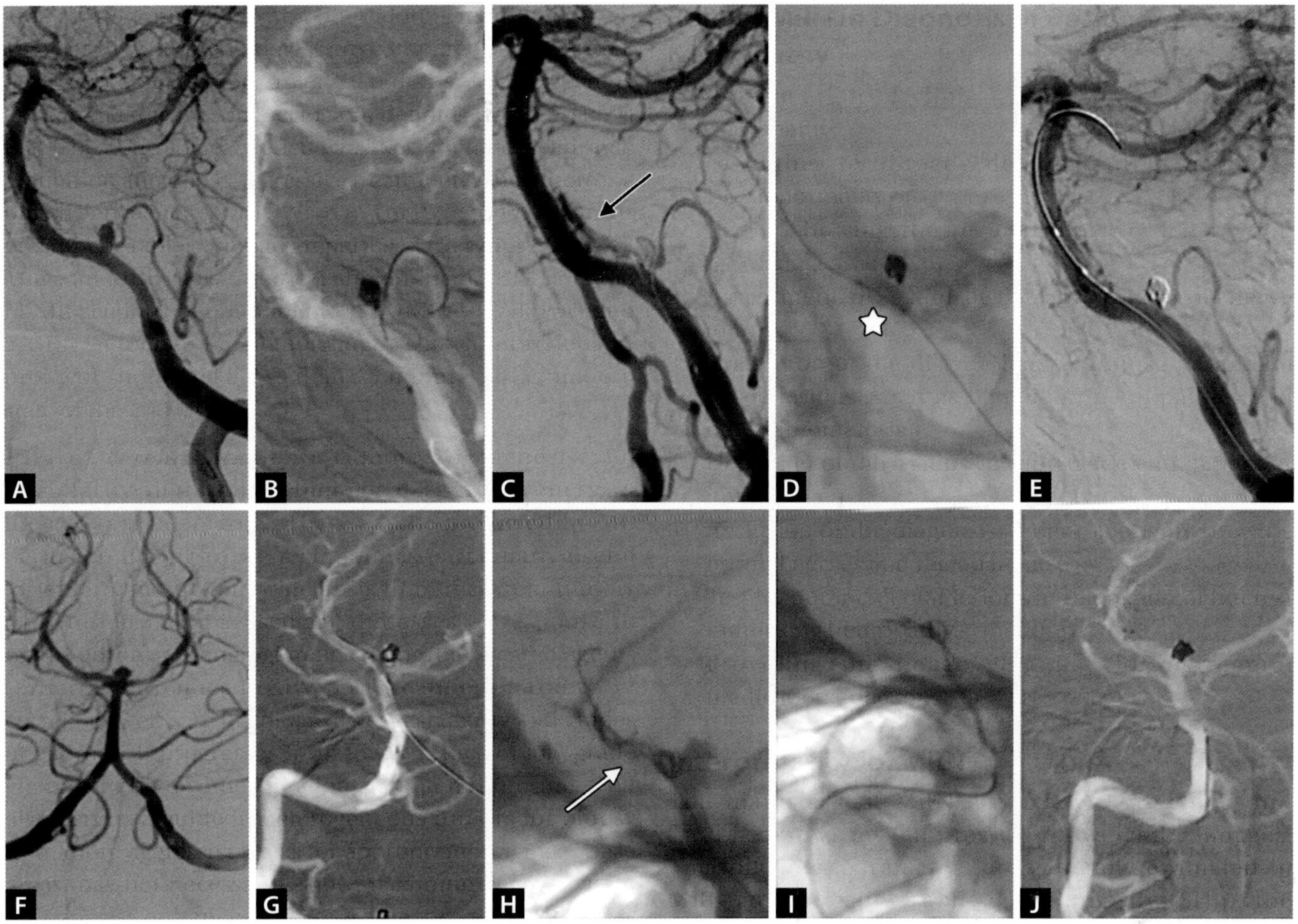

Figs. 8A to J: Complications: Intraprocedural aneurysmal rupture. LVA angiogram (A) reveals PICA aneurysm which was coiled with protection of PICA (B). Check angiogram postcoiling (C) shows leak in vicinity of aneurysm (black arrow) suggestive of aneurysmal rupture. Heparin was reversed and balloon inflated across neck of aneurysm (* in D). Control angiogram (E) shows control of contrast extravasation and complete obliteration of aneurysm.
Coil migration: RVA angiogram (F) shows basilar top aneurysm. Initially balloon assisted coiling was attempted (G). After deflation of balloon (H) detached coil migrated into right PCA (white arrow). It was subsequently retrieved via solitaire stent (I). Finally stent-assisted coiling (J) was done.

retrieval is not possible, the loop of coil should be plastered against the vessel wall by placement of intracranial stent.[58]

Stretched Coil

Stretching of a coil is potentially disastrous complication. It requires prompt recognition and remedy. Stretched coil should be suspected if the coil is not responding one-to-one under fluoroscopy with hand movements at the groin, or if difficulty is encountered in repositioning of the coil.

In this situation, the coil and microcatheter should be retrieved together as a single unit from the patient. However if the coil cannot be retrieved, it should be stretched as long as possible and positioned either into the external carotid artery or descending thoracic aorta to prevent distal arterial migration. Patient should be kept anticoagulated overnight in the NICU and given an antiplatelet agent. Within span of 6–8 weeks the stretched coil becomes endothelized.

Intraprocedural Rupture of Aneurysm

Intraoperative aneurysm rupture is the most dreaded complication can occur due to fragile nature of the aneurysm wall **(Figs. 8A to E)**. It usually occurs either during aneurysmal microcatheterization or coil placement.[59] When this occurs, there is a rapid severe elevation of the blood pressure.

Given very high mortality with this complication, it is of utmost importance to quickly secure the aneurysm and control blood extravasation into subarachnoid space. Circulating systemic heparin must be immediately reversed with protamine [1 mL (10 mg) protamine per 1000 units of circulating heparin], so that the ACT is less than 150 seconds. If the patient has been placed on dual antiplatelets, an attempt at reversal of platelet inhibition should be made with the infusion of platelets. The blood pressure should also be lowered immediately by pharmaceutical means in an attempt to prevent any further extravasation of blood.[60,61]

If a balloon is present within the parent vessel, this should be carefully positioned and inflated at aneurysmal neck and aneurysm rapidly packed with additional coils. If the microcatheter is within the subarachnoid space, the operator must not panic and remove the microcatheter. Coiling should be performed from the subarachnoid space into the aneurysm.

After the aneurysm is secure, CT of the head should be immediately performed to assess for hydrocephalus and the need for placement of a ventriculostomy catheter.

Rupture of Vessel

Arterial perforation by either microcatheter or microguide wire is rare. This rupture may be self-limiting and seal off spontaneously, or may lead to life-threatening hemorrhage particularly in patients premeditated on antiplatelets. If angiographic leak or life-threatening hemorrhage is identified, permanent occlusion of the vessel may be life-saving. A liquid embolic agent or coils can be used for this purpose.[62]

Intraprocedural Thromboembolism

A thromboembolic event is probably the most common complication related to endovascular management of an aneurysm. To prevent thrombus formation during the procedure patients are fully anticoagulated so that the ACT range is between 250 and 300 seconds.

If there is evidence of clot formation with or without distal embolization on angiogram, most interventionists prefer local infusion of a glycoprotein IIa/IIIb inhibitor (Abciximab) at site of thrombus formation. At authors' institution, abciximab is administered intra-arterially through the microcatheter at a dose of 2 to 4 mg over 10 to 20 minutes. In case of small emboli with resultant stasis is noted in distal cerebral vasculature, the neuroanesthetic should be asked to escalate the blood pressure in attempt to clear distal emboli and augment pial collaterals. Abciximab has also been shown to be effective in ruptured aneurysms, with no increased risk of bleeding complications.[63]

ANEURYSM TREATMENT COILING VS CLIPPING: WHERE DO WE STAND?

Treatment of intracranial aneurysms is based on their exclusion from the intracranial circulation to prevent bleeding, which can be achieved by surgical or endovascular techniques. In past neurosurgical clipping of the aneurysmal neck was the only effective method of treating a cerebral aneurysm, however with advent of detachable coils by Guglielmi in 1992 endovascular treatment has swiftly transformed into being the primary therapeutic option.

We present couple of studies to bring in the perspective how both the treatment modalities fare when compared to each other.

International Subarachnoid Aneurysm Trial (ISAT)

About 23.7% patients allocated to endovascular treatment were dependent or dead at 1 year compared with 30.6% allocated to neurosurgical treatment ($p = 0.0019$). The relative and absolute risk reductions in dependency or death after allocation to an endovascular versus neurosurgical treatment were 22.6% (95% CI 8.9–34.2) and 6.9% (2.5–11.3), respectively. In patients with a ruptured intracranial aneurysm, for which endovascular coiling and neurosurgical clipping are therapeutic options, the outcome in terms of survival free of disability at 1 year is significantly better with endovascular coiling.[64]

Barrow Ruptured Aneurysm Trial (BRAT)

Poor outcome (mRS score > 2) was observed in 33.7% of the patients assigned to aneurysm clipping vis-à-vis 23.2% of the patients assigned to coil embolization (OR 1.68, 95% CI 1.08–2.61; $p = 0.02$). One year after treatment, a policy of intent to treat favoring coil embolization resulted in fewer poor outcomes than clip occlusion.[65]

From the above-mentioned studies it becomes that clinical results with endovascular treatment are better as compared to surgical counterparts. Note should be made that there was higher percentage of patient with complete aneurysm obliteration following surgery in contrast to endovascular coiling. Consequently more patients from endovascular arm required retreatment, however difference in risk of rebleed was statistically insignificant.

With advancement in interventional neuroradiology tools and techniques, complete aneurysmal obliteration is more routinely achieved. There is change in clinical practice favoring endovascular procedure over microsurgical clipping as first choice of treatment in large number of institutes. Although a policy of intent to treat favoring coil embolization resulted in fewer poor outcomes at 1 year, it remains important that high-quality surgical clipping be available as an alternative treatment modality. Treatment of aneurysm needs to tailored for each given case and thereby it is imperative for a centers to offer both treatment modalities

ENDOVASCULAR TREATMENT OF CEREBRAL VASOSPASM

Cerebral vasospasm following aneurysmal SAH is a delayed, reversible narrowing of the intracranial vasculature that occurs most commonly 4–14 days after aneurysmal SAH and can lead to permanent ischemic injury.

Cerebral vasospasm should be suspected in any patient with SAH who develops new onset neurological deficit not attributable to any other cause like seizure, hydrocephalus or hematoma. Patients with Fisher grade 3 SAH have the highest risk of developing symptomatic vasospasm.[66] Transcranial ultrasonography (TCD) can reliably predict the presence of significant cerebral vasospasm when the flow velocities are greater than 200 cm/s or there is a rapid rise in flow velocities as compared to baseline values. Angiography remains gold standard in diagnosing vasospasm. Greater than 50% narrowing in vessel caliber is defined as severe vasospasm, and 25% to 50% narrowing in vessel caliber is defined as mild vasospasm. Plain CT can reveal developing rounded hypodensities, whereas CT perfusion can identify ischemic area at risk of infarction.[67]

Prophylaxis and Medical Treatment for Cerebral Vasospasm

Expectant treatment for cerebral vasospasm following aneurysmal SAH is controversial and varies among institutions. Triple-H (hypervolemia, hypertension, and hemodilution) therapy has been a mainstay of vasospasm treatment for years. Calcium channel blockers, magnesium, HMG-CoA reductase inhibitors (statins), fasudil, thrombolytics and endothelial receptor antagonists have all been used in attempts to prevent and treat vasospasm.[58]

At authors' institute short acting calcium channel blocker namely nimodipine is used as primary pharmacological drug against vasospasm. Drug is given at dose 1 mg (5 mL)/hour as continuous IV infusion and subsequently changed to oral nimodipine tablets 60 mg/4 hourly. The drug is continued at least up to 21 days post SAH. All effort is made to maintain mean blood pressure in range around 90–100 mm Hg, once the aneurysm has been secured. We will emphasize more on endovascular management of cerebral vasospasm.

Endovascular treatment with intra-arterial (IA) infusion of a vasodilator or balloon angioplasty is indicated in patients with symptomatic vasospasm refractory to medical therapy to prevent neurologic deficits referable to the vascular territory of the angiographic vasospasm.

INTRA-ARTERIAL VASODILATOR INFUSION

Calcium Channel Antagonists

Nimodipine is a short acting dihydropyridine derivative, which has proven systemic efficacy in cerebral vasospasm.[68] Nimodipine is administered by diluting 2–6 mg (5 mL = 1 mg) with 75–100 mL of normal saline **(Figs. 9A to D)**. Diluted drug is then administered at a slow continuous infusion over 30–45 minutes. In authors practice maximum dose has never been greater than 6 mg per artery. The main complications of nimodipine include hypotension and bradycardia. It is imperative to maintain blood pressure during and after the procedure. Other CCBs that can be used are verapamil and nicardipine.[69]

Inodilators

Milrinone is a phosphodiesterase III inhibitor that affects cyclic adenosine monophosphate (cAMP) pathways with both inotropic and vasodilatory effects. At authors institution milrinone is administered as slow infusion in 1:4 dilution over 10–20 minutes. Dose ranges from 2–4 mg per artery. Milrinone is now becoming drug of choice at many institutions owing to its no significant effect on blood pressure. Due to its positive inotropic action, potential adverse effect includes tachycardia and arrhythmias. Other phosphodiesterase inhibitor is papeverine.[70,71]

It is important to understand that these drugs have short duration of action, hence repeat procedures are a rule. Patient will generally require multiple session in addition to medical therapy for successfully overcoming period of vasospasm.

TRANSLUMINAL BALLOON ANGIOPLASTY

Contrary to chemical angioplasty (intra-arterial vasodilation), which is more effective for distal arterial spasm, balloon angioplasty is preferred for proximal vessel spasm. Inflammatory changes mediating smooth muscle contraction, changes in the linkage of the protein matrix, and collagen deposition in the vessel wall have all been implicated as a possible cause of blood vessel narrowing in SAH.[72,73]

Transluminal balloon angioplasty (TBA) acts by stretching the vessel wall, leading to morphologic and functional changes in the smooth muscle fibers, resulting in impairment of contractility. At a cellular level it has been shown that there is fragmentation of the collagen matrix and flattening of the endothelial cells, resulting in permanent restoration of vessel diameter.

The typical location for balloon angioplasty is supraclinoid ICA, basilar artery, intradural vertebral artery,

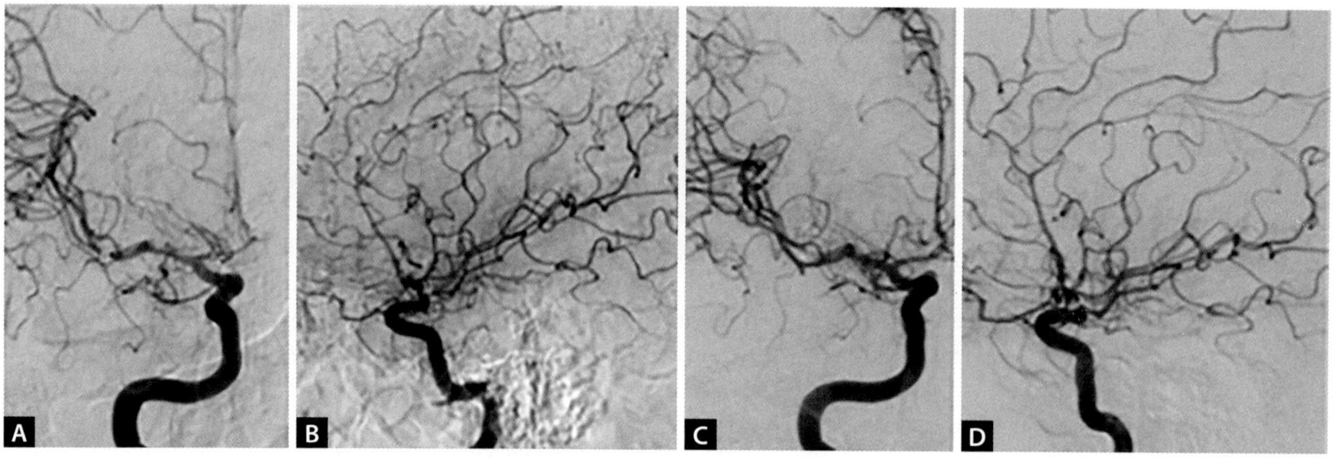

Figs. 9A to D: Intra-arterial nimodipine for vasospasm: RICA angiogram (A and B) in postcoiling case show decreased caliber of right supraclinoid ICA, A1 ACA and M1 MCA with attenuation of their distal branches. Postnimodipine infusion (C and D) there is marked improvement in caliber of proximal as well as distal arteries.

A1 ACA and M1 MCA. Balloon angioplasty is generally avoided in vessel with diameter less than 2 mm. Commonly used balloons are either compliant or extra compliant like Hyperglide (eV3) or Secptor (Microvention). Care must be followed when negotiating across the stenotic segment to avoid inadvertent dissection. While perform balloon angioplasty care should be taken not to overinflate, given relatively large volume of these balloons.[58]

Transluminal balloon angioplasty itself has some potential significant risks. These most serious one include vessel rupture and arterial dissection. These balloons can be flow limiting and may cause thrombus formation with resultant stroke. Finally, there is risk of reperfusion injury by restoration of blood flow in ischemic vascular territory.

FOLLOW-UP AND MONITORING

All patients who have undergone an endovascular procedure undergo check angiogram to confirm the aneurysm status after 3–6 months following primary procedure. Aneurysm can re grow secondary to coil compaction, extension of arterial dissection, continued dual antiplatelets or de novo new aneurysm formation. Small neck compactions can be followed up on serial angiograms, whereas larger recurrences require repeat procedure. Follow-up angiogram also assumes importance in modulating and down stepping antiplatelet agent once aneurysm/parent artery is healed. It has been shown that stable occlusions at 6 months, will rarely show recurrences.

CONCLUSION

Advancement in endovascular techniques has revolutionized the treatment of intracranial aneurysm. With further refinement of interventional tools, majority of the aneurysms today can be treated via endovascular route. Clear understanding of the disease, treatment options, available equipment/hardware, possible complications and requirement for follow-up is important is ensuring overall success for any given endovascular procedure is an patient.

ACKNOWLEDGMENT

The author acknowledges Dr Nishchint Jain, DM resident in the Department of Neuroimaging and Interventional Radiology, AIIMS, New Delhi for active involvement and helping in writing the chapter.

REFERENCES

1. Nakagawa T, Hashi K. The incidence and treatment of asymptomatic, unruptured cerebral aneurysms. J Neurosurg. 1994;80:217-23.
2. Winn HR, Jane JA Sr, Taylor J, et al. Prevalence of asymptomatic incidental aneurysms: review of 4568 arteriograms. J Neurosurg. 2002;96:43-9.
3. Krishna H, Wani AA, Behari S, et al. Intracranial aneurysms in patients 18 years of age or under, are they different from aneurysms in adult population? Acta Neurochir. 2005;147:469-76.
4. Kanaan I, Lasjaunias P, Coates R. The spectrum of intracranial aneurysms in pediatrics. Minim Invasive Neurosurg. 1995;38:1-9.
5. Stehbens WE. Etiology of intracranial berry aneurysms. J Neurosurg. 1989;70:823-31.
6. TerBrugge K. Aneurysm in the pediatric population. Rivista di Neuroradiologia. 1998;11(Suppl 1):54-5.
7. Swietaszczyk C, Maciaczyk J, Tafil-Klawe M, et al. What is the origin of cerebral aneurysms? Przegl Lek. 2004;61:115-9.
8. Strother CM, Graves VB, Rappe A. Aneurysm hemodynamics: an experimental study. Am J Neuroradiol. 1992;13:1089-95.

9. Foutrakis G, Yonas H, Sclabassi R. Saccular formation in curved and bifurcating arteries. Am J Neuroradiol. 1999;20:1309-17.
10. Malek AM, Alper SL, Izumo S. Hemodynamic shear stress and its role in atherosclerosis. JAMA. 1999;282:2035-42.
11. Kondo S, Hashimoto N, Kikuchi H, et al. Cerebral aneurysms arising at nonbranching sites. An experimental Study. Stroke. 1997;28:398-403.
12. Schievink WI. Genetics of intracranial aneurysms. Neurosurgery. 1997;40:651-63.
13. Torner JC. Epidemiology of subarachnoid hemorrhage. Semin Neurol. 1984;4:354-69.
14. Krog M, Almgren B, Eriksson S. Vascular complications in the Elhers-Danlos syndrome. Acta Chir Scand. 1983;149:279-82.
15. Bromberg JEC, Rinkel GJ, Algra A, et al. Subarachnoid haemorrhage in first and second degree relatives of patients with subarachnoid haemorrhage. BMJ. 1995;311:288-9.
16. Schievink WI, Schaid DJ, Michaels VV, et al. Familial aneurysmal subarachnoid hemorrhage: a community-based study. J Neurosurg. 1995;83:426-9.
17. Shinton R, Beevers DG. Meta-analysis of relation between cigarette smoking and stroke. BMJ. 1989;298:789-94.
18. Juvela S, Hillbom M, Numminen H, et al. Cigarette smoke and alcohol consumption as risk factors for aneurysmal subarachnoid hemorrhage. Stroke. 1993;24:639-46.
19. Batjer HH, Kopitnik TA, Giller GA, et al. Surgery for paraclinoid carotid artery aneurysms. J Neurosurg. 1994;80:650-8.
20. Day AL. Aneurysms of the ophthalmic segment: a clinical and anatomical analysis. J Neurosurg. 1990;72:677-91.
21. Endo S, Nishijima M, Nomura H, et al. A pathological study of intracranial posterior circulation dissecting aneurysms with subarachnoid hemorrhage: report of three autopsied cases and review of the literature. Neurosurgery. 1993;33:732-8.
22. Bonneville F, Sourour N, Biondi A. Intracranial aneurysms: an overview. Neuroimaging Clin N Am. 2006;16:371-82.
23. Anson JA, Lawton MT, Spetzler RF. Characteristics and surgical treatment of dolichoectatic and fusiform aneurysms. J Neurosurg. 1996;84:185-93.
24. Schnee CL, Flamm ES. Unusual aneurysms. Neuroimaging Clin N Am. 1997;7:803-18.
25. Corr PD, Wright M, Handler LC. Endocarditis-related cerebral aneurysms: radiologic changes with treatment. AJNR Am J Neuroradiol. 1995;16:745-8.
26. Kurino M, Kuratsu J, Yamaguchi T, et al. Mycotic aneurysm accompanied by aspergillus granulomas: a case report. Surg Neurol. 1994;42:160-4.
27. DiMaio S, Mohr G, Dufour JJ, et al. Distal mycotic aneurysm of the AICA mimicking intracanalicular acoustic neuroma. Can J Neurol Sci. 2003;30:388-92.
28. Holmes B, Harbaugh RE. Traumatic intracranial aneurysms: a contemporary review. J Trauma. 1993;35:855-60.
29. Amirjamshidi A, Rahmat H, Abbassioun K. Traumatic aneurysms and arteriovenous fistulas of intracranial vessels associated with penetrating head injuries occurring during war: principles and pitfalls in diagnosis and management. J Neurosurg. 1996;84:769-80.
30. Proust F, Callonec F, Bellow F, et al. Tentorial edge traumatic aneurysm of the superior cerebellar artery. Case report. J Neurosurg. 1997;87:950-4.
31. Wiebers DO, Whisnant JP, Huston J III, et al. International Study of Unruptured Intracranial Aneurysms Investigators. Unruptured intracranial aneurysms: natural history, clinical outcome, and risks of surgical and endovascular treatment. Lancet. 2003;362:103-10.
32. Kallmes DF, Layton K, Marx WF, et al. Death by nondiagnosis: why emergent CT angiography should not be done for patients with subarachnoid hemorrhage. Am J Neuroradiol. 2007;28:1837-8.
33. Schellinger PD, Richter G, Kohrmann M, et al. Noninvasive angiography (magnetic resonance and computed tomography) in the diagnosis of ischemic cerebrovascular disease. Techniques and clinical applications. Cerebrovasc Dis. 2007;24(Suppl 1):16-23.
34. Willinsky RA, Taylor SM, TerBrugge K, et al. Neurologic complications of cerebral angiography: prospective analysis of 2,899 procedures and review of the literature. Radiology. 2003;227:522-8.
35. Villablanca JP, Rodriguez FJ, Stockman T, et al. MDCT angiography for detection and quantification of small intracranial arteries: comparison with conventional catheter angiography. Am J Roentgenol. 2007;188:593-602.
36. McKinney AM, Palmer CS, Truwit CL, et al. Detection of aneurysms by 64-section multidetector CT angiography in patients acutely suspected of having an intracranial aneurysm and comparison with digital subtraction and 3D rotational angiography. Am J Neuroradiol. 2008;29:594-602.
37. Hacein-Bey L, Provenzale JM. Current imaging assessment and treatment of intracranial aneurysms. Am J Roentgenol. 2011;196:32-44.
38. Wardlaw JM, White PM. The detection and management of unruptured intracranial aneurysms. Brain. 2000;123(Pt 2):205-21.
39. Mallouhi A, Felber S, Chemelli A, et al. Detection and characterization of intracranial aneurysms with MR angiography: comparison of volume-rendering and maximum-intensity-projection algorithms. Am J Roentgenol. 2003;180:55-64.
40. Hunt WE, Hess RM. Surgical risk as related to time of intervention in the repair of intracranial aneurysms. J Neurosurg. 1968;28(1):14-20.
41. Report of World Federation of Neurological Surgeons Committee on a Universal Subarachnoid Hemorrhage Grading Scale. J Neurosurg. 1988;68:985-6.
42. Adams HP Jr, Kassell NF, Torner JC, et al. Early management of aneurysmal subarachnoid hemorrhage: a report of the Cooperative Aneurysm study. J Neurosurg. 1981;54:141-5.
43. Cognard C, Weill A, Castaings L, et al. Intracranial berry aneurysms: angiographic and clinical results after endovascular treatment. Radiology. 1998;206:499-510.

44. Hasan D, Vermeulen M, Wijdieks EFM, et al. Management problems in acute hydrocephalus after subarachnoid hemorrhage. Stroke. 1989;20:747-53.
45. Rhoney DH, Tipps LB, Murry KR, et al. Anticonvulsant prophylaxis and timing of seizures after aneurysmal subarachnoid hemorrhage. Neurology. 2000;55:258-65.
46. Spiotta AM, Hussain MS, Sivapatham T, et al. The versatile distal access catheter: the Cleveland Clinic experience. Neurosurgery. 2011;68:1677-86.
47. Hauck EF, Tawk RG, Karter NS, et al. Use of the outreach distal access catheter as an intracranial platform facilitates coil embolization of select intracranial aneurysms: technical note. J Neurointerv Surg. 2011;3:172-6.
48. Park MS, Stiefel MF, Fiorella D, et al. Intracranial placement of a new, compliant guide catheter: technical note. Neurosurgery. 2008;63:E616-7.
49. Khaghany K, Al-Ali F, Spigelmoyer T, et al. Efficacy and safety of the Perclose Closer S device after neurointerventional procedures: prospective study and literature review. Am J Neuroradiol. 2005;26:1420-4.
50. Moret J, Cognard C, Weill A, et al. Reconstruction technic in the treatment of wide-neck intracranial aneurysms. Long-term angiographic and clinical results. Apropos of 56 cases. J Neuroradiol. 1997;24:30-44.
51. Aletich VA, Debrun GM, Misra M, et al. The remodeling technique of balloon-assisted Guglielmi detachable coil placement in wide-necked aneurysms: experience at the University of Illinois at Chicago. J Neurosurg. 2000;93:388-96.
52. Blanc R, Piotin M, Mounayer C, et al. Direct cervical arterial access for intracranial endovascular treatment. Neuroradiology. 2006;48:925-9.
53. Fiorella D, Kelly ME, Albuquerque FC, et al. Curative reconstruction of a giant midbasilar trunk aneurysm with the pipeline embolization device. Neurosurgery. 2009;64:212-7.
54. Kallmes DF, Ding YH, Dai D, et al. A new endoluminal, flow-disrupting device for treatment of saccular aneurysms. Stroke. 2007;38:2346-52.
55. Kallmes DF, Ding YH, Dai D, et al. A second-generation, endoluminal, flow-disrupting device for treatment of saccular aneurysms. Am J Neuroradiol. 2009;30:1153-8.
56. Fiorella D, Woo HH, Albuquerque FC, et al. Definitive reconstruction of circumferential, fusiform intracranial aneurysms with the pipeline embolization device. Neurosurgery. 2008;62:1115-20.
57. Nelson PK, Lylyk P, Szikora I, et al. The pipeline embolization device for the intracranial treatment of aneurysms trial. AJNR Am J Neuroradiol. 2011;32:34-40.
58. Gemmete JJ, Pandey AS, Chaudhary N, et al. Endovascular management of intracranial aneurysms. In: Quinones-Hinojosa A (Ed). Schmidek and Sweet Operative Neurosurgical Techniques: Indications, Methods, and Results, 6th edition, Vol. 1. Elsevier; 2012. pp. 1019-27.
59. Doerfler A, Wanke I, Egelhof T, et al. Aneurysmal rupture during embolization with Guglielmi detachable coils: causes, management, and outcome. Am J Neuroradiol. 2001;22:1825-32.
60. Hirai T, Suginohara K, Uemura S, et al. Management of aneurysm perforation during Guglielmi electrodetachable coil placement. Am J Neuroradiol. 2002;23:738-9.
61. Ricolfi F, Le Guerinel C, Blustajn J, et al. Rupture during treatment of recently ruptured aneurysms with Guglielmi electrodetachable coils. Am J Neuroradiol. 1998;19:1653-8.
62. Wada H, Piotin M, Boissonnet H, et al. Carotid rupture during stent-assisted aneurysm treatment. Am J Neuroradiol. 2004;25:827-9.
63. Kwon OK, Lee KJ, Han MH, et al. Intra-arterially administered abciximab as an adjuvant thrombolytic therapy: report of three cases. Am J Neuroradiol. 2002;23:447-51.
64. Molyneux A, Kerr R, Stratton I, et al. International Subarachnoid Aneurysm Trial (ISAT) of neurosurgical clipping versus endovascular coiling in 2143 patients with ruptured intracranial aneurysms: a randomised trial. Lancet. 2002;360:1267-74.
65. McDougall CG, Spetzler RF, Zabramski JM, et al. The Barrow Ruptured Aneurysm Trial. Clinical article. J Neurosurg. 2012;116:135-44.
66. Macdonald LR, Weir B. Epidemiology. In: Cerebral Vasospasm. San Diego (CA): Academic Press; 2001. pp. 17-43.
67. Sloan MA, Alexandrov AV, Tegeler CH, et al. Therapeutics and Technology Assessment Subcommittee of the American Academy of Neurology. Assessment: transcranial Doppler ultrasonography: report of the Therapeutics and Technology Assessment Subcommittee of the American Academy of Neurology. Neurology. 2004;62(9):1468-81.
68. Pickard JD, Murray GD, Illingworth R, et al. Effect of oral nimodipine on cerebral infarction and outcome after subarachnoid haemorrhage: British aneurysm nimodipine trial. BMJ. 1989;298:636-42.
69. Biondi A, Ricciardi GK, Puybasset L, et al. Intra-arterial nimodipine for the treatment of symptomatic cerebral vasospasm after aneurysmal subarachnoid hemorrhage: preliminary results. Am J Neuroradiol. 2004;25:1067-76.
70. Macdonald RL, Weir BK, Young JD, et al. Cytoskeletal and extracellular matrix proteins in cerebral arteries following subarachnoid hemorrhage in monkeys. J Neurosurg. 1992;76:81-90.
71. Pennings FA, Albrecht KW, Muizelaar JP, et al. Abnormal responses of the human cerebral microcirculation to papaverin during aneurysm surgery. Stroke. 2009;40:317-20.
72. Zubkov YN, Nikiforov BM, Shustin VA. Balloon catheter technique for dilatation of constricted cerebral arteries after aneurysmal SAH. Acta Neurochir (Wien). 1984;70:65-79.
73. Zwienenberg-Lee M, Hartman J, Rudisill N, et al. Effect of prophylactic transluminal balloon angioplasty on cerebral vasospasm and outcome in patients with Fisher grade III subarachnoid hemorrhage: results of a phase II multicenter, randomized, clinical trial. Stroke. 2008;39:1759-65.

CHAPTER 11

Endovascular Management of Arteriovenous Malformations

Ajay Kumar, Niranjan Khandelwal, Shallesh B Gaikwad, Chirag Kamal Ahuja, Vivek Gupta

INTRODUCTION

Brain arteriovenous malformations (bAVMs) are uncommon vascular lesions with arteriovenous shunting and a prevalence of about 0.2%–0.8% in general population per year.[1] Classification of arteriovenous malformations AVMs is based on the type of primary defects, such as arterial, arteriovenous, capillary and venous **(Table 1)**. For each of them, different effects on the remaining vascular system can be encountered. Spetzler's classification incorporates the size of the AVM, the pattern of venous drainage, and the "eloquence" of the regions of the brain adjacent to the AVM.[2] Objective assessment of surgical risk is the major aim of this classification, and the risk derived is compared to the assumed natural history of all AVMs as a group.

Brain AVMs are an abnormal connection between the arteries and veins through dysplastic plexiform network of vessels with shunting of blood from arterial to venous side.[3] In the past 15 years, there is a lot of improvement in the understanding of bAVMs, their natural history, angioarchitecture, imaging techniques and available treatment modalities. bAVMs can be asymptomatic and incidental finding on imaging or may present clinically with headache, spontaneous ICH (58%), seizures (34%) and neurological deficits (8%).[4-14]

Most common presentation of symptomatic bAVMs is with spontaneous intracranial hemorrhage and the high risk predisposing factors are associated aneurysms, deep venous drainage, deep or posterior fossa location and associated venous stenosis.[15-17] According to large studies by Kim et al.[18] and Gross et al.[19] annual rupture risk for unruptured bAVM was 1.3–2.2% and for ruptured bAVM was 4.5–4.8%. Another important clinical presentation is focal or generalized seizures.[20] The exact etiology for

Table 1: Primary classification of the brain arteriovenous malformations (Berenstein and Lasjaunias).

Arteriovenous shunts
Single Micro AV shunts (mAVM or mAVF) Macro AV shunts (compartmented nidus ormAVF)
Multiple (nonfamilial) Systemic (Wyburn-Mason) Nonsystemic (multiple separate niduses or separated compartment within one nidus)
Multiple (familial) Systematized (Rendu-Osler-Weber) Nonsystematized (multiple separate niduses with or without AVF)
Associated vascular variants Arterial or venous
Secondary vascular changes Angiogenesis, kinking and dolichoid vessels Arterial aneurysms, venous ectasias and pouches Venous and arterial stenoses and thrombosis
External carotid supply Shunting (remote) Arterial and venous collateral circulation Pseudoaneurysms (hematomas)
Secondary morphological changes Hydrocephalus, cerebral atrophy, cavities Perivascular ischemia, calcification Bone hypertrophy
Associated vascular tumors

seizures in bAVMs is still unclear. However, some authors propose the role of venous hypertension for seizures.[21,22] The patients with bAVM in temporal location (strong correlation), cortical involvement, larger size and younger age group are at high risk to present with seizures.[23,24] Contrary to this patients with associated aneurysms and posterior fossa location of bAVMs were seen to have less risk for seizures.[25] The occurrence of neurological deficits is rare. The basic mechanism responsible for this is local ischemia/hypoxia either due to arterial steal or venous hypertension.[26,27]

ANGIOARCHITECTURE/COMPONENTS OF BRAIN ARTERIOVENOUS MALFORMATION

Morphologically AVMs are one of the most complex pathological condition. The central component of AVMs is abnormal/dysplastic tangle of vessels replacing the normal capillary network known as nidus. The nidus can be compact or diffuse depending upon its spread in relation to brain parenchyma. Compact nidus **(Figs. 1A to D)** usually does not have intervening normal brain parenchyma, thus, easier for microsurgery, radiosurgery or embolization. Diffuse nidus **(Figs. 2A to F)** usually have intervening brain parenchyma which poses difficulty in the management by any available treatment modalities.

Another important component of the AVM are arterial feeders. They can be single, multiple and en-passage, latter two poses difficulty in management. However, single feeder are associated with high risk of hemorrhages.[28] Terminal arterial feeders ends into the nidus and are easier for embolization or microsurgery. On the contrary, pseudoterminal feeders supply the normal brain parenchyma distally **(Figs. 3A to I)** and indirect feeders are the smaller branches of major and significant vascular channels that pose great challenge for microsurgery or embolization with high risk of thromboembolic complications and ischemic events

Venous drainage pattern is also equally important for prognostication and management strategies. There can be three patterns of venous drainage—superficial, deep and combined. bAVMs draining into superficial venous system are responsible for less hemorrhagic complications and also associated with better prognosis and management. Apart from venous pattern, the presence of venous stenosis is associated with higher risk of hemorrhage, seizures and neurological deficits.[29]

Along with its complex anatomical morphology another factor peculiar for AVMs is their dynamic nature. Depending on the blood flow rate across the AVM nidus, they can be classified into low, intermediate or high flow lesions. High blood flow rate AVMs poses great difficulty for management by embolization or microsurgery and are also associated with high incidence of failed radiosurgery.

Aneurysms associated with bAVMs are one of the most common causes of spontaneous hemorrhage. Depending up on the location, the aneurysms are classified as pre-nidal/flow related **(Figs. 4A to D)**, nidal/intra and peri-nidal **(Figs. 5 to 7)** and post-nidal/venous varices . Unruptured feeder artery aneurysm (pre-nidal) usually do not warrant any treatment and are believed to regress after nidal obliteration. The aneurysms on any location if responsible for the hemorrhage requires urgent microsurgical resection or embolization on emergent basis to prevent rebleed.[30] Aneurysms unrelated to bAVMs, i.e. in different vascular territory or contralateral hemisphere can be treated as per management strategies for aneurysms.

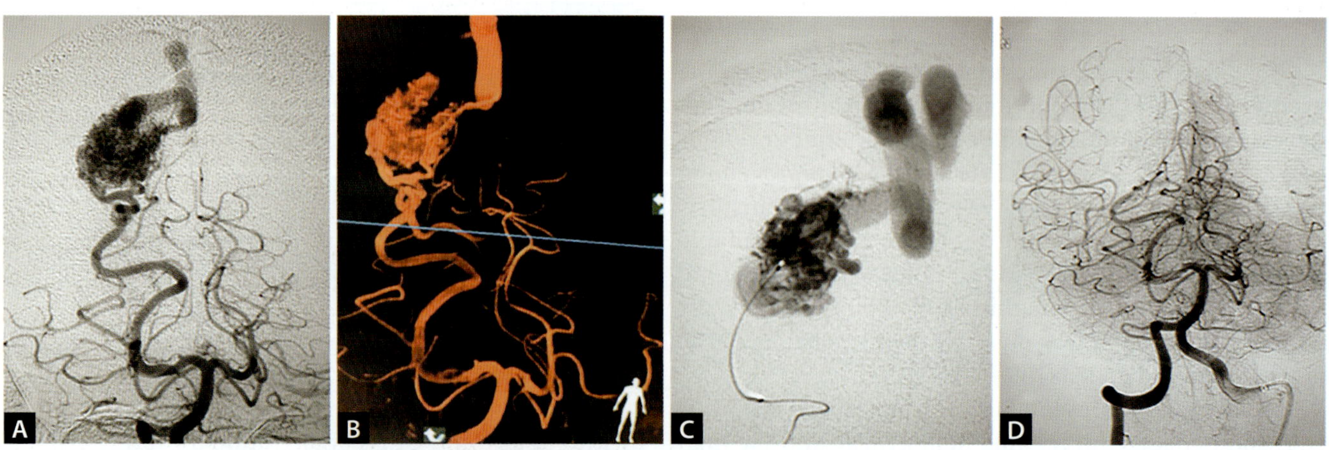

Figs. 1A to D: A 27-year-old male presented with severe headache and disorientation and diagnosed to have compact AVM nidus in right parieto-occipital region. Diagnostic DSA with 3-DRA images accurately shows the nidus with PCA feeders and superficial venous drainage (A and B). Complete obliteration of nidus was achieved using PHIL and detachable tip microcatheters (C and D).

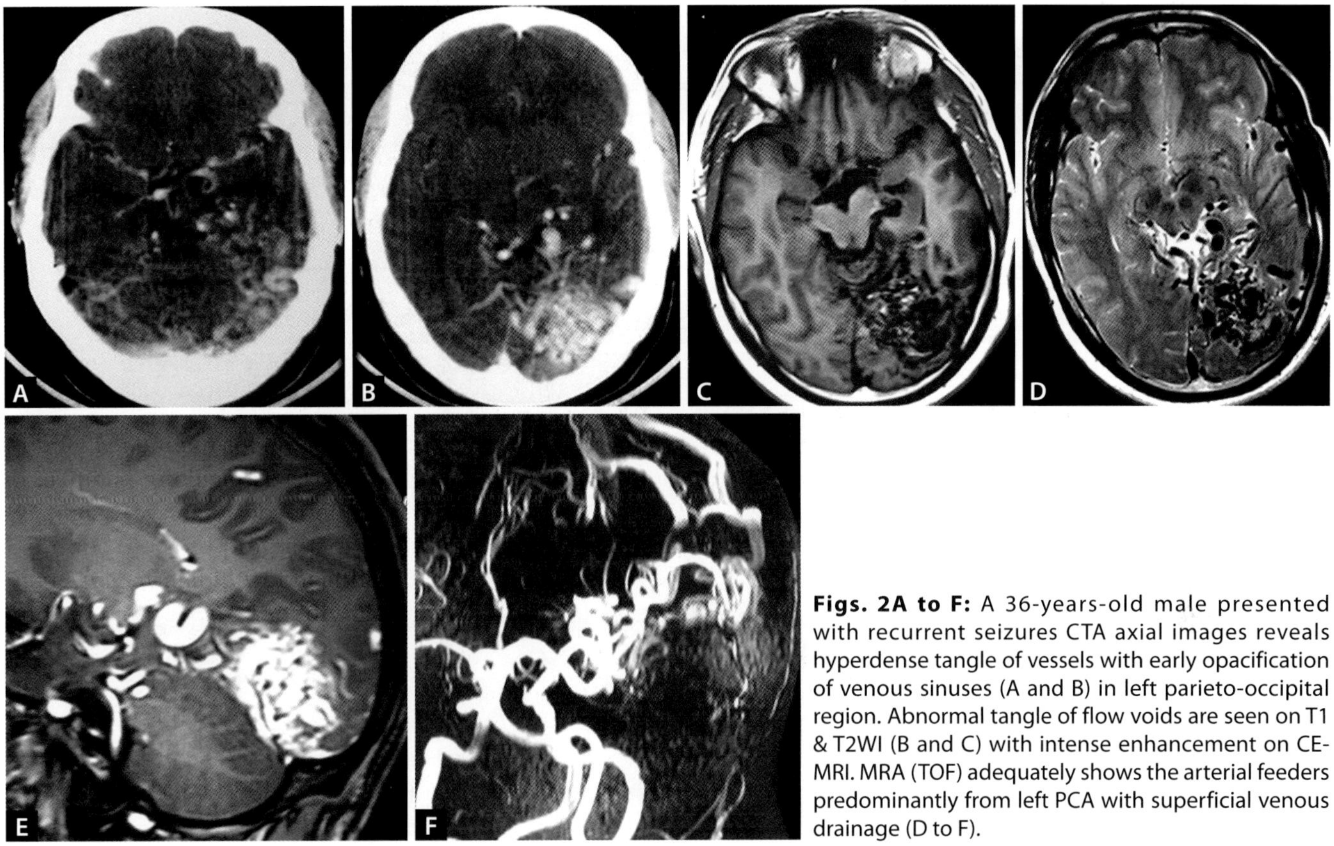

Figs. 2A to F: A 36-years-old male presented with recurrent seizures CTA axial images reveals hyperdense tangle of vessels with early opacification of venous sinuses (A and B) in left parieto-occipital region. Abnormal tangle of flow voids are seen on T1 & T2WI (B and C) with intense enhancement on CE-MRI. MRA (TOF) adequately shows the arterial feeders predominantly from left PCA with superficial venous drainage (D to F).

GRADING/CLASSIFICATION OF BRAIN ARTERIOVENOUS MALFORMATION

The treatment strategies for the bAVM are still unclear and complex in terms of prognostication and choice of available modalities. The Spetzler-Martin (SM) scale (2) is one of the most used and accepted grading system for the treatment planning and prognostication of bAVMs. However, it was developed only for the patients planned for treatment by microsurgical resection.[31] In the recent past advent of newer treatment modalities, i.e embolization and radiosurgery has opened new possibilities in the management protocols of bAVMs with or without rupture. Also with the advent of new embolic materials and endovascular hardware there is an increasing and established role of endovascular management either stand alone or adjunctive to micro or radiosurgery. Apart from the variables used in the SM grading, other components of AVM such as number and diameter of arterial pedicles and draining veins, vascular eloquence and presence of arteriovenous fistulous component also plays important role for the management planning by radiosurgery or embolization. Newer grading scales proposed by Demetrius et al.,[31] Bell et al.[32] and Buffalo Score of AVM[33] are described in **Tables 2 to 5**. All of these grading scales have point system for different characteristics of AVM and the grade of the AVM can be calculated by adding them up. Higher the scores suggest poorer prognosis and difficulty in management.

IMAGING EVALUATION OF BRAIN ARTERIOVENOUS MALFORMATIONS

Computed tomography (CT) is usually the first line of investigation for the symptomatic bAVMs. Depending upon the findings on non-contrast or contrast-enhanced CT scan the patients can be further evaluated by MRI and digital subtraction angiography (DSA). The primary diagnosis of bAVM can be easily made on CECT and MRI. However, for exact treatment planning, prognostication and follow-up imaging CEMRI and DSA plays important role. bAVMs can represent as incidental imaging finding in the patients of headache and other neurological symptoms undergoing cross-sectional imaging.

Computed Tomography

Noncontrast CT is usually the first investigation in the symptomatic patients. It has high sensitivity for

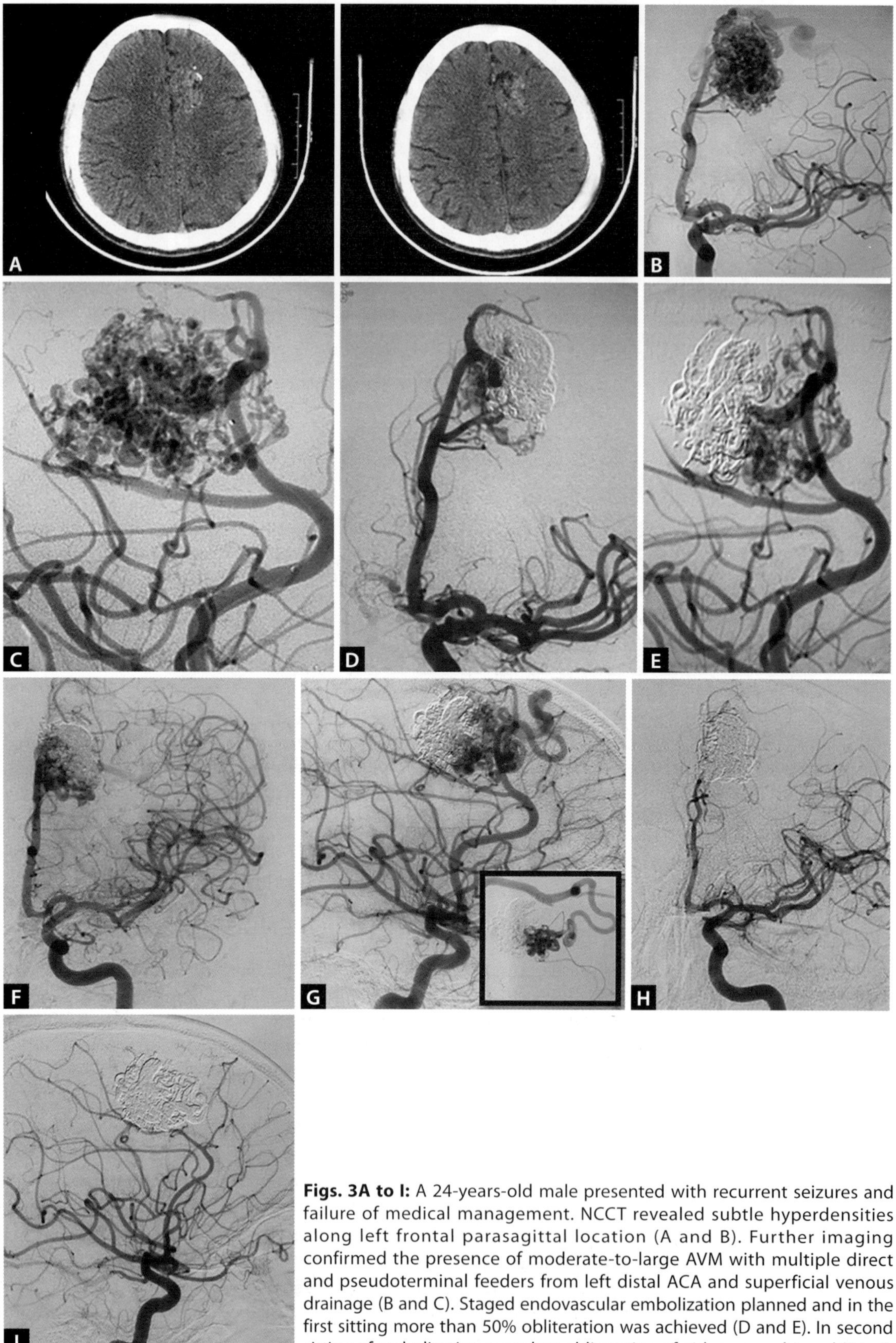

Figs. 3A to I: A 24-years-old male presented with recurrent seizures and failure of medical management. NCCT revealed subtle hyperdensities along left frontal parasagittal location (A and B). Further imaging confirmed the presence of moderate-to-large AVM with multiple direct and pseudoterminal feeders from left distal ACA and superficial venous drainage (B and C). Staged endovascular embolization planned and in the first sitting more than 50% obliteration was achieved (D and E). In second sitting of embolization complete obliteration of nidus was achieved (F to I).

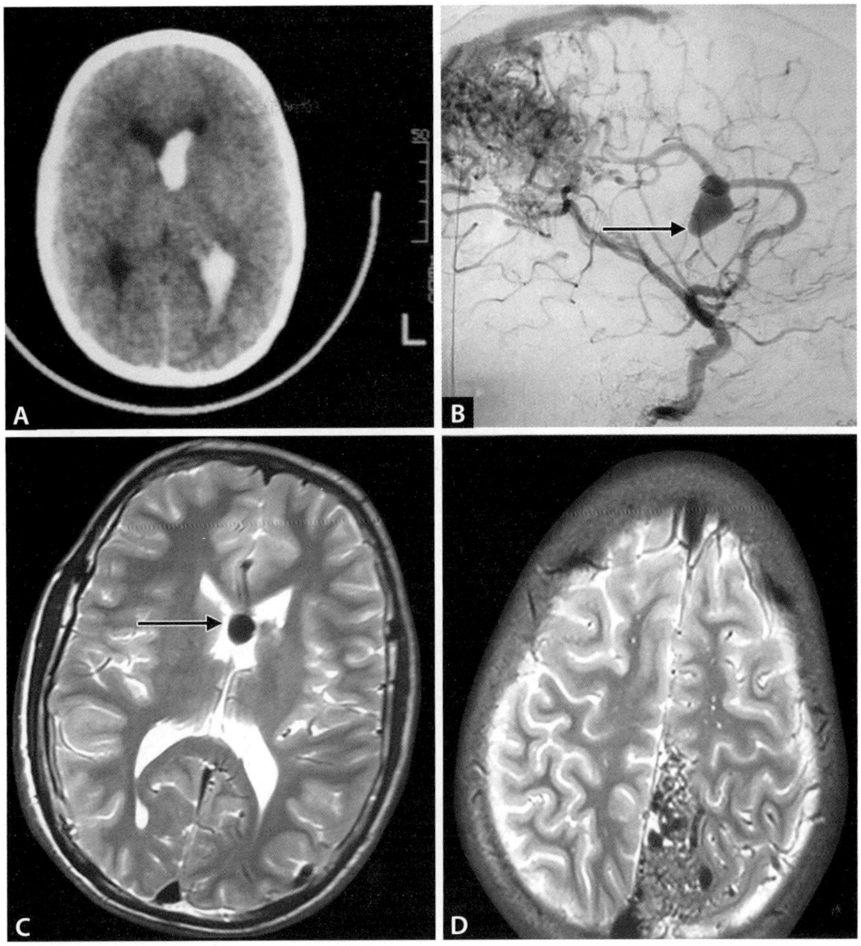

Figs. 4A to D: A 17-year-old male presented with severe headache. NCCT shows left IVH (A) with Axial T2WI of MRI depicting pre-nidal aneurysmal flow void projecting into ventricle also confirmed on diagnostic DSA (arrow) along with distal parieto-occipital AVM nidus on both modalities (B to D).

detecting hemorrhage, infarct[34-36] and hyperdensities due to calcification and slow flowing tangle of vessels **(Figs. 3A and B)**. With the advent of multislice technology CT angiography (CTA), thin slice isometric multiplanar imaging can help diagnose the bAVMs with high sensitivity and specificity **(Figs. 2A and B)**. Different bAVM features as-evaluation of arterial feeders, AVM nidus and draining veins can also be assessed easily on CTA. CTA also provides a very good noninvasive imaging tool for the future treatment planning either by microsurgery, embolization or radiosurgery especially in the patients where MRI is contraindicated. There is sufficient literature suggesting that CTA is comparable to DSA in the terms of sensitivity (83.6-100%) and specificity (77.2%-100%) for making the diagnosis and evaluating the other features of bAVMs.[37,38]

4D-CTA is the multiphasic dynamic CTA acquisition algorithm. It is able to diagnose almost all bAVMs however there is suboptimal evaluation of angioarchitecture when compared to DSA. It appears promising noninvasive tool for treatment planning and follow-up imaging for patients of bAVM treated by any of the available modalities.[39]

Magnetic Resonance Imaging

Recent advances in the techniques and acquisition sequences places MRI as key imaging modality for the diagnosis and detailed evaluation of bAVM characteristics. In the pediatric and other patients where the radiation and contrast nephropathy are serious considerations MR imaging plays the central role for the evaluation of suspected brain vascular lesions. The bAVM can be diagnosed as an abnormal tangle of flow voids on basic MR T1W, T2W and FLAIR sequences. The associated hemorrhage and calcification can also be diagnosed on basic sequences along with susceptibility weighted imaging (SWI). MR angiography (time of flight-TOF) gives an adequate idea about the arterial feeders and draining veins **(Figs. 2C to F)**. In the meta-analysis by Josephson et al.[38] MRA was suggested to have high sensitivity (95%, CI

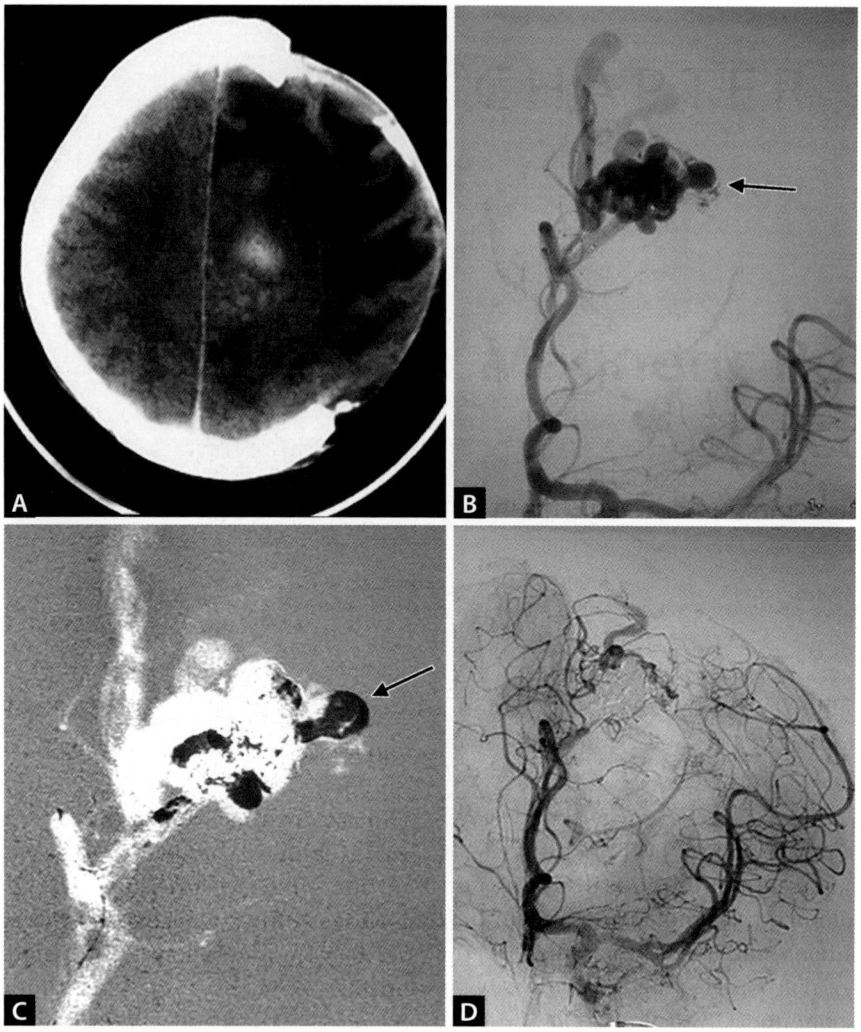

Figs. 5A to D: A 18-year-old male had history of sudden unconsciousness with right hemiparesis, large ICH diagnosed on NCCT, undergone emergency decompression craniotomy (A). CTA revealed compact AVM nidus with perinidal aneurysm (arrow) (B). Endovascular embolization with curative intention was performed to obliterate nidus and aneurysm using onyx and 1.5 cm detachable tip Apollo microcatheter (C). Check run post-embolization shows complete obliteration of nidus and aneurysm (D).

0.80-1.00) and specificity (95%, CI 0.97-1.00) for diagnosis of bAVMs. Even with available advanced MR sequences, there are still some limitations like detecting small arterial feeders (<1 mm), associated aneurysms and AVMs with smaller nidus (<10 mm).[40-42] There is an increasing role of functional MR imaging (fMRI) in the treatment planning and prognostication of the patients presented with symptomatic bAVMs. The findings of fMRI can guide a neurosurgeon for microsurgery, selection of the arterial feeders for neurointerventionist and safe ROI marking during radiosurgery.[43]

Digital Subtraction Angiography

DSA serves as the gold standard imaging modality for the diagnosis and evaluation of bAVMs because of its peculiar ability to assess the dynamicity and role of specific feeder in the AVM nidus. It provides the highest degree of special and temporal resolution.[44-47] The points of concern are its invasive nature, need of operator expertise and experience, radiation risks, use of contrast and risk of some serious vascular and neurological complications.[48] Complete and adequate DSA can accurately evaluate almost all anatomical components (arterial feeder, aneurysms, nidus, shunts, collaterals, draining veins and venous abnormalities) of bAVM.[12,14]

THERAPEUTIC OPTIONS

The treatment of diagnosed bAVM depends upon whether it is symptomatic or asymptomatic and if symptomatic presented with hemorrhage or not. In the present scenario

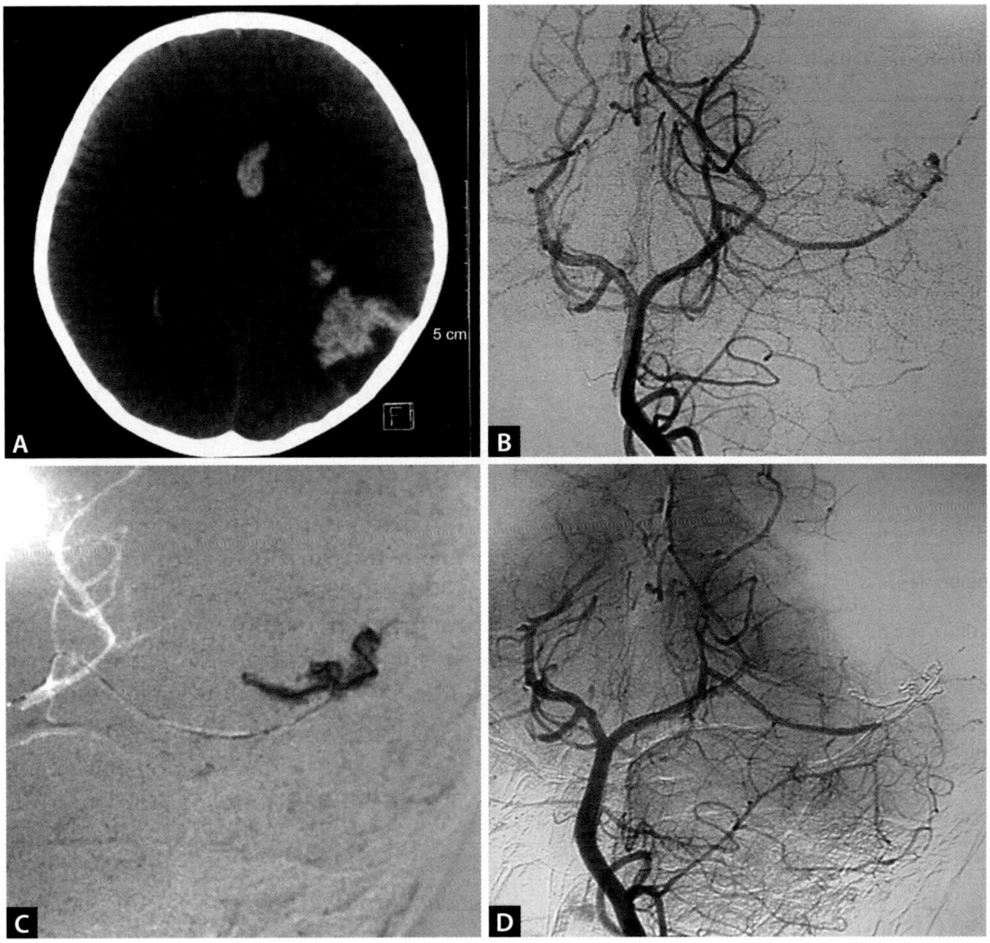

Figs. 6A to D: A 3-year old female presented with sudden loss of consciousness, NCCT revealed (A) revealed left parietal ICH with associated IVH. Diagnostic DSA shows small AVM nidus with intranidal aneurysm and having feeder from left posterior cerebral artery (B). patient taken for endovascular embolization on urgent basis with curative intention, complete obliteration of AVM nidus and aneurysm was achieved (C and D) using onyx 18.

the management options for diagnosed bAVMs include medical management, microsurgery, embolization, radiosurgery and/or combined therapy. The main aim of either modality is to prevent hemorrhage and to ameliorate the symptoms.[23]

Microsurgery

Neurosurgical resection of the bAVM whenever possible remains the only definitive cure. The major aims of microsurgery include complete resection of nidus, evacuation of associated hematoma if present; avoid injury to normal brain parenchyma and careful ligation of the true arterial feeders and draining veins. However indications for the definitive resection are reserved for smaller and superficially located nidus away from eloquent brain parenchyma. Larger complex AVMs requires adjunctive embolization to decrease the size, intra operative hemorrhage and to eliminate weak point in AVM.[23]

Radiosurgery

Radiosurgery as primary modality is usually performed in the patients having high risk for surgery, deep or eloquent location and smaller lesion without weak points. Recent studies suggests that the patients with smaller volumes nidus < 12 cm^3 have better treatment outcomes.[49] There are many limiting factors in radiosurgery as radiation necrosis, no significant change in the annual risk of hemorrhage during latency period in comparison with natural history of bAVM and long term cyst formations.[50,51]

ENDOVASCULAR INTERVENTION

Currently the management of bAVM is a multidisciplinary approach and endovascular management serves as an

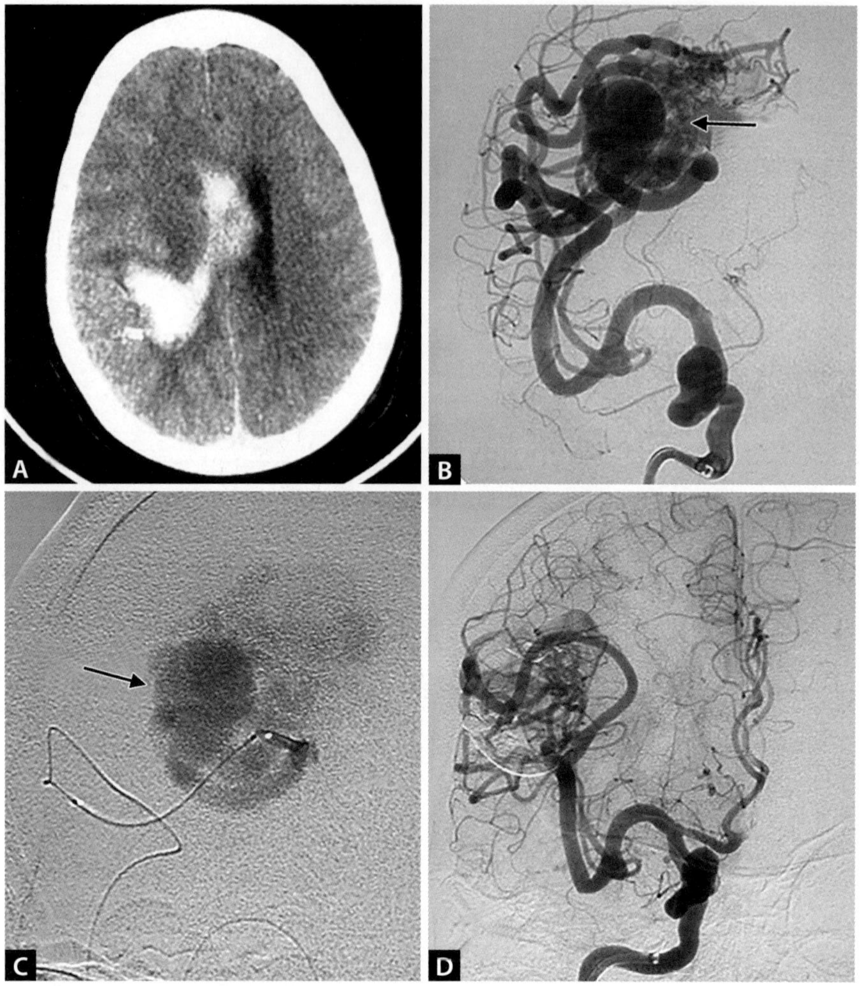

Figs. 7A to D: A 50-year-old female presented with sudden severe headache, vomiting and loss of consciousness. NCCT shows large right parietal ICH with extension into lateral ventricle (A). CTA elsewhere revealed AVM with a large perinidal aneurysm (arrow) on the MCA feeder close to nidus (B). Endovascular embolization was planned using onyx and detachable tip micro-catheter (C) adjunct to radiosurgery with the aim to obliterate the aneurysm and decrease the size of AVM nidus. Post embolization check run (D) shows obliteration of aneurysm and part of nidus.

Table 2: Spetzler-Martin grading scale for AVMs.

Characteristic	*Number of points assigned*
Size of AVM	
Small (<3 cm)	1 point
Medium (3–6 cm)	2 points
Large (> 6 cm)	3 points
Location	
Non-eloquent site	0 points
Eloquent site*	1 point
Pattern of venous drainage	
Superficial only	0 points
Deep component	1 point

*Sensorimotor, language, visual cortex, hypothalamus, thalamus, internal capsule, brainstem, cerebellar peduncles or cerebellar nuclei

Table 3: AVM embocure score (Demetrium et al.).

Value	*Definition*	*Scoring value*
Size	Size of AVM nidus	1 (<3 cm) 2 (3–6 cm) 3 (>6 cm)
Arterial pedicles	Number of arterial pedicles feeding AVM	1 (1–3 pedicles) 2 (4–6 pedicles) 3 (>6 pedicles)
Draining veins	Number of draining veins	1 (1–3 draining veins) 2 (4–6 draining veins) 3 (>6 draining veins)
Vascular eloquence	Emergence of small and short arterial pedicles from parent vessel whose injury/occlusion would cause severe neurologic complications	0 (non-eloquent) 1 (eloquent)

Table 4: Endovascular grading scale (Bell et al.).

Feature and value	*Points*
No. of feeding arteries	1
<3	2
≥3, <6	3
≥6	
Eloquence of adjacent areas	
Noneloquent	0
Eloquent	1
Presence of arteriovenous fistula component	
No AVF	0
AVF	1

Table 5: Buffalo score of AVM.

Graded feature	*Points assigned*
Number of arterial pedicles	
1 or 2	1
3 or 4	2
5 or more	3
Diameter of arterial pedicles	
Most >1 mm	0
Most ≤1 mm	1
Nidus location	
Noneloquent	0
Eloquent	1

AVM grade = (number) + (diameter) + (nidus location)

important central role for the same. With the advent of newer techniques, better imaging machines, endovascular hardware and embolic materials, the role of endovascular management is increasing. The endovascular management can be used as a standalone "curative" treatment to eliminate AVMs in selected cases, "palliative" to improve symptoms in cases of larger complex AVMs, "targeted" embolization for eliminating intranidal aneurysms and fistulous components and "adjunct" to radio or microsurgery for larger and complex bAVMs.

Curative Embolization

About 10–20% of patients can be expected to have complete cure by embolization alone using n-butyl cyanoacrylate.[52] Currently with the advent of newer EVOH based embolizing material (onyx and squid) there is significant increase in total obliteration rates up to 51% of all bAVMs. The best results with obliteration rates up to 96% can be achieved in selected cases.[53,54] Most of these AVMs are small in size, with only few feeding arteries **(Figs. 1, 3, 5 and 6)**.

Preoperative Embolization

Preoperative embolization facilitates surgical treatment by reducing the arteriovenous shunt, decreasing the size of feeding arteries and veins and reducing blood loss.[55] High flow direct arteriovenous shunts and areas of the AVM with associated aneurysms should be targeted by embolization. Deep lenticulostriate or posterior cerebral feeder, that may be difficult to access surgically, can also be embolized.

Pre-radiosurgery Embolization

A combination of embolization and radiosurgery may be used for treating AVMs. Embolization can reduce the size of the AVM nidus, making the lesion more amenable to radiosurgery. Areas of nidus that contain aneurysm should be fully embolized to allow added protection from hemorrhage during 1–3 years latency period after treatment before an AVM is cured by radiation **(Figs. 7A to D)**. The fistulous components also needs to be meticulously diagnosed prior to radiosurgery to prevent the failure of treatment as fistulous components are believed to be resistant to radiation treatment.[56,57]

Palliative Embolization

The main aim of the palliative embolization in complex large untreatable bAVMs is to reduce the risk of hemorrhage due to weak points, to diminish the flow across nidus and to further decrease venous hypertension. It is increasingly being realized that potentially reducing the AVM nidus with elimination of fistulous communications effectively accomplishes longer uneventful time period and in many it may ensure a full and unconstrued life.[58,59] Long-term follow-up angiographic studies have shown even the residual lesion in many AVMs to progressively thrombose.

Staging Embolization

Staging embolization is usually done in large malformations or when the delay is expected to let a small feeder enlarge in order to facilitate future catheterization. By staging occlusion of a large AVM, the hemodynamic consequences of rapid elimination of a large shunt are avoided. Normal pressure perfusion breakthrough phenomena are less likely to occur and the ultimate goal is achieved without avoidable risks of embolization **(Figs. 3A to I)**.

ENDOVASCULAR HARDWARE

For the endovascular management of bAVM, the hardware to be used are microcatheters (flow related, wire-guided and detachable tip), micro guidewire having longer soft portion unlike wires used for aneurysm treatment and liquid embolic agents (Glue, Onyx, Squid and PHIL). Comparison of the different available liquid embolic agents are given in **Table 6**.

Flow-dependent Catheters

A major advance in the recent past has been the development of the Magic catheter (Balt, Montmorency, France), a variable stiffness design with extremely soft and flexible distal segments. The proximal segment is 3 French, whereas the distal segment varies from 1.8, 1.5 to 1.2 French sizes. In moderate to high flow AVMs Magic or other flow-dependent catheter can be positioned easily within the AVM nidus. Newer catheters come with hydrophilic coating that facilitates rapid, atraumatic and distal catheterizations. Liquid adhesives and thrombi are less likely to adhere to these coated catheters.[60,61] Ultraflow and Marathon (Micro Therapeutics, Inc., Irvine, CA) are also promising micro catheters for AVM cannulation.

Guidewire Dependent Catheters

These include Baltacci (Balt), Tracker-10 (Boston Scientific Target, CA) and Prowler (Cordis Neurovascular, USA). These catheters are available with hydrophilic coating.

Detachable Tip Microcatheters

With the advent of newer detachable tip catheters, the risk of catheter entrapment has been eliminated, hence there is significant increase in the occlusion rate of AVM nidus as per recent literature. In these microcatheters distal 1.5–3 cm segment is detachable from the main micro catheter. Two major available important microcatheters are Apollo Onyx Delivery Micro Catheter (Micro Therapeutics, Inc., Irvine, CA) and Sonic (Balt, Montmorency, France).

EMBOLIC AGENTS

Acrylic Glue

N-butyl-cyanoacrylate (glue) was the main embolic agent for the treatment of bAVM in past. It is readily available and cheap. For visualization and radio-opacity it is mixed with oil based contrast agent lipiodol or tantalum powder. The rate of polymerization, viscosity and penetration depends upon the ratio of its mixture with lipiodol which can be from 10% to >90%. Higher percentage of glue is used for the larger fistulous components. As the rate of polymerization of glue when it comes in contact of ions is very much high, especially with higher concentrations the risk of catheter entrapment is high. The rate of injection of glue is always moderate to high. The catheter must be primed with 5% dextrose to prevent ionic substances from causing premature polymerization in the catheter **(Figs. 8A and B)**.

Onyx/Squid

With the introduction of non-adhesive ethylene vinyl alcohol copolymer embolic agent, onyx (Ev3, Irvine, California), complete obliteration of small and intermediate-sized bAVMs is possible with low complication rate. Onyx consists of EVOH, dissolved in DMSO and mixed with tantalum powder for radio-opacity. When the material comes in contact with an aqueous solution, it precipitates and forms a soft spongy polymer cast. It is available in ready to use vials of 1.5 ml in 3 different viscosities, onyx 18, 20 and 34. The vials must be placed on a mixer and shaken for at least 20 minutes

Table 6: Characteristics of Liquid embolic agents.

	N-butyl -2 cyanoacrylate (Glue) (Trufil; codman neurovascular)	***Ethylene-vinyl alcohol copolymer with dimethyl sulfoxide (Onyx, eV3 Inc)***	***Precipitating Hydrophobic Injectable Liquid (PHIL; Microvention California)***
Availability	Easy	Few places	Near future
Cost	Cheap	Expensive	Expensive
Concentration	Desired	Few specified	Few specified
Compatibility	Most of the catheters	Few selected catheters (For DMSO)	Few selected catheters (For DMSO)
Preparation	With lipiodol	Agitated >20 min	Instant ready to use
Priming	5% dextrose	DMSO	DMSO
Radio-opacity	Lipiodol	Tantalum/Physical form	Iodine chemically bonded
Adhesiveness	High (Depends on concentration)	Low	Low
Polymerization	Depends on conc	Low	Low
Rate of injection	Usually fast	Slow/Fast	Slow/Fast

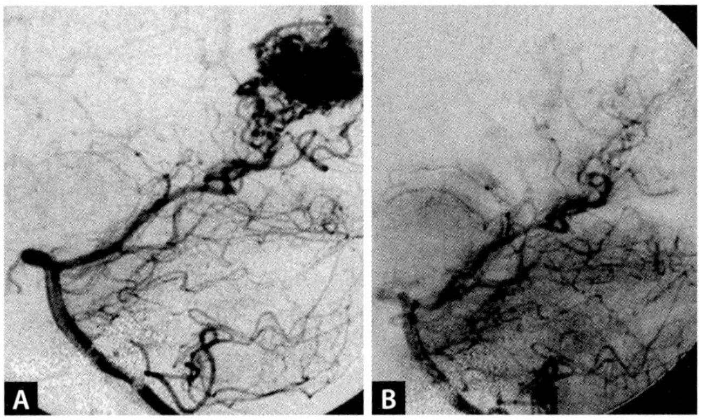

Figs. 8A and B: (A) Lateral view of the left vertebral artery shows an occipital AVM. The AVM was embolized with 33% mixture of N-butyl cyanoacrylate and lipoidol; (B) Post- embolization angiogram shows complete ablation of the nidus.

to obtain a homogenous solution.[62] Another EVOH based liquid embolic agent SQUID (emboflu, Switzerland) is also available in different concentrations as SQUID 12, 12LD, 18 and 18LD. The micro catheter needs to be primed with DMSO before using Onyx/SQUID **(Figs. 3, 5 to 7)**.

Precipitating Hydrophobic Injectable Liquid (PHIL)

Recently a newer nonadhesive embolic agent PHIL (Precipitating Hydrophobic Injectable Liquid, Micro-Vention, Tustin, California) was introduced. It is a copolymer dissolved in dimethyl-sulfoxide (DMSO), with chemically bonded iodine for radio-opacity. The PHIL liquid embolic system consists of a sterile, prefilled, 1.0 mL syringe of PHIL liquid embolic agent, a sterile, prefilled 1.0 mL syringe of DMSO, and micro catheter hub adaptors. In comparison with conventionally available EVOH based embolic agents which uses the physical form of tantalum powder for radio-opacity and hence needs to be agitated for 20 minutes, this embolic agent is ready to be used. Another concern with earlier embolic agents were high radio-opacity and streak artefacts due to tantalum powder which hampers the visualization of residual AVM components on follow-up imaging. It is believed that radio-opacity of PHIL is less in comparison with the tantalum powder and lipiodol **(Figs. 1A to D)**.

Other Embolic Agents

Microcoils: Detachable microcoils are used for the treatment of high risk/ruptured prenidal or intranidal aneurysms. Another important use of detachable microcoils is to decrease the flow across larger arteriovenous shunts where there is high risk of significant distal migration of liquid embolic agents leading to serious complications.

Complications of AVM Embolization

Complications may occur during or after the procedure itself. These include (i) thromboembolic stroke,(ii) arterial injury producing hemorrhage, (iii) arterial and venous occlusions, (iv) pulmonary embolism. Thrombotic occlusion of normal vessels can be treated by judicious usage of intravenous heparin or intra-arterial thrombolytic agents, such as urokinase. Injecting glue or deploying a coil can treat arterial rupture. Large parenchymal hematomas may be evacuated surgically. After every embolization procedure, a cranial computed tomography must be done to exclude various potential complications at its nascent stage and to obtain a status document. All patients should be closely monitored in an intensive care unit for minimum 24 hours after the procedure to allow for rapid and early intervention for these complications.

DURAL ARTERIOVENOUS FISTULAE

Dural arteriovenous fistulae (DAVFs) are abnormal vascular connections located within the walls of dural sinus or adjacent cortical vein.[63] There is growing evidence to suggest that DAVFs are acquired lesions.[64] The proposed contributing factors are middle ear and intracranial infections, trauma, surgery, and following dural sinus thrombosis.[64] Although the cause and effect relationship between dural sinus thrombosis and DAVF appears well established, it does not exclude other mechanisms for the development of an arteriovenous shunt because most cases of dural thrombosis do not result in a dural fistula.

Classification

Djindjian et al.[64] defined four types, with type 1 draining via the ipsilateral sinus, type 2 draining toward the contralateral sinus, type 3 draining via cortical veins and type 4 with venous ectasia. This classification system allows one to predict the severity of the presenting symptoms and the risk of intra-parenchymal hemorrhage. Modified classification by Cognard has also been proposed (See-appendix—E). Up to 42% of DAVFs with cortical venous drainage were associated with hemorrhage in a series reported by Castaigne.[65]

Radiological Evaluation

Plain skull radiography can sometimes demonstrate enlargement of middle meningeal grooves. CT scan may demonstrate parenchymal edema related to venous hypertension, or intracranial hemorrhage and thrombus in sinus. Contrast-enhanced CT scan can demonstrate serpiginous enhancing parenchymal tubular structures representing the transmedullary veins without any parenchymal nidus. MR imaging may demonstrate brain edema **(Figs. 9A to C)**, infarction and dilated veins.[66] However, CT and MR imaging can both completely miss low grade DAVFs without dilated cortical veins (Djindjian type 1). Selective arteriography **(Figs. 10A to F)** remains the gold standard for the detection and characterization of DAVFs. Bilateral external carotid, internal carotid and vertebral artery studies are mandatory for comprehensive analysis.

Therapeutic Options

Patients with visual loss, hemorrhage or infarction and those with cortical venous drainage require prompt therapy. Djindjian type I fistulae on the other end, can be followed conservatively without treatment.

Compression Therapy

Patients with DAVFs located in the posterior sigmoid or transverse sinus without severe symptoms or high risk angiographic features are ideal candidates for manual compression of the ipsilateral feeding occipital artery behind the mastoid bone.[67]

Transarterial Embolization

Superselective embolization of the ECA feeder vessels to a DAVF can be an effective treatment for certain cases.[68] A variety of agents are available to embolize DAVFs including polyvinyl alcohol (PVA) particles, liquid adhesive agents, such as NBCA. Proximal occlusion of a feeding artery should be avoided because (i) the fistula usually acquires arterial supply from a neighboring

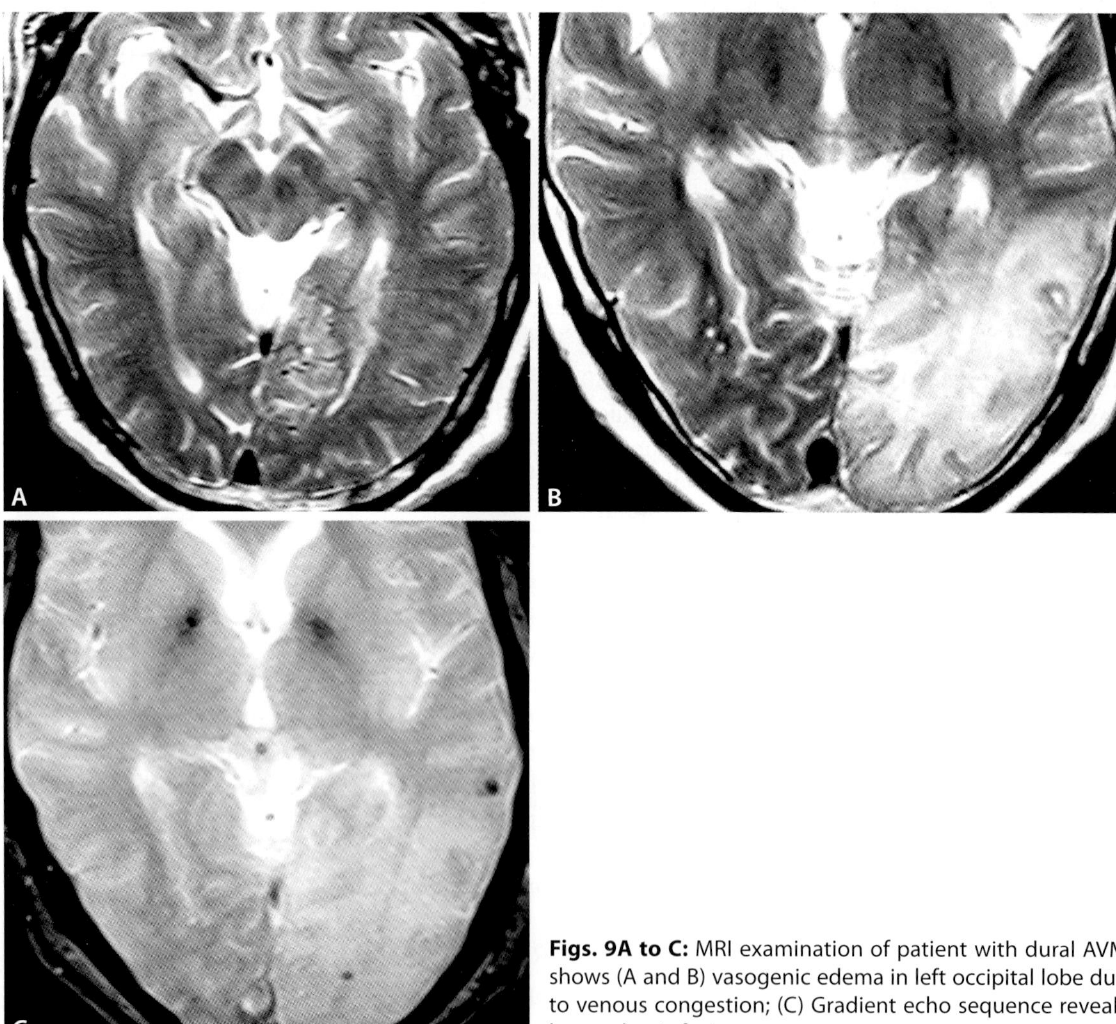

Figs. 9A to C: MRI examination of patient with dural AVM shows (A and B) vasogenic edema in left occipital lobe due to venous congestion; (C) Gradient echo sequence reveals hemorrhagic foci.

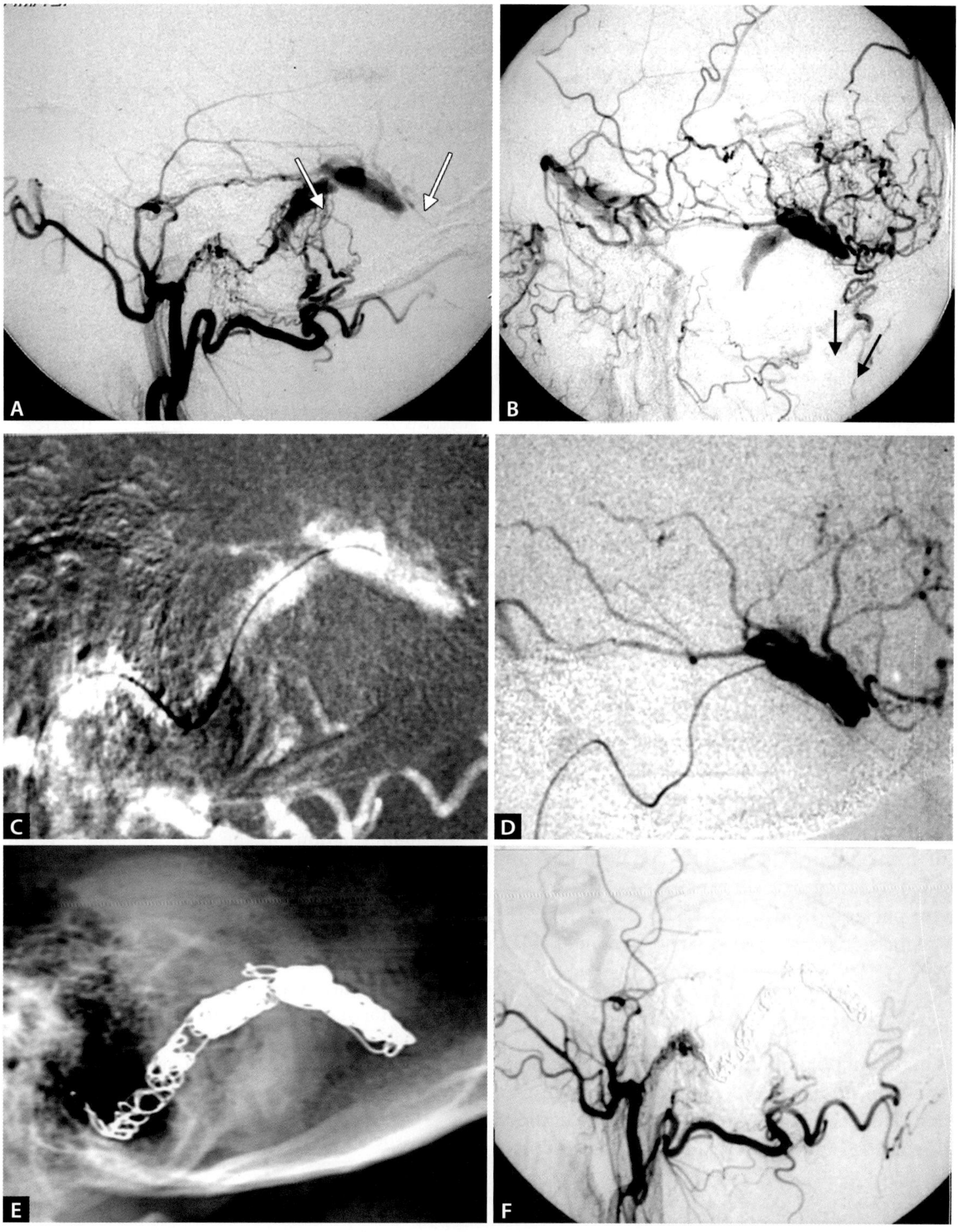

Figs. 10A to F: (A) LECA lateral projection shows occlusion of lateral sinus with dural AVF fed by ECA branches; (B) Venous phase with cortical venous reflux. Transvenous occlusion of dural AVFs. Roadmap image (C) showing position of microcatheter in the sigmoid sinus. Angiogram; (D) obtained with microcatheter; (E) Complete packing of the sigmoid sinus with coils; (E) Postembolization ECA angiogram; (F) Showing occlusion of the dural AVF.

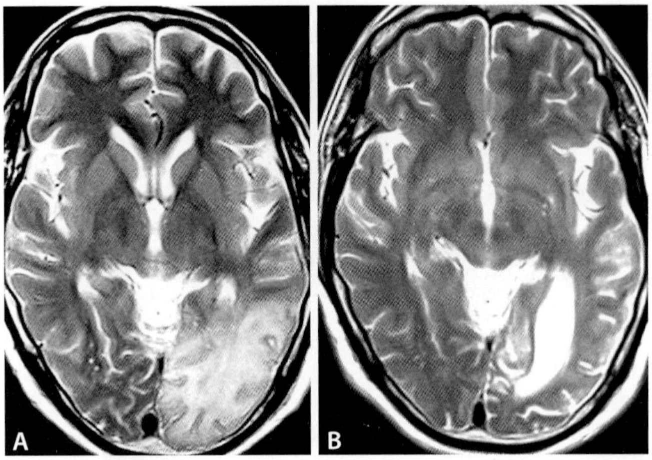

Figs. 11A and B: MRI (A) Pre-embolization and (B) post-embolization as in Figures 11.9A to C with significant resolution of edema in the occipital lobe.

collateral vessel and (ii) it interferes with future access when it is needed.

Transvenous Embolization

This method enables placement of coils via a transvenous route under direct fluoroscopic guidance to achieve closure of difficult DAVFs. Development of newer and softer delivery catheters have permitted transfemoral access to the venous drainage of many DAVFs allowing coil packing.[69] Only those patients with cortical venous drainage (Djindjian's type 3) should be treated by transvenous route if the sinus is not being used for significant venous drainage of normal brain. Platinum fibered thrombogenic coils with slightly larger diameter than that of the sinus is preferred for packing the fistulous sinus. Follow-up MRI may show regression of brain parenchymal changes **(Figs. 11A and B)**.

Preoperative Embolization

The combination of preoperative arterial and subsequent surgical excision of the DAVF has been shown to be effective in treating complex lesions.[70] Particulate embolic materials are used 1–2 days before the surgical excisions.

CONCLUSION

The endovascular management plays the central role in multimodal treatment strategies of the brain AVMs. Recent advancement in the available angiography machines (flat panel biplane DSA suites), endovascular hardware in the form of detachable tip microcatheters, non-adhesive newer liquid embolic agents and improved skills and experience has presented new possibilities in the treatment of these complex dynamic brain lesions. Ongoing research and increasing literature suggests that endovascular embolization of bAVMs provides safe and effective management options.

ACKNOWLEDGMENTS

The authors acknowledge Dr Vivek Agarwal (DM), resident in the Neuroradiology Division, Department of Radiodiagnosis, PGIMER, Chandigarh for his support in image archival and editing of chapter.

REFERENCES

1. Berenstein A, Lasjaunias P. Surgical Neuro-angiography. New York: Springer-Verlag; 1992. pp.1-266.
2. Spetzler RF, Martin NA. A proposed grading system for arteriovenous malformations. J Neurosurg. 1986; 65:476-83.
3. Dorothea S, Raul G, Sean D L. Endovascular treatment of intracranial arteriovenous malformation. Neurosurg Clin N Am. 2009;20:399-418.
4. Brown RD Jr, Wiebers DO, Torner JC, et al. Frequency of intracranial hemorrhage as a presenting symptom and subtype analysis: a population-based study of intracranial vascular malformations in Olmsted Country, Minnesota. J Neurosurg. 1996; 85:29–32.
5. Brown RD Jr, Wiebers DO, Forbes G, et al. The natural history of unruptured intracranial arteriovenous malformations. J Neurosurg. 1988; 68:352-7.
6. Graf CJ, Perret GE, Torner JC. Bleeding from cerebral arteriovenous malformations as part of their natural history. J Neurosurg. 1983;58:331-7.
7. Arteriovenous Malformation Study Group. Arteriovenous malformations of the brain in adults. N Engl J Med 1999;340:1812-8.
8. Stapf C, Mast H, Sciacca RR, et al New York Islands AVM Study Collaborators. The New York Islands AVM Study: design, study progress, and initial results. Stroke. 2003;34:e29-e33.
9. Hartmann A, Mast H, Mohr JP, et al. Morbidity of intracranial hemorrhage in patients with cerebral arteriovenous malformation. Stroke. 1998;29:931-4.
10. Hoh BL, Chapman PH, Loeffler JS, et al. Results of multimodality treatment for 141 patients with brain arteriovenous malformations and seizures: factors associated with seizure incidence and seizure outcomes. Neurosurgery. 2002;51:303-9.
11. Stapf C, Mast H, Sciacca RR, et al. Predictors of hemorrhage in patients with untreated brain arteriovenous malformation. Neurology. 2006;66:1350-5.
12. da Costa L, Wallace MC, Ter Brugge KG, et al. The natural history and predictive features of hemorrhage from brain arteriovenous malformations. Stroke. 2009;40:100-5.
13. Hofmeister C, Stapf C, Hartmann A, et al. Demographic, morphological, and clinical characteristics of 1289 patients with brain arteriovenous malformation. Stroke. 2000;31:1307-10.

14. Stapf C, Labovitz DL, Sciacca RR, et al. Incidence of adult brain arteriovenous malformation hemorrhage in a prospective population-based stroke survey. Cerebrovasc Dis. 2002;13:43-6.
15. Kim H, Al-Shahi Salman R, McCulloch CE, et al. MARS Coinvestigators. Untreated brain arteriovenous malformation: patientlevel meta-analysis of hemorrhage predictors. Neurology. 2014;83:590-7.
16. Gross BA, Du R. Natural history of cerebral arteriovenous malformations: a meta-analysis. J Neurosurg. 2013;118: 437-43.
17. Abecassis IJ, Xu DS, Batjer HH, et al. Natural history of brain arteriovenous malformations: a systematic review. Neurosurg Focus. 2014;37:E7.
18. Kim H, Al-Shahi Salman R, McCulloch CE, et al. MARS Coinvestigators. Untreated brain arteriovenous malformation: patientlevel meta-analysis of hemorrhage predictors. Neurology. 2014;83:590-7.
19. Gross BA, Du R. Natural history of cerebral arteriovenous malformations: a meta-analysis. J Neurosurg. 2013;118: 437-43.
20. Ross J, Al-Shahi Salman R. Interventions for treating brain arteriovenous malformations in adults. Cochrane Database Syst Rev. 2010:CD003436.
21. Fierstra J, Conklin J, Krings T, et al. Impaired peri-nidal cerebrovascular reserve in seizure patients with brain arteriovenous malformations. Brain. 2011;134(pt 1): 100-9.
22. Krings T, Hans FJ, Geibprasert S, et al. Partial "targeted" embolisation of brain arteriovenous malformations. Eur Radiol. 2010;20:2723-31.
23. Derdeyn CP, Zipfel GJ, et al. Management of brain arteriovenous malformations A scientific statement for healthcare professionals from the American Heart Association/ American Stroke Association. Stroke. ahajournals 2017;48.
24. Galletti F, Costa C, Cupini LM, et al. Brain arteriovenous malformations and seizures: an Italian study. J Neurol Neurosurg Psychiatry. 2014;85:284-8.
25. Jiang P, Lv X, Wu Z, et al. Characteristics of brain arteriovenous malformations presenting with seizures without acute or remote hemorrhage. Neuroradiol J. 2011;24:886-8.
26. Mast H, Mohr JP, Osipov A, et al. "Steal" is an unestablished mechanism for the clinical presentation of cerebral arteriovenous malformations. Stroke. 1995;26:1215-20.
27. Higgins JN, Kirkpatrick PJ. Stenting venous outflow gives symptomatic improvement in a patient with an inoperable brainstem arteriovenous malformation. Br J Neurosurg. 2013;27:698-700.
28. Lv Xianli, Wu Z et al. Angioarchitectural Characteristics of Brain Arterivenous Malformations with and without haemorrhage. World Neurosurgery. 2011; 76,1/2: 95-99.
29. Alexander MD, Cooke DL, Nelson J, et al. Association Between Venous Angioarchitectural Features of Sporadic Brain Arteriovenous Malformations and Intracranial Hemorrhage. AJNR. Am J Neuroradiol. 2015;36(5):949-52.
30. Ranmos SK, Gardenghi B. Aneurysms Associated with Brain Arteriovenous Malformations. AJNR. 2016;37;1966-71.
31. Lopes DK, et al. Arteriovenous malformation embocure score: AVMES. J Neurointerv Surg. 2016;8(7):685-91.
32. Bell DL, Leslie-Mazwi TM, Yoo AJ, et al. Application of novel brain arteriovenous malformation endovascular grading scale for trans arterial embolization. Am J Neuroradiol. 2015; 36(7): 1303-9.
33. Dumont TM, Kan P, Snyder KV, Hopkins LN, Siddiqui AH, Levy EI. A proposed grading system for endovascular treatment of cerebral arteriovenous malformations: Buffalo score. Surg Neurol Int. 2015;6:3.
34. Byyny RL, Mower WR, Shum N, et al. Sensitivity of noncontrast cranial computed tomography for the emergency department diagnosis of subarachnoid hemorrhage. Ann Emerg Med. 2008;51:697-703.
35. McCormack RF, Hutson A. Can computed tomography angiography of the brain replace lumbar puncture in the evaluation of acute-onset headache after a negative noncontrast cranial computed tomography scan? Acad Emerg Med. 2010;17:444-45.
36. Brazzelli M, Sandercock PA, Chappell FM, et al. Magnetic resonance imaging versus computed tomography for detection of acute vascular lesions in patients presenting with stroke symptoms. Cochrane Database Syst Rev. 2009:CD007424.
37. Delgado Almandoz JE, Schaefer PW, et al. Diagnostic accuracy and yield of multidetector CT angiography in the evaluation of spontaneous intraparenchymal cerebral hemorrhage. Am J Neuroradiol. 2009;30:1213–122.
38. Josephson CB, White PM, Krishan A, et al. Computed tomography angiography or magnetic resonance angiography for detection of intracranial vascular malformations in patients with intracerebral haemorrhage. Cochrane Database Syst Rev. 2014;9:CD009372.
39. Willems Peter WA, Taeshineetanakul et al. The use of 4D-CTA in the diagnostic work-up of brain arteriovenous malformations. Neuroradiology. 2012; 54:123-31.
40. Gross BA, Frerichs KU, Du R. Sensitivity of CT angiography, T2-weighted MRI, and magnetic resonance angiography in detecting cerebral arteriovenous malformations and associated aneurysms. J Clin Neurosci. 2012;19:1093-5.
41. Hadizadeh DR, Kukuk GM, Steck DT, et al. Noninvasive evaluation of cerebral arteriovenous malformations by 4D-MRA for preoperative planning and postoperative follow-up in 56 patients: comparison with DSA and intraoperative findings. Am J Neuroradiol. 2012;33:1095-101.
42. Machet A, Portefaix C, Kadziolka K, et al. Brain arteriovenous malformation diagnosis: value of time-resolved contrastenhanced MR angiography at 3.0T compared to DSA. Neuroradiology. 2012;54:1099–108.
43. Gallagher TA, Nair VA, Regner MF, et al. Characterizing the relationship between functional MRI–derived measures and clinical outcomes in patients with vascular lesions. Neurosurg Focus. 2013;34:E8.
44. Prestigiacomo CJ, Niimi Y, Setton A, et al. Three-dimensional rotational spinal angiography in the evaluation and

treatment of vascular malformations. Am J Neuroradiol. 2003;24:1429-35.
45. Neuropathology Group. Medical Research Council Cognitive Function and Aging Study. Pathological correlates of late-onset dementia in a multicentre, community-based population in England and Wales: Neuropathology Group of the Medical Research Council Cognitive Function and Ageing Study (MRC CFAS). Lancet. 2001;357:169-75.
46. Kakizawa Y, Nagashima H, Oya F, et al. Compartments in arteriovenous malformation nidi demonstrated with rotational three-dimensional digital subtraction angiography by using selective microcatheterization. J Neurosurg. 2002;96:770-4.
47. Gailloud P, Oishi S, Carpenter J, et al. Three-dimensional digital angiography: new tool for simultaneous three-dimensional rendering of vascular and osseous information during rotational angiography. Am J Neuroradiol. 2004;25:571-3.
48. Alexander MD, Oliff MC, Olorunsola OG, et al. Patient radiation exposure during diagnostic and therapeutic interventional neuroradiology procedures. J Neurointerv Surg. 2010;2:6-10.
49. Ding D, Yen CP, Starke RM, Xu Z, Sun X, Sheehan JP. Outcomes following single-session radiosurgery for high-grade intracranial arteriovenous malformations. Br J Neurosurg. 2014;28:666-674.
50. Bollet MA, Anxionnat R, Buchheit I, et al. Efficacy and morbidity of arc-therapy radiosurgery for cerebral arteriovenous malformations: a comparison with the natural history. Int J Radiat Oncol Biol Phys. 2004;58:1353-63.
51. Ding D, Yen CP, Starke RM, et al. Outcomes following single-session radiosurgery for high-grade intracranial arteriovenous malformations. Br J Neurosurg. 2014;28: 666-74.
52. Yu SC, Chan MS, Lam JM, et al. Complete obliteration of intracranial arteriovenous malformation with endovascular cyanoacrylate embolization: initial success and rate of permanent cure. Am J Neuroradiol. 2004;25:1139-43.
53. Saatci I, Geyik S, Yavuz K, et al. Endovascular treatment of brain arteriovenous malformations with prolonged intranidal Onyx injection technique: long-term results in 350 consecutive patients with completed endovascular treatment course. J Neurosurg. 2011;115:78-88.
54. Van Rooij WJ, Jacobs S, Sluzewski M, et al. Curative embolization of brain arteriovenous malformations with onyx: patient selection, embolization technique, and results. AJNR Am J Neuroradiol. 2012;33:1299-304.
55. Jafar JJ, Davis AJ, Berenstein A, et al. The effect of embolisation with N-butyl cyanoacrylate prior to surgical resection of cerebral arteriovenous malformations. J Neurosurg. 1993;78:60-69.
56. Krings T, Hans FJ, Geibprasert S, et al. Partial "targeted" embolisation of brain arteriovenous malformations. Eur Radiol. 2010;20:2723-31.
57. Brown RD Jr, Wiebers DO, Forbes GS. Unruptured intracranial aneurysms and arteriovenous malformations: frequency of intracranial hemorrhage and relationship of lesions. J Neurosurg. 1990;73:859-63.
58. Batjer HH, Devous MD Sr, Seibert GB, et al. Intracranial arteriovenous malformation: relationships between clinical and radiographic factors and ipsilateral steal severity. Neurosurgery. 1988;23:322-32.
59. Kusske JA, Kelly WA. Embolization and reduction of the "steal" syndrome in cerebral arteriovenous malformations. J Neurosurg. 1974;40:313-21.
60. Kallmes DF, McGraw JK, Evans AJ, et al. Thrombogenicity of hydrophilic and non-hydrophilic microcatheters and guiding catheters. Am J Neuroradiol. 1977;18:1243-51.
61. Mathis JM, Evans AJ, DeNardo AJ, et al. Hydrophilic coatings diminish adhesion of glue to catheter. An in vitro simulation of NBCA embolisation. Am J Neuroradiol. 1997;18:1087-91.
62. Rooij WJ, Jacobs S, et al. Curative Embolization of Brain Arteriovenous Malformations with Onyx: Patient Selection, Embolization Technique, and Result. Am J Neuroradiol. 33:1299-304.
63. Choudhary MY, Sachdev VP, Cho SH, et al. Dural arteriovenous malformations of the major venous sinuses. An acquired lesion. Am J Neuroradiol. 1982;3:13-9.
64. Djindjian R, Cophignon J, Theron J. Embolisation by superselective arteriography from the femoral route in neuroradiology: Review of 60 cases, technique, indications, complications. Neuro-radiology. 1973;6:20-26.
65. De Marco KJ, Dillon W, Halbach VV, et al. Dural arteriovenous fistulas: Evaluation with MR imaging. Radiology. 1990;175:193-9.
66. Halbach VV, Higashida RT, Heishima GB, et al. Dural fistulas involving the transverse and sigmoid sinuses: Results of treatment in 28 patients. Radiology. 1987;163:443-7.
67. Vinuela F, Fox AJ, Debrun GM, et al. Spontaneous carotid-cavernous fistulas: Clinical radiological and therapeutic considerations: Experience with 20 cases. J Neurosurg. 1984;60:976-84.
68. Halbach VV, Higashida RT, Hieshima GB, et al. Transvenous embolisation of dural fistulas involving the cavernous sinus. Am J Neuroradiol. 1989;10:377-84.
69. Barnwell SL, Hallbach VV, Higashida RT, et al. Complex dural arteriovenous fistulas: Results of a new combined neuro-surgical and inter-ventional neuroradiology treatment in 16 patients. J Neurosurg. 1989;71:352-8.
70. Panagiotopoulos V, Gizewski E, Asgari S, et al. Embolization of Intracranial Arteriovenous Malformations with Ethylene-Vinyl Alcohol Copolymer (Onyx). Am J Neuroradiol. 2009;30:99-106.

CHAPTER 12

Carotid-cavernous Fistulas

Chirag Kamal Ahuja, Vivek Gupta, Ajay Kumar, Niranjan Khandelwal

INTRODUCTION AND HISTORICAL PERSPECTIVE

Carotid-cavernous fistula (CCF), as the name suggests, is an abnormal communication between the carotid arteries [internal carotid artery (ICA) and/or external carotid artery (ECA)] and the cavernous sinus (CS).[1] It is of two types- direct and indirect. CCF was one of the earliest neurological entities that was recognized and understood by neurophysicians dating back two centuries. Taveras first described it in 1811. Due to unavailability of precise tools to reach the specific site of fistula at that time, it was treated by common carotid ligation for the first time in 1837 followed by internal carotid artery (ICA) ligation in 1847. Dandy and Jefferson are considered pioneers in the surgical treatment of CCFs in the early twentieth century. However, due to proximal occlusion techniques, there was significantly increased incidence of recurrence due to retrograde collateral flow from ophthalmic artery as well as ECA branches. This also resulted in arterial steal resulting in distal ischemia and visual loss. It took decades of thinking in this regard. As a corrective measure, Adson advocated occlusion of ophthalmic artery in addition to ICA (1942). Simultaneously, procedure of muscle embolization of the fistula was also attempted by Brooks[2] with variable results. 1971 marked the modern era of endovascular access routes when Prolo and Hanberry successfully occluded CCFs with *non-detachable balloons* which sacrificed the ICA. Serbinenko's method (1974) of using detachable balloons was a game-changer as it preserved the ICA with complete fistula closure.[3] Latex detachable balloons were subsequently used by Debrun with good ICA patency rates. Mullan achieved fistula closure by cavernous sinus packing with still better ICA patency rates.[4] After the introduction of detachable platinum coils by Guglielmi,[5] cavernous sinus coiling became the standard of care giving excellent results. CCF treatment still evolved further with the availability of liquid embolic material in recent times which can be combined with platinum coils.

ETIOLOGY AND PATHOGENESIS

CCFs can either occur spontaneously, which are more often of the indirect variety (fed by ECA branches), or following closed head trauma associated with basal skull fracture/rupture of cavernous carotid aneurysm (which leads to direct communication of the ICA with the ipsilateral cavernous sinus[CS], hence referred to as direct type). Other causes of direct CCFs are collagen vascular disorders (Ehlers-Danlos syndrome, Osteogenesis imperfecta, etc.), arterial dissections, direct surgical trauma (iatrogenic), fibromuscular dysplasia, etc.[6,7] Congenital direct CCFs are extremely rare, and only a few cases have been reported.[8] Combined Direct Indirect CCFs have abnormal communication between dural branches of the ICA and/or ECA with the CS. Their etiology is not clear, but they have been noticed following pregnancy, sinusitis, trauma, localized surgical procedures and cavernous sinus thrombosis.

Direct CCFs are postulated to develop secondary to bony fractures which tear the cavernous ICA from its dural attachment or due to shearing strain resulting from sudden change in inertia secondary to acceleration/deceleration.[9] The latter occurs due to fixity of the ICA between the foramen lacerum and anterior clinoid process. Another school of thought contests this hypothesis debating that fractures are not a feature in all CCF cases. These proponents believe that these lesions arise as a result of increased intraluminal pressure of ICA which may occur abruptly as a result of neck flexion or twisting injury which gets transmitted to the weakest arterial point resulting in its rupture within the cavernous sinus.[10] Traumatic CCFs occur mostly in C4 segment of the intracavernous ICA followed by the C3, C2 and C5 segments. Direct CCFs occur more commonly in younger patients. The other mechanism of traumatic CCF is direct injury. A penetrating wound from a bullet, gunshot shrapnel, pellets, a transorbital stab, or a surgical procedure could result in a lesion of the intracavernous ICA.[11,12] Iatrogenic CCFs have been reported as complications of many procedures, including transsphenoidal surgery,[13] microcompression of the Gasserian ganglion[14] and endovascular procedures in which the ICA is perforated with a Fogarty catheter[15] or a guidewire.[16]

The precise pathogenesis of indirect CCFs is controversial. Some authors believe that they arise from rupture of thin-walled dural arteries that normally traverse the CS.[17] Others have proposed that these fistulae are, in fact, collateral anastomoses following cavernous sinus thrombosis that develop in patients prone to venous thrombosis.[18] This partially explains the increased frequency of such fistulae in women, especially in post-partum state.

CLINICAL SYMPTOMATOLOGY

Clinical features of CCFs are similar in nature in both direct and indirect fistulae, except that symptoms and signs are less severe in indirect CCFs because of slow flow shunts. The clinical manifestations of CCFs can be predicted based on the presence of structures in the cavernous sinus and the venous drainage of the sinus. The neural involvement (III, IV, V1, V2, VI) may cause ophthalmoparesis due to involvement of cranial nerves in varying combinations. The symptoms may range from palsy in one gaze (lateral rectus palsy) to complete ophthalmoplegia. With respect to the dominant venous drainage, the symptoms are predominantly localized to the respective drainage site. Venous drainage towards the orbit produces proptosis, chemosis, and arterialization of scleral veins **(Figs. 1A to D)**. The resultant venous hypertension, mass effect, and hemorrhage produce ocular and orbital symptoms. The neural paresis may be exacerbated by thickening of extraocular muscles secondary to venous congestion. The onset of symptoms may be significantly delayed after the onset of trauma and may begin abruptly. Sudden rupture of a cavernous carotid aneurysm has been postulated as a cause, the injury of which would have occurred during trauma. Dominant venous drainage to the inferior petrosal sinus leads to aural symptoms especially tinnitus. Contralateral cavernous sinus drainage through intercavernous anastomosis causes similar symptoms localizing to the other eye. In about 5% of the patients, high venous flow may be retrogradely transmitted to the cortical veins resulting in life-threatening hemorrhages. There may occur brainstem venous congestion resulting in altered consciousness including various other cerebellar symptoms. Another type of symptom which is commonly seen with high-flow direct CCFs is downstream ischemia e.g. transient ischemic attacks (TIA) due to steal of blood away from the intracranial circulation. Even myelopathy due to spinal venous drainage of the fistula is reported.[19] Most direct CCFs are acquired, secondary to trauma, including iatrogenic trauma, or rupture of an intracavernous aneurysm.

Indirect CCFs do not present with abrupt onset of fulminant symptoms due to lesser quantity of shunted blood. A typical patient is a middle aged female presenting with slowly progressive history of orbital pain, congestion and some degree of restriction of movements. Congestion may not be easily noticeable and hence referred to as 'white-eyed shunt'.[20] There may be increased intraocular pressure with new onset glaucoma. Posterior draining sinus may present as tinnitus. The clinical course may be waxing-waning and some fistulae may occlude due to spontaneous thrombosis. The nature of symptoms including vision loss may not be significantly different between the two groups.[21] However the abruptness and quantum of the symptoms are definitely higher in the direct variety.

Differential diagnosis: The following need to be considered when the patient presents with ocular signs and symptoms—thyroid disease, idiopathic orbital inflammation (pseudotumor), orbital cellulitis, orbital neoplasms, cavernous sinus thrombosis, Tolosa Hunt syndrome, conjunctivitis, scleritis, episcleritis, etc.

ANATOMY OF INTRACAVERNOUS INTERNAL CAROTID ARTERY AND CAVERNOUS SINUS

Before embarking upon treatment, it is very important to have a thorough knowledge and understanding of the

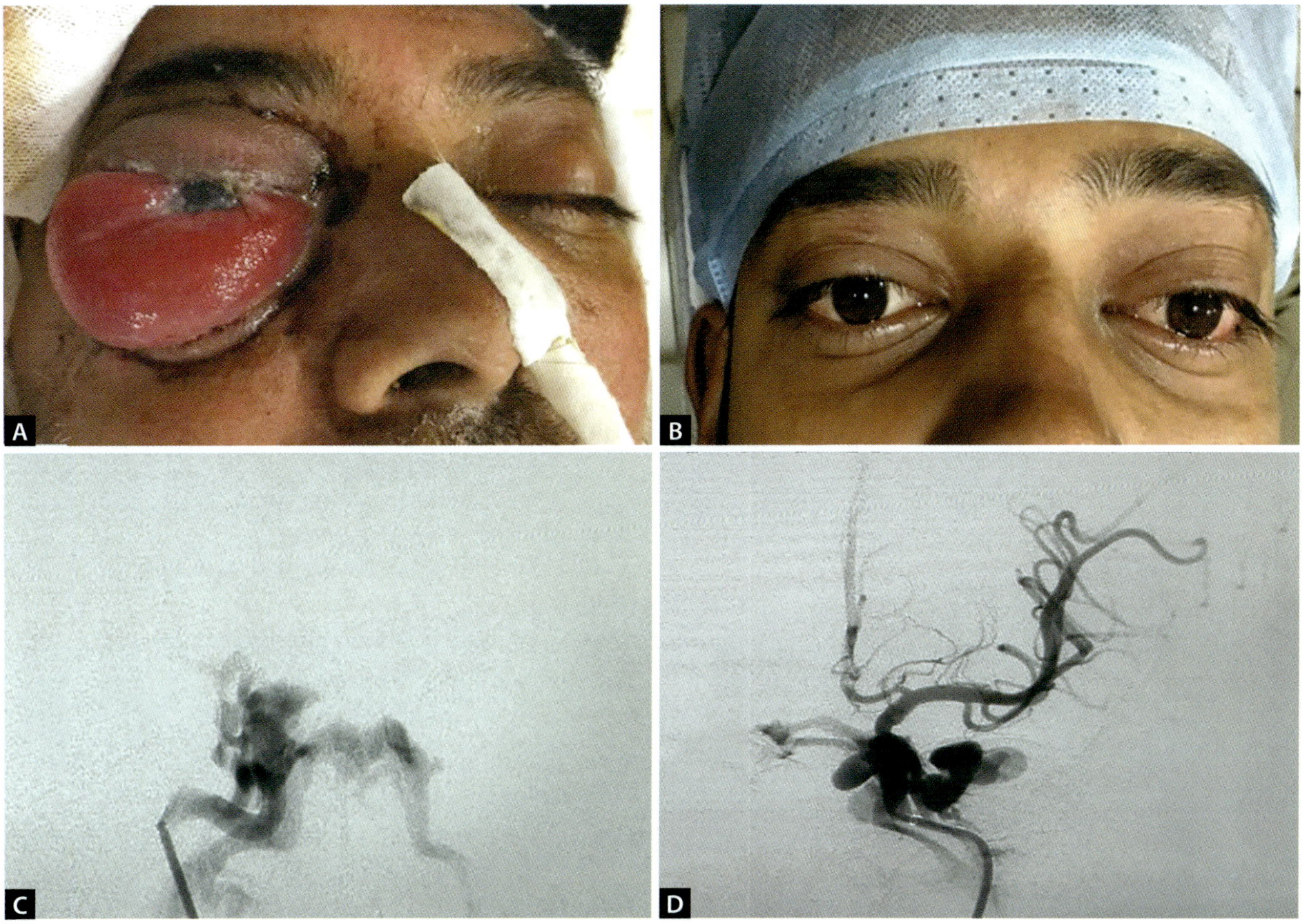

Figs. 1A to D: Clinical photograph depicting variable degree of post-traumatic proptosis—severe (A) and mild (B) and the corresponding ICA run showing high flow (C) and low flow states (D).

anatomy of the internal carotid artery (ICA) and cavernous sinus (CS).

The cavernous ICA, as the name suggests, runs within the cavernous sinus. The ICA enters the cavernous sinus by piercing the dura as it exits the petrous carotid canal at the skull base across the foramen lacerum. It subsequently has intrasinus course during its cavernous segment beyond which it pierces the dura to enter the subarachnoid space adjacent to the anterior clinoid process. The cavernous ICA can be subdivided into five segments:[22,23] posterior vertical segment (C5), first posterior genu (C4), horizontal segment (C3), second anterior genu (C2) and the ascending vertical segment (C1) **(Fig. 2)**. Meningohypophyseal artery arises near junction of C5 and C4. Meningohypophyseal artery branches supply the posterior pituitary, cavernous sinus, clival dura and cranial nerves III to VI. The inferolateral trunk arises from C4 segment and supplies the dura of the cavernous sinus and cranial nerves III, IV, V and VI.

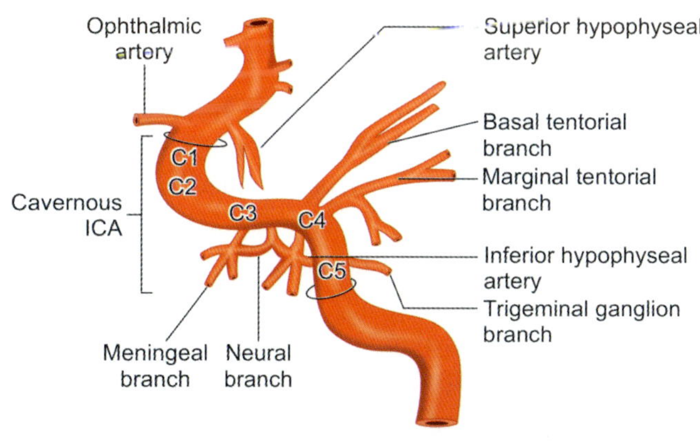

Fig. 2: Pictorial depiction of the segments (C1 to C5) of the cavernous ICA alongwith its branches.

The CS is stuated on either side of the sella turcica and is formed by the folds of the dura. It is not a single venous pouch but is compartmentalized in to smaller caverns, the three main ones being the (i) anteroinferior compartment in relation to the superior and inferior ophthalmic veins and the pterygoid plexus; (ii) the posterosuperior compartment in relation to the superficial middle cerebral

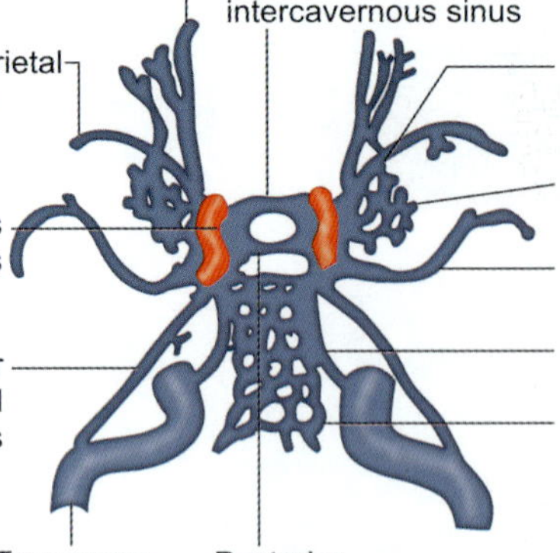

Fig. 3: Pictorial representation of the cavernous sinus anatomy with its drainage connections and tributaries.

vein, the inferior and superior petrosal sinuses, and the contralateral CS through the intercavernous sinus; and (iii) a medial compartment. The CS receives blood flow from the superficial middle cerebral vein, the middle meningeal vein, and the superior and inferior ophthalmic veins. It drains through the superior and inferior petrosal sinuses and the pterygoid plexus **(Fig. 3)**. In the case of a CCF, arterial blood enters the CS at high pressure and flow. The main efferent pathways of this arterialized blood are the inferior petrosal sinus (IPS) and the superior ophthalmic vein (SOV) which are responsible for the patients symptoms.

CLASSIFICATION

CCFs are classified to maintain homogeneity in nomenclature and to prognosticate the disease status. Carotid-cavernous fistulas can be classified based on three criteria:

I. Based on etiopathogenesis—into spontaneous or traumatic fistulae
II. Based on hemodynamics of blood flow—into high-flow or low-flow fistula
III. Based on angiographic appearance and feeders—into direct or indirect (dural) fistulae.

Based on angiographic findings, Barrow et al.[24] classified CCFs into 4 types: (i) A, (ii) B, (iii) C, and (iv) D.

Type A fistulae—direct shunts between the ICA and the CS. They are usually high-flow fistulae, frequently post-traumatic, may also occur spontaneously from rupture of an intracavernous aneurysm. Type A fistulae have been further divided into three types based on size of fistula[25] on ICA injection.

Small size: Both anterior cerebral artery (ACA) and middle cerebral artery (MCA) opacified on ICA injection **(Fig. 1D)**.

Medium size: Either ACA or MCA opacified.

Large size: None of the two opacified **(Fig. 1C)**.

Types B, C and D are indirect (dural) shunts, which usually occur spontaneously and generally have slow flow.

Type B: Fistulae between the meningeal branches of the ICA and CS.

Type C: Dural shunts between the meningeal branches of the ECA and the CS.

Type D: Between the meningeal branches of both ICA and ECA and CS.

CCFs have also been classified based on the venous drainage pattern:[26]

Type 1: CCFs with posterior/inferior drainage only.

Type 2: Posterior/inferior and anterior drainage.

Type 3: Anterior drainage only.

Type 4: Retrograde drainage into cortical veins with/without other drainage channels.

Type 5: Direct connection between the ICA and CS.

RADIOLOGICAL EVALUATION

A thorough clinical history and examination often helps us in reaching at a diagnosis of CCF.

The following modalities can be utilized for diagnosis and as part of pre-intervention work-up.

CT Scan

The findings concern the effects rather than the fistula itself. Proptosis is noted on the affected side. There is engorgement of ophthalmic veins alongwith extraocular muscle congestion. A markedly enhancing cavernous sinus, often varicose, is seen bulging outward **(Fig. 4)**. Associated soft-tissue and bony injuries (fractures) may also be seen in the acute stage.[27] CT angiography demonstrates the dilated cavernous sinus. However the rent is often not visible.

MRI

The sensitivity of MRI in diagnosing CCF is reasonably high.[28] The features of proptosis, dilated superior ophthalmic vein, orbital congestion, prominent CS point to CCF **(Figs. 5A to C)**. It also helps us in identifying the

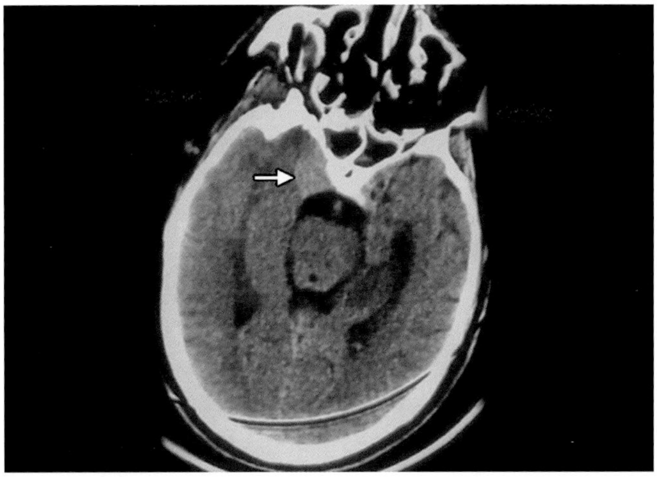

Fig. 4: Axial CT scan shows a prominent right cavernous sinus (arrow) as a manifestation of traumatic CCF.

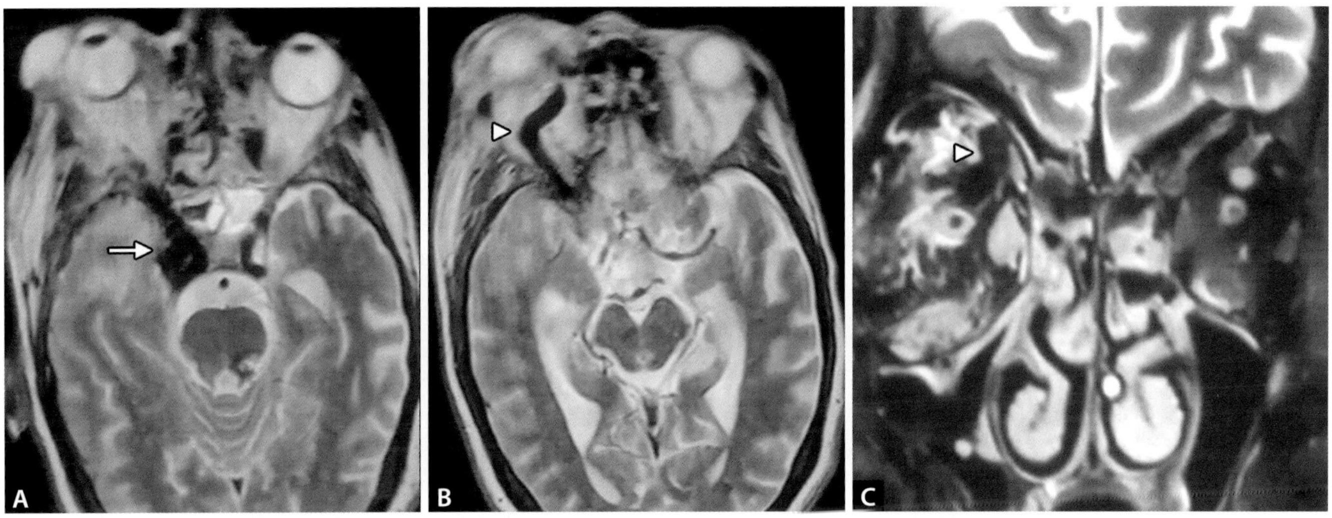

Figs. 5A to C: Axial T2 (A and B) and coronal T2-weighted (C) images demonstrating the dilated cavernous sinus (white arrow) and superior ophthalmic vein (arrowhead) in a case of direct caroticocavernous fistula. Note the proptosis, extraocular muscle enlargement and orbital congestion. Note the left superior cerebellar peduncle hemorrhagic contusion.

sequelae of trauma in traumatic fistulae like cerebral contusions, hemorrhages, etc. MRA shows prominent CS and its draining veins (better seen in direct CCF).

Digital Subtraction Angiogram (DSA)

DSA is the gold standard in the diagnosis of carotico cavernous fistula. However it is an invasive modality. Moreover with the advent of multidetector CT scanners and the technique of dynamic CT and MR angiography, DSA is hardly required as just a diagnostic modality. When performed, it demonstrates the CCF and differentiates between a direct and an indirect type. Bilateral ICAs, ECAs and the vertebral arteries must be injected to assess exact site of fistula, its venous drainage and hemodynamic effects. Dangerous angiographic findings include pial venous reflux **(Figs. 6A and B)** and giant CS varix extending intradurally because such signs indicate a higher likelihood of venous rupture and intracerebral or/and subarachnoid hemorrhage. Sometimes in high flow fistula, it becomes very difficult to visualize the ICA rent. We may do a high frame acquisition during ICA injection which may show the fistula in the early frames. However, in a significant subset of cases still, the fistula site remains elusive. A couple of maneuvers have been described which can aid us in identifying the ICA rent.

1. *Mehringer-Hieshima maneuver*: In this maneuver, the ipsilateral common carotid artery (CCA) is compressed manually while taking the ICA run. This prevents the

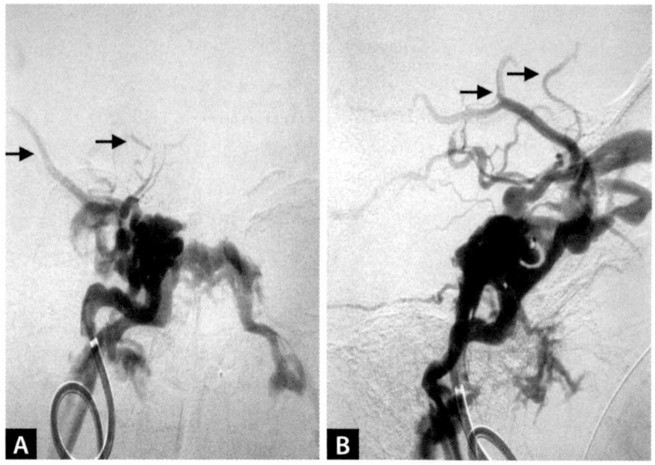

Figs. 6A and B: Digital subtraction angiogram frontal (A) and lateral (B) projection showing a high flow direct CCF with non-visualization of the anterior and middle cerebral arteries. A large quantity of blood is being shunted into the cavernous sinus and its drainage routes. Note the poor visualization of the ICA rent and significant cortical venous reflux (arrows) which demand urgent treatment.

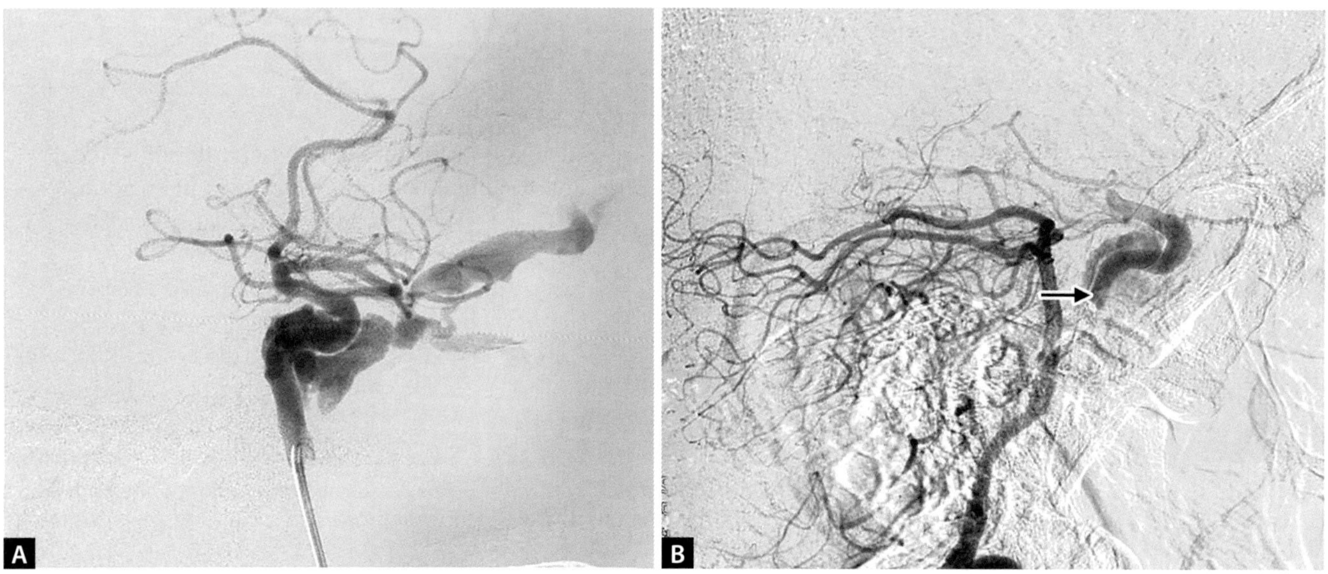

Figs. 7A and B: Frontal ICA (A) and lateral verterbal; (B) angiograms in a direct CCF displaying the cavernous sinus opacification simultaneously as that of the internal carotid artery with poor delineation of the rent. Huber maneuver demonstrating the site of rent (arrow) through retrograde flow into the ICA through the posterior communicating artery.

diluting affect of blood coming from below through the CCA and helps in increasing the chance of fistula identification.

2. *Huber/Alcock maneuver*: Herein, manual compression of ipsilateral CCA is done while taking the dominant vertebral artery run.[29] Contralateral ICA run also serves the same purpose. In this case, the blood flows retrogradely from the basilar to involved ICA through the posterior communicating artery or from the contralateral ICA through the anterior communicating artery and lines the outline of the involved ICA and hence the rent **(Figs. 7A and B)**.

In addition, other tests are often performed prior to embolization procedure which include visual acuity, intraocular pressure measurement, fundoscopy and gonioscopy.

INDICATIONS OF TREATMENT

The indications for treatment depends on a number of factors like the patient's general physical condition, severity of the symptoms and the fistula anatomy as the latter decides the treatment modality. As a general rule, type A fistulae almost always require treatment as they rarely resolve spontaneously. Definite indications for treatment are progressive visual loss, uncontrolled glaucoma, intolerable headache/bruit/tinnitus, enlargement of the fistula, epistaxis or signs of cerebral ischemia.[30] Another strong indication is presence of cortical venous reflux which indicates an increased tendency for subarachnoid or parenchymal hemorrhage.

Controversy still exists over the natural history and treatment of indirect CCFs. Several authors have reported that many of these patients will have alleviation of symptoms from spontaneous thrombosis with time, and therefore, treatment should not be instituted. Although indirect dural CCFs tend to be low flow and low-pressure lesions as compared to direct CCFs, follow-up with serial ophthalmologic examinations have shown progressive visual deterioration in such patients. Current recommendation in patients with dural CCFs without rapidly progressive visual deterioration, evidence of abnormal cortical venous drainage, hypoxic ocular changes involving the retina and optic nerve or ischemic keratopathy, is to give a trial of manual carotid artery jugular vein compression therapy first. If patients do not respond to this therapy and continue to have symptoms of visual disturbance, headache, diplopia, and chemosis, then embolization therapy is warranted.

TREATMENT OPTIONS

As discussed in the opening section, the treatment of direct CCF has evolved tremendously over the last century. There are 3 basic methods to manage such patients—conservative, endovascular and surgical. The type of fistula determines the choice of treatment.

Conservative treatment may be attempted in slow flow indirect type fistulae and involves subjecting the patient to a trial of carotid compression.[31] The procedure involves manual occlusion of the affected carotid with opposite hand for 10 seconds three times an hour while the patient is awake. The occlusion time is gradually increased. This maneuver is proposed to induce thrombosis and fistula closure subsequently. Complete resolution of symptoms has been reported in 2–34% of indirect CCF patients. Even without thrombosis, a large number of patients experience significant improvement with conservative treatment alone.

The previous surgical techniques of ligation and proximal embolization have gone out of repute due to the significant risks involved. *Surgical treatment*, in fact, is reserved in only those patients who donot respond to endovascular means.

Endovascular treatment remains an excellent minimally invasive technique which has shown consistently good results over a period of time. The main goal of the treatment is to occlude the fistula without compromising the parent artery. Both arterial and venous access routes are available, the former has been shown to offer less complications. In polytrauma patients with CCF, the more life-threatening injuries should be addressed prior to embarking upon the fistula closure surgery. Before the surgery is planned and executed, the patients are invariably administered steroid to take care of the inflammation. Additionally, pharmacological treatment is advised for raised intraocular pressure.

ENDOVASCULAR MANAGEMENT

Because the diagnosis is clinical, angiography is usually reserved as the first step of the therapeutic procedure. Local anesthesia with mild sedation is preferred to allow test occlusion of the ICA, but general anesthesia may be necessary in children and uncooperative patients. Anticoagulation is obtained with heparin bolus of 3-5,000 units, followed by 1,000 units every hour in an adult.

The CS is characterized by early filling, which may obscure detection of the shunt; hence, an ICA angiogram with high-speed imaging is necessary. Injection into the vertebral artery (VA) in the lateral view demonstrates retrograde flow into ICA through the posterior communicating artery, moving toward the CCF, if there is a complete arterial steal. If not, compression of the ICA during injection of the VA enhances retrograde flow into the ICA and reveals the exact location of the shunt as described in the previously described maneuvers **(Figs. 7A and B)**. The size of the CS is also an important consideration. Chronic CCFs show progressive enlargement of the CS making the procedure more difficult. Alternatively, a small CS does not necessarily mean easy selective occlusion. Because a small CS corresponds to a small rent and balloon catheterization in such cases may be difficult. Hence, coils may be preferable. The coils can be deployed either through the arterial or through the venous route and the CS is packed close to the rent so that the fistula is obliterated. There have also been reports of stent assisted coiling and covered stents **(Figs. 8A to G)** for fistula closure.[32,33] These options were chosen in cases where the fistula is large or the exact site of the rent is not clear.

The success rates of endovascular management have continued to improve over the last few decades

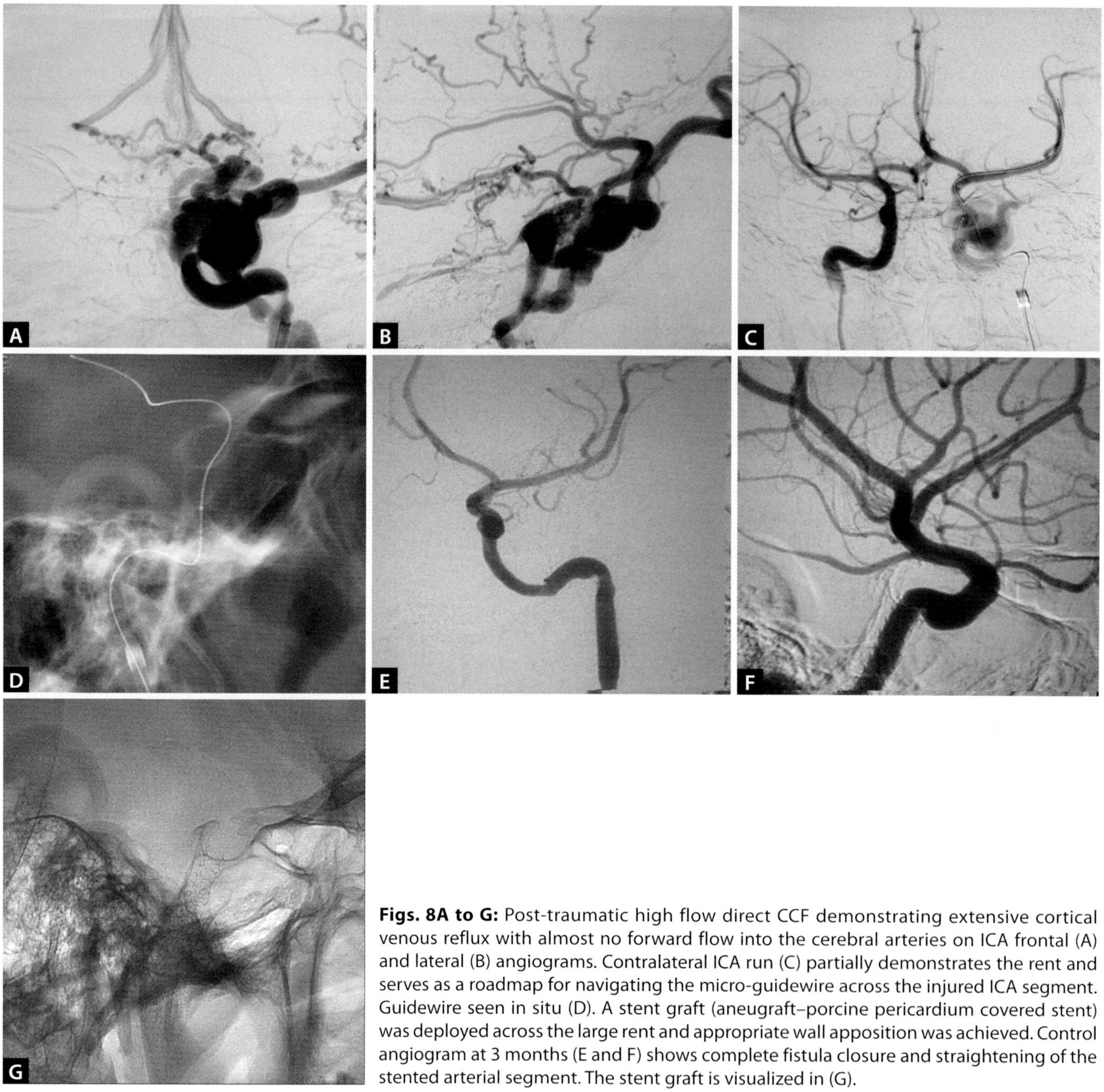

Figs. 8A to G: Post-traumatic high flow direct CCF demonstrating extensive cortical venous reflux with almost no forward flow into the cerebral arteries on ICA frontal (A) and lateral (B) angiograms. Contralateral ICA run (C) partially demonstrates the rent and serves as a roadmap for navigating the micro-guidewire across the injured ICA segment. Guidewire seen in situ (D). A stent graft (aneugraft–porcine pericardium covered stent) was deployed across the large rent and appropriate wall apposition was achieved. Control angiogram at 3 months (E and F) shows complete fistula closure and straightening of the stented arterial segment. The stent graft is visualized in (G).

as more experience and expertise has been gained in the field of interventional neuroradiology. Still, as with any neurovascular procedure, complications may occur which include thromboembolic and ischemic events due to catheter, balloon or coil manipulation, injury to the blood vessel, or inadvertent balloon detachment, pseudoaneurysm formation due to balloon deflation or migration and alteration of arterial flow resulting in hemorrhage, edema, or worsening of ocular symptoms.

Tools and Hardware

The tools currently available for use in endovascular treatment include detachable balloons, coils, stents, balloon catheters (for directing microcatheter and coils across the rent), flow diverters, liquid embolics, particles and vascular micoplugs. The optimal and widely practiced treatment of CCFs is embolization by detachable balloons or coils. Since the year 1974 when Serbinenko first reported the use of detachable balloons for occlusion of

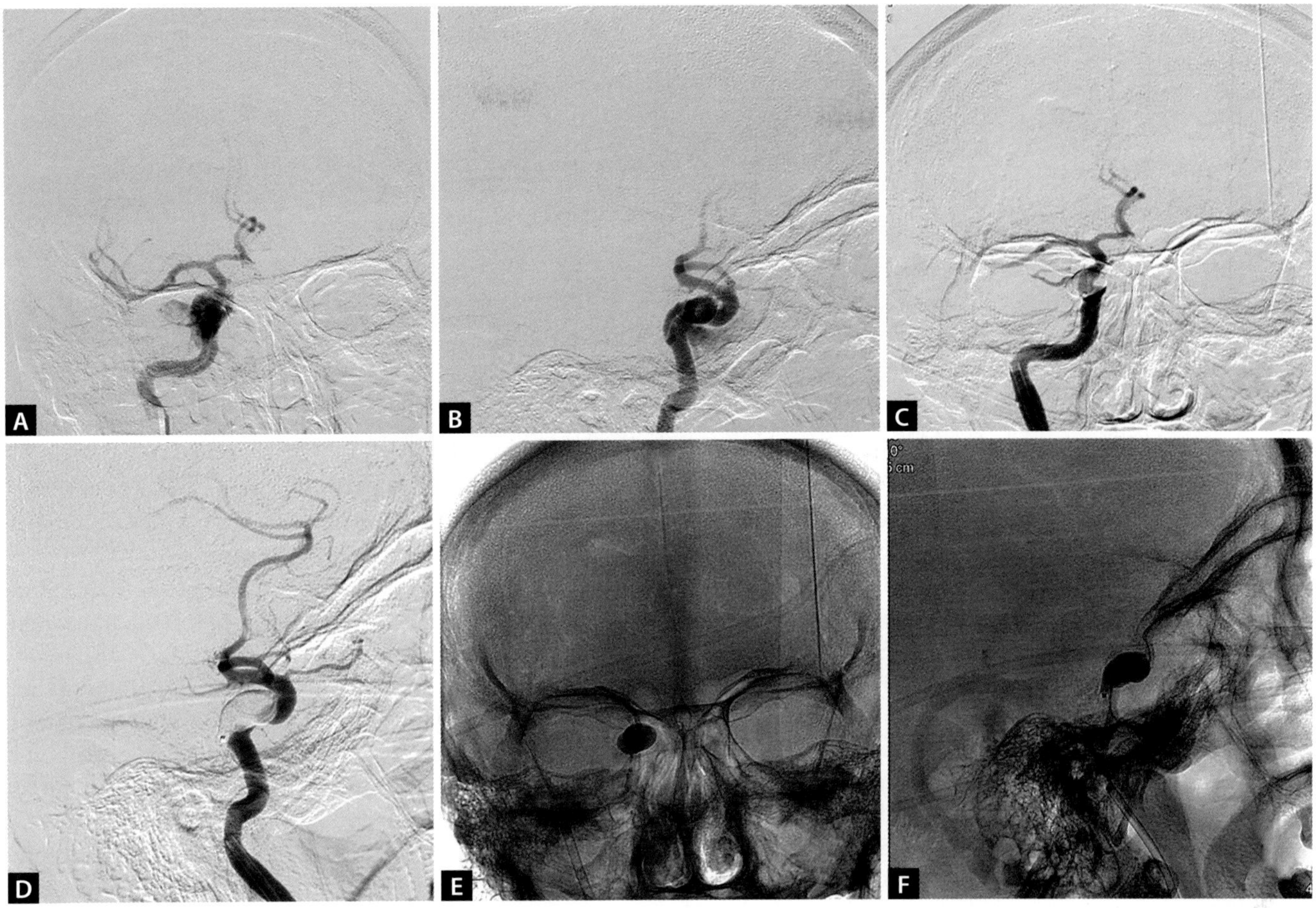

Figs. 9A to F: Post-traumatic low flow CCF treated with detachable balloon. Pre- (A and B) and post-embolization (C and D) angiograms displaying fistula closure. The hyperdense balloon is visualized partially within the cavernous sinus across the ICA rent (E and F).

these fistulae, we have come a long way in devising other embolic agents which are more convenient to use and associated with less complication rates. Of the embolic agents currently available to us in the neurointerventional armamentarium, liquid embolic agents such as N-butyl cyanoacrylate (NBCA) are rarely indicated, whereas particulate agents are not suited to the occlusion of the large arteriovenous shunt of a direct CCF, but have been used for treatment of type B, C, D fistulae.

Extensively used since their inception, balloons are the favored devices for treatment of CCFs[34] because in medium-sized CCFs (which constitute the majority of these fistulae), a single balloon can occlude the rent while entirely sparing the ICA **(Figs. 9A to F)**. Nycomed-Ingenor (Paris, France) and Balt (Monomorency, France) manufactured latex balloons, some with a self-sealing valve (Gold valve) and others without it. Some interventionists prefer the silicone balloon (Interventional Therapeutics, San Francisco, CA, USA). Most of these balloons were mounted over a microcatheter and a few older ones had to be secured with a hand-made ligature. These balloons are detached by giving traction over the microcatheter. Balloons were available in various sizes and volumes ranging from 0.1 mL to 3 mL.

Metallic coils come in various sizes and shapes and are mostly platinum based, a biocompatible, radiopaque, and nonferromagnetic material. They can be pushed through a microcatheter and on exiting resume their original circular or/helical shape. Some delivery systems allow coils to be retracted into the microcatheter if placement is unsatisfactory. The Guglielmi detachable coils (GDC) (Boston Scientific) are electrically detached **(Figs. 10A to D)**. Coils with controlled detachment, such as GDC, should be used when inadequate placement has a risk of occluding the ICA whereas mechanically detachable coils (MDC), interlocking detachable coils (IDC) or regular coils (cheaper, more thrombogenic and less time-consuming) can be used when there is little risk of migration, as is the case in most transvenous occlusions or in assorted type B, C and D fistulae. In recent times, liquid embolic

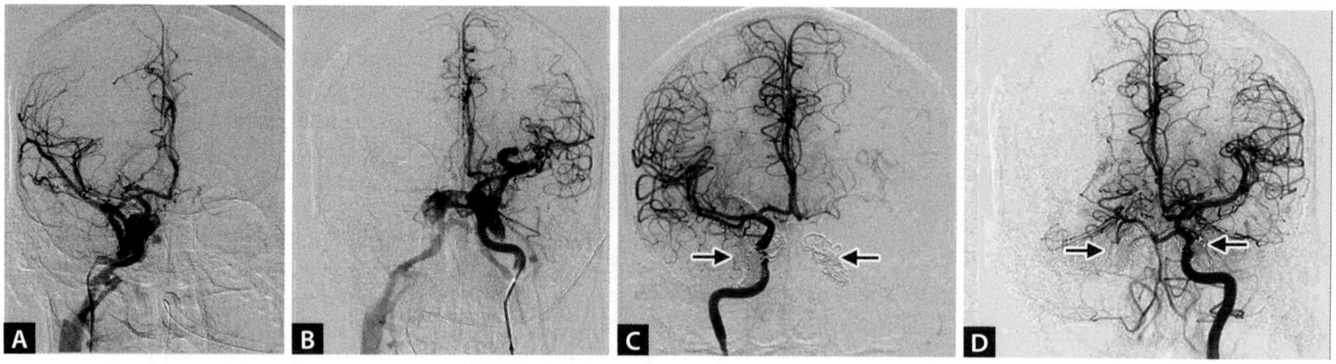

Figs. 10A to D: Bilateral traumatic direct CCF treated with endovascular coil embolization. Pre- (A and B) and postembolization (C and D) angiograms revealing complete fistula closure. Note the arrows pointing towards the coil mass.

agents like nBCA and 'Onyx', a polymer which precipitates upon contact with blood has been used successfully by some authors both by transarterial as well as transvenous approach.[35-39] Particles like gelfom and polyvinyl alcohol can be used in slow flow indirect fistulae where venous washout is very slow. Flow diverters have been deployed across the rent by few authors[40] with reasonable results.

Transarterial Embolization

Most direct CCFs can be treated by placing a detachable balloon/coils transarterially, through the rent in the ICA wall, and then selectively into the CS, obstructing the fistula while preserving ICA flow. Occasionally, the rents in the ICA are multiple or very large, necessitating carotid occlusion. In children, navigating large size balloons is difficult and hence coil embolization perhaps is preferable.

Procedure: A transfemoral guiding catheter of suitable size (6–9 F) is positioned in the ipsilateral ICA through which the wire/balloon mounted microcatheter or a coaxial assembly is introduced. In a patient with a previously ligated carotid artery, the direct arterial route to the CCF is unavailable, but arterial access is still possible by direct puncture of the cervical ICA or through the anterior or posterior communicating artery.[41] The balloon is guided into the CCF by pushing the microcatheter and, if necessary, by slightly inflating and deflating the balloon to benefit from the preferential flow into the CCF. Once the balloon is in the CS, it is progressively inflated while performing frequent angiographic controls until the CCF is occluded. If there is mild or no ICA stenosis, the balloon is detached, either by gentle traction or by coaxial detachment **(Figs. 9A to F)**. Many large series have described the use of balloons by transarterial approach in CCF with excellent results.[42-44] These series show similar positive results after transarterial balloon embolization of direct CCFs. Overall, cure was obtained in 85–90%, with ICA patency preserved in 59–80% and neurologic complications in 4–5%, of which 2% were permanent. When the CS is large, several balloons may be needed. If coils have been decided to be placed in the CS, the microcatheter tip is guided into the CS and coiling started once a stable position of the tip is reached **(Figs. 10A to D)**. At times when the rent is not easily discernible or it is large, a balloon catheter (hyperglide, scepter C, etc.) may need to be used to outline the parent artery lumen and the rent and for guiding the microcatheter across the rent. Liquid embolic (onyx) may be used at times to complete the CS occlusion by placing the balloon across the rent in the parent artery so that there is no reflux into the ICA and subsequent stroke. Occasionally, there can be extensive skull base fractures leading to CCF on both sides **(Fig. 10A to D)**. In such instances, both the ICAs are individually accessed and the fistulae are embolized by either coils or balloons.

Occasionally, selective balloon occlusion of the CCF is not possible, and the ICA must also be occluded **(Figs. 11A to I)**. ICA occlusion is also mandated when the fistula persists or recurs. A 30-minute balloon test occlusion (BTO) should be done first except in cases of complete cerebral steal from the CCF. Next, both the ICA and the CCF must be occluded, and one must avoid occluding the ICA without occluding the CCF as well. The safest way is to occlude the ICA beyond and proximal to the carotid rent by either detachable balloons or coils. Occlusion of the CCF can be confirmed before balloon detachment by vertebral angiography with a catheter through the contralateral femoral artery. With CCF occlusion, there will be no retrograde flow through the posterior communicating artery into the ICA toward the CCF. When there is extensive damage to the blood vessel with active hemorrhage or a rapidly expanding hematoma of the soft tissues, it is usually not possible to preserve the parent vessel. In these instances, test occlusion across or distal to the tear should

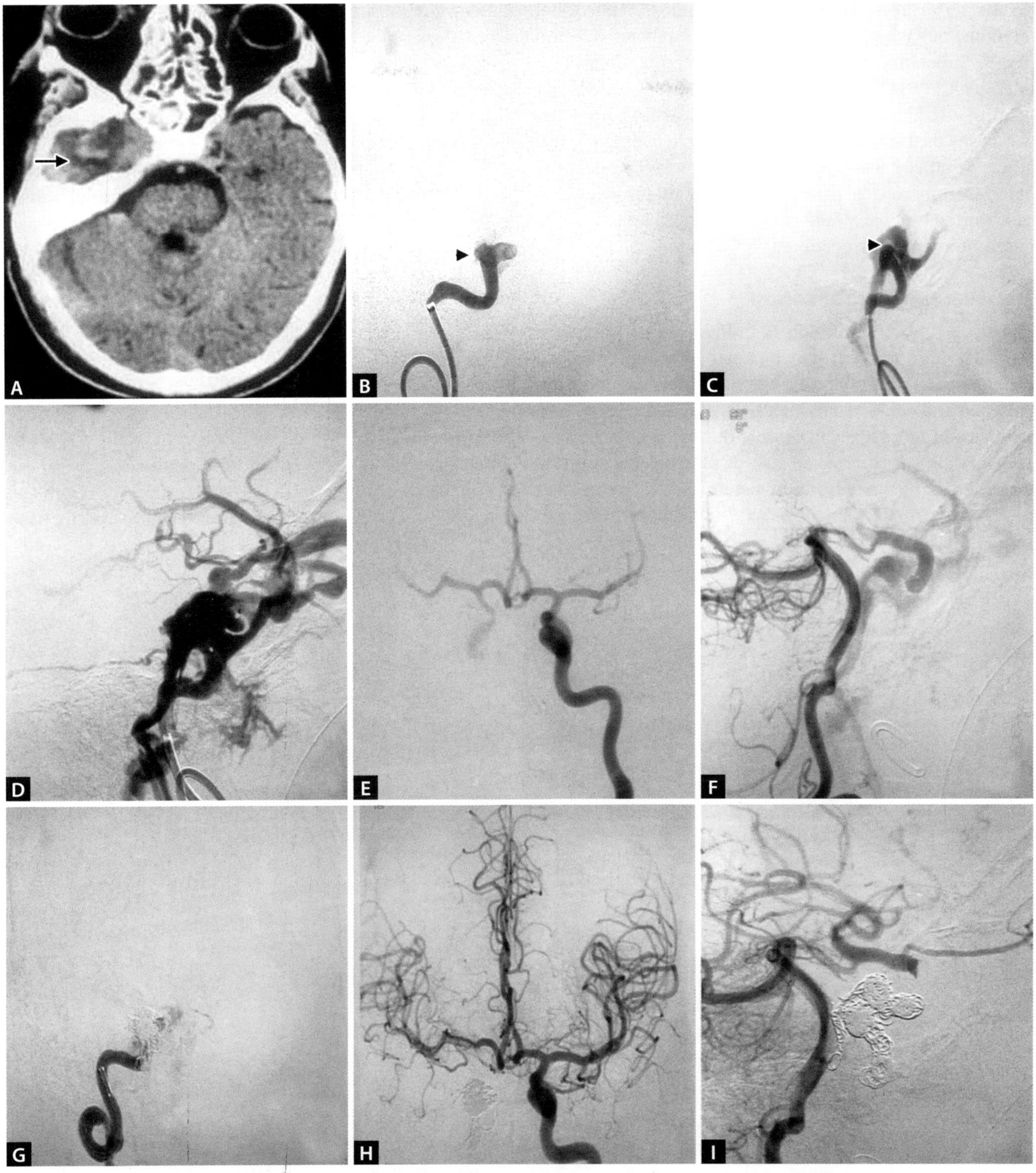

Figs. 11A to I: Post-traumatic high flow direct CCF (Barrow type A) showing the temporal contusion (arrow) on computed tomography. Frontal (B) and lateral (C) angiograms demonstrating a large ICA rent (arrowheads) with significant cortical venous reflux and poor downstream cerebral arterial blood flow (D). Contralateral ICA (E) and vertebral angiograms (F) help in delineating the fistula. Endovascular coiling was attempted but there was constant high flow into the cavernous sinus. Balloon test occlusion was performed and the patient was subjected to parent artery occlusion (PAO) (using the sandwich technique across the ICA rent) once the test was tolerated well. Control angiograms following PAO obtained from the ipsilateral ICA (G), contralateral ICA (H) and vertebral artery (I) showed no fistula opacification with good distal flow in the MCA through the anterior and posterior communicating arteries.

first be performed, if possible, to determine the individual tolerance of each patient to occlusion of a major cerebral vessel. Subsequently it may be sacrificed if the patient tolerates the BTO. The presence of underlying persistent primitive trigeminal artery (PTA) has been noticed in two cases of traumatic CCF at our centre over the last 5 years. Whether it was a coincidental finding or it made the patient prone to CCF is debatable. The anatomy in such cases has to be clearly delineated before embarking on the neurointervention procedure **(Figs. 12A to J)**.

Transvenous Embolization

The transvenous approach is indicated only after the transarterial approach fails because of a higher risk of venous rupture and hemorrhage.[45] Because the veins are enlarged and subjected to high flow, they are weaker than arteries and more likely to rupture during catheterization. There is also an increased risk of placing the embolic material at a distance from the fistula itself or redirecting flow into cortical veins. The CCF is accessed through one of its draining veins, generally the IPS **(Figs. 13A to L)** or the ophthalmic vein, whichever seems the easiest to catheterize on the initial angiogram. For IPS access, a guiding catheter is placed into the internal jugular vein at the level of the jugular bulb from a transfemoral venous access or direct cervical jugular puncture. A second possibility is to approach via the superior ophthalmic vein (SOV) and the angular vein from a transfemoral catheterization or if necessary, from a surgically exposed ophthalmic vein.[46] Once the microcatheter has reached the CS, it is guided toward the CCF. Embolization begins with blockage of the venous drainage of the CS, starting with the cortical draining veins if present. Coils are the embolic agent of choice for transvenous embolization, but balloons can be used, if access permits.

Parent Artery Reconstruction

There are instances when the artery needs to be reconstructed. The aim is to exclude the CCF from the circulation. For this purpose, covered stents may be used

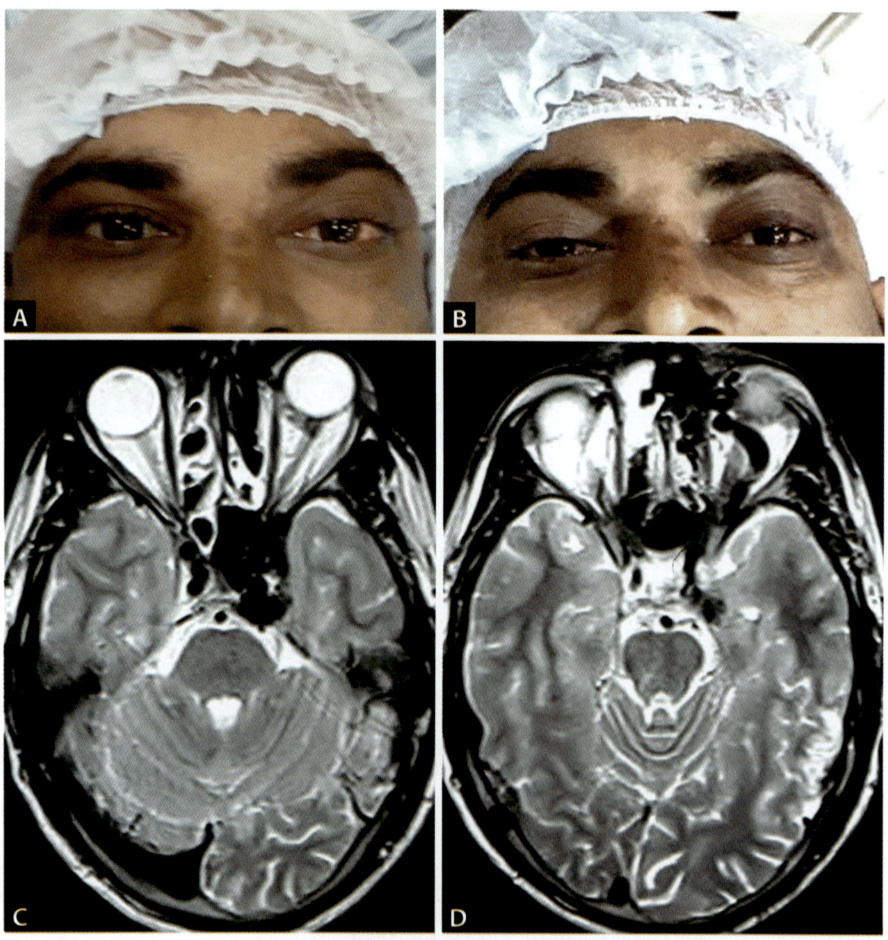

Figs. 12A to D

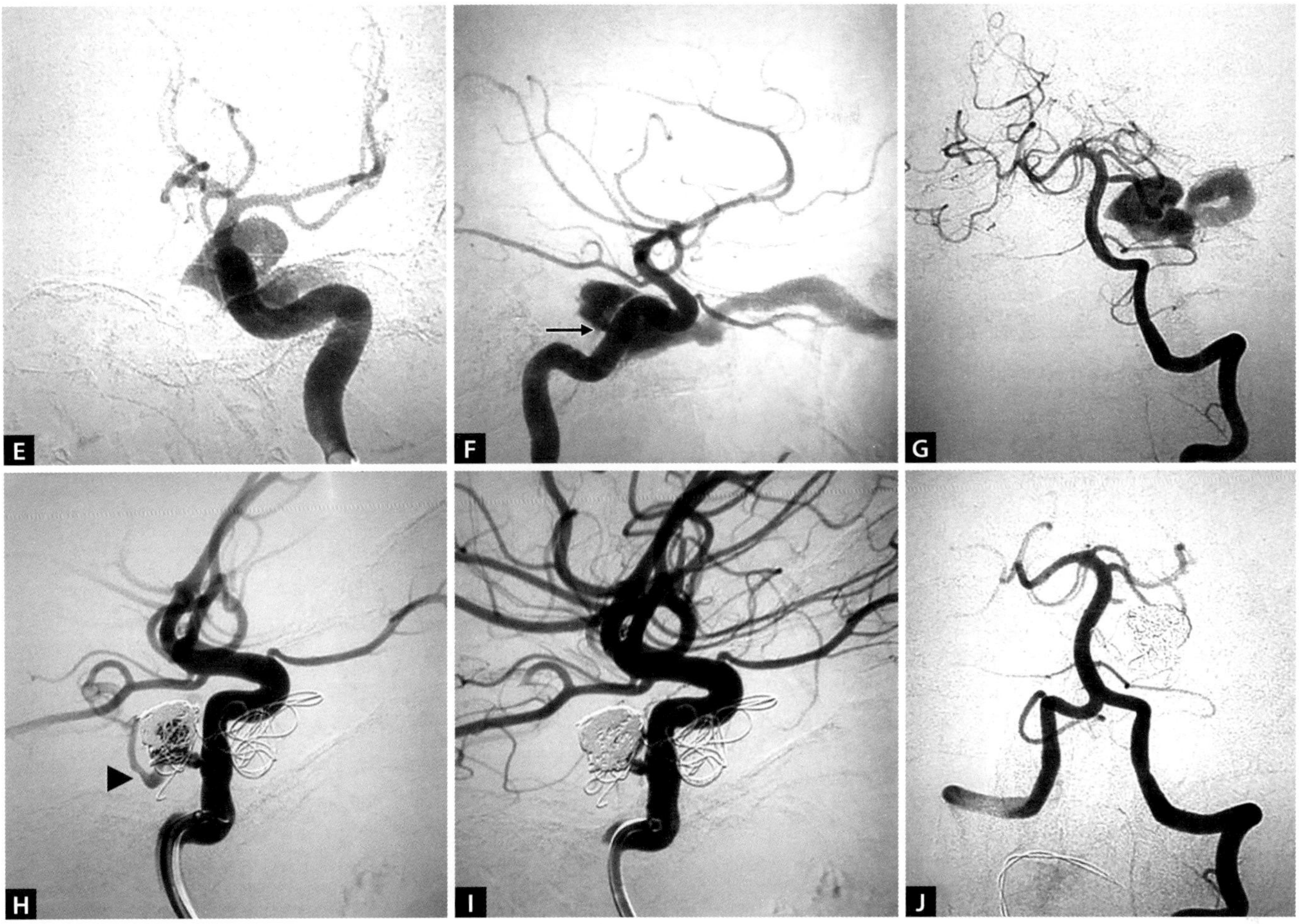

Figs. 12E to J

Figs 12A to J: Clinical photograph of a patient with traumatic trigeminocavernous fistula prior to (A) and following embolization (B) shows good clinical response. Axial T2-weighted images (C and D) demonstrating the bulky left cavernous sinus with dilated superior ophthalmic vein. Frontal (E) and lateral (F) ICA runs demonstrating the opacification of the cavernous sinus through a small stump (arrow) arising from the C5 segment. Verterbal artery run (G) similarly demonstrates the arterial channel arising from the distal basilar trunk and leading to the cavernous sinus. Following partial coiling of the cavernous sinus close to the rent (H), the persistent trigeminal artery is better visualized (arrowhead). Control angiograms following complete embolization show complete fistula closure with only small stumps on the ICA as well as basilar trunk side (I and J).

(Figs. 8A to G). However, dedicated neurovascular covered stents are currently not available. Carotid stent grafts are stiff and not easily maneuverable across the carotid siphon. They find use when there is no other option and artery needs to be preserved. Apart from covered stents, there has been description of deployment of flow diverters with coils/in isolation with favorable results.

Follow-up

The fistula may not be fully embolised. Some angiographic residual flow, if present, is not an indication for an attempt at achieving complete angiographic cure. The goal of treatment is to alleviate the patient's symptoms and not offer a complete cure on angiogram. Follow-up DSA may be done after 3–4 months if there is no significant improvement in patient's symptoms.

CONCLUSION

Interventional neurovascular techniques continue to be at the helm and form the preferred mode of treatment for CCF. The goal of therapy is to occlude the fistulae involving the carotid artery with preservation of the parent vessel. Endovascular coil embolization is the current technique of choice.

ACKNOWLEDGEMENT

The authors acknowledge Dr NK Mishra, former author of this chapter for integral contribution in the revised chapter.

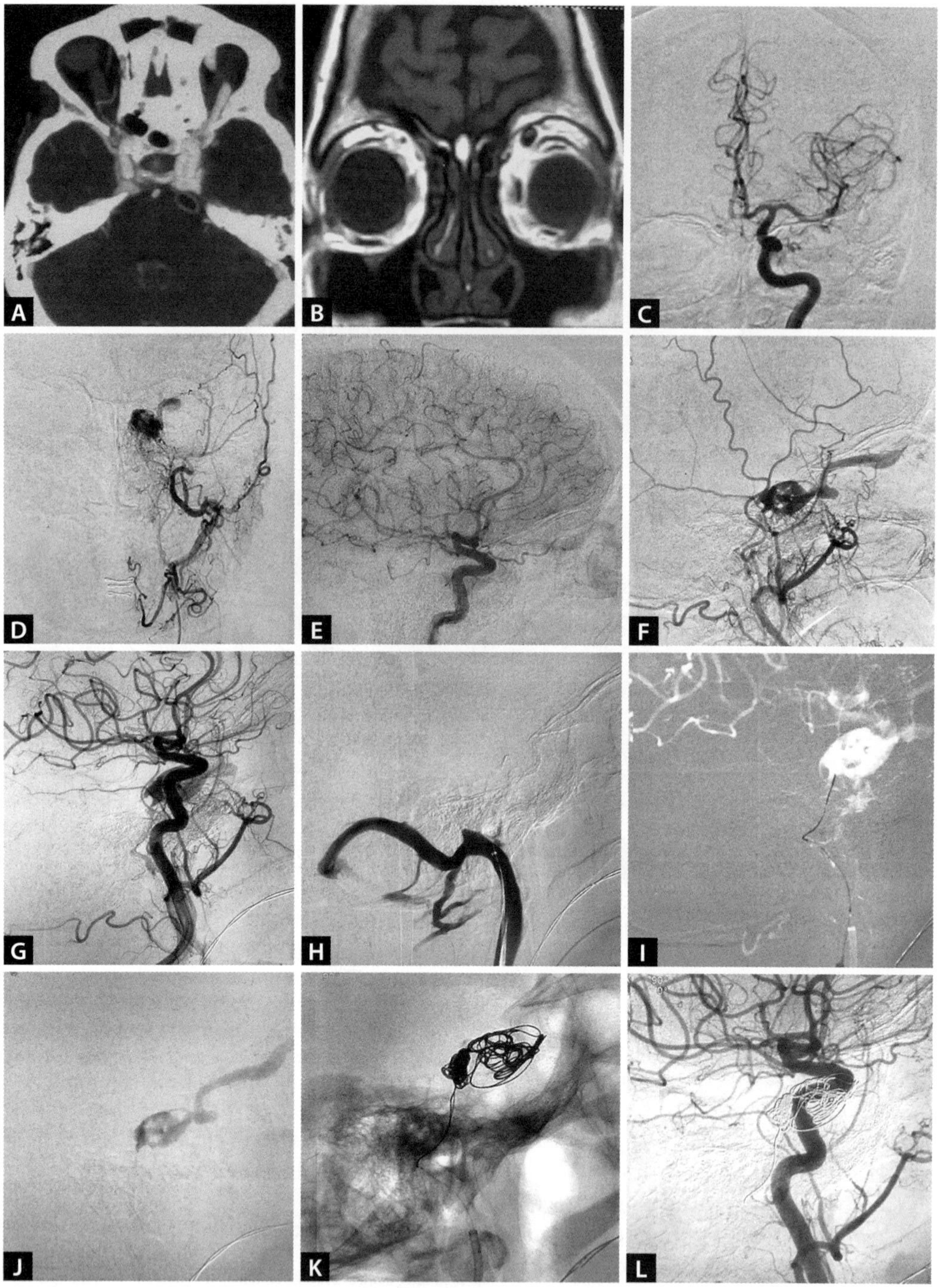

Figs. 13A to L: A middle aged female patient presented with long-standing orbital congestive changes. CT angiography (A) shows bulky left cavernous sinus and dilated SOV which was confirmed on coronal T1-weighted MRI (B). Left ICA injection (C and E) shows faint cavernous sinus opacification. The external carotid artery injection demonstrates the venous opacification clearly (D and F), Diagnosis of Barrow type D CCF was made and the patient was subjected to coil embolization through the transvenous route. Preprocedure common carotid angiogram (G) and internal jugular venogram (H) helped in guiding the microcatheter (I). Cavernous sinogram (J) showing the dilated SOV. Progressive coiling of the sinus was done (K) resulting in complete fistula closure as demonstrated on control CCA injection (L) following the procedure.

REFERENCES

1. Pool JL. Carotid-Cavernous Fistula. Arch Neurol. 1967; 16(1):111.
2. Hamby WB. Carotid Cavernous Fistula, Springfield, IL: Charles C Thomas, 1966.
3. Serbinenko FA. Balloon catheterization and occlusion of major cerebral vessels. J Neurosurg. 1974;41:125-45.
4. Mullan S. Treatment of carotid-cavernous fistulas by cavernous sinus occlusion. J Neurosurg. 1979;50:131-44.
5. Guglielmi G, Viñuela F, Briganti F, et al. Carotid-cavernous fistula caused by a ruptured intracavernous aneurysm: endovascular treatment by electrothrombosis with detachable coils. Neurosurgery. 1992;31:591-7.
6. Hirai T, Korogi Y, Goto K, et al. Carotid-cavernous sinus fistula and aneurysmal rupture associated with fibromuscular dysplasia: a case report. Acta Radiol. 1996;37: 49-51.
7. Mitsuhashi T, Miyajima M, Saitoh R, et al. Spontaneous carotid-cavernous fistula in a patient with Ehlers-Danlos syndrome type IV—case report. Neurol Med Chir (Tokyo) 2004;44:548-53.
8. Yamamoto T, Asai K, Lin YW, et al. Spontaneous resolution of symptoms in an infant with a congenital dural caroticocavernous fistula. Neuroradiology. 1995;37:247-9.
9. Parkinson D. Transcavernous repair of carotid cavernous fistula: case report. J Neurosurg. 1967;26:420-4.
10. Helmke K, Kruger O, Laas R. The direct carotid-cavernous fistula: a clinical, pathoanatomical, and physical study. Acta Neurochir. 1994;127:1-5.
11. Lasjaunias P, Berenstein A. Surgical Neuroangioraphy, Springer-Verlag; 1987. pp. 175-234.
12. Bullock R, Van Dellen J. Acute carotid-cavernous fistula with retained knife blade after transorbital stab wound. Surg Neurol. 1985;24:555-8.
13. Ahuja A, Guterman LR, Hopkins LN. Carotid cavernous fistula and false aneurysm of the cavernous carotid artery: complications of transsphenoidal surgery. Neurosurgery. 1992;31:774-9.
14. Revuella R, Nathal E, Balderrama J, et al. External carotid artery fistula due to microcompression of the gasserian ganglion for relief of trigeminal neuralgia. Case report. J Neurosurg. 1993;78:499-500.
15. Flandroy P, Lenelle J, Collignon J, et al. Carotid cavernous fistula associated with Fogarty catheter angioplasty. Am J Neuroradiol. 1988;9:1242.
16. Barr JD, Mathis JM, Horton JA. Iatrogenic carotid-cavernous fistula occurring after embolization of a cavernous sinus meningioma. Am J Neuroradiol. 1995;16:483-5.
17. Newton TH, Hoyt WF. Dural arteriovenous shunts in the region of the cavernous sinus. Neuroradiology. 1970;1: 71-81.
18. Taniguchi RM, Goree JA, Odom GL. Spontaneous carotid-cavernous shunts presenting diagnostic problems. J Neurosurg. 1971;35:384-91.
19. Narita Y, Watanabe Y, Hoshino T, et al. Myelopathy due to large veins draining recurrent spontaneous caroticocavernous fistula. Neuroradiology. 1992;34:433-5.
20. Acierno MD, Trobe JD, Cornblath WT, Gebarski SS. Painful oculomotor palsy caused by posterior-draining dural carotid cavernous fistulas. Arch Ophthalmol. 1995;113:1045-9.
21. Grumann AJ, Boivin-Faure L, Chapot R, et al. Ophthlamologic outcome of direct and indirect carotid cavernous fistulas. Int Ophthalmol 2012;32:153-9.
22. Rhoton AL Jr, Inoue T. Microsurgical approach to the cavernous sinus. Clin Neurosurg. 1989;37:391-439.
23. Dolenc VV. Direct microsurgical repair of intracavernous vascular lesions. J Neurosurg. 1983;58:824-31.
24. Barrow DL, Spector RH, Braun IF, et al. Classification and treatment of spontaneous carotid-cavernous sinus fistulas. J Neurosurg 1985;62:248-56.
25. Chi CT, Nguyen D, Duc VT, et al. Direct traumatic carotid cavernous fistula: angiographic classification and treatment strategies. Study of 172 cases. Interv Neuroradiol. 2014;20(4):461-75.
26. Thomas AJ, Chua M, Fusco M, et al. Proposal of Venous Drainage-Based Classification System for Carotid Cavernous Fistulae With Validity Assessment in a Multicenter Cohort. Neurosurgery. 2015;77(3):380-5.
27. Chung JW, Chang KH, Han MH, et al. Computed tomography of cavernous sinus diseases. Neuroradiology. 1988;30(4):319-28.
28. Uchino A, Hasuo K, Matsumoto S, et al. MRI of dural carotid-cavernous fistulas: comparisons with postcontrast CT. Clin Imaging. 1992;16:263-8.
29. Huber P. A technical contribution of the exact angiographic localization of carotid cavernous fistulas. Neuroradiology. 1976;10:239-41.
30. Halbach VV, Hieshima GB, Higashida RT, et al. Carotid-cavernous fistulae: indications for urgent treatment. Am J Roentgenol. 1987;149:587-93.
31. Higashida RT, Hieshima GB, Halbach VV, et al. Closure of carotid cavernous sinus fistulae by external compression of the carotid artery and jugular vein. Acta Radiol Suppl. 1986;369:580-3.
32. Archondakis E, Pero G, Valvassori L, et al. Angiographic follow-up of traumatic carotid cavernous fistulas treated with endovascular stent graft placement. Am J Neuroradiol 2007;28(2):342–7.
33. Tiewei Q, Ali A, Shaolei G, et al. Carotid cavernous fistulas treated by endovascular covered stent grafts with follow-up results. Br J Neurosurg. 2010;24:435-40.
34. Debrun G, Lacour P, Vinuela F, et al. Treatment of 54 traumatic carotid-cavernous fistula. J Neurosurg. 1981;55: 678-92.
35. Arat A, Cekirge S, Saatci I, et al. Transvenous injection of Onyx for casting of the cavernous sinus for the treatment of a carotid- cavernous fistula. Neuroradiology. 2004;46:1012-5.
36. Wakhloo AK, Perlow A, Linfante I, et al. Transvenous n-butyl-cyanoacrylate infusion for complex dural carotid cavernous fistulas: technical considerations and clinical outcome. Am J Neuroradiol. 2005;26:1888-97.
37. Baccin CE, Campos CM, Abicalaf R, et al. Traumatic carotid-cavernous fistula: endovascular treatment with Onyx and coils. Interv Neuroradiol. 2005;11:363-7.

38. Luo CB, Teng MM, Chang FC, et al. Transarterial balloon-assisted n-butyl-2-cyanoacrylate embolization of direct carotid cavernous fistulas. Am J Neuroradiol. 2006;27:1535-40.
39. Suzuki S, Lee DW, Jahan R, et al. Transvenous treatment of spontaneous dural carotid-cavernous fistulas using a combination of detachable coils and Onyx. Am J Neuroradiol. 2006;27:1346-9.
40. Iancu D, Lum C, Ahmed ME, et al. Flow diversion in the treatment of carotid injury and carotid-cavernous fistula after transsphenoidal surgery. Interventional Neuroradiology. 2015;21(3):346-50.
41. Garcia-Cervigon E, Bien S, Laurent A, et al. Treatment of a traumatic carotid cavernous fistula: vertebro-basilar approach after surgical occlusion of the internal carotid artery. Neuroradiology. 1988;30:355-7.
42. Lewis AK, Tomsick TA, Tew JM Jr. Management of 100 consecutive direct carotid-cavernous fistulas. results of treatment with detachable balloons. Neurosurgery. 1995; 36:239-45.
43. Higashida RT, Halbach VV, Tsai FY, et al. Interventional neurovascular treatment of traumatic carotid and vertebral artery lesions: results in 234 cases. Am J Roentgenol. 1989;153:577-82.
44. Kendall B. Results of treatment of arteriovenous fistulae with the Debrun technique. Am J Neuroradiol. 1983;4:405-8.
45. Halbach VV, Higashida RT, Hieshima GB, et al. Transvenous embolization of direct carotid-cavernous fistulas. Am J Neuroradiol. 1988;9:741-7.
46. Quinones D, Duckwiler G, Gobin YP, et al. Embolization of dural cavernous fistulas via superior ophthalmic vein approach. Am J Neuroradiol. 1997;18:921-8.

CHAPTER 13

Central Nervous System Infections

Sapna Singh, Gaurav S Pradhan, Anju Garg, Anjali Prakash

INTRODUCTION

Despite advancements in antibiotic therapy, infections of the central nervous system continue to be a major cause of mortality and morbidity. The brain, its surrounding membranes and the subarachnoid space provide an anatomic and functional barrier to the spread of pathogens. However, there are certain structural peculiarities of the central nervous system (CNS).

The factors that account for a unique response of CNS to microorganisms include:

a. Absence of true lymphatics
b. Absence of capillaries in the subarachnoid space.
c. Presence of diploic and emissary veins which provide a direct intercommunication between the intra- and extra-cranial venous system.
d. Differences in the vascular supply between grey and white matter.
e. Deficiency of immunoglobulin and complement making cerebrospinal fluid an excellent culture medium for bacterial growth.

CRANIAL MENINGES AND EXTRA-AXIAL SPACES

The osseous and membranous coverings, that is the pachymeninx (dura) and the leptomeninges (pia-arachnoid), the blood brain and the blood cerebrospinal fluid (CSF) barriers protect the brain from direct spread of infections and disease processes. The pachymeninx or the duramater is a thick tough structure composed of dense connective tissue. The outer layer is highly vascularized and is not of true meningeal origin while the inner dural layer is derived from the meninx. The falx cerebri, the falx cerebelli, tentorium cerebelli are all reflections of the true inner layer of the cranial dura mater.[1] The leptomeninges are constituted by the arachnoid and piamater. The arachnoid is closely apposed to the inner layer of the dura while the piamater covers the cerebral sulci and fissures and carries a vast network of vessels. While the normal parietal duramater is not normally visualized on imaging studies, the normal falx cerebri and tentorium cerebelli may be seen on a normal T1- and T2-weighted MR image as a thin membrane. The epidural space is the space between the dura and the inner table of the skull while subdural space is between the dura and the arachnoid. The subdural space is a potential space containing bridging veins and arachnoid villi. The arachnoid is separated from the pia by the subarachnoid space which contains the CSF.

In normal meninges, enhancement is seen as a thin, markedly discontinuous rim covering the surface of the brain and is most prominent parasagittally. This enhancement is primarily in the dura.[2,3] Thin, linear, well-demarcated and symmetric enhancement may sometimes be seen in the sulci because of enhancing veins.[4] Abnormal meningeal enhancement is asymmetrical, longer and continuous, extends deep into the base of the sulci and is not as sharply demarcated as normal meningeal enhancement **(Table 1)**.

Meningeal enhancement present on more than three contiguous MR images is considered abnormal.[6]

Table 1: Differences between normal and abnormal meningeal enhancement.[5]

Normal meningeal enhancement	*Abnormal meningeal enhancement*
Symmetric	Asymmetric
Sharply demarcated	Not well-demarcated
Thin and smooth	Thick, irregular or nodular
Short and discontinuous	Long and continuous
Superficial	Extends deep into the base of sulci
No enhancement in suprasellar cisterns	Enhancement may be seen in suprasellar cisterns
No enhancement of ventricular walls	Enhancement in ventricular walls may be seen

On contrast administration, short segments of enhancing duramater can be visualized on normal MR imaging. Pachymeningeal or dural enhancement occurs along the calvarial contours while enhancement along the cerebral and cerebellar sulci and fissures constitutes leptomeningeal or the pial subarachnoid type of enhancement. Enhancement along the brainstem is always of the pial subarachnoid space type. A pachymeningeal or dural enhancement may result from intracranial hypotension, transient postoperative changes, following lumbar puncture, infections, sarcoidosis and even metastasis. Leptomeningeal enhancement which has a gyriform or serpentine appearance is usually associated with meningitis, neoplastic disease and inflammatory diseases (e.g. sarcoidosis).[7] Normal cranial nerves never enhance within the subarachnoid space. Any enhancement of the cranial nerves is always abnormal.

The various infectious agents can be classified as bacterial, viral, parasitic and fungal.

BACTERIAL/PYOGENIC INFECTIONS

Bacteria can reach meninges either by hematogenous route, local extension, direct implantation of micro-organisms which is usually due to trauma or by transmission along cranial nerves. Rarely, the infection may be iatrogenic in nature as during cranial surgery or when microbes are introduced with a lumbar puncture needle.

Causative Organisms

The causative bacteria vary according to the age of patient. *Escherichia coli* and group B streptococci are the most common organisms in neonates, Haemophilus influenzae prevails in infants and children, while Neisseria meningitides is most commonly encountered in adolescents and young adults. *Streptococcus pneumoniae* and Listeria monocytogenes are the commonest organisms in the elderly. Eighty percent of the reported cases of meningitis are caused by *H. influenzae, N. meningitides* and *S. pneumoniae.*[8,9] *Klebsiella* and anaerobic bacteria constitute the causative organisms in immunosuppressed or immunocompromised patients.

Pathophysiology

The earliest changes in meningitis begin in the meningeal and cerebral capillaries. The permeability of the blood brain barrier increases resulting in vasogenic edema. The inflammatory mediators in the meningeal exudate and parenchymal hypoxia contribute to cytotoxic edema.[10] The meningeal inflammation then spreads through the basal subarachnoid cisterns and over the cerebral hemispheres which may cause thrombosis of the superficial pial arteries and veins with consequent infarction and resultant focal signs, such as hemiparesis, dysphasia and visual field deficits. The accumulation of inflammatory basilar exudate along the course of nerves through the subarachnoid space results in cranial nerve palsies with the III, VI and VIII cranial nerves being most commonly involved.

Further spread of the inflammation results in ventriculitis which further spreads to involve the walls of the leptomeningeal veins and eventually the substance of the brain resulting in focal meningoencephalitis.

PYOGENIC MENINGITIS

Clinical Features

The clinical findings include headache, photophobia, neck stiffness, irritability and loss of consciousness. The typical triad is of fever, neck stiffness and altered mental status with nearly 100% of patients having one of the three symptoms.[11,12] The cerebrospinal fluid in pyogenic meningitis is turbid with a marked decrease in glucose (<40 mg %) and a marked increase in the protein value (>250 mg %). There is marked pleocytosis with a predominance of polymorphonuclear leukocytes/neutrophils.

Imaging

Cross sectional imaging is neither sensitive nor specific for the detection of meningitis.[13] The role of neuroimaging in meningitis is to identify complications, rule out mimics of meningitis and increased intracranial pressure before lumbar puncture. The earliest positive finding may be slight hyperattenuation with sulcal effacement on a non-contrast CT scan but it may be subtle resulting in a false negative scan. On a fluid attenuated inversion recovery sequence (FLAIR), abnormal hyperintensity may be seen in the sulci due to increased protein content but this again is not a specific finding for meningitis.[14] The sulcal hyperintensity on a FLAIR sequence may be also caused by subarachnoid hemorrhage, CSF pulsations, acute stroke, motion or magnetic susceptibility artifacts and even leptomeningeal carcinomatosis and is hence non-specific **(Table 2)**.[15]

In early meningitis, no abnormality may be detected on imaging. The positive findings on imaging seen later in the course of the disease include leptomeningeal enhancement, enhancement along the fissures or sulci secondary to the presence of brain swelling and inflammatory exudates **(Figs. 1A and B)**. Postcontrast MR imaging is more sensitive than CT in detection of abnormal leptomeningeal enhancement and easily differentiates basal cisternal enhancement from vessels in the region of Circle of Willis. Owing to the inner table of the skull seen as a signal void on MR imaging, enhancement over the cerebral convexities is better seen on MR as compared to CT scanning. Postcontrast T1-weighted magnetization transfer (MT) imaging is superior to the conventional T1-weighted images in detecting meningeal enhancement.[16] A differentiation between infective and neoplastic enhancement is important as the two may appear similar on imaging studies. A diffuse, thin, regular sheet like enhancement over the brain surface suggests an inflammatory aetiology whereas an irregular, nodular enhancement favors a neoplastic cause.[4]

Table 2: Causes of sulcal hyperintensity on FLAIR.[15]

• Subarachnoid hemorrhage
• Meningitis
• Susceptibility/flow artifacts
• CSF metastasis
• Stroke
• Pial angioma
• High inspired oxygen
• Ruptured dermoid

Diffusion Tensor Imaging in the Diagnosis of Meningitis

DTI is a relatively new MR imaging technique which provides tissue microstructural information. Fractional anisotropy (FA) and mean diffusivity (MD) are the most commonly used DTI derived metrics. Increased FA values have been reported in both enhancing and non-enhancing cortical regions in pyogenic meningitis.[17,18] The high FA values have been attributed to the diffuse inflammatory activity in meningitis. The orientation of the inflammatory cells in the pia arachnoid causes the high FA values. The high FA values may be used as a surrogate marker of inflammatory molecules in meningitis and DTI has been found to be superior to postcontrast T1W images in the diagnosis of meningitis.

COMPLICATIONS OF BACTERIAL MENINGITIS

There are several complications or alternative manifestations of bacterial meningitis. These are:

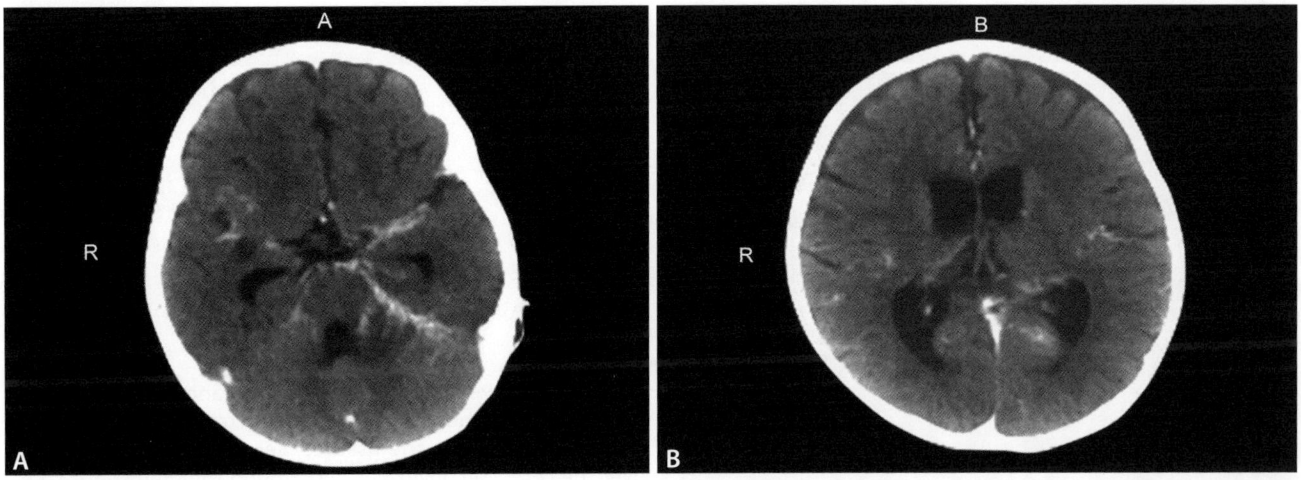

Figs. 1A and B: CECT axial scans of the cranium revealing irregular, shaggy enhancement along the tentorium, the basal cisterns and Sylvian fissures with dilated temporal horns and early hydrocephalus—pyogenic meningitis.

1. Hydrocephalus, 2. Extra-axial fluid and pus collections, 3. Cerebritis and abscess, 4. Central nervous system infarction, 5. Cranial nerve involvement, and 6. Ventriculitis.

Hydrocephalus

Hydrocephalus occurs more commonly in children and adults and occurs due to the inflammatory debris blocking the flow and resorption of the CSF.[19] This occurs more commonly at the level of the arachnoid villi. Obstruction at the level of the cerebral aqueduct or the foraminal outflow of the lateral or fourth ventricles due to exudates may also result in hydrocephalus **(Figs. 2A to C)**.[20] A focal parenchymal lesion which compresses ventricular drainage is classified as an extraluminal obstructive type.

The hydrocephalus that develops in cases of meningitis may be irreversible at times inspite of medical treatment, for example, in cases of pneumococcal meningitis, copious amounts of the capsular polysaccharide of the organism produce a gelatinous exudate that leads to arachnoid fibrosis and chronic adhesive arachnoiditis.[21]

Extra-axial Fluid and Pus Collections

Both sterile and infected extra-axial collections may be associated with meningitis. A sterile subdural effusion or hygroma is the most common collection and occurs due to irritation of the pachymeninx by the infectious agent or its products or due to inflammation of the subdural veins with resultant increase in protein and fluid within the subdural space[22] **(Fig. 3)**. Subdural effusions may occur in the H. influenzae meningitis, are usually bilateral and crescent shaped. No specific treatment is required for the effusions, these usually resolve with specific therapy against the infectious agent.[23]

Subdural Abscess/Empyema

Ten to fifteen percent of subdural empyemas are a complication of meningitis. The most common location of subdural empyemas is the cerebral convexities and the interhemispheric fissure. Unenhanced CT scan reveals a crescentic or lentiform extra-axial fluid collection that is slightly denser than cerebrospinal fluid. An overlying

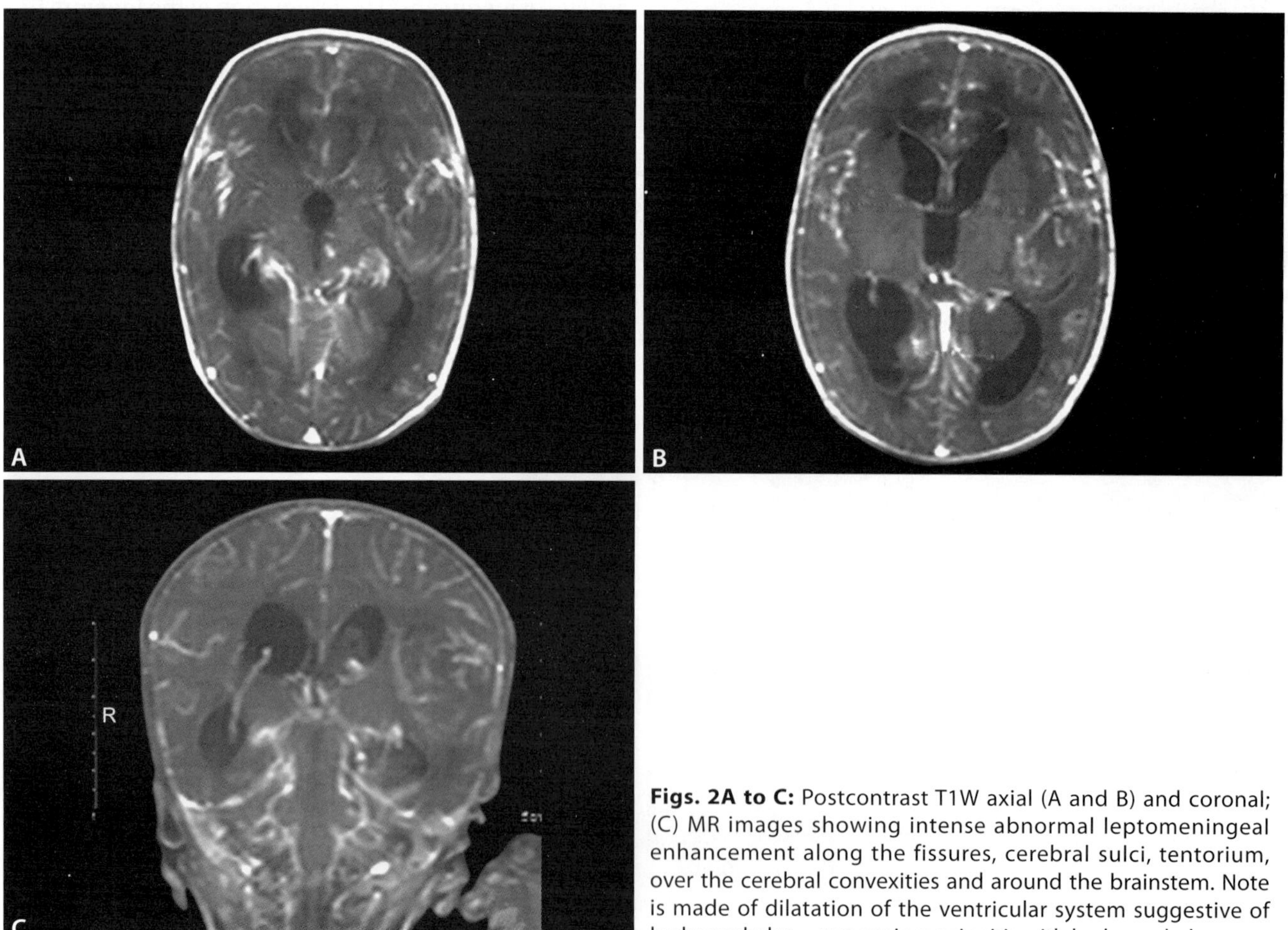

Figs. 2A to C: Postcontrast T1W axial (A and B) and coronal; (C) MR images showing intense abnormal leptomeningeal enhancement along the fissures, cerebral sulci, tentorium, over the cerebral convexities and around the brainstem. Note is made of dilatation of the ventricular system suggestive of hydrocephalus—pyogenic meningitis with hydrocephalus.

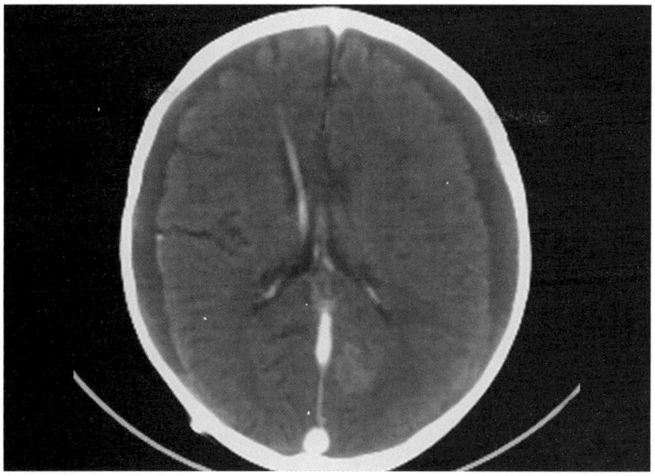

Fig. 3: CECT axial scan of the cranium showing bilateral crescent-shaped concavoconvex extra-axial fluid collections isodense to the cerebrospinal fluid in the parietal region. VP shunt is seen in situ—subdural effusions.

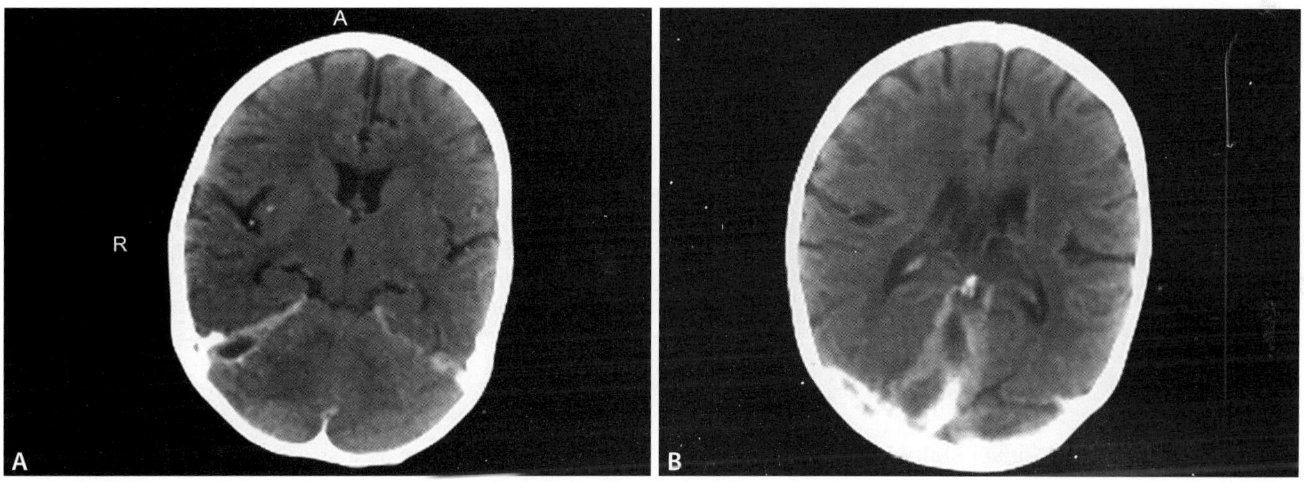

Figs. 4A and B: Contrast-enhanced axial CT scans reveal extra-axial collections along the tentorium and the interhemispheric fissure. The collections are crescent shaped with an enhancing rim—Subdural empyemas.

peripheral rim of enhancement of varying thickness is identified after intravenous contrast administration **(Figs. 4A and B)**. This rim represents an inflammatory membrane of granulation tissue on the leptomeningeal surface bordering the empyema. Hypodensity with/without contrast enhancement of the adjacent brain parenchyma may also be seen secondary to thrombophlebitis of the bridging draining veins crossing the subdural space resulting in venous occlusion and venous infarction of the involved brain.[24]

MR imaging is considered the modality of choice in the evaluation of subdural empyema.[25] In cases where the findings on CT scanning are equivocal, MR imaging helps differentiate between aseptic subdural effusions and infected subdural empyemas by virtue of the relatively shortened T1 relaxation times of purulent fluid in comparison with otherwise normal cerebrospinal fluid signal within a sterile subdural effusion. Subdural effusions are low-protein collections that are isointense relative to cerebrospinal fluid whereas empyemas are more proteinaceous and have higher MR imaging signal intensities than that of normal cerebrospinal fluid. After intravenous contrast administration, the internal and the external inflammatory membranes of subdural empyemas enhance on MR imaging **(Figs. 5A to C)**. The external membrane often is not appreciated on CT scanning because the adjacent radiodense skull obscures the contrast enhancement. When present concomitant parenchymal changes of edema and venous infarction are best visualized on T2-weighted or contrast-enhanced

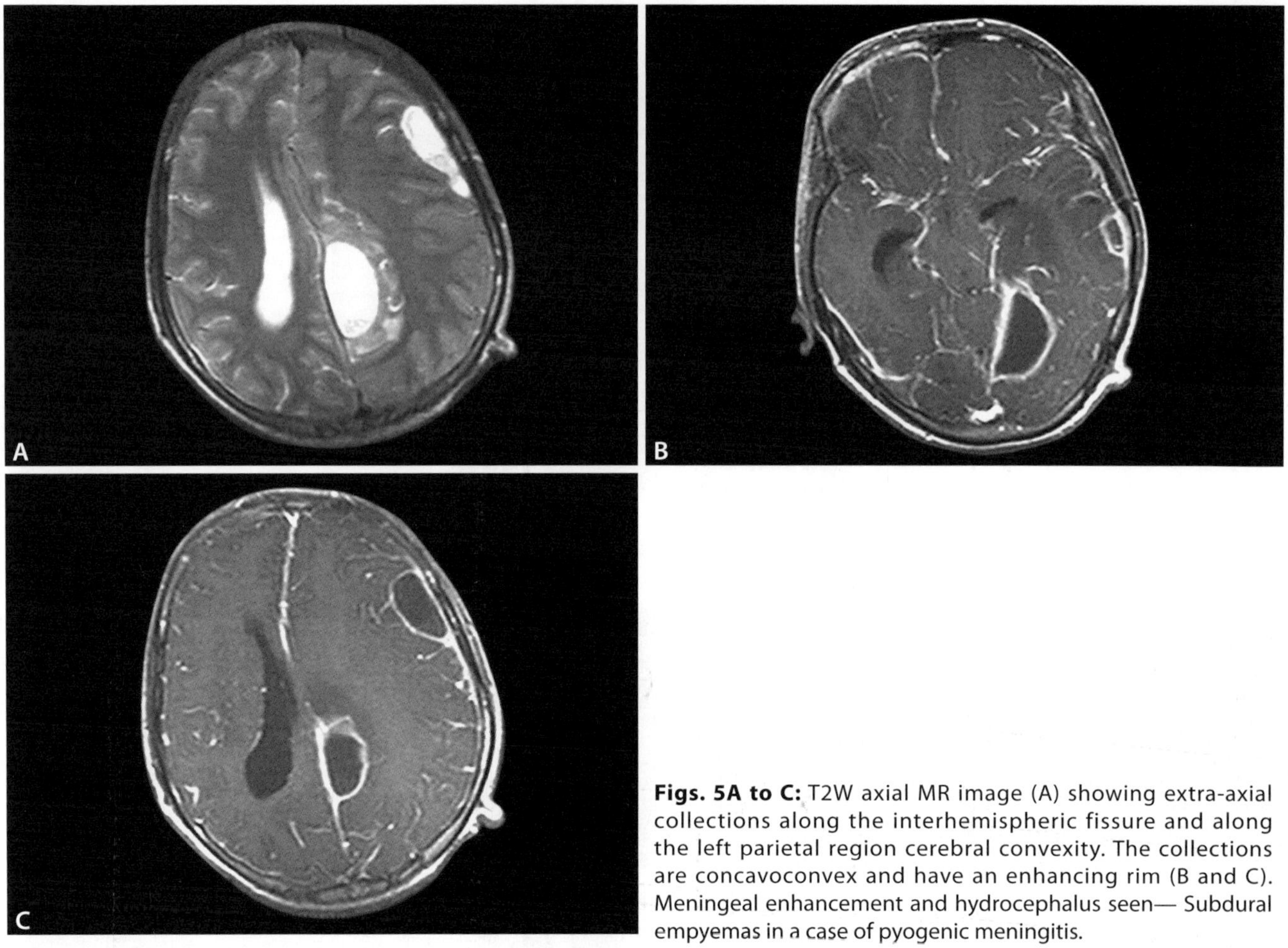

Figs. 5A to C: T2W axial MR image (A) showing extra-axial collections along the interhemispheric fissure and along the left parietal region cerebral convexity. The collections are concavoconvex and have an enhancing rim (B and C). Meningeal enhancement and hydrocephalus seen— Subdural empyemas in a case of pyogenic meningitis.

T1- weighted images. The most helpful imaging technique to identify an empyema is diffusion-weighted imaging (DWI). Empyemas are very bright on DWI unlike effusions that are dark or only mildly bright **(Figs. 6 and 7)**. Empyemas need to be drained surgically.[26]

Epidural Abscess/Empyema

Epidural abscess associated with meningitis is most frequently seen in cases that result from direct extension of infection from an external source. In infants the extra-axial collections can be visualized on sonography as well. As in cases of subdural empyema, the CT density or MR signal intensity within the collection is usually higher than that of normal cerebrospinal fluid. The involved dura mater is thickened and shows marked enhancement after intravenous contrast administration. The dura itself can be detected on MR as a hypointense medial rim separating the fluid collection from the underlying brain parenchyma. The underlying brain parenchyma is usually normal because the dura acts as a strong barrier against further intracranial dissemination. Advanced or untreated cases, however, may eventually spread to the overlying brain by way of retrograde infectious thrombophlebitis.

Cerebritis and Abscess

Cerebritis is an area of acute inflammation in the brain parenchyma which is poorly defined. Though there is an increased permeability of the local blood vessels, there is no neovascularity or angiogenesis. If untreated, cerebritis progresses to abscess formation. A pyogenic brain abscess is a focal area of parenchymal infection containing pus in the center and vascularized collagenous capsule in the periphery.[27]

Brain abscesses can occur by direct extension or hematogenous route. A contiguous focus of infection is usually the cause for a brain abscess, e.g. an abscess in the temporal lobe or cerebellum is the result of chronic otitis media.[28] Chronic sinusitis, untreated dural tears, infections

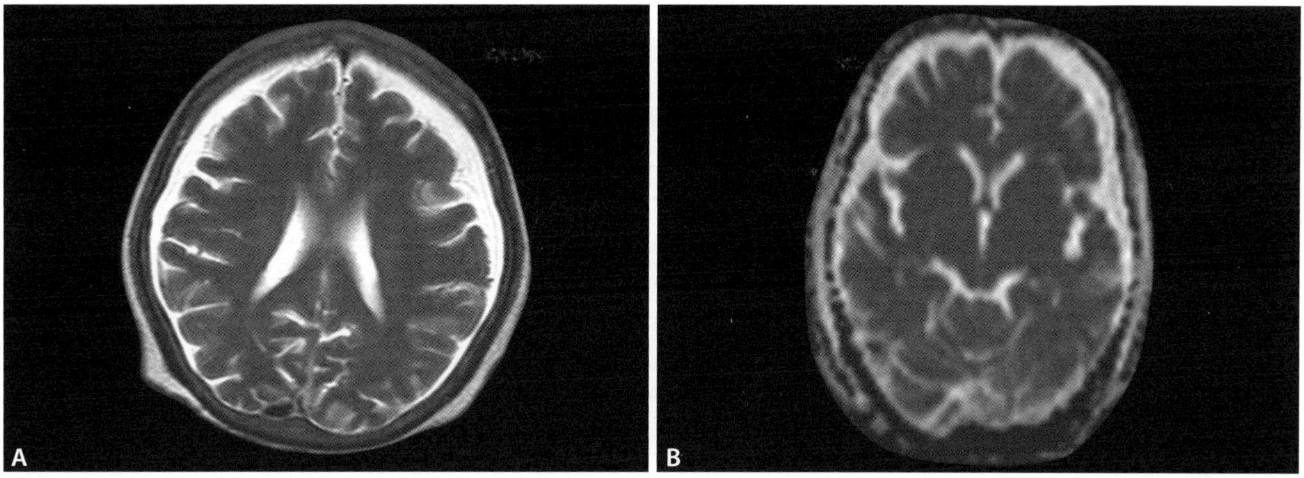

Figs. 6A and B: Axial T2W MR image (A) showing bilateral subdural effusions isointense to the CSF. Diffusion-weighted MR image (B) reveals no restricted diffusion.

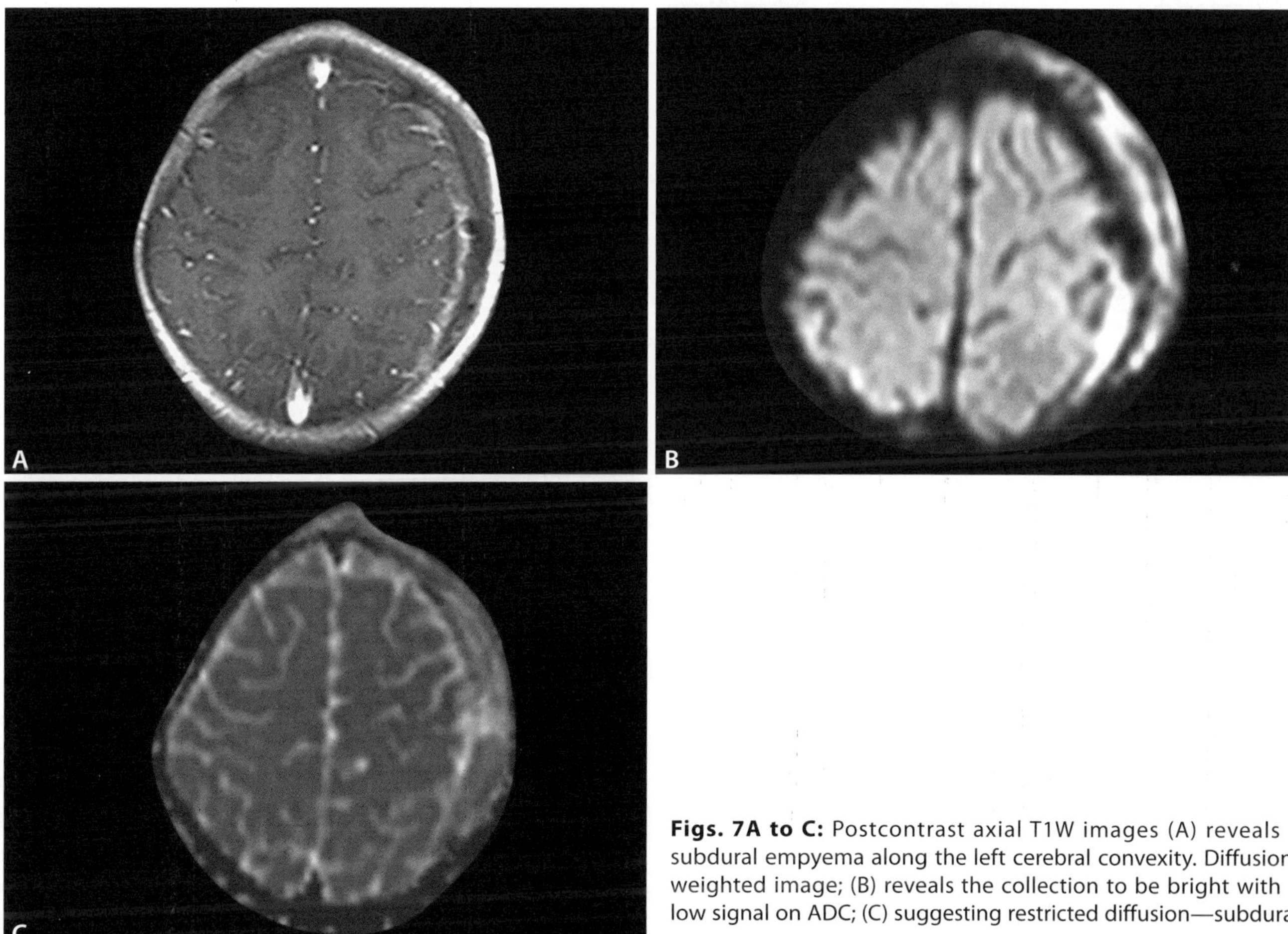

Figs. 7A to C: Postcontrast axial T1W images (A) reveals a subdural empyema along the left cerebral convexity. Diffusion-weighted image; (B) reveals the collection to be bright with a low signal on ADC; (C) suggesting restricted diffusion—subdural empyema.

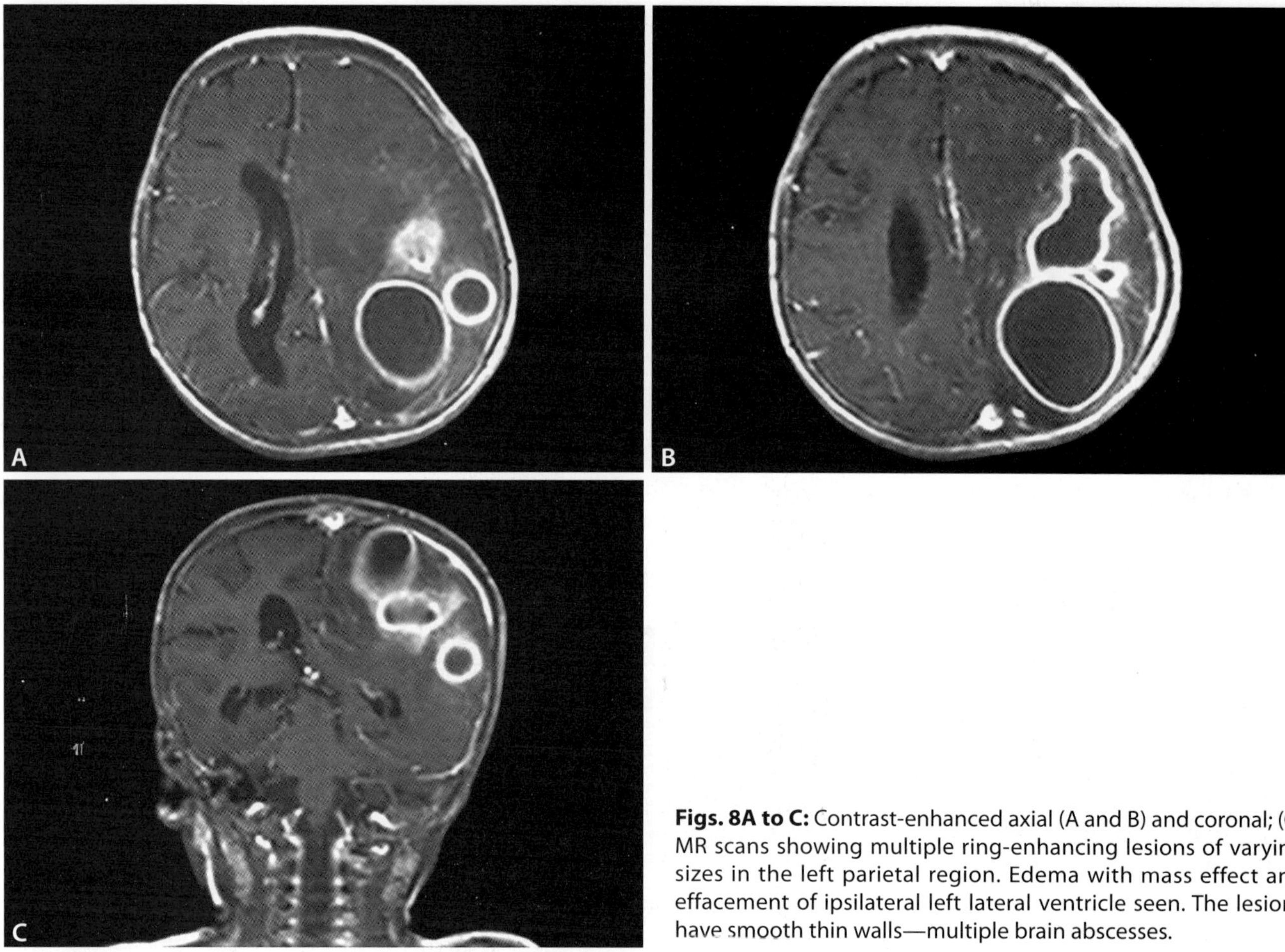

Figs. 8A to C: Contrast-enhanced axial (A and B) and coronal; (C) MR scans showing multiple ring-enhancing lesions of varying sizes in the left parietal region. Edema with mass effect and effacement of ipsilateral left lateral ventricle seen. The lesions have smooth thin walls—multiple brain abscesses.

about the face and scalp and dental sepsis constitute the other causative factors for a direct spread. Direct spread occurs through involvement of bone or via emissary veins which are valveless.

The source of a hematogenous brain abscess may be a congenital cyanotic right to left shunt or pulmonary AVM, bacterial endocarditis, pulmonary abscess or intra-abdominal infections[29] **(Figs. 8A to C)**. Hematogenous brain abscesses have a distant focus of infection and show the following features:

- Multiple and multiloculated rather than solitary.
- Location at the corticomedullary junction/gray white matter junction.
- Poor encapsulation.
- Distribution along the middle cerebral artery (MCA)
- High mortality.

About 30% of brain abscesses are reported to be cryptogenic. Brain abscesses may occur secondary to trauma and neurosurgery. Diabetes mellitus, intravenous drug abuse, alcoholism, immunosuppression are the other predisposing factors. In infants and children, congenital malformations, such as meningomyelocele, encephalocele, ectodermal defects are the usual predisposing factors.

The evolution from cerebritis to abscess formation is a continuum. Four stages are involved—the stages of early cerebritis, late cerebritis, early capsule and late capsule formation.[30] In the first 4–5 days, that is, the early cerebritis stage, the organism grows within the parenchyma. The neutrophils migrate to the involved region to destroy the bacteria and edema occurs due to the opening of the blood brain barrier **(Figs. 9A to C)**. Punctate foci of hemorrhage may occur during this stage. Coalescence of the small areas of necrosis to produce a large necrotic focus results in the late cerebritis stage which is seen 7–10 days later. Satellite lesions surrounding the main abscess are seen during this stage. Development of a fibrous capsule to wall off the infection constitutes the early capsule stage which occurs 10–14 days later. Fibroblasts forming the collagenous capsule, liquefaction of central necrotic area and persistence of edema characterize this early capsule

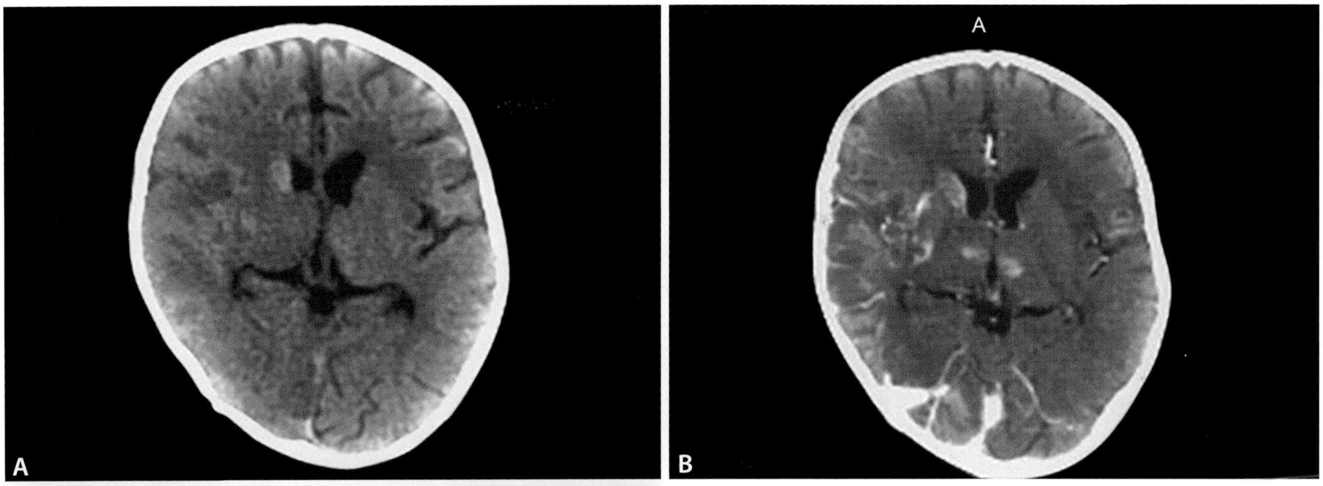

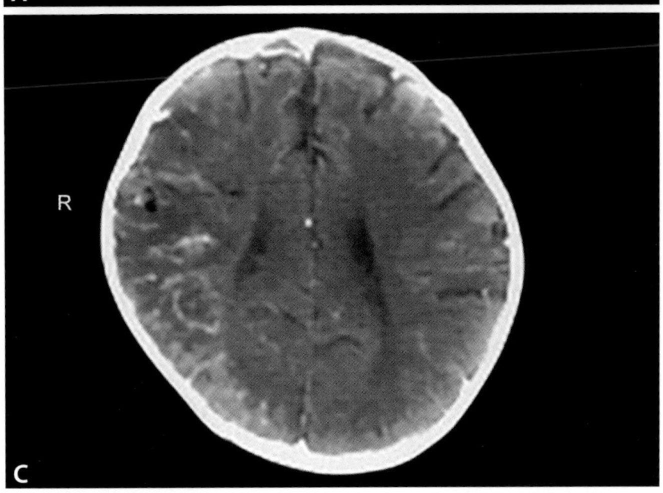

Figs. 9A to C: Noncontrast axial scan of the cranium (A) showing an ill-defined hypodensity in the right parietal region with evidence of postcontrast gyriform enhancement; (B and C)— cerebritis.

stage.[31] In the late capsule stage (>14 days) a gliotic reaction develops at the outer margin of the abscess and there is a decrease in the surrounding edema. It might take 2 weeks to several months for cerebritis to progress to a mature abscess depending on the host's immune response, virulence of the organism and several other factors.

Imaging

In the early stages of cerebritis, a localized hypoattenuation may be seen on a noncontrast CT with variable enhancement on the postcontrast scans. If enhancement is present it is nodular or ring like. When a capsule forms, a round or ovoid area of low density with ring enhancement is seen. The necrotic center of a mature abscess typically shows a low signal on T1 and high signal on T2-weighted MR images while the abscess capsule is typically low signal on the T2-weighted images[32] **(Figs. 10A to F)**. The various constituents of the capsular rim- like collagen, the paramagnetic free radicals produced by the actively phagocytosing macrophages and hemorrhage—account for its marked hypointensity on T2-weighted images. On postcontrast scans enhancement of the capsular rim occurs. The ring enhancement is usually thin and smooth measuring less than 5 mm in thickness. A poorer vascular supply of the white matter as compared to the grey matter of the brain accounts for the thinner medial/ventricular margin of the abscess cavity which may rupture with resultant daughter abscesses in the white matter or ventricle. Daughter abscesses are seen as smaller ring enhancing lesions adjacent to the parent abscess **(Figs. 11A and B)**. Vasogenic edema surrounding the abscess cavity is seen as a surrounding hypointensity on a T1 and hyperintensity on T2W images. Mass effect may be seen **(Figs. 12A and B)**.

Differentiation of a brain abscess from a necrotic neoplasm on imaging can be achieved by the fact that an abscess has a thin, smooth enhancing rim while a neoplasm has an irregular, nodular wall **(Figs. 13A to C)**. The collagen capsule being less developed on

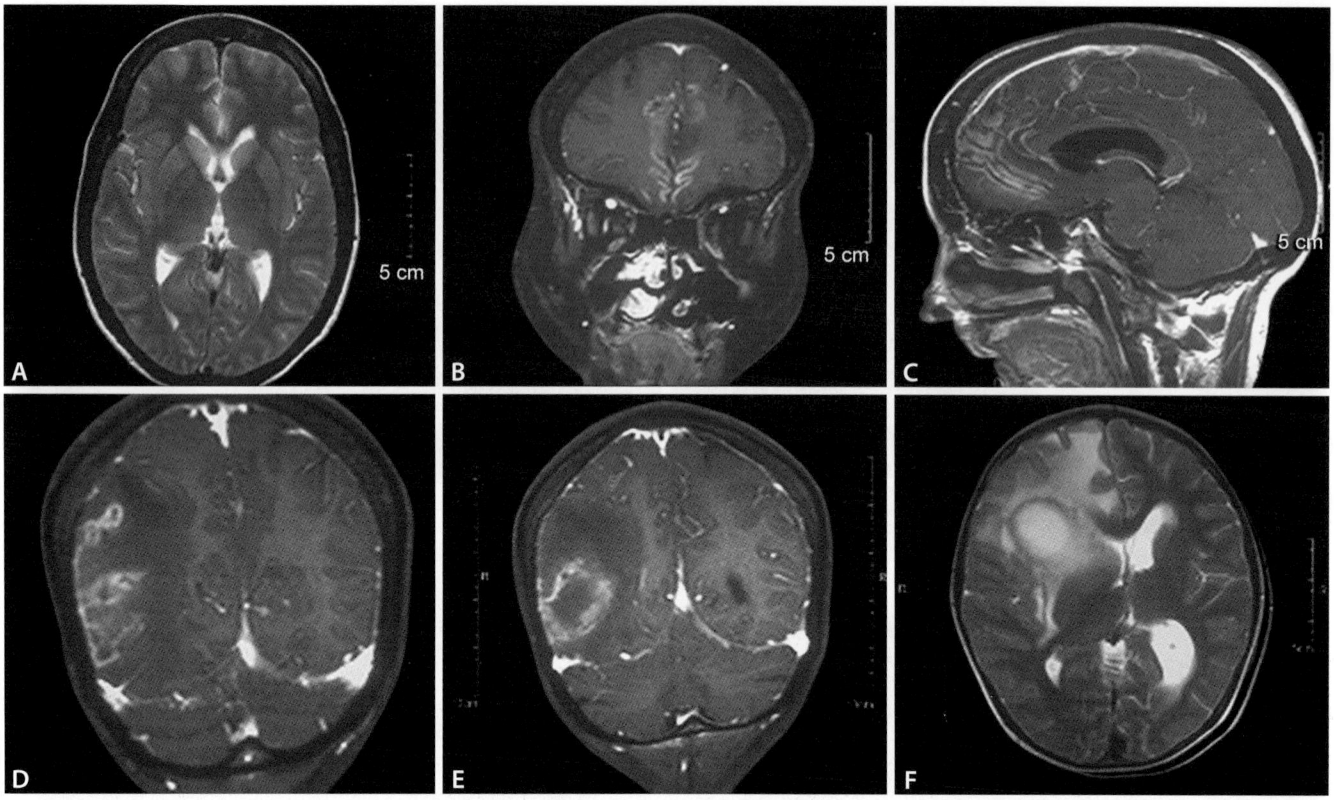

Figs. 10A to F: Axial T2W MR image (A) reveals an ill-defined hyperintense signal in the right parietal region. Postcontrast images; (B to D) reveal an irregular gyriform enhancement in the adjacent brain parenchyma—early cerebritis stage. MR image; (E) shows walling of the infection in the late cerebritis stage. Axial T2W MR image; (F) shows the stage of abscess formation with a hyperintense center and a hypointense rim of the collagenous capsule.

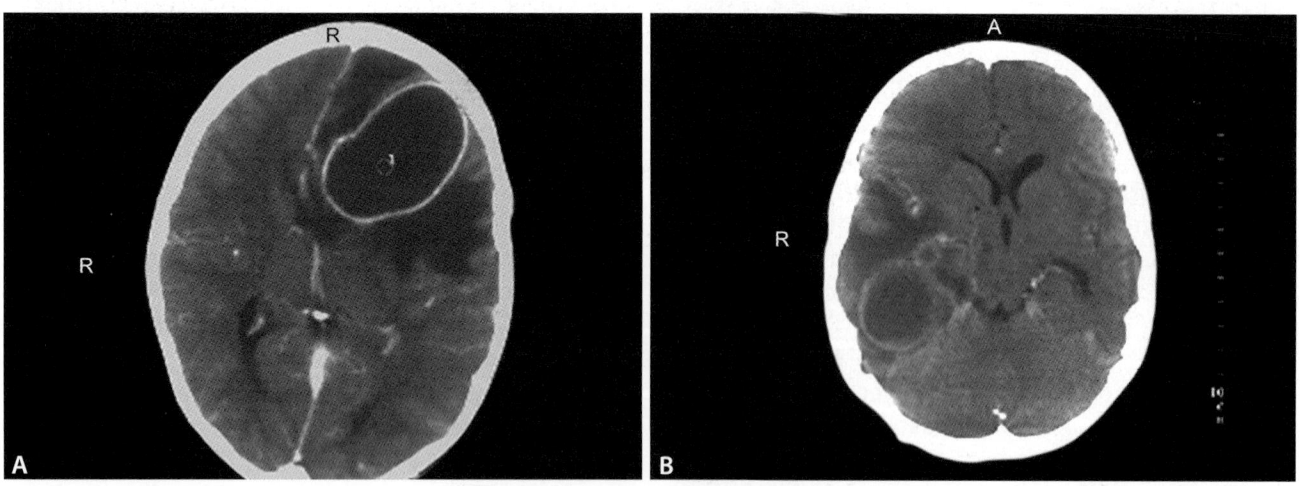

Figs. 11A and B: CECT axial scans of the cranium showing a large ring-enhancing lesion with smooth thin walls in a left parafalcine location with extensive vasogenic edema causing effacement of the ipsilateral frontal horn and midline shift to the contralateral side. Adjacent smaller enhancing rings are also seen in another case—brain abscess with daughter abscesses.

the medial/ventricular side of an abscess, presence of daughter abscesses, presence of extra-axial collections, ependymal/meningeal enhancement are features that help differentiate an abscess from a necrotic neoplasm.[33]

MR spectroscopy reveals various amino acid peaks like succinate (at 2.4 ppm), leucine, isoleucine, valine (at 0.85 ppm), glycine (3.5 ppm), alanine (at 1.5 ppm) in case of pyogenic brain abscess. Metabolites like acetate

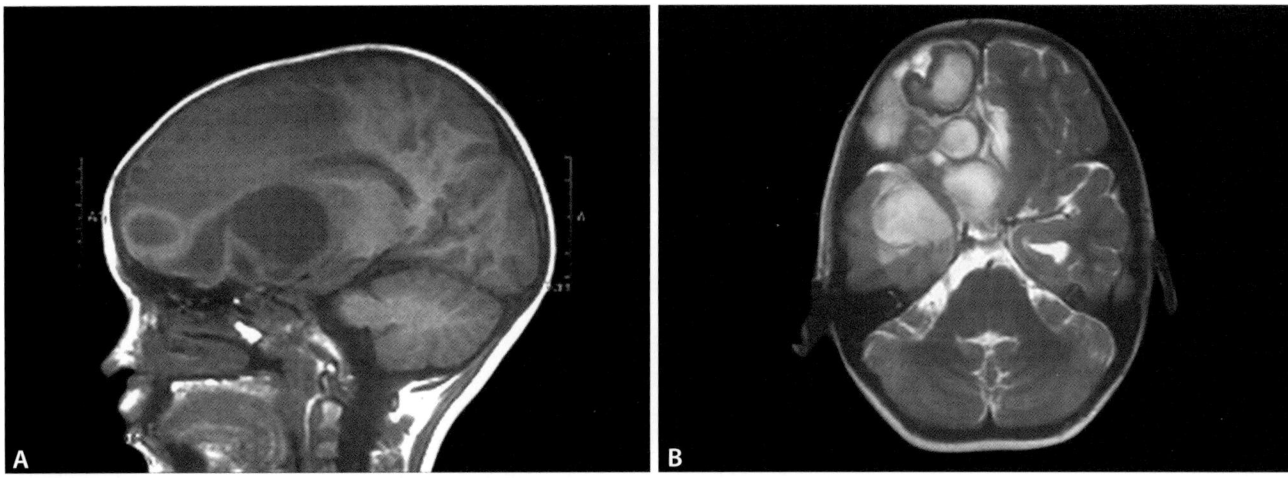

Figs. 12A and B: T1W sagittal (A) and T2W axial; (B) MR images showing multiple lesions having a hypointense center on T1 and hyperintense center on T2W images with perilesional edema. The collagenous capsule of the lesions is iso to slightly hyperintense on T1 and hypointense on T2W images. Mass effect on the ipsilateral ventricular system with dilatation of the contralateral temporal horn is seen—multiple brain abscesses.

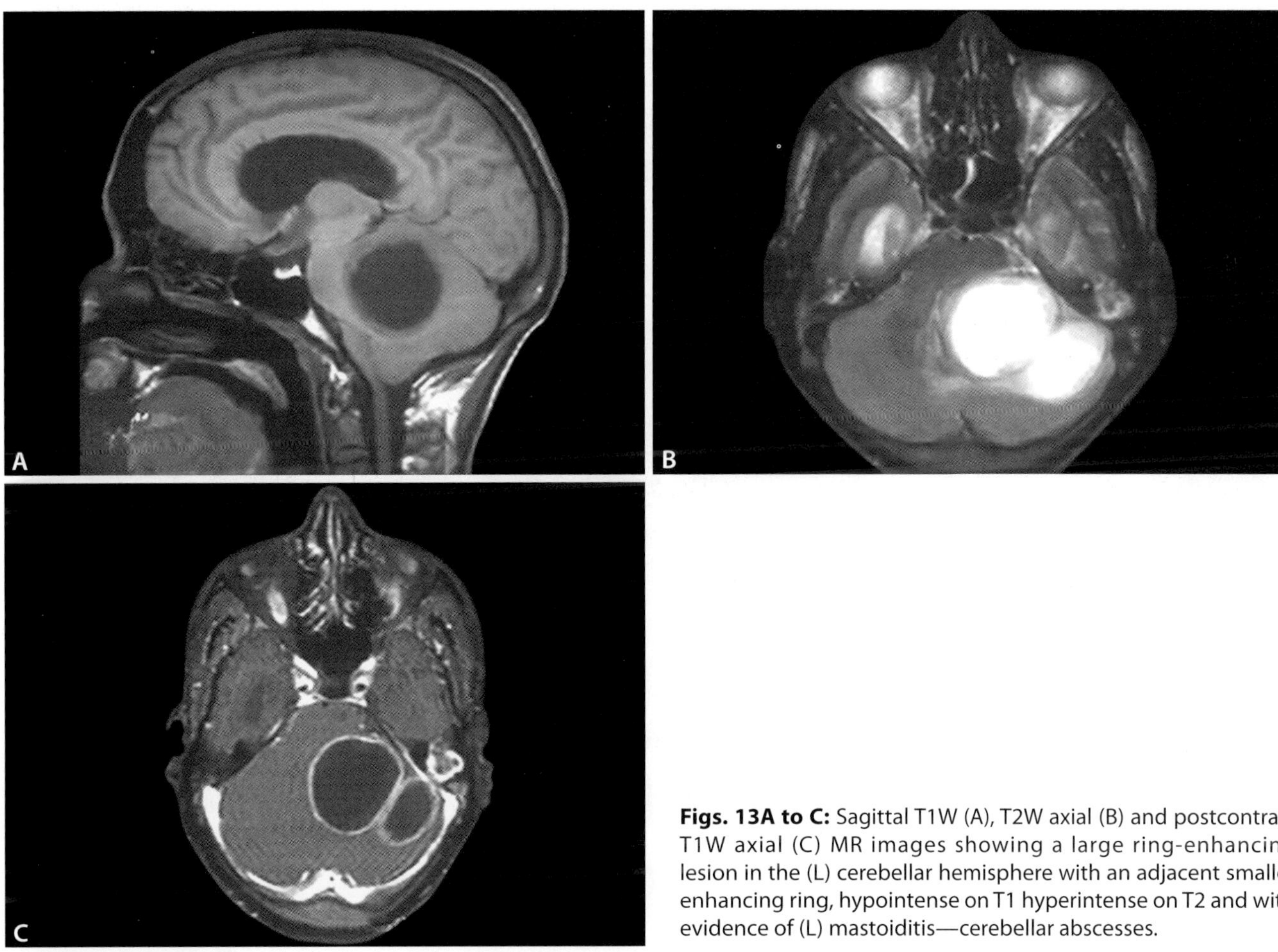

Figs. 13A to C: Sagittal T1W (A), T2W axial (B) and postcontrast T1W axial (C) MR images showing a large ring-enhancing lesion in the (L) cerebellar hemisphere with an adjacent smaller enhancing ring, hypointense on T1 hyperintense on T2 and with evidence of (L) mastoiditis—cerebellar abscesses.

and succinate are of bacterial origin while others result due to death and degeneration of inflammatory cells and exudate.[34,35] A large amount of proteolytic enzymes are produced by the dead and degenerating inflammatory cells that degrade the proteins to free amino acids. Lactate/lipid peak may be seen in an abscess at 1.3 ppm owing to anaerobic glycolysis. The presence of amino acid peak is considered specific of an abscess and is not seen in a cystic neoplasm.[36]

On diffusion-weighted MR images, the high cellularity and viscosity of pus in an abscess impedes water mobility resulting in a restricted pattern of diffusion with consequent low ADC values.[37] Low ADC values are not observed in cystic necrotic tumors helping in the differentiation of an abscess from cystic neoplasm[38] **(Figs. 14A to D)**. The reported sensitivity of diffusion-weighted imaging in differentiating an abscess from other pathologies is 72–95% while the specificity ranges from 96–100%.[39]

On diffusion tensor imaging (DTI), brain abscess cavity shows regions of increased fractional anisotropy (FA) and low mean diffusivity (Dav) while cystic tumours and neurocysticercosis shows low fractional anisotropy (FA) and high diffusivity (Dav).[40] Dynamic susceptibility contrast perfusion MRI can also help to distinguish an abscess from a neoplasm as an abscess has lower rCBV values compared to a neoplasm. The lower rCBV values are attributed to the presence of mature collagen and decreased neovascularity in an abscess as compared to a neoplasm.[41]

Multiple Brain Abscesses Secondary to Septic Emboli

The causes for septic emboli include cyanotic heart disease, intravenous drug abuse, bacterial endocarditis, etc **(Figs. 15A to C)**. Small septic emboli may lead to occlusion of small arteries and arterioles while the larger

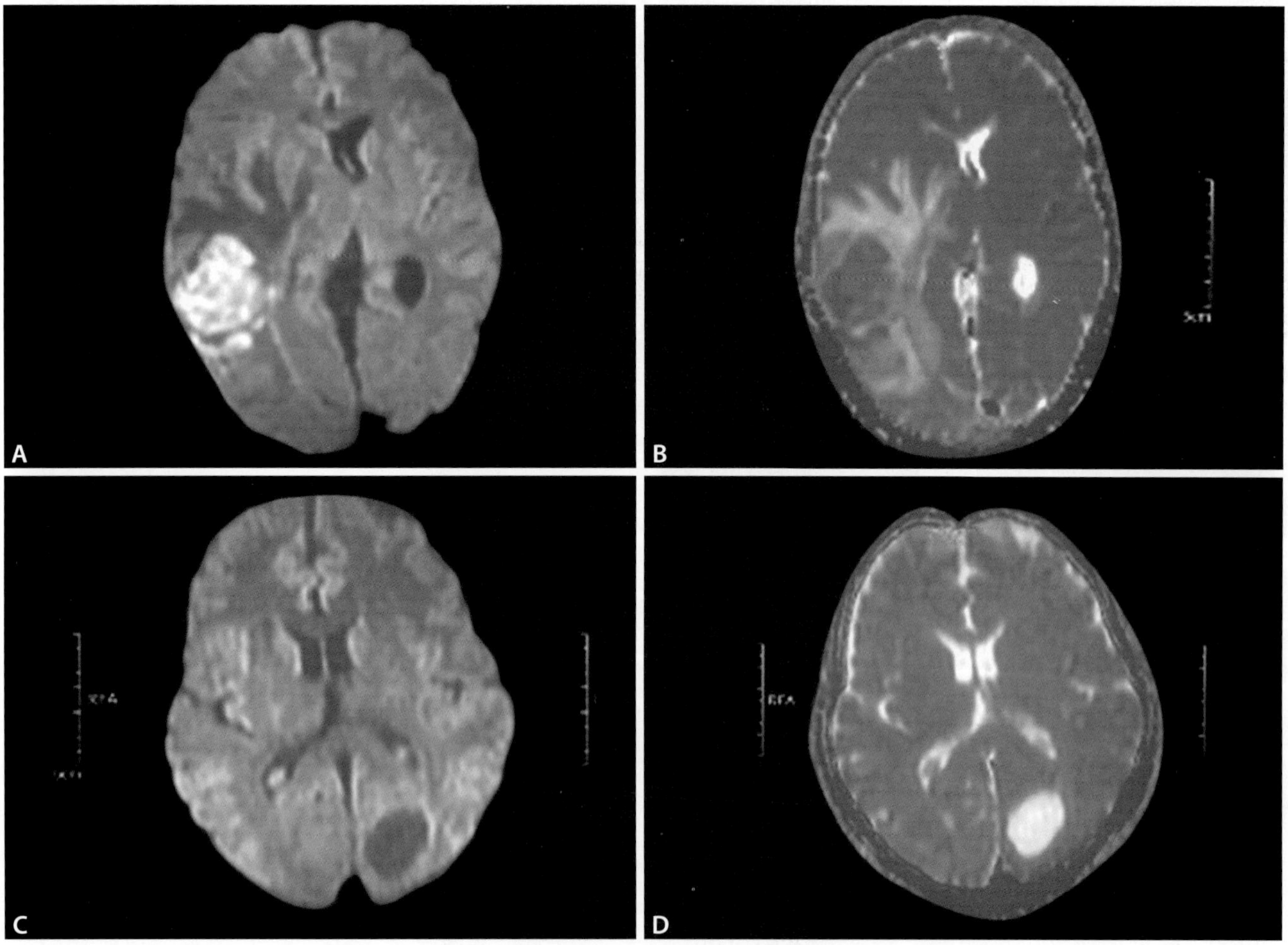

Figs. 14A to D: Bright signal on diffusion-weighted images b-1000 (A) and low signal on ADC map; (B) seen in a cerebral abscess while low signal seen on DW images; (C) and high signal on ADC map; (D) seen in a necrotic neoplasm.

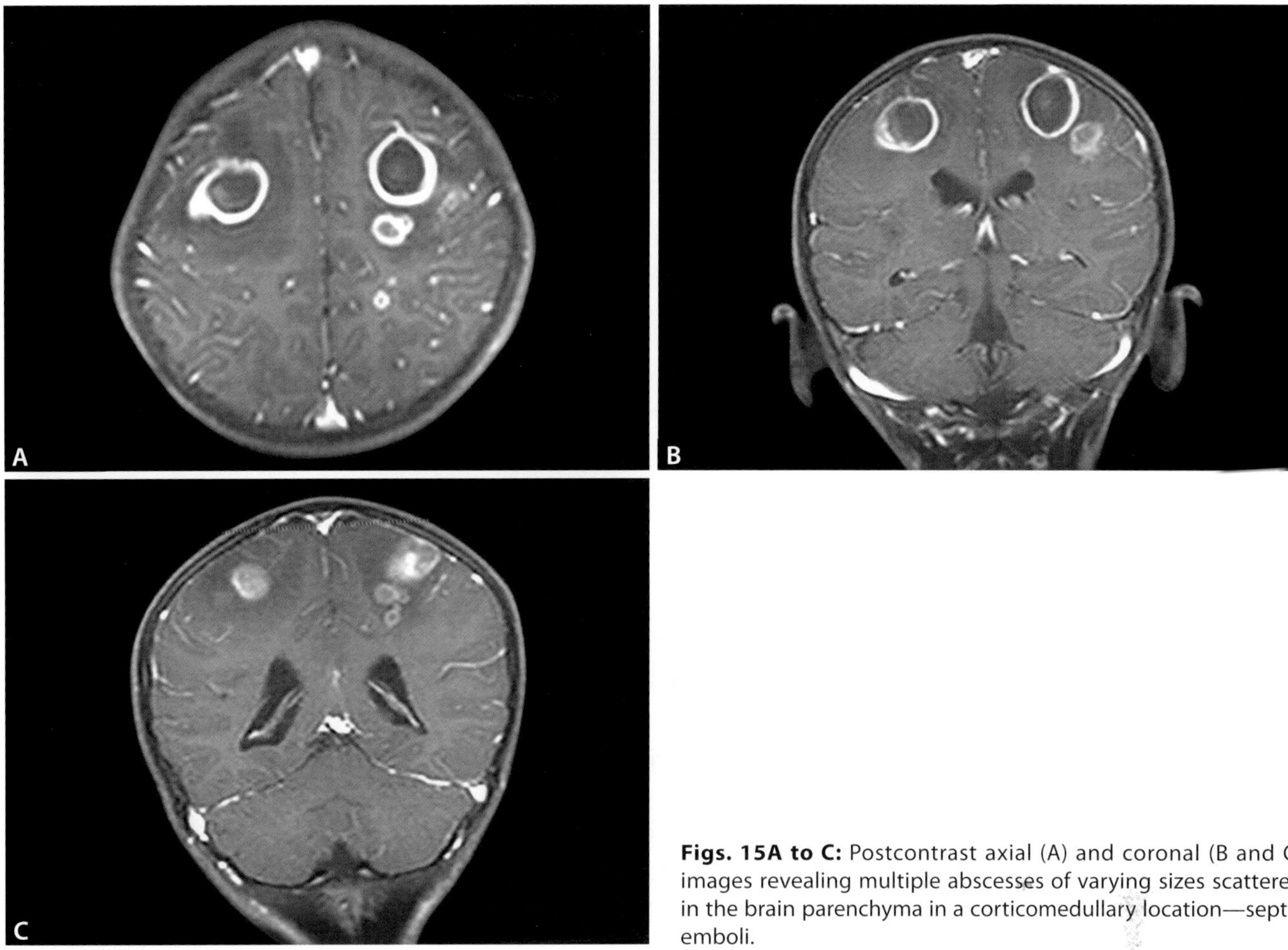

Figs. 15A to C: Postcontrast axial (A) and coronal (B and C) images revealing multiple abscesses of varying sizes scattered in the brain parenchyma in a corticomedullary location—septic emboli.

ones may cause hemispheric infarction **(Figs. 16A to D)**. Mycotic aneurysms usually involve peripheral branches of intermediate to small cerebral arteries. The presence of parenchymal and subarachnoid bleed in a patient of abscess/infection should suggest mycotic aneurysm which should be ruled out on MR angiography.[33]

Central Nervous System Infarction

Central nervous system infarction associated with meningitis occurs because of inflammation-induced arterial spasm or because of direct inflammation of the walls of arteries and arterioles resulting in an infectious arteritis. Most infarcts occur in the basal ganglia secondary to involvement of the penetrating lenticulostriate arteries. Large arterial branch occlusions seen in some instances can result in cortical infarction. Cortical veins or dural venous sinuses may also be involved with resultant venous thrombosis and venous infarction of involved central nervous system tissues.[42,43] Venous infarcts are usually bilateral and multiple, involve non arterial territories and tend to occur in the convexities. Areas of hemorrhage are seen in about 25% of cases. On angiography, the spectrum of cerebrovascular changes associated with advanced cases of meningitis and arteritis include:[42,44]

1. Narrowing and spasm of the major arteries at the base of the brain, such as the supraclinoid portion of the internal carotid artery and the A1 and M1 segments of the anterior and middle cerebral arteries.
2. Irregularities or focal aneurysmal dilatations of medium-sized cerebral arteries.
3. Occlusions of the distal branches of the middle cerebral artery with or without retrograde flow.
4. Focal, abnormal parenchymal (i.e. gyral) blush.
5. Marked prolongation of circulation time.
6. Early venous filling.
7. Thrombosis of cortical veins, dural venous sinus or both.

Cranial Nerve Involvement

This occurs due to direct inflammation of the nerve or pressure caused on the nerve by the exudates with

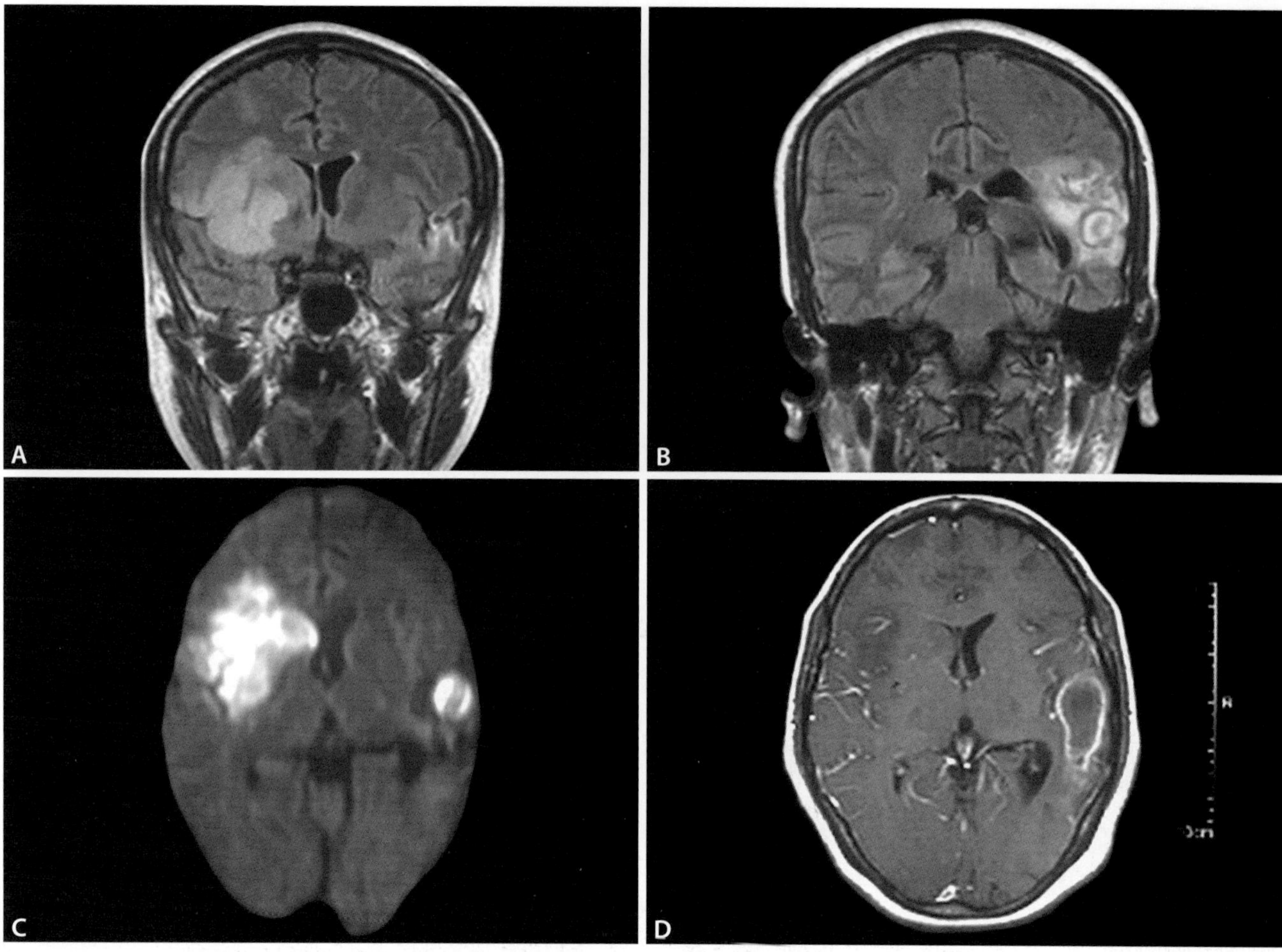

Figs. 16A to D: FLAIR coronal (A and B), diffusion-weighted (C) and postcontrast T1W axial (D) MR images showing an area of signal alteration in the distribution of the right MCA territory showing a restricted pattern of diffusion suggestive of infarct. Another lesion showing perilesional edema, a restricted pattern of diffusion and ring enhancement is seen in the left parietal region suggestive of an abscess—septic emboli.

resultant stretching. The commonest nerve to be involved is the VIIIth cranial nerve or vestibulocochlear nerve with hearing loss seen in about 30% cases.[5] Hearing loss is usually bilateral, permanent and *Streptococcus pneumoniae* is the commonest causative organism.[45] Other involved nerves include the facial, oculomotor and the optic nerve. Transient palsies of the optic and abducens nerves may be seen due to raised intracranial pressure.

Ventriculitis

Involvement of the cerebral ependyma leads to ventriculitis. Rupture of a parenchymal abscess into the ventricular system, ventricular catheter placement or meningitis may all cause ventriculitis. Cranial sonography is a useful imaging modality for the diagnosis of ventriculitis. Ventricular dilatation, irregular and echogenic ependyma, intraventricular debris are the common findings seen. Intraventricular adhesions and septae seen in about 10% of patients with meningitis are better picked up on sonography than CT. CT and MR may reveal ventricular dilatation, intraventricular debris and periventricular edema seen as hyperintense signal along the ventricular margin on T2W images. Entrapment of portions of ventricles may occur due to adhesions and septae which may result in segmental dilatation. On contrast administration there is diffuse enhancement of the ventricular margin **(Figs. 17A and B)**. Another finding associated with ventriculitis is choroid plexitis. A swollen choroid plexus with ill-defined margins and enhancement on contrast administration constitute the imaging findings[46] **(Figs. 18A and B)**. No calcifications are seen in cases of ventriculitis resulting from pyogenic meningitis unlike those from viral infection. Diffusion weighted images reveal presence of restricted diffusion in the intraventricular debris.

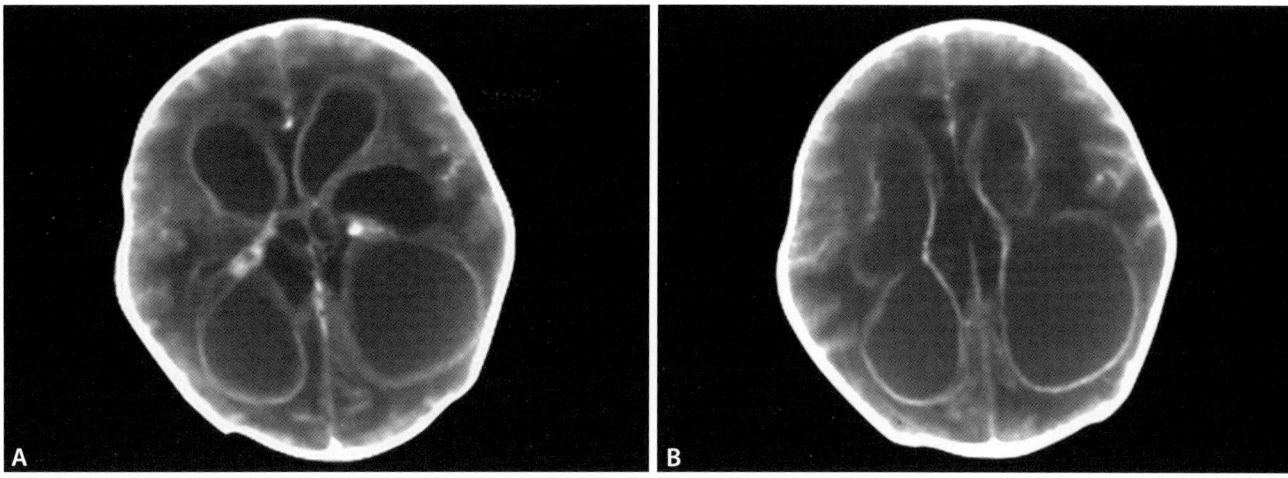

Figs. 17A and B: CECT axial scans of the cranium showing massive dilatation of the ventricular system with transependymal edema with diffuse enhancement along the ventricular walls—ventriculitis.

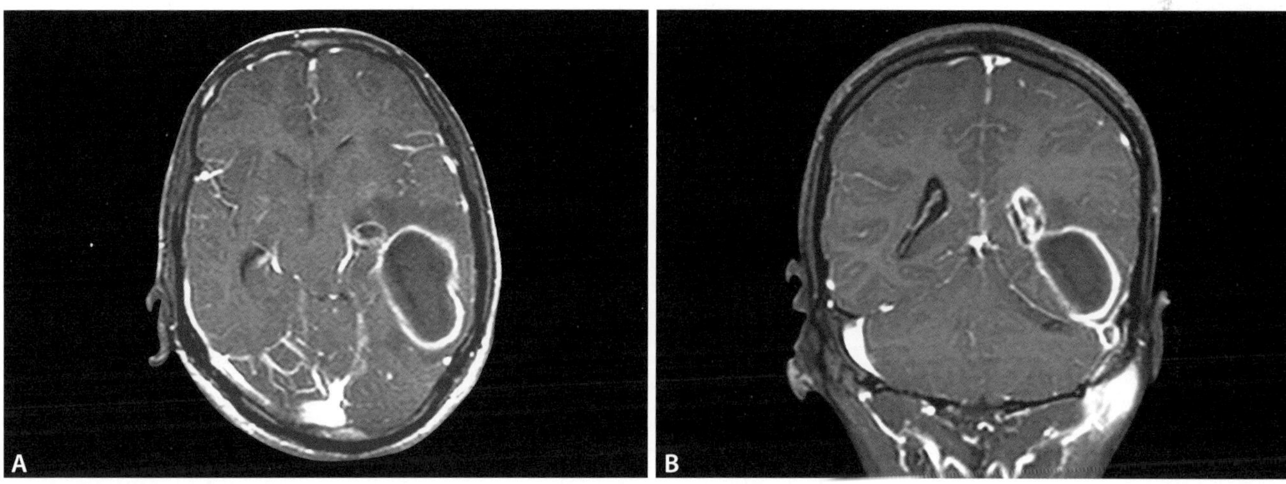

Figs. 18A and B: Contrast enhanced axial (A) and coronal; (B) MR images revealing a large brain abscess in the left parieto-occipital region with enhancing choroid plexus of the left lateral ventricle s/o choroid plexitis. Note is also made of sigmoid sinus thrombosis of the left side and an abscess in the neck (B).

Recurrent Meningitis

Recurrence is seen in about 16% cases of meningitis, the commonest cause is an occult cerebrospinal fluid leak or fistula and the commonest causative organisms include streptococci and gram-negative bacilli[47] **(Figs. 19A to C)**.

GRANULOMATOUS INFECTION

TUBERCULOSIS

The causative organism is *Mycobacterium tuberculosis* which is a slowly dividing facultative intracellular pathogen that has plagued mankind for thousands of years and continues to be the cause of 1.7 million of deaths per year. About 9 million cases of TB are reported every year.[48] The unique feature of this organism to hide and divide in the macrophages (doubling time 15–20 hours) poses a diagnostic challenge and makes administration of therapeutic regimens difficult and time consuming. This is further complicated by the emergence of HIV infection, AIDS and by the multidrug resistant variety. About 5–10% of all patients with tuberculosis and up to 20% of patients with AIDS related tuberculosis have CNS involvement.[49,50]

Pathogenesis

A two step model for the pathogenesis of CNS TB includes: 1. The bacteria reach the oxygen rich CNS via the hematogenous route from a distant focus, e.g. in lungs to establish a subpial or subependymal focus of infection called

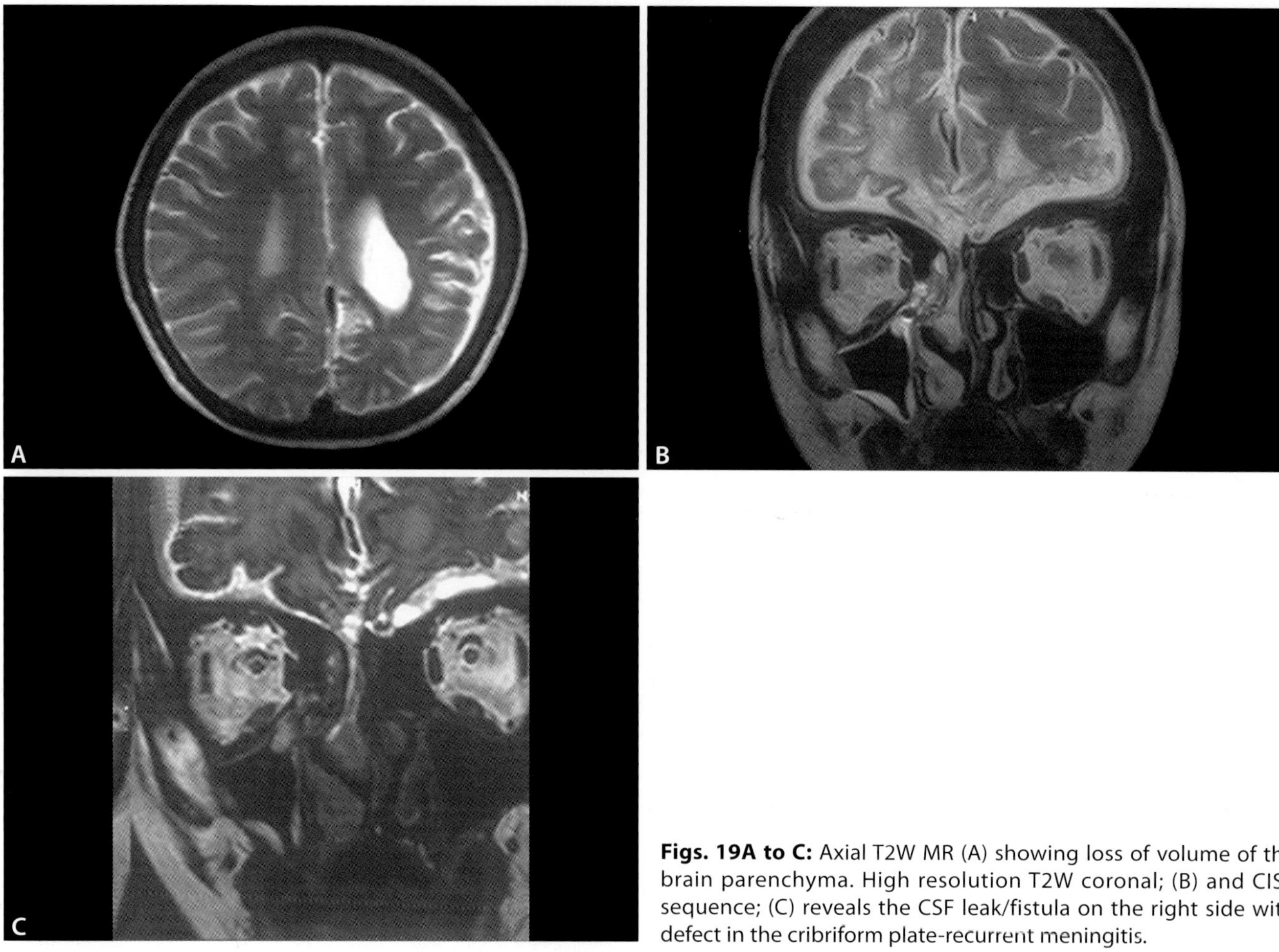

Figs. 19A to C: Axial T2W MR (A) showing loss of volume of the brain parenchyma. High resolution T2W coronal; (B) and CISS sequence; (C) reveals the CSF leak/fistula on the right side with defect in the cribriform plate-recurrent meningitis.

the "Rich" focus.[51] 2. The Rich focus may rupture into the subarachnoid space or into the ventricular system leading to meningitis.[52] The basal spaces are filled with gelatinous exudates containing chronic inflammatory cells, fibrin and hemorrhage.[53] An initial nonspecific inflammatory response (tuberculous cerebritis) may occur in the beginning. This may then result in granuloma formation. A tuberculous focus may develop into a tuberculoma or abscess in the absence of adequate host immunity.

Tuberculous Meningitis (TBM)

Meningeal tuberculosis is the most common presentation of CNS TB and is seen most frequently in children and adolescents. Children are most vulnerable and more frequently affected by TBM due to their poor immune response to contain bacteria within the lungs. The infection disseminates hematogenously from a distant focal point and the meningeal involvement usually occurs due to rupture of the Rich focus in the subarachnoid space. The primary subpial exudate from the discharging Rich focus is located in the inferomedial surface of the frontal, the anteromedial surface of the temporal lobes, the superior aspect of the cerebellum and the floor of the fourth ventricle. From these sites it disseminates to the interpeduncular cisterns enveloping the optic nerves at the optic chiasma and to the anterior part of the pontomesencephalic cisterns, the ambient cisterns, the suprasellar cisterns and onto the Sylvian fissures. In the later stages, the leptomeningeal process extends to the convexities and to the ependymal surfaces of the ventricles. Within the lateral ventricles, a similar exudate often covers the choroid plexus resulting in choroid plexitis. The exudates surround meningeal and cortical blood vessels inciting inflammation and vasculitis, obstruction of the CSF pathways and obliterative endarteritis leading to infarction.[54]

Clinical Manifestations

Malaise, lassitude, low-grade fever and intermittent headache characterize the insidious prodrome of tuberculous meningitis. The most common clinical manifestation occurs with fever, headache, nausea, vomiting, photophobia and neck stiffness. Cranial nerve palsies of third, fourth and sixth nerves are common. Meningismus, confusion and long tract signs can accelerate into seizures, hemiparesis, hemiplegia, stupor and coma. Cerebrospinal fluid analysis demonstrates lymphocytosis, increased protein levels and decreased glucose level. Identification of *M. tuberculosis* in cerebrospinal fluid by acid-fast methods is achieved in 90% of cases, however, a negative result does not preclude treatment, if there is strong clinical or radiologic evidence of tuberculous disease.

Imaging

Non contrast CT may show obliteration of the basal cisterns by isoattenuating or hyperattenuating exudates. Plaque-like dural thickening may be seen. On contrast administration basal cisternal enhancement is seen **(Figs. 20A and B)**. The objective criteria for abnormal basal enhancement in TBM include:[55]

1. *Contrast filling the cisterns*: The CSF spaces that surround the normal vascular enhancement are obliterated by the contrast medium.
2. *Linear enhancement*: A linear enhancement that is seen in more than two contiguous slices is abnormal as the MCA is too small to be seen in its full horizontal length in more than one slice or as a continuous line.
3. *Double and triple lines*: Two or three lines seen represent enhancement of meninges along the middle cerebral artery.
4. *Y sign*: Pure vessel enhancement is never seen as a Y while meningeal enhancement at the junction of the suprasellar and middle cerebral artery cistern produces the Y.
5. *Ill-defined edge*: The normal vessels always show a sharply marginated enhancement while meningeal enhancement is ill-defined.
6. *Infundibular recess of third ventricle*: No vessel lies in the region and any enhancement along the posterior aspect of the infundibular recess of the 3rd ventricle in suprasellar cistern is abnormal and meningeal.
7. *Join the dots sign*: Vessels in the Sylvian sulcus are seen as separate dots on cross-section. When the dots are joined by linear enhancement it is abnormal.
8. *Nodular enhancement*: Normal meningeal enhancement is smooth and sharply marginated so nodular enhancement is always abnormal.
9. *Asymmetry*: Asymmetry aids recognition of abnormal basal enhancement.

Basal exudative meningitis may extend to the convexities, Sylvian fissures and the tentorium. The Sylvian fissures is a very common site of involvement by tuberculous meningitis.[56] Hydrocephalus may be seen in 45–87% of patients at the time of diagnosis and indicates a poor prognosis.[57,58] Ependymitis may be seen as linear enhancement along the ventricular margin. Infarction is demonstrated on CT as areas of hypoattenuation with loss of gray white matter differentiation. The triad of basal meningeal enhancement, hydrocephalus and infarct increases the specificity of the diagnosis of TBM.

Owing to its multiplanar imaging capability, greater soft tissue contrast and lack of bone artifacts, gadolinium enhanced MR is superior to CT in the detection of meningeal disease and associated parenchymal abnormalities.[59,60] Characteristic thick or nodular enhancement in

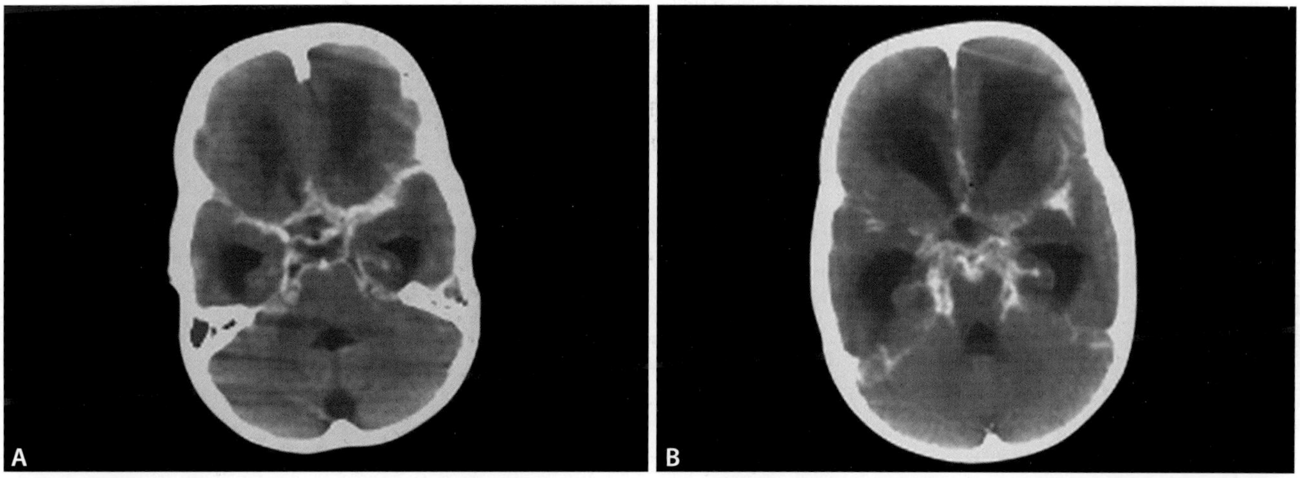

Figs. 20A and B: CECT axial scans of the cranium showing dense meningeal enhancement along the basal cisterns, tentorium and the Sylvian cisterns with evidence of hydrocephalus and periventricular ooze—tubercular meningitis.

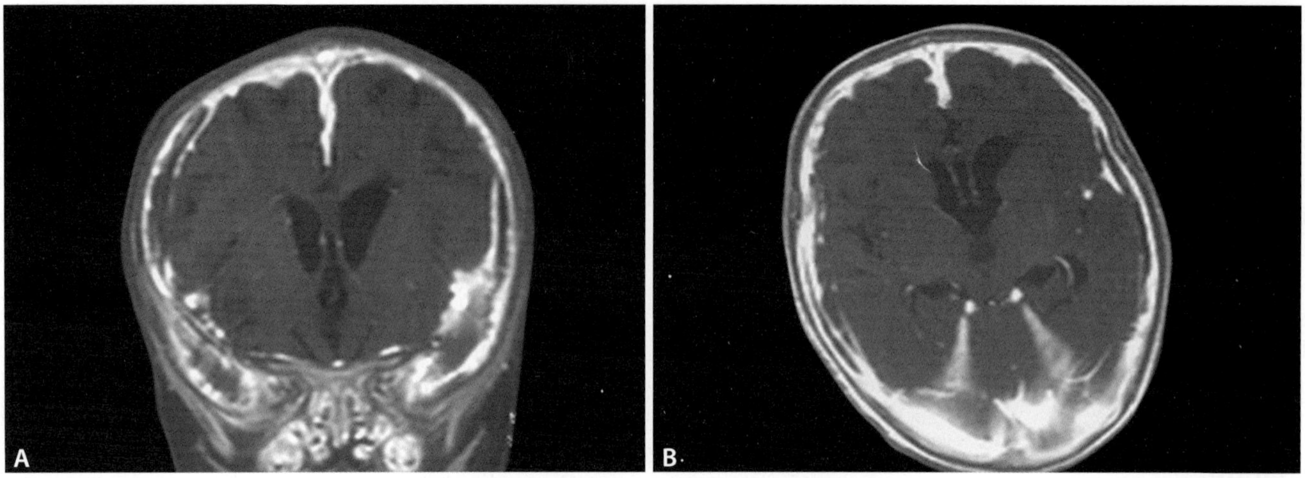

Figs. 21A and B: Postcontrast T1W axial (A) and coronal (B) MR images showing diffuse meningeal enhancement along the cerebral convexities, tentorium and the basal cisterns with hydrocephalus—tubercular meningitis.

the basal cisterns is seen in TBM **(Figs. 21A and B)**. Recent advances in neuroimaging of tubercular meningitis.

Magnetization Transfer (MT)

The quantification of MT ratio (MTR) helps in predicting the cause of meningitis. It has been used to differentiate TBM from other causes of meningitis. The abnormal meninges show a hyperintense signal on the precontrast T1 weighted MT images and enhance further on the post contrast T1-weighted MT images. The MTR of the meninges in TBM is lower than that of fungal and pyogenic meningitis but higher than that in viral meningitis.[61] The visibility of the meninges on a pre contrast MT image and low MTR is diagnostic of TBM and differentiates it from other causes of meningitis. It is the high lipid content of the tuberculous bacilli that accounts for the low MTR in TBM.

Ex Vivo Protein MR Spectroscopy

High resolution ex vivo MRS of CSF has shown presence of lactate, acetate, and sugars along with signals from cyclopropyl rings (–0.5 to + 0.5 ppm) and phenolic glycolipids (7.1 and 7.4 ppm) in tubercular meningitis. These metabolites have not been observed with pyogenic meningitis.[33]

COMPLICATIONS OF TUBERCULAR MENINGITIS

Hydrocephalus, cranial neuropathies, focal infarction, focal atrophy and syringobulbia are the complications associated with tubercular meningitis.

Hydrocephalus

Communicating hydrocephalus is more common in tuberculous meningitis than the obstructive type.[62,63] The exudates become thick, adhesive, gelatinous and fibrotic blocking the basal cisterns and CSF circulation and resorption with resultant hydrocephalus. A focal parenchymal lesion may cause mass effect on the cerebral aqueduct or the fourth ventricular foramina causing obstructive variety of hydrocephalus.[64] There may be entrapment of the ventricle by granulomatous ependymitis. A complex type of hydrocephalus can be seen in TB with a combination of communicating (defective absorption) and non-communicating (obstructive) hydrocephalus. It is important to determine the site and type of obstruction because of impending cerebral herniation in case of obstruction and also to determine the optimum treatment option. CSF flow studies done on MR imaging provide qualitative and quantitative information of CSF flow, which help in differentiating the type of hydrocephalus and provides information about the CSF dynamics.

Vasculitis

Intracranial vasculitis, which occurs as a complication of tuberculous meningitis, causes neurological deficits in these patients. In can occur due to a direct invasion of the vessel by the microorganism or extension of adjacent arachnoiditis. It is usually the small arteries or veins that are involved which undergo fibrinoid degeneration resulting in spasm or thrombosis of vessels leading to bland or hemorrhagic infarction. The most commonly involved regions are the basal ganglia, thalamus and internal capsule due to the involvement of the small

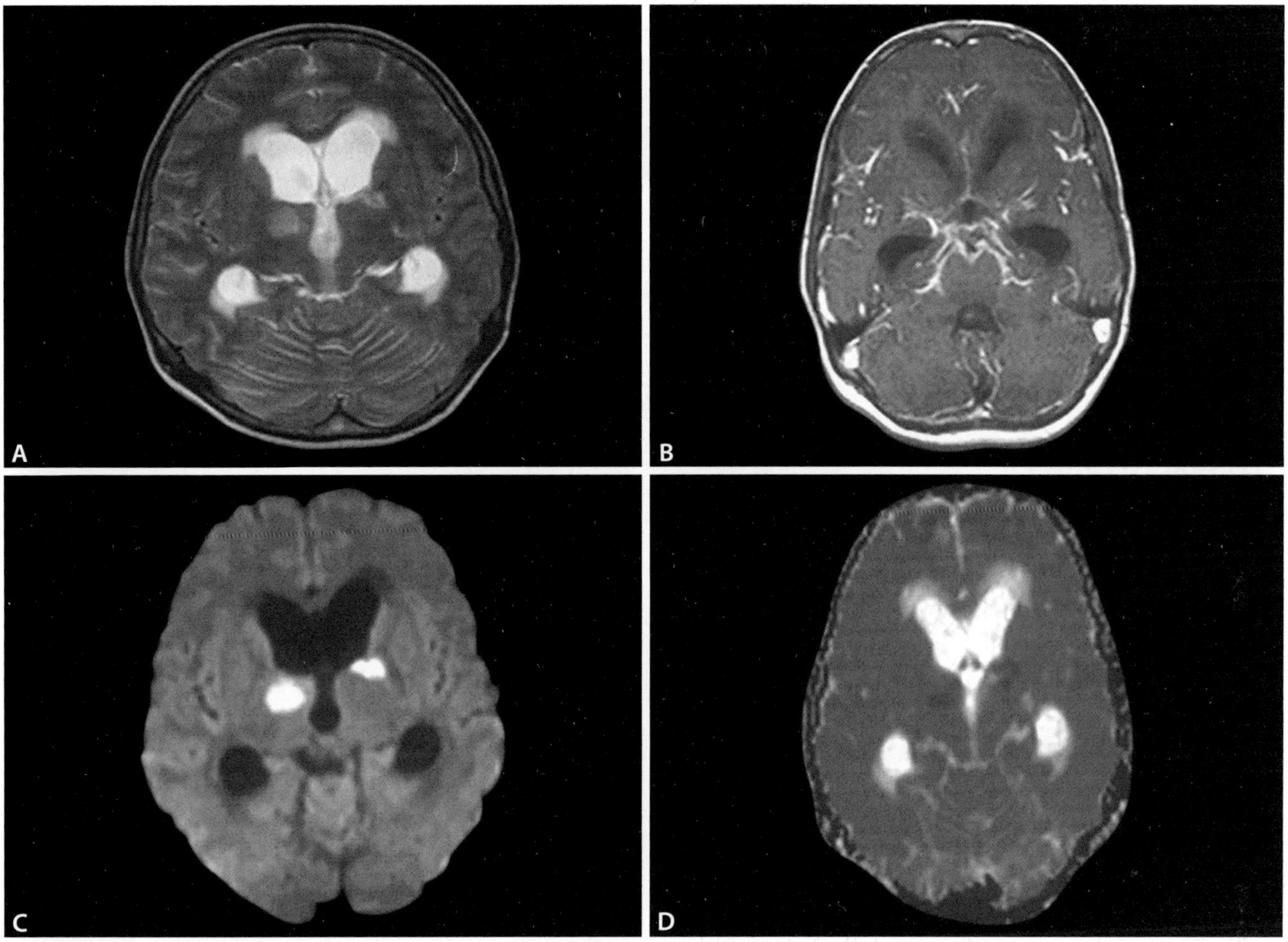

Figs. 22A to D: T2W axial (A), T1W postgadolinium axial; (B) diffusion-weighted; (C) and ADC; (D) MR images showing basal cisternal enhancement with hydrocephalus and periventricular ooze suggestive of tubercular meningitis. Areas of signal alteration noted in bilateral basal ganglia showing hyperintense signal on T2W images and increasing hyperintensity on b1000 with hypointensity on ADC maps—bilateral basal ganglia infarcts (vasculitis) in tubercular meningitis.

perforating branches supplying these regions, particularly the lentriculostriate and thalamoperforating arteries.[65] These vessels perfuse the so called "medial tuberculous zone". Vasculitic infarcts are usually bilateral in nature **(Figs. 22A to D)**.

CT shows these vasculitic infarcts as hypoattenuating areas while MR images show them as areas of hyperintense signal with a restricted pattern of diffusion on DW MR images.

Cranial Neuropathies

They can occur in 17–40% of patients with CNS TB.[66] The II, III, IV, VI and VII nerves are the most commonly affected cranial nerves in tuberculous meningitis. A vascular compromise may result in ischaemia of the nerve or there may be nerve entrapment caused by the exudates.[67] A direct mass effect on the nerve within the subarachnoid space by a tuberculoma or direct involvement of the cranial nerve nuclei in the brain may be the other causative factors. A permanent loss of function of the nerves can be explained by the fibrotic changes that occur in the late stage. Contrast enhancement may be seen at entry/exit zone of the involved nerve suggesting its involvement. The entire nerve may be thickened and show enhancement.[68] Neuritis/perineuritis may improve with treatment while palsies due to involvement of brainstem nuclei usually do not, hence localization of the cause of cranial nerve involvement is important as it helps in prognostication.

TUBERCULAR PACHYMENINGITIS

Tubercular pachymeningitis can be focal or diffuse. The focal form is known as tuberculoma en plaque and it may mimic other dural based masses like meningioma. On imaging it is hyperdense on non-contrast CT, isointense to brain on T1W image, hypo to isointense on T2W images and shows homogenous enhancement with contrast administration.[69] In the setting of TB elsewhere in the body and a pachymeningeal abnormality, this form should be suspected as it responds well to antitubercular treatment.

PARENCHYMAL TUBERCULOSIS

Parenchymal form of tuberculosis includes tuberculomas, miliary TB, abscess, TB encephalopathy and focal tubercular cerebritis.

TUBERCULOMAS

These usually occur secondary to an infective focus elsewhere in the body and are more common in the pediatric age group than adults. Tuberculomas may occur anywhere in the cerebral hemispheres in the basal ganglia, brainstem or the cerebellar hemispheres. The location is usually corticomedullary junction or periventricular owing to a hematogenous route of dissemination.[70] Tuberculomas can be small or large in size, they can be solitary or multifocal in nature. Rare sites of tuberculomas include the cavernous sinuses, sphenoid sinus, sella turcica, the hypophysis and mastoid air cells.[71,72]

The CT appearance may vary from isodense to hyperdense solid enhancing lesions to ring enhancing lesions with central area of necrosis in cases of caseating granulomas **(Figs. 23A to C)**. A central area of calcification surrounded by a rim of enhancement called the 'target sign' is highly suggestive of a tuberculous infection.[73]

MR features of tuberculomas vary depending on the nature of the granuloma-whether it is non-caseating, caseating with a solid center or caseating with central liquefaction. Non caseating granuloma shows hypointense signal on T1 and hyperintense signal on T2-weighted images. On contrast administration, there is homogenous enhancement of the lesion. Caseating granulomas with a solid centre appear hypointense on T1 and markedly hypointense on T2-weighted images. These granulomas are highly cellular, the compressed glial tissue and

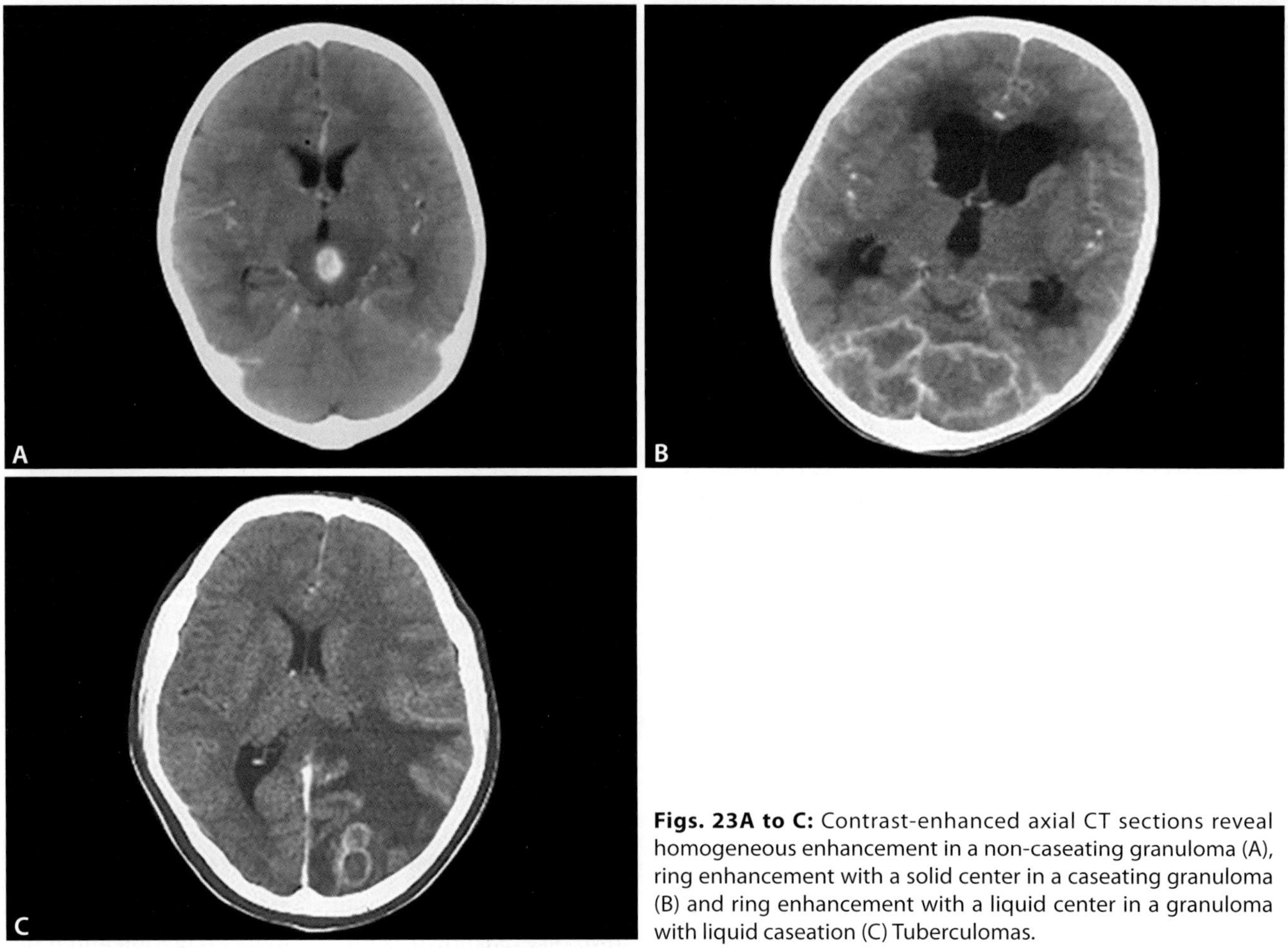

Figs. 23A to C: Contrast-enhanced axial CT sections reveal homogeneous enhancement in a non-caseating granuloma (A), ring enhancement with a solid center in a caseating granuloma (B) and ring enhancement with a liquid center in a granuloma with liquid caseation (C) Tuberculomas.

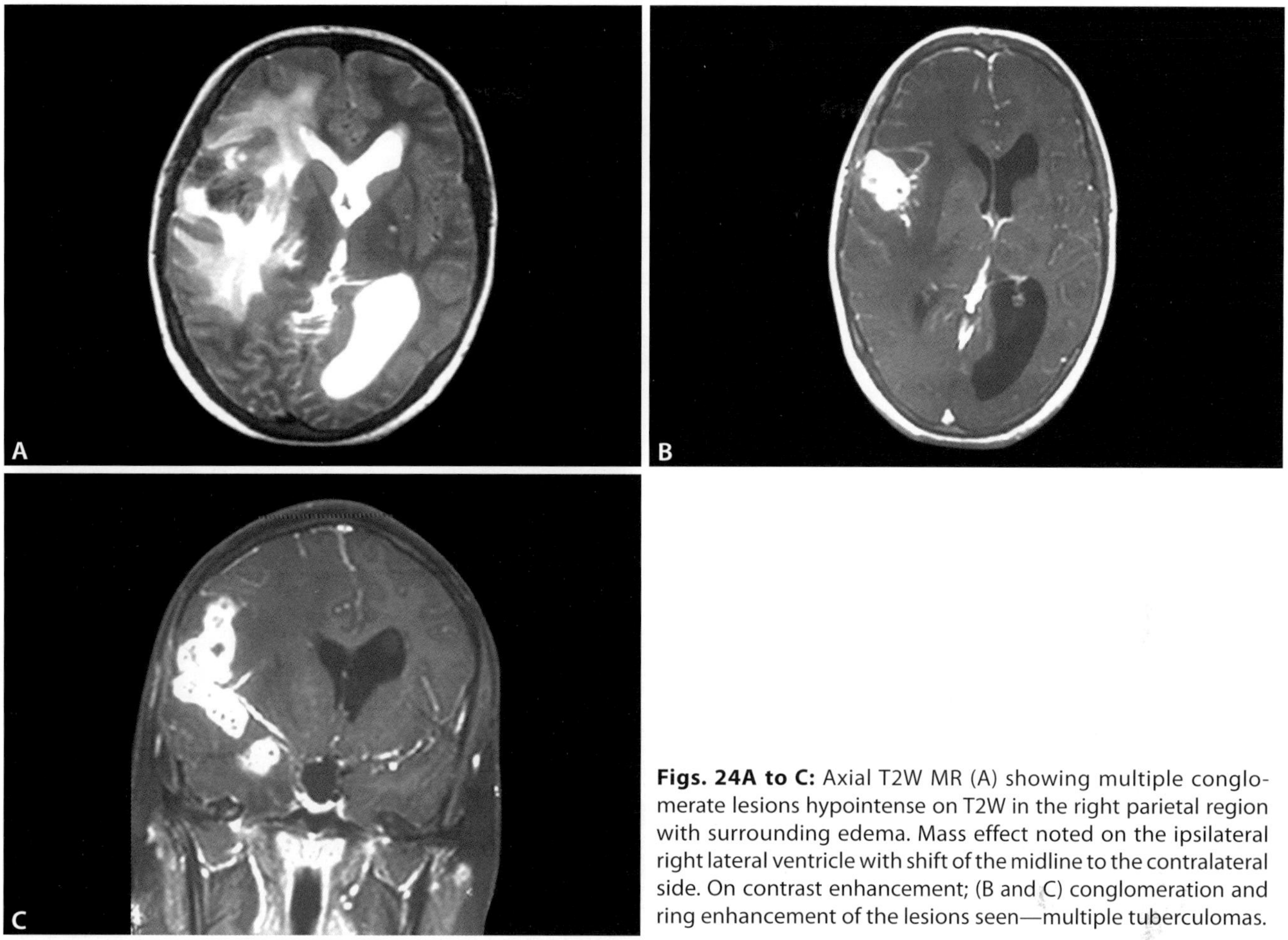

Figs. 24A to C: Axial T2W MR (A) showing multiple conglomerate lesions hypointense on T2W in the right parietal region with surrounding edema. Mass effect noted on the ipsilateral right lateral ventricle with shift of the midline to the contralateral side. On contrast enhancement; (B and C) conglomeration and ring enhancement of the lesions seen—multiple tuberculomas.

granulation tissue in the central core accounting for the cellular density and the marked hypointensity[74] **(Figs. 24A to C)**. Granulomas with central liquefaction show a peripheral hypointense rim on T2 weighted images. The low signal intensity of the capsule is due to the collagen content. Extensive edema and mass effect can be seen around the granuloma specially in the early stages of formation. Rim enhancement on postcontrast images is typically seen[75] **(Figs. 25 and 26)**.

MT Imaging

Precontrast MT T1-weighted images detect the tuberculomas better than conventional spin echo (CSE) images. Lesions which are isointense on both T1 and T2-weighted images may remain undetected and are called CSE invisible lesions. These lesions are detectable on MT images because of the lower transfer magnetization in tuberculomas as compared to the surrounding parenchyma making these lesions visible[61,76] **(Figs. 27A and B)**. Also lower MT ratios are obtained from the outer rim as compared to the inner core. The high lipid content of the tuberculomas contributes to the lower MTR of these lesions.

MR Spectroscopy

Prominent lipid peak at 0.9 and 1.3 ppm is seen in the case of tuberculomas owing to the presence of caseous material[76] **(Figs. 28A and B)**. Differentiation from metastasis and glioma can be achieved by the presence of elevated choline peak in these lesions compared to tuberculomas which show only a prominent lipid peak.

Dynamic contrast-enhanced MRI (DCE MRI) has been performed in tuberculomas and the relative cerebral blood volume rCBV has been correlated with their cellular and necrotic components.

Diffusion Tensor Imaging (DTI)

A decrease in fractional anisotropy (FA), linear anisotropy (CL) and planar anisotropy (CP) while an increase in spherical anisotropy (CS) has been reported in the case

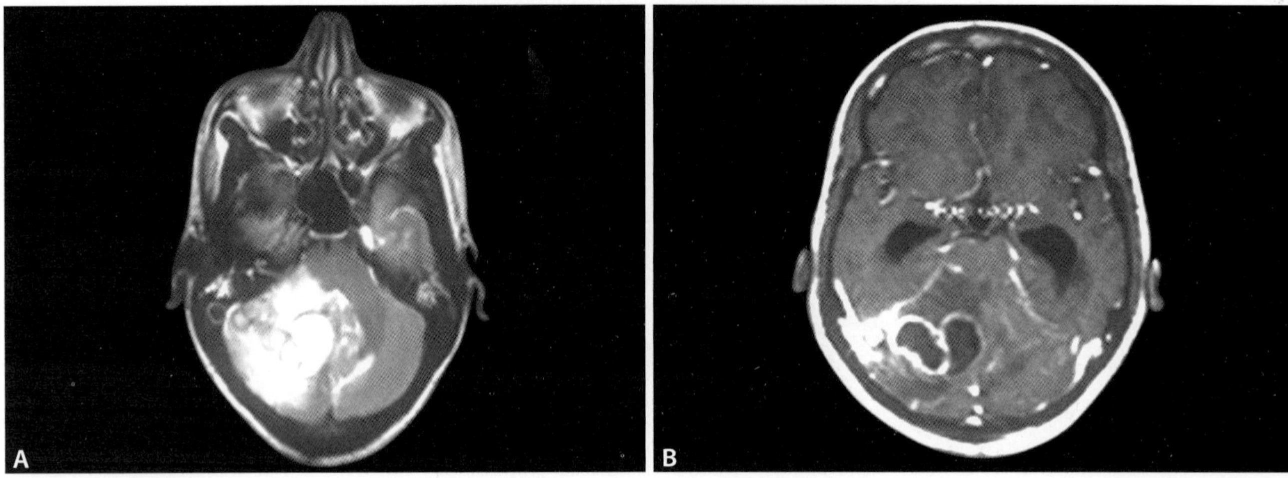

Figs. 25A and B: Axial T2W (A) and postcontrast T1W; (B) axial images showing conglomerate round lesions in the right cerebellar hemisphere with surrounding edema. There is attenuation of the fourth ventricle and obstructive hydrocephalus. The lesions show ring enhancement—tuberculomas posterior fossa.

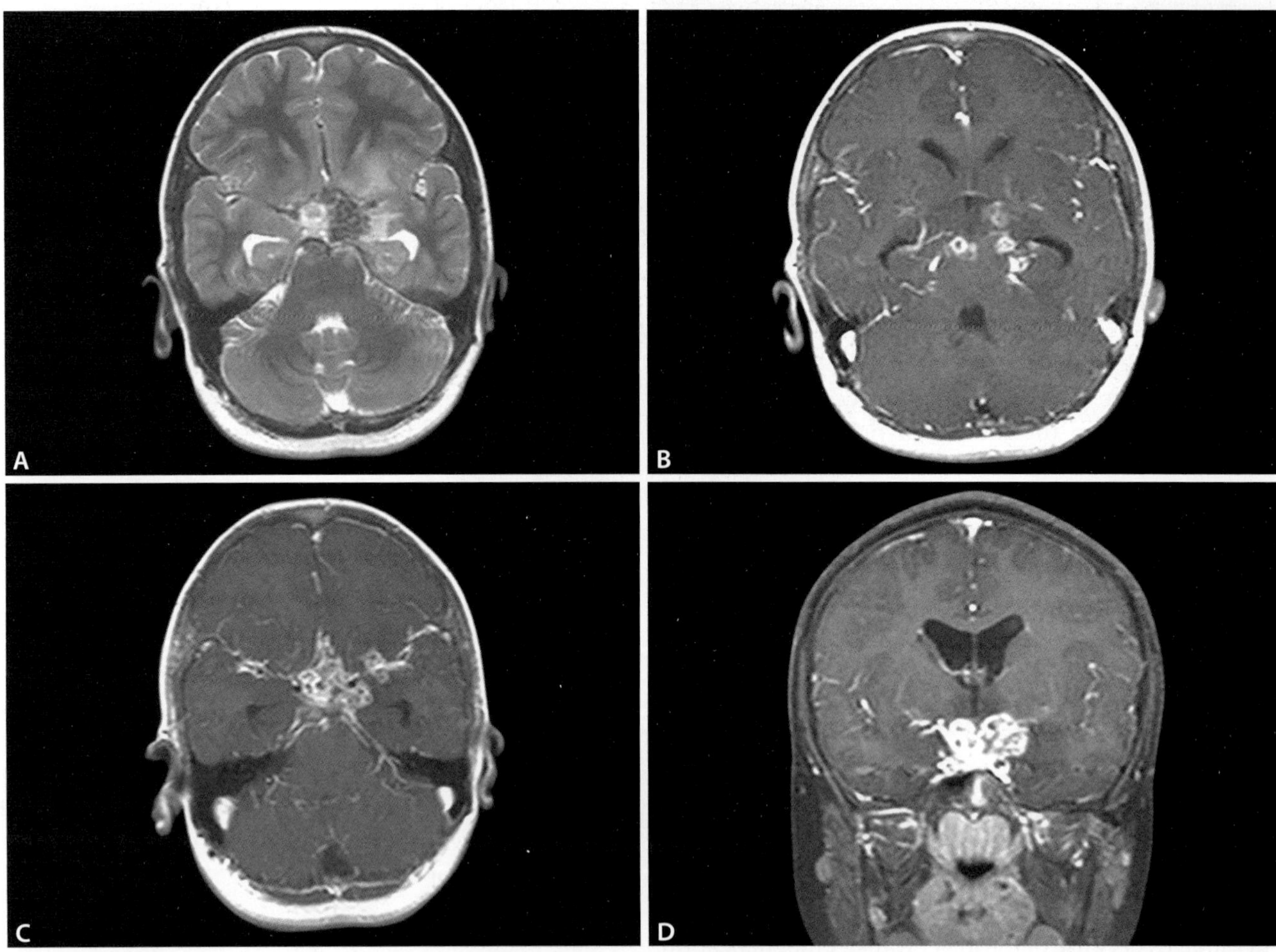

Figs. 26A to D: Axial T2W (A) and postcontrast axial; (B and C) and postcontrast coronal images; (D) reveal multiple conglomerate ring enhancing lesions in the suprasellar cisterns with encasement of the optic chiasma—multiple tuberculomas.

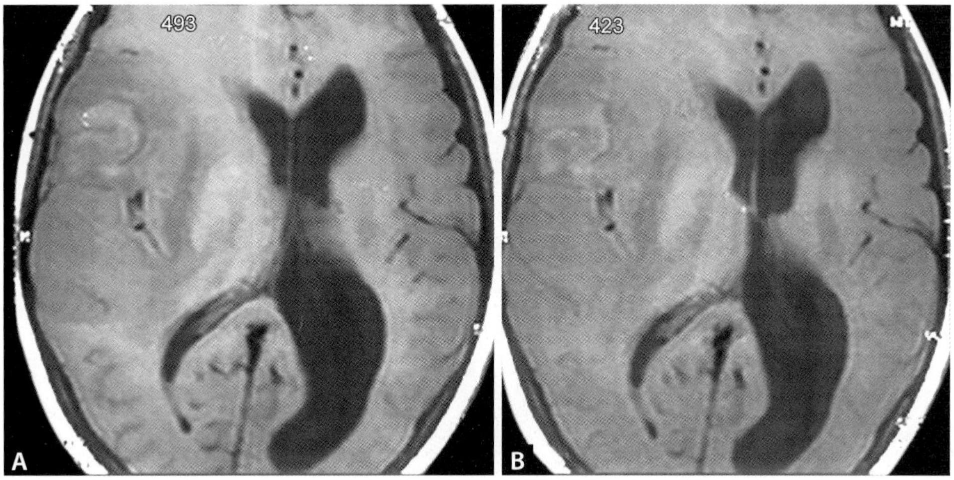

Figs. 27A and B: Values taken on axial T1W without MT (A) and with MT; (B) reveal a MT ratio of 14%—multiple tuberculomas with low MT ratio.

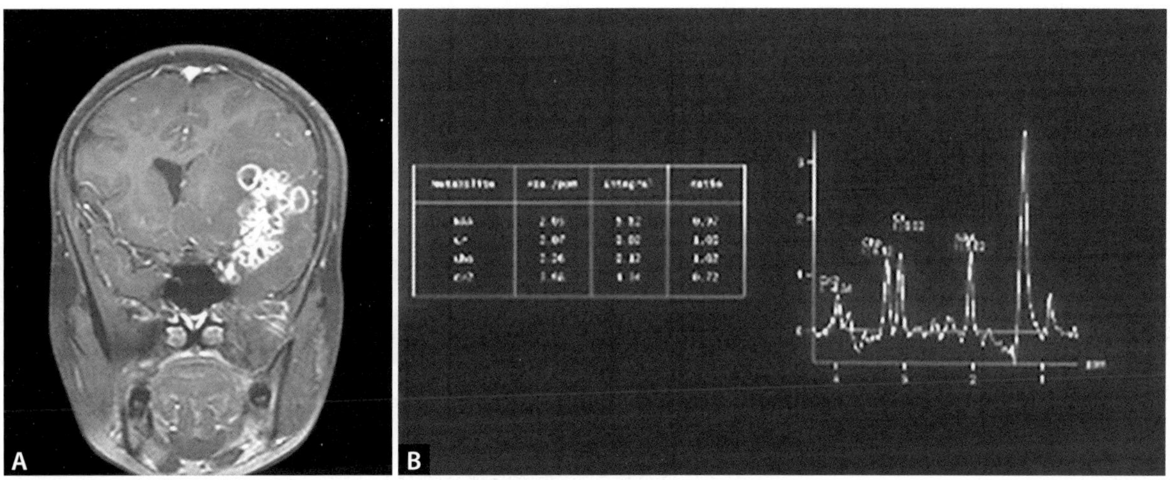

Figs. 28A and B: MR spectroscopy image (B) showing a prominent lipid peak at 1.3 ppm in the multiple conglomerate ring-enhancing lesions (A) Tuberculomas.

of tuberculomas. These parameters show an increase with antitubercular therapy and hence can be used as a means to follow-up the disease.[77]

DISSEMINATED TUBERCULOMAS (MILIARY TB)

Small granulomas (<5 mm) showing high or low signal on T2-weighted images diffusely infiltrating the brain parenchyma form the imaging pattern in disseminated disease[78] **(Figs. 29A to D)**. Gadolinium enhanced MR images which show the lesions as round areas of intense enhancement are best to depict the lesions. These lesions are clearly seen on MT T1W images and MT imaging helps to define the disease load.

TUBERCULOUS ABSCESS

A tuberculous abscess is more common in the elderly or immunocompromised patients and is often indistinguishable from a pyogenic brain abscess or a caseous tuberculoma. Presence of a purulent center rich in tubercle bacilli and absence of giant cell epitheloid granulomatous reaction in the wall distinguishes a tuberculous abscess from a granuloma. According to the Whitner criteria for tuberculous abscess, there should be macroscopic evidence of abscess formation within the brain parenchyma and the abscess wall should have vascular granulation tissue containing acute and chronic inflammatory cells and tubercle bacilli on histology.[79,80]

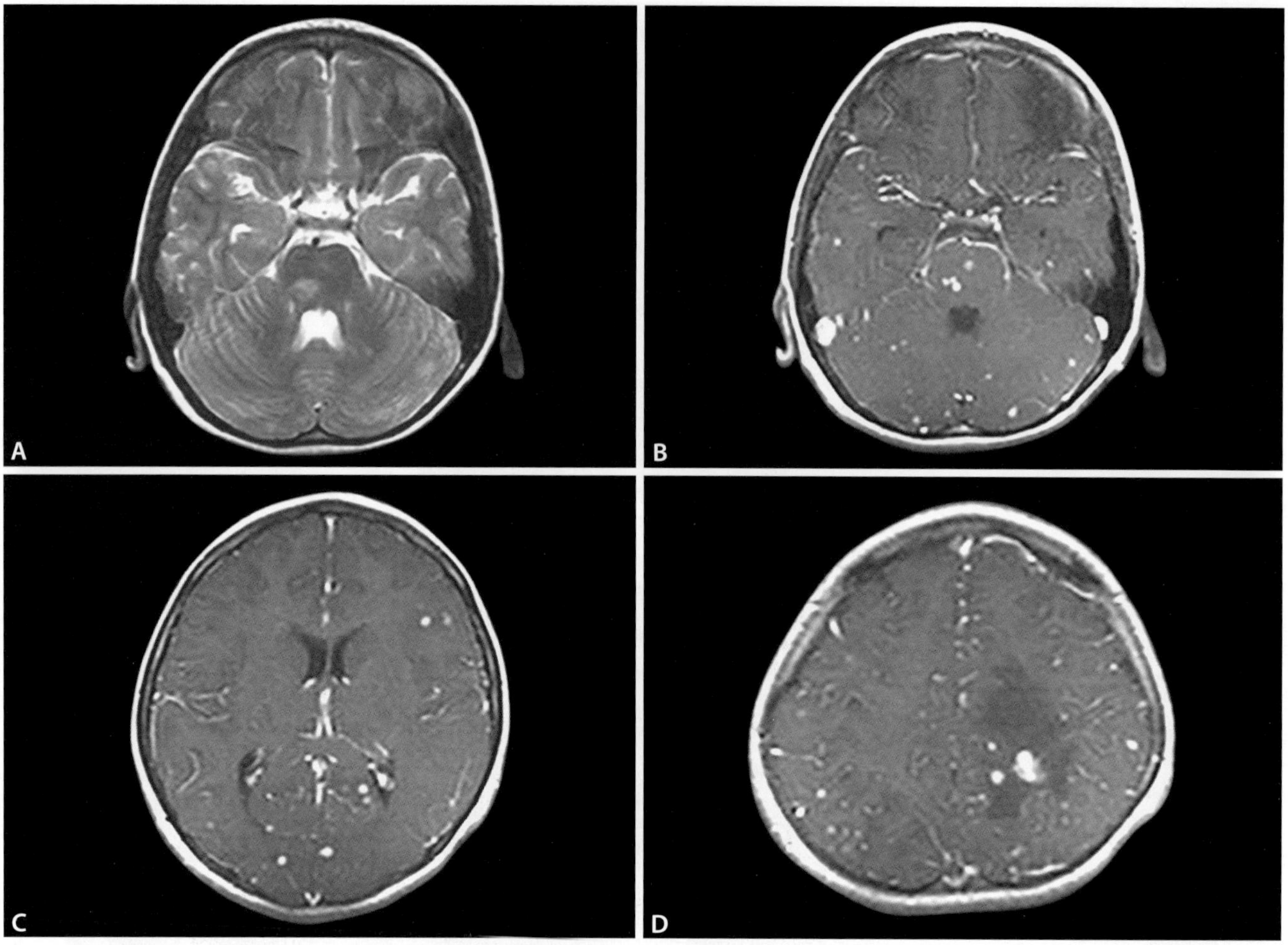

Figs. 29A to D: T2W axial MR image (A) showing lesions in the pons, cerebellum with a hyperintense signal. Postcontrast axial images; (B to D) showing intensely enhancing small granulomas in the cerebellum, pons and the cerebral hemispheres. The lesions are numerous and small in size— disseminated tuberculomas.

These occur in less than 10% of patients with CNS TB. On imaging, these are large in size (>3 cm), are multiloculated with smooth, thin enhancing wall, with mass effect and peripheral edema.[81] These are usually solitary with diffusion-weighted imaging showing restricted pattern of diffusion due to the presence of pus[82] **(Figs. 30A and B)**. Differentiation from a pyogenic brain abscess can be done with the help of MR spectroscopy and magnetization transfer MR imaging.[83] A lower magnetization transfer ratio (MTR) in a tubercular abscess as compared to a pyogenic abscess owing to the presence of lipid due to a large number of tubercle bacilli helps in differentiation.[76] Also the presence of amino acid peak (leucine, isoleucine, valine) at 0.9 ppm due to the presence of proteolytic enzymes in a pyogenic brain abscess and absence of amino acid peak in a tubercular abscess further aids in the differentiation. A tubercular abscess may show lipid, lactate and phosphoserine on MR spectroscopy[76] **(Figs. 31A to G)**.

TB ENCEPHALOPATHY

This form usually occurs in infants, pre-school and school age children following pulmonary tuberculosis. It occurs because of an immunologic mechanism with a type IV hypersensitivity reaction to the tuberculous protein mediated by the T lymphocytes. Pathologically, there is loss of myelin, decrease in the oligodendroglia and increase in the astrocytes. There is onset of perivascular demyelination. Imaging shows a diffuse cerebral edema which may be unilateral or bilateral seen as a T2 hyperintense signal. Death usually occurs within 1–2 months of the onset despite antitubercular treatment.[84]

FOCAL TUBERCULOUS CEREBRITIS

This entity has specific clinical, radiologic and histologic manifestations. On histology, multiple caseating and non-caseating granulomas, exudates, Langerhans giant cells and reactive parenchymal changes are seen.[85] A focal

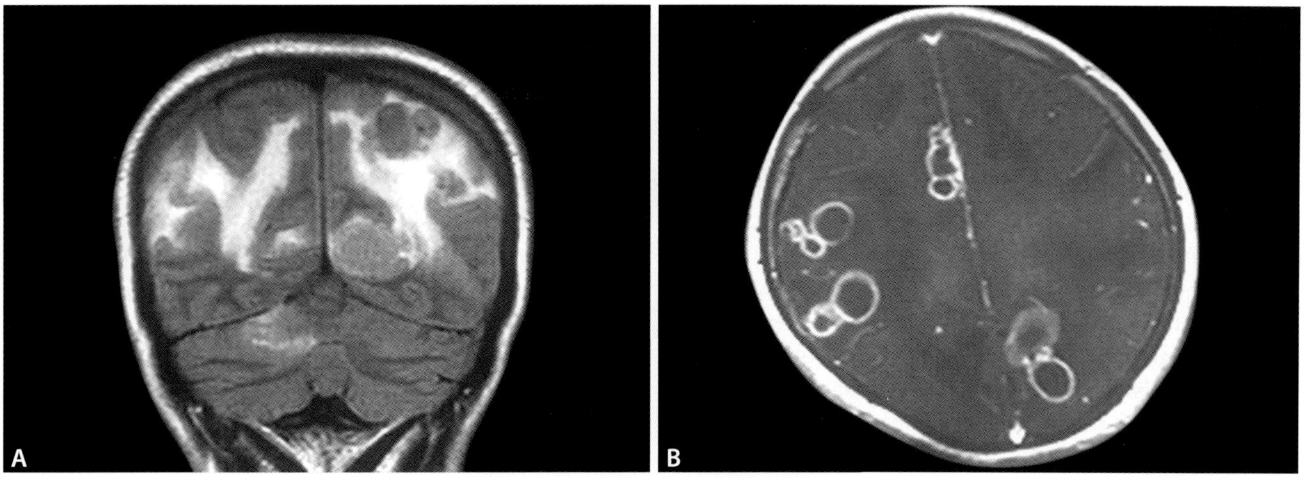

Figs. 30A and B: FLAIR coronal (A) and postcontrast axial; (B) images reveal multiple multiloculated lesions with smooth, thin walls seen in bilateral cerebral hemispheres with perilesional edema—multiple tuberculous abscesses.

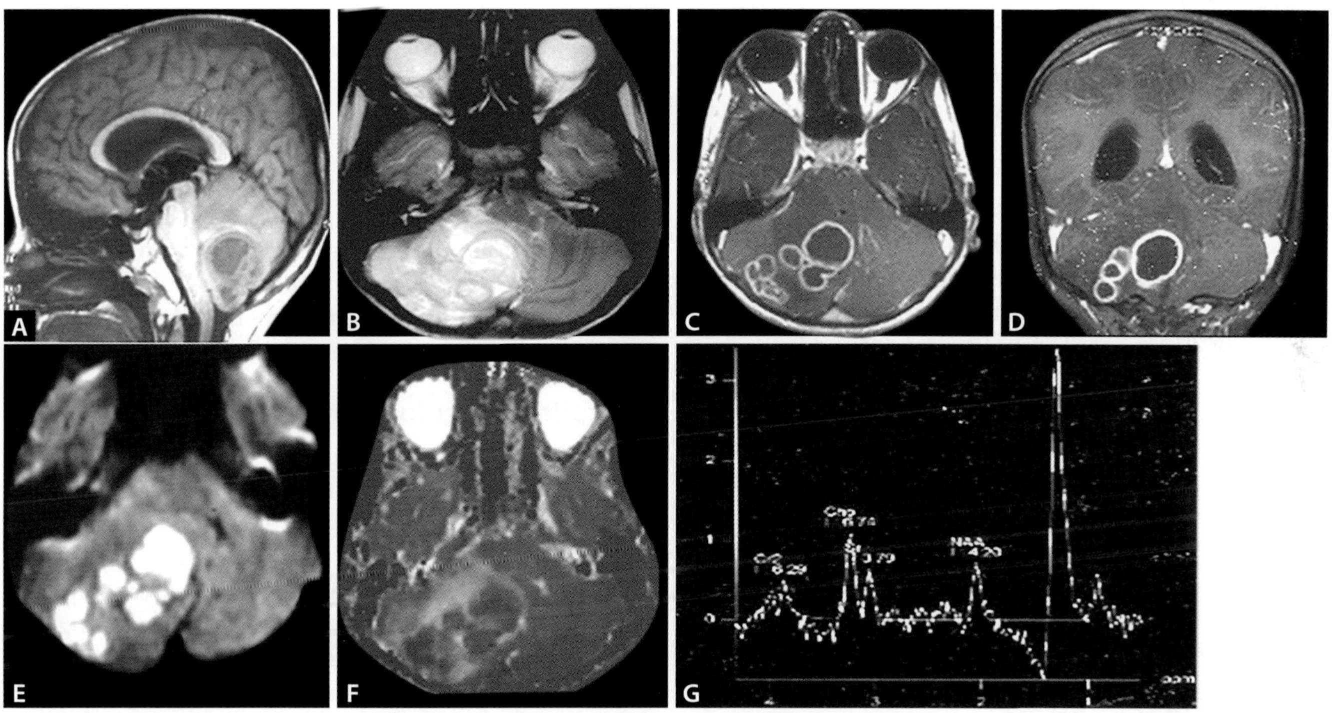

Figs. 31A to G: Sagittal T1W (A), axial T2W (B) postcontrast axial; (C and D) images reveal multiple multiloculated ring-enhancing lesions in the posterior fossa with extensive perilesional edema. Diffusion-weighted images; (E and F) reveal restricted pattern of diffusion. MR spectroscopy; (G) shows a prominent lipid at 1.3 ppm—multiple tuberculous abscesses.

gyriform pattern of enhancement is seen on both CT and MR in this entity on imaging.[86]

CNS TB AND AIDS

Tuberculous infections of CNS in AIDS patients follows a rapidly progressive course. Infarction, meningeal enhancement and parenchymal disease are more common in patients with TB who are also HIV infected. However, the differential diagnosis in AIDS patients must include other opportunistic infections and primary or metastatic lymphoma of the CNS.

NEUROSARCOIDOSIS

Involvement of the CNS in sarcoidosis is seen in about 15% of patients. Non caseating granulomas are the histologic hallmark of sarcoidosis. The patterns of CNS involvement by sarcoidosis include—parenchymal, leptomeningeal and meningoencephalitis. The commonest form is leptomeningeal (seen in 40% cases) which is characterized by a circumscribed involvement of the optic chiasma, hypothalamus, the pituitary gland and the floor of the third ventricle. A diffuse involvement and enhancement of the leptomeninges may also be seen, involvement of the cortical sulci, perivascular spaces and basal cisterns distinguish it from dural disease. Postcontrast T1-weighted images are the best to depict the diffuse thickening and enhancement of the leptomeninges. Multiple cranial nerves may also be involved in neurosarcoidosis, the commonest being the facial and optic nerves. A unilateral or bilateral involvement of the cranial nerves can occur which may involve the optic chiasma or the infraorbital portion of the optic nerves.[87] Involvement is usually seen as diffuse thickening and enhancement of the nerves on imaging. The differential diagnosis of this form includes lymphoma and tuberculosis.

Dural involvement by sarcoidosis can be either focal or diffuse. The focal masses appear to be low signal on the T2-weighted images and may mimic a calcified meningioma or very cellular dural metastasis.

The parenchymal form is characterized by multiple granulomas scattered diffusely in the brain parenchyma, iso to hypointense on T1, hyperintense on T2W images and showing intense homogenous enhancement. There is usually little or no perilesional edema around the lesions which resolve significantly following steroid treatment. Another form of parenchymal involvement is multiple periventricular white matter lesions which do not show any contrast enhancement and mimic lesions of multiple sclerosis or those seen in vascular disease. These lesions occur due to involvement of small arteries in the white matter by sarcoidosis.

The meningoencephalitis form is the rarest form and is characterized by nodular and meningeal enhancement. This enhancement usually extends into the parenchyma through the Virchow-Robin spaces.

FUNGAL INFECTIONS OF THE CENTRAL NERVOUS SYSTEM

Fungi are a distinct group of pathogenic organisms which may exist either as yeast form (*Candida, Cryptococcus, Histoplasma, Coccidioides, Torulopsis*) or hyphal form (*Aspergillus, Mucormycosis, Pseudallescheria*). The yeast form or the single celled form being smaller in size usually spreads hematogenously to present as meningitis or granulomas while the hyphal form being the larger form usually involves the parenchyma resulting in cerebritis or encephalitis. Vasculitis, vascular occlusion, septic infarction and aneurysm formation may occur due to invasion of small or medium sized arteries by the large mycelial forms, formed by the coalescence of the yeast or hyphal form.

ASPERGILLOSIS

Aspergillosis is an opportunistic infection which usually involves immunocompromised patients.[88] The predominant form is the hyphal form and this fungus exists in soil, water or decaying vegetation.

The mode of entry is by inhalation of the fungal spores. The infection is initially confined to the pulmonary tree with a resultant hypersensitivity reaction. When the host's defence mechanism are weak a hematogenous dissemination in the body with involvement of the CNS may occur.[89] CNS involvement is in the form of vasculitis/vasculopathy, brain abscess or granuloma formation. A rhinocerebral form may rarely occur caused by the direct extension of disease in the nasal cavity and paranasal sinuses.[90]

MR imaging reveals a characteristic "target like pattern" on the T2W images. *Aspergillus* lesions show a characteristic central hyperintensity surrounded by a peripheral hypointensity. The hypointense signal is attributed to increased iron due to fungal elements, hemorrhage and ferromagnetic metals like calcium and manganese resulting from fungal metabolism.[91]

Vasculitis/Vasculopathy

Aspergillus is angioinvasive. The invasive nature of the aspergillosis accounts for the vascular occlusion with resultant infarction which is often hemorrhagic. Focal microhemorrhages occur because of the production of the enzyme elastase by the fungus which digests the internal elastic lamina of arteries. Weakening and digestion of the walls leads to the formation of a mycotic aneurysm. Amongst the fungal infections, aspergillosis is the commonest cause of a mycotic aneurysm. The presence of subarachnoid hemorrhage or mycotic aneurysm formation in immunocompromised patients with suspected fungal infection should prompt instillation of appropriate antifungal therapy.[92] *Aspergillus* has an affinity for the origins of small perforating arteries with consequent sterile infarctions in the basal ganglia, corpus callosum, and thalamus. Thus, infarction of the corpus callosum is highly suggestive of aspergillus infection as this is not the site for pyogenic or thromboembolic infarction.[93] The sterile infarct gets converted into septic infarct as direct extension of fungal elements into the surrounding

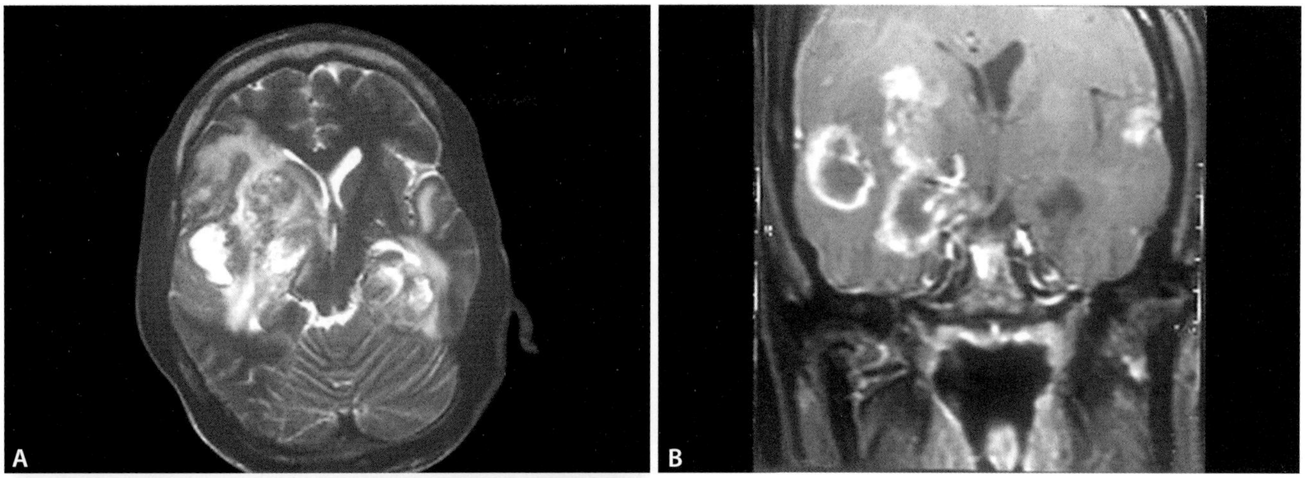

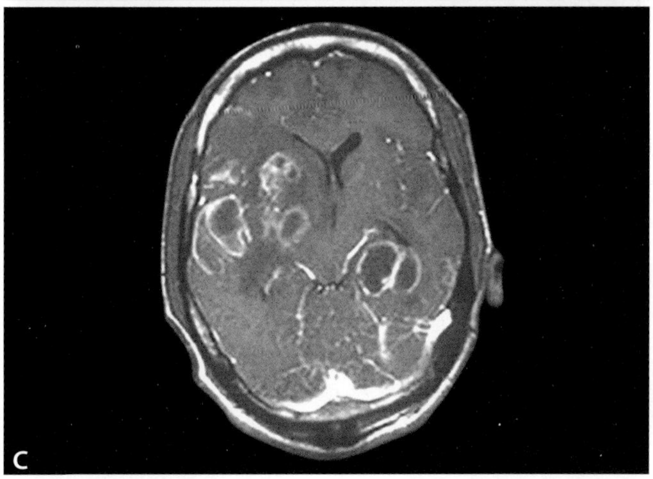

Figs. 32A to C: T2W axial (A) postcontrast T1W coronal; (B) and postcontrast axial; (C) MR images showing multiple ring or nodular enhancing lesions in the right basal ganglia, right parietal and left temporal regions. Extensive perilesional edema is seen around the lesions causing mass effect and shift of the midline of the contralateral side. The lesions have irregular and crenated margins —CNS aspergillosis.

brain parenchyma occurs when breakdown of brain tissue occurs at sites of infarction.

Cerebritis and abscess formation can occur when the host defense mechanism tries to encapsulate the offending organism **(Figs. 32A to C)**. A restricted pattern of diffusion is seen in an *Aspergillus* abscess due to the high cellularity and viscosity of the pus material.[94] A typical pattern of restricted diffusion "the ring pattern" is seen in *Aspergillus* with the lesion center being hypointense on DWI and the lesion periphery being hyperintense on DWI. Postcontrast scans reveal weak or no enhancement which is an important diagnostic clue. Capsule formation from chronic inflammation and production of granulation tissue can contribute to the weak ring enhancement seen in some cases. A crenated border and non enhancing intracavitary projections also help to differentiate a fungal from a pyogenic or tubercular abscess. The demonstration of α-trehalose peak on MR spectroscopy (3.6–3.8 ppm) in fungal abscess also helps in the differentiation. Meningitis and ventriculitis may manifest as hydrocephalus on imaging and ependymal enhancement is distinctly uncharacteristic.

Rhinocerebral form occurs when infection spreads from the orbit, the paranasal sinuses or base of the skull to the brain. The sinuses have a low signal on both T1- and T2-weighted images owing to the presence of paramagnetic metals within the infectious mass and show evidence of contrast enhancement.[95]

CRYPTOCOCCAL INFECTION

Cryptococcosis is the commonest fungal infection to involve the CNS and the most frequently identifiable fungal infection in AIDS patients.[96] Caused by the fungus *Cryptococcus neoformans*, it is more commonly seen in men (80%). This may be attributed to the fungus thriving in soil contaminated with pigeon droppings and a greater occupational exposure to the fungal spores in men. Inhalation of spores leads to pulmonary disease which is usually subclinical. In the pulmonary tree, the organism forms a highly resistant polysaccharide capsule which may be related to the high carbon dioxide tension present in the lungs. From the lungs, the organism may lodge in the intrathoracic lymph nodes and remain dormant. Any weakening of the host's immune system leads to a reactivation with dissemination occurring to the CNS predominantly. The propensity of CNS dissemination is accounted by the absence of anticryptococcal factors in the CSF as compared to serum.[97] Also, the polysaccharide capsule of the fungus is resistant to phagocytosis and confers protection against the host's inflammatory response.

Imaging

On CT, cerebral atrophy and hydrocephalus may be the only positive findings.[98] *Cryptococcus* often causes meningeal disease which is usually basal in location but may not be detected on the postcontrast scans owing to the inability of the host to mount a cell mediated immune response. Hydrocephalus may also not be seen in the immunocompromised patients due to the lack of inflammatory leptomeningeal reaction and paucity of adhesions. Thus imaging findings are often lacking in immunocompromised patients on CT scans.

On MRI, the positive imaging findings include dilated Virchow Robin spaces and cryptococcomas. Dilated Virchow Robin spaces are seen as foci isointense to the CSF, less than 3 mm in size, bilateral and symmetric with a predilection for the basal ganglia and thalamus. These foci are not associated with any mass effect, perilesional edema or contrast enhancement[99] **(Figs. 33A to C)**. These spaces may coalesce producing gelatinous pseudocysts. The perivascular spaces get filled with fungi and mucoid gelatinous material produced by the capsule of the organism. Gelatinous pseudocysts have a classic "soap bubble" appearance and are most commonly seen in the basal ganglia, thalamus and midbrain. These pseudocysts may show restricted diffusion owing to the gelatinous content.

Invasion of the brain parenchyma may result in the formation of chronic granulomas or cryptococcomas.

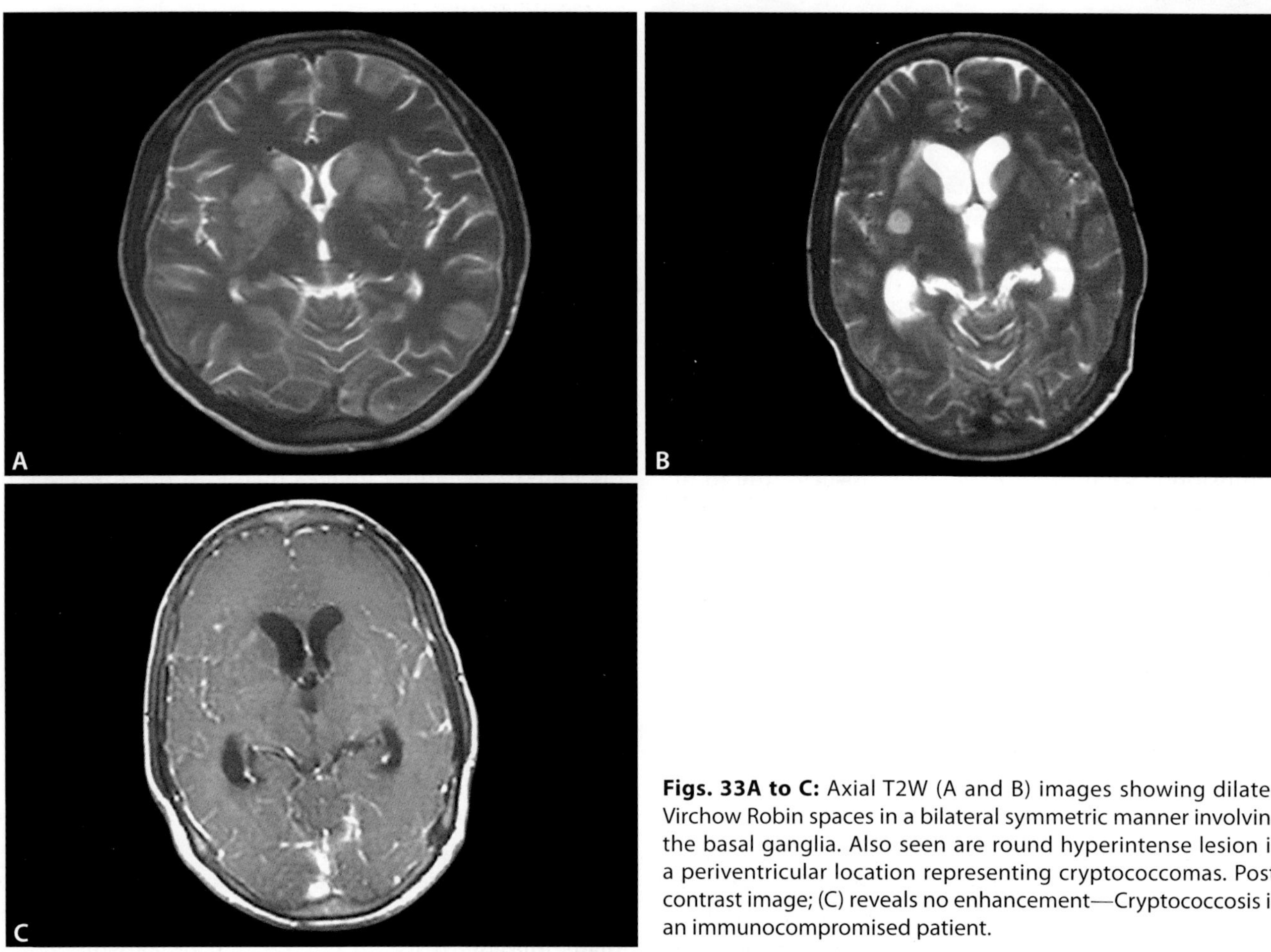

Figs. 33A to C: Axial T2W (A and B) images showing dilated Virchow Robin spaces in a bilateral symmetric manner involving the basal ganglia. Also seen are round hyperintense lesion in a periventricular location representing cryptococcomas. Post-contrast image; (C) reveals no enhancement—Cryptococcosis in an immunocompromised patient.

Cryptococcomas are low to intermediate signal on T1 and high signal on T2W images. No enhancement is seen in the immunocompromised/AIDS patients but in the immunocompetent patient some degree of enhancement may be seen. A double dose technique may show the lesions better. These granulomas have also been reported along the ependyma of the choroid plexus and this finding if seen is considered highly specific for cryptococcosis.[100]

MR Spectroscopy in Cryptococcomas

High levels of MR visible α-trehalose have been reported from cryptococcomas. This helps in an early and correct diagnosis and in differentiation from mitotic lesions. Trehalose is a disaccharide found in the fungal wall and identification of multiple signals between 3.6 and 3.8 ppm adds specificity to the diagnosis.[81]

A rare pattern of involvement is multiple miliary enhancing nodules in the parenchyma or leptomeninges suggestive of granuloma formation. Another uncommon pattern is the involvement of the spinal cord which may be seen as high signal on T2 with or without enhancement.

Diagnosis of cryptococcal infection is easier than other fungal infections because of the following reasons:

1. The yeast can be seen in the CSF
2. Immunologic tests for antigen in blood and CSF are highly sensitive.
3. Infection has a unique appearance on histology.

The diagnosis is usually made by India ink preparation or by fungal culture of CSF.

MUCORMYCOSIS

It is the most aggressive of all fungal infections and those with diabetes are at increased risk. A triad of diabetic ketoacidosis, naso-orbital infection and meningoencephalitis is highly suggestive of the diagnosis. Though diabetes compromises 70% of all cases, sepsis, chronic renal failure, severe chronic diarrhea, severe dehydration constitute the other predisposing factors. Immunocompromised patients or those with a history of renal transplant are also at increased risk.[101] Two forms of the disease are recognized—the rhinocerebral form and the hematogenous form.

Imaging

The rhinocerebral form, which is the more common form occurs when the sinus infection extends into the CNS. The organism may spread via the perivascular and perineural channels through the cribriform plate into the frontal lobe or through the orbital apex into the cavernous sinus[102] **(Figs. 34A to F)**. Direct invasion of the arteries with consequent thrombosis and infarction can occur. The internal carotid artery and the basilar artery may be involved by thrombus formation **(Figs. 35A to C)**. MRI shows nonspecific inflammatory changes involving the paranasal sinuses and the orbits similar to *Aspergillus* infection. The sinuses have a low signal on T2W images owing to the presence of paramagnetic metals like calcium, manganese, magnesium, iron within the fungal mass. A "black turbinate" sign has been describe in mucormycosis.[103] It refers to the non-enhancing mucosa on MRI suggesting infarction of the invaded mucosa. Meningitis may occur in the rhinocerebral form or with central skull base involvement resulting from direct extension of infection.

The hematogenous form is less common and is usually seen in patients with malignancies and intravenous drug abusers. The vascular changes seen are arteritis, ischaemia changes, bland or haemorrhagic infarction and aneurysm formation.[104]

CANDIDIASIS

Candidiasis is caused by *Candida albicans* species. These fungi lack a sexual cycle and reproduce by budding or fission. Pseudohyphae predominate though rarely true hyphae may form. The fungus is present as a part of the normal intestinal flora. *Candida* infection occurs when there are disturbances in equilibrium that normally exists within the intestinal flora, such as following antibiotic therapy, chemotherapy and hematologic conditions such as thrombocytopenia. Indwelling catheters, intravenous drug abuse with resulting candidal endocarditis are the other predisposing factors. HIV infection with low CD4 counts (<135 mm^3) is another risk factor. Preterm, low birth infants are particularly susceptible to acquire the infection. The infections may be acquired in utero, during passage through an infected genital tract or postnatally. In the disseminated/systemic form of candidiasis the kidneys are the most common affected organs followed by the central nervous system which is involved in about 50% cases.

Imaging

The imaging hallmark is microabscesses which are defined as <3 mm small ascesses diffusely scattered in the brain parenchyma **(Figs. 36A and B)**. Other imaging manifestations include macroabscesses, meningitis, meningoencephalitis, granuloma formation, ependymitis, ischaemia, infarction or mycotic aneurysm formation.[105]

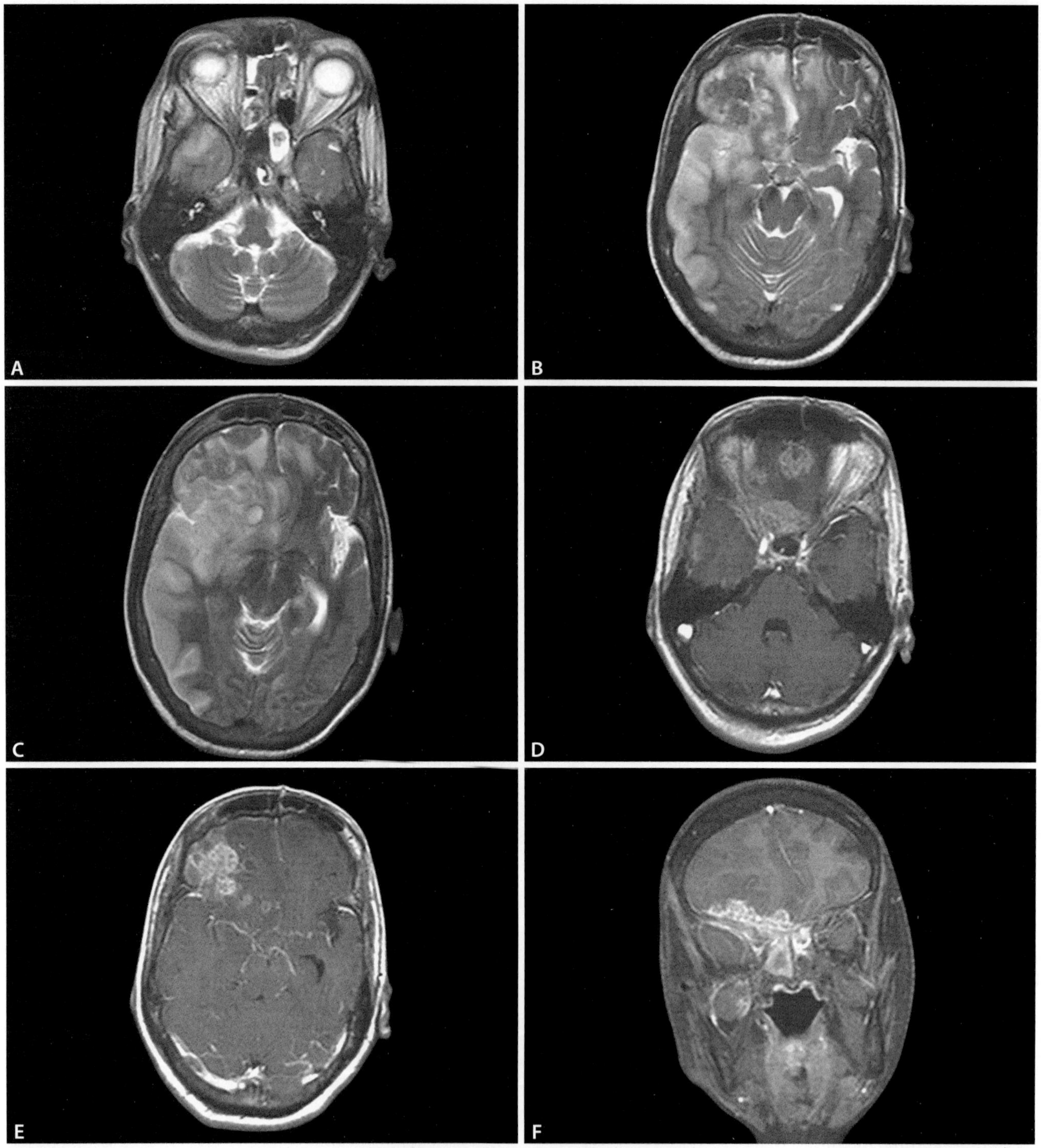

Figs. 34A to F: Axial T2W (A to C) images reveal a large area of signal alteration in the right frontotemporoparietal region with mass effect and gyral swelling. Postcontrast; (D to F) images reveal ring enhancing lesions in the basifrontal region, the lesions are hypointense on T2W images. Evidence of sinusitis seen which shows a low signal on T2W images.

Early diagnosis is essential as CNS involvement warrants a different therapy. Fluconazole along with Amphotericin B leads to better prognosis.

COCCIDIOIDOMYCOSIS

The causative organism *Coccidioides immitis*, is a dimorphic yeast found in the soil. The spores produced

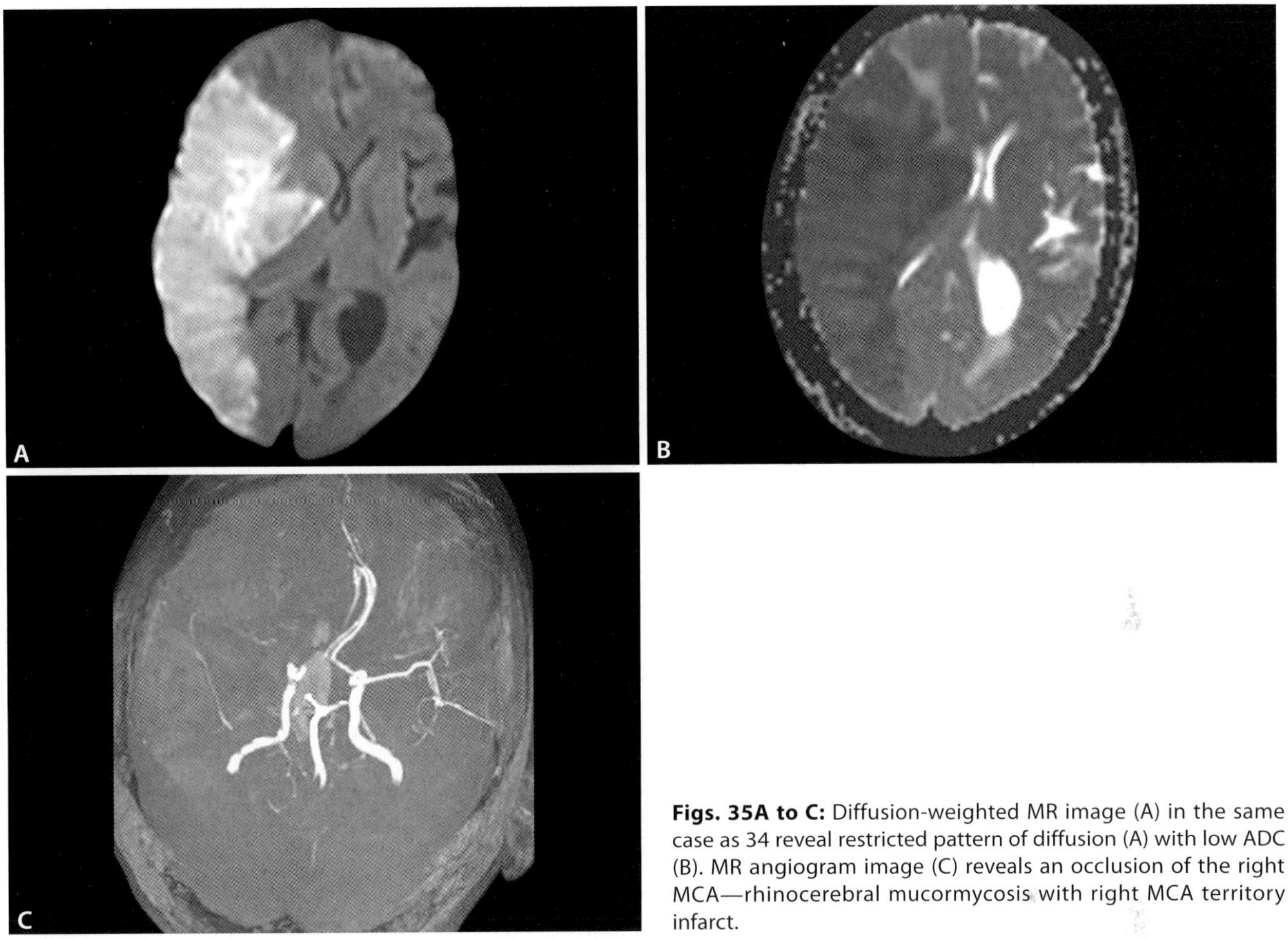

Figs. 35A to C: Diffusion-weighted MR image (A) in the same case as 34 reveal restricted pattern of diffusion (A) with low ADC (B). MR angiogram image (C) reveals an occlusion of the right MCA—rhinocerebral mucormycosis with right MCA territory infarct.

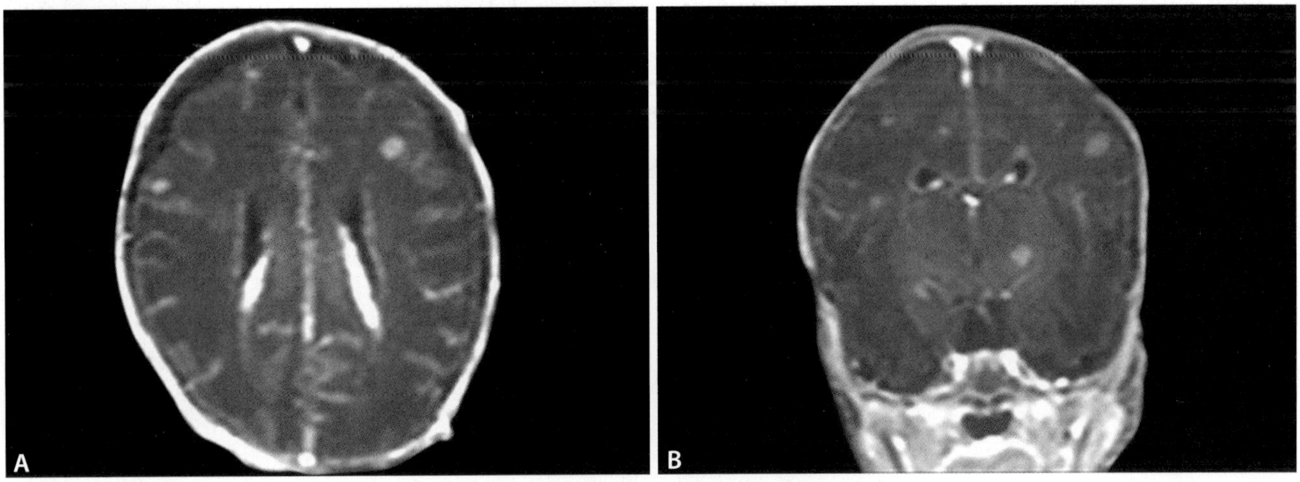

Figs. 36A and B: Postcontrast axial images showing multiple microabscesses and nodular enhancing lesions in bilateral cerebral hemispheres—Candidiasis.

by this organism are called anthroconidia. These spores are extremely resilient and virulent and may lie dormant in the soil for long periods. Activities like farming and construction may cause a dispersal of the spores which may then be inhaled by the humans resulting in a subclinical upper respiratory inection. An immunocompromised state, diabetes and pregnancy may act as risk factors for dissemination of the infection. The most common CNS manifestation is meningitis which may be associated with cerebritis and hydrocephalus. Granuloma and abscess formation may be the other manifestations with multiple granulomas resembling miliary tuberculosis.[106] Vascular complications can be seen in about 40% of patients with meningitis and include arteritis and infarction. Aneurysm formation and subarachnoid hemorrhage resulting from rupture of the aneurysm are the other manifestations of this infection.

HISTOPLASMOSIS

The most common mode of entry is inhalation of airborne spores. The lung are therefore the most common organ affected and CNS involvement usually occurs in immunocompromised host resulting from a hematogenous spread.

The radiologic findings are similar to other fungal infections such as meningitis, encephalitis, brain abscess and histoplasmoma (granuloma) formation. A miliary pattern and vasculitis has also been described.[107,108] Definitive diagnosis can be achieved by CSF analysis or by brain biopsy.[109]

NOCARDIOSIS

Nocardia asteroides is actually a bacterial pathogen found in the soil but has traditionally been included in medical mycology. Patients with diabetes, immunocompromised patients, those with a pre-existing pulmonary disease or collagen vascular disease are at increased risk. As the infection is airborne, the primary site of involvement is the lungs and brain involvement occurs secondary to hematogenous spread seen in about 25% of cases. Multiple brain abscesses is the imaging hallmark of the disease. Contrast enhanced CT scan or MRI may show multiple or mutiloculated ring enhancing lesions.

PARASITIC INFECTIONS

NEUROCYSTICERCOSIS

Cysticercosis is the commonest parasitic disease in humans caused by the worm Taenia solium. It is the most common cause of acquired epilepsy throughout the world. Humans are the definitive host when infected with adult tapeworm and the intermediate host when infected with the larval stage/cysticercus. Thus taeniasis is the term used for infection by the adult tapeworm while cysticercosis is an infection by the larval stage. Infected humans excrete the gravid proglottids or eggs in the feces which are ingested by the pig. Pigs acquire cysticercosis as the larva migrate via the circulatory system and get embedded in the muscle where they may persist for many years. Taeniasis is acquired when humans ingest undercooked meat or raw flesh of an infected animal. Humans can also get infected by the larval stage when they accidentally consume T. solium eggs. Once the eggs reach the small intestine, they penetrate the intestinal mucosa to enter the bloodstream and can reach any organ of the body to form cysts. Cysts can be found in the skin, muscles, eyes, heart, and the CNS where they cause neurocysticercosis **(Figs. 37A to D)**.

Clinical Features

CNS involvement occurs in 60–90% of cases with cysticercosis.[110] Patients may be asymptomatic with the neurocysticerci discovered incidentally on imaging. When symptomatic, headache, seizure, diplopia, visual field deficits are the most common neurologic manifestations. At times patients may present with focal neurological deficits and stroke.[111]

Four patterns of cysticercosis in the CNS are recognized-parenchymal, intraventricular, spinal, subarachnoid or a combination of these.

Parenchymal Cysticercosis

The cysts are seen in the parenchyma and basal ganglia owing to the rich vascular supply of these areas. These cysts are usually less than 10 mm in size as the compliance of the brain parenchyma prevents excessive growth of the vesicles.

Escobar classified the cysts into four pathologic states[112] **(Figs. 38A to D)**. In the vesicular stage the larva is seen as a small marginal nodule projecting into a small cyst containing clear fluid. On imaging the vesicular stage is seen as a clearly marginated cyst with thin imperceptible walls with CSF signal intensity and a discrete eccentrically located scolex within. A "dot in a hole" or a "target" appearance may be seen owing to the presence of the scolex which has a soft tissue attenuation or signal intensity distinct from the cyst fluid. No perilesional edema is seen. No contrast enhancement is seen at this stage as there is no immune response by the host.

In the next stage, that is the colloidal vesicular stage, the larva begins to degenerate. This may occur from effects of therapy or from natural death of the scolex with associated disruption of the cyst wall. There is a decrease in the size of the cyst, the cyst fluid becomes turbid, the wall becomes perceptible and thick. There is evidence of

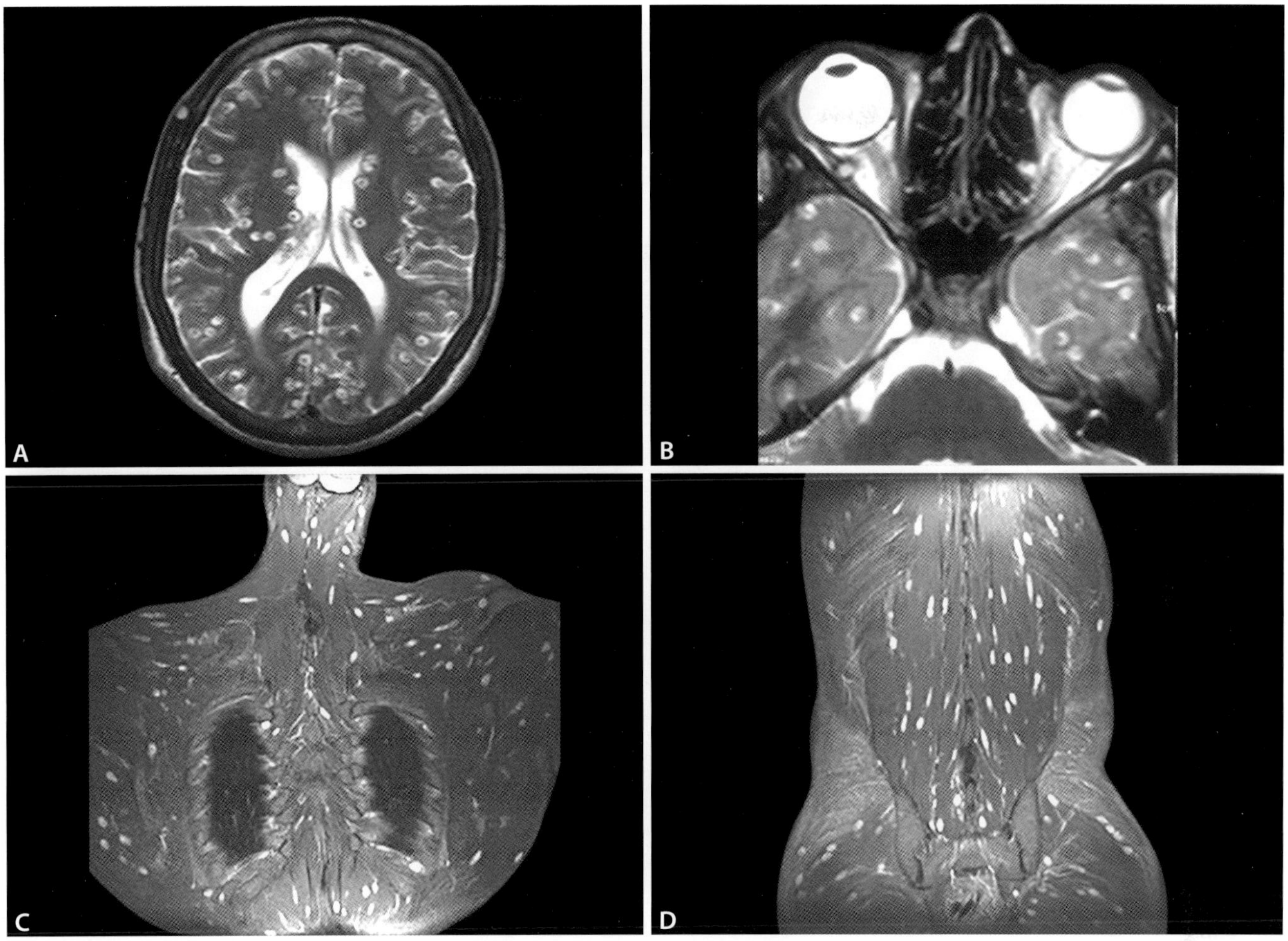

Figs. 37A to D: Axial T2W (A and B) images showing multiple small lesions hyperintense on T2W in both cerebral hemispheres, right lateral rectus muscle in the orbit. STIR coronal images (C and D) reveal lesions in the muscles—multiple cysticerci.

substantial perilesional edema and contrast enhancement of the cyst wall owing to the inflammatory reaction caused by the degeneration of the larva.[113] On the postcontrast T1W images, a pattern of ring enhancement is seen. The late colloidal vesicular stage is characterized by thick and irregular cyst wall, retraction, moderate perilesional edema and absence of scolex.

The third stage, that is the granular nodular stage, is characterized by further retraction and thickening of the cyst wall with a coarse mineralized scolex. There is near complete resorption of the cyst fluid, the capsule is thick and collagenous and there is a marked decrease in the amount of perilesional edema in this stage.

The fourth or final stage is the nodular calcified stage in which there is shrinkage of the lesion and it is completely mineralized.[114] No perilesional edema or contrast enhancement is seen. On imaging a calcified nodule or a focal area of gliosis is seen. Magnetization transfer ratio (MTR) helps in the differentiation of T2 hypointense lesions of cysticercus (granular nodular stage) from that of tuberculoma. Cysticercus larvae have higher protein and amino acid content and result in higher magnetization transfer ratio as compared to tuberculomas.

On imaging, the cysticercus cysts may be seen in various stages and in transition from one stage to another as the evolution is a dynamic process and no abrupt change occurs from one stage to another. An encephalitic form of cysticercosis can be seen in the pediatric population. This form is characterized by multiple small enhancing lesions along with diffuse cerebral edema[115] **(Figs. 39A to C)**. The increased vascularity and capillary endothelial proliferation adjacent to the cysts accounts for the lesions showing contrast enhancement. The sequelae of the encephalitic form is seen as multiple punctate calcifications scattered in the brain parenchyma representing the nodular calcified stage of the disease.

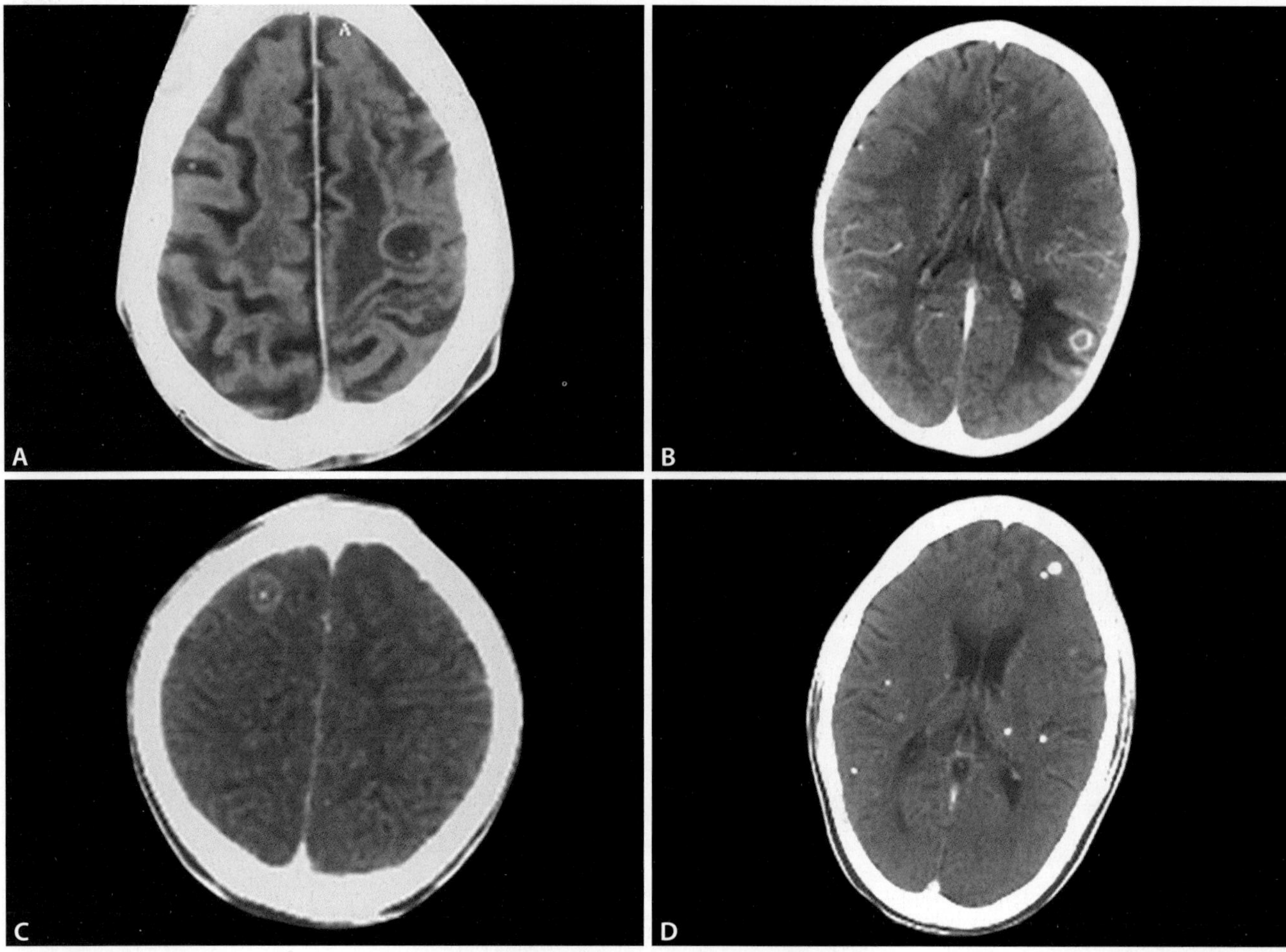

Figs. 38A to D: Contrast-enhanced axial CT (A) showing a cyst with fluid similar to CSF attenuation with an eccentrically located scolex in the left parietal region with no contrast enhancement/edema—vesicular stage. Axial CT scan; (B) showing a ring-enhancing lesion with perilesional edema in left parieto-occipital region colloid vesicular stage. CECT axial image; (C) showing a cyst with thick capsule with calcific nodule with no edema—granular nodular stage. CECT axial images; (D) showing calcific foci in bilateral hemispheres—nodular calcified stage.

The cysticercus lesion needs to be differentiated from a tuberculoma on imaging **(Table 3)**.

Intraventricular Cysticercosis

The intraventricular form usually occurs in isolation and is not associated with cysts elsewhere. These are seen most commonly in the fourth ventricle followed by the lateral and third ventricle. These cysts may migrate from one ventricle to another. Obstructive hydrocephalus occurs when the cyst gets entrapped in the aqueduct of Sylvius obstructing the ventricular outflow. Multiple cysts are rare and if found are usually seen in the lateral ventricles.

On imaging, the intraventricular cyst is seen as a high signal intensity mural nodule outlined by the CSF on T1-weighted and FLAIR images.[117] CISS sequence (constructive interference in the steady state) is the best sequence to demonstrate the intraventricular cysticercosis as the cyst wall is clearly delineated on this sequence **(Figs. 40A and B)**. Sagittal T1-weighted imaging is helpful in differentiating a fourth ventricular cysticercus from a dilated fourth ventricle and in showing aqueductal obstruction.

MR imaging is helpful in the preoperative locatization of the cyst and in detecting granular ependymitis seen as ring like or nodular enhancement.[118] The diagnosis of granular ependymitis is important as all these patients require a shunt even after surgical removal of the cyst. Intraventricular cyst may migrate within the ventricular system or into the basal cisterns or subarachnoid space from the ventricles.

Subarachnoid Cysticercosis

The subarachnoid or racemose variety of cysticercosis is seen within the cortical sulci, gyri or within the basal

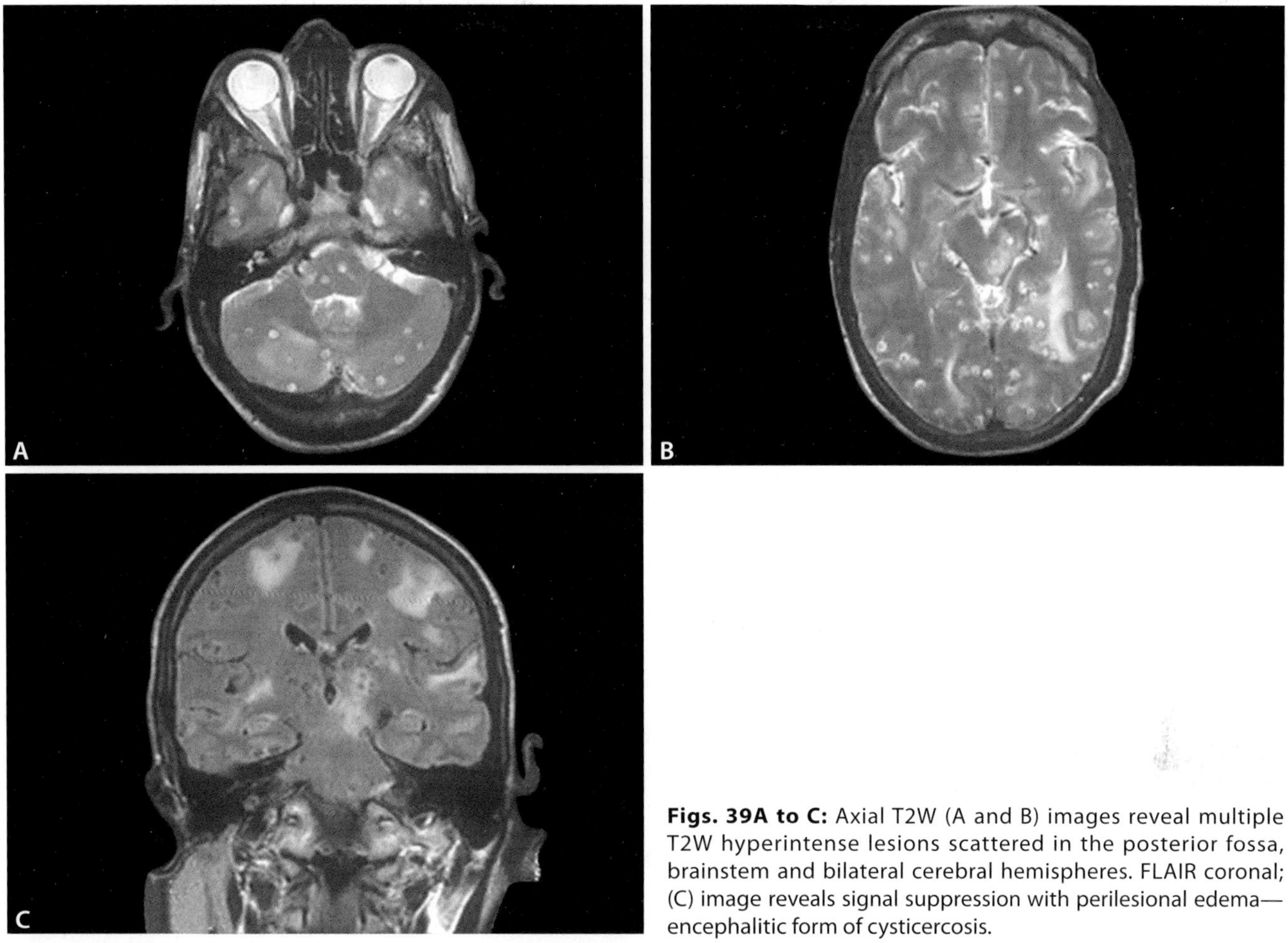

Figs. 39A to C: Axial T2W (A and B) images reveal multiple T2W hyperintense lesions scattered in the posterior fossa, brainstem and bilateral cerebral hemispheres. FLAIR coronal; (C) image reveals signal suppression with perilesional edema—encephalitic form of cysticercosis.

Table 3: Differences between neurocysticercosis (NCC) and tuberculomas on imaging.[116]

Neurocysticercosis	***Tuberculoma***
Usually <20 mm in size, cystic	>20 mm in size, solid
Regular in outline	Has an irregular outline
Mild-to-moderate perilesional edema	Extensive/marked perilesional edema
No midline shift seen	Midline shift may be seen
An eccentric scolex may be seen	No scolex seen
May be single/multiple	Usually multiple, may show conglomeration
T2 hyperintense lesions with complete signal suppression on FLAIR sequence	Caseating granulomas with solid centre are hypointense on T2W images. Those hyperintense on T2W images do not show complete signal suppression on FLAIR images
No lipid peak on MR spectroscopy	Lipid peak seen on MRS
High MTR because of protein content	Low MTR because of lipid content

cisterns. Those in the basal cisterns attain a large size owing to the lack of pressure from the adjacent brain parenchyma and characteristically lack a mural nodule. Many theories have been postulated to explain the absence of the scolex in the racemose variety. While Martinez has suggested that the racemose variety is an arrested form in the development of the cyst with the scolex never being formed some have suggested that a disordered proliferation of the cyst wall in the racemose variety accounts for the lack of the scolex.[114,118] A lack of encapsulation in the basal cisterns as compared to the parenchymal forms also has been suggested in the etiopathogenesis. On imaging, large multiple, multilobulated cysts in a basal cisternal location, isointense to the CSF on all sequences, with lack of a mural nodule and leptomeningeal enhancement characterize the racemose variety **(Figs. 41A to C)**.

Cysts located at the cortical sulci are usually small while those located in the Sylvian fissures may grow to large sizes similar to echinococcus infection.

Basilar leptomeningitis, arachnoiditis, mass effect, communicating hydrocephalus and vasculitis may

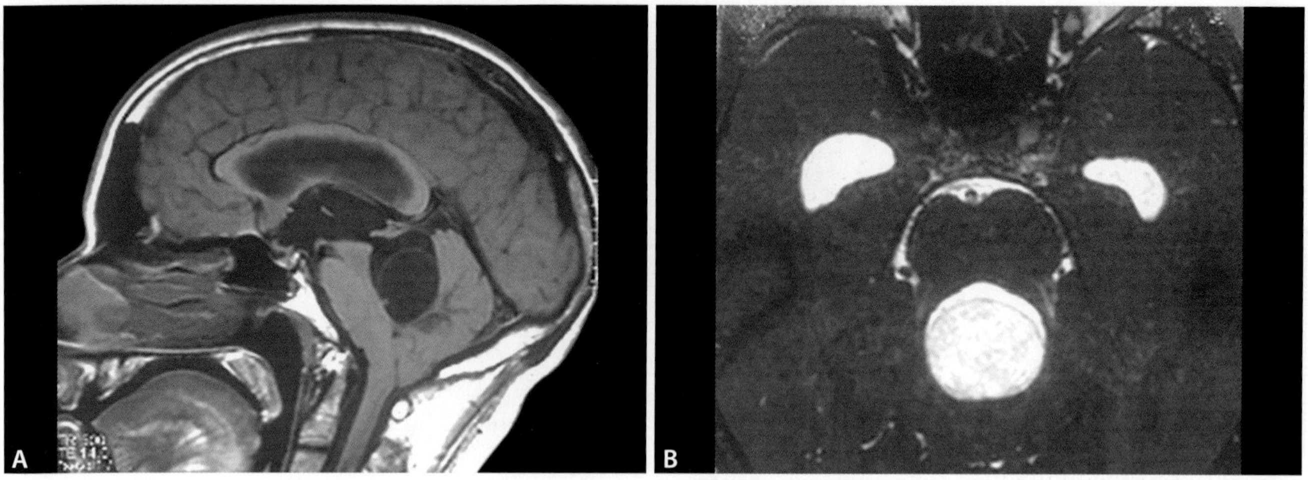

Figs. 40A and B: Sagittal T1W (A) and CISS axial; (B) MR images showing a cystic lesion with signal intensity almost similar to CSF in the fourth ventricle with resultant obstructive hydrocephalus—intraventricular cysticercus.

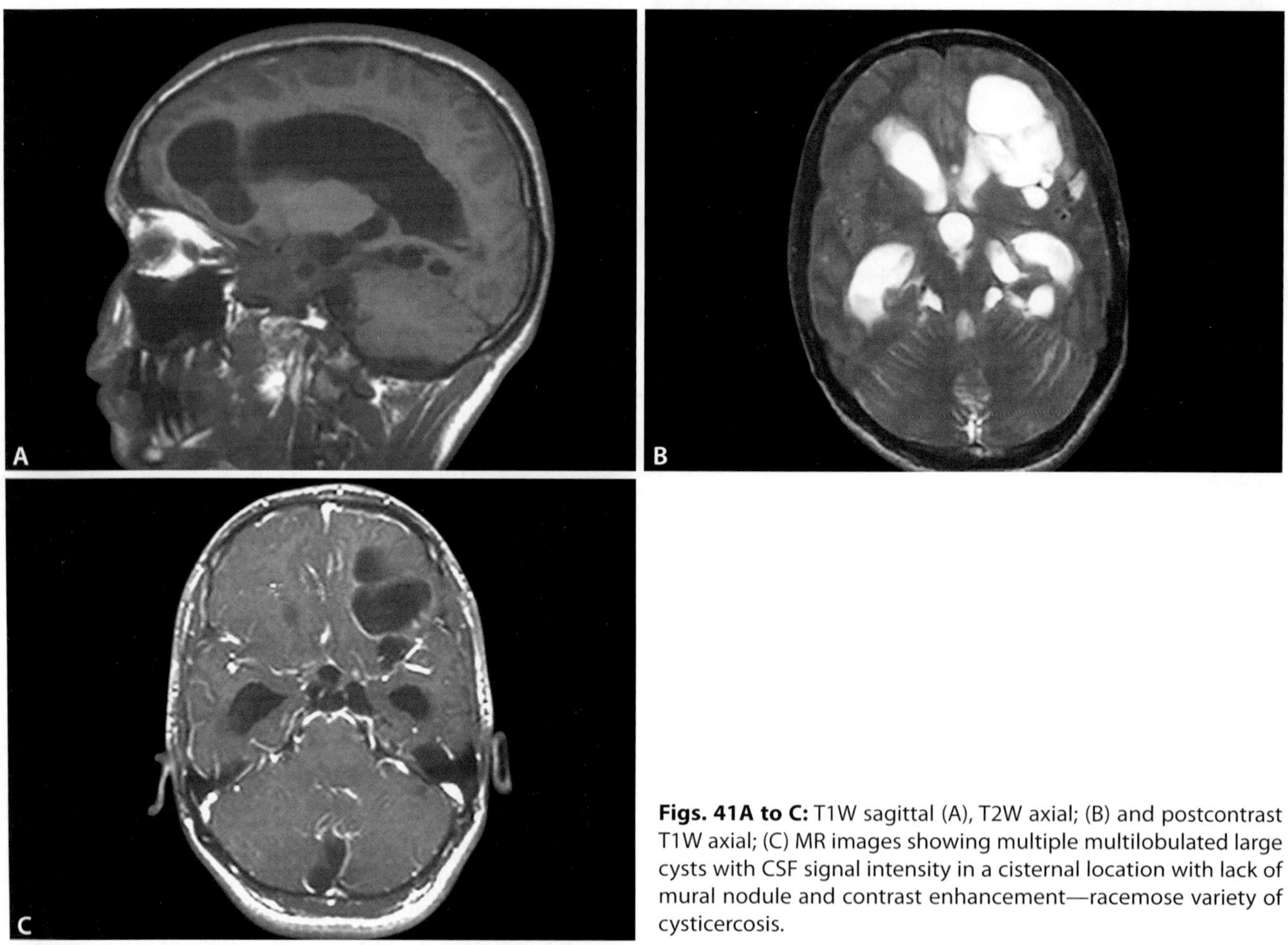

Figs. 41A to C: T1W sagittal (A), T2W axial; (B) and postcontrast T1W axial; (C) MR images showing multiple multilobulated large cysts with CSF signal intensity in a cisternal location with lack of mural nodule and contrast enhancement—racemose variety of cysticercosis.

occur in the subarachnoid variety owing to an intense inflammatory response. The walls of the arteries are invaded by inflammatory cells leading to vasculitis and proliferative endarteritis.

Spinal Cysticercosis

Spinal cysticercus appears as a cystic mass compressing the spinal cord, that is, as an intradural extramedullary cyst or as arachnoiditis.

Orbital Disease

The lesions may involve the globe or the extraocular muscles. The parasitic cysts may be seen in the choroid/retina, in the subconjunctival region. In the muscles, it is the muscle belly which is usually involved and the appearance is that of one or more cysts ("peas in a pod" appearance).

TOXOPLASMOSIS

Toxoplasma gondii is a parasite well known throughout the world. The definitive host is the cat and other Felidae. After ingestion, the organism develops in the epithelial cells of the intestine to form schizonts, gametocytes and oocytes which are shed in the cat's feces. The cat excretes the oocytes for approximately 2 weeks after the primary insult. Human consumption of undercooked, infected meat or contact with infected cat feces can lead to human infection.

Most toxoplasmosis infections in immunocompetent individuals are subclinical or mildly symptomatic. A minimal number of patients develop symptoms that resemble infectious mononucleosis (i.e. fever, chills, headache, tender lymphadenopathy and fatigue). Rarely, symptoms may be severe and include a maculopapular rash, hepatitis, encephalomyelitis or myocarditis.

Toxoplasmosis is a major cause of encephalitis in AIDS patients. In patients with HIV infection, Toxoplasma encephalitis results in a progressive and often fatal encephalitis if untreated.[119]

Pathologically, parenchymal toxoplasma lesions have three distinct zones: A central zone which is avascular, contains few organisms and demonstrates coagulative necrosis; an intermediate zone which is engorged with blood vessels containing numerous free extracellular and intracellular organisms and has fewer areas of necrosis. The outermost is the peripheral zone with few vascular changes and more encysted organisms with little necrosis. Inflammatory reaction is most intense in the intermediate zone. There is endothelial cell swelling and proliferation with cuffing of venules by lymphocytes, plasma cells and macrophages. *Toxoplasma* lesions do not have capsules. When leptomeningitis is present it only involves the meninges directly adjacent to the areas of encephalitis. Although small vessel thrombosis and necrosis are characteristically associated with lesions, arteritis of large vessels is absent.

Imaging

On noncontrast CT, toxoplasma encephalitis characteristically appears as multiple areas of hypodensity. There is a predilection for the basal ganglia (in 75 to 88%) and the corticomedullary junction and lesions may involve the posterior fossa. Lesions vary in size from less than 1 cm to over 3 cm and there is surrounding mass effect and edema of variable degree. Hemorrhage is uncommon and the presence of hyperattenuating lesions on a non-contrast CT should suggest an alternative diagnosis like lymphoma.

Postcontrast CT demonstrates ring or nodular enhancement **(Figs. 42A to D)**. Ring enhancement is more common with central hypodensity. The rings are usually thin and smooth but may be thick and irregular especially in the larger lesions. Double-dose delayed technique (using 200 mL of intravenous contrast by bolus/drip infusion with delayed scanning at 1 hour) has been found to be extremely effective in detection of these lesions. Double-dose delayed technique permits maximal enhancement and the central portion of ring lesions of toxoplasma may fill in on delayed scans.

The radiologic appearance correlates well with the pathologic findings, with the central hypodensity corresponding to the region of avascular coagulative necrosis. The enhancing ring corresponds to the intermediate zone of intense inflammation and the peripheral zone may appear as edema on neuroimaging studies. Pathologic-radiologic correlation has revealed that the pathologic extent of these lesions is often greater than the area of contrast enhancement evident on CT.

MR imaging reveals multiple ring and nodular enhancing lesions with a predilection for the basal ganglia and the corticomedullary junction of the cerebral hemispheres. There is some amount of perilesional edema and mass effect. Multiplicity of the lesions is a characteristic imaging finding. On the T2-weighted images, a "concentric target sign" may be seen which is central T2 hypointensity surrounded by alternate concentric bands of hyper and hypointensity. A small enhancing nodule along the lesion margins constitutes an "eccentric target" sign on the post-contrast scans and is considered virtually diagnostic of

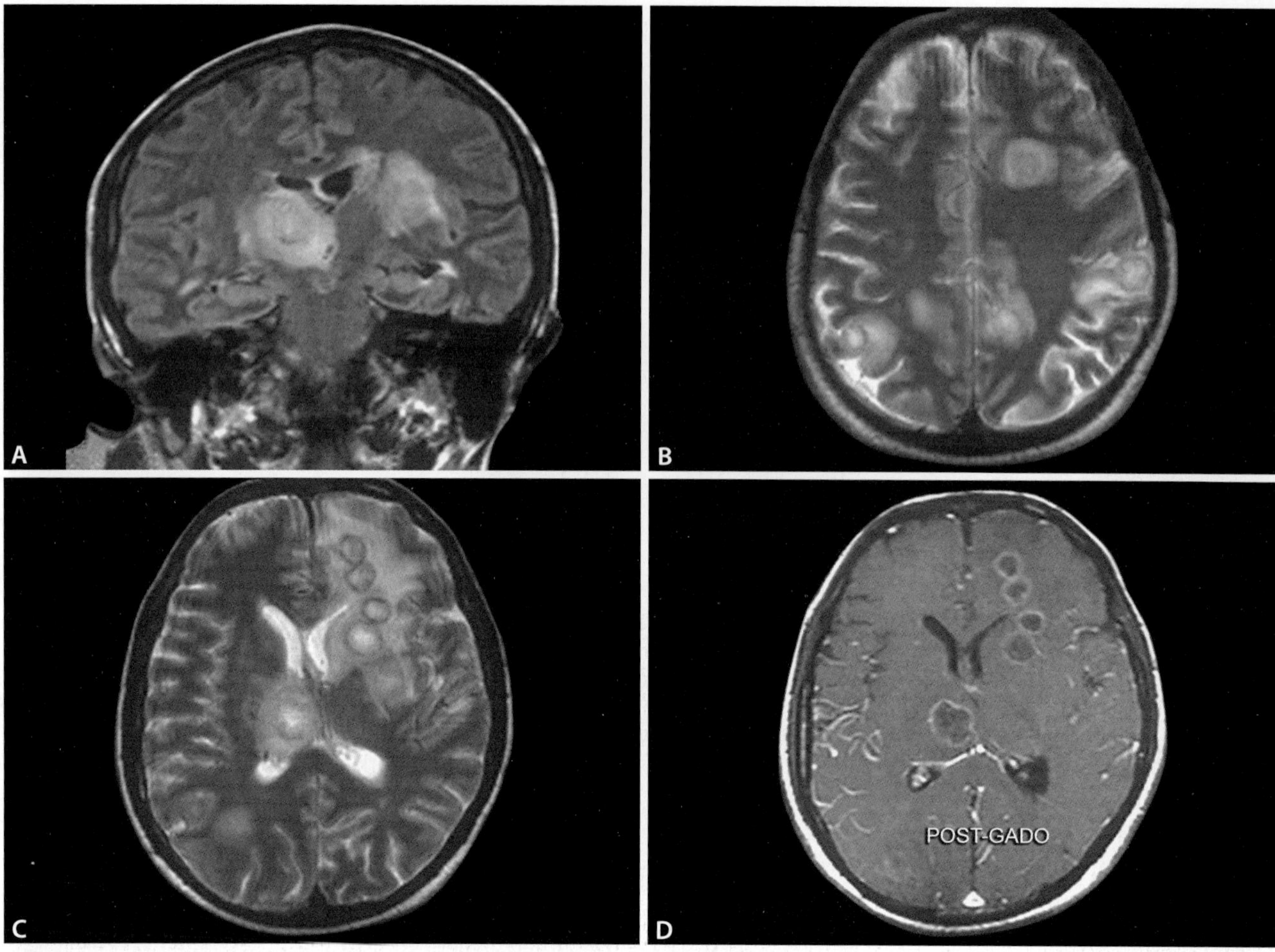

Figs. 42A to D: FLAIR coronal (A), T2W axial (B and C) MR images showing multiple lesions in bilateral basal ganglia, left frontoparietal region and right thalamus seen as isointense signal surrounded by a hypointense rim and high signal intensity edema giving the typical 'target' sign. Postcontrast T1W axial (D) MR image reveals ring or nodular enhancement in the lesions—toxoplasmosis.

toxoplasmosis[120] **(Figs. 43A to H)**. This sign is caused by a leash of inflammatory vessels entering the lesion. This sign is seen in 30% cases but is 95% specific.

Differentiation of Toxoplasmosis from CNS Lymphoma

It is important to differentiate between the two owing to the difference in treatment and prognosis. A periventricular location in contact with the ventricular/ependymal surface with evidence of subependymal spread and ventricular encasement favours the diagnosis of lymphoma while toxoplasmosis has a predilection for the basal ganglia and the corticomedullary junction. An "eccentric target" sign, absence of corpus callosal or leptomeningeal involvement and marked edema favour the diagnosis of toxoplasmosis while a T2 hypointensity favours the diagnosis of lymphoma. Lymphoma being highly cellular shows a restricted pattern of diffusion while toxoplasmosis does not.[121] On MR spectroscopy an elevated choline peak is seen in lymphomas while toxoplasmosis shows a suppression of all major metabolites with a lipid lactate peak owing to anaerobic glycolysis. An increased uptake on PET imaging favours the diagnosis of lymphoma over toxoplasmosis. Also toxoplasmosis responds to medical treatment while lymphoma does not. If toxoplasmosis is suspected on the basis of clinical and neuroimaging findings, anti-toxoplasma therapy should be given for 2–3 weeks as an empirical treatment. An interval decrease in the size of the lesion is considered to be a sufficient proof for the diagnosis and therapy to be continued. A stable or increasing size of lesion may indicate an alternative diagnosis like lymphoma. Also perfusion MR studies show a much higher regional cerebral blood volume in lymphoma as compared to toxoplasma lesions. The differences are summarized in **Table 4**.

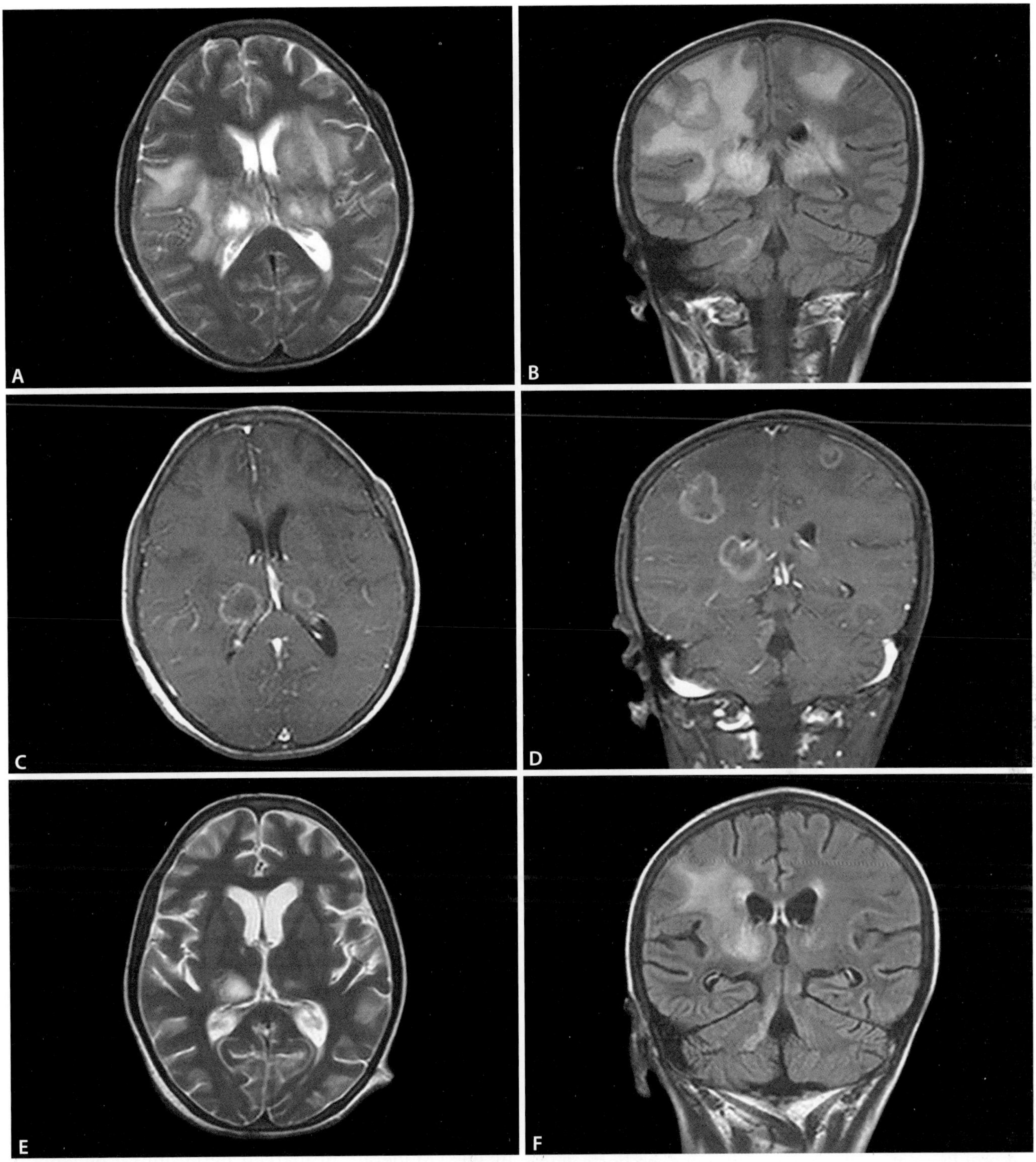

Figs. 43A to F

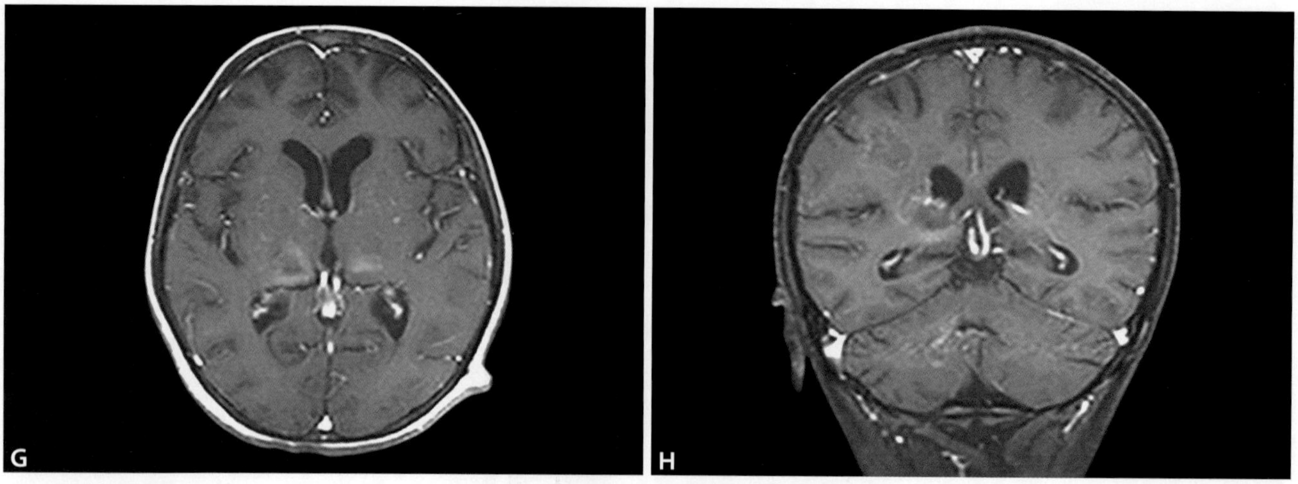

Figs. 43G and H

Figs. 43A to H: MR images in a case of toxoplasmosis before treatment (A to D) and after treatment (E to H) with sulpha drugs reveals a decrease in the number and size of lesions, a decrease in the amount of perilesional edema and degree of contrast enhancement. An 'eccentric target sign' is well seen in the pretreatment image (D) Toxoplasmosis.

Table 4: Differences between toxoplasmosis and CNS lymphoma.

Toxoplasmosis	*Lymphoma*
Predilection for basal ganglia and corticomedullary junction	Periventricular location in contact with ventricular/ ependymal lining
Lesions are T2 hyperintense	Lesions are T2 hypointense
Ring/nodular enhancement of lesions	Subependymal enhancement, ventricular encasement seen
Corpus callosum not involved	Corpus callosum usually involved
Concentric target or eccentric target signs seen	Absent
No restricted diffusion	Restricted diffusion on DWI
No uptake on PET	↑ uptake on PET imaging
High regional cerebral blood flow on perfusion imaging not seen	Higher regional cerebral blood flow on perfusion imaging seen
Lipid lactate peak on MRS	Choline peak on MRS
Responds to medical treatment	No response to medical treatment

HYDATID DISEASE

The causative organisms are *Echinococcus granulosus* and multilocularis. Humans are intermediate hosts with the definitive host being the dog. Human infection occurs by contact with the definitive host (dog) or by drinking or eating contaminated water or vegetables.

Hydatid disease involves the liver (75%) and the lungs (15–20%) most commonly. CNS involvement is rare and occurs in about 5% cases.[122]

Imaging

The cysts in *E. granulosus* are usually solitary, unilocular and located in the parietal lobe. On imaging, these are seen as large, unilocular cysts with well defined, smooth, thin wall. The cyst fluid is isointense to the CSF on all imaging pulse sequences **(Figs. 44A to D)**. No perilesional edema is seen. No contrast enhancement is usually seen unless the cyst becomes secondarily infected.[123] The capsule of the cyst is seen as a hypointense rim on the T2-weighted images surrounding the hyperintense lesion.[124]

Spinal hydatid cysts are seen in less than one percent of cases and are of five types—intramedullary, intradural, extramedullary, extradural, vertebral and paravertebral. The cysts may occur paravertebrally and then invade the vertebral column and spinal cord. Symptoms usually result from compression of the spinal cord or nerve roots.

E. Multilocularis grows by external budding causing progressive infiltration of the brain parenchyma with resultant multilobulated cystic structure. On imaging these are seen as heterogenous solid, partially solid or cystic masses with calcification. Owing to the calcification, these are hypointense on both T1- and T2-weighted images. Moderate to marked perilesionsal oedema is seen. The enhancement may be heterogenous, ring-like, nodular and cauliflower.[125] Thus oedema and calcification in the wall help it to be distinguished from *E. granulosus*. MR spectroscopy may reveal an elevated succinate level in addition to elevated acetate, glycine and lactate, thus differentiating it from neoplasms.[126] Also, the presence

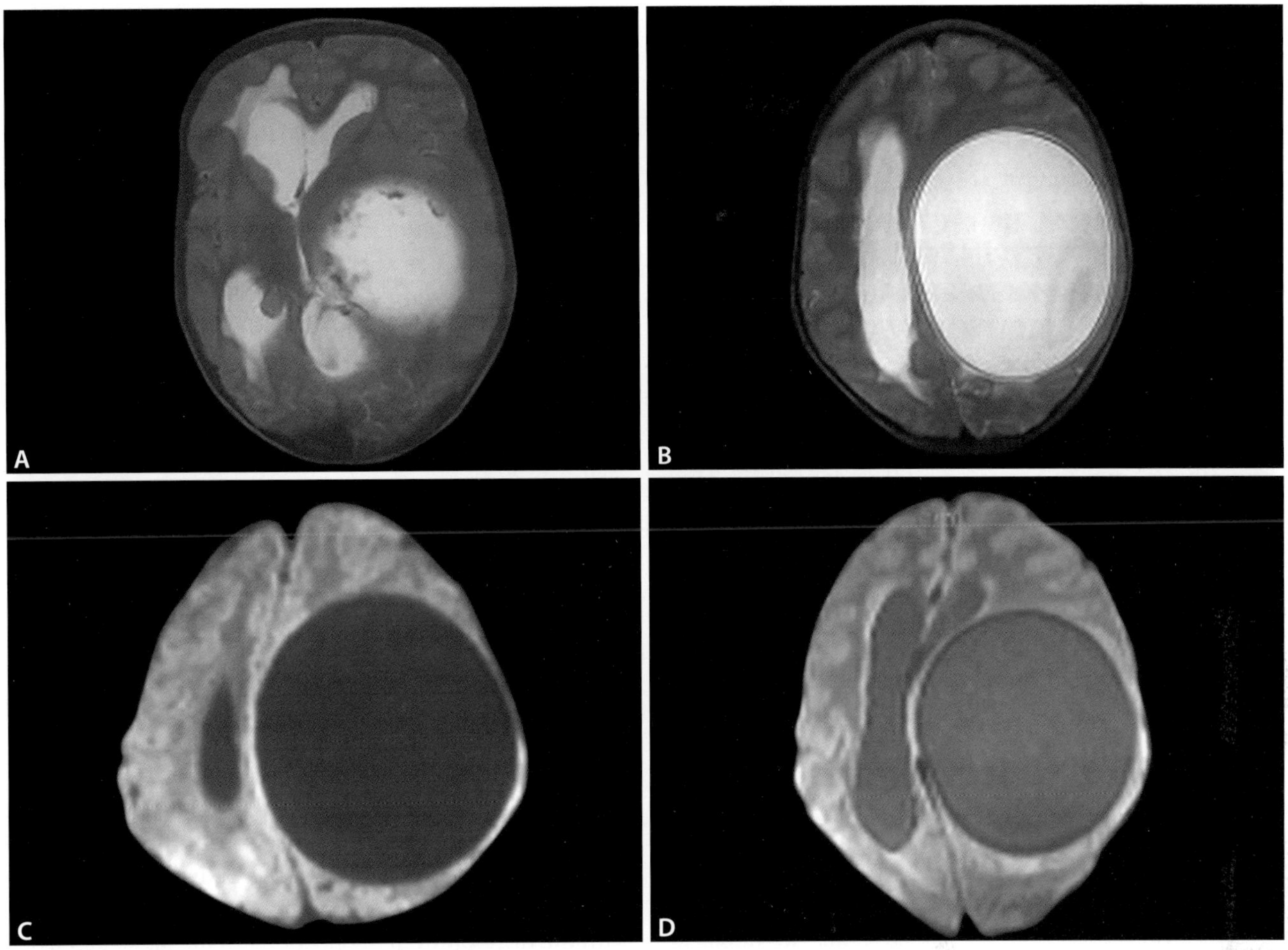

Figs. 44A to D: T2W axial (A and B), T1W axial (C) and proton density (D) MR images showing a large well-defined, smooth, thin walled, homogeneous cystic lesion isointense to cerebrospinal fluid on all pulse sequences with no significant edema. Few daughter cysts are seen in the periphery of the large cystic lesion—hydatid cyst.

of multiloculated cystic lesions in the liver help it to be differentiated from neoplastic lesions.

CEREBRAL MALARIA

Malaria is caused by the protozoan parasite *Plasmodium. Plasmodium falciparum* infection is one of the most deadly infections. Sequestration of infected erythrocytes in the microcirculation may cause cerebral malaria in 2% of the cases. This may manifest as encephalopathy or coma and is associated with a mortality rate of 15–25%.[127]

MR imaging may reveal cortical infarcts and non-specific white matter hyperintensity on T2-weighted imaging. T2 hyperintense lesions may be seen involving the splenium of the corpus callosum. Hemorrhagic infarctions and multiple punctate petechial hemorrhages may be seen at the gray-white matter junction or in the deep white matter.[128,129]

GRANULOMATOUS AMOEBIC ENCEPHALITIS

Amoeba are free living protozoa. Many of these organisms are non pathogenic but some may cause devastating infection in the CNS, e.g. *Acanthamoeba* and *Balamuthia* species.[130] These infections are seen in the immunocompromised patients and clinical presentation is with headache, altered mental state and focal neurologic deficits. Imaging findings are non specific and may mimic other encephalitis or acute disseminated encephalomyelitis or toxoplasmosis.[131]

PRIMARY AMOEBIC MENINGOENCEPHALITIS

Naegleria fowleri (brain-eating worm) is found in warm fresh water bodies and is thermophilic. Infection is acquired in humans via the nasal cavity following a swimming or diving activity.[132] It is extremely aggressive and usually results in death. Neuroimaging studies are non-specific and a very high index of suspicion is required for the diagnosis.

VIRAL INFECTIONS

HERPES SIMPLEX ENCEPHALITIS (HSV-1) ENCEPHALITIS/ACUTE INFECTIVE ENCEPHALITIS

HSV-1 is the cause of 95% of all herpetic encephalitis.[133] A fulminant haemorrhagic meningoencephalitis, it is the most common cause of fatal encephalitis. High grade fever, an altered mental state, diminished level of consciousness and focal neurologic deficits characterize the clinical picture.

HSV-1 occurs due to reactivation of latent infection. The trigeminal ganglion is the most common site of reactivation. A retrograde transmission of the infection along the trigeminal nerve to the brainstem results in pontine infection/rhomboencephalitis.

The herpes virus has a predilection for the inferomedial temporal lobes, the insular cortex and the cingulate gyrus.[134] There is a relative sparing of the basal ganglia, a finding that helps to distinguish this disease process from other encephalitis. The occipital cortex, external capsule and the cerebral convexity may also be involved. Infection is unilateral to begin with but soon involves the contralateral side to become a bilateral process. This "sequential bilaterality" is virtually diagnostic of herpes encephalopathy **(Figs. 45A and B)**.

Imaging

CT scan may show symmetric areas of hypodensity involving the limbic system, at times hemorrhagic foci may be seen. Hemorrhage seen in the appropriate clinical setting is highly suggestive of herpes infection.[135] MR images reveal areas of signal alteration in the temporal lobes, inferior frontal lobes, insular cortex and cingulate gyrus **(Figs. 46A to C)**. The signal alteration is seen as hypointense signal on T1 and hyperintense signal on T2-weighted images. There is usually involvement of both grey and white matter. The changes may be seen as early as 48 hours after the onset of symptoms. A gyriform pattern of enhancement seen on the postcontrast scans suggest disease progression.[136] Focal petechial hemorrhages are also better detected on MR imaging as areas of blooming on gradient echo sequences. MR is the modality of choice not only for an early diagnosis but also to monitor response to treatment in cases of herpes encephalitis.

Diffusion-weighted MR Imaging (DWI)

DWI may show the abnormalities much before the conventional MR images **(Figs. 47A to D)**. DWI may reveal a larger number of lesions and more extensive lesions than seen on conventional images and this modality can be used to monitor response to treatment. Facilitated diffusion with high ADC values is seen later consistent with the development of encephalomalacia.

MR Spectroscopy

A decrease in NAA levels and an increase in choline levels represents the loss of structural/functional activity

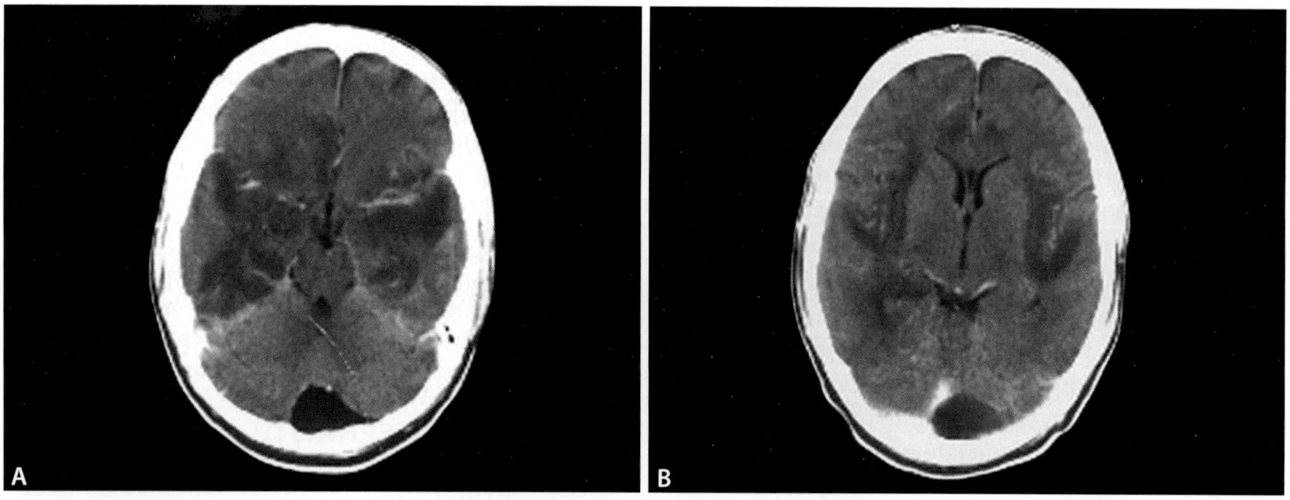

Figs. 45A and B: CECT axial scans of the cranium showing bilateral symmetric areas of hypodensity involving the inferomedial temporal lobes,insular cortex and the cingulate gyrus with sparing of the basal ganglia—herpes encephalitis.

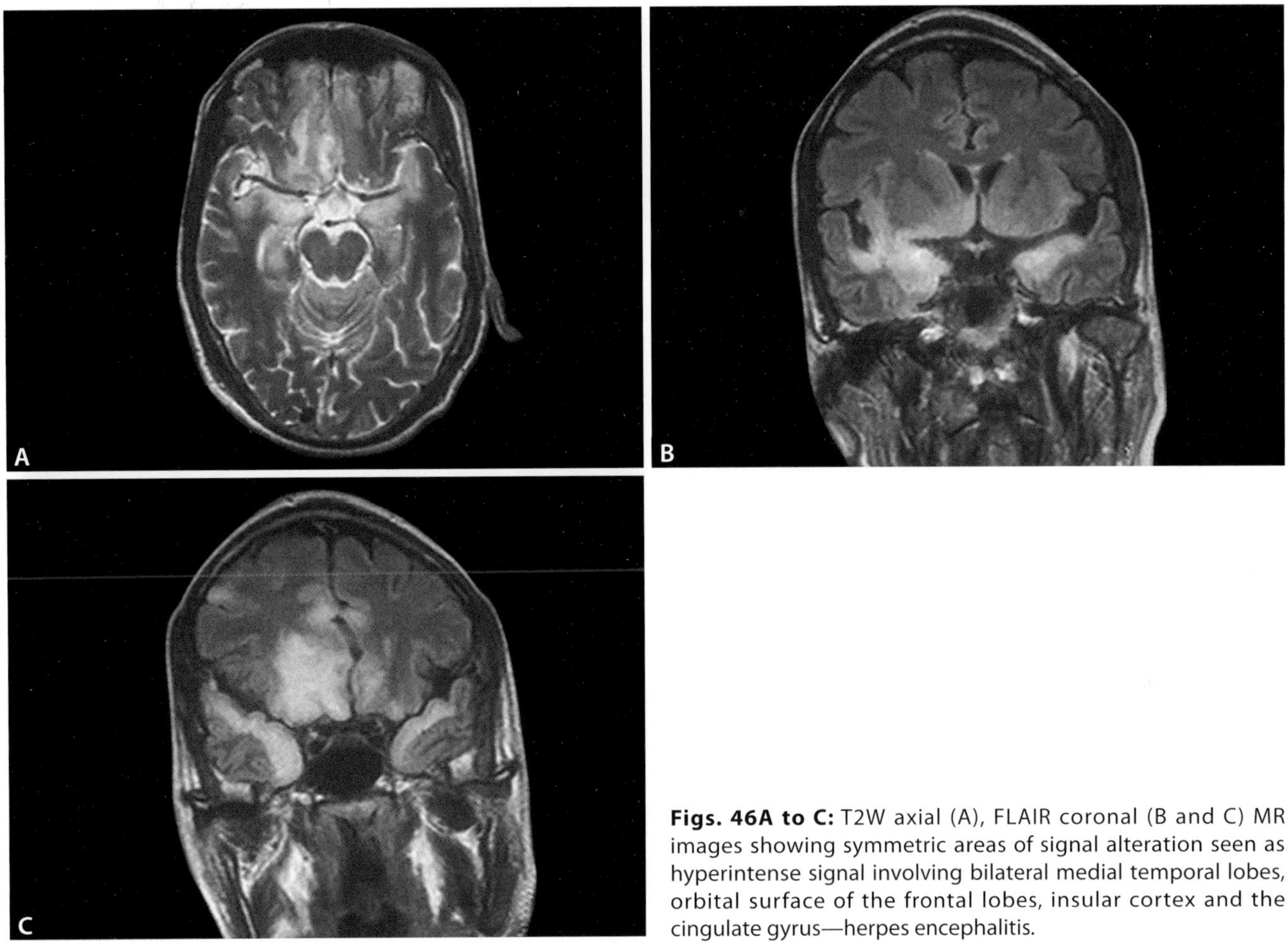

Figs. 46A to C: T2W axial (A), FLAIR coronal (B and C) MR images showing symmetric areas of signal alteration seen as hyperintense signal involving bilateral medial temporal lobes, orbital surface of the frontal lobes, insular cortex and the cingulate gyrus—herpes encephalitis.

of the neurons between 2–17 weeks after the onset of the disease. Spectroscopy can be used to predict progression and prognosticate the disease process. An increase of Cho/Cr along with a progressive decrease in NAA/Cr occurs in cases with neurological sequelae in the form of demyelination or neuronal dysfunction.

Differential Diagnosis

Limbic encephalitis has a more protracted and subacute onset (weeks to months). The imaging findings may be indistinguishable from herpes encephalitis. History of an extracranial primary carcinoma and neuronal antibodies in the CSF and serum favor the diagnosis of limbic encephalitis.

HHV-6 encephalitis—This shows an exclusive involvement of one or both medial temporal lobes. Extratemporal involvement and petechial hemorrhages as seen with HSE are not seen with this form.[136,137]

MOLLARET MENINGITIS

It is a rare syndrome seen in young females caused by herpes simplex type 2 virus. It is characterized by recurrent episodes of aseptic meningitis with each episode presenting with fulminant high grade fever, severe headache and signs of meningitis. It can be diagnosed by polymerase chain reaction analysis of CSF. No specific imaging findings are described.[138]

VARICELLA ZOSTER ENCEPHALITIS

Varicella Zoster virus which causes chickenpox (Varicella) and shingles (Zoster) can involve the CNS. The most common manifestation is meningitis with encephalitis being the second most common. In children this infection may present with acute cerebellar ataxia. Diffuse cerebellar swelling with hyperintensity on FLAIR images may be seen on imaging in children. MR may show multiple deep white matter hyperintensities in cases of vasculopathy. Granulomatous angitis involving small cerebral arteries may occur. Cerebral infarction and aneurysm formation may be seen.[139]

JAPANESE ENCEPHALITIS (JE)

JE usually occurs as epidemics in Asian countries specially during the summer season. The clinical presentation is

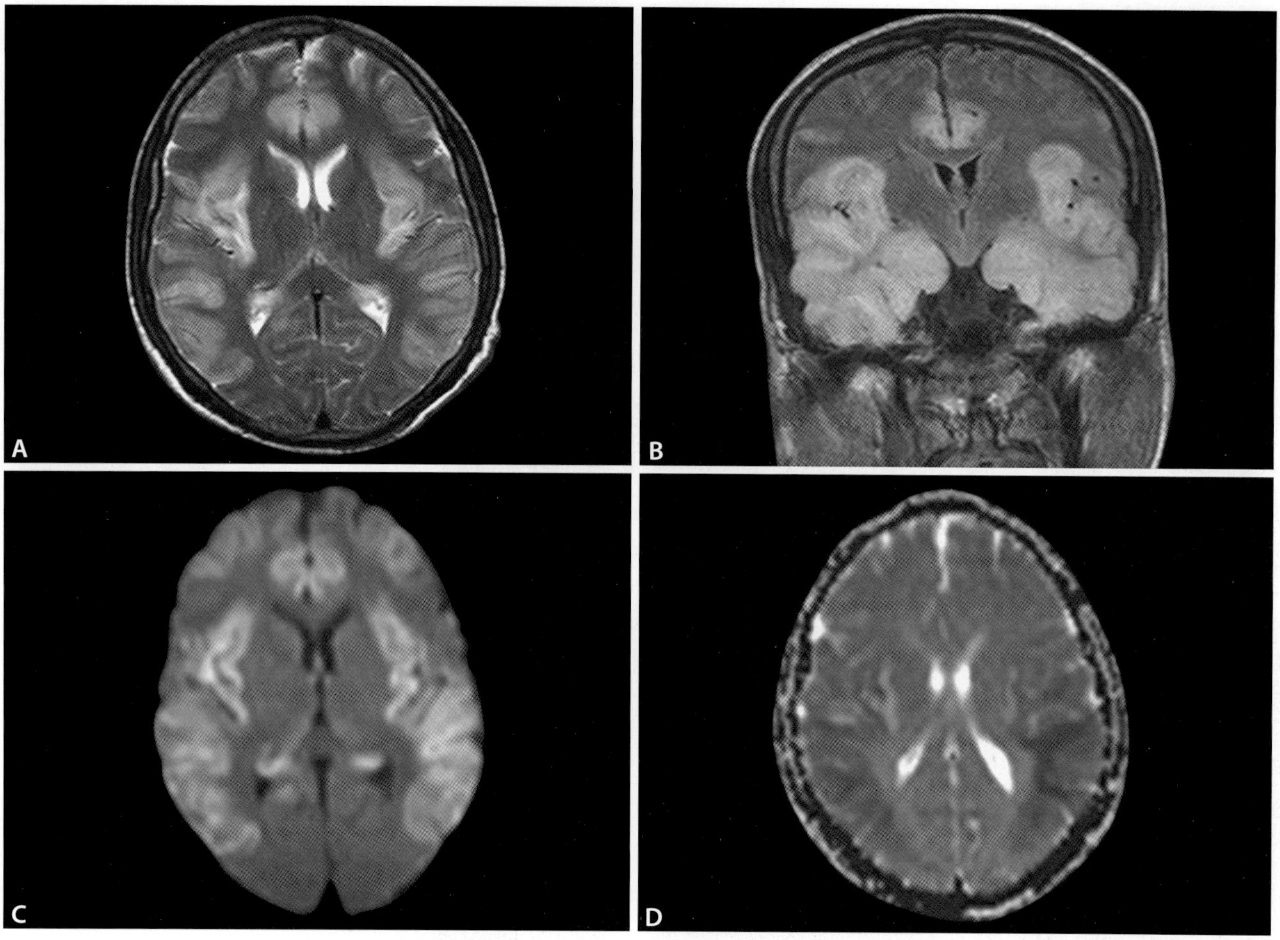

Figs. 47A to D: Axial T2W (A) and FLAIR coronal; (B) MR images showing diffuse gyral swelling and areas of signal alteration involving the cingulate gyrus, bilateral insular cortex, bilateral medial temporal lobes and parieto-occipital regions. The areas show evidence of restricted diffusion; (C and D)—herpes encephalitis.

fever, dystonia, tremors, rigidity, seizures often progressing to coma. Seizures are more common in the pediatric population. The disease is a diffuse meningoencephalitis involving both gray and white matter of the cerebral hemispheres, brainstem, cerebellum, basal ganglia and thalamus. The spinal cord may also be diffusely enlarged particularly the anterior and lateral column.

Imaging

Bilateral and symmetric areas of signal alteration are seen in the thalamus and basal ganglia. This is seen as a hyperintense signal on T2W images and hypointene signal on T1W images. Involvement of the basal ganglia and thalami may occur as an isolated finding without involvement of other regions[140] **(Figs. 48A to C)**. Isolated involvement of the substantia nigra may also be seen. Rarely foci of hemorrhage may occur in the involved regions. Minimal or no enhancement is seen on the post contrast scans. MR spectroscopy shows a decrease in NAA peak, an elevated choline peak at 3.22 ppm and a lactate peak at 1.33 ppm. A definitive diagnosis is established on serology by demonstrating a fourfold rise in antibody titre. However, presence of lesions in the thalamus, basal ganglia and substantia nigra in a patient presenting with encephalitic illness from an endemic zone of JE strongly suggests the diagnosis.

A co-existence of neurocysticercosis and JE has been noted.[141] The reason behind this has been stated to be multiple common factors in the etiopathogenesis of the two disorders. Pigs are the intermediate hosts of *Taenia solium* and act as amplifiers of the JE virus. Common endemicity of the two illnesses caused by poor socioeconomic status, poor hygienic conditions as well as malnutrition is the other factor. The changes of JE have been found to be more pronounced on the side of the cyst and hence NCC may act as an amplifier/modulator of JE.

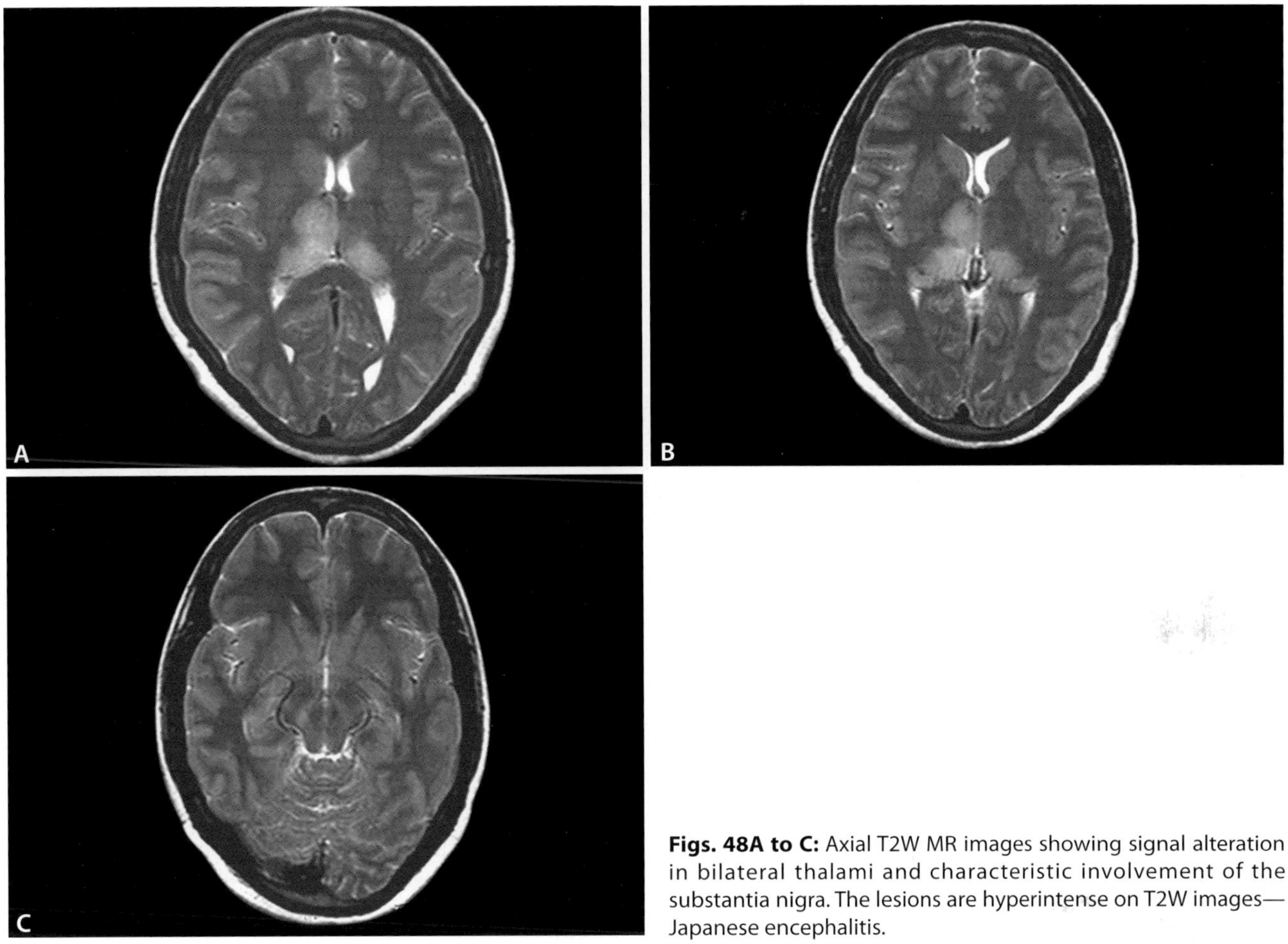

Figs. 48A to C: Axial T2W MR images showing signal alteration in bilateral thalami and characteristic involvement of the substantia nigra. The lesions are hyperintense on T2W images—Japanese encephalitis.

Japanese encephalitis needs to be differentiated from herpes encephalitis because antiviral therapy is very effective for herpes while treatment for JE is usually supportive **(Figs. 49A to C)**.

MEASLES ENCEPHALITIS

Measles is caused by the rubeola virus and is an acute highly contagious infection. Three syndromes have been described

Acute Measles Encephalitis (AME)

It is an autoimmune process and presents as renewed fever in patients recovering from measles. A wide variety of neurological symptoms—seizures, altered mental status and focal neurologic signs may be seen during the convalescence period. Though the measles virus is absent during this phase demyelination, hemorrhage, necrosis and vascular damage characterize this phase.

Subacute Sclerosing Panencephalitis (SSPE)

SSPE develops secondary to a previous measles infection early in childhood. The virus remains dormant and becomes active after a decade or so to manifest as SSPE which is invariably fatal.[142] The onset is with mild alterations in behavior in a previously healthy child, followed by myoclonic jerks which become increasingly frequent followed by dementia and coma. The average age of onset is from 9–13 years. An immature immune system that fails to destroy the virus completely has been stated to be the cause for the dormant partially degraded virus that remains in the CNS.

On MR imaging the white matter lesions of SSPE are seen as a predominant involvement of the subcortical white matter with a predilection for the posterior parietal, occipital and temporal region. Lesions may also be seen in the brainstem and cerebellum. The lesions are seen as hypointense signal on T1 and hyperintense signal on

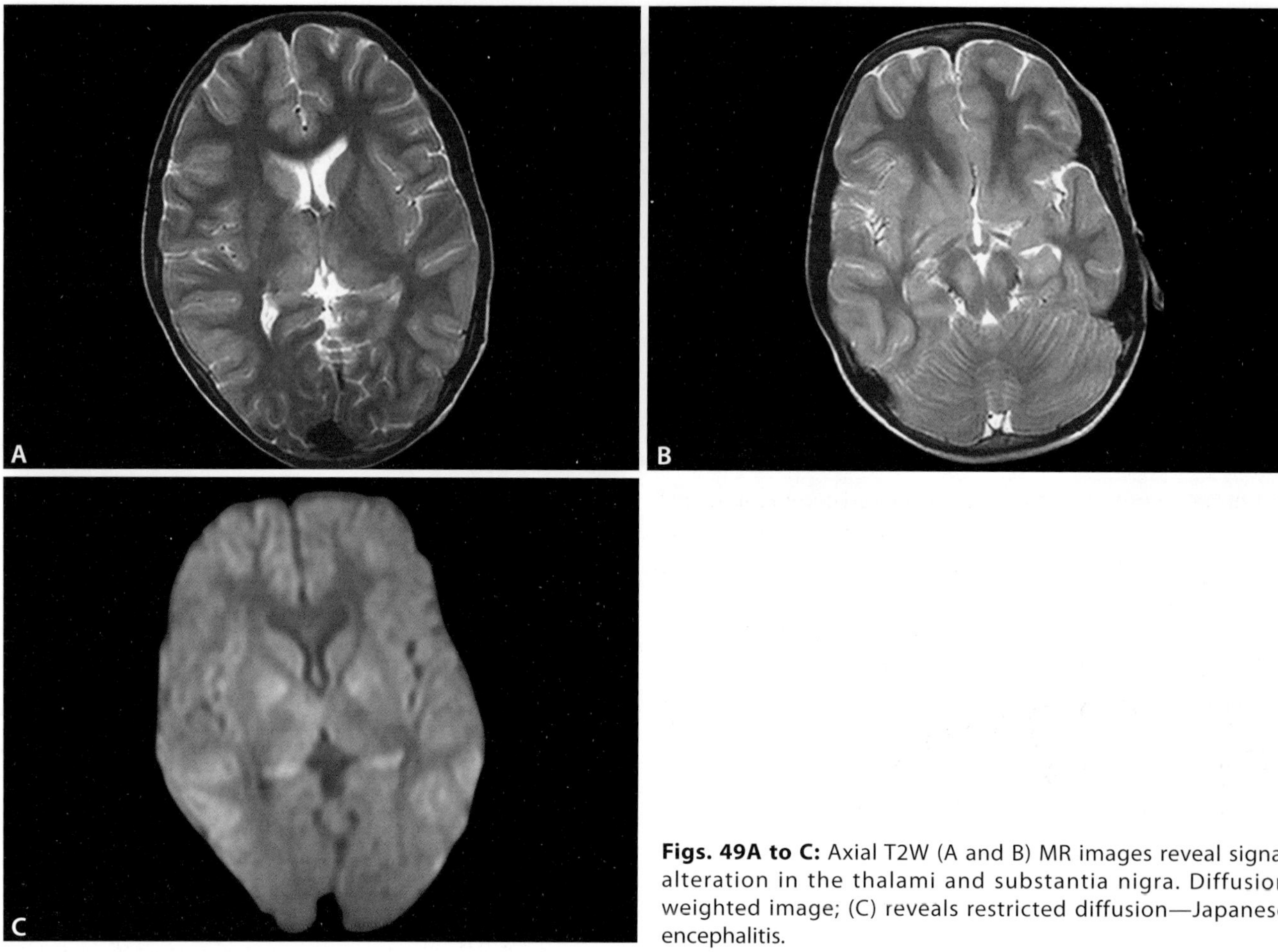

Figs. 49A to C: Axial T2W (A and B) MR images reveal signal alteration in the thalami and substantia nigra. Diffusion weighted image; (C) reveals restricted diffusion—Japanese encephalitis.

T2W images. Diffuse atrophy of the cortex, atrophy of the brainstem and ventricular dilatation may be seen. In long standing disease and severe disease, involvement of the basal ganglia may be seen.

Subacute Measles Encephalitis

This form occurs in an immunocompromised patient with a latent period of 1–7 months. The onset is subacute with a more rapid evolution. However seizures rather than myoclonic jerks is what differentiates SME from SSPE.

MRI shows areas of signal alteration involving the occipital cortical and subcortical regions with some enhancement on the post contrast study.

RABIES ENCEPHALOMYELITIS

It is a fulminant disease and is invariably fatal once clinical symptoms develop. It is caused by a neurotropic RNA virus, the virus being abundant in the saliva of the infected animal which is usually the dog. The virus gets deposited in the bite wounds, replicates in the muscle tissues of the wound and then infects motor neurons. It then gains entry into the CNS via retrograde flow.[143] The rabies virus has a predilection for the brainstem, thalami and hippocampi. An ill-defined hyperintense signal may be seen on the T2W images in these regions. No enhancement or haemorrhage is seen, features that differentiate it from other viral encephalitis.

RASMUSSEN'S ENCEPHALITIS

Rasmussen's encephalitis is a childhood disease. A viral infection or autoimmune disease involving glutamate receptors with glutamine toxicity have been postulated in the etiopathogenesis. The child presents with severe epilepsy and progressive neurologic deficits. Seizures are usually of the partial motor seizure type and tend to be intractable. The intractable nature of the seizure may make hemispherectomy necessary, if medical therapy is ineffective. The disease tends to affect one hemisphere although bilateral involvement has also been reported.

Early in the disease process, CT and MRI findings may be normal. MRI may reveal focal and progressive atrophy of a hemisphere and hyperintensity in white matter and putamen on T2-weighted images. PET imaging using FDG-18 may show decreased hemispheric activity.

PRION INFECTIONS—CREUTZFELDT-JAKOB DISEASE

Creutzfeldt-Jakob Disease (CJD) is caused by a slow unconventional virus or prion. Prions are proteinaceous infectious particles that contain little or no nucleic acid and evoke no inflammatory response. The age of onset is between 40–80 years with survival being less than a year from the onset of symptoms. Patients typically present with dementia accompanied by confusion and cerebellar ataxia.

CJD is a human spongiform encephalopathy as spongiform changes are seen in the cortical and subcortical gray matter histologically. There is loss of neurons and gliosis. White matter is relatively spared, rarely Wallerian degeneration may be seen. No inflammatory changes are seen.

Imaging Findings

CT of these patients is either normal or diffuse cerebral atrophy may be seen. MRI shows bilateral and symmetric areas of signal alteration in the corpus striatum, that is the putamen and caudate nucleus. No mass effect and no enhancement of the lesion is seen. Lesions may also be seen in the thalamus, basal ganglia, cortical gray matter and occipital lobes. Diffusion weighted images help in an early diagnosis as these show the involved regions as areas of restricted diffusion. DWI has emerged as the most sensitive sequence for the diagnosis of human prion disease. The combined use of FLAIR and DWI improves diagnostic accuracy to 90%.[144] The findings include a restricted diffusion in the cortex, caudate nucleus, putamen and thalamus with a distribution pattern that does not correspond to arterial circulation.[145] Diffuse cerebral atrophy is another characteristic imaging finding that ensues, so rapidly as to result in the formation of subdural hygromas. MR spectroscopy shows decreased levels of NAA reflecting neuronal loss.

ACQUIRED IMMUNODEFICIENCY SYNDROME (AIDS) AND ITS RELATED CNS INFECTIONS

Human immunodeficiency virus (HIV) is a retrovirus that causes AIDS. Two subtypes are recognized HIV-1 and 2. HIV is a neurotropic virus and the commonest pathogen in AIDS patients. Over 40% of untreated AIDS patients develop neurologic manifestations of the disease either by direct invasion of the CNS by HIV virus or by several opportunistic infections like toxoplasmosis, cytomegalovirus, cryptococcosis, progressive multifocal leukoencephalopathy, etc.

CNS infection in AIDS includes:[146]

- HIV encephalitis—most common (60%).
- Toxoplasmosis—commonest opportunistic infection (20–40%).
- Cryptococcosis (5%).
- Progressive multifocal leukoencephalopathy (PML) (1–4%).

Others:

- Tuberculosis (2–18%)
- Neurosyphilis (1–3%)
- Varicella zoster (< 1%)
- CMV encephalitis

HIV ENCEPHALITIS

It is the commonest CNS infection seen in AIDS patients. AIDS dementia complex is seen in 15–20% of HIV patients inspite of highly active antiretroviral therapy (HAART) and usually occurs with CD4 counts of less than 200 cells/µl.[147] it manifests clinically as a progressive dementia characterized by cognitive, behavioural and motor deterioration culminating in death if left untreated.

The lesions are present in the white matter to begin with and progress to involve the cortex and gray matter. Brainstem, cerebellum and spinal cord may also be involved. Demyelination, gliosis, myelin pallor, infiltration with multinucleate giant cells may be seen on pathology.

Imaging

CT may show diffuse cerebral atrophy only. MR is more sensitive in detecting the lesions. MR not only shows diffuse cerebral atrophy but bilateral and symmetric areas of signal alteration involving the deep periventricular white matter and centrum semiovale. The signal alteration is in the form of diffuse, symmetric, confluent areas of hypointensity on T1W and hyperintensity on the T2W images[148] **(Figs. 50A and B)**. No mass effect or contrast enhancement is seen. Gray matter is typically spared initially. The hyperintense lesions correspond to foci of demyelination and vacuolation and the extent of the lesions is proportionate to the neurologic deterioration seen. The frontal lobes are the most common sites to be affected and FLAIR sequence is excellent in the depiction of white matter disease.

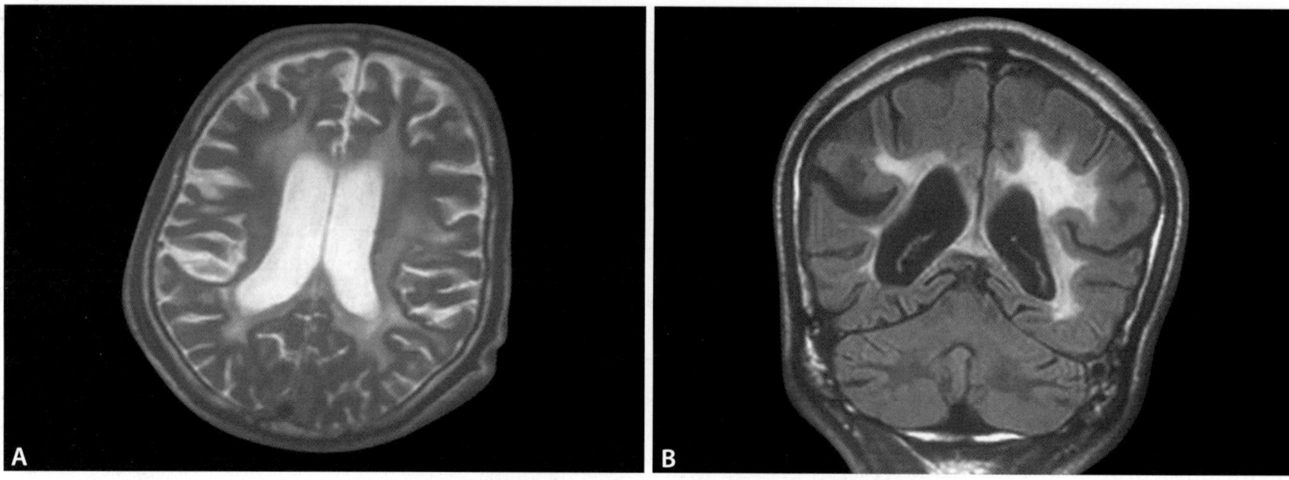

Figs. 50A and B: Axial T2W (A) and FLAIR coronal; (B) MR images showing a bilateral diffuse periventricular white matter hyperintensity with sparing of the gray matter with diffuse cerebral atrophy—HIV encephalitis.

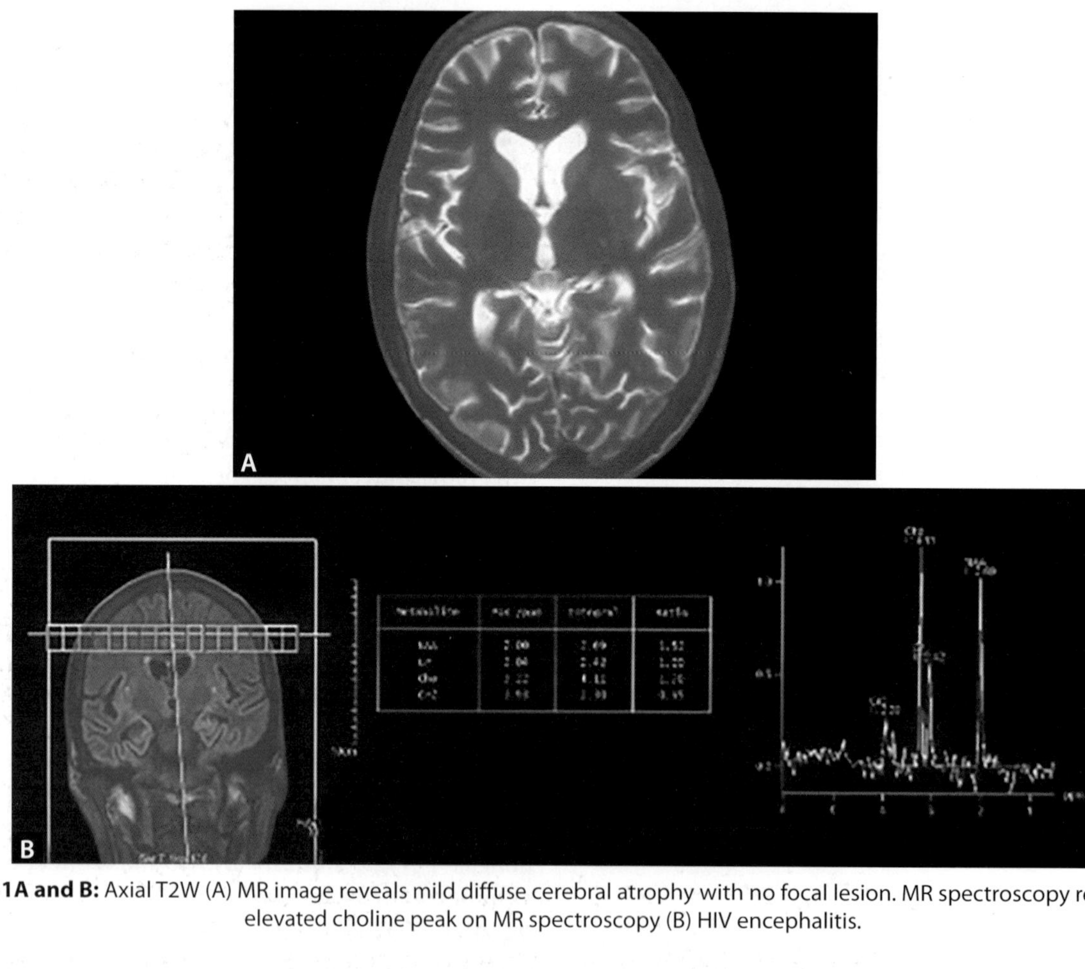

Figs. 51A and B: Axial T2W (A) MR image reveals mild diffuse cerebral atrophy with no focal lesion. MR spectroscopy reveals an elevated choline peak on MR spectroscopy (B) HIV encephalitis.

MR spectroscopy may reveal metabolic abnormality much before the morphological changes in the form of a decreased NAA and elevated choline peak reflecting neuronal loss and presence of gliosis, macrophages and lymphocytes[149] **(Figs. 51A and B)**. Elevated myoinositol (MI) may be seen early in infection and occurs due to the gliosis. MRS is helpful not only in an early diagnosis of HIV encephalitis but also in monitoring response to treatment.

Magnetization transfer ratio is abnormal in asymptomatic patients and hence can also be used for an early diagnosis. SPECT has also been used in patients suspected of HIV encephalitis, and shows uptake defects in the brain.

Diffusion tensor imaging demonstrates a decrease in both fractional anisotropy and mean diffusivity in the cerebral white matter. This correlates with the neurological findings and DTI picks up changes much before changes are seen on conventional MR.[150]

PROGRESSIVE MULTIFOCAL LEUKOENCEPHALOPATHY (PML)

Earlier PML was stated to be seen in immunodeficient states like lymphoproliferative disorders, non-tropical sprue, Whipple's disease, autoimmune disorders and those treated with chemotherapy. However, the strong association of PML with AIDS has now been recognized and 55–85% cases of PML are now attributable to AIDS alone.[151] PML occurs in about 50% of patients of AIDS.

A papovavirus is the causative agent. The JC (John Cunningham) virus, a human polyomavirus, belongs to the papova family of CNS viruses and causes a relentlessly progressive demyelinating disorder. The virus establishes a latency in the bone marrow, kidneys and the CNS becoming reactivated with profound immunosuppressed states or various immunosuppressive drugs such as efalizumab for psoriasis and natalizumab for multiple sclerosis. PML develops in patients of HIV when the CD4 counts are usually below 100.

The target cell for the JC virus is the oligodendrocyte. Cytolytic destruction causes loss of myelin as the primary function of the oligodendrocyte is to form and maintain the myelin sheath. Electron microscopy reveals intranuclear inclusions within the oligodendrocyte corresponding to the JC virus particle (called the spaghetti and meatball appearance), foci of demyelination which enlarge and coalesce over time.[152]

Clinical features of PML are loss of memory, altered mental status, cognitive and speech disturbances, personality change, seizures, headache, vertigo and aphasia. Death occurs within a year of the onset of symptoms.

Imaging

MR is more sensitive than CT in the detection of PML lesions specially for the posterior fossa lesions. The extent and number of lesions are better picked on MR than CT scans. Solitary/multifocal well-demarcated asymmetric lesions are usually seen which are hypointense on T1 and hyperintense on T2-weighted images. It is the subcortical white matter that is predominantly involved with sparing of the deep periventricular white matter **(Fig. 52)**. The lesions become more confluent with disease progression. No mass effect or contrast enhancement is seen. Rarely a faint and peripheral enhancement may be seen.[153] PML lesions usually involve the posterior fossa which is involved in about one third cases with the most common site being the middle cerebellar peduncles. The subcortical lesions follow the gray-white matter interface giving rise to a "scalloped appearance"

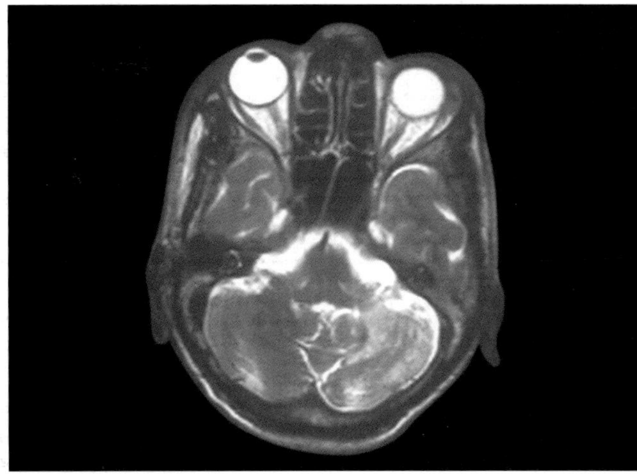

Fig. 52: Axial T2W image in a HIV patient shows a predominantly subcortical lesion in the posterior fossa with no mass effect and along the gray-white matter interface—PML.

The PML lesions need to be differentiated from HIV encephalitis.[152,153] While HIV encephalitis is usually bilateral and symmetrical, PML is multifocal and asymmetric. HIV encephalitis involves the deep periventricular white matter while PML lesions are subcortical in location. "Scalloped" appearance and clear demarcations of the lesions on a T1 weighted image favours the diagnosis of PML. HIV encephalitis presents with global cognitive disturbances while PML presents with a focal motor or sensory deficit. PML shows a marked reduction in the MT ratio as compared to HIV encephalitis which is useful in differentiating between the two **(Table 5)**.

In a minority of patients with PML, the institution of HAART can precipitate an immune reconstitution inflammatoty response (PML-IRIS) following recovery of the immune function.[154] PML-IRIS is an acute inflammatory response at the site of the CNS lesions and results in a worsening of the neurological symptoms. Lesions of PML-IRIS may show mass effect and heterogenous enhancement. Thus it is important to consider the clinical context before ruling out PML on seeing an enhancing lesion.

Table 5: Differences between HIV encephalitis and progressive multifocal leukoencephalopathy (PML).

HIV encephalitis	*PML*
Presents with global cognitive disturbances	Presents with a focal motor/ sensory deficit
Bilateral and symmetric	Multifocal and asymmetric
Deep periventricular white matter predominantly involved	Subcortical white matter predominantly involved
Not well-defined/sharply defined on T1W images	Well-defined and sharply marginated on T1W images
Scalloped appearance not seen	Scalloped appearance of lesions
Mild reduction of MT ratio	Marked reduction of MT ratio due to its demyelinating nature

Diffusion-weighted imaging of PML lesions shows a core of low signal intensity with high ADC values while the periphery has a high signal on DWI with low ADC values suggesting restricted diffusion at the more leading edges of the lesion. DWI may thus be used not only for diagnosis but also for monitoring response to HAART and may predict the risk of PML-IRIS.[155,156]

MR spectroscopy demonstrates decreased NAA, increased choline, increased lactate more in the core of the lesion than the leading edge of the lesion where the degree of neuronal loss is less advanced.

NEUROSYPHILIS

The causative organism is Treponema pallidum. It can enter the CNS during primary or secondary syphilitic infection with neurosyphilis developing in 5–10% of untreated cases.[157] The disease became rare after the introduction of penicillin but there has been an emergence again due to the AIDS pandemic. The latent period for different types of syphilis is different. It is <2 years for meningeal, 5–7 years for vascular, 10–20 years for general paresis and 15–20 years for tabes dorsalis. The onset is much earlier in patients with HIV and early forms (meningeal, vascular) may predominate over late forms. The clinical manifestations may range from asymptomatic to headache, confusion, cranial nerve palsies, dementia and focal neurological deficits.

A positive CSF VDRL is specific for neurosyphilis, not very sensitive while a CSF antibody testing is less specific but very sensitive. Histopathology reveals arteritis of the medium and large vessels (Huebner's arteritis). The MCA territory and the perforating vessels are the most commonly involved. Gummas which are granulomas with central necrosis and non-specific white matter lesions may be seen.

Imaging

The imaging findings depend on the form of the disease. Syphilitic meningitis may be thick and nodular like other granulomatous diseases. Vascular neurosyphilis is characterized by medium and large vessel infarcts seen as hyperintense areas showing restricted diffusion in the MCA territory or in the basal ganglia and brainstem because of perforating vessel disease. Angiographic findings may show alternating stenosis and dilatations of vessels within the circle of Willis giving them a beaded appearance. Non-specific white matter changes may be seen as hyperintense foci on T2-weighted images in the deep periventricular and subcortical white matter.

Syphilitic cerebral gummas are usually seen as cortical or dural based mass lesions isointense on T1 and hyperintense on T2 W images mimicking meningioma and dural based metastasis. On contrast administration homogenous enhancement of the lesions may be seen with focal meningeal enhancement adjacent to the lesion. Surrounding vasogenic edema with or without mass effect is seen.[158]

Other findings include leptomeningeal enhancement and cranial neuritis typically of the second and eighth cranial nerves. Bilateral involvement of the medial temporal lobes mimicking herpes encephalitis has also been described.

CYTOMEGALOVIRUS ENCEPHALITIS/ CMV ENCEPHALITIS

Cytomegalovirus is a herpes virus that lies latent in the majority of the population and gets reactivated when the host defense mechanisms are weak. Patients with AIDS (CD4 < 50) and those with renal transplant are at the maximum risk of opportunistic infection.[159] Neurologic manifestations may be acute or chronic meningoencephalitis, cranial neuropathies, vasculitis, retinitis, myelitis, brachial plexus neuropathy and peripheral neuropathy. The risk of developing encephalitis increases 10 fold in patients with CMV retinitis. The infection is often unrecognized or subclinical in AIDS patients and CMV often co-exists with other lesions like toxoplasmosis and cryptococcosis.

Two forms of CMV encephalitis are recognized-microglial nodular encephalitis and ventriculoencephalitis. The microglial nodular encephalitis has an extremely rapid and quick course, causes cranial nerve palsies, disorientation and serum electrolyte imbalance such as hyponatremia. The cytomegalovirus ventriculoencephalitis form presents with confusion and lethargy which has a progressive downward course resulting in coma and death in a matter of weeks. This form is a subacute necrotizing infection of the ependyma and subependyma.

The pathologic hallmark of CMV is the "owl's eye", an enlarged cell with a distended nucleus. The cell contains viral inclusion bodies and is surrounded by a halo giving a characteristic appearance.

Imaging

CT is not sensitive in the detection of CMV encephalitis and may show atrophy with low attenuation areas in the periventricular white matter. MR is more sensitive in detecting the changes and may show focal or diffuse areas of high signal on T2W images in the periventricular white matter similar to HIV encephalopathy. An ependymal T2 hyperintensity accompanied with an ependymal and subependymal enhancement on the post-contrast scans is suggestive of CMV infection. Diffusion weighted images may reveal a restricted pattern of diffusion along the ependyma and subependyma which again is diagnostic.[160] A thickened enhancing choroid/retina seen on the fat suppressed post-contrast MR images is suggestive of CMV retinitis which occurs in about 20–40% of the AIDS population.

IMMUNE RECONSTITUTION INFLAMMATORY SYNDROME (IRIS)

This is a T-cell mediated encephalitis that occurs in the setting of treated HIV or autoimmune disease like multiple sclerosis. Several different pathogens have been identified in the setting of IRIS. The most common are JC virus (PML-IRIS), tuberculosis (TB-IRIS) and fungal infections especially cryptoccus (crypto IRIS). There may be a natalizumab associated PML IRIS in patients of multiple sclerosis. Two forms are recognized:

- *Unmasking IRIS*: This occurs when a previously unrecognized opportunistic infection manifests with antiretroviral therapy.
- *Paradoxical IRIS*: This occurs when a patient who has been treated for a recent opportunistic infection deteriorates after initiation of antiretroviral therapy.

The most common presentation of neuro IRIS is clinical deterioration inspite of rising CD4 counts and lower viral loads in a newly treated HIV patient. Patients with neuro IRIS may die within days to weeks, the mortality from PML-IRIS being more than 40%.[161]

Imaging

TB IRIS patients may develop florid TB pseudoabscesses (TB gone wild) and extensive enhancements in the basal cisterns. Bizarre looking parenchymal masses and progressively enlarging enhancing lesions are suggestive of PML-IRIS. This condition needs to be differentiated from non-IRIS associated opportunistic infection as IRIS requires steroids to halt the inflammatory process while non IRIS opportunistic infections require immune restoration.[162] Contrast enhancement with mass effect is highly suggestive of IRIS and should be kept in mind in a patient of PML who shows sudden deterioration following HAART therapy.

DIFFERENTIAL DIAGNOSIS OF RING ENHANCING LESIONS IN THE BRAIN

Various CNS infections, such as an abscess, tuberculoma, neurocysticercus, toxoplasma, cryptococcomas present as ring enhancing lesions. Various other lesions like metastasis, demyelinating plaque, lymphoma also present as ring enhancing lesions in the brain parenchyma. The differential of ring enhancing lesions in the brain are enumerated in **Table 6**.

CONGENITAL INFECTIONS

Congenital infections, as the name implies, are infections acquired in utero through the transplacental route or during birth. Infections acquired during the first 4 weeks of life are called neonatal infections. TORCH is an acronym for the congenital infections—Toxoplasmosis, Others (Syphillis, HIV), Rubella, Cytomegalovirus (CMV) and Herpes simplex virus (HSV) type 2. While others occur via the transplacental route, herpes is most commonly an ascending infection.

TOXOPLASMOSIS

Congenital toxoplasmosis occurs when infection is acquired antenatally. Transplacental infection rates increase with increasing trimester with the infection rate being 20% in the first trimester and 60% in the third trimester.[164] Hydrocephalus, bilateral chorioretinitis and intracranial calcifications form the typical triad found in infants with congenital toxoplasma encephalitis. Mortality rates range from 1 to 5% and children with neurologic symptoms at birth who survive usually have long-term sequelae including developmental delay and seizures.

Toxoplasmosis infection is multifocal and scattered. US, CT and MR scans most often demonstrate calcifications that can involve the periventricular regions, basal ganglia or cerebral cortex **(Figs. 53A and B)**. The size of the calcification has been correlated with the duration of infection. A larger size of the calcification is seen in

Table 6: Ring-enhancing lesions in the brain parenchyma: Differential diagnosis.[163]

Differential diagnosis	CT	MRI							PET
		T1	T2	Post-contrast	DW1	ADC	MRS	MT Ratio	
IMMUNOCOMPETENT									
Neurocysticercosis	Thin regular ring enhancement with eccentric dot sign	Core is hypointense	Core hyperintense with hypointense rim	Ring enhancement, smooth outline	Core dark	High	Variable	Higher due to protein and amino acid	No increased uptake
Tuberculoma with central liquefaction	Irregular outline of ring enhancement	Core is hypointense	Core is hyperintense with hypointense rim	Ring enhancement, irregular outline	Bright due to restriction	Low	Lipid peak	Lower	No increased uptake
Pyogenic brain abscess	Ring-enhancing lesion with thinner medial/ventricular margin, smooth thin rim, satellite lesions and perilesional edema	Hypointense	Hyperintense	Smooth, thin ring enhancing lesion with thinner medial margin, satellite lesions, edema	Bright	Low	Amino acids, acetate and succinate peaks	Higher than tuberculoma	May show increased uptake
Metastasis	Hypodense lesions with rim enhancement, extensive perilesional edema	Hypointense	Hyperintense, extensive edema	Thick rim or nodular enhancement	Dark	High	Suppressed NAA and elevated choline		Increased uptake
Demyelinating/tumefactive plaque	Open ring enhancement/incomplete ring	Hypointense	Hyperintense	Open-rim enhancement thinner at the cortical side	Acute-Bright Chronic-Dark	Acute-low Chronic-High	Decreased NAA, glutamate peak may be seen	Decreased	Variable depending on phase
IMMUNOCOMPROMISED									
Fungal brain abscess	Hyperdense lesions with thick ring enhancement	Hypointense, show blooming on SWI	Hyperintense core with hypointense rim	Thick rim enhencement	Bright, in an intracavitary projection	Low in projection	Elevate choline peak, suppressed NAA, alpha trehaose at 3.6–3.8 ppm	Higher than tuberculoma	Increased uptake
Toxoplasmosis	Ring enhancement wit central hypodensity	Isointense, predilection for basal ganglia and corticomedullary junction	Central T2 hypointensity surrounded by alternte bands of hyper and hypointensity	Ring and nodular enhancement with perilesional edema, eccentric target sign	Dark	Higher than lymphoma	Lipid and lactate peaks	–	No increased uptake

Contd...

Contd...

Differential diagnosis	*CT*	*MRI*							*PET*
		T1	*T2*	*Post-contrast*	*DW1*	*ADC*	*MRS*	*MT Ratio*	
Lymphoma	Isodense with ring enhancement	Hypo-intense, predilection for periventricular location/ ependymal surface	Hypo-intense, lesion crosses the corpus callosum	Intense enhancement, subependymal enhancement and ventricular encasement	Bright	Low	↓ NAA ↑ Choline	–	Increased uptake

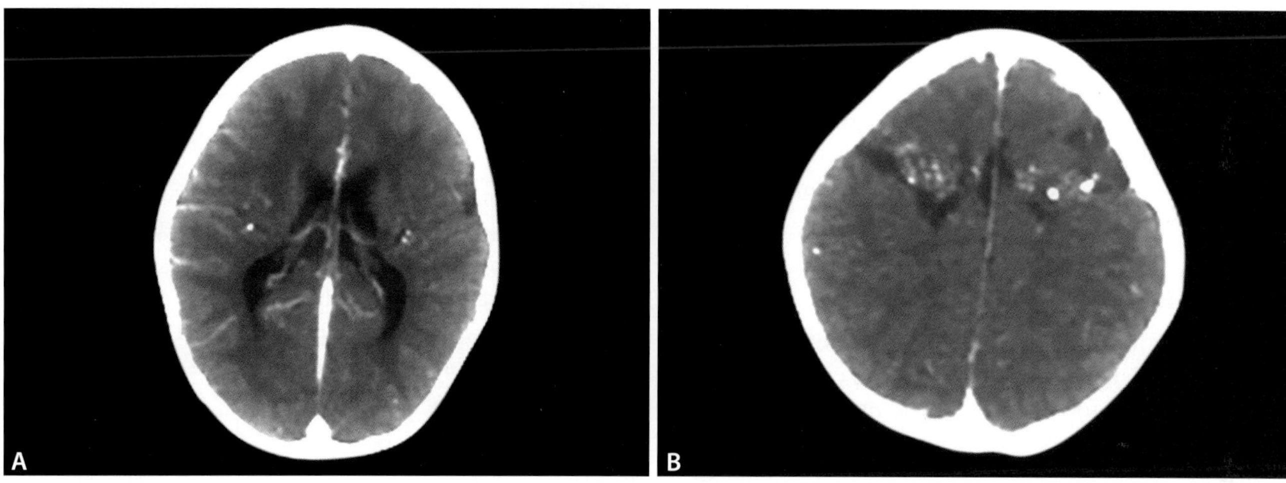

Figs. 53A and B: Axial CT sections reveal areas of gliosis with calcification seen in the periventricular regions and peripheral cerebral tissue—congenital toxopasmosis.

the first and second trimester infections. Hydrocephalus, when present, is secondary to aqueductal stenosis and often has a characteristically marked expansion of the atria and occipital horns resulting from associated tissue loss.[165] Toxoplasmosis causes necrosis but does not result in migrational anomalies. Nonspecific findings include atrophy, encephalomalacia, hydranencephaly or microcephaly.

SYPHILIS

Maternal syphilis poses a threat to the fetus regardless of the stage of the maternal infection. It can result in spontaneous abortion, stillbirth, nonimmune hydrops, premature delivery and perinatal death. Forty percent of congenitally infected infants die during the perinatal period.

Approximately 33% of congenitally infected infants have disseminated infection at birth. Clinical signs of disseminated infection characteristically include long bone periostitis. Other signs consist of hepato-splenomegaly, jaundice, skin rash, persistent rhinitis, lymphadenopathy, meningitis and hydrocephalus. The late manifestations of congenital syphilis appear after 2 years of age. These include orodental, facial and skin deformities, sensorineural hearing loss, hydrocephalus, mental retardation, seizures and hemiplegia.[166]

Cranial imaging findings may show hydrocephalus and enhancement of the leptomeninges. This may extend through the meningeal vessels and the cortical perforators to involve the brain parenchyma and appear on imaging as an enhancing parenchymal mass. Infarction may occur, attributed to the accompanying arteritis or less commonly phlebitis. The cerebral infarction most often involves the middle cerebral artery (MCA) distribution.

RUBELLA

The risk of rubella infection is maximum during the first trimester. Congenital rubella syndrome is characterized by hepatosplenomegaly, congenital heart disease (PDA, pulmonary artery stenosis), growth retardation, ocular abnormalities (cataract, pigmentary retinopathy), jaundice, rash, sensorineural hearing loss and meningoencephalitis. An entity in which the brain is formed but is markedly diminished in size called "microcephalia vera" has also been reported in rubella. Microcephaly in rubella is not caused by a destructive process but is related to an inhibition of progenitor cell multiplication by rubella virus resulting in insufficient generation of astroglia and neurons.

Imaging

Ultrasonography may show nonspecific findings of subependymal cysts in the caudate nucleus and subthalamic regions or echogenic foci in the basal ganglia representing mineralizing vasculitis. CT may show microcephaly and parenchymal calcifications while deep and subcortical white matter lesions, delayed myelination may be seen on MR. Cerebellar hypoplasia and neuronal migration anomalies have been reported.

CYTOMEGALOVIRUS (CMV)

CMV is the commonest cause of congenital infection with CNS involvement seen in about 70% cases. The virus has a predilection for the periventricular subependymal germinal matrix layer. Necrosis of this region followed by calcification accounts for the periventricular calcification seen in these cases. Other sites of involvement include the cerebral cortex, white matter, brainstem, spinal cord and the cerebellum. Disorders of neuronal migration (polymicrogyria, heterotopia), microcephaly, hydranencephaly and porencephaly may also occur. Long term sequelae such as visual deficits, mental retardation, hearing loss and seizures may occur. CMV is the leading cause of nonhereditary deafness in children.

Imaging

Microcephaly with egg shell periventricular calcification is the imaging hallmark of CMV infection[167] **(Fig. 54)**. On sonography, hypoechoic periventricular ring like zones followed by bilateral periventricular calcifications is specific for CMV. Intracranial calcification is seen in about 40% cases and is typically located in the periventricular areas but may also be seen in the basal ganglia, cortical and subcortical regions. Calcifications are best seen on CT while parenchymal abnormalities like encephalomalacia, migrational anomalies (polymicrogyria, lissencephaly, pachygyria, heterotopia), ventricular enlargement, delayed myelination and subependymal periventricular cysts are better seen on MRI.

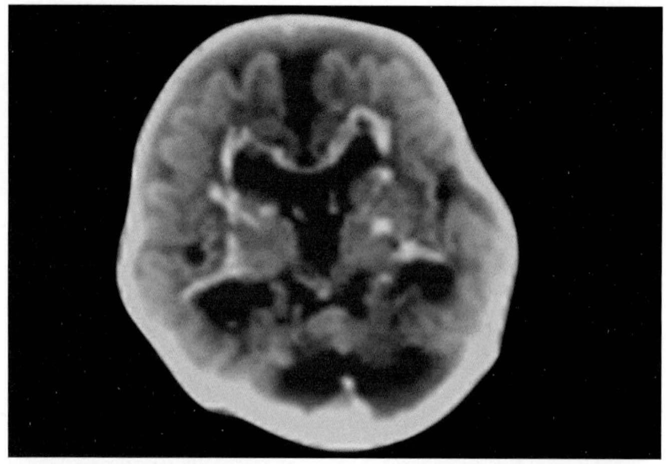

Fig. 54: Noncontrast CT scans of the cranium of a newborn showing hydrocephalus and extensive periventricular calcification. Also seen is calcification in bilateral basal ganglia—CMV.

The major differential diagnosis of CMV is congenital toxoplasmosis. The calcifications in CMV are generally periventricular while those of toxoplasmosis tend to be peripheral. Microcephaly is seen in CMV while macrocephaly is seen in toxoplasmosis **(Figs. 55A and B)**. Anomalies or cortical development are common in CMV but rare in toxoplasmosis.

HERPES SIMPLEX VIRUS (HSV)

HSV is the second most common TORCH infection. In contrast to other TORCH infections most of the HSV infection in neonates are not strictly congenital but occur in the perinatal period. These result from exposure to HSV type 2 genital lesions of the mother at the time of vaginal birth. On CT hypodense lesions may be seen in the periventricular white matter. Finger like areas of increased attenuation within the cortical grey matter along with increased white matter lucency have been attributed to the increased blood flow from cortical infection and has been described as a characteristic imaging finding occurring in the first 3 weeks after presentation. With disease progression, focal necrosis, cystic encephalomalacia, parenchymal calcification and diffuse cerebral atrophy may ensue.

HIV

Mother-to-child transmission of HIV can occur in utero, intrapartum during birth and postpartum via breast milk. The transplacental route accounts for most pediatric AIDS cases and is the major route of infection in infants.

Pathologically multinuclear giant cells and microglial nodules are seen in the basal ganglia, brainstem and the

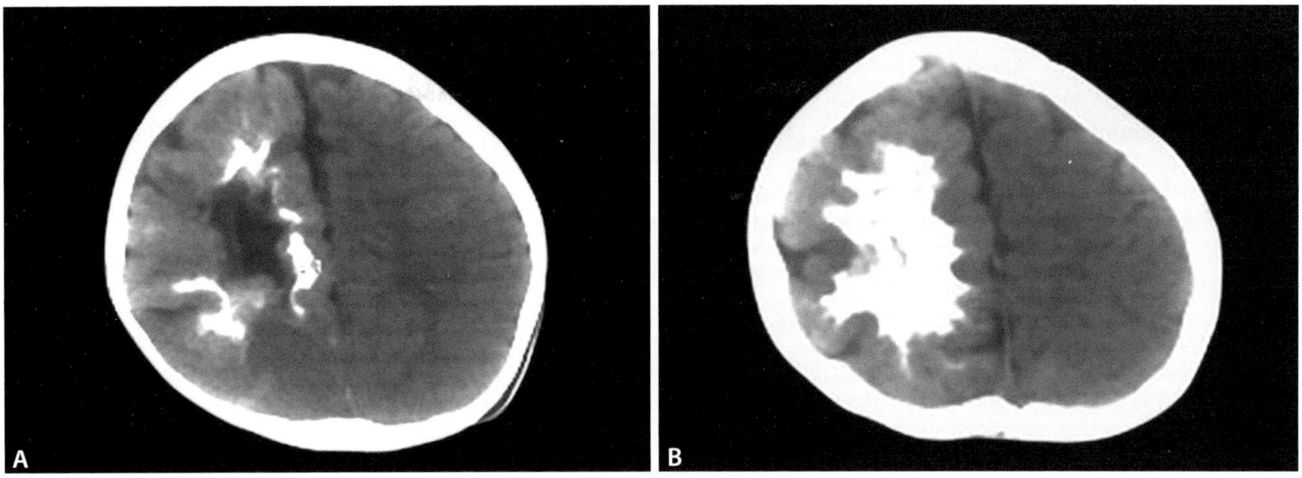

Figs. 55A and B: Axial section CT reveal microcephaly with egg shell periventricular calcification (A) and intraparenchymal coarse chunky calcification; (B) Congenital CMV.

white matter. Perivascular inflammation, demyelination and calcification may be seen, most commonly in the basal ganglia. The infants may be asymptomatic at birth and then develop chronic symptoms over months which include developmental delay, microcephaly, spastic paraparesis and ataxia. However, unlike adults, opportunistic infections like toxoplasmosis and tuberculosis are not seen in the congenital variety.

Imaging

CT may show diffuse cerebral atrophy associated with bilateral low attenuation areas in the white matter with no mass effect or edema. Bilateral and symmetrical calcifications can be seen in the basal ganglia as a result of vasculitis in which calcium is deposited in and around the small vessels. Calcifications may also occur in the white matter and cerebellum. Rarely haemorrhage may occur in cases where there is severe thrombocytopenia.

MR imaging reveals diffuse atrophy and abnormalities of the white matter. These include delayed myelination and areas of increased signal in the peripheral white matter on proton-density and T2-weighted images without associated mass effect. Cortical spinal tract degeneration and demyelination are also seen in children.

CONCLUSION

The imaging findings seen in CNS infections are variable and challenging. A knowledge of the common patterns seen in the various CNS infections may enable the radiologist to suggest a diagnosis or arrive at a differential diagnosis in equivocal cases. The clinical picture and laboratory testing are of vital importance in making a definitive diagnosis and guiding therapy.

REFERENCES

1. Meltzer CC, Fukui MB, Kanal E, et al. MR imaging of the meninges. Radiology. 1996;20:297-308.
2. Kanamalla US, Ibarra RA, Jinkins JR. Imaging of cranial meningitis and ventricles. Neuroimag Clin N Am. 2000;10:309-31.
3. Farn JW, Mirowitz SA. MR imaging of the normal meninges: Comparison of contrast enhanced patterns on 3D gradient echo and spin echo images. Am J Roentgenol. 1994;162:131-5.
4. Sze G, Soletsky S, Bronen R, et al. MR imaging of the cranial meninges with emphasis on contrast enhancement and meningeal carcinomatosis. Am J Neuroradiol. 1989;10:965-75.
5. Mohan S, Jain KK, Arabi M, et al. Imaging of meningitis and ventriculitis. Neuroimag Clin N Am. 2012;22:557-83.
6. Quint DJ, Eldevik OP, Cohen JK. Magnetic resonance imaging of normal meningeal enhancement at 1.5T. Acad Radiol. 1996;6:463-8.
7. Smirniotopoulos JG, Murphy FM, Rushing EJ, et al. Patterns of contrast enhancement in the brain and meninges. Radiographics. 2007;27:525-51.
8. Hakan T, Ceran N, Erdem I, et al. Bacterial brain abscesses: an evaluation of 96 cases. J Infect. 2006;52:359-66.
9. Xaio F, Tseng MY, Teng LJ, et al. Brain abscess:clinical experience and analysis of prognostic factors. Surg Neurol. 2005;63:442-9.
10. Tunkel AR, Scheld WM. Pathogenesis and pathophysiology of bacterial meningitis. Clin Microbiol Rev. 1993;6:118-36.
11. Ashwal S. Neurologic evaluation of the patient with acute bacterial meningitis. Neurol Clin. 1995;13:549-77.
12. Van de Beek D, de Gans J, Spanjaard L, et al. Clinical and prognostic factors in adults with bacterial meningitis. N Engl J Md. 2004;351:1849-59.
13. Shih RY, Koeller KK. Bacterial, fungal and parasitic infections of the central nervous system:Radiologic-pathologic correlation and historical perspectives. Radiographics. 2015;35:1141-69.

14. Parmer H, Sitoh YY, Anand P, et al. Contrast enhanced FLAIR imaging in the evaluation of infectious leptomeningeal diseases. Eur J Radiol. 2006;58:89-95.
15. Stuckey SL, Goh TD, Heffernan T, et al. Hyperintensity in the subarachnoid space on FLAIR MRI. Am J Roentgenol. 2007;189:913-21.
16. Runge VM, Wells JW, Williams NM, et al. Detectability of early brain meningitis with magnetic resonance imaging. Invest Radiol. 1995;30:484-95.
17. Trivedi R, Malik GK, Gupta RK, et al. Increased anisotropy in neonatal meningitis: an indicator of meningeal inflammation. Neuroradiology. 2007;49:767-75.
18. Yadav A, Malik GK, Trivedi R, et al. Correlation of CSF neuroinflammatory molecules with leptomeningeal cortical subcortical white matter fractional anisotropy in neonatal meningitis. Mag Reson Imaging. 2009;27:214-21.
19. Cabral DA, Flodmark O, Farrell K, et al. Prospective study of computed tomography in acute bacterial meningitis. J Pediatr. 1987;111:201-5.
20. Castillo M. Imaging of meningitis. Semin Roentgenol. 2004;39:458-64.
21. Smith RR. Neuroradiology of intracranial infection. Paediatr Neurosurg. 1992;18:92-104.
22. Rabe EF. Subdural effusion in infants. Paed Clin North Am. 1967;14:831-50.
23. Sze G, Zimmerman RD. The magnetic resonance imaging of infections and inflammatory diseases. Radiol Clin North Am. 1988;26:839-59.
24. Zimmerman RD, Leeds NE, Danziger A. Subdural empyema: CT findings. Radiology. 1984;150:417-22.
25. Weingarten K, Zimmerman RD, Becker RD, et al. Subdural and epidural empyemas: MR imaging. Am J Roentgenol. 1989;152: 615-21.
26. Wong AM, Zimmerman RA, Simon EM, et al. Diffusion weighted MR imaging of subdural empyema in children. Am J Neuroradiol. 2004;25:1016-21.
27. Mathisen GE, Johnson JP. Brain abscess. Clin Infect Dis. 1997;25:763-79.
28. Saez-Llorens XJ, Umana MA, Odio CM, et al. Brain abscess in infants and children. Ped Infect Dis J. 1989;8:449-58.
29. Strong AJ, Ingham HR. Brain abscess. Br J Hosp Med. 1983;30:396-403.
30. Enzmann DR, Britt RH, Placone R. Staging of human brain abscess by computed tomography. Radiology. 1983;146:703-8.
31. Brit RH, Enzmann DR. Clinical stages of human brain abscesses on serial CT scans after contrast infusion: CT, neuropathological and clinical correlation. J Neurosurg. 1983;59:972-89.
32. Haimes AB, Zimmerman RD, Morgello S, et al. MR imaging of brain abscesses. Am J Neuroradiol. 1989;152:1073-85.
33. Whiteman MLH, Bowen BC, Post MJD, et al. Intracranial infection. In Magnetic resonance imaging of the brain and spine SW atlas, New York: Lippincott Raven. 1996;706-66.
34. Dev R, Gupta RK, Poptani H, et al. Role of in vivo proton magnetic resonance spectroscopy in the diagnosis and management of brain abscess. Neurosurgery. 1998;42: 37-43.
35. Demaerel P, Hecke PV, Oostende SV, et al. Bacterial metabolism shown by magnetic resonance spectroscopy. Lancet. 1997;344:1197-202.
36. Martinez-Perez I, Moreno A, Alonso J, et al. Diagnosis of brain abscess by magnetic resonance spectroscopy: Report of two cases. J Neurosurg. 1997;86:708-13.
37. Desprechins B, Stadnik T, Koerts G, et al. Use of diffusion weighted MR imaging in differential diagnosis between intracerebral necrotic tumors and cerebral abscesses. Am J Neuroradiol. 1999;20:1252-7.
38. Ebisu T, Tanaka C, Umeda M, et al. Discrimination of brain abscess from necrotic or cystic tumors by diffusion weighted echo planar imaging. Mag Reson Imaging. 1996;14:1113-6.
39. Lai PH, Hsu SS, Ding SW, et al. Proton magnetic resonance spectroscopy and diffusion-weighted imaging in intracranial cystic mass lesions. Surg Neurol. 2007;68:S25-36.
40. Gupta RK, Hasan KM, Mishra AM, et al. High fractional anisotropy in brain abscesses versus other cystic intracranial lesions. Am J Neuroradiol. 2005;26:1107-14.
41. Holmes TM, Petrella JR, Provenzale JM. Distinction between cerebral abscesses and high grade neoplasms by dynamic susceptibility contrast perfusion MRI. AJR. 2004;183:1247-52.
42. Crain MR, Yuh WT, Greene GM, et al. Cerebral ischaemia: Evaluation with contrast enhanced MR imaging. Am J Neuroradiol. 1991;12:631-9.
43. Harris TM, Edwards MK. Meningitis. Neuroimaging. Clin N Am. 1991;1:39-56.
44. Raimondi AJ, Rocco C. Cerebral angiography in meningococcal inflammatory diseases in infancy and childhood: a study of thirty five cases. Neurosurgery. 1978;3:37-44.
45. Beijen J, Casselman J, Joosten F, et al. Magnetic resonance imaging in patients with meningitis induced hearing loss. Eur Arch Otorhinolaryngol. 2009;266:1229-36.
46. Barloon TJ, Yuh WT, Knepper LE. Cerebral ventriculitis: MR findings. J Comput Assist Tomogr. 1990;14:272-5.
47. Durand ML, Calderwood SB, Weber DJ, et al. Acute bacterial meningitis in adults: A review of 493 episodes. N Eng J Med. 1993;328:21-8.
48. World Health Organization, Global Tuberculosis Control 2014. Geneva, Switzerland: WHO;2014. Available at: http://apps.who.int/iris/bitstreah/10665/137094/1/9789241564809_eng.pdf
49. Bernaerts A, Vanhoenacker FM, Parizel PM, et al. Tuberculosis of the central nervous system:overview of neuroradiological findings. Eur Radiol. 2003;13:1876-90.
50. Berenguer J, Moreno S, Laguna F, et al. Tuberculous meningitis in patients infected with human immunodeficiency virus. N Engl J Med. 1992;326:668-72.
51. Rich AR, McCordock HA. Pathogenesis of tubercular meningitis. Bull John Hopkins hosp. 1933;52:5-13.
52. Dastur DK, Manghani DK, Udani PM. Pathology and pathogenic mechanisms in neurotuberculosis. Radiol Clin North Am. 1995;33:733-52.
53. Leonard JM, Des RP. Tuberculous meningitis. Infect Dis Clin North Am. 1990;4:769-87.

54. Dastur DK, Lalitha VS, Udani PM, et al. The brain and meninges in tuberculous meningitis-gross pathology in 100 cases and pathogenesis. Neurol India. 1970;18:86-100.
55. Przybojewski S, Andronikou S, Wilmshurst J. Objective criteria to determine the presence of abnormal basal enhancement in children with suspected Tuberculous Meningitis. Pediatr Radiol. 2006;36:687-96.
56. Klingensmith WC, Datu J. Tuberculous meningitis of the sylvian fissure. Clin Nucl Med. 1978;3:315-7.
57. Trautmann M, Kluge W, Otto HS, et al. Computed tomography in CNS tuberculosis. Eur Neurol. 1986;25:91-7.
58. de Castro CC, de Baros NG, Campos ZM, et al. CT scans of cranial tuberculosis. Radiol Clin North Am. 1995;33:753-69.
59. Chang KH, Han MH, Roh JK, et al. Gd-DTPA enhanced MR imaging in intracranial tuberculosis. Neuroradiology. 1990;32:19-25.
60. Gupta RK, Gupta S, Singh D, et al. MR imaging and angiography in tuberculous meningitis. Neuroradiology. 1994;36:87-92.
61. Gupta RK, Kathuria MK, Pradhan S. Magnetization transfer MR imaging in central nervous system tuberculosis. Am J Neuroradiol. 1999;20:867-75.
62. Jamieson DH. Imaging intracranial tuberculosis in childhood. Paediatr Radiol. 1995;25:165-70.
63. Kioumehr F, Dadsetan MR, Rooholamini SA, et al. Central nervous system tuberculosis: MRI. Neuroradiology. 1994;36:93-6.
64. Rovira M, Romero F, Torrent O, et al. Study of tuberculous meningitis by CT. Neuroradiology. 1980;19:137-41.
65. Wallace RC, Burto EM, Barrett FF, et al. Intracranial tuberculosis in children: CT appearance and clinical outcome. Paed Radiol. 1991;21:241-6.
66. Torres C, Riascos R, Figueroa R, et al. Central Nervous System Tuberculosis. Top Mag Reson Imaging. 2014;23:173-89.
67. Gupta RK, Kumar S. Central nervous system tuberculosis. Neuroimaging Clin N Am. 2011;21:795-814.
68. Silverman IE, Liu GT, Bilaniuk LT, et al. Tuberculous meningitis with blindness and perichiasmal involvement on MRI. Ped Neurol. 1995;12:65-7.
69. Praharaj SS, Sharma MC, Prasad K, et al. Unilateral meningeal thickening: a rare presentation of tuberculous meningitis. Clin Neurol Neurosurg. 1997;99:60-2.
70. Gupta RK, Kohli A, Gaur V, et al. MRI of the brain in patients with miliary pulmonary tuberculosis without symptoms or signs of central nervous system involvement. Neuroradiology. 1997;39:699-704.
71. Altunbasak S, Baytok V, Alhan E, et al. Suprasellar tuberculoma causing endocrinologic disorders and imitating craniopharyngioma. Paediatr Neurosurg. 1995; 23:328-31.
72. Esposito V, Fraioli B, Ferrante L, et al. Intrasellar tuberculoma: Case report. Neurosurgery. 1987;21:721-3.
73. Bargallo J, Berenguer J, Garcia-Barrionuevo J, et al. The "target sign" is it a specific sign of CNS tuberculoma? Neuroradiology. 1996;38:547-50.
74. Salgado P, Del Brutto OH, Talamas O, et al. Intracranial tuberculoma: MR imaging. Neuroradiology. 1989;31:299-302.
75. Shah GV. Central nervous system tuberculosis imaging manifestations. Neuroimaging Clin North Am. 2000; 10:355-74.
76. Gupta RK, Vatsal DK, Husain N, et al. Differentiation of tuberculous from pyogenic brain abscesses with in vivo proton MR spectroscopy and magnetization transfer MR imaging. Am J Neuroradiol. 2001;22:1503-9.
77. Trivedi R, Saksena S, Gupta RK. Magnetic resonance imaging in central nervous system tuberculosis. Indian J Radiol Imaging. 2009;19:256-65.
78. Patkar D, Narang J, Yanamandala R, et al. Central Nervous System Tuberculosis Pathophysiology and Imaging Findings. Neuroimag Clin N Am. 2012;22:677-705.
79. Whitener DR. Tuberculous brain abscess. Report of a case and review of literature. Arch Neurol. 1978;35:148-55.
80. Farrar DJ, Fiangan TP, Gordon NM, et al. Tuberculous brain abscess in a patient with HIV infection: case report and review. Am J Med. 1997;102:297-301.
81. Luthra G, Parihar A, Nath K, et al. Comparative evaluation of fungal, tubercular and pyogenic brain abscesses with conventional and diffusion MR imaging and proton MR spectroscopy. AJNR Am J Neuroradiol. 2007;28: 1332-8.
82. Gupta RK, Prakash M, Mishra AM, et al. Role of diffusion weighted imaging in differentiation of intracranial tuberculoma and tuberculous abscess from cysticercus granuloma—a report of more than 100 lesions. Eur J Radiol. 2005;55:384-92.
83. Saxena S, Prakash M, Kumar S, et al. Comparative evaluation of magnetization transfer contrast and fluid attenuated inversion recovery sequences in brain tuberculoma. Clin Radiol. 2005;60:787-93.
84. Sheller JR, Des Prez RM. CNS tuberculosis. Neurol Clin. 1986;4:143-58.
85. Garcia-Monco JC. Central nervous system tuberculosis. Neurol Clin. 1999;17:737-59.
86. Ahluwalia VV, Sagar GD, Singh TP, et al. MRI Spectrum of CNS tuberculosis. JIACM. 2013;14:83-90.
87. Post MJ, Quencer RM, Tabei SZ. CT demonstration of sarcoidosis of the optic nerve, frontal lobes and falx cerebri. Case report and literature review. Am J Neuroradiol. 1982;3:523-6.
88. Khoo TK, Sugai K, Leong TK. Disseminated aspergillosis. Am J Clin Pathol. 1966;45:697-703.
89. Young RC, Bennett JE, Vogel CL, et al. Aspergillosis. The spectrum of disease in 98 patients. Medicine. 1970;49: 147-73.
90. Ostrow TD, Hudgins PA. Magnetic resonance imaging of intracranial fungal infections. Magn Reson Imaging. 1994;6:22-31.
91. Cox J, Murtagh FR, Wilfrong A, et al. Cerebral aspergillosis MR imaging and histopathologic correlation. Am J Neuroradiol. 1992;5:1489-92.
92. Ashdown BC, Tien RD, Felsberg GJ. Aspergillosis of the brain and paranasal sinuses in immunocompromised patients: CT and MR imaging findings. Am J Roentgenol. 1994;162:155-9.

93. DeLone DR, Goldstein RA, Petermann G, et al. Disseminated aspergillosis involving the brain: distribution and imaging characteristics. AJNR Am J Neuroradiol. 1999;20:1597-604.
94. Gabelmann A, Klein S, Kern W, et al. Relevant imaging findings of cerebral aspergillosis on MRI: a retrospective case based study in immunocompromised patients. Eur J Neurol. 2007;14:548-55.
95. Zinreich SJ, Kennedy DW, Malat J, et al. Fungal sinusitis: diagnosis with CT and MR imaging. Radiology. 1988; 169:439-44.
96. Mathews VP, Alo PL, Glass JD, et al. AIDS-related CNS cryptococcosis: Radiologic—pathologic correlation. Am J Neuroradiol. 1992;13:1477-86.
97. Igel HJ, Bolande RP. Humoral defense mechanisms in cryptococcosis: substances in normal human serum, saliva and cerebrospinal fluid affecting the growth of Cryptococcus neoformans. J Inf Dis. 1966;116:75-83.
98. Cornell SH, Jacoby CJ. The varied computed tomographic appearance of intracranial cryptococcosis. Radiology. 1982;143:703-7.
99. Andreula CF, Burdi N, Carella A. CNS cryptococcosis in AIDS: spectrum of MR findings. J Comput Assist Tomogr. 1993;17:438-41.
100. Offiah CE, Naseer A. Spectrum of imaging appearances of intracranial cryptococcal infection in HIV/AIDS patients in the anti-retroviral therapy era. Clin Radiol. 2016;71:9-17.
101. Blitzer A, Lawson W, Meyers BR, et al. Patient survival in paranasal sinus mucormycosis. Laryngoscope. 1980;90:635-48.
102. Bergstrom L, Hemenway WG, Barnhart RA. Rhinocerebral and otologic mucormycosis. Ann Oto Rhino Laryngol. 1970;79:70-81.
103. Safder S, Carpenter JS, Roberto TD, et al. The "Black Turbinate" Sign: an early MR imaging finding of nasal mucormycosis. Am J Neuroradiol. 2010;31:771-4.
104. Morduchowicz G, Shmueli D, Shapira Z, et al. Rhinocerebral mucormycosis in renal transplant recipients. Rev Infect Dis. 1986;8:441-6.
105. Lipton SA, Hickey WF, Morris JH, et al. Candidal infection in the central nervous system. Am J Med. 1984;76:101-8.
106. Castro S, Bernardes I. Coccidioidal cerebral abscess with peripheral restricted diffusion. J Neuroradiol. 2009;36:162-4.
107. Stone JH, Pomper MG, Hellmann DB. Histoplasmosis mimicking vasculitis of the central nervous system. J Rheumatol. 1998;25:1644-8.
108. Go JL, Kim PE, Ahmadi J, et al. Fungal Infections of the central nervous system. Neuroimaging Clin North Am. 2000;10:409-25.
109. Mathur M, Johnson CE, Sze G. Fungal infections of the Central Nervous System. Neuroimag Clin N Am. 2012; 22:609-32.
110. Stepien L. Cerebral cysticercosis in Poland: clinical symptoms and operative results in 132 cases. J Neurosurg. 1962;19:505-13.
111. Keane JR. Death from cysticercosis: Seven patients with unrecognized obstructive hydrocephalus. West J Med. 1984;140:787-9.
112. Sotelo J, Del Brutto OH, Penagos P, et al. Comparison of therapeutic regimen of anticysticercal drugs for parenchymal brain cysticercosis. J Neurol. 1990;237: 69-72.
113. Chang KH, Lee JH, Han MH, et al. The role of contrast enhanced MR imaging in the diagnosis of neurocysticercosis. Am J Neuroradiol. 1991;12:509-12.
114. Martinez HR, Rangel Guerra R, Gonzalez J, et al. MR imaging in neurocysticercosis. A study of 56 cases. Am J Neuroradiol. 1989;10:1011-9.
115. Noujaim SE, Rossi MD, Rao SK, et al. CT and MR imaging of neurocysticercosis. AJR Am J Roentgenol. 1999;17: 1485-90.
116. Sharma BB, Sharma S. Neurocysticercosis (NCC) vs central nervous system (CNS) tuberculoma in children: Dilemma over clinicoradiological diagnosis? Open J Pediatr. 2016;6: 245-51.
117. Zee CS, Segall HD, Boswell W, et al. MR imaging of neurocysticercosis. J Comput Assist Tomogr. 1988;12:927-34.
118. Zee CS, Segall HD, Apuzzo ML, et al. Intraventricular cysticercal cysts: further neuroradiologic observations and neurosurgical implications. Am J Neuroradiol. 1984; 5:727-30.
119. Ramsey RG, Gean AD. Neuroimaging of AIDS central nervous system toxoplasmosis. Neuroimaging Clin North Am. 1997;7:171-86.
120. Kumar GG, Mahadevan A, Guruprasad AS, et al. Eccentric Target Sign in Cerebral Toxoplamosis-neuropathological correlate to the imaging feature. J Magn Reson Imaging. 2010;31:1469-72.
121. Camacho DL, Smith JK, Castillo M. Differentiation of toxoplasmosis and lymphoma in AIDS patients by using apparent diffusion coefficients. Am J Neuroradiol. 2003;24:633-7.
122. Coates R, von Sinner W, Rahm B. MR imaging of an intracerebral hydatid cyst. AJNR Am J Neuroradiol. 1990;11:1249-50.
123. Turgut M, Benli K, Eryilmaz M. Secondary multiple intracranial hydatid cysts caused by intracerebral embolism of cardiac echinococcosis: an exceptional case of hydatidosis. J Neurosurg. 1997;86:714-8.
124. Nurchi G, Floris F, Montaldo C, et al. Multiple cerebral hydatid disease: case report with magnetic resonance imaging study. Neurosurg. 1992;30:436-8.
125. Senturk S, Oguz KK, Soylemezoglu F, et al. Cerebral alveolar echinococcosis mimicking primary brain tumours. Am J Neuroradiol. 2006;27:420-2.
126. Kohli A, Gupta RK, Poptani H, et al. In vivo proton magnetic resonance spectroscopy in a case of intracranial hydatid cyst. Neurology. 1995;45:562-4.
127. Mohanty S, Taylor TE, Kampondeni S, et al. Magnetic resonance imaging during life: the key to unlock cerebral malaria pathogenesis? Malar J. 2014;13:276.
128. Nickerson JP, Tong KA, Raghavan R. Imaging cerebral malaria with a susceptibility weighted MR sequence. Am J Neuroradiol. 2009;30:85-6.
129. Gupta S, Patel K. Case series: MRI features in cerebral malaria. Indian J Radiol Imaging. 2008;18:224-6.
130. Alkhunaizi AM, Dawamneh MF, Banda RW, et al. Acanthamoeba encephalitis in a patient with systemic

lupus treated with rituximab. Diagn Microbiol Infect Dis. 2013;75:192-4.
131. Ranjan R, Handa A, Choudhary A, et al. Acanthamoeba infection in a interhemispheric ependymal cyst: a case report. Surg Neurol. 2009;72:185-9.
132. Mayer PL, Larkin JA, Hennessay JM. Amoebic encephalitis. Surg Neurol Int. 2011;2:50.
133. Corey L, Spear PG. Infection with herpes simplex viruses. N Eng J Med. 1986;314:749-57.
134. Weiner LP, Fleming JO. Viral infections of the nervous system. J Neurosurg. 1984;61:207-24.
135. Baringer JR. Herpes simplex infections of the nervous system. Neurol Clin. 2008;26:657-74.
136. Noguchi T, Yoshiura T, Hiwatashi A, et al. CT and MRI findings of human herpes virus 6-associated encephalopathy: comparision with findings of herpes simplex virus encephalitis. AJR Am J Roentgenol. 2010;194:754-60.
137. Soares BP, Provenzale JM. Imaging of herpes virus infections of the CNS. Am J Roentgenol. 2016;206:39-48.
138. Prandota J. Mollaret meningitis may be caused by reactivation of latent cerebral toxoplasmosis. Int J Neurosco. 2009;119:1655-92.
139. Gliden D, Cohrs RJ, Mahalingam R, et al. Varicella zoster virus vasculopathies: diverse clinical manifestations, laboratory features, pathogenesis and treatment. Lancet Neurol. 2009;8:731-40.
140. Handique SK, Das RR, Barman K, et al. Temporal lobe involvement in Japanese encephalitis: problems in differential diagnosis. Am J Neuroradiol. 2006;27:1027-31.
141. Singh P, Kalra N, Ratho RK, et al. Coexistent neurocysticercosis and Japanese B encephalitis: MR imaging correlation. Am J Neuroradiol. 2001;22:1131-6.
142. Kipps A, Dick G, Moodie JW. Measles and the central nervous system. Lancet. 1983;2:1406-10.
143. Laothamatas J, Hemachudha T, Mitrabhakdi E, et al. MR imaging in human rabies. Am J Neuroradiol. 2003;24: 1102-9.
144. Ukisu R, Kushihashi T, Tanaka E, et al. Diffusion weighted MR imaging of early stage Creutzfeldt-Jacob disease: typical and atypical manifestations. Radiographics. 2006;26:S191-204.
145. Zeidler M, Sellar RJ, Collie DA, et al. The pulvinar sign on magnetic resonance imaging in variant Creutzfeldt-Jacob disease. Lancet. 2000;355:1412-8.
146. Smith AB, Smirniotopoulos JG, Rushing EJ. Central nervous system infections associated with human immunodeficiency virus infection: radiologic-pathologic correlation. Radiographics. 2008;28:2033-58.
147. McArthur JC, Haughey N, Gartner S, et al. Human immunodeficiency virus associated dementia: an evolving disease. J Neurovirol. 2003;9:205-21.
148. Post MJ, Tate LG, Quencer RM, et al. CT, MR and pathology in HIV encephalitis and meningitis. Am J Roentgenol. 1988;151:373-80.
149. Jarvik JG, Lenkinski RE, Grossman RI. Proton MR spectroscopy of HIV infected patients: characterization of abnormalities with imaging and clinical correlation. Radiology. 1993;186:739-44.
150. Pomara N, Crandall DT, Choi SJ, et al. White matter abnormalities in HIV-1 infection: a diffusion tensor imaging study. Psychiatry Res. 2001;106:15-24.
151. Major EO, Amemiya K, Tornatore CS, et al. Pathogenesis and molecular biology of progressive multifocal leukoencephalopathy, the JC virus induced demyelinating disease of the human brain. Clin J Microbiol Rev. 1992; 5:49-73.
152. Sahraian MA, Radue EW, Eshaghi A, et al. Progressive multifocal leukoencephalopathy: a review of the neuroimaging features and differential diagnosis. EJ Neurol. 2012;19:1060-9.
153. Arbusow V, Strupp M, Pfister HW, et al. Contrast enhancement in progressive multifocal leukoencephalopathy: a predictive factor for long term survival. J Neurol. 2000; 247:306-8.
154. Muller M, Wandel S, Colebunders R, et al. Immune reconstitution inflammatory syndrome in patients starting antiretroviral therapy for HIV infection: a systematic review and meta-analysis. Lancet Infect Dis. 2010;10:251-61.
155. Ohta K, Obara K. Lesion extension detected by diffusion weighted magnetic resonance imaging in PML. J Neurol. 2001;248:809-11.
156. Bergui M, Bradac GB, Oguz KK, et al. Progressive multifocal leukoencephalopathy: diffusion-weighted imaging and pathological correlations. Neuroradiology. 2004;46:22-25.
157. Clark EG, Danbolt N. The Oslo study of the natural history of untreated syphilis; an epidemiologic investigation based on a restudy of the Boeck-Bruusgaard material; a review and appraisal. J Chronic Dis. 1955;2:311-44.
158. Brightbill TC, Ihmeidan IH, Post MJ, et al. Neurosyphilis in HIV-positive and HIV-negative patients: neuroimaging findings. Am J Neuroradiol. 1995;16:703-11.
159. Arribas JR, Storch GA, Clifford DB, et al. Cytomegalovirus encephalitis. Ann Intern Med. 1996;125:577-87.
160. Seok JH, Ahn K, Park HJ. Diffusion MRI findings of cytomegalovirus-associated ventriculitis: a case report. Br J Radiol. 2011;84:e179-e81.
161. Tan K, Roda R, Ostrow L, et al. PML-IRIS in patients with HIV infection: clinical manifestations and treatment with steroids. Neurology. 2009;72:1458-64.
162. Marzocchetti A, Di Giambenedetto S, Cingolani A, et al. Reduced rate of diagnostic positive detection of JC virus DNA in cerebrospinal fluid in cases of suspected progressive multifocal leukoencephalopathy in the era of potent antiretroviral therapy. J Clin Microbiol. 2005;43:4175-7.
163. Garg RK, Sinha MK. Multiple ring-enhancing lesions of the brain. J Postgrad Med. 2010;56:307-16.
164. Bale JF Jr, Murph JR. Congenital infections and the nervous system. Pediatr Clin North Am. 1992;39:669-90.
165. Diekler C, Dusser A, Dulae O. Congenital toxoplasmosis: clinical and neuroradiologic evaluation of the cerebral lesions. Neuroradiology. 1985;27:125-30.
166. Griffith BP, Booss J. Neurologic infections of the fetus and newborn. Neurol Clin. 1994;12:541-64.
167. Becker LE. Infections of the developing brain. Am J Neuroradiol. 1992;13:537-49.

CHAPTER 14

Imaging of White Matter Disease

Anjali Prakash, Jyoti Kumar, Swati Gupta, Gaurav S Pradhan

INTRODUCTION

The white matter is primarily composed of myelinated axons and support elements, i.e. oligodendrocytes, astrocytes, microglia, and blood vessels. The myelin sheath is formed by the oligodendrocyte. Each oligodendrocyte extends over several cell processes around one or more neighboring axons, forming few segmental myelin sheaths. The myelin sheath is the major structural element in white matter, comprising approximately 50% of the dry weight of the adult brain; thus primary white matter diseases are considered to be diseases affecting myelin and oligodendrocytes. Neuroglial cells, i.e. oligodendrocytes and astrocytes are primarily responsible for the maintenance of the white matter by providing structural and nutritional support of neurons and regulating the extracellular environment. These cells are also important for guiding the migrating neurons during development and are involved in repair of the nervous system.

White matter disease is caused by a pathologic process that prevents the normal formation and maintenance of myelin or that selectively destroys the oligodendrocyte and/or myelin sheath. The disruption of myelin interrupts the efficient transmission of the axonal action potentials, which in turn may be clinically expressed as a neurological deficit. Any process, including metabolic injury or ischemia, that changes the chemical composition of myelin will result in a less stable structure that is more susceptible to injury.[1,2]

White matter diseases may be categorized as inherited or acquired or as demyelinating and dysmyelinating. Primary demyelinating diseases are characterized by loss of normally formed myelin with relative preservation of axons; Multiple sclerosis is the prototype of primary demyelinating disease. Secondary demyelination is demyelination associated with a known etiology or a systemic disorder and with destruction of both axons and myelin. It consists of a group of entities with very diverse etiologies, pathogenesis, clinical presentation and distribution of lesions.[2,3] Dysmyelination is a pathological process characterized by defective formation/maintenance of normal myelin. Many of these disorders or leukodystrophies have a known genetic basis, others however are poorly understood.

Demyelinating Disease: Classification based on Etiology

Autoimmune Causes

- *Multiple sclerosis:*
  - Classic Charcot type
  - MS Variants
  - Acute-Marburg type
  - Diffuse cerebral sclerosis-Schilder type
  - Concentric sclerosis-Balo type
- Neuromyelitis optica-Devic disease
- Acute disseminated encephalomyelitis (ADEM) Classic (acute disseminated encephalomyelitis)
- Hyperacute (acute hemorrhagic leukoencephalitis)

Associated with Infectious Agents and/or Vaccination

- Progressive multifocal leukoencephalopathy (PML)
- Human immunodeficiency virus (HIV) encephalopathy

- Lyme disease
- Subacute sclerosing panencephalitis (SSPE)
- Progressive rubella panencephalitis.

Associated with Vascular Causes

- Small vessel disease
- Cerebral amyloid angiopathy
- CADASIL
- Primary angiitis of the CNS
- Susac syndrome
- Neuro lupus-SLE

Associated with Toxic Metabolic Causes

- Central pontine myelinolysis
- Posterior reversible encephalopathy syndrome (PRES)
- Marchiafava–Bignami disease
- Wernicke encephalopathy
- Vitamin B_{12} deficiency
- Postradiation white matter injury
- Necrotizing leukoencephalopathy following chemotherapy
- Solvent vapor abuse leukoencephalopathy (SVAL)

IMAGING OF WHITE MATTER DISEASES

Magnetic resonance imaging (MRI) has become the standard and, in most instances, the only acceptable imaging modality and it is proven to be far superior to computed tomography (CT) in detecting and demonstrating the extent of abnormality within intracerebral and extracerebral white matter. Conventional MRI is proven to be sensitive for detecting lesions and their changes. However, it is not able to characterize and quantify the tissue damage within and outside these lesions. With the advent of newer MR techniques, including magnetization transfer (MT) imaging, ^{1}H-MR spectroscopy, and diffusion weighted imaging, the ability to detect and characterize disease has increased significantly.[4-6]

Multiple Sclerosis

Multiple sclerosis (MS) is a chronic inflammatory-demyelinating disorder of the CNS characterized pathologically by multifocal areas of demyelination with loss of oligodendrocytes and astroglial scarring. Axonal loss is now being recognized as an important pathological feature.[4] Although the etiology is not clearly understood, MS is considered to be a result of an autoimmune mediated process in which environmental factors (such as exposure to EBV virus) act on genetically susceptible individuals. A strong association with HLA-DR2 class II has been identified. Some authors have proposed a theory of 'Chronic cerebrospinal venous insufficiency' as a cause for MS. It implicates an abnormal CNS venous outflow as a cause of MS.[7-9]

Epidemiology: Multiple sclerosis is one of the most common neurological disorders in the world and the commonest cause of chronic non-traumatic neurological disorders of young adults in the developed world. The prevalence rates of MS have been reported to vary by continent and geographical latitude. The condition is of high prevalence (>30 per 100,000) in northern parts of Europe and North America; medium prevalence (5–30 per 100,000) in southern Europe and southern United States; and Central and South America (10–20 per 100,000); and low prevalence (<5 per 100,000) in Asia and South America.[10] The risk of MS increases in first-order relatives of patients with clinically definite MS as compared to the general population. The presentation of MS typically differs between Asian and western populations. In Asian patients, the opticospinal type of MS is more frequent, an older age group (>35 years of age) is affected, fewer cases are positive for oligoclonal bands and the CSF protein concentration is higher.[11]

The disease onset is usually between 20–40 years of age. Incidence of MS is low in childhood and in the elderly. It is twice as common in females, often with a more favorable prognosis compared to when it affects men. The clinical manifestations of MS are highly variable, but an attack of neurologic dysfunction (e.g., optic neuritis, incomplete transverse myelitis, brain stem or cerebeller syndrome), also referred to as a **clinically isolated syndrome (CIS)**,[12-14] heralds the onset of the disease in approximately 90% of patients. **CIS** is the first episode of neurologic symptoms typical of an MS relapse in a person not known to have MS symptoms, which depend on lesion location and extent of tissue destruction. It ranges from mild to severe. Common symptoms of an MS exacerbation (relapse or attack) include numbness, tingling, weakness, impaired balance, blurred vision, double vision, vertigo, and bladder or bowel dysfunction. Patients accumulate disability as a result of incomplete recovery from acute exacerbations and/or gradual disease progression.

The clinical course of MS is variable with varying plaque location and disease progression over time. A number of patterns of longitudinal disease presentation have been described.[4] The most common (70% of cases) is a **relapsing-remitting pattern** There is usually an acute episode of worsening, with complete recovery later on ,followed by a relapsing-remitting course. Many of these patients enter a phase where there is only progression of the disease, called **secondary progressive pattern** In some patients there is no clear cut period of remission and the disease follows a progressive course right from the onset—the **primary progressive MS (PPMS)**. Primary progressive MS comprise a minority (10%) of cases. Another variant is called **progressive relapsing MS** which follows a course like PPMS but there are clear acute relapses which may or may not show recovery. In 15–50% of cases, patients have **benign multiple sclerosis** defined as patients who remain functionally active for over 15 years.[15,16]

Radiologically isolated syndrome (RIS)—this subset of patients have MR findings suggestive of MS, but without related symptoms and have a normal neurological examination. One third will develop MS within 5 years whereas 2/3rd will show imaging progression. Patients of RIS who have cervical cord lesions or cortical lesions have a greater likelihood of conversion to MS.[17]

Pathology of MS: Demyelination occurs in discrete perivenular foci, termed plaques, which range in size from a few millimeters to a few centimeters. Each lesion goes through three pathological stages. The early acute stage (active plaque) is of active myelin breakdown. The plaques appear pink and edematous. The subacute stage is characterized by pale colored plaques with abundant macrophages. The chronic stage (inactive plaque) is characterized by gliosis with associated volume loss and plaque becoming grey in color.[18]

Diagnosis of Multiple Sclerosis

Multiple Sclerosis is primarily diagnosed clinically. The criteria for establishing the diagnosis are based on three main principles:

1. Demonstration of demyelinating lesions disseminated in space (DIS)
2. Demonstration of demyelinating lesions disseminated in time (DIT)
3. Exclusion of alternative explanation for the clinical presentation.

The various investigations required apart from clinical history and lack of viable alternative diagnosis, are the presence of oligoclonal bands in CSF, immunoglobulin (IgG) in serum, abnormal visual evoked potentials and MR imaging.[19,20]

MR imaging is the most important paraclinical tool in diagnosing and monitoring MS.[21,22] It was formally included in the clinical workup of patients suspected to have MS in 2001. Acquisition protocols vary widely. A simple protocol recommended is given in **Table 1**.

Table 1: Recommended sequences—MRI of multiple sclerosis.

Conventional MR sequences used in MS
• Fast spin echo T2 W and PD weighted—axial Specially for posterior fossa • FLAIR—axial and sagittal Better visualization of periventricular lesion due to suppression of CSF • Non-contrast T1 Hypointensity of white matter-black hole-axonal loss in chronic plaque • Contrast T1 Enhancement indicates disruption of blood-brain barrier, indicates inflammation • Diffusion-restriction—acute plaque • Scans for comparison must be technically adequate and positioned using specific landmarks
MR findings in multiple sclerosis—brain
• Focal white matter lesion Hyperintense on T2 in following location **Periventricular**—ovoid lesion on axial, triangular on sagittal, often perpendicular to ventricular surface **Callososeptal interface** **Juxtacortical/cortical** **Infratentorial** • Enhancement and diffusion restriction in acute lesion • T1 hypointensity-Acute-excessive edema, chronic-black hole • Basal ganglia and thalamus-T2 hypointensity-iron deposition • Brain atrophy
MRI characteristics of spinal cord lesions typical of MS
• Unequivocal hyperintensity on T2-weighted sequences and visible in two planes (e.g. axial and sagittal) • Size at least 3 mm but less than two vertebral segments in length • Occupy only a part of the cord in cross-section • Focal (i.e. clearly delineated and circumscribed on T2-weighted sequences) • Little or no cord swelling

MR Imaging of Multiple Sclerosis

Distribution and Characteristics of Lesion in the brain and spine

The characteristic lesion demonstrated on MRI is the cerebral or spinal plaque and is seen as a T2 hyper intense lesion **(Figs. 1A and B)**. The plaque consists of a discrete region of demyelination with relative preservation of axons. Active demyelination presents as areas of moderate T1 prolongation with mildly indistinct margins due to associated edema. Older plaques are smaller, more sharply defined and lower in signal intensity on T1W1.[23]

Multiple sclerosis plaques have a propensity to affect specific regions of the brain-periventricular white matter, callososeptal interface along the inferior surface of the corpus callosum, cortico-juxtacortical regions and the infratentorial regions. MS plaques are usually round to ovoid in shape, few millimeters to more than a centimeter in diameter **(Figs. 2A and B)**.

Periventricular lesions are oriented perpendicular to the outer surface of the lateral ventricle surrounding the medullary veins that radiate centripetally away from the lateral ventricle. These are the **Dawson's fingers**. These abut the ependymal surface unlike the nonspecific white matter hyperintensities (WMHs) **(Figs. 3 and 4)**.

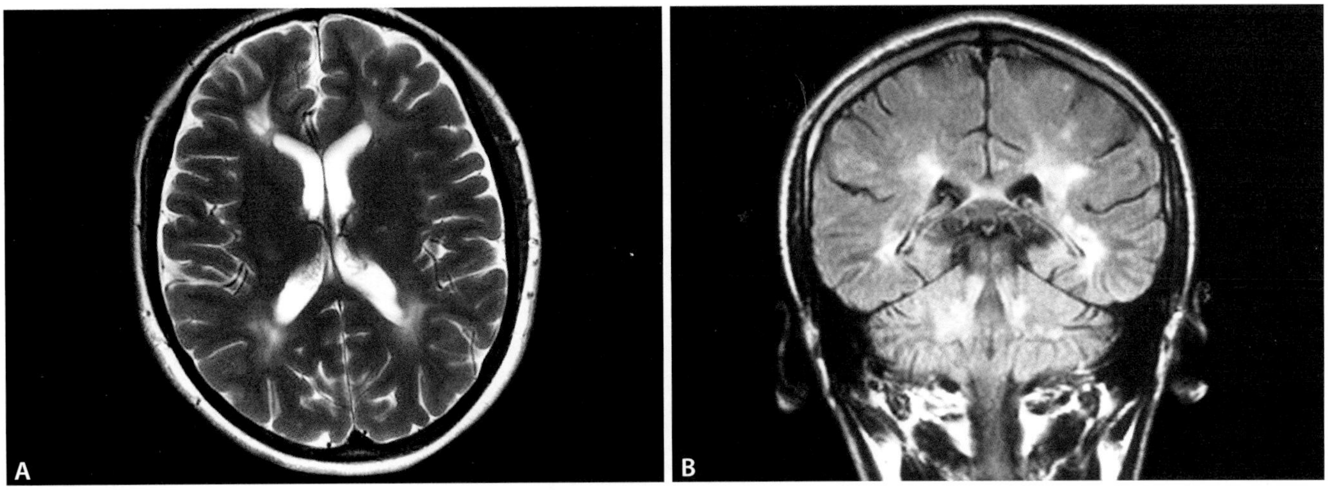

Figs. 1A and B: T2W-axial (A) Multiple periventricular hyperintensities seen in a case of multiple sclerosis. In another case, changes are seen in the periventicular location and brachium pontis on FLAIR coronal image (B).

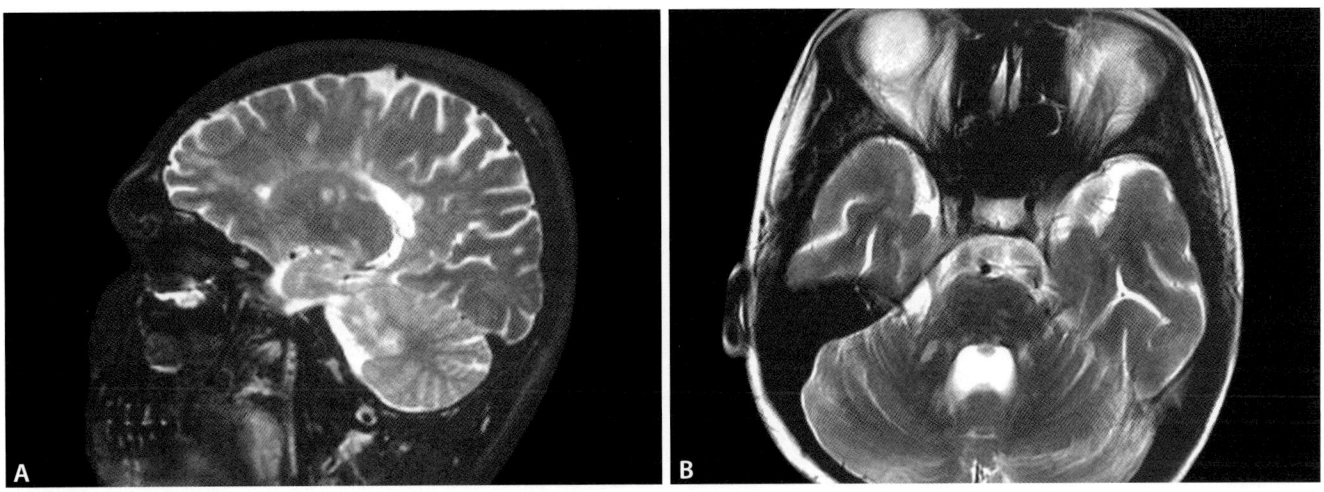

Figs. 2A and B: Hyperintense striations are seen in the corpus callosum, middle cerebeller peduncles. T2W sagittal (A), multiple plaques in the brainstem on T2W axial (B) image—a case of multiple sclerosis.

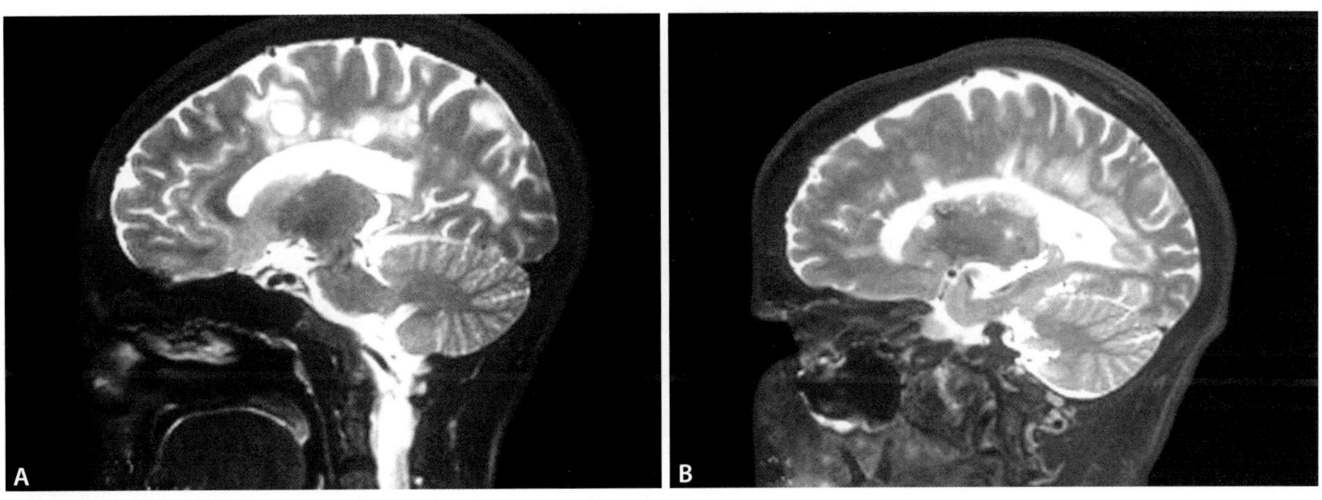

Figs. 3A and B: Sagittal T2W images show multiple plaques in the body and splenium of corpus callosum and callosal-septal interface with periventricular extension into centrum semiovale 'Dawson's fingers'.

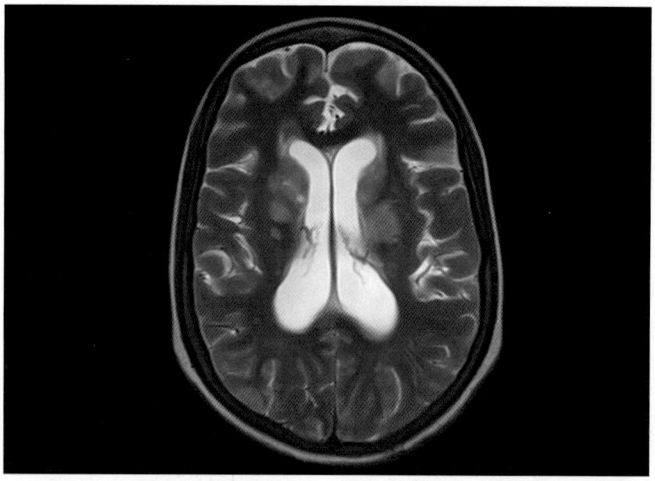

Fig. 4: T2W axial image-multiple hyperintense lesions in the periventricular location, extending almost at a right angle from and touching the ventricular surfaces.

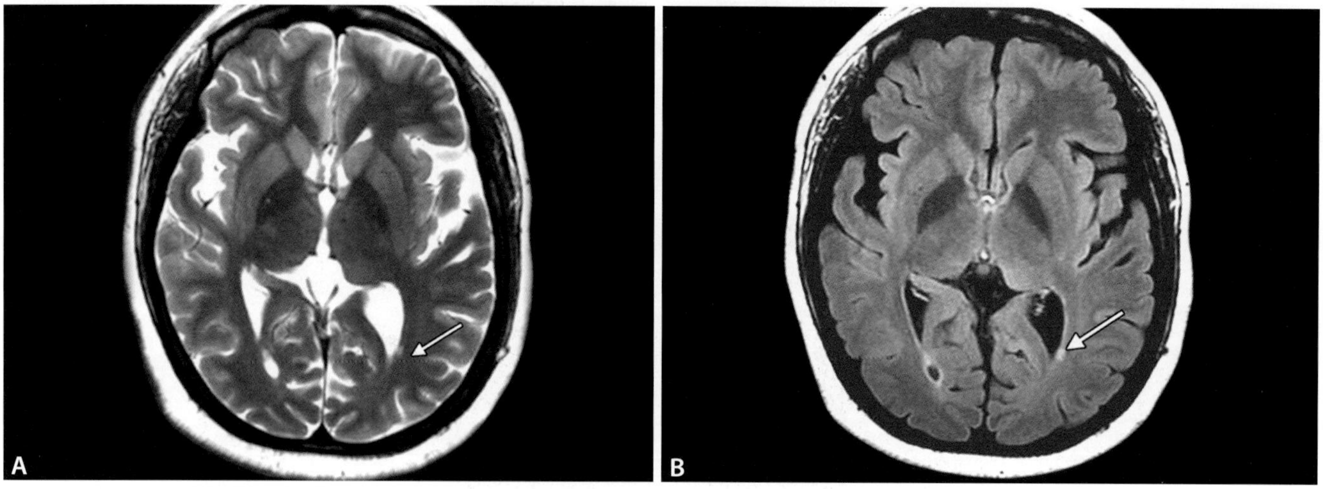

Figs. 5A and B: A small hyperintense focus touching the ventricular surface on T2W axial (A), better delineated on the FLAIR axial image (B).

Focal involvement of periventricular white matter in anterior temporal lobe is also typical for MS, rarely seen in other white matter disorders.[23] Small periventricular lesions are best appreciated using FLAIR sequence as it suppress the CSF and makes them more conspicuous **(Figs. 5A and B)**.

The **corpus callosum** is a region that is especially vulnerable to demyelination in MS, possibly due to its intimate neuroanatomic relationship to the lateral ventricular roofs and to small penetrating vessels. Presence of focal areas of high signal intensity on long TR images in the inferior aspect of the corpus callosum at the junction of the corpus callosum and the septum pellucidum (callosal-septal interface) **(Fig. 6)** is highly sensitive and specific for MS. This area is spared in white matter disease of ischemic origin due to rich collateral supply. In early disease these are focal and discrete and produce the 'dot and dash appearance', best seen on sagittal T2-weighted images **(Fig. 7)**.[24,25] On T1-weighted images callososeptal interface may have multiple small hypointense lesions (Venus necklace) or the corpus callosum may merely appear thinned.

Juxtacortical lesions involve the subcortical 'U fibers' seen in a majority of patients with MS. These are best appreciated on FLAIR sequences **(Figs. 8A and B)**. Cortical lesions are now recognized in early MS and may precede appearance of classic plaque. These are associated with cognitive impairment and can only be appreciated on 3D double inversion recovery sequence and higher magnetic fields.[26-28]

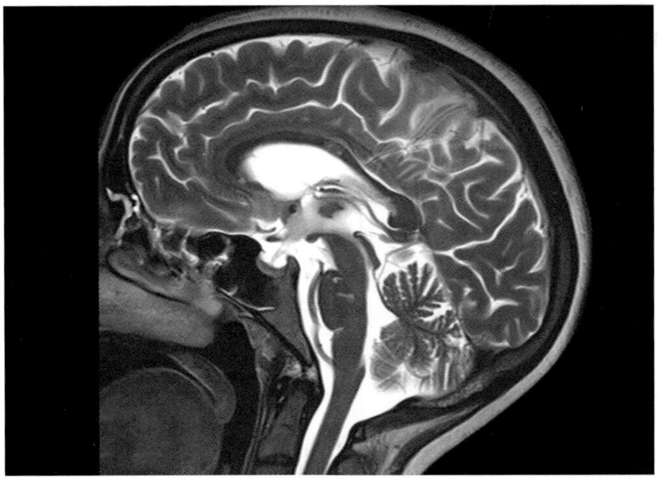

Fig. 6: T2 sagittal FLAIR image shows small plaques in the corpus callosum at the callososeptal interface, periventricular region and in the pons.

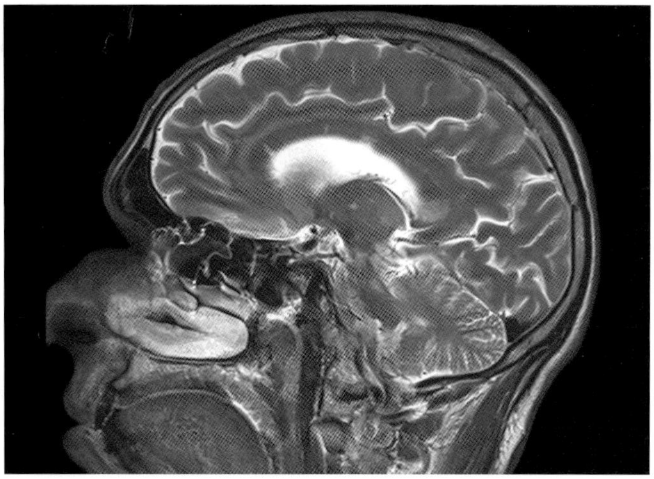

Fig. 7: 'Dot and dash'-small focal and discrete lesions in the corpus callosum in a patient of MS.

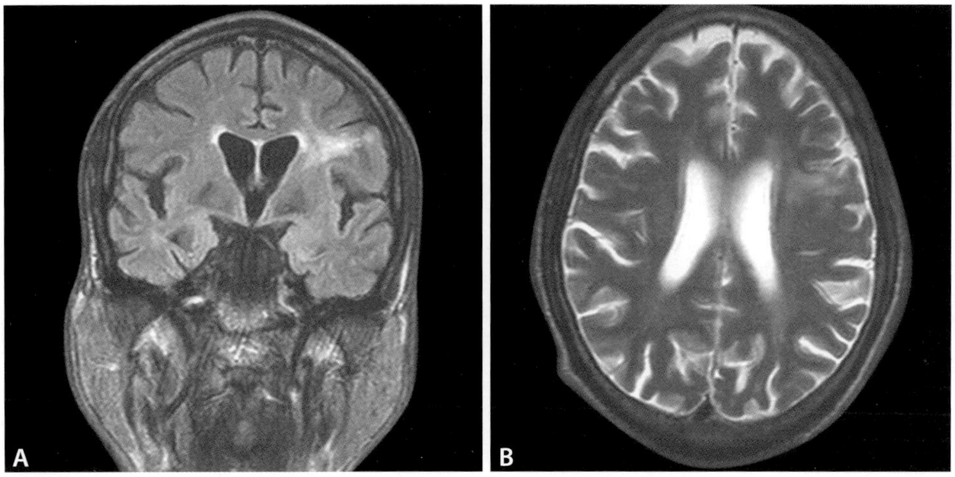

Figs. 8A and B: Juxtacortical lesion in a case of MS better appreciated on FLAIR image (A), than the T2 W image (B).

In the **infratentorial compartment**, lesions involve the floor of the fourth ventricle, middle cerebellar peduncle and the brainstem **(Fig. 9)**. Contiguous with cisternal or ventricular spaces, these may be seen as patchy, confluent to solitary well defined paramedian lesions or just as a discrete line along the ependymal surface. This peripheral location helps to differentiate them from focal areas of ischemia and infarction where the central white matter tracts are involved. PD/T2 FSE sequences are recommended over SE/FLAIR to image the posterior fossa in patients with MS.

Spinal cord lesions are reported in a high percentage (30–40%) of cases with clinically isolated syndromes and in up to 90% of patients in definite MS.[29] The cervical cord is mostly affected; the lesions are less than 1 or 2 vertebral segments in cranio-caudal dimension, are well defined and occupy less than 50% of cross-sectional area of the cord in axial plane **(Figs. 10A and B)**. The lesion involves the peripheral white matter, the lateral and posterior white matter columns. An acute spinal cord plaque may produce mild to moderate mass effect and some cord swelling, though extensive swelling of the cord is uncommon. Active lesions may enhance. The involvement of the spinal cord varies with lesions being multifocal in relapsing remitting MS. Extensive, diffuse abnormalities and cord atrophy are seen in secondary progressive subtype, while there may be more extensive involvement of cord as compared to brain in PPMS.[30,31]

Optic neuritis may be the only presentation in the initial stage of MS. It is a clinical diagnosis and MR imaging is not required to make the diagnosis. In patients who present initially with optic neuritis, many clinicians believe

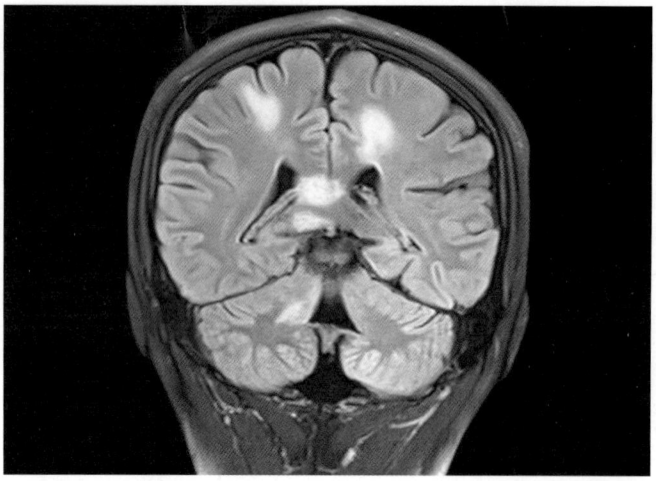

Fig. 9: In a patient of multiple sclerosis multiple T2 hyperintense lesions are seen in corpus callosum, juxtacortical and infratentorial location. Lesion in the middle cerebral peduncle is touching the ventricular surface on coronal FLAIR image.

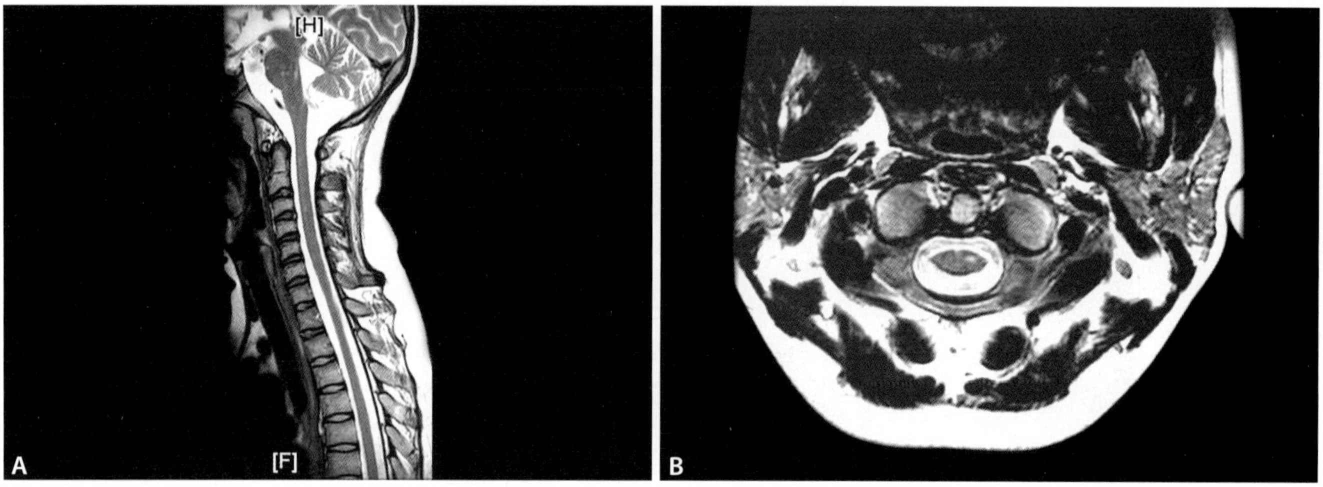

Figs. 10A and B: T2W sagittal (A) and axial (B) A tiny speck of hyperintensity is seen in the left lateral aspect of the spinal cord at C3 level. Note that the cord is of normal caliber-MS.

that the role of MR is to exclude the rarely found alternative cause of the clinical symptomatology aside from optic neuritis and to detect the presence of intracerebral lesions that may indicate MS. Coronal fat saturated T2 images are sensitive to depict signal alteration in optic neuritis. Optic nerve may be thickened, hyperintense and may show intense contrast enhancement. In MS, the optic nerve may show signal abnormalities in the absence of acute attacks of optic neuritis. A positive brain MR at the time of optic neuritis may provide diagnostic criteria for possible MS, if negative, it suggests a low risk for MS.[32]

Atrophy of the brain and spinal cord are seen in patients with multiple sclerosis. This is more severe in progressive form of disease but may also occur early in the disease. Atrophy is an important predictor for development of physical disability. It involves both gray and white matter **(Figs. 11A and B)**. **Basal ganglia** hypointensity is seen in 10–20% of chronic cases and represents heavy metal deposition.

Contrast-enhanced imaging is routinely used to assess inflammatory activity. In the acute inflammatory phase, the lesion may disrupt blood-brain barrier, leading to gadolinium enhancement, which may last for a variable time. Disease activity seen as enhancement is detected more frequently than clinical evaluation of relapses, indicating that most enhancing lesions remain clinically silent. The **enhancement pattern** may be variable within and between patients **(Fig. 12)**.[33,34] This is suggestive of a heterogenous pathology related to host response. MS plaques may show transient enhancement

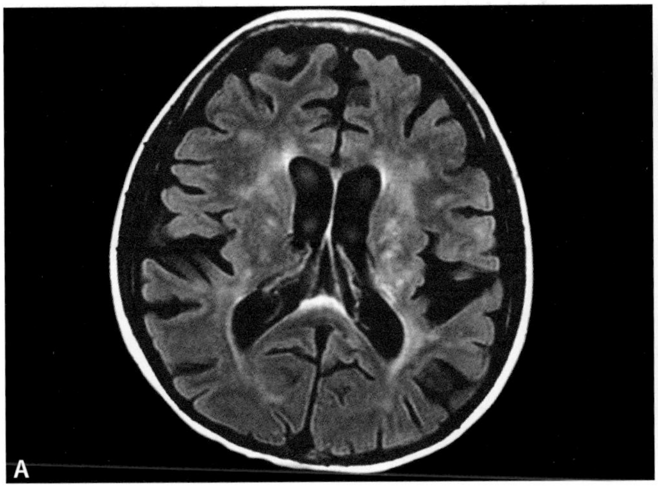
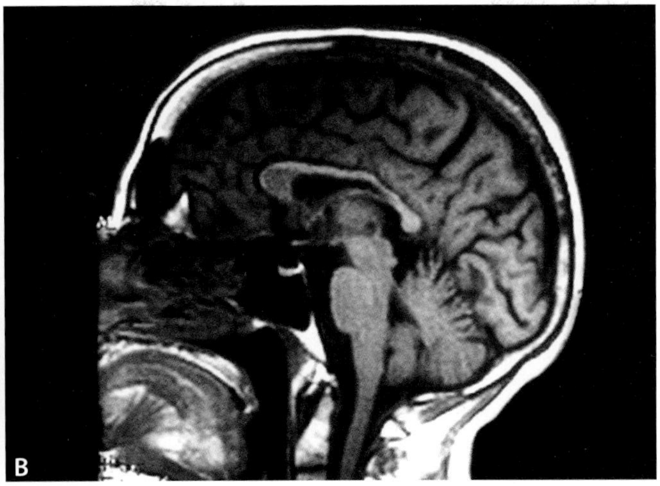

Figs. 11A and B: Diffuse cerebral atrophy along with plaques is noted in a case of MS on FLAIR axial image (A), atrophy of the corpus callosum is noted in another case -T1 axial image (B).

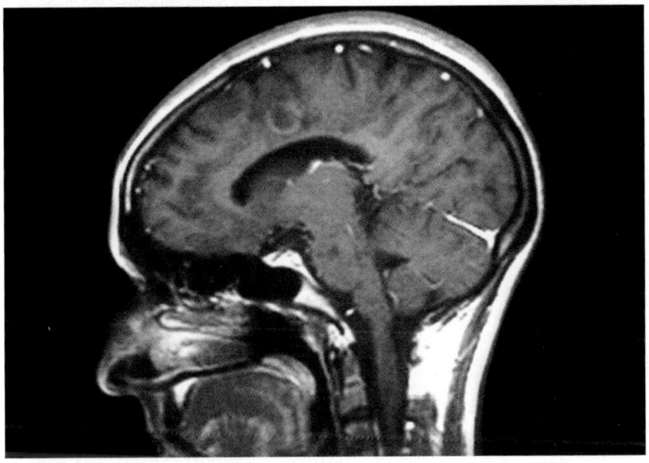

Fig. 12: Contrast-enhanced TIW MR image shows rim enhancement of a plaque, suggesting activity.

in acute and relapsing stages of disease. This may be punctate, rim or nodular. Incomplete rim (horseshoe) pattern of enhancement with the open border facing the cortex or basal ganglia in acute stages is a pointer towards inflammatory demyelinating pathology, contrasting to a complete ring in abscess or tumors. Enhancement usually disappears within 6 months; earlier with steroid administration. Persistence of enhancement should be treated with caution as a point against the diagnosis of MS.

Contrast enhancement may be used to add specificity to the finding of multiple hyperintensities on T2-weighted images, because the finding of enhancing along with nonenhancing lesions is seen in MS. In relapsing remitting and secondary progressive MS, enhancement is seen during relapses and correlates with clinical activity. However in PPMS, enhancement does not match the clinical deterioration. High dose of gadolinium and a long post injection delay increase sensitivity in detecting enhancement, especially in the spinal cord.[35]

Acute or Chronic MS

Acute as well as chronic MS plaques appear hyperintense on PD and T2WI reflecting increased water content with edema, inflammation, demyelination, gliosis and axonal loss being the underlying pathology. Larger lesions may depict a very hyperintense center surrounded by less hyperintense periphery and variable amounts of perilesional edema. Acute MS lesions tend to be larger with fuzzy margins. As resolution occurs they become smaller and more sharply defined, reflecting reduction of edema and inflammation. T2 hyperintensity shrinks over a period of time leaving a smaller lesion which may remain unchanged over years. As the disease progresses the T2 lesion number and volume of T2 lesion increases and is called **T2 load**. This increases in absence of or due to poor response to treatment. The T2 burden is an important measure of abnormal tissue.[36–38]

Most of the MS plaques are hypo- or iso-intense on T1-weighted imaging. These are called '**black holes**' and in acute cases these black holes become iso-intense in a few months, whereas the persisting or chronic black holes correlate with severe demyelination and axonal destruction **(Figs. 13A and B)**.[39] These T1 black holes have relatively reduced MTR, elevated diffusion coefficient and reduced NAA, also indicative of more severe focal injury. Chronicity of T1 hypointense lesion is also based on lack of contrast enhancement **(Figs. 14A and B)**. A T1 hypointense lesion that shows contrast enhancement is an acute lesion, hypointensity being attributable to edema.

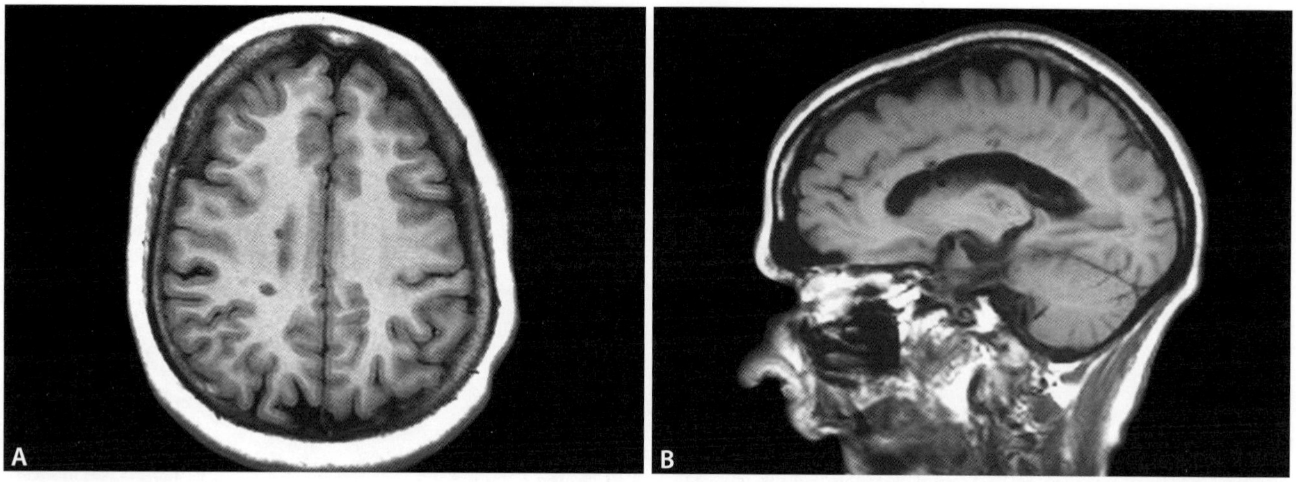

Figs. 13A and B: T1W axial image (A) and sagittal image (B) Hypointense well demarcated lesions in right periventricular region and corpus callosum- T1 'black hole'.

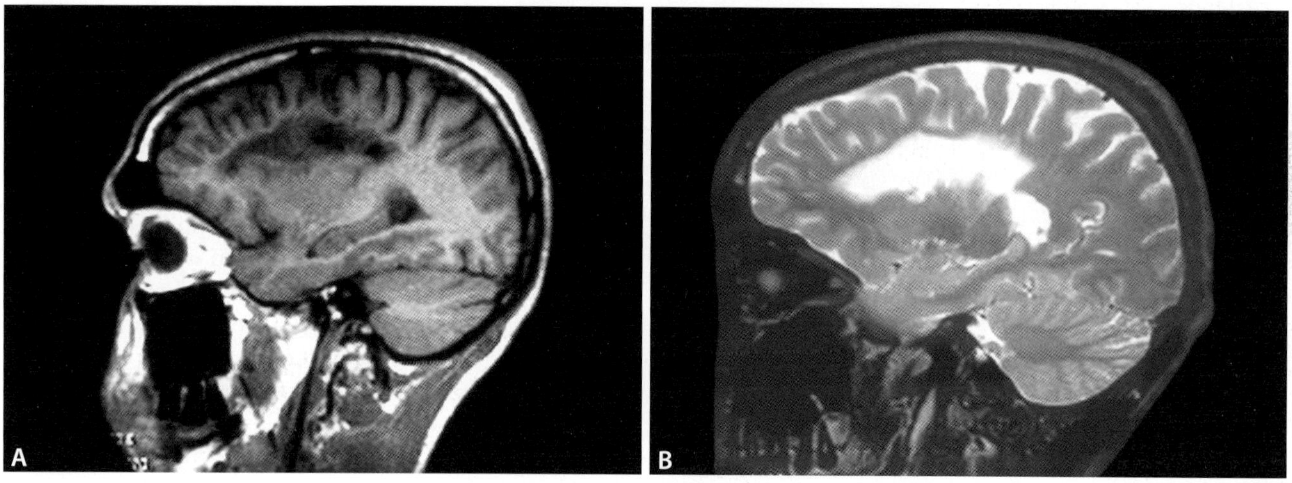

Figs. 14A and B: Sagittal T1W MR image (A) shows confluent areas of decreased signal intensity in the periventricular regions and along the callosal-septal interface. Sagittal T2W image (B) shows the same lesions to be hyperintense.

A faint peripheral rim of hyper-intensity may surround these T1 hypointensities giving a beveled appearance. T1 hypointensity is an independent predictor of atrophy, disability and disease progression.

Advanced MR techniques in multiple sclerosis: Subtle pathological changes have been described in normal appearing white matter (NAWM) and normal appearing gray matter (NAGM).[40] These represent a significant component of the disease burden and require advanced MR techniques for detection of the same.

Magnetization transfer imaging—is sensitive to the macromolecular environment of cell membrane and tissue. Decreased MTR (magnetization transfer ratio) is noted in NAWM in patients of MS in the absence of visible T2 lesions **(Figs. 15A to F)**. A decrease in MTR parallels enhancement of the lesion, a marker of inflammation. Post treatment these values increase.[41–44]

Diffusion tensor imaging—increased diffusivity is a nonspecific finding and is seen in focal MS lesions and in normal appearing brain tissue in contrast to reduced diffusivity characteristic for cerebral infarction. Acute plaques may be associated with restricted diffusion **(Figs. 16A to F)**. Decreased fractional anisotropy is seen in focal MS lesions. Various studies have correlated damage to a particular white matter tract on DTI with patient symptomatology.[44–51]

MR proton spectroscopy—an alteration in various metabolites has been shown on spectroscopy in both the demyelinating plaque and in NAWM and NAGM. NAA-N acetyl aspartate, a neuronal marker is reduced in focal lesions and in NAWM, the decrease being more pronounced in chronic disease **(Figs. 17A to C)**. Choline, a marker of cell turnover can be increased in acute plaque. Myoinositol and creatine are markers of gliosis and can

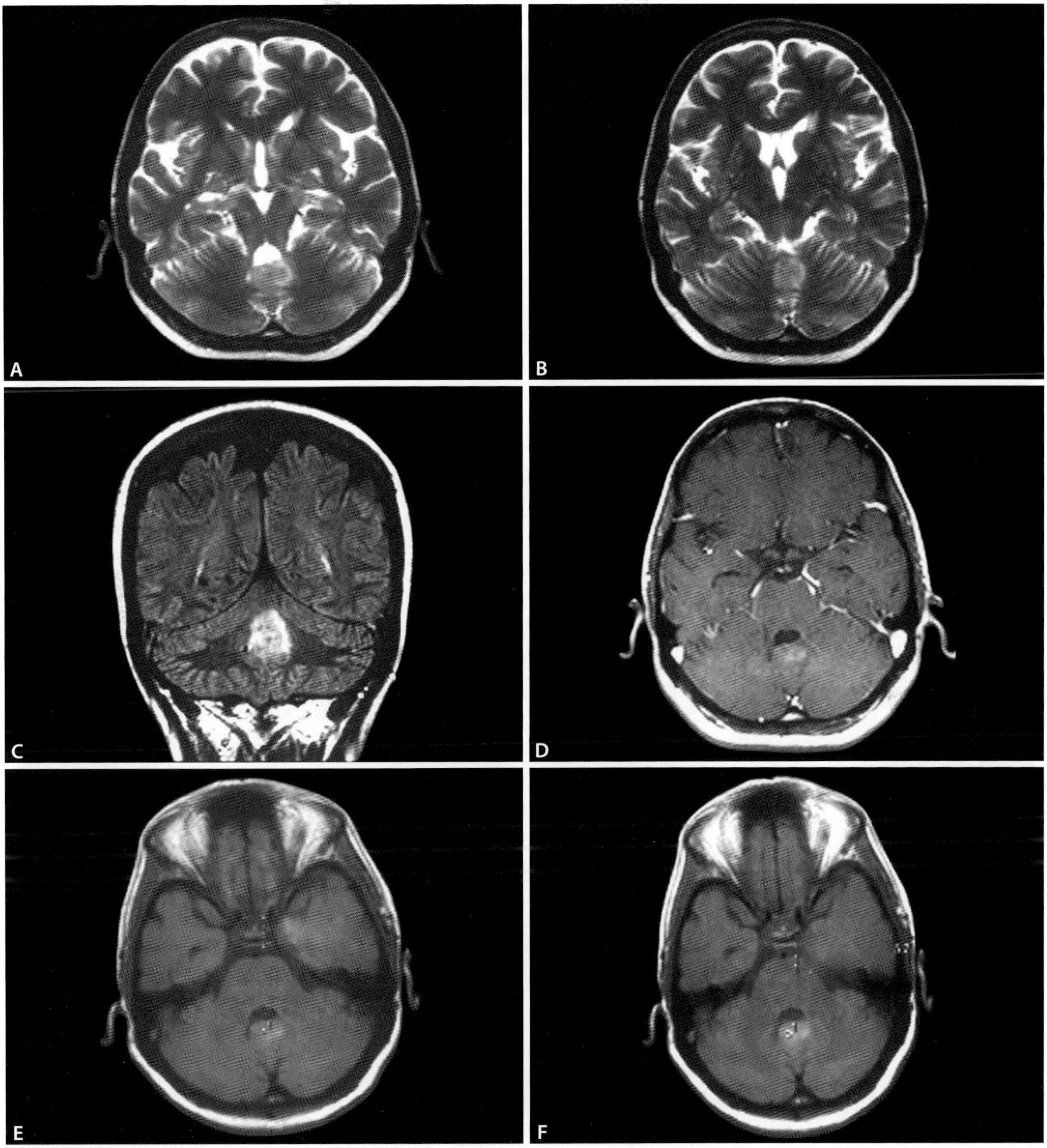

Figs. 15A to F: Axial T2WI (A and B) and coronal flair image (C): Poorly marginated hyperintense lesion seen in cerebellar vermis. Small hyperintense areas also seen in periventricular white matter around left frontal horn. The lesion in the vermis shows patchy inhomogenous enhancement (D). Axial T1W without MT (E) and with MT (F) MTR = 15%. Multiple sclerosis-acute plaque.

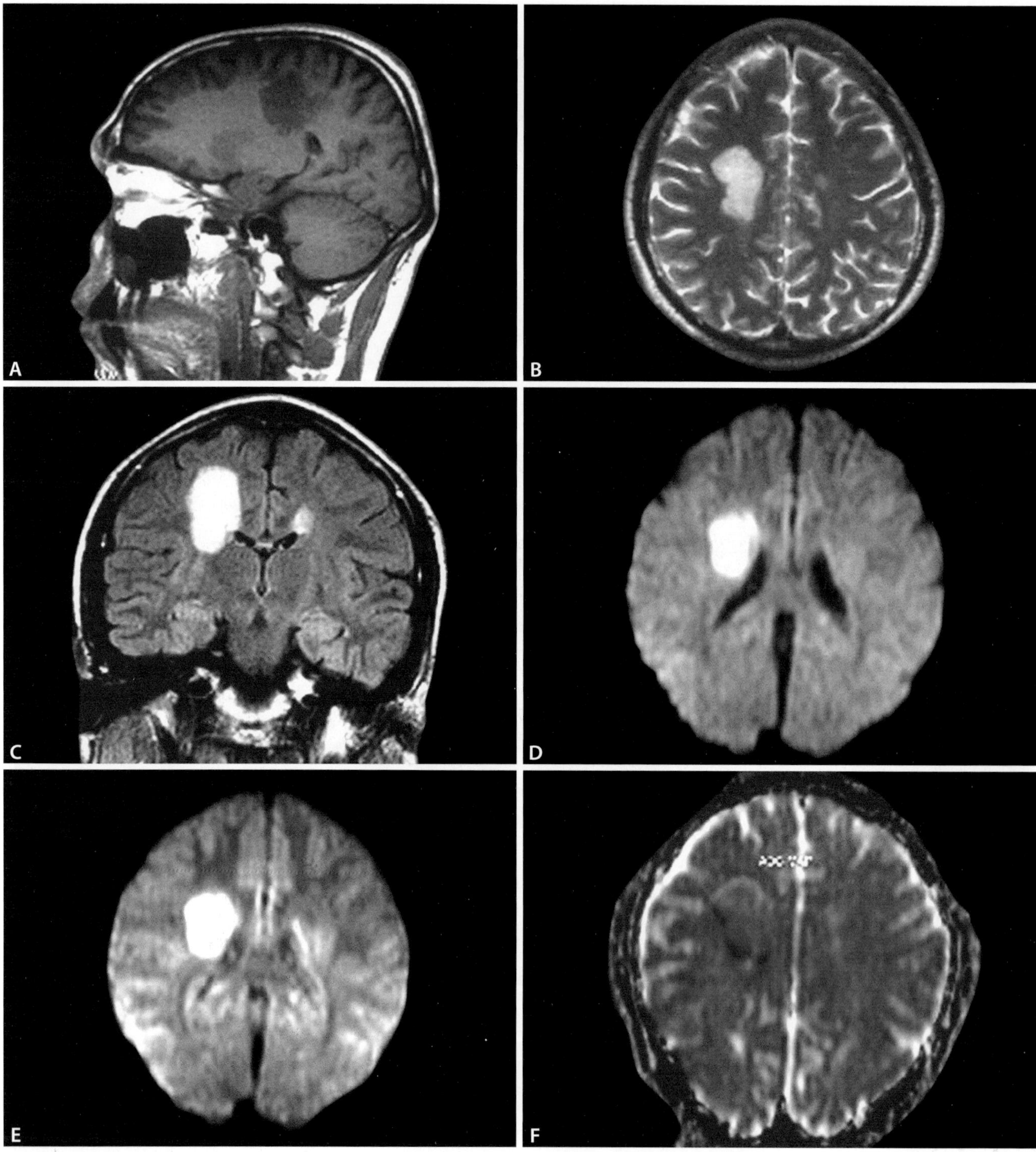

Figs. 16A to F: In a case of multiple sclerosis sagittal T1W image (A) shows a large well-defined hypointense lesion in the region of right centrum semiovale which is hyperintense on axial T2W (B). Another small hyperintense focus is also seen in left centrum semiovale region. Coronal FLAIR image (C) shows the lesions to be of high signal intensity. Diffusion-weighted image reveals the lesion to be hyperintense on 'b' = 500. (D) The lesions show increase in signal intensity on 'b' = 1000 DWI (E) ADC map (F) reveals restricted diffusion within the lesions.

be increased in acute white matter lesion. Glutamate, an excitatory neurotransmitter increases in focal white matter lesions and in NAWM.[44,52–55]

Functional MR Imaging—studies have shown cortical re-organization on fMRI in patients with MS that varies with stage of disease and correlates with specific

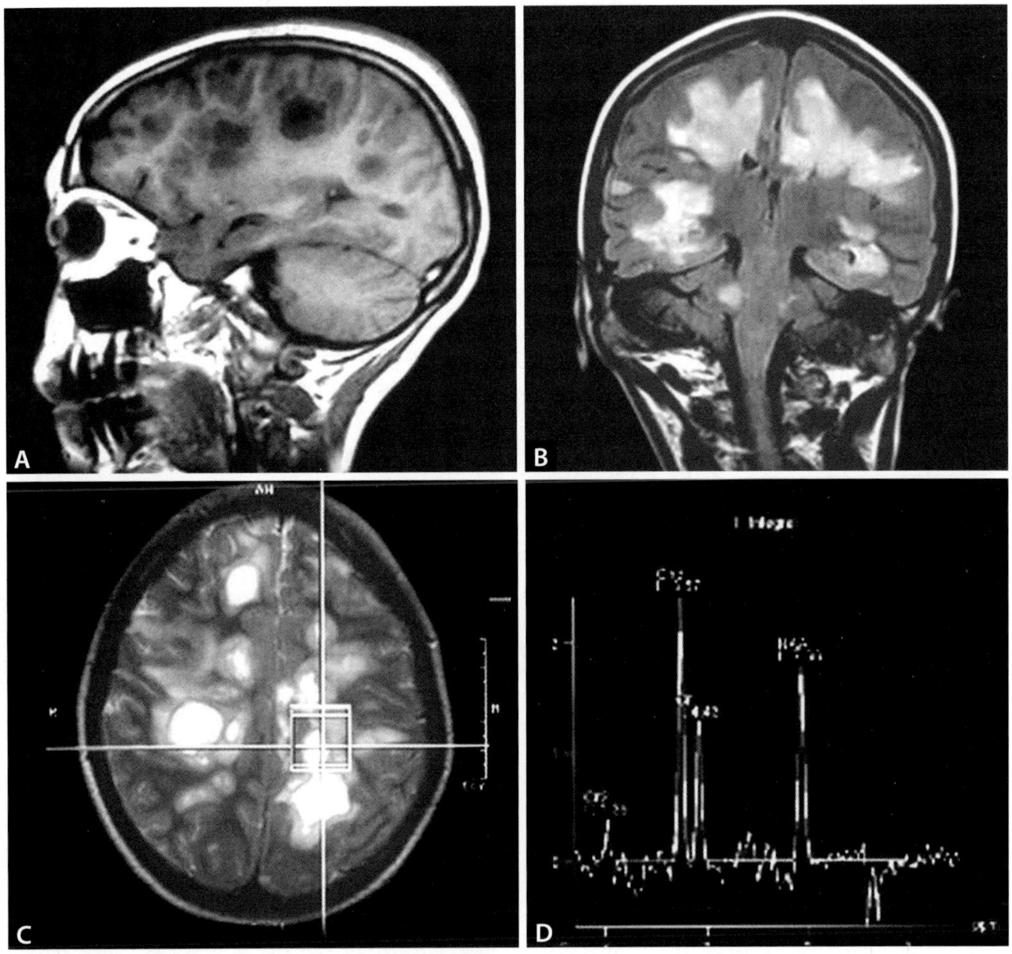

Figs. 17A to D: Sagittal T1W (A) shows multiple well-defined hypointense lesions in the deep as well as subcortical white matter in the frontoparieto-occipital regions. Lesions also shows typical 'beveled' or 'lesion within lesion' appearance. FLAIR coronal image (B) and T2 axial image (C) shows multiple hyperintense lesions which appear confluent in the fronto-parieto-occipital white matter. MR spectroscopy (D) reveals reduction of NAA level with marked elevation of choline level and reversal of Cho/Cr ratio. Doublet lactate peak is also noted.

symptoms. Brain plasticity has also been demonstrated, explaining the discordance seen between MR findings and patient symptomatology.[56,57]

MR perfusion imaging—Alterations in cerebral perfusion have been seen in patients of MS with increase in CBV in acute lesions, decreased perfusion reflecting microvascular change or injury is detected in NAWM, with increased perfusion preceding development of a new lesion. The reduction in relative CBF and CBV has been shown to correlate with cognitive impairment.[58]

Double inversion recovery (DIR): a new sequence that suppresses both CSF and white matter signal and offers better delineation of the plaques especially in the cortical gray matter.[44,52–55]

7T MRI—Ultra-high Field MR Imaging

One of the main advantages of high field imaging is the high signal intensity to noise ratio, the lesion detection improves, as does the potential to detect cortical lesions. The enhanced T2 effects are also beneficial for perfusion, diffusion and functional MR imaging. Increased detection of cortical abnormalities is seen with the use of ultra high field MR. The perivenular location of the MS plaque has been delineated with high sensitivity on 7T MRI using susceptibility weighted imaging (SWI), this is called the **central vein sign.**[21,44,28] Increased proportion of this finding in the brain may differentiate MS from other neurological diseases such as small vessel disease, migraine SLE etc.

Myelin water imaging: This technique utilizes multiple T2 echoes during a single acquisition. Based on different echo times (TE), it separates the more slowly relaxing intra/extracellular water compartment from the more rapidly relaxing water trapped between myelin sheaths. The myelin water fraction (MWF) describes the ratio of the myelin water to total water, MWF has been found to be reduced in white matter of patients with MS and also in NAWM.[44,59]

Diagnostic Criteria for Diagnosis of MS

Several criteria have been developed to integrate MR imaging into clinical evaluation to achieve earlier and more accurate diagnosis.

McDonald diagnostic criteria for multiple sclerosis are clinical, radiographic, and laboratory criteria used in the diagnosis of multiple sclerosis. The criteria are named after **Ian McDonald** (1933–2006), a New Zealander neurologist, who devised the original criteria with his international colleagues in 2001. They were originally introduced in 2001,[60] and were revised in 2005,[61] 2010,[62] 2016 (by MAGNIMS[63]) and most recently in 2017.[64]

These criteria apply to individuals experiencing a typical clinically isolated syndrome—CIS. A MS attack (also called as relapse or exacerbation) is defined by McDonald criteria as a patient having reported or objectively observed event typical of an acute inflammatory demyelinating event in the CNS, with a duration of at least 24 hours, without fever or signs of infection. **The criteria are based on demonstration of dissemination in space (DIS), dissemination in time (DIT) and absence of any other viable alternative diagnoses.**

Dissemination in Space on MRI

Dissemination in space requires ≥1 T2-hyperintense lesions (≥3 mm in long axis), symptomatic and/ or asymptomatic, that are characteristic of multiple sclerosis in two or more of the four following locations: periventricular (≥1 lesion, unless the patient is over the age of 50 in which case it is better to seek a higher number of lesions), cortical/juxtacortical, infratentorial, spinal cord **(Fig. 18)**.

T2-hyperintense lesions of the optic nerve, such as those in a patient presenting with optic neuritis, are not counted in the 2017 revised McDonald criteria.

Dissemination in Time

- A new T2-hyperintense or gadolinium-enhancing lesion when compared to a previous baseline MRI scan (irrespective of timing).
- Simultaneous presence of a gadolinium-enhancing lesion and a non-enhancing T2-hyperintense lesion on any one MRI scan **(Figs. 19A to C)**.

McDonald Criteria 2017: The following changes were made:

- In patients with a typical clinically isolated syndrome and clinical or MRI demonstration of dissemination in

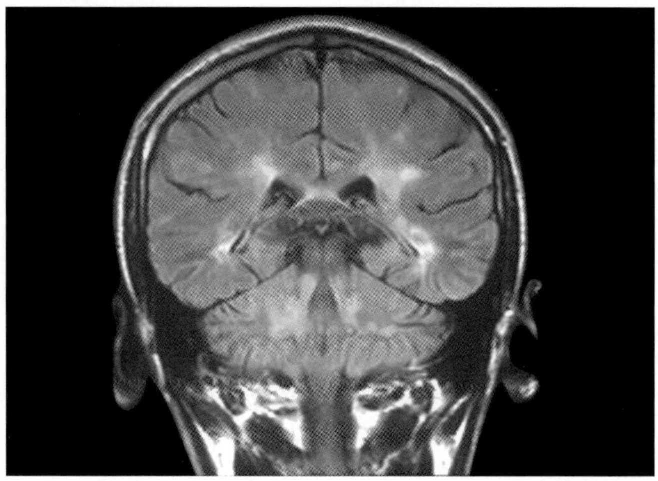

Fig. 18: Coronal FLAIR image depicts multiple hyperintense lesions (>1) in multiple locations-juxtacortical. periventricular and infratentorial-Dissemination in space in MS.

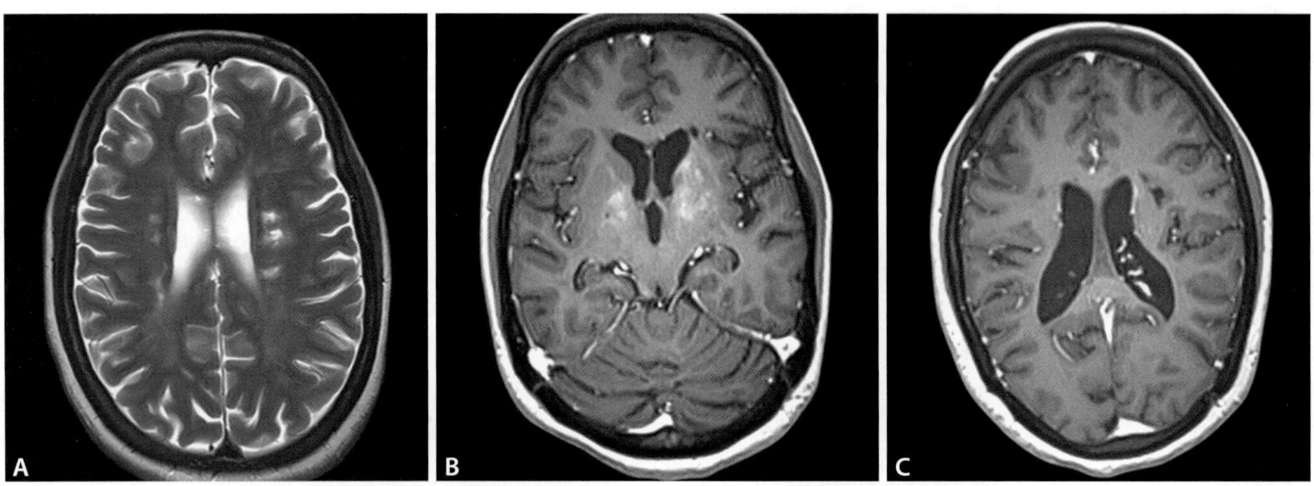

Figs. 19A to C: T2W axial image (A), Postcontrast T1WI images (B and C) show enhancing and nonenhancing foci in the same patient—dissemination in time in MS.

space, the presence of CSF-specific oligoclonal bands allows a diagnosis of multiple sclerosis.

- Symptomatic lesions can be used to demonstrate dissemination in space or time in patients with supratentorial, infratentorial, or spinal cord syndrome;
- Cortical lesions can be used to demonstrate dissemination in space.

The new criteria are expected to speed up the diagnosis of MS, thus enabling early initiation of therapy. In addition, chances of misdiagnosis of MS are expected to reduce. A summary of the criteria is given in the **Table 2**.

Primary Progressive Multiple Sclerosis

The McDonald criteria also defines the diagnosis of primary progressive multiple sclerosis (PPMS). The diagnosis requires:

- ≥1 year of disability progression which can be determined either prospectively or retrospectively with two of the following:
  - ≥1 T2-hyperintense lesions characteristic of multiple sclerosis in one or more of the following regions: periventricular, cortical or juxtacortical, or infratentorial.

Differential Diagnosis of MS Lesion on MR

The differential diagnosis of lesions with increased signal on T2-weighted images is large. These may be normal variants or truly not primary demyelinating processes, but may simulate MS on MR imaging.

1. **Normal anatomical structures** may potentially mimic MS lesions. Ependymitis granularis represent small areas of denuded ependyma within the lining of the

Table 2: McDonald criteria for the diagnosis of MS (2017).

• ***Requires elimination of more likely diagnoses*** • ***Requires demonstration of dissemination of lesions in the central nervous system in space and time***	
Clinical presentation	***Additional criteria to make MS diagnosis***
...in a person who has experienced a typical attack/CIS at onset	
• 2 or more attacks and clinical evidence of 2 or more lesions; OR • 2 or more attacks and clinical evidence of 1 lesion with clear historical evidence of prior attack involving lesion in different location	None. DIS and DIT have been met.
• 2 or more attacks and clinical evidence of 1 lesion	DIS shown by *one* of these criteria: • Additional clinical attack implicating different CNS site • 1 or more MS-typical T2 lesions in 2 or more areas of CNS: periventricular, cortical, juxtacortical, infratentorial or spinal cord
• 1 attack and clinical evidence of 2 or more lesions	DIT shown by *one* of these criteria: • Additional clinical attack • Simultaneous presence of both enhancing and non-enhancing MS-typical MRI lesion, or new T2 or enhancing MRI lesion compared to baseline scan (without regard to timing of baseline scan) • CSF oligoclonal bands
• 1 attack and clinical evidence of 1 lesion	DIS shown by *one* of these criteria: • Additional attack implicating different CNS site • 1 or more MS-typical T2 lesions in 2 or more areas of CNS: periventricular, cortical, juxtacortical, infratentorial or spinal cord AND DIT shown by *one* of these criteria: • Additional clinical attack • Simultaneous presence of both enhancing and non-enhancing MS-typical MRI lesions, or new T2 or enhancing MRI lesion compared to baseline scan (without regard to timing of baseline scan) • CSF oligoclonal bands
...in a person who has steady progression of disease since onset	
1 year of disease progression (retrospective or prospective)	DIS shown by at least *two* of these criteria: • 1 or more MS-typical T2 lesions (periventricular, cortical, juxtacortical or infratentorial) • 2 or more T2 spinal cord lesions • CSF oligoclonal bands

Abbreviations: DT: Dissemination in time; CNS: Central nervous system; CSF: Cerebrospinal fluid; DIS: Dissemination in space; T2 lesion: Hyperintense lesion on T2-weighted MRI.

lateral ventricles adjacent to anterolateral angles of the frontal horns with a small amount of CSF seepage adjacent to tips of frontal horns. This should not be confused with periventricular plaque **(Fig. 20)**.

2. **The Virchow Robin spaces** are invaginations of the subarachnoid space into the brain associated with leptomeningeal vessels. These spaces enlarge with age and hypertension as vessels within the space become more ectatic, termed "etat crible".[65] Dilated perivascular spaces occur in characteristic locations, typically in basal ganglia (inferior portion) around the atria, near the anterior commissure, in corona radiata, centrum semiovale and in peri insular region **(Fig. 21)**. They follow the intensity of cerebrospinal fluid. The FLAIR/PDWI sequences are most suited at discriminating perivascular spaces from white matter lesions because the perivascular spaces are isointense to CSF, whereas MS and other lesions are hyperintense.
3. **Ischemic white matter lesions/small vessel ischemic changes**: Incidental white matter hyperintensities are seen commonly in the elderly. The prevalence ranges from 11–21% in adults aged around 64 yrs to 94% at 82 yrs of age.[66] Foci of hyperintense signal on T2-weighted images, frequently found in subcortical or periventricular white matter in elderly are smoother than the smaller, lobulated ovoid MS lesions **(Figs. 22A to C)**. Corpus callosum and spinal cord involvement is not seen in ischemic changes. MR detects all these changes, but all are not clinically significant. Most lesions are age related, but careful analysis of diffusion images is required to detect acute ischemia.
4. **Vasculitis**: MS lesions can mimic lesions from vasculitides such as SLE.

   MS may involve gray matter in 5–10%. MR is unable to definitively distinguish between these etiologies, although the presence of cortical lesions is suggestive of vasculitis. Therefore, the clinical history, the presence of systemic symptoms, results of laboratory studies and a positive angiogram, all help to differentiate these entities.
5. **Migraine**: Signal abnormalities may be seen in the centrum semiovale, frontal subcortical matter which can extend into deeper white matter at the level of basal ganglia.[67]
6. **ADEM**: This acute demyelinating disease that occurs after a viral infection or a recent immunization bears many similarities to MS in initial clinical presentation, pathological findings and MR appearance. ADEM is a monophasic illness unlike MS. The differences are tabulated in **Table 3**.
7. **Trauma**: Traumatic shear injuries that result from torsional stresses on white matter fiber tracts that occur at the time of high speed acceleration/deceleration brain injury may produce signal abnormalities at gray white matter junction, brainstem and corpus callosum-locations similar to MS. The clinical history of closed head injury plus the presence of associated punctuate hemorrhages clinch the diagnosis.

Treatment of multiple sclerosis: The aim of treatment is twofold: to curtail progression (disease-modifying agents) and to provide symptomatic relief. Immunosuppressant and immunomodulatory drugs are used, and studies have shown a significant decrease in relapse rate and reduction of brain lesion accumulation when therapy is started early.[68-71] Steroids, interferon, monoclonal antibodies and stem cell therapy are all used in the treatment.

There are certain complications, related to treatment.

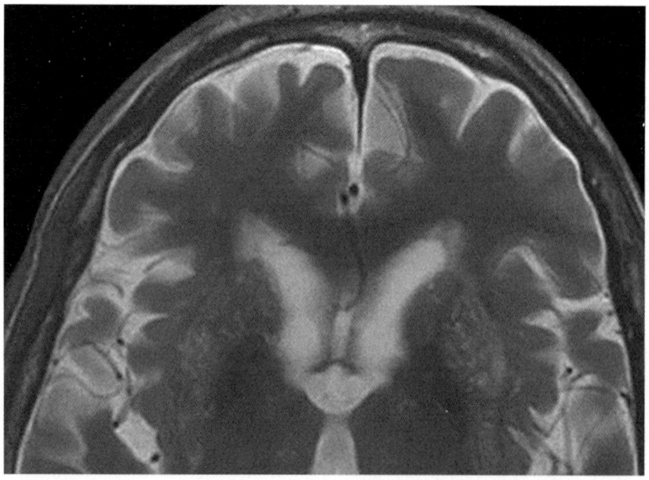

Fig. 20: T2W axial image–Ependymitis granularis at the tips of frontal horns.

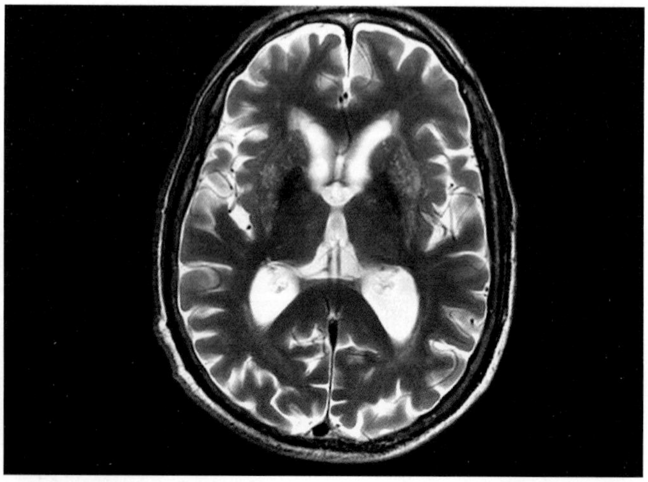

Fig. 21: Virchow-Robin spaces appreciated as multiple pinpoint hyperintense foci in the basal ganglia region on T2W axial image.

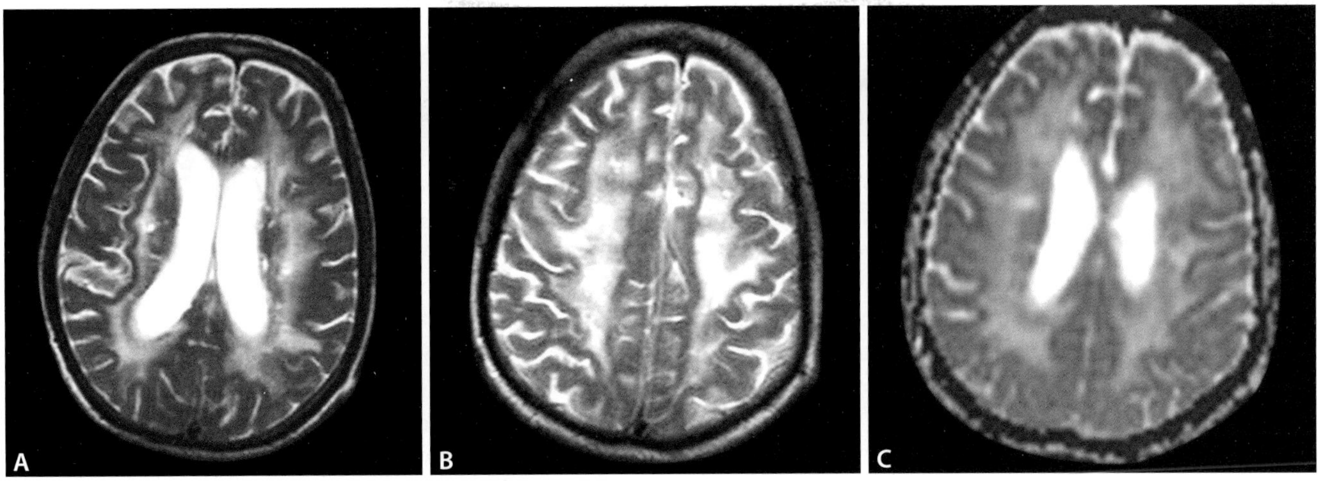

Figs. 22A to C: Extensive confluent periventricular and deep white matter hyperintensities on T2WI (A and B) which show facilitated diffusion on ADC map (C) Ischemic changes in an elderly hypertensive patient.

Table 3: Differences between multiple sclerosis and ADEM.

Feature	*MS*	*ADEM*
Age	>10 years	<10 years
Sex	Female preponderance	No sex predominance
Preceding illness	Usually no	Yes
Encephalopathy	No	Yes
Optic neuritis	Unilateral and common	Bilateral rare
Spinal cord involvement	Partial	Extensive with cord swelling
MRI	Periventricular, callosal	Cortical, deep gray matter Thalamic
T1 black hole	Seen	Not seen
Lesion of different ages	Seen	Not seen
T2 hyperintense lesions	Well circumscribed	Fuzzy margins
Size of lesion-large	Rare	Common
CSF	Oligoclonal bands	Lymphocytosis and increased proteins
Follow up	New lesions	Monophasic

Progressive multifocal leukoencephalopathy (PML) is seen in patients treated with natalizumab with positive JC virus serology. PML-IRIS, a complication of cessation of natalizumab or treatment for natalizumab-related PML are treated with plasma exchange or immunoabsorption.

Idiopathic Inflammatory Demyelinating Disorders (IIDDs)[72]

They represent a spectrum of CNS disorders that can be differentiated on the basis of severity, clinical course, lesion distribution as well as imaging, laboratory and pathological findings. The spectrum of IIDDs includes monophasic, multiphasic and progressive disorders. The lesions can be localized or multifocal/diffuse variants.

Differential diagnosis—multiple sclerosis
Multifocal T2/FLAIR hyperintensities
• Normal variants-ependymitis granularis, Virchow Robin spaces
• ADEM
• Lyme disease
• Vasculitis- and age related ischemic changes
• Susac syndrome
• CNS manifestations of antiphospholipid syndrome
• Marchiafava Bignami disease (corpus callosum lesion)
Solitary 'tumefactive' MS
• Neoplasm (GBM, metastasis)
• PML/PML-IRIS in natalizumab treated MS
Spinal lesions
• Transverse myelitis
• Spinal tumor

MS is considered the most representative of IIDDs, with others considered as variants or a borderline form of MS. These are classified on clinical presentation, neuro-imaging and CSF abnormalities.

1. *Fulminant/Acute IIDDs*: Marburg, Schilder, Balo's concentric sclerosis considered as MS variants.
2. *Monosymptomatic IIDDs*: Isolated optic neuritis
3. *IIDDs restricted to a particular geographic distribution*: Neuromyelitis optica and isolated transverse myelitis

Marburg disease is an acute fulminant disorder with a monophasic rapid progressive course seen in young adults. Mortality is early within weeks or months due to brainstem involvement. It is often preceded by febrile illness and hence is also considered a fulminant form of ADEM. Imaging shows multifocal disseminated involvement with large T2 lesions, which may coalesce and show large cavitating lesions with incomplete ring enhancement.[72]

Schilder disease—myelinoclastic diffuse sclerosis: It is a rare disorder seen in children and young adults. It presents as aphasia and with psychiatric symptoms. There is no prior history of fever or vaccination. MR shows large ring enhancing lesions in both hemispheres, sometimes symmetric and located preferentially in parieto-occipital regions.[72] The lesion rim may show restricted diffusion. Dramatic response, both clinically and on imaging may be noted on administration of steroids. The differential diagnosis includes tumefactive MS, pyogenic abscess, metastasis and glioblastoma.

Balo's concentric sclerosis is a rare aggressive variant of MS seen usually in young adult males. Disease may show a rapid downhill progression or remain relatively benign. The pathological hallmark is concentric ring of myelin destruction and repair in centrum semiovale and corona radiate, resembling an onion ring. MR imaging reflects the same as alternating bands of differing signal intensities (hyper-iso-hypointense) on T2 images. The outer rim or advancing edge of demyelination shows restricted diffusion and may enhance on contrast administration. The center of the lesion may not show layering due to massive demyelination.[72]

Tumefactive or Pseudotumoral IIDDs[73-79]: Tumefactive demyelinating lesion is an acute tumor-like demyelination in which patients present with large (>2 cm) lesions, usually solitary but may be multiple. The solitary lesion is sometimes referred to as **monofocal acute inflammatory demyelination (MAID)**.

The clinical abnormalities in such patients are variable; Focal neurological deficits, seizures may be seen or the symptoms may be very slight even in a patient with a massive lesion. In some instances, there may be a rapid downhill course.

Tumefactive demyelination is most frequently encountered in women, usually young middle age (average onset at 37 years of age). It is not post infective, unlike ADEM. Patients who present with solitary tumefactive demyelinating lesion (TDL) develop MS infrequently though patients with multiple sclerosis can develop similar large tumefactive plaques.

Imaging

MRI: Large demyelinating (T2/FLAIR hyperintense) lesion with relatively less mass effect and edema is seen centered on the white matter and may involve subcortical U fibers. Various patterns have been described-diffusely infiltrative, mega cystic or large 'Balo' like lesion. Half of the TDLs show enhancement, usually in the form of an open ring and the incomplete part of the ring faces the gray matter side of the lesion Low relative cerebral blood volume (CBV) is found in TDLs compared to high grade gliomas. Diffusion imaging shows increase in ADC values similar to necrotic neoplasms. Proton spectroscopy shows an increase in choline and lactate.

Differential Diagnosis

The main imaging differential is a glioma: Clinical and radiological features to differentiate tumor from tumefactive demyelinating lesion are nonspecific. An incomplete ring of enhancement, relative lack of mass effect, and perilesional edema with a lower CBV on perfusion imaging may point towards demyelinating pathology. Biopsy is often required to differentiate the two.

Neuromyelitis Optica (Devic Disease)[80–91]

Neuromyelitis optica (NMO), also known as **Devic disease** and, more recently, **NMO spectrum disorder**, is a severe demyelinating disease of idiopathic nature, possibly of autoimmune etiology. It is caused by autoantibody to the aquaporin-4 water channel. These are found in astrocytes and are related to conduction of water through cell membrane. The antibodies target the region where blood-brain barrier is weakest—the spinal cord and optic nerve. Devic disease was initially considered a variant of MS but is now recognized as a distinct disease.

Epidemiology

Neuromyelitis optica is found in patients somewhat older than those with MS, with an average age of presentation being 41 years, although it can be seen in children and elderly. There is an even stronger female predilection (F:M 6.5:1) than MS. NMO is seen in Asian, Indian and African population.

Clinical Presentation

NMO presents as blindness or paraplegia due to optic neuritis and myelitis which may occur synchronously or metachronously. Optic neuritis is usually bilateral, that some patients present with unilateral optic nerve involvement. It follows a relapsing course though occasionally it may be a monophasic illness.

There is a specific biomarker of the disease, NMO-Immunoglobulin G, which has 90% specificity and 70–90% sensitivity. NMO-IgG is negative in almost all cases of MS and other autoimmune disease.

Criteria have been proposed to diagnose NMO **(Table 4)**. The NMO spectrum includes recurrent longitudinal extensive myelitis, bilateral simultaneous or recurrent optic neuritis. Asian optic-spinal MS, optic neuritis or myelitis associated with lesions in areas like hypothalamus, brainstem and myelitis/optic neuritis associated with systemic autoimmune disease.

Imaging

- **Myelitis**: Cervical spinal cord is usually affected. Involvement of three or more contiguous vertebral segments is seen and is called as longitudinally extensive spinal cord lesion. This pattern differs from MS, with involvement being more extensive in NMO. Central part of cord is involved unlike the peripheral part of the cord in MS **(Figs. 23A and B)**. A heterogeneous appearance of the cord on axial T2 images, described as "bright spotty "lesions may help to differentiate NMO from MS. The lesion appears hypointense on T1WI. Patchy cloud-like enhancement is seen along with thin ependymal enhancement. On sagittal images, lens like enhancement may be seen.

Table 4: NMO diagnostic criteria.

Essential/required
• Optic neuritis
• Acute myelitis
Plus two or more supportive criteria
• Disease onset MR imaging non-diagnostic for MS
• Contiguous spinal cord lesions on MR ≥3 vertebral segments
• NMO-IgG seropositivity

- **Optic neuritis:** Optic nerves appear hyperintense and swollen on T2-weighted sequences and show enhancement. Bilateral optic nerve involvement and extension of the abnormal signal posteriorly as far as the chiasm is particularly suggestive of NMO **(Fig. 24)**. In the chronic stage, there is atrophy of optic nerve.
- **Brain** was initially thought to have no abnormality in NMO but it has been shown that asymptomatic abnormalities may be present in a majority of patients. The lesions are present in areas with high concentration of aquaporin 4-the periependymal region abutting the ventricles, periaqueductal gray matter, hypothalamus and medial thalamus, dorsal pons and medulla. Corpus callosum may also be affected with preferential involvement of splenium; with lesions being larger, edematous and heterogeneous compared to MS. Multiple lesions with heterogeneous signal seen in corpus callosum leads to a marbled appearance. Punctuate lesions resembling MS may be present. Involvement of corticospinal tracts has been seen in a subset of patients. Large hemispheric white matter lesions that respond to steroids are seen in children and in patients from the Far East and Africa. NMO does not involve the cerebral cortex.

Differential Diagnosis

The differential diagnosis depends upon the clinical presentation, and in classic cases, the diagnosis can be made with a degree of confidence.

1. For patients with spinal cord involvement, the differential is that of a longitudinally extensive spinal cord lesion which includes idiopathic transverse myelitis.

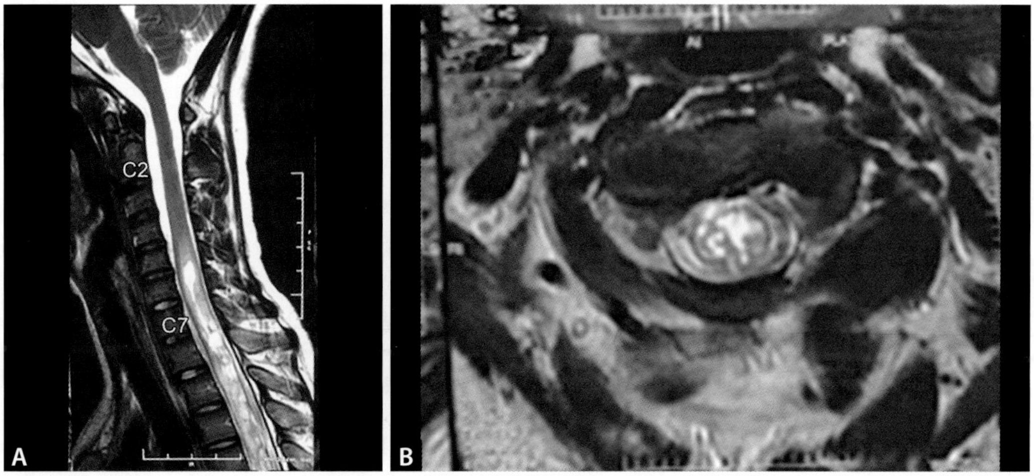

Figs. 23A and B: (A) T2W sagittal image of cervicodorsal spine-long segment hypertintensity seen in cervicodorsal cord in a case of neuromyelitis optica. (B) T2W axial image of the spinal cord shows heterogenous hyperintense signal with involvement of entire cross-section of cord in a case of NMO.

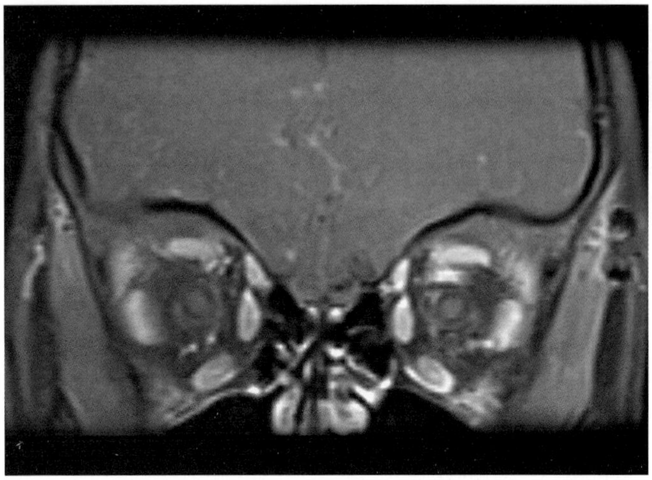

Fig. 24: T1W Post-contrast coronal image with fat saturation shows thickened and enhancing optic nerves on both sides (NMO).

2. Involvement of the cerebral white matter and corpus callosum has a broad differential depending on the pattern, but the most important differential is Multiple sclerosis. It is important to distinguish NMO from MS as the treatment not only is different but treating a patient with NMO with MS-specific therapies (e.g. beta-interferon or natalizumab) can actually lead to its exacerbation.

Imaging features that favor the diagnosis of NMO over MS are the distribution of lesions—periaqueductal location, absent perivenular orientation of periventricular lesions (Dawson's fingers are not seen in NMO), more extensive involvement of the corpus callosum, larger, more confluent lesions and enhancement of brain lesions that does not show incomplete ring pattern and NMO does not involve the cortical gray matter unlike MS.

Treatment and Prognosis

Treatment of NMO is with immunosuppression (e.g. Anti-CD20 monoclonal antibody rituximab) being the main stay. Patients who relapse have a poorer prognosis with increase in the incidence of blindness and paraplegia.

NMO spectrum disorders
Neuromyelitis optica—Devic disease/syndrome
Other NMO spectrum disorders
• Recurrent longitudinal extensive myelitis
• Bilateral simultaneous/recurrent optic neuritis
• Asian optic—spinal MS
• Optic neuritis or myelitis + specific brain lesions
• Optic neuritis or myelitis + systemic autoimmune disease.

White Matter Diseases Associated with Infections

Viral Encephalitides

The acute encephalitides may be secondary to a known causative agent or may be an autoimmune response to a nonspecific viral illness or vaccination. In such cases, the cerebral hypersensitivity reaction causes the observed clinical and pathologic state, whether the initial offending antigen is a virus, foreign protein, or autoantigen.

Conversely, there are patients with diminished immunity in whom a virus, which normally cannot gain a foothold in the central nervous system, propagates unchecked and results in demyelination.

The glial and neuronal cells may be directly infected or destroyed, as seen in acute encephalomyelitis (ADEM) in which a virus is not isolated from the brain. The subacute encephalitides (i.e. subacute sclerosing panencephalitis and PML) refer to direct infections of the brain that last for months or years and become reactivated years after the primary infections.

ACUTE DEMYELINATING ENCEPHALOMYELITIS

It is also called para-infectious encephalomyelitis. It is triggered by an infection, such as upper respiratory viral infection, measles, mumps or post vaccination for rabies, yellow fever. It is considered as immune mediated myelin destruction. Patients present within a few days or 3 weeks after viral illness/vaccination with fever, headache and decreased level of consciousness varying from lethargy to coma, seizure, and multifocal neurologic symptoms such as hemiparesis, cranial nerve palsies, and movement disorders; behavioral changes like depression, delusions, and psychosis may dominate the symptoms. Unlike multiple sclerosis, symptoms are more systemic rather than focal.

Epidemiology

Acute demyelinating encephalomyelitis (ADEM) presents in children or adolescents (usually younger than 15 years of age). However, cases have been reported in all ages. Winter and spring seasonal peaks in the presentation have been observed in some studies, underlining the upper respiratory infection etiology. Less than 5% of all ADEM cases follow an immunization. Unlike many other demyelinating diseases (e.g. multiple sclerosis or neuromyelitis optica), ADEM has no female predilection.[92]

Pathology

ADEM is thought to occur from cross-reactivity in immunity to viral antigens, triggering a subsequent autoimmune attack on the CNS. In approximately half of confirmed cases, Anti-MOG (myelin oligodendrocyte glycoprotein) immunoglobulin G antibodies can be identified. The pathological hallmark is perivenular inflammation with limited sleeves of demyelination.

Clinical Diagnosis

The diagnosis is clinical. CSF shows lymphocytosis and may show an increase in myelin basic protein. Anti MOG IgG antibodies may be detected. Majority of patients recover completely, while 20% show residual impairment. Mortality ranges from 10–25 %. Various patterns of disease evolution have been described.[72,88,93]

Monophasic ADEM is the most common pattern, although, within the episode, individual lesions may be of varying stages of evolution, with different lesions maturing over a number of weeks. In 10% of cases, relapse within the first three months is encountered. Rarely it may show a waxing-waning course over a few months.

Recurrent ADEM is characterized by a second episode occurring more than 3 months after the initial illness and involving the same anatomical area as the original illness.

Multiphasic ADEM—when the subsequent illness involves a different anatomical region.

Progression of ADEM to multiple sclerosis is not uncommon, and has been reported in up to 35% of cases. As fever and infection are well-known triggers for multiple sclerosis, a history of recent infection is identified in clinically isolated syndrome (CIS).

Imaging

Non-contrast CT is usually normal. On administration of contrast punctate lesions with ring enhancement may be seen.

MRI is usually abnormal but normal scans or a delay in appearance of findings may be seen. Clinical improvement often precedes resolution of the MR abnormality, which may continue to evolve while symptoms are regressing. Follow-up MR commonly demonstrates marked decrease in the size and number of lesions, and complete resolution of disease may be seen in response to steroids. No new lesions should appear on MR approximately 6 months from the start of the disease.

Lesions are usually multiple and bilateral but asymmetrical **(Figs. 25A to C)**. ADEM can involve both brain and spine, gray and white matter. T2/FLAIR hyperintensities are seen in the brain parenchyma typically situated in the subcortical location; the thalami and brainstem can also be involved. The size of the lesion may vary from small punctate foci to flocculent cotton ball lesions with poorly defined fuzzy margins **(Figs. 26A and B)**. Large confluent lesions **(Figs. 27A and B)** or occasionally a solitary lesion may be seen. Mass effect is mild, less than expected for the size of involvement. The deep gray matter is usually involved in ADEM **(Figs. 28A and B)**. Corpus callosal involvement can be seen but it does not affect the undersurface, unlike MS. Enhancement may be variable ranging from minimal or intense. Larger 'tumefactive' lesions display incomplete horse shoe enhancement like MS **(Figs. 29A to E)**. Cranial nerves may also enhance in ADEM. Absence of enhancement does not exclude the diagnosis Myelitis is seen in only in 1/3rd of patients. Spinal cord lesion may appear

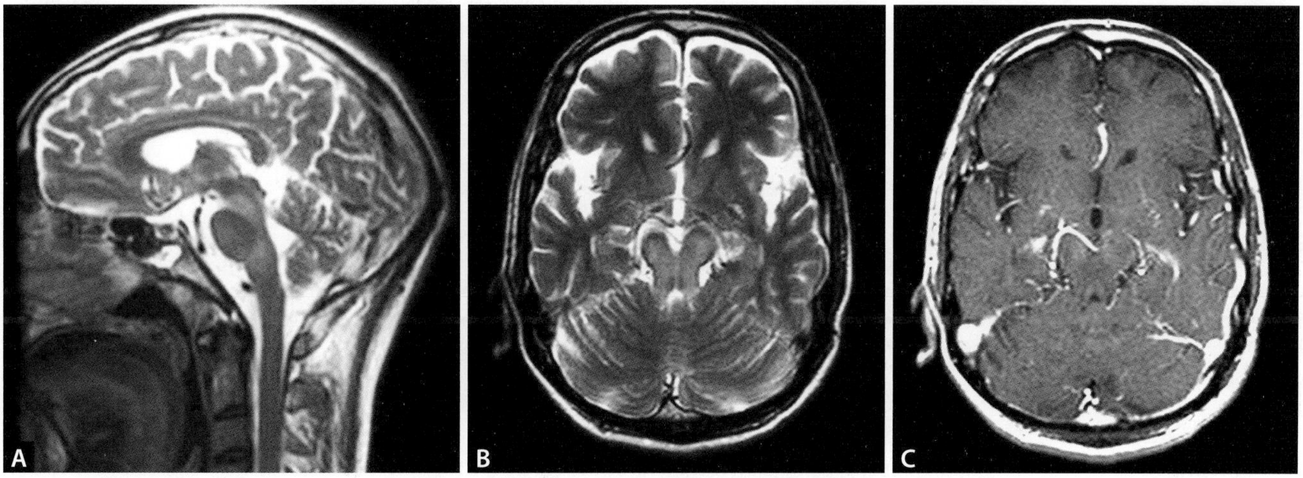

Figs. 25A to C: Hyperintensities seen in brainstem on T2W sagittal (A) T2W axial (B) images with subtle enhancement on T1W post contrast image (C) Brainstem encephalitis

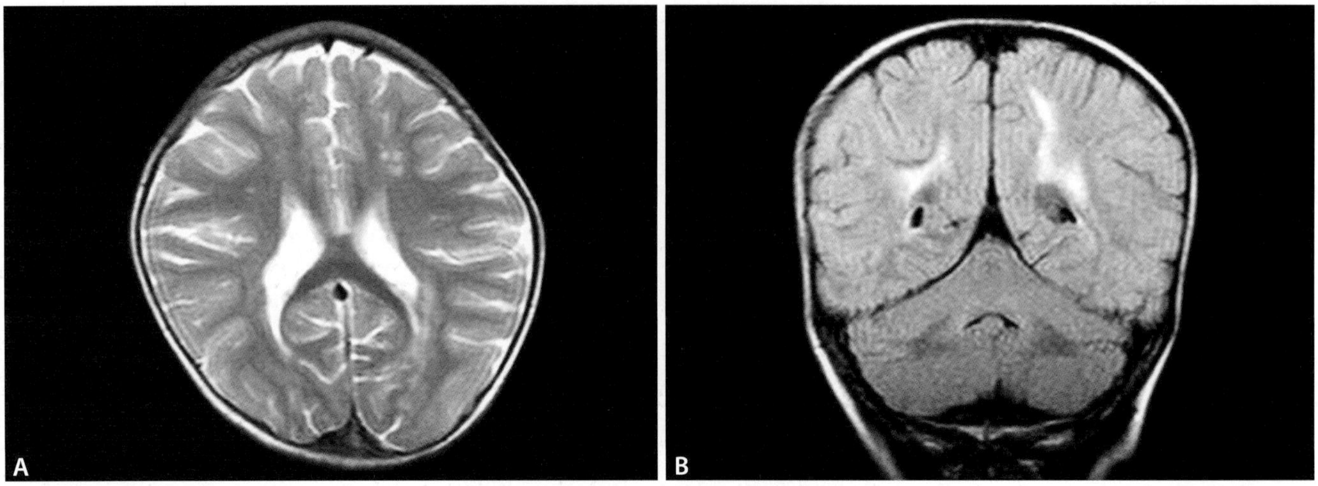

Figs. 26A and B: History of viral illness symmetrical white matter hyperintensities seen in T2W axial (A) and FLAIR coronal (B) image in a case of ADEM

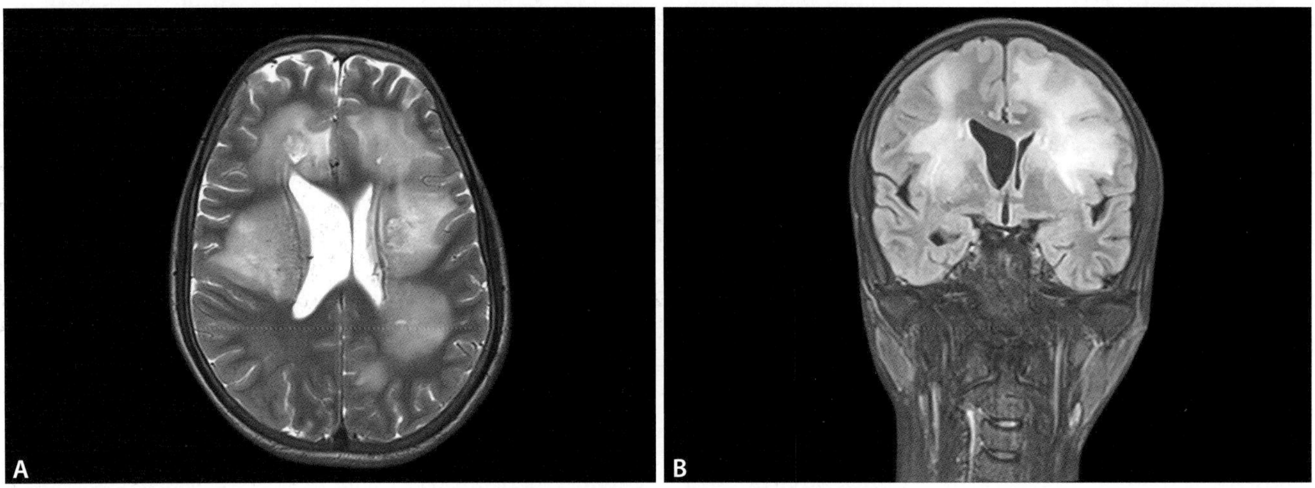

Figs. 27A and B: Large confluent hyperintensities seen bilaterally in a patient of ADEM in T2 axial (A) and coronal FLAIR (B) Image.

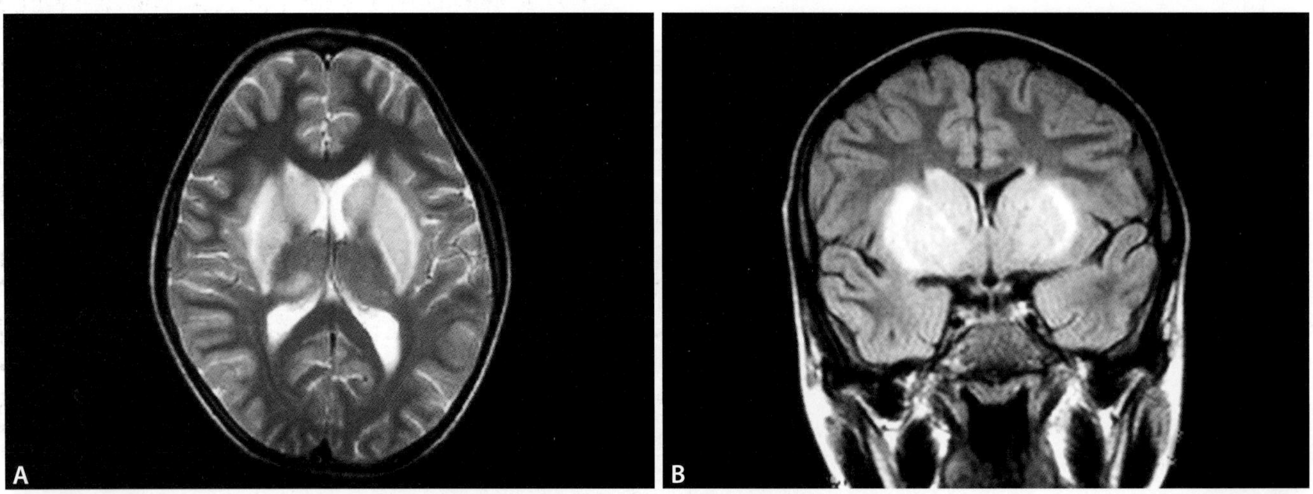

Figs. 28A and B: ADEM with predominant basal ganglia involvement. T2W axial (A) and FLAIR coronal (B) image in a patient with recent history of rabies vaccination show hyperintensity in both basal ganglia, right thalamus and cerebral peduncles. Hyperintense foci also seen in subcortical white matter with mild attenuation of right frontal horn.

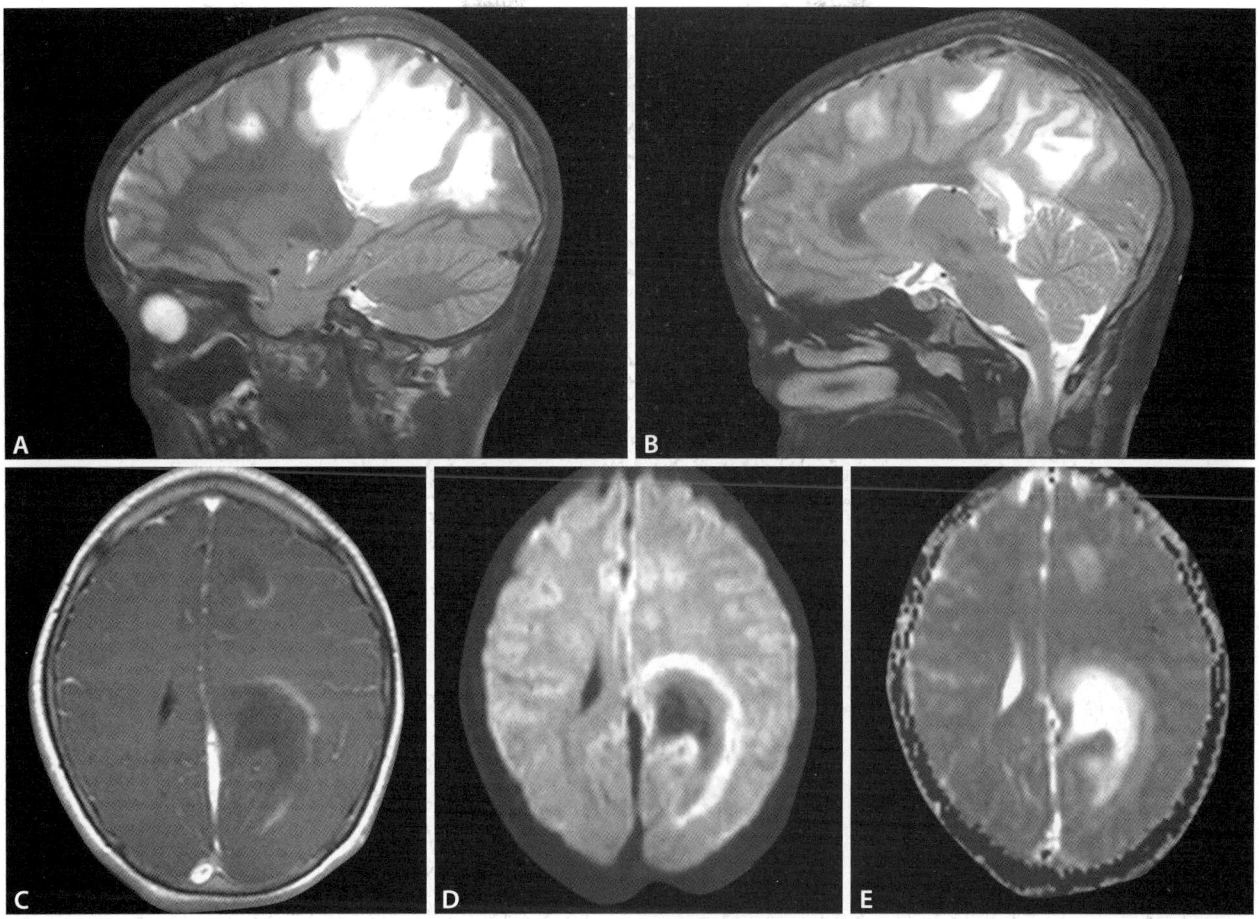

Figs. 29A to E: Large tumefactive demyelinating foci are seen in the subcortical location and in corpus callosum (A and B), open ring type of enhancement is seen on post-contrast T1W1 (C) with peripheral restricted diffusion (D and E) acute demyelination in a case of postviral ADEM.

as a swollen confluent lesion resembling transverse myelitis **(Fig. 30)**. Isolated spinal cord lesion without supratentorial involvement is rare.

Severe acute lesions may show restricted diffusion which can be seen as peripherally restricted diffusion; the center of the lesion, although high on T2 and low on T1, does not show restriction on DWI. A nonspecific appearance is seen on proton spectroscopy of a low NAA peak and an elevated lactate peak **(Figs. 31A to C)**.

A rare variant of ADEM is **Acute Infantile bilateral striatal necrosis which** is characterized by enlarged hyperintense basal ganglia, caudate nucleus and internal/external capsules.

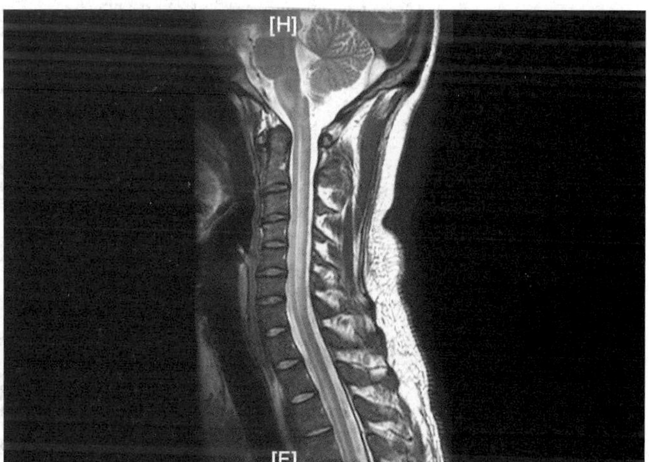

Fig. 30: ADEM-T2W sagittal image shows multilevel involvement of the cord with hyperintensity and mild swelling of the cord.

Treatment

Treatment consists of methylprednisolone, with immunoglobulin and cyclophosphamide reserved for patients refractory to steroids. Complete recovery within one month is the most common outcome (50–60%), with sequelae (most commonly seizures) seen in a significant proportion of cases (20–30%).

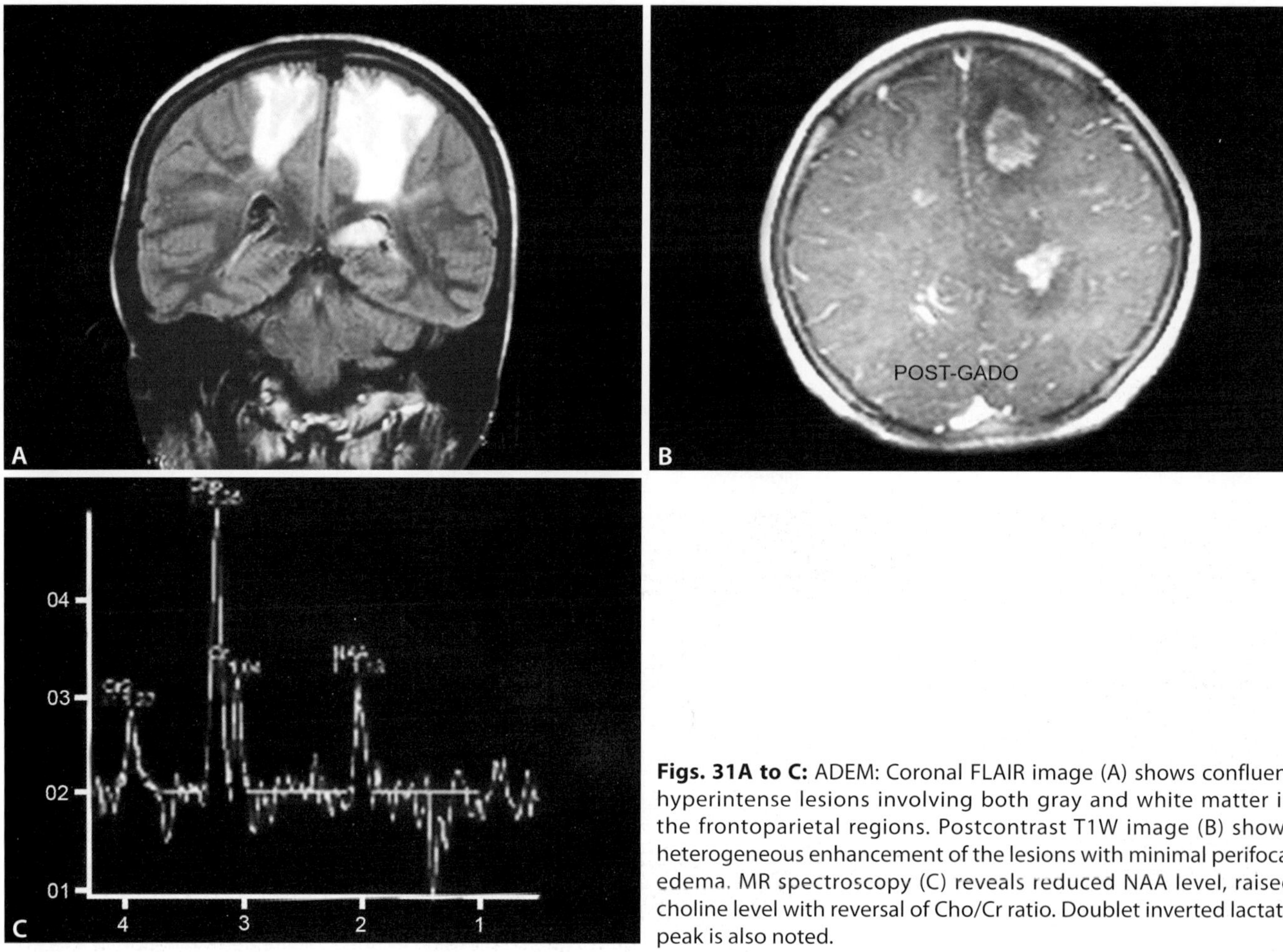

Figs. 31A to C: ADEM: Coronal FLAIR image (A) shows confluent hyperintense lesions involving both gray and white matter in the frontoparietal regions. Postcontrast T1W image (B) shows heterogeneous enhancement of the lesions with minimal perifocal edema. MR spectroscopy (C) reveals reduced NAA level, raised choline level with reversal of Cho/Cr ratio. Doublet inverted lactate peak is also noted.

Differential Diagnosis

- Multiple Sclerosis and variants—the major differentiating features are tabulated in **Table 3**.
- Susac syndrome
- Acute necrotizing encephalitis of childhood—it is a rare condition seen in children less than 4 years of age. Bilateral thalamic involvement hemorrhage, cavitation and post contrast enhancement is seen.
- Acute Hemorrhagic Leukoencephalitis.

ACUTE HEMORRHAGIC LEUKOENCEPHALITIS

Acute hemorrhagic leukoencephalitis (AHLE), also known **Acute hemorrhagic encephalomyelitis (AHEM)**, or **Weston-Hurst syndrome**, is a very rare form of demyelinating disease. AHLE is a severe fulminant form of ADEM. Histologically it differs from ADEM and is considered as a separate entity. History of flu like illness often precedes the neurological deterioration.[94]

Epidemiology

It is typically seen in young patients, though all ages are affected. Patients present with fever, neck stiffness and progressive neurological deficits, often leading to coma and death in a few days. There is no gender predilection.

Pathology

It is an autoimmune reaction to myelin protein. The brain shows multifocal areas of acute perivascular demyelination and hemorrhage confined to cerebral white matter with strict sparing of the subcortical U fibers. There is marked cerebral edema and congestion, often with herniation with punctate hemorrhages within the cerebral white matter, not infrequently necrotic. Typically, there is no involvement of the spinal cord.

Imaging

MR-T2* imaging is essential for diagnosis. Hemorrhages are a key finding in AHLE which can range from large, confluent hemorrhages or microbleeds seen on SWI **(Figs. 32A and B)** with extensive mass effect and significant edema. Multifocal, punctate, linear areas of blooming are seen in corpus callosum and extend to the full thickness of hemispheric white matter to subcortical U fibers **(Figs. 33A to C)**. The cortical grey matter is usually spared. About 50% show variable enhancement. Multifocal scattered or confluent hyperintensities of cerebral white matter are seen on T2/FLAIR images but these are non-specific findings.[94]

Treatment and Prognosis

Acute hemorrhagic leukoencephalitis is associated with a very poor prognosis. It is well known to demonstrate an initial good response to steroids with subsequent new onset of symptoms and devastating outcome.

Differential Diagnosis

- **ADEM**: It has a less fulminant course and does not demonstrate characteristic lobar/perivascular hemorrhages of AHLE.
- **Acute necrotizing encephalopathy**: This is a rare complication of viral infection influenza A, B, herpes virus. There are bilateral symmetrical lesions in thalami, internal capsule and tegmentum.[95]
- The petechial hemorrhages seen in AHLE are also seen in other diseases, such as diffuse vascular injury, fat emboli,

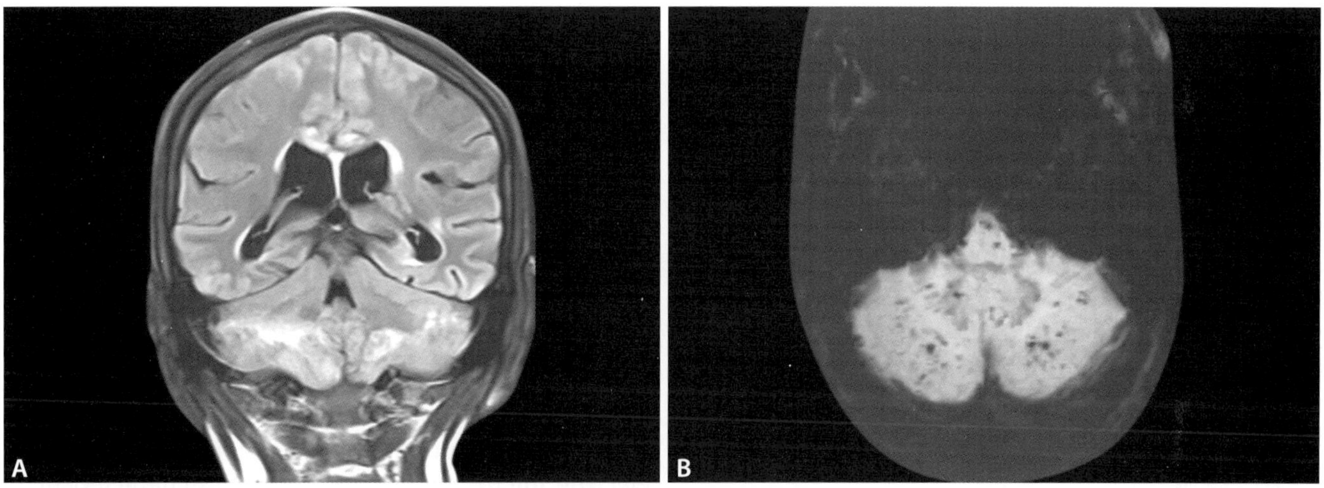

Figs. 32 A and B: FLAIR Coronal (A), SWI (B)-Hemorrhagic foci are seen in the cerebeller hemispheres in a case of AHLE. Note is also made of supratentorial involvement.
Abbreviations: AHLE: Acute hemorrhagic leukoencephalitis

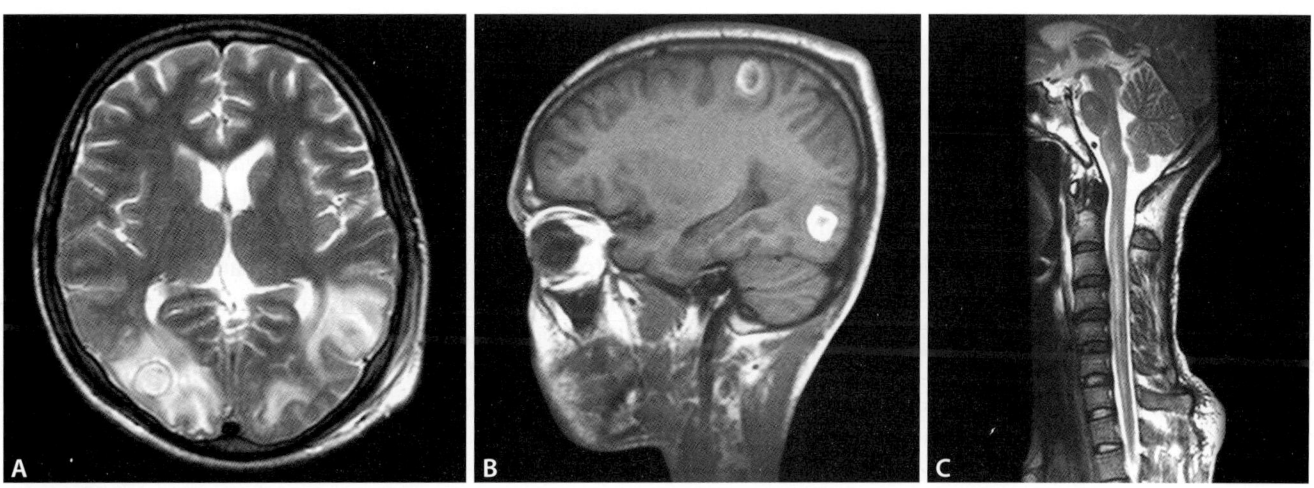

Figs. 33A to C: Hyperintensities are seen in parieto-occipital region bilaterally seen on T2W axial (A), with foci of hemorrhage, appreciated on T1W sagittal (B) Mild swelling of the cord with hyperintense signal seen on T2W sagittal (C) hemorrhagic leukoencephalitis.

thrombocytic purpura, sepsis, vasculitis, haemorrhagic viral fever, malaria and rickettsial disease.

- **Acute fulminant MS (Marburg)**: This does not have clinical features of fever and leukocytosis seen in AHLE and no haemorrhages are seen.

Subacute Sclerosing Panencephalitis

Subacute sclerosing panencephalitis (SSPE) results from a slow infection reactivated after an episode of measles. Clinical features include behavioral changes with progressive myoclonus, ataxia, and seizures. SSPE usually progresses to death in 6 months to 6 years.

Imaging

MRI shows subcortical white matter hyperintensities and extensive symmetrical diffuse periventricular white matter changes, followed by an end stage appearance of marked cerebral atrophy.

Progressive Rubella Panencephalitis

Progressive Rubella Panencephalitis (PRP) is a neurological disorder which may occur in a child with congenital rubella. It is a slow viral infection of the brain characterized by chronic encephalitis, usually manifesting between 8–19 years of age. It is believed to be due to a persistence or reactivation of rubella virus infection. It has an insidious onset with subtle changes in behavior and declining school work, later developing neurological symptoms, develops progressive spasticity, ataxia and seizures. Progressive rubella panencephalitis is characterized pathologically by widespread demyelinating changes in the brain with extensive involvement in the basal ganglia and brainstem. On MRI cerebral atrophy with demyelinating lesions are seen.

Progressive Multifocal Leukoencephalopathy (PML)[96–102]

It is a demyelinating disease secondary to an opportunistic viral infection by the JC virus (John Cunningham virus), a member of the papovaviridae family. This virus is ubiquitous with latent persistence in kidney and cerebrum. In patients who are immunocompromised, JC virus becomes neurotropic with infection and lysis of oligodendrocytes which leads to failure of myelin production. PML is seen in three clinical contexts:

- PML due to immunocompromised state
- *PML-s-IRIS*: Simultaneous development of Immune Reconstitution Inflammatory Syndrome (IRIS) and PML due to immune reconstitution
- *PML-d-IRIS*: Immune reconstitution worsens preexisting PML.

Epidemiology

Progressive multifocal leukoencephalopathy has a strong association with immunosuppressed states, particularly AIDS, where it typically develops in patients with CD4 counts of 50–100 cells/μL. PML is also seen in patients of collagen vascular disease, in post-transplant patients on immunosuppression, chemotherapy with rituximab for hematological malignancies and patients of multiple sclerosis on natalizumab. PML is one of the classic conditions encountered in immune reconstitution inflammatory syndrome. Patients with idiopathic CD4 lymphocytopenia, systemic lupus erythematosus, cirrhosis, pregnancy have also been diagnosed with PML.

Clinically, PML typically presents with an insidious onset. The most common presenting complaints are motor weakness, followed in frequency by altered mental status, visual disturbances and gait abnormalities. Untreated, it is fatal; with the institution of highly active antiretroviral therapy (HAART) survival improves. PML in natalizumab treated MS cases has high mortality rate.

Pathology

There are multifocal demyelinating plaques involving the subcortical U fibers with sparing of the cortical ribbon and the deep gray matter. The most significant finding is the presence of intranuclear inclusion bodies, which on electron microscopy are viral particles characteristic of papovavirus.

Imaging

Imaging suggests the diagnosis in patients of HIV/AIDS, and is confirmed by presence of JCV antigen in CSF.

The **classic MR appearance of PML** is multifocal areas of ill-defined high signal intensity on long TR sequences within the subcortical white matter. Any lobe may be involved by PML, but the frontal and parieto-occipital locations are most common and thus correlate well with the symptoms of homonymous hemianopia, focal neurologic deficit, and altered mentation. Lesions may be initially small in size but usually progress to larger areas of involvement. A multifocal distribution pattern is seen, which may be unilateral but is more often bilateral and asymmetric **(Fig. 34)**. There is an absence of mass effect. Hemorrhage is uncommon.

The subcortical lesions follow the gray-white interface, resulting in a "scalloped" appearance due to the involvement of subcortical U fibers. This relative sparing

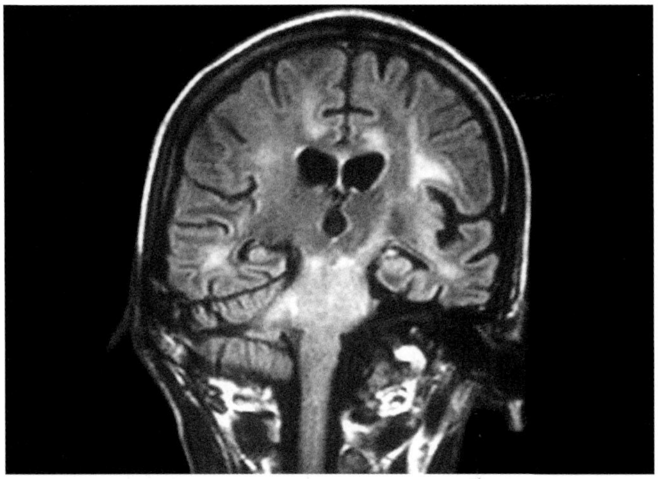

Fig. 34: Coronal FLAIR image: Patchy, asymmetrical white matter hyperintensities predominantly involving subcortical white matter in left cerebral hemisphere. Similar hyperintensities are also seen in pons and midbrain. Diffuse cerebral atrophy is also noted—PML.

of cortical ribbon is called the **"heart of the gyrus"** sign. Individual gyri are thickened by edema of central white matter with conspicuous sparing and margination of the overlying cortical ribbon.

In classical PML there is no significant contrast enhancement which is attributable to the paucity of perivenous inflammation. When enhancement is present, it is faint and peripheral. However ring enhancement is noted in cases of **immune reconstruction inflammatory syndrome (IRIS)** in PML related to natalizumab therapy. On T1-weighted images, PML lesions are usually hypointense to parenchyma and fairly well-demarcated, although early lesions may be isointense. In contrast, HIV-related demyelination is usually isointense on T1-weighted images and is often inapparent.

In advanced PML, smaller, very hyperintense foci may be seen within and surrounding the hyperintense confluent lesion denoting spongy nature of the lesion. There is relatively less mass effect. Acute lesions show diffusion restriction. DTI shows reduced fractional anisotropy suggestive of disorganised white matter structure. Perfusion studies show a decrease in rCBV as compared to normal white matter reflecting its avascular nature.

Differential Diagnosis

- HIV encephalopathy—More symmetric involvement and sparing of subcortical U fibres. The differences are enumerated in **Table 5**.
- Other opportunistic infections—Toxoplasmosis and CMV. Toxoplasmosis is mass like, CMV causes ependymitis and ventriculitis.

Table 5: Differences between HIV dementia and PML.

	HIV Dementia	*PML*
Clinical presentation	Memory loss and mental slowing	Focal neurological signs
Course	Several months	Weeks to months
MR findings	Bilateral symmetrical periventricular hyperintensities on T2WI, normal-to-mild hypointensity on T1WI. No enhancement/ mass effect	Focal, unilateral or asymmetrical, multifocal subcortical white matter hyperintensity on T2WI. Mild-to-severe hypointensity on T1WI. Usually no enhancement/mass effect

Human Immunodeficiency Virus Encephalopathy[103–105]

Neurologic manifestations are the initial manifestations of AIDS in 7 to 20% of patients. White matter changes in HIV have a varied etiology, though may show similar appearance. These can be the result of the primary effects of HIV or due to opportunistic infections (such as cytomegalovirus, toxoplasmosis, JC virus that cause PML and fungi), neoplasms (lymphoma), vascular disease or may be a result of associated metabolic and nutritional disorders.

CNS involvement in AIDS can manifest as acute encephalopathy, subacute encephalitis, acute and chronic meningitis, vacuolar myelopathy and peripheral neuropathy. Among these various forms, subacute encephalitis is most frequently associated with cerebral white matter disease.

HIV-associated dementia (HAD) previously called as **AIDS dementia** complex, corresponds to a neurological clinical syndrome seen in patients with HIV infection. The associated imaging appearance is generally referred to as **HIV encephalopathy (HIE)**. HAD, HIE are part of the spectrum of HIV-associated neurocognitive disorders (HANDs). Typically, HIV encephalopathy occurs in patients with advanced immunosuppression and with coexistent systemic diseases.

HIV virus is not only lymphotrophic, but also neurotropic. It replicates in multinucleated giant cells within the central nervous system, resulting eventually in demyelination. This demyelination is characterized by little edema and a lack of inflammation.

The clinical syndrome of HAD comprises of a combination of cognitive, behavioral and motor dysfunction like gait disturbance and tremors. Patients present with inattention and reduced concentration, apathy and dulling of personality, psychomotor slowing, marked motor slowing and ataxia. Prognosis is poor with fatality seen within a year.

Imaging features of HIV encephalopathy, whether by CT or MR, tends to lag behind the pathologic involvement. Generalized atrophy is the most common abnormality that is nonspecific, with a predominantly central distribution. With more severe involvement, CT shows symmetric white matter hypodensity, usually seen bifrontally. There is no contrast enhancement or mass effect. On MR there is greater sensitivity with various patterns seen on T2 and proton density weighted images. These include punctate foci of signal hyperintensity, larger focal and diffuse areas of hyperintensity, and less well-defined patchy areas of hyperintensity. Symmetrical diffuse lesions in periventricular white matter and within the centrum semiovale suggest underlying HIV infection **(Figs. 35A and B)**. There is relative sparing of subcortical region and posterior fossa. Multifocal confluent lesions or diffuse symmetric high signal intensity in the periventricular and deep white matter may be seen as the disease progresses **(Figs. 36A and B)**. Bilateral symmetric increased signal intensity on the long TR sequences has been described in the basal ganglia (caudate and putamen) and thalamus and may also involve the brainstem. Follow-up MR studies after the institution of highly active antiretroviral therapy in patients with the AIDS dementia complex have shown regression or stabilization of signal abnormalities on MR.

A range of decreased MT ratios in areas of high signal intensity as compared with control subjects has been shown. Abnormal MT ratios have also been found in the normal appearing white matter of HIV-positive patients in patients with both PML and HIV encephalopathy. Proton MR spectroscopy studies have shown decreased NAA/Cr,

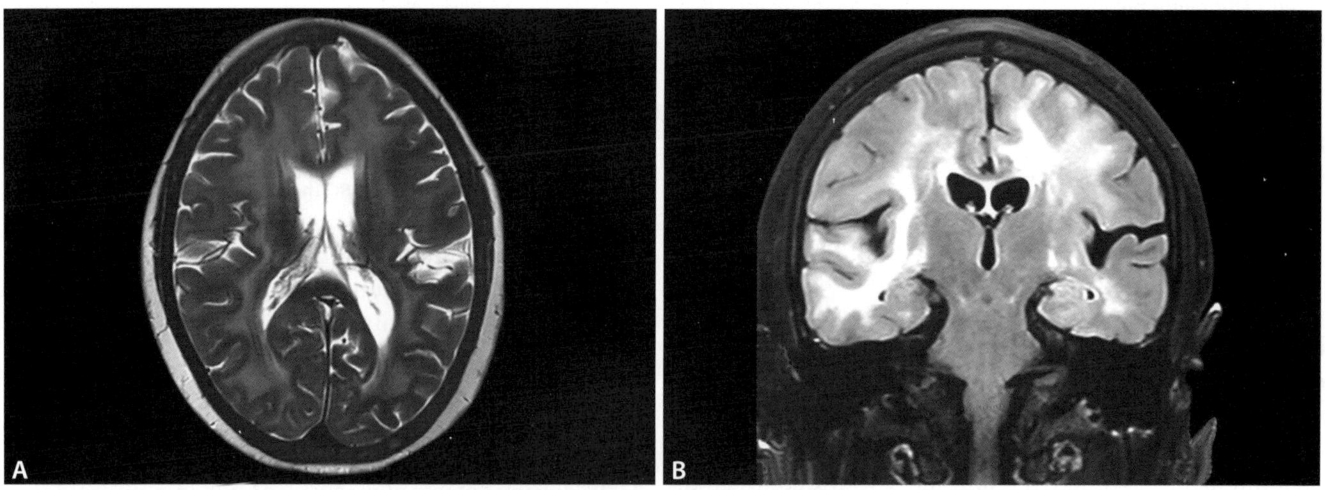

Figs. 35A and B: Axial T2WI (A), Coronal FLAIR images (B) show bilateral symmetrical hyperintensities in the periventricular white matter in a case of AIDS-HIV encephalopathy.

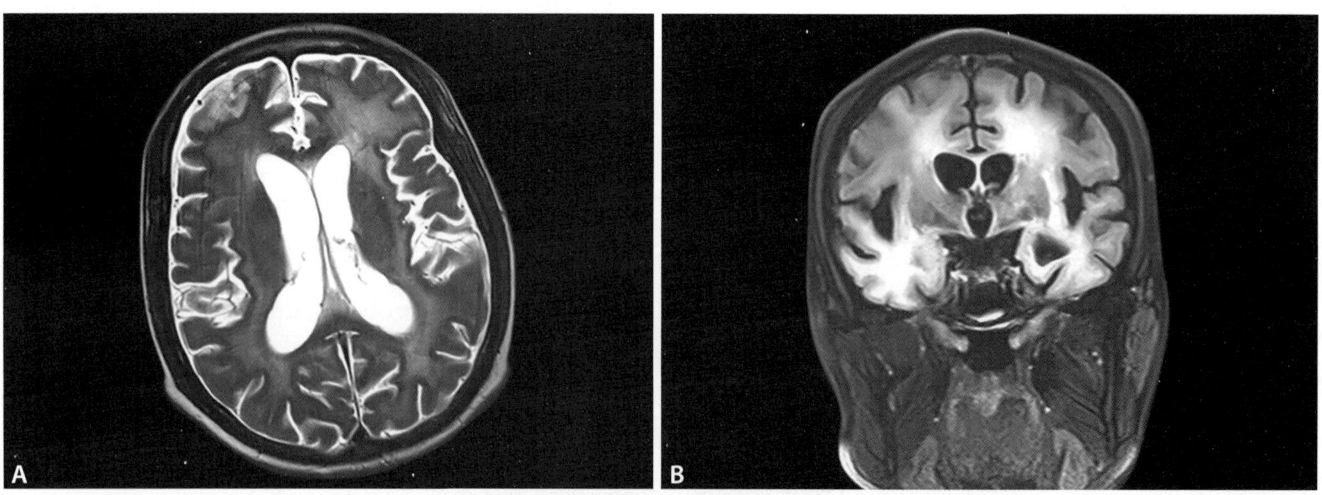

Figs. 36A and B: T2W axial image (A) and coronal FLAIR images (B) show bilateral symmetrical hyperintensities in the centrum semiovale with cerebral atrophy in a case of HIV dementia.

increased levels of choline, and the presence of lactate in normal appearing white matter and regions of white matter with signal abnormality.

LYME DISEASE/LYME NEUROBORRELIOSIS (LNB)

Borreliosis is a multisystem inflammatory reaction caused by a spirochete *Borrelia burgdorferi*. It is transmitted by tick bite and is the most common vector borne disease in the US. Patients initially present with target like rash and flu like syndrome. This is followed by neurological and cardiac abnormalities seen weeks to months later.

Imaging

Multiple T2/FLAIR small (2–8 mm) white matter hyperintensities are seen in the subcortical ,periventricular location and Corpus callosum. Variable enhancement is seen. Leptomeningeal enhancement has also been described in LNB. Lyme disease mimics MS due to similarity of site involvement. Cranial nerve involvement most commonly of CN VII, followed by CN III and V is a feature of LNB. Unilateral disease is more common. The altered nerves show uniform contrast enhancement. Spinal cord involvement in rare but may be seen.[106]

Differential Diagnosis

- *Multiple sclerosis*: Involves periventricular white matter. Cranial nerve enhancement is less common in MS. Leptomeningeal enhancement is not seen in multiple sclerosis.
- *Susac syndrome*: Sensorineural hearing loss is a key feature in Susac syndrome.

White Matter Diseases Associated with Vascular Causes

It can be divided into six broad categories[107]

Type 1: Arteriosclerotic type

Type 2: Cerebral amyloid angiopathy

Type 3: Inherited vasculopathies CADASIL, MELAS (mitochondrial myopathy lactic acidosis, stroke-like episodes)

Type 4: Inflammatory vasculitis—CNS vasculitis encompasses a heterogeneous group of inflammatory disorders that primarily affect the small leptomeningeal and parenchymal blood vessels of the same. Primary angitis of the central vascular system (PACVS), Susac syndrome, connective tissue disorders such as systemic lupus erythematosus and Sjogren syndrome.

Type 5: Venous collagenosis

Type 6: Others—related to radiation.

Type 1: Small vessel disease related to arteriosclerosis: Small vessel disease is the commonest cause of white matter disease and leads to cognitive and physical disability. Multiple nonspecific small hyperintensities seen on T2W/FLAIR involving white matter in subcortical location and deep gray matter are the most frequent presentation of vasculitis. Nonspecific white matter changes range from periventricular caps and rims [periventricular white matter lesions (PVWMLs)] to deep white matter punctuate patchy or confluent lesions. There is a difference in etiology and clinical presentation of white matter lesions. Smooth PVWMLs are due to ependymal loss or differing degrees of myelination in adjacent fiber tracts. These are thought to have a nonischemic origin. Irregular PVWMLs are associated with atherosclerosis. Cerebral microhemorrhages are small (<5 mm) areas of blooming seen on T2*/susceptibility weighted imaging. These are usually not seen on CT or other MR sequences. In patients with chronic hypertension they are found in deep gray matter. Brain atrophy is another manifestation of small vessel disease.

An international task force has drafted a consensus classifying small vessel disease as white matter hyperintensities (WMHs), recent small subcortical infarcts, lacunes, microbleeds and brain atrophy.[108]

White matter hyperintensities (WMHs), are commonly seen in patients above 60 years of age usually in frontal and parietal regions. WMH are further rated as focal, beginning confluent, diffuse confluent, and are seen in basal nuclei, corona radiata and centrum semi ovale—the area of vascular end zones. There is a correlation between WMHs with cognitive, behavioral, gait and urinary impairment.

Recent small subcortical infarcts also known as acute lacunar infarcts are defined as infarcts less than 20 mm. These occur in the territory of perforating arterioles. These acute lacunar infarcts may develop into lacunas which are round/ovoid cavities of 3–15 mm, following CSF signal intensity. Alternately these may develop into WMHs or disappear.

Binswanger's disease (subcortical arteriosclerotic encephalopathy): Binswanger disease, described in 1894 is a demyelinating disease equally affecting men and women generally more than 55 years old. It is associated with hypertension and lacunar infarction.[109] Patients may have acute stroke followed by declining mental status or slow insidious mental status change with psychiatric disturbance, seizures, urinary incontinence and gait changes. MR reveals broad regions of high signal intensity in the white matter of frontal, parietal and occipital regions extending into the centrum semiovale **(Figs. 37A and B)**. The U fibers are spared. Binswanger disease differs from multinfarct dementia because of its distinctive white matter involvement and absence of consistent focal stroke like symptoms.

Type 2: Cerebral amyloid angiopathy (CAA): CAA is one of the manifestations of amyloid disease of the brain. It is caused by accumulation of amyloid protein in the media and adventitia of cerebral small vessels (cortical and leptomeningeal arteries). It shows a preferential involvement of occipital and frontal regions. Advancing age predisposes to the development of CAA; a hereditary form is also known which presents earlier. Patients are usually normotensive. Amyloid disease is typically seen after 55 years of age. There is no gender predilection. Cerebral amyloidosis is not related to systemic amyloidosis.

Gross pathology shows the presence of lobar, corticosubcortical and cortical haemorrhages of different age and sizes. Signs of previous subarachnoid haemorrhage are also seen. The fragility of the vessels due to deposition of amyloid and subsequent inflammation underlines the propensity to bleed and the chronic cerebral hypoperfusion being the cause for leukoencephalopathy.[110]

Imaging

CT: Lobar hematoma with variable peripheral edema is seen. Multiple irregular confluent hyperintensities are noted along with cerebral atrophy; atraumatic convexal subarachnoid hemorrhage may be seen.

MRI: Hematoma is noted which displays age related signal intensity. Focal white matter hyperintensity may be seen. T2* (GRE, SWI) sequences demonstrate multifocal punctate areas of blooming in leptomeninges. Cortex and subcortical white matter, basal ganglia and cerebellum are relatively spared. The microbleeds associated with CAA lack mass effect, peripheral edema and there is no enhancement, differentiating it from hemorrhagic metastasis. Microbleeds that are associated with hypertension involve basal ganglia, a site not favored by CAA. The radiological findings (Boston criteria) [111] can suggest the diagnosis, but can be confirmed only on postmortem examination.

Type 3: Cerebral autosomal dominant arteriopathy with subcortical infarcts and leukoencephalopathy (CADASIL):[111-114] CADASIL is an inherited non-arteriosclerotic small vessel disease related to mutation in chromosome 19. It is transmitted in an autosomal dominant pattern. It has a prevalence of 2–4 per 100,000, has no gender predilection. It is seen in the 3rd–4th decade of life with young adults presenting with migraines, recurrent ischemic stroke and progressive cognitive impairment.

Imaging

WMHs are noted in the 3rd decade in the temporal pole, a location not seen in other microvascular disease. This progress to involve posterior temporal, frontal and parietal regions, basal nuclei and thalamus. Subcortical U fibers can be involved External capsule and corpus callosum are also involved, these locations being important pointers to the diagnosis of CADASIL. Microbleeds and extension with WMHs are seen as the patient ages.

Type 4: Primary angitis of the central nervous system (PACNS):[115-117] PACNS is a rare idiopathic vasculitis of the brain and spinal cord. It is seen in the 5th–6th decade.

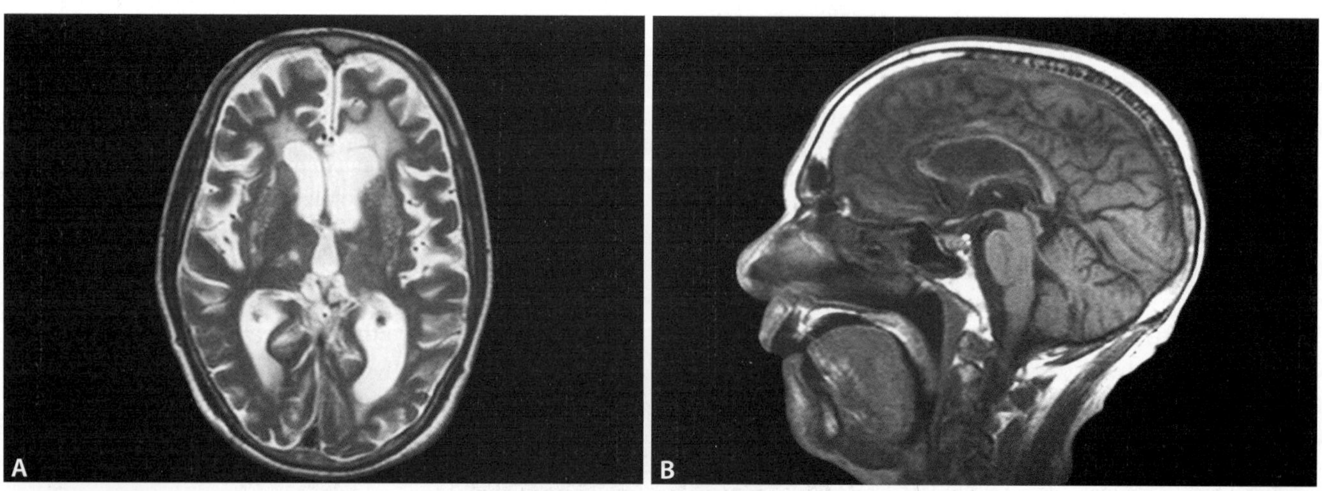

Figs. 37A and B: T2W axial image (A) and T1 sagittal image (B). Binswanger's disease. MRI demonstrates bilateral patchy hyperintensities extending from the subcortical region to the ventricular margins. Few lacunar infarcts are seen with evidence of cerebral atrophy.

Patients present with headache and encephalopathy, stroke and hemorrhages are seen occasionally. CSF is abnormal in majority of the cases, showing elevated inflammatory markers and raised proteins.

Imaging

MRI is abnormal in more than 90% patients and shows multiple cortical, subcortical infarcts, WMHs, hemorrhages, parenchymal and leptomeningeal enhancement. A normal MR study rules out PACNS. Reversible central vasoconstriction syndrome (RCVS) mimics PACNS in its clinical presentation of severe headache, but has normal CSF analysis. Brain biopsy may be required for the diagnosis.

Type 4: Inflammatory Vasculitis

Susac syndrome:[118-124] This is a recently recognized small vessel disease affecting young adults (20–40 years) with a female predominance. Described by **John O Susac,** an American neurologist and neuro-ophthalmologist and his colleagues, it is a vasculitis produced due to antiendothelial antibodies to specific neural vessels. The immune attack causes endotheliopathy that involves cochlea, retina and brain with microinfarcts in these locations.

Patients present with a triad of acute or subacute encephalopathy manifested in a broad spectrum of symptoms, e.g. memory impairment, confusion, behavioral disturbances, ataxia, dysarthria, paranoid psychosis, and headaches, sensorineural hearing loss at low and medium frequencies and visual loss (due to branch retinal artery occlusion). The course is usually self limiting but it may have a relapsing remitting course. It is also known as retino-cochleal-cerebral vasculopathy, RED-M (retinopathy, encephalopathy and microangiopathy) or SICRET (small infarcts of cochlear retinal and encephalic tissue).

Imaging

MRI: Corpus callosum is involved in almost all cases and is considered pathognomic. The middle of the corpus callosum (body and splenium) is involved, without involvement of the callosal undersurface unlike in MS. The roof of the corpus callosum is also frequently involved, resulting in "icicle" or linear "spoke" lesions that look to hang from the roof of the corpus callosum. Lesions have been described as "snow ball" and may involve the entire width of corpus callosum. As the disease progresses lesions become hypointense on T1 (black holes) and there may be atrophy of the corpus callosum signifying severe damage. The lesions are best appreciated on a sagittal view.

Multiple small microinfarcts are seen in the periventricular and deep white matter, centrum semiovale, brain stem as T2/FLAIR hyperintensities. A "string of pearls" appearance due to punctate microinfarcts involving the internal capsule has been described. Contrast enhancement is seen in acute stage. T2 shine through may be seen on DWI.

Differential Diagnosis

- *MS*: callososeptal interface is involved in multiple sclerosis
- *ADEM/Lyme disease*: Middle layer of corpus callosum is not involved. ADEM is usually preceded by viral illness or vaccination.
- Vasculiltis and thromboembolic infarcts—corpus callosum is rarely affected.
- Transient lesions of the splenium—these are seen in many conditions, with sudden stoppage of medication in epileptics being among them. There is no contrast enhancement and restricted diffusion is seen.

SYSTEMIC LUPUS ERYTHEMATOSUS[125-127]

Systemic lupus erythematosus (SLE) is a multisystem autoimmune disorder, affecting respiratory, cardiovascular, gastrointestinal, genitourinary, musculoskeletal and central nervous system when it is termed CNS Lupus or neuropsychiatric SLE (NPSLE).

The peak age of onset is 2nd to 4th decade with female preponderance. Diagnostic criteria have been established by the American College of Rheumatology and include malar rash, renal disease, arthritis, scoliosis etc. NPSLE manifests as psychosis, stroke, epilepsy, headache and cognitive abnormalities.

Imaging

MR may be normal or may show varied abnormality. Multiple small subcortical and deep white matter hyperintensities on T2/FLAIR, cerebral atrophy, infarction, are seen. Diffuse cortical, brainstem lesions and lesions in basal ganglia may be seen and are indicative of vasculitis. Transient enhancement, restricted diffusion and increased perfusion may be seen in acute cases. Dural venous sinus or cortical/deep venous thrombosis may be seen. The **presence of multifocal infarcts and migratory edematous areas are suggestive of CNS lupus.**

Differential diagnosis: Multifocal subcortical and deep white matter hyperintensities are seen in a host of other conditions—arteriosclerosis, multiple sclerosis, susac syndrome, Lyme disease and primary angiitis, etc.

BEHÇET DISEASE

It is a multisystemic, vascular inflammatory disease of unknown origin. Neurological involvement is noted in about a half of these cases and is called Neuro Behçet's disease.[128]

Clinically Behçet's presents as neurocuteneous syndrome, recurrent oral, genital ulcers, aphthous stomatitis, uveitis and arthralgia.

Imaging

MRI: Brainstem and specifically cerebral peduncles are involved in 50% of cases. Other sites of involvement are thalamus, basal ganglia. Circular, linear foci of T2/FLAIR hyperintensities are noted with minimal mass effect and mild to moderate contrast enhancement.

Differential diagnosis: MS, sarcoid and neoplasm form the major differential of Behçet's disease. Oligoclonal bands are not seen in Behçet's disease. Skin lesions are generally absent in sarcoidosis and ACE levels may be elevated in sarcoidosis. Biopsy may be required to differentiate widespread form of Behçet's from gliomatosis/lymphoma. Similar lesions, such as Behçet's are seen in systemic inflammatory diseases such as SLE, antiphospholipid syndrome and Sjögren's disease. Skin lesions are noted in these, but oral and genital ulceration is not seen.

WHITE MATTER DISEASES ASSOCIATED WITH TOXIC METABOLIC CAUSES

Osmotic Demyelination Syndrome (ODS)

Osmotic demyelination syndrome is the new terminology for what was earlier called central pontine myelinosis and/or extra pontine myelinosis. It is seen in hypoosmolar states, where the oligodendrocytes are vulnerable to osmotic changes. It has been considered a pontine lesion, but typically there is extrapontine involvement as well. Isolated pontine involvement is seen in 50% of cases. In 30% of cases there is concomitant extra pontine involvement. In 20–25% of patients white matter demyelination is exclusively extrapontine in the basal ganglia and with hemispheric involvement.[129-132]

Pathology

On gross examination, the classic pontine lesion is seen as triangular or butterfly lesion of symmetric gray discoloration along the midline of the basis pontis. There is edematous demyelination of the central ventral pons, with characteristic sparing of the tegmentum. A rim of normal white matter surrounds the area of demyelination. It is believed that the grid arrangement of descending and crossing tracts in the pons or its vulnerable vascularity leads to the characteristic focality of the lesion.

Clinical features: It is a rare disorder, seen usually in middle aged patients with slight male predominance. The most common cause is rapid correction of hyponatremia, a condition noted in chronic alcoholics or in the setting of malnutrition. Patients on cyclosporine, post liver transplant are also predisposed for electrolyte disturbance. There may be comorbidities such as renal, adrenal or paraneoplastic syndromes predisposing to ODS. The condition is also associated with diabetes and anorexia in paediatric patients. ODS may also be seen in normonatremic patients and independent of changes in sodium level. Clinically osmotic demyelination syndrome presents in a biphasic pattern. The first phase is usually attributable to the underlying electrolyte abnormality, with patients being acutely encephalopathic. Following rapid reversal of this abnormality, the patient transiently improves before progressing onto the classic osmotic demyelination syndrome features 2–3 days later. When pontine involvement is prominent, clinical features consist of pseudobulbar palsy, dysthermia, dysphagia. Patients may recover completely or progress to coma and death.

The clinical diagnosis is often difficult and recognition of the entity on imaging by the radiologist often prompts a search for electrolyte abnormalities by the physician.

Imaging

CT: Hypo density may be seen in the affected areas.

MRI: Is the modality of choice. It is initially normal on routine sequences. DWI shows restricted diffusion in acute ODS in the lower pons, seen within 24 hours of onset of quadriplegia **(Figs. 38A and B)**. This area shows T2 hyperintensity followed by T1 hypointensity. The characteristic appearance is a symmetric round to oval area of T2 hyperintensity within the base of the pons **(Figs. 39A and B)**. These changes may take up to two weeks to be seen. Peripheral pons as well as corticospinal tracts and transverse fibres are spared leading to a classic trident shaped appearance **(Figs. 40A and B)**. Similar hyperintensity may be seen in basal ganglia, midbrain and subcortical white matter. Usually there is no enhancement but moderate enhancement may be seen in subacute cases.

Differential Diagnosis

- Pontine infarcts are usually asymmetric and involve the surface of pons in basilar perforating artery infarcts.
- Demyelinating disease: MS may involve pons but lesion is usually asymmetric and may show additional lesions in sites such as callososeptal interface.
- Pontine glioma: seen in children and young adults.

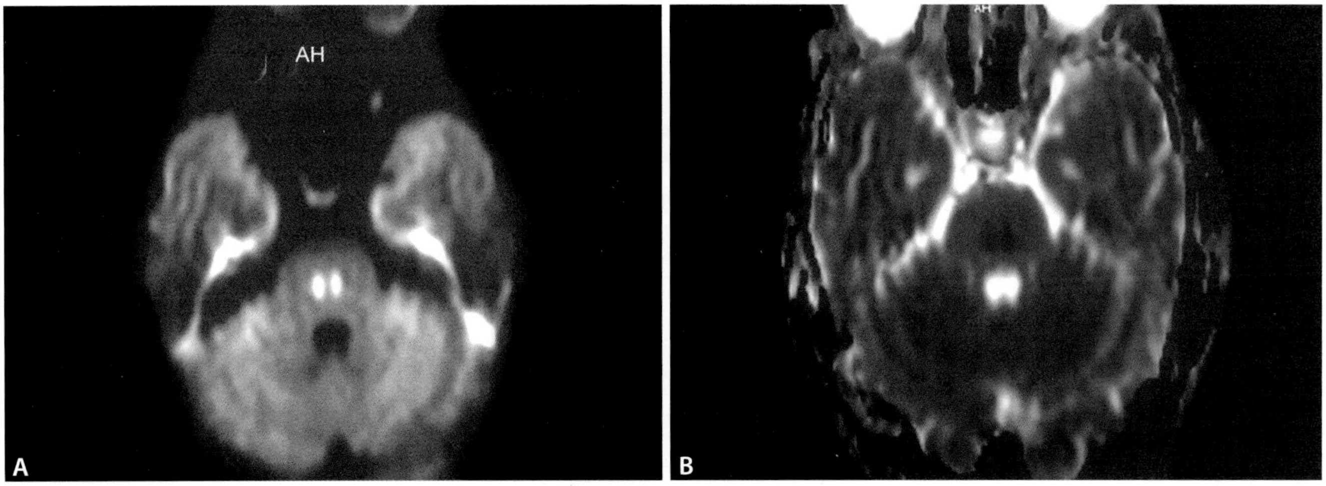

Figs. 38A and B: DWI in a suspected case of osmotic demyelination syndrome—restricted diffusion seen in pons signifying acute demyelination.

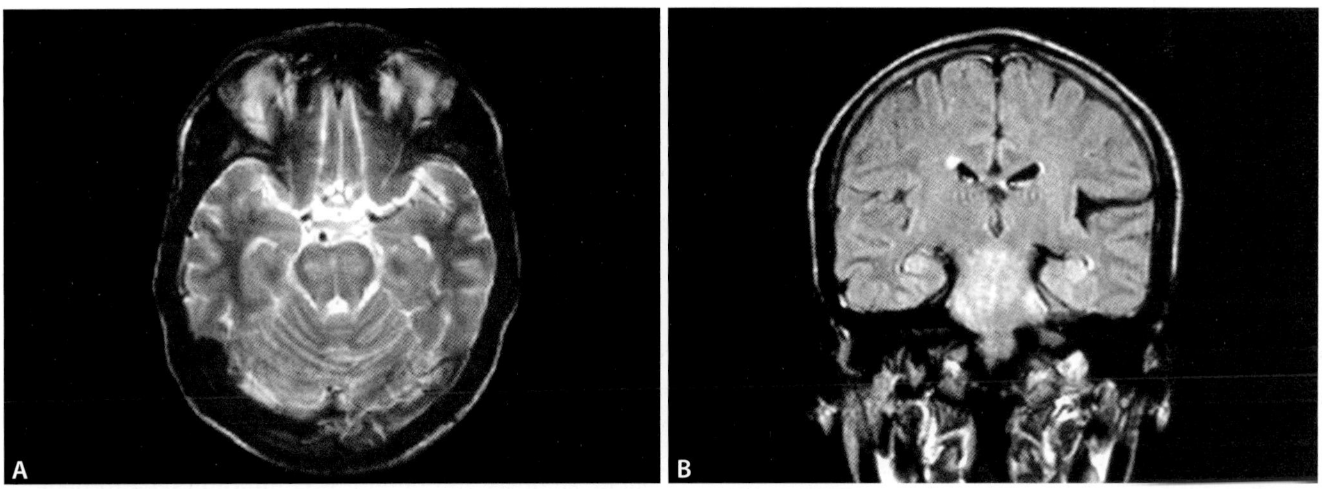

Figs. 39A and B: T2W axial image (A) shows increased signal intensity within the midpons, with surrounding rim of normal-appearing pontine parenchyma. Coronal FLAIR image (B) shows patchy area of hyperintensity in the pons—central pontine myelinolysis.

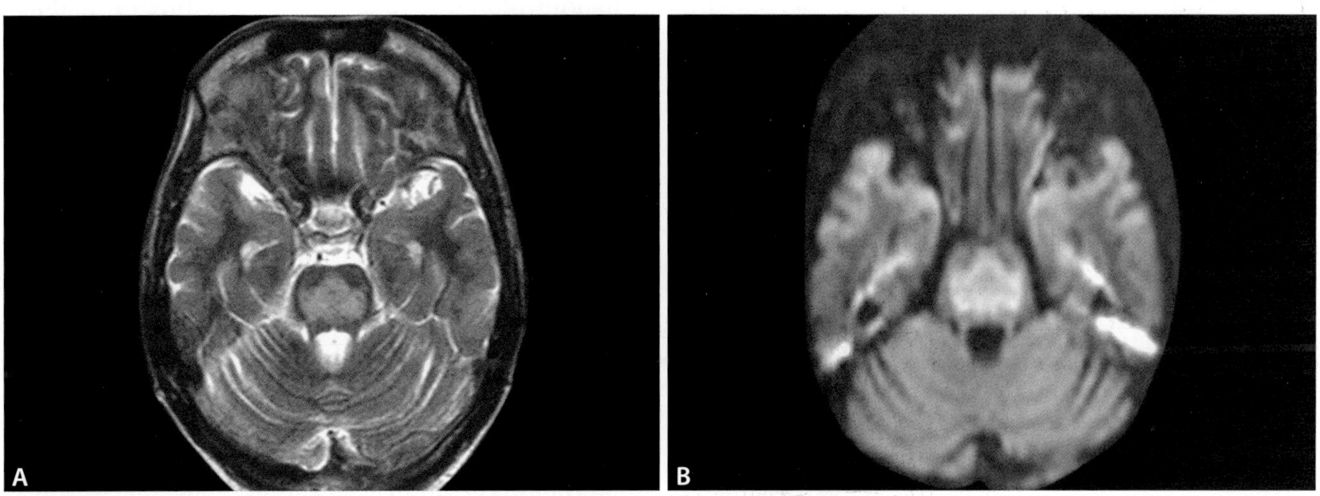

Figs. 40A and B: Trident-shaped hyperintensities T2 axial image (A) in the pons with restricted diffusion on DWI (B) in a case of ODS.

- PRES: can involve pons but does not spare the peripheral white matter.
- Wilson's disease and mitochondrial disorders- may mimic ODS in basal ganglia but pons is rarely involved in Wilson's disease and mitochondrial disorders.

Acute Hypertensive Encephalopathy/ Posterior Reversible Encephalopathy Syndrome (PRES)[133–137]

Hypertension with failed cerebral autoregulation, blood-brain barrier disruption and vasogenic edema are considered the cause for this entity. It was initially described in pre-eclampsia and an acute hypertensive crisis. Other conditions such as thrombotic hemolytic anemia, disseminated intravascular coagulation, use of certain drugs, immunosuppressive therapy have all been implicated.

Patients usually present with single short, grandmal seizure, headache and visual disturbances. Majority of patients have an elevated blood pressure. PRES can also occur in the absence of hypertension or mild hypertension. Severe PRES is a life-threatening complication, if not recognized and treated. PRES usually resolves completely with little or no residual abnormality with rapid institution of treatment. In rare cases disabilities may persist.

Imaging

PRES, as the name implies shows preferential involvement of the parieto-occipital lobes (85–95%) Posterior circulation has comparatively less sympathetic innervation than anterior and hence is less protected from the vasoconstriction mechanism. The frontal lobes are involved in 75–77% of cases and cerebellar involvement is noted in 50–55%.

CT shows subtle patchy cortical/subcortical hypodensity in the parieto-occipital lobes/watershed zones/ cerebellum. PRES associated hemorrhages are seen rarely.

MR: shows the classic findings of bilateral parieto-occipital hypointensities on T1 and hyperintensities on T2W/FLAIR. Patchy enhancement may be seen. As the edema is vasogenic and not cytotoxic, DWI is negative except in atypical cases and in children. There is a decrease in rCBV on perfusion MR **(Figs. 41A to D)**.

In atypical PRES: There is Involvement of frontal lobes, cortical watershed zones, Basal ganglia, brainstem and cerebellum. Rare site of PRES is spinal cord **(Figs. 42A and B)**.

Differential Diagnosis of PRES

- *Acute cerebral ischemia/infarction*: DWI is positive in infarction. Bilateral PCA distribution infarcts are rare in absence of basilar top thrombosis.
- *Vasculitis*: The lesions in vasculitis are more random and less symmetric.
- *Hypoglycemia*: Affects the parieto-occipital region. Clinical findings of hypoglycemia and lack of hypertension can be used to differentiate the two conditions.
- *Thrombotic microangiopathies*: The distinction may be difficult and is based on clinical/laboratory findings.
- *Reversible cerebral vasoconstriction syndrome*: Convexal subarachnoid hemorrhage may be seen but has a limited distribution to a few sulci.

Ethanol-related Diseases

Chronic Alcoholism

Ethanol adversely affects the vascular, glial and neural tissues and causes myelin degeneration. Nonspecific deep white matter and periventricular demyelinating lesions are seen on MR imaging of chronic alcoholics. Demyelination is the main pathological finding in Marchiafava-Bignami disease and most constant in Wernicke disease.[138]

Wernicke Encephalopathy[139,140]

Wernicke-Korsakoff syndrome: named after Carl Wernicke, a German neurologist and psychiatrist and Sergei Sergeievich Korsakoff, a Russian neuropsychiatrist.

It is related to thiamine deficiency which results in lactic acidosis. Although it is commonly seen in patients with alcohol dependence, nearly 50% of cases occur in non-alcoholics. The underlying pathogenesis in all cases is malnutrition due to any cause resulting in thiamine deficiency.

The classical triad of presentation is ocular dysfunction, ataxia, and altered mentation. Untreated, it is fatal and rapid intravenous thiamine replacement can prevent sequelae.

Imaging

MR: In acute phase T2/FLAIR hyperintensity is noted in affected areas—mammillary bodies (which show symmetrical involvement) around the third ventricle, medial thalami, the tectal plate and periaqueductal gray matter. DWI demonstrates diffusion restriction in the involved areas. Strong uniform enhancement of mammillary bodies is pathognomic of Wernicke encephalopathy.

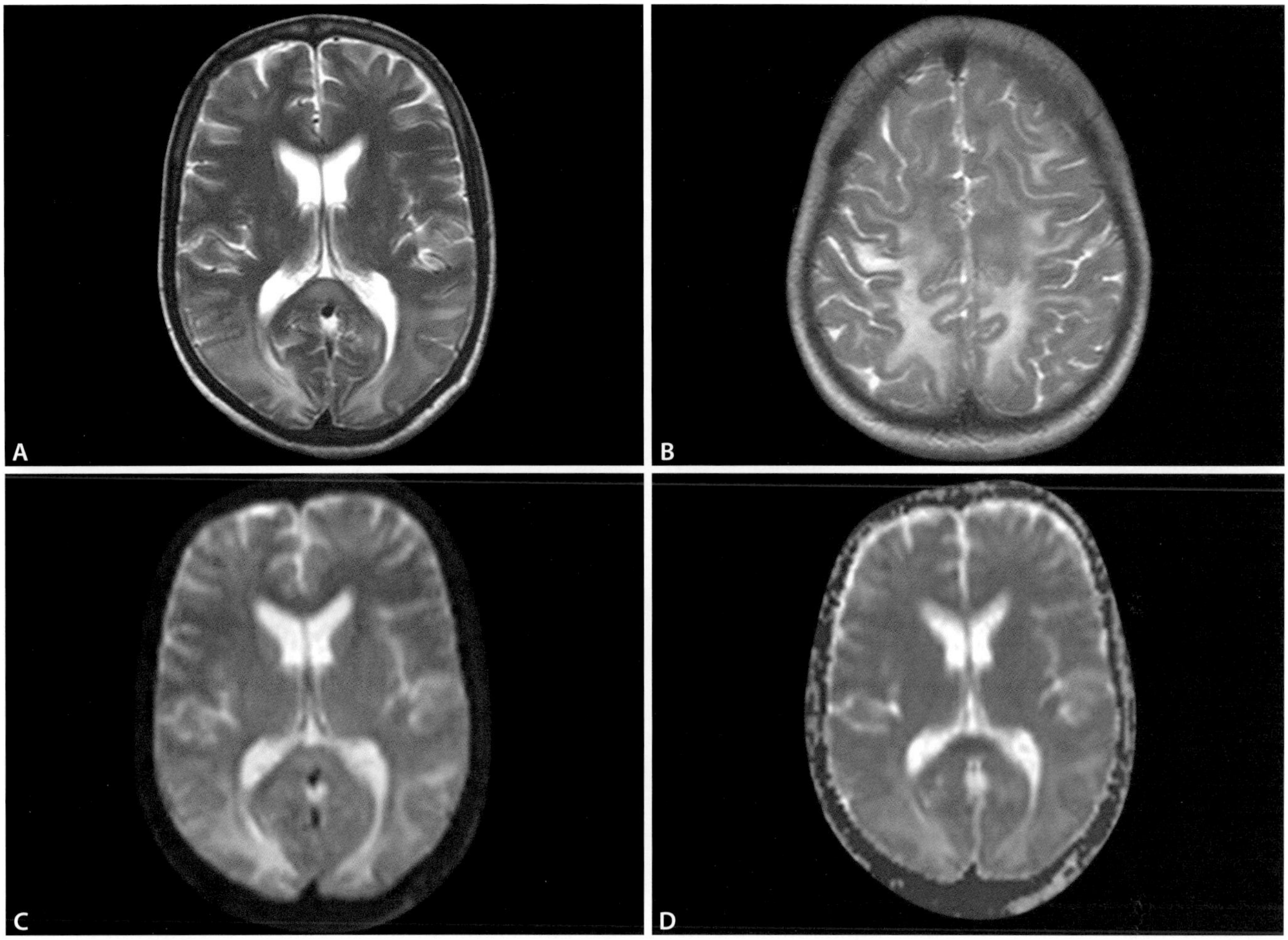

Figs. 41A to D: Bilateral symmetrical hyperintensity in the parieto-occipital region on T2W axial images (A and B). No restricted diffusion seen in DWI (C) and ADC map (D)—a case of PRES.

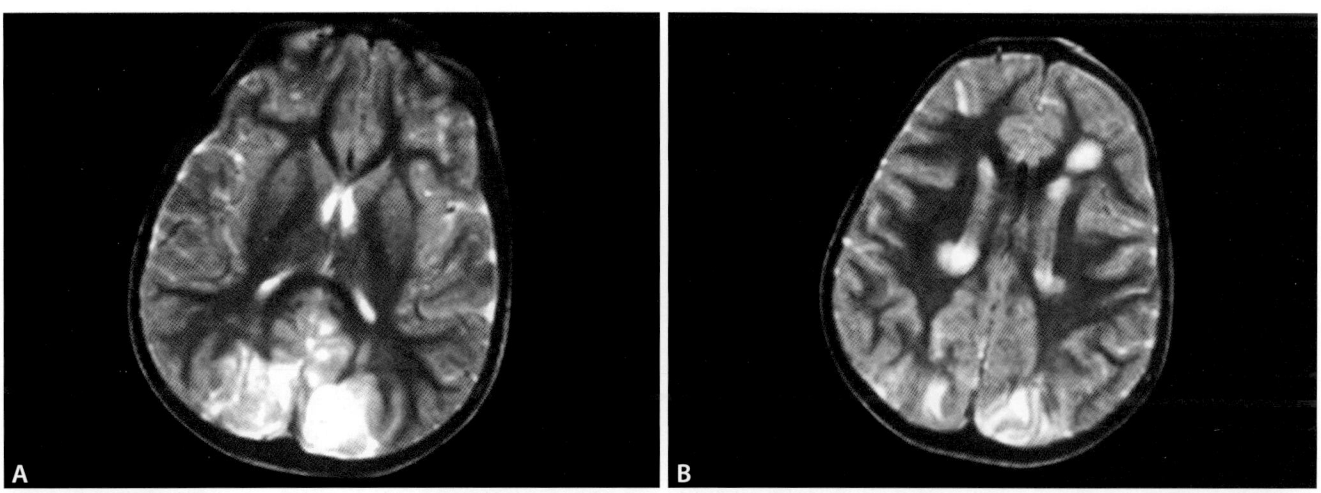

Figs. 42A and B: PRES-due to hypertension T2 axial image (A) Typical bilateral symmetric high signal intensity is seen within the occipital white matter with mild swelling of the overlying cortex. Symmetric high signal intensity within the subcortical white matter in frontal-parietal regions (B).

Differential Diagnosis

- Medial thalamic and midbrain involvement is seen in artery of percheron infract but it does not involve the mammillary bodies.
- Leigh disease-mammillary bodies are not invoved.

Marchiafava-Bignami Disease

Marchiafava-Bignami disease (MBD): The disease was originally described in Italian alcoholic patients addicted to crude red wine consumption by Italian pathologists Ettore Marchiafava and Amico Bignami. It is characterized by toxic demyelination of the corpus callosum and frequently, extends to the centrum semiovale. In more recent years, it has been described in other population groups and poorly nourished non-alcoholics. Pathologically, the myelin loss may be striking and accompanied by axonal degeneration. Acute deterioration is common.[141,142]

Imaging

In the acute stage of the disease, the corpus callosum shows diffuse swelling and high signal intensity on the long TR images. In the chronic stage, diffuse atrophy of the corpus callosum and focal necrosis may be seen in the genu, body, or splenium of the central portion of the corpus callosum **(Figs. 43A and B)**. Focal hypointensity on T2-weighted images within the corpus callosum has been described, which has been speculated to represent either hemosiderin deposits or lipid-laden macrophages. MR imaging studies have shown that lesions may also be found in the hemispheric white matter. Two cases of MBD have been reported in which FLAIR and diffusion-weighted imaging studies revealed symmetrical hyperintense lesions in the cerebral cortex, particularly in the lateral-frontal regions, in addition to the callosal lesions, which suggests an association of diffuse cortical lesions such as Morel's laminar sclerosis with MBD.

Differential Diagnosis

- Multiple sclerosis-clinical history is different.
- Diffuse axonal injury-involving corpus callosum-history of trauma
- Transient lesions of the splenium of the corpus callosum-related to epilepsy and cessation of anti-epileptic medication.

Subacute Combined Degeneration of the Spinal Cord

Vitamin B_{12} (cobalamin) deficiency may affect the central or peripheral nervous system but mainly involves the spinal cord. Subacute combined degeneration (SCD) refers to demyelination and vacuolation found in the posterior and lateral columns of the spinal cord. Patients present with parasthesias, tingling of hands and feet which evolves to ataxic paraplegia and spasticity. Vitamin B_{12} deficiency is a result of pernicious anemia, gastric bypass surgery and malabsorption syndrome.

Imaging

SCD affects the dorsal and lateral columns of the cord and shows increased signal intensity of the affected cord on T2-weighted sequences **(Figs. 44A and B)**.[143] This symmetric bilateral high signal within the cord is referred

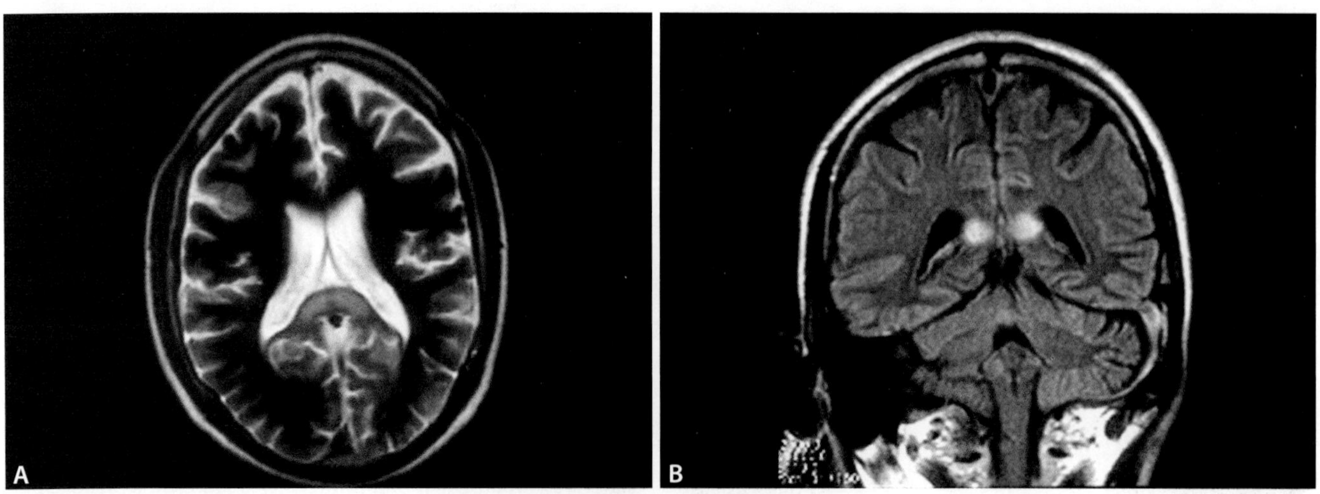

Figs. 43A and B: Demyelination seen in the splenium of corpus callosum in an alcoholic patient on T2W axial image (A) and coronal FLAIR image (B)—a case of Marchiafava-Bignami disease.

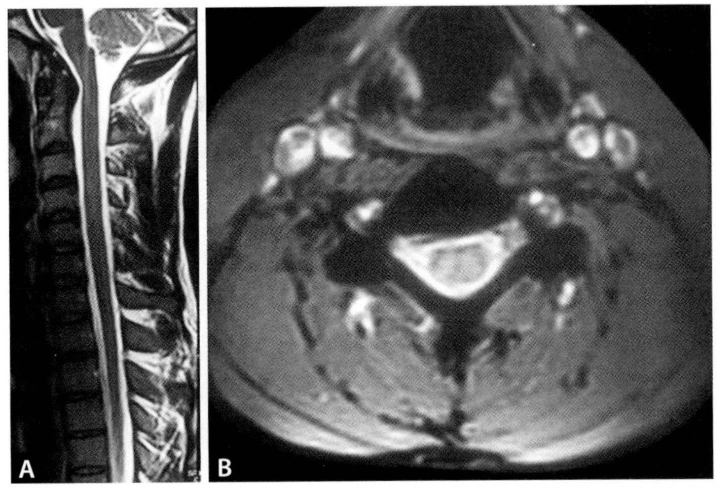

Figs. 44A and B: Subacute combined degeneration of the spinal cord (B_{12} deficiency). Sagittal and axial T2W images (A and B) show mild expansion of the cord and increased signal within the dorsal columns of cervical spinal cord.

to as inverted V sign.[144] Mild expansion of the cord may be seen, and mild contrast enhancement has been described. There is typically a continuous long segment of signal abnormality confined to the dorsal columns, which may help distinguish this entity from other demyelinating lesions found in the cord that appear patchy in distribution.

Vacuolar myelopathy seen in patients with AIDS may appear similar on imaging, and therefore the clinical history plays an important role in distinguishing these entities. Imaging findings in SCD may resolve after treatment with vitamin B_{12}. MR findings in the brain may reveal areas of high signal intensity on the T2-weighted images in the cerebral white matter that may also resolve after treatment with vitamin B_{12}.

White Matter Diseases Associated with Physical/Chemical Agents or Therapeutic Procedures

There are numerous toxic agents that selectively affect the central nervous system. Specific toxins affect specific vulnerable regions of the brain.

RADIATION INJURY[145-149]

Radiation induced injury to the brain is usually caused by whole brain radiation and with doses of up to 30–40 Gy. Associated chemotherapy adds to the risk of radiation injury. It is divided into early and late changes.

Acute radiation injury occurs days to weeks after radiation. This is now rare with use of modern radiation protocols; there can be no changes seen on imaging or transient white matter edema may be seen.

Early radiation injury is noted within 6 months of therapy. Patients may present with cognitive impairment, somnolence. Confluent periventricular hyperintensity is noted which is indicative of transient demyelination. These changes often resolve.

Late delayed injury is seen after 6 months and produce irreversible glial loss noted as necrotizing leukoencephalopathy in deep white matter **(Figs. 45A and B)**. U fibres and corpus callosum are spared. Mass effect and variable enhancement may be seen. The changes depend on total dose of radiation, field size, frequency of dosage and concominant chemotherapy. Various tissues of CNS are affected with oligodendrocytes being most sensitive.

Radiation also predisposes to long term sequlae-vasculopathy (results in ischemic strokes and a moya moya pattern of vasculitis), mineralizing microangiopathy (calcification can be seen in bilateral basal ganglia and subcortical white matter), radiation induced vascular malformation (RIVM)—capillary telangiectasia or cavernomas can be formed. Pediatric patients are at an increased risk. Radiation induced neoplasm are rare, most common being meningioma.

Solvent Vapor Abuse Leukoencephalopathy-Toluene

It is a colorless liquid found in glue, paints and thinner. It is sniffed, huffed or inhaled from a plastic bag. It affects the cerebral white matter and optic nerves. Imaging abnormalities are seen only after several years of abuse. T2/FLAIR hyperintensities are seen in the deep periventricular white matter, centrum semiovale and subcortical areas **(Figs. 46 and 47)**.[150]

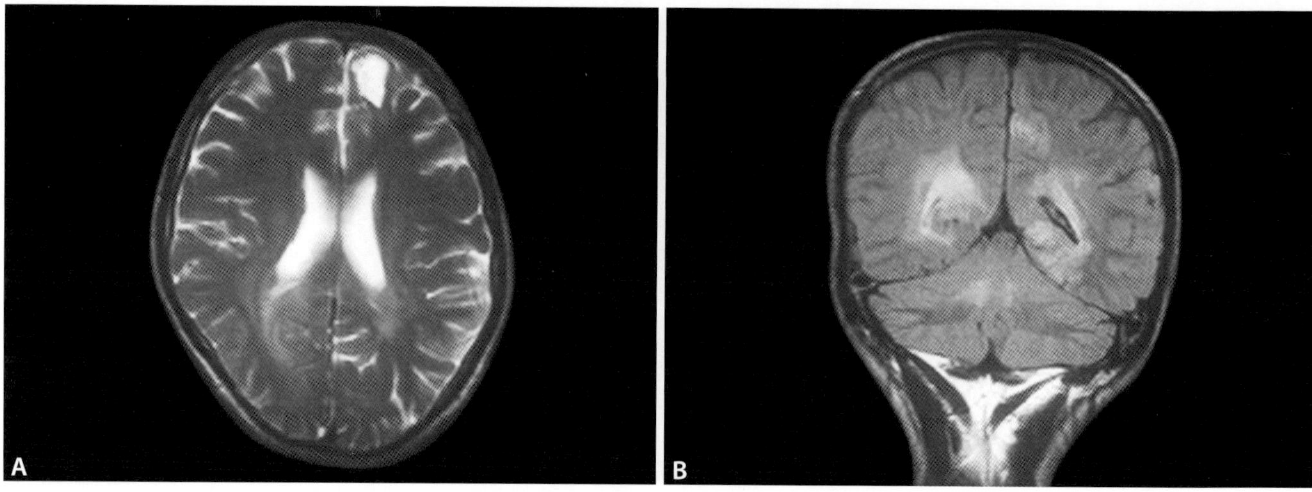

Figs. 45A and B: Demyelination following radiotherapy for left frontal lobe astrocytoma. Axial T2W (A) and coronal FLAIR (B) reveal gliosis in left frontal region with poorly marginated subtle hyperintensity in parieto-occipital regions and in the cerebellum.

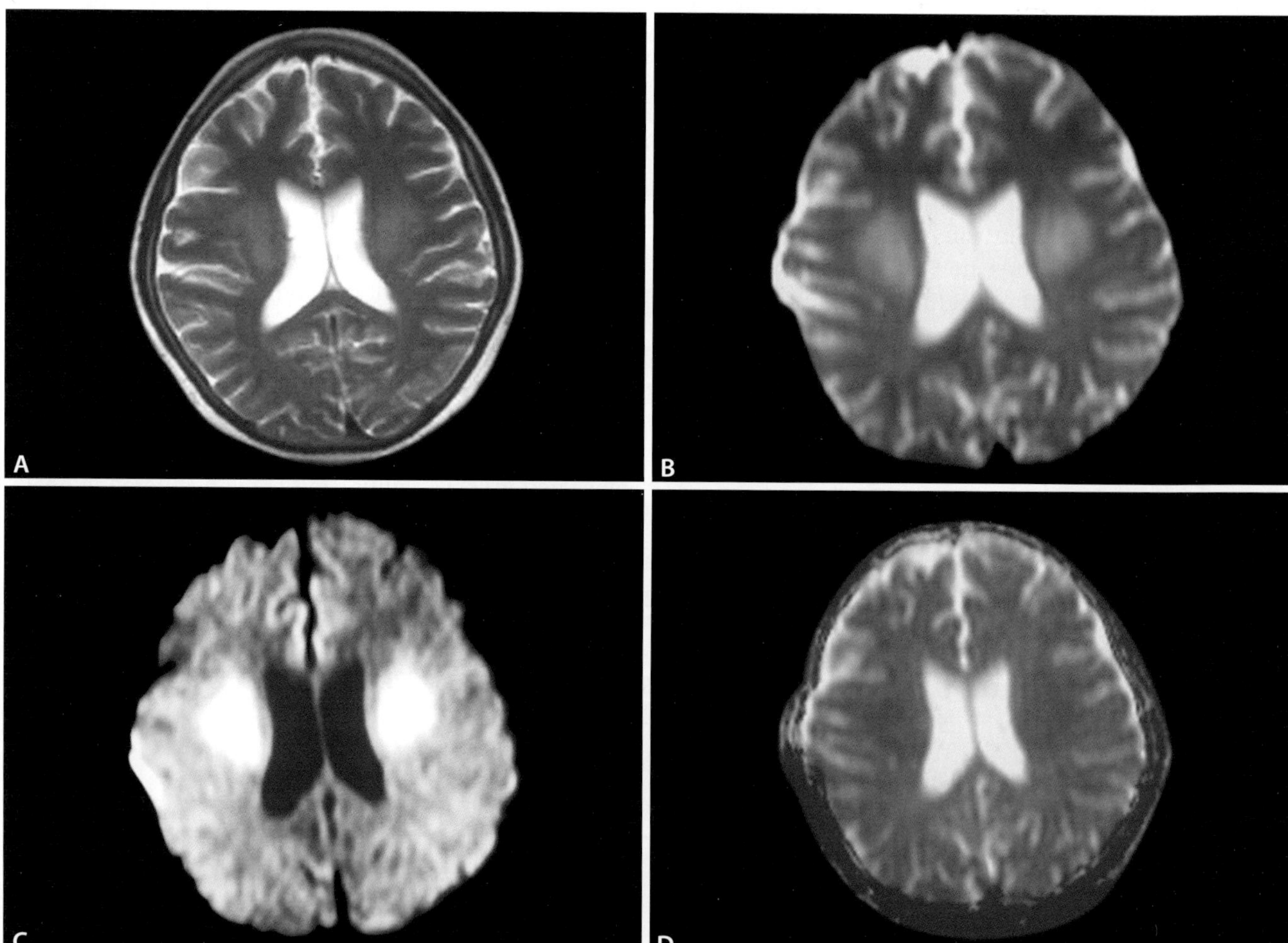

Figs. 46A to D: MRI T2 axial image (A) shows hyperintensity in periventricular deep white matter. There is increase in hyperintensity with increase in b values, b = 500 (B) b = 1000 (C) on ADC maps (D) restricted diffusion is seen—toxic demyelination.

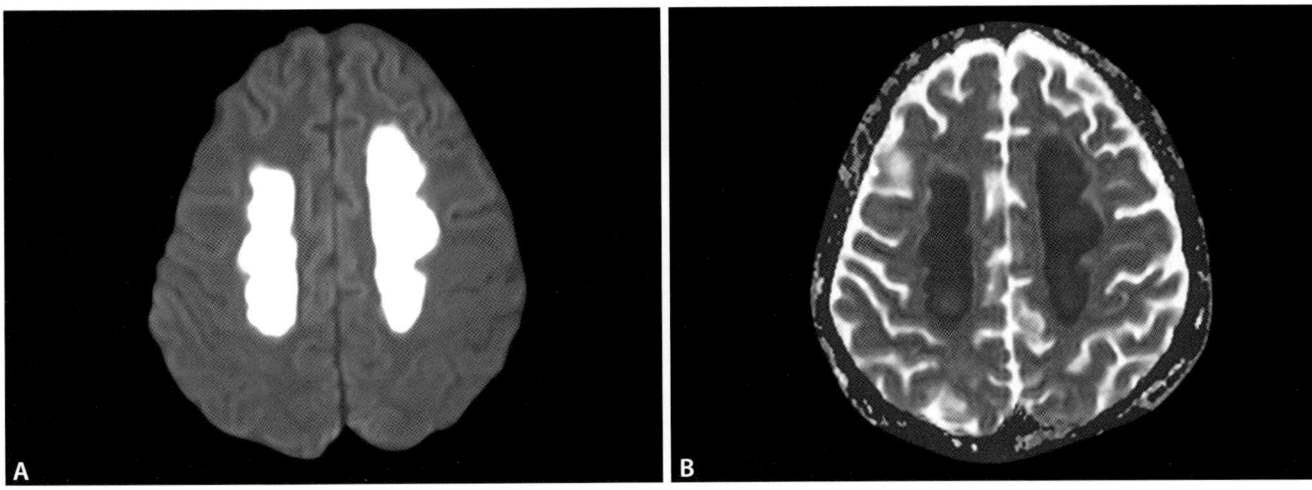

Figs. 47A and B: DWI shows restricted diffusion in centrum semiovale in a case of toxic demyelination. Cb = 1000 (A), ADC map (B).

Chemotherapy

Various chemotherapeutic drugs such as methotrexate, cytarabine, vincristine have CNS toxicity.

Imaging finding of CNS toxicity include:

Posterior reversible encephalopathy syndrome (PRES)—findings are often atypical with involvement of cerebellum, brainstem and basal ganglia and diffusion restriction with enhancement.

Leukoencephalopathy—confluent T2/FLAIR hyperintensities are seen in periventricular white matter, especially with methotrexate.

Cocaine

Cocaine is sniffed, inhaled or injected. The effects are vascular with patients presenting with spontaneous hemorrhagic strokes due to hypertension. Nearly half of these are associated with rupture of preexisting aneurysm or underlying vascular malformation. Acute hypertensive encephalopathy-PRES may also be seen.

Differential diagnosis

- Underlying vascular malformation—unexpected parenchymal hemorrhage in a young adult/middle aged should raise the possibility of drug abuse.
- Embolic infarcts due to heart disease or vasculitis due to any cause (infection, autoimmune, collagen) may appear similar.

Methanol Poisoning

Ingestion of spurious alcohol or accidental ingestion of solvents containing methanol leads to metabolic acidosis due to its metabolite formic acid. It is characterized by headache, visual disturbances and can lead to coma and death. Putamen shows hyperintensity on T2WI **(Figs. 48A and B)**.

Carbon Monoxide Poisoning

It is colorless odorless gas. Poisoning can occur by accident or intentional ingestion. CO attaches to hemoglobin to form carboxyhemoglobin, reducing its ability to transport oxygen. CO poisoning causes headache, tinnitus, dizziness, loss of consciousness.

Imaging

MR: CO poisoning causes bilateral pallidal necrosis, extending into lenticular nuclei and caudate nuclei which appear hypointense on T1 and hyperintense on T2. There may be involvement of subcortical white matter. Diffusion restriction in basal ganglia may be seen. In patients who survive, the lesions show cavitation and cerebral atrophy. A delayed leukoencephalopathy with extensive bilateral symmetrical confluent areas of hyperintensity on T2/FLAIR may be seen.

Differential Diagnosis: CO Poisoning

- Hypoxic ischemic encephalopathy. HIE affects the entire basal ganglia and hippocampus, rarely only globus pallidus.
- Organophosphorus poisoning- bilateral hemorrhagic pallidal necrosis.
- Wilson disease—involves basal ganglia, midbrain, pons and dentate nucleus.
- Leigh disease affects younger patients; here brainstem and putamen lesions are more common.

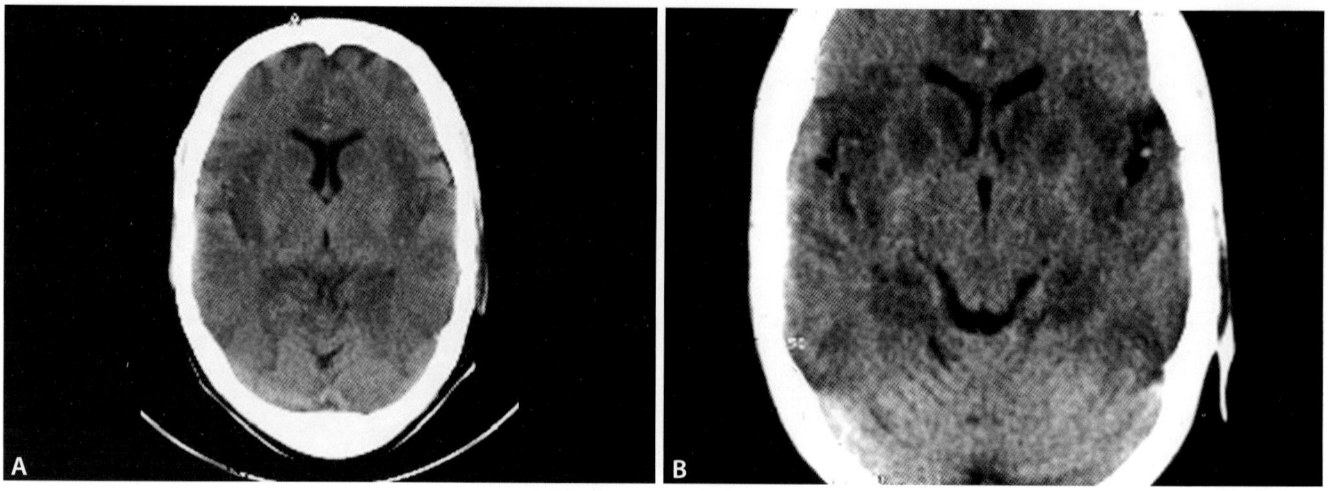

Figs. 48A and B: CT scan in a patient with methanol poisoning shows hypodensities within bilateral basal ganglia, subcortical white matter, and insular cortex.

- JE-encephalitis preferentially involves the basal ganglia and thalamus.
- Creutzfeldt-Jakob disease—affects caudate nucleus, anterior basal ganglia and cortex. Posteromedial thalamic involvement (pulvinar) is common in CJD and rare in CO poisoning.

Heavy Metal Poisoning

This usually occurs as an occupational health hazard. Manganese poisoning occurs in people working in mining industry or in patients receiving total parenteral nutrition. Manganese gets deposited in basal ganglia and is seen as bilateral global pallidal hyperintensity on T1W images. T2 signal is normal. Mercury poisoning affects people in miners or fish consumers who eat fish from contaminated waters. Mercury accumulates in cerebellar vermis and visual cortex and appears hypointense on T1, iso to hypointense on T2-weighted images.

Amphetamine and Derivatives

There are addictive substances which lead to a short lived feeling of euphoria, increased energy and alertness due to blockage of reuptake of catecholamines. Vascular events such as ischemia, hemorrhage and leukoencephalopathy are noted.[151-153]

Methamphetamine (MA/METH/CRYSTAL) results in both ischemic strokes and hemorrhage. Chronic users show cerebral atrophy, more marked in frontal lobe with nonspecific white matter hyperintensites.

MDMA (Ecstasy)—this is a party drug and causes arterial constriction, vasculitis with acute infarcts.

Benzodiazepine—is frequently prescribed to treat anxiety, insomnia. Overdose can lead to hypoxic encephalopathy, hemorrhagic ischemic strokes.

CONCLUSION

Focal white matter hyperintensities pose a diagnostic challenge as the cause may vary from infectious, inflammatory, neoplastic to nonspecific WMH. A systematic imaging approach including age, history, clinical findings, and pattern of distribution of lesion, enhancement pattern and the use of various MR sequences can help to reach a diagnosis.

REFERENCES

1. Rao, Zimmerman RA (Eds). Cranial MRI and CT (4th edn). New York: Mc Graw Hill; 1999.
2. Nusbaum AO, Kar Ming Fung, Atlas SW. White matter diseases and inherited metabolic disorders. In: Scott W, Atlas (Eds). Magnetic Resonance Imaging of the Brain and Spine (3rd edn). Philadelphia: Lippincott Williams and Wilkins; 2002.
3. Suzuki K, Armao D, Stone JA, et al. Demyelinating diseases, leucodystrophies, and other myelin disorders. Neuroimaging Clin North Am. 2001;11:1.
4. Lakhanpal SK, Maravilla KR. Multiple sclerosis. In: Stark DD, Bradley WG (Eds). Magnetic Resonance Imaging, 3rd ed. St Louls Mo: Mosby; 1999. pp. 1379-402.
5. Jacobs I, Kinkel WR, Polachini I, et al. Correlations of nuclear magnetic resonance imaging, computerized tomography, and clinical profiles in multiple sclerosis. Neurology. 1986;36:27-34.
6. Fillipi M. In vivo characterization of multiple sclerosis and other white matter diseases using magnetic resonance based techniques. Neurology. 2001;248:1019-29.

7. Garaci FG, Marzialis S, Meschini A, et al. Brain haemodynamic changes associated with chronic cerebrospinal venous insufficiency are not specific to multiple sclerosis and do not increase its severity. Radiology. 2012;265(1):233-9.
8. Flynn KC, Flynn Lc, Moster ML. Current thoughts on chronic cerebrospinal venous insufficiency in multiple sclerosis. Curr Opin Ophthalmol. 2011;22(6):463-7.
9. Ghezzi A, Comi G, Federico A. Chronic cerebrospinal venous insufficiency and multiple sclerosis. Neurol Sci. 2011;32(1):17-21.
10. Koch-Henriksen N, Sørensen PS. The changing demographic pattern of multiple sclerosis epidemiology. Lancet Neurol. 2010;9(5):520-32.
11. Fujihara K, Onk BK. MS across continents: challenging our knowledge of MS in Asia and the middle East - Report from 2nd MS Forum Pan - Asian Conference, 19-20 November.
12. Swanton JK, Rovira A, Tintore M, et al. MRI criteria for multiple sclerosis in patients presenting with clinically isolated syndromes: a multicentric retrospective study. Lancet Neurol. 2007;6:677-86.
13. Achten E, Deblaere K. Health technology assessment on the use of magnetic resonance imaging (MRI) and computed tomography (CT) in the diagnosis of multiple sclerosis (MS) and clinically isolated syndromes CIS. European Journal of Radiology. 2008;65:211-3.
14. Montalban X, Tintore M, Swanton J, et al. MRI criteria for MS in patients with clinically isolated syndromes. Neurology. 2010;74(5):427-34.
15. Inglese M. Multiple sclerosis: new insights and trends. AJNR. 2006;27:954-7.
16. Ge Y. Multiple sclerosis: the role of MR imaging. Am J Neuro Radiol. 2006;27:1165.
17. Granberg T, Martola J, Kristoffersen-Wiberg M, et al. Radiologically isolated syndrome. Incidental magnetic resonance imaging findings suggestive of multiple sclerosis-a systemic review. Mult Scler. 2013;19(3):271-80.
18. Sarbu N, Shih RY, Jones RV, et al. White matter diseases with radiologic-pathologic correlation. Radiographics. 2016;36(5):1426-47.
19. Gold Man MD, Cohen JA. Multiple sclerosis. In: Rakel RE, Bope ET (Eds). Conn's Current Therapy. Philadelphia: Elsevier Saunders; 2005. pp. 1057-66.
20. Kornienko VN, Pronin IN. Diagnostic Neuroradiology. Springer Verlag; 2008.
21. Fillipi M, Evangelou N, Kangarlu A, et al. Ultrahigh field MR imaging in multiple sclerosis.J Neurol Neurosurg Psychiatry. 2014;85(1):60-6.
22. Fazekas F, Barkhof F, Filippi M, et al. The contribution of magnetic resonance imaging to the diagnosis of multiple sclerosis. Neurology. 1999;53:448-56.
23. Jackson JA, Leake DR, Schneiders NJ, et al. Magnetic resonance imaging in multiple sclerosis: Results in 22 cases. Am J Neuroradiol. 1985;6:171-6.
24. Gean Marton AD, Venzina LG, Marton KI, et al. Abnormal corpus callosum: a sensitive and specific indicator of multiple sclerosis. Radiology. 1991;180:215-21.
25. Lisanti CJ, Asbach P, Bradley WG. The ependymal 'Dot-Dash' sign. An MR imaging finding of early Multiple sclerosis. AJNR. 2005;26:2033-6.
26. Roosendaal SD, Moraal B, Pouwels PJW, et al. Accumalation of cortical lesions in MS: relation with cognitive impairment. Mult Scler. 2009;15(6):708-14.
27. Filippi M, Rocca MA,Calabrese M, et al. Intracortical lesions: relevance for new MRI siagnostic criteria for multiple sclerosis. Neurology. 2010;75(22):1988-94.
28. de Graaf WL, Kilsdonk ID, Lopez-Soriano A, et al. Clinical application of multi contrast 7T MR imaging in multiple sclerosis: increased lesion detection compared to 3 T confined to gray matter. Eur Radiol. 2013;23(2):528-40.
29. Filippi M, Rocca MA. MR imaging of multiple sclerosis. Radiology. 2011;259(3):659-81
30. Edwards MK, Farlow MR, Stevens JC. Cranial MR in spinal cord MS: diagnosing patients with isolated spinal cord symptoms. Am J Neuroradiol. 1986;7:1003-5.
31. Thielen KR, Miller GM. Multiple sclerosis of the spinal cord: magnetic resonance appearance. J Comput Assist Tomogr. 1996;20:434-8.
32. Smith RR, Edwards MK, Farlow MR, et al. Imaging of optic neuritis using STIR MR. Am J Neuroradiol. 1989;10:905(abstr).
33. Miller DH, Barkhof F, Nauta JJ. Gadolinium enhancement increases the sensitivity of MRI in detecting disease activity in multiple sclerosis. Brain. 1993;116:1077-94.
34. Tas MW, Barkhol F, Van Walderveen MA, et al. The effect of gadolinium on the sensitivity and specifig of MR in the initial diagnosis of multiple sclerosis. Am J Neuro Radiol. 2005;26:2316-9.
35. Silver NC, Good CD, Barker GJ, et al. Sensitivity of contrast enhanced MRI in multiple sclerosis. Effects of gadoliniumdose, magnetisation transfer contrast and delayed imaging. Brain. 1997:120(pt 7):1149.
36. Rovira A, Leon A. MR in the diagnosis and monitoring of multiple sclerosis: an over view. European Journal of Radiology. 2008;67:409-14.
37. Simon JH. Update on multiple sclerosis. Radial Clin N Am. 2006;44:79-100.
38. Lane B. Leucoencephalopathies and demyelinating disease. In: Haaga JR (Ed). Computed Tomography and Magnetic Resonance Imaging of the Whole Body (5th edn), Mosby: Elsiever; 2009.
39. Van Walderveen MA, Kamphorst W, Scheltens P, et al. Histopathologic correlates of hypointense lesions on T1 - weighted spin - echo MRI in multiple sclerosis. Neurology 1998;50:1282-8.
40. Allen IV, Mc Quaid S, Mirakhur M, et al. Pathological abnormalities in the normal appearing white matter in multiple sclerosis. Neurol Sci. 2001;22:141-4.
41. Bozzali M, Rocca MA, Iannucci G, et al. Magnetization transfer histogram analysis of the cervical cord in patients with multiple sclerosis. Am J Neuroradiol. 1999;20:1803-8.
42. Van Buchem MA, McGowan JC, Kolson DL, et al. Quantitative volumetric magnetization transfer analysis in multiple

sclerosis: Estimation of macroscopic and microscopic disease burden. Magn Reson Med. 1996;36:632-6.
43. Loevner LA, Grossman RI, Cohen J, et al. Microscopic disease in normal - appearing white matter on conventional MR images in patients with multiple sclerosis: Assessment with magnetization— transfer measurements. Radiology. 1995;196:511-5.
44. Bischof A, Caverzasi E, Cordano C, et al. Advances in imaging Multiple sclerosis. Semin Neurol. 2017;37:538-54.
45. Bammer R, Augustin M, Strasser Fuchs S, et al. Magnetic resonance diffusion tensor imaging for characterising diffuse and focal matter abnormalities in multiple sclerosis. Magn Reson Med. 2000;44:583-91.
46. Basser PJ, Pierpaoli C. Microstructural and physiological features of tissues elucidated by quantitative - diffusion - tensor MRI. J Magn Reson. 1996;111:209-19.
47. Pierpaoli C, Jezzard P, Basser PJ, et al. Diffusion tensor MR imaging of the human brain. Radiology. 1996;201:637-48.
48. Bammer R, Fazekas F. Diffusion imaging in multiple sclerosis. Neuroimag Clin North Am. 2002;12(1):71-106.
49. Nusbaum AO, Tang CY, Wei T, et al. Whole – brain diffusion MR histograms differ between MS subtypes. Neurology. 2000;54:1421-7.
50. Pagani E, Bammer R, Horsfield MN, et al. Diffusion MR imaging in Multiple sclerosis. Technical aspects and challenges. AJNR. 2007;28:411-20.
51. Nusbaum AO, Lu D, Tang CY, et al. Quantitative diffusion measurements in focal multiple sclerosis lesions: Correlation with appearance on T1-weighted MR images. Am J Roentgenol. 2000;175:821-5.
52. Davie CA, Hawkins CP, Barker GJ, et al. Serial proton magnetic resonance spectroscopy in acute multiple sclerosis lesions. Brain. 1994;117:49-58.
53. Arnold DL, Mathews PM, Francis GS, et al. Proton magnetic resonance spectroscopic imaging for metabolic characterization of demyelinating plaques. Ann Neurol. 1992;31:235-41.
54. De Stefano N, Bartolozzi ML, Guidi L, et al. Magnetic resonance spectroscopy as a measure of brain damage in multiple sclerosis. J Neurol Sci. 2005;233:203-8.
55. Tartaglia MC, Narayanan S, De Stefano N, et al. Choline is increased in prelesional normal appearing white matter in multiple sclerosis. J Neurol. 2002;249:1382-90.
56. Fillipi M, Rocca MA, Mezzapesa DM, et al. Simple and complex movement. Associated functional MRI changes in patients at presentation with clinically isolated syndromes suggestive of multiple sclerosis. Hum Brain Mapp. 2004;21:108-17.
57. Filippi M, Rocca MA, Mezzapesa DM, et al. A functional MRI study of cortical activations associated with object manipulation in patients with MS. Neuro Image. 2004;21:1147-54.
58. Law M, Saindane AM, Ge Y, et al. Microvascular abnormality in relapsing – remitting multiple sclerosis: perfusion MR imaging findings in normal appearing white matter. Radiology. 2004;231:645-52.
59. Laule C, Leung E, Lis DK, et al. Myelin water imaging in multiple sclerosis: quantitative correlations with histopathology. Mult Scler. 2006;12(06):747-53.
60. Mc Donald WI, Compston A, Edan G, et al. Recommended diagnostic criteria for multiple sclerosis: guidelines from the international panel on the diagnosis of multiple sclerosis. Ann Neurol. 2001;50:121-7.
61. Polman CH, Reingold SC, Edan G, et al. Diagnostic criteria for multiple sclerosis: 2005 revisions to the McDonald criteria. Ann Neurol. 2005;58:840-6.
62. Polman CH, Reingold SC, Banwell B, et al. Diagnostic criteria for multiple sclerosis: 2010 revisions to the McDonald criteria. Ann Neurol. 2011;69(2):292-302.
63. Filippi M, Rocca MA, Ciccarelli O, et al. MRI criteria for the diagnosis of multiple sclerosis: MAGNIMS consensus guidelines. The Lancet. Neurology. 2016;15 (3):292-303.
64. Thompson AJ, Banwell BL, Barkhof F, et al. Diagnosis of multiple sclerosis: 2017 revisions of the McDonald criteria. The Lancet. Neurology. 2017;17(2)162-73.
65. Kwee RM, Kwee TC. Virchow-Robin spaces at MR Imaging. Radiographics. 2007;27:1071-86.
66. Galluzzi S, Lanni C, Pantoni L, et al.White matter lesions in the elderly: pathophysiological hypothesis on the effect on brain plasticity and treseve. J Neurol Sci. 2008;273(1-2):3-9.
67. Igarashi H, Sakai F, Kan S, et al. Magnetic resonance imaging of the brain in patients with migraine. Cephalagia. 1991;11:69-74.
68. Berger JR. Functional improvement and symptom management in multiple sclerosis: clinical efficacy of current therapies. Am J Manag Care. 2011;17(Suppl 5):S146-S153.
69. Brust JC. Current diagnosis & Treatment in Neurology. McGraw-Hill Medical; 2006.
70. McNamara C, Sugrue G, Murray B, et al. Current and emerging therapies in multiple sclerosis: implications for the radiologist, Part 1-mechanisms, efficacy, and safety. AJNR. 2017;38(9):1664-71.
71. McNamara C, Sugrue G, Murray B, et al. Current and emerging therapies in multiple sclerosis: implications for the radiologist, Part 2-surveillance for treatment complications and disease progression. AJNR. 2017;38(9):1772-80.
72. Canellas AR, et al. Idiopathic inflammatory -demyelinating diseases of the central nervous system. Neuroradiology. 2007;49(5):393-409.
73. Cha S, Pierce S, Knopp EA, et al. Dynamic contrast-enhanced T2*-weighted MR imaging of tumefactive demyelinating lesions. AJNR Am J Neuroradiol. 2001;22 (6): 1109-16.
74. Dagher AP, Smirniotopoulos J. Tumefactive demyelinating lesions. Neuroradiology. 1996;38(6): 560-5.
75. Given CA, Stevens BS, Lee C. The MRI appearance of tumefactive demyelinating lesions. Am J Roentgenol. 2004; 182 (1):195-9.
76. Masdeu JC, Moreira J, Trasi S, et al. The open ring. A new imaging sign in demyelinating disease. J Neuroimaging. 1996;6(2):104-7.

77. Paley RJ, Persing JA, Doctor A, et al. Multiple sclerosis and brain tumor: a diagnostic challenge. J Emerg Med. 1989;7(3):241-4.
78. Saindane AM, Cha S, Law M, et al. Proton MR spectroscopy of tumefactive demyelinating lesions. Am J Neuroradiol. 2002;23(8):1378-86.
79. Fallah A, Banglawala S, Ebrahim S, et al. Case Series: tumefactive demyelinating lesions: a diagnostic challenge. Can J Surg. 2010;53(1):69-70.
80. Eckstein C, Saidha S, Levy M. A differential diagnosis of central nervous system demyelination : beyond multiple sclerosis. J Neurol. 2012;295(5):801-16.
81. Wingerchuk DM, Lennon VA, Pittock SJ, et al: Revised diagnostic criteria for neuromyelitis optica. Neurology. 2006;66(10):1485-9.
82. Barnett Y, Sutton IJ, Ghadiri M, et al. Conventional and advanced imaging in neuromyelitis optica. Am J Neuroradiol. 2013. doi:10.3174/ajnr.A3592.
83. Chang KH, Lyu RK, Chen CM, et al. Distinct features between longitudinally extensive transverse myelitis presenting with and without anti-aquaporin 4 antibodies. Mult. Scler. 2013;19 (3):299-307.
84. Bruna Garbugio Dutra, Antônio José da Rocha, Renato Hoffmann Nunes, et al. Neuromyelitis optica spectrum disorders: spectrum of MR imaging findings and their differential diagnosis. RadioGraphics. 2018;38(1):169-93.
85. Lu Z, Zhang B, Qiu W, et al. Comparative brain stem lesions on MRI of acute disseminated encephalomyelitis, neuromyelitis optica and multiple sclerosis. PLoS One 2011;6(8):e22766.
86. Barnett Y,Sutton IJ,Ghadiri M, et al.Conventional and advanced imaging in neuromyelitis optica. Am J Neuroradiol. 2014;35(8):1458-66.
87. Huh SY, Min JH, Kim W, et al. The usefulness of brain MEI at onset in the differentiation of multiple sclerosis and seropositive neuromyelitis optica spectrum disorders. Mult Scler. 2014;20(6):695-704.
88. Rovira A, Sastre-Garriga J, Auger C, et al. Idiopathic inflammatory diseases of the brainstem. Semin Ultrasound CTMR. 2013;34(2):123-30.
89. Sahraian MA, Radue EW, Minagar A. Neuromyelitis optica: clinical manifestations and neuroimaging features. Neurol Clin. 2013;31(1):139-52.
90. Yonezu T, Ito S, Mori M, et al. "Bright spotty lesions" on spinal magnetic resonance imaging differentiates neuromyelitis optica from multiple sclerosis. Mult Scler. 2014;20(3):331-7.
91. Kister I, Herbert J, Zhou Y, et al. Ultra high field MR (7T) imaging of brain lesions in neuromyelitis optica. Mult Scler INT. 2013;2013:398259.
92. Tenembaum SN. Disseminated encephalomyelitis in children. Clin Neurol Neurisyrg. 2008;110(9):928-38.
93. DeSanto J, Ross JS. Spine infection/inflammation. Radiol Clin North Am. 2011:49(1):105-27.
94. Lee HY, Chang KH, Kim JH, et al. Serial MR imaging findings of acute hemorrhagic leukoencephalitis: a case report. Am J Neuroradiol. 2005;26(8):1996-9.
95. Wong AM, Simon EM, Zimmerman RA, et al. Acute necrotizing encephalopathy of childhood: correlation of MR findings and clinical outcome. Am J Neuroradiol. 2006; 27(9): 1919-23.
96. Mark AS, Atlas SW. Progressive multifocal leucoencephalopathy in patients with AIDS: appearance on MR images. Radiology. 1989;173:517-21.
97. Mader I, Herrlinger U, Klose U, et al. Progressive multifocal leucoencephalopathy: analysis of lesion development with diffusion weighted MRI. Neuroradiol. 2003;45:717-21.
98. Lanska DL. Epidemiology of human immunodeficiency virus dementia. Semin Neurol. 1999;19:105-11
99. Thurnber MM, Thurnber SA, Fleischmann D, et al. Comparison of T2-weighted and fluid - attenuated inversion - recovery fast spin echo MR sequences in intracerebral AIDS - associated disease. Am J Neuroradiol. 1997;18:1601-9.
100. Dousset V, Armand JP, Lacoste D. Magnetization transfer study of HIV encephalitis and progressive multifocal leucoencephalopathy. Am J Neuroradiol. 1997;18:895-901.
101. Berger JR, Major EO. Progressive multifocal leucoencephalopathy. Semin Neurol. 1999;19:223-33.
102. Bag AK, Curé JK, Chapman PR, et al. JC virus infection of the brain. AJNR Am J Neuroradiol. 2010;31 (9):1564-76.
103. Clifford DB, Ances BM. HIV-associated neurocognitive disorder. Lancet Infect Dis. 2013;13(11): 976-86.
104. Smith A, Smirniotopoulos J, Rushing E. Central nervous system infections associated with human immunodeficiency virus infection: radiologic-pathologic correlation1. Radiographics. 2008;28(7):2033-58.
105. Barker PB, Lee RR, McArthus JC. AIDS dementia complex: evaluation with proton MR spectroscopic imaging. Radiology. 1995;195:58-64.
106. Hildenbrand P, Craven DE, Jones R, et al. Lyme neuroborreliosis: manifestations of a rapidly emerging zoonosis. Am J Neuradiol. 2009;30(6):1079-87.
107. Wardlaw JM, Smith EE, Bissels GJ, et al. Neuroimaging standards for research into small vessel disease and its contribution to ageing and neurodegeneration. Lancet Neurol. 2013;128:822-38.
108. Schmidt R, Schmidt H, Haybaeck J, et al. Heterogenity in age related white matter changes. Acta Neuropathol (Berl). 2001;122(2):171-85.
109. Gallasi R, Morrreale A, Montagna P, et al. Binswanger's disease and normal pressure hydrocephlus. Arch Neurol. 1991;48:1156-9.
110. Biffi A, Greenberg SM. Cerebral amyloid angiopathy: a systematic review. J Chin Neurol. 2011;7(1):1-9.
111. Knudsen KA, Rosand J, Karluk D, et al. Clinical diagnosis of cerebral amyloid angiopathy: validation of the boston criteria. Neurology. 2010;74(17):1346-50.
112. Tournier-Lasserve E, Iba Zizen MT, Romero N, et al. Autosomal dominant syndrome with stroke like episodes and leucoencephalopathy. Stroke. 1991;22:1297-302.
113. Chabriat H,Vahedi K, Iba-Zizen MT, et al. Clinical spectrum of CADASIL: a study of 7 families-cerebral autosomal

dominant arteriopathy with subcortical infarcts and leukoencephalopathy. Lancet 1995;346(8980):934-9.

114. Singhal S, Rich P, Markus HS. The spatial distribution of MR imaging abnormalities in cerebral autosomal dominant arteriopathy with subcortical infarcts and leukoencephalopathy and their relationship to age and clinical features. Am J Neuradiol. 2005;26(10):2481-7.
115. Salavari C, Brown RD Jr, Calamia KT et al. Primary central venous system vasculitis: analysis of 101 patients. Ann Neurol. 2007;62:442-51.
116. Abdel Razek AAK, Alvarez H, et al. Imaging spectrum of CNS vasculitis. Radiographics. 2014;34(4):873-94.
117. Birnbaum J, Hellmann DB. Primary angiitis of the central nervous system. Arch Neurol. 2009;66(6):704-9.
118. Susac JO. Susac's syndrome. Am J Neuroradiol. 2004;25 (3):351-2.
119. Demir MK. Case 142: Susac syndrome. Radiology. 2009;250 (2):598-602.
120. Susac JO, Hardman JM, Selhorst JB. Microangiopathy of the brain and retina. Neurology. 1979;29(3):313-6.
121. Gross M, Eliashar R. Update on Susac's syndrome. Curr Opin Neurol. 2005;18(3):311-4.
122. Saenz R, Quan AW, Magalhaes A, et al. MRI of Susac's syndrome. Am J Roentgenol. 2005;184(5):1688-90.
123. Susac JO, Egan RA, Rennebohm RM, et al. Susac's syndrome: 1975-2005 microangiopathy/autoimmune endotheliopathy. J Neurol Sci. 2007;257(1-2):270-2.
124. Buzzard KA, Reddel SW, Yiannikas C, et al. Distinguishing Susac's syndrome from multiple sclerosis. Journal of Neurology. 2015;262(7):1613-21.
125. Goh YP, Naidoo P, Ngian GS. Imaging of systemic lupus erythematosus. Part I: CNS, cardiovascular, and thoracic manifestations. Clinical Radiology. 2013;68(2):181-91.
126. Lalani TA, Kanne JP, Hatfield GA, et al. Imaging findings in systemic lupus erythematosus. Radiographics: a review publication of the Radiological Society of North America, Inc. 24(4):1069-86.
127. Luyendijk J, Steens SC, Ouwendijk WJ et al. Neuropsychiatric systemic lupus erythematosus: lessons learned from magnetic resonance imaging. Arthritic Rheum. 2011;63(3):722-32.
128. Noel N, Hutié M, Wechsler B, et al. Pseudotumoural presentation of neuro-Behcet's disease: case series and review of literature. Rheumatology (Oxford). 2012; 51(7):1216-25.
129. Gerard D, Healy ME, Hesselink JR. MR demonstration of mesencephalic lesions in osmotic demyelination syndrome (central pontine myelinolysis). Neuroradiology. 1987;29:582-84.
130. Lampl C, Yazdi K. Central pontine myelinolysis. Euro Neurol. 2002;47:3-10.
131. King JD, Rosner MH. Osmotic demyelination syndrome. Am J Med Sci. 2010;339(6):561-7.
132. De Souza A, Desai PK. More often striated myelinosis than pontine? A consecutive series of patients with osmotic demyelination syndrome. Neurol Res. 2012;34(3):262-71.
133. Engelter ST, Petrella JR, Alberts MJ, et al. Assessment of cerebral microcirculation in a patient with hypertensive encephalopathy using MR perfusion imaging. Am J Roentgenol. 1999;173: 1491-3.
134. Senger AR, Gupta RK, Dhanuka AK, et al. MR imaging, MR angiography, and MR spectroscopy of the brain in eclampsia. Am J Neuroradiol. 1997;18:1485-90.
135. Fugate JE, Claassen DO, Cloft HJ, et al. Posterior reversible encephalopathy syndrome: associated clinical and radiological findings. Mayo Clin Proc. 2010;85(50:427-32.
136. Ni J, Zhou LX, Hao HL, et al. the clinical and radiological spectrum of posterior reversible encephalopathy syndrome. A retrospective series of 24 patients. J Neuro Imaging. 2011;21(3):219-24.
137. Bartynski WS. Posterior reversible encephalopathy syndrome, Part 1: fundamental imaging and clinical features. AJNR. 2008;29(6):1036-42.
138. Geibprasert S, Gallucci M, Krings T. Alcohol induced changes in the brain as assessed by MRI and CT, Eur Radiol. 2010;20(6):1492-501.
139. Zuccoli G, Gallucci M, Capellades J, et al. Wernicke encephalopathy: MR findings at clinical presentation in twenty-six alcoholic and nonalcoholic patients. Am J Neuroradiol. 2007;28 (7):1328-31.
140. Zuccoli G, Pipitone N. MR imaging: an increasingly important tool in the early diagnosis of Wernicke encephalopathy. Am J Neuroradiol. 2012;33(6): E92.
141. Arbelaez A, Pajon A, Castillo M. Acute Marchiafava Bignami disease: MR findings in two patients. Am J Neuroradiol. 2003;24:1955-7.
142. Johkura K, Naito M, Naka T. Cortical involvement in Marchiafava Bignami disease. Am J Neuroradiol. 2005; 26:670-3.
143. Ravina B, Loevner LA, Bank W. MR findings in subacute combined degeneration of the spinal cord: a case of reversible cervical myelopathy. Am J Roentgenol. 2000; 174(3):863-5.
144. Kumar A, Singh AK. Teaching neuroimage: inverted V sign in subacute combined degeneration of spinal cord. Neurology. 2009;72(1):e4.
145. Chan Y, Leung S, King AD, et al. Late radiation injury to the temporal lobes: Morphologic evaluation at MR imaging. Radiology. 1999;213:800-7.
146. Greene-Schloesser D, Robbins ME, Peiffer AM, et al. Radiation induced brain injury: a review. Front Oncol. 2012;2:73.
147. Vázquez E, Delgado I, Sánchez-Montañez A, et al. Side effects of oncologic therapies in the paediatric central nervous system: update on neuro imaging findings. Radiographics. 2011;31(4):1123-39.

148. Chowdhary A, Spence AM, Sales L, et al. Radiation associated tumours following therapeutic cranial radiation. Surg Neurol Int. 2012;3:48.
149. Brown MS, Stemmer SM, Simon JH, et al. White matter disease induced by high-dose chemotherapy: longitudinal study with MR imaging and proton spectroscopy. Am J Neuroradiol. 1998;19:217- 21.
150. Rosenberg NL, Kleinschmidt-DeMasters BK, Davis KA, et al. Toluene abuse causes diffuse central nervous system white matter changes. Ann Neurol. 1988;23:611.
151. Tamrazi B, Almast J. Your brain on drugs: imaging of drug related changes in central nervous system. Radiographics. 2012;32(3):701-19.
152. De Smet K, De Maeseneer M, Talebian YA, et al. Bilateral globus pallidus infarcts in ecstasy use. JBR-BTR. 2011;94(2):93-201.
153. Geibprasert S, Gallucci M, Krings T. Addictive illegal drugs: structural neuroimaging. Am J Neuroradiol. 2010; 31(5):803-8.

CHAPTER 15

Imaging of Epilepsy

Shailesh B Gaikwad, Anuj Prabhakar

INTRODUCTION

As per the International League Against Epilepsy, an epileptic seizure is defined as "a transient occurrence of signs and/or symptoms due to abnormal excessive or synchronous neuronal activity in the brain". Epilepsy is a disease involving the central nervous system that is characterized by any of the following features:

1. Atleast 2 seizures that are unprovoked and occur within 24 hours of each other.
2. One unprovoked seizure and a probability of further seizures similar to the general recurrence risk after 2 unprovoked seizures, occurring over the next 10 years.
3. Diagnosis of an epilepsy syndrome.[1]

The disease afflicts all age groups and socioeconomic strata. It has a significant impact on the quality of life of most patients. The incidence of epilepsy in children varies from 50 to 100 cases per 100,000 persons per year. The highest incidence occurs in the first year of life.[2] Brain imaging is an important part of epilepsy management. Conservative treatment with antiepileptic drugs fails to control seizures in up to one third of the patients. Surgery is helpful in such cases. Presurgical imaging is essential to localize the lesions.

All populations of epilepsy patients do not require imaging. Imaging is useful in the following subsets:[1]

1. Focal seizures that can be localized to a particular part of the brain based on the characteristics of the seizure, abnormalities on the electroencephalogram (EEG), history or examination.
2. Abnormalities in neurological examination like focal deficits, neurocutaneous syndromes or syndromes associated with cerebral malformations.
3. Developmental regression, delay or arrest in children.
4. Children with clinical features suggestive of symptomatic generalized epilepsy syndromes like early Lennox-Gastaut syndrome or infantile spasms.
5. Children younger than two years of age (Those suffering from febrile seizures are to be excluded).
6. Atypical course of seizures.
7. Raised intra cranial pressure.
8. History of status epilepticus.

Imaging is not indicated in:

1. Patients with primary generalized epilepsy
2. Typical absence epilepsy (petit mal)
3. Juvenile myoclonic epilepsy
4. Patients with benign partial epilepsy with either centrotemporal or occipital spikes.
5. Children with simple febrile convulsions.

Rapid advances in the field of imaging have lead to a large number of different imaging techniques that may be utilized to evaluate of a patient with seizure disorder. Imaging techniques may be used to evaluate either the functional or structural substrates of the disease. MRI with nuclear imaging is the main stay of epilepsy imaging nowadays. The primary role of imaging is to detect any form of structural abnormality that might be responsible for seizures.

MRI PROTOCOLS

Patients suffering from chronic epilepsy need to be evaluated using specific imaging protocols which must be tailored to best demonstrate the structural and functional abnormalities. Imaging must be preferably performed at 3T field strength as the image clarity, spatial resolution and contrast resolution are better as compared to 1.5 Tesla MRI scanners.[3] Axial T2, volumetric 3DT1 and 3D FLAIR sequences covering the whole brain are acquired. In order to evaluate temporal lobe sclerosis additional FLAIR and inversion recovery sequences are acquired in the coronal oblique plane that is perpendicular to the hippocampus. The slice thickness in these coronal oblique sections is kept to a minimum (2–3 mm). The entire hippocampus including the head, body and tail must be imaged. Gradient recalled echo and susceptibility weighted imaging are useful to identify small foci of calcification or hemosiderin deposition. Other sequences that may be included in the protocol are diffusion tensor imaging (DTI) and 3D double inversion recovery (DIR). 3D DIR sequence is very sensitive for cortical abnormalities. Non-contrast perfusion imaging using pseudo continuous or continuous arterial spin labeling (ASL) is also performed. If a tumor is considered as the cause of epilepsy, a post contrast 3D T1-weighted fast spin echo sequence must be performed to look for enhancement. Specialized sequences like T2* relaxometry and spectroscopy may be performed if necessary.

Structural Lesions in Chronic Epilepsy

The histological findings in patients undergoing surgery for temporal lobe epilepsy reveal mesial temporal sclerosis (50–70%) to be the commonest abnormality, with tumors, developmental abnormalities of neuronal migration and cortical organization, vascular malformations and post-traumatic, inflammatory or ischemic gliosis being found less frequently. A non-specific or normal histological examination is found in 10–25%.

Mesial Temporal Lobe Epilepsy

Mesial temporal lobe epilepsy occurs due to lesions involving the temporal lobe. Hippocampal sclerosis (HS) is the most common pathology affecting the mesial temporal lobe. This is characterized by gliosis and neuronal loss involving the hippocampus. Neuronal pathways undergo reorganization which leads to formation of epileptogenic focus.[4] Hippocampal sclerosis may be associated with a preceding insult like childhood febrile seizures, trauma during birth, perinatal insults, encephalitis. It is the commonest cause of intractable epilepsy. Surgical resection of the anterior temporal lobe and hippocampus has good results in such patients and renders up to 90% of these patients seizure-free. HS affects older children and young adults. Clinically, most patients present with aura and complex partial seizures

The two primary MRI findings of HS are hippocampal atrophy (usually recognized by asymmetry in the case of unilateral atrophy) **(Figs. 1A to C)** and increased T2 signal intensity of the hippocampus.[5] Atrophy of the fornix, mammillary body and widening of the choroid fissure on the ipsilateral side are seen. Other secondary imaging features include temporal horn dilatation, ipsilateral atrophy of the temporal lobe, poor gray-white matter differentiation in the parahippocampus and loss of hippocampal signal on T1-weighted images. These secondary features help in improving the diagnostic confidence when used in conjunction with the primary findings. They may be seen in 40–60% of the cases. However, individually they are not reliable signs. HS does not enhance on post contrast imaging.

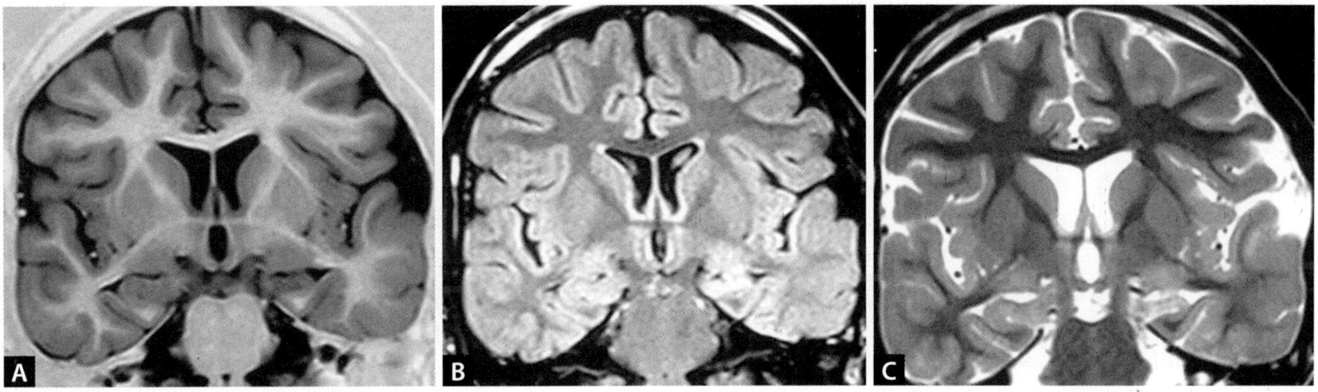

Figs. 1A to C: Mesial temporal sclerosis on the left side. (A) STIR sequence with reverse window setting showing loss of volume; (B) FLAIR; and (C) (T2W) sequences showing hyperintense signal in the ipsilateral hippocampus.

DWI shows hyperintensity of the involved hippocampus with increased diffusivity on ADC. Spectroscopy shows reduced NAA in the epileptogenic site without any change in choline or creatinine. The reduction in NAA may be seen in the surrounding extrahippocampal and extratemporal regions also.

MR scans done for hippocampal sclerosis may show association with other potentially epileptogenic extrahippocampal abnormalities such as cortical dysgenesis. These are termed as dual pathologies and have been observed in approximately 15% cases undergoing epilepsy surgery. The presence of dual pathologies denotes a poor surgical outcome.

The sensitivity and specificity, for detection of HS using optimized imaging protocols is high (93% and 83%, respectively).[6] Bilateral hippocampal abnormalities **(Fig. 2)** or subtle lesions may be difficult to diagnose. These patients may require volumetric analysis, T2 relaxometry, or MR spectroscopy (increased glutamate ratio). Ictal and interictal single photon emission tomography is used as a complimentary tool **(Fig. 3)**.

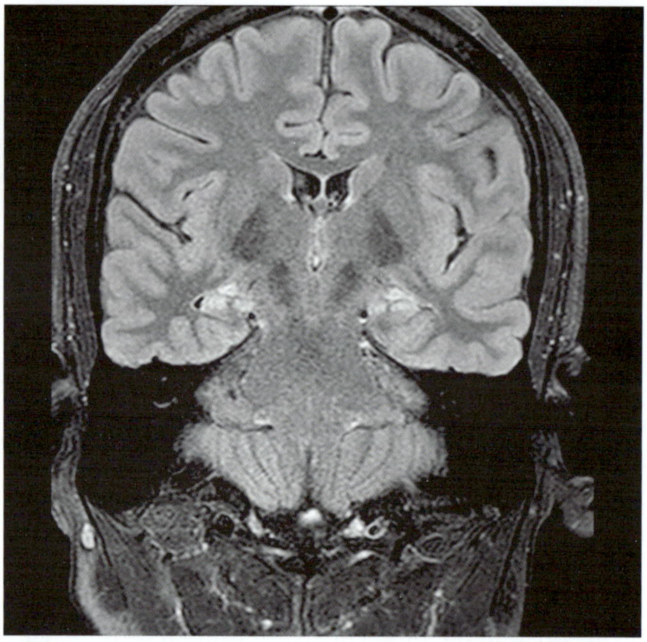

Fig. 2: Volume loss and increased signal alterations in both the hippocampus suggesting bilateral MTS.

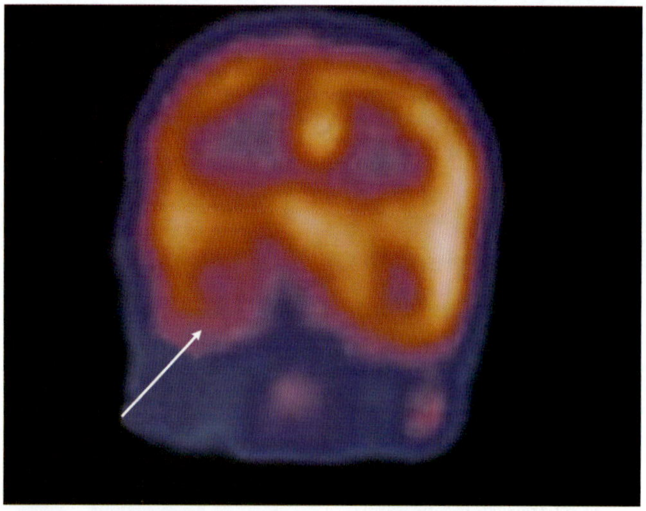

Fig. 3: SPECT (Interictal) shows reduced perfusion in the right mesial temporal lobe.

MRI IN MALFORMATIONS OF CORTICAL DEVELOPMENT

Disorders of cortical organization and neuronal migration are commonly found in young pediatric epilepsy patients. They are the cause of infantile spasms in up to 40% of the children. Developmental disorders, as a group of epileptogenic abnormalities, are being increasingly recognized with the routine use of MRI during evaluation of investigate patients suffering from refractory epilepsy. The evaluation of these malformations requires close attention to the gray matter, gray-white matter interface, white matter and the periventricular region. Small lesions may require volumetric data acquisition with subsequent 3D reconstruction. Development malformations of the cortex may be classified as:[7]

Group I: Malformations secondary to abnormal cell proliferation or apoptosis

- Microcephaly
- Megalencephaly
  - Polymicrogyria and megalencephaly
- Cortical dysgeneses with abnormal cell proliferation
  - Cortical tubers
  - Focal cortical dysplasia 2b
  - Hemimegalencephaly

Group II: Malformations secondary to abnormal cell migration

- Heterotopia
- Lissencephaly pattern
  - Agyria
  - Pachygyria
  - subcortical band heterotopias
- Subcortical heterotopias and sublobar dysplasia
  - Large focal collections of neurons in deep white matter
- Cobblestone malformation
  - Congenital muscular dystrophies

Group III: Malformations secondary to abnormal post-migrational development

- Polymicrogyria
- Schizencephaly
- FCD (type 1, 3)
- Post-migrational microcephaly.

Focal Cortical Dysplasia

Focal cortical dysplasia (FCDs) are localized areas of malformed gray matter that is not neoplastic. FCDs are a common cause of medically refractory epilepsy in both children and adults. Surgical resection has become an important management option in these patients. However, refractory epilepsy is not seen in all patients harboring an FCD.

Based on the imaging, clinical and histopathological findings FCDs are classified into three types:

Type 1: An isolated lesion showing abnormal layering of the involved cortex that shows persistence of vertical developmental micro columns (type 1a) or the loss of horizontal hexalaminar structure (type 1b). Both patterns of abnormal layering in the cortex may also be seen simultaneously (type 1c). There are no dysmorphic neurons or balloon cells in type 1 FCDs **(Fig. 4A)**.

Type 2: These are also isolated lesions that show both abnormal cortical layering and dysmorphic neurons. Type 2A FCDs **(Fig. 4B)** do not have balloon cells while type 2B **(Fig. 4C)** FCDs show balloon cells.

Type 3: This refers to FCD associated with other lesions. This is considered as a post-migrational disorder secondary to an insult. The cytoarchitectural abnormalities described above may occur along with hippocampal sclerosis (FCD type 3a), epilepsy associated tumors (FCD type 3b), vascular malformations (FCD type 3c) or other epileptogenic lesion (FCD type 3d) acquired in childhood **(Fig. 4D)**.

FCD may be seen as areas of cortical thickening with loss of the normal gray-white interface, T2/FLAIR hyperintense signal, and focal atrophy. FCD type 1a may mild hemispheric hypoplasia without any other visible signal alteration. In many patients MRI may be normal. Mild focal cortical thickening abnormalities in the shape of the gyrus and deep sulci may also be seen.

FCD type 2 presents with a gradient of morphologic changes; ranging from dysplastic lesions that can be easily identified by conventional MRI techniques to minor structural abnormalities, like small areas of discrete cortical thickening and/or blurring of the gray-white-matter interface that often go unrecognized. Sometimes it shows subtle hyperintense T2 signal in the subcortical and deep white matter. FCD type 2a may show only mild

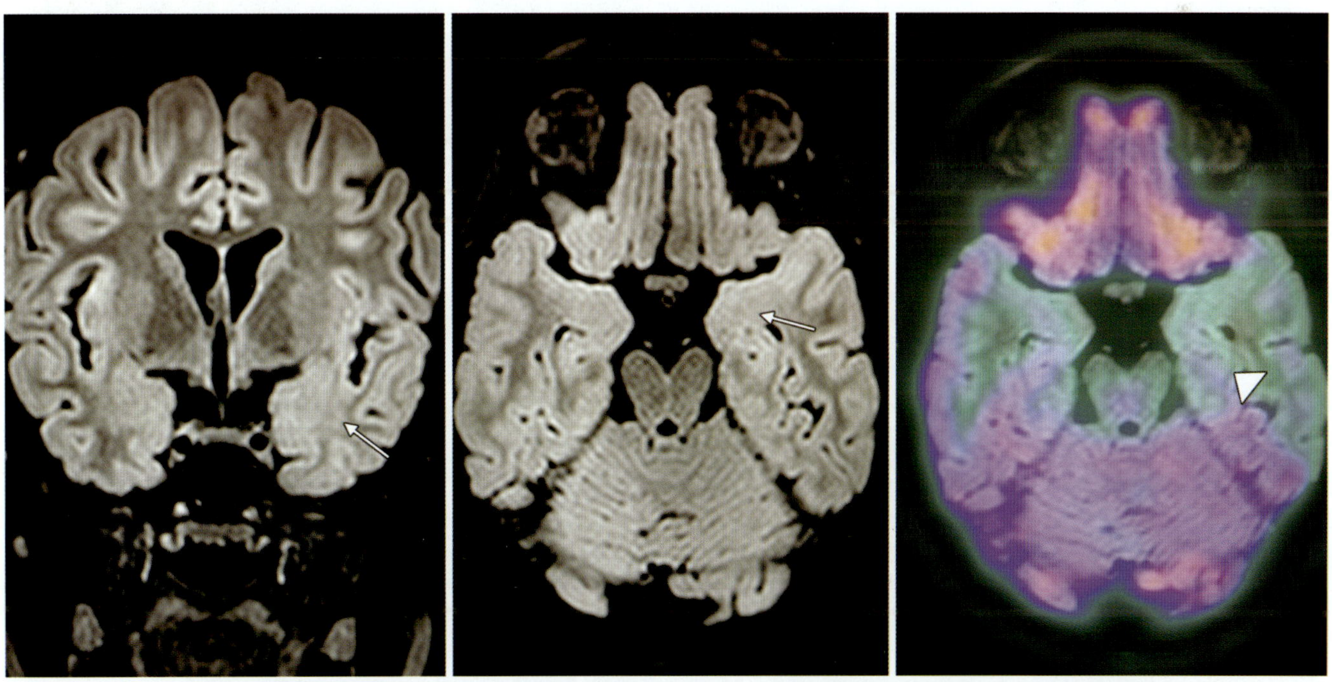

Fig. 4A: FCD type 1: Coronal and axial FLAIR images of patient show hypoplasia of left anterior temporal lobe with blurring of gray-white interface and subtle white matter hyperintensity (arrows). PET-MR fusion shows decreased uptake of tracer within left temporal lobe (arrowhead) as compared to right side.

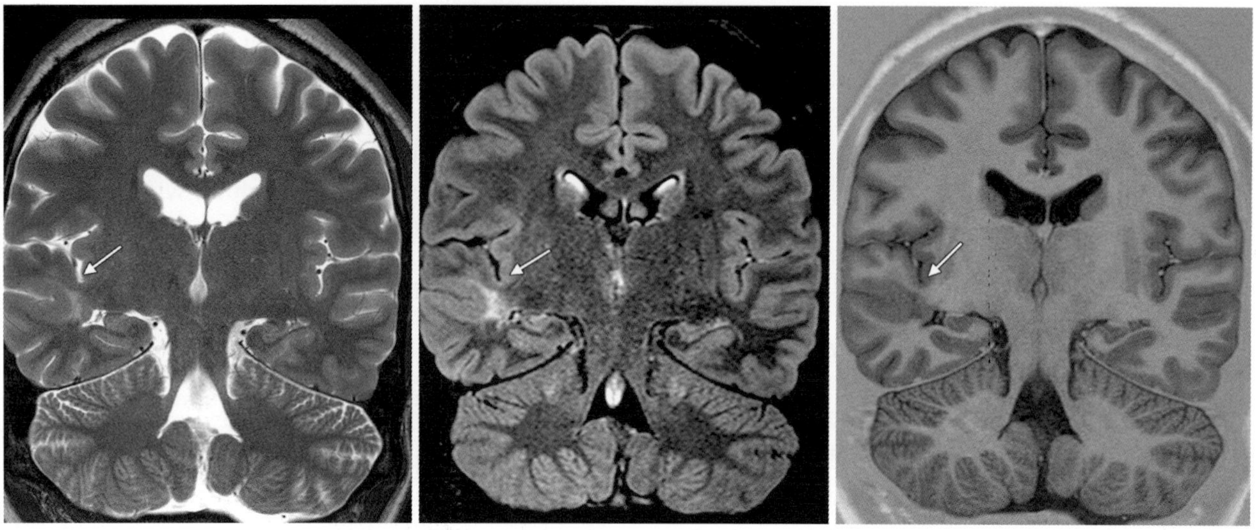

Fig. 4B: FCD type 2A: Oblique coronal T2, FLAIR and IR images of patient show cortical thickening, blurring of gray-white interface and subcortical hyperintensity along right superior temporal sulcus (arrows).

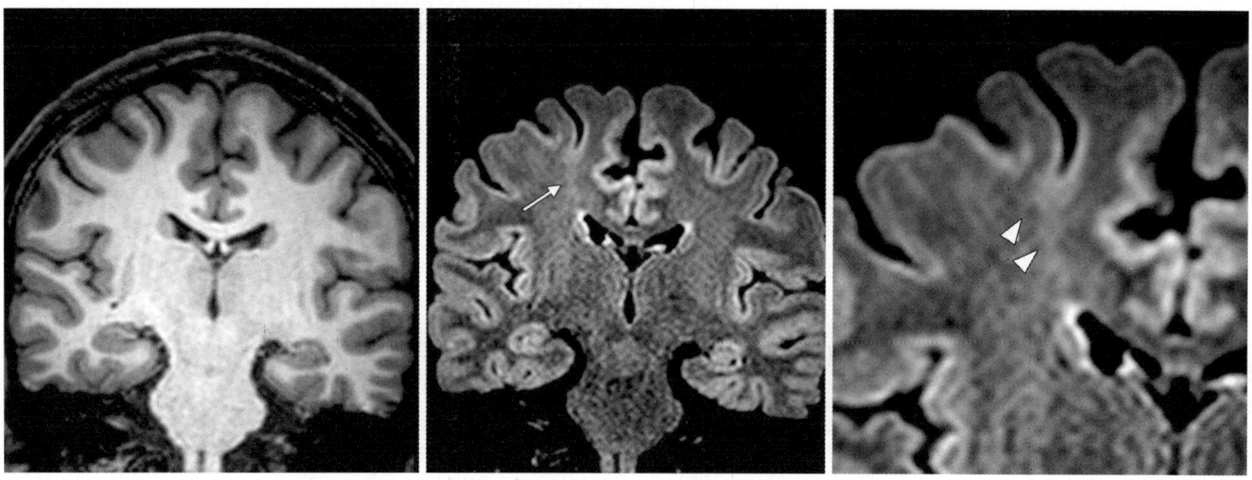

Fig. 4C: FCD type 2B: Coronal T1 and FLAIR images of patient show blurring of gray-white interface and subcortical hyperintensity along right superior frontal sulcus. Increased FLAIR signal tapering from gray-white interface to superolateral margin of right lateral ventricle (arrowheads), typical transmantle sign.

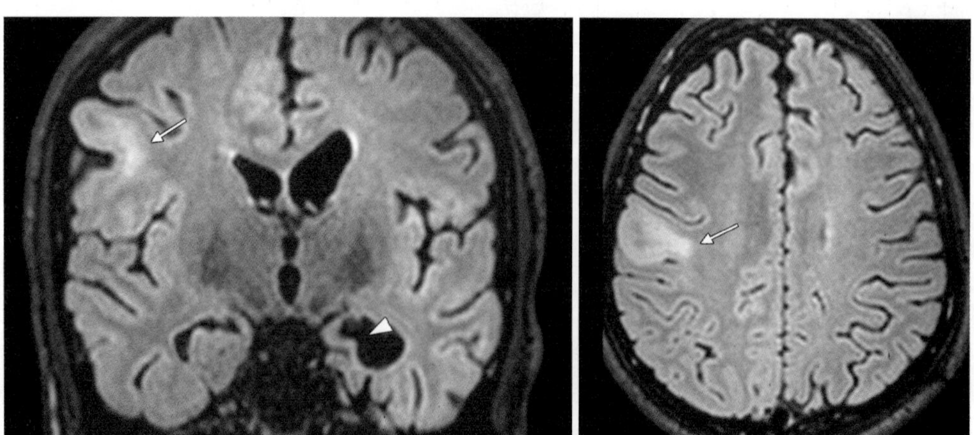

Fig. 4D: FCD type 3D: Coronal and axial FLAIR images reveal cortical thickening, blurring of gray white interface and subcortical hyperintensity along right inferior frontal sulcus (arrows) s/o FCD with left MTS (arrowhead).

discrete changes and without FLAIR hyperintense signal. FCD type 2b shows areas of localized cortical thickening on MRI, blurring of the gray-white-matter differentiation and wedge shaped T2 FLAIR hyperintensity in the subcortical white matter extending to the ependymal surface of ipsilateral ventricle (transmantle sign) **(Fig. 4C)**. Sometimes the lesion may be localized only to bottom of the sulcus. There is no contrast enhancement.The lesions have increased diffusivity and decreased fractional anisotropy values. NAA: Cr ratio is decreased with elevated Myoinositol on MR spectroscopy. Perfusion (rCBV) is normal or reduced.[8]

Other Disorders of Neuronal Migration and Cortical Organization

Hemimegalencephaly is characterized by hamartomatous growth that may affect either the entire cerebral hemisphere or a part of it. The involved hemisphere shows enlargement with white matter hyperintensity, ipsilateral ventricular enlargement, heterotopias and thickened cortex. It may be associated with areas of heterotopia, polymicrogyria, pachygyria, FCD, and gliosis.[8]

Nodular heterotopia may be periventricular or subcortical depending upon the location of the ectopic neuron clusters. These nodules contain clusters of mature neurons and glial cells that do not show well-defined lamellar organization. These follow gray matter on all sequences and do not enhance on contrast administration.[8]

Classic lissencephaly incorporates the agyria-pachygyria spectrum. It often has a genetic origin and may be gender linked. This anomaly is characterized by a reduction in the number of sulci and gyri. This manifests as shallow sulci with large gyri and cortical thickening. Near complete absence of sulci with smoothening of the cortex is seen in classical lissencephaly. Subcortical laminar heterotopia (band heterotopia) is characterized by a band of ectopic gray matter that lies below the cortex with intervening normal white matter.[8]

Polymicrogyria most commonly affects the perisylvian region and is a common cortical developmental malformation. It is characterized by a large number of small, prominent convolutions with shallow intervening sulci. The abnormal small gyri give the appearance of thickened cortex on standard thick sections. Polymicrogyria may be associated with other lesions such as callosum agenesis, may or may not lead to epilepsy, and in those patients with epilepsy the seizures are often well controlled with medication.

Schizencephaly refers to CSF containing transcerebral cleft connecting pial and ependymal surfaces, usually lined by polymicrogyric cortex. The lips of the cleft may be closely apposed (closed lip schizencephaly) or widely separated (open lip schizencephaly).

Hypothalamic hamartomas occur due to abnormalities of neuronal migration. These are located between the infundibular stalk and the mammillary body in the tuber cinereum. Pedunculated and sessile subtypes are seen. The pedunculated lesions project into the suprasellar cistern while the sessile lesions arise from the floor of third ventricle and extend into its lumen. Gelastic seizures (ictal laughing fits) are commonly associated with this lesion. The lesions are isointense to normal gray matter on T1-weighted images and iso to hyperintense on FLAIR/T2-weighted images. They do not show any post contrast enhancement.

The imaging algorithm of patients with suspected cortical maldevelopment should include high resolution volume acquisition, high resolution coronal T2 and FLAIR images. Multiplanar reconstructions, thin coronal IR protocols are helpful. Dedicated pulse sequences that generate high gray and white matter contrast are needed with high spatial resolution to detect subtle development malformation. High spatial resolution can be achieved by using the SPGR sequence, use of phased array surface coils and homogenous high field strength magnets.

TUMORS

Brain tumors may cause up to 1–2% of all seizures and 4–6% of partial seizures. Temporal lobe tumors are often slow growing and include gliomas, oligodendrogliomas, dysembryoplastic neuroepithelial tumors (DNETs), and gangliogliomas.

DNETs are known to be associated with partial complex seizures that have an intractable course. Neuroimaging typically shows predominantly cortical-based, well-demarcated lesion, usually in the temporal lobe or parieto-occipital region. The lesion is hypodense compared to white matter on CT **(Fig. 5)**, hypointense on T1WI and hyperintense on T2WI **(Fig. 6)** with variable enhancement following contrast administration. Lack of peritumoral edema and mass effect on midline structures, triangular pattern of distribution and presence of septations are frequently observed.[5] Some lesions may appear as an enlarged gyrus, producing a soap bubble appearance at the cortical margin.[9] Calcification (20%) and scalloping of inner table of skull may be seen **(Fig. 5)**.

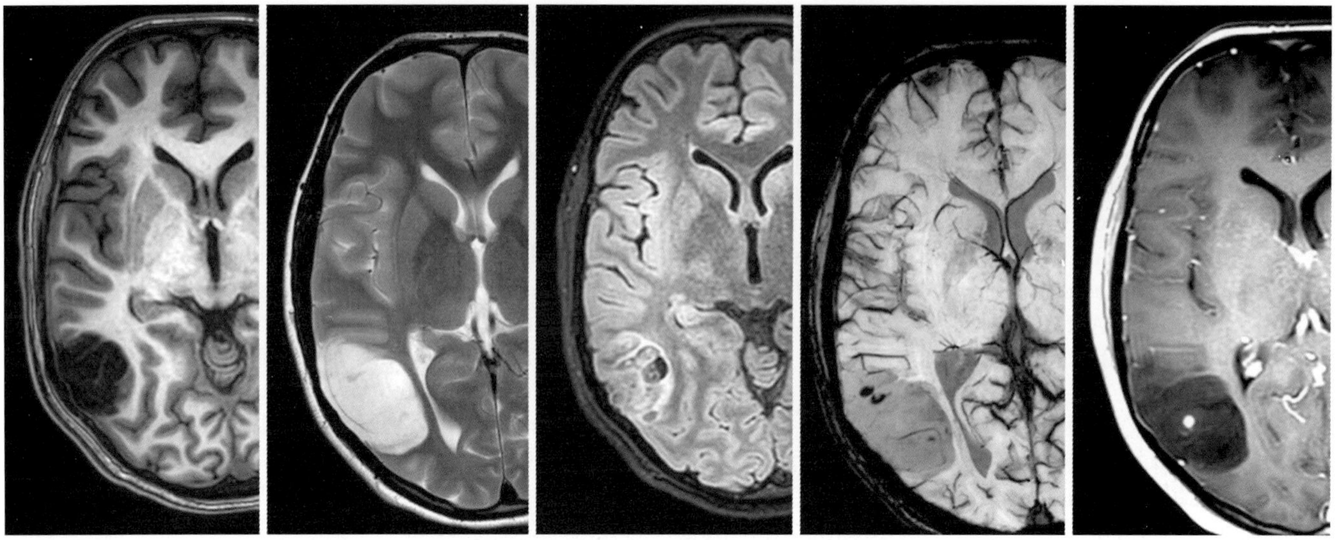

Fig. 5: DNET: T1, T2, FLAIR, SWI and T1 PC show a well-defined cortical-based lesion having "bubbly" appearance in T2 and FLAIR with cystic areas within. SWI shows focal calcification. There is a nodular area of enhancement on the T1 PC image. Note adjacent bone remodeling and no edema.

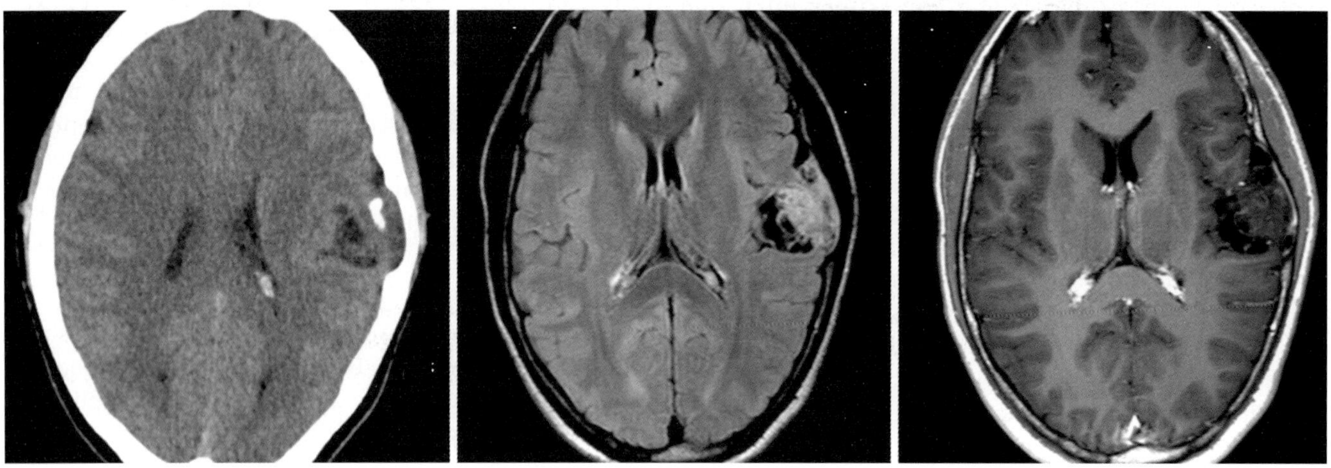

Fig. 6: Ganglioglioma: CT, FLAIR and T1 PC images show a cortical-based solid cystic lesion with calcification. Adjacent bone remodeling is seen. There is no post-contrast enhancement.

Gangliogliomas, the most frequently occurring mixed glioneuronal tumors of the CNS, are more common in the pediatric group and patients usually present with seizures. The temporal lobes are the most common site. Gangliogliomas are characterized on CT scans as hypodense lesions with calcification and a variable contrast enhancement pattern. The MR findings **(Fig. 6)** are nonspecific; the lesions may be iso- to hypointense on T1WI and hyperintense on T2WI.[10] Contrast enhancement was reported in 44% of one series and may have either a nodular rim or solid enhancement pattern **(Fig. 7)**.

Oligodendrogliomas involve the cortex or the sub-cortical region. They are T1 hypointense, T2/FLAIR hyperintense and show variable enhancement. Foci of increased T1 signal representing intratumoral hemorrhage may be seen. Calcifications are common and may be ring-shaped, shell-like, or nodular **(Fig. 7)**. Dual abnormalities which are usually due to a combination of HS and either glioma, heterotopia or vascular abnormalities, may be present in 8–22% of patients.

Vascular Malformations

Intractable epilepsy due to vascular malformations may be seen in 2–3% of patients. Arteriovenous malformations (AVMs) have are seen on MRI as a cluster of abnormal round or linear signal voids. Cavernous hemangiomas

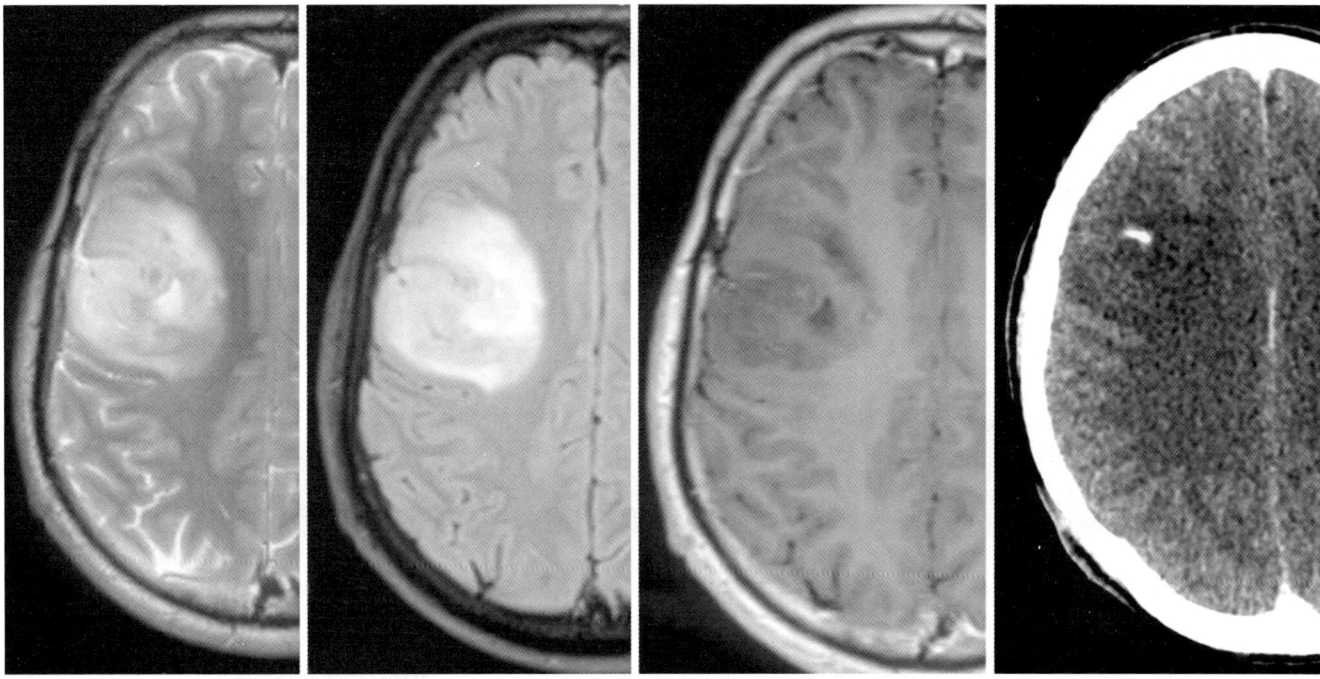

Fig. 7: Oligodendroglioma: T2, FLAIR, T1 PC images show non-enhancing T2/FLAIR hyperintense, T1 hypointense lesion involving gray and white matter with heterogeneity; CT shows a focal calcification.

have a higher epileptogenic potential as compared to AVMs.[11] This may be secondary to the greater degree of reactive gliosis in these lesions. Cavernous hemangiomas are seen as circumscribed lesions with a central heterogeneous area of mixed signal intensity secondary to presence of methemoglobin, deoxyhemoglobin and foci of calcification. A complete hemosiderin ring that is hypointense on T2-weighted imaging is seen **(Fig. 8)**. Vascular malformations that are superficial in location with surrounding T2-hyperintensity are more likely to cause seizures as compared to deeper lesions.

Other Lesions Associated with Epilepsy

Insults like trauma, infection or infarction lead to cortical encephalomalacia and gliosis. These lesions may act as epileptogenic foci and are well delineated on MRI. Destructive lesions are also an important source of childhood seizures. Smooth porencephalic cavities form in patients who suffer from an insult during the first 6 months of gestation these cavities are not lined by gliosis. on the other hand, perinatal, post-natal or late gestational injury leads to focal or generalized encephalomalacia. Tuberculomas and cysticercosis are also commonly identified causes of epilepsy in developing countries. MRI may demonstrate the various stages in development of the non-calcified neurocysticercosis lesions. Children with neurocutaneous syndromes, such as Sturge-Weber syndrome **(Figs. 9A and B)** and tuberous sclerosis, are also prone to develop epilepsy.

Congenital infections, like the TORCH group (toxoplasmosis, rubella, cytomegalovirus and herpes simplex), may produce intractable seizures, Lennox-Gastaut syndrome and infantile spasms. Cytomegalovirus infection may also lead to neuronal migration abnormalities.

Rasmussen's encephalitis is chronic encephalitis generally progressive in nature and is characterized by seizures that are refractory to medical treatment. Radiological findings of stable or progressive hemispheric atrophy on serial imaging in a setting of intractable epilepsy with progressive hemiparesis may help to establish the diagnosis **(Figs. 10A to D)**.

Epilepsy occurs in about 20% of children with diplegic and dystonic cerebral palsy, whereas the incidence is 50–80% in the hemiplegic and quadriplegic forms.

ADVANCES IN EPILEPSY IMAGING AND MANAGEMENT

Reformatted Images

3D volume data, usually T1-weighted inversion recovery sequences (IR, SPGR, MPRAGE, etc.) and 3D FLAIR are

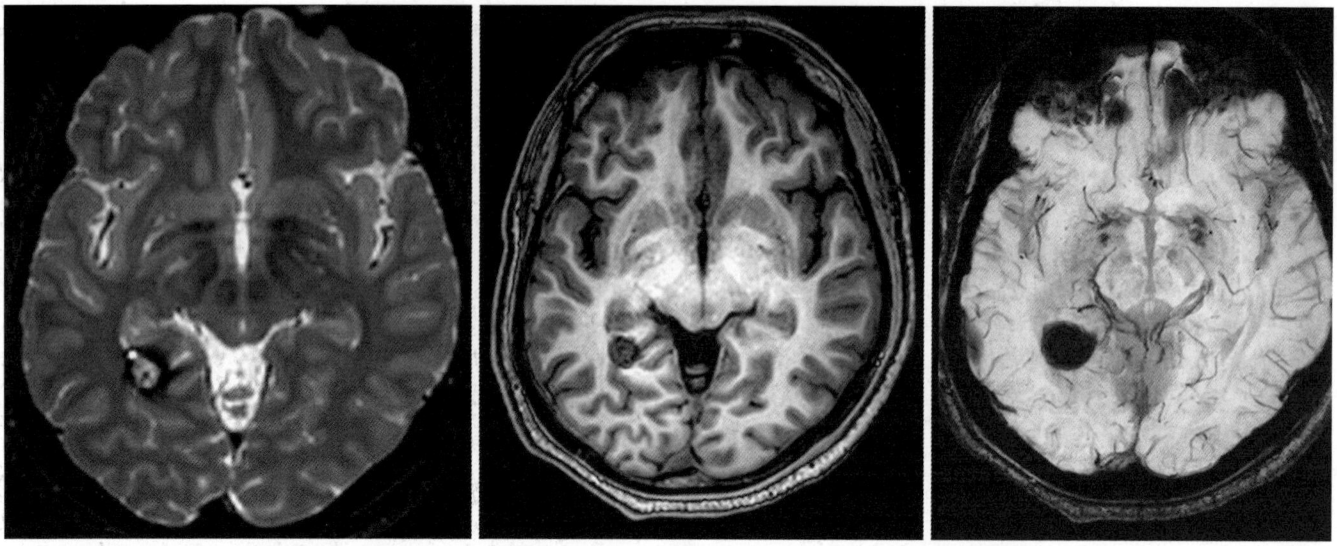

Fig. 8: Cavernoma: T2, T1 and SW images show right temporo-occipital lesion with heterogeneous hyperintense core and a complete hypointense rim. The lesion shows "blooming" on SWI. Core of the lesion is hyperintense due to methemoglobin.

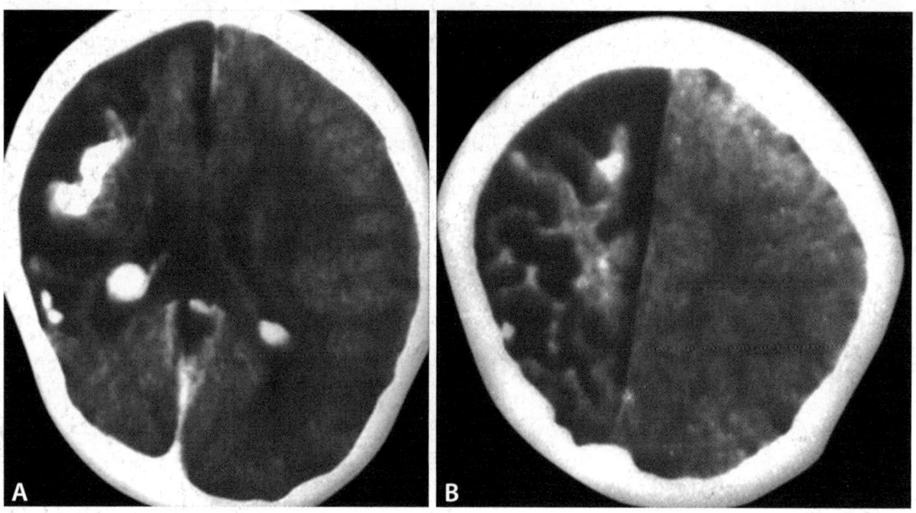

Figs. 9A and B: Sturge-Weber syndrome involving right hemisphere with typical tram-track calcification and ipsilateral atrophy.

acquired as thin sections (<1.5 mm) can be reconstructed in any desired plane using multi-planar (MPR) and curved-planar (CPR) reconstructions. CPR **(Fig. 11)** is a very useful tool for picking up subtle lesions especially those of focal cortical dysplasias and for clarifying "abnormal" appearing areas on the routine orthogonal sequences.[12]

Quantitative MR Imaging

Volume estimation (MR volumetry) of hippocampi is an established method in epilepsy evaluation.[13] Now, many more techniques of quantitative MR imaging are available, all of them mostly utilizing T1-weighted 3D volume acquisitions. One method is by classifying tissues into categories such as gray matter, white matter, and cerebrospinal fluid, and then segmenting various structures by using manual or automated segmentation techniques, such as artificial neural networks and 3D model-based segmentation techniques. Using this method, volumetric neocortical measurements may provide an objective way to evaluate the extent of resection and its relation to surgical results.

Another method is voxel-based morphometry, which involves a voxel-wise comparison of the local "concentration" of signal intensity between two groups. Voxel-based morphometry has been used to demonstrate neocortical gray matter reduction, on the same or the contralateral side of seizure focus, and for demonstrating

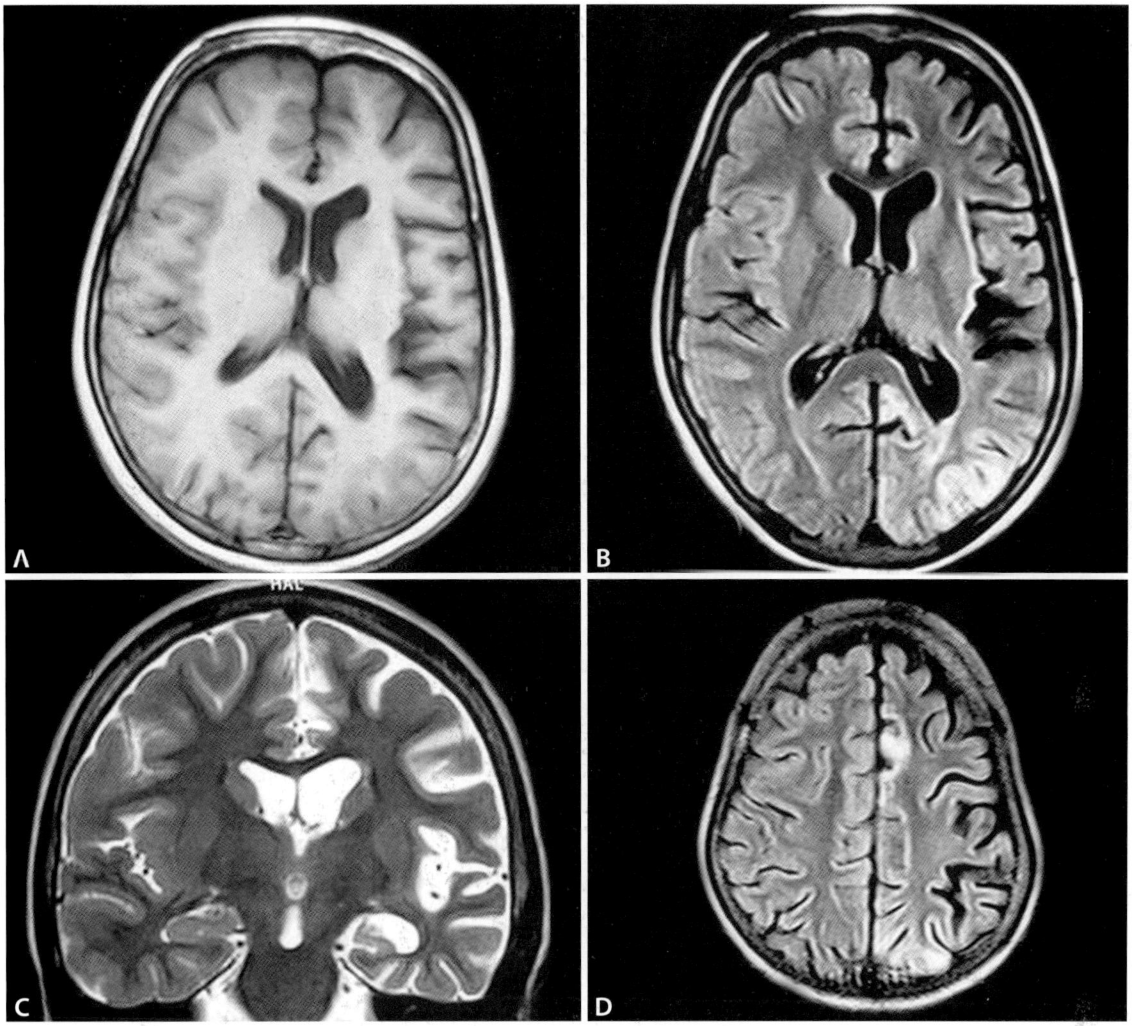

Figs. 10A to D: MRI (A) TIW; (C) T2W (coronal); (B and D) FLAIR axial, Rasmussen's encephalitis involving left hemisphere with areas of high signal and atrophy.

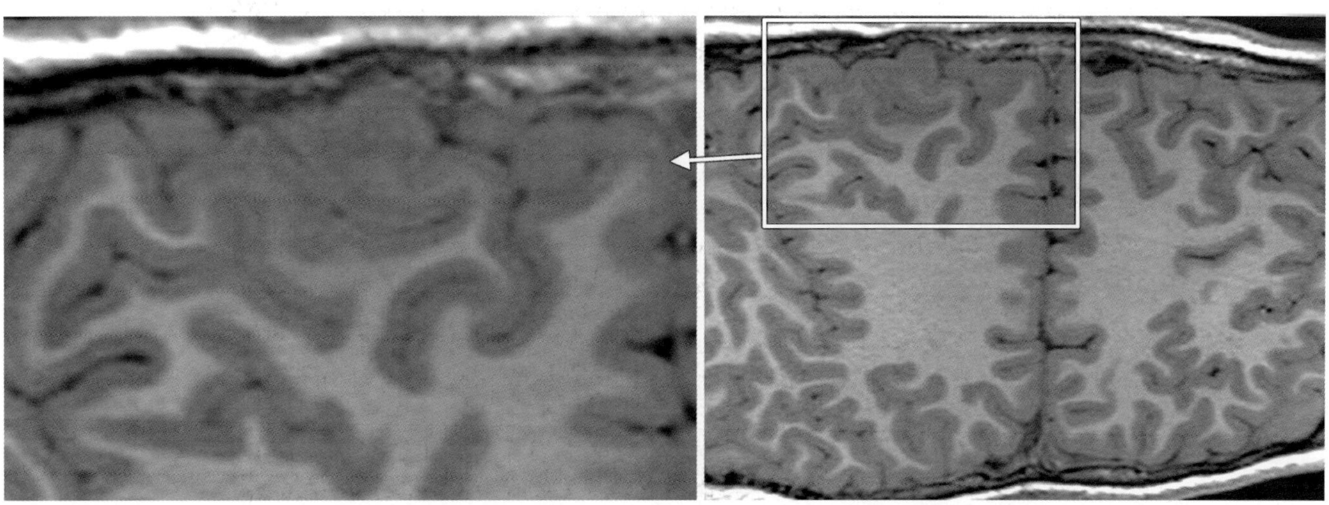

Fig. 11: Curved planar reconstruction of subtle right frontal cortical dysplasia; such lesions are virtually undetectable in routine sequences but well shown on CPR images because they get "opened up".

abnormalities in brain parenchyma beyond the visualized lesions. Texture analysis of the 3D T1-weighted images performed using voxel-wise operators has been used to assess focal cortical dysplasias. Voxel-wise operators have been used to model gray matter thickness, to quantify the gray matter–white matter interface to detect its blurring, and to model hyperintense T1-weighted signals within gray matter through intensity measurement of a voxel relative to the threshold intensity between gray and white matter.

Magnetic Resonance Spectroscopy

Magnetic resonance spectroscopy (MRS) is a non-invasive method of evaluating brain metabolites. The role of MRS is in aiding lateralization, detecting bilateral abnormalities and identifying metabolic abnormalities in epileptogenic areas **(Figs. 12A to C)**.[13] Usually, proton (1H) spectroscopy is performed, and can be used to measure N-acetyl aspartate (NAA), choline (Cho) and creatine (Cr) in vivo. Other metabolites useful in epilepsy evaluation are lactate (Lac), myoinositol (mI), and Glutamine and Glutamate (Glx). Both absolute and relative values can be obtained, with neuronal loss reducing NAA levels and gliosis/astrocytosis increasing Cr and Cho levels. Use of the NAA/Cho+Cr signal intensity ratio has been advocated as possibly the simplest and single most useful index of spectroscopic abnormality. Lactate may be raised especially when imaged soon after seizures, and indicate altered metabolism. Myoinositol is raised when there is gliosis and usually reflects irreversible damage to the parenchyma. Glx concentration in gray matter reflects the glutamate concentration in glutamatergic neurons and can be increased even when structural MRI is normal and other metabolite levels are normal on MRS. Abnormal NAA ratios have also been found contralateral to the seizure focus side, which reversed in patients who became seizure free after surgery. Reduction in NAA may relate to neuronal and glial dysfunction rather than absolute neuronal cell loss. In extratemporal epilepsy, the ability of MRS to lateralize seizure focus is less. In a study of patients with frontal lobe epilepsy, MR spectroscopy results enabled lateralization of the seizures in 50% of cases.

T2 Relaxometry (Mapping)

This provides an objective measure of T2 relaxation time. The T2 time is elevated in mesial temporal sclerosis, and abnormal T2 relaxometry is significantly associated with intractable epilepsy. T2 values are elevated ipsilateral to seizure focus, contralateral to seizure focus (to a lesser degree) as well as non-temporal tissues distant from the seizure focus site **(Figs. 13A and B)**.[14]

Diffusion Tensor Imaging

Diffusion tensor imaging (DTI) studies the motion of water at the voxel level and can provide quantitative and reproducible data, e.g. mean diffusivity and fractional anisotropy, to assess the structural integrity of brain tissue. Imaging the preferential direction of water diffusion in the brain allows us to visualize the major white matter tracts and deduce the fundamental basis of cerebral networks. Thus, the effect of epilepsy syndromes on these pathways and the consequences of various therapies can be assessed with this technique. The anisotropy of diffusion in the brain depends on concentration of macromolecules, organelles, density of nerve fibers and glia, fiber diameter, and myelination. In white matter, anisotropy is a result of the parallel structure of axons and their myelin sheaths.

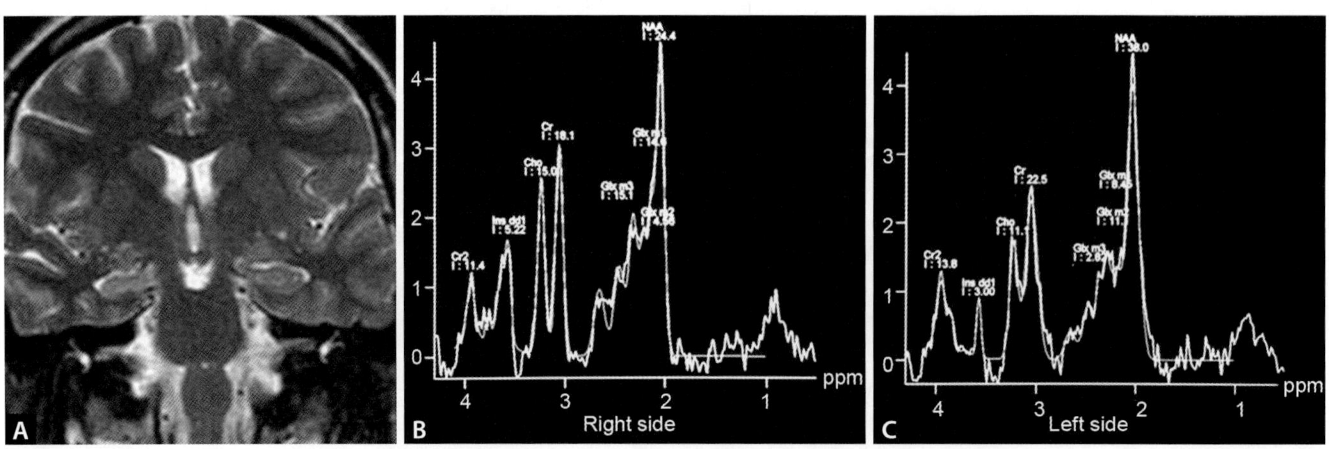

Figs. 12A to C: Role of MRS: Minimally increased T2 hyperintensity of right hippocampus (A) but significantly increased Glx/NAA ratio (1.4) of right hippocampus (B) as compared to left side (0.59) (C).

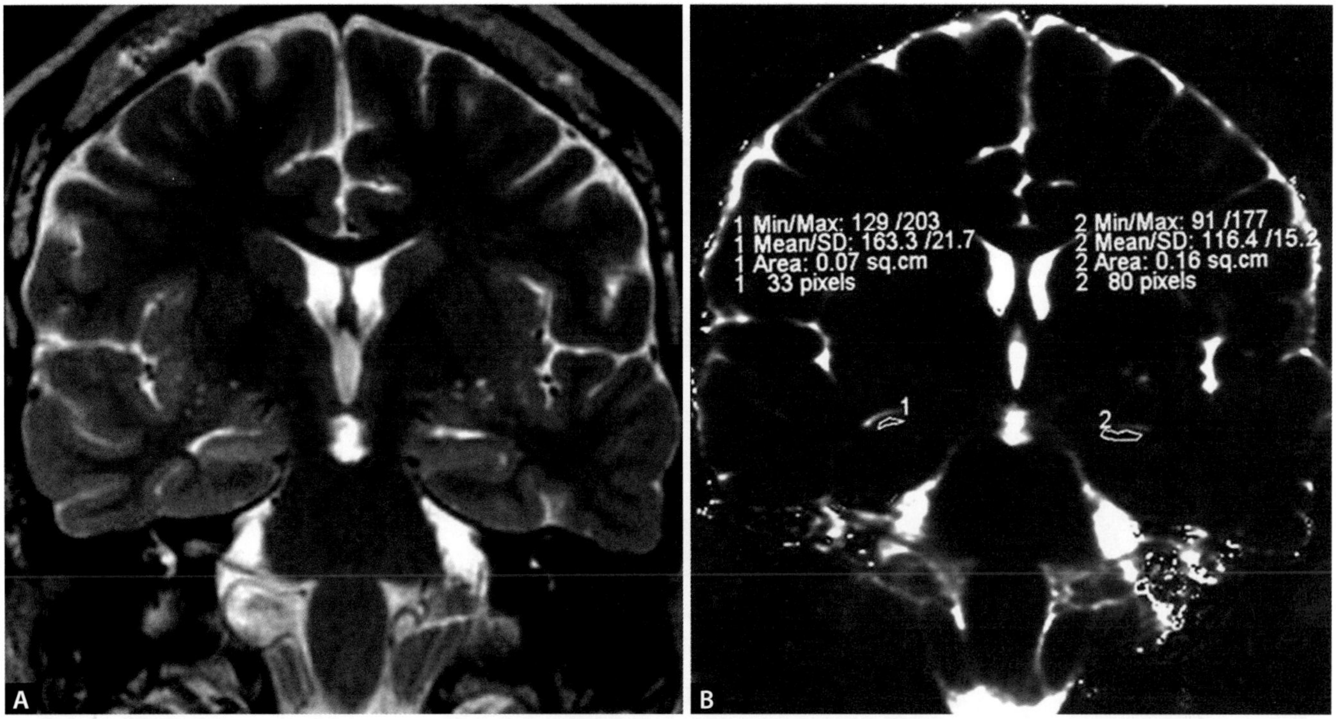

Figs. 13A and B: Role of T2 relaxometry: Minimally increased T2 hyperintensity of right hippocampus on T2WI (A) but significantly increased T2 value (B).

Water can diffuse freely along the long axis of the fibers rather than perpendicular to the fiber orientation. Lesions that disrupt the microstructural environment, lead to changes in the anisotropy of the involved brain tissue. This commonly results in reduced anisotropy and increased mean diffusivity.

Diffusion studies can be done in both ictal/peri/postictal and interictal periods.

Ictal/peri-/postictal studies: Seizures generally result in early postictal depression, followed by normalization, and then transient or chronic elevation of mean diffusivity. The early decline in diffusivity in prolonged seizures is due to cytotoxic edema. Vasogenic edema also has been reported in subcortical white matter. Seizures can trigger breakdown of the blood–brain barrier, which, together with local vasodilatory effects, can give rise to vasogenic edema as well as an increase in intercellular space and diffusivity. Excitotoxic mechanisms eventually lead to cell lysis and death, which result in increased extracellular space and increased diffusion. Diffusion changes often are more widespread, possibly indicating involved networks and secondary spread.

Interictal studies: Diffusivity is increased in diseased hippocampi whether they show increased T2/FLAIR signal or not, or whether they show volume changes or not. Anisotropy also is abnormal in hippocampal sclerosis, but to a lesser magnitude than mean diffusivity changes. Studies of normal appearing tissue have demonstrated bilateral and extratemporal abnormalities, indicative of structural or functional abnormalities that may extend beyond the seizure onset zone. Diffusion tensor imaging also is sensitive to neocortical pathologies that underlie epilepsy. Areas of increased mean diffusivity and decreased fractional anisotropy correlate with abnormalities identified on visual inspection of conventional MRI and also often identify areas of pathology that appear normal on standard MRI. Both diffusion tensor imaging measurements and stereo electroencephalographic recordings have found good spatial concordance between epileptiform activity and diffusivity abnormalities.

Tractography

Diffusion tensor imaging enables the non-invasive in-vivo delineation of white matter tracts **(Figs. 14A to D)**. There are various clinical scenarios were tractography is helpful. Meyers loop is the part of the optic radiation that passes anteriorly into the anterior temporal lobe and then sweeps back along the lateral wall of the ventricle to reach the

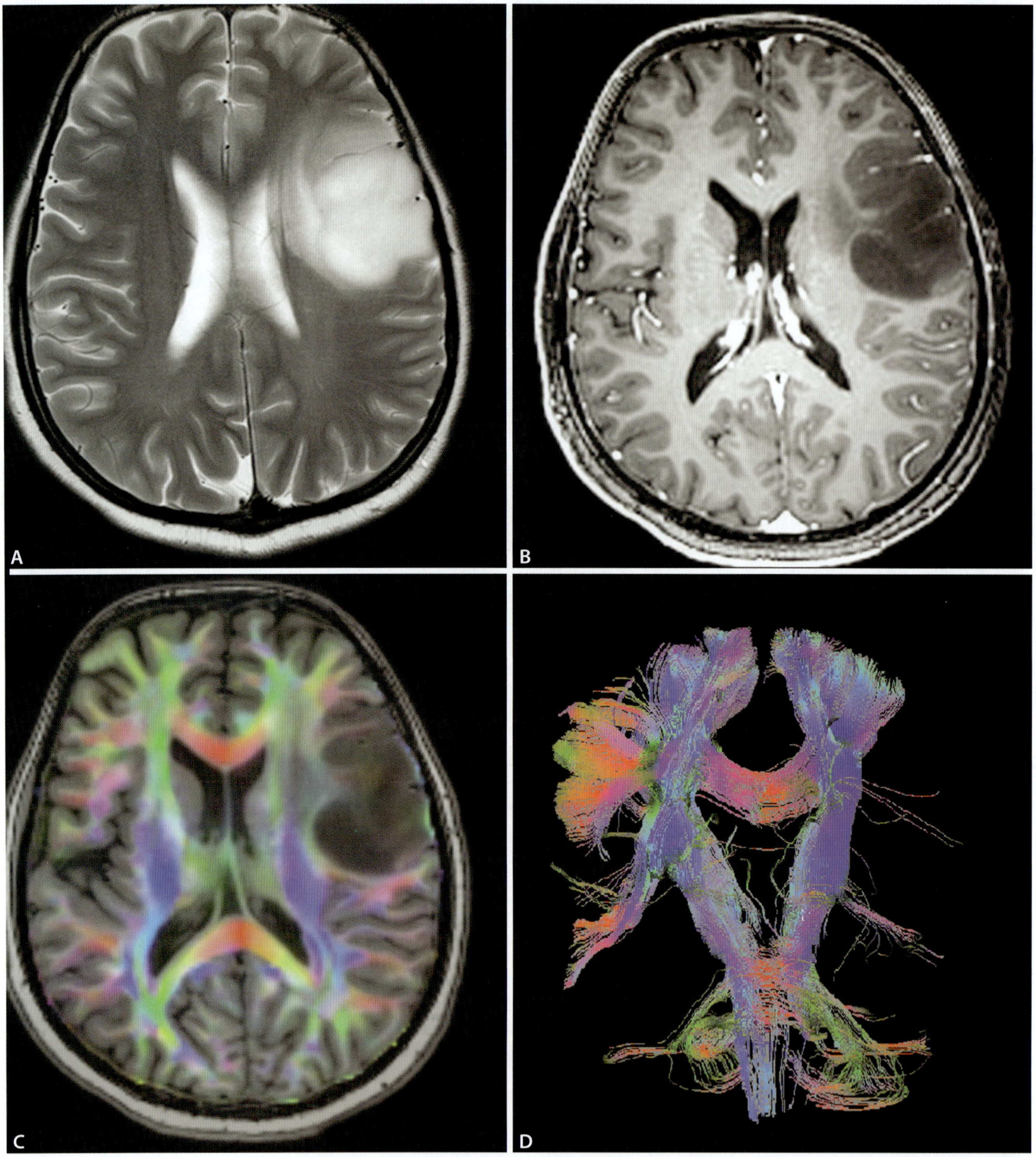

Figs. 14A to D: T2 (A), post-contrast T1-weighted (B) images in a 24-year-old female who presented with 3 episodes of seizures, show a non-enhancing T2 hyperintense low grade glioma in the left frontal region. Axial T1/DTI fused image (C) and reconstructed tractography volume image (D) shows infiltration, thinning and displacement of tracts in the left frontal white matter as compared to the right side.

occiput. Injury to the loop during anterior temporal lobe resection can cause a visual field deficit. Preoperative delineation of the Meyers loop can predict the risk of a visual field defect and thus assist with surgical planning. Similarly, evaluation of the corticospinal tracts and the arcuate fasciculus may be performed if resection of an adjacent lesion is necessary.[15]

Functional MR

Temporal lobe epilepsy (TLE) may be associated with disturbance of language and memory functions. These may be further impaired by anterior temporal lobe resection. Anterior temporal lobe resection in the speech-dominant hemisphere is followed by significant language deficits in up to 40% of patients and often by a decline in verbal memory as well. The main application of functional MR in clinical practice is preoperative localization of the motor strip, language localization and identifying memory laterality in the temporal lobe. While planning surgery for hippocampal sclerosis localization and lateralization of the language and memory functions is essential to minimize the risk of postsurgical deficits and to prognosticate the patients.

Language

Functional MRI (fMRI) is an essential tool that is used to evaluate the language networks in epilepsy patients. Tasks that activate Broca's area and Wernicke's area are performed by the patient during acquisition of the fMRI. A box car design is commonly used in clinical practice. In this technique discrete blocks of rest and activation follow each other. Various paradigms that may be used include verbal fluency, verb generation, word generation, sentence completion and picture naming. A lateralization index (LI) can be calculated for selected areas of activation in frontal, parietal and temporal lobes. LI is quantitative measure of language dominance (right/left/bilateral). It helps is identifying the dominant lobe for language function and in decision making prior to surgery. Traditionally the Wada test was used for language lateralization. However, the Wada test is invasive and in not available widely. Language lateralization on fMRI has been seen to correlate with results from the intracarotid amobarbital test in 80–90% of patients.[15]

Various studies have shown that the left hemisphere is dominant for language in right handed individuals. Atypical language dominance is seen more in ambidextrous or left handed individuals.[16,17] Individuals who have structural lesions in the left temporal lobe and are left dominant for language are more likely to show atypical language lateralization on fMRI as compared to those with right hemisphere epilepsy suggesting reorganization of the language network. In the absence of reorganization there is a higher risk of postsurgical deficit. Atypical language lateralization in the Wernicke's area is more common in patients with temporal lobe epilepsy. On the other hand, anterior language areas are more likely to be affected in frontal lobe epilepsy (**Figs. 15A to C**). When cortical resection is essential close to eloquent language cortex,

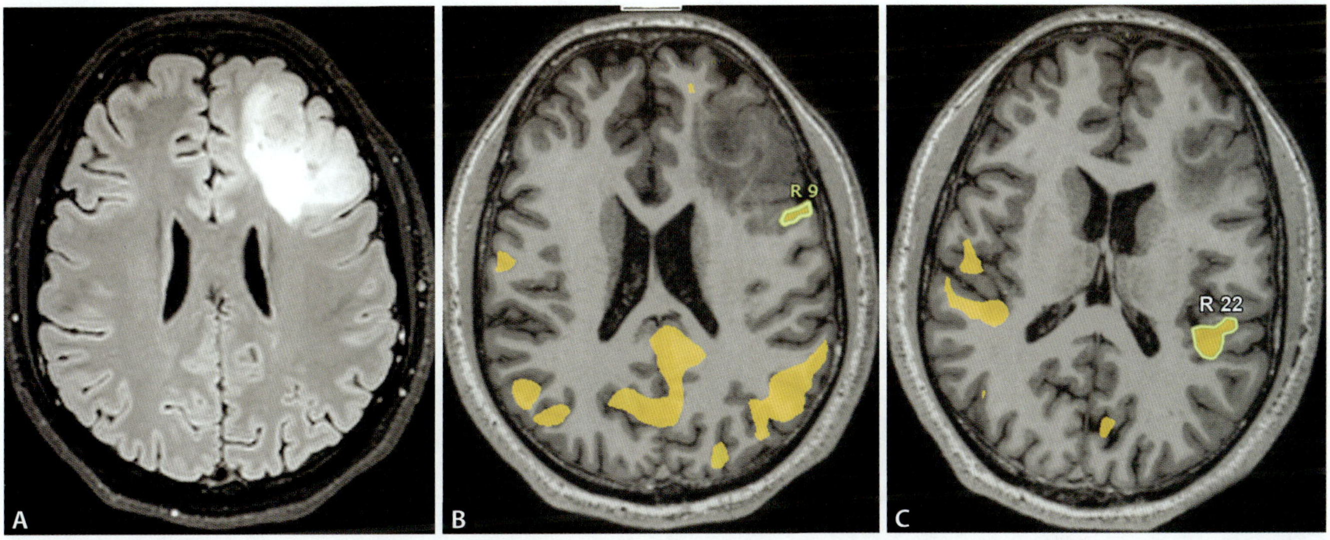

Figs. 15A to C: Preoperative imaging in a 35-year-old patient, who presented with focal seizures and headache. Axial FLAIR (A) image shows a hyperintense lesion in the left frontal cortical and subcortical regions. Fused T1/BOLD fMR images for language paradigm in axial plane (B and C) show that the Broca's area (ROI in B) has been displaced posteriorly, while the Wernicke's area (ROI in C) is normal in location.

electrocortical stimulation or awake resections are necessary as fMRI is not an adequate modality to mapping the entire eloquent area. Cortical language function can also be localized with transcranial magnetic stimulation and the results fused with the individual's MRI scan.[15]

Episodic Memory

Temporal lobe epilepsy is commonly associated with memory impairment. Temporal lobe surgery can cause further worsening of memory. Activations for verbal memory are seen in bilateral temporal, parietal, and frontal lobes. More activation in the left hippocampus during word encoding has been correlated with better verbal memory in left temporal lobe epilepsy patients. Verbal memory has been seen to decline in 1/3rd of patients after left temporal lobe resection.

Greater right hippocampus activation for face encoding correlates with better visual memory in right temporal lobe epilepsy patients. Visual memory also declines in 1/3rd of right temporal lobe resection patients. Reorganization of networks for verbal and visual memory encoding may occur in hippocampal sclerosis. This suggests that the brain may compensate to some extent for the impaired function of the involved hippocampus.[15]

Motor Function

Motor function can be evaluated in fMRI using finger and foot tapping tasks. Identification of the primary motor cortex is essential prior to surgical resection of lesions in this area and when planning for intracranial electrode implantations **(Figs. 16A and B)**.[15]

Resting State and Connectivity

fMRI studies of functional connectivity using resting state fMRI can be used to investigate the pathophysiological basis of epileptic networks. This may help in predicting the surgical outcome in future. The potential clinical benefit for resting state fMRI has not been established.

Positron Emission Tomography

Interictal FDG-PET is used in presurgical evaluation of intractable epilepsy. It helps to lateralize the epileptogenic focus. Glucose hypometabolism is seen. Although it is widespread, the site of ictal onset is usually located at the area of the most severe hypometabolism within the larger volume. Interictal FDG-PET hypometabolism, when correlated with MR imaging, EEG and clinical data, can be used to lateralize the side of seizure onset,

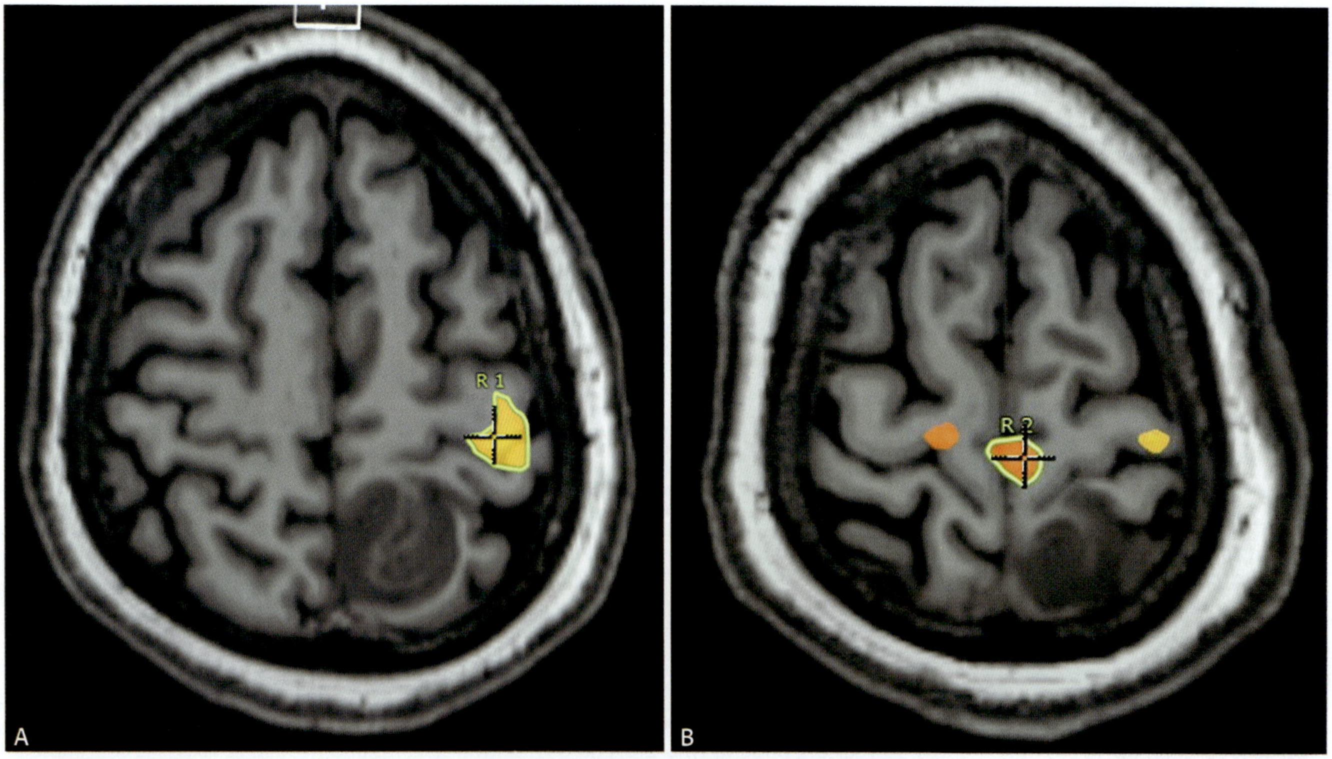

Figs. 16A and B: Fused T1/BOLD fMR images for finger tapping (A) and foot movement (B), show activity in the premotor cortex (ROIs in A and B) that is away from the left parietal lesion.

prognosticate the patient for the degree of seizure control after surgery and also help in deciding the placement of intracranial electrodes. Patients in whom the epilepsy focus is localized to the neocortex FDG–PET scans show a large hypometabolic area on interictal imaging, including areas like thalamus and basal ganglia ipsilateral to the involved neocortical site. Also, when a lesion is identified on imaging, the hypometabolic area in the involved neocortex is often much larger than the structural abnormality. The area of hypometabolism, excluding the site of MR imaging-visible structural lesion, usually contains the electrophysiologically defined ictal onset zone. The absence of hypometabolism does not rule out focal epilepsy. Although regional hypometabolism suggests that epileptic discharge may begin within that region, multiple other areas of ictus onset beyond the hypometabolic cortex are not ruled out. It has been seen that severity of hypometabolism in the temporal lobe, correlates with postsurgical outcome for seizure control.

Other PET receptor ligands that have been utilized in the evaluation of epilepsy are ^{11}C-flumazenil/^{18}F-flumazenil and α-^{11}C-methyl-L-tryptophan. In a recent study of patients who suffer from intractable focal epilepsies, decreased ^{11}C-flumazenil uptake was noted in the temporal piriform cortex. This was associated with an increase in the seizure frequency. Increased α-^{11}C-methyl-L-tryptophan uptake has been used to identify the epileptogenic focus in tuberous sclerosis patients with multiple.[15]

Single-Photon Emission Computed Tomography (SPECT)

The main role of SPECT studies is as a problem-solving tool. SPECT can localize the site of seizure onset in cases where other imaging modalities are not diagnostic and the physician is unable to identify the epileptogenic site via other non-invasive means also **(Figs. 17A to C)**. The SPECT studies evaluate changes in CBF. Commonly used radiopharmaceuticals include technetium-99m hexamethylpropyleneamine oxime or technetium-99m bicisate. Both of these have rapid first-pass brain extraction. Maximum uptake is achieved 30–60 seconds after IV injection. The SPECT images can be acquired up to 4 hours after the injection therefore combined ictal and interictal examination are performed. The ictal SPECT examination will localize the site of seizure as an area of focal hyperperfusion. The epileptogenic zone will show focal hypoperfusion on the interictal SPECT. The diagnostic yield of ictal SPECT is superior to interictal SPECT alone. Interictal SPECT imaging serves as a reference for evaluation of the ictal SPECT images. Interictal SPECT alone has poor sensitivity with a high false-positive rate in mesial temporal lobe epilepsy. It also has a low diagnostic yield in patients suffering from extratemporal seizures. ictal SPECT imaging has poorer spatial resolution as compared to PET scans. Following image acquisition, the coregistered and normalized interictal images can be subtracted from the ictal images and then coregistered with high-resolution MR images with the aid of computer software. ("subtraction ictal SPECT coregistered to MR imaging" also known as SISCOM). This technique has been shown to reliably indicate the location of the seizure focus, and is superior to visual analysis.

Magnetoencephalography

Magnetoencephalography (MEG) (magnetic source imaging) is a non-invasive modality used in localization of epilepsy **(Figs. 18A to D)**. MEG measures the extracranial changes in the magnetic field that occur perpendicular to the direction of current flow in the apical dendrites. This means that MEG is capable of measuring flow of current tangential to the scalp. This corresponds to activation within the sulci. One of the main advantages of MEG over EEG is that the magnetic fields are not affected by the varying conductivity of the intervening structures like bone and scalp. The spikes that are recorded on MEG have been shown to correlate with invasive monitoring. As MEG records signal from the surface of the brain, it is well suited toward evaluation of neocortical epilepsy. In children who have normal MRI or subtle MR findings, MEG results have been found to predict surgical outcome. Also, in patients who suffer from recurrent seizures after unsuccessful epilepsy surgery, MEG helps in localizing the site of postsurgical epileptiform discharge. This is possible as MEG is affected to a lesser degree by the postoperative changes, cranial defects and gliotic changes. MEG is unable to identify epileptiform discharge from deep areas such as the medial temporal lobe. MEG can also help in pediatric epilepsy by mapping the eloquent cortex. MEG directly measures the electrophysiological changes due to the underlying neuronal activity and has higher temporal resolution compared to fMR.

CONCLUSION

Significant advances have occurred in the presurgical evaluation of epilepsy. It is now possible to utilize multimodality imaging to identify small lesions in the brain. Further advances in MR imaging, for example, 7T MRI scanners will increase the diagnostic accuracy in difficult cases.

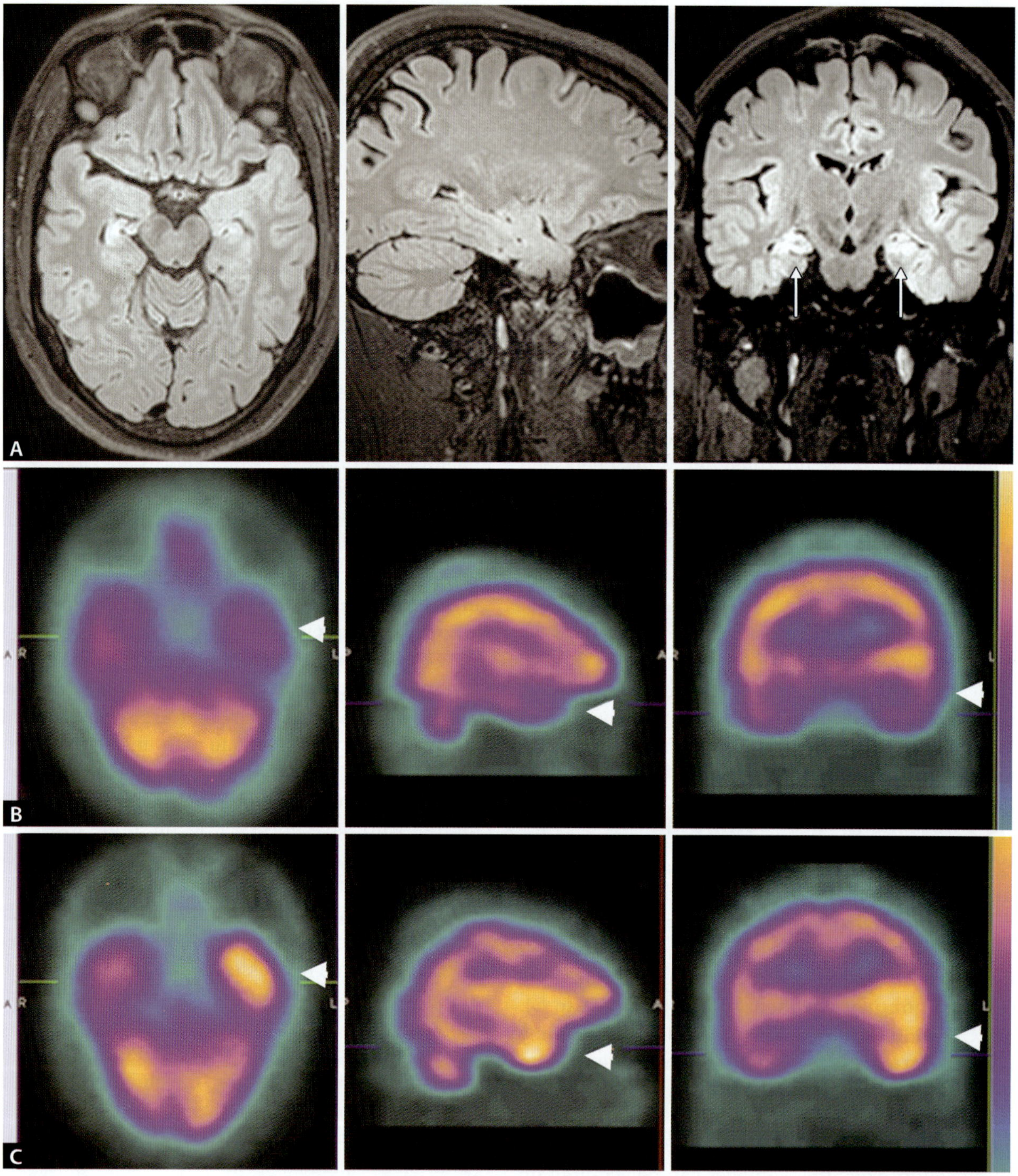

Figs. 17A to C: FLAIR MRI (A) and Tc-99m ECD SPECT images (B and C) in a 30-year-old male suffering from complex partial seizures show bilateral hippocampal sclerosis (arrows, A) with interictal hypoperfusion (arrowheads, B) and ictal hyperperfusion (arrowheads, C) in the left temporal lobe, suggesting that the epileptogenic focus is localized to the left temporal lobe. *Courtesy*: Dr Madhavi Tripathi, Department of Nuclear Medicine, All India Institute of Medical Sciences, New Delhi, India.

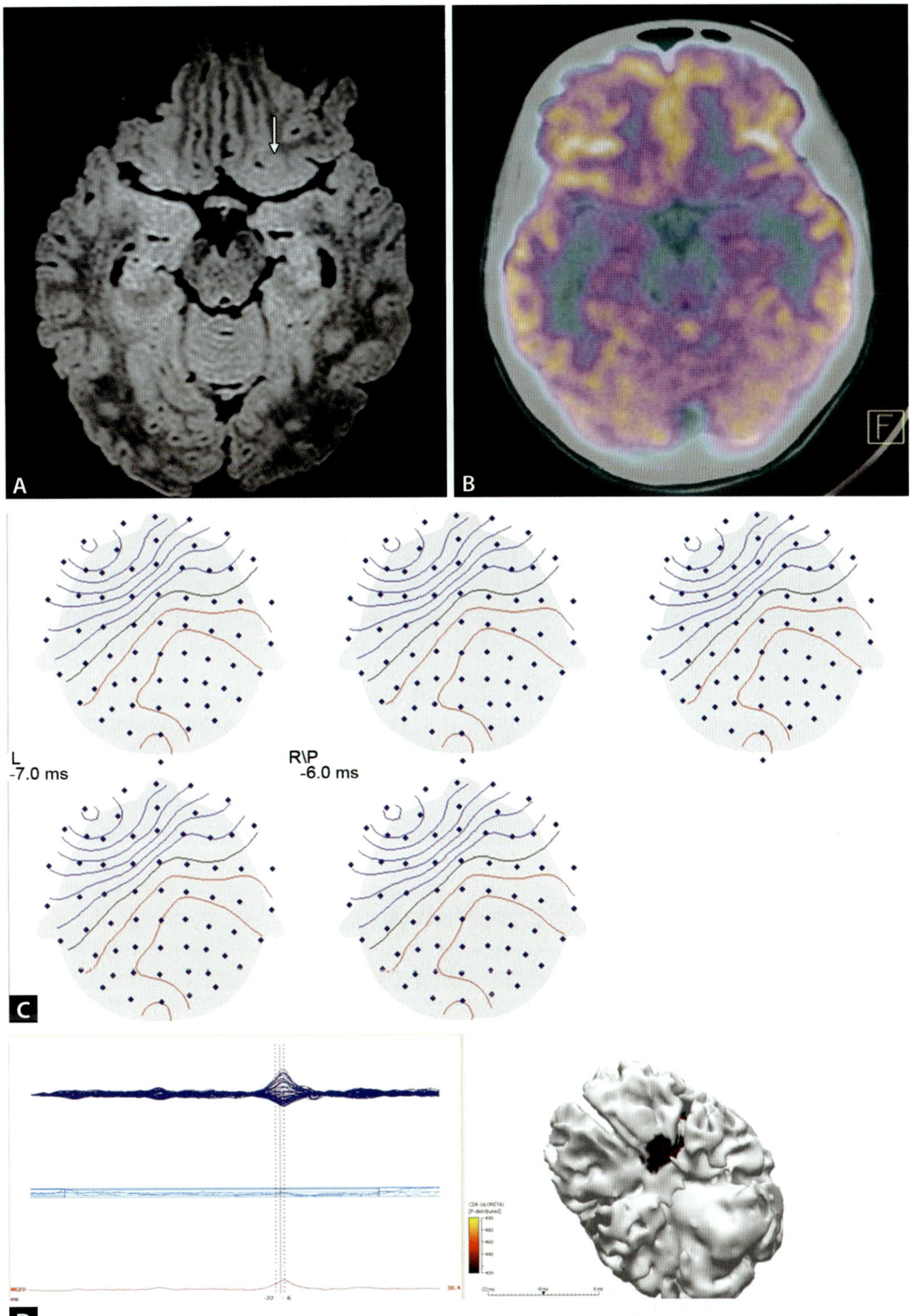

Figs. 18A to D: Axial FLAIR (A) image shows subtle cortical thickening in the left basifrontal region with loss of gray-white matter differentiation (arrow). Interictal SPECT (B) shows hypoperfusion in this region. MEG current maps (C) and MEG analysis using CURRY Neuroimaging platform (D) also show localization in the left basifrontal region.
Courtesy: Dr Manjari Tripathi, incharge MEG center; AIIMS-DBT.

REFERENCES

1. Fisher RS, van Emde Boas W, Blume W, et al. Epileptic seizures and epilepsy: definitions proposed by the International League Against Epilepsy (ILAE) and the International Bureau for Epilepsy (IBE). Epilepsia. 2005;46(4):470-2.
2. Nagae LM, Lall N, Dahmoush H, et al. Diagnostic, treatment, and surgical imaging in epilepsy. Clin Imaging. 2016;40(4):624-36.
3. Chavakula V, Cosgrove G. Imaging for epilepsy surgery. Semin Neurol. 2017;37(05):580-8.
4. Cendes F, Andermann F, Gloor P, et al. Atrophy of mesial structures in patients with temporal lobe epilepsy: cause or consequence of repeated seizures? Ann Neurol. 1993;34:795-801.
5. Berkovic SF, Andermann F, Olivier A, et al. Hippocampal sclerosis in temporal lobe epilepsy demonstrated by magnetic resonance imaging. Ann Neurol. 1991;29: 175-82.
6. Lee DH, Gao FQ, Rogers JM, et al. MR in temporal lobe epilepsy: analysis with pathologic confirmation. Am J Neuroradiol. 1998;19(1):19-27.
7. Osborn A. Commissural and cortical maldevelopment. In: Osborn's Brain Imaging, Pathology, and Anatomy, 1st edition. Canada: Amirsys; 2013. pp. 1083-113.
8. Cendes F, Theodore WH, Brinkmann BH, et al. Neuroimaging of epilepsy. In: Handbook of Clinical Neurology [Internet]. Elsevier; 2016 [cited March 1, 2018]. pp. 985-1014. Available from http://linkinghub.elsevier.com/retrieve/pii/ B978044453486600051X.
9. Fernandez C, Girard N, Paz Paredes A, et al. The usefulness of MR imaging in the diagnosis of dysembryoplastic neuroepithelial tumor in children: a study of 14 cases. Am J Neuroradiol. 2003;24:829-34.
10. Zentner J, Wolf H, Ostertun B, et al. Ganglio-gliomas: clinical, radiological, and histopathological findings in 51 patients. J Neurol Neurosurg Psychiatry. 1994;57:1497-502.
11. Casazza M, Broggi G, Franzini A, et al. Supratentorial cavernous angiomas and epileptic seizures: preoperative course and postoperative outcome. Neurosurgery. 1996;39:26-32.
12. Bastos AC, Comeau RM, Andermann F, et al. Diagnosis of subtle focal dysplastic lesions: curvilinear reformatting from three-dimensional magnetic resonance imaging. Ann Neurol. 1999;46:88-94.
13. Li LM, Caramanos Z, Cendes F, et al. Lateralization of temporal lobe epilepsy (TLE) and discrimination of TLE from extra-TLE using pattern analysis of magnetic resonance spectroscopic and volumetric data. Epilepsia. 2000;41:832-42.
14. Bernasconi A, Bernasconi N, Caramanos Z, et al. T2 relaxometry can lateralize mesial temporal lobe epilepsy in patients with normal MRI. NeuroImage. 2000;12(6):739-46.
15. Duncan JS, Winston GP, Koepp MJ, et al. Brain imaging in the assessment for epilepsy surgery. Lancet Neurol. 2016;15(4):420-33.
16. Knecht S, Deppe M, Dräger B, et al. Language lateralization in healthy right-handers. Brain. 2000;123(1):74-81.
17. Szaflarski JP, Binder JR, Possing ET, et al. Language lateralization in left-handed and ambidextrous people: fMRI data. Neurology. 2002;59(2):238-44.

CHAPTER 16

Imaging of Supratentorial Brain Tumors

Shailesh B Gaikwad, Ajay Garg

INTRODUCTION

Brain tumors in adults comprise a diverse group of neoplasms that vary in their behavior depending on such factors as cell of origin, site of occurrence, morphology and pattern of spread. The annual incidence of primary intracranial neoplasms is estimated to be 12.3 people per lac population and it is increasing in frequency, however, prognosis of these patients has improved considerably due to recent advances in diagnostic techniques, microneurosurgery, chemotherapy and radiotherapy. Central to the efficacy of these techniques, however, is the ability of the neuroradiologist to diagnose and interpret the growth pattern of these tumors.

This chapter describes various types of brain tumors of supratentorial region in adults with emphasis on imaging features, various modalities used in diagnosis, pitfalls in diagnosis, effect of radiotherapy and important recent advances in imaging of brain tumors. Embryonal tumors have been discussed in chapter on infratentorial brain tumors.

CLASSIFICATION OF SUPRATENTORIAL BRAIN TUMORS (2016)

Classifying brain tumors is valuable, but the conceptual basis for such complex scheme is controversial. The putative histogenic or "cell-of-origin-approach" classification proposed by Bailey and Cushing has been most widely used. In 1993, the WHO ratified a new comprehensive classification of neoplasms affecting the central nervous system.[1]

In 2016 update to WHO brain tumor system classification first time gave the concept of integrated diagnosis taking into consideration the light microscopy findings and molecular genetics[2] **(Table 1)**. The molecular genetics have been found to predict prognosis better than histological grading. Several previously described entities such as gliomatosis cerebri, primitive neuroectodermal tumor have been removed.

DIFFUSE ASTROCYTIC AND OLIGODENDROGLIAL TUMORS

Diffuse astrocytomas and oligodendrogliomas are of different genetic profiles. Diffuse astrocytomas are IDH positive or IDH negative. The term 'NOS' is used when genetic profiling is not done or not available. ODG have genetic hallmark of IDH mutant and 1p/19q co-deletion.[2] IDH mutant gliomas have better prognosis than IDH wild gliomas. Anaplastic astrocytoma, IDH-wild has worse prognosis than GBM, IDH-mutant.

Diffuse Astrocytoma, IDH-mutant/ IDH-wildtype/NOS

These are low-grade WHO grade II gliomas. Genetically they are IDH mutant or wild but negative for 1p-19 q co-deletion. Diffuse astrocytomas constitute 25 to 30% of all cerebral gliomas with peak incidence in fourth decade. These astrocytomas have an inherent tendency for anaplastic transformation. Diffuse fibrillary astrocytoma occurring in the cerebral hemispheres is most common. They are most common in frontal lobe.

Table 1: Classification of brain tumor[2]

1. *Diffuse astrocytic and oligodendroglial tumors*: • Diffuse astrocytoma, IDH-mutant/IDH-wildtype/NOS • Anaplastic astrocytoma, IDH-mutant/IDH-wildtype/NOS • Glioblastoma, IDH-mutant/IDH-wildtype/NOS • Diffuse midline glioma, H3 K27M-mutant • Oligodendroglioma, IDH-mutant and 1p/19q-codeleted/ NOS • Anaplastic oligodendroglioma, IDH-mutant and 1p/19q-codeleted/NOS • Oligoastrocytoma, NOS
2. *Other astrocytic tumors*: • Pilocytic astrocytoma • Subependymal giant cell astrocytoma • Pleomorphic xanthoastrocytoma • Anaplastic pleomorphic xanthoastrocytoma
3. *Ependymal tumors*: • Subependymoma • Myxopapillary ependymoma • Ependymoma (papillary/ clear cell/ tanycytic) • Anaplastic (malignant) ependymoma
4. *Other gliomas*: • Chordoid glioma of third ventricle • Angiocentric glioma • Astroblastoma
5. *Choroid plexus tumors*: • Choroid plexus papillomas • Atypical choroid plexus papillomas • Choroid plexus carcinoma
6. *Neuronal and mixed neuronal-glial tumors*: • Dysembryoplastic neuroepithelial tumors (DNETs) • Gangliocytoma • Ganglioglioma • Anaplastic ganglioglioma • Dysplastic gangliocytoma of cerebellum • Desmoplastic infantile astrocytoma and ganglioglioma • Papillary glioneuronal tumor • Rosette-forming glioneuronal tumor • Diffuse leptomeningeal glioneuronal tumor • Central neurocytoma • Extraventricular neurocytoma • Paraganglioma
7. *Pineal regional tumors*: • Pineocytoma • Pineal parenchymal tumor of intermediate differentiation • Pineoblastoma • Papillary tumor of the pineal region
8. *Embryonal tumors*: • Medulloblastomas, WNT-activated/ SHH-activated/ group 3/ group 4 • Embryonal tumors with multilayered rosettes, C19MC-altered/ NOS • CNS neuroblastoma
9. *Tumors of cranial and paraspinal nerve*: • Schwannoma (Cellular/Plexiform) • Melanotic schwannoma • Neurofibroma (Atypical/Plexiform) • Malignant peripheral nerve sheath tumors

Contd...

Contd...

10. Meningioma
11. *Mesenchymal, non-meningothelial tumors*: • Solitary fibrous tumor/ hemangiopericytoma • Hemangioblastoma • Ewing's sarcoma
12. *Lymphomas*: • Diffuse large B-cell lymphoma of the CNS • Immunodeficiency-associated CNS lymphoma
13. *Histiocytic tumors*: • Langerhans cell histiocytosis • Erdheim-Chester disease • Rosai-Dorfman disease
14. *Germ cell tumors*: • Germinoma • Embryonal carcinoma • Yolk sac (endodermal sinus) tumors • Choriocarcinoma • Teratoma (mature/ immature) • Mixed germ cell tumors
15. *Tumors of the sellar region*: • Craniopharyngioma • Granular cell tumor of the sellar region • Pituicytoma • Spindle cell oncocytoma
16. Metastatic tumors

Imaging Features

The tumor is hypodense on noncontract CT, hypointense to isointense on T1W and hyperintense on T2W MR imaging **(Figs. 1A to D)**. Enhancement patterns following contrast administration are variable, however, the majority of these tumors demonstrate only minimal and inhomogeneous enhancement. Calcification may be found in 15–20% cases. Up to 10% of diffuse astrocytomas have T2-hyperintense lesion which show more than 50% signal suppression on FLAIR image, a sign known as 'T2-FLAIR mismatch" specific for 1p/19q noncodeleted tumors **(Figs. 2A to C)**.[3]

Necrosis is not found, but may have cystic degeneration. Edema and hemorrhages are rare.

Progressive malignant transformation is characterized by progressive increase in tumoral necrosis, intratumoral hemorrhage, peritumoral edema and appearance of contrast enhancement. On SWI, areas of susceptibility foci secondary to hemorrhagic foci are usually not seen. On MR perfusion, rCBV values are low.

Anaplastic Astrocytoma, IDH-mutant/ IDH-wildtype/NOS

Anaplastic astrocytomas are mixed density/intensity masses with areas of necrosis and cyst formation; blood

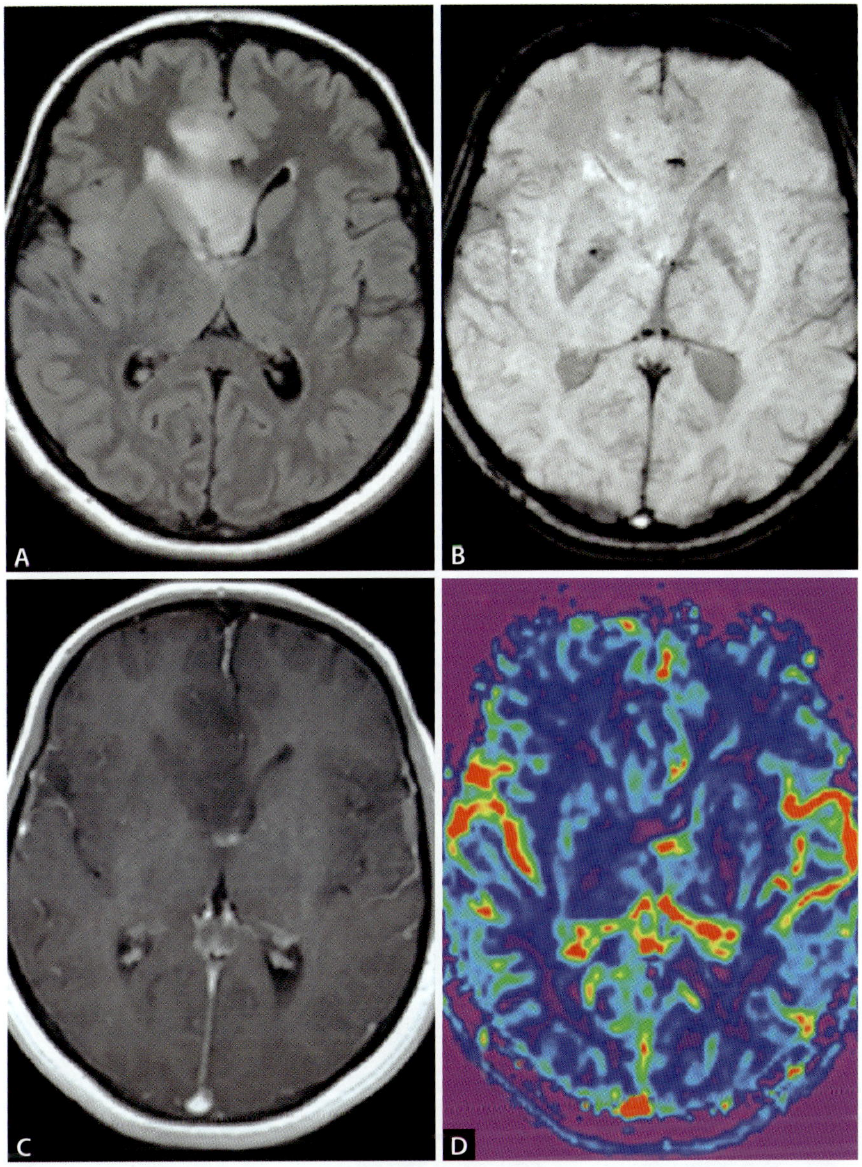

Figs. 1A to D: Diffuse astrocytoma: Axial flair (A) shows a well-defined hyperintense lesion in right frontal lobe and adjacent corpus callosum. No hemorrhagic foci are seen on SWI (B). Following contrast administration, no enhancement is noted (C). on DSC perfusion, rCBV maps show low perfusion (D).

products from hemorrhage may also be seen, although this is more common in glioblastoma. Mild vasogenic edema of adjacent white matter, mass effect, and more intense irregular enhancement following contrast administration is usually observed. When foci of anaplasia are separated by more low-grade components of the tumor, post-contrast scans may demonstrate multiple separate foci of necrosis or enhancement, thus, mimicking metastatic disease or multifocal glioma. On perfusion MRI, these tumors show increased rCBV compared with diffuse astrocytoma **(Figs. 3A to D)**.[4] On MR spectroscopy, increased choline, decreased NAA and decreased myo-inositol is present.

Glioblastoma, IDH-mutant/ IDH-wildtype/NOS

Glioblastoma represent 15–20% of all primary brain neoplasms, and 50% of all astrocytomas. Previously glioblastomas were known as glioblastoma multiforme, but recent WHO classification has dropped the 'multiforme' and these tumors are referred merely as glioblastomas.

Glioblastoma are genetically and imaging phenotypically heterogeneous tumors. The peak incidence is between the ages of 45 and 55 with definite male preponderance. Traditionally glioblastomas have been

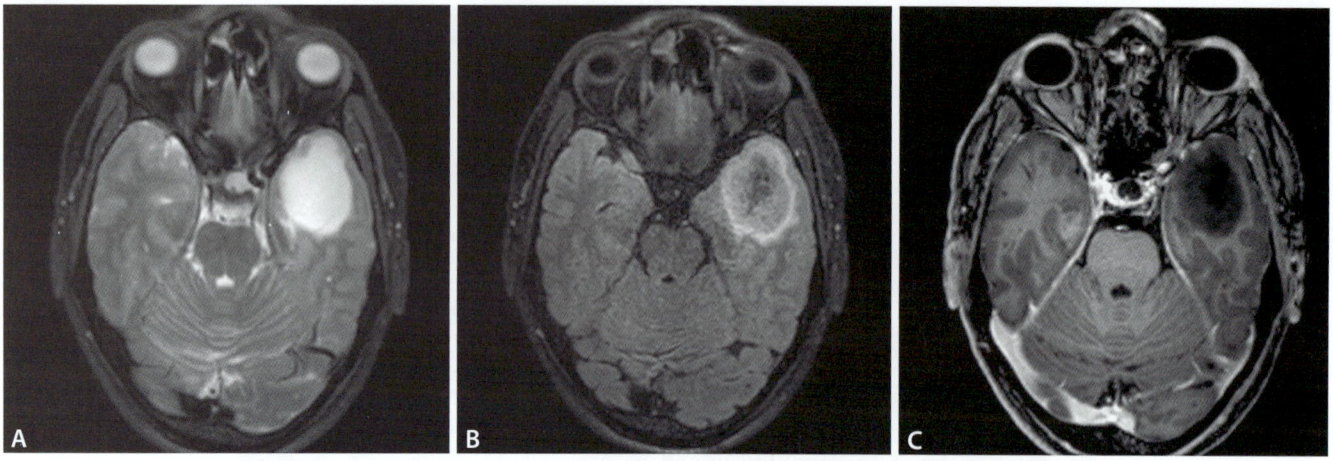

Figs. 2A to C: Diffuse astrocytoma in left temporal lobe: The lesion is brightly hyperintense on T2-WI (A) and partial suppression of signal on FLAIR (B): T2-FLAIR mismatch/ No contrast enhancement is seen (C).

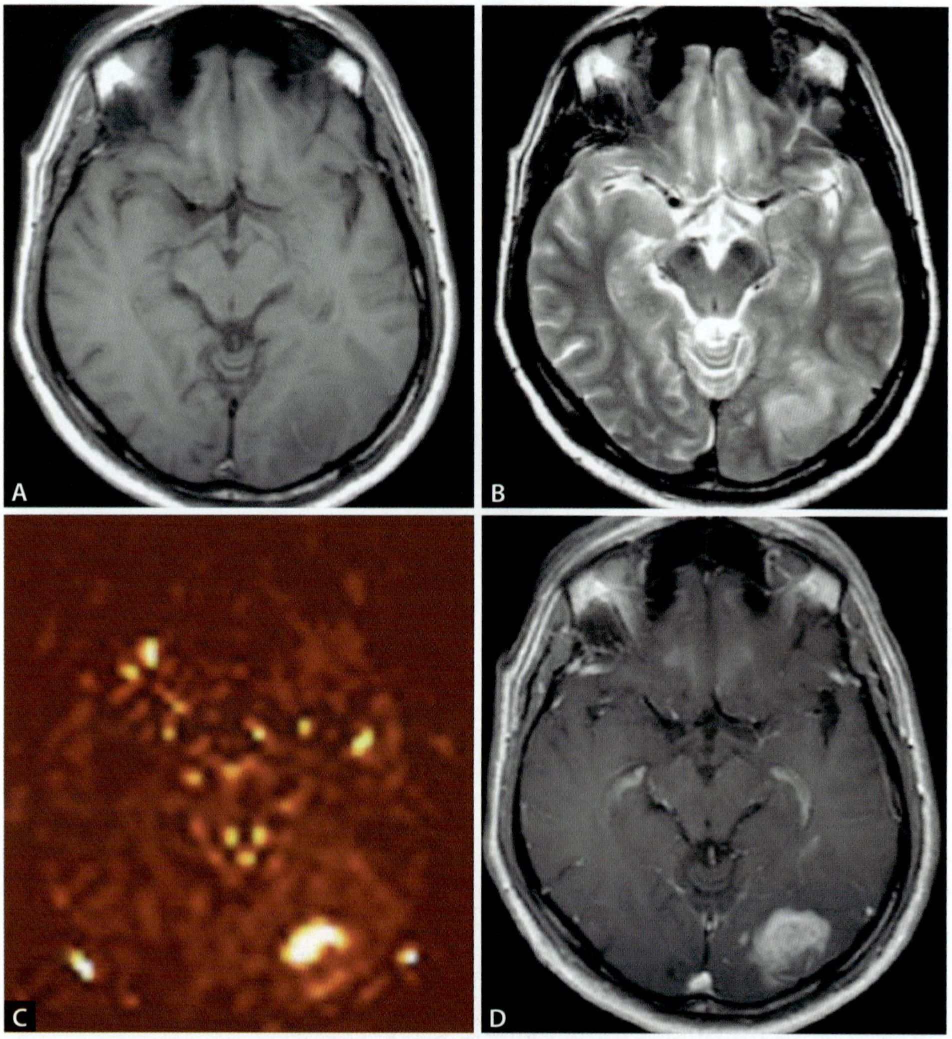

Figs. 3A to D: Anaplastic astrocytoma: Axial T1-WI (A) and T2-WI (B) show a left occipital ill-defined lesion, which shows high perfusion in ASL (C) and enhances heterogeneously following gadolinium administration (D).

divided into primary (90%) and secondary (10%); the former arising de novo whereas the later developed from a pre-existing low-grade glioma. Most of the secondary glioblastoma are IDH-mutant, occur at younger age and almost always MGMT methylated. The primary glioblastoma are almost invariably IDH-wild, occur at the older age and have worse prognosis. If IDH status is not known or indeterminate, diagnosis of glioblastoma NOS should be made. Glioblastoma has a predilection for the cerebral white matter especially frontal and temporal lobes and frequently infiltrates into the adjacent lobes and deep structures, such as the corpus callosum. Glioblastoma is an aggressive tumor which spreads locally along the white matter tracts or the ependymal lining of the ventricles into the leptomeninges resulting in seeding of the subarachnoid space. Distant metastasis to lungs, liver and bone have also been reported.

Imaging Features

Marked intratumoral inhomogeneity is a frequent feature, with focal areas of necrosis or cyst formation producing hypointensity on T1WI and hyperintensity on T2W images **(Figs. 4A to D)**. Focal areas of acute hemorrhage or hemosiderin deposition are often best seen on GRE images, but may produce areas of marked hypointensity on T2WI and less commonly hyperintensity on T1-WI. Identification of blood products may help to differentiate glioblastoma from anaplastic astrocytoma which show bleeds less frequently. SWI are extremely sensitive for detecting blood products. Calcification is rare in de novo primary glioblastomas and are more commonly seen in secondary glioblastoma. Invasion of the cortex, leptomeninges and dura may occur.

Enhancement is almost always seen and usually in the form of thick irregular rim or nodular enhancement

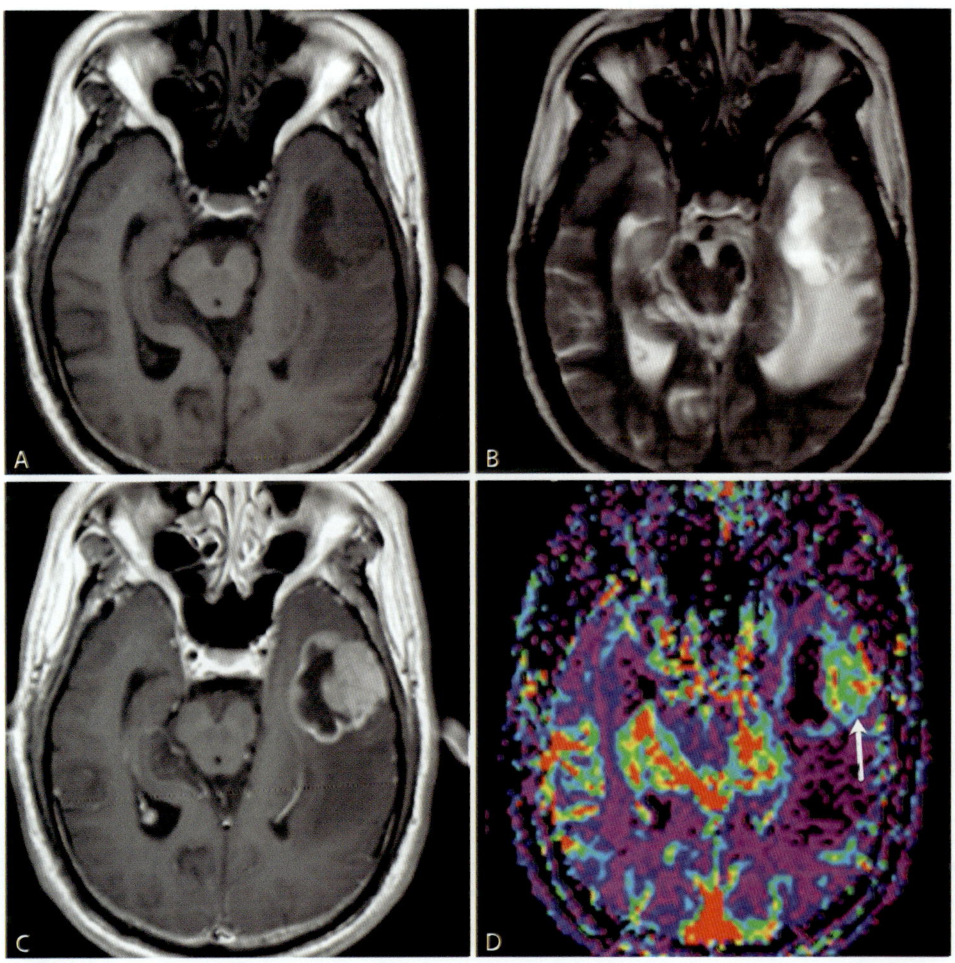

Figs. 4A to D: Glioblastoma: Axial T1-WI (A) and T2-WI (B) show a left temporal nodular ring-lesion with perilesional edema. The mass enhances avidly with central necrosis (C). On DSC perfusion rCBV maps, perfusion is high in the solid component of the mass (D).

surrounded by peritumoral T2- and FLAIR hyperintensity which represents region of tumor cell infiltration and vasogenic edema both in varying proportions **(Figs. 4A to D)**. On angiography large mass with striking tumor blush, contrast stasis and pooling in bizarre vascular channels is noted.

Multiple glioblastomas are also occasionally seen. These have been ascribed to either multifocal origin (when there is a microscopic connection between various foci of the tumor) or a multicentric origin (when there are no connections between the tumors).

Advanced MR imaging techniques like diffusion, perfusion and spectroscopy provide complimentary physiologic information. DWI provide the measure of water diffusion in a voxel. High grade gliomas tend to have areas of high cellularity so lower ADC values. ADC values as a marker of glioma should be interpreted cautiously because of inherent and quite remarkable tissue heterogeneity associated with gliomas. ADC threshold value of 1185 × 10^{-6} mm^2/s sensitivity (97.6%) and specificity (53.1%) in the discrimination of high-grade (WHO grade III & IV) and low-grade (WHO grade II) gliomas.[5]

MR perfusion imaging evaluate tumor angiogenesis and permeability of blood-brain barrier, which may be predictive of the tumor grade and higher malignant histology **(Fig. 4)**.[6] MR spectroscopy provide metabolic information. One must remember that regional tumor heterogeneity may influence conventional and advanced MRI findings.

Diffuse Midline Glioma, H3 K27M-mutant

In 2016 update of the WHO CNS tumor classification, diffuse midline glioma, H3 K27M-mutant is a new entity characterized by a diffuse growth pattern, and a midline location (e.g., thalami, brainstem, spinal cord, and other midline structures, including the third ventricle, hypothalamus, and pineal region) **(Figs. 5A to C)**.[2] The majority of these tumors are high-grade astrocytomas with high proliferative potential.[7,8]

Oligodendroglioma, IDH-mutant and 1p/19q-codeleted/NOS

Oligodendroglioma (ODG) constitutes 5–20% of all cerebral gliomas. IDH-mutation and 1p/19q-codeletion are genetic signature of ODG. The peak age incidence is in the fifth and sixth decades.

Imaging Features

On CT, this tumor appears as a heterogeneous hemispheric mass involving the cortex, usually located in the frontal lobe. The mass is hypo-isodense relative to the gray matter; heavy streaky, ribbon like calcification is seen in 70 to 90% of tumors **(Figs. 6A to C)**. Hemorrhage is present in about 20% of cases with mild edema. Scalloping of inner table of the calvarium is other feature in about 17% of cases. Although cysts are frequent, necrosis or gross hemorrhage may also be rarely seen. Mild to moderate heterogeneous enhancement after contrast administration is common. Most are high grade at time of diagnosis. Contrast enhancement does not necessarily reflect malignant transformation, as in astrocytic tumors. On MR, the tumors have heterogeneously hyperintense signal on T2-WI and typically have indistinct borders **(Figs. 7A to C)** compared to homogenously hyperintense T2 signal and sharp border seen in astrocytomas **(*see* Figs. 2A to C)**.[9]

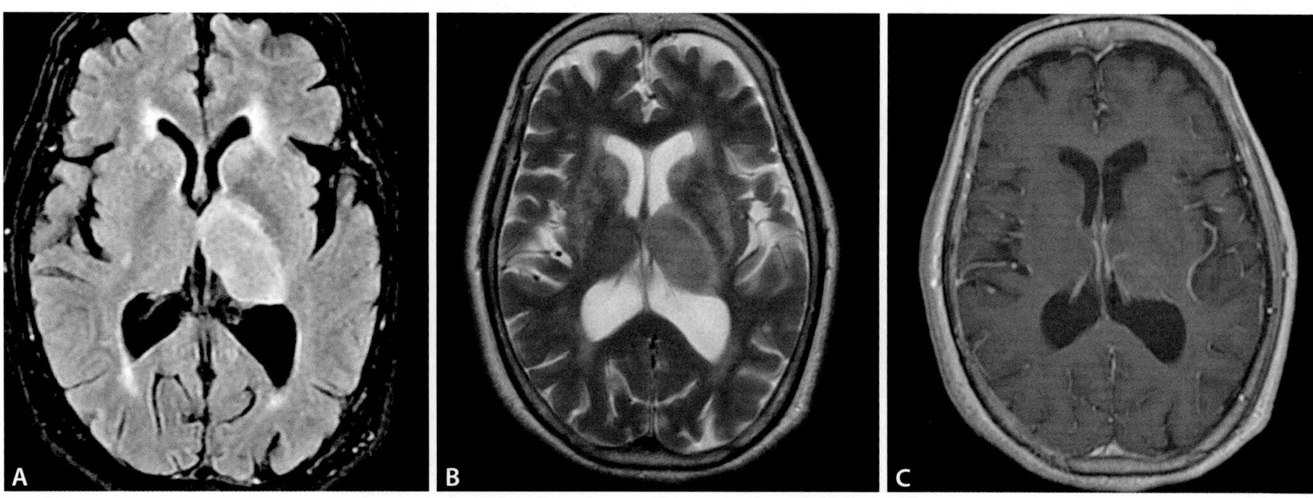

Figs. 5A to C: Thalamic glioma: Axial flair (A) and T2-WI (B) show a left thalamic mass, which shows patchy enhancement following contrast administration (C).

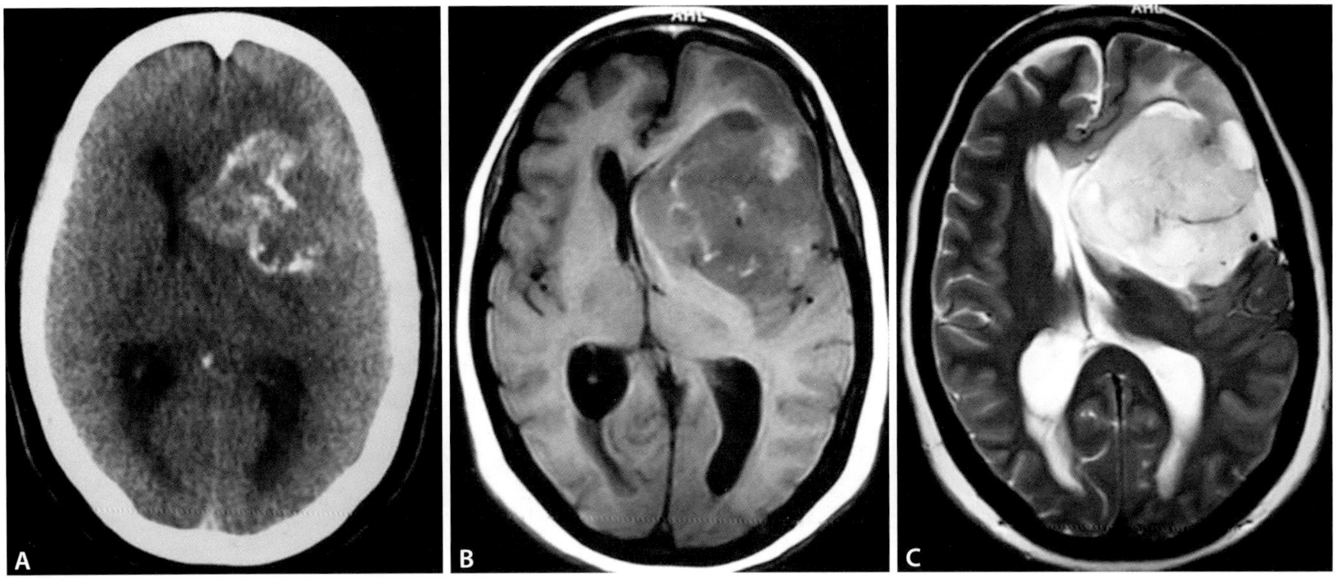

Figs. 6A to C: Oligodendroglioma: NCCT (A) shows a left frontal deep white matter and basal ganglion mass with calcification. The mass is predominantly hypointense on T-WI (B) with foci of high signal intensity and heterogeneously hyperintense on T2-WI (C). Minimal perilesional edema is seen.

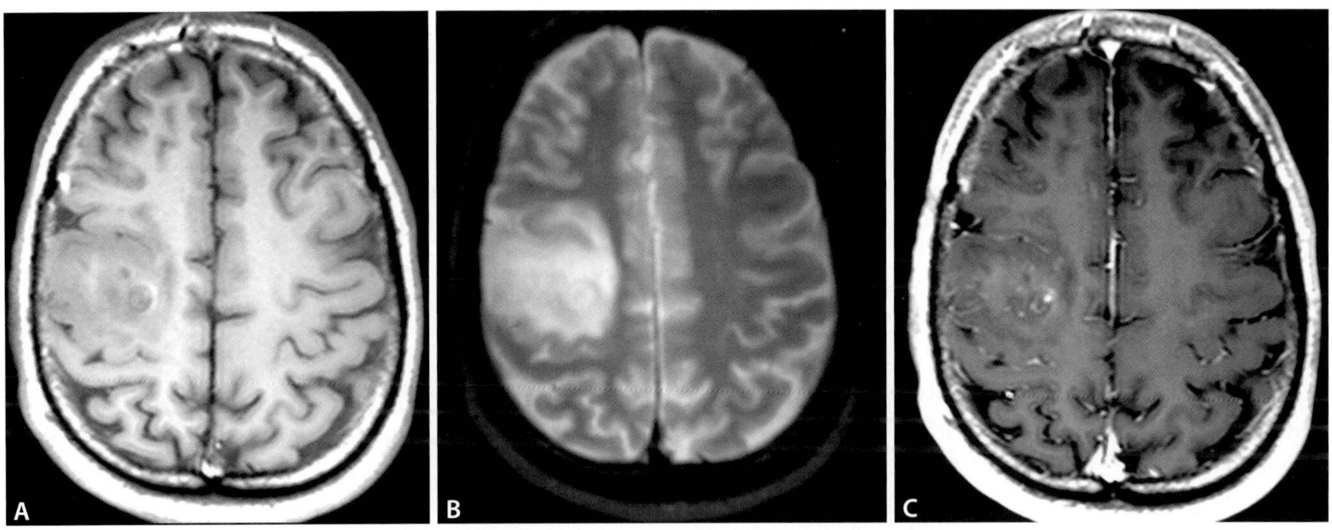

Figs. 7A to C: Anaplastic oligodendroglioma: Axial T1-Wi (A) and T2-WI (B) show a right frontal cortical-subcortical mixed signal intensity lesion which show patchy enhancement (C)

Anaplastic Oligodendroglioma, IDH-mutant and 1p/19q-codeleted/ NOS

Anaplastic ODG are characterized by more enhancement and increased rCBV values.

OTHER ASTROCYTIC TUMORS

Pilocytic Astrocytoma

These are slow growing WHO grade I CNS neoplasms. It usually presents in the first two decades.[10] These tumors are generally located around the optic chiasma-hypothalamus and optic nerve in the supratentorial region. Cerebral hemispheric pilocytic astrocytomas are rare and present later beyond 20 years of age.

Most PA have BRAF-KIAA1549 fusion gene mutation which is associated with better prognosis.[11] They lack IDH and TP53 mutations. These tumors have strong association with NF1.

Imaging Features

Hemispheric pilocytic astrocytomas present either as a well-defined cystic mass with enhancing mural nodule

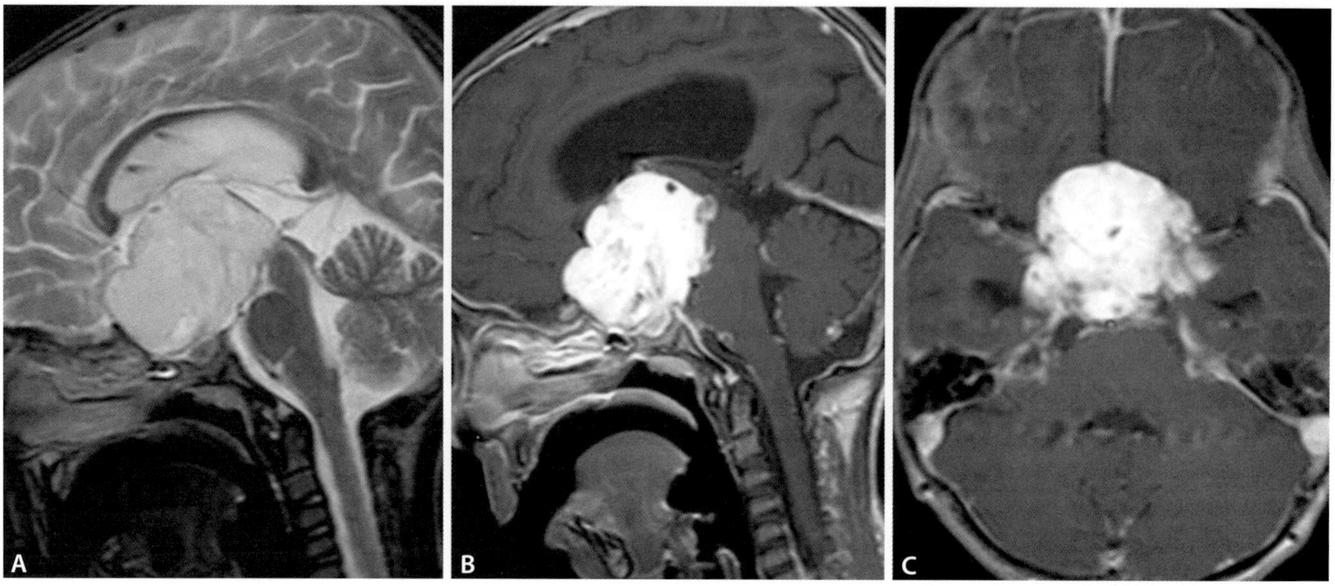

Figs. 8A to C: Chiasmal-hypothalamic pilocytic astrocytoma: Sagittal T2-WI (A) shows a hyperintense mass in Chiasmal-hypothalamic region which shows intense contrast enhancement in sagittal (B) and axial (C) T1-WI.

or solid enhancing lesion on CT and MRI **(Figs. 8A to C)**. About 10% of pilocytic astrocytomas are calcified.

Despite their benign nature, they show intense enhancement and show wide range of choline values in MR spectroscopy. They have low rCBV ratio (<1.5) and characteristic signal intensity curve which overshoots baseline during recovery caused by massive contrast leakage into interstitial space.[12] Angiography demonstrates an avascular mass with displacement of the normal vessels.

Subependymal Giant Cell Astrocytoma

Subependymal giant cell astrocytoma (SGCA) are slow-growing WHO grade I CNS tumors. They are seen in 10 to 15% of patients with tuberous sclerosis complex (TSC). SGCAs probably arise from subependymal nodules in the ventricular wall of patients with tuberous sclerosis.[13] They usually become symptomatic before 20 years of age. These tumors are characteristically located in a lateral ventricle near the foramen of Monro.

Imaging Features

On CT scan, SGCA appears as focal partially calcified mass, iso- attenuated to slightly hypo-attenuated intraventricular mass **(Figs. 9A and B)**. Contrast enhancement is strong but heterogeneous. This enhancement do not distinguish a SGCA from a subependymal nodule, which may also enhance.[14] Growth over serial imaging or symptomatic hydrocephalus may help to differentiate SEGA from subependymal nodule.[15] Co-existing lesions of tuberous sclerosis are usually present. On MR, the tumor exhibits mixed signal intensities on both T1 and T2WI.

Pleomorphic Xanthoastrocytoma (Noninvasive, WHO Grade II)

Pleomorphic Xanthoastrocytoma (PXA) is tumor of children and young adults and usually present with seizures.

Temporal and frontal lobe of young adult is the most common site of involvement. Marked cellular pleomorphism may be noted at histology. In 2016 WHO CNS Tumor classification update, anaplastic PXA (WHO grade III) has been added as separate entity.[2]

Imaging Features

On CT PXAs are typically seen as superficially located solid enhancing nodule, frequently associated with a peripheral eccentric cyst component (50-60%) **(Figs. 10A and B)**.[16] These slow-growing tumor may cause scalloping of overlying calvarium. On MRI, these tumors appear of mixed signal intensity on T1WI. On T2WI both the cystic component and solid components are hyperintense.[17] Peritumoral edema is variable and may be mild to moderate.[18] The solid component shows homogeneous enhancement after intravenous contrast administration **(Figs. 11A to D)**. Extension to leptomeningeal surfaces is present in over 70% of cases.[17] One third may undergo malignant transformation.

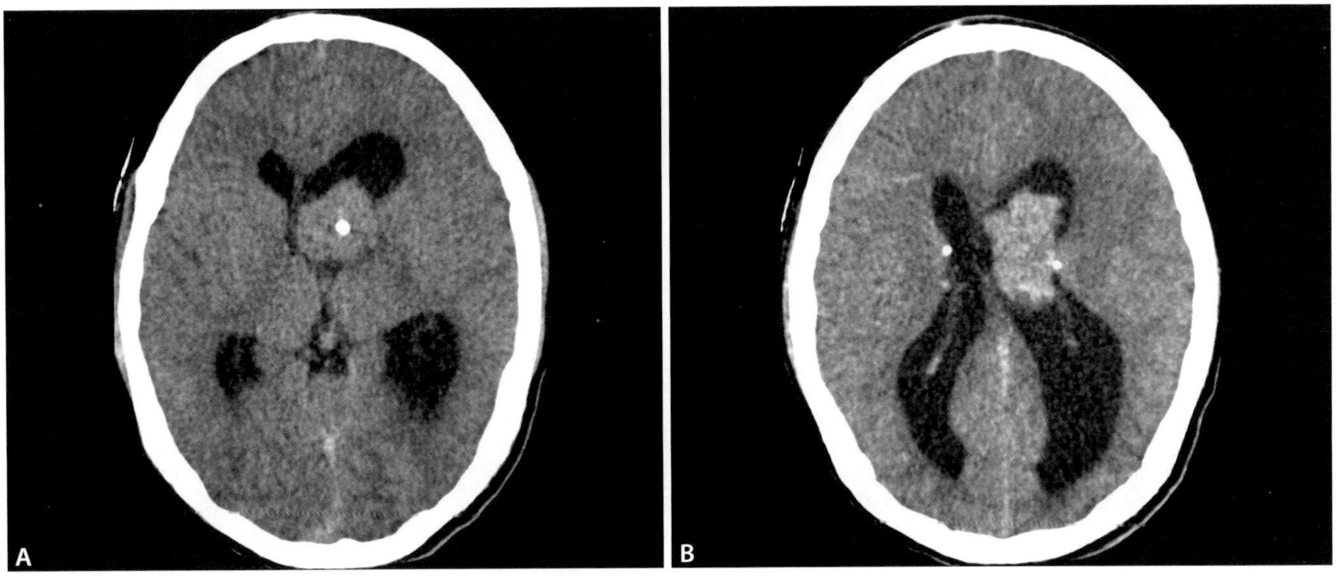

Figs. 9A and B: CECT (A and B) show a enhancing mass in region of left foramen of Monro with focal calcification. Also note multiple calcified subependymal nodules (B) along left lateral ventricle suggestive of tuberous sclerosis.

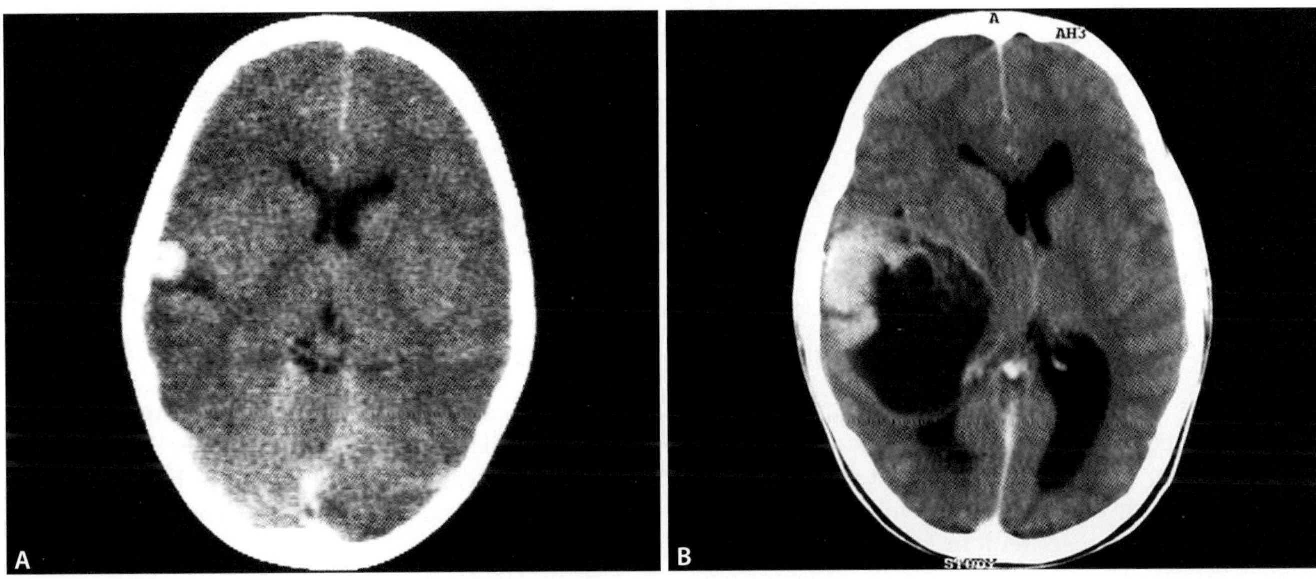

Figs. 10A and B: Pleomorphic xanthoastrocytoma. CECT (A) show a enhancing nodule abutting pial surface in right temporal lobe with minimal edema. Three years later, follow-up CECT scan (B) show significant increase in the size of the lesion with cystic component and mass-effect.

EPENDYMAL TUMORS

Subependymoma

Subependymomas are another variant of ependymoma with a significant astroglial component to the tumor; however, they still have characteristic ependymal features. They occur most frequently in the frontal horn of lateral ventricle and inferior fourth ventricle. They are multiple and slow growing. They are common in middle aged and elderly patients.

Imaging Features

On CT and MRI subependymoma, appears as a non-enhancing mass similar to brain with focal areas of cystic degeneration and hemorrhage.[19]

Ependymoma

Ependymomas constitute 2 to 6% of all gliomas. Peak age range is 1–5 years for intraventricular lesions but second small peak occurs in mid-thirties for supratentorial

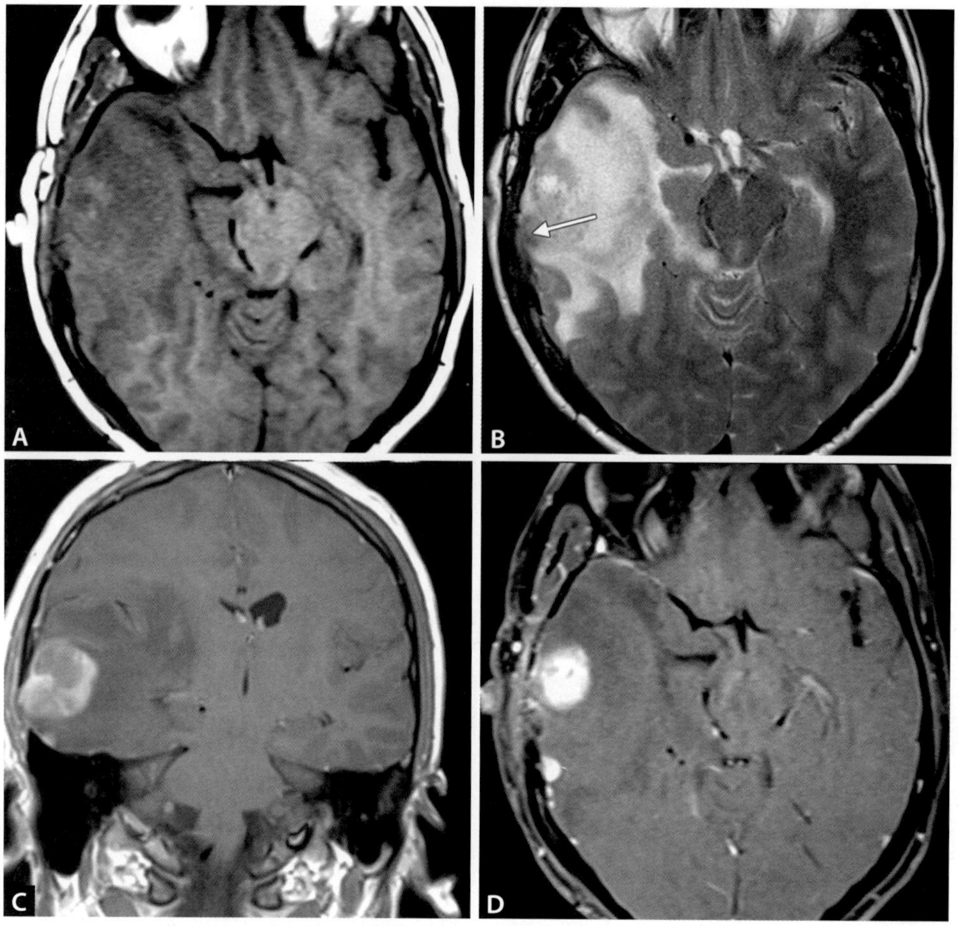

Figs. 11A to D: Pleomorphic xanthoastrocytoma: Axial T1-Wi (A) and T2-WI (B) show a mixed signal intensity lesion in right temporal lobe with marked perilesional edema and focal scalloping of overlying bone (arrow in B). The mass enhances avidly (C and D) with enhancement of adjacent leptomeninges (arrow in D).

masses. Only 40% of ependymomas are supratentorial where parenchymal location is more common than intraventricular site. It is believed that subependymal neural glia may extend into adjacent white matter leading to ependymal cell rests remote from the ventricular lining.[20] Extraventricular ependymomas are larger than intraventricular ependymomas at time of presentation.

Imaging Features

Ependymomas are multilobulated, well-demarcated, frequently calcified masses that are either intraventricular or juxtaventricular in supratentorial region. On noncontrast CT, ependymomas are isodense with dense punctate calcification in about 50% and hemorrhage may occur.[21] There is mild to moderate enhancement following contrast administration varying from homogenous to inhomogeneous or rim enhancement.[22] On MRI **(Figs. 12A and B)**, the solid component of ependymoma appear hypo- to isointense on T1WI and hyperintense on T2WI. Calcification can be less conspicuous than on CT, whereas cysts and small hemorrhagic foci are better demonstrated on MRI. When calcification, necrosis or blood products are present the tumor appears heterogeneous.[13]

CHOROID PLEXUS TUMORS

Choroid Plexus Papilloma

Choroid plexus papilloma (CPP) are uncommon benign WHO grade I neoplasm. They are commonly seen in children less than 5-year of age and rare in adults. They have predilection for the trigone of lateral ventricle in children and the fourth ventricle in adults.[23]

Imaging Features

On CT, CPP appears as a mottled mass which is isodense to hyperdense on noncontrast scans and usually show homogeneous enhancement. Intratumoral fine, speckled calcification is seen in about 25% of cases. On MRI

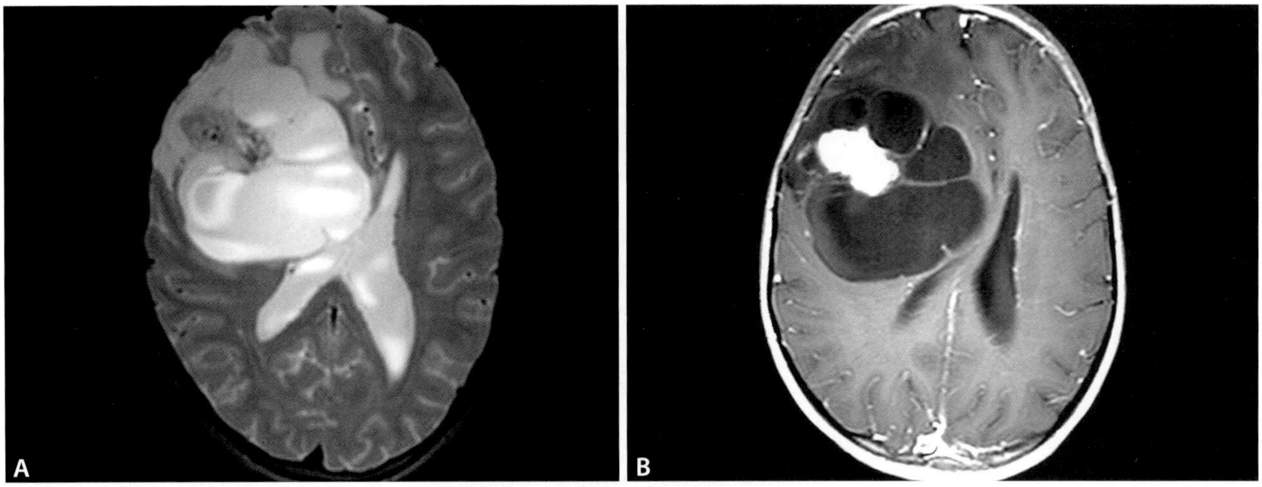

Figs. 12A and B: Ependymoma: Axial T2-WI (A) shows a solid-cystic mass in right juxtaventricular region. The solid portion enhances intensely with contrast (B).

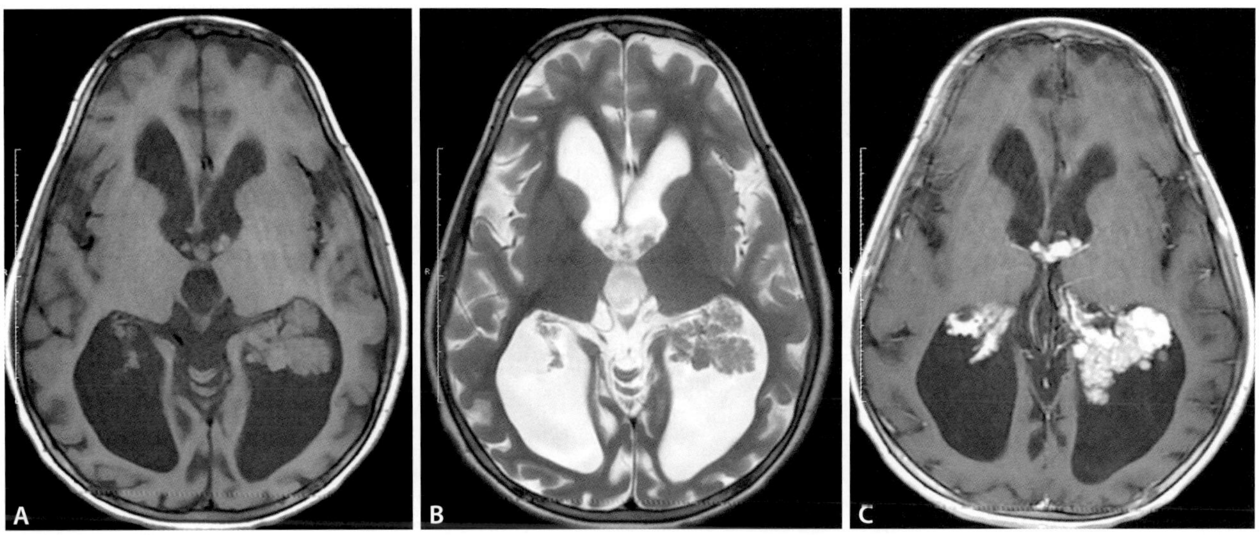

Figs. 13A to C: Choroid plexus papilloma: Axial T1-WI (A) and T2-WI (B) show frond-like intraventricular lesion in both lateral ventricles (left larger than right) with hydrocephalus. The lesions are isointense in T1-WI (A) and T2-WI and enhances intensely with contrast (C).

(Figs. 13A to C), CPPs show lobulations at the peripheral margin (frond-like morphology), masses usually are isointense to brain on T1WI and iso to slightly hyperintense on T2WI. Calcification is not normally appreciated on spin echo pulse sequences. They enhance intensely and homogeneously. Many choroid plexus tumors are attached by a vascular pedicle to the choroid plexus.

All ventricles usually enlarge with trigonal CPPs. Hemorrhage and cyst formation may be seen.

Choroid Plexus Carcinoma

Choroid plexus carcinoma may be difficult to differentiate from CPP on imaging or even on histopathology unless evidence of brain invasion is seen. They occur almost exclusively in young children. Compared to CPP, they show heterogeneous enhancement.

NEURONAL AND MIXED NEURONAL-GLIAL TUMORS

Dysembryoplastic Neuroepithelial Tumor

Dysembryoplastic neuroepithelial tumors (DNET) are benign (WHO grade 1), slow growing mixed glioneuronal tumor. The arise from either cortical or deep gray matter. Children and young adults are commonly affected and present with intractable epilepsy. The "specific glioneuronal element" is characteristic pathological feature. Association cortical dysplasia in seen in up to 80%

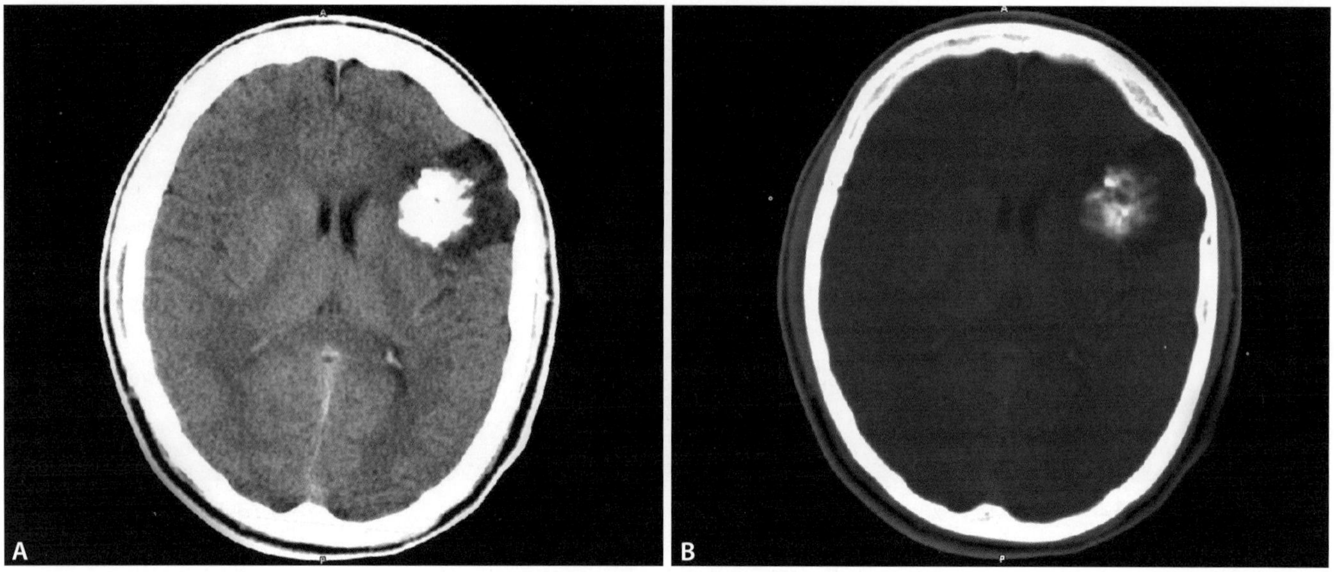

Figs. 14A and B: Dysembryoplastic neuropithelial tumor (DNET): Axial CT (A) shows mixed density lesion in left frontal lobe. The medial portion of lesion is calcified; the lateral portion is hypodense causing scalloping of overlying bone (B). Note that no perilesional edema or commensurate mass effect is seen.

of cases. Temporal lobe is most common location followed by frontal lobe and caudate nucleus.

Imaging Features

These tumors are hypodense on CT scan, but are slightly denser than CSF. Contrast enhancement or calcification is reported in 20% of cases **(Figs. 14A and B)** MR scans show focal intracortical lesion most commonly located in the temporal lobe.[24] The tumor is hypointense on T1 and hyperintense on T2WI with well demarcated margins and lacks peritumoral edema **(Figs. 15A to D)**. The lesion often follows gyriform pattern. The mass effect is not commensurate with the size of the lesion. Compared with ganglioglioma, DNET is less likely to show enhancement and calcification and 'bubbly' appearance is not seen in ganglioglioma.

Ganglioglioma

Gangliogliomas are usually benign WHO grade I CNS tumors. This tumor has a very high prevalence in patients with chronic epilepsy. It is most common in temporal lobe followed by frontal, parietal and occipital lobes. Grossly and at histology it has been found to be frequently associated with cortical dysplasia. Typically it manifests with cyst and solid enhancing nodule **(Figs. 16A to C)** or a solid mass expanding overlying gyrus. Calcification is found in about 30–40% of cases. Solid non-calcified portion show enhancement in approximately 50% cases.

Central Neurocytoma

Central neurocytoma are WHO grade II intraventricular tumor. They generally occur at young age (range of 17 to 53 years).

Imaging Features

Central neurocytoma appears as inhomogeneous, partially calcified (typically punctate in over 50%) mass; typically located in the lateral ventricles adjacent to the foramen of Monro with broad attachment to the septum pellucidum. Most of the tumors, esp, large one contain multiple small cysts and areas of hemorrhage. Ventricular dilation is present in most cases. They show mild-moderate enhancement **(Figs. 17A to C)**. If appropriate staining with immunohistochemical examinations is not performed the lesion will be mistaken for an oligodendroglioma. IDH mutation and 1p/19q co-deletion, genetic signature of oligodendroglioma, are absent.

PINEAL REGION TUMORS

Pineal Germinoma and Teratoma

These account for 55% of all pineal tumors. They are described together as they have common imaging features. On CT, these tumors appear as slightly hyperdense masses which surround and engulf a calcified pineal gland **(Figs. 18A to D)**. On CECT, intense and uniform enhancement

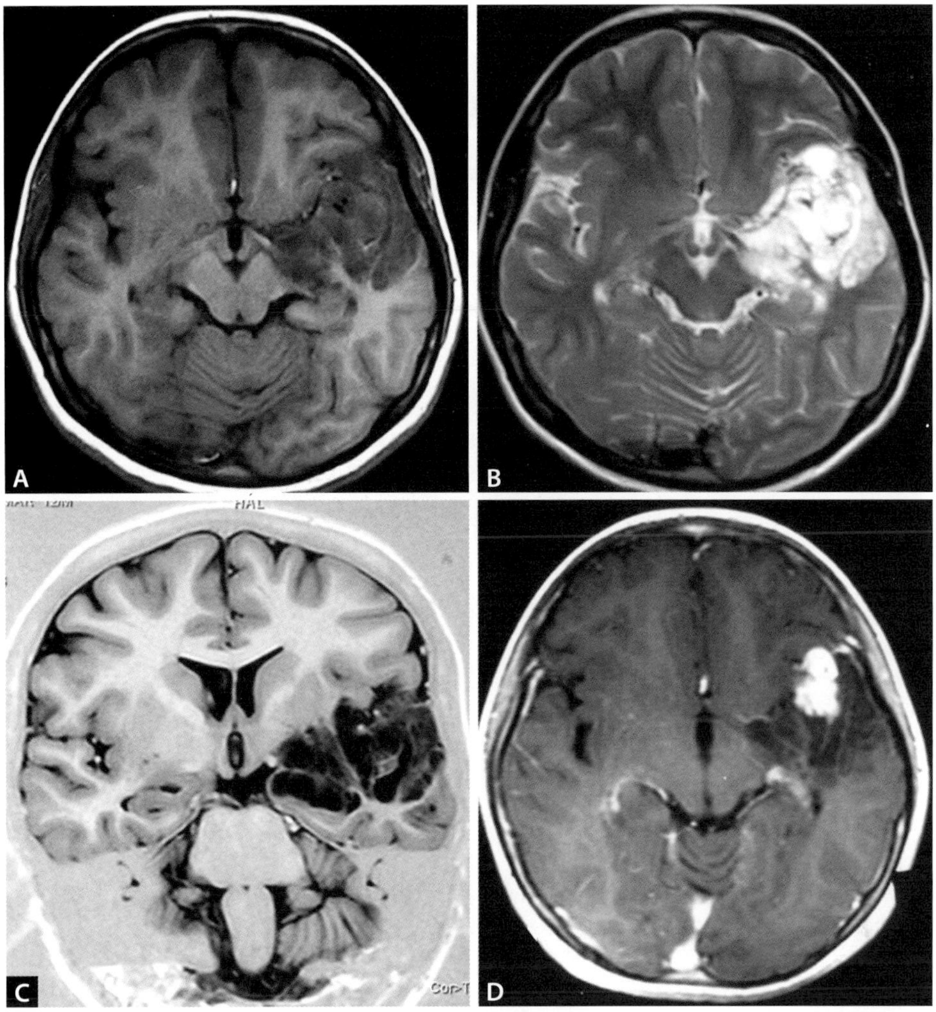

Figs. 15A to D: DNET-MRI: Axial T1-WI (A), T2-WI (B) and coronal T1-IR image (C) show a cortical-based lesion in left temporal lobe. The lesion is hypointense on T1-WI (A) and T1-IR image (C) and hyperintense on T2-WI (B) and is following gyriform pattern. Note that no perilesional edema or commensurate mass effect is seen. The anteromedial portion of lesion enhances with contrast (D).

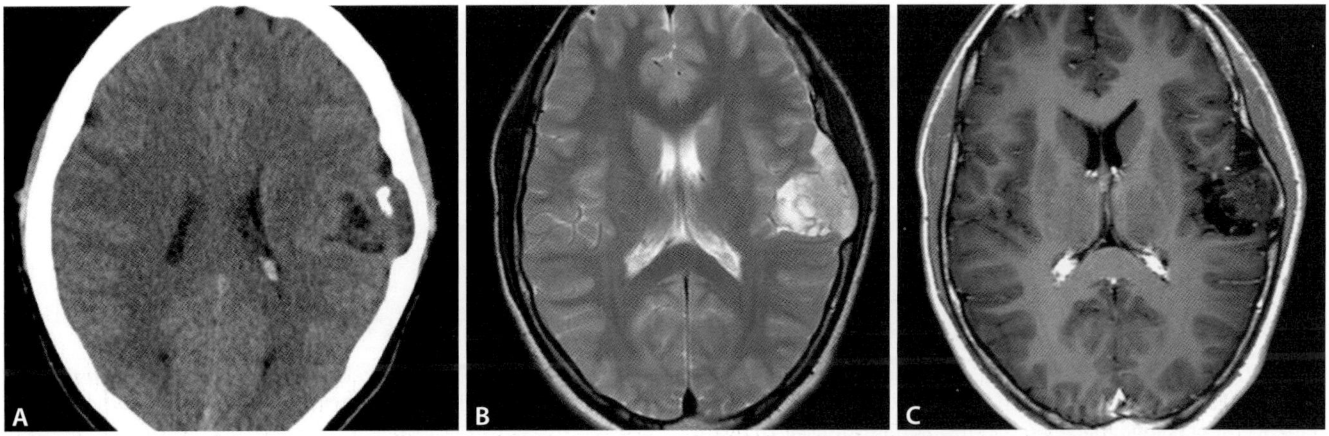

Figs. 16A to C: Ganglioglioma: CECT (A) and T2-WI (B) show a solid-cystic lesion in left temporal lobe. On CT, the mass is having focal calcification and causing scalloping of overlying skull. Minimal enhancement is seen following contrast administration (C).

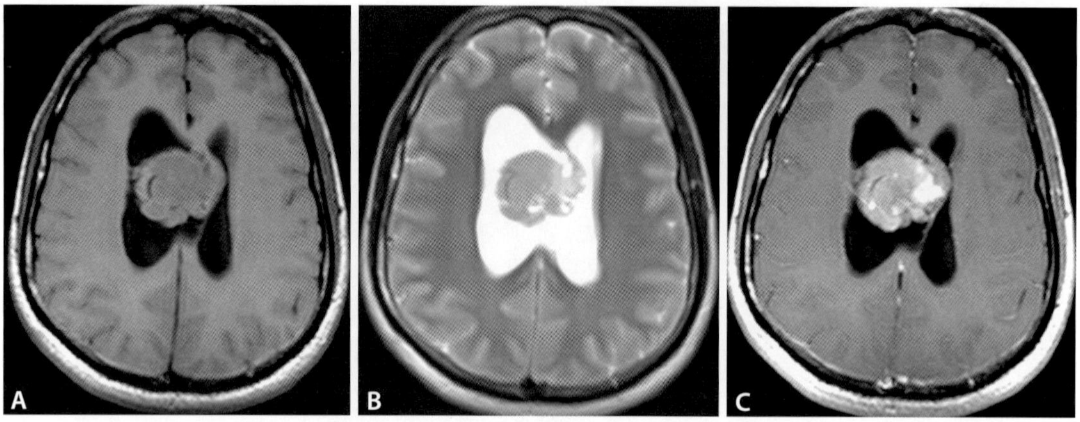

Figs. 17A to C: Central neurocytoma: Axial T1-WI (A) and T2-WI (B) show a intraventricular lesion in right lateral ventricle. The lesions are isointense in T1-WI (A) and T2-WI and enhances heterogeneously with contrast (C).

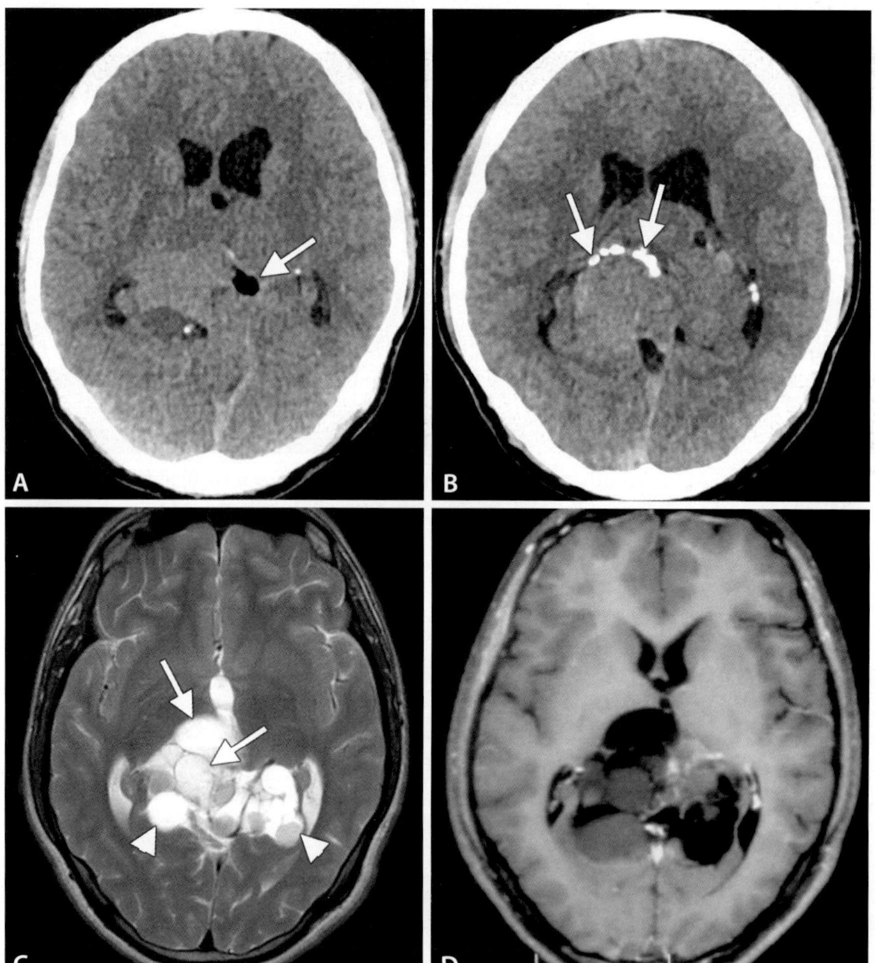

Figs. 18A to D: Pineal teratoma: CECTs (A and B) show a mixed-signal intensity lesion in pineal region with foci of fat density (arrow in A) and calcifications (arrows in B). On MRI, T2-WI (C) shows multiple cysts of varying signal intensity (arrows and arrowheads). No enhancement is seen following contrast administration (D).

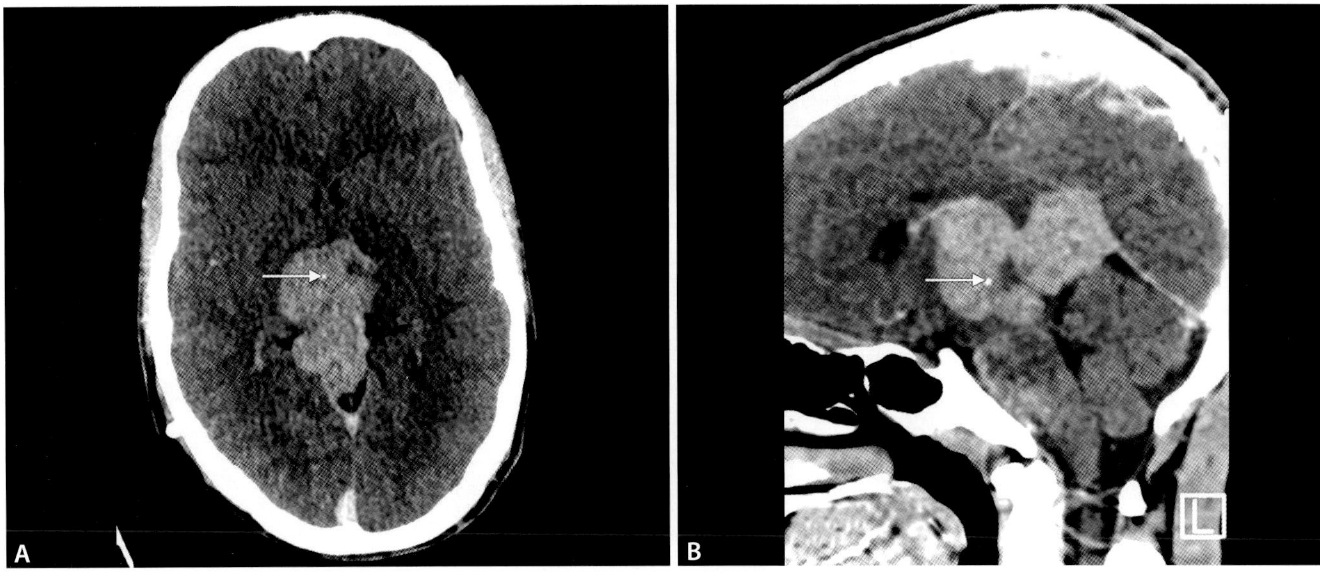

Figs. 19A and B: Pineal germinoma. Axial (A) and reconstructed coronal (B) CT show a homogeneously enhancing pineal mass lesion engulfing pineal calcification (arrow in A and B).

is seen in germinomas **(Figs. 19A and B)**. They often have secondary implants in the third ventricular recesses. Diffuse ependymal and subarachnoid spread is common. Teratoma may have heterogeneous appearance because of calcification. On MRI, the germinoma is isointense with cortex on all pulse sequences, and appears homogeneously hyperintense on post Gd T1WI.

Pineal Cell Tumors

Pineal parenchymal tumors represent less than 15% of all pineal region tumors. These are of two types: (i) Pineocytoma, and (ii) Pineoblastoma.

Pineocytoma

Pineocytomas are uncommon slow growing, WHO grade I tumors accounting for only 0.4–1% of all primary brain tumors. Average age of presentation is 34 years. Unlike other pineal neoplasms there is no male predominance.

Imaging features: They generally appear as well-circumscribed mass with less than 3 cm size. The mass is iso- to hyperdense on NCCT, iso to hypointense on T1WI and hyperintense on T2WI.[25] Following contrast administration, characteristically intense homogenous enhancement is seen. Like other pineal parenchymal tumors, pineal calcification is displaced peripherally. Small cystic tumors may resemble benign pineal cysts on imaging studies.

Pineoblastoma

Pineoblastomas are uncommon malignant WHO grade IV tumors, typically found in young children with slight female predilection.

Imaging features: On imaging, pineoblastoma appear as large (>4 cm) irregular mass, hyperdense on NCCT, iso to hypointense on T1 and isointense on T2. The diffusion is restricted due to high cellularity.[25] Area of cyst formation and necrosis may be present. The tumor shows intense heterogeneous enhancement. Leptomeningeal spread may be present in 45% of cases **(Figs. 20A to E)**.[25]

TUMORS OF CRANIAL AND PARASPINAL NERVE

Schwannomas and neurofibromas are the commonest tumors arising from the cranial nerves.

Schwannoma (Cellular/Plexiform)

Schwannomas account for 6–8% of primary brain tumors. They are seen in the fourth to sixth decades. These tumors are most commonly seen in relation to VIIIth cranial nerve. The Vth, VIIth IIIrd and VIth cranial nerves are the other nerves which can be affected. On CT, they appear as sharply delineated masses. Smaller lesion show homogeneous enhancement, while larger lesions appear heterogeneous. On MRI 60% of the tumors appear hypointense on T1WI and 34% are isointense. On

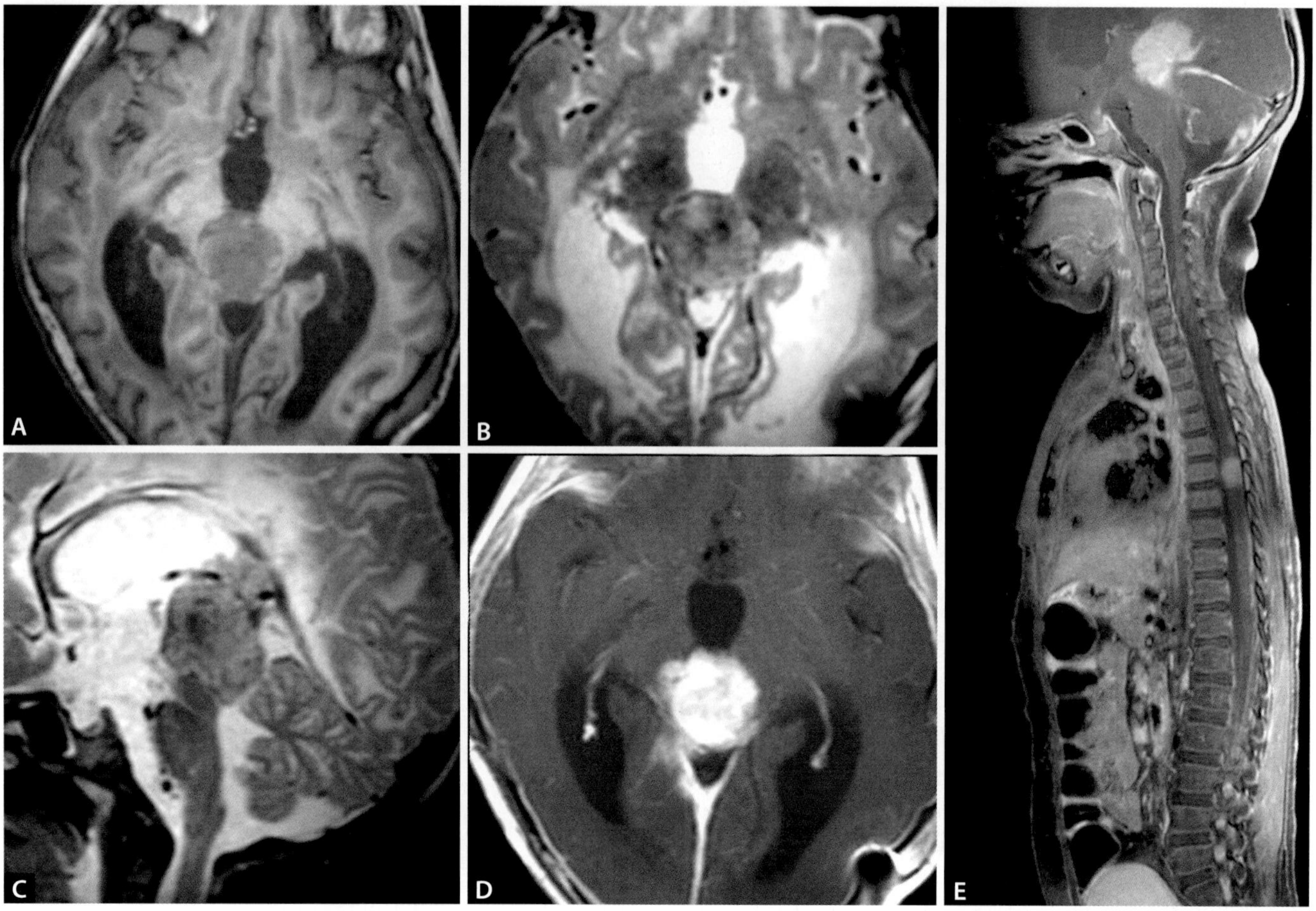

Figs. 20A to E: Pineoblastoma: Axial T1-WI (A), T2-WI (B) and sagittal T2-WI (C) show a large ill-defined pineal region mass. The lesions are isointense in T1-WI (a) and T2-WI and enhances intensely with contrast (D), Sagittal T1-WI (E) of spine show multiple leptomeningeal deposits suggestive of CSF dissemination.

T2WI these tumors are hyperintense. They enhance after contrast administration.

Neurofibroma (Atypical/ Plexiform)

Neurofibromas are uncommon tumors affecting the cranial nerves, except when associated with the constellation of lesions of neurofibromatosis type I. They are encountered in any age group and predominantly affect cutaneous and spinal nerves. In the head and neck the ophthalmic division of the Vth nerve is commonly affected.

On CT, these tumors are poorly delineated. These are infiltrative lesions which shows homogeneous enhancement. On MR they are isointense with muscle on T1WI and hyperintense to muscle on T2WI. Unlike schwannomas they enhance moderately after contrast enhancement.

TUMORS OF THE MENINGES

Meningioma

Meningiomas form 15% of all intracranial tumors, predominantly occurring in 40 to 60 yrs age group with definite female predominance (M:F = 1:2 to 1:4). Most frequent sites are parasagittal (25%) convexity (20%), sphenoid ridge (15–20%), olfactory groove (5–10%), parasellar (5–10%), and posterior fossa (10%). Rarely meningiomas may occur at extracranial sites such as nose, sinus, and orbit (1%). Atypical meningiomas are more common in children than in adults and likely to be malignant than those in adults, and are frequently associated with neurofibromatosis.

Multiple meningiomas have been reported in up to 10% of cases.

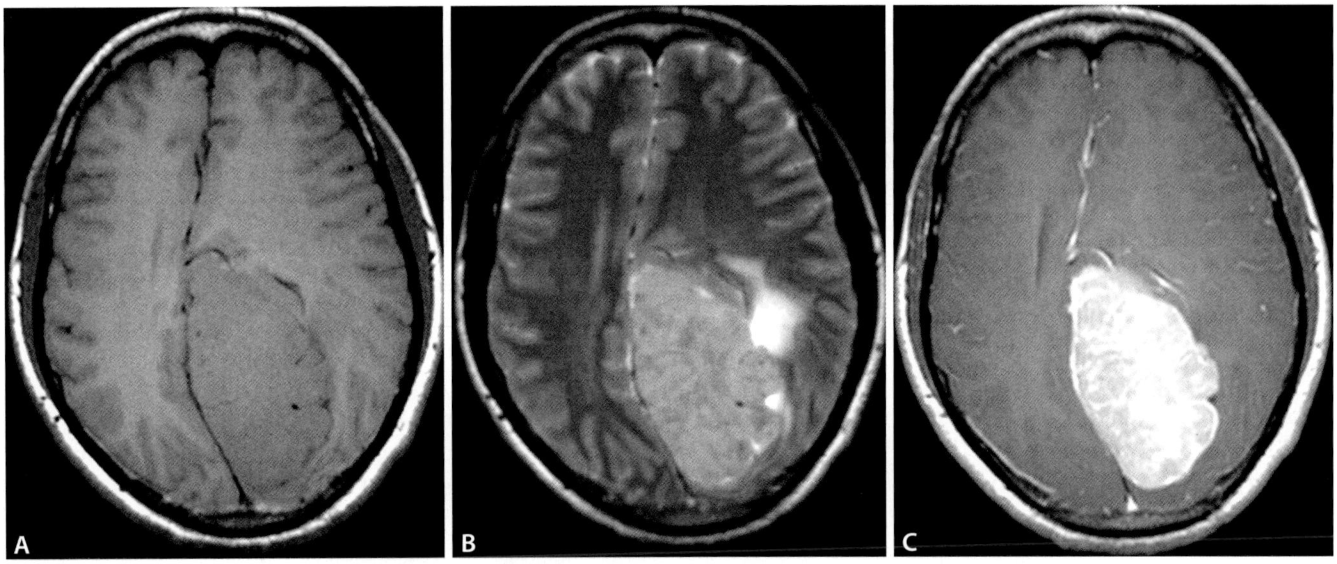

Figs. 21A to C: Meningioma: Axial T1-WI (A) and T2-WI (B) show a large extra-axial left parafalcine mass. The lesions are isointense in T1-WI (A) and T2-WI and enhances intensely with contrast (C).

Imaging Features

On plain films hyperostosis or erosion of overlying bone, enlarged vascular grooves, tumor calcification and pneumosinus dilatans indicate presence of a meningioma.

On angiography dual vascular supply is common (dural to the central and pial to the periphery of the tumor). Sunburst pattern of enlarged dural feeders in the tumor is characteristic along with prolonged vascular homogeneous stain.

On CT meningiomas are hyperdense in 75% of cases, 90% enhance intensely and uniformly and 20–30% calcify. In 60% of cases peritumoral edema is encountered. Hemorrhage occurs in about 5% of cases. Degenerative parenchymal cysts and trapped arachnoid cysts between the meningioma and adjacent brain may occasionally be found.

On MRI meningiomas exhibit typical features of extra axial tumors. Gray white matter "buckling" or displacement, a cleft or pseudocapsule of CSF and vessels surrounding the mass separating it from brain characterize the extraaxial location of these tumors. The presence of a "dural tail" in 60% of cases on contrast enhanced MRI is highly suggestive but not pathognomonic of meningioma.

It is seen as homogeneously enhancing dural thickening extending from the margin of the meningioma and may be due either to extension of the tumor or to reactive change in the dura. MR imaging is superior to CT in assessing vascular encasement, particularly of the internal carotid arteries in lesions around the skull base. It is also superior in assessing the patency of the venous sinuses, notably the sagittal sinus, which may be invaded by parafalcine meningiomas. 95% of meningiomas show enhancement which is usually homogenous and intense **(Figs. 21A to C)**. Meningiomas tend to be isointense with gray matter on all pulse sequences. Thirty percent to 40% are mildly hypointense on T1WI and mildly hyperintense on T2WI.

Intraventricular meningiomas are usually in the lateral ventricle but can manifest in the third and fourth ventricles. They arise from the arachnoidal cap cell rest within the stroma of the choroid plexus. Although large majority of meningiomas have characteristic imaging features, there are at times lesions that mimic meningiomas. These include schwannomas, gliosarcomas, metastasis, dural vascular malformations associated with venous ectasia, fungal masses and extramedullary hematopoiesis in the skull vault.

MESENCHYMAL, NON-MENINGOTHELIAL TUMORS

Solitary Fibrous Tumor/Hemangiopericytoma

Solitary fibrous tumors/hemangiopericytoma are rare dural masses, histologically identical to solitary fibrous tumors found elsewhere. In the 2016 update to the WHO classification of brain tumors, solitary fibrous tumors of the dura and hemangiopericytomas are considered to be one entity with variable morphology. They are composed of spindle cells thought to be of mesenchymal origin. They usually occur in middle-aged individuals and symptoms depend on the size of the mass and its location.

On imaging, these tumors appear as extra-axial well circumscribed solid masses with intense contrast enhancement thereby mimicking meningiomas **(Figs. 22A to D)**. They are iso-hypointense on T2WI which may suggest diagnosis.

On MRI, these tumors are well-circumscribed, lobular, homogeneously enhancing masses with broad dural attachments that may be indistinguishable from meningioma.[26]

Ewing's Sarcoma

Primary CNS Ewing sarcoma are rare lesions that involve the CNS by extension from dura, bone, or paraspinal soft tissue. The peak incidence is in adolescence.

LYMPHOMA

Primary Lymphoma of the CNS

These tumors account for 1 to 2% of all primary CNS neoplasms. The incidence of these tumors is rising rapidly in both AIDS and non-AIDS patients. Peak incidence is in sixth decade in immunocompetent and in the third decade in immunocompromised patients. Primary malignant lymphoma is a non-Hodgkin's lymphoma that occurs in the brain in the absence of systemic involvement.

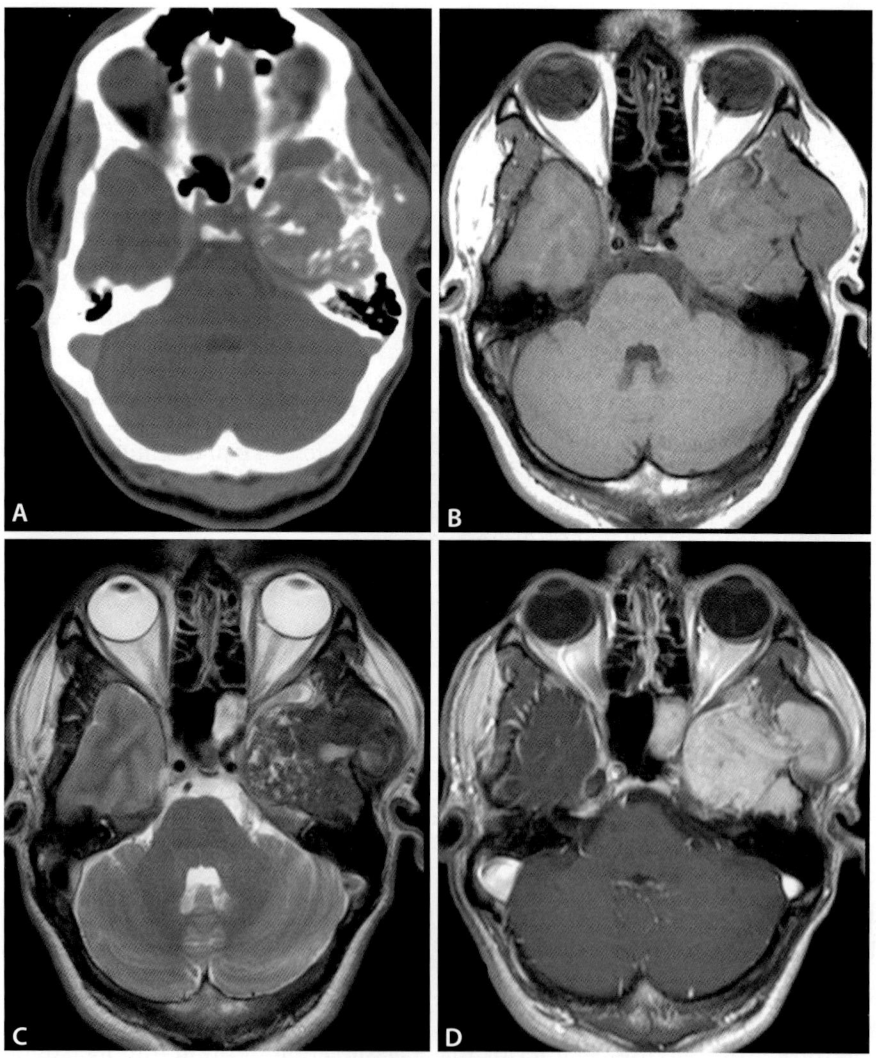

Figs. 22A to D: Solitary fibrous tumor: CT bone window (A), axial T1-WI (B) and T2-WI (C) show extra-axial lesion involving left temporal bone. The mass has foci of calcification and extending to scalp. The lesions are isointense in T1-WI (B) and markedly hypointense on T2-WI (C) and enhances intensely with contrast (D).

CNS lymphoma typically involves deep white matter in the periventricular area (frontal and parietal lobes, basal ganglia, thalami, hypothalamus, and corpus callosum). Believed to arise from periadventitial cells of penetrating arterioles.[27]

Imaging Features

On NCCT, primary CNS lymphomas appear as isodense lesions in two third of cases and hyperdense in remaining one third cases. They may be solitary or multiple in as many as 50% **(Figs. 23A to F)** Have a propensity to extend across the corpus callosum into the opposite hemisphere. Vasogenic edema is usually minimal. Enhancement is homogeneous **(Figs. 23A to F)** in 70% of cases, in AIDS or posterior fossa lesions; ring enhancement is seen in 20% of cases. Calcification is not seen, and hemorrhage is uncommon. On MRI, lymphomas tend to be isointense to gray matter in all spin echo sequences.[28] Intravascular or infiltrative lymphomas may be markedly hyperintense on T2-WI. Restricted diffusion and low ADC value on DWI is due to its high cellularity and restricted diffusion matches T2 abnormality. Lymphomas show dense and homogenous enhancement in most immunocompetent patients; ependymal and perivascular enhancement suggest lymphoma. Necrosis, hemorrhage and inhomogeneous or ring enhancement are features of lymphoma in immunodeficiency patients, but may be seen in EBV-positive tumors in immunocompetent patients.[28] Infiltrative and intravascular lymphomas may not enhance.

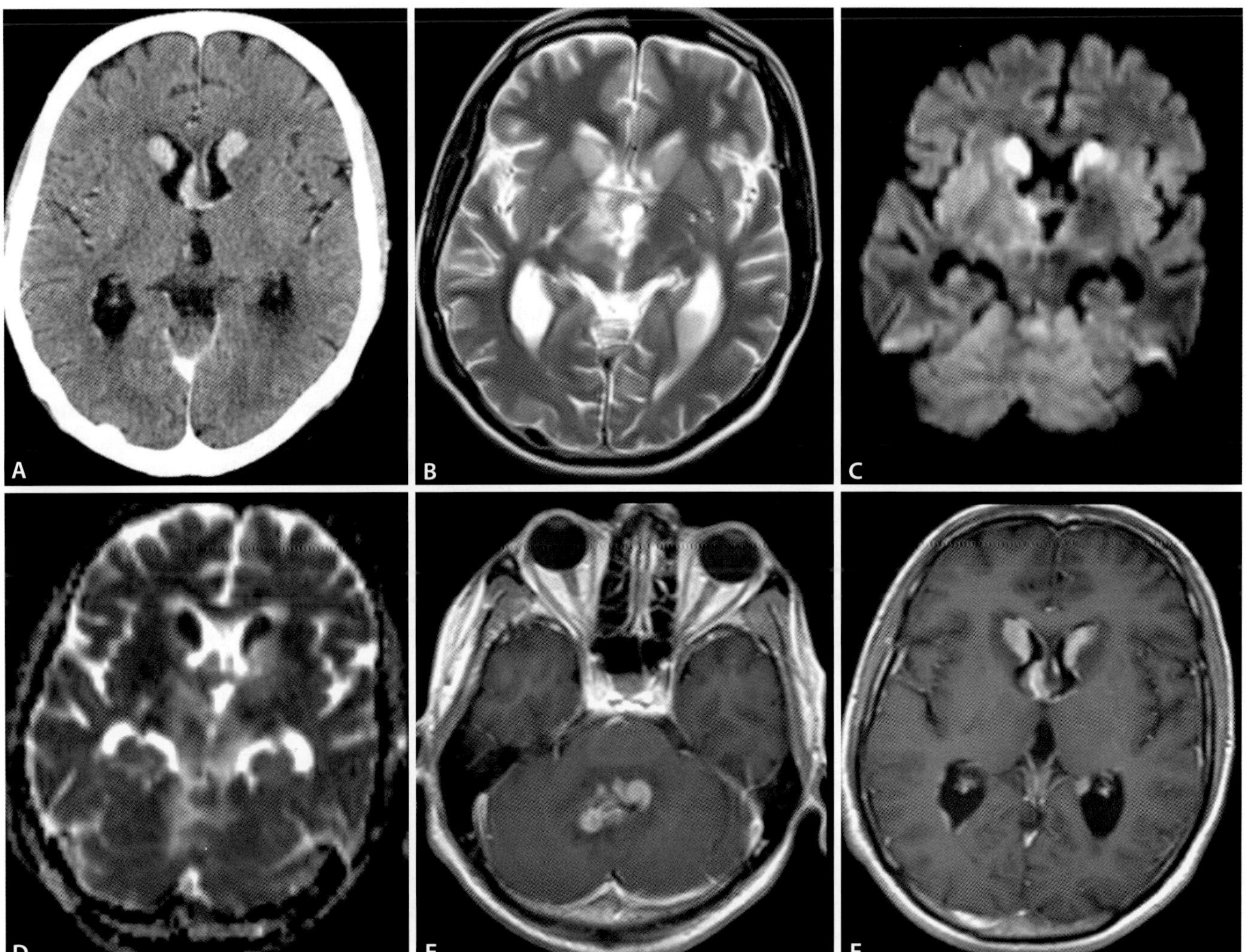

Figs. 23A to F: Primary CNS lymphoma: CECT (A) shows multiple enhancing periventricular lesions. These lesions are isointense on T2-WI (B), bright on diffusion trace image (C), dark on ADC maps (D) and enhancing with contrast (E and F). The lesions are distributed in both supratentorial and infratentorial compartment.

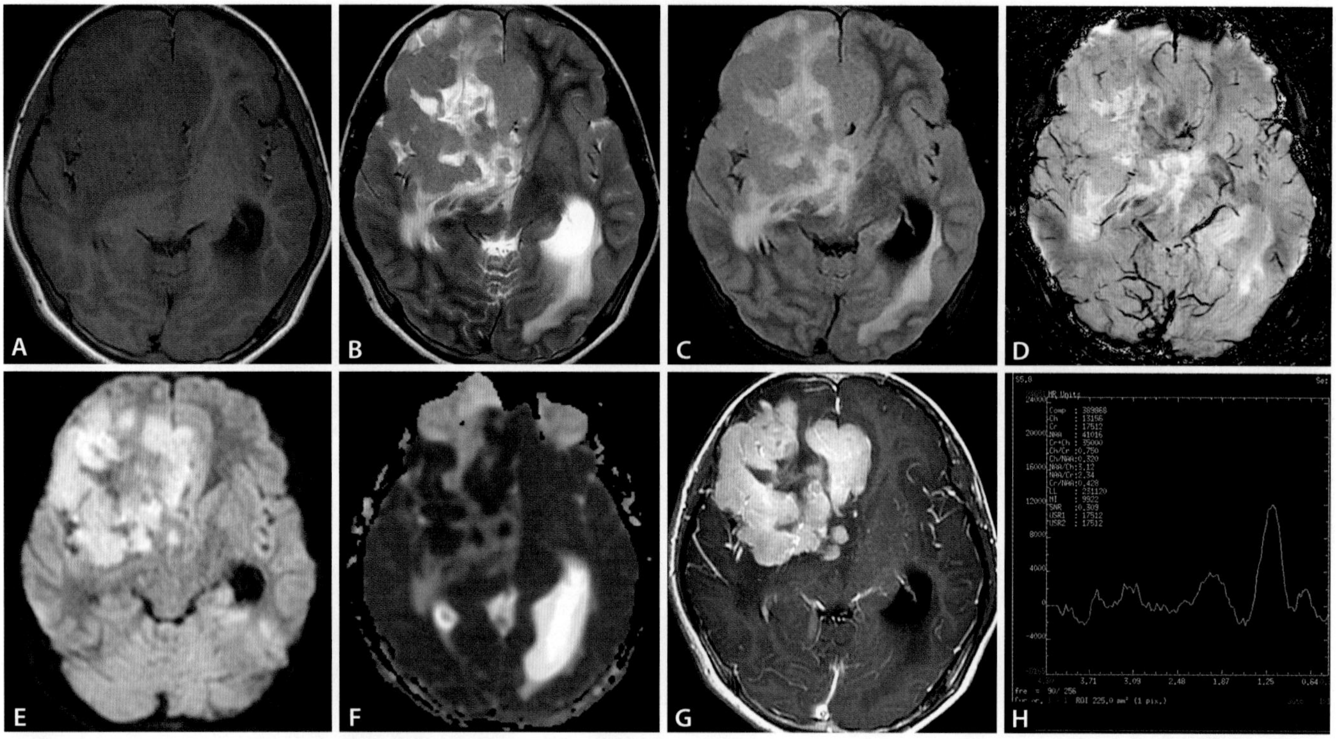

Figs. 24A to H: Primary CNS lymphoma. Large T1 (A) and T2 (B) isointense lesion with perilesional edema is present in right frontal lobe (C). No foci of hemorrhages are seen on SWI (D). The lesion is bright on diffusion trace image (E), dark on ADC maps (F) and is enhancing with contrast (G). On MRS from the solid enhancing portion, lipid is seen (H).

MR spectral pattern of lymphomas is similar to malignant brain tumors and reveal elevated signals of lipid, lactate, and choline and reduced NAA, creatinine, and myo-inositol signals. Presence of lipids in solid enhancing tumor suggest lymphoma **(Figs. 24A to H)**.[29] MRS can help in differentiating lymphoma from toxoplasmosis, which typically has elevated lactate and lipid signals but absence of the other metabolites in MR.

Differentiation of lymphoma and primary high-grade glial neoplasm is possible using multimodal imaging. Lymphoma tends to have a lower ADC, lower FA and typically lower rCBV. Rarely rCBV in lymphomas may be high, but low ADC values in matching areas of T2 abnormalities and contrast enhancement, and lipid in solid enhancing region help to clinch the diagnosis. Lymphoma tends to show higher rCBV compared with toxoplasmosis.

Cerebral lymphomas are highly radiosensitive and respond dramatically to steroid therapy. Following steroid treatment, restricted diffusion may not be seen.

Immunodeficiency-associated CNS lymphoma

Immunodeficiency-associated CNS lymphoma is seen in organ transplant recipients, patients with congenital immunodeficiency syndrome and patients with AIDS. Incidence of AIDS-related lymphomas is decreasing in patient who receive antiretroviral therapy.[30] Pattern is modified somewhat in AIDS-related lymphoma. Multiplicity seems to be more common. Lymphomas exhibit more aggressive behavior and readily outgrow their blood supply. As a result, central necrosis and ring enhancement are often seen in lymphomatous masses in AIDS patients.

METASTATIC TUMORS

Intracranial metastases may be either parenchymal or extra-axial. Extra-axial metastasis may be epidural, dural or leptomeningeal.

Epidural metastases are nearly always associated with adjacent osseous metastases with spread to the epidural space.

Parenchymal Metastases

Intra-axial metastasis form 13 to 41% of all intra-cranial tumors. Common primary tumors which metastasize to brain are from the lung, breast, melanoma, gastrointestinal tract, and kidney.

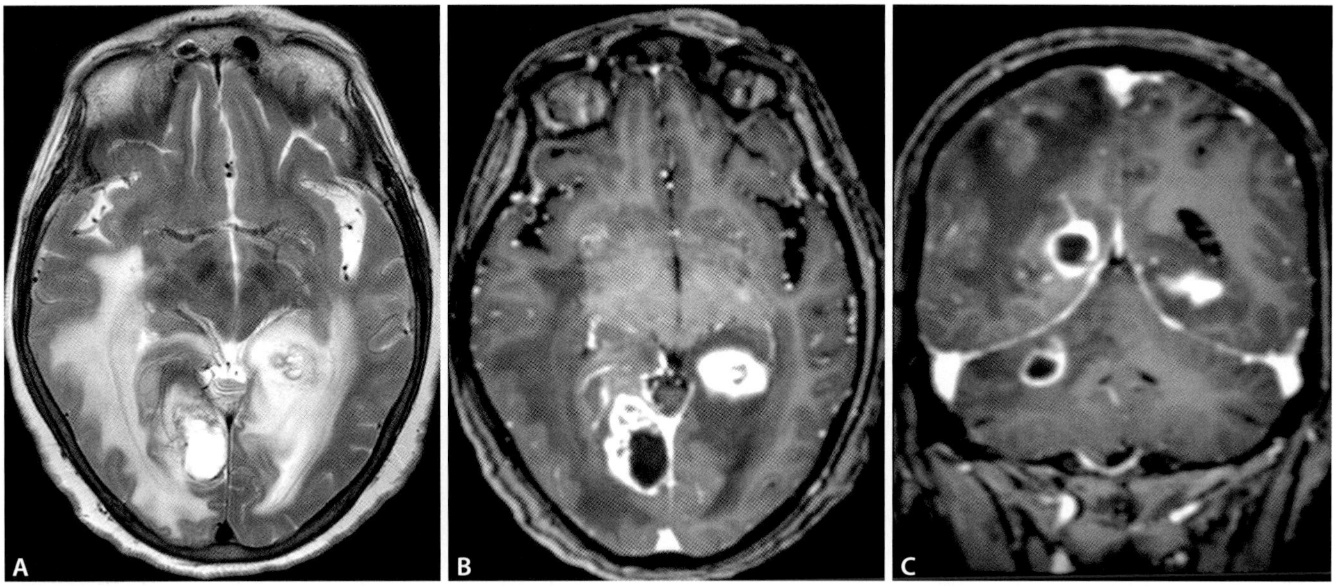

Figs. 25A to C: Metastases. T2-WI (A) shows ring lesions in both occipital lobes with marked edema. These lesions enhances with contrast (B and C). Another ring-enhancing lesion is seen in right cerebellar hemisphere.

More than 60 to 70% metastases are multiple. Solitary (30-40%) are associated with lung and renal carcinomas. Metastases can occur at any site; however, most common site is the gray-white matter junction. The cause of this preferential location is related to abrupt reduction of the diameter of arterioles at this point causing arrest of tumor emboli at this location.

Imaging Features

On NCCT, metastases are usually hypodense and occasionally isodense. Hyperdensity is common and may be due to hemorrhage–especially in secondaries from Choriocarcinoma, melanoma and renal carcinoma, tumor cellularity or contents (melanoma or mucin secreting tumors) and rarely calcification.

Typically, disproportionate and extensive vasogenic edema exists with metastases. CECT reveals cortical metastases and metastases in the white matter that are less than 1 cm in diameter as intense homogenous nodular or ring enhancement with central non-enhancing area caused by cystic degeneration or necrosis. The blood-brain barrier does not exist for metastatic lesions because they recruit their own vascular supply. Contrast-enhanced MRI is the most sensitive modality for detecting cerebral metastases. Metastases are usually hypointense to gray matter and enhance following contrast administration **(Figs. 25A to C)**.

Typical MR spectroscopic features for secondary neoplasms include elevated signals of lipid, lactate, and choline and reduced or absent NAA signal. Primary neoplasms have the propensity to infiltrate surrounding brain tissue; interrogation of areas outside the enhancing portion of the lesion has proved to be promising. The ADC values of metastatic lesions are variable and overlap with those of primary neoplasms. However, it is possible to separate metastasis from primary brain neoplasm by measuring ADC values in the peritumoral regions. Peritumoral diffusion-tensor imaging tends to show lower ADC values in regions of peritumoral "edema" compared with those seen with metastatic disease. Perfusion parameters of metastatic lesions tend to overlap with those of high-grade neoplasms, probably because of their similarity in the degree of angiogenesis. One possible feature that might allow differentiation between secondary and primary neoplasms is that metastatic lesions have lower rCBV measurements outside their enhancing portion, compared with those of the more infiltrative primary neoplasms.

Leptomeningeal Metastases

Leptomeningeal metastases are commonly seen in leukemia, lymphoma, carcinoma of breast, and lung and melanoma. Few primary brain tumors also have leptomeningeal spread pattern like GBM, ependymomas and pineoblastomas. The arachnoid membrane usually provides a barrier to leptomeningeal and parenchymal spread from the dura.

Leptomeningeal involvement is graded as follows:

Type A: Tumor deposited in leptomeninges.

Type B: Minor infiltration into the cortex.

Type C: Edema associated with invasion into the parenchyma.

Type D: invasion into perineural spaces which at times can simulate a benign neurogenic tumor such as-schwannomas.

Imaging Features

Contrast enhanced MR imaging is a more sensitive study than CT and may demonstrate abnormal meningeal enhancement, diffuse or irregular plaque like or nodular deposits along the cortical surface or cisterns.

Dural Metastases

Isolated dural metastases are rare, usually associated with skull lesions and are secondary to hematogenous spread. Sometime solitary focal dural metastases may mimic meningioma. Most common sites of primary are breast, lung, and kidney.

Calvarial Metastases

CT is still believed by many to be the most sensitive modality for detection of bony calvarial metastases, however, MRI with contrast is superior for detecting subtle intradiploic lesions, for delineating lesion extent and determining involvement of underlying dura or brain. Most common primaries which metastasize to the calvarium are breast followed by lungs, prostate and lymphoma.

CONCLUSION

Supratentorial brain tumors are a diverse group of neoplasms and in this chapter most common neoplasm are covered with stress on their imaging features. There are few recent advanced techniques like diffusion and perfusion MR imaging, MR spectroscopy and positron-emission tomography. These techniques are still evolving and certainly helpful in solving diagnostic dilemmas.

REFERENCES

1. Kleihues P, Burger PC, Scheithauer BW. The new WHO classification of brain tumours. Brain Pathol. 1993;3(3):255-68.
2. Louis DN, Perry A, Reifenberger G, et al. The 2016 World Health Organization Classification of Tumors of the Central Nervous System: a summary. Acta Neuropathol. 2016;131(6):803-20.
3. Lasocki A, Gaillard F, Gorelik A, et al. MRI Features Can Predict 1p/19q Status in Intracranial Gliomas. American Journal of Neuroradiology. 2018.
4. Cha S. Update on brain tumor imaging: from anatomy to physiology. Am J Neuroradiol. 2006;27(3):475-87.
5. Hilario A, Ramos A, Perez-Nunez A, et al. The added value of apparent diffusion coefficient to cerebral blood volume in the preoperative grading of diffuse gliomas. Am J Neuroradiol. 2012;33(4):701-7.
6. Law M, Yang S, Babb JS, et al. Comparison of cerebral blood volume and vascular permeability from dynamic susceptibility contrast-enhanced perfusion MR imaging with glioma grade. Am J Neuroradiol. 2004;25(5):746-55.
7. Aihara K, Mukasa A, Gotoh K, et al. H3F3A K27M mutations in thalamic gliomas from young adult patients. Neuro Oncol. 2014;16(1):140-6.
8. Buczkowicz P, Bartels U, Bouffet E, et al. Histopathological spectrum of paediatric diffuse intrinsic pontine glioma: diagnostic and therapeutic implications. Acta Neuropathol. 2014;128(4):573-81.
9. Johnson DR, Diehn FE, Giannini C, et al. Genetically Defined Oligodendroglioma Is Characterized by Indistinct Tumor Borders at MRI. Am J Neuroradiol. 2017;38(4):678-84.
10. Collins VP, Jones DT, Giannini C. Pilocytic astrocytoma: pathology, molecular mechanisms and markers. Acta Neuropathol. 2015;129(6):775-88.
11. Hawkins C, Walker E, Mohamed N, et al. BRAF-KIAA1549 fusion predicts better clinical outcome in pediatric low-grade astrocytoma. Clin Cancer Res. 2011;17(14):4790-8.
12. Li HM, Hsu SS, Wang JS, et al. Cerebral pilocytic astrocytoma with spontaneous intracranial hemorrhage in adults. J Chin Med Assoc. 2008;71(11):587-93.
13. Shepherd CW, Scheithauer BW, Gomez MR, et al. Subependymal giant cell astrocytoma: a clinical, pathological, and flow cytometric study. Neurosurgery. 1991;28(6):864-8.
14. O'Callaghan FJ, Martyn CN, Renowden S, et al. Subependymal nodules, giant cell astrocytomas and the tuberous sclerosis complex: a population-based study. Arch Dis Child. 2008;93(9):751-4.
15. Rovira A, Ruiz-Falco ML, Garcia-Esparza E, et al. Recommendations for the radiological diagnosis and follow-up of neuropathological abnormalities associated with tuberous sclerosis complex. J Neurooncol. 2014;118(2):205-23.
16. Crespo-Rodriguez AM, Smirniotopoulos JG, Rushing EJ. MR and CT imaging of 24 pleomorphic xanthoastrocytomas (PXA) and a review of the literature. Neuroradiology. 2007;49(4):307-15.
17. Yu S, He L, Zhuang X, et al. Pleomorphic xanthoastrocytoma: MR imaging findings in 19 patients. Acta Radiol. 2011;52(2):223-8.
18. Moore W, Mathis D, Gargan L, et al. Pleomorphic xanthoastrocytoma of childhood: MR imaging and diffusion MR imaging features. Am J Neuroradiol. 2014;35(11):2192-6.
19. Spoto GP, Press GA, Hesselink JR, et al. Intracranial ependymoma and subependymoma: MR manifestations. Am J Roentgenol. 1990;154(4):837-45.
20. Koeller KK, Sandberg GD, Armed Forces Institute of P. From the archives of the AFIP. Cerebral intraventricular

neoplasms: radiologic-pathologic correlation. Radiographics. 2002;22(6):1473-505.
21. Yuh EL, Barkovich AJ, Gupta N. Imaging of ependymomas: MRI and CT. Childs Nerv Syst. 2009;25(10):1203-13.
22. Yanaka K, Kamezaki T, Kobayashi E, et al. MR imaging of diffuse glioma. Am J Neuroradiol. 1992;13(1):349-51.
23. Smith AB, Smirniotopoulos JG, Horkanyne-Szakaly I. From the radiologic pathology archives: intraventricular neoplasms: radiologic-pathologic correlation. Radiographics. 2013;33(1):21-43.
24. Reiche W, Feiden W, Eymann R, et al. Dysembryoplastic neuroepithelial tumor-Neuroradiologic findings in common and uncommon sites. International Journal of Neuroradiology. 1997;3(5):428-34.
25. Dumrongpisutikul N, Intrapiromkul J, Yousem DM. Distinguishing between germinomas and pineal cell tumors on MR imaging. Am J Neuroradiol. 2012;33(3):550-5.
26. Pekala JS, Gururangan S, Provenzale JM, et al. Central nervous system extraosseous Ewing sarcoma: radiologic manifestations of this newly defined pathologic entity. Am J Neuroradiol. 2006;27(3):580-3.
27. Jack CR, Jr., O'Neill BP, et al. Central nervous system lymphoma: histologic types and CT appearance. Radiology. 1988;167(1):211-5.
28. Haldorsen IS, Espeland A, Larsson EM. Central nervous system lymphoma: characteristic findings on traditional and advanced imaging. Am J Neuroradiol. 2011;32(6):984-92.
29. Brandao LA, Castillo M. Adult Brain Tumors: Clinical Applications of Magnetic Resonance Spectroscopy. Magn Reson Imaging Clin N Am. 2016;24(4):781-809.
30. Diamond C, Taylor TH, Aboumrad T, et al. Changes in acquired immunodeficiency syndrome-related non-Hodgkin lymphoma in the era of highly active antiretroviral therapy: incidence, presentation, treatment, and survival. Cancer. 2006;106(1):128-35.

CHAPTER 17

Imaging of Infratentorial Tumors

Ajay Garg

INTRODUCTION

The infratentorial tumors include tumors arising from the brain parenchyma (cerebellum and the brainstem), the cranial nerves, the meninges, or the bone. In addition, head and neck neoplasm can extend into the infratentorial compartment.

In children, 48% of primary intracranial neoplasms are infratentorial in location while in adults infratentorial tumors are uncommon.[1] In pediatric infratentorial neoplasms, medulloblastomas and cerebellar astrocytomas account for one-third each; brainstem gliomas represent another one-fourth and ependymomas account for one-eighth of neoplasms.[1] In adults, most of the infratentorial neoplasms are extra-axial in location; vestibular schwannoma is the most common neoplasm followed by meningioma and epidermoid. Among the intra-axial infratentorial neoplasms in adults, metastases are most common followed by hemangioblastoma and glioma.[2]

Magnetic resonance imaging (MRI) is the imaging modality of choice for the assessment of infratentorial neoplasms as it has better soft tissue contrast, multi-planar imaging capability, and potential to provide complementary physiologic information with diffusion-weighted images (DWI), perfusion MRI and susceptibility-weighted images (SWI).[2] Computed tomography (CT) has better sensitivity to detect subtle calcifications within tumors. Once a mass is identified, it must be localized to the intra-axial or the extra-axial compartment. Extra-axial masses typically have well-defined margins, displace normal brain structures causing enlargement of the ipsilateral cistern and have a Cerebrospinal fluid (CSF)-vascular cleft between an the mass and the adjacent normal brain. On the other hand, intra-axial masses lack such clear cut demarcation and blend into the normal brain; and compress sulci and cisterns.

CLASSIFICATION OF INFRATENTORIAL TUMORS BASED ON TOPOGRAPHY

The diagnostic algorithm to differentiate various infratentorial lesions is most easily formulated using the neuroanatomic classification as a starting point. Then imaging characteristics help to narrow down the differential diagnoses **(Table 1)**.

CEREBELLAR HEMISPHERE AND VERMIS

Medulloblastoma

Medulloblastoma (MB) is a malignant primitive ectodermal tumor and is the most common infratentorial tumor in children, accounting for one-third of childhood pediatric tumors. About three-quarters of MBs occur in children 5–15 years old. In adults, though much less common, MBs usually occur in the 3rd and 4th decades of life. MBs are typically midline infratentorial tumors and the most common location is in the region of the vermis and the inferior medullary velum. Cerebellar hemispheric MBs are less frequent and occur primarily in adults. Approximately 80% of patients with MB present with features of raised intracranial pressure. CSF seeding occurs in 10–30% of patients with MB.

Table 1: Classification of infratentorial tumors based on topography and age.

Location	*Age-group*	*Tumor*
Cerebellar hemisphere and vermis	Pediatric	Medulloblastoma, ependymoma, astrocytoma, atypical teratoid/rhabdoid tumor
	Adult	Metastasis, hemangioblastoma, dysplastic cerebellar gangliocytoma, medulloblastoma
Brainstem	Pediatric	Diffuse midline glioma
	Adult	Diffuse midline glioma, GBM
Cerebellopontine angle	Pediatric	Atypical teratoid/rhabdoid tumor, medulloblastoma, ependymoma
	Adult	Vestibular Schwannoma, meningiomas, epidermoid, arachnoid cyst, endolymphatic sac tumor
Fourth ventricle	Pediatric	Medulloblastoma, ependymoma
	Adult	Choroid plexus papilloma, epidermoid, subependymoma

Pathology

Histologically MBs are classified as classic; nodular or desmoplastic; MB with extensive nodularity; or as anaplastic/large cell variants. Over the past 5 years, considerable advances have been made in understanding MB biology[3] and the 2016 WHO update has incorporated histological and molecular schemes into the classification of MBs.[4,5] Based on genomic characterization, MBs can be subdivided into 4 distinct molecular subgroups: wingless (WNT), sonic hedgehog (SHH), group 3, and group 4. These molecular subgroups are more predictive of clinical behavior and outcome than the tumor histology (classic or "variants") or the clinical staging system.[3,4] Distribution of the different molecular subtypes between adult MB (50–60% SHH subgroup, 20–30% group 4 and 10–15% WNT) and pediatric MB (50–60 % group 3 tumors, 10–30% group 4 tumors, 10–15% WNT and 10–15% SHH) are significantly different.[6]

Imaging

Most pediatric MBs arise in the cerebellar vermis and often extend into the roof of the fourth ventricle and the brain stem. On imaging, MB appears as a well-circumscribed fourth ventricular mass. On CT scan, MBs are isodense to hyperdense due to their high cellularity **(Figs. 1A and B)** and show variable enhancement after contrast administration.[7] Approximately 20% of MBs have intratumoral calcification **(Fig. 1B)**. Cystic and necrotic degeneration are most commonly found in adult MBs.

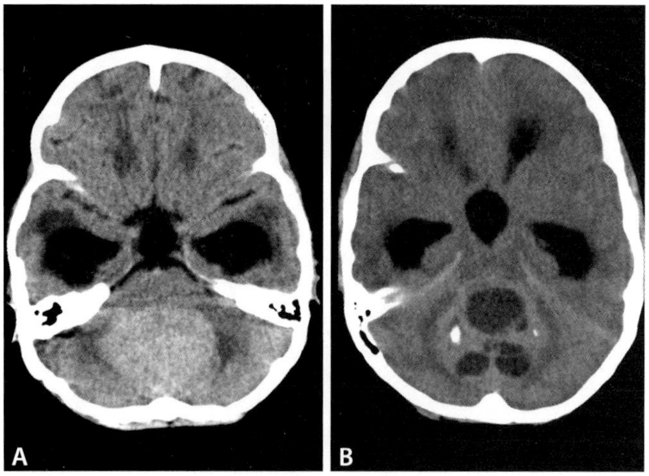

Figs. 1A and B: Medulloblastoma: NCCT shows a hyperdense midline mass (A) and midline isodense mass (B) with cystic areas and calcifications.

On MRI, typically they are hypointense to isointense on T1- and T2-WI; and show avid contrast enhancement **(Figs. 2A to F)**. The tumors are mostly homogeneous, although some display T2 heterogeneous signal due to the presence of intratumoral cysts, hemorrhage, calcification and necrotic foci.[7] MBs show evidence of restricted diffusion (bright on DWI and dark on ADC maps) in their solid components presumably due to their high cellularity and high nucleus-to-cytoplasm ratio **(Fig. 2D)**[8] Post-gadolinium brain and the spine MR imaging may show evidence of leptomeningeal metastatic spread in 33% of cases at the time of diagnosis or during the course of the disease **(Figs. 3A to C)**.[7] At MR spectroscopy, MBs characteristically show taurine, detectable at short TE, and a high choline peak.[9]

Compared to pediatric MBs, adult MBs are more likely to be located in cerebellar hemispheres and have an atypical presentation with more hyperintense signal on T1-WI, more hypointense signal on T2-WI and inhomogeneous contrast enhancement.[10]

Recently, there have been attempts to predict the molecular subtype of MBs based on imaging phenotype; a new emerging field of imaging known as radiogenomics. This is quite helpful when advanced molecular subtyping is not available. Wingless-type-subgroup MBs are likely to be off-midline tumors arising from the dorsal brain stem and cerebellum around the foramen of Luschka **(Figs. 4A to C)**.[11] This subtype of MBs may present as an isolated CP angle mass, a mass in region of foramen of Luschka or as a midline fourth ventricle mass. These tumors are

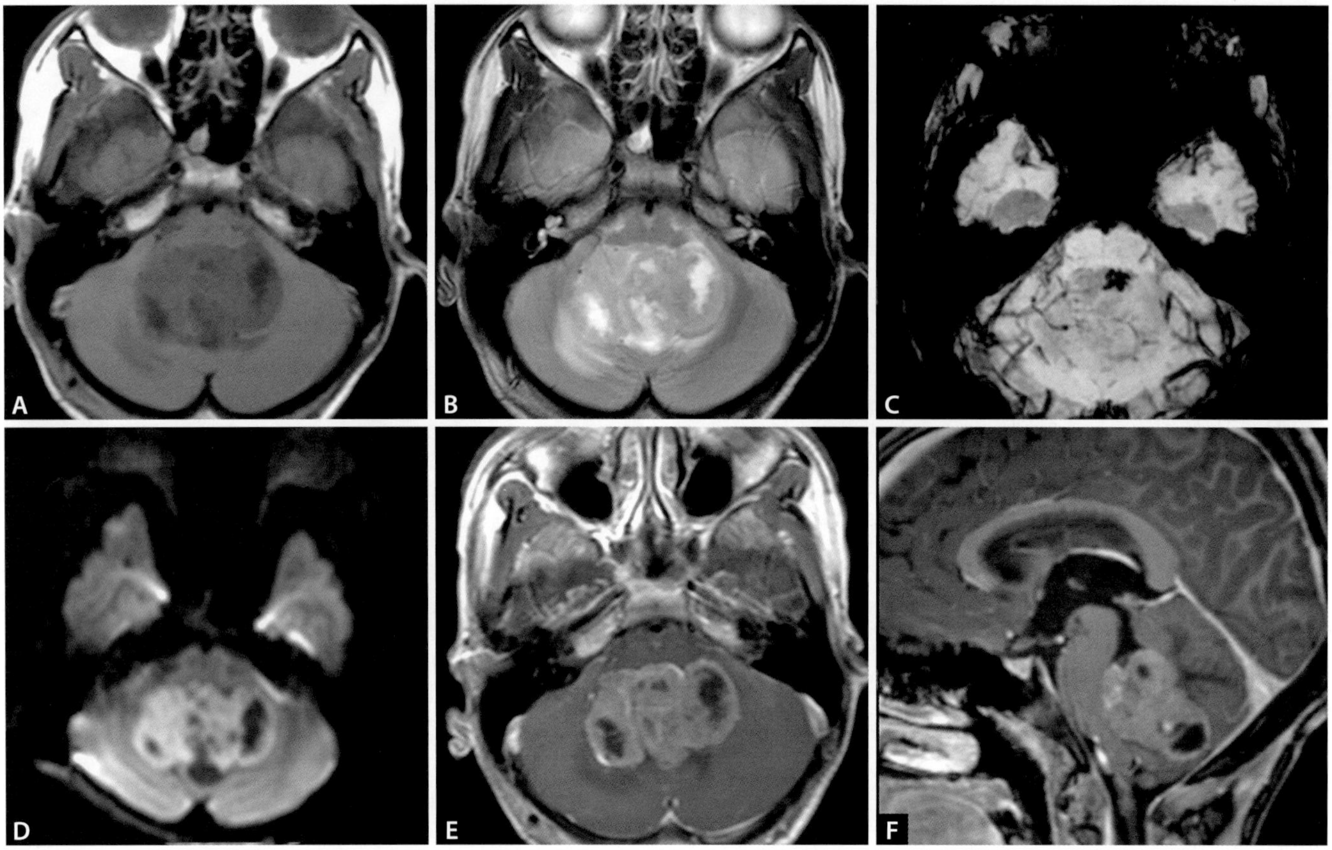

Figs. 2A to F: Medulloblastoma: MR scans show a midline vermian mass which is iso-hypointense on T1WI (A) and iso-hyperintense on T2WI (B) having foci of susceptibility on SWI (C). The mass is hyperintense on DWI (D) and hypointense on ADC maps (E) suggesting restricted diffusion. Postgadolinium axial (E) and sagittal (F) T1WI show intense enhancement of the mass.

likely to contact the dorsal brainstem. SHH subgroup of MBs typically occurs in adults and appear as off-midline intracerebellar tumors without any contact with the brainstem **(Figs. 4A to C)**. Group 3 MBs are likely to present as midline intraventricular tumors esp. in children with small tumor size and prominent enhancement. In addition, diffuse leptomeningeal spread at the time of first presentation is also more likely to occur in Gp 3 MBs **(Figs. 5A to D)**. Group 4 MBs are likely to present as midline intraventricular tumors which show no or minimal enhancement **(Figs. 6A to F)**.

Ependymoma

Ependymomas are an infrequent group of glial tumors that typically arise from ependymal cells in supratentorial, infratentorial and spinal cord regions. Ependymomas are common tumors in children, comprising 10% of pediatric CNS neoplasms and 15% of infratentorial tumors. The peak age at presentation is 1–5 years, with a smaller peak in adults in their fourth decade. Nearly two-thirds of intracranial ependymomas are present in the infratentorial compartment, arising from the ependymal lining of the fourth ventricle and the foramina of Luschka. Supratentorial lesions can be either intraventricular, typically in the lateral ventricles; or parenchymal. Approximately 60% of these tumors develop infratentorially, 30% supratentorially and 10% in the spinal cord.[12] Infratentorial ependymomas usually present with symptoms of raised intracranial pressure.[13] Cranial nerve palsies are also common, especially involving cranial nerves VI to X.

Pathology

Ependymomas are glial tumors arising from the ependymal lining of the ventricles and the central canal. The WHO classifies ependymal tumors into four types: (1) ependymoma (grade II), which include variants such as cellular, papillary, epithelial, clear-cell and mixed; (2) anaplastic ependymoma (grade III), (3) subependymoma (grade I), and (4) myxopapillary ependymoma (grade I).

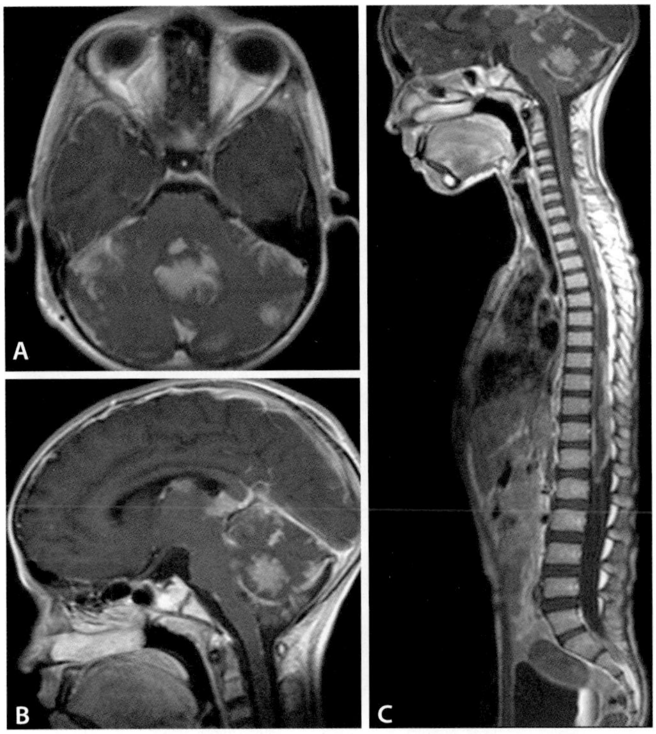

Figs. 3A to C: Type 3 Medulloblastoma with leptomeningeal spread: Axial (A) and sagittal (B) T1WIs of brain reveal patchy enhancement within a midline mass and enhancement of the leptomeningeal deposits in bilateral CPA cisterns and cerebellar sulci. Sagittal T1WI (C) of spine show diffuse leptomeningeal deposits in the spinal subarachnoid spaces.

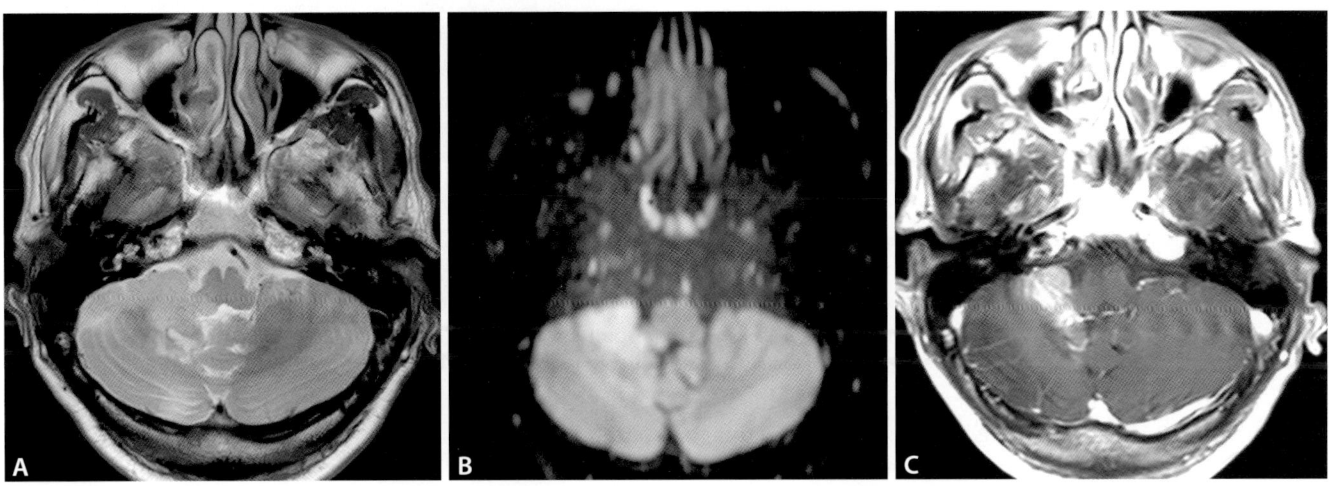

Figs. 4A to C: WNT Medulloblastoma: Axial T2WI (A) shows characteristic location in CPA cistern/foramen of Luschka region with involvement of dorsal brainstem, restricted diffusion DWI (B) and intense enhancement following contrast (C).

Anaplastic ependymomas have a greater incidence of leptomeningeal spread at the time of diagnosis and have poorer prognosis.

Typical gross pathology shows a well-defined lobulated mass with areas of calcification, hemorrhage, and cysts. The tumor cells usually form ependymal rosettes, which are diagnostic but not always present.

Comprehensive genomic studies have divided infratentorial ependymomas into 2 prognostcially different subgroups, PF-A and PF-B.[14] The poor prognostic subgroup (group A), found predominantly in infants, exhibited a CpG island methylator phenotype and transcriptional silencing of the polycomb repressive complex 2, leading to repressed expression of differentiation genes.[14]

Imaging

At CT, ependymomas appear as irregular and lobulated heterogeneous midline intraventricular masses with calcification (up to 45%).[15] At MRI, they appear heterogeneous with T1 hypointensity, T2 iso/hyperintensity and

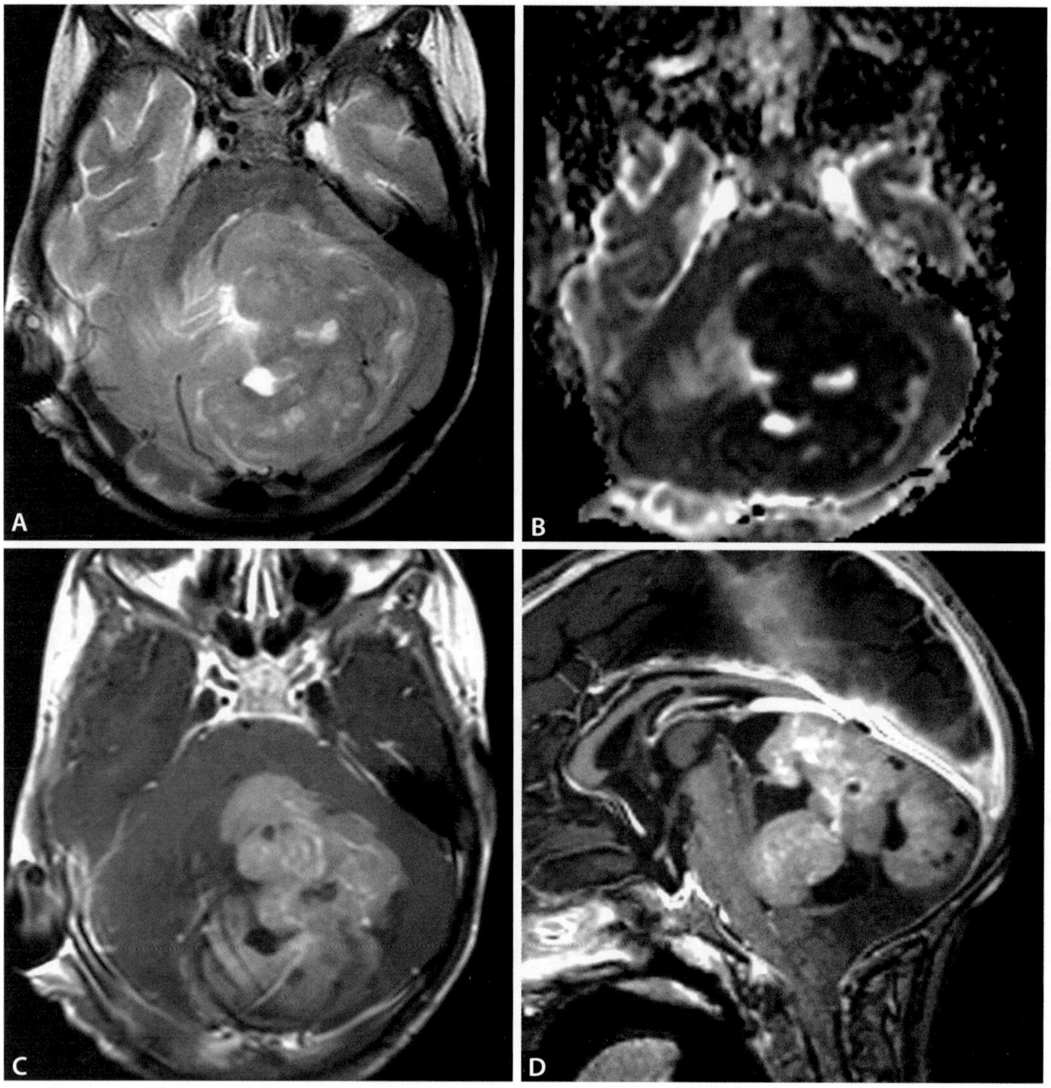

Figs. 5A to D: SHH Medulloblastoma: Hemispheric cerebellar tumor isointense on T2WI (A), hypointense on ADC maps (B) and avidly enhancing in axial (C) and sagittal (D) post-gad T1WIs.

iso-to-hyper FLAIR signal intensity **(Figs. 7A and B)** due to presence of calcification, hemorrhage and cystic changes within the tumor. Following contrast administration they usually show intense mixed heterogeneous enhancement **(Figs. 7C and D)**; however, rarely, ependymomas do not enhance.[16] The presence of calcifications within a lobulated heterogeneous fourth ventricular mass is highly suggestive but not diagnostic of ependymoma. Diffuse leptomeningeal spread is seen in less than 10% of patients at diagnosis when ependymoblastomas (ETANTR) are excluded.[17]

On DWI, ADC of ependymomas is generally intermediate between that of pilocytic astrocytomas and MBs,[18] however, ADC values are not completely reliable in differentiation between various infratentorial parenchymal masses. On Dynamic Susceptibility Contrast (DSC) perfusion MRI, ependymomas typically have markedly elevated perfusion (rCBV) and marked leakiness of contrast with poor return to baseline presumably due to presence of fenestrated blood vessels and an insufficient blood-brain barrier.[19] This behavior, although very characteristic of ependymomas, is not entirely pathognomonic and also may be demonstrated in other tumors, such as embryonal tumors.[20]

Typically, ependymomas show tumor extension through the fourth ventricular outflow foramina; however, this feature is not entirely pathognomonic, as some MBs may also extend through the fourth ventricular exit foramina.[21] The extensions through the foramina in MBs is more bulbous and have more restricted diffusion

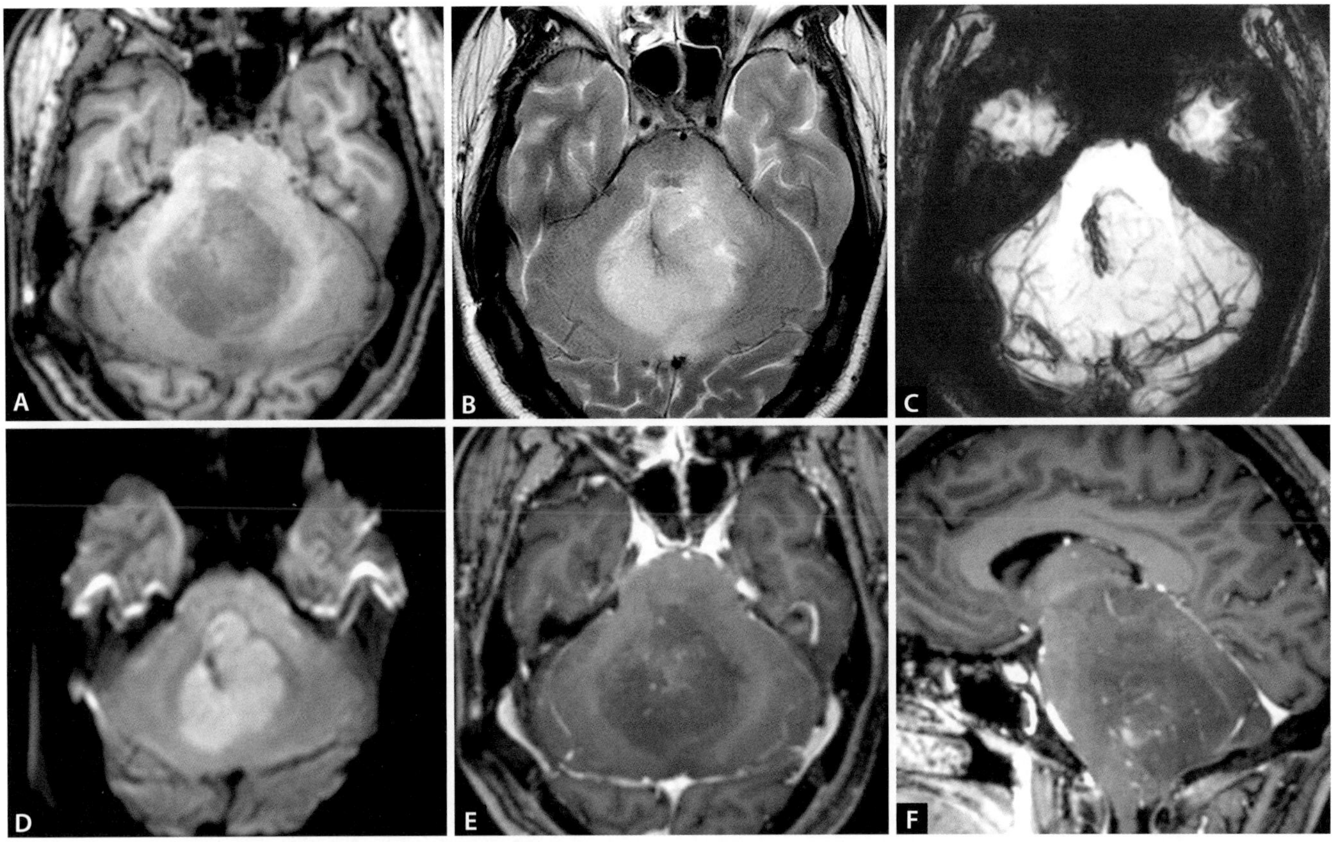

Figs. 6A to F: Type 4 Medulloblastoma: MR scans show a midline vermian mass which is iso-hypointense on T1WI (A), iso-hyperintense on T2WI (B), having foci of susceptibility on SWI (C) and hyperintense on DWI (D). Postgadolinium axial (E) and sagittal (F) T1WI show minimal enhancement of the mass.

compared to the thin tongues of tissue and intermediate diffusion in ependymomas. Rarely, ependymoma can present as an isolated mass within the cerebellopontine angle, presumably arising from the rests of ependymal cells.

Proton MR spectroscopy typically demonstrates elevated high myo-inositol (MI) levels in classic grade II ependymomas.[22,23]

Treatment for EPN to this date remains maximal-safe surgical resection followed by adjuvant radiotherapy in order to reduce the likelihood of recurrence in the tumor bed.[24] The survival rates have seen limited improvement (~80%) in the last decade, with survivors suffering from the debilitating side effects of radiation induced severe neurocognitive impairment and other radiation-induced complications.

Cerebellar Pilocytic Astrocytoma

Pilocytic astrocytomas (PA) are well-defined, slow growing, WHO Grade I tumors of CNS arising from astrocytic precursor cells. They typically present between 5 and 15 years of age. They generally arise from the cerebellum (60%), hypothalamus-optic chiasma region, brain stem and less commonly from cerebral hemispheres. Classically, cerebellar astrocytoma manifests with waxing and waning headache, truncal ataxia, dysdiadochokinesia are other cerebellar signs. They have an excellent prognosis with 90% of patients having a 10-year survival after total resection.

Pathology

PAs may be vermian or hemispheric in origin. Grossly, the cerebellar PA is usually sharply circumscribed, with a very narrow zone of microscopic infiltration. Approximately 50% of tumors are cystic with an enhancing mural nodule. Enhancement of the cyst wall is possible, but is not pathognomonic.[25] Nearly 40% of tumors are mixed solid with cystic or necrotic components and the rest are purely solid mass lesions. The tumor is supplied by capillaries that lack a complete blood-brain barrier (BBB). It has open tight junction in the endothelial cells with fenestration and therefore differs from low grade astrocytoma. This fact and

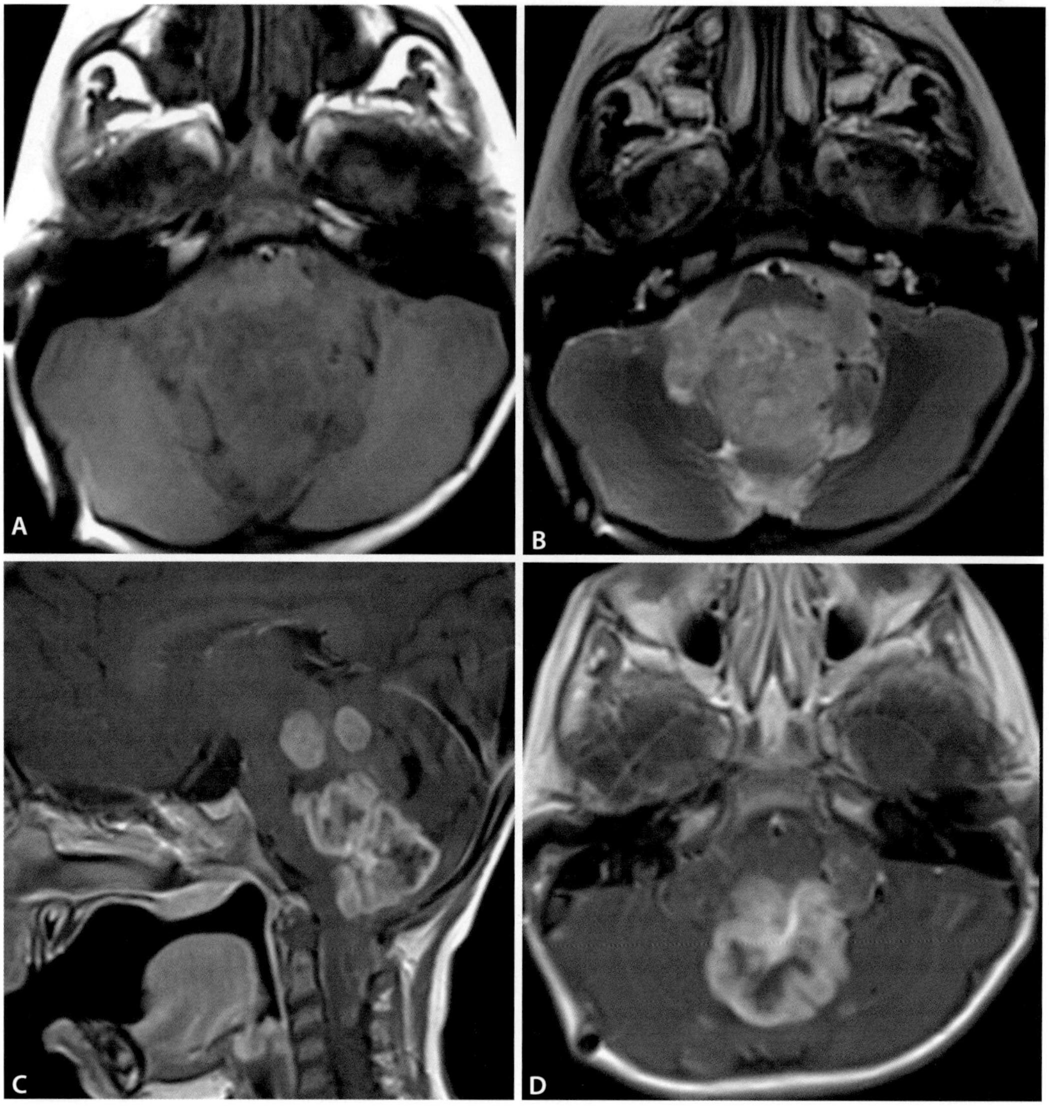

Figs. 7A to D: Ependymoma: Axial T1WI (A) and T2WI (B) show a heterogeneous mass filling the fourth ventricle. Post-gadolinium sagittal (C) and axial (D) T1WI demonstrate heterogeneous enhancement. The tumor is creeping anteriorly through foramen of Luschka into CPA cisterns and posteriorly through foramen of Magendie into upper cervical canal.

the lack of BBB is the cause of both intense enhancement, as well as the source of production of the proteinaceous fluid that accumulates in the "cyst" of the tumor.

Imaging

Classically, cerebellar PA appears as a cystic mass with an enhancing mural nodule **(Figs. 8A to C)** or a mixed solid-cystic mass **(Figs. 9A to D)**. Solid portion is hypointense on T1WI (higher than CSF intensity) and hyperintense on T2W1 and show variable enhancement **(Figs. 9A to D)**. Typically diffusion is facilitated in the solid enhancing portion of the tumor in comparison to MB and AT-RT. Peritumoral edema and intratumoral calcifications are usually absent. Hemorrhage can be present but rare **(Figs. 9A to D)**.

MR spectroscopy is quite tricky. Choline is typically very high in pilocytic tumors, despite the benign clinical course for tumors of this type.[22] In addition, Lipids and lactate are also usually demonstrated in the spectra of PAs. Despite being low grade (grade I tumors), PAs may present with high blood volumes on MR perfusion studies. This finding is not related to aggressiveness in these lesions.

Atypical Teratoid/Rhabdoid Tumor

CNS AT/RTs are highly malignant neoplasms which account for 1–3% of all primary CNS tumors in the pediatric

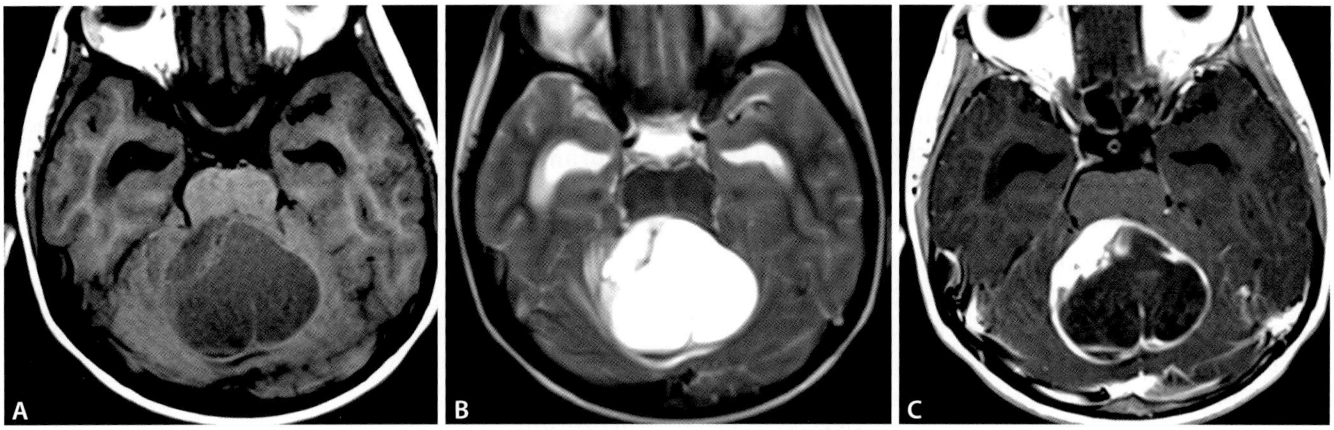

Figs. 8A to C: Cystic cerebellar astrocytoma: Axial T1WI (A) and T2WI (B) show a cystic mass with a mural nodule. The mural nodule is hypointense on T1WI (A) and hyperintense on T2WI (B). Following contrast administration, both the mural nodule and cyst wall enhance intensely (C). Note that no vascular flow-voids are seen in and around the mural nodule.

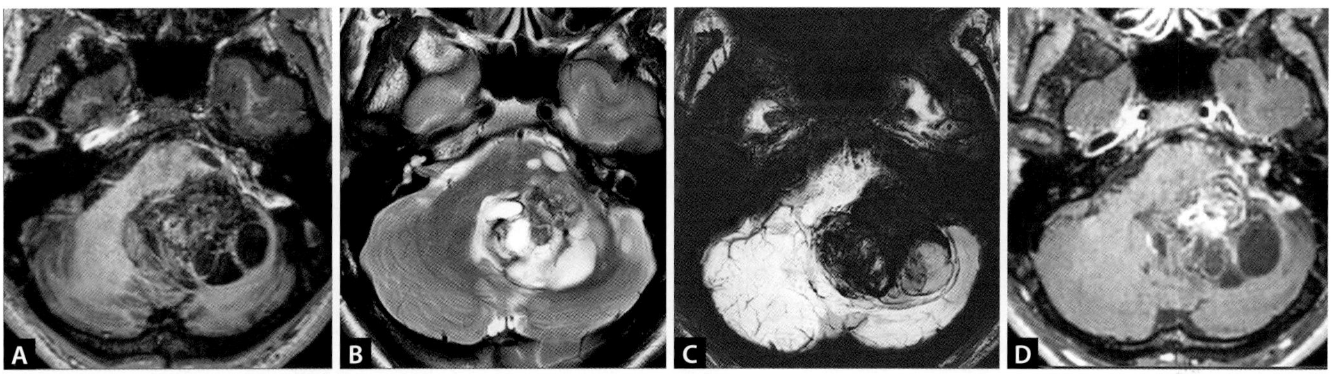

Figs. 9A to D: Solid-cystic cerebellar astrocytoma: Axial T1WI (A) and T2WI (B) show a heterogeneous mass in left cerebellum. On SWI (C), evidence of hemorrhage is seen within the mass. Following contrast administration, the mass shows heterogeneous enhancement (D). Note that no vascular flow-voids are seen in and around the mural nodule.

population and 6.7% of all primary CNS tumors in children less than 3 years of age.[26,27] Although by definition they contain rhabdoid cells, ATRTs have widely divergent cell populations, including mesenchymal, epithelial, glial, and neuronal cell lines accounting for the "teratoid" descriptor.[28] About two-thirds of ATRTs occur in the cerebellum, typically in the cerebellopontine angle, with invasion of the surrounding structures. About one-fourth are supratentorial and 8% are multifocal.[29] The primary AT-RT of the brain can present between 1 month to 12 years of age (average age 24.5 months), and have with a male predominance (M:F, 3:1).[29]

Pathology

Histologically, ATRTs are characterized by rhabdoid cells and are similar to that of other small round blue cell tumors; up to 70% also contain cell fields typical of a primitive neuroectodermal tumor. Necrosis and a high MIB-index are common.

Nearly all ATRTs demonstrate bi-allelic inactivation of SMARCB1 (or INI1) on chromosome 22, whereas a very small percentage show inactivation of SMARCA4 (or BRG1).[30] Having one of these genetic alterations is now formally required for diagnosis.[4]

Imaging

On imaging, lesions are usually large at presentation, with moderate- to- marked surrounding edema. On CT, these tumors are hyperdense or mixed density lesions attributed to the presence of areas of necrosis, cyst formation, hemorrhage and calcification[31] and show varying pattern of enhancement following contrast administration.[32] On MR, they are T1-hypointense, T2-iso to hypointense with restricted diffusion and inhomogeneous enhancement **(Figs. 10A to F)**. These imaging findings overlap with those described for MBs and are likely secondary to high cell density and high nucleus-to-cytoplasm ratio. Diffuse leptomeningeal dissemination is common, hence the spine should also be imaged. MRS shows elevated Cho, reduced NAA and a prominent lipid peak.

The main differential diagnosis for posterior fossa ATRT is MB and both show restricted diffusion. If a posterior fossa tumor occurs in a child less than 3 years of age, located off-midline, has intratumoral blood products and extends to the CPA, it is more likely to be an AT-RT than a MB.[33] Very young children presenting with cranial nerve deficits and masses involving the CPA with restricted diffusion are more likely to have an ATRT.[34]

Hemangioblastoma

Hemangioblastomas are uncommon, slow-growing tumors of CNS (WHO grade 1) that occur in the cerebellum (83–86%), brainstem (2–5%), spinal cord (3–13%) and cerebrum (1.5%).[35] They may occur either sporadically (75%) or as a manifestation of von Hippel-Lindau (VHL) disease in 25% along with retinal angioma, renal cell carcinoma, adrenal pheochromocytoma, as well as benign cysts in the lungs, liver, kidneys, and pancreas. The hemangioblastomas in VHL disease develop at an earlier age and are often multifocal in 20%.

Pathology

Hemangioblastomas typically appear as well-demarcated masses with smooth margins. The tumor can be either

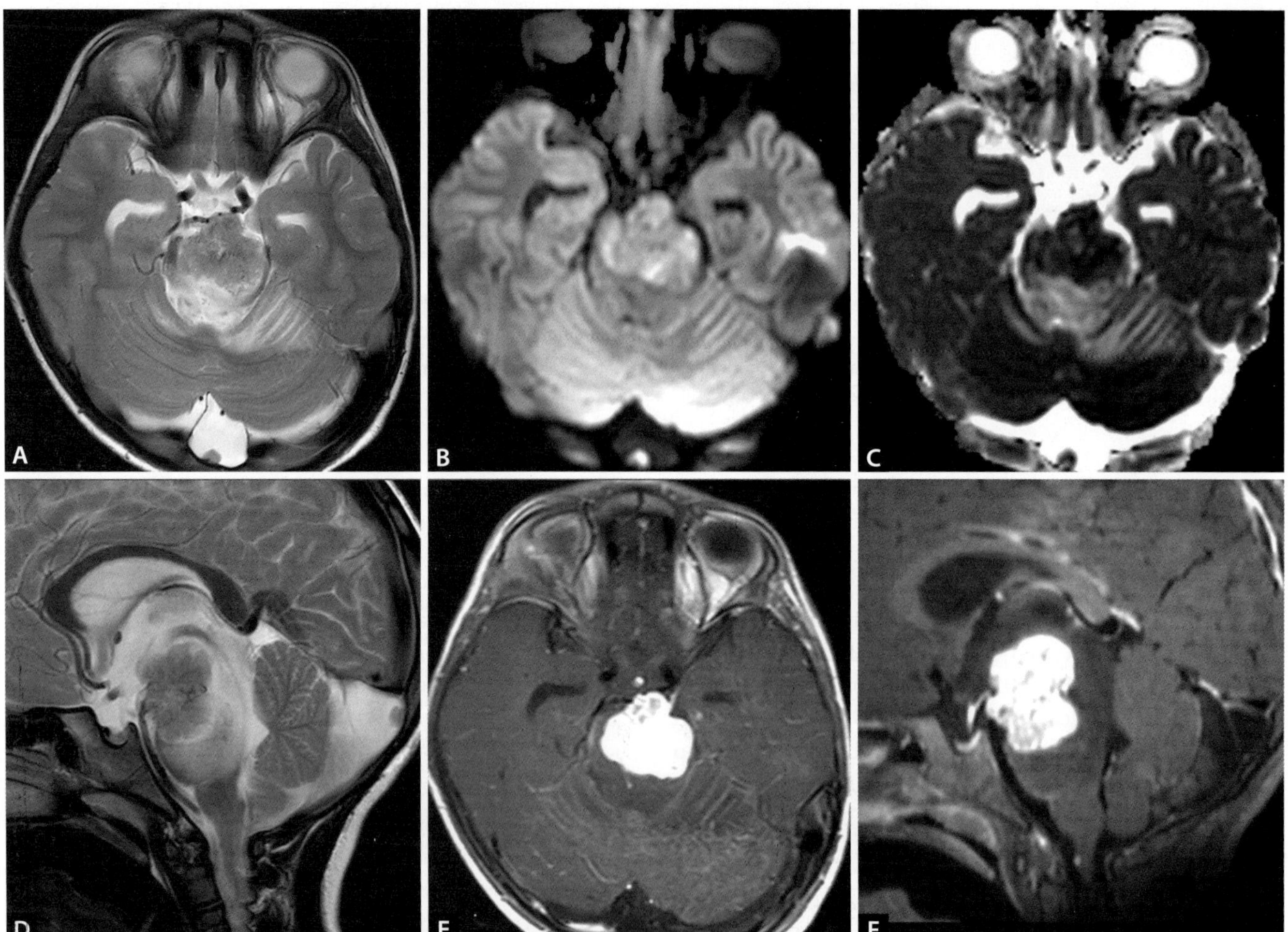

Figs. 10A to F: ATRT. A well-defined prepontine mass is seen without any plane between the tumor and the brainstem. The mass is isointense on axial (A) and sagittal (D) T2WI, bright on DWI (B) and dark on ADC maps (C) suggesting restricted diffusion. Post-gad axial (E) and sagittal (F) images show avid contrast enhancement of the mass.

entirely solid (40%) or cystic with a hypervascular enhancing mural nodule with prominent blood vessels (60%). VHL-associated and some sporadic hemangioblastomas are caused by inactivation of the VHL tumor suppressor gene, located on chromosome 3p.

Imaging

On NCCT, hemangioblastoma typically appears as a well-defined, either entirely solid or hypodense cystic lesion with an iso-hyperdense mural nodule. Solid hemangioblastomas appear hyperdense on NCCT and show strong homogeneous enhancement. The iso-hyperdense mural nodule abuts the pial surface and shows strong homogeneous contrast enhancement.

On MRI the cystic component of hemangioblastoma is either iso- or slightly hyperintense relative to CSF on T1WI and hyperintense on T2WI.[35] The nodule is T1 hypointense, T2 hyperintense and enhances avidly following gadolinium administration **(Figs. 11A to D and Figs. 8A and B)**. Vascular flow-voids may be present within and at the periphery of the tumor **(Figs. 11C and D)**. The peritumoral edema is usually minimal or absent. Perfusion MR imaging reveals high rCBV ratios in these lesions (around 11), values significantly higher than those of metastases (around 5) and pilocytic astrocytomas.[36] Cerebral angiography is reserved for preoperative tumor embolization and shows dilated feeding arteries and a prolonged tumoral blush corresponding to the solid portion.[37] The other differential diagnosis of a cyst with enhancing mural nodule in the infratentorial compartment is pilocytic astrocytoma which generally occurs at a younger age, is not associated with intratumoral flow-voids and show less increase in rCBV and permeability.

Metastases

Metastases are the most common infratentorial intra-axial neoplasms in the adult population. They are usually well-defined round masses, often with nodular or ring enhancement (due to central necrosis). Multiple masses are usually seen and help to confirm the diagnosis.

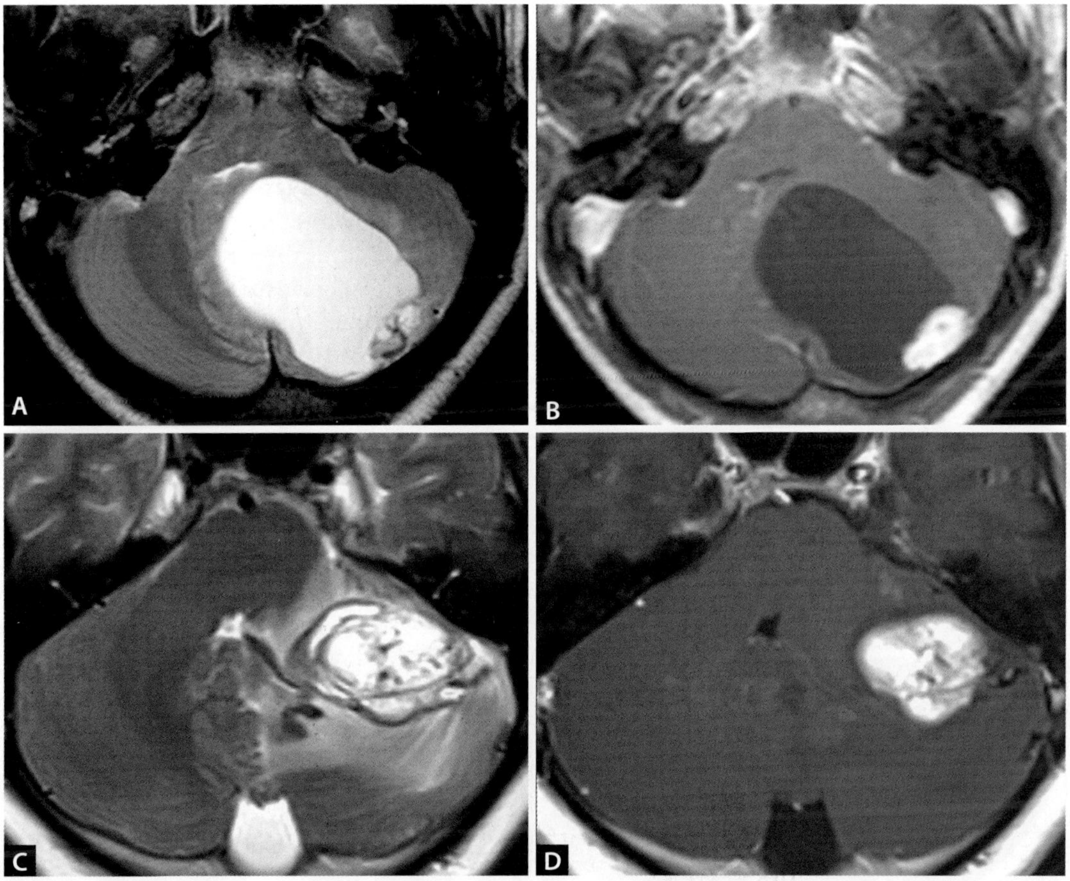

Figs. 11A to D: Hemangioblastoma: Axial T2 (A) and post-gad T1(B) show a cystic hemangioblastoma with enhancing mural nodule and vascular flow-voids within the mural nodule (A). Axial T2 (C) and post-gad T1 (D) show a solid hemangioblastoma with intense enhancement, multiple vascular flow-voids and perilesional edema.

However, even if solitary, the lesion is still more commonly metastasis than a primary intracranial neoplasm. In adults, lung and breast carcinoma account for the majority of metastatic disease, followed by melanoma, renal cell carcinoma, thyroid carcinoma, and gastrointestinal malignancies. Unknown primaries account for 10–15% of patients with brain metastases.

Imaging

Metastases are typically hypodense on CT; they are hypointense on T1WI and hyperintense on T2WI; and show varying pattern of enhancement **(Figs. 12A and B)**. Most metastases have considerable surrounding edema. Metastases with increased T1 signal intensity before contrast administration include melanoma, renal cell carcinoma, lung carcinoma, choriocarcinoma, and gastrointestinal adenocarcinoma (because of the presence of mucin).[38] Metastases with areas of hemorrhage and calcification have variable signal on T2WI. MR spectroscopy shows significantly elevated choline and very low NAA (the presence of NAA in many metastases represents contamination from adjacent tissues due to partial averaging).[39] Lactate and lipids are usually high. The tissues surrounding the enhancing mass usually are normal by spectroscopy (unlike high grade gliomas).

Dysplastic Cerebellar Gangliocytoma

Dysplastic cerebellar gangliocytoma, also known as Lhermitte-Duclos disease, is a rare entity characterized by focal thickening of the folia and loss of normal cerebellar cortical architecture.[40] There is debate as to whether this abnormality is a hamartoma, a malformation or a tumor; if neoplastic, it corresponds to WHO grade I.[41,42] Patients generally present with headache and hydrocephalus. The median age of presentation is in the 4th decade. Most adults, but not children, with dysplastic gangliocytoma have PTEN (phosphatase and tensin homolog) germline mutations.[43] LDD patients should be evaluated carefully to rule out Cowden syndrome, because Cowden syndrome patients have a high incidence of multisystemic cancers and other diseases including breast cancer (25%–50%), nonmedullary thyroid cancer (3%–10%), and endometrial adenocarcinoma (5%–10%).[44] Nowadays, Lhermitte-Duclos disease and Cowden syndrome are included in PTEN hamartoma tumor syndrome (PHTS).

Pathology

Histologically, there is reduced cerebellar white matter and presence of abnormal hypertrophic ganglion cells that superficially resemble Purkinje cells.

Imaging

On CT scan, the lesions are typically hypodense but may be isodense.[42] Calcification may occur but is uncommon.[42] On MRI, the lesion is seen as a focal cerebellar mass typically involving one hemisphere with a highly characteristic folial pattern (also described as laminated, corduroy, lamellar, or striated) **(Fig. 13A)**. The central core of T1 hypointensity and T2 hyperintensity corresponds to the inner molecular layer, widened granular cell layer, and loss of central white matter within the folia; whereas the outer thinner layer on MR images (T1 isointense, T2 iso- to hypointense) corresponds to the outer molecular layer and the leptomeninges.[45] Typically these lesions do not enhance **(Fig. 13B)**.[45] Rarely enhancement may be seen presumably secondary to venous proliferation in the outer

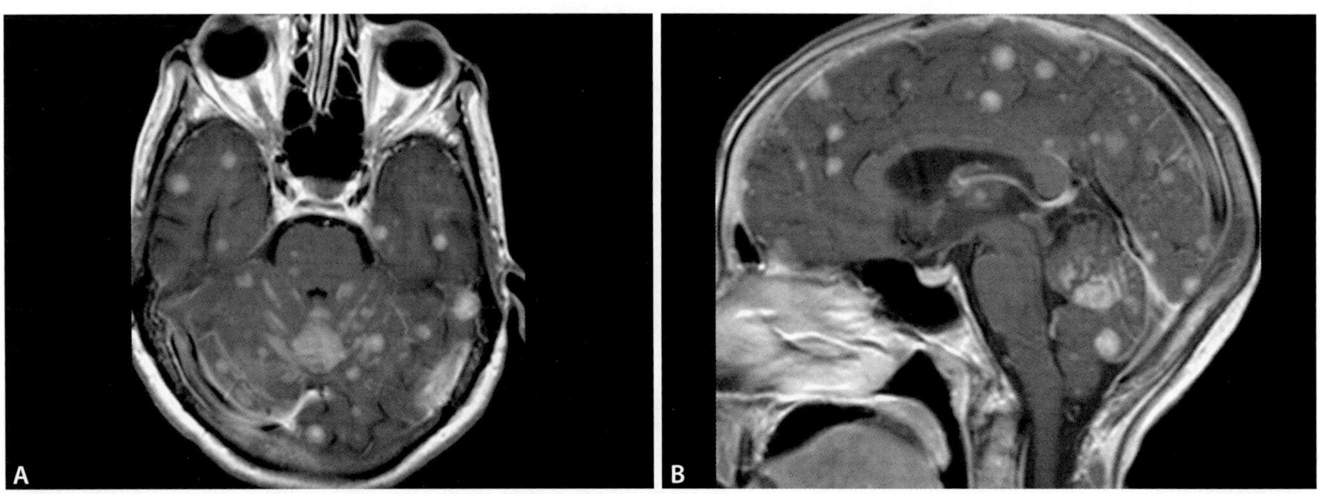

Figs. 12A and B: Metastases: Axial (A) and sagittal (B) T1WIs show multiple enhancing nodules throughout the brain parenchyma.

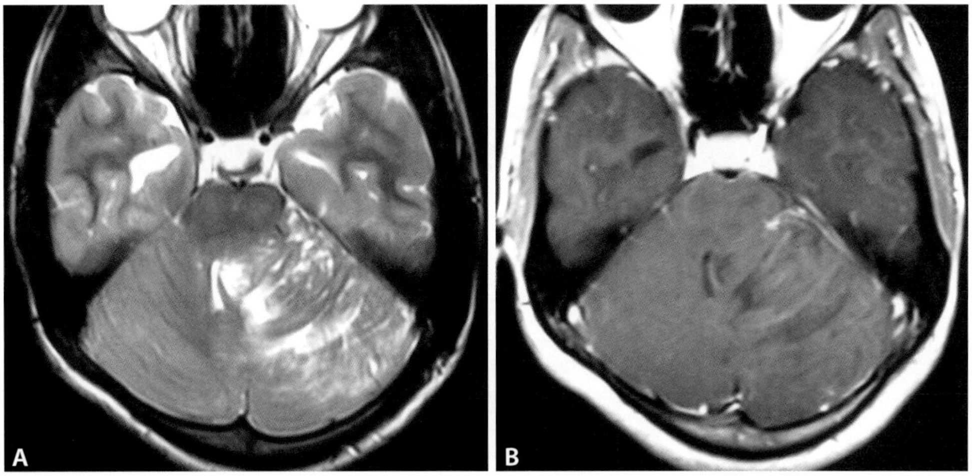

Figs. 13A and B: Dysplastic cerebellar gangliocytoma: (A) Axial T2WI shows a cerebellar mass with a striped appearance, composed of alternating hyperintense and isointense bands associated with compression on the 4th ventricle; (B) Contrast-enhanced axial T1WI shows mild enhancement of the mass.

portions of the cerebellar cortex and prominent draining veins.[46]

Treatment of symptomatic dysplastic gangliocytoma of the cerebellum is surgical resection.

Embryonal Tumor with Multilayered Rosettes C19MC-Altered

A new entity, embryonal tumor with multilayered rosettes (ETMR) C19MC-altered, was recently described in children younger than 4 years.[4] The term, primitive neuroectodermal tumor (PNET), has been removed and they are classified according to the presence of amplification of the C19MC region on chromosome 19 (19q 13.42). The presence of C19 MC amplification results in a diagnosis of ETMRs (ETMR-C19MC-altered). In its absence, the tumor is called ETMR-NOS.

These are usually large masses, more than 5 cm in size at the time of presentation in the supratentorial compartment, but may also be found in the infratentorial compartment. They are well-delineated masses with absent or minimal peritumoral edema despite their large size.[47-49] Typically they are heterogeneous isodense to hyperdense masses on CT. Calcifications are seen in 70% of cases.[49] On MRI, the signal on T1/T2 is variable due to the presence of blood products, calcifications, and cystic changes. FLAIR shows areas of necrosis (hyperintense) and cystic components (hypointense).[47] On diffusion-weighted imaging, the tumor shows restricted diffusion presumably due to its high cellularity and nucleus-to-cytoplasm ratio.[47] The solid components demonstrate avid heterogeneous contrast enhancement.[49] Perfusion MRI shows increased relative cerebral blood volume.[49] ETMRs develop subarachnoid dissemination in 40% of cases; thus, the entire neuroaxis should be imaged. The presence of metastases changes management, requiring chemotherapy and increased radiation dose.[47,49] Prognosis is dismal despite radiation therapy.

BRAINSTEM AND CERVICOMEDULLARY JUNCTION

Brainstem Gliomas

Brainstem gliomas are a heterogeneous group of tumors that differ significantly in their growth characteristics, histology, and response to therapy. They represent 10–20% of pediatric CNS tumors and three-fourths of these occur before 20 years of age.[50] In adults, they represent less than 2% of brain tumors and usually occur in younger adults and tend to be of low grade (WHO I or II).

The majority (85%) are composed of high-grade fibrillary gliomas, which arise predominantly in the pons and less frequently in the medulla. There is no sex predilection, and children between 7 and 10 years of age are commonly affected. Multiple cranial nerve palsies, pyramidal tract signs, ataxia and nystagmus are the usual presentation. Except in tectal gliomas, hydrocephalus is uncommon in brain stem gliomas. Diffuse pontine gliomas have the worst prognosis.[51]

Pathology

Brainstem gliomas can be divided into the diffuse brainstem glioma and focal glioma (including dorsal exophytic, tectal, and cervicomedullary).[52]

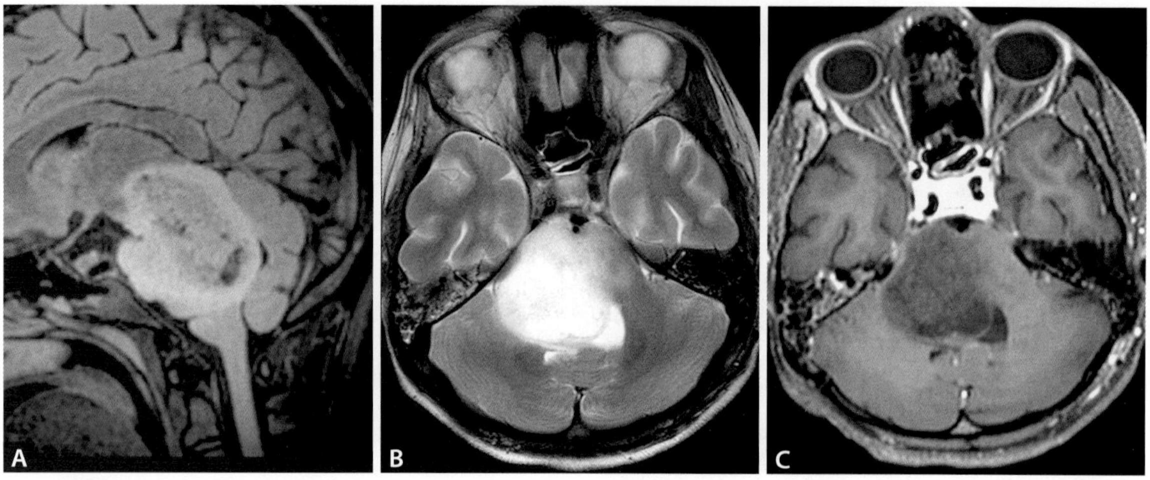

Figs. 14A to C: Diffuse midline glioma: Sagittal FLAIR (A) and axial T2WI (B) show diffuse pontine glioma causing expansion of pons and basilar artery encasement. No definite enhancement is seen following gadolinium administration (C).

Recent molecular studies have revealed that diffuse brainstem gliomas in children most likely harbor a highly specific point mutation, K27M, in histone 3.3, 3.2, or 3.1.3–7. In the revised 2016 update of the WHO brain tumor classification, these neoplasms constitute a new entity termed as diffuse midline glioma, H3 K27M-mutant characterized by a diffuse growth pattern, and a midline location (e.g., thalami, brainstem, spinal cord, and other midline structures, including the third ventricle, hypothalamus, and pineal region).[4] The majority of histone H3 K27M-mutant tumors are high-grade astrocytomas with high proliferative potential,[53,54] often with contiguous extension of tumor from the brainstem into the thalami and upper cervical spinal cord.[4,54] Most of these tumors have poor prognosis but exceptions have been reported.

Imaging

MR imaging is useful for diagnosis and localization of the tumor. Diffuse brainstem glioma appears as poorly defined T1 hypointense and T2 hyperintense regions **(Figs. 14A to C)**.[55] Intratumoral heterogeneity is occasionally present, but cysts are not common. The signal changes may extend into the cerebellum and/or the adjacent brainstem. There is often exophytic spread laterally and ventrally with basilar artery encasement. An undulating ventral border of the brainstem on sagittal image may be an indirect clue to the presence of the mass lesion. Contrast enhancement has been reported in approximately one-half of the cases and is often focal and nodular (**Fig. 14C**). Areas of restricted diffusion may be present, indicating higher cell density and providing targets for biopsy. No significant differences are seen in the characteristics of enhancement, infiltration, or peritumoral edema in patients with Diffuse pontine glioma with or without the histone H3 K27M mutation.[56]

Focal brainstem gliomas are often well circumscribed and sometimes markedly exophytic. Exophytic component is readily identified on MR, due to its multiplanar imaging capability. The dorsally exophytic lesions are grossly multicystic and often enhance intensely **(Figs. 15A and B)**. The presence of enhancement has not been correlated reliably with type or grade of malignancy.[51] The other subtypes of focal gliomas are tectal plate glioma **(Figs. 16A and B)** and cervicomedullary glioma **(Figs. 17A and B)**.

Ganglioglioma

Ganglioglioma (GG) is another diagnostic consideration for tumors located in the brainstem and upper cervical cord. Infratentorial GGs are less common than supratentorial GGs.[57]

On imaging, infratentorial GGs are typically infiltrative and expansile solid masses with dorsal predominant "paintbrush" enhancement.

Infratentorial GGs are difficult to resect completely and have poor progression-free survival and high mortality, in comparison to supratentorial GGs.[58]

CEREBELLOPONTINE ANGLE AND INTERNAL AUDITORY CANAL

Lesions of the cerebellopontine angle (CPA) are frequent and represent 6–10% of all intracranial tumors. Vestibular schwannomas and meningiomas are the two most frequent lesions and account for approximately 85–90% of all CPA tumors.

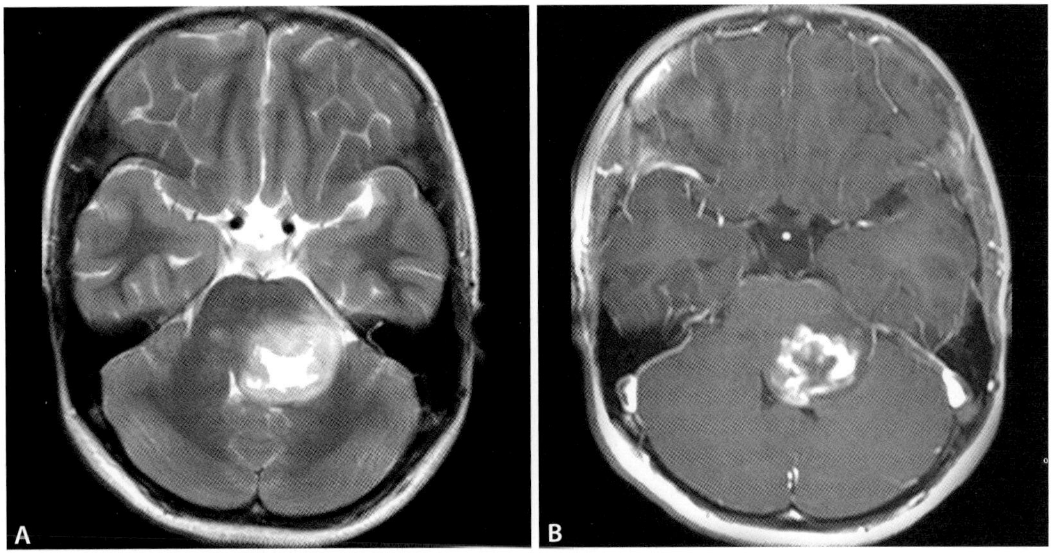

Figs. 15A and B: Dorsal exophytic pontine glioma: Axial T2WI (A) shows a hyperintense lesion with central necrosis arising from left brachium pontis and compressing fourth ventricle. The mass shows enhancement around central necrosis (B).

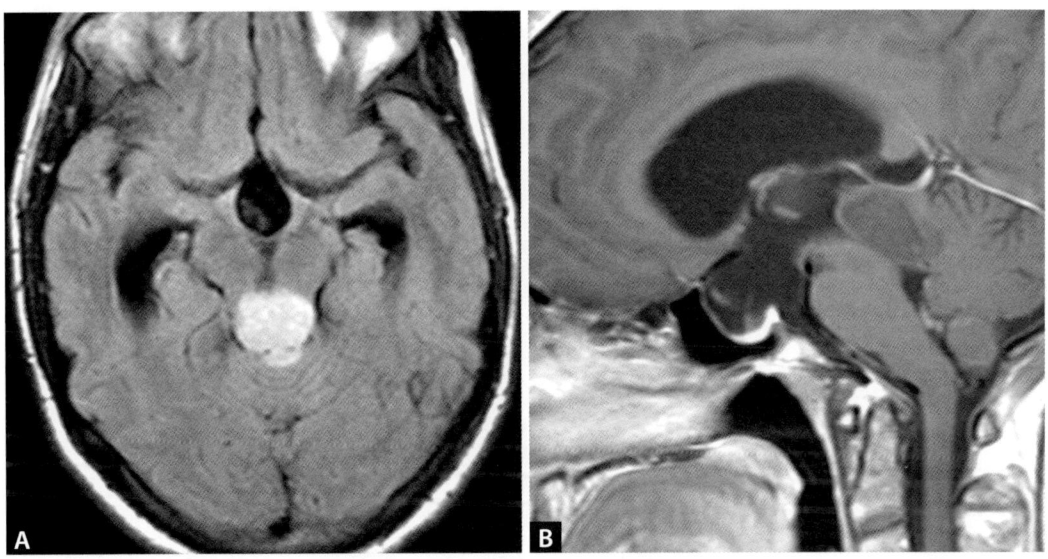

Figs. 16A and B: Tectal plate glioma: Axial flair (A) image shows thickening and hyperintensity in the region of tectal plate, compressing the aqueduct and causing proximal hydrocephalus. No enhancement is seen following gadolinium administration (B).

Vestibular Schwannomas

Vestibular schwannomas are Schwann cell-derived tumors that account for nearly 8% of intracranial tumors in adults and 80 to 90% of tumors of the cerebellopontine angle (CPA). Typically they present with adult-onset unilateral sensorineural hearing loss or tinnitus.[59] Bilateral vestibular schwannomas are pathognomonic for neurofibromatosis type 2 (NF2) **(Figs. 18A and B)**. These are generally benign and slow growing tumors with rare malignant degeneration when associated with NF-1.

Pathology

Vestibular schwannomas arise from perineural elements of the Schwann cell and are similar in pathology to other peripheral schwannomas. Histologic examination of schwannomas reveal compact Antoni Type A tissue and loose textured, often cystic, Antoni Type B tissue.

Imaging

On imaging, vestibular schwannomas are seen as enhancing CPA mass lesions with variable extension

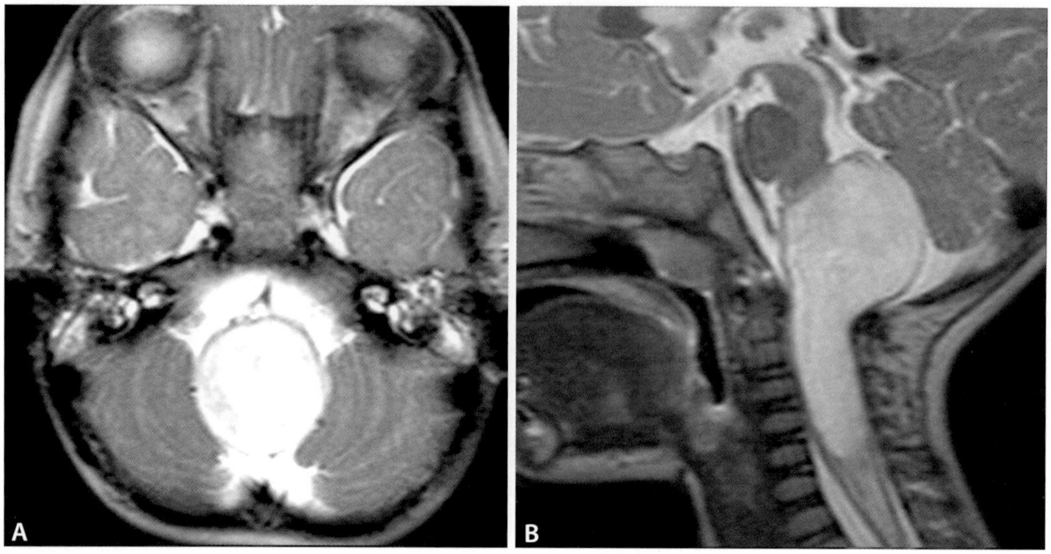

Figs. 17A and B: Cervicomedullary glioma: Axial (A) and sagittal T2WI (B) images show an expansile well-defined mass lesion involving medulla and upper cervical spinal cord.

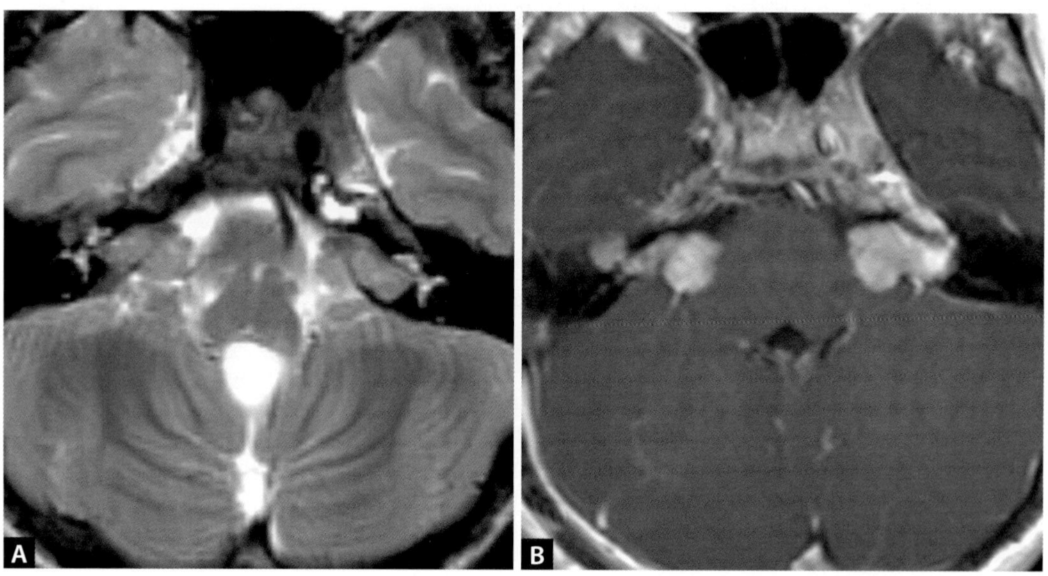

Figs. 18A and B: Schwannomas: A patient of neurofibromatosis 2 with bilateral acoustic schwannomas and right facial nerve schwannoma in region of geniculate ganglion. These lesions are isointense on T2WI (A) and shows homogenous enhancement on contrast administration (B).

into the internal auditory canal in most cases, resulting in the description of an "ice-cream cone" tumor. The intracanalicular component often causes widening of the porus acusticus resulting in the trumpeted IAM sign in up to 90% of cases. Purely extracanalicular tumors only abutting the porus acusticus are less common (~20%) and present late with features of mass effect rather than hearing loss. Generally, a small "CSF cap" is present between the intracanalicular component and the cochlea. Sometimes these tumors extend laterally into the middle ear through the cochlea (transmodiolar) or the vestibule (transmacular). Rarely small tumors are limited to the vestibule (intravestibular) or the cochlea (intracochlear) or both (vestibulocochlear).[60]

Degree of IAC widening and the tumor extent ventral and caudal to the IAC on NCCT can predict postoperative hearing loss.[61]

The low T2 acoustic schwannomas have a predominance of the Antoni Type A tissue. Large tumors have predominant Antoni Type B tissue and appear heterogeneous secondary

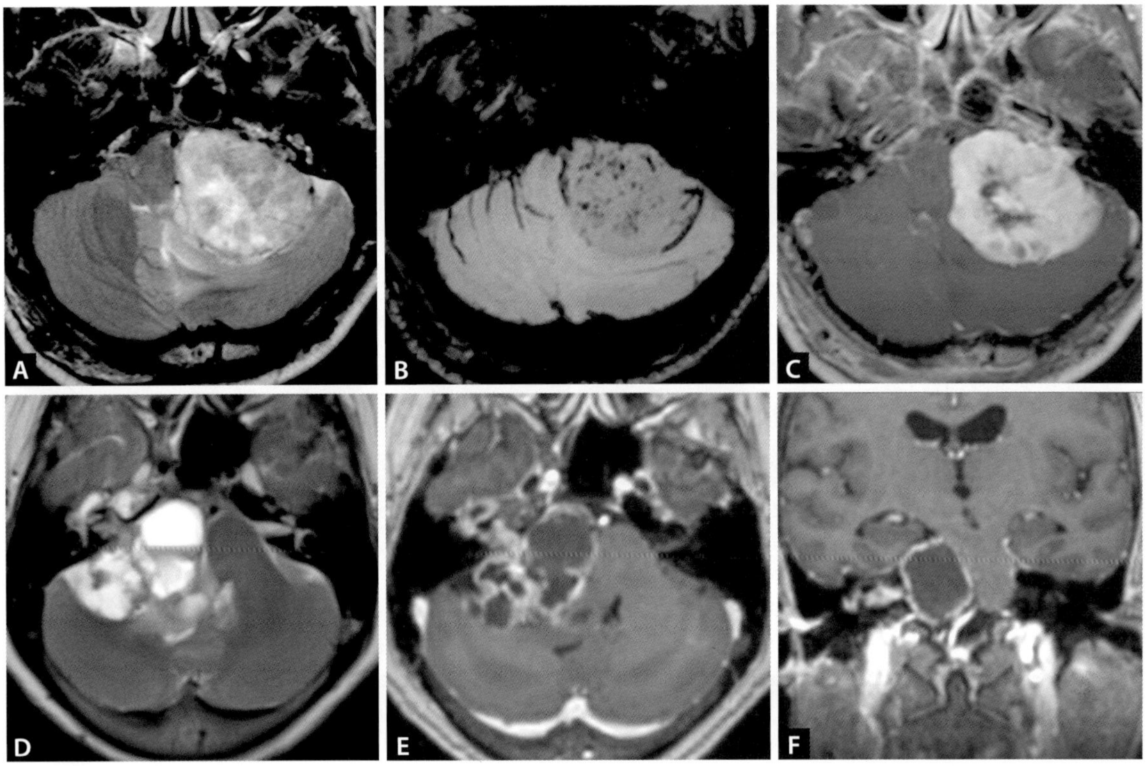

Figs. 19A to F: Acoustic Schwannomas: Axial T2 (A) image shows an iso-hyperintense CPA mass with extension into IAC, areas on susceptibility on SWI (B) and heterogeneous enhancement (C). Cystic acoustic schwannomas with multiple septations and fluid-fluid levels on T2WI (D), extension into IAC and heterogeneous enhancement (E and F).

to presence of regions of internal necrosis/cyst formation **(Figs. 19A to F)**. Peritumoral cysts are also associated (7 to 10%) with large lesions-believed to be secondary to elevation and deformation of the leptomeninges. Since the IAC is involved (80%), flaring of the porous acusticus, expansion of the IAC, and an acute angle with the dura can be seen. In vestibular schwannomas, the vestibule may have a low T2 signal intensity, presumably due to increased protein concentration in the perilymph (but not in patients who have CPA meningiomas). Some patients who have vestibular schwannomas larger than 2 cm in diameter demonstrate a tiny area of hyperintensity in the dorsal brain stem on T2WIs at the lateral angle of the fourth ventricular floor. This may represent degeneration of the vestibular nucleus and should not be confused with infarction.

Small tumors typically show homogeneous enhancement, whereas larger lesions more often have heterogeneous enhancement due to presence of hemorrhage and cystic areas. Occasionally, vestibular schwannomas show extension into the cochlea and "dural tails" of enhancement.

The major treatment options for patients with a vestibular schwannoma are surgery, radiation therapy, and observation.

Meningiomas

Meningiomas are extra-axial neoplastic lesions arising from arachnoidal cap cells. Approximately, 10% of all intracranial meningiomas arise in the infratentorial compartment. They are the second most common CPA tumor and account for 10% of CPA masses. They usually arise from the posterior petrous surface or the underside of the tentorium **(Figs. 20A and B)**.

Imaging

On NCCT, meningiomas are frequently hyperdense. Focal areas of calcification are present in up to 25% of cases. A dural tail, the presence of bony reaction, and an obtuse angle with the dura, as well as the centre of the lesion being located away from the IAC, suggest meningioma. Relatively T2 hypointense signal is characteristic of most meningiomas, especially the transitional and fibroblastic varieties.[62] Necrosis and cystic degeneration are uncommon with meningiomas and help to differentiate them from schwannomas **(Figs. 20A and B)**. On SWI, presence of susceptibility foci secondary to hemorrhage suggest schwannoma rather than meningioma. Rarely, meningiomas may originate within the internal auditory

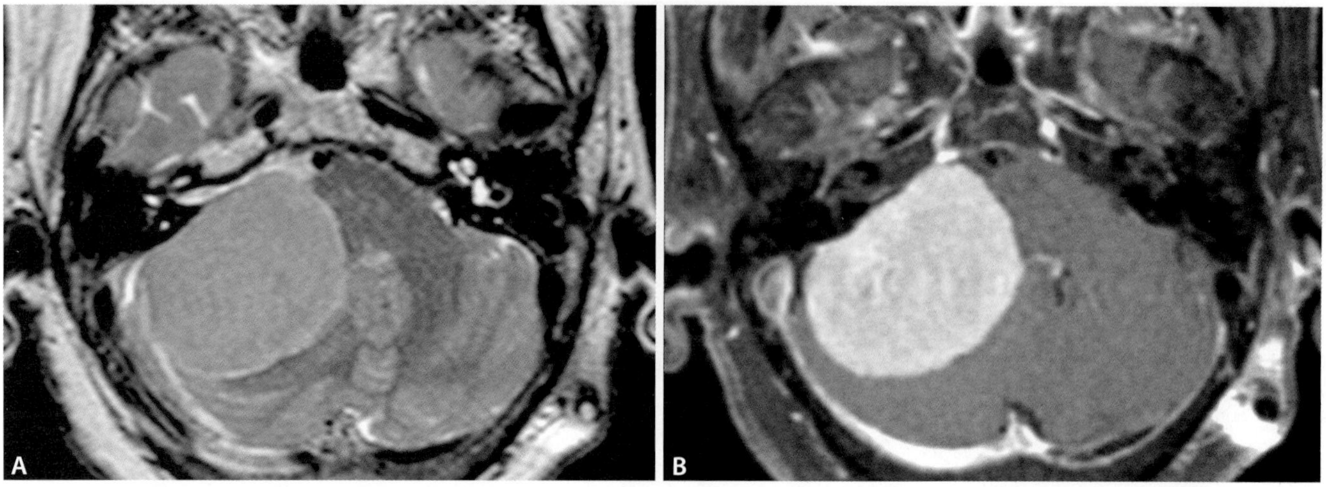

Figs. 20A and B: Meningioma: Extra-axial CPA mass with broad dural base, isointense T2 signal (A) and avid contrast enhancement (B).

canal, or even within the labyrinth. CPA meningioma may extend into the IAC, however canal is often not widened. The presence of a dural tail is suggestive but not pathognomonic of meningioma.

Epidermoid and Dermoid

Epidermoid and dermoid are generally believed to be congenital/ developmental masses rather than neoplastic, arising from ectodermal heterotopia. Both cysts have stratified squamous epithelium inner lining, with dermoids having additional mesodermal elements such as hair, sebaceous and sweat glands.

Epidermoids are slightly more common than dermoids and account for 3–7% of CPA masses. They grow very slowly via desquamation and therefore present late in adults despite their congenital etiology. They may become quite large before becoming symptomatic. The CPA is the most common location, followed by the parasellar region.

Imaging

At CT, most epidermoids are non-enhancing hypodense lesions with calcification in up to 25% of cases. Most epidermoids are isointense to CSF on both T1 and T2WI **(Figs. 21A to F)** due to presence of cholesterol in its solid/ crystalline state rather than the liquid state. The latter would result in bright T1 signal. The adamantinomatous craniopharyngioma typically contains this type of cholesterol; epidermoids rarely do.[63] Epidermoids often have a lamellated appearance secondary to surface desquamation. Most epidermoids do not enhance, although some minimal rim enhancement occurs in approximately 25% of cases. Malignant transformation of an epidermoid (squamous cell carcinoma) is rare and shows a significant enhancement. The rare "white epidermoid" is an interesting variant that is hyperdense at CT, hyperintense on T1WI, and hypointense on T2WI. This may be explained by high protein content, hemorrhage or the presence of saponified keratinized debris, and as indicated previously, cholesterol in the liquid state. When epidermoids are hyperintense on T1WI, then they need to be differentiated from dermoids and lipomas. Chemical shift artefact is absent in epidermoids and also a fat saturation pulse sequence will suppress the high signal of dermoids and lipomas, but not of epidermoids.

On FLAIR sequence, epidermoid cysts have mixed iso- to hyperintense signal with poor demarcation **(Fig. 21C)**. On DWI, epidermoids are hyperintense due to restricted diffusion (low ADC), while arachnoid cysts are hypointense due to increased diffusion (high ADC). DWI signal is also useful for detecting postoperative residual epidermoid.[64] The lamellated appearance and the tendency to insinuate rather than displace the surrounding structures are characteristic features of epidermoid.

Like epidermoid cysts, dermoid cysts are congenital ectodermal inclusions but are extremely rare, far less common than epidermoid cysts. Dermoids are midline lesions, occurring in the parasellar, frontobasal region or infratentorial compartment (vermis or fourth ventricle). Dermoids on CT are essentially fat density, extra-axial midline masses that do not enhance on contrast administration. They may be associated with bone defect in nasofrontal or occipital region that indicates the presence of a dermal sinus tract. CT is essential for detection of the calvarial defect, while MR delineates the tumor better. Unruptured cysts are hyperintense, similar to fat on T1WIs

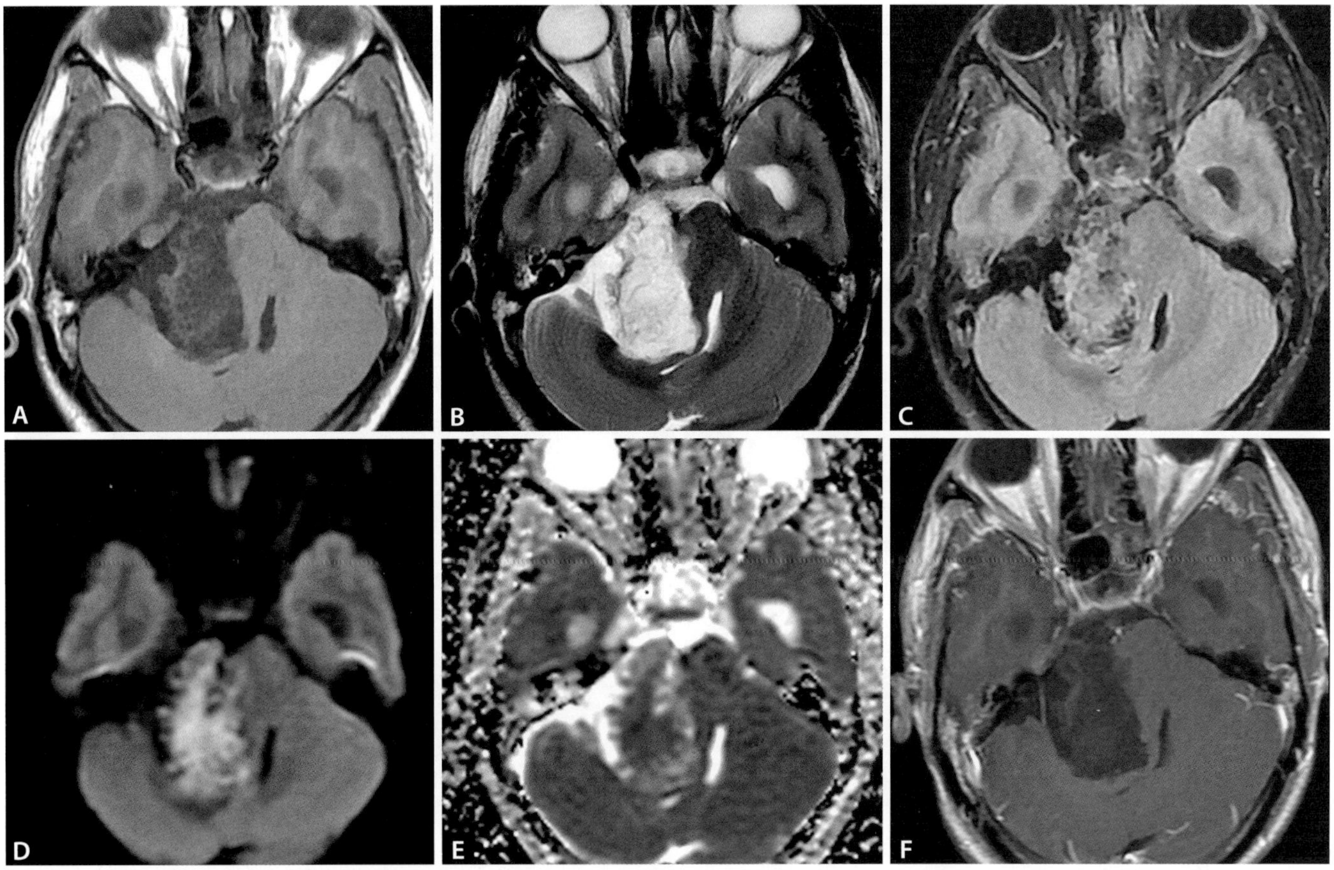

Figs. 21A to F: Epidermoid: MR scans show an extra-axial right CPA mass which is hypointense on T1WI (A) and hyperintense on T2WI (B). The mass has little internal heterogeneity on FLAIR images (C); bright on DWI (D) and dark on ADC images (E). No enhancement is seen following gad administration (F).

and are heterogeneous on T2WI. Chemical shift artefact is present similar to lipomas. However, dermoids are less lobulated than lipomas, and displace blood vessels and neural structures, in contrast to encasement of these structures by lipomas. Growth can lead to rupture of the cyst, causing a chemical meningitis. Imaging findings vary. Fat-like leptomeningeal and intraventricular deposits are diagnostic of a ruptured dermoid cyst.[65]

Arachnoid Cyst

Arachnoid cysts are congenital, benign, intra-arachnoid CSF filled lesions.[65] Mostly these are supratentorial lesions and about 70% are present in the middle cranial fossa[66] anterior to the temporal poles. Infratentorial arachnoid cysts account for only 10% of arachnoid cysts and a vast majority of these are located in the CPA. Typically arachnoid cysts are asymptomatic. However they can compromise cranial nerve functions by stretching them or rarely present with spontaneous or traumatic intracystic hemorrhage.[67]

Imaging

At neuroimaging, arachnoid cyst is hypodense on CT and follows CSF signal intensity on all MRI sequences including DWI, and do not enhance after gadolinium administration **(Figs. 22A to D)**. Complete suppression of signal intensity on FLAIR sequence and the lack of diffusion restriction differentiate arachnoid cyst from epidermoid cyst **(Figs. 22A to D)**.[68]

Facial Nerve Schwannomas

Schwannomas may arise anywhere along the course of the facial nerve from the CPA to the stylomastoid foramen. The facial nerve schwannoma arising in the IAC or CPA may be difficult to differentiate from vestibular schwannoma.[69] The presence of enhancing component extending along the labyrinthine segment of the facial nerve to the geniculate ganglion suggests the diagnosis of a facial nerve schwannoma over a vestibular schwannoma.[70]

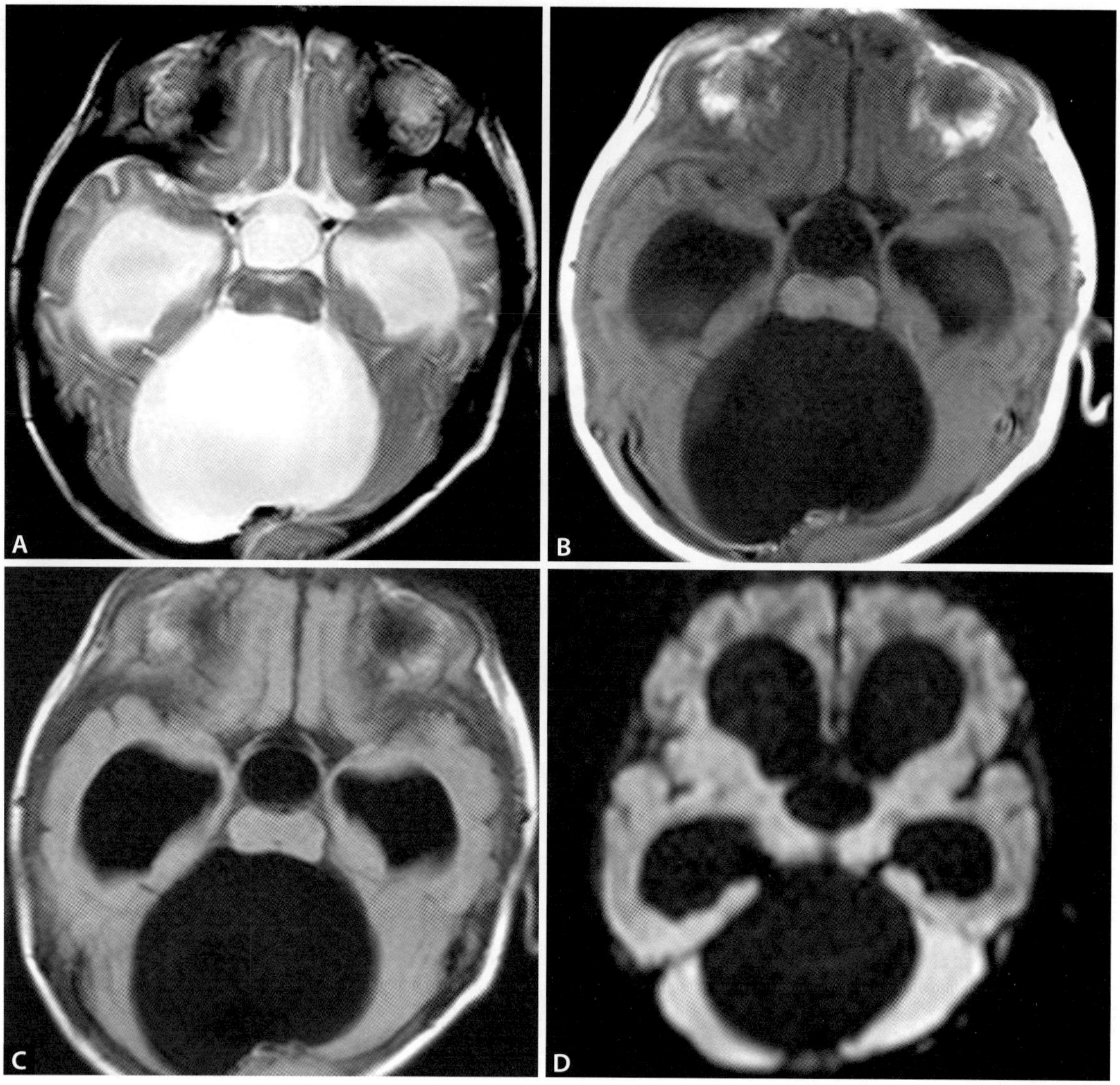

Figs. 22A to D: Arachnoid cyst: Axial T2WI shows a well-defined extra-axial cyst in superior cerebellar cistern which is isointense to the CSF on T1WI (A), T2WI (B) and Flair (C). The lesion is dark on DWI (D) suggesting increased diffusion.

Cerebellopontine Angle/Internal Auditory Canal Lipomas

Lipomas represent mesodermal inclusions and are rare CPA/IAC lesions. Characteristically, these lesions are hyperintense on T1-WI and show signal suppression on fat-sat images. These should not be mistaken for retained pantopaque (iophendylate) dye when clinical history of previous myelogram may suggest diagnosis.

Metastatic Disease

CPA metastatic disease is rare and may be leptomeningeal or parenchymal (brainstem, cerebellum). Meningeal metastases may be diffuse, nodular or mass-like. Parenchymal lesions are exophytic brainstem or cerebellar hemispheric lesions mimicking CPA masses. With large lesions, it may be difficult to differentiate meningeal from parenchymal metastases. Breast and lung are the most common sources of primary tumors.

Primary Parenchymal Neoplasms

Primary parenchymal neoplasms such as MB, astrocytoma, and ependymoma may rarely have an exophytic component and appear as an isolated CPA mass. One must evaluate different MR sequences in multiple planes to establish an intra-axial component to clinch the diagnosis.

Endolymphatic Sac Tumor

Endolymphatic sac tumors arise from the endolymphatic sac located in the distal portion of the vestibular aqueduct and are papillary adenomatous tumors. These tumors are frequent in von Hippel–Lindau disease,[71] but may also occur sporadically. At CT, the tumor causes destruction of the retrolabyrinthine petrous bone, has geographic or moth-eaten margins, and intratumoral spiculated or reticulated bone **(Fig. 22A)**.[72] At MR imaging, these tumors are heterogeneous on both T1 and T2WIs with foci of hyperintensity due to subacute hemorrhages and hypointensity due to calcification or hemosiderin.[73] Presence of T1- and T2-hyperintense blood-filled cysts and protein-filled cysts may suggest the diagnosis **(Figs. 23A to D and 20A and B)**. Enhancement is heterogeneous after gadolinium administration. Vascular flow-voids are seen within the tumor or peritumoral region in tumors more than 2 cm in size.[74]

FOURTH VENTRICLE

Choroid Plexus Papillomas

Choroid plexus papillomas (CPPs) and choroid plexus carcinomas (CPCs) originate from choroid plexus epithelium. They constitute 5% of supratentorial pediatric tumors and less than 1% of all primary intracranial neoplasms. CPPs are most frequent in the first year of life, and present with hydrocephalus. CPCs make up 30–40% of choroid plexus tumors and occur mostly during the first 5 years of life. Focal neurologic deficit resulting from adjacent brain invasion is a frequent presentation of CPC. Male predominance is seen for both the tumors.

Pathology

The common site of origin for CPP is the lateral ventricles; third and fourth ventricles are rarely involved in children. Fourth ventricle is the commonest site of adult CPP. CPPs are well-defined lobulated masses and cause enlargement of the involved ventricles. Foci of small hemorrhages and calcification may be found. Anaplastic papillomas, frequently invade the brain, and are difficult to differentiate from carcinomas. Metastasis through CSF pathways is common for both anaplastic papillomas and carcinomas.

Imaging

CPP are typically isodense to hyperdense on NCCT with occasional foci of calcification **(Figs. 24A and B)**.

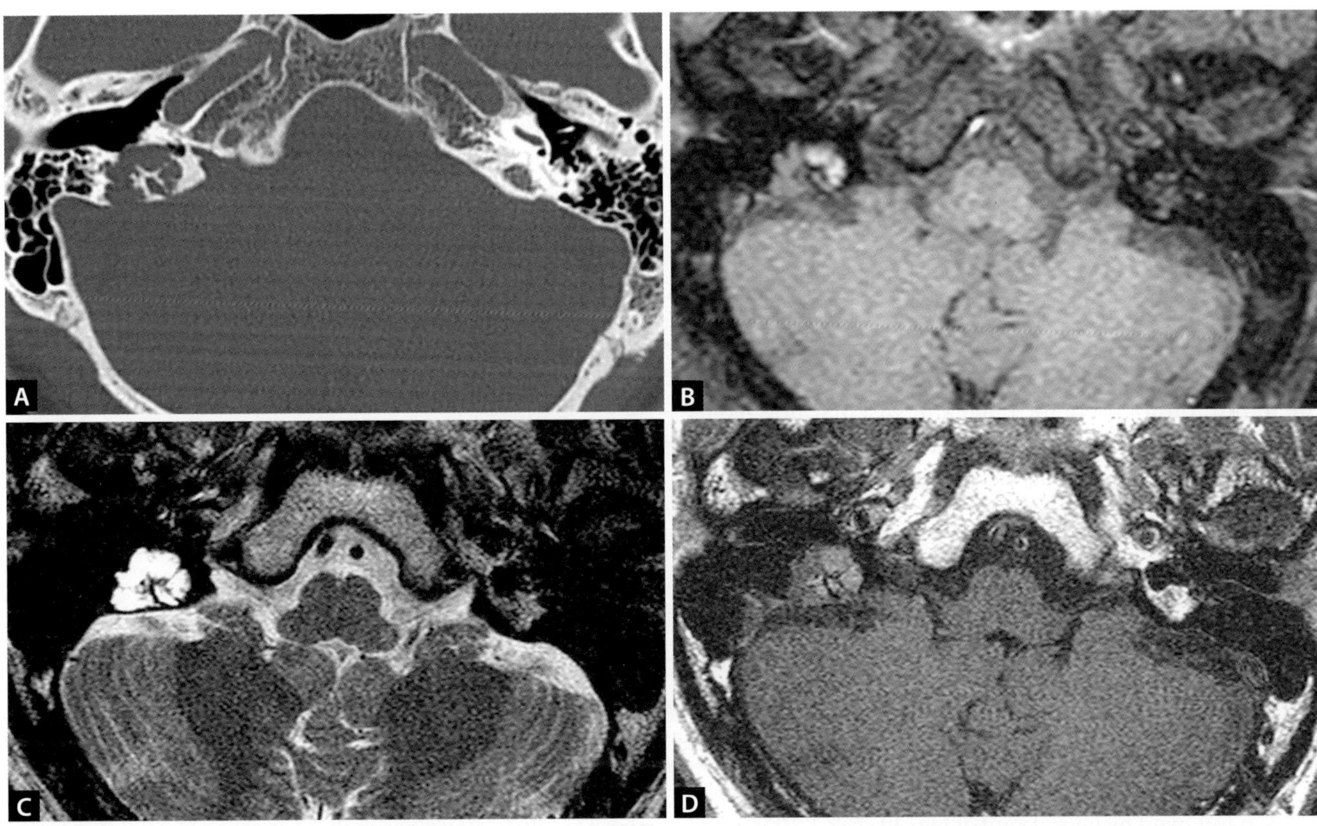

Figs. 23A to D: Endolymphatic sac tumor: Axial CT scan (A) shows a well-defined retrolabyrinthine mass in right petrous bone with intratumoral bony spicules. The mass is heterogeneously hyperintense on fat-saturated T1-WI (B) and T2-WI (C) and shows heterogeneous enhancement (D).

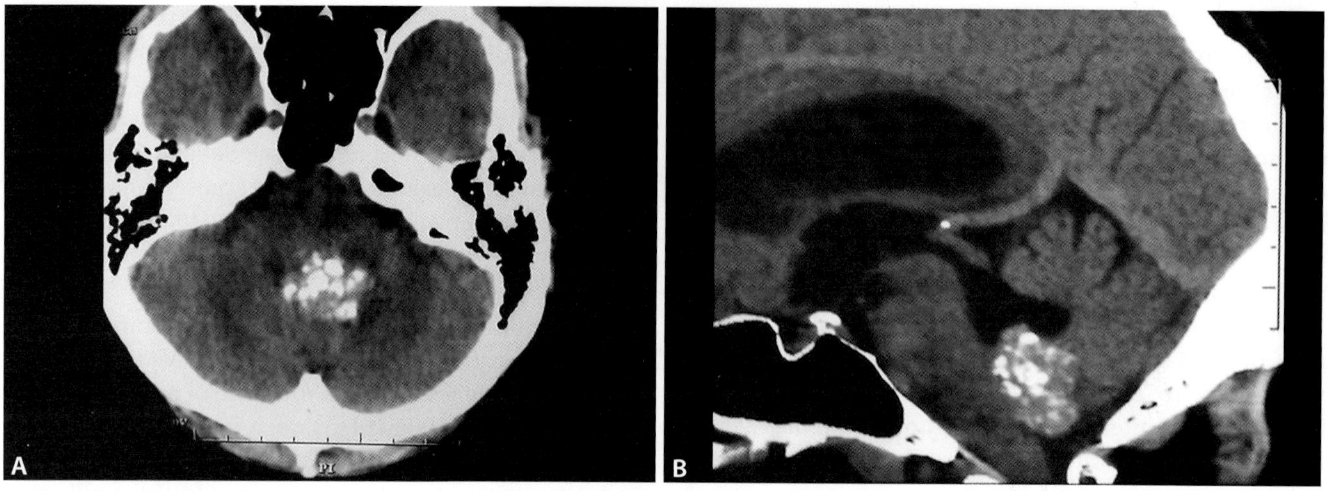

Figs. 24A and B: Choroid plexus papilloma—CT. Axial (A) and reformatted sagittal (B) NCCT scan images show a partially calcified mass in the inferior fourth ventricle.

Homogenous enhancement is seen following intravenous contrast. Anaplastic CPPs invade the ependyma and grow into the surrounding white matter, producing vasogenic edema. They are more irregular in outline and closely resemble CPCs.

Choroid plexus carcinomas are much more aggressive than papillomas, irregular in contour, mixed density on pre-contrast study and show variable enhancement. Cysts and hemorrhage are frequent. They almost always grow through the ventricular wall into the brain with associated edema.

At MRI, CPPs are homogeneous or heterogeneous cauliflower-like tumors. They are usually iso/hypointense on both T1 and T2WI and show avid contrast enhancement, unless the tumor is highly calcified **(Figs. 25A to D)**. Heterogeneous tumors contain areas of low signal intensity due to calcifications, foci of high signal intensity due to intratumoral hemorrhage and vascular flow-voids secondary to feeding vessels.[75] Hydrocephalus is usually associated with CPP; it may be partially explained by CSF hypersecretion by the tumor, but also by fourth ventricle obstruction when the tumor is located in the infratentorial compartment.[76]

Subependymoma

Subependymomas are rare, benign (WHO grade I), slow-growing intraventricular tumors. They usually occur in middle-aged and older individuals with a mean age of 50 years. Fourth ventricle (30-60%) is the most common location followed by lateral ventricles (40–75%).[77] They are commonly identified as an incidental finding. They usually present with hydrocephalus based on critical location and size.[77] Calcifications, hemorrhages and/or micro-vascular proliferation may be present.

Imaging

Imaging findings of subependymoma vary with the location. On CT, fourth ventricular subependymomas demonstrate variable density with calcifications (50–100%) and enhancement (62–92%) in most cases.[77] On the other hand, lateral ventricle subependymomas are more often hypodense, usually do not enhance and less likely to have calcifications (less than 10% of cases).

MRI of fourth ventricular subependymoma demonstrates its origin from the floor of the fourth ventricle and almost always has extension through the foramina of Luschka or Magendie. They are T1 hypo-isointense, T2 iso-hyperintense and almost always demonstrate heterogeneous enhancement. No paraventricular extension is seen in subependymomas, unlike other ventricular tumors.[78] These tumors are very hypometabolic in 18F-FDG PET, which is believed to be secondary to their low cellular density and slow growth.[79]

Rosette-forming Glioneuronal Tumor (RGNT)

RGNT of the fourth ventricle is a rare, benign, mixed neuronal-glial primary brain tumor primarily affecting young adults.[80] It is recognized as a distinct entity since the 2007 WHO Classification of Tumors of the Central Nervous System.[81] RGNT often occupies the fourth ventricle but occasionally it shows cerebellar (vermian) invasion or may involve the aqueduct.[82] Rare extraventricular locations have been reported, including the cerebellar hemispheres,

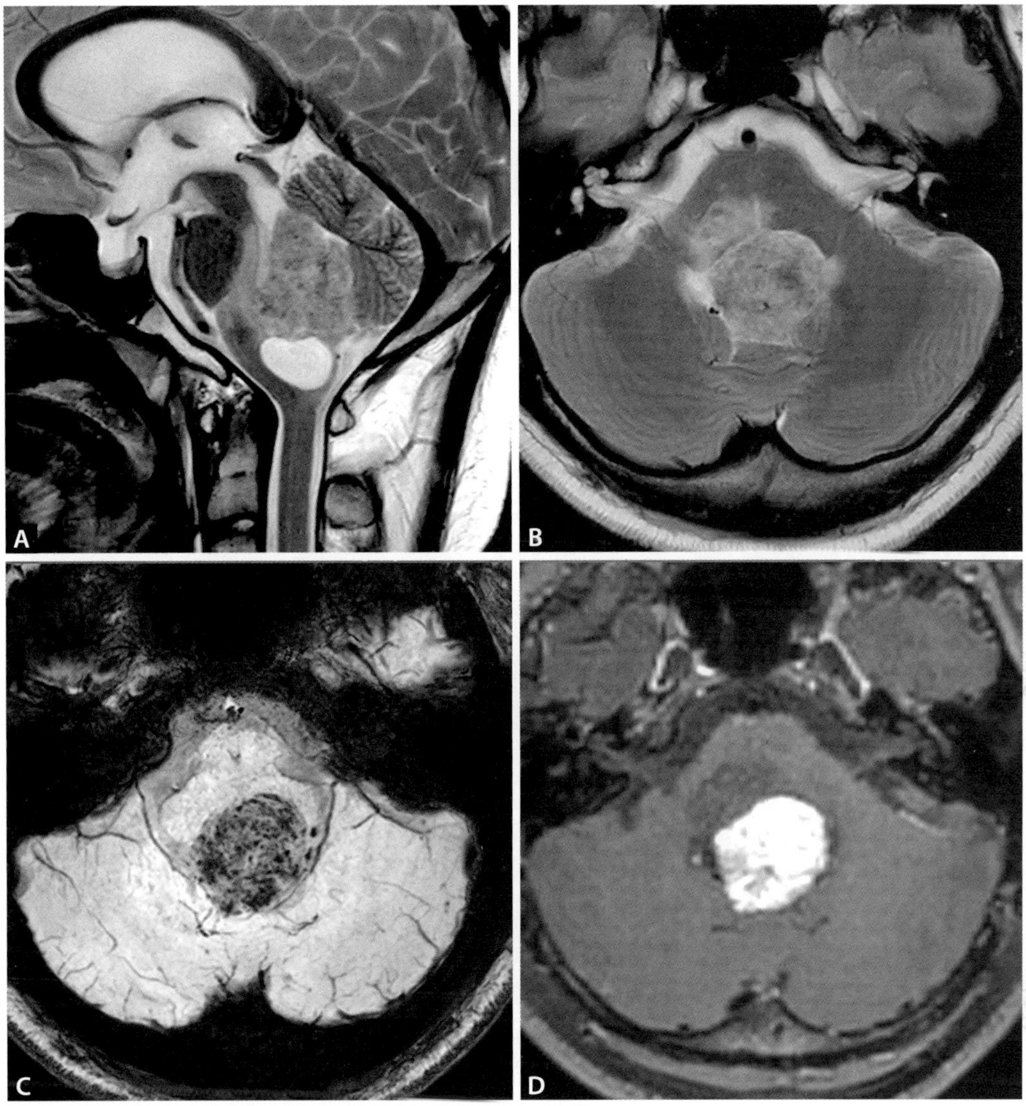

Figs. 25A to D: Choroid plexus papilloma—MRI: Sagittal (A) and axial (B) T2-WI show fourth ventricle iso-hypointense mass with hydrocephalus. The mass has foci of susceptibility signal on SWI (C) and shows intense enhancement (D).

cerebellopontine angles, pineal gland, tectum, thalami, third ventricle, optic chiasm, spinal cord, and a recent case in the septum pellucidum.[80] Symptoms are nonspecific and include headache, gait disturbances, vertigo, and visual disturbances, which develop over months to years. The tumor may be incidentally discovered.[82]

Pathology

The defining histopathological feature is a mixed population of neurocytes organized in pseudorosettes and pilocytic astrocytes. Unlike pilocytic astrocytomas, rosette-forming glioneuronal tumors do not harbor alterations in *BRAF*; some may harbor mutations in *PIK3CA* or *FGFR1*.[83,84]

Imaging

RGNT is mostly an enhancing tumor that can display solid, cystic, or mixed features on brain MRI. RGNT is usually T1 isointense or hypointense and T2 hyperintense without any restricted diffusion **(Figs. 26A to F)**. Intratumoral hemorrhage and calcifications (25%) may occur. The diagnosis of RGNT should be considered when a cystic neoplasm of the fourth ventricle/superior vermis is encountered in an adult. RGNT may expand the cortex and involve underlying white matter or be deeply situated abutting the ventricles.

These tumors are usually curable by surgical resection, although rare cases of tumor dissemination throughout the ventricular system have been described.

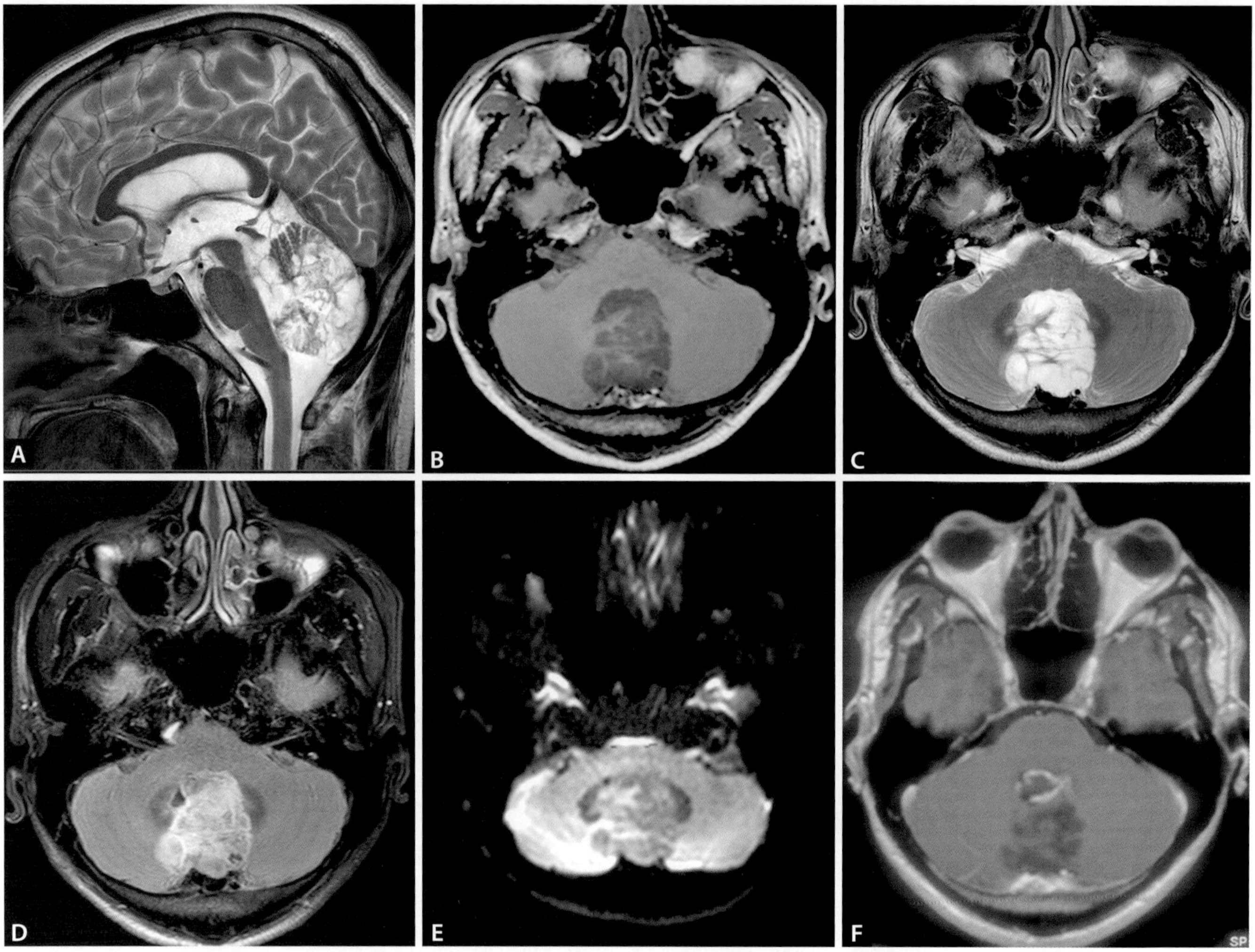

Figs. 26A to F: Rosette-forming glioneuronal tumor (RGNT): Sagittal T2-WI (A) shows a midline vermian lesion with extension into the 4th ventricle. The lesion is hypointense on axial T1-WI (B), hyperintense on axial T2- (C) and FLAIR (D) images. Note any absence of vasogenic edema. No diffusion restriction is seen on DWI image (E). Post-contrast T1W axial image (F) shows minimal enhancement.

CONCLUSION

Many neoplastic lesions can occur in the infratentorial compartment of brain. In order to make an accurate diagnosis, radiologists must answer several essential questions: (1) Whether the patient is an adult or a pediatric patient? (2) Whether the tumor is intra-axial or extra-axial? (3) What are the imaging characteristics of the tumor? Apart from the CT scan and conventional MR sequences, advanced MR imaging protocols like DWI, SWI, perfusion and MRS may help to clinch the diagnosis.

REFERENCES

1. Harwood-Nash DC. Primary neoplasms of the central nervous system in children. Cancer. 1991;67(S4):1223-8.
2. Lizak PF, Woodruff WW. Posterior fossa neoplasms: multiplanar imaging. Semin Ultrasound CT MR. 1992;13(3):182-206.
3. Taylor MD, Northcott PA, et al. Molecular subgroups of medulloblastoma: the current consensus. Acta Neuropathol. 2012;123(4):465-72.
4. Louis DN, Perry A, Reifenberger G, et al. The 2016 World Health Organization Classification of Tumors of the Central Nervous System: a summary. Acta Neuropathol. 2016;131(6):803-20.
5. Wataya T, Hamasaki M, Taylor MD. Molecular subgrouping and characterization analysis of medulloblastomas in a cohort of Japanese patients. No Shinkei Geka. 2015;43(2):117-25.
6. Kool M, Korshunov A, Remke M, et al. Molecular subgroups of medulloblastoma: an international meta-analysis of transcriptome, genetic aberrations, and clinical data of WNT, SHH, Group 3, and Group 4 medulloblastomas. Acta Neuropathologica. 2012;123(4):473-84.
7. Koeller KK, Rushing EJ. From the archives of the AFIP: medulloblastoma: a comprehensive review with radiologic-pathologic correlation. Radiographics. 2003;23(6):1613-37.

8. Kotsenas AL, Roth TC, Manness WK, et al. Abnormal diffusion-weighted MRI in medulloblastoma: does it reflect small cell histology? Pediatr Radiol. 1999;29(7):524-6.
9. Moreno-Torres A, Martinez-Perez I, Baquero M, et al. Taurine detection by proton magnetic resonance spectroscopy in medulloblastoma: contribution to noninvasive differential diagnosis with cerebellar astrocytoma. Neurosurgery. 2004;55(4):824-9; discussion 9.
10. Beier D, Kocakaya S, Hau P, et al. The Neuroradiological Spectra of Adult and Pediatric Medulloblastoma Differ: Results from a Literature-based Meta-analysis. Clin Neuroradiol. 2016.
11. Patay Z, DeSain LA, Hwang SN, et al. MR Imaging Characteristics of Wingless-Type-Subgroup Pediatric Medulloblastoma. Am J Neuroradiol. 2015;36(12): 2386-93.
12. Pajtler KW, Witt H, Sill M, et al. Molecular Classification of Ependymal Tumors across All CNS Compartments, Histopathological Grades, and Age Groups. Cancer Cell. 2015;27(5):728-43.
13. Allen JC, Siffert J, Hukin J. Clinical manifestations of childhood ependymoma: a multitude of syndromes. Pediatr Neurosurg. 1998;28(1):49-55.
14. Witt H, Mack SC, Ryzhova M, et al. Delineation of two clinically and molecularly distinct subgroups of posterior fossa ependymoma. Cancer Cell. 2011;20(2):143-57.
15. Tortori-Donati P, Fondelli MP, Cama A, et al. Ependymomas of the posterior cranial fossa: CT and MRI findings. Neuroradiology. 1995;37(3):238-43.
16. Furie DM, Provenzale JM. Supratentorial ependymomas and subependymomas: CT and MR appearance. J Comput Assist Tomogr. 1995;19(4):518-26.
17. Vanuytsel L, Brada M. The role of prophylactic spinal irradiation in localized intracranial ependymoma. Int J Radiat Oncol Biol Phys. 1991;21(3):825-30.
18. Rumboldt Z, Camacho DL, Lake D, et al. Apparent diffusion coefficients for differentiation of cerebellar tumors in children. Am J Neuroradiol. 2006;27(6):1362-9.
19. Uematsu Y, Hirano A, Llena JF. Electron microscopic observations of blood vessels in ependymoma. No Shinkei Geka. 1988;16(11):1235-42.
20. Brandao LA, Young Poussaint T. Posterior Fossa Tumors. Neuroimaging Clin N Am. 2017;27(1):1-37.
21. Blaser SI, Harwood-Nash DC. Neuroradiology of pediatric posterior fossa medulloblastoma. J Neurooncol. 1996;29(1):23-34.
22. Brandao LA, Poussaint TY. Pediatric brain tumors. Neuroimaging Clin N Am. 2013;23(3):499-525.
23. Harris LM, Davies N, Macpherson L, et al. The use of short-echo-time 1H MRS for childhood cerebellar tumours prior to histopathological diagnosis. Pediatr Radiol. 2007;37(11):1101-9.
24. Merchant TE, Li C, Xiong X, et al. Conformal radiotherapy after surgery for paediatric ependymoma: a prospective study. Lancet Oncol. 2009;10(3):258-66.
25. Fernandez C, Figarella-Branger D, Girard N, et al. Pilocytic astrocytomas in children: prognostic factors—a retrospective study of 80 cases. Neurosurgery. 2003;53(3):544-53; discussion 54-5.
26. Arslanoglu A, Aygun N, Tekhtani D, et al. Imaging findings of CNS atypical teratoid/rhabdoid tumors. Am J Neuroradiol. 2004;25(3):476-80.
27. Jin B, Feng XY. MRI features of atypical teratoid/rhabdoid tumors in children. Pediatr Radiol. 2013;43(8):1001-8.
28. Fuller CE. All things rhabdoid and SMARC: An enigmatic exploration with Dr. Louis P. Dehner. Semin Diagn Pathol. 2016;33(6):427-40.
29. Rorke LB, Packer R, Biegel J. Central nervous system atypical teratoid/rhabdoid tumors of infancy and childhood. J Neurooncol. 1995;24(1):21-8.
30. Hasselblatt M, Gesk S, Oyen F, et al. Nonsense mutation and inactivation of SMARCA4 (BRG1) in an atypical teratoid/rhabdoid tumor showing retained SMARCB1 (INI1) expression. Am J Surg Pathol. 2011;35(6):933-5.
31. Zuccoli G, Izzi G, Bacchini E, et al. Central nervous system atypical teratoid/rhabdoid tumour of infancy. CT and MR findings. Clin Imaging. 1999;23(6):356-60.
32. Agranovich AL, Ang LC, Griebel RW, et al. Malignant rhabdoid tumor of the central nervous system with subarachnoid dissemination. Surg Neurol. 1992;37(5): 410-4.
33. Koral K, Gargan L, Bowers DC, et al. Imaging characteristics of atypical teratoid-rhabdoid tumor in children compared with medulloblastoma. Am J Roentgenol. 2008;190(3):809-14.
34. Katz JS, Peruzzi PP, Pierson CR, et al. Cerebellopontine angle tumors in young children, displaying cranial nerve deficits, and restricted diffusion on diffusion-weighted imaging: a new clinical triad for atypical teratoid/rhabdoid tumors. Childs Nerv Syst. 2017;33(5):833-8.
35. Lee SR, Sanches J, Mark AS, et al. Posterior fossa hemangioblastomas: MR imaging. Radiology. 1989;171(2): 463-8.
36. Hakyemez B, Erdogan C, Bolca N, et al. Evaluation of different cerebral mass lesions by perfusion-weighted MR imaging. J Magn Reson Imaging. 2006;24(4):817-24.
37. Abo-Al Hassan A, Ismail M, Panda SM. Pre-operative endovascular embolization of a cerebellar haemangioblastoma. A case report. Med Princ Pract. 2006; 15(6):459-62.
38. Isiklar I, Leeds NE, Fuller GN, et al. Intracranial metastatic melanoma: correlation between MR imaging characteristics and melanin content. Am J Roentgenol. 1995;165(6):1503-12.
39. Smith JK, Castillo M, Kwock L. MR spectroscopy of brain tumors. Magn Reson Imaging Clin N Am. 2003;11(3):415-29, v-vi.
40. Nagaraja S, Powell T, Griffiths PD, et al. MR imaging and spectroscopy in Lhermitte-Duclos disease. Neuroradiology. 2004;46(5):355-8.
41. Nowak DA, Trost HA. Lhermitte-Duclos disease (dysplastic cerebellar gangliocytoma): a malformation, hamartoma or neoplasm? Acta Neurol Scand. 2002;105(3):137-45.

42. Koeller KK, Henry JM. From the archives of the AFIP: superficial gliomas: radiologic-pathologic correlation. Armed Forces Institute of Pathology. Radiographics. 2001;21(6):1533-56.
43. Zhou XP, Marsh DJ, Morrison CD, et al. Germline inactivation of PTEN and dysregulation of the phosphoinositol-3-kinase/Akt pathway cause human Lhermitte-Duclos disease in adults. Am J Hum Genet. 2003;73(5):1191-8.
44. Mester J, Eng C. Cowden syndrome: recognizing and managing a not-so-rare hereditary cancer syndrome. J Surg Oncol. 2015;111(1):125-30.
45. Kulkantrakorn K, Awwad EE, Levy B, et al. MRI in Lhermitte-Duclos disease. Neurology. 1997;48(3):725-31.
46. Awwad EE, Levy E, Martin DS, et al. Atypical MR appearance of Lhermitte-Duclos disease with contrast enhancement. AJNR Am J Neuroradiol. 1995;16(8):1719-20.
47. Chawla A, Emmanuel JV, Seow WT, et al. Paediatric PNET: pre-surgical MRI features. Clin Radiol. 2007;62(1): 43-52.
48. Prasad AN. Supratentorial PNET in a young child. Indian J Pediatr. 2011;78(5):613-5.
49. Borja MJ, Plaza MJ, Altman N, et al. Conventional and advanced MRI features of pediatric intracranial tumors: supratentorial tumors. Am J Roentgenol. 2013;200(5):W483-503.
50. Jallo GI, Biser-Rohrbaugh A, Freed D. Brainstem gliomas. Childs Nerv Syst. 2004;20(3):143-53.
51. Fischbein NJ, Prados MD, Wara W, et al. Radiologic classification of brain stem tumors: correlation of magnetic resonance imaging appearance with clinical outcome. Pediatr Neurosurg. 1996;24(1):9-23.
52. Fisher PG, Breiter SN, Carson BS, et al. A clinicopathologic reappraisal of brain stem tumor classification. Identification of pilocystic astrocytoma and fibrillary astrocytoma as distinct entities. Cancer. 2000;89(7):1569-76.
53. Aihara K, Mukasa A, Gotoh K, et al. H3F3A K27M mutations in thalamic gliomas from young adult patients. Neuro Oncol. 2014;16(1):140-6.
54. Buczkowicz P, Bartels U, Bouffet E, et al. Histopathological spectrum of paediatric diffuse intrinsic pontine glioma: diagnostic and therapeutic implications. Acta Neuropathol. 2014;128(4):573-81.
55. Lee BC, Kneeland JB, Walker RW, et al. MR imaging of brainstem tumors. Am J Neuroradiol. 1985;6(2):159-63.
56. Aboian MS, Solomon DA, Felton E, et al. Imaging Characteristics of Pediatric Diffuse Midline Gliomas with Histone H3 K27M Mutation. Am J Neuroradiol. 2017;38(4):795-800.
57. Lindsay AJ, Rush SZ, Fenton LZ. Pediatric posterior fossa ganglioglioma: unique MRI features and correlation with BRAF V600E mutation status. Journal of Neuro-Oncology. 2014;118(2):395-404.
58. Chassot A, Canale S, Varlet P, et al. Radiotherapy with concurrent and adjuvant temozolomide in children with newly diagnosed diffuse intrinsic pontine glioma. Journal of Neuro-Oncology. 2011;106(2):399-407.
59. Moffat DA, Ballagh RH. Rare tumours of the cerebellopontine angle. Clin Oncol (R Coll Radiol). 1995;7(1):28-41.
60. Mafee MF, Lachenauer CS, Kumar A, et al. CT and MR imaging of intralabyrinthine schwannoma: report of two cases and review of the literature. Radiology. 1990;174(2):395-400.
61. Matthies C, Samii M, Krebs S. Management of vestibular schwannomas (acoustic neuromas): Radiological features in 202 cases - Their value for diagnosis and their predictive importance. Neurosurgery. 1997;40(3):469-81.
62. Swartz JD. Lesions of the cerebellopontine angle and internal auditory canal: diagnosis and differential diagnosis. Semin Ultrasound CT MR. 2004;25(4):332-52.
63. Ben Hamouda M, Drissi C, Sebai R, et al. Atypical CT and MRI aspects of an epidermoid cyst. J Neuroradiol. 2007;34(2):129-32.
64. Dechambre S, Duprez T, Lecouvet F, et al. Diffusion-weighted MRI postoperative assessment of an epidermoid tumour in the cerebellopontine angle. Neuroradiology. 1999;41(11):829-31.
65. Osborn AG, Preece MT. Intracranial cysts: radiologic-pathologic correlation and imaging approach. Radiology. 2006;239(3):650-64.
66. Wester K. Peculiarities of intracranial arachnoid cysts: location, sidedness, and sex distribution in 126 consecutive patients. Neurosurgery. 1999;45(4):775-9.
67. Ikeda H, Deinsberger W, Boker DK. Retroclival arachnoid cyst presenting with spontaneous intracystic haemorrhage—case presentation. Acta Neurochir (Wien). 2000;142(11):1317-8.
68. Dutt SN, Mirza S, Chavda SV, et al. Radiologic differentiation of intracranial epidermoids from arachnoid cysts. Otol Neurotol. 2002;23(1):84-92.
69. Bonneville F, Sarrazin JL, Marsot-Dupuch K, et al. Unusual lesions of the cerebellopontine angle: a segmental approach. Radiographics. 2001;21(2):419-38.
70. Kertesz TR, Shelton C, Wiggins RH, et al. Intratemporal facial nerve neuroma: anatomical location and radiological features. Laryngoscope. 2001;111(7):1250-6.
71. Jensen RL, Gillespie D, House P, et al. Endolymphatic sac tumors in patients with and without von Hippel-Lindau disease: the role of genetic mutation, von Hippel-Lindau protein, and hypoxia inducible factor-1alpha expression. J Neurosurg. 2004;100(3):488-97.
72. Lo WW, Applegate LJ, Carberry JN, et al. Endolymphatic sac tumors: radiologic appearance. Radiology. 1993;189(1):199-204.
73. Baltacioğlu F, Ekinci G, Türe U, et al. MR imaging, CT, and angiography features of endolymphatic sac tumors: report of two cases. Neuroradiology. 2014;44(1):91-6.
74. Mukherji SK, Albernaz VS, Lo WW, et al. Papillary endolymphatic sac tumors: CT, MR imaging, and angiographic findings in 20 patients. Radiology. 1997;202(3):801-8.
75. Shin JH, Lee HK, Jeong AK, et al. Choroid plexus papilloma in the posterior cranial fossa: MR, CT, and angiographic findings. Clin Imaging. 2001;25(3):154-62.

76. Pencalet P, Sainte-Rose C, Lellouch-Tubiana A, et al. Papillomas and carcinomas of the choroid plexus in children. J Neurosurg. 1998;88(3):521-8.
77. Chiechi MV, Smirniotopoulos JG, Jones RV. Intracranial subependymomas: CT and MR imaging features in 24 cases. AJR Am J Roentgenol. 1995;165(5):1245-50.
78. Nishio S, Morioka T, Mihara F, et al. Subependymoma of the lateral ventricles. Neurosurg Rev. 2000;23(2):98-103.
79. Mineura K, Shioya H, Kowada M, et al. Subependymoma of the septum pellucidum: characterization by PET. J Neurooncol. 1997;32(2):143-7.
80. Sharma P, Swain M, Padua MD, et al. Rosette-forming glioneuronal tumors: a report of two cases. Neurol India. 2011;59(2):276-80.
81. Hsu C, Kwan G, Lau Q, et al. Rosette-forming glioneuronal tumour: imaging features, histopathological correlation and a comprehensive review of literature. Br J Neurosurg. 2012;26(5):668-73.
82. Kumar M, Samant R, Ramakrishnaiah R, et al. Rosette-forming glioneuronal tumor of the fourth ventricle. Radiol Case Rep. 2013;8(1):740.
83. Ellezam B, Theeler BJ, Luthra R, et al. Recurrent PIK3CA mutations in rosette-forming glioneuronal tumor. Acta Neuropathol. 2012;123(2):285-7.
84. Gessi M, Moneim YA, Hammes J, et al. FGFR1 mutations in Rosette-forming glioneuronal tumors of the fourth ventricle. J Neuropathol Exp Neurol. 2014;73(6): 580-4.

CHAPTER 18

Sellar and Parasellar Lesions

Paramjeet Singh, Chirag Kamal Ahuja, Niranjan Khandelwal

INTRODUCTION

Pituitary gland plays a central role in body growth, metabolism and reproductive functions. It is an anatomically complex area where a number of neoplastic, infectious, inflammatory, developmental and vascular pathologies can occur. Pathological lesions of sellar and parasellar region can have profound clinical/endocrinological as well as neurological consequences. The diagnosis often needs multidisciplinary approach using ophthalmological, endocrine, neurological and radiological methods. Cross sectional imaging by computed tomography (CT) and magnetic resonance imaging (MRI), especially the latter, have expanded our understanding of the structure and pathology of this region.

NORMAL ANATOMY AND APPLIED PHYSIOLOGY

The key to imaging interpretation of sellar/parasellar pathology lies in a thorough knowledge of the complex anatomy of nervous, bony, vascular and meningeal structures located in and around this region **(Figs. 1A and B)**. While sella has clearly defined landmarks, the parasellar area includes all structures bordering it.

The sella-turcica is a spherical depression in the superior surface of the sphenoid bone bounded by the sphenoid sinus anteroinferiorly, the paired cavernous sinuses laterally, the suprasellar cisterns and its contents, diaphragma sellae and hypothalamus superiorly and the dorsum sella and brainstem posteriorly.

The cortical bone of sella varies from few microns to several millimeters in thickness, depending upon the degree of pneumatization of the sphenoid sinus. The carotid artery forms a groove on the posterosuperior wall of the sphenoid sinus. The wall between the artery and the sinus may be very thin, even absent in up to one-third of patients, thus making it vulnerable to injury during trans-sphenoidal surgery. Localized defects in its bony cortex or asymmetry of the sellar floor are common.[1] The bony sella is invested by a reflection of dura, the outer layer of which lines the floor while the inner layer forms a diaphragm at the roof (diaphragma sellae). A central opening in the diaphragm allows the pituitary infundibulum to pass into the sella. Anteriorly, the sellar floor is continuous with the tuberculum sellae and limbus sphenoidale. The dorsum sella demarcates the posterior sellar border.

Cavernous sinuses are two multiseptated, symmetrically paired parasellar venous sinuses with a straight or slightly convex outer wall. The two layers of dura form the roof, outer wall and inner wall of the sinuses. The lateral walls of the cavernous sinuses from superior to inferior contain the cranial nerves III, IV as well as first and second divisions of the Vth nerve (V1 and V2) **(Fig. 2)**. The VIth nerve passes through the sinus below the internal carotid artery (ICA). The ICA has a variable course within the sinus; however, a more medial location of the artery is a normal variation and is surgically important. The artery may actually indent the gland at times and the distance between the arteries may be as little as 4 mm. The ICA exits the sinus at level of anterior clinoid process

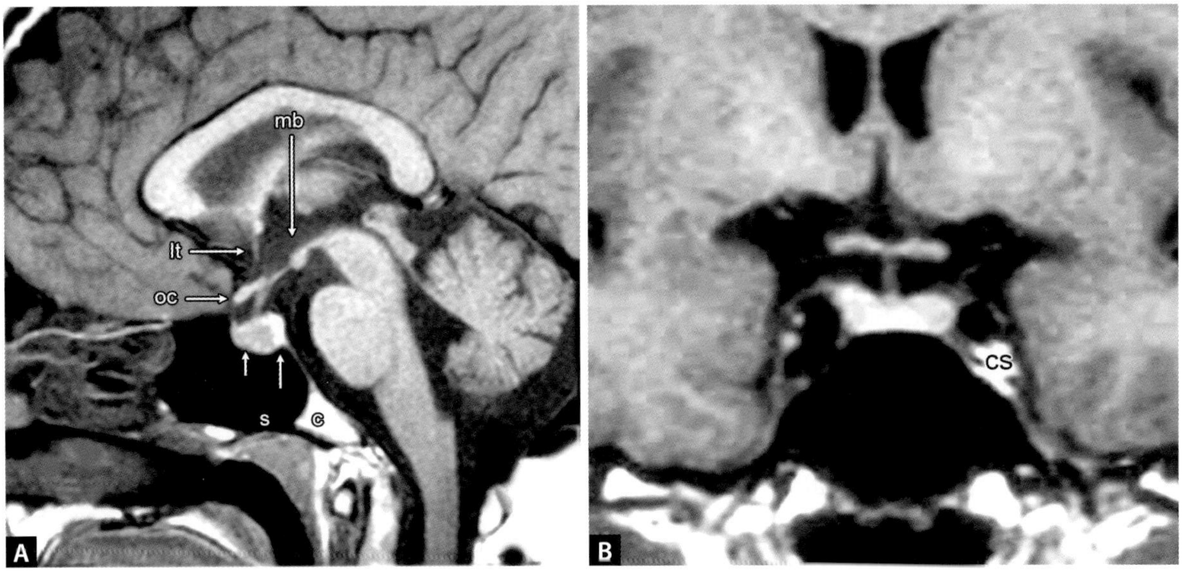

Figs. 1A and B: Normal sellar anatomy: T1-weighted (A) sagittal and (B) coronal images showing adenohypophysis (short arrow), posterior pituitary bright spot (long arrow), infundibulum, mammillary body (mb), sphenoid sinus (s), clivus (c), optic chiasma (oc), cavernous sinus (CS) and lamina terminalis (lt). Tuber cinerium is the ridge of tissue between mammillary body and infundibulum.

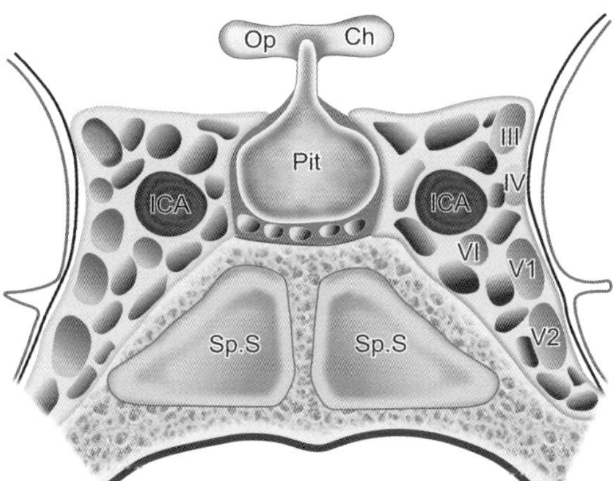

Fig. 2: Pictorial representation of the coronal view of the sella and parasellar (cavernous sinus) region depicting the anatomy and relationship of various structures.
Abbreviations: ICA: Internal carotid artery; Op.Ch.: Optic chiasma; Pit: Pituitary gland; Sp.S: Sphenoid sinus; III, IV, V1, V2 and VI represent the respective cranial nerves.

to give off its supracavernous branches. Meckel's cave housing the Gasserian ganglion lies at the posterior part of the cavernous sinus. The third division of Vth nerve (V3) passes inferior from here to foramen ovale.

The suprasellar cistern is a six pointed expansion of the subarachnoid space containing the optic nerves, optic chiasma and the tracts, circle of Willis and the pituitary infundibulum. The optic chiasma lies 4–6 mm posterosuperior to the tuberculum sellae, however, it may be directly above it (prefixed) or lie more posteriorly above the dorsum sella (postfixed). These variations are important for surgeons. The optic and infundibular recesses are downward invaginations of the third ventricle in relation to its floor.

The hypothalamus is a layer of tissue extending from the anterior commissure to the posterior commissure and forms the floor and the lateral walls of the third ventricle. The inferior ridge of the tissue from the optic chiasma anteriorly to the paired mammillary bodies posteriorly is called the tuber cinereum. At the lateral margins of the hypothalamus are the optic tracts and the sulci of temporal lobes. The hypothalamus consists of multiple nuclei regulating temperature, water balance, drinking behavior and sexual activity. The hypothalamus and the pituitary gland are functionally and physiologically interlinked contiguous structures and often referred to as the hypothalamic-pituitary-axis (HPA). Release of pituitary hormones is mediated by the hypothalamus. Oxytocin and vasopressin are synthesized in hypothalamus and transported to the posterior pituitary.

The pituitary gland is composed of two anatomically and functionally distinct lobes: the anterior lobe (adenohypophysis) and the posterior lobe (neurohypophysis) **(Figs. 1A and B)**. The anterior lobe comprises 75% of the volume of the gland and consists of pars tuberalis, pars intermedia and pars distalis which develop from Rathke's pouch. Pars intermedia which lies between the adeno and neurohypophysis, is a vestigial structure and common site for developmental cysts. The anterior lobe of pituitary is isointense to brain on both T1 and T2WI.[2] It secretes growth hormone (GH), adrenocorticotropic hormone (ACTH), prolactin (PRL), thyroid stimulating hormone (TSH), luteinizing hormone (LH) and melanocyte-stimulating hormone (MSH). The anterior lobe shares a common blood supply with hypothalamus via the hypophyseal portal system, the pathway by which hypothalamic releasing hormones reach this structure. Alternately the hypophyseal arteries, branches of internal carotid supply the stalk and posterior lobe. The venous drainage is to ipsilateral cavernous sinus predominantly and then to petrosal sinuses.

The posterior lobe develops as a downward projection from the neuroectoderm at the base of the brain and along with infundibular stalk, supraoptic and paraventricular hypothalamic nuclei forms the neurohypophysis. Oxytocin and vasopressin synthesized in the hypothalamus are transported to and stored in the posterior pituitary. The posterior lobe appears as a bright spot on T1-weighted images (T1WI) in midline along the dorsum of the sella.[2,3] The anterior lobe of pituitary gland is larger and rounded and appears hyperintense like posterior lobe in newborns and becomes isointense by 4–6 months of life.[3-5]

The dimensions of pituitary gland are extremely variable, particularly its height. The gland undergoes significant changes in size and shape throughout life and this fact must be kept in mind when assessing it for abnormality. A useful guide to the gland's height in relation to age is the "Elster's rule" of 6, 8, 10, 12 **(Table 1)**.[3] On an average, it is 12 mm in width and 8 mm in anteroposterior diameter. The maximal height is achieved in adolescent girls and during pregnancy. The pituitary stalk tapers inferiorly and has thickness of 2 mm. It should not exceed the width of the basilar artery or a maximum of 4 mm.

IMAGING MODALITIES

Currently MRI is the examination of choice for sellar and parasellar pathology due to its superior soft tissue contrast, multiplanar capability and lack of ionizing radiation. This allows better demonstration of pathology, relationship of lesions with surrounding structures and tissue differentiation. CT, though less frequently used is a useful examination particularly for showing calcification, bony destruction and surgically relevant bony anatomy (sphenoid septae and pneumatization). Digital subtraction angiography (DSA) is helpful for vascular lesions and to show vascularity of tumors. However, due to its invasive nature, it is hardly used nowadays and instead has been replaced by CT and MR angiographic techniques. In central Cushing's disease, if no adenoma is visible in MRI, inferior petrosal sinus venous sampling may help in lateralizing a microadenoma to guide selective surgical resection.

Plain Radiography

Plain radiography is infrequently requested these days for diagnosing sellar and parasellar pathology. If indicated, lateral view of the skull centered on the sella is the single most important view **(Fig. 3A)**.

The radiographic size of the sella **(Table 2)**[6] in itself is not a sensitive indicator of pituitary gland abnormalities unless distinctive changes of erosion and other bony abnormalities are seen. The empty sella may itself lead to enlargement of size.[1]

The cortical line of sella called lamina dura is a pencil-sharp thin line. When sella becomes enlarged due to intrasellar tumor, it becomes rounded (ballooning; **Fig. 3B**) and extends forward underneath the anterior clinoid processes. The undercutting of the clinoid processes and intact dorsum sella in these cases results in a closed type of sella, characteristic of intrasellar pathology. Posteriorly the loss of lamina dura is first seen at the junction of base of the dorsum and sellar floor. Large intrasellar masses, however, can cause complete destruction of dorsum. Double flooring of sella may also be seen due to intrasellar masses or can be a normal variant. In contrast early involvement of tip of the dorsum or its complete destruction favors a suprasellar mass (open sella from above, **Fig. 3C**).

Suprasellar calcification is seen in cases of craniopharyngioma, meningioma, clival chordoma and vascular lesions. Meningiomas, in addition, may show hyperostosis

Table 1: Elster's rule for pituitary gland height on MRI.

Age	*Maximum allowable height (mm)*
Infants and children (either sex)	6
Men and postmenopausal women	8
Women of childbearing age	10
Women in late pregnancy and postpartum	12

Table 2: Sellar dimensions on plain radiograph.

Anteroposterior diameter	17 mm (range 5–16 mm)
Depth	13 mm
Width	16 mm (range 10–15 mm)
Area on lateral view	130 sq mm
Volume	1092 cubic mm (mean 599 cubic mm)

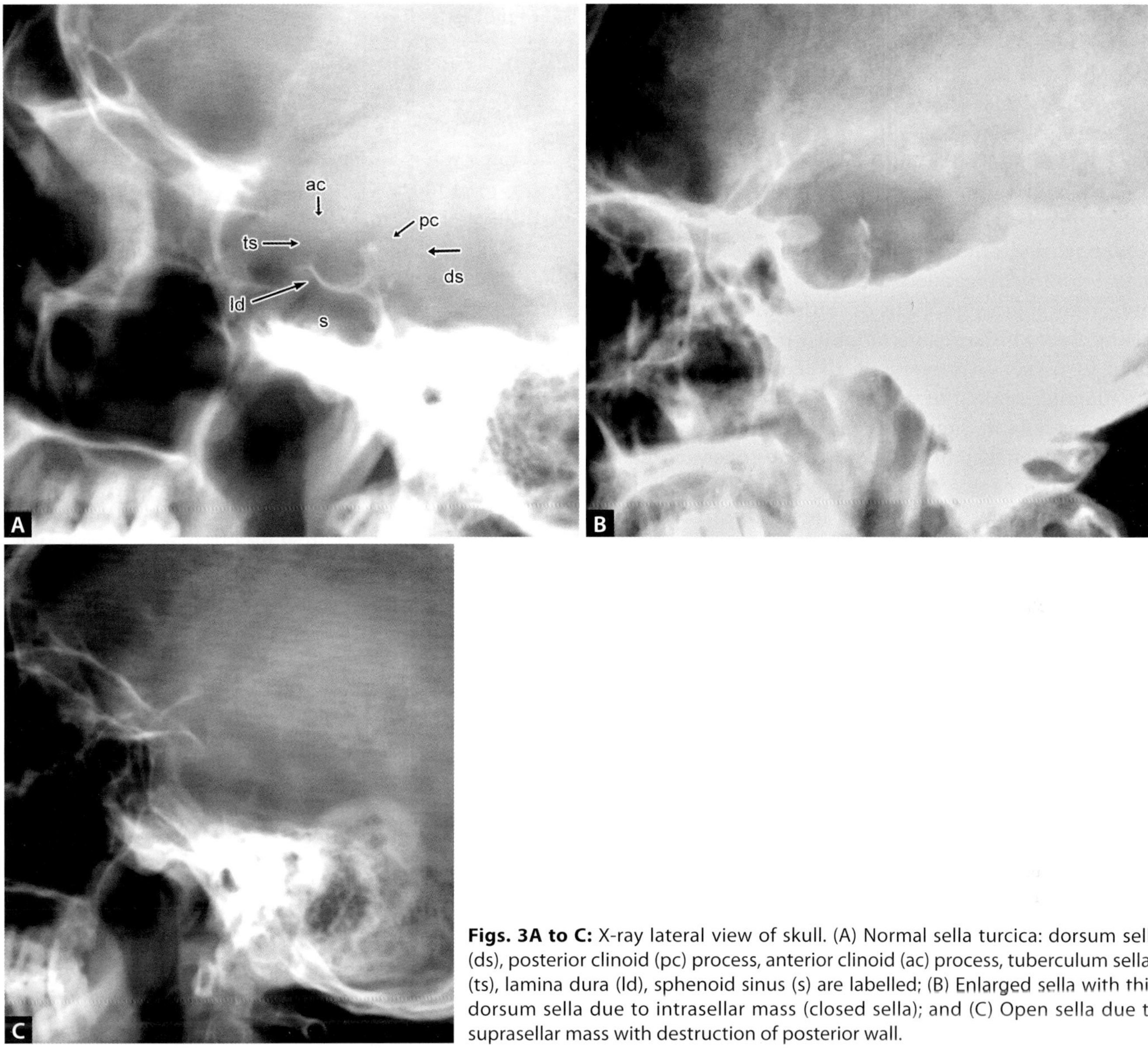

Figs. 3A to C: X-ray lateral view of skull. (A) Normal sella turcica: dorsum sella (ds), posterior clinoid (pc) process, anterior clinoid (ac) process, tuberculum sellae (ts), lamina dura (ld), sphenoid sinus (s) are labelled; (B) Enlarged sella with thin dorsum sella due to intrasellar mass (closed sella); and (C) Open sella due to suprasellar mass with destruction of posterior wall.

of the sphenoid bone. Rarely, adenomas may also show calcification on plain radiographs.

Computed Tomography

Computed tomography of sella used to be performed in coronal plane by taking thin (2 mm sections) perpendicular to the sellar floor using high radiation flux. Additional axial sections were required for larger lesions. With the advent of multidetector CT, volumetric data acquisition can be performed and submillimeter thickness excellent quality images can be reconstructed in any plane. Dynamic scanning consists of sequential CT sections obtained at a single level every few seconds after a bolus of contrast which leads to progressive enhancement of the sellar tissue and provides information about differential enhancement of various components helping in the diagnosis of various lesions.

Magnetic Resonance Imaging

The objective of MR is to obtain high contrast spatially resolved images with reasonable signal to noise ratio (SNR). Requirements for spatial detail are to be balanced against SNR and imaging time penalty. It is important to identify the gland separate from the lesion if possible.

Coronal and sagittal sections are preferred and acquired using a small FOV (16 × 20 cm), thin slices (3 mm) and high resolution matrix (256 × 512) using T1 spin echo and to a lesser extent T2 fast spin echo sequences. Both dynamic and routine postcontrast images as well as delayed scanning after 30–60 minutes may be combined in one study for optimal imaging. A dose of 0.05–0.1 mmol/kg of gadolinium (Gd) compound is usually adequate.[5] A 3-dimensional Fourier transformation gradient echo or fast spin echo sequence may be used for dynamic study. After injecting a bolus of contrast, 6–8 consecutive sets of coronal images are obtained covering the entire gland (3–5 sections) every 10–12 seconds. Differential rate of enhancement of the normal pituitary from small adenomas help in identifying the latter. Fat suppression is particularly useful in evaluation of postoperative sella. 3 Tesla (MR) imaging has potential for higher resolution imaging particularly for cranial nerves and cavernous sinus, but with penalty of susceptibility artifacts in this region caused by bone air interface.[7]

PATHOLOGY OF THE SELLAR AND PARASELLAR REGION

The lesions in this area may arise from the pituitary gland, infundibulum, adjacent brain, bone, dura, leptomeninges, blood vessels, cranial nerves and the extracranial structures such as nasopharynx and sphenoid sinus. These may be categorized depending on their location (intrasellar, suprasellar and parasellar), the age groups affected, the structures involved (pituitary gland, infundibulum, hypothalamus, cavernous sinus, etc.), predominant tissue character (cystic or solid) or etiology (traumatic, neoplastic, inflammatory, vascular, etc.). The following classification is a rough guide to commonly encountered pathologies, however, there may be considerable overlap with many of the lesions affecting more than one region, structure or age group **(Table 3)**.

TUMORS

Pituitary Adenoma

Adenomas arise from the adenohypophysis and are classified by size and hormonal activity; features that determine their clinical presentation. They are the most common tumors of the sellar and parasellar region in adults and constitute 10–15% of all intracranial neoplasms.[8] By definition, adenomas measuring less than 10 mm are called microadenomas while the larger ones are termed macroadenomas. In general, hormonally active lesions are discovered at a smaller size due to endocrinopathy and consequent clinical symptoms. Nonfunctioning adenomas are usually large at the time of diagnosis when they produce symptoms due to mass effect on surrounding structures. Approximately three-fourths of adenomas show signs of hormone excess while the rest are nonfunctioning tumors.[8] Sometimes these nonfunctioning lesions may be discovered incidentally (Incidentalomas). Clinically silent adenomas have been demonstrated in 10% of asymptomatic volunteers.[9] The rest may produce symptoms by compressing adjacent structures, causing various symptoms, i.e. visual field defects (bitemporal hemianopia) due to optic chiasma compression, hypopituitarism due to compression of pituitary gland, cranial nerve deficits due to lateral extension into cavernous sinuses, hydrocephalus/CSF rhinorrhea due to third ventricular obstruction, or rarely, diabetes insipidus due to mass effect on hypothalamus.

Types of Adenomas

Prolactinomas are the most common functioning adenomas comprising 50% of all adenomas.[5] These tumors clinically present with amenorrhea, galactorrhea and infertility in females and loss of libido and impotence in males. Serum PRL level is usually greater than 100 ng/mL (normal 20 ng/mL). In case serum PRL level is greater

Table 3: Sellar and parasellar lesions.

Intrasellar masses	Physiological and pathological hyperplasia, micro and macroadenomas, non-neoplastic cyst, craniopharyngioma, meningioma
Suprasellar mass (child)	Craniopharyngioma, hypothalamic glioma, germinoma, arachnoid cyst, tuber cinereumhamartoma
Suprasellar mass (adult)	Macroadenoma, meningioma, aneurysm, metastasis, epidermoid/dermoid
Cystic lesions	Craniopharyngioma, arachnoid cyst, epidermoid, pituitary abscess
Infundibular masses (child)	Pituitary hypoplasia, histiocytosis, germinoma, leukemia
Infundibular masses (adult)	Hypophysitis, sarcoidosis, metastasis/lymphoma, pituicytoma
Parasellar lesion (tumors)	Metastasis, meningioma, schwannoma, lymphoma, chordoma, osteocartilaginous tumors, nasopharyngeal carcinoma, plasmacytoma
Parasellar lesions (vascular and inflammatory)	Sarcoidosis, histiocytosis, infections, fungal, non-fungal, cavernous sinus thrombosis, cavernous sinus hemangioma, aneurysm, caroticocavernous fistula, Tolosa-Hunt syndrome

than 200 ng/mL, the cause is nearly always a pituitary adenoma.[10] ACTH secreting adenomas produce early symptoms when they are small,[5] often measuring 1-2 mm in size and thus are difficult to diagnose. However, an ectopic source of ACTH secretion must also be kept in mind in a patient with hypercortisolism. GH secreting tumors are macroadenomas as they are diagnosed late in the course of disease. They produce acromegaly in adults and gigantism in children. Rarely adenomas arise from the thyrotrophs (TSH secreting) or gonadotrophs (FHS and/or LH secreting). In addition, 10% of secreting adenomas are plurihormonal,[8] the most common combination being the PRL-GH producing adenoma.

Imaging of Adenomas

Imaging is indicated both to confirm the existence of an adenoma and to define its size and location for appropriate surgical or medical therapy. MRI is the preferred modality, though CT is also useful. Reported sensitivity and specificity of noncontrast MRI and contrast enhanced CT are roughly equal varying from 50% to 90%.[3] However, there is no large blinded prospective study comparing CT and MRI in the same group of patients.[5] Overall, T1WI are more reliable for detection of adenomas. The addition of Gd enhancement increases the detection rate of microadenomas by 10%. Postcontrast dynamic acquisition allows evaluation of temporal changes in signal intensity in intrasellar structures and adds additional 5–20% sensitivity over the nondynamic studies for detection of microadenomas (particularly small ACTH secretors and those which are isointense).[10] Signal intensity increases more rapidly and to a greater degree in normal pituitary gland than in microadenoma, however, 3–5 minutes following the contrast administration the signal of the normal gland and the adenoma may become identical **(Fig. 4)**. The maximum contrast difference between the normal gland and the microadenoma occurs at about 30–60 seconds when the distinction between normal pituitary and the adenoma is the best. Microadenomas also demonstrate a slower washout of accumulated contrast that may cause them to appear hyperintense on delayed images (>20 minutes postcontrast). With modern state-of-the-art MRI equipments, more than 90% adenomas should be picked up.[5] The prescribed protocol should be high resolution plain scan which if negative should be followed by contrast-enhanced magnetic resonance imaging consisting of both dynamic scanning and regular postcontrast scan. Certain studies have shown that if the conventional and dynamic contrast imaging is combined with an additional 3D volumetric interpolated breath-hold examination, a spoiled-gradient echo 3D T1 sequence (SGE), the accuracy of identifying microadenomas increases significantly.[11] Parasellar extension and invasion of the base of skull are also accurately shown on MRI with dynamic T1 and heavily T2-weighted sequences proving the best. CT scores over MRI in showing subtle cortical involvement, however, this may not be surgically important.[5]

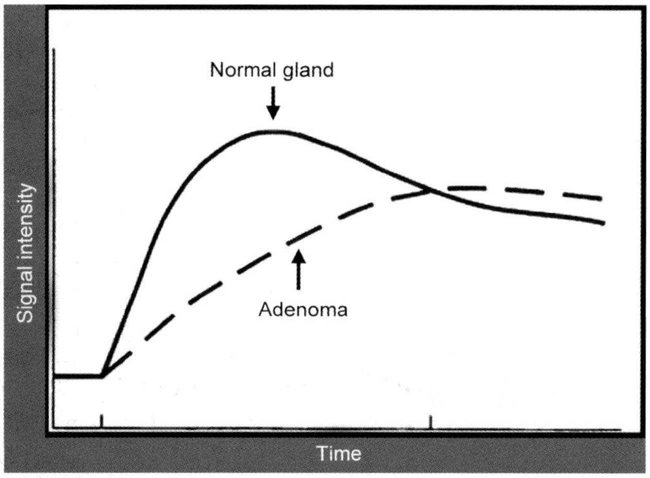

Fig. 4: Enhancement pattern of adenoma and normal pituitary gland shown as time intensity curve. Early and higher degree of enhancement of normal pituitary versus lower and delayed uptake of contrast by the adenoma is noted. After sometime they become isointense as contrast washes out from gland. Later on adenoma may appear hyperintense.

Microadenomas (<10 mm in size) typically appear hypointense compared to the normal adenohypophysis on T1WI (80–90%)[5] and iso to hyperintense on T2WI **(Figs. 5A and B)**. The signal intensity of adenomas and normal gland are comparable to the grey and white matter of the temporal lobe respectively on T1WI. They may sometimes appear hyperintense on T1WI. This is attributable to hemorrhage. Occasionally they may be isointense and can only be detected on enhanced scans (particularly dynamic study) where they stand out as hypointense areas within the enhancing gland **(Figs. 6 and 7)**. On contrast-enhanced CT (CECT) adenomas are seen as discrete, hypodense regions within the enhancing gland **(Fig. 8)**. Imaging has little to offer for differentiating different types of microadenomas; however, the PRL and GH secreting adenomas tend to be located more laterally in the gland and ACTH and gonadotropin secretors tend to be more central **(Figs. 5 and 6)**.[12] Indirect signs for the presence of adenoma include enlargement of gland and a bulge in the gland outline. Tilt of the pituitary stalk and asymmetry of the sellar floor though helpful signs may sometimes occur physiologically due to developmental asymmetry of the brain or stalk insertion. Inferior petrosal sinus

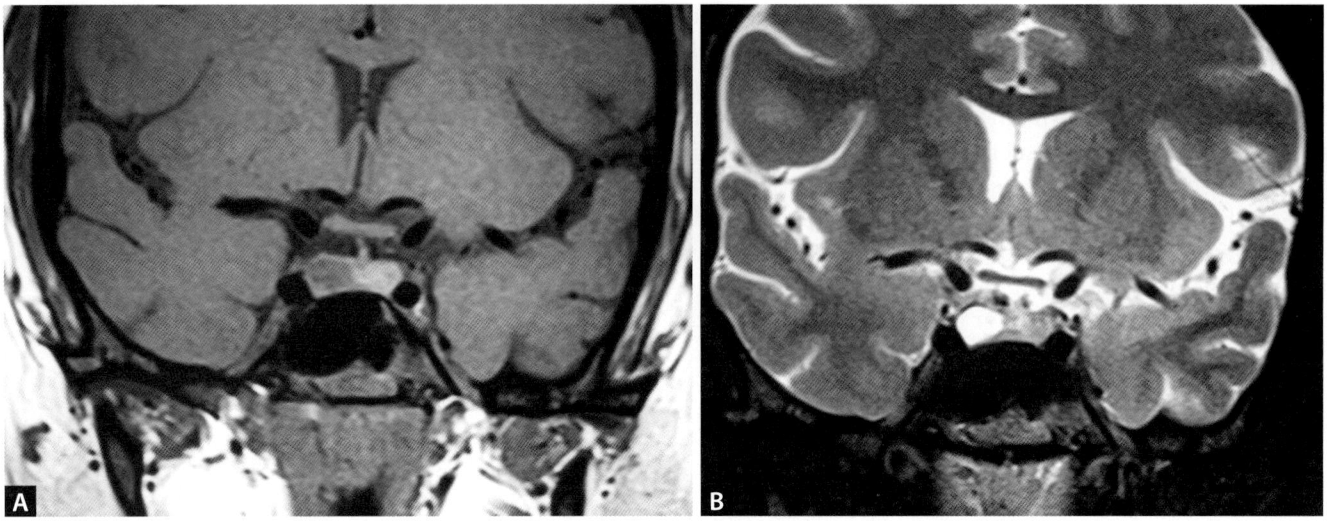

Figs. 5A and B: Prolactin secreting pituitary adenoma : T1-weighted coronal image shows hypointense microadenoma on right aspect of the gland (A). Adenoma appears hyperintense on T2WI (B).

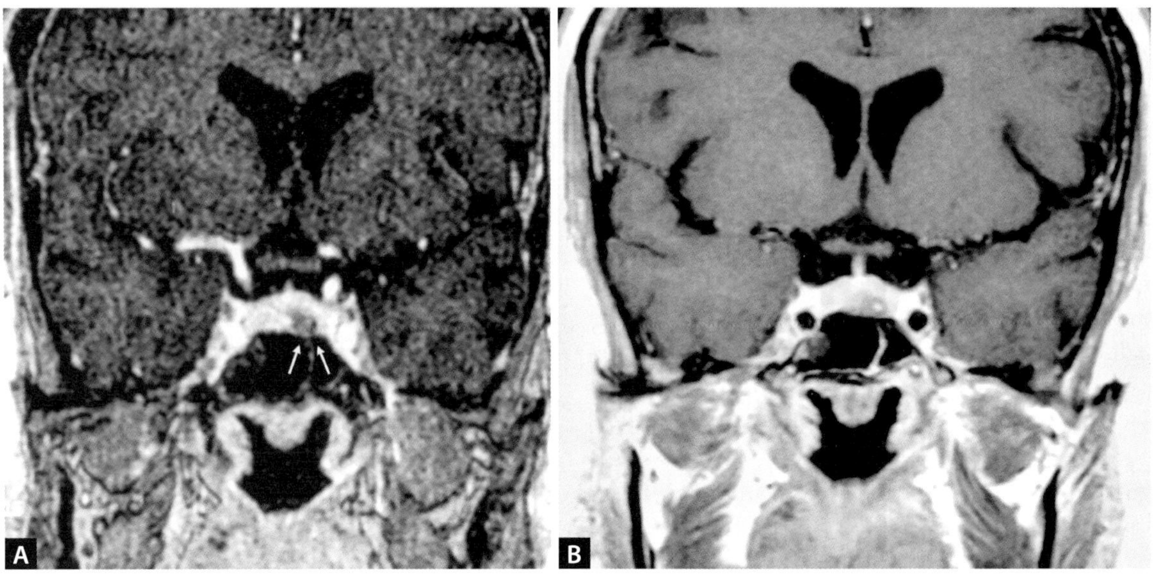

Figs. 6A and B: Dynamic CEMR (A) showing a small ACTH secreting adenoma in the central part of the gland (arrows) which is mostly isointense to rest of the gland on routine CEMR, however, a small central area shows higher uptake of contrast on this delayed image (B).

sampling may be extremely useful for localizing adenoma and distinguishing Cushing's disease from ectopic ACTH secretion and autonomous adrenal disease when imaging fails to show the site of adenoma. Lateralization of the lesion to either half of the pituitary gland is also possible. However, in larger lesions, lateralization may not be accurate due to venous drainage occurring in either direction i.e. both cavernous sinuses.[13,14]

Macroadenomas (>10 mm), being larger, are easier to diagnose. They usually enlarge the sella, erode the sphenoid sinus, encroach upon the suprasellar cistern and may displace the chiasma **(Figs. 9A to D)**. Solid adenomas enhance uniformly, while others may show heterogeneous hypodense areas within it on CECT. Macroadenomas are frequently hyperintense on T2WI. Hyperintense macroadenomas may be soft and necrotic while hypointense lesions may be more fibrous; a finding that may be of help to the surgeon.[5] Apparent diffusion coefficient values on diffusion-weighted imaging may be higher in softer variety.[15] Hemorrhage and necrosis are common particularly following bromocriptine therapy, majority of these being subclinical.[4] In large lesions, residual pituitary tissue may not be visible. Most microadenomas enhance late as compared to the

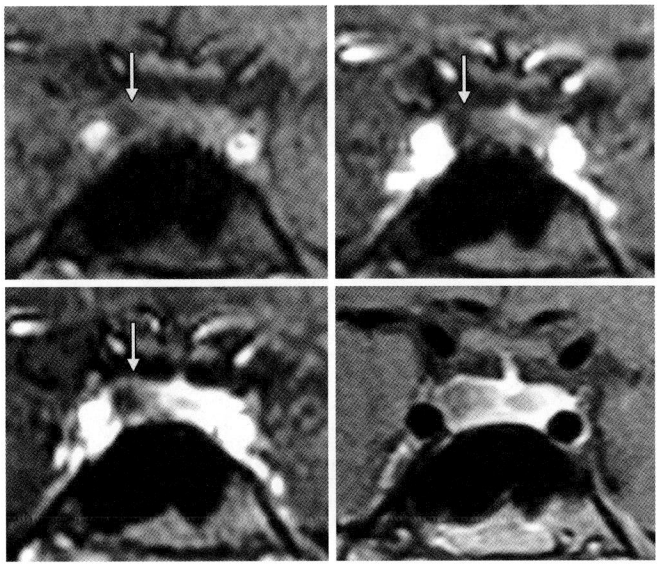

Fig. 7: Consecutive four frames of dynamic CEMR shows progressive enhancement of pituitary gland leading to better definition of microadenoma on the right aspect (arrows). Delayed frame (lower right corner) shows progressive fill in of adenoma.

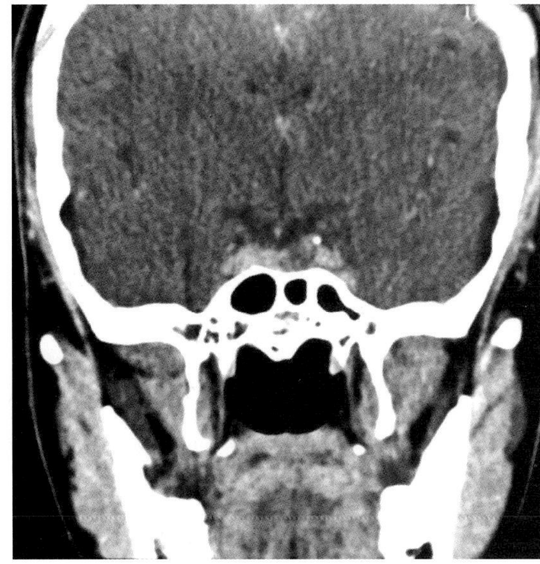

Fig. 8: Adenoma: CECT scan shows a relatively hypodense adenoma within intensely enhancing normal gland.

adenohypophysis while macroadenomas enhance early. This reflects the difference in their blood supply. With suprasellar extension, the adenomas acquire a typical "figure-of-eight", appearance.

Early cavernous sinus involvement by adenoma is often difficult to diagnose. The most reliable signs of cavernous sinus invasion are encasement of cavernous carotid arteries, presence of tumor lateral to them, delayed enhancing soft tissue in sinus, a lateral bulge of the outer dura and a serum PRL level of 1,000 ng/mL or more (in case of prolactinomas) **(Figs. 10A and B)**.[3,5] In one study MDCT was found to better delineate the lateral margin of tumor.[15]

MR has been shown to be useful in precisely demonstrating the cavernous sinus invasion. Many grading schemes have been proposed to prognosticate the effect of cavernous sinus extension on the surgical outcomes of these patients. Knosp grading has been widely used and has proven to show good correlation with outcomes.[16] The grading is defined by the relation of carotid lines with the limits of invasion **(Fig. 11)**. These lines pass through supra- and intracavernous parts of ICA in coronal view. There are medial, median and lateral carotid lines. Micko et al.[17] partially revised the classification by bifurcating grade 3 into A and B (marked (*) in **Table 4**). A new classification scheme was proposed by Edal et al.[18] wherein they classified the adjoining invasion in all three planes which was called the SIPAP (superior inferior parasellar anterior posterior) grading.

Atypical Presentations of Adenomas

Their blood supply being marginal, pituitary adenomas may present acutely with infarction and hemorrhage; a condition called *pituitary apoplexy*. However, these events may be silent and only detected at pathology or imaging.[19] Hemorrhage/infarction may be spontaneous or following bromocriptine therapy (in more than half of the treated patients). The gland may show areas which appear hyperdense on noncontrast CT, dark on T2WI (acute blood) or bright on T1WI (subacute blood) **(Figs. 12A and B)**. Massive hemorrhage may have subarachnoid/intracerebral extension. Diffusion imaging may show restriction.[20]

Although pituitary adenomas are generally benign slow growing neoplasms, *malignant variants* exist. These tend to infiltrate dura, bone and surrounding structures. As histology and imaging do not allow distinction between the two, the presence of metastatic disease is the only definite clue to diagnosis.[7]

The term *invasive pituitary adenomas* represent an intermediate part of the spectrum. These infiltrate surrounding structures but grow slowly and by definition do not cause metastasis.

An aggressive subtype of ACTH producing adenoma is seen in Nelson's syndrome, a condition in which the adenoma enlarges in the absence of regulatory mechanisms after bilateral adrenalectomy.[9]

Ectopic adenomas can arise from infundibulum or in suprasellar cistern from pars tuberalis.

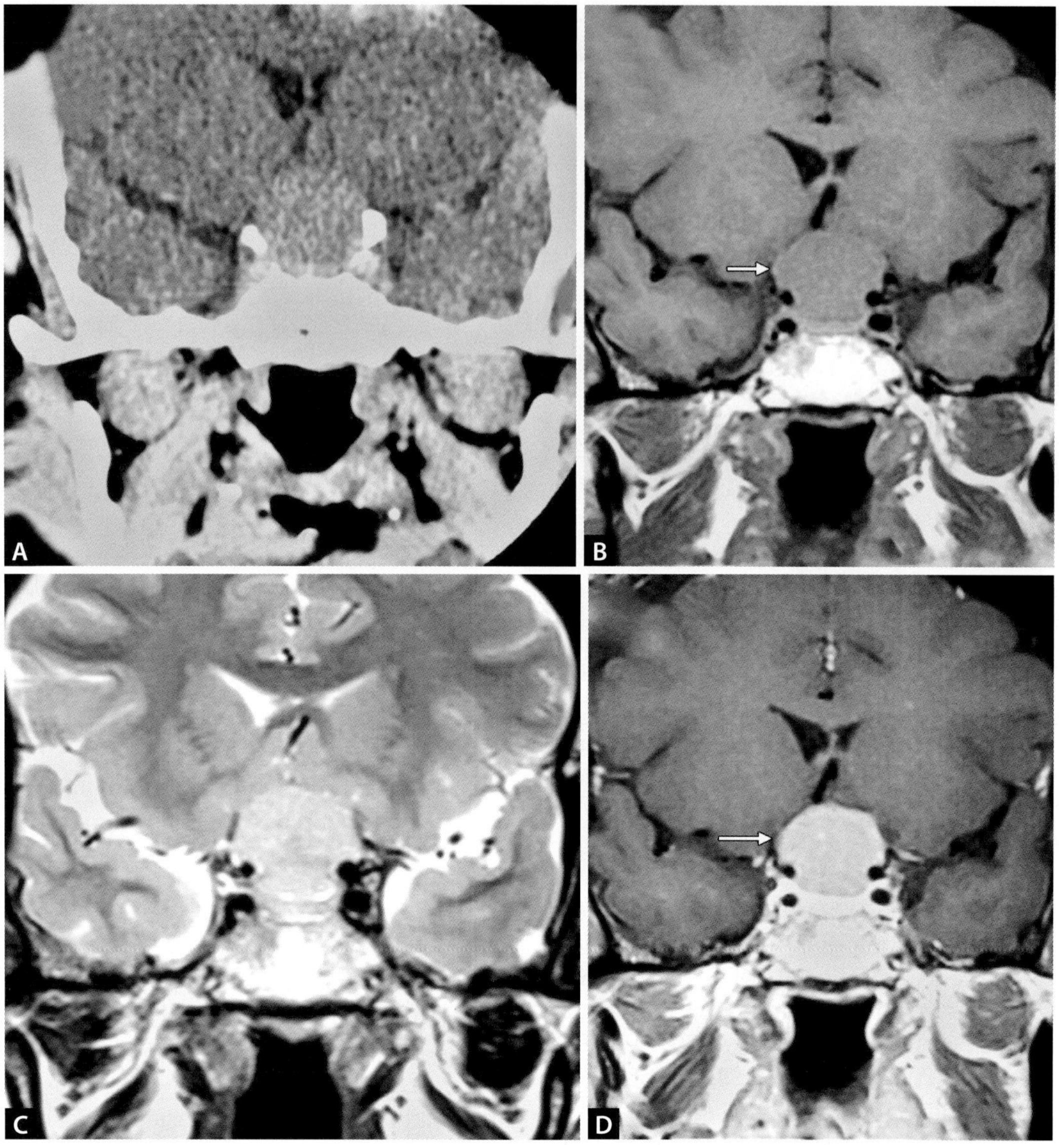

Figs. 9A to D: Coronal sections: CECT (A), T1-weighted, T2-weighted and gadolinium enhanced T1-weighted MR images (B to D) show a solid enhancing macroadenoma with suprasellar extension. The optic chiasma is stretched superiorly (arrow).

Postoperative Sella

It may be difficult to differentiate residual/recurrent tumor from scarring and a variety of graft materials in the post-operative bed, i.e. fat, gelfoam, muscle, etc. Gadolinium-enhanced scan may be helpful in such cases. It is recommended that postoperative scanning be done 4–6 months after surgery to allow resorption of gelfoam, hemorrhagic material and debris.[21] Comparison with preoperative scans, progressive growth of lesion and correlation with endocrinological markers are important. Development of empty sella, CSF leaks and sinusitis are some of the sequel of surgery.[22] Positron emission tomography potentially appears useful for assessing tumor response to therapy and for differentiating postsurgical changes from recurrent tumors.

Craniopharyngioma

These are benign, slowly growing, locally invasive, hormonally inactive lesions accounting for 2–4% of all intracranial lesions. They are derived from Rathke's pouch. Twenty percent of craniopharyngiomas may be purely intrasellar, while 80% have their epicenter in the suprasellar cistern.[5] Rarely, they may be intraventricular or infrasellar. There is a bimodal age distribution, majority of lesions

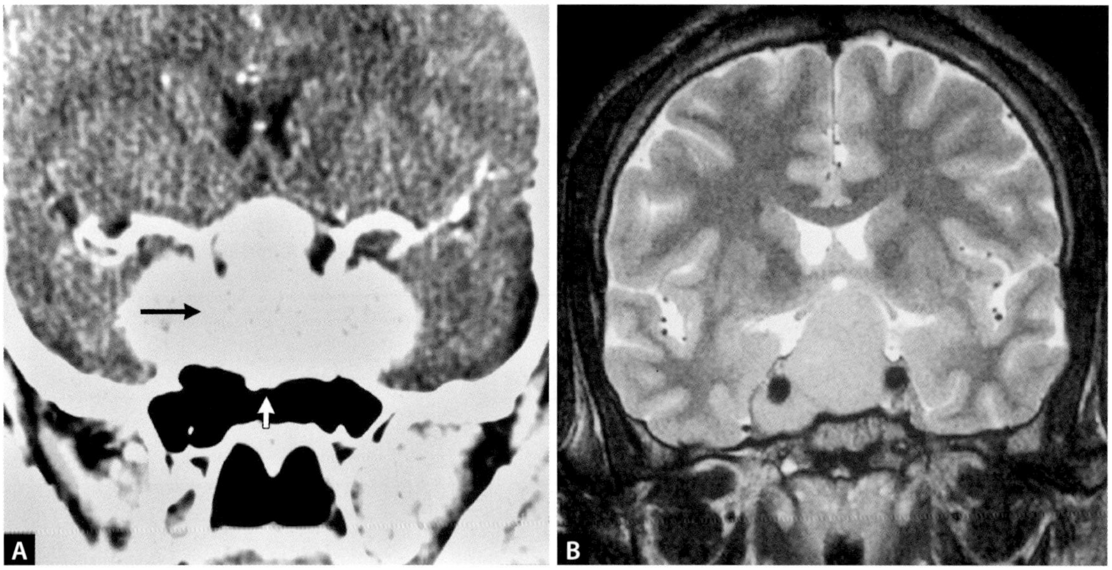

Figs. 10A and B: CECT coronal section: (A) Lobulated relatively homogenous macroadenoma with involvement of cavernous sinuses on both sides. Encasement of carotid vessels (black arrow) and erosion of floor of sella (white arrow) can be noted. MR coronal T2 image (B) showing extension of the adenoma into right cavernous sinus.

presenting in the 5–10 years age group with a second small peak in 6th decade.[10] The children usually have features of raised intracranial pressure while visual disturbances and endocrinopathy are the usual presentation in 70–90% of adults. There are two histological subtypes of the lesions-adamantinomatous and papillary types. They are distinct in terms of clinical presentation, imaging features and treatment outcome.[23]

The more common classic form is adamantinomatous type, usually seen in children. They are almost always cystic with small solid component which frequently calcifies (80% cases). Characteristically, these tumors appear as a combination of hypodense (cystic) and hyperdense (calcified) areas on CT. The solid portion appears isodense/isointense to brain on CT and MRI. The cyst fluid contains wet keratin, cholesterol crystals, proteinaceous fluids, hemorrhages and necrotic debris and is likened to *motor oil*. Such cysts appear extremely bright on both T1 and T2-weighted images **(Figs. 13A and B)**. The other cysts may be slightly hyperintense to CSF on T1WI, more so, on FLAIR and may show peripheral enhancement. CT is useful for showing calcification, particularly if the tumor is only a small solid calcified nodule, which may be totally overlooked on MRI **(Figs. 14A to E)**. The adamantinomatous type is more likely to be locally invasive, encase vessels, cause surrounding gliosis and may recur after surgery. Contrast enhancement of the solid portions of the tumor may be seen.[5] Papillary variety

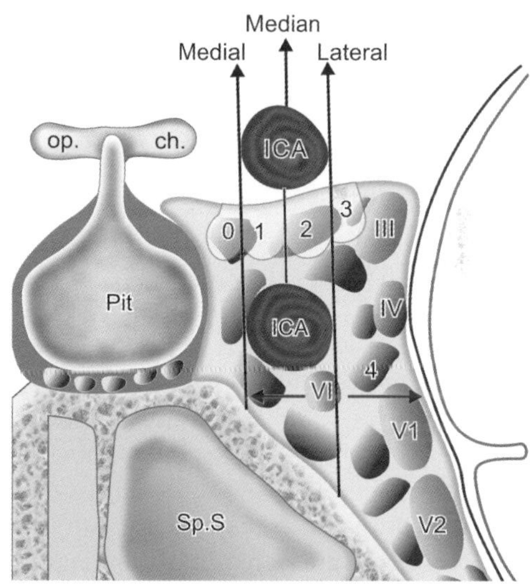

Fig. 11: Pictorial representation of the coronal view of the sella and parasellar (cavernous sinus) region depicting the demarcation of the sinus into three compartments by imaginary medial, median and lateral lines. The numerals 0, 1, 2, 3 and 4 represent the grade of adenoma extension according to Knosp scheme (detailed discussion in the text and table).

of craniopharyngioma seen in adults are solid, often located within third ventricle and do not calcify. They are encapsulated and easily removable and hence have a lesser tendency to recur.[22] Craniopharyngiomas cause fibroinflammatory adhesions with surrounding tissues and tend to recur after surgery.

Table 4: Knosp grading system for demonstrating invasion of cavernous sinus by pituitary macroadenoma.

Grade	*Cavernous sinus extension*
0	Adenoma does not extend beyond the medial carotid line
1	Adenoma extends beyond the medial line, but does not reach the median line, so-called "intracarotid" line
2	Tumor extends beyond the median line, but does not extend beyond or tangent to the lateral line
3	Tumor extends beyond the lateral line
3A*	The tumor extends lateral to the lateral tangent of the intracavernous and supracavernous ICAs into the **superior** CS compartment
3B*	The tumor extends lateral to the lateral tangent of the intracavernous and supracavernous ICAs into the **inferior** CS compartment
4	Tumor totally wraps around the intracavernous carotid artery

* Micko et al. revision of Grade 3 into A and B.

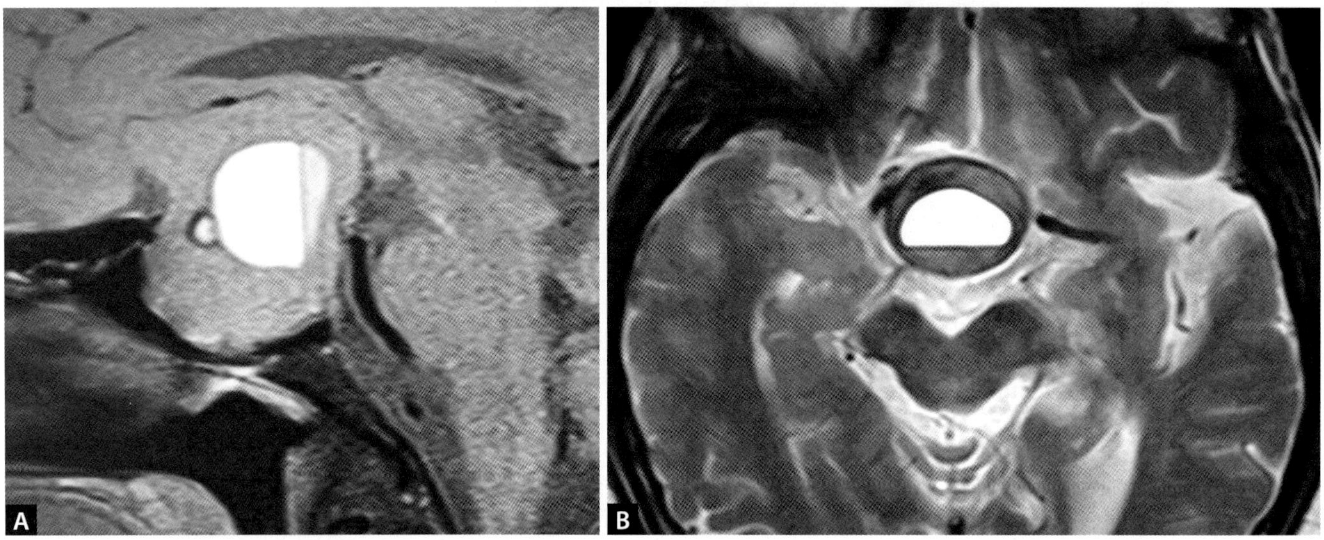

Figs. 12A and B: Pituitary apoplexy: T1-weighted sagittal section: Macroadenoma with bright signal with fluid-fluid level within the tumor representing subacute blood (A). T2WI reveals hyperintense blood with a fluid level showing shading in the dependent portions due to settled red blood cells (B).

Pituicytoma

These arise from pituicyte, a glial cell in neurohypophysis and infundibulum and are also called granular cell tumors and myoblastoma. The location is usually posterior intrasellar with suprasellar extension. Size ranges from 1 mm to 2 mm to 4 cm. On CT a hyperdense sellar/suprasellar mass is seen which enhances homogenously. On T1WI, the lesion is iso to hypointense with absent bright spot and on T2 it is usually heterogeneous.[3-5]

Meningioma

Ten percent of meningiomas occur in sellar and parasellar region. The site of origin is commonly tuberculum sella, the other locations being clinoid processes, the dorsum, medial sphenoid wing and cavernous sinuses. Tumors originating from optic sheath, olfactory groove and planum sphenoidale may also extend into supra/parasellar regions.[5] They are slow growing lesions causing mass effect, i.e. visual loss, ophthalmoplegia or proptosis due to venous congestion at the orbital apex.

On MRI, they are usually isointense to grey matter on T1WI. T2WI images show isointensity in 50% and hyperintensity in 30–40%.[10] Meningiomas show bright contrast enhancement on both CT and MRI **(Figs. 15A and B)**. It is important to differentiate meningioma from adenoma as the surgical approach varies in the two. MR signal intensity and enhancement pattern do not allow this differentiation. However, morphological features like a broad base with dural tail, hyperostosis rather than erosion, calcification (better shown on CT, **Figs. 16A and B**), a cleft demarcating the lesion from brain and

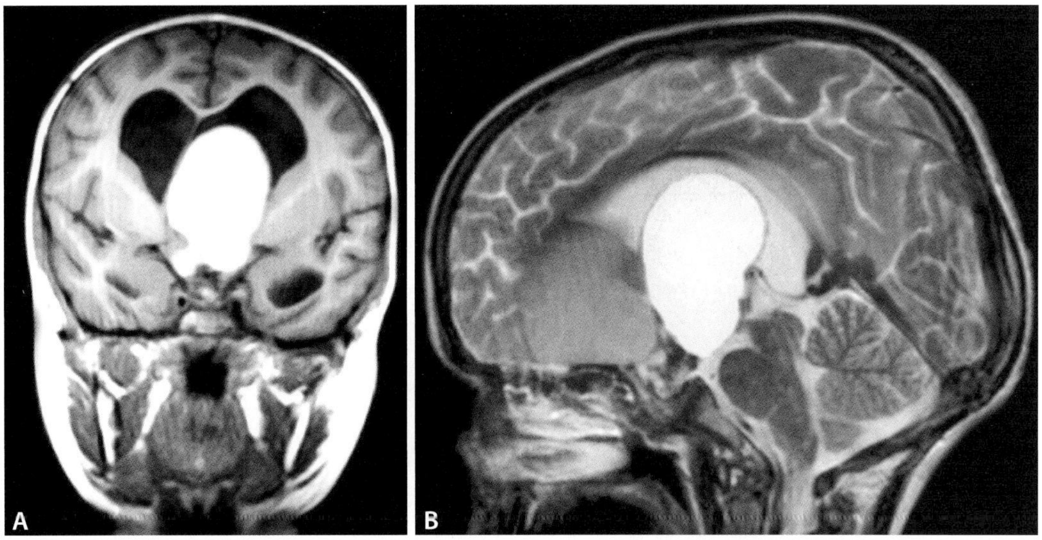

Figs. 13A and B: Craniopharyngioma: Hyperintense motor oil cyst on T1 coronal (A) and T2 sagittal (B) MR sections. Differing T2 signal in the cysts can be seen on T2 section (B) with low signal calcification in the immediate suprasellar area.

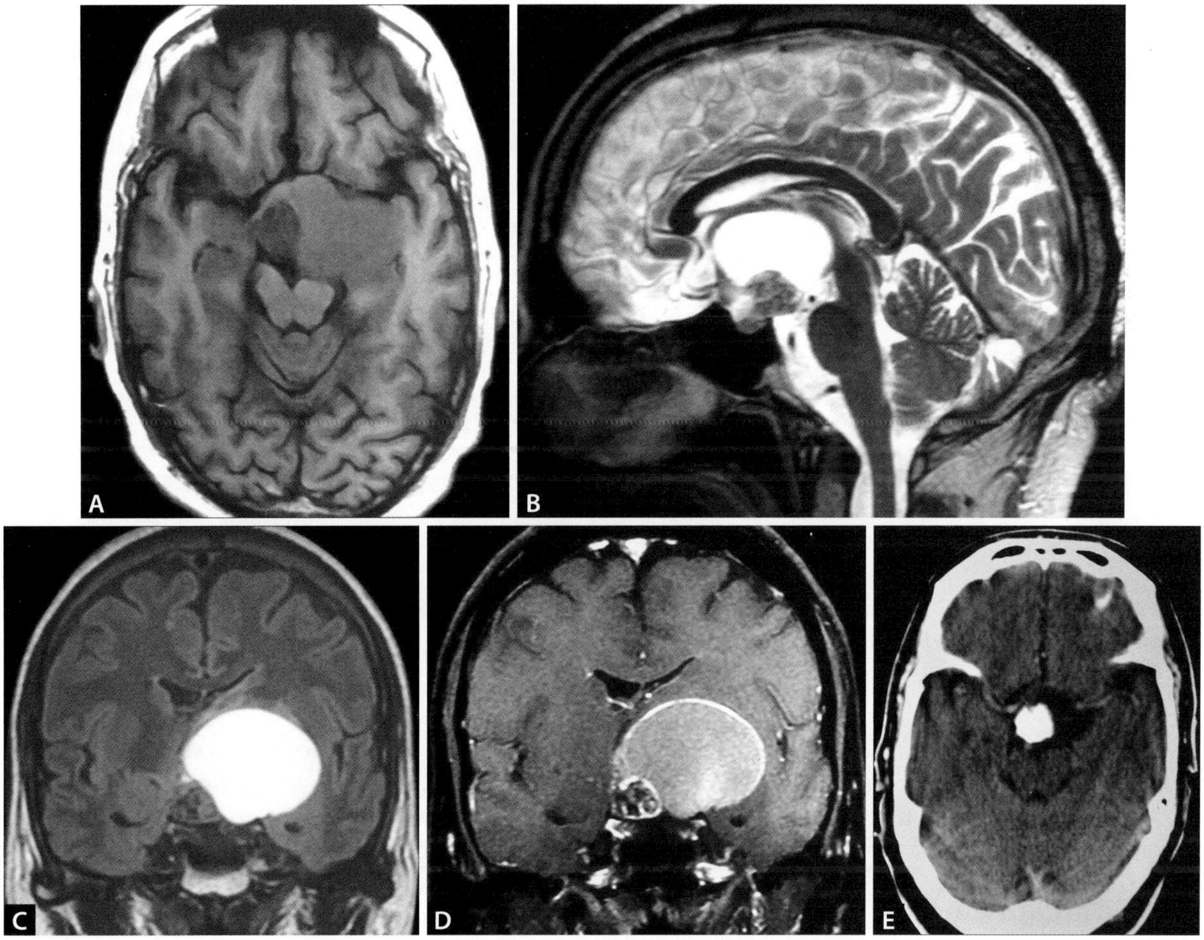

Figs. 14A to E: Craniopharyngioma: Axial T1WI (A) and sagittal T2WI (B) show cystic and solid suprasellar mass. Coronal FLAIR (C) shows high signal of the cyst compared to CSF. Enhanced T1WI (D) shows peripheral enhancement of the cyst but calcification is difficult to comment upon which is clearly shown on axial CT (E).

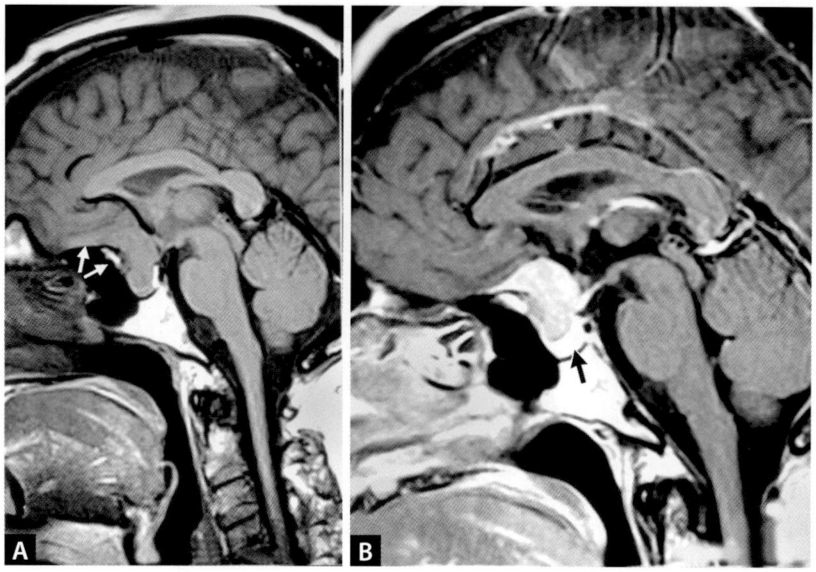

Figs. 15A and B: Tuberculum sellae meningioma: T1 sections before (A) and after (B) contrast administration. The broad dural-based tumor is nearly isointense to pituitary gland before contrast but can be easily differentiated from it on early postcontrast images as the gland enhances to a greater degree (arrows).

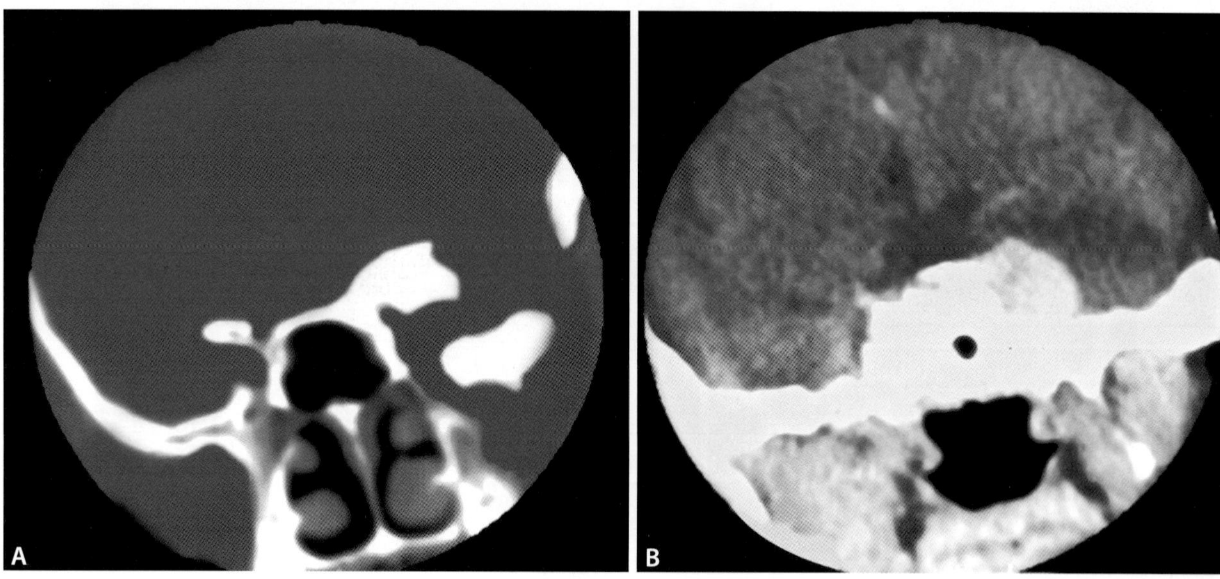

Figs. 16A and B: Anterior clinoidal meningioma. (A) Coronal CT bone window and (B) soft tissue window shows hyperostosis of the left anterior clinoid process (A) and associated soft tissue component of the mass (B).

pituitary gland, greater propensity for arterial encasement and normal sized sella favor a diagnosis of meningioma. ^{31}P-spectroscopy may show higher phosphate monoester in meningioma vis-à-vis adenoma.

Germinoma and Teratoma

Twenty percent of these germ cell tumors may be seen in suprasellar cistern or pituitary fossa in children and young adults.[24] They may arise here or may be metastatic lesions from a pineal tumor. There is no sex predilection unlike pineal tumors, which have a strong male predominance. Patients present with endocrinopathy, visual field defects, hydrocephalus, etc. as is common to all suprasellar neoplasms. However, diabetes insipidus is the earliest symptom due to invasion of hypothalamus.

Germinomas tend to be large noncapsulated solid lesions, centered on or behind stalk that infiltrate into surrounding structures. They are homogenous lesions

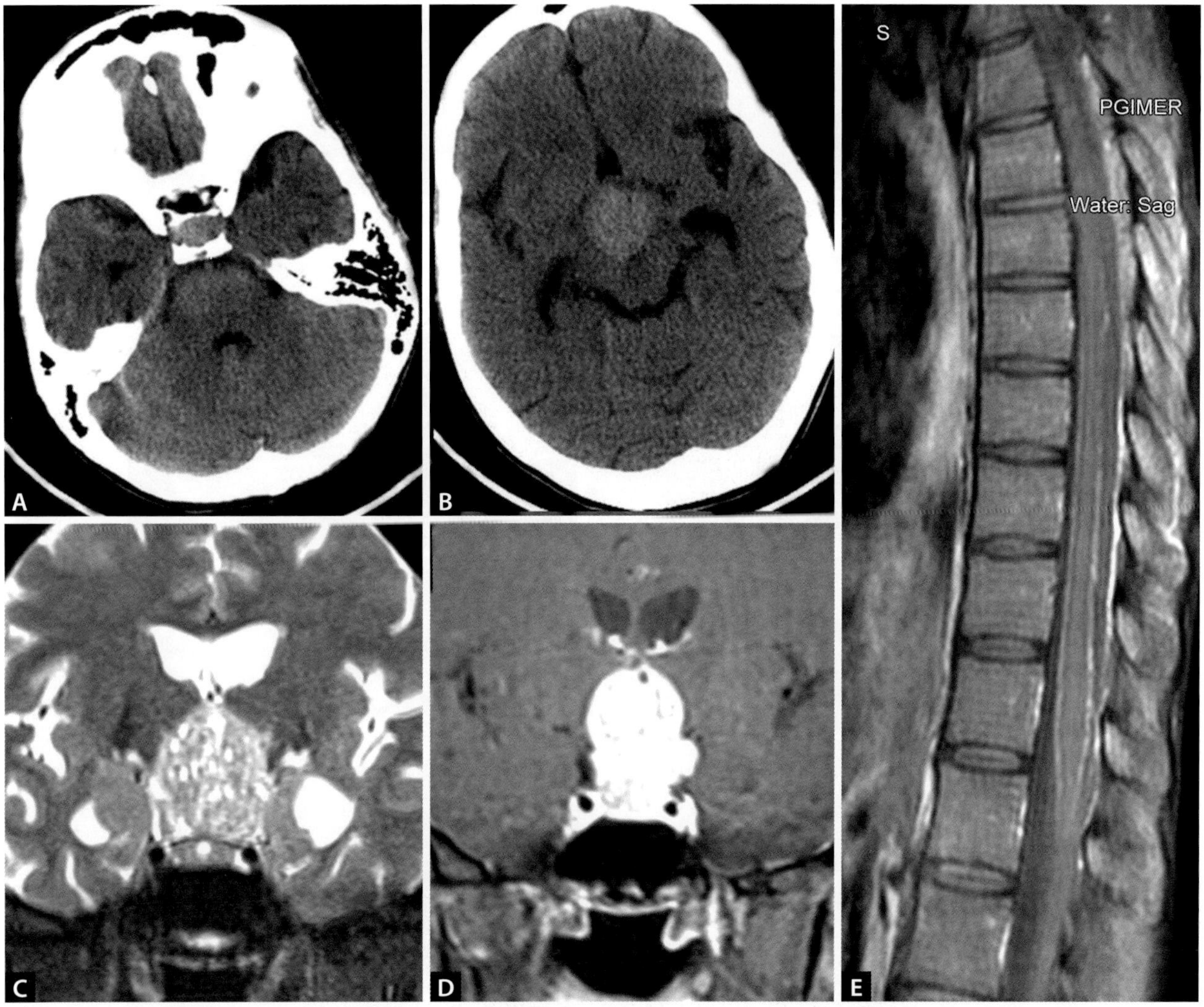

Figs. 17A to E: Suprasellar germinoma: A young girl presenting with hypopituitarism was evaluated with noncontrast CT (A and B) which revealed hyperdense sellar-suprasellar mass. Craniospinal MR confirmed the lesion with T2 hypo to isointensity (C) and moderate postcontrast enhancement (D). There was CSF spread in the spinal canal as demonstrated by leptomeningeal enhancement in the dorsal spine (E). She responded to radiotherapy.

without cystic components (unlike craniopharyngioma). On CT they are hyperdense like lymphoma **(Figs. 17A and B)**. On MRI, they are slightly hypointense on T1 and hyperintense on T2WI **(Fig. 17C)**. They show strong contrast enhancement on CT/MRI **(Figs. 17D)**. There is also a high tendency of CSF dissemination **(Fig. 17E)**. The posterior pituitary bright spot is often absent. Teratomas show evidence of fat or calcification and are more heterogeneous.[5,24]

Dermoid and Epidermoid Tumors

These are slow growing benign inclusion tumors due to trapping of ectodermal cells during neural tube closure.[25]

Epidermoids are five times more common than dermoids and usually are parasellar in location; the second most common site in the head after the CP angles. They are seen in adults of 20–40 years of age. Dermoids are more common in children,[26] tend to occur in the midline and in posterior fossa but may occur in the suprasellar cistern. Epidermoid cysts are composed of desquamated keratin while the dermoids contain dermal appendages. Both show slow growth, tend to insinuate in the available space and produce symptoms by compression of the adjacent structures. Rarely, chemical meningitis may occur due to rupture. Epidermoids appear heterogeneous and slightly hyperdense to CSF on CT and usually slightly hyperintense to CSF on T1WI **(Figs. 18A to D)**. They rarely enhance but occasionally calcify peripherally.[26,27] FLAIR and diffusion images **(Figs. 18A to D)** are extremely useful in showing these lesions as is CT cisternography.

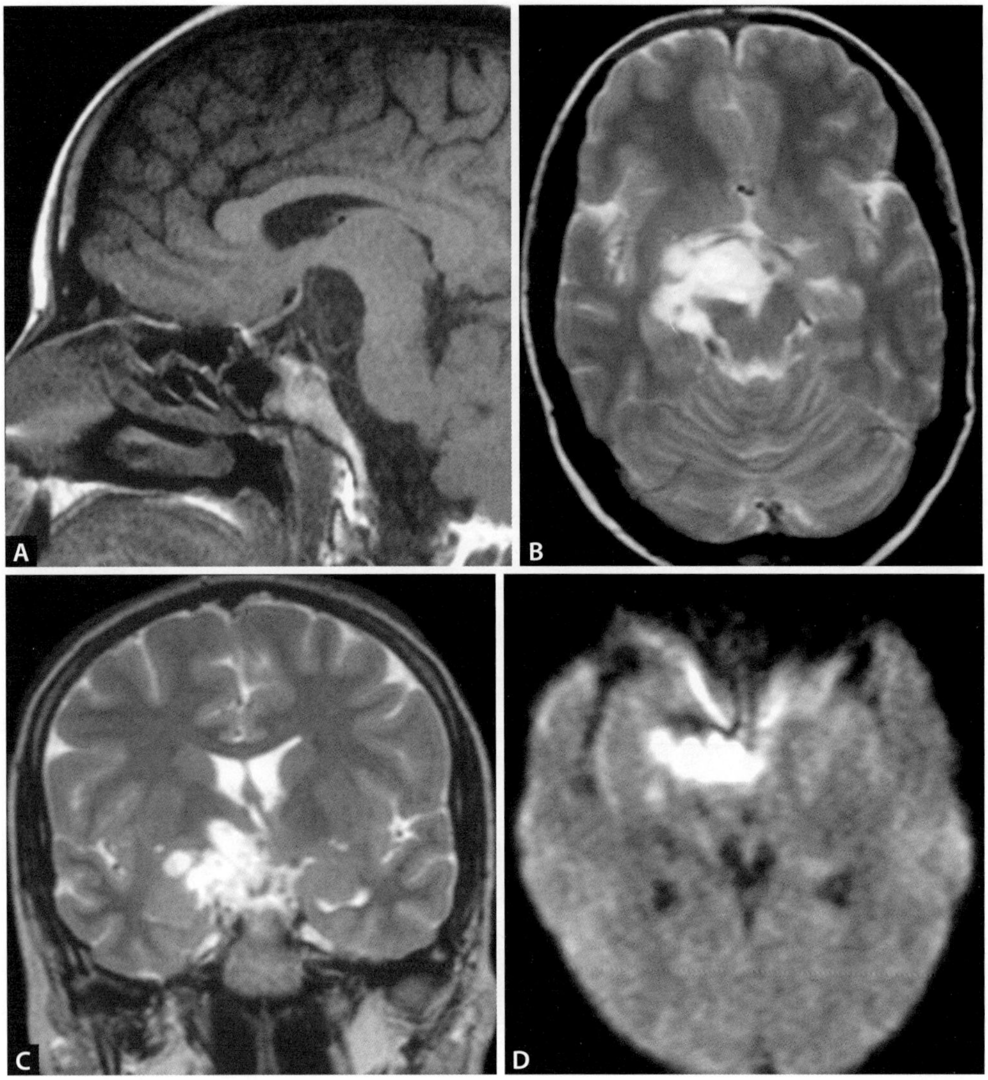

Figs. 18A to D: Suprasellar epidermoid appearing slightly hyperintense compared to CSF on T1WI (A), extremely bright like CSF on T2WI (B and C) with a lobulated outline and shows bright signal on diffusion image (D).

Dermoids are more heterogeneous and often show fat density (fat fluid levels sometimes) or calcification. Fat droplets may be visualized in the subarachnoid space in ruptured dermoids. However, epidermoids, dermoids and other purely cystic lesions may be indistinguishable on imaging.

Chiasmatic/Hypothalamic Glioma

Seventy five percent of these tumors occur in first decade of life. This diverse group of neoplasms often present with different behavior and response to therapy and are referred to together as chiasmatic-hypothalamic gliomas. The site of origin is often difficult to decide, as the lesions are usually large when detected and are infiltrative in nature. Neurofibromatosis 1 (NF-1) is present in 20–50% patients with opticochiasmatic lesions. The chiasmatic lesions tend to infiltrate the hypothalamus leading to hypothalamic dysfunction and hydrocephalus. They also tend to infiltrate along the optic tracts, hence the importance of imaging the entire brain.[28] The tumors confined to the chiasma can be differentiated from optic neuritis by clinical presentation or resolution of neuritis on steroids.[5,10,29]

The lesions appear isointense to brain on T1WI and hyperintense on T2WI **(Figs. 19A to D)**. Calcification and hemorrhages are not seen but cystic component can occur. Contrast enhancement is seen in 50% lesions. Lack of serial growth and enhancement differentiate benign hamartomatous NF lesions from glioma.

Hypothalamic gliomas are aggressive and present with hypothalamic dysfunction. Diencephalic syndrome

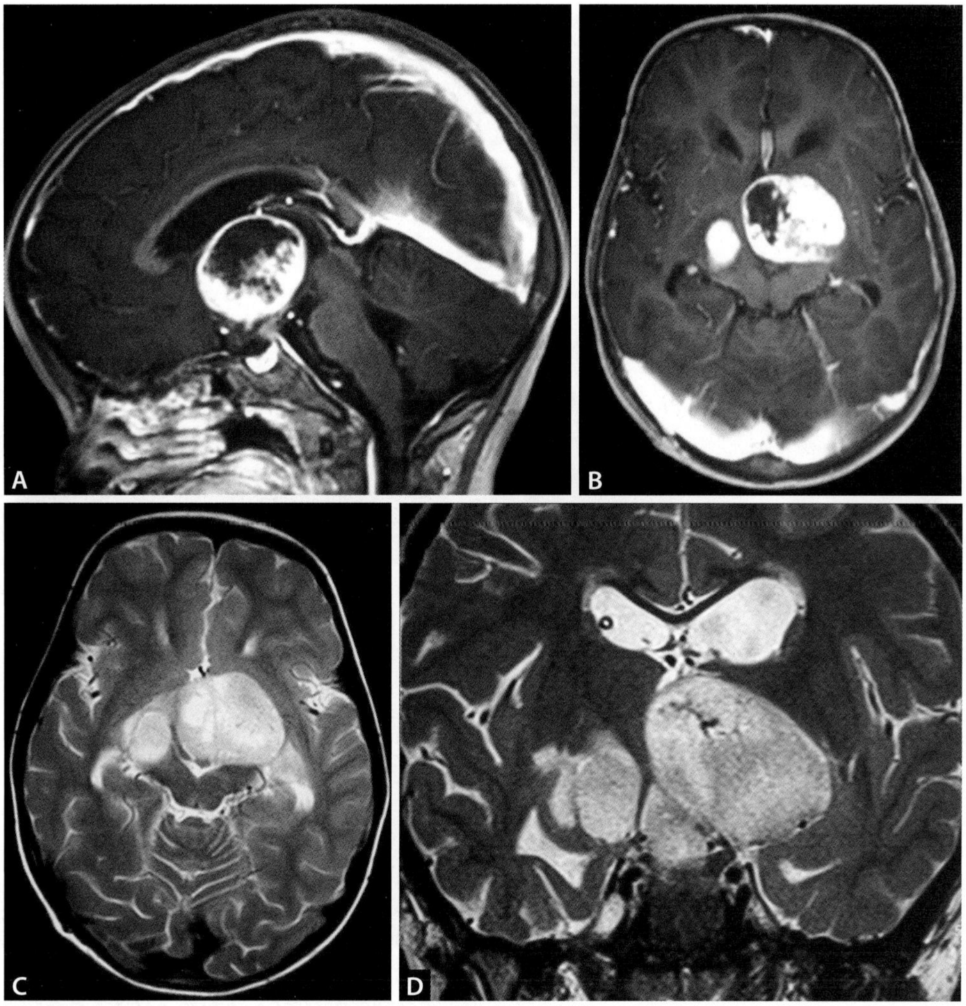

Figs. 19A to D: Hypothalamic glioma: The lobulated suprasellar mass shows moderate enhancement on postcontrast T1WI (A and B), is hypertense on T2WI (C) and is seen to extend along B/L optic tracts (D).

almost always indicates this diagnosis and refers to a clinical state of cachexia in an alert/euphoric child who often has a good appetite.

In general, chiasma/hypothalamic lesions are more aggressive compared to the optic nerve lesions. Lesions arising above 20 years and below 5 years of age also show a more aggressive behavior compared to those arising between 5 years and 20 years.[28] Similarly sporadic lesions also are more aggressive.

Schwannoma

Parasellar schwannomas most commonly arise from branches of Vth nerve. The lesions present with sensory deficit, problems of mastication, facial pain or diplopia. Imaging shows asymmetry and expansion of cavernous sinus. They are encapsulated lesions isointense to brain on T1WI and bright on T2WI. They are isodense on CT and enhance strongly. Larger tumors may be heterogeneous with a tigroid appearance. The 3rd to 6th nerve schwannomas follow the course of respective nerves but are rare lesions.

The dumb-bell configuration of Vth nerve schwannoma[30] straddling the petrous apex is characteristic but less common than a Meckel's cave or posterior fossa mass **(Figs. 20A and B)**.

SKULL BASE LESIONS

Primary, secondary and metastatic tumors of the skull base can involve the parasellar area. The primary lesions include chondroma, chondrosarcoma and plasmacytoma. Secondary tumors are often from nasopharynx and paranasal sinuses. Common metastasis comes from lung, breast and prostate primaries. These are difficult to differentiate from chordoma.

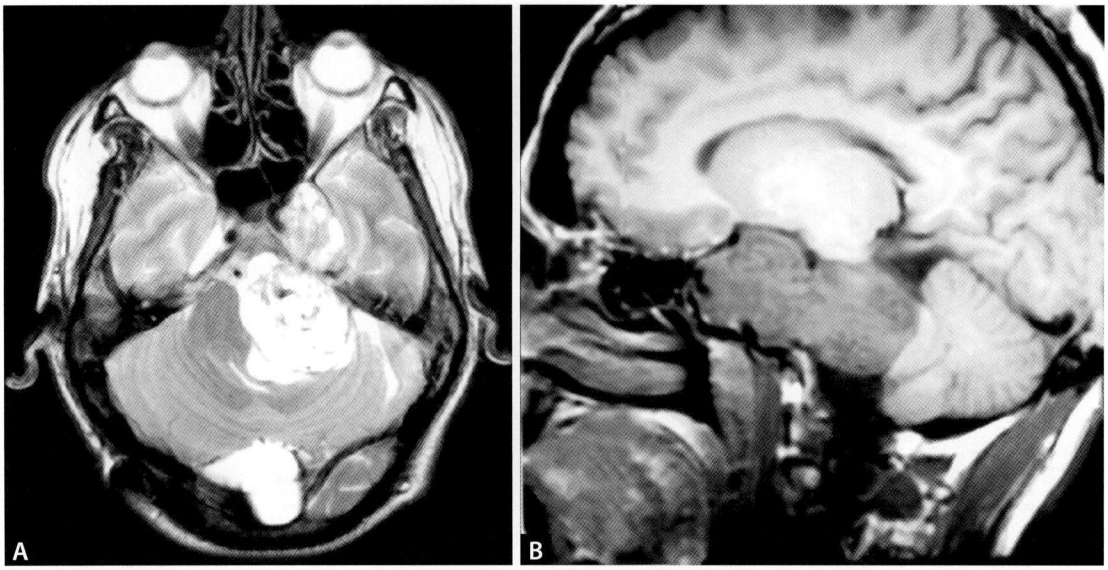

Figs. 20A and B: Schwannoma: (A) T2-weighted axial section shows characteristic hyperintense Vth nerve tumor straddling the petrous apex and expanding the left cavernous sinus; (B) T1 sagittal image of another patient shows extension of tumor from posterior to middle cranial fossa.

Chordoma

They are locally malignant tumors derived from notochordal remnants; 35% of them arise in the clivus (spheno-occipital synchondrosis) though occasionally they may present in Meckel's cave and petrous bone. Mean age of presentation is 20–40 years though no age is exempt. Imaging shows lobular lesions iso to hypointense on T1WI and heterogeneous on T2WI replacing the clival marrow **(Figs. 21A to C)**.[31] They appear hyperintense on postcontrast studies with septations of fibrous connective tissue. CT shows a destructive mass with fragments of bone and calcification. Localization of the epicenter of the lesion within the clivus and identification of normal or displaced pituitary gland differentiates chordomas from invasive adenomas.[25]

Metastasis

Anterior lobe dysfunction or diabetes insipidus in a patient with known malignancy (carcinomas of lung, GI tract, breast, leukemia/lymphoma and skull base tumors) may indicate pituitary metastasis.[32] However, most of these lesions are detected on autopsy. Presumably, most patients succumb to advanced disseminated malignancy before these lesions produce symptoms. The routes of spread may be hematogenous, by CSF seeding or by direct extension.

Imaging may show an enhancing intrasellar, suprasellar or combined lesion. Although difficult to differentiate from adenoma by imaging, endocrinopathy in a patient with known malignancy, rapid growth/disproportionate invasion and destruction of surrounding structures by a small-sized lesion, a dumbbell shape with constriction at diaphragm in a normal sized sella, associated brain edema and enhancement and thickening of infundibulum suggest the diagnosis of metastasis **(Figs. 22A to C)**.[32]

CONGENITAL AND METABOLIC ABNORMALITIES OF PITUITARY GLAND

Some miscellaneous pathologies of pituitary gland have been grouped here. These either have a developmental basis of origin or are acquired in nature but often have endocrinological and surgical implications.

Developmental Anomalies of Pituitary Gland

Persistent hypophyseal canal is a rare congenital anomaly of a skull base defect (craniopharyngeal canal) extending from sellar floor to the nasopharynx (incidence 0.42%). There can be nasopharyngeal extension of the gland, associated hamartomas[33] or duplication of pituitary gland/stalk. The findings on X-ray and CT can be a spur and two widely separated fossae. A duplicated basilar artery with widely separated carotids may be seen. On MRI, thickened tuber cinereum and third ventricular floor (due to tubo-mammillary fusion, **Figs. 23A and B**) or two glands and stalk can be identified. Associated anomalies with larger craniopharyngeal canals include callosal dysgenesis,

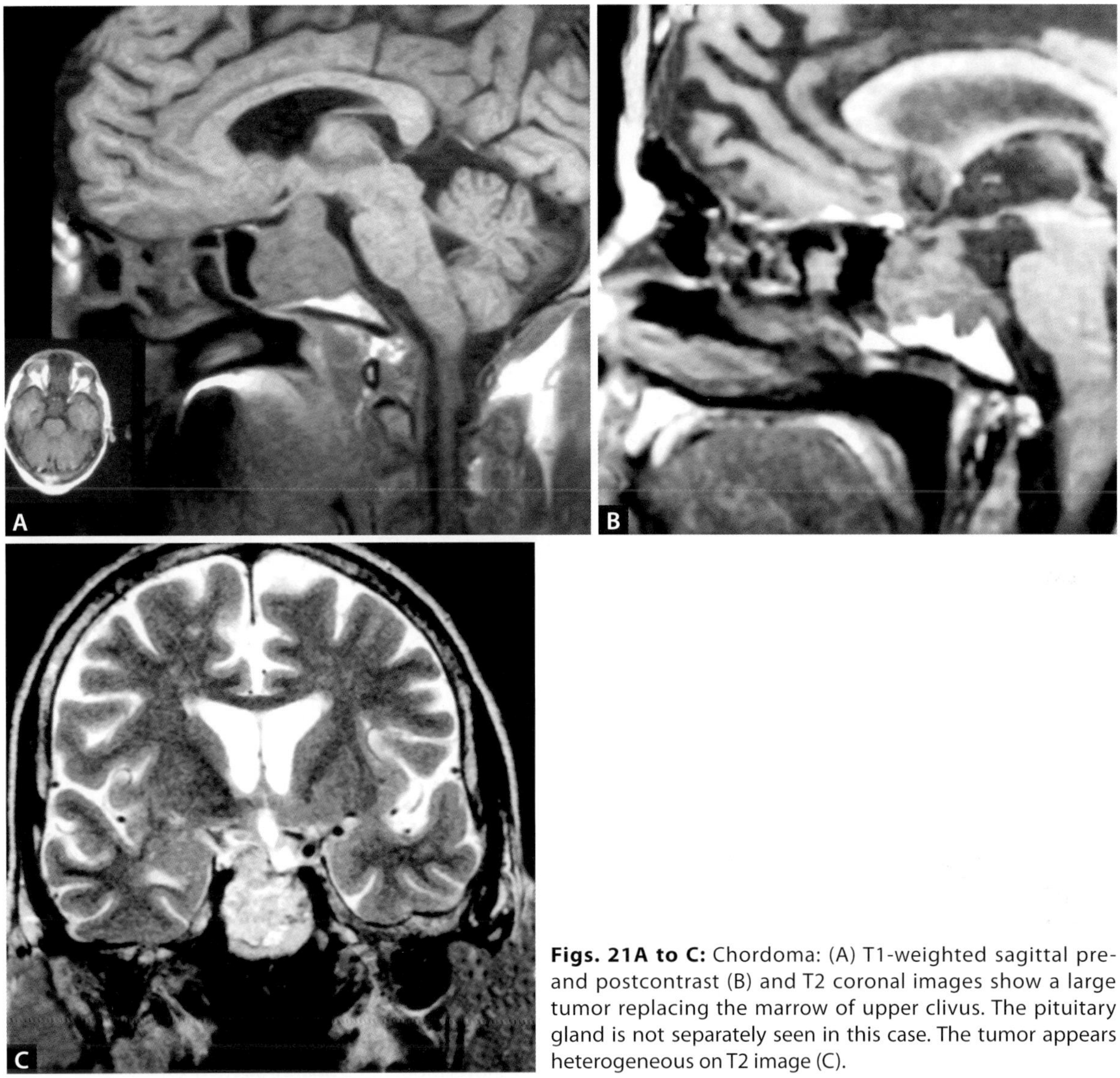

Figs. 21A to C: Chordoma: (A) T1-weighted sagittal pre- and postcontrast (B) and T2 coronal images show a large tumor replacing the marrow of upper clivus. The pituitary gland is not separately seen in this case. The tumor appears heterogeneous on T2 image (C).

facial dysmorphism and defects (i.e. frontonasal dysplasia) and various degrees of transsphenoidal meningoencephaloceles presenting as nasopharyngeal masses.

Pituitary Hypoplasia and Congenital Pituitary Deficiency Disorders

This group of deficiency disorders are recognized clinically by growth failure, short stature and occasionally by other anterior pituitary hormone deficiencies.[34] There may be a history of birth trauma, anoxia or associated anomalies of development of midline structures suggestive of a development lesion. The findings are a small pituitary fossa and kissing carotids on CT. On MRI absent or thread like stalk, small adenohypophysis (less than 2 mm high) and ectopic bright spot can be seen **(Figs. 24A and B)**. Associated abnormalities include Chiari I, absent septum pellucidum, ocular and frontal lobe dysgenesis. Absence stalk correlates with multiple hormonal deficiencies and truncated or thin stalk is seen more frequently in isolated GH deficiency.[34] MRI abnormalities may help determine the severity of congenital hormone deficiency syndromes.

Empty Sella

A thin diaphragm, a sellae and a large hiatus in it are responsible for invagination of CSF space into sella leading to empty sella and compression of the gland (primary empty sella). Empty sella may be secondary to surgery and

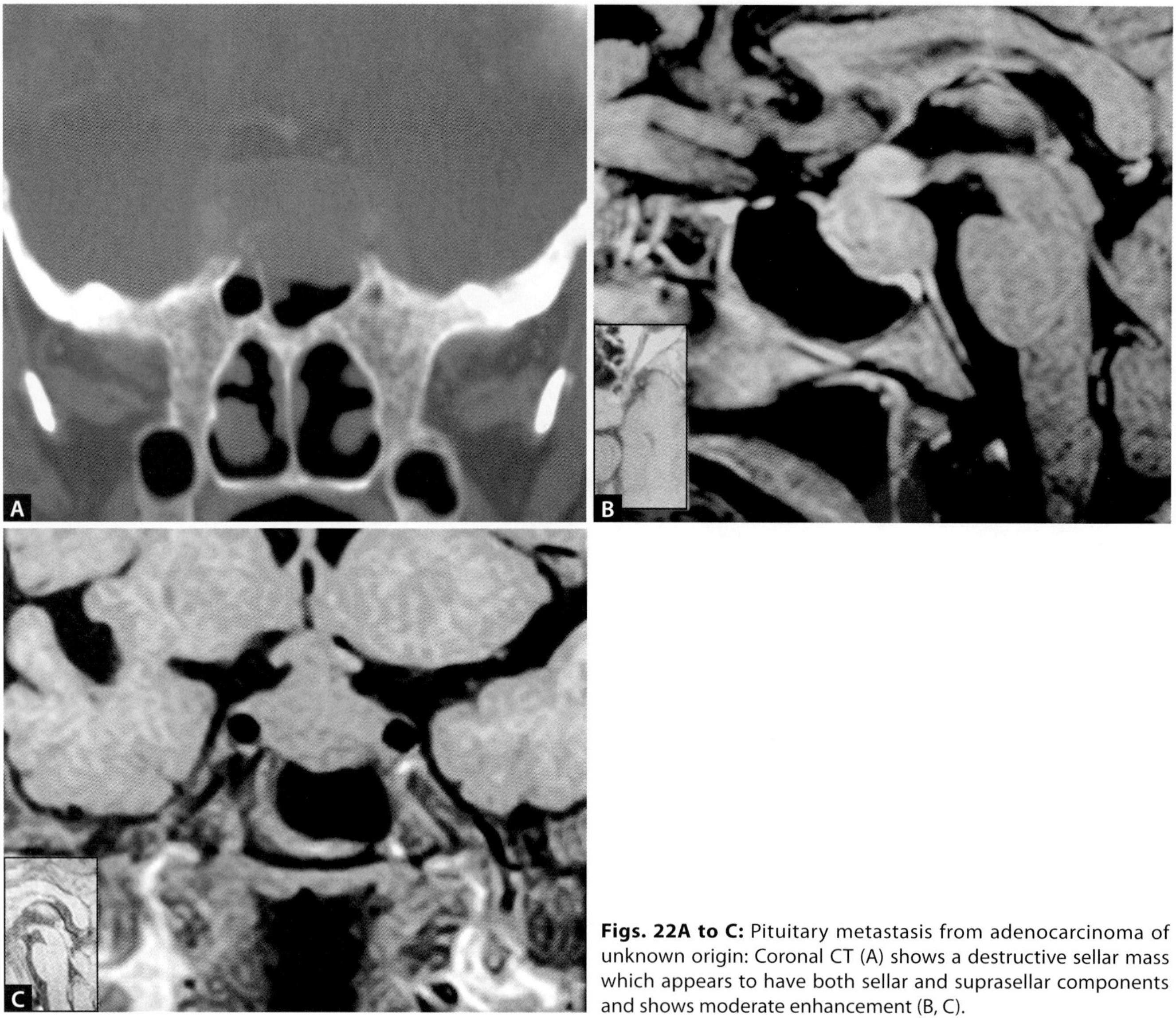

Figs. 22A to C: Pituitary metastasis from adenocarcinoma of unknown origin: Coronal CT (A) shows a destructive sellar mass which appears to have both sellar and suprasellar components and shows moderate enhancement (B, C).

postpartum necrosis too **(Fig. 25)**. This finding may be seen normally in older patients. The symptoms are nonspecific and include memory loss, dizziness and headache. Severe cases may present with CSF rhinorrhea, endocrinopathy or visual field loss due to herniation of optic chiasma into the sella. Imaging typically reveals invagination of suprasellar cistern into the sella compressing the gland against the floor. Typical central position of the infundibulum is a useful sign to rule out a cystic lesion in the suprasellar region.[5]

Diabetes Insipidus

This condition results from lack of ADH. In non-nephrogenic diabetes insipidus, destruction of the ADH producing hypothalamic nuclei, the hypothalamic receptors or the proximal stalk may disrupt the transport of vasopressin via the pituitary stalk to the neurohypophysis. Trauma and operative procedures together account for 50% of cases. Suprasellar/intrasellar neoplasms and granulomatous/inflammatory processes are the other major causes. One-third of all cases are, however, idiopathic.[5,35] The role of imaging in nontraumatic cases is to rule out suprasellar or intrasellar pathology. Stalk transection may be demonstrated on MR.[35] The other consistent observation is lack of visualization of the posterior pituitary bright spot on T1WI irrespective of the cause of diabetes insipidus **(Table 5, Fig. 26)**.[34-36] This bright signal in the posterior lobe is a normal finding due to neurovesicles containing vasopressin in axonal endings

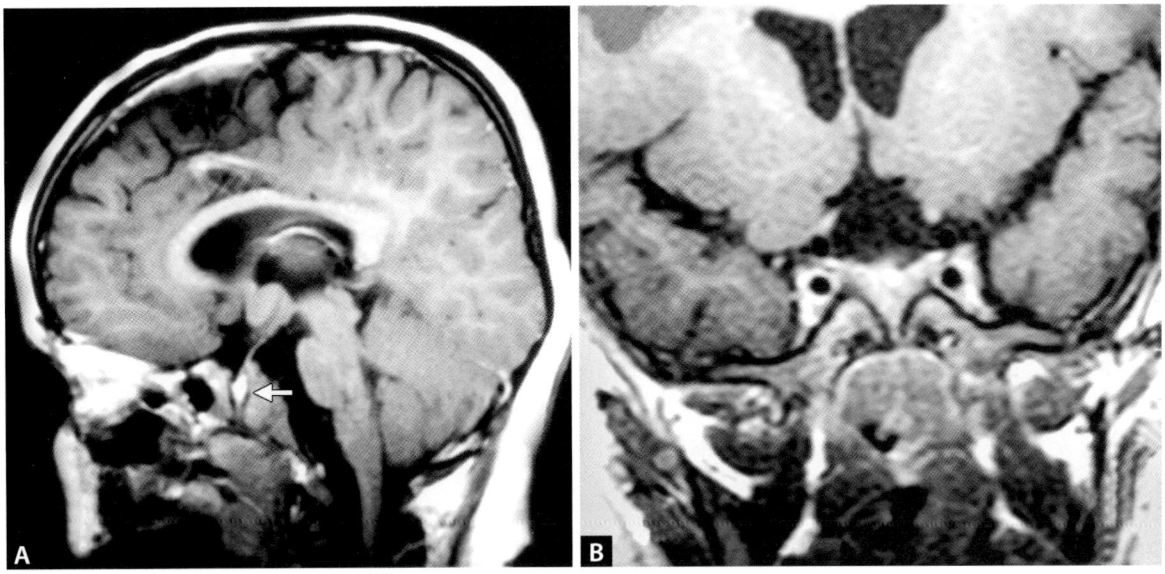

Figs. 23A and B: Persistent craniopharyngeal canal. (A) T1 sagittal and (B) coronal sections. A defect in the sellar floor, inferior location of pituitary gland (arrow in A), tubo-mammillary fusion and wide separation of carotid arteries can be observed.

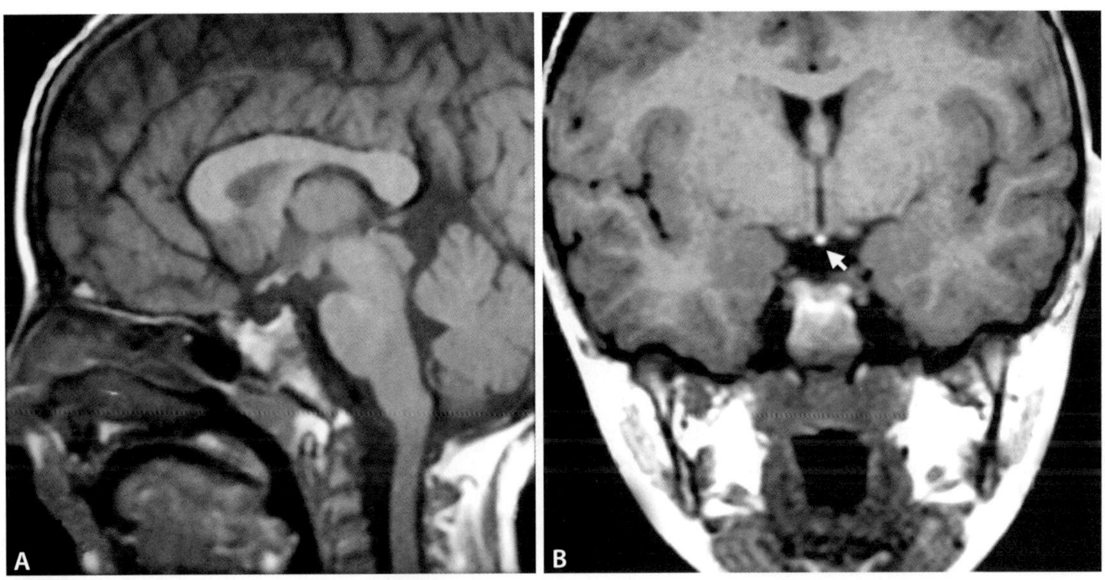

Figs. 24A and B: Pituitary hypoplasia in a child with retarded growth. T1 sagittal image (A) shows a small pituitary gland, absent stalk and ectopic bright spot near the hypothalamus [better seen on coronal T1 image (B) arrow].

seen in 60–98% of normal scans.[2] However, it is important to perform a high resolution thin contiguous section imaging of the gland to avoid false positive results. Patients with psychogenic polydipsia have a normal bright posterior pituitary as their hypothalamic-neurohypophyseal axis is intact.[35]

Hemochromatosis

Gonadotrophs are particularly susceptible to iron deposition and their dysfunction is reflected in the clinical picture. T2-weighted MR images showing an abnormally dark pituitary gland is the only means of showing iron overload in the pituitary tissue.[37]

TUMOR-LIKE LESIONS

Pituitary Hyperplasia

Physiological enlargement of the gland can be seen normally (*see* **Table 1**). Glandular enlargement can also be seen in response to exogenous estrogens, extrapituitary

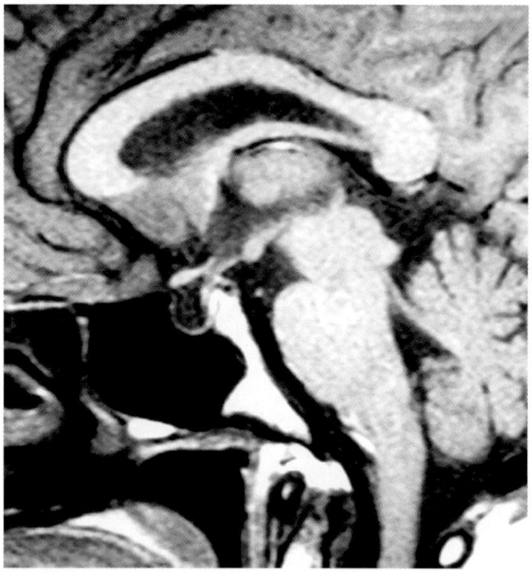

Fig. 25: Empty sella: Pituitary gland is not visualized on this T1 sagittal image, secondary to postpartum necrosis. The stalk is seen extending to the floor.

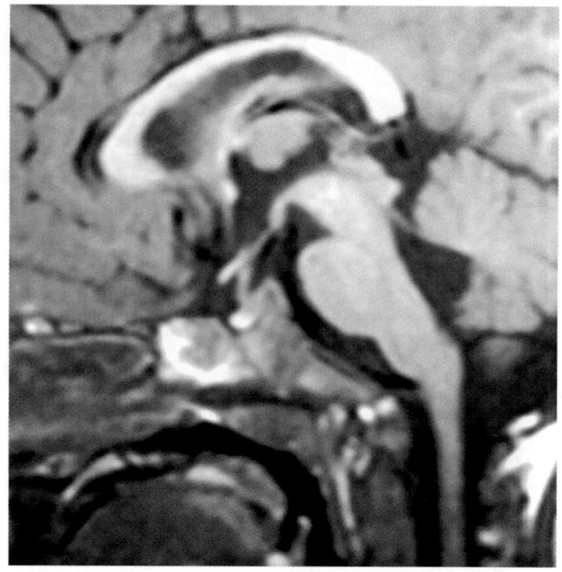

Fig. 26: Diabetes insipidus in a child: Absence of pituitary bright spot on T1 sagittal image with a normal stalk and no other demonstrable intra/suprasellar pathology.

Table 5: Central diabetes insipidus.

Etiology
• Trauma or surgery—50% of cases
• Idiopathic—25% of cases
• Craniopharyngioma
• Hypothalamic glioma
• Germinoma
• Granulomatous disease

hormonally active neoplasms and in end organ failure like primary hypothyroidism due to thyrotroph hyperplasia **(Fig. 27)**. Imaging shows an enlarged homogenously enhancing gland with convex superior margin (size >10–15 mm).

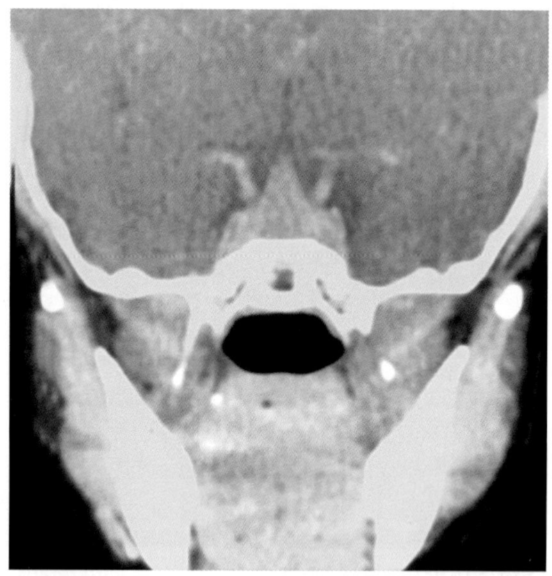

Fig. 27: Pituitary hyperplasia: Diffuse enlargement of the gland on CECT coronal section in a patient of hypothyroidism.

Arachnoid Cysts

Arachnoid cysts are frequent incidental findings in anterior or middle cranial fossae with 15% being juxtasellar.[38] They are usually developmental lesions due to lack of fenestration of membrane of Liliequist. They may also be acquired secondary to adhesions (due to arachnoiditis, trauma and hemorrhage). They are often asymptomatic but may present with hydrocephalus, hypopituitarism or seizures.

Both MRI and CT show a well-defined, nonenhancing cystic lesion with or without remodeling of skull base **(Figs. 28A and B)**. Differential diagnoses include an enlarged third ventricle, craniopharyngioma, epidermoid, Rathke'sand ependymal/parasitic cysts. Enhancement and calcification are usually seen in craniopharyngioma, while signal intensity greater than CSF on T1/proton images and less rounded shape are hallmarks of epidermoid cysts. FLAIR and diffusion images characteristically show epidermoids as bright lesions. Arachnoid cysts may extend into the sella and need to be differentiated from empty sella. The key to diagnosis lies in the location of the pituitary stalk which will be displaced in case of arachnoid cyst. The differentiation from other cystic suprasellar lesions may be impossible without histology.[39]

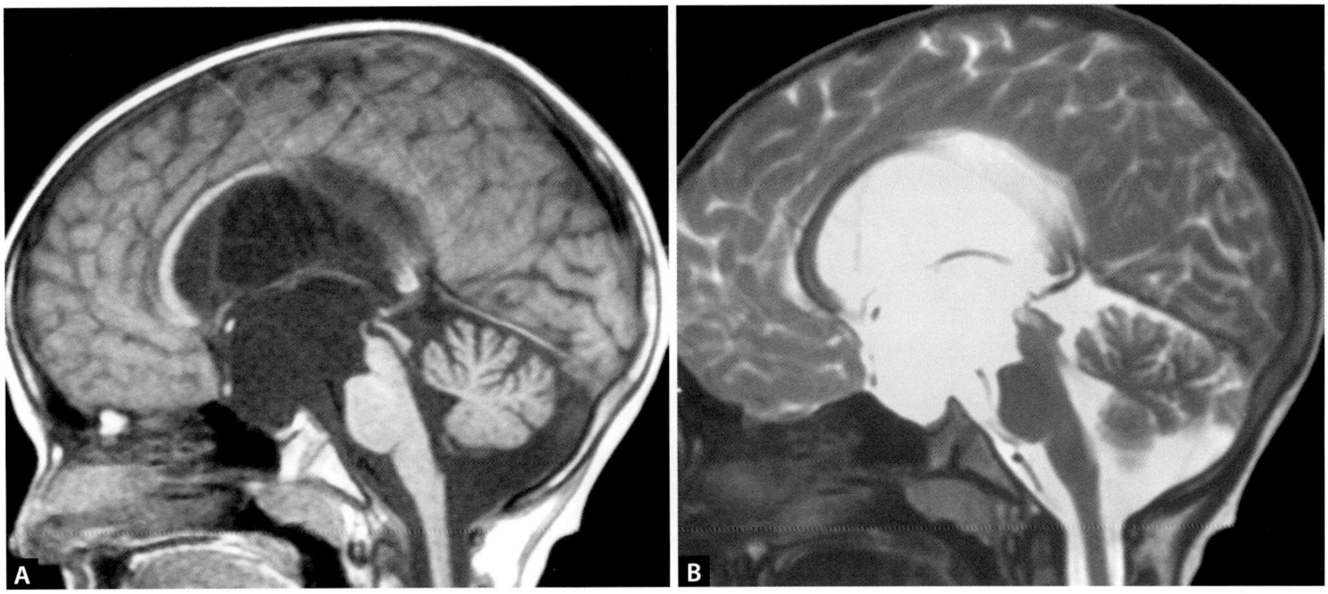

Figs. 28A and B: Arachnoid cyst: T1 and T2 sagittal MR images. The cyst appears hypointense on T1 and hyperintense on T2. The sella is normal with normal pituitary gland.

Rathke's Cleft Cysts

This is a common incidental finding at autopsy (11.3% incidence).[40] They form as a result of failure of Rathke's pouch to completely regress. They occasionally become symptomatic due to compression of adjacent structures. The cyst may contain mucoid, serous or cellular debris.[41] Most of the lesions are small, located within the gland in midline or may be large, suprasellar anterior to the stalk and compress pituitary, infundibulum or chiasma.

The imaging findings depend on cyst contents. Mucoid contents may appear hyperintense on T1 and T2WI, thus indistinguishable from craniopharyngiomas. Serous cysts will have features of typical benign cysts (CSF-like intensity) **(Figs. 29A and B)**. Cellular debris may sometimescause a diagnostic problem.[5] However, the lesions only show a faint rim of enhancement. Lack of solid nodular enhancement is a useful differentiating point from necrosed adenomas and along with lack of calcification from craniopharyngiomas.[3,5,25]

Tuber Cinereum Hamartoma

These are slow growing non-neoplastic heterotopias arising from the tuber cinereum (region between infundibulum and the mammillary bodies).[42] These patients present commonly with precocious puberty [secretion of luteinizing hormone-releasing hormone (LHRH)] and rarely with gelastic seizures (limbic lobe involvement) and mental impairment. On imaging they are sessile, nonenhancing, noncalcified, pedunculated, solid masses isointense to grey matter on T1 and T2WI but may be bright on T2WI **(Figs. 30A to D)**. Clinical history, location and morphology allow a straightforward diagnosis.

INFECTIVE CONDITIONS

Acute infections of hypothalamus and pituitary are rare. Pyogenic, viral, parasitic and tubercular infections, syphilis, candida, toxoplasma and cryptococcosis may affect these structures. A rare but well-described infective pathology is a pituitary bacterial abscess which can occur by hematogenous or direct spread. Infections in up to 30% cases arise in pre-existing lesions like adenoma, craniopharyngioma and Rathke's cleft cyst.[43] Abscesses are ring enhancing hypodense lesions on CT or appear as hypointense masses on T1WI showing bright signal on T2WI images. They are difficult to distinguish from other lesions, particularly adenoma and a diagnosis is rarely made preoperatively.[44] Infections in the parasellar region are more common than sellar infections and are usually part of disseminated disease or secondary to sinus infection. Basal meningitis affects this region in tuberculosis and other granulomatous infections. Tuberculosis is a common cause of meningitis and frequently shows thick basal exudates, infundibular involvement, hydrocephalus and brain infarction. Rarely tuberculosis can affect pituitary gland and but isolated tuberculomas or abscesses in the suprasellar cisterns are

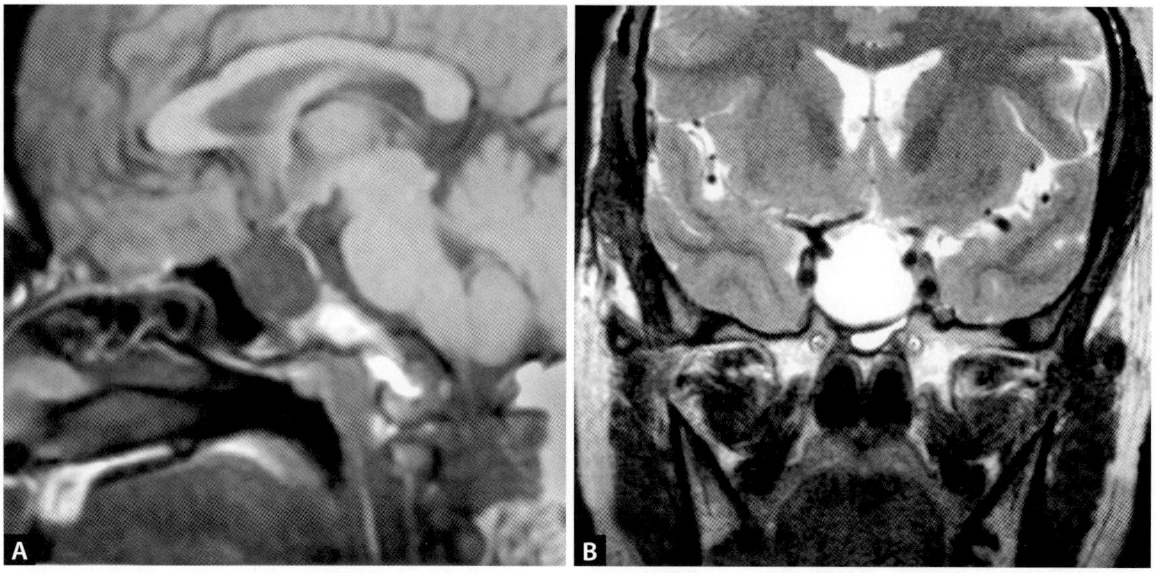

Figs. 29A and B: Rathke's cleft cyst: T1 sagittal (A) and T2 coronal (B) MR images. The cyst appears hypointense on T1 and hyperintense on T2 (like CSF). The sella is enlarged and stalk pushed posteriorly.

not uncommon in our setting **(Figs. 31A to D)**. Infections of cavernous sinus spread from a periorbital or paranasal source via the veins. Enhanced scans best show these lesions.

Fungal Infection

Increasing incidence of chronic indolent (granulomas) or fulminant fungal infection of sellar/parasellar region has been observed primarily as part of invasive rhinonasal disease by *Aspergillus* and mucormycosis. Immune compromised and diabetic patients are particularly prone. Paranasal sinus disease with headache, meningitis, altered sensorium, skull base/cavernous sinus or orbital apex syndromes should raise this possibility. Sellar/parasellar area, orbital apex area may show T1/T2 isointense enhancing soft tissue often with concurrent PNS, parapharyngeal space and middle cranial fossa disease **(Figs. 32A and B)**. There may be associated carotid artery aneurysm, brain infarctions, abscesses and orbital involvement.

INFLAMMATORY/GRANULOMATOUS CONDITIONS

Langerhans Cell Histiocytosis

Formerly called histiocytosis X, this is a group of diseases characterized by proliferation of histiocytes.[5] There are unifocal and multifocal forms of this disease. The unifocal disease shows solitary lytic bone lesion. This form spares the hypothalamic pituitary axis. The multifocal form of the disease is recurring, chronic, aggressive and presents in children with classical triad of diabetes insipidus, exophthalmos and lytic bone lesions (Hand-Schüller-Christian disease) due to granulomas in the hypothalamus and pituitary gland.

Computed tomography and MRI show thickening and enhancement of the infundibulum and hypothalamus **(Figs. 33A to D)**.[45] The posterior pituitary bright spot may be absent. The lesions are hyperintense on T2WI.[5] Differential diagnosis includes other suprasellar granulomas. Characteristic bone lesions and classical clinical picture aid in diagnosis of histiocytosis.

Lymphocytic Hypophysitis

This is noninfectious inflammatory process of auto-immune etiology affecting woman in late pregnancy or early postpartum period. The patient may present with severe hypopituitarism or with failure of lactation, headache, visual disturbances, etc. The condition regresses spontaneously with steroids. Pathologically, there is lymphocytic infiltration of the adenohypophysis or less commonly infundibulo-neuohypophysis or a combination of both. Imaging will show an intensely enhancing mass with or without extrasellar component. A thick nontapered enhancing stalk can be seen **(Figs. 34A to C)** as well as diaphragma sellae involvement (periglandular component). Seventy-five percent patients show loss of bright spot. Hence both pre- and

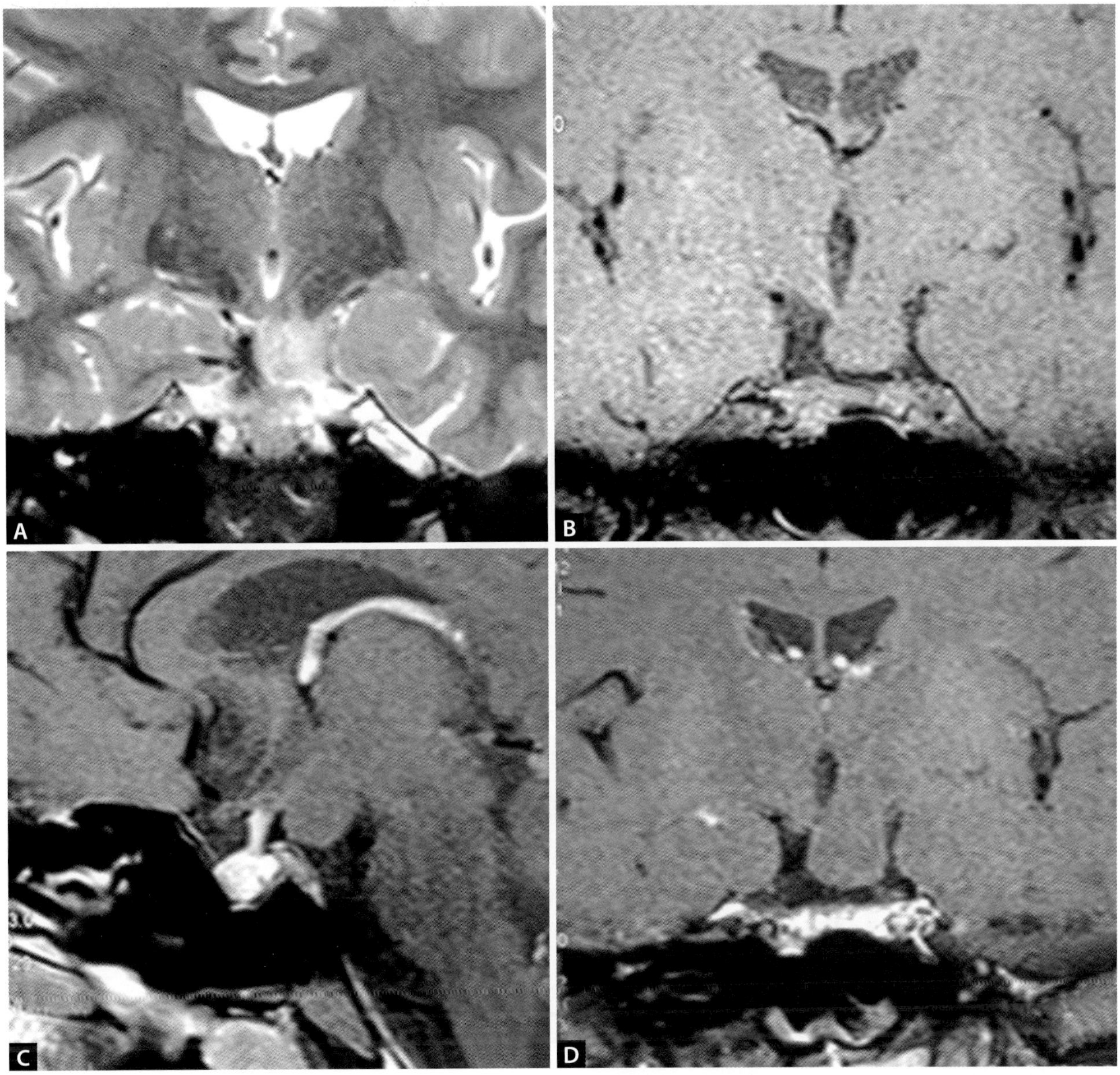

Figs. 30A to D: Tuber cinereum hamartoma: Coronal T2 (A) and T1 (B) weighted images reveal a sessile lesion (isointense to grey matter) typically located between mammillary body and infundibulum of pituitary gland. Gadolinium enhanced sagittal (C) and coronal (D) sections show no significant enhancement.

postcontrast scans are important. It is differentiated from Sheehan's syndrome by lack of hemorrhage. Physiological enlargement of gland in pregnancy rarely exceeds 12 mm in height and does not show any extrasellar enhancing component.[46] Granulomatous giant cell hypophysitis in middle aged people is another idiopathic inflammatory condition of sellar structures.

Sarcoidosis

This multisystem granulomatous lesion involves the meninges and tracks along perivascular spaces.[47] Five percent patients show neurological findings—frequently cranial nerve palsy and diabetes insipidus. However, since any part of the CNS may be involved, clinical features vary.

Basal meningeal involvement is common in neurosarcoid and best seen on CECT and CEMR.[47] Multiple small nodular or large mass like enhancing lesions or distortion, thickening and enhancement of meninges and cranial nerves may be seen. The pituitary gland infundibulum and hypothalamus may be involved. Multiple scattered parenchymal lesions also suggest a diagnosis of neurosarcoid.[5]

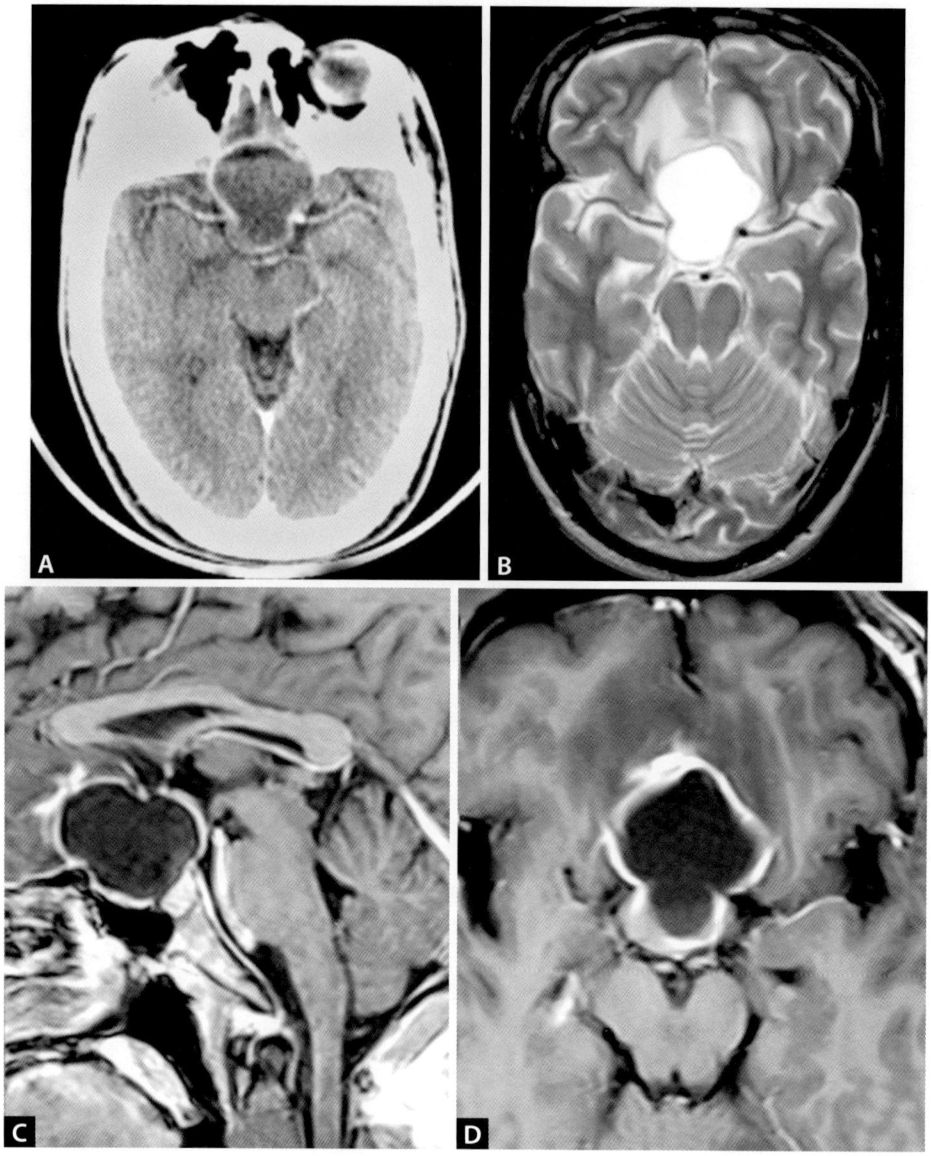

Figs. 31A to D: CECT axial (A), MR T2 axial (B), CE MR sagittal and axial (C and D) images show a surgically proven suprasellar tubercular abscess. Note the fluid intensity center, smooth peripheral rim enhancement (C and D) and associated edema in brain (B) indicating an inflammatory lesion.

Differential diagnosis is with other granulomatous lesions. Presence of systemic disease in 60% of cases, steroid responsiveness, localized or generalized basal meningeal disease with scattered parenchymal nodules aid in diagnosis of sarcoidosis.

Tolosa-Hunt Syndrome

It is an idiopathic steroid responsive inflammatory lesion of the cavernous sinus causing painful ophthalmoplegia and visual defects. The condition can have recurrent attacks with remissions and is steroid responsive. It is a granulomatous inflammation pathologically similar to orbital pseudotumor which can cause periarteritis of carotid artery. Imaging findings of asymmetric enlargement of cavernous sinus, enhancing soft tissue in the orbital apex and prepontine cistern have been described **(Figs. 35A and B)**. The soft tissue typically shows isointensity to muscle on T1 and to fat on T2-weighted images.[48] Similar intensity patterns are also shared by lymphomas, meningiomas and sarcoidosis.

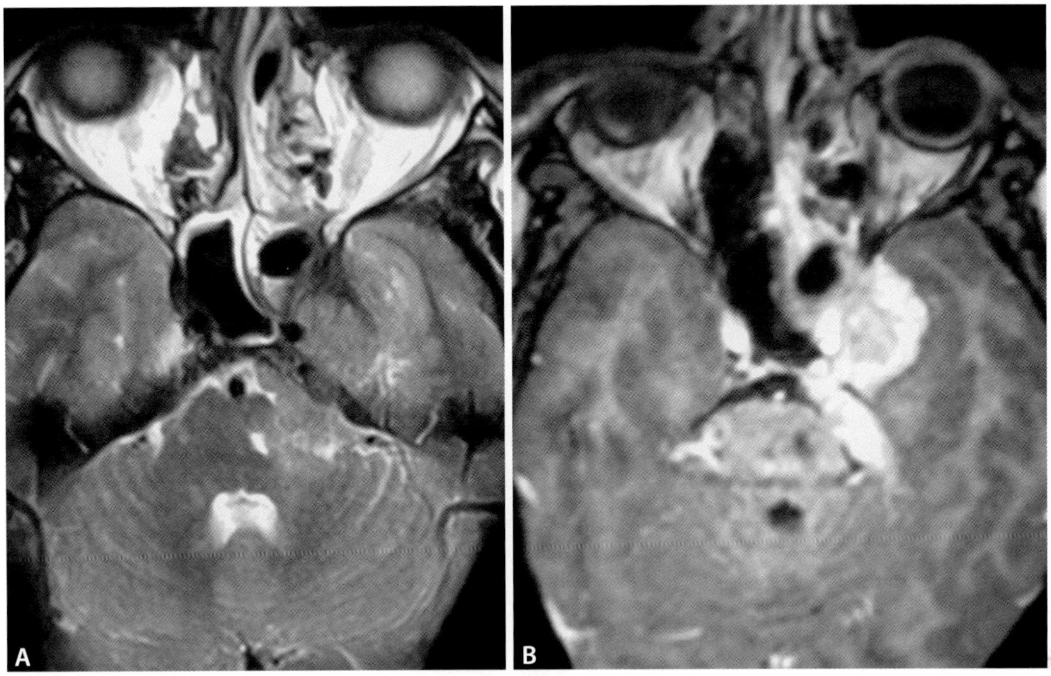

Figs. 32A and B: Fungal sinusitis with intracranial extension. Axial T2 (A) and gadolinium enhanced T1 (B) images showing spheno-ethmoid sinusitis with left parasellar and cavernous sinus invasion. Posterior extension into the prepontine and cerebellopontine angle cistern is also noted.

VASCULAR LESIONS

Aneurysms and Vascular Loops

Critical to diagnose, intracavernous and supraclinoid internal carotid aneurysms present as juxtasellar masses. The area is the most common site of giant aneurysms. These may project into the sella and show contiguity with vascular structures, flow void on MRI, strong contrast enhancement and can be easily picked up by CT/CT angiography. Partially thrombosed aneurysms may cause diagnostic difficulty but lamellated thrombus, flow characteristics including artifacts in phase encoding direction, surrounding blood products in various stages of evolution, etc. are distinctive findings of aneurysms on MRI **(Figs. 36A to C)**.[49]

Carotid Cavernous Fistula and Vascular Malformations

A fistulous communication between the carotid artery and the cavernous sinus may present as a pulsatile parasellar lesion due to enlarged arterialized cavernous sinus. Patients present with chemosis, proptosis and visual loss. Presence of flow artifacts, enlarged cavernous sinus and superior ophthalmic vein suggest the diagnosis which is confirmed on an angiographic study. Digital subtraction angiography shows immediate opacification of the cavernous sinus on internal carotid artery (ICA) injection with communication at the level of the cavernous segment of ICA **(Fig. 37A)**. This fistulous communication can be embolized by either detachable balloon or coils **(Fig. 37B)**. Extra-axial cavernous malformations rarely present in supra/parasellar area and should be suspected if an atypical mass with T2 hyperintensity is seen. Cavernous sinus hemangiomas classically show intense T2 hyperintensity with T hypointensity and brilliant enhancement on gadolinium administration **(Figs. 38A to C)**. Dynamic contrast enhanced images show progressive centripetal enhancement of the lesion.

Sheehan's Syndrome

This is a syndrome of postpartum pituitary necrosis in complicated deliveries with clinical and imaging features similar to pituitary apoplexy in the acute phase.[50] However, there is no sellar mass and circulatory disturbances lead to hemorrhage and necrosis of a vulnerable hyperplasic gland secondary to pregnancy related changes.[5,50] The end result may be an empty sella.

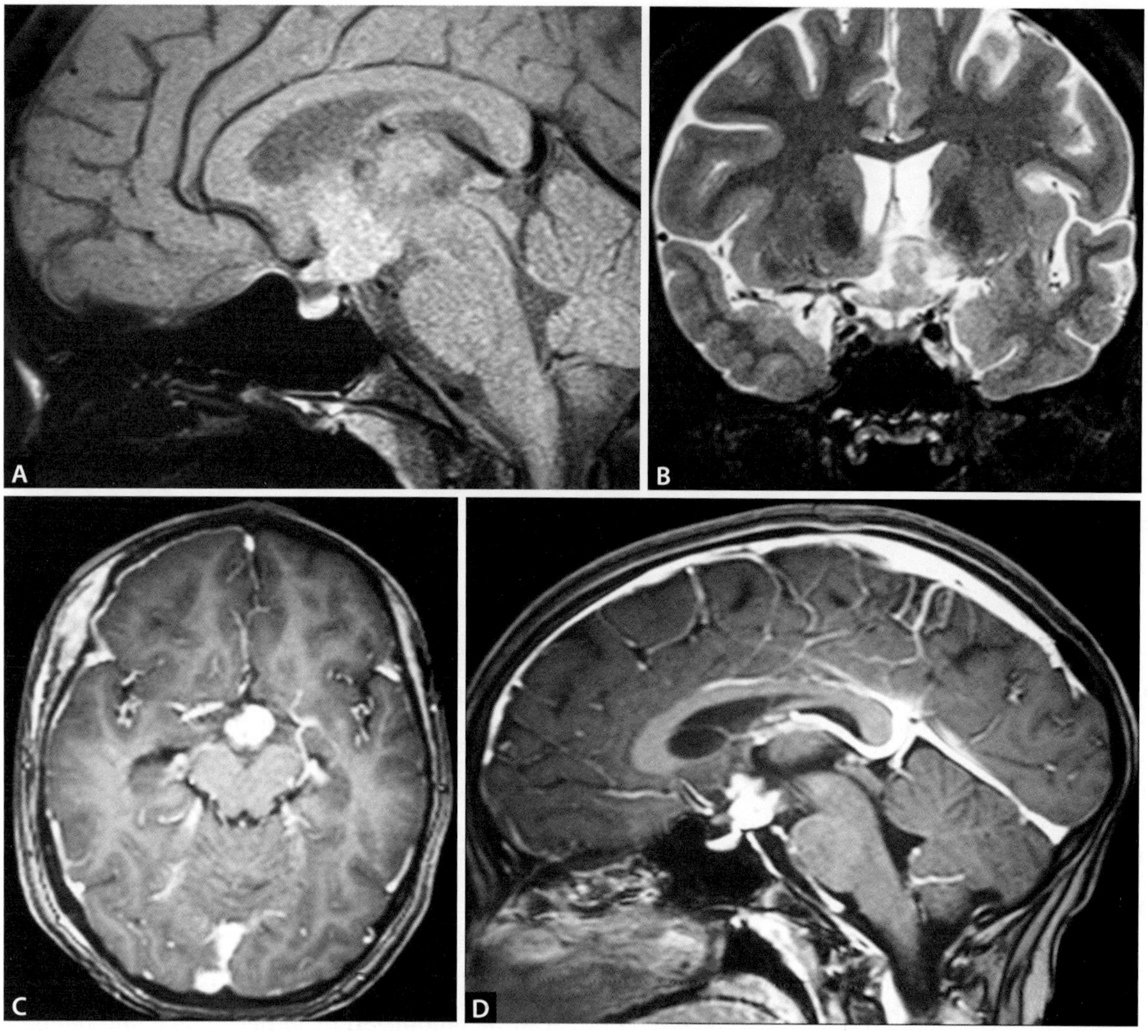

Figs. 33A to D: Langerhan's cell histiocytosis: Sagittal T1 WI (A) and coronal T2 WI (B) shows isointense thickening of hypothalamus and infundibulum which is showing strong enhancement (C and D). A bone lesion may be noted in the right frontal area (C).

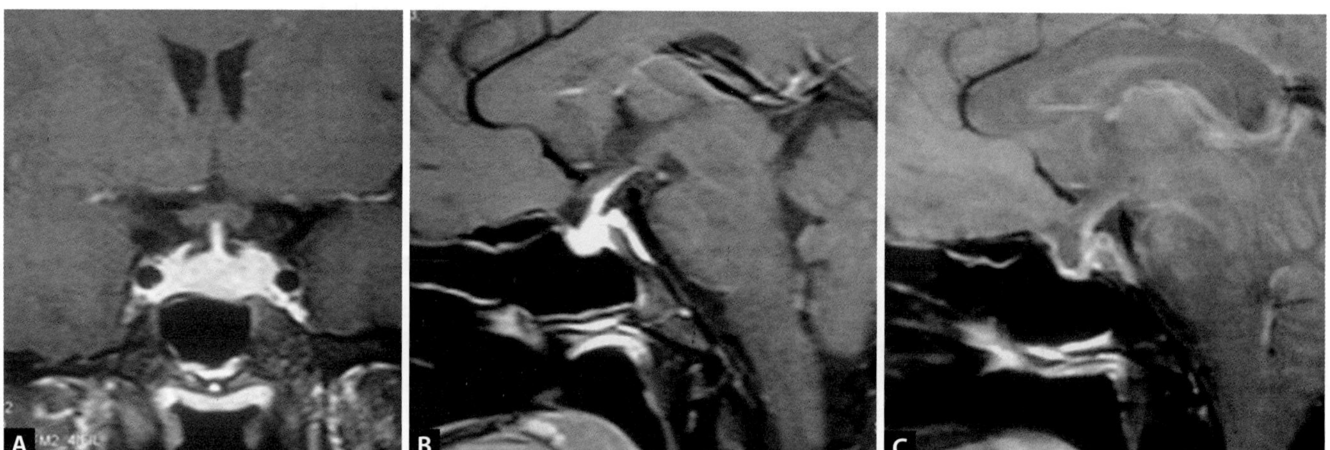

Figs. 34A to C: Lymphocytic hypophysitis: Increased bulk of the hypophysis is seen with soft tissue extension into bilateral parasellar region. Note that the arc of contact with carotid artery is approx 150° (A). Sagittal MR section (B) demonstrating the same with infundibular thickening and retroclival extension. Follow-up MR (C) following pulse steroid therapy reveals marked reduction in the bulk of abnormal tissue.

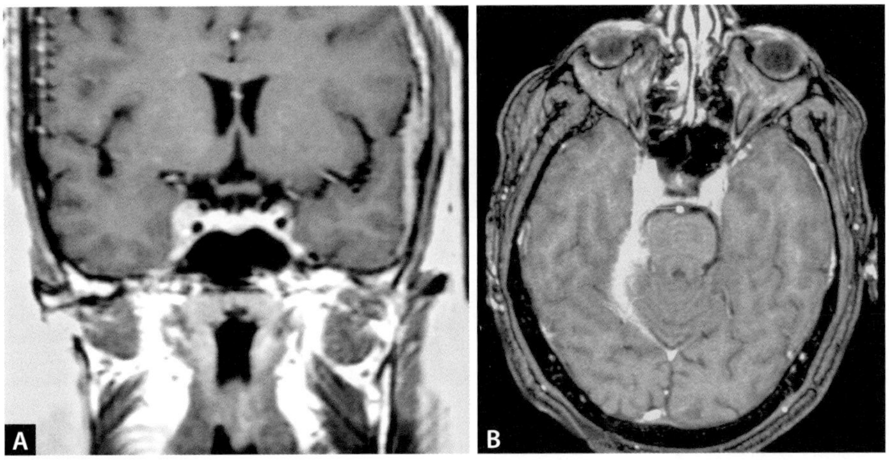

Figs. 35A and B: Tolosa-Hunt syndrome: Contrast enhanced T1 coronal (A) and axial GRE image (B) shows abnormal enhancing soft tissue in the region of right cavernous sinus, extending into the tentorium cerebelli in a patient with headache.

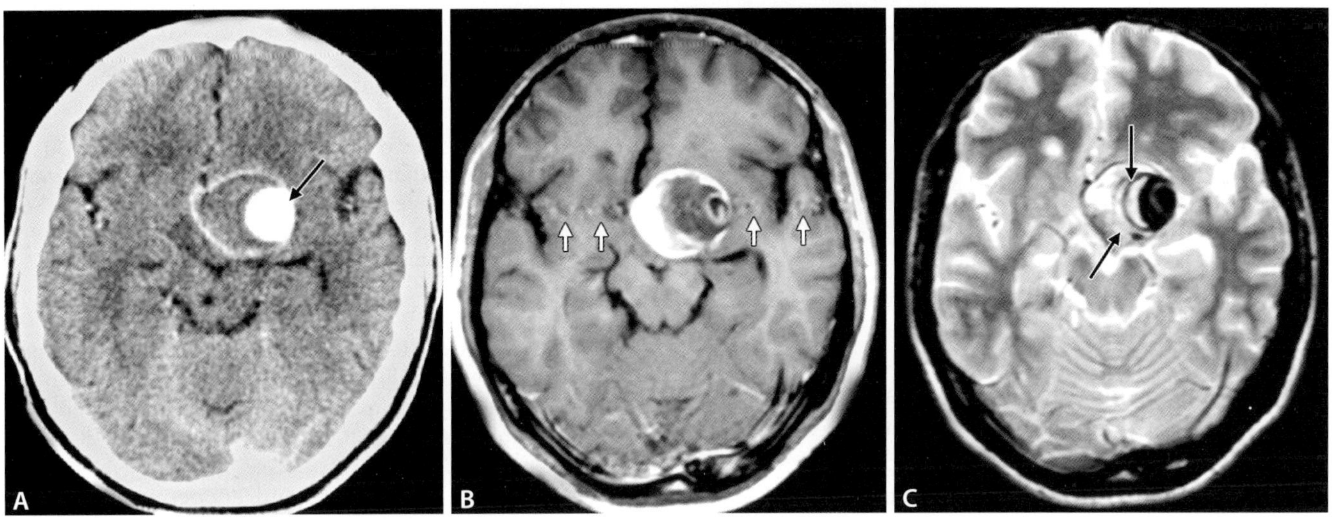

Figs. 36A to C: Axial sections CECT (A), T1 SE (B) and T2 FSE (C) show partly thrombosed suprasellar aneurysm arising from left ICA bifurcation. Note layered thrombus (arrows in C) and patent lumen on the left side of the lesion which enhances on CECT (arrow in A). Note pulsation artifacts in phase direction (arrows in B).

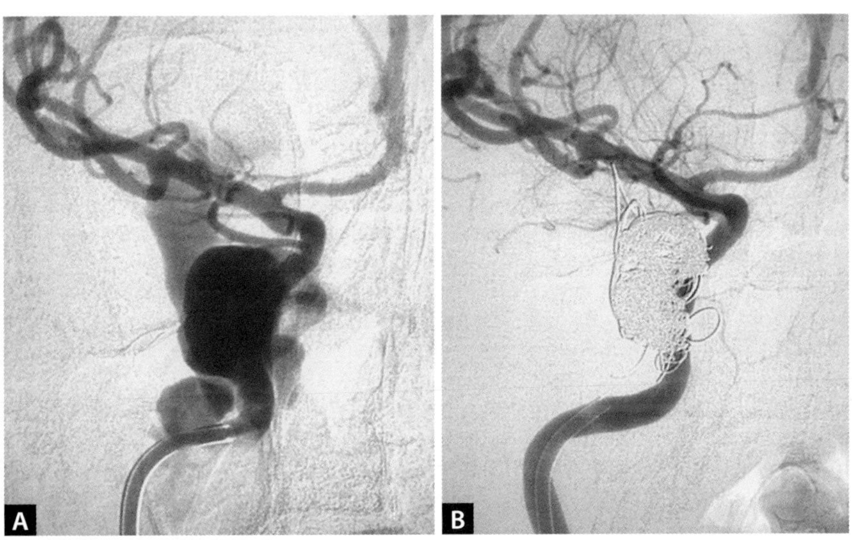

Figs. 37A and B: Caroticocavernous fistula (CCF): Digital subtraction angiogram (DSA) of the right internal carotid artery (A) demonstrating immediate opacification of the cavernous sinus through the cavernous ICA segment. Post coil embolization (B) DSA showing complete fistula closure.

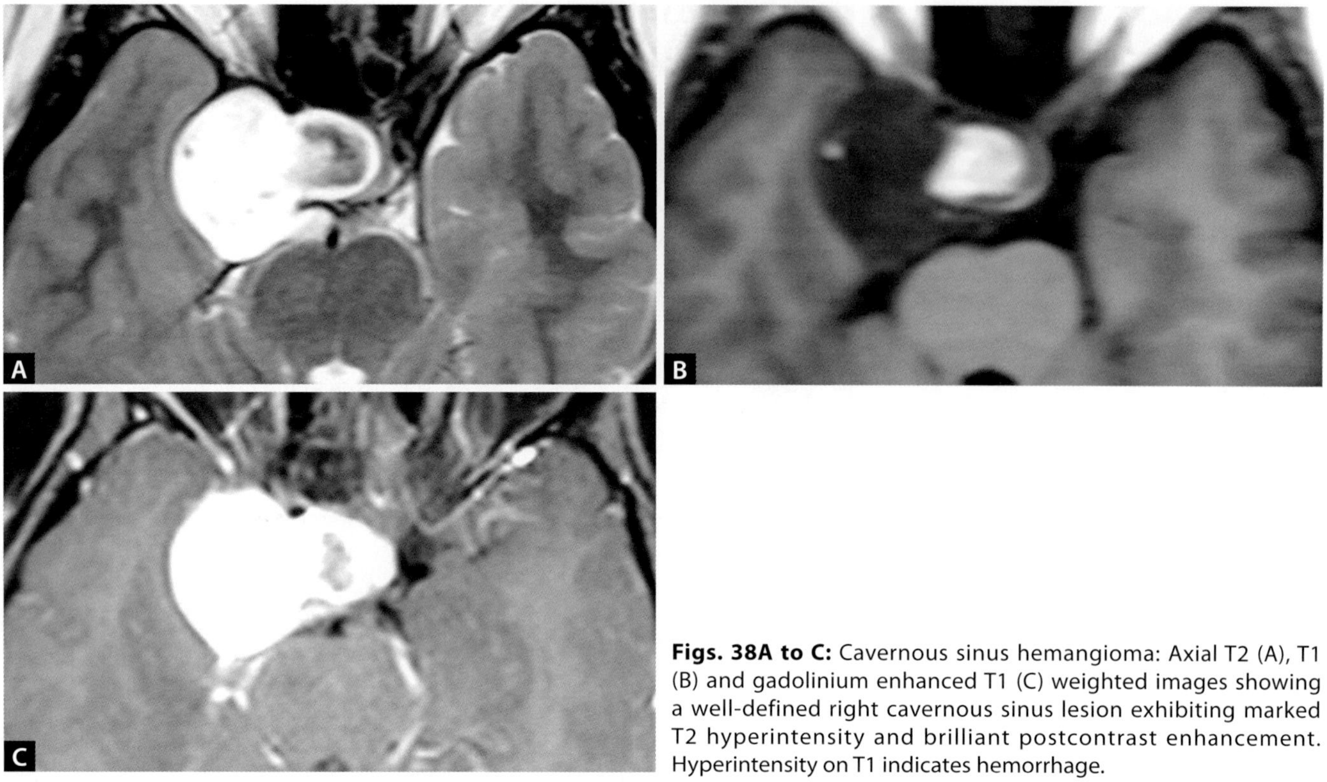

Figs. 38A to C: Cavernous sinus hemangioma: Axial T2 (A), T1 (B) and gadolinium enhanced T1 (C) weighted images showing a well-defined right cavernous sinus lesion exhibiting marked T2 hyperintensity and brilliant postcontrast enhancement. Hyperintensity on T1 indicates hemorrhage.

CONCLUSION

Though a small zone spatially, the sellar region harbours many structures and hence many pathologies related to these structures. A thorough understanding of its anatomy and structures in its vicinity is of prime importance in formulating an appropriate diagnosis of pathologies in this region. MR has transformed the evaluation of sellar lesions and currently forms the backbone of sellar evaluation. An optimal utilization of the MR techniques helps us in understanding the disease process better. A good correlation of anatomy, clinical symptomatology and imaging (MR) evaluation often clinches the diagnosis.

REFERENCES

1. Latchaw RE, Roppole HMN. Radiographic evaluation of the normal sellaturcica and the pituitary gland. In: Radiology Diagnosis Imaging Intervention, Volume 3. Philadelphia: JB Lippincott Co.; 1986. pp. 1-7.
2. Fujisawa I, Asato R, Nishimura K, et al. Anterior and posterior lobes of pituitary gland, assessment by 1.5T MR imaging. J Comput Assist Tomogr. 1987;11(2):214-20.
3. Elster AD. Imaging of sella: anatomy and pathology. Semin Ultrasound CT MR. 1993;14(3):182-94.
4. Cox TD, Elster AD. Normal pituitary gland: changes in shape, size and signal intensity during the 1st year of life at MR imaging. Radiology. 1991;179(3):721-4.
5. Symons SP, Aviv RI, Montanera WJ, et al. The sella turcica and parasellar region. In: Atlas SW (Ed). Magnetic Resonance Imaging of the Brain and Spine, 5th edition. Philadelphia: Lippincott Williams and Wilkins; 2016. pp. 1120-92.
6. Pressman BD. Pituitary Imaging. Endocrinol Metab Clin North Am. 2017;46:713-40.
7. Pinker K, Ba-Ssalamah A, Wolfsberger S, et al. The value of high field MRI (3T) in the assessment of sellar lesions. Eur J Radiol. 2005;54(3):327-34.
8. Kovacs K, Horvath E, Asa SL. Classification and pathology of pituitary tumors. In: Wilkins RH, Rengachary SS (Eds). Neurosurgery. New York: McGraw-Hill; 1985. pp. 834-42.
9. Hall WA, Lunciano MG, Doppman JL, et al. Pituitary magnetic resonance imaging in normal human volunteers: occult adenomas in general population. Ann Int Med. 1994;120(10):817-20.
10. Go JL, Rajamohan AG. Imaging of the sella and parasellar region. Radiol Clin North Am. 2017;55(1):83-101.
11. Grober Y, Grober H, Wintermark M, et al. Comparison of MRI techniques for detecting microadenomas in Cushing's disease. J Neurosurg. 2017;28:1-7.
12. Schwartzberg DG. Imaging of pituitary gland tumors. Semin Ultrasound CT MR. 1992;13(3):207-23.
13. Zampetti B, Grossrubatscher E, Dalino Ciaramella P, et al. Bilateral inferior petrosal sinus sampling. Endocr Connect. 2016;5(4):R12-25.
14. Bonnelli FS, Huston J, Carpenter PC, et al. Adreno-corticotropic Hormone-dependent Cushing's syndrome:

sensitivity and specificity of inferior petrosal sinus sampling. Am J Neuroradiol. 2000;21(4):690-6.
15. Pierallini A, Caramia F, Falcone C, et al. Pituitary macroadenomas: preoperative evaluation of consistency with diffusion-weighted MR imaging-initial experience. Radiology. 2006;239(1):223-31.
16. Knosp E, Steiner E, Kitz K, et al. Pituitary adenomas with invasion of the cavernous sinus space. A magnetic resonance imaging classification compared with surgical findings. Neurosurgery. 1993;33:610.
17. Micko AS, Wöhrer A, Wolfsberger S, et al. Invasion of the cavernous sinus space in pituitary adenomas: endoscopic verification and its correlation with an MRI-based classification. J Neurosurg. 2015;122:803-11.
18. Edal AL, Skjödt K, Nepper-Rasmussen HJ. SIPAP: a new MR classification for pituitary adenomas. Suprasellar, infrasellar, parasellar, anterior and posterior. Acta Radiol. 1997;38:30-6.
19. Miki Y, Kanagaki M, Takahashi JA, et al. Evaluation of pituitary macroadenomas with multidetector-row CT (MDCT): comparison with MR imaging. Neuroradiology. 2007;49(4):327-33.
20. Ostrov SG, Quencer RM, Hoffman JC, et al. Hemorrhage within pituitary adenomas: how often associated with pituitary apoplexy syndrome? Am J Roentgenol. 1989;153(1):153-60.
21. Rogg JM, Tung GA, Anderson G, et al. Pituitary apoplexy: early detection with diffusion-weighted MR imaging. Am J Neuroradiol. 2002;23(7):1240-5.
22. Steiner E, Knosp E, Herold CJ, et al. Pituitary adenomas, findings of postoperative MR imaging. Radiology. 1992;185(2):521-7.
23. Crotty TB, Sheithauer BW, Young WF, et al. Papillary craniopharyngiomas: a clinico-pathological study of 48 cases. J Neurosurg. 1995;83(2):206-14.
24. Jellinger K. Primary intrasellar germ cell tumors. Acta Neuropathol. 1973;25(4):291-306.
25. Chong BW, Newton TH. Hypothalamic and pituitary pathology. Radiol Clin North Am. 1993;31(5):1147-53.
26. Conley FK. Epidermoid and dermoid tumor: clinical features and surgical management. In: Wilkins RG, Rengachary SS (Eds). Neurosurgery. New York: McGraw-Hill; 1985. pp. 668-70.
27. Takeuchi J, Handa HM, Nagata I. Suprasellar germinoma. J Neurosurg. 1978;49(1):41-8.
28. Hua F, Asato R, Miki T, et al. Differentiation of suprasellar non-neoplastic cysts from cystic neoplasms by Gd-DTPA MRI. J Comput Assist Tomogr. 1992;16(5):744-9.
29. Alshail E, Rutka JT, Becker LE, et al. Opticochiasmatic hypothalamic glioma. Brain Pathol. 1997;7(2):799-806.
30. Yuh WT, Wright DC Barloon TJ, et al. MR imaging of primary tumors of trigeminal nerve and Meckel's cave. Am J Roentgenol. 1988;151(3):577-82.
31. Sze G, Uichanco LS, Brant-Zawadzki MN, et al. Chordomas: MR Imaging. Radiology. 1988;166(1 Pt 1):187-91.
32. Schubiger O, Haller D. Metastasis to the pituitary hypothalamic axis. An MR study of 7 symptomatic patients. Neuroradiology. 1992;34(2):131-4.
33. Kizilkilic O, Yalcin O, Yildirim T, et al. Hypothalamic hamartoma associated with craniopharyngeal canal. Am J Neuroradiol. 2005;26(1):65-7.
34. Fahrendorf G, Bramswig J, Bals-Pratsch M. MR findings in patients with idiopathic panhypopituitarism. Rofo. 1990;152(5):550-5.
35. Tien R, Kucharczyk J, Kucharczyk W. MR imaging of the brain in patients with diabetes insipidus. Am J Neuroradiol. 1991;12(3):533-42.
36. Fujisawa I, Nishimura K, Asato R, et al. Posterior lobe of pituitary in diabetes insipidus: MR findings. J Comput Assist Tomogr. 1987;11(2):221-5.
37. Fujisawa I, Morikawa M, Nakano Y, et al. Hemochromatosis of pituitary gland, MR imaging. Radiology. 1988;168:213-4.
38. Wiener SN, Pearlstein AE, Eiber A. MR imaging of intracranial arachnoid cysts. J Comput Assist Tomogr. 1987;11(2):236-41.
39. Gentry LR, Smoker WR, Turski PA, et al. Suprasellar arachnoid cysts: 1. CT recognition. Am J Neuroradiol. 1986;7(1):79-86.
40. Teramoto A, Hirakawa K, Sanno N, et al. Incidental pituitary lesions in 1,000 unselected autopsy specimens. Radiology. 1994;193(1):161-4.
41. Kucharczyk W, Peck WW, Kelly WM, et al. Rathke cleft cysts: CT, MR imaging and pathological features. Radiology. 1987;165(2):491-5.
42. Boyko OB, Curnes JT, Oakes WJ, et al. Hamartomas of tuber cinereum CT, MR and pathological findings. Am J Neuroradiol. 1991;12(2):309-14.
43. Domingue JN, Wilson CB. Pituitary abscesses. Report of seven cases and review of literature. J Neurosurgery. 1977;46(5):601-8.
44. Dutta P, Bhansali A, Singh P, et al. Pituitary abscess: report of four cases and review of literature. Pituitary. 2006;9(3):267-73.
45. Tien RD Newton TH, McDermott MW, et al. Thickened pituitary stalk on MR images in patients with diabetes insipidus and Langerhans cell histiocytosis. Am J Neuroradiol. 1990;11(4):703-8.
46. Ahmadi J, Meyers GD, Segall HD, et al. Lymphocytic adenohypophysitis: contrast-enhanced MR imaging in five cases. Radiology. 1995;195(1):30-4.
47. Sherman JL, Stern BJ. Sarcoidosis of the CNS: comparison of unenhanced and enhanced MR images. Am J Neuroradiol. 1990;11(5):915-23.
48. Yousem DM, Atlas SW, Grossman RI, et al. MR imaging of Tolosa-Hunt syndrome. Am J Neuroradiol. 1989;10(6):1181-4.
49. Atlas SW, Mark AS, Fram EK, et al. Vascular intracranial lesions: applications of gradient echo MR Imaging. Radiology. 1988;169(2):455-61.
50. Sheehan HL, Stanford JP. The pathogenesis of postpartum necrosis of the anterior lobe of the pituitary gland. Acta Endocrinol. 1961;37:479-510.

CHAPTER 19

Intraventricular Lesions

Chirag Kamal Ahuja, Paramjeet Singh, Niranjan Khandelwal

INTRODUCTION

The ventricular system forms an important compartment of the brain with cerebrospinal fluid (CSF) playing the major role of hemodynamic regulation, lubrication and scavenging. It may harbor many different lesions, some of which can be native to it while others may infiltrate from surrounding structures and some even from distant areas through CSF pathways. Intraventricular (IV) lesions can be congenital, inflammatory/infective, traumatic or neoplastic.[1,2] Categorization of IV lesions can often be challenging, especially of the larger ones, as many of these arise in the paraventricular region and efface or grow into the adjoining ventricle. Native IV lesions are fewer in number. There is a predilection of certain lesions for specific age groups and locations. Diagnosis of an IV lesion thus should involve a comprehensive evaluation of the patient's age and clinical symptomatology in addition to imaging findings.[1,3] Tumors constitute the major bulk of intraventricular lesions, though contributing less than 10% of all intracranial tumors.[4] In this chapter, IV lesions are described according to their location within various parts of ventricular system with particular emphasis on the more common lesions.

IMAGING MODALITIES

1. ***Plain skull radiograph***: This may demonstrate calcification within the lesion and evidence of raised intracranial tension. Associated features of syndromic disorders can be seen at times, e.g. cyst-like or sclerotic bone lesions in tuberous sclerosis.
2. ***Plain and contrast enhanced computed tomography (CT)***: CT may aid in lesion characterization and confirm or refute the presence of calcification. Multi detector computed tomography (MDCT) may help in better localization through its multiplanar capability with the help of volumetric data acquisition.
3. ***Conventional ventriculography/CT ventriculography***: These investigations have become obsolete with the advent of magnetic resonance imaging (MRI).
4. ***Magnetic resonance imaging***: It has transformed the way we look at intracranial lesions with its exquisite resolution and multiplanar capability.
5. ***Angiography***: Indicated in vascular malformations and for angioembolization.

A sound understanding of the ventricular lesions requires a thorough knowledge of the anatomy and physiology of the ventricular system. Thus, a brief overview of the ventricles is presented before discussing the various intraventricular lesions.

ANATOMY AND PHYSIOLOGY OF VENTRICULAR SYSTEM

The ventricular system (*Latin*: ventriculus = cavity) is constituted by two lateral and two median ventricles, the latter referred to as the third and fourth ventricles **(Fig. 1A)**. They are lined by ependymal cells and are filled with CSF which has free communication with each other as well as with the extra-axial cisternal spaces through the fourth ventricular outflow tracts. The CSF is

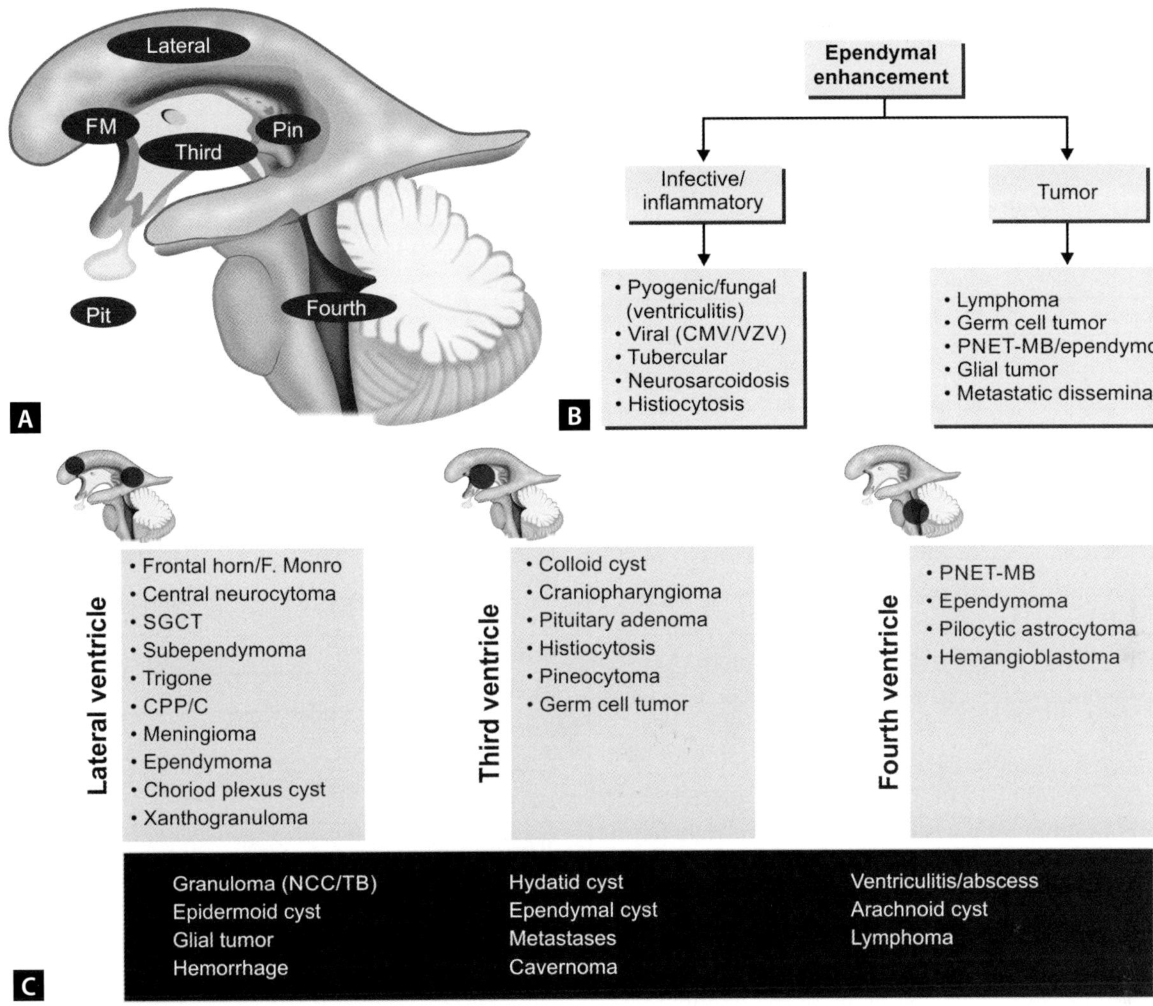

Figs. 1A to C: (A) Pictorial diagram of the relationship of the ventricular system with important adjoining structures; (B) Differentials of ependymal enhancement; (C) Distribution of the lesions according to location within the ventricular system. The reverse black box represents lesions common to all ventricles.

Abbreviations: CMV: Cytomegalovirus; CPP/C: Choroid plexus papilloma/carcinoma; FM: Foramen of Monro; Pin: Pineal gland; Pit: Pituitary gland; NCC: Neurocysticercosis; PNET-MB: Primitive neuroectodermal tumor-medulloblastoma; SGCT: Subependymal giant cell tumor; TB: Tuberculoma; VZV: Varicella-Zoster virus.

produced by the choroid plexus (composed of specialized ependymal cells surrounding a core of capillaries and loose connective tissue) by the process of ultrafiltration and active secretion and flows with a pressure gradient through the ventricles and cisterns before being absorbed by the arachnoid granulations situated in relation to the dural venous sinuses. The lesions in the ventricles can thus, arise per se from within or adjacent to the ventricles or may spread secondarily via CSF or be of hematogenous origin, the latter being extremely rare. Most commonly the lesions are neoplastic in origin, with inflammatory and developmental ones being relatively uncommon. Some lesions can present in the form of diffusely spreading ependymal enhancement along the ventricular margins. These can be either of infective/inflammatory etiology or of neoplastic origin **(Fig. 1B)**. The various intraventricular lesions are described based on their location within the respective ventricles **(Fig. 1C)**. The lesions which are common to all ventricles and can be seen in any of them are mentioned in the box below in the Figure 19.1C. Common lesions in children and adults are tabulated in **Tables 1 and 2**.

Lateral Ventricular Lesions

Neoplasms constitute the major bulk of lateral ventricular lesions.[4] Intraventricular neoplasms constitute one-tenth of all central nervous system (CNS) neoplasms.[1,2] About half of these in adults and one-fourth in children are found

Table 1: Intraventricular lesions in children.

Lateral ventricle
• Choroid plexus papilloma/carcinoma
• Astrocytoma (low grade)
• Giant cell astrocytoma
• primitive neuroectodermal tumor (PNET)
Foramen of Monro
• Subependymal giant cell astrocytoma
• Astrocytoma
Third ventricle
• Craniopharyngioma
• Astrocytoma
• Histocytosis
• Germinoma
Fourth ventricle
• Astrocytoma
• Ependymoma
• Medulloblastoma

Note: Cysticercal cyst, hydatid cyst, granuloma (TB) can occur in any ventricle.

Table 2: Intraventricular lesions in adults.

Lateral ventricle
• Astrocytoma
• Meningioma
• Central neurocytoma
• Subependymoma
• Choroid plexus cyst/xanthogranulomas
• Metastasis
Foramen of Monro
• Astrocytoma
• Central neurocytoma
• Subependymal giant cell astrocytoma
Third ventricle
• Colloid cyst
• Extrinsic masses
• Metastasis
Aqueduct
• Hemorrhage
• Glioma
Fourth ventricle
• Epidermoid
• Arachnoid cyst
• Metastasis

Note: Cysticercal cyst; hydatid cyst, granuloma (TB) can occur in any ventricle particularly during the first two years of life. CPP is a benign tumor but carcinomatous degeneration occurs in up to 20% of patients. The usual presenting symptoms are related to hydrocephalus and increased intracranial pressure.

in the lateral ventricles.[5] The frequency and the type of tumor differs in different parts of the lateral ventricle (e.g. frontal horn, body, atrium, occipital horn). These tumors originate from the cells located within/in the vicinity of the ventricles. The ependymal cells lining the ventricles are the precursors of ependymomas. There is a subependymal plate composed of glial cells just beneath the ependymal lining from which the subependymomas are postulated to arise. Glial cells along with residual neuronal precursor cells line the septum pellucidum from which the central neurocytomas arise. Primary tumors of the choroid plexus (choroid plexus papilloma and carcinoma) originate from the cells of the vascular choroid plexus epithelium. The choroid plexus also contributes to the hematogenous deposition of various metastases. Meningiomas are thought to arise from the trapped arachnoid cap cells forming the arachnoid granulations. There can be secondary ventricular involvement by contiguous extension of lesions from the adjoining brain parenchyma. Apart from neoplasms, the lateral ventricle may harbor a number of developmental, inflammatory and infective lesions, e.g. ependymal cyst, neurocysticercus, hydatid cyst, extension of pyogenic abscess, etc.

In children, intraventricular neoplasms occur more often in the trigone, primarily because certain tumor types that favor the trigonal region have a predilection for occurring in children. Choroid plexus tumors are one of the most common lesions of the lateral ventricle in young children, and the majority occur within the trigone. Ependymomas and low grade astrocytomas [e.g. pilocytic astrocytomas and subependymal giant cell astrocytomas (SGCAs)] occur in the anterior body/trigonal region in older children and young adults. Intraventricular meningiomas typically occur in the trigonal region in older adults. Two non-neoplastic lesions that frequently present as trigonal lesions are choroid plexus cysts and xanthogranulomas, both of which are incidentally detected, benign, typically asymptomatic and are often bilateral. The former are epithelial lined cysts located in the glomus that can be seen in neonates. The latter are choroid plexus masses that typically occur in adults but are occasionally found in children.[6]

Choroid Plexus Tumors

Choroid plexus tumors (CPTs) account for a fifth of all neoplasms occurring in infancy and about 2–4% of all pediatric tumors.[7,8] Half of all arise in relation to the ventricular trigone while the rest occur in relation to the fourth (40%) and third ventricle (10%). Children often present with lateral ventricular masses while adults have an equal distribution between both lateral and fourth ventricles. Syndromic association is also seen sometimes with Aicardi and Li-Fraumeni syndromes. Based on histology, they are divided into choroid plexus papilloma (CPP) (WHO grade I), atypical variant of CPP (WHO grade II) and choroid plexus carcinoma (WHO grade III).

Choroid plexus papilloma and its atypical variant: It is the most common tumor occurring in the lateral ventricles in the first decade. Their incidence and distribution corresponds to that of all CPTs, mentioned above.[7] Bilateral tumors are rare, accounting for 3–4% of all CPPs. In children, as previously stated they occur more commonly in the atrium of the lateral ventricles in contrast to adults, where these are more frequently seen in the fourth ventricle. On CT the tumor is seen as a well-defined, frond-like mass which is iso or mildly hyperdense to brain. Calcification is seen within the tumor in about 25% cases **(Fig. 2)**. There is usually homogeneous and intense enhancement following contrast administration. Diffuse hydrocephalus involving dilatation of all the ventricles occurs which is usually attributed to the overproduction of CSF. The ventricular system can also be asymmetrically dilated due to decreased CSF absorption secondary to obstruction of arachnoid granulations following repeated hemorrhage and ependymitis. On MR the tumor is hypo to isointense on T1WI and iso to hyperintense to T2WI[7] **(Figs. 3A to D)**. There is intense homogeneous enhancement after gadolinium administration though heterogeneous enhancement can also be seen when tumor outgrows its blood supply **(Fig. 3D)**. Flow voids can sometimes be seen. Choroid plexus papillomas can transform into carcinomas in 5–15% of cases.[9]

Choroid plexus carcinoma: In comparison to papillomas, choroid plexus carcinomas tend to have a more irregular contour. They typically show heterogeneous pattern of enhancement (reflecting necrosis), invasion of surrounding brain and rapid spread along CSF pathways.[10] There is invariably presence of hydrocephalus **(Figs. 4A to D)**. MR spectroscopy demonstrates a high choline peak with elevated lactate.[11]

Astrocytoma

It usually arises in the tissues around the ventricle and invades the lateral ventricle secondarily. The most common site is the thalamus where it can develop into a large mass

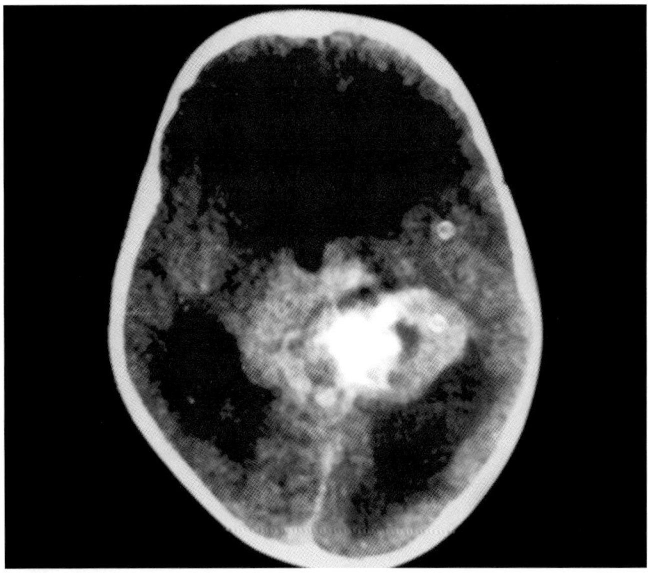

Fig. 2: Choroid plexus papilloma: Plain CT shows hyperdense mass with calcification in the atrium of left lateral ventricle with hydrocephalus.

within the lateral ventricle. The presenting symptoms and signs are dependent on the location and degree of brain infiltration. On CT, the low grade astrocytoma is seen as a poorly marginated low density mass. There is usually minimal mass effect or edema around the lesion. It shows little or no contrast enhancement. The anaplastic astrocytoma and glioblastoma have heterogeneous appearance due to areas of hemorrhage, necrosis or cyst formation[12] **(Figs. 5A and B)**. Surrounding white matter edema is more common and there are thick, irregular areas of contrast enhancement. MRI is helpful in the evaluation of degree of differentiation of the astrocytoma. The low grade astrocytoma has a signal pattern lower than normal brain parenchyma. The high grade gliomas and glioblastomas show varied signal intensity with areas of necrosis, hemorrhage, cyst formation and peripheral thick heterogeneous enhancement. MR perfusion and spectroscopy help us to grade the gliomas better with hyperperfusion and significantly raised Choline levels indicative of a higher grade.

Subependymal Giant Cell Tumor

Subependymal giant cell tumor (SGCT) is a circumscribed glioneuronal tumor typically larger than 1 cm, which occurs almost exclusively in patients with tuberous sclerosis (TS). Rarely, it has been reported from patients without manifestations of TS, though these cases may represent somatic mosaicism of the TS gene. It is a slow growing tumor and is discovered either during the course

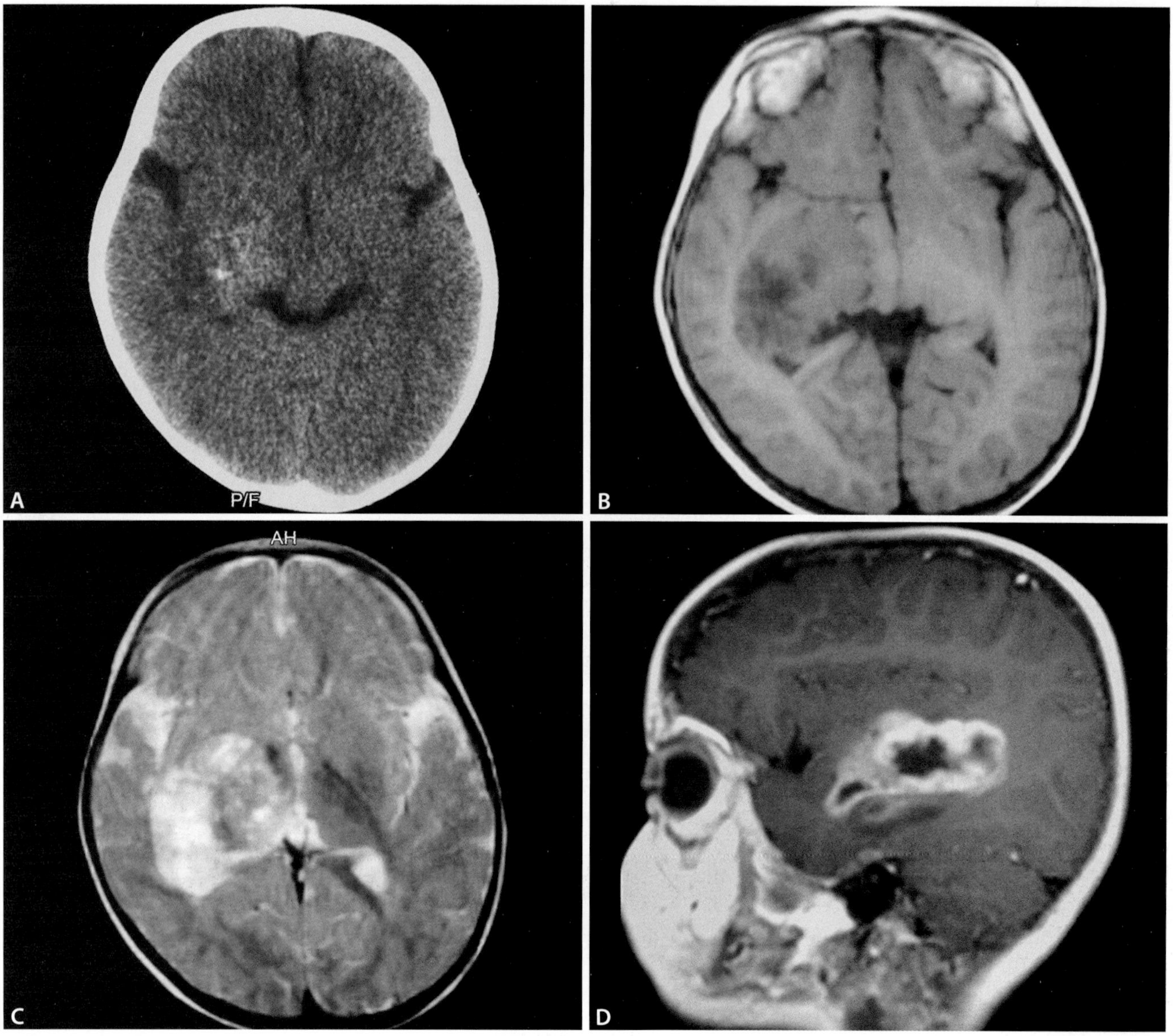

Figs. 3A to D: Choroid plexus papilloma: Noncontrast CT (A) shows presence of a relative hyperdense mass with calcific foci in the right temporal lobe which is confirmed to be intraventricular on MRI (B to D) and located in the temporal horn of the right lateral ventricle with peripheral solid enhancement.

of routine studies in patients with TS or because it causes obstructive hydrocephalus. Rarely, it undergoes malignant change and becomes aggressive. It usually arises in the region of foramen of Monro but can occur anywhere in the ventricles. SGCT occurs in 10–15% of patient with TS before the age of 20 years in addition to subependymal nodules which are much more commonly seen in these patients **(Figs. 6A and B)**. On CT, SGCT appears as a well-defined mass which is iso to hypodense to cerebral parenchyma. Foci of calcification are common. On MRI, the mass is hypo- to isointense on T1WI and iso- to hyperintense on T2WI with prominent enhancement after IV gadolinium injection.[13] SGCAs are treated only when there is evidence of growth, progressive hydrocephalus, new focal neurologic deficit or symptoms of raised intracranial pressure. Surveillance is recommended every 2 years for patients with TSC2 mutation and every 3 years for the ones with TSC1 mutation, preferably with MRI. Annual follow-up is suggested after SGCT has been diagnosed.

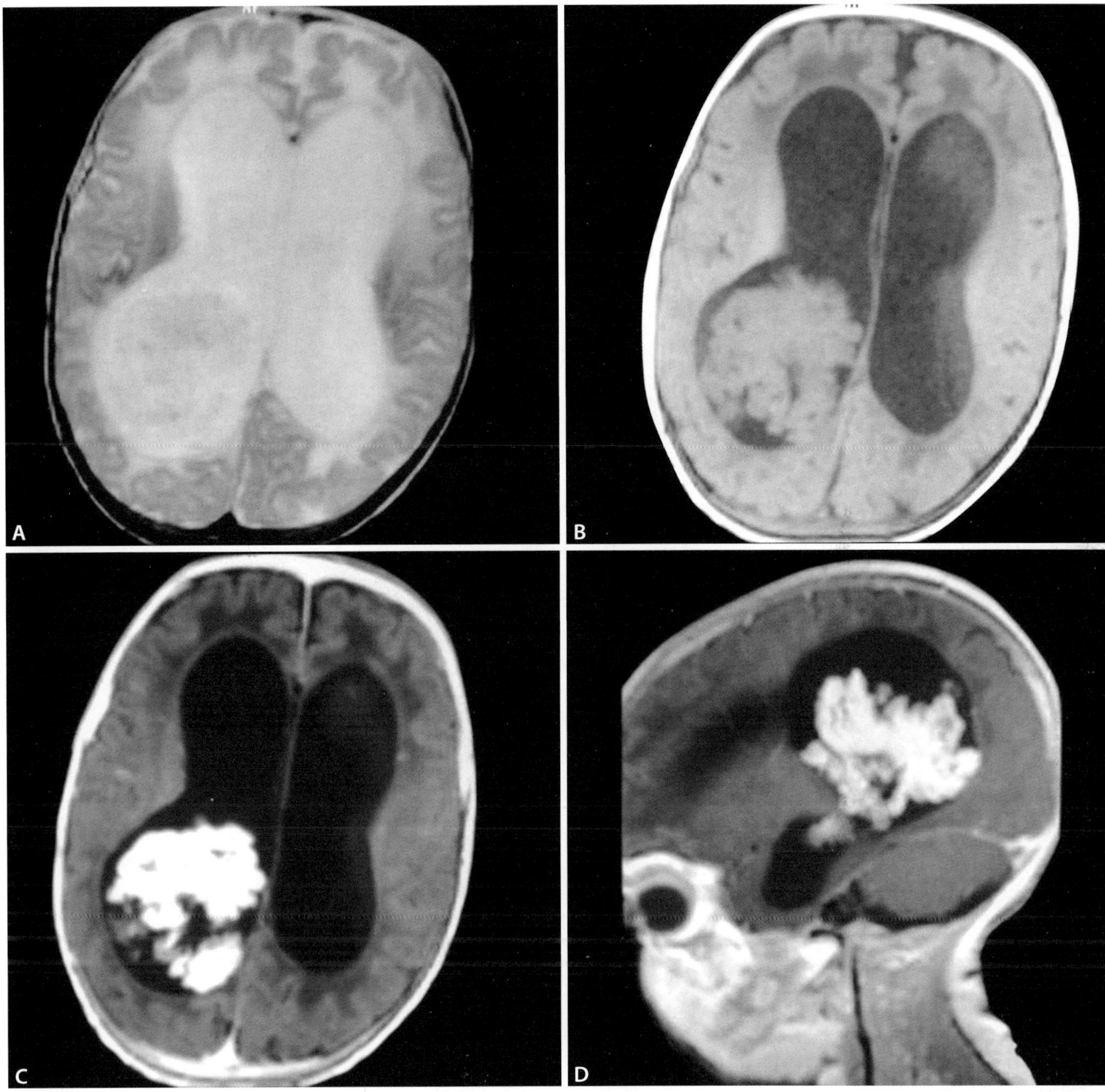

Figs. 4A to D: Choroid plexus carcinoma: Axial T2WI (A), T1WI (B), post-contrast axial (C) and sagittal (D) T1W images revealing a lobulated intensely enhancing right lateral ventricular choroid plexus based mass causing hydrocephalus.

Ependymoma

Ependymomas constitute 3–5% of intracranial tumors.[4] These are commonly seen in children in the posterior fossa (60%) and have a predilection for males. Supratentorial ependymomas are seen in 30–40% cases and are usually parenchymal (>50%). Extraventricular lesions are proposed to arise from embryonic rests of ependymal tissue trapped in the developing cerebral hemisphere. When intraventricular, they usually arise in the trigone of lateral ventricle. They have a variety of histologic patterns varying from well differentiated to aggressive, poorly differentiate ones.[14] The clinical presentation is variable ranging from headache, seizures to focal neurological deficits and are often delayed till these tumors grow into the ventricular system. On CT, ependymomas are iso- to hypoattenuating, may show cystic component (70%),

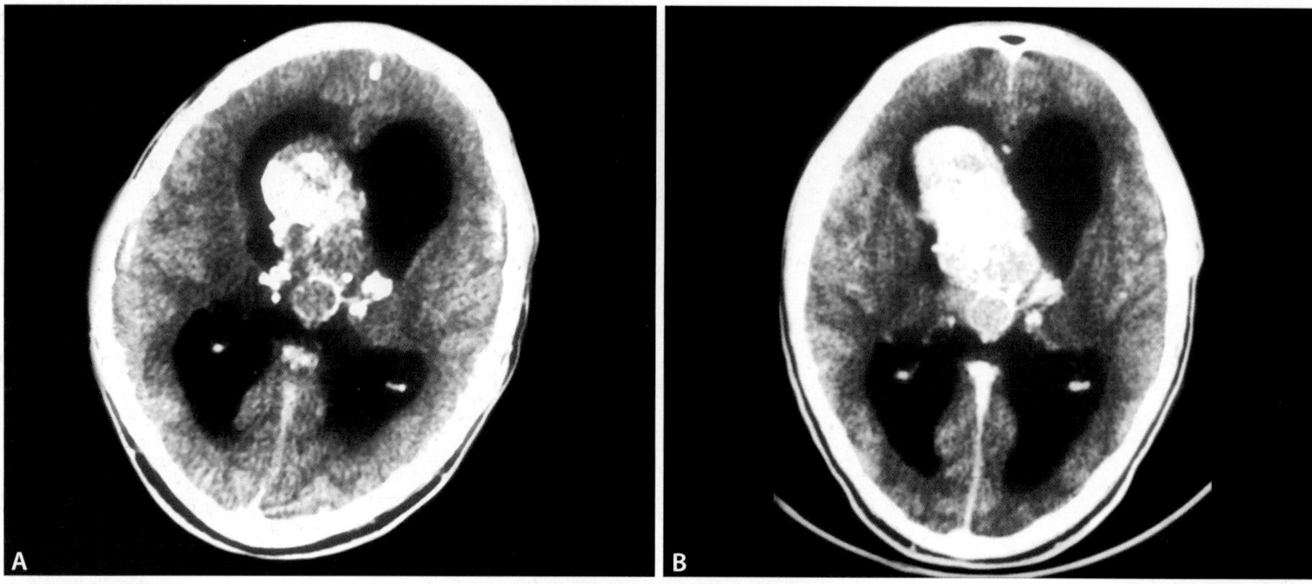

Figs. 5A and B: Astrocytoma: Plain (A) and contrast (B) CT show intensely enhancing heterogeneous mass with dense calcification occupying the frontal horn and body of right lateral ventricle.

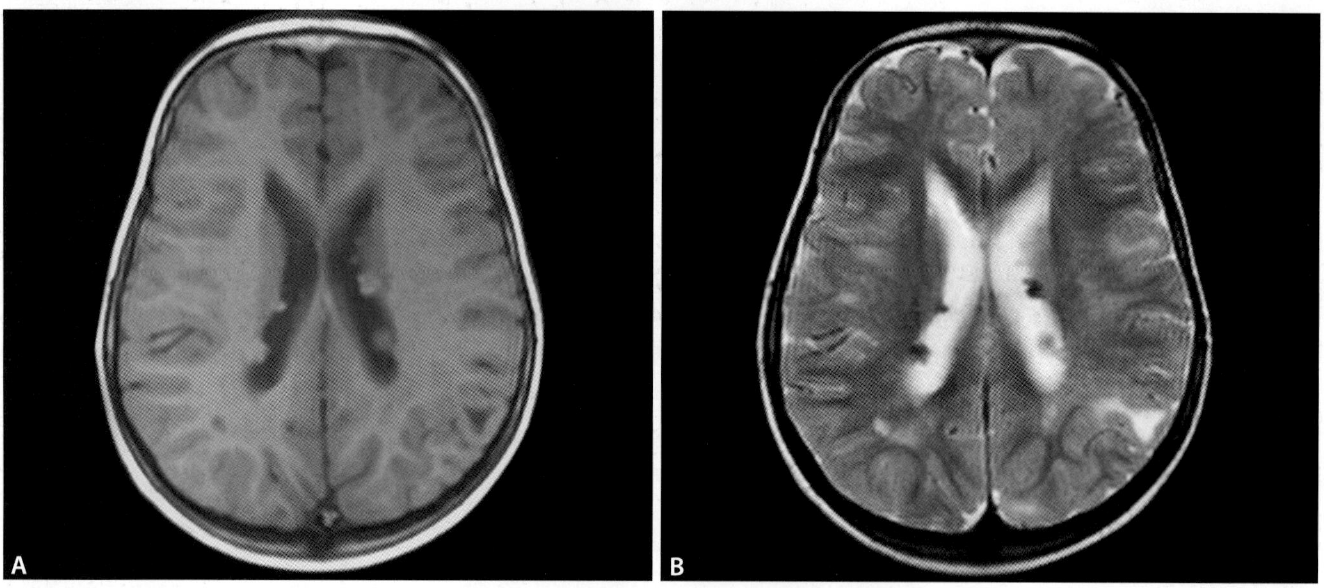

Figs. 6A and B: Subependymal nodules in tuberous sclerosis: Axial T1WI (A) and T2WI (B) in a patient of tuberous sclerosis shows presence of multiple small subependymal nodules.

calcification (50%) and rarely hemorrhages. The solid component is iso dense to brain parenchyma with bright enhancement with contrast administration.[15] On MRI, the tumor is iso- to hypointense on T1WI and hyperintense on T2WI. There is usually heterogeneity due to areas of hemorrhage, necrosis and calcification **(Figs. 7A to D)**. With gadolinium administration there is usually moderate to intense enhancement. Diffusion restriction may be seen in highly cellular areas of the tumor. Vasogenic edema may occur in the adjoining white matter. Although ependymoma is a benign tumor, it has a high recurrence rate and can spread through CSF pathways. Thus, imaging of the entire craniospinal axis should be performed at presentation and follow-up.

Meningioma

Intraventricular meningioma is an uncommon tumor and constitutes 0.5–3% of all intracranial tumors.[4] It is more

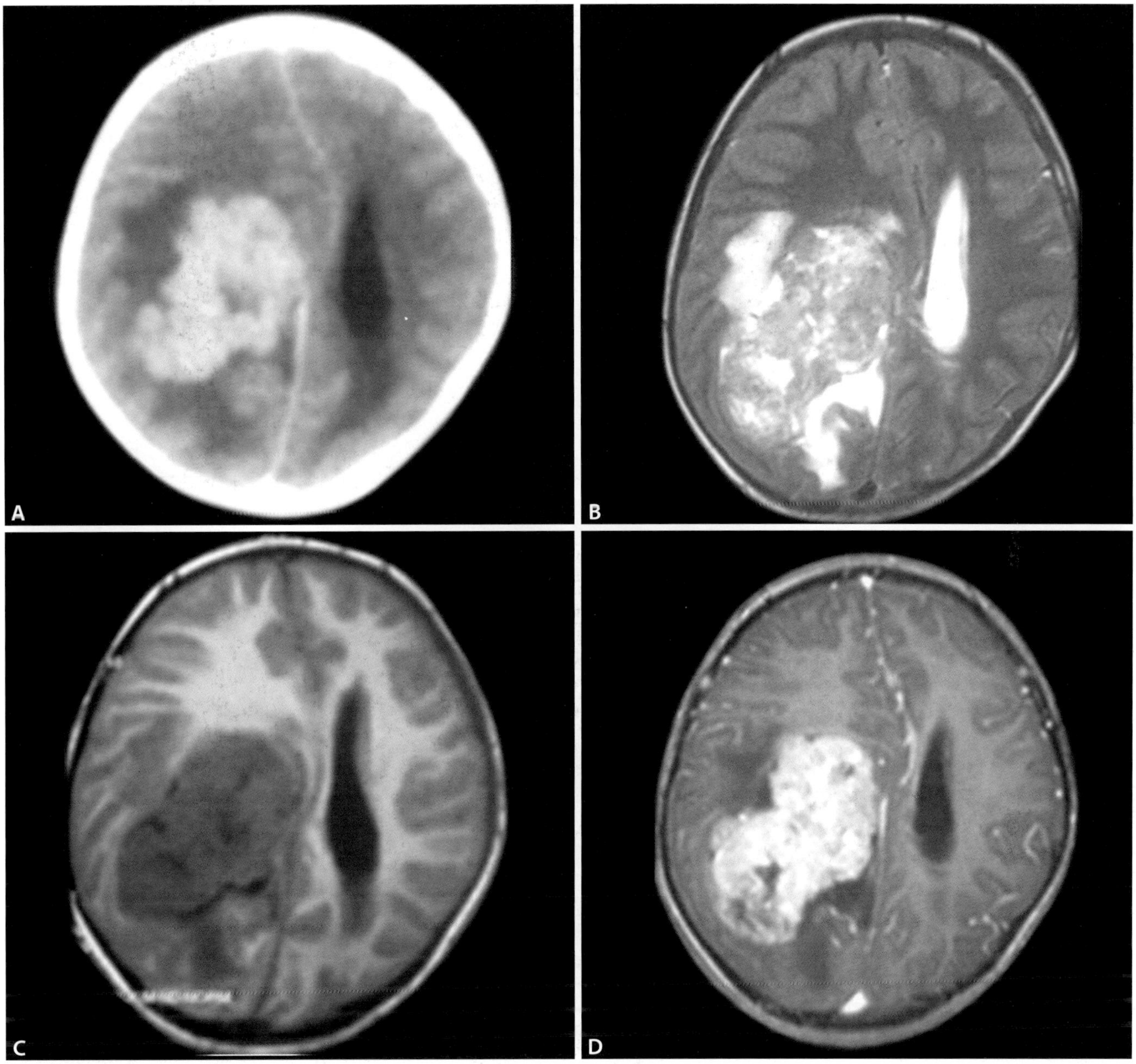

Figs. 7A to D: Ependymoma: Axial CT (A) depicting the lobulated moderately enhancing right lateral ventricular mass with adjoining parenchymal edema. Axial T2WI (B), T1WI (C) and contrast-enhanced T1WI (D) demonstrating the lesion character-heterogeneous T2 hyperintense, T1 hypointense with moderate enhancement.

common in adult females. It is a benign tumor (WHO grade I) rising from the arachnoid cap cells trapped within the choroid plexus. Although rare, the meningiomas in children are more frequently intraventricular and malignant, show equal incidence in both sexes and are usually associated with neurofibromatosis 2. The lateral ventricle particularly the atrium, is the most common site (80%) followed by third (15%) and fourth (5%) ventricles.[16]

On CT, meningioma appears as a sharply defined, globular mass, iso to hyperdense to brain parenchyma. Calcification is seen in 40–50% cases. It shows diffuse intense enhancement with contrast **(Fig. 8A).** There may be localized or diffuse ventricular dilatation, depending on obstruction to CSF flow. On MRI, it is isointense (60%) or hypointense (40%) on T1WI and isointense (50%) or hyperintense (50%) on T2WI **(Figs. 8B and C).**

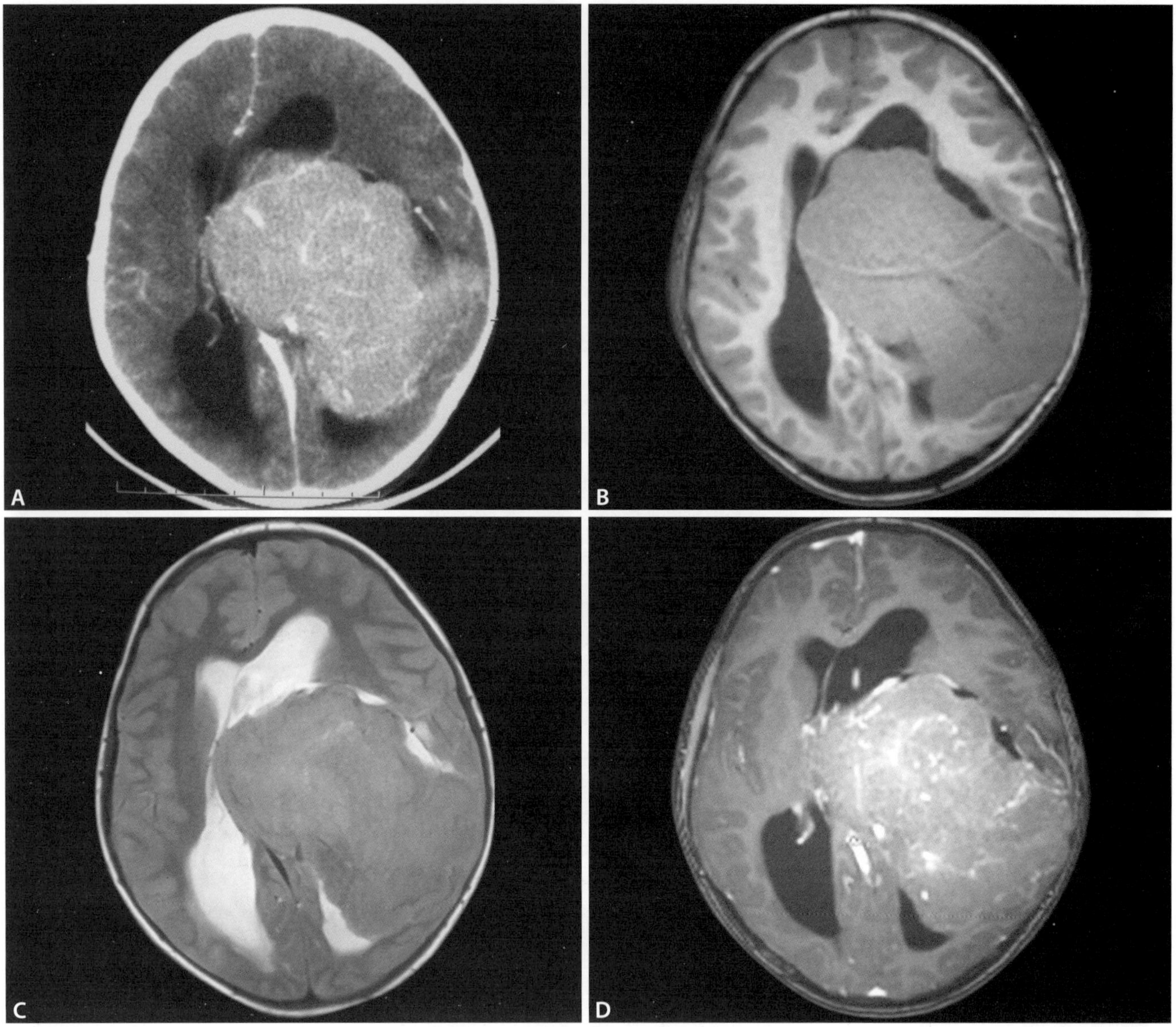

Figs. 8A to D: Intraventricular meningioma: CECT (A) shows a well-defined moderately enhancing globular mass in the atrium/body of the left lateral ventricle which is hypointense on T1WI (B), isointense on T2WI (C) with intratumoral vascularity on post contrast T1WI (D). Note the mass effect with mild contralateral midline shift.

There is usually homogeneous and moderate to intense enhancement with IV gadolinium administration **(Fig. 8D)**. Diffusion restriction may be observed in some lesions reflecting high cellular density. High vascularity on perfusion MR is often appreciated with mean rCBV values >3.[17] There is persistence of contrast material within the tumor interstitium due to deficiency of blood brain barrier. Proton MR spectroscopy reveals a high choline peak[16] with markedly low NAA and creatine levels. Presence of alanine (doublet at 1.4 ppm) and high levels of glutamate, if seen, are reasonably specific.[18]

Metastases

Intraventricular metastases can develop either due to dissemination by blood (hematogenous route) or CSF. The blood borne metastasis most often involves the choroid plexus in the ventricles due to its direct relationship with the systemic blood supply. The common primary tumors with intraventricular metastases are bronchogenic, breast, renal cell and colon carcinoma in adults and Wilm's tumor, retinoblastoma and neuroblastoma in children.[19] On CT or MRI the choroid plexus metastasis shows expansion of choroid plexus with marked contrast enhancement.

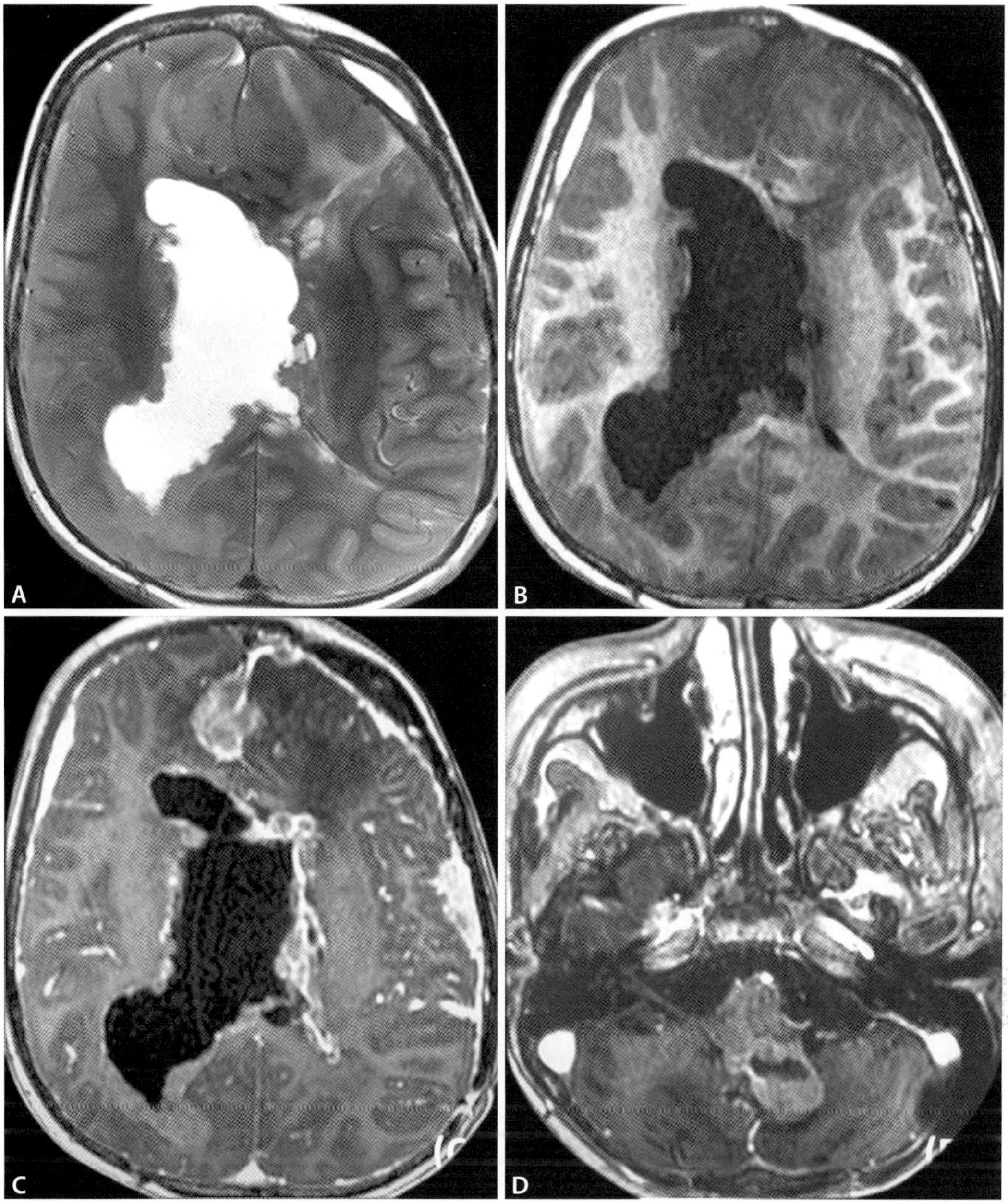

Figs. 9A to D: Transependymal and CSF spread of medulloblastoma: Axial T2WI (A), T1WI (B) and post-contrast T1WI (C) revealing diffuse nodular ependymal enhancement with sulcal deposits. Axial post contrast T1WI (D) showing the primary lesion in relation to the fourth ventricle.

Dynamic susceptibility contrast imaging (DSCI) may show elevated rCBV values (>3) in hypervascular tumors (renal and thyroid carcinomas).

The paraventricular spread of tumor can occur along CSF pathways to ventricular ependymal lining and leptomeninges. There may also be infiltration of the subependymal space by a sheet of tumor cells. Such a spread can occur in both primary CNS and systemic malignancies. Malignant astrocytomas are the commonest tumor to show CSF spread followed by ependymomas, medulloblastomas **(Figs. 9A to D)**, pineal tumors and choroid plexus papillomas.[4] The sites involved in order of frequency, are the lateral ventricles, the fourth ventricle, aqueduct and third ventricle. Metastatic deposits are often seen in the recesses such as ventricular horns, supraoptic and interpeduncular recesses of the third ventricle. On CT, these lesions are seen as discrete, iso to hyperdense nodular or sheet like having subependymal rim surrounding

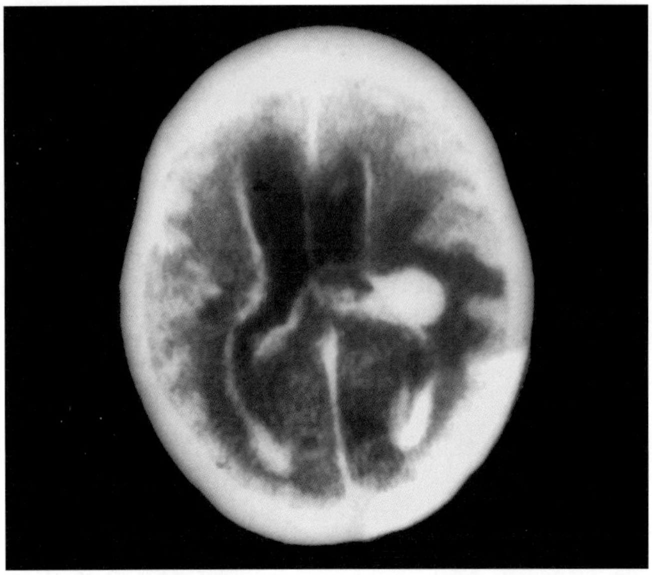

Fig. 10: Metastasis: CECT shows diffuse ependymal enhancement and hyperdense nodule in the left paraventricular region with edema in a patient patient of carcinoma thyroid.

a part or the entire ventricle **(Fig. 10)**. On MRI, they appear hypointense on T1WI and hyperintense on T2WI. Melanoma metastasis differs in being hyperintense on T1WI and isointense on T2WI.

Primary CNS Lymphoma

It constitutes 1–1.5% of all primary CNS tumors. There is a male sex predilection and peak incidence is in fifth and sixth decades. There is a sharp rise in the incidence over the past decades with the increasing spread of AIDS.[20] Most primary CNS lymphomas are of the non-Hodgkin's type. Lymphoma rarely presents as a purely intraventricular mass and generally exhibits diffuse subependymal spread (12%). Most commonly, it is seen as well-defined nodular lesion in the subependymal region. There may be extension along the perivascular Virchow-Robin spaces. The imaging findings are reflective of the high cellularity and nucleocytoplasmic ratio in addition to features of blood-brain barrier disruption **(Figs. 11A to F)**. On CT, it appears as iso- to hyperattenuating lesion showing homogeneous or rarely ring-like contrast enhancement. On MRI, it shows variable signal pattern, often isointense on all spin echo sequences **(Figs. 11A and B)**; high cellularity gives a hypointense signal on T2WI. Occasionally it can be hyperintense on T1WI. It shows diffusion restriction **(Fig. 11D)** with low ADC values. Contrast enhancement is usually homogenous **(Fig. 11C)** and bright.[4] MR spectroscopy reveals high choline with low NAA **(Fig. 11E)**. Mean curve analysis of the perfusion data demonstrates blood-brain barrier breach with the curve over-shooting the baseline **(Fig. 11F)**.

Central Neurocytoma

Central neurocytoma is a well-differentiated benign (WHO grade II) intraventricular tumor of neuroepithelial origin, first described in 1982.[21] It is a rare tumor, constituting 0.1%–0.5% of all primary tumors of the CNS and occurs in adults (2nd to 5th decades). The site of origin is usually at or near the midline at the base of the septum pellucidum and usually in close proximity to foramen of Monro. It is quite large at presentation and usually presents due to symptoms of raised intracranial pressure and obstructive hydrocephalus. Neurocytomas are gray friable lesions having solid as well as cystic components, often with amorphous calcification (50%).[22] Gross total excision is usually curative though recurrence is known. Overall it has a good prognosis. Previously these tumors were erroneously classified as "intraventricular oligodendrogliomas (ODGs)" due to their resemblance to ODGs on histopathology. The presence of pineocytomatous rosettes allows their differentiation from ODGs. On CT, they appear as iso to slightly hyperdense masses with cystic changes (giving bubbly appearance) and foci of calcification. Mild to moderate enhancement with contrast is seen. On MRI, the tumor shows heterogeneous pattern and there is variable (moderate to strong) enhancement following IV gadolinium administration[22] **(Figs. 12A to D)**. The presence of glycine (3.55 ppm) on MR spectroscopy[23] may help in differentiating it from other similar tumors like ependymoma, subependymoma and oligodendrogliomas. Other differential like heterotopic gray matter can be excluded as the latter neither shows enhancement nor calcification. Meningiomas can be differentiated based on their posterior location in the atrium of lateral ventricle as are choroid plexus tumors.

Subependymoma

It is a rare benign (WHO grade I) tumor seen in middle-aged and elderly patients. The common site of occurrence is in frontal horn of lateral ventricle or in the caudal fourth ventricle.[24] It typically appears as a well-defined lobular mass. On CT, it appears as an iso- or hypodense lesion with minimal or no enhancement. Calcification is seen occasionally. On MRI, subependymoma is homogeneously hypo to isointense on T1WI and mildly hypointense on T2WI **(Figs. 13A to D)**. Contrast enhancement is typically absent to mild.[24]

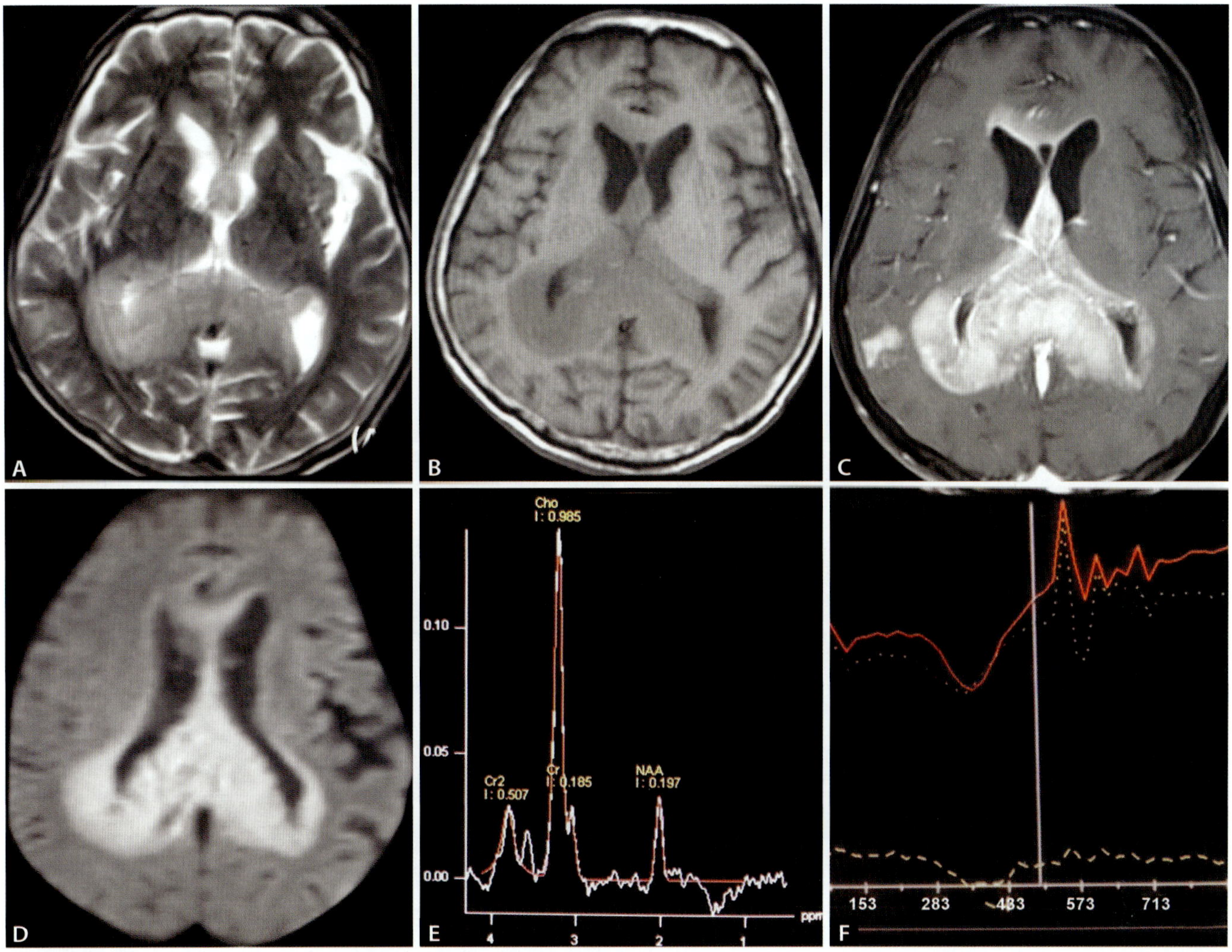

Figs. 11A to F: Primary CNS lymphoma: Multiparametric MR depicting the extensive subependymal spread of the lymphomatous lesion having T2 hyperintense (A), T1 hypointense (B), moderate enhancing (C) nature with diffusion restriction (D). MR spectroscopy reveals high choline (E) with upshoot above baseline on mean curve analysis of DSCI due to T1 effect (F).

Vascular Malformations

Arteriovenous malformations (AVMs) and cavernous angiomas can have some component within the ventricle, particularly those arising in the basal ganglia and thalamus. Lateral ventricle is the most common to be involved but they can occur in any part of the ventricular system.[25] On CT these lesions are seen as heterogeneous areas, with or without calcifications. On contrast administration, abnormal vessels are seen as tortuous high density structures. MRI is superior to CT in demonstrating the feeding vessels the nidus and the serpiginous draining veins which appear as flow voids both on T1WI and T2WI. Digital subtraction angiography (DSA) is the confirmatory study which shows all aspects of the vascular malformations. Four dimensional (4D) CT angiography has been proven to be a noninvasive modality giving excellent details, without the ill-effects of DSA. Subependymal AVMs can be difficult to treat surgically. They are prone to rupture **(Figs. 14A to D)**. Endovascular embolization of the nidus is a minimally invasive method of treating these lesions. Gamma knife radiotherapy can also be offered to these patients.

Intraventricular blood-fluid levels can occur in cases of intraventricular hemorrhage secondary to rupture of saccular aneurysms or arteriovenous malformations. Other important causes are Moyamoya disease and systemic coagulopathies. Fluid-fluid levels can be seen in severe cases of ependymitis, meningitis or as a result of rupture of parenchymal abscess into the ventricles.

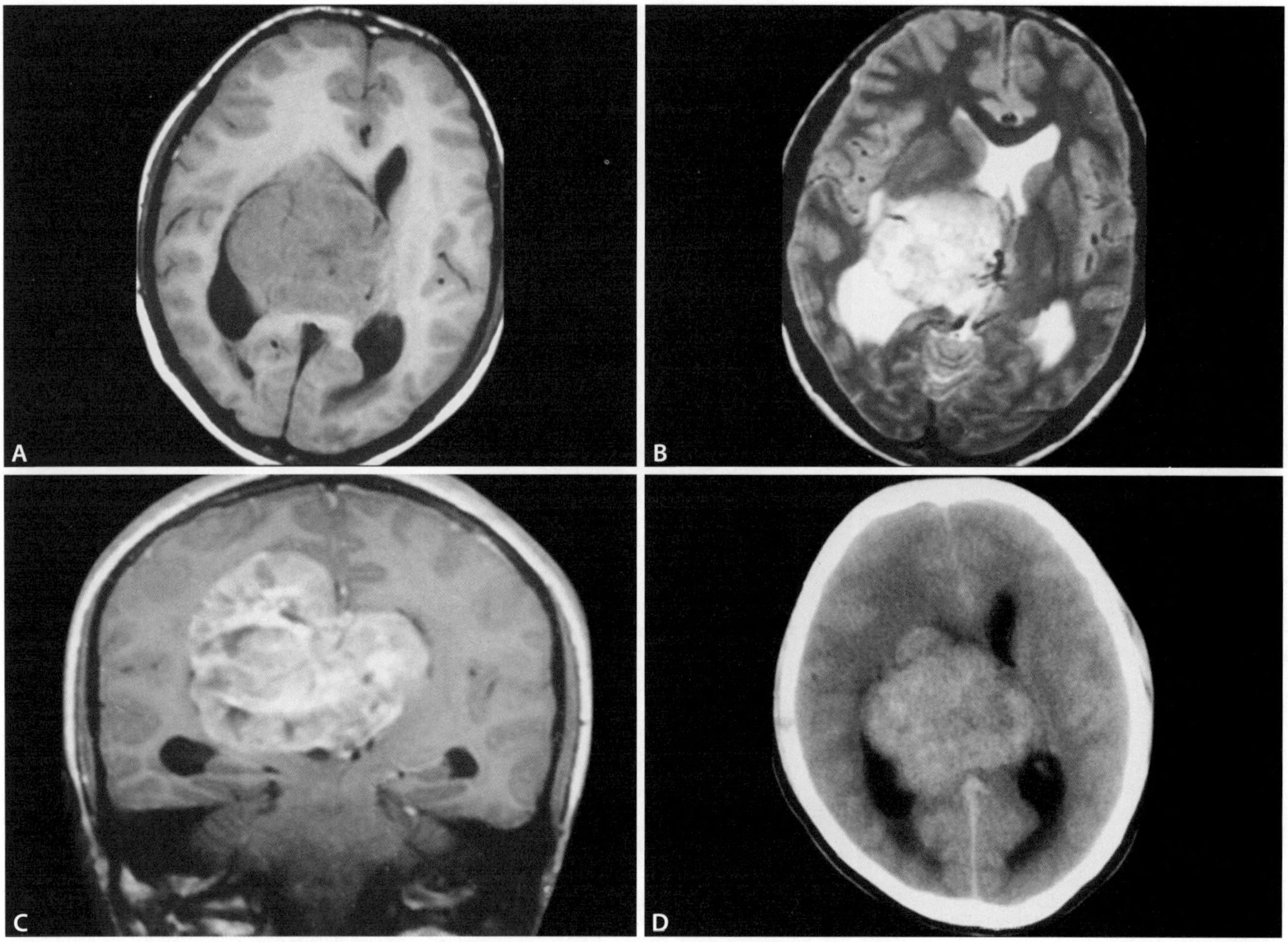

Figs. 12A to D: Central neurocytoma: (A) T1 MR image shows intraventricular solid mass attached to septum pellucidum. The tumor shows heterogeneous signal on T2WI (B) and intense contrast enhancement following IV gadolinium (C). (D) CECT shows enhancing intraventricular tumor.

Choroid Plexus Cysts and Xanthogranulomas

Xanthogranulomas are usually discovered incidentally. They are symptomatic only when they cause obstruction at foramen of Monro. Cysts show low density on CT with signal characteristics similar to CSF on MRI.[26] They lack contrast enhancement and show diffusion restriction on DWI. Xanthogranulomas are dense on CT and may show flecks of calcification. The center is often of low attenuation due to fat content. On MRI, these are well-defined partially cystic masses that appear hypo or isointense on T1WI and iso to hyperintense on T2WI and show contrast enhancement.[27]

Sometimes parasitic cysts can also be encountered in the lateral ventricles[28] which may cause obstruction to the CSF flow and may present as hydrocephalus, e.g. neurocysticercosis (NCC) **(Figs. 15A and B)**, hydatid cyst **(Fig. 16)**.

Dermoids

These are uncommon lateral ventricular lesions. On CT, the dermoids are hypodense (fat containing) with presence of calcification. On MRI, the dermoid shows hyperintense foci of fat and areas of signal loss due to calcification on T1WI **(Figs. 17A to C)**. Heterogeneous hyperintensity is noted on T2WI. Contrast enhancement is typically none to mild. Dermoids may show intraventricular rupture with distant spread of fat through CSF. This can lead to chemical meningitis or obstructive hydrocephalus due to blockage of CSF pathways.

Third Ventricular Masses

In children, hydrocephalus is the most common feature of 3rd ventricular masses. The endocrine and visual disturbances are uncommon. Diencephalic syndrome

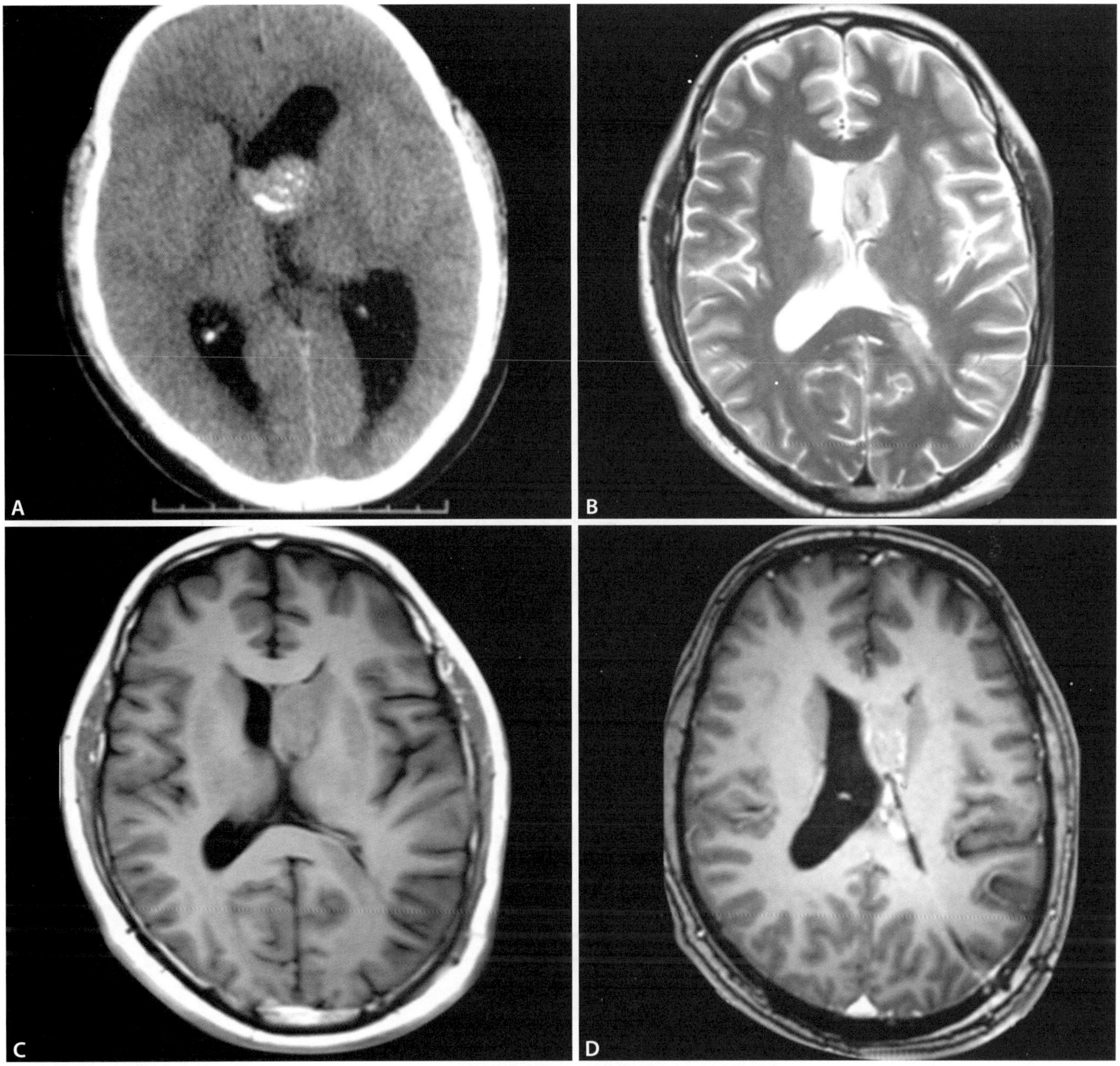

Figs. 13A to D: Subependyoma: Hyperdense (A) left frontal ventricular nodular lesion. Axial T2WI (B), T1WI (C) and gadolinium enhanced T1WI (D) showing T2 iso/hyperintensity, T1 isointensity with mild enhancement.

which comprises hyperkinesis and alertness associated with emaciation in infants is the only specific syndrome described with hypothalamic gliomas. In adults mental and behavioral changes, particularly increasing apathy, are common. Depending on the parts of the ventricle involved these tumors can be further categorized as anterior or posterior 3rd ventricular masses.

Anterior Third Ventricular Masses

Colloid Cyst

They arise from the roof of the 3rd ventricle at the level of foramen of Monro. They are round to oval lesions and vary in size from few millimeters to several centimeters in diameter. They represent 15–20% of all IV lesions and occur

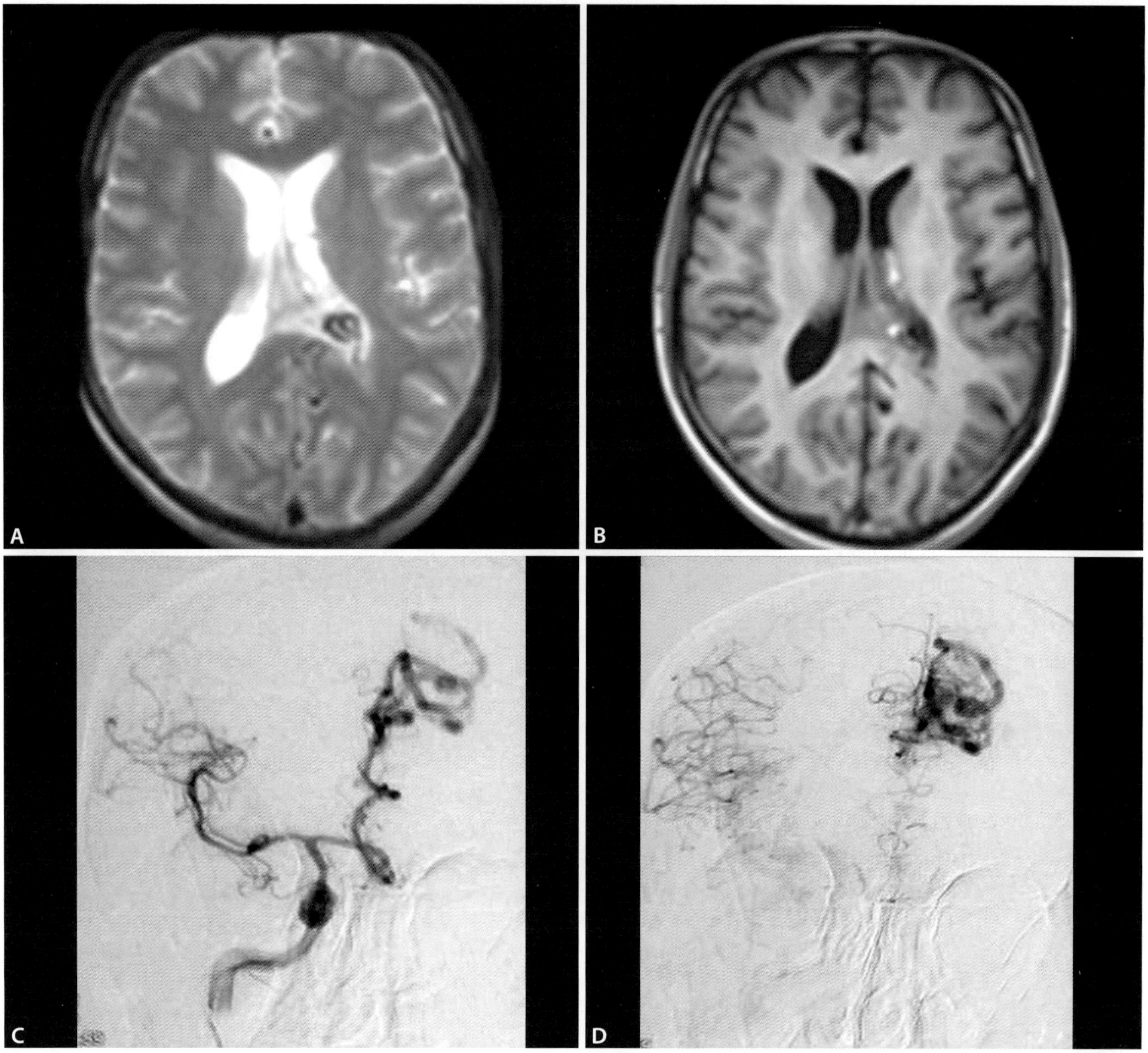

Figs. 14A to D: Arteriovenous malformation (AVM): Axial T2WI (A) and T1WI (B) demonstrating left ventricular hemorrhage (mixed signal on T1 and T2). Cerebral DSA frontal (C) and lateral (D) projections depicting the AVM nidus in left parietal lobe as the cause of bleed.

in 3rd to 5th decades of life.[29] Less than 2% of colloid cysts occur in children. Symptoms of intermittent obstruction are common and sudden death due to acute obstruction has been reported.[30] It arises from endoderm rather than ectoderm which is morphologically similar to bronchial and nasal cavity epithelium. On CT, colloid cysts are well encapsulated, homogeneously hyperdense masses (due to intrinsic proteinaceous content) which show little or no contrast enhancement (**Fig. 18A**). There may be dilatation of lateral ventricles which can be asymmetrical. Hydrocephalus can also be intermittent.[30] Calcification is not a feature. On MR, the signal characteristics of colloid cysts vary widely.[28] The most common appearance is a mass that is hyperintense on T1WI and hypointense on T2WI though it can be isointense on both T1 and T2WI (**Figs. 18B to D**). Rim enhancement following contrast can be observed. CSF flow artifacts at foramen of Monro can mimic colloid cysts (pseudotumor) on MRI and should be

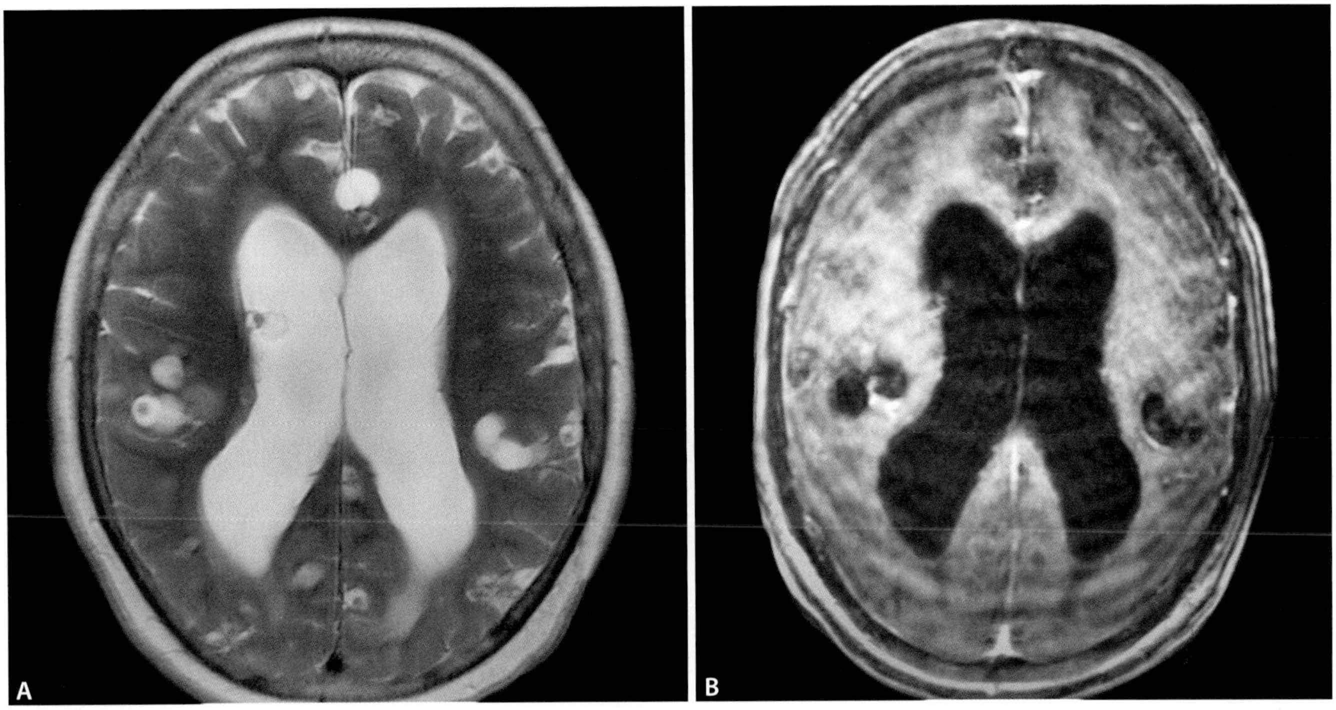

Figs. 15A and B: Neurocysticercosis: Axial T2WI (A) and post-contrast T1WI (B) showing multiple cystic lesions scattered in both cerebral hemispheres with one lodged in the right ventricular ependyma. Note the presence of scolices.

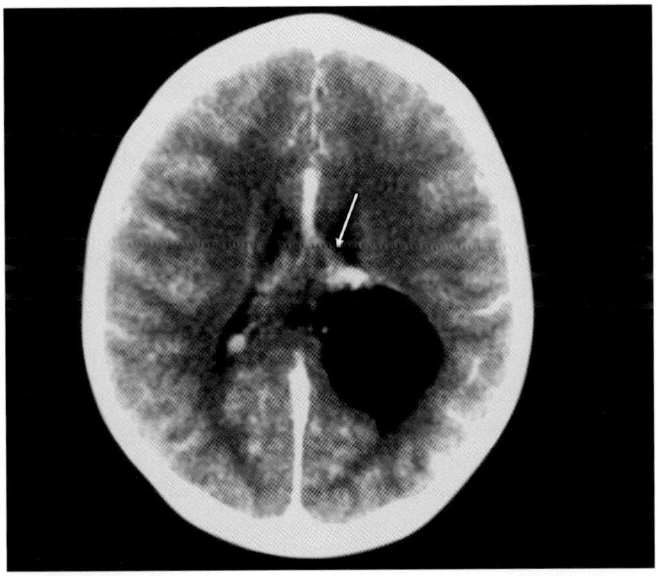

Fig. 16: Hydatid cyst: CECT shows well-defined cystic lesion in the trigone of left lateral ventricle with anteriorly displaced choroid plexus (arrow).

kept in mind while evaluating these lesions.[30] Currently available heavily T2-weighted imaging (e.g. CISS, FIESTA, etc.) helps in better delineating the lesion location and morphological details.

Astrocytoma

In children, the most common type of astrocytoma that arises primarily from ventricular wall is juvenile pilocytic astrocytoma.[31] This differs from the one which arises in cerebellum in that, it rarely shows cystic component. Astrocytoma arising in the hypothalamic or chiasmatic region may extend into the third ventricle. Visual field defects are often the presenting complaints and endocrine disturbances occur late in the course of the disease. Growth hormone deficiency is the earliest endocrine abnormality. Hydrocephalus due to the tumor is rare. Pathologically, it is a low grade-glioma but is usually not resectable. Role of biopsy is controversial and it is often advocated when the clinical or imaging features are peculiar and suggest a different type of tumor.[28] On noncontrast CT, the tumor is iso to hypodense and shows variable enhancement after IV contrast administration. Calcification and cyst formation are rare. The anatomy is better evaluated on MRI which can show thickened optic chiasm, the floor and walls of the 3rd ventricle with extension of the lesion along the optic tracts. Sometimes, it becomes difficult to distinguish it from craniopharyngioma. Diffusion tensor imaging is important in such cases which reveal altered tensor values along the optic pathways in case of astrocytomas.

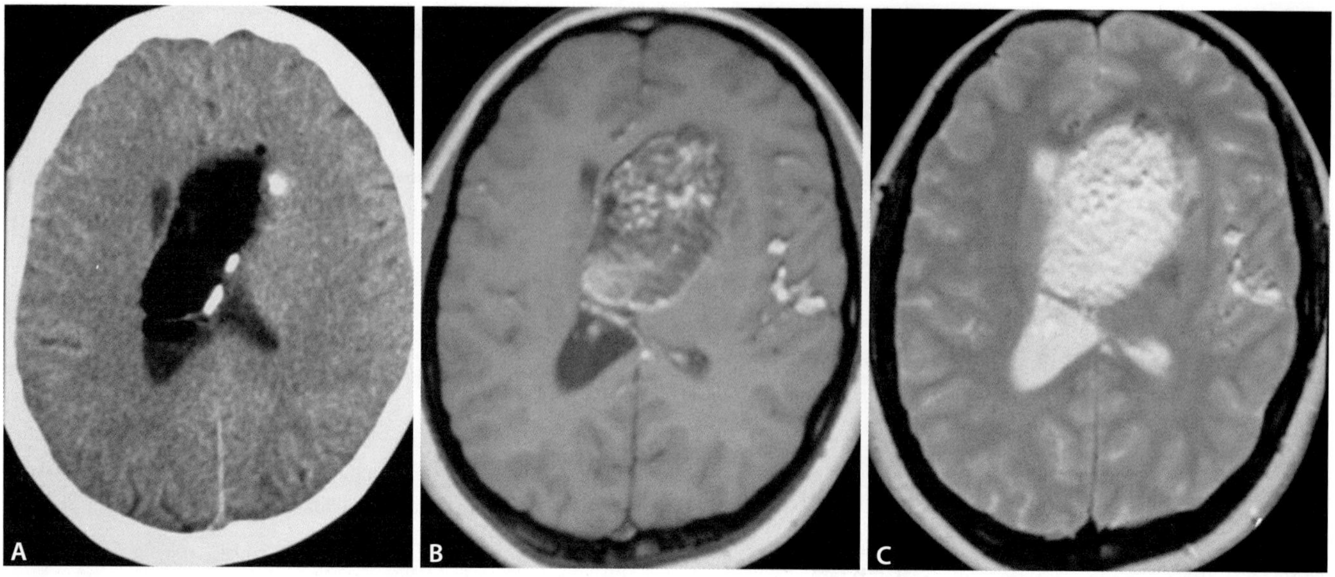

Figs. 17A to C: Dermoid: Axial CT (A), T1WI (B) and T2WI (C) showing the fat containing (CT hypodense and T1 hyperintense) left lateral ventricle mass with presence of eccentric calcification causing foramen of Monro obstruction and contralateral lateral ventriculomegaly.

Ependymoma

It is rare in the third ventricle. The imaging features are similar to those as seen in other areas.[15]

Germinoma

The tumor that occurs solely in the 3rd ventricle is called "ectopic pinealoma" and rarely occurs in association with the posterior third ventricular germinoma. The clinical triad includes visual loss, loss of libido and diabetes insipidus. Histologically, this tumor resembles seminoma and dysgerminoma. The tumor has the potential to spread via CSF pathways and therefore CSF analysis for tumor cells can be helpful in obtaining diagnosis in some patients.[32]

On noncontrast CT, the germinoma appears as an iso to hyperdense mass with indistinct tumor boundaries. Calcification is rare. It shows uniform enhancement on contrast injection. The tumor shows similar character on MRI with homogeneous enhancement following IV gadolinium administration. Germinomas are very sensitive to radiotherapy **(Figs. 19A to D)**.

Metastases

Isolated metastasis into the 3rd ventricle is very rare and almost always associated with other cerebral metastasis. The imaging features are variable. Most commonly it is hyperdense or hyperintense relative to normal brain with significant edema surrounding the tumor. It shows either a solid or ring-like enhancement following contrast administration. Contrast-enhanced magnetic resonance (CEMR) is the most sensitive modality for defining both the presence and location of metastatic lesions.[4]

Craniopharyngioma

Primary third ventricular craniopharyngioma is extremely rare and is almost always an extension of the craniopharyngioma from the sellar-suprasellar region. There are two peaks of occurrence; the first in young children less than 15 years and the second in the 5th–6th decades. The clinical presentation is growth disturbance and visual field defects in children, and behavioral change or memory disturbance in adults. On CT the tumor shows solid and cystic components in majority of patients. The solid component shows contrast enhancement particularly in children. Calcification is seen in almost all patients in childhood while it is seen in up to 50% of cases in adults. MRI may show T1 hyperintense cyst (motor oil appearance) with heterogeneous enhancement of the solid component **(Fig. 20A to C)**.

Epidermoid and Dermoids

These are uncommon tumors encountered in the anterior 3rd ventricle.[33] They usually present due to obstructive hydrocephalus. On CT, the epidermoid appears as hypodense lesion which does not enhance with contrast

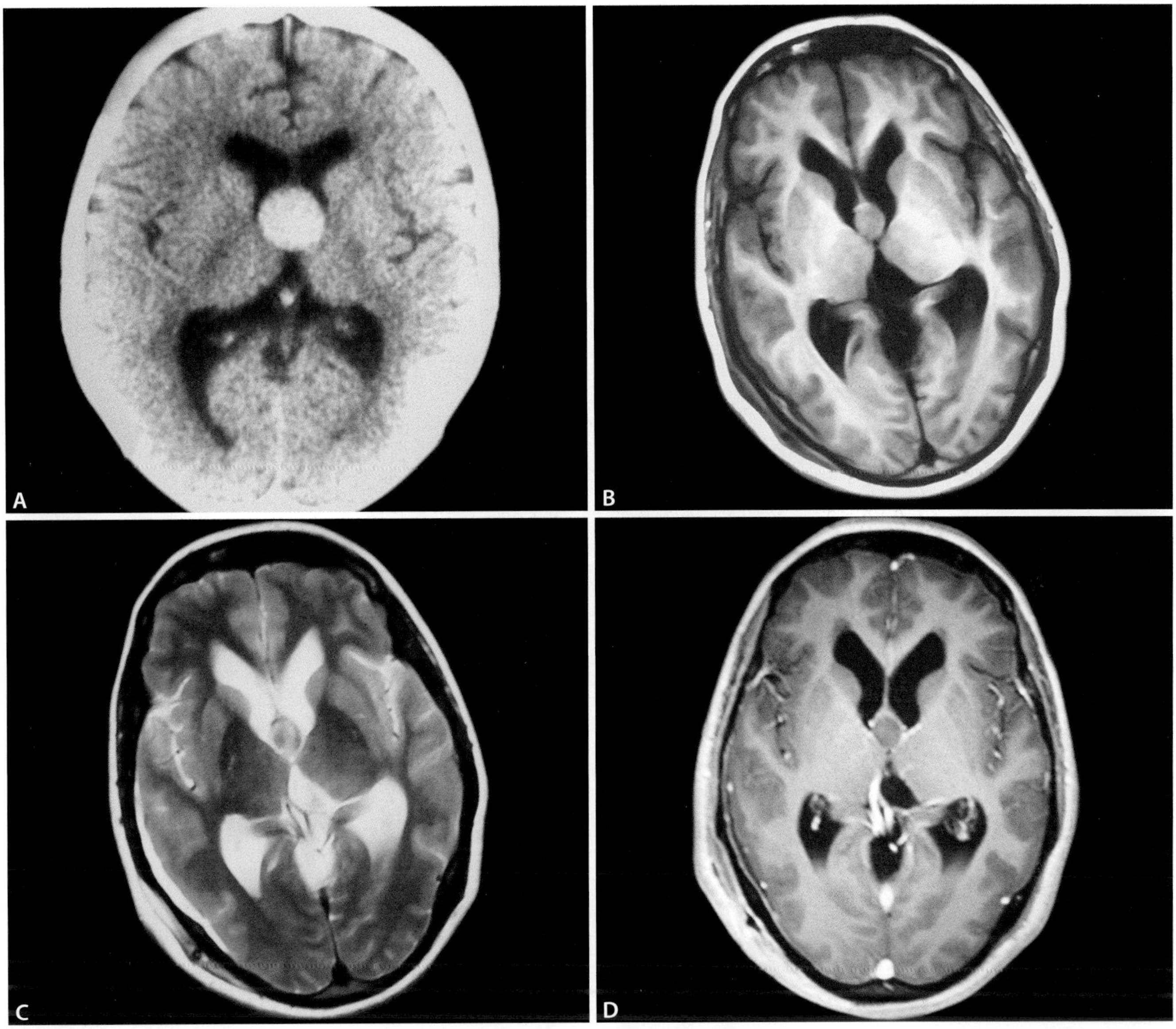

Figs. 18A to D: Colloid cyst: Plain CT (A) shows a homogenously hyperdense midline non enhancing globular lesion in the foramen of Monro. MRI in another patient shows a similar lesion which is isointense to gray matter on T1 (B) as well as T2 (C) Weighted sequences showing no post contrast enhancement (D).

administration. Dermoid usually shows the presence of fat and calcification. On MRI, the epidermoid shows signal characters similar to CSF while the dermoid shows hyperintense foci of fat and areas of signal loss due to calcification on T1WI. Both these lesions characteristically displace the brain parenchyma around it rather than invading it. The epidermoid classically shows diffusion restriction **(Figs. 21A to D)**.

Cysticercosis

Intraventricular cysticercosis presents with repeated attacks of meningitis in children and with hydrocephalus in adults. The diagnosis should always be suspected in an endemic area. It is seen in 20–25% of all neurocysticercosis, most commonly in 4th ventricle, foramen of Monro and lateral ventricle **(Figs. 22A and B)**. It can be difficult to diagnose on CT because it shows similar attenuation like CSF. MR is the best imaging modality and T2WI clearly shows the hyperintense cyst in the ventricular wall. It can be of the racemose variety at times and sometimes is not readily differentiated from a tuberculoma. Unilocular cystic forms may often show an eccentric hypointense nodule suggestive of scolex within the cyst on thin

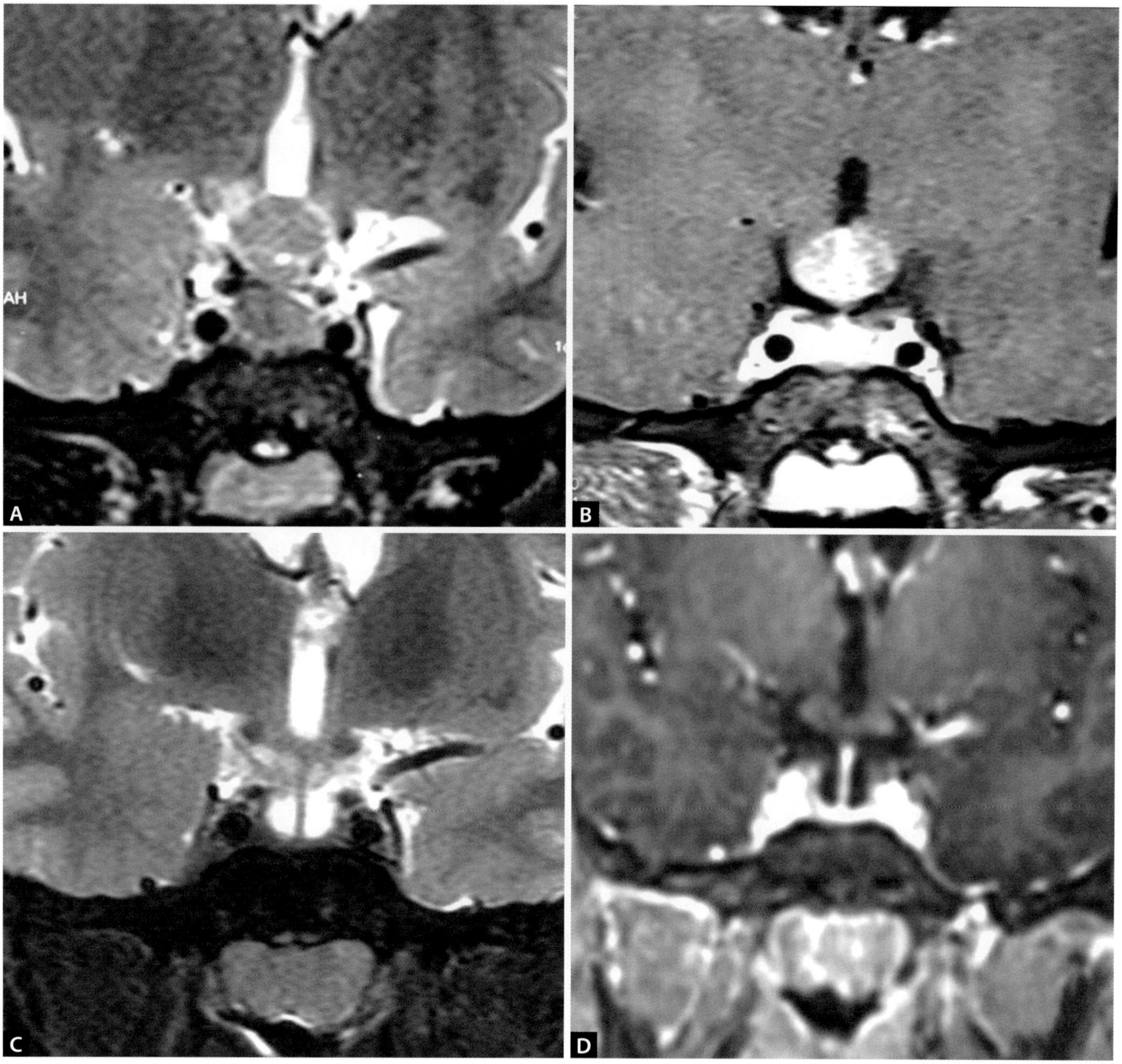

Figs. 19A to D: Third ventricular/suprasellar germ cell tumor. Coronal T2WI (A) and post-contrast T1WI (B) showing the T2 isointense homogeneously enhancing third ventricular floor lesion. Corresponding sections (C and D) show complete lesion resolution following radiotherapy.

T2-weighted sequences [e.g. constructive interference in steady state (CISS)] as previously discussed.

Pituitary Tumor

Pituitary tumors when large can invade the anterior third ventricle and present as anterior third ventricular masses. They can also cause compression of optic pathways. The diagnosis is usually straight forward. There is enlargement and erosion of sella with suprasellar extension.

Posterior Third Ventricular Masses

A variety of structures in and around the posterior third ventricle, including the pineal gland can be the origin of these tumors. The tumors can be astrocytoma of all grades, ependymomas, germinomas, meningiomas, vascular malformations, pineal tumors, metastasis or primary lymphomas. Regardless of the origin, these masses cause obstructive hydrocephalus due to compression of the posterior third ventricle or aqueduct and abnormal

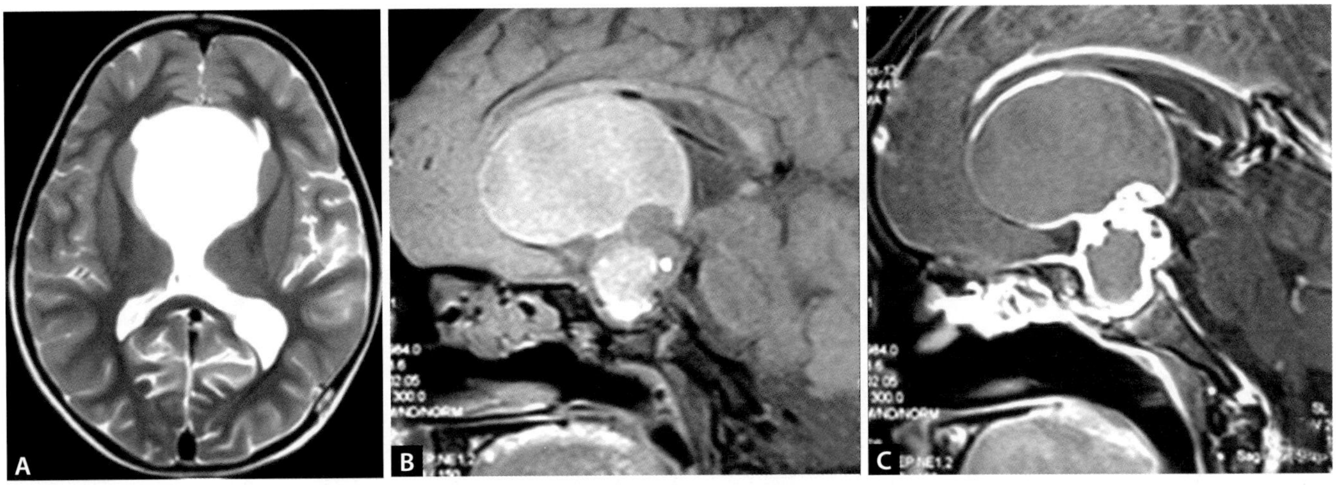

Figs. 20A to C: Craniopharyngioma: Large suprasellar lesion invading the anteroinferior third ventricle as shown on axial T2WI (A), sagittal pre (B) and post-contrast (C) T1W images. Note the T1 hyperintense signal in the cyst (motor oil appearance) with peripheral enhancement.

eye movements from pressure on, or infiltration of the pretectal area (e.g. Parinaud's syndrome).[28,30,33]

Glial Tumors

Astrocytomas comprise 25% of the mass lesions in the posterior third ventricle. Other gliomas like ependymomas, oligodendrogliomas, or glioblastomas can also occur in this area. There is no significant age or sex predilection. The imaging features are similar to those occurring in other areas of brain.

Germinoma

Germinoma is more common in posterior than anterior 3rd ventricle. It is common in young males and causes precocious puberty. It may lead to Parinaud's syndrome and hydrocephalus. On CT and MRI, it appears as well demarcated, homogeneous soft tissue mass and shows uniform enhancement after IV contrast administration. There is no calcification within the tumor. The tumor spreads through CSF pathway and responds to radiotherapy. Therefore, after obtaining tissue diagnosis (either by stereotactic or open biopsy) the entire neuroaxis should be irradiated.

Teratoma

Mature teratomata are well-differentiated benign tumors with a malignant potential. They are well encapsulated and show no evidence of infiltration of surrounding structures. On CT, teratomas show areas of fat attenuation and calcification or ossification. The solid portion can show some degree of contrast enhancement. On T1WI the fat in the teratoma appears hyperintense. Signal loss due to calcific foci can be seen on both T1WI and T2WI.

Pineoblastoma

It resembles other primitive neuroectodermal tumors (PNETs) (e.g. medulloblastoma) histologically. It is an infiltrative tumor and presents with obstructive hydrocephalus or Parinaud's syndrome. On CT, it appears hyperdense and enhances homogeneously and brightly following IV contrast injection. On MRI, it is hypo or isointense on T1WI and hyperintense on T2WI. Small areas of necrosis, hemorrhage, cyst formation or calcification can be seen. There is typically brilliant enhancement on gadolinium injection. It also shows spread along CSF pathways like germinoma and therefore the entire craniospinal axis should be imaged in such patients.[32]

Pineocytoma

Pineocytoma differs from pineoblastoma in that it contains more differentiated tumor cells and is not as infiltrative (**Figs. 23A to C**). It can cause hydrocephalus and the imaging features are similar to those of pineoblastoma.[32]

Vascular Masses

Arteriovenous malformations and cavernous angiomas, both can occur in the third ventricle.[25] They present on CT as brilliantly enhancing lesions consisting of serpiginous channels. MRI shows these lesions without contrast

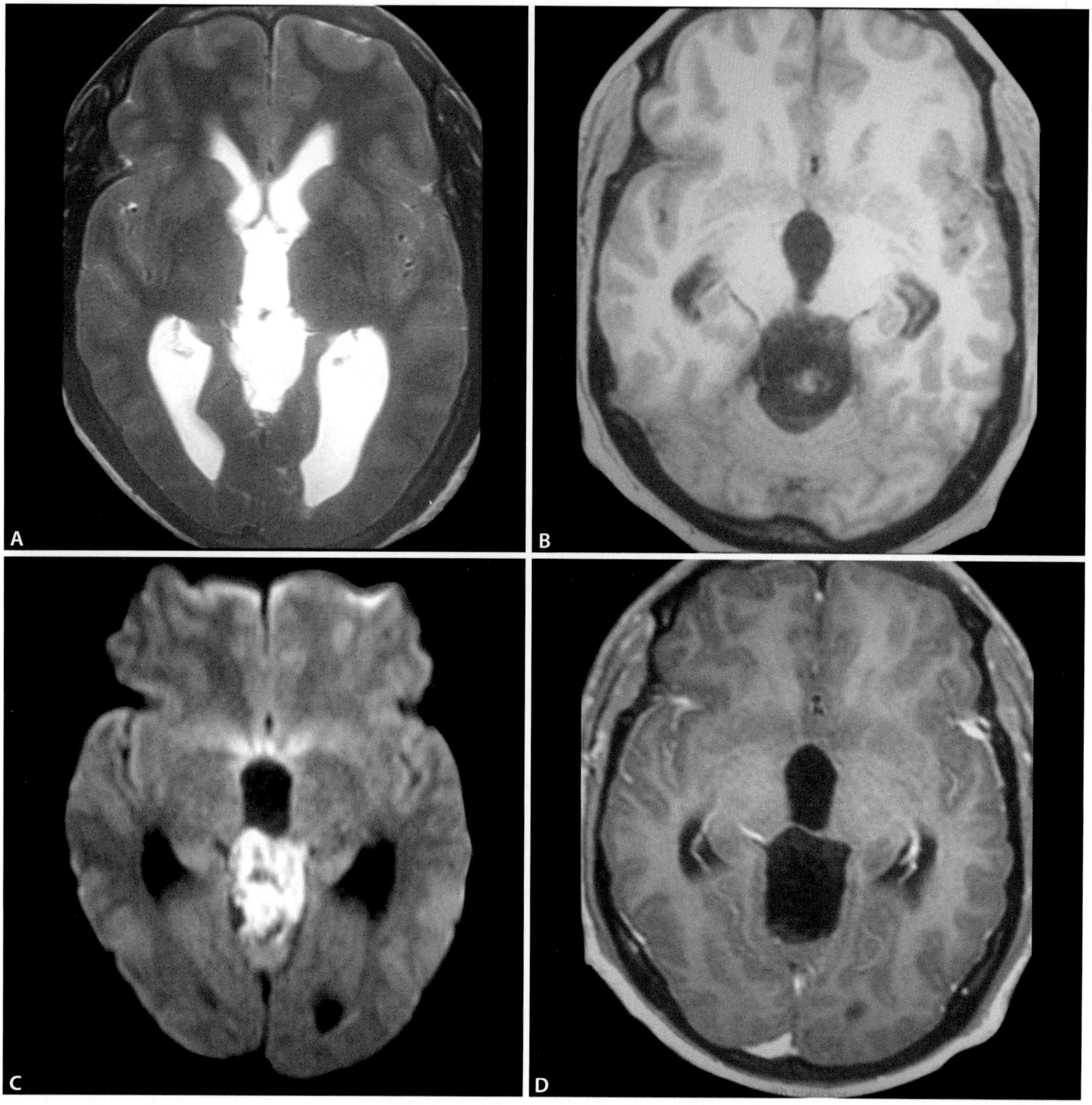

Figs. 21A to D: Third ventricular epidermoid cyst: Axial T2WI (A), T1WI (B) showing posterior third ventricular cyst with intense diffusion restriction (C). No post-contrast enhancement seen (D).

injection as serpiginous cluster of signal void seen in a cluster. MR angiography can be useful in delineating the feeding artery or draining veins. Angiography is the definitive investigation and it is almost always required preoperatively. When the feeders are located in surgically inaccessible sites, angioembolization can be attempted as a definitive treatment. Cavernous angiomas classically appear as lobulated "popcorn" shaped lesions having heterogeneous T1 and T2 signal with intense blooming on susceptibility weighted images **(Figs. 24A to C)**.

Fourth Ventricular Masses

Primary fourth ventricular neoplasms are common in children but rare in adults. The pediatric tumors are

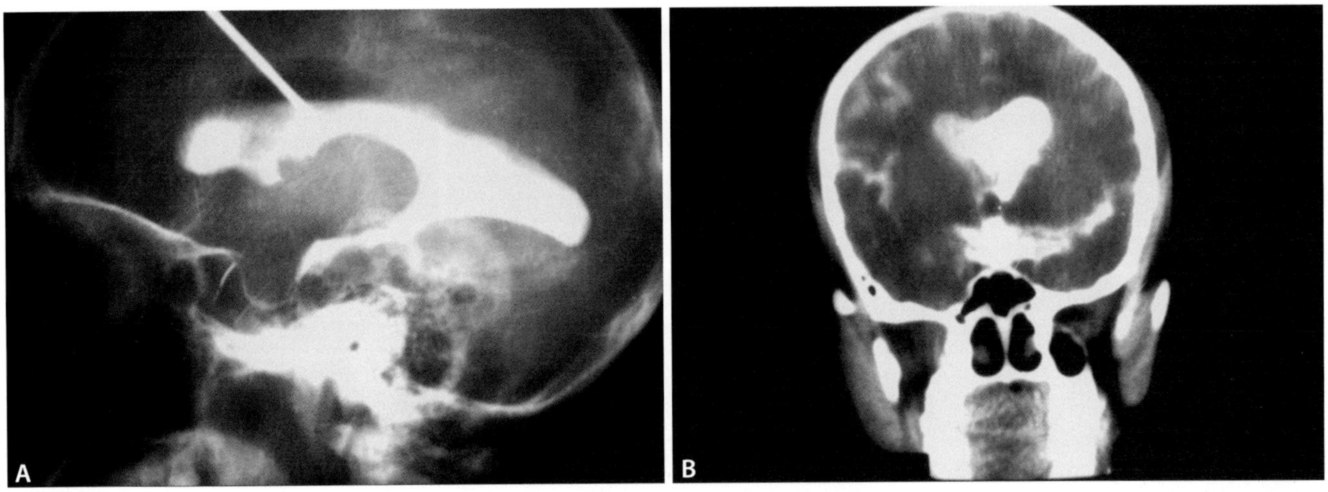

Figs. 22A and B: Cysticercosis: Lateral contrast ventriculogram (A) shows well-defined filling defect at foramen of Monro (B) CT ventriculogram confirms the cystic lesion.

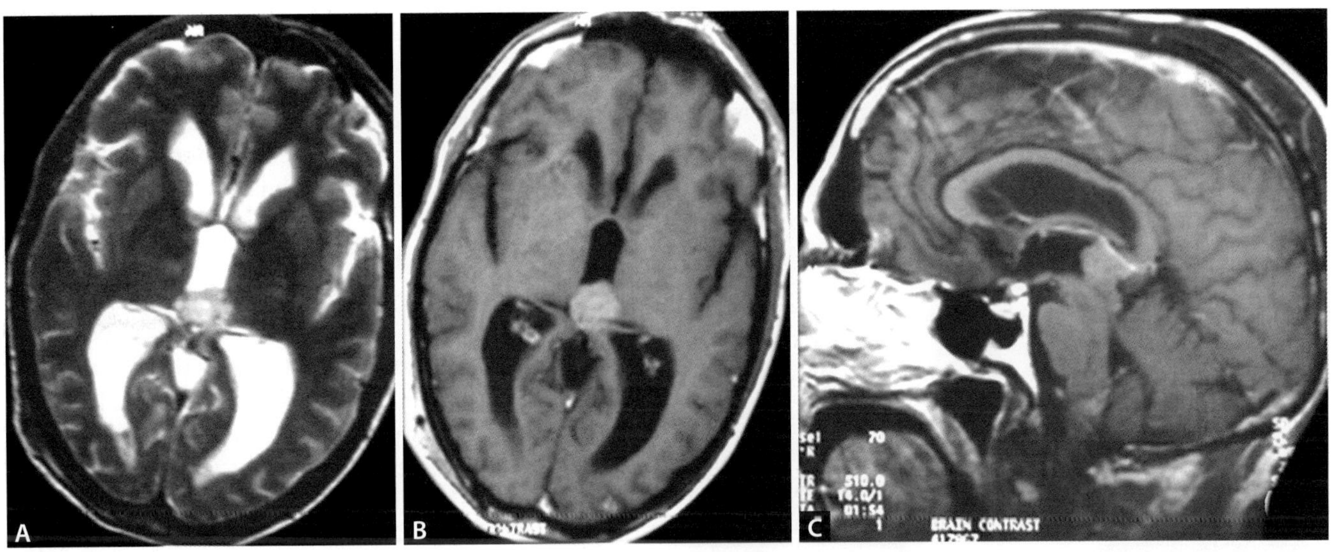

Figs. 23A to C: Pineocytoma: Axial T2WI (A), gadolinium enhanced axial (B) and sagittal (C) T1W images showing the posterior third ventricular lesion. Note the origin of the lesion from the pineal gland on sagittal image.

cerebellar astrocytoma, medulloblastoma, ependymoma and choroid plexus papilloma.[34] In adults, metastases are the most common fourth ventricular neoplasm. Other tumors, such as choroid plexus papilloma, epidermoid, dermoid and hemangioblastomas **(Fig. 25)** are rare. Subependymoma occur in caudal fourth ventricle near the obex. Non-neoplastic masses like arachnoid cysts, vascular malformation, cysticercosis, inflammatory cysts are occasionally seen within the fourth ventricle **(Figs. 26A to C)**. Partially exophytic masses may cause sudden loss of consciousness due to CSF obstruction referred to as Bruns syndrome.[35]

Cerebellar Astrocytoma

It is the most common posterior fossa neoplasm and constitutes 25% of all fourth ventricular neoplasms in children.[34] Histologically majority of the tumors are of pilocytic type. It usually originates from the vermis and extends anteriorly into the fourth ventricle. Rarely, the tumor arises primarily within the ventricle itself. The child usually presents with enlarging head and features of raised intracranial tension due to obstructive hydrocephalus. On CT, the tumor appears as a large lesion with solid (40%) or cystic (60%) components. The cystic mass shows a mural nodule. The nodule is always solitary and isodense

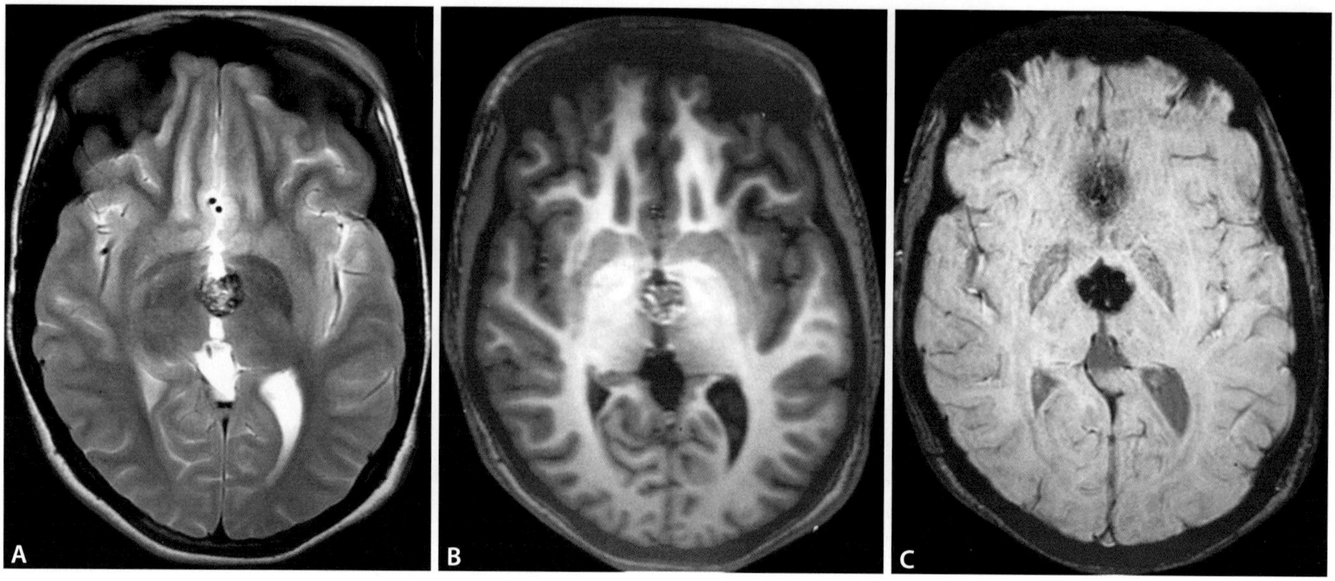

Figs. 24A to C: Third ventricular cavernoma: Axial T2WI (A) and T1WI (B) depicting the third ventricular ependymal "popcorn" lesion with blooming on susceptibilty weighted image (C).

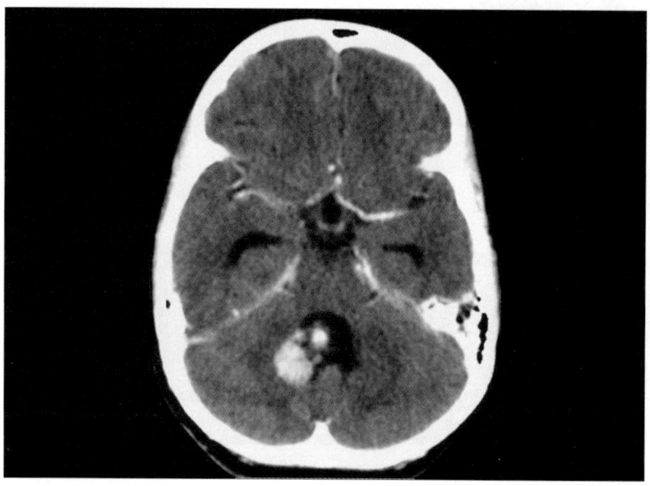

Fig. 25: Fourth ventricular cerebellar hemangioblastoma: Contrast-enhanced CT demonstrating the presence of a cystic lesion with enhancing mural nodule in the fourth ventricle.

with cerebellum on noncontrast scans. The nodule may or may not be calcified. On contrast administration the nodule shows intense, homogeneous enhancement which does not extend beyond the contour of the cyst. The cyst in unilocular and its walls apart from the site of nodule shows no enhancement. This distinguishes it from necrotic astrocytoma in which the cyst is multilocular, has ill-defined mural nodule, the tumor blush extends beyond the contour of the cyst and entire circumference of the cyst wall and the intervening septa also enhance.[36] The solid astrocytoma is round to oval, iso to hyperdense with nearly homogeneous dense contrast enhancement. On MRI, the appearance is similar with cystic component being hypo to isointense on T1WI and hyperintense on T2WI. The mural nodule shows intense enhancement with IV gadolinium **(Figs. 27A and B)**.

Medulloblastoma

This primitive neuroectodermal tumor is the second most common posterior fossa tumor constituting one fourth of all posterior fossa tumors in children. Ninety percent of these lesions originate in the inferior vermis and fill the fourth ventricle. The tumor shows dissemination along the CSF pathways in 60–100% cases. This is usually thickest at the skull base and within the sylvian fissures. Spinal cord metastases are also common (12–40%). Dorsal and lumbosacral region is seeded most commonly and the deposits are often multiple. Systemic metastases (15%) can also occur in bones (86%), peritoneum (via shunt) (43%), lymph nodes (30%), and in lung and liver (7%).

On CT, medulloblastoma is usually seen as a large, mildly hyperdense, midline solid mass arising from the inferior vermis. The tumor bulges anteriorly into the fourth ventricle and may extend into adjacent cisterns. Rarely, calcification, hemorrhage and necrosis are seen. On contrast, it shows moderate degree of homogeneous enhancement **(Fig. 28A)**. Typical appearance is seen in only one-third of cases. Cystic changes (65%), isodense mass on plain CT (3%) and absent contrast enhancement (3%) are also encountered. On MR, the

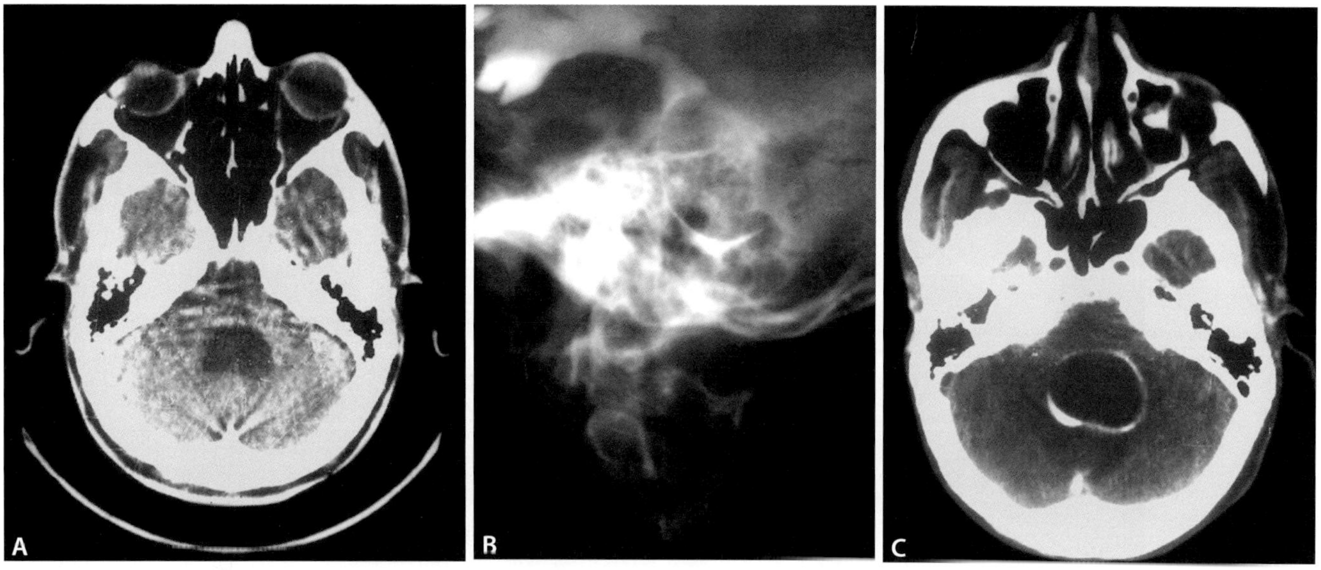

Figs. 26A to C: Fourth ventricular cysticercosis: (A) CECT shows dilation of the 4th ventricle, (B) lateral contrast ventriculogram shows well-defined filling detect in the 4th ventricle and (C) CT ventriculogram confirms the findings.

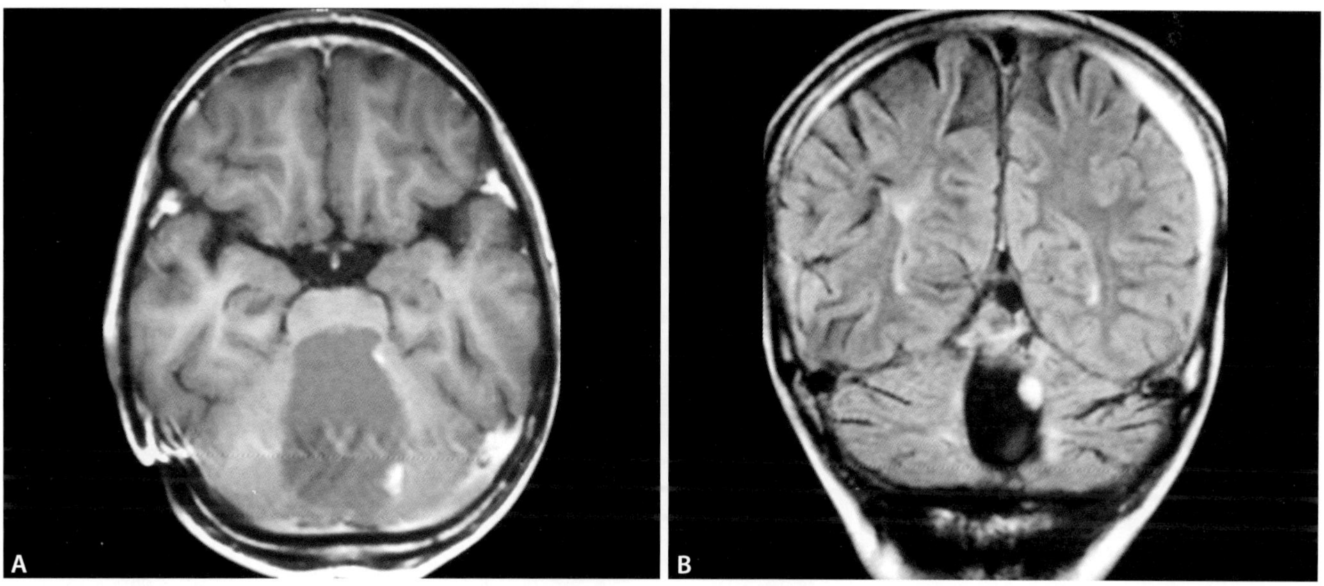

Figs. 27A and B: Pilocytic astrocytoma: MRI brain showing a large posterior fossa cystic mass with enhancing mural nodule.

typical medulloblastoma fills the fourth ventricle and extends inferiorly through foramen of Magendie into the cistern magna. It appears hypointense on T1WI and shows variable signal pattern on T2WI. Moderate enhancement is typical after IV gadolinium injection **(Figs. 28B and C)**. Due to high tumor cellularity it may show diffusion restriction with low apparent diffusion coefficient (ADC) values **(Fig. 28D)**. Other fourth ventricular tumors like ependymoma and astrocytomas can often be differentiated from it on MRI based on this finding. Hydrocephalus is seen in up to 85% cases.[34]

Ependymoma

It is the third most common fourth ventricular tumor in children. Nearly 50% of posterior fossa ependymomas are located in the fourth ventricle. On CT, the mass is midline and situated within an expanded fourth ventricle and often shows calcification (50%). There is usually moderate enhancement on contrast administration **(Fig. 29A)**. The mass typically extends outward into cerebellopontine cisterns or into the cisterna magna through the fourth ventricular exit foramina **(Figs. 29B and C)**. Hydrocephalus is nearly always seen. The tumor exhibits

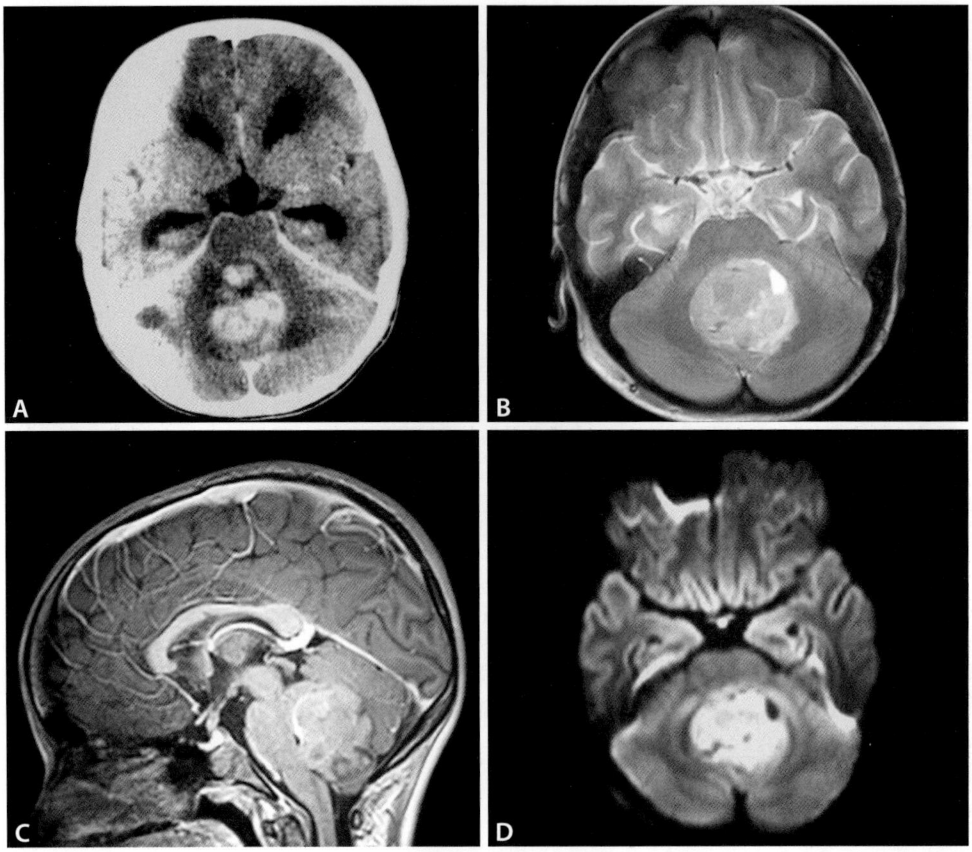

Figs. 28A to D: Medulloblastoma: CECT (A) shows a heterogeneously enhancing fourth ventricular mass. MRI (B and C) in another patient shows a similar mass in the fourth ventricle showing diffusion restriction (D) indicating high tumor cellularity.

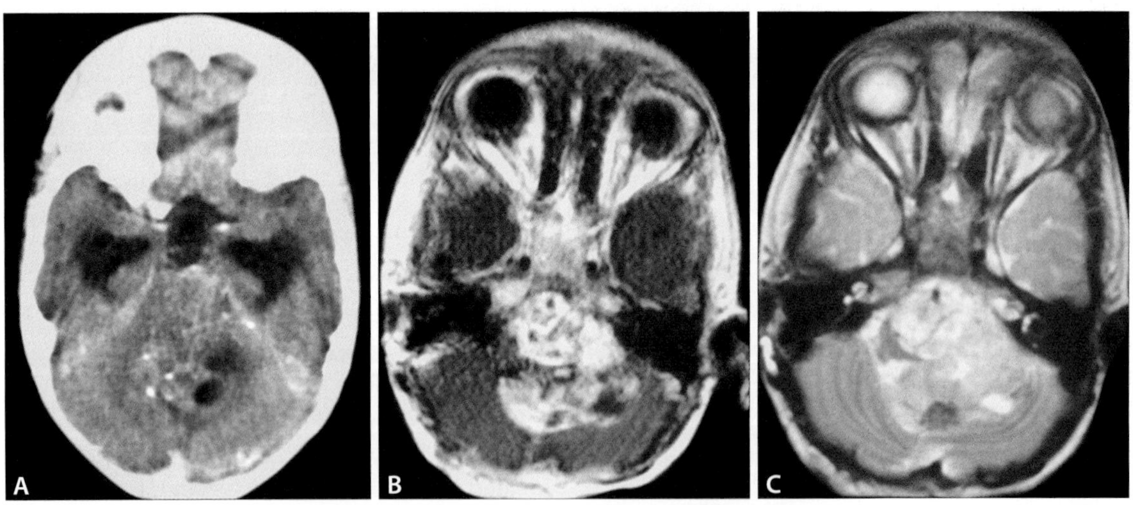

Figs. 29 A to C: Ependymoma: CECT (A) showing an ill-defined heterogeneously enhancing fourth ventricular tumor with presence of calcification. MRI (B and C) showing "plasticity" of the tumor with extension through the fourth ventricular outlet foramina into the adjacent cisternal spaces.

similar morphology on MRI as hypo to isointense signal on T1WI and intermediate to hyper intense signal on T2WI with heterogeneous post-contrast enhancement.[24]

Table 3 highlights the important points of differences between the most common posterior fossa tumors in childhood.

Table 3: Differences between common posterior fossa tumors in children.

Tumor characteristics	*Astrocytoma*	*Medulloblastoma*	*Ependymoma*
CT	Hypodense	Hyperdense	Isodense
Calcification	~10%	10–15%	40–50%
T1WI	Iso/hypo	Iso/hypo	Iso/hypo
T2WI	Hyper	Iso	Iso/hyper
Post gadolinium	Nodule enhances	Moderate	Mild
Cyst formation	Very common	Rare	Common
Transforaminal spread	No	No	Yes
CSF seeding	Rare	Yes (15–40%)	No

Brainstem Gliomas

They are the fourth most common posterior fossa tumors in children.[34] About 70% of gliomas in the brainstem are of high grade. The low grade gliomas typically show a dorsal exophytic component that grows into the fourth ventricle. It involves the pons (54%) but can extend inferiorly into medulla, superiorly into thalamus and midbrain and posterolaterally along cerebellar peduncles into cerebellar hemispheres. The imaging features are similar as described in other areas.

CONCLUSION

Intraventricular lesions are histologically distinct but residentially similar lesions. A distinct understanding of their clinical behavior including presenting age, typical location and morphological description is required for reaching at a correct set of differential diagnosis.

REFERENCES

1. Tien RD. Intraventricular mass lesion of the brain: CT and MRI findings. Am J Roentgenol. 1991;157:1283-90.
2. Waldron JS, Tihan T. Epidemiology and pathology of intraventricular tumors. Neurosurg Clin N Am. 2003;14:469-82.
3. Jelinek J, Smirniothopoulos JG, Parisi JE, et al. Lateral ventricular neoplasms of the brain: differential diagnosis based on clinical, CT and MR findings. Am J Neuroradiol. 1990;11:567-74.
4. Agarwal A, Kanekar S. Intraventricular tumors. Semin Ultrasound CT MR. 2016;37:150-8.
5. Seçer HI, Düz B, Izci Y, et al. Tumors of the lateral ventricle: the factors that affected the preference of the surgical approach in 46 patiens. Turk Neurosurg. 2008;18:345-55.
6. Zuccaro G, Sosa F, Cuccia V, et al. Lateral ventricle tumors in children: a series of 54 cases. Childs Nerv Syst. 1999;15:774-85.
7. Wolff JE, Finlay JL. Choroid plexus tumors. In: Carroll WL, Finlay JL (Eds). Cancer in Children and Adolescents. Sudbury, Mass: Jones & Bartlett; 2009. p. 299.
8. Paulus W, Brandner S. Choroid plexus tumors. In: Louis DN, Ohgaki H, Wiestler OD, Cavenee WK (Eds). WHO Classification of Tumours of the Central Nervous System. Lyon, France: IARC; 2007. pp. 82-5.
9. Coates TL, Hinshaw DB, Peckman N. Pediatric choroid plexus papillomas. MR, CT and pathologic correlation. Radiology. 1989;173:818.
10. Meyers SP, Khademian ZP, Chuang SH, et al. Choroid plexus carcinomas in children: MRI features and patient outcomes. Neuroradiology. 2004;46:770-80.
11. Horská A, Ulug AM, Melhem ER, et al. Proton magnetic resonance spectroscopy of choroid plexus tumors in children. J Magn Reson Imaging. 2001;14(1):78-82.
12. Castillo M, Scatiff JH, Bouldin TW, et al. Radiologic-pathologic correlation: intracranial astrocytoma. Am J Neuroradiol. 1992;13:1609-16.
13. Kumar R, Singh V. Subependymal giant cell astrocytoma: a report of five cases. Neurosurg Rev. 2004;27:274-80.
14. Zamora C, Huisman TA, Izbudak I. Supratentorial tumors in pediatric patients. Neuroimaging Clin N Am. 2017;27: 39-67.
15. Swartz GP, Zimemerman RA, Bilaniuk LT. Computed tomography of intracranial ependymoma. Radiology. 1982;143:97-101.
16. Darwish B, Munro I, Boet R, et al. Intraventricular meningioma with drop metastases and subgaleal metastatic nodule. J Clin Neurosci. 2004;11:787-91.
17. Holvek A, Grand S, Boini S, et al. Dynamic susceptibility contrast-enhanced MRI evaluation of cerebral intraventricular tumors: preliminary results. J Neuroradiol. 2010;37:269-75.
18. Vuckovic N, Kozic D, Vulekovic P, et al. MR and MRS characteristics of intraventricular meningioma. J Neuroimaging. 2010;20:294-6.
19. Koeller KK, Sandberg GD; Armed Forces Institute of Pathology. From the archives of the AFIP. Cerebral intraventricular neoplasms: radiologic-pathologic correlation. Radiographics. 2002;22(6):1473-505.
20. Cordoliani YS, Derosier C, Pharaboz C. Primary cerebral lymphoma in patients with AIDS: MR findings in 17 cases. AJR. 1992;159:841-7.

21. Kerkovský M, Zitterbart K, Svoboda K, et al. Central neurocytoma: the neuroradiological perspective. Childs Nerv Syst. 2008;24:1361-9.
22. Kim DG, Chi JG, Park SH. Intraventricular neurocytoma: clinicopathological analysis of seven cases. J Neurosurg. 1992;76:759-65.
23. Shah T, Jayasundar R, Singh VP, et al. MRS characterization of central neurocytomas using glycine. NMR Biomed. 2011;24(10):1408-13.
24. Spoto GP, Press GA, Hesselink JR, et al. Intracranial ependymoma and subependymoma: MR manifestations. Am J Neuroradiol. 1990;11:83-91.
25. Miyagi Y, Mannoji H, Akaboshi K. Intraventricular cavernous malformation associated with medullary venous malformation. Neurosurgery. 1993;32:461-4.
26. Nakase H, Morimoto T, Sakaki T. Bilateral choroid plexus cysts in the lateral ventricles. Am J Neuroradiol. 1991;12:1204-5.
27. Gaskill SJ, Saldivar V, Rutman J, et al. Giant bilateral xanthogranulomas in a child: a case report. Neurosurgery. 1992;31:114-7.
28. Vandesteen L, Drier A, Galanaud D, et al. Imaging findings of intraventricular and ependymal lesions. J Neuroradiol. 2013;40(4):229-44.
29. Lach B, Scheithauer BW, Gregor A, et al. Colloid cyst of the third ventricle: a comparative immunohistochemical study of neuraxis cyst and choroid plexus epithelium. J Neurosurg. 1993;78:101-11.
30. Peraud A, Illner A, Rutka JT. Intraventricular congenital lesions and colloid cysts. Neurosurg Clin N Am. 2003;14:607-19.
31. Waggenespack GA, Guinto FC Jr. MR and CT of masses of the anterosuperior third ventricle. Am J Roentgenol. 1989;152:609-14.
32. Smirniotopopulos JG, Rushing EJ, Mena H. Pineal region masses: differential diagnosis. Radiographics. 1992;12:577-96.
33. Smith AB, Smirniotopoulos JG, Horkanyne-Szakaly I. From the radiologic pathology archives: intraventricular neoplasms: radiologic-pathologic correlation. Radiographics. 2013;33(1):21-43.
34. Maroldo TV, Barkovich AJ. Pediatric brain tumors. Semin Ultrasound CT MR. 1992;13:412-48.
35. Krasnianski M, Müller T, Stock K, et al. Bruns syndrome caused by intraventricular tumor. Eur J Med Res. 2008:13;179-81.
36. Favre J, Deruaz JP, de Tribolet N. Pilocytic cerebellar astrocytoma in adults: case report. Surg Neurol. 1993;39:360-4.

CHAPTER 20

Imaging of the Temporal Bone

Vivek Gupta, Niranjan Khandelwal

INTRODUCTION

The temporal bone forms the segment of the cranium which separates the middle cranial fossa from the posterior cranial fossa. It contains the organs of hearing and equilibrium and is in direct relation with the temporal lobe. A number of important vascular and neural structures traverse through this bone.

A number of radiographic views are available which include the standard lateral view of skull, the Towne's view, Law's projection and its modifications, and the Stenver's view. However, with the advent of modern cross-sectional imaging modalities now the X-ray evaluation of the temporal bone has become obsolete. Computed tomography (CT) has revolutionized the imaging of the temporal bone because it is with this modality that axial, coronal and sagittal sections of the dense bone could be obtained and is the mainstay in the imaging of the temporal bone. Reconstructions in virtually any plane is made possible with the advent of multi-detector spiral CT. Magnetic resonance imaging (MRI) essentially complements CT, because of its excellent soft tissue contrast; but the osseous and air-containing structures are suboptimally imaged with this modality.

COMPUTED TOMOGRAPHY TECHNIQUE

Typically, a high resolution matrix (512 × 512) with thin sections (0.6–1.5 mm) and a field of view of 15–20 cm is employed for high resolution imaging in a bone algorithm. Newer high resolution multi-detector spiral imaging can generate isotropic voxels for multiplanar reconstruction making the need for multiple series with direct imaging in several planes unnecessary.

Planes for acquiring (or reconstructing) images are described in relation to the zero degree baseline which is the line extending between the external auditory canal and the inferior orbital rim on a lateral scout film **(Fig. 1)**.[1]

Computed tomography images are usually acquired or displayed in axial or coronal planes. Axial images are

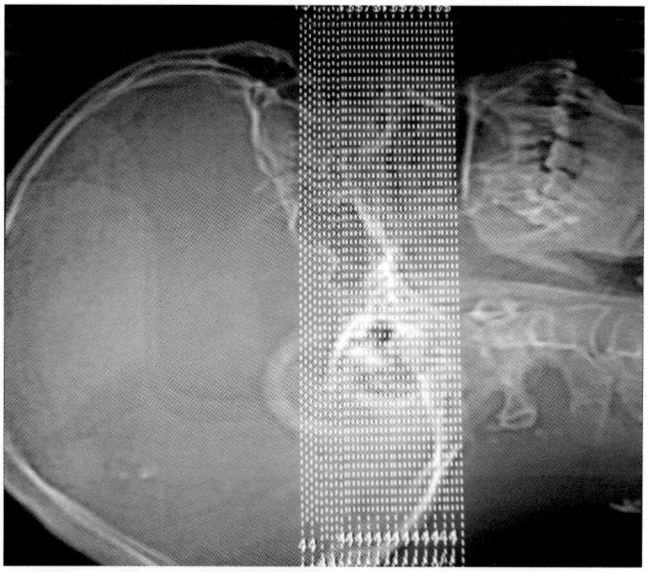

Fig. 1: Lateral topogram with planning for acquiring axial section through the temporal bone.

acquired in a plane rotated 30° superior to this baseline which is parallel to the lateral semicircular canal, beginning at or just above the external auditory meatus. This section will partly show the basal turn of the cochlea and the round window niche. Sections just above the basal turn of the cochlea will show the incudostapedial region and turns of the cochlea. Sections superior to these will pass through the vestibule and lateral semicircular canal. The internal auditory meatus is visualized at this level, as are the head of malleus and short process of the incus. All three segments of the facial nerve canal can be identified, though the descending portion of the canal appears in cross-section just behind the middle ear cavity. Crura of the stapes can be visualized but the oval window is not adequately demonstrated in these sections **(Figs. 2A to J)**.

Reconstructed coronal images from axial section are oriented 90° to the baseline. With the advent of volumetric data it is no longer required to obtain direct coronal acquisition. However, in the older scanners where volumetric acquisitions are not possible, direct coronal sections are acquired with patient in supine or prone positions. Sections can be acquired with neck extended to the maximum. The plane is approximately 105° to 120° the baseline which is perpendicular to the lateral semicircular canal. In patients who cannot extend the neck, modified coronal sections can be obtained in a plane parallel to the clivus which is 70° to the baseline.

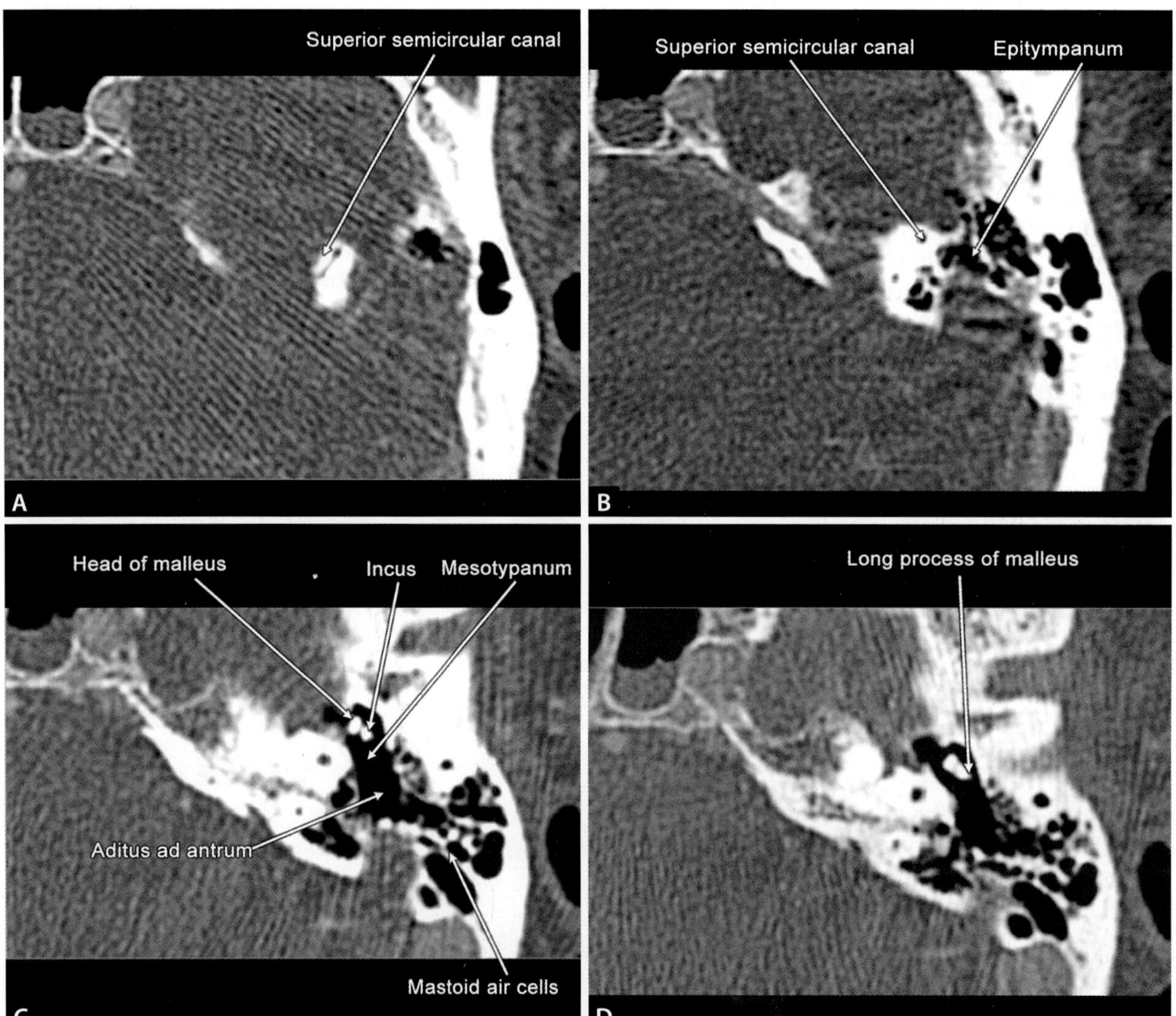

Figs. 2A to D

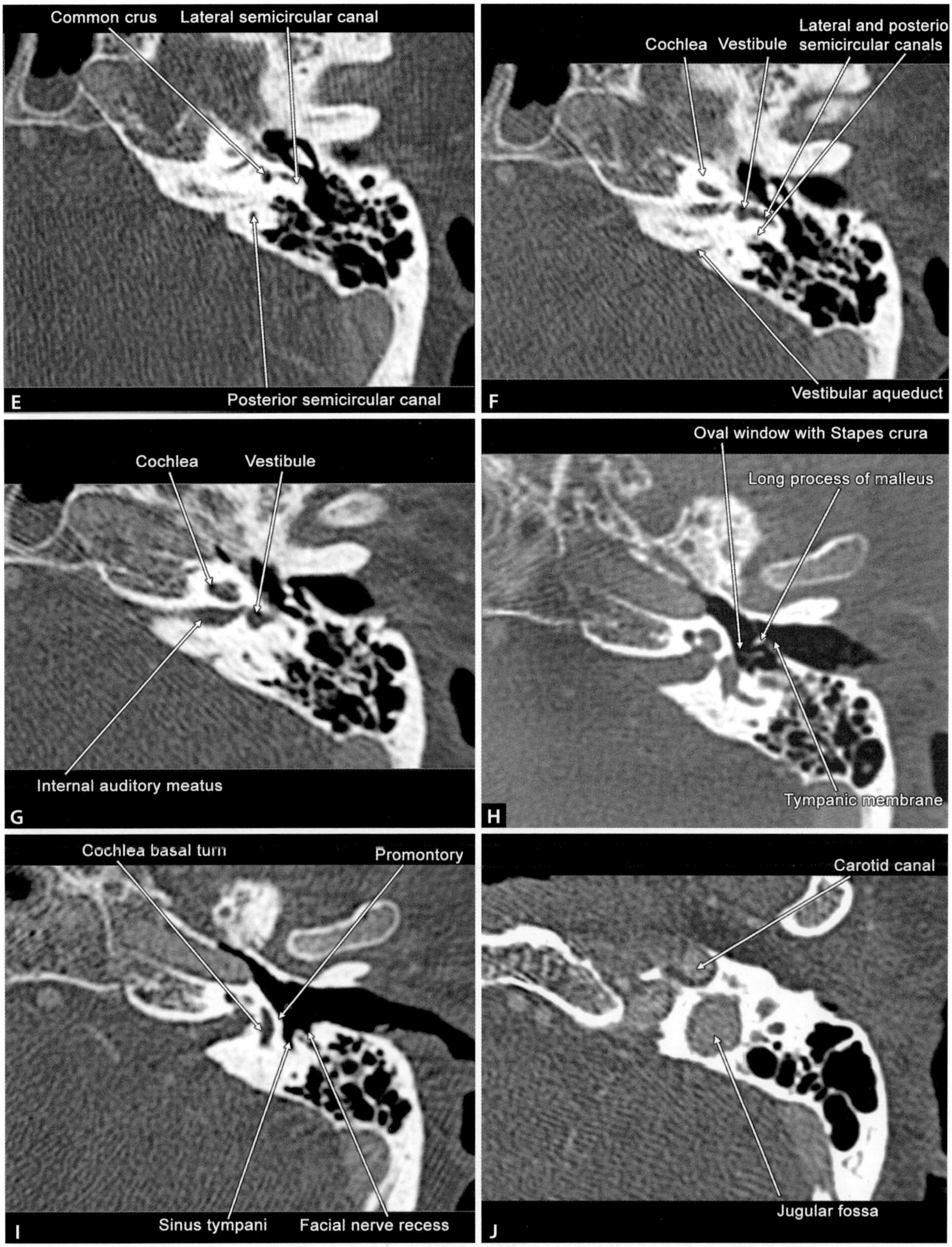

Figs. 2E to J

Figs. 2A to J: Normal anatomy of temporal bone. Axial high-resolution computed tomography (HRCT) section through the temporal bone superior to inferior.

Coronal sections begin at the level of the carotid canal. The coil of the cochlea forms the bulge of promontory with the oval and round window niches superior and inferior to it. The malleusis best seen in this section. Further posteriorly the vestibule and the semicircular canals can be identified and the internal auditory meatus is well seen in this section. The pyramidal eminence is present at this level, which shows the most prominent segment of the lateral semicircular canals, between the facial recess and sinus tympanicum. The descending facial canal and jugular foramen can be identified in the posterior most sections **(Figs. 3A to C)**.

Sagittal, oblique or curved projections can be reconstructed to obtain images in the plane of the long axis of the temporal bone or in planes parallel to specific areas of interest such as the facial nerve canal. 3D surface reconstructions of the temporal bone or the inner ear structures can be generated to allow studies on models thus obtained.

MAGNETIC RESONANCE IMAGING

Magnetic resonance imaging (MRI) examination is directed towards imaging of fluid containing spaces in the temporal bone, vascular structures and their pathologies and the adjacent brain parenchyma. Basic MR protocols have been recommended[2] which include: (i) whole brain/head imaging, (ii) high resolution fluid space imaging, (iii) high resolution T1-weighted contrast enhanced imaging with or without fat suppression and (iv) MR angiography.[3]

Routine brain survey includes noncontrast and contrast enhanced T1WI, T2WI fast-echo sequence and a fluid attenuation inversion recovery (FLAIR) sequence. These sequences are especially useful in delineating brainstem demyelination or tumor. Sequences like FLAIR can also be used to differentiate hemorrhage from fat. Three-dimensional constructive interference in steady state (3D CISS) sequence is in routine use these days. Since it is a heavily T2 weighted sequence it is especially useful in imaging of structures surrounded by fluid-like seven-eighth nerve complex and membranous labyrinth. It is a 3D sequence and images in any plane can be generated **(Fig. 4A)**. It is important to understand the detailed anatomy and relationship of VII-VIIIth cranial nerve complex once they enter the internal acoustic meatus. On the axial plane the VIIth cranial nerve is anterior to the VIIth cranial nerve in their cisternal segment. Within the IAC, the facial nerve is antero-superior, cochlear nerve is antero-inferior, superior vestibular nerve is posterosuperior and the inferior vestibular nerve is posteroinferior. These relationships are best studied in sagital-oblique plane as shown in **Figure 4B**.

Some authors used another new sequence of 3D variable-flip-angle fast-spin-echo (3D VFA FSE) to image the membranous labyrinth. This technique can be used

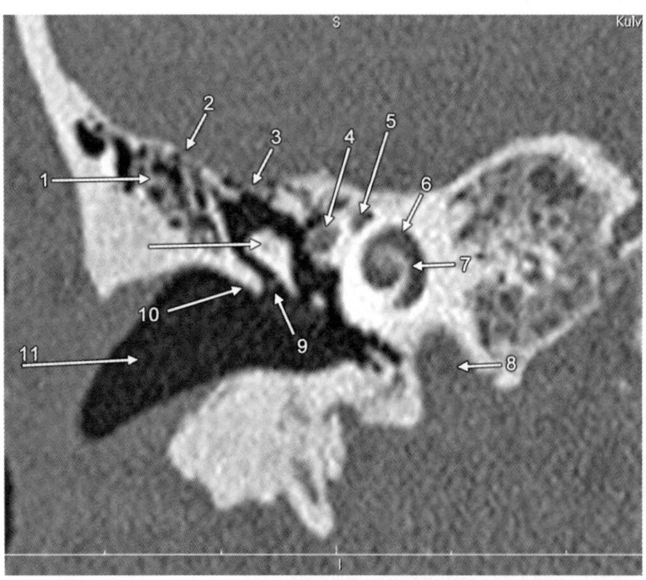

Fig. 3A: Coronal CT image shows: (1) Mastoid air cells; (2) Tegmen mastoideum; (3) Tegmen tympani; (4) Tympanic segment of facial nerve; (5) Labrynthine segment of facial nerve; (6) Basal turn of cochlea; (7) Interscalar septum; (8) Carotid canal; (9) Lateral malleal ligament; (10) scutum; (11) External auditory canal.

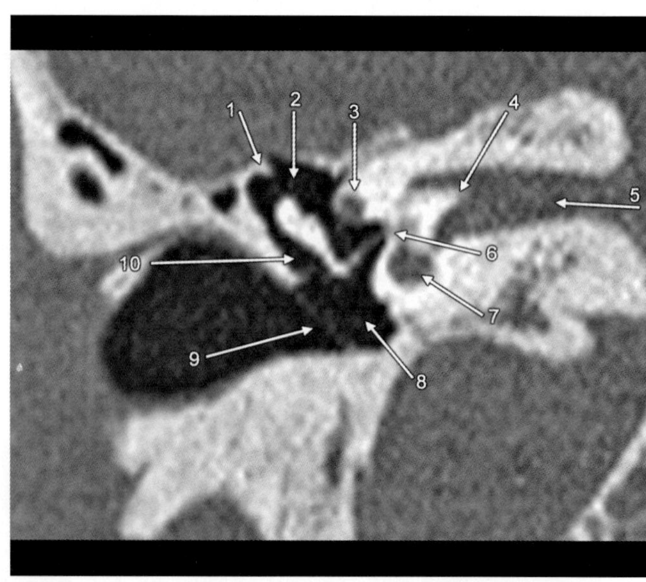

Fig. 3B: Coronal HRCT image. (1) Tegmen tympani; (2) Epitympanum; (3) Tympanic segment of facial nerve; (4) Crista falciformic; (5) Internal auditory canal; (6) Oval window; (7) Vestibule; (8) Hypotympanum; (9) Tympanic membrane; (10) Prussak space.

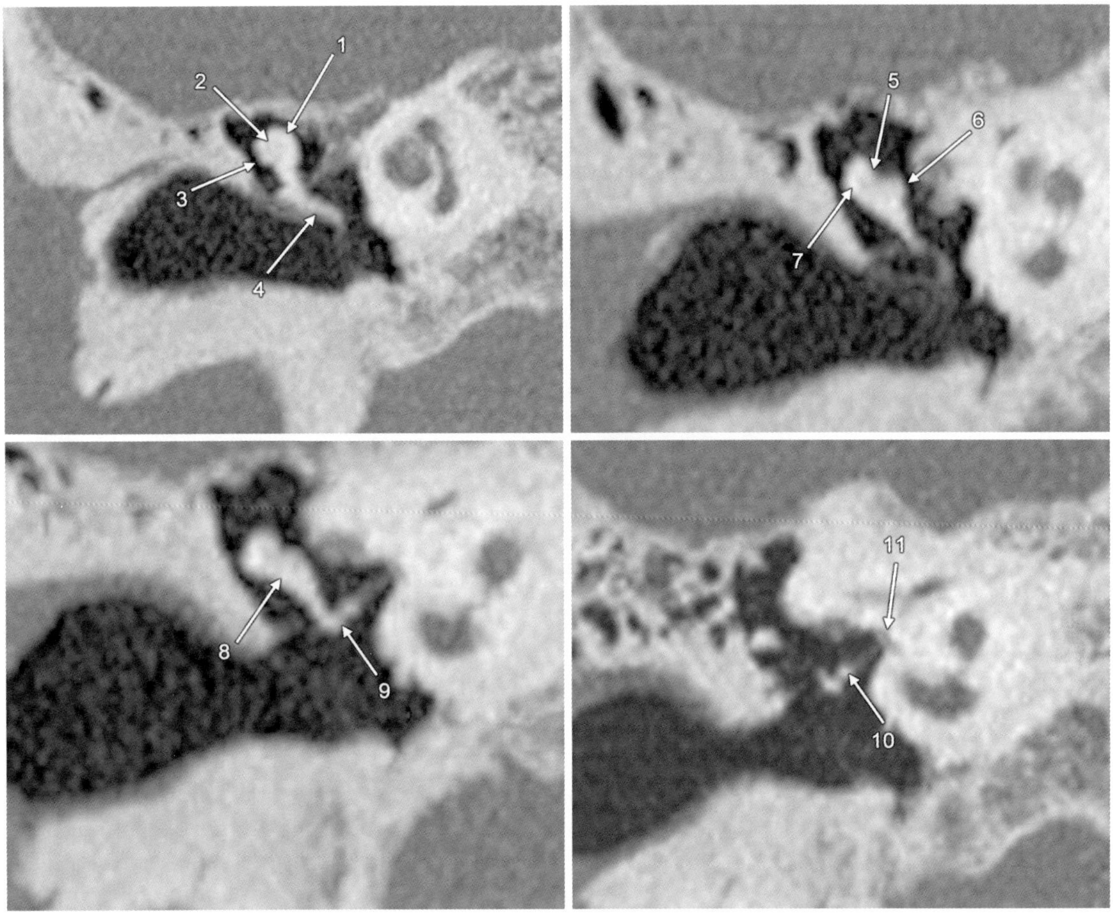

Fig. 3C: Ear ossicles as seen on coronal cuts: (1) Head of Malleus; (2) Malleo-incudo joint; (3) Incus; (4) Handle of Malleus; (5) Articulating surface of Incus; (6) Short limb of Incus; (7 and 8) Body of Incus; (9) Long limb of Incus; (10) Head of Stapes; (11) Oval window.

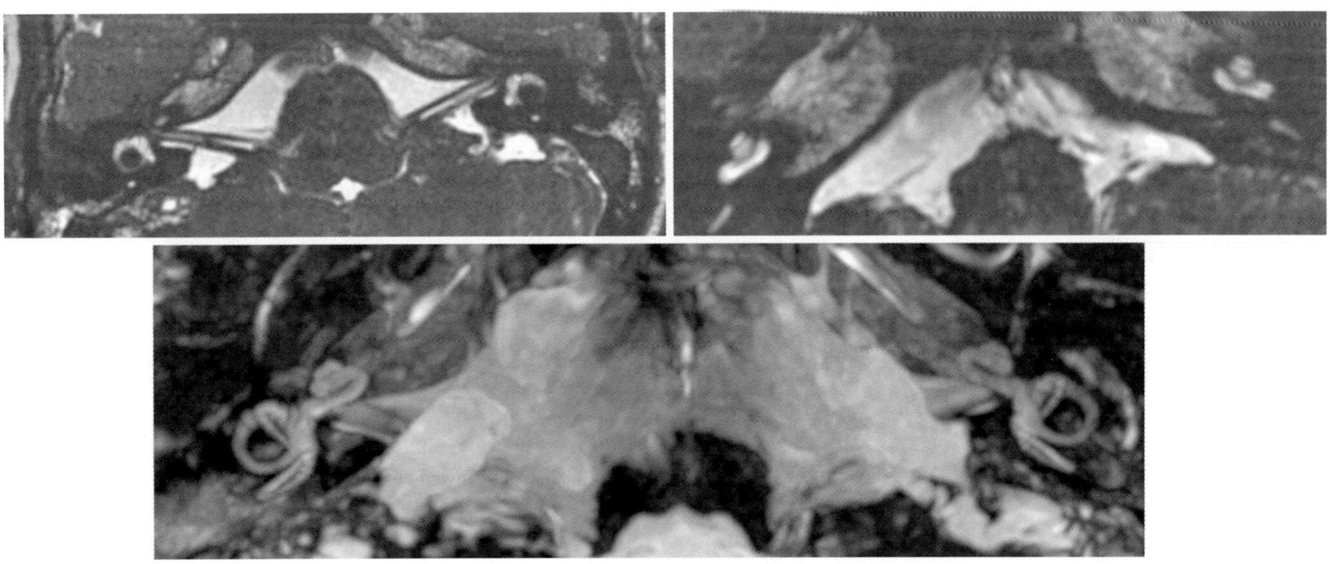

Fig. 4A: Maximum intensity projection (MIP) image of 3D-CISS sequence showing detailed anatomy of inner ear-cochlea (C), vestibule (V), semicircular canals (SC) and VII-VIII cranial nerves (CN).

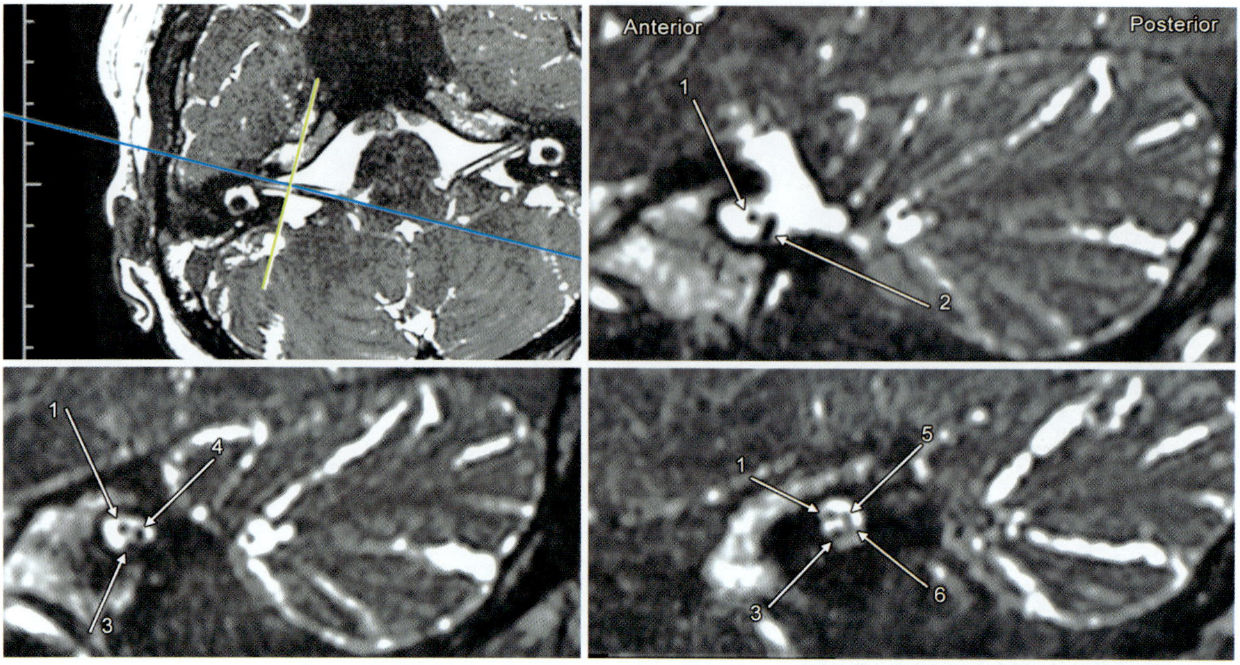

Fig. 4B: (1) Facial nerve; (2) Vestibullo-cochlear nerve; (3) Cochlear nerve; (4) Vestibular nerve; (5) superior vesibular nerve; (6) Inferior vestibular nerve.

clinically to reduce susceptibility artifacts and image blurring which may be a problem when small field-of-view (FOV) is used to image temporal bone with sequences which are heavily T2 weighted.[4]

High resolution T1W contrast enhanced images are acquired using a three-dimensional Fourier transformation (3DFT) technique. Fluid spaces have low signal intensity and nerves have higher signal intensity on this sequence. This sequence is ideal for identification of subtle changes, such as those seen in vestibulitis or in demonstrating small vestibular tumors. Magnetic resonance angiography is specifically indicated to assess structures around the jugular foramen and internal acoustic meatus and consists of sequence for visualization of arteries and veins in relation to the temporal bone.

CONGENITAL ANOMALIES OF THE TEMPORAL BONE

Congenital anomalies of the temporal bone can be divided into two groups: those involving the external and middle ears and those involving the inner ear. This division can be explained on the basis of development of the temporal bone. The external and middle ear develop from the first and second branchial arches, the first branchial groove and the adjacent mesenchyme. The inner ear develops from the pars optica which develops from auditory vesicle and the adjacent mesenchyme.[2,5,6]

Anomalies of the External and Middle Ear

The external auditory canal may be stenotic or atretic. Both stenosis and atresia of the canal can be associated with small auricles, a condition which is termed as microtia **(Figs. 5A and B)**. Stenosis of the external auditory canal can be diffuse, involving the entire length of the canal, or it can be focal. Severe stenosis of the external auditory canal may be associated with an acquired cholesteatoma due to trapping of epithelial debris in the medial end of the canal.

Bony atresia of the external auditory canal (EAC) is due to aplasia of the tympanic ring. It can be complete or partial, and can be unilateral or bilateral. The canal is replaced by a bony plate called the atresia plate. This anomaly is associated with the fusion of the ossicles with the atresia plate. The neck of malleus is the common segment which fuses with the plate. In certain instances, there may be absence of the short process of the malleus. The middle ear cleft is usually narrow and may be filled with mesenchymal remnants which appear as soft tissue densities similar to fluid on HRCT **(Fig. 6)**.

Anomalous development of the middle ear may be associated with EAC stenosis or atresia. Maldevelopment of the ossicles, their fusion or hypoplasia may be seen. These are associated with anomalous course of the facial nerve or position of the sigmoid sinus. Isolated ossicular abnormalities are rarely seen without coexisting external ear abnormalities. The long process of the incus and stapes are commonly involved in such situations.[6]

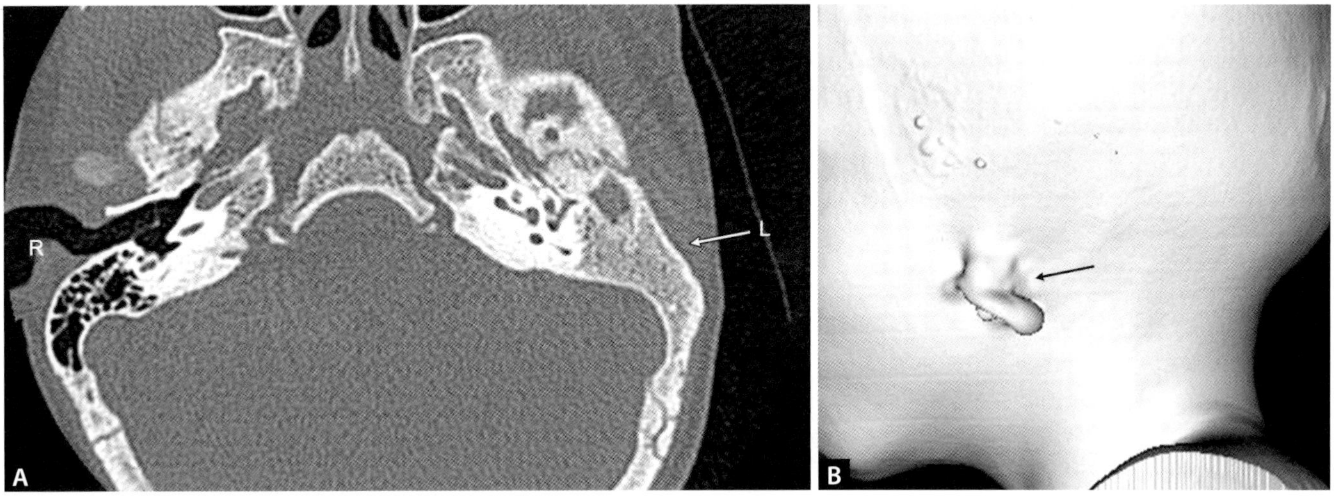

Figs. 5A and B: Axial HRCT section showing left external auditory canal atresia (white arrow) and associated microtia (black arrow).

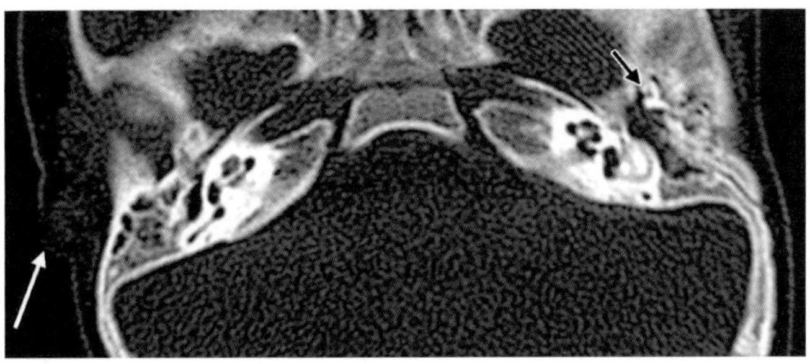

Fig. 6: Axial HRCT section showing the thick atresia plate on the left side (black arrow). The ossicular mass is fixed with the atresia plate. On the right side also the EAC is atretic and rudimentary external ear (white arrow) is seen.

Inner Ear Abnormalities

Inner ear abnormalities affect the cochlea, semicircular canals, vestibule and the vestibular/cochlear aqueducts. Radiologically, it is not possible to diagnose the anomalies of the membranous labyrinth because the overlying bony labyrinth may be normal. Amongst the congenital abnormalities of the inner ear, malformation of the semicircular canals is the commonest. Of these, the lateral semicircular canal malformation is most frequent. The most common form of congenital malformation is hypoplasia of the semicircular canal which leads to compensatory enlargement of the vestibule. Aplasia of the semicircular canals is one of the associations of the CHARGE syndrome. A notable recently described anomaly is semicircular canal dehiscence which causes pressure or sound induced vertigo.

Cochlear anomalies are numerous and Jackler et al. have attempted to classify them on the basis of stages of arrested development during organogenesis.[7] According to this classification the cochlear abnormalities can be grouped as follows.

Complete Labyrinthine Aplasia or Michele Aplasia

In this the inner ear is replaced by a small, single, cystic, cavity or several small cavities. This condition on imaging may look like *labrynthitis obliterans*. However, in latter condition since the labyrinth is formed completely but is secondarily obliterated the bulge of promontory as seen on CT is present. The distinction between these two conditions is important because cochlear implant is contraindicated in aplasia.[8]

Common Cavity

A large cystic cavity without any internal architecture is formed due to poor development of cochlea and bony labyrinth. This is associated with poor differentiation of membranous labyrinth as well resulting in severe to profound hearing loss.

Cochlear Aplasia

In this the cochlea fails to form and the other elements of the inner ear may also be malformed.

Cochlear Hypoplasia

This represents a small rudimentary cochlear bud associated with a normal or malformed vestibule and semicircular canal. On CT the height of cochlea is around 6 mm as compared to normal height of about 12–13 mm. Membranous differentiation is affected to a variable degree and is reflected in degree of hearing loss.

Incomplete Partition or Dilatational Defects

This includes the *Mondini's defect.* In Mondini's defect the basal turn of the cochlea is formed, however, the middle and apical turns are replaced by a common cavity or cloaca.[9,10]

Thus instead of having 2.5 turns there are 1.5 turns of the cochlea. It is commonly associated with enlarged vestibular aqueduct; stapes footplate deformity and modiolar defects **(Figs. 7A and B)**. Cystic cochlea lacking all interscalar septae and modiolus has been referred to as *pseudo-Mondini malformation* or cystic cochleovestibular malformation.[11]

Imaging of cochlear implant: cochlear implant is used to restore hearing in select indications of sensorineural deafness. It involves the implantation of the electrode of the cochlear implant in the inner ear. This is achieved via mastoid route, into the middle ear and through the facial recess into the widened round window. The electrode is inserted into the cochlea for about 1½ turn. Pre-procedure, imaging involves the HRCT for evaluation of the bony structures and MRI for establishing the integrity of the hearing pathway including the cochlear nerve. Post-procedure the position of the electrode can be assessed by HRCT evaluation **(Figs. 8A to D)**.

Congenital Dilatation of the Vestibular Aqueduct

Congenital dilatation of the vestibular aqueduct is the most common cause of congenital sensorineural deafness. Enlargement of the aqueduct to 1.5–2 mm is diagnostic of this condition. This entity is often associated with Pendred syndrome characterized by euthyroid goiter and sensorineural hearing loss.

Narrowed vestibular aqueducts less than 0.5 mm are associated with Ménière's disease. Congenital enlargement of cochlear aqueduct may occur. This leads to abnormal perilymph pressure which results in CSF leaks from the oval window during stapedectomy, the eponymous "Stapes Gushers".

Vestibular Anomalies

Most common is absence or dysplasia of lateral semicircular canals.

Internal auditory canals (IAC) may be stenosed or atretic. This is associated with absent cranial nerve VIII. The IAC can be partitioned into two or more separate channels by bony septae.[5]

Vascular Anomalies

Aberrant course of the carotid artery is an important vascular congenital anomaly. The normal carotid canal extends vertically and then horizontally anteroinferior to the cochlea. When the course of the artery is aberrant, the lateral wall of the carotid canal is absent and the canal lays posteroinferior to the cochlea. Therefore, the carotid artery protrudes into the anterior middle ear and has a more lateral and tortuous course than a normal artery.[5]

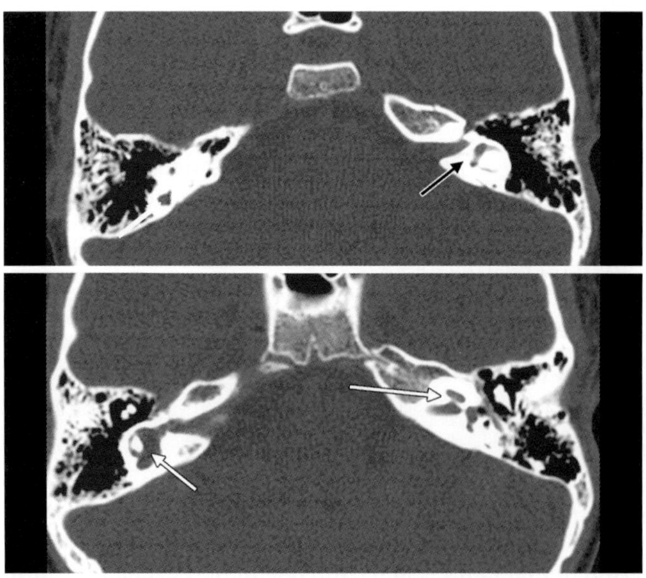

Fig. 7A: Mondini's defect: Axial HRCT images showing dilated vestibule and a large common cavity (white arrows) on right side with absence of cochlear turns. On left side, vestibule (black arrow) and cochlear turn is seen well (long white arrow).

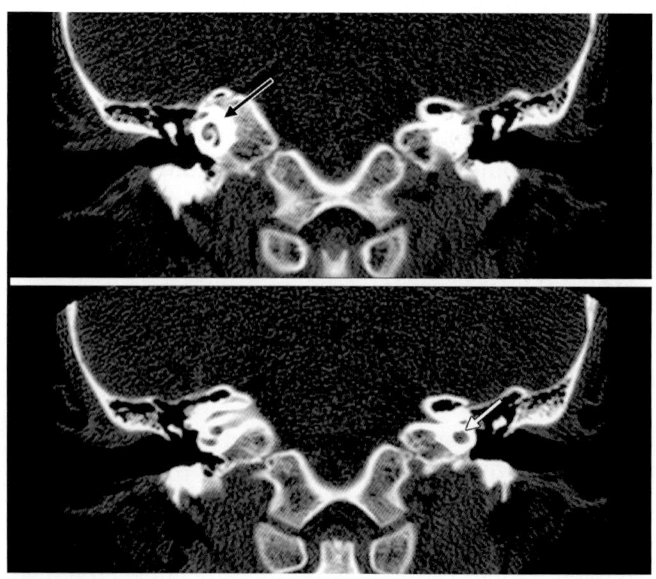

Fig. 7B: Mondini defect: Coronal images showing absence of middle and apical turns of cochlea (white arrow). Note mode of normal cochlear turn on opposite side (black arrow).

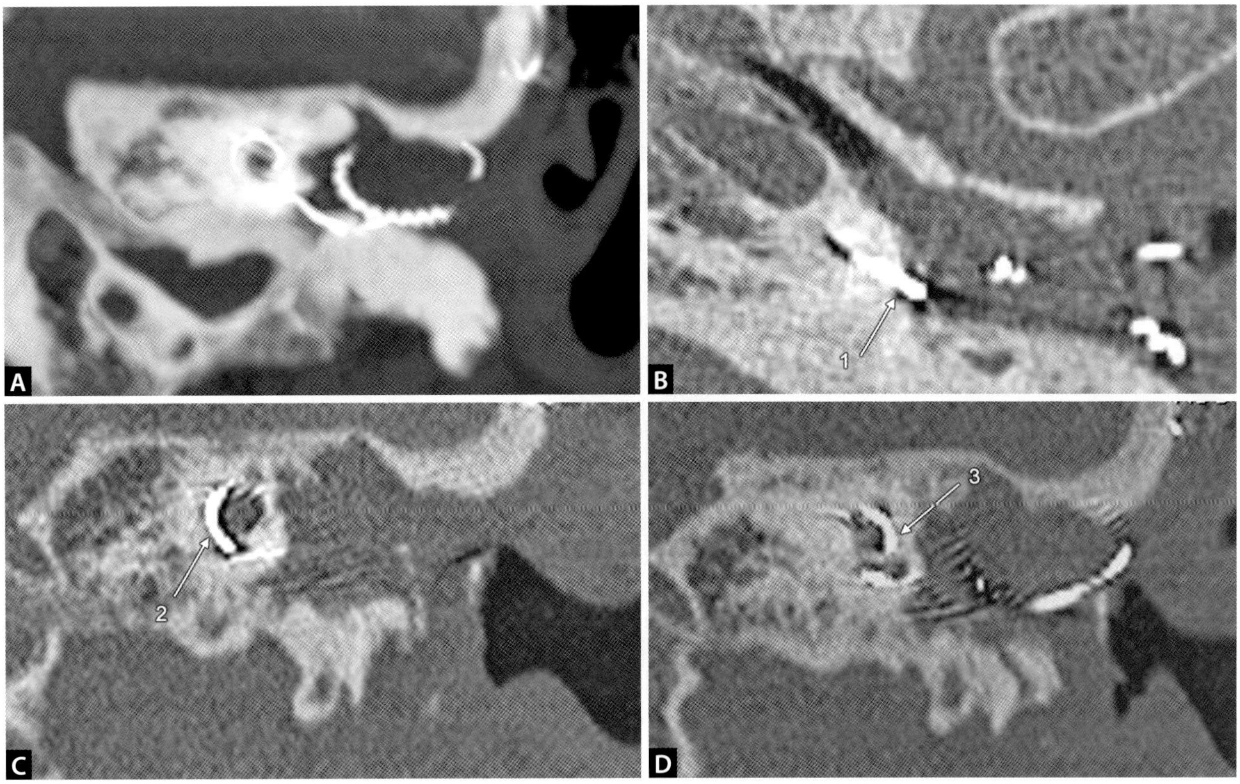

Figs. 8A to D: Coronal MIP (A), axial (B) and coronal (C and D) images of HRCT post-cochlear implant. Electrode is seen entering the round window (1) and further into the cochlear basal turn (2) and outer turn (3).

A persistent stapedial artery is an uncommon vascular anomaly. The artery branches from the infracochlear carotid artery and enters the tympanic facial canal via the stapedial obturator foramen. It usually enlarges the canal and exits the canal at the geniculate ganglion to become the middle meningeal artery.[3-5]

Jugular bulb dehiscence or jugular diverticula are venous abnormalities and are described in the sections on pulsatile tinnitus.

Temporal Bone Fractures

Plain X-ray examination is inadequate in demonstrating temporal bone fractures. In a study, only 17–30% of fractures could be demonstrated on plain X-rays.[12] Diagnosis of fractures is primarily done by CT. MR examination is supplementary in evaluation of temporal bone fractures and is used to evaluate associated intracranial pathologies, e.g. hemorrhage or contusions in the adjacent brain.[12]

Computed tomography examination of the temporal bone consists of routine surveys of the temporal bone by 5 mm thick sections, followed by high resolution scan for assessing the petromastoid complex.[12,13] Fractures of the squamous temporal bone can be easily identified on routine scans. The petromastoid fractures are identified on HRCT and are of two types: longitudinal and transverse.

Fractures of the petromastoid that are parallel to the long axis of the petrous bone are called longitudinal fractures **(Fig. 9)**. There are two subtypes—anterior and posterior.[13] The anterior subtype involves the tegmen, glenoid fossa and facial nerve together with the squamous temporal bone. The posterior subtype involves the facial nerves, ossicular chain and mastoid. The fractures line passes through the mastoid or along the external auditory canal which is the path of least resistance. The inner ear structures are usually spared, however, as the fracture line passes through the middle ear, there is high incidence of ossicular disruption, the incudostapedial joint being the most common. Tympanic membrane perforation occurs frequently when there is involvement of the external auditory canal. Although, the principle fracture line runs parallel to the longitudinal axis of petrous pyramid, orthogonal fractures convert this seemingly simple injury into more complex lesions. Facial paralysis is found in 10–20% of patients but usually has delayed presentation and is often incomplete.

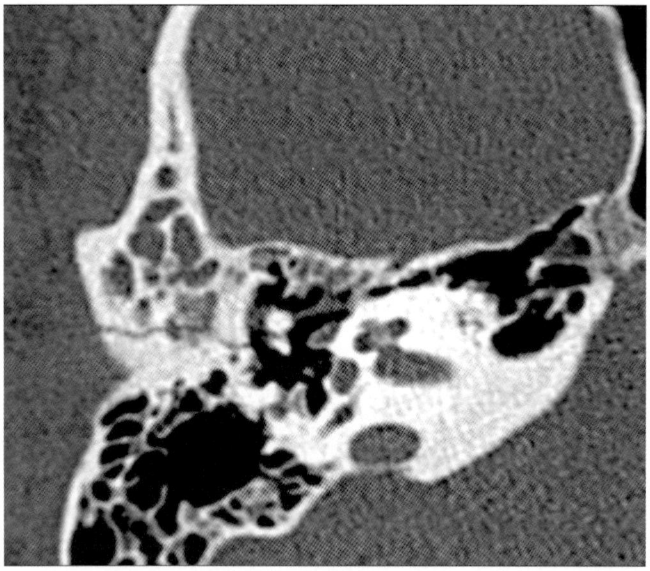

Fig. 9: Longitudinal fracture of the left temporal bone on axial HRCT. The fracture line runs in the long axis of the petrous bone. Ossicular chain was not disrupted and the mastoid air cells are filled with blood which appears as soft tissue density.

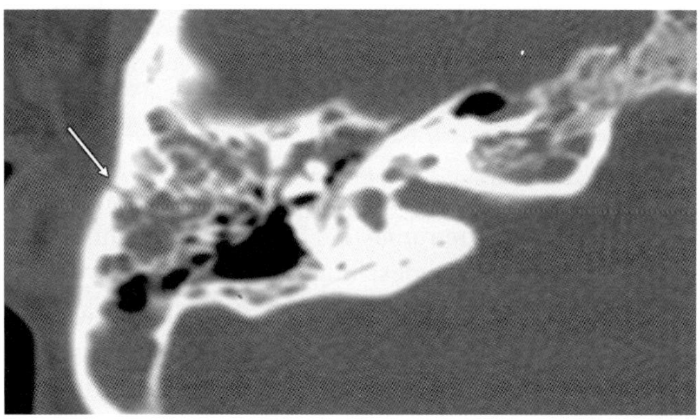

Fig. 10: Axial HRCT section shows a transverse fracture. The fracture line causes disruption of the ice cream cone configuration of the middle ear ossicles. Note blood (soft tissue) in the middle ear and mastoid.

Transverse fractures are less common than longitudinal petromastoid fractures. They occur perpendicular to the long axis of the petrous ridge **(Fig. 10)**. The etiology of these injuries is thought to be due to a force from the occiput towards the temporal bone and hence is associated with multiple fractures of the skull base. They are of two types, medial or lateral, depending upon the relative position of the fracture line in relation to the arcuate eminence. These fractures commonly involve the bony labyrinth. A 50% of patients may have facial paralysis. The facial nerve can be transected and the resulting deficit can be permanent.[14,15] The bony labyrinth, vestibule and internal auditory canal may be involved resulting in severe vertigo and sensorineural deafness. Complications associated with fractures, such as CSF rhinorrhea or otorrhea, merit an aggressive attempt either by cisternography or noncontrast MR to delineate the site of CSF leak so that attending sequelae can be avoided.[14]

Some authors have proposed a new system of classifying temporal bone fractures as "otic capsule sparing versus otic capsule violating". They believe that this system can be better in predicting the clinical outcome of these fractures.[16]

Inflammatory Diseases of the Temporal Bone

The CT is undoubtedly superior to demonstrate bony abnormalities along with detection and localization of soft tissue masses in inflammatory conditions of the temporal bone. However, MRI offers improved characterization of the soft tissue lesions associated with infections.

Inflammatory Conditions of the External Ear

Otitis externa: It can be diagnosed easily and treated adequately by topical antimicrobial therapy. However, in necrotizing or malignant otitis externa (MOE), imaging studies are required to delineate the extent and spread of the disease. This condition is typically seen in elderly diabetic patients. The most common organism causing MOE is *Pseudomonas*. The infection begins at the junction of the bony and cartilaginous segment of the EAC.[17]

In the early stage, CT shows abnormal contrast enhancement in the region of the external auditory canal. In the late phase, there is increase in the soft tissue thickness with bony destruction **(Fig. 11)**. The aggressive inflammation may rapidly extend into the parapharyngeal space, infratemporal fossa, middle and inner ear, and intracranially in the extradural space. The temporomandibular joint and retroauricular region may be involved. VI, VII, IX, X and XII cranial nerve palsies have been described. Extradural spread in the cranium may lead to sigmoid sinus thrombosis. MRI better shows changes in soft tissue and involvement of the retrocondylar fat pad on MRI has been proposed as an early diagnostic finding in patients being evaluated for MOE.[18]

Differential diagnosis includes basal cell carcinoma, squamous carcinoma, adenoid cystic carcinoma, or metastases.

External ear cholesteatoma: It arises due to periostitis of the bony canal. The sequestrum resulting from the periostitis embeds into the canal wall and grows through the

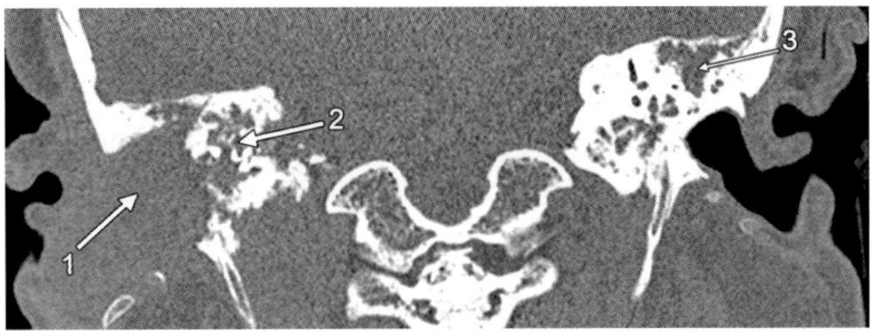

Fig. 11: Right malignant otitis externa causing destruction of the entire external auditory canal with presence of soft tissue (1) at its place with extention and destruction of the mastoid portion of the temporal bone (2). Note is made of the left mastoiditis (3).

Table 1: External autditory canal inflammatory conditions.

EAC cholesteatoma	Unilateral, rare, old age, pain and discharge	Soft tissue with erosions
Ketosis obturans	Bilateral, younger age, pain and conductive loss	Soft tissue with widened EAC but no erosions
Malignant otitis externa	Old age, immune-compromised, severe pain and discharge	Soft tissue with extensive bone destruction

epidermis to form a cholesteatoma. CT is primarily used to assess the bony erosion and in planning surgical approach. *Keratosis obturans* is a painful condition in which a plug of keratin obstructs the external auditory canal. It is a usually seen in middle aged adults and presents bilaterally. Bone erosion extending into the mastoid or middle ear is similar to the pattern seen with congenital cholesteatomas.[19]

Salient clinical and imaging features of impotant EAC inflammatory conditions are summarized in **Table 1**.

Inflammatory Condition of the Middle Ear

Otitis media: It is the term given to inflammation of the middle ear. It can be acute or chronic in nature.

Acute otitis media: The most common causative organisms of acute otitis media are *Streptococcus pneumoniae*, *Haemophilus influenzae*, and *Moraxella catarrhalis*. The term acute otomastoiditis denotes infection of the middle ear and mastoid. Acute otomastoiditis is diagnosed on CT as opacification of middle ear and mastoid cells with or without air fluid levels. The bony septae within the mastoid and the mastoid cortex are preserved when there is destruction and/or resorption of bony septate, the term coalescent otomastoiditis is used. Subperiosteal abscesses may form when the retained pus in a closed mastoid erodes through the mastoid cortex. Bezold's abscess is the term given to an abscess formed in the soft tissue of neck when pus discharges from the tip of the affected mastoid. Perisinus, extradural, or parenchymal abscesses can form when the medial cortex of mastoid is breached. A fistula between the external auditory canal forms when pus discharges spontaneously from a breach in the anterior cortex of the mastoid **(Fig. 12)**.

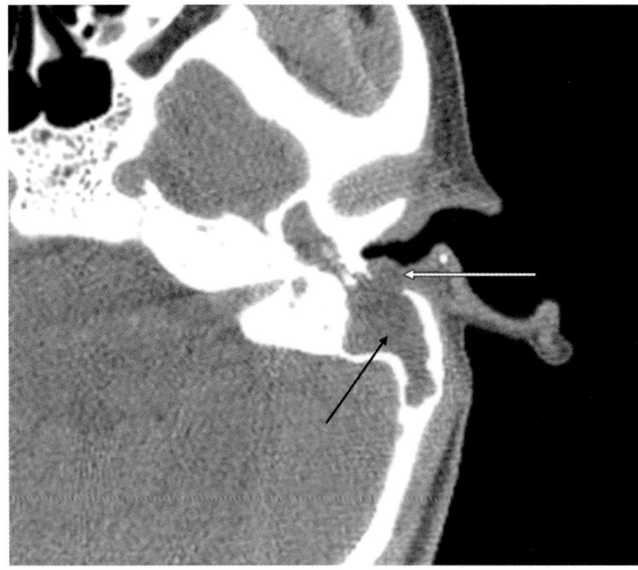

Fig. 12: Complicated acute otomastoiditis. There is evidence of coalescent otomastoiditis (black arrow) with fistulous communication between external auditory canal and mastoid antrum (white arrow).

Chronic otits media: Acute otitis media frequently progresses to chronic otitis media. It causes either effusion or formation of granulation tissue. If not diagnosed or treated, complications of chronic otits media may result. Inflammatory effusion in the middle ear associated with chronic otitis media is also termed as serous otitis. Presence of air-fluid level in two orthogonal planes helps in diagnosing this condition. However, in many patients opaque middle ear may be present rendering it difficult to diagnose this condition.

Granulation tissue: It is a common finding in chronic otitis media and is diagnosed when debris is present in the middle ear cavity or in mastoid. On CT, it has variable density and on MRI it usually enhances. However, there is absence of any bony changes or mass effect on both these modalities **(Fig. 13)**.

Cholesterol granulomas: It is a type of granulation tissue which needs separate mention as this entity can be mistaken for a vascular mass otoscopically owing to its hemorrhagic component. It is formed due to foreign body

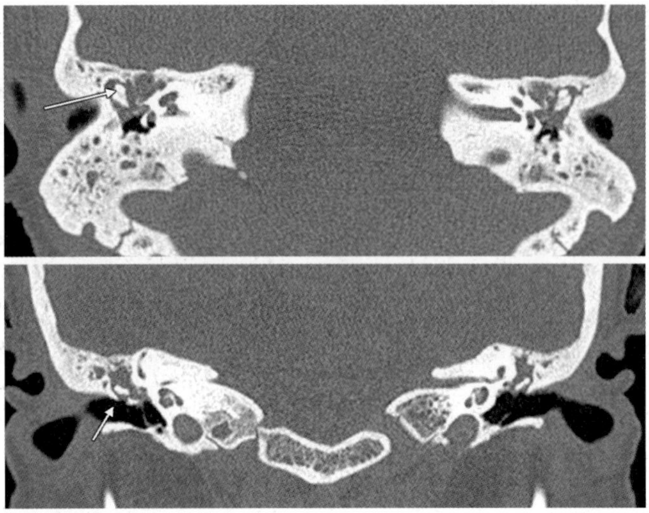

Fig. 13: Bilateral CSOM: soft tissue in the epitympanum likely granulation tissue on both sides without erosion of the ossicles (long arrow) or the scutum (short arrow).

Table 2: Inflammatory lesion of the middle ear on MRI.

Lesion	T1WI	T2WI	Post-contrast T1WI	DWI
Granulation tissue	Dark	Bright	Present	No
Cholesterol granuloma	Bright	Bright	No	Variable
Cholesteatoma	Dark	Bright	No	Yes

response to the cholesterol crystals in the middle ear. Since it is a type of granulation tissue, the features of mass effect are absent which helps to differentiate it from vascular tumors. Also, presence of history of chronic otitis media helps in the diagnosis.

On MRI, it is hyperintense on all pulse sequences because of extracellular methemoglobin. It can occur anywhere in the middle ear; other common location is petrous apex where it can be seen even without history of chronic otitis media.

The main differentiating features of various important inflammatory lesions seen in middle ear on MR imaging is given in **Table 2**.

COMPLICATIONS

The important complications of otitis media are tympanic membrane retraction, acquired cholesteatomas and ossicular fixation and erosions.

Acquired Cholesteatomas

They are collections of keratinous debris from an ingrowth of stratified squamous epithelium through a perforated

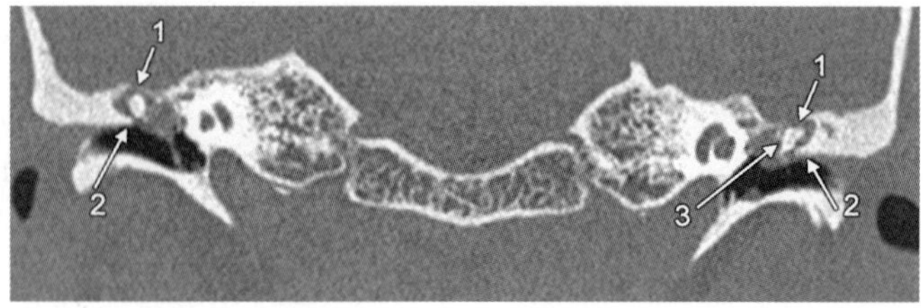

Fig. 14: Case of bilateral acquired cholesteatomas with erosion of Tegmen tympani (1), erosion of scutum (2) and erosion of ossicles (3).

tympanic membrane. Acquired cholesteatomas are of inflammatory etiology and are of two types. The more common variety arises from the pars flaccida of the tympanic membrane and the second variety arises from the pars tensa of the tympanic membrane. The former are called attic cholesteatomas and the latter are called sinus cholesteatomas.[20,21]

The CT features of cholesteatomas are a nondependent soft tissue mass in typical locations with or without erosions of surrounding bony structures.[22] Attic cholesteatomas are best demonstrated on coronal section while the sinus cholesteatomas are easily identifiable on axial or coronal sections **(Fig. 14)**.

Complete radiographic evaluation of cholesteatomas should include a description of the location of the soft tissue mass, presence of erosion of the margins of the middle ear cavity, status of the ossicular chain and presence of anatomic variants which might affect the surgical approach to the middle ear cavity.[23]

On MRI, the cholesteatomas are hypointense on T1WI and hyperintense on T2WI. They usually do not exhibit any contrast enhancement. However, the peripheral enhancing rim may be seen occasionally. Some authors have advocated delayed MR imaging in cases where differentiation from inflammatory or granulation tissue is doubtful. MRI after 45 minutes following contrast injection may show continued enhancement of inflammatory or granulation tissue and not in cholesteatomas. Also, diffusion weighted imaging has a role as cholesteatomas are hyperintense on $b = 1000/m^2$. In diffusion non-EPI turbo spin echodiffusion sequences give better signal to noise ratio than conventional EPI sequences.[24,25]

The complications of cholesteatomas are disabling and at times life-threatening because there is risk of infection spreading intracranially giving rise to meningitis, otogenic abscesses and sinovenous thrombosis. Ossicular destruction is the most common complication of cholesteatomas.[26,27] The long process of the incus is the most common segment of the ossicular chain which is

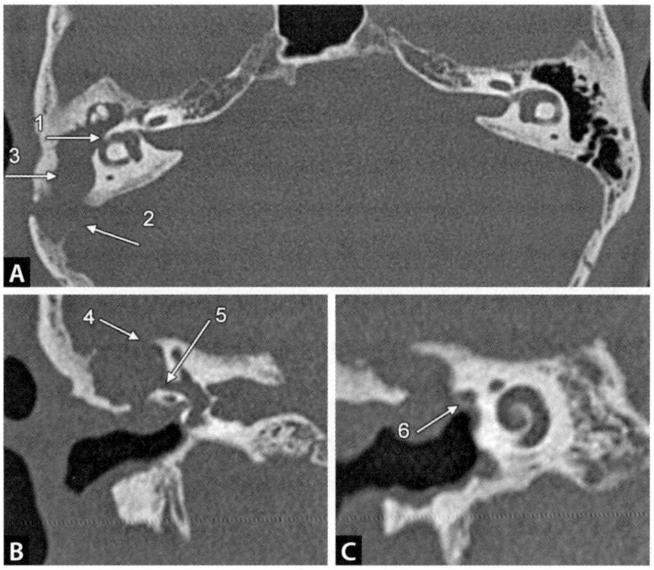

Fig. 15A to C: Right CSOM with cholesteatoma: Axial (A) and coronal (B and C) HRCT sections of patient showing fistula between middle ear and lateral semicircular canal (1 and 5) and almost complete erosion of the sinus plate (2) and tegmen tympani (4). Almost the entire mastoid air cells and epitympanum is filled with soft tissue (3). Additionally, there is dehiscence of bony canal of facial nerve in its tympanic segment (6).

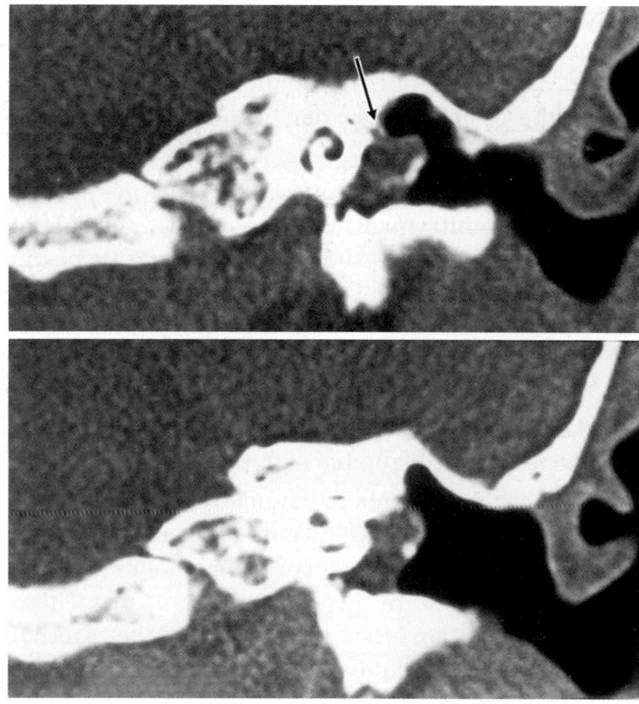

Fig. 16: Facial canal dehiscence due to cholesteatoma: The coronal HRCT shows the facial canal is exposed and the cholesteatoma is adherent to it (arrow).

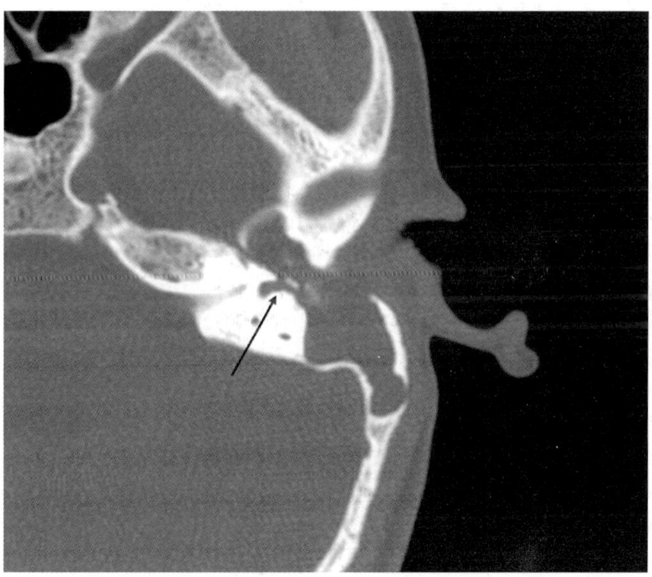

Fig. 15D: Cholesteatoma leading to fistula between lateral semicircular canal and the middle ear cavity (arrow).

affected. The other serious complications which should be evaluated are the presence of labyrinthine fistula which occurs when the bone over the lateral semicircular canal is eroded. This diagnosis can be made with confidence when the soft tissue mass is in direct opposition with membranous portion of the labyrinth **(Figs. 15A to D)**.[27]

The facial nerve canal which may be focally dehiscent in normal individual is another important structure which is frequently eroded by aggressive cholesteatomas. Soft tissue masses abutting the horizontal segment of the facial canal with the presence of erosion and with the clinical evidence of facial palsy, suggests that the facial nerve that has been involved by the inflammatory process, is of importance **(Fig. 16)**. Erosion of either the tegmen tympani and the sigmoid sinus plate is a setting for spread of infection into the intracranial cavity.[27,28]

OTHER COMPLICATIONS

In children, noncholesteatomatous inflammatory processes affecting the middle ear occur due to eustachian tube obstruction from nasopharyngeal lymphoid hypertrophy. These conditions are broadly termed as tubotympanic diseases. Middle ear effusion, chronic otitis media, granulation tissue, postinflammatory ossicular erosions and ossicular fixation are sequelae encountered in this condition. Middle ear effusions are seen as fluid/soft tissue opacities in the middle ear cavity. There are no erosions of the ossicles. Noninflammatory effusion may be due to a pressure phenomenon and can be seen in patients after air travel in poorly pressurized aircraft.[29]

Ossicular erosions can rarely occur with uncomplicated otitis media. The long process of the incus is commonly affected. Erosions appear as punched out small lytic area on the ossicles. Ossicular fixation occurs due to postinflammatory fibrosis.

Gradenigo's syndrome is a manifestation of petrous apicitis when purulent otitis media is associated with ipsilateral lateral rectus palsy and pain along distributions of the 6th cranial nerve. But the classical presentation of this syndrome is seldom seen. The pathology is explained on the basis of irritation of the 6th cranial nerve as it travels beneath the petroclinoid ligament and irritation of the gasserian ganglion by the inflammatory process in the petrous apex due to disruption of the bony cortex.[29]

Antral cholesteatomas are less common than those found within the middle ear and are diagnosed when a larger than normal smooth walled cavity containing nondependent soft tissue densities are seen within the antrum. These cholesteatomas then erode anteriorly into the external canal or involve the petrous apex via the facial canal.[29]

Inflammatory Conditions of the Inner Ear

Labyrinthitis is the term used to describe inflammation of the membranous labyrinth. Viruses are the most common etiologic agents. But it may also be due to bacterial, luetic or of autoimmune origin. Tuberculous labyrinthitis has also been described.[29]

Labyrinthitis can also be classified as tympanogenic, meningogenic, hematogenic and post-traumatic.

Tympanic labyrinthitis occurs when infection from the middle ear spread to the labyrinth via the oval or round windows, or via a labyrinthine fistula. The latter is commonly associated with cholesteatoma. Infections can travel into the inner ear following surgery and are termed iatrogenic tympanogenic labyrinthitis.

Meningogenic labyrinthitis occurs when infection spreads along CSF spaces via the internal auditory canal or cochlear aqueduct. Labyrinthitis is usually bilateral.

Hematogenic labyrinthitis is caused due to spread of infection by the bloodstream. Viruses, e.g. measles and mumps; syphilis and tuberculosis and other bacterial infections spread by this route.

Post-traumatic labyrinthitis can also occur as a complications of trauma.

Bilateral labyrinthitis leads to profound sensorineural deafness. CT is usually normal in acute and subacute labyrinthitis. Ossification of the fluid-filled labyrinth spaces in late chronic phase appears as areas of increased densities. The best method of diagnosis is by contrast enhanced MR. On the enhancement of cochlea or vestibule is pathognomic for labrynthitis. MR contrast enhanced T1W images show moderate to intense enhancement within the normal fluid-filled structures of the inner ear. Some authors have also advocated use of FLAIR postcontrast images for diagnosing this enhancement.[30]

Usually viral conditions causes subtle contrast enhancement and bacterial especially pneumococcal labrynthitis causes intense enhancement.

A sequela of labyrinthitis is **fibrous obliterans** followed by **labyrinthitis ossification**. It is also called sclerosing labyrinthitis or chronic labyrinthitis.[29] Most common cause of labyrinthitis ossificans is suppurative bacterial labyrinthitis. This condition can also be associated with viral labyrinthitis, advanced otosclerosis, trauma, occlusion of labyrinthine artery, leukemia or following labyrinthectomy. Following suppurative labyrinthitis inflammation leads to fibroblast proliferation within the labyrinth. These fibroblasts differentiate into osteoblasts which lead on to osteoneogenesis and deposition of bone in the labyrinth. The most common site to see fibrosis and new bone formation is the basal turn of the cochlea near the round window niche. Dense sclerosis due to new bone formation is best appreciated on CT. Fibro-osseous changes can be appreciated on high resolution T2W MR images where the normal hyperintense fluid signal intensity of the labyrinth is replaced by intermediate or low signal from the encroaching fibro-osseous material.

It is important to distinguish the changes of labyrinthitis ossifications in the cochlear and pericochlear regions. The cochlear labyrinthitis ossification makes cocheal implantation difficult. A cochlear implant is a multicomponent electronic device which directly stimulates the auditory fibers in cochlea to provide auditory information. Typically the components include a microphone, a speech processor, a transmitter, a receiver and a stimulator. The stimulator wire is placed in the cochlea through the round window to directly stimulate the spiral ganglion cells and the cochlear axons. Placement of a cochlear implant is most effective in patients less than 2 years of age with profound sensorineural hearing impairment in whom hearing aids are not effective or beneficial. Prior to implantation a high resolution temporal bone CT or high resolution T2 MRI study is required to assess the changes in and around the bony labyrinth. Labyrinthine aplasia is an absolute contraindication for an implant. Cochlear labyrinthitis ossificans is a relative contraindication presumably because it can hinder the placement of the stimulator. Other relative contraindications include conditions which may influence the surgical approach, such as aberrant course of the facial nerve, otomastoiditis, fenestral and cochlear otosclerosis and the aberrant course of the internal carotid artery. An ipsilateral brainstem infarct detected on MR scanning of the brain would also be a contraindication for cochlear implantation.[31]

RADIOLOGICAL EVALUATION OF VASCULAR TINNITUS AND VASCULAR TYMPANIC MEMBRANE

Vascular tinnitus is a common complaint pertaining to the ear. The term tinnitus refers to rhythmic sound heard by the patient. This sound may or may not be synchronous with the radial pulse. Nonpulsatile synchronous tinnitus is usually associated with muscular dysfunction, such as myoclonus of the tensor tympani muscle or the palatal muscles. Synchronous tinnitus, also referred to as pulsatile tinnitus is the condition which is of radiological significance. It is classified as objective or subjective. By objective pulsatile tinnitus, authors refer to the tinnitus which is audible to the observing physician as well as the patient, and subjective tinnitus is one which is audible only to the patient. Tinnitus may be caused by extrinsic causes, such as muscular or vascular diseases, or may be due to intrinsic pathologies like vestibulocochlear dysfunction.[31,32]

Causes of Pulsatile Tinnitus[33]

- *Normal vascular variants:*
  - *Arterial variants*: Aberrant/laterally displaced carotid artery, persistent stapedial artery, persistent trigeminal artery, anomalous artery in the stria vascularis of the cochlea
  - *Venous variants*: Large jugular bulb, large emissary veins, idiopathic venous tinnitus, jugular bulb diverticulum.
- *Pathological vascular causes:*
  - *Arterial causes*: Carotid artery dissection, aneurysms of the petrous carotid/anterior communicating artery aneurysms, atherosclerosis, fibromuscular dysplasia, arteritis.
  - *Arteriovenous vascular causes:* Glomustympanicum/glomus jugulare AVMs intracranial arteriovenous malformation, e.g. cerebral AVMs, dural AV fistulas and direct AV fistulas, otosclerosis, Paget's disease of bone, miscellaneous vascular tumors, such as hemangiomas, jugular meningiomas histiocytosis and cholesterol granulomas.
  - *Venous causes:* Pregnancy, anemia, thyrotoxicosis, hypertension, transverse sinus stenosis.

Normal Vascular Variants

Aberrant position of the internal carotid artery is thought to be due to abnormal regression of the cervical ICA during embryogenesis resulting in opening of and enlargement of collateral arteries, such as the anastomosis between the carotid tympanic artery anastomosis between the caroticotympanic artery and the inferior tympanic artery. The aberrant artery, therefore, courses through the middle ear over the cochlear promontory to join the horizontal carotid canal via a dehiscence in the carotid plate. The findings on HRCT are characteristic in that the posterior carotid plate is absent and that the horizontal part of the carotid canal appears to merge with the lateral cochlear promontory. Variations of the jugular bulb include a very high riding jugular bulb. This normal variant is associated with well-defined bony margins of the jugular foramen. When the caroticojugular plate is deficient, the condition is termed as dehiscent jugular bulb. Jugular bulb diverticulum is a finger like extension of the jugular bulb in the cephalad direction. Ecstatic loops of AICA/PICA or tortuous course of vertebral artery going into the internal auditory meatus may cause tinnitus due to compression on the VIII nerve complex **(Figs. 17A and B)**.

Pathological Vascular Causes

Arterial Causes

Dissection of the internal carotid artery can be spontaneous or traumatic. Angiographic appearances include intimal flaps, with or without occlusion. MRI will show loss of flow void which suggest occlusion of the artery. If there is intraluminal hemorrhage, a hyperintense signal will be observed in the affected artery. Petrous carotid aneurysms and AVMs can be detected on digital subtraction angiography (DSA). Atherosclerosis of the carotid artery at times produces pulsatile tinnitus. Atherosclerotic plaques may produce turbulence of carotid flow which manifests as pulsatile tinnitus. Fibromuscular dysplasia (FMD) is a segmental noninflammatory, nonatheromatous vasculopathy. It is seen in 0.5–0.6% of carotid angiograms and autopsies. It is a disease which affects medium-size muscular arteries. Vertebral and renal arteries can also be affected apart from the extracranial arteries. It is associated with intracranial berry aneurysms. Middle-aged females are most commonly affected. Unlike atherosclerotic

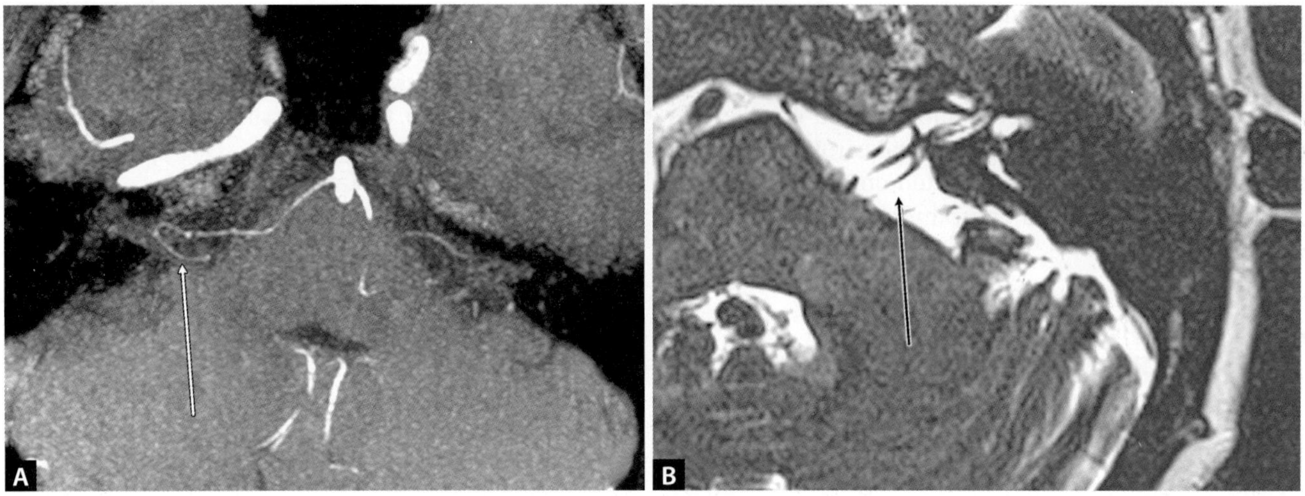

Figs. 17A and B: Axial magnetic resonance angiography (MRA) and CISS images showing loops of AICA in the right and left IAC, respectively (arrows).

plaques fibromuscular dysplasia affects the cervical internal carotid arteries at the level of the first two cervical vertebrae. Hence, these patients generally present with symptoms of vascular tinnitus more frequently unlike those with atherosclerosis. The classical angiographic appearance of FMD is the string of beads appearance which is seen in 85% of patients. Successful treatment of FMD by transluminal angioplasty has been reported.[34,35]

Arteriovenous Causes

The diagnosis of cerebral AVMs and dural AV fistulas and direct AV fistulas depends upon the clinical presentation apart from that of pulsatile tinnitus **(Figs. 18A and B)**. Angiography is the gold standard in demonstration of the vascular lesions which may be partly delineated on CT scans and MRI. Paget's disease and otosclerosis are representative bony pathologies associated with neovascularization and AV shunting, resulting in pulsatile tinnitus.[32]

Amongst the group of arteriovenous causes, paragangliomas or glomus tumors are the typical lesions which require radiographic evaluation.[32] Glomus tumors of the temporal bone are the most common neoplastic cause of pulsatile tinnitus and vascular tympanic membrane. Tumors commonly involve the jugular bulb and/or the tympanic cavity. CT scan will help to delineate whether the lesion is confined within the tympanic cavity or involves the jugular bulb. If the lesion is confined within the tympanic cavity, no further investigation is required **(Figs. 19A and B)**. If the lesion is seen to extend to involve the jugular foramen and beyond, CT examination is continued up to the carotid bifurcation to see the complete extent of the lesion and to rule out multicentricity. An MR examination will help in assessing the involvement of internal jugular vein. On MR high resolution T1WI, a flow void pattern can be appreciated. On post-contrast T1WI, intense enhancement is seen. Post-contrast MR angiography shows relatively low signal of the tumor with high signal intensity spots inside due to high flow in feeding vessels **(Fig. 20)**.

Venous Tinnitus

Venous tinnitus unlike arterial tinnitus is heard as a continuous murmur accentuated during systole. It is caused by turbulent flow in the venous structures around the ear. It is usually heard on the side of the dominant jugular vein which is usually on the right side. A venous hum is physiological and can be elicited in an 80% of pregnant women and in the lower jugular vein in 50% of normal individuals. Venous tinnitus is also observed in patients of thyrotoxicosis, anemia and hypertension.[32]

Venous tinnitus may be the presenting symptom of intracranial hypertension. It is believed that tinnitus in conditions of raised intracranial tension is related to CSF pressures and compression of dural sinuses by transmitted intracranial arterial pulsations. Raised intracranial hypertension can manifest as pulsatile tinnitus as well. Conditions, such as aqueduct stenosis, Chiari I malformation, pneumocephalus and idiopathic intracranial hypertension can present with tinnitus which can be the role symptoms of the underlying pathology.

Venous tinnitus can also be caused by stenosis of the transverse sinuses. This can be idiopathic and unrelated to dural arteriovenous fistula. A large or exposed jugular bulb or laterally placed sigmoid sinus also has been associated with venous tinnitus.[32]

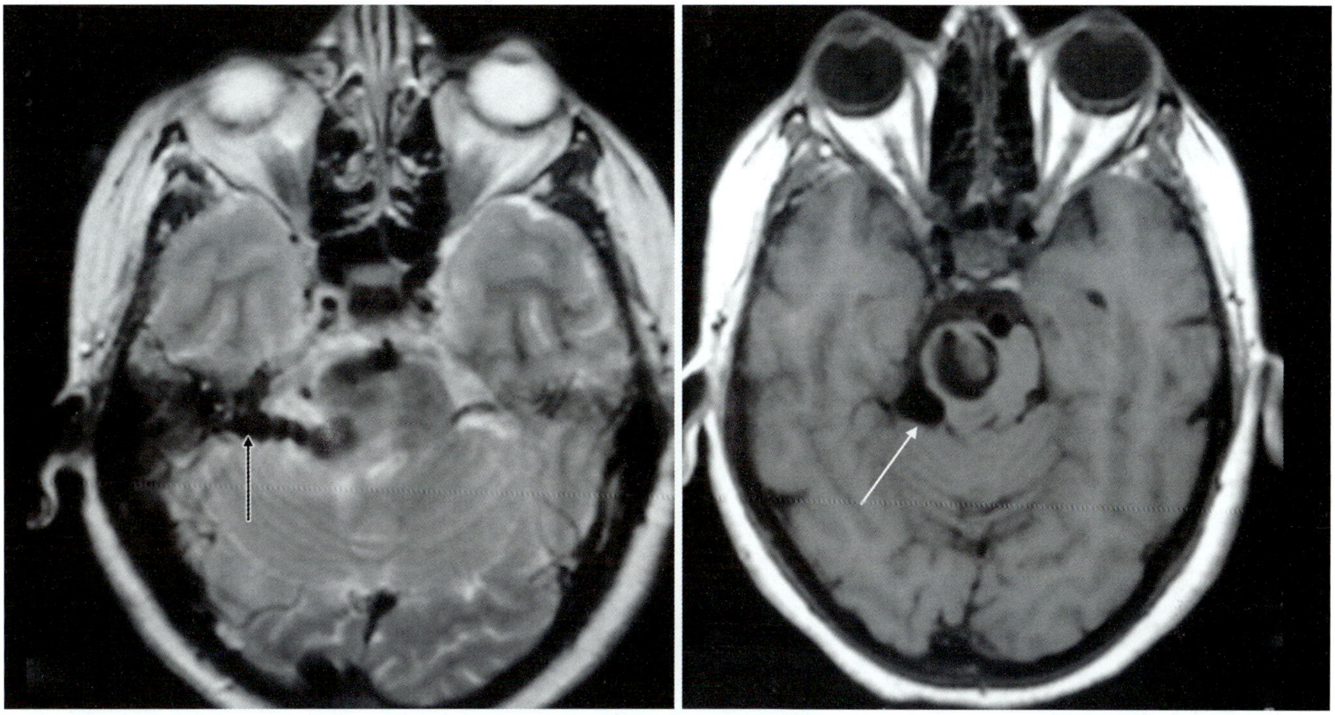

Fig. 18A: Dural AVM as cause of tinnitus: MR T2- and T1WI showing multiple flow voids in the right CP angle region and in pre- and perimesencephalic cistern.

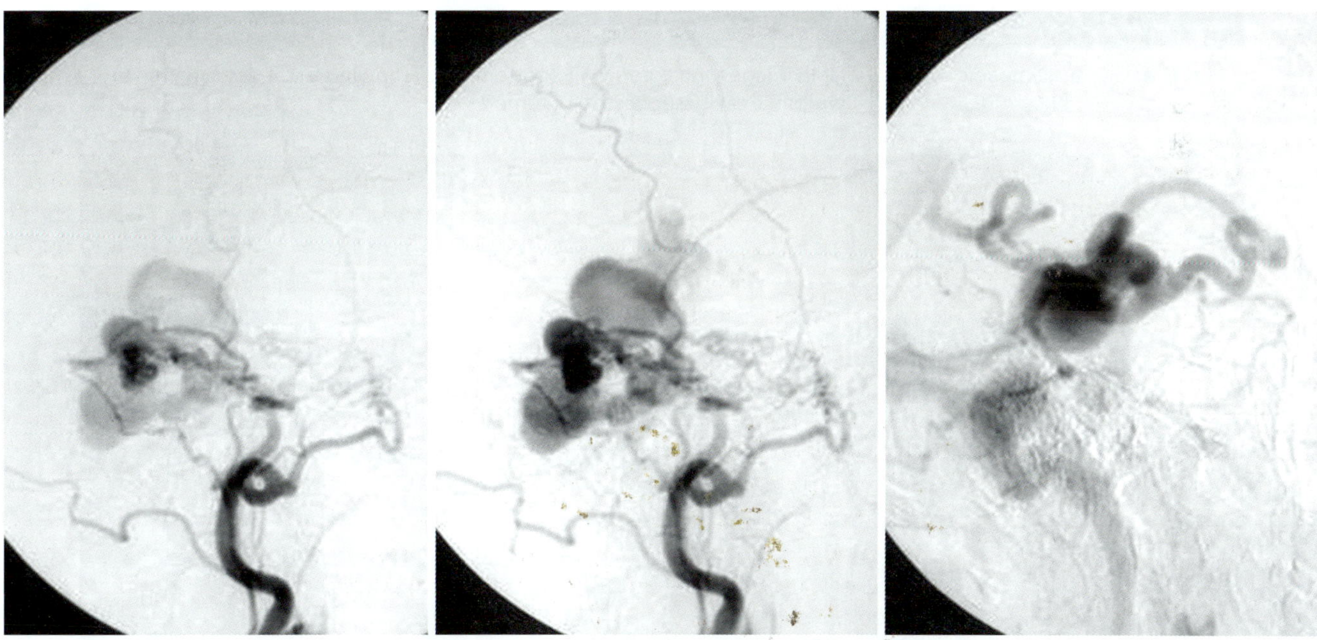

Fig. 18B: DSA images of the same showing a dural AVM being fed by branches of right external carotid artery and draining through ecstatic veins into ipsilateral sigmoid sinus and internal jugular vein (IJV).

Otosclerosis

Otosclerosis represents foci of spongy vascular haversian bone in the ivory like endochondral bone of the otic capusle.[36] Otosclerosis is bilateral in up to 90% of patients. It is of two types: cochlear and fenestral. The cochlear variety is rare and presents with sensorineural deafness. CT is the modality of choice in diagnosing this entity. CT diagnosis of cochlear otosclerosis is based upon locating variable sized

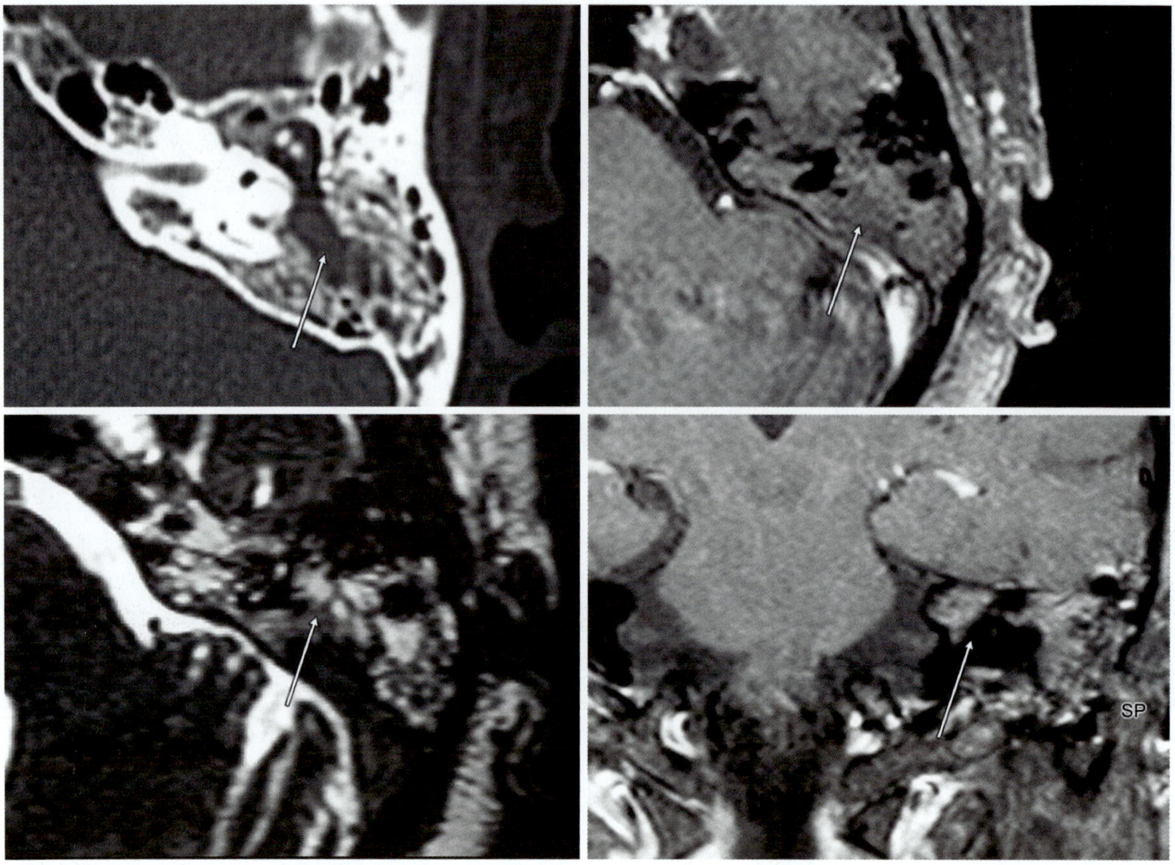

Fig. 19A: Glomus tympanicum: Axial CT, MR images and coronal MR (bottom right) showing a soft tissue within the tympanic cavity suggestive of tumor.

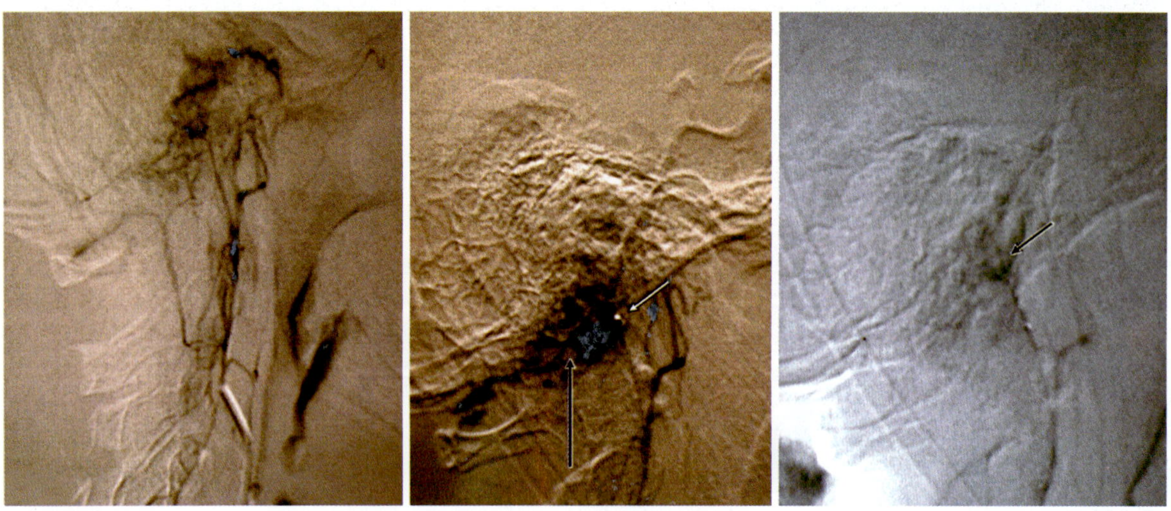

Fig. 19B: Glomus tympanicum: DSA images showing blush in the region of middle ear on ascending pharyngeal artery injection (left), microcatheter injection (tip shown by white arrow) showing intense localized tumor blush (large black arrow) and absence of blush after preoperative embolization (small black arrow).

regions of demineralization. On HRCT, cochlear otosclerosis appears as radiolucent foci in a pericochlear distribution. In very severe cases there is a hypodense ring surrounding the cochlea giving a "double ring sign". In chronic cases mixed dense and lucent foci can be seen around the bony labyrinth. Fenestral otosclerosis presents as similar lesion but they are

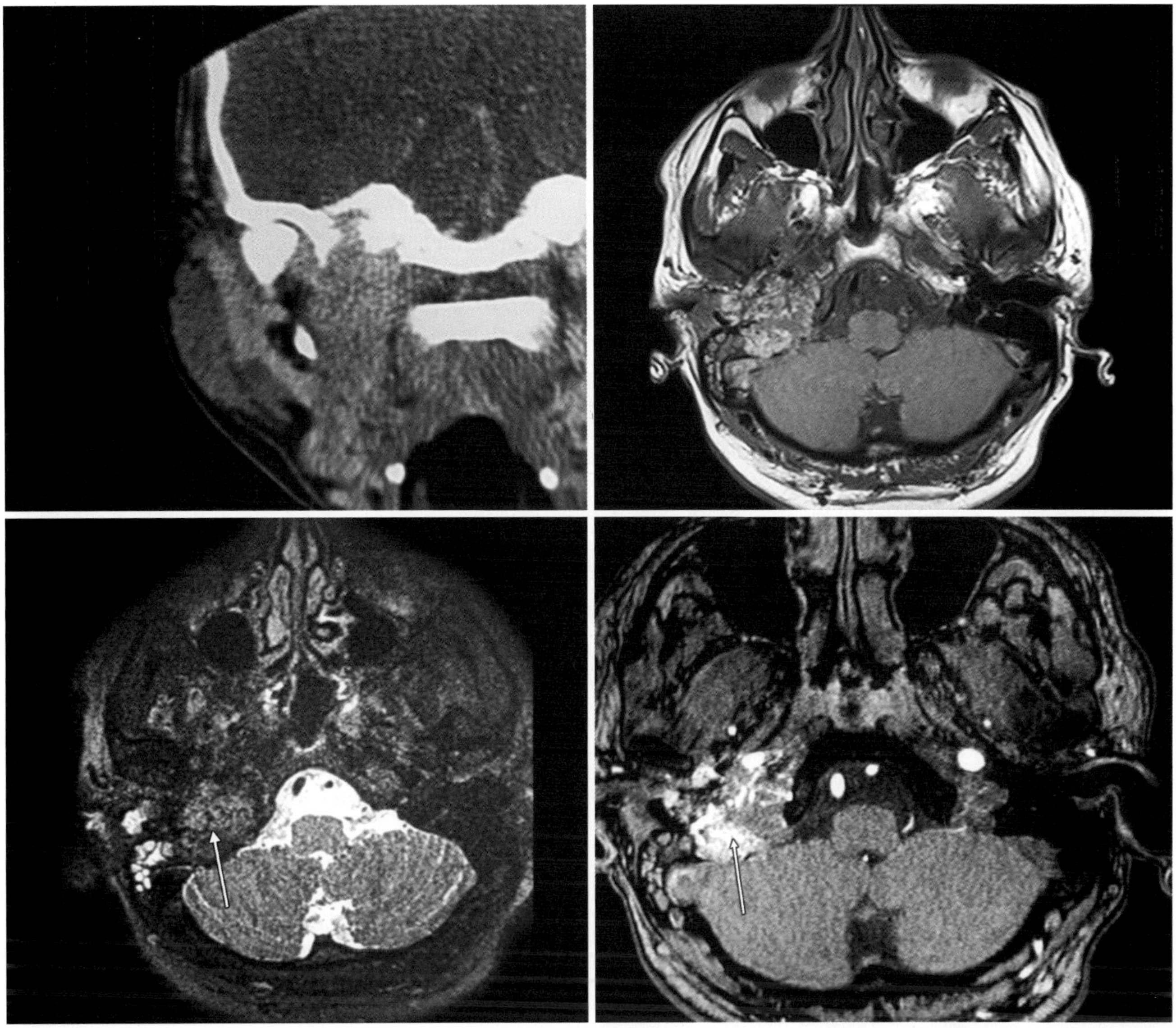

Fig. 20: Glomus jugulare: Contrast-enhanced axial CT, T1WI, T2WI, contrast MRA. All images showing a large mass lesion in the right jugular fossa with typical features of glomus tumor. Note hypointense flow voids on T2WI (black arrow) which are better seen as bright areas on contrast MRA (white arrow).

clustered around the oval and round windows. Fenestral otosclerosis may coexist with cochlear lesions. MR findings of otosclerosis include a ring of intermediate signal intensities in the pericochlear and perilabyrinthine regions on T1WI. Postcontrast T1WI may reveal enhancing pericochlear foci which represent active lesions not detected on HRCT. T2WI may not be useful as early lesions may be missed and chronic lesions may only appear as subtle pericochlear high signal areas. It is important to distinguish cochlear otosclerosis from labyrinthitis ossificans. Labyrinthitis ossificans present as bony encroachment of the membranous labyrinths with progressive loss of the fluid-filled spaces of the labyrinth, unlike otosclerosis which presents as erosions around the labyrinth. Both the conditions are relative contraindication for placement of cochlear implants and are therefore important differential diagnoses.

Fenestral otosclerosis is more common than cochlear otosclerosis. Involvement of the oval window results in stapediovestibular compromise. Plaques of bone formation are present anterior to the oval window and are best seen in the axial HRCT sections. Axial sections also demonstrate narrowing of the oval window, thickening of the stapedial footplate and the annular ligament complex, best seen in the coronal HRCT sections. Prior to surgery, the radiological examination by HRCT is done by taking overlapping sections preferably on a helical scanner.

The position of the facial nerve, presence of ossicular fixation, position of jugular vein and internal carotid artery should be meticulously recorded. Differential diagnosis of fenestral otosclerosis include oval window tympanosclerosis and osteogenesis imperfecta.[37]

DYSPLASTIC CONDITIONS OF THE TEMPORAL BONE

Fibrous dysplasia, osteogenesis imperfecta, Paget's disease and progressive diaphyseal dysplasia are some of the other dysplastic conditions that affect the temporal bone.

Fibrous dysplasia is a disease characterized by progressive replacement of bone marrow by a mixture of disorganized bone matrix and fibrous tissue. CT scan is diagnostic and shows increased bone volume with a ground-glass appearance. Cystic, sclerotic and pagetoid appearance have been described. The cystic lesions contain more fibrous tissue and appear less dense that the predominantly bone containing dense sclerotic variety. Pagetoid variety of fibrous dysplasia contains both fibrous and osseous tissues.[38]

On MR high signal intensity on T1- and T2-weighted spin echo images with strong post-contrast images indicate acute phase of fibrous dysplasia.[39]

Paget's disease is a chronic condition of bone characterized by two phases: the osteolytic phase which is due to resorption of bone by osteoclasts and the osteosclerotic phase where there is increased new bone formation. The new bone is hard and dense **(Fig. 21)**. The petrous apex is the first segment to be affected and the otic capsule is the last to be affected. The calvarium is invariably involved and its characteristic appearance clinches the diagnosis.[38]

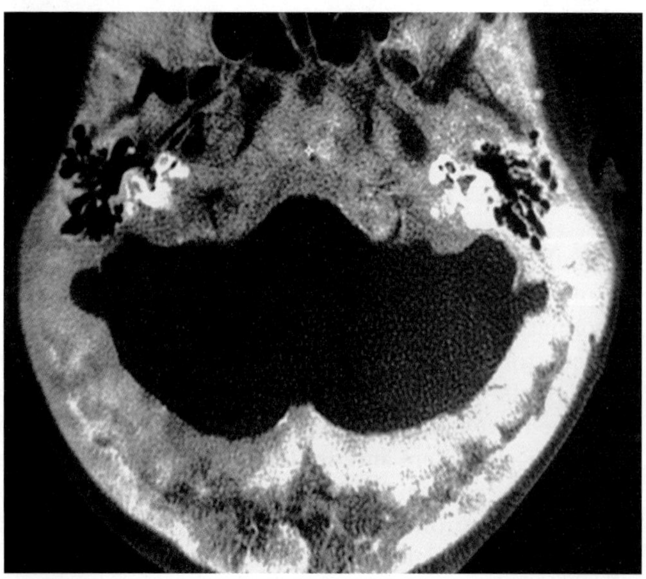

Fig. 21: Paget's disease involving the temporal bone. The bony labyrinth can be partly seen in the mass of thick bone. Both internal auditory canals are obliterated.

Tumors of the Temporal Bone

Primary bone tumors of the temporal bone are numerous and can be classified as carcinomas, sarcomas, metastases, benign epithelial lesions, hematological malignancies and histiocytosis.[40]

Neurogenic tumors of the temporal bone are commonly schwannom as associated with the facial nerve. Hemangiomas and congenital cholesteatomas are other common tumors associated with the temporal bone.[40]

Facial schwannomas can occur in the geniculate, tympanic or mastoid segments of the facial nerve; the geniculate segment being the most frequently involved segment. Symptoms of the tumors depend on the site of involvement hearing loss is present in approximately 70% of cases, followed by slowly progressive facial palsy in nearly 50% of cases.[37] Tumors distally beyond the stylomastoid foramen appear as asymptomatic masses in the neck. Geniculate ganglion schwannomas are the most common variety and they grow silently into the middle cranial fossa until they cause sensorineural deafness or facial nerve dysfunction. Facial schwannomas in the CP angle or internal auditory meatus present with sensorineural deafness.

Facial nerve schwannomas appears as sausage-shaped lesions along the course of the facial nerve with smooth erosion of the facial canal depending on the location of the lesion. Geniculate ganglion lesions cause smooth enlargement of the geniculate fossa, tympanic schwannomas project into the middle ear and the mastoid lesions appears as tubular lesions in the mastoid air cells.

On HRCT, they appear as soft tissue density lesions along the facial nerve. On T1WI, they are intermediate to low intensity lesion which are hyperintense on T2WI. There lesion show uniform contrast enhancement **(Fig. 22)**.

The list of tumors which may present with slowly progressive facial nerve palsy include hemangiomas, hamartomas, meningiomas and epidermoids. In elderly patients spread of parotid carcinomas upward along the facial nerve also needs to be ruled out.

Hemangiomas were considered to be rare tumors of the facial nerve, however, are now considered to be as common as facial neuromas.[41] These subset of tumors along with vascular malformations are termed intratemporal benign vascular lesions (IBVT). These tumors tend to invade the nerve rather than compress it and present with hemifacial spasm and facial palsy. On CT scan, their presence can be

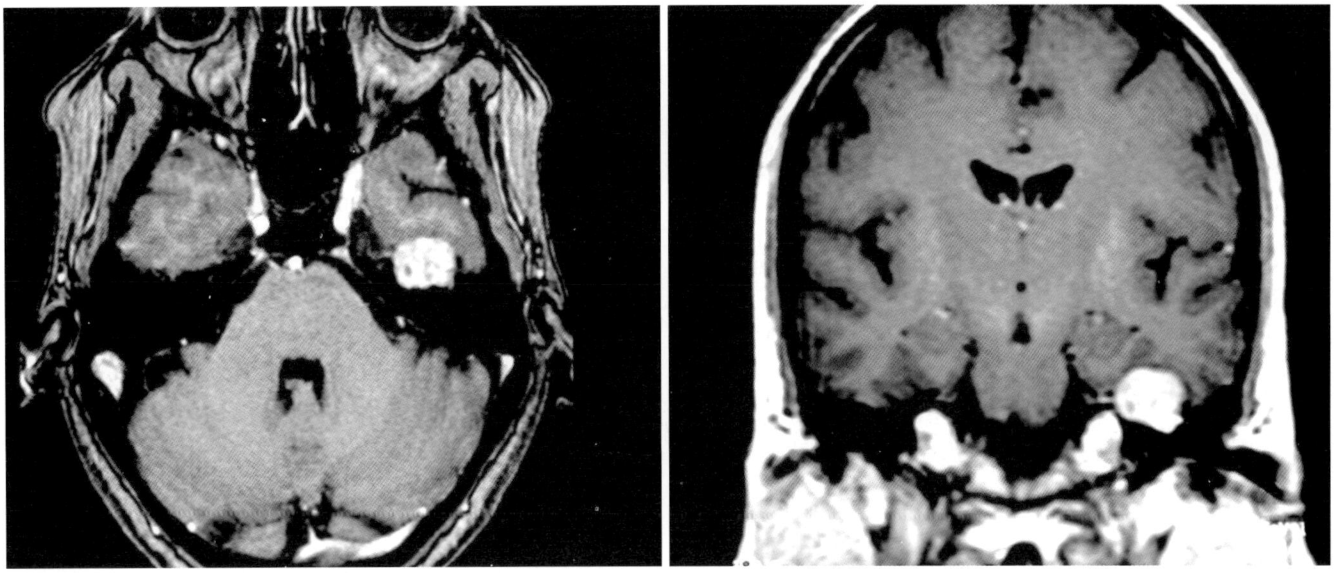

Fig. 22: Facial schwannoma: Axial and coronal contrast-enhanced T1W sections showing the lesion as a uniformly hyperintense lesion consistent with a geniculate facial schwannoma.

inferred by gas cisternography when in the labyrinthine and geniculate ganglion regions, these tumor cause erosions which are irregular with indistinct margins, give a reticular or "honeycomb" pattern to the eroded bone.[38] Since enhancement after contrast renders them isodense to surrounding bone, this is unnecessary with CT scan. On MRI these lesions are exquisitely delineated. They are isointense to mildly hyperintense on T2WI and markedly hyperintense on T1WI.

Congenital cholesteatoma or epidermoid cysts of the EAC appear as sharply defined mixed density lesions on CT. The core of the lesion may appear hypodense. On MRI, they are hypointense on T1WI images and hyperintense on T2W. These lesions can be also seen in the petrous apex, tympanic cavity or supralabyrinthine region.[41]

Common tumors of the bony external auditory canal are osteoma, and exostoses.[41] Osteoma of the external auditory canal is rare benign lesions which appears as dense pedunculated bony outgrowths from the external auditory canal. They are incidental lesions appearing similar to exostosis which are broad-based expanded bony lesions at or medial to the isthmus of the external auditory canal. Ceruminomas are glandular tumors arising from the apocrine seromucous glands or ectopic salivary gland of the external auditory canal. These are locally invasive tumor and are best treated by en bloc resection. Squamous cell carcinomas are by far the most common malignant tumor of the canal. Lesions appear as aggressive lytic areas of destruction of the walls of bony canal with contiguous spread into the middle ear cavity, temporomandibular joint, parotid gland, or carotid canal. A mass in the external auditory canal which aggressively destroys the adjacent bone suggests the presence of a squamous cell carcinoma. A noncontrast HRCT is the imaging modality of choice to assess the extent of bone destruction. Contrast-enhanced MR may be required for large lesions involving adjacent structures, such as the temporomandibular joint and parotid gland **(Fig. 23)**.[42]

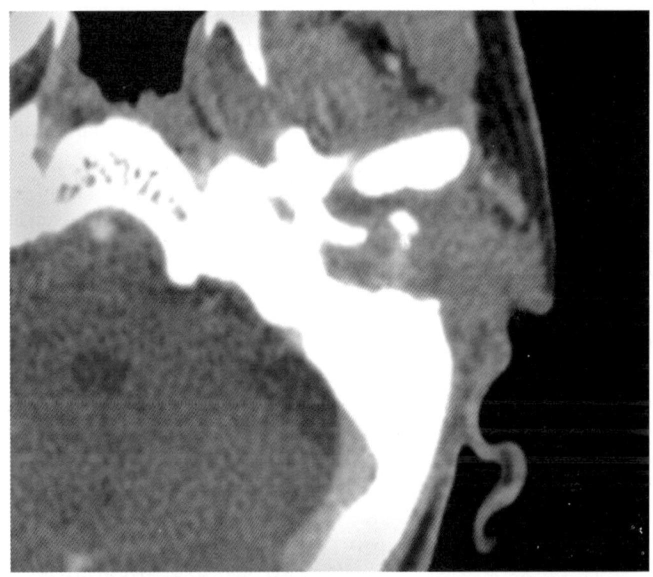

Fig. 23: Squamous cell carcinoma of the external auditory canal: Soft tissue mass fills the canal with partial destruction of the posterior wall of the canal.

REFERENCES

1. Brogan M, Chakeres DW. Computed tomography and magnetic resonance imaging of the normal anatomy of the temporal bone. Semin Ultrasound CT MR. 1989;10:178-94.
2. Eelkema EA, Curtin HD. Congenital anomalies of the temporal bone. Semin Ultrasound CTMR. 1989;10:195-212.
3. Chakeres DW, Augustyn MA. Temporal bone imaging. In: Som PM, Curtin HD (Eds). Head and Neck Imaging, 4th edition. St. Louis Mo: Mosby Year Book; 2003. pp. 1093-108.
4. Lane JI, Witte RJ, Bolster B, et al. State of the Art: 3T Imaging of the Membranous Labyrinth. Am J Neuroradiol. 2008;29:1436-40.
5. Romo LV Casselman JW, Robson CD. Temporal bone congenital anomalies. In: Som PM, Curtin HD (Eds). Head and Neck Imaging, 4th edition. St. Louis: Mosby Year Book; 2003. pp. 1109-72.
6. Swatz J, Faerber EN. Congenital malformations of the external and middle ear: High resolution CT findings of surgical import. Am J Roentgenol. 1985;144:501-6.
7. Jackler RK, Lusford WM, House WF. Congenital malformation of the inner ear. A classification based on embryogenesis. Laryngoscope. 1987;97:2-14.
8. Parry DA, Booth T, Roland PS. Advantages of magnetic resonance imaging over computed tomography in preoperative evaluation of pediatric cochlear implant candidates. Otol Neurotol. 2005;26:976-82.
9. Curtin HD, Vignaud J, Bar D. Anomaly of the facial canal in a Mondini malformation with recurrent meningitis. Radiology. 1982;144:335-41.
10. Curtin HD. Facial nerve canal. In: Vignaud J, Jordin C, Rosen L (Eds). The ear diagnostic imaging CT scanning, tomography and magnetic resonance. Paris: Masson; 1986.pp. 318-33.
11. Rodriguez K, Shah RK, Kenna M. Anomalies of the middle and inner ear. Otolaryngol Clin North Am. 2007;40:81-96.
12. Exadoktylos AK, Sclabas GM, Nuyens M, et al. The clinical correlation of temporal bone fractures and spiral computed tomographic scans: A prospective and consecutive study at a level 1 trauma center. J Trauma. 2003;55:704-6.
13. Swartz JD. Temporal bone trauma. Semin in Ultrasound; CT, MR. 2001;22:219-28.
14. Alvi A, Bereliani A 4th. Trauma to the temporal bone: Diagnosis and management of complications. J Craniomaxillofac Trauma. 1996;2:36-48.
15. Darrouzet V, Duclos JY, Liguoro D, et al. Management of facial paralysis resulting from temporal bone fractures: Our experience of 115 cases. Otolaryngol Head Neck Surg. 2001;125:77-84.
16. Little SC, Kesser BW. Radiographic classification of temporal bone fractures: clinical predictability using a new system. Arch Otolaryngol Head Neck Surg. 2006;132:1300-4.
17. Guy RL, Wylie E, Hickey A, et al. Computed tomography in malignant external otitis. Clin Radiol. 1991;43:166-70.
18. Kwon BJ, Han MH, Oh SH, et al. MRI findings and spreading patterns of necrotizing external otitis: is a poor outcome predictable? Clin Radiol. 2006;61:495-504.
19. Shire JR, Donegan JO. Cholesteatoma of the external auditory canal and keratosis obturans. Am J Otol. 1986;7:361-4.
20. Swartz JD, Goodman RS, Russel KB, et al. High resolution computed tomography of the middle ear and mastoid. Part II: Tubotympanic disease. Radiology. 1983;148:455-9.
21. Swartz JD. Cholesteatoma of the middle ear: diagnosis, etiology and complications. Radiol Clin North Am. 1984;22:15-35.
22. Cody DTR. The definition of cholesteatoma. In: McCabe BF, Sade JM Abramson M (Eds). Cholesteatoma. First International Conference. Birmingham, Ala: Aesculpius Publishers Inc; 1977. pp. 6-9.
23. Sade J. Pathogenesis of attic cholesteatoma: The metaplasia theory. In: McCabe BF, Sade J, Abramson M (Eds). Cholesteatoma. First International Conference, Birmingham, Ala: Aesculpins Publishers Inc; 1977. pp. 6-9.
24. Vercruysse JP, De Foer B, Pouillon M, et al. The value of diffusion-weighted MR imaging in the diagnosis of primary acquired and residual cholesteatoma: a surgical verified study of 100 patients. Eur Radiol. 2006;16:1461-7.
25. De Foer B, Vercruysse J-P, Pouillon M, et al. Value of high-resolution computed tomography and magnetic resonance imaging in the detection of residual cholesteatomas in primary obliterated mastoids. Am J Otolaryngol. 2007;28:230-34.
26. Holliday RA. Inflammatory diseases of temporal bone: Evaluation with CT and MR. Semin Ultrasound CT MR. 1989;10: 213-35.
27. Johnson DW, Hinshaw DB Jr, Hasso AN, et al. Computed tomography of local complications of temporal bone cholesteatomas. J Comput Assist Tomogr. 1985;9:519-23.
28. Watts S, Flood LM, Clifford K. A systematic approach to interpretation of computed tomography scans prior to surgery of middle ear cholesteatoma. J Laryngol Otol. 2000;114:248-53.
29. Nemzek WR, Swartz JD. Temporal bone inflammatory disease. In: Som PM, Curtin HD (Eds). Head and Neck Imaging, 4th edition. St. Louis MO: Mosby Year Book; 2003. pp. 1173-242.
30. Sugiura M, Naganawa S, Teranishi M, et al. Three-dimensional fluid attenuated inversion recovery magnetic resonance imaging findings in patients with sudden sensorineural hearing loss. Laryngoscope. 2006;116:1451-4.
31. Witte RJ, Lane JI, Driscoll CL, et al. Pediatric and adult cochlear implantation. Radiographics. 2003;23:1185-200.
32. Lo WWM, Marcel Maya M. Vascular tinnitus. In: Som PM, Curtin HD (Eds). Head and Neck Imaging, 4th edition. St. Louis MO: Mosby Year Book; 2003. pp. 1361-74.
33. Remley KB, Coit WE Harnsberger HR. Pulsatile tinnitis and vascular tympanic membrane: CT, MR and Angiographic Findings. Radiology. 1990;174:383-9.
34. Dufour JJ, Lavigne F, Plante R, et al. Pulsatile tinnitus and fibromuscular dysplasia of the internal carotid. J Otoclaryngol. 1985;14:293-5.

35. Hasso AN, Bird CR, Zinke DE, et al. Fibromuscular dysplasia of the internal carotid artery: Percutaneous transluminal angioplasty. Am J Roentgenol. 1981;136:955-60.
36. Lippy WH, Berenholz LP, Burkey M. Otosclerosis in the 1960s, 1970s, 1980s and 1990s. Laryngoscope. 1999;109:1307-9.
37. Osamu S, Curtin HD, Harro AN, Swartz JD. Otosclerosis and dysplasias of the temporal bone. In: Som PM, Curtin HD (Eds). Head and Neck Imaging Bone, 4th edition. St Louis: Mosby Year Book; 2003. pp. 1245-73.
38. Hullar TE, Lustig LR. Paget's disease and fibrous dysplasia. Otolaryngol Clin North Am. 2003;36:707-32.
39. Casselman JW, De Jonge I, Neyt L, et al. MR in craniofacial fibrous dysplasia. Neuroradiology. 1993;35:234-7.
40. Fisch U, Ruttner J. Pathology of intratemporal tumours involving the facial nerve. In: Fisch U (Ed): Facial Nerve Surgery. Birmingham, Ala: Aesculpius; 1977. pp. 448-56.
41. Marcel Maya M, Lo WWM, Kouvanlikaya. Tumours of the temporal bone and the cerebellopontine angle. In: Som PM, Curtin HG (Eds). Head and Neck Imaging, 4th edition. St Louis MO: Mosby Year Book; 2003. pp. 1275-360.
42. Pulec JL, Deguine C. Squamous cell carcinoma of the external auditory canal. Ear Nose Throat J. 2004;83:9.

CHAPTER 21

Imaging of the Globe and Orbit

Sanjay Sharma, Smriti Hari, Deep Narayan Srivastava, Kumble S Madhusudhan

INTRODUCTION

Radiological evaluation of orbital pathology presents a diagnostic challenge. The aetiologies are diverse and clinical input is often necessary to narrow the diagnostic possibilities. Cross-sectional imaging plays a vital role in detection and evaluation of the disease, supplementing the clinical and ophthalmologic examination in providing information beyond fundoscopy. In this chapter, the imaging features of the more common adult and childhood orbital pathologies are discussed.

NORMAL ANATOMY

The orbit is a lopsided, pear-shaped cavity, wide anteriorly and narrow posteriorly formed by seven interconnecting bones with the optic canal analogous to the stem of the pear. The central axis of the orbit lies approximately 25° to the sagittal plane. It consists of roof, floor, lateral and medical walls and the apex. The roof of the orbit is composed of the orbital process of the frontal bone anteriorly and lesser wing of the sphenoid posteriorly. The lateral wall of the orbit is formed by the greater wing of the sphenoid posteriorly and by the zygomatic process of the frontal bone and frontal process of the zygomatic bone anteriorly. The medial wall of the orbit is formed posteriorly by the lamina papyracea of the ethmoid bone and anteriorly by the lacrimal bone. The floor of the orbit is composed essentially of the orbital plate of the maxilla and is limited posterolaterally by the inferior orbital fissure. The infraorbital groove runs on the orbital floor to reach the infraorbital foramen. Superior orbital fissure is a comma-shaped opening bounded by the greater wing of sphenoid inferolaterally and the lesser wing superomedially. It provides a large communication between the orbit and middle cranial fossa via the cavernous sinus allowing the spread of tumor or inflammation between these two compartments. The inferior orbital fissure lies between the floor and greater wing of sphenoid. It communicates with the pterygopalatine fossa and masticator space. The optic canal lies above and medial to the fissure and is separated from it by the optic strut that connects lesser wing to the body of the sphenoid. The lacrimal gland lies in the lacrimal fossa, a recess of frontal bone anterolaterally within the orbit.

The globe is surrounded by three tissue layers: (1) sclera and cornea, (2) uveal tract (choroids, iris and ciliary body), and (3) retina. The lens and iris divide the globe into anterior and posterior chamber. Optic nerve is about 5 cm long and divided into four segments: intraocular, intraorbital, intracanalicular and intracranial. The subarachnoid space between the dura and pia covering the optic nerve is continuous with the suprasellar cistern. The six extraocular muscles comprise of four recti and two oblique muscles. Thick orbital fascial septum situated anterior to the globe divides preseptal (anterior skin and subcutaneous) from the postseptal (more posterior orbit) compartment.

Radiographic Views

Standard projections for the bony orbit include posteroanterior (PA), lateral and optic foramen view.

The patient could be either seated or semi prone. The *PA projection (occipito-frontal)* is obtained with 20° caudad tilt, with the central beam existing at the nasion. In this view, the innominate line is seen crossing the greater wing of sphenoid on the temporal side of the orbit. It has no true anatomical counterpart. For the *lateral view* the mid sagittal plane of the skull is placed parallel to the image receptor with the beam centered at a point 2.5 cm posterior to the outer canthus. In the true lateral projection, the floor of the anterior cranial fossa is superimposed. For *optic foramen view* (Rhese projection), the head rests on cheek, nose and chin, with orbit in center, in a manner that orbitomeatal line is perpendicular, keeping the mid sagittal plane at an angle of 53° to the image receptor, and the orbitomeatal line is raised at 35° from the horizontal. Beam is centered 7.5 cm superior and 7.5 cm posterior to the upper external auditory meatus, emerging at the center of orbit under examination. These orbital radiographs are now less commonly requested. An orbital radiograph is now mainly needed to exclude metallic foreign body prior to MRI.

Ultrasound

It is a widely available non-invasive diagnostic modality for evaluation of ocular and orbital pathology. It is particularly useful in the evaluation of intraocular lesions, especially when the media is opaque. It is useful in differentiating cystic from solid lesions. However, it is limited by the lack of visualization of more deeply placed intraorbital lesions. Both A and B-mode scans are used. A-mode scan is particularly popular with the ophthalmologists. B-mode scan of the globe is done with 7.5–10 MHz, whereas orbit proper is scanned with 5–7.5 MHz transducer. It is carried out after applying coupling gel over the closed eyelids. Both the anterior and posterior chambers of the eyeball are echo-free with the lens present between the two. Posterior to the globe, the echogenic fat is seen with central hypoechoic band representing the optic nerve sheath complex. Colour Doppler evaluation can be combined with the B-scan to evaluate the blood flow in tumors and vascular lesions, or spectral trace obtained from superior ophthalmic vein in patients with carotico-cavernous fistula. Preliminary studies show that the contrast enhanced harmonic imaging could become a powerful tool in the evaluation of perfusion in ocular tumors.[1] Ultrasound biomicroscopy (UBM) uses approximately 50 MHz transducer to produce exceptionally detailed two dimensional gray scale images of the anterior chamber.

Computed Tomography

The newer generation multidetetor row computed tomography represents an important modality offering the advantages of shorter acquisition times, reduced motion artifacts, isotropic resolution, and excellent multiplanar image reconstruction. In addition, postprocessing of axial volumetric data now allows sophisticated 3D volume rendered images that allowing better understanding of the pathology. It provides excellent anatomic detail of the eyeball, extraocular muscles, optic nerve and retrobulbar fat, etc. Volumetric acquisition is routinely performed in contiguous thin (2–3 mm) axial plane,and displayed both in soft tissue and bone windows. The plane of axial orbital imaging is parallel to the infraorbitomeatal line. Intravenous contrast is routinely administered except in the setting of trauma, foreign body or thyroid ophthalmopathy.

Magnetic Resonance Imaging

Magnetic resonance imaging (MRI) has gained wide-spread acceptance because of its greater sensitivity in characterizing the orbital pathologies with direct multiplanar imaging, higher soft tissue resolution, use of fat suppressed sequences with or without contrast enhancement, T2-weighted images, combined head and surface coils and increasingly faster data acquisition. FLAIR (Fluid Attenuation Inversion Recovery) sequence may be used to suppress the CSF hyperintensity for better evaluation of optic nerve. Compared to CT, MRI has a greater versatility in detecting concomitant intracranial abnormalities. Vitreous body appears aslow intensity on T1 and high intensity on T2-weighted images. Optic nerve and its coverings are hypointense on T1 weighted images and surrounded by high intensity retrobulbar fat. Cerebrospinal fluid (CSF) surrounding the optic nerve can be seen as low intensity sleeve around the optic nerve on T1 and high signal on T2-weighted images. The intracanalicular and intracranial parts of the optic nerve are well evaluated because of lack of bone artifacts. Sequences and plane of imaging must be tailored to suit the clinical requirement. Spin echo T1 and T2-weighted, thin (3 mm) section contiguous (or with small interslice gap) images are acquired in axial, coronal and/or even oblique planes. Applications of MRI are still evolving. Although CT provides good anatomical delineation of structures, MRI has been found to have distinct advantages over CT in certain conditions, e.g. evaluation of hemorrhagic and vascular pathology without the requirement of intravenous contrast, periorbital and orbital apex pathologies. However, it limited by relatively long imaging time and higher cost.

PATHOLOGICAL CONDITIONS

Lesions of the orbit can be broadly subdivided into two groups: Ocular (limited to the globe) and orbital (rest of the

Table 1: A guide to differential diagnosis.

	Pathological conditions		
Anatomical compartment	***Common***	***Uncommon***	***Rare***
Intraconal	Optic neuritis, Papilloedema	Meningioma, Sarcoidosis	Lymphoma, Hemangioma
Optic nerve	Apical fractures affecting optic nerve Optic glioma, Inflammatory pseudotumor	Metastases	
Others	Cavernous hemangioma, Pseudotumor, Varices	Lymphangioma, Neurofibroma Lymphoma, Metastasis	Hemangiopericytoma Yolk sac tumor, Chondrosarcoma
		Capillary hemangioma	Granular cell myoblastoma
Extraconal	Capillary hemangioma, Dermoid Lymphoma, Rhabdomyosarcoma	Neurofibroma, Metastases	Fibrous histiocytoma
Preseptal space	Cutaneous conditions (Xanthelesma etc.), Basal cell cancer	Capillary hemangioma, Dermoid, Lymphoma, Neurofibromas, fibroma	Metastasis, Melanoma
Subperiosteal space	Mucocele, Fractures, PNS neoplasms Abscess, Osteoma, Metastases, Dermoid, Epidermoid, Rhabdomyosarcoma, Menigioma,	Craniofacial dysplasia Fibrous dysplasia, Wegener's granulomatosis Pagets disease, Plasmacytoma	Histiocytosis, Sphenoid dysplasia Encephalocele, Bone tumors Osteopetrosis
Lacrimal gland	Inflammatory pseudotumor, Dacryoadenitis, Abscess	Lymphoma, Dermoid, Sarcoid Pleomorphic adenoma, Carcinoma Sjögren's syndrome	Wegener's granulomatosis, Miculicz syndrome, Metastases
Orbital apex and Cavernous sinus	Pituitary adenoma, Meningioma, Empty sella, Craniopharyngioma, Arachnoid cyst, Optic chiasm glioma	Metastases, Tolosa Hunt syndrome, Carotico-cavernous fistula	
Muscles	Endocrine orbitopathy, Myositis, Inflammatory pseudotumor	Metastases, Wegener's granulomatosis, Acromegaly, Myoblastoma, Lithium therapy	
Globe	Foreign body, Retinal/Choroidal detachment, Scleritis, Uveitis	Retinoblastoma, Melanoma, Metastases	Lymphoma, Hemangioma, PHPV, Coats' disease, Norie's disease, Osteoma, Medulloepithelioma

orbit excluding globe). The orbital lesions can be further subdivided according to their predominant location in respective spaces. A knowledge of the compartmental localization of the pathological process helps to limit the differential diagnoses **(Table 1)**.[2,3]

OCULAR LESIONS

These comprise a broad spectrum of diseases which include ocular detachment, vitreous hemorrhage, benign and malignant tumors (retinoblastoma, malignant melanoma, choroidal metastases), Coats' disease, persistent hyperplastic primary vitreous (PHPV), intraocular foreign body, parasitic infestation (the commonest being cysticercosis) and congenital anomalies of the eyeball.

Ocular Detachments

Three potential spaces exist-posterior hyaloid space, subretinal space and suprachoroidal space. Only under pathological conditions, when accumulation of fluid or hemorrhage occurs, do these spaces become visible and distinguishable on imaging **(Table 2)**.[4] *Posterior hyaloid detachment* occurs with physiological liquefaction of vitreous in elderly, myopia, PHPV or trauma. It presents on imaging as a fluid-fluid level. *Retinal detachment* is seen as a thin membrane attached to the optic nerve head posteriorly and ora serrata anteriorly, often assuming V or Y shaped appearance due to lifting of retinal leaves by subretinal fluid or hemorrhage. Partial detachment may be seen as a localized area of elevated retina. On CT, mild or focal retinal detachment may not be detected. Any choroidal lesion may produce retinal detachment. It is commonly seen in retinoblastoma in children and neoplasms like malignant melanoma or choroidal hemangioma in adults. *Choroidal detachment* occurs in two distinct forms viz, serous or hemorrhagic, each with different imaging appearances, even though the etiology of both may be similar. It may occur after intraocular

Table 2: Diagrammatic representation of ocular detachments.

Posterior hyaloid detachment	***Retinal detachment***	***Choroidal detachment***	
		Hemorrhagic	***Serous***
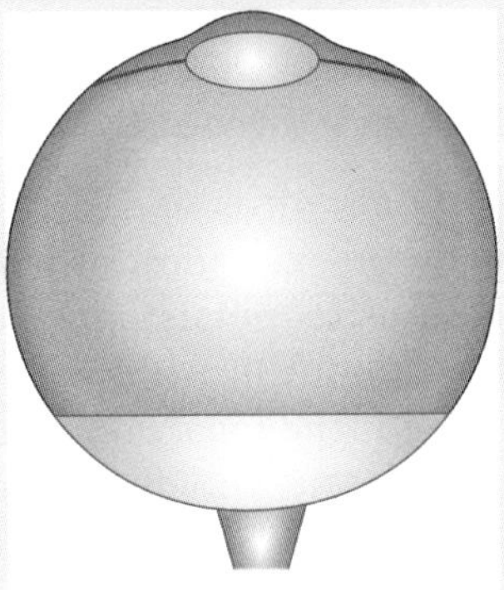	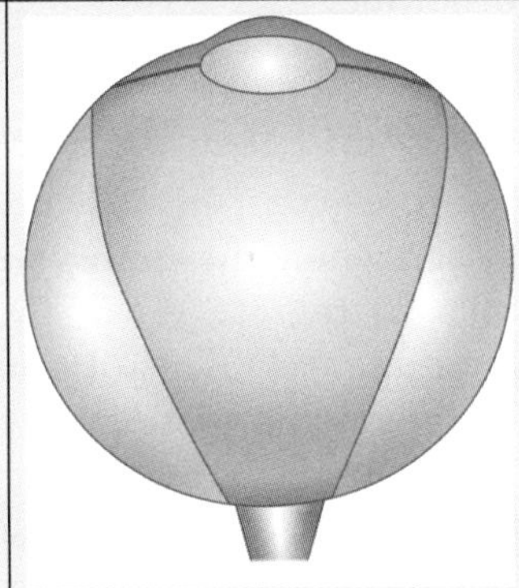	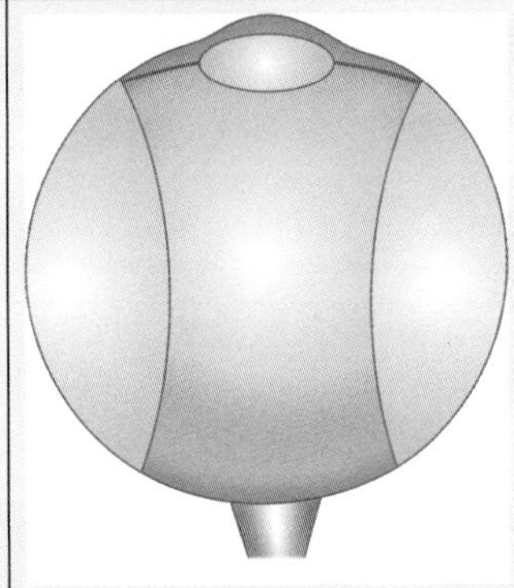	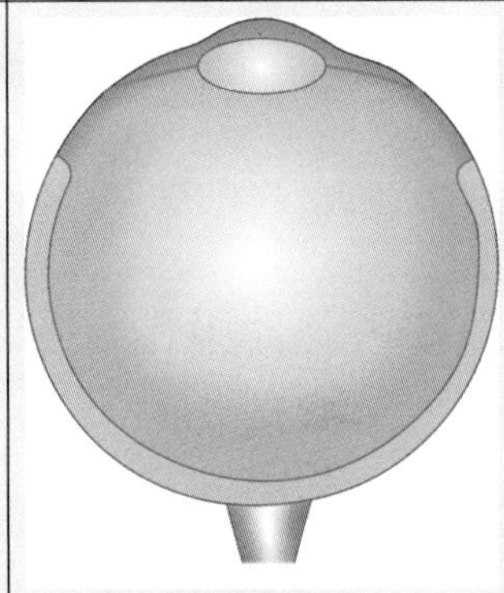
Adults: Macular degeneration *Children*: PHPV	• Subretinal hemorrhage • Choroidal lesion	• Trauma • Intraocular surgery	Ocular hypotony
Fluid-fluid level	• Macular degeneration • Trauma • V-shaped with apex at optic disk	• Contusion • Choroidal inflammation Lentiform	Crescent or Ring

surgery, penetrating ocular injury, or inflammatory disorders. Hemorrhagic detachment presents as a lens like configuration, caused by the fixation of choroid by the posterior ciliary vessels. Serous detachment is characterized by a crescent or ring shape, essentially due to ocular hypotony.

Vitreous Hemorrhage

The vitreous is normally clear and echo-free on ultrasound (US). Vitreous hemorrhage is seen especially in patients with diabetic retinopathyand trauma. On ultrasound acute hemorrhage is seen as scattered, low amplitude echoes on US, which subsequently becomes highly echogenic. Estimation of the extent of vitreous hemorrhage is important to know the prognosis for spontaneous clearing, and planning for vitrectomy in the event of its non-clearance. Normal vitreous is of low attenuation on CT scan but in the presence of vitreous hemorrhage it becomes diffusely hazy.

Retinoblastoma

It is the most common, highly malignant, intraocular tumor of childhood. Over 90% affect children less than 5 years with no sex prediliction. Most common presentation is leucocoria (60%) followed by strabismus (20%). In 25–33% patients the disease is bilateral and represents autosomal dominant pattern of genetic transmission. In bilateral cases there is frequently a family history.[5] Three growth patterns are described: (1) Endophytic- anterior tumor growth from retina into vitreous cavity (simulating endophthalmitis), (2) Exophytic tumor growth into subretinal space, producing secondary retinal detachment (simulating coats' disease), (3) Diffuse tumor growth along the retina appearing as a placoid mass (simulating inflammatory and hemorrhagic conditions). This rare form presents diagnostic difficulties because of its lack of calcification and occurrence outside the typical age group.[6]

Ophthalmoscopy allows diagnostic confirmation of even the smallest tumors, however ultrasound evaluation is complimentary. On US, retinoblastomas are seen as intraocular masses of varying size and mixed echogenicity located in the coats of the eyeball with calcification seen in upto 90%.[7,8] The detection of calcification is an important diagnostic criterion. Tumors that are non-calcified may be of low to medium reflectivity. CT scanning better depicts subtle calcification **(Fig. 1)**, delineation of its soft tissue component and intraorbital and/or intracranial extension. However, it is no longer considered a primary modality for the diagnosis of retinoblastoma owing to the radiation risks in small children. On the other hand, MRI has now evolved as a standard tool in the diagnostic assessment of tumor stage (optic nerve spread and extra ocular extension) **(Figs. 2 and 3)** and intracranial involvement. It is also useful in its follow up and differentiating it from other causes of leucocoria. The echoplanar diffusion weighted imaging (DWI) has the benefit of assessing the diffusivity in retinoblastoma, potentially aiding the improved diagnosis of tumors and its follow up on treatment[9] **(Figs. 3A and B)**. However, with its insensitivity to field inhomogeneity and high spatial resolution, the 3D turbo field echo (TFE) with diffusion-sensitized driven-equilibrium (DSDE) MRI technique has been recently shown to better assess the diffusivity in retinoblastomas without geometrical distortion.[10]

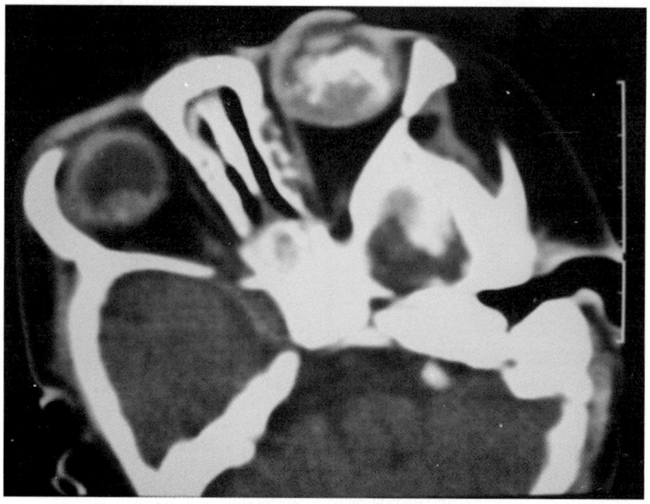

Fig. 1: Retinoblastoma: NCCT shows bilateral calcified intraocular soft tissue masses.

Persistent Hyperplastic Primary Vitreous

The persistent hyperplastic primary vitreous (PHPV) arises when the embryonic hyaloid vascular system fails to regress normally leading to persistence of abnormal segments of primary vitreous. It is primarily unilateral and presents at birth. It is the most common lesion closely resembling retinoblastoma. On ultrasound doppler and MRI a triangular retrolental band of soft tissue extends along the Cloquet's canal from the posterior surface of crystalline lens to the posterior pole of the globe **(Figs. 4A to D)**. It may demonstrate moderate or no enhancement on the administration of intravenous contrast. Computed tomography may demonstrate gravitational layering of high attenuation fluid in retrohyaloid or subrential space, possibly resulting from the presence of hemorrhage or

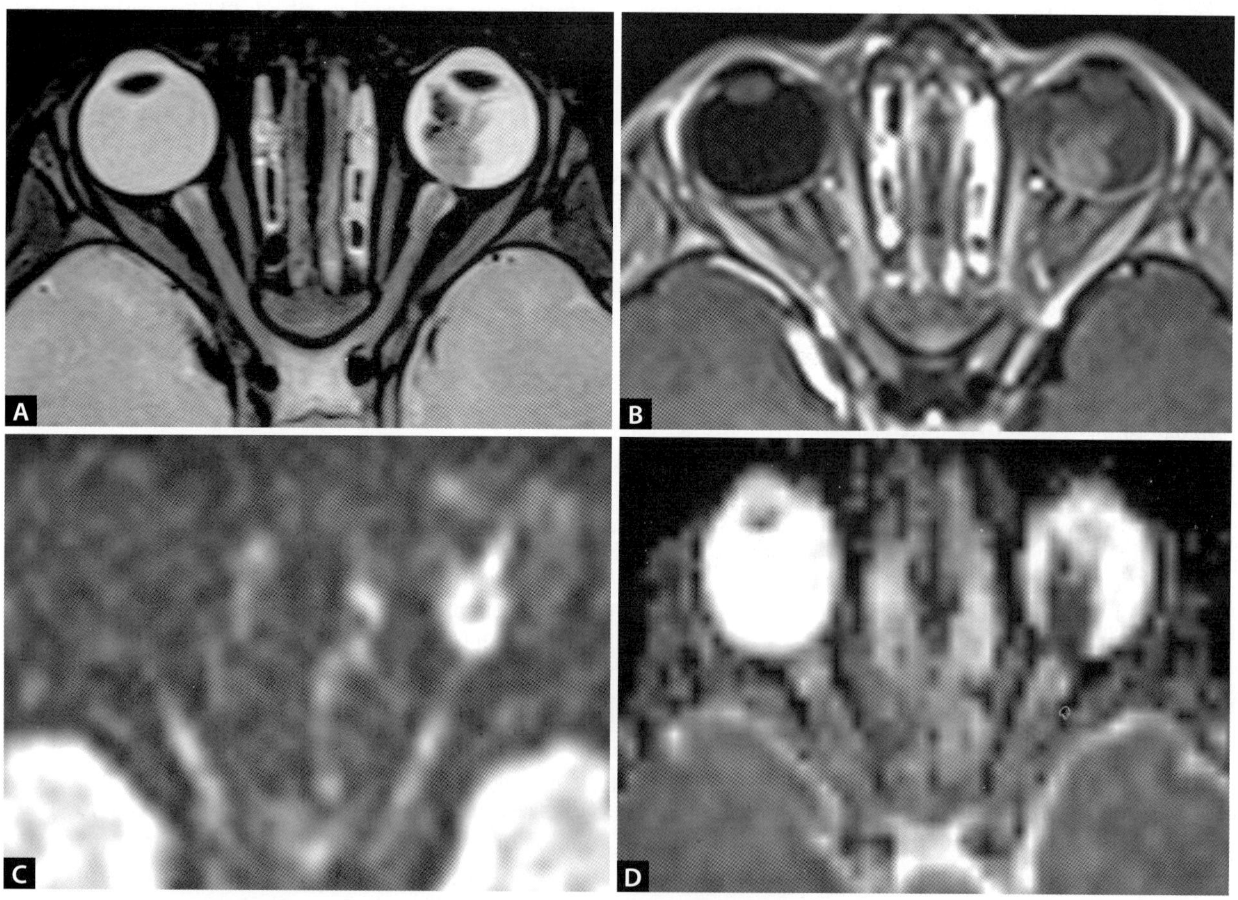

Figs. 2A to D: Retinoblastoma: Left intraocular mass is hypointense on T2WI (A) and shows moderate enhancement (B). It exhibits diffusion restriction (C, DWI and D, ADC map). The optic nerve is not involved.

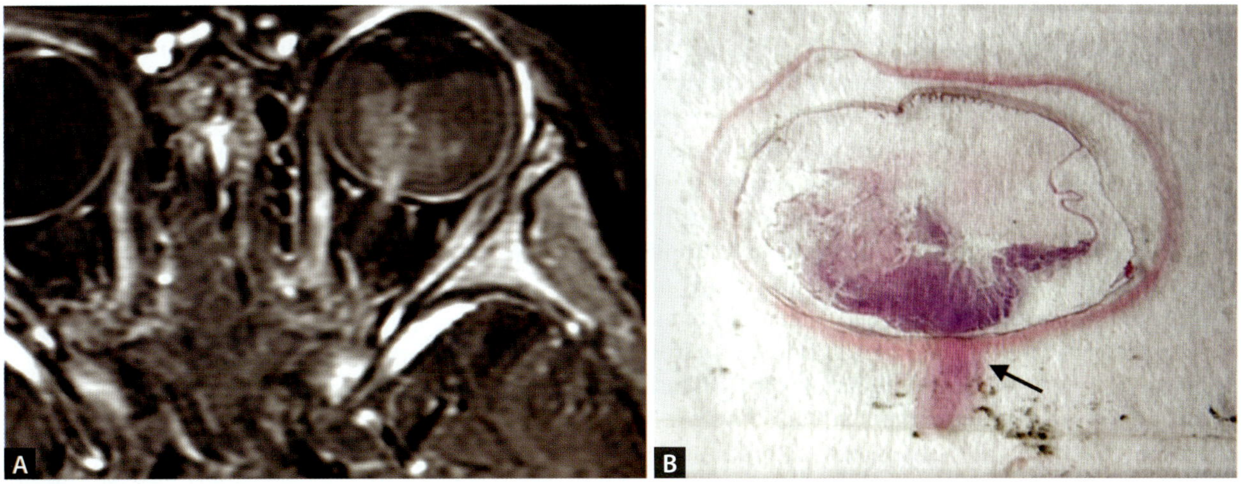

Figs. 3A and B: Retinoblastoma involving the left globe (in another child) (A and B). Postcontrast MRI image (A) shows moderate tumor enhancement and postlaminar optic nerve involvement for about 2 mm. Whole mount enucleation specimen (B) confirms early the optic nerve spread (arrow).

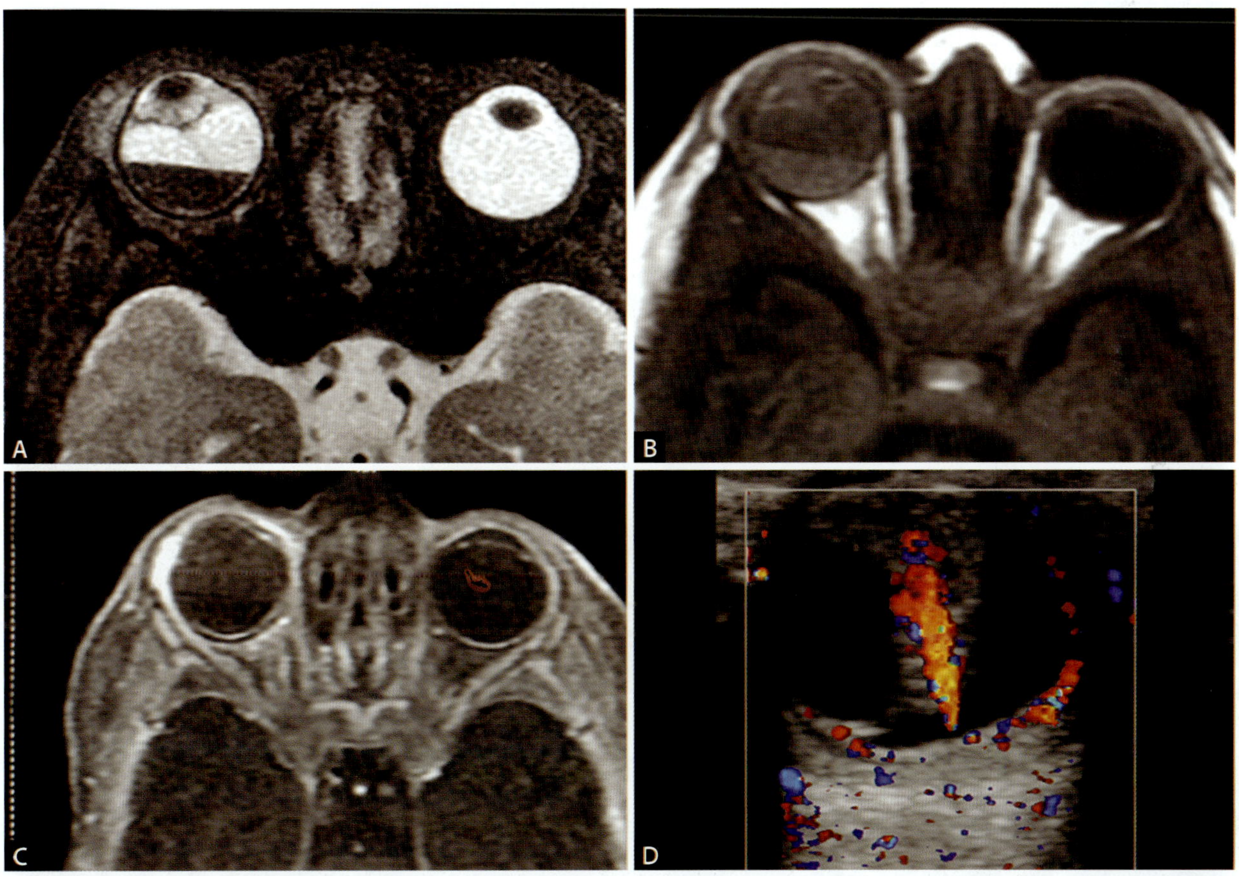

Figs. 4A to D: Persistent hyperplastic primary vitreous (right): Axial T2W (A) MRI shows a triangular retrolental opacity with an intraocular linear channel representing embryonic vascular remnant. T1W pre (B) and postcontrast © image shows no mass. Note the posterior hyaloid detachment seen as a fluid-fluid level. Ultrasound Doppler (D) shows a patent vascular channel (another patient).

serosanguineous material. The affected eyeball is often small. Absence of intraocular calcification often helps to differentiate PHPV from retinoblastoma.

Although sensitivity of MRI in detecting calcification is inferior to CT, it represents the most important imaging modality in the evaluation and staging of retinoblastoma.

This is due to its high soft tissue contrast resolution, enabling simultaneous assessment of spread along the optic nerve and intracranial involvement. Retinoblastoma appears as slightly hyperintense compared to vitreous on T1 and PD weighted images, with patchy low signal intensity on T2W images.[11] It exhibits moderate to marked contrast enhancement best appreciated in the fat suppressed sequences. The involvement of the optic nerve is best assessed in the postcontrast T1-weighted fat suppressed images and compared with the normal side. It best differentiates patients of retinoblastoma from other causes of leucocoria viz, PHPV and Coats' disease. Less commonly retinal detachment, endophthalmitis, toxocariasis, late stages of retinopathy of prematurity (ROP), choroidal hemangioma, retinal hamartoma, etc. may also be considered.

Coats' Disease

Coats' disease is a primary idiopathic vascular anomaly of the retina, characterized by telangiectasis. The telangiectatic vessels cause leakage of serum and lipid with accumulation of a lipoproteinaceous exudate in the retina and subretinal space. It is almost always unilateral and occurs in boys aged 6–8 years, older than those who have retinoblastoma. It does not generally become symptomatic until retinal detachment occurs, which finally leads to central vision loss and painful glaucoma.

At the early stages the diagnosis is reliably established by Ophthalmoscopy, and CT or MRI provide little additional information. Diagnostic imaging is helpful at a more advanced stage when retinal detachment occurs and is seen on US and CT **(Figs. 5A and B)**. Absence of intraocular calcification does not differentiate Coats' disease from unilateral non-calcifying retinoblastoma. MRI is superior to CT in distinguishing Coats disease from retinoblastoma.[12] The most significant finding on T1, PD and T2-weighted images is the identification of homogenous hyperintensity of subretinal fluid caused by high protein content in comparison to the vitreous body of the opposite eye. Detached V-shaped retina may be seen having a low signal on both T1 and T2-weighted images. Detached retina may show enhancement after intravenous gadolinium, but the subretinal fluid does not. In contrast, retinoblastoma is inhomogenous, moderately hyperintense mass on T1W and PD images, but with hypointense areas on the T2W images. Tumor mass in retinoblastoma shows moderate to marked enhancement after contrast administration in contrast to subretinal fluid in Coat's disease.[13]

Uveal Malignant Melanoma

It is the commonest primary malignant intraocular tumor of adults. The incidence of disease increases with age with mean age at 53 years.[14] The specific diagnostic US, CT and MRI criteria include: collar button (mushroom) shaped intraocular mass which is broad based towards the coats of the eyeball with its dome projecting into the vitreous body. Associated retinal detachment may be seen in a large percentage of patients. Further, choroidal excavation dueto replacement of the choroids by the tumor mass may also be seen.

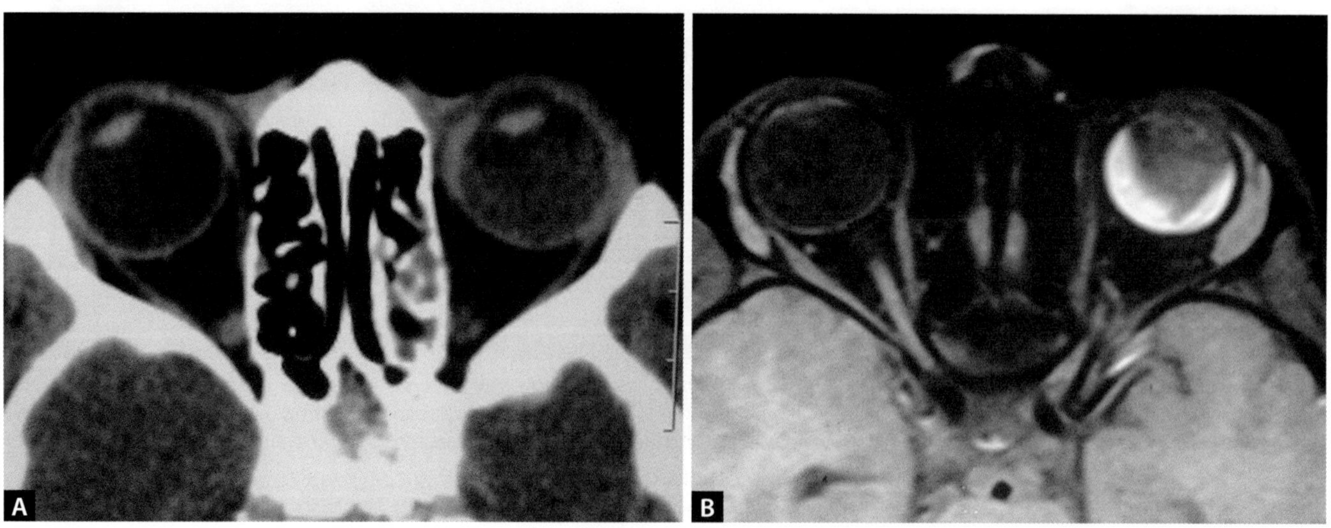

Figs. 5A and B: Coats' disease (L): Axial CT (A) and T1W MRI (B) show sub-retinal hemorrhage in the small left globe in a 8-year-old boy. Note that there is no mass or calcification.

Ultrasound Doppler imaging may show marked vascularity. MRI is the imaging technique of choice. On MRI the tumor is seen as hyperintense on T1W and hypointense on T2W images **(Figs. 6A and B)**. This unique signal of melanin is due to shortening of both T1 and T2 relaxation times. The factors associated with a poor prognosis include: older patients (60 years), large tumor base diameter, location in anterior uvea and cilliary body, and extraocular extension.[15]

The sites of metastasis include liver, lungs, bone, kidneys and brain.

Choroidal Metastases

The choroid is the most common site of carcinoma metastatic to the eye. The metastatic carcinomas of the choroids are subretinal masses located mainly in the posterior part of the fundus. They are frequently associated with serous retinal detachment. These are relatively flattened or placoid masses and may be multiple. In contrast to the uveal melanoma, these tumors may occur bilaterally or be multifocal and affect both the eyes in about one-third of cases. The common sites of primary tumors are lung, breast, prostate, etc.

Foreign Body

Foreign bodies represent ophthalmic emergencies and require thorough evaluation. It is mandatory to localize a foreign body to define appropriate treatment. Plain radiograph may show presence of radiopaque foreign body. A circular radiopaque marker is sutured to the surface of the eye. Lateral and posteroanterior views are obtained with marker in place to allow reliable measurements. CT is however, the modality of choice for detection of intraorbital foreign bodies, associated brain injuries or facial fractures. In case of wooden foreign body, fresh wood is usually hyperdense on CT whereas dry wood is hypodense, sometimes even indistinguishable from intraorbital fat or air.[16] Glass foreign bodies are hyperdense but without typical streak artifacts of metallic foreign body **(Fig. 7)**. MRI can be useful to differentiate foreign body (generally hypointense) and orbital fat. The patients with suspected metallic-ferromagnetic intraorbital foreign bodies must never be exposed to the high field MRI. A preliminary plain radiograph is customary to exclude its presence. US may be helpful in evaluation of radiolucent intraocular foreign bodies. In addition, the presence of vitreous hemorrhage and retinal detachment may also be assessed. However, in general, US has no significant role in the detection of intraorbital foreign bodies.

Parasitic Infestation

Cysticercosis cellulosae is the most common intraocular parasitic infestation. On US, it is seen as a ring-shaped lesion with a dense nodule representing the scolex **(Fig. 8)**. Cysticerci are usually seen adjacent to the coats of the eyeball. Associated retinal detachment may be seen.[17] CT scan demonstrates the scolex as a pin-head area of increased attenuation. The cyst wall, however, is not seen, presumably due to very low attenuation difference between the fluid in the cyst, vitreous and wall of the cysticercus cellulosae.

Congenital Anomalies

Congenital anophthalmos is a rare condition characterized by absence of globe(s) due to failure of development

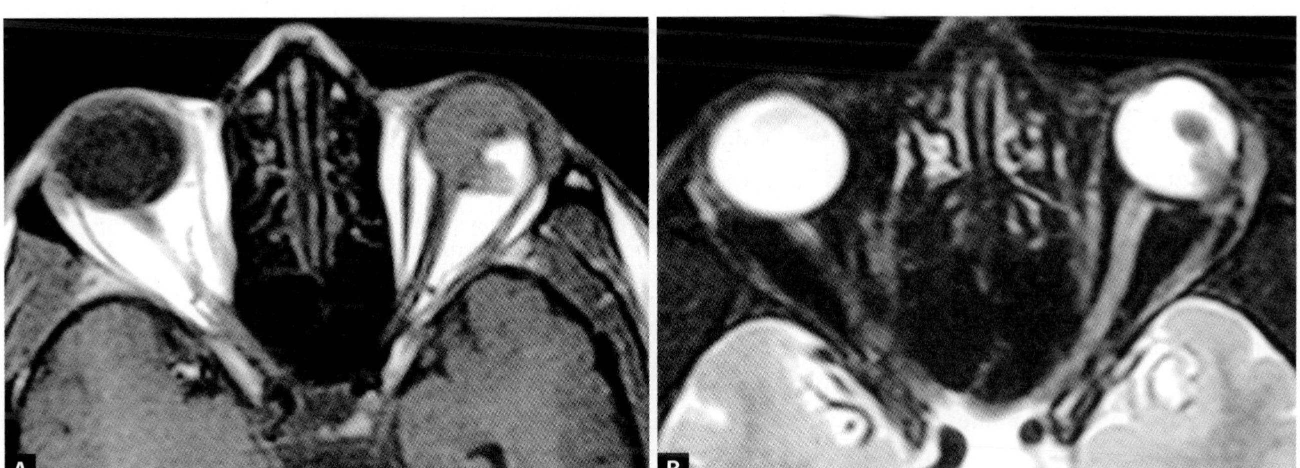

Figs. 6A and B: Uveal melanoma involving left globe. MR axial images (A) and (B), showing that the lesion is typically hyperintense on T1W (A) and hypointense on the T2W fat suppressed (B) images.

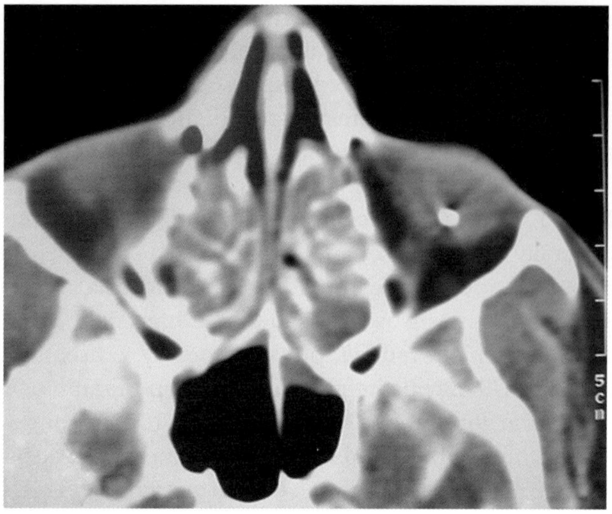

Fig. 7: Foreign body: Metallic intraocular foreign body within the left globe. Note incidental ethmoid sinusitis.

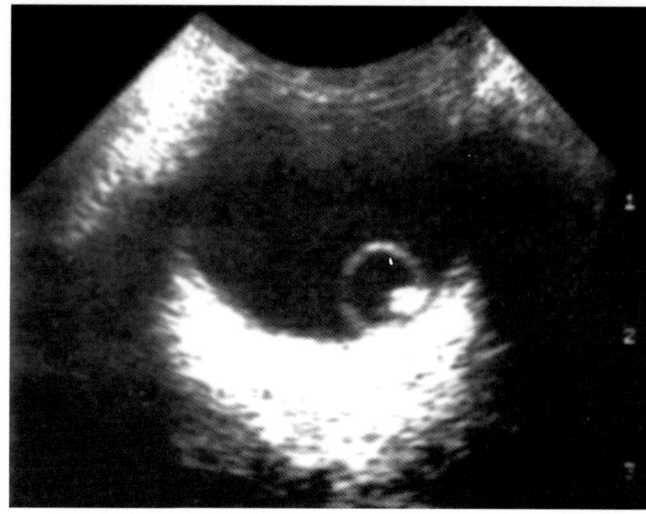

Fig. 8: Intraocular cysticercus: Ultrasound image showing a cyst with a scolex within the left eyeball.

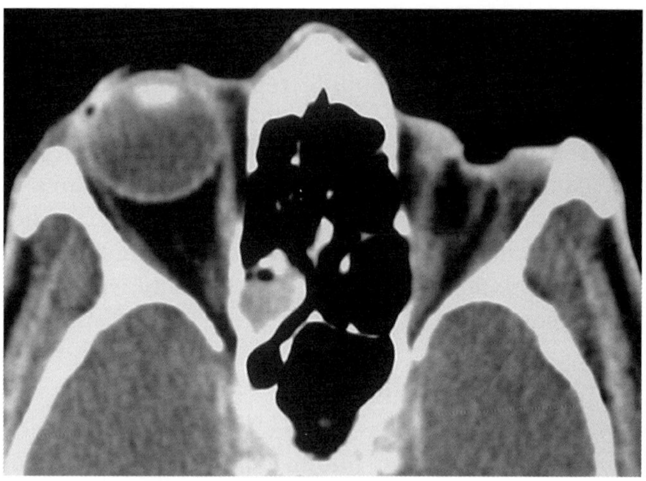

Fig. 9: Anophthalmia (L): Axial CT image shows absence of left globe. Note the intact extraocular muscles, atrophic optic nerve and relatively small bony orbit.

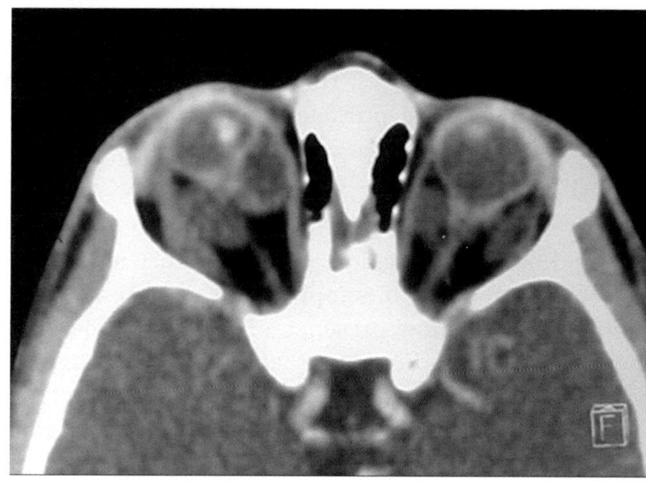

Fig. 10: Bilateral colobomatous cysts: Axial CT shows a bilateral microphthalmia and multiple variable sized intraorbital cysts. The right lens is densely calcified.

of the optic vesicle **(Fig. 9)**. No eye is visible on inspection. Extraocular muscles may be well developed. *Microphthalmos* is characterized by a unilateral small eye. This is either isolated or found associated with other craniofacial anomalies. It may be accompanied by a *colobomatous cyst* as a manifestation of failure of the closure of the embryonic optic fissure **(Fig. 10)**. This cyst is generally located inferior to globe and may be a cause of rapidly worsening proptosis mimicking neoplasia.

When congenital anomalies are present, the role of imaging is to rule out associated intracranial abnormalities, or to identify extraocular muscles in a patient who may have to undergo surgery for microphthalmos. However, when anophthalmos is suspected, the presence of cryptophthalmos (eye covered with a layer of skin), a colobomatous cyst or retinoblastoma must be ruled out. When colobomatous cyst is suspected, an orbital cephalocele must always be excluded to choose an appropriate surgical approach.

ORBITAL LESIONS

These can be discussed under the following broad categories: tumors, developmental cysts, inflammatory lesions, endocrine exophthalmos, parasitic infestations, vascular lesions and trauma.

ORBITAL TUMORS

Hemangioma

It could be either capillary or cavernous in type. Both are different lesions differing in clinical presentation, location and age of presentation.

Capillary hemangioma: These are the commonest intraorbital tumors of childhood. They are usually extraconal, situated in the superomedial quadrant with associated cutaneous malformation over the face. They present at birth, grow rapidly in the first year of life and usually regress by 7–10 years of age. They most commonly arise anteriorly, are unencapsulated and less well-defined than the cavernous forms. Intraconal extension also sometimes occurs. On imaging they are slightly hypodense on CT, iso- to hyperintenseon T1 and moderately hyperintense on T2W MR images. Signal intensity is determined by the amount of fibrosis, calcification and hemosiderin deposition after hemorrhage. Flow voids may be identified within and on the surface on T2W images, which is a helpful distinguishing feature from lymphangioma. A prominent arterial supply is usually demonstrable from external or internal carotid circulation.[13]

Cavernous hemangioma: They are commonest intraorbital tumors in adults, occurring mainly in the 4th and 5th decade of life. Although they usually occur as isolated intraconal masses, these may extend into the extraconal space, may be entirely extraconal or multiple. These are well encapsulated tumors and tend to be round to oval in shape. Histologically, they are composed of large, dilated, vascular channels (sinusoid-like spaces) lined by thin attenuated endothelial cells.[10] They contain relatively stagnant blood and the walls forming the vascular spaces produce large interfaces resulting in either hyperechoic or mixed hypo- and hyperchoic appearance on US. On CT they appear well demarcated, smoothly marginated, homogeneous, rounded, ovoid or lobulated soft tissue masses of increased density with a variable degree of contrast enhancement owing to slow intratumoral circulation. Uncommonly phleboliths may be seen. They are normally iso- to hypointense on T1 and homogeneously hyperintense on T2W image, showing marked enhancement that becomes homogeneous in delayed phase **(Figs. 11A to C)**.[19] Depending upon size of the lesion, orbital bony expansion may occur. They usually spare the orbital apex.

Lymphangioma

These lesions are unencapsulated and represent hamartomas. Large majority of these lesions are extraconal in location, however these often cross anatomic compartments. They usually present during early childhood. Usual presentation is that of sudden proptosis caused by hemorrhage. On CT and MRI, lymphangiomas appear as irregularly marginated, multilobulated, poorly defined lesions that may be heterogenous and enhance partially. MR is more specific than CT in identifying blood products and showing various components of lymphangioma **(Figs. 12A and B)**. Ultrasound is useful to evaluate the internal architecture of lymphangioma, especially as intralesional sclerotherapy of its macrocystic variants is now becoming an increasingly popular and effective treatment.[20,21]

Lacrimal Gland Tumors

Pleomorphic adenoma (benign mixed tumor) is the most common benign epithelial tumor of the lacrimal gland. The peak age of incidence is between 25 years and 40 years. It is painless and typically develops over many years. These are slow growing and may show fossa formation in the superolateral part of the bony orbit. Most involve the orbital part of the gland and are seen as well defined masses with rounded configuration, displacing and deforming the globe. The tumor is surrounded by a pseudocapsule formed by compressed adjacent tissue and reactive fibrosis. It should be excised without a preceding biopsy and within its pseudocapsule to prevent the risk of recurrence and malignant degeneration. Malignant transformation occurs into an *adenoid cystic carcinoma (malignant mixed tumor)* and is stated to be around 20%. The other primary lacrimal gland tumor is *mucoepidermoid carcinoma*. The morphological criteria on MRI are same as those of CT (smooth outline, round to oval). The tumor is of low signal intensity on T1 and high signal intensity on the T2-weighted images, and frequently heterogeneous. Imaging alone can not distinguish benign from malignant lesions. The presence of calcification and bone destruction suggests malignancy **(Fig. 13)**. Contrast enhancement is moderate to intense. Compared to the globular configuration of the lacrimal gland tumors, the inflammatory or lymphomatous masses show a flattened appearance. Further, in the latter lesions there is almost equal involvement of the palpebral and orbital part of the lacrimal gland.[2]

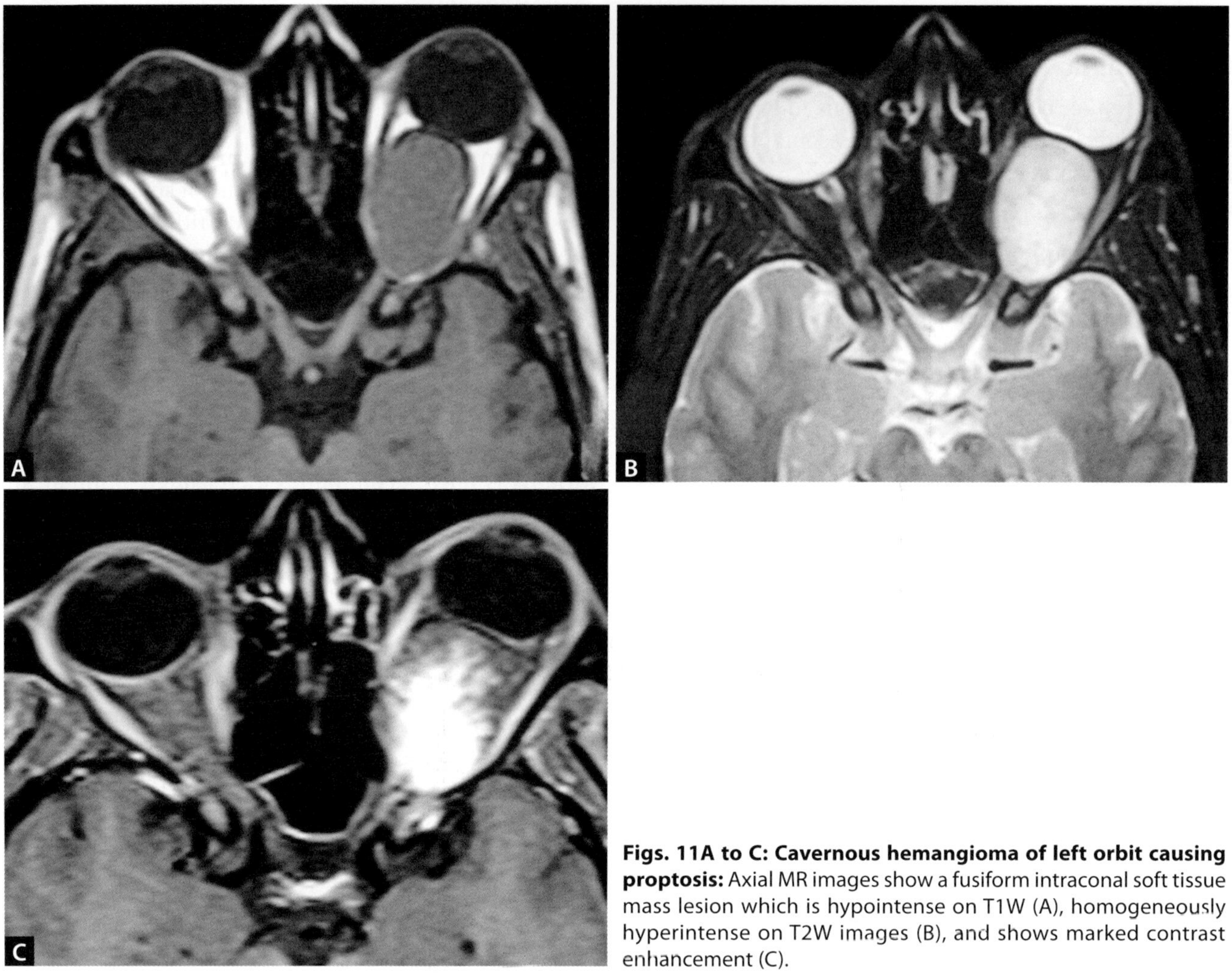

Figs. 11A to C: Cavernous hemangioma of left orbit causing proptosis: Axial MR images show a fusiform intraconal soft tissue mass lesion which is hypointense on T1W (A), homogeneously hyperintense on T2W images (B), and shows marked contrast enhancement (C).

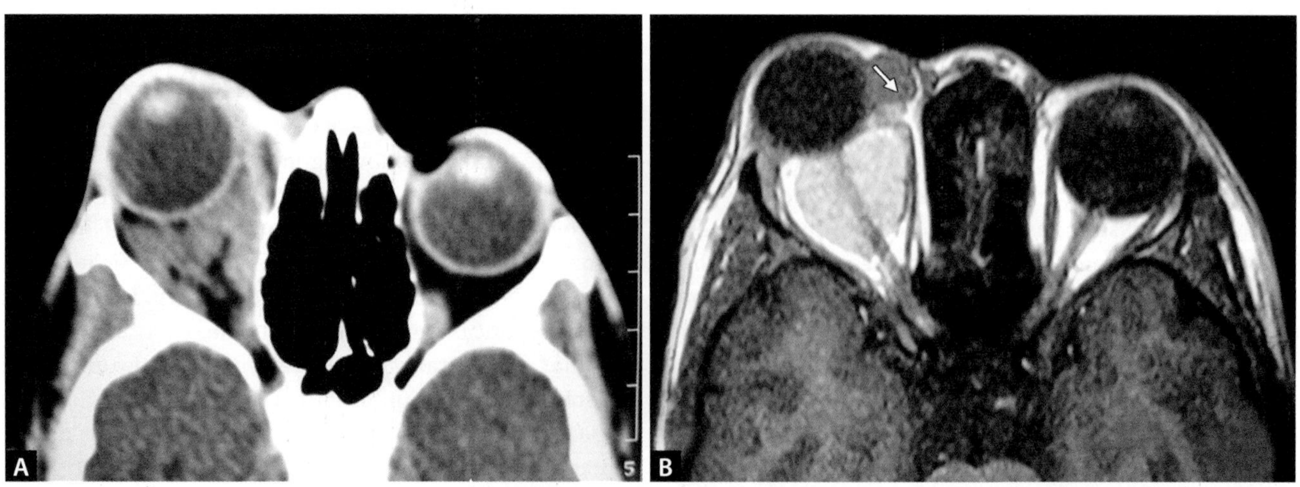

Figs. 12A and B: Lymphangioma, right side causing proptosis: Axial CECT (A) and MR image (B), Ill-defined retrobulbar mass involving both intra- and extraconal compartments (A). Axial T1W MR image (another patient), with intraconal mass with small extraconal extension on the nasal aspect. Note that mass is hyperintense and shows fluid-fluid level (arrow) suggesting hemorrhage.

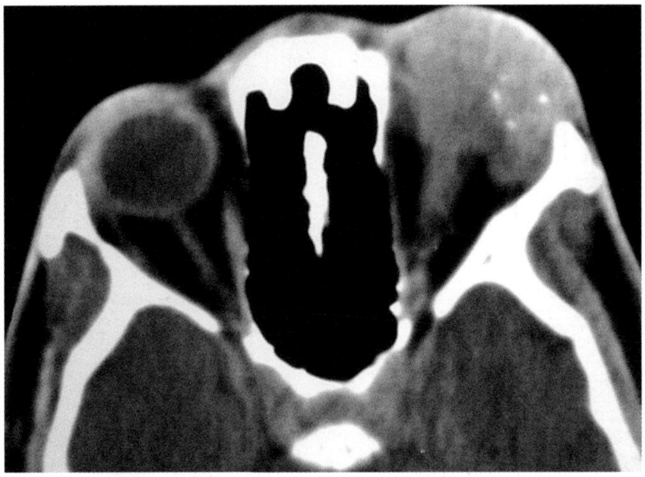

Fig. 13: Malignant mixed tumor of the left lacrimal gland: CECT shows soft tissue mass with calcific foci and remodeling of the adjacent bony lacrimal fossa.

Optic Nerve Glioma

This is the commonest childhood tumor affecting the optic nerve with a female preponderance and largely indolent course. A high association of visual pathway gliomas with neurofibromatosis, amounting to over 50% in some series, has been noted.[22] Two types of neurofibromatosis type I (Von Recklinghausen's disease) and type II (bilateral acoustic neuromas), have been recognized as distinct disorders, each having a different chromosome linkage.[23] Bilateral optic nerve glioma is almost always a manifestation of neurofibromatosis. The adult form of the tumor is aggressive and associated with high mortality. Fifty percent of those presenting in adulthood will have optic nerve and chiasmatic involvement.[24]

US, CT or MRI may reveal tubular, fusiform or saccular enlargement of the optic nerve **(Fig. 14A)**. Tortuosity of the optic nerve, if seen, goes in favor of optic nerve glioma in contrast to rather straight course of thickened optic nerve in optic nerve sheath meningioma. Contrast enhancement is less intense in optic nerve glioma as compared to optic nerve sheath meningioma. Calcification may be rarely present. MRI permits a better demonstration of involvement of intracanalicular and intracranial part of the nerve **(Figs. 14B to D)** and is a modality of choice. Proton density and T2W images demonstrate homogeneous high signal intensity of the affected nerve compared to the low signal of unaffected contralateral optic nerve. Contrast enhancement is variable.

Meningioma

Second most common tumor of the optic nerve sheath complex is meningioma. These are more common in women and frequently occur in middle age. Symptoms depend on the site of involvement within the orbit and the size of tumor. Orbital meningiomas can be divided into 3 types, sphenoid wing meningioma with extension into the orbit, optic nerve sheath meningioma, and those arising de-novo from arachnoid cell rests in the orbit.

Sphenoid wing meningioma: It often results in marked hyperostosis and expansion of the bone. The tumor may extend into the orbit, anterior and middle cranial fossa or extracranially to the temporal fossa. Mass effect from the hyperostotic reaction as well as the soft tissue component compromises the orbital volume causing proptosis. Plain radiography may show sclerosis and thickening of the sphenoid wing. CT and MRI are useful in demonstrating the contiguity between the orbital and intracranial components of orbital meningioma. CT features of a typical meningioma include a well defined smooth outlined mass showing marked contrast enhancement, contiguity with adjacent dura and hyperostosis of adjacent bones **(Fig. 15)**. Bone destruction by an aggressive meningioma may mimic a metastatic or other malignant tumor.

Optic nerve sheath meningioma: Meningioma of the optic nerve sheath arise from arachnoid cells of the dural covering the optic nerve. They are bilateral in about five percent cases, usually associated with NF type 2, radiotherapy or meningiomatosis.[25] These commonly cause diffuse enlargement of the optic nerve sheath complex resulting in a tubular, fusiform or saccular appearance. The difference in density between the tumor and the optic nerve results in a tram track appearance on axial imaging. On the coronal imaging this appears as a 'doughnut sign'. It sign is not specific and has also been described in optic neuritis and pseudotumor. The tumor is isointense to the optic nerve on T1- and T2-weighted images although it may be of low signal intensity on T1 and high signal intensity on T2-weighted images.[26] Fat saturated gadolinium enhanced T1W images provide best lesion demonstration. They usually exhibit marked enhancement following intravenous contrast administration **(Figs. 16A and B)**. Calcification is a common feature of the optic nerve sheath meningiomas and may appear diffuse, coarse or punctuate. The calcification may be tubular in shape along the optic nerve sheath **(Fig. 17)**.

Meningioma arising from arachnoid cells rests within the orbit: This type is very rare and does not show any characteristic features but is seen as an orbital mass located in any part of the orbit.

Rhabdomyosarcoma

Orbit is the most common location of RMS in children, with 40% of all head and neck tumors occurring here. It

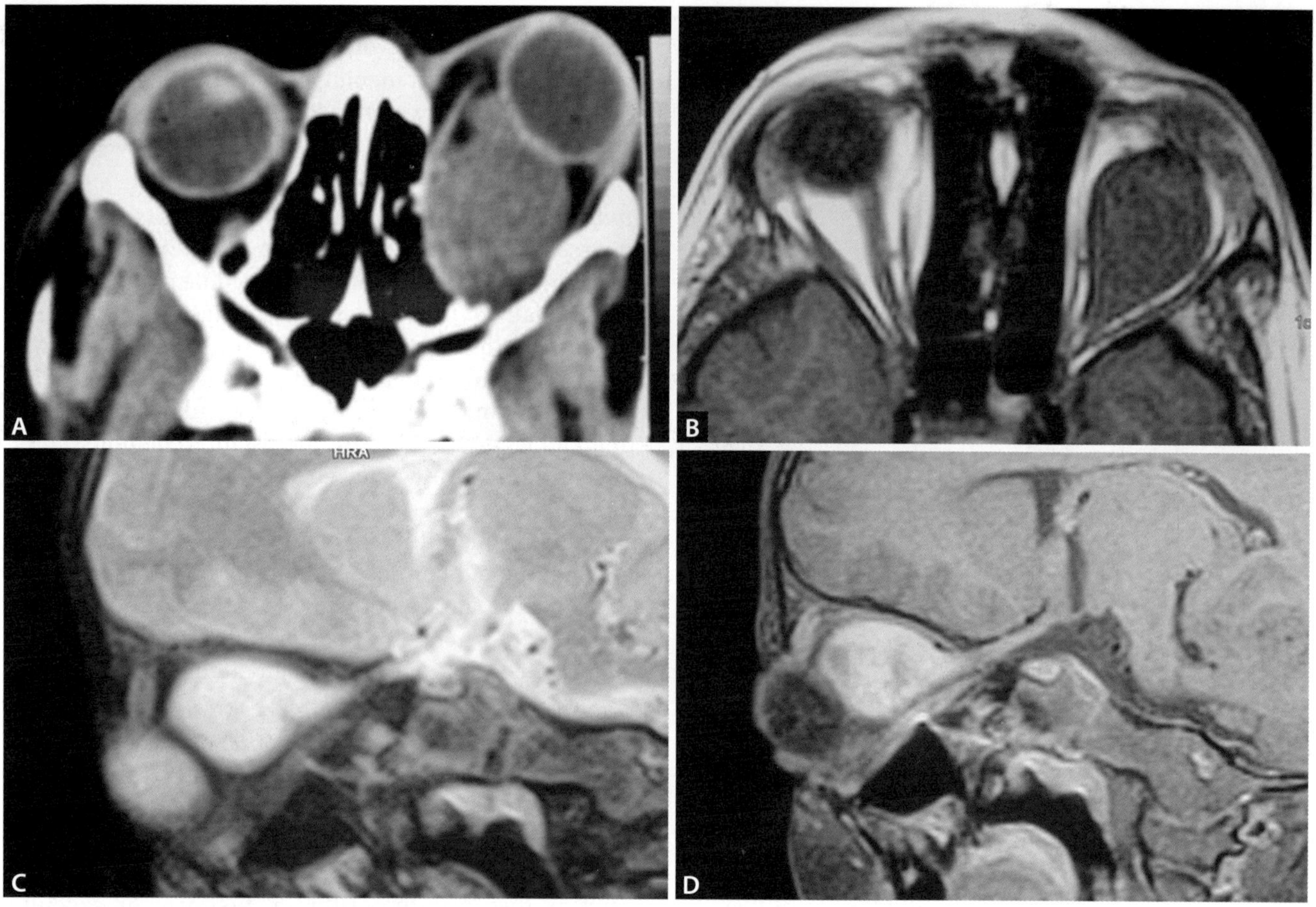

Figs. 14A to D: Optic nerve glioma (L): Axial CT (A) shows fusiform intraconal mass causing proptosis and bony expansion. MRI (B, Axial T1W; C, sagittal T2W; D, sagittal postcontrast) shows that the mass is not separate from optic nerve. It is hypointense on T1WI, hyperintense seen on T2WI and shows enhancement.

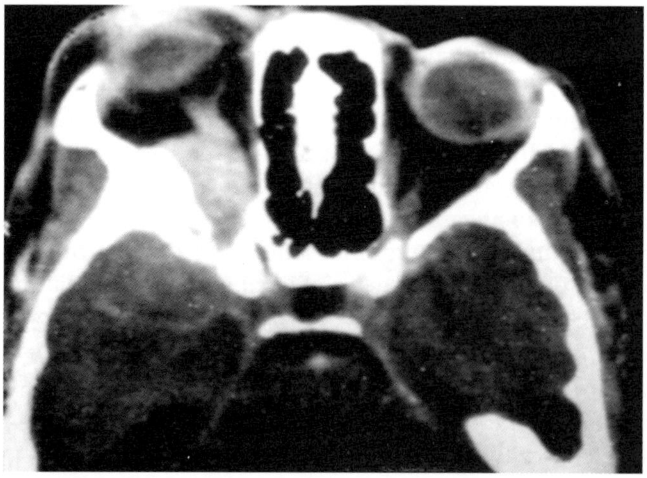

Fig. 15: Sphenoid wing meningioma right orbit: Axial CT scan showing thickening of the greater wing of sphenoid with soft tissue component in the orbit and middle cranial fossa. Right optic nerve appears pushed medially and infiltrated.

is the most common primary orbital malignancy of childhood. The mean age of onset is approximately 6 years. The usual clinical presentation is the rapidly progressive painless proptosis and displacement of the globe or motility disturbance. It is invariably unilateral. The tumor arises in the orbit from extraocular muscles and generally occupies both intra- and extraconal compartments. These are aggressive bone destroying and bone pushing lesions. The most common site of rhabdomyosarcoma (RMS) is considered to be superonasal quadrant of the orbit. Of the head and neck sites, the orbital RMS has a better prognosis presumably because of paucity of lymphatics and confinement by the bony orbit. CT provides information regarding the location, extent of the mass **(Fig. 18)** and presence of bone destruction if any. It is low- to intermediate signal on T1 and bright on T2W images. It exhibits significant contrast enhancement that is more prominent on the fat suppressed images.

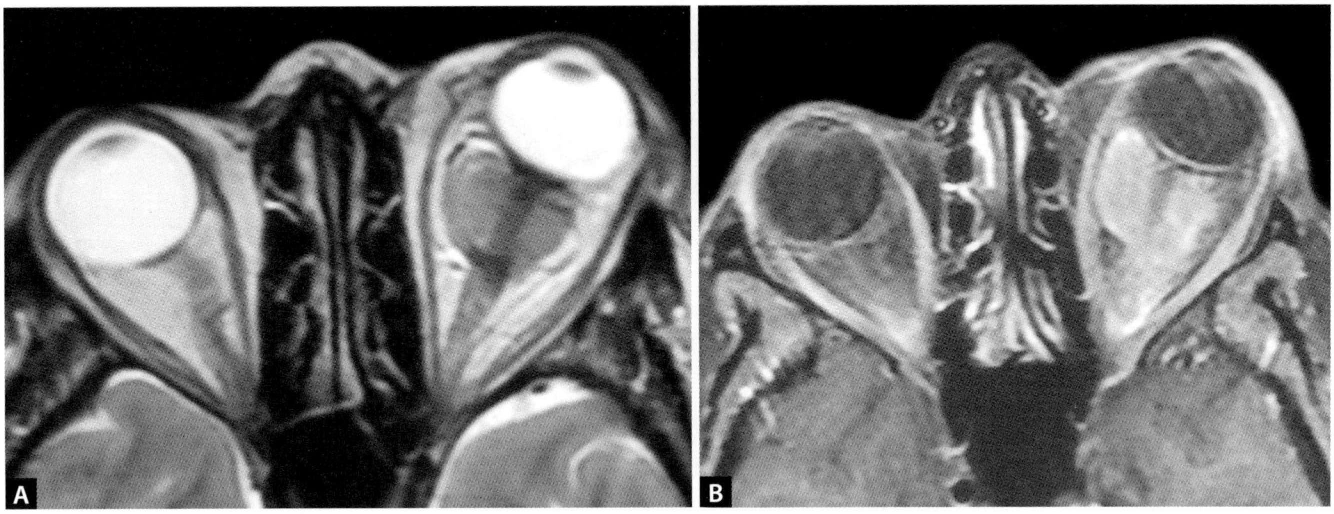

Figs. 16A and B: Optic nerve sheath meningioma (L): Axial MRI images that show the mass is hypointense on T2W (A) and shows bright enhancement on T1W postcontrast images (B). It is seen to be centered around the optic nerve.

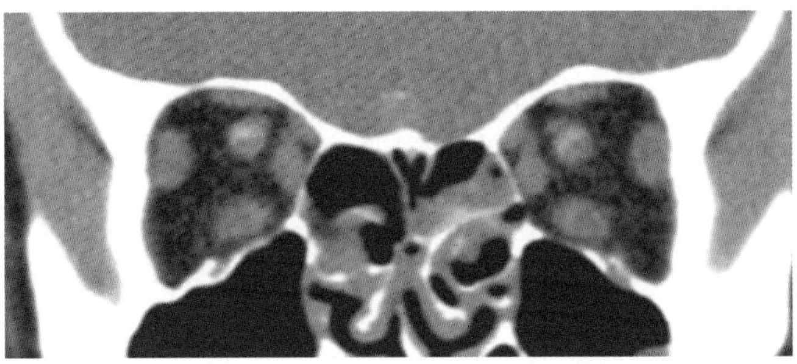

Fig. 17: Bilateral optic nerve sheath meningioma: Ring calcification (Donought sign) of the optic nerve sheaths consistent with neurofibromatosis Type 2.

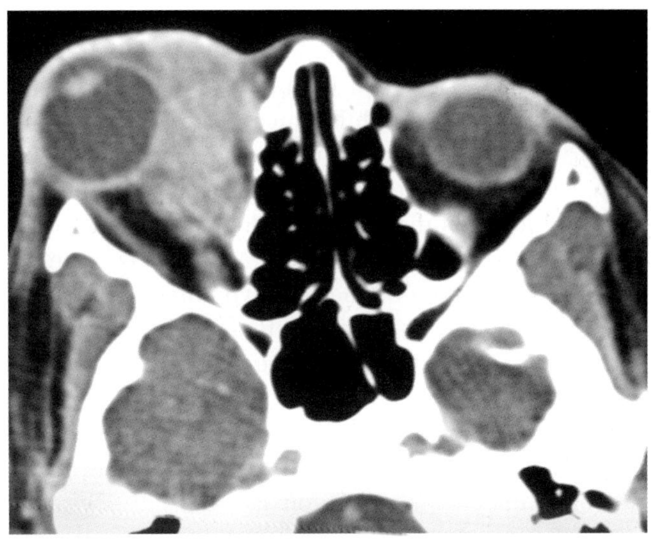

Fig. 18: Rhabdomyosarcoma: Axial CECT showing enhancing soft tissue swelling along the medial quadrant on the right. The mass has both intra- and extraconal components and is causing proptosis.

Lymphoma

Orbital lymphomas are homogeneous masses of relatively high density and sharp margins more often seen in the anterior portion of the orbit **(Fig. 19)**, retrobulbar area, superior orbital compartment or lacrimal gland. Generally the lesions mold themselves to pre-existing structures such as globe, optic nerve and the bony orbit without eroding the bone or enlarging the orbit.

Majority of orbital lymphomas will eventually have systemic disease, usually non-Hodgkin's lymphomas (NHL). However, rarely will a patient with NHL have orbital involvement during course of their illness. Presentation is usually in adults in the 6th to 7th decade. The signal characteristics are determined by cell packing. It may be low on T1 or and T2-weighted images when packing is dense, or high on T2 where packing is less dense. It shows restriction of diffusion on MRI owing to its marked cellularity. Contrast enhancement is variable. Bilateral orbital masses should raise a suspicion of lymphoma. It may have an appearance identical to that of orbital pseudotumor. Orbital lymphoma responds both to chemotherapy and radiotherapy.[26]

Schwannoma/Neurofibroma

These tend to be extraconal, share similar appearances and nerve involvement and therefore considered together. Schwannoma is more common and comprises upto 6% of orbital masses.[26] Both are benign and slow

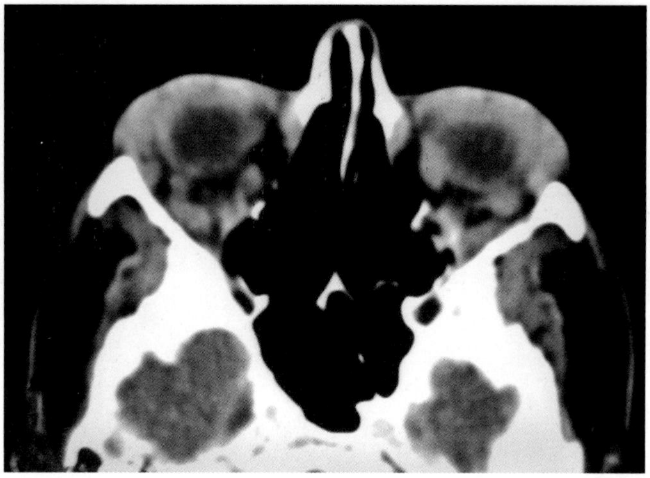

Fig. 19: Lymphoma: Axial CECT of a patient with known systemic Non-Hodgkin's lymphoma shows secondary orbital involvement in form of bilateral preseptal homogeneously enhancing soft tissue swelling.

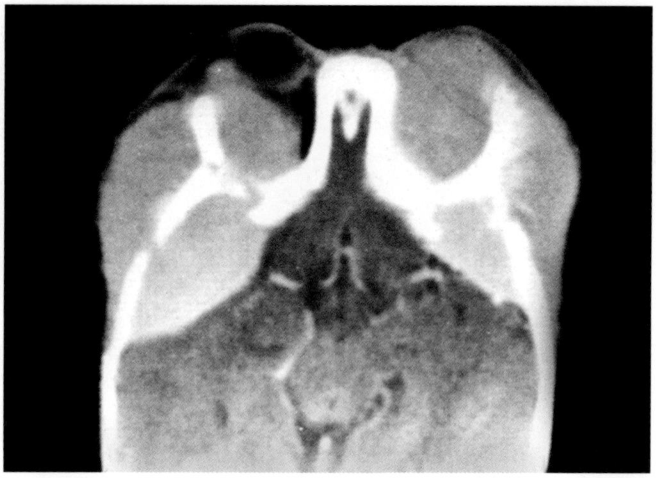

Fig. 20: Metastatic neuoroblastoma: CT shows soft tissue masses occupying both orbits extending into the middle cranial and superficial temporal fossae. The bones show destructive changes and sclerotic bony spiculation.

growing presenting more commonly in adults except neurofibromatosis. Most commonly affected are the sensory branches of ophthalmic division of trigeminal nerve accounting for their superior position in the orbit. Painless proptosis is the commonest presentation. Imaging depends upon the histological characteristics of the schwannomas with Antoni A tumors being more uniform than Antoni B. They are hypointense on T1 and hyperintense on T2-weighted images. Both enhance with contrast. The benign nature of these lesions lead to expansion of bony orbit and remodeling. Plexiform neurofibroma are associated with hypoplasia of the greater wing of sphenoid, and macrophthalmia in neurofibromatosis.[1] Neurofibromas may be distinguished by calcification that is rare in schwannomas.[26]

Orbital Metastases

Orbital metastases are relatively rare. Simultaneous brain metastases may occur in two-thirds, of patients with orbital metastasis. The spread to the orbit may occur by direct extension or through blood borne metastases from a distant primary. In adults, metastases occur from breast, lung, prostate, stomach, etc. In children, the primary sites include neuroblastoma, Ewing's sarcoma and leukemia. The gross morphological pattern of orbital metastatic tumors is variable. These may be infiltrative and poorly defined or may produce a well defined mass. Neuroblastoma is the most common tumor to metastasize to the orbit in infants and young children and bilateral lesions are seen in about 40% of these children.[27] The lesions often show rapid progression with bony and soft tissue components. The bony orbit may be focally or diffusely involved. Bone changes consist of permeative sclerosis, irregular spiculated appearance or irregular destruction **(Fig. 20)**.

Developmental Cysts

The most frequent developmental cyst involving the orbit is the dermoid cyst. These cysts are believed to arise from ectodermal elements that get entrapped in developing sutures of the orbital bones. These are most frequently located in the superolateral quadrant of the orbit. Dermoid cysts are lined by keratinizing squamous ephithelium. They contain adnexal structures such as hair and sebaceous glands which contain keratinacious debris and fatty substance **(Fig. 21)**. Contents of dermoid cysts are oily due to presence of secretion of sebum from the sebaceous glands. The slow enlargement of dermoid cysts produces bony changes by expansion and pressure erosion, with thinning and scalloping of adjacent bones. These cysts are usually well marginated, oval, lobulated or dumb bell shaped lesions with cystic or solid components. Specific diagnosis of dermoid cyst can be made when a fat fluid level is demonstrated.

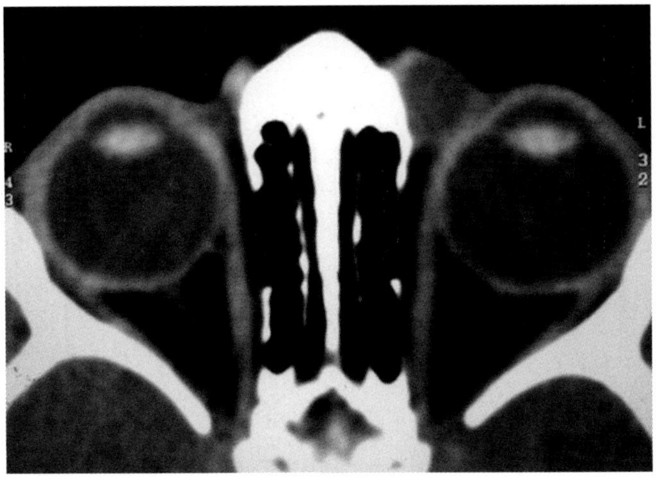

Fig. 21: Inner angular dermoid (L): Axial NCCT image shows a low density (HU-40) mass in relation to the left medial canthus.

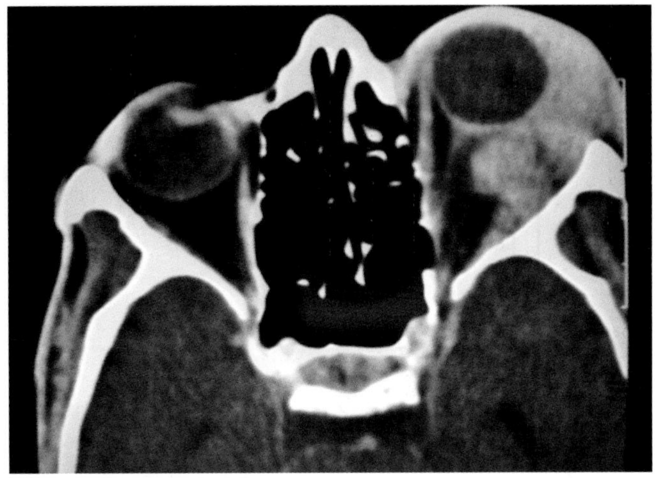

Fig. 22: Pseudotumor: Axial CECT showing a moderately enhancing ill-defined transcompartmental mass involving the left orbit, centered at the lacrimal gland extending to the retrobulbar area and preseptal soft tissues causing proptosis.

INFLAMMATORY LESIONS

Pseudotumor

Pseudotumor (idiopathic orbital inflammation) is the commonest inflammatory lesion of the orbit. It usually occurs in the middle age and is characterized by the classic triad of proptosis, pain and impaired ocular motility. Children may have constitutional symptoms leading to false diagnosis of orbital cellulitis. It is usually unilateral. Diagnosis is made after exclusion of other pathologies like Wegener's granulomatosis, sarcoid, systemic lupus erythematosus, polyarteritis nodosa, rheumatoid arthritis, lymphoproliferative disorders and metastasis. Associated disorders include fibrosing mediastinitis, retroperitoneal and hepatic fibrosis, Reidel's thyroiditis and cholangitis. Depending upon the site involved, they show varied presentation, the most common being the myositic form in which the affected muscle is enlarged and ill-defined right up to its insertion. The other presentations include lacrimal gland involvement, retrobulbar anteriorly located mass (Tenon's space), posteriorly located mass (apical involvement), focal well circumscribed mass in any part of the orbit, diffuse mass occupying whole of the orbit and multifocal masses involving various intraorbital structures or lacrimal gland **(Fig. 22)**. Sclerosing form presents in a chronic progressive form and is resistant to treatment. Imaging features on CT and MRI are nonspecific. These exhibit some contrast enhancement. It is hypointense to fat on T1 and iso- to hypointense on T2W images. This appearance may help to distinguish pseudotumor from true tumors.[28]

IgG4-related Orbital Disease

This entity is now considered distinct from the orbital pseudotumor. It commonly causes painless swelling of the lacrimal gland(s), extraocular muscles, orbital fat, infraorbital nerve, lacrimal apparatus and lids. It is a systemic condition in which the lesions rich in IgG4+ plasma cells could be present multiple other organs. On MRI the lesions are isointense on T1WI, hypointense on T2WI and enhance following gadolinium administration.[29] FDG-PET imaging is often used for systemic evaluation to locate distant or clinically silent disease.[30] Nearly half of IgG4-related orbital disease (IgG4-ROD) patients will have systemic involvement.[31] There is a well known association between bilateral IgG4-ROD and systemic disease.[32]

Endocrine Orbitopathy

Graves' ophthalmopathy usually affects middle aged women. It may precede systemic disease. It usually causes bilateral muscle enlargement, involving most commonly the inferior rectus followed by the medial rectus muscle and superior rectus complex. Isolated lateral rectus involvement is rare and prompts consideration of alternative diagnoses. There may be increase in volume of intraorbital fat. This combination of extraocular muscle enlargement and increased intraorbital fat produces proptosis. Optic nerve compression due to apical crowding is rare. Muscle belly rather than the insertion is involved **(Figs. 23A and B)**. The tendinous involvement is more

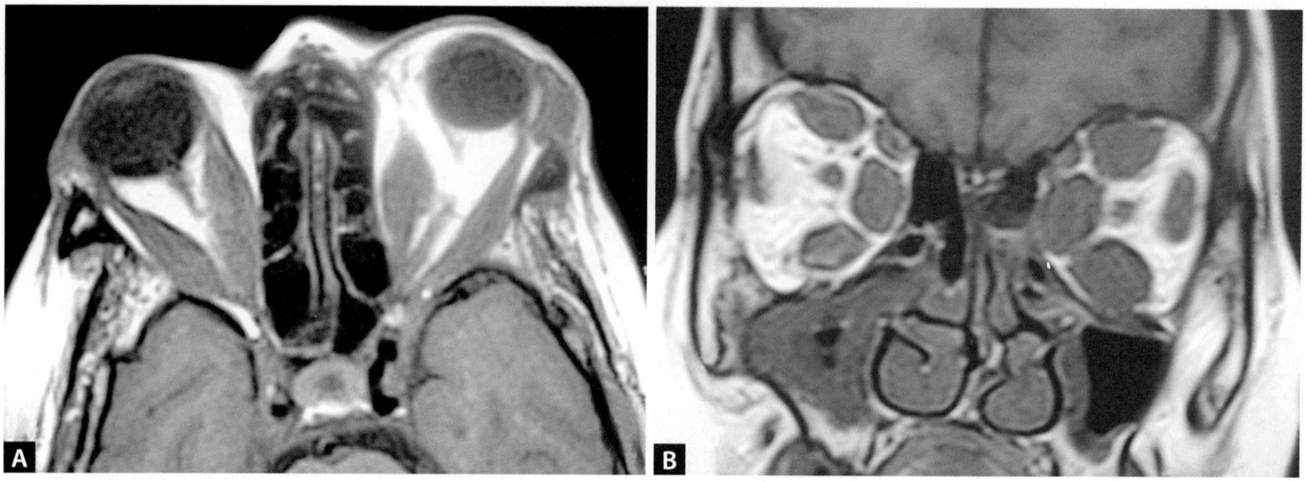

Figs. 23A and B: Endocrine exophthalmos: Axial (A) and coronal (B) T1W MR images show thickening of the bellies of extraocular muscle of both orbits, sparing the tendinous insertions.

suggestive of a pseudotumor. Imaging appearances can be efficiently diagnosed and monitored by with CT, especially in the coronal plane.[26]

Parasitic Cysts

Cysticercosis is the most common parasitic infestation of the orbit. Commonly cysticerci affect the muscles of the orbit resulting in muscle thickening due to inflammatory reaction. In addition, a cystic area representing the cysticercus cellulosae and a nodule representing scolex may be seen **(Fig. 24)**. Muscle thickening due to cysticercus may be confused with a pseudotumor or vice versa.

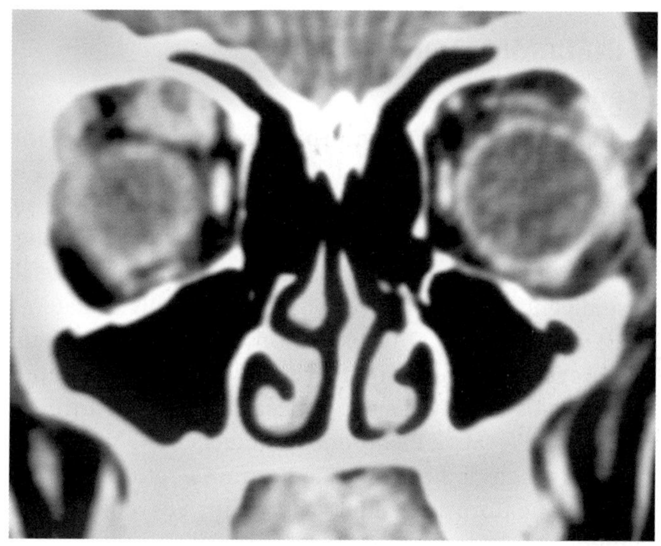

Fig. 24: Orbital myocysticercus: Coronal CT showing a cyst with a scolex and thickened superior rectus muscle in the right orbit.

VASCULAR LESIONS

Caroticocavernous Fistula

The fistulous communication occurs between the carotid siphon and cavernous sinus (direct), or between meningeal branches of internal or external carotid artery and dural veins (indirect) in the vicinity of the carvernous sinus producing congestion of the orbit and globe, pulsatile exophthalmos, bruit and eventually glaucoma and visual loss. It may occur secondary to trauma or spontaneously. Pulsating exophthalmos is the most frequent presenting symptom. CT and MRI depict signs of orbital venous hypertension with an enlarged superior ophthalmic vein and extraocular muscles **(Fig. 25A)**. MRI shows a signal void and in the cavernous sinus superior ophthalmic vein due to arterial flow. The cavernous sinus is enlarged. Digital subtraction arteriography not only demonstrates the fistulous communication **(Fig. 25B)**, but also allows interventional neuroradiological procedures using detachable balloon and/or coil embolization to occlude the site of fistula.

Orbital Varices

True orbital varices are congenital venous malformations in which the afferent and efferent vessels are veins. Most common clinical feature of congenital orbital varices is intermittent proptosis that increases on leaning forward, coughing or straining. US shows dilated intraorbital veins usually with slow flow. On CT and MRI, the varix is seen as a lobulated soft tissue mass that usually tapers towards the apex and increases in size during Vasalva maneuver.

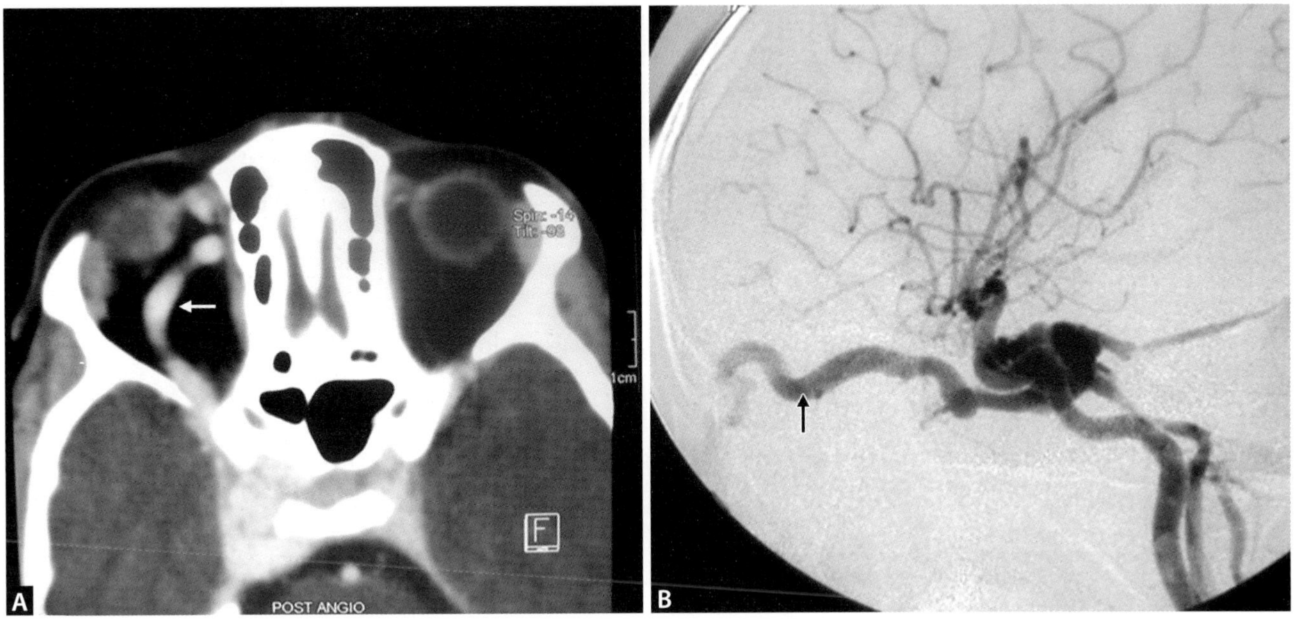

Figs. 25A and B: Traumatic caroticocavernous fistula: CECT (A) and right internal carotid angiogram (B) shows dilated superior ophthalmic vein (white arrow) and prominent right cavernous sinus on CT. Angiogram shows direct communication between the internal carotid artery and cavernous sinus with retrograde filling of dilated superior ophthalmic vein (black arrow).

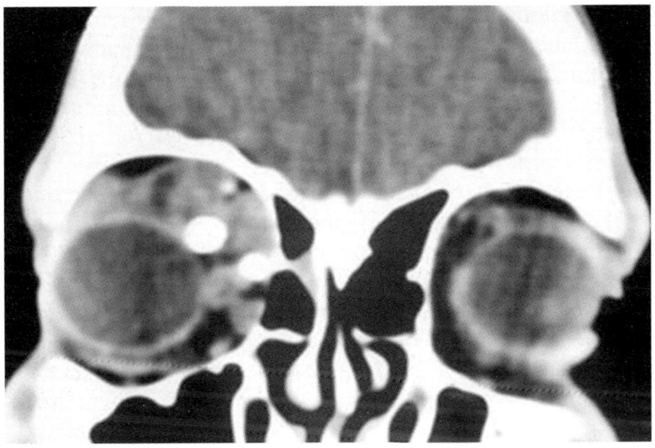

Fig. 26: Orbital varices: Coronal CT image shows tortuous vascular channels with phleboliths superomedial to the right globe.

Calcified phleboliths may be seen in some patients **(Fig. 26)**. MRI depicts the varix as a signal void if associated with rapidly flowing blood. Spontaneous thrombosis is common and the signal intensity depends on the age of thrombus. Orbital phlebography is now considered redundant to define the varices.

Osseous Lesions

Bones of the orbit may be involved by dysplasias, primary or metastatic bone tumors, etc. Fibrous dysplasia typically presents during the first two decades of life. It represents both arrested and altered maturation of bone. Alterations in the bone maturation result in replacement of normal bone with immature bone and fibrous stroma. The bone is markedly expanded, encroaches upon and distorts the adjacent structures, e.g. orbits and paranasal sinuses. Lesions of fibrous dysplasia are generally diffusely sclerotic, having a ground glass appearance but may be heterogeneous. Most patients with orbital fibrous dysplasia present with unilateral proptosis. Plain radiography shows characteristic expanded, sclerotic bone often with ground glass appearance. CT better demonstrates these features and exact extent of the lesion **(Figs. 27A and B)**.

Trauma

The orbit may be injured directly or indirectly, both with blunt or penetrating trauma. Injury to the globe may occur as an isolated event. Soft tissue swelling often obscures direct clinical evaluation of the globe. Plain film evaluation of the orbit remains the initial imaging modality; however the lack of soft tissue detail limits its utility for treatment planning. CT is the method of choice in diagnosing traumatic lesions involving the orbit. It shows both bony and soft tissue details, and more clearly defines the location and orientation of displaced bony fragments, foreign bodies and air. A commonly encountered intraorbital fracture, the so called blow out fracture **(Fig. 28)**, occurs when direct blunt force is applied

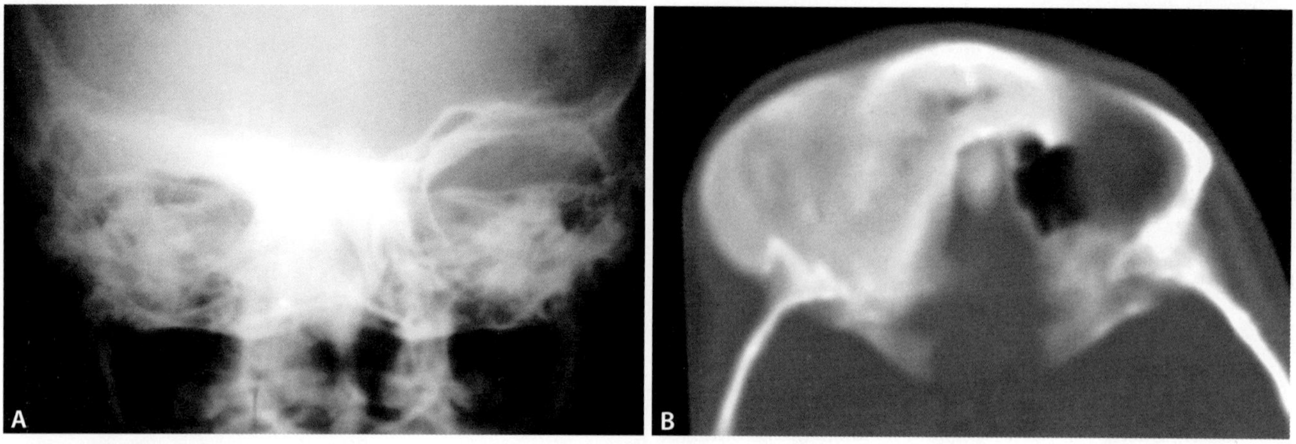

Figs. 27A and B: Fibrous dysplasia: (A) Frontal orbital radiograph showing sclerosis of the right orbital and frontonasal region; (B) Axial CT (bone window) shows ground glass haze of the involved bones.

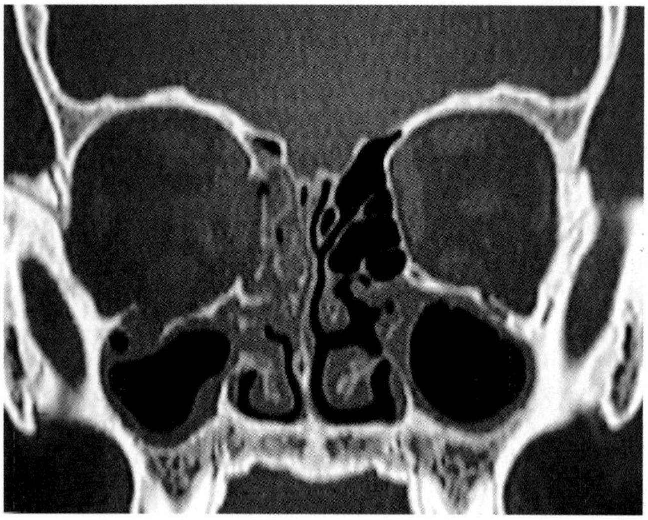

Fig. 28: Blow out fracture: Coronal CT image (bone window) shows fracture of the medial wall and floor of the right orbit. There was no extraocular muscle entrapment on the soft tissue window (not shown).

to the globe and orbit with disruption of the orbital wall. The floor or medial walls are most often fractured with the orbital rim remaining intact. In patients with optic nerve injury following trauma, thin sections of CT may delineate the injured nerve, apical bony fragments and adjacent hematoma for crucial preoperative assessment. MRI may be complementary to CT scanning in certain patients particularly with injuries involving the globe or optic nerve.[33]

A variety of other injuries occur involving globe, ranging from rupture, dislocation of lens, and vitreous/retrohyloid/ or retro-ocular hematoma. CT provides exact localization of metallic foreign bodies without risk of their dislocation. MRI is contraindicated in the presence of a metallic foreign body but may be useful in detection and localization of a nonmetallic foreign body.[34] Retained foreign bodies may lead to granuloma or abscess formation.

REFERENCES

1. Schlotmann K, Koelwel BF, Hackenberg MD, Gabel VP, Scholmerich J. High frequency contrast harmonic imaging of ophthalmic tumor perfusion. Am J Radiol. 2005;184:574-78.
2. Hosten N, Bornfeld N (Eds). Imaging of the globe and orbit: A guide to differential diagnosis. New York: Thieme Stuttgart, 1998.
3. Mafee MF, Putterman A, Valvassori GE, Campos M, Capek V. Orbital space occupying lesions: Role of computed tomography and magnetic resonance imaging. RCNA. 1987;25:520-59.
4. Muller-Forell WS, Pitz S. Orbital Pathology. In: Muller-Forell WS (Ed). Imaging of orbital and visual pathway pathology. Heidelberg. 2002. pp. 147-340.
5. Zimmerman RA, Bilaniuk LT. Computed tomography in the evaluation of patients with bilateral retinoblastomas. J Comput Tomogr. 1979;3:251-57.
6. Haik BG, Saint Louis L, Smith ME, Ellsworth RM, Abramson OH, Cahill P, Deck M, Coleman J. Magnetic resonance imaging in evaluation of leucokoria. Ophthalmology. 1985;92:1143-52.
7. Vashisht S, Goulatia RK, Dayal Y, Bhargava S. Retinoblastoma: A CT study. IJRI 1986;40:17-21.
8. Char DH, Hedges TR, Norman D. Retinoblastoma. Ophthalmology. 1984;91:1347-59.
9. de Graaf P, Pouwels PJ, Rodjan F, Moll AC, Imhof SM, Knol DL, Sanchez E, van der Valk P, Castelijns JA. Single-shot turbo spin-echo diffusion weighted imaging for retinoblastoma: initial experience. Am J Neuroradiol. 2012;33(1):110-8.
10. Hiwatashi A1, Togao O1, Yamashita K1, Kikuchi K1, Yoshikawa H2, Obara M3, Honda H1. Br J Radiol. 2016;89(1067):20160074. Epub 2016 Sep 16.

11. Mafee MF. The eye. In: Som PM, Curtin HD (Eds). Head and Neck imaging (4th edn.) St. Louis: Mosby. 2003;2:441-527.
12. De Potter P, Shields CL, Shields JA, Flanders AE. The role of magnetic resonance imaging in children with intraocular tumors simulating lesions. Ophthalmology. 1996;103:1774-83.
13. De Potter P, Shields JA, Shields CL, Flanders AE. The role of MRI in children with intra-ocular tumors and simulating lesions. Ophthalmology. 1996;103:1774-83.
14. De Potter P, Shields JA, Shields CL. MRI of the eye and orbit. Philadelphia: Lippincott, 1995.
15. Damato BE, Paul J, Foulds WS. Risk factors of residual and recurrent uveal melanoma after transscleral local resection. Br J Ophthalmol. 1996;80:102-08.
16. Glatt HJ, Custer PL, Barrett L, Sator K. Magnetic resonance imaging and computed tomography in a model of wooden foreign bodies in the orbit. Ophthalm Plast Reconstr. 1990;6:108-14.
17. Kumar A, Verma L, Jha SN, Tiwari HK, Khosla PK. Ultrasonic evaluation of intraocular cysticercosis. Afro-Asian Jour of Ophthalmology. 1989;55:55-6.
18. Ruchman MC, Stefanyszn MA, Flangagan JC, et al. Orbital tumors. In: Gonzalez CA, Becker MH, Flanagan JC (Eds). Diagnostic Imaging in Ophthalmology, New York: Springer - Verlag. 1986. pp. 201-38.
19. Bilaniuk LT. Orbital vascular lesions—role of imaging. Radiol Clin North Am Imaging Ophthal II; 1999;169-83.
20. Barnacle AM, Theodorou M, Maling SJ, Abou-Rayyah Y. Sclerotherapy treatment of orbital lymphatic malformations: a large single-centre experience. Br J Ophthalmol. 2016;100(2):204-8. doi: 10.1136/bjophthalmol-2015-306657. Epub 2015 Jun 17.
21. Patel KC, Kalantzis G, El-Hindy N, Chang BY. Sclerotherapy for orbital lymphangioma—case series and literature review. In Vivo. 2017;31(2):263-6.
22. Bternn J, Jacobiec FA, Housepian EM. The architecture of optic nerve gliomas with and without neurofibromatosis. Arch Ophth. 1980;98:505-11.
23. National Institutes of Health Consensus development. neurofibromatosis. Arch Neural. 1988;45:545-78.
24. Hollander MD, Fitzpatrick M, O'Connor SG, Flanders AE, Tartaglino LM. Optic gliomas. RCNA. 1999;37:59-71.
25. Hodes JE, Sanders M, Patel P, Patchell RA. Radiosurgical management of meningiomas. Stereotact Funct Neurosurg. 1996;6:15-18.
26. Aviv RI, Miszkiel K. Orbital Imaging - Part 2. Intraorbital pathology. Clin Radiol 2005;60:288-307.
27. Rootman J, Chan KW. Neuroblastoma: In rooman J (Ed). New York: JB Lippincott. Diseases of the Orbit. 1988;25.
28. Mombaerts I, Schlingermann RO, Goldschmeding R, Koorneef L. Are systemic corticosteroids useful in the management of orbital pseudotumors? Ophthalmology. 1996;103:521-8.
29. Toyoda K, Oba H, Kutomi K et al. MR imaging of IgG4-related disease in the head and neck and brain. Am J Neuroradiol. 2012;33(11):2136-9.
30. Masaki Y, Kurose N, Umehara H. IgG4-related disease: a novel lymphoproliferative disorder discovered and established in Japan in the 21st century. J Clin Exp Hematop. 2011;51:13-20.
31. McNab A, McKelvie P. IgG4-related ophthalmic disease. Part II: Clinical Aspects. Ophthal Plast Reconstr Surg. 2015;31(3):167-78.
32. Wu A, Andrew NH, McNab AA, Selva D. Bilateral IgG4-related ophthalmic disease: a strong indication for systemic imaging. Br J Ophthalmol. 2016;100:1409-11.
33. Rothman M. Orbital trauma. Seminars in US, CT and MRI 1997;18:437-97.
34. Wilson WB, Dreisbach JN, Lattin DE, Stears JC. Magnetic resonance imaging of non metallic foreign bodies. Am J Ophthal. 1988;105: 612-7.

CHAPTER 22

Imaging of the Paranasal Sinuses

Vivek Gupta, Niranjan Khandelwal

INTRODUCTION

Nose and paranasal sinuses (PNS) are affected by a wide variety of diseases and to diagnose them understanding of the anatomy and physiology of this region is necessary. PNS have been described in ancient text by many people like description of maxillary sinuses by Leonardo da Vinci and of ethmoid air cells by Galen. Later, X-rays remained the mainstay in diagnosing the diseases of the sinuses for many years. Presently the technology has evolved to a point where a virtual tour of the sinuses can be taken to see normal structures and abnormalities. The present chapter deals with all aspects of PNS, from embryology, to development and normal variations followed by infections, inflammations, benign and malignant conditions.

PARANASAL SINUS EMBRYOLOGY

Paranasal sinuses start developing from the primitive choana. At 25–28 weeks of gestation, three projections arise from the lateral wall of the nose and serve as the beginning of the development of PNS. The anterior projection forms the agger nasi. The inferior (maxilloturbinate) projection forms the inferior turbinate and maxillary sinus. The superior projection (ethmoidoturbinate) forms the ethmoidal air cells and their corresponding drainage channels. The middle meatus invaginates laterally to form the embryonic infundibulum and uncinate process and the embryonic infundibulum grows superiorly to form the frontal recess area. The frontal sinus may develop as a direct continuation of embryonic infundibulum and frontal recess superiorly during the 16th week. It can also develop by upward migration of anterior ethmoidal air cells to penetrate the inferior aspect of the frontal bone between its outer and inner tables. The maxillary sinuses are the first to be seen on plain X-rays and are usually aerated at birth. They increase in size till the age of 14 years. The ethmoid sinuses are also aerated at birth but are rarely visible on plain X-rays. They rapidly expand till the age of 4 years with a spurt of growth during adolescence. The ethmoid sinuses are thus a site of infection in childhood sinusitis. The pneumatization of the sphenoid sinus begins by age 2 years.

Its growth is slower than other PNS. Pneumatization of frontal sinuses occurs last and is not visualized before 6 years. They grow to adult size by 12–14 years. The osteomeatal complexes (OMCs) are fully developed at birth. The development of sinuses is influenced by dentition.

IMAGING MODALITIES AND TECHNIQUE OF EVALUATION

Conventional Radiography

Standard radiography of the PNS usually consists of four views: (i) Lateral view, (ii) Caldwell view, (iii) Water's view, and (iv) Submentovertex (SMV) or base view. The lateral view demonstrates the frontal, maxillary and sphenoid sinuses. The Caldwell view shows the frontal sinuses and posterior ethmoid air cells. The Water's view shows

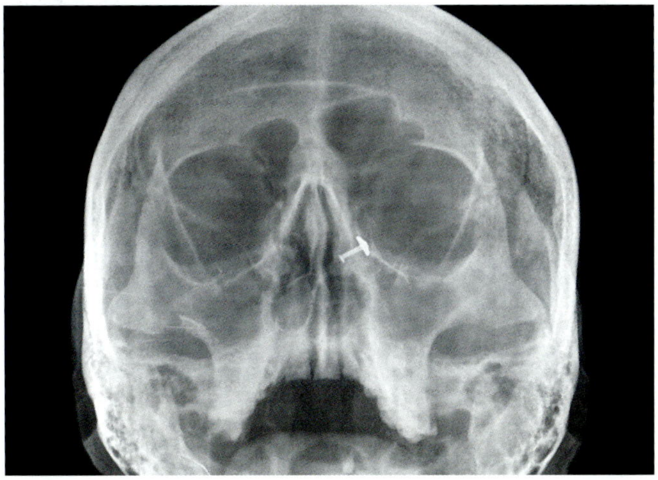

Fig. 1: Plain X-ray (Water's view) showing complete opacification of the bilateral maxillary sinuses.

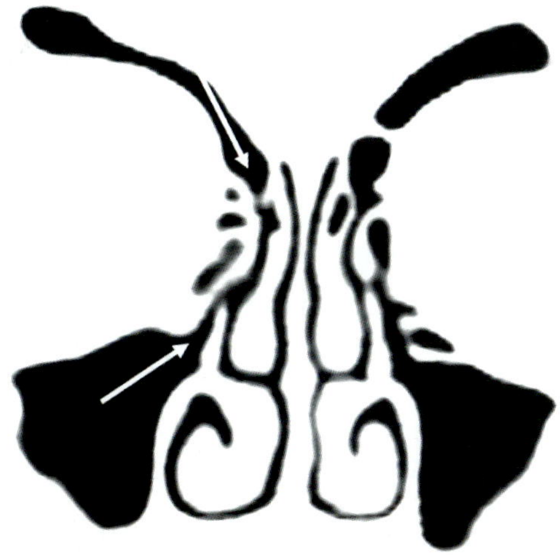

Fig. 2: Paranasal sinuses seen in lung window with clear depiction of osteomeatal complex (OMC) and frontal recess (arrow).

the maxillary sinuses, anterior ethmoid air cells, inferior orbital rims and orbital floors. The submentovertex view evaluates the sphenoid sinus as well as the anterior and posterior walls of the frontal sinuses.

The findings which are suggestive of bacterial sinusitis on the X-rays are mucoperiosteal thickening, air-fluid level and complete opacification of the sinus **(Fig. 1)**. The X-rays thus have been used based upon above findings as a screening tool for sinusitis. However, there are many studies which question the sensitivity of plain X-rays.[1-3] One such study compared three views (Caldwell, lateral and Water's) with CT scans of the PNS (3 × 3 mm coronal sections). They found that sensitivity was 57–62% and specificity 88% when the X-rays were interpreted by radiologists and were 48–67% and 75–100%, respectively when interpreted by emergency medicine staff members. The wide variation in sensitivity and specificity and interobserver variations makes X-ray evaluation a poor modality even as a screening tool.[4]

Computed Tomography

Computed tomography (CT) is the modality of choice in the evaluation of the PNS and adjacent structures.

Present generation of CT scanners have obviated the need to scan twice in axial and coronal plan. Now, volumetric axial scans of the PNS can be one in matter of few seconds and can then be reconstructed automatically into coronal and sagittal orientations. Also, both bone and soft tissue images are reconstructed by the systems.

Positions (if multislice CT is available and thin reconstruction can be done and direct scanning in coronal plane may not be done).

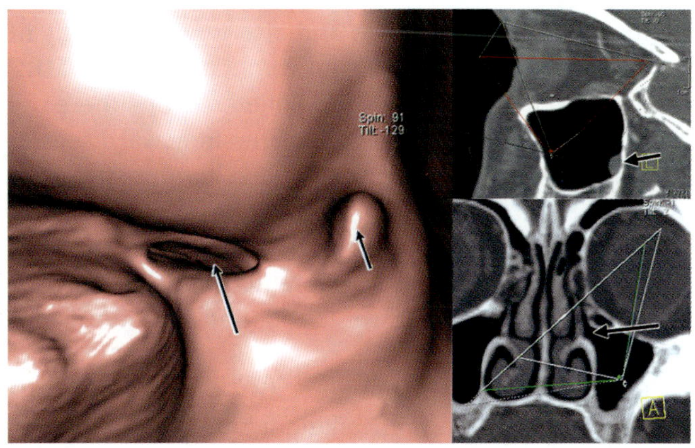

Fig. 3: Virtual sinoscopic image obtained on a 16-slice scanner showing maxillary ostium and infundibulum (long arrows) and a small maxillary polyp (short arrows) on VR, sagittal and coronal images.

The anatomy is best evaluated in the bone window. The osteomeatal complex may further be studied in lung window **(Fig. 2)** to see for patency of the OM complex and other draining pathways. Since the coronal images closely resemble the view of endoscopy which is frequently employed for diagnosis and treatment. These images are preferred more over axial images. Now, with the advent of contiguous data acquisition, it has become possible to see the sinus anatomy in coronal plane in 3D.[5]

With the improvement in post-processing software and isotropic voxel image acquisition, it is now possible to obtain virtual endoscopic images of the sinus on CT **(Fig. 3)**. In a study exploring this aspect, virtual sinoscopy was done in patients and compared with preoperative fiberoptic endoscopy and intraoperative findings.

Significant correlation was found between the findings on virtual sinoscopy, preoperative endoscopy and intraoperative findings.[6]

Sagittal reconstruction adds to the information, especially drainage pathway of sphenoid sinus and posterior ethmoid sinuses and the spread of pathology through them.

Contrast enhancement is not routinely done in the evaluation of sinus pathologies like sinusitis or polyposis. However, it is used if differentiation between inflammation and neoplasms is to be done and if intracranial spread is suspected.

MAGNETIC RESONANCE IMAGING

Magnetic resonance imaging (MRI) has not gained much importance when it comes to routine evaluation of sinonasal diseases, especially sinusitis. There are many reasons for that, bony outlines are not well visualized, sinuses filled with chronic inspissated secretions appear as normally aerated sinuses and also fungal sinusitis in a sinus may give normal signal void like of air on MRI. However, in spite of above mentioned reasons there are certain indications or role of MRI in the sinonasal diseases. MRI has a very important role in evaluating spread of pathology into brain and orbits. Due to its superior soft tissue resolution it can detect even minimal extension into these areas. Also, it is able to differentiate reliably between mucosal hypertrophy, chronic retained secretions and mucoceles.

Postcontrast MRI images are also helpful in differentiating tumors from inflammations. Inflammations enhance peripherally and the tumors show central enhancement.

In a recent randomized study, CT and MRI were compared. They found that Lund–Mackay staging of sinus disease by MRI is closely correlated to corresponding staging based on CT. MRI does not significantly overstage or overclassify patients with sinus disease.[7]

MRI is also particularly suited for the evaluation of the skull base and posterior fossa as these areas are inadequately imaged by CT due to beam hardening artifacts.[8-10]

Routine MRI studies include both coronal and axial images. Sagittal scans are also obtained to image the pathology in planes which are nearly parallel to the axial planes, e.g. palate, orbital floor and skull base. Routine sequences include proton density images (PDI), T1WI and T2WI. Fat suppressed enhanced T1 WI should be routinely employed for evaluation of complicated sinusitis or for suspected neoplastic disease especially when there is orbital or skull base extension or involvement.[11]

NORMAL ANATOMY AND ANATOMIC VARIATIONS[12-14]

Normal Anatomy

Description of the anatomy of this region involves nasal structures, PNS and their draining pathways. In these three areas the delineation of the drainage pathways is most important as their patency or blockage holds the key for treatment.

Nasal Structures

The nasal septum is a midline structure composed of both bone and cartilaginous tissue. Its deviation can cause partial obstruction in the nasal cavities unilaterally or on both sides depending on its shape. The lateral nasal wall has three projections: (i) superior, (ii) middle and (iii) inferior turbinates. These structures divide the nasal cavity into three air passages: (i) superior, (ii) middle, and (iii) inferior meatus.

The inferior turbinate is the lower most projections arising from the lateral nasal bone and extending into the nasal cavity and running posteriorly toward the nasopharynx. These turbinates are frequently enlarged in deviated nasal septum or allergic rhinitis.

The nasolacrimal duct (NLD) is a small tubular structure which runs along the lateral nasal wall and opens into the inferior meatus underneath the inferior turbinate. The NLD runs within a bony canal formed by the maxilla, lacrimal apparatus and inferior turbinate bones.

The middle turbinate lies above the inferior turbinates. Anterosuperiorly, the middle turbinate attaches to the skull base just lateral to the cribriform plate. In its middle third it turns coronally and laterally to insert on the lamina papyracea and posteriorly to the roof of ethmoidal complex. The basal lamella is the portion of the middle turbinate where it attaches to the ethmoid complex and divides it into anterior and middle sinus complex **(Figs. 4 and 5)**.

Draining Pathways

Anterior draining pathways: The OMC is the term given to anterior draining pathways and consists of air passages between the frontal, anterior ethmoid and maxillary sinuses.

The components of the OMC include the frontal recess, ethmoid infundibulum, hiatus semilunaris and middle meatus. The frontal sinus, drain via *frontal recess* which is hourglass shaped structure. The frontal recess affords mucociliary drainage of the frontal and anterior ethmoidal sinuses into the middle meatus.

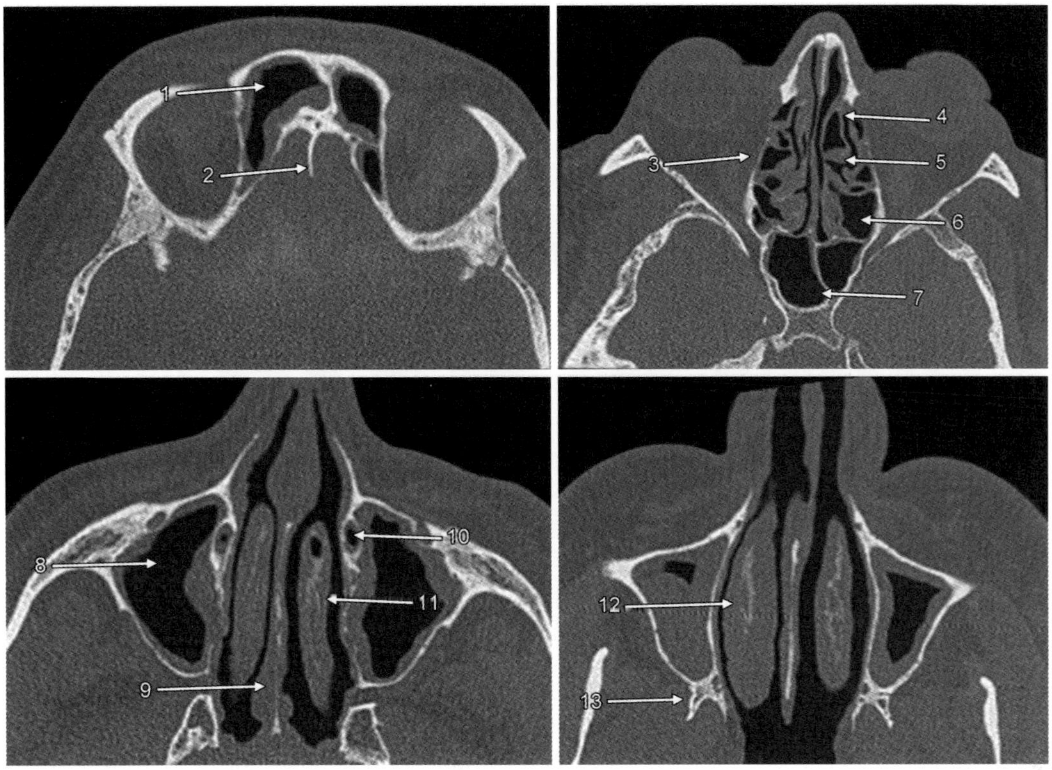

Fig. 4: Axial anatomy: (1) Frontal sinus; (2) Crista galli; (3) Lamina papyracea; (4) Ant ethmoid cells; (5) Middle ethmoid cells; (6) Post-ethmoid cells; (7) Sphenoid sinus; (8) Maxillary sinus; (9) Nasal septum; (10) Nasolacrimal duct; (11) Inferior turbinate; (12) Middle turbinate; (13) Pterygoid plates.

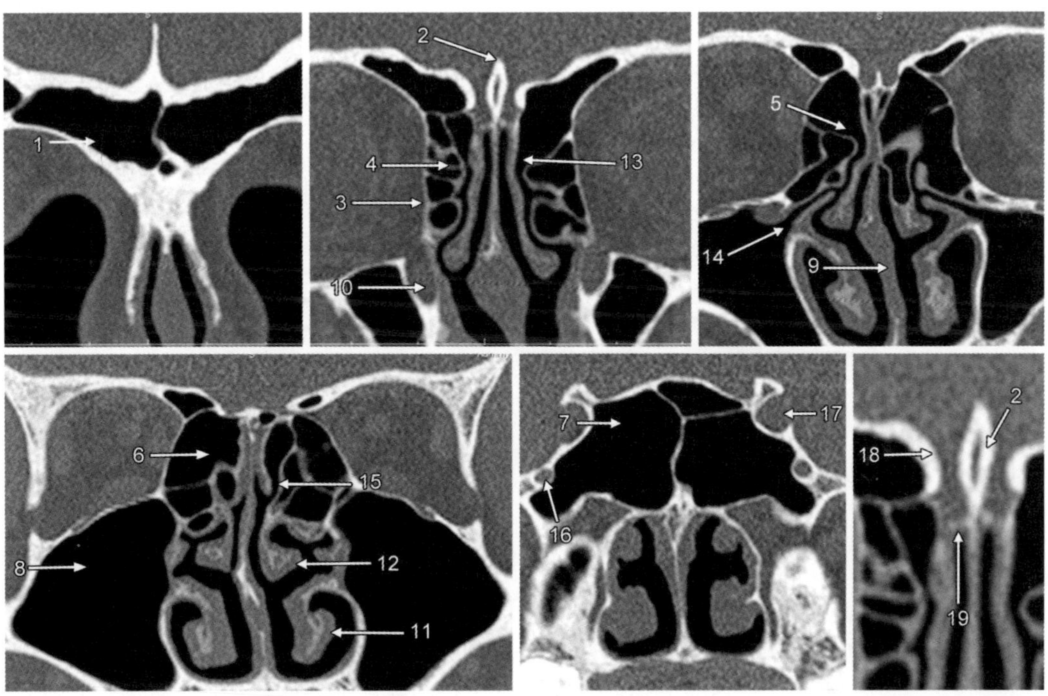

Fig. 5: Coronal anatomy: (1) Frontal sinus; (2) Crista galli; (3) Lamina Papyracea; (4) Anterior ethmoid cells; (5) Middle ethmoid cells; (6) Postethmoid cells; (7) Sphenoid sinus; (8) Maxillary sinus; (9) Nasal septum; (10) Nasolacrimal duct; (11) Inferior turbinate; (12) Middle turbinate; (13) Frontal recess; (14) Infundibulum; (15) Superior turbinate; (16) Optic nerve; (17) Internal carotid artery; (18) Fovea ethmoidalis; (19) Lamina Cribrosa.

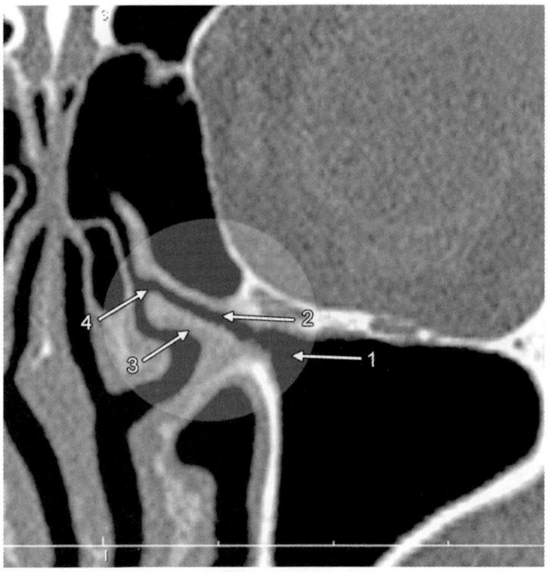

Fig. 6: Osteomeatal complex: (1) Maxillary osteum; (2) Infundibulum; (3) Uncinate process; (4) Hiatus semilunaris.

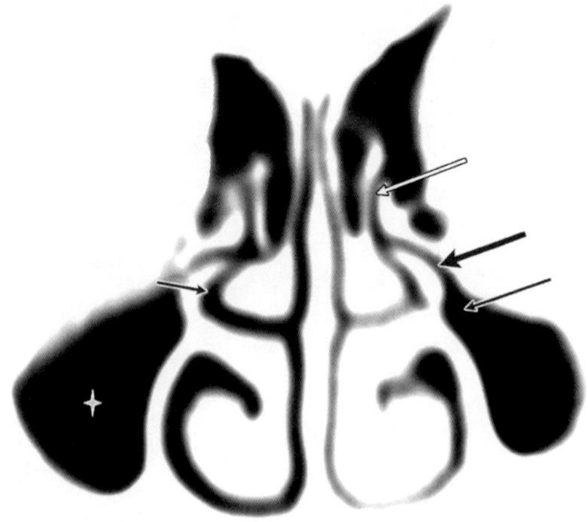

Fig. 7: Coronal section showing anterior draining pathway including frontal recess (white arrow), maxillary ostium (thin black arrow), infundibulum (thick black arrow), middle meatus (short black arrow) and maxillary sinus (star).

The middle meatus is an air space lateral to the middle turbinate and medial to the uncinate process and *ethmoid bulla* (they are largest aerated cells of the anterior ethmoidal complex). The *uncinate process* is a superior extension of the medial maxillary sinus wall. Anteriorly, the uncinate process fuses with the *agger nasi cells* (term given to the most anterior cells in the anterior ethmoidal sinus complex) and the posterior wall of the nasolacrimal duct. Superiorly the uncinate process has a free edge that is separated from the ethmoid bulla by a crevice termed the *hiatus semilunaris*. This hiatus communicates with *ethmoidal infundibulum* which is a short channel starting from the maxillary ostium and leading into middle meatus and is bordered laterally by lamina papyracea and medially by uncinate process **(Figs. 6 and 7)**.

The inferior meatus contains the opening of the drainage channel of the NLD.

Posterior draining pathways: It consists of draining pathway of sphenoid and posterior ethmoidal sinuses. The sphenoid sinus drains via an ostium located in its anterosuperior wall. It leads into *sphenoethmoidal recess* which drains the sphenoid sinus along with posterior ethmoidal complex into the superior meatus. This recess lies between anterior sphenoid sinus wall and posterior wall of ethmoid sinus air cells **(Figs. 8A and B)**.

Most of the above-mentioned structures are adequately visualized in coronal plane except for the sphenoethmoidal recess which is seen in sagittal or axial planes.

Anatomic Variations

Certain anatomic variations are common and important. They are frequently associated with chronic inflammatory disease. These variants can obstruct the air passages and thus can give rise to recurrent sinus infections. The most common variations are described in brief.

Concha Bullosa

This is an aerated middle turbinate. It enlarges to obstruct the middle meatus or even the infundibulum **(Fig. 9)**. It may be unilateral or bilateral. Since the concha is lined with the same mucosa as the rest of the nasal cavity, these cells can suffer the same inflammatory disorders experienced in the PNS. The other normal structures which can be pneumatized are the anterior clinoid processes in conjunction with an extensively pneumatized sphenoid sinus. The crista galli can be pneumatized and may predispose to formation of a mucocele.

Nasal Septum Deviation

It can be asymmetric. The curved septum may compress the middle turbinate laterally and thus narrow the middle meatus. Bony spurs associated with septal deviation may obstruct the OMC.

Paradoxical Middle Turbinate

The middle turbinate may project laterally rather than medially, thus narrowing the middle meatus.

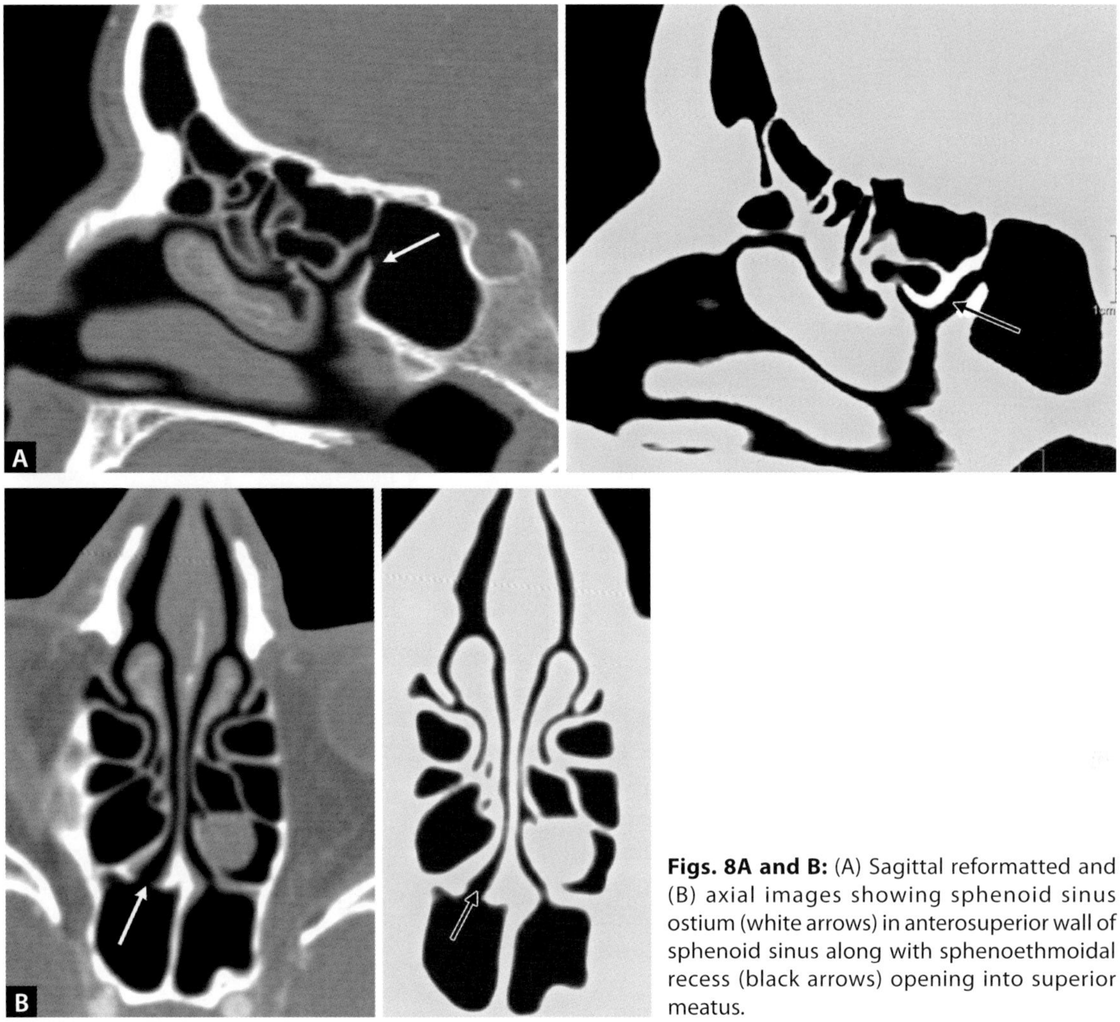

Figs. 8A and B: (A) Sagittal reformatted and (B) axial images showing sphenoid sinus ostium (white arrows) in anterosuperior wall of sphenoid sinus along with sphenoethmoidal recess (black arrows) opening into superior meatus.

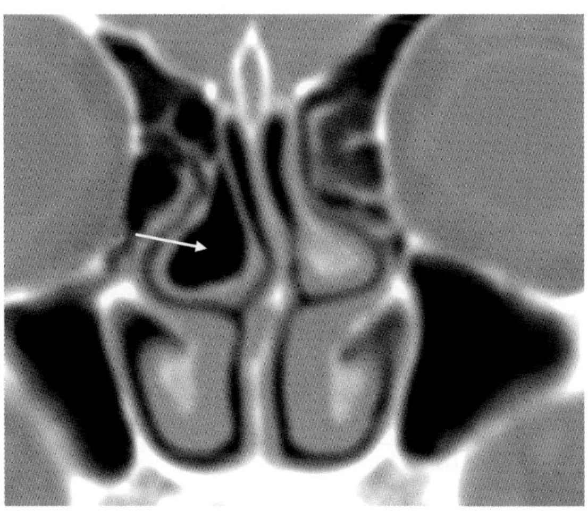

Fig. 9: Concha bullosa (arrow) causing partial obstruction of the middle meatus. Note left DNS.

Variations in the Uncinate Process

The superior "free" edge of the uncinate process may be: (i) deviated medially to obstruct the middle meatus and (ii) inclined laterally to compromise the infundibulum. Fusion with the medial orbital wall may endanger the orbital contents while an uncinectomy is being done.

Haller cells are infraethmoid air cells which extend along the roof of the maxillary sinus. Haller cells may contribute to narrowing of the infundibulum **(Fig. 10)**.

Onodi cells are lateral and posterior extensions of the posterior ethmoid air cells. They extend close to the optic nerves as they exit the orbits **(Fig. 11)**.

Prominent ethmoid bulla is the largest of the ethmoid air cells, and may enlarge to narrow or obstruct the middle meatus and infundibulum **(Fig. 12)**.

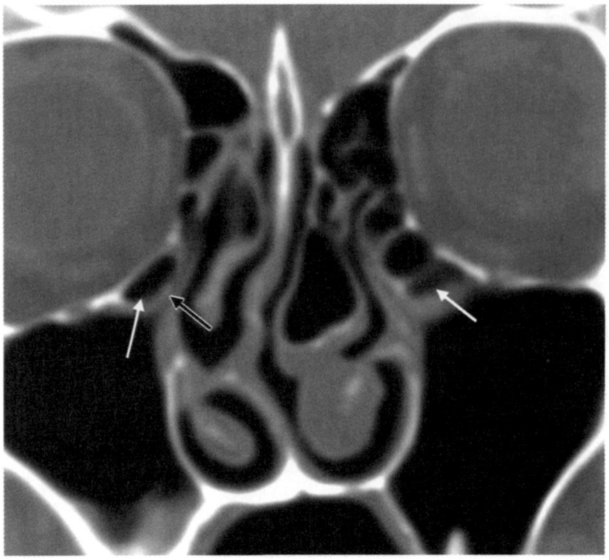

Fig. 10: Coronal CT image showing Haller cells (white arrows) along the roof of the maxillary sinus medially, causing narrowing of the infundibulum (black arrow).

SINONASAL REPORTING

It has been observed that the radiology reports of PNS are not very relevant to the operating ENT surgeons before FESS in cases of sinusitis. This is mainly because radiologists are not very well versed about the anatomical variations and or danger points encountered by the surgeon during the FESS. Thus, it becomes imperative that the radiologists learn about these points and report carry the relevant information.

The points to be included include the information about:

1. Cribriform plate
2. Lamina papyracea
3. Onodi cells
4. Sphenoid sinus pneumatization pattern
5. Ethmoid sulcus

Cribriform plate adjoining the crista galli has Olfactory fossa. Its superior boundary is marked by Fovea ethmoidalis, lateral boundary by Lateral lamella, inferior boundary by lamina cribrosa and medial by crista galli. The deeper the olfactory fossa, more is the chance of injury to the lateral lamella. Since it's the thinnest portion of anterior skull base and its breech can cause CSF rhinorrhea and infections, its status and depth of olfactory fossa needs to be reported **(Fig. 13A)**. Lamina payracea again is very this bony separation between nasal cavity and the orbits. Maintaining its integrity is important during FESS. If it's medially deviated it may get injured during ethmoidectomy. Also, it has close relation with uncinated process.

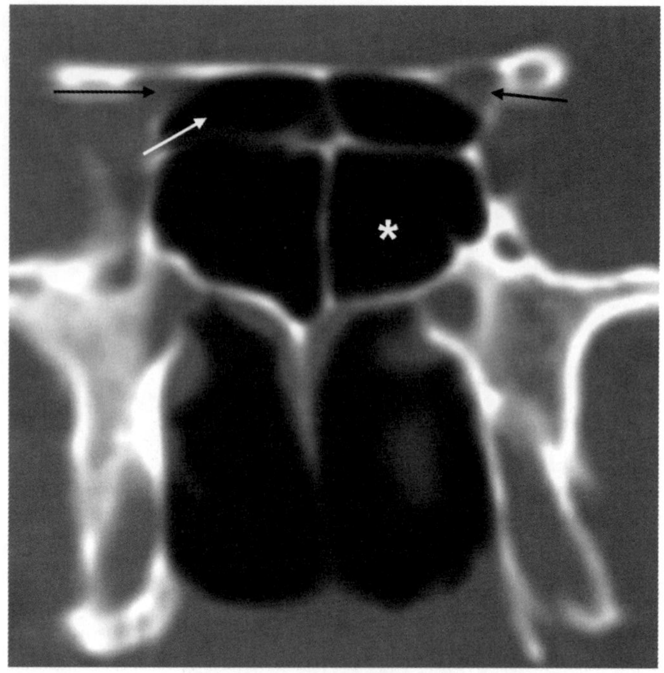

Fig. 11: Coronal CT at the level of sphenoid sinus (asterisk), showing Onodi cells (white arrow) lying superior to the sphenoid sinuses and in close relation to optic nerves (black arrows).

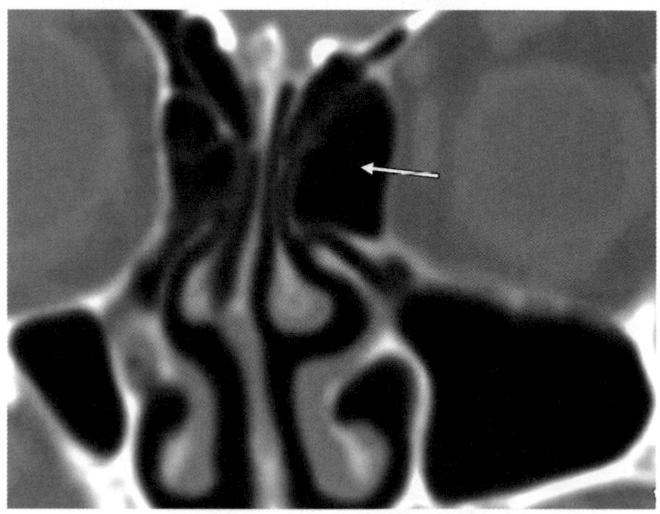

Fig. 12: Ethmoid bulla (arrow) seen on the left side.

Onodi cells, are important to report since optic nerve may be passing through it. During posterior ethmoidectomy surgeon may enter these mistaking them for posterior ethmoid cells and nerve injury may result.

Sphenoid sinus lateral wall has intimate relation to the cavernous segment of ICA and optic nerve. Over pneumatization may make the wall thin and chance of inadvertent ICA or optic nerve injury **(Fig. 13B)**.

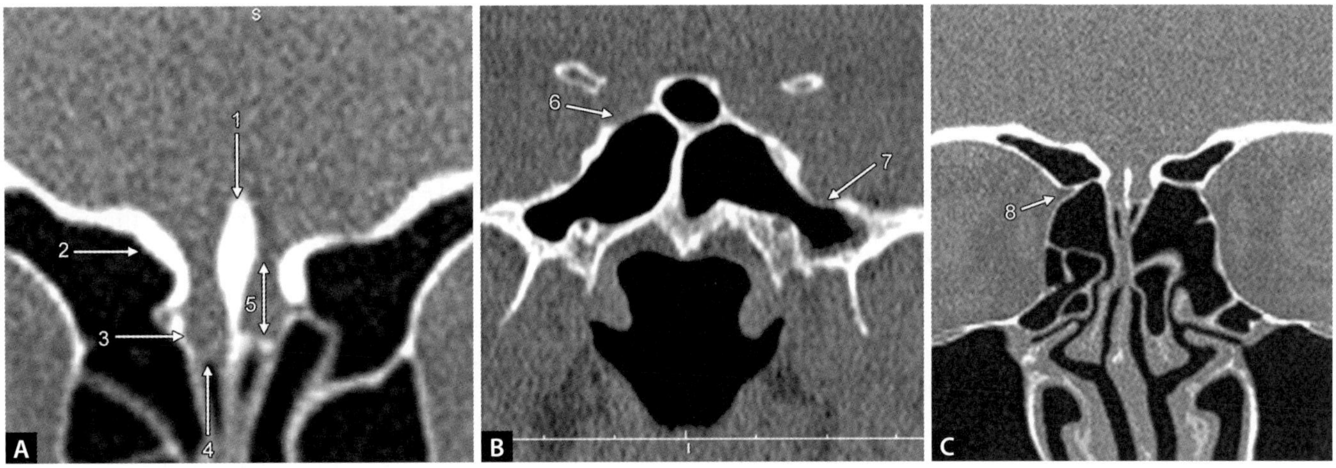

Fig. 13A to C: (A) Olfactory fossa bound by fovea ethmoidalis (2), lateral lamella (3), lamina cribrosa (4), crista galli (1), Depth of the fossa (5); (B) Optic nerve (6) and internal carotid artery (7) relation to the sphenoid sinus; (C) Ethmoidal notch (8).

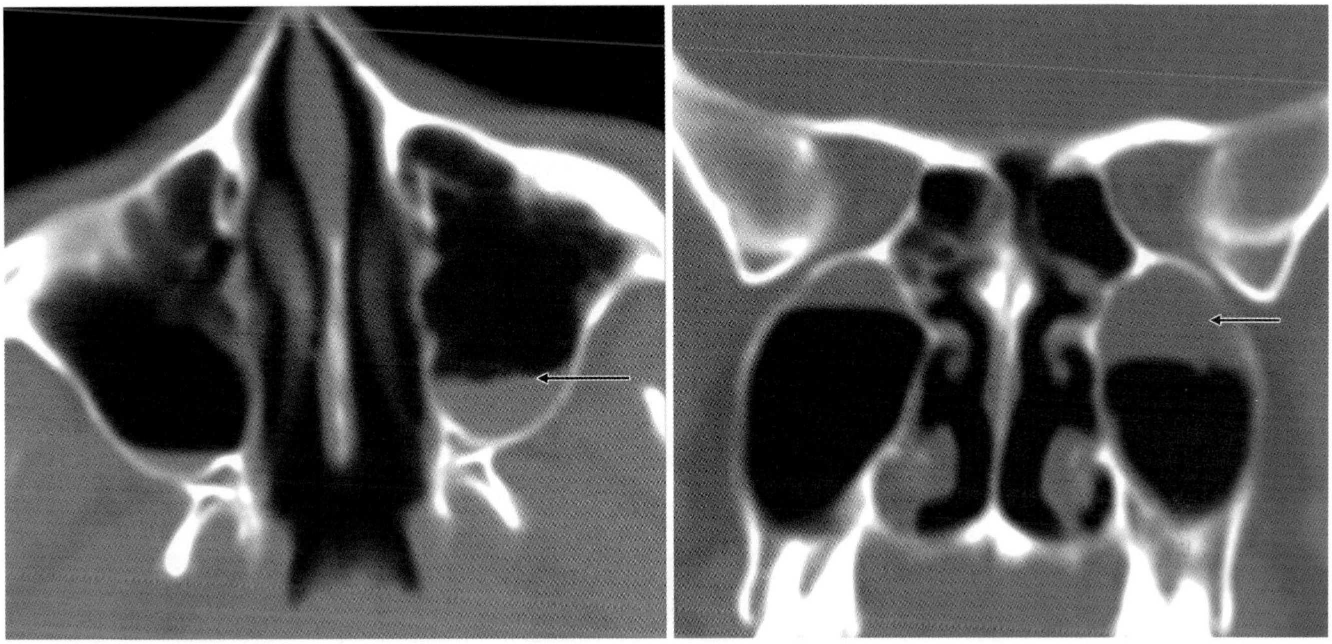

Fig. 14: Axial and coronal CT images showing air-fluid levels (arrows) seen in the dependent position.

Lastly, anterior ethmoid artery, a branch of ophthalmic artery lies at supero-medial margin of the orbit at the level of anterio ethmoid air cells. Pneumatization of air cells above and below the sulcus may lead to arterial injury during ethmoidectomy **(Fig. 13C)**.[15,16]

INFLAMMATORY SINUS DISEASE

Acute Sinusitis

Inflammatory sinus is usually caused by superinfection in a previously obstructed sinus. The previously inflamed mucosa becomes edematous leading to obstruction of the ostium of the sinus. Secretions from the sinuses accumulate and form a good culture medium for bacterial pathogens. Viral infections rarely cause sinusitis.[17]

The hallmark of acute sinusitis is an air fluid level on plain X-rays or CT **(Fig. 14)**. It may be associated with shadows of thickened mucosa or may be represented by an opaque sinus. The findings are nonspecific and one of the important differential diagnoses is the presence of fluid in the sinus due to hemorrhage following trauma.

Chronic Sinusitis

Chronic inflammation of the PNS occurs either due to recurrent inflammatory episodes or due to an indolent inflammatory process. Patients usually have a chronic history of headache, retrobulbar pain and may have had previous surgeries which have failed to give relief.[18,19]

Both CT and MRI are used to assess chronic inflammation. However, CT is better in pretherapeutic planning before functional endoscopic sinus surgery (FESS).[20]

MRI can be done post-FESS to see therapeutic response, complications and in patients where dental filling cause artifact obscuring the anatomical details.[21] A recent report in which sinusitis scoring system was used on both CT and MRI images did not find any overstaging or understaging on MRI images. Thus, there is a possibility where MRI may still be used in patients likely to be managed conservatively.[7]

In chronic sinusitis the mucosa is hypertrophic. Polypoid changes can occur with areas of atrophy and fibrosis. If there is superadded acute inflammation due to infections or allergy the mucosa will thicken. It is essential to note the number of sinuses involved and the degree of mucosal thickening within them **(Fig. 15)**.

Sinus secretions in the acute state have a density ranging 10–25 HU, which is slightly higher than water but less than muscle. As the condition becomes chronic, the secretions become more mucoid and CT attenuation values range between 30 HU and 60 HU, and the density equals that of muscle.

Hyperdense secretions on CT may be due to four main causes:[11] (i) inspissated secretions, (ii) fungal sinusitis, (iii) hemorrhage in sinus, and (iv) calcification chronic bacterial sinusitis may occasionally results in a hyperdense sinus on CT, particularly in patients who have very long-standing disease with coexisting cystic fibrosis. The hyperdense sinus often corresponds to the hypointense sinus on T2W MRI images. On MRI, intensity of secretion depend on the relative contrast of water and mucous. The high water content is reflected as low intensity on T1WI and high intensity on T2WI. On MRI appearances of chronic inflammatory sinus secretions vary with the protein content. The intensity on T1WI progressively decreases with the increase in protein content while the intensity on T2WI progressively increases till the protein content is 25% of the secretion following which the intensity decreases till the protein content is 40% of the secretion. This is because all the free water is eliminated from the secretion and macromolecular protein to protein binding occurs. Thus, four intensity patterns on MRI for sinus secretions have been described.[22]

1. Hypointense on T1WI and hyperintense on T2WI in most liquid form (total protein concentration < 9%).
2. Hyperintense on T1WI and hyperintense on T2WI in mild to moderately proteinaceous form (total protein concentration 20–25%).
3. Hyperintense on T1WI and hypointense on T2WI in a highly proteinaceous form (total protein concentration 25–28%).
4. Hypointense on T1WI and hypointense on T2WI when secretion are in a nearly solid (total protein concentration >28%).

On CT scans, the inspissated chronic secretions appear as bright densities whereas on T1WI and T2WI the sinuses show signal voids similar to air. Enhancement of sinuses after gadolinium administration helps diagnose chronic

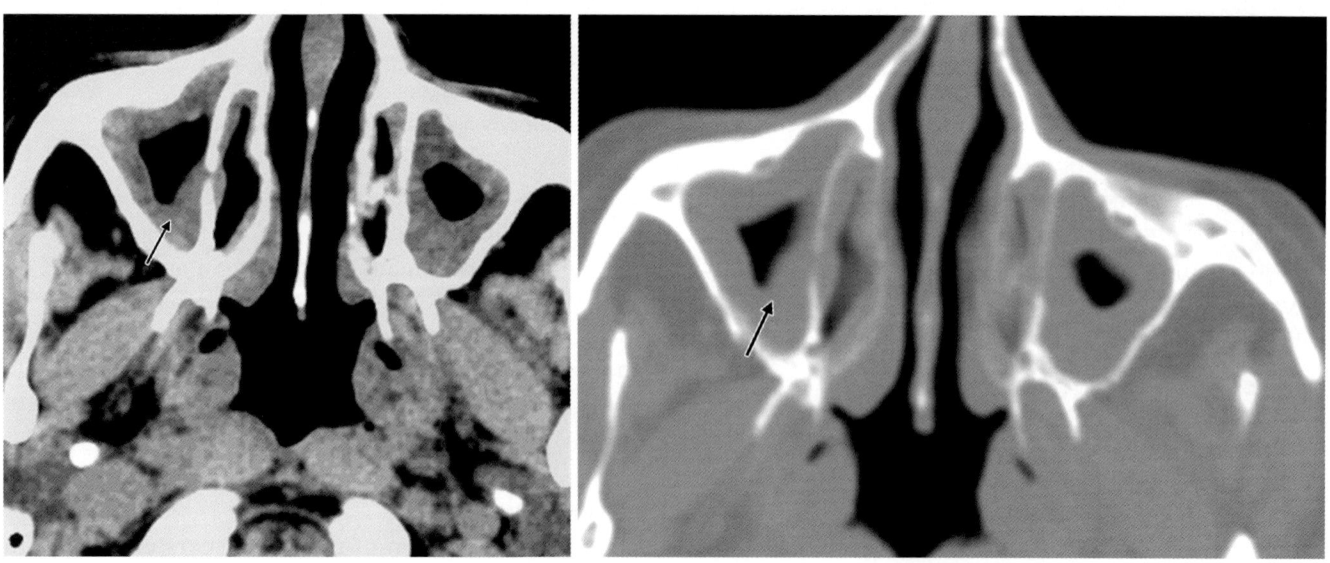

Fig. 15: Axial sections showing diffuse mucosal hypertrophy (arrows) without any significant change in the bones.

sinusitis (**Figs. 16A and B**). CT however remains the modality of choice, as it shows both soft tissue and bony changes, and is cost effective and easily available.[22]

As the chronic inflammation becomes indolent, changes in the facial bones become evident and these are best seen on CT scans. These include thickening of the facial bones adjacent to the inflamed mucosa and progressive sclerosis in these bones. These changes are due to increased vascularity due to chronic inflammation. Rarely, osteomyelitis may supervene with areas of sequestration and bony rarefaction.

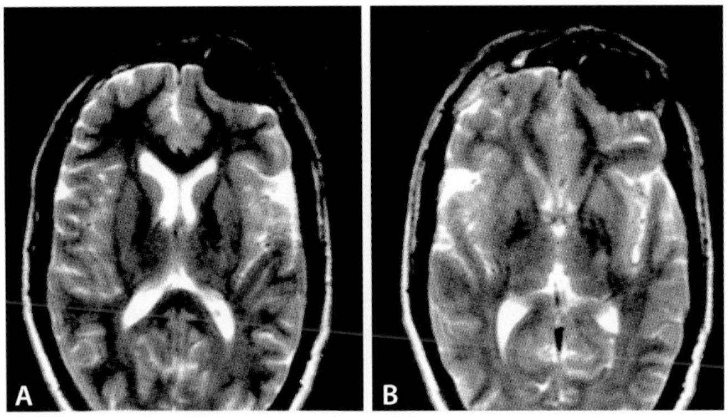

Figs. 16A and B: (A) Axial T2WI showing featureless well pneumatized, hypointense frontal sinuses in a diagnosis case of chronic sinusitis; (B) Peripheral rim enhancement of walls of the sinus and enhancement of inspissated secretions characterize the chronic inflammation in these T1W sections.

Five patterns of chronic inflammation in the sinuses given by Sonkens et al.[20] give an important insight into the importance of imaging the anterior and posterior draining pathways described before. According to them the patterns are as follows:

1. *Infundibular pattern:* In this the disease is limited to maxillary sinus and corresponding infundibulum and can occur due to mucosal thickening, polyp in that location or Haller cells. Rest of the sinuses are normal.
2. *Osteomeatal unit pattern:* In this the obstruction is in the middle meatus thus causing obstruction and changes in frontal sinus, anterior and middle ethmoid sinus and maxillary sinus. Cause may be mucosal thickening, polyps, concha bullosa, deviated septum or nasal tumor (**Fig. 17**).
3. *Sphenoethmoidal recess pattern:* In this the spheno-ethmoid recess is blocked and changes seen only in ipsilateral sphenoid and posterior ethmoid air cells (**Fig. 18**).

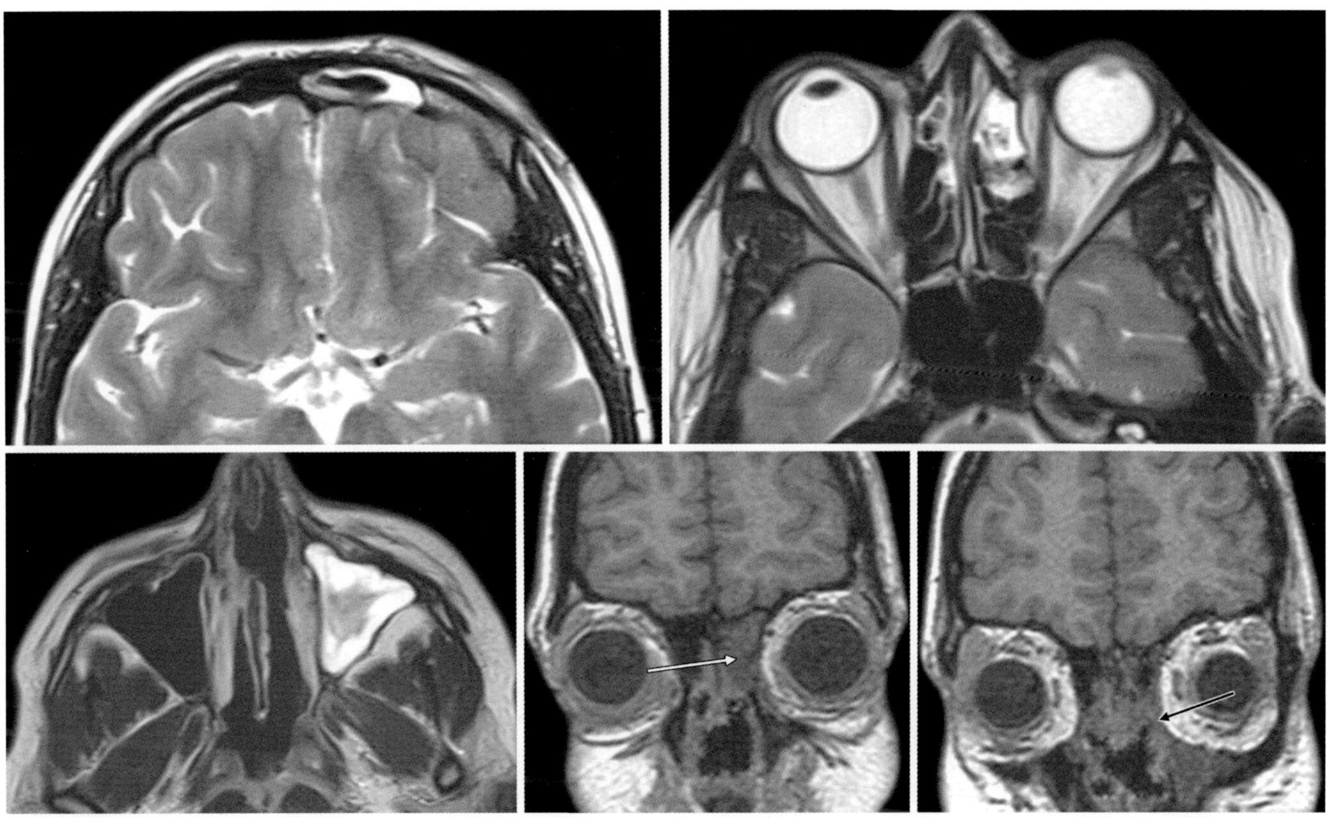

Fig. 17 : Osteomeatal pattern of obstruction with involvement of all left sided anterior sinuses due to obstruction at the frontal recess (white arrow) and left OM complex (black arrow).

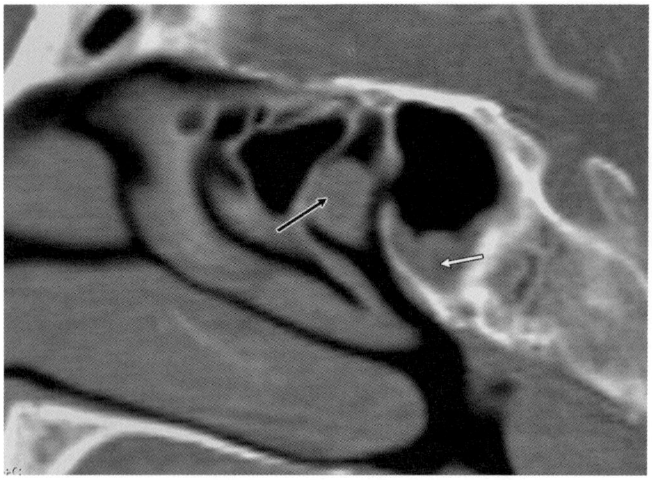

Fig. 18: A polyp in posterior ethmoid (black arrow) is causing partial obstruction of the sphenoethmoid recess causing sphenoid sinusitis (white arrow).

4. *Sinonasal polyposis pattern:* In this both the nasal cavities and the sinuses are filled with polyps and the resultant chronic inflammatory changes are a mix of above three patterns **(Fig. 19)**.
5. *Sporadic/Unclassified pattern:* When no specific kind of obstruction is seen and when mucocele, retention cysts or postoperative changes are there.

Classifying disease under one of these headings can help a surgeon to plan FESS as the rationale behind endoscopic sinus surgery is to restore the flow of sinus secretion via their natural pathways. To revise the anatomy and to systematically read PNS CTs, it is important the following structures are identified first:

- Frontal sinus
- Frontal recess
- Agger nasi cells
- Ethmoid roof
- Ethmoid bulla
- Basal or grand lamella
- Sinus lateralis
- Uncinate process
- Infundibulum
- Maxillary sinus
- Middle meatus
- Nasal septum and nasal turbinates
- Posterior ethmoid sinus
- Sphenoid sinus

Following this evaluation, the orbits and any normal variations are studied. The third step in evaluation involves study of the bony outline of the orbits and to observe areas of erosion or bone thickening.[17]

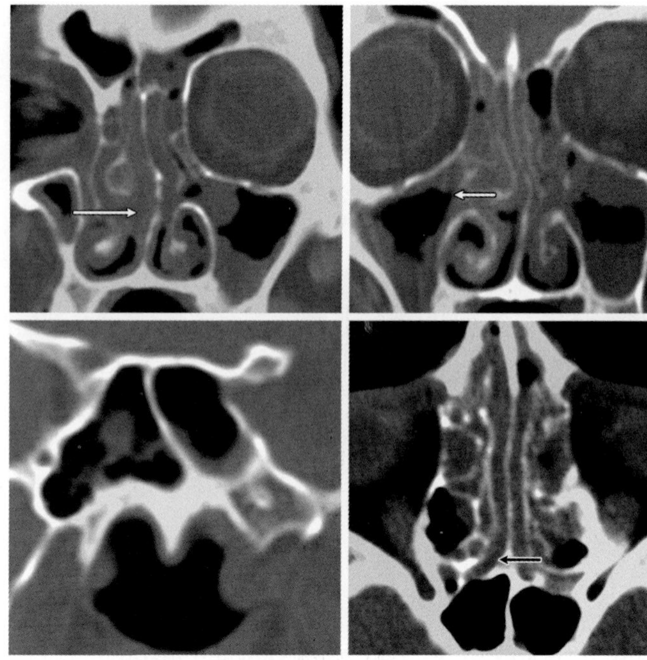

Fig. 19: Extensive nasal polyposis (long white arrow) causing obstruction of anterior (short white arrow) and posterior (black arrow) drainage pathways causing pansinusitis.

Post-FESS Scanning

Postoperatively, neither CT nor MRI is accurate in distinguishing fibrosis from inflammation. Both enhance and appear as mucosal thickening. CT is the study of choice in the acute setting of orbital complications after FESS, which usually occurs within 48 hours after surgery. CT is reliable in diagnosing an orbital hematoma, assessing for optic nerve compression or inadvertent resection and also for planning therapy to relieve increased intraorbital pressure.

Mucocele

Mucocele is a term used for those expanded and remodeled sinuses which are obstructed and contain secretions.[17] About 66% of the mucoceles occur in the frontal sinus, 25% in the ethmoid sinuses and 10% in the maxillary sinus. Sphenoidal mucoceles are rare. When infected a mucocele is termed as a mucopyocele. Radiographically, the sinus is airless, expanded and filled with soft tissue shadows **(Fig. 20A)**. CT appearance is that of an expanded sinus with intact walls, containing mucoid soft tissue densities.[23] The sinus may be remodeled **(Fig. 20B)**. It is essential to note the expanding wall of the sinus and its encroachment upon the orbit, intracranial space, nasal cavities and pterygopalatine fossa, all of which contain important neural and vascular structures.[23,24] MRI

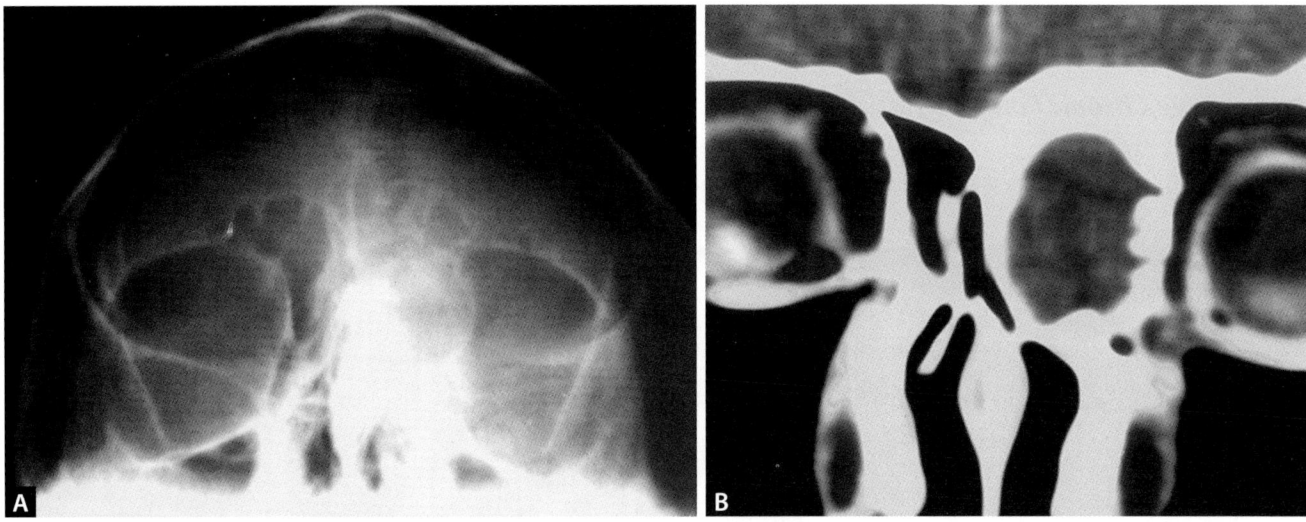

Figs. 20A and B: Mucocele of the ethmoid sinus: (A) Plain X-ray Water's view shows an expanded and opaque left ethmoid sinus; (B) Coronal non-contrast CT shows the expanded sinus containing soft tissue densities. The wall of the sinus are thickened but are intact.

appearance depends on the nature of the secretion within the mucocele as in chronic sinusitis. MRI can detect the interface of mucocele with intracranial or intraorbital structures. A peripheral rim enhancement pattern is seen on MRI which is useful for distinguishing mucocele and obstructed secretions form neoplasms such as inverted papillomas on malignancies which may also remodel bone but show solid enhancement[25] **(Figs. 21A and B)**.

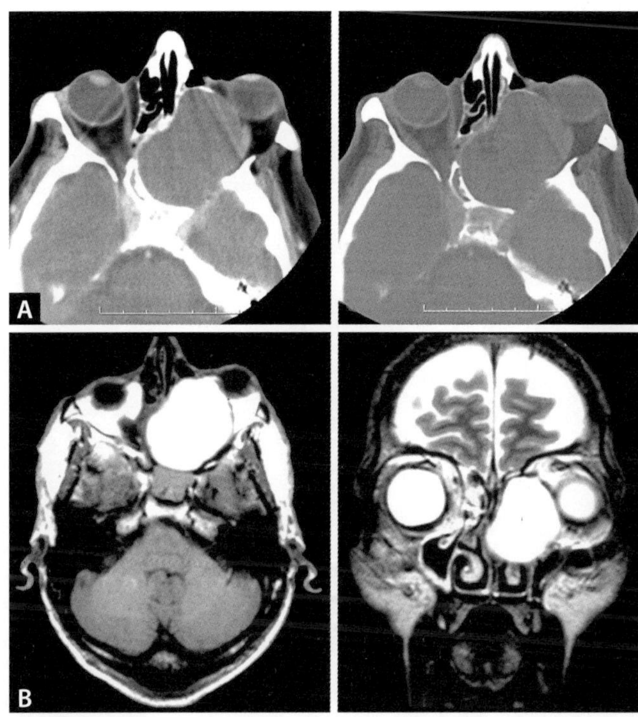

Figs. 21A and B: (A) Left-sided ethmoidal mucocele encroaching on the left orbit. Left globe is proposed; (B) T2W MRI axial and coronal sections of the same patient showing hyperintense fluid contents of the mucocele.

Fungal Sinusitis

It may be classified as: (i) allergic fungal rhinosinusitis, (ii) invasive fungal sinusitis, and (iii) noninvasive chronic fungal sinusitis.

Allergic Fungal Rhinosinusitis

It occurs as an allergic response to fungal elements in atopic patients. On CT, diffuse mucosal thickening involving multiple sinuses is present. Within the sinus there may be central hyperdense content and peripheral hypodensity. On MRI the central content is usually hypointense on both T1WI and T2WI. Sinus may be expanded with its walls remodeled or rarified **(Fig. 22)**. Bony destruction is usually not seen. Calcification is also a common finding in fungal infections especially with aspergillosis. Central or fine punctate pattern of calcification is characteristic of fungal infection. Many patients may have polyps.

Invasive Fungal Sinusitis

This usually occurs in immunosuppressed individuals and may occur by invasion by the fungus colonizing the sinuses in setting of chronic sinusitis or by inhalation of fungal spores. *Mucor, Aspergillus* or *Fusarium* are the common fungi causing invasive form of sinusitis. On CT, it cause opacification of the sinuses due to mucosal hypertrophy and secretions but the course is fulminant. Also, the bony wall is destroyed early in the course of disease with spread of infection directly into orbits, cavernous sinuses or brain **(Figs. 23A and B)**.

Noninvasive Chronic Fungal Sinusitis

Noninvasive chronic fungal sinusitis or mycetomas may be seen in sinus cavities as a noninvasive ball of fungus which is hyperdense on CT, does not change position on changing head position and may have calcifications. They are usually found in setting of chronic non-resolving sinusitis.

The final diagnosis of the type of fungus however, rests with the pathologist.[17,18,26]

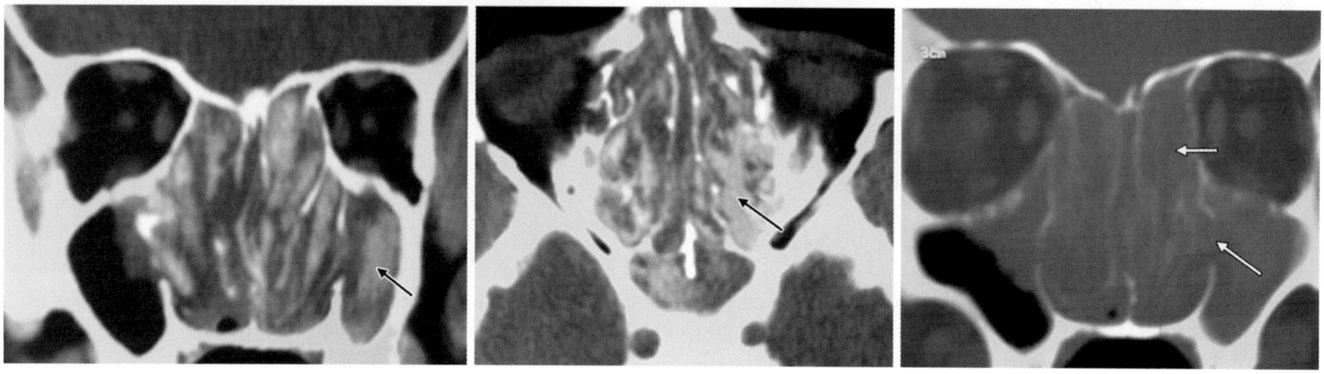

Fig. 22: Allergic fungal rhinosinusitis (AFRS) CT images coronal and axial showing diffuse nasal and sinus mucosal thickening with hyperdensities (black arrows) causing expansion and blockage of the sinuses. On bone window, the ethmoid lamellae and sinus walls are remodeled and eroded (white arrows).

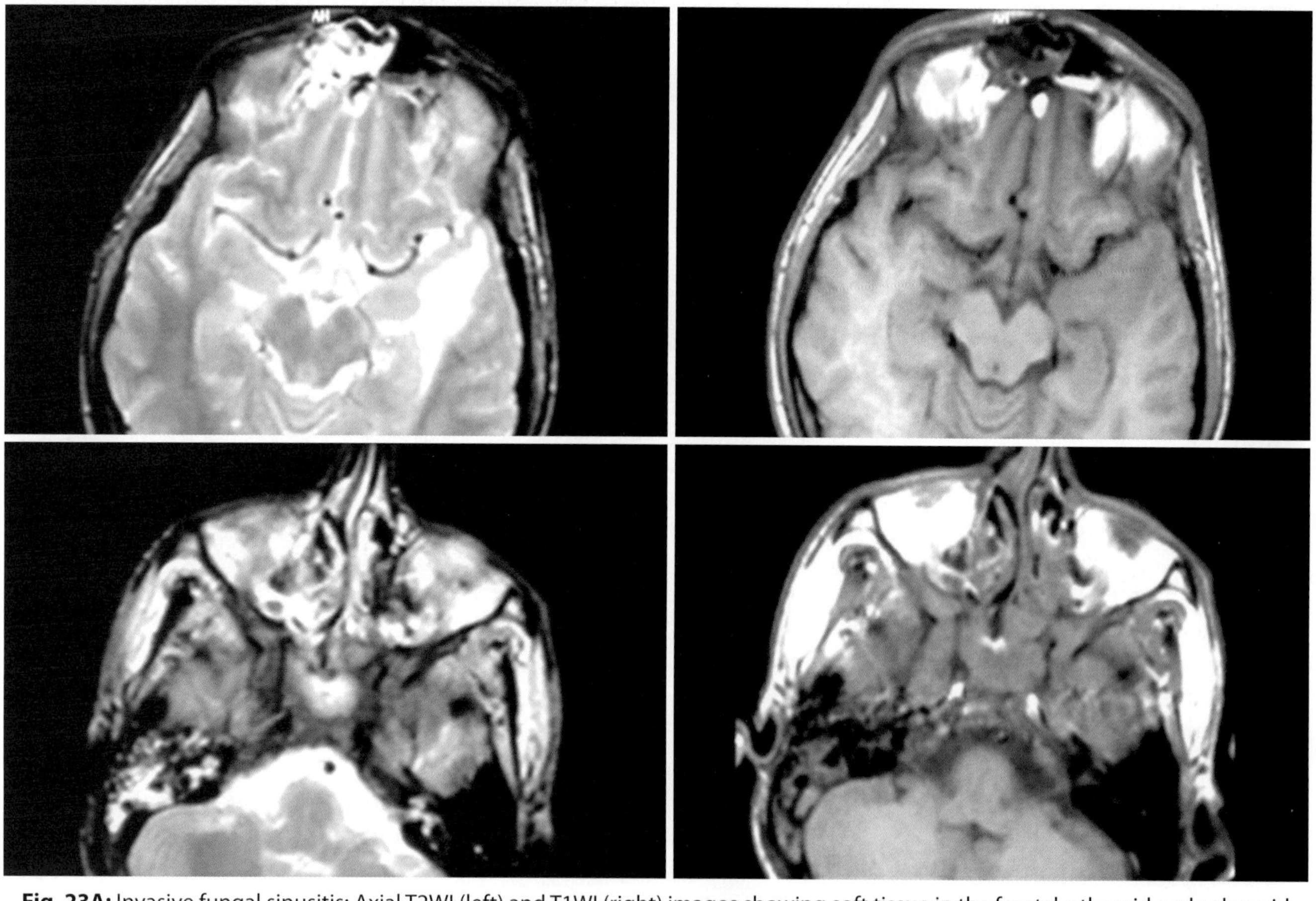

Fig. 23A: Invasive fungal sinusitis: Axial T2WI (left) and T1WI (right) images showing soft tissue in the frontal, ethmoid and sphenoid sinuses which are isointense on T1WI and hyperintense on the T2WI.

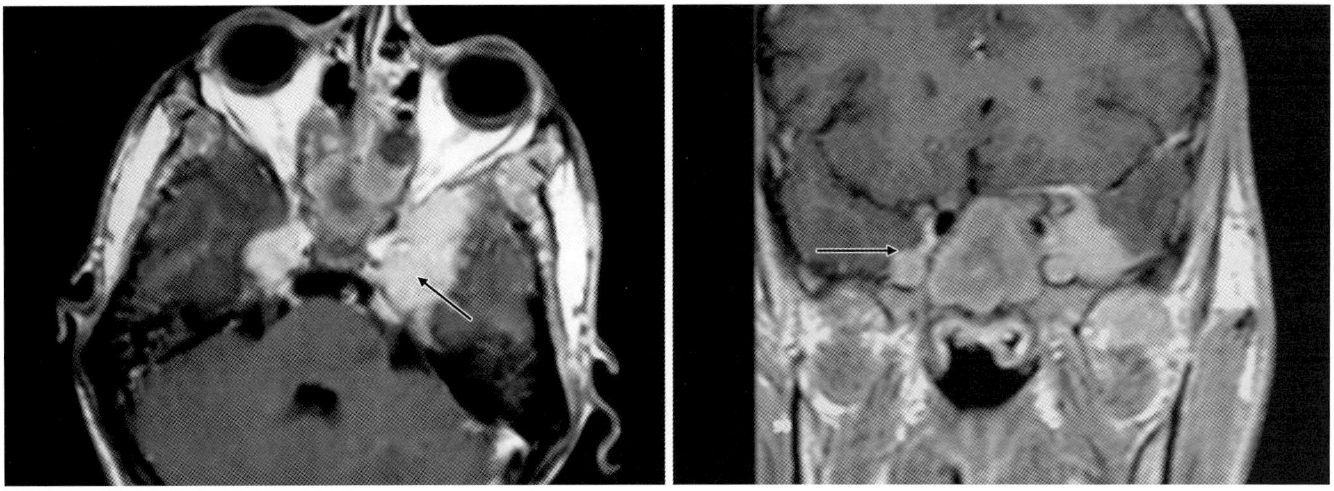

Fig. 23B: Invasive fungal sinusitis: Postcontrast T1WI axial and coronal showing intense enhancement and contiguous extension of the soft tissue from the sinuses into the bilateral cavernous sinuses and temporal lobe (arrows).

GRANULOMATOUS DISEASES

Actinomycosis,[27] tuberculosis,[28] syphilis, leprosy,[29] rhinoscleroma, rhinosporidiosis, sarcoidosis, Wegener's granulomatosis, midline granuloma, leishmaniasis and yaws are some of the chronic granulomatous diseases which affect the PNS and nasal fossa. As a group, these conditions cause nonspecific findings which include focal erosions and soft tissue masses **(Fig. 24)**. Often the sinuses are filled with fluid-like densities which on multiple examinations are un changing. Involvement of the nasal septum either with erosions or soft tissue thickening is a pointer to such conditions like leprosy **(Fig. 25)**, Wegener's granulomatosis or granulomas due to cocaine abuse. In one study of 28 patients of Wegener's granulomatosis following features were observed—bony destruction, mainly of the nasal cavity, maxillary sinuses and mastoid cells; sclerosing osteitis, mainly of the maxillary sinuses; bony thickening, mainly of the maxillary sinuses and mastoid cells and mucosal thickening, mainly of the maxillary sinuses. Although these findings were seen frequently still they are nonspecific and need clinicopathologic correlation.[30]

Polyps and Cysts

Polyps appear as well defined dome-shaped homogeneous lesions. If multiple, they trap secretions between their crevices. On CT scan they appear as well defined lobulated lesions, sometimes extending into the nasal cavities **(Fig. 26)**. On MRI, they are of varying intensity depending upon the degree of desiccation within the polyp.

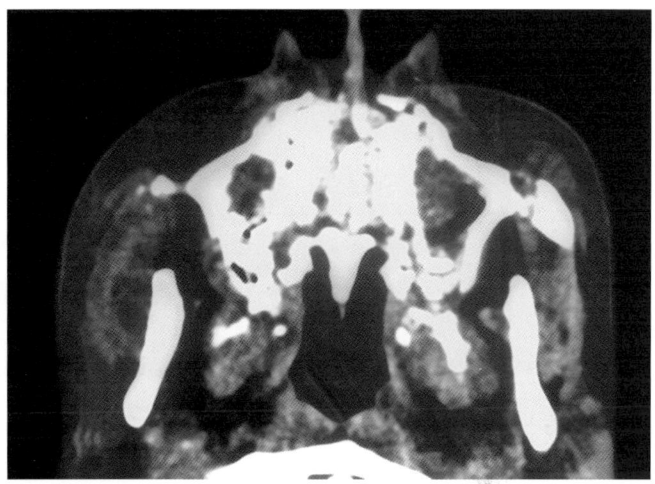

Fig. 24: Actinomycosis of the hard palate and adjacent maxillary antrum. Fragmentation of the palate is present with accompanying soft tissue densities in the maxillary antrum. Similar soft tissues invade the premaxilla and the columella of the nose.

Diagnosis on imaging may be problematic sometimes because the lesion, although benign, may demonstrate aggressive bony destruction on CT. The findings suggestive of polyposis include enlargement of sinus ostia, rounded masses within the nasal cavity, expanded sinuses or portions of the nasal cavity **(Figs. 27A and B)** thinning of bony trabeculae, and less commonly, erosive bone changes at the anterior aspect of skull base.[11] Retention cysts occur due to obstruction of ducts of the glands in the mucosa. They can be either serous or mucinous. They are indistinguishable from polyps and have similar appearances on CT and MRI.[11,17]

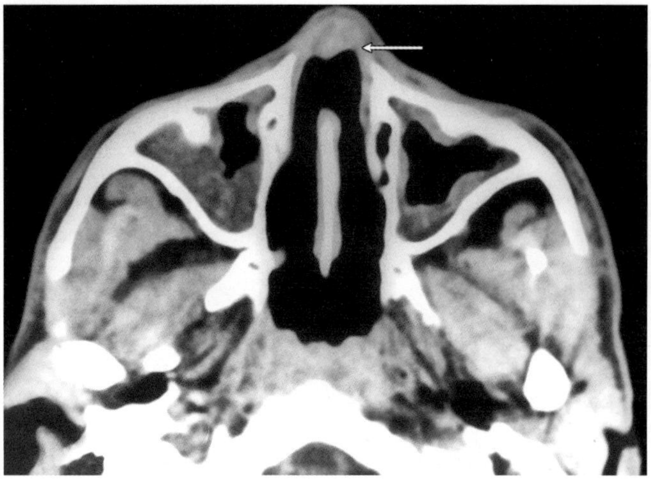

Fig. 25: Leprosy: Destruction of the nasal bones (arrow) and a perforated nasal septum are characteristic changes of lepromatous leprosy.

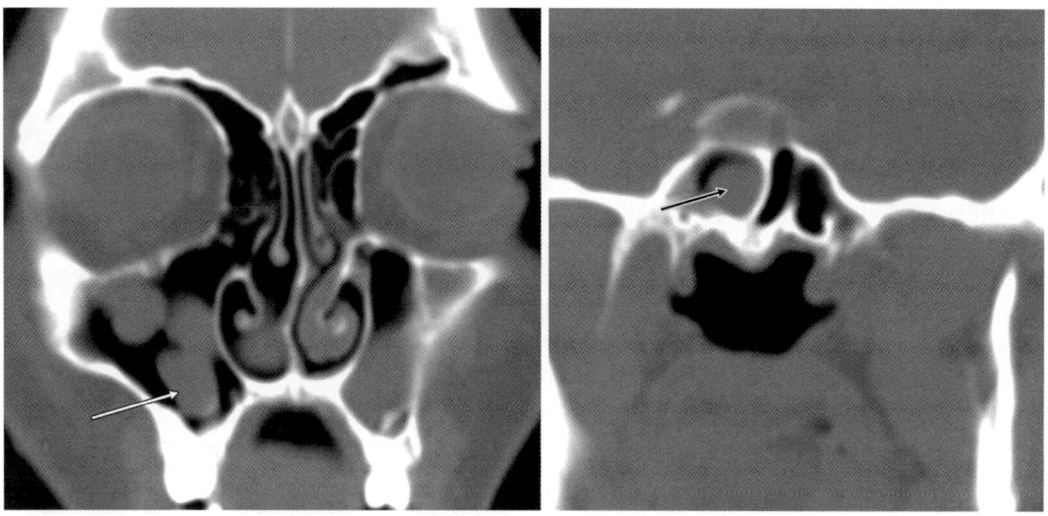

Fig. 26: Multiple polyps in the maxillary sinus (white arrow) and in the sphenoid sinus (black arrow).

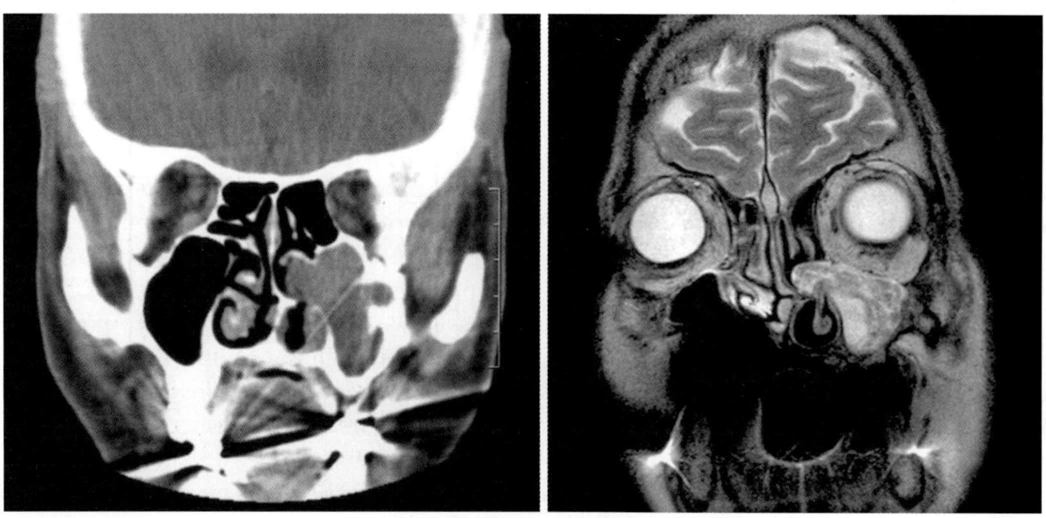

Fig. 27A: Coronal CT image and T2WI MRI image of a left antrochoanal polyps, showing the heterogeneous intensity of the polyps, which widens the ostia enters the nasal cavity and expand the sinus.

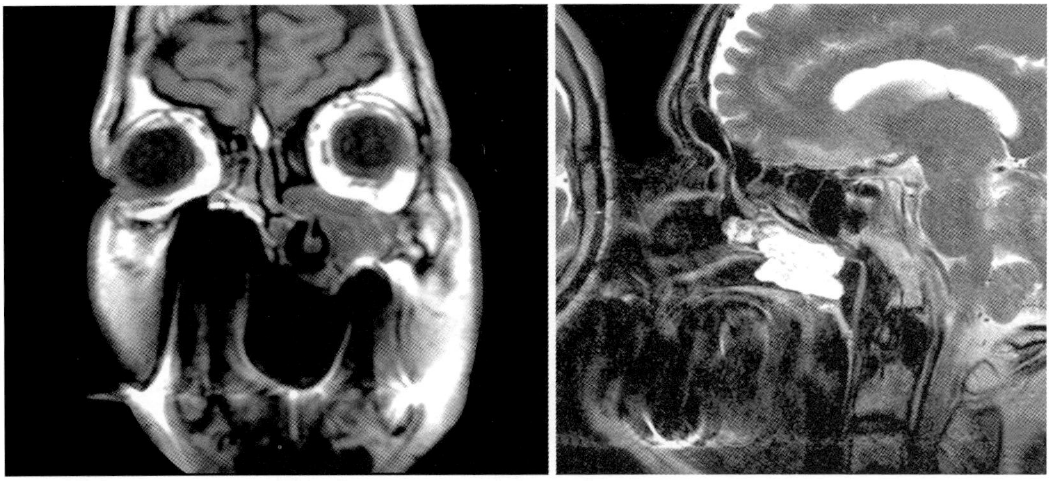

Fig. 27B: Coronal T1WI and sagittal T2WI showing the change in single characterization of the polyps and its extent up to the posterior choana.

NEOPLASTIC LESIONS OF THE PARANASAL SINUSES

Neoplastic lesions of the paranasal sinus are either of epithelial or nonepithelial origin.

Epithelial Tumors of the PNS

Epithelial tumors are further subdivided into two groups:
1. Tumors of epithelial origin
2. Tumors of salivary gland origin

Tumors of epithelial origin include:
- Papillomas
- Squamous cell carcinoma
- Adenocarcinoma

Tumors of salivary gland origin include:
- Pleomorphic adenoma
- Adenocystic carcinoma
- Acinic cell carcinoma
- Mucoepidermoid carcinoma

Squamous cell carcinomas are the most common epithelial neoplasms of the PNS. They constitute up to 63% of malignancies of this region.[31,32]

Maxillary sinus (25–58%) is most commonly involved followed by ethmoid (10%) and sphenoid and frontal sinuses (1%). The nasal cavity is the site of origin in 25–35% of cases. The industrial workers involved in the production of nickel, chromium, isopropyl alcohol, radium, mustard gas and wooden furniture are at an increased risk to develop this malignancy. Chronic sinusitis and polyposis may predispose to squamous cell carcinomas probably believed to be related to the squamous cell metaplasia of the respiratory mucosal lining of the sinuses.[33,34] Squamous cell carcinoma is twice as common in men than women and occurs in the 6th and 7th decades.[34] Unilateral facial pain and purulent nasal discharge are the most common presenting features of sinonasal carcinoma. Epistaxis and nasal obstruction are other presenting symptoms. If the sphenoid sinus is involved cranial neuropathy may be encountered.

The hallmark of imaging malignancies of the sinonasal cavity is bony destruction, seen in approximately 80% of scans of sinonasal squamous cell carcinomas at initial presentation.[11] Squamous cell carcinomas are hypointense on T2WI and should be distinguished from inflammations which are hyperintense on T2WI. Inspissated inflammatory secretions appear increasingly hypointense on T2WI; however, they retain their homogeneity in contrast to the typical heterogeneous signal intensity of malignant neoplasms.

Maxillary sinus carcinomas appear as destructive lesions which transgress the bony confines **(Fig. 28)** of the sinus and involve the ethmoid sinus, pterygopalatine fossa and infratemporal fossa. Orbital invasion is present in nearly two-thirds of the patients followed by invasion of the pterygopalatine and infratemporal fossa in one-third of the patients. The ethmoid sinus and cheek are involved in roughly a quarter of the patients.[31]

Ethmoid cell carcinomas **(Fig. 29A)** appear as destructive lesions which spread through the fovea ethmoidalis and cribriform plate into the anterior cranial fossa; and from the posterior ethmoidal cells into the middle cranial fossa via the superior orbital fissure. Orbital involvements by the carcinomas of the PNS are of some prognostic importance because of considerable morbidity following radiation therapy. These patients may then develop cataract, keratitis and optic nerve atrophy.

Both CT and MRI scans are complementary in assessing the presence, extent and progress following therapeutic intervention. CT scanning is of prime importance, because it is helpful in evaluation of soft tissues, sinus cavities and more importantly involvement of the bones. The posterior wall of the maxillary sinus, the pterygoid plate, pterygopalatine fossa, the cribriform plate, the orbital walls, the sphenoid sinuses, the fossa ethmoidalis and the posterior wall of the frontal sinus are the areas which are of importance because the breach due to the malignant process of any of these structures would indicate the spreads of the lesion beyond the PNS.[35,36]

Squamous cell carcinomas show little contrast enhancement. However, contrast administration is necessitated in CT evaluation of these tumors because it

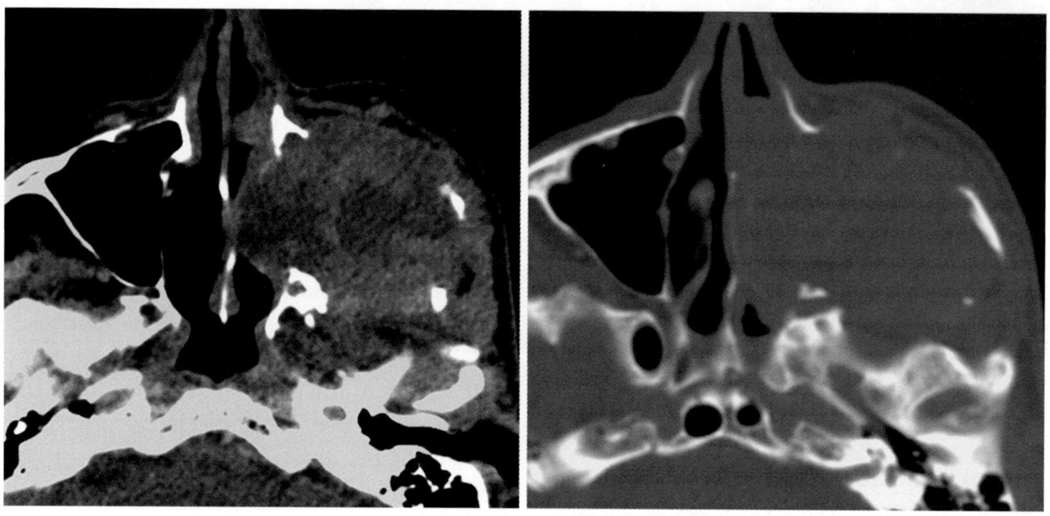

Fig. 28: Squamous cell carcinoma of the right maxillary sinus: Noncontrast CT scan shows soft tissue mass of intermediate attenuation with central necrosis filling the right antrum. The lesion extends beyond the bony walls of the sinus, bone window setting show extensive lytic destruction of the walls.

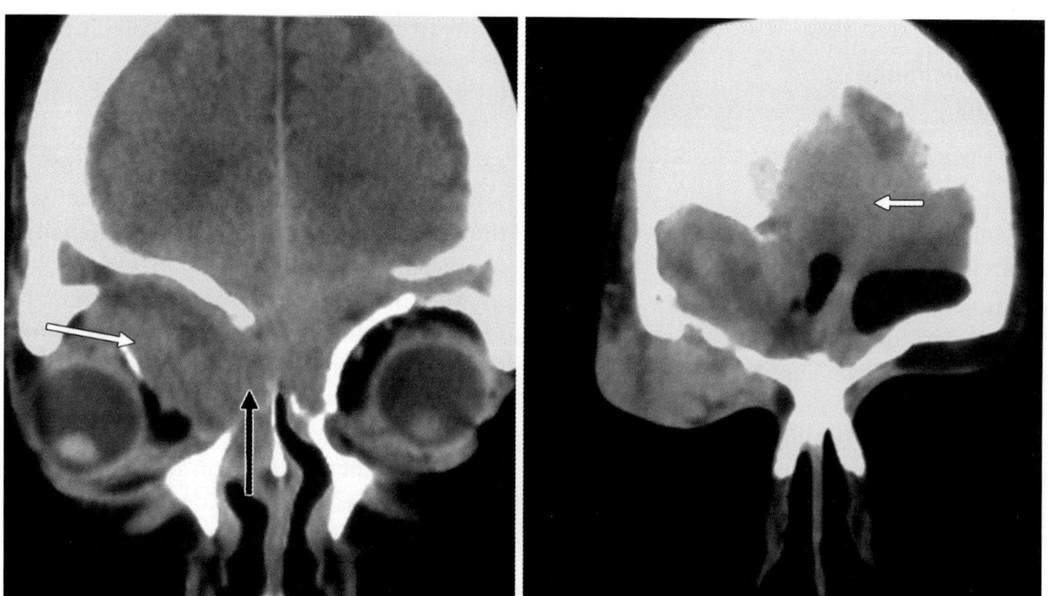

Fig. 29A: Coronal CT showing extensive enhancing ethmoidal soft tissue mass (black arrow) completely filling the sinus with frank bony destruction and extension into right orbit (long white arrow) and frontal sinuses (short white arrow).

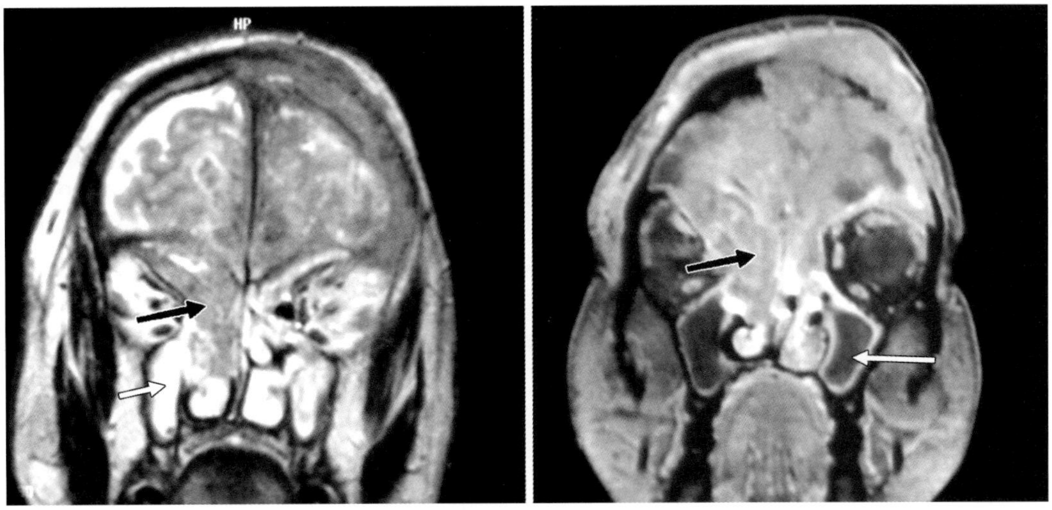

Fig. 29B: Coronal MRI images showing mass to be isointense on T2WI which enhances on post contrast images (black arrows). MRI show extensive lesion with aggressive behavior infiltrating into the right orbit, frontal sinuses and frontal bone diploe. Also seen are intensely bright maxillary sinuses (short white arrow) on T2WI which do not enhance suggestive of postobstructive changes. Note normal thin mucosal enhancement of maxillary sinuses (long white arrow).

can help to differentiate: (i) fluid from areas of necrosis, (ii) involvement of normal structures from tumors especially in the orbit, and (iii) to delineate intracranial extent of the tumor.[37]

Limitations of CT scan include inability to distinguish between inspissated and retained secretions from tumors, detect involvement of the periorbital structures especially the lamina papyracea and the adjacent structures, and to differentiate soft tissues involvement by tumors versus swelling due to edema.

On MRI, inflammatory tissue and retained secretions can be differentiated with some degree of confidence from tumors as the latter have a higher water content and thus appear to be of high intensity on T2WI and low intensity on T1WI **(Fig. 29B)**. Discontinuous dural enhancement without intervening hypointense epidural margination favors neoplastic invasion.

No dural enhancement and enhancing tissue over 5 mm thick imply neoplasm over reactive changes.[11]

Chow et al.[36] have characterized carcinoma of the nasal cavity and PNS, and have stated that: (1) They are highly cellular tumors with little free water and thus have low to intermediate signal intensity on T1WI and T2WI. They appear as masses of homogeneous signal intensities. (2) Instances where subacute to chronic hemorrhages have appeared within the masses, these will appear as well-defined areas of intermediate to high signal intensities on T1 and T2WI. (3) Necrotic areas within the tumor appear as areas of low to intermediate signal intensities on T1WI and high intensity on T2WI. (4) Intracranial spread of the tumor tends to be broad based and flat despite destruction of the skull base. This is in contrast to the contained, highly polypoidal intracranial surfaces of benign processes like papillomas and polyps. MRI scans with contrast is useful because Gd-DTPA enhancement of tumors is less intense than enhancement of mucosa. In cases where sinuses are obstructed due to inflammation with presence of tumor, mucosal enhancement helps differentiate the obstructed sinus from tumor invasion. The extent of tumor enhancement is directly proportional to the vascularity of the tumor. Gd-DTPA enhancement is also helpful in detecting intracranial extension.

In a study comparing CT and MRI to evaluate extension of tumor, there was no significant difference in staging by either modality. Errors occurred in both modalities and it has been generalized that MRI is more accurate than CT in evaluation of large bony structures and soft tissues, while CT scores over MR in imaging and evaluating fine bony structures.[7] Diffusion weighted MR imaging may help in differentiating malignant lesions from benign lesion. In one study apparent diffusion coefficient (ADC) values of the tumors were found to be significantly lower than benign lesions. Also, the ADC values were inversely related to the lesions cellularity.[38] In an another study of 55 patients, the mean ADC value of nasal and paranasal sinus malignant lesions were significantly different from that of benign lesions. Also, there was a significant ADC difference between carcinoma and sarcoma as well as between well differentiated and poorly differentiated malignancies.[39]

Imaging is also important in the assessment of operability of sinonasal tumors. There are the following five general criteria for non-resectability:[32]

1. Distant metastases
2. Optic chiasm invasion
3. Extensive cerebral involvement
4. Bilateral carotid infiltration
5. Very poor general health.

Papillomas arise from the pseudociliated columnar epithelium of the nasal cavity and PNS. They are of three types:

1. Fungiform papillomas
2. Inverted papillomas
3. Cylindric cell papillomas.

Fungiform papillomas constitute 50% of papillomas. The nasal septum is the most common site for fungiform papillomas. They have a verrucous appearance and are not premalignant.

Inverted papillomas constitute 47% of papillomas. They are also called endophytic papillomas. They are unilateral, arise from the lateral nasal wall near the middle turbinate and tend to invade the antrum and ethmoids **(Fig. 30)**. They have a propensity to recur after local resection. They appear typically hyperintense on T2WI. Three to twenty-four percent show malignant transformation.

On MRI, the lesion is typically isointense to muscle on T1WI and is isointense to hypointense on T2WI. A crenated or convoluted enhancement is typical.

Recurrences may be distinguished from postoperative thickening by dynamic enhanced MRI. Recurrent inverted papillomas have earlier and greater enhancement than granulation tissue.

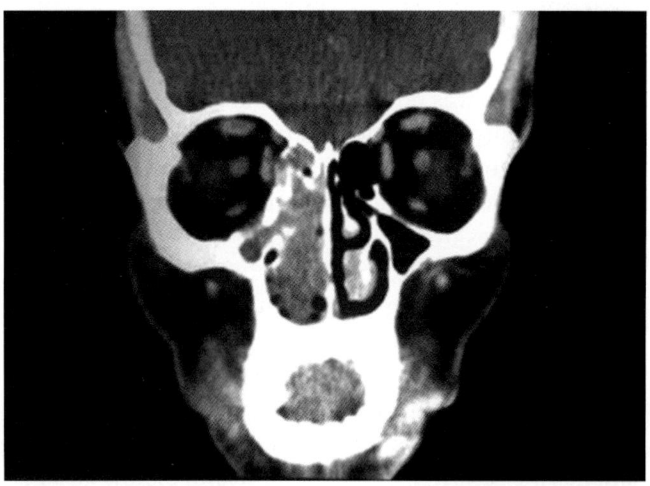

Fig. 30: Inverted papilloma of the right antrum and ethmoids: Non-contrast CT scan shows a hyperdense soft tissue lesion in the right ethmoid and nasal cavity extending into the right antrum. The middle turbinate is destroyed and the septum shows focal erosion. The floor and medial wall of the orbit is eroded at places.

Staging classification for inverted papillomas was proposed by Krause which was later modified by Cannady.[40] The modified Krause staging are as follows:

A. Inverted papilloma (IP) confined to the nasal cavity, ethmoid sinus, or medial maxillary wall.
B. Inverted papilloma with involvement of any maxillary wall (other than the medial wall) or frontal sinus or sphenoid sinus.
C. Inverted papilloma with extension beyond the PNS.

The significance of the staging is that, Stage A lesions may need only endoscopic resection while the more radical approaches reserved for stage B or C lesions.

Cylindric cell papillomas are the rarest of the papillomas and arise from the lateral nasal wall. Imaging findings are nonspecific, lesions vary in appearance as polypoid masses in the nasal cavity to expansile masses causing invasion of adjacent sinuses. Bony margins of nasal cavity are remodeled. Nasal septum is intact.[40,41]

Epithelial Tumors of Glandular Origin

These lesions originate in the minor salivary glands and constitute 10% of all sinonasal tumors. These glands can occur anywhere within the sinonasal cavity; however, the most common site of these glands is within the palate and therefore these lesions can extend into the PNS and nasal cavity from this location. The histological types of tumors in this group are:

- Adenoid cystic carcinoma
- Adenocarcinoma
- Pleomorphic adenomas
- Mucoepidermoid carcinoma
- Acinic cell carcinoma

Amongst these the adenoid cystic carcinoma are the most frequent tumors. This lesion typically causes destruction and remodeling of bone. Adenoid cystic carcinoma characteristically shows perineural and intraneural spread.[17] *Adenocarcinoma* is the name given to the heterogeneous group of neoplasm which does not fit into the classical feature of salivary tumor. They can be subclassified into various morphological subgroups such as mucinous, nonmucinous, clear cell, papillary, tubular and "intestinal type" tumors. These tumors expand bony margins and appear as relatively benign lesions on CT and MRI. High-grade adenocarcinoma invades and destroys bony margins whereas low grade tumors push the margins of bone ahead of them. High-grade adenocarcinomas appear to be of intermediate signal intensity on T2WI because of ill-defined glandular formation and severe nuclear pleomorphism. Low-grade adenocarcinoma appears to have higher signal intensity on T2WI because the cells form small, compact, uniformly glandular patterns.

NONEPITHELIAL TUMOR OF PARANASAL SINUSES

Nonepithelial tumors of the PNS and nasal cavity could be of soft tissue origin (e.g. angiofibroma, hemangioma, hemangiofibroma, hemangiopericytoma), bony/ cartilaginous/ odontogenic tissues (e.g. fibrous dysplasia, chondromas myxomas), neuroectodermal origin (e.g. schwannomas and neurofibromas).

Developmental tumors (dermoids, teratomas), metastatic tumors (from the kidneys, lung and GI tract) are also classified into this group. Since this classification contains a wide variety of tumors only common lesions will be described in this section.

Angiofibroma

It is a benign, but locally invasive highly vascular, nonencapsulated neoplasm of the PNS. These tumors always originate near the pterygopalatine fossa. Patients are almost exclusively adolescent males between the ages of 10–20 years. The tumor spreads into the maxillary, ethmoid and sphenoid sinus and also into the infratemporal fossa and nasal cavity. These are highly vascular tumors and are supplied from the internal maxillary and ascending pharyngeal arteries. It can invade the orbit through the inferior orbital fissure or have an intracranial extension via the superior orbital fissure, pterygoid canal and foramen rotundum. On plain X-rays the characteristic sign of anterior bowing of the posterolateral wall of the maxillary sinus **(Fig. 31)** widening of thepterygopalatine fossa and soft tissue density filling the nasopharynx and sphenoid sinus are pathognomonic of this lesion. On plain CT these tumors appear to be slightly isohyperdense on plain scans and show intense enhancement following contrast administration. On dynamic CT the enhancement shows an early peak which characterizes the highly vascular nature of the tumor.

On MRI, these lesions appear as a mass of low to intermediate signal intensity on T1WI and PDI and as intermediate to high signal intensity on T2WI and gradient echo scans. Multiple flow voids within the mass represent vessels within the lesion. There is marked enhancement noted after Gd-DTPA administration **(Fig. 32)**. Imaging studies are required to assess the extent of the tumor, especially when intracranial and intraorbital spread is present.[42] Angiography is necessary to demonstrate: (i) the feeding vessels, (ii) to assess cross circulation from contralateral evaluation of intracranial aneurysms (ECA), and (iii) to assess feeding from the internal carotid artery in cases of intracranial spread and for preoperative embolization. The latter is helpful in reduction of blood loss during surgery.[43]

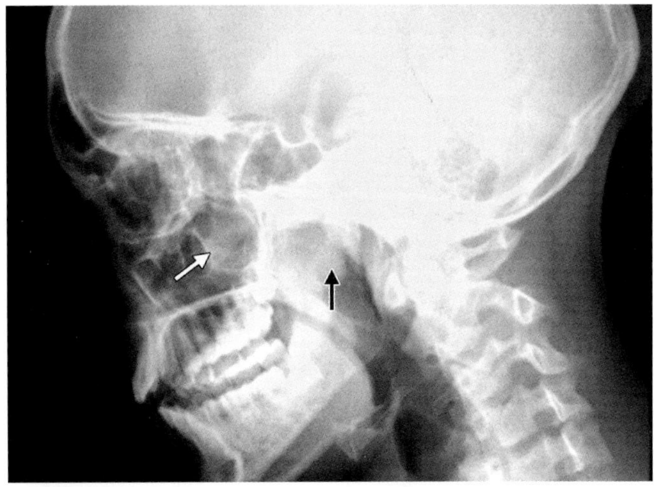

Fig. 31: Angiofibroma lateral X-ray of skull showing anterior bowing (white arrow) of the posterolateral wall of the maxillary sinus due to the angiofibroma (black arrow).

Lymphomas

Forty-seven percent of non-Hodgkin's lymphomas are found in the head and neck; 90% of these are in the cervical lymph nodes. Though the nasopharyngeal region surrounded by the Waldeyer's ring is a potential site of lymphoma, actual involvement of the sinonasal cavity is rare. Lymphomas arising in the nose and PNS are of the non-Hodgkin's type and are seen in cases of disseminated lymphoma. They occur with or without nodal disease. Lesions may be mistaken for sinusitis, polyposis and granulomatous processes. Clinically they may be confused with infection, granulomatous or nonlymphomatous neoplastic processes. On CT and MRI they are seen as bulky masses which show moderate enhancement. The osseous changes include remodeling, expansion, erosion and infiltration of the sinus walls. Primary lymphoma of the paranasal sinus is uncommon. In a study of seven patients of primary maxillary lymphomas, it was found that periantral soft tissue infiltration was the most consistent finding seen in all the patients with some degree of lytic or permeative bony destruction. Mucosal thickening may be mild or in the form of a mass.[44]

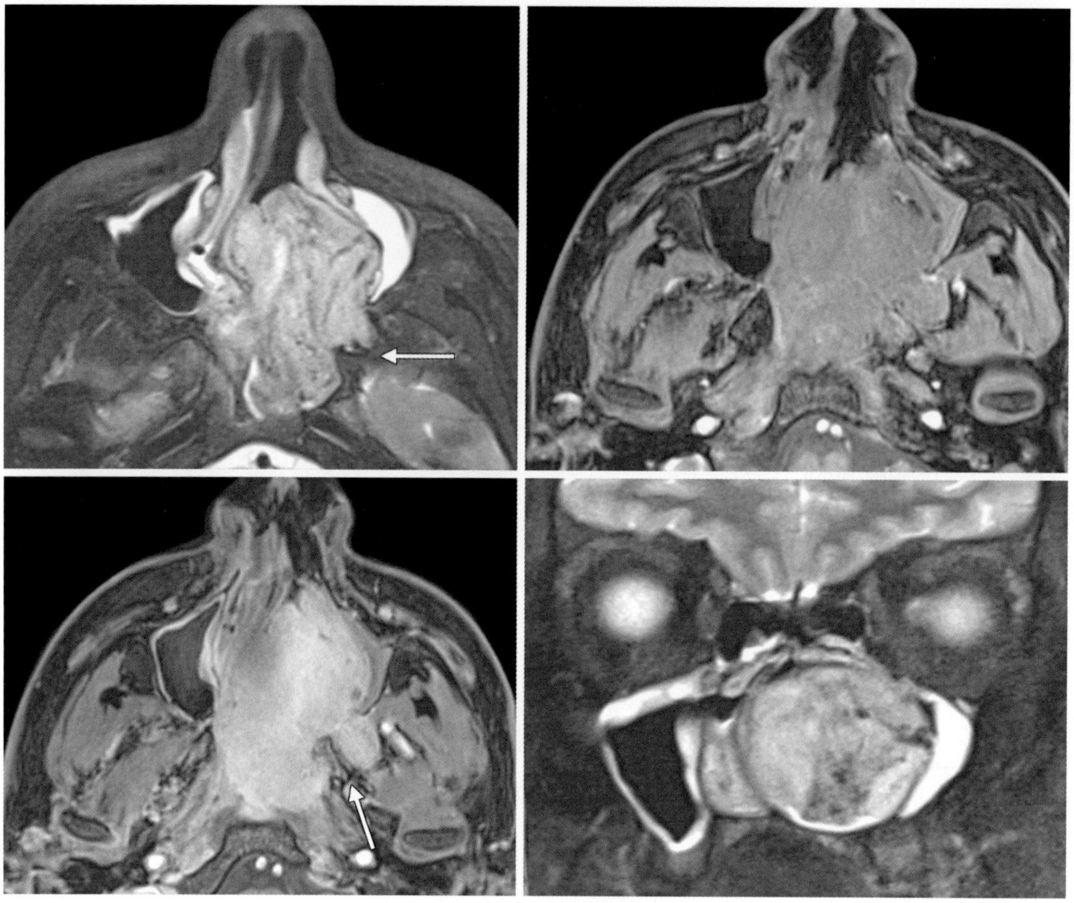

Fig. 32: Nasopharyngeal angiofibroma originating near the pterygopalatine fossa (white arrows) and extending posteriorly into nasopharynx and anteriorly into nasal cavity.

Plasmacytoma

Plasma cell neoplasm can be grouped into multiple myeloma, solitary plasmacytoma of bone and extramedullary plasmacytoma (EMP). Of these EMP are the plasma cell tumors which are predominantly seen in the sinonasal region. Only 5% of multiple myeloma cases present with sinonasal lesions. EMP accounts for 20% of plasma cell neoplasm. It is confined to soft tissue and there is no generalized bone involvement or systemic manifestation. It may arise in the sinonasal cavity and nasopharynx, sphenoid sinus, petrous ridge, base of skull and clivus.

Plasmacytoma of the sinonasal tract appears on CT as a well-defined expansile mass. There is associated bone erosion or remodeling. These tumors show moderate to marked enhancement after contrast administration.

On MRI, T1WI reveal a mass of low to intermediate signal intensity and moderate contrast enhancement and T2WI show intermediate to high signal intensity.[43]

Rhabdomyosarcoma is the most common soft tissue sarcoma. Thirty-five to forty-five percent of rhabdomyosarcoma occurs in the head and neck. It primarily affects infants and children. Peak incidence is in the 2–5 years age group with a second peak between 15 years and 19 years of age. Forty-three percent of cases are under 5 years, and 78% of cases are under the age of 12 years. Histopathologically, they are classified as embryonal, differentiated or alveolar. Embryonal rhabdomyosarcoma is the most common type and arises from primitive muscle cells. They have a potential for metastases to lymph nodes. The alveolar rhabdomyosarcoma occurs in older patients in the age range of 15–25 years. The diagnosis of these two types is difficult. Differentiated rhabdomyosarcoma is the least frequent and most easy to diagnose by histopathology. CT findings are of homogenous soft tissue density mass with moderate enhancement. MRI findings are those of a mass of intermediate signal intensity on all sequences. Bone destruction or remodeling is usually seen.

Olfactory Neuroblastoma (Olfactory Neuroepithelioma/Esthesioneuroblastoma)

It is a rare tumor of neuroectodermal origin that arises from the neural crest. It is located in superior nasal fossa and presents as a polypoid tumor which bleeds profusely when biopsied.

Age incidence has characteristically 2 peaks, the first during 11–22 years and the second in the 50–60 years age group.

Both contrast enhanced CT and MRI are required in the preoperative assessment of these patients to assess intracranial extension into the frontal lobe and dural involvement.

CT imaging shows a homogenous mass with moderate to marked enhancement **(Fig. 33)**. On MRI, they are hypointense to brain on T1WI and hyperintense to brain on T2WI. Sometimes, they may be in homogenous with areas of cystic degeneration. Calcification within these tumors is reported.[10,35,36]

Neurogenic Tumors

Peripheral nerve sheath tumors can be of three types: (i) schwannomas, (ii) neurofibromas, and (iii) neurogenic sarcomas. These tumors usually arise from sensory nerves. In the sinonasal cavity, neurogenic tumors arise from the first and second division of trigeminal nerve and from the autonomic nerves. The olfactory nerve has no Schwann cells. So these tumors cannot arise from this site. Schwannomas are encapsulated, benign, slow growing masses. They are in frequent in nasal cavity, being found in the nasal fossa, maxillary and ethmoidal sinuses. They can be completely excised from the nerve from which they originate.

On CT they appear as well defined, homogenous masses with moderate enhancement after contrast administration. They may be inhomogeneous as well as cystic in appearance occasionally.

On MRI, schwannomas show low to intermediate signal intensity on T1WI and high signal on T2WI with moderate to marked enhancement after contrast administration. They may show varied signal characteristics depending on their histologic patterns and the presence or absence of cystic as well as cholesterol degeneration. Presence of aggressive bone destruction should be considered as an indication of malignant transformation.[45]

Neurofibromas

Neurofibromas are benign, nonencapsulated nerve sheath tumors. These are seen in the constellation of tumor of neurofibromatosis or Von Recklinghausen's disease.

They have a variable appearance on CT with areas of fatty infiltration and cystic degeneration. Bone remodeling is seen rather than aggressive bone destruction **(Figs. 34A and B)**. On MRI they are usually nonhomogeneous with an intermediate T1WI signal intensity and a higher T2WI signal intensity.[46]

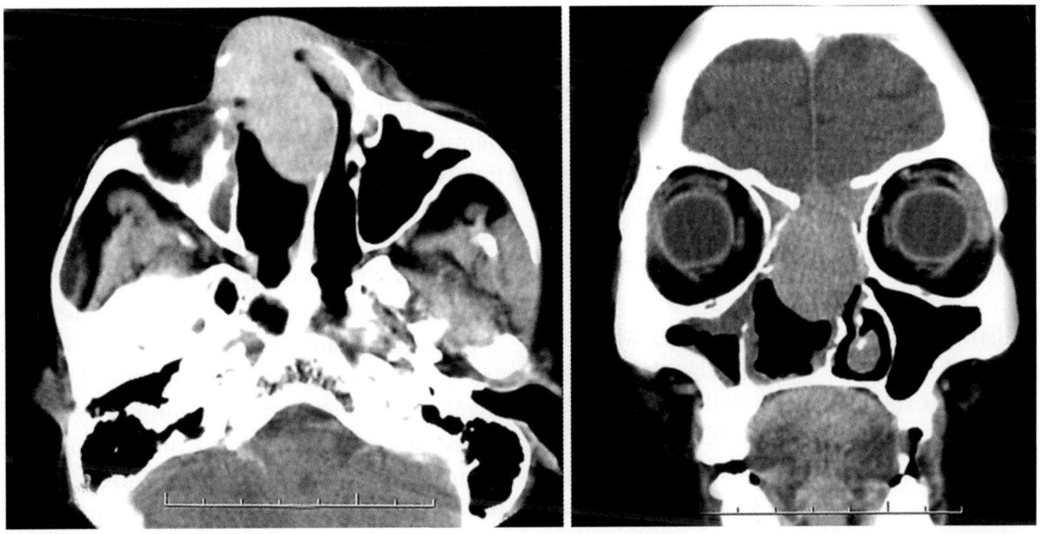

Fig. 33: Olfactory neuroblastoma: Axial and coronal contrast-enhanced CT section showing a uniformly enhanced mass in the right nasal cavity extending from the superior nasal fossa up to the inferior turbinate, the thinned out nasal septum bulges to the left. There is erosion of the right fovea ethmoidalis and the cribriform plate.

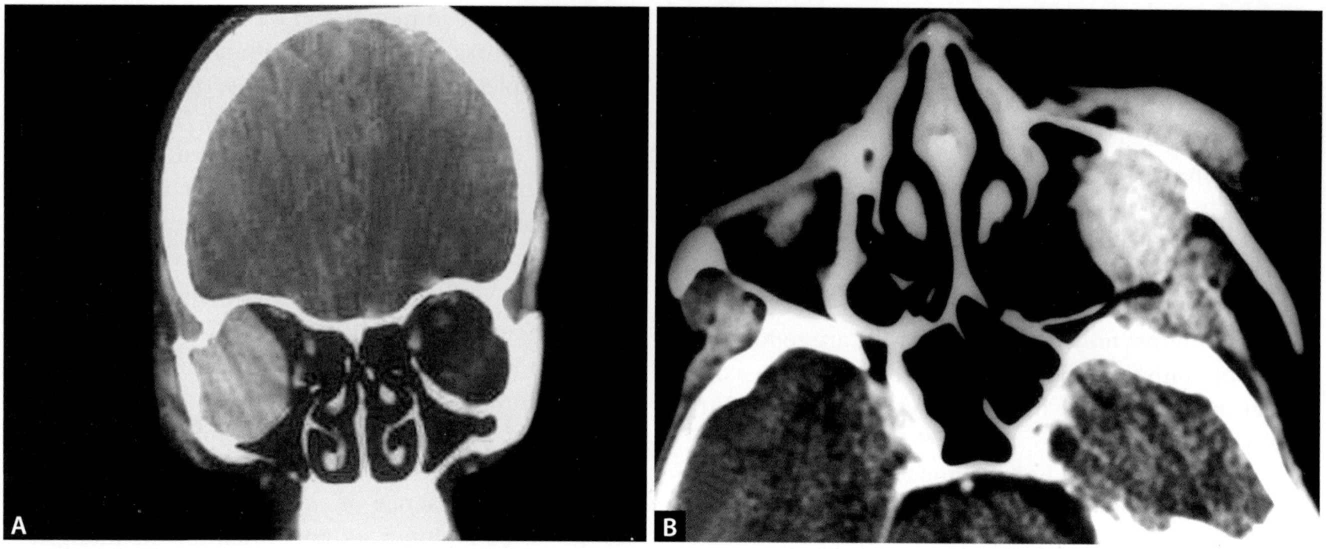

Figs. 34A and B: (A) Axial; and (B) Coronal contrast enhanced scan for a neurofibroma. A homogeneous hyperdense soft tissue mass is present in the right temporal quadrants of the left orbit. The orbital walls are remodeled and the lesion projects into the right maxillary antrum and the cheek.

FIBROSSEOUS LESIONS OF CRANIOFACIAL BONES[47,48]

Fibrosseous lesions of craniofacial bones constitute 25% of nonepithelial neoplasm of this region. They are a varied group of pathologic conditions which are difficult to classify. A common denominator to all these lesions is the replacement of the bone with a benign fibrous tissue containing various amounts of mineralized (calcified) structures.

Osteoma

Osteomas are benign lesions which are commonly seen in the skull and facial bones. These tumors are small usually solitary. These are located within the sinus cavity. The most common sinus affected is the frontal sinus followed by ethmoid, maxillary and sphenoid sinus. They are usually silent lesions and found incidentally on plain X-rays. Their radiopacity is determined by the amount of mature bone within them. On CT scans they are seen to arise from the sinus wall. The cancellous bone and fibrous matrix can be distinguished on CT **(Fig. 35)**. On MRI they may be undetected due to absence of any signal from their bony matrix. Multiple osteomas of the skull and mandible are seen in patients of Gardner syndrome. Osteomas may obstruct the outflow of the frontal sinus. Cerebrospinal fluid (CSF) rhinorrhea may be associated with these tumors.

Fibrous dysplasia is an idiopathic skeletal disorder in which medullary bone is replaced by a dysplastic fibrosseous tissue which is composed of woven type of bone with few osteoclasts. Osteoblasts are typically absent except near the area of transition to normal bone. Some authors consider it to be a hamartomatous malformation that presumably results from an idiopathic arrest in the maturation of bone at the woven bone stage.

It is a condition of young adults affecting males and females equally. It can occur at one skeletal site (monostotic) or at multiple sites (polyostotic). Seventy percent of cases are of the monostotic variety, rest being polyostotic. Monostotic fibrous dysplasia does not progress to the polyostotic form of the disease. The process may involve the facial bones, skull bones or both. Polyostotic fibrous dysplasia may be associated with endocrinopathies (3–5% of all cases). This disease if accompanied by skin pigmentations (Café au lait spots) ipsilateral to osseous involvement, and precocious puberty in girls is referred to as Albright's syndrome. Other endocrine disorders that have been identified include hyperparathyroidism, Cushing's syndrome, hyperthyroidism and acromegaly.

The common site in the facial skeleton is the maxilla and mandible amounts to 12% cases of fibrous dysplasia. The most common presentation is with a painless bony swelling causing facial asymmetry. Visual compromise can occur when the sphenoethmoidal complex is involved. Hearing disturbances are present when the temporal bone is involved. The radiographic appearance of fibrous dysplasia is that of diffuse areas of sclerosis termed as ground glass appearance. The affected bones are wide and thick. The lesions if large do not have sharply defined

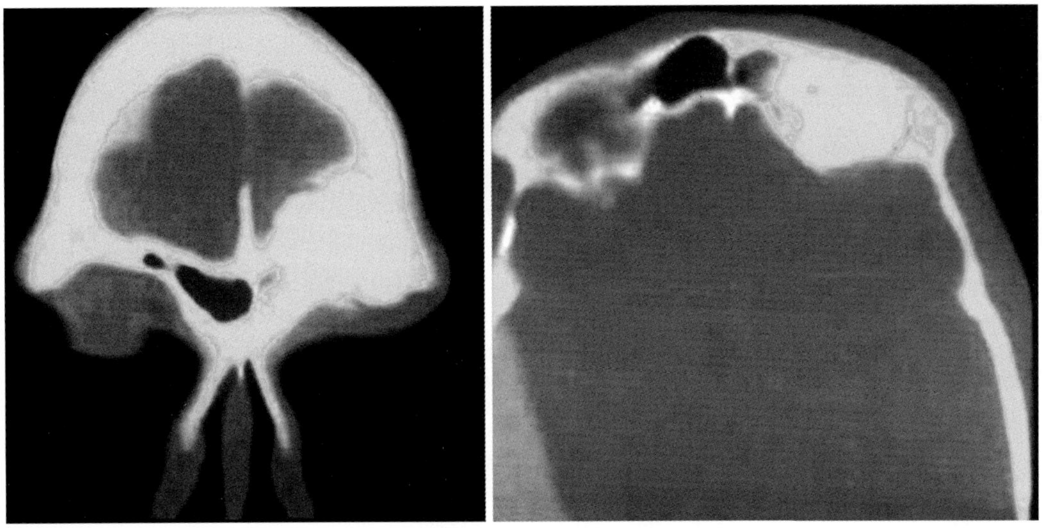

Fig. 35: Osteoma of the left frontal sinus. Axial and coronal CT scans showing a dense bony lesion of the left sinus occupying much of the sinus cavity leaving only a thin rim of air around it.

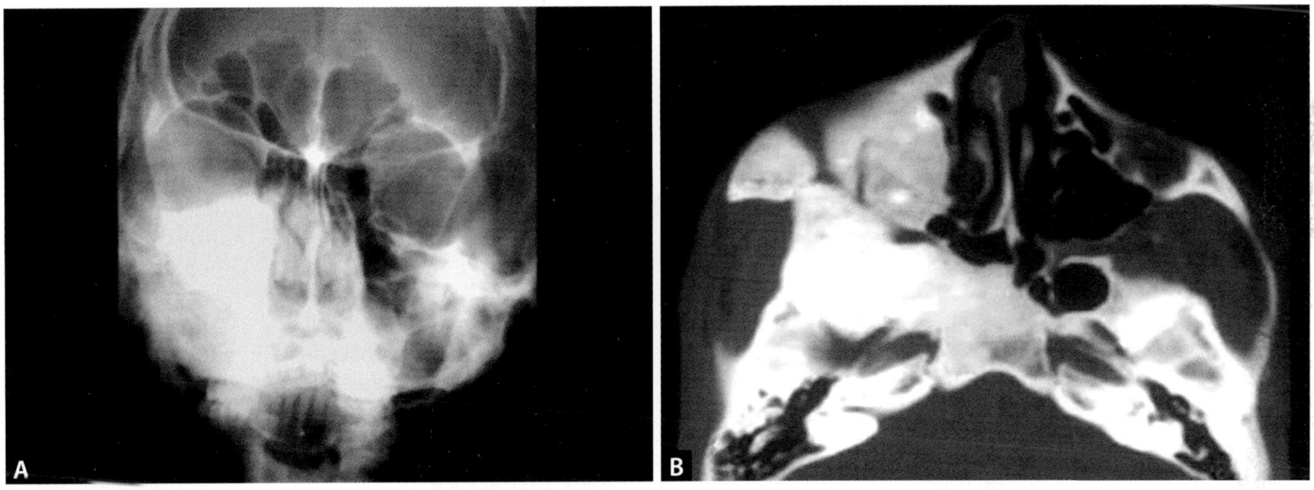

Figs. 36A and B: (A) Fibrous dysplasia: Plain X ray of the skull PA view shows the typical ground glass appearance of the expanded bones of the right side of the face. Note the dimensions of the right orbit are reduced; (B) Axial CT shows the expanded and dense right maxilla, zygoma and sphenoid bones. The right maxillary sinus and the right side of the sphenoid sinus are obliterated. There is relative sparing of the nasal cavities and ethmoids with distortion of the facial contour.

margins. CT appearance of fibrous dysplasia is that of an expanded bone of heterogeneous density. CT attenuation depends on the amount of fibrous tissue and bone present in the affected region **(Figs. 36A and B)**.

On MRI, fibrous dysplasia exhibits an intermediate signal on T1WI and PDWI and heterogeneous hypointense signal on T2WI. With Gd-DTPA the lesions may show moderate to marked contrast enhancement.

Ossifying Fibroma

Ossifying fibroma is a well circumscribed fibrous tumor which ossifies in time. Ossification begins from the periphery of the tumor and progresses to the core. The newly formed bone is of the woven type initially and later matures into lamellar bone. On CT, lesions appear somewhat similar to fibrous dysplasia but have larger areas of unossified fibrous tissues **(Fig. 37)**. They may be indistinguishable from lesions of fibrous dysplasia on histopathological studies. However, these lesions tend to be more aggressive than fibrous dysplasia as they grow inward to involve the orbits nasal cavities and the sinus, leaving the surface contours of bones intact.

Paget's Disease

Paget's disease affects patients above the age of 50 years. Involvement of the spine calvarium is common and seen

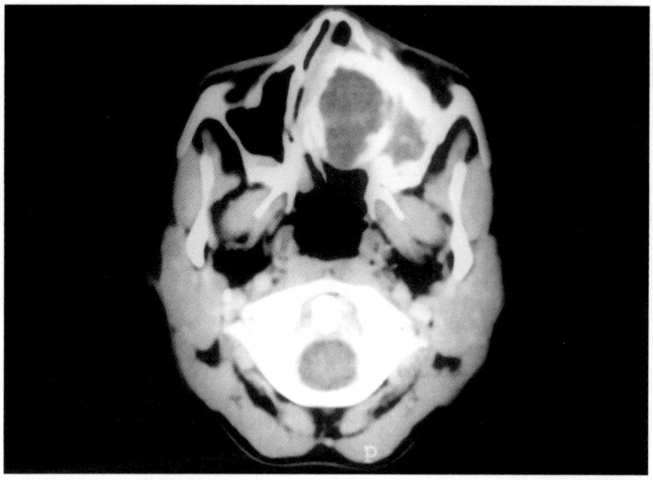

Fig. 37: Ossifying fibroma of the left maxilla: The core of the lesions isodense to muscle, the peripheral zone shows a well ossified structure. The lesion expands toward the median plane, and the facial contour is relatively preserved as compared to fibrous dysplasia (above).

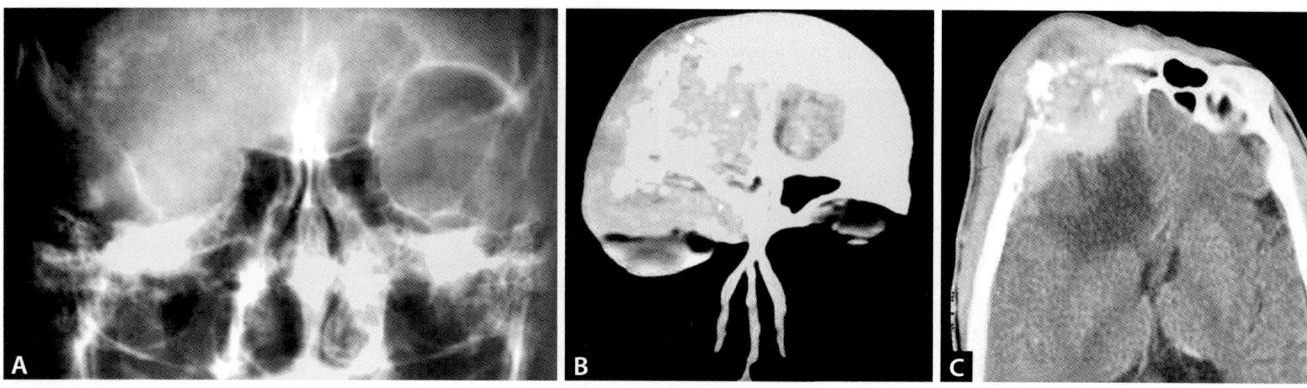

Figs. 38A to C: Metastases from carcinoma gallbladder: (A) Detail from X-ray skull shows a soft tissue density lesion causing destruction of the right and superior orbital rim and the bony outline of the right frontal sinus; (B) Coronal contrast enhanced sections show destruction of the frontal bone; (C) Axial sections of the study showing intracranial extension as well as involvement of the soft tissues of the forehead.

in 76% and 65% of cases respectively. Involvement of the facial skeleton is rare. When the sinonasal cavity and orbits are affected signs of neurovascular compromise can develop.

Metastatic lesions to the PNS arise from primaries form the kidneys, lung, breast and GI tract.[49,50] Uncommon primary malignancies metastasizing to the PNS are from the cervix and liver. Clinical presentation is not unlike primary PNS carcinomas as are the imaging findings. Metastases from the breast, lung, GI tract, distal genitourinary tract are aggressive lesions which destroy bony boundaries **(Figs. 38A to C)**. Secondaries from melanoma and renal cell carcinoma appear as enhancing lesions which remodel and destroy sinonasal walls. Multifocal erosion lesions with normal bone are suggestive of metastatic disease; however, a solitary metastatic lesion has nonspecific imaging findings.[11]

REFERENCES

1. Williams JW, Roberts L, Distell B, et al. Diagnosing sinusitis by X-ray: is a single waters view adequate? J Gen Intern Med. 1992;7(5):481-5.
2. McAlister WH, Lusk R, Muntz HR. Comparison of plain radiographs and coronal CT scans in infants and children with recurrent sinusitis. Am J Roentgenol. 1989;153(6):1259-64.
3. Lazar RH, Younis RT, Parvey LS. Comparison of plain radiographs, coronal CT, and intraoperative findings in children with chronic sinusitis. Otolaryngol Head Neck Surg. 1992;107(1):29-34.
4. Burke TF, Guertler AT, Timmons JH. Comparison of Sinus X-rays with computed tomography scans in acute sinusitis. Acad Emerg Med. 1994;1(3):235-9.
5. Gotwald TF, Zinreich SJ, Corl F, et al. Three-dimensional volumetric display of the nasal ostiomeatal channels and paranasal sinuses. Am J Roentgenol. 2001;176(1):241-5.
6. Bisdas S, Verink M, Burmeister HP, et al. Three-dimensional visualization of the nasal cavity and paranasal sinuses

clinical results of a standardized approach using multislice helical computed tomography. J Comput Assist Tomogr. 2004;28:661-9.
7. Lin HW, Bhattacharyya N. Diagnostic and staging accuracy of magnetic resonance imaging for the assessment of sinonasal disease. Am J Rhinol Allergy. 2009;23(1):36-9.
8. Lloyd GAS, Lund VJ, Phelps PD, et al. Magnetic resonance imaging in the evaluation of nose and paranasal sinus disease. Br J Radiology. 1987;60(718):957-68.
9. Vogl JJ, Mack MG, Juergens M, Stark M, et al. MR diagnosis of head and neck tumours: comparison of contrast enhancement with triple dose gadodiamide and standard dose gadopentate dimeglumine in the same patient. Am J Roentgenol. 1994;163(2):425-32.
10. Oliverio PJ, Benson ML, Zeinrich SJ. Update on imaging for functional endoscopic surgery. Otolarynaging, 4th editiongol Clin North Am. 1995;28(3):585-608.
11. Grossman RI, Youserm DM. Sinonasal disease. In: Grossman RI, Yousem DM (Eds). Neuroradiology: the Requisites, 2nd edition. Philadelphia: Mosby; 2003.
12. Zeinrich SJ, Albayrams S, Benson ML, et al. Sinonasal cavities: the osteomeatal complex and functional endoscopic surgery. In: Som PM and Curton HD (Eds). Head and Neck Im. St. Louis Mosby-Year Book, 2003.
13. Mafee MF. Preoperative Imaging: anatomy of nasal ethmoid complex for functional endoscopic sinus surgery. Radiologic Clin North Am. 1993;31(1):1-20.
14. Som PM, Brandwein MS. Sinonasal cavities: inflammatory diseases. In: Som PM, Curton HD (Eds). Head and Neck Imaging, 14th edition. St Louis: Mosby Year Book; 2003.
15. Hoang JK, Eastwood JD, Tebbit CL, et al. Multiplanar sinus CT: a systematic approach to imaging before functional endoscopic sinus surgery. Am J Roentgenol. 2010;194(6):W527-36.
16. O'Brien WT Sr, Hamelin S, Weitzel EK. The Preoperative Sinus CT: Avoiding a "CLOSE" Call with Surgical Complications. Radiology. 2016;281(1):10-21.
17. Som PM, Curtin HD. Chronic inflammatory sinonasal disease including fungal infection. The role of imaging. Radiologic Clin North America. 1993;31(1):33-44.
18. Babbel R, Harnsberger HR, Nelson B, et al. Optimization of techniques in screening CT of the sinuses. Am J Neuroradiol. 1991;12(5):849-54.
19. Som PM, Curtin HD. Sinuses. In: Stark DD, Bradley WG (Jr) (Eds). Magnetic Resonance Imaging, 2nd edition. St. Louis: Mosby Year Book; 1992. pp. 1113-34.
20. Sonkens JW, Harnsberger HR, Blanch GM, et al. Hunt S. The impact of screening sinus CT on the planning of functional endoscopic sinus surgery. Otolaryngol Head Neck Surg. 1991;105(6):802-13.
21. Hahnel S, Ertl-Wagner B, Tasman AJ, et al. Relative value of MR imaging as compared with CT in the diagnosis of inflammatory paranasal sinus disease. Radiology. 1999;210(1):171-6.
22. Som PM, Dillon WP, Fullerton GD, et al. et al. Chronically obstructed sinus secretions: observations on T1 and T2 shortening. Radiology. 1989;172(2):515-20.
23. Perugini S, Pasquini U, Menichelli F, et al. Mucoceles in the paranasal sinuses involving the orbit CT signs in 43 cases. Neuroradiology. 1982;23(3):133-9.
24. Osborn AG, Johnson L, Roberts TS. Sphenoidal mucoceles with intracranial extension. J Comput Assist Tomogr. 1979;3(3):335-8.
25. Lanzieri CF, Shah M, Kraun D, et al. Use of gadolinium enhanced MR imaging for differentiating mucoceles from neoplasm in the paranasal sinuses. Radiology. 1991;178(2):425-8.
26. Centono RS, Bentson JR, Mancuso AA. CT scanning in rhinocerebral mucormycosis and aspergillosis. Radiology. 1981;140(2):383-9.
27. Kingdom TT, Tami TA. Actinomycosis of the nasal septum in a patient infected with HIV. Otolaryngol Head and Neck Surgery. 1994;71:675-7.
28. Bath AP, O'Flynn P, Gibbin KP. Nasopharyngeal tuberculosis. J Laryngol Otol. 1992;71:675-7.
29. Sharma VK, Bapuraj JR, Kumar B, et al. Computed tomographic surgery of paranasal sinuses in lepromatous leprosy. International Journal of Leprosy. 1998;66(2):201-7.
30. Lohrmann C, Uhl M, Warnatz K, et al. Sinonasal computed tomography in patients with Wegener's granulomatosis. J Comput Assist Tomogr. 2006;30(1):122-5.
31. Sakai S, Fuchilate H, Hamasaki Y. Treatment policy of maxillary sinus carcinoma. Acta Otolaryngol (Stockh). 1976;82(3-4):172-81.
32. Lund VS, Howard DJ, Lloyd GAS. CT evaluation of paranasal sinus tumor for craniofacial resection. Br J Radiol. 1983;56(667):439-46.
33. Barnes L, Verbin RS, Gnepp DR. Disease of the nose, paranasal sinuses and nasopharynx. In: Barnex L (Ed). Surgical Pathology of the Head and Neck. New York: Marcel Dekker Inc; 1985. pp. 403-51.
34. Momose KJ, Weber ALM, Goodman M, et al. Radiological aspects of inverted papilloma. Radiology. 1980;134(1):73-9.
35. Lund VS, Howard DJ, Loyd GAS, et al. Magnetic resonance imaging of paranasal sinus tumor for craniofacial resection. Head Neck. 1989;11(3):279-83.
36. Chow JM, Leonetti JP, Mafee MF. Epithelial tumours of the paranasal sinuses and nasal cavities. Radiological Clinics of North America. 1993;31(1):61-73.
37. Hunink MGM, de Slegte RGM, Gerritsen GJ, et al. CT and MR assessment of tumours of the nose and paranasal sinuses, the nasopharynx and parapharyngeal space using ROC methodology. Neuroradiology. 1990;32(3):220-5.
38. White ML, Zhang Y, Robinson RA. Evaluating tumors and tumorlike lesions of the nasal cavity, the paranasal sinuses, and the adjacent skull base with diffusion-weighted MRI. J Comput Assist Tomogr. 2006;30(3):490-5.
39. Razek AA, Sieza S, Maha B. Assessment of nasal and paranasal sinus masses by diffusion-weighted MR imaging. J Neuroradiol. 2009;36(4):206-11.
40. Cannady SB, Batra PS, Sautter NB, et al. New staging system for sinonasal inverted papilloma in the endoscopic era. Laryngoscope. 2007;117(7):1283-7.

41. Yousem DM, Fellows DW, Kermedy DW, et al. Inverted papilloma evaluation with MR imaging. Radiology. 1992;185(2):501-5.
42. Bryan RN, Serrons RB, Horowitz BL. Radiographic management of juvenile angiofibroma. AJNR. 1981;2(2):157-66.
43. Mafee MF. Nonepithelial tumours of the paranasal sinuses and nasal cavity: role of CT and MR imaging. Radio Clin North Am. 1993;31(1):75-90.
44. Yasumoto M, Taura S, Shibuya H, et al. Primary malignant lymphoma of the maxillary sinus: CT and MRI. Neuroradiology. 2000;42(4):285-9.
45. Derdeyn CP, Moran CJ, Wippold FJ, et al. MRI of esthesioneuroblastoma. JCAT. 1994;18(1):16-21.
46. Jellquist HB, Lundgren J. Neurogenic sarcoma of the sinonasal tract. J Laryngo Otol. 1991;105(3):186-90.
47. Mohammadi-Araghi H, Haery C. Fibrosseous lesions of the craniofacial bones. Radiologic Clinics of North America. 1993;31(1):121-34.
48. Rao VM, EI-Noueam KJ. Sinonasal imaging. Radiol Clin North Am. 1998;36(5):921-39.
49. Som P, Norton K, Shugar J, et al. Metastatic hypernephroma to the head and neck. AJNR. 1987;8(6):1103-6.
50. Marchke DA, Mc Culloch TM, Nerad JA. Prostate cancer metastatic to the orbit. Ann Otol Rhinol Laryngol. 1996;105(1):70-1.

CHAPTER 23

Imaging of the Neck Spaces

Rashmi Dixit, Sapna Singh, Radhika Batra, Alpana Manchanda

The neck has a complex anatomy where many critical structures are compartmentalized into a small space. It is divided into various spaces and compartments by arrangement of the superficial and deep layers of the cervical fascia on the basis of pioneering work by anatomists. With the advent of cross-sectional imaging radiologists, clinicians and surgeons have adopted the spatial organization of the head and neck into fascial compartments.

A systematic approach and a sound grasp of this anatomic organization is essential in approaching neck masses. It is important to localize the space of origin or the epicenter of the lesion, which helps generate a differential diagnosis based upon the contents characteristic of each space. Alongwith imaging techniques, clinical history, physical examination and laboratory studies have a very important complementary role to help arrive at the correct diagnosis.[1,2]

This chapter presents a discussion of the various spaces of the neck alongwith the differential diagnosis relevant to that space according to its anatomical contents. Some lesions that are specific to a neck space are discussed alongwith the description of the space and lesions that may be common to various spaces are discussed later in the chapter.

The neck can be divided into two portions anatomically—**suprahyoid and infrahyoid neck**. The suprahyoid neck is the region of the neck that extends from the skull base superiorly to the hyoid bone inferiorly. The infrahyoid neck extends from the hyoid bone superiorly to the thoracic inlet inferiorly.

IMAGING MODALITIES

Plain radiographs were once the mainstay of diagnosis. Fractures, cervical spine abnormalities, airway compromise and calcification are well seen on plain radiographs. Soft tissue radiographs of the neck in the lateral position are used to delineate mass lesions but soft tissue interfaces are often not visualized optimally. Fistulous or sinus tracts are seen on **contrast examinations**.

Ultrasonography performed with a high frequency probe is excellent for visualization of superficial lesions and helps in differentiating solid from cystic lesions. It can also be used to evaluate the vessels of the neck and provides guidance for fine needle aspiration. Sonography is particularly useful in the pediatric age group.

Cross-sectional imaging with **computed tomography** and **magnetic resonance imaging** has greatly extended our understanding of this region. The entire head and neck region from the base of skull to the thoracic inlet is scanned with computed tomography (CT) or magnetic resonance imaging (MRI). Contrast-enhanced studies are performed to assess the vascularity of the lesion and opacify the arteries and veins. High quality three dimensional reconstructions are useful in evaluating the extent of the lesion. Dynamic maneuvers during the scans are possible due to rapid acquisition by multislice scanners. Such maneuvers include:

a. Phonation (for better visualization of laryngeal ventricle).
b. Modified valsalva (for better visualization of the pyriform sinuses, postcricoid region and the gingivobuccal tumors).

c. Puffed cheek technique (to assess buccal and gingival mucosal involvement and other deeper involvement of oral vestibule).

CT perfusion imaging is a dynamic contrast enhanced technique for quantitative assessment of tissue microcirculation and is a noninvasive tool for the evaluation of microcirculatory changes associated with head and neck carcinomas.[3] A significant increase in blood flow (BF), blood volume (BV) and permeability surface area product alongwith a reduction in mean transit time (MTT) have been found in malignant tumors of head and neck. It can also be used for monitoring treatment response.

While imaging neck spaces on MRI, a combined head and neck coil is used for a comprehensive evaluation of the entire extracranial head and neck evaluating all the nodal masses, a second primary neoplasm and perineural tumor spread. In addition to the conventional contrast-enhanced MR, diffusion-weighted imaging (DWI) may also be performed. DWI is sensitive for detection of tumor recurrence after treatment and also helps in accurate lymph node staging.[4]

Similar to perfusion CT, **dynamic perfusion MRI** offers the potential of visualizing the tumor vascularity. Echo-planar imaging (EPI) or a volumetric interpolated breath-hold examination (VIBE) sequence are used and mean signal intensity versus time curves are plotted. Parameters such as peak time (in seconds), peak enhancement (percent baseline) and washout slope estimate can be obtained.

Proton magnetic resonance spectroscopy (MRS) is another promising technique wherein data can be acquired on the same scanner and with the same coils. Single voxel spin (SVS) echo sequence can be used and it allows detection of the choline signal which is increased in neoplastic tissue. Metastatic nodal disease also shows a higher choline concentration.[5]

PET-CT is useful for assessment of head and neck cancers. It helps to evaluate successful treatment of neoplasms, differentiate between tumor and scar and enables precise localization of the tumor. It also facilitates guided biopsy and allows accurate tissue sampling.[6]

FASCIAL LAYERS OF THE NECK

There are two layers of fascia in the neck, the superficial and deep layers **(Flowchart 1)**. The **superficial cervical fascia** is a thin layer that is comprised mainly of loose areolar connective tissue and adipose tissue. It extends from the head to the thorax and the shoulders to the axilla. It contains the platysma, muscles of facial expression, cutaneous nerves, blood vessels, and lymph nodes.

The **deep cervical fascia (DCF) or fascia colli** is divided into 3 layers **(Figs. 1A and B)**:

Flowchart 1: Cervical fascial layers.

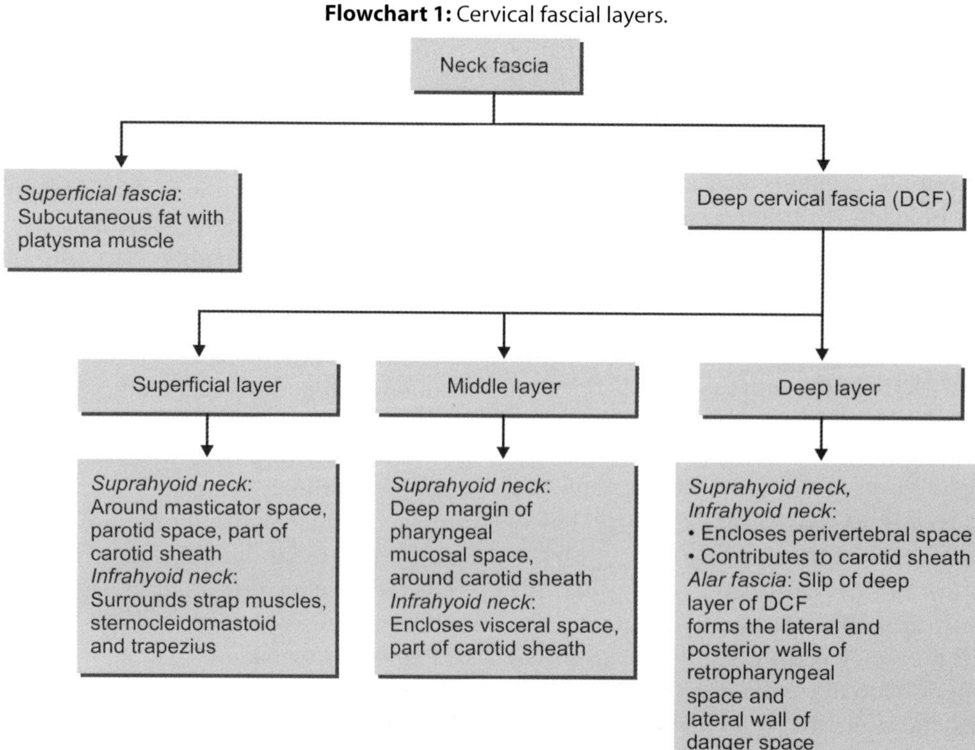

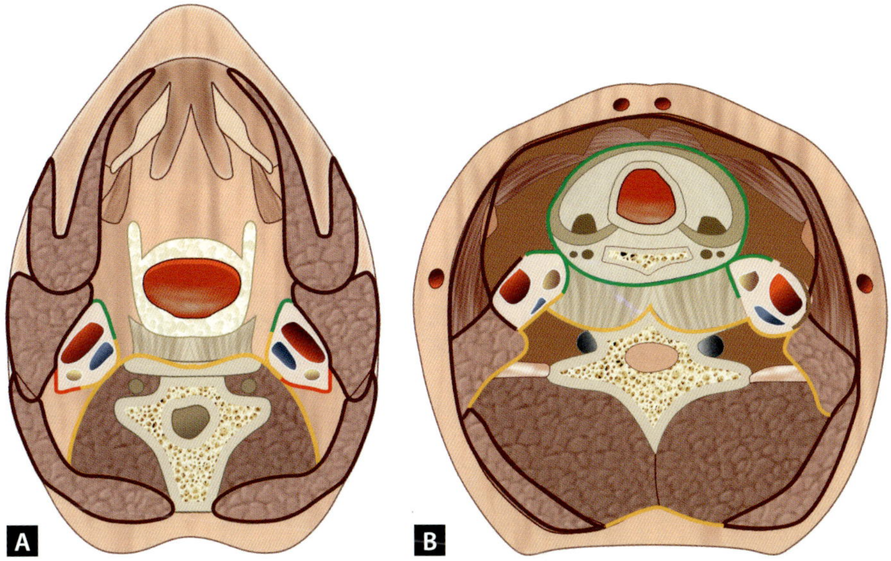

Figs. 1A and B: Deep cervical fascia in suprahyoid (A) and infrahyoid (B) neck in axial plane; superficial layer of deep cervical fascia is outlined in red, middle layer of deep cervical fascia is outlined in green and deep layer of deep cervical fascia is outlined in orange color.

The superficial or investing layer of deep cervical fascia is the layer that lies between the superficial cervical fascia and the neck muscles. Anteriorly, it is attached to the hyoid bone and superiorly to the inferior border of the mandible, the mastoid process, the superior nuchal line, and the external occipital protuberance. It invests all the superficial structures of the neck.[7] It splits to enclose the sternocleidomastoid and trapezius muscles and merges posteriorly with the ligamentum nuchae. It splits again between the angle of the mandible and the mastoid process to enclose the parotid gland. Inferiorly, it is attached to the spine and acromion of the scapula, the clavicle, and the manubrium.[8]

The spaces enclosed are: (i) masticator space **(Figs. 2A and B)** (ii) parotid space **(Figs. 3A and B)** (iii) submandibular **(Fig. 4)** and sublingual spaces **(Figs. 5A and B)**.

The middle layer of deep cervical fascia—The extent of this layer ranges from the skull base superiorly to the mediastinum inferiorly and anteriorly from the hyoid bone to the thoracic inlet. It has two divisions: the muscular and visceral. The muscular division encloses the strap muscles—the sternohyoid, sternothyroid, omohyoid, and thyrohyoid. It blends with the superficial layer of deep cervical fascia over the sternocleidomastoid muscle. The visceral division, also known as the *buccopharyngeal fascia* in the suprahyoid neck, encloses the pharynx, larynx, esophagus, trachea, thyroid, parathyroid glands, periesophageal lymph nodes and the recurrent laryngeal nerve. Posteriorly this layer attaches to the prevertebral fascia and fuses with the investing fascia at the lateral margins of the infrahyoid muscles.[9]

The spaces enclosed are: (i) pharyngeal mucosal space **(Figs. 6A and B)** (ii) parapharyngeal space **(Figs. 7A and B)** (iii) retropharyngeal space **(Figs. 8A and B)** and (iv) buccal space.

The deep layer of deep cervical fascia surrounds the deep muscles of the neck and the cervical vertebrae. It extends from the skull base into the mediastinum (to the third thoracic vertebra, it fuses in the midline with the anterior longitudinal ligament in front of T3 vertebral body) and has two divisions: the alar and prevertebral layers. The alar layer contributes to the posterior and lateral walls of the retropharyngeal space and bridges the transverse processes of the vertebrae. The prevertebral layer encircles the paraspinal muscles: the longus colli and longus capitis muscles; the anterior, middle, and posterior scalene muscles; and the levator scapulae. The brachial plexus trunks, phrenic nerve, cervical plexus, vertebral artery and vertebral vein are also surrounded by the prevertebral fascia with the cervical sympathetic trunk fixed into the anterior part of the fascia.[9] The spaces enclosed extend through the suprahyoid and infrahyoid neck. These are the (i) carotid space **(Fig. 9)** (ii) retropharyngeal space (iii) danger space (iv) perivertebral space **(Fig. 10)** and (v) the posterior cervical space **(Fig. 11)**.

Within the infrahyoid neck the three layers of DCF form two additional spaces (i) visceral space **(Figs. 12A and B)** and (ii) the anterior cervical space. **Table 1** lists the various spaces of the neck.

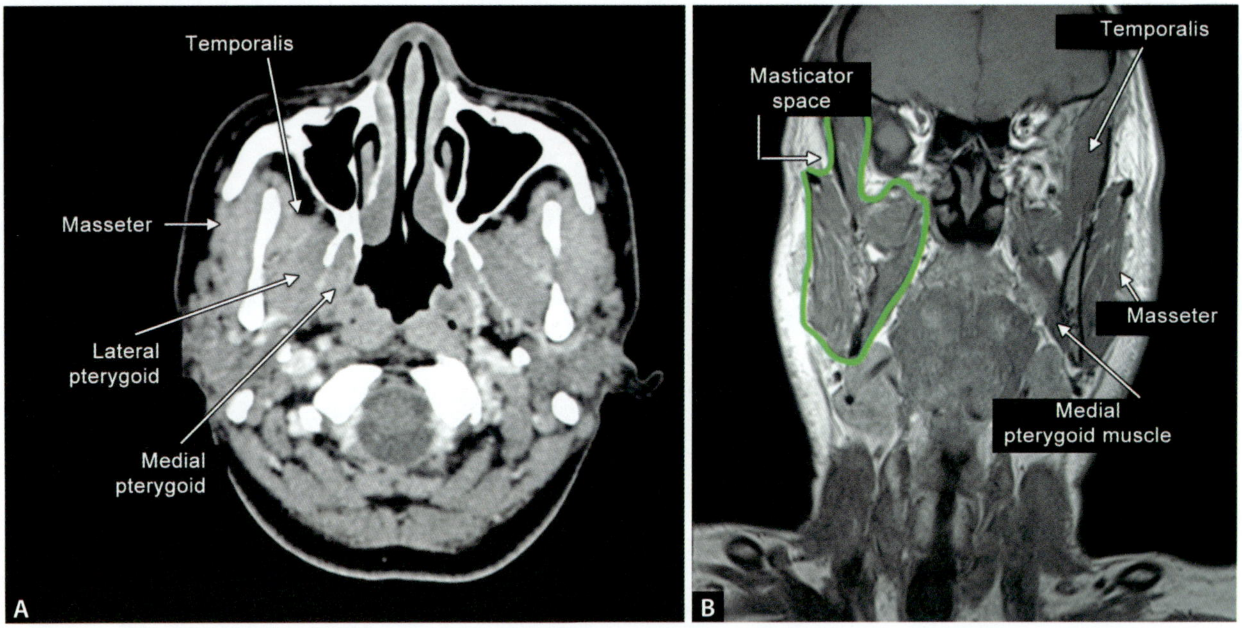

Figs. 2A and B: Axial CECT (A) and coronal T1W MR (B) images show the masticator space containing muscles of mastication and ramus of mandible.

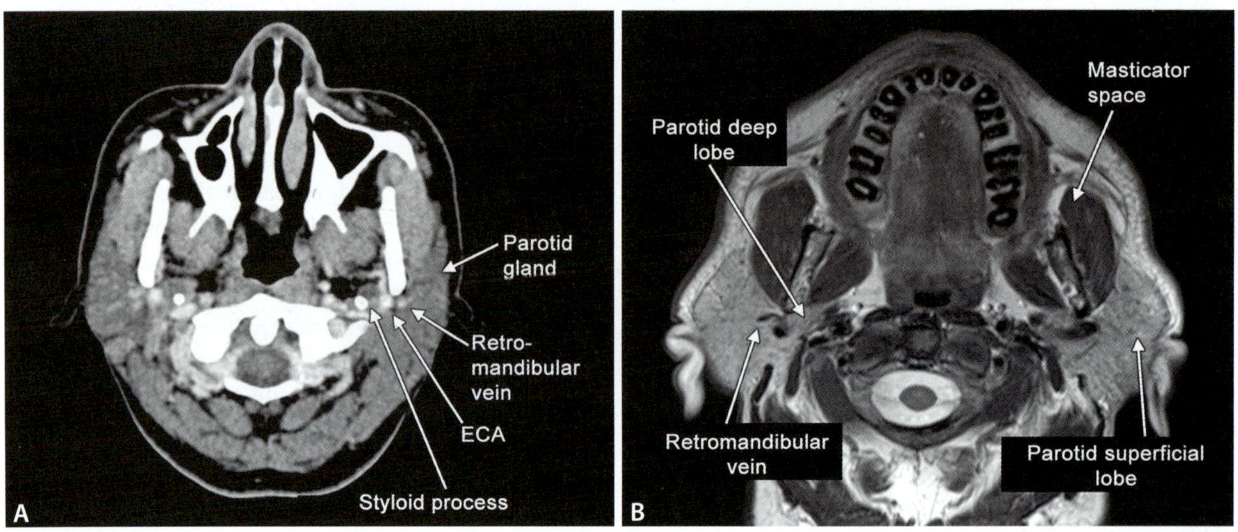

Figs. 3A and B: Axial CECT (A) and axial T2W MR (B) images show the parotid space containing superficial and deep lobes of parotid gland, ECA and retromandibular vein.

Table 1: Spaces of the suprahyoid and infrahyoid neck **(Figs. 13A to D)**.

Suprahyoid neck	***Infrahyoid neck***	***Spaces spanning entire neck***
• Masticator space • Parotid space • Submandibular space • Sublingual space • Pharyngeal mucosal space • Parapharyngeal space • Buccal space	• Visceral space • Anterior cervical space • Posterior cervical space	• Retropharyngeal space • Danger space • Perivertebral space • Carotid space

MASTICATOR SPACE

These are paired spaces located in the anterolateral aspect of suprahyoid neck. The superficial layer of DCF splits to enclose the muscles of mastication and forms the borders of this space. The masticator space (MS) extends inferiorly to the attachment of the medial pterygoid and masseter muscles to the mandible. Its superomedial margin is at the skull base and includes soft tissues inferior to the foramen ovale. Therefore, any malignancy involving the MS can extend to the cavernous sinus via retrograde perineural

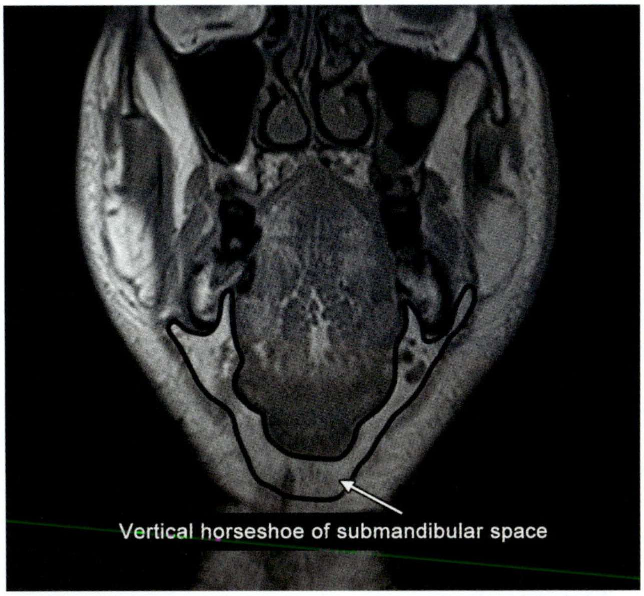

Fig. 4: Coronal T1W MR image showing the submandibular space.

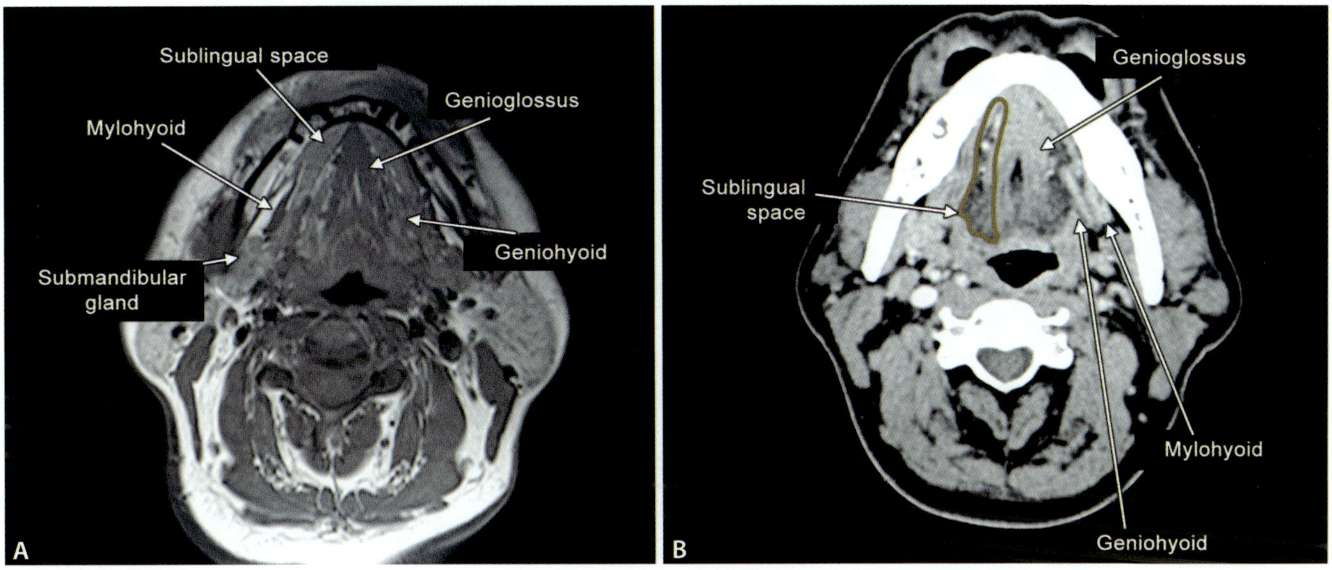

Figs. 5A and B: Axial T1W MR (A) and axial CT (B) sections show the normal sublingual space (outlined in brown color in B).

extension along the mandibular division of trigeminal nerve (V3).

The **contents (Table 2)** of this space are, therefore, the muscles of mastication (medial and lateral pterygoid muscles, masseter and temporalis), posterior body and ramus of mandible, pterygoid venous plexus and V3 and its branches.[1] **(*see* Figs. 2A and B)**.

The most common **lesions** in the masticator space are dental tumors, cysts and abscesses. Other lesions include osteomyelitis **(Figs. 14A and B)**, nerve sheath tumors, lipomas, vascular lesions such as hemangiomas, lymphatic malformations and rarely pseudoaneurysms. Mandibular and soft tissue sarcomas **(Figs. 15A and B)** can also arise in the masticator space including rhabdomyosarcoma in children.

Mandibular nerve denervation atrophy of the muscles of mastication on one side makes the opposite normal side look like pseudolesion. Accessory parotid gland may appear as a lesion over the surface of masseter muscle. Unilateral or bilateral masseteric hypertrophy may also appear as a pseudomass.[10]

The masticator space is divided by a transaxial plane passing through the notch between coronoid and condyloid process. Disease above this plane is classified

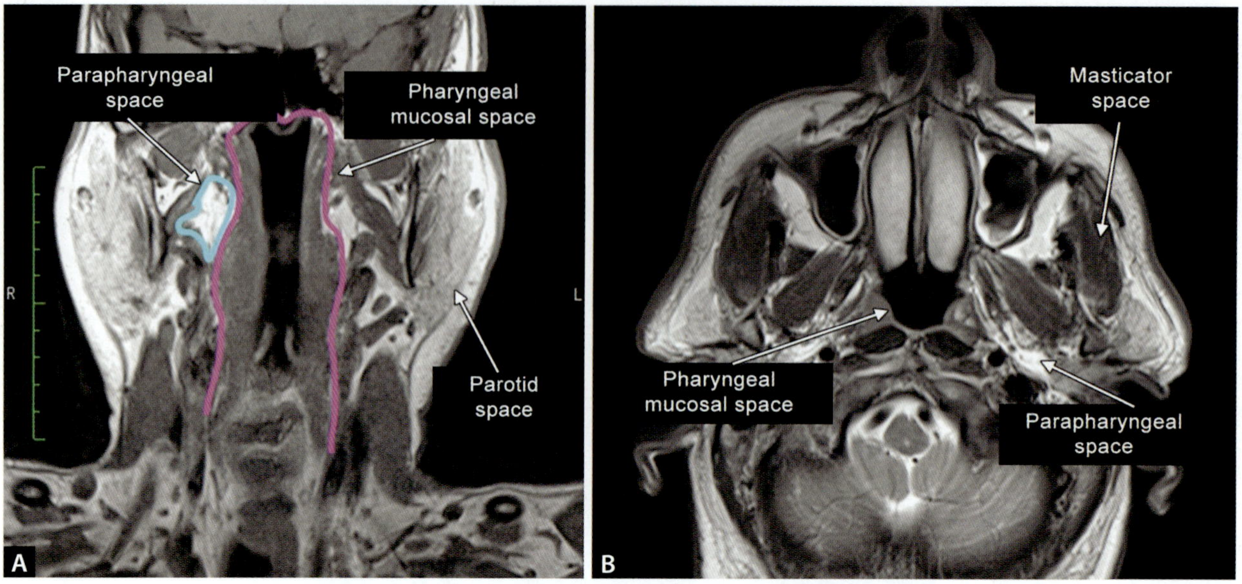

Figs. 6A and B: Coronal T1W (A) and axial T2W (B) MR images show the normal pharyngeal mucosal space (outlined in pink) that extends from the nasopharynx to the hypopharynx, the parapharyngeal space (outlined in light blue) lies lateral to the pharyngeal mucosal space.

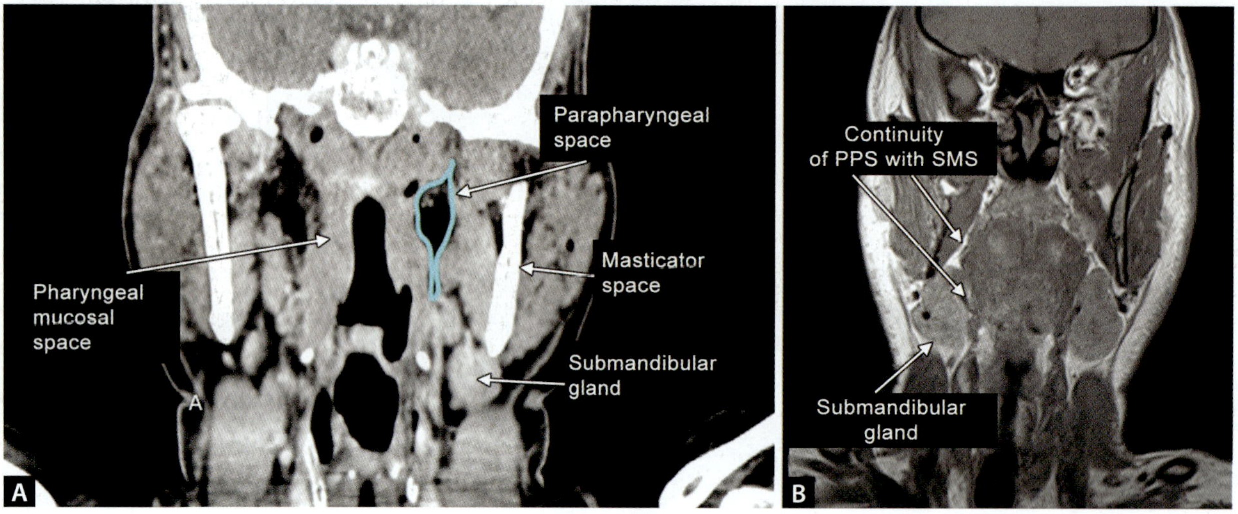

Figs. 7A and B: Coronal CECT (A) and coronal T1W MR (B) images depict the fat containing parapharyngeal space in the lateral aspect of suprahyoid neck, continuity of the parapharyngeal space with the submandibular space is seen in B.

as 'supranotch' and below it as 'infranotch' disease. The supranotch compartment includes the lateral pterygoid muscle, tendon of temporalis and upper two-thirds of the pterygoid plates. The infranotch compartment includes the bulk of masseter, medial pterygoid muscle and lower part of the pterygoid plates. This classification is relevant in evaluation of disease spread in oral squamous cell carcinomas. In oral carcinomas, spread of disease above or below the notch has an implication on resectability and good results have been reported in patients with extension of disease below the notch. Therefore, description of disease extension according to this classification by radiologists is useful as infranotch masticator space disease is resectable.[11]

Infratemporal Fossa Versus Masticator Space

Radiologists are familiar with the masticator space while surgeons commonly use the term infratemporal fossa (ITF). However, there is a difference between the two. The ITF contains the medial and lateral pterygoid muscles, the mandibular division of the trigeminal nerve (V3),

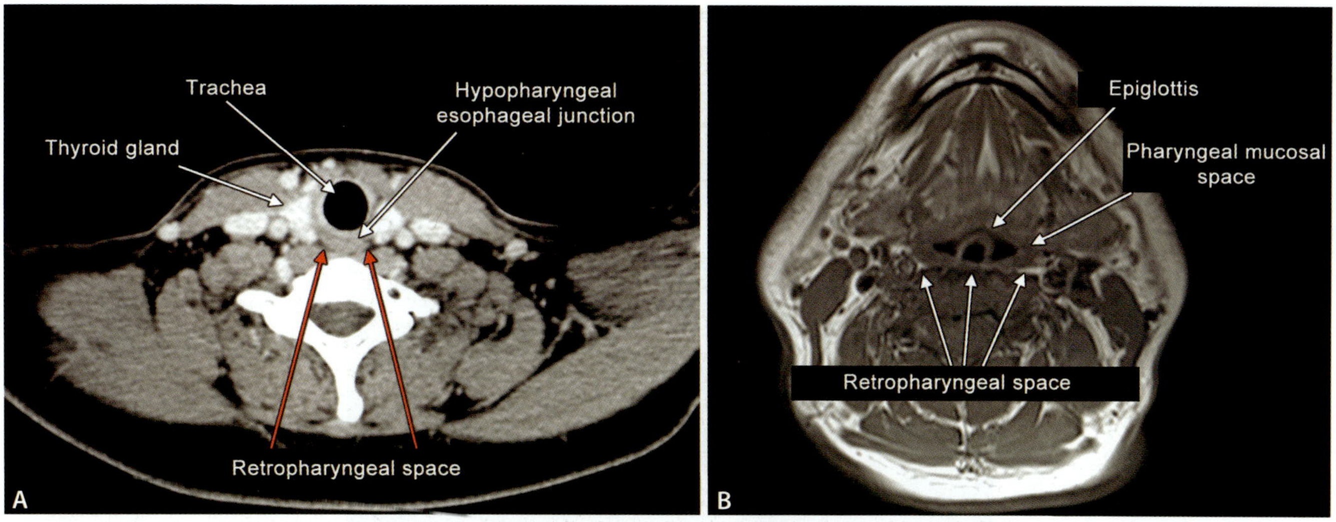

Figs. 8A and B: Axial CECT (A) and axial T1W MR (B) images show the fat-filled retropharyngeal space in posterior midline of neck; the carotid space lies lateral and the pharyngeal mucosal space lies anterior to the retropharyngeal space.

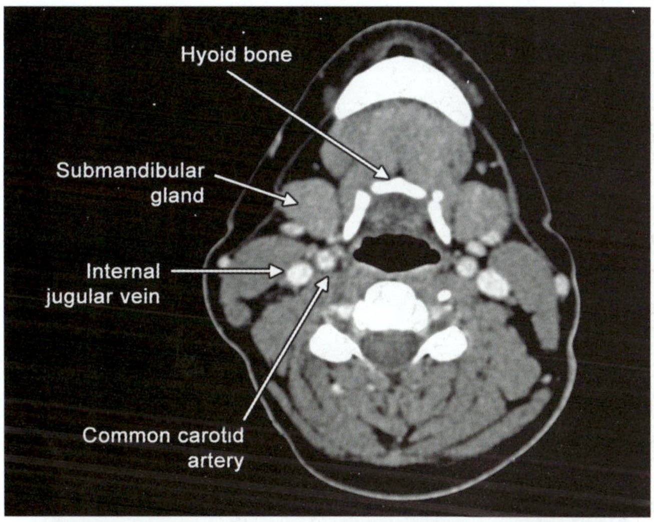

Fig. 9: Axial CECT image shows the carotid space containing the common carotid artery and internal jugular vein with the common carotid artery seen medial to the internal jugular vein.

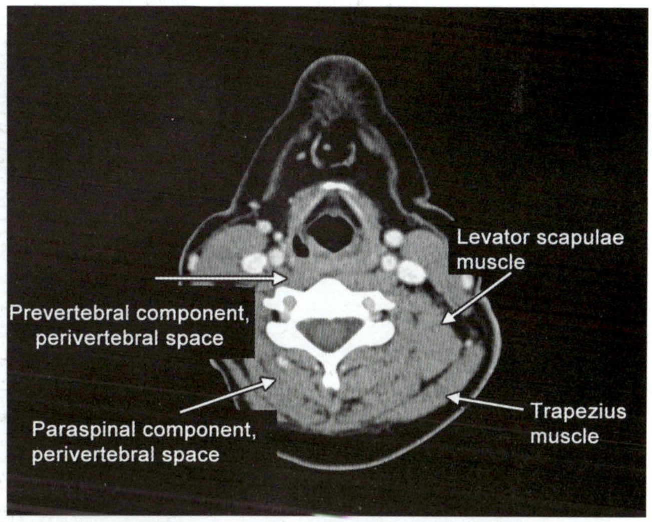

Fig. 10: Axial CECT image shows the two components of the perivertebral space: prevertebral and paraspinal components.

chorda tympani branch of facial nerve, otic ganglion, internal maxillary artery and pterygoid venous plexus. It lies medial to the inner surface of the vertical ramus of the mandible and the zygomatic arch and is not lined by fascia. The ITF contains much of the MS (except masseter), the retroantral buccal fat and the medial part of prestyloid parapharyngeal space (PPS)[11] **(Fig. 16)**.

Its anterior boundary is formed by the posterior surface of the maxilla and the inferior orbital fissure; posterior boundary by the mastoid and tympanic portions of the temporal bone; and superior boundary by the inferior surfaces of the greater wing of the sphenoid and the squamous portion of the temporal bone. The infratemporal fossa communicates with the temporal fossa cranially. The lateral boundary of the infratemporal fossa is formed by the zygomatic arch and ascending ramus of the mandible.[12]

Medially it is bounded by the sphenoid pterygoid process, lateral portion of the clivus, first cervical vertebra and inferior surface of the petrous portion of the temporal bone.[12,13] The lateral lower limit is at the insertion of the medial pterygoid to the mandible and the inferior boundary is the superior limit of the posterior belly of the digastric muscle.

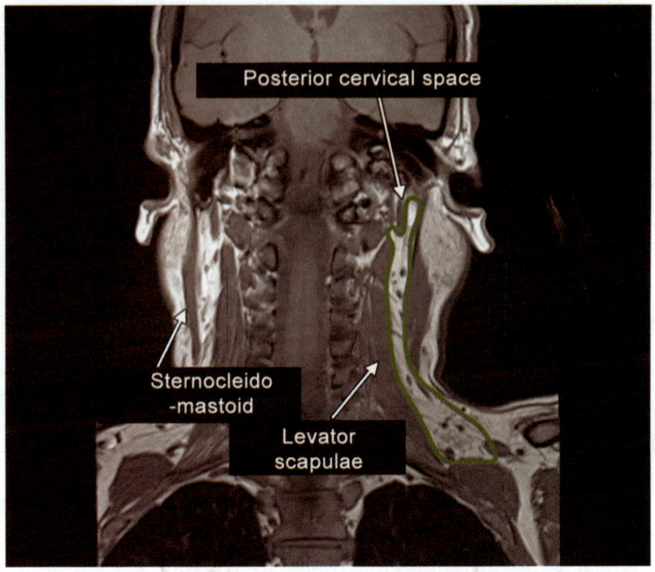

Fig. 11: Coronal T1W MR image shows the posterior cervical space deep to the sternocleidomastoid muscle.

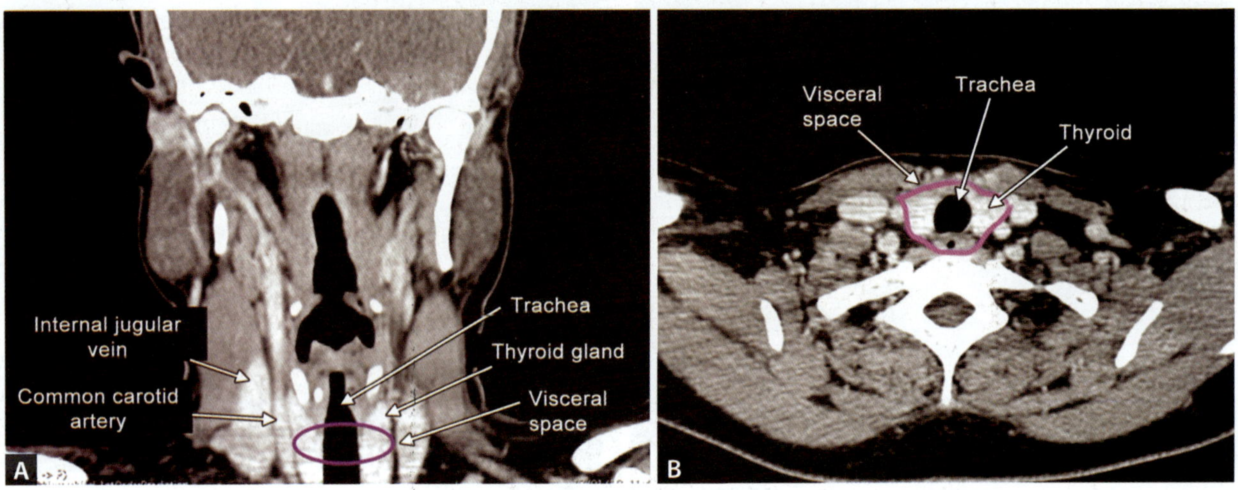

Figs. 12A and B: Coronal (A) and axial (B) CECT images depict the visceral space in midline infrahyoid neck (outlined in purple).

Table 2: Contents and lesions of the masticator space.

Contents
• Muscles of mastication • Ramus and posterior body of mandible • Mandibular nerve and its branches from foramen ovale to mandibular canal • Internal maxillary artery and its branches
Lesions
• *Mandible:* Odontogenic abscess, osteomyelitis, primary jaw lesions, metastases, myeloma • *Muscles of mastication:* Benign and malignant, e.g. hemangiomas and sarcomas, benign masseteric hypertrophy, denervation atrophy, metastases, myositis ossificans • Lymphoma • *Mandibular branch of trigeminal nerve:* Neurogenic tumors, perineural spread of tumor • *Secondary extension into MS:* Spread of malignancy from oropharynx or retromolar trigone, inferior extension of intracranial or skull-base lesions

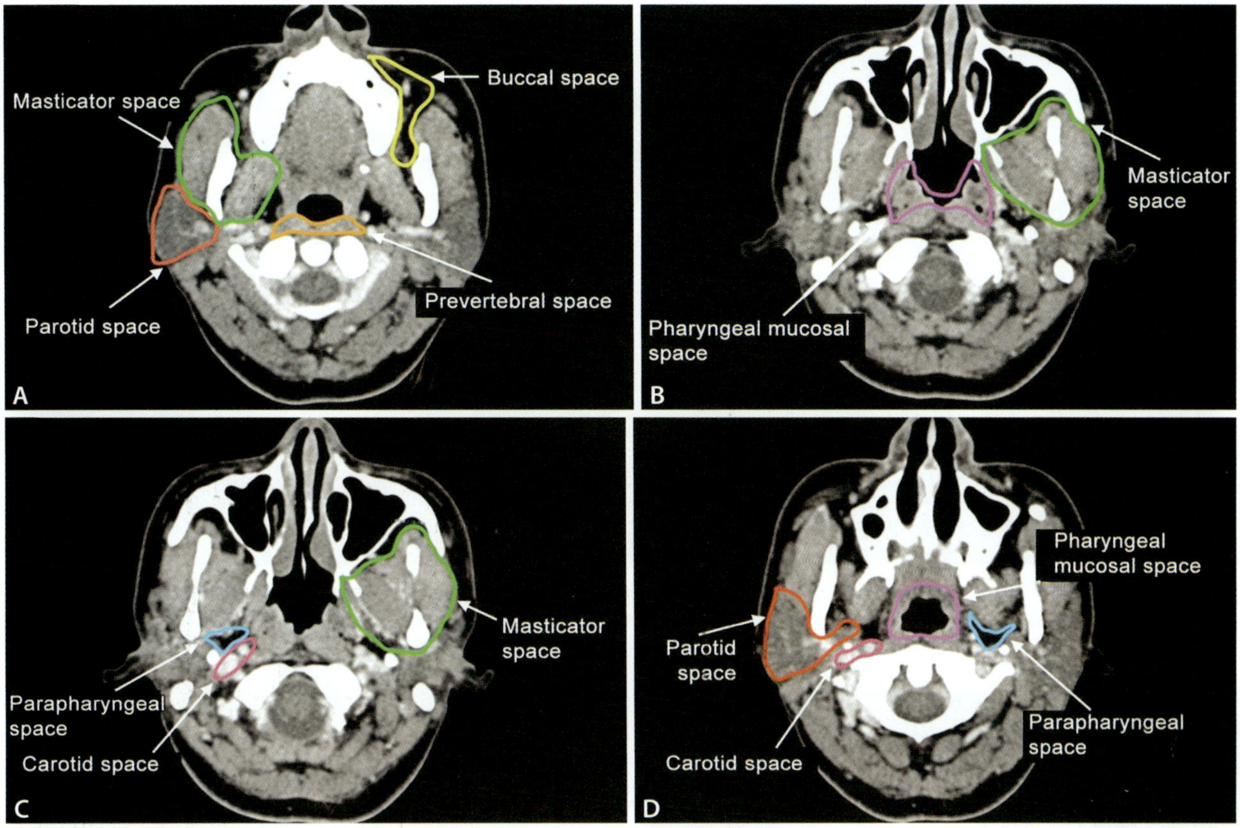

Figs. 13A to D: Axial CECT images (A and B) show the various spaces of the neck; masticator space (outlined in green), parotid space (outlined in red), buccal space (outlined in yellow), prevertebral space (outlined in orange) and pharyngeal mucosal space (outlined in pink). Axial CECT images (C and D) show the important spaces including the pharyngeal mucosal space (outlined in pink), parotid space (outlined in red), masticator space (outlined in green) and carotid space (outlined in deep pink); surrounding the parapharyngeal space (outlined in light blue).

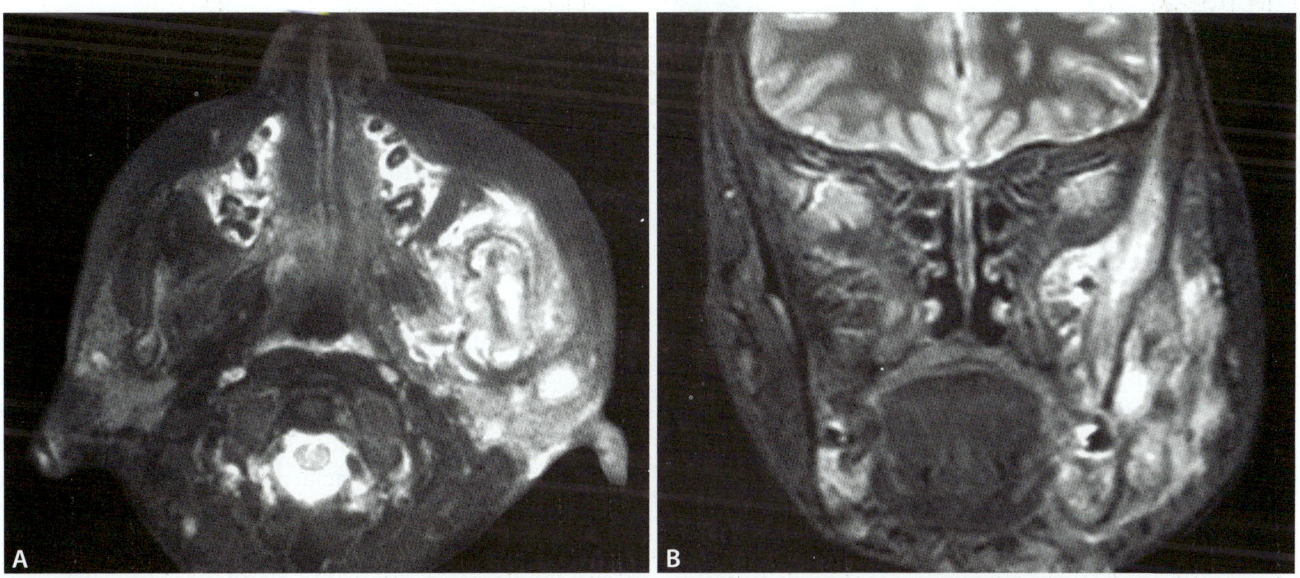

Figs. 14A and B: Axial (A) and coronal (B) fat sat T2W MR scans reveal destruction and altered signal of the left hemimandible with soft tissue edema involving muscles of mastication—Osteomyelitis of mandible secondary to odontogenic infection.

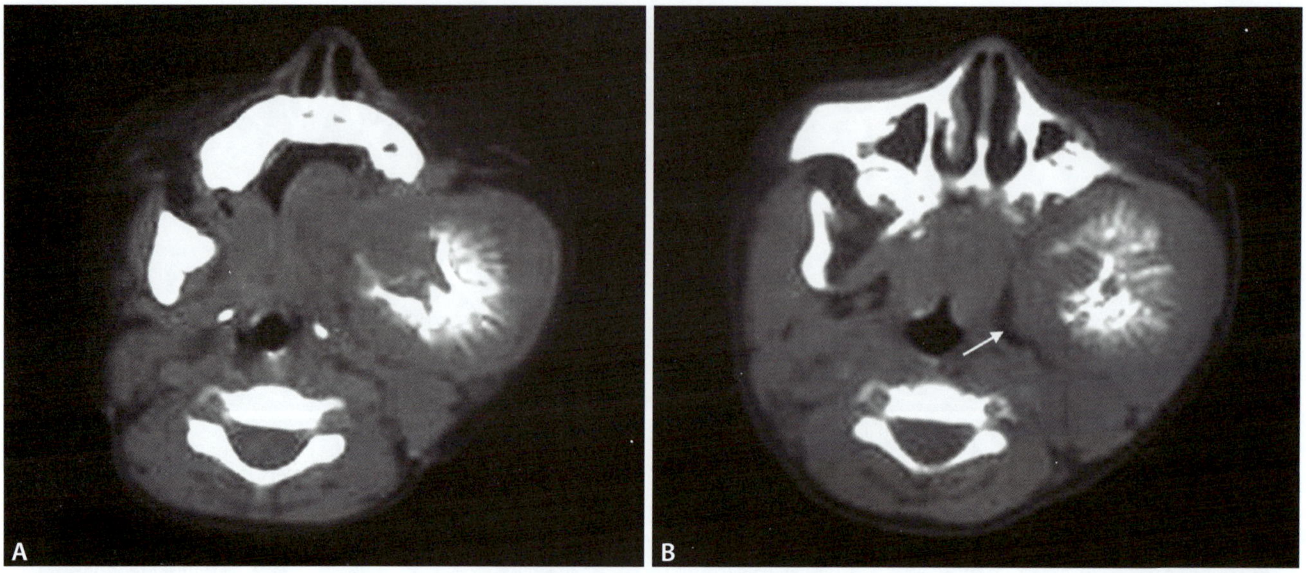

Figs. 15A and B: Axial CT scans showing an expansile lytic lesion with spiculated periosteal reaction involving the left hemimandible with a large soft tissue mass, note posteromedial displacement of parapharyngeal fat (arrow in B)—Osteogenic sarcoma of the mandible.

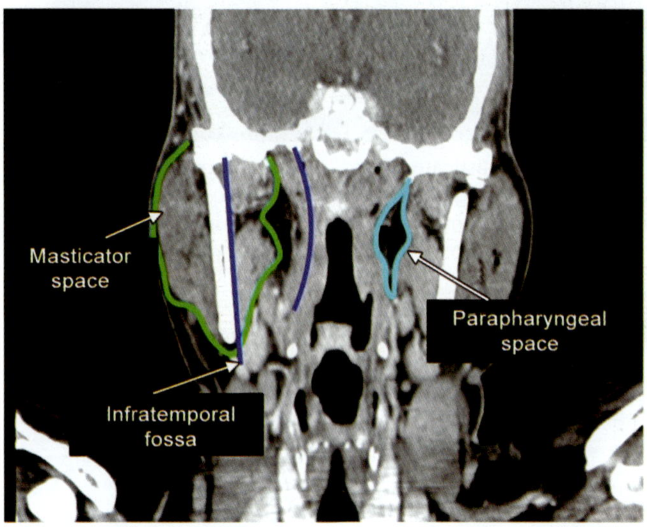

Fig. 16: Coronal CT section shows the relation between the infratemporal fossa (outlined in dark blue), masticator space (outlined in green) and parapharyngeal space (outlined in light blue); note that the infratemporal fossa does not have an anatomical floor.

The ITF communicates with the orbit through the inferior orbital fissure, with the middle cranial fossa through the foramina ovale and spinosum, and with the pterygopalatine fossa through the pterygomaxillary fissure.

The incidence of masticator space infections, usually of odontogenic origin is much more common while abscesses in the ITF are uncommon.[14] This is because infective disease processes, especially abscesses tend to be initially confined to fascial lined spaces, while malignancy more commonly spreads across fascial boundaries and hence involvement of the components of a larger compartment like the ITF is more common. Bone erosion is more common with neoplasia than with infections.

The venous drainage of the ITF is by the pterygoid venous plexus, which also anastomoses with the cavernous sinus, ophthalmic veins and pharyngeal venous plexus. Therefore, infection in the ITF can extend to involve the orbit and cavernous sinus.

PAROTID SPACE

These are paired lateral spaces in the suprahyoid neck enclosed by the superficial layer of deep cervical fascia. The parotid space (PS) extends from external auditory canal and mastoid tip superiorly to below the angle of mandible. The parapharyngeal space is medial to the parotid space and the masticator space is anterior to it. The posterior belly of digastric muscle separates the upper part of parotid space from carotid space.

The **contents (Table 3)** of this space are the parotid gland, facial nerve, retromandibular vein, branches of the external carotid artery and lymph nodes. The facial nerve divides the parotid gland into superficial and deep lobes **(*see* Figs. 3A and B)**. The facial nerve lies just lateral to the retromandibular vein and maybe difficult to localize on routine imaging, therefore the retromandibular vein is a useful landmark to divide the gland into superficial and deep lobes.

Table 3: Contents and lesions of the parotid space.

Contents
• Parotid gland • Intraparotid lymph nodes • Facial nerve and its branches • Branches of external carotid artery • Retromandibular vein
Lesions
• *Salivary gland neoplasms:* Pleomorphic adenoma, Warthin's tumor, mucoepidermoid carcinoma, adenoid cystic carcinoma, oncocytoma [most parotid tumors are benign (80%) and around 20–25% are malignant] • *Neoplasms (nonsalivary):* Hemangioma, lipoma • *Vascular malformation:* Venolymphatic malformation • *Infectious/Inflammatory:* Parotiditis, parotid abscess, cellulitis, radiation sialadenitis, lymphoepithelial cysts • First branchial cleft anomaly • *Lymph nodes:* Metastases from skin malignancy (SCC), non-Hodgkin's lymphoma, melanoma • *Facial nerve:* Neurogenic tumors, perineural extension of tumor

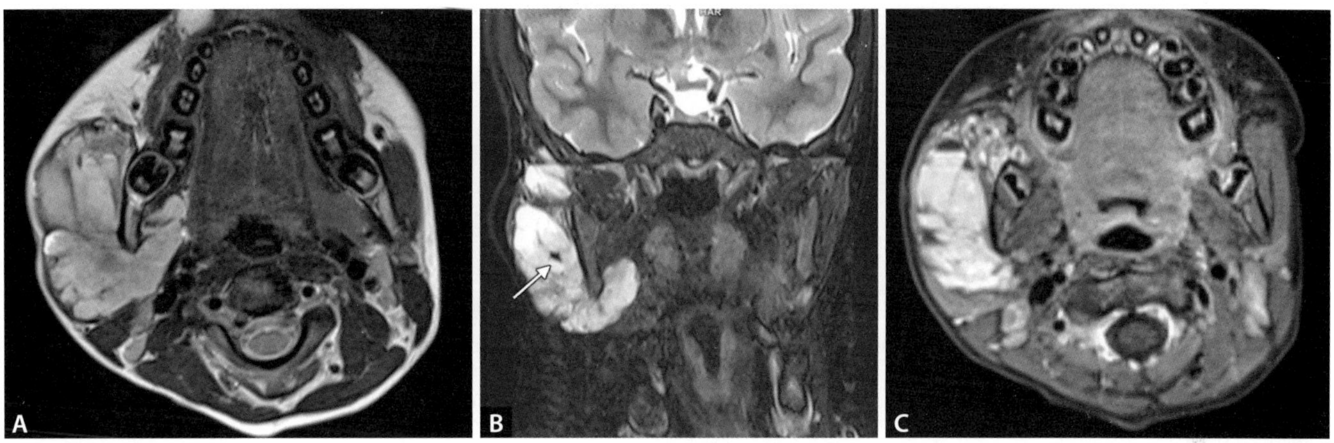

Figs. 17A to C: Axial T2W (A), Coronal STIR (B) and axial postcontrast (C) images depict a lobulated lesion involving the superficial and deep lobes of parotid gland, appearing hyperintense on T2W and STIR images with near homogeneous postcontrast enhancement. A phlebolith is seen in the lesion (arrow in B)—Venous malformation of parotid gland.

It is important to determine whether a lesion is intraparotid or extraparotid. If 50% or more of the lesion's circumference is surrounded by parotid tissue, it is considered as intraparotid. Intraparotid masses of the deep lobe displace the parapharyngeal fat medially and widen the stylomandibular tunnel.[1,15] Identification of a fat plane between the lesion and the parotid indicates a parapharyngeal space site of origin whereas direct continuity of the mass to the gland indicates a deep lobe parotid origin. It is important to recognize intraparotid lesions of the tail region as excision of these lesions may cause facial nerve injury.

Lesions in the parotid space include benign tumors such as pleomorphic adenomas, Warthin's tumors and less commonly, malignant tumors. The parotid gland may be involved by inflammatory pathology. In children, 50% of parotid lesions are hemangoimas. Other lesions include venous malformations **(Figs. 17A to C)**, calculi, lymphoepithelial lesions associated with HIV, lipomas, first branchial cleft cysts **(Figs. 18A to E)** and rarely schwannomas (from facial nerve).

Tumors of the parotid gland—Majority of the parotid tumors are **benign** (up to 80%). The commonest benign tumor is *pleomorphic adenoma* which is also known as benign mixed tumor. It is commonly seen in middle aged females. Pleomorphic adenoma appears hypoechoic on ultrasound. On CT, it shows smoothly marginated or lobulated surface with homogeneous contrast enhancement. As the size increases, pleomorphic adenoma appears more heterogeneous with foci of necrosis and areas of calcification within **(Figs. 19A and B)**. It shows very high signal on T2WI, low signal on T1WI

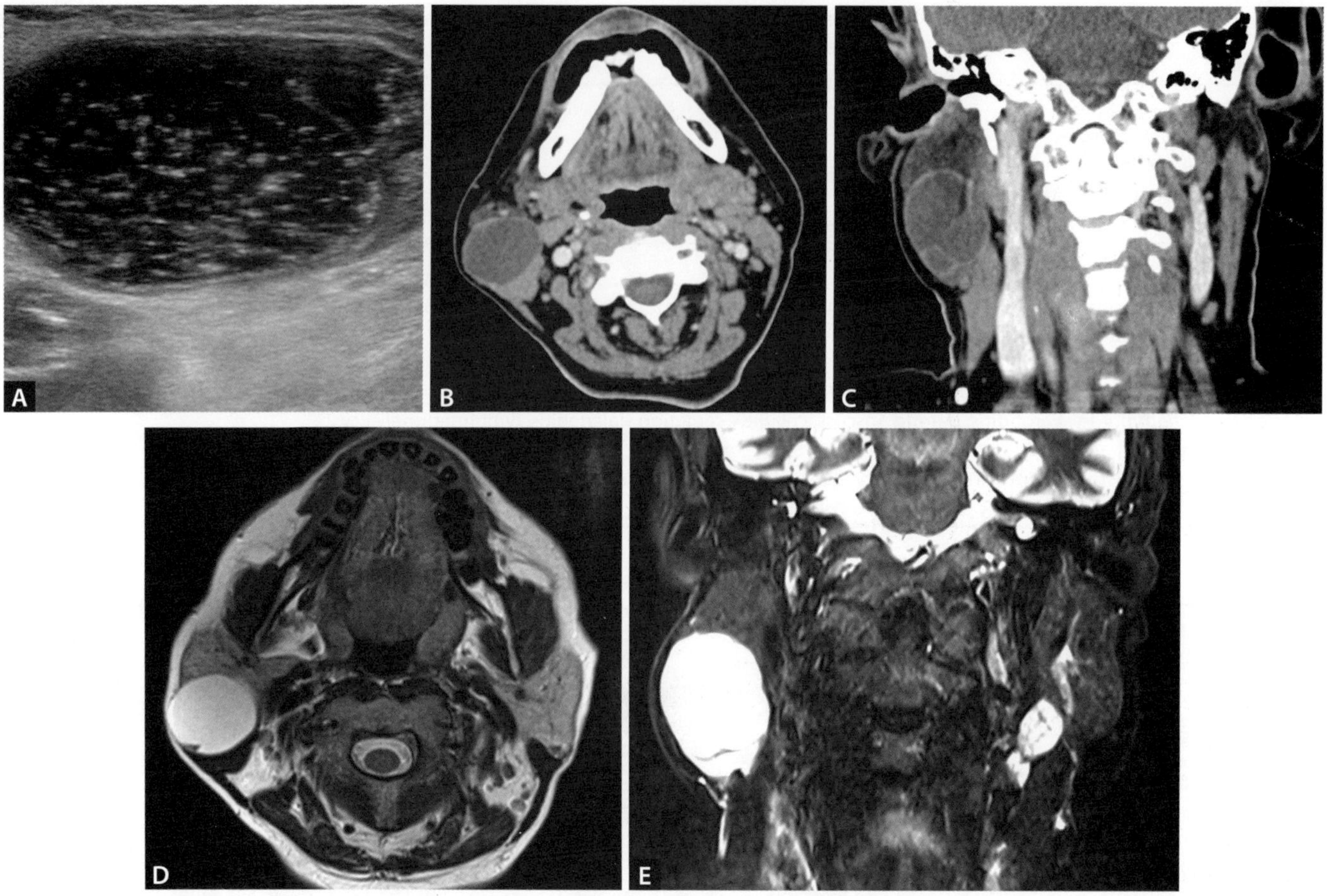

Figs. 18A to E: USG (A), axial and coronal (B and C) CECT images show a well-demarcated cystic lesion in the right parotid gland showing multiple internal echoes on USG and few thin septations within, on CECT images. Axial T2W and coronal STIR (D and E) images show a hyperintense lesion with few septations within in right parotid gland—Histopathology proven first branchial cleft cyst in a young patient.

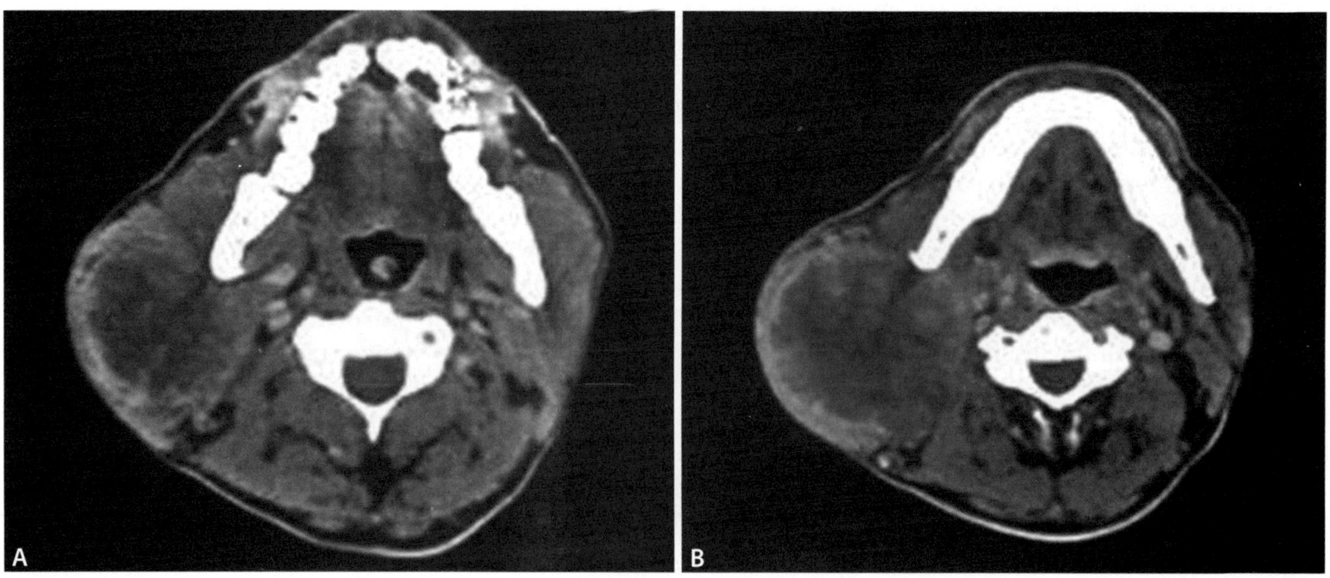

Figs. 19A and B: Axial CECT scans show a large, well-encapsulated, hypodense mass in the superficial lobe of the right parotid gland involving the deep lobe and causing displacement of the masseter and sternocleidomastoid muscles. No bony destruction or lymphadenopathy seen—Pleomorphic adenoma of the parotid gland.

and homogeneous postcontrast enhancement on MRI. The lesions are excised as they are associated with risk of malignant degeneration and also for cosmetic reasons. Complete excision is essential as residual tumor can create daughter lesions that are difficult to resect.

Warthin's tumors can present as multifocal masses and are well defined cystic lesions. They often present as slow growing masses in older men. On ultrasound, they show multiple small anechoic areas within. Cystic content of the lesion increases with the size of the lesion. Warthin's tumors are well defined solid cystic structures located in the superficial lobe of parotid or tail region. They may show a mural nodule which is strongly suggestive of the diagnosis. Warthin's tumors appear hypointense on T2WI and show variable enhancement.

Oncocytoma is a rare benign parotid tumor, no specific imaging features are seen on CT and ultrasound, but they show well defined contours on T1WI and appear isointense to the parotid tissue on postcontrast T1WI categorizing it as a "vanishing lesion". *Schwannomas* arising from facial nerve appear as solid enhancing masses that may show cystic degeneration as the size enlarges. Benign tumors are not associated with facial nerve palsy.[16]

Malignant lesions of the parotid include *mucoepidermoid carcinoma* (commonest primary malignancy of the parotid) and *adenoid cystic carcinoma*. Mucoepidermoid carcinoma appears as a well circumscribed hypoechoic lesion with cystic areas within on ultrasound. On CT, enhancement of the solid component is seen and calcification may be present. Mucoepidermoid carcinoma shows areas of low signal intensity on T2WI and may not be seen on postcontrast scans as it appears similar to adjacent parotid tissue. High grade lesions show poorly defined margins, local infiltration and nodal spread **(Figs. 20A to C)**.

Adenoid cystic carcinoma shows low signal intensity on T1WI and moderate signal intensity on T2WI, aggressive appearance increases with tumor grade. It has greatest propensity for perineural spread among head and neck cancers and is associated with poor long-term prognosis **(Figs. 21A to C)**.

Sialadenitis—Various conditions can cause inflammatory changes in the salivary glands including infections, ductal obstruction due to calculi or tumor, facial trauma, radiotherapy and autoimmune diseases. Patients present with facial swelling and pain. During the acute phase imaging demonstrates enlargement of the gland with increased enhancement on CT and MRI. Unilateral *infectious sialadenitis* is often due to bacterial infections **(Fig. 22)**.

Bilateral involvement of the glands is seen in viral infection, radiotherapy, HIV infection or autoimmune diseases such as Sjögren's disease and sarcoidosis. Viral sialadenitis is most commonly caused by mumps (*paramyxovirus*). Radiation sialadenitis is seen in patients who receive I-131 therapy for thyroid disease or patients who receive external beam radiotherapy. The glands are swollen, edematous and hypodense in acute phase. In the chronic phase the glands become small and fibrotic, hyperdense on noncontrast-enhanced computed tomography (NCCT) and show increased enhancement on contrast-enhanced CT (CECT).

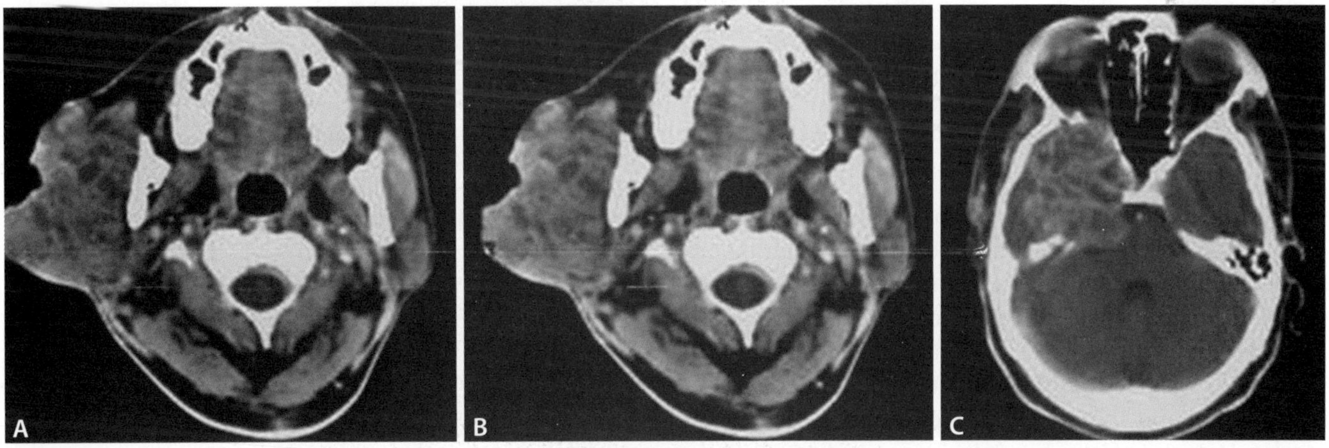

Figs. 20A to C: Axial CECT scans show a poorly demarcated ulcerating heterogeneous mass involving the right parotid gland with infiltration of the masseter and sternocleidomastoid muscles (A), multiple hypodense areas s/o necrosis are seen within (B), Intracranial extension into the middle cranial fossa, the right cerebellopontine angle and erosion of the greater wing of the sphenoid bone is also seen (C) mucoepidermoid carcinoma of the parotid gland.

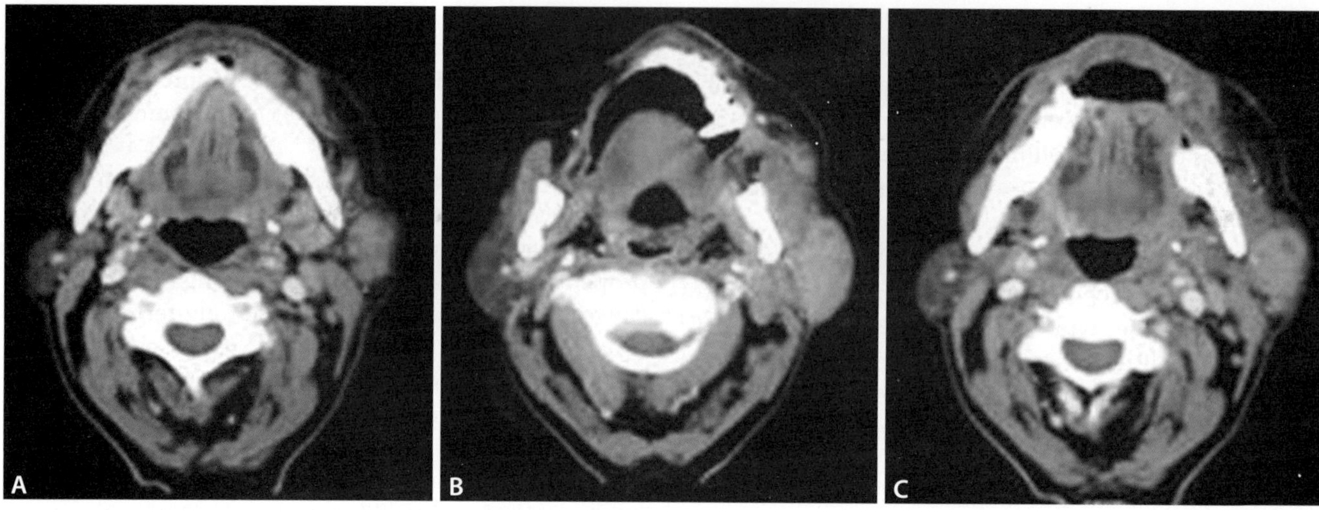

Figs. 21A to C: Axial CECT scans showing an enhancing heterogeneous mass involving both the superficial and deep lobes of the parotid gland (A and B) with loss of planes seen with masseter muscle (C) adenoid cystic carcinoma of the parotid.

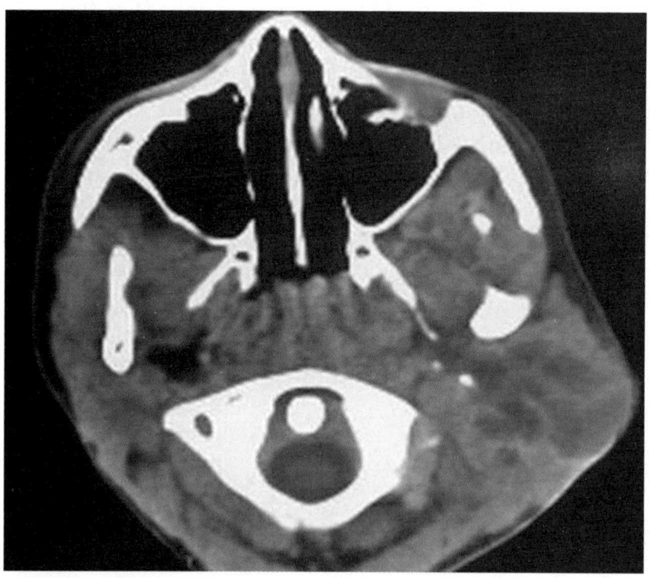

Fig. 22: Axial CECT scan showing enlarged left parotid gland with ill-defined, irregularly marginated hypodense areas within showing mild peripheral rim enhancement—Parotid gland abscess.

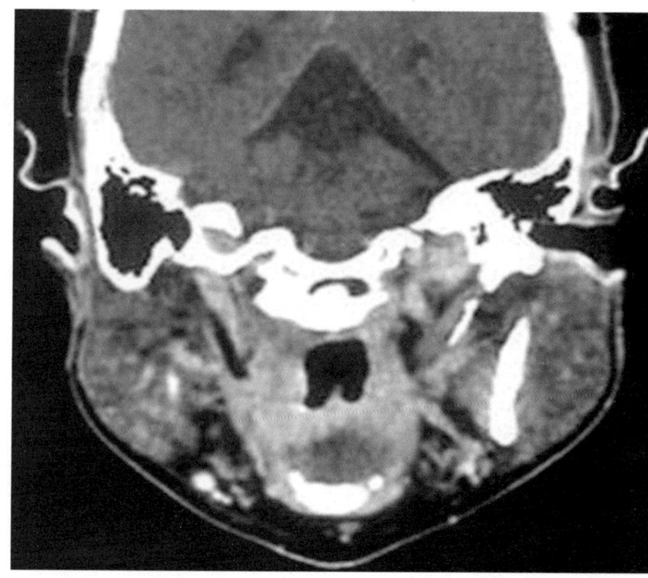

Fig. 23: Coronal CECT image shows enlarged parotid glands bilaterally with heterogeneous appearance of the parenchyma—in a case of granulomatous parotitis.

Sjögren's disease affects female patients in fourth to fifth decades. Acute cases are similar to viral sialadenitis but chronic disease causes atrophic glands with heterogeneous stippled attenuation, multiple small parotid cysts and intraglandular sialoliths. These patients are at a risk of developing lymphoma. A lesion that is hyperenhancing, T2 hypointense and shows restricted diffusion is concerning for development of lymphoma.[17]

Multiple *granulomatous diseases* including tuberculosis, fungal infections and Wegner's granulomatosis can involve the glands with focal or diffuse involvement[18] **(Fig. 23)**.

SUBMANDIBULAR SPACE

The submandibular space (SMS) is a superficial space located inferior to the mylohyoid muscle and above the hyoid bone. It is a vertical horseshoe shaped space and communicates posteriorly with sublingual space and with inferior parapharyngeal space at the posterior margin of the mylohyoid muscle **(*see* Fig. 4)**.

The **contents (Table 4)** of the submandibular space are the anterior belly of digastric muscle, superficial portion of the submandibular gland, submandibular and submental lymph nodes, facial artery and vein, inferior loop of hypoglossal nerve and fat.

Lesions—Metastatic lymphadenopathy from squamous cell carcinoma of tongue and floor of mouth is the most common lesion of the submandibular space. Other lesions include lymphoma, adenitis, obstructed submandibular duct, salivary gland tumors, spread from odontogenic infections. In children, the most common lesion is second branchial cleft cyst. Congenital and developmental lesions also include thyroglossal cyst, hemangioma, lymphatic malformation, dermoid/ epidermoid and diving ranula.

Dermoid cysts are composed of epithelial elements but dermoids have skin appendages in contrast to epidermoid. Majority of the cervical dermoid cysts occur in the midline or in paramedian location and are mostly present at birth. They are seen more often in the submandibular space than floor of mouth. Dermoid cysts do not move with swallowing unlike thyroglossal duct cysts. On CT fatty internal elements, mixed density fluid and calcification can be found in dermoid cysts. The admixture of fat globules with fluid can give rise to the typical *sac of marbles* appearance of dermoid cyst.

Table 4: Contents and lesions of the submandibular space.

Contents
• Anterior belly of the digastric muscle • Superficial portion of the submandibular gland • Submandibular and submental lymph nodes • Facial artery and vein • Fat • Inferior loop of the hypoglossal nerve
Lesions
• *Lymph nodes:* Metastatic disease (most commonly from SCC), lymphoma, adenitis • *Submandibular gland:* Obstructed submandibular duct, salivary gland tumors (around 40–50% of submandibular gland tumors are malignant) • *Infection/Inflammation (usually spread from odontogenic infection):* abscess, Ludwig's angina, diving ranula • *Congenital/developmental:* Thyroglossal duct cyst, hemangioma, lymphatic malformation, dermoid/epidermoid, second branchial cleft cyst

Sialolithiasis—Approximately 80-90% of salivary gland calculi occur in the submandibular gland and only 10% in the parotid gland. They may be intraglandular or intraductal and can be visualized well on sonography. Associated sialectasia may also be well seen on sialography or sonography. Mucocele formation may also result as a complication of sialolithiasis. The most common cause of salivary inflammatory lesions is calculus disease, especially in the submandibular space **(Figs. 24A and B)**, due to the upward secretion of the more mucinous, viscous, and alkaline saliva. Also, the opening of the Wharton's duct (the main salivary duct of the submandibular gland) is narrower than the diameter of the duct.

Calculus disease causes painful glands and is often associated with fever. CT imaging is preferred to MRI for identification of calculi. MR is useful for detecting mandibular infection (osteomyelitis) and to differentiate between cellulitis/myositis and abscess. MRI demonstrates an enhancing submandibular gland and offers the advantage of MR sialography. Fat infiltration or gland size reduction, compared to the healthy side in MRI may also indicate chronic disease with sialadenitis.

Tumors, such as pleomorphic adenomas can also arise in the submandibular glands **(Figs. 25A and B)**,

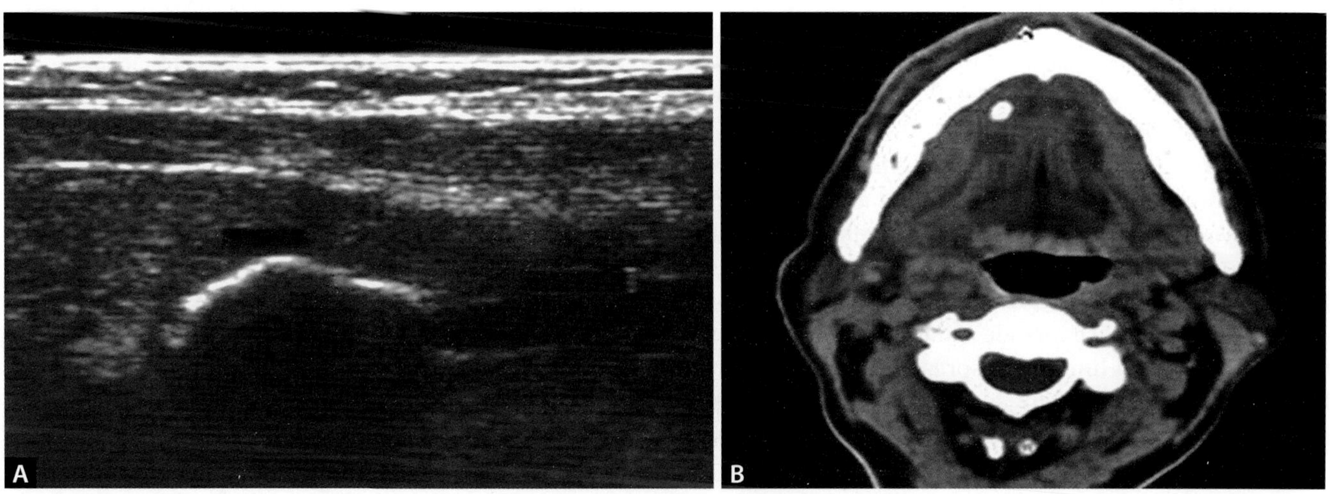

Figs. 24A and B: USG showing a dilated right submandibular gland duct with a calculus within (A) a calculus is seen in the floor of the mouth anteriorly in a paramedian location on axial CT scan (B) calculus in Wharton's duct.

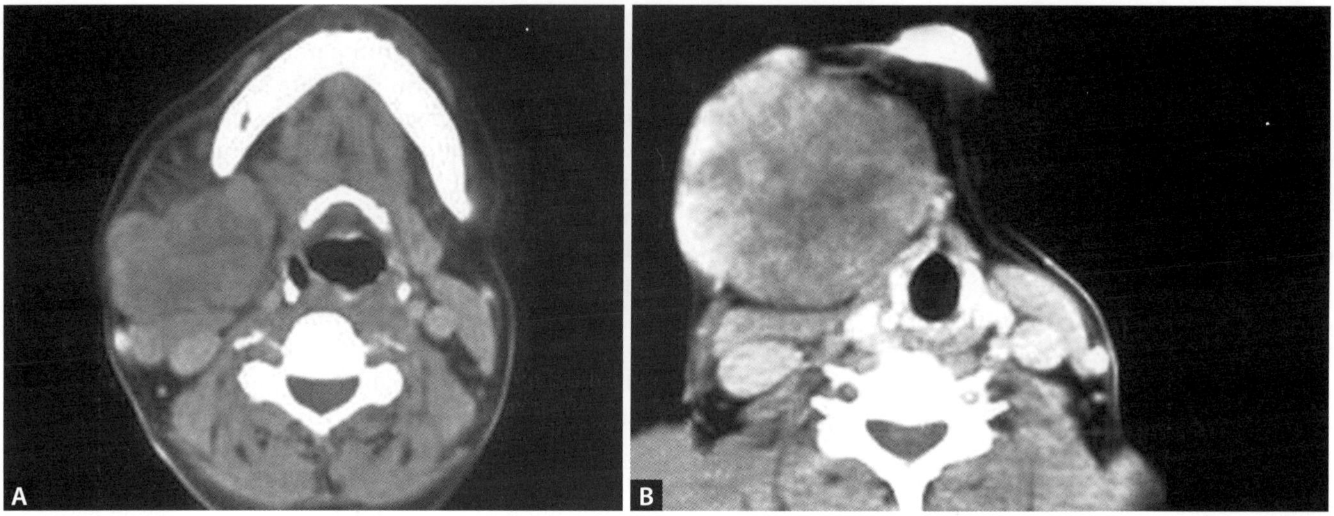

Figs. 25A and B: Axial CECT scans showing a bulky heterogeneous mass with patchy contrast enhancement in the right submandibular gland (A) causing displacement of the sternocleidomastoid muscle and attenuation of the right carotid sheath (B) pleomorphic adenoma of the submandibular gland.

the imaging features have been discussed in the section on parotid tumors. Adenoid cystic carcinoma is the most common malignant tumor arising from the submandibular gland.

SUBLINGUAL SPACE

It is a tea cup-shaped space located on both sides of the tongue lying superomedial to the mylohyoid and lateral to the midline geniohyoid-genioglossus muscle complex.[19] The mylohyoid sling is formed by the paired mylohyoid muscles, arising from the inner surface of the mandible to insert onto the posterior aspect of the hyoid bone. Medially the paired muscles insert into a fibrous median raphe, forming a muscular sling. The mylohyoid muscle sling separates the sublingual space (SLS) from the right and left submandibular spaces and the midline submental space. The SLS is however continuous with the SMS behind the posterior edge of mylohyoid.

The **contents (Table 5)** of the sublingual space are fat, the anterior extension of the hypoglossal muscle, hypoglossal nerve, lingual artery and vein, sublingual gland and ducts, deep portion of submandibular gland and lymph nodes **(*see* Figs. 5A and B)**. The common **lesions** of the sublingual space include squamous cell carcinoma from the epithelial lining and spread from odontogenic infections. Metastatic lymphadenopathy from squamous cell carcinomas also involves the sublingual space. Other lesions include minor salivary gland tumors, neurogenic tumors, ranula, obstructed submandibular gland duct, dermoid and epidermoid.

Table 5: Contents and lesions of the sublingual space.

Contents
• Fat • Muscles (anterior extension of the hyoglossus muscle) • Hypoglossal nerve • Lingual nerve • Lingual artery and vein • Sublingual gland and ducts • Deep portion of the submandibular gland and duct • Lymph nodes
Lesions
• *Epithelial lining:* SCC—generally secondary spread • *Salivary gland:* Ranula, obstructed submandibular duct, minor salivary gland tumors • *Infection (usually spread from odontogenic infection):* Abscess, Ludwig's angina • *Lingual/hypoglossal nerve:* Neurogenic tumor • *Congenital/developmental:* Lingual thyroid, thyroglossal duct cyst hemangioma, lymphatic malformation, dermoid/epidermoid

Epidermoid cysts typically involve the floor of the mouth incorporating the sublingual, submandibular spaces and the root of the tongue.[20] Epidermoid cysts are composed of epithelial elements and are of fluid density with little or no complex features.

Ranula is an inflammatory lesion of the sublingual space. It is actually a mucous retention cyst that may result from an obstructed sublingual or minor salivary gland or from trauma or retained secretions that may lead to rupture of acini. A ranula usually results from trauma or inflammation of the salivary glands, however rare congenital ranulas have also been described. It may herniate into the submandibular or lower parapharyngeal space through the mylohyoid muscle and evolve into a plunging ranula **(Figs. 26A to C)**. A plunging ranula has a distinct *"tail sign"* within the sublingual space with the bulk of the cyst seen in the submandibular space. Ranula shows high fluid attenuation on CT, the cyst wall may enhance depending upon presence of infection. On MRI, it appears hyperintense on T2WI and may show high signal on T1WI due to high protein content **(Figs. 27A to D)**.

Floor of the Mouth versus Sublingual Space

The floor of the mouth is a term commonly used in surgical literature It is a horizontally aligned U-shaped space situated in the part of the oral cavity lying beneath the tongue. For surgical planning, the floor of the mouth is defined as the space between the mucosal surface and the mylohyoid sling and comprising both structures. Thus, according to the surgical definition, the sublingual space is a part of the floor of mouth. However, in most radiology literature the mylohyoid muscle sling is considered to be

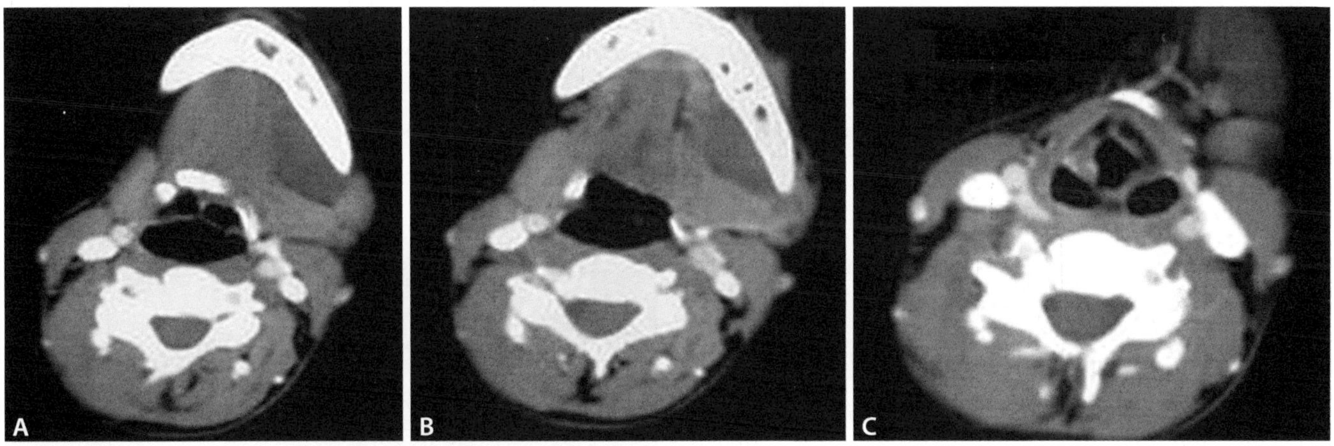

Figs. 26A to C: Axial CECT scans revealing an oval, well-defined hypodense lesion with cystic attenuation and smooth walls in the sublingual space on the left side (A and B) extending around the mylohyoid muscle into the submandibular space posteriorly (C) Plunging ranula.

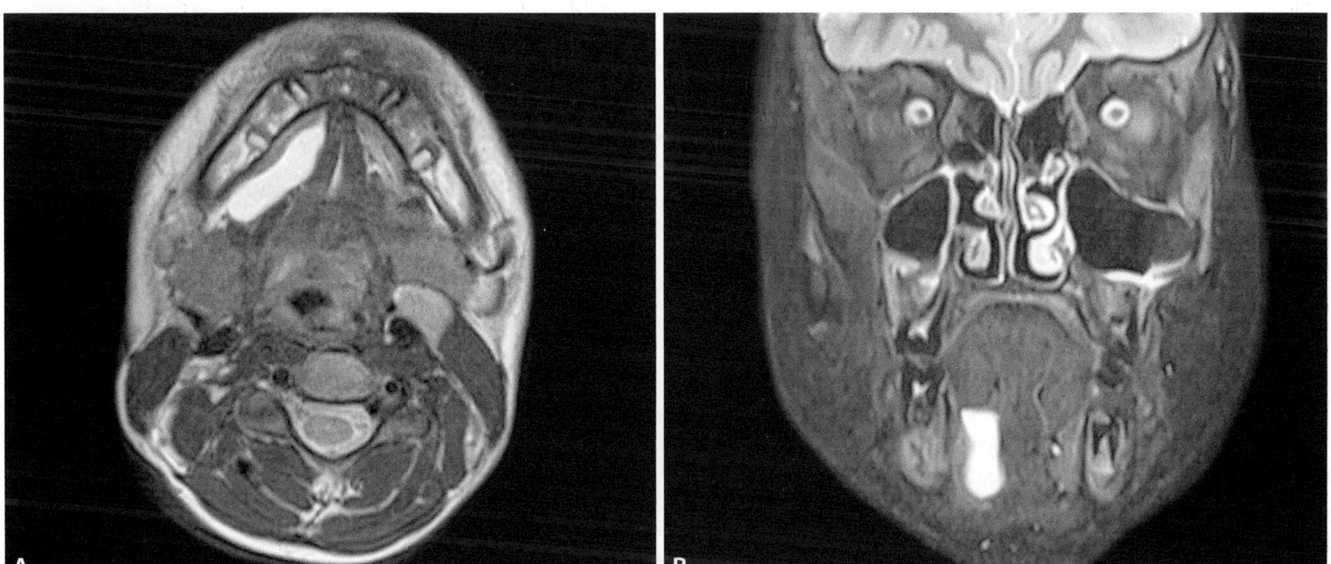

Figs. 27A and B

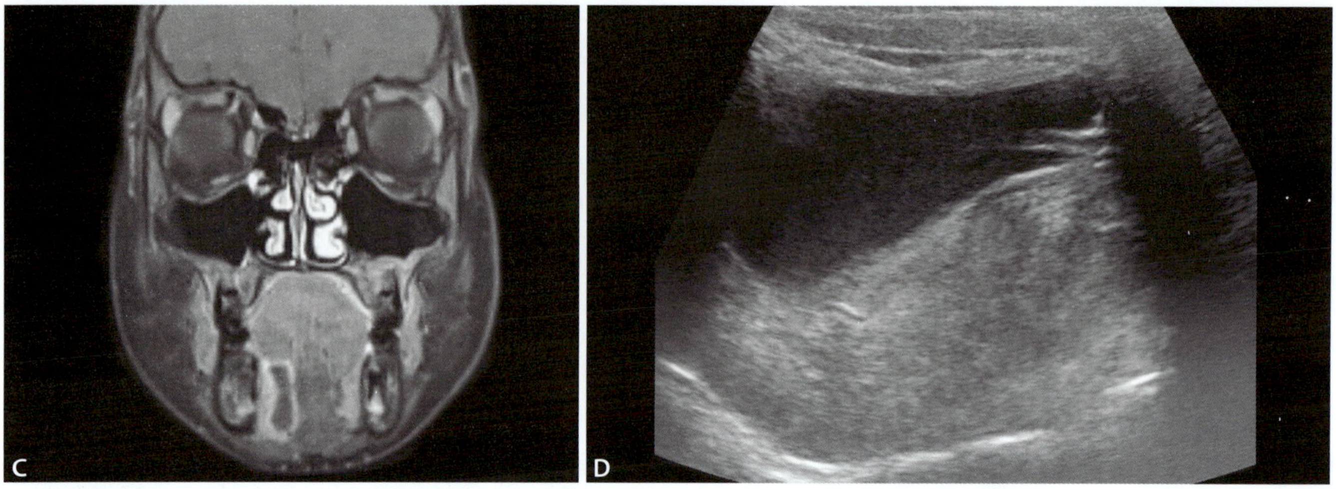

Figs. 27C and D

Figs. 27A to D: Axial T2W (A), coronal STIR (B), coronal postcontrast T1W (C) and USG (D) images show a cystic lesion in the right sublingual space. It appears markedly hyperintense on T2W and STIR images (A and B) and shows peripheral enhancement (C). On USG (D), it is seen as an anechoic lesion in the sublingual space— Infected simple ranula.

synonymous with the floor of mouth and sublingual space is considered as a separate compartment.[19]

PHARYNGEAL MUCOSAL SPACE

The pharyngeal mucosal space (PMS) abuts the skull base along the superior/posterior aspect of the nasopharyngeal roof superiorly and extends to the level of the hypopharynx inferiorly.[16] It is divided into nasopharyngeal, oropharyngeal, and hypopharyngeal segments. The nasopharynx is the part that lies posterior to the nasal choanae and extends from the vault of pharynx superiorly to the soft palate inferiorly. The oropharynx lies posterior to base of tongue, inferior to soft palate and superior to the superior aspect of epiglottis. The hypopharynx lies inferior to the superior aspect of the epiglottis and superior to the cricoid cartilage **(Fig. 28)**.

The retropharyngeal space is posterior to PMS and parapharyngeal space is lateral to it. The middle layer of the deep cervical fascia borders the lateral and posterior deep margins of the PMS, but it is not a truly encircled fascial space as there is no fascia along the surface.

Accurate identification of pathology within the PMS is largely related to the imaging appearance, site of origin, and its effect on the PMS airway. Clinicians can assess the surface of the pharyngeal mucosal surface well, therefore clinical examination and impressions are useful for image interpretation. Asymmetry in the PMS may be misinterpreted as a tumor. A mass which is primary to the PMS will have its center medial to parapharyngeal space, push the parapharyngeal fat from medial to lateral and will disrupt the normal PMS mucosal and submucosal architecture.

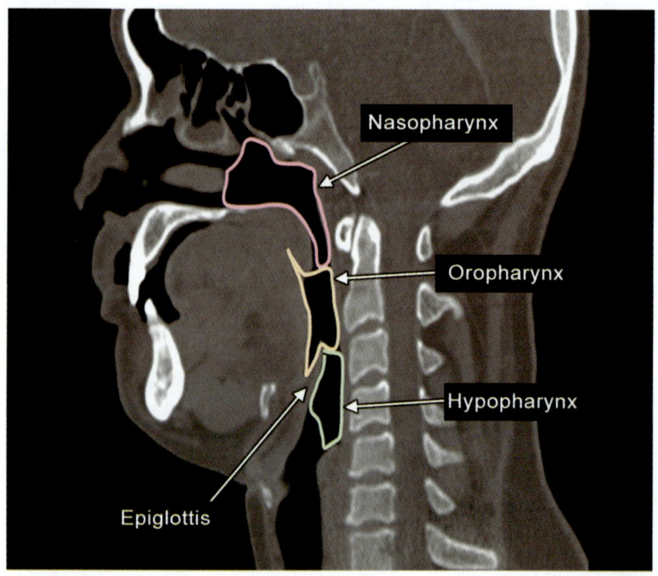

Fig. 28: Sagittal CT image shows the division of the pharyngeal mucosal space into the nasopharynx, oropharynx and hypopharynx.

The **contents (Table 6)** of this space are the mucosal surface of the pharynx, pharyngeal lymphatic ring and minor salivary glands. **Lesions**—Squamous cell carcinoma (SCC) is the most common malignancy in this location. Cross-sectional imaging helps in guiding treatment

Table 6: Contents and lesions of the pharyngeal mucosal space.

Contents
• Mucosal surface of the pharynx • Pharyngeal lymphatic ring (adenoids, palatine, and lingual tonsils) • Minor salivary glands contained in the submucosa in highest concentration within the hard and soft palate
Lesions
• *Malignant tumors:* Nasopharyngeal carcinoma, oropharyngeal carcinoma (palatine and lingual tonsil), non-Hodgkin lymphoma, minor salivary gland carcinoma • *Inflammatory lesions:* Tonsillar lymphoid hyperplasia, pharyngitis or postradiation change • *Infectious causes:* Tonsillar or peritonsillar abscess • *Musculoskeletal tumors:* Rhabdomyosarcoma, chordoma • *Miscellaneous:* Thornwaldt cyst

decisions in SCC by characterizing the extent of the mass deep to the mucosal surface, invasion into the adjacent spaces and assessing nodal spread. The relationship between the PMS and base of skull is important in the setting of nasopharyngeal carcinoma as it has a propensity for early intracranial spread primarily because of its proximity to the foramen lacerum. Tumors can invade through the foramen's cartilaginous floor and travel along the ICA to invade the cavernous sinus. Nasopharyngeal carcinoma may also spread via perineural tumor spread into the skull base and cavernous sinus. The evaluation of the extent of disease is important for planning of radiotherapy.

Thornwaldt's cyst is a congenital cyst that is seen in the midline in the posterior PMS and is lined by pharyngeal mucosa.[20] Focal adhesion of pharyngeal mucosa to the notochord results in a nasopharyngeal diverticulum. Majority of these cysts are seen as incidental findings on head MRI and the peak incidence is between 15 and 30 years. The patient becomes symptomatic when the intracystic pressure rises consequent to infection with anaerobic bacteria.

CT scan reveals a well-circumscribed, thin-walled cyst located in the midline in posterior nasopharyngeal mucosal space lodged between the prevertebral muscles. Attenuation of the cyst increases as the protein content increases with infection and may mimic a soft tissue mass. On MR the cyst has a T1 signal intensity, which increases from low to high with increasing protein content. The SI is high on T2W images.

Acute tonsillitis is one of the commonest infections that occurs in the pharyngeal mucosal space, especially in young adults. The common causes include viral (*Epstein Barr virus*) and bacterial (*Staphylococcus aureus and Streptococcus species*) infections. The diagnosis is usually clinical and imaging is only required in severe cases to evaluate the extent of disease and associated complications such as presence of abscess. On CT and MRI, acute tonsillitis is seen as enlargement and increased enhancement of the palatine tonsils which may approximate in the oral cavity. A striated enhancement pattern within the tonsils may be seen on postcontrast scans with parallel hypodense streaks within representing edema, cellular debris and trapped fluid. This should not be confused with abscess formation, which requires surgical drainage. Focal hypodense central areas in the tonsils without discernable rim enhancement are also not amenable to drainage.[17]

Abscesses related to tonsillitis may be (i) *peritonsillar abscess* (more common) (ii) *true tonsillar abscess*. In peritonsillar abscess, inflammatory fluid extends into the peritonsillar space. This can result in cellulitis or abscess formation in the parapharyngeal, masticator and retropharyngeal spaces. Peritonsillar abscess can cause airway narrowing by causing midline deviation of the tonsil. In true tonsillar abscess area of liquefaction is contained within the gland and shows rim enhancement.

It is essential to differentiate between *cellulitis* and *abscess* formation as cellulitis can be treated medically and an abscess needs surgical intervention. On CT imaging, abscesses appear as peripherally enhancing, single or multiloculated, low-density masses that conform to fascial spaces. They appear hyperintense on T2WI. Cellulitis can easily spread to adjacent fascial spaces. If a diagnosis of cellulitis is made and the patient shows no response to appropriate antibiotic therapy, a second examination should be performed to ensure that an abscess cavity has not formed.

Lemierre syndrome consists of IJV thrombosis following a primary oropharyngeal infection with development of distal septic emboli, most commonly to the lungs. As imaging findings often precede positive blood cultures, radiologists play an important role in early diagnosis of this entity. *Fusobacterium necrophorum* is almost always the causative organism. Contrast enhanced CT reveals tonsillar and peritonsillar edema and abscess associated with primary site of infection with IJV thrombosis and thrombophlebitis. The infection can spread into the retropharyngeal and perivertebral spaces.[21]

Juvenile nasal angiofibroma is the commonest benign yet locally invasive, noncapsulated, vascular, mesenchymal tumor of the nasopharynx occurring almost exclusively in adolescent boys with mean age of presentation at 15 years. The most common presenting symptom is nasal speech due to nasal obstruction or severe recurrent epistaxis. It is thought to arise near the sphenopalatine foramen at the junction between the nose and the nasopharynx at the root of the medial pterygoid plate. Extra-nasopharyngeal spread is not uncommon at the time of presentation and this occurs to the retroantral region via the pterygopalatine fossa and anterior displacement of the posterior wall of antrum is commonly seen. Lateral extension to the infratemporal fossa occurs through the pterygomaxilla fissure. It may also spread to the orbit through the inferior orbital fissure, to the cavernous sinus and middle cranial fossa through the superior orbital fissure. Inferiorly it can bulge into the oropharynx and oral cavity. Invasion of the sphenoid sinus may be seen in up to two-third of cases implying an internal carotid artery supply whereas the lesion is typically supplied by the ipsilateral internal maxillary and ascending pharyngeal arteries **(Figs. 29A to C)**.

On CT and MR images juvenile angiofibroma appears as a soft tissue mass of variable size. It may be visualized as a small nodule within the sphenopalatine foramen striding the choana or a large, locally aggressive growth extending in any or a combination of directions. Erosion of the pterygoid lamina on CT is probably a pathognomonic sign. On unenhanced CT scans the tumor appears isodense, on MR it displays intermediate signal on T1W and bright signal intensities on T2W images. The extent of the tumor and its characteristics are best evaluated on contrast enhanced scans. Postcontrast scans show intense enhancement with punctate areas of signal void indicating the highly vascular stroma **(Figs. 30A to D)**. The following imaging based grading system of juvenile angiofibroma has been proposed.

Grade I: Tumor confined to nasopharynx.

Grade II: Tumor extending into pterygopalatine fossa or masticator space.

Grade III: Tumor extending into orbit or intracranially.

The high tumor vascularity contraindicates biopsy and preoperative embolization is necessary.

PARAPHARYNGEAL SPACE

The parapharyngeal space (PPS) is located in the suprahyoid neck and is a symmetric crescent-shaped space situated lateral to the pharynx. It is an anatomic recess that was historically separated into the prestyloid and retrostyloid spaces by the tensor veli palatini,[22] styloid process, and associated musculature and ligaments. The anteriorly situated prestyloid compartment is deep to the MS and lateral to the pharyngeal mucosa and medial to the deep lobe of the parotid gland. The posteriorly situated retrostyloid compartment contains the carotid sheath and its contents. The retrostyloid space is now considered a separate carotid space.

The PPS extends from the skull base up to the hyoid bone, however, fusion of the fascial layers and muscle sheaths near the angle of the mandible limits the inferior extent of the PPS. It is encircled by layers of investing fascia laterally, separating it from the MS and PS and by the buccopharyngeal and prevertebral fascia, medially and posteriorly. The PPS does not have a fascial barrier anteriorly and is continuous with the submandibular and sublingual spaces. The lack of anterior border allows the spread of disease from the PPS along the

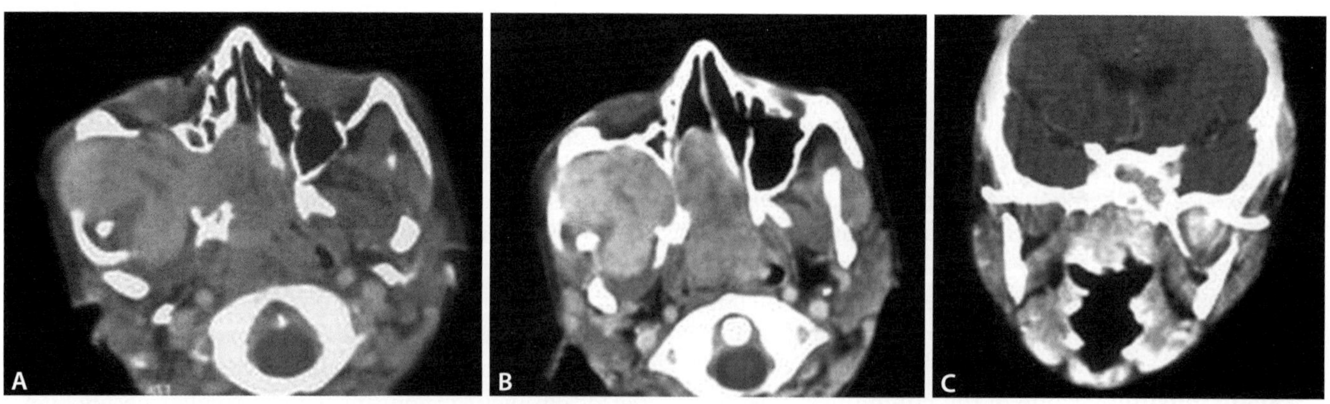

Figs. 29A to C: Axial CECT (A and B) and coronal (C) scans showing a large enhancing mass in the nasopharynx extending anteriorly in the nasal cavity pushing the nasal septum medially and encroaching upon/obliterating the contralateral nasal cavity. Widening of the pterygopalatine fossa and anterior bowing of the intact posterior maxillary antral wall is seen. Lateral extension through the pterygomaxillary fissure into the infratemporal fossa is seen. Coronal scan (C) reveals erosion of the floor of the sphenoid sinus with intrasinus extension and erosion of the root of the medial pterygoid plate. No intracranial extension seen—Juvenile nasopharyngeal angiofibroma.

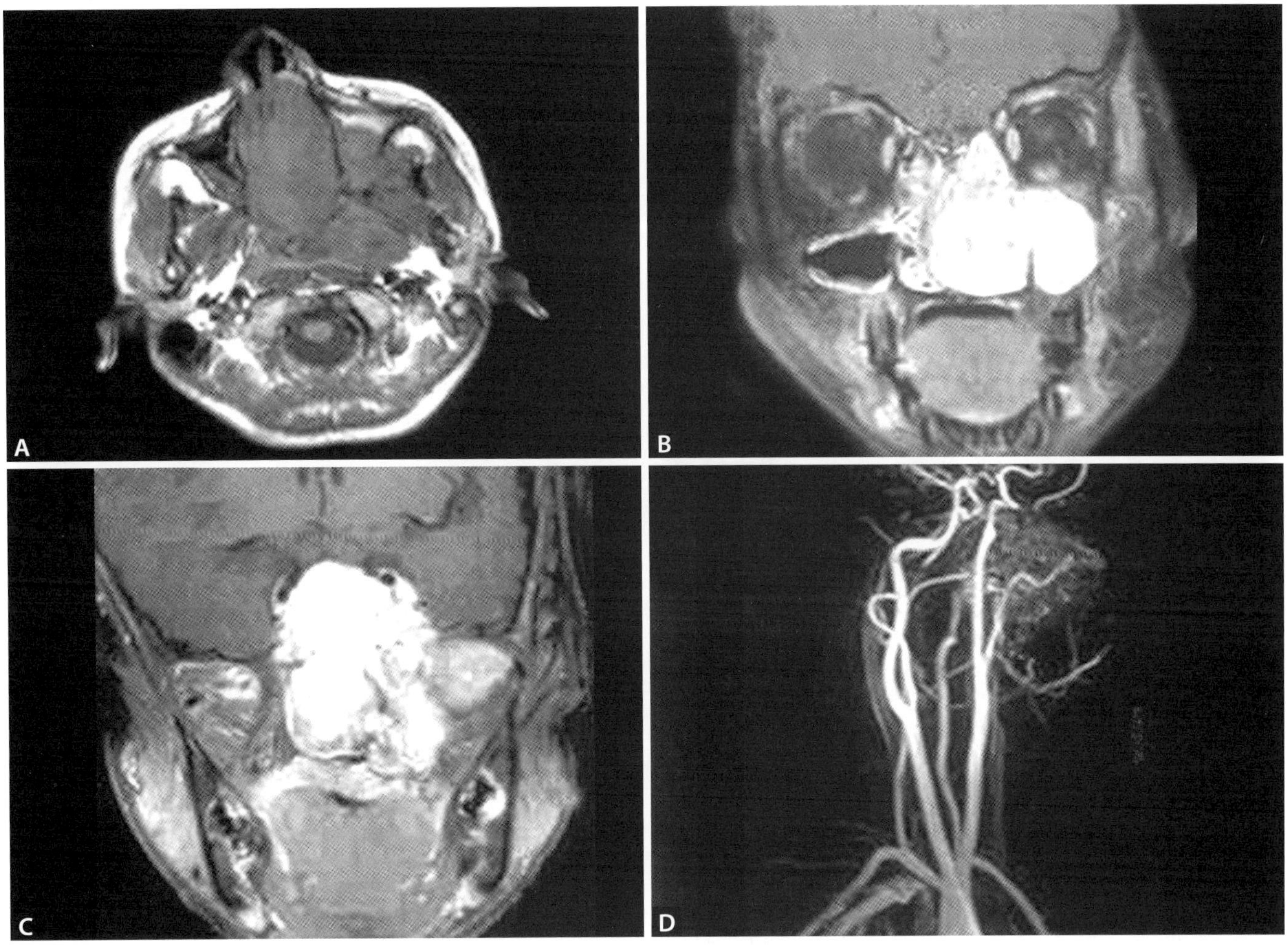

Figs. 30A to D: Axial T1W (A), coronal postcontrast T1W (B and C) MR images showing an intensely enhancing lobulated mass in the nasopharynx, the nasal cavity, the pterygopalatine fossa, the infratemporal fossa with erosion of the pterygoid lamina. Extension into the extraconal space of the left orbit, ethmoids and the left maxillary sinus is seen. Superior extension into the sphenoid sinus, and the left cavernous sinus is noted. MR angiogram images (D) show multiple prominent arterial channels suggestive of feeders from branches of left ECA— Juvenile nasopharyngeal angiofibroma.

pterygomandibular raphe, which connects the medial pterygoid plate to the lingual surface of the mandible along the posterior margin of the mylohyoid muscle. PPS lesion may present as a mass at the angle of mandible **(*see* Figs. 7A and B)**.

Contents—The PPS contains predominantly fat which can be easily differentiated from other tissue types on imaging. It also contains vascular structures including the maxillary and ascending pharyngeal artery and the pterygoid venous plexus.

Lesions—Primary masses of the PPS are rare, the source is likely minor salivary gland ectopic rests and the commonest tumor arising from these rests is a benign mixed tumor. Identification of a fat plane completely surrounding the lesion localizes the mass to the PPS **(Fig. 31)**.

The importance of PPS is its conspicuity on CT and MRI as well as its direction of displacement by mass lesions of the surrounding suprahyoid neck spaces.

This provides confirmation as to the origin of surrounding pathology as the adjacent mass lesions displace the PPS in specific directions **(Table 7)**.

BUCCAL SPACE

It is situated lateral to the buccinator muscle; medial to the zygomaticus major and anterior to the masseter. The posterior extension of the buccal space is the retroantral fat pad that reaches up to the anterior margin of the masticator

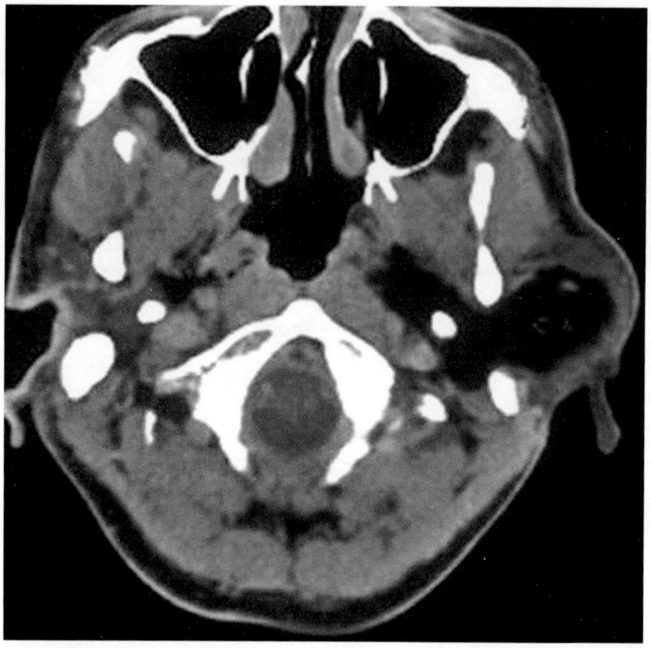

Fig. 31: Axial CECT image showing a well-defined non-enhancing hypodense mass having fat attenuation values within (– 90 HU) in the left parapharyngeal space. The lesion is seen extending superficially between the styloid process and the ramus of the mandible displacing the parotid gland laterally—parapharyngeal lipoma.

Table 7: PPS fat displacement pattern by lesions in different neck spaces.

Location of Lesion	***Displacement***
Pharyngeal mucosal space	Parapharyngeal fat displaced posterolaterally and styloid displaced posteriorly
Masticator space	Parapharyngeal fat displaced posteromedially and styloid displaced posteriorly
Carotid space	Parapharyngeal fat and styloid displaced anteriorly
Parotid space	Parapharyngeal fat displaced anteromedially
Retropharyngeal space	Parapharyngeal fat displaced anterolaterally and styloid displaced anteriorly

space. The buccal space (BS) does not have complete fascial coverings. It is separated from the subcutaneous tissues of the face by the plane formed by the superficial muscles of facial expression and the investing fascia.

The **contents** of the BS include adipose tissue, minor salivary gland tissue, parotid duct, lymph nodes, facial vein, facial and buccal artery, buccal branch of the cranial nerve VII, buccal division of V3.[22] The differential diagnosis for the **lesions** that can occur in this space include SCC (direct extension or nodal metastases), lymphoma, minor salivary gland tumors, lipoma, hemangioma, sarcoma, sebaceous cyst, obstructed duct, cellulitis and abscesses.

RETROPHARYNGEAL SPACE

The retropharyngeal space (RPS) is a midline space bordered anteriorly by the visceral fascia and posteriorly by the prevertebral fascia. It extends from the skull base superiorly to the T3 vertebral level inferiorly. In the suprahyoid neck, the PMS is anterior to the RPS while in the infrahyoid neck, hypopharynx and cervical esophagus are anterior to it. The carotid space is lateral to RPS in the suprahyoid and infrahyoid neck **(*see* Figs. 8A and B)**. The alar fascia, which is a thin fascial layer, divides the RPS into two compartments: the anterior and posterior. The posterior compartment is the *"danger space".* The RPS and danger space cannot be differentiated on imaging.[10] Disease from the RPS can spread into the mediastinum via the danger space.

Contents—The RPS contains mainly fat and retropharyngeal lymph nodes, also known as the nodes of Rouviere (lymph nodes are found only in the suprahyoid RPS).

Retropharyngeal **pathologies** include edema, cellulitis and abscess. Secondary extension into the RPS may result from direct extension of squamous cell carcinoma, tortuous carotid artery, lipoma, hemangioma, diskitis and osteomyelitis from the prevertebral space. Lymph nodal enlargement can be due to reactive adenopathy, suppurative adenitis, metastatic adenopathy and lymphoma. Inflammatory conditions such as IJV thrombosis and longus colli tendinitis can cause edema of the RPS.

A mass in the RPS pushes the prevertebral muscles posteriorly whereas a mass in the prevertebral space lifts the prevertebral muscles anteriorly **(Figs. 32A and B)**. Nodal mass in lateral RPS may mimic a lesion in the carotid space. It is located medial to the carotid space and causes posterolateral displacement of the same.

CAROTID SPACE

These are paired tubular spaces extending along the suprahyoid and infrahyoid neck. Superiorly, the sheath of the carotid space (CS) extends up to the jugular foramen and inferiorly to the aortic arch. Anteriorly, it is bordered by the styloid process and parapharyngeal space, laterally by the anterior belly of the diagastric muscle and parotid space and medially by the lateral aspect of

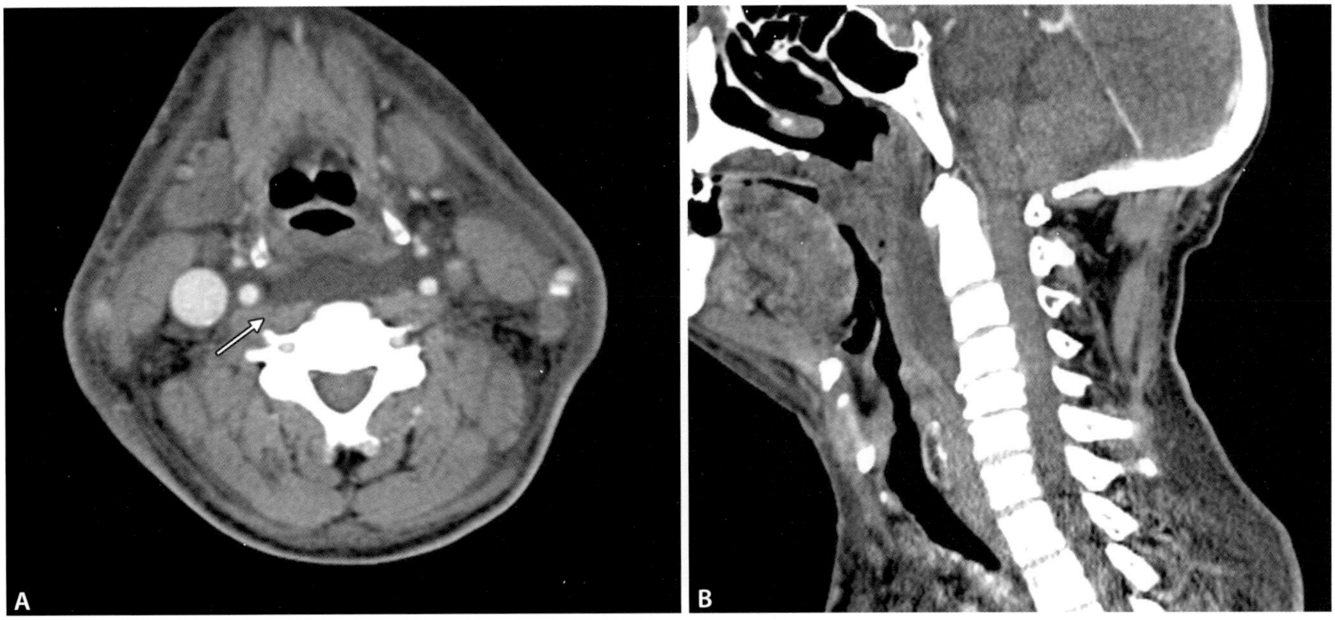

Figs. 32A and B: Axial (A) and sagittal (B) CECT images show a hypodense collection in the retropharyngeal space. Note the posterior displacement of prevertebral muscles (arrow in A), localizing the collection to the RPS.

the retropharyngeal space. The CS has nasopharyngeal, oropharyngeal, cervical, and mediastinal segments. In the suprahyoid neck, the RPS is medial, perivertebral space is posterior, PS is lateral and PPS space is anterior to the CS while in the infrahyoid neck, the visceral space and RPS are medial, perivertebral space is posterior, anterior cervical space is anterior and posterior cervical space is lateral to the CS.

The **contents (Table 8)** of the suprahyoid carotid space include the internal carotid artery (ICA), internal jugular vein (IJV), cranial nerves IX to XII and sympathetic plexus. The contents of the infrahyoid carotid space include the common carotid artery (CCA), internal jugular vein and vagus nerve (X) (***see* Fig. 9**).

A lesion primary to the CS is epicentered within the area of CCA/ICA-IJV and posterior to the PPS. It causes anterior displacement of the PPS fat. In addition to anterior displacement of PPS fat, lesions in the nasopharyngeal segment of CS displace the styloid process anterolaterally and lesions in the oropharyngeal segment displace the posterior belly of digastric muscle laterally.

Masses within the CS may arise from or compress the cranial nerves within the space, most commonly detected if cranial nerve X is involved. Glomus jugulare paraganglioma, schwannoma and meningioma[16] are lesions that involve the jugular fossa, therefore, the skull base must be assessed carefully. Displacement of structures within the CS can help as a differentiating factor. Vagal schwannoma and a sympathetic schwannoma have similar imaging appearances but a vagal schwannoma divides the ICA and IJV whereas a sympathetic schwannoma causes displacement of both structures anteriorly.

Table 8: Contents and lesions of the carotid space.

Contents
• Carotid artery • Internal jugular vein (IJV) • CNs IX, X, XI, XII and sympathetic chain • Lymph nodes (lateral to carotid space, disease can spread to carotid space).
Lesions
• *Vascular pathology:* Carotid artery—aneurysm, dissection, arteritis; Jugular vein—thrombosis and thrombophlebitis • *Mass lesions:* Neurogenic tumors and paragangliomas • *Lymph nodes:* Neoplastic or inflammatory causes • *Neoplastic causes:* Contiguous or from perineural spread of tumor

Lesions—The commonest pathology in the carotid space is enlarged lymph nodes. Vascular pathology can arise from internal carotid artery or internal jugular vein and includes vessel tortuosity, thrombosis/phlebitis, pseudoaneurysm, dissection and stenosis. Flow related phenomenon of IJV may mimic thrombosis or schwannoma on imaging.

Paragangliomas are slow growing hypervascular tumors arising from neural crest derivatives. They occur at multiple levels within the carotid space including the carotid bifurcation (carotid body tumors), along the nodose ganglia of vagus nerve (glomus vagale tumors) and along the nerves supplying the jugular bulb (glomus jugulare tumors).[23]

Glomus jugulare tumors may present with pulsatile tinnitus. *Glomus vagale* and carotid body tumors often present as a pulsatile neck mass which may be multiple in 3–5% of cases. The nonchromaffin paragangliomas can occur as multifocal lesions especially in patients with a family history of these tumors. Therefore, a study of both the right and the left carotid regions is necessary in these patients. Small tumors are ovoid or spherical while large tumors have a pear or dumb-bell shape with smooth contours.

Paragangliomas are highly vascular tumors that enhance intensely on CT **(Figs. 33A and B)** and MR. On MR these tumors have an intermediate signal intensity on all sequences. Areas of necrosis or hemorrhages give rise to a nonhomogeneous appearance. MRI may also show the typical *'salt and pepper' appearance*. This is present due to multiple serpiginous vascular channels that produce the dark 'pepper'and small hemorrhages that produce focal hyperintensities on T1 the 'salt' appearance. On diffusion weighted MR imaging paragangliomas may show low ADC values, therefore, when dealing with lesions showing lower ADC value in head and neck region, the possibility of paraganglioma should be ruled out before giving a diagnosis of malignancy, especially for those lesions without typical conventional MRI features.[24] Post contrast studies are helpful in identifying small tumors and synchronous lesions. They can be differentiated from schwannomas and neurofibromas on dynamic imaging. Dynamic scanning after 20-25 seconds of contrast injection reveals a sharp filling peak and a rapid washout after 150 seconds.[25] Schwannomas on the other hand do not show early enhancement but enhance intensely in scans obtained after 60 seconds. Angiography may be done in patients with equivocal lesions and for therapeutic embolization. Digital subtraction angiography and reformatted CT angiography/magnetic resonance angiography in case of carotid body tumors show a hypervascular mass splaying the internal and external carotids—the classic *"lyre sign"*.

Glomus jugulare tumor may cause variable erosion of the jugular foramen **(Figs. 34A to E)** and typically produces a permeative pattern of destruction in contrast to a neurofibroma or schwannoma which has a scalloped appearance.

The other differential diagnoses of these vascular lesions include metastasis from primary malignancies like hypernephroma, papillary thyroid carcinomas and melanoma and rare lesions such as extramedullary plasmacytomas, angiosarcomas and

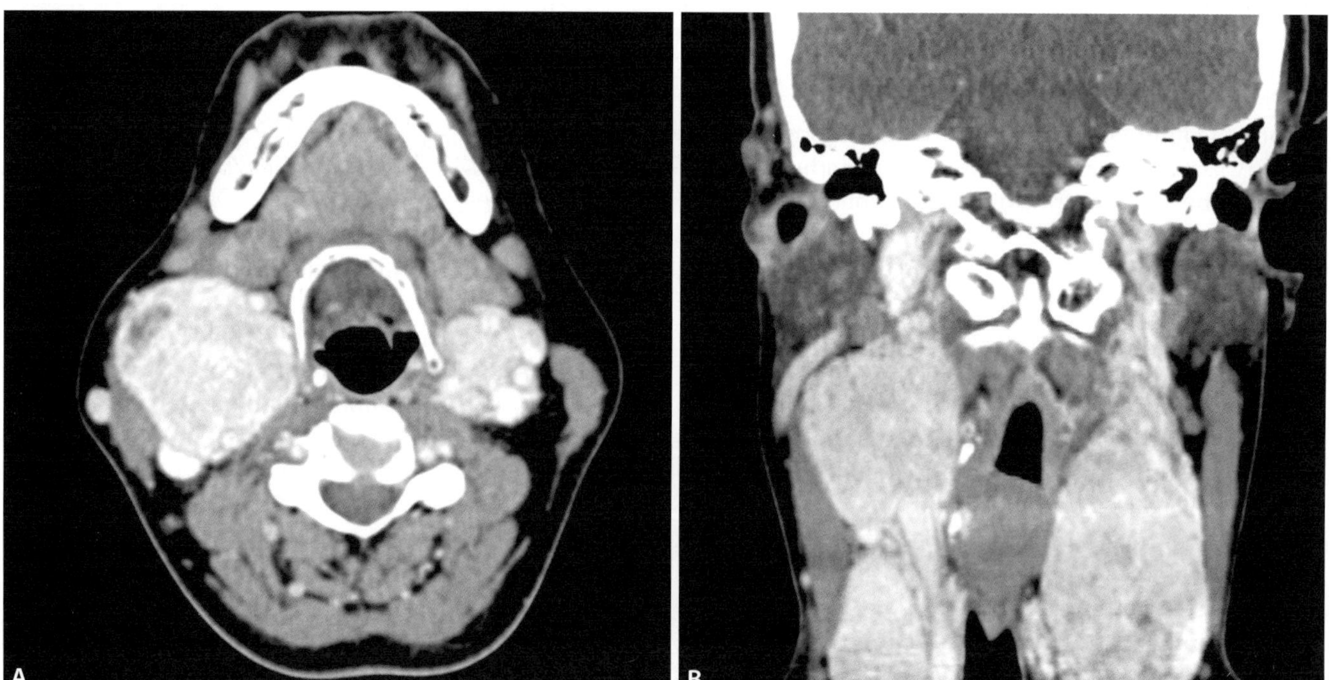

Figs. 33A and B: Axial (A) and coronal (B) CECT images show two well-marginated, hyperenhancing solid lesions with lobulated outline in the carotid space on each side—Bilateral paragangliomas.

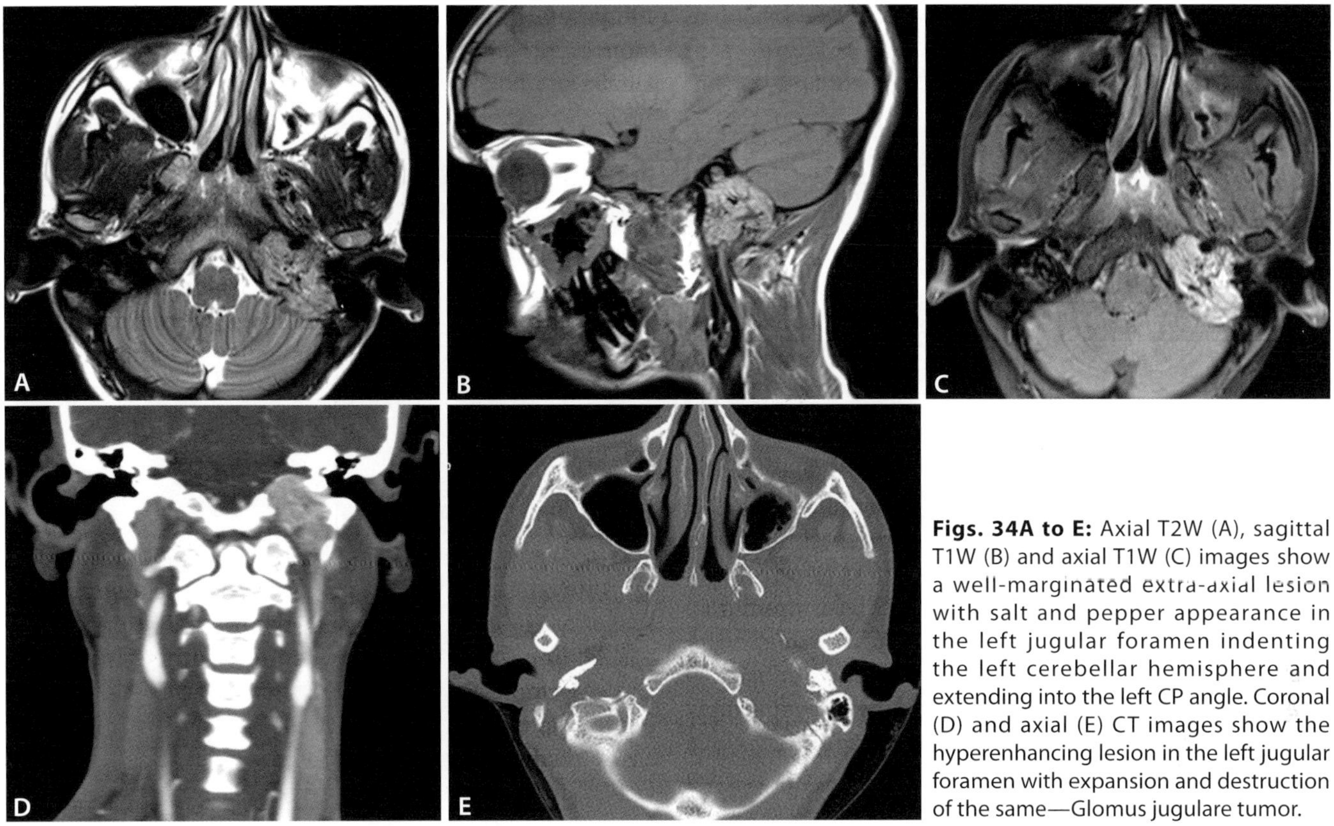

Figs. 34A to E: Axial T2W (A), sagittal T1W (B) and axial T1W (C) images show a well-marginated extra-axial lesion with salt and pepper appearance in the left jugular foramen indenting the left cerebellar hemisphere and extending into the left CP angle. Coronal (D) and axial (E) CT images show the hyperenhancing lesion in the left jugular foramen with expansion and destruction of the same—Glomus jugulare tumor.

hemangiopericytomas. Some hemangiomas may have a similar imaging appearance with flow voids. A key feature for the differential diagnosis is the lack of displacement of adjacent vessels.

Surgical resection is the treatment of choice with preoperative embolization because it decreases operative blood loss.

Neurogenic tumors are the most common carotid space lesions.[26] They can also occur in the masticator space, the parapharyngeal space and rarely the parotid space. The vagus, hypoglossal, or cervical roots may be involved. Two types of tumors (1) *schwannomas* and (2) *neurofibromas* can arise from the nerves in the carotid space.

Schwannomas are the most common tumors originating from the Schwann cells surrounding the nerves. Most commonly the tumor arises from the vagus nerve and less commonly the glossopharyngeal nerve, the ventral and dorsal cervical nerve roots, the cervical sympathetic chain, and the brachial plexus.

A tumor originating from the *vagus nerve* manifests as a mass in the anterior triangle and displaces the internal or common carotid artery anteromedially and the internal jugular vein posterolaterally whereas a tumor arising from the *cervical nerve roots* manifests as a mass in the posterior triangle which may extend into one of the neural foramina of the cervical spine. *Sympathetic chain tumors* demonstrate a constant relationship with the longus colli muscles and lesions of the cervical sympathetic chain as they grow and expand, tend to push the common carotid, or internal and external carotids, anteriorly. *Brachial plexus schwannomas and neurofibromas* in the infrahyoid neck often displace the anterior scalene muscle anteriorly.

Schwannomas are well-encapsulated tumors that do not contain neural or collagen tissue but consists of cellular and myxoid components. The presence of these two components differentiates it from a neurofibroma. On CT the tumor is isodense to muscle and displays enhancement. The internal carotid artery is displaced anteriorly and laterally. Hypodense areas due to cystic changes are visualized in 20% of tumors. Fluid-fluid levels may be seen in schwannomas and they must then be differentiated from lymphatic malformations. The fusiform shape is well visualized on sagittal and coronal planes. On MRI the tumor appears hypointense on T1W and hyperintense on T2W. The T2 relaxation time decreases with increasing cellularity of the lesion **(Figs. 35A to D)**.

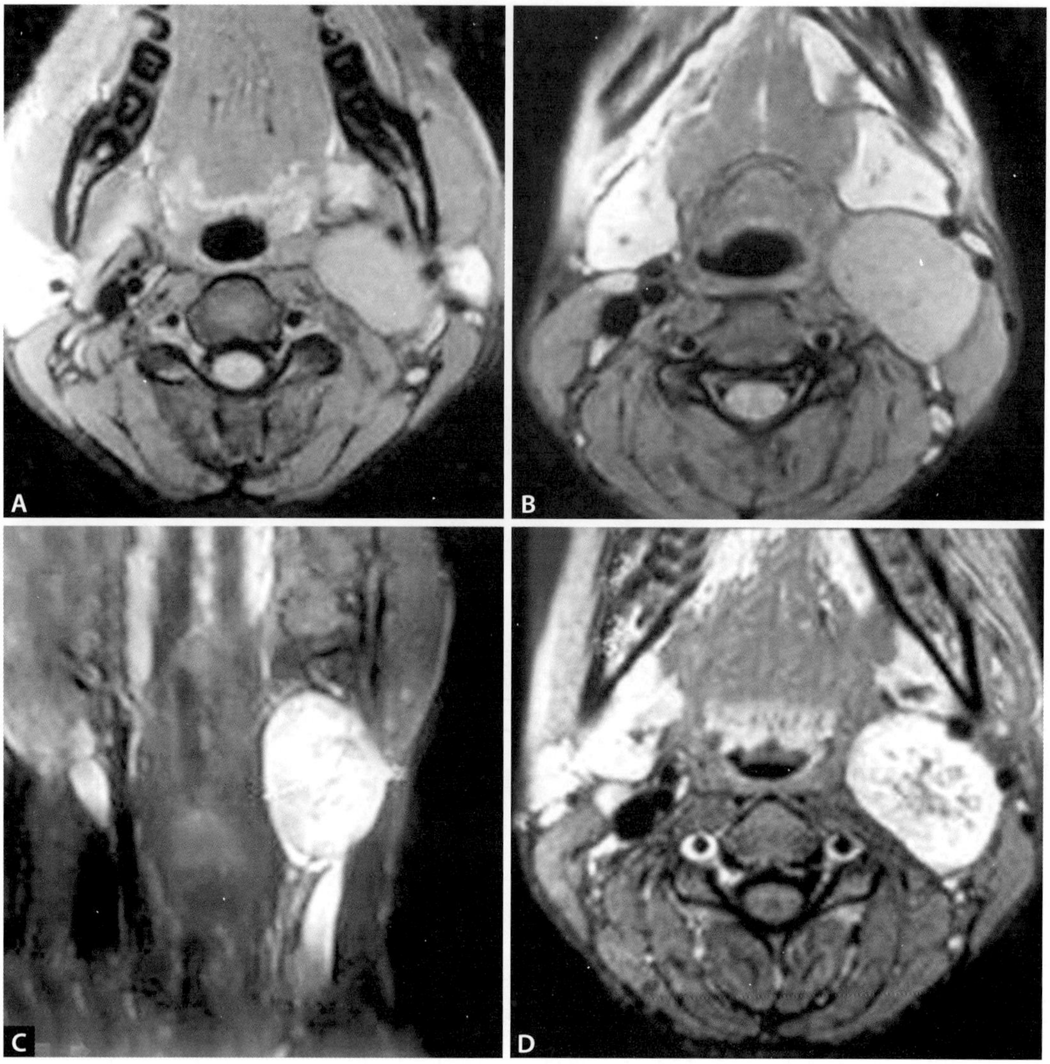

Figs. 35A to D: Axial T1W (A and B), coronal STIR (C) and axial postcontrast T1W (D) MR images showing an oval well-marginated lesion in the left carotid space displacing the ICA, ECA anterolaterally with attenuation of the IJV. The lesion is hyperintense with cystic areas on STIR images and shows intense contrast enhancement—Schwannoma.

Avascular schwannomas can be differentiated from paragangliomas due to the absence of flow voids but vascular schwannomas have identical imaging features to paragangliomas. Dynamic scans can reveal the true nature of the lesion and differentiate it from hypervascular lesions. The enhancement of the schwannomas is seen at least two minutes after contrast injection and depicts the equilibrium phase of the contrast agent and the poor venous drainage of the tumor in contrast to paragangliomas which show a rapid filling and rapid wash out.

Neurofibromas are the second type of neurogenic tumors arising in the CS. In contrast to schwannomas these are noncapsulated and contain all elements of the nerve of origin and are continuous with it.[27] Circumferential compression of the involved nerve is seen which is diffusely penetrated by tumor elements and symptoms depend on the nerve involved. Around 10% of patients of neurofibromas have neurofibromatosis and malignant transformation is more common in this group.

The imaging features are dependent on the underlying histology. On CT neurofibromas show low attenuation due to lipid rich schwann and fat cells scattered in the tumor and there is no appreciable contrast enhancement. The low density (near water) on CT is characteristic **(Figs. 36A and B)**. Neurofibromas appear identical to avascular schwannomas on MRI. They have a low SI on T1W and high SI on T2W images with variable enhancement **(Figs. 37A to D)**.

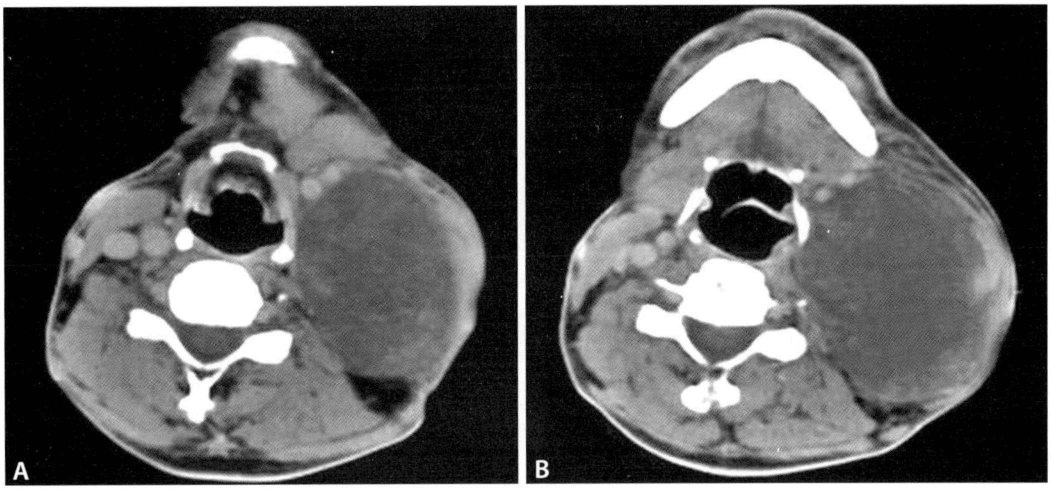

Figs. 36A and B: Axial CT scans showing a large well-encapsulated lesion in the left carotid space with displacement of carotid vessels anteriorly. (A) The lesion has a homogeneous low density and shows no significant enhancement (B) Neurofibroma.

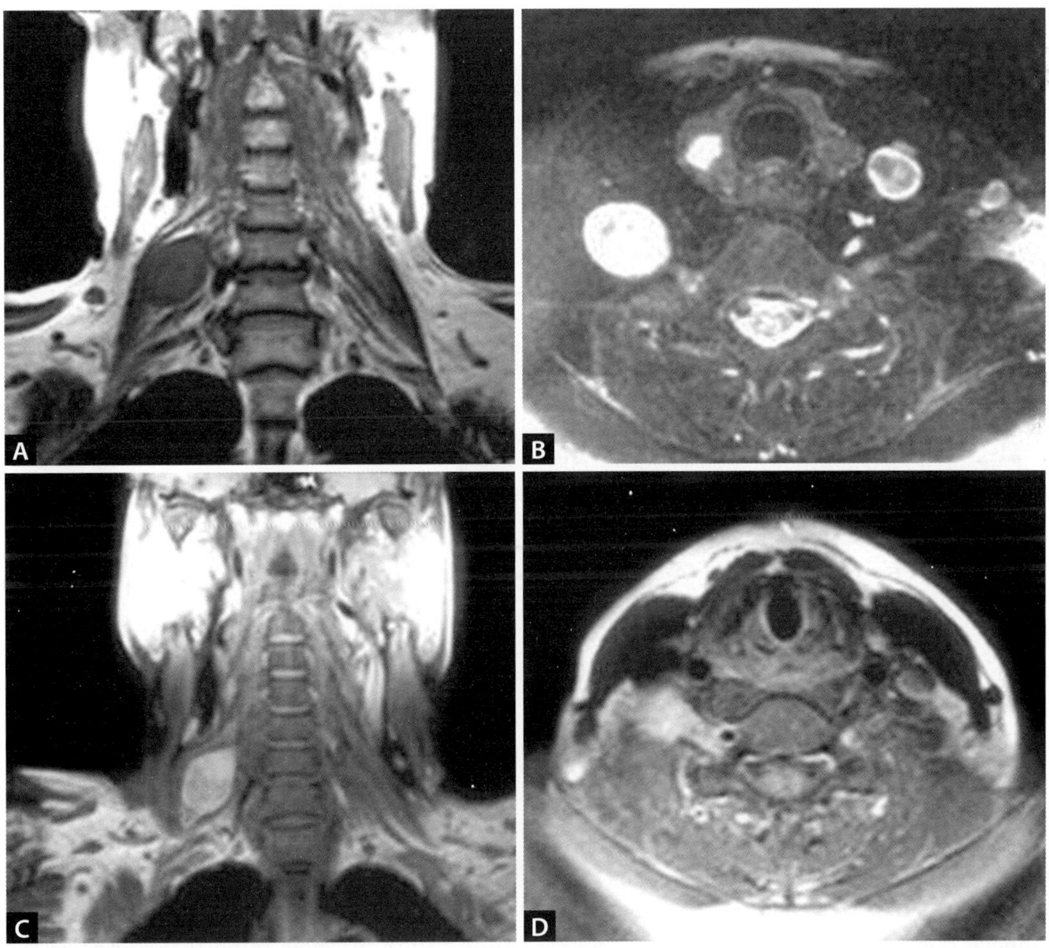

Figs. 37A to D: Coronal T1W (A), axial STIR (B), coronal (C) postcontrast and axial (D) postcontrast T1W MR images showing a well-marginated oval lesion in the right carotid space causing anterior displacement of the carotid vessels. The lesion is hypointense on T1, hyperintense on STIR with homogeneous contrast enhancement. Continuity with an enhancing nerve is best seen on the postcontrast coronal images and extension into the right neural foramen is seen—Neurofibroma.

Differentiation between Neurofibromas and Schwannomas

The imaging appearance of peripheral nerve sheath tumors depends on the histologic composition of the tumors and it may not be possible to differentiate between neurofibromas and schwannomas on imaging. However, certain imaging findings may be helpful in distinguishing the two. Neurofibromas may be seen at any age whereas schwannomas most commonly present between 20 and 50 years of age with occasional occurrences in childhood. Neurofibromas are characteristically asymptomatic whereas schwannomas are often associated with pain and tenderness. The pain may be localized or radicular in nature with associated paresthesias. A characteristic finding of neurofibromas is the *"target sign"*. On MRI an area of relatively hypointense central signal with peripheral hyperintense signal is seen on T2-weighted sequences, which is characteristic. NCCT may also be very useful, neurofibromas being hypodense on noncontrast scans as opposed to schwannomas.

Aneurysm of the ICA can present as a mass lesion of the neck. Helpful characteristics for differentiation of aneurysm from schwannomas or other rare tumors are the peripheral calcification and the obliteration of the ICA lumen. CT and MR angiography (MRA) can confirm the diagnosis of aneurysm.

PERIVERTEBRAL SPACE

The perivertebral space (PVS) is a cylindrical space surrounding the vertebral column and extends from the skull base to the coccyx. It is bounded by the deep layer of deep cervical fascia. It consists of the *prevertebral space* and *paraspinal space. Prevertebral space* is situated directly behind the retropharyngeal space. The carotid space is anterolateral to the prevertebral space and the posterior cervical space is lateral to it. *Paraspinal space* lies deep to posterior cervical space and posterior to the transverse processes of cervical spine.[21] **(*see* Fig. 10)**

The **contents** of the perivertebral space include prevertebral muscles (longus collis and capitis), scalene muscles, brachial plexus roots, phrenic nerve, vertebral artery and vein and vertebral bodies which lie in the prevertebral PVS. The paraspinal muscles, posterior elements, vertebral column and the proximal aspect of the brachial plexus lie in the paraspinal PVS. The anterior deep layer of deep cervical fascia is tenacious and infections or tumors of the PVS are redirected into the epidural space by this fascia.

The **pathologies** in this space include osteophytes, osteomyelitis, benign and malignant mesenchymal tumors, calcific tendinitis, primary bone tumors, metastases, diskitis, anterior disk herniation, aneurysm, lymphoma, and direct extension of carcinoma of the nasopharynx. The commonest malignancy of the prevertebral space in children is a rhabdomyosarcoma.

Vertebral body involvement is a conclusive sign of prevertebral space involvement. A mass in the prevertebral space proper has its center in the vertebral body or prevertebral muscles and displaces the prevertebral soft tissue. Therefore, a primary prevertebral space mass causes anterior displacement of the RPS and posterior wall of visceral space and lateral displacement of the carotid sheath. A mass from the paraspinal portion has its center in the paraspinal musculature or posterior elements of the vertebrae and displaces the paraspinous muscles and posterior cervical space fat outwards away from the spine.

Prevertebral abscesses represent a significant portion of PVS pathology. Etiologies include tubercular spondylitis, pyogenic osteomyelitis and postoperative infections.

In *tuberculous spondylitis* the inflammation is centered at the disk space which is often associated with partial destruction of the anterior aspect of the vertebral body. This is usually associated with a large paraspinal soft tissue mass that may show calcification **(Figs. 38A and B)**.

Pyogenic vertebral body osteomyelitis presents at the disk space with decreased height, subchondral bony erosions and fragmentation of the vertebral body without well-defined margins. Extension into the epidural space may be seen with both tubercular and pyogenic infections.

Longus colli tendinitis is a condition that needs to be differentiated from infections, it is an inflammatory response to the rupture of calcium hydroxyapatite deposits within the longus colli tendon. Calcification is seen at the longus capitis-colli tendinous insertions usually at C1-C2 levels and is best visualized on CT. Edema is seen in the adjacent retropharyngeal space.[21] On MRI, the calcification appears hypointense and does not enhance. Enlargement of muscle bellies can be seen in longus colli tendinitis, however, presence of the striated appearance of the muscle helps differentiate it from a neoplasm. Absence of lymphadenopathy and preserved bony structures helps differentiate this condition from infectious disease.

INFRAHYOID NECK

This is the region of the neck which extends from the hyoid bone to the thoracic inlet. It is divided into the visceral space, carotid space, retropharyngeal space, posterior cervical space, anterior cervical space and perivertebral space.

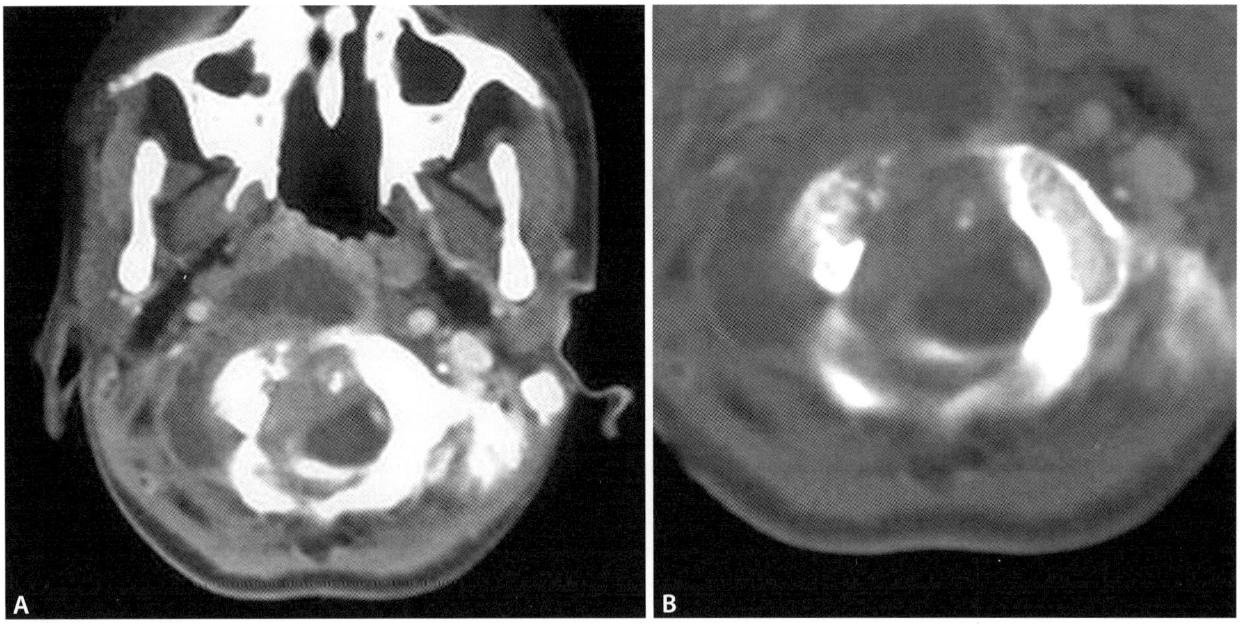

Figs. 38A and B: Axial CECT scans showing erosion of the basiocciput, right lateral mass of atlas and the dens with a large prevertebral and paravertebral collection. Note the anterior displacement of prevertebral muscles due to the collection. Caries C1, C2 with prevertebral abscess.

VISCERAL SPACE

It is a cylindrical space in the neck in midline enclosed by middle layer of deep cervical fascia. The visceral space (VS) is the largest space of the infrahyoid neck (***see* Figs. 12A and B**). The anterior cervical spaces are situated lateral to the visceral space, carotid spaces are posterolateral and the retropharyngeal space is posterior to it.

The **contents** of the visceral space are the larynx, trachea, hypopharynx, esophagus, thyroid and parathyroid glands. The recurrent laryngeal nerve is found in this space. The level VI group of lymph nodes including the paratracheal, prelaryngeal and pretracheal nodes and the infrahyoid strap muscles are also found in this space.

The **pathologies** that can arise in this space can arise from the larynx—laryngocele, squamous cell carcinoma; esophagus—esophageal diverticula, thyroid—colloid cyst, goiter, thyroid carcinoma, thyroglossal cyst; parathyroid—parathyroid adenoma; lymph nodes—metastases and lymphoma.

ANTERIOR CERVICAL SPACE

This is a small space situated in the anterolateral aspect of the neck and contains only fat. The anterior cervical space (ACS) lies lateral to the visceral space and anterior to the carotid space **(Fig. 39)**.

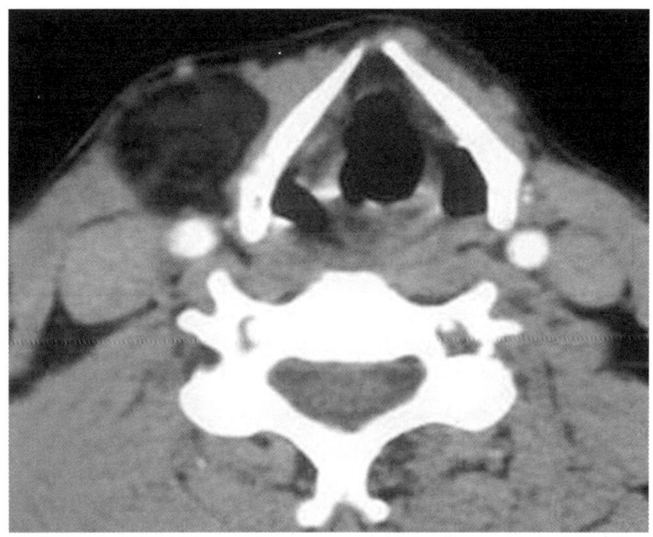

Fig. 39: Axial CECT scan showing a well-defined soft tissue density lesion of fat attenuation values in the anterior cervical space—lipoma.

POSTERIOR CERVICAL SPACE

Posterior cervical space (PCS) is a fat-containing space situated in the posterolateral aspect of the neck and extends from posterior mastoid tip to the clavicle. It lies between the superficial and deep layers of deep cervical fascia. The contents of this space include fat, accessory

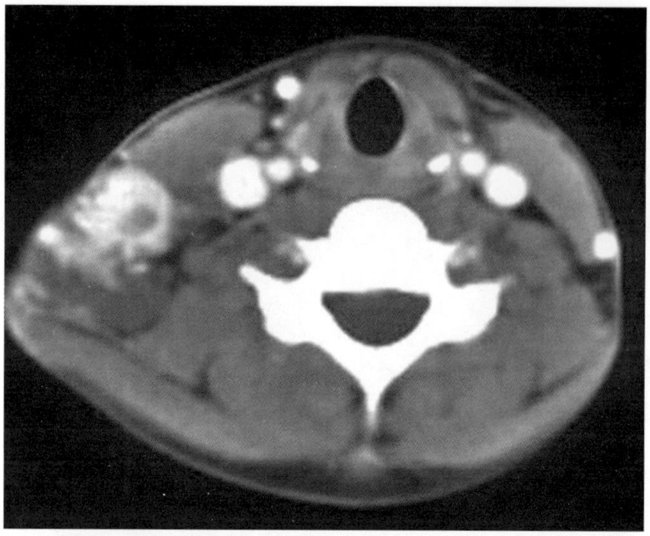

Fig. 40: Axial CECT image shows an ill-defined soft tissue density lesion with intense enhancement posterior to the sterno-cleidomastoid muscle on the right side—Hemangioma.

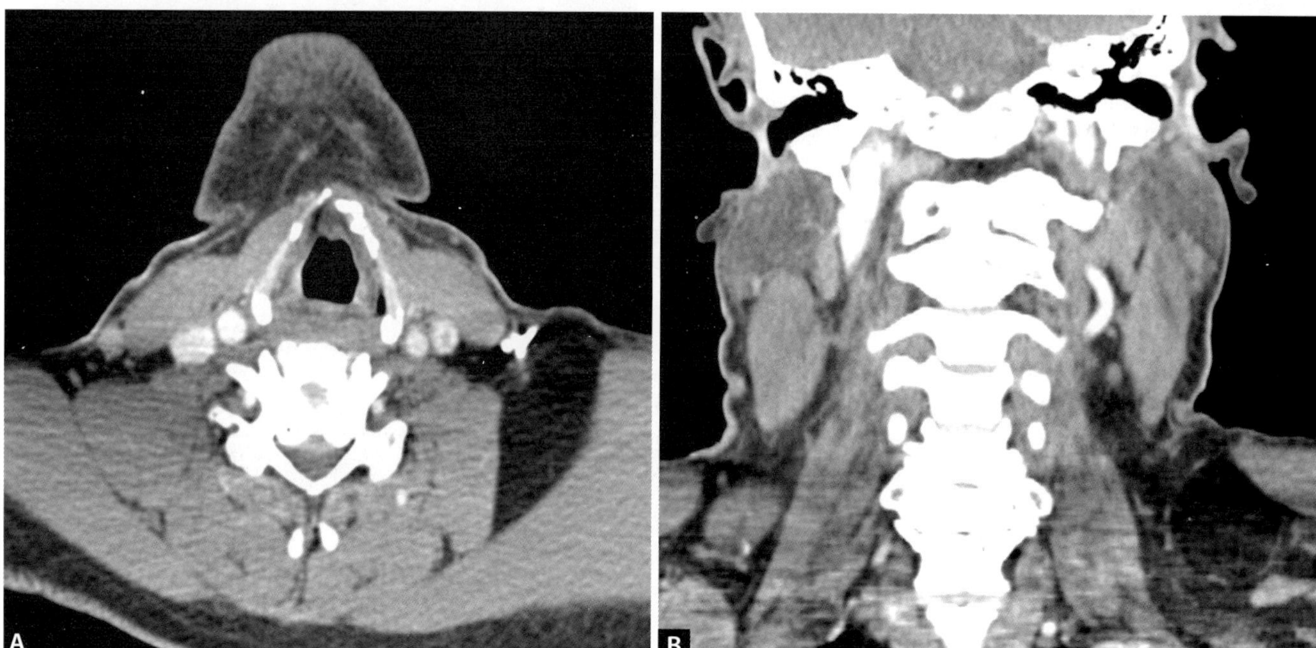

Figs. 41A and B: Axial (A) and coronal (B) CECT images show a hypodense lesion of fat density in the posterior cervical space—Lipoma.

nerve (cranial nerve XI), spinal accessory lymph nodal chain, pre-axillary brachial plexus and dorsal scapular nerve.

The *posterior triangle* is the region of the neck posterolateral to the sternocleidomastoid muscle and anteromedial to the trapezius muscle. It is divided by the inferior belly of omohyoid muscle into *occipital and subclavian triangles. Occipital triangle* forms majority of the PCS and its boundaries are formed by the sternocleidomastoid muscle anteromedially, trapezius muscle posterolaterally and inferior belly of omohyoid muscle inferiorly. It contains fat, cranial nerve XI, dorsal scapular nerve and spinal accessory nodes. The *subclavian triangle* is the smaller portion of the PCS, it is bound by inferior belly of omohyoid superiorly, sternocleidomastoid anteromedially and trapezius posterolaterally. It contains the third portion of subclavian artery and cervical brachial plexus.[10]

A mass lesion primary to the PCS must be centered within the fat of PCS. It displaces the CS anteromedially, elevates sternocleidomastoid muscle and flattens deeper perivertebral space structures **(Figs. 40 and 41)**.

LESIONS COMMON TO DIFFERENT NECK SPACES

Branchial Cleft Anomalies

Branchial cleft anomalies are thought to arise because of incomplete obliteration of a portion of the branchial apparatus. A **first branchial cleft cyst** arises from the residual embryonic tract that extends from the external auditory canal (EAC) through the parotid gland to the submandibular region and is of two types. Preauricular location is seen with type 1 cysts while type 2 is periparotid extending from the EAC to the angle of the mandible.

Approximately 95% of branchial cleft anomalies are related to the second branchial cleft, it also represents the second most commonly encountered congenital neck mass after thyroglossal duct cyst. The **second branchial anomaly** may cause fistulas **(Figs. 42A to C)**, sinuses or cysts. It can occur anywhere from the tonsillar fossa to the supracalvicular region. Bailey classified second branchial cleft cysts into four types. Type I are most superficial and lie along the anterior surface of the sternocleidomastoid muscle just deep to the platysma. Type II are seen along the anterior surface of the sternocleidomastoid muscle, lateral to the carotid space and posterior to the submandibular gland.[28] Type III cysts are seen to extend medially between the bifurcation of the internal and external carotid arteries. Type IV is seen in the PMS.

Imaging findings include low echogenicity on US, low attenuation on CT, and variable signal on MR imaging. Thickened enhancing walls are seen on cross-sectional imaging if infection is present.

Third and fourth branchial cleft cysts are rare. Most third branchial cleft cysts are situated posterior to the sternocleidomastoid muscle. Fourth branchial cleft anomalies are usually sinus tracts which arise from the pyriform sinus through the thyrohyoid membrane and descend into the mediastinum.

LESIONS OF VASCULAR ORIGIN

Vascular lesions of the head and neck are common and classified according to system the described by Mulliken and Glowacki[29] into two groups i.e. *vascular malformations*, which have normal endothelial cell turnover and *vascular tumors*, with high endothelial cell turnover. Since vascular malformations are not neoplastic, their growth is proportional to body size. Evaluation of the imaging characteristics and clinical presentation is important for correct diagnosis and providing appropriate treatment. There has been confusion with various terms in the past (such as cavernous hemangioma, which actually represent venous vascular malformations), it is important to use more consistent terminology **(Table 9)**.

Capillary Malformations

Head and neck capillary malformations (CMs) present as a "port wine stain" cutaneous lesion following the dermatomal pattern of the trigeminal nerve in up to 43% of patients. About 3% of patients may have Sturge-Webber syndrome, the association is higher when trigeminal dermatomal pattern is seen.[30,31]

Table 9: New and old terminology for vascular lesions.

New	*Old*
Hemangioma	Capillary hemangioma
Capillary malformation	Port wine stain
Venous malformation	Cavernous hemangioma
Lymphatic malformation	Lymphangioma, cystic hygroma

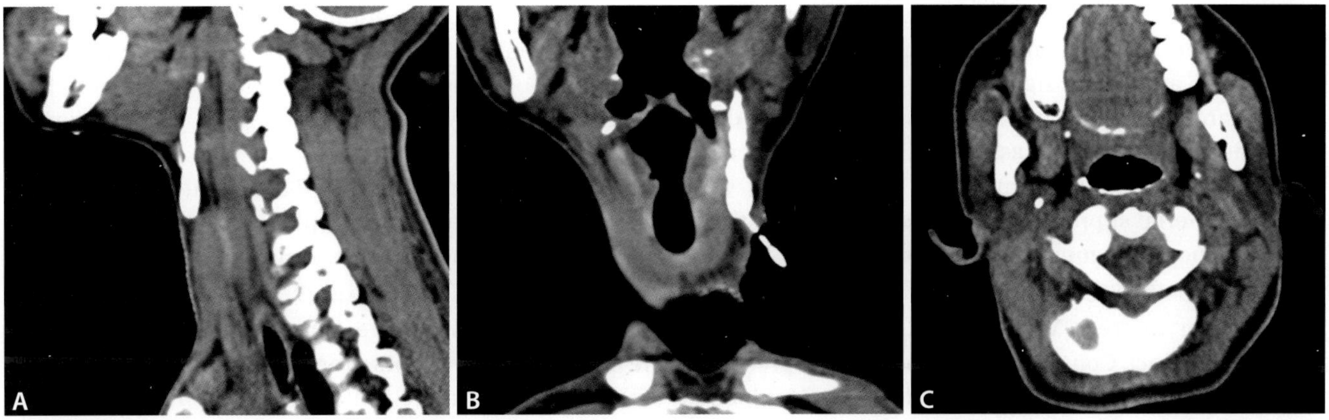

Figs. 42A to C: Sagittal (A), coronal (B) and axial (C) images from CT sinogram show a contrast-filled tract in the left side of the neck with internal opening in the tonsillar fossa, pooling of contrast is seen in the pharynx (C) second branchial cleft fistula.

Diagnosis is usually made based on clinical characteristics but imaging can be useful in patients with Sturge-Weber syndrome or with equivocal clinical presentation. Differentials of CMs include superficial hemangioma, venous malformation, and arteriovenous malformation.

CMs are usually located in the dermis and appear isoechoic on high resolution sonography.[32] Doppler signal can be identified in nearly 30%. MRI or CT can be used to evaluate for suspected Sturge-Weber and can also help in the differentiation of CMs from other vascular lesions, which commonly extend deeper into the tissues, may involve bony structures, and have more internal flow. CMs can become darker and more apparent with time in many patients. In these cases, the treatment of choice is laser therapy.

Venous Malformations (VM)

They often present with facial deformity and pain secondary to local inflammatory changes or compressive effects. Up to 50% of head and neck VMs are seen at birth and are soft bluish masses that enlarge with dependent positioning, compression of the ipsilateral jugular vein, and Valsalva maneuvers. Differential diagnosis of VMs includes hemangioma, arteriovenous malformation, mixed vascular malformations, and dermoids.

The hallmark of VMs is the presence of phleboliths, which can be seen in up to 48% of cases.[33,34] On US, they are hypoechoic and heterogeneous with phleboliths appearing hyperechoic alongwith acoustic shadowing. Doppler flow may be seen in up to 37%. Bone changes can include osteolysis, demineralization, hypoplasia, and cortical thickening best seen on CT alongwith phleboliths and variable enhancement. MRI clearly delineates the spatial extent of the lesion. VMs are generally isointense on T1, hyperintense on T2W and show a heterogeneous enhancement pattern after contrast administration. Phleboliths appear as signal voids on both T1WI and T2WI. Rarely, magnetic resonance venography is done when there is suspicion of associated intracranial venous anomalies. On angiography, these lesions have slow flow and arterial supply is often not definitely identified. On direct percutaneous injection, contrast can be seen pooling in dilated venous channels.

Decision to treat VMs depends on the size and functional impact. Conservative management is preferred, if possible. Treatment generally includes percutaneous sclerotherapy with ethanol or sodium tetradecyl sulfate (Sotradecol) with majority of patients being cured or having significant improvement. If the lesion is large and difficult to delineate, sclerotherapy is used in combination with reconstructive surgery. Care should be taken in determining the dose of ethanol given during treatment, particularly when VMs have prominent draining veins as diffuse VMs with high-flow communication to conducting veins or adjacent arteries have increased risk of systemic toxicity and lesion recurrence. Recurrence has been noted to occur in up to 35% of patients.

Lymphatic Malformations (LM)

These generally present as a soft, colorless mass with 70–80% of cases occurring in the head and neck, this being the commonest site in the body. Up to 90% of these lesions are diagnosed by 2–5 years.[35] There are 2 types of LMs, macrocystic (> 1 cm) and microcystic (< 1 cm) groups. Microcystic LMs are more common and present later than macrocystic LMs, which are mostly present at birth. Macrocystic lesions commonly arise below the mylohyoid in the anterior or posterior triangles of the neck (previously called cystic hygromas). Microcystic LMs generally occur above the mylohyoid in the oral/perioral region and the parotid gland (previously called lymphangiomas).

Differential diagnosis includes venous malformations, mixed malformations, and cystic lesions such as branchial cleft cysts, and thyroglossal duct cysts.

On US, LMs are usually anechoic, microcystic variants appearing hyperechoic; Doppler flow is distinctly uncommon. On CT, these lesions are seen as a low density cystic mass which may be uniloculated or multiloculated and may be poorly circumscribed. In macrocystic lesions with previous internal hemorrhage or infection fluid–fluid levels can be identified **(Figs. 43A and B)**. Simple LMs show absence of contrast enhancement. On MRI, LMs are hypointense on T1WI, hyperintense on T2WI, with no contrast enhancement unlike VMs. Macrocystic LMs show a septated cystic mass appearing T1 hypointense to isointense often heterogeneous due to proteinaceous fluid with fluid-fluid levels. On the other hand, microcystic LMs appear as diffuse hypointensity on T1-weighted imaging and diffuse hyperintensity on T2-weighted imaging. MRI is valuable in preoperative planning and determining lesion extent because LMs can engulf and encase adjacent structures.

LMs located in life-threatening areas such as retropharyngeal LMs require prompt treatment otherwise treatment indications are similar to other VMs. Sclerotherapy is the most common treatment for macrocystic LMs. Microcystic LMs are less responsive to

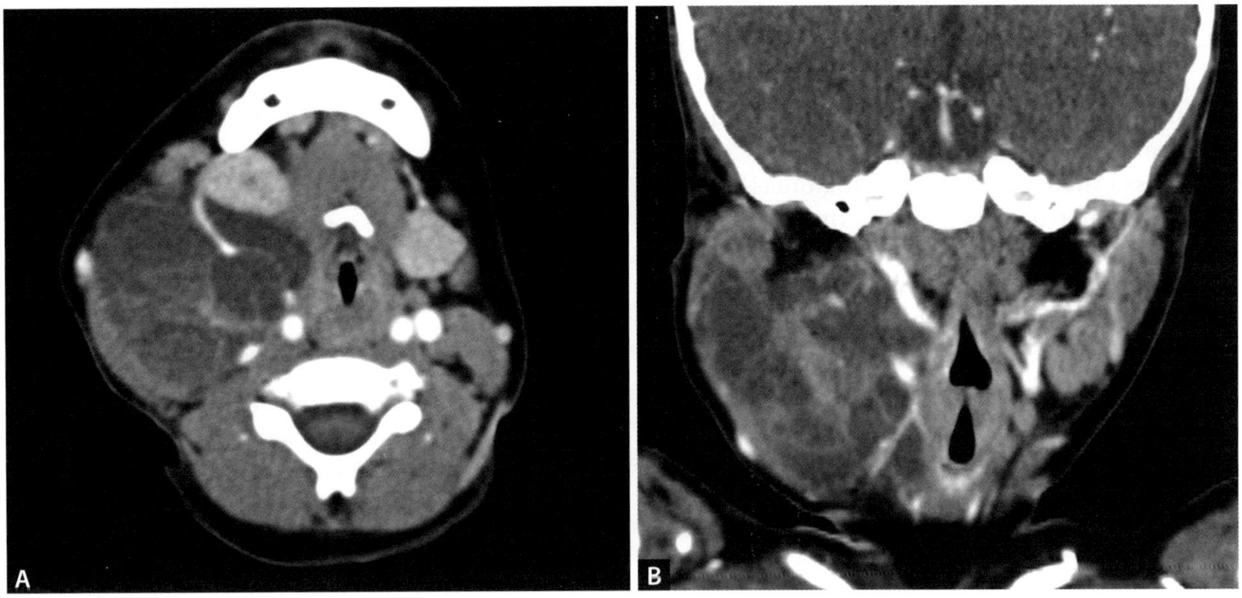

Figs. 43A and B: Axial (A) and coronal (B) CECT images show a multiloculated hypodense cystic lesion involving multiple spaces of the neck, displacing the submandibular gland anteriorly and carotid sheath structures posteromedially—Macrocystic lymphatic malformation (cystic hygroma).

therapy and are typically managed conservatively unless symptomatic, threaten vital structures or for aesthetic reasons. Surgery is the preferred first-line treatment. Whatever the therapy, recurrence rates can be high (especially in microcystic lesions) and more than one procedure is often required.

Arteriovenous Malformations

Arteriovenous malformations (AVMs) are composed of arteries and veins that directly communicate through a central nidus. The lesions are present at birth in 40% of cases but AVMs of the head and neck generally present later in childhood or in adolescence often with cosmetic deformity, skin discoloration, an underlying pulsatile bruit, pain, bleeding, or ulceration.[36] Differential considerations include HM and VM. Color Doppler US helps to characterize these lesions as high flow showing high systolic and diastolic flow, prominent arteriovenous shunting and arterialization of venous flow. CT shows large, dilated, serpiginous enhancing structures, often indistinguishable as arterial or venous in origin. Skeletal involvement, not uncommon, is an additional CT finding.

MRI is integral to determining lesion extent and soft tissue involvement. AVMs are seen as tangled mesh of dilated arteries and veins demonstrating flow void on T1W and T2W echo imaging and hyperintense signal on T2W gradient echo imaging and angiography, indicating rapid flow. T1W postcontrast images demonstrate contrast enhancement of multiple vessels with early venous enhancement, AVMs lack enhancement of adjacent soft tissue. Angiography helps in determining extent of the lesion as well as in directing therapeutic embolization. Treatment includes surgical resection, embolization, or combined therapy.

VASCULAR TUMORS

Hemangiomas

Hemangiomas (HM) are benign vascular neoplasms occurring most commonly in the head and neck region. They are divided into *infantile* and *congenital types*. Congenital hemangiomas are further divided into *noninvoluting congenital hemangiomas* (NICH) and *rapidly involuting congenital hemangiomas* (RICH).[36] Infantile hemangiomas (IH) present present postnatally usually by 6 weeks and represent 70% of all hemangiomas. Congenital HMs (30%) are present at birth.

HMs appear as a well-circumscribed mass with variable or heterogeneous echogenicity on gray scale US. They display high vascular flow on Doppler particularly in the proliferative phase seen as flow vessels in and around the mass, with the arterial feeder showing increased color flow, high Doppler shift and low resistance. On NCCT, HMs are isoattenuating to muscle making them difficult to delineate. They however, enhance avidly (especially in the proliferative phase). On MRI, HMs are isointense to slightly hyperintense on T1WI, hyperintense on T2WI, (often being mildly hyperintense to surrounding muscles) with avid contrast enhancement. Adjacent serpiginous flow voids can be seen. MR angiography (MRA) is useful when posterior fossa malformations hemangiomas—arterial anomalies—cardiac defects-eye abnormalities—sternal cleft and supraumbilical raphe syndrome is suspected. In this syndrome, hemangiomas present alongwith cerebral vascular anomalies and other abnormalities. MRA helps to visualize arterial stenosis, agenesis and aneurysms. On catheter angiography, high flow, an arterial blush, and persistent tissue staining is seen.

HM are usually small and self-involuting, hence the first step in therapy is expectant management. When cosmetically bothersome or if associated with compromised function of important structures intervention may be required. The first line of therapy is systemic propranolol, which leads to improvement in 97% of cases, significant improvement mostly occurring during the first week of therapy. In unresponsive cases treatment modalities include surgery, laser therapy, intralesional steroids, or chemotherapeutic agents.

MASSES OF MESENCHYMAL ORIGIN

Lipomatous tumors such as lipoma, lipoblastoma, and liposarcoma are the most common cervical neoplasms of mesenchymal origin. They usually manifest as painless masses, occurring most commonly in the midline of posterior neck or the posterior triangle. Cervical lipoblastoma typically presents as a rapidly growing mass.[37] Liposarcoma is one of the most frequent malignant soft tissue tumors in adults. It should be suspected whenever a large (5 cm) fat containing soft tissue tumor is found especially when it is clinically associated with pain and rapid growth. Well-differentiated liposarcoma displays a hypodense fat density (<–20 HU) mass on CT; the tumor shows signal intensities similar to those of subcutaneous normal fat on MR images. Poorly differentiated liposarcoma displays tissue density on CT and appears hypointense on T1-weighted images, hyperintense on T2-weighted MR images and shows intense early enhancement on dynamic acquisition contrast-enhanced images. Ill-defined borders and nonfatty heterogeneous contents indicate the high probability of malignancy. Other sarcomas that may be present are rhabdomyosarcoma, fibrosarcoma, osteosarcoma, chondrosarcoma, malignant fibrous histiocytoma, leiomyosarcoma, alveolar soft part sarcoma and synovial sarcoma. The imaging findings of these entities frequently are nonspecific.

CERVICAL LYMPHADENOPATHY

Understanding cervical lymph node anatomy, drainage pathways, and common abnormalities is central to interpretation of lymph node pathology. Clinical information along with location-specific approach and knowledge of lymph node morphology in various disease processes can further refine the differential diagnosis.

Cervical lymph nodes can be classified based on anatomic location or described with neoplastic processes using the formal *American Joint Committee on Cancer's (AJCC)* criteria.[10,38] The former differs from the latter in that it includes all lymph nodes and not just those important for surgical planning. Anatomically, various groups and chains of lymph nodes are described. These include:

- **Submental group**: Inferior to the anterior mandible.
- **Submandibular group**: Near the submandibular glands at the angles of the mandible.
- **Parotid lymph nodes**: The intraglandular nodes and within the fascia circumscribing the parotid space.
- **Preauricular nodes**: Within the subcutaneous tissues anterior to the external auditory canal
- **Postauricular nodes**: Posterior to the external auditory canal
- The **retropharyngeal space lymph nodes**: Medial RPS nodes situated in the paramedian RPS and the lateral RPS nodes situated lateral to the prevertebral muscles and medial to the internal jugular vein and internal carotid artery in the lateral RPS.
- The **facial lymph nodes** include multiple nodes named according to location, e.g. mandibular nodes superficial to the mandible, buccinator nodes in the subcutaneous tissues of the cheek, infraorbital nodes below the orbits, the malar nodes at the malar eminence, and the zygomatic nodes anterior to the zygomatic arch.
- The **occipital nodes** within the subcutaneous tissues posteroinferior to calvarium.
- The major nodal chains within the neck can be thought of as 3 linear chains of lymph nodes forming a triangle on each side of the neck. The **internal jugular chain** lies anteriorly surrounding the IJV from the skull base to the thoracic inlet. Posteriorly, the **spinal accessory chain** runs along the spinal accessory nerve in the posterior cervical space. The **transverse cervical chain** lies along the transverse cervical artery in the supraclavicular fossa and connects the inferior portion of internal jugular and spinal accessory chain.
- The **anterior cervical group** includes the prelaryngeal, pretracheal and paratracheal chains. The prelaryngeal

chain is midline and superficial. The pretracheal chain lies in the superficial fascia of the neck external to the strap muscles following the external jugular vein in its course. The paratracheal chain runs in the tracheoesophageal groove in the visceral space of the infrahyoid neck.

Cervical lymph nodes can also be categorized by surgical levels used for cancer treatment planning. These include 7 levels based on surgical landmarks while for imaging, radiologic landmarks are used **(Table 10)**.

Some lymph nodes are not included in the AJCC's surgical classification but are relevant in patient care. These include the parotid, retropharyngeal, occipital, and facial nodal groups.

The term *supraclavicular lymph nodes* is commonly used, however, it is not a defined nodal group and includes parts of both levels IV and VB. Supraclavicular nodes should be identified as they are important in cancer staging. *Virchow node* is a named lymph node that lies within the left supraclavicular fossa.[39]

Table 10: American Joint Committee on Cancer classification of cervical lymph nodes based on level and location **(Figs. 44 to 47)**.

Level I **Ia**: Submental—between anterior bellies of digastric below mandible **Ib**: Submandibular—lateral to anterior bellies of digastric and anterior to submandibular gland
Level II: Anterior cervical lymph node chain. Lymph nodes in the internal jugular chain from the skull base to the level of the hyoid bone. **IIa**; Nodes anterior, medial, or lateral to the internal jugular vein **IIb**: Nodes posterior to the internal jugular vein with a fat plane between the node and the vessel, nodes anterior to posterior edge of sternocleidomastoid
Level III: Nodes along the internal jugular chain between the hyoid bone and the cricoid cartilage
Level IV: Nodes along the lower IJV, from inferior margin of cricoid cartilage to supraclavicular fossa
Level V: Nodes in posterior cervical space corresponding to SAC, lie posterior to posterior margin of sternocleidomastoid in coronal plane **Va**: Level V nodes from the skull base to lower border of cricoid cartilage **Vb**: Level V nodes from lower border of cricoid cartilage to the supraclavicular fossa
Level VI: Nodes in the visceral compartment from the hyoid bone superiorly to the superior aspect of manubrium inferiorly, includes prelaryngeal, pretracheal, paratracheal, tracheoesophageal nodes
Level VII: Nodes in the superior mediastinum, between the carotid arteries, extending from superior margin of manubrium to innominate vein.

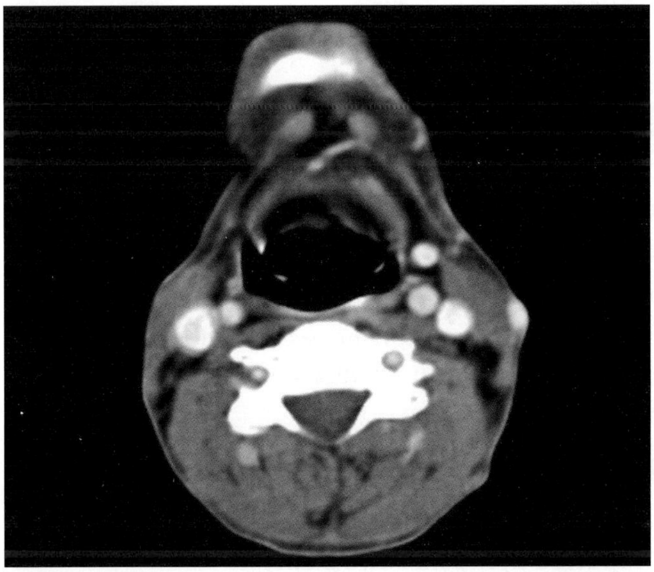

Fig. 44: Axial CECT image showing submental lymph nodes, the nodes are seen between the anterior bellies of digastric, below the mandible (level Ia).

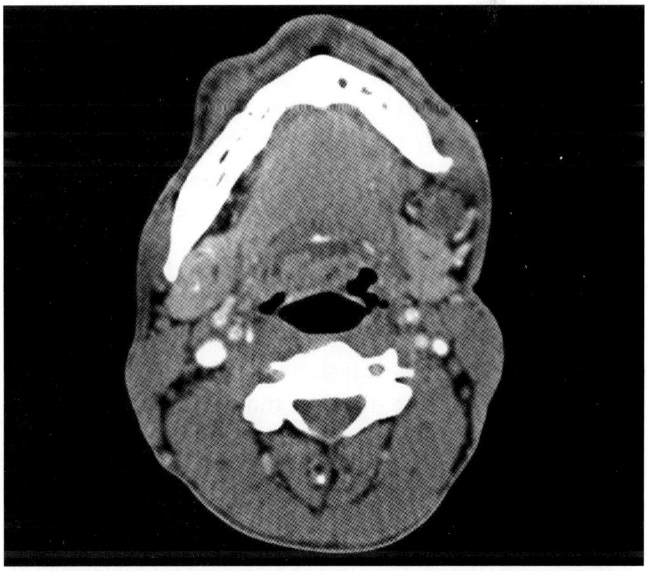

Fig. 45: Axial CECT image shows enlarged necrotic level Ib lymph node (anterior to the submandibular gland) on left side.

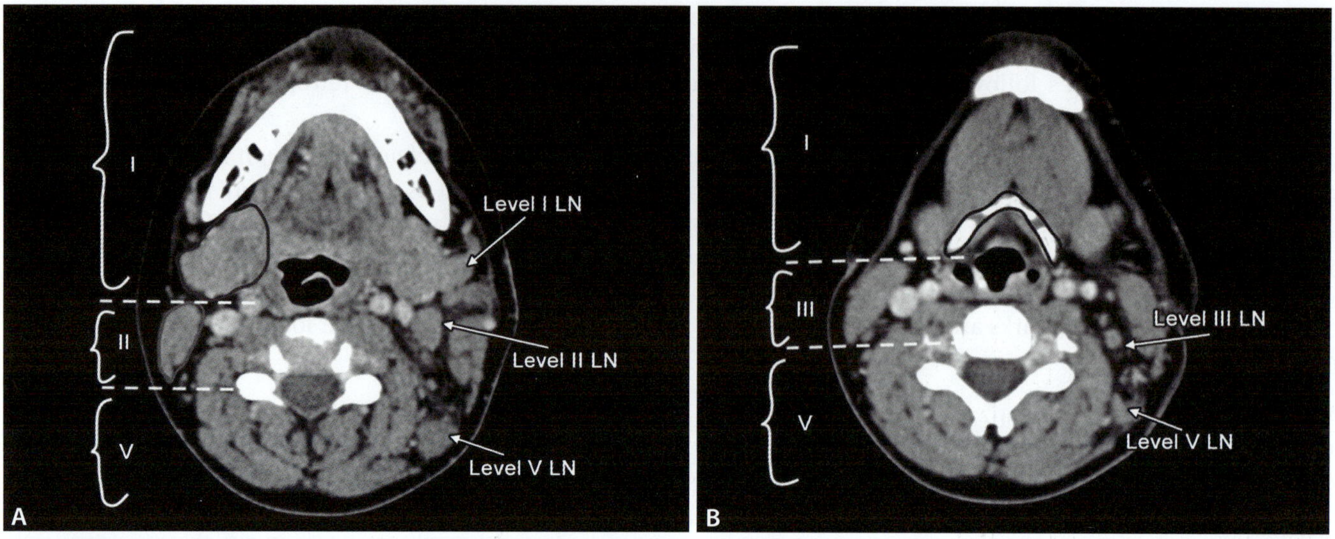

Figs. 46A and B: Axial CECT images show enlarged level I, II, III and V lymph nodes on left side in a known case of lymphoma. Level I lymph nodes are anterior to the submandibular gland, level II are posterior to the submandibular gland and level V are posterior to the sternocleidomastoid.

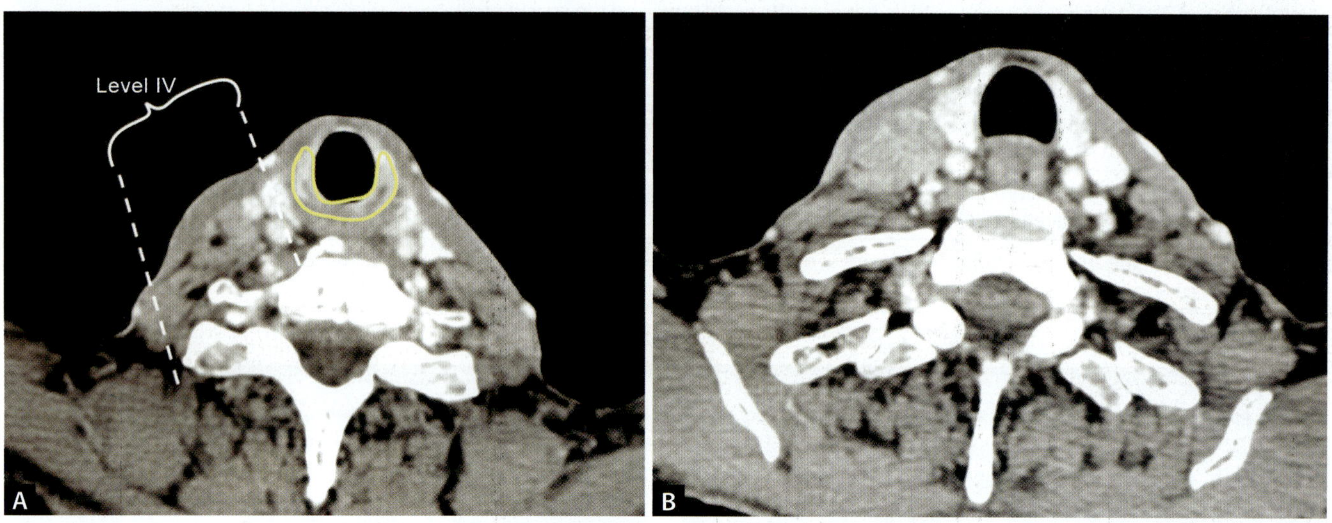

Figs. 47A and B: Axial CECT image shows enlarged level IV lymph nodes on right side in a known case of carcinoma larynx, level IV lymph nodes are seen between the inferior margin of the cricoid to supraclavicular fossa.

In evaluation of a neck mass, it is important to differentiate between lymph nodes and other pathologies such as congenital cystic lesions, inflammatory/infective diseases or neoplastic diseases that can mimic a lymph node **(Figs. 48A to C)**. Normal lymph nodes have a central fatty hilum which is continuous with surrounding cervical fat and reniform shape. Lymph node enlargement criteria include a long diameter of more than 15 mm for level I or II nodes, > 8 mm for retropharyngeal nodes and > 10 mm for other cervical nodes. However, up to 50% of the nodes with malignant deposits measure <5 mm in size.[40] Thus, other important features that should be considered while assessing lymph nodes include configuration, homogeneity, enhancement, fatty hilum and surrounding fat planes.

MORPHOLOGICAL CHARACTERISTICS OF LYMPH NODES

Reactive Lymphadenopathy

Reactive lymph nodal enlargement occurs in response to an antigen or infiltration. It can be acute or chronic and

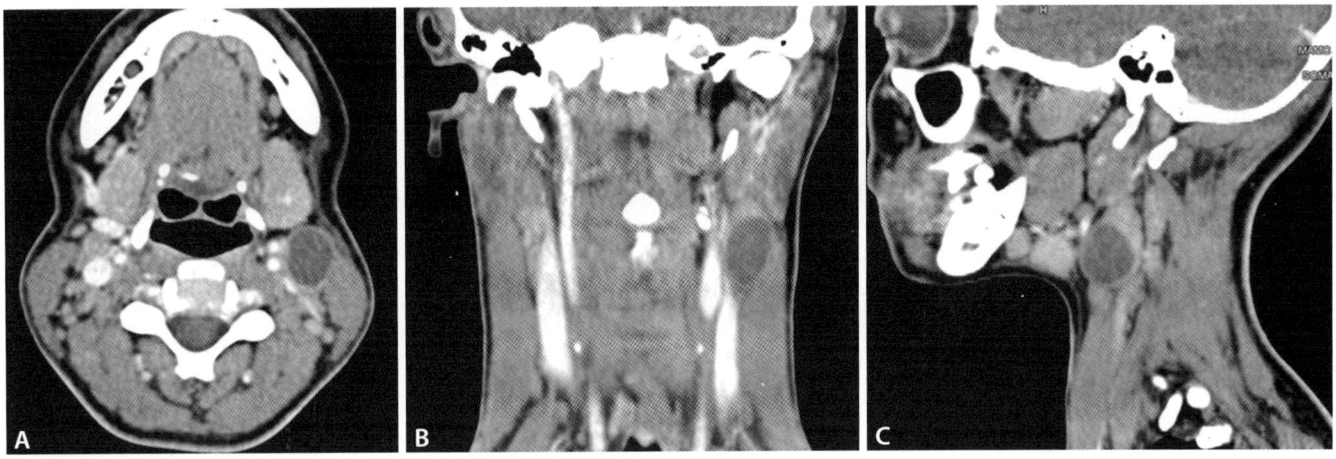

Figs. 48A to C: Axial (A), coronal (B) and sagittal (C) CECT images show a necrotic lymph node posterior to the posterior margin of submandibular gland (level II) on left side in a follow-up case of squamous cell carcinoma oral cavity. Note the near cystic appearance of the node.

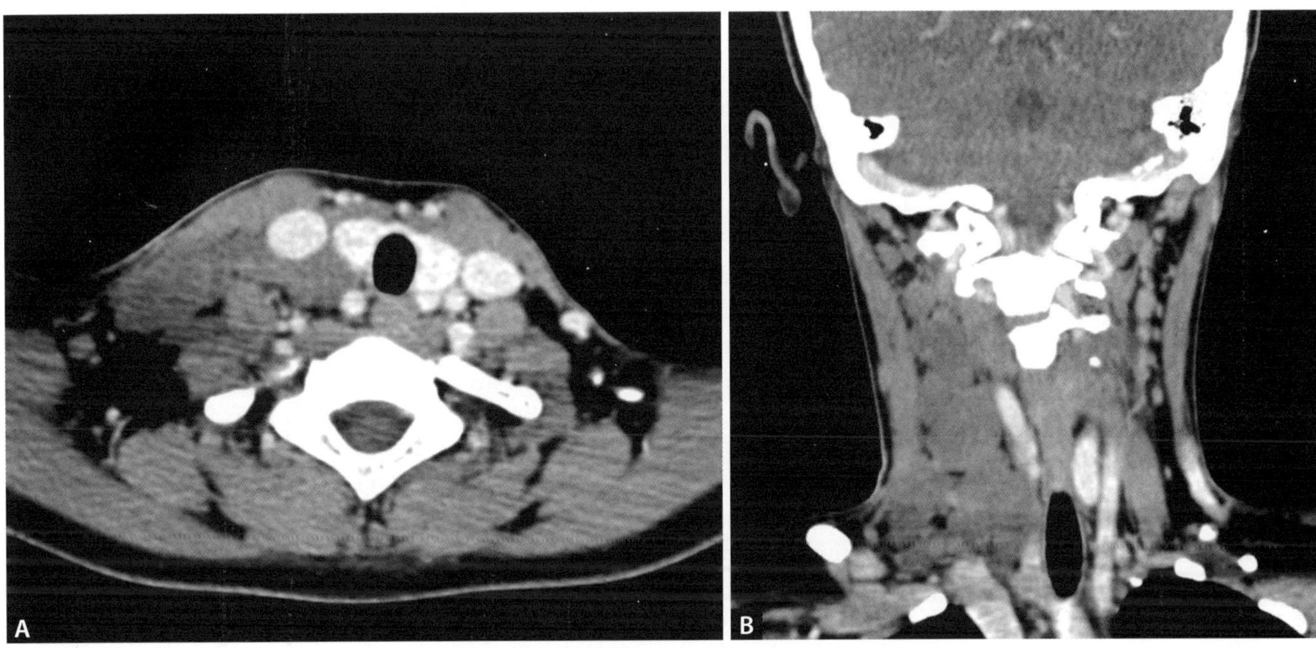

Figs. 49A and B: Axial (A) and coronal (B) CECT images show multiple enlarged necrotic lymph nodes (levels II, III, IV, V) on right side, showing conglomeration—Tubercular lymphadenopathy.

localized or generalized. The causes include drugs, foreign antigens, chemicals and infectious agents. Lymph nodes are enlarged with preserved reniform shape and show mild enhancement with enhancing linear markings. Reactive lymphadenopathy is commonly seen in children following upper respiratory tract infections.

Necrotic Lymphadenopathy

Necrotic lymph nodes show central necrosis due to inadequate vascular supply and can be seen with metastatic disease and necrotizing granulomatous disease like tuberculosis **(Figs. 49A and B)**. The frequency of nodal necrosis increases with metastatic nodal size. Therefore, the detection of nodal necrosis in isolation is most helpful if the necrotic nodes are less than 10 mm and there are no other abnormal nodes.

Contrast enhanced CT shows low central density. On MR, central low signal intensity is seen on T1WI with central hyperintensity on T2WI. Diffusion-weighted imaging can show diffusion restriction, and low apparent diffusion coefficient (ADC) values ($<1.0 \times 10^3$ mm^2/s) can be seen within malignant nodal disease, similar to primary site ADC values. Contrast enhanced MR imaging shows low signal intensity with no enhancement in the central aspect with surrounding enhancement of the part of the lymph nodes that have increased vascular supply. US reveals decreased central echogenicity with increased through transmission, similar to suppurative nodal disease.[41]

If a suspected necrotic lymph node is detected a consideration of tuberculosis and metastatic disease should be kept in mind. Age and smoking history should be taken into account, although some cancers, such as human papillomavirus positive (HPV1) squamous cell carcinomas can occur in younger adults without a smoking history.[42] These are most frequently found in the oropharynx and may be associated with necrotic nodal disease which may mimic cysts.

Suppurative lymph nodes are pus-containing lymph nodes and are also referred to as adenitis, acute lymphadenitis, or intranodal abscess and are commonly seen in children and young adults. The retropharyngeal, jugulodigastric, and submandibular group of lymph nodes are commonly involved. The nodes show similar characteristics as that of necrotic nodes and appear oval to round, cystic and often have poorly defined margins; stranding of the surrounding fat and subcutaneous tissue may be seen. Clinical history may be useful to differentiate between necrotic and suppurative lymphadenopathy.

Calcified Lymphadenopathy

Calcified lymph nodes can be seen with infection, granulomatous disease, or metastatic disease and are best evaluated with CT. Bone windows can help assess the extent of calcification and the configuration. The most important causes of calcified lymph nodes in the neck are tuberculous adenitis **(Fig. 50)** and thyroid cancer, especially metastatic papillary thyroid carcinoma. The configuration of the calcifications within the nodes is similar to the calcifications in the primary lesion helping in determining the site of origin. Lymph nodal calcification may also be seen postradiotherapy.

Matted Lymphadenopathy

It is a confluence of nodes that may be associated with surrounding fluid or inflammatory changes. They can be seen with infectious disease such as tuberculosis or metastatic disease. In squamous cell carcinomas, matted lymph nodes are associated with poor prognosis independent of T classification, HPV status, epidermal growth factor or smoking status.

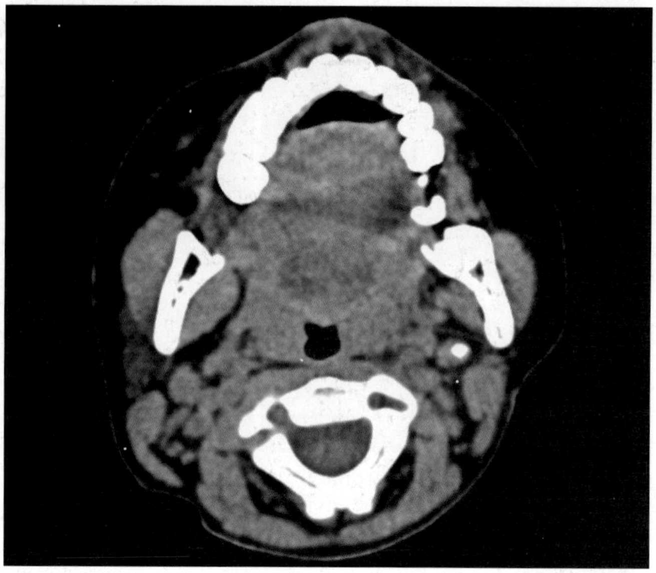

Fig. 50: Axial CT image shows cervical lymph node with a calcific focus within on left side (level II) in a known case of tuberculosis on treatment.

Diffuse Lymphadenopathy

Diffuse lymphadenopathy can be seen with infection, generalized systemic disease or neoplasms. Viral, bacterial sepsis and human immunodeficiency virus adenopathy can cause diffuse nodal involvement. Metastatic disease from lung, breast, kidney and melanoma can metastasize to the head and neck. Non-Hodgkin lymphoma and Hodgkin lymphoma can also cause diffuse cervical lymphadenopathy **(Figs. 51A to D)**. Lymphomas are usually homogeneous on CT and show variable degree of enhancement. On MRI, lymphomas are hypointense to isointense on T1WI and hyperintense on T2WI compared with muscle.

There are a few rare diseases that affect the cervical lymph nodes. *Castleman disease* is a benign lymphoproliferative disorder. Involvement of one or multiple nodal groups can be seen with more than 90% of neck lesions being unifocal.[43] Contrast enhanced CT shows moderate to marked homogenous enhancement. On MRI the nodes are hypointense or isointense on T1WI and hyperintense on T2WI. Branching striations that are hypointense on T2WI are suggestive of Castleman disease, although this is a rare finding.

Kimura disease is another disease of lymph node enlargement also known as eosinophilic lymphogranuloma or eosinophilic hyperplastic lymphogranuloma. It presents with painless unilateral cervical lymphadenopathy or subcutaneous nodules. Parotid or submandibular

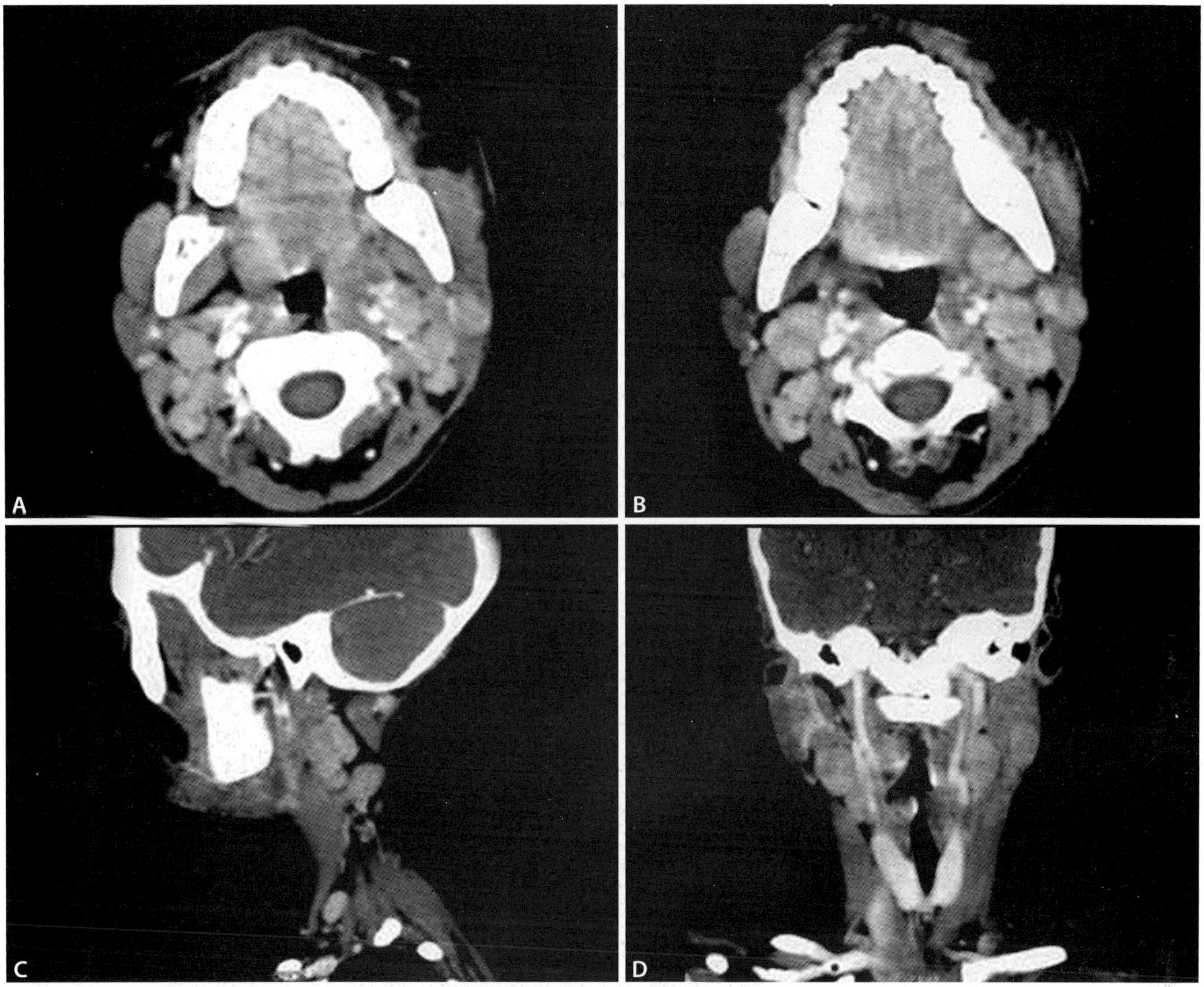

Figs. 51A to D: Axial (A and B) sagittal (C) and coronal (D) CECT scans of the neck revealing multiple varying sized round to spherical discrete lymph nodes along bilateral internal jugular veins, posterior triangle of neck and submandibular spaces s/o mitotic etiology—lymphoreticular malignancy.

gland involvement must be present, although the lacrimal gland is rarely involved.

Kikuchi disease, or Kikuchi-Fujimoto disease, is a rare, benign, self-limited disease associated with tender, regional cervical lymphadenopathy and is accompanied by mild fever and night sweats.

Rosai-Dorfman disease, or sinus histiocytosis with massive lymphadenopathy, is another very rare, benign process with proliferation of hematopoietic cells and fibrous tissue often presenting in the head and neck region. Symmetric, painless and bilateral cervical adenopathy is seen.[39]

CONCLUSION

A sound understanding of the anatomy of the spaces and contents of the suprahyoid and infrahyoid neck alongwith a systematic approach is essential for detection and characterization of neck lesions. Alongwith clinical data this helps in accurate diagnosis and providing better care for patients.

REFERENCES

1. Bannister LH, Berry MM, Collins P, Dyson M, Dussek JE, Ferguson MWJ. Grays Anatomy. Churchill Livingston: Edinburg, 1995.

2. Carlson GW. Surgical anatomy of the neck. Surgical Clinics North Am. 1993;73:837.
3. Faggioni L, Neri E, Bartolozzi C. CT Perfusion of head and neck tumors: how we do it. AJR. 2010;194:62-9.
4. Chawla S, Kim S, Wang S, et al. Diffusion-weighted imaging in head and neck cancers. Future Oncology. 2009;5(7): 959-75.
5. Bisdas S, Baghi M, Huebner F, et al. In vivo proton MR spectroscopy of primary tumors, nodal and recurrent disease of extracranial head and neck. Eur Radiol. 2007;17:251-7.
6. Fukui MB, Blodgett TM, Snyderman CH, et al. Combined PET-CT in the head and neck. Radio Graphics. 2005;25(4):913-30.
7. Cummings C, Flint P. Cummings otolaryngology—Head and Neck Surgery, 5th edition, revision. Philadelphia: Mosby Elsevier; 2010. pp. 201-8.
8. Brown W, Gleeson M. Scott-Brown's Otolaryngology, Head and Neck Surgery. 7th edition. London: Hodder Arnold; 2008.
9. Warshafsky D, Goldenberg D, Kanekar SG. Imaging anatomy of deep neck spaces. Otolaryngol Clin N Am. 2012;45:1203-21.
10. Harnsberger HR, Glastonbury CM, Michael MA, et al. Diagnositc Imaging. Head and Neck. Salt Lake City (UT): Amirsys Publishing, 2011.
11. Arya S, Rane P, D'Cruz A. Infratemporal fossa, masticator space and parapharyngeal space: can the radiologist and surgeon speak the same language? Otorhinolaryngol Clin: Int J. 2012;4(3):125-35.
12. Oliver ER, Gillespie MB. Deep neck space infections. In: Paul WF, Bruce H, Valerie JL (Eds). Cummings Otolaryngology Head and Neck Surgery (4th edition). Philadelphia, PA: Elsevier Mosby 2005; pp. 202-03.
13. Standring S. Infratemporal and Pterygopalatine Fossae and Temporomandibular Joint. In: Strandring S (Ed). Gray's Anatomy: The Anatomical Basis of Clinical Practice, 14th edition. Churchill Livingstone: Elsevier 2011; p. 527.
14. Tovi F, Hertzanu Y, Noyek AM. Infections of the infratemporal fossa: Imaging/clinical correlations. J Otolaryngol. 1991;20(Suppl 3):1-11.
15. Mukherji SK, Castillo M. A simplified approach to spaces of the suprahyoid neck. Radiol Clin North Am. 1998; 36(5):761-80.
16. Gamss C, Gupta A, Chazen JL, et al. Imaging evaluation of the suprahyoid neck. Radiol Clin N Am. 2015;53:133-44.
17. Brucker JL, Gentry LR. Imaging of head and neck emergencies. Radiol Clin N Am. 2015;53:215-52.
18. Rastogi R, Bhargava S, Mallarajapatna GJ, et al. Pictorial essay: salivary gland imaging. Indian J Radiol Imaging 2012;22:325-33.
19. La'Porte SJ, Juttla JK, Lingam RK. Imaging the floor of the mouth and the sublingual space. RadioGraphics. 2011; 31:1215-30.
20. Meuwly JY, Lepori D, Theuman N. Multi modality imaging evaluation of the paediatric neck: techniques and spectrum of findings. Radiographics. 2005;25:931-48.
21. Mills MK, Shah LM. Imaging of the perivertebral space. Radiol Clin N Am. 2015;53:163-80.
22. Meesa IR, Mukherji SK. A simplified approach to the spaces of the suprahyoid neck. Appl Radiol. 2017;46(4):6-14.
23. Win T, Lewin JS. Imaging characteristics of carotid body tumors. Am J Otol. 1995;16:325-8.
24. Yuan Y, Shi H, Tao X. Head and neck paragangliomas: diffusion weighted and dynamic contrast enhanced magnetic resonance imaging characteristics. BMC Medical Imaging. 2016;16:12.
25. Som PM, Brandwein-Gensler MS. Anatomy and pathology of the salivary glands. In: Som PM, Curtin HD (Eds). Head and Neck Imaging, 5th edition. Elsevier Mosby; 2011; pp.2449-609.
26. Colreavy MP, Lacy PD, Hughes J. Head and neck schwannomas—a 10 year review. J Laryngol Otol. 2000;114: 119-24.
27. Chung CJ, Armfield KB, Mukherji SK. Cervical neurofibromas in children with NF-I. Pediat Radiol. 1999-2000;29:353-6.
28. Turkington JRA, Paterson A, et al. Neck masses in children. BJR. 2005;78:75-85.
29. Mulliken JB, Glowacki J. Hemangiomas and vascular malformations in infants and children: a classification based on endothelial characteristics. Plast Reconstr Surg. 1982;69(3):412-22.
30. Hennedige AA, Quaba AA, Al-Nakib K. Sturge-Weber syndrome and dermatomal facial port-wine stains: incidence, association with glaucoma, and pulsed tunable dye laser treatment effectiveness. Plast Reconstr Surg. 2008;121(4):1173-80.
31. Enjolras O, Riche MC, Merland JJ. Facial port-wine stains and Sturge-Weber syndrome. Pediatrics. 1985;76(1):48-51.
32. Eivazi B, Fasunla AJ, Hundt W, et al. Low flow vascular malformations of the head and neck: a study on brightness mode, color coded duplex and spectral Doppler sonography. Eur Arch Otorhinolaryngol. 2011;268(10):1505-11.
33. Berenguer B, Burrows PE, Zurakowski D, et al. Sclerotherapy of craniofacial venous malformations: complications and results. Plast Reconstr Surg. 1999;104(1):1-11.
34. Aspestrand F, Kolbenstvedt A. Vascular mass lesions and hypervascular tumors in the head and neck. Characteristics at CT, MR imaging and angiography. Acta Radiol. 1995; 36(2):136-41.
35. Mathur NN, Rana I, Bothra R, et al. Bleomycin sclerotherapy in congenital lymphatic and vascular malformations of head and neck. Int J Pediatr Otorhinolaryngol. 2005;69(1):75-80.
36. Mulligan PR, Prajapati HJS, Martin LG, Patel TH. Vascular anomalies: classification, imaging characteristics and implications for interventional radiology treatment approaches. Br J Radiol. 2014;87:20130392.
37. Brodsky JR, Kim DY, Jiang Z. Cervical lipoblastoma. Case report review of literature and genetic analysis. Wiley Periodicals. 2007;1055-60.
38. Edge SB, Byrd DR, Compton CC, et al. Lymphoidneoplasms. AJCC Cancer Staging Manual. 7th edition. Salt Lake City (UT): Springer; 2010. p. 599-615.

39. Eisenmenger LB, Wiggins RH. Imaging of head and neck lymph nodes. Radiol Clin N Am. 2015;53:115-32.
40. Chong V. Cervical lymphadenopathy: what radiologists need to know. Cancer Imaging. 2004;4(2):116-20.
41. King AD, Tse GM, Ahuja AT, et al. Necrosis in metastatic neck nodes: diagnostic accuracy of CT, MR imaging, and US. Radiology. 2004;230(3):720-6.
42. Goldenberg D, Sciubba J, Koch WM. Cystic metastasis from head and neck squamous cell cancer: a distinct disease variant? Head Neck. 2006;28(7):633-8.
43. Liang J, Newman JG, Frank DM, et al. Cervical unicentric Castleman disease presenting as a neck mass: case report and review of the literature. Ear Nose Throat J. 2009; 88(5):E8.

CHAPTER 24

Thyroid Imaging

Alpana Manchanda, Anju Garg, Jyoti Kumar, Rashmi Dixit

INTRODUCTION

The thyroid is a bilobed butterfly or bow-tie shaped gland located anteriorly in the lower neck. Under or over production of thyroid hormones leading to thyroid dysfunction is relatively common; with blood biochemistry, ultrasonography and radionuclide scintigraphy being the mainstay of investigation and management. Lesions of the thyroid gland arise from a variety of conditions which are usually benign, but may be due to malignancy in a minority. Increasing use of high resolution ultrasonography and cross-sectional imaging like CT and MR Imaging has led to a significant increase in the detection of incidental thyroid lesions. Imaging, especially high resolution ultrasonography is highly sensitive in detecting small nodules, calcifications, septations and cysts, as well as guiding fine needle aspiration (FNA) biopsies and has a major role in the differentiation of a benign lesion from a malignant one.[1]

EMBRYOLOGY

The thyroid gland develops from median and lateral anlages. The median anlage arises in the midline of the oropharynx during the fourth to fifth gestational week and gives rise to follicular thyroid tissue, which secretes hormones. The lateral anlages are thought to arise from the ultimobranchial bodies, which in turn are derived from the fourth and fifth branchial pharyngeal pouches. They give rise to the parafollicular C cells which secrete calcitonin. Fusion of the median and lateral anlages occurs by tenth week *in utero* resulting in the bilobed form of the gland.[2]

The thyroid gland originates embryologically in the foramen caecum at the base of the tongue, and migrates to its final location in the anterior lower neck. Knowledge of the typical course of the thyroid primordium during embryologic development is important in understanding the various locations in the path where ectopic thyroid tissue can be found. From its origin at the foramen caecum, the thyroid primordeum first courses anterior to the hyoid bone then loops inferior and posterior to the hyoid and then descends anterior to the thyrohyoid membrane, thyroid cartilage and trachea into the orthotopic location in the infrahyoid neck.[3] This course of descent is represented by the remnant thyroglossal duct, which normally involutes by the 8th week of gestation along which residual thyroid tissue may be found. Descent beyond the normal results in a mediastinal component of the thyroid gland.

Very rare and unusual locations of ectopic thyroid tissue which may be detected within the neck and mediastinum are intralaryngeal, pre-laryngeal, intrapharyngeal, intra-esophageal, intratracheal, intrapericardial, intracardiac, etc. A large majority of mediastinal thyroids are retrosternal extensions of large goiters in the neck.[4]

ANATOMY

The thyroid gland is located in the lower anterior neck in the infrahyoid compartment. It is bounded by the strap muscles anteriorly and the second to fourth tracheal rings and the longus colli muscle posteriorly. The gland is made up of two lobes located lateral to the trachea, each with a superior and inferior pole. The right and left lobes are joined at the midline in front of the trachea by a thin bridge of thyroid tissue called isthmus at the junction of middle and lower one thirds of the gland. The normal dimensions of each lobe of the thyroid is less than 5 × 2 × 2 cm in longitudinal, transverse and anterior-posterior dimension respectively. The gland size varies with patient age, sex and weight and normal weight is between 15 and 35 g. The average thyroid volume in males is 19.6 mL while in females it is 18.6 mL.

An accessory lobe, the pyramidal lobe, may be present in 10–40% of normal population. It originates from the isthmus or the medial aspect of either lobe and extends superiorly along the course of the distal thyroglossal duct.[5] The pyramidal lobe can be regularly seen in younger patients. But it undergoes progressive atrophy in adulthood and becomes invisible.[6] The pyramidal lobe is most commonly recognized in patients with Graves' disease because it is enlarged and easily identified on nuclear scintigraphy.

The thyroid gland is enveloped by portions of the deep cervical fascia which attach the thyroid gland to the larynx and trachea. As a result, the thyroid gland moves with the larynx during swallowing. The entire thyroid gland is in the neck above the level of the clavicles. Sufficient enlargement of the thyroid gland results in its extension to outside the normal volume of the thyroid bed. It grows caudally into the pretracheal space and may even extend to lie in the retrosternal region, anterior to the common carotid arteries and the internal jugular veins. In this location, the thyroid enlargement is referred to as a retrosternal or substernal goiter.

The thyroid gland has a rich vascular supply, being derived from the paired superior and inferior thyroid arteries which are braches of external carotid arteries and the thyrocervical trunk respectively. The thyroidca ima is an inconstant vessel which when present arises directly from the aortic arch and helps supply the inferior thyroid gland. The venous drainage of the thyroid gland is via the superior and middle thyroidal veins which empty into internal jugular vein, and an inferior vein which drains into the innominate vein. The thyroid is innervated by the tenth cranial nerve (vagus) and the cervical sympathetic neural plexus.

ENDOCRINOLOGY

The primary function of the thyroid gland is to synthesize hormones that play a vital role in the regulation of metabolic functions. Triiodothyronine (T_3) and thyroxin (T_4) are two hormones synthesized within the thyroid. They are released from the thyroid in response to a feedback mechanism with the pituitary-hypothalamic axis. The secretion of thyroid hormones is mediated by thyrotropin-stimulating hormone (TSH) secreted by the anterior pituitary gland. Pituitary secretion of TSH, is in turn regulated by thyrotropin-releasing hormone (TRH) secreted by the hypothalamus. T_3 is three to four times more active physiologically than T_4. T_4 is synthesized entirely within the gland while 80–95% of T3 is synthesized by peripheral conversion of T_4. **Table 1** shows the normal reference range of thyroid hormones.

Table 1: Normal reference ranges of thyroid hormones.

Thyroid hormones		*Normal range*
Thyroxin	T_4	4.5–12.0 µg/dL
Triiodothyronine	T_3	90–200 ng/dL
Thyroid-stimulating hormone	TSH	0.4–4.5 µIU/mL
Free T_4 (0.03% of T_4)	FT_4	0.7–1 6 ng/dL
Free T_3 (0.4% of T_3)	FT_3	230–420 ng/L

Calcitonin is a hormone produced by the parafollicular (C cells) of the thyroid gland in response to high calcium levels in the bloodstream and helps in regulating calcium and phosphate levels in the blood.

CLINICAL MANIFESTATIONS OF THYROID DISEASE

The spectrum of symptoms of thyroid disease is varied and the clinical manifestations are due to an increased or decreased function of the thyroid gland. **Hyperthyroidism** refers to a sustained thyroid hyperfunction with increase in synthesis and release of thyroid hormone. **Thyrotoxicosis** refers to a clinical syndrome that develops when circulating levels of T_4 and T_3 are markedly increased (TSH is usually suppressed). It is manifested by a multitude of symptoms including warmth, increased heat loss, weight loss, myopathy and increased appetite. Cardiac manifestations are more common in older patients and include tachycardia, palpitations, arrhythmias and cardiomegaly.

Thyrotoxicosis associated with hyperthyroidism is most frequently seen with Graves' disease (autoimmune thyroiditis) but may also be seen in toxic multinodular goiter (MNG) or a hyperfunctioning adenoma. Thyrotoxicosis not associated with hyperthyroidism (low radioactive iodine uptake) may be related to inflammatory thyroid disease or ectopic thyroid tissue (ovarian strumii).

Thyroid storm may present as a clinical emergency in patients with unrecognized or inadequately treated thyrotoxicosis. It is characterized by hypertension, tachycardia and fever and if unrecognized, may result in death.

Thyroid ophthalmopathy is most commonly seen in Graves' disease and hyperthyroidism. It is more common in women and presents with proptosis secondary to enlargement of the extraocular muscles. A characteristic feature is enlargement of the muscle bellies with sparing of the tendinous insertions. The common patterns of extraocular muscle involvement are enlargement of inferior rectus muscle alone, enlargement of inferior rectus and medial rectus muscles, and enlargement of all of the muscles.[7] Relative sparing of the lateral rectus muscle is usually seen and isolated involvement of this muscle should raise the suspicion of a different disease process such as myositis or pseudotumor.

Hypothyroidism refers to a decrease in synthesis of thyroid hormone (serum TSH is high, while T_3 and T_4 levels are low). Primary hypothyroidism may be secondary to structural or functional derangements of the thyroid gland. In adults it most often results from processes that destroy thyroid tissue such as autoimmune disease or ^{131}I treatment. In children it may be related to enzyme deficiencies, defects in organification or congenital anomalies such as lingual thyroid or thyroid agenesis.

Enlargement of the thyroid gland is most commonly seen in multinodular goiter with other causes of enlargement being neoplastic and inflammatory processes. Many of the secondary manifestations of thyroid disease are frequently responsible for the clinical presentation in patients. The most common effect of glandular enlargement is compression of the adjacent structures such as trachea and esophagus which may result in respiratory distress and dysphagia. Similarly, there may be compression and displacement of the jugular vein and carotid artery. The recurrent laryngeal nerve travels in the tracheoesophageal groove and thyroid lesions that extend to this area may present with vocal cord paralysis.

IMAGING

Plain Radiographs

Soft tissue radiographs of the neck in anteroposterior (AP) and lateral projections show the enlarged thyroid in the pretracheal location, associated calcification within the mass and deviation and narrowing of trachea. The tracheal shift or deviation is appreciated in the AP view while the degree of narrowing is assessed on the lateral view **(Figs. 1A and B)**. This information is important to the anesthetist for intubation prior to surgery. Plain X-rays of the neck and upper chest also demonstrate retrosternal extension of a thyroid mass, and any associated bony destruction.

Nuclear Scintigraphy

Nuclear scintigraphy provides excellent functional information about the thyroid because the radionuclides

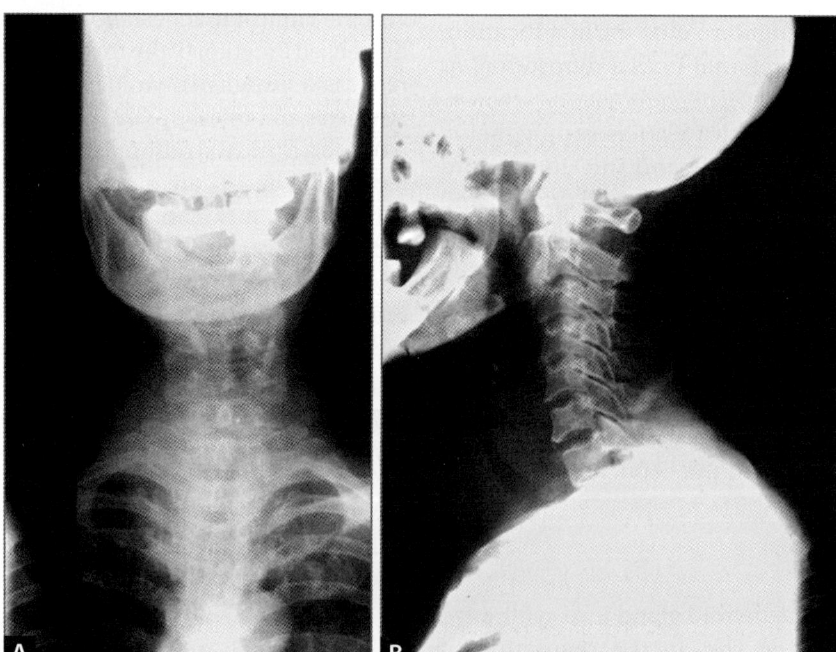

Figs. 1A and B: Plain radiographs (A) Anteroposterior; and (B) Lateral view of the neck show a soft tissue opacity in the right lower neck with tracheal deviation to the left with increase in prevertebral space suggestive of retrotracheal extension. Significant narrowing of the trachea is seen opposite C_5-C_6 intervertebral disc space.

used to image the gland do so by utilizing some step of hormone synthesis within the thyroid. Thyroid scintigraphy is a reflection of the functional as well as physiological state of the gland and provides information that cross-sectional imaging such as USG, CT or MRI lack. The major role of scintigraphy is in the evaluation of patients with abnormal thyroid function tests, especially hyperthyroidism. It can ascertain if the cause of hyperthyroidism is a diffuse process such as Graves' disease or an autonomously functioning nodule. A patient with hyperfunctioning nodule once identified on scintigraphy does not require tissue sampling.

Scintigraphy of a focal thyroid lesion in euthyroid patients determines if the lesion is "hot" (more uptake than the normal thyroid gland), warm (some activity but not as much as the normal gland) or cold (little or no uptake). A functioning "hot" lesion has an extremely low incidence of malignancy, while the reported risk of malignancy of a non-functioning "cold" lesion ranges from 5% to 25%. The majority (~95%) of the nodules are cold, and advancements in other imaging modalities, especially ultrasonography, has resulted in scintigraphy being less utilized in the evaluation of focal thyroid nodules.[8]

Table 2 lists the various radionuclides used in thyroid imaging.[2,5,8-11]

Nuclear imaging is done with a gamma scintillation camera. The normal thyroid gland shows homogeneous radionuclide uptake and distribution while the isthmus may show slightly less activity than the thyroid lobes.

Thyroid uptake reflects the percentage of the dose given to the patient that is accumulated within the thyroid gland corrected for radioactive decay. Normal 24 hours uptake ranges from 10 to 30%. Several medications and iodine-containing contrast agents used for imaging may temporarily interfere with the organification of iodine, altering radioactive iodine uptake measurements for as long as 6 weeks. The uptake of radioactive iodine may be reduced to one half of the expected one week following the injection of iodinated contrast agent for a CT scan. Also, in more than one third of patients with underlying thyroid disease, temporary changes in thyroid function can occur following injection of iodinated contrast agent.

Table 2: Various radionuclides with their indications used in thyroid imaging.

Radionuclide with half life	*Indication*	*Route of administration*	*Time of imaging after administration*	*Remarks*
^{99m}Tc pertechnetate $t_{1/2}$ = 6.02hr	Preferred for anatomical evaluation	Intravenous	20 minutes	• Higher dose can be administered. • Permits higher resolution.
^{123}I $t_{1/2}$ = 13.6 hr	• For obtaining 24-hour thyroid iodine uptake. • Gives true assessment of diffuse/focal regions of uptake	Oral	4–24 hours	• Shorter half-life resulting in lower radiation • Better resolution
^{131}I	• In whole body scan. *Diagnostic*: (i) Post-thyroidectomy patients in the operative bed; (ii) To assess for recurrent/distant metastasis; (iii) To detect ectopic thyroid tissue such as struma ovarii. • It is preferred for imaging substernal thyroid as it has high radiation energy (36 KeV) • *Diagnostic and therapeutic*: In the evaluation and treatment of patients with thyroid cancer that concentrate iodine	Oral	24–72 hours	• Limited spatial resolution requires 2–3 sittings for 24 hour scintigraphy. • Is subject to the effects of diet and medicine
^{18}FDG-PET $t_{1/2}$ = 110 minutes	• In the follow-up of patients treated for thyroid cancer due to increased glucose metabolism by malignant tumors. • In metastatic thyroid tumors that do not concentrate radioiodine In the evaluation of patients with rising thyroglobulin levels following thyroidectomy	Intravenous		

Hence, if cross-section imaging is necessary in a patient undergoing nuclear scans with iodinated radionuclides, one should perform a CT scan after nuclear scintigraphy, or go for MR imaging instead of CT or perform a non-contrast CT.

Medications which interfere with thyroid function should be withdrawn for adequate period of time prior to nuclear scanning.

Ultrasonography

The superficial location of the thyroid allows excellent visualization and evaluation of its normal anatomy and pathologic condition by high-resolution real-time gray-scale sonography. As a result it plays an important role in the diagnostic evaluation of thyroid diseases. The advents of high resolution ultrasound and FNA biopsy have decreased the indications for radionuclide thyroid scanning. Ultrasonography is generally the first choice for the evaluation of thyroid morphology because of its sensitivity for small nodule detection. The spatial resolution achieved by ultrasound is of the order of 0.5–1 mm, not achieved by any other imaging method.[6]

Technique

Real-time ultrasound of the thyroid gland is usually performed with high-resolution linear array transducers ranging from 7.5 to 15 MHz.[6] These allow excellent visualization of not only the superficial portions of the gland but also evaluate the deeper structures posteriorly to the level of the spine. With the patient in supine position, the neck is mildly hyperextended and the thyroid gland is imaged in its entirety in both the transverse and longitudinal planes. A small pad placed under the shoulders provides a better exposure of the neck especially in patients with a short, stocky built. Imaging of the lower poles can be improved by asking the patient to swallow, which momentarily raises the thyroid gland in the neck. The carotid arteries and jugular veins are posterior and lateral to the thyroid lobes respectively and provide excellent anatomic landmarks during the examination. The entire gland, including the isthmus, must be examined. The examination should also extend laterally to include the region of the carotid artery and jugular vein to identify enlarged jugular chain lymph nodes, superiorly to visualize submandibular adenopathy, and inferiorly to define any pathologic supraclavicular lymph nodes.

The sternohyoid and omohyoid muscles are seen as thin, hypoechoic bands anterior to the thyroid gland **(Figs. 2A and B)**. The sternocleidomastoid is seen as a larger oval band that lies lateral to the thyroid gland. The longus colli is an important anatomic landmark that is located posterior to each thyroid lobe, in close contact with the prevertebral space. The recurrent laryngeal nerve and the inferior thyroid artery pass in the angle between the trachea, esophagus and the thyroid lobe. On longitudinal scans, the recurrent laryngeal nerve and inferior thyroid artery may be seen between the thyroid lobe and esophagus on the left and the thyroid lobe and longus colli muscle on the right. The esophagus may be seen laterally more on the left side than in the midline and is identified by its target appearance in the transverse plane.

Appearance

Normal thyroid parenchyma has homogeneous medium to high-level echoes that makes detection of focal cystic hypoechoic thyroid lesions possible. The more hypoechoic a focal lesion is relative to the normal thyroid gland, the higher the likelihood of malignancy. The capsule of the thyroid gland is identifiable by ultrasound and appears as a thin, hypoechoic line that bounds the thyroid lobes. Measurement of the dimensions of the thyroid lobe is an important part of ultrasound examination if diffuse thyroid pathology is suspected.[1] In adults, the mean longitudinal dimension (length) varies from 40 to 60 mm and the mean anteroposterior dimension (depth) is between 13–18 mm. The mean thickness of the isthmus is 4–6 mm. Among the linear parameters, anteroposterior diameter is the most precise and relatively independent measurement that is remarkably constant among individuals. When it is greater than 2 cm, it is suggestive of underlying thyroid pathology that is not sonographically visible, and when it is above 2.5 cm it is considered grossly abnormal.[12]

Ultrasound is an accurate method to use in calculating thyroid volume. Thyroid volume measurements may be useful for determining the size of the goiter, to assess the need for surgery, to permit calculation of the dose of iodine ^{131}I needed for treating thyrotoxicosis and to evaluate the response to suppression treatments. The most common mathematical method to calculate thyroid volume is based on the ellipsoid formula with a correction factor (length × width × thickness × 0.52 for each lobe). By this method the mean estimated error is around 15%.[13] The normal volume in adults ranges from 12 to 15 ± 3 mL. Thyroid volume is found to be larger in patients living in regions of iodine deficiency, and in patients who have acute hepatitis or chronic renal failure, while a smaller volume is seen in patients who have chronic hepatitis or have been treated with thyroxine or radioactive iodine.[6]

The thyroid gland is one of the most vascular organs of the body. The rich vascularity of the gland can be very well

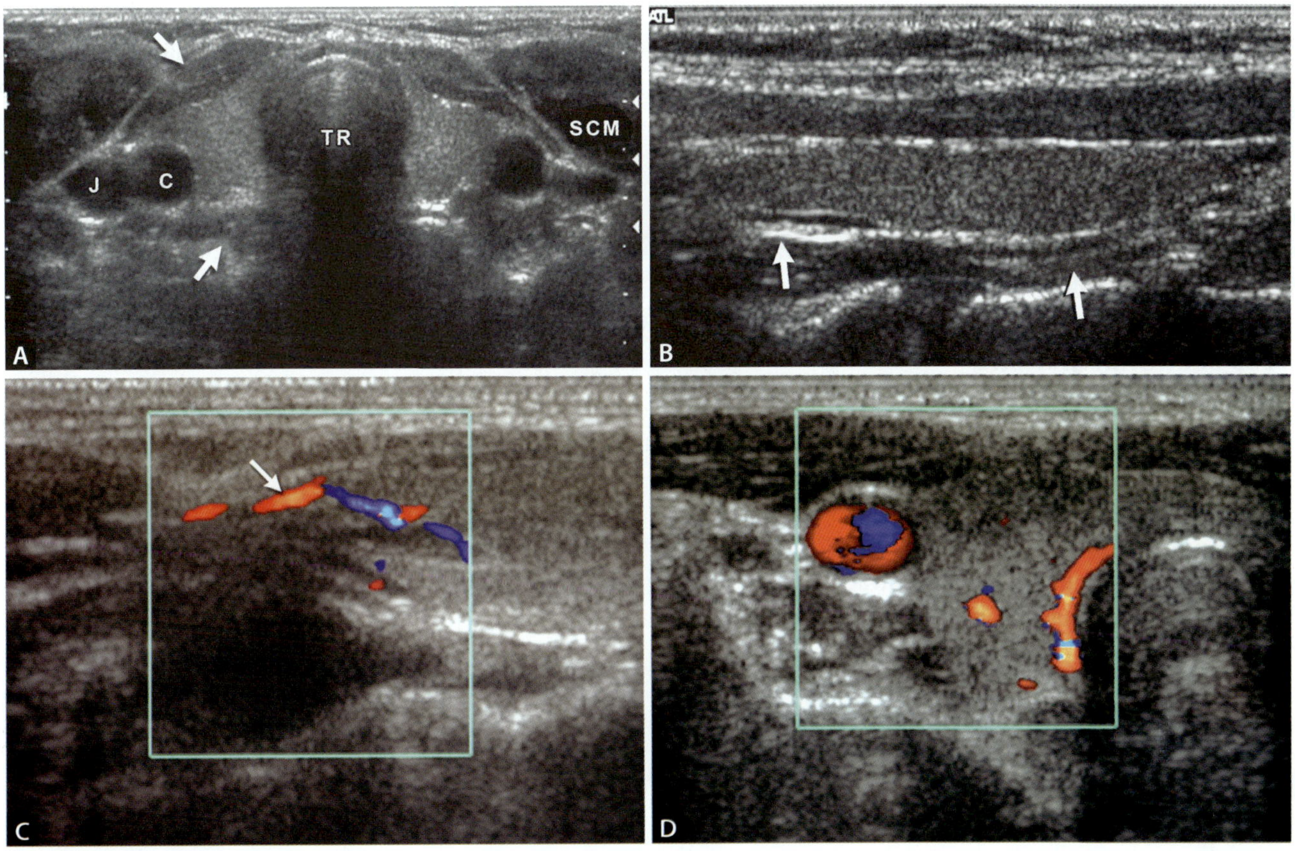

Figs. 2A to D: (A) High-resolution sonogram of the normal thyroid gland in transverse section shows homogeneous high level echoes of the parenchyma. The right and left lobes are connected by the isthmus in front of the trachea (TR). The common carotid artery (C) and internal jugular vein (J) are seen posterolaterally in relation to each lobe. The strap muscles are anterior to the thyroid gland while the longus colli is located posterior to each thyroid lobe (arrows).' (B) Longitudinal scan showing the thin linear sonolucent recurrent laryngeal nerve (arrow) posterior to the left lobe of the thyroid. CDFI showing the vascularity of the thyroid gland being supplied by (C) superior thyroid artery and (D) inferior thyroid artery.
Abbreviation: SCM: Sternocleidomastoid muscle.

seen on Doppler. The superior thyroid artery and vein are found at the upper pole of each lobe. The inferior thyroid vein is found at the lower pole, and the inferior thyroid artery is located posterior to the lower third of each lobe **(Figs. 2C and D)**. Normally the peak systolic velocities in the major thyroid arteries are 20–40 cm/sec and 15–30 cm/sec in intraparenchymal arteries. These are the highest velocities found in blood vessels supplying superficial organs.[13]

Ultrasound also provides guidance for performing FNA/biopsy thereby obviating the need for an expensive, long and often nondiagnostic workup of a palpable nodule. Evaluation of retrotracheal and mediastinal lesions is difficult by ultrasound because of acoustic shadowing from overlying air or bone.[14] Another limitation of ultrasound is in evaluating for extension of thyroid disease into the soft tissues of the neck or chest.[15]

US Elastography

Ultrasound elastography (USE) is a noninvasive ultrasound based technology which has been developed to evaluate tissue stiffness objectively. It is analogous to manual palpation which is a basic and important method of assessment of thyroid nodules, wherein malignant nodules tend to be harder than benign ones. Conventional ultrasound does not provide any information corresponding to hardness of a nodule. Ultrasound elastography using the technique of **strain elastography** evaluates the degree of distortion of a tissue when an external force is applied and is based on the principle that when compressed, softer parts deform easily compared to harder parts. Elastography has been found to be useful in differentiating malignant from benign thyroid nodules, because malignant nodules are harder than benign nodules as well as surrounding adjacent parenchyma and deform less and exhibit less strain (change in size or shape in response to external compression or stress). **Shear wave or ARFI** (acoustic radiation force impulse) **elastography** is used to evaluate elasticity of tissues quantitatively with stiffer the tissue, the greater is the shear wave velocity (SWV), expressed in m/s. Shear wave elastography has been extensively used in the differentiation of malignant from benign thyroid nodules and also in the evaluation of various diffuse thyroid pathologies.[16]

Cross-sectional Imaging

CT and MR imaging not only provide better delineation of lesions within the thyroid, but also play a critical role in the detection of lymph node metastasis as well as extension of thyroid disease to adjacent tissues in the neck and mediastinum **(Figs. 3A and B)**. Specifically, invasion of paraspinal musculature, esophagus, trachea and carotid sheath structures may be assessed.[17] Cross-sectional imaging is also useful for the evaluation of recurrent disease following treatment of thyroid cancer.

For CT and MR examination, patients are scanned in the supine position with the neck mildly hyperextended when possible, with quiet breathing and suspended swallowing. Contiguous 5 mm thick axial sections are obtained from the level of the base of the tongue superiorly and extend inferiorly into the superior mediastinum to include the aortic arch. When small lesions are being evaluated thin sections (1–3 mm) may be obtained.[15]

On CT the normal thyroid gland is typically seen at or just below the level of the cricoid cartilage.[18] It appears on noncontrast CT as two wedge shaped structures of homogeneous attenuation on either side of the trachea, connected by a narrow isthmus. The normal thyroid gland because of its iodine content has a density of approximately 80 to 100 Hounsfield units on noncontrast CT. It enhances homogenously following intravenous administration of iodinated contrast **(Figs. 4A and B)**. While iodinated contrast may provide additional information about lesions within the thyroid, such contrast will alter radioactive iodine uptake measurements for up to 6 weeks following the study. MR is superior to CT in this regard as MR contrast (gadolinium) does not interfere with iodine uptake or organification by thyroid and hence, may be used in conjunction with scintigraphy.

The role of MR imaging of thyroid has expanded with the development of dedicated surface coils. MRI is best performed with a dedicated surface coil centred over the thyroid gland. Using a surface coil with small field of view allows greater signal to noise ratios and higher resolution than the standard body or head coil. Nodules as small as 4mm size can be detected.[8] Multiple pulse sequences are obtained including non-contrast sagittal, coronal and axial T1-weighted images, as well as axial fast spin-echo T2-weighted images with the application of fat saturation. As the lesions may be hyperintense and fat in the neck is hyperintense on T1W and T2W images, fat suppression is necessary to increase the conspicuity of the lesion.[8]

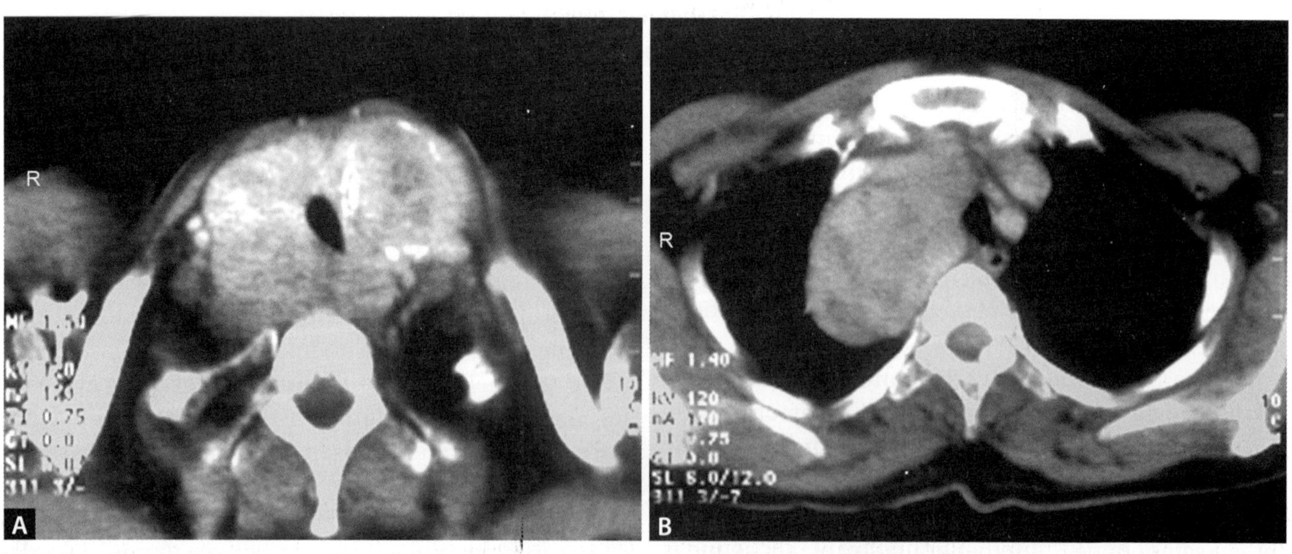

Figs. 3A and B: (A) CECT shows enlarged, heterogeneous enhancement of both lobes of thyroid (R > L) with attenuation of tracheal airway. Bilateral carotid sheaths are displaced laterally by the thyroid. However, fat planes are well maintained; (B) Mass shows retrosternal extension.

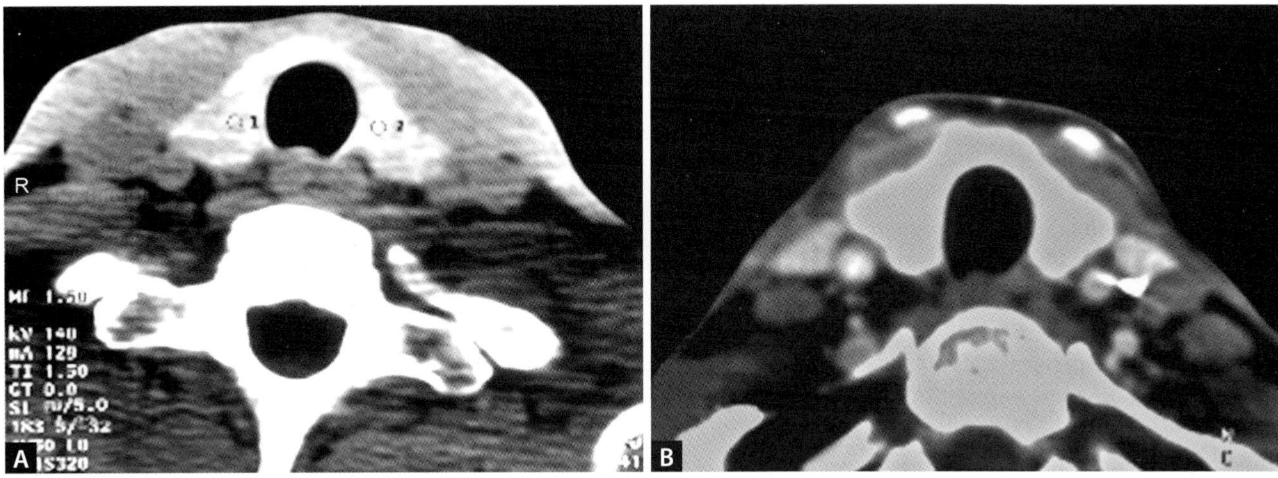

Figs. 4A and B: Axial noncontrast and contrast-enhanced sections through the lower neck show the normal thyroid gland with homogeneous enhancement on postcontrast images with normal relation and enhancement of the carotid arteries and jugular veins.

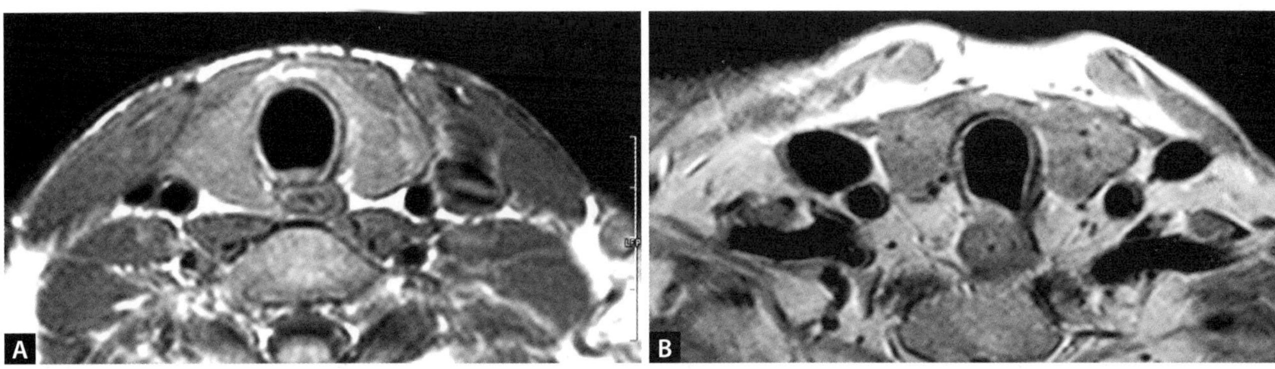

Figs. 5A and B: Normal thyroid gland on MR imaging: Unenhanced axial T1- and T2-weighted MR images show the normal appearance of the thyroid gland which is homogeneously hyperintense to the neck musculature. The vessels, carotid artery and jugular vein are seen as signal void posterolateral to the lobes of thyroid.

Following intravenous contrast administration (0.1 mmol/kg), axial T1-weighted images with fat saturation are usually acquired. On T1-weighted images, normal thyroid gland shows homogeneous signal intensity slightly greater than that of the neck musculature. On T2-weighted images, the thyroid gland is hyperintense relative to the neck musculature **(Figs. 5A and B)**. The normal gland enhances diffusely and homogeneously following contrast administration.

MR imaging provides excellent depiction of the internal parenchyma of the thyroid gland as well as relationship with adjacent structures in the neck and thoracic inlet. It is useful in identifying metastasis to regional nodes, however it is not effective in differentiating benign from malignant causes of lymphadenopathy.[19] MR has also been used to differentiate postoperative recurrence from scar tissue in patients of thyroid carcinoma. On T2-weighed images, postoperative recurrent mass is usually of medium to high signal intensity while scar tissue in the operative bed usually reveals low signal intensity.[20] However, postoperative edema, infection or hemorrhage may simulate a recurrent tumor. MR imaging has been recommended in conjunction with ^{131}I radioisotope scanning for confusing postoperative cases.[21]

PATHOLOGY OF THE THYROID GLAND

Developmental Anomalies

Abnormal development or aberrant caudal descent of the thyroid gland results in a variety of congenital anomalies. Arrest of descent can occur anywhere from the tongue down to the lower neck. The anatomic course of the embryologic thyroid tissue provides a road map for the possible locations of thyroglossal duct cyst and ectopic thyroid as these masses typically occur in lingual, suprahyoid and infrahyoid locations.[3]

Lingual Thyroid

Complete failure of descent of the thyroid gland results in a lingual thyroid at the base of the tongue, in midline. It is the most common type of functioning ectopic thyroid tissue accounting for as much as 90% of reported cases.[3] In such cases up to 75% of patients have no functioning thyroid tissue in the neck.[5] If the tissue at the base of the tongue is not recognized as thyroid and resected, the patient may become acutely and severely hypothyroid.[8]

Nuclear imaging plays a major role in establishing the diagnosis of a lingual thyroid gland as well as determining whether there is normal functioning thyroid tissue in the neck. However, a normal thyroid gland can trap majority of the radionuclide due to which it may be difficult to identify small ectopic rests.[3] On noncontrast CT, lingual thyroid is hyperdense due to its iodine content and on MR imaging it has high signal intensity on T1-weighted and T2-weighted images compared to the tongue musculature with avid enhancement following contrast administration **(Figs. 6A to C)**.

Overdescent of the thyroid may result in ectopic thyroid in the lower neck or mediastinum. Scintigraphy using 99Tc pertechnetate or ^{123}I should be performed when ectopic thyroid is suspected. Other developmental anomalies of the thyroid gland include agenesis or hemiagenesis of one lobe with normal formation of the contralateral lobe and isthmus. In rare occasions, thyroid tissue may be found in remote locations, such as within the heart and within ovarian teratomas (struma ovarii).[5]

Thyroglossal Duct Cyst (TDC)

Incomplete degeneration of the thyroglossal duct (it normally involutes during the eighth to tenth week) may result in a persistent fistulous tract or a thyroglossal duct cyst along the path of migration of the thyroid. **Figure 7** is the schematic representation for the course of thyroglossal duct. Thyroglossal duct cysts are anterior midline cystic neck masses and are commonly occurring congenital masses. They may occur anywhere along the course of the duct but typically occur at or above the hyoid bone. About 15% of thyroglossal duct cysts are at the hyoid bone level, 20% at suprahyoid level and 65% are in infrahyoid location, splaying the strap muscles or are embedded deep within them.[3] Suprahyoid cysts are more likely to be in midline while infrahyoid lesions are paramedian in location.[22] When large, these cysts are detected clinically. Vertical motion of the mass with swallowing or tongue protrusion is highly suggestive of thyroid origin. Small thyroglossal duct cysts are usually occult clinically and may be recognized only when they are secondarily infected or traumatized, or noted incidentally on imaging studies of the neck performed for unrelated reasons.[15] They usually present before 20 years of age and occur four to five times more frequently in females than males.[17]

Imaging Features

Being superficial, thyroglossal duct cyst (TDC) are easily assessed by ultrasound which is the initial investigation of choice. On sonography, they have typical features of a cyst. They may also show internal echoes when the contents are proteinaceous or get infected. On cross-sectional imaging, uncomplicated thyroglossal cysts are usually well demarcated. Sagittal reconstruction on CT and sagittal MR imaging can help in the detection of TDC and ectopic thyroid tissue as these two masses

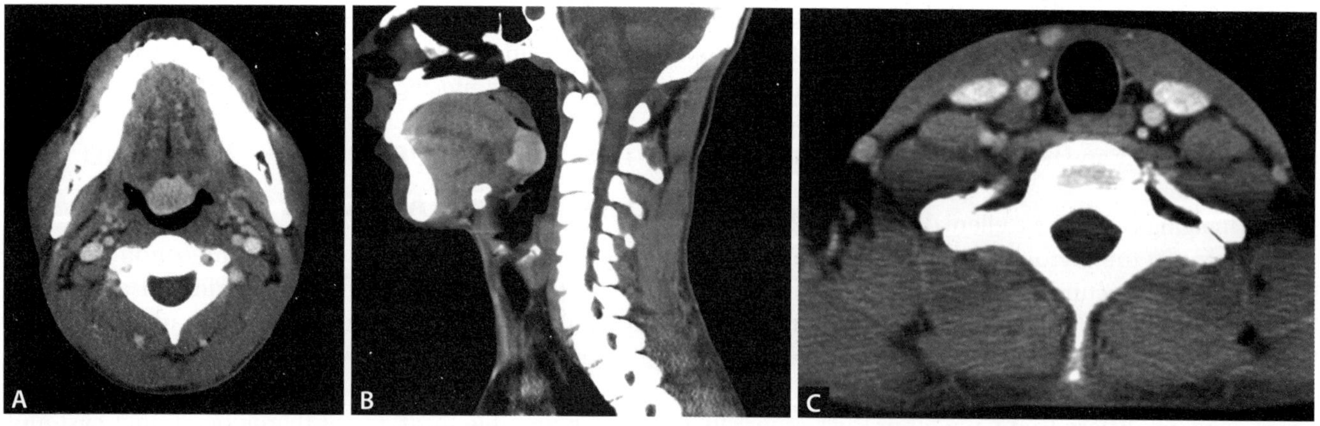

Figs. 6A to C: (A and B) Axial and sagittal CECT of the neck shows a well-defined homogeneous markedly hyperdense tissue at the base of the tongue in the midline; (C) Axial CT of the lower neck reveals absence of normal thyroid tissue in the neck. Findings consistent with **lingual thyroid**.

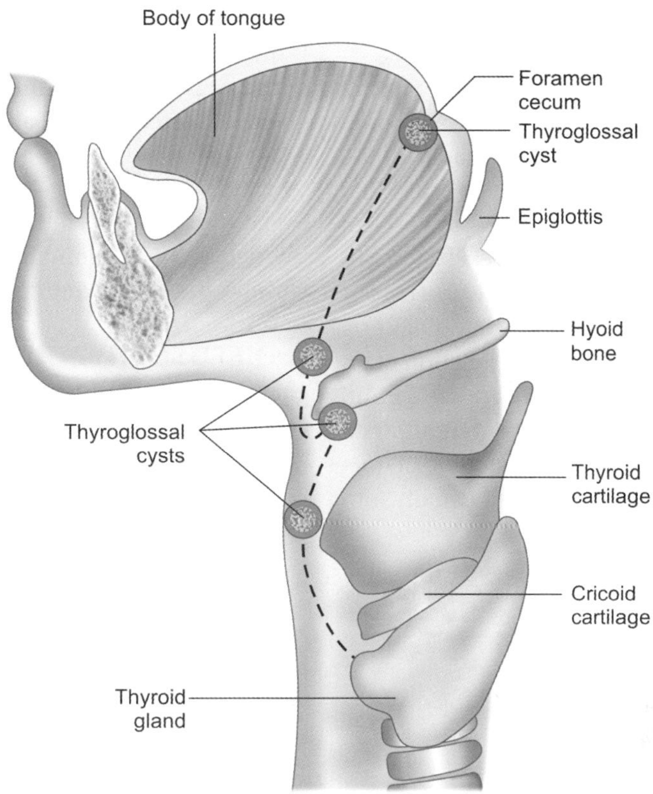

Fig. 7: Schematic diagram showing the course of thyroglossal duct and possible locations of thyroglossal duct cysts from foramen cecum to anterior lower neck.

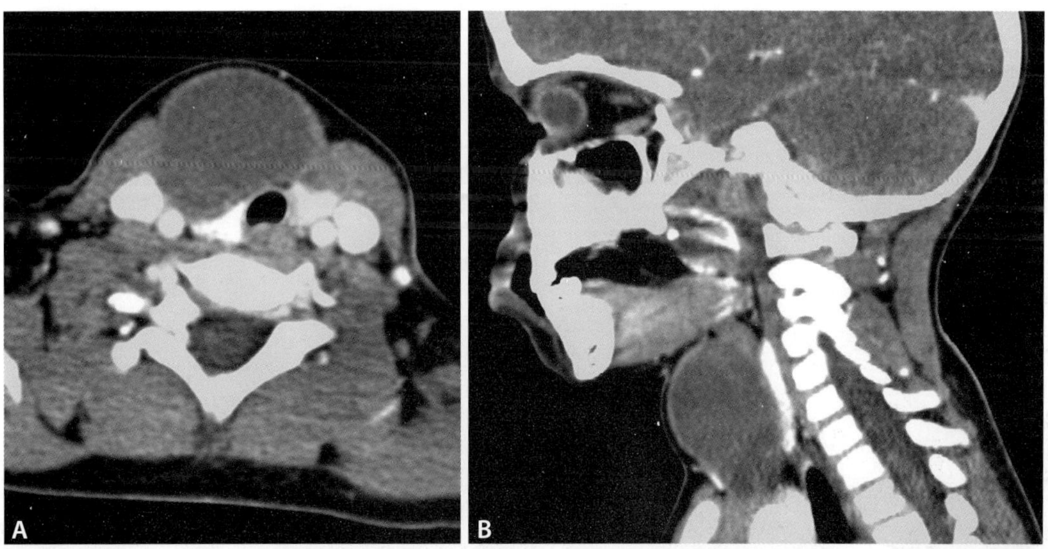

Figs. 8A and B: Contrast-enhanced axial CT with sagittal reformation in a 10-year-old child shows a well-defined, rounded lesion of fluid attenuation in the lower neck in the midline anterior to and abutting the right lobe of thyroid: **Thyroglossal duct cyst**.

are typically midline.[3] On CT they are isodense to water **(Figs. 8A and B)**, however, they may be hyperdense when there is high protein content. On MR the intensity is like CSF on T1-weighted and T2-weighted images. If the contents are proteinaceous, cysts become hyperintense on T1-weighted images, but remain intermediate to hyperintense on T2-weighted scans.[15] Enhancement is uncommon in thyroglossal duct cysts unless it has been traumatized or infected. Then, a peripheral rim enhancement or internal septations may be seen.

Nuclear scintigraphy is usually not necessary in the evaluation of thyroglossal duct cysts. Cross-sectional imaging is usually not needed in children because of the clinical presentation of painless midline neck mass that moves on swallowing. Ultrasonography helps to confirm the normal position of the thyroid before surgery. CT or MR is usually performed preoperatively in cases of suspected thyroglossal duct cyst in adults to confirm the diagnosis and to exclude other nodal masses. It is the location of an infrahyoid thyroglossal duct cyst in the strap muscles, and not its signal or attenuation characteristics that allows a definitive diagnosis on imaging.[17] Rarely, thyroglossal duct cysts may undergo malignant degeneration, usually into papillary carcinoma.

On imaging, carcinoma in a TDC should be considered if there is soft tissue in a midline cystic mass associated with irregular calcification, along with a normal thyroid gland. An infected TDC also shows increased density and a thickened wall. A congenital dermoid cyst can appear as a cystic midline mass but can be differentiated from a TDC if fat is detected within the lesion. Also, unlike a thyroglossal duct remnant, a dermoid tumor is usually not closely related to the strap muscles.

DIFFUSE THYROID DISEASE

Several thyroid diseases are characterized by diffuse rather than focal enlargement of the gland. Goiter is the term for the generalized enlargement of the gland and may be seen with hyperthyroidism or hypothyroidism **(Figs. 9A to D)**.

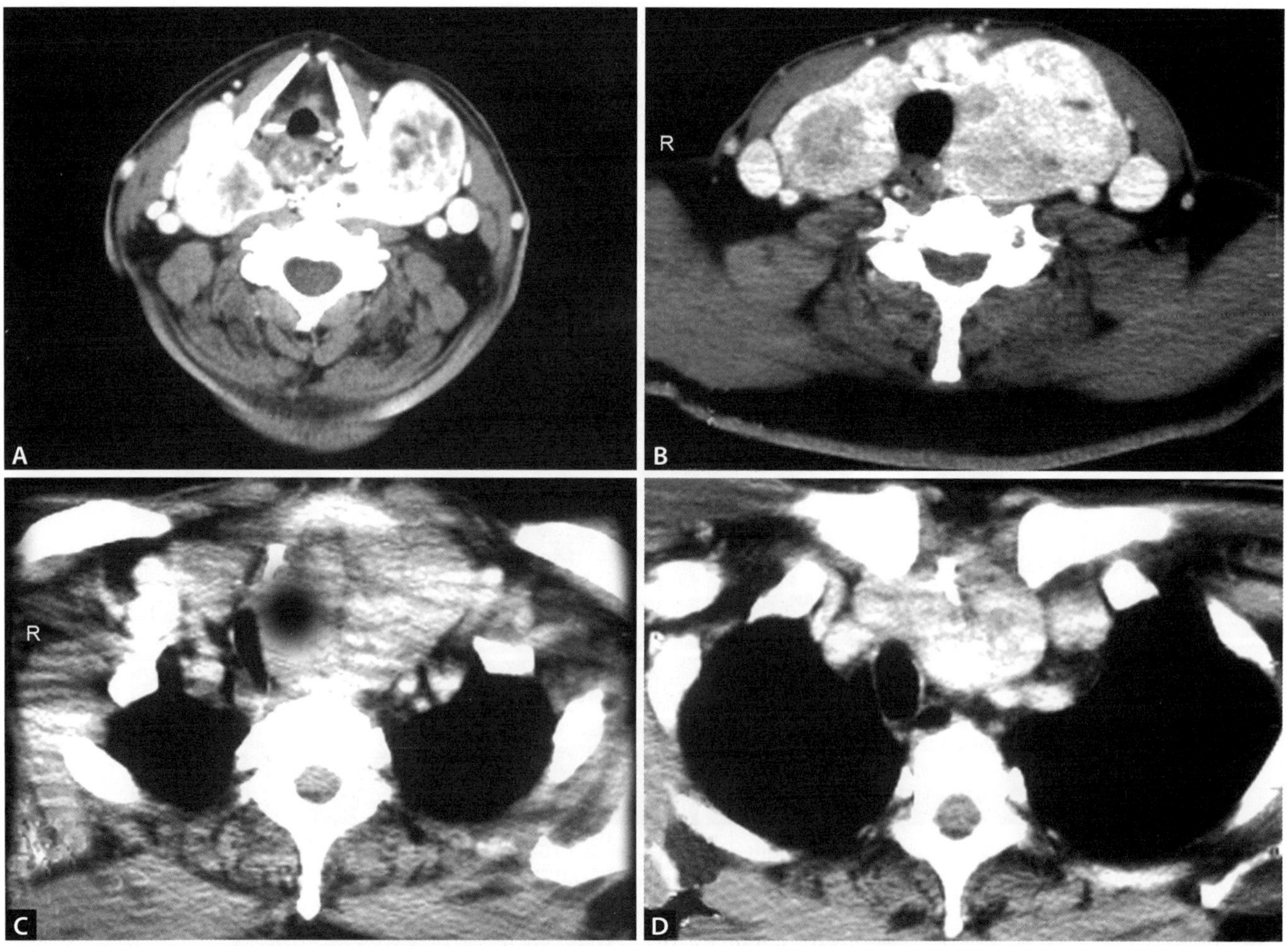

Figs. 9A to D: (A and B) CECT showing a densely enhancing thyroid with multiple hypodense nodules in both lobes and isthmus of thyroid. It is seen to extend posteromedially in the retrolaryngeal region; (C and D) The left lobe of thyroid is markedly enlarged, causing attenuation and complete deviation of the trachea to the right. Foci of calcification and necrosis are seen in the gland which extends below the medial end of both clavicles: **Multinodular goiter**.

Table 3: Diffuse thyroid diseases.

• Diffuse nontoxic goiter (Adenomatous or colloid goiter)
• Diffuse toxic goiter (Graves' disease)
• Chronic lymphocytic thyroiditis (Hashimoto's disease)
• Silent painless thyroiditis
• Acute suppurative thyroiditis
• Subacute granulomatous thyroiditis (de Quervain disease)

Thyroiditis is infiltration of the thyroid gland with inflammatory cells which may be seen in a disease group of autoimmune, inflammatory and infectious processes. Thyroiditis may be acute and self-limiting or chronic and progressive. Specific conditions commonly produce diffuse enlargement such as chronic autoimmune lymphocytic (Hashimoto's) thyroiditis, colloid or adenomatous goiter and Graves' disease. **Table 3** lists the various diffuse thyroid diseases. Diagnosis of these conditions is usually made on the basis of clinical presentation and laboratory findings of thyroid function, and occasionally by FNAC. Sonography is seldom required and when performed it is the thickness of the isthmus which facilitates the recognition of diffuse thyroid enlargement. The isthmus which is normally only a few millimeters (2–4 mm) thick in anteroposterior dimension, may be up to 1 cm or more in thickness with diffuse thyroid disease.[13]

Each of the types of thyroiditis enumerated has distinctive clinical and laboratory features. Imaging is not important in the initial workup of these patients as the findings in them are usually not distinguishable from other thyroid pathology such as goiter or a neoplastic lesion. However, imaging is useful in patient follow-up and monitoring of the disease.

Diffuse Nontoxic Goiter

Diffuse nontoxic goiter represents diffuse, non-nodular enlargement of the thyroid associated with a euthyroid state. There are two stages in its development. The first stage is hyperplasia characterised by diffuse glandular enlargement and hyperemia. The second stage is colloid involution, which occurs when a euthyroid state is maintained. Over time, most simple goiters progress to multinodular goiters, which may remain nontoxic or may induce thyrotoxicosis.[2] When 10% or more of the local population has goiter, it is referred to as endemic goiter. These are seen in iodine poor areas, usually away from oceans, with high incidence of goiter as well as anaplastic carcinoma of the thyroid. However, once iodine is introduced in the diet, the incidence of goiter and anaplastic carcinoma decreases while that of papillary carcinoma increases.[8]

Imaging Features

On ultrasonography, a simple goiter appears as diffuse enlargement of the thyroid gland with uniform or variable echogenicity. A heterogeneous appearance may be seen on CT/MRI due to the presence colloid, blood products, calcification or fibrosis in the gland.

Graves' Disease (Diffuse Toxic Goiter)

Graves' disease is a common diffuse abnormality of the thyroid gland and is usually biochemically characterized by hyperfunction (thyrotoxicosis). It is the most common of the autoimmune disorders, with a peak incidence in the third to fourth decades of life, having a female preponderance. Although Graves' disease is autoimmune, it is not really a thyroiditis as it does not have a significant inflammatory component.

In Graves' disease, thyroid autoantibodies bind to the thyrotropin receptor on the follicular cells, stimulating them as though TSH triggered the receptor. This results in constant autonomous function of the thyroid, which results in hyperthyroidism. The diagnosis in confirmed by serological tests for specific autoimmune markers which are elevated.

There is marked enlargement of the thyroid gland without focal nodules. The gland shows diffuse hyperplasia of the follicular epithelial cells with depletion of colloid. Pyramidal lobe may be enlarged. Graves' disease is associated with other autoimmune diseases of the thyroid such as Hashimoto's thyroiditis.[8]

Imaging Features

Radionuclide scintigraphy may be helpful in evaluating patients with suspected Graves' disease and also differentiating it from acute thyroiditis. In Graves' disease, the gland is diffusely enlarged, shows intense homogeneous radiotracer uptake which may be up to 80% in 24 hours (normal is 10–30%). Also, there is concordance between clinical thyrotoxicosis and increased radionuclide uptake in Graves' disease. In contrast, in the acute phase of thyroiditis, though the patient is clinically hyperthyroid, the radionuclide uptake in markedly low (as low as 10%). The uptake generally returns to normal if the gland recovers and the patient becomes euthyroid.

On ultrasound, the gland is diffusely enlarged with a smooth lobular contour. The echotexture is homogeneous without discrete nodules but patchy areas of altered echotexture may be present due to numerous, large intraparenchymal vessels.[6] The parenchyma may be isoechoic or diffusely hypoechoic because of extensive lymphocytic infiltration.

Color Doppler sonography often demonstrates a hypervascular pattern referred to as "thyroid inferno", indicating an acute stage of the process, the severity of which tends to parallel the patient's degree of hyperthyroidism.[8] Spectral Doppler often shows peak systolic velocities to exceed 70 cm/sec which is the highest velocity found in thyroid disease **(Figs. 10A to C)**. Studies have shown that Doppler analysis can be used to monitor therapeutic response in patients with Graves' disease.[23] A significant decrease in flow velocities in the superior and inferior thyroid arteries after medical treatment has been reported.

The CT and MR imaging findings in Graves' disease are nonspecific with the enlarged gland showing intense enhancement. Even though there is an overall increase in iodine content in the gland, the iodine concentration is decreased, due to which the CT density is actually decreased in Graves' disease. Following treatment, the density values may not return to normal.[8]

As the management of Graves' disease and subacute thyroiditis is different, it is important to differentiate the two. The treatment of patients with Graves' disease involves medication to treat the secondary manifestations of hyperthyroidism, radioactive ablation of the thyroid gland or even surgery if necessary, while thyroiditis is treated conservatively with medicines for symptomatic relief.

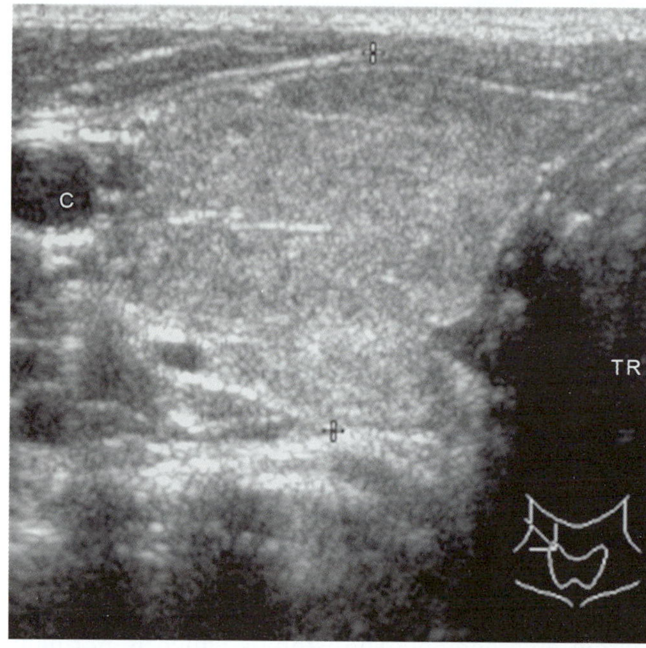

Fig. 10A: High-resolution ultrasound showing mildly enlarged right lobe of thyroid gland (AP diameter 2.27 cm) in a patient of **Graves' disease**.
Abbreviations: C: Common carotid artery; TR: Trachea.

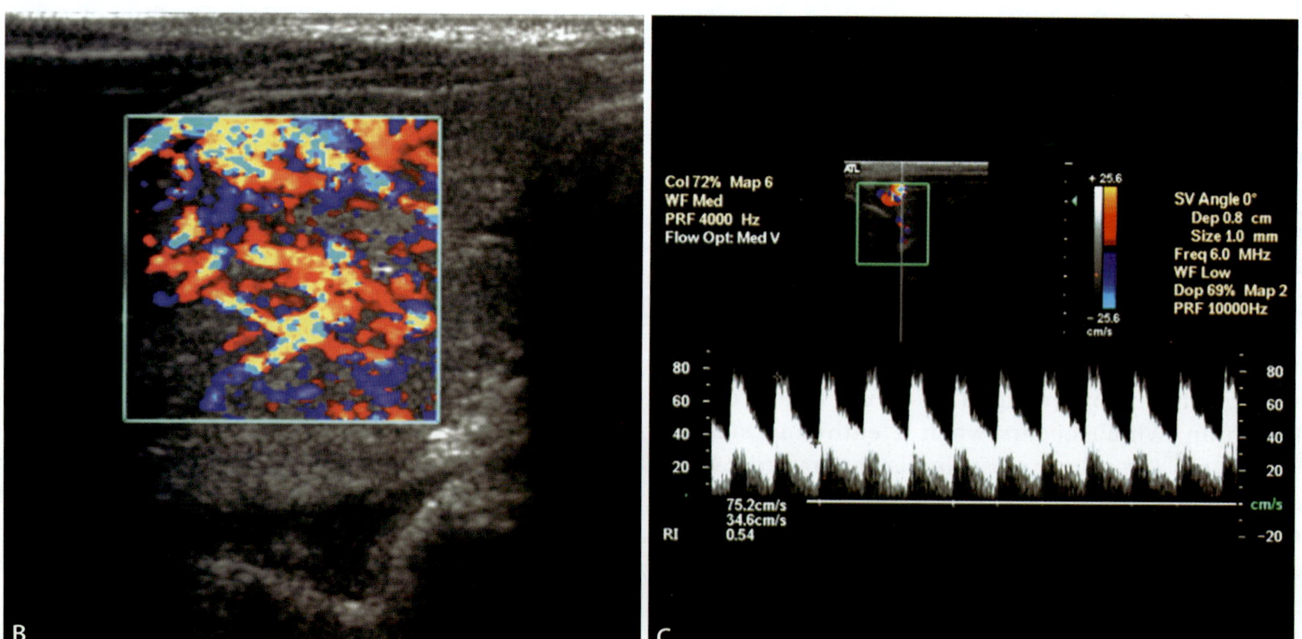

Figs. 10B and C: (B) CDFI showing significantly increased intraglandular vascularity in a patient of Graves' disease: Thyroid inferno; (C) Spectral Doppler of the same showing markedly increased peak systolic velocity (75 cm/s).

Chronic Autoimmune Lymphocytic (Hashimoto's) Thyroiditis

Hashimoto's thyroiditis is the most common type of thyroiditis and occurs when patients develop antibodies to their own thyroglobulin. As the disease is an autoimmune process, its diagnosis is based on serology. Antibody titers are usually elevated. It typically occurs as a painless, diffuse enlargement of the gland in young or middle aged women, but in later stages the thyroid may be atrophic.[8] It is often associated with hypothyroidism. It may also be seen in children in whom it is the most common thyroiditis.[5]

Imaging Features

Scintigraphy does not show any typical pattern in Hashimoto's thyroiditis. The uptake of radioiodine or ^{99m}Tc pertechnetate is most commonly heterogeneous and patchy and may be uniformly increased or mildly to severely decreased.[5]

Ultrasonography demonstrates a spectrum of findings in chronic lymphocytic thyroiditis, depending on the duration and severity of disease. The typical appearance is a diffuse, coarsened echotexture, more hypoechoic than the normal thyroid gland. In patients with mild or previously undetected chronic lymphocytic thyroiditis, the gland may be normal with multiple small discrete, irregular hypoechoic micronodules. These nodules range from 1 to 6 mm in diameter and are highly suggestive of chronic lymphocytic thyroiditis with this appearance called "micronodulation"[24] **(Figs. 11A and B)**.

The sonographic appearance of micronodulation has been described to have a positive predictive value of 94.7% in the diagnosis of chronic thyroiditis.[6] Histologically, the micronodules represent lobules of thyroid parenchyma that have been infiltrated with lymphocytes and plasma cells. These lobules are surrounded by multiple linear echogenic fibrous septations which may give the parenchyma a 'pseudolobulated' appearance. Cervical lymphadenopathy may often be present at the lower pole of the thyroid. Both benign and malignant thyroid nodules may co-exist with chronic lymphocytic thyroiditis and FNA is often necessary to establish the diagnosis.

The vascularity on color Doppler imaging is normal or decreased in most patients with the diagnosis of Hashimoto's thyroiditis **(Fig. 11C)**. CT shows an inhomogeneous appearance, while on MR imaging T2-weighted images may show areas of increased signal intensity. Following contrast administration, there may be regions which enhance more than the remainder of the gland.

Ultrasound may be used to follow patients with Hashimoto's thyroiditis to detect occult malignancy. This is because like other autoimmune disorders there is an increased risk of malignancy of non-Hodgkin's lymphoma of the thyroid. Thyroid lymphoma may produce solitary or multiple focal hypoechoic lesions or diffuse disease that may be difficult to distinguish from Hashimoto's thyroiditis. Sonographic features which raise the suspicion of malignancy in Hashimoto's thyroiditis are a large or infiltrating hypoechoic nodule, nodule with microcalcification, development of respiratory obstructive symptoms and/or cervical lymphadenopathy.[8]

The CT and MR imaging findings of thyroiditis are non-specific and hence these are not routinely performed.

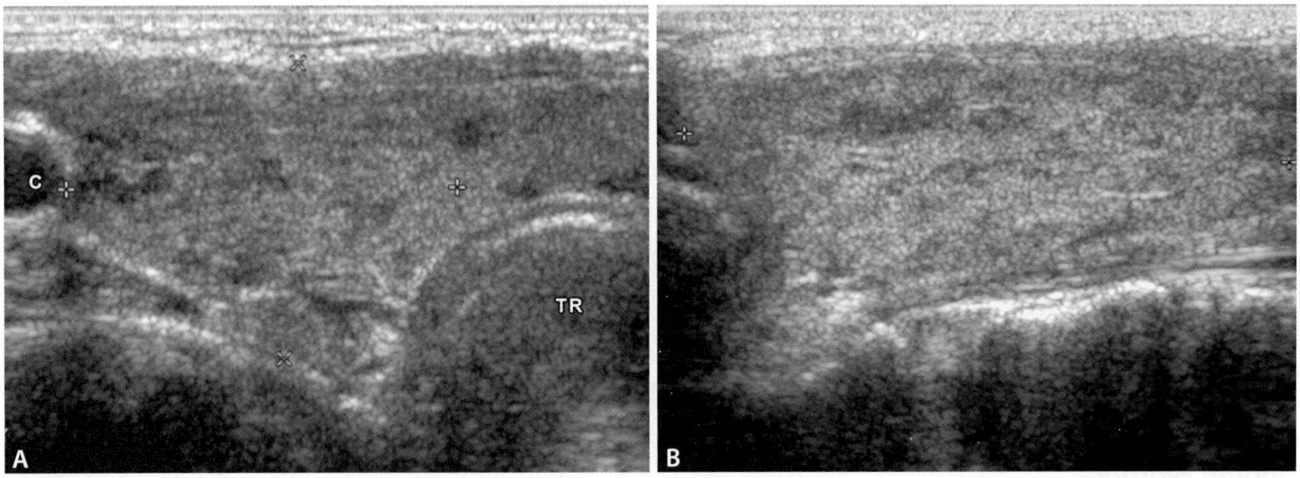

Figs. 11A and B: High-resolution sonography of the right lobe of thyroid showing ill-defined hypoechoic foci scattered in the parenchyma. Isthmus measures 5 mm in A-P dimension FNAC: **Lymphocytic thyroiditis.**
Abbreviations: C: Common carotid artery; TR: Trachea.

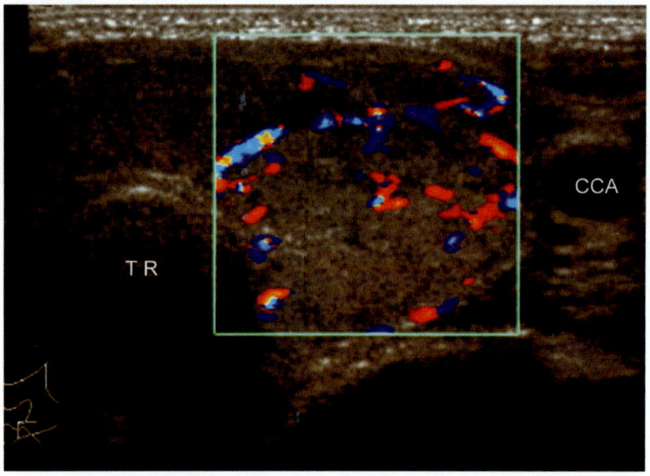

Fig. 11C: CDFI shows normal vascularity in the left lobe of thyroid. *Abbreviation*: FNAC: **Lymphocytic thyroiditis**.

The end stage of chronic thyroiditis is atrophy when the gland becomes small with poorly-defined margins and heterogeneous echotexture due to progressive fibrosis. Blood flow signals are absent. Occasionally, discrete nodules may develop when FNAC is needed to establish the diagnosis.[13]

Silent Painless Thyroiditis and Postpartum Thyroiditis

These are two different types of subacute lymphocytic thyroiditis which are usually self-limiting. Patients may present with goiter, thyrotoxicosis and antithyroid antibodies. When the inflammatory process occurs in the absence of pregnancy, it is termed painless thyroiditis. Postpartum thyroiditis typically occurs 4-6 weeks following delivery in up to 5% of postpartum women and may recur with subsequent pregnancy.[5] It usually resolves after transient hypothyroidism, though some patients may progress to chronic lymphocytic thyroiditis.

Acute Suppurative Thyroiditis

It is an uncommon disease which results from seeding of the thyroid gland by bacterial infection and usually affects children, immunocompromised or debilitated patients. The infection usually develops in the perithyroidal soft tissues. As the disease progresses, focal abscesses may develop. Adjacent soft tissues in the neck may be obliterated due to associated myositis and cellulitis.[25]

Imaging Features

On ultrasound, an abscess is seen as an ill-defined, hypoechoic, heterogeneous mass with internal debris with or without septa or gas. Adjacent inflammatory nodes are often present. On cross-sectional imaging, the affected portion of the gland is enlarged and appears heterogeneous. As thyroid abscesses are rare, any time it occurs in a child, the possibility of a third or fourth branchial cleft cyst must be excluded. On CT, one must rule out a fistula from the pyriform sinus as an etiology of the thyroiditis.[8]

Subacute Granulomatous Thyroiditis (de Quervain's disease)

It is a spontaneously remitting inflammatory disease that usually occurs following a viral upper respiratory tract infection. The peak incidence is in the second to fifth decades of life. Diagnosis is clinical ,with imaging not done routinely.

Imaging Features

Sonographically the gland may appear enlarged and hypoechoic, with normal or decreased vascularity. On noncontrast CT the gland is slightly enlarged with a lower than normal attenuation. Scintigraphy shows a low radioactive iodine uptake that usually reverts to normal as the patient returns to a euthyroid state.

Invasive Fibrous Thyroiditis (Riedel's Struma)

It is the rarest type of inflammatory thyroid disease that is characterized by a fibrosing reaction which destroys the thyroid and extends into the adjacent soft tissues of the neck. The cause of Riedel's thyroiditis is unknown. It is mainly seen in women and usually occurs in the fourth to seventh decades of life presenting with stridor, dysphagia and vocal cord paralysis from recurrent laryngeal nerve involvement. It is the only benign thyroid disease that may cause a recurrent laryngeal nerve paralysis, as the fibrosing reaction encases the nerve. Some cases may be associated with mediastinal or retroperitoneal fibrosis as well as sclerosing cholangitis.[8]

Imaging Features

Ultrasonographic appearance of Riedel's thyroiditis may mimic anaplastic thyroid carcinoma when there is extrathyroid extension of the inflammatory process with encasement of adjacent vessels.[13] This requires an open biopsy to distinguish the two conditions. On ultrasound the thyroid may be hypoechoic and on CT the involved thyroid may be hypodense compared to the normal thyroid. The characteristic MR appearance includes decreased signal

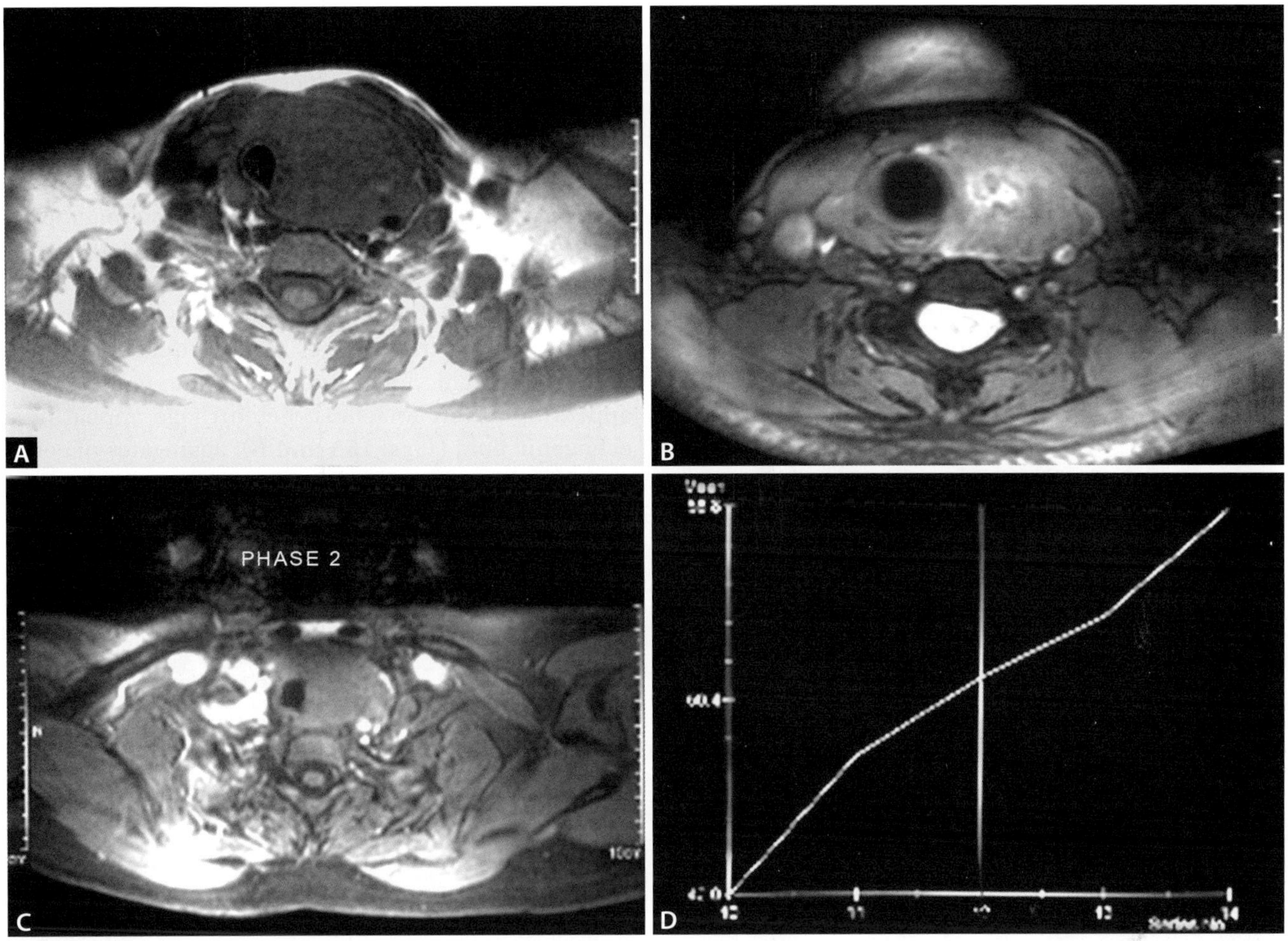

Figs. 12A to D: (A) Axial T1W image shows an iso to mildly hypointense nodule in the left lobe and isthmus which is iso to mildly hyperintense on T2W sequence; (B) It is causing tracheal attenuation and displacement to the right with compression of the left CCA and IJV. (C) The lesion is showing mild homogeneous contrast enhancement; (D) The time signal intensity curve reveals a slow persistently rising curve suggestive of a benign etiology.
Abbreviation: FNAC: **Riedel's thyroiditis**.

intensity on T1-weighted and T2-weighted images, believed to correspond to fibrosis, as well as infiltration of adjacent soft tissues in the neck **(Figs. 12A to D)**.[26] It may spread to encase neck vessels and may obliterate tracheo-esophageal groove.

Miscellaneous Thyroid Conditions

Other inflammatory but rare thyroid conditions include tuberculosis, sarcoidosis, fungal diseases, and opportunistic organisms, especially in patients with acquired immunodeficiency syndrome (AIDS). Amyloidosis and hemochromatosis may replace thyroid parenchyma and may cause decreased signal intensity on T2-weighted MR images.[22] Radiation received from external beam or radioactive iodine therapy may lead to fibrosis and atrophy of the thyroid gland.

NODULAR THYROID DISEASE

Nodular thyroid disease is characterized by the presence of one or more palpable or nonpalpable nodules within the substance of the thyroid gland.[27] Etiology of nodular thyroid disease includes iodine deficiency (endemic), hereditary familial forms and poor utilization of iodine as a result of medication. Approximately 80–85% of nodular thyroid disease is due to hyperplasia of the gland, with women being effected three times more than men.[1] Adenomas and carcinomas are responsible for the rest of the nodular thyroid pathology.

Multinodular Goiter

Multinodular goiter (MNG) is the most common benign pathology of the thyroid with multiple nodules in the thyroid resulting in an enlarged gland. Glandular enlargement may be asymmetric, involving one lobe more than the other, with or without involving the isthmus. Thyroid goiters may extend substernally and into the anterior mediastinum.

It is characterized by nodularity, focal hemorrhage, focal calcifications, cyst formation, and scarring. Pathologically, the nodules are referred to as hyperplastic, adenomatous or colloid nodules. They appear as complex cystic masses representing colloid, mixed with areas of hemorrhage and necrosis. Dystrophic calcification is a common feature of multinodular goiter and is typically multiple, large and coarse.

Imaging Features

On sonography, multinodular goiter appears as an enlarged gland with multiple nodules of different sizes. Most hyperplastic or adenomatous nodules appear isoechoic compared to the normal thyroid parenchyma, with a thin peripheral hypoechoic halo **(Fig. 13)**. Less commonly, a sponge like or honeycomb pattern is seen **(Fig. 14)**. An ultrasound feature for a benign thyroid nodule that has been described is a "spongiform appearance". This term is used for a nodule containing macrocystic components occupying more than half of the entire volume and has been found to be specific, especially in combination with the feature of isoechogenicity.[28]

The degenerative changes in the nodule are reflected in the sonographic appearance with serous or colloid fluid appearing purely anechoic; hemorrhage appearing as echogenic fluid **(Figs. 15A and B)**; aggregates of colloid typically seen as bright echogenic foci with comet-tail artefacts. Calcification occurring due to the degenerative

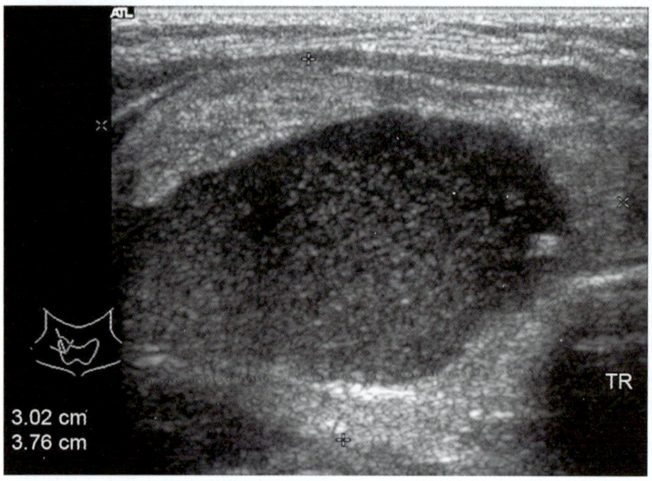

Fig. 13: High-resolution sonography showing a well-defined oval cystic lesion in the right lobe of thyroid with internal echoes within: **Benign nodule**.

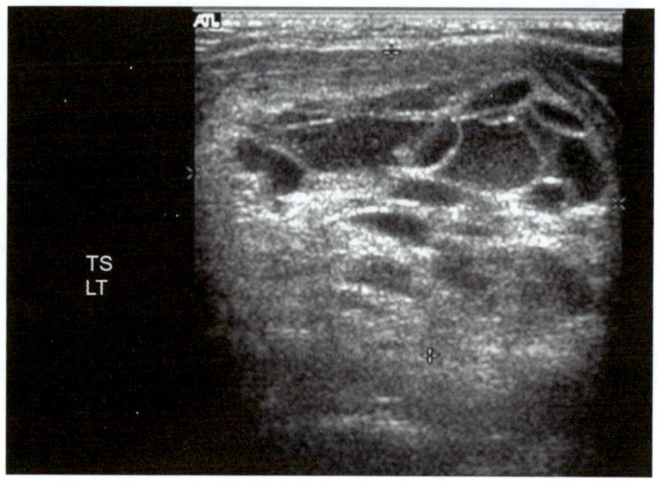

Fig. 14: High-resolution sonography of the left lobe of thyroid reveals a well marginated, multiseptated, cystic lesion. *Abbreviation*: FNAC: **Colloid goiter**.

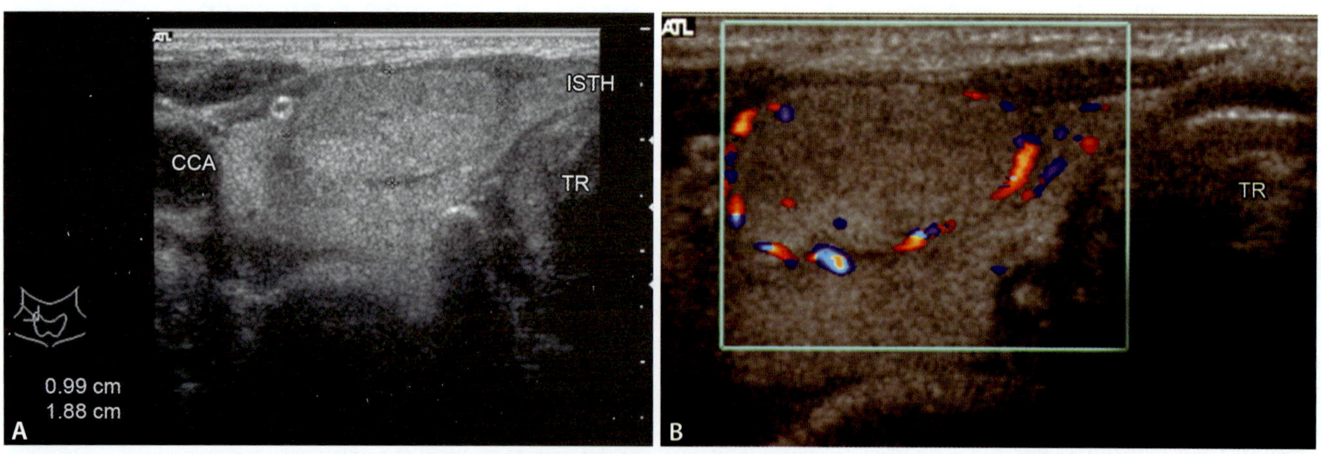

Figs. 15A and B: (A) High resolution sonography of the right lobe of thyroid reveals an oval, well-defined isoechoic nodule with thin sonolucent halo around it: Hyperplastic nodule. (TR—trachea, CCA—Common carotid artery); (B) CDFI of a hyperplastic nodule in the right lobe reveals peripheral vascularity.

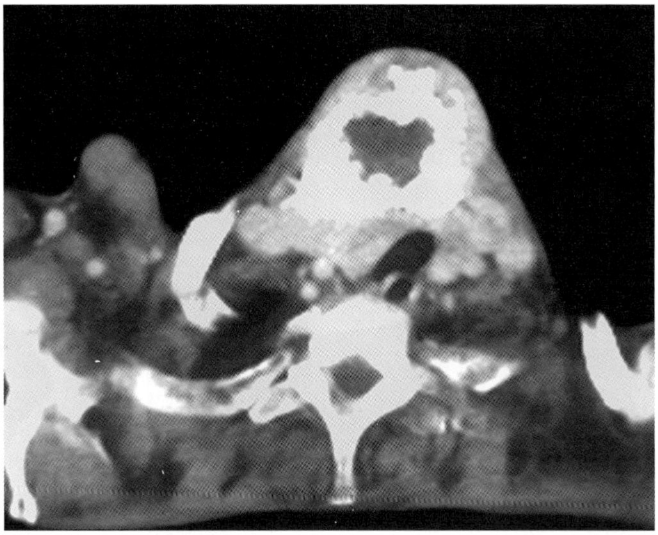

Fig. 16: CT scan showing a nodule in the isthmus of thyroid gland with dense peripheral calcification. Histopathology showed **colloid goiter**.

process may be thin peripheral 'egg shell' type or coarse, seen as highly reflective foci with posterior shadowing scattered throughout the gland.[6]

On CT, the gland is asymmetric in multinodular goiter with multiple low-density areas that reflect regions of hemorrhage, cyst formation, or necrosis. Focal regions of hyperdensity are common, reflecting calcifications, hemorrhage, or colloid. Peripheral or egg-shell-like calcification is considered to be the most reliable feature of a benign nodule, but it is seen only in a small percentage of benign nodules **(Fig. 16)**.[13] On MR imaging, multinodular goiter may show a spectrum of appearances. On T1-weighted images, multiple foci of high signal intensity may represent cysts containing colloid or hemorrhage. On T2-weighted images, diffuse heterogeneity is present **(Figs. 17A to D)**.[2] The individual nodules in MNG enhance intensely with contrast on both CT and MRI.[4] Secondary manifestations of goiter such as compression and displacement of the trachea, esophagus and adjacent vessels are best assessed by CT or MR Imaging, which also depict retrosternal and mediastinal extension, if any.

BENIGN NEOPLASMS

Thyroid Adenoma

Thyroid adenomas are true benign neoplasms distinctly separate from the adjacent thyroid parenchyma and encased by a fibrous capsule. They may be functioning or nonfunctioning, but are usually solitary and non-functioning and are most commonly detected in young and middle-aged adults. They are usually less than 3 cm in diameter, have well-defined margins, and may involute, become cystic or may develop internal hemorrhage, necrosis, calcification or fibrosis **(Figs. 18A and B)**.[9]

Benign follicular adenoma is a true thyroid neoplasm that is characterized by compression of adjacent tissues and fibrous encapsulation. Various sub-types of follicular adenoma include the fetal adenoma, Hürthle cell adenoma and embryonal adenoma, each distinguished according to the character and pattern of cell proliferation.

Imaging Features

Most thyroid adenomas are hyperechoic or isoechoic at sonography. Almost 50% of adenomas are isoechoic, but they are often visible because of their hypoechoic peripheral halo.[29] The halo is due to fibrous capsule and blood vessels which can be readily seen by color Doppler imaging. On CT an adenoma may appear solid, or cystic when it has an degenerated. On T2-weighted MR images thyroid adenomas are typically of increased signal intensity, but are often heterogeneous.

FNA cannot generally distinguish follicular adenoma from follicular carcinoma as they have similar cytological features. Only on histopathological examination it is possible to differentiate an adenoma from a carcinoma based on the criteria of vascular and capsular invasion.[29]

MALIGNANT NEOPLASMS

Malignant thyroid neoplasms constitute the most common endocrine cancer.[5] Thyroid carcinoma arises both from follicular and parafollicular C cells. Malignant potential and behavior range from low grade (papillary carcinoma) to aggressive (anaplastic carcinoma). The for major histologic types of thyroid carcinoma includes papillary, follicular, medullary and anaplastic types.

Papillary and follicular carcinomas (including the Hurthle cell variant of follicular carcinoma) are known as differentiated thyroid carcinomas (DTC). They are the most common and account for 88% and 8% respectively of all thyroid malignancies.[30] They originate from the follicular epithelial cells and have an excellent prognosis with 10-year survival rates of greater than 95% and 85% respectively.[31]

Papillary Carcinoma

Papillary carcinoma is the most common type of thyroid cancer. It is a low grade malignancy occurring most commonly in females. They occur in any age with a peak most commonly seen in the third and seventh decade.

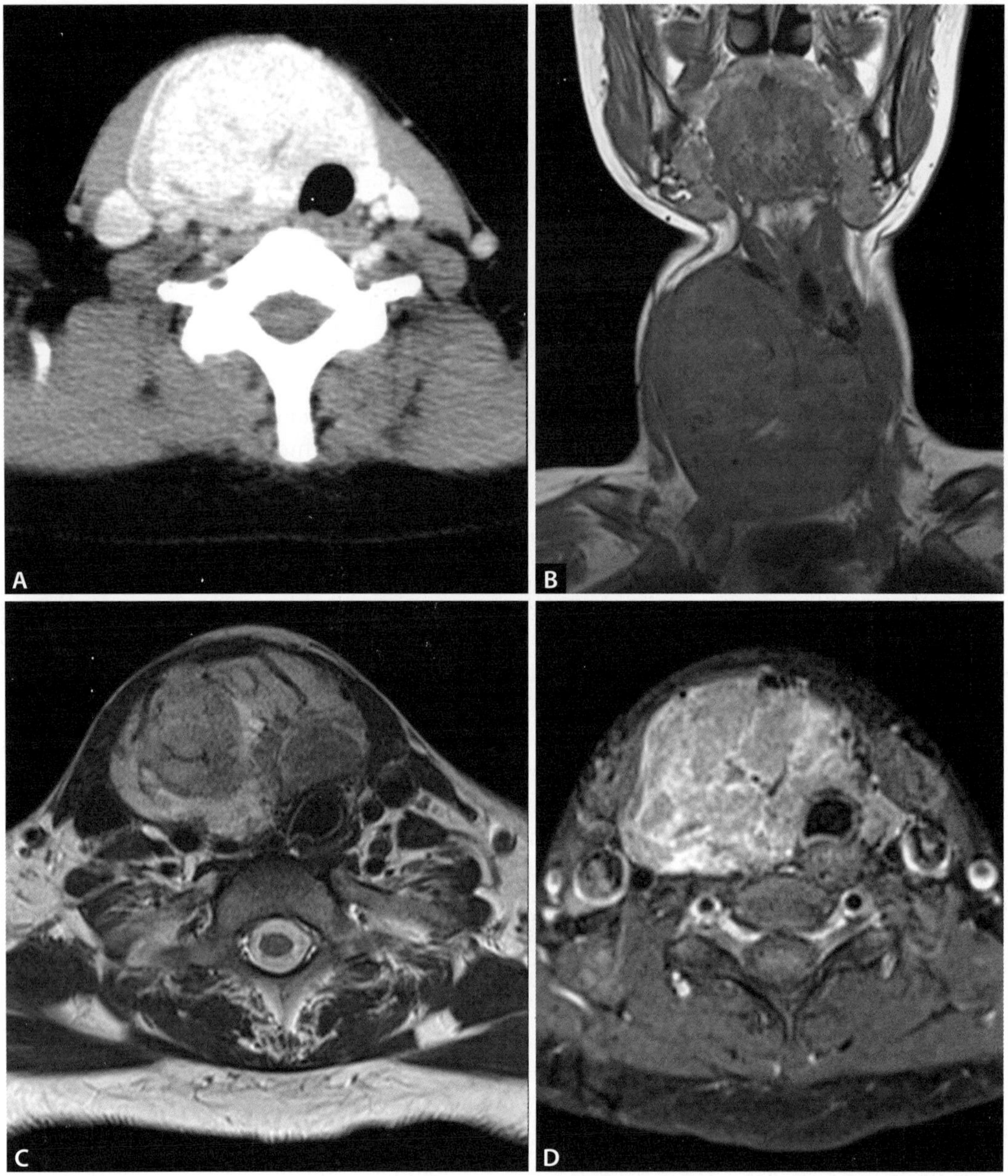

Figs. 17A to D: (A) CECT Neck shows markedly enlarged right lobe of thyroid. (B) Coronal T1W and (C) axial T2W images show a well-defined nodule hypointense on T1 and heterogeneously hyperintense on T2W image showing (D) heterogeneous contrast enhancement: **Goiter**.

Histologically, papillary carcinoma may have a spectrum of findings and may be purely papillary, mixed papillary and follicular, or completely follicular. Frequently, papillary carcinoma is multifocal and microscopic in the thyroid gland and is thought to represent intraglandular lymphatic spread rather than multiple synchronous tumors. Papillary carcinoma is associated with risk factors such as exposure to ionizing radiation, especially childhood head and neck irradiation, family history of thyroid cancer.[31]

Imaging Features

Ultrasound is very useful in the evaluation of papillary carcinomas as a high percentage of them are occult and multicentric. Sonographically, 90% of papillary carcinomas are hypoechoic and rarely of mixed or isoechoic echotexture.[32] Fine, punctate, intralesional microcalcifications (Psammomatous) are considered characteristic of papillary carcinomas. Microcalcification are the result of deposition of calcium in Psammoma

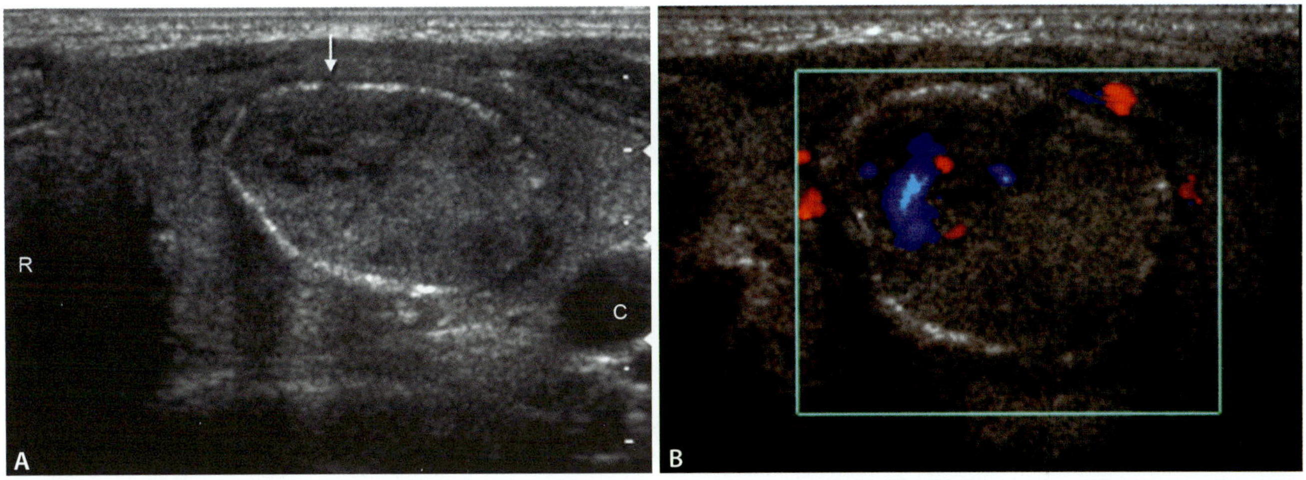

Figs. 18A and B: (A) Ultrasound of the left lobe of thyroid showing a well-defined, hypo- to isoechoic nodule with thin peripheral rim of calcification (arrow): **Thyroid adenoma**; (B) Color Doppler imaging shows both central and peripheral vascularity in a left lobe thyroid adenoma.

bodies, which are infarcted papilla that take up calcium into the dying cells. Papillary carcinomas are typically centrally vascularized lesions with a chaotic vascular pattern. The irregular vascularization is caused by stenosis, occlusions, aneurysms or arteriovenous shunts of the tumor vessels.[32] Cystic papillary carcinoma, a rare variant consists of a predominantly cystic lesion associated with protruding, mural, solid, hypervascular tissue (excrescences) and microcalcifications **(Fig. 19)**.[33]

Papillary carcinoma has the highest incidence of all the thyroid malignancies for cervical lymph node spread, seen in up to 50% of cases **(Figs. 20A to D)**.[5] However, this does not appear to effect the prognosis. Metastatic lymph nodes are not uncommonly normal in size and may be calcified, cystic, hemorrhagic or may contain colloid.[34] Cystic nodal metastasis are characterized by a thin or imperceptible wall and can be mistaken for benign cysts. They occur in the neck almost exclusively in association with papillary thyroid carcinoma, but occasionally may occur in nasopharyngeal carcinomas.[13] Cystic nodes are different from the necrotic nodes frequently seen with metastatic squamous cell carcinoma that have central low density but retain a thick rind of residual lymphatic tissue.[5] In most cases, cystic nodal metastasis show a thickened outer wall, internal nodularity and septations, whereas in younger patients they may appear purely cystic.[35]

Regional nodal metastasis from thyroid cancer occur in the lateral cervical lymph chains (levels II-IV) and central compartment (level VI) in the majority of cases. Occasionally, metastasis may occur in retropharyngeal nodes, usually in the setting of recurrent disease.[8] Hence, any lymph node seen in a patient with papillary carcinoma should raise the suspicion of metastatic disease because of the high rate of lymphatic spread. This is especially true if the node enhances, as these tumours are highly vascular.

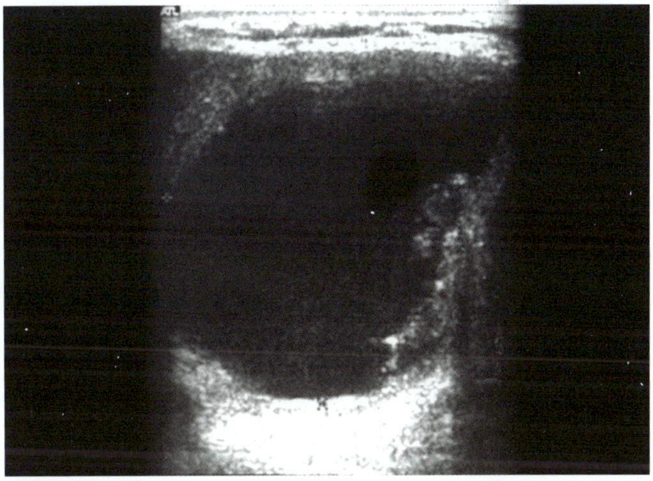

Fig. 19: T-S of right lobe of thyroid on ultrasound showing a predominantly cystic mass with eccentric mural nodularity, punctate calcification: Cystic papillary carcinoma.

Hematogenous spread to the lungs, bones and central nervous system may occur, but this is less common (around 5%) especially in the absence of nodal disease. As papillary carcinomas concentrate radioiodine, scanning with ^{131}I following thyroidectomy may be valuable in detecting residual/recurrent thyroid disease in the operative bed of the neck as well as in detecting distant metastasis. Subsequently treatment with ^{131}I may be instituted. The prognosis for papillary thyroid carcinoma is excellent, with a 20-year survival rate of over 90%.[5]

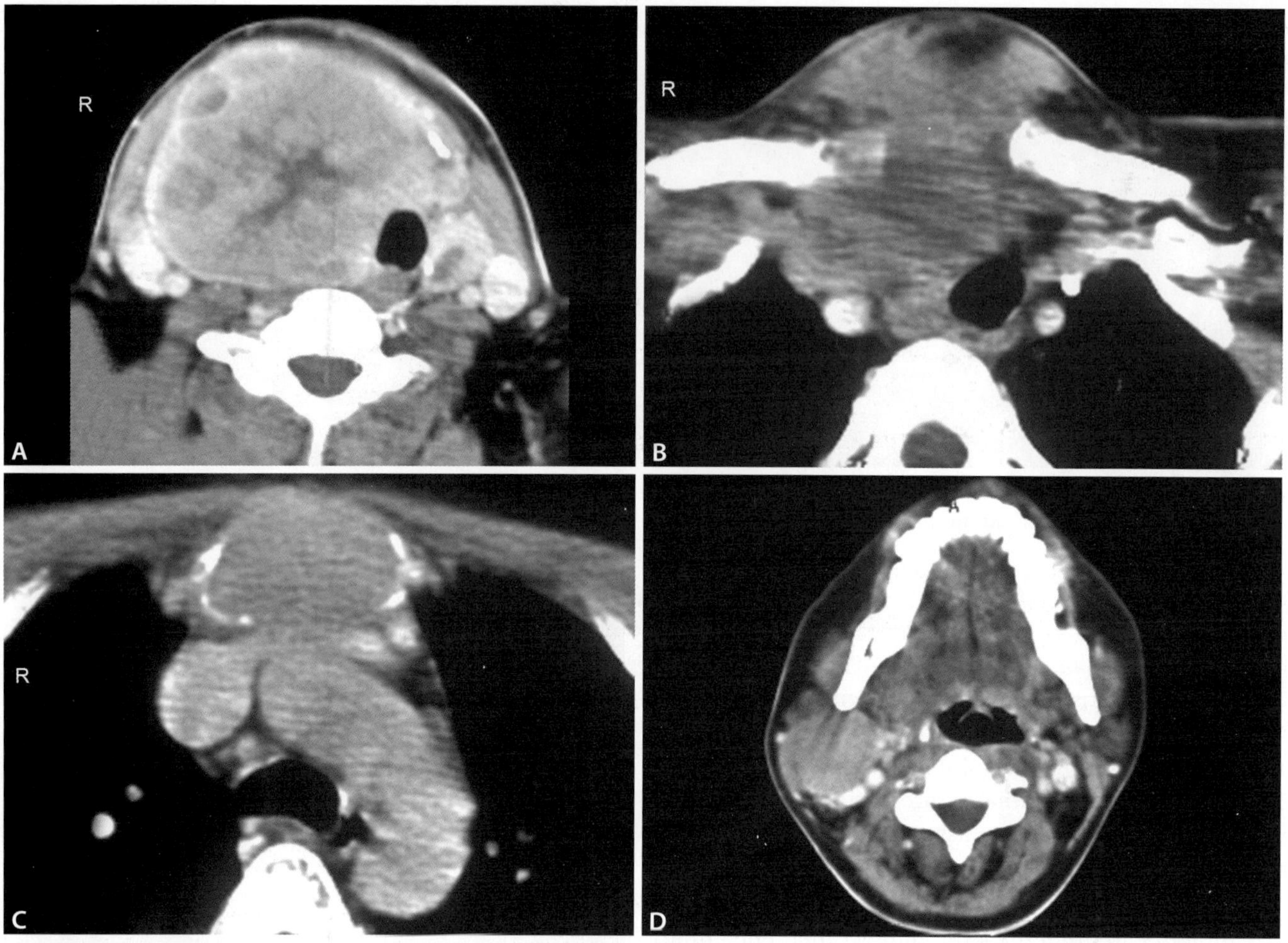

Figs. 20 A to D: (A and B) CECT neck showing a large, heterogeneously enhancing mass in the right lobe and isthmus of thyroid causing contralateral displacement of trachea and ipsilateral displacement of carotid sheath vessels. A curvilinear peripheral focus of calcification is seen in the mass along with a small hypodense lesion in the left lobe. CT sections through the upper chest reveals extension of the mass into the thorax with destruction of medial end of right clavicle and (C) expansile lytic destruction of the manubrium. (D) A well-circumscribed metastatic node is seen along the right internal jugular vein: **Papillary carcinoma**.

Follicular variant of papillary thyroid carcinoma (FVPTC) is the second most common variant of thyroid carcinoma after papillary thyroid carcinoma (PTC), accounting for nearly 9–50% of all papillary carcinomas. Sonographic features of FVPTC have been found to be different from the conventional PTC by being larger in size, more round to ovoid than tall in shape, isoechoic or hypoechoic with a hypoechoic halo and the absence of calcification; i.e. having more benign sonographic features. FVPTC have been reported to have a lower incidence of lymph node metastasis and capsular invasion as well as higher rates of lung and bone metastasis as compared to conventional PTC.[36]

Follicular Carcinoma

True follicular carcinomas of the gland comprise 5% of all thyroid tumors. They are well-differentiated or moderately differentiated, relatively low-grade malignancies that are reportedly more commonly seen in the setting of iodine deficiency. They are usually solitary and slightly more aggressive than papillary carcinomas if vascular invasion is present. Women are affected 2–3 times more often than men, with slightly older age group involvement than papillary carcinoma.

There are two variants of follicular carcinoma that differ greatly in histology and clinical course.[13] In the *minimally invasive* form, the tumor often exhibits a capsule indicative of a better prognosis and only the histologic demonstration of focal invasion of blood vessels of the fibrous capsule permits differentiation from follicular adenoma. The *widely invasive* follicular carcinomas are not well encapsulated, and invasion of the vessels and adjacent thyroid is more easily demonstrated. Both the variants of follicular carcinoma tend to spread via blood stream rather than via lymphatics. Distant metastases to bone, lung, brain and liver are more likely than metastases to cervical lymph nodes.

Imaging Features

Follicular carcinoma resemble follicular adenoma on imaging. Ultrasonography of follicular carcinomas demonstrates a hypoechoic mass in approximately 45% of cases and an isoechoic mass in the remainder.[22] Although the diagnosis is strictly histologic, the presence of a nodule with ill-defined borders, heterogeneous internal echoes, a thick irregular capsule, tortuous intranodal and perinodal vessels and sonographic evidence of vascular and extracapsular invasion raises the possibility of malignancy of the tumor.[1]

Power Doppler sonography has been found to be more sensitive and reliable than velocity mode color Doppler sonography in depicting the vascular pattern of intranodular and perinodular vessels, thereby aiding in the differentiation of malignant and benign thyroid nodules.[37] Most of the follicular carcinomas have been found to have a central flow with a moderate increase of intranodular vascularization on Power Doppler sonography (PDS). In contrast, follicular adenomas have been shown to have a predominant peripheral rim of color flow on PDS. However, power Doppler characteristics cannot be used to rule out malignancy as 20% of malignant nodules have been found to have peripheral flow. *Color flow imaging* can show the hemodynamic features of neovascularization such as the presence of penetrating feeding arteries, thereby enabling the differentiation between *follicular adenoma and carcinoma* to be made. The vascularity of each nodule by power Doppler has been graded 0 to 4, in increasing order of flow.

Grade 0—nodule with no visible flow
1—peripheral flow only
2—peripheral with small amount of central flow
3—peripheral with extensive internal flow
4—nodule with central flow only

CT and MR demonstrate a solid mass not dissimilar to papillary carcinoma and are useful for demonstrating invasion of adjacent structures, extension into mediastinum and cervical lymphadenopathy. Like papillary carcinoma, follicular cancers concentrate iodine, and ^{131}I imaging may be useful in the follow-up of these patients. Prognosis for follicular carcinoma is poorer than that for papillary carcinoma. The 5-year survival rate for encapsulated variants is around 90%, while invasive variants have a poorer prognosis.[5]

Hurthle Cell Neoplasms of the Thyroid

Hurthle cell neoplasms (HCN) are poorly understood thyroid tumors and considered variants of follicular thyroid neoplasms. Some consider them distinct from other follicular neoplasms or consider that they should be classified as a sub group of papillary thyroid carcinomas.[38] They represent 3% of thyroid carcinomas. They are also known as oncocytic or oxyphilic neoplasms and are defined as tumors consisting of at least 75% Hürthle cells and a paucity of colloid cells which are thyroglobulin producing epithelial cells. These cells are present in both non-neoplastic and neoplastic thyroid lesions.

Hürthle cell neoplasms have been reported to have a wide spectrum of sonographic appearances from predominantly hypoechoic to hyperechoic lesions and from peripheral blood flow with no internal flow to extensively vascularized lesions. The differentiation between benign and malignant HCNs (adenoma from carcinoma) has been found to be beyond the resolution of sonography and FNAC and diagnosis can only be made by pathological evaluation of resected tumors.

Medullary Carcinoma

Medullary carcinomas of the thyroid are relatively uncommon, and are derived from the parafollicular C cells, which are of neural crest origin. Approximately 80–90% of medullary carcinomas secrete calcitonin which is used as a sensitive indicator of tumor presence and volume. Those medullary carcinomas that do not produce calcitonin have a poorer prognosis. They have a higher mortality rate than well-differentiated papillary and follicular malignancies. Medullary carcinomas are usually solitary lesions. They may invade locally, may spread to regional cervical lymph nodes and may result in hematogenous spread. Distant metastasis most commonly occur to lungs, bones and liver.

Medullary carcinomas occur sporadically, but a familial link is seen in approximately 15% of adult patients.[22] They are inherited as an autosomal dominant trait and comprises a component of the multiple endocrine neoplasia (MEN) syndromes, types IIA and IIB, which include medullary thyroid carcinoma and adrenal phaeochromocytomas. The disease is multicentric and/or bilateral in about 90% of the familial cases.

Imaging Features

On ultrasonographic examination, medullary carcinomas are typically hypoechoic, although focal calcification may cause echogenic foci both at the primary site and within metastatic lymph nodes. The calcifications tend to be

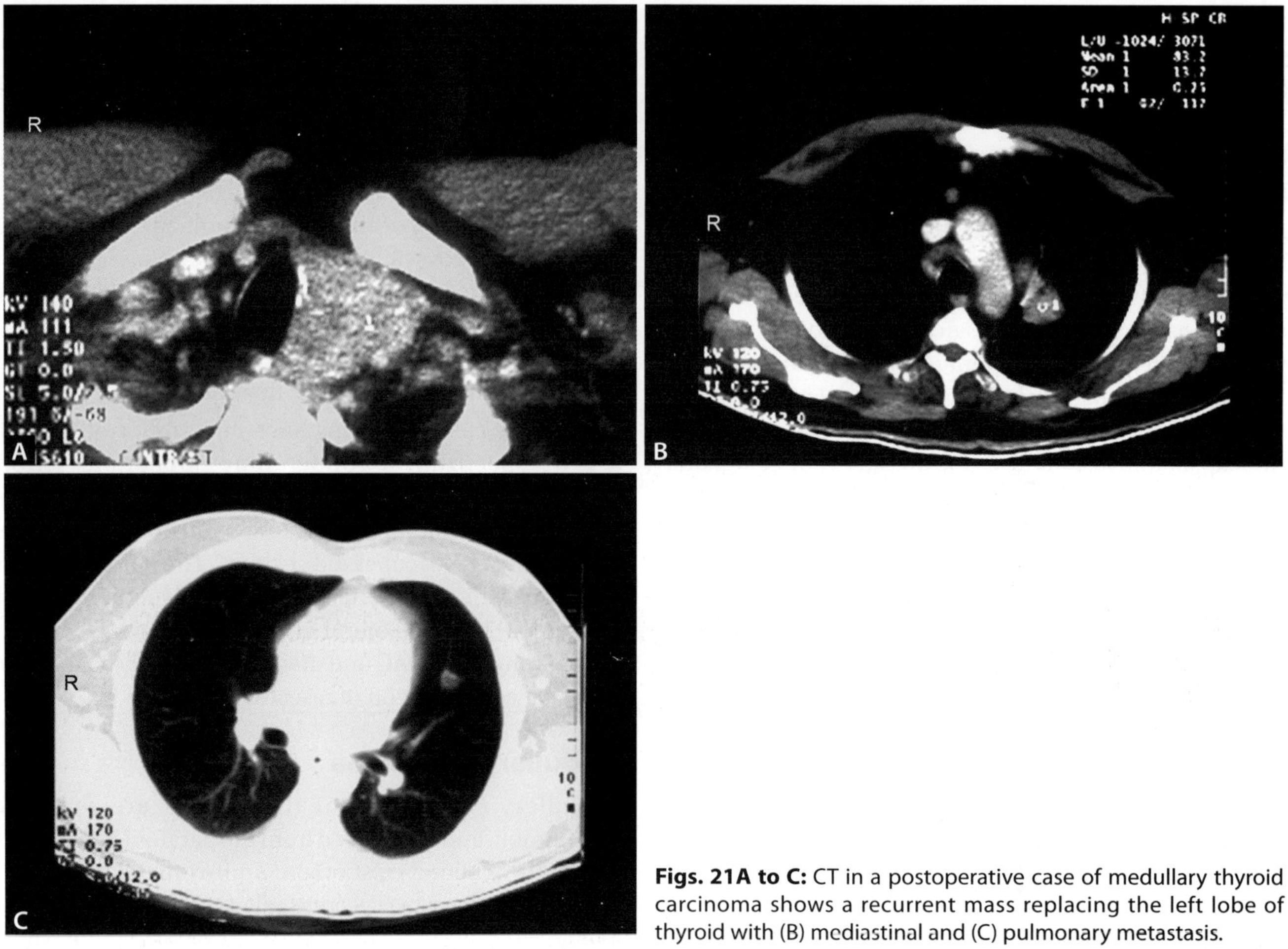

Figs. 21A to C: CT in a postoperative case of medullary thyroid carcinoma shows a recurrent mass replacing the left lobe of thyroid with (B) mediastinal and (C) pulmonary metastasis.

more coarse than the calcifications of typical papillary carcinoma. CT and MRI demonstrate a solid mass, are helpful in displaying surgical anatomy and adjacent lymphadenopathy; malignant lymph nodes being seen in approximately 50% of cases **(Figs. 21A to C)**.[9] Unlike papillary and follicular subtypes, medullary carcinoma does not concentrate radioiodine. However, radionuclide specific for neuroendocrine tissue such as ^{131}I meta-iodobenzylguanidine (MIBG) has been used with some success to evaluate primary as well as metastatic medullary thyroid carcinoma.[5]

The prognosis for medullary thyroid cancer is variable. Patients with thyroid cancer in the setting of MEN type IIB tend to have very aggressive tumors that frequently occur at a young age. In contrast, those in association with MEN type IIA have favorable outcomes. The reported 5-year survival rates are around 75%.

Anaplastic Carcinoma

Anaplastic carcinoma of the thyroid is a highly aggressive and rapidly fatal tumor usually presenting in elderly women. It accounts for less than 2% of all thyroid cancers and is often inoperable at presentation. Anaplastic thyroid carcinomas are often associated with papillary or follicular carcinoma. They are more prone to aggressive local invasion of the neck muscles and blood vessels, instead of lymphatic spread. They commonly occur in patients with long standing goiter. These cancers grow rapidly, and compress and invade the aerodigestive tract and vessels.

Imaging Features

On ultrasound, anaplastic carcinomas are usually hypoechoic and often encase or invade blood vessels and neck muscles. Often these tumors cannot be adequately examined by ultrasound because of their large size. On CT, calcification and necrosis are seen in approximately 60 and 75% cases respectively.[39] CT and MR imaging of the neck usually demonstrate more accurately the extent of the disease **(Figs. 22A to D)**. Anaplastic carcinomas do not concentrate radioiodine. Of all the thyroid cancers, anaplastic thyroid cancers carry the worst prognosis, with a 5-year mortality rate of more than 95%.[13]

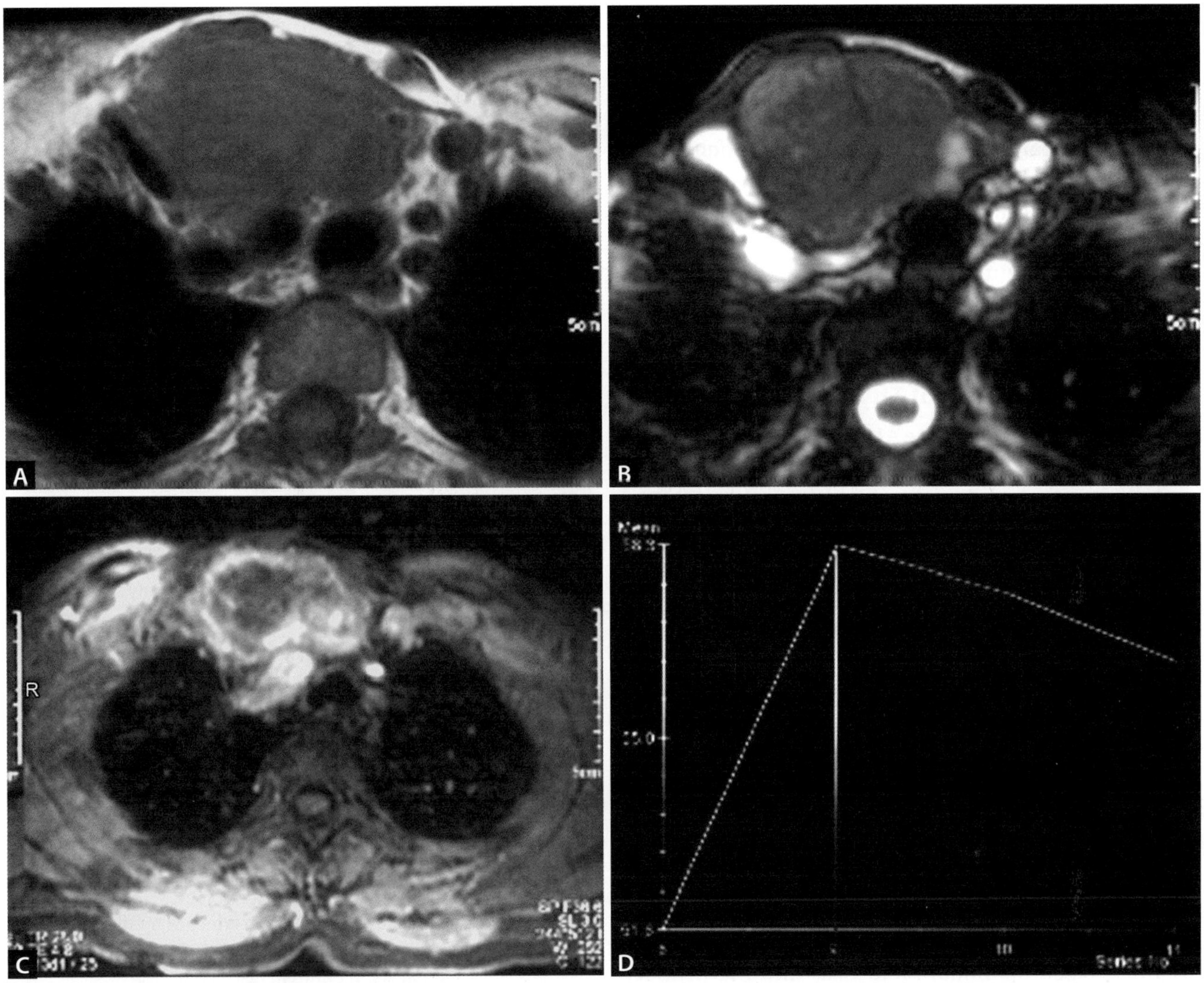

Figs. 22A to D: (A and B) T1W and T2W axial images show a hypodense mass in the right thyroid lobe causing deviation of trachea to the left. The mass is causing attenuation and splaying of the strap muscles anteriorly and great vessels posterolaterally; (C) Postcontrast image reveals heterogeneous, intense peripheral enhancement; (D) The time signal intensity curve shows a rapid uptake and washout of contrast: **Anaplastic carcinoma**.

Primary Lymphoma

Primary lymphoma of the thyroid gland is uncommon. It usually presents in elderly women with a long history of goiter. Patients with Hashimoto's thyroiditis have an increased incidence of developing lymphoma of the thyroid, which is usually of the non-Hodgkin's type.[40]

Patients usually present with a rapidly enlarging thyroid mass and symptoms of obstruction related to compression of the aerodigestive tract.

Imaging Features

Lymphoma typically appears as a solitary, hypoechoic, lobulated mass on sonography with significant enlargement of the gland. The adjacent parenchyma may be heterogeneous due to associated chronic lymphocytic thyroiditis.[13] These tumors are hypodense on CT.[50] On MRI, lymphoma is often hyperintense on T2-weighted images and isointense to normal thyroid on T1-weighted images.[41] It enhances less compared to other thyroid tumours.[42] Imaging including MR imaging, cannot reliably distinguish lymphoma from thyroiditis in patients with Hashimoto's thyroiditis.[43] While lymphoma is typically cold on iodine and technetium nuclear scintigraphy, it may show increased uptake on gallium scans.[5] The prognosis is highly variable and depends on the stage of the disease. The 5-year survival rate may range from nearly 90% in early-stage to less than 5% in advanced, disseminated disease.[13]

Metastatic Disease

Metastases to the thyroid gland are relatively rare. The thyroid is a hypervascular organ and the site of haematogenous metastases most commonly secondary to melanoma, carcinoma of the kidney, bronchus and breast **(Fig. 23)**. The appearance of metastatic lesions is nonspecific and may be multifocal.[44] On ultrasound, the echotexture is nonspecific, metastasis from hypernephroma being hypervascular on color Doppler sonography. Metastatic disease should be considered when histology of a resected thyroid mass is atypical.

Preoperative Staging of Thyroid Carcinoma

Thyroid cancer is staged by the AJCC / TNM staging system based on the size/extent of the tumor(T), spread to nearby lymph nodes (N) and the spread to distant sites(M). The extent of local invasion can involve the trachea, larynx, pharynx/esophagus, vascular structures (mainly carotid arteries) and inferiorly up to mediastinum.[45] **Tables 4 and 5** illustrate the TNM staging and the eighth edition of the AJCC/TNM staging system for thyroid carcinomas.

Preoperative workup involves ultrasonography to detect multifocal disease and lymphadenopathy. CT and MRI are performed if local invasion is suspected.

Evaluation of Nodal Metastasis on CT/MRI

Papillary carcinoma and medullary thyroid carcinoma are the most common thyroid cancers that metastasise to lymph nodes while nodal metastasis are uncommon in follicular carcinoma. Papillary and medullary carcinoma may first present as nodal metastasis and the primary thyroid nodule may not be seen on CT or MRI due to their small size. Features which suggest that a nodal mass is of primary thyroid origin are its cystic composition,[45]

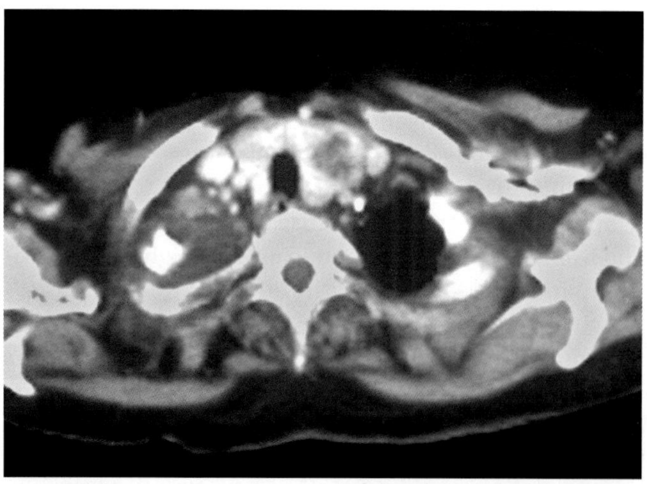

Fig. 23: CT scan in a known case of carcinoma breast showing a hypodense nodule in the left lobe of thyroid.
Abbreviation: FNAC: **Metastatic adenocarcinoma**.

Table 4: TNM Definitions for Papillary, Follicular, Poorly Differentiated, Hürthle Cell, and Anaplastic Thyroid Carcinomas.[45]

	Definition of primary tumor (T)
T category	***T criteria***
TX	Primary tumor cannot be assessed
TO	No evidence of primary tumor
T1	Tumor < 2 cm in greatest dimension limited to the thyroid
T1a	Tumor < 1 cm in greatest dimension limited to the thyroid
T1b	Tumor> 1 cm but < 2 cm in greatest dimension limited to the thyroid
T2	Tumor > 2 cm but < 4 cm in greatest dimension limited to the thyroid
T3	Tumor > 4 cm limited to the thyroid or gross extrathyroidal extension invading only strap muscles
T3a	Tumor > 4 cm limited to the thyroid
T3b	Gross extrathyroidal extension invading only strap muscles (sternohyoid, sternothyroid, thyrohyoid, or omohyoid muscles) from a tumor of any size
T4	Includes gross extrathyroidal extension into major neck structures
T4a	Gross extrathyroidal extension invading subcutaneous soft tissues, larynx, trachea, esophagus, or recurrent laryngeal nerve from a tumor of any size
T4b	Gross extrathyroidal extension invading prevertebral fascia or encasing carotid artery or mediastinal vessels from a tumor of any size
	Definition of regional lymph node (N)
N category	***N criteria***
NX	Regional lymph nodes cannot be assessed
NO	No evidence of regional lymph nodes metastasis
NOa	One or more cytologic or histologically confirmed benign lymph node
NOb	No radiologic or clinical evidence of locoregional lymph node metastasis
N1	Metastasis to regional nodes
N1a	Metastasis tc level VI or VII (pretracheal, paratracheal, or prelaryngeal/Delphian, or upper mediastinal) lymph nodes; this can be unilateral or bilateral disease
N1b	Metastasis to unilateral, bilateral, or contralateral lateral neck lymph nodes (levels I, II, III, IV, or V) or retropharyngeal lymph nodes
	Definition of distant metastasis (M)
M category	***M criteria***
M0	No distant metastasis
M1	Distant metastasis

Table 5: Staging protocol for thyroid cancer: **Eighth edition of the AJCC/TNM staging system.**[45]

Differentiated thyroid cancer				
Age at diagnosis	***T stage***	***N stage***	***M stage***	***Stage group***
<55 yrs	Any T	Any N	M0	I
	Any T	Any N	M1	II
>55 yrs	T1	N0/NX	M0	I
	T1	N1	M0	II
	T2	N0/NX	M0	I
	T2	N1	M0	II
	T3a/T3b	Any N	M0	II
	T4a	Any N	M0	III
	T4b	Any N	M0	IVA
	Any T	Any N	M1	IVB

Anaplastic thyroid cancer			
T stage	***N stage***	***M stage***	***Stage group***
T1-T3a	N0/NX	M0	IVA
T1-T3a	N1	M0	IVB
T3b	Any N	M0	IVB
T4	Any N	M0	IVB
Any T	Any N	M1	IVC

calcification, intense enhancement or proteinaceous/hemorrhagic content. Lymphatic drainage from the thyroid is extensive and various nodal stations or groups at the highest risk of metastasis are:[45]

- *Central compartment*: Level VII (upper mediastinal lymph nodes)
- *Lateral nodal groups*: Levels II – IV
- Delphian node (or prelaryngeal node) involvement in papillary thyroid cancer is predictive of advanced nodal disease as patients are nine times more likely to have lateral nodal involvement.
- *Lower paratracheal nodes*: Level VI
- Retropharyngeal and retroesophageal nodes

Nodal morphology rather than size criteria should be used when assessing metastatic disease because up to 61% of nodal metastasis maybe < 10 mm in size. **Table 6** depicts the rate of lymph nodal spread and morphological characteristics of lymph nodes of thyroid carcinomas.

MRI has been reported to have an accuracy of 86–94% in detecting local invasion.[4,31] The following findings are suggestive of local invasion on CT /MRI.

- >90° encasement of thyroid cartilage
- 90–180° or more contact with circumference of trachea or esophagus
- Deformity of lumen of trachea, focal mucosal irregularity and thickening—suggestive of tracheal invasion while soft tissue within trachea is highly reliable sign of tracheal invasion
- Invasion of recurrent laryngeal nerve (RLN) which is seen as effacement of fatty tissue in the tracheopharyngeal groove
- Circumferential encasement of common carotid artery to 270° has been reported to increase the sensitivity and specificity on MRI to 100% and 88% respectively

The presence of vascular and prevascular space invasion (T4b) precludes the patient from any curative surgery.

Table 6: Lymph node characteristics in various types of thyroid carcinomas.

Type of thyroid cancer	***Rate of LN metastasis***	***Lymph nodes morphology***
Papillary carcinoma	>75%	Foci of calcification, cystic/necrotic change, increase attenuation (hemorrhage/thyroglobulin)
Anaplastic and medullary carcinoma	>50%	Necrotic change ++
Follicular carcinoma	<20%	Lower incidence of morphological changes in LN

Treatment

Except anaplastic carcinoma, treatment involves total or near total thyroidectomy, central nodal resection and radionuclide ablation.

Recurrent Thyroid Cancer

Rates of recurrence of thyroid cancer range from 7–14%. Patients undergoing thyroidectomy for thyroid cancer require long-term follow-up as in 1/3rd of cases recurrence can occur after more than 10 years after treatment.[46] The most common site of recurrence is the neck mainly to lymph nodes. Recurrence in the chest may be in the form of pulmonary metastasis which are often tiny, i.e. miliary and have an indolent course. Bone metastasis are also common and are seen as expansile lytic metastasis.

Follow up relies on clinical evaluation, TSH monitoring to ensure suppression and serum thyroglobulin measurement (calcitonin levels for medullary thyroid carcinoma). Serum thyroglobulin is used as a marker for recurrent or residual differentiated thyroid cancer. When its levels are increased, neck ultrasound and ^{131}I or ^{123}I scintigraphy is typically obtained. Scintigraphy may be negative in 50–80% of patients when it represents progression to dedifferentiated thyroid cancer. Then, MRI or PET CT has a role in localizing tumor for surgery as well as nodal disease. FDG-PET is frequently positive when radio iodine uptake is negative, and vice versa, as radio-iodine negative tumor represents dedifferentiated disease. A pitfall of PET CT is that thyroid nodal metastasis may be missed because of their small size. However, distant metastasis to lungs and bone can be recognized on PET CT.[31]

DIFFERENTIATION OF BENIGN AND MALIGNANT THYROID NODULES

High Resolution Gray Scale Ultrasonography

In the past few years, advancements in high resolution gray scale sonography has led to the development of certain ultrasound criteria for differentiating benign from malignant thyroid nodules.[28] Ultrasound features which are predictive of malignant thyroid nodules are:

1. Taller than wide shape
2. Spiculated/irregular margin
3. Markedly hypoechogenic nodule
4. Predominantly solid composition
5. Presence of microcalcification in a predominantly solid nodule (3 fold risk)
6. Macrocalcification in a solid nodule (2 fold risk)
7. Absence of a halo
8. Intranodular vascularity

A taller than wide shape is very specific for differentiating malignant thyroid nodules from benign ones as malignant nodules grow across tissue planes while benign nodules grow parallel to normal tissue planes. A spiculated margin is suggestive of malignancy while an ill defined margin can be seen in both benign and malignant nodules. The reason for an ill defined margin in benign thyroid nodules is that benign nodules are known to be incompletely encapsulated and can also merge with normal tissue. On the basis of echogenicity, there has been a considerable overlap in the echogenicity of benign and malignant thyroid nodules. Marked hypogenicity has been suggested to be a more specific and a more reliable criteria for diagnosing a malignant thyroid nodule than hypogenicity in a broader sense. This is because 50% of the benign nodules and majority of malignant thyroid nodules are found to be hypoechoic.

As regards calcification within a thyroid nodule, it has been found that the presence of microcalcification in a predominantly solid nodule was found to increase the risk of cancer three-fold, while coarse macrocalcifications increase cancer risk two fold compared with predominantly solid nodules without any calcification. There is no clear size criteria for determining whether a calcification is a micro- or macrocalcification, but a cut off of 1 mm has been suggested. Microcalcifications correspond pathologically to calcified psammoma bodies that are typical of papillary carcinoma. Macrocalcifications or coarse calcifications are related to fibrosis and degeneration. Benign nodules have a coarse calcification, especially with a long standing disease. Studies have shown that a combination of the above ultrasound findings provide a better diagnostic accuracy in predicting malignancy in a thyroid nodule than the presence of only one finding.

Various newer imaging techniques have been used in studies for differentiating benign from malignant thyroid nodules.

US Elastography

Various studies have shown significant difference in the SWV of benign and malignant nodules with malignant nodules having a median SWV of 3.0 m/s and benign nodules 2.06 m/s in a study in 2012. ARFI imaging achieved a specificity of 95% using a cut-off of 3 m/s.[47,48] **Figures 24 and 25** depict gray scale images and corresponding shear wave velocities (SWV) of a benign and malignant thyroid nodule.

The use of US- elastography has been found to be a promising technology that can assist in the differential diagnosis of thyroid cancer and in the selection of nodules suitable for FNAC.

Contrast-enhanced Ultrasound for Evaluation of Thyroid Nodules

Contrast-enhanced ultrasound (CEUS) is a noninvasive ultrasound technique that provides macro- and micro-visualization of tissues studied and can assess blood perfusion of thyroid nodules. Zhang et al. assessed the utility of contrast enhanced ultrasound in the evaluation of thyroid nodules. It was found that the enhancement pattern was different in benign and malignant lesions. In all 104 nodules were scanned with real-time grey-scale pulse inversion harmonic US imaging following intravenous injection of 1.2 ml bolus of SonoVue. Scanning for at least 3 minutes was done and enhancement patterns were classified into one of the 4 patterns—homogeneous, heterogeneous, ring enhancing, and no-enhancement. Ring enhancement was found to correlate highly with benign lesions while heterogeneous enhancement was helpful for detecting malignant lesions.[49]

Diffusion-weighted MR Imaging (DW- MRI)

In recent years, diffusion-weighted MR imaging of thyroid nodules has been performed with the aim of differentiating

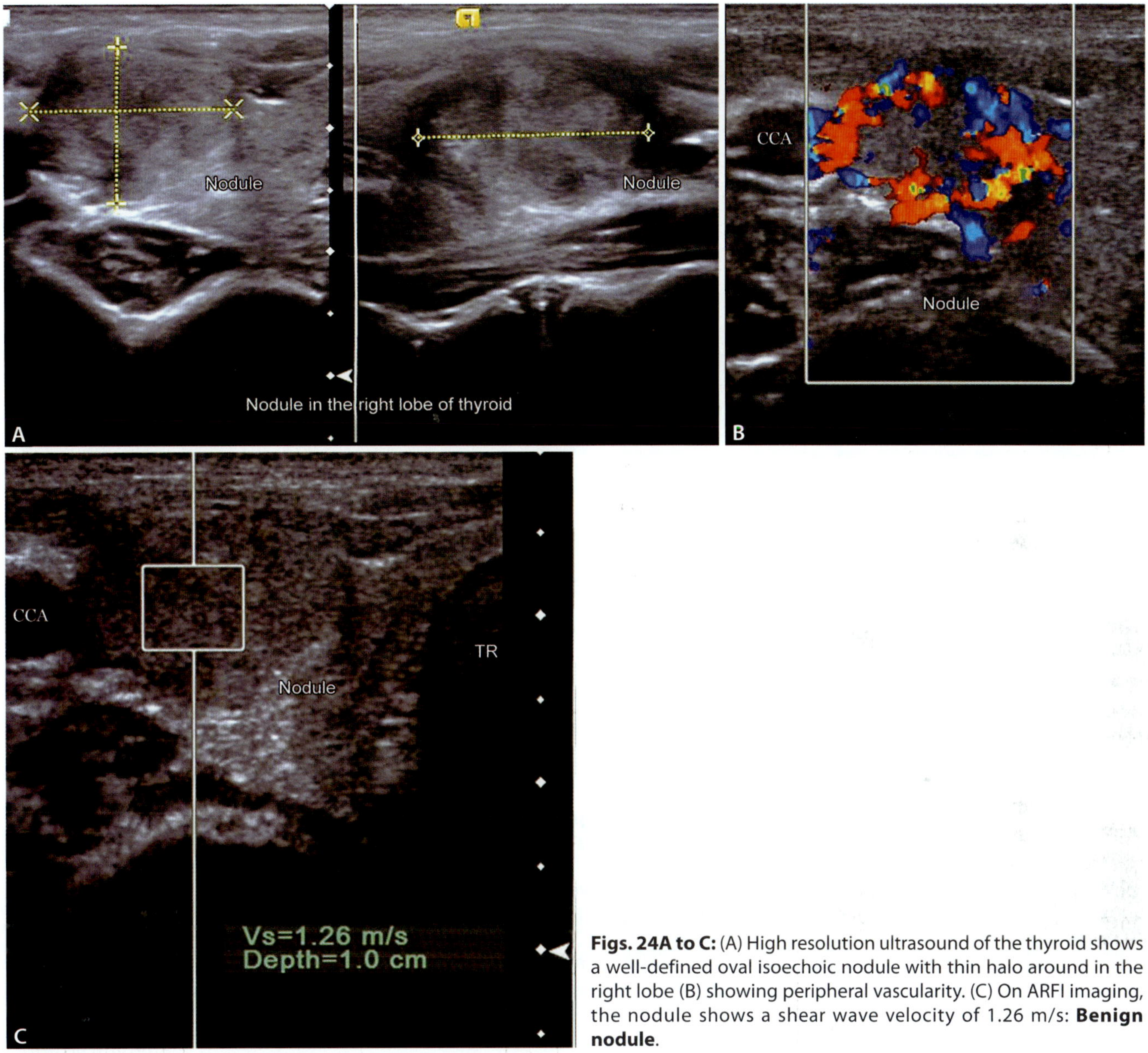

Figs. 24A to C: (A) High resolution ultrasound of the thyroid shows a well-defined oval isoechoic nodule with thin halo around in the right lobe (B) showing peripheral vascularity. (C) On ARFI imaging, the nodule shows a shear wave velocity of 1.26 m/s: **Benign nodule**.

benign from malignant thyroid nodules. A significant difference in the ADC values of benign and malignant thyroid nodules has been reported, with all benign thyroid nodules having higher mean ADC values compared with malignant nodules. The mean ADC values of malignant solitary thyroid nodules was found to be $0.73 \pm 0.19 \times 10^{-3}$ mm^2/sec and of benign nodules was $1.8 \pm 0.27 \times 10^{-3}$ mm^2/sec.[50] The difference in the ADC values of thyroid nodules is based on the difference in cellularity and histopathologic features of benign and malignant thyroid nodules. Malignant thyroid nodules have increased cellularity and enlarged nuclei as compared with benign ones. This reduces the extracellular matrix and the diffusion space of water protons in the extracellular areas, with a resultant decrease in the ADC values.

Approach to Incidental Thyroid Nodules Detected on Imaging

Incidental thyroid nodules (ITN) or thyroid incidetalomas are one of the most common findings on imaging studies which include the neck. ITN is defined as a nodule identified on an imaging study that was not previously

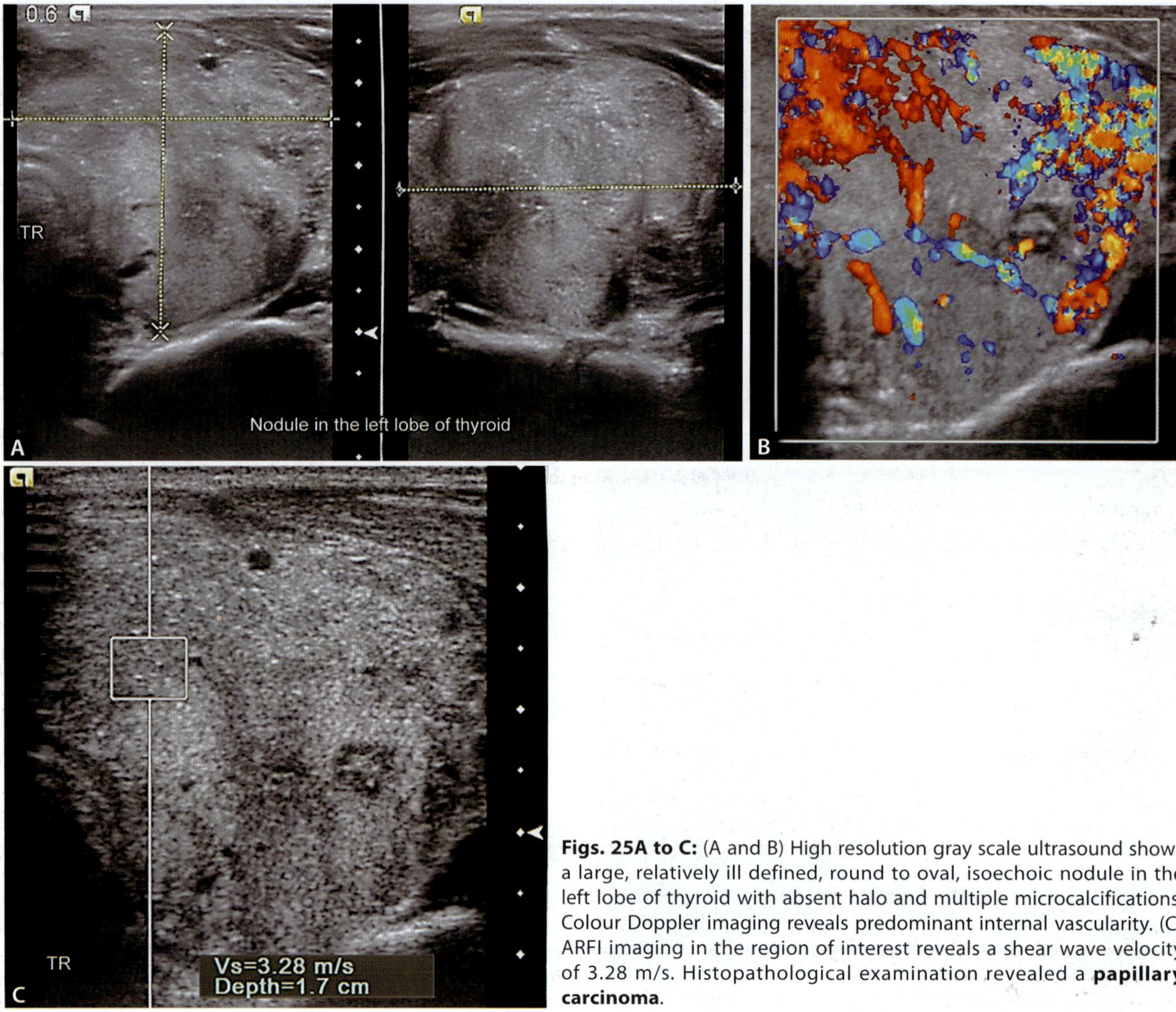

Figs. 25A to C: (A and B) High resolution gray scale ultrasound shows a large, relatively ill defined, round to oval, isoechoic nodule in the left lobe of thyroid with absent halo and multiple microcalcifications. Colour Doppler imaging reveals predominant internal vascularity. (C) ARFI imaging in the region of interest reveals a shear wave velocity of 3.28 m/s. Histopathological examination revealed a **papillary carcinoma**.

detected or suspected clinically. They are seen in 20–67% of ultrasound studies, up to 25% of contrast enhanced CT scan of the chest and 16–18% of CT and MRIs of the neck.[51]

The malignancy rate of an individual nodule has been found to be low, ranging from 0–9% with a rate as low as 1.2% according to a recent population based case control study[R]. Also, most thyroid cancers are not aggressive in nature, due to which most patients with small thyroid cancers are seen to die with, rather than from, thyroid cancer. There are no reliable signs to indicate that a thyroid nodule detected incidentally on CT and MRI is benign or malignant in the absence of frank local invasion.

If an incidental thyroid nodule has been detected on CT or MRI of the neck, the next investigation is ultrasound due to the higher spatial resolution and better characterization of nodules by sonography.

According to a largest recent retrospective study, the only useful sonographic signs of malignancy reported were microcalcification, solid compostion and a size >2 cm having odds ratios of 8.1, 4.0 and 3.6 respectively.[46]

Due to variability in reporting of ITN on CT and MR imaging, a 3 tiered system of risk categorization for thyroid nodules has been proposed based on patient age, nodule size and suspicious imaging findings as given in **Table 7**.[31,46] A recent study has shown a 46% reduction in ITN work-up with a 3-tiered system compared to a 1 cm size as cut-off size.

Table 7: The 3-tiered system of risk categorization for thyroid nodules detected by CT, MRI or PET.

Category	*Criteria for Categorization*	*Suggested Workup/ Recommendation*
Risk Category 1: Highly suspicious for malignancy	• PET avid thyroid nodule • *Suspicious lymphadenophathy • Extrathyroid spread with or without signs of vocal cord palsy on side of nodule • Lung metastasis	Recommend FNA for nodule of any size
Risk Category 2: Indeterminate with risk factors of young age	• **High risk history • Age < 35 years	Recommend USG if ≥ 1 cm in adults Consider USG workup for any size in pediatric patients
Risk Category 3: Indeterminate without risk factors	• Age ≥ 35 years	Consider USG workup if ≥ 1.5 cm

***Suspicious LN**
- > 10 mm short axis (except jugulodigastric which can be up to 15 mm in short axis diameter)
- Nodes with calcification, cystic component or irregular margins

****High Risk history**
- History of cancer in one or more relatives
- History of external beam radiation as child, ionizing radiation in childhood/adolescence, previous hemithyroidectomy with thyroid cancer, MEN2/Familial MTC (medullary carcinoma thyroid), associated gene mutation, calcitonin >100 pg/mL

Recommendations for Incidental Thyroid Nodules Detected on CT, MR Imaging and PET Scan (Flowcharts 1 to 3)[51]

With focal metabolic activity in the thyroid on FDG-PET:dedicated thyroid ultrasound and FNA of the PET avid lesion, if the patient has normal life expectancy

Focal activity on other nuclear medicine scans: dedicated thyroid ultrasound if the patient has normal life expectancy

Approach to a Patient with Thyroid Nodule/Nodules

Evaluation of a patient with thyroid nodule consists of *clinical assessment* with complete history, physical examination focussing on the thyroid and for any enlarged cervical lymph nodes. This is followed by *diagnostic evaluation* consisting of

1. High resolution ultrasound of the thyroid
2. Thyroid scintigraphy

Flowchart 1: incidental thyroid nodule detected on CT/MRI

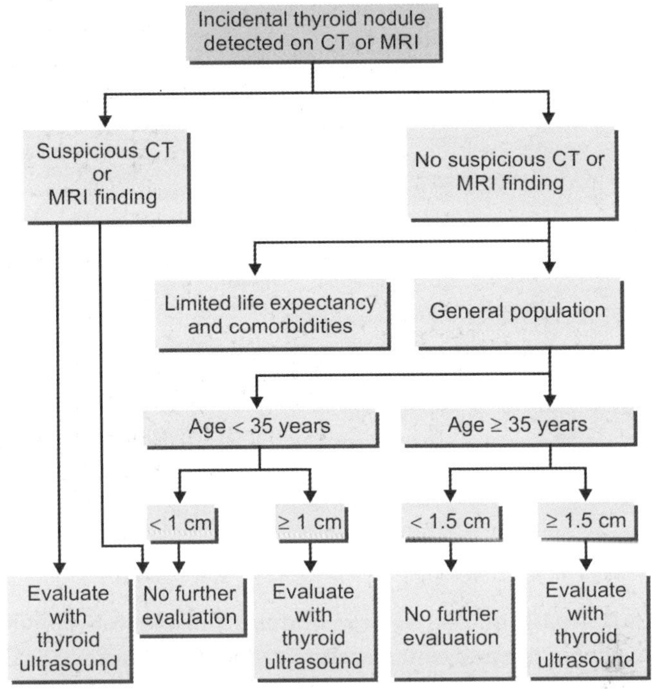

Flowchart 2: incidental thyroid nodule detected on ultrasound for extrathyroidal structures

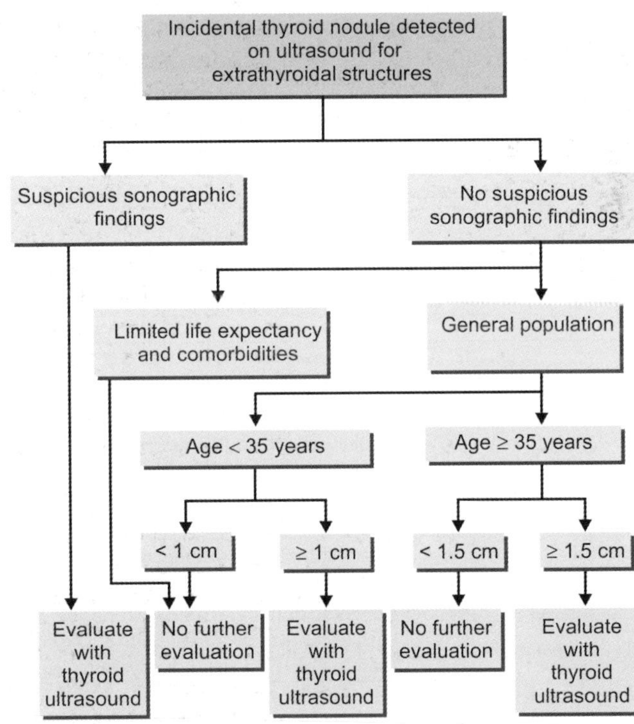

Recommendation: for ITN detected on CT, MRI or extrathyroidal ultrasound
Age < 35 yrs: Dedicated thyroid ultrasound if nodule ≥ 1 cm with no suspicious findings on CT or MRI, with patient having normal life expectancy
Age > 35 yrs: Dedicated thyroid ultrasound if nodule ≥1.5 cm with no suspicious imaging findings, with patient having normal life expectancy

Flowchart 3: Incidental thyroid nodule detected on 18FDG-PET and other nuclear medicine scans

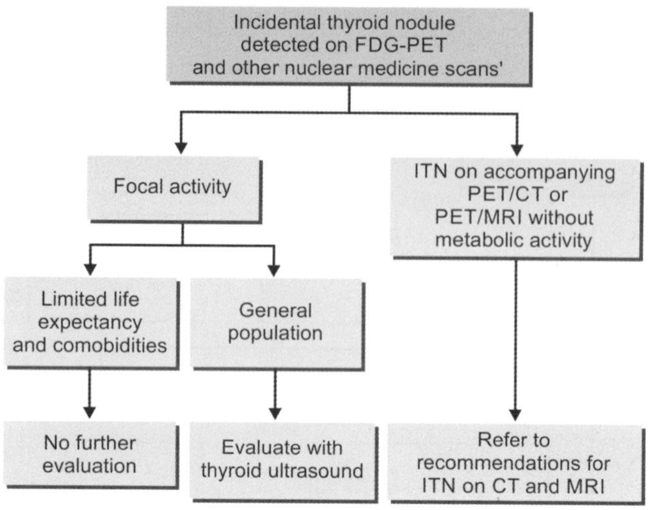

3. CT/MRI in case of large nodules/masses to evaluate spread to adjacent structures and for any retrosternal extension
4. FNA (fine needle aspiration) biopsy

Estimation of *serum thyrotropin (TSH)* is the initial evaluation. A low or subnormal TSH is suggestive of hyperthyroidism and requires a *thyroid scintigraphy* with ^{99m}Tc pertechnetate or ^{123}I to determine the functional status of the nodule. If serum TSH is normal or elevated, a radionuclide scan should not be performed as initial evaluation. In the setting of a low TSH, a nodule appears hot or hyperfunctioning and cytological evaluation is not required as hyperfunctioning nodules rarely harbour malignancy.

All patients with a nodular thyroid detected clinically should be evaluated with high resolution *ultrasound* to (a) confirm the presence of a mass, (b) determine if it is of thyroidal origin, (c) assess if it is solitary or multiple, (d) characterise the nodule's pattern on the basis of its sonographic characteristics, (e) evaluate for any suspicious cervical lymph nodes whenever a nodule shows features suspicious of malignancy, (f) provide guidance for FNA biopsy.

The American Thyroid Association (ATA) have formulated guidelines for the assessment of thyroid nodules so as to improve inter-and intra-departmental consistency in the assessment of nodules on sonographic evaluation and to facilitate communication with referring clinicians. The ATA guidelines have been last updated in 2015. The recommendations regarding which nodules should undergo fine needle aspiration are based on size and suspicious sonographic features of the nodules. These have been given in **Table 8**.

Fine needle aspiration is an accurate, costeffective investigation and plays an essential role in the evaluation of patients with thyroid nodules. It helps in reducing the number of unnecessary thyroid surgeries in patients with benign nodules and triages patients with thyroid cancer to appropriate surgery. Thyroid nodules which are clinically palpable generally undergo FNA without image guidance. The ATA guidelines recommend ultrasound-guided FNA for those nodules which are: (1) nonpalpable, (2) predominantly cystic, (3) located posteriorly in the thyroid,

Table 8: ATA (2015) guidelines for assessment of thyroid nodules: Sonographic Patterns, Estimated Risk of Malignancy, and Fine-Needle Aspiration Guidance for Thyroid Nodules.[52]

Sonographic pattern	*USG features*	*Estimated risk of malignancy, %*	*Nodule cut-off size (largest dimension)*
High suspicion	Solid hypoechoic nodule or solid hypoechoic component of a partially cystic nodule with one or more of the following features: irregular margins (infiltrative, microlobulated), microcalcifications, taller than wide shape, rim calcifications with small extrusive soft tissue component, evidence of ETE	>70–90	FNA recommended for ≥1 cm
Intermediate suspicion	Hypoechoic solid nodule with smooth margins without microcalcifications, ETE*, or taller than wide shape	10–20	FNA recommended for ≥ 1 cm
Low suspicion	Isoechoic or hyperechoic solid nodule, or partially cystic nodule with eccentric solid areas, without microcalcification, irregular margin or ETE, or taller than wide shape.	5–10	FNA recommended for ≥ 1.5 cm
Very low suspicion	Spongiform or partially cystic nodules without any of the sonographic features described in low, intermediate, or high suspicion patterns	<3	FNA to be considered for ≥2 cm Observation without FNA is also an option
Benign	Purely cystic nodules (no solid component)	<1	No biopsy

*ETE—extrathyroid extension

Flowchart 4: Algorithmic approach for evaluation of a patient with thyroid nodule.

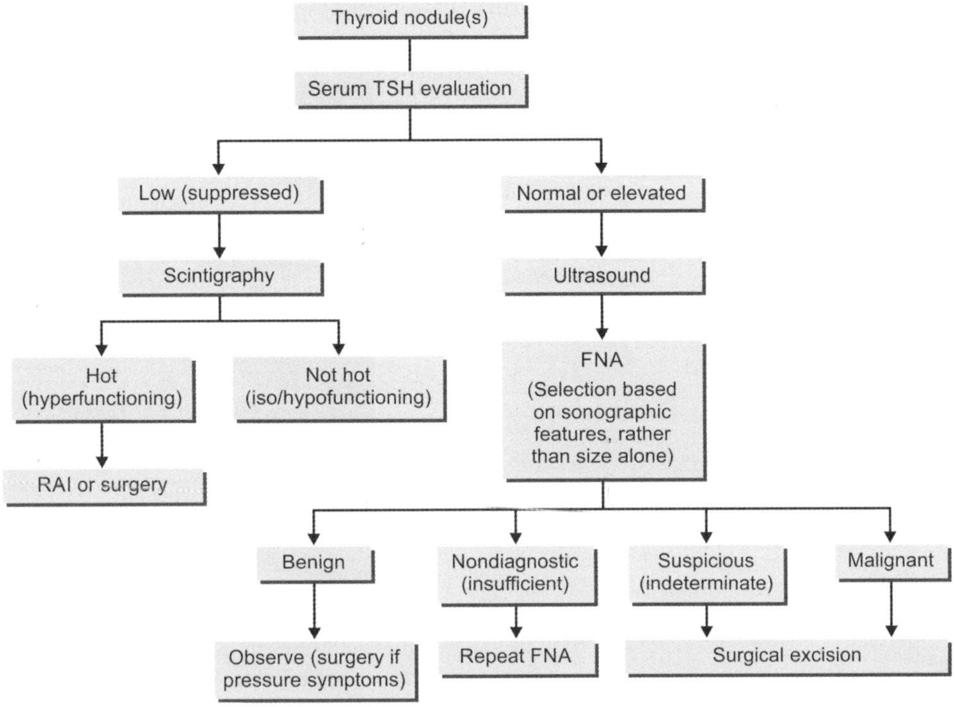

(4) require a repeat biopsy when a palpation-guided FNA yields an inadequate sample.

The FNA recommendations apply to both solitary and multiple nodules as both have similar risk for malignancy. The sonographic features are considered a better indicator than size in determining which nodule or nodules merit FNA in a multinodular gland.

Guidelines for differentiated thyroid carcinoma (especially papillary)—these may frequently be multifocal, with multiple nodules requiring FNA to ensure appropriate surgical planning. When one suspicious malignant nodule is identified sonographically, a careful assessment to rule out another such nodule is essential as the management for single <1 cm papillary thyroid carcinoma is lobectomy while bilateral cancers require total thyroidectomy.

Flowchart 4 depicts the algorithmic approach to a patient with thyroid nodule [53]

THYROID ULTRASOUND REPORTING LEXICON = THYROID IMAGING REPORTING AND DATA SYSTEM (TIRADS)

Ultrasound is the most commonly used imaging modality for the evaluation of thyroid nodules, with nodules being detected in at least 60% of the population who undergo ultrasonography. However, the percentage which are malignant are relatively low, ranging from 1.6–12%. The sonographic findings described are often not specific in differentiating benign from malignant nodule, and a fine nodule aspiration (FNA) or surgery is required for a definitive diagnosis.

Since 2009, several professional organizations such as the ATA (American Thyroid Association) and the SRU (Society of Radiologists in Ultrasound) felt that the terms used to describe thyroid nodules were poorly defined and inconsistent. They proposed ultrasound based risk stratification to identify which nodules were suspicious and would require a biopsy and sonographic follow-up and which could be safely left alone. This came to be called the Thyroid Imaging, Reporting and Data System (TIRADS), modelled on the BIRADS system of breast imaging. However, these TIRADS classifications came from individual institution, hence; the American College of Radiology (ACR) convened committees to (i) provide recommendation for reporting incidental thyroid nodules (ii) develop a set of standard terms (lexicon) for ultrasound reporting and (iii) propose a TIRADS on the basis of the lexicon.

The White Paper of the ACR-TIRADS Committee was first published in 2015 which describes the consensus process and the resultant lexicon. Ultrasound elastography, though a promising technique for evaluation of thyroid lesions is not incorporated into the ACR-TIRADS.

Table 9: Ultrasound categories of thyroid nodules based on ACR-TIRADS lexicon.

Ultrasound categories	*Score*
Composition (Choose 1)	
• Cystic or almost completely cystic	0
• Spongiform	0
• Mixed cystic and solid	1
• Solid or completely solid	2
• Cannot be determined due to calcification	2
Echogenicity (Choose 1)	
• Anechoic	0
• Hyper or isoechoic	1
• Hypoechoic (compared to parenchyma)	2
• Very hypoechoic (compared to strap muscles)	3
• Cannot be determined	1
Shape (Choose 1)	
• Wider than tall	0
• Taller than wide	3
Margin (Choose 1)	
• Smooth	0
• Ill-defined	0
• Lobulated or irregular	2
• Extrathyroidal extension	3
• Cannot be determined	0
Echogenic FOCI (Choose 1)	
• None or large comet tail artifact (>1 mm)	0
• Macrocalcification	1
• Peripheral (rim) calcification	2
• Punctate echogenic foci (<1 mm)	3

Table 9 depicts the standard lexicon of the categories of ultrasound features of nodules and the score assigned to them based on their sonographic features.[54]

Points are assigned for all the sonographic features of a nodule, with additional points being awarded to a nodule with a more suspicious feature **(Fig. 26)**. Hence, higher the cumulative score, higher is the TR (thyroid reporting) level and likelihood of malignancy. If multiple nodules (≥4) are present, then, four of the nodules with the highest score are to be scored, reported and followed-up. These need not be the largest nodules.

The ACR-TIRADS does not provide a grade for "normal thyroid gland". The ACR white paper of 2015 which developed a lexicon from descriptive reports has been updated.

The ACR-TIRADS white paper of 2017 is a stratified scoring system rather than relying on a pattern-based system. **Table 10** gives the ACR-TIRADS scoring and classification of nodules based on the TIRADS lexicon and recommendation for FNA or follow-up ultrasound based on a nodule's ACR-TIRADS level and its maximum diameter.[55]

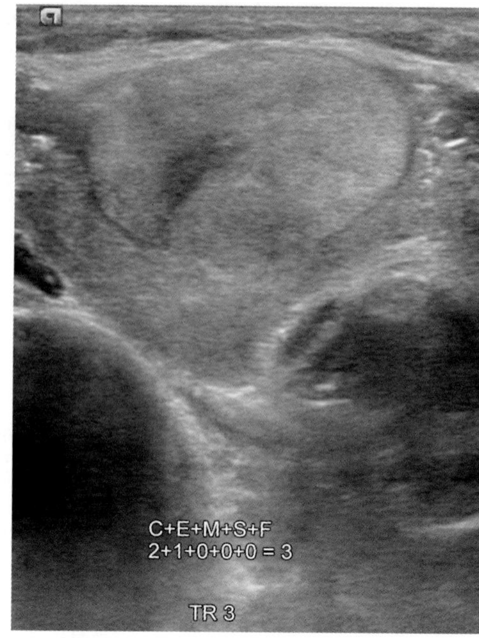

Fig. 26: A well-defined solid (Score 2), isoechoic nodule (Score 1) with smooth margins (Score 0), wider than tall (Score 0) with no echogenic foci within (Score 0) seen in the left lobe of thyroid: **TR3 nodule**.

Table 10: TIRADS scoring and classification.

Scoring	*TIRADS*	*Recommendations for FNA*	*Follow-up ultrasound*
0 points	TR 1	Benign, No FNA	—
2 points	TR 2	Not suspicious, No FNA	—
3 points	TR 3	Mildly suspicious FNA if ≥2.5 cm, Follow-up if ≥1.5cm	At 1,3, 5 years
4–6 points	TR 4	Moderately suspicious FNA if ≥1.5 cm, Follow-up if ≥1.0 cm	At 1, 2, 3 and 5 years
>7 points	TR 5	Highly suspicious FNA if ≥1.0 cm Follow-up if ≥0.5 cm	Every year up to 5 years

- ACR-TIRADS recommends FNAC of suspicious lesions (TR 3 – TR 5) with the above size criteria.
- If there are multiple nodules, two of the highest ACR-TIRADS grades should be sampled rather than the two largest.
- Internal enlargement of a nodule on follow-up is considered significant if there is an increase of 20% and 2 mm in two nodules, or a 50% increase in volume.
- Imaging can stop at 5 years if there is no change in size of the nodule

REFERENCES

1. Senchenkov A, Staren ED. Ultrasound in head and neck surgery: Thyroid, parathyroid and cervical lymph nodes. Surg Clin N Am. 2004;84:973-1000.

2. Pawa S, Chowdhury V. Thyroid and parathyroid imaging. In: Berry, Chowdhury, Suri (Eds). Diagnostic Radiology - Advances in Imaging Technology (1st edition); Jaypee; 2000.
3. Zander DA, Smoker RK. Imaging of ectopic thyroid tissue and thyroglossal duct cyst. Radiographics. 2014;34:37-50.
4. Kabala JE. Computed tomography and magnetic resonance imaging in diseases of the thyroid and parathyroid. European Journal of Radiology. 2008;66:480-92.
5. Loevner LA. Thyroid and parathyroid glands: Anatomy and pathology. In: Som PM, Curtin HD (Eds). Head and Neck Imaging (4th edn) Vol 2 Mosby; 2003.
6. Solbiati L, Charboneiu JW, Cantisani V, et al. The Thyroid Gland. In: Rumack CM, Levine D (Eds). Diagnostic Ultrasound. 5th Edition, Volume 1, Elsevier 2013; pp. 691-731.
7. Villadolid MC, Yokoyama N, Izumi M, et al. Untreated Graves' disease patients without clinical ophthalmology demonstrate a high frequency of extraocular muscle (EOM) enlargement by magnetic resonance. J Clin Endocrinal Metab. 1995;80(9):2830-33.
8. Loevner LA. Anatomy and Pathalogy of the Thyroid and Parathyroid glands. In: Som PM, Curtin HD (Eds). Head and Neck Imaging, Volume 1. 5th Edition, Mosby Elsevier 2012, 2611-77.
9. Yousem DM. Parathyroid and thyroid imaging. Neuroimaging Clinics of North America. 1996;6(2):435-59.
10. Feine U, Leitzenmayer R, Hanke J, et al. Fluore 18 - FDG and I131 uptake in thyroid cancer. J Nucl Med. 1996;37: 1468-72.
11. Wang W, Larson SM, Fazzari M, et al. Prognostic value of 18F fluorodeoxyglucose positron emission tomographic scanning in patients with thyroid cancer. J Clin Endocrinol Metab. 2000;85:1107-13.
12. Bruneton JN, Livraghi T, Viateau-Poncin J. Thyroid gland. In: Bruneton JN (Ed). Applications of Sonography in Hand and Neck Pathology. Berlin Springer-Verlag. 2002; pp. 1-66.
13. Solbiati L, Charboneau JW, Osti V, et al. The thyroid gland 735-770 Vol I Part IV. In: Rumack CM, Wilson SR, Charboneau JW (Eds). Diagnostic Ultrasound, 3rd edition. Elsevier; 2005.
14. Hopkins CR, Reading CC. Thyroid and parathyroid imaging. Seminars in US, CT and MRI. 1995;16:279-95.
15. Loevner LA. Imaging of the thyroid gland. Seminars in US, CT and MRI. 1996;17:539-62.
16. Moon HJ, Sung JM, Kim EK, et al. Diagnostic performance of gray-scale US and elastography in solid thyroid nodules. Radiology. 2012;262(3):1002-13.
17. Gotway MB, Higgins CB. MR imaging of the thyroid and parathyroid glands. Magn Reson Imaging. 2000;8(1): 163-82.
18. Vogi Thomas, Bisdas Sotirios. Cervical Adenopathy and Neck Masses in CT and MRI of the Whole Body: Haaga John R, Dogra Vikram S, Forsting Michael et al (Eds), Fifth Edition Vol I, Mosby Elseiver: 2009; pp. 639-69.
19. Dooms GC, Hricak, Moseley ME, et al. Characterisation of lymphadenopathy by magnetic resonance relaxation times: Preliminary result. Radiology. 1985;691-97.
20. Auffermann W, Clark OH, Thurnher S, et al. Recurrent thyroid carcinoma. Characteristics on MR images. Radiology. 1988;168:753-7.
21. Yousem DM, Scheff AM. Thyroid and parathyroid gland pathology: Role of imaging. Otolaryn Clin N Am. 1995;28(3): 621-49.
22. Larson TC, Smith MM, Chong WK, Martin WH. Thyroid and parathyroid glands in CT and MR imaging of the whole body. In: Haaga JR, Lanzieri CF, Gilkeson RC (Eds). 4th edition Vol I, Mosby. 2003; pp. 663-90.
23. Castagnone D, Rivolta B, Rescalli S, et al. Colour Doppler sonography in Graves' disease: Value in assessing activity of disease and predicting outcome. AJR 1996;66:203-07.
24. Yeh HC, Futterweit W, Gilbert P. Micronodulation: Ultrasonographic sign of Hashimoto's thyroiditis. J Ultrasound Med. 1996;15:813-9.
25. Kawanaka M, Sugimoto Y, Suehiro M, et al. Thyroid imaging in a typical case of acute suppurative thyroiditis with abscess formation due to infection from a persistent thyroglossal duct. Ann Nucl Med. 1994;8(2):159-62.
26. Fontan JP, Carballido FC, Felipe FP, et al. Case report. Riedel's thyroiditis: US, CT and MR evaluation. J Comput Assist Tomogr. 1993;17:324-5.
27. Gharib H. Changing concepts in the diagnosis and management of thyroid nodules. Endocrinol Metab Clin North Am. 1997;26:777-800.
28. Won-Jin Moon, So Lyung Jung, Jeong Hyun Lee, et al. Benign and Malignant Thyroid Nodules: US Differentiation - multicentre retrospective study. Rad. 2008;247(3): 763-70.
29. Gritzmann N, Koischwitz D, Rettenbacher T. Sonography of the thyroid and parathyroid glands. RCNA. 2000;38(5): 1131-45.
30. Saeedan MB, Aljohani IM, Elnaas ST. Thyroid Computed tomography imaging: Pictorial review of variable pathologies. Insights imaging. 2016;7(4):601-17.
31. Hoang JK, Branstetter IV, Glastonbury CM. Imaging of thyroid carcinoma with CT and MRI. Cancer Imaging. 2013;13(1)128-39.
32. Reading CC, Charboneau JW, Hay ID et al. Sonography of Thyroid Nodules: a "classic pattern" diagnostic approach. Ultrasound Q. 2005;21:157-65.
33. Hatabu H, Kasagi K, Yamamoto K, IIda Y, et al. Cystic papillary carcinoma of the thyroid gland. Clin Rad. 1991; 43:121-24.
34. Som PM, Brandwein M, Lidov M, et al. The varied appearance of papillary carcinoma cervical nodal disease: CT and MR findings. AJNR. 1994;15:1129-38.
35. Wunderbaldinger P, Harisinghani MG, Hahu PF, et al. Cystic lymph node metastases in papillary thyroid carcinoma. AJR. 2002;178:693-7.
36. Kim Dae Sik, Kim Ji-hoon, Na Dong Gyu, et al. Sonographic features of follicular variant papillary thyroid carcinomas in comparison with conventional papillary thyroid carcinoma. J Ultrasound Med. 2009;28:1685-92.
37. Miyakawa M, Onoda N, Etoh M et al. Diagnosis of thyroid follicular carcinoma by the vascular pattern and

velocimetric parameters using high resolution pulsed and power Doppler ultrasonography. Endocrine Journal. 2005;52(2):207-12.
38. Maizhin ZV, Wiseman SM, Vora P, et al. Hurthle cell neoplasms of the thyroid: sonographic appearance and Histologic characteristics. J Ultrasound Med. 2008;27: 751-7.
39. Takashima S, Morimoto S, Ikezoe J, et al. CT evaluation of anaplastic thyroid carcinoma. AJR. 1990;154:1079-85.
40. Takashima S, Ikezoe J, Morimoto S, et al. Primary thyroid lymphoma: evaluation with CT. Radiology. 1988;168:765-8.
41. Shibata T, Noma S, Nakano Y, Konishi J. Primary thyroid lymphoma: MR appearance. J Comput Assist Tomogr. 1991;15:629-33.
42. Nakahara H, Noguchi S, Murakami N, et al. Gadolinium enhanced MR imaging of thyroid and parathyroid masses. Radiology 1997;202:765-72.
43. Ohnishi T, Noguchi S, Murakami N, et al. MR imaging in patients with primary thyroid lymphoma. Am J Neuroradiol. 1992;13(4):1196-98.
44. Eftekhari F, Peuchot M. Thyroid metastases: Combined role of ultrasonography and fine needle aspiration biopsy. J Clin Ultrasound. 1989;17:657-62.
45. Perrier ND, Brierley JD, Tuttle RM. Differentiated and anaplastic thyroid carcinoma: major changes in the American Joint Committee on Cancer Eighth edition Cancer staging manual. CA Cancer J Clin. 2017;0(0)1-8.
46. Hoang JK, Sosa JA, Nguyen XV, Galvin PL, Oldan JD. Imaging Thyroid disease: Updates, Imaging approach, and management pearls. Radiol Clin N AM. 2015;53:145-61.
47. Zhan J, Diao XH, Chai QL, et al. Comparative study of acoustic radiation force impulse imaging with real-time elastography in differential diagnosis of thyroid nodules. Ultrasound Med Biol. 2013;39(12):2217-25.
48. Liu, BJ, Li DD, Xu Hx, et al. Quantitative shear wave velocity measurement on acoustic radiation force impulse elastography for differential diagnosis between benign and malignant thyroid nodules: a meta analysis. Ultrasound Med Biol. 2015;41(12):3035-42.
49. Zhang B, Jiang YX, Lin J B et al. Utility of contrast enhanced ultrasound for evaluation of thyroid nodules. Thyroid. 2010; 20(1):51-7.
50. Abdek Razek AAK, Sadak AG, Kombar OR, et al. Role of apparent diffusion coefficient values in differentiation between malignant and benign solitary thyroid nodules. AJNR. 2008;29:563-8.
51. Hoang JK, Langer JE, Middleton WD et al. Managing Incidental Thyroid Nodules Detected on Imaging: White paper of the ACR Incidental Thyroids Committee. J Am Col Radiol. 2015;12:143-50.
52. Haugen BR, Alexender EK, Bible KC, et al. 2015 American Thyroid Association Management Guidelines for Adult Patients with Thyroid Nodules and Differentiated Thyroid Cancer: The American Thyroid Association Guidelines Task Force on Thyroid Nodules and Differentiated Thyroid Cancer. Thyroid. 2016;26(1):1-133.
53. Bahn Rebecca S, Castro Regina M. Approach to the patient with nontoxic multinodular goitre. J Clin Endocrinol Metab. 2011;96(5):1202-12.
54. Grant EG, Tessler FN, Hoang JK et al. Thyroid Ultrasound Reporting Lexicon: White Paper of the ACR Thyroid Imaging, Reporting and Data System (TIRADS) Committee. J Am Coll Radiol. 2015;12(12 Pt A):1272-9.
55. Tessler FN, Middleton WD, Grant EC, et al. ACR Thyroid Imaging, Reporting and Data System (TI-RADS): White Paper of the ACR TI-RADS Committee. J Am Coll Radiol 2017;14(5):587-595.

CHAPTER 25

Malignancies of Upper Aerodigestive Tract

Mukesh Kumar Yadav, Ankur Goyal, Ashu Seith Bhalla, Sanjay Sharma

Malignancies of the upper aerodigestive tract (UADT) include a wide range of tumor locations and histology. Majority (~90%) are squamous cell carcinoma (SCCA) or its variants like lymphoepithelioma (carcinoma with lymphoid stroma), spindle cell carcinoma, verrucous carcinoma (low grade) and undifferentiated carcinoma (high grade).[1] Other malignancies include lymphoma, sarcoma and tumors of minor salivary glands. Risk factors for the development of SCCA of the head and neck include tobacco and alcohol use, human papillomavirus or Epstein-Barr virus infection, immunosuppression by HIV infection or transplantation, poor oral hygiene and radiation exposure. The mucosa of oral cavity is derived from ectoderm and tends to be involved by well-differentiated SCCA while the mucosa of pharynx is derived from endoderm and tends to be affected by aggressive SCCA. With declining tobacco use, there has been a steady decline in the incidence of malignancies of the UADT; however, the incidence of human papilloma virus (HPV) associated SCCA of the oropharynx has been rising. In certain cancer registries of the country, oral cancer has surpassed lung cancer to become the commonest malignancy in males.

Computed tomography (CT) and magnetic resonance imaging (MRI) are the primary imaging modalities in head and neck cancers. Most head and neck cancers are diagnosed clinically and primary role of imaging is to define the stage of malignancy. The most recent guidelines for TNM (Tumor, Node, Metastasis) staging are included in the eighth edition of the American Joint Committee on Cancer (AJCC) Staging Manual, published in 2017.[2,3] The indications of imaging are listed in **Table 1**. The commonly used cross-sectional imaging examination is CT/MRI from the skull base to aortopulmonary window; however, for metastatic work-up in advanced disease, whole body positron emission tomography (PET) is employed. Treatment decisions are mainly based on imaging findings. For accurate interpretation of the imaging, the radiologists should be familiar with locoregional anatomy, spread pattern and clinical behavior of the tumors, various treatment modalities and post-treatment imaging appearances. Imaging modalities like ultrasound and CT also enable radiology-guided interventions, especially in sampling of equivocal lesions.

Malignancies of the upper aerodigestive tract shall be discussed under the following headings:
- Oral cavity
- Nasopharynx
- Oropharynx

Table 1: Role of imaging in head and neck malignancies.

• Staging of the lesion (local extent, nodal status and detection of metastases)—most common indication
• Identifying the lesion in case of clinically occult primary
• Detecting synchronous lesions
• Documenting the local extent of the lesion
• Image-guided interventions (sampling)
• Assessment of response to chemotherapy and radiotherapy
• Follow-up and surveillance of patients

- Hypopharynx
- Larynx
- Cervical lymph nodes
- Miscellaneous neoplasms
- Post-treatment imaging

ORAL CAVITY

Oral cavity is separated from oropharynx by soft palate, anterior tonsillar pillars and the circumvallate papilla of the tongue. SSCA of oral cavity cancers is more common in males than in females. Very High incidence is observed in India.[4] This is mainly attributed to tobacco and betel chewing. Oral cavity cancer is the most common cancer in males in Ahmedabad and Bhopal. In west, lip is the most common site of oral cancer; followed by oral tongue, floor of mouth, lower alveolus-gingiva, upper alveolus-hard palate and buccal mucosa in that order.[5] In India, gingiva-alveolar, buccal mucosa and tongue cancers are more common. Following are the different sites in oral cavity where malignancy can arise:

- Floor of mouth
- Tongue (excluding the base)
- Lip
- Gingivo-alveolus
- Buccal mucosa
- Hard palate
- Retromolar trigone

Floor of Mouth

Floor of mouth is a space bounded superiorly by under surface of the tongue, laterally by inner mandibular gingiva on both sides and inferiorly by mylohyoid muscles. Paired genioglossus-geniohyoid muscle complex, separated by lingual septum, are located in the central part of floor of mouth and these form the imaging landmark of floor of mouth on axial images **(Figs. 1A and B)**. Hyoglossus muscle can be seen in posterolateral part of floor of mouth where it lies medial and parallel to the mylohyoid. Lingual artery and the hypoglossal nerve are located in the fat medial to hyoglossus muscle. Other contents of floor of mouth include submandibular ducts, sublingual glands and lymph nodes. The space inferior to the mylohyoid muscle is outside the floor of mouth and it is called submandibular space.

Squamous cell carcinoma (SCCA) of floor of mouth commonly arise within 2 cm of anterior midline. With local spread, medially it may involve geniohyoid and genioglossus muscle complex, laterally it involves mylohyoid muscle and subsequently the gingiva and mandible **(Figs. 1A and B)**. Submucosal spread may involve lingual neurovascular bundle, sublingual gland and tongue base. Involvement and obstruction of the submandibular duct leads to enlargement of the ipsilateral submandibular gland.

Oral Tongue

Oral tongue is a muscular structure and consists of two halves which are separated by a midline septum. Intrinsic tongue muscles arranged in various planes and these are not identified separately on imaging. Extrinsic muscles anchor the tongue to floor of mouth and these are named as per their origin and insertion sites. These include genioglossus-geniohyoid muscles near anterior

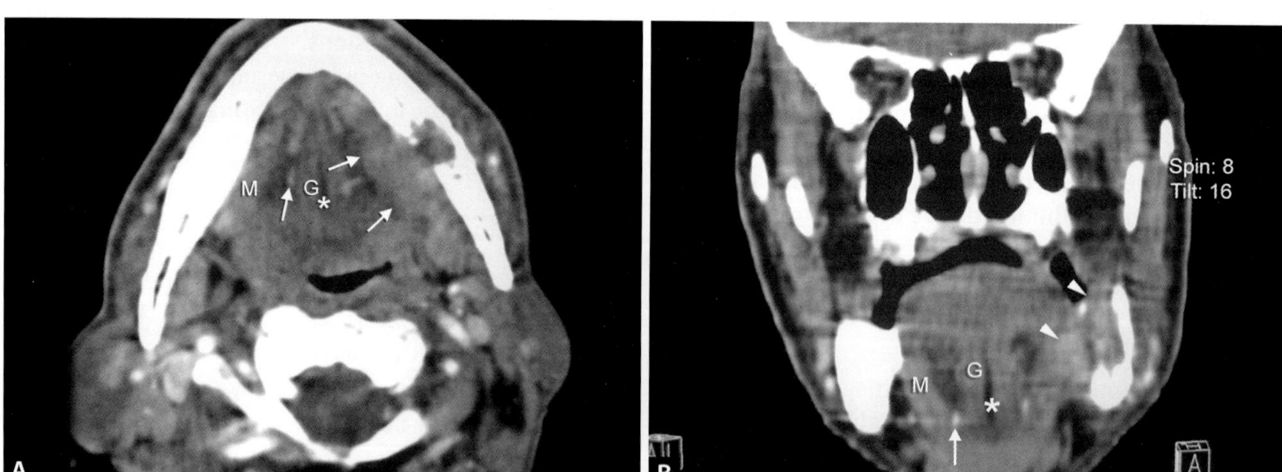

Figs. 1A and B: Carcinoma of floor of mouth: Axial (A) and coronal (B) CT show large mass in left floor of mouth (arrowheads) involving mylohyoid and inner cortex of mandible. It is not involving the lingual neurovascular bundle. Normal lingual septum (asterisk), contralateral genioglossus geniohyoid muscle (G), neurovascular bundle surrounded by fat (arrow), and mylohyoid muscles (M).

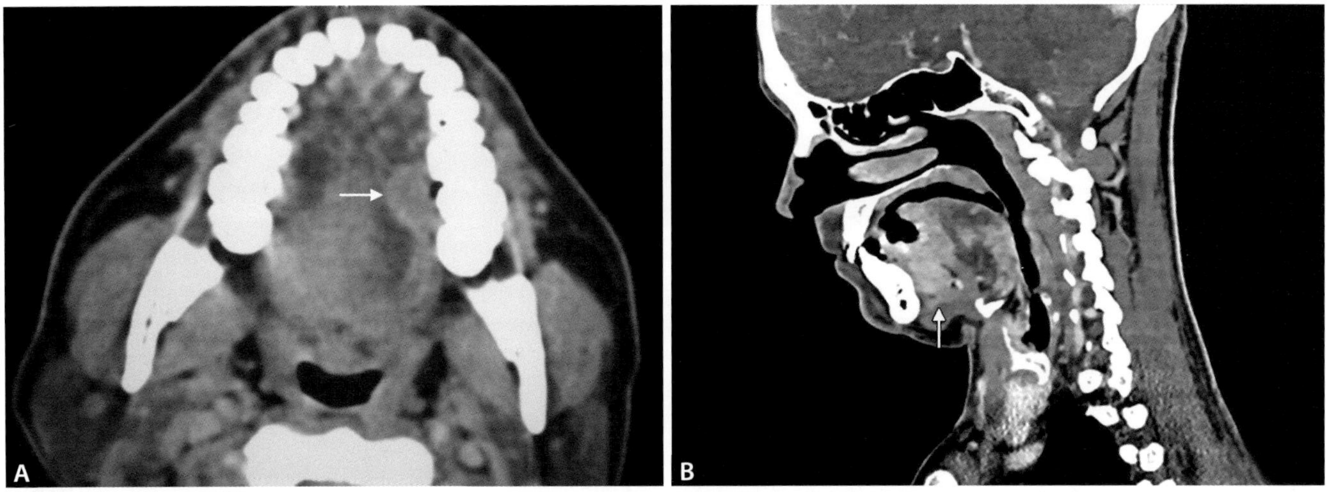

Figs. 2A and B: (A) Carcinoma of tongue: CT shows small mass (arrow) located at the left lateral margin of oral tongue; (B) CECT coronal reformatted images showing enhancing mass involving right lateral border in anterior half of the tongue. It is infiltrating the floor of mouth.

lingual septum and hyoglossus-styloglossus muscles in posterolateral part. SCCA of oral tongue usually arise in middle and posterior third of the tongue at lateral margin or under surface of the tongue **(Figs. 2A and B)**. Early tumors remain localized to the intrinsic muscle of the tongue unilaterally. With local spread, it involves the midline lingual septum and extends across it. Large tumors involve extrinsic muscle of the tongue and floor of mouth. Tumors of posterior part of oral tongue may extend into base of tongue, anterior tonsillar pillar or mandible. On imaging it should be determined if the tumor has crossed the midline lingual septum, extended anywhere outside intrinsic tongue muscles and whether mandible is eroded **(Figs. 3A to D)**. Tongue is richly supplied with lymphatics and large number of patients already have lymph node metastases at the time of initial presentation.[1]

Lip

The lip consists of orbicularis oris muscle. It is covered with thin layer of squamous epithelium. The inside lining of the lip is buccal mucosa. Dry lip is the transition between skin and buccal mucosa. SSCA of the lip most commonly arise at vermilion border of the lip and invade underlying musculature. Subsequently, it may involve buccal mucosa, gingiva and the maxilla or mandible **(Figs. 4A to C)**.

Gingivo-alveolus

Gingiva is the mucosal lining of the alveolar processes of mandible and maxilla. Laterally the gingiva is continuous with buccal mucosa. Medially, the upper gingiva is continuous with mucosa of hard palate while the lower gingiva is continuous with floor of mouth. Tumors arising from gingiva have different patterns of spread depending on whether it is arising from lower or upper gingiva. Lower gingival tumors involve and erode alveolar process of mandible. Lateral spread leads to involvement of the buccal mucosa while with medial or inner aspect spread, these involve floor of mouth. Upper gingival tumors involve mucosa of the hard palate on medial aspect and buccal mucosa on lateral aspect. With further spread, upper gingival tumors involve maxillary alveolar process, hard palate and floors of the maxillary sinus and the nasal cavity **(Figs. 5A and B)**. Coronal images are valuable to assess these areas. Bone involvement makes oral cavity cancer T4 tumor, however, early erosion of tooth socket by a gingival cancer is an exception. With posterior spread, gingivoalveolar tumors involve retromolar trigone and then extend to the masticator space.[6]

Buccal Mucosa

Buccal mucosa is the lining of cheek, inner surface of lips and it is continuous with gingiva via upper and lower gingiva-buccal sulci. Most cancers arise on lateral or buccal surface of the buccal mucosa on the background of leukoplakia. Small tumors are difficult to visualize on imaging. Large tumors are diffuse or ulceroinfiltrative and there spread pattern is similar to gingiva-alveolar tumors **(Fig. 6)**.

Hard Palate

Primary SCCA of hard palate are rare and most are extensions from upper gingival tumors. Primary tumors

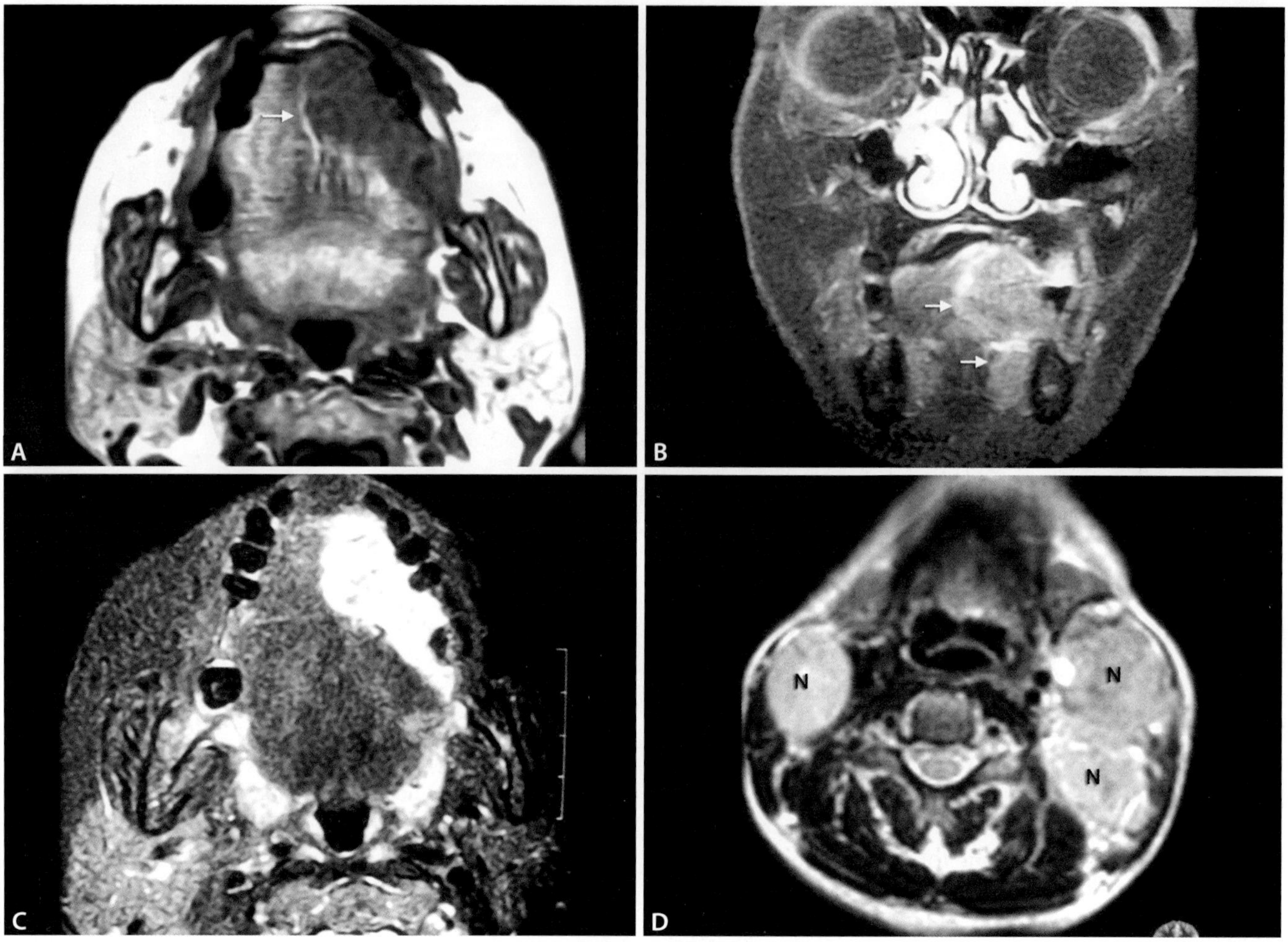

Figs. 3A to D: Carcinoma of tongue: MRI shows large mass in left half of oral tongue on T1-weighted (A) and fat suppressed T2-weighted (B) axial images. It abutting and displacing the midline lingual septum (arrows). Fat suppressed contrast-enhanced T1-weighted coronal image (C) shows invasion of lingual septum and extension into floor of mouth. T2-weighted axial image at more caudal level (D) shows multiple bilateral enlarged cervical lymph nodes (N).

of hard palate are usually adenocarcinoma of minor salivary gland. These tumors have propensity for early bone erosion and perineural extension along greater and lesser palatine nerves to pterygopalatine fossa, foramen rotundum and the cavernous sinus.[7]

Retromolar Trigone

Retromolar trigone (RMT) is a small triangular areas posterior to the last molar. Primary SCCA of RMT rare and most are extensions of buccal mucosa or gingival tumors. RMT is important because of its strategic location. The pterygomandibular raphe is a band of connective tissue that lies beneath the mucosa of RMT. It extends from hamulus of medial pterygoid plate superiorly to the posterior aspect mylohyoid groove on mandible inferiorly. Pterygomandibular raphe forms a junction of oral cavity, oropharynx and infratemporal fossa. Hence, once the tumor reaches RMT, it gets access to various critical areas. With posterior extension, the tumors enter infratemporal fossa and involve medial or lateral pterygoid muscles. Medially, the tumor may spread to tonsils via superior constrictor muscles **(Fig. 6)**. Superior tumor spread along the pterygomandibular raphe involves skull base and nasopharynx, while inferior spread occurs to the floor of mouth. Mandibular cortex is in close proximity of the mucosa of RMT and hence it is eroded early in cases with tumor at RMT. Inferior alveolar nerve also lies here and can get involved resulting in perineural tumor spread.

Staging of Oral Cavity Cancers

Staging of oral cavity cancers is based on TNM system of AJCC **(Table 2)**. In the eighth edition, T-stage takes into

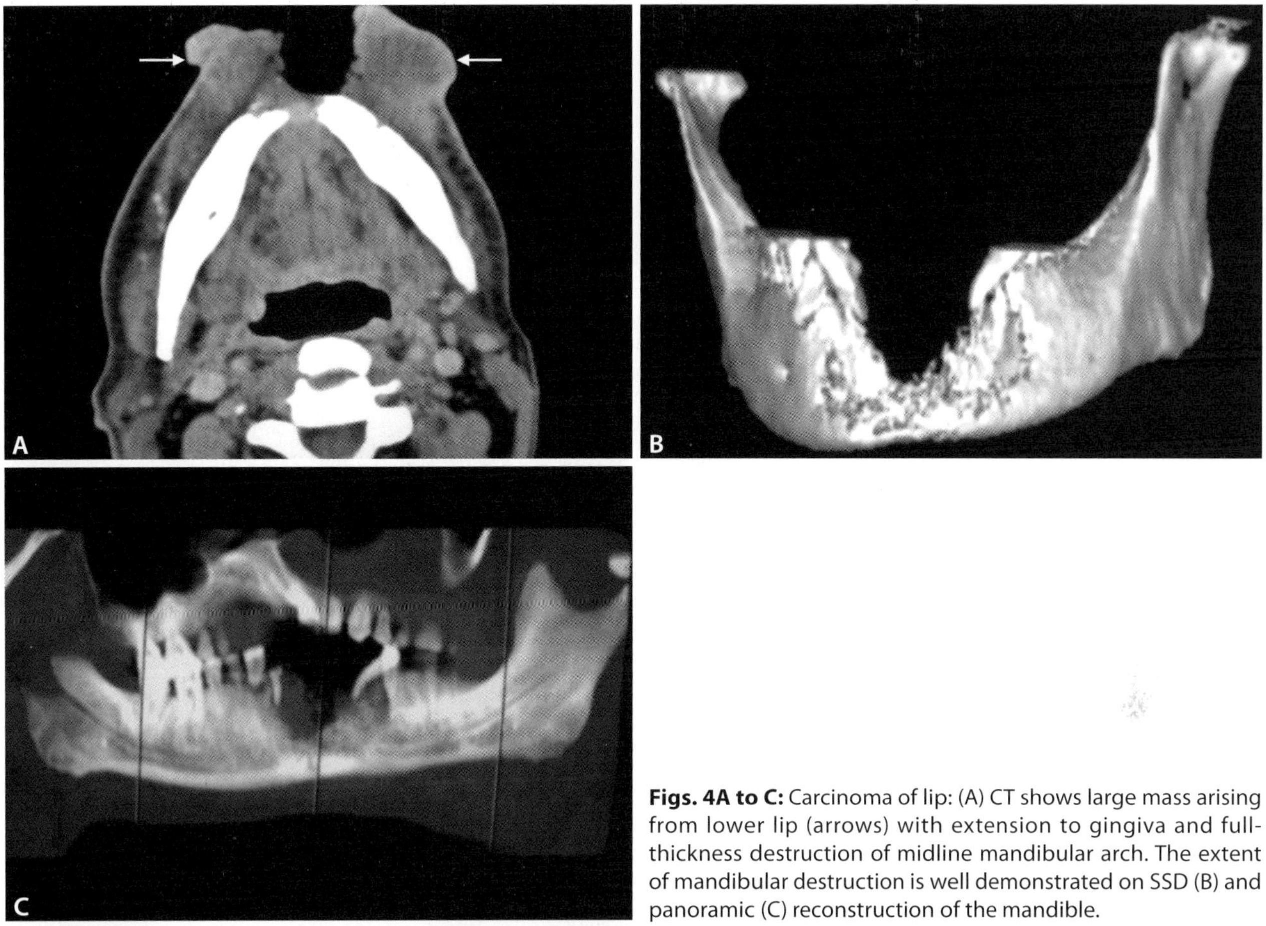

Figs. 4A to C: Carcinoma of lip: (A) CT shows large mass arising from lower lip (arrows) with extension to gingiva and full-thickness destruction of midline mandibular arch. The extent of mandibular destruction is well demonstrated on SSD (B) and panoramic (C) reconstruction of the mandible.

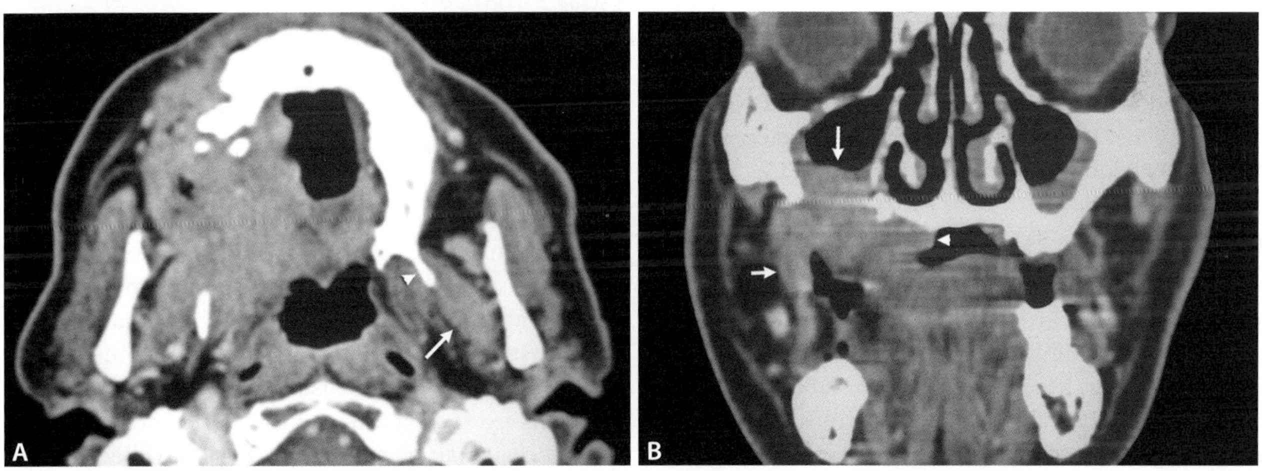

Figs. 5A and B: Carcinoma of upper alveolus: (A) CT shows large tumor arising from and destroying right upper alveolus with extension to masticator space. There is destruction of lateral pterygoid plate and invasion and enlargement of lateral pterygoid muscle which can be appreciated if compared with normal contralateral pterygoid plate (arrowhead) and lateral pterygoid muscle (arrow); (B) Coronal image shows extension of tumor to buccal mucosa with thickening of buccinators muscle (small arrow), hard palate (arrowhead) and destruction of floor of the maxillary sinus (large arrow).

account the depth of invasion in addition to the size.[2,3] It may be noted that the depth of invasion is different from the tumor thickness since the former does not include the exophytic component, rather assesses only the deep invasion. N stage depends on site and size of the lymph nodes. Another point that has been added in the

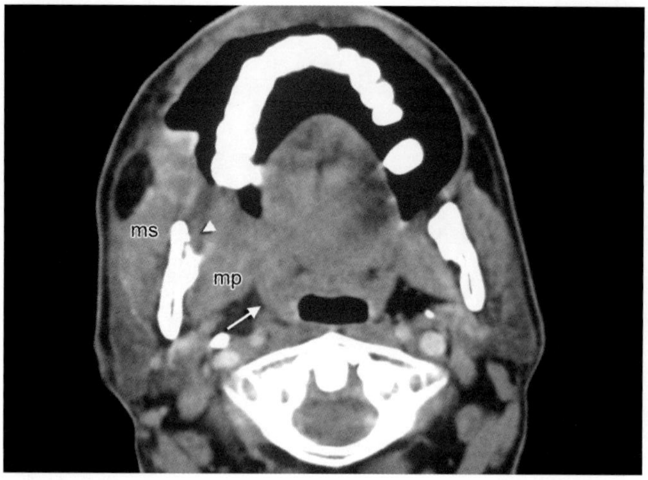

Fig. 6: Carcinoma of buccal mucosa: CT with puffed-cheek maneuver shows polypoid mass in right buccal mucosa. It is extending into right retromolar trigone with erosion of ramus the mandible (arrowhead). There contiguous invasion of pharyngeal wall (arrow), medial pterygoid (mp) and masseter (ms) muscles.

Table 2: Staging of oral cavity cancers: Overview.

T1	Tumor ≤ 2 cm and ≤ 5 mm depth of invasion (DOI)
T2	Tumor ≤ 2 cm and DOI 5–10 mm OR Tumor 2–4 cm and DOI ≤ 5 mm
T3	Tumor > 4 cm or DOI > 10 mm
T4	Advanced local disease
	Moderately advanced: T4a: Invasion of bone, maxillary sinus, extrinsic tongue muscles, skin of the face OR lip tumor involving inferior alveolar nerve, floor of mouth OR tumor with bilateral tongue involvement and/or DOI > 20 mm *Note*: Superficial bone erosion in tooth socket by gingival primary is not T4
	Very advanced: T4b: invasion of masticator space, pterygoid plates, skull base or internal carotid artery (ICA) encasement
N1	Metastasis to single Ipsilateral lymph node (LN) up to 3 cm in greatest dimension, No extranodal extension (ENE)
N2	Sigle/Multiple lymph nodes up to 6 cm
	N2a: Ipsilateral single LN 3–6 cm, No ENE
	N2b: Ipsilateral multiple LNs up to 6 cm, No ENE
	N2c: Contralateral or B/L LNs up to 6 cm, No ENE
N3	*N3a*: Lymph node > 6 cm, No ENE
	N3b: Any sized LN with clinically overt ENE present
M0	No distant metastases
M1	Distant metastases
Stage 1	T1, N0
Stage 2	T2, N0
Stage 3	Up to T3 or N1
Stage 4	T4, N2, N3 and M1

recent N-staging system is the extranodal spread. Most of the studies on extranodal extension (ENE) of the disease are based on pathological evaluation and imaging (both CT and MRI) are not very reliable. Thus, clinically overt ENE refers to unambiguous cases there is involvement of overlying dermis, invasion of adjacent soft tissues, tethering to adjacent structures or clinical evidence of nerve involvement.[3] Imaging may suggest ENE based on the presence of ill-defined nodal margins and irregularity of the capsule of the node.

Eighth edition of AJCC includes both the pathological / surgical staging as well as clinical stage (based on clinical examination, endoscopy, biopsy and imaging).

Imaging Modalities

CT and MRI are the primary imaging modalities. The role of the imaging in oral cavity cancers is not for the diagnosis but to evaluate extent of the tumor and lymph node involvement. Mere demonstration of the tumor on CT or MRI should not lead to satisfaction and possible overlooking of the important positive and negative imaging findings. Both CT and MRI perform similar in evaluation of most oral cavity cancers. MRI is better for assessment of soft tissue extension of the tumor, however, CT is more accurate for assessment of the bone erosions and lymph node involvement.[8] MRI takes much longer time than CT. Sometimes, this may be problematic, especially in patients with large oral cavity tumors as there is constant pooling and swallowing of the saliva. This degrades the MRI quality.[9] MRI must be performed with contrast enhancement. However, a non-contrast, non-fat suppressed axial sequence is essential to evaluate tumor margins and bone invasion. MRI is a preferred modality in cancer of the oral tongue and floor of mouth as small tumors at these locations may not be visualized on CT. Demonstration and extent evaluation of these tumors better on MRI.[10] MRI is also useful when any oral cavity tumor is extending into the RMT and invasion of other structures, such as pterygoid muscles, is equivocal on CT.[9,11]

SCCA of oral cavity do not enhance significantly when compared with adjacent soft tissues. Hence, small tumors may not be visualized. *Puffed-cheek maneuver* during CT help to identify small tumors which may be seen as asymmetric mucosal thickening, ulceration or the mass **(Fig. 6)**. It also separates buccal mucosa and gingiva and hence, helps to locate the tumor to gingival or buccal side, identify the involvement of upper or lower GB sulcus and submucosal tumor extension beyond it. Bone erosions upstage the oral cavity cancers to T4. These require extensive surgery and mandibular or maxillary resection. Type and extent of the bone resection is also determined by imaging findings. CT images reconstructed with sharp kernel and viewed on bone window are essential to detect and define the extent of bone erosions in oral cavity cancers. 3D reconstruction, MPRs and dental CT software with panoramic and real size zoom CT images provide important information to facilitate surgical decisions (***See* Figs. 4B and C**). Coronal images are useful to evaluate hard palate and any tumor extension to the maxillary sinus or floor of the nasal cavity **(Fig. 5)** and hence, these must be assessed in any tumor involving upper gingiva or hard palate.[5]

Oral cavity tumors involving RMT require extensive surgery. Invasion of masticator muscles upstage the tumor to T4 and any involvement of pterygoid muscles must be carefully looked for on imaging. Clinically, presence of trismus is highly specific for the masticator space involvement. Although, limited medial pterygoid involvement at its lower insertion can be resected, tumors involving pterygoid plates or lateral pterygoid muscle are unresectable.

In tumors of oral tongue and floor of mouth, involvement of ipsilateral neurovascular bundle, tumor extension across midline lingual septum and its relationship with contralateral neurovascular bundle must be carefully evaluated on imaging. Any deep invasion along mylohyoid muscle, bone involvement or posterior extension into the base of tongue or deep neck spaces must also be determined.

Treatment

Although small oral cavity cancers are amenable to radiotherapy, surgery is the primary treatment modality. Early oral cavity tumors are not detected on CT and clinical assessment determines the extent of wide local excision. Tumors involving bone or RMT require extensive surgery. Tumor abutting the mandible or with small superficial erosion are subjected to marginal resection in which bony continuity is maintained. With deeper or marrow invasion, segmental resection of the mandible and reconstruction with titanium plate is done. Myocutaneous flap or free flap is used to fill the defect.[12] The decision of marginal versus segmental resection as well as extent of the segmental resection of the mandible depends on imaging findings. Tumors involving upper alveolus or the hard palate require partial maxillectomy.

Floor of mouth cancers are treated with wide local excision using combined transoral and cervical approach. Mandibulotomy is required for tumor extending posteriorly in the base of tongue.[5]

Carcinoma of the tongue with small superficial tumor is treated with wide local excision or radical radiotherapy. Large tumors are treated with partial glossectomy (ipsilateral neurovascular bundle involvement) or total glossectomy (lingual septum and contralateral neurovascular bundle involvement). The latter is functionally crippling and concurrent chemoradiotherapy may be consideredas an alternative.[1]

NASOPHARYNX

Nasopharynx is a cuboid midline fibromuscular structure suspended from the skull base. It is bounded superiorly by sphenoid sinus and clivus, laterally by parapharyngeal spaces posteriorly by prevertebral muscles and anteriorly by nasal choanae. Nasopharynx continues inferiorly into the oropharynx. Two recesses can be normally identified on lateral wall of the nasopharynx; the posterosuperior recess is called the fossa of Rosenmuller. Anterior recess is the site for opening of eustachian tube. It enters in nasopharynx through a defect in pharyngobasillar fascia and this defect is a potential channel for spread of nasopharyngeal cancer to parapharyngeal spaces. Beneath the posterior mucosal surface of nasopharynx lie retropharyngeal and prevertebral spaces. Retropharyngeal lymph nodes are located in retropharyngeal space and these are usually the first lymph nodes to be involved in nasopharyngeal carcinoma.

Nasopharyngeal Carcinoma

Nasopharyngeal carcinoma is most common in China and Southeast Asian countries. In India, it as an uncommon tumor with national age averaged rate of less than 1 case per 100,000 per year, however, much higher incidence is found in some parts of North-East India.[4] Nasopharyngeal carcinoma is more common in males. It usually involves middle aged people but children and adolescents are also frequently affected. Pathological majority of nasopharyngeal carcinomas are undifferentiated and highly aggressive tumors and they have strong association with EBV infection. Unlike most other head and neck sites, well differentiated squamous cell carcinoma is rare in nasopharynx.

Most patients with nasopharyngeal carcinoma present with painless upper cervical nodal mass. Nasal obstruction, epistaxis and otitis media are other presenting symptoms. Facial pain is found in patients with nerve involvement and sore throat in those with oropharyngeal spread. Patients with advanced tumors may also have headache, proptosis, trismus, cranial nerve palsies or painful neck movements.[1] Fiberoptic examination shows tumor in roof or lateral wall of nasopharynx, however, early lesions may not be visible.

Most nasopharyngeal carcinomas arise in fossa of Rosenmuller and spread via submucosal route. Invasion of palatal muscles (levator and tensor veli palatine) occurs early. Dysfunction of these muscles affects normal opening mechanism of eustachian tube. The opening may also be directly obstructed by the tumor. Hence, it commonly results into serous otitis media. On imaging, early nasopharyngeal carcinoma may not be demonstrated or seen as nonspecific bulge or obliteration of fossa of Rosenmuller. Others are seen as mildly enhancing mass confined to nasopharynx **(Fig. 7)**. Advanced tumors then extend along all direction. Lateral spread to parapharyngeal space is the most common direction of spread **(Figs. 8 and 9)**. Subsequently, it involves pterygoid muscles. Tumor involvement of these masticator muscles is prone for mandibular nerve involvement and perineural intracranial extension through the foramen ovale. This is the most common route for intracranial extension in nasopharyngeal carcinoma.[13] Tumor spread in posterior direction involves retropharyngeal space and then prevertebral muscles. In advanced cases, vertebral bodies may also be destroyed. Posterolaterally, the tumors may involve carotid artery and posterosuperiorly, the jugular fossa and posterior cranial fossa. With direct superior spread of nasopharyngeal carcinoma, the tumor erodes skull base in the region of sphenoid sinus, clivus and petrous apex **(Fig. 9C)**. Anterior spread of nasopharyngeal carcinoma extends into nasal cavity, maxillary sinus. From the upper part of nasal cavity, the tumor may extend into pterygopalatine fossa and orbit. Once tumor reaches orbital apex, it can easily gain intracranial access to middle cranial fossa via superior orbital fissure.

Nasopharyngeal carcinoma has very high propensity for cervical lymph node involvement. Up to 75% of the patients have nodal metastases, often bilateral, at presentation.[14] Distant metastases are also common than in other head and neck cancers and these usually occur in bone, lung and liver.[15]

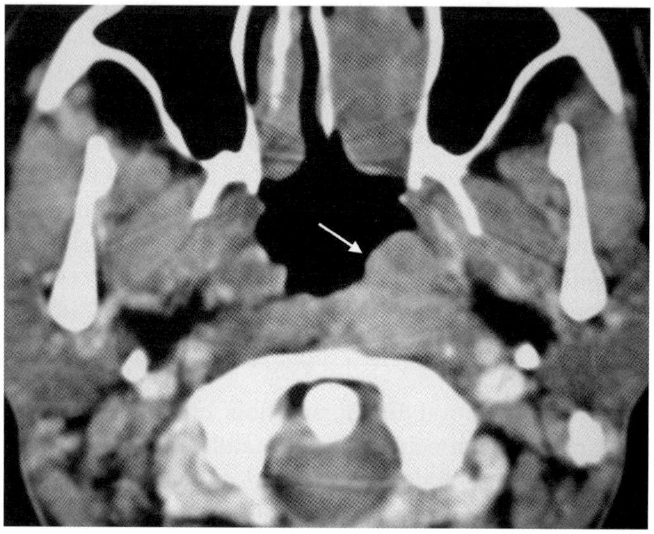

Fig. 7: Carcinoma of nasopharynx: CT shows mildly enhancing mass confined to left posterolateral aspect of nasopharynx.

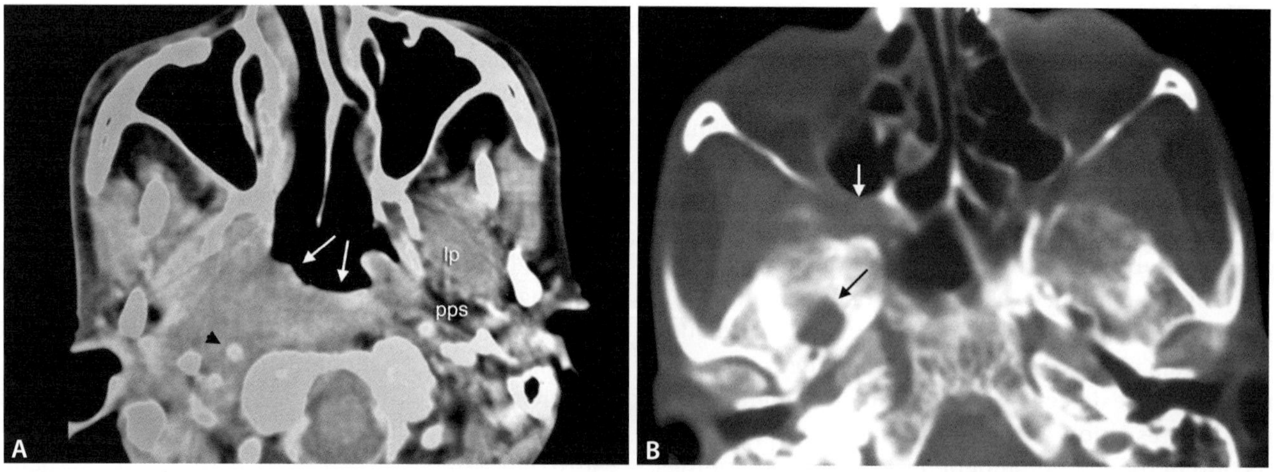

Figs. 8A and B: Carcinoma of nasopharynx. (A) CT shows a large nasopharyngeal mass (arrows) extending to retropharyngeal space, obliteration of right parapharyngeal fat space and invasion of right lateral pterygoid muscle. Normal left parapharyngeal space (pps) and lateral pterygoid muscle (lp) are well seen. The tumor is also encasing ipsilateral internal carotid artery (arrowhead); (B) Bone window at the level of skull base shows widening of the right pterygopalatine fossa (white arrow) and foramen ovale (black arrow) suggestive of perineural extension of the tumor.

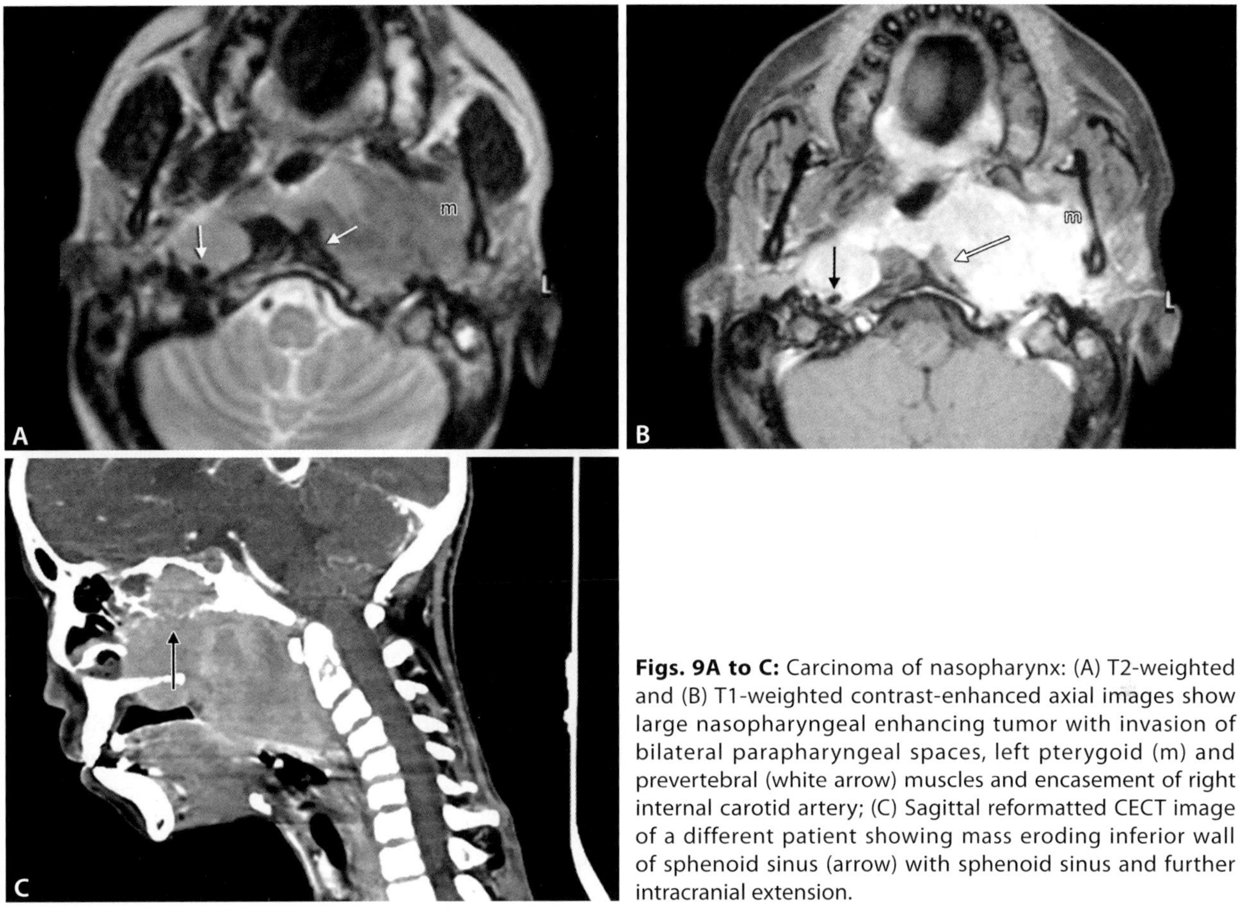

Figs. 9A to C: Carcinoma of nasopharynx: (A) T2-weighted and (B) T1-weighted contrast-enhanced axial images show large nasopharyngeal enhancing tumor with invasion of bilateral parapharyngeal spaces, left pterygoid (m) and prevertebral (white arrow) muscles and encasement of right internal carotid artery; (C) Sagittal reformatted CECT image of a different patient showing mass eroding inferior wall of sphenoid sinus (arrow) with sphenoid sinus and further intracranial extension.

Staging of Nasopharyngeal Carcinoma

Eighth edition TNM staging by AJCC is used **(Table 3)**. T1 tumors are confined to oro-nasopharynx and/or nasal cavity. T2 extend into parapharyngeal tissues. T3 tumors have bony invasion. T4 tumors are those with intracranial extension or involvement of cranial nerves, orbit, hypopharynx, parotid or beyond the lateral pterygoid muscles. Cervical lymph nodal staging for nasopharyngeal carcinoma is different from that of oral cavity cancers. Nodal size of 6 cm is used to differentiate N1 and N2 nodes in nasopharyngeal carcinoma, unlike the criteria of 3 cm for oral cavity cancers.

Imaging Features

Thin section CECT with axial and coronal reconstruction and sharp kernel bone window images are useful. For MRI, pre- and post-contrast fast spin echo sequences are obtained. Both fat suppressed and non-fat suppressed images need to be evaluated. Both CT and MRI are equivalent in staging of nasopharyngeal carcinoma. CT is superior in evaluation of bony erosion and lymph node involvement while MRI better shows perineural

Table 3: Staging of nasopharyngeal carcinoma: Overview.

T1	Limited to nasopharynx or extends to oropharynx and/or nasal cavity
T2	Parapharyngeal extension and/or involvement of pterygoid, and/or pre-vertebral muscles
T3	Bone invasion (skull base, cervical vertebra, pterygoid plate, paranasal sinuses)
T4	Intracranial extension or involvement of cranial nerves, orbit, hypopharynx, parotid or extension lateral to lateral pterygoid muscles
N1	Ipsilateral cervical LN up to 6 cm (above caudal border of cricoid cartilage) Any side retropharyngeal LN up to 6 cm
N2	Bilateral cervical LN up to 6 cm (above caudal border of cricoid cartilage)
N3	LN more than 6 cm or caudal to caudal border of cricoid cartilage
M0	No distant metastases
M1	Distant metastases
Stage 1	T1, N0
Stage 2	Up to T2, N1
Stage 3	Up to T3, N2
Stage 4	T4, N3 and M1

intracranial spread along maxillary or mandibular nerves. Along the nerves, it further extends to cavernous sinus and Meckel's cave. The diagnosis of nasopharyngeal carcinoma in children is often made late on because of presence of benign adenoid hypertrophy. It should be remembered that nasopharyngeal carcinoma can occur in children. If any asymmetry of the nasopharyngeal mass is observed, a careful search for any tumor spread outside the nasopharynx should be made on imaging as this suggests the correct diagnosis.[16]

Treatment

Radiotherapy is the standard treatment of nasopharyngeal carcinoma as surgery is not feasible. Patients with advanced disease also receive concurrent chemotherapy. Apart from the nasopharynx, radiation field also includes skull base, infratemporal fossa and adjoin parts of nasal cavity, sinuses and oropharynx. The margin of the radiation field is modified as per the tumor extension into specific areas. 3D CT based conformal treatment planning is normally used. Bilateral neck nodes irradiation up to clavicle is also required in all cases.

OROPHARYNX

Oropharynx extends from soft palate superiorly to the vallecula inferiorly. Anterior margin is a plane formed by soft palate, anterior tonsillar pillars and the circumvallate papilla of the tongue. Posterior pharyngeal wall forms the posterior limit of oropharynx. Laterally, the oropharynx has anterior tonsillar pillar (palatoglossus muscle), posterior tonsillar pillar (palatopharyngeus muscle) and the lymphoid tissue in between these, called as palatine or faucial tonsils. Parts of the oropharynx are soft palate, posterior pharyngeal wall, tonsils and the base of the tongue. Most cancers are SCCA. In India, it is an uncommon malignancy with the national age averaged rate is less than 1.3 per 100,000 per year, except in some parts of North-East India, where higher incidence has been observed.[4] Other tumors of oropharynx include lymphoma involving the Waldeyer's ring, adenocarcinoma, lymphoepithelioma and sarcoma. Submucosal spread of the tumors is common and hence, endoscopy tends to underestimate the tumor spread. Extent assessment and therapeutic decisions are normally based on imaging findings.

Carcinoma of Tonsil

Superficial and small tonsillar tumors, especially those located in the tonsillar fossa may not be visible on CT. Other may just show suspicious tonsillar asymmetry.

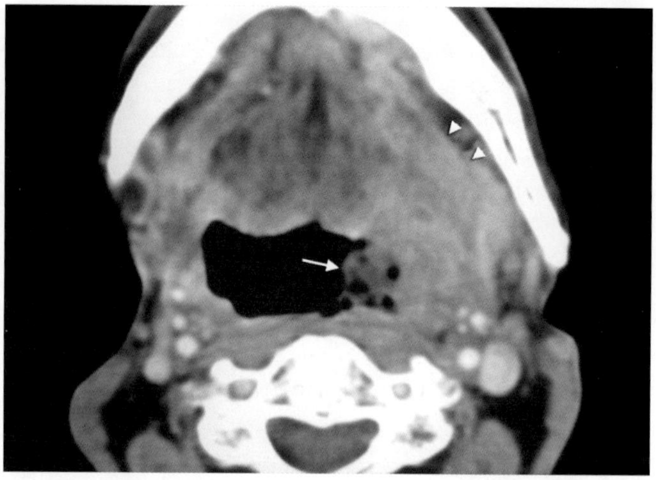

Fig. 10: Carcinoma of tonsil: CT shows ulcerated left tonsillar mass (arrow) with parapharyngeal and base of tongue invasion which is further extending floor of mouth and involving mylohyoid muscle (arrowheads).

Larger tumors are seen as ulcerated or infiltrative masses with enhancement similar to normal tonsil on CT[9] **(Fig. 10)**. Fat suppressed post-contrast MRI improves the tumor delineation. Tumors arising from mucosa overlying anterior tonsillar pillar spread along underlying palatoglossus muscle. Superior spread and involvement of the soft palate is common. Subsequently hard palate may also be involved. With further superior spread, tonsillar tumors involve nasopharynx and reach the skull base. Anterior spread of the tumor involves retromolar trigone and pterygomandibular raphe, pterygoid and buccinators muscles. Inferior spread involves the base of the tongue. Posterior tonsillar pillar is rarely a site of origin of SCCA and most are extensions from anterior pillar or tonsillar fossa tumors. The spread is similar; however, inferiorly these may extend to aryepiglottic folds the thyroid cartilage. Tumors arising at the tonsillar fossa between two tonsillar pillars frequently remain occult and may present with cervical nodal metastases. Deep tumor invasion through superior constrictor muscle into the parapharyngeal space and then to the skull base is common with tonsillar fossa tumors.[5]

Carcinoma of Soft Palate

Most are SCCA however minor salivary gland type adenocarcinomas (minor salivary gland tumors) are also common, especially in posterior part of soft palate. Soft palate SCCAs are usually well-differentiated or low grade tumors among all pharyngeal cancers and behave more like oral cavity cancers. Carcinomas of the soft palate arise at oral surface and nasopharyngeal surface is rarely involved. Early tumors are difficult to visualize on axial images although it may be seen as asymmetrical thickening of the soft palate **(Fig. 11A)**. Coronal and sagittal CT or MRI is essential to evaluate the tumors involving soft and hard palate **(Figs. 12A and B)**. Soft palate carcinoma commonly spread in anteriorly to hard palate or laterally to tonsillar pillars. Advanced tumors involve nasopharynx, parapharyngeal spaces and the skull base **(Fig. 11B)**.

Carcinoma of Base of Tongue

Posterior-one third of the tongue is called base of tongue. It is the vertically oriented part of the tongue that extends from triangular circumvallate papilla superiorly to the vallecula inferiorly. Lingual tonsils, a lymphoid tissue, lie beneath the mucosa of base of tongue and vallecula and appears isodense to muscles. Most SCCA of base of tongue arise on its lateral aspect. Small cancers of the base of tongue often remain occult and present with neck node metastases **(Figs. 13A and B)**. These may not be clearly visualized on CT or MRI, primarily because of poor contrast enhancement of the tumor, dense muscles of the tongue, isodense lingual tonsils and absence of well-defined fat planes in this region. Larger tumors are seen as asymmetric or bulky contours **(Fig. 14)**. Earliest

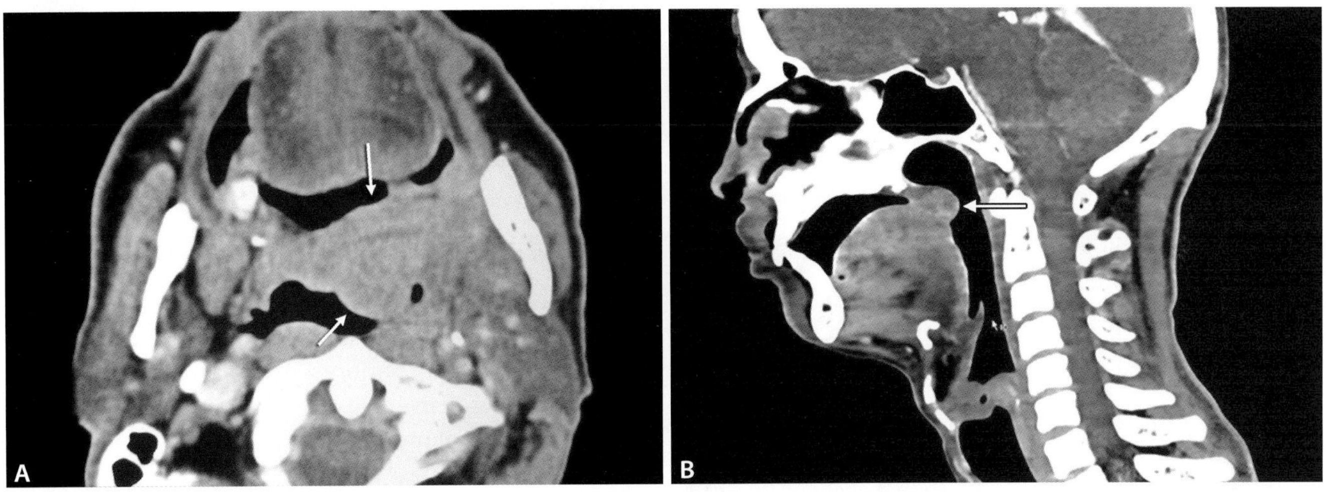

Figs. 11A and B: Carcinoma of soft palate: (A) CT shows the tumor as asymmetric bulky thickening of the soft palate on left side (arrows) with left parapharyngeal extension and invasion of left medial pterygoid muscle; (B) Sagittal reformatted image of another patient showing bulbous enlargement of posteroinferior part of soft palate with mild heterogeneous enhancement (arrow).

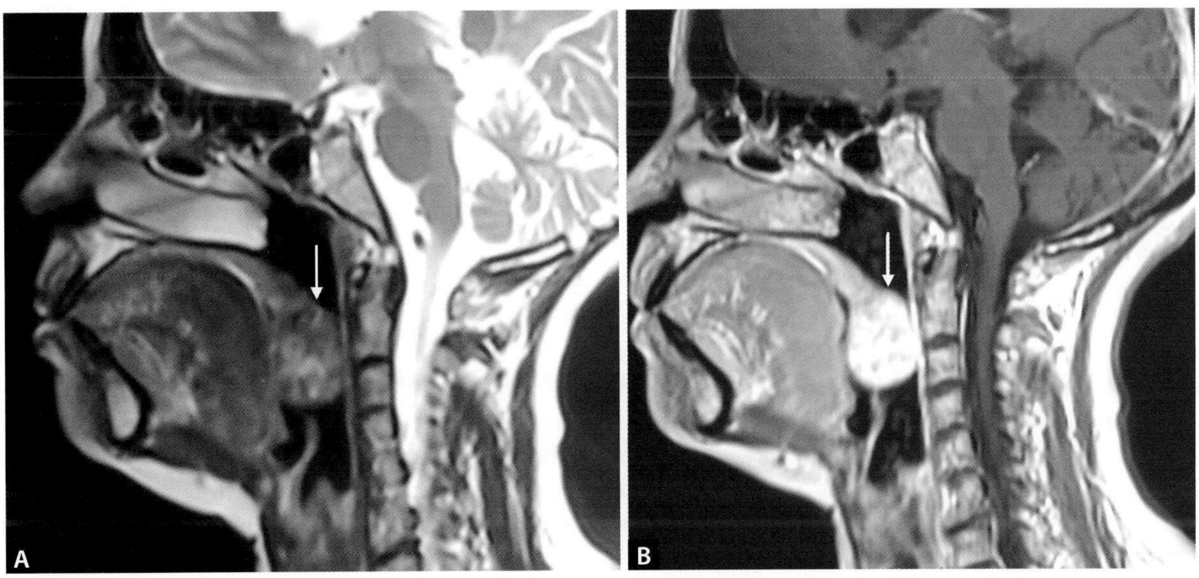

Figs. 12A and B: Carcinoma of soft palate: (A) T2-weighted and (B) contrast-enhanced T1-weighted sagittal images show small enhancing tumor (arrows) arising from and limited to the soft palate.

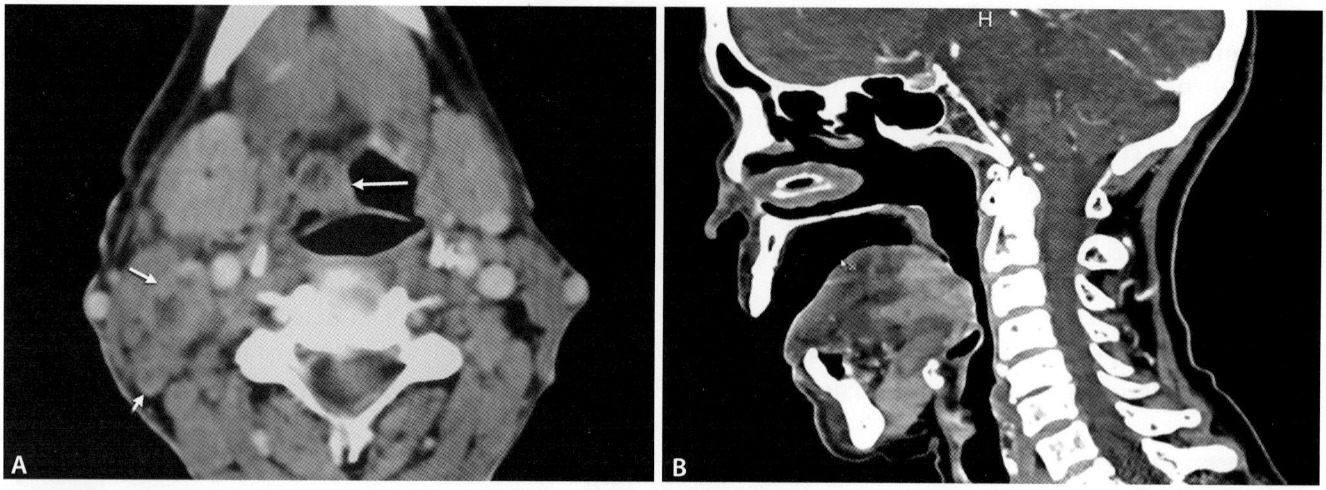

Figs. 13A and B: Carcinoma of base of tongue: (A) CT of the patient presenting with left cervical lymphadenopathy shows multiple enlarged necrotic right level II lymph nodes (small arrows). The primary tumor seen in right vallecula (large arrow) was detected on CT; (B) Sagittal image of a different patient showing enhancing mass in posterior third of tongue.

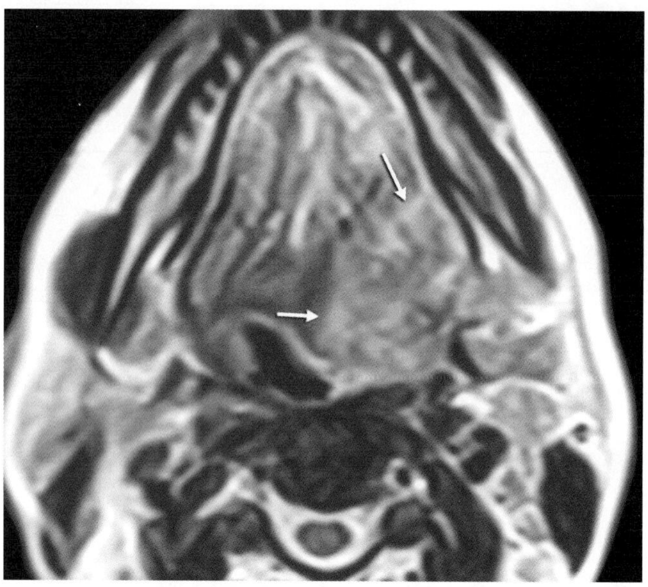

Fig. 14: Carcinoma of base of tongue: T2-weighted MR image shows large tumor in base of tongue on left side with extension to the floor of mouth (arrows).

tumor extension occurs inferiorly to vallecula, which is in anatomical continuity with base of tongue, and then below it into the pre-epiglottic space. Lateral spread form vallecula extends deep into the neck spaces and then rapidly extends to styloid muscles. With further growth to the prestyloid area, it may encase internal carotid artery. Anterior spread of base of tongue carcinoma involves floor of mouth. Obliteration of fat planes around lingual neurovascular bundle is highly suggestive of its encasement and perineural and perivascular spread of the tumor. In base of tongue carcinomas, medial spread across the midline or lateral spread to tonsils are uncommon and occur late in the course of the disease.

Because of the rich lymphatic supply of the tongue and advanced disease stage when patients become symptomatic, most patients of carcinoma of base of tongue have extensive and often bilateral cervical lymph node metastases at presentation.

Staging and Treatment of Carcinoma of Oropharynx

In the latest staging system **(Table 4)**, a new classification has been introduced for HPV-positive oropharyngeal cancers.[4] This was the need of the hour because of their biologically distinct behavior as well as differences in clinical care and surveillance. HPV-positive oropharyngeal cancers are positive on p16 immunostaining and have better prognosis.

Although early tumors of tonsils or soft palate can be resected with intraoral approach, radical radiotherapy is the primary treatment modality for oropharyngeal tumors. Advanced tumors require concurrent chemoradiotherapy.[1]

HYPOPHARYNX

Hypopharynx is the part of upper aerodigestive tract which lies below and continuous with the oropharynx. Hypopharynx extends from the level of hyoid bone superiorly to the level of inferior margin of the cricoid cartilage. Hypopharynx continues below as the cervical esophagus. Parts of hypopharynx are posterior pharyngeal wall, bilateral pyriform sinuses and the post-cricoid

Table 4: Staging of oropharyngeal cancers.

T1	Tumor ≤ 2 cm	
T2	Tumor 2–4 cm	
T3	Tumor > 4 cm OR extension to upper surface of epiglottis	
T4	Advanced local disease	
	For p16 negative cancers: Invasion of larynx, extrinsic muscle of the tongue, medial pterygoid, hard palate, or mandible	
	For p16 positive cancers: *Moderately Advanced T4a: Tumor invades the larynx, extrinsic muscle of the tongue, medial pterygoid, hard palate, or mandible* *Very advanced T4b: invasion of lateral pterygoid muscle, pterygoid bone, lateral nasopharynx, skull base or ICA encasement*	
	For p16 positive tumors	*For p16 negative tumors*
N1	Single/multiple Ipsilateral LNs up to 6 cm	Single ipsilateral LN up to 3 cm, No ENE
N2	Bilateral LNs up to 6 cm	Sigle/Multiple lymph nodes up to 6 cm
		N2a: ipsilateral single LN 3–6 cm, No ENE
		N2b: ipsilateral multiple LNs up to 6 cm, No ENE
		N2c: contralateral or B/L LNs up to 6 cm, No ENE
N3	LN> 6 cm	N3a: LN> 6 cm, No ENE
		N3b: LN with clinically overt ENE
M0	No distant metastases	
M1	Distant metastases	
Stage	*For p16 positive tumors*	*For p16 negative tumors*
Stage 1	Up to T2, N1	T1N0M0
Stage 2	Up to T3, N2	T2N0M0
Stage 3	Up to T4 or N3	Up to T3 or N1
Stage 4	M1	T4 or N2 or M1 (further subdivided into A, B and C)

region. The posterior wall of hypopharynx is continuous with posterior wall of oropharynx. Pyriform sinuses are lateral air distended recess created by aryepiglottic folds. Each pyriform sinus is triangular in shape having medial, anterior and lateral walls. The apex or lower tip of the pyriform sinus lies at the level of true vocal cords. At the level of cricoid cartilage, posterior parts of two pyriform sinuses merge to form the post cricoid region of the hypopharynx. Postcricoid region forms the pharyngo-esophageal junction.

Carcinoma of hypopharynx is more common in males. In India, it is more common than naso- or oropharyngeal carcinoma, with age averaged rate ranging from 1 to 6.3 cases per 100,000 per year.[4] Much higher incidence is found in some parts of North-East India, where it is the second most common cancer in males. SCCAs of hypopharynx spread submucosally, often remain clinically silent for long and majority of the patients already have cervical lymph node metastases at presentation.

Carcinoma of Posterior Wall of Hypopharynx

Carcinomas arising at posterior wall of hypopharynx most commonly spread superiorly and inferiorly with submucosal infiltration. With superior spread, these extend into the oropharynx and may also involve posterior tonsillar pillars. Inferior spread involves post-cricoid region and the esophagus. Rarely, the tumor may spread posteriorly into the prevertebral space.

Carcinoma of the Pyriform Sinus

Most SCCA of hypopharynx arise at the pyriform sinus. Apart from endoscopic evaluation, carcinoma of the pyriform sinus can also be demonstrated with barium swallow **(Fig. 15)**. CT or MRI is required for assessment of submucosal extent of the tumor. Adequate distension of the pyriform sinus is essential during imaging. A collapsed pyriform sinus may simulate the tumor and on the other hand, a documented tumor may not apparent on CT or MRI.[5]

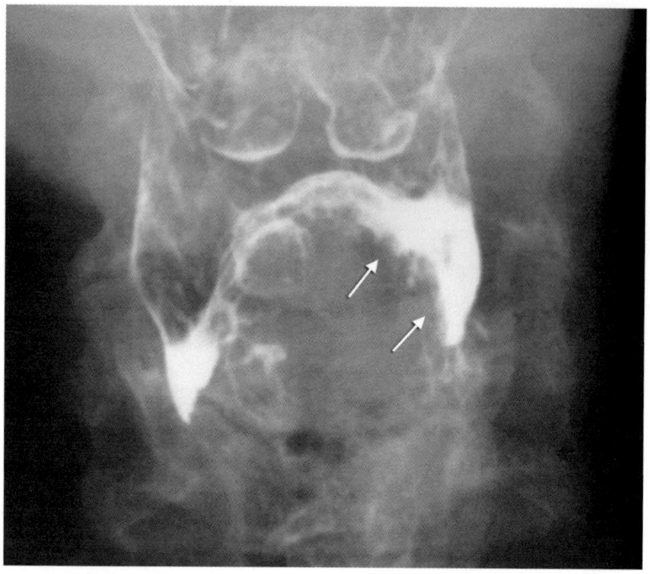

Fig. 15: Carcinoma of pyriform sinus: Barium swallow shows irregularity and narrowing of left pyriform sinus (arrows).

Carcinoma of pyriform sinus is seen on CT or MRI as homogenous masses with submucosal spread. Commonly spread in anatomical contiguity into the posterior pharyngeal wall, medially to aryepiglottic fold or inferiorly into the postcricoid region. Tumors on medial aspect of the pyriform sinus involve aryepiglottic fold and then along with it, spread to false vocal cords, paraglottic space and arytenoids cartilage **(Figs. 16A to C)**. With further growth, these may involve epiglottis, pre-epiglottic space and the base of the tongue. Posterior spread of the carcinoma of pyriform sinus involves postcricoid region or posterior pharyngeal wall **(Fig. 17)**. With further posterior submucosal growth along the posterior pharyngeal wall, the tumor extends across the midline to involve contralateral pyriform sinus.

Carcinoma of the Postcricoid

Carcinomas arising at the postcricoid are uncommon. It usually occurs in patients with Plummer-Vinson syndrome

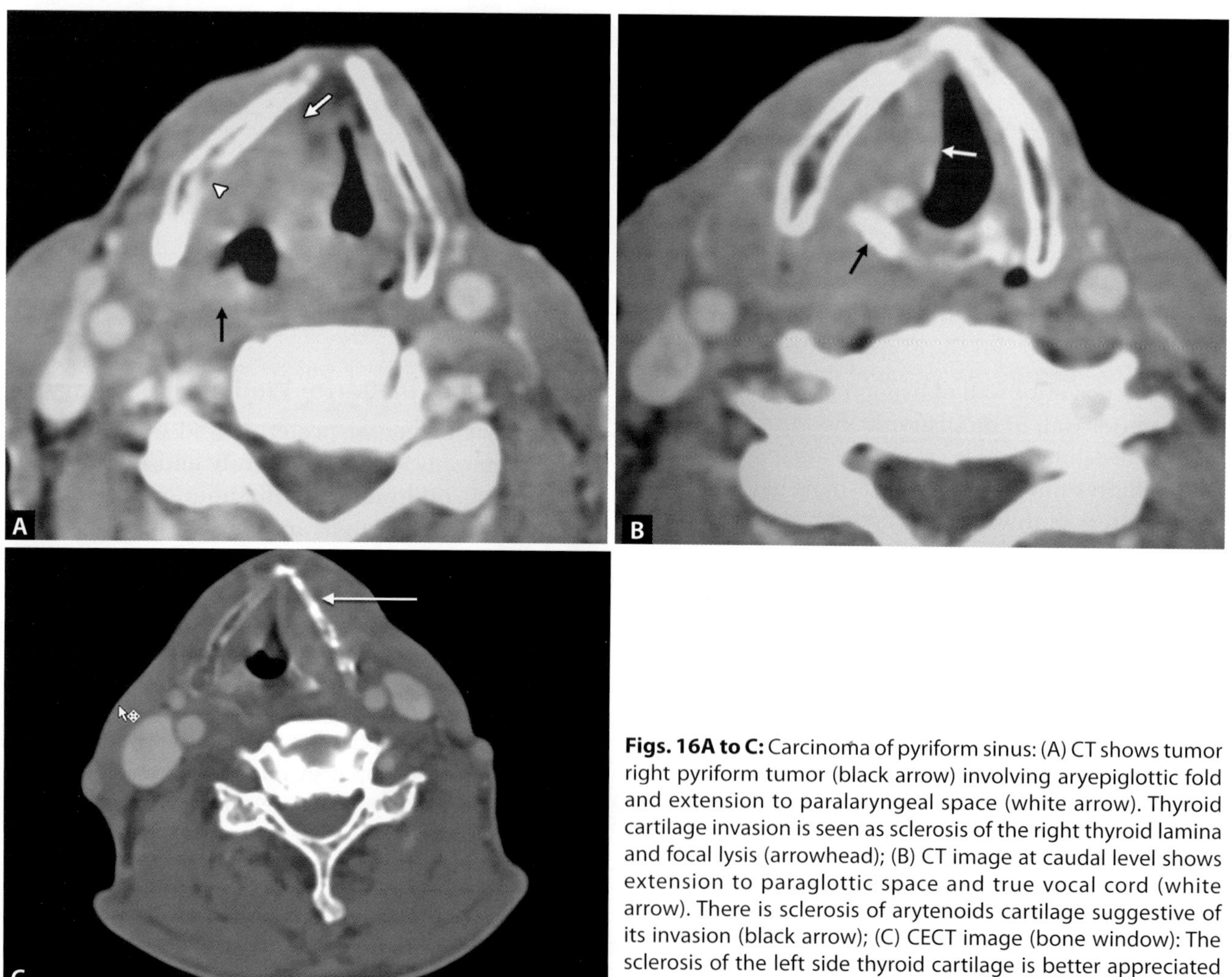

Figs. 16A to C: Carcinoma of pyriform sinus: (A) CT shows tumor right pyriform tumor (black arrow) involving aryepiglottic fold and extension to paralaryngeal space (white arrow). Thyroid cartilage invasion is seen as sclerosis of the right thyroid lamina and focal lysis (arrowhead); (B) CT image at caudal level shows extension to paraglottic space and true vocal cord (white arrow). There is sclerosis of arytenoids cartilage suggestive of its invasion (black arrow); (C) CECT image (bone window): The sclerosis of the left side thyroid cartilage is better appreciated on bone window image (white arrow).

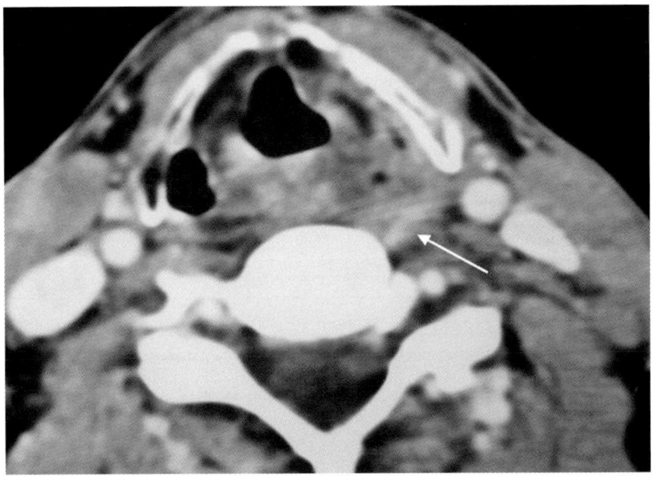

Fig. 17: Carcinoma of pyriform sinus: CT shows left pyriform sinus tumor involving posterior pharyngeal wall and prevertebral muscles (arrow).

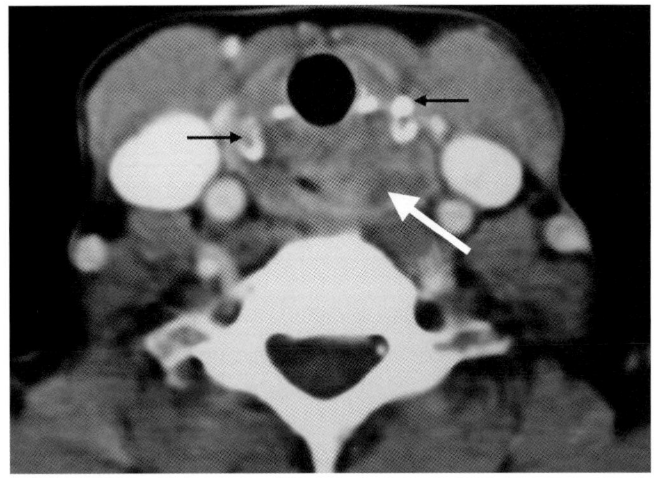

Fig. 18: Carcinoma of postcricoid: CT shows postcricoid tumor (white arrow) with anterior extension to glottis with invasion and sclerosis of cricoid and arytenoids cartilages (black arrows).

(dysphagia, weight loss, iron deficiency anemia and cervical esophageal web). Carcinoma of the postcricoid cause concentric wall thickening and narrowing of the hypopharyngeal lumen. Because of the close anatomical proximity, these usually spread to posterior part of the larynx and involve arytenoids and cricoid cartilages **(Fig. 18)**. Inferior extension of the carcinoma of postcricoid involves cervical esophagus.

Treatment

Radical radiotherapy is the preferred modality of treatment for low volume carcinomas of hypopharynx. Others are treated with surgery and this may include wide local excision and partial or total laryngo-pharyngectomy. Type of the surgery depends on extent of the tumor as depicted on imaging. In hypopharyngeal cancers; important points that need to be determined on imaging include location and submucosal extent of the tumor, extension across the midline, lower margin of the tumor, involvement of apex of the pyriform sinus, cartilage erosion and invasion of prevertebral muscles. Tumor involving apex of the pyriform sinus lies close to true vocal cords and it has high probability of involvement of cricoid and arytenoid cartilages and paraglottic space. Hence, such tumors require total laryngo-pharyngectomy. Tumors involving postcricoid or cervical esophagus also require esophagectomy in addition to total laryngo-pharyngectomy. Advanced tumors of hypopharynx are treated with combination of chemotherapy and radiotherapy.

LARYNX

Larynx is made up of mucosal surface and supporting cartilage skeleton. True vocal cords divide larynx into supraglottic, glottis and subglotic compartments. Supraglottis extends from vallecula superiorly to the laryngeal ventricle (space between false and true vocal cords) inferiorly.

Supraglottic larynx includes epiglottis, aryepiglottic folds, false cords and arytenoids process of the arytenoids cartilage. Superior part of the epiglottis has free margins and lower lateral margins have mucosal folds extending from it to the arytenoids cartilages. These are aryepiglottic folds. Inferior continuation of aryepiglottic folds are false vocal cords. Glottic larynx is composed of pair of true vocal cords and cartilages. True vocal cords extend from arytenoid cartilages posteriorly to the anterior commissure. Anterior commissure is composed of mucosa only and measures less than 1 mm on imaging. Arytenoid cartilage is articulated inferiorly to cricoid cartilage and the cricoarytenoid joint allows the movements of the true vocal cords. Subglottic larynx extends from inferior surface of true vocal cords to inferior margin of cricoid cartilage.

Larynx also has several muscles grouped into extrinsic and intrinsic muscles. Extrinsic muscles are elevators of larynx (stylohyoid, mylohyoid, thyrohyoid and digastric) and depressors of larynx (sternothyroid, sternohyoid and omohyoid). Intrinsic muscles are located in vocal cords and adjacent to it and these muscles provide vocal and airway control. Supraglottic and subglottic larynx have rich lymphatic supply, however, glottis has sparse lymphatics.

Carcinoma of larynx is primarily related to smoking. In India, the age averaged rate ranges from 1.4 to 7.5 cases per 100,000 per year.[4] It is the second most common cancer in males in Delhi. Carcinoma of the larynx includes supraglottic, glottic and subglottic cancers. Involvement of both supraglottic and glottis is termed as transglottic cancer. There is separate AJCC tumor staging system for each compartment as outlined in **Table 5**. Nodal staging is same in all.

Table 5: Staging of carcinoma of larynx: Overview.

T stage	***Supraglottic tumors***
T1	Limited to one subsite (structure), normal vocal cord mobility
T2	Involvement of more than one subsites or extension outside supraglottis (vallecula, base of tongue, piriform sinus). Vocal cords not fixed
T3	Limited to larynx with fixed vocal cords Any extension to pre-epiglottic space or postcricoid or paraglottic space or inner cortex of thyroid cartilage
T4	*T4a Moderately advanced*: Involvement of outer cortex of thyroid cartilage or extralaryngeal spread (e.g., trachea, soft tissues of the neck including deep extrinsic muscle of the tongue, strap muscles, thyroid, or esophagus)
	T4b Very advanced: Extends to prevertebral space, encases carotid artery, or invades mediastinal structures
T stage	***Glottic tumors***
T1	Limited to one (T1a) or both (T1b) vocal cords with preserved mobility of vocal cords
T2	Extension to supraglottic or subglottis or impaired vocal cord mobility
T3	Limited to larynx with fixed vocal cords or invasion of paraglottic space or inner cortex of thyroid cartilage
T4	*T4a Moderately advanced*: Involvement of outer cortex of thyroid cartilage or extralaryngeal spread (e.g. trachea, cricoid cartilage, soft tissues of the neck including deep extrinsic muscle of the tongue, strap muscles, thyroid, or esophagus)
	T4b Very advanced: Extends to prevertebral space, encases carotid artery, or invades mediastinal structures
T stage	***Subglottic tumors***
T1	Limited to subglottis
T2	Involvement of vocal cords, not fixed
T3	Limited to larynx, vocal cords fixed or invasion of paraglottic space or inner cortex of thyroid cartilage
T4	*T4a Moderately advanced*: Involvement of outer cortex of thyroid cartilage or extralaryngeal spread (e.g. trachea, cricoid cartilage, soft tissues of the neck including deep extrinsic muscle of the tongue, strap muscles, thyroid, or esophagus)
	T4b Very advanced: Extends to prevertebral space, encases carotid artery, or invades mediastinal structures
N	***Stage***
N1	Single ipsilateral LN up to 3 cm, No ENE
N2	Sigle/Multiple lymph nodes up to 6 cm
	N2a: Ipsilateral single LN 3–6 cm, No ENE
	N2b: Ipsilateral multiple LNs up to 6 cm, No ENE
	N2c: Contralateral or B/L LNs up to 6 cm, No ENE
N3	*N3a*: LN> 6 cm, No ENE
	N3b: LN with clinically overt ENE
M	***Stage***
M0	No distant metastases
M1	Distant metastases
Stage grouping	
Stage 1	T1, N0
Stage 2	T2, N0
Stage 3	Up to T3 or N1
Stage 4	T4a or N2 (4a), T4b or N3 (4b) and M1 (4c)

Supraglottic Carcinoma

These may arise from any mucosal surface of the supraglottic larynx but epiglottis is the most common site of origin. Early tumors of epiglottis are often seen on imaging as midline, well-defined enhancing nodules. With further spread, epiglottic tumors may spread superiorly to vallecula and base of tongue and laterally to aryepiglottic folds, false vocal cords and paralaryngeal fat deep to false vocal cords. Anterior extension of epiglottic tumors involves fat in pre-epiglottic space **(Figs. 19 and 20)**. Early tumors arising from aryepiglottic folds or false cords are also exophytic and confined to the fold of origin. Such early lesions are also called as marginal tumors. With medial or lateral spread, these involve epiglottis and pyriform sinus respectively **(Fig. 21)**.

Any supraglottic carcinoma can directly extend to glottis and involve true vocal cords. The glottic involvement may be anteriorly to anterior commissure or posteriorly to involve cricoarytenoid joint; the later results in fixity of the cord. Further inferior spread to subglottis however, is prevented till late by a fibrous barrier, known as conus elasticus. It extends from cricoid cartilage to medial margins of true vocal cords. Cartilage invasion by supraglottic carcinoma is also a late feature.

In supraglottic carcinoma, deep extension beneath the mucosa is underestimated clinically and can be detected only on imaging. Important submucosal spaces that need to be evaluated on imaging include pre-epiglottic space anterior to epiglottis and paralaryngeal spaces lateral to aryepiglottic folds and false cords **(Figs. 19 and 20)**. These spaces normally contain fat and hence tumor invasion of these spaces can be seen as partial or complete obliteration of fat. Paralaryngeal fat is also continuous with paraglottic space lateral to true vocal cords and via this route; supraglottic cancers can directly involve true vocal cords. Pre-epiglottic space also has rich and bilateral lymphatic drainage and tumors involving this space have high probability of bilateral neck node metastases.

Glottic Carcinoma

True vocal cords are the most common site of laryngeal carcinoma. Most glottis carcinoma arise along the anterior free margin of the true vocal cords. Small lesions result in thickening of the vocal cord on imaging and large lesions may be seen as bulky masses **(Fig. 22)**. With anterior spread, glottis carcinoma readily involves anterior commissure. From here, it may spread to contralateral vocal cord or extend along tendon of the anterior commissure to thyroid cartilage where this tendon is attached. This results in early thyroid cartilage invasion **(Fig. 23C)**. Glottic carcinoma may also arise at the commissure. Posterior extension of the glottis carcinoma involves interarytenoid region (posterior commissure) and cricoarytenoid joint. Glottic carcinoma superiorly spread to ventricle and false vocal cords. It may also extend inferiorly to subglottic region, although it is relatively uncommon **(Figs. 23A and B)**.

Subglottic Carcinoma

Carcinoma primarily arising at subglottic larynx is rare and most are extensions of glottic or supraglottic carcinomas **(Figs. 23A to C)**. Primary subglottic carcinoma is seen as circumferential mucosal thickening of the subglottis.

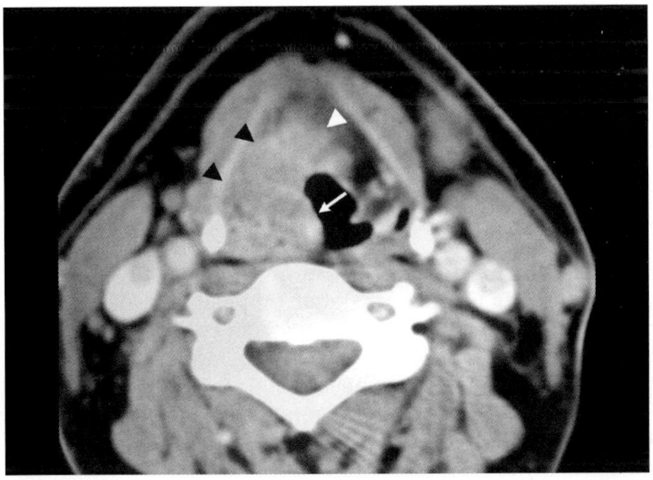

Fig. 19: Supraglottic carcinoma: CT shows epiglottic tumor involving aryepiglottic fold (arrow), paralaryngeal space (black arrowheads) and pre-epiglottic space (white arrowhead).

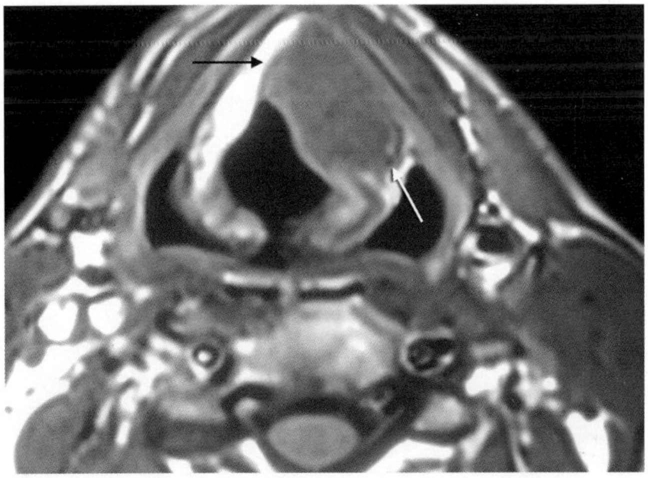

Fig. 20: Supraglottic carcinoma: T1-weighted axial MR image shows hypointense epiglottic tumor extending into and obliterating pre-epiglottic (black arrow) and paralaryngeal (white arrow) spaces.

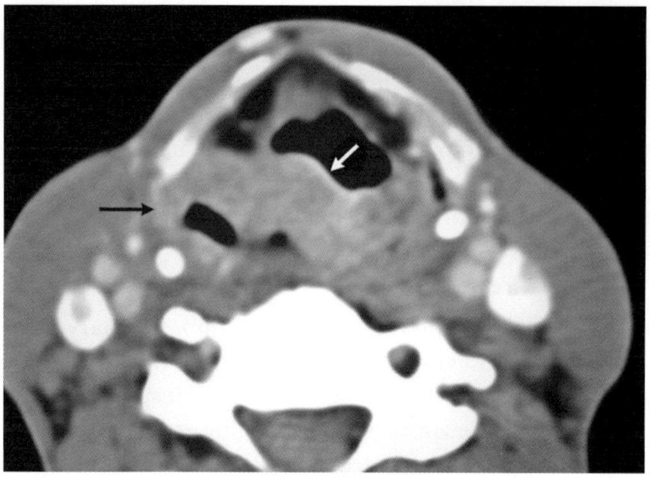

Fig. 21: Supraglottic carcinoma: CT shows right aryepiglottic tumor (white arrow) with extension to the pyriform sinus (black arrow).

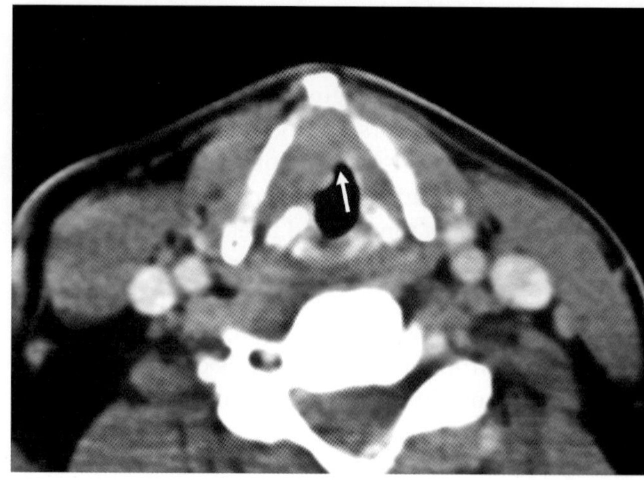

Fig. 22: Glottic carcinoma: CT shows tumor in right true vocal cord with extension to anterior commissure (arrow).

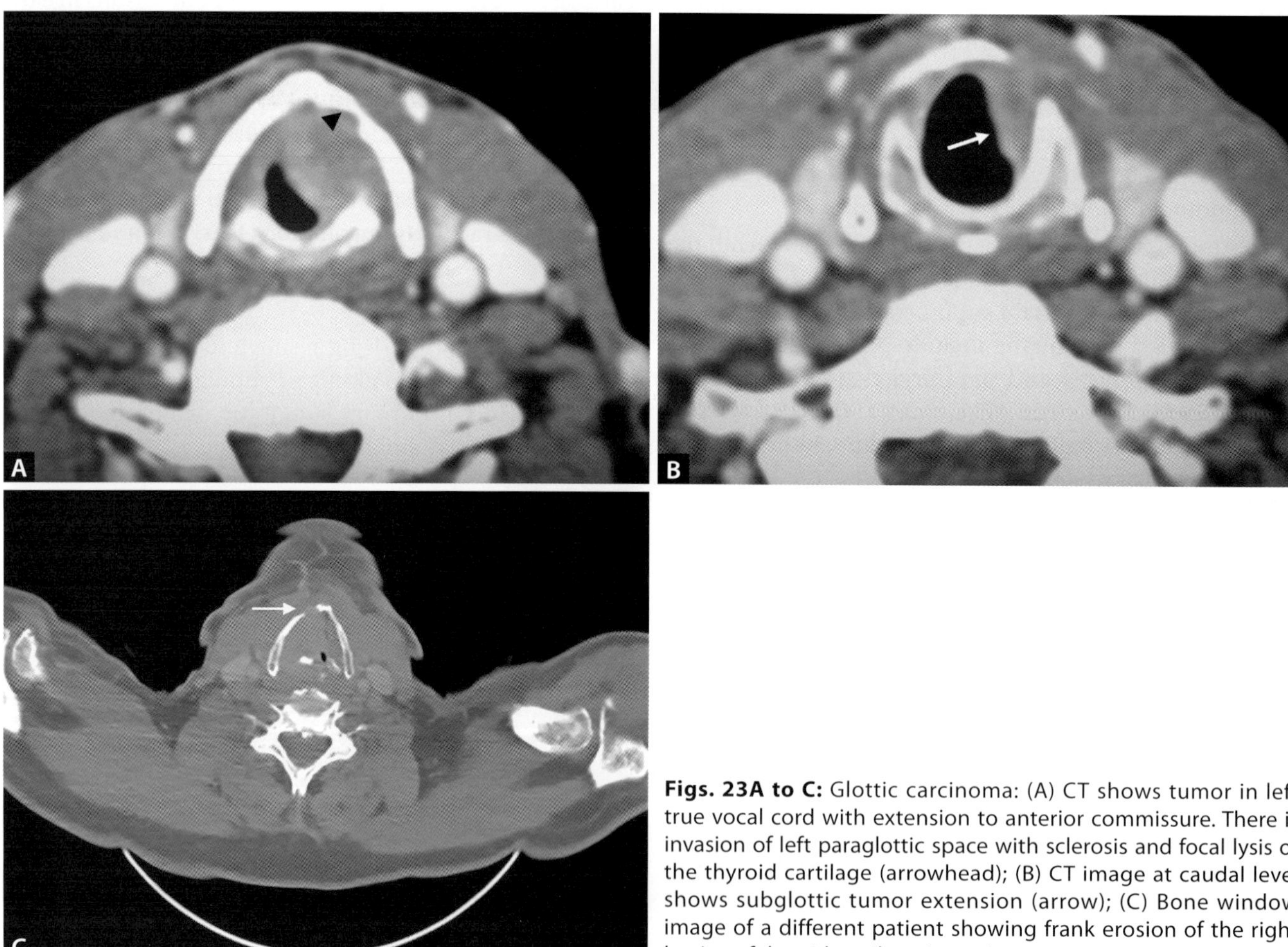

Figs. 23A to C: Glottic carcinoma: (A) CT shows tumor in left true vocal cord with extension to anterior commissure. There is invasion of left paraglottic space with sclerosis and focal lysis of the thyroid cartilage (arrowhead); (B) CT image at caudal level shows subglottic tumor extension (arrow); (C) Bone window image of a different patient showing frank erosion of the right lamina of thyroid cartilage (arrow).

Because of the close proximity, cricoid cartilage invasion occurs early. It may also spread superiorly to involve glottis.

Imaging Protocol

Contrast-enhanced CT or MRI is used for pre-treatment evaluation of the laryngeal carcinoma. Thin section CT images are normallyobtained from the level of skull base to thoracic inlet in a planeparallel to ventricle of the larynx. Ventricle is best seen on the lateral topograms. During scanning, quite breathing is ensured to keep vocal cords away. Breath hold, swallowing or phonation is to be avoided by the patient as it opposes the medial margins of the cord. MRI is performed using dedicated neck coil, short duration sequences and phase encoding gradients in AP direction in order to avoid pulsation artefacts arising from great vessels of the neck. Most laryngeal cancers enhance well on contrast enhanced MR sequences and well demarcated. It is important to note that both CT and MRI may not depict early mucosal cancers.

On CT or MRI, location and size of the tumor should be defined. Any tumor extension to adjacent segments or fat containing spaces, invasion of soft tissues of the neck, exolaryngeal structures or laryngeal cartilage should be documented.

Cartilage Invasion

Cartilage invasion by laryngeal cancers precludes the treatment with radiotherapy as response to radiation is poor in such lesions, chances of recurrence are very high and it may also induce radiation necrosis of the cartilage.[17] If no other contraindication, extensive surgery is the only option in such tumors. Because of this, cartilage invasion upstages all laryngeal cancers to T4. Cartilage invasion cannot be detected on endoscopy and it must be carefully evaluated on imaging. In adults, normal thyroid, arytenoids and cricoid cartilages have both purely cartilaginous as well as ossified areas with cortex and marrow. However, the pattern of ossification is quite variable in thyroid cartilage and hence, it is the most difficult cartilage to assess for invasion.[18]

On CT, cartilaginous part has soft tissue density while ossified part has bony cortex and medulla. Sclerosis of the cartilage (caused by inflammatory and osteoblastic activities of the tumor) is the earliest CT sign of cartilage invasion, although its specificity is variable. Erosion or frank destruction of the cortex develop subsequently and these are more specific indicators of cartilage invasion by the tumor[19] **(Figs. 16 and 23)**. Presence of tumor on both sides of the cartilage is a reliable CT indicator of cartilage invasion; however, it is seen only in advanced cases. On MRI, non-ossified cartilage has low to intermediate signal intensity on both T1- and T2-weighted images and it does not enhance. Ossified cortex has very low signal intensity while the marrow is hyperintense. Non-ossified cartilage invaded by tumor is hyperintense on T2-weighted images, similar to the tumor signal intensity. Tumor invaded marrow of ossified cartilage appear hypointense on plain T1-weighted images. On contrast administration, the involved part of the cartilage enhances, similar to the tumor. Specificity of MRI for cartilage invasion is lower as abnormal signal intensity or enhancement may also be caused by peritumoral inflammation and edema without actual tumor invasion of the cartilage. However, if these MR abnormalities are absent, cartilage invasion can be reliably excluded on MRI.[18]

Treatment

Radical (definitive) radiotherapy is the preferred treatment for supraglottic carcinomas, as it offers better functional preservation. Patients with early tumor stage, small (< 6 mL) tumor volume, as assessed on imaging, and absence of cartilage invasion have high chances of cure with radiotherapy.[20] In unfavorable situations, surgery is preferred. Most are amenable to supraglottic laryngectomy. It is a voice preserving procedure and consists of removal of all endolaryngeal structures above the ventricle, including false vocal cords, aryepiglottic folds, epiglottis and hyoid bone. Tumors involving true vocal cords or the cartilage are treated with supracricoid laryngectomy and for advanced tumors, total laryngectomy is required. Cord fixation is an indirect evidence of cricoarytenoid joint involvement. It upstages the tumor to T3 and precludes voice preserving surgery in all laryngeal cancers.

Radiotherapy is also the preferred modality for definitive treatment of early glottic carcinomas as it allows voice preservation.[21] Hemilaryngectomy is the usual surgical procedure early glottic cancers in which affected true vocal cord, ipsilateral false vocal cord and adjacent thyroid cartilage is removed. Supracricoid laryngectomy is performed if there is imaging evidence of invasion of anterior or posterior commissure, contralateral true vocal cord, false vocal cord or paraglottic fat invasion. Patients with advanced tumors may be given neoadjuvant chemotherapy and if they respond well, radiotherapy is subsequently considered. Non-responders may be offered surgery. Supraglotic or glottic tumors which do not respond or recur after radiotherapy are also subjected to salvage surgery.

CERVICAL LYMPH NODES

Cervical lymph node metastasis is the most important prognostic factor in the outcome of patients with carcinoma of head and neck. Regardless of the primary tumor, presence of a metastatic cervical lymph node reduces the 5-year survival by 50% and presence of contralateral lymph node further reduces it to 25%.[22] Risk of distant metastases also depend on the lymph node status; distant metastases are rare in patients with N0 or N1 nodes, but the incidence is above 30% in patients with N3 nodes or any node below the level of thyroid notch.[1]

Site and size of the primary tumor, density of lymphatics in that area, neurovascular infiltration and the histological tumor grade determine the risk of cervical lymph nodes metastases in SCCA of the upper aerodigestive tract. Well lateralized tumors spread to ipsilateral nodal stations. Lesions at the midline or carcinoma of the nasopharynx and tongue, even if well lateralized, may have bilateral lymphadenopathy. AJCC classification is the most widely used system for nomenclature and communication of cervical lymph node locations. It divides the cervical lymph nodes into seven stations on each side **(Table 6)**.

Imaging

Evaluation of cervical lymph nodes is important in patients with head and neck carcinomas as it assesses the prognosis and help to select the appropriate management. Imaging can identify up to 20% of clinically silent metastatic cervical lymph nodes and thus help to choose most appropriate management.[23] Imaging normally use size criteria; lymph node measuring more than 10 mm in short axis or more than 15 mm in long axis are considered to be involved **(*See* Fig. 3D)**. A group of three or more nodes measuring 8-10 mm in tumor drainage area can also be considered involved. Central necrosis in a non-enlarged lymph node, as seen on contrast enhanced CT or MRI is also suggestive of nodal metastasis **(*See* Figs. 13A and B)**. Inaccuracies are common in imaging diagnosis of cervical lymph node metastases. About 16% of CT or MRI negative patients actually have lymph node metastases while 50% patients with imaging positive lymph nodes have no metastases.[24]

Table 6: Cervical lymph nodes classification.

Level	*Site*	*Imaging landmarks*
I	Submental and submandibular LN	Anterior to submandibular gland, above hyoid
II	Upper jugular	Skull base to hyoid, submandibular gland to posterior margin of sternocleidomastoid
III	Mid jugular	Hyoid to cricoid
IV	Lower jugular	Cricoid to clavicle
V	Posterior triangle	Posterior to sternocleidomastoid
VI	Anterior visceral	Between carotid arteries
VII	Superior mediastinal	Below sternal notch

Perinodal tumor extension is a poor prognostic indicator. Although, it is pathological finding, gross or macroscopic perinodal spread can be seen on CT as a thick, enhancing rim with infiltration of surrounding fat. Such patients have ten times higher chances of recurrence. Invasion of internal carotid artery by nodal mass is also a grave prognostic finding; as such patients cannot be salvaged. On imaging, artery is considered to be invaded if more than 270 degree of the circumference is surrounded by the tumor on CT.

CT and MRI performed for primary tumor evaluation should always include area from skull base to the thoracic inlet. CT is more accurate than MRI, both for detection of metastatic lymph nodes as well as for assessment of perinodal extension.[23] Ultrasound of the neck is generally superior to both CT and MRI in evaluation of cervical lymph nodes, although some found similar accuracies.[25] Apart from the size criteria, various morphological abnormalities seen on ultrasound in enlarged or non-enlarged lymph nodes are also suggestive of metastatic involvement. These include rounded shape, loss of fatty hilum, focal cortical thickening, focal or diffuse hypoechoic areas suggestive of tumor deposits and cystic areas suggestive of necrosis **(Fig. 24)**. Power Doppler may also provide additional findings. A normal lymph node usually shows hilar perfusion. The metastatic lymph nodes may show obliterated hilar vessel, mixed vascularity in entire lymph node or peripheral hypervascularity[26] **(Figs. 24 and 25)**. However, many of these abnormal sonographic features are difficult to demonstrate in small, non-enlarged lymph nodes. In order to improve the negative predictive value of neck ultrasound in clinically N0 neck, smaller size criteria (6 or 7 mm) along with other morphological features can be used. Abnormal nodes are subjected to ultrasound guided FNAC or biopsy. This procedure is very accurate and it can correctly stage the cervical lymph nodes in up to 95% of patients with head and neck carcinoma.[27,28] Newer imaging techniques like contrast enhanced ultrasonography, MRI with superparamagnetic contrast agent, diffusion weighted MRI and PET-CT may prove helpful in doubtful cases and to detect metastases in subcentimetric lymph nodes.[29] Sentinel lymph node mapping may also be useful in detection of occult cervical lymph node metastases.[30,31]

Management

Both surgery and radiotherapy are effective in management of cervical lymph nodes. Surgical neck dissection is performed either simultaneously with

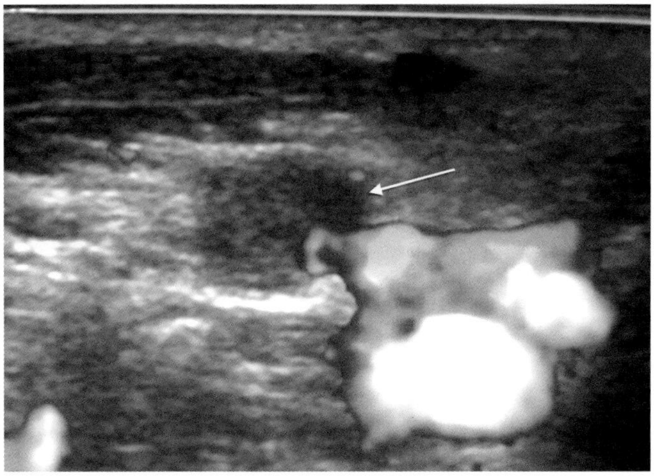

Fig. 24: Cervical lymphadenopathy: Ultrasound of the neck in a patient with tongue carcinoma of pyriform sinus shows a non-enlarged cervical lymph node with obliteration of hilar vessel and peripheral hypoechoic deposit (arrow) suggestive of metastatic involvement.

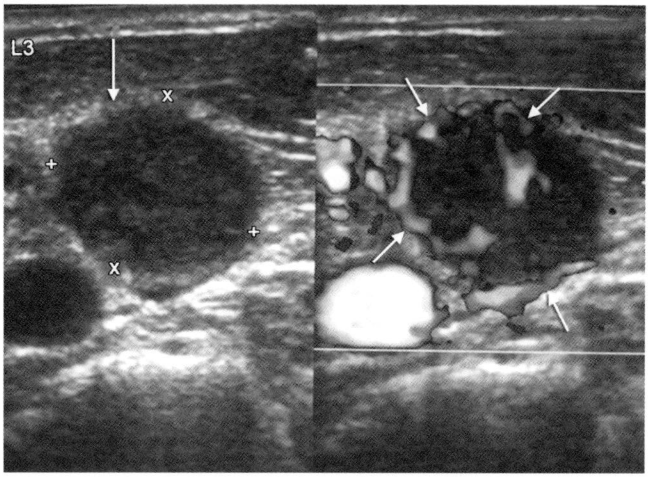

Fig. 25: Cervical lymphadenopathy: Ultrasound of the neck in patient with supraglottic carcinoma shows rounded hypoechoic cervical lymph node (arrow) with fine nodular hypoechoic deposits. Power Doppler shows increased peripheral vascularity (arrows). These features are suggestive of metastatic involvement of the lymph node.

surgery of primary tumor or electively for patients treated with radiotherapy. This procedure is both diagnostic (for pathological N staging) as well as curative. In a radical neck dissection, superficial and deep cervical fascia with enclosed level I to V lymph nodes are removed along with sternocleidomastoid and omohyoid muscles, internal jugular vein, spinal accessory nerve and the submandibular gland. In modified neck dissection, depending on the type, one or more of these structures are spared. Selective neck dissection is the term used when only selected lymph node levels are removed.[1]

Exact type of management depends on risk, i.e. site as well as pre-treatment T and N stage of the tumor. In clinically N0 neck, patients with small tumors of oral cavity have minimal risk and hence may require follow-up only. With small tumors from intermediate risk sites (oropharynx, larynx) partial neck treatment (selective neck dissection or radiotherapy) may be considered. Some centres use ultrasound of the neck (with or without ultrasound guided FNAC) in clinically N0 patients. If these investigations are negative, no neck treatment is given.[32] Any tumor in high risk areas (nasopharynx, tongue and pyriform sinus) or T4 tumors at any site are subjected to entire neck management; surgery or radiotherapy. In patients with clinically N1 or unilateral N2 lymph nodes, ipsilateral modified neck dissection is performed. If positive, radiotherapy is given to control contralateral subclinical nodes.[1] Patients with advanced nodal disease require both radical neck dissection and radiotherapy, frequently combined with chemotherapy. Lymph nodes which persist or recur after radiotherapy are also treated with surgery.

Cervical Lymphadenopathy with Carcinoma of Unknown Primary Site (CUPS)

Patients frequently present with enlarged cervical lymph nodes positive for squamous cell carcinoma pathologically but with occult primary tumor. In these patients, primary can be located anywhere in head and neck however, nasopharynx, tonsil and base of tongue are the usual primary sites of occult cancer.[33,34] Thorough clinical examination, pan endoscopy and imaging may demonstrate primary site **(*See* Fig. 13A and B)**. Location of the lymph node also gives a clue to the likely primary site. Level I nodes are more likely from oropharyngeal or oral tumors while level V are more likely from nasopharyngeal carcinoma. Bilateral lymph nodes raise the suspicion for base of tongue cancers. If the tumor is not visualized on endoscopy and imaging, blind biopsies of nasopharynx or any suspicious site and sometimes, ipsilateral tonsillectomy is performed. If lower cervical or supraclavicular lymph nodes are involved, a lung cancer must also be excluded with CT of the chest. However, despite extensive work-up, the site of origin may remain obscure in up to 50% of patients.[1,34] In all CUPS, the T-stage is taken as T0. For EBV-related disease, N-classification follows that of nasopharyngeal cancers and for HPV-positive disease, N-stage is same as that of p16 positive oropharyngeal carcinomas. In the remaining lesions, N-staging is similar to that of oral cavity cancers and takes into account extranodal extension.

Distant Metastases and Second Primary Tumors

Distant metastases are rare in early, node negative head and neck cancers and hence, routine work up for distant metastases is not required. A chest X-ray may be sufficient. The risk of distant metastases mainly depends on the nodal status as described above. Nasopharyngeal carcinoma has higher risk of distant metastases as compared to other head and neck cancers. Lung is the most common site of distant metastases; other sites are liver and bones. Patients with T4, N3 or any lymph node enlargement below thyroid should be considered for chest CT or PET-CT.[1,35] Patients with SCCA of head and neck also have 10% risk (up to 15% for tonsil or base of tongue cancers) of having second malignancy, either synchronous or metachronous.[7] It may develop in head and neck or elsewhere, such as lung and esophagus.[36]

POSITRON EMISSION TOMOGRAPHY-COMPUTED TOMOGRAPHY

As for other malignancies, positron emission tomography-computed tomography (PET-CT) is increasingly being utilized in head and neck cancers. Normal physiological uptake of FDG is common in lymphoid tissues of Waldeyer's ring, salivary glands and to some extent, mucosa of soft plate and gingiva.

PET is more likely to demonstrate a small tumor in upper aerodigestive tract than CT or MRI and hence, it is frequently used for the search of the tumor in patients presenting with cervical nodal metastases from occult primary. It identifies the primary in up to 70% of patients with occult primary; however, its sensitivity is lower for tonsil and base of tongue carcinomas.[37] In diagnosed cases, CT or MRI is sufficient for local staging and PET does not have a role.[38] PET detects more lymph node metastases than CT.[39] **(Fig. 26)**. However, less than 5 mm lymph nodes cannot be evaluated with PET and hence, it cannot exclude nodal metastases in neck. If distant metastatic work up is indicated, PET is useful to detect metastases as well as synchronous second primary tumors.

PET is highly accurate in detection of recurrences after treatment, both at the primary tumor site and the lymph nodes. PET should not be performed at least for 10 weeks after completion of treatment in order to avoid false positive results from post-treatment changes. After radiotherapy of neck nodes, persistent lymph nodes are worrisome. PET can differentiate between fibrotic and diseased lymph nodes in such situation. Thus, surveillance endoscopies and planned neck dissection can be avoided in PET negative patients.[40]

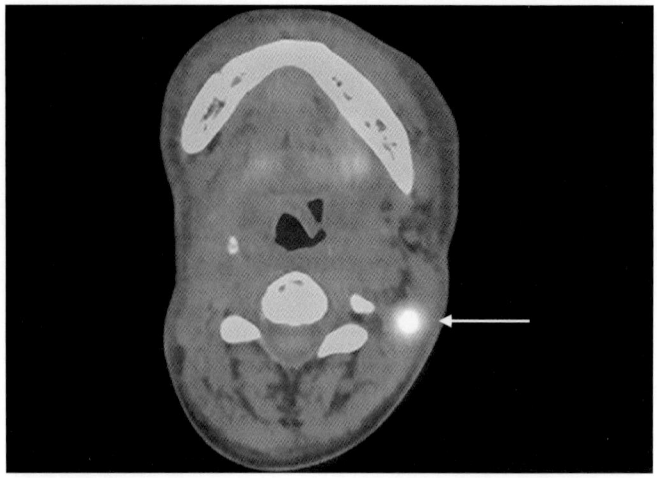

Fig. 26: Follow-up case of nasopharyngeal carcinoma. Small lymph node on left side of neck showing intense uptake on FDG PET (arrow) suggesting metastatic lymph node recurrence.

MISCELLANEOUS TUMORS

Minor Salivary Gland Tumors

These tumors arise in minor salivary glands which are normally located in buccal mucosa, tongue, floor of mouth and oropharynx, apart from sinonasal cavities. Adenoid cystic carcinoma is the most common type and others include mucoepidermoid carcinoma, adenocarcinoma, pleomorphic adenoma and mixed malignant tumors. Minor salivary gland tumors occur in elderly in fifth or sixth decade. Soft palate is the most common site where the incidence is equal to SCCA. Imaging appearances of salivary gland tumors are similar to SCCA; however, cervical lymph node involvement is uncommon.

Adenoid cystic carcinoma is characterized by extensive local invasion and its propensity for perineural spread. Perineural tumor spread is seen on CT as widening of pterygopalatine fossa and foramen rotundum (V2) or that of foramen ovale (V3). V2 involvement is more common in tumors at palate or nasopharynx while V3 involvement is more common with tumors located in oral cavity **(Figs. 8 and 27)**. Direct visualization of nerve involvement is unusual on CT. Contrast-enhanced MRI is more accurate to evaluate perineural spread and intracranial extension and should be performed in all cases of adenoid cystic carcinoma. Mucoepidermoid carcinoma may show cystic areas or calcification within it.

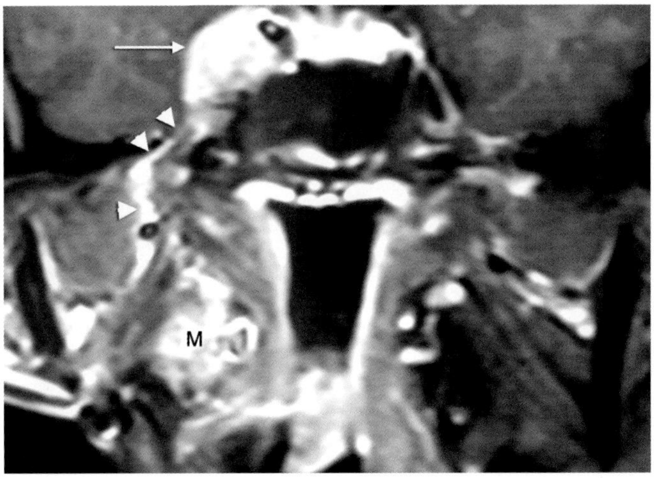

Fig. 27: Perineural tumor extension: Coronal contrast-enhanced T1-weighted MRI of a patient with oral cavity adenoid cystic carcinoma shows tumor invasion of right pterygoid muscles (M) with perineural extension seen as enhancement of thickened mandibular nerve (arrowheads) extending through the foramen ovale to cavernous sinus (arrow).

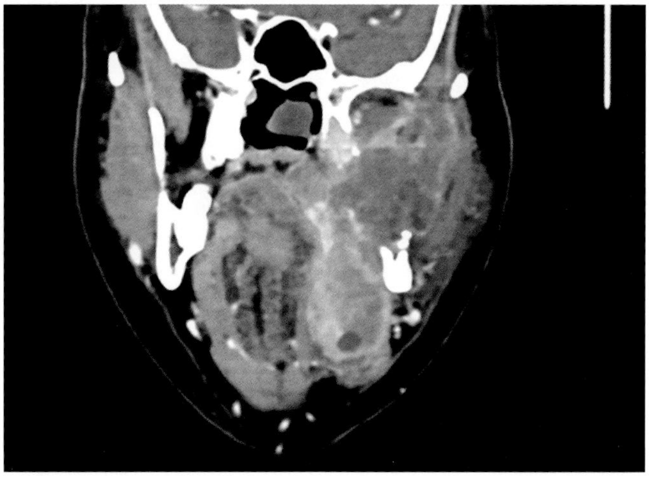

Fig. 28: Coronal reformatted image of a biopsy proven rhabdomyosarcoma patient showing large heterogeneously enhancing locally infiltrating mass lesion with extension into masticator space, parapharyngeal space as well as infratemporal fossa.

Rhabdomyosarcoma

Rhabdomyosarcoma is the rare malignancy which can involve any part of the body. About 30% of rhabdomyosarcoma occur in head and neck with orbit and nasopharynx as the most common sites. These usually occur in young children but can also affect adolescents and young adults.

On imaging, nasopharyngeal rhabdomyosarcoma appear similar to SCCA. These are seen as large aggressive locally infiltrating tumors with variable contrast enhancement **(Fig. 28)**. Tumor extension to sinuses and skull base erosion are the common findings.[5]

Lymphoma

Both Hodgkin's lymphoma (HL) and non-Hodgkin's lymphoma (NHL) can involve cervical lymph nodes and imaging cannot differentiate between nodes of HL and NHL. Lymphoma is the most common diagnosis in young patients presenting with unilateral enlarged neck nodes. Extranodal lymphoma in head and neck is usually NHL and it is more common in elderly. Waldeyer's ring is the most common extranodal site. Other sites of extranodal head and neck lymphoma include sino-nasal cavities, orbit, salivary glands and thyroid.[41] CT is the preferred modality for imaging evaluation of lymphoma and it should also include chest, abdomen and pelvis for baseline staging.

Waldeyer's ring is the lymphoid collection in pharyngeal mucosal space and it consists of nasopharyngeal tonsil (adenoids), palatal (oropharyngeal) tonsils and lingual (base of tongue) tonsils. Large number of patients are asymptomatic. Others have clinical symptoms similar to naso- or oropharyngeal SCCAs and include sore throat, nasal obstruction or hearing loss due to obstruction of eustachian tubes. Unlike SCCA, mucosa over the lesion is usually normal. On imaging, Waldeyer's ring lymphomas are seen as homogenous, mildly enhancing masses which tend to diffusely involve all walls of nasopharynx and spread in exophytic fashion to fill the nasopharynx, nasal cavity or oropharynx **(Figs. 29A and B)**. Invasion of deep structures is absent or minimal.[42] Associated cervical lymphadenopathy is non-necrotic. Primary lymphomas of larynx and oral cavity are extremely rare and have nonspecific imaging findings, similar to SCCA.[43]

POST-TREATMENT IMAGING

Recurrences are detected on endoscopy or imaging. Most recurrences of head and neck cancers appear within 2–3 years which may be local, nodal or both **(Fig. 30)**. Treatment of local recurrence is chemo-radiotherapy. Surgery may be used to resect the nodal recurrence or recurrent tumor confined to nasopharynx. Both surgery and radiotherapy alter the normal imaging appearance of the neck and familiarity with post-treatment changes is essential for accurate response assessment and to prevent misinterpretation of post-treatment changes as residual or recurrent disease.

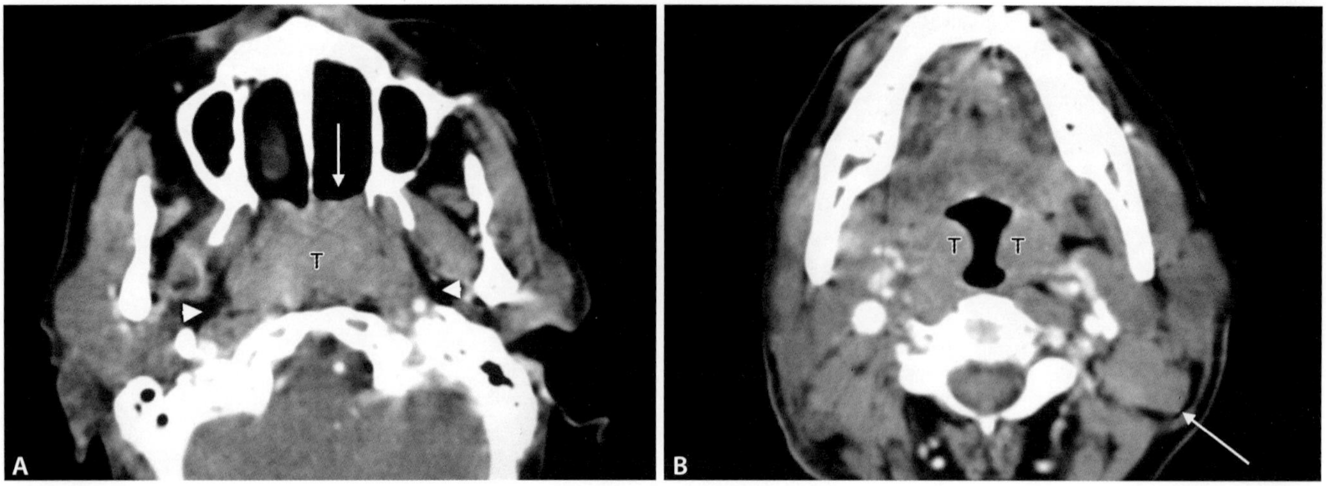

Figs. 29A and B: NHL of Waldeyer's ring: (A) CT shows large homogeneous mass filling entire nasopharynx (T) and extending into the nasal choanae (arrow). Note that bilateral parapharyngeal spaces are not involved (arrowheads) in spite of a large nasopharyngeal tumor; (B) CT image at caudal level shows smooth homogeneous enlargement of both tonsils (T) and enlarged left cervical lymph node (arrow).

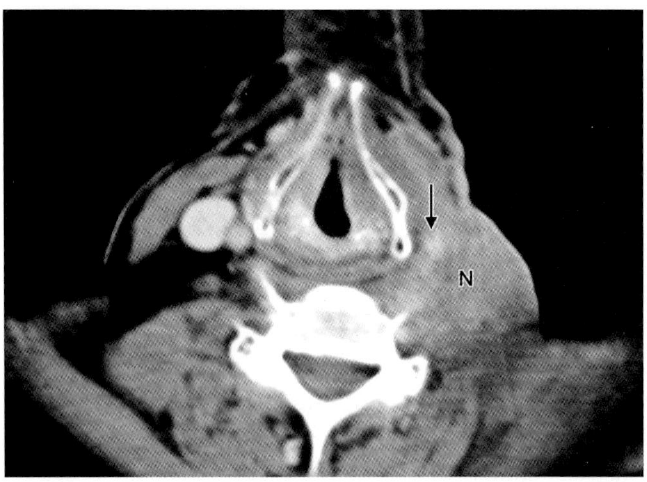

Fig. 30: Lymph nodal recurrence: Follow-up CT of a treated patient of supraglottic carcinoma shows a large ill-defined necrotic left side cervical nodal mass (N) with encasement of the carotid artery. Note the absence of internal jugular vein and the sternocleidomastoid muscle on left side secondary to the modified neck dissection which was performed for the neck treatment.

Post-radiotherapy Neck

Radical (definitive) radiotherapy is the preferred treatment modality for pharyngeal and laryngeal cancers and it involves delivery of high radiation doses. Radiotherapy results in edema and fibrosis and it affects all areas of pharynx, larynx and superficial soft tissues of the neck included in radiation field. Acute effects of radiotherapy are characterized by inflammation, increased capillary permeability of small vessels and lymphatics and interstitial edema. Clinically, acute treatment sequels like sore throat, xerostomia (due to atrophy of salivary glands), mucositis and nausea are common. After 4–6 months, there is sclerosis and fibrosis of the connective tissues, obliteration of small vessels and lymphatics and resolution of the edema. Degree of these changes depends on the total radiation dose. On imaging, thickening of the skin and platysma muscle, enhancement of the mucosa and salivary glands as well as increase density and trabecular thickening of subcutaneous fat is seen in most patients 3 to 4 months after completion of radiotherapy[44] **(Fig. 31)**. In naso-oropharynx, there is thickening of posterior pharyngeal wall and edema of the retropharyngeal space. These changes may resolve or persist for several months. In larynx, radiotherapy also causes symmetric thickening of epiglottis, aryepiglottic folds, and false vocal cords. Such thickening is uncommon in glottis and subglottis. These radiotherapy changes gradually resolve to variable extent.[45]

Imaging is required to assess the response to the treatment and for follow-up in patients treated with radiotherapy. A baseline post-treatment scan is obtained 3–4 months after completion of radiotherapy. The post-treatment changes and edema have attenuations less than that of muscles and the appearance remain stable on serial imaging. Any high density or enhancing mass or progressively enlarging mass is suspicious for residual or recurrent tumor. Differentiation of recurrence form fibrosis may sometimes be difficult on CT. MRI is useful in such situations but only if the scar is mature, as both tumor and the immature scar tissue are T2 hyperintense

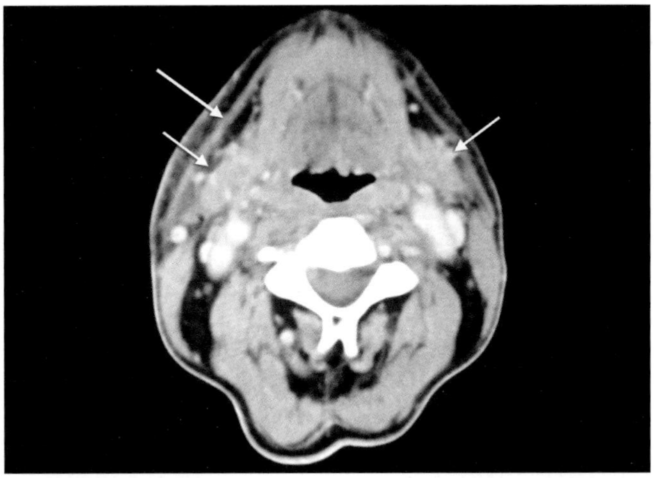

Fig. 31: Post-radiotherapy neck: CT shows diffuse increased density and trabeculations of subcutaneous fat, thickening of skin and platysma muscles (large arrow), atrophy of submandibular salivary glands (small arrows) and symmetric thickening of the pharyngeal wall.

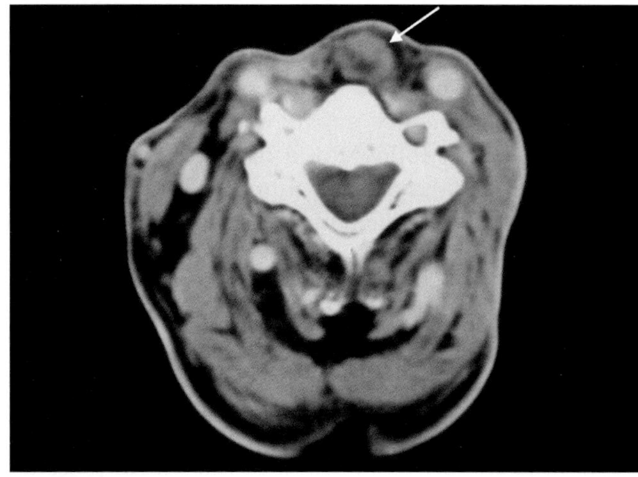

Fig. 32: Post-laryngectomy neck: CT scan after total laryngectomy shows absence of larynx with rounded contour and anterior subcutaneous bulging of the esophagus (arrow).

and show contrast enhancement on MRI.[46] Diffusion-weighted MRI, perfusion CT and PET-CT may help in differentiating residual/recurrent tumor from post therapy changes. Nasopharyngeal carcinoma is highly radiosensitive tumor and near complete resolution of the tumor is expected after radiotherapy. Persistent, moderately thick nasopharyngeal wall beyond 6 months increases the risk of relapse.[47] In hypopharynx and larynx, near complete resolution of the tumor indicates successful local control whereas less than 50% shrinkage of the tumor or persistent mass measuring more than 1 cm is suspicious for residual disease and biopsy is required. Other cases are indeterminate and require clinical examination and follow-up imaging to determine the stability.[48]

Late Effects of Radiotherapy

Long-term radiation complications include brain necrosis in temporal lobes, trismus due to fibrosis of masticator muscles and atrophy of salivary glands. Uncommon complications of radiotherapy include soft tissue necrosis and osteochondronecrosis. These may occur during radiotherapy or several months after radiotherapy. It may be seen as sclerosis, fragmentation and sloughing of the cartilage or bone, osteomyelitis and fistula formation.[49] On imaging, these findings cannot be reliably differentiated from recurrent tumor. Biopsy is required and if it is negative, a close imaging follow-up is necessary.[18]

Radiation induced tumors are rare and occur several years, at least 5 years, later. Sarcoma is the usual radiation induced tumor. Osteosarcoma is the most common bone sarcoma while malignant fibrous histiocytoma is the most common soft tissue sarcoma. Other radiation induced tumors include meningioma, glioma, thyroid tumors, chondrosarcoma, malignant peripheral nerve sheath tumor and squamous cell carcinoma. Heterogeneous well enhancing mass with bone destruction seen in radiation field, after a latency period of at least 5 years is a useful clue to the diagnosis of radiation induced sarcoma.[50]

Postoperative Neck

Variety of surgical procedures may be employed for the treatment of pharyngeal tumors. Anatomical alterations and depend on type and extent of surgical resection and this information should be available for interpretation of postoperative scans. Postoperative pharyngeal wall is typically thin and smooth. Myocutaneous flap reconstructions are seen as fatty, bulky areas. Neck dissection is a common procedure for the management of cervical lymph nodes and exact postoperative appearance depends on the type of neck dissection procedure.

In total laryngectomy, entire larynx with thyroid and cricoid cartilages and hyoid bone are removed. With no anterior firm structures, pharynx and esophagus are more anteriorly located and appear prominent **(Fig. 32)**. With supraglottic laryngectomy, glottis, cricoid cartilage and contralateral thyroid cartilage are retained. The pharynx is more distended and if not resected, hyoid bone may be seen at the same level as glottis. After hemilaryngectomy, ipsilateral vocal cord, arytenoids cartilage and part of the thyroid cartilages can be seen missing on CT.

Acute postoperative changes (granulation and immature scar tissue) show contrast enhancement on CT and MRI and cannot be differentiated from residual tumor. These changes resolve subsequently. Similar to the post-radiotherapy follow-up, a baseline postoperative scan is obtained and used to compare with subsequent follow-up scans. Recurrent tumor is suspected if there is a progressively enlarging or enhancing mass at the primary tumor site or at the resection margin or appearance of a new lymph node **(*See* Fig. 29A and B)**.

REFERENCES

1. Mendenhall WM, Werning JW, Pfister DG. Treatment of head and neck cancers. In: DeVita VT, Lawrence TS, Rosenberg SA (Eds). Cancer: Principles and Practice of Oncology. 8th edition, Philadelphia, Lippincott Williams and Wilkins 2008;799-877.
2. Huang SH, O'Sullivan B. Overview of the 8th Edition TNM Classification for Head and Neck Cancer.Curr Treat Options Oncol. 2017;18(7):40.
3. Lydiatt WM, Patel SG, O'Sullivan B, Brandwein MS, Ridge JA, Migliacci JC, Loomis AM, Shah JP. Head and Neck cancers-major changes in the American Joint Committee on cancer eighth edition cancer staging manual. CA Cancer J Clin. 2017;67(2):122-37.
4. National Cancer Registry Program three year report of PBCRs 2012-2014. Report of population based cancer registries, Indian Council of Medical Research, New Delhi, 2016
5. Mukherji SK, Fatterpekar G, Chong VF. Malignancies of the oral cavity. In: Brag DG, Rubin P, Hricak H (Eds). Oncologic Imaging, 2nd edition, Philadelphia, WB Saunders Co. 2002; 202-31.
6. Kimura Y, Sumi M, Sumi T et al. Deep extension from carcinoma arising from gingival: CT and MR imaging features. AJNR 2002:23;468-72.
7. Ginsberg LE, DeMonte F.Imaging of perineural tumor spread from palatal carcinoma. AJNR 1998;22:14-7.
8. Imaizumi A, Yoshino N, Yamada I, et al. A potential pitfall of MR imaging for assessing mandibular invasion of squamous cell carcinoma in the oral cavity. AJNR 2006;27:114-22.
9. Stambuk HE, Karimi S. Oral cavity and oropharynx tumors. Radiol Clin N Am 2007;45:1-20.
10. Campbell RSD, Baker E, Chippindale AJ, et al. MRI T staging of squamous cell carcinoma of the oral cavity. Radiological pathological correlation. Clin Radiol. 1995;50:533-40.
11. Wiener E, Pautke C, Link TM, et al. Comparison of 16 slice MSCT and MRI in the assessment of squamous cell carcinoma of oral cavity. Eur J Radiol. 2006;24:4371-6.
12. Deo SVS, Purkayastha J, Das DK, et al. Reconstruction of complex oral defects using bi-paddle pectoralis major flap-technical modifications and outcome in 54 patients. Indian Journal of Otolaryngology and Head and Neck Surgery 2003; 55:1-9.
13. Sham JST, Cheung YK, Choy D. Cranial nerve involvement and base of skull erosion in nasopharyngeal carcinoma. Cancer 1996;68:422-7.
14. Chong VFH, Fan YF, hoo JBK. MRI features of cervical nodal metastases in metastatic disease. Clin Radiol. 1996;51:103-8.
15. Sham JST, Cheung YK, Chan FL. Nasopharyngeal carcinoma: patterns of skeletal metastases. Br J Radiol. 1990;63:202-07.
16. Stambuk HE, Patel SG, Mosier KM, et al. Nasopharyngeal carcinoma: recognizing the radiographic features in children. AJNR 2005;26:1575-9.
17. Castelijns JA, Becker M, Hermans R. The impact of cartilage invasion on treatment and prognosis of laryngeal cancer. Eur Radiol. 1996;6:156-69.
18. Yousem DM, Tufano RP. Laryngeal imaging. Radiol Clin N Am 2004;14:611-24.
19. Baker M, Zbarin P, Delavelle J, et al. Neoplastic invasion of the laryngeal cartilage: Reassessment of criteria for diagnosis at CT. Radiology 1997;203:521-32.
20. Mancuso AA, Mukerji SK, Schmalfuss I, et al. Preradiotherapy computed tomography as a predictor of local control in supraglottic carcinoma. J Clin Oncol 1999;17:631-7.
21. Mendenhall WM, Werning JW, Hinerman RW, et al. Management of T1 and T2 glottic carcinoma. Cancer 2004;100:1786-9.
22. Som PM. Detection of metastases in cervical lymph nodes: CT and MR criteria and differential diagnosis. AJR 1992;158: 961-9.
23. Som PM, Brandwein MS. Lymph nodes. In: Som PM, Curtin HD (Eds). Head and Neck Imaging. 4th edition. St Louis, Mosby 2003;1865-934.
24. Curtin H, Ishwaran H, Mancuso A, et al. Comparison of CT and MR imaging in staging of neck metastases. Radiology 1998;207:123-30.
25. Casteljins JA, Van Den Brekel MW, Mukherji SK, Lameris JS. Ultrasound of the neck. In: Som PM, Curtin HD (Eds). Head and Neck Imaging. 4th edition. St Louis, Mosby 2003;1935-53.
26. Ahuja A, Ying M. Sonography of neck lymph nodes. Clin Radiol. 2003;58:359-66.
27. Knappe M, Louw M, Gregor KT. Ultrasonography guided fine needle aspiration for the assessment of cervical metastases. Arch Otolaryngol Head Neck Surg. 2000;126:1091-6.
28. DeBondt RB, Nelemans PJ, Hofman PA, et al. Detection of lymph node metastases in head and neck cancer: meta-analysis comprising US, USFNAC, CT and MR imaging. Eur J Radiol. 2007;64:266-72.
29. Sigal R, Vogl T, Casselman J, et al. Lymph node metastases from head and neck squamous cell carcinoma: MR imaging with ultra small superparamagnetic iron oxide particle—results of a phase III multicenter clinical trial. Eur Radiol. 2002;12:1104-13.
30. Ross GL, Soutar DS, Gordon MD, et al. Sentinel node biopsy in head and neck cancer: preliminary results of a multicenter trial. Ann Surg Oncol 2004;11:690-6.

31. King AD. Mutlimodality imaging of head and neck cancers. Cancer Imaging. 2007;7:S37-S46.
32. Nieuwenhuis EJ, Castelijns JA, Pijpers R, et al. Wait and see policy for the N0 neck in early stage oral and oropharyngeal squamous cell carcinoma using ultrasonographically guided cytology: is there a role for identification of sentinel node? Head Neck 2002;24:282-9.
33. Schmalbach CE, Miller FR. Occult primary head and neck carcinoma. Curr Oncol Rep 2007;9:139-46.
34. Cianchetti M, Mancuso AA, Amdur RJ, et al. Diagnostic evaluation of squamous cell carcinoma metastatic to cervical lymph nodes from an unknown head and neck primary site. Laryngoscope 2009;119:2348-54.
35. Loh KS, Brown DH, Baker JT, et al. A rational approach to pulmonary screening in newly diagnosed head and neck cancer. Head Neck 2005;27:990-94.
36. Erkal HS, Mendenhall WM, Amdur RJ, et al. Synchronous and metachronous squamous cell carcinomas of the head and neck mucosal sites. J Clin Oncol 2001;19:1358-61.
37. Dong MJ, Zhao K, Lin XT, et al. Role of fluorodeoxyglucose PET versus fluorodeoxyglucose PET/computed tomography in detection of unknown primary tumor: meta-analysis of the literature. Nucl Med Commun. 2008;29:791-802.
38. Dammann F, Horger M, Berg MM, et al. Rational diagnosis of squamous cell carcinoma of head and neck region: comparative evaluation of CT, MRI and 18FDG PET. AJR 2005;184: 1326-31.
39. Syed R, Bomanji JB, Nagabhushan N, et al. Impact of combined 18F-FDG PET/CT in head and neck tumors. Br J Cancer 2005;92:1046-50.
40. Isle MG, McConkey C, Mehanna. A systematic review and meta- analysis of the role of positron emission tomography in the follow- up of head and neck squamous cell carcinoma following radiotherapy or chemotherapy. Clin Otolaryngol. 2008;33: 210-22.
41. Aiken AH, Glastonbury C. Imaging Hodgkin and non-Hodgkin lymphoma in head and neck. Radiol Clin N Am. 2008;46:363-78.
42. King AD, Lei KI, Richards PS, et al. Non-Hodgkin's lymphoma of the nasopharynx. CT and MR imaging. Clin Radiol. 2003;58:621-25.
43. King AD, Yeun EH, Lei K, et al. Non-Hodgkin lymphoma of the larynx: CT and MR imaging findings. Am J Neuroradiol. 2004;25:12-15.
44. Mukherji SK, Mancuso AA, Kotzur IM, et al. Radiographic appearance of the irradiated larynx. Radiology 1994;193: 141-48.
45. Curtin HD. The larynx. In: Som PM, Curtin HD (Eds). Head and Neck Imaging. 4th edition. St Louis, Mosby 2003;1595-1698.
46. Chong VHF, Fan YF. Detection of recurrent nasopharyngeal cancer. CT vs MR imaging. Radiology 1997;202:453-70.
47. Luo D, Zhou C, Li E, et al. Post radiation CT changes and recurrent nasopharyngeal carcinoma. Chin Med J. 2008;121: 916-22.
48. Hermans R, Parneljer FA, Mancuso AA, et al. Laryngeal or hypopharyngeal squamous cell carcinoma: can follow up CT after definitive radiation therapy be used to detect local failure earlier than clinical examination alone? Radiology 2000;214: 683-87.
49. Hermans R. Imaging of mandibular osteoradionecrosis. NeuroimagClin N Am 2003;13:597-604.
50. Makimoto Y, Yamamoto S, Takano H, et al. Imaging finding of radiation sarcoma of head and neck. Br J Radiol 2007;790-7.

CHAPTER 26

Imaging of Skull Base Lesions

Atin Kumar, Manisha Jana, Priyanka Naranje, Ashu Seith Bhalla

INTRODUCTION

In general, skull base is inaccessible to clinical evaluation. Hence, the clinicians are dependent on the radiological assessment of this region for planning treatment and surgical approach.[1] However, the radiologist needs to be familiar with the complex anatomy of the skull base and also the correct imaging protocols so as to enable him to correctly diagnose and accurately delineate the lesions involving it.

ANATOMICAL DIVISION[2]

When viewed from above, the floor of the calvaria appears to be divided into three naturally contoured regions: (1) the anterior, (2) middle and (3) posterior cranial fossae. However, when viewed from below, the margins between the three fossae are indistinct.

- The anterior skull base is the part of base of skull lying anterior to a line that follows the tuberculum sella, the anterior clinoid processes, the posterior margins of the lesser sphenoid wings and the anterior and superior rim of the greater sphenoid wings.
- The part behind this line is the middle skull base which in turn is separated from the posterior skull base by a line following the spheno-occipital synchondrosis medially and the petroclival synchondrosis and the superior ridge of the petrous and mastoid bones posteriorly and laterally **(Fig. 1)**.

In this chapter, we will discuss the relevant radiological anatomy and the lesions involving each division of skull base separately. However, there may be some lesions like those arising from tissues common to all skull base compartments such as bone, meninges and sinuses which can involve any of the divisions or may diffusely involve the skull base. Some lesions may simultaneously involve more than one division.

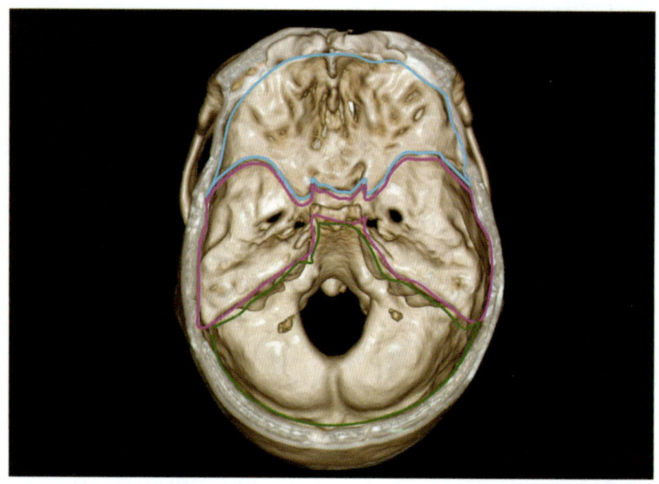

Fig. 1: Surface shaded display CT reconstruction of skull base as viewed from top shows division of skull base into anterior compartment (outlined by blue), middle compartment (outlined by pink) and posterior compartment (outlined by green).

IMAGING TECHNIQUES AND THEIR ROLE

Conventional radiographs of the skull base done in earlier decades have now given way to cross-sectional imaging by

CT and MRI. The cross-sectional imaging techniques are useful for localizing the lesion, narrowing the differential diagnosis based on the site of origin, pattern of growth and the imaging features of a given lesion, correctly delineating the lesion margins and its relation to surrounding structures so as to enable treatment planning and are also helpful for follow up of these patients.[3]

CT and MR have a complimentary role in the imaging of skull base and are often used together.[4] CT is the technique of choice for delineation of fine bony details, especially the thin cortical margins of the skull base neurovascular foramina. CT is highly specific in diagnosis of neoplastic as well as non-neoplastic bone lesions, can distinguish aggressive from a benign lesion by delineating the pattern of bone involvement and can depict calcification better than MR. Infectious processes, malignant neoplasms and aggressive rapidly growing lesions lead to permeative and erosive pattern of bone involvement whereas benign slow-growing lesions cause bone expansion and remodeling with cortical thinning.

CT studies of the skull base should be acquired on a multidetector CT scanner with minimum 0.5 mm reconstruction. An acquisition in the axial plane with reconstructions in other planes (coronal and sagittal) should be done. The images should be reconstructed in both soft tissue and high resolution bone algorithm. Contrast imaging should be done in case of evaluation of mass lesions to best assess tumor vascularity, margins, relation to adjacent structures and to obtain perfusion studies which may help to differentiate benign from malignant conditions. Contrast-enhanced images should be evaluated in soft tissue algorithm. However, contrast administration may be obviated if the CT is being done as an adjunct to contrast enhanced MR evaluation.

MR imaging is more sensitive than CT to assess the soft tissue component. It is the modality of choice to detect the intracranial extent including invasion of the dura, leptomeninges, cranial nerves and brain parenchyma. MR imaging is also good for detecting perineural and perivascular spread and bone marrow involvement. Utility of CT and MRI in evaluation of skull base lesions is summarized in **Table 1**.

MR protocol **(Box 1)** should include 3D sequences of a T1-weighted without fat saturation, T2-weighted with fat saturation and balanced steady-state free precession (CISS).[5] The images should be obtained with small field of view, high resolution and isotropic resolution. It should be remembered that skull base has multiple interfaces and hence is extremely susceptible to artifacts from tissue inhomogeneity. Therefore, fat suppression may be a problem sometimes. Contrast administration is required for evaluation of infections, tumors and cranial nerve assessment. A 3D T1-weighted VIBE sequence with fat saturation and 3D CISS sequence should be obtained after contrast. Angiography has a limited role in evaluation of vascular lesions and hypervascular tumors.[6,7] At our institute it is mainly reserved for interventional procedures like embolization of hypervascular tumors such as juvenile nasopharyngeal angiofibromas, paragangliomas, hemangiopericytomas, etc. Positron emission imaging with FDG is useful in differentiating residual/recurrent neoplasm from post-treatment changes in the follow-up of skull base tumors.

Table 1: Utility of CT and MRI in evaluation of skull base lesions.

CT	*MRI*
Fine bony details	Assessment of soft tissue component
Walls of skull base neurovascular foramina	Intracranial extension; Invasion of dura, leptomeninges cranial nerves, brain parenchyma
Pattern of bone destruction	Detecting perineural and perivascular spread
Depiction of calcification	Bone marrow involvement

Box 1: MRI protocol for skull base.

Precontrast:
- T1 axial and coronal
- T2 axial and coronal
- 3D T1W sequence without fat suppression (VIBE)
- 3D T2W sequence with fat suppression (STIR SPACE)
- 3D steady-state free precession imaging (CISS)

Postcontrast:
- 3D T1W sequence with fat suppression (VIBE with FS)
- 3D CISS

ANTERIOR SKULL BASE

Anatomy

The anterior skull base forms the bottom of the anterior skull, i.e. the floor of the anterior cranial fossa. It is formed by the roof of the nasal cavity and the ethmoid sinuses in the median plane with the roof of the orbits on either side of the median plane. It extends from the posterior wall of the frontal sinus anteriorly to the lesser wing of sphenoid bone posteriorly. The roof of the nasal cavity is formed by the thin cribriform plate of the ethmoid bone which has multiple small perforations transmitting olfactory nerves from the nasal mucosa to the olfactory bulb **(Fig. 2)**. Fracture of this plate (most commonly at the lateral lamella where the anterior ethmoidal artery enters

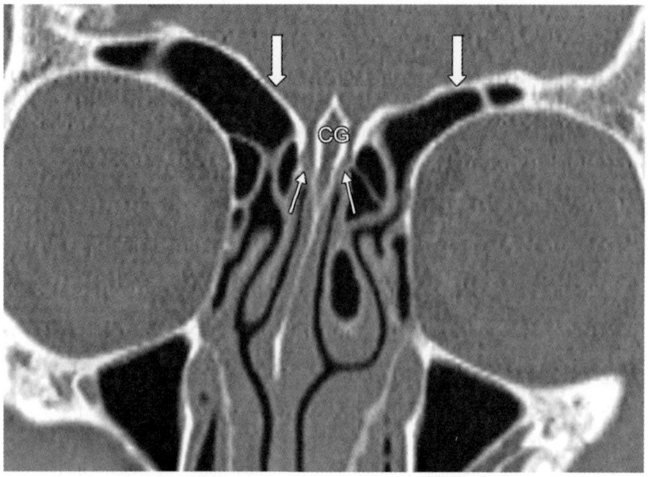

Fig. 2: Coronal CT image of anterior skull base. Crista Galli (CG), cribriform plate (thin arrows), orbital plate of frontal bone (block arrows).

the skull base) either by trauma or by instrumentation during functional endoscopic sinus surgery is a common cause for cerebrospinal fluid (CSF) leaks. The orbital plate of the frontal bone forming the roof of the orbits is comparatively thick and sturdy and relatively resistant to erosions.

Pathology

The anterior skull base may be involved by number of pathologies **(Table 2)** arising from the bones of the skull base proper, exocranially from the sinonasal mucosa, olfactory mucosa and orbit, intracranially from the meningeal coverings, or from the vessels and nerves passing through this region including the olfactory nerve. The involvement can also be secondary to trauma (fractures) or congenital defects leading to cephaloceles. Most of the tumors presenting in this region show similar radiological features. Hence, it is often very difficult to differentiate between them based on radiology and not possible to give specific diagnosis. The role of imaging should be to comment upon the lesion resectability, bony involvement, invasion of meninges and brain parenchyma, and extension into the orbit and into the neurovascular structures, including the cavernous sinuses. The dural involvement is evident radiologically as thickness of more than 5 mm or nodular thickening whereas brain parenchymal involvement is evident as edema with or without contrast enhancement.[8] Orbital involvement occurs most often through the lamina papyracea. The strong periorbita resists intraorbital invasion for long. However periorbital breach requires orbital exenteration.

Table 2: Anterior skull base lesions.

Lesions arising from below	
Sinonasal lesions	• Esthesioneuroblastoma
	• Squamous cell carcinoma
	• Adenocarcinoma
	• Adenoid cystic carcinomas
	• Melanoma
	• Lymphoma
	• Sarcomas
	• Juvenile nasopharyngeal angiofibroma
	• Mucocele
	• Other miscellaneous lesions: • Sinonasal polyposis, osteomyelitis, fungal sinusitis GPA
Orbital lesions	• Lacrimal gland tumors
	• Neurogenic tumors, lymphoma, sarcomas, metastases
Lesions arising from above	
	• Olfactory groove meningioma
	• Schwannoma
	• Encephalocele
Lesions of the proper skull base	
	• Trauma and CSF leak
	• Osteoma

Abbreviations: GPA: Granulomatosis polyangiitis; CSF: Cerebrospinal fluid.

Involvement of the orbital apex also has serious prognostic implications: tumor reaching orbital apex can also extend into middle cranial fossa via the superior orbital fissure and surgical excision in this region usually requires sacrificing of optic nerve and eye. The nasal cavity and sinus tumors commonly extend across skull base to involve the anterior cranial fossa. In contrast the orbital tumors are rarely seen to breach the orbital roof to involve the anterior cranial fossa.

Lesions Arising from Below

Sinonasal Lesions

Esthesioneuroblastoma: Also known as olfactory neuroblastomas as they arise in olfactory epithelium. They are similar to other neural crest tumors like neuroblastomas, PNET and small cell lung carcinomas.[9] They have bimodal age distribution affecting in second and fifth decades of life.[10] They appear hyperdense on plain CT and show homogenously enhancing solid mass in the roof of the nasal cavity with possible destruction of the cribriform

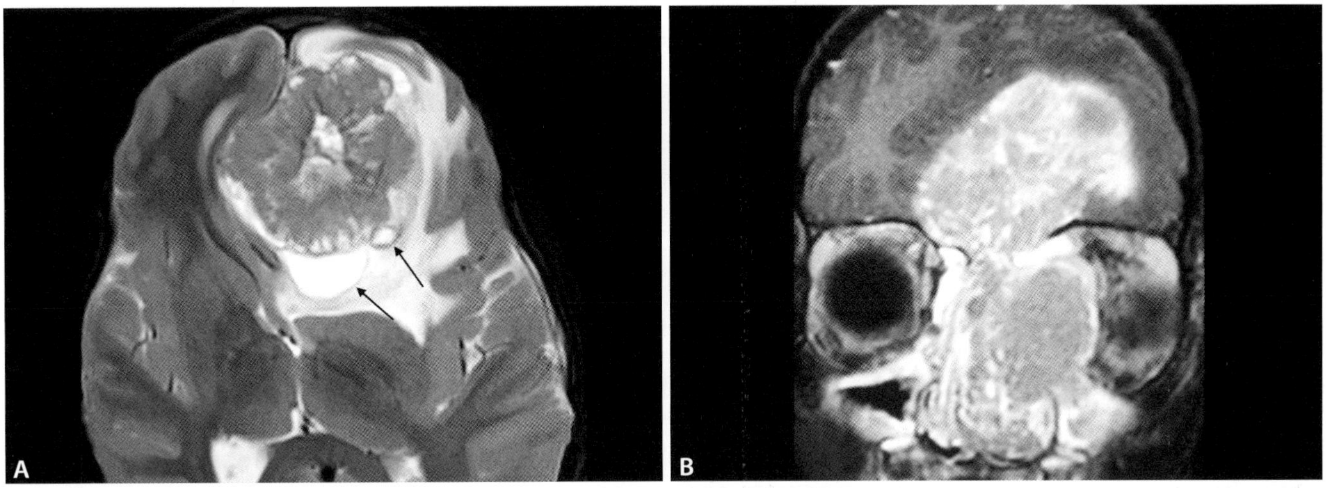

Figs. 3A and B: *Esthesioneuroblastoma*: (A) T2W axial MRI showing a large isointense intracranial extra-axial mass lesion with presence of T2W hyperintense cysts at tumor—brain interface (arrows); (B) Coronal contrast enhanced MR image reveals avid contrast enhancement of the mass.

plate and intracranial extension **(Figs. 3A and B)**. They show intermediate signal intensity on T1- and T2-weighted images on MRI. Larger lesions with intracranial extension may show a specific feature of peripheral tumor cysts at the margins, especially at the interface with brain parenchyma.[11] Calcification may also be seen.

Squamous cell carcinoma: Most common epithelial neoplasm of this region. Average age at presentation is 50 years with male predominance.[9] They are aggressive lesions showing bone destruction, intermediate T2 signal (high cellularity), necrosis and hemorrhage and homogeneous contrast enhancement (slightly less than normal mucosa). Contrast enhancement differentiates it from mucoceles which do not enhance.

Adenocarcinoma: Seen in elderly males. It is difficult to differentiate them radiologically from the more common squamous cell carcinomas but in general, the adenocarcinomas show a less aggressive pattern of bone involvement evident as remodeling and thinning rather than permeative bone destruction.

Adenoid cystic carcinomas: These tumors arise from minor salivary glands of the hard palate with spread to involve the paranasal sinuses. They are slow but steady growing lesions which have a strong propensity for perineural spread, trigeminal nerve involvement being most common in this region. These tumors exhibit T2 prolongation with areas of remodeling and destruction.

Melanoma: Presents from fifth to eighth decade with equal preponderance in men and women. Radiological features include bone remodeling, intense contrast enhancement and areas of T1 hyperintensity due to melanin or hemorrhage.

Lymphoma: B cell lymphoma involves paranasal sinuses and presents as bulky expansile mass eroding bones and adjacent soft tissues. T cell lymphoma involves the midline nasal septum with aggressive features of bone destruction in excess of involvement of soft tissues. The differential diagnosis includes granulomatous polyangitis (GPA) and cocaine abuse.

Sarcomas: Rhabdomyosarcoma (pediatric age group), Ewing's sarcoma and chondrosarcoma can also rarely involve the sinonasal region.

Juvenile nasopharyngeal angiofibroma: They are benign, highly vascular tumors seen in adolescent males. They arise in the nasopharyngeal region from primitive vascular tissue at sphenopalatine foramen. They are aggressive tumors which infiltrate through foramens and fissures to involve the orbits and intracranial compartment. They involve central skull base more often than anterior skull base.

Mucocele: It is a benign lesion occurring in sinonasal region with frontal sinus more commonly involved than the ethmoidal sinuses. It is formed by obstruction of sinus ostium with resultant expansion of the sinus with secretions. CT confirms the diagnosis. MR may show peripheral enhancement on contrast administration.

Other miscellaneous lesions: Sinonasal polyposis, osteomyelitis, fungal sinusitis **(Figs. 4A to D)**, GPA may also extend to involve the anterior skull base after having origin from the sinonasal region.

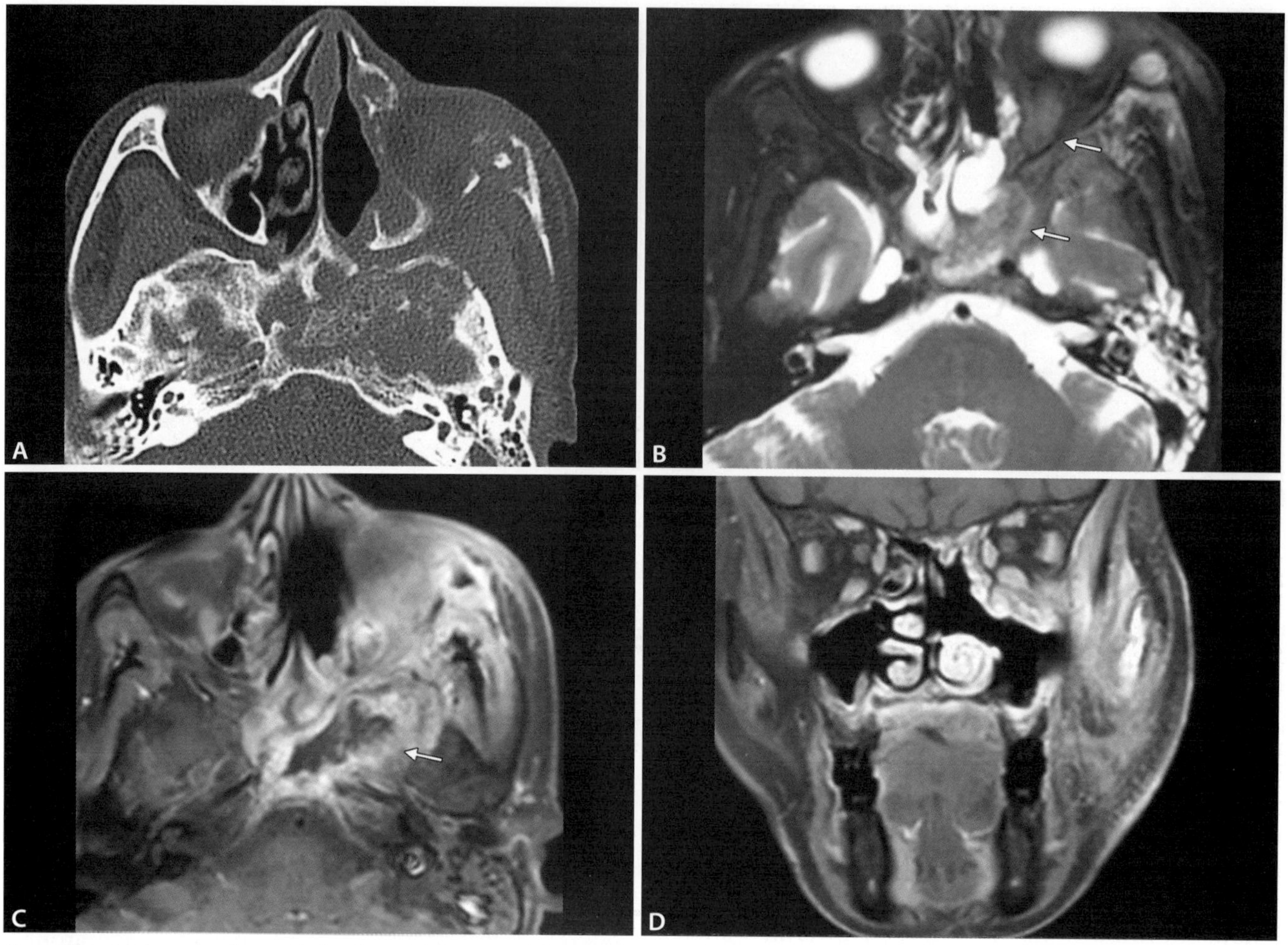

Figs. 4A to D: Invasive fungal infection with intracranial extension: Axial CT bone window (A) image shows destruction of the left sphenoid wing, left zygoma and left lateral nasal wall. T2-weighted (B) axial MR image reveals a hypointense mass in left orbital apex and cavernous sinus location (arrows). Contrast-enhanced T1-weighted axial (C) and coronal (D) MR images show a heterogeneous peripheral enhancement of the lesion, and destruction of left side superior and middle turbinates.

Orbital Lesions

Lacrimal gland tumors: They appear as mass lesions in the superolateral compartment of the orbit anteriorly. They may cause erosion of the orbital roof with subsequent extension into the anterior cranial fossa.

Other tumors: Rarely neurogenic tumors, lymphoma, sarcomas, leukemic deposits (chloroma) **(Figs. 5A to D)**, metastases arising in orbits may also extend to involve anterior skull base.

Lesions Arising from Above

Olfactory groove meningioma: It is the most common intracranial lesion affecting the anterior skull base from above. Radiologically, they appear as well-circumscribed, T1 and T2 isointense, intensely enhancing extra-axial masses with dural tail, with or without calcification **(Fig. 6)**. They may extend exocranially through the cribriform plate. They may also produce characteristic reactive bony sclerosis in the adjacent bone.

Schwannoma: It is a rare tumor at this region which arises from olfactory nerve or from meningeal branch of fifth cranial nerve. On imaging it appears as a benign well-defined lesion with intense contrast enhancement and is difficult to differentiate from olfactory groove meningioma.

Encephalocele: Frontal meningoencephaloceles are rare congenital anomalies that are divided into sincipital and basal types. The sincipital meningoencephaloceles are located anteriorly and are extranasal masses (nasofrontal, nasoethmoidal or nasoorbital) while basal meningoencephaloceles are located posteriorly and

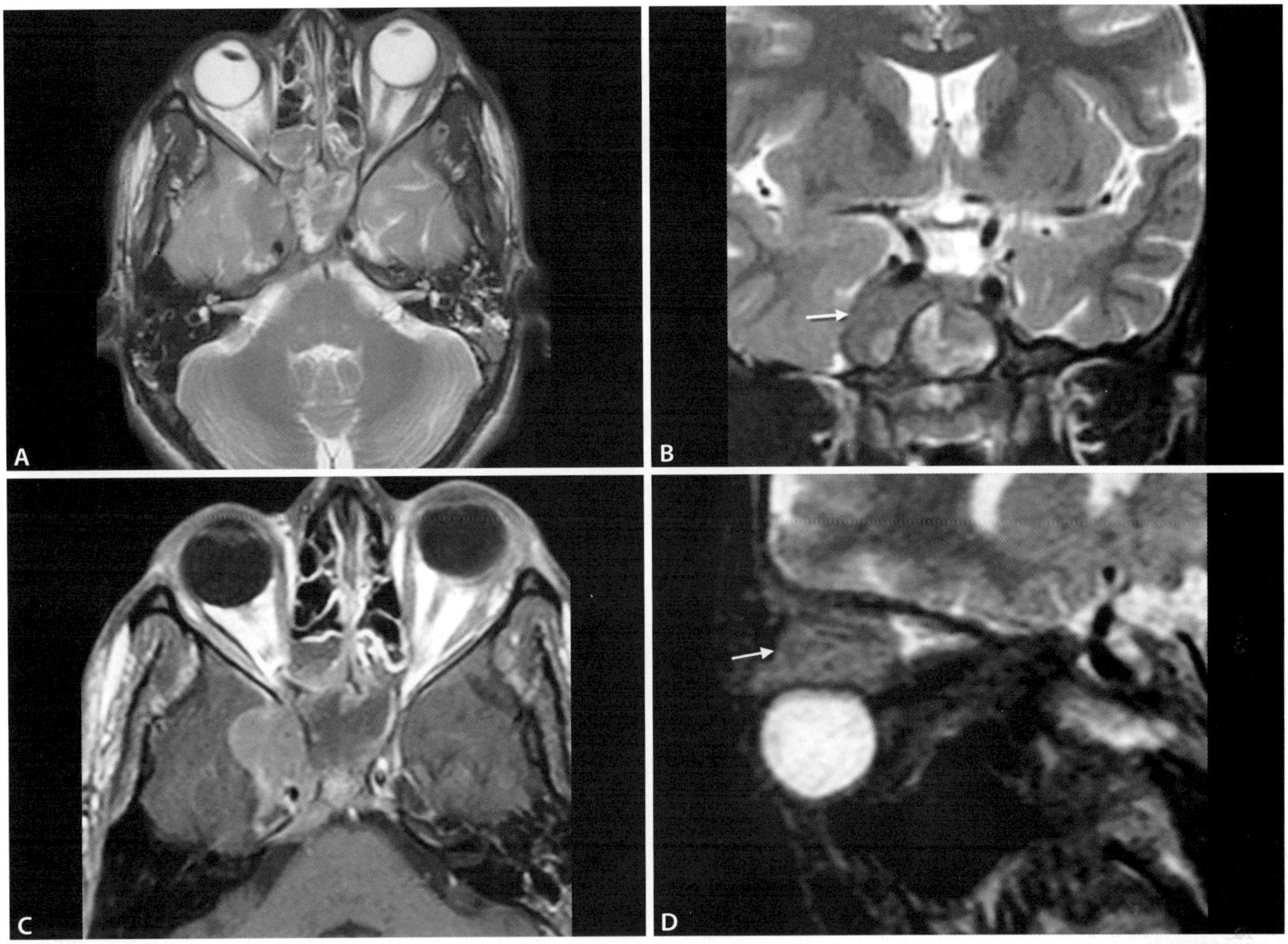

Figs. 5A to D: Chloroma in a 40-year-old lady with AML: Axial (A) and coronal (B) T2W MR images show hypointense mass involving right cavernous sinus and parasellar region (arrow). T1W postcontrast MR image (C) shows avid contrast enhancement. Sagittal T2W image (D) of the orbit reveals another deposit (arrow) in the left lacrimal fossa having the same signal intensity.

usually occur in ethmoid/sphenoid region.[12-14] Imaging by CT or MR help to confirm the diagnosis by noting the skull base defect and the contents of the mass **(Figs. 7A and B)**. Meningoceles have fluid following CSF signal intensity on all sequences while cephaloceles have brain parenchyma following gray matter signal. Correct diagnosis should avert a biopsy.

Lesions of the Proper Skull Base

Trauma and cerebrospinal fluid leak: At the anterior skull base there is dense adhesion of the dura to the bone. Hence fractures of the anterior skull base (most commonly of cribriform plate, fovea ethmoidalis or posterior table of frontal sinus)[15] after trauma also cause dural tear leading to complications of CSF rhinorrhea **(Figs. 8A to C)**, pneumocephalus **(Figs. 9A to C)** and brain herniation. Olfactory nerve injury is also known complication of anterior skull base trauma. Thin section high resolution CT can detect the small defect. Anatomical classification of frontabasal fractures are divided into three types.[16,17] Detailed description of it is beyond the scope of this chapter. MRI with cisternography enables differentiating the contents of the herniated tissue. In doubtful cases CT cisternography after intrathecal contrast injection or radionuclide cisternography may help.

Osteoma: Osteomas are benign bone tumors found most commonly in membranous bones of skull and face, commonly within frontal and ethmoidal sinuses. They can be diagnosed on radiograph and confirmed on CT.

MIDDLE SKULL BASE

Anatomy

The middle cranial fossa is limited by the greater wings of sphenoid bone anteriorly and the anterior surface

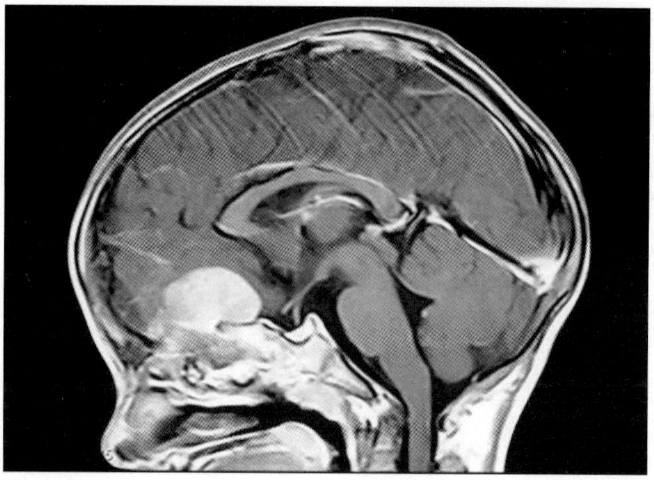

Fig. 6: *Meningioma*: Postcontrast T1-weighted sagittal MR image shows a homogeneously enhancing dural-based mass at the floor of anterior cranial fossa.

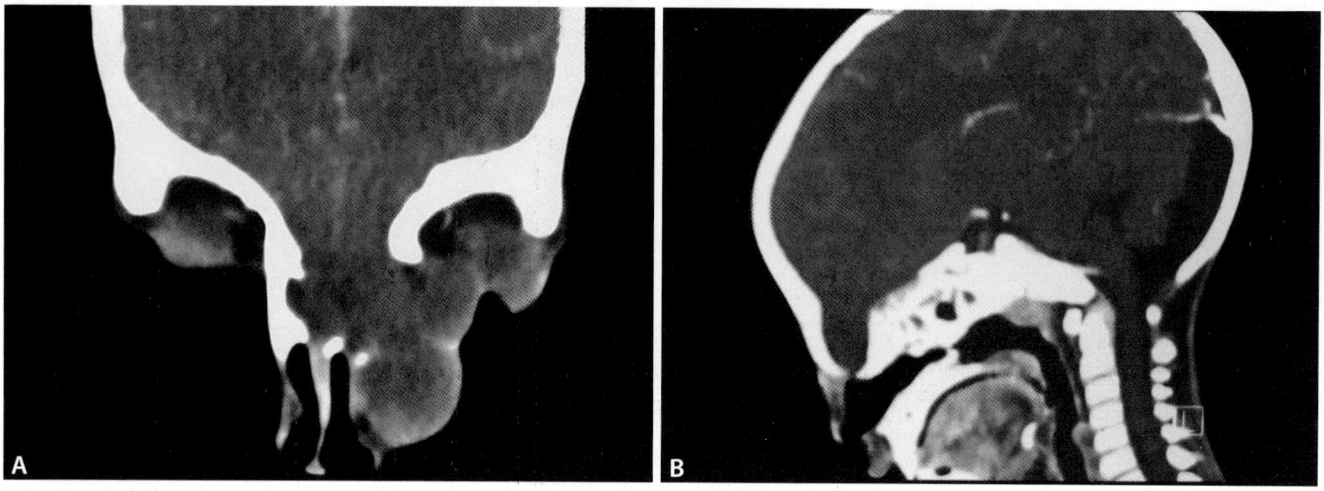

Figs. 7A and B: *Cephalocele*: Coronal MPR (A) and sagittal MPR (B) images of CT show a defect in the floor of anterior skull base on left side with herniation of brain parenchyma downwards.

of the petrous bone posteriorly. Cavernous sinus within the sphenoid body forms the medial border whereas the squamous temporal bone forms the lateral border. Sella turcica is a large depression in the body of the sphenoid bone and the sphenoid sinus lies below the sella turcica. The clivus forms the posteromedial boundary. The middle cranial fossa has multiple openings of foramens and fissures which are best demonstrated on CT **(Figs. 10A and B)**. The optic canal passes through the lesser wing of the sphenoid bone to open posteriorly into the middle cranial fossa and transmits the optic nerve and the ophthalmic artery. The superior orbital fissure lies between the lesser wing of sphenoid bone superiorly and greater wing inferiorly and is bordered medially by the sphenoid body. It transmits cranial nerves III, IV, V1, and V2 and the superior ophthalmic vein from the cavernous sinus posteriorly to the orbit anteriorly. Foramen rotundum lies inferior to the superior orbital fissure and transmits the cranial nerve V2 from the cavernous sinus posteriorly to the pterygopalatine fossa anteriorly. The vidian canal, lying between the sphenoid body and the pterygoid process, transmits the vidian nerve and the vidian artery between the foramen lacerum and pterygopalatine fossa. The foramen ovale lies in the posterolateral part of the greater wing and transmits cranial nerve V3 from the middle cranial fossa to the masticator space. The foramen spinosum is a smaller foramen located just posterolateral to foramen ovale and transmits the middle meningeal artery. The cavernous sinus contains the carotid artery and the cranial nerve VI within it and cranial nerves III, IV,

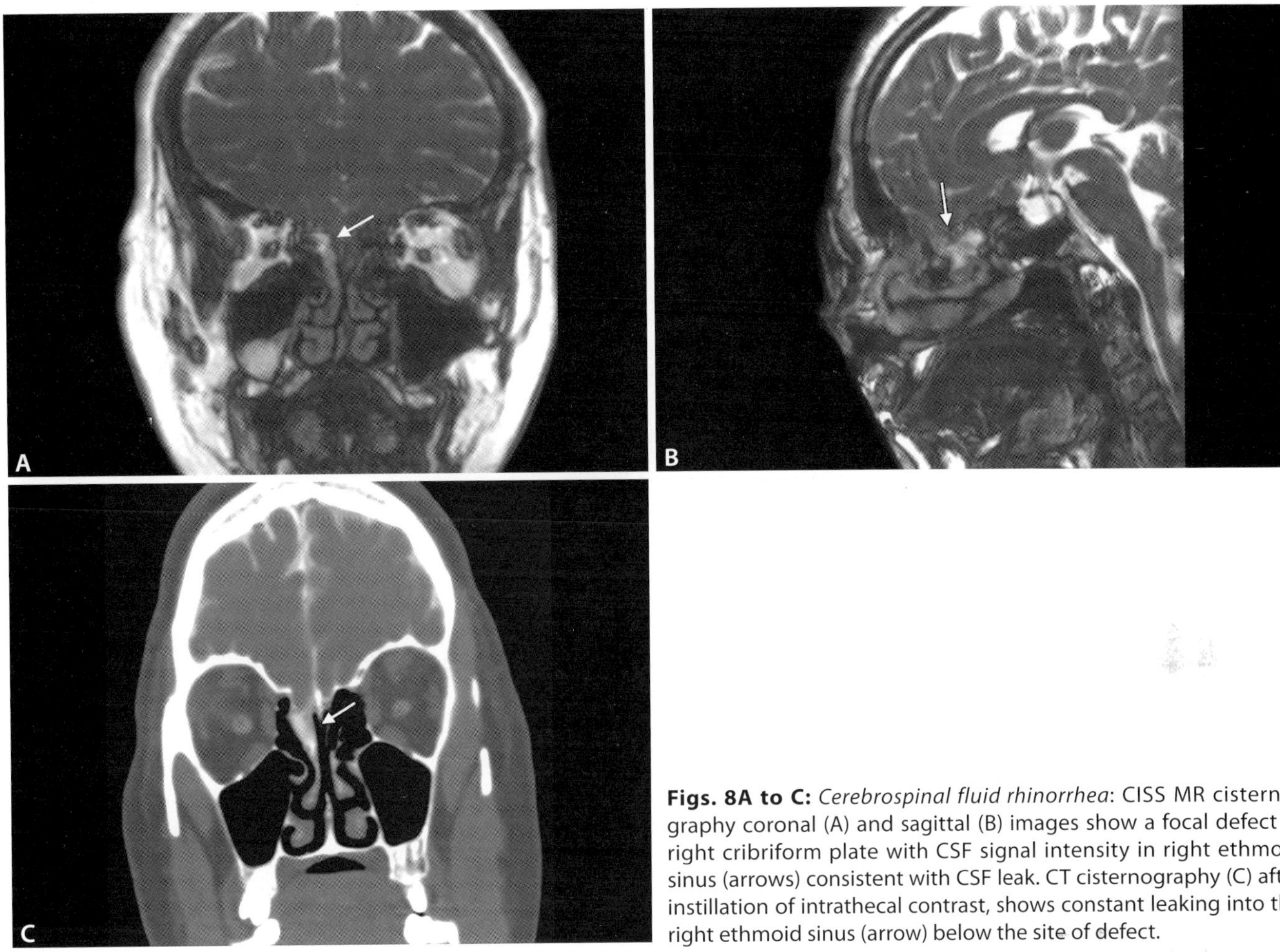

Figs. 8A to C: *Cerebrospinal fluid rhinorrhea*: CISS MR cisternography coronal (A) and sagittal (B) images show a focal defect in right cribriform plate with CSF signal intensity in right ethmoid sinus (arrows) consistent with CSF leak. CT cisternography (C) after instillation of intrathecal contrast, shows constant leaking into the right ethmoid sinus (arrow) below the site of defect.

V1 and V2 (from superior to inferior) enclosed within the dural leaflet of its lateral wall.

Pathology

The middle skull base may be affected by lesions arising from skull base proper, from the intracranial compartment or from the extracranial compartment. It may also be involved by systemic conditions.

The lesions may extend into the middle cranial fossa from below through the existing foramina in the sphenoid bone or by direct erosion. Spread through these foramina is clinically evident by involvement of the nerves passing through them and is radiologically evident as widening of these foramina. Difference in size of more than 4 mm between the two foramen ovale is considered as abnormal. Foramen spinosum size of more than 5 mm or size difference of more than 2 mm from contralateral side is considered abnormal. It is important to radiologically comment upon involvement of structures which act as contraindications for surgical resection which are summarized in **Box 2**.[18] Imaging signs of cavernous sinus invasion by any mass are described in **Box 3**. Or the purpose of radiologically narrowing down the differential diagnosis of the lesions involving the central skull base, it is useful to subdivide the central skull base into midline sagittal (medial to petroclival fissure), off-midline parasagittal (between petroclival fissure and foramen ovale) and lateral compartments (lateral to foramen ovale) **(Table 3)**.

Midline Sagittal Central Skull Base Lesions

It comprises lesions arising from sphenoid body, sphenoid sinus, clivus, sella turcica and nasopharynx.

Sphenoid mucocele: As previously described in the frontal and ethmoid sinuses, the sphenoid mucoceles occur due to obstruction of its drainage. It presents as expansion of the sinus with thinning of walls with contained fluid within it which may show T1 hyperintensity on MR due

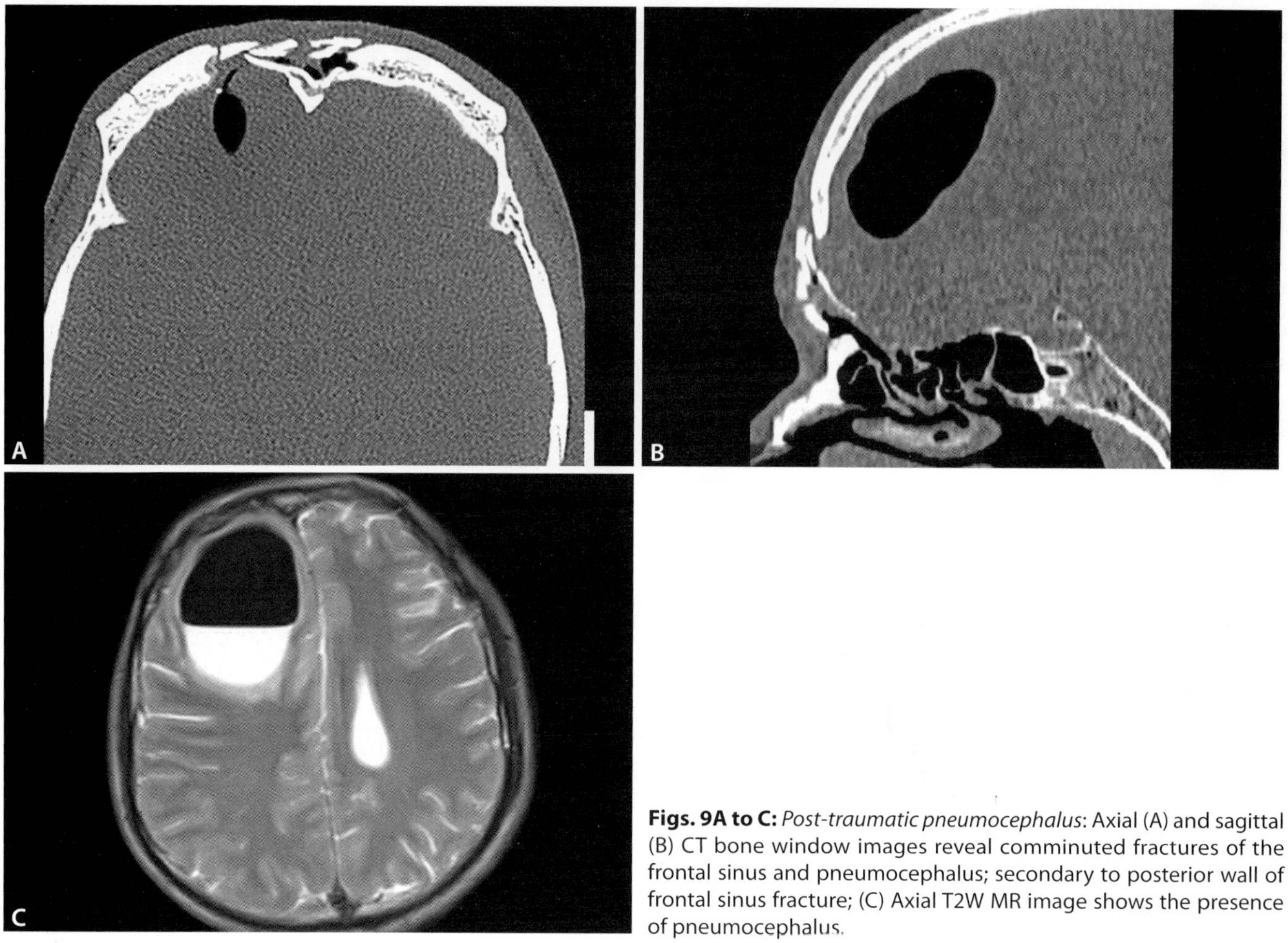

Figs. 9A to C: *Post-traumatic pneumocephalus*: Axial (A) and sagittal (B) CT bone window images reveal comminuted fractures of the frontal sinus and pneumocephalus; secondary to posterior wall of frontal sinus fracture; (C) Axial T2W MR image shows the presence of pneumocephalus.

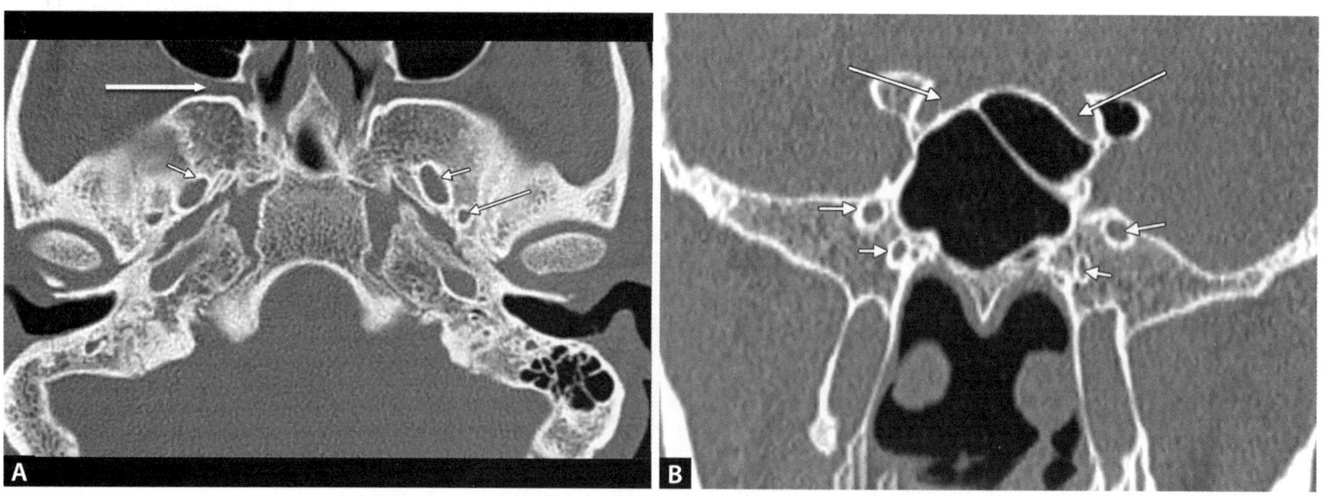

Figs. 10A and B: Axial (A) and coronal (B) CT sections through central skull base show foramen ovale (arrows), foramen spinosum (long arrow) and pterygopalatine fossa (block arrow). Coronal CT image (B) reveals foramen rotundum (arrows), vidian canal (short arrows), and optic foramen (long arrows).

Box 2: Invasion of following structures is contraindications for surgical resection.

- Cavernous sinus
- Bilateral optic nerves or optic chiasm involvement
- Nasopharynx
- Prevertebral fascia
- Lateral or superior wall of sphenoid sinus

Box 3: Signs of cavernous sinus invasion.[19,20]

- Loss of contrast enhancement
- Bulging of lateral sinus wall
- Compression, stenosis, encasement of cavernous carotid artery

Table 3: Middle skull base lesions.

Midline sagittal (medial to petroclival fissure) • Sphenoid mucocele • Clival chordoma • Pituitary macroadenoma • Craniopharyngioma • Meningiomas • Encephaloceles • Nasopharyngeal infections and nasopharyngeal carcinoma
Off-midline parasagittal (between petroclival fissure and foramen ovale) • Peripheral nerve sheath tumors • Perineural spread • Juvenile nasopharyngeal angiofibroma • Cavernous sinus lesions • Chondroid tumors
Lateral compartments (lateral to foramen ovale) • Meningioma • Temporomandibular joint (TMJ) lesions

to high protein content. It does not enhance except for a thin enhancing rim of mucosa **(Figs. 11A to D)**. This differentiates it from the rare squamous cell carcinomas originating in the sphenoid sinus.

Clival chordoma: It is a benign locally invasive neoplasm presenting as expansile lytic lesion with aggressive pattern of bone destruction. It is best seen as replacement of normal bone marrow on T1-weighted MR images with erosion of its cortical margins and heterogeneously hyperintense on T2-weighted images **(Figs. 12A to C)**. It commonly shows areas of hemorrhage, calcification and cystic degeneration. Lobulated pattern of contrast enhancement has been described as a typical feature.[21] The differential diagnosis includes plasmacytoma, metastases and chondrosarcoma.

Pituitary macroadenoma: Pituitary macroadenomas cause expansion of sella and invade the cavernous sinuses laterally with encasement of the carotid artery. The invasive adenomas may also breach the floor and grow into the sphenoid sinus.[22] The best diagnostic clue is a lesion in the sphenoid bone with the pituitary fossa bulging downwards into the lesion and simulating an empty sella **(Figs. 13A and B)**.

Craniopharyngioma: Craniopharyngiomas are benign neoplasms arising from remnants of pharyngohypophyseal canal or Rathke's pouch and hence can be seen anywhere from the nasopharynx to hypothalamus. They appear as cystic or mixed lesions with calcification and show contrast enhancement of the solid part **(Figs. 14A and B)**. MRI may show T1 hyperintensity of the cystic component due to proteinaceous content.

Meningiomas: In the sellar and parasellar region, the meningiomas arise from planum sphenoidale, tuberculum sella, diaphragm sella or the clinoid processes. Radiological features include a solid T1 and T2 isointense intensely enhancing mass with broad base towards dura, with or without dural tail. The pituitary gland may be seen separately compressed by the mass. Associated findings include pneumosinus dilatans (increased pneumatization of the sphenoid sinus) and hyperostosis with upward blistering of the planum sphenoidale and tuberculum sella. Differential diagnosis includes other causes of dural thickening and enhancement, such as sarcoid, carcinomatous meningitis, lymphoma and granulomatous disease.

Encephaloceles: Encephaloceles or meningoceles may occur into the sphenoid bone or more anteriorly between the ethmoid and sphenoid bones **(Figs. 15A and B)**. CT and MR can show the bony defect with herniated contents.

Other miscellaneous lesions: Nasopharyngeal infections and nasopharyngeal carcinoma may spread from below to involve the midline sagittal central skull base.

Parasagittal Central Skull Base Lesions

It comprises lesions arising from the cavernous sinus, cranial nerves traversing the neural foramina, the greater sphenoid wing and the petroclival synchondrosis.

Peripheral nerve sheath tumors: Schwannomas and neurofibromas can arise from any cranial nerve, most commonly from the trigeminal nerve. Schwannomas show hypointensity on T1-weighted images and intermediate to high signal on T2-weighted MR images with necrosis and intense heterogeneous enhancement after contrast. They remodel the adjacent bone and may cause neural foramina widening if involving the nerve traversing

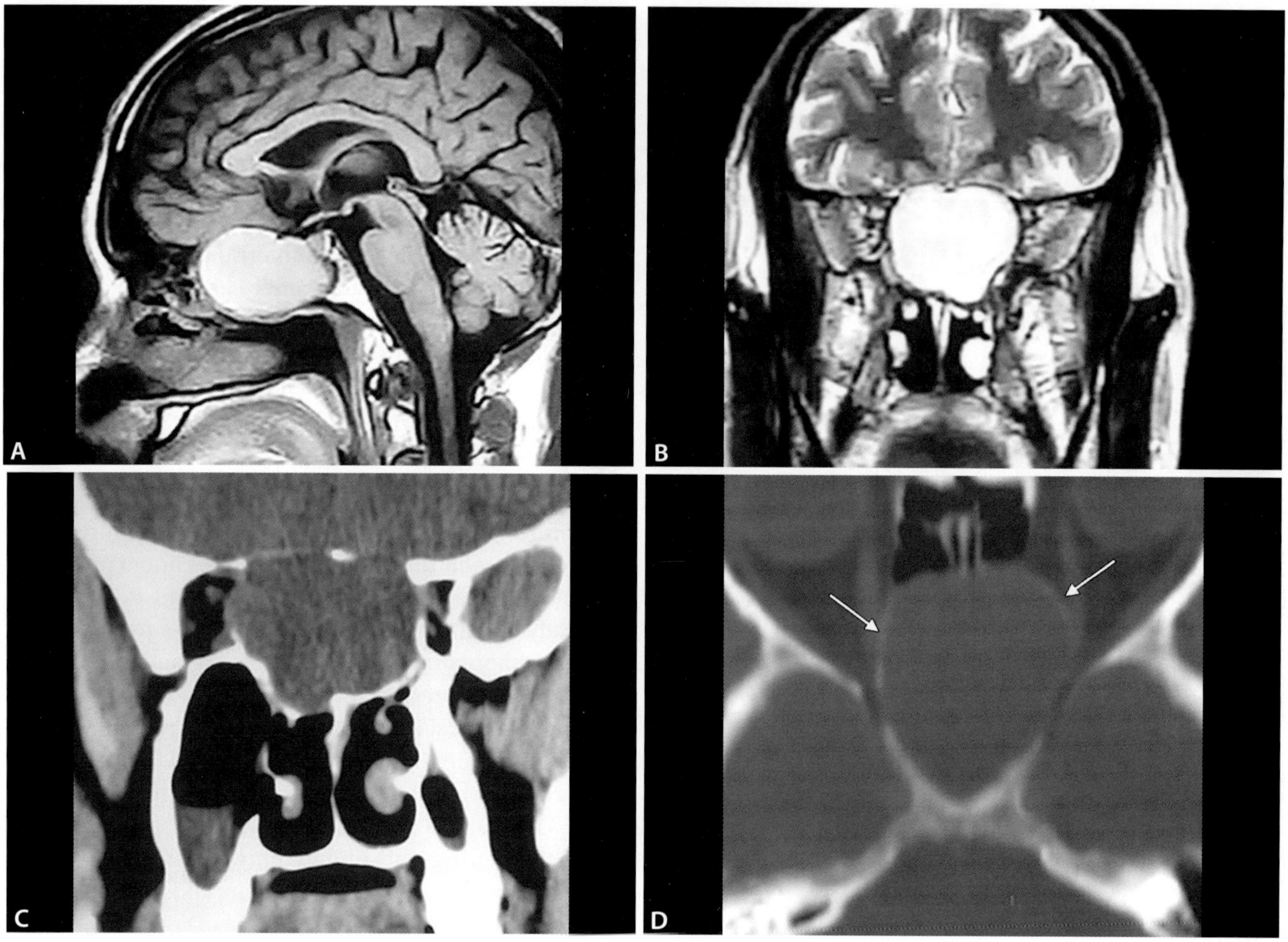

Figs. 11A to D: *Sphenoid mucocele*: T2-weighted sagittal (A) and coronal (B) MR images show expanded fluid-filled sphenoid sinus. Coronal CT soft tissue window reformatted image (C) and axial bone window image (D) reveal bony expansion and thinning (arrows) of sphenoid sinus walls.

through it. Neurofibromas are more aggressive infiltrative lesions which spread diffusely along peripheral branches and show ill-defined borders.[23] Tumors of the trigeminal nerve often appear as dumbbell-shaped tumors with a middle cranial fossa component within cavernous sinus and posterior cranial fossa component within the Meckel's cave **(Figs. 16A and B)**. Vidian nerve neurofibromas present as soft tissue masses expanding the vidian canal from foramen lacerum posteriorly to pterygopalatine fossa anteriorly.

Perineural spread: Cranial nerve involvement may be secondary to spread of various malignancies or infectious/inflammatory conditions along the course of the nerve.[24,25] It is commonly seen with squamous cell carcinoma of head and neck region, salivary gland malignancies (most common adenoid cystic carcinoma) and hematological malignancies. MR detects early perineural spread in the form of thickening of nerve, enhancement of nerve and effacement of neuroforaminal fat. Similar features may be seen in neuritis due to infectious conditions like herpes simplex and CMV. CT scan is less sensitive than MR and detects perineural spread in the form of enlargement of the neural foramina, effacement of foraminal fat or indirectly through denervation atrophy of the muscles supplied by the particular nerve.

Juvenile nasopharyngeal angiofibroma: As already discussed in the section of anterior skull base, the angiofibroma has propensity to insinuate through various

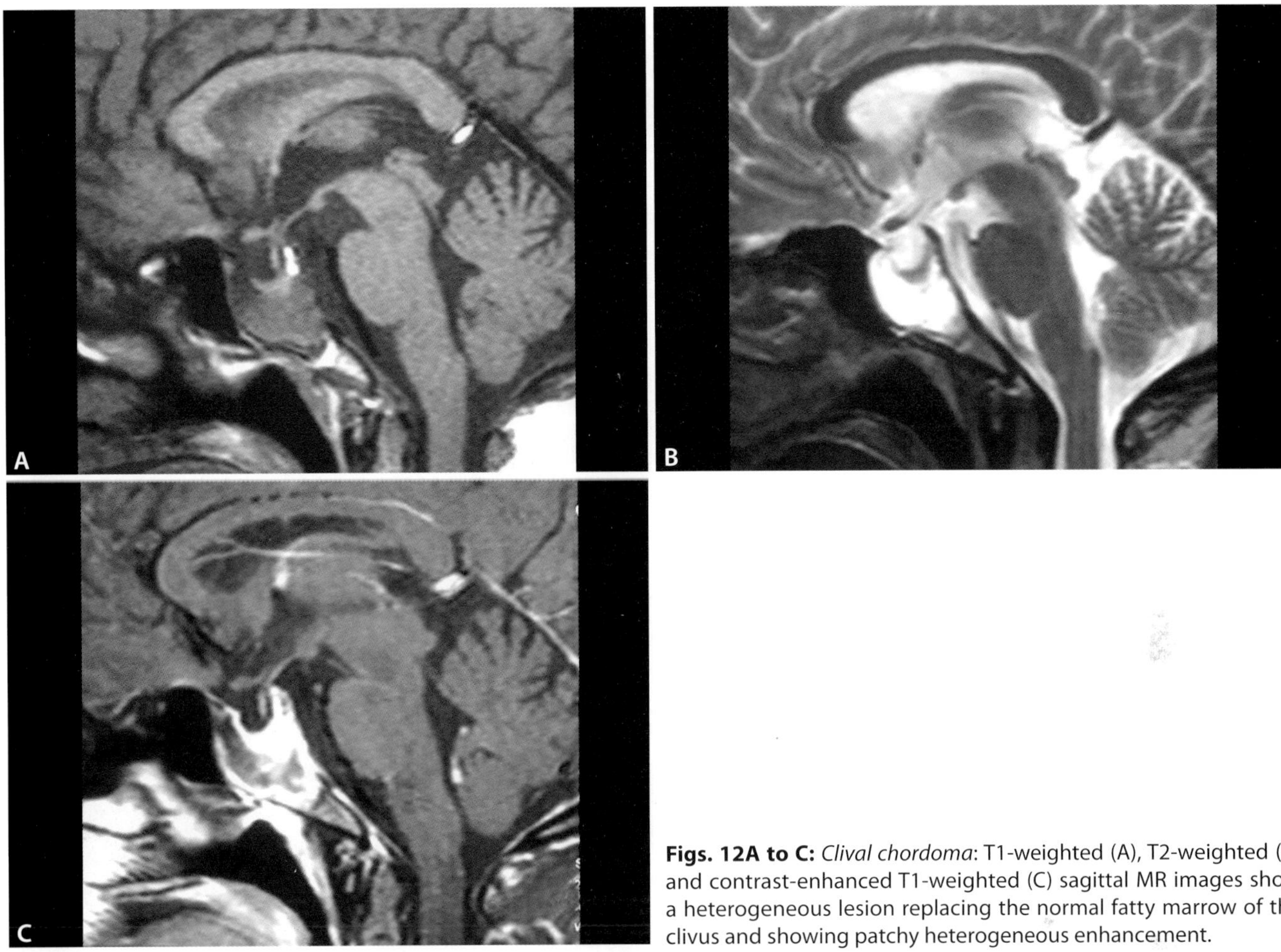

Figs. 12A to C: *Clival chordoma*: T1-weighted (A), T2-weighted (B) and contrast-enhanced T1-weighted (C) sagittal MR images show a heterogeneous lesion replacing the normal fatty marrow of the clivus and showing patchy heterogeneous enhancement.

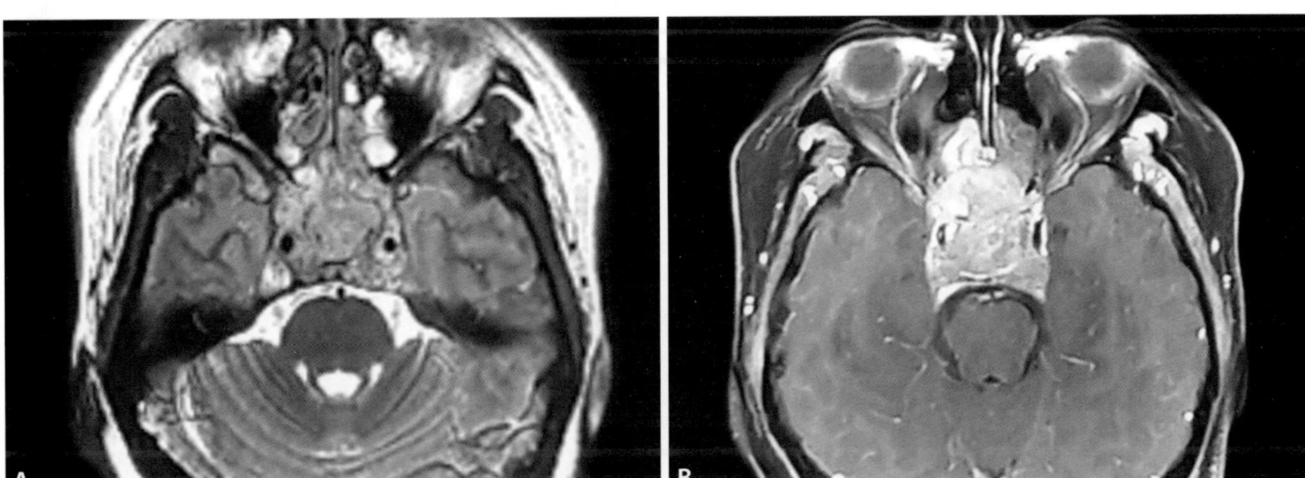

Figs. 13A and B: *Invasive pituitary adenoma*: T2W (A) and postcontrast (B) axial MR images of the sellar region show a soft tissue mass filling the sella, with extension into bilateral cavernous sinuses.

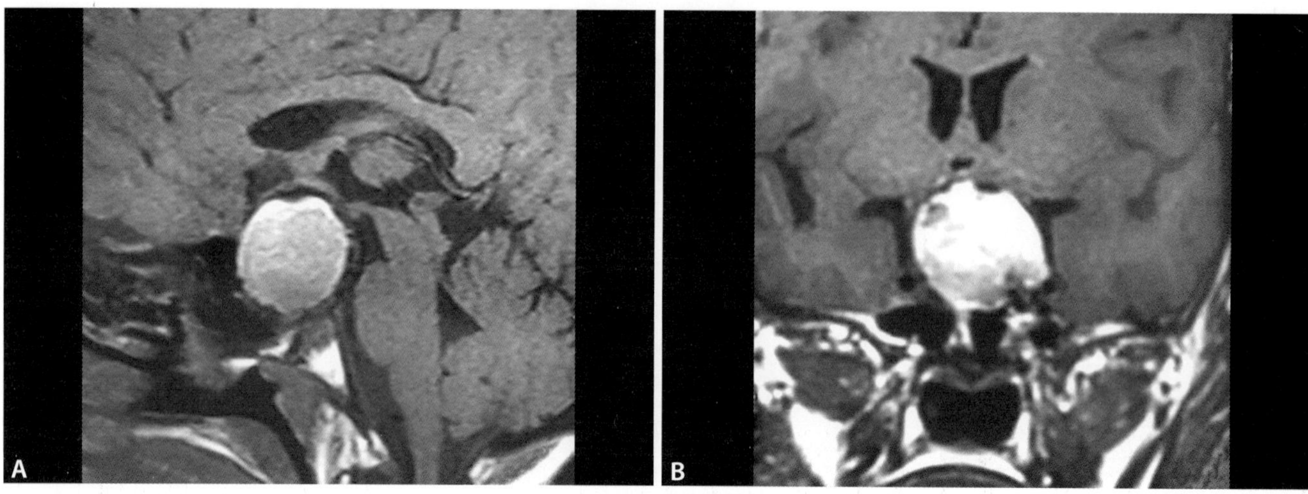

Figs. 14A and B: *Craniopharyngioma*: T1W sagittal (A) and coronal (B) MRI shows a hyperintense mass lesion in the sellar and suprasellar region extending into the sphenoid sinus.

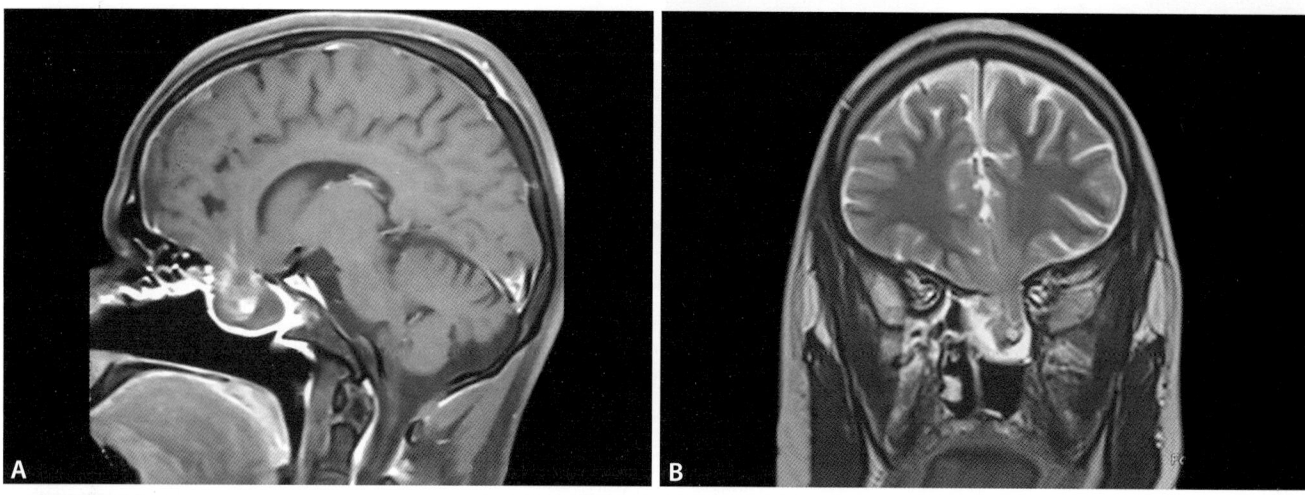

Figs. 15A and B: *Sphenoid encephalocele*: T1W sagittal (A) and T2W coronal (B) MRI show herniation of brain parenchyma into the spheno ethmoid region.

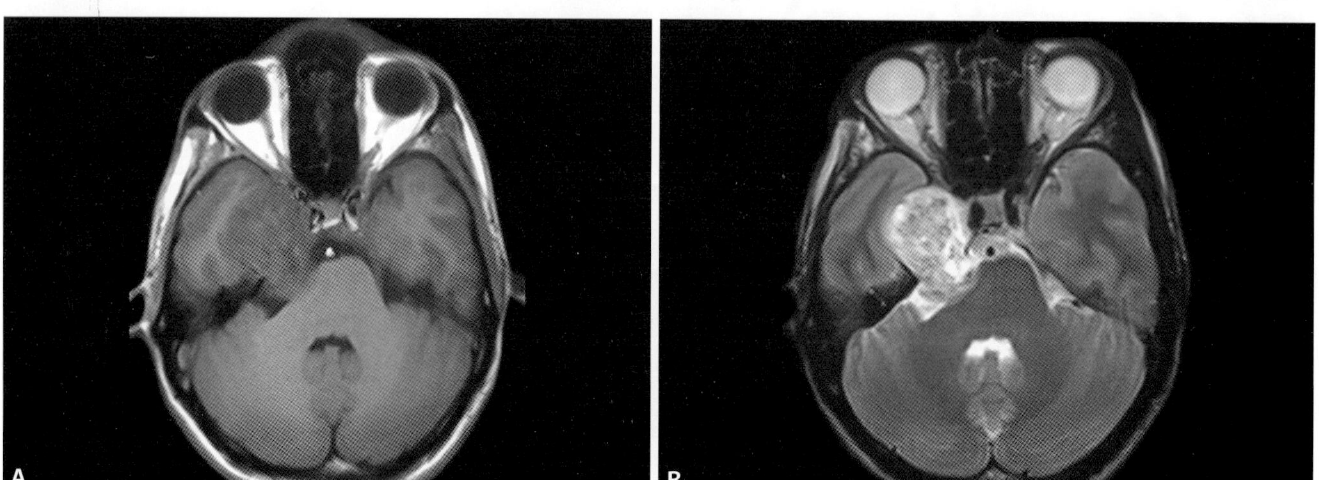

Figs. 16A and B: *Trigeminal schwannoma*: T1-weighted (A) and T2-weighted (B) axial MR images show a dumbbell-shaped heterogeneous mass lesion involving the right cavernous sinus and extending into posterior cranial fossa through the Meckel's cave.

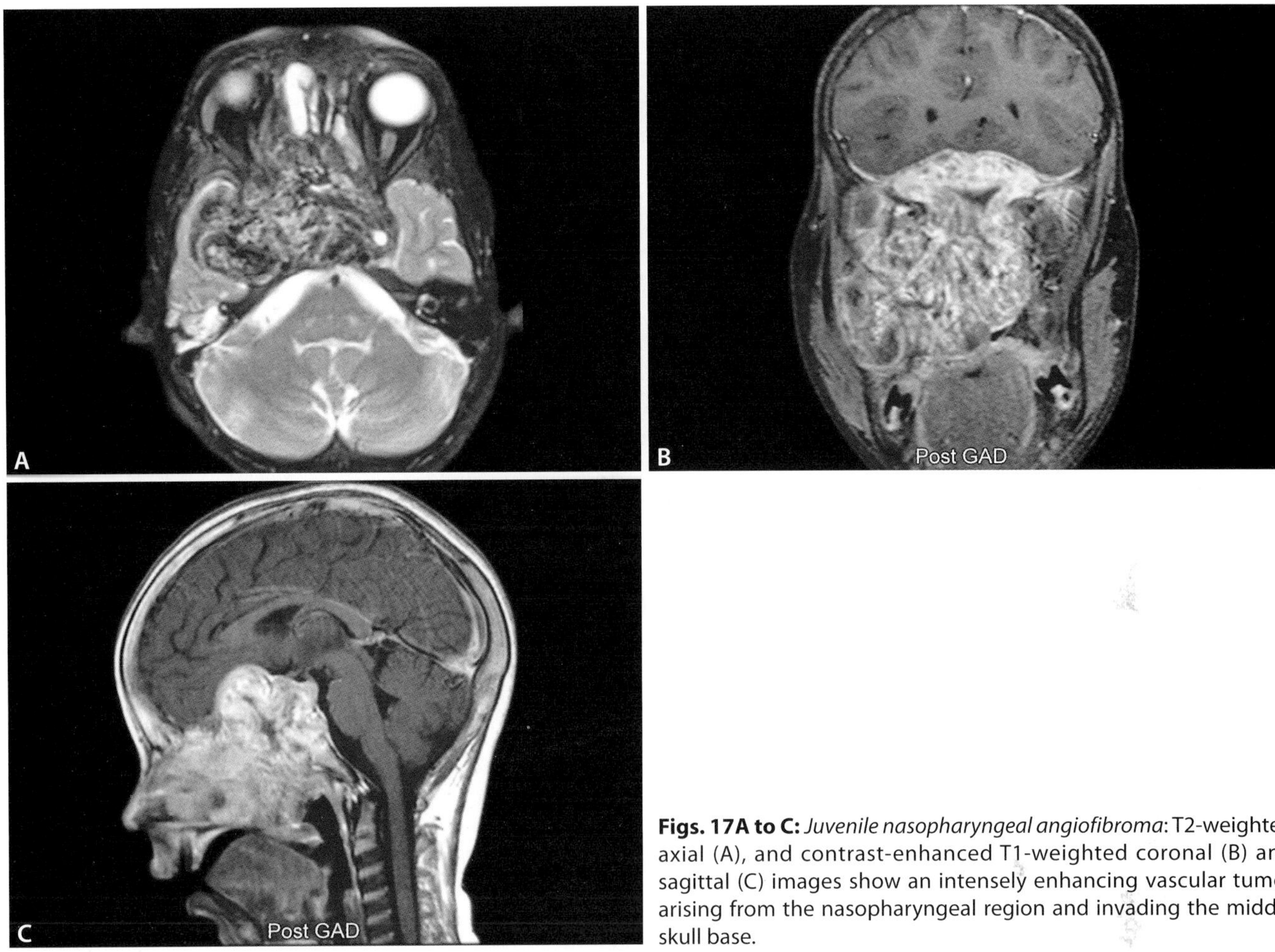

Figs. 17A to C: *Juvenile nasopharyngeal angiofibroma*: T2-weighted axial (A), and contrast-enhanced T1-weighted coronal (B) and sagittal (C) images show an intensely enhancing vascular tumor arising from the nasopharyngeal region and invading the middle skull base.

foramina into the skull. It extends into the parasagittal central skull base from the pterygopalatine fossa through the foramen rotundum or the vidian canal and into the orbit through the inferior orbital fissure. They are highly vascular tumors and show 'salt and pepper' pattern on MRI with intense post-contrast enhancement **(Figs. 17A to C)**. Preoperative embolization of these tumors has a significant role in decreasing the hemorrhage and surgical morbidity.

Cavernous sinus lesions: The cavernous sinus may be involved by spread of pyogenic or fungal infections originating from paranasal sinuses, nasopharynx and orbits. It will show enlargement of cavernous sinus with or without thrombosis. The cavernous sinus may be involved in addition to orbital apex by inflammatory pseudotumor (Tolosa Hunt syndrome). It is seen on MRI as low signal intensity soft tissue mass on T1- and T2-weighted images which enhances on contrast images and occupies the orbital apex with extension into the cavernous sinus. Cavernous sinus enlargement may also be seen in vascular lesions including carotico-cavernous fistulas, aneurysms and hemangiomas and in meningiomas of the cavernous sinus.

Chondroid tumors: Chondromyxoid fibromas and chondrosarcomas arise from petroclival synchondrosis. CT depicts the characteristic chondroid type of calcification. Marked high signal intensity on T2-weighted MR images is also a characteristic feature **(Figs. 18A to C)**.

Lateral Central Skull Base Lesions

It comprises lesions arising from the lateral aspect of temporal bone, temporomandibular joint and far lateral aspect of greater sphenoid wing.

Meningioma: Meningiomas commonly arise from the greater sphenoid wing. They may be either en plaque or classic globular. The characteristic MR features include T1 and T2 low signal intensity with intense contrast enhancement and dural tail **(Figs. 19A to D)**.

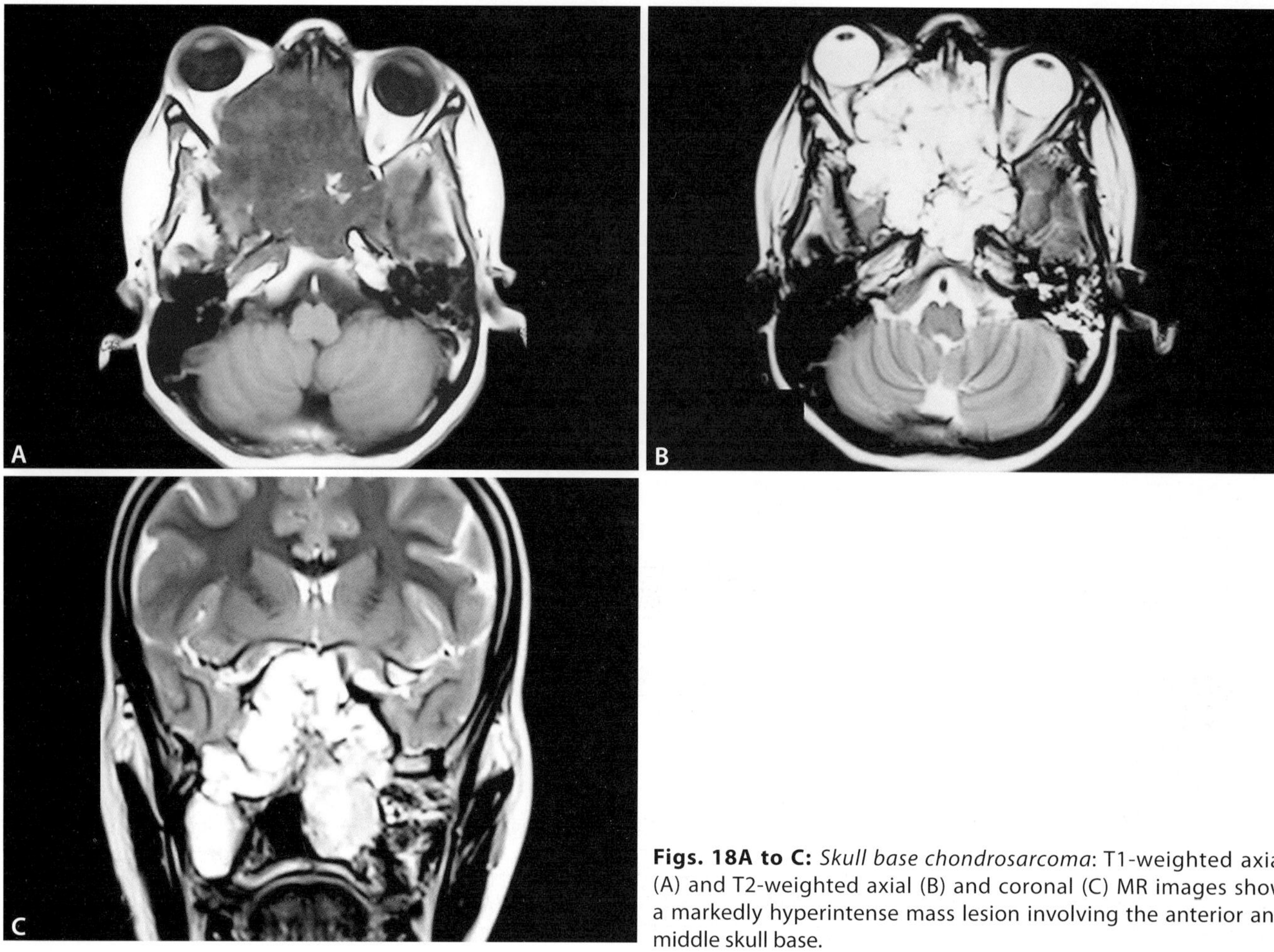

Figs. 18A to C: *Skull base chondrosarcoma*: T1-weighted axial (A) and T2-weighted axial (B) and coronal (C) MR images show a markedly hyperintense mass lesion involving the anterior and middle skull base.

Temporomandibular joint (TMJ) lesions: TMJ infections and tumors including pigmented villonodular synovitis may appear as mass lesions in the region of lateral central skull base.

POSTERIOR SKULL BASE

Anatomy

The posterior cranial fossa extends from the posterior surface of the clivus to the foramen magnum. The posterior skull base consists of the petrous and mastoid parts of the temporal bone and the squamous and condylar portions of the occipital bone. The jugular foramen lies between the petrous temporal and occipital bones and lies lateral to the hypoglossal canal. The foramen has oblique course through the skull base. It is divided by a fibrous or bony septum into a smaller anteromedial compartment (pars nervosa) and a larger posterolateral compartment (pars vascularis). Cranial nerve IX and inferior petrosal sinus pass through the pars nervosa and cranial nerves X and XI along with jugular vein and posterior meningeal artery pass through the pars vascularis. The foramen magnum lies within the occipital bone.

Pathology

Lesions involving the posterior skull base can be categorized according to the site of origin into jugular fossa lesions, petrous apex lesions and foramen magnum lesions **(Table 4)**.

Jugular Foramen Lesions

Glomus jugulare paraganglioma: They are the most common tumors of this region, seen mostly in women in fifth and sixth decades. They are often multiple. It usually arises in the pars vascularis but may extend to involve the pars nervosa. CT shows a permeative 'moth eaten' pattern of bone destruction which distinguishes it from the nerve

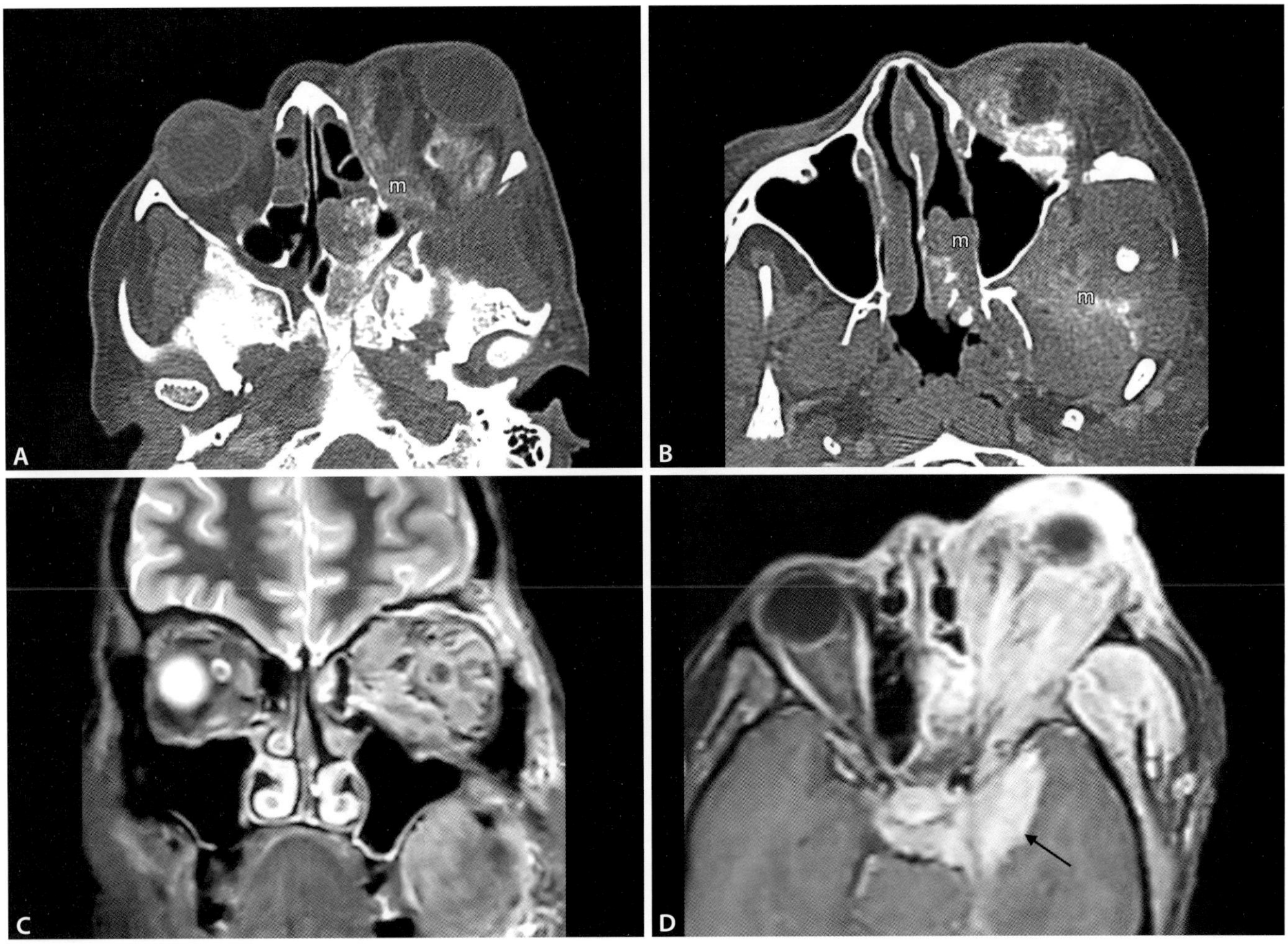

Figs. 19A to D: *Left sphenoid wing meningioma*: Axial CT bone window images (A and B) reveal mass (m) with amorphous calcification involving left infratemporal fossa, left ethmoid air cells and left orbit. T2W coronal MR image (C) shows the mass to be isointense with hypointense areas. Postcontrast T1W image (D) shows avid contrast enhancement of the extracranial soft tissue along with extension to the left cavernous sinus (arrow).

Table 4: Posterior skull base lesions.

Jugular foramen lesions
• Glomus jugulare paraganglioma
• Nerve sheath tumors
• Lesions extending into the jugular foramen
• Jugular bulb pseudolesion
• Large or high riding jugular bulb
Petrous apex lesions
• Nonaggressive cystic expansile lesions
• Aggressive appearing solid lesions
Foramen magnum lesions
• Chordoma Chondrosarcoma
• Neurogenic tumors
• Infections and inflammatory processes of the CV junction

sheath tumors of this region which produce smooth and scalloped erosions.[26] MR shows the characteristic 'salt and pepper' appearance due to multiple vascular flow voids and foci of subacute hemorrhage interspersed within the lesion. These tumors show intense enhancement on contrast administration. It is important to comment upon the extension into the tympanic cavity if present (glomus jugulotympanicum) as it changes the surgical approach **(Figs. 20A and B)**. Preoperative embolization can significantly reduce the surgical morbidity and mortality.

Nerve sheath tumors: Schwannomas and neurofibromas can arise from the cranial nerves traversing the jugular foramina. As described earlier, they tend to cause smooth bone erosions and remodeling rather than frank destruction. On CT they may appear as slightly low attenuation masses due to their rich lipid content. The schwannomas usually show intense postcontrast enhancement with intratumoral cysts in up to 25% of cases but the neurofibromas show variable enhancement.[27] It is radiologically difficult to differentiate between the two.

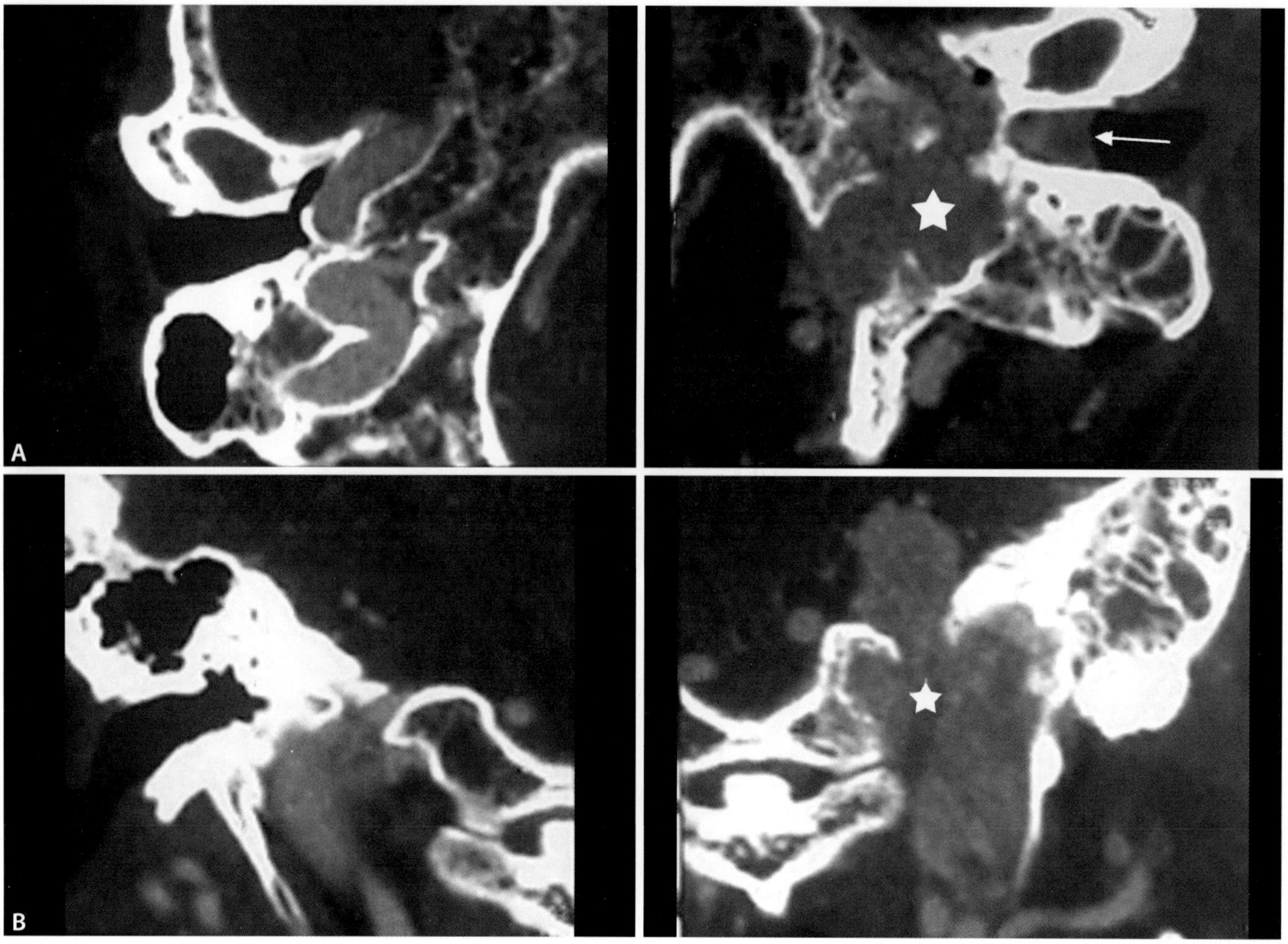

Figs. 20A and B: *Glomus jugulotympanicum*: Axial (A) and Coronal (B) CECT images reveal a hypervascular mass (stars) involving left jugular fossa, middle ear cavity and extending into left external auditory canal (arrow). Note the associated bone destruction.

Lesions extending into the jugular foramen: Perineural spread from malignancies of oral cavity and pharynx can extend to involve the jugular fossa. Glomus vagale arising from the cranial nerve X in the lower part may extend up into the jugular foramen causing its expansion. Infections and inflammatory processes arising from adjacent structures like mastoiditis, otitis media and malignant otitis externa can spread to involve the jugular foramen by eroding the intervening bone and may lead to venous thrombosis.

Jugular bulb pseudolesion: Abnormal high signal intensity on T1-weighted MR images within the jugular bulb is commonly seen due to the complex flow pattern within a normal jugular bulb. It may be mistaken for a pathology like glomus tumor. It needs to be correctly identified to prevent unnecessary further intervention. It can be recognized as the 'lesion' is not evident on T2-weighted images and MR venogram depicts a normal patent jugular bulb.[28]

Large or high riding jugular bulb: Normal variation in size and symmetry of the jugular bulbs is common with right side being dominant. It should not be mistaken for pathology as there is no bony erosion. High riding jugular bulb is defined as a jugular bulb roof extending above the level of inferior margin of the basal turn of the cochlea or the inferior tympanic annulus.[29,30] They are also more common on right side. It may be associated with dehiscence of the superior jugular plate leading to protrusion of the bulb superolaterally into the posterior hypotympanum. It is important to identify these anatomical variations before any surgery for the middle ear or CP angle lesion.

Petrous Apex Lesions

Nonaggressive cystic expansile lesions: Cholesterol granuloma forms secondary to obstruction of a pneumatized air cell with subsequent hemorrhage and cholesterol deposition. It has a characteristic MR appearance of being hyperintense on both T1- and T2-weighted images.[27] CT shows expansion of the bony cortex. No enhancement is seen in the central part. Petrous carotid artery aneurysm can also lead to an expansile lesion in this region with thinning of the walls of the carotid canal. The MR signal changes are dependent upon amount of thrombus within it. Contrast enhancement (if not thrombosed) can differentiate it from cholesterol granuloma. Mucoceles **(Figs. 21A and B)** and arachnoid cysts may also be rarely seen in the region of petrous apex presenting as cystic expansile lesions.

Aggressive appearing solid lesions: Cholesteatomas of the petrous apex are seen as expansile lesions with variable degree of bone destruction.[31] They do not enhance on contrast administration. When no bony destruction is present, they may mimic cholesterol granuloma but can be differentiated on MR wherein the cholesteatomas show low to intermediate signal on T1-weighted images in contrast to cholesterol granuloma which shows high signal on T1-weighted images. Cholesteatoma may also show restricted diffusion.[32] Infection of the petrous apex may be seen in the form of petrous apicitis or a true petrous apex osteomyelitis. The former is caused by extension of otitis media into a pneumatized petrous apex and causes classical Gradenigo's syndrome: triad of otitis media/mastoiditis, severe facial pain in cranial nerve V1 distribution and ipsilateral cranial nerve VI palsy. Imaging shows opacification of petrous air cells with bony erosion and destruction and enhancement of entire petrous apex including the dura on postcontrast MR. Petrous apex osteomyelitis occurs secondary to direct medial extension of malignant otitis externa into a nonpneumatized petrous apex. CT shows bone erosions with sclerosis and MR shows replacement of the normal fatty marrow with enhancement.

Foramen Magnum Lesions

Mass lesions extending into the foramen magnum may have origins from the following structures:

- Bony lesions arising from the clivus-like chordoma and chondrosarcoma which can extend into the foramen magnum causing compression of the medulla and cervical cord.
- Tumors arising from the nerves (neurogenic tumors) and the covering meninges (meningiomas).
- Bony tumors arising from atlas and axis vertebra.
- Infections and inflammatory processes of the CV junction like rheumatoid arthritis and tuberculosis. RA shows evidence of erosion of the dens with pannus causing encroachment of the spinal canal. Tuberculosis will show destruction of the dens with adjacent soft tissue/collections and peripheral enhancement.

DIFFUSE/NON-SITE-SPECIFIC SKULL BASE LESIONS

Skull base may be affected by a variety of systemic conditions, bone tumors, fibro-osseous lesions or infections which are not site-specific and may involve any part of the skull base from anterior to posterior.

Metastases: They usually involve bones with high marrow content so are most commonly seen in the skull base in the region of petrous apex, clivus and sphenoid triangle. They

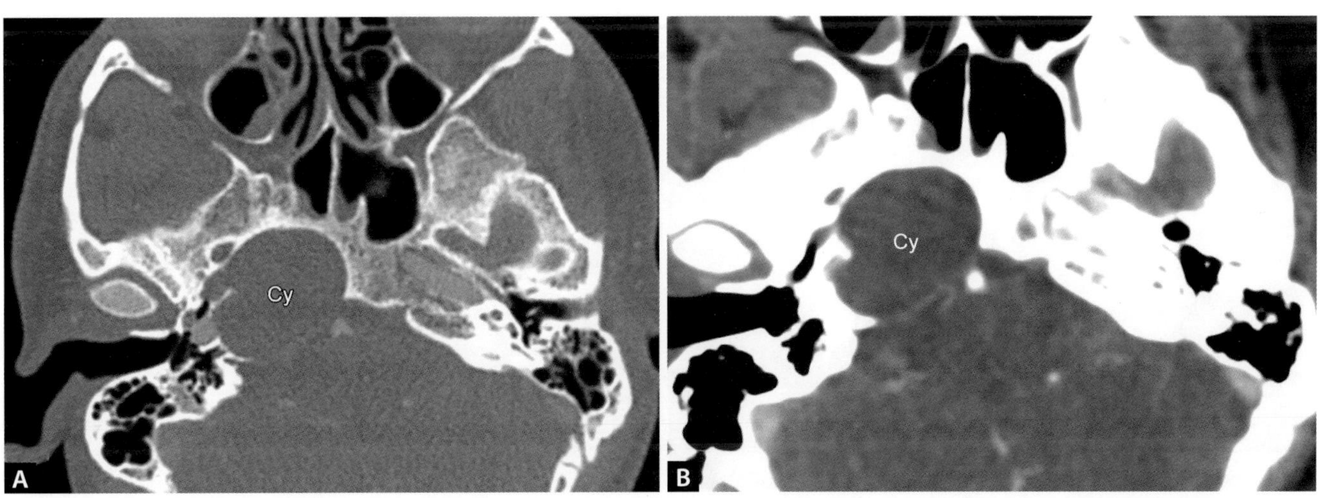

Figs. 21A and B: *Petrous apex mucocele*: NCCT axial bone window (A) and soft tissue window (B) images reveal exapansile low attenuation cystic focal lesion (Cy) at right petrous apex with well corticated scalloped margins.

may be lytic (breast, lung, kidney, thyroid and multiple myeloma), sclerotic (prostate) or mixed (breast).[33] CT is the preferred modality to detect them. Diffuse metastases may be difficult to differentiate from Paget's disease or other fibro-osseous conditions.

Fibrous dysplasia: It is a fibro-osseous lesion arising from skull base seen in children and adolescents. The medullary bone gets replaced by fibro-osseous tissue. CT is the imaging modality of choice for making the correct diagnosis. It initially shows coalescent cystic spaces in the initial phase which progress to the characteristic 'ground glass' appearance with a thin cortical rim and finally a sclerotic late phase **(Figs. 22A and B)**. It shows marked contrast enhancement in the active phase and is nonenhancing in the quiescent phase.[34] CT and MR are also helpful for exact extent of the lesion including depicting the encroachment of the foramina. It appears as low signal intensity lesion on both T1- and T2-weighted images. The lesion spares the cortical bone which helps to differentiate it from Paget's disease.

Paget's disease: It is seen in adults after 40 years of age. It causes diffuse thickening of the cortical bone and radiologically is seen as bone expansion and sclerosis with coarse bony trabeculae. There is usually associated involvement of skull vault and of the otic capsule which also helps it to differentiate from fibrous dysplasia **(Figs. 23A and B)**.[20]

Skull base osteomyelitis: Osteomyelitis of the central skull base is a potentially life-threatening rare condition. Headache may be the only symptom and cranial nerve palsies present later. It is usually seen in patients with underlying diseases such as diabetes mellitus, chronic inflammatory sphenoid sinus disease, corticosteroid use or HIV infection. The diagnosis is difficult to make clinically and therefore is often delayed. The source of infection of the central skull base can be hematogenous or contiguous spread from nearby infective process.

The invasive fungal sinonasal infections tend to spread to medial part of central skull base (region of clivus) whereas the otogenic infections and odontogenic infections tend to spread to the lateral aspects of central skull base (region of pterygoid plates and sphenoid wings).[35]

MDCT signs of osteomyelitis are medullary expansion, cortical destruction, periosteal reaction and sclerosis **(Figs. 24A and B)**. The signs of the source of infection may also be noted such as sinonasal disease, otomastoiditis and mandibular osteomyelitis. Soft tissue mass like lesions and fluid colllections may be seen. Surrounding masticator muscles edema (myositis) and overlying fat cellulitis may also be seen. MRI can depict the extent of involvement in the adjacent soft tissues and intracranial extensions with better resolution **(Figs. 25A to D)**. Bony involvement can be seen as T2 hyperintensity and T1 hypointensity within the clival bone, adjacent soft tissue infiltration with obliteration of normal fat planes, abnormal soft tissue in the cavernous sinus, internal carotid artery narrowing or occlusion, abnormal meningeal enhancement and local cerebritis or venous ischemia, abnormal marrow signal intensity around the skull foramina and abnormal soft tissue infiltrating adjacent fat planes.

Tissue sampling is often required for definite diagnosis.

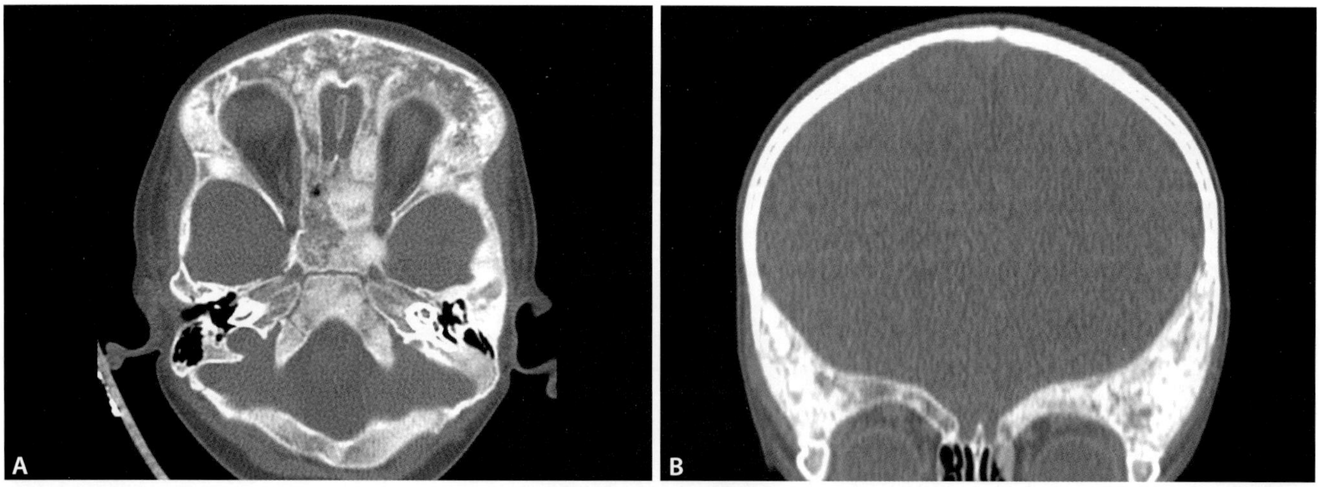

Figs. 22A and B: *Fibrous dysplasia*: Axial (A) and coronal (B) CT images show diffuse involvement of skull base with the characteristic "ground-glass" appearance.

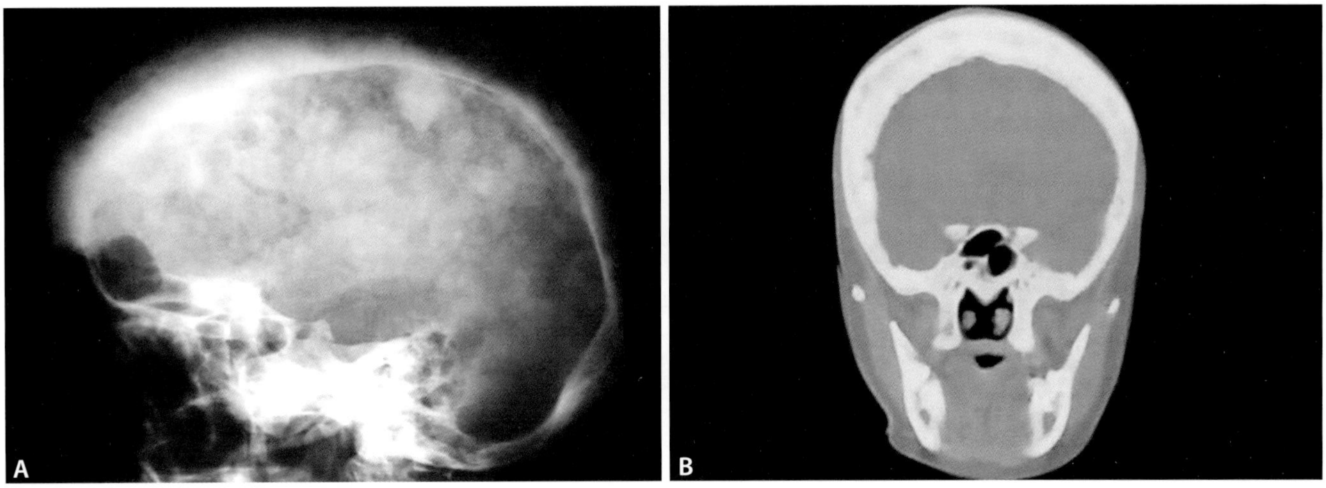

Figs. 23A and B: *Paget's disease*: Lateral skull radiograph (A) and coronal (B) MPR CT images show sclerosis and expansion of the skull bones with involvement of the vault.

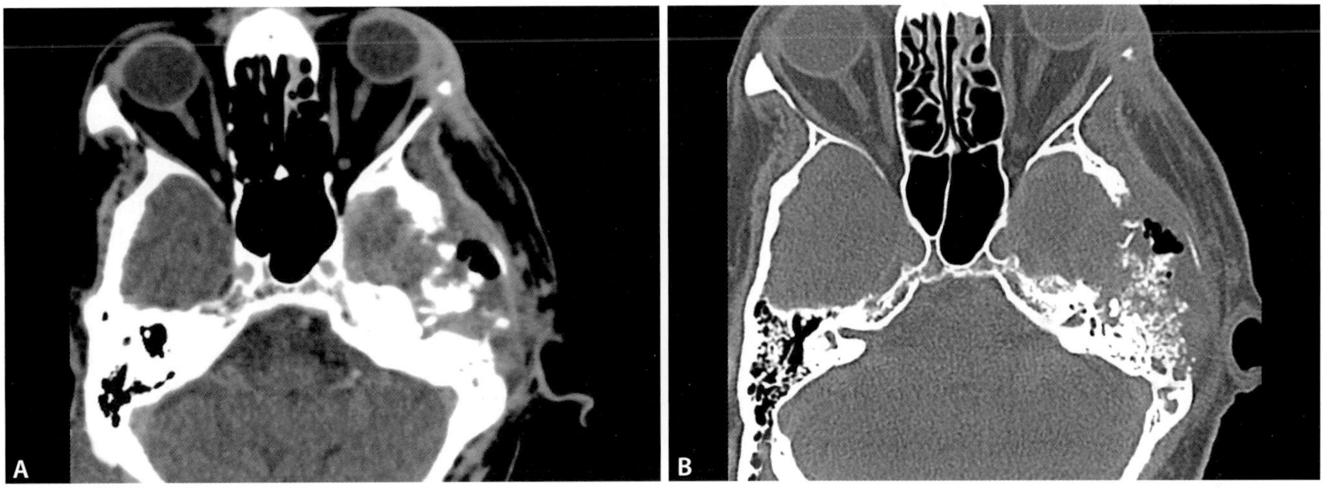

Figs. 24A and B: *Skull base pyogenic osteomyelitis*: Axial CT soft tissue (A) and bone (B) window images reveal permeative lytic bone destruction involving left petrous and mastoid temporal bone, with adjacent soft tissue. Another focus of bone destruction is noted in left lateral orbital wall.

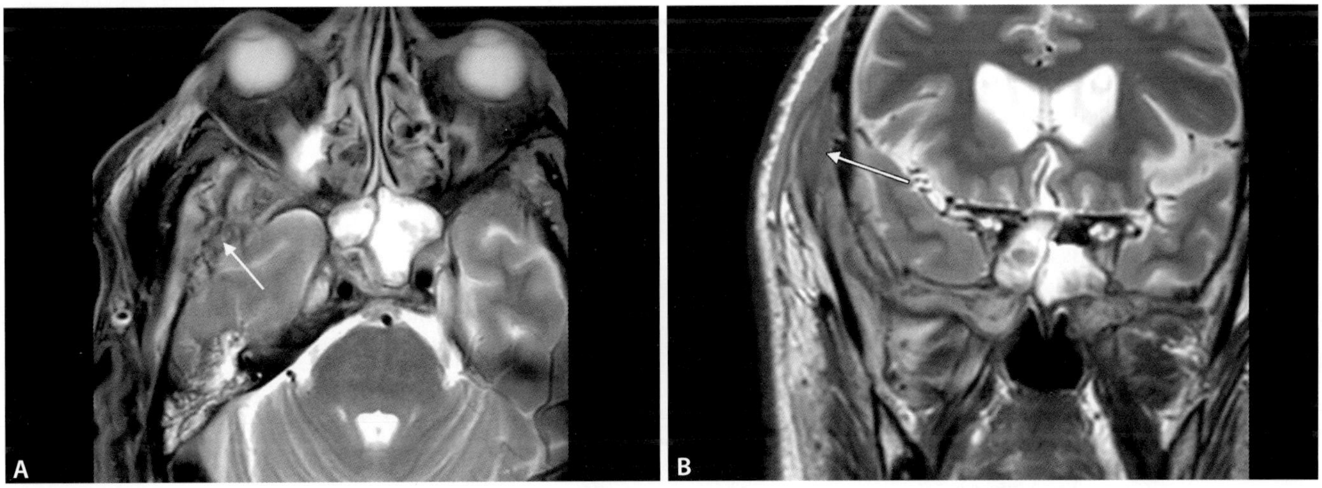

Figs. 25A and B

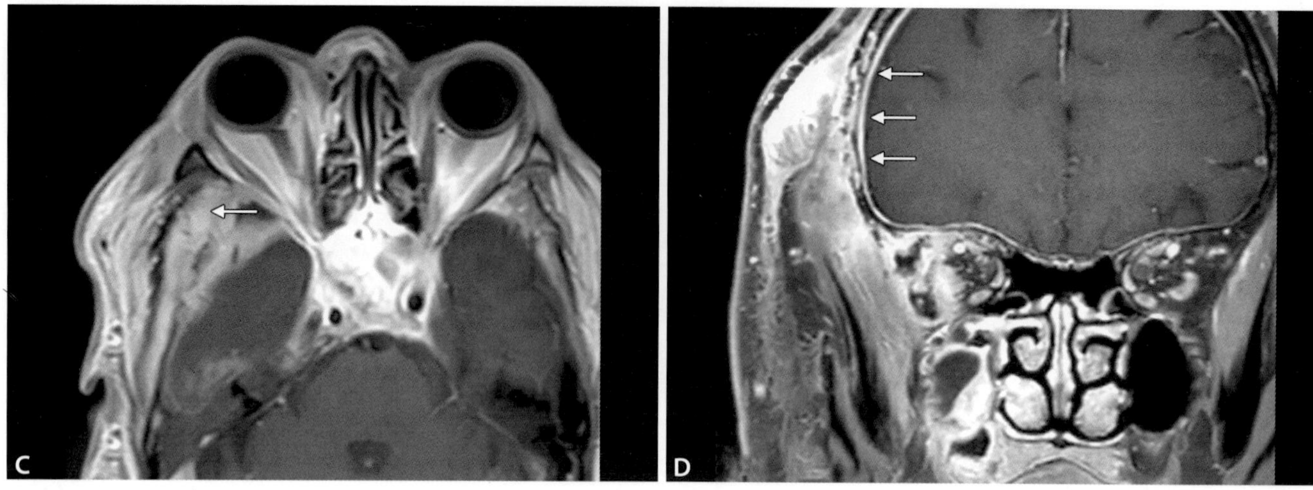

Figs. 25C and D

Figs. 25A to D: *MRI in Skull base pyogenic osteomyelitis*: Axial (A) and coronal (B) T2W MR images reveal soft tissue thickening and hyperintensity (arrows) involving right temporal fossa, and altered marrow signal intensity involving right greater wing of sphenoid. Postcontrast T1W images (C and D) show avid contrast enhancement of the soft tissue along the bone (arrows) as well as soft tissues in right orbit and temporal fossa.

CT and MRI are also helpful in assessing the complications in the form of cranial neuropathy, cavernous sinus thrombosis. septic cavernous sinus thrombosis, meningeal and brain parenchymal extension, epidural and petroclival abscesses.

Miscellaneous conditions: Osteopetrosis may cause thick and sclerotic skull base appearance with increased tendency to fracture. In children, eosinophilic granuloma may cause punched-out lytic lesions in the skull base. Primary bone tumors like osteosarcoma and osteoblastoma may arise from skull base bones.

CONCLUSION

CT and MRI are the mainstay of evaluation of skull base. MR is more sensitive for evaluation of the soft tissue component, characterization of lesions and their extent whereas CT compliments it by better depicting the fine bony details and the neurovascular foramina. Often, both imaging modalities are used in conjunction. Since the list of lesions involving the skull base is huge, dividing the skull base into three compartments with further subdivision into smaller areas helps in narrowing down the differential diagnosis significantly.

REFERENCES

1. Ginsberg LE, Pruett SW, Chen MY, Elster AD. Skull-base foramina of the middle cranial fossa: reassessment of normal variation with high-resolution CT. Am J Neuroradiol. 1994;15(2):283-91.
2. Policeni BA, Smoker WR. Imaging of the skull base: anatomy and pathology. Radiol Clin North Am. 2015;53(1):1-14.
3. Durden DD, Williams DW, 3rd. Radiology of skull base neoplasms. Otolaryngol Clin North Am. 2001;34(6):1043-64, vii.
4. Borges A. Skull base tumours part I: imaging technique, anatomy and anterior skull base tumours. Eur J Radiol. 2008;66(3):338-47.
5. Blitz AM, Aygun N, Herzka DA, Ishii M, Gallia GL. High resolution three-dimensional MR imaging of the skull base: compartments, boundaries, and critical structures. Radiol Clin North Am. 2017;55(1):17-30.
6. Som PM, Curtin HD. Head and Neck Imaging, Skull Base, 4th edition. St. Louis: Mosby Year Book; 2003.
7. Atlas SW. Magnetic resonance imaging of the brain and spine, 3rd edition. Philadelphia: Lippincott Williams & Wilkins; 2002.
8. Parmar H, Gujar S, Shah G, Mukherji SK. Imaging of the anterior skull base. Neuroimaging Clin N Am. 2009;19(3):427-39.
9. Vrionis FD, Kienstra MA, Rivera M, Padhya TA. Malignant tumors of the anterior skull base. Cancer Control. 2004;11(3):144-51.
10. Morita A, Ebersold MJ, Olsen KD, Foote RL, Lewis JE, Quast LM. Esthesioneuroblastoma: prognosis and management. Neurosurgery. 1993;32(5):706-14; discussion 14-5.
11. Som PM, Lidov M, Brandwein M, Catalano P, Biller HF. Sinonasal esthesioneuroblastoma with intracranial extension: marginal tumor cysts as a diagnostic MR finding. AJNR Am J Neuroradiol. 1994;15(7):1259-62.
12. Kennard CD, Rasmussen JE. Congenital midline nasal masses: diagnosis and management. J Dermatol Surg Oncol. 1990;16(11):1025-36.
13. Rahbar R, Resto VA, Robson CD, Perez-Atayde AR, Goumnerova LC, McGill TJ, et al. Nasal glioma and

encephalocele: diagnosis and management. Laryngoscope. 2003;113(12):2069-77.
14. Adil E, Robson C, Perez-Atayde A, Heffernan C, Moritz E, Goumnerova L, et al. Congenital nasal neuroglial heterotopia and encephaloceles: an update on current evaluation and management. Laryngoscope. 2016;126(9):2161-7.
15. Kienstra MA, Van Loveren H. Anterior skull base fractures. Facial Plast Surg. 2005;21(3):180-6.
16. Manson PN, Stanwix MG, Yaremchuk MJ, Nam AJ, Hui-Chou H, Rodriguez ED. Frontobasal fractures: anatomical classification and clinical significance. Plast Reconstr Surg. 2009;124(6):2096-106.
17. Garg A, Prabhakar A. Anterior skull base lesions: Imaging in Clinico Radiological Series: Sinonasal Imaging, 1st edition. New Delhi: Jaypee; 2018.
18. Curtin HD, Chavali R. Imaging of the skull base. Radiol Clin North Am. 1998;36(5):801-17, v-vi.
19. Fischbein NJ, Kaplan MJ. Magnetic resonance imaging of the central skull base. Top Magn Reson Imaging. 1999;10(5):325-46.
20. Borges A, Casselman J. Imaging the cranial nerves: Part I: methodology, infectious and inflammatory, traumatic and congenital lesions. Eur Radiol. 2007;17(8):2112-25.
21. Lufkin R, Borges A, Villablanca P. Teaching atlas of head and neck imaging, 1st edition. New York: Thieme; 2000.
22. Casselman JW. The skull base: tumoral lesions. Eur Radiol. 2005;15(3):534-42.
23. Borges A, Casselman J. Imaging the cranial nerves: part II: primary and secondary neoplastic conditions and neurovascular conflicts. Eur Radiol. 2007;17(9):2332-44.
24. Williams LS. Advanced concepts in the imaging of perineural spread of tumor to the trigeminal nerve. Top Magn Reson Imaging. 1999;10(6):376-83.
25. Borges A. Imaging of the central skull base. Neuroimaging Clin N Am. 2009;19(3):441-68.
26. Ong CK, Fook-Hin Chong V. Imaging of jugular foramen. Neuroimaging Clin N Am. 2009;19(3):469-82.
27. Carvalho GA, Tatagiba M, Samii M. Cystic schwannomas of the jugular foramen: clinical and surgical remarks. Neurosurgery. 2000;46(3):560-6.
28. Chong VF, Khoo JB, Fan YF. Imaging of the nasopharynx and skull base. Magn Reson Imaging Clin N Am. 2002;10(4):547-71, v.
29. Overton SB, Ritter FN. A high placed jugular bulb in the middle ear: a clinical and temporal bone study. Laryngoscope. 1973;83(12):1986-91.
30. Kawano H, Tono T, Schachern PA, Paparella MM, Komune S. Petrous high jugular bulb: a histological study. Am J Otolaryngol. 2000;21(3):161-8.
31. Robert Y, Carcasset S, Rocourt N, Hennequin C, Dubrulle F, Lemaitre L. Congenital cholesteatoma of the temporal bone: MR findings and comparison with CT. Am J Neuroradiol. 1995;16(4):755-61.
32. Aikele P, Kittner T, Offergeld C, Kaftan H, Huttenbrink KB, Laniado M. Diffusion-weighted MR imaging of cholesteatoma in pediatric and adult patients who have undergone middle ear surgery. Am J Roentgenol. 2003;181(1):261-5.
33. Weber AL. Imaging of the skull base. Eur J Radiol. 1996;22(1):68-81.
34. Chong VF, Khoo JB, Fan YF. Fibrous dysplasia involving the base of the skull. Am J Roentgenol. 2002;178(3):717-20.
35. Shama SA. Osteomyelitis of the central skull base: otogenic and odontogenic sources. Multidetector CT study. The Egyptian Journal of Radiology and Nuclear Medicine. 2012;43(4):519-26.

CHAPTER 27

Maxillofacial Imaging: Imaging of Cysts, Tumors and Tumor-like Conditions of the Jaw

Ashu Seith Bhalla, Smita Manchanda, Atin Kumar, Chandan Jyoti Das

Maxillofacial imaging represents a diverse area of radiology and includes imaging of dental caries, periodontal tissues, periapical tissues, dental restorations, implants, developmental abnormalities, cysts and tumors, trauma, salivary glands and temporomandibular joints. The application of advanced imaging modalities for these diseases has lead to increased involvement of radiologists in this field. This chapter will focus on evaluation of cysts, tumors and tumor-like conditions of the jaw.

IMAGING MODALITIES

Plain Radiography

Plain radiography remains the mainstay investigation in the evaluation of jaw lesions despite the availability of modern imaging modalities. These radiographs may be intraoral or extraoral **(Table 1)**.

Table 1: Plain radiographs in maxillofacial imaging.

Plain radiographs
Intraoral: • Periapical • *Occlusal view:* – *Anterior maxilla*: Upper standard maxilla – *Posterior maxilla*: Upper oblique – *Buccolingual expansion of mandible*: Lower 90° occlusal – *Anterior mandible*: Lower 45° (or anterior) occlusal – *Posterior mandible*: Lower oblique
Extraoral: • *Mandible*: Oblique-lateral, PA view • *Maxilla*: Water's view OPG/Panoramic radiography

Intraoral radiographs **(Figs. 1A and B)** present a detailed view of the teeth and periapical region, however are not useful for lesions larger than 3 cm because of the small film size.[1] Intraoral radiographs include periapical view, which shows individual teeth and tissues around the apices. Two to four teeth are seen in each image with detailed information about the teeth and surrounding alveolar bone. Occlusal radiography refers to a radiographic technique wherein the image receptor (film or digital phosphor plate) is placed in the occlusal plane. Various occlusal views are used depending upon the region of interest. These include the upper standard maxilla for anterior maxilla, upper oblique for posterior maxilla, lower 90° occlusal for evaluating buccolingual expansion of mandible, lower 45° (or anterior) occlusal for anterior mandible and lower oblique for posterior mandible.[2]

Extraoral radiographs **(Figs. 2A and B)** are primarily used for the larger lesions and to evaluate the skull and facial structures. Commonly used extraoral radiographs include the oblique-lateral view.

Extraoral radiographs were predominantly used before the development of panoramic equipment. In recent years though, due to limitations of panoramic radiographs this view is still useful. Posteroanterior view of the jaw (PA mandible) shows posterior parts of the mandible. It is not suitable however for showing the facial skeleton including maxilla due to superimposition of the base of skull. An occipitomeatal or Water's view may be used for this purpose.[2]

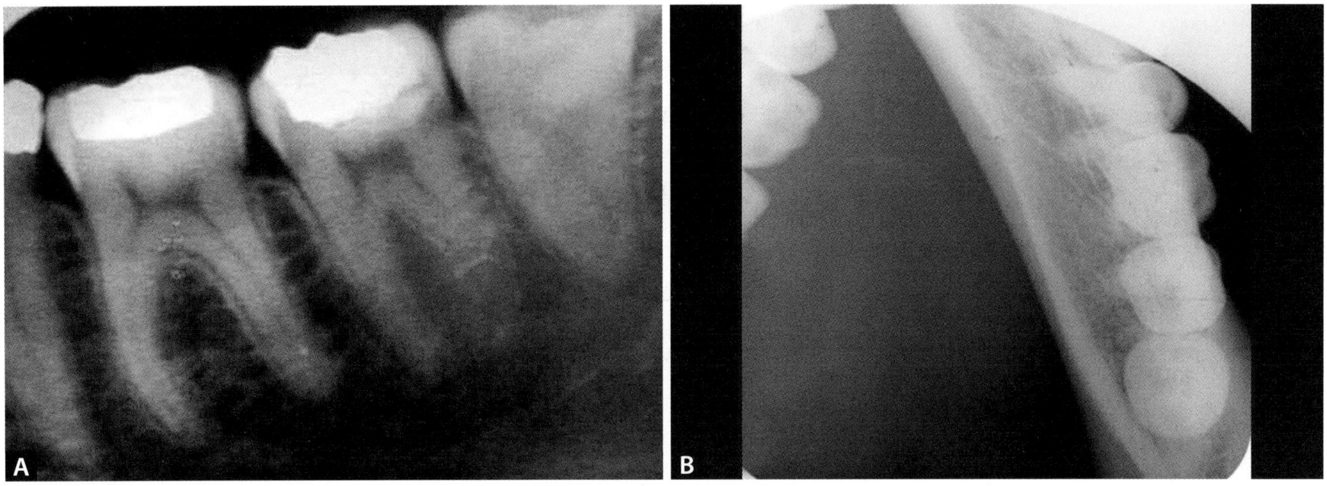

Figs. 1A and B: Intraoral radiographs: (A) Periapical view of mandibular molars showing detailed view of three teeth with periapical and interdental tissues; (B) Lower oblique occlusal view demonstrating the posterior mandible. This view is also used for evaluating submandibular gland calculi.

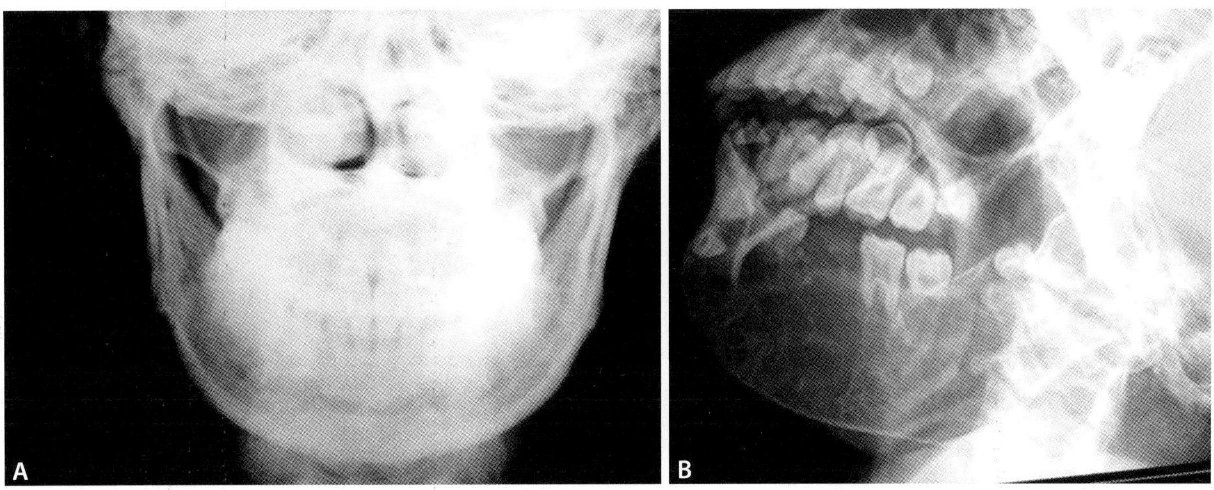

Figs. 2A and B: Extraoral radiographs: (A) Anteroposterior view demonstrating the posterior part of the mandible, while the (B) lateral oblique view shows almost the entire hemimandible, except the midline well. Patient in (B) has an odontogenic myxoma.

Orthopantomography (OPG)/Panoramic radiography or dental panoramic tomography **(Fig. 3)** is a special technique, for evaluating a broad area with relatively low radiation dose. It is also beneficial for patients who are unable to open their mouths.[1,2] It is an extraoral radiographic technique, which is popular because it is used to examine the upper and lower jaws on a single film and it involves low radiation doses. A number of panoramic systems have been developed that generate tomographic sections of various facial structures such as mid face, orbit, temporo mandibular joints, mandible, and paranasal sinuses.

The major drawback of the technique is that since the resultant film is a sectional radiograph produced by moving equipment, therefore like all other forms of tomography only structures within the section will be in focus. In panoramic imaging, the section or focal trough is nearly horseshoe-shaped aligning to the shape of the dental arches. Image quality is less compared to that obtained using intraoral radiography, irrespective of the image receptor used.[2] Various ghost images and technical artifacts because of patient rotation maybe seen.

Computed Tomography

After plain radiography computed tomography (CT) is the primary modality used in the evaluation of cystic or tumorous jaw lesions. CT is useful in determining the complete topography of these lesions. It aids in evaluating

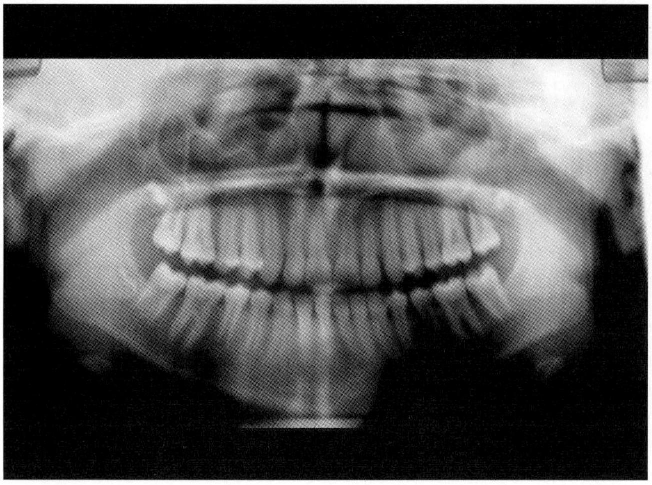

Fig. 3: Panoramic radiograph giving a global view of upper and lower jaws as well as the temporomandibular joints.

integrity of the bony margins of the lesion, its matrix, proximity of the lesion to vital structures and soft tissue extension.[3] Multislice CT technique using multidetector CT (MDCT) has now become the new standard in radiological imaging, including in head and neck imaging. Because of the shorter examination time due to faster scans, motion artifacts are reduced. Due to the thin-slicing and nearly isotropic multiplanar reconstruction (MPR), examination in only one plane is necessary with MDCT, saving both time and radiation exposure. Various 3D processing and advanced evaluation tools can be used in maxillofacial imaging, as elsewhere in the body **(Table 2)**. Some techniques, which are peculiar to the evaluation of this region, are highlighted.

Dental CT Reformatting Programs

Dental reformatting programs were basically developed for the preoperative evaluation of dental implants. These are however finding increasing application in the evaluation of a variety of dental and periodontal diseases including cysts and tumors. Dental CT programs are reconstruction techniques that use thin axial images (up to 1 mm) of the mandible and maxilla to reformat a series of multiple cross-sectional and panoramic images **(Figs. 4A to C)**. The axial images should be acquired parallel to the alveolar ridge. The cross-sectional images are used for preoperative implant assessment. The measurements obtained help to determine the size of the implant to be used. The numerous cross-sectional images obtained can be intimidating and need to be closely correlated with the markings on the base axial and reconstructed panoramic image.[4] The panoramic reconstructions are immensely useful in the evaluation of maxillofacial tumors and

Table 2: Computed tomography in maxillofacial imaging.

Base acquisition: 0.6 mm
Reconstructions: • Standard axial 3 mm in soft tissue and bone windows • Multiplanar reconstructions (MPR): axial, coronal and sagittal planes • Mininmum intensity projections (MIP) • Volume rendered techniques (VRT)
CECT: For all cysts/ tumors
Dental CT Reformatting Programs: Panoramic, Paraxial
Cone-beam CT

cysts. Similar to panoramic radiography the relationship of the lesion to the roots of teeth is demonstrated. The relationship to mandibular canal and maxillary antra is exquisitely demonstrated.

Cone-Beam CT

Also referred to as digital volume tomography cone-beam CT is a low dose CT technology developed specifically for use in dental and maxillofacial region. This equipment uses a cone-shaped X-ray beam vs the fan-shaped beam used in conventional CT. An image intensifier or amorphous silicon flat panel is used as detector. The equipment rotates around the patient acquiring a cylindrical or spherical volume in one rotation. The time taken is approximately 20–40 seconds. The X-ray beam typically has high kV (90–110 kV) pulsed beam to reduce soft tissue absorption. The technique has a small voxel size and hence has high spatial resolution. The computer softwares allow multiplanar reconstruction in axial, coronal and sagittal planes. The advantages of the technique are its low radiation dose, relatively low cost, multiplanar reconstruction and its compatibility with implant and cephalometric planning software. The disadvantage is the need for patient to remain absolutely stationary for 20–40 seconds. Also the soft tissues are not imaged in detail, dental fillings produce streak artifacts and interpretation of panoramic images needs care.[2]

Magnetic Resonance Imaging

Magnetic resonance imaging (MRI) is useful to differentiate cysts from tumors and for evaluating infiltration of the malignant tumors into the bone and surrounding soft tissues, especially for detecting early bone marrow changes of the jaw. However, the differentiation between cysts and tumors requires a contrast-enhanced study.[5]

MRI, unlike CT has the advantage of minimal artifacts caused by heavy metals used for dental fillings. Its major

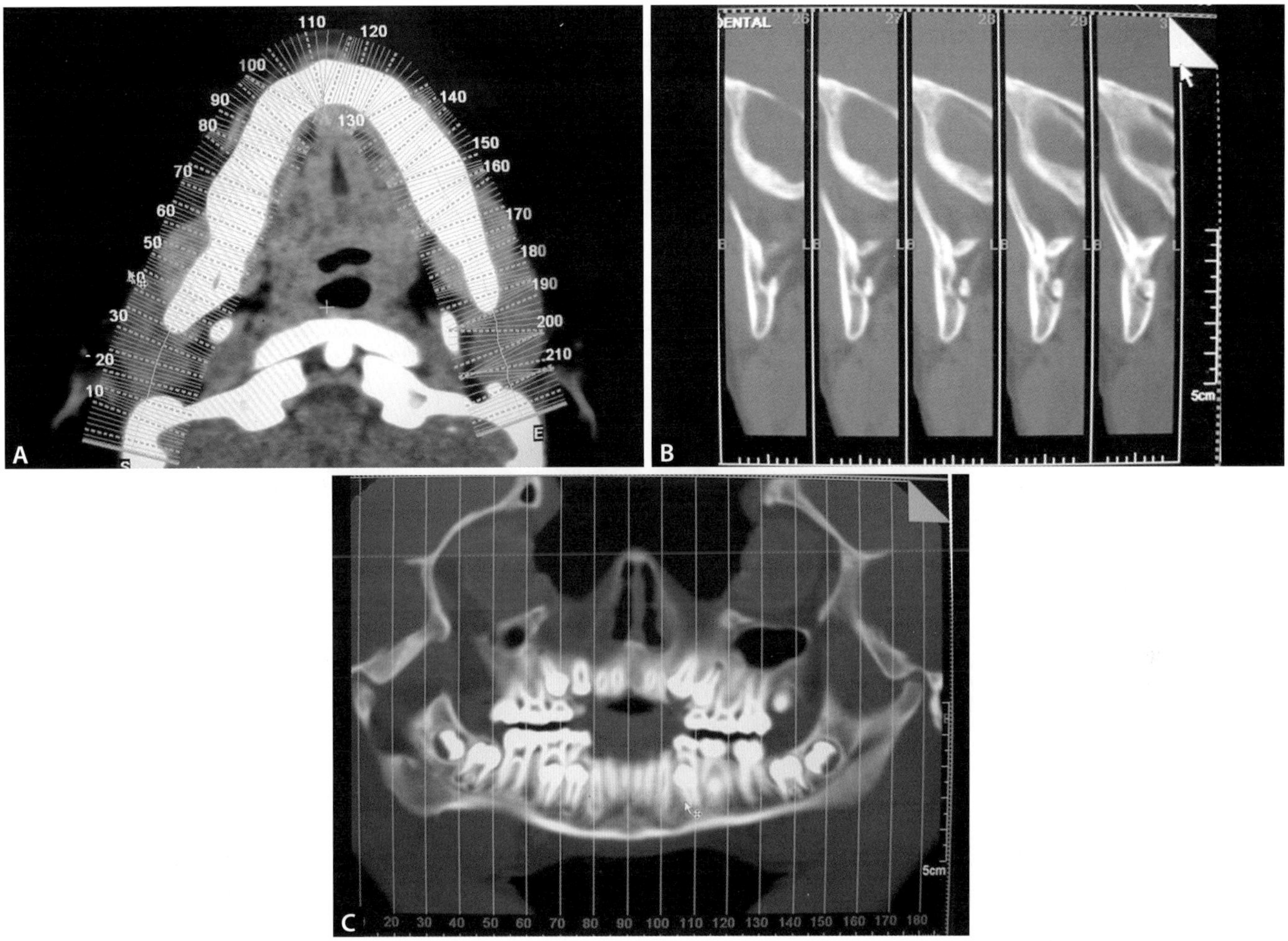

Figs. 4A to C: Dental CT reformatting program: (A) Axial-base image showing planning of the cross-sectional images; (B) Para-axial cross-sectional images used for planning and measurements of implants; (C) Panoramic reconstruction simulating a panoramic radiograph.

drawback, however, is lack of signal from cortical bone. Hence, it is not effective in identifying calcified portion of the tumor and the cortex of the bone. MR imaging is ideal for the assessment of bone marrow, subtle cortical erosion, and the extent of extraosseous soft tissue component. However, CT remains superior to MRI for the detection of bone destruction and calcification.

MR signal intensities have also been used for evaluating MRI features of cysts of the oral and maxillo-mandibular region **(Figs. 5A to D)**.

Diffusion weighted imaging[6] also has a key role to play in the differentiation of unilocular cystic lesions. It is difficult to differentiate cystic ameloblastoma from keratocystic odontogenic tumor (OKC) on CT and conventional MR sequences. However, OKC **(Figs. 5A to D)** has highly viscous contents and its cystic component shows restricted diffusion (values $< 2 \times 10^{-3}$ mm^2 s^{-1} suggestive of OKC).[6]

The superior contrast resolution of MRI helps in the accurate delineation of tumor extent. In addition, the use of a T1-weighted 3D sequence (ultrafast gradient echo) with integrated fat saturation (e.g. VIBE) can accurately demonstrate the inferior alveolar neurovascular bundle. Suppression of the fatty marrow improves the contrast between the neurovascular structures and the surrounding bone. *The reconstructed panoramic image **(Figs. 6A and B)*** is an effective alternative to panoramic MDCT images and can be used in patients with contraindications to MRI.[6,7] **Table 3** summarizes the suggested MRI protocol in maxillofacial imaging.[6,7]

CLASSIFICATION

The primary lesions involving the jaw may be either odontogenic or nonodontogenic. Odontogenic cysts and tumors develop during or after the formation of teeth.

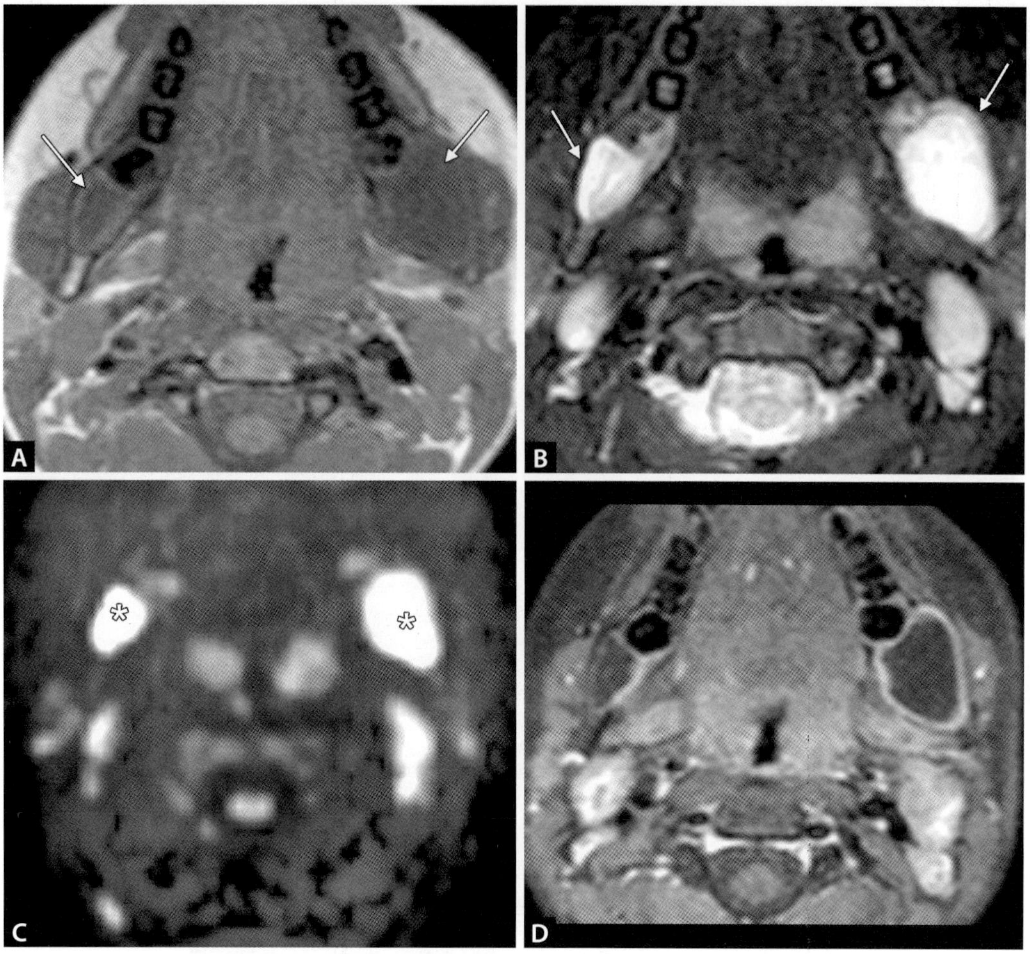

Figs. 5A to D: Multiple odontogenic keratocysts MRI: Axial T1WI (A) shows two small, well-defined hypointense lesions in rami of both hemimandible (arrows). These are hyperintense on T2WI (B) and show diffusion restriction in DWI image b value 800 (asterisks in C). Axial postcontrast T1WI (D) reveals mild enhancement of wall of the lesions.

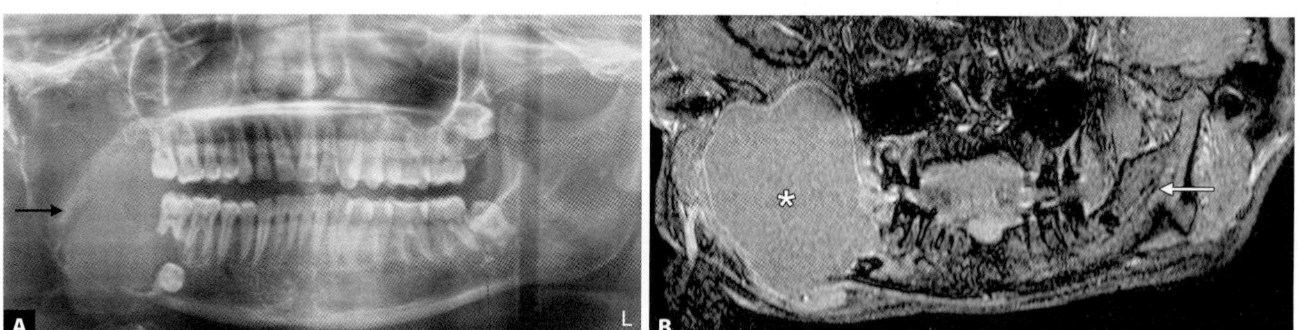

Figs. 6A and B: Ameloblastoma: (A) Panoramic radiograph showing large expansile multilocular lesion in the ramus of the right hemimandible (black arrow); (B) Curved multiplanar reformatted image after gadolinium administration shows a hypointense lesion (asterisk) in the right hemimandible with destruction of the right canal. The left inferior alveolar canal was normal (arrow).

These lesions could be either cystic or solid and benign or malignant with varying degrees of destructive potential. Most odontogenic maxillomandibular lesions are benign, but some may exhibit aggressive behavior locally.

Secondary involvement of the jaw is seen in neoplastic or inflammatory process involving the soft tissues adjoining the jaw, hematogenous metastases, or part of a systemic disease.[8-10]

Table 3: Suggested MRI protocol in maxillofacial imaging.

Precontrast sequences: • Axial T1WI • Axial T2WI, Coronal and Sagittal T2FSWI
Postcontrast sequences: • Post gad axial, coronal T1WI • T1-weighted FS 3D sequence (e.g. VIBE)
Special sequences: Diffusion (b values 0, 500 and 1000)
Advanced reconstructions: Curved MPR (panoramic image)

In 2017, the 4th edition of the World Health Organization Classification of Head and Neck tumors was published with a number of significant changes.[11,12] The common lesions seen in the maxillofacial region are summarized in **Table 4**.

CLINICAL FEATURES

Usually asymptomatic in the early period, many lesions are incidentally seen on plain radiographs. Most common symptoms are swelling and pain. Swelling may be either intraoral or outside resulting in facial asymmetry. Presence of paresthesia indicates mandibular canal involvement, and is common in malignant lesions. Other presentations include tooth displacement or mobility. Few lesions may present with bleeding or with signs and symptoms of secondary infection. The symptoms have no correlation with benign or malignant disease process.[10]

RADIOLOGICAL FEATURES/APPROACH

Maxillomandibular lesions have a wide range of pathologic descriptions but with similar imaging characters. Many of these lesions have a cyst-like radiographic appearance and can be indistinguishable on imaging. Patient age at presentation, history, and location within the mandible, its internal architecture, border contour, and effect of the lesion on contiguous structures are all taken into consideration before reaching the possible diagnosis. At times, it is difficult to make a definitive diagnosis without biopsy and the role of imaging in such cases is to define the extent and malignant potential. Imaging should help narrow the differential diagnosis and help in guiding patient treatment. Detailed description of the lesion aids in arriving at the differential diagnosis and is also imperative in mapping its extent. The radiological report should detail the features as described in **Table 5**.

ANATOMICAL LOCATION

Some lesions have a predilection for particular sites, whereas others can occur anywhere in the jaw. Systemic disorders (metabolic or endocrine) should be considered if all structures of maxillofacial region appear involved.[1,9]

Table 4: Common odontogenic and maxillofacial lesions[11,12]

Cystic lesions *Inflammatory cysts* • Radicular cyst • Inflammatory collateral cysts *Developmental cysts* • Dentigerous cyst • Odontogenic keratocyst (OKC) • Gingival cyst • Nasopalatine duct cyst • Primordial cyst
Solid lesions ***Odontogenic tumors*** *Benign odontogenic tumors* • *Epithelial*: – Ameloblastoma – Adenomatoid odontogenic tumor – Calcifying epithelial odontogenic tumor • *Mesenchymal*: – Odontogenic myxoma/myxofibroma – Cemento-ossifying fibroma – Cementoblastoma • *Mixed epithelial and mesenchymal*: – Ameloblastic fibroma – Odontoma *Malignant odontogenic tumors* • Odontogenic carcinomas • Odontogenic sarcomas • Odontogenic carcinosarcoma *Bone and cartilage tumors* • *Benign*: – Osteoblastoma – Chondroblastoma – Osteoma – Osteoid osteoma – Chondroma – Chondromyxoid fibroma • *Malignant*: – Osteosarcoma – Chondrosarcoma – Mesenchymal chondrosarcoma **Fibro- and chondro-osseous lesions** • Osteochondroma • Ossifying fibroma • Fibrous dysplasia • Cemento-osseous dysplasia **Miscellaneous lesions** • Simple bone cyst • Aneurysmal bone cyst • Central giant cell granuloma • Cherubism • Solitary plasmacytoma

Site

In the mandible, majority of the lesions occur in posterior part of mandible or angle as this region has more vascularity. Lesions having a propensity for the anterior

Table 5: Key radiologic descriptors for maxillofacial lesions.

1. *Anatomical location*: - Site - Relation to dentition - Relation to mandibular canal
2. Size
3. Shape
4. Density and Internal architecture
5. Outline/definition/margin
6. *Effect on surrounding structures*: - Teeth - Bone - Soft tissues

mandible include: periapical cemental dysplasia, florid cemento-osseous dysplasia, odontoma, simple bone cyst, central hemangioma, central giant cell granuloma and brown tumor. Midline maxilla may be involved by an incisive canal cyst, central giant cell granuloma, simple bone cyst or hemangioma. Stafne's cyst is typically located inferior to the mandibular canal in posterior mandible (below 3rd molar).

Relation to Dentition

Involvement of only one tooth or a specific part of the tooth is suggestive of odontogenic lesion. For instance, radicular dental cysts develop at the apices of nonvital teeth, whereas dentigerous cysts develop at the crown **(Figs. 7A and B)**. Cementomas occur at the apex of vital teeth.

Non-odontogenic lesions generally have no specific relationship to the dentition or can involve the bone around two or more teeth.

Relation to Mandibular Canal

Relationship of the lesion to the inferior alveolar canal also indicates the origin of the lesion. Lesions above the canal are probably odontogenic, whereas those involving the canal or below it are usually non-odontogenic.

SIZE

Size of a lesion can be expressed in centimeters in two dimensions on a single view (along the axis of the lesion and an axis perpendicular to it). Size may also be expressed in terms of landmarks, e.g. the overlying teeth or mandibular canal. In central lesions it must be mentioned if these cross the midline. Size of the lesion does not help in differentiation between benign and malignant. Some lesions however are typically small (2–3 cm, e.g. Stafne's cyst), while others may assume very large sizes (e.g. ameloblastoma).[2]

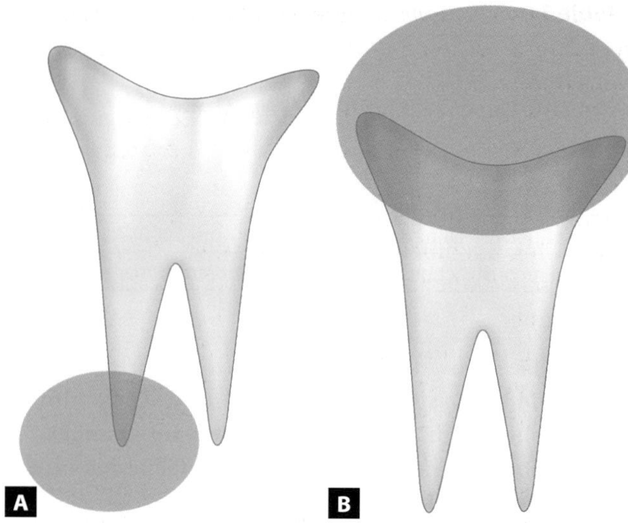

Figs. 7A and B: Relationship of cysts to teeth: (A) Periapical lesions: The differential diagnosis of lesions in this location include periapical granuloma, radicular cyst abscess, osteomyelitis, simple bone cyst and periapical cemento-osseous dysplasia; (B) Pericoronal lesions include dentigerous cyst (commonest), ameloblastoma (unicystic), odontogenic keratocyst, calcifying odontogenic cyst (rare).

SHAPE

Shape of a lesion is described as being oval, round, scalloped (or undulating) or irregular. Shape of a lesion may help in the diagnosis, e.g. a radicular cyst is round and unilocular. Odontogenic, keratocyst is oval, growing along the long axis of the mandible. Unequal growth results in scalloped margins. Simple bone cyst typically has irregular margins as it arches between roots of teeth. Irregular margins also suggest an infective or malignant lesion. Whether the lesion is uni or multilocular may also be described under shape of the lesion.[2]

DENSITY AND INTERNAL ARCHITECTURE OF LESION

Radiographically, jaw lesions are often classified according to their radiographic densities on plain radiographs. They can be described as having either a radiolucent, radiopaque or mixed appearance relative to the density of adjacent bone.

The *radiolucent lesions* can be further divided as being well circumscribed or poorly circumscribed.

Well-defined radiolucent lesions include periapical cyst, dentigerous cyst, odontogenic keratocyst, ameloblastoma, simple bone cyst, central giant cell granuloma.

Poorly-circumscribed radiolucent are acute osteomyelitis, primary bone neoplasm and secondary bone neoplasms.

Radiopaque lesions include odontoma, torus, osteoma, osteochondroma, cementoblastoma, and late stages of fibrous dysplasia.

Mixed density lesions are fibrous dysplasia, ossifying fibroma, cemento-osseous dysplasia, chronic osteomyelitis, osteosarcoma.[1,2]

Analysis of internal structure of the lesion is also helpful in narrowing the differential diagnosis, i.e. describing the lesion as being either unilocular/multilocular/honeycomb appearance, thin/thick internal bony trabaculae. Multilocular odontogenic lesions include ameloblastoma and odontogenic myxoma; while non-odontogenic lesions include central giant cell granuloma, hemangioma and rarely aneurismal bone cyst.

The cyst/tumor may be uniformly radiolucent or have calcific radiodensities within or have a ground-glass appearance or be uniformly radiodense. Lesions may also have internal cementum (amorphous calcification) or identifiable dental tissue (dentine or enamel).

OUTLINE/DEFINITION/MARGINATION

In general, lesions with well-defined borders are usually benign, whereas lesions with ill-defined borders represent aggressive, inflammatory or neoplastic processes. A well-defined outline may be further detailed as being punched-out (sharp with no surrounding bone reaction), corticated (surrounding radiopaque bone), sclerotic (non-uniform radiopaque boundary) or encapsulated (surrounding radiolucent line). Similarly a poorly defined margin may blend imperceptibly with the surrounding bone or show "moth-eaten" margins.[2] A benign cyst with secondary infection may mimic a more aggressive lesion.

EFFECT ON SURROUNDING STRUCTURES

The effect of the lesion on surrounding structures, i.e. teeth, bone and soft tissue also needs to be evaluated **(Figs. 8A and B)**.

Teeth

Benign lesions typically cause displacement of teeth without resorption. However, long standing, benign but locally aggressive lesions can cause tooth resorption. Inflammatory and malignant lesions also cause resorption. When lesions occur in young patients, they can result in delayed eruption or disrupted development (abnormal shape or density) of teeth. Loss of lamina dura may also be seen. Malignant lesions may rapidly grow down the periodontal ligament resulting in initial widening and later disruption of lamina dura.[1,2]

Surrounding Bone

Bone expansion in all four directions should be noted, i.e. buccal, lingual, inferior and superior. Areas of cortical perforation should be recorded in the report as they help in guiding management decisions. For mandibular lesions, the thickness and integrity of the inferior cortex is important. On the other hand, for maxillary lesions the superior involvement, i.e. floors of the maxillary antrum, nasal cavity and orbit need to be commented upon. Cortical perforation is seen in aggressive inflammatory or malignant lesions. However, focal areas of cortical break may also be seen in benign lesions causing massive osseous expansion, e.g. aneurysmal bone cyst. MDCT with multiplanar reconstruction is superior to plain radiography in this regard.

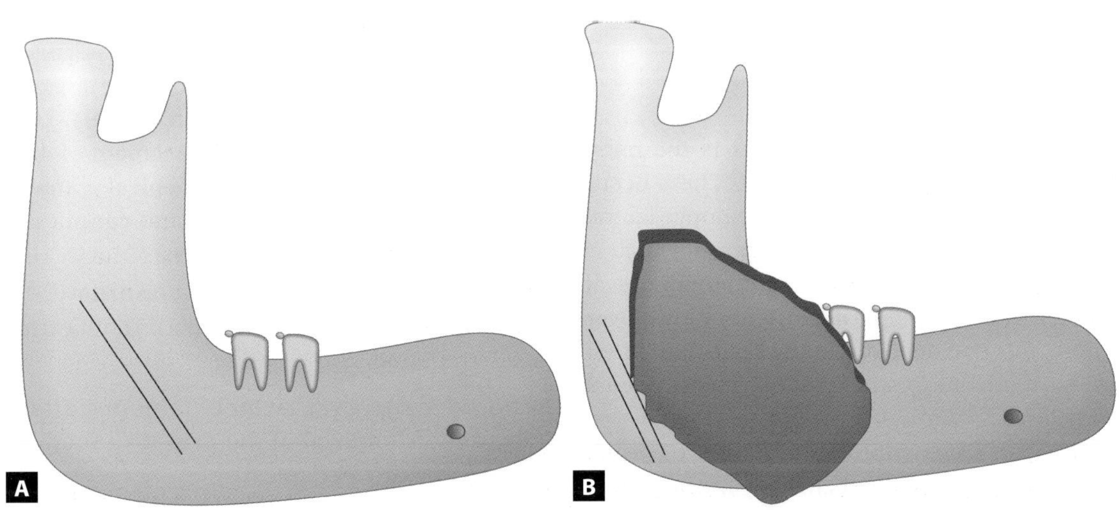

Figs. 8A and B: Effect on surrounding structures (A) normal mandible, (B) an expansile aggressive cystic lesion causing displacement of the inferior alveolar canal and erosion of the roots of overlying teeth, as well as tooth displacement.

Table 6: Common radiolucent lesions of the maxillofacial region.

Well defined				***Poorly defined***		
Jaw cysts		Solid Lesions/ Tumors		Osteomyelitis	Tumors	
Odontogenic	Non-odontogenic	Odontogenic	Non-odontogenic		Odontogenic	Non-odontogenic
• Radicular cyst • Dentigerous cyst • Odontogenic keratocyst	• Nasopalatine duct cyst • Simple bone cyst • Aneurysmal bone cyst	• Ameloblastoma • Ameloblastic fibroma	• Central giant cell reparative granuloma • Eosinophilic granuloma • Hemangioma • AVM		• Odontogenic carcinoma • Malignant ameloblastoma	• Oteosarcoma • Chondrosarcoma • Fibrosarcoma • Lymphoreticular malignancies

Involvement or displacement of inferior dental canal and mental foramen needs to be evaluated. Erosion of the cortex indicates involvement. Widening of the inferior alveolar canal may be seen in lesions of vascular and neurogenic origin. Presence of sclerosis or subperiosteal reaction aid in arriving at a diagnosis. Periosteal reaction indicates inflammatory or malignant lesions.

Surrounding Soft Tissues

Extent of soft tissue involvement in aggressive lesions should be detailed including the muscles involved, i.e. masseters and pterygoids.

The further description of the maxillofacial lesions is on the basis of the predominant radiographic appearance (radiolucent, mixed density or radiopaque).

Table 6 summarizes the common radiolucent lesions of the maxillofacial region.

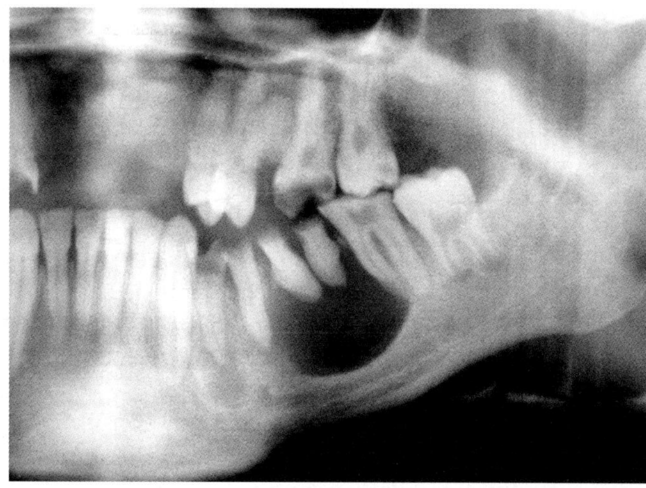

Fig. 9: Radicular cyst: Panoramic radiograph showing a round, well-defined, smooth, unilocular radiolucent lesion located in the periapical region of a grossly carious first molar tooth.

WELL-DEFINED RADIOLUCENT LESIONS

Jaw Cysts

Odontogenic Cysts

Radicular cyst: Radicular (periapical) cyst is the most frequently seen cyst of the jaw (about 70%).[2] These occur at the apex of a non-vital tooth, particularly upper lateral incisors. A radicular cyst is an inflammatory cyst which is the last step in a chain of events resulting from periapical inflammation secondary to pulpal necrosis in a tooth. Over a period of time, this cyst develops in the bone at the root apex of a carious tooth due to proliferation of the epithelial cell rests of Malassez.[2,10]

Commonly seen in asymptomatic adults between 20 and 50 years of age. These cysts usually measure less than 1 cm, although sizes up to 3 cm may be seen. Plain radiographs reveal round, unilocular, radiolucent lesions in the periapical region with defined, smooth margins and surrounded by a thin rim of cortical bone. There is usually associated caries. The cyst may displace adjacent teeth or rarely cause mild root resorption **(Fig. 9)**. The cyst may cause buccal expansion or displacement of the maxillary antrum. Radicular cysts and periapical granulomas have a similar imaging morphology, and cannot always help distinguish a granuloma from a cyst.[2,9,10,13]

Treatment consists of enucleation of the cyst lining and endodontic obturation (root canal). Tooth extraction may be also required.

Residual cyst: Cyst, which remains after surgical intervention/removal of the causative root. Thus, most residual cysts are periapical cysts.

Dentigerous cyst: Dentigerous (follicular) cyst is the most common type of non-inflammatory odontogenic cyst.[14]

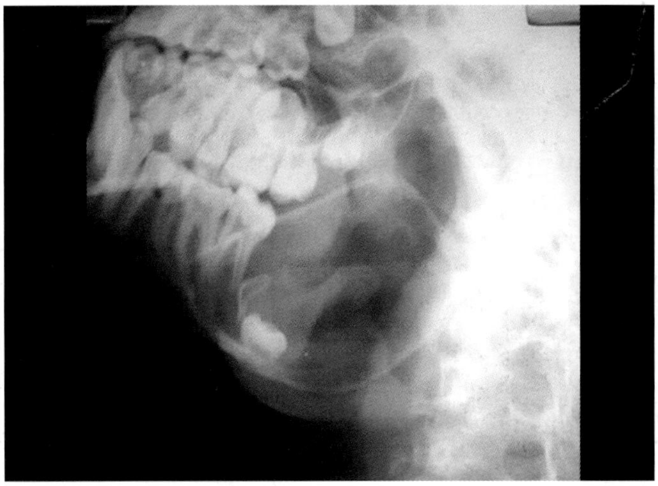

Fig. 10: Dentigerous cyst: Lateral oblique view of mandible show a large expansile, well-defined, ovoid, unilocular, radiolucent lesion surrounding the crown of an unerupted last molar tooth.

Impacted tooth is seen with associated pericoronal lucency. It forms within the lining of the dental follicle when fluid accumulates between the enamel epithelium and the crown of the developing or unerupted tooth. Usually seen in adolescents and young adults, and patients are typically pain free.

On imaging, dentigerous cysts appear as well-defined, round or ovoid, smooth, well-defined, well-corticated, uniformly radiolucent, unilocular lesions. These typically are located around the crowns of unerupted teeth, usually third molars and envelope the crown symmetrically **(Fig. 10)**. The roots of the involved teeth are often outside the lesion. The adjoining teeth are displaced and resorbed in about half the cases.[2] They may be large in size and can extend up into the ramus with mandibular expansion. Buccal or medial expansion can be extensive in large cysts causing facial asymmetry or antral displacement. The characteristic features of this lesion are its marked, relatively asymptomatic, expansion and its potential to displace or resorb adjacent teeth.[2,10]

Extremely large dentigerous cysts simulate odontogenic keratocyst or ameloblastoma as they may have undulating borders. Rarely, an untreated cyst may develop an ameloblastoma within its lining referred to as a mural ameloblastoma. However, malignant tranformation is extremely rare.

Treatment includes removal of the entire cyst and associated tooth extraction.

Odontogenic keratocyst: Odontogenic keratocysts (OKC) has been restored to odontogenic cysts by the WHO Classification[11,12] of Head and Neck Tumors (4th edition) and rejects the previous terminology of Keratocystic odontogenic tumor (KOT). These are believed to arise from the epithelium of dental lamina rather than the normal tooth.[2] The cyst is lined by a parakeratinized lining epithelium and the lumen contains "cheesy" material. Daughter cysts are found outside the primary lesion. Only curettage as the treatment has high recurrence rate of any odontogenic cyst because of the presence of daughter cysts outside the primary lesion.[15] Hence the preferred treatment for these lesions is surgical enucleation, with wide bone margins.

OKC are relatively uncommon and represent approximately 5–15% of all jaw cysts.[10] The age range of these lesions is very variable with the peak during the 2nd to 4th decades of life. Multiple lesions are associated with the basal cell nevus syndrome (Gorlin-Goltz syndrome).

On imaging, OKC may be seen anywhere in the maxilla or the mandible but are most commonly located in the posterior body and ramus of the mandible. OKC are characteristically oval in shape extending along the body of the mandible with relatively little mediolateral expansion. These lesions usually appear as a unilocular, lucent lesions but may be multilocular. Their borders are smooth, scalloped, well-defined and corticated. They are often associated with an impacted tooth **(Figs. 11 and 12)**. Although odontogenic keratocysts in some cases may arise in the lining of primordial cysts without a tooth, while at times they include the crown of the last molar. Such lesions are indistinguishable from dentigerous cysts on radiography. OKC may show aggressive growth compared to other odontogenic cysts and may have undulating borders and a multilocular appearance simulating ameloblastomas. Odontogenic keratocysts may cause cortical thinning. Adjacent teeth are usually displaced, and occasionally resorbed.[15]

On MRI **(*See* Figs. 5A to D)**, odontogenic keratocysts have an intermediate to high signal intensity on T1W images and heterogeneous low to high signal intensity on T2W images. On contrast administration OKC show thin rim enhancement unlike tumors such as ameloblastoma, which have solid components. Diffusion restriction of the contents of the cyst is characteristic for OKC.[16]

Primordial cyst: Primordial cyst is an uncommon cystic lesion, which develops instead of a tooth. Cystic degeneration of the dental follicle before completion of odontogenesis results in primordial cyst. These are well-defined, non-expansile, well-defined radiolucent lesions without an associated tooth.[9]

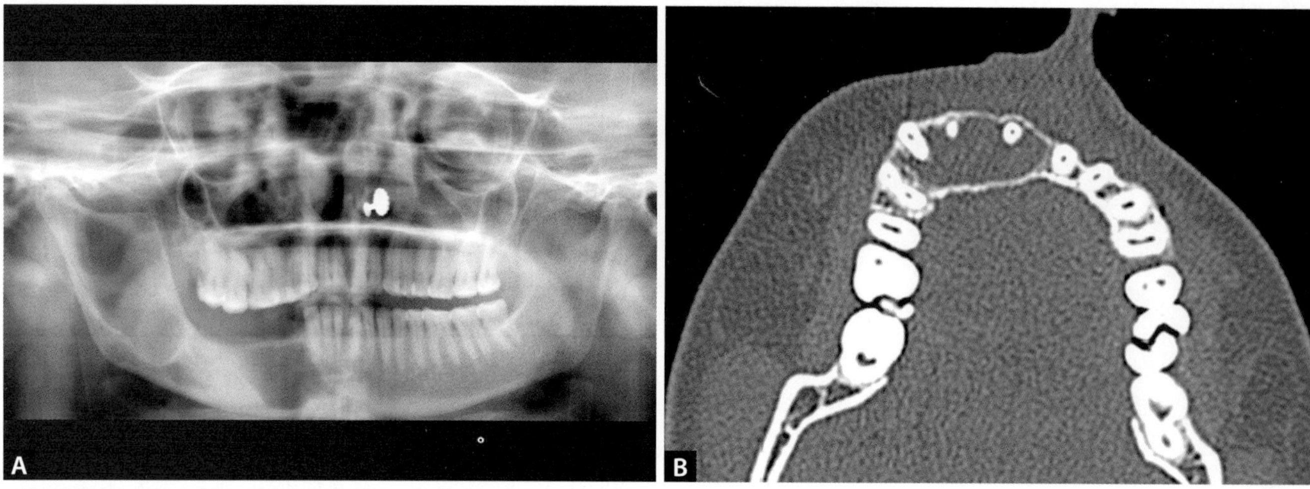

Figs. 11A and B: Odontogenic keratocyst: (A) Panorax view of a young adult shows an oval, smooth, well-corticated, unilocular cyst located in the posterior body and ramus of the mandible, extending along the body of the mandible with relatively little mediolateral expansion. Another lesion is present in the body of the mandible on the right side; (B) Axial CT scan of a different patient shows the characteristic ovoid disposition of an OKC with minimal buccolingual expansion.

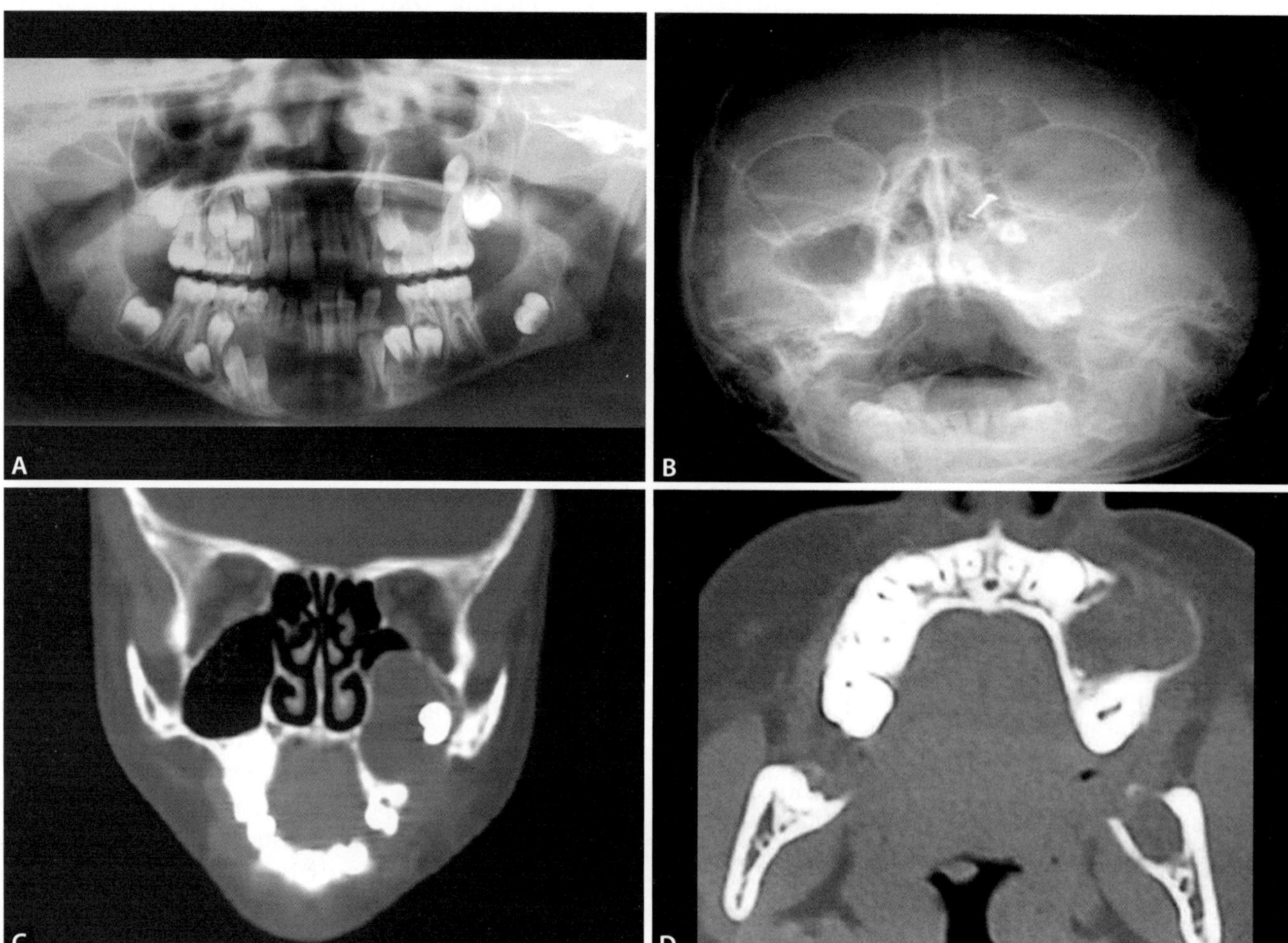

Figs. 12A to D: (A) Panorex view of a 12 years old girl with past history of curettage for an OKC shows multiple, recurrent lesions; (B) Water's view shows cranial displacement of a left-sided tooth with apparently opaque maxillary antrum; (C) Coronal CT scan shows a large maxillary cyst displacing and encasing a molar tooth. The maxillary antrum is compressed;[9] (D) Axial CT section reveals both the maxillary and mandibular lesions.

Non-odontogenic Cysts

Nasopalatine duct cyst: A nasopalatine duct cyst (also known as incisive canal cyst) is a non-odontogenic developmental cyst or fissural cyst arising from epithelial remnants of the nasopalatine duct.[16] It is located in the midline in anterior maxilla. It is the commonest nonodontogenic cyst. They are most frequently found at middle age (4th to 6th decades). Their size is variable from 6 mm to several centimetres.[2] These cysts are usually asymptomatic, but at times complain of a swelling in the palate or discharge of mucoid material.

On imaging, they appear as round, ovoid or heart-shaped, well-defind lucent lesion in the anterior maxilla. The margin is well-defined, smooth and a dense rim of cortical bone is often seen along the periphery. The lesion may displace the roots of the central incisor teeth.

Nasolabial or nasoalveolar cyst: This lesion too is considered likely to be a fissural cyst arising adjacent to the apex of the incisors just beneath the lip. It may scallop the anterior cortex of the maxilla.[16]

Simple bone cyst: A traumatic (simple) bone cyst is an intraosseous pseudocyst because it lacks an epithelial lining. Its cause is not known, though some believe that it develops in response to trauma. These lesions are usually asymptomatic, discovered incidentally in children or young adult.[2,10] They are rare lesions and are usually treated by curettage.

Usually seen in the mandible, particularly anteriorly in the molar/premolar region. On radiography, these appear as typically unilocular, lucent defects between the roots of teeth and with scalloped margins. Mild expansion with cortical thinning may be seen. There is minimal or no displacement of adjacent teeth.

Aneurysmal bone cyst: These lesions are rare in the mandible and show imaging characteristics similar to aneurysmal bone cysts elsewhere in the skeleton **(Figs. 13A to D)**.[17]

Lingual salivary gland inclusion defect: Lingual salivary gland inclusion defect (Stafne's cyst) is a well-defined lucent lesion found on the lingual surface of the posterior body of the mandible. These are usually asymptomatic and seen as incidental findings. On imaging, the appearance is of an oval lucent area just above the inferior border of the mandible and below the mandibular canal. Typical location is anterior to the angle of the jaw and posterior to the third molar **(Fig. 14)**. The border of the defect may be surrounded by an opaque line.[10] No treatment except follow-up is required as it represents an extension of the aberrant lobe of the submandibular gland fat.

Tumors or Tumor-like Conditions

Odontogenic Tumors

Ameloblastoma: Ameloblastomas are benign epithelial neoplasms which arise from various sources of odontogenic epithelium, and constitute about 10% of odontogenic tumors. These tumors show locally aggressive but non-metastasizing behavior. Ameloblastomas may arise from the epithelial lining of dentigerous cysts and are then referred to as mural ameloblastomas.[18]

Ameloblastomas typically present in the 3rd to 5th decades of life but may be seen in younger patients. Patients generally present with a slow-growing, painless mass.[2,10]

Although solid on pathology they are radiolucent on plain radiographs. Most ameloblastomas (about 80%) occur in the ramus and posterior body of the mandible.[11] They have a variable imaging appearance. Typically the lesions are multilocular with distinct internal septae. The closest differential of such lesions is OKC. Lesions may assume a "honeycomb" or "soap-bubble" appearance. Less commonly, ameloblastoma may be unilocular. Their margins are smooth, scalloped, well-defined and corticated but with significant expansion. However, large tumors may have cortical perforation, especially on the lingual side with infiltration of adjacent soft tissues.[2,10] The adjacent teeth are often resorbed, displaced and loosened. Erosion of the roots of adjacent teeth is unique to ameloblastoma and indicates its aggressive nature **(Figs. 15 and 16)**.[9] However, only histopathologic findings can help confirm benignity and the absence of carcinomatous change.[19] Few (about 15%) of ameloblastoma may be unilocular. This form may envelop the crown of a tooth resembling a dentigerous cyst,[1,2] or occasionally the apex of a tooth **(Figs. 17A to D)**.

On CT, ameloblastoma reveal a mixed appearance with cystic areas of low attenuation with iso attenuating solid regions. On MRI, the solid component of the lesion show enhancement on Gd-T1WI and diffusion restriction **(Figs. 18A to D)**.[19,20]

Treatment of ameloblastoma depends on the extent of adjacent tumor infiltration. Either localized removal of the lesion with wide margins or en bloc resection would be performed.

Ameloblastic fibroma: Ameloblastic fibroma are rare benign mixed odontogenic tumors arising from both odontogenic epithelium and connective tissue of

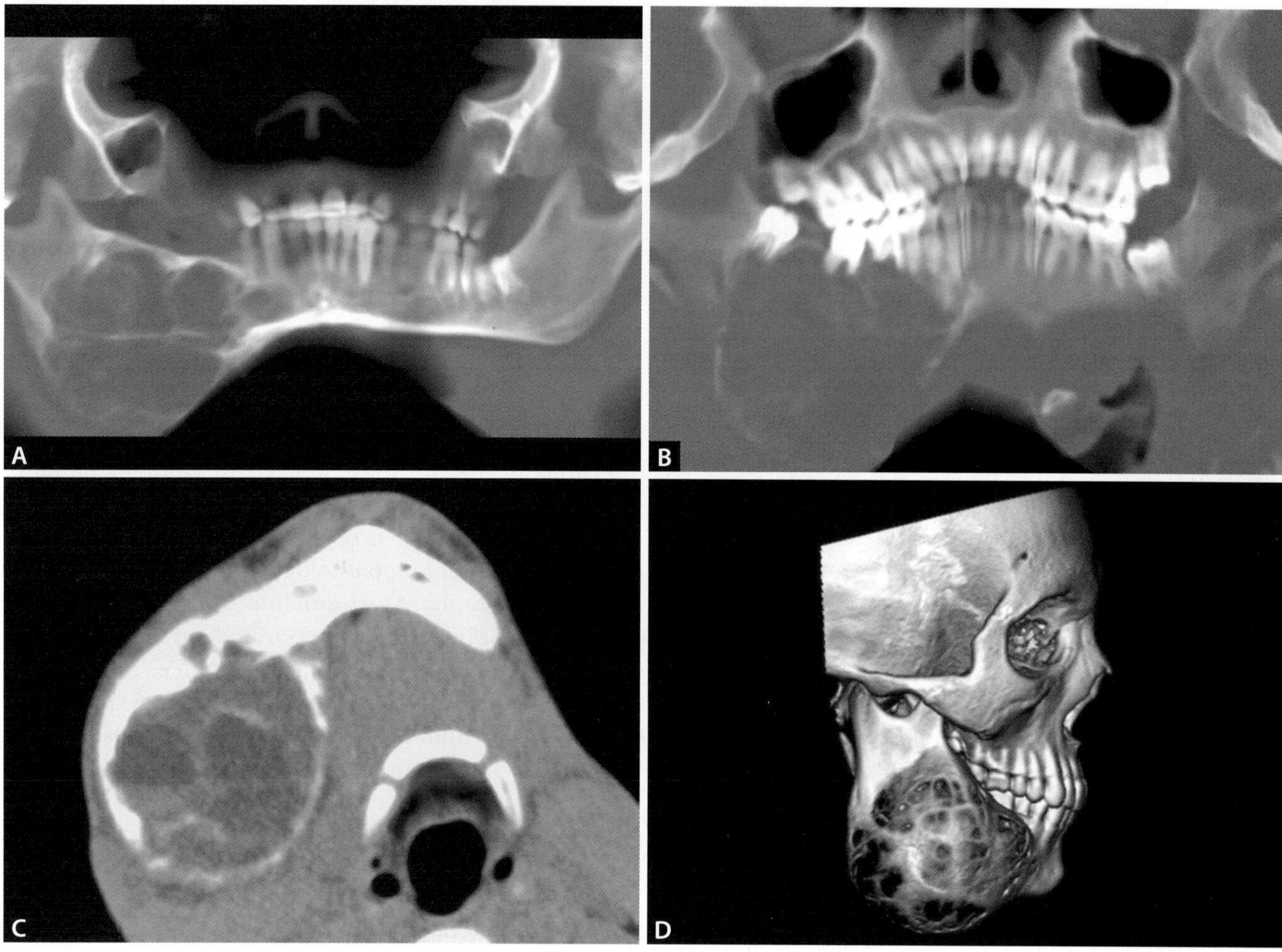

Figs. 13A to D: Aneurysmal bone cyst: Posterior to anterior panoramic CT reconstructions (A and B) show a markedly, expansile multilocular radiolucent lesion involving the right hemimandible. Significant cortical thinning is present; (C) Axial CT scan reveals characteristic multiple fluid-fluid levels; (D) VRT image illustrates the expansile, multilocular character of the lesion.

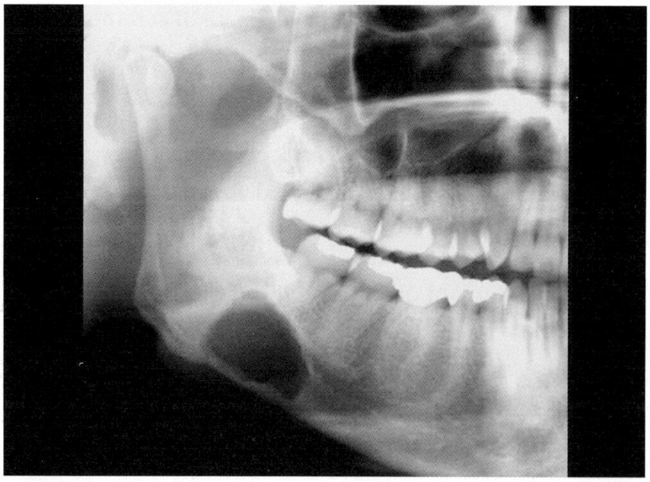

Fig. 14: Stafne's cyst: Lateral oblique view of mandible shows an ovoid, well-defined area of lucency located just above the inferior border of the mandible, anterior to the angle of the jaw and inferior to the mandibular canal.

developing tooth. On imaging, these tumors closely resemble ameloblastomas, but occur in a younger age group (children and adolescents).[2,9]

Non-Odontogenic Lesions

Central giant cell granuloma: Central giant cell granuloma (giant cell reparative cyst) typically occurs in adolescents and young adults. This lesion represents a reactive process rather than a true neoplasm. Histologically, it is composed of fibrous tissue, areas of hemorrhage, reactive bone formation and osteoclast-like giant cells.[2] The histologic appearance is similar to that of brown tumor of hyperparathyroidism.[1,21]

These lesions are typically located in the anterior mandible or maxilla, with a tendency to cross the midline. The radiographic appearance is of a radiolucent, multilocular lesion with thin internal septae or sometimes

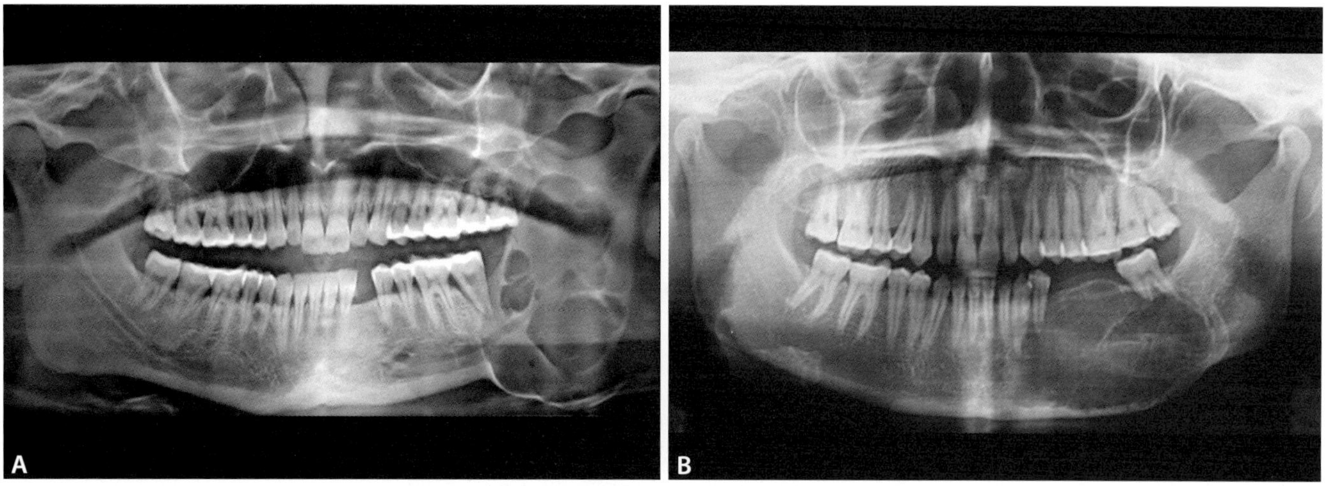

Figs. 15A and B: Ameloblastoma: (A and B) Panoramic radiographs of two different adult patients showing multilocular, expansile, smooth, radiolucent lesions located in the ramus and posterior body of mandible adjacent root resorption is seen in (B).

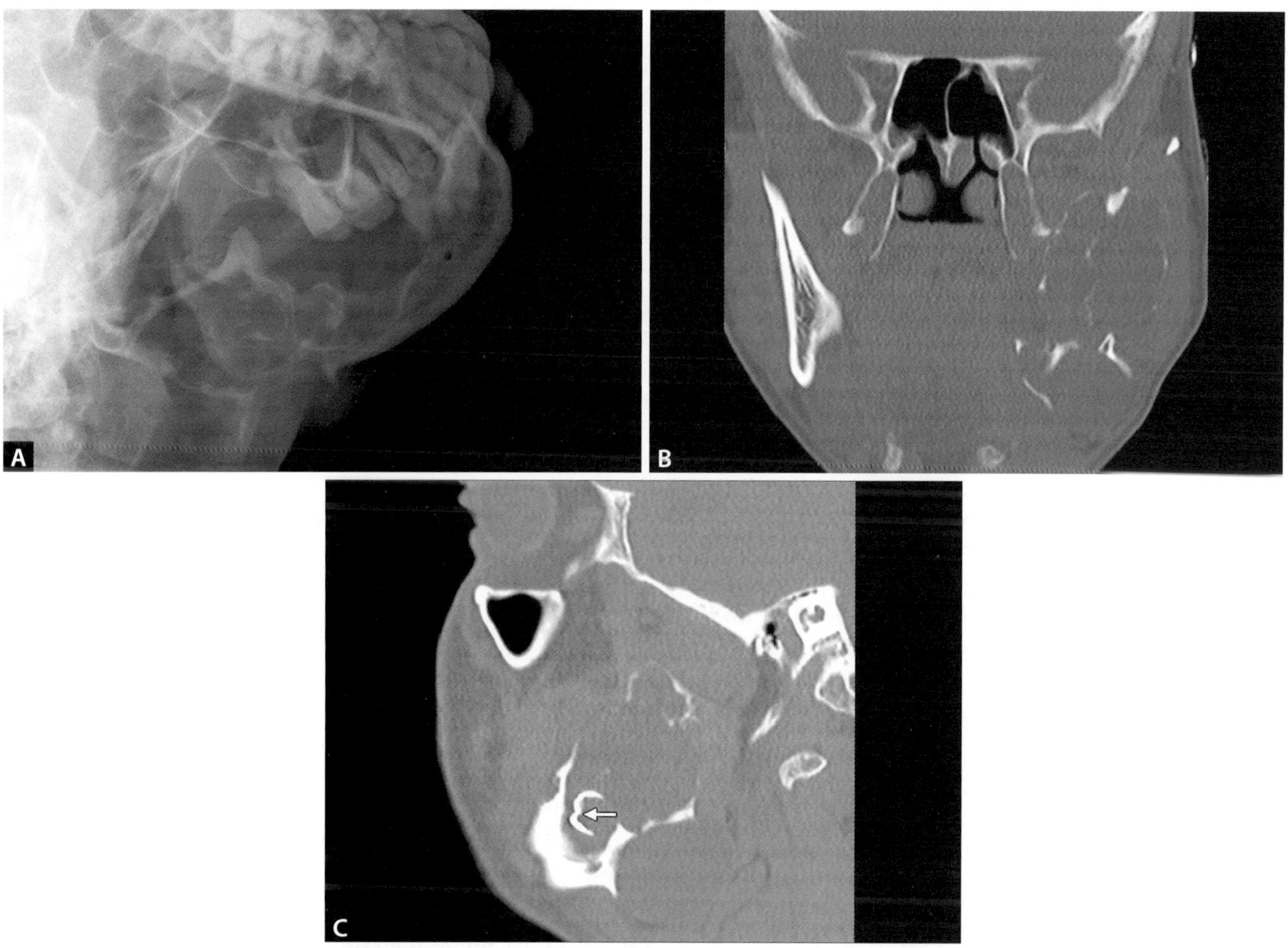

Figs. 16A to C: Ameloblastoma: Lateral oblique view of mandible (A), coronal CT scan (B) and sagittal CT section (C) showing an expansile, multilocular radiolucent lesion with multiple areas of cortical perforation. The lesion encases a tooth (arrow) (while the overlying teeth are largely missing).

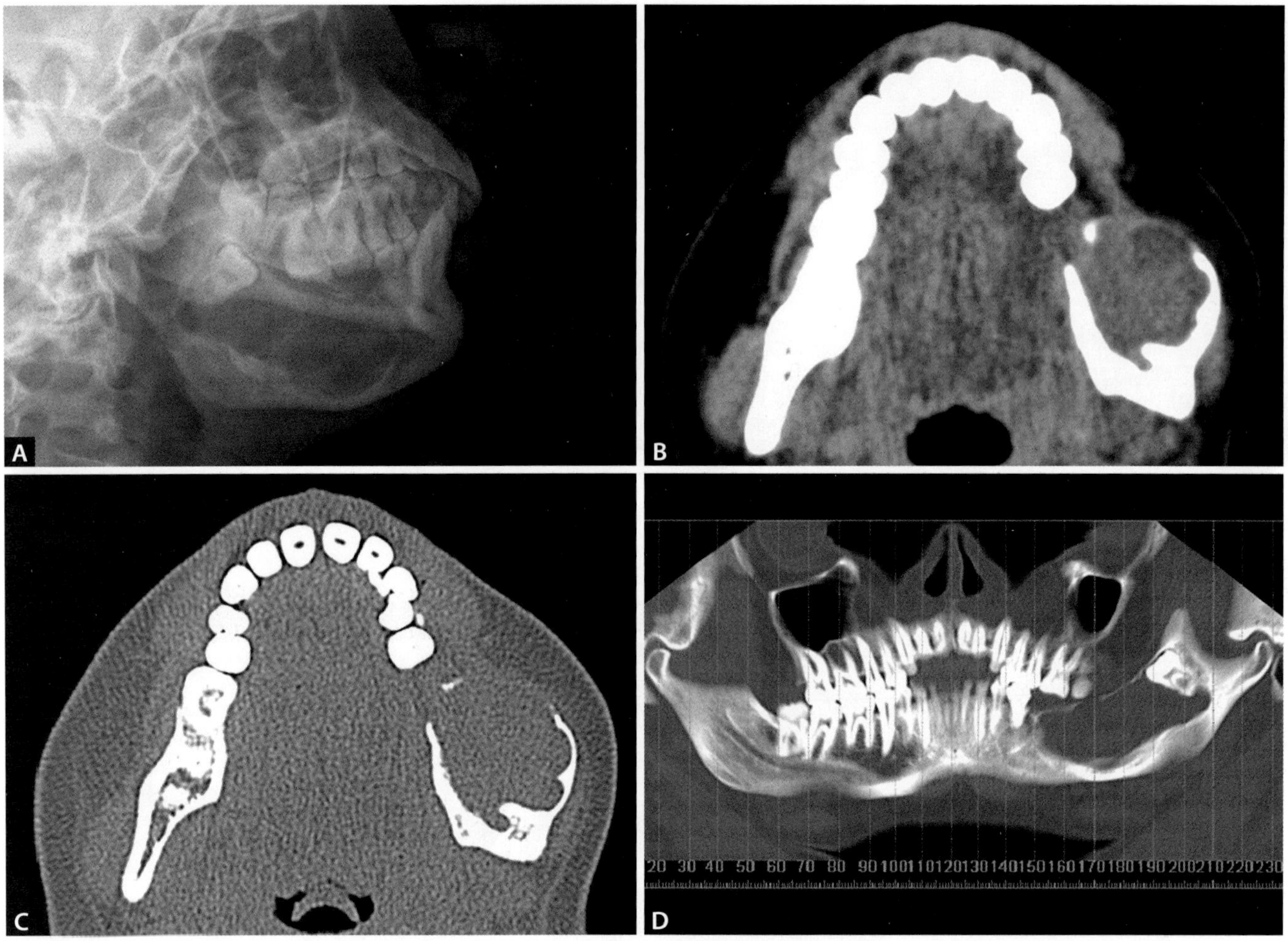

Figs. 17A to D: Unicystic ameloblastoma: Lateral oblique view of mandible (A) shows an ovoid well-defined, radiolucent lesion with scalloped borders involving the body and ramus of mandible, encasing an unerupted last molar. Axial CT soft tissue window (B) shows the solid appearance of the lesion, while bone window (C) illustrates areas of cortical perforation. CT panoramic reconstruction (D) exquisitely demonstrates the lesion.

"honey-comb" appearance.[22] Usually well defined because of slow growth, ill-defined borders may be seen in more aggressive lesions. There is uneven osseous expansion causing scalloped borders **(Figs. 19A and B)**. Adjoining teeth are often displaced and less commonly resorbed. On imaging and histopathology, brown tumors of hyperparathyroidism can appear identical.[1,2,10]

Eosinophilic granuloma: Eosinophilic granuloma is a benign form of Langerhans'cell histiocytosis, and usually occurr in children or young adults. Multiple or solitary lesions may be seen. Lesions are smooth, well-defined, radiolucent **(Fig. 20)**. Associated floating teeth may be seen due to loss of peri-odontal bone support.[1,2]

Intraosseous hemangioma: Hemangioma is a rare benign tumor. It is regarded as a developmental malformation (hamartoma), rather than a true neoplasm. It commonly presents in adolescents either with swelling or bleeding. On radiology, these appear as expansile radiolucent lesions with multilocular or "honey-comb" appearance. The thickened trabeculae within the lesion may also give a "spoke-wheel pattern". These often cause displacement of adjacent structures with root resorption **(Fig. 21)**. It is important to suggest the diagnosis on radiology due to their potential to cause bleeding.[2,9]

Arteriovenous malformation: Arteriovenous malformations refers to abnormal, direct communication between arteries and veins. In the jaw, most lesions occur in the ramus and posterior body of the mandible. These lesions have a potential for causing massive hemorrhage, and extraction of a tooth adjacent to an arteriovenous malformation may result in lethal bleeding. On radiology **(Figs. 22A to C)**, arteriovenous malformations appear

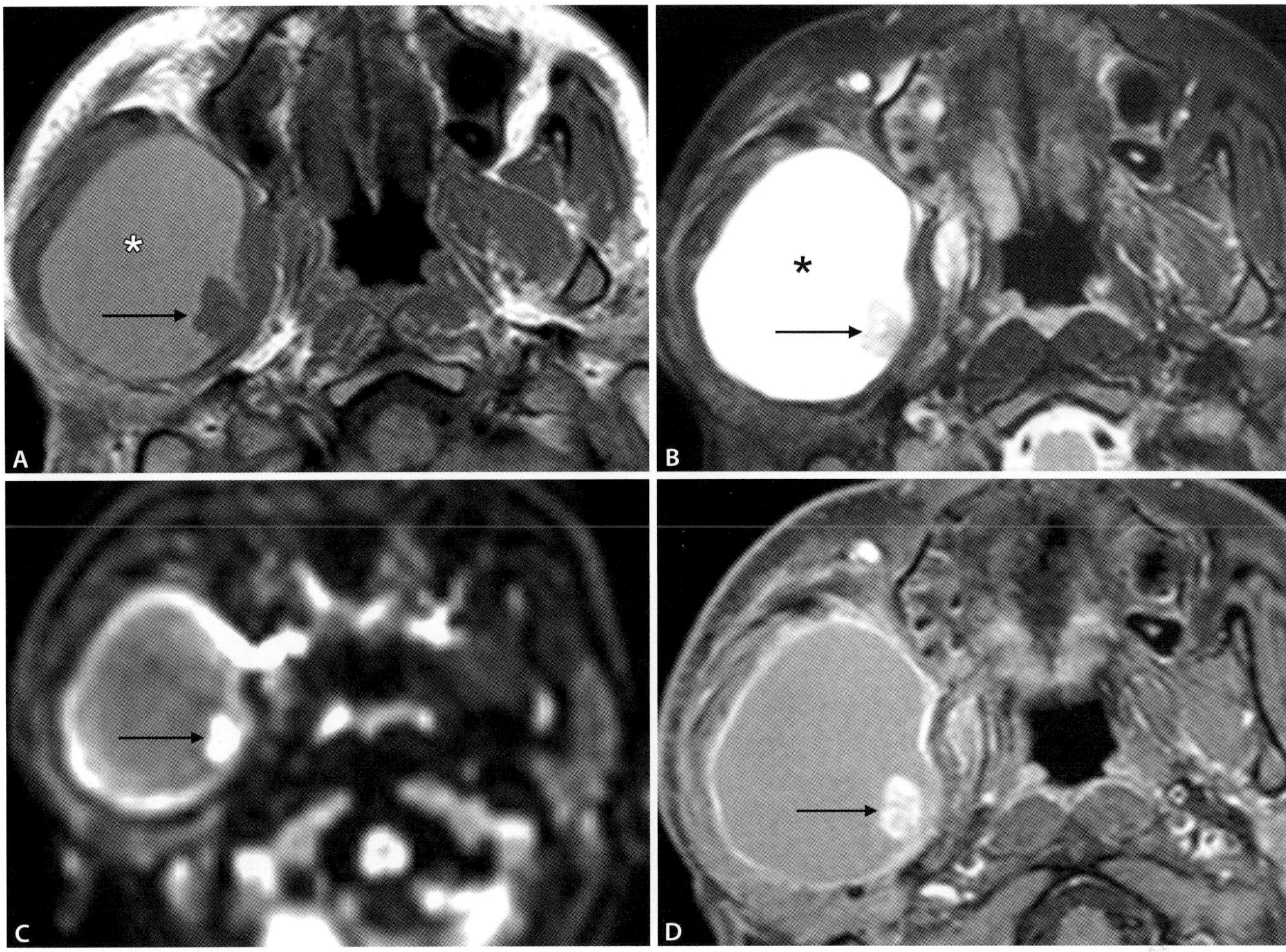

Figs. 18A to D: Ameloblastoma MRI (same patient as in Figs. 6A and B): Axial T1WI (A) and T2WI (B) show a large, well-defined cystic mass with hyperintense contents in ramus of mandible (asterix). Note the small eccentric mural nodule (arrows in A and B) showing diffusion restriction (arrow in C) in DWI image b value 800 (C). Axial postcontrast T1WI (D) reveals enhancement of wall of the lesion and the mural nodule (arrow).

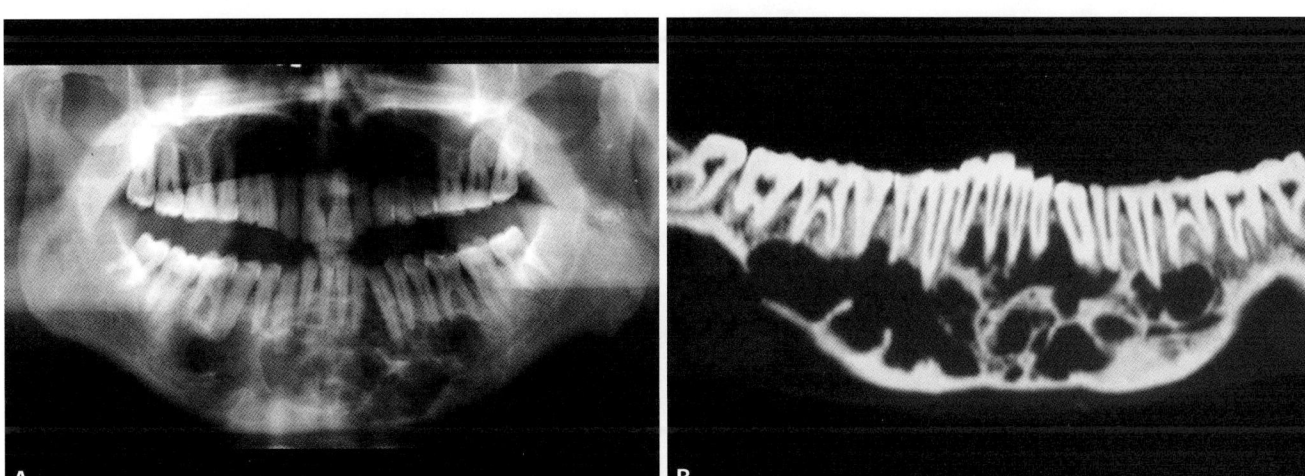

Figs. 19A and B: Central giant cell granuloma: Panoramic radiograph (A) and CT panoramic reconstruction (B) show a radiolucent, multilocular lesion with internal septae characteristically located in the anterior mandible, crossing the midline. Adjoining teeth are displaced, not resorbed.

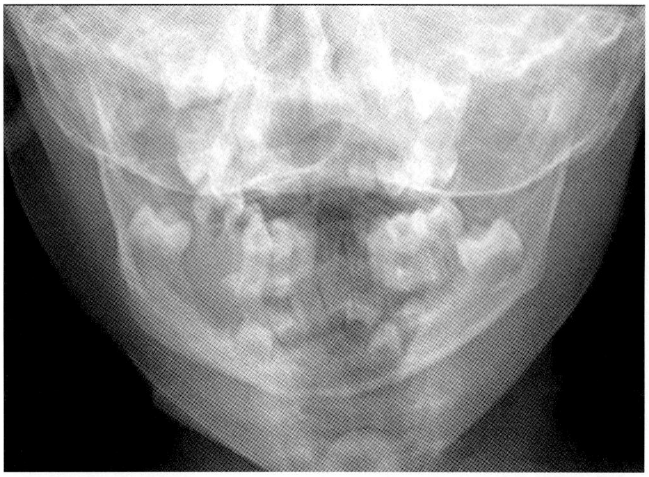

Fig. 20: Eosinophilic granuloma: Panoramic radiograph of a young boy showing a smooth, well-defined lytic lesion involving the right hemimandible.

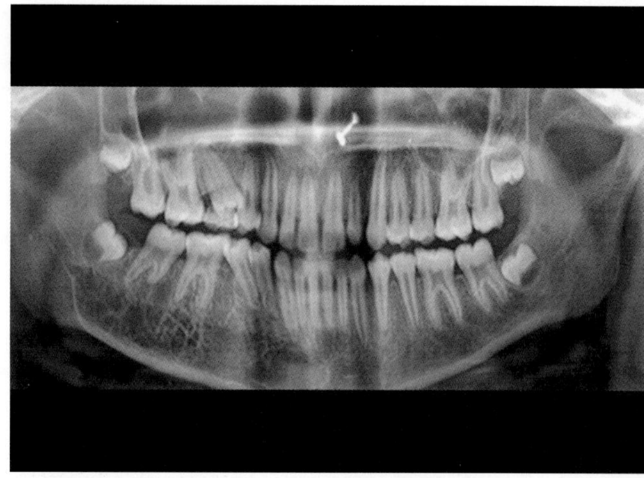

Fig. 21: Hemangioma: A multilocular, mildly expansile radiolucent lesion is seen involving the right hemimandible of a young female. There is displacement of the overlying roots.

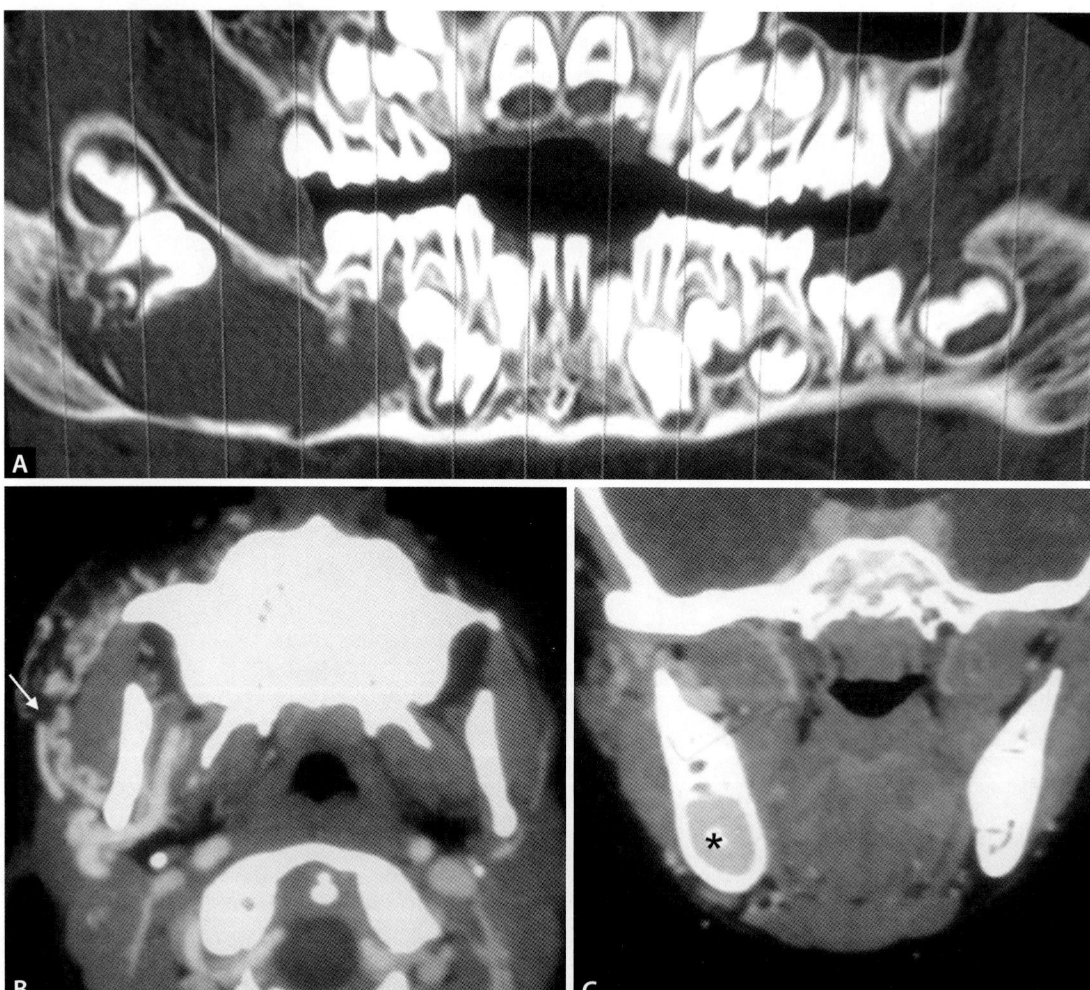

Figs. 22A to C: Arteriovenous malformation: (A) Panoramic CT reconstructed image shows well-defined, expansile lytic lesion in the body and ramus of right hemimandible. CECT axial image (B) shows multiple, tortuous vessels in the mandibular space (arrow) and coronal image (C) shows the large, intraosseous ectatic varix (asterix).

radiolucent due to resorption of the adjacent bone. The lesions may be multilocular.[10] They may appear well defined, cyst-like or have erosive margins simulating a malignancy. Angiography is required to confirm the diagnosis and determine its extent and dynamics.

RADIOLUCENT LESIONS WITH ILL-DEFINED MARGINS

Osteomyelitis

While periapical infection causing granuloma and cyst formation is common; osteomyelitis of the jaw bone is rare. It ranges from acute or chronic suppurative to sclerosing osteomyelitis.

Acute suppurative osteomyelitis has no significant early imaging findings. When present, the appearance is of ragged, patchy or moth-eaten areas of radiolucency, with or without subperiosteal reaction.[2]

Chronic osteomyelitis on the other hand has radiolucent and radiopaque areas and is hence characterized as mixed density lesion. Subperiosteal new bone formation, particularly along lower border of mandible or sequestra may be seen **(Figs. 23 and 24)**.[2,18,23]

Sclerosing osteomyelitis occurs in low-grade infections with bone deposition occurring along the osseous cortex and trabeculae.[9]

Malignant Tumors

The majority of carcinomas of the mandible are secondary to invasion from the adjoining buccal mucosa **(Figs. 25A and B)**.

Primary Tumors

Odontogenic

Primary odontogenic malignancies are rare and include odontogenic carcinoma and malignant ameloblastoma. Malignant ameloblastoma are very rare and presence of metastases establishes this diagnosis. Few cases of carcinomatous transformation of OKCs have also been reported.[9]

Non-odontogenic Tumors

Various non-odontogenic solid malignant tumors occur in the jaws. Sarcomas such as chondrosarcoma, osteosarcoma, lèiomyosarcoma, and fibrosarcoma can occur.

Osteosarcoma: Amongst these osteosarcoma is the commonest, and generally occurs in young adults under 30 years of age. Based on radiological appearance osteosarcomas can be divided into osteolytic, osteosclerotic and mixed lytic-sclerotic types.[2] The osteolytic type presents with an ill-defined, unilocular, ragged area of radiolucency, with no neoplastic new bone formation. The sclerotic and mixed forms on the other hand have variable internal radiopacity with cortical perforation and periosteal reaction, occasionally producing the classical "sun-burst" pattern. Both forms are associated with "spiking" resorption with or without loosening of teeth.[2,9]

Other malignat non-odontogenic primary tumors include chondrosarcoma **(Figs. 26A to C)** and fibrosarcoma.

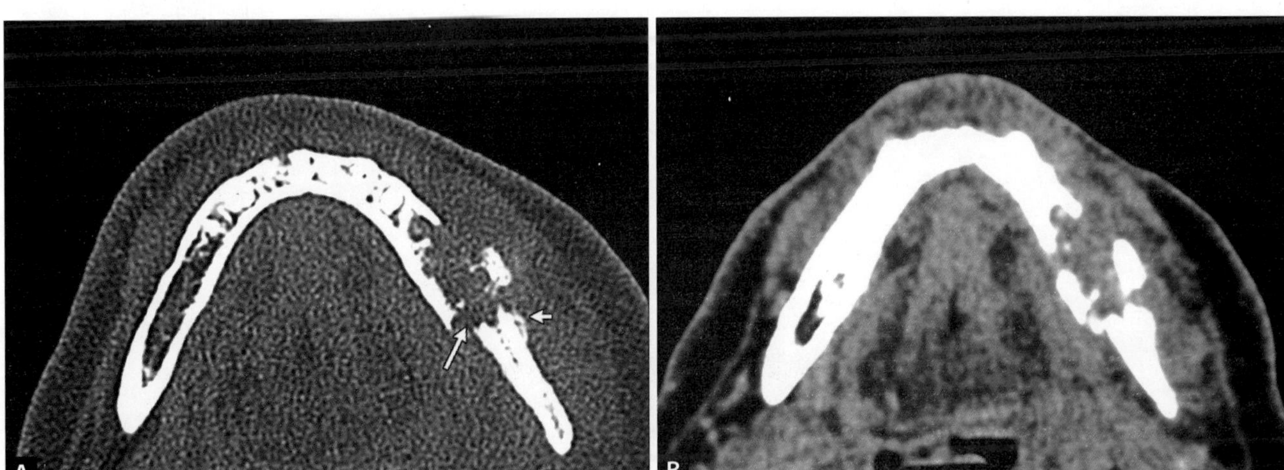

Figs. 23A and B: Osteomyelitis: Axial CT scan bone window (A) reveals an irregular lytic defect involving the ramus of left mandible with subtle periosteal reaction (arrow) and pathological fracture (long arrow). Soft tissue window (B) reveals associated inflammation.

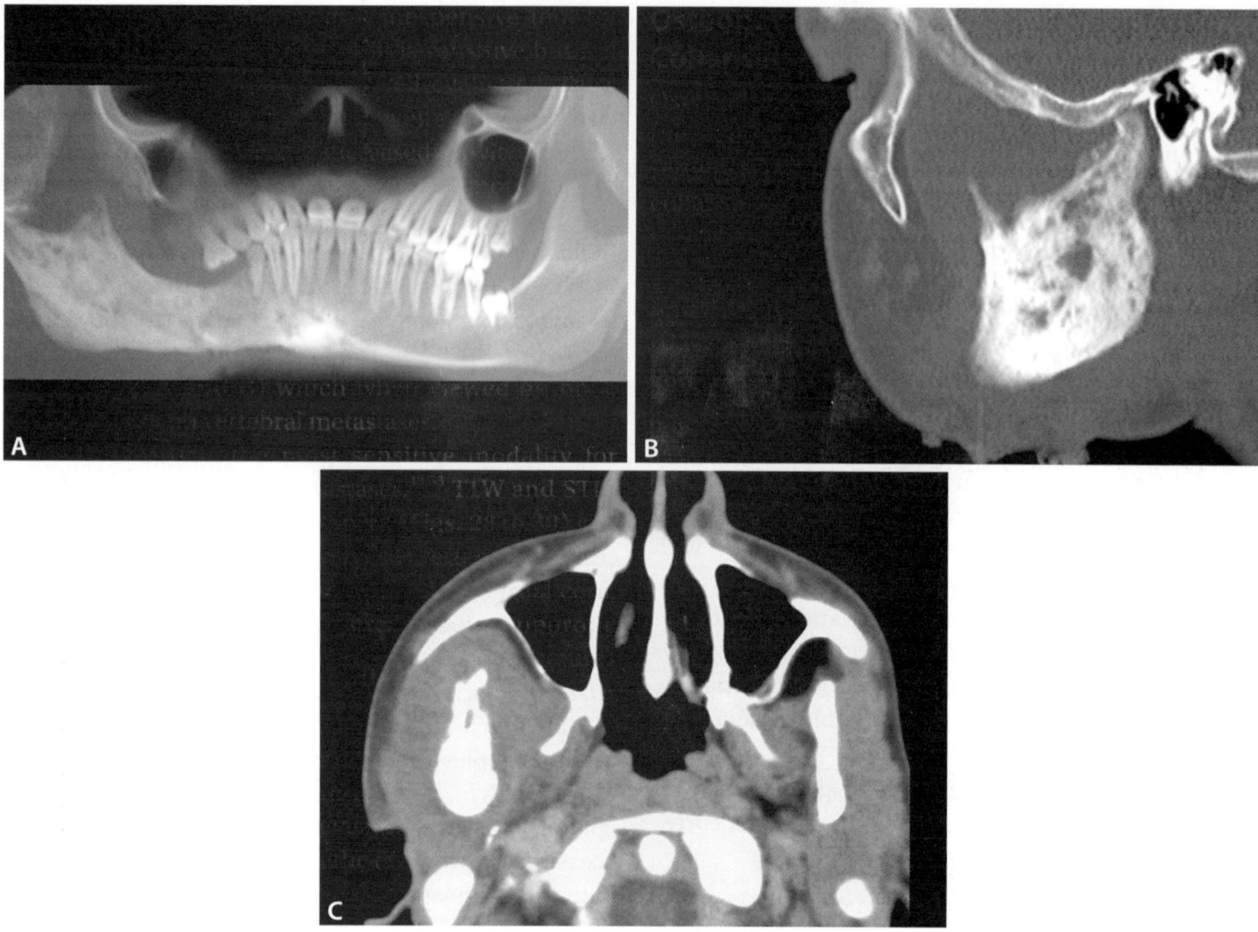

Figs. 24A to C: Chronic osteomyelitis: Panoramic radiograph (A) and MDCT (B and C) showing a mixed density lesion diffusely involving the right mandible, with irregular areas of areas of lysis and sclerosis. Subtle periosteal reaction is also present. Significant soft tissue swelling of muscles of mastication seen.

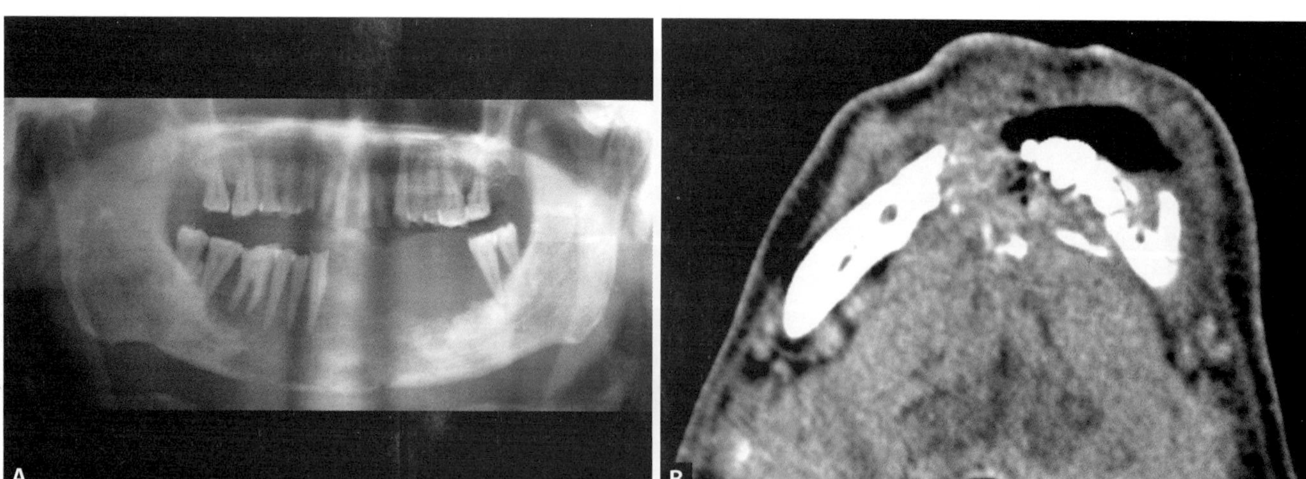

Figs. 25A and B: Carcinoma lower alveolus: Panoramic radiograph (A) of an elderly man showing a bulky soft tissue on the left side of the mouth with extensive, ill-defined, permeative destruction of the mandible; (B) CT scan of a different patient revealing an ulcerated buccal mucosa growth with irregular mandibular destruction.

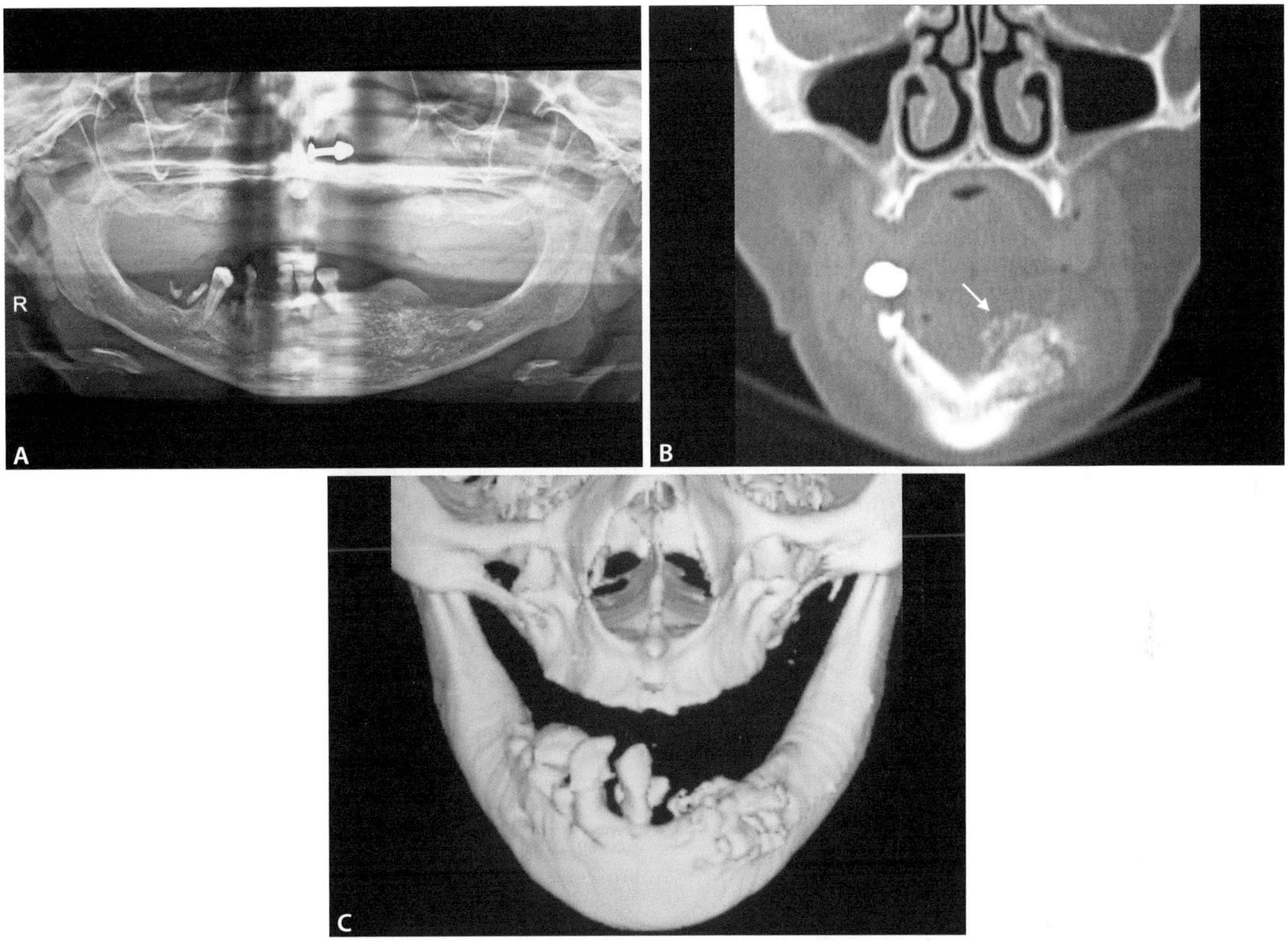

Figs. 26A to C: Chondrosarcoma: Panoramic radiograph (A) of an elderly female with a soft tissue swelling overlying the body of left mandible, and a subtle underlying mixed-density lesion. Coronal CT section (B) reveals chondroid pattern of calcification (arrow), cauliflower-like appearance seen on the VRT image (C).

Lymphoreticular malignancies: Lymphoma and leukemia ususlly present as ill-defined osteolytic lesions of varying sizes. Multiple myeloma may also involve the mandible, with or without the typical "punched-out" lesions. The ovoid radiolucent lesions show no osseous expansion but may erode the mandibular cortex **(Fig. 27)**.[9] Patients with multiple myeloma may thus present with "chin numbness" due to involvement of the inferior alveolar nerve.[24]

Metastases: Metastatic disease often involves the jaw, particularly the posterior body and angle of mandible, these being most vascular. Metastasis to the mandible is four times more common than metastasis to the maxilla.[9] Commonly ill-defined radiolucent lesions, blastic metastases may also be seen. The most common primary sites of origin include kidney, lung, and breast.

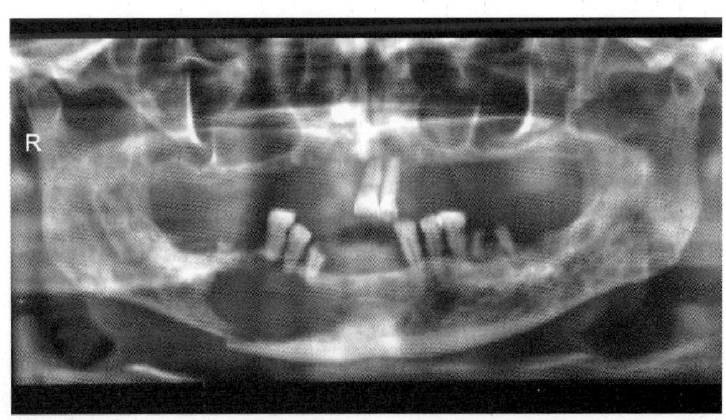

Fig. 27: Multiple myeloma: Panoramic radiograph of an elderly male showing loss of bone density, multiple oval to round rardiolucent lesions scattered throughout and a large lesion in the fracture.

MIXED-DENSITY LESIONS

Table 7 summarizes the common mixed density lesions of the maxillofacial region.

Table 7: Common mixed density lesions of the maxillofacial region.

Odontogenic	*Non-odontogenic*
Odontogenic myxoma	Osteoblastoma
Calcifying epithelial odontogenic tumor	Ossifying fibroma
Ameloblastic fibro-odontoma	Fibrous dysplasia
Adenomatoid odontogenic tumor	Focal cemento-osseous dysplasia
	Osteoradionecrosis

Odontogenic Lesions

Several benign odontogenic tumors have variable degree of calcification within and present as lesions of variable radiopacity.

Odontogenic Myxoma

Odontogenic myxoma is an uncommon benign neoplasm originating from mesenchymal odontogenic tissue. This tumor has a slight predilection for maxilla. They typically present in young adults and are usually painless. The lesion can be locally aggressive. Unerupted teeth may be associated.

On radiology, odontogenic myxoma typically appear as multilocular radiolucent lesions with fine internal septae giving the so called "tennis-racquet" appearance. Foci of irregular calcification are frequently present within the tumor. Teeth may be displaced with or without root absorption **(Figs. 28A and B)**.[2,10] Treatment is attempt to complete surgical resection because the tumor is infiltrative with high recurrence rates.[10]

Calcifying Epithelial Odontogenic Tumor

Calcifying epithelial odontogenic tumor (Pindborg tumor) is a rare odontogenic tumor seen in adults, located in molar/premolar region of the mandible. It is composed of epithelial cells in a fibrous stroma. It is a radiolucent lesion with few scattered calcific densities. Most tumors are associated with the crown of an impacted tooth. The radiodensities are most evident around the crown, giving it the "driven snow" appearance.[2,9]

Ameloblastic Fibro-odontoma

Ameloblastic fibro-odontoma has been questioned in current WHO classification and is believed to be a variant of odontoma. It has a distinct radiographic appearance of a radiolucent lesion, often associated with an unerupted tooth, and contains enamel or dentine seen as multiple radiopacities **(Figs. 29A and B)**. It may affect children too.[2]

Adenomatoid Odontogenic Tumor

Adenomatoid odontogenic tumor is a rare tumor that is typically seen in young adults, especially girls and young women. Majority are found in the anterior maxilla. The tumors appear as well-defined radiolucent lesions with punctate (snowflakes) calcifications. These tumors can often surround an unerupted tooth, typically more apically on the root than dentigerous cysts.[9]

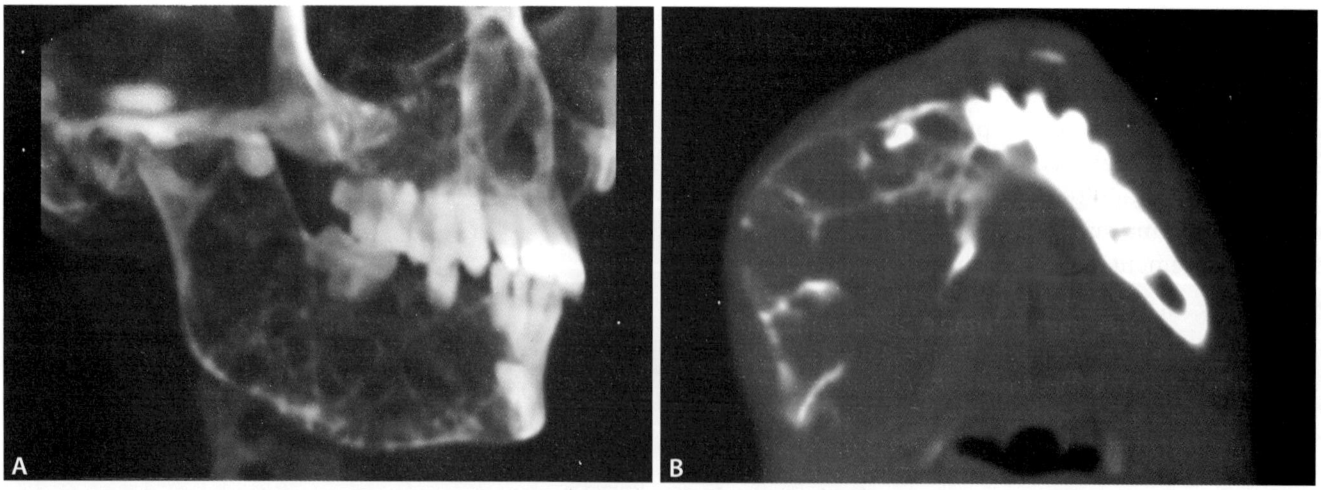

Figs. 28A and B: Odontogenic myxoma: VRT image (A) and axial CT scan (B) of a young male reveal an expansile, multilocular lesion with internal septae involving the right body and ramus of mandible. The last molar is displaced cranially. The overlying teeth are splayed with no root resorption.

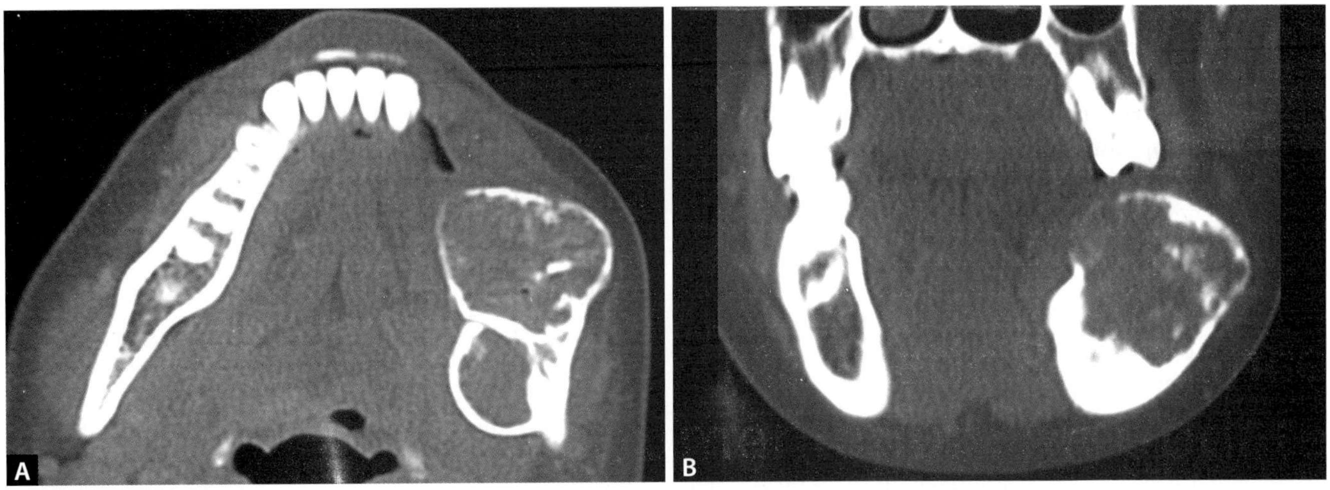

Figs. 29A and B: Ameloblastic fibro-odontoma: MDCT axial (A) and coronal (B) of an adult female showing a septated expansile predominantly radiolucent lesion with calcific densities along its periphery and ill-defined radiodensity scattered centrally. Biopsy revealed the lesion as ameloblastic fibro-odontoma.

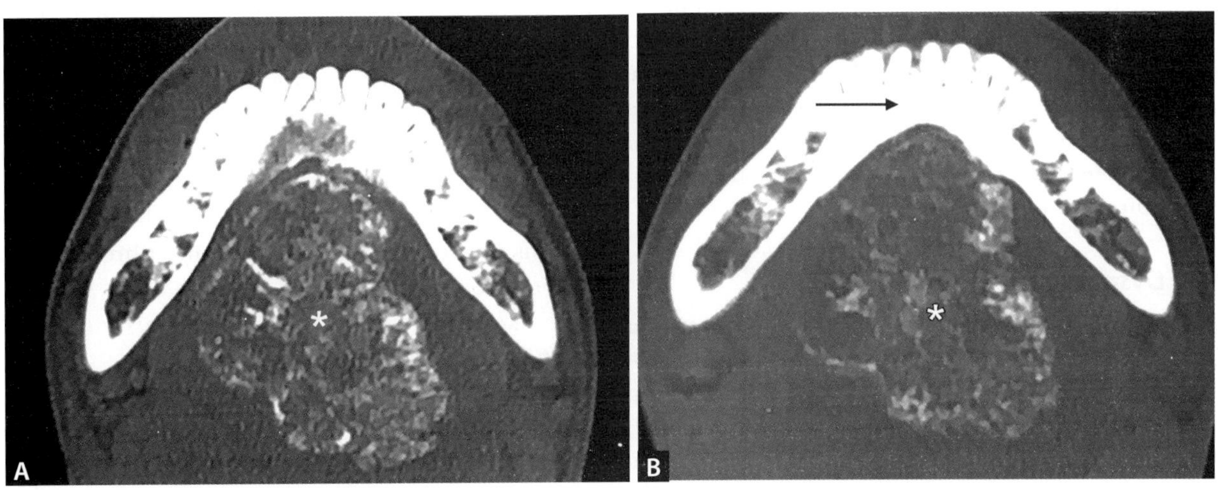

Figs. 30A and B: Osteoblastoma. Axial CT images (A and B) of an adolescent male showing a large, expansile, mixed-density lesion in the floor of mouth (asterix in A and B). Note the sclerosis (arrow in B) along the inner margin of the mandible in the midline: the nidus and cause of recurrence in case of incomplete removal.

Non-Odontogenic Lesions

Mixed density lesions including chronic osteomyelitis, osteogenic sarcoma and metastases have been previously detailed. *Osteoblastoma* is a rare entity, which can also present as a mixed density or sclerotic lesion.

Osteoblastoma

Osteoblastoma is a rare benign tumor, which infrequently involves the jaws. It is usually either periosteal or medullary and not cortical. The mandible is more commonly affected than the maxilla with most lesions occurring in the body of the mandible. The age group most commonly affected is between 5 and 30 years of age.[25] Lesion is usually of mixed density, however radiolucent and radiopaque lesions have also been described. They are well-circumscribed lesions, usually <12 cm in diameter with internal sclerotic matrix.[26] The associated cortical sclerosis represents the nidus **(Figs. 30A and B)** and should be resected to ensure complete removal.

Other mixed density lesions are benign fibro-osseous lesions, which are discussed below.

Ossifying Fibroma

Ossifying fibroma, previously also known as cemento-ossifying or cementifying fibroma is a fibro-osseous lesion containing fibrous tissue with varying amounts of bony trabeculae. It is typically an encapsulated, well-circumscribed lesion. These lesions grow slowly and symmetrically with resultant bone expansion and facial asymmetry. In the tooth-bearing region, there are two clinicopathologic variants of ossifying fibroma: the odontogenic cemento-ossifying fibroma and the nonodontogenic ossifying fibroma. The juvenile ossifying fibroma variants (trabecular and psammatoid variants) typically occur in the 2nd–4th decades with a female preponderance.[2] Juvenile ossifying fibromas occur in younger patients, can be locally destructive and have a greater tendency to recur.[10]

Ossifying fibroma most commonly affects the posterior mandible, but maxilla is also a less common site. On imaging, early lesions are radiolucent, in the intermediate stage gradually increasing internal, coalescing calcified patches are seen and in the late stages the lesion is predominantly radiopaque.[2,10] The radiopaque lesions may be demarcated from the surrounding bone by a radiolucent line. There is osseous expansion in all dimensions with downward bowing of the inferior mandibular cortex. The adjoining teeth are usually displaced. The differential diagnosis of the lesion varies according to its extent of calcification **(Figs. 31A to C)**. Recurrence of conventional ossifying fibroma is uncommon.

Fibrous Dysplasia

Fibrous dysplasia usually presents in adolescents or young adults. Maxilla (especially posterior maxilla) is more commonly affected than the mandible. The adjoining bones such as zygoma and sphenoid may also be involved. The lesions initially appear radiolucent and gradually become opaque resulting in the classical "ground-glass" appearance **(Figs. 32A and B)**. There is bucco-lingual expansion with encroachment or obliteration of the maxillary sinus. The adjoining teeth are displaced and associated loss of lamina dura may be seen. Involvement of adjoining bones and skull base aids in the diagnosis.[2,18]

Cemento-osseous Dysplasia

Cemento-osseous dysplasia is a clinicopathologic variant of the spectrum of benign fibro-osseous lesions. These lesions arise exclusively in the tooth-bearing regions of the jaw bones and include three conditions: Periapical osseous dysplasia, focal osseous dysplasia (periapical cementoma), florid osseous dysplasia. These lesions are radiolucent initially (fibrous tissue) and gradually become mixed-density (mineralized tissue). These lesions are generally incidental, asymptomatic radiographic findings. Most variants are localized, small, discrete lesions, more common in the mandible. Florid osseous dysplasia however manifests as diffuse, multi-quadrant mixed lucent-opaque lesions in both the mandible **(Fig. 33)** and the maxilla. The periapical form is characteristically seen as small 5–6 mm lesion at the apices of lower incisor teeth. The teeth are typically viable. Differential diagnosis includes apical periodontitis for small, discrete lucent lesions (carious teeth) and ossifying fibroma for larger lesion.[2,10]

Osteoradionecrosis

Post-radiation therapy, osteoradionecrosis can manifest years later. Imaging appearance varies depending on radiation dose and duration. As with bone elsewhere,

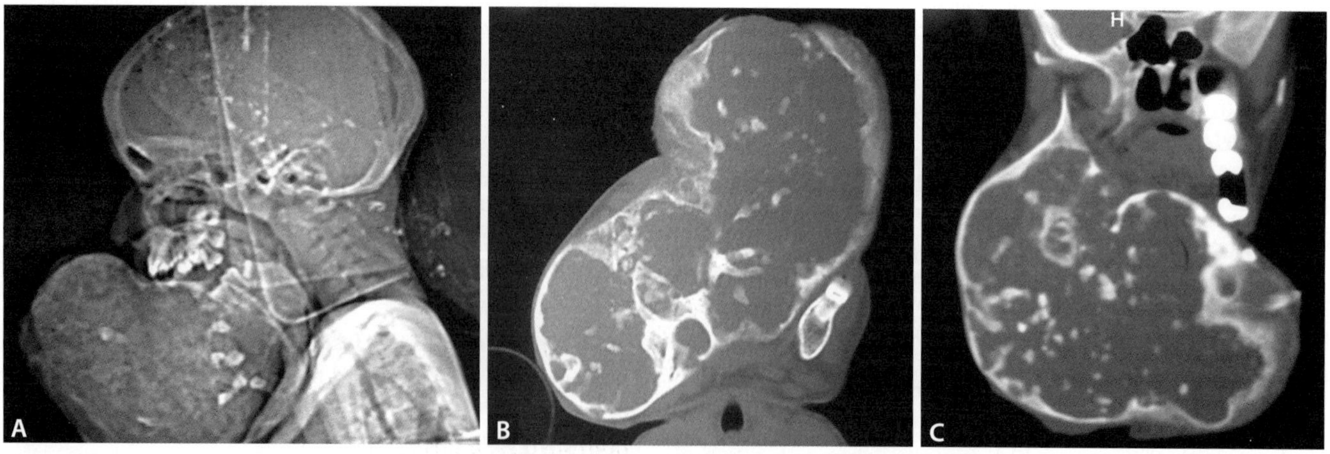

Figs. 31A to C: Juvenile ossifying fibroma: CT scout film (A) of a 10 years old male patient reveals a huge mixed-density lesion with caudal displacement of the teeth, involving the mandible; Axial (B) and coronal (C) CT images reveal coalescing radiodensities within. There is massive expansion with bowing of the inferior mandibular cortex, but no thinning. Patient subsequently underwent a difficult resection and reconstruction.

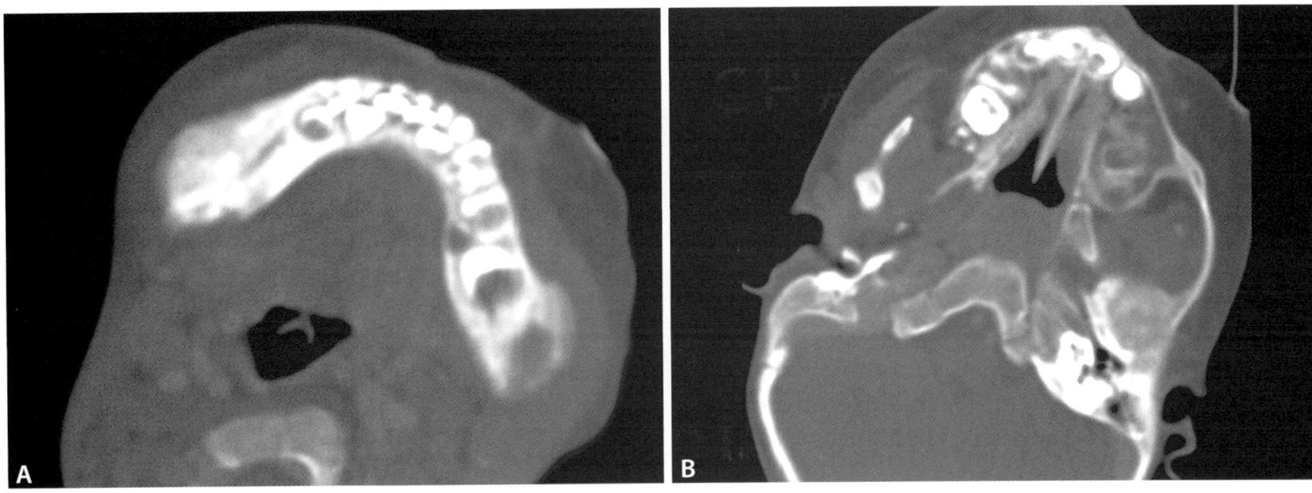

Figs. 32A and B: Fibrous dysplasia: (A) Axial MDCT of a 4-year-old girl showing expansion of the mandible with characteristic "ground-glass" opacity. A more cranial section (B) reveals involvement of the left temporal bone.

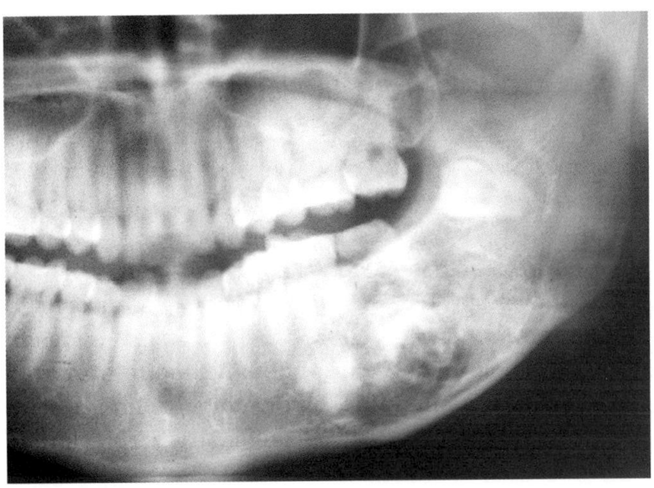

Fig. 33: Cemento-osseous dysplasia: Part of a panoramic radiograph showing a mixed-density lesion in the left hemimandible containing amorphous areas of calcification.

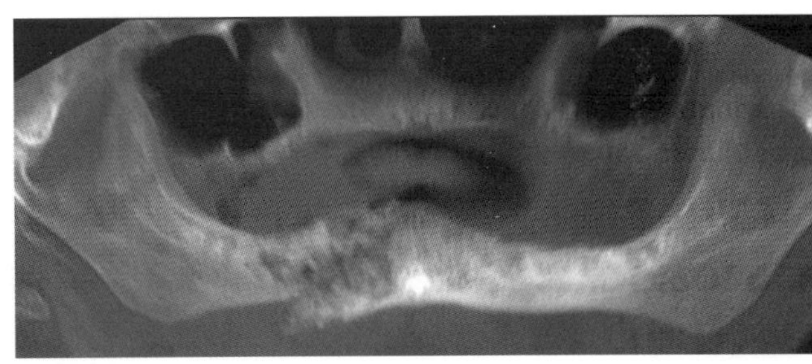

Fig. 34: Osteoradionecrosis of the mandible. Panoramic reconstructed image of CECT face of a 50-year-old male patient of carcinoma tongue (postsurgery and postradiotherapy). Mixed lytic sclerotic density in body of right hemimandible with pathological fracture. Sclerosis is also seen in the body of left hemimandible.

radiation results in endothelial cell death and vessel thrombosis. Mixed lytic sclerotic areas are seen with ill-defined borders and enlarged trabecular spaces **(Fig. 34)**. Sequestered bone may be identified within the lesion.[9]

RADIOPAQUE LESIONS

Table 8 summarizes the radiopaque lesions of the maxillofacial region.

Table 8: Common radiopaque lesions of the maxillofacial region.

Odontogenic	*Non-odontogenic*
Odontomes	Osteoma
Cementoblastoma	Chondroma
	Osteochondroma
	Torus

Odontogenic Lesions

Odontomes

Odontome is an odontogenic hamartomatous malformation composed of any or all odontogenic tissues in various states of differentiation. It is the most common odontogenic "tumor" (67% of cases).[27]

There are two types of odontomas: complex and compound. Complex odontomes are made of multiple, irregular masses of dental tissue (amorphous calcifications on plain radiographs). Compound odontome contains multiple teeth or toothlike structures. The miniature tooth shape are surrounded by a radiolucent line. Compound odontomes are more common. Most lesions are 1–3 cm in size and may cause malpositioning, impaction or resorption of adjacent teeth. The differential diagnosis of the amorphous odontomes includes focal cemento-osseous dysplasia and adenomatoid odontogenic tumor.[2,10,18]

Cementoblastoma

Cementoblastoma is a rare odontogenic tumor characterized by formation of cementum like tissue in relation to root of a tooth in patients less than 25 years of age. It is characteristically found in association with the apex of the first mandibular molar. These measure up to 2–3 cm. The lesion appears as a round, well-demarcated opaque round or irregular, sunburst mass with a thin radiolucent rim ("golf-ball" appearance) **(Figs. 35A and B)**.[2] It is attached to the root of the tooth, which is often obscured. However, the periodontal ligament space is obscured by the lesion unlike in condensing osteitis.

Non-Odontogenic Lesions

Osteoma

Osteomas are slow growing, benign osseous tumors occurring most often in 10–40 years age group.[8] These lesions are found on the skull or facial skeleton. Gardner's syndrome is commonly associated with multiple osteomas. Osteomas may be located within the medullary bone (endosteal) or on the surface (periosteal) **(Figs. 36A and B)**. There are two main types—compact and cancellous. The compact form consists of dense lamellae of bone (ivory osteoma), while the cancellous form comprises of bone trabaculae.[2]

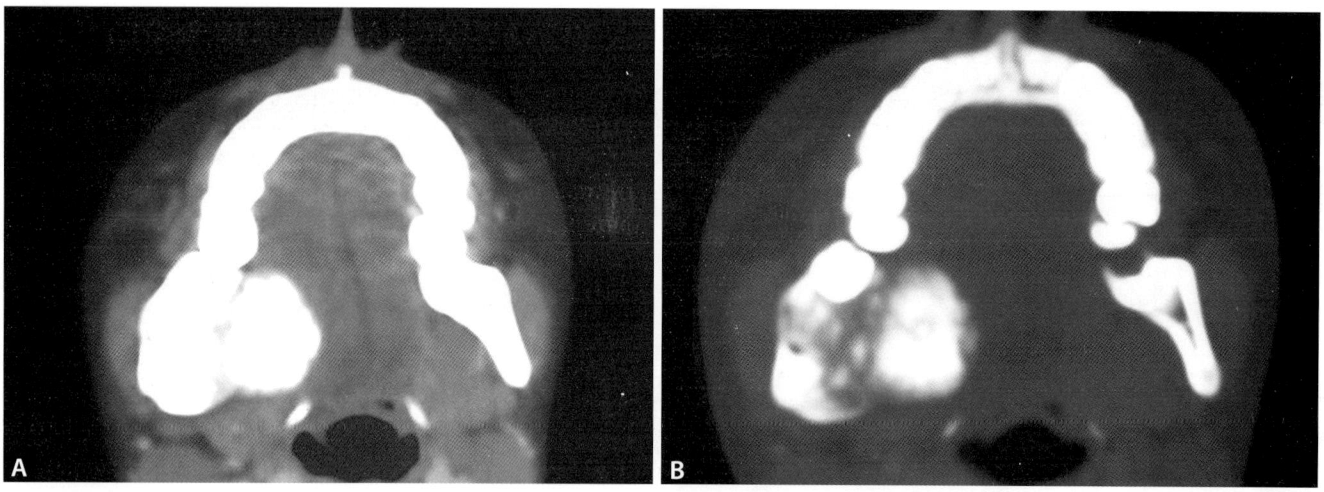

Figs. 35A and B: Cementoblastoma: Soft tissue (A) and bone window (B) of axial CT scan of 10 years old girl showing a round, well-demarcated, round, irregular, sunburst radiopaque mass closely related to the adjoining tooth. Biopsy revealed a cementoblastoma.

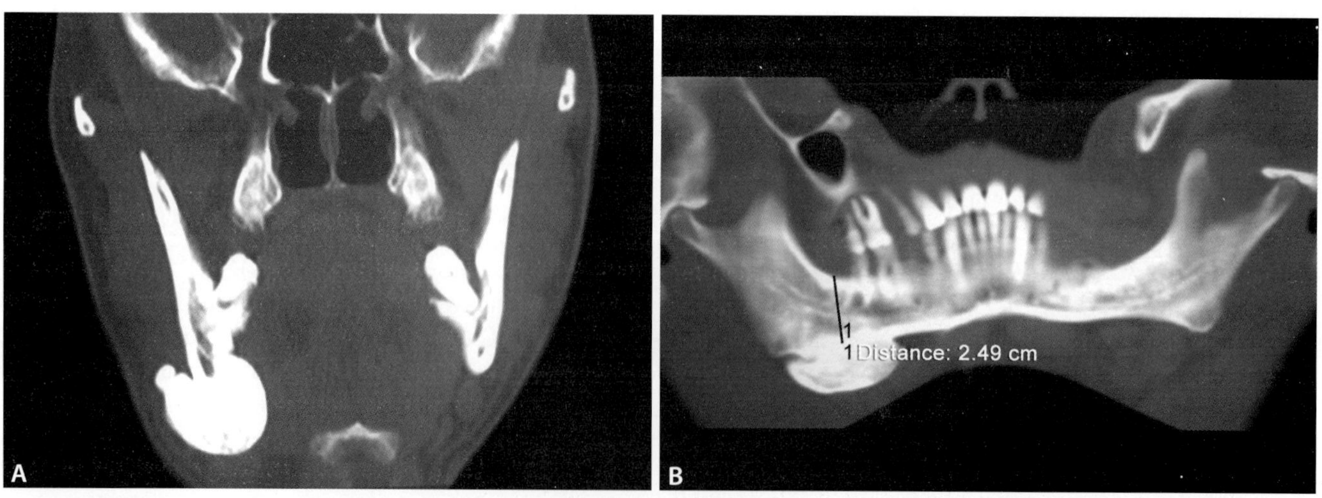

Figs. 36A and B: Periosteal (surface) osteoma: Coronal CT (A) and panoramic CT reconstruction (B) of a young male reveal a well-defined radiodense surface outgrowth at the angle of the mandible.

Chondroma and Osteochondroma

Chondromas and osteochondromas are rare jaw lesions, seen in the region of the condylar head or coronoid process of the mandible. Lesions involving the condylar head cause mandibular deviation to the opposite side and elongation of the face on the affected side.[8] Mushroom-shaped enlargement with restricted mouth opening occurs in lesions involving the coronoid process.[8] On imaging, osteochondromas appear as regular- or irregular-shaped areas of varying radiographic opacity contiguous with the cortex of the involved bone. The imging morphology is well delineated with CT with 3D reconstructions.[8]

Torus (Exostoses)

Exostoses are developmental abnormalities, which are small irregular overgrowths of bone and are often bilateral. Torus mandibularis is seen on lingual aspects of premolar/molar region of mandible. Torus palatinus is seen on either side of midline on posterior aspect of the hard palate. Usually, two views are required to delineate the lesions.[2]

CONCLUSION

Although the list of tumor and tumor-like lesions in the jaw appears intimidating, familiarity with common lesions and a systematic approach would aid us in often arriving at the diagnosis. In several instances, only a differential diagnosis can be proffered necessitating a biopsy.

REFERENCES

1. Neyaz Z, Gadodia A, Gamanagatti S, et al. Radiographical approach to jaw lesions. Singapore Med J. 2008;49(2):165-77.
2. Whaites E (Ed). Essentials of Dental Radiography and Radiology, 4th edition. Churchill Livingstone: Elsevier; 2007.
3. Bodner L, Bar-ziv J, Kaffe I . CT of cystic jaw lesions. J Comput Assist Tomogr. 1994;18(1):22-6.
4. Abrahams JJ, Hayt MW, Rock R. Dental CT reformatting programs and dental imaging. In: Som PM, Curtin HD (Eds). Head and Neck Imaging, 4th edition. Missouri, USA: Mosby; 2003. pp. 907-18.
5. Kaneda T, Tohru M. Benign odontogenic tumors of the maxilla and the mandible. Neuroimaging Clin N Am. 2003;13:495-507.
6. Srinivasan K, Bhalla AS, Sharma R, et al. Diffusion-weighted imaging in the evaluation of odontogenic cysts and tumours. Br J Radiol. 2012;85:e864–e870.
7. Srinivasan K, Seith A, Gadodia A, et al. Evaluation of the inferior alveolar canal for cysts and tumors of the mandible—comparison of multidetector computed tomography and 3-dimensional volume interpolated breath-hold examination magnetic resonance sequence with curved multiplanar reformatted reconstructions. J Oral Maxillofac Surg. 2012;70:2327-32.
8. DelBalso AM. An approach to the diagnostic imaging of jaw lesions, dental implants, and the temporomandibular joint. Radiol Clin North Am. 1998;36(5):855-90.
9. Dunfee BL, Sakai O, Pistey R, et al. Radiologic and pathologic characteristics of benign and malignant lesions of the mandible. RadioGraphics. 2006;26:1751-68.
10. Scholl RJ, Kellett HM, Neumann DP, et al. Cysts and cystic lesions of the mandible: clinical and radiologic-histopathologic review. RadioGraphics. 1999;19:1107-24.
11. Speight PM, Takata T. New tumour entities in the 4th edition of the World Health Organization Classification of Head and Neck tumours: odontogenic and maxillofacial bone tumours. Virchows Arch. DOI 10.1007/s00428-017-2182-3.
12. El-Naggar AK, Chan JKC, Grandis JR, et al. WHO Classification of Head and Neck Tumours, 4th edition. IARC, Lyon; 2017. pp. 204-6.
13. Weber AL. Imaging of cysts and odontogenic tumors of the jaw. RCNA Radiol Clin North Am. 1993;31:101-20.
14. Mourshed F. A roentgenographic study of dentigerous cysts. Oral Surg Oral Med Oral Pathol. 1967;51:54-61.
15. Oikarinen VJ. Keratocyst recurrences at intervals of more than 10 years: case reports. Br J Oral Maxillofac Surg. 1990;28:47-9.
16. Hisatomi M, Asaumi JI, Konouchi H, et al. MR imaging of epithelial cysts of the oral and maxillofacial region. Eur J Radiol. 2003;48:178-82.
17. Roychoudhury A, Rustagi A, Bhatt K, et al. Aneurysmal bone cyst of the mandible: report of 3 cases. J Oral Maxillofac Surg. 2009;67(9):1996-2004.
18. Weber AL, Kaneda T, Scrivani SJ, et al. Jaw: Cysts, tumors, and nontumorous lesions. In: Som PM, Curtis HD (Eds). Head and Neck Imaging, 4th edition. USA: Mosby; 2003.
19. Minami M, Kaneda T, Yamamoto H, et al. Ameloblastoma in the maxillomandibular region: MR imaging. Radiology. 1992;184(2):389-93.
20. Kaneda T, Minami M, Kurabayashi T. Benign odontogenic tumors of the mandible and maxilla. Neuroimaging Clin N Am. 2003;13(3):495-507.
21. Horner K. Central giant cell granuloma of the jaw: a clinico-radiological study. Clin Radiol. 1989;40:622-26.
22. Murphey MD, Nomikos GC, Flemming DJ, et al. Imaging of giant cell tumor and giant cell reparative granuloma of bone: radiologic-pathologic correlation. RadioGraphics. 2001:21:1283-309.
23. Hudson JW. Osteomyelitis of the jaws: a 50-year perspective. J Oral Maxillofac Surg. 1993;51(12):1294-301.
24. Witt C, Borges AC, Klein K, et al. Radiographic manifestations of multiple myeloma in the mandible: a retrospective study of 77 patients. J Oral Maxillofac Surg. 1997;55(5):450-3.
25. Mardaleishvili K, Kakabadze Z, Machavariani A. Benign osteoblastoma of the mandible in a 12-year-old female: a case report, Oncol Lett. 2014;6:2691-4.
26. Manjunatha BS, Sunit P, Amit M, et al. Osteoblastoma of the jaws: report of a case and review of literature. Clin Pract. 2011;4:e118.
27. Regezi JA, Kerr DA, Courtney RM. Odontogenic tumors: an analysis of 706 cases. J Oral Surg. 1978;36:771-8.

CHAPTER 28

Craniovertebral Junction Anomalies

Niranjan Khandelwal, Vivek Gupta

INTRODUCTION

The craniovertebral junction (CVJ) anatomically denotes the occiput, the first (atlas) and second cervical (axis) vertebral segments, their articulations and connecting ligaments.[1] This is a complex transition between the skull and the upper cervical spine, and the brain and the spinal cord respectively. Collectively, these structures surround and protect the cervicomedullary junction and lower cranial nerves. A knowledge of bony anatomy, embryology and biomechanics of the CVJ helps to understand various anomalies associated with CVJ.[2]

ANATOMY AND EMBRYOLOGY

Skeletal Anatomy (Figs. 1A to D)

Foramen Magnum and the Occiput

The occiput which surrounds the foramen magnum consists of three parts: (1) The squamosal portion (supra-occiput) situated in the dorsal aspect of foramen magnum, (2) The basi-occiput or clival portion located anterior to the foramen magnum, and (3) The condylar part (exo-occiput) that joins the clival parts and the squamosal.[3,4]

Atlas

It is dissimilar to the other cervical vertebrae because it is ring shaped and lacks a vertebral body and spinous process. It consists of two thick lateral masses which are located at the anterolateral part of the ring. A short anterior arch connects it in the front and the long posterior arch at the back. The lateral mass of atlas consists the superior and the inferior articular facets which articulate with occipital condyles and the superior apophysis of the atlas respectively.

It is a ring with pivot-like structure and contains the odontoid process or dens, body of axis, lateral masses, posterior arch and a bifid spinous process. The odontoid process projects cephalad from its articulation with the axis body. The oval facet on the ventral odontoid surface articulates with the dorsal surface of the anterior atlas arch. In the dorsal aspect of the dens is a transverse groove over which the transverse ligament of the atlas passes.[3-5]

The superior and inferior apophysis of the atlas and the superior apophysis of the axis are unique from the rest in that they are located ventral to the spinal nerve exits. The atlantoaxial complex is unique among the intervertebral articulations on account of the horizontal orientation of its lateral facet joints, pivot-like atlantodental articulation and special ligamentous support (alar ligaments and transverse or cruciate ligament).

Ligamentous Anatomy (Figs. 2A and B)

The occipito-atlantoaxial ligaments are arranged in four layers. The most anterior layer is the superior extension of anterior longitudinal ligament known as anterior atlanto-occipital membrane that it attaches to the anterior arch of the atlas. The second layer is formed by the alar ligament and the apical ligament. The paired alar ligaments connect the odontoid with the lateral masses and the occipital

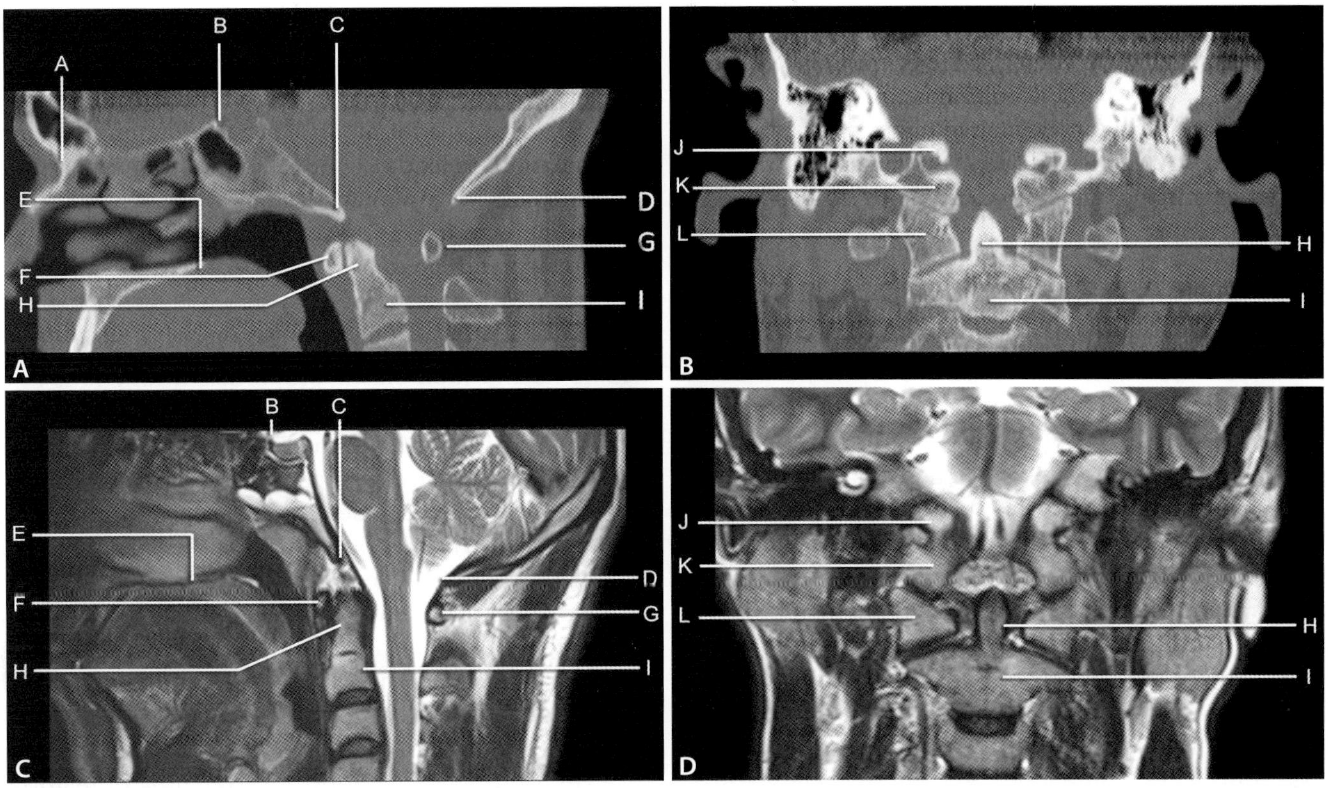

Figs. 1A to D: Normal landmarks of craniovertebral junction (CVJ): Midsagittal (A) computed tomography (CT); (B) T2-weighted magnetic resonance (T2W MR) and coronal; (C) CT; (D) T2W MR. (A, nasion; B, tuberculum sella; C, basion (anterior margin of foramen magnum); D, opisthion (posterior margin of the foramen magnum); E, posterior margin of the hard palate; F, anterior arch of atlas; G, posterior arch of atlas; H, odontoid process; I, body of axis; J, jugular tubercles; K, occipital condyles; L, lateral atlas masses).

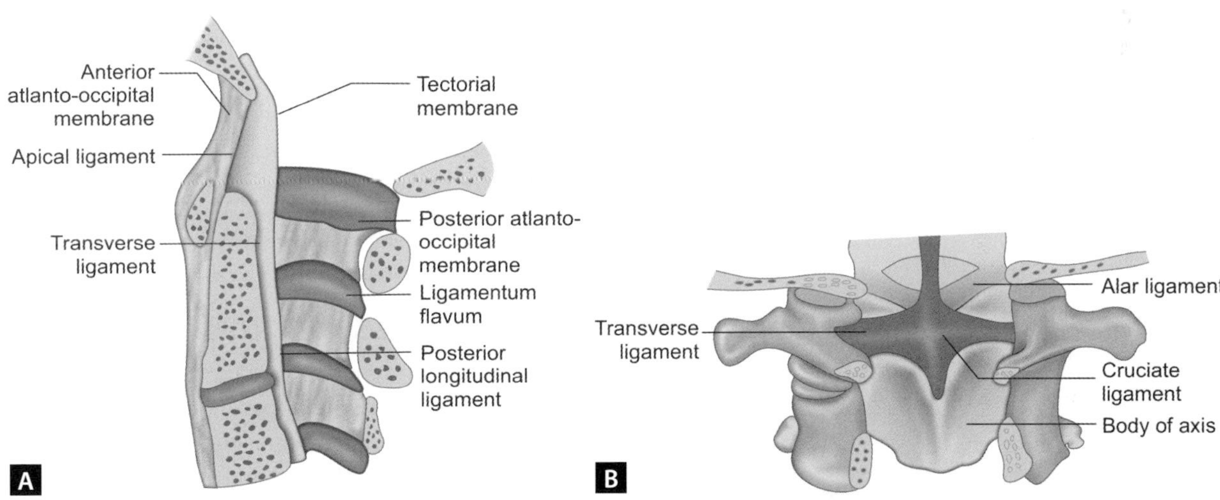

Figs. 2A and B: Ligamentous anatomy of craniovertebral junction.

condyles. The small apical ligament extends from the tip of the odontoid to the foramen magnum. The cruciate ligament forms the third layer and is seen immediately dorsal to the odontoid process. The transverse portion of the cruciate ligament or the transverse ligament connects both lateral masses of the atlas and passes dorsal to the odontoid, keeping it pressed forward against the anterior arch of the atlas. The most posterior layer is formed by the tectorial membrane which is a superior continuation of the posterior longitudinal ligament.[3-7]

The muscles attached to the cranio-vertebral complex assist in stabilization of the spine and initiate as well as maintain movement of the joints. There is no vascular communication between the base of dens and body of axis. This is important in understanding the etiology of Os odontoideum and formation of a sequestrum with type II odontoid fracture.

Embryology

The bony cranial base is developed by a process of endochondral ossification. The bones of the CVJ are developed from four occipital sclerotomes and the first two cervical sclerotomes. The first two occipital sclerotomes form the basiocciput. The third occipital sclerotome forms the exoccipital bone that forms jugular tubercles. The key sclerotome is the fourth occipital sclerotome termed the pro-atlas. It forms the anterior tubercle of the clivus, the apical cap of the dens, anterior margin of the foramen magnum, occipital condyles, lateral atlantal masses and the superior portion of the posterior arch of the atlas. The first spinal sclerotome forms the anterior arch of atlas, posterior and inferior portion of the C1 arch, odontoid process. The second cervical sclerotome forms the rest of the axis vertebra **(Fig. 3)**.[3-7]

There are two sources of blood supply. First, anterior and posterior descending vessels arise from the vertebral arteries and pass in front and behind the axis and odontoid process. They anastomose in the apical arcade in the region of the alar ligament. These vessels supply small perforators to the body of the axis and odontoid process. Second, the anterior descending artery as well as the apical arcade receives contributions from the carotid and occipital arteries. Lymphatic drainage is primarily into the retropharyngeal lymph nodes, and then into the upper jugular deep cervical chain. Thus, a retrograde infection may affect the synovial lining of the CVJ complex.

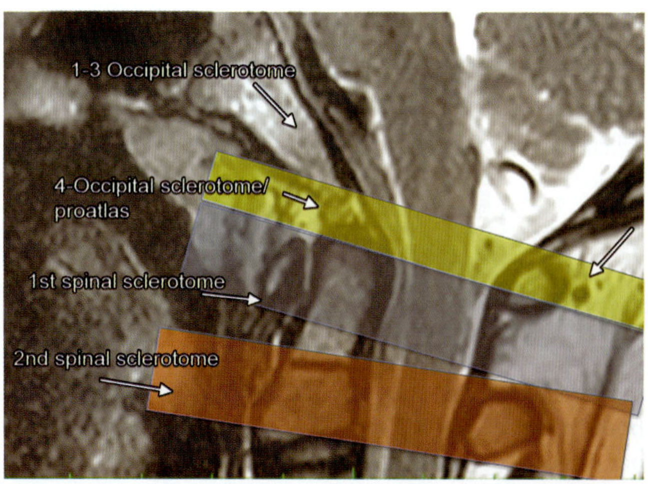

Fig. 3: Occipital and spinal sclerotomes and the development of the CVJ components.

BIOMECHANICS

Relative motion of the occipitoatlantoaxial region is controlled by the geometry of the surfaces as well as the ligaments and their elastic properties. It functions as a single unit, and the complex allows the necessary range of motion while providing support to the head. Nodding or yes-yes movements occur at the atlanto-occipital joints. Rotatory or no-no movements occur at atlantoaxial joints **(Figs. 4A and B)**. Both occipitoatlantal and atlantoaxial articulations are involved in flexion and extension. The average range of this motion at the occipitoatlantal joint is 13–15°. An additional 10° of motion occurs in the atlantoaxial articulation. Flexion is limited by the tectorial membrane and by contact between the dens and occipital basion.

Extension is restricted by the stretching of tectorial membrane and by bony contact between opisthion and posterior arch of atlas. In the normal adult less than 3 mm of anteroposterior translation occurs between the dens and anterior ring of atlas. This measurement may be up to 5 mm in children younger than 8 years of age. If the transverse component of cruciate ligament ruptures with intact alar ligament, up to 5 mm of displacement may occur.

Rotation of the craniovertebral complex occurs only at the atlantoaxial joint. The articular surfaces of atlantoaxial complex are convex with horizontal orientation so as to allow maximal mobility. Atlantoaxial joint rotation varies from 37° to 42°.[8]

CLINICAL PRESENTATION

In most cases, the symptoms of the pathologic conditions affecting the CVJ become apparent after the compromise of these neural structures. Signs and symptoms are diverse and usually have a subtle beginning; they arise fairly late, progress slowly, remain stationary, and rarely relapse. It may be in the form of dysfunction of the brainstem, cervical spinal cord, cranial nerves, cervical nerve roots or the vascular supply to these structures. Myelopathy is the most common neurological deficit.[2] Sensory abnormalities may be related to posterior column involvement. Lower cranial nerve dysfunction is seen in 20% of children with basilar invagination.[9] Vascular symptoms occur in 15% patients.

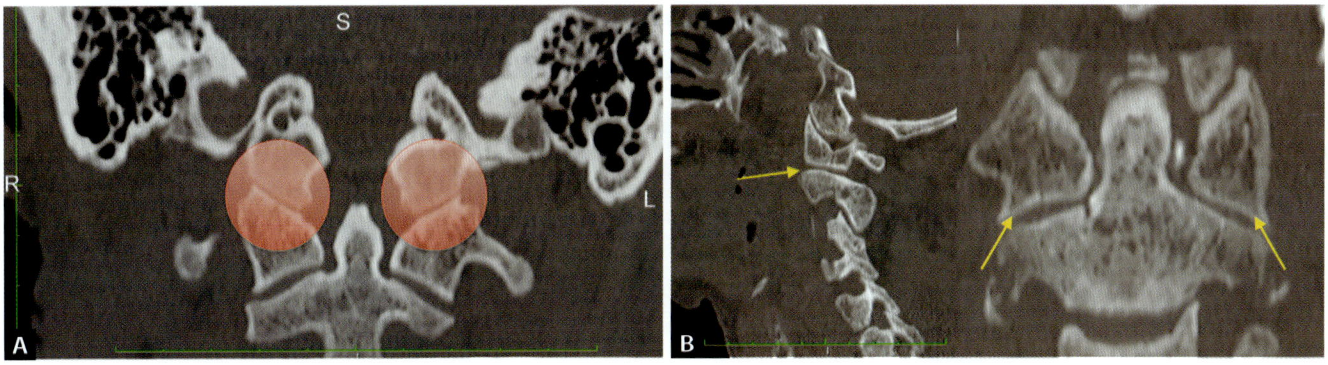

Figs. 4A and B: (A) Atlanto-occipital joint; and (B) Atlanto-axial joint.

Neck pain is present in 85% patients typically described as originating in the suboccipital area with radiation to the vertex.[9]

CRANIOMETRY (TABLES 1 AND 2)

Craniometry of the CVJ usesaseries of lines, planes and angles to define the normal anatomic relationships of the CVJ[10] **(Figs. 5A and B)**. These measurements were initially defined on plain X-rays but are now extrapolated to NCCT saggital and coronal images.

CLASSIFICATION OF CVJ ANOMALIES[11,12]

Congenital Anomalies and Malformations of the Craniovertebral Junction

- *Malformations of the occipital sclerotomes including proatlas*:
  - Clivus segmentation anomalies
  - Proatlas remnants around foramen magnum
  - Condylar hypoplasia
  - Assimilation of atlas
- *Malformation of atlas*:
  - Assimilation of atlas
  - Atlantoaxial fusion
  - Aplasia of atlas arches
- *Malformation of axis*:
  - Irregular atlantoaxial segmentation
  - Dens dysplasias
- Ossiculum terminale persistens
- Os odontoideum
- *Hypoplasia-aplasia*:
  - Segmentation failure of C2-C3

Developmental and Acquired Abnormalities of the CVJ

- Abnormalities at the foramen magnum. Foraminal stenosis (e.g. achondroplasia)
- Secondary basilar invagination (e.g. Osteogenesis imperfecta, Hadju-Cheney, Paget's disease, osteomalacia, rickets, rheumatoid arthritis)
- *Atlantoaxial instability*:
  - Down syndrome
  - Ehlers-Danlos syndrome
  - *Errors of metabolism*: Morquio's, Hurlers
  - Trauma
  - *Infection*: Tuberculosis
  - *Inflammatory*: Rheumatoid arthritis, Reiter's syndrome
  - *Tumor*: Osteoblastoma, eosinophilic granuloma, chordoma, neurofibromatosis, metastasis
- Miscellaneous, e.g. Conradi-Hünermann syndrome, fetal warfarin syndrome, fibrous dysplasia
- *Spontaneous atlantoaxial rotatory subluxation*: Grisel syndrome

INCIDENCE

Craniovertebral junction anomalies are seen all over the world, but are common in our country. Exact incidence of these anomalies is not known. In a study over a period of 12 years, they were responsible for 3.03% of total admissions to the neurology wards.[9] They were the single major cause of cervical cord compression, accounting for nearly half the cases. Therefore, in every patient presenting with high cervical cord compression in our country, the diagnosis of CVJ anomalies must be excluded. Majority of patients are between 11 and 40 years, although the defect is present since birth. There is a male preponderance. Onset is usually gradual. The most common precipitating factor is in the form of trivial trauma to the neck either by a fall or by carrying heavy loads at the back of head.[2,9] Recurrent throat infection and fever may lead to hyperemia and laxity of ligament causing dislocations.

In a recent study of 70 patients with bony CVJ anomalies in our institute, the most common presenting symptom

Table 1: Craniometric lines in lateral view.

Synonyms	*Definition*	*Normal measurement*	*Implications*
Wackenheim's line (Clivus canal line)	Line drawn along clivus into cervical canal	Odontoid tip is ventral and tangential to this line	Odontoid process transects the line in basilar invagination or forward position of skull
Chamberlain's line (Palato-occipital line)	Joins posterior pole of hard palate to opisthion	Tip of dens 1 ± 3.6 mm below this line	Odontoid process bisects the line in basilar invagination
McRae's line (Foramen magnum line)	Joins anterior and posterior edges of foramen magnum (Basion to opisthion)	Tip of dens does not exceed this line	When effective sagittal diameter is <20 mm, neurological symptoms occur (Foramen magnum stenosis)
McGregor's line (Basal line)	Hard plate to the lowest point of occipital bone	Tip of dens should not exceed 5 mm above the line	Line position varies with flexion + extension hence not important
Height index of Klauss	Distance between tip of dens and tuberculum torcula line	40–41 mm	<30 mm seen in basilar invagination
Spinolamellar line (Spinous interlaminar line)	Line drawn from interoccipital ridge above and down along the fused spinous process of C2 and C3	Should intersect posterior arch of atlas	If atlas is fused, posterior arch is anterior to the line, posterior compression of spinal cord may occur
Boogard's line	Joins nasion to opisthion	Basion below this line	Altered in basilar impression
Atlanto temporo-mandibular index	Joins superior edge of anterior arch of atlas to the highest point of temporomandibular interspace	30 + 9 mm	<10 mm in basilar invagination
Basion odontoid index (Whooley)	Joins basion to the trip of odontoid process	5 mm in adults up to 10 mm in children (in neutral position)	Measurements altered in both flexion and extension
Basal angle	Angle between the lines drawn from nasion to tuberculum sellae and tuberculum sellae to basion	124–142°	Widening is called platy-basia
Bull's angle (Atlantopalatine angle)	Angle formed by joining the hard palate posteriorly and the line joining mid points of anterior and posterior arches of atlas	<10°	>13° in basilar invagination (BI) 10–13° : tendency to BI
Boogard's angle	Angle between McRae's line and line drawn from dorsum sellae to basion along the plane of clivus	122°	>135° in basilar invagination

Table 2: Craniometric lines and angles in anteroposterior view.

Synonyms	*Definition*	*Normal*	*Implications*
Fishgold digastric line (Biventer line)	Joins the fossae for digastric muscles on undersurface of skull (Just medial to mastoid process)	Dens tip should not project above this line. Central axis of dens should be perpendi cular to the line	Corresponds to McRae's line on lateral view: may be oblique in unilateral condylar hypoplasia: oblique odontoid suggest paramedian abnormality
Fishgold bimastoid line	Line connecting tips of mastoid process	Runs across atlantooccipital joints, line is 10 mm below digastric line	Odontoid tip may be the line
Schmidt-Fischer angle	Angle of axes of atlanto-occipital joints	124–127° should be measured in plane dens on tomography	Angle is wider in condylar hypoplasia

was cervical pain and stiffness (77%) and majority of the patients were in second decade. The common neurological sign was involvement of pyramidal tract (70%). Multiple anomalies are frequently seen. A study of 82 patients with CVJ anomalies in our institute showed congenital atlantoaxial dislocation (AAD) to be the most common (56%) anomaly followed by multiple anomalies (48.8%) the common combinations being AAD with occipitalization of C1, basilar invagination with Chiari malformation and basilar invagination with occipitalization of C1.[13]

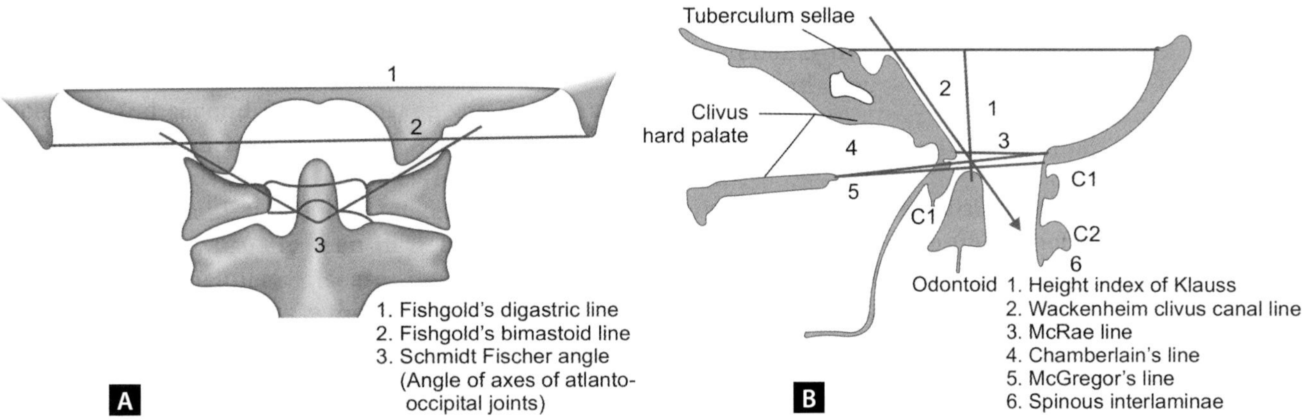

Figs. 5A and B: Various craniometric lines in (A) lateral and (B) anteroposterior views.

NEURORADIOLOGIC INVESTIGATIONS

- *Conventional radiography*:
  - Translateral view of skull including the upper cervical spine (neutral, flexion and extension). These give the points of references for various radiological base lines and angles in assessing atlanto-odontoid distance, anomalies of dens and arches of atlas and axis vertebrae and the soft tissues of neck.
  - Open mouth view—additionally detects dens anomalies and its lateral displacement.
- *Conventional tomography (AP and lateral)*: It defines the CVJ relationship and dimensions (rarely done).
- *Noncontrast CT*: Axial sections show arches of atlas, lateral masses, atlanto-odontoid distance, position of dens and canal diameters. Structures within the canal are indistinguishable without the use of subarachnoid contrast. CT helps to make definitive diagnosis of atlantoaxial rotatory fixation and spatial appreciation of bony fragments in relation to foramen magnum.
- *Three-dimensional CT and reconstruction images*: It helps in understanding the spatial relationships of complex skeletal and traumatic pathology and makes it possible to make a definitive and comprehensive radiographic diagnosis, without additional radiation exposure or significant modification of scanning technique. Little literature is available about its potentials in evaluating CVJ.
- *Conventional MRI*: It provides multiplanar images and is especially helpful in evaluating the brainstem, spinal cord, cerebellar tonsils, syringohydromyelia, cervicomedullary kink and hydrocephalus, etc.
- *Dynamic MRI*: It attempts to combine the advantages of plain films, CT and conventional MRI together. A study conducted in this institute on the role of dynamic MRI in evaluating the CV-Junction abnormalities in 25 patients revealed the diagnosis of mobile AAD, dynamic nature of spinal canal narrowing and variability in cord compression with changing position of the neck.[14] In neutral position, 81% patients had some degree of canal narrowing out of which 16% patients showed increase in canal narrowing on flexion with half of them having direct cord compression which was not detected in neutral position. Thus, dynamic MRI was able to detect cases where surgical intervention was needed as the cord was being compressed in one of the physiological positions. Dynamic MRI of CVJ attempts to give information regarding the dynamic nature of CVJ abnormalities along with the established advantages of MRI like excellent soft tissue visualization and multiplanar capability. The knowledge of dynamic nature of cord compression is important in planning the management of these abnormalities.

A combination of MRI and either standard radiography or CT is ideal in evaluating most of the CVJ anomalies. In all techniques of investigations, dynamic flexion and extension studies are essential to assess the stability and angular osseous relationships and to provide information related to their reducibility and position of fixation. A recent study was conducted in this institute to compare the role of plain radiographs, linear tomograms, axial noncontrast computed tomography (NCCT) and 3D CT in flexion and extension for CVJ anomalies. It was found that the most common radiological abnormality was bony atlas anomalies (86.7%) followed by AAD (80%) and multiple anomalies (50%). Three-dimensional CT was found either equivalent or superior to plain X-rays and tomograms except in the assessment of foramen magnum dimensions.

SPECIFIC CONDITIONS

Basilar Invagination

It is a developmental defect implying prolapse of the vertebral column into the skull base **(Fig. 6)**. There is a distinct developmental defect of the chondrocranium, often associated with other anomalies of the notochord in the region of the CVJ such as occipitalization of atlas **(Figs. 7A to E)** and Klippel-Feil syndrome.[2] Basilar invagination is also associated with anomalies of development of the epicaudal neuroaxis such as Chiari malformations, syringobulbia and syringomyelia in about 25–30% of cases. Two types of basilar invagination are recognized.[7] In the anterior variety, there is shortening of the basiocciput and the clivus is short and horizontally oriented known as Basi-occiput hypoplasia **(Fig. 8)**. In the paramedian variety, there is hypoplasia of the exoccipital bones and dorsal displacement of the clivus, which is otherwise of normal length.

Basilar impression refers to secondary or acquired forms of basilar invagination due to softening of the bone as occurs in hyperparathyroidism, rickets, osteomalacia, Paget's disease, Hurler's syndrome, osteogenesis imperfecta, etc. Traumatic basilar impression has also been reported.[15,16] Inflammation and infection producing bone destruction with or without ligamentous instability may also cause basilar impression, e.g. rheumatoid arthritis, tuberculosis, etc. In this anomaly, all three parts of the occipital bone (basiocciput, exoccipital bone, and supraoccipital bone) are deformed. There is abnormal rostral location of clivus-atlas-odontoid complex within the foramen magnum.

Platybasia refers only to an abnormally obtuse basal angle. It is not a measure of basilar invagination, although it may be associated with invagination **(Figs. 9A and B)**. There are no symptoms or signs associated with platybasia alone.

Assimilation of Atlas

Assimilation of atlas represents the most cephalic blocked vertebra encountered in the spine. It is defined as a failure of segmentation between the atlas and skull and occurs in 0.25% of the population.[17] It may be bilateral, unilateral, segmental, or focal **(Figs. 10A and B)**. In most instances, atlas assimilation occurs in association with other abnormalities such as basilar invagination and Klippel-Feil syndrome. Associated congenital anomalies present in 20% of patients, include incomplete clefting of the nasal cartilage, cleft palate, congenital external ear deformities, cervical ribs hypo-spadiasis and urinary tract anomalies.[18]

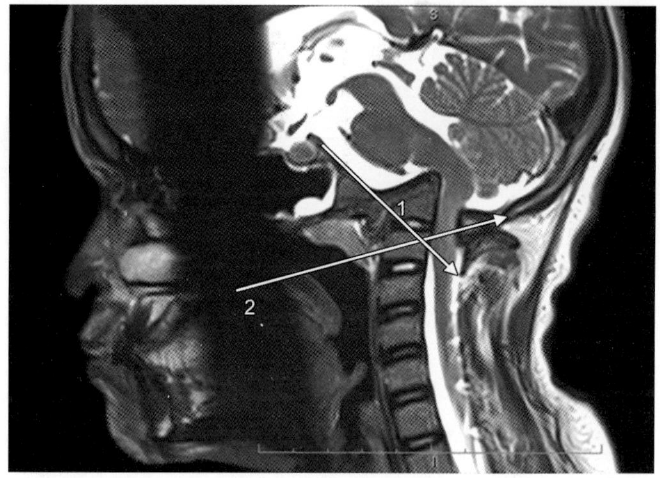

Fig. 6: Basilar invagination with odontoid tip crossing both the clivus-canal line (1) and McGregor's line (2).

A combination of assimilation of the atlas and segmentation failures between the second and third cervical vertebrae results in progressive laxity of the atlantoaxial joint with development of luxation between the atlas and axis in childhood in about 50% of cases. The progressive proliferation of granulation tissue due to instability leads to irreducible compression.

Atlas Arch Anomalies

The most common anomaly in this group is posterior rachischisis, which is present in 4% of the autopsy specimens of adults.[19] Majority of these are midline in location (97%). Posterior arch rachischisis has been reported in 70% of children with myelomeningoceles. It may be associated with atlantoaxial instability.[18]

Congenital defects of the posterior arch of atlas may also be discovered as incidental findings.[7]

Anterior arch rachischisis is very rare and occurs only in 0.1% adult autopsy specimens. It is almost invariably encountered with posterior rachischisis, in case of which the term "split atlas" is applied[20] **(Figs. 11A and B)**.

Malformations of atlas may be confused with Jefferson fracture.[19,21] CT may help in differentiating the two entities. Margins of developmental cleft are smooth with an intact cortical edge with no abnormal soft tissue, whereas fractures have jagged edges or are comminuted and generally associated with soft tissue swelling.[22]

Dens Dysplasias

The odontoid tip normally lies approximately at the level of the superior margin of the anterior arch of atlas. Hypoplasia of the odontoid process **(Figs. 12A to C)** predisposes to atlantoaxial instability, injuries and rheumatoid complications. A hypertrophic odontoid may be viewed

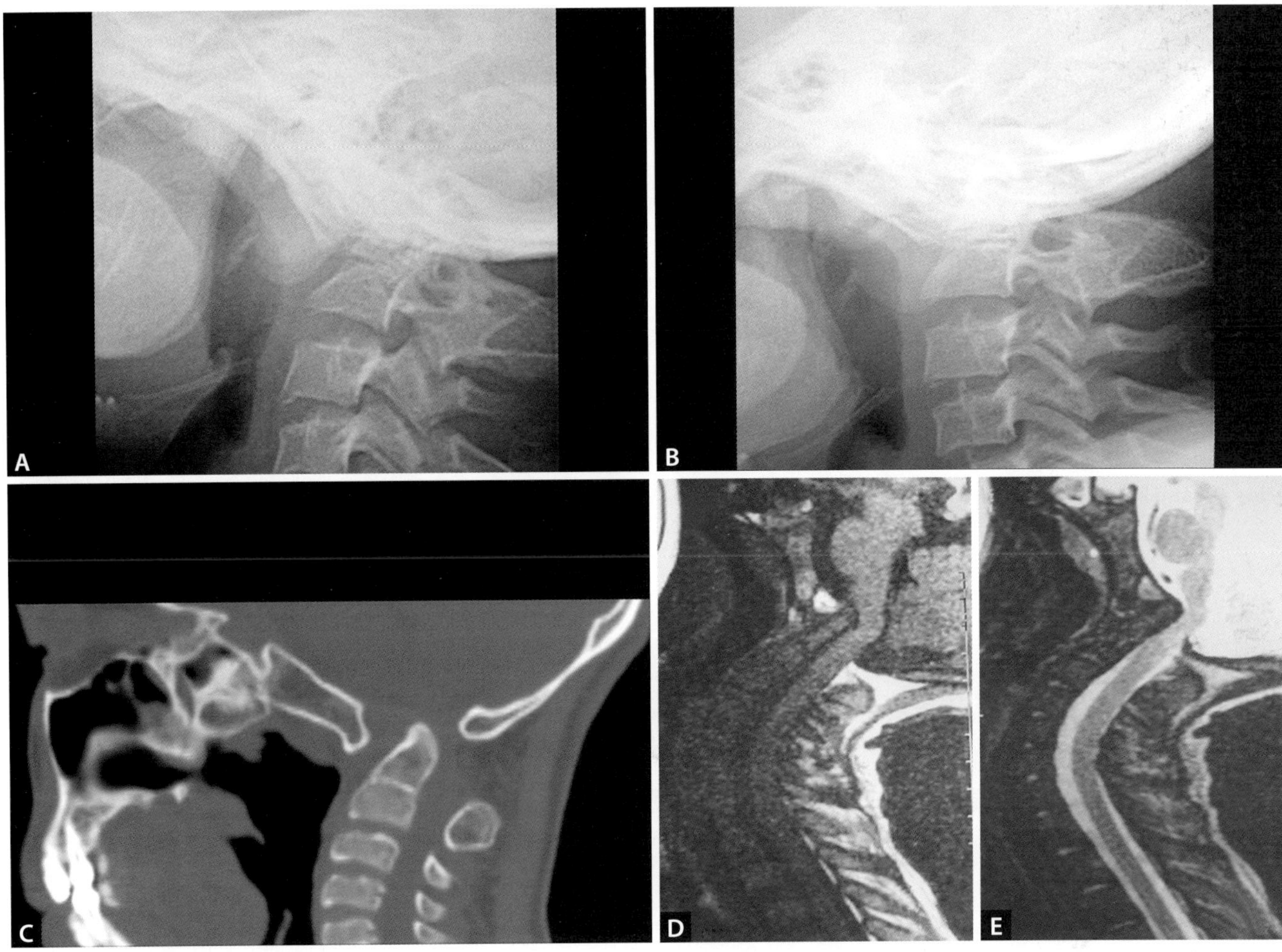

Figs. 7A to E: Basilar invagination: (A and B) Lateral cervical X-ray in extension and flexion shows high placed odontoid with narrowed spinal canal. Also note the assimilation of atlas; (C) Noncontrast CT midsagittal maximum intensity projection (MIP) confirms the high placed odontoid and complete assimilation of atlas; (D) T1W and (E) T2W sagittal images show the compression at the cervicomedullary junction.

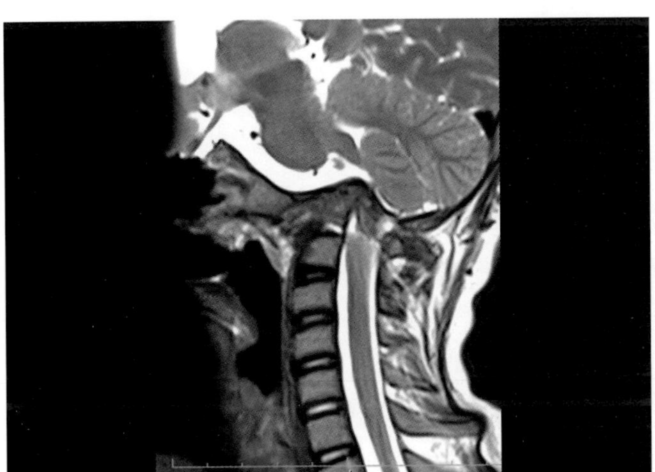

Fig. 8: Basilar invagination (BI) with basi-occiput hypoplasia—clivus is short and clivus-canal angle is typically less than 150°.

as manifestations of the occipital vertebra. Significant vascular compromise on stretching and distortion of the vertebral artery may occur with odontoid dysplasias.

Os Terminale

It refers to the nonfused terminal part of the odontoid derived from the centrum of the IVth occipital sclerotome. This apical segment is usually about 12 mm in length, but can be very small. In case of disruption at the interface and if AAD occurs, the remaining part of the odontoid may compress the cervicomedullary region.

Os Odontoideum

This denotes an independent bone seen cranial to the axis in place of the dens, which is hypoplastic. Its most common location is in the position of the normal odontoid

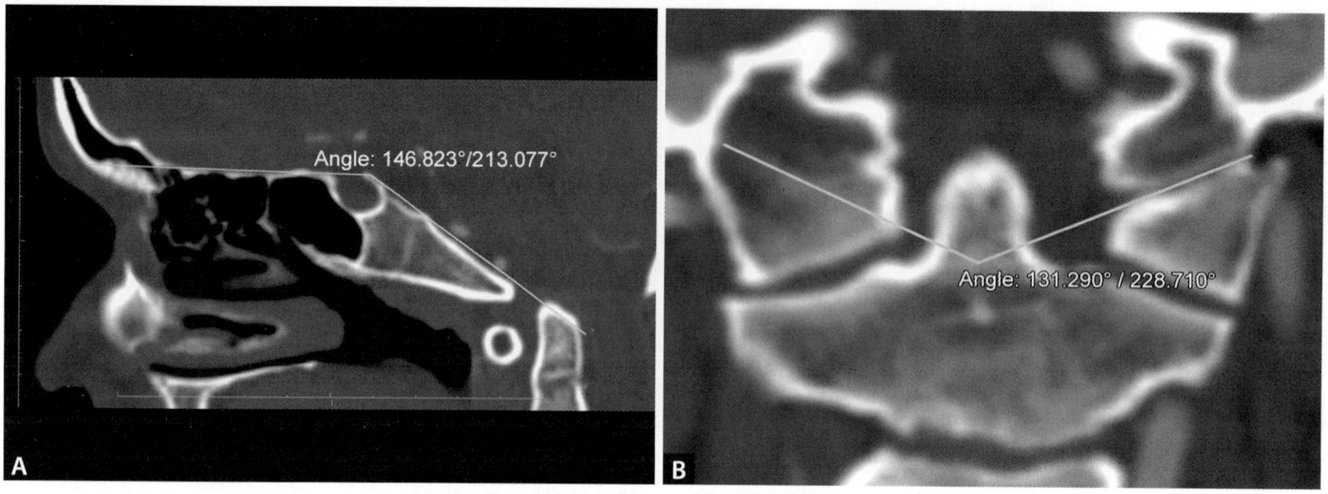

Figs. 9A and B: Platybasia may be associated with: Basilar invagination, cord symptoms, clivus-canal angle becomes acute (<150°), Welcher basal angle > 140°.

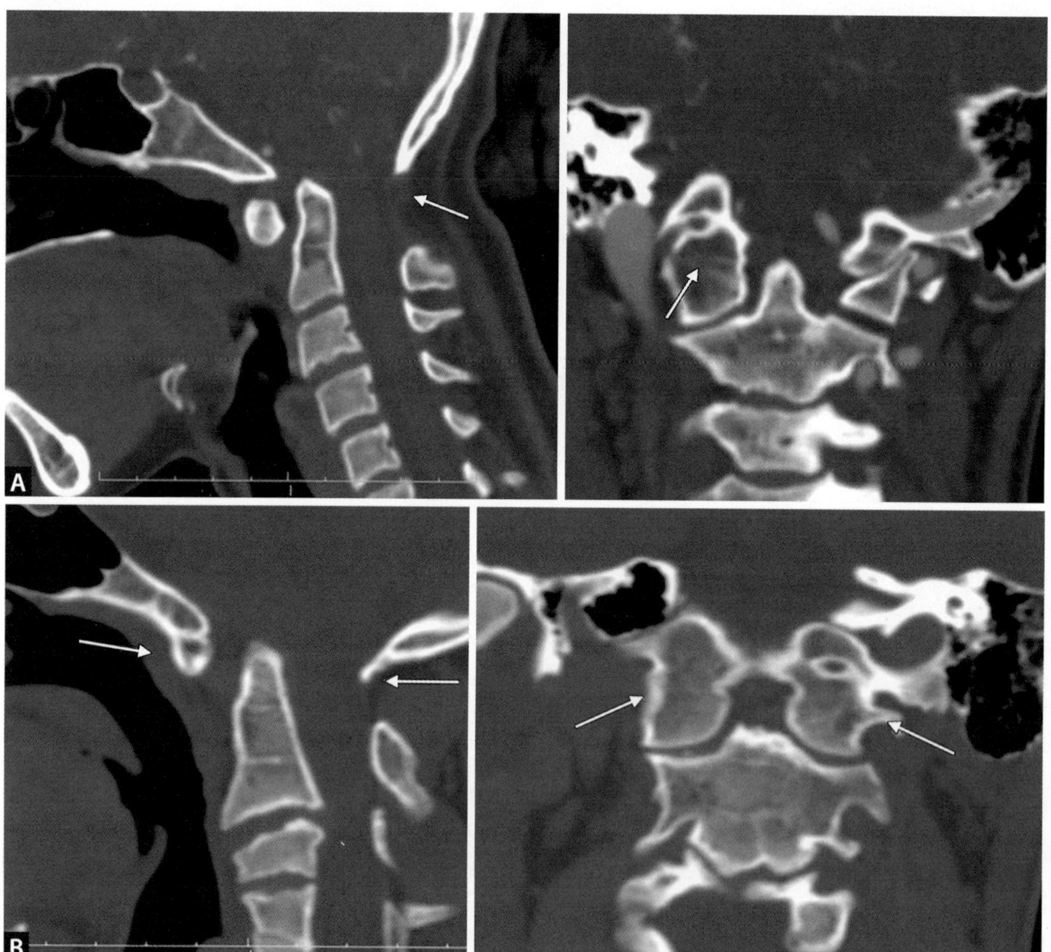

Figs. 10A and B: Assimilation of Atlas: Partial assimilation of C-1 With occiput (A). Note (arrows) pointing fusion of posterior arch with occiput and right lateral mass with occipital condyle. Complete assimilation (B) showing fusion of both anterior and posterior arch and lateral masses with occiput.

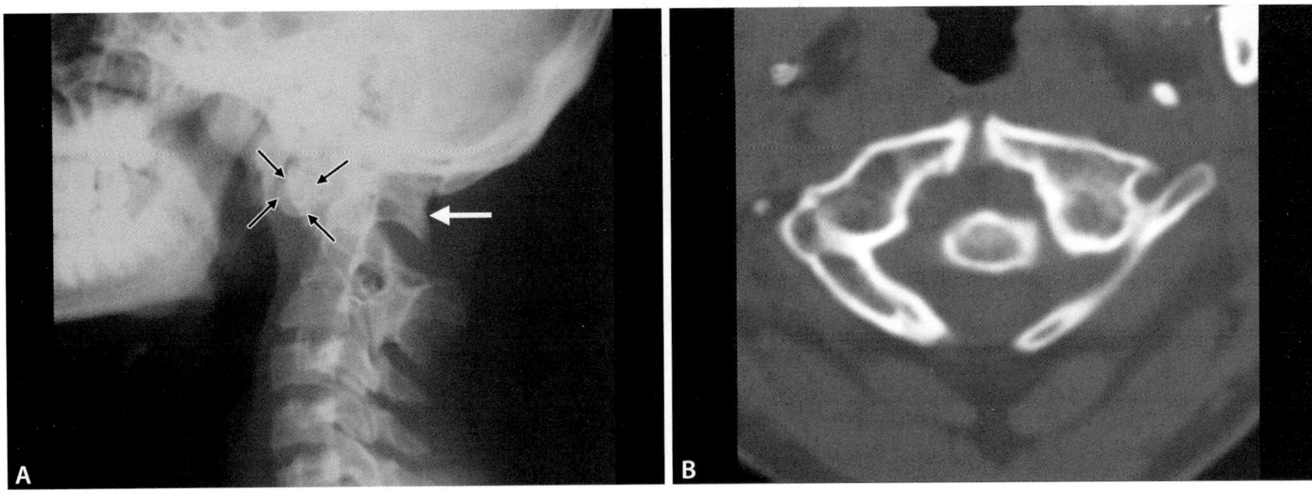

Figs. 11A and B: Split atlas: (A) Lateral cervical radiograph shows rounded, hypertrophic anterior arch of atlas without typical cortication (thin arrows) and two posterior atlas arches without visualization of a spinolaminar line (thick arrow); (B) NCCT image show presence of clefts in both anterior and posterior arch of atlas.

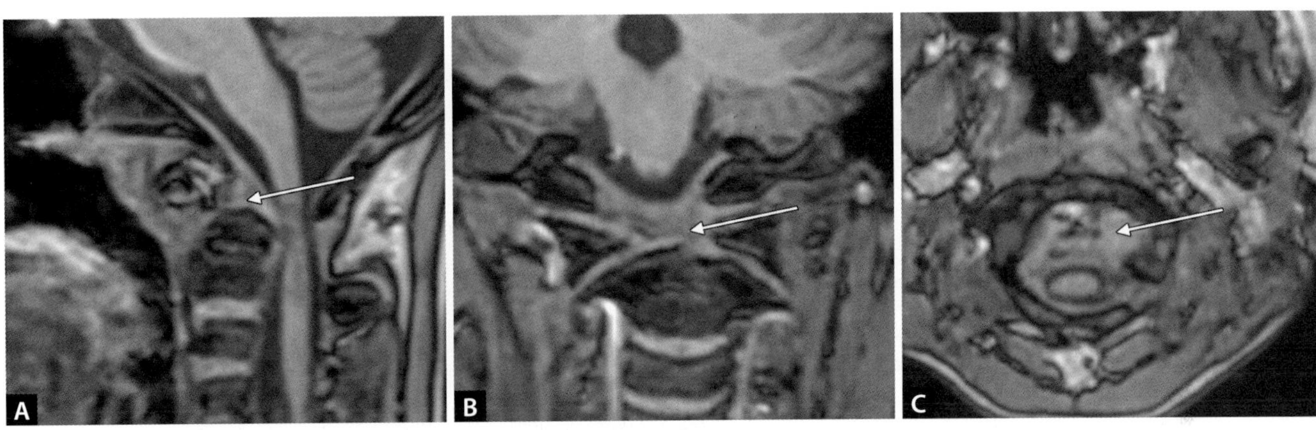

Figs. 12A to C: Odontoid hypoplasia—the odontoid process is barely seen and the attachments for the apical and alar ligaments are absent.

tip or near the base of the occiput in the area of foramen magnum, where it may fuse with the clivus. This leads to incompetence of the cruciate ligaments and atlantoaxial instability.[7] Hypertrophy of the anterior arch of C1 is often associated with Os odontoideum **(Figs. 13A to D)**. There are two hypotheses postulated congenital and traumatic in the causation of Os odontoideum. The weight of the current evidence now points to a traumatic etiology in the majority of cases of Os odontoideum.[23]

Two types of Os odontoideum are described: *Dystopic* and *Orthotopic*. In the orthotopic variety, the Os lies in the position of normal dens and moves in unison with the atlas and axis.

In the dystopic variety, the Os lies near the basion or may be fused with the occipital bone and moves in unison with the clivus. The anterior arch of the atlas is hypertrophied and the posterior arch is often hypoplastic. In the orthotopic Os odontoideum, the transverse component of the cruciate ligament is functional as there is movement in unison with atlas and axis. The incidence of Os odontoideum is increased in patients with Down's syndrome, spondyloepiphyseal dysplasia, or Morquio's syndrome. It is important to differentiate Os odontoideum from type II odontoid fracture. CT is the best modality to distinguish these two entities. In Os odontoideum, the upper margin of the body of axis is convex and may be associated with hypertrophy of anterior arch of atlas seen as enlargement, convex posterior border and increased cortical thickness **(Fig. 14A)**.

In odontoid fracture, the upper margin of axis is flattened with sharp uncorticated margin and normal appearing anterior arch **(Fig. 14B)**.[24,25]

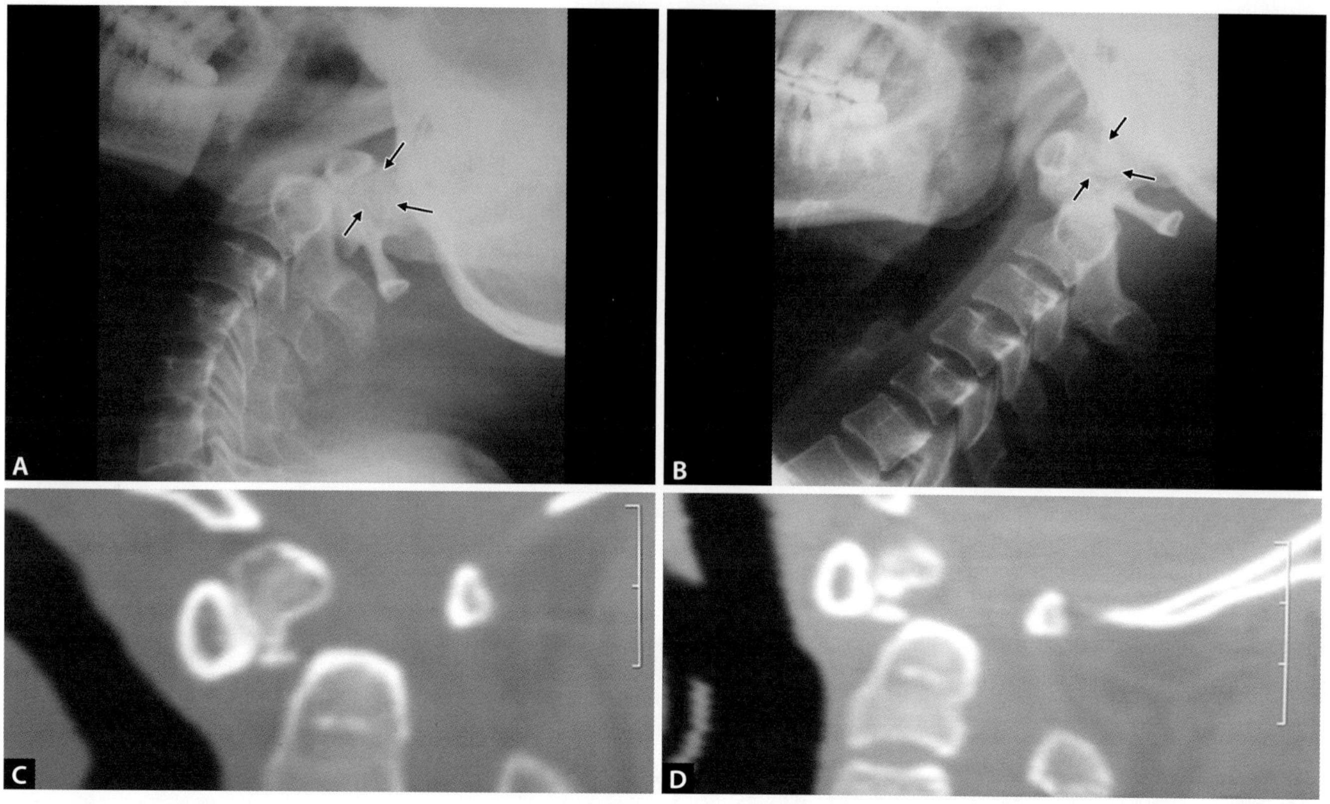

Figs. 13 A to D: Os odontoideum: (A and B) Lateral plain radiographs of craniovertebral junction (CVJ) in extension and flexion show the presence of hypoplastic odontoid process and presence of independent osseous structure (arrows) posterior to anterior arch of atlas; (C and D) Sagittal reconstruction CT image confirm the presence of well corticated smooth Os odontoideum and hypertrophied anterior arch of C1. Note a small bony fragment inferior to the Os odontoideum.

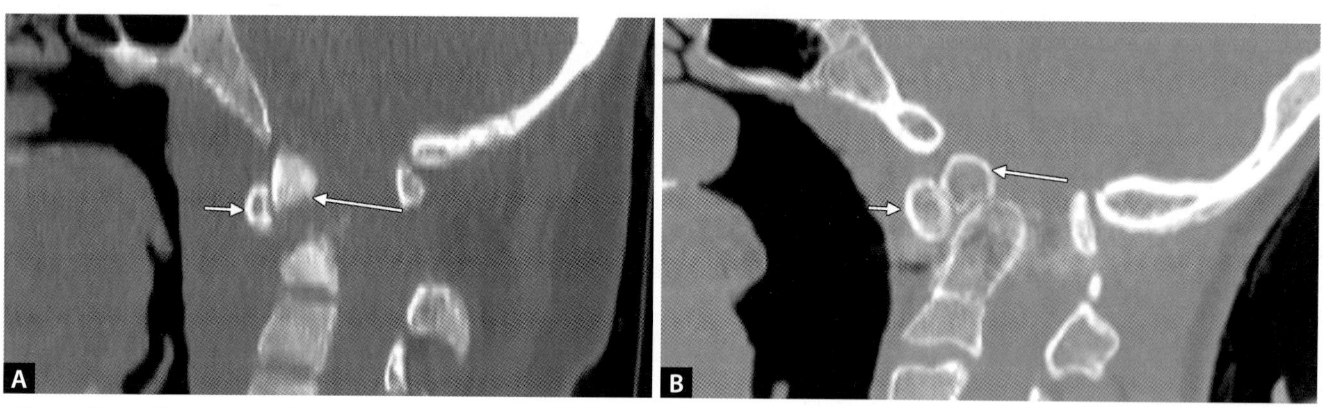

Figs. 14A and B: Odontoid fracture (A) and Os odontoideum (B). Small arrows showing normal anterior arch (A) and hypertrophied arch (B); Long arrows showing fracture with no cortex (A) and well corticated surface is Os (B).

Atlantoaxial Instability

Stability at atlantoaxial area is dependent on integrity of osseous, ligamentous and muscle complex. Instability of atlantoaxial joint can be documented by lateral cervical radiographs done in flexion and extension. The diagnosis of rupture of transverse ligaments and AAD is purely radiological. An atlas dens interval of more than 4 mm in children and more than 3 mm in adults is diagnostic. If more than 5 mm motion of anterior atlantoaxial interval is present, conclusive evidence of instability exists.

The 10–20% of children with Down's syndrome have atlantoaxial instability radiologically, and only 18%

of them are symptomatic. AAI or occipitoatlantoaxial dislocations have been reported with upper respiratory tract infection, mastoiditis, partotitis, tuberculosis, gout, seronegative arthropathy, rheumatoid arthritis and following tonsillectomy, adenoidectomy,[19] mastoidectomy and cardiac surgeries.[26]

Classification of AAI

Group I: AAI in combinations with occipitalization of atlas, fusion of C2 and C3. Odontoid is displaced posteriorly.

Group II: AAI due to incompetence of odontoid process (maldevelopment)

Type I: Os odontoideum

Type II: Ossiculum terminale

Type III: Agenesis of odontoid base

Type IV: Agenesis of apical segment Type

V: Agenesis of odontoid.

Group III: Odontoid is seen dislocated posteriorly. There is no abnormality of C1 or odontoid.

Dynamic studies (Flexion and extension) are important not only for the diagnosis but also for the management, i.e. whether the instability is fixed or mobile.[27]

Inflammatory, Arthritic and Infectious Disorders

The most common disorder in this category is rheumatoid arthritis (RA). Other disorders include psoriatic and osteoarthritis, synovial cysts and calcium pyrophosphate deposition disease (CPPD), etc.

Infectious diseases with CVJ involvement are rare and include tuberculosis and fungal infections.

In RA, cervical spine is clinically affected in 44–88% of patients.[28] Three types of abnormalities are seen: (1) AAI (25%), (2) upward migration of odontoid process or cranial settling (8–16%) and (3) rheumatoid granulation tissue or pannus formation around the odontoid process (10–30%). In cranial settling, there is erosion and compression of lateral masses of C1, downward displacement of anterior arch with cranial rotation of posterior arch of C1 resulting in upward migration of dens. The AP diameter of the cervical canal is reduced causing compression. MRI is the imaging modality of choice for the evaluation of rheumatoid pannus. The rheumatoid pannus can be of three types, i.e. hypervascular, hypovascular or fibrous types. On T2W images the hypervascular pannus is hyperintense, whereas hypovascular and fibrous pannus show intermediate and low signal intensity respectively. The hypervascular pannus and the rheumatoid joint effusion, both of which are hyperintense on T2W images can be differentiated by presence of early intense contrast enhancement in hypervascular pannus on dynamic postcontrast studies **(Figs. 15A to E)**. The hypovascular pannus shows delayed enhancement whereas fibrous type of pannus shows no enhancement on postcontrast images **(Figs. 16A to C)**.[29]

Calcium pyrophosphate crystal deposition disease which frequently involves the joints in the appendicular skeleton, has a predilection for anterior atlantoaxial joint. The transverse ligament is usually the site of involvement with presence of retro-odontoid soft tissue. The radiographic findings are usually subtle. The NCCT images show retro-odontoid calcifications and the MRI shows the retro-odontoid soft tissue that is hypointense on both T1W and T2W images with the disruption of transverse ligament at times.[30]

Tuberculosis of atlantoaxial region accounts for less than 1% of all case of spinal tuberculosis.[31] Local neck pain tenderness and restriction of neck movements are the cardinal features.

The disease is divided into three stages:

1. *Stage I*: Retropharyngeal abscess AAD/AAI
   Normal bony architecture
2. *Stage II*: Retropharyngeal abscess ± AAD mild bony destruction
3. *Stage III*: Retropharyngeal abscess ± AAD gross bony destruction

Myelo-CT or MR demonstrates the characteristic radiographic appearance of bony destruction of C1–C2 with increased prevertebral soft tissue.

TRAUMA

As discussed, the continuity of the craniocervical biomechanical is dependent on the integrity of the skull base, atlas, and axis and their attaching ligaments. Initially, most of the trauma patients undergo conventional radiography. However NCCT is now the mainstay in imaging of the trauma for bone and high resolution MRI for the soft tissue. Trauma can cause fractures of clivus, C-1, C-2 vertebrae either in isolation or in combinations. An abnormal distance between the dens or posterior axial line and the basion suggests failure or insufficiency of the alar ligaments, tectorial membrane, or both. Increased atlantoaxial distance, which should be less than 4 mm in children under 9 years of age and less than 3 mm in adults, points to injury of the transverse ligament. On the open-mouth view of the CVJ, the lateral masses of

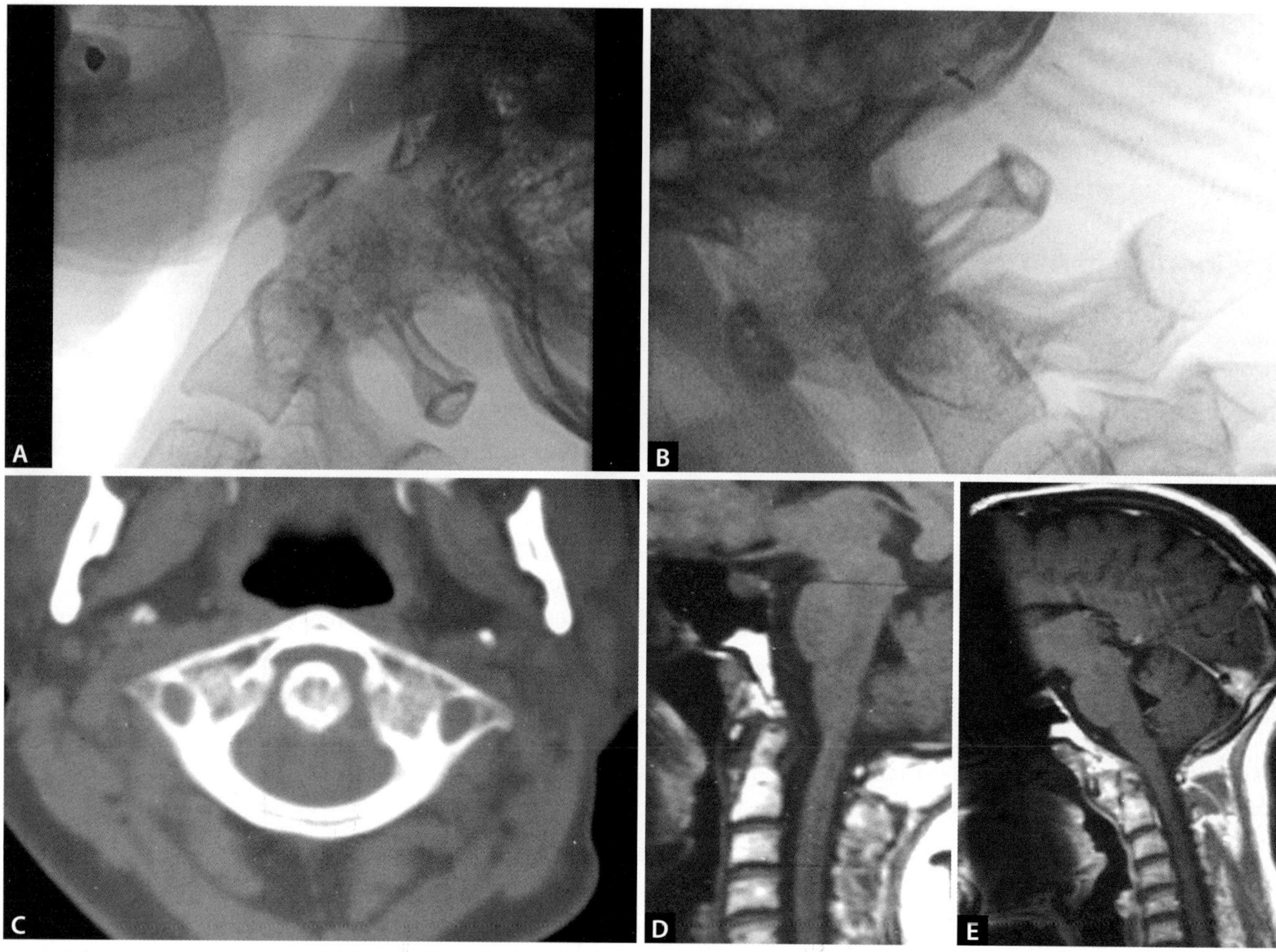

Figs. 15A to E: Rheumatoid arthritis of the CVJ: (A and B) Lateral cervical X-rays show minimally increased predental interval in extension position which is more marked in flexion position; (C) CT axial image showing the increased anterior atlantoaxial distance and erosions of odontoid process; (D) Sagittal spin echo precontrast and (E) postcontrast T1W images showing presence of predental hypointense soft tissue that is showing intense postcontrast enhancement.

C1 should align exactly with the lateral margins of C2 vertebra. CT with sagittal and coronal reformatted images permits optimal detection and evaluation of fracture and subluxation. The atlanto-occipital and atlantoaxial articulations should be congruent on both coronal and sagittal reformatted images. Fractures of the tip of the dens or of the occipital condyles may be associated with alar ligament insufficiency. Subarachnoid hemorrhage and epidural hematoma may accompany injuries to the craniocervical junction.[32]

The most common bone involved in the fractures of this region is odontoid process. Conventionally, its fractures are classified into three types—Type-I, if there is avulsion of the tip **(Fig. 17)**; Type-II, if there is fracture of the body of the odontoid process **(Figs. 18A to E)** and Type-III if the odontoid process is fractured along with base of C-2.

Magnetic resonance imaging of the cervical spine with fat-suppressed gradient-echo T2W or STIR sequences can display an increased signal intensity in the atlantoaxial and atlanto-occipital joints, craniocervical ligaments, prevertebral soft tissues, and the spinal cord **(Figs. 19A and B)**. Axial gradient-echo MRIs may be prominently useful in assessing the integrity of the transverse atlantal ligament.[33,34]

Conventional radiography and CT findings in AAD include prevertebral soft-tissue swelling, C1-C2 dislocation or subluxation, and widening of the C1-C2 facets. MRI findings consist of prevertebral, interspinous, or nuchal ligament edema as well as facet widening or fluid, possible epidural hematoma, and increased signal intensity of the spinal cord on T2W or STIR images. The various types of CVJ injuries is been discussed elsewhere in this book.

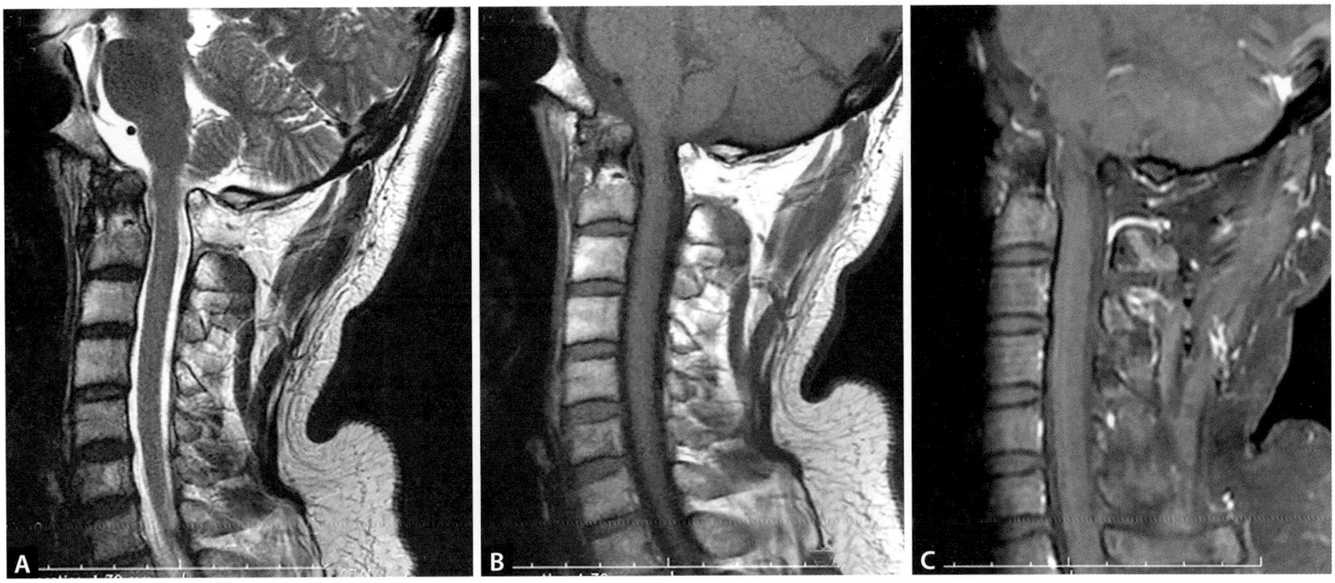

Figs. 16A to C: Chronic RA with hypointense soft tissue at the CVJ without any enhancement.

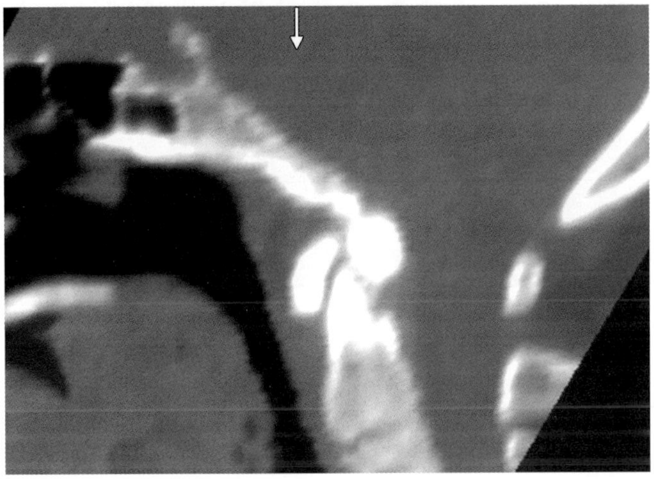

Fig. 17: Type-I odontoid fracture with avulsion fracture of the tip of the odontoid process.

SYNDROMES INVOLVING THE CVJ[35]

Klippel-Feil Syndrome

The classic triad consists of a low posterior hairline, short neck and limitation of neck movement. The syndrome is associated with fused vertebrae (usually C2-3 and C5-6 interfaces), hemivertebra, spina bifida occulta and scoliosis. Along with the vertebral segmentation anomalies, many CVJ anomalies are often present including basilar invagination, atlanto-occipital assimilation, odontoid hypoplasia platybasia, and Chiari I malformation. Associated congenital anomalies include urogenital anomalies, otological anomalies, cleft palate, etc. Syndactyly, Sprengel's shoulder and absence of ulna are common **(Figs. 19A and B)**.

Down Syndrome

Down syndrome or trisomy 21, the most frequent of the chromosomal disorders, is frequently complicated by atlanto- occipital instability (61%) as well as atlantoaxial instability (9–30%). Other observed osseous abnormalities comprise of persistent synchondroses, posterior C1 rachischisis and Os odontoideum.

Arnold-Chiari Malformation

The Arnold-Chiari malformations (ACM), type I through III, are a group of disorders characterized by increasing degrees of hindbrain dysgenesis. Each may be associated with deformities of the CVJ.

Chiari I Malformation

In cases with this disorder the vermis, fourth ventricle and medulla are normal or very slightly deformed. Elongated pointed peg-like cerebellar tonsils are displaced inferiorly through the foramen magnum into the upper cervical spinal canal. A syrinx is present in 20–40% of all patients with Chiari I, which increase to 60–90% in symptomatic patients.

Osseous anomalies are seen in 25% patients in the form of basilar invaginations (25–50%) Klippel-Feil anomaly (5–10%) **(Figs. 20A to C)** and atlanto-occipital assimilation (1–5%).[20]

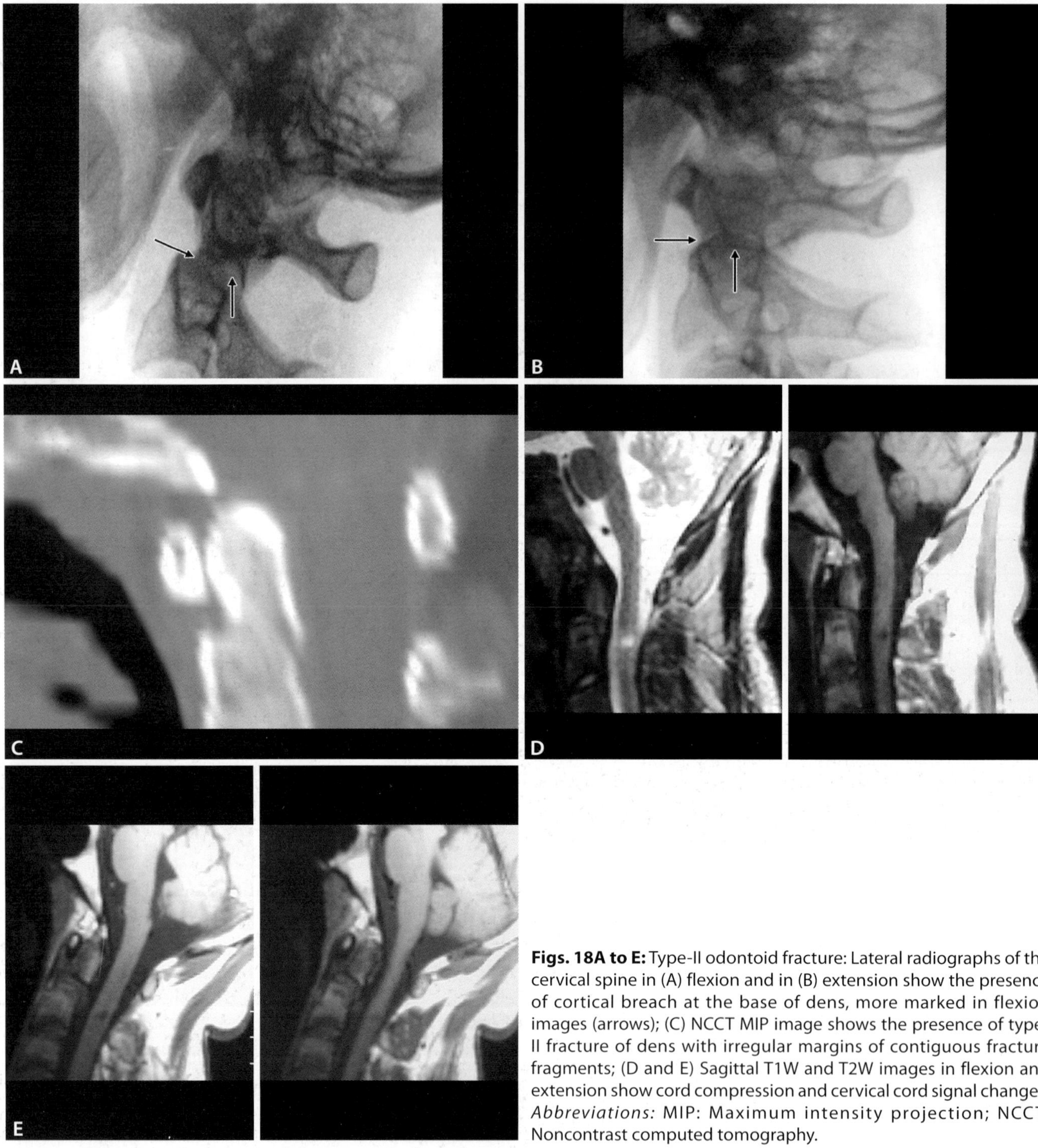

Figs. 18A to E: Type-II odontoid fracture: Lateral radiographs of the cervical spine in (A) flexion and in (B) extension show the presence of cortical breach at the base of dens, more marked in flexion images (arrows); (C) NCCT MIP image shows the presence of type-II fracture of dens with irregular margins of contiguous fracture fragments; (D and E) Sagittal T1W and T2W images in flexion and extension show cord compression and cervical cord signal changes. *Abbreviations:* MIP: Maximum intensity projection; NCCT: Noncontrast computed tomography.

Presently research is being done to better understand the cause of syrinx formation in patients where there is no direct cord compression. For this researchers have used phase-contrast line MRI to calculate and study CSF flow across Foramen Magnum. During cardiac systole the CSF goes down the spinal canal across the F Magnum and during diastole the reverse happens. This occurs due to relative increase and decrease of the cerebral blood vessels during the cardiac cycle which affects the CSF flow. It has been observed that in majority of these patients there is abnormality of this normal CSF flow **(Fig. 21)**.[36-38]

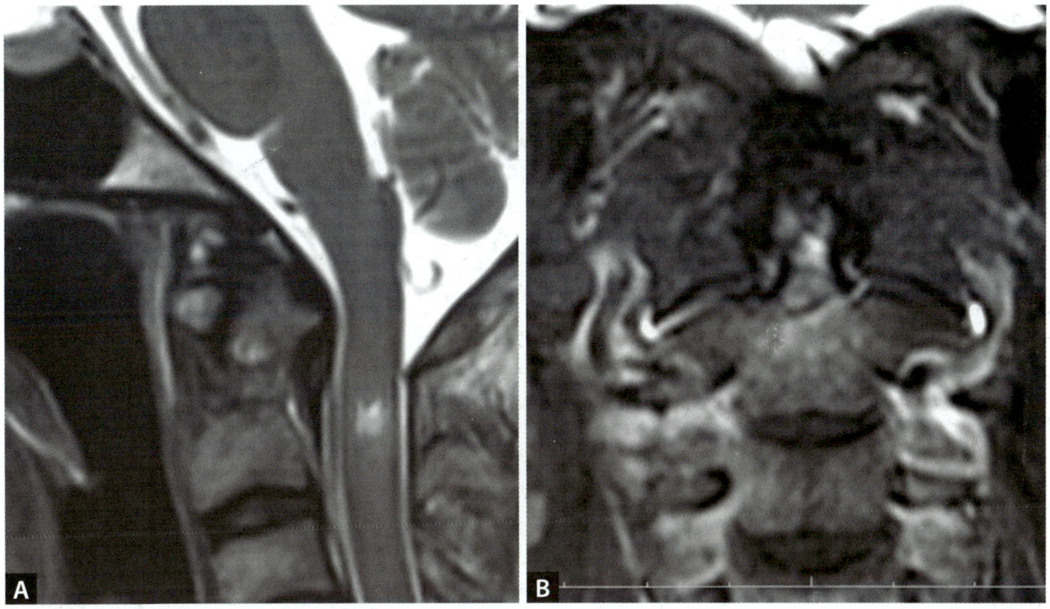

Figs. 19A and B: Type-II fracture showing cord contusion on T2WI and marrow edema on the STIR image.

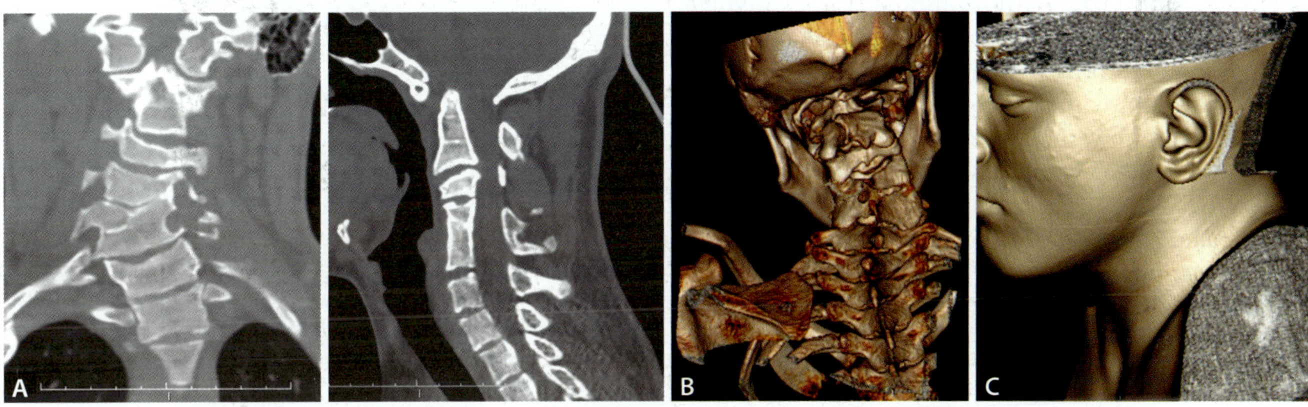

Figs. 20A to C: Klippel-Feil syndrome: Young patient showing multiple vertebral anomalies (A), Sprengel's shoulder (B), and short neck (C).

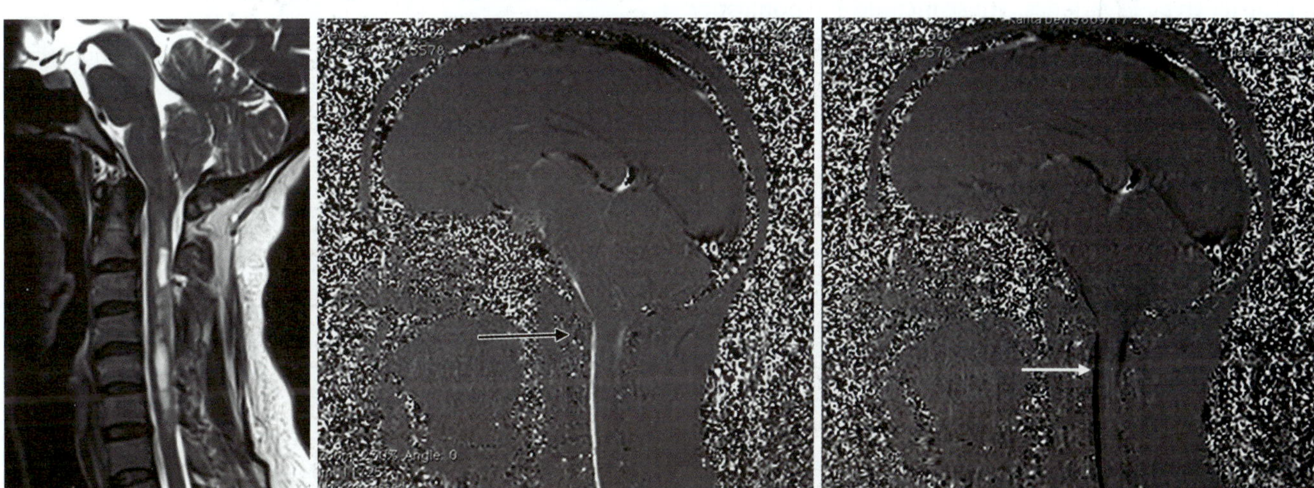

Figs. 21: Arnold Chiari Type-I with syrinx: Phase-contrast cine MRI showing downward (black arrow) and upward flow of the CSF (white arrow).

Chiari II Malformation

This is characterized by herniation of the inferior portions of the vermis, fourth ventricle and medulla into the spinal canal, kinking and displacing normal structures. It is associated with small posterior fossa, low lying transverse sutures, concave clivus and petrous ridges and fenestrate falx. The other associations include myelomeningocele (95–100%), hydrocephalus (90%) syringohydromyelia (50–90%) and segmentation anomalies (<10%).

Chiari III Malformation

This is defined as herniation of the hindbrain associated with occipital encephalocele in combination with many of the features of the Chiari II malformation. MR is the best modality to visualize the various anomalies of ACM.

Achondroplasia

Achondroplasia is the most common of the short-limbed dwarfisms. The radiographic abnormalities involve the regions in which the growth and development occur primarily through enchondral ossification. The foramen magnum is constricted and has a distinct tear drop configuration with obliteration of the surrounding subarachnoid space. Other CVJ abnormalities include odontoid dysplasia, basiocciput hypoplasia, decrease in the basal angle and thickening of the posterior rim of the foramen magnum.

Mucopolysaccharidoses

Mucopolysaccharidoses are inherited lysosomal storage disorders. Abnormalities at the CVJ are a major cause of morbidity and mortality especially in Morquio (type IV) and Hurler (type I) varieties. These include a hypoplastic/dysplastic odontoid process, ligamentous instability, soft-tissue thickening around the dens, and compression of the cord by the posterior atlas arch. The soft-tissue mass around the dens is typically hypointense or isointense on T1W and hypointense on T2W MRIs which may represent nonossified fibrocartilage.

Osteogenesis Imperfecta

Osteogenesis imperfecta, is a hereditary disorder which is the result of a defect in collagen production leading to osteoporosis. Pathology at the CVJ is most commonly seen in type IV, with a prevalent in the range of rare to 25%. The osteoporotic bones result in repetitive microfractures causing infolding of the occipital condyles with elevation of the clivus and the posterior cranial fossa, accompanied by an upward migration of the cervical spine into the foramen magnum (basilar impression).

SUMMARY

There has been renewed interest in the CVJ anomalies with the growth of 3D CT and magnetic resonance. Both the acquired and congenital pathologies are readily diagnosed using these modalities. MR in association with either plain X-rays or 3D CT would be ideal in the evaluation of CVJ anomalies.

REFERENCES

1. Johnson MH, Smoker WR. Lesions of the craniovertebral junction. Neuroimaging Clin N Am. 1994;4:599-17.
2. Menezes AH. Bony anomalies of the craniovertebral junction. In: Pang D (Ed): Disorders of Paediatrics Spine. Raven Press, New York. 1995. pp. 97-100.
3. Menezes AH, Traynelis VC. Anatomy and biomechanics of normal craniovertebral junction (a) and biomechanics of stabilization (b). Childs Nerv Syst. 2008;24:1091-100.
4. Smoker WR. Craniovertebral Junction: Normal anatomy, craniometry, and congenital aomalies. Radiographics. 1994;14:255-7.
5. Menezes AH. Craniocervical developmental anatomy and its implications. Childs Nerv Syst. 2008;24:1109-22.
6. Martin MD, Bruner HJ, Maiman DJ. Anatomic and biomechanical considerations of the craniovertebral junction. Neurosurgery. 2010;66:2-6.
7. Menezes AH. Congenital and acquired abnormalities of the craniovertebral junction. In Youmans Neurological Surgery. WB Saunders. 1996;4:1035-89.
8. Penning L. Normal movements of the cervical spine. AJR. 1978;130:317-26.
9. Sambasivan M. Anatomy of the craniovertebral anomalies. Progress in Clinical Neurosciences. 1988;1:81-100.
10. Dolan KD. Cervicobasilar relationships. RCNA. 1977;15: 155-66.
11. Rao VR, Gupta AK. Imaging of craniovertebral anomalies. Progress in Clinical Neurosciences. 1989;2:229-56.
12. Menezes AH. Craniovertebral junction database analysis: incidence, classification, presentation, and treatment algorithms. Childs Nerv Syst. 2008;24:1101-8.
13. Chopra JS, Sawhey IM, Kak VK, et al. Analysis of 82 cases of craniovertebra anomalies. Br J Neurosurg. 1988;2:455-63.
14. Gupta V, Khandelwal N, Mathuria SN, et al. Dynamic magnetic resonance imaging evaluation of craniovertebral junction abnormalities. J Comput Assist Tomogr. 2007;31:354-9.
15. Dilorenzo N, Fortuna A, Guidetti B. Cranio-vertebral junction malformation: clinico-radiological findings, long-term results and surgical indication in 63 cases. Neurosurgery. 1982;57:603-8.
16. Kuroiwa T, Tanabe H, Hasegawa T. Traumatic basilar impression. Surg Neurol. 1995;44:31-2.

17. Mc Rae DL, Barnum AS. Occipitalization of the atlas. AJR. 1953;70:23-46.
18. Smoker WR. Congenital anomalies of the cervical spine. Neuroimaging Clinics of North America. 1995;5:427-49.
19. Dyste GN, Menezes AH. Symptomatic Chiari malformation: an analysis of presentation, management and long-term outcome. J Neurosurg. 1989;71:159-68.
20. Zonneveld FW, Lobregt S, Meulen JC, et al. Three dimensional imaging in craniofacial surgery. World J Surg. 1989;13:328-42.
21. Wackenheim A. Occipitalization of the vertebral part and vertebralization of the dorsal part of atlas with insufficiency of the transverse ligament. Neuroradiology. 1982;24:45-7.
22. Gehweiler JA, Daffner RH, Robert SL. Malformation of the atlas simulating the Jefferson fractures. AJNR. 1983;4:187-90.
23. Babak A, Gosselin MP, Fehlings MJ. Os Odontoideum: etiology and surgical management. Neurosurgery. 2010;66:22-31.
24. Holt RG, Helms CA, Munk PL, et al. Hypertrophy of C1 anterior arch: useful sign to distinguish OS odontoideum from acute dens fracture. Radiology. 1989;173:207-9.
25. Menezes AH. Os odontoideum pathogenesis dynamics and management. Paed Neurosurg. 1988;8:133-45.
26. Onerci M, Ogretmenoglu O, Ozcan OE. Atlanto-axial subluxation after tonsillectomy and adenoidectomy. Otolanyg Head Neck Surg. 1997;116:271-3.
27. Gupta SK, Khosla VK, Sharma BS, et al. Cranio-vertebral junction anomalies–PGI Chandigarh experience, In the proceedings of "Cranio-vertebral junction anomalies. The Indian experience". In: Jain VK, Behari S (Eds). 1998. pp. 176-8.
28. Foster HE, Carins RA, Burnell RH. Atlantoaxial subluxation in children with seronegative enthesiopathy and arthropathy syndrome. J Rheumatol. 1995;22:548-51.
29. Stiskal MA, Neuhold A, Szolar H, et al. Rheumatoid arthritis of the craniocervical region by MR Imaging: detection and characterization. AJR. 1995;165:585-92.
30. Kakitsubata Y, Boutin RD, Theodorou DJ, et al. Calcium pyrophosphate dihydrate crystal deposition in and around the atlantoaxial joint: association with type 2 odontoid fractures in nine patients. Radiology. 2000;216:213-9.
31. Khandelwal N, Khosla VK, Malik N, et al. Tuberculous atlanto-axial dislocation. Neuroradiology (Supp). 1991;33:1060-8.
32. Anastasia VD, Alexander B, Julian A, et al. Radiologic spectrum of craniocervical distraction injuries. Radiographics. 2000;20:S237-50.
33. Warner J, Shanmuganathan K, Mirvis SE, et al. Magnetic resonance imaging of ligamentous injury of the cervical spine. Emerg Radiol. 1996;3:9-15.
34. Dickman CA, Memourian A, Sonntag VK, et al. Magnetic resonance imaging of the transverse atlantal ligament for the evaluation of atlantoaxial instability. J Neurosurg. 1991;75:221-7.
35. Smoker WR, Khanna G. Imaging the craniocervical junction. Childs Nerv Syst. 2008;24:1123-45.
36. Linge SO, Haughton V, Løvgren AE, et al. CSF flow dynamics at the craniovertebral junction studied with an idealized model of the subarachnoid space and computational flow analysis. Am J Neuroradiol. 2010;31(1):185-92.
37. Linge SO, Mardal KA, Haughton V, et al. Simulating CSF flow dynamics in the normal and the Chiari I subarachnoid space during rest and exertion. Am J Neuroradiol. 2013 Jan;34(1):41-5.
38. Ozsoy KM, Oktay K, Cetinalp NE, et al. The role of cine flow magnetic resonance imaging in patients with Chiari 0 malformation. Turk Neurosurg. 2018;28(2):251-6.

CHAPTER 29

Endovascular Management of Craniofacial Vascular Lesions

Ajay Kumar, Niranjan Khandelwal, Chirag Kamal Ahuja

INTRODUCTION

Craniofacial vascular lesions comprise a wide variety of lesions ranging from vascular malformations, arterial and venous injuries to vascular tumors. Due to their heterogeneity, no standardized categorization or classification exists. The workup of these lesions includes an elaborate evaluation of the clinical symptomatology, astute physical examination and appropriate imaging assessment. Magnetic resonance imaging (MRI) currently forms the gold standard for the evaluation of these lesions. Minimally invasive techniques of endovascular and percutaneous interventions have transformed the way these lesions are being treated currently. Interventional radiology can potentially offer cure in certain lesions like slow flow venous malformations, lymphovenous malformations and traumatic vascular injuries. In other lesions like high flow arteriovenous malformation and hypervascular tumors, embolization may be performed prior to surgical excision. The current chapter will discuss these lesions under the heads tabulated in **Table 1**.

Table 1: Classification of craniofacial vascular lesions.

• *Hypervascular tumors (tumors with significant vascularity)*: – Juvenile nasopharyngeal angiofibroma (JNA) – Paraganglioma – Meningioma – Esthesioneuroblastoma, etc.
• *Vascular malformation*: – Arterial with or without fistula – Capillary – Capillarovenous – Venous – Lymphangiomas – Hemolymphangiomas
• *Vascular tumors*: – Hemangiomas 1. Capillary 2. Cavernous – Hemangiopericytoma – Hemangioendothelioma – Kaposi's sarcoma – Angiosarcoma

Embolization Techniques

Embolization of hypervascular tumors and arteriovenous malformations (AVMs) in the head and neck is a well-established therapeutic modality. Preoperative embolization reduces intraoperative blood loss, shortens surgical time and decreases surgical morbidity and mortality. Furthermore, intraoperative hemorrhage renders incomplete resection of a lesion with an increased risk of recurrence. Embolization as the sole treatment of AVM can be either curative or palliative for symptoms such as pain or mass effect. Treatment of craniofacial vascular lesions assumes a special importance because of their close relationship with the vital structures. Surgical procedure is sometimes extensive and causes esthetic changes and loss of function of important structures. Endovascular interventional techniques offer an alternate mode of treatment either as a definitive therapy or as an adjunct to conventional surgical techniques.[1]

Recent advances in the technology of catheters and guidewire systems have allowed superselective catheterization and targeted embolization. Direct access to many head and neck lesions is possible through percutaneous and intraoral routes and embolization can be carried out under fluoroscopic guidance.[2,3] Injection of the embolic agent with a microcatheter wedged into the nidus may lead to permanent devascularization of an AVM without risk of ischemia of the adjacent normal tissue. Cross-sectional imaging modalities like US and CT have led to further advancement by providing accurate guidance. Open MR units with real time MR imaging (MR fluoroscopy) and availability of MR compatible needles will further increase the scope of treatment in lesions that are poorly visualized by other imaging modalities.

EMBOLIC AGENTS

The choice of embolic agent depends upon the goal of the procedure, the extent of selective catheterization and angioarchitecture of the lesion. These are divided into solid particles or liquid agents by their physical characteristics and into absorbable, nonabsorbable or cytotoxic agents by their biological behaviors **(Table 2)**.[4]

Gelfoam and avitene are collagen-based materials that are reabsorbable and recanalization of the embolized vessel usually occurs within 7–21 days. Gelfoam can be powdered to fine particles to embolize capillary or precapillary bed of tumors whereas the more proximal vessels are embolized by larger particles. It is mixed with contrast medium to allow direct visualization of the embolized vascular bed. It is readily available and easy to use. It is suitable for temporary embolization (e.g. epistaxis, traumatic arterial hemorrhage) and for preoperative tumor embolization to reduce blood loss. But the only shortcoming with gelfoam is that the sizes of particles are not homogeneous.

Table 2: Embolic agents commonly used in head and neck embolization.

Absorbable (biodegradable) • Gelfoam powder/particles • Autologous clot
Nonabsorbable (particulate) • Polyvinyl alcohol foam/particles (PVA) • Detachable balloons/metallic coils
Nonabsorbable (liquids) • Isobutyl 1-2 cyanoacrylate (IBCA) • N-butyl cyanoacrylate (NBCA) • Onyx
• Cytotoxic agents • Ethanol (95%) • Chemotherapeutic agents

Polyvinyl alcohol (PVA) particles are similar to collagen-based agents in that they may be mixed with contrast material, injected through the catheter and carried by blood flow into the distal vascular bed. They are nonabsorbable but their irregular shape allows some recanalization. The latter property undermines its advantage as permanent embolic agents especially in AVMs and arteriovenous fistulas (AVFs) where permanent occlusion is essential. It is available in 150–1,000 μm sizes and is suitable in preoperative devascularization. On the contrary to gelfoam, their size is precise and homogeneous.

Detachable balloons and metallic coils are used for the occlusion of large vessels and aneurysms. Detachable balloons can be of silicone or latex type. These can be deflated, repositioned or removed prior to final deployment and therefore offer flexibility in usage. Metallic coil is available in almost any shape and size with or without attached fibers to increase thrombogenicity and can also be custom made. Electrolytically and mechanically detachable coils may also allow repositioning or removal prior to deployment. However, these materials have little role in preoperative devascularization and may even be contraindicated.[4]

Liquid embolizing materials like isobutyl-2-cyanoacrylate (IBCA), n-butyl cyanoacrylate (n-BCA) and ethanol are becoming more popular because they can cause permanent occlusion of the vessels and are easy to handle. NBCA glue is liquid embolic material of choice as it is easily available, cheap, easy to handle and can be prepared in desired concentration (as contrast to onyx). The dangerous drawback is the high risk of catheter entrapment due to its fast polymerization.

Ethanol is a suitable agent when tissue necrosis in addition to devascularization is required specially in venous malformation,[5] in malignant or aggressive tumors. Chemoembolization is an attractive method because of its ability to provide very high concentrations of cytotoxic drugs at the site of tumor which may eliminate the systemic side effects. Time released microcapsules have been developed which have a very promising role in both hypervascular and hypovascular tumors.[4]

Onyx is a less adhesive liquid embolic agent containing ethylene vinyl alcohol copolymer, dimethyl sulfoxide (DMSO) and tantalum. The advantage of onyx is that it is less adhesive and can be injected slowly for a prolonged duration through intra-arterial and direct percutaneous access. Onyx first forms an embolic cast within the vascular structures and then, unlike n-BCA, permeates with each injection following the path of least resistance. This leads to embolization of large area in single sitting through single feeder.

The disadvantages of onyx are high cost, catheter entrapment due to proximal reflux, pain and discomfort during injections and skin discoloration.[6]

PRETHERAPEUTIC EVALUATION

Multidisciplinary approach is the key to optimize the analysis and treatment strategy related to the management of a specific case. A detailed clinical examination and presurgical evaluation is essential. Contrast enhanced CT/MRI provides information regarding the lesion, bone and soft tissue extension and extension to orbit or cavernous sinus.[4]

Doppler examination prior to embolization may be performed whenever it is possible. It gives information about flow dynamics (high/low flow), arterial or venous pattern, lesion architecture and presence of AVFs. It helps in the decision making for percutaneous approach and postembolization follow-up.

Dedicated diagnostic angiography and its detailed evaluation is the most important exercise prior to any attempt at intervention. Superselective catheterization where ever necessary should be performed. These steps determine the contribution of individual vessels to the lesion, ascertain the compartmentalization within the lesion and identify potentially dangerous anastomosis between the vessels supplying the lesion and the internal carotid or vertebral arteries. Determination of compartmentalization is important as different compartments function as hemodynamically independent units. Provocative testing is used to obtain information regarding the adequacy of collateral circulation in cases where it is planned to sacrifice a major vessel or inadvertent occlusion of major vessel is apprehended during the embolization procedure. Provocative testing in the region of interest can be performed by injection of lidocaine through the microcatheter prior to embolization. Lidocaine without preservative (e.g. methylparaben) is used. If the test demonstrates a deficit, then either more superselective catheter position or an embolic material that occludes vessels larger than the vasa nervosa should be used (150–200 μm).[7] A combination of clinical neurologic examination, electroencephalography (EEG) monitoring and blood flow imaging such as positron emission tomography (PET), xenon CT and single-photon emission computerized tomography (SPECT), can be employed to evaluate tolerance of vessel occlusion.[8] Stump pressure monitoring of the vessel proximal to the one planned to be occluded and hypotensive challenge have also been advocated during test occlusion.

IMPORTANT ANATOMIC CONSIDERATIONS

Transarterial embolization in external carotid artery (ECA) territory has major role in endovascular management of epistaxis, skull base tumors and arteriovenous malformation. It appears safe during endovascular embolization in ECA territory than in internal carotid artery (ICA) territory; however there are potential anastomotic routes which can cause significant neurological complication such as blindness or cranial nerve palsies. There are three important regions along skull base which constitute potential anastomoses between ECA and ICA system. The orbital, the petrocavernous and the upper cervical region.

The branches of internal maxillary artery have anastomoses with ophthalmic and petrocavernous ICA. Branches of both ascending pharyngeal and occipital artery have anastomoses with the vertebrobasilar system. Most of these anastomotic channels may not be visualized on routine catheter angiography but may start filling during the course of embolization.

During embolization procedures the penetration capacity of particles (Gelfoam and PVA) is dependent on size. In general, the size of these nonvisualized anastomotic vessels are 50–80 μm therefore particles that are >160 μm will not penetrate these channels. Liquid embolic materials (NBCA and onyx) can open and enter small anastomotic channels and therefore should be used with increased caution. Knowledge of potential anastomotic routes and proper choice of embolic material are crucial to avoid embolic complication to brain and cranial nerves.[9]

POSTEMBOLIZATION CARE

It includes the routine care following diagnostic angiography. Cerebral and/or ophthalmic complications may occur in 0.5–1% of cases and require rigorous treatment like in acute stroke. Postembolization soft tissue swelling occurs within 24 hours and usually resolves spontaneously in a few days; corticosteroids, postural drainage or IV diuretics may help. Skin necrosis, if occurs in skin that is going to be part of the resection, needs no special attention; in other areas grafting may be needed. The need for follow-up angiography will depend upon individual primary problems **(Table 3)**.[10]

NASOPHARYNGEAL ANGIOFIBROMAS

It is the most common benign nasopharyngeal tumor. It occurs almost exclusively in adolescent males, and is rarely reported in females and adults. It is highly vascular, locally

Table 3: Various lesions amenable to embolization.

• *Preoperative devascularization*: – Nasopharyngeal angiofibroma – Paraganglioma – Meningioma – Schwannoma – Esthesioneuroblastoma – Hypervascular metastatic tumor – Hypervascular soft tissue/bony tumor
• *Definitive therapy*: – Hemangioma – AVM/AVF – Aneurysm/Pseudoaneurysm – Epistaxis

invasive and extends into the surrounding compartments like infratemporal fossa, orbit or cranium. The common presenting symptoms are nasal obstruction and recurrent epistaxis. Cross-sectional imaging (CT and MR) demonstrates the complete extent of the tumor. MR is superior to CT because of its ability to demonstrate the extent of local invasion and intracranial extension. Diagnosis is usually made based on clinical features and imaging findings; biopsy is contraindicated because of the risk of uncontrollable bleeding.

Intrasellar, intracavernous and extra cavernous-intracerebral extension is evaluated using a frontal transorbital projection. Late phase of internal carotid angiogram verifies the patency of cavernous sinus. Surgical removal of tumor is the best therapeutic option, but the limiting factors are intraoperative bleeding, the size of tumor and intracranial extension. Embolization and radiotherapy have been used in such situations as an adjunct to surgery or as a definitive therapy. In view of the risk of secondary neoplastic induction in young patients, radiotherapy is usually reserved for bilateral cavernous sinus involvement, failure of embolization and in situation where adequate surgical or therapeutic angiographic team is not available.

Preoperative embolizations 24–48 hours prior to surgery significantly reduces intraoperative blood loss resulting in better surgical removal.[11,12] The goal of endovascular therapy is to occlude the capillary bed and to devascularize the tumor. Routinely, bilateral external carotid and internal carotid angiograms with cross-compression are performed to evaluate the angioarchitecture of the tumor. The next step involves selective catheterization and embolization of external carotid artery (ECA) feeders to the tumor, starting from the most distal one to avoid the loss of access due to subsequent spasm. In general, distal internal maxillary artery (IMA) is embolized first followed by the accessory meningeal, the ascending pharyngeal and the ascending palatine arteries. Sequential catheterization and embolization of feeding vessels from the opposite side is also done in almost all cases, in the same order.[13] Embolization is performed with gel foam powder or PVA particles (200–250 μm) so as to pack the tumor bed **(Figs. 1A to E)**. This is followed by larger gelfoam particles for temporary occlusion of the feeding artery. This secondary embolization produces a transient devascularization of the region adjacent to the tumor, as well as, augmentation of the distal thrombosis within the tumor itself. Intracranial extension or large nonresectable tumors may require the use of liquid agents, e.g. NBCA, alcohol or transient or definitive occlusion of ICA siphon.[14] Direct puncture of the tumor through intraoral or transmandibular route followed by embolization with ethanol or NBCA has been a recent advancement **(Figs. 2A to F)**.

Nasopharyngeal angiofibroma (NAF) has high recurrence rate of 30% or more. Embolization in these patients is feasible only if surgical ligation or prior embolization has not blocked the vascular access. These patients are generally managed by surgery or by radiotherapy.

PARAGANGLIOMA

Paragangliomas (PGs) arise from paraganglion or glomus bodies that form part of the chemoreceptor system. It is also called glomus tumor, chemodectoma, nonchromaffin PG and neurocristopathic tumor. It can be located within or adjacent to the temporal bone (glomus tympanicum and glomus jugulare), carotid bifurcation (carotid body tumor), X cranial nerve (glomus vagale). Laryngeal, nasopharyngeal or orbital PG has been described.

Carotid body tumor and glomus jugulare are the most common PGs encountered in clinical practice. The peak age of presentation is in the 5th decade with a female preponderance (F:M = 2.5–3:1). It is a benign encapsulated neoplasm but can be locally invasive. Familial inheritance of autosomal dominant pattern has also been described. The 30% of the familial forms have multicentric disease which is more common in carotid (15%) and vagal (10%) tumors. Temporal glomus tumors are rarely multicentric (2%) and rarely malignant (3%). Incidence of malignancy is high in carotid (10–15%), vagal (10%) and laryngeal tumors (18%).[4,10]

Pathologically, PG shows sinusoidal stroma with compartments which behave like hemodynamically independent units. The clinical symptomatology is related to the location of the tumor. The tympanic PGs present with pulsatile tinnitus, conductive deafness, VIII cranial N palsy

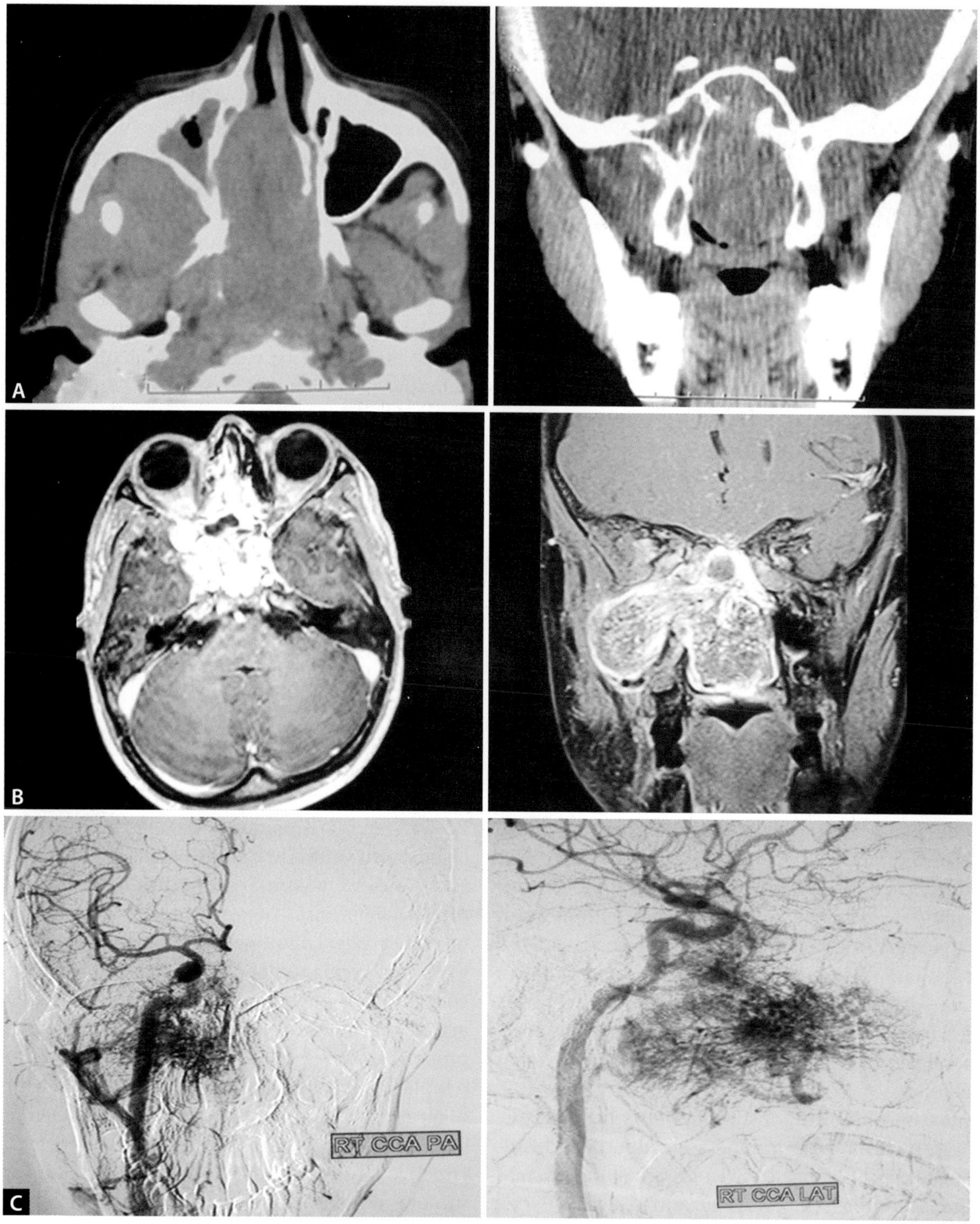

Figs. 1A to C: Nasopharyngeal angiofibroma: (A) CECT axial and coronal sections show large nasopharyngeal mass with bone destruction; (B) T1W axial and coronal postcontrast images show intensely enhancing large nasopharyngeal mass with extensions; (C) Right common carotid angiogram show large nasopharyngeal hypervascular mass with tumor blush supplied predominantly by internal maxillary artery (IMA) and partially by internal carotid artery.

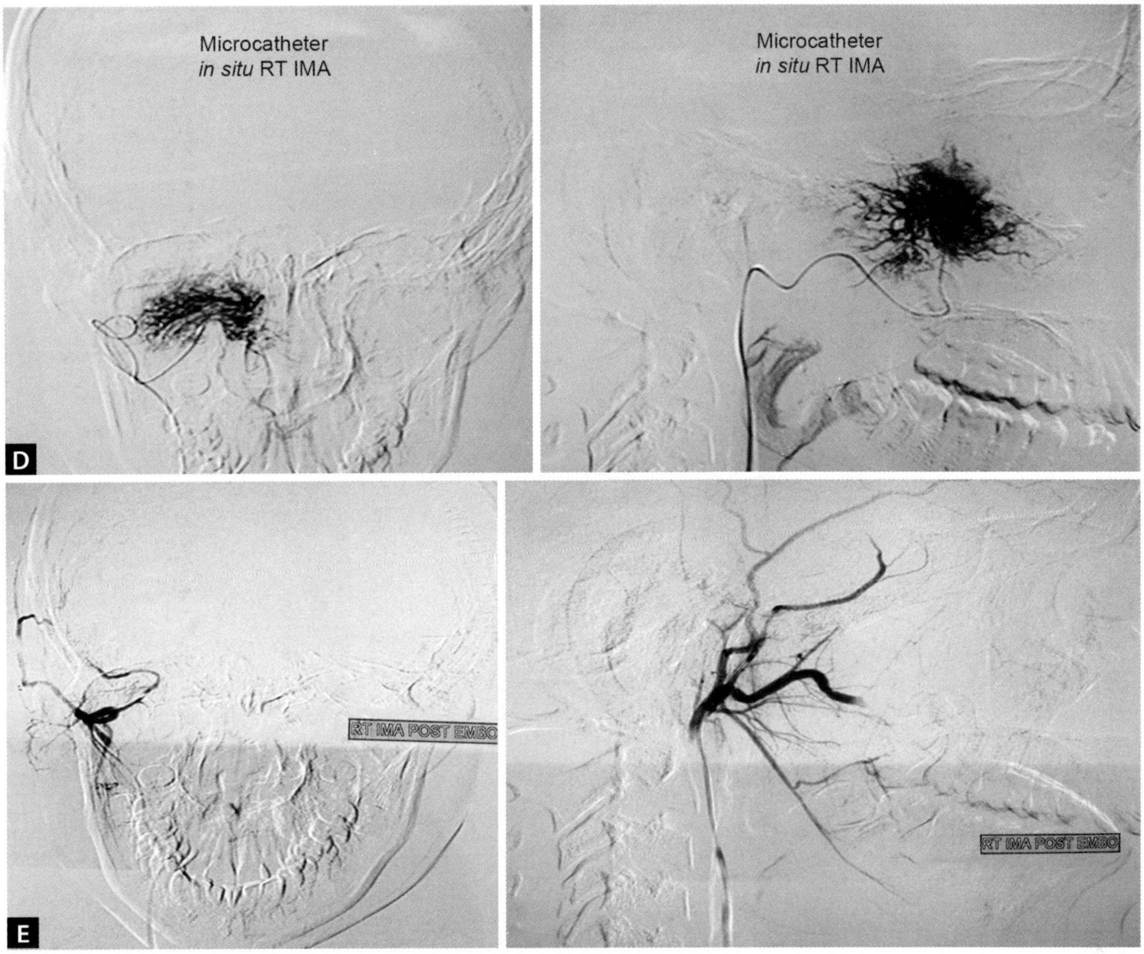

Figs. 1D and E: (D) Superselective right IMA angiogram reveals the tumor blush; Preoperative superselective IMA embolization with PVA particles (200–250 µm) was done and postembolization angiogram (E) frontal and lateral projections show almost complete obliteration of tumor bed supplied by IMA.

or reddish/bluish bulging of the tympanic membrane. Jugular PGs present with jugular foramen syndrome (Vernet syndrome) which includes paralysis of IX, X and XI cranial nerves. Carotid and vagal PGs present as pulsatile neck masses with or without cranial nerve involvement.

Computed tomography and MRI are usually required to assess the extent of lesion and to rule out other masses mimicking these tumors. On CECT, PGs show a typical intense blush. On MR, the flow void of small vessels within the tumor gives typical pepper pot appearance. Angiography is the most specific diagnostic technique and should always be performed before biopsy is attempted. Typical angiographic features include moderate enlargement of the feeding arteries, an early intense parenchymal blush and rapid venous filling **(Figs. 3A to D)**. In the temporal bone PG, the arteries that should be studied selectively are ipsilateral vertebral, internal carotid, distal ECA, posterior auricular, occipital and bilateral ascending pharyngeal arteries. The late phase of dominant vertebral injection is also necessary for visualization of venous pattern. In cervical PG, the arteries that should be studied selectively are ipsilateral vertebral, proximal ICA, facial, lingual, superior laryngeal, carotid body artery, ascending cervical, inferior laryngeal and bilateral ascending pharyngeal arteries. Vagal PG displaces ICA anteromedially whereas carotid PG displaces the ICA posterolaterally.[4]

Embolotherapy is a safe and efficient method to devascularize these tumors preoperatively. It can be used as the sole therapy for inoperable tumors in order to achieve stabilization of growth. In most cases, particulate agents (PVA 140–150 µm) are used to occlude the capillary bed followed by large gel foam particles to promote distal thrombosis **(Figs. 3A to D)**. Liquid agents are used only in the treatment of inoperable tumors and when optimal

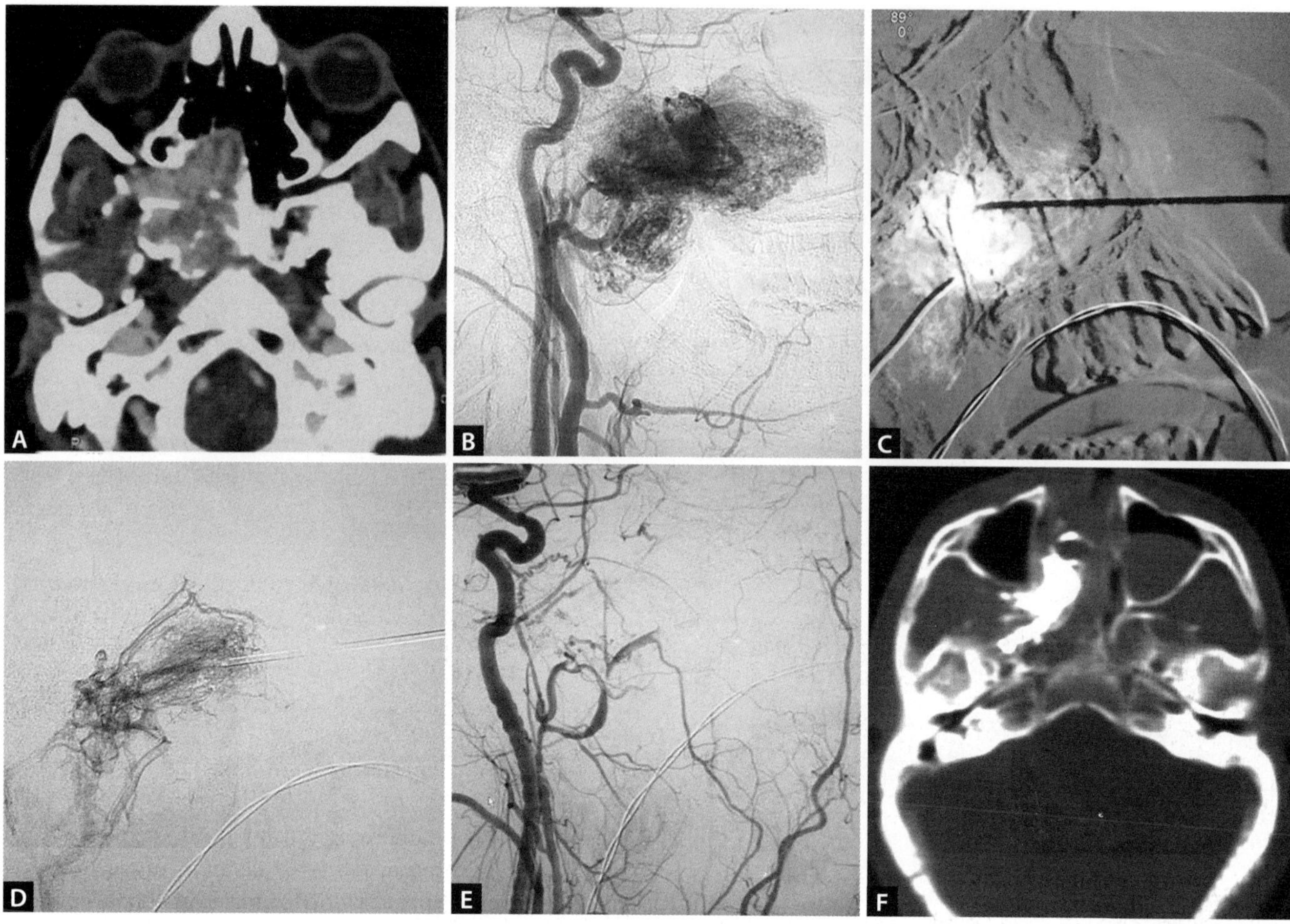

Figs. 2A to F: Juvenile nasopharyngeal angiofibroma: Axial contrast-enhanced CT (A) demonstrating the hypervascular nasopharyngeal mass with significant vascularity from branches of right external carotid artery as revealed on DSA (B). Percutaneous transnasal lesion puncture was done under guidance of "smart-mask" (C) followed by a nidogram (D). 60% mixture of n-butyl cyanoacrylate glue was injected under fluoroscopic guidance. Control DSA (E) showing complete lesion embolization. CT scan (F) following the procedure shows hyperdense lipiodol mixed glue within the tumor mass.

flow control can be achieved. ICA may be sacrificed where there is encasement of ICA or petrous apex involvement. Provocative testing should be performed prior to such procedures. Those tumors which are supplied by AICA/PICA are usually not amenable to embolization.[15] Embolization can be associated with neurological complications. Ascending pharyngeal artery embolization with liquid agents almost always results in lower cranial nerve palsy and the patient should be informed about the same, prior to the procedure.

Endovascular embolotherapy is considered to be the sole method of preoperative embolization for carotid body tumors. However, recent literature documents that direct percutaneous embolization offers much more important devascularization than endovascular route. The endovascular embolization is often not complete and successful due to high vascularity and numerous tiny feeders from both ECA and ICA system which are not feasible for catheterization even with latest microcatheters. Secondly, there is increased risk of stroke and cranial nerve palsies due to reflux of embolic material into ICA and vertebrobasilar system. Complete devascularization can be achieved using percutaneous embolization with NBCA glue or onyx combined with endovascular microballoon occlusion that offer protection of internal carotid system. Percutaneous onyx appears to be promising than glue.[16,17]

CRANIOFACIAL VASCULAR ANOMALIES

These are complex lesions due to abnormal vasculature and are broadly categorized into vascular malformations and vascular tumors. The original classification of vascular anomalies was given by Mulliken and Glowacki.[18] It was easy to interpret and was used intensively in the clinics but did not correlate with the origin of these lesions. After a

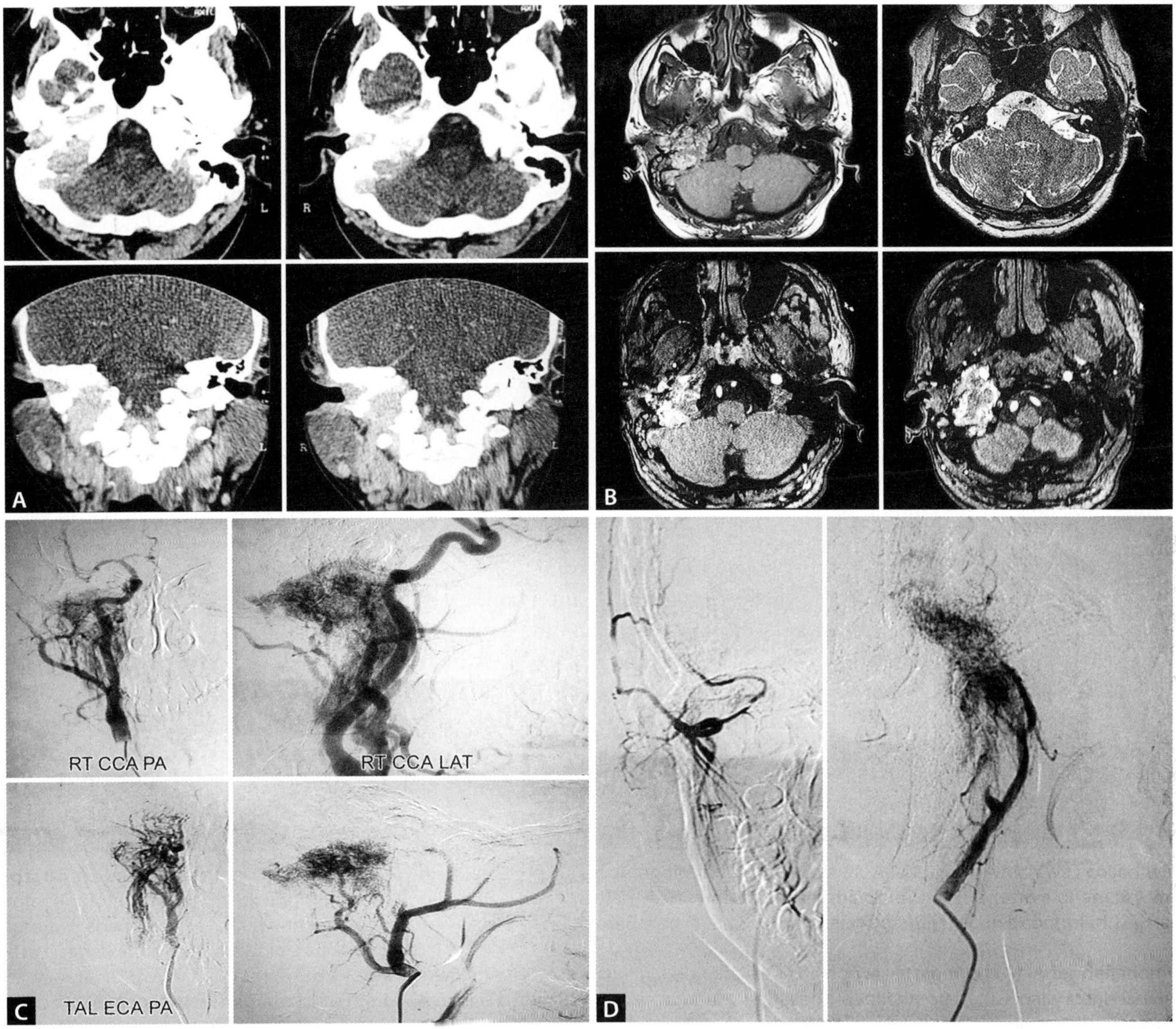

Figs. 3A to D: Paraganglioma: (Glomus jugulare) (A) CECT shows brightly enhancing right CP angle mass with bony petrous destruction; (B) T1, T2WI and GRE MR images revealing hypervascular lesion; (C) Selective CCA and ECA injections reveal dense-tumor blush; (D) Selective right ECA and superselective ascending pharyngeal angiogram reveal significant reduction of tumor blush following embolization.

Table 4: 2014 ISSVA classification of vascular anomalies.

Vascular tumors			***Vascular malformations***	
Benign	***Locally aggressive***	***Malignant***	***Simple***	***Combined***
Infantile hemangioma	Kaposiform hemangioendothelioma	Angiosarcoma	Capillary malformation (C)	CVM, CLM
Congenital hemangioma	Retiform hemangioendothelioma	Epithelioid hemangioendothelioma	Lymphatic malformation	LVM, CLVM
Tufted hemangioma	PILA, Dabska tumor		Venous malformation (VM)	CAVM
Spindle-cell hemangioma	Composite hemangioendothelioma		Arteriovenous malformation (AVM)	CLAVM
Epithelioid hemangioma	Kaposi's sarcoma		Arteriovenous fistula	
Pyogenic granuloma				

series of expert meetings and an intensive understanding of the pathological processes, the International Society for the Study of Vascular Anomalies (ISSVA) came out with the latest classification in 2014 **(Table 4)**.[19]

Vascular Tumor

Hemangiomas

These are benign tumors of endothelial cells and are of two types: capillary and cavernous hemangioma. Capillary hemangiomas are seen in infants and children. They may involute with time. The cavernous hemangiomas are seen in adults and do not exhibit involution. The capillary hemangiomas show strong female predominance (M:F = 1:5) and are present at birth in approximately 30% of patients. They show an initial phase of rapid growth (first 6 months) followed by gradual involution by 7–8 years in more than 95% of patients. Active therapy to increase the rate of involution is indicated in selected patients with functional impairment (orbital, oral, subglottic), complications (hemorrhage, congestive heart failure, hypoprothrombinemia), and in extremely large lesions. Therapeutic embolization has a definite role in these patients as complementary to the natural involutive process.

The angiographic features of capillary hemangioma are mass effect, an organized pattern of arterial supply from adjacent arteries with drainage into dilated superficial veins that empty into normal veins, and parenchymal stains which are often lobulated. AV shunting may be present. Non-involutive cavernous hemangiomas of adults typically appear as soft tissue masses on angiography, and occasionally parenchymal blush and filling of vascular spaces may occur in the late venous phase **(Figs. 4A to C)**.

Vascular Malformations

These are formed by a combination of abnormal capillary, arterial, venous or lymphatic channels with or without shunt. They are almost always present at birth. They are neither proliferative nor potentially involutive. They may remain dormant for years and may result in facial deformity, discoloration or disturbances in orofacial function. They may bleed following trivial trauma or infection. They can exhibit rapid growth with excessive pain. Arteriovenous shunting may sometime result in congestive heart failure.[20]

Vascular malformations of the head and neck often involve multiple contiguous anatomic spaces and encase critical neurovascular structures, making

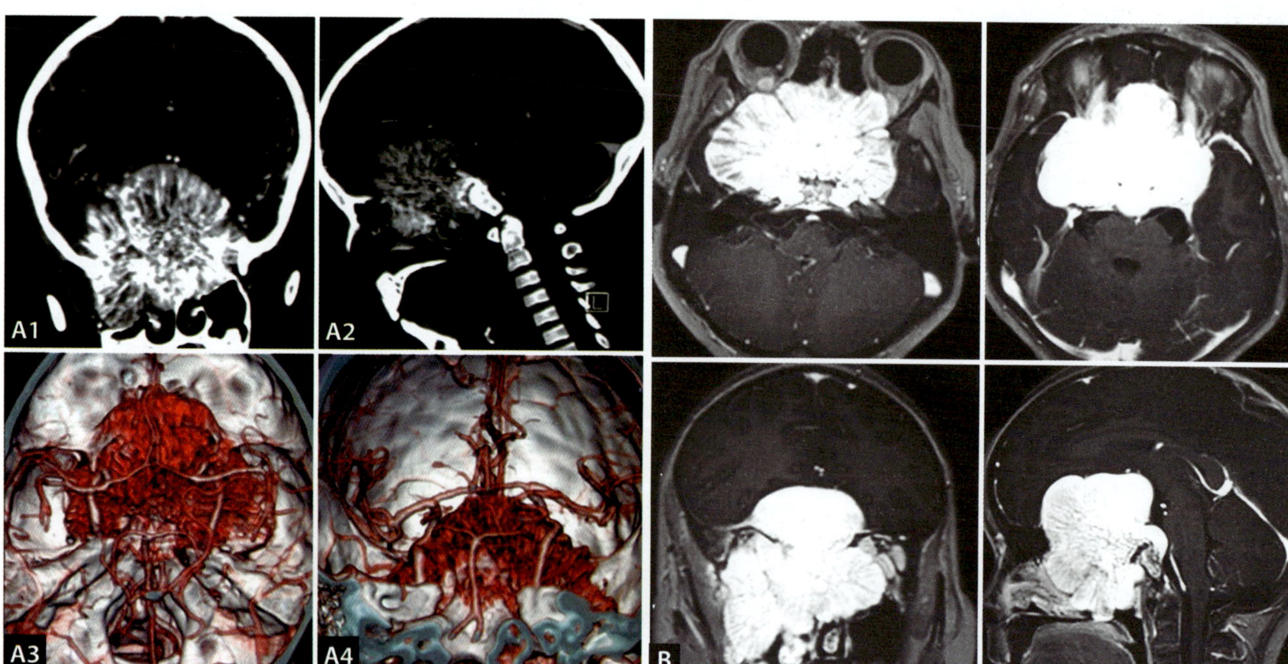

Figs. 4A and B: (A1 and A2) CT coronal and sagittal reformatted images showing abnormal rarefaction, trabeculation of skull base predominantly the sphenoid bone; (A3 and A4) CT angiogram VR images cranial and coronal views show large hypervascular base of skull lesion; (B) Postcontrast axial, coronal and sagittal T1W images reveal intense enhancement with intracranial and sinonasal extension.

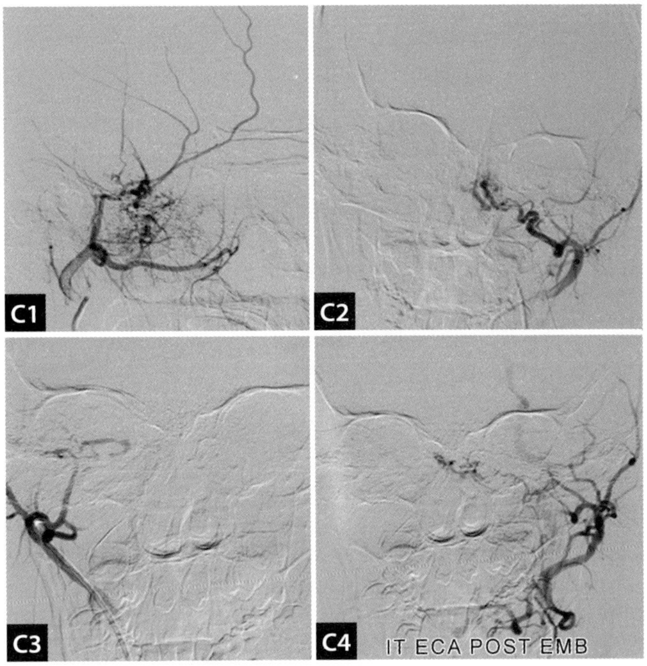

Fig. 4C: (C1 and C2) Primary intraosseus cavernous hemangioma of skull base. Bilateral selective internal maxillary artery angiogram shows tumor blush in early arterial phase with persistence in delayed phase. Postembolization internal maxillary check angiogram shows absence of tumor blush.

surgical treatment difficult and often unsuccessful. The great majority of vascular lesions in children are treated conservatively until their complete regression or till maxillofacial maturity is reached. Emergency evaluation is required for subglottic or eyelid hemangiomas, hemorrhagic episodes, severe consumption coagulopathy or heart failure. Angiography is required in cases where therapeutic intervention is planned.

From a therapeutic perspective, one of the most important differentiating characteristics of vascular malformations is their classification as "high-flow" or "low-flow" based on findings at physical examination **(Table 5)**, imaging, or both.[20,21] High-flow lesions are those that contain arteriovenous fistulas (AVFs) and slow flow lesions are those which lack any significant AVFs. MRI is an excellent noninvasive imaging technique for classification of vascular malformations, and it is often used to help therapeutic decision making and to provide follow-up after embolotherapy.[22] High-flow vascular malformations, which produce signal voids on wspin echo (SE) images and high-signal-intensity flow-related enhancement on flow- compensated gradient-echo images, are often treated with embolization via a transarterial approach.[21,23] High-flow lesions are treated by occlusion at the site of fistulous

Table 5: Schobinger classification of arteriovenous malformation.

Stage	*Features*
I	Cutaneous blush/warmth
II	Bruit, audible pulsations, expanding lesion
III	Pain, ulceration, bleeding, infection
IV	Cardiac failure

connection with permanent embolic agents **(Figs. 5 to 7)**. Tissue adhesives (NBCA) are used in small fistulas. Platinum coils or detachable balloons are preferred in large fistulas. Alcohol has also been used but the variability in the level of occlusion is a significant problem with this agent. Without superselective catheterization of the nidus, transarterial embolization often results in occlusion of arteries proximal to the arteriovenous connection and of the collateral vessels that are supplied via the rich arterial network that frequently is recruited. Many times combined endovascular and surgical approaches are used to treat these lesions.

Alternatively, low-flow vascular malformations, which appear predominantly bright on T2-weighted SE images, without evidence of flow void are often successfully treated by a direct percutaneous sclerotherapy using sodium tetradecyl sulfate or alcohol. Slow flow venous malformations can be superficial (subcutaneous or submucosal) or deep (within muscle, bone, etc.). In the superficially located lesions, direct percutaneous puncture is done followed by fluoroscopic-guided injection of contrast material to delineate the exact extent of lesion **(Figs. 8A to C)**. This is followed by embolization using liquid embolic agent such as ethanol. Care is taken to avoid extravasation especially in lesions adjacent to cranial nerves. Large lesion often requires multiple sittings.

Aneurysms

Aneurysms can involve common carotid artery, ICA, ECA, or their branches or vertebral arteries. These aneurysms occur most frequently in the ICA, followed by the vertebral artery and least frequently in the ECA and its branches. Among extradural ICA aneurysms, cavernous segment is most commonly affected (80%) and they are often giant aneurysms. ICA aneurysms are either developmental or traumatic; atherosclerotic and mycotic aneurysms are uncommon. ECA and vertebral artery aneurysms are mostly traumatic. The patients may present with TIA, epistaxis, expanding neck mass, cranial nerve palsies or they may be asymptomatic.

These aneurysms, particularly those near skull base like petrous/cavernous part of ICA are difficult to treat

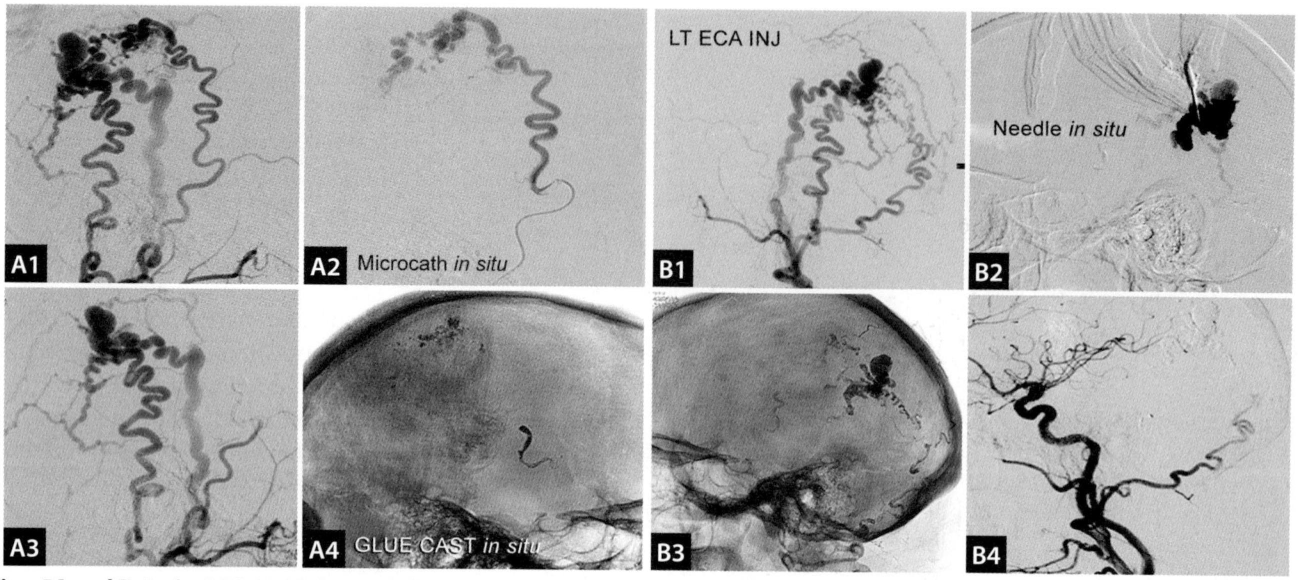

Figs. 5A and B: Scalp AVM: (A1) Selective left ECA injection shows dilated tortuous superficial temporal artery branches supplying a large complex AVM with cirsoid aneurysms; (A2) Superselective STA angiogram; (A3) ECA check angiogram after superselective embolization using 50% NBCA glue through STA feeder shows embolization of anterosuperior component of AVM; (A4) Glue cast in the AVM nidus and arterial feeder. Second sitting percutaneous glue embolization; (B1) Post first sitting selective left ECA injection shows superficial temporal and occipital artery branches supplying residual AVM; (B2) Percutaneous intranidal AVM angiogram; (B3) Large glue cast in AVM nidus and distal arterial feeders after percutaneous injection of 60% glue; (B4) Postembolizations CCA check angiogram reveals complete obliteration of AVM nidus and distal most arterial feeders.

by surgery due to limited access. They are, however, amenable to endovascular therapy with high cure rates. Pretherapeutic evaluation with CTA/MRA is often required to assess the size of aneurysm, the complete extent of trauma and associated complications if any.

There are two approaches of embolization: selective occlusion of the aneurysms and parent artery occlusion. Selective occlusion is the treatment of choice in saccular aneurysms having a narrow neck, which helps to contain the occlusion device within the aneurysm. This is achieved by using conventional fibered platinum coils or the electrolytically detachable coil (e.g. GDC). Fresh traumatic pseudoaneurysms, however, are too fragile to tolerate such manipulation of aneurysms and therefore require parent artery occlusion. Fusiform aneurysms and wide necked saccular aneurysms are also treated by occlusion of parent artery. The occlusion of parent artery is achieved by using detachable balloon (silicone or latex) in large arteries and platinum coils in smaller arteries. The aneurysm is usually trapped by placing a balloon at or just distal to the neck of the aneurysm and another balloon proximal to the first balloon. Caution is taken in preserving circulation to vital tributaries like ophthalmic artery while embolizing ICA aneurysms and PICA while embolizing vertebral aneurysms. Large ICA pseudoaneurysms can also be treated safely with use of covered stent **(Figs. 9A to C)**. A combined surgical and endovascular approach may sometimes be required when provocative testing confirms major functional loss. In these patients, a surgical bypass graft to the distal vessels may be performed in an accessible region, followed by endovascular occlusion of the diseased segment.

MISCELLANEOUS LESIONS

Meningiomas are hypervascular tumors which usually derive their blood supply from dural branches of ECA. A significant contribution can also be from intracranial circulation. Surgery is the treatment of choice in these lesions and embolization is only performed preoperatively for allowing easy resection. Embolization is warranted only in those meningiomas which are at surgically inaccessible sites, e.g. skull base. Small particle (PVA) embolization of tumor bed is done followed by devascularization by embolizing the feeding artery using larger particles like gel foam. The embolization procedure is restricted to external carotid artery branches only.

Occasionally other vascular masses like schwannomas, esthesioneuroblastomas, soft tissue tumor and hypervascular metastatic tumors require embolization.

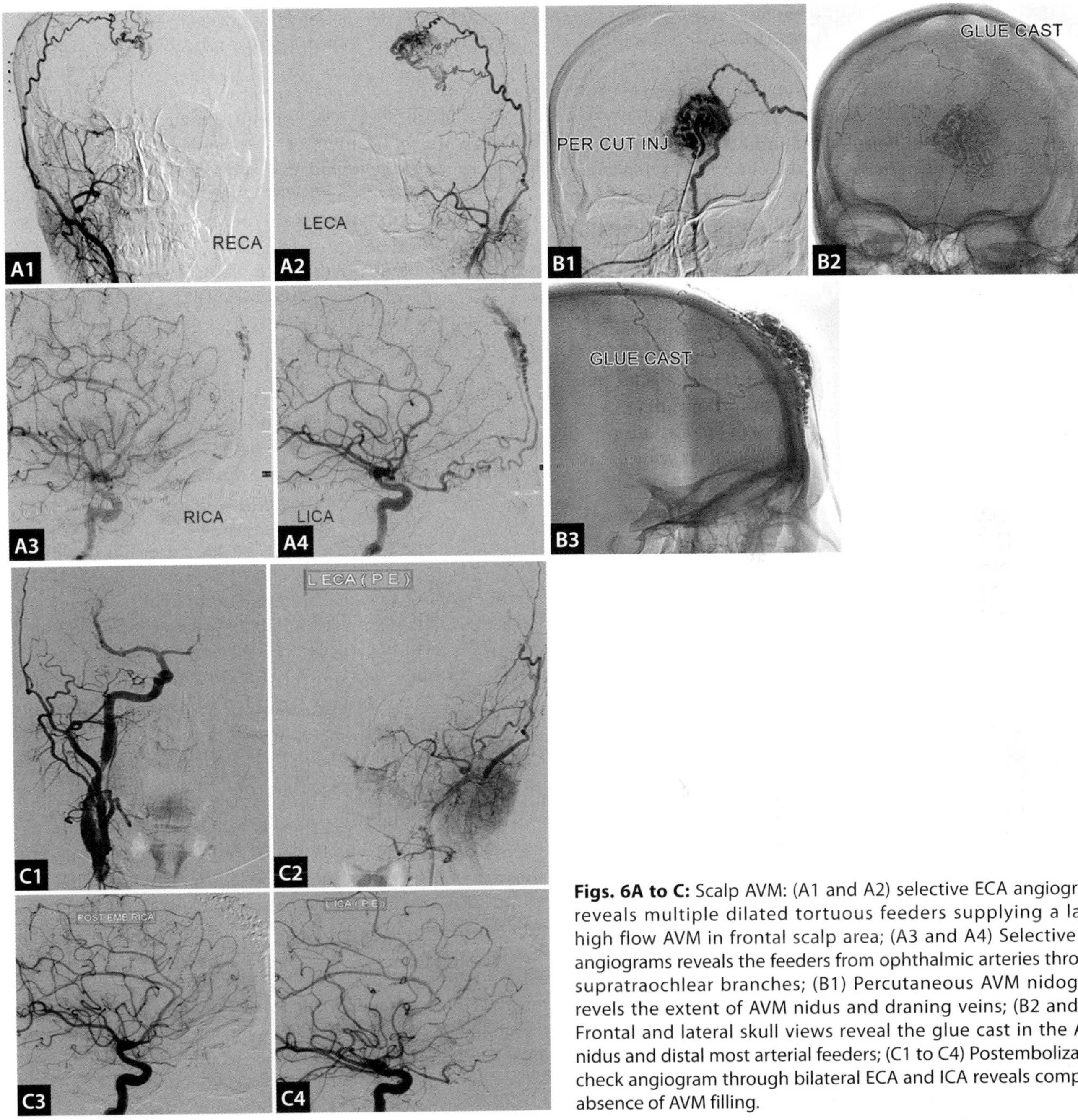

Figs. 6A to C: Scalp AVM: (A1 and A2) selective ECA angiograms reveals multiple dilated tortuous feeders supplying a large high flow AVM in frontal scalp area; (A3 and A4) Selective ICA angiograms reveals the feeders from ophthalmic arteries through supratraochlear branches; (B1) Percutaneous AVM nidogram revels the extent of AVM nidus and draning veins; (B2 and B3) Frontal and lateral skull views reveal the glue cast in the AVM nidus and distal most arterial feeders; (C1 to C4) Postembolization check angiogram through bilateral ECA and ICA reveals complete absence of AVM filling.

The principle of embolization is similar to that employed for meningiomas.

Epistaxis

Epistaxis is usually self-limiting. However, sometimes, it can be severe and life threatening requiring emergency treatment. Such severe epistaxis usually follows facial trauma, iatrogenic complication, aneurysms rupture, neoplasm, coagulopathies and vascular malformations such as hereditary hemorrhagic telangiectasias. Immediate management includes hemodynamic stabilization, nasal packing with or without electrocautery of bleeding vessels. When these measures fail to control bleeding, angiography and embolization are indicated. The failure rate of surgical ligation of internal maxillary artery (IMA) is as high as 10–15% as the source of bleeding can be elsewhere. Angiography, however, can identify the exact source of bleed and can assist in embolization. Even when the exact

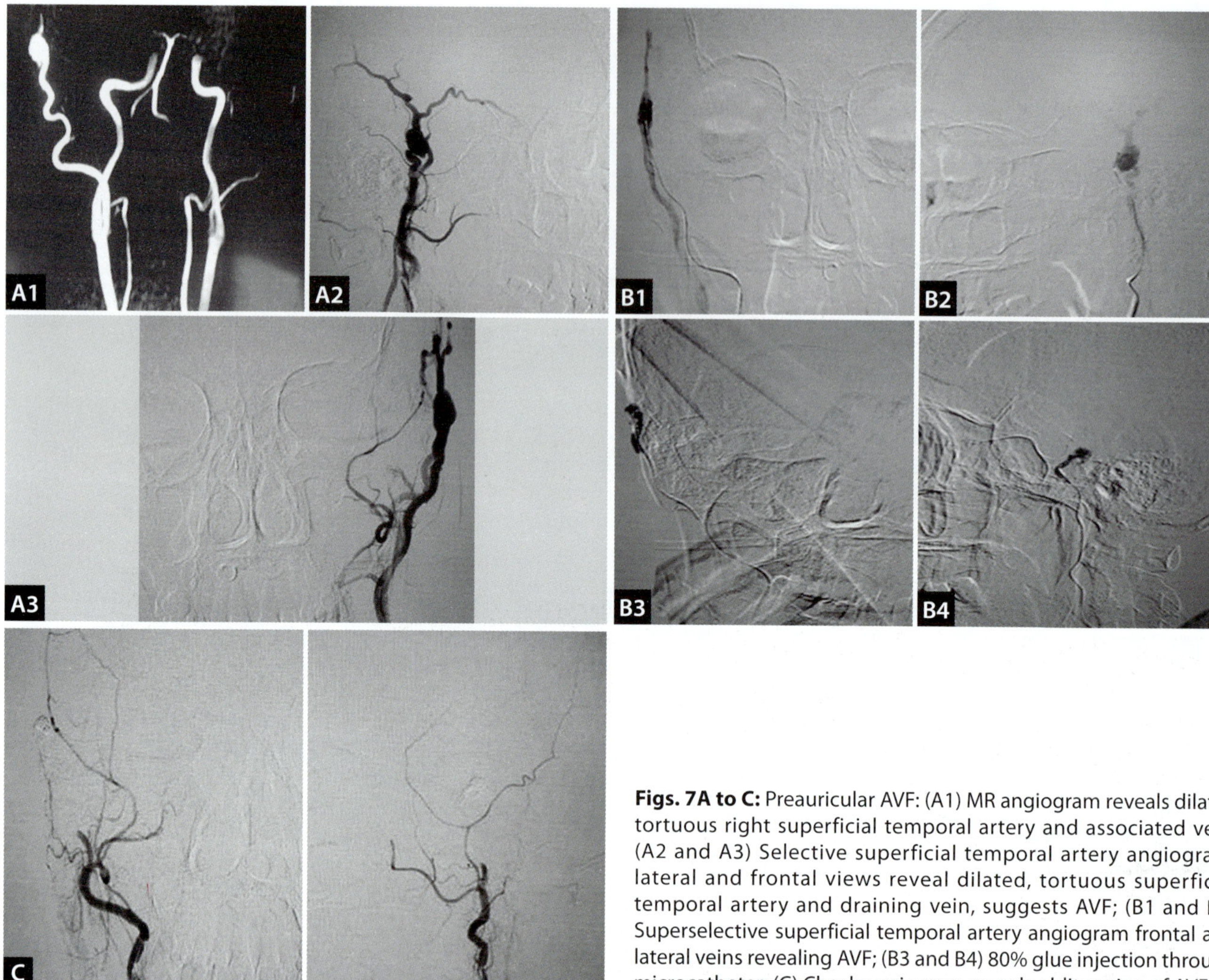

Figs. 7A to C: Preauricular AVF: (A1) MR angiogram reveals dilated tortuous right superficial temporal artery and associated vein; (A2 and A3) Selective superficial temporal artery angiogram, lateral and frontal views reveal dilated, tortuous superficial temporal artery and draining vein, suggests AVF; (B1 and B2) Superselective superficial temporal artery angiogram frontal and lateral veins revealing AVF; (B3 and B4) 80% glue injection through microcatheter; (C) Check angiogram reveals obliteration of AVF.

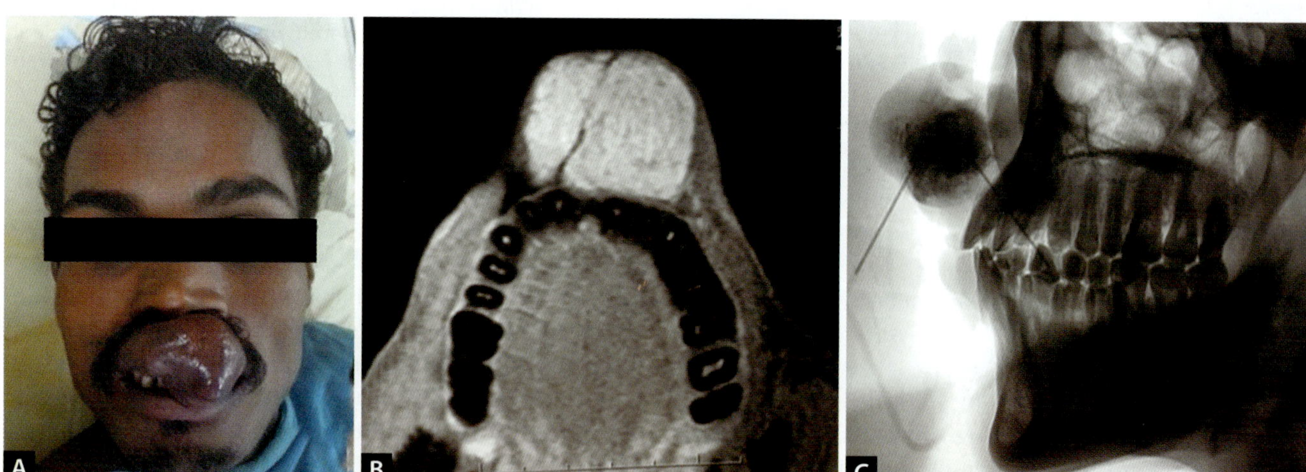

Figs. 8A to C: Lip venous malformation: Clinical photograph (A) showing a large upper lip venous malformation. Axial T1W FS (B) image revealing the well-circumscribed exophytic hyperintense upper lip lesion. Fluoroscopy image (C) demonstrating the percutaneous puncture of the lesion followed by sclerosant injection.

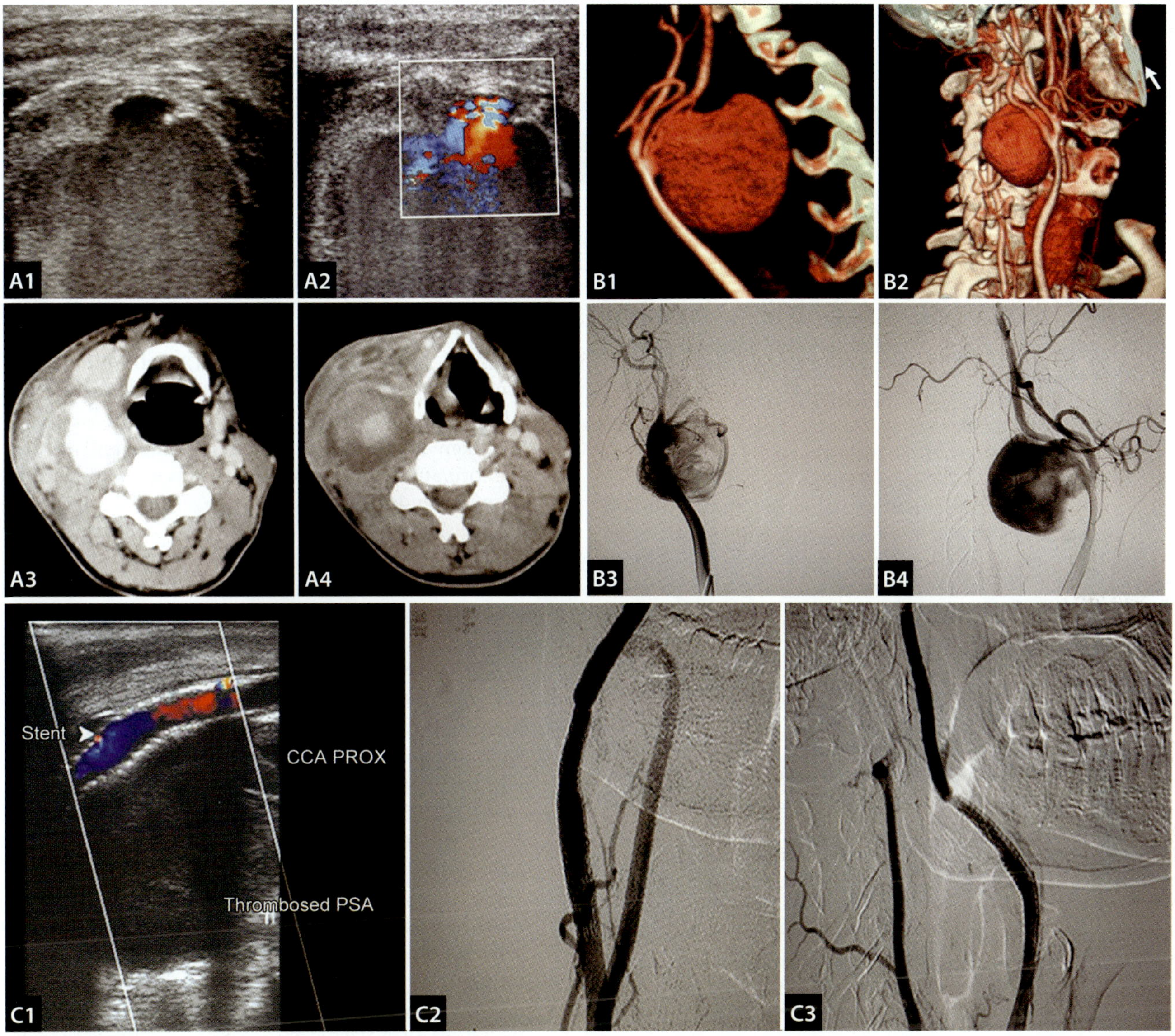

Figs. 9A to C: Post-tonsillar biopsy ICA pseudoaneurysm: (A1 and A2) Doppler images reveal large intimal ICA defect with pseudoaneurysm; (A3 and A4) Axial CECT neck sections showing the ICA pseudoaneurysm; (B1 to B4) CT and digital substraction angiogram revealing large pseudoaneurysm arising from proximal ICA; (C1) Post-ICA stenting (covered stent) Doppler USG study reveals absence of flow into the pseudoaneurysm; (C2 and C3) Anteroposterior and lateral angiogram reveals opacification of ICA with obliteration of pseudoaneurysm.

site of bleeding is not identified angiographic embolization of the arterial territory of the clinically affected mucosa is usually effective in controlling epistaxis. Super-selective catheterization is done followed by embolization using platinum coils or tissue adhesives (NBCA).[24]

SUMMARY

Endovascular treatment through intra-arterial or percutaneous approach is a safe and cost-effective nonsurgical therapeutic option for the treatment of a variety of non-neoplastic and neoplastic vascular lesions in the craniofacial region. It can be used as a definitive treatment or as an adjunct to surgery. The strategy for selecting the route of embolization and embolic material should be based on clinical and angiographic characteristics. The ongoing improvement in the technique, microcatheters, guidewires and safe embolic agents have widened the scope of endovascular procedures.

REFERENCES

1. Dion JE. Endovascular treatment of cervicocerebral aneurysms. Semin Intervent Radiol. 1994;11:37-63.
2. Cil BE, Vargel I, Geyik S, et al. Venous vascular malformations of the craniofacial region: preoperative embolization with direct percutaneous puncture and N-butyl cyanoacrylate. Br J Radiol. 2008;81:935-9.
3. Dabus G, Linfante I, Benenati J, et al. Interventional management of high-flow craniofacial vascular malformations: a database analysis and review of the literature. J Neurointerv Surg. 2017;9(1):92-6.
4. Lasjaunias P, Berenstein A. Craniofacial vascular lesions. In: Surgical Neuroangiography. Berlin: Springer Verlag; 1989. pp. 19-45.
5. Horbach SE, Lokhorst MM, Saeed P, et al. Sclerotherapy for low-flow vascular malformations of the head and neck: a systematic review of sclerosing agents. J Plast Reconstr Aesthet Surg. 2016;69(3):295-304.
6. Arat A, Cil BE, Vargel I, et al. Embolization of high flow craniofacial vascular malformations with onyx. AJNR. 2007;28:1409-14.
7. Horton JA, Kerber CW. Lidocaine injection into external carotid branches: provocative test to preserve cranial nerve function in therapeutic embolization. AJNR. 1986;7:105-8.
8. Ebra SM, Horton JA, Latchaw RE, et al. Balloon test occlusion in the internal carotid artery with stable xenon/CT cerebral blow flow imaging. AJNR. 1988;9:533-7.
9. Geibprasert S, Pongpech S, Armstrong D, et al. Dangerous extracranial intracranial anastomoses and supply to cranial nerves: vessels the neurointerventionalist needs to know. AJNR. 2009;30:459-68.
10. Jensen ME. Endovascular treatment of vascular pathology of the head and neck. Semin Intervent Radiol. 1994;11:22-36.
11. Marshall AH, Bradely PJ. Management dilemmas in the treatment and follow-up of advanced juvenile nasopharyngeal angiofibroma. ORL. 2006;68:273-8.
12. Tan G, Ma Z, Long W, et al. Efficacy of preoperative transcatheter arterial embolization for nasopharyngeal angiofibroma: a comparative study. Cardiovasc Intervent Radiol. 2017;40(6):836-44.
13. Davis KR. Embolization of epistaxsis and juvenile nasopharyngeal angiofibroma. AJNR. 1986;7:953-62.
14. Introcaseo JH, Rusell EJ. Interventional neuro-radiologic treatment of head and neck lesions Otolaryng. Clin N Am. 1995;28:563-84.
15. Smith JD, Harvey RN, Darr OA, et al. Head and neck paragangliomas: a two-decade institutional experience and algorithm for management. Laryngoscope Investig Otolaryngol. 2017;2(6):380-9.
16. Firat A, Aytekin C, Boyvat F, et al. Multidisciplinary approach to carotid body paraganglioma: preoperative percutaneous embolization and surgical resection. Turkish Neurosurgery. 2003;13:81-4.
17. Wanke I, Jackel MC, Goericke S, et al. Percutaneous embolization of carotid paragangliomas using solely onyx. AJNR. 2009;30:1594-7.
18. Mulliken JB, Golwacki J. Hemangiomas and vascular malformations in infants and children: a classification based on endothelial characteristics. Plast Reconstr Surg. 1982;69:412-20.
19. Wassef M, Blei F, Adams D, et al.; ISSVA Board and Scientific Committee. Vascular anomalies classification: recommendations from the International Society for the Study of Vascular Anomalies. Pediatrics. 2015;136(1):e203-14.
20. O'Donovan JC, Donaldson JS, Morello FP, et al. Symptomatic hemangiomas and venous malformations in infants, children, and young adults: treatment with percutaneous injection of sodium tetradecyl sulfate. AJR. 1997;169:723-9.
21. Meyer JS, Hoffer FA, Barnes PD, et al. Biological classification of soft-tissue vascular anomalies: MR correlation. AJR. 1991;157:559-64.
22. Yakes WF, Haas DK, Parker SH, et al. Symptomatic vascular malformations: ethanol embolotherapy. Radiology. 1989;170:1059-66.
23. Widlus DM, Murray RR, White RI, et al. Congenital arteriovenous malformations: tailored embolotherapy. Radiology. 1988;169:511-6.
24. Strutz J, Schermacher M. Uncontrolled epistaxis. Arch Otolaryn Head Neck Surg. 1990;116:697-7.

CHAPTER 30

Imaging of Head Trauma

Shivanand Gamanagatti, Atin Kumar, Arun Kumar Gupta, Surabhi Vyas

Traumatic brain injury (TBI) is one of the major causes of mortality and morbidity in the world's population.[1] According to National Center for Injury Prevention and Control, approximately 2% of the entire population of the world currently suffers from disabilities caused by TBI.[2] The etiologies of head trauma vary with the patient age. In the elderly individuals, accidental falls are the most common causes whereas in young individuals, the motor vehicle crashes are common culprits. In children, abuse and neglect are common reasons.

Traumatic brain injury (TBI) is not a single "one and done" event. TBI is an ongoing series of pathophysiologic reactions that extends from the moment of injury for days, months, or even years in to the future. Acute TBI is just the initial triggering insult.

TBI CLASSIFICATION

Broad Classification

- *Primary lesions*: Are the direct result of trauma (Already occurred at the time of presentation)
- *Secondary lesions*: As complications of primary lesions (preventable)
  - *Acute and subacute*: Include cerebral edema, ischemia, and brain herniation
  - *Chronic*: Hydrocephalus, the cerebrospinal fluid (CSF) leak, leptomeningeal cyst, and encephalomalacia.

According to Location of Lesions

- *Intra-axial*: Cortical contusions, intracerebral hematoma, axonal shearing injuries, gray matter injury, and vascular injury
- *Extra-axial*: Epidural, subdural, subarachnoid, and intraventricular hemorrhage.

According to Mechanism

- Open (penetrating)
- Closed (blunt)

According to Clinical Severity (According to Glasgow Coma Scale)[3]

- Minor GCS : 15
- Mild GCS : 13–14
- Moderate GCS : 9–12
- Severe GCS : 3–8

Marshall CT Classification of Head Injury (HI)[4]

A 6 category scheme to classify head injury (HI) based on initial CT scan. It was published in the Journal of Neurosurgery by Lawrence Marshall and colleagues in 1991. It was based on their experience in the pilot phase of the Traumatic Coma Data Bank (TCDB).[5]

An increase in mortality was noted with increasing grade of diffuse injury.

Categories

Diffuse Injury—Type I:
- No CT visible intracranial pathology.

Diffuse Injury—Type II:
- Cisterns present with midline shift 0-5 mm
- No high- or mixed-density lesion > 25 cc.

Diffuse Injury—Type III (swelling):
- Cisterns compressed or absent with midline shift 0-5 mm
- No high- or mixed-density lesion > 25 cc.

Diffuse Injury—Type IV (shift):
- Midline shift > 5 mm
- No high- or mixed-density lesion > 25 cc.

Evacuated Mass Lesion—Type V:
- Any lesion surgically evacuated.

Non-evacuated Mass Lesion—Type VI:
- High- or mixed-density lesion > 25 cc.

This classification grades the severity of the injury as follows: I = normal, II = diffuse injury, III = diffuse injury with swelling, IV = diffuse injury with shift, V = mass lesion surgically evacuated, and VI = mass lesion not operated.

GOALS OF NEUROIMAGING

- To detect the presence of injuries that may require immediate surgical or procedural intervention.
- To detect the presence of injuries that may benefit from early medical therapy.
- To determine the prognosis of patients to tailor rehabilitative therapy or help with family counseling.

IMAGING TECHNIQUES

Plain Radiographs

Skull X-rays are poor predictors of intracranial pathology and should not be performed to evaluate adult TBI.[6-8] Lack of abnormality on skull films does not exclude major intracranial injury.[9] Patients who are at high risk for acute intracranial injury must be imaged by CT. The "scout view" that is obtained with all CT exams can be used as a "pseudo skull film" **(Fig. 1).** Twenty- five percent of cases with fatal injuries do not demonstrate a skull fracture, although the incidence of intracranial hematomas in patients who have skull fractures is much higher than in those who do not. It is often implied that many skull X-ray films are taken because of medicolegal considerations rather than clinical necessity.[6-8]

Computed tomography (CT), CT is the modality of choice in acute HI. It is easily available, fast, and compatible with equipment for monitoring of vital functions and artificial ventilation. If image is spoiled by motion artifacts, then it is possible to repeat selectively several slices without much time constraints. The acquired CT images can be visualized in bone, soft tissue, and varying window widths (adequate to diagnose subdural hemorrhages) without contrast administration to reveal intra-axial, extra-axial injuries and bone fractures.[10] In addition, CT is usually superior to MR in revealing skull fractures and radiopaque foreign bodies.

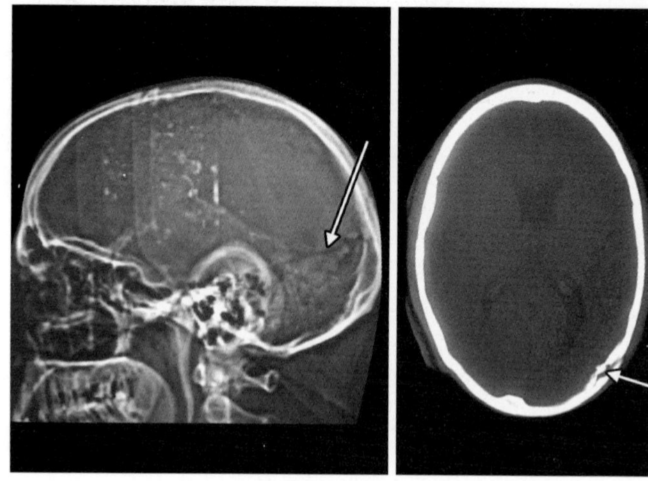

Fig. 1: Lateral topogram (Scout view) of skull obtained during CT scan of head showing linear fracture of parietal bone (arrow) and axial CT section in bone window confirming the presence of fracture in left posterior parietal bone (arrow).

The Goal of Imaging is to Identify Treatable Injuries to Prevent Secondary Damage

With modern CT scanners, contiguous 3 or 5-mm sections from the skull base to the vertex can be obtained in less than 10 minutes. Thinner 1- or 2.5 mm sections are used to evaluate the orbits, maxillofacial structures, and skullbase. With recent advances in multidetector CT (MDCT), thin cross-sectional slices can be performed which allowed for high-quality three-dimensional reconstruction. Thinner slices also improve the diagnostic accuracy of CT in the evaluation of maxillofacial, orbital, and temporal bone fractures. Intravenous contrast administration should not be performed because it can both mask and mimic underlying hemorrhage.

CT images must be reviewed using multiple windows and levels. A narrow window width (W: 80, L: 40) is used to evaluate the brain. A slightly wider window width (W: 150, L: 75) is used to exaggerate contrast between extra-axial blood and the adjacent skull. An even wider window (W: 2500, L: 500) is used to evaluate the osseous structures **(Figs. 2A to C)**.[9]

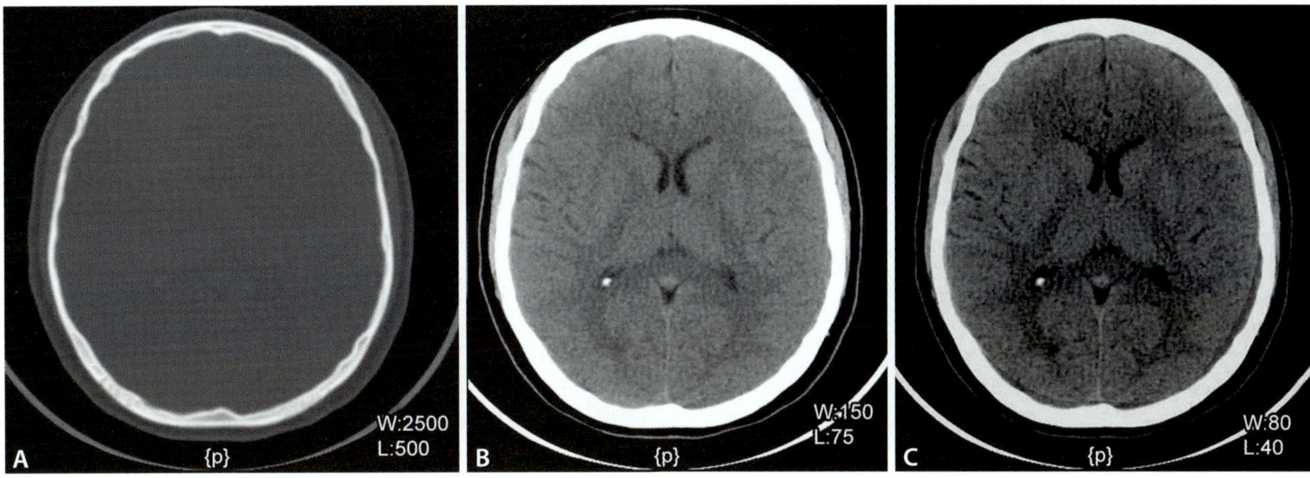

Figs. 2A to C: Axial CT images of brain (A to C) to show various window values used to view the CT images.

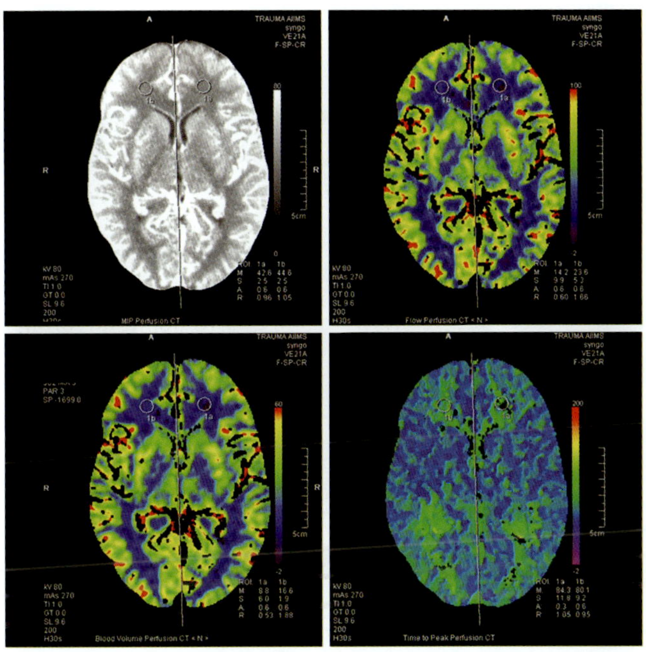

Fig. 3: Axial CT perfusion images showing the various parameters (time to peak, blood volume and flow rate) used to define regional brain perfusion alterations.

Perfusion CT (Fig. 3) affords insight into regional brain perfusion alterations due to head trauma, with the major advantages of being able to depict regional heterogeneity. Perfusion CT also offers prognostic information with respect to functional outcome, even as early as at the time of admission. Patients with altered brain perfusion might be considered for more aggressive and early treatment to prevent intracranial hypertension, whereas patients with preserved brain perfusion might benet from less invasive treatment. It might allow clinicians to distinguish between patients with preserved autoregulation (or pseudoregulation) and those with impaired autoregulation.[10,11]

Magnetic resonance imaging (MRI) is recommended for patients with acute TBI when the neurologic findings cannot be explained by CT. MR is also the modality of choice for subacute or chronic injury. MR is usually comparable to CT in the detection of an acute epidural and subdural hematoma.[12,13] However, MR is more sensitive to subtle extra-axial collections, nonhemorrhagic lesions, brainstem injuries, and subarachnoid hemorrhage (SAH) when using fluid-attenuated inversion recovery (FLAIR).[14,15]

Fluid-attenuated inversion recovery imaging improves the conspicuity of focal gray matter abnormalities (e.g. contusions), white matter abnormalities, shear injuries, and SAH by eliminating (or "nulling") the bright cerebrospinal fluid signal **(Fig. 4A)**. Sagittal and coronal FLAIR images are particularly helpful in the detection of diffuse axonal injury (DAI) involving the corpus callosum and the fornix, two areas that are difficult to evaluate on routine T2-weighted images.

Gradient-echo/Susceptibility weighted imaging (SWI) is highly sensitive to local magnetic inhomogeneity caused by the presence of blood. Hemosiderin, a breakdown product of blood, is ferromagnetic. The presence of hemosiderin alters the local magnetic susceptibility of tissue, resulting in areas of signal loss on gradient-echo T2*-weighted images **(Fig. 4B)**. Because hemosiderin can persist indefinitely, its detection on gradient-echo T2*-weighted images allows for improved evaluation of remote injury. However, due to the inherent inhomogeneity adjacent to the paranasal sinuses and mastoid air cells, gradient-echo images are limited in

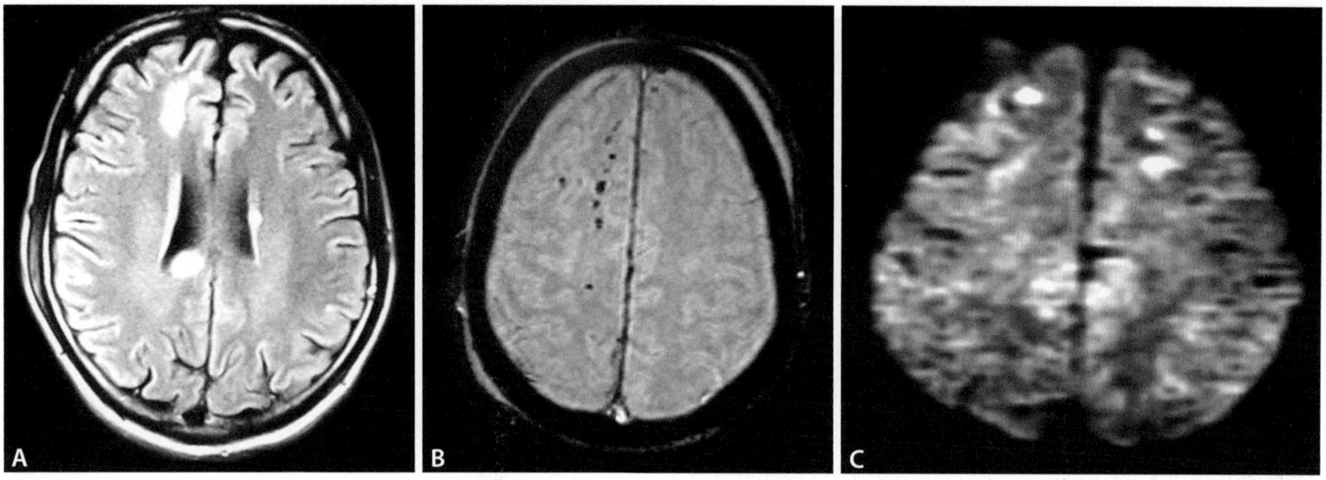

Figs. 4A to C: Axial MR images of brain to show the advantages of various MR sequences in detection of different intra-axial lesions (A) FLAIR sequence improves the conspicuity of focal gray matter abnormalities (e.g. contusions), white matter abnormalities; (B) Gradient echo sequence can detect many hemorrhagic foci because of better sensitivity to blood products; (C) DWI sequence improves detection of DAI because of superior sensitivity to foci of acute shearing injury.

the evaluation of cortical contusions of the inferior frontotemporal lobes.[16,17]

Diffusion-weighted imaging (DWI), which measures the random motion of water molecules in brain tissue, has improved the evaluation of TBI. Through its superior sensitivity to foci of acute shearing injury, DWI has especially improved detection of DAI **(Fig. 4C)**. DWI reveals more DAI lesions than fast spin-echo T2-weighted or gradient-echo T2*-weighted images in patients imaged within 48 hours of injury. The apparent diffusion coefficient (ADC), which measures the magnitude of water diffusion averaged over a three-dimensional space, is often reduced in acute DAI. The fractional anisotropy (FA), which measures the preferential motion of water molecules along the white matter axons, is frequently reduced in chronic DAI. Tissue anisotropy is exploited in the new technique of diffusion tensor imaging (DTI).[18-20]

Angiography: Contrast angiography has been the gold standard for diagnosis of vascular lesions. However, MRI, MRA, and CT angiography (CTA) are also growing in use and capability to provide the same information. Unlike conventional angiography that only images the lumen of blood vessels, MRA and CTA can provide information about the arterial walls. CTA offers better resolution and fewer flow-related artifacts than MRA. In addition CT and MRI also provide information about the adjoining brain parenchyma **(Fig. 5)**.

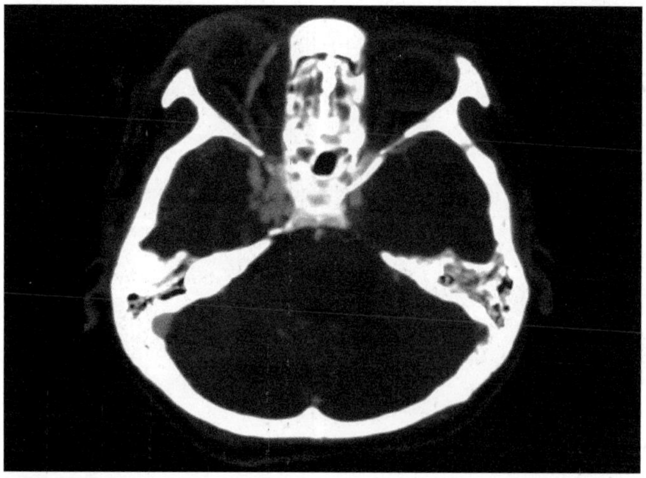

Fig. 5: CT angiography image showing lobulated and enlarged right cavernous sinus with abnormally dilated superior ophthalmic vein suggestive of carotid-cavernous fistula.

1. Clinical predictors of traumatic neurovascular injuries include a high-velocity mechanism, low Glasgow Coma Scale score, high injury severity score, mandible fracture, complex skull fractures, basilar skull fractures (including carotid canal fractures), scalp degloving, any type of cervical spine injury, and/or TBI with thoracic injuries, and/or thoracic vascular imaging, as well as in patients with penetrating neck injury (class I recommendation).
2. CTA should include arch of aorta till the circle of Willis for all patients with suspected vascular trauma.
3. Significant percentage of traumatic neurovascular injuries is treated by interventional procedures such as coil embolization, stent placement with a less morbidity and mortality.

Advanced Neuroimaging Techniques

Advanced neuroimaging techniques such as diffusion tensor imaging, blood oxygen level dependent (BOLD) functional MRI, spectroscopy and perfusion imaging are useful in recognizing any abnormality in patients with TBI when conventional NCCT and MR imaging findings are normal. These techniques also help in prognostication of patients with intractable symptoms. However, there is no sufficient data available in literature for routine clinical use of these advanced neuroimaging techniques.

Summary of Imaging Recommendations

Modality of sequence	*Head injury Indication*	*Recommendation*
NCCT head CT	First line acute mild, moderate and severe TBI	Class I
NCCT head CT	Repeat Assessment in Acute TB1 with neurologic deterioration	Class I
NCCT head CT	Judicious use in pediatric mild TB1	Class I
NCCT head CT	Repeat assessment of mild TBI with negative initial NCCT	Class III
CTA of brain	Suspected vascular trauma	Class IIa
Brain MRI without contrast	Acute or subacute TBI, initial or follow/up NCCT is negative with unexplained neurologic findings	Class I
T2* & SWI MRI	Acute, early subacute and chronic stages of DAI	Class IIa
Brain MRI with contrast	Can aid in visualizing subacute brain contusion	Class IIb
Advanced Neuroimaging	Mild TB1 with negative conventional CT and MRI	Class IIb

Evidence-based Guidelines for Imaging Patients with Head Injury

Suggested guidelines for acute neuroimaging in adult patient with mild TBI (Glasgow Coma Scale score 13–15):[21]

If GCS 13–15, CT recommended if patient has any one of the following:

- *High risk*:
  - GCS remains <15 at 2 hours after injury
  - Suspected open or depressed skull fracture
  - Any clinical sign of basal skull fracture
  - Two or more episodes of vomiting
  - Aged 65 years or older
- *Medium risk*:
  - Possible loss of consciousness
  - Amnesia for period before impact, of at least 30-minute time span
  - Dangerous mechanism (pedestrian versus motor vehicle, ejected from motor vehicle, fall from greater than 3 feet or five stairs)
  - Any transient neurologic deficit
  - Headache, vomiting

  If GCS of 15, patient can be discharged without CT scan if:
- *Low risk*:
  - GCS remains 15
  - No loss of consciousness or amnesia
  - No neurologic/cognitive abnormalities
  - No headache, vomiting

Suggested guidelines for acute neuroimaging in adult patient with severe TBI (GCS 3–8): [21]

- CT scan patient with severe TBI as soon as possible to determine if require surgical intervention.
- If initial scan is normal, but patient has neurologic deterioration, repeat CT scan or consider MRI as soon as possible.
- If initial scan is abnormal, but patient status is unchanged, repeat CT scan within 24–36 hours to determine possible progressive hemorrhage or edema requiring surgical intervention, particularly if initial scan showed:
  - Any intracranial hemorrhage
  - Any evidence of diffuse brain injury
- If initial scan is abnormal, repeat CT scan or consider MRI as soon as possible if GCS worsens
- Consider MRI within first few days if:
  - Suspect secondary injury such as focal infarction, diffuse hypoxic-ischemic injury or infection.

Imaging Guidelines for Pediatric Head Injury

CT Algorithm for Children <2 years

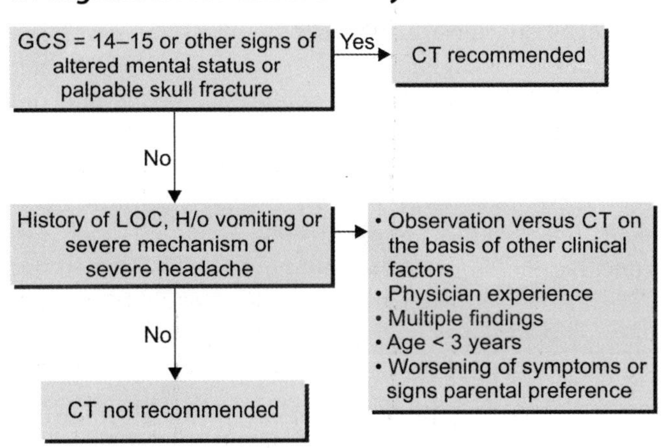

CT Algorithm for Children >2 years

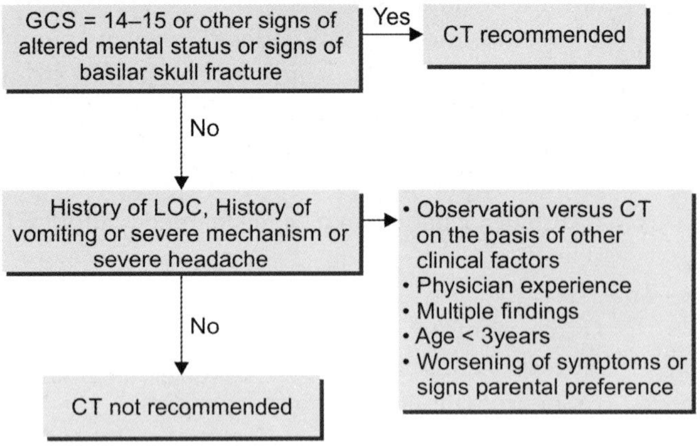

IMAGING FINDINGS

Scalp Injury

While interpreting CT scans of head trauma, begin by looking at the extracranial structures for evidence of soft-tissue injury and/or radio-opaque foreign bodies. Scalp injury provides a reliable indication of the site of impact.

Types of Scalp Injury

- Simple soft-tissue lacerations
- Subgaleal hematoma
- Cephalohematoma
- Residual foreign bodies

The subgaleal hematoma is the most common manifestation of scalp injury **(Fig. 6)**. It is seen as focal soft-tissue swelling located beneath the subcutaneous fibrofatty tissue and above the temporalis muscle and calvarium.[9,23]

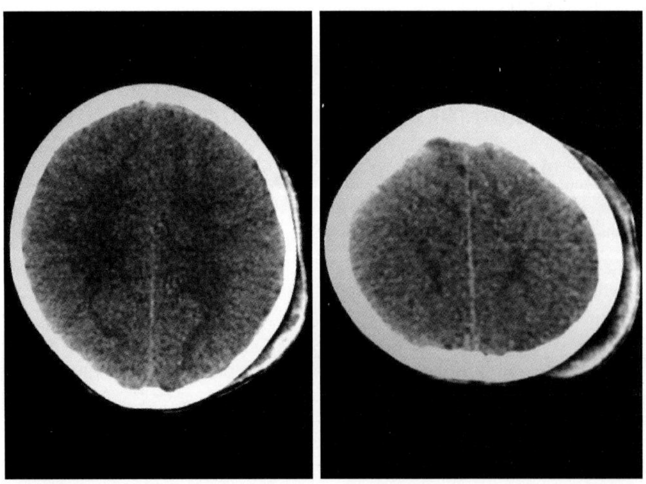

Fig. 6: Axial CT section of brain showing focal soft-tissue swelling located beneath the subcutaneous fibrofatty tissue in left temparoparietal region suggestive of scalp hematoma.

Skull Fractures

Types of Skull Fractures

- Linear
- Depressed
- Compound

Non-displaced linear fractures of the calvarium may be difficult to detect on CT when the fracture plane is parallel to the plane of section. Also, isolated linear skull fractures **(Fig. 7A)** usually do not require treatment unless they are associated with an epidural hematoma.

However, the depressed and compound skull fractures are easily detectable on CT **(Figs. 7B and C)**, which require surgical intervention. Depressed skull fractures may be associated with an underlying contusion; therefore, it is important to have careful look at the subjacent parenchyma **(Fig. 7C)**.

Recommendations

Thin reconstructions (1 mm) and use of bone algorithm is recommended for the evaluation of fractures in the skull base, orbit or facial bones. Thin sections are helpful for evaluating the degree of comminution and depression of bone fragments. MDCT with 3D reconstruction such as volume rendered algorithms can display complex fractures very clearly.[9,23]

Temporal Bone Fractures

When to suspect temporal bone fractures?

- Presence of pneumocephalus,
- Opacification of the mastoid air cells, and
- Fluid in the middle ear cavity should raise the suspicion of a temporal bone fracture.

Thin-sections (1 to 1.5 mm) in axial plane and coronal 3D reconstructions in bone algorithm is recommended for the evaluation of temporal bone fractures.

Types of Temporal Bone Fractures[22] (Figs. 8A and B)

- Longitudinal
- Transverse
- Mixed

Fractures are classified depending on the orientation of fracture line relative to the long axis of the petrous bone. Longitudinal fractures parallel the long axis of the petrous pyramid, and transverse fractures are perpendicular to the long axis of the petrous bone.

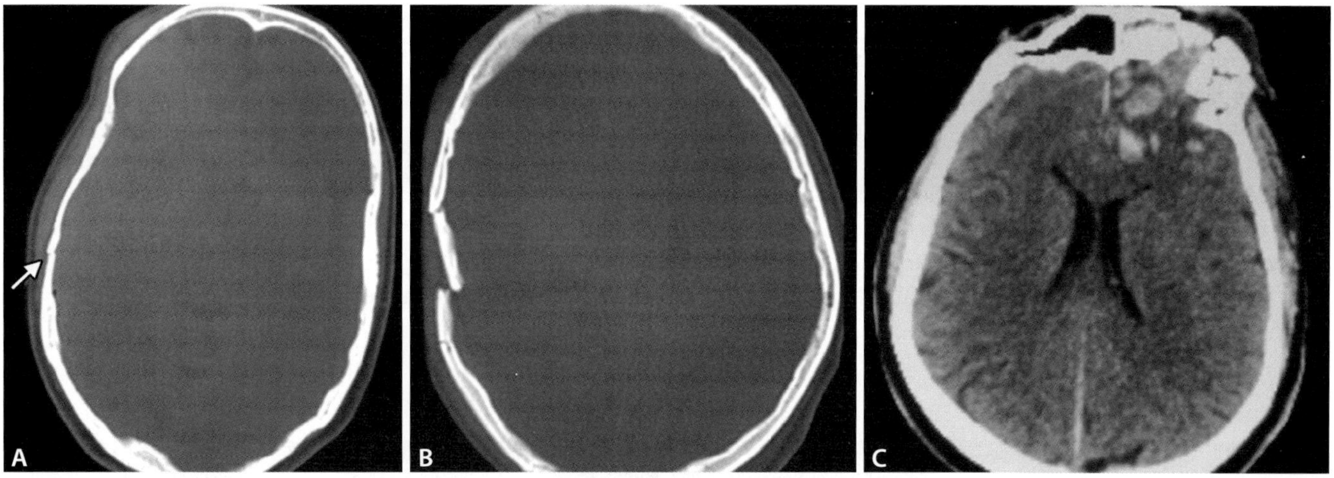

Figs. 7A to C: Axial CT sections to show various types of skull fractures: (A) Linear fracture (arrow); (B) Depressed fracture; (C) Compound fracture.

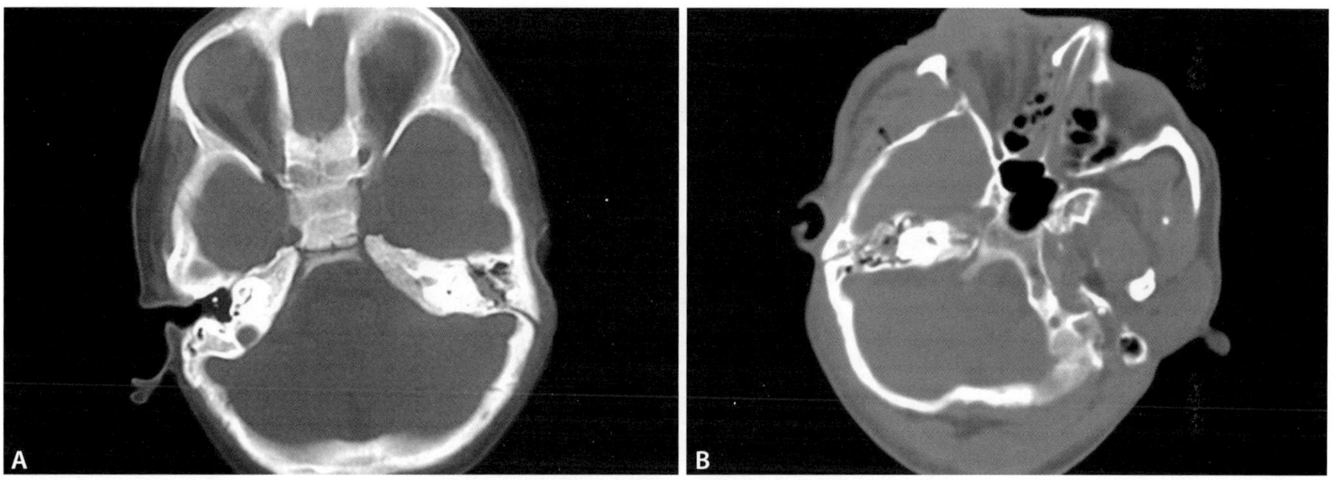

Figs. 8A and B: Thin-CT sections (1 mm) in axial plane in bone algorithm showing temporal bone fractures: (A) Transverse fracture; and (B) Longitudinal fracture.

Longitudinal temporal bone fractures represent more than 70% of temporal bone fractures.[20] The line of force runs roughly from lateral to medial **(Fig. 8B)**. A fracture line may extend through the facial nerve canal, thereby damaging the facial nerve, designated as cranial nerve (CN) VII. Complications include conductive hearing loss from dislocation or fracture of the ossicles, otorhinorrhea from CSF leak, and facial nerve palsy.

Transverse temporal bone fractures typically result from trauma to the temporal or parietal region and commonly involve fractures of the temporal squamosa or parietal bone. Fracture line passes through the vestibulocochlear apparatus and can cause sensorineural hearing loss and equilibrium disorders **(Fig. 8A)**. Transverse fractures also commonly injure CN VII, because their path often takes them close to the nerve's labyrinthine segment.

Mixed or complex temporal bone fractures involve a combination of fracture planes. They typically result from severe crushing blows to the skull. Patients with mixed temporal bone fractures have a high incidence of associated intracranial injury.

PRIMARY HEAD INJURY LESIONS

Extra-axial Injury[9,23]

- Epidural hematoma
- Subdural hematoma
- Subarachnoid hemorrhage
- Intraventricular hemorrhage

Epidural Hematoma (EDH)

Blood collects in the potential space located between the inner table of the skull and the dura. The developing hematoma dissects the dura from the inner table of the skull, forming an ovoid mass that displaces the adjacent brain. Majority of the EDH are due to arterial hemorrhage and most commonly affected artery is the middle meningeal artery, due to the fracture in the squamous part of temporal bone. In children, EDH can occur due to stretching or tearing of meningeal arteries without fracture. Venous EDHs are less common and can occur due to rupture of venous sinuses.[9,23]

Imaging Features

On CT, the acute EDH appears as a well-defined, hyperdense, biconvex, extra-axial collection **(Fig. 9A)**. It is usually associated with an overlying skull fracture **(Fig. 9B)**. Mass effect with sulcal effacement and midline shift is frequently seen. Because the EDH is located in the potential space between the dura and inner table of the

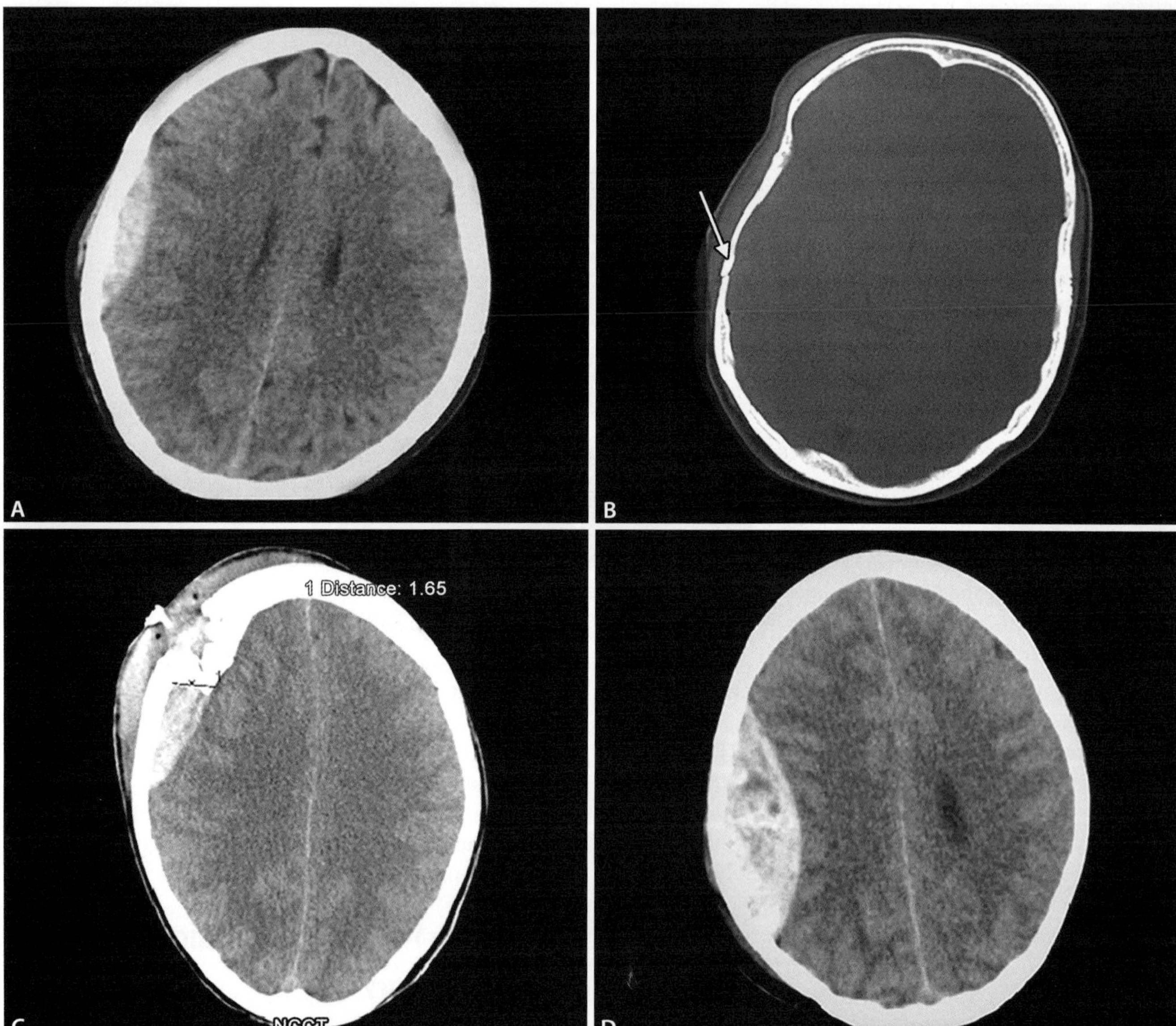

Figs. 9A to D: Axial CT images showing features of extradural hematoma: (A) A well-defined, hyperdense, biconvex, extra-axial collection associated with overlying skull fracture (arrow) (B), presence of low-attenuation areas within the hyperdense hematoma called "swirl sign" (D), diameter of hematoma >1.5 cm is an indication for surgery (C).

skull, it rarely crosses cranial sutures because theperiosteal layer of the dura is firmly attached at sutural margins. However, at the vertex, where the periosteum that forms the outer wall of the sagittal sinus is not tightly attached to the sagittal suture, the EDH can cross midline.[9,23]

Ominous sign: An imaging finding that predicts rapid expansion of an arterial EDH is the presence of low-attenuation areas within the hyperdense hematoma (the so-called "swirl sign"), represents active bleeding **(Fig. 9C)**.[24]

Management[25]

Conservative treatment is persued if:

- Volume of EDH < 30 cm^3
- Midline shift < 5 mm
- Diameter of lesion <1.5 cm

Potential indications for surgery are:

- Size > 1.5 cm **(Fig. 9D)**
- Active bleeding
- Pending herniation
- Corresponding neurological deficit.

In the presence of swirl sign, patient should be carefully monitored for signs of herniation due to expanding hematoma.[24]

Classic Acute Epidural Hematoma
Terminology Blood between dura and skull
Etiology • Skull fracture: 90–95% • Arterial source: 90% (middle meningeal artery) • Venous source: 10%
Pathology • Unilateral, supratentorial (90%) • Dura stripped away from skull • Usually does not cross sutures (exception children) • Does not cross sites of dural attachment
Clinical • 1-4% of head trauma • Most common young adults • M:F = 4:1 • Classic lucid interval in 50% only • Delayed presentation is common • Low mortality of recognized and treated • Small EDHs managed conservatively
Imaging • Hyperdense lens-shaped (biconvex) • *Swirl sign*: Ongoing bleed

Subdural Hematomas (SDH)

Blood collects in between the inner dural layer and the arachnoid. The hematoma dissects in-between these two layers because these layers are not firmly attached, hence SDH are frequently seen along the entire hemispheric convexity from the anterior falx to the posterior falx.

SDHs are generally venous in origin. They usually arise from laceration of bridging cortical veins during sudden head deceleration. SDHs are commonly seen in elderly due to prominent extra-axial space (resulting from cerebral atrophy), which allows an increased motion between the brain parenchyma and the calvarium. Other causes of the SDH include rapid decompression of obstructive hydrocephalus, and injury to pial vessels and pacchionian granulations.[9,23,25]

Imaging Features

On CT, the acute SDH are seen as hyperdense (50–60 HU), homogenous, crescent-shaped, extra-axial collection **(Fig. 10A)**. Most are supratentorial and located along the convexity. They are also frequently identified along the falx and tentorium **(Figs. 11A and B)**.

The density of SDH will progressively decrease due to protein degradation within the hematoma **(Figs. 10A to C)**. Rebleeding during courseof a SDH appears as heterogenous attenuation on CT, due to mixture of fresh blood and partially liquid hematoma **(Figs. 12A and B)**. A sediment level or "hematocrit effect" may be seen either from rebleeding or in patients with clotting disorders. The chronic SDH has a low-attenuation value similar to, but slightly higher than, CSF **(Fig. 10C)**.

Challenges During Interpretation[9,23]

1. It can be difficult to distinguish from prominent subarachnoid space in patients with cerebral atrophy. In these patients, intravenous contrast administration can be helpful by demonstrating an enhancing capsule or displaced cortical veins.
2. A small thin convexity SDH can be difficult to appreciate adjacent to the hyperdense skull unless the images are viewed with a "wide window" **(Fig. 13A)**.
3. During the transition from acute to the chronic SDH, an isodense phase occurs, usually between 1 and 3 weeks after the acute event, depending on the patient's hematocrit level, clotting capability, and presence or absence of rebleeding. Recognition of indirect imaging findings **(Fig. 13B)**, such as effacement of sulci, displacement of gray matter with white matter "buckling," and midline shift **(Fig. 14)** on a non-contrast CT scan can avoid this common pitfall.

SDH Evolution on MRI

The MR appearance of a SDH also evolves over time, depending on the biochemical state of hemoglobin

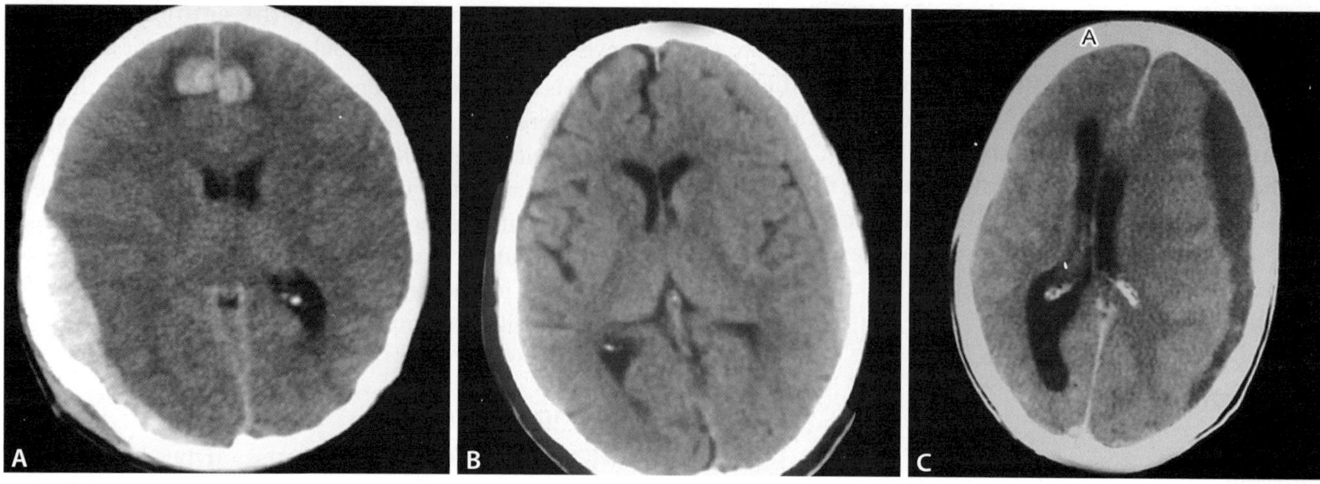

Figs. 10A to C: Axial CT images showing various stages of subdural hematoma: (A) Acute SDH seen as hyperdense (50–60 HU), homogeneous, crescent-shaped, extra-axial collection; (B) Subacute SDH seen as isodense (30–40 HU), homogeneous, crescent-shaped, extra-axial collection; (C) Chronic SDH seen as hypodense (10 HU) extra-axial collection.

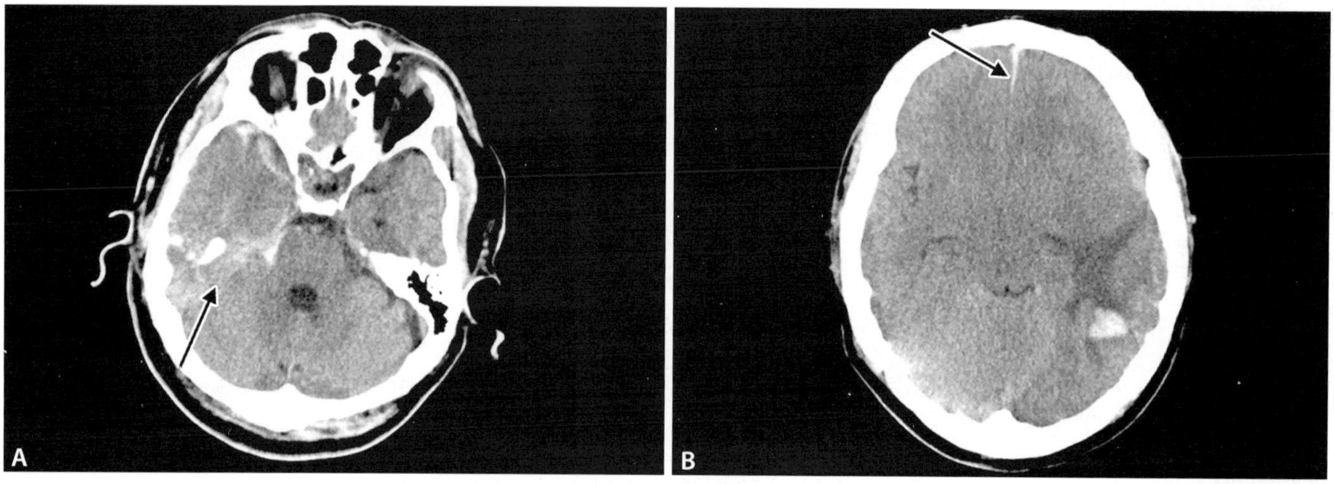

Figs. 11A and B: Axial CT section to show SDH along tentorium (arrow) (A) and along falx (arrow) (B).

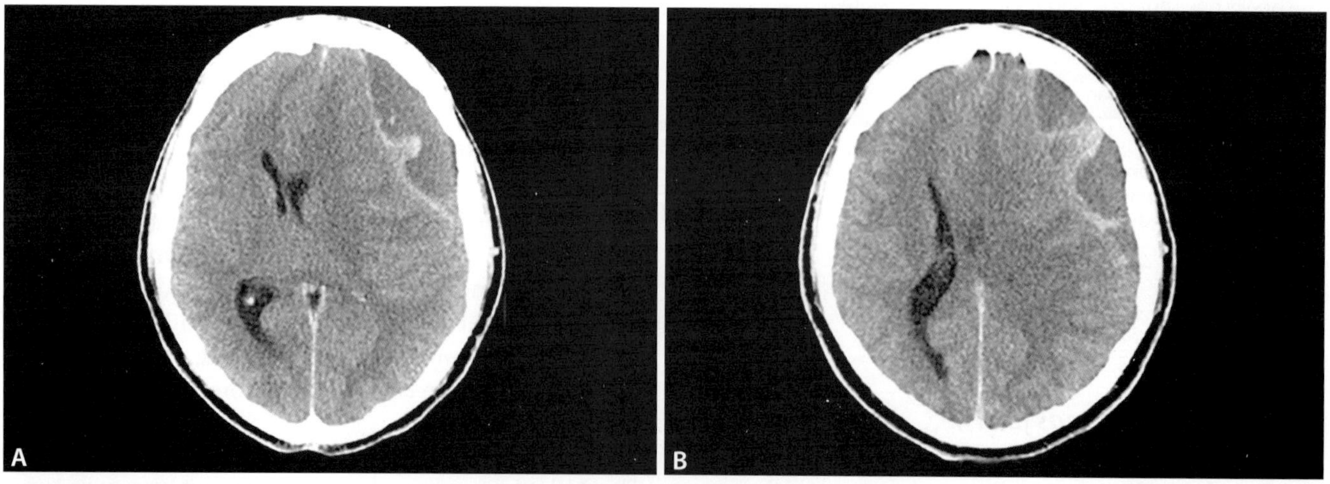

Figs. 12A and B: Axial CT section showing heterogeneous attenuation SDH in left frontoparietal region, due to mixture of fresh blood and partially liquefied hematoma due to rebleeding during course of a SDH.

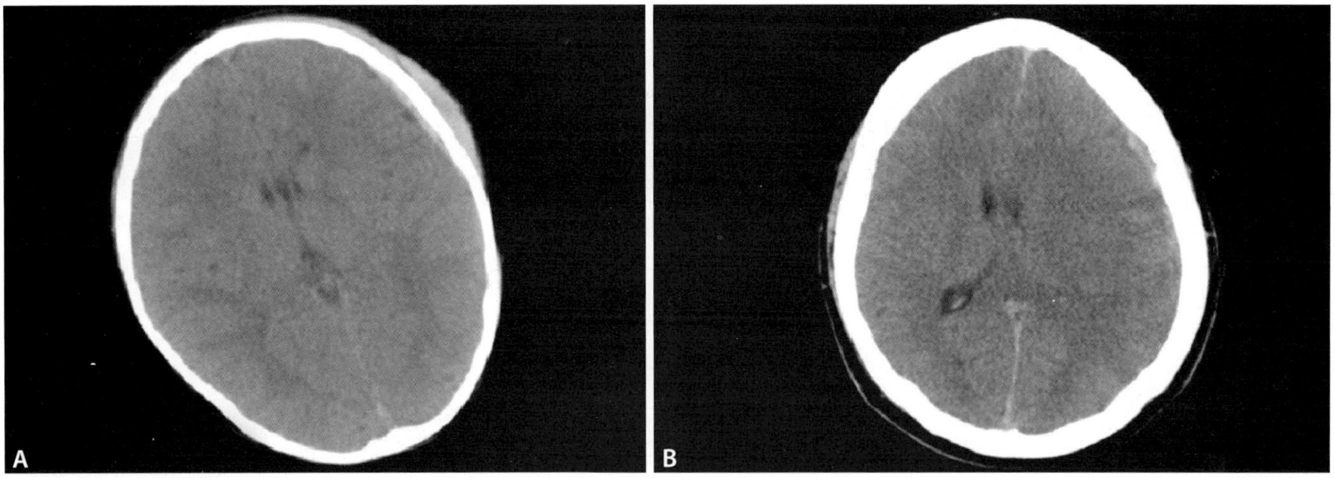

Figs. 13A and B: Axial CT images to show technical difficulties in interpretation of SDH: (A) A small thin convexity SDH can be difficult to appreciate adjacent to the hyperdense skull unless the images are viewed with a "wide window"; (B) identification of isodense phase of SDH diificult unless one should look at indirect imaging findings, such as effacement of sulci, displacement of gray matter with white matter "buckling," and midline shift on a non-contrast CT scan to avoid this common pitfall.

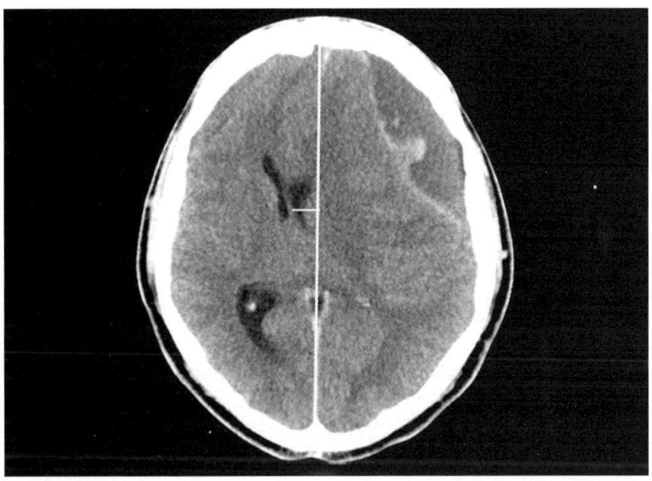

Fig. 14: Axial CT image at the level of septum pellucidum to show technique of measurement of midline shift. Draw a line joining a bone protrusion is located in the anterior section of the skull; (the falx cerebri extends from this point) and another bony protrusion in posterior section of the skull (falx cerebri ends at this point). Another line is drawn perpendicular to the former line from septum pellucidum that gives the exact amount of midline shift.

(Table 1). The acute SDH is isointense to brain on T1-weighted and hypointense on T2-weighted images. During the subacute phase, when the subdural hematoma may be isodense or hypodense on CT scans, T1-weighted images demonstrate high signal intensity due to the presence of methemoglobin in the subdural collection. The chronic SDH appears hypointense on T1-weighted and hyperintense on T2-weighted images relative to normal brain. The signal intensity of chronic SDH is slightly higher than CSF signal intensity on T1-weighted, FLAIR, and proton-density T2-weighted imaging. Because of its multiplanar capability, MR is useful in identifying convexity and vertex hematomas that might not be detected on axial CT scans because of the similar attenuation of the adjacent bone.[9,23,26]

Traumatic Subarachnoid Hemorrhage

Traumatic subarachnoid hemorrhage (SAH) can result from:

- The disruption of small pial vessels;

Table 1: Temporal evolution of ICH.

Biochemical form	*Clinical stage*	*Approximate time of appearance*	*Intensity on T1WI*	*Intensity on T2WI*
OxyHg in RBCs	Hyperacute	Immediately to first several hours	Isointense	Hyperintense
DeoxyHg in RBCs	Acute	Hours to days	Iso to hypointense	Hypointense
MetHg in RBCs	Early subacute	First several days	Hyperintense	Hypointense
Extracellular MetHg	Subacute to chronic	Days to months	Hyperintense	Hyperintense
Ferritin and Hemosiderin	Remote	Days to indefinitely	Hypointense	Hyperintense

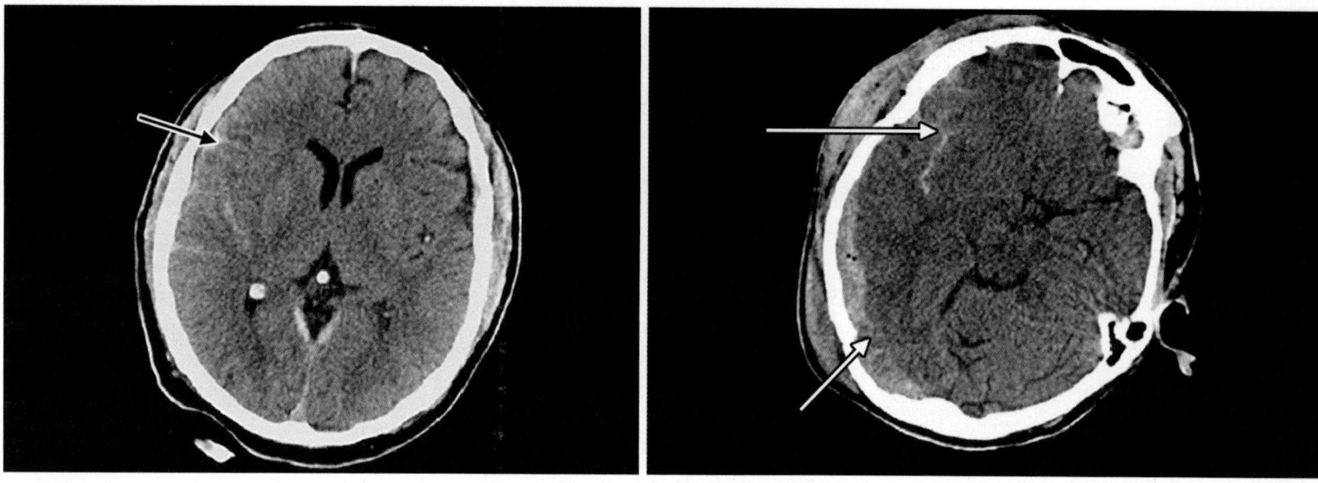

Fig. 15: Axial CT sections showing linear or serpentine areas of high attenuation that confirming to the morphology of the cerebral sulci and sylvian cisterns (Black arrow). *Note*: There is associated SDH along the right occipital region (white arrows).

- Extension into the subarachnoid space by a contusion or hematoma; or
- Diffusion of intraventricular hemorrhage.

SAH is very common with TBI, but it rarely causes mass effect. On CT, SAH appears as linear or serpentine areas of high attenuation that conform to the morphology of the cerebral sulci and cisterns **(Fig. 15)**. Common sites for SAH include the sylvian and interpeduncular cisterns. sometime, "effacement" of sulci due to the presence of intrasulcal SAH may be the only imaging clue of the presence of SAH. In patients who are found unconscious after an unwitnessed event, the detection of SAH in key cisterns (basilar, sylvian, and circle of Willis) may indicate a ruptured aneurysm, rather than trauma. In such cases, contrast-enhanced CT angiography is recommended as the next step in the patient evaluation **(Figs. 16A and E)**.

MR Imaging of SAH

Acute subarachnoid hemorrhage may be more difficult to detect on conventional MR than on CT because it can be isointense to brain parenchyma on routine T1- and T2-weighted images. However, FLAIR has been shown to be more sensitive than CT in detecting acute subarachnoid hemorrhage.[14] Subacute subarachnoid hemorrhage may be better appreciated on MR because of its high signal intensity when the blood is isointense to CSF on CT. Chronic hemorrhage on MR scans may show hemosiderin staining in the subarachnoid space, which appears as areas of decreased signal intensity on T1- and T2-weighted sequences ("superficial hemo-siderosis"). Hemosiderins are best detected on gradient-echoT2*- weighted images. SAH may lead to communicating hydrocephalus by impeding CSF resorption at the level of arachnoid villi.[9,14,15,23]

Subdural Hemorrhage

Acute SDH (aSDH)
• Second MC traumatic extra axial hemorrhage (SAH>SDH>EDH)
• Crescentic blood collection between dura and arachnoid
  – Supratentorial (95%). bilateral (15%)
  – SDH cross sutures
  – SDH do not cross dural attachments
• CT
  – Hyperdense (60%)
  – Mixed (40%)
  – Isodense acute SDH (anemia—coagulopathy)

Subacute SDH (sSDH)
• Clot organizes. lyses forms neomembranes
• CT
  – Density decreases (1–2HU/day)
  – Isodense with cortex in 7–10 days
  – Look for displaced "dots" of CSF under SDH
  – Gray-white interface "buckled" inward
  – Displaced cortical veins seen on CECT
• MRI
  – Signal varies with clot age
  – R2* and SWI shows bloom ing

Chronic SDH (cSDH)
• Serosanguineous fluid
  – Hypodense on NCCT
  – Rehemorrhage (5–10%)
  – Loculated blood pockets with fluid-fluid levels

Traumatic intraventricular hemorrhage (IVH) can also occur by one of three mechanisms.

- Rotationally induced tearing of subependymal veins along the surface of the ventricles.
- Direct extension of a parenchymal hematoma into the ventricular system.

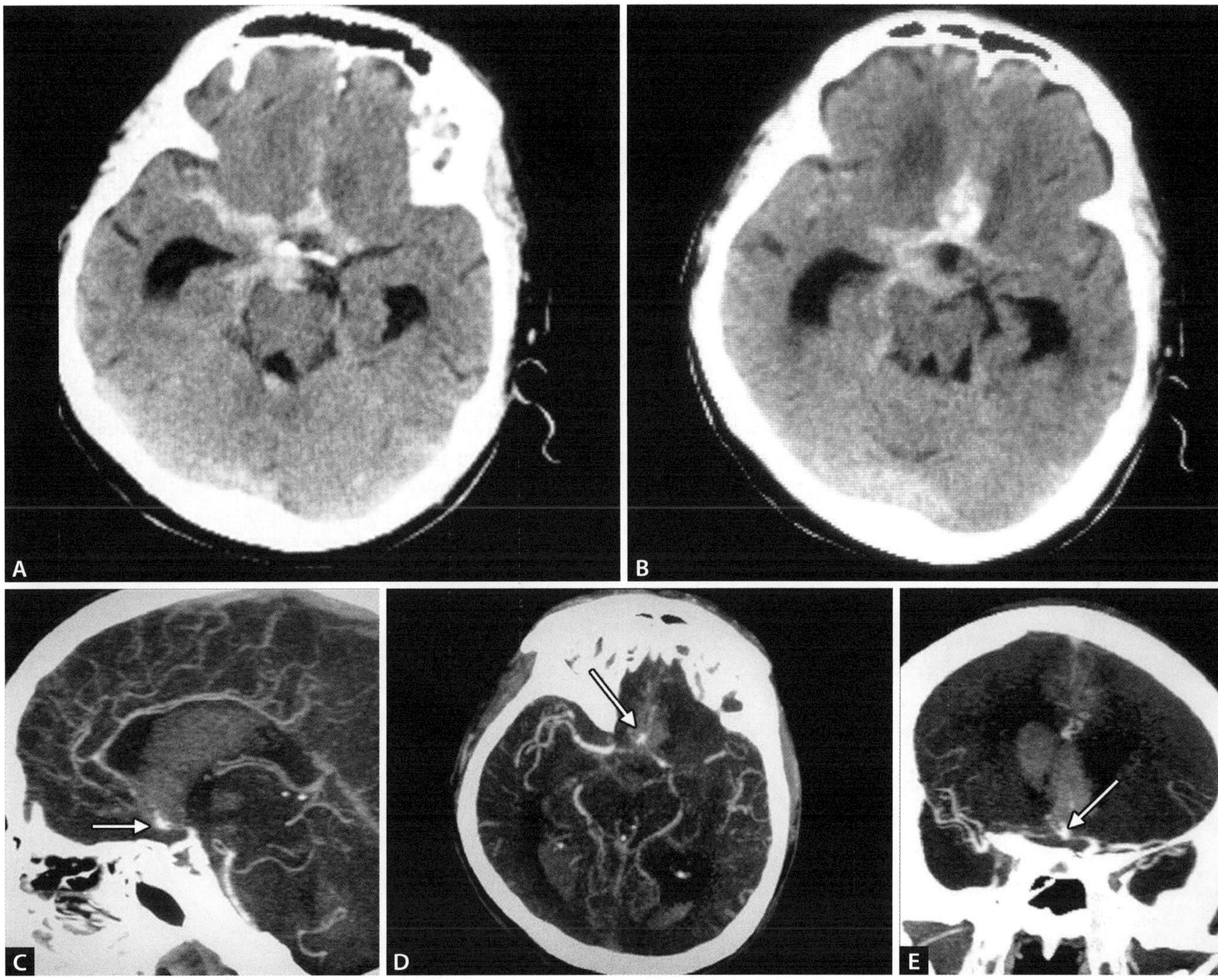

Figs. 16A to E: NCCT axial sections showing subarachanoid hemorrhage in basal cisterns (A and B), 3D reformation of CT angiography showing ACoM pseudoaneurysm responsible for subarachanoid hemorrhage (C to E).

- Retrograde flow of SAH into the ventricular system via the fourth ventricular outflow foramina (the reverse mechanism in which IVH can extend into the subarachnoid space).

Patients with IVH are at risk for developing both communicating and non-communicating hydrocephalus secondary to obstruction at the level of the arachnoid villi or aqueduct, respectively. They are also at risk of ependymitis from the irritant effects of the blood. On CT, IVH usually appears as CSF-hyperdense fluid level, layering within the ventricular system **(Fig. 17A and B)**. Certainly, tiny collections of increased density layering in the occipital horns may be the only clue to IVH. Occasionally, the IVH may appear "tumefactive" as a cast within the ventricle.[9,23]

Intra-axial Injury

Diffuse axonal injury (DAI) results from rotational acceleration and deceleration forces that produce shearing deformations of brain tissue. Clinically, DAI is characterized by loss or severe impairment of consciousness beginning at the moment of direct impact. DAI in the chronic stage may result in overwhelming cognitive and psychiatric problems.

MRI is clearly superior to CT for detecting DAI, and therefore, provides increased success at explaining neurologic deficits after trauma and predicting long-term outcome. Newer imaging methods, such as DWI and DTI with 3D tractography, have shown potential in improving the detection of white matter injury in both acute and chronic DAI.[26-28]

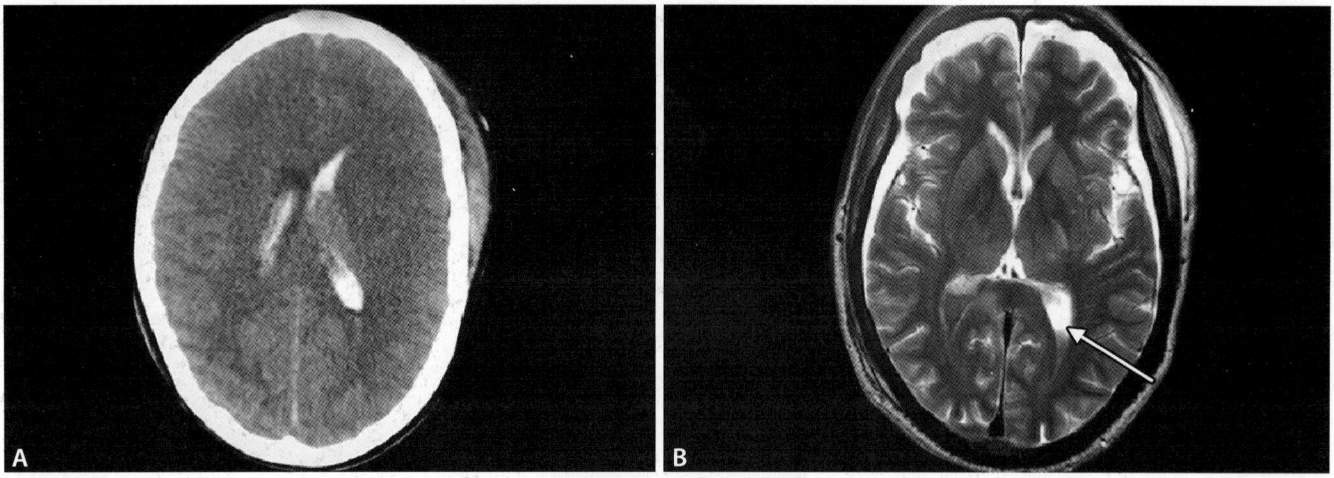

Figs. 17A and B: Axial CT and MR sections to show appearances of IVH. (A) Hyperdense (blood) within the bilateral lateral ventricles, (B) CSF-blood fluid level (hyper-hypo intense) layering within the ventricular system (arrow).

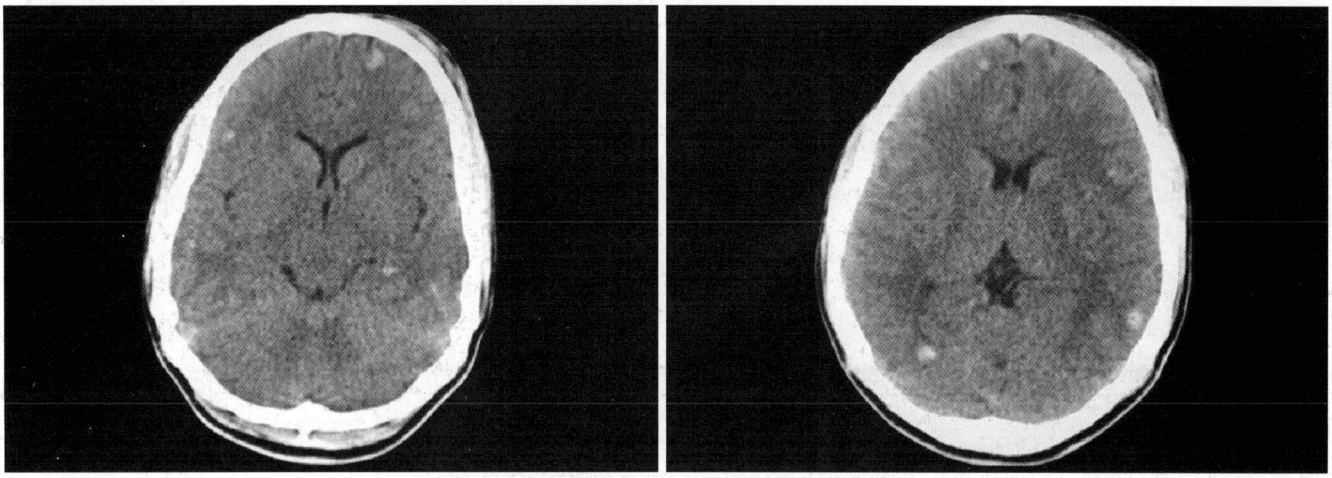

Fig. 18: Axial CT images showing multiple, small, petechial hemorrhages at the gray–white junction of the cerebral hemispheres suggestive of DAI.

CT is mostly limited to depicting the small focal hemorrhages associated with axonal shearing injury. Common findings include small, petechial hemorrhages at the gray-white junction of the cerebral hemispheres **(Fig. 18)** and corpus callosum. Unfortunately, only about 20% of DAI lesions contain sufficient hemorrhage to be detectable on CT.

Because of better sensitivity to blood products, gradient-echo T2*-weighted MR demonstrates more DAI lesions than CT **(Fig. 19A)**.[16] Spin-echo T2-weighted MR techniques, especially FLAIR imaging, can detect many nonhemorrhagic foci of DAI but still underestimate the true extent of traumatic white matter damage. On MR, nonhemorrhagic DAI lesions appear as multiple small foci of increased signal on T2-weighted images, DWI images **(Fig. 19B)** and as decreased signal on T1-weighted images within the white matter. Petechial hemorrhage causes a central hypointensity on T2-weighed images and hyperintensity on T1-weighted images as a result of intracellular methemoglobin in the subacute stage.

The conspicuity of DAI on MR eventually diminishes as the damaged axons degenerate and the edema resolves. Residual findings may include nonspecic atrophy, gliosis, or hemosiderin staining, which can persist indefinitely on gradient-echo T2*-weighted images.

The location of the DAI tends to correlate with the severity of the trauma.[26-28]

- **Grade I DAI:** Involves only the peripheral gray–white junctions of the lobar white matter. The parasagittal regions of the frontal lobes and periventricular

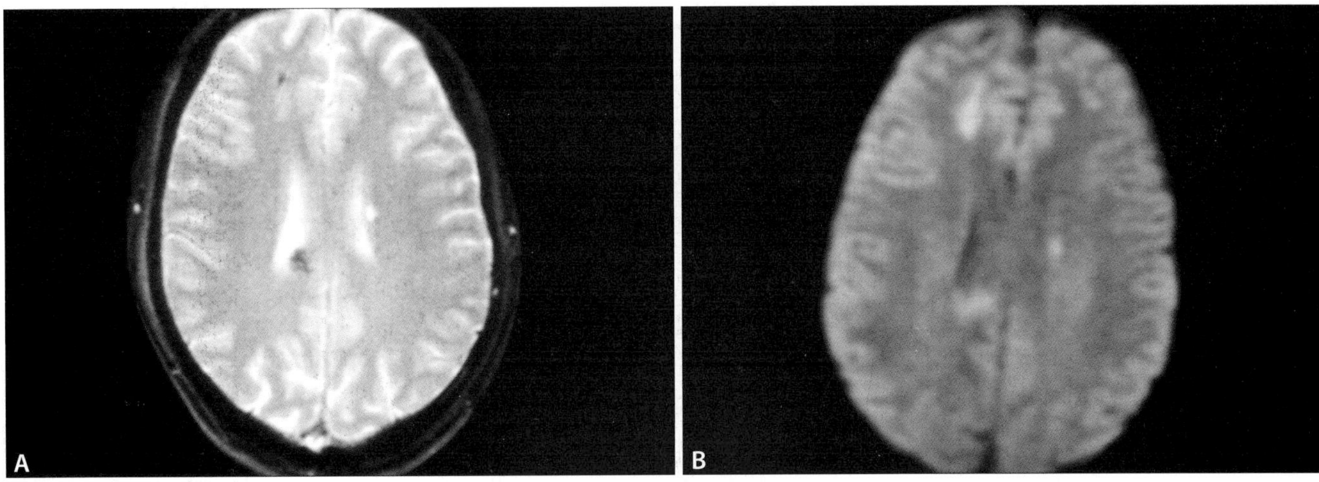

Figs. 19A and B: Axial MR images showing features of DAI: (A) Gradient echo sequence showing hypointense foci in carpus callosum and in right frontal lobe (sensitive to detect hemorrhagic DAI lesions due to sensitivity to blood products); (B) DWI image showing multiple small foci of increased signal in both cerebral hemisphere and in corpus callosum (sensitive to detect additional nonhemorrhagic DAI lesions).

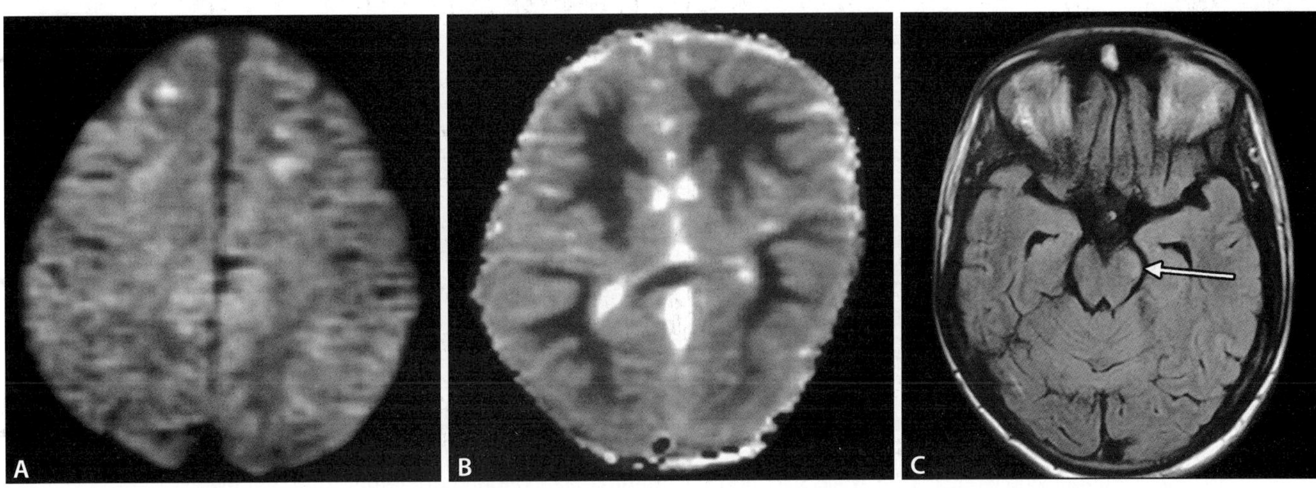

Figs. 20A to C: MR images to show types of DAI lesions: (A) Lesions seen at peripheral gray-white junctions of the lobar white matter; (B) Lesions involve both the lobar white-matter as well as the corpus callosum; (C) Lesions involve dorsolateral midbrain (brainstem, arrow).

regions of the temporal lobes are commonly affected **(Fig. 20A)**.

- **Grade II DAI:** Involves both the lobar white-matter as well as the corpus callosum, particularly the posterior body and splenium. The corpus callosum is susceptible to DAI because the falx prevents displacement of the cerebral hemispheres **(Fig. 20B)**.
- **Grade III DAI:** Dorsolateral midbrain (brainstem), in addition to the lobar white matter and corpus callosum are affected **(Fig. 20C)**.

Diffuse Vascular Injury: Diffuse vascular injury (DVI) signifies the most severe form of the diffuse axonal injury range. Most of these patients with DVI do not reach hospital or live long ample of time for imaging.

In patients who get imaging done, most conspicuous finding is diffuse brain swelling with effaced sulci and small ventricles. Sometime few small foci of hemorrhage in the white matter and basal ganglia may be identified.

Cortical contusion is a focal brain lesion primarily involving superficial gray matter, with relative sparing of the underlying white matter. Regions of the brain that are in close contact with the rough surface on the inner skull table are commonly affected. These areas include the orbitofrontal and temporal lobes, and less so, the parasagittal convexity. The temporal lobes above the petrous bone or posterior to the greater sphenoid wing, and the frontal lobes above the cribriform plate, planum sphenoidale, and lesser sphenoid wing are commonly affected **(Figs. 21A and B)**. Contusions are associated with a better prognosis than DAI, unless they are accompanied by brainstem injury or significant mass effect. Contusions can also occur at the margins of depressed skull fractures **(Fig. 22)**. The cerebellum is involved less than 10% of the time.[9,23,29]

On CT, non-hemorrhagic contusions are difficult to detect initially until the development of associated edema. Hemorrhagic contusions are more easily identified and appear as foci of high attenuation within superficial gray matter. They may be surrounded by larger areas of low attenuation from the associated vasogenic edema. As the contusion evolves, the characteristic "salt and pepper" pattern of mixed areas of hypodensity and hyperdensity becomes more apparent. Contusions with severe mass effect may require surgical decompression to prevent secondary injury.[9,23]

On MRI, contusions appear as ill-defined areas of variable signal intensity on both T1- and T2-weighted images, depending on the age of the lesions. They are limited to the surface and often have a "gyral" morphology. Hemosiderin from an old contusion leads to decreased signal intensity on T2- and especially T2*-weighted images, especially at higher field strengths. The signal loss can persist indefinitely and serves as an important marker of prior hemorrhage.[29]

The **intracerebral hematoma** is the most common cause of clinical deterioration in patients who have experienced a lucid interval after the initial injury. In

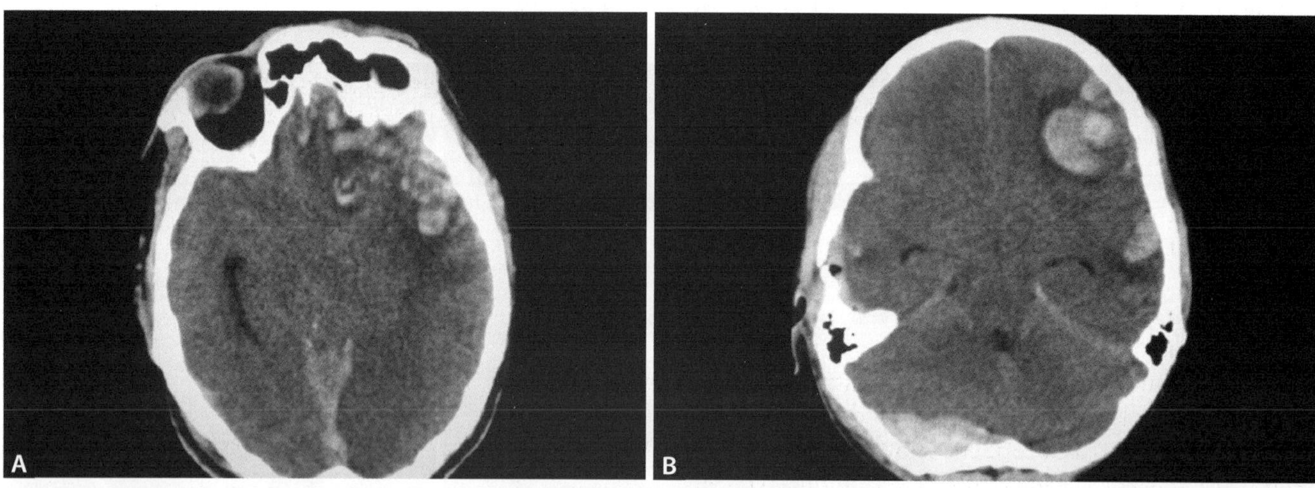

Figs. 21A and B: Axial CT sections showing contusions in orbitofrontal lobe (A), temporal lobe (B) involving the superficial gray matter sparing the underlying white matter. *Note*: SDH along tentorium (A) and along right temporo-occipital regions (B).

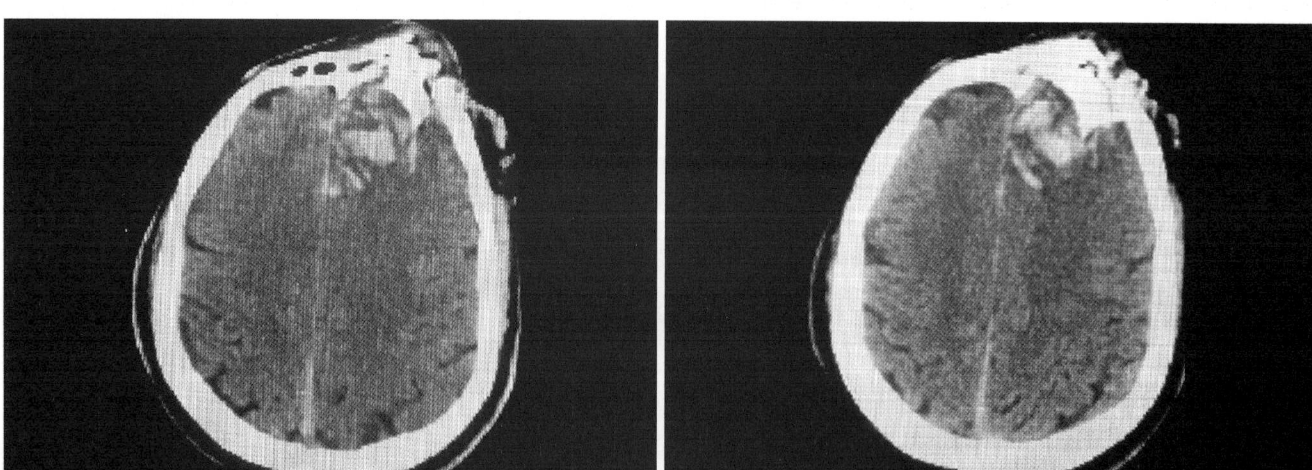

Fig. 22: Axial CT sections showing cerebral contusion in left frontal lobe associated with compound skull fracture.

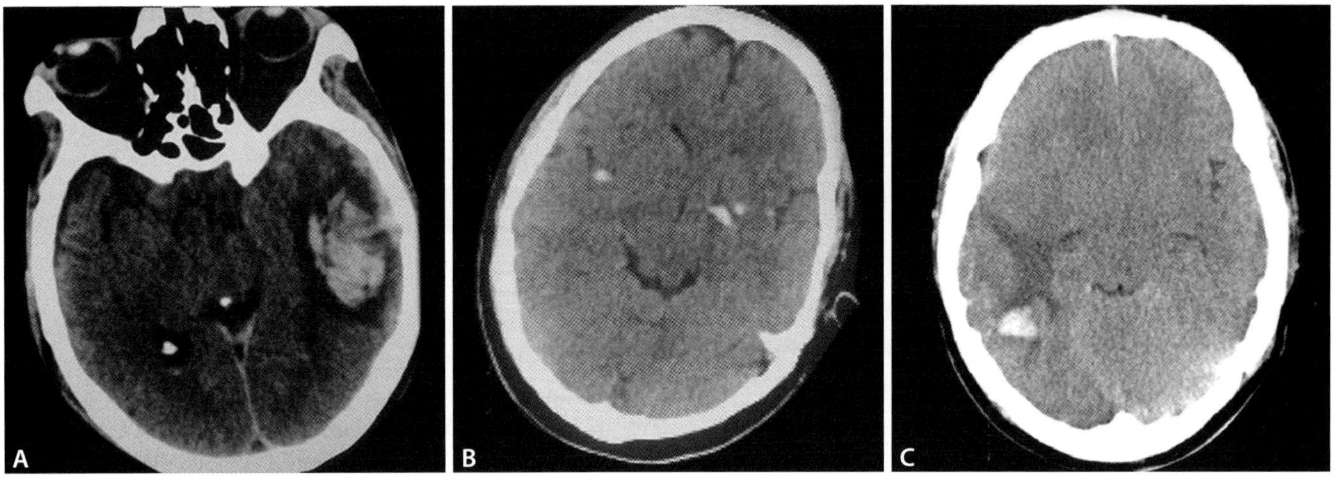

Figs. 23A to C: Axial CT sections showing intracerebral hematomas in left temporal lobe (A); basal ganglia (B); and temporo-occipital lobe (C).

contrast to the common contusion described above, the intracerebral hematoma is due to shear-induced hemorrhage from the rupture of small intraparenchymal blood vessels. Because the bleeding occurs into areas of relatively normal brain, intracerebral hematomas tend to have less surrounding edema than cortical contusions. Most traumatic intracerebral hematomas are located in the frontotemporal white matter **(Figs. 23A to C)**. Involvement of the basal ganglia has been described; however, hemorrhage in basal ganglia should alert the radiologist that an underlying hypertensive bleed may be the culprit. Intracerebral hematomas are often associated with skull fractures and other primary neuronal lesions, including contusions and DAI, especially in patients who are unconscious at the time of injury. Symptoms typically result from the mass effect associated with an expanding hematoma. Indeed, delayed hemorrhage is a common cause of clinical deterioration during the first several days after head trauma.[9,23] It is important to differentiate benign hemorrhage from intratumoral hemorrhage **(Table 2)**.

Brain laceration happens when severe injury disrupts the pia mater and factually tears the underlying brain apart. It is usually seen in infants and children due to head trauma associated with child abuse. A "burst lobe" is the most severe form of brain laceration, where in the affected lobe is completely disrupted with surrounding large hematoma formation.

Table 2: Intratumoral hemorrhage versus benign intracranial hematomas.

Intratumoral hemorrhage	*Benign hemorrhage*
Markedly heterogeneous, related to:	Shows expected signal intensities of acute, subacute or chronic blood, depending on stage of hematoma
• Mixed stages of blood	
• Debris-fluid (intracellular-extracellular blood) levels	
• Edema + tumor + necrosis with blood	
Identification of nonhemorrhagic tumor component	No abnormal nonhemorrhagic mass
Delayed evolution of blood breakdown products	Follows expected orderly progression
Absent, diminished, or irregular ferritin/hemosiderin	Regular complete ferritin/ hemosiderin rim
Persistent surrounding high intensity on long TR images (i.e. tumor/edema) and mass effect, even in late stages	Complete resolution of edema and mass effect in chronic stages

Subcortical (Deep Brain) Injury

Subcortical injuries (SCIs) are traumatic intra-axial lesions that affect deep brain structures such as the brainstem, basal ganglia, thalami, and ventricles. These represent severe form of shear injuries that interrupt axons, tear penetrating blood vessels, and damage the choroid plexus of the lateral ventricles. SCIs are the third most common parenchymal brain injury, after cortical contusions and DAI. On imaging, initial scans may show subtle abnormalities with dramatic increase of findings on follow-up scans. Typical findings include diffuse brain edema with punctate hemorrhages in the deep gray nuclei and midbrain. Bleed within ventricles and choroid plexus are form and may form a "cast" of the lateral ventricles. This condition has to be differentiated from Duret hemorrhage that occur due to descending transtentorial herniation.

Duret hemorrhages are typically located within the center of midbrain, whereas SCIs are located dorsolateral.

Pneumocephalus: Pneumocephalus refers to presence of air within the intracranial cavity. In this condition, gas can be found anywhere within any compartment, including blood vessels.

Intracranial air is not normal finding, however it can be an expected and routine finding after brain surgery.

Tension pneumocephalus is a collection of intracranial gas under pressure that causes mass effect on the brain manifests with neurologic deterioration.

Patients with pneumocephalus may be asymptomatic or present with nonspecific headache. Very rarely, neurologic deficit and consciousness disturbances are observed. Most intracranial air resolves spontaneously within a few days after trauma or surgery. Occasionally, air collections increase and may require evacuation with duraplasty especially in case of tension pneumocephalus. On Imaging intracranial air may be seen in any compartment, i.e. epidural, subdural, subarachnoid, intraventricular, or intraparenchymal. It conforms to the shape of that compartment. Pneumocephalus is usually seen in subdural space, and the most common site is frontal location.

Pneumocephalus
Terminology • Air in any intracranial compartment • *Tension pneumocephalus*:   – Air under pressure>>>neurologic deterioration
Etiology • Surgery (MC) • Trauma (8–10%) • Spontaneous (defect in sinus)

Location
• *Epidural*:
  – Unilateral, biconvex
  – May cross midline
  – Does not move with change of position
• *Subdural*:
  – Confluent, Crescentic
  – Bilateral
  – Changes with head position
  – Does not cross midline
• *Subarachanoid*:
  – Discrete spots and dots in sulci, cisterns
• *Intraventricular*:
  – Usually air-fluid levels. frontal horns
• *Intraparenchymal*:
  – Confluent, well delineated
Imaging Features
• CT
  – Extremely hypodense (-1000 HU)
• MRI
  – Signal void
  – Prominent blooming on GRE
  – Alternating dark holes + /- concentric bright rings

Vascular Injury

Vascular injuries are mentioned here because they are causes of both intra- and extra-axial injuries, including the cause of hematomas and subarachnoid hemorrhages. Traumatic vascular injuries include arterial dissection, pseudoaneurysm, and arteriovenous fistula. Arterial injuries are usually related to skull base fractures. Most often injured artery is the internal carotid artery, especially at sites of fixation, where it enters the carotid canal at the base of the petrous bone, and at its exit from the cavernous sinus beneath the anterior clinoid process.

MR findings of vascular injury include: (a) presence of an intramural hematoma, which is best seen on T1-weighted with fat suppression; (b) intimal flap with dissection and (c) absence of a normal vascular flow void secondary to slow flow or occlusion. An associated parenchymal infarction supplied by the injured vessel may also be seen. Conventional angiogram remains the gold standard for confirmation and delineation of the vascular dissection and may also show spasm or pseudoaneurysm formation **(Figs. 24A to F)**. However, magnetic resonance angiography and MDCT angiography serve as important screening tools in the evaluation of patients with suspected vascular injury.[30]

The acquired **carotid cavernous fistula (CCF)** typically results from full-thickness arterial injury. The injury leads to communication between the cavernous portion of the internal carotid artery and the surrounding venous plexus, resulting in venous engorgement of the cavernous sinus **(Figs. 25 and 26)** and its draining branches namely the ipsilateral superior ophthalmic vein and inferiorpetrosal sinus. Skull base fractures, especially those involving the sphenoid bone, should alert the radiologist to search for associated cavernous carotid injury. Another cause of CCF is the rupture of a cavernous carotid aneurysm. On imaging, CCF can present as an enlarged superior ophthalmic vein, cavernous sinus, and/or petrosal sinus. Other findings include proptosis, preseptal soft-tissue swelling, and extraocular muscle enlargement. The findings may be bilateral because venous channels connect the cavernous sinuses. Again, definitive diagnosis often requires selective carotid angiography with rapid filming to demonstrate the site of communication. Patients can present with findings weeks or even months after the initial trauma.[31] Therefore, a CCF can be overlooked if a detailed clinical history and ophthalmic examination is notperformed.

Types of CCF[31]

Type A: Direct shunt between ICA and cavernous sinus.
Type B: Fistula between meningeal branches of ICA and cavernous sinus.

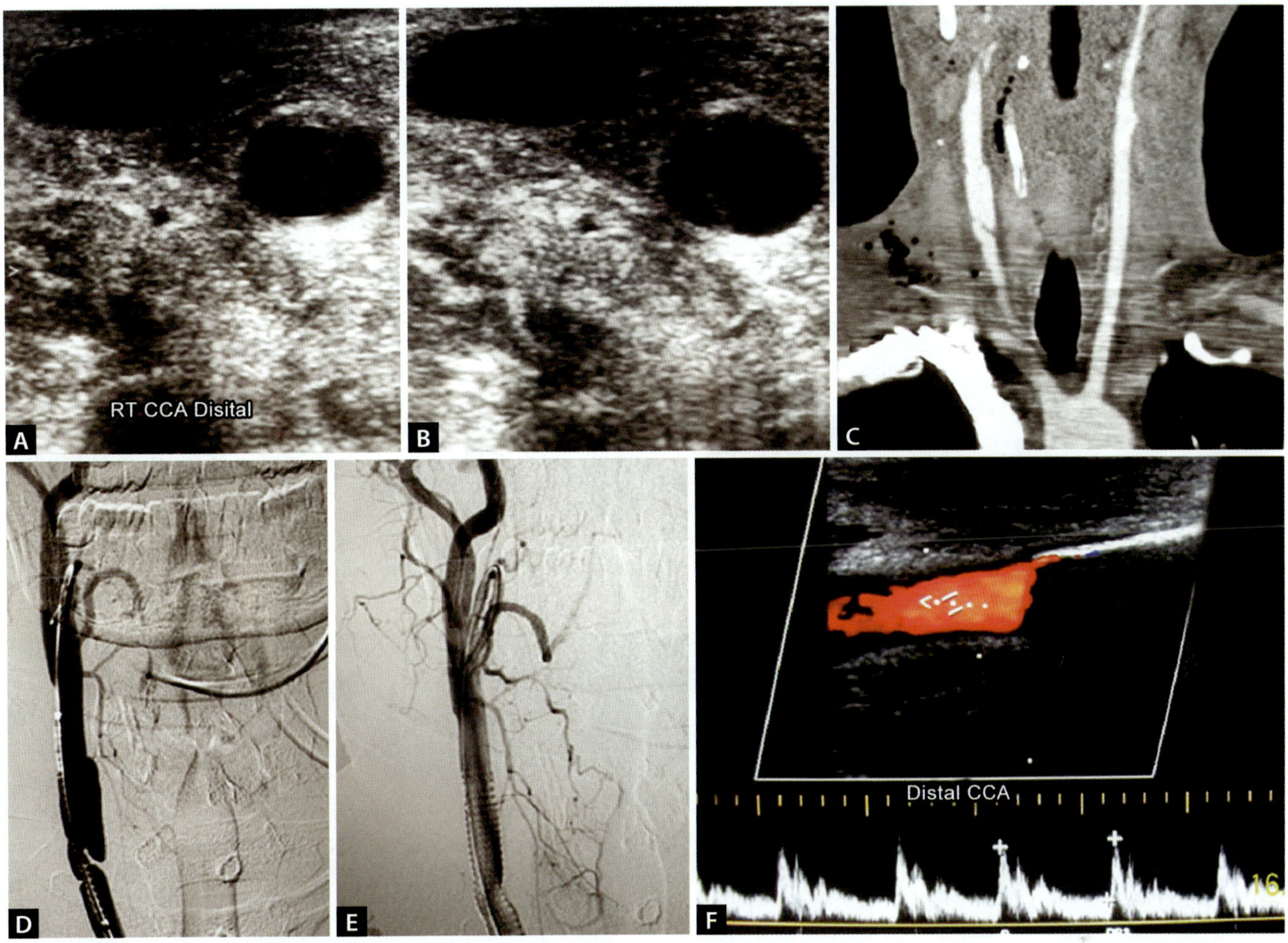

Figs. 24A to F: A case of post-traumatic carotid artery dissection with pseudoaneurysm formation: (A and B) ultrasound images showing intimal flap with dissection; (C) MDCT angiography image better delineation of the vascular dissection and also pseudoaneurysm formation (D) conventional DSA confirming the dissection and pseudoaneurysm formation; (E) DSA image following stent graft insertion to cover the dissection showing complete closure of the dissection flap and patent carotid artery lumen; (F) Follow-up Doppler image showing normal flow through carotid artery and obliteration of dissection flap.

Type C: Fistula between meningeal branches of ECA and cavernous sinus.

Type D: Fistula between meningeal branches of both ICA and ECA and cavernous sinus.

Treatment of CCF[31]

Direct CCFs rarely undergo spontaneous resolution and, without treatment, eventually cause loss of vision in 80–90% of cases from central retinal vein occlusion or glaucoma.

Endovascular management is the treatment of choice. Direct CCF can be effectively treated by using different therapeutic alternatives such as detachable balloons and detachable coils, alone or in combination with N-butyl-2-cyanoacrylate (n-BCA) or Onyx. Stents have also been used in an attempt to improve preservation of the parent artery while still occluding the fistula.

Indirect fistulas can be cured successfully by transarterial embolization if the blood supply is solely from the ECA territory. Otherwise, the transvenous approach appears to have a higher rate of success with these low-flow indirect lesions, probably due to the decreased resistance imparted upon the small-bore catheters while navigating through tortuous anatomy.

Another traumatic vascular injury is the **dural fistula**, usually caused by laceration of the middle meningeal artery with resultant meningeal artery to meningeal vein fistula formation. The dural fistula generally drains via the meningeal veins; therefore, they rarely lead to the formation of an EDH. Patients are often asymptomatic or present with nonspecific complaints such as tinnitus.

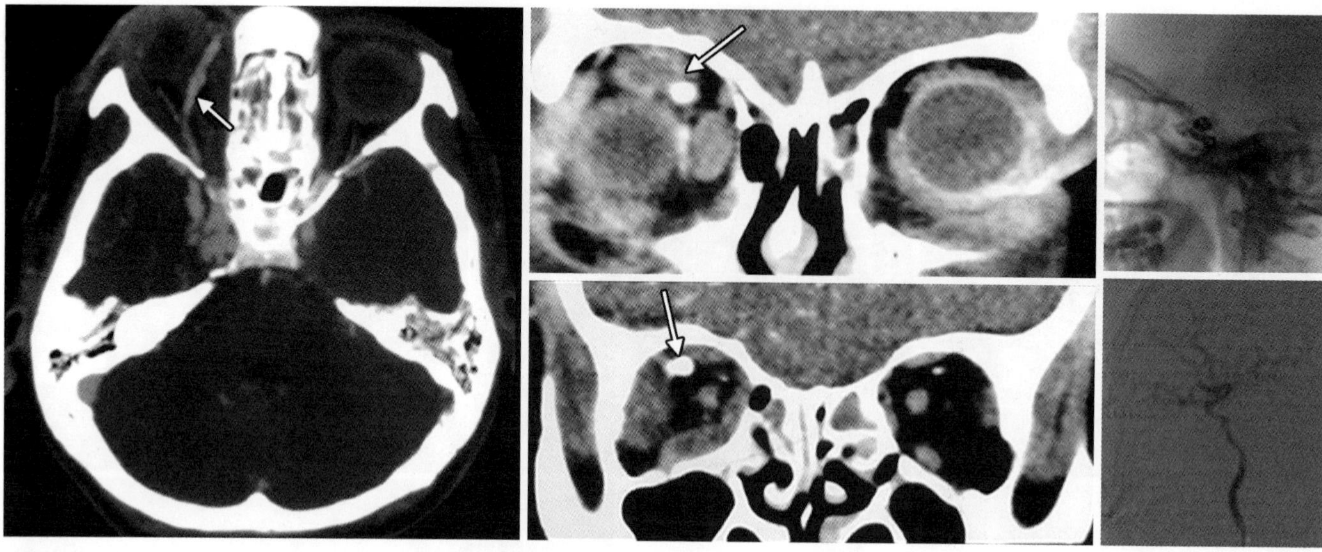

Fig. 25: CT angiography images showing enlarged and lobulated right cavernous sinus with dilated superior ophthalmic vein (arrows) suggestive of carotid cavernous fistula, treated by detachable coils.

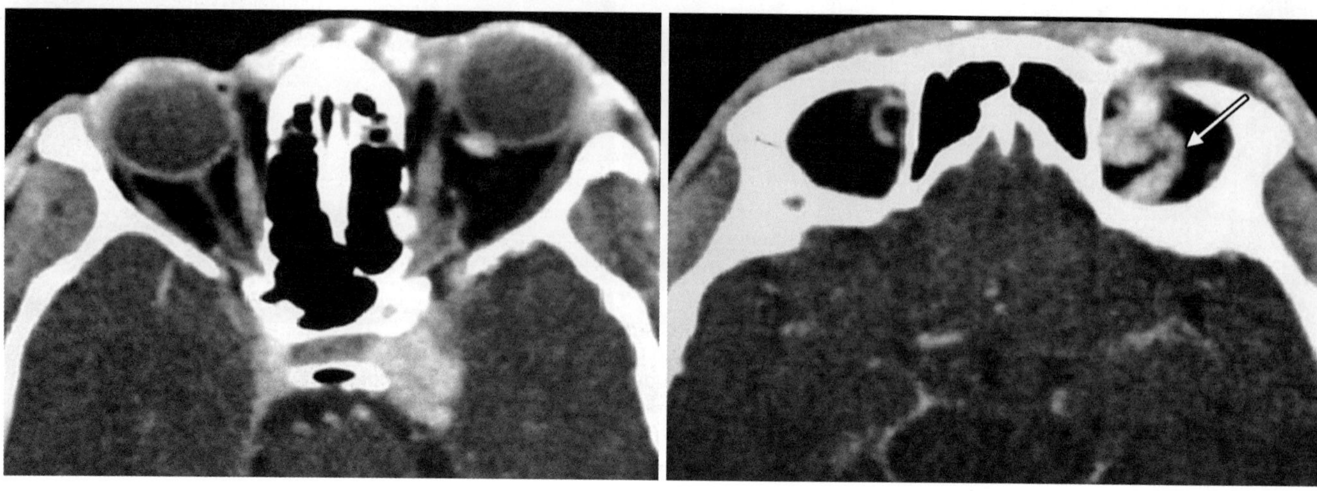

Fig. 26: CT angiography images showing enlarged and lobulated left cavernous sinus with dilated superior ophthalmic vein (arrow) suggestive of carotid cavernous fistula.

SECONDARY HEAD INJURY

Acute Secondary Changes

1. **Diffuse Cerebral Swelling (edema)** results from

- Increase in cerebral blood volume (hyperemia),
- Vasogenic edema, or
- An increase in tissue fluid (cytotoxicedema).

Imaging features of cerebral edema include effacement of the cerebral sulci and cisterns, compression of the ventricles and loss of gray-white differentiation. The cerebellum and brainstem are usually spared in cerebral edema and may appear hyperdense (On CT) relative to the affected cerebral hemispheres **(Fig. 27)**.

2. **Brain herniation** occurs secondary to mass effect produced by other causes.[9,23]

There are three types of herniation **(Figs. 28A to D):**

1. Subfalcine
2. Uncal
3. *Transtentorial:*
   - Descending
   - Ascending

Subfalcine herniation is the most common form of herniation.

Imaging features include displacement of the cingulate gyrus across the midline under the falx cerebri, compression of the ipsilateral ventricle due to mass effect

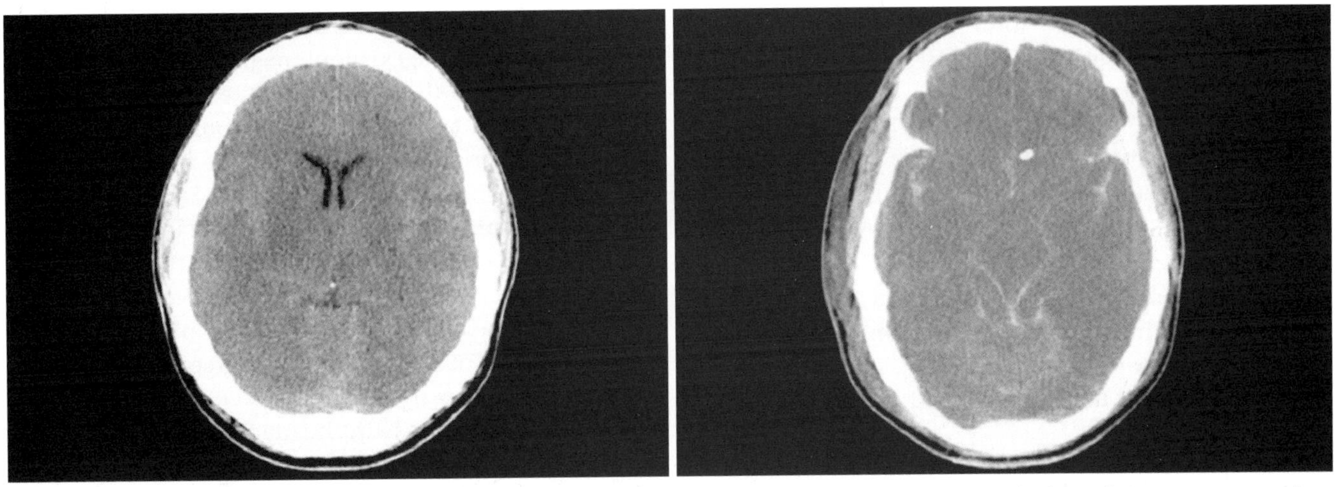

Fig. 27: Axial CT images showing features of diffuse cerebral edema such as effacement of the cerebral sulci and cisterns, compression of the ventricles and loss of gray-white differentiation with relative sparing of cerebellum.

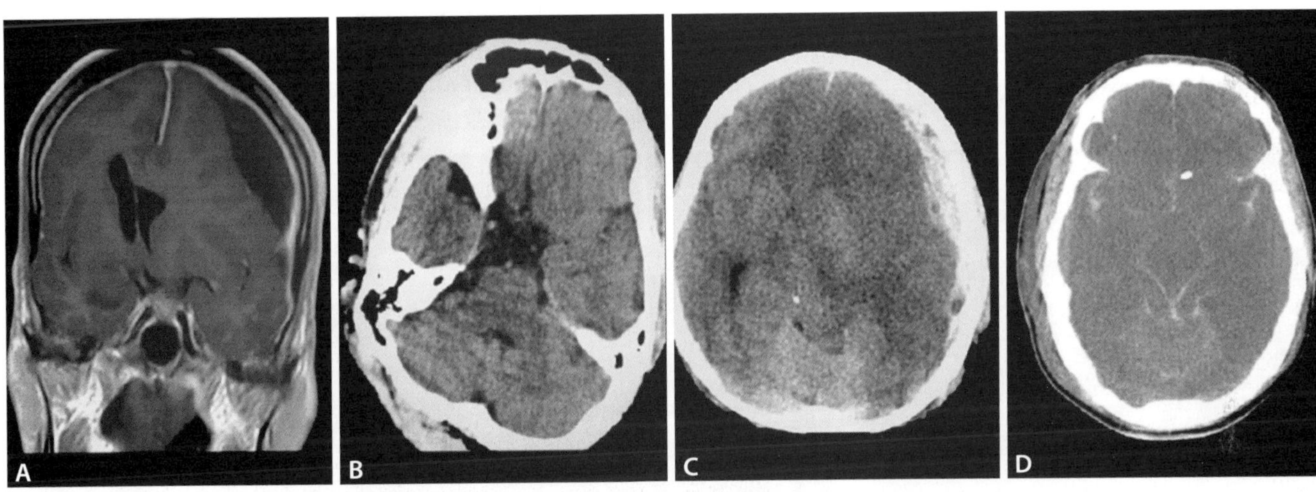

Figs. 28A to D: Axial CT images showing various types of brain herniations: (A) Subfalcine herniation; (B) Uncal herniation; (C) Downward transtentorial; and (D) Ascending transtentorial herniation.

and enlargement of the contralateral ventricle due to obstruction of the foramen of Monro **(Fig. 28A)**. Due to such displacement, there will be trapping of the callosomarginal branches of the ACA, which may lead to ACA infarction.

Uncal herniation: Imaging features include displacement of the medial temporal lobe over the free margin of the tentorium, effacement of the ambient and lateral suprasellar cisterns. In severe cases, displacement can cause compression of the contralateral cerebral peduncle against the tentorium (Kernohan's notch), leading to peduncular infarction or hemorrhage.

Transtentorial herniation can occur either in upward or downward direction.

Upward herniation typically occurs with large posterior fossa hematomas that displace portions of the cerebellum and vermis through the tentorial incisura. The mass effect of the hematoma can also cause downward herniation of the cerebellar tonsils through the foramen magnum.

Downward herniation of the cerebrum manifests as effacement of the suprasellar and perimesencephalic cisterns. Inferior displacement of the pineal calcification is an additional imaging clue for the presence of downward herniation.

3. **Infarction or ischemia** can complicate TBI as a result of increased intracranial pressure or mass effect on cerebral vasculature by herniation or hematoma. In addition to ACA infarction secondary to the subfalcine herniation described above, uncal herniation and tonsillar herniation can cause ischemia in the territory

of the posterior cerebral artery and the posterior inferior cerebellar artery distributions, respectively **(Fig. 29)**.

Chronic Secondary Changes

1. **Traumatic hydrocephalus** occurs secondary to impaired CSF resorption at the level of the arachnoid villi or secondary to obstruction of the cerebral aqueduct and 4th ventricular outflow by SAH or IVH. Mass effect from cerebral herniation or a hematoma can also cause non-communicating hydrocephalus via compression of the aqueduct and ventricular outflow foramina **(Fig. 30)**.[9,23]
2. **Encephalomalacia** is a common, but nonspecific, sequelae of prior parenchyma injury. It may be clinically asymptomatic, but it can also be a potential seizure focus. On CT, the imaging appearance consists of an area of low attenuation with volume loss. It typically follows CSF signal intensity on both CT and MR, except for the areas of gliosis, which appears as low intensity on T1- and high intensity on T2-weighted images. If on imaging encephalomalacia is seen within the orbitofrontal (especially the gyrus rectus) and anteroinferior temporal lobes then it is characteristically due to remote traumatic injury **(Fig. 31)**.
3. **Cerebrospinal fluid (CSF) leak** occurs when there is an osseous and dural defect at the skull base, with direct communication of the subarachnoid space to the extracranial space, usually a paranasal sinus. Recognition of the leak site and source and appropriate treatment are necessary to avoid rhinorrhea or otorrhea, low-pressure headaches, and meningitis, known complications of CSF leak.[32,33]
   - **CSF otorrhea** occurs when there is communication between the subarachnoid space and middle ear in association with a ruptured tympanic membrane.
   - **CSF rhinorrhea** occurs when there is communication between the subarachnoid space and the paranasal sinuses.

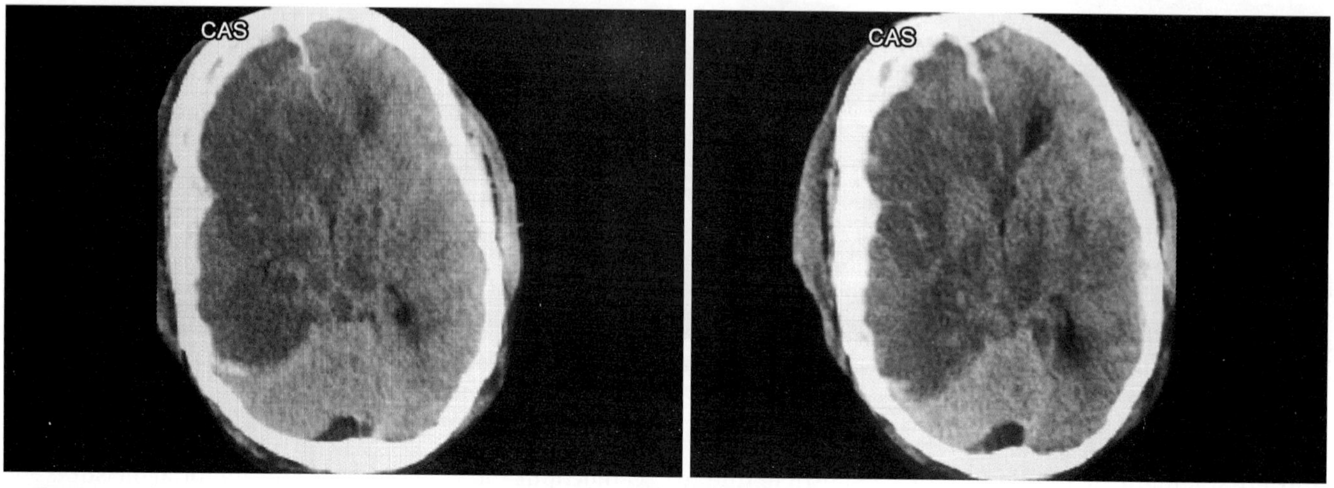

Fig. 29: Axial CT images showing almost near complete infarction of right cerebral hemisphere secondary to increased intracranial pressure following head injury.

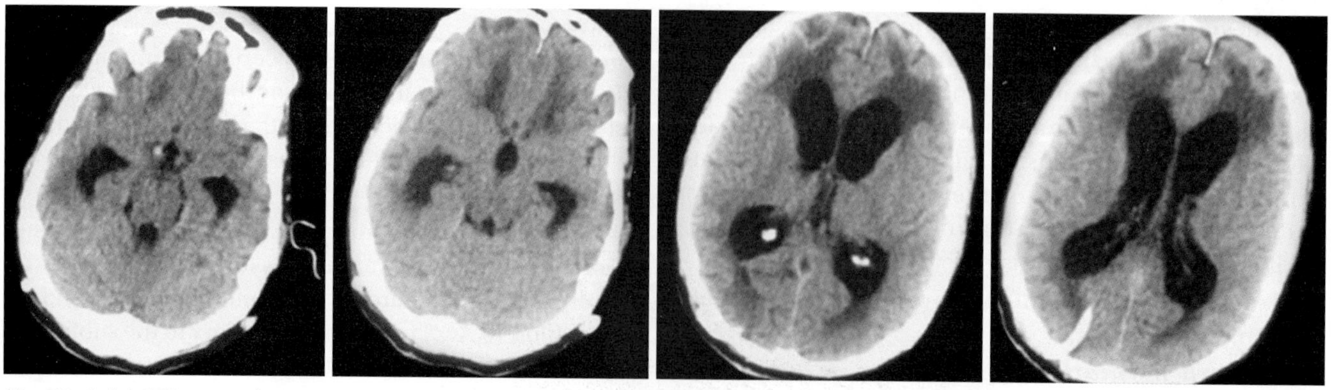

Fig. 30: Axial CT images showing communicating hydrocephalus with periventricular ooze in follow-up scan as a complication of SAH.

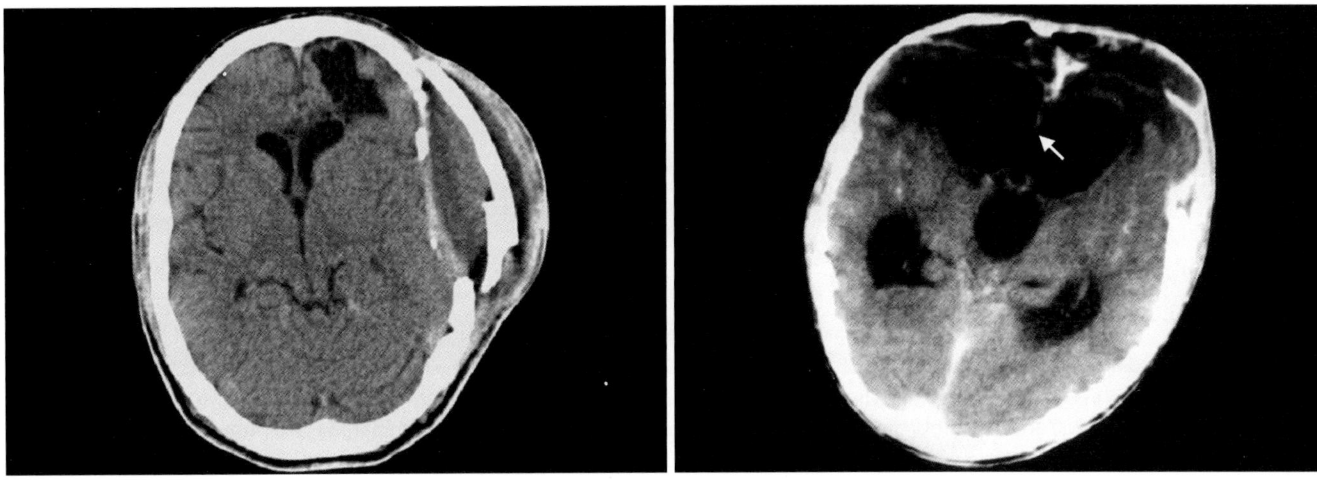

Fig. 31: Axial CT images showing areas of gliosis with exvacuodilatation of ventricles suggestive of encephalomalacia, sequelae of prior parenchyma injury.

About 80% of post-traumatic CSF leaks occur within the first 48 hours after injury, and 95% will manifest within the first 3 months. A small subset of patients will present with rhinorrhea or meningitis decades after the trauma.

Imaging[32,33]

The goals of imaging are

- To confirm the diagnosis
- Evaluate for an underlying cause,
- Localize and characterize the defect site prior to surgical repair, and
- Exclude an associated meningocele at the defect.

Since small skull base defects are now routinely repaired with nasal endoscopy, accurate localization is imperative. CSF leaks are often difficult to localize and a variety of nuclear medicine and cross-sectional computed tomographic and magnetic resonance imaging techniques have been applied to diagnose, localize, and characterize skull base defects responsible for leakage of CSF. So far there has been no imaging "gold standard" for the diagnosis of CSF leak.

CT Imaging

The use of CT for evaluation of skull base defects has become a mainstay in the workup of CSF fistula, due to its ability to resolve osseous structures. With the advent of modern thin-section and multidetector CT scanners, smaller defects are visualized with a reported sensitivity as high as 92% and specificity of 100%. The CT findings suggestive of a CSF leak include a skull base bone defect and an air-fluid level or opacification of the contiguous sinus. In the evaluation of temporal bone CT scans, a unilaterally opacified mastoid and middle ear, in the presence of a tegmen defect or fracture through an inner ear structure, is consistent with CSF fistula.

MR imaging techniques offer noninvasive methods of imaging a CSF leak and are indicated to assess possible encephalocele or meningoencephalocele. Herniation of brain parenchyma or meninges through the bone defect may be difficult to differentiate from obstructed secretions on CT scans but is obvious on MR images **(Fig. 32)**.

CT Cisternography

CT cisternography is being used widely for evaluating a possible CSF fistula. This technique traditionally involves obtaining thin-section coronal and axial CT images in both prone and supine positions through the region of interest (maxillofacial or temporal region) both before and after intrathecal contrast material. Approximately 3–10 mL of an iodinated nonionic low-osmolar contrast agent is administered by means of lumbar puncture, and the patient is placed in a Trendelenburg position to opacify the basal cisterns, followed by CT imaging after administration of contrast material. Manoeuvres that provoke an active leak, such as sneezing or head hanging, are performed prior to the CT portion of cisternography. Postcontrast images are then compared with the precontrast images. A positive result involves the presence of a skull base defect and contrast opacification within the sinus, nasal cavity, or middle ear.

MR cisternography typically involves heavily T2-weighted fast spin-echo sequences with fat suppression

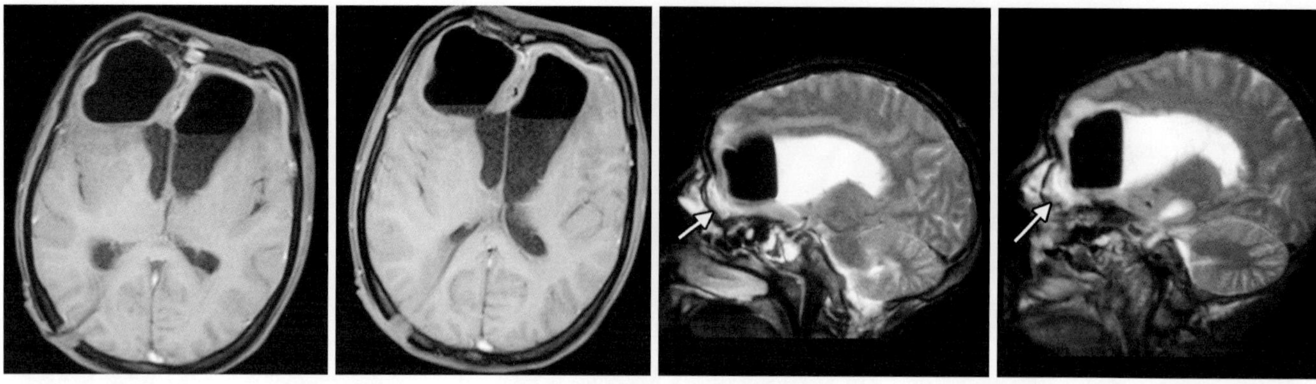

Fig. 32: MR images in multiple planes showing herniation ofbrain parenchyma through the bone defect in anterior cranial fossa (arrows) and air-cerebrospinal fluid level suggestive of communication with paranasal sinuses.

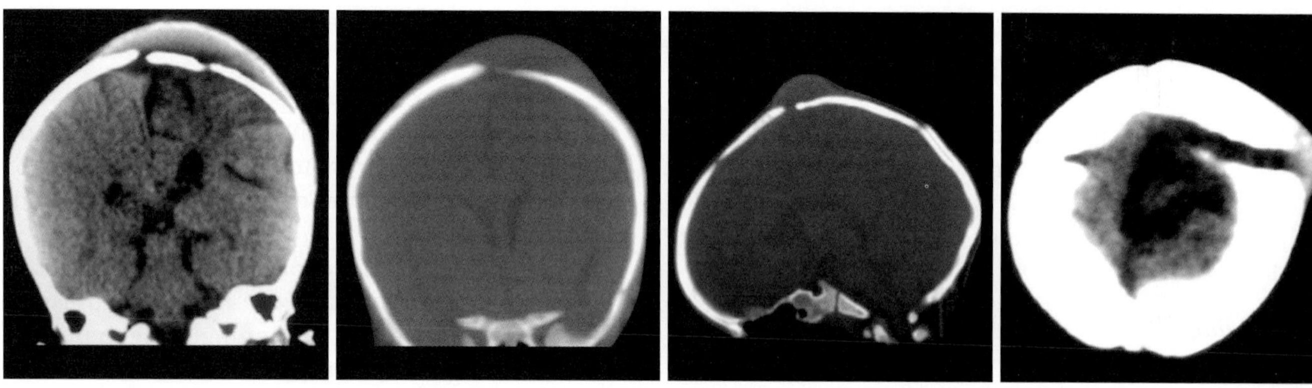

Fig. 33: CT images showing features of leptomeningeal cyst (growing fracture) as evidenced by herniation of subarachanoid space though the fracture line into subcutaneous tissue with underlying encephalomalacia, focal ventricular enlargement.

and subtraction of the adjacent background tissue signal to enhance conspicuity of the fistulous tract, or CSF column. The fast spin-echo sequences have decreased susceptibility artifacts at the air-bone interface of the skull base, compared with conventional T2-weighted imaging. Images are generally obtained in coronal, axial, and sagittal planes, and, similar to conventional MR, the finding of a contiguous CSF column communicating from the subarachnoid space to the extracranial space and/or the herniation of brain parenchyma and/or meninges, extracranially heralds a positive examination.

4. **The leptomeningeal cyst or "growing fracture"** is usually seen children and are accompanied by tear in the dura in association with a calvarial defect.[34]

Leptomeningeal cysts are usually delayed complications of skull fractures, although they occasionally occur within weeks of trauma. Since the infant skull is highly malleable, the margins of pediatric skull fractures are often inwardly displaced at the time oftrauma. Depressed, or transiently depressed, fractures can easily lacerate the underlying dura and severely contuse the adjacent brain. The pia-arachnoid membrane (and occasionally swollen, edematous cortex) can herniate through the dural tear and prevent apposition and healing of the dura. CSF pulsations subsequently fill and enlarge the subarachnoid pouch that extends through the fracture line. The pulsations eventually widen the dural defect and expand the fracture margins. This results in a leptomeningeal cyst that extends from the subarachnoid space into the subgaleal space. CSF pulsations tend to erode the inner table more than the outer one, giving rise to "beveled" edges. The margins of the fracture often show marked resorption and saucerization.

The term "growing fracture" refers to interval widening of the space between the fracture margins on successive skull radiographs or CT scans. CT scans obtained after the development of the leptomeningeal cyst often reveal posttraumatic encephalomalacia, focal ventricular enlargement, and porencephaly because of the prior associated brain injury **(Fig. 33)**.[35]

CONCLUSION

The main aim of imaging in the management of head trauma is to identify treatable injuries so as to prevent secondary brain damage. CT remains the modality of choice in the evaluation of acute head injury, because it is fast, is widely available, and can easily accommodate life-support and monitoring equipment. CT can accurately identify acute hemorrhages, mass effect, midline shift, hydrocephalus, ischemia, and herniation. An advance in CT methods such as CT perfusion offers prognostic information with respect to functional outcome, even as early as at the time of admission. MRI should be used as a problem solving modality and is indicated for patients with acute TBI when the neurologic findings cannot be explained by CT. MRI is also the modality of choice for subacute or chronic injury. An advance in MR methods, such as diffusion-weighted imaging, has improved the neuroradiological evaluation of traumatic brain injury and offers a better understanding of the pathophysiological manifestations of head trauma.

REFERENCES

1. MacDorman MF, Minino AM, Strobino DM, et al. Annual summary of vital statistics—2001. Pediatrics 2002;110(6):1037-52.
2. National Center for Injury Prevention and Control. Injury Fact Book 2001-2002. Atlanta, GA: Centers for Disease Control and Prevention; 2001.
3. Teasdale G, Jennett B. Assessment of coma and impaired consciousness: a practical scale. Lancet 1974;13:81-4.
4. Marshall LF, Marshall SB, Klauber MR, et al. A new classification of head injury based on computerised tomography. J Neurosurg 1991;75(Suppl):S14-20.
5. Kunitz SC, Gross C. A National Traumatic Coma Data Bank. Proc Annu Symp Comput Appl Med Care. 1980;2:1333-9.
6. Bell RS, Loop JW. The utility and futility of radiographic skull examination for trauma. N Engl J Med. 1971;284(5):236-9.
7. Hackney DB. Skull radiography in the evaluation of acute head trauma: a survey of current practice. Radiology. 1991;181(3): 711-14.
8. Masters SJ. Evaluation of head trauma: efcacy of skull lms. Am J Roentgenol. 1980;135(3):539-47.
9. Zee CS, Go JL. CT of head trauma. Neuroimaging Clin North Am. 1998;8(3):525-39.
10. Metting Z, Rödiger LA, Stewart RE, et al. Perfusion computed tomography in the acute phase of mild head injury: regional dysfunction and prognostic value. Ann Neurol. 2009;66(6):809-16.
11. Wintermark M, van Melle G, Schnyder P, et al. Admission perfusion CT: prognostic value in patients with severe head trauma. Radiology. 2004;232(1):211-20.
12. Gentry LR, Godersky JC, Thompson B, et al. Prospective comparativestudy of intermediate-eld MR and CT in the evaluation of closed head trauma. Am J Roentgenol. 1988;150(3):673-82.
13. Orrison WW, Gentry LR, Stimac GK, et al. Blinded comparison of cranial CT and MR in closed head injury evaluation. Am J Neuroradiol. 1994;15(2):351-6.
14. Noguchi K, Ogawa T, Seto H, et al. Subacute and chronic subarachnoid hemorrhage: diagnosis with fluid-attenuated inversion-recovery MR imaging. Radiology. 1997;203(1):257-62.
15. Woodcock RJ Jr, Short J, Do HM, et al. Imaging of acute subarachnoid hemorrhage with a fluid-attenuated inversion recovery sequence in ananimal model: comparison with non-contrast-enhanced CT. Am J Neuroradiol. 2001;22(9):1698-1703.
16. Akiyama Y, Miyata K, Harada K, et al. Susceptibility-weighted magnetic resonance imaging for the detection of cerebral microhemorrhage in patients with traumatic brain injury. Neurol Med Chir (Tokyo) 2009;49(3):97-9.
17. Topal NB, Hakyemez B, Erdogan C, et al. MR imaging in the detection of diffuse axonal injury with mild traumatic brain injury. Neurol Res. 2008;30(9):974-8.
18. Le TH, Mukherjee P, Manley GT, et al. Automated detection of traumatic white matter injury using voxel-based morphometry of diffusiontensor images: a 3T study with parallel imaging. American Society of Neuroradiology 43rd Annual Meeting, May 23-27, 2005, Toronto, On tario, Canada, Paper 374.
19. Huisman TA, Sorensen AG, Hergan K, et al. Diffusion-weighted imaging for the evaluation of diffuse axonal injury in closed head injury. J Comput Assist Tomogr. 2003;27(1):5-11.
20. Liu AY, Maldjian JA, Bagley LJ, et al. Traumatic brain injury: diffusion-weighted MR imaging ndings. Am J Neuroradiol. 1999;20(9):1636-41.
21. Medina LS, Blackmore CC, Evidence based imaging of Traumatic Brain injury. Evidence-Based Imaging: Optimizing Imaging in Patient Care. Springer Science+Business Media, Eds. New York; 2006.
22. Gentry LR. Temporal bone trauma. Neuroimaging Clin North Am. 1991;1:319-40.
23. Gean AD, Kates RS, Lee S. Neuroimaging in head injury. New Horiz. 1995;3(3):549-61.
24. Al-Nakshabandi NA. The swirl sign. Radiology. 2001;218(2):433.
25. Loftus CM. Neurosurgical Emergencies, 2nd edition. Thieme Medical Publishers, New York; 2008.
26. Arfanakis K, Haughton VM, Carew JD, et al. Diffusion tensor MR imaging in diffuse axonal injury. Am J Neuroradiol. 2002;23(5):794-802.
27. Le TH, Mukherjee P, Henry RG, et al. Diffusion tensor imaging with three-dimensional ber tractography of traumatic axonal shearing injury: an imaging correlate for the posterior callosal "disconnection" syndrome: case report. Neurosurgery. 2005;56(1):189.
28. Adams JH, Graham DI, Gennarelli TA, et al. Diffuse axonal injury in non-missile head injury. J Neurol Neurosurg Psychiatry. 1991;54(6):481-3.

29. Hesselink JR, Dowd CF, Healy ME, et al. MR imaging of brain contusion: a comparative study with CT. Am J Neuroradiol. 1988;150:1133-42.
30. Gentry LR. Head trauma. In: Atlas SW (Ed). Magnetic Resonance Imaging of the Brain and Spine, 2nd edition. Philadelphia: PA, Lippincott-Raven; 1996.pp.611-47.
31. Tjoumakaris SI, Jabbour PM, Rosenwasser RH. Neuroendovascular management of carotid cavernous fistulae. Neurosurg Clin N Am. 2009;20(4):447-52.
32. Bullock R, Soares D. Current imaging of cerebrospinal fluid leaks. West Indian Med J. 2009;58(4):362-6.
33. Lloyd KM, DelGaudio JM, Hudgins PA. Imaging of skull base cerebrospinal fluid leaks in adults. Radiology. 2008;248: 725-36.
34. Husson B, Pariente D, Tammam S, el al. The value of MRI in the early diagnosis of growing skull fracture. Pediatr Radiol. 1996;26(10):744-7.
35. Poussaint TY, Moeller KK. Imaging of pediatric head trauma. Neuroimaging Clin N Am. 2002;12(2):271-94.

CHAPTER 31

Imaging of Facial Trauma

Ajay Kumar, Vivek Gupta, Paramjeet Singh

INTRODUCTION

Imaging of facial trauma requires a thorough knowledge of the regional anatomy and precise imaging techniques. These are required to restore the facial skeleton and prevent disfigurement. The facial skeleton has been described as a honeycomb structure of varying thickness and form, which are protected superficially by strong plate-like bone, so that the deepest and most delicate structures are well protected.

Classification of facial fracture was first described by Rene Le Fort in 1901.[1] He performed a series of macabre cadaveric experiments and described the three facial fractures which bear his name, the concept of which was based on three major levels of inherent facial weakness through which the fracture lines run. Le Fort method of classifying facial fracture was essentially a clinical one. The palpation of fracture margins, the instability of fractured segment, crepitus and plain X-rays provided the indirect evidence of the location of the injury.

The diagnosis of fracture was refined further with the help of plain X-rays and the conventional tomograms. However, the major drawback of this mode of investigation was that it overlooked the evaluation of soft tissues which is also an important aspect in the management of facial fracture.[2]

Computed tomography (CT) scanning not only visualizes the bony injury, but also provided insight into injury of the soft tissues. It also helped to give panoramic access to the entire facial skeleton from its most superficial surface to the intricate depth. The availability of high-spatial resolution and thin-section scanning added to the improvement of diagnosis of lesions of the orbits and its contents, nasoethmoidal region and fractures in children.[3,4] The need for reclassifying facial fractures was thus necessary and in 1980 Gentry et al. gave an extended concept in the imaging of fractures of this region.[5,6]

IMAGING TECHNIQUES

The maxillofacial region represents a complex area for diagnosis especially when it is injured. Most patients with acute maxillofacial trauma do not cooperate for radiographic evaluation and often the situation is further hampered due to associated severe life-threatening injuries, such as injuries to the cervical spine.[7] Tailored radiographic projections and imaging techniques are required to assess the injuries. A systematic approach is thus essential so that all the fractures are delineated and the soft-tissue injuries are adequately demonstrated.

Plain radiography has been the first line of investigation. However, the complexity of the modern high-velocity injuries, the precision required in the diagnosis of fractures as well as the demanding legal aspects of facial injuries highlight the inadequacy and inherent limitations of plain radiography alone as the imaging tool.[8]

Noncontrast CT scan is the modality of choice for the complete evaluation of the osseous and soft-tissue component of facial fractures, the brain and dura. Both axial and coronal sections are done to provide the clinician a complete insight of orientation of fractured segments. Patient cooperation is essential to do direct coronal sections. However, with helical CT overlapping axial acquisitions can be used to reconstruct two- and three-dimensional (3D) views of the facial skeleton. 3D reconstructions are especially useful in treatment planning. This technique enables the surgeon to have a global assessment of the injuries, to locate bony fragments and their relationships when several sites are involved. It enables optimal presurgical planning, indicates the anatomical areas involved and determines the number of fracture lines where miniplates are to be affixed. The display of information in orthogonal planes enhances the perception of malocclusion and comminution and directs the appropriate therapeutic approach. 3D-volumetric evaluation can provide area measurements and volume changes. Measurements of bony landmarks on 3D reconstructions are qualitatively accurate for planning surgery and evaluation of the treatment.[9-12] Dual energy CT (DECT) has shown to be effective in producing significantly improved images in the presence of metal artifacts by using metal suppression techniques.[13]

Although standard CT scanners with three-dimensional dataset are routinely used for maxillofacial trauma, it exposes the patient to a higher radiation dose.[14] A dental CT scanner based on cone beam CT (CBCT) is becoming more popular in diagnosis and treatment planning for maxillofacial trauma because of less radiation dose and its ability to produce accurate three-dimensional imaging.[15,16] As expected, CBCT offers lower radiation dose compared with standard CT machines: the integral absorbed radiation dose of radiation was less than one-fifteenth that of spiral CT when the exposure condition of the latter was optimized.[17] The radiation dose from CBCT was significantly lower than the lowest dose from conventional CT in terms of effective dose and dose to the lens.[17] Moreover, because of its smaller size, it is possible to install the CBCT scanner in the operative room or physicians' clinic itself which enables the treating physician to assess the adequacy of surgery and immediate appropriate measures for correction.[18] Although the CBCT has found to produce excellent bony details which is comparable to conventional CT, the soft tissue resolution is low because of its inherent low contrast resolution. Hence if soft tissue evaluation is intended, either conventional CT or MRI should be considered.[18]

Magnetic resonance imaging (MRI) has a limited role to play in the assessment of facial fractures since it does not visualize bone directly. MRI is especially helpful in the following situations: (a) in differentiating blood from inflammatory reactions and edema fluid especially, if MRI is performed after 48 hours of trauma. In this situation, such an investigation is directed by those groups of surgeons who wait for several days after trauma before surgical correction as they believe soft-tissue injury will subside and surgery becomes easier, and (b) imaging of injured orbit and its contents can also be better performed on MRI. These fractures of bony orbit can themselves be diagnosed by recognition of the fat invaginating into adjoining paranasal sinuses.[19] MRI is also risky in patients with roadside accidents as there is always risk of metallic foreign body deep inside.

FACIAL BUTTRESSES AND REGIONAL CLASSIFICATION OF INJURIES[5,6]

Le Fort determined the predictable lines of least resistance through which fracture lines run. The forces, which generated these fractures, were small as compared to those of modern day high-velocity injury. Hence, the injuries, which we encounter now-a-days, incorporate the Le Fort fractures together with complex fractures with multiple fracture lines. In keeping with the general concept of plate-like structures, which constitute the facial skeleton; the current analysis of fracture is based on the concept of anatomical buttresses **(Figs. 1 to 4)**.[9]

There are two sagittal buttresses described, on each side of the face. The medial sagittal buttress extends from the maxillary alveolus up to the lateral wall of pyriform aperture and into the medial orbital wall. This buttress comprises of lower maxilla, frontal process of maxilla, lacrimal bone and nasal process of frontal bone. This forms a medial supportive pillar on each of the midline and is termed as the nasomaxillary buttress. The lateral sagittal buttress is formed on each side by the lateral wall of maxilla, body of zygoma orbital process of frontal bone in lateral orbital wall. This is termed as the zygomaticomaxillary buttress. A third buttress called the pterygomaxillary buttress extending from the posterior maxillary alveolus towards the pterygoid plates has also been described.[9] The sagittal group of buttresses also includes a median strut formed by nasal septum. These sagittal buttresses are reinforced by three horizontal buttresses formed by: (1) the floor of the anterior cranial fossa, (2) the orbital floor and zygomatic arches, and (3) the hard palate respectively.

The above two groups of facial supports are in turn strengthened by two conceptualized coronal buttresses. They are called the anterior-coronal buttress and the posterior-coronal buttress. The anterior buttress comprises of the anterior wall of frontal and maxillary sinuses, the nasofrontal process, the zygomaticofrontal buttress and the anterior maxillary alveolar arch. The posterior-coronal

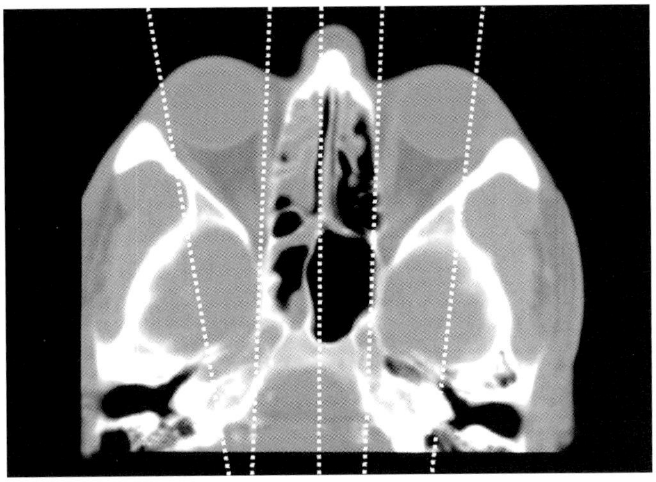

Fig. 1: Axial computed tomography (CT) section at the level of orbits, optic foramen and sphenoid sinus. The midline sagittal strut, parasagittal strut and the lateral sagittal struts are indicated.

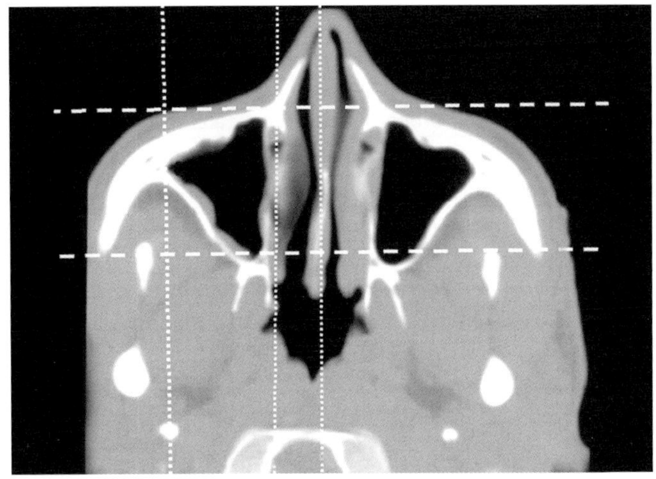

Fig. 2: Axial computed tomography (CT) section at the level of maxillary sinuses with the condyles and pterygoid plates. The anterior and posterior coronal buttress (dashed line) together with the right sagittal buttress (dotted line) are indicated.

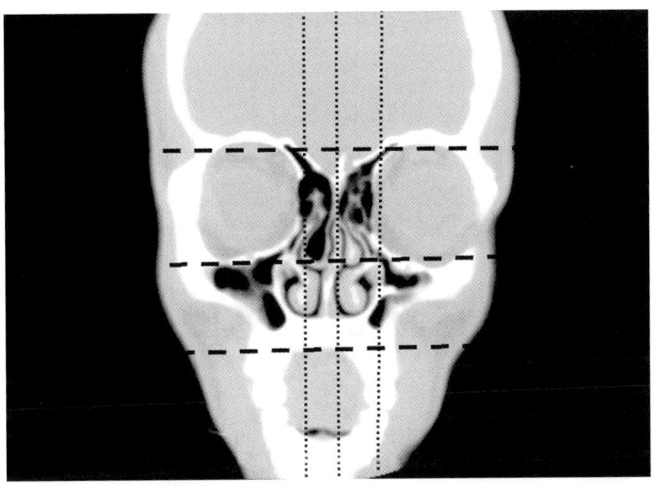

Fig. 3: Coronal computed tomography (CT) section at the level of orbits showing the superior, middle and inferior horizontal struts aligned along the orbital plates, inferior orbital margin and the alveolus. In addition, the position of the sagittal struts are indicated.

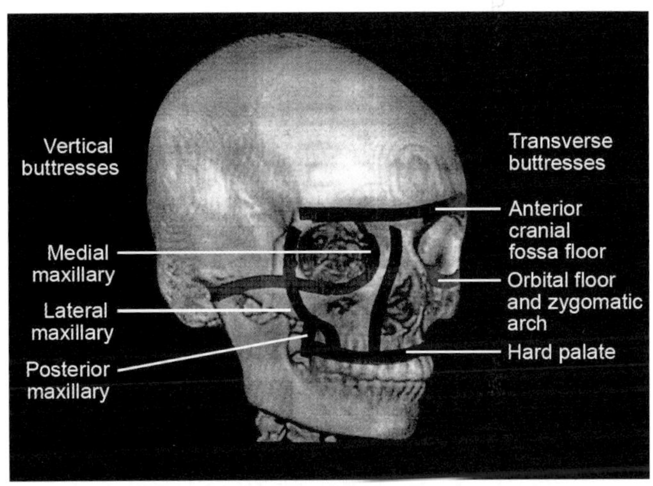

Fig. 4: Diagrammatical representation of facial buttresses system.

buttress comprises of two bilaterally symmetrical walls of maxillary sinus and the pterygoid plates.

Importance of Facial Buttresses[20]

- Buttresses have sufficient bone thickness to accommodate metal screw fixation
- Buttresses are all linked either directly or through another buttress
- Transverse buttresses reduction restores the facial width and vertical reduction restores the facial height
- Buttresses reduction establishes a functional support for teeth and globes.

Table 1 summarizes the components of the facial struts.

CLASSIFICATION OF MAXILLOFACIAL FRACTURES

Facial fractures can be classified by type, location or extension and complexity of the fractures. A detailed system under these different systems is depicted in **Table 2**.

It is evident from **Table 2**, that no single system can describe the complex morbid anatomy of the facial

Table 1: Components of the facial struts.

Superior horizontal	Cribriform plate, ethmoid sinus roof, orbital roof
Middle horizontal	Orbital floor, zygomatic arch
Inferior horizontal	Palate/maxillary alveolus
Midline sagittal	Nasal septum, Vomer
Parasagittal	Medial orbital wall, medial maxillary sinus wall, lateral maxillary alveolus
Lateral sagittal	Lateral orbital wall, lateral maxillary sinus wall
Anterior coronal	Nasal arch, anterior and posterior walls of the frontal sinus, anterior wall of the maxillary sinus, anterior maxillary alveolus
Posterior coronal	Posterior aspect of the maxillary sinus, pterygoid plate

fractures. This is especially true for high-velocity accidents where the injury force acts from multiple directions on the face grossly distorting the anatomy. The traditional and oldest accepted classification of facial fractures of Le Fort merits mention in the modern context. High-impact facial fractures, such as those in automobile accidents, are so extensive and complicated that so-called "pure" Le Fort fractures are unusual. The Le Fort classification can be reworked in the newer framework of buttresses as summarized in **Table 3**. The Le Fort fractures, therefore, can be incorporated in the fractures of the midface **(Figs. 5 and 6)**.

The complexities of the midfacial fractures including Le Fort III need a special mention at this point. These injuries result in distortion of the anatomy in midface causing severe post-traumatic deformities. It is also important to realize that these fractures are often associated with severe intracranial, orbital and paranasal sinus injuries which need special concern in the treatment protocol.[9]

Regional Facial Fractures

Frontal Sinus Fractures

They can result from extensions from calvarial fractures into the frontal sinus or due to direct blows to the forehead. The fractures are described in relation to the anterior and posterior walls of the sinus. The anterior wall of the sinus is most commonly involved resulting in hemorrhage or edema. The sinus appears opaque on plain radiographs. The fracture is best appreciated on lateral views of the skull. They may be obscured on the standard posteroanterior (PA) and Water's projections. CT scan is very helpful to delineate the fractured segments in cases of comminuted fractures **(Figs. 7 and 8)**. It is also

Table 2: Classification of maxillofacial fractures.

Traditional Le Fort classification		• Le Fort I • Le Fort II • Le Fort III
Based on the type of fracture		• Closed (simple) • Open (compound) • Green stick • Comminuted • Undisplaced • Displaced
Based on location of fracture	*Upper third of the face*	• Frontal sinuses (glabella) • Supraorbital ridge • Frontal bone
	Middle third of the face	• Nasal bones and septum • Naso-orbital area • Zygoma • Zygomatic arch • Orbital floor • *Maxilla*: – Transverse (Le Fort I) – Pyramidal (Le Fort II) – Craniofacial dysjunction (Le Fort III)
	Lower third of the face (mandible)	• Alveolar process • Symphysis • Body • Angle • Ascending ramus • Coronoid process • Condyle • Temporomandibular joint region
Based on the extent of fracture line		• Limited fracture • Transfacial fracture

Table 3: The Le Fort classification.

Type	***Structures involved***	***Strut***
Le Fort I	• Anterior, lateral and medial walls of the maxillary sinuses • Nasal septum • Pterygoid plate	• Parasagittal • Lateral sagittal • Anterior coronal • Midline sagittal • Posterior coronary
Le Fort II	• Nasion (nasal bones, arch, or nasofrontal suture) • Medial orbital wall, lacrimal bone • Orbital floor • Anterior maxillary wall • Lateral maxillary wall • Pterygoid plate	• Anterior coronal • Parasagittal • Middle horizontal • Anterior coronal • Lateral sagittal • Posterior coronal
Le Fort III	• Nasion (nasal bones, arch, or nasofrontal suture) • Medial orbital wall, lacrimal bone • Lateral orbital wall • Zygoma • Pterygoid plate	• Anterior coronal • Parasagittal • Lateral sagittal • Middle horizontal • Posterior coronal

helpful to localize injury to the posterior wall of the sinuses and the adjacent orbital palate.

Fractures of the posterior wall of the frontal sinus may result in pneumocephalus. They may also present with cerebrospinal fluid (CSF) rhinorrhea due to tears in the dura of the anterior cranial fossa. Noncomminuted fractures of the frontal sinus involving the anterior wall may be managed conservatively or by relatively simple surgical procedures to restore the contour of the forehead, whereas the more complex comminuted fracture may at times require cranialization of the sinus.[9]

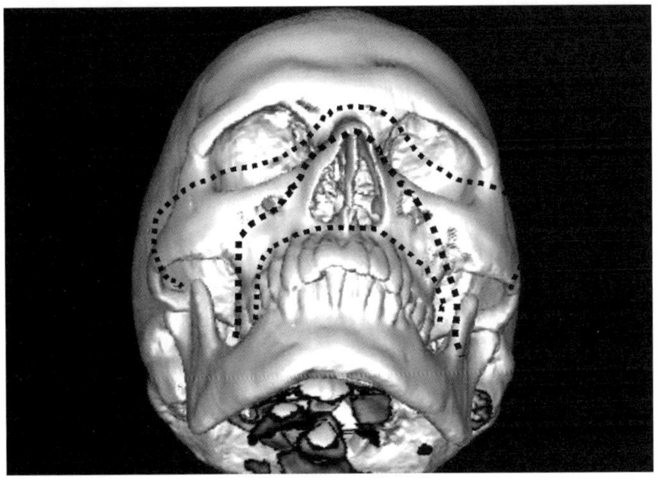

Fig. 5: Fracture lines in the Le Fort I, II and III fractures.

Recognizing nasofrontal outflow tract injuries on CT is of utmost importance as injury to the outflow tract can lead to formation of frontal mucocele and creation of an anaerobic environment leading to subsequent osteomyelitis and possible intracranial extension leading to brain abscess. Such injuries should be strongly suspected on CT if there is involvement of the base of the frontal sinus, the anterior ethmoids, or both.

Nasal Fractures

Nasal bone fractures are amongst the most common facial fractures. About half of these, fractures are isolated nasal pyramid fractures. It is important to differentiate nasal

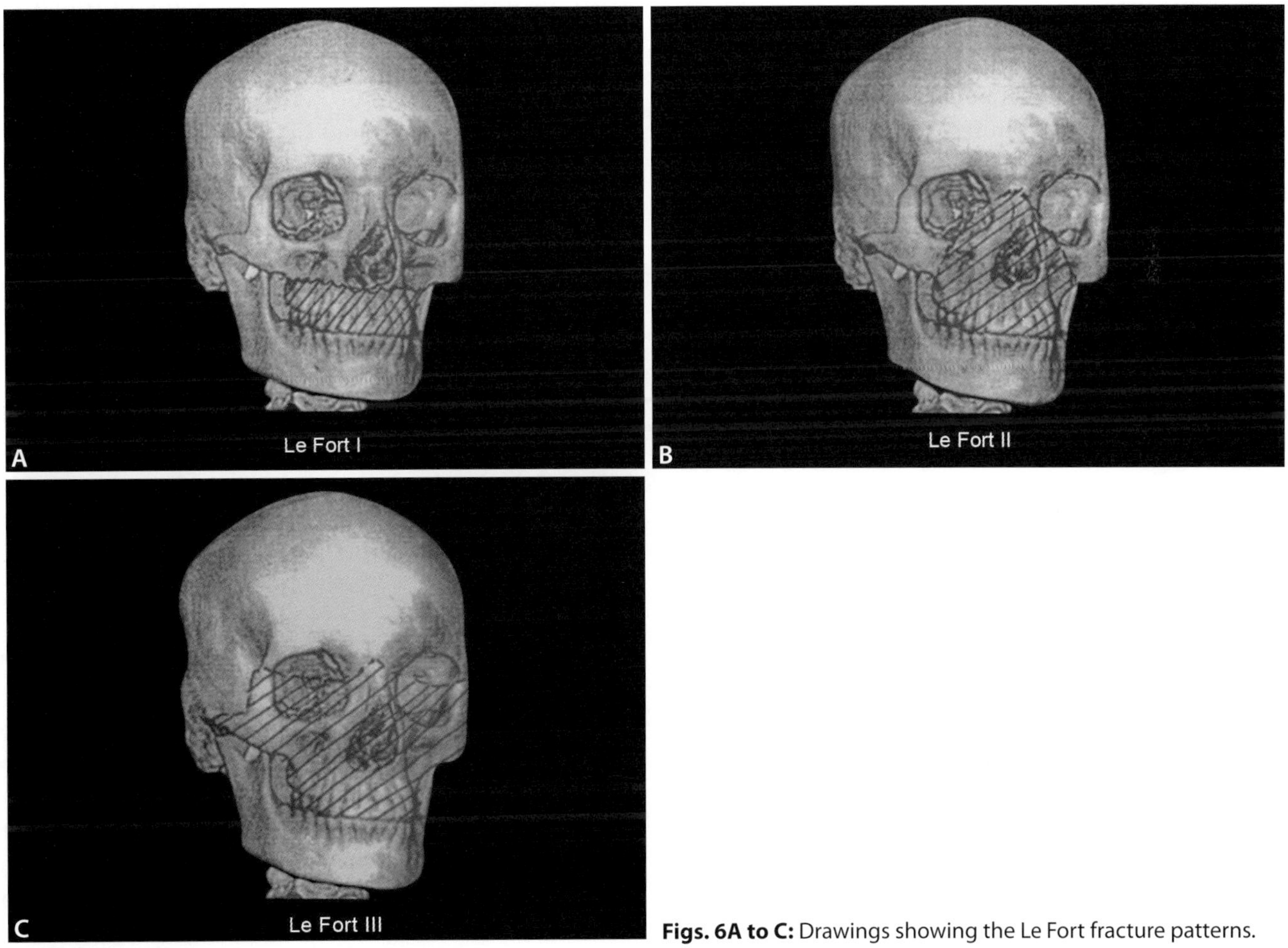

Figs. 6A to C: Drawings showing the Le Fort fracture patterns.

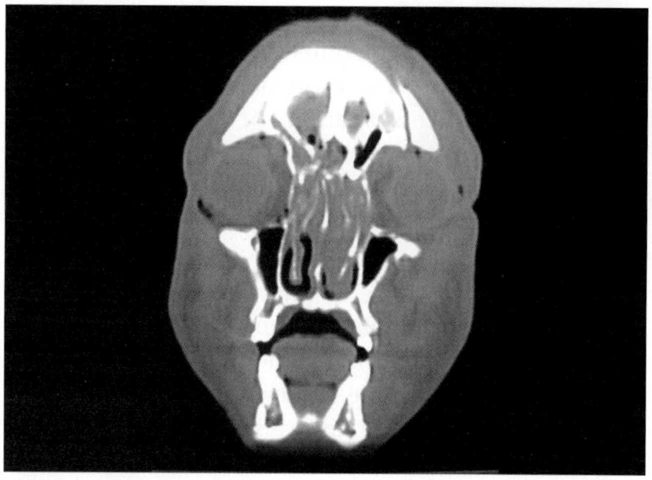

Fig. 7: Computed tomography (CT) three-dimensional coronal reconstruction image shows slightly displaced fracture of left frontal and ethmoid fractures with soft-tissue densities and air specks in orbit and sino-nasal cavities.

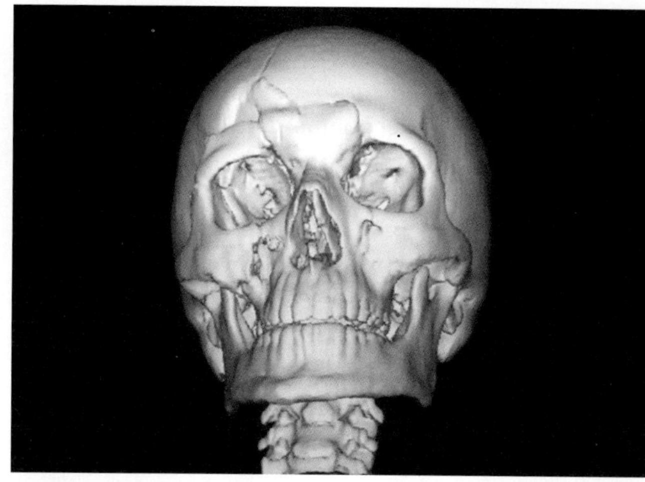

Fig. 8: Three-dimensional volume-rendered image (VRT) reconstruction showing fracture of frontal bone involving superior fracture of frontal bone involving superior orbital margins with right inferior orbital rim fracture.

cartilage injuries from nasal bone injuries. Cartilage injuries result from lateral blows to the nose. The nasal cartilages may be depressed with fracture of the ipsilateral nasal bone. Early detection of cartilage injuries is essential as they are often associated with a hematoma which needs to be evacuated. Nasal bone fractures result from anterior blows to the nose **(Figs. 9A to D)**. Such low-velocity injuries result in fractures of the lower third of the nasal bones which are thin. Typically, the nasoethmoid margin is intact.[9]

Central Midface Fractures

The central midface fractures include the naso-orbito-ethmoidal (NOE) fractures, isolated fractures of the maxillary alveolar process and hard palate, and the Le Fort fractures **(Figs. 9 and 10)**.[9]

Naso-orbito-ethmoidal fractures: They result from a direct impact to the bridge of the nose resulting in fractures of the nasal bones, nasal septum, ethmoid sinuses, frontal process of the maxilla, lamina papyracea, lacrimal bone and the cribriform plate. The NOE fractures are complex because they can be associated with intracranial and orbital injuries and a head and face CT scan is warranted. The floor of the anterior cranial fossa may be fractured in continuation with these structures. The latter fracture may tear the dura resulting in CSF leaks. NOE injuries are divided in three groups according to the degree of injury to the medial canthal attachment using the Manson classification **(Table 4)**.[21] The classification is important from treatment point of view as the most important factor determining the need for surgical correction in NOE fractures is the stability of the bone to which the medial canthal tendon attaches which is generally the anterior aspect of medial orbital wall.[22] In addition, the nasolacrimal canal injury is a frequent association of NOE fractures and should be clearly mentioned in CT report as the patients may be asymptomatic in early period but later may develop epiphora or recurrent dacrocystorhinitis.[22]

Isolated fractures of the maxillary alveolus and hard palate: They result from a direct upward blow to the mandible which pushes the mandible into the maxilla. The fracture can injure the teeth which can be displaced or devitalized. The hard palate is fractured in the parasagittal plane along the palatine process of the maxilla which is the weakest plane of the hard palate. An axial or oblique blow to the chin or a direct injury to the upper jaw results in these type of fractures.

Le Fort Fractures

- *Le Fort type I fractures*: These fractures extend through the lower nasal septum, inferior walls of the maxillary sinuses and pterygoid plates. This results in palate being displaced posteriorly and malocclusion. There is associated hemorrhage in the maxillary sinuses.
- *Le Fort type II fractures*: These are characterized by fractures through the root of the nose, the lacrimal bones and medial orbital walls, thence on to the floor of the orbits, zygomaticomaxillary suture and the

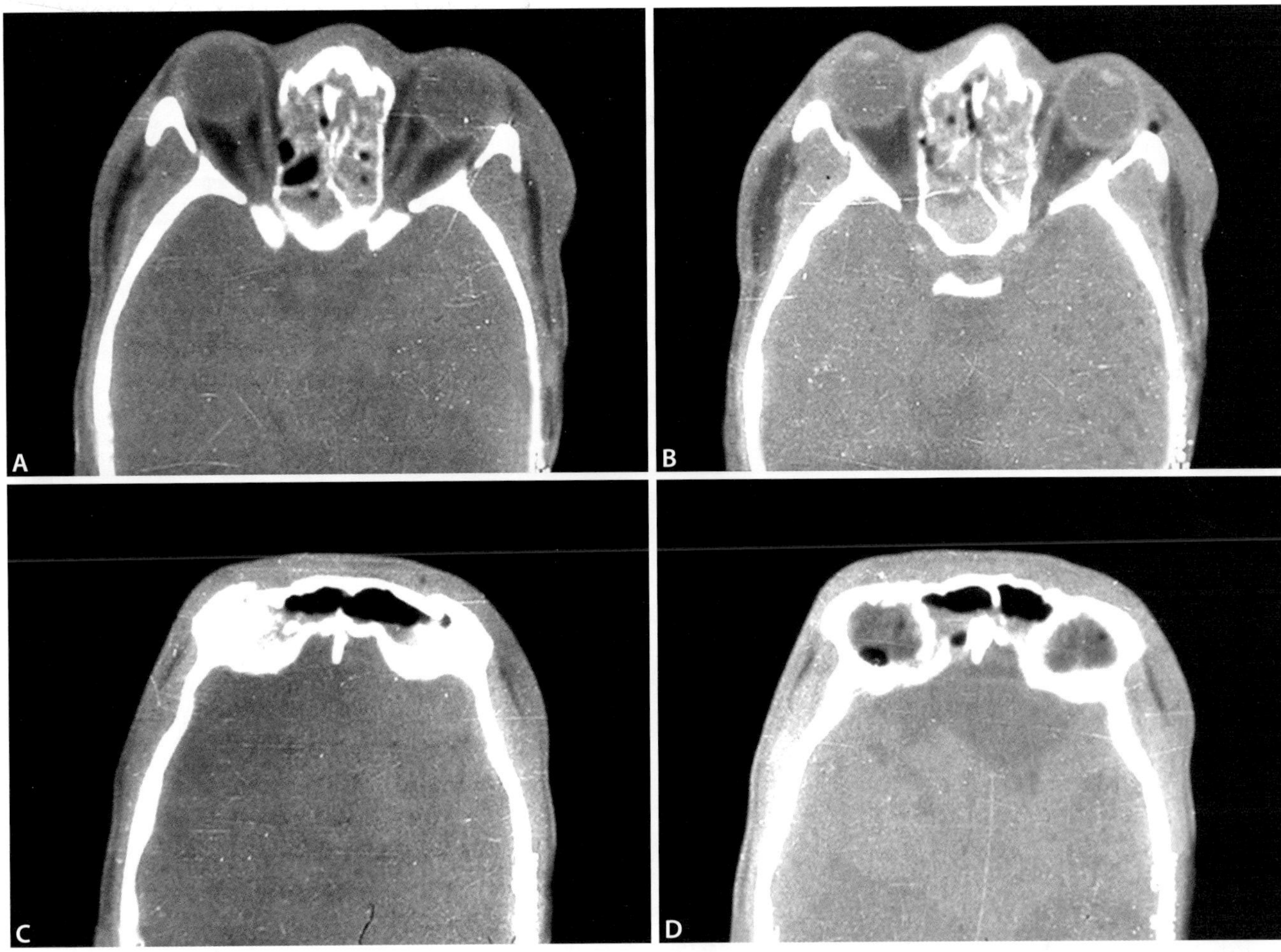

Figs. 9A to D: Fracture nasal bones as a result of a direct blow to the bridge of the nose resulting in a depression. Note the accordion-like collapse of the ethmoid bones and a concomitant fracture of the anterior wall of the frontal sinus containing blood.

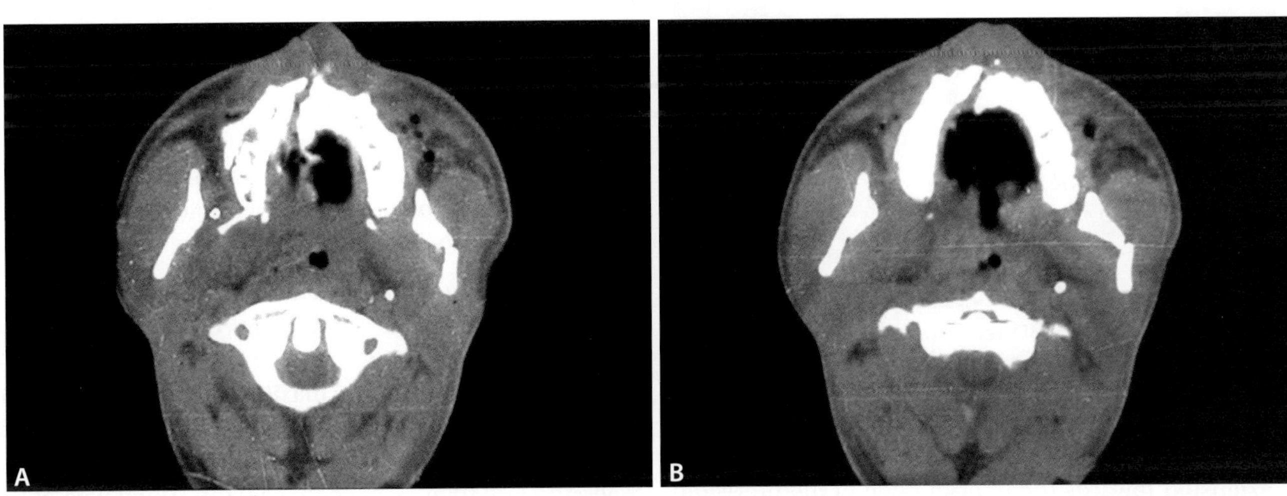

Figs. 10A and B

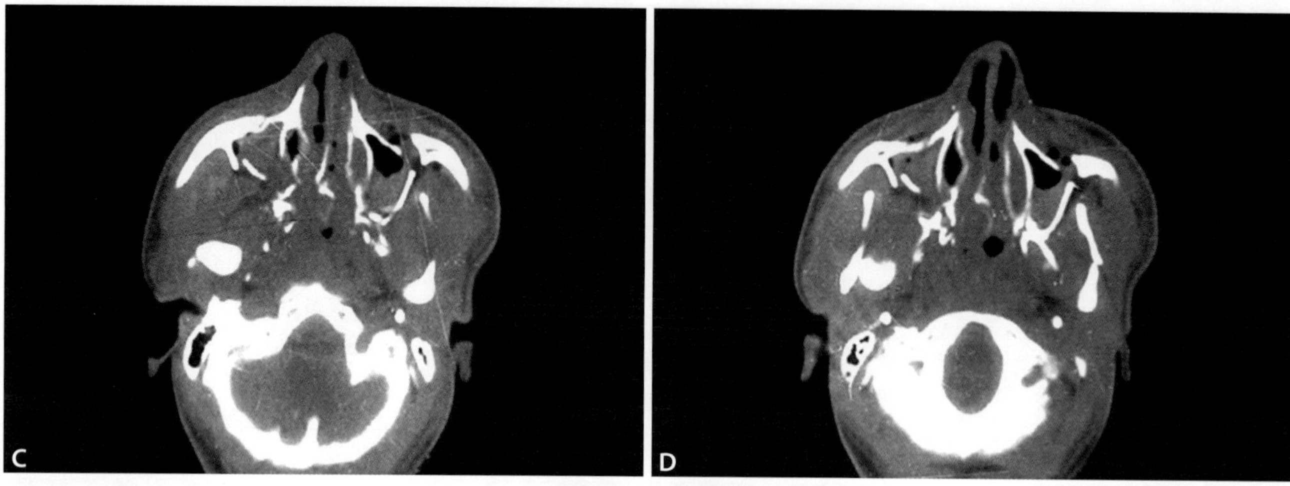

Figs. 10C and D

Figs. 10A to D: Fracture of the hard palate through the plane of the right palatine foramen as a component of a Le Fort II fracture. Note the fracture of both maxillae.

Table 4: Manson classification of naso-orbito-ethmoidal fractures.

Type 1	Single fragment (most common)
Type 2	Comminuted with intact insertion of medial canthal tendon
Type 3	Comminuted with lateral displacement or avulsion of medial canthal ligament (uncommon)

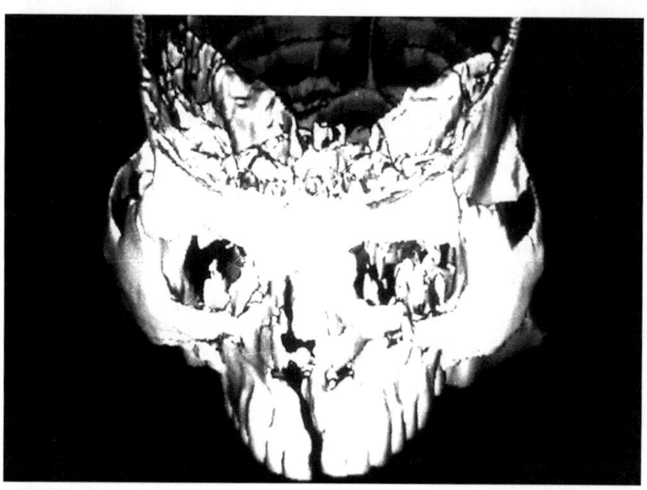

Fig. 11: Three-dimensional (3D) reconstruction of the same patient of Figure 6 showing the involvement of the superior alveolus.

anterior wall of the maxilla. There may be posterior extension towards the inferior edge of the pterygoid plates **(Figs. 9 to 11)**.

- *Le Fort type III fractures*: These fractures include the entire gamut of injuries included in Le Fort type II fractures with extension into the lateral orbital walls and zygoma. This results in the separation of the entire facial skeleton from the skull base.

There are numerous components in the Le Fort fractures that make classification difficult; however, each of the Le Fort fractures has at least one unique component that is easily recognizable. Therefore, first recognize the unique component as: fracture of lateral margin of nasal fossa indicates Le Fort I, inferior orbital rim (Le Fort II) and zygomatic arch (Le Fort III). Secondly confirm the presence of other fractures which is suspected Le Fort plane.[23] Patient with higher grade Le Fort injuries more frequently need surgical airway. Le fort III injuries have higher chance of requiring neurosurgical intervention and may need immediate intensive care unit (ICU) care.[24]

Lateral Midface Fractures

They include the trimalar (zygomatic) fractures, fractures of the zygomatic arch and the zygomaticomaxillary/zygomaticomandibular fractures. The blowout fractures of the orbits are also included in the fractures of this region.[9]

Trimalar or zygomatic fractures: They are so termed because they involve three bony connections of the zygomatic bone namely with the: (1) lateral orbital wall, (2) zygomatic bone and (3) maxilla. The fracture line runs from the lateral orbital wall down to the inferior orbital fissure, along the orbital floor and anterior maxillary wall. The line then turns to involve the lateral wall of the maxilla to end at or near the inferior orbital fissure. These fractures are the second most common fractures of the facial skeleton, the first being fractures of the nasal bone **(Fig. 12)**.

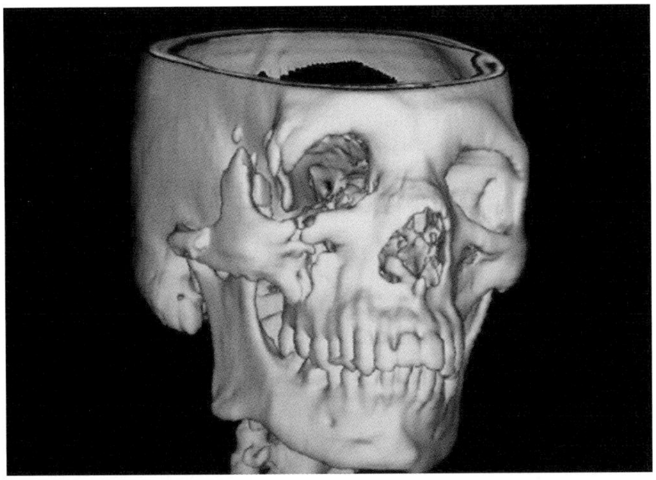

Fig. 12: Trimalar fracture of right zygomatic bone showing three fracture lines which characterize this fracture.

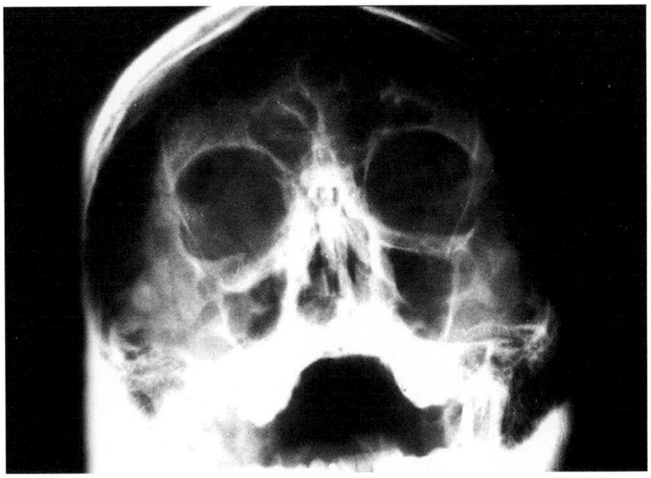

Fig. 13: Blow out fracture of the right orbit showing the fracture of the inferior margin of the orbit in the Walter's view.

Zygomaticomaxillary fractures: They include a maxillary component to the zygomatic fracture which includes the hard palate and the pterygoid plates.

The zygomaticomandibular fractures: They include fractures of the mandibular condyle or coronoid process in addition to the zygomatic fracture outlined above.[9]

Blowout Fractures of the Orbit

Injuries to the orbital margins result in blowout fractures. Typically, injuries result due to an object larger than orbit. The force of the injury results in the transmission of the vector to the orbital floor. The floor is fractured in the middle third close to the infraorbital canal. Rarely, the inferior orbital rim is fractured resulting in the so-called impure blowout fracture. Herniation of the orbital fat, inferior rectus and inferior oblique muscle into the maxillary antrum may result. Rarely, the fractured fragments may protrude into the orbit impinging on the inferior rectus complex or into the globe **(Figs. 13 to 15)**.[25-27]

Medial wall fractures of the orbit: Imaging is crucial in recognizing these fractures which are often overlooked. CT evaluates these fractures which have been classified into four types:

1. Type 1 confined to the medial wall of the orbit
2. Type 2 fracture involves the medial orbital wall and the contiguous floor of the orbit
3. Type 3 is a fracture of the medial wall, orbital floor and the malar bones
4. Type 4 includes medial wall fractures associated with complex midface fractures **(Figs. 13 to 17)**.[23]

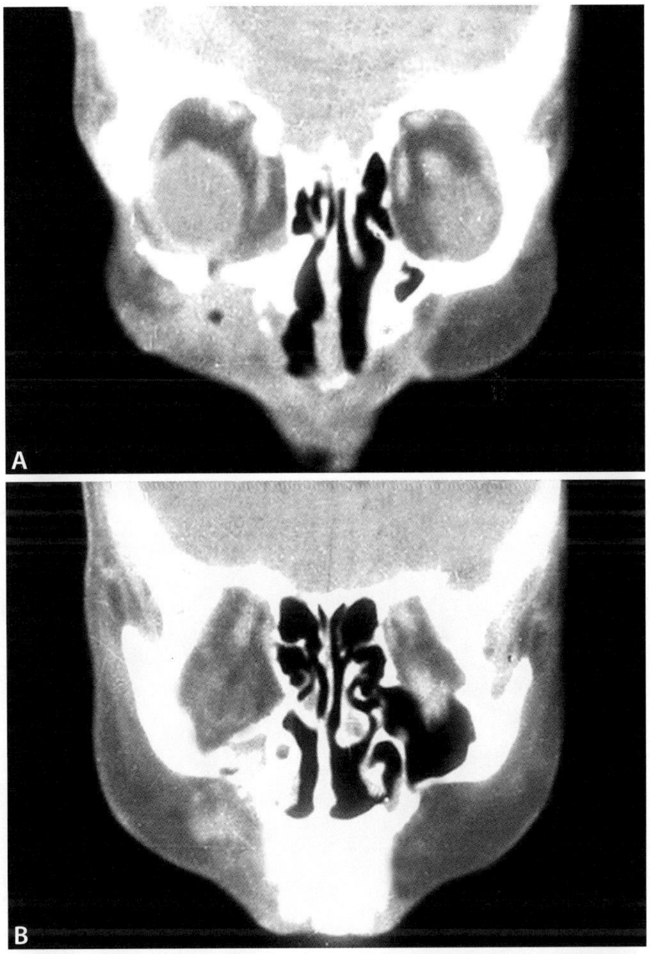

Figs. 14A and B: Coronal computed tomography (CT) sections showing the fracture line along the inferior orbital rim and inferior displacement of the globe.

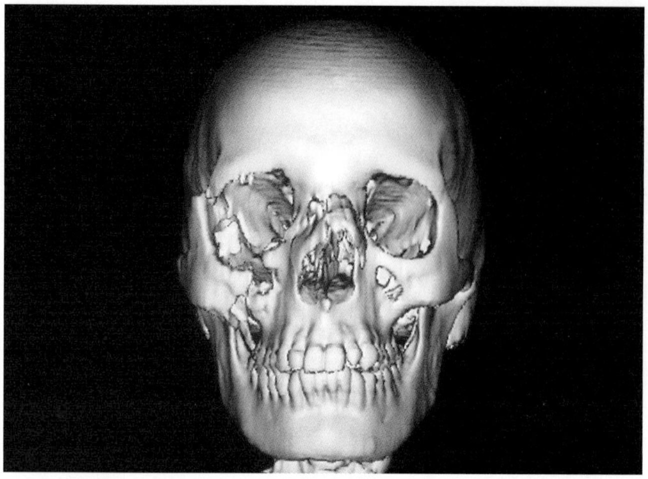

Fig. 15: Three-dimensional (3D) volume-rendered technique (VRT) reconstruction image reveals right orbital fracture involving inferolateral wall (zygomatic bone) with lateral displacement resulting in increased orbital volume.

An interesting area and often neglected in routine assessment of facial trauma is the nasoethmoidal region and nasolacrimal canal and fossa. Thin coronal and axial CT sections are essential to image this region. Fractures of this region should be specifically looked for in the medial blow in fractures of the orbit and complications due to this injury avoided.[25,26]

The different types of orbital fractures are also associated with soft tissue injury, injuries to different intraocular structures and the optic nerve which are discussed in the Chapter 21.

Mandibular Fractures

Fractures of the mandible are classified according to the site of fracture. They are fractures of the: (a) condyle, (b) coronoid process, (c) angle and body, (d) ramus, and (e) midline fracture of the mandible. This U-shaped bone is likely to fracture at two sites, since it is firmly held at its

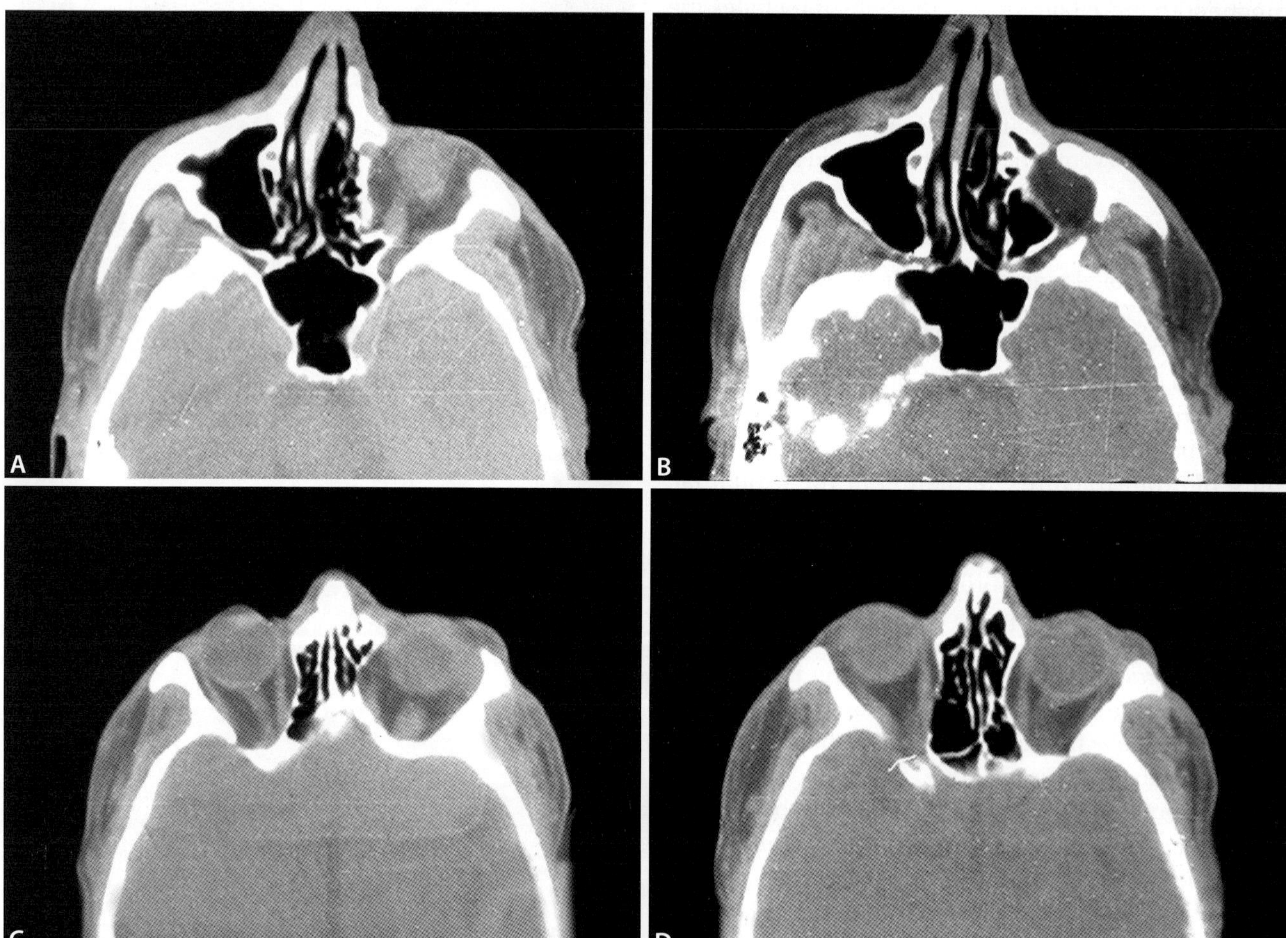

Figs. 16A to D: Fracture of the medial wall of the left orbit. The thin lamina papyracea is bowed medially with a resulting increase in the orbital volume. A fracture of the floor of the orbit is present in this axial computed tomography study.

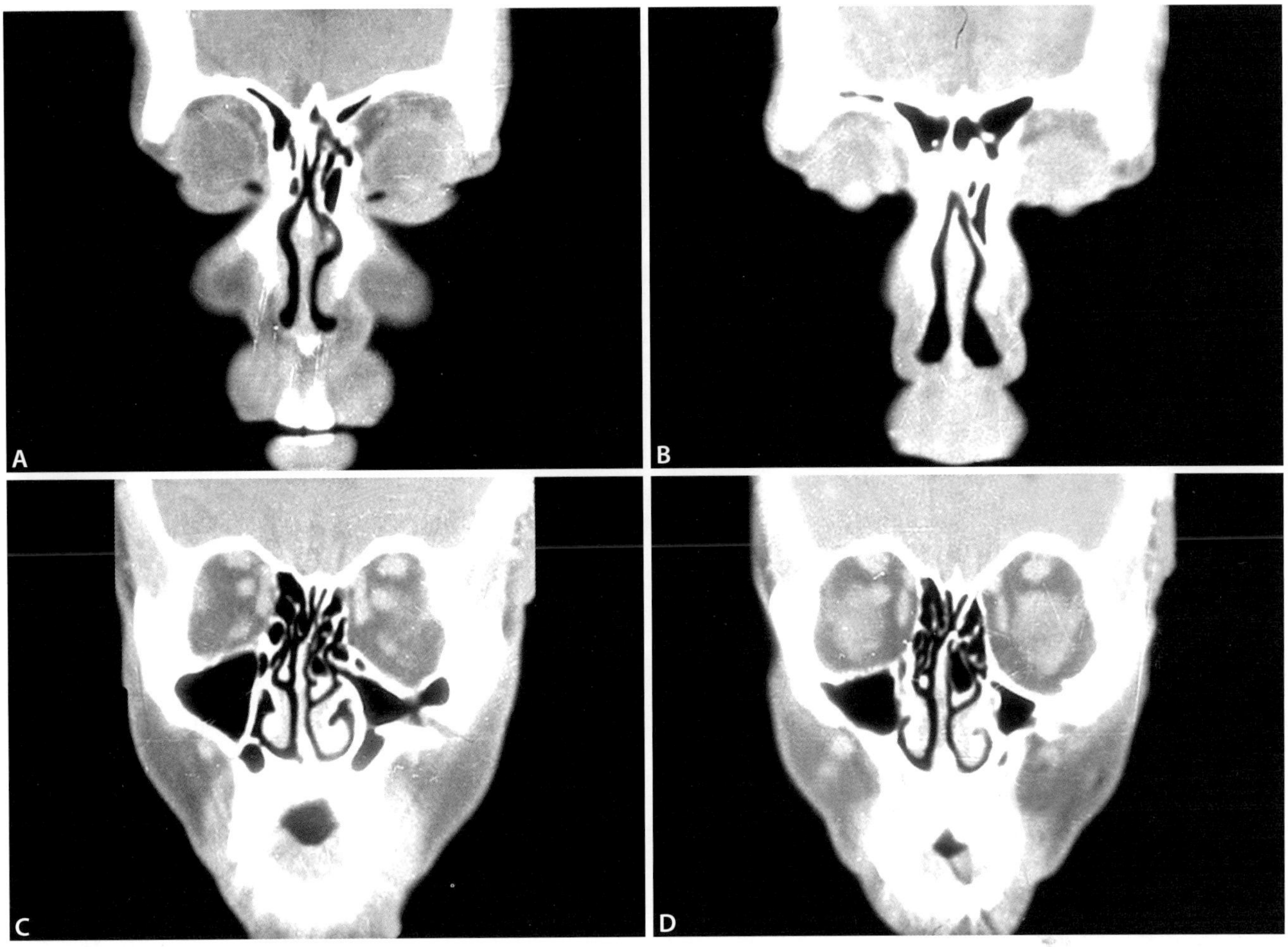

Figs. 17A to D: Coronal computed tomography (CT) section of the above patient (Fig. 9), showing the subtle increase in orbital volume. The medial wall fracture cannot be fully appreciated as is the fracture along the orbital floor.

ends by the capsules of the temporomandibular joints. Fracture of the neck of the condyle of the mandible is most commonly followed by those of the ramus and body **(Figs. 18A and B)**.

The initial radiological investigation for assessment of a mandibular fracture is a panoramic view of the mandible. This investigation will give most of the information regarding the sites of the fractures; however, it may be difficult to obtain in uncooperative patients. In the latter situation, PA views of the skull with oblique views for the mandible are suitable alternatives. Radiological investigations may be tailored to demonstrate fractures at specific site, e.g. intraoral dental views may be required to demonstrate fractures of the teeth and alveolar processes; Towne's view of the skull may be needed to show fractures of the neck of the condyle and rotated PA views may be required to show fractures of the ramus.

Coronal CT scan and 3D reconstructions may be required to demonstrate undisplaced fractures of the ramus and condyle of the mandible.

Skull Base Fractures

The skull base comprises of 7 bones, the paired frontal and temporal bones, and the unpaired ethmoid, sphenoid, and occipital bones. It is divided into anterior, central, and posterior regions, which form the floor of the anterior, middle, and posterior cranial fossae. The skull base fractures are associated with myriad of complications which are summarized in **Table 5**.

Anterior skull base fractures: The anterior skull base, formed by the frontal and ethmoid bones, separates the anterior and inferior frontal lobes and olfactory structures within the anterior cranial fossa from the orbits

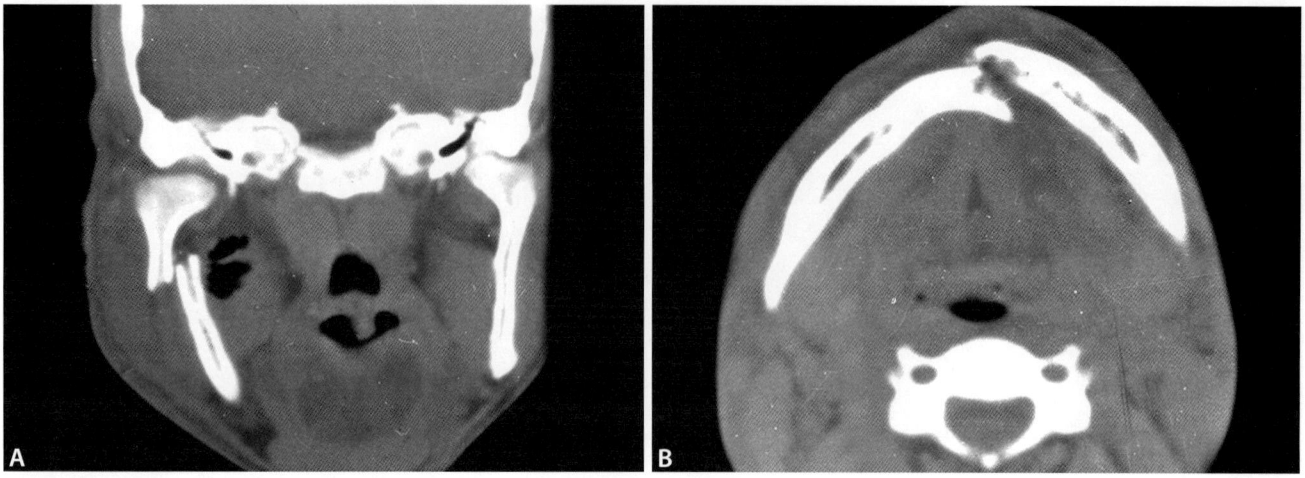

Figs. 18A and B: Fractures of the mandible: (A) Coronal computed tomography (CT) section shows fracture of the right condylar process; and (B) The axial CT section shows the concomitant fracture of the body of the mandible.

Table 5: Complications associated with skull base fractures.

Site of fracture	*Complications*
Anterior skull base fractures	• CSF leak and Meningoencephalocele • Orbital injury • Anosmia (due to CN I injury) • Frontal contusions/hemorrhage
Central skull base fractures	• Vascular injury (Internal carotid artery or basilar trunk)—psedouaneurysm, dissection, laceration or transection, carotid-cavernous fistula and other dural arteriovenous fistula • Nerve injury- CN II, III, IV, V, VI injury, Horner syndrome • Multicompartmental intraparenchymal hemorrhage/contusion, diffuse axonal injury • CSF leak • Anterior middle cranial fossa epidural hemorrhage
Posterior skull base fractures	• Vertebrobasilar injury • Venous vascular injury causing thrombosis • Lower cranial nerve injuries (CN IX to XII) • CVJ and cervical spine injuries
Posterolateral skull base fractures	• Vascular injury (ICA) • Nerve injury-CN VII & VIII injury • CN VII and VIII injuries

Abbreviations: CSF: Cerebrospinal fluid; CN: Cranial nerve; CVJ: Craniovertebral junction; ICA: Internal carotid artery.

and the sinonasal cavity. Direct frontal trauma often results in anterior skull base fractures, so-called fronto-basal injuries, with the "frontal" component of fractures involving the upper facial third (frontal bone/sinus and superior orbital rim), while the "basal" component of fracture involving the anterior skull base (cribriform plate, ethmoid roofs, and planum sphenoidale).[27] Complications associated with the anterior skull base fractures include orbital injury, CSF leak, meningoencephalocele formation, anosmia (due to cranial nerve olfactory nerve injury) and frontal lobe contusions.[28]

Central skull base fractures: The central skull base, formed by the sphenoid and anterior temporal bones, separates the pituitary gland (within the sella), the cavernous sinuses (including the carotid artery and cranial nerves), the Meckel cave, and the temporal lobes superiorly from the sphenoid sinus anteriorly and inferiorly, and the extracranial soft tissues deep to the skull base inferiorly, including the masticator, parotid, parapharyngeal, and pharyngeal mucosal spaces. Transverse fractures in a coronal plane through the central skull base are common and are usually the result of high velocity lateral impact to the lateral frontal bone, zygoma, temporal, or parietal bone.[27] Extension of frontobasal fractures from frontal impact can occur in a sagittal or oblique fashion through the central skull base with involvement of the sella and sphenoid sinus, and, in some cases, the temporal bone.[28] The management of central skull base fractures are based on the associated complications and it is generally associated with a variety of potentially lethal complications. Associated intracranial injuries like multicompartmental intraparenchymal hemorrhages, contusions and diffuse axonal injuries are common as these are associated with high velocity injury. Injury to the greater wing of sphenoid often causes anterior middle cranial fossa epidural hematoma and are believed to be due to venous injury in sphenoparietal sinus.[29] CSF leaks can occur in association with sphenoid bone fracture although less common than frontobasal fractures.[30] Vascular injuries are most frequently encountered and most dreaded complications of central skull base fractures. Blunt cerebrovascular injury is reported in approximately

1% of all head and facial traumas, with risk increased to 8.5% in the setting of basilar skull fractures.[31-33] The internal carotid arteries are most prone to be involved because of its course through the central skull base and cavernous sinus. However, the basilar trunk is also prone to injury because of its vertical retroclival course.[28] The most common fractures associated with vascular injuries are clival fractures, fractures through the sella/sphenoid sinus, orbital apex fractures, petrous ridge fractures, and occiput and occipital condyle fractures. The vascular injuries include arterial dissection, pseudoaneurysm formation, frank transection or laceration, incarceration (entrapment within fracture line) and dural arteriovenous fistula formation, most notably carotid-cavernous fistula. Cranial nerve injuries may be associated in case of involvement of cavernous sinuses.

Posterior skull base fractures: The posterior skull base is formed by the posterior temporal bone and the occipital bone, and separates the posterior fossa structures, including the cerebellum and brainstem, from the extracranial soft tissues: the posterior nasopharynx, retropharyngeal space, carotid space, and perivertebral space. Most posterior cranial fossa fractures occur as a result of a lateral and/or posterior blow to the occiput, and involve the occipital bone with frequent extension to the petrous temporal bone.[28] Potential complications include associated intraparenchymal hemorrhage and contusions including cerebellar involvement, sigmoid or transverse sinus thrombosis, dural arteriovenous fistula and lower cranial nerve injuries and CSF otorrhea in temporal bone fractures.[28] Associated injury to craniovertebral junction or cervical spine are also frequently encountered.[29]

PEDIATRIC FACIAL FRACTURES

Pediatric patients with facial fractures require a different approach than adults. It has been stressed in literature that routine radiographs may underestimate the most trivial injury. Hence, a CT scan is advocated for complete assessment. A high index of suspicion of maxillofacial trauma should always be maintained, especially in children with multiple traumas. The varying degree of ossification and pediatric dentition will affect the CT images and hence CT parameters should be specifically tailored for children. There are many features of pediatric facial bones which influence radiological features of facial trauma. Pediatric facial bones are elastic and do not fracture as easily as adult bones. The thick elastic periosteum prevents bone displacement resulting in greenstick fractures **(Figs. 19 and 20)**. In pediatric trauma, the fracture of orbital roof is most common and there is strong correlation between the orbital hematomas and orbital roof/naso-orbital ethmoid fractures.[34] Healing of facial fractures is faster in pediatric patients than adults requiring shorter periods of immobilization. Moreover, if the treatment is delayed, the fractures fragments heal and become fixed which prevents any further reduction. Dental deformities or delayed dentition may result, if the growth centers are involved. Since children have fewer teeth to place splints, the treatment plans need to be modified and wire ligatures used frequently in adult fractures are contraindicated, especially in children below 2 years of age.[35]

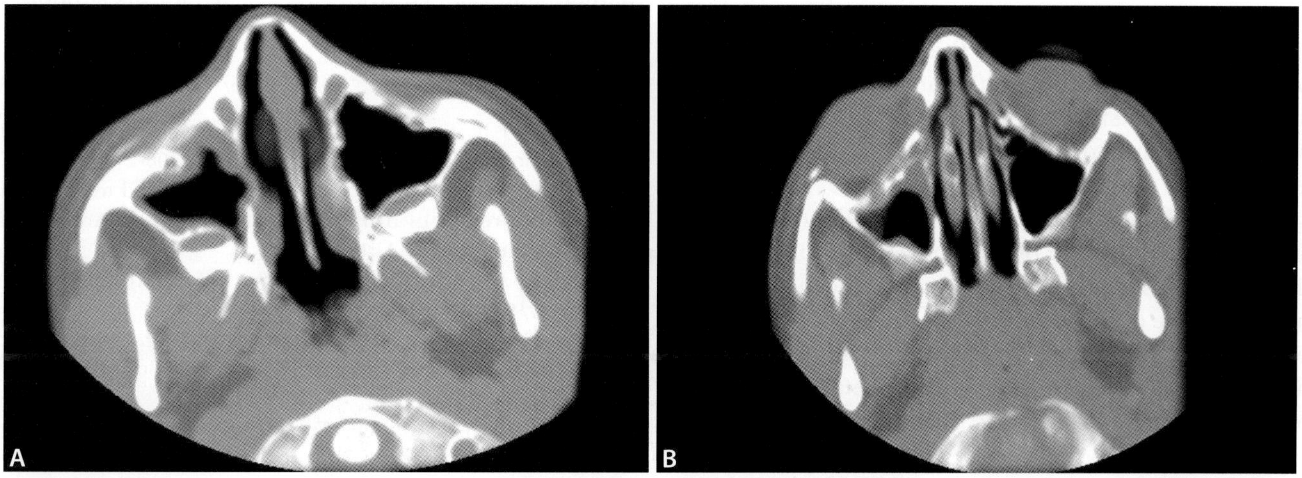

Figs. 19A and B: Pediatric facial fractures: Fracture of the inferior and lateral margins of the right orbit in a 6-year-old girl. The fracture appears as a subtle depression in the orbital outline.

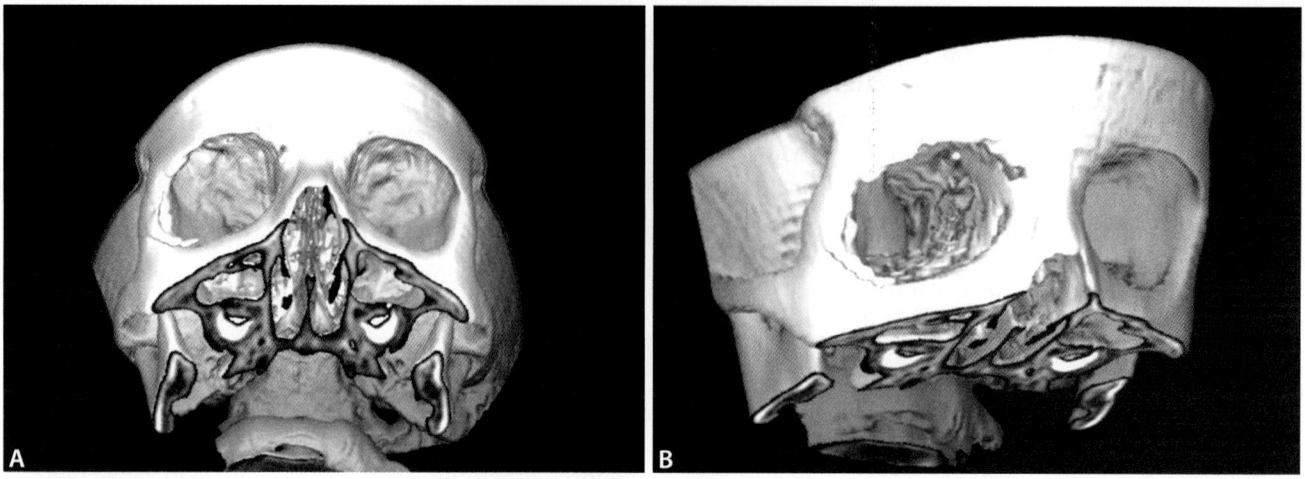

Figs. 20A and B: Three-dimensional (3D) reconstruction of the axial computed tomography (CT) of the patient in Figure 15. The fracture line in clearly demonstrated in the reconstructed views.

CLINICAL ASPECTS OF MAXILLOFACIAL IMAGING

There have been major changes in the concepts of surgical management of facial fractures in the last decade. Modern principles of reconstructive surgery lay stress on extensive subperiosteal dissection, exposure of all fracture lines open reduction and rigid fixation. Internal fixation is done by the extensive use of miniplates or microplates with screw. Complex internal fixation schemes using wire sutures and wire suspensions have become obsolete. The use of tissue adhesives, such as N-butyl cyanoacrylate for fixing small thin fragments of bone, have been a novel advance.[9,36,37]

Imaging of a patient with maxillofacial injury should be so complete that the surgeon has a clear delineation of the location of fractures, direction and amount of displacement, and the location of anatomic landmarks (keys) that will help restore the preinjury position of bone.[38] The regional classification reflects upon the increasing sophistication in the operative management of patients. Surgeons require specific information to accomplish their task in restoring the geometrical symmetry of the face, e.g. in the midfacial fracture. The surgeon would want to restore the vertical dimension of the face in a Le Fort injury which would mean restoration of at least one of the four major buttresses in that region. Together with the corrected dental deformities and mandibular fractures, if any, the preinjury position of the face can be restored. Therefore, the radiologist should understand the morbid anatomy and present to the surgeon both an axial and coronal evaluation so that vertical buttresses can be clearly delineated. In the Le Fort injuries, skull base fractures merit special mention and their presence can influence the prognosis of a seemingly innocuous superficial fracture.[9]

Amongst the more serious complications of facial fractures is infection of the fracture line. Any fracture may be considered to be infected, if the fracture line crosses the alveolus, nasal cavity or any of the paranasal sinuses; or if there is a communication with the associated soft-tissue wound. Demonstration of these fracture lines and fragments should be done with clarity to aid surgical approach to the fractures.[26]

ACKNOWLEDGMENTS

The authors acknowledge Dr Nirmaly Ray, DM resident in the Neuroradiology Division of Department of Radiodiagnosis, PGIMER, Chandigarh for his support in editing of chapter.

REFERENCES

1. Le Fort R. Etude experimental sur les fractures de la machoire superieure. Rev Chir. 1901;25:208-27.
2. Stanley RB. Use of intraoperative computed tomography during repair of orbitozygomatic fractures. Arch Facial Plast Surg. 1999;1(1):19-24.
3. Zilkha A. Computed tomography in facial trauma. Radiology. 1982;144(3):545-8.
4. Bartlett SP, DeLozier JB. Controversies in the management of pediatric facial fractures. Clin Plastic Surg. 1992;19(1):245-58.
5. Gentry LR, Manor WF, Turski PA, et al. High-resolution CT analysis of facial struts in trauma: 1. Normal anatomy. AJR. 1983;140(3):523-32.

6. Gentry LR, Manor WF, Turski PA, et al. High-resolution CT analysis of facial struts in trauma: 2. Osseous and soft-tissue complications. AJR. 1983;140(3):533-41.
7. Beirne JC, Butler PE, Brady FA. Cervical spine injuries in patients with facial fractures: a 1-year prospective study. Int J Oral Maxillofac Surg. 1995;24(1 Pt 1):26-9.
8. Manson PN. Facial injuries the face—part 1. In: Joseph GM (Ed). Plastic Surgery. Philadelphia, PA, USA: WB Saunders; 1990. pp. 867-89.
9. Som PM, Brandwein MS. Facial fractures and postoperative findings. In: Som PM, Curtin HD (Eds). Head and Neck Imaging, 5th edition. St Louis, MO: Mosby; 2011. pp. 374-438.
10. Lill W, Solar P, Ulm C, et al. Reproducibility of three-dimensional CT-assisted model production in the maxillofacial area. Br J Oral Maxillofac Surg. 1992;30(4): 233-6.
11. Cavalcanti MG, Haller JW, Vannier MW. Three-dimensional computed tomography landmark measurement in craniofacial surgical planning: experimental validation in vitro. J Oral Maxillofac Surg. 1999;57(6):690-4.
12. Chen WJ, Yang YJ, Fang YM, et al. Identification and classification in Le Fort type fractures by using 2D and 3D computed tomography. Chin J Traumatol. 2006;9(1): 59-64.
13. Coupal TM, Mallinson PI, McLaughlin P, et al. Peering through the glare: using dual-energy CT to overcome the problem of metal artefacts in bone radiology. Skeletal Radiol. 2014;43(5):567-75.
14. Cavalcanti MG, Rocha SS, Vannier MW. Craniofacial measurements based on 3D-CT volume rendering implications for clinical applications. Dentomaxillofac Radiol. 2004;33(3):170-6.
15. Guerrero ME, Jacobs R, Loubele M, et al. State-of-the-art on cone beam CT imaging for preoperative planning of implant placement. Clin Oral Investig. 2006;10(1):1-7.
16. van Steenberghe D, Naert I, Andersson M, et al. A custom template and definitive prosthesis allowing immediate implant loading in the maxilla: a clinical report. Int J Oral Maxillofac Implants. 2002;17(5):663-70.
17. Brisco J, Fuller K, Lee N, et al. Cone beam computed tomography for imaging orbital trauma—image quality and radiation dose compared with conventional multislice computed tomography. Br J Oral Maxillofac Surg 2014; 52(1):76-80.
18. Parmar HA, Ibrahim M, Mukherji SK. Optimizing craniofacial CT technique. Neuroimaging Clin N Am. 2014;24(3):395-405.
19. Zimmerman R, Bilaniuk L, Hackney D, et al. Paranasal sinus hemorrhage: evaluation with MR imaging. Radiology. 1987;162(2):499-503.
20. Hopper RA, Salemy S, Sze RW. Diagnosis of midface fractures with CT: what the surgeon needs to know. Radiographics. 2006;26(3):783-93.
21. Manson PN, Markowitz B, Mirvis S, et al. Toward CT-based facial fracture treatment. Plast Reconstr Surg. 1990;85(2):202-12.
22. Uzelac A, Gean AD. Orbital and facial fractures. Neuroimaging Clin N Am. 2014;24(3):407-24.
23. Rhea JT, Novelline RA. How to simplify the CT diagnosis of Le Fort fractures? AJR. 2005;184(5):1700-5.
24. Bagheri SC, Holmgren E, Kademani D, et al. Comparison of the severity of bilateral Le Fort injuries in isolated midface trauma. J Oral Maxillofac Surg. 2005;63(8):1123-9.
25. Schultz RC, Elbel WR. Facial bone fractures. In: Stark RB (Ed). Plastic Surgery of the Head and Neck, Part 3. Philadelphia, PA, USA: Churchill Livingstone; 1987. p. 1039.
26. Burn JS, Chung CH, Oh SJ. Pure orbital blowout fractures: new concepts and importance of medial orbital blowout fracture. Plast Reconstr Surg. 1999;103(7):1839-49.
27. Pelton RW, Rainey AM, Lee AG. Traumatic subluxation of the globe into the maxillary sinus. AJNR. 1998;19(8): 1450-1.
28. Baugnon KL, Hudgins PA. Skull base fractures and their complications. Neuroimaging Clin N Am. 2014;24(3): 439-65.
29. Gean AD, Fischbein NJ, Purcell DD, et al. Benign anterior temporal epidural hematoma: indolent lesion with a characteristic CT imaging appearance after blunt head trauma. Radiology. 2010;257(1):212-8.
30. Lin DT, Lin AC. Surgical treatment of traumatic injuries of the cranial base. Otolaryngol Clin North Am 2013;46(5): 749-57.
31. Berne JD, Cook A, Rowe SA, et al. A multivariate logistic regression analysis of risk factors for blunt cerebrovascular injury. J Vasc Surg. 2010;51:57-64.
32. Mundinger GS, Dorafshar AH, Gilson MM, et al. Blunt-mechanism facial fracture patterns associated with internal carotid artery injuries: recommendations for additional screening criteria based on analysis of 4,398 patients. J Oral Maxillofac Surg. 2013;71(12):2092-100.
33. Feiz-Erfan I, Horn EM, Theodore N, et al. Incidence and pattern of direct blunt neurovascular injury associated with trauma to the skull base. J Neurosurg. 2007;107(2): 364-9.
34. Chapman VM, Fenton LZ, Gao D, et al. Facial fractures in children: unique patterns of injury observed by computed tomography. J Comput Assist Tomogr. 2009;33(1): 70-2.
35. Kim DB, Sacapano M, Hardesty RA. Facial fractures in children. West J Med. 1997;167(2):100.
36. Venkatramu NK, Khandelwal N, Bapuraj JR, et al. Evaluation of 3DCT in maxilla-facial trauma: surgical correlation (work-in- progress). Ind J Radiol Imag. 1997;7(2): 97-102.
37. Schierle HP, Hausamen JE. Modern principles in treatment of complex injuries of the facial bones. Unfallchirurg. 1997; 100(5):330-7.
38. Laine FJ. Maxillofacial trauma. In: Haaga JR, Lanzieri CF, Sartoris DJ, Zerhonni EA (Eds). Computed Tomography and Magnetic Resonance Imaging of the Whole Body, 3rd edition. St Louis, MO: Mosby; 1994. p. 388.

CHAPTER 32

Imaging of Acute Spinal Trauma

Sameer Vyas, Niranjan Khandelwal, Paramjeet Singh

INTRODUCTION

Imaging in acute spinal trauma plays a pivotal role for the diagnosis and treatment of patients by delineating extent, classification and severity of the osseous and ligamentous injury. Spinal trauma occurs with an annual incidence of approximately 15–40 cases per million.[1] It commonly results from motor vehicle accident (most commonly), fall from height, penetrating and sports injuries.[1,2] Most studies had shown a bimodal age distribution and is more common in young adults (approx 80%, <40 years) with a male predominance (80–85%).[3] Spinal cord injuries are seen in about 10–14% of spine fractures and dislocations. The incidence of neurological damage varies with the site of injury (fractures or dislocations), and is seen in approximately 40% of cervical spine, in about 10% of thoracic spine and about 4% of thoracolumbar junction injuries. However, there are no associated fractures or dislocations in about 10% spinal cord injuries. Imaging plays a crucial role in the evaluation of the acutely traumatized patient by providing information that allows timely and appropriate management, thus reducing the morbidity and mortality.

IMAGING INDICATIONS OF THE TRAUMATIC SPINE

Most of the patients presenting with blunt spinal trauma even minor are subjected to radiographs of the spine because of the significant morbidity and mortality associated with the spinal trauma. It is very important to answer these two questions before performing any radiological investigation, Is imaging necessary? And if yes, what is appropriate imaging technique? Several clinical trials have been carried out for improving guidelines and to standardize clinical practice, to help clinicians or radiologists to properly screen and use plain radiographs, to reduce the workload of emergency department and cost of imaging.[2-4] Two clinical decision rules have been developed for the cervical spine injuries. The first rule developed was National Emergency X-Radiography Utilization Study (NEXUS) Low-Risk Criteria (NLC), which tested a five-part decision rule to predict patients with a spinal injury.[4] The NLC concluded that radiography after blunt C-spine trauma is unnecessary, if patients satisfy all five of the following **low-risk criteria**: absence of midline cervical spine tenderness, normal level of alertness, no evidence of intoxication, no abnormal neurologic findings, and no painful distracting injuries. Due to the low specificity of NLC, the Canadian C-spine rule (CCR) was developed subsequently based upon clinical questions. It stated that **low-risk patients** (ambulatory, without midline tenderness or immediate onset of pain, able to attain sitting position, victims of simple rear- end motor vehicle crashes) do not require imaging if they can actively turn their heads 45° in both directions. Similar clinical criteria have been evaluated in the thoracic and lumbar spine. Imaging is however indicated when high risk factors are identified in these patients. These high risk factors are summarized in **Table 1**.

Table 1: Canadian C-spine Rule high-risk criteria.

High-risk criteria of CCR
• Age greater than 65 years • Dangerous mechanism of injury (e.g. fall from height >1 metre, high speed motor vehicle accident) • Paresthesia in extremities
Further high-risk criteria
• Altered mental status • Multiple fractures • Drowning or diving accidents • Significant head or facial injury • Rigid spinal disease (i.e. ankylosing spondylitis, DISH)

The American college of radiology appropriateness criteria for suspected spine trauma highlights the following points:

- No imaging is required in patients having low risk criteria by NLC/CCR.
- In adults with high risk criteria by NLC/CCR, MDCT is the investigation of choice. The entire spine is usually imaged due to high prevalence of non contiguous multiple injuries.
- However, in children up to 14 years of age radiography is the imaging method of choice due to high radiation dose by a CT scan. Recommended views for cervical spine are: AP, lateral and open mouth and for thoracolumbar spine are AP and lateral.
- MR imaging is method of choice when spinal cord injury, cord compression and/or ligament injury is suspected especially in obtunded patients.
- MRI is also considered in patients with persistent neck pain showing no evidence fracture on CT scan.[5]

Advanced imaging techniques are incorporated more frequently for evaluation of spinal trauma in older patients. It is because the elderly patients undergo a different injury pattern due to associated osteopenia, degenerative changes and ankylosed spinal segments. Low energy mechanism is a common cause of spinal fractures especially in cervical spine. In addition, spinal cord injury is seen in over 20% of cases. CT is excellent to define the full extent of osseous injury; however MRI should also be performed in this subset of patients due to higher incidence of spinal cord and ligamentous injury.[6]

IMAGING MODALITIES

The various imaging modalities for imaging spinal trauma are plain radiograph, tomography, myelography, computed tomography (CT) and magnetic resonance imaging (MRI).[7,8] It is very important to decide the optimal imaging method for the spinal trauma patients depending upon the merits and limitations of each modality.

Plain Radiography

In the current scenario, radiographs are not usually obligatory prior to the CT for acute spinal trauma because a normal radiograph does not exclude an injury and hence a CT is eventually performed if the clinical suspicion of injury is high. Recent studies have shown that MDCT is more effective in identification of thoracolumbar injuries as compared to plain X-ray.[30] The same fact is also supported by the ACR appropriateness criteria as already discussed. However, plain films, is commonly used in the initial evaluation of a patient with spinal trauma. The first and most important radiograph in spinal trauma is the lateral view with cross-table technique.[9,10] This has been reported to be positive in 70–90% of cases. The standard additional views are anteroposterior (AP) open mouth for cervical spine, AP view for thoracic spine and AP and oblique views for lumbosacral spine injury. The most important addition in the routine views of cervical trauma patients has been the cervical trauma oblique view.[11] This is obtained with patient supine and X-ray tube is angled 30–40° from horizontal. This view more often provides a clear visualization of C1 to T1 with an additional 15° cranial tube tilt. A traditional "swimmer's view" is obtained only if "trauma oblique view" is inadequate.[11] The "swimmer's view" usually needs a change in patient's position and is contraindicated in a high suspicion of cervicothoracic injury and is not helpful in obese or muscular patients. The use of flexion-extension radiographs is controversial and can be performed if there is a question of the ligamentous injury. However, they should be performed only in conscious patients who are able to cooperate and only active motion should be applied. Limitations of plain radiography include inability to detect subtle undisplaced fractures, to visualize upper cervical (C1, C2) and cervicothoracic junction and to evaluate nonosseous injuries. At present, CT has replaced plain x-ray as the initial modality for evaluation of spinal trauma at many level 1 trauma centers across the world.[12]

The use of tomography in the evaluation of acute spinal trauma is obsolete with the advent of CT, especially multidetector CT (MDCT). Disadvantages of tomography include need to change position of the patient for lateral tomography and high radiation dose as compared to CT. The role of myelography has significantly reduced since the advent of CT and MRI. It is an invasive procedure and has limited role in present scenario, i.e. patients with contraindication to MRI. There are contrast-related complications and risk of arachnoiditis. Myelography may still be indicated in the evaluation of nerve root avulsions or suspected dural tears.

Computed Tomography

Multidetector CT is the preferred imaging modality for evaluating blunt spinal trauma patients.[13-16] The high quality multiplanar reformations in different planes in MDCT have markedly improved the detection of varied spinal abnormalities like abnormal intervertebral distance, abnormal angulations, subluxations and dislocations which were not well-visualized in axial CT plain radiography or tomography. The advantages of MDCT include larger area coverage, short scanning time, thinner slices and better reconstructions. Thin contiguous axial sections are acquired in helical mode at the site of interest. Other advantages of CT include the ability to assess the spinal canal and impingement by osseous fragments, optimal visualization of vertebral injuries, soft tissue abnormality and associated disk prolapse and imaging without changing patient's position. The disadvantages of CT include incomplete evaluation of horizontal fractures and displacements in the sagittal plane. Multiplanar and three-dimensional (3D) reconstructions help in the evaluation of vertebral alignment and horizontal fractures.[17,18] The spatial information and relationship in complex fractures is better appreciated on 3D images **(Figs. 1A and B)**. Limitations of the CT in spinal trauma include radiation exposure and inability to assess spinal cord injury.

Magnetic Resonance Imaging

The role of MRI in acute spinal trauma is fully established especially in the evaluation of spinal cord, both in correlating the appearances of the spinal cord with the level of neurologic deficit and in identification of parameters predictive of neurologic outcome.[19-22] It is the investigation of choice for assessing injuries to the soft tissue structures including posterior ligamentous complex, spinal cord, intervertebral disks and adjacent muscles. **(Fig. 2)**. Thus, no contraindications assumed, an immediate MR imaging is warranted if CT/neurological symptoms suggest an injury to the neural/ligamentous structures.

According to ACR appropriateness criteria, MRI of spine combined with CT is appropriate in the setting of acute spinal trauma if NEXUS or CCR criteria are met and clinical/imaging (X-ray/CT) findings are suggestive of:

- Myelopathy
- Ligamentous injury
- Mechanically unstable spine

The radiographic or CT findings which suggest ligamentous injury include findings like spondylolisthesis, widening of facet joints/interspinous space or asymmetric disk space widening.

MRI is also used for prognosticating the injury by differentiating the hemorrhagic and non-hemorrhagic cord injury as the former is associated with poorer prognosis.

Both T1- and T2-weighted sequences with a spin echo technique in axial, sagittal and coronal planes are helpful in the assessment of the spinal injury. A spine surface coil

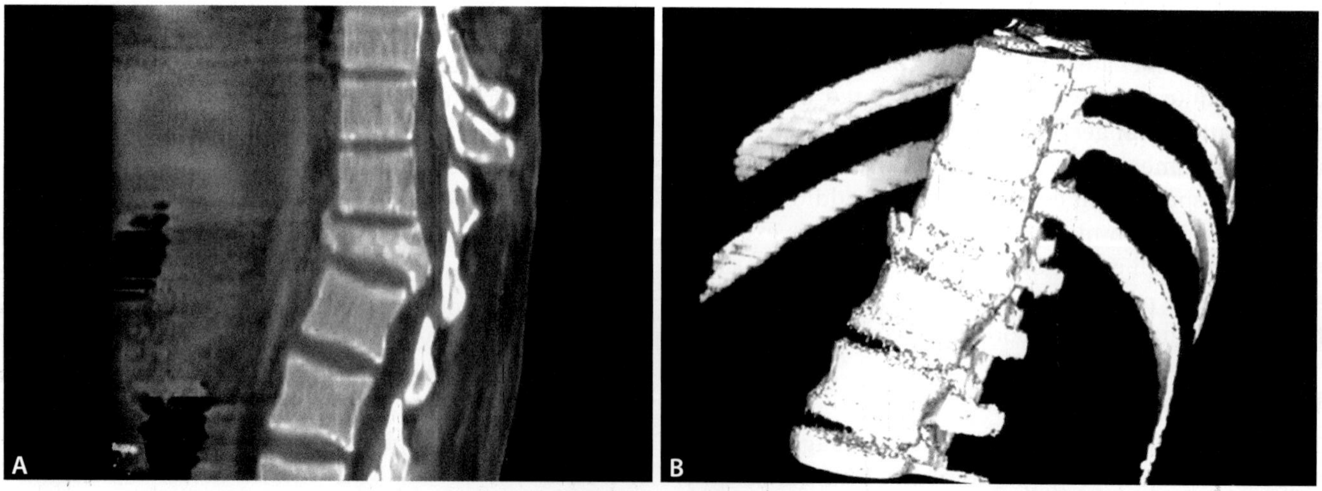

Figs. 1A and B: (A) Sagittal reformation of MDCT showing fracture fragments and posterior displacement; (B) 3D CT demonstrating the fractured vertebra.

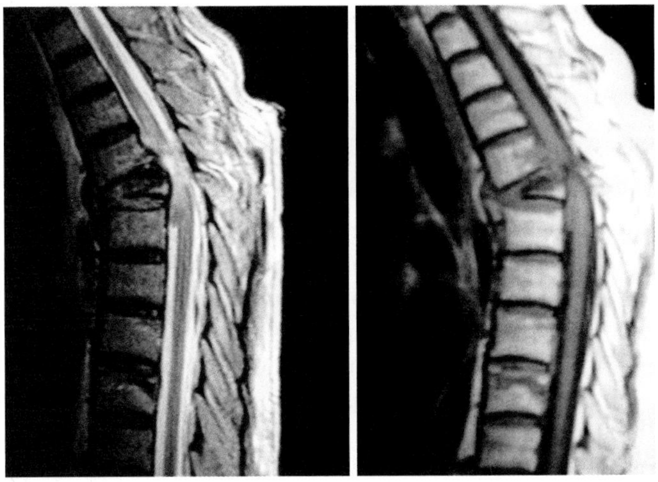

Fig. 2: Sagittal T2- and T1WI MR showing burst fracture of midthoracic vertebra with retropulsed fractured fragment and associated cord changes.

is used to improve resolution. T1-weighted images are helpful in the assessment of bony element abnormality while T2-weighted images are more useful for assessment of spinal cord. Cord contusions manifest as hyperintense foci on T2-weighted images and are iso- to hypointense on T1-weighted images. Gradient echo images help to identify the hemorrhagic cord contusions which have prognostic significance. Short tau inversion recovery (STIR) and T2 fat sat images are sensitive for detection of marrow edema which is seen in acute fractures but not in chronic fractures. Appearance of cord hemorrhage varies with the age of hematoma. Patients with predominant edema or contusions show neurological improvement whereas cord hemorrhage has a poor outcome.

Ideally MRI should be done within 72 hours of injury. It is because during this period edema gives T2 hyperintense signal which in turn increases the conspicuity of the ligaments. Later on as the edema subsides, the sensitivity of MRI for detection of injury also reduces.[23]

In addition, the long-term sequelae of spinal cord trauma such as cord transaction, traumatic syrinx, myelomalacia and meningocele are well-delineated with MRI.

The details of MRI imaging for assessing nonosseous injury will be discussed later in this chapter.

The disadvantages of magnetic resonance as compared to CT include its relative inferiority for demonstration of osseous anatomy and fractures and failure to detect the posterior element fractures. In addition, MRI is expensive, not readily available, and patient support and ventilator system should be magnetic resonance compatible.

Advances in Magnetic Resonance Imaging

Diffusion weighted imaging: Post traumatic spinal canal hematoma, though rare, occurs most commonly in cervical spine due to the injury to the epidural venous plexus. Depending on the age of the hematoma, sometimes it becomes difficult to differentiate it from the epidural fat. Hoch et al. have shown that hematoma has fairly obvious hyperintensity on diffusion trace images due to echo planar imaging (EPI) signal artifact.[24] They also show diffusion restriction due to gelatinous nature of the evolving hematoma. It has also been shown that if the cord shows T2 hyperintensity along with low ADC value in acute epidural hematoma, patient may suffer from irreversible compressive cord damage.[25] Role of DWI has also been studied in patients with SCINA as discussed later. Use of DWI is however limited by distortion of the image due to magnetic field inhomogeneity and susceptibility changes due to bones and ligaments of the spine. In addition there is physiologic motion of the cord secondary to respiratory and cardiac motion which further degrades the quality of image.

Diffusion tensor imaging: Diffusion tensor imaging assesses the integrity of the white matter tracts in the spinal cord and can detect very early changes in spinal cord injury which are not seen on conventional MR images. Shamuganathan et al. revealed that whole cervical spine DTI parameters in patients with cervical cord contusions were significantly lower and the VR was higher as compared to healthy controls.[26] Greater decrease in ADC and RA values was seen at the site of injury. Thus DTI can be used to document the true extent of injury which otherwise appears normal on conventional imaging. They also concluded that change in DTI parameters correlated with the severity of cord injury and can be used for predicting the severity of cord injury and monitoring recovery following treatment.

CLASSIFICATION OF SPINAL TRAUMA

The spinal trauma can be classified according to the level of injury, severity of injury, mechanism of injury and stability versus instability.[7]

Level of Injury

Cervical spine injury is most common (40–60%) due to excessive mobility and lack of supporting structures. Thoracic spine injury is less common (20%) as the stability is provided by thoracic cage whereas lumbar spine injury is seen in about 20–30%. Most of the thoracic and lumbar injuries are seen at thoracolumbar junction (60% between D12 and L2) as there is transition from immobile to mobile segment and orientation of facet joints from coronal to sagittal. Multilevel injury is seen in about 5–20%.

Severity of Injury

Spinal trauma is minor, when associated with no neurological symptoms and the patient is alert and able to cooperate. Trauma is major, when associated with neurological deficits and the patient is unconscious as well as having multisystem trauma.

Mechanism of Injury

Flexion, extension, rotation, compression, distraction or shear forces may produce damage in isolation or in combination. Ligaments are resistant to compression or distraction but are vulnerable to rotation or shear forces. But the osseous end plates fail when pure compressive or tensile forces are applied to the vertebra. Thus, pure compression or distraction produces fracture whereas rotatory or shear forces result in dislocations.

- Flexion injury results in anterior wedging, vertebral body fractures, posterior longitudinal ligament (PLL) interspinous ligament disruption.
- Hyperextension injury causes fractures of posterior element, anterior longitudinal ligament (ALL) rupture and subluxations. It is common in C-spine.
- Vertical compression (axial load) injury causes burst/compression fractures, lateral element fractures. It is seen in diving and jumping injury.
- Rotation-shearing injury results in lateral mass fracture and facet subluxation.

Stable versus Unstable Fracture

Spinal injuries which can withstand stress without progressive deformity and neurological damage are referred as stable injuries as compared to the injuries where spine is not able to maintain integrity and further damage to spinal cord or nerve root cannot be avoided are reefed to as unstable injuries. Dennis et al. introduced the concept of three columns of spine and concluded that instability requires disruption of at least two of these columns.[27] Anterior column is formed by anterior half of vertebral body, anterior longitudinal ligament and anterior annulus. Middle column is formed by posterior half of the body, posterior longitudinal ligament and posterior annulus. Posterior column is formed by posterior bony complex (pedicles, lamina, articular processes and spinous process) and the posterior ligamentous complex (facet joint capsule, ligamentum flavum, interspinous and supraspinous ligaments). Signs of instability on imaging include widened interspinous distance, increased facet joint distance, disk space narrowing, focal angulation of greater than 11°, vertebral body compression of more than 25% and subluxation of greater than 3.5 mm.

RADIOLOGICAL INTERPRETATION OF SPINAL TRAUMA (ABCS)

The radiographic signs of trauma are as follows:

- *A-Alignment:* Disruption of lines, focal kyphoscoliosis, rotation of spinous process, increased interpedicular distance and vertebral listhesis.
- *B-Bone integrity:* Fracture, anterior wedging, cortical buckling, disrupted posterior vertebral line and disrupted C2 ring.
- *C-Cartilage:* Interspinous/facet joint widening, increased/decreased disk spaces and vacuum phenomenon.
- *S-Soft tissue:* Widening of pre-/paravertebral soft tissue.

NEW RADIOLOGICAL CLASSIFICATION SYSTEMS

The newer classification systems like subaxial injury classification (SLICS) and thoracolumbar injury classification and severity score (TLICS) have included neurologic status of the patient and integrity of posterior ligamentous complex for grading the status of the patient **(Table 2)**. It is contrary to the old radiological classification systems which only considered the location and morphology of the fracture. These newer classifications (TLICS and SLICS) are based on a scoring system that also provides a therapeutic recommendation toward surgical or conservative management. In addition MR imaging has found its way into these classification system which includes evaluation of the posterior ligamentous complex.[5]

CERVICAL SPINE INJURY

Cervical spine injuries occur predominantly at two levels. One-third fractures occur at the level of C2, and one half at the level of C6 or C7. The most frequent mechanism of injury is flexion, followed by extension, vertical compression and rotation. Injuries of the cervical spine can be divided into injury of upper (C1-C2) and lower (C3-C7) cervical spine.

Upper Cervical Spine Injuries

The upper cervical spine differs both anatomically and functionally from the remainder of the spine. The primary motion is rotation. The bony ring of C1 lacks a body and spinous process and its articulation with C2 is circular and flat. This unique anatomy results in a set of injuries. Upper

Table 2: Thoracolumbar injury classification and severity score.

Morphology	0 1 2 3 4	No abnormality Compression Burst fracture Rotation/translation Distraction	Radiograph/CT/MRI
Posterior ligamentous complex	0 2 3	Intact Suspected/indeterminate Injured/disrupted	MRI*
Neurologic status	0 2 2 3 3	Intact Root injury Complete cord/conus medullaris injury** Incomplete cord/conus medullaris injury Cauda equina syndrome	Physical examination
Score	<=3 4 >= 5	Nonoperative treatment Consider conservative or surgical therapy Operative treatment	

*The most reliable sign of PLC injury are disruption of the low-signal intensity black stripe on sagittal T1/T2 WI, fluid in the facet capsules or edema in the interspinous regions.
**Contrary to expectation, a higher score (3 points) is allocated to incomplete cord injury and cauda equina syndrome because these patients may experience better outcome from surgical decompression than patients with complete spinal cord injury.

cervical spine injuries can be divided into dislocations of the cervical spine (occipitoatlantoaxial injuries) and fractures of C1 or C2. Occipitoatlantoaxial injuries occur as atlanto-occipital dislocation or atlantoaxial subluxation.

Atlanto-occipital Dislocation

Traumatic atlanto-occipital dislocation is a rare but fatal injury as it is often associated with spinomedullary transection. The mechanism of the injury is hyperextension and distraction. Plain radiography shows retropharyngeal soft tissue swelling, anterior displacement of basion from its normal position superior to odontoid (distance >12.5 mm on lateral film) and malalignment between spinolaminar line of C1 and posterior margin of foramen magnum. CT demonstrates the above findings clearly particularly with the reformatted images. MRI helps to delineate cord transection that is often associated **(Figs. 3A and B)**.

Atlantoaxial Injuries

Post-traumatic atlantoaxial subluxation is a rare injury. Tears of the transverse ligament or avulsion fractures at the site of insertion allow anterior displacement of C1 relative to C2. The normal distance between dens and posterior margin of C1 in adults is less than 3 mm (less than 5 mm in children). It widens abnormally in flexion. Plain films in flexion and extension or conventional tomography is most helpful in detecting subluxation. Rotatory atlantoaxial dislocation (AAD) may occur following minor trauma or it may develop spontaneously following upper respiratory tract infection. The atlas is rotated more than 45° and the facets are often locked.

Anteroposterior open mouth view shows eccentrically placed dens and no movement following cranial rotation. CT in both resting positions and with maximum rotation to contralateral side is the optimal method of evaluation. There is no change in relationship of C1 and C2 with contralateral rotation in rotatory dislocation whereas in normal healthy subjects or patients with torticollis, the deformity is corrected.

Fractures of the Atlas (C1)

A variety of C1 ring fractures have been described but the most common is that involving posterior arch as it is compressed between the occiput and posterior arch of C2 in extension. Gehweiler and colleagues classified it into five types:

1. *Type I*—fracture of the anterior arch
2. *Type II*—fracture of the posterior arch
3. *Type III*—combined fracture of the anterior and posterior arch (Jefferson fracture)
4. *Type IV*—fracture of lateral mass
5. *Type V*—fracture of transverse process

Axial compression of C1 results in Jefferson fracture that consists of ipsilateral disruption of both the anterior and posterior arches and it may be unilateral or bilateral. The patient is neurologically intact unless the transverse ligament is disrupted. Plain film or CT shows soft tissue swelling, anterior/posterior arch fracture and lateral displacement of lateral masses of atlas relative to C2.

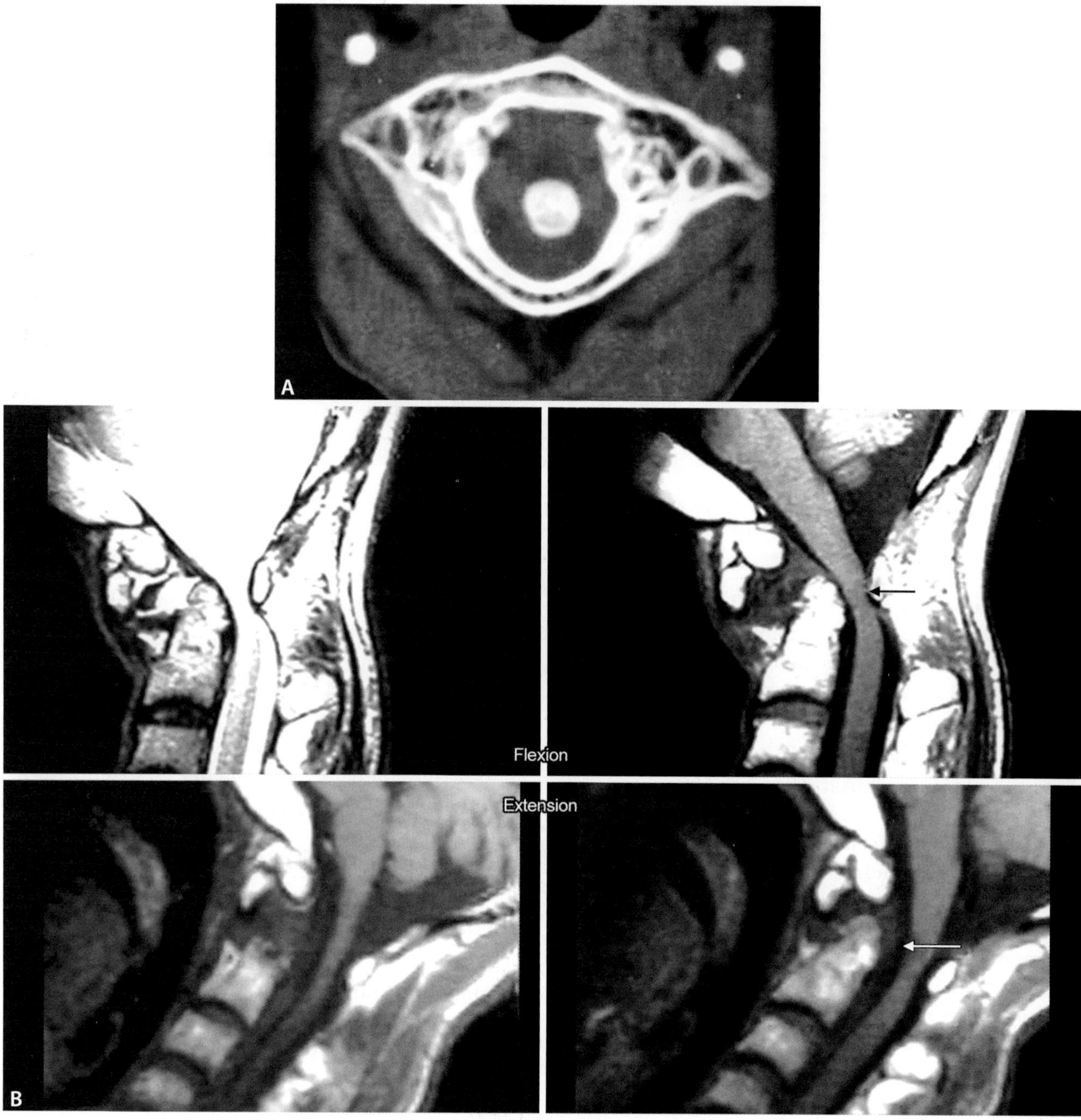

Figs. 3A and B: (A) Axial CT showing posteriorly dislocated odontoid process with anterior compression of cord; (B) Sagittal MRI T1 and T2WI in flexion and extension confirm AAD as well as cord compression (maximum in flexion).

Vertebral artery injury can be associated with atlas fracture (most commonly with Type V fracture).

Fractures of the Axis (C2)

The Anderson and d'Alonzo classification of odontoid fractures is based on fracture location and has both therapeutic and prognostic significance **(Fig. 4)**. Type I fractures are oblique fractures through the tip of the dens secondary to avulsion of alar ligament (stable). Type II fracture occurs at the junction of dens and body of C2 (nonunion is as high as 36%). Type III is horizontal fracture through the C2 vertebral body (frequently displaced).

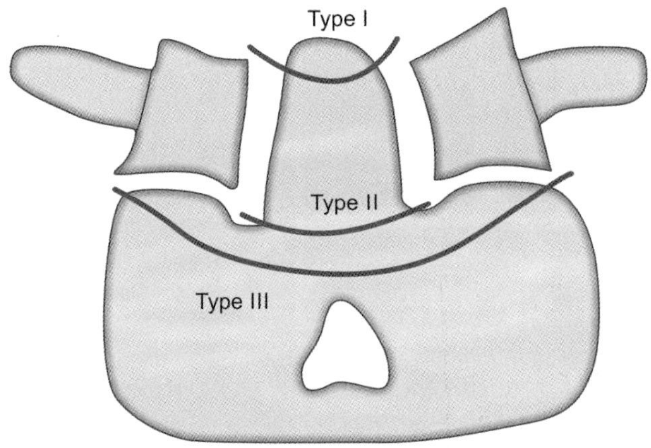

Fig. 4: The Anderson and d'Alonzo classification of odontoid fractures.

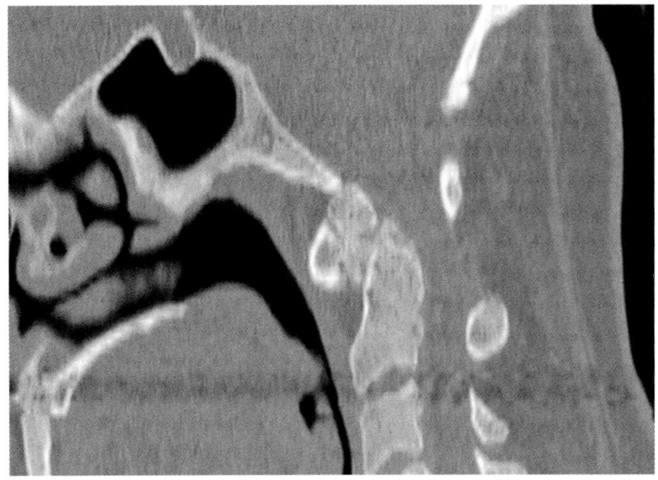

Fig. 5: Sagittal multidetector CT (MDCT) reformation showing fracture of the C2 with anteriorly displaced odontoid.

Odontoid fractures are best evaluated by open mouth AP view. Since these fractures are mostly horizontal, CT with sagittal and coronal reformats is useful for their detection and characterization.

The most characteristic injury of C2 is the Hangman's fracture that includes bilateral avulsion of neural arches from the vertebral body. In reality this fracture usually involves the pars interarticularis and is referred to as traumatic spondylolisthesis and accounts for 4–7% of all cervical spine fractures. It is classified into three subtypes. Type I is a minimally displaced fracture, Type II is associated with more displacement with involvement of adjacent disk, and Type III includes bilateral facet dislocation with anterior displacement and angulations **(Figs. 5 and 6)**. The lateral view of the cervical spine demonstrates the fracture in more than 90% of patients. There is anterior subluxation of C2 vertebral body and retrolisthesis of the posterior elements of C2 relative to C3. CT is necessary to detect Type I fracture as well as vertebral foramen involvement.

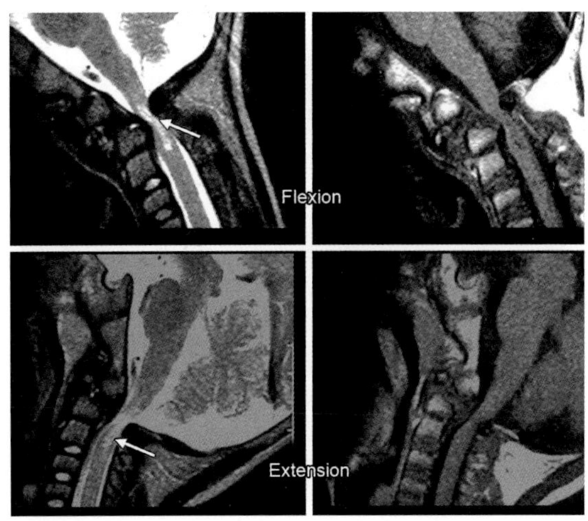

Fig. 6: Sagittal T1- and T2WI in flexion and extension shows Type II odontoid fracture with cord compression and abnormal T2 cord signal (arrows).

Lower Cervical Spine Injury (C3-C7)

The most frequent mechanism of lower cervical spine injury is flexion and hyperextension.

Flexion injuries are the most common accounting for 50–80% of all cervical spine injuries.[28] C4-C7 vertebrae are affected most commonly **(Figs. 7 and 8)**. Simple wedge compression fracture may involve one or more anterior vertebral bodies without concomitant injury to the posterior vertebral body or posterior bony elements. The clay shoveler's fracture is an oblique fracture of the spinous process of C6 or C7 resulting from avulsion by the supraspinous ligament. The unstable flexion injuries include hyperflexion sprain, bilateral articular facet lock and flexion tear drop fracture. The hyperflexion sprain is a ligamentous injury with disruption of posterior ligamentous complex. Radiographic features are focal hyperkyphosis, mild anterior listhesis, widened apophyseal and interspinous space and narrowed anterior disk space. The facet joint may be subluxated. Flexion/extension views as well as delayed images after resolution of muscle spasm are often helpful. Bilateral facet lock is secondary to disruption of posterior and middle columns. This injury is recognized easily on lateral film as anterior subluxation with "bow-tie" sign (oblique position of facet and articular masses). On CT facet dislocation is recognized

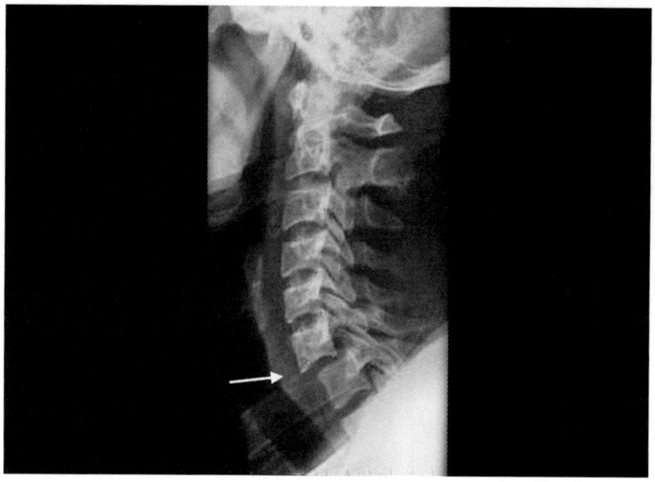

Fig. 7: Lateral view of the C-spine showing anterolisthesis of C6 over C7 with widening of prevertebral space (arrow).

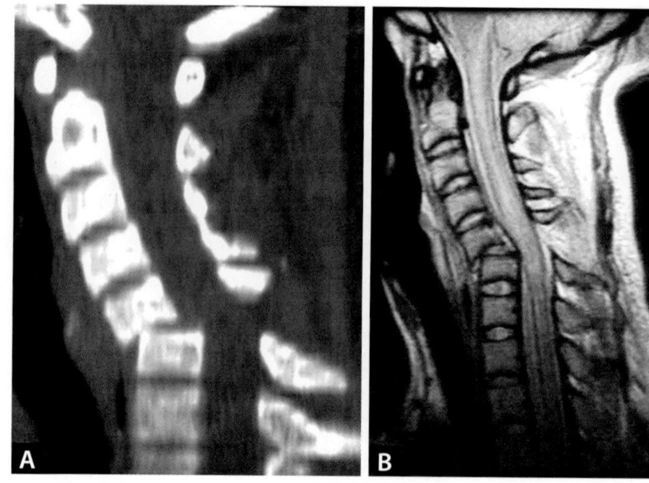

Figs 8A and B: (A) CT sagittal reformation showing fracture dislocation of C5 with anterior displacement; (B) Sagittal T2WI confirms the fracture-dislocation but additionally demonstrates cord injury.

by the "naked" facet sign where articular surfaces of the apophyseal joints are no longer in apposition.

Flexion tear drop fracture results in acute anterior cord syndrome due to disruption of anterior and posterior ligamentous structures as well as intervertebral disk and apophyseal joints. Radiographically, there is a triangular fragment from anteroinferior corner of the vertebral body (the tear drop), widening of interspinous and interfacet spaces, posterior disk space narrowing, fracture of lamina and focal kyphosis.

Hyperextension injuries include wide spectrum of injuries that may be radiologically occult. In patients with neurologic damage and normal radiographs, hyperextension injury should be suspected. The injuries include hyperextension tear drop fracture, spinal cord injuries secondary to impingement and ligamentous sprain. MRI is the optimal method for evaluation of spinal cord impingement in these patients **(Fig. 9)**.

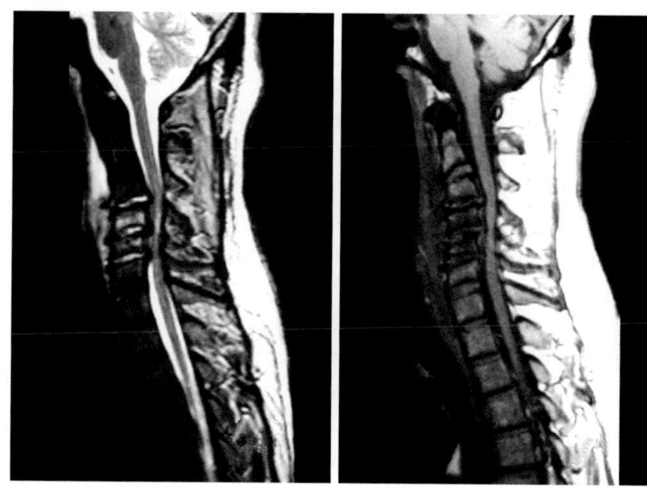

Fig. 9: Sagittal T2- and T1WI in showing altered curvature with marrow signal of the midcervical vertebrae. In addition, cord changes are also seen in the form of abnormal T2 cord signal.

THORACOLUMBAR SPINE INJURY

Most of the fractures in the adult thoracic and lumbar spine occur near the thoracolumbar junction, about 60% are found between T12 and L2 and about 90% are located between T11 and L4. The increased susceptibility to injury at thoracolumbar junction is due to loss of the stabilizing effect of the ribs and thoracic musculature, change of thoracic kyphotic curve to lumbar lordotic curve and change in orientation of the articular facet joints from the thoracic coronal to lumbar sagittal plane. The thoracolumbar injuries have been classified into hyperflexion compression (wedge) fractures, burst fractures, flexion-distraction (chance type fracture or lap seat-belt type) and fracture-dislocation.

Compression or Wedge Fracture

It is the most common type of injury of the thoracolumbar spine comprising approximately 48% of all fractures. The mechanism of injury is hyperflexion of the spine with the axis of rotation located in the center of the intervertebral disk and represents failure of the anterior column. Flexion compression injuries result in anterior wedge fractures **(Figs. 10 and 11)**. Depression of anterior column is usually

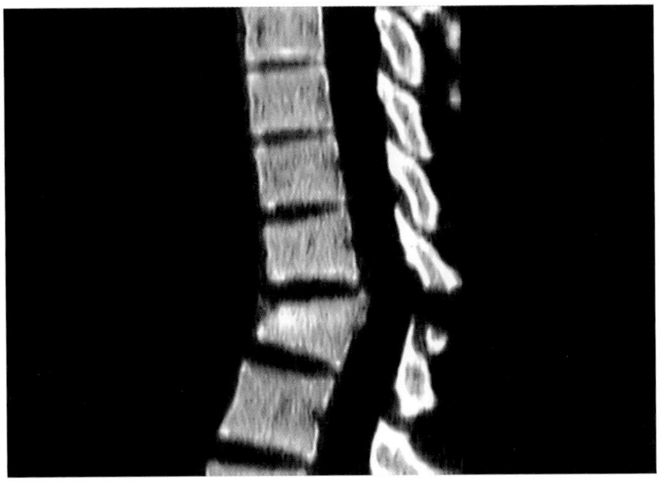

Fig. 10: Sagittal multidetector CT (MDCT) reformat showing wedge fracture of the L1.

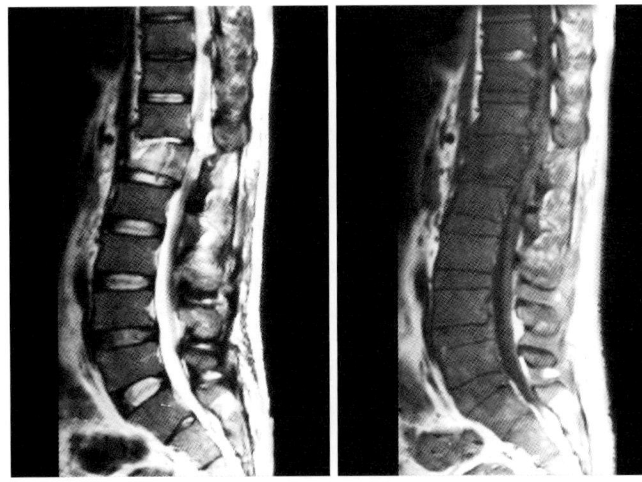

Fig. 11: Sagittal T2- and T1WI showing wedge fracture with altered marrow signal of L1 vertebra.

less than 50% of focal vertebral height and is usually most prominent at superior endplate. A greater than 50% loss of anterior vertebral body height is frequently associated with posterior ligamentous injury and/or subluxation/dislocation of facet joints. Plain radiograph shows anterior wedging of the vertebral body with or without fracture of anterior bony cortex. Height of posterior bony cortex and interpedicular distance is maintained. In general, anterior vertebral height more than 2 mm shorter than posterior vertebral height indicates a fracture.

Burst Fracture

It comprises approximately 14% of all spinal fractures. The mechanism of injury is axial compression of the vertebral body and represents failure of both the anterior and middle columns. The fractures are usually unstable and frequently associated with neurological deficit **(Figs. 12 to 14)**. Plain radiograph shows a decrease in the height of vertebral body (anterior and posterior), displacement of bony fragment in the spinal canal and vertical fractures involving the pedicle/laminae/spines. Two signs namely posterior bow sign and vanishing line sign have been described recently to diagnose burst fractures. Normally, the posterior cortex is seen as thin white line concave posteriorly. Posterior bow sign occurs when the posterior cortex is deformed and becomes convex. This represents the most posterior aspect of retropulsed fragment. Vanishing line sign occurs when the dorsal cortex is displaced so far back that is no longer visible and becomes obscured by the posterior elements.

Computed tomography is clearly the best way to evaluate burst fractures. The findings include comminuted fracture of the vertebral body (greatest near the superior aspect), disruption of posterior vertebral body, fracture fragments in the spinal canal and fractures of posterior elements with or without disruption of apophyseal joint. Sagittal or 3D reconstruction clearly shows the retropulsed fracture fragment and the unstable spine. MRI may show the cord changes like cord contusion/hemorrhage, compression of cord as well as soft tissue hematoma/contusion.

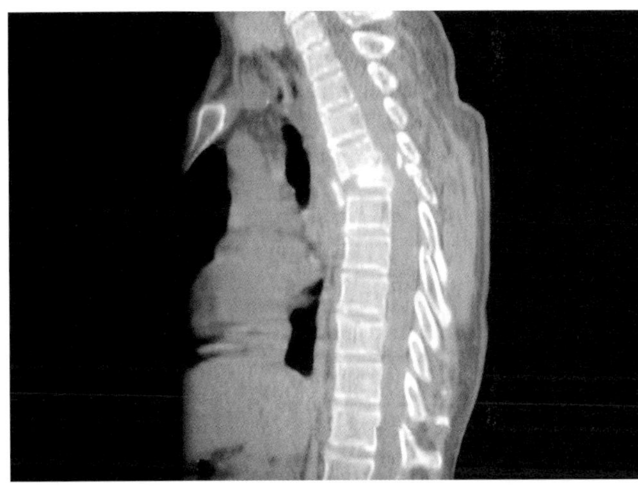

Fig. 12: Sagittal MDCT reformat showing burst fracture of the D5.

Lap Seat-belt Type Fracture or Chance Fracture

The most common variant of flexion-distraction injuries of thoracolumbar spine is the "seat-belt type injury".

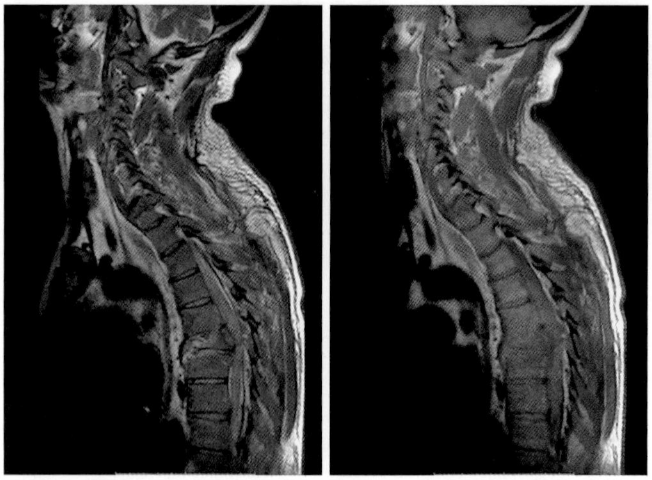

Fig. 13: Sagittal T2- and T1WI showing burst fracture of D6 vertebra with posterior displacement. Note associated ligamentous disruption and cord edema.

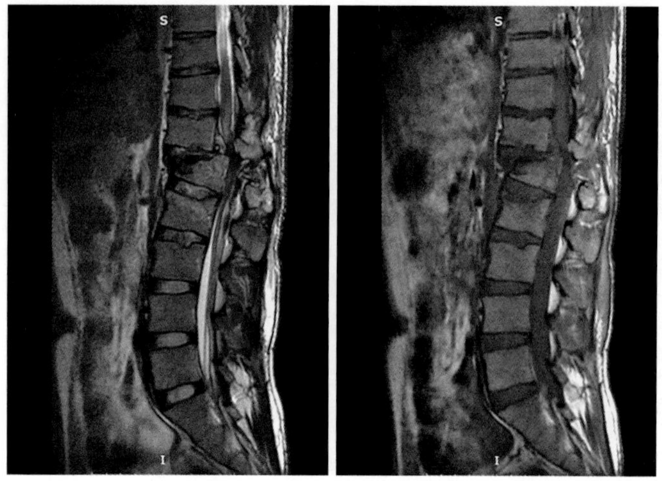

Fig. 15: Sagittal T2WI and T2WI MR images show unstable fracture involving all three columns with associated cord edema.

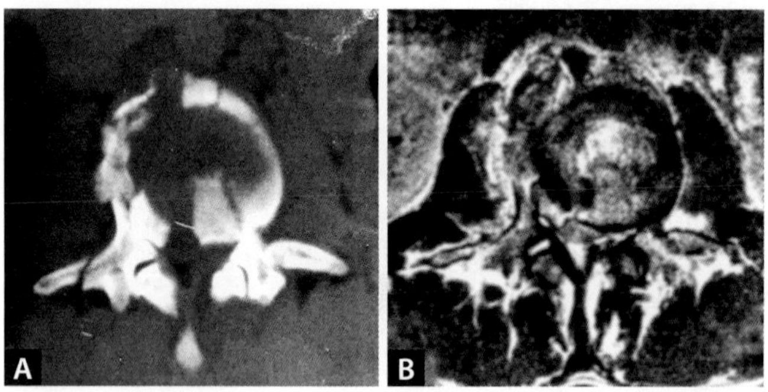

Figs. 14A and B: (A) Axial CT; (B) Axial T2WI magnetic resonance show burst fracture of L1 vertebra with narrowing of canal, cord contusion and prevertebral hematoma.

It represents 10% of all spinal fractures and has a high frequency of neurological deficits. The mechanism of injury is hyperflexion with distraction of the posterior spinal elements and the axis of rotation is located more anteriorly at anterior abdominal wall in contrast to compression or wedge fracture. It is frequently but not always the type of injury associated with the use of lap seat-belt. It represents failure of both posterior and middle columns.

Three subtypes of seat-belt type injury have been described. Horizontal disruption pattern may either involve posterior bony elements (Type I chance fracture) or posterior ligaments (Type II Smith fracture). In the third type, the annulus fibroses is torn allowing for subluxation. Plain radiograph shows increase in the distance between the spinous process and horizontal fractures of lamina, pedicles and posterior aspect of vertebral body. There may be apparent increase in the height of the posterior aspect of body or widening of disk space. MDCT with sagittal reconstruction may demonstrate the nature and extent of the injury.

Fracture Dislocation

It comprises approximately 15% of all spinal injuries. The injuries result from violent complex shearing force and there is disruption of all three spinal columns which causes gross instability. There is anterior dislocation with severe hyperflexion injuries and facet joints may be dislocated with flexion rotation injuries **(Fig. 15)**. Plain radiograph shows displacement of vertebral bodies, multiple fractures, locking of articular processes and compression of vertebrae below. CT demonstrates fracture dislocation very clearly as these are recognized by "double rim" sign and "naked facet" sign. When the inferior facet of superior vertebra and superior facet of inferior vertebra are displayed on different images, the facet joint is said to be disrupted and the sign is called "naked facet sign". Reconstructed images demonstrate the degree of canal compromise.

NONOSSEOUS INJURY

Nonosseous injuries in the spinal trauma include injury to spinal cord, intervertebral disk, ligaments and nerve roots.[30,31] In addition, there is formation of spinal epidural hematoma and tears of dura in major spinal trauma.

Spinal Cord Injuries

Spinal cord injuries (SCI) can result directly from spinal trauma (fracture or dislocations) or indirectly from

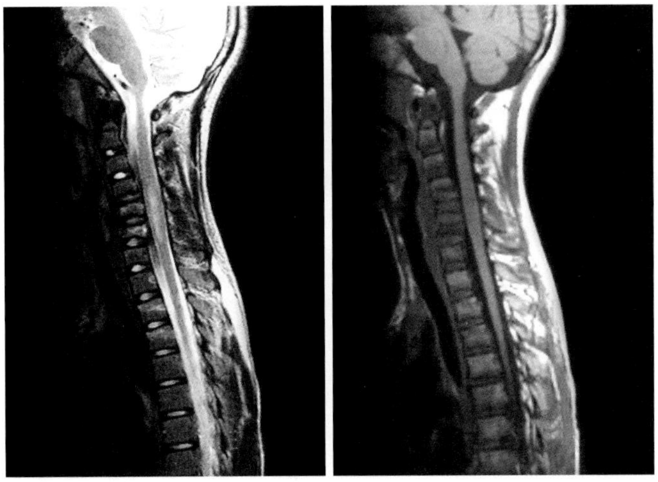

Fig. 16: Sagittal T2 and T1WI showing increased signal intensity within the cervical spinal cord representing intramedullary edema.

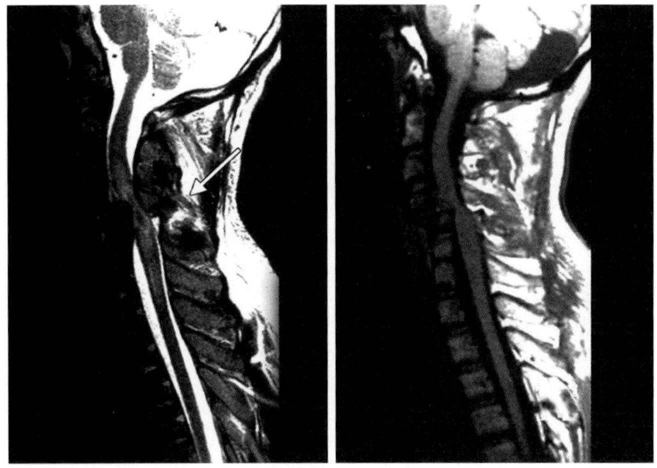

Fig. 17: Sagittal T2- and T1WI demonstrate unstable fracture with fracture-dislocation of C4-C5 vertebrae. Extensive abnormal cord signal on T2 WI are consistent with cord contusion. Note also mode of interspinous ligament injury (arrow).

compression by displaced bony fragment, hematoma or disk material, or ischemia from damage or impingement of the spinal arteries. MRI can depict the exact location, extent and severity of the injury and cord changes (edema or hemorrhage) **(Figs. 16 and 17)**. Patients with minimal cord changes on MRI have the best outcome followed by those with cord edema.[29]

For assessment of SCI, the best MRI sequences are axial and sagittal T2W and T2*GRE images. The most common MRI finding of SCI are hyperintensity on T2WI involving the cord suggestive of edema and hypointensity on T2/GRE indicating hemorrhage. Presence of hemorrhage on MRI is the most important imaging finding associated with poor prognosis, probably explained by the acceleration of the injury cascade due to the presence of iron that potentiates lipid peroxidation. Other findings of prognostic significance are extent of cord hematoma or edema and cord compression by extra-axial hematoma **(Fig. 17)**. In addition, very early detection of spinal cord damage is possible with diffusion-weighted MRI. Resolution of spinal cord edema as demonstrated on follow-up MRI often will correlate with (limited) neurologic improvement. An entity which is more frequently described in elderly patients with hyperextension injury is 'acute traumatic central cord syndrome' in which the patient experiences disproportionately severe upper extremity motor weakness along with bladder dysfunction and sensory loss below the level of injury. This happens due to associated extensive degenerative changes in the elderly patients. The osteophytes or buckled ligamentum flavum along with narrowed spinal canal may result in injury to the central gray matter along with injury to the central portion of the corticospinal tract of the spinal cord.

Intervertebral Disk Injury

It is seen as widening or asymmetric narrowing of disk space, relative hyperintensity of one disk on T2WI, frank protrusion of disk material into the epidural space and dorsal displacement of PLL and epidural venous plexus **(Fig. 18)**.

Disc herniations are commonly seen in association with vertebral fracture dislocation and hyperextension injuries. These are caused due to injury to the annulus fibrosus with resultant herniation of the nucleus pulposus. It is important to identify the disk herniation as undetected herniation can later cause new/worsening cord injury which can result in progressive neurological deficits. Radiologically, however, it is difficult to differentiate a traumatic versus non traumatic disk herniation as appearance is the same. The presence of other post traumatic lesions as the same level can help in differentiating the two entities.

Ligamentous Injury

Spinal ligaments are very essential to maintain the normal vertebral alignment and integrity. Presence of ligamentous injury can convert a stable single column fracture into unstable two column fracture. Recently the TLICS and SLICS classification system have also taken into account the status of the posterior ligamentous complex. Normal ligament of the spine shows low signal intensity in all the sequences. The ligamentous injury can be partial or complete and depends on the mechanism of injury. The partial tear/sprain are the most common variety.

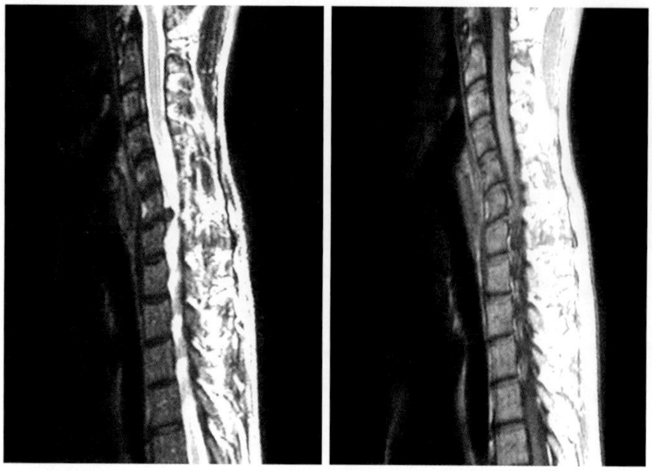

Fig. 18: Sagittal T2- and T1WI showing protrusion of C6-C7 disk into the epidural space with significant neural compromise.

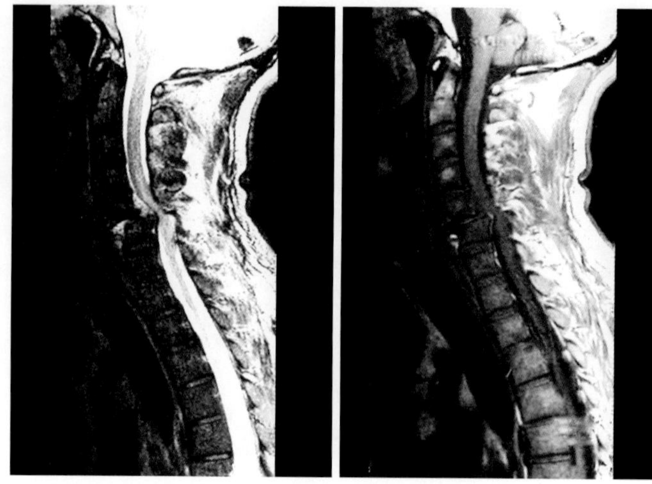

Fig. 19: Sagittal T2- and T1WI showing fracture-dislocation of C5-C6 with discontinuity in the ligaments (ALL and PLL).

Partial tears are visualized as areas of abnormally high signal areas on T2/STIR images which occur due to associated edema/hemorrhage. Complete tears are seen as complete lack of continuity of fibers associated with increased signal on T2/FLAIR. Hyperextension injuries result in damage to the anterior column ligaments with or without involvement of the ligaments of posterior column depending on the severity of the injury. Conversely, injury to the posterior column ligaments occur on hyperflexion injuries.[23]

ALL and PLL injuries are seen as focal disruption of the hypointense signal on all the sequences **(Fig. 19)** with associated soft tissue edema best seen on STIR. Injury to the ligamentum flavum is best seen in parasagittal image and is usually associated with posterior element fractures. Injuries to the supraspinous/interspinous ligaments are seen as increased signal in the interspinous space and tip of the spinous process especially on STIR sequence.

Epidural and Subdural Hemorrhage

It is a common finding in trauma patient and symptoms depend on the location as well as the severity of compression of the spinal cord. Surgical evaluation is necessary for a favorable outcome. In some scenarios; it becomes difficult to exactly localize the compartment of hemorrhage to epidural or subdural space. 'Curtain sign' may help in differentiating the two if the hematoma is localized anteriroly in the spinal cord. Normally the dura is attached to the posterior longitudinal ligament by the Trolard ligament. Thus the epidural hemorrhage may lift the dura except anteriorly in mid line. Accordingly a subdural hemorrhage will show negative curtain sign.[25]

Nerve Root Avulsion

It is usually seen in cervicothoracic location due to greater degree of mobility of the cervical spine. Complete avulsion of the nerve root can result in pseudomeningocele formation which is pathological collection of CSF. These collections are in communication with the physiological CSF space, however are not covered by dura. These injuries can be easily seen on high resolution T2W sequence e.g, CISS (constructive interference in steady state) or FIESTA (fast imaging employing steady-state acquisition).

Vascular Injury

The incidence of the vascular injury in blunt trauma patients is less than 1%.[2] Vascular injuries should be looked for in patients with otherwise unexplained neurologic deficits, and patients with severe blunt trauma to the neck.[2] Vertebral arteries are more commonly involved as compared to carotid arteries in patients with neck trauma. There is risk of cerebral and cerebellar infarctions especially when the injury is bilateral. Following are the risk factors for vascular injury according to the Denver screening criteria in patients with neck injury:

- C1 to C3 fracture
- Fracture extending into foramen transversarium
- Cervical spine subluxation
- Facial fractures Le fort II and III
- Base of the skull fracture involving the carotid canal

- Expanding neck hematoma
- Diffuse axonal injury

DSA is the gold standard investigation but it carries a minor risk of stroke itself (risk of ~0.5%). CT Angiography is a fast, high resolution technique and is a preferred investigation for detecting vascular injury. A recent clinical review revealed sensitivity of CTA in detecting vertebral artery injury (VAI) to be around 99%.[23]

MR Angiography is also proven to be a valid technique for detecting vascular injury. Most of the vascular injury can be seen as loss of flow void on spin echo sequences associated with wall irregularity. In addition intramural hematoma can be seen as T1 hyperintense periarterial rim with flow void in the patent lumen. This T1 hyperintensity is imparted by the T1 shortening effect of methaemoglobin. In equivocal cases further evaluation can be done by CTA/DSA. However in context of polytrauma patients MRA can be unsuitable due to long scan time as well as safety challenges within the scanning environment.

SUBACUTE AND CHRONIC INJURIES

In the subacute phase following spinal cord injury, MRI often reveals hyperintense signal on T2WI in the white matter tracts above (dorsal columns) and below (lateral columns) the injury level. This Wallerian degeneration is first noticeable on MRI approximately 1 month after trauma. Approximately 1–3 weeks following cord injury, a subacute progressive ascending myelopathy occasionally can be seen, presenting as an enlarged cord with high signal on T2WI several segments superior to the original injury site.

Late sequelae of spinal cord injury include progressive enlargement of an intramedullary or extramedullary cyst, progressive myelomalacia, tethering and adhesions and/or cord atrophy.

Post-traumatic syringomyelia: It develops after severe spinal cord injury and is fusiform intramedullary cystic cavitation with an incidence of 3.5–4.3%. Contrary to hydromyelia which is pathologic dilatation of the central canal, it is not lined by ependyma. The pathogenesis of post traumatic syringomyelia is multifactorial and symptoms depend on the location and extent. Arachnopathic scarring plays an important role in its development. Due to altered CSF flow, the lesion may ascend up later, even years after initial insult and can lead to worsening of the neurological status. High resolution T2-weighted images (like CISS) have a role to assess the arachnoid adhesions which facilitate in planning surgical procedures. The disturbance of CSF circulation can also be detected using modern sequences like ECG gated phase contrast imaging which can detect and quantify the altered dynamics of CSF flow.[30]

SPINAL CORD INJURY WITHOUT RADIOGRAPHIC ABNORMALITY

Spinal cord injury without radiographic abnormality (SCIWORA) is defined as "clinical symptoms of traumatic myelopathy with no radiographic or CT features of spinal fracture or instability.[32] Almost 6–19% of spinal injury in children comprises of SCIWORA compared to 9-14% in adults. [32] SCIWORA is most common in children less than 8 years of age probably due to greater head size, weaker neck muscles and higher elasticity of vertebral ligaments. In addition the facet joints are more horizontally oriented which in turn increase the susceptibility to injury. The specific biomechanics of the vertebral column allows for a greater physiological range of motion of the spine without association with fracture. During the excessive motion of the spine, there is temporary occusion of the vertebral artery which leads to ischemic injury to the cord.

In adults SCIWORA mostly occurs as a result of hyperextension forces (e.g. rear end car accident). It is commonly associated with underlying degenerative changes and the level of injury to the cord corresponds to the location of these degenerative changes. Venous congestion in the compressed cord is also believed to be an additional factor.

The most typical presentation of SCIWORA is upper extremity weakness more severe than the lower extremity weakness. MRI is the investigation of choice of spinal cord. Edema **(Fig. 20)** and hemorrhages can be seen using T2 and GRE sequences. The appearance of the hemorrhage on MR will depend on the age of bleed. Bone marrow edema can also be assessed on STIR sequence that cannot be seen on CT. A number of patients however have normal MRI of the spinal cord but have neurological symptoms. Such patients should be classified as SCIWNA (spinal cord injury without neuroimaging abnormality).[32] In this subset of patients advanced imaging like DWI, DTI can provide vital information. Szwedowski et al have shown that patients with SCIWNA revealed hyperintense signal on DWI in the areas corresponding to cord injury. In addition DTI can assess the white matter integrity in spinal cord. However the quality of images may be degraded by artifacts due to breathing or pulsatile motion of CSF. In a study conducted in the institute comprising forty patients, SCIWORA contributed to 12% of cases of spinal cord injury.

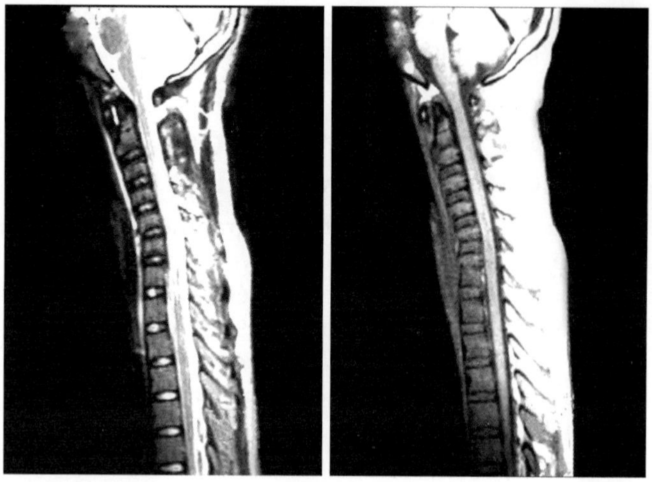

Fig. 20: Sagittal T2- and T1WI demonstrate abnormal cord signal on T2WI suggest cord edema, however, there is no evidence of bony injury.

Whiplash Injury

The term "whiplash" refers to a wide variety of soft tissue neck injuries resulting from multiple causes.[2] Commonly the injury follows a forced hyperextension-hyperflexion of the spine. It can result from rear-end vehicle collision and side- or front-impact collisions. The injury has a wide variety of nonspecific clinical presentations. Common symptoms include neck pain or stiffness, paresthesia, upper extremity pain, jaw pain, and headache. Plausible causes are muscle tears, ligamentous injuries, perineural scarring, discogenic and joint disease, and fractures. Plain radiograph may show abnormal soft tissue or vertebral alignment. CT helps to exclude the presence of fractures or dislocations. MRI is helpful in demonstrating lesion of the ligaments, disks, spinal cord, prevertebral soft tissue and muscles.

OSSEOUS VARIANTS THAT MAY SIMULATE INJURY[33]

Variants of the Atlas (C1)

- *Atlantal clefts:* Most commonly occurs at posterior synchondrosis, however can be seen anywhere within the C1 ring. They occur due to non fusion of ossification center. These clefts show smooth corticated margin differentiating it from fracture. An anterior midline cleft can be formed due to failure of anterior ossification center to form or a bipartite anterior ossification center.
- A normal *groove* is seen along the posterolateral aspect of atlas on both the sides which transmits the vertebral artery and suboccipital nerve (C1). These structures are normally covered by posterior atlantooccipital membrane. Occasionally this membrane can become partially calcified and give an appearance of an apparent bony fragment. On complete ossification, an osseous ring is formed which is known as arcuate foramen.

Variants of the Axis (C2)

Ossific densities cranial to odontoid process: Persistent os terminale, Os odontoideum.

- *Persistent os terminale:* it is a normal secondary ossification center that fuses to the odontoid process by 12 years of age. However, there can be non fusion and is seen as a well corticated ossicle abutting the odontoid tip.
- *Os odontoideum:* It can be mistaken for dens fracture. It has a sclerotic and well corticated margin. It is also associated with hypertrophy of anterior arch of C1. An os odontoideum also has a larger gap between the os and the odontoid process. It usually does not exhibit the expected contour of the upper odontoid process.

Anterior Subluxation of C2 on C3

It is usually seen in children less than 8 years of age. It is caused due to ligamentous laxity and a horizontal orientation of the facet joint.

Variants of C3 through L5 Verterba

- *Anterior wedging of cervical vertbera:* It is a normal finding in young population and is most prominent at C3 level. A difference in height of up to 3 mm between anterior and middle aspects of the vertebral body is considered normal. It should not be confused with compressed fracture.
- *Single linear osseous defect through foramen transversarium:* It likely represents a developmental cleft. A fracture involving the transverse foramen or any ring like structure will likely involve 2 or more locations and are usually displaced fractures. An isolated defect of the transverse foramen is unlikely to be a fracture.
- *Limbus vertebra:* It is due to herniation of disk material between the ring apophysis and the vertebral body. It most commonly occurs in lumbar spine in anterosuperior aspect and is seen as a small triangular bony fragment with smooth corticated margin.
- *Clefts* may occur at several locations due to non fusion of synchondrosis. It may involve pars interarticularis, pedicle, lamina etc.

SUMMARY

There is significant change in imaging spinal trauma over the recent years with advancement in CT (multidetector CT) and MRI technology. When the clinical suspicion of spinal injury is high, MDCT is performed, as it is faster, more accurate and needs less patient mobilization than radiography. MDCT is an excellent modality in detecting the osseous abnormalities (especially posterior element fractures), spinal alignment and assessment of stability. Early and accurate diagnosis of spinal injury is crucial in better patient management and prevention of neurological deterioration. However, plain radiography remains usually the initial screening modality as it is readily available, portable and inexpensive. MRI is best imaging modality for detection of spinal cord changes (edema and hemorrhage), extradural lesions (disk herniation and epidural hematoma), ligamentous injury and characterizing spinal fractures.

ACKNOWLEDGMENT

The authors acknowledge Dr Shashank Raj, DM resident in the Neuroradiology Division of Department of Radiodiagnosis, PGIMER, Chandigarh for his support in editing of chapter.

REFERENCES

1. Kaji A, Hockberger R. Imaging of spinal cord injuries. Emerg Med Clin North Am. 2007;25:735-50,ix.
2. Bagley LJ. Imaging of spinal trauma. Radiol Clin North Am. 2006;44:1-12.
3. Lali HS, Fehlings MG. Epidemiology, demographics and pathophysiology of acute spinal cord injury. Spine. 2001;26:2-12.
4. Tins B, Cassar-Pullicino V. Controversies in "clearing" trauma to the cervical spine. Semin Ultrasound CT MR. 2007;28:94-100.
5. Wolf M, Weber MA. Neuroimaging of the Traumatic Spine. Magn Reson Imaging Clin N Am. 2016;24(3):541-61.
6. Shah LM, Ross JS. Imaging of spine trauma. Neurosurgery. 2016;79(5):626-42.
7. Pathria MN, Petersirge CA. Spinal trauma. Radiol Clin North Am. 1991;29:847-65.
8. Heinemann U, Freund M. Diagnostic strategies in spinal trauma. Eur J Radiol. 2006;58:76-88.
9. Dalinka MK, Boorstein JM, Zlatkin MB. Computed tomography of musculoskeletal trauma. Radiol Clin North Am. 1989;27:933-43.
10. Kaye JJ, Nance EP. Thoracic and lumbar spine trauma. Radiol Clin North Am. 1990;28:361-77.
11. Abel MS. The exaggerated supine oblique view of the cervical spine. Skeletal Radiol. 1982;8:213-9.
12. Gamanagatti S, Rathinam D, Rangarajan K, et al. Imaging evaluation of traumatic thoracolumbar spine injuries: radiological review. World J Radiol. 2015; 7(9):253-65.
13. Murphey MD, Batnitzky S, Bramble JM. Diagnostic imaging of spinal trauma. Radiol Clin North Am. 1989;27: 855-72.
14. Rabassa AE, Guinto FC, Crow WN, et al. CT of the spine: value of reformatted images. Am J Roentgenol. 1993;161:1223-7.
15. Gonzalez-Beicos A, Nunez DB. Role of multidetector computed tomography in the assessment of cervical spine trauma. Semin Ultrasound CT MR. 2009;30:159-67.
16. Bensch FV, Koivikko MP, Kiuru MJ, et al. Measurement of spinal canal narrowing, interpedicular widening, and vertebral compression in spinal burst fractures: plain radiographs versus multidetector computed tomography. Skeletal Radiol. 2009;38:887-93.
17. Blackmore CC, Mann FA, Wilson AJ. Helical CT in primary trauma evaluation of the cervical spine: an evidence-based approach. Skeletal Radiol. 2000;29:632-9.
18. Siberstein M, Tress BM, Hennessy O. A comparison between MRI and CT in acute spinal trauma. Australas Radiol. 1992;36:192-7.
19. Provenzale J. MR imaging of spinal trauma. Emerg Radiol. 2007;13:289-97.
20. Demaerel P. Magnetic resonance imaging of spinal cord trauma: A pictorial essay. Neuroradiology. 2006;48: 223-32.
21. Mhuircheartaigh NN, Kerr JM, Murray JG. MR imaging of traumatic spinal injuries. Semin Musculoskelet Radiol. 2006;10:293-307.
22. Geck MJ, Yoo S, Wang JC. Assessment of cervical ligamentous injury in trauma patients using MRI. J Spinal Disord. 2001;14:371-7.
23. Kumar Y, Hayashi D. Role of magnetic resonance imaging in acute spinal trauma: a pictorial review. BMC Musculoskelet Disord. 2016;17:310.
24. Hoch MJ, Rispoli J, Bruno M, et al. Clinical utility for diffusion MRI sequence in emergency and inpatient spine protocols. Clin Imaging. 2017;45:37-50.
25. Endo T, Suzuki S, Inoue T, et al. Prediction of neurological recovery in spontaneous spinal epidural hematoma using apparent diffusion coefficient values. Spinal Cord. 2014; 52(10):729-33.
26. Shanmuganathan K, Gullapalli RP, Zhuo J, et al. Diffusion tensor MR imaging in cervical spine trauma. Am J Neuroradiol. 2008; 29(4):655-9.
27. Dennis F. The three column spine and its significance in the classification of acute thoracolumbar spinal injuries. Spine. 1983;8:817-31.
28. Jelly LM, Evans DR, Easty MJ, et al. Radiography vs spinal CT in the evaluation of cervicothoracic junction injuries in polytrauma patients who have undergone intubations. Radiographics. 2000;20:251-9.
29. Tewari MK, Gifti DS, Singh P, et al. Diagnosis and prognostication of adult spinal cord injury without

radiographic abnormality using magnetic resonance imaging: Analysis of 40 patients. Surg Neurol. 2005;63: 204-9.
30. Van Goethem JW, Maes M, Ozsarlak O, et al. Imaging spinal trauma. Eur Radiol. 2005;15:582-90.
31. Sundgren PC, Philipp M, Maly PV. Spinal trauma. Neuroimaging Clin N Am. 2007;17:73-85.
32. Szwedowski D, Walecki J. Spinal Cord Injury without Radiographic Abnormality (SCIWORA)—Clinical and Radiological Aspects. Pol J Radiol. 2014;79:461-4.
33. Carr RB, Fink KR, Gross JA. Imaging of trauma: Part 1, Pseudotrauma of the spine—osseous variants that may simulate injury. Am J Roentgenol. 2012;199(6): 1200-6.

CHAPTER 33

Spinal Neoplasm

Ajay Garg

INTRODUCTION

Spinal neoplasms include a wide range of lesions in the spinal cord, the surrounding dural spaces and the spine. Location of the tumor is the most important feature in establishing the differential diagnosis for a spinal lesion, followed by patient's age and gender. Due to the insidious onset of frequently vague symptoms in most spinal neoplasms, clinical presentation is not of much help.

MRI is the imaging modality of choice for evaluation of spinal tumors; helps to classify tumors as intramedullary, intradural-extramedullary or extradural, which is the first step in tumor characterization. Apart from localization, additional imaging features like presence of hemorrhage, degree of edema, extent of the lesion, diffusion characteristics and the enhancement pattern help to narrow down differential diagnosis. This chapter will address the clinical, pathological and imaging characteristics of various spinal tumors to help the reader make a reasonable differential diagnosis.

CLASSIFICATION OF LESIONS

Spinal tumors are classified according to their site of origin into intramedullary, intradural-extramedullary (IDEM) and extradural tumors. This classification provides a convenient and meaningful framework to approach the majority of spinal tumors. Some spinal tumors such as lymphoma have the tendency to traverse these compartments and may not follow this classification.

Intramedullary Tumors

Single: Ependymoma, myxopapillary ependymoma, astrocytoma, ganglioglioma, hemangioblastoma, subependymoma, paraganglioma
Multiple: Hemangioblastomas, metastases, lymphoma

Intradural-extramedullary Tumors

Single: Meningiomas, nerve sheath tumors, intradural metastases, lymphoma/leukemia, paraganglioma

Multiple: Any of the preceding except paraganglioma

Extradural Tumors

Single: Aneurysmal bone cyst, giant cell tumor, osteoblastoma, osteochondroma, chordoma, chondrosarcoma, chondroblastoma, metastasis, hemangioma, solitary plasmacytoma, lymphoma Multiple: Metastatic disease, hemangiomas, multiple myeloma, lymphoma

Epidural lesions: Angiolipoma and angiomyolipoma, epidural lipomatosis, lymphoma.

INTRAMEDULLARY TUMORS

Intramedullary spinal cord tumors account for about 4–10% of all CNS tumors and are rare. These tumors include both glial tumors (ependymoma, astrocytoma and ganglioglioma) and nonglial tumors (such as hemangioblastoma, paraganglioma, lymphoma and metastases).

Intramedullary neoplasms are most often slow-growing masses with vague, nonspecific symptoms. The most frequent presenting symptoms of intramedullary cord tumors are dull, aching back pain and weakness.[1] The pain usually localizes to the involved spinal levels and often worsens at night when lying down.[2] Upper extremity weakness with arm and neck pain is seen with cervical lesions. Sensory levels, spasticity, and gait disturbances predominate with thoracic lesions. Tumors of the lumbar region and conus medullaris present with back pain, radicular symptoms, and bowel and bladder dysfunction. Symptoms tend not to be relieved with rest. Valsalva maneuver frequently amplifies the symptoms.[1] Because of the non-specific nature of symptoms, the clinical diagnosis of intramedullary neoplasms is often delayed.

Ependymomas

Ependymomas are the most common intramedullary neoplasms in adults and generally occur in the cervical region.[3] These are slightly more common in women of 40–50 years of age. Patients with NF2 have increased incidence of these tumors. Most cord ependymomas are of low grade, classified as either WHO grade I or grade II; malignant cord ependymomas are quite rare.[4]

The symptoms are chronic and consist mainly of pain, myelopathy and radiculopathies. Occasionally, these ependymomas may bleed and produce subarachnoid hemorrhage or hematomyelia, thus producing acute symptoms.

Characteristically, ependymomas have slow growth. So, they compress rather than infiltrate the adjacent spinal cord tissue. Thereby, they have a good cleavage plane that helps in surgical resection.[4] Since these lesions arise from the ependymal cell lining of the central canal, they tend to be central in location.

On MRI, ependymomas are typically central well-circumscribed lesions and tend to produce symmetric spinal cord expansion. Ependymomas typically have both solid and cystic components. The solid component is iso- to hypointense on T1WI and hyperintense on T2WI **(Figs. 1A to C)**. Cysts can be intratumoral or peritumoral (polar). Intratumoral cysts are located within the solid tumor and should be resected along with the tumor as they may contain neoplastic cells.[5] Peritumoral (polar) cysts on the other hand, occur at the superior or the inferior aspects of the tumor and do not need resection as they do not contain neoplastic cells.[4] Similar cysts are also seen with astrocytomas, hemangioblastomas and gangliogliomas and are not specific for ependymomas. Ependymomas

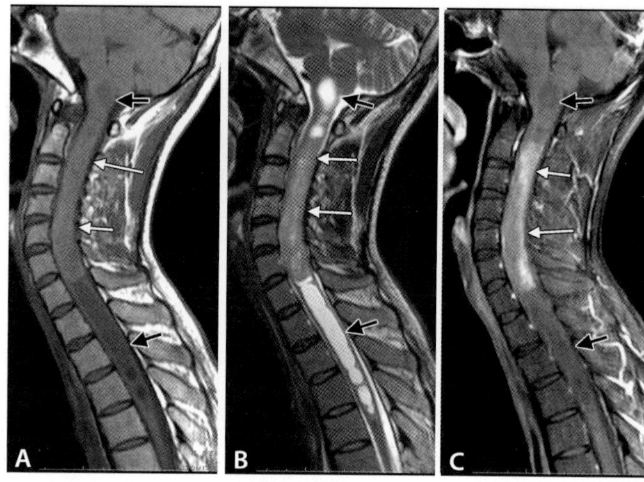

Figs. 1A to C: Cervical intramedullary ependymoma. Sagittal T1WI (A) and T2WI (B) show extensive cord enlargement from medulla to D4 level. Except for a cranial and caudal cyst-like area (black arrows in A and B), the mass (white arrows) is nearly isointense relative to the normal spinal cord. Contrast-enhanced sagittal T1WI (C) shows homogeneous enhancement of the oval mass (white arrows, C) extending from C2 to C6. The cranial and caudal cysts (black arrows) show no enhancement of cyst wall suggesting benign cysts.

show variable contrast enhancement (homogeneous or heterogeneous), but some degree of enhancement is usually seen.[4] In addition, 20% of spinal ependymomas may show a hypointense rim at the periphery of the tumor on T2-WI known as "cap sign", which is related to hemosiderin deposition from intratumoral hemorrhage **(Figs. 2A to C)**.[6] When present, this sign is highly suggestive of an ependymoma.

DTI and DT-FT may show displacement rather than interruption of fiber tracts which confirms the noninfiltrative growth pattern of spinal ependymomas. Unlike in adults, differentiating ependymomas from pilocytic astrocytomas in children by using DTI and DT-FT is difficult.[7]

Clear tumor margins, more uniform enhancement and central location are differentiating features of ependymomas from other intramedullary spinal cord tumors.[3]

Leptomeningeal CSF spread is rarely seen in spinal ependymomas, but when present, it is more commonly associated with higher-grade tumors.

The prognosis in spinal ependymoma depends on the grade of the tumor, degree of surgical resection, and presence or absence of leptomeningeal spread. The 5-year survival rate is approximately 85% when gross total resection is done and approximately 57% with less than suboptimal resection.[8]

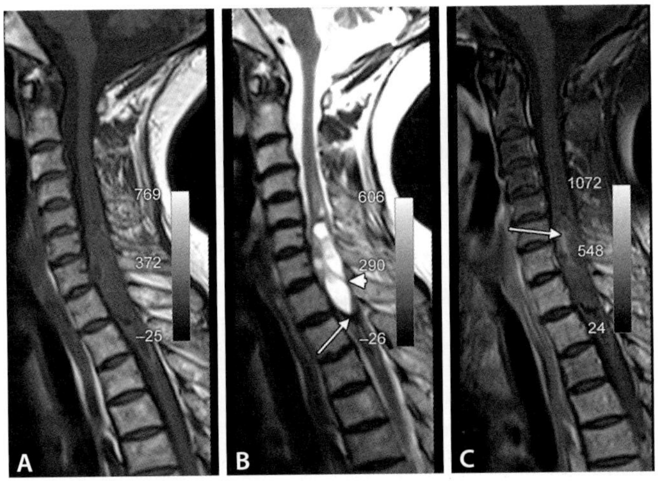

Figs. 2A to C: Cervical intramedullary ependymoma. MR imaging reveals a well-defined intramedullary mass extending from C6-D2 with mild cord expansion. The mass is iso-hypointense on T1WI (A) and has mixed intensity on T2WI (B). Note fluid-fluid level within the lesion (arrowhead in B) and hypointense hemosiderin cap at the distal extent of the lesion (arrow in B). Sagittal T1WI (C) shows faint heterogeneous enhancement (arrow).

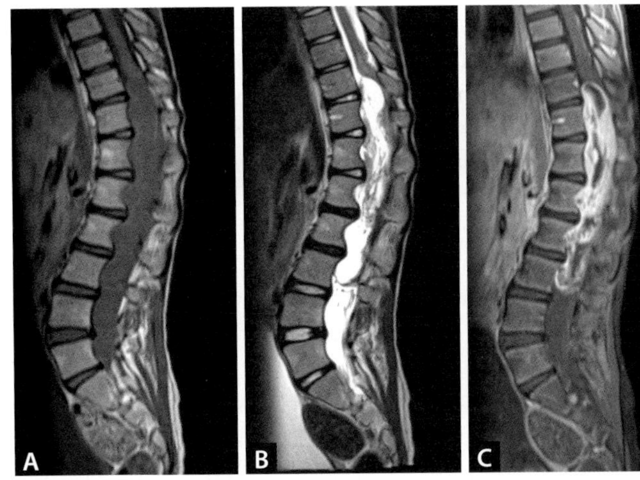

Figs. 3A to C: Myxopapillary ependymoma: Sagittal T1WI (A) shows an intradural lesion extending from D10-L3 spinal canal, causing canal expansion with scalloping of posterior margins of vertebral bodies. The mass is of mixed intensity on T2WI (B) and shows intense heterogeneous enhancement (C).

Myxopapillary Ependymoma

Myxopapillary ependymomas typically occur at the conus medullaris, cauda equina or the terminal filum level and are the most frequent type of ependymomas in these locations.[9] They tend to occur in the fourth decade of life in adults and rarely between 10 and 13 years of age in the pediatric population. They typically manifest with lower back ache, leg pain, sacral pain, weakness or sphincter dysfunction.

These are believed to arise from the ependymal glia of the filum terminale. Rarely, they are extradural in location, presumably arising from the coccygeal medullary vestige at the distal portion of the neural tube.[10] Multiple lesions may be present in about 14–43% of cases.[9,10] Despite being WHO grade I lesions, CSF dissemination occurs occasionally.

Myxopapillary ependymomas are characteristically lobulated, soft, sausage-shaped masses that are often encapsulated. These are typically T1 isointense and T2 hyperintense relative to the spinal cord **(Figs. 3A to C)**. Occasionally, they are T1 and T2 hyperintense presumably secondary to mucin content or hemorrhage. These tumors may show superficial siderosis which is not specific, as it has been reported with other highly vascular spinal tumors. Typically, these show homogeneous enhancement, however may enhance heterogeneously depending the amount of intratumoral hemorrhage. Larger lesions tend to expand the spinal canal (resulting in posterior scalloping of the vertebral bodies) and may extend out of the neuroforamina.

The differential diagnoses of a mass arising in the filum terminale are ependymoma, astrocytoma, nerve sheath tumor, metastases, paraganglioma and hemangioblastoma.

Subependymoma

Subependymoma is a WHO grade I glioma which is a variant of CNS ependymomas.[11,12] It is believed to arise from tanycytes (from the Greek word tanyos—to stretch), cells that bridge the pial and ependymal layers.[11] These tumors present with a slowly progressive clinical course. Pain is the most common symptom, while sensory and motor dysfunctions are less common.

At MR imaging, they appear as well-defined tumors causing fusiform dilatation of the spinal cord. They are located eccentrically within the cord[11] unlike central location of other ependymomas. Enhancement is seen in approximately 50% of cases and non-enhancing tumors present as diffuse symmetric spinal cord enlargement.[11] Edema may or may not be present around the tumor. It may be possible to differentiate ependymomas from subependymomas solely on the basis of MRI findings alone.[11] Rarely, a spinal subependymoma may present as an intradural extramedullary mass lesion, probably arising from leptomeningeal heterotopic glial cells.[13]

Astrocytomas

Astrocytomas arise from the astrocytic glial cells of the spinal cord and represent approximately 30% of spinal cord tumors. They are the most common intramedullary tumors in children and are second only to ependymomas in adults. The cervicomedullary junction and the cervicothoracic cord are the most common locations, although rarely holocord presentation may occur. Most of the spinal cord astrocytomas arise sporadically, although there is an association with NF 1, particularly for WHO grade 1 pilocytic astrocytomas.

A total of 80%–90% of all spinal cord astrocytomas are low grade and include both fibrillary astrocytomas (WHO grade 2) and pilocytic astrocytomas (WHO grade 1). Most of higher grade tumors consist of anaplastic astrocytomas (WHO grade III), whereas glioblastomas (WHO grade IV) of the cord are uncommon.[4] Spinal cord astrocytomas tend to infiltrate the cord and are, therefore, difficult to resect completely. Hence they have a poor prognosis.[4]

On MR imaging, astrocytomas are classically eccentric within the cord, which demonstrates asymmetric cord expansion. Lesions are usually multisegmental and span fewer than 4 vertebral levels.[2] Pilocytic astrocytomas tend to demonstrate discrete margins, whereas high-grade astrocytomas usually have poorly defined tumor margins due to their infiltrative nature. Tumors can show areas of necrotic-cystic degeneration (60% of cases), can have a "cyst with mural nodule" appearance, or can be structurally solid (about 40% of cases). The solid components are iso- to hypointense on T1WIs and hyperintense on T2WIs **(Figs. 4A to E)**, whereas necrotic-cystic components display higher relaxation times on T1 and T2WIs. The pattern of enhancement can be focal nodular, patchy or diffuse inhomogeneous. The enhancing portions of the tumor do not necessarily define its margins. Up to 30% of intramedullary astrocytomas do not show enhancement.[14] Like ependymomas, they can have intratumoral or polar cysts but hemorrhage is uncommon and, therefore, a "cap sign" is usually absent.[4]

An acute cord lesion in patients with multiple sclerosis (MS) may be virtually indistinguishable from an astrocytoma. MS lesions, however, generally appear more homogeneous than astrocytomas and typically demonstrate a surrounding rim of normal cord intensity, which is less common in astrocytomas.

In adults, DTI and DT-FT often assist in differentiating ependymomas, which displace white matter tracts, versus astrocytomas, which tend to disrupt white matters tracts

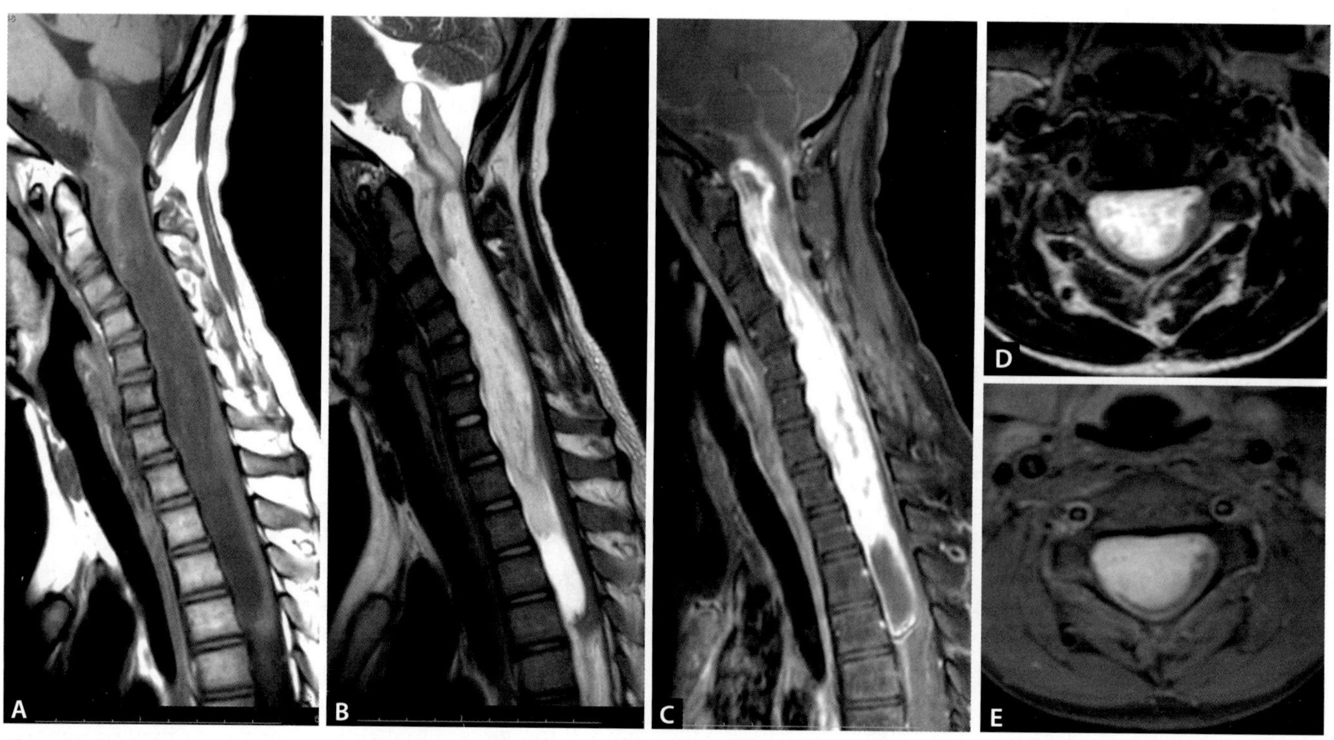

Figs. 4A to E: Astrocytoma in a 7-year-old boy. Long segment intramedullary mass lesion in seen extending from lower medulla to T4 vertebral level. The mass is predominantly hypointense on sagittal T1WI (A), hyperintense on sagittal T2WI (B) and show intense enhancement on post-gad sagittal T1WI (C). Axial T2WI (D) and post-gad axial T1WI (E) show eccentric location of the tumor.

due to their infiltrative growth pattern. Unfortunately, DTI is less reliable in differentiating these tumors in children because most pediatric astrocytomas are pilocytic, which tend to be circumscribed with discrete margins.[7,15] Non etheless, DTI and DT-FT can still aid preoperative assessment in these patients by determining the degree of resectability. Tumors that displace white matter tracts have well-defined margins and often can be treated with gross total or subtotal resection supplemented with adjuvant chemotherapy.[16] Infiltrative or disruptive patterns indicate a tumor of higher grade, which may preclude resection. These tumors are treated with adjuvant chemotherapy and radiation therapy.

Gangliogliomas

Gangliogliomas are slow-growing benign tumors that are composed of ganglion cells and glial elements.[4] They are the second most common intramedullary tumor following astrocytoma in the pediatric age group (15% of cases). Children between age 1 and 5 years are most commonly affected, like in the case of pilocytic astrocytomas. These neoplasms most commonly occur in the cervical and upper thoracic spinal cord, and occasionally extend up to the medulla. Gangliogliomas tend to be longitudinally extensive occupying an average length of 8 vertebral segments, compared with an average of 4 vertebral segments in length in ependymomas and astrocytomas.[17] Gangliogliomas are perhaps the second most common tumor after astrocytomas to have a holocord distribution. Like astrocytomas, gangliogliomas tend to be eccentrically located within the spinal cord. These tumors tend to have a low malignant potential, but they have a significant propensity for local recurrence.

On imaging, calcification is probably the single most suggestive feature of gangliogliomas. In the absence of gross calcification, the MR imaging appearance of gangliogliomas is highly variable, but certain imaging features may suggest the diagnosis. Gangliogliomas have a mixed signal intensity on T1WI, presumably due to the presence of a dual cell population composed of ganglion cells and glial elements.[17] They are usually T2 hyperintense. Perilesional edema is not as common as seen with ependymomas or astrocytomas. The gangliogliomas usually show patchy enhancement and cord surface enhancement.[17] Tumoral cysts are more common in gangliogliomas than in astrocytomas or ependymomas.[18] Gangliogliomas usually show chronic bony changes, including scoliosis and erosions due to their relatively slow growth; these are rarely seen with ependymomas or astrocytomas.[17]

Surgical resection is the treatment of choice with an excellent 5-year survival rate of 89% following surgical resection.[19]

Atypical Teratoid/Rhabdoid Tumors

Spinal atypical teratoid/rhabdoid tumors (ATRTs) are highly cellular malignant neoplasms of uncertain origin and are very rare. Most cases are seen in children who are less than 24 months old.[20] They may be either intramedullary or intradural extramedullary.

Imaging findings of ATRTs are heterogeneous and variable because of variable degrees of necrosis, hemorrhage, and calcification, mimicking their intracranial counterparts.[21] They show T2 iso-hypointensity and diffusion restriction presumably secondary to the hypercellularity of these tumors.[22] They enhance heterogeneously with gadolinium.[21] Cord expansion and edema are common findings. Diffuse leptomeningeal spread may occur and may be present at the time of diagnosis; therefore, imaging of the entire neuroaxis should be done. Prognosis is poor, and most patients die within 1 year.[23]

Treatment is variable, including surgical resection and/or debulking, chemotherapy, and radiation therapy.[2]

Hemangioblastomas

Hemangioblastomas are benign (WHO grade I) vascular neoplasms of unknown cell origin and account for 1.6 to 6.4% of spinal tumors.[24] Although most of these tumors (75%) are intramedullary, they may involve the intradural space or even be extradural.[4] The thoracic spinal cord is most frequently involved, followed by the cervical spinal cord. Most spinal hemangioblastomas occur sporadically, but approximately one-third to one-half of cases are associated with von Hippel-Lindau (VHL) syndrome.[25] These neoplasms are slow growing and may present with sensory changes, pain, and motor dysfunction.

MR features of spinal hemangioblastomas vary depending on the size of the tumor.[24] Small (10 mm or less) hemangioblastomas are mostly T1 isointense, T2 hyperintense, avidly enhancing and are located at the surface of the spinal cord, most frequently on it is the posterior aspect. Large hemangioblastomas are T1 and T2 heterogeneous, likely to have associated vascular flow-voids and show heterogeneous enhancement.[24] **(Figs. 5A to C)**. A hemangioblastoma larger than 24 mm is usually accompanied by vascular flow-voids on MR images. On MRI, a tumor is not likely to be a hemangioblastoma if it is 25 mm or more in size without

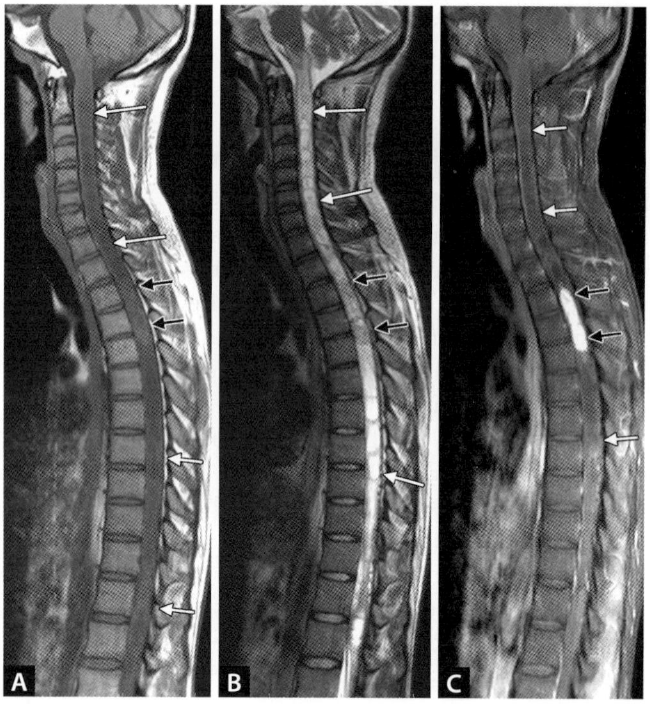

Figs. 5A to C: Hemangioblastoma: Sagittal T1WI (A) and Sagittal T2WI (B) show a long-segment syrinx (white arrows) in the cervicodorsal cord. Post-gad sagittal T1WI (C) shows an intensely enhancing pial based lesion (black arrows) at D3-D4 level.

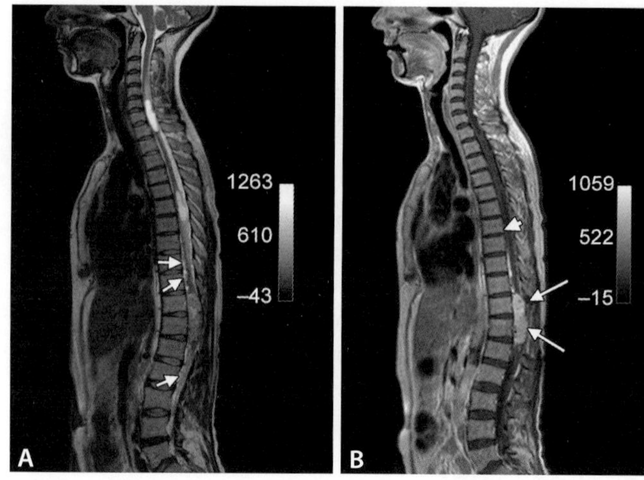

Figs. 6A and B: VHL with multiple hemangioblastomas. Sagittal T2WI (A) and post-gad T1WI (B) show cystic hemangioblastomas with enhancing mural nodules (arrowhead in B) in cervicodorsal cord and middorsal cord. In addition, a solid enhancing hemangioblastoma (arrows in B) with multiple intradural flow-voids (arrows in A) is seen in the region of the conus.

associated vascular flow-voids.[24] Syrinx associated with a spinal hemangioblastoma is usually more extensive than those seen with ependymomas or astrocytomas.[25] When no cystic component is present, extensive edema is typically found. Multiple hemangioblastomas are typically found in patients with von Hippel- Lindau disease **(Figs. 6A and B)** and this necessitates screening of the entire spine and brain. Hemangioblastomas are surgically treated with maximal safe resection.

Key imaging features include a focal pial or subpial enhancing nodule with an intraspinal cyst and enlarged vascular flow voids **(Figs. 6A and B)**.

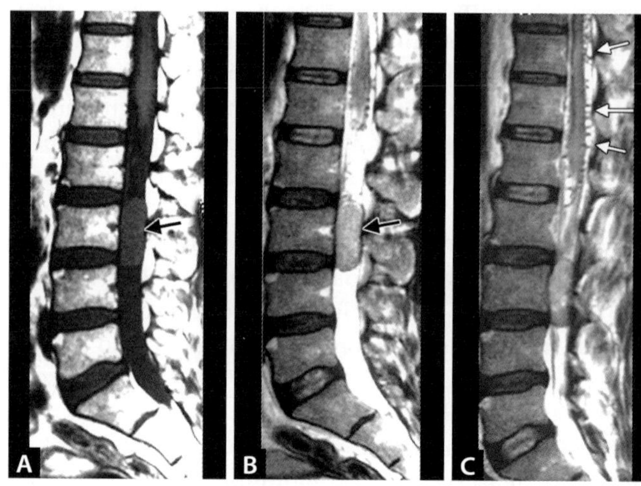

Figs. 7A to C: Paraganglioma: Sagittal T1WI (A) and T2WI (B and C) of the lumbosacral spine show an intradural isointense mass at L3 vertebral level. Note multiple vascular flow-voids in the intradural space.

Paraganglioma

Although spinal paragangliomas are rare, they are the third most common primary tumor to arise in the filum terminale (after ependymoma and astrocytoma). On MR imaging, these lesions generally appear as a well-circumscribed mass that is T1 isointense and T2 iso- to hyperintense **(Figs. 7A to C)**.[26,27] Hemorrhage is common (third most common after ependymoma and hemangioblastoma) and a low- signal-intensity rim (cap sign) may be seen on T2WI. After Gd- DTPA administration, heterogeneous and intense enhancement is seen virtually always.[27] Multiple punctate and serpiginous vascular flow-voids may be seen within and around these tumors.[26,27] Associated syringohydromyelia has been reported in some cases.[26]

Intramedullary Lymphoma

Lymphoma of the spine is usually caused by secondary involvement of the CNS from non-Hodgkin's lymphoma (NHL), often presenting with epidural or meningeal disease. Primary spinal cord lymphoma is exceedingly rare, accounting for 1–3% of primary central nervous system lymphoma (PCNSL) which itself constitutes only 1% of all NHLs.[4]

Intramedullary lymphoma can present as a solitary or a multifocal poorly defined enhancing mass. Unlike in the brain, most of the reported cases of spinal cord lymphoma have high signal intensity on T2-weighted images.[2] Multifocality is a characteristic of intramedullary spinal lymphoma, with more than 50% of the cases having multiple sites of involvement, including intracranial lesions. The presence of diffusion restriction can suggest areas of compact cellularity and may provide targets for biopsy.[28] There is no associated syringomyelia. Secondary intramedullary lymphoma of the spinal cord **(*see* Figs. 10A to C)** is more common in the cervical and thoracic regions, whereas primary intramedullary spinal cord lymphoma favours both cord and conus regions.[29,30]

Intramedullary Metastases

Intramedullary spinal cord metastases are rare. But, with increasing use of MR imaging, they are being encountered with increasing frequency. These represent approximately 2% of all metastases to the central nervous system; they usually involve the cervical cord. The most common source of intramedullary metastases is lung cancer (>50% of cases). Other primary malignancies include breast cancer, melanoma, lymphoma, leukemia, renal cell cancer, and colorectal cancer.[31] Rarely, intramedullary spinal cord metastasis may be an initial presentation of the malignancy.[4]

Spinal cord metastases are typically small, less than 1.5 cm, enhancing lesions which are spherical or ovoid in configuration, with extensive surrounding edema.[4]

Associated syrinxes, cystic change and hemorrhage are rare and the presence of these findings make the diagnosis of metastasis unlikely.[32] Recently described "rim" and "flame" patterns of enhancement can also be helpful in determining primary vs metastatic disease. Rykken et al.[33] have described the presence of "rim" and "flame" signs, which are more common in cord metastases than primary cord lesions, with sensitivity and specificity of 40% and 97%, respectively. The rim sign is defined as complete or partial rim enhancement more intense than the central portion **(Figs. 8A to C)**. The flame sign is characterized as an ill-defined flame-shaped region of enhancement superior and/or inferior to an otherwise well-defined enhancing lesion **(Figs. 8A to C)**.

INTRADURAL EXTRAMEDULLARY TUMORS

Intradural extramedullary tumors are located in the spinal subarachnoid space and include benign lesions (such as meningiomas and schwannomas) and metastatic lesions.

Meningiomas

Meningiomas are neoplasms that arise from the meninges of the spinal cord. Spinal meningiomas have a strong female predominance with a peak incidence in the fifth and sixth decades.[34] Childhood meningiomas are rare,

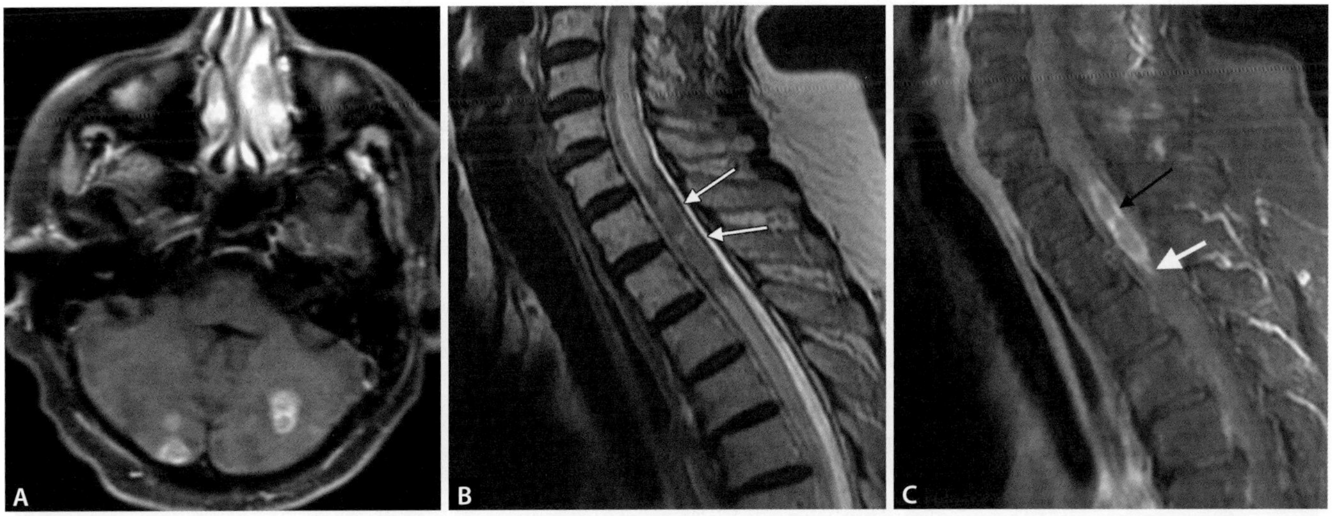

Figs. 8A to C: Intramedullary metastases: A 68-year-old lady with metastatic breast carcinoma. Axial post-gad T1WI (A) shows multiple cerebellar metastases. MR imaging of the cervical spine shows an intramedullary spinal cord metastasis at C7-D1 sagittal T2W (B) and post-gad T1W fat-suppressed (C) images. Note the enhancing intramedullary mass with a thin rim of more intense enhancement (rim sign; black arrow, C) as well as the ill-defined flame-shaped regions of enhancement at the inferior margins of the mass (flame sign; white arrow, C).

commonly of the clear-cell histologic subtype and tend to be more aggressive with higher rates of recurrence and metastasis.[35] Multiples spinal meningiomas are seen in patients with NF-2. Most meningiomas are intradural and only 10% are extradural or dumbbell tumors. Most spinal meningiomas are found in the thoracic spine, followed by the craniocervical junction and the lumbar region.[34] Although most thoracic and lumbar meningiomas are based on the posterior dura, craniocervical ones may be anterior or posterior in location.[36]

Typically, these lesions are well circumscribed, isointense to spinal cord on both T1- and T2WI; and display intense homogeneous enhancement following gadolinium administration **(Figs. 9A to C)**.[34] A dural tail may be present which could be secondary to tumor spread or reactive changes in the dura adjacent to the tumor. If they are densely calcified, they show low signal on both T1- and T2WI. CT may show intratumoral calcifications and this finding may aid in distinguishing between meningiomas and nerve sheath tumors, which do not contain calcifications.[36] Occasionally, spinal meningiomas have a plaque-like configuration and may encircle the cord. Meningiomas are primarily treated with surgical resection.

Nerve Sheath Tumors

In this category, most authors include neurofibromas and schwannomas. Strictly speaking, only schwannomas are nerve sheath tumors because neurofibromas arise from proper nerve fascicles. Regardless of this distinction, nerve sheath tumors are the most common spinal tumor. Schwannomas are the most common tumors, while neurofibromas generally occur in association with neurofibromatosis (especially NF-1). Like all nerve sheath tumors (in the absence of NF-1), these tumors tend to arise from sensory nerves (posteriorly in the spine) (Bell Magendie law). Approximately 50% of nerve sheath tumors are intradural-extramedullary (dumbbell-shaped) in location and 50% are purely extradural.[37] Malignant degeneration of neurofibromas may occur in patients with NF-1, but schwannomas rarely undergo malignant transformation.

Neurofibromas and schwannomas present similarly on imaging. They usually are round or fusiform, well-defined masses that can expand the neural foramina (due to extension into the extradural space), erode the undersurface of the ribs, and cause posterior vertebral body scalloping, which is best seen with CT. On MRI, both masses show isointense T1 and hyperintense T2 signal

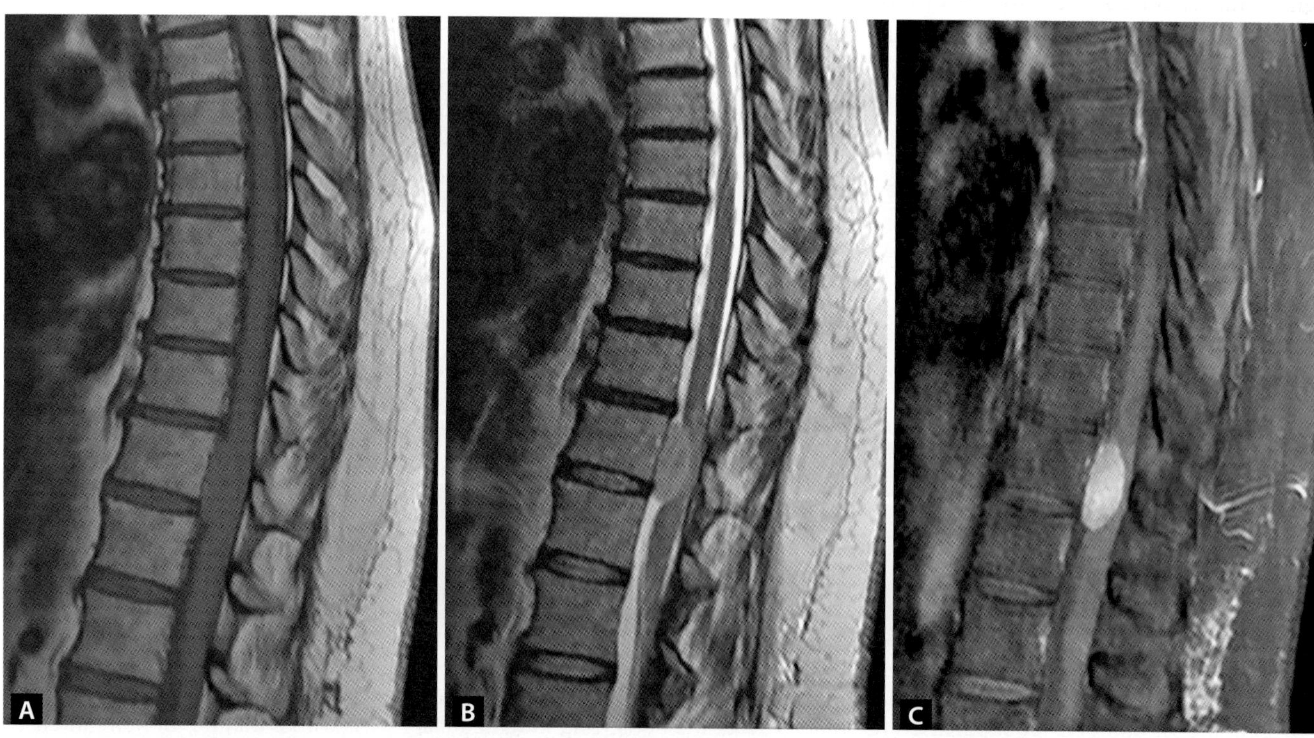

Figs. 9A to C: Meningioma: Sagittal T1WI (A) and T2WI (B) of the dorsal spine show an isointense extramedullary intradural mass anterior to the cord. The lesion shows intense enhancement (C) following contrast injection.

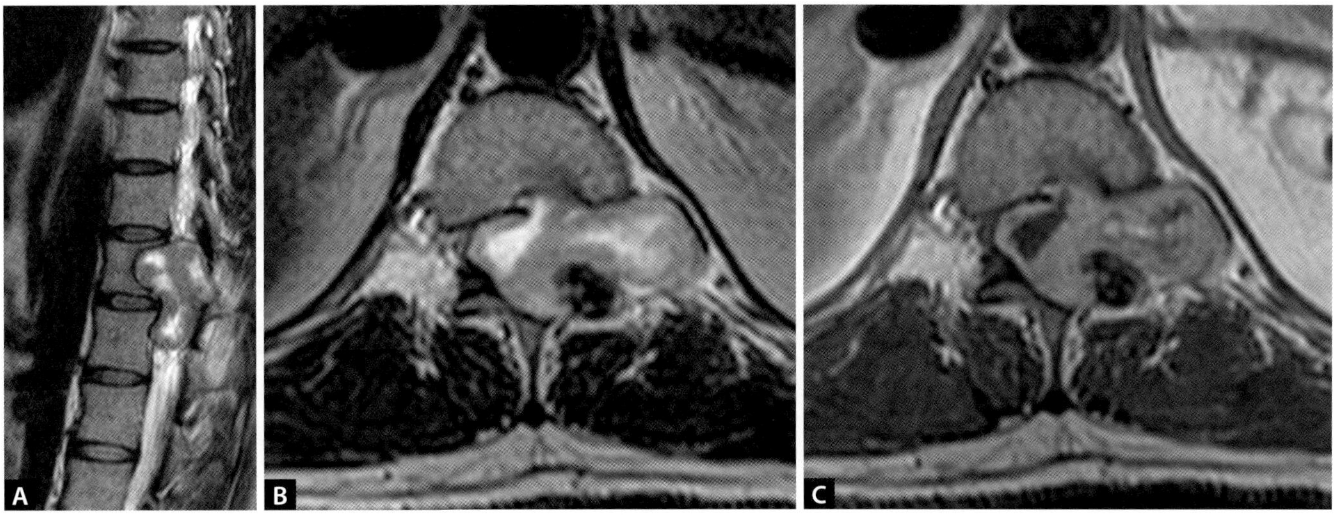

Figs. 10A to C: Nerve sheath tumor. Sagittal T2WI (A) and axial T2WI (B) of the spine show an isohyperintense extramedullary intradural mass with extradural extension through left neural foramina. The mass shows heterogeneous enhancement following gad administration (C).

(Figs. 10A to C). However, schwannomas especally large lesions may be heterogeneous on T2WI because of the mixture of Antoni A and B histologies and the presence of necrosis. Sometimes neurofibromas have a central area of lower T2 signal surrounded by peripheral T2 hyperintense signal probably due to a dense central area of collagenous stroma. This is referred to as the "target sign".[38] Localized neurofibromas demonstrate a focal mass, whereas plexiform lesions are multilobulated, often fusiform, masses that extend along nerve fascicles. Plexiform neurofibromas diffusely thicken the involved nerves and consist of numerous smaller lesions.[39] Neurofibromas are bright on short tau inversion recovery (STIR) images. Whole-body MR imaging with STIR is suggested to aid in the assessment of total tumor burden.[40] Schwannomas may hemorrhage and undergo cystic or fatty degeneration, but these findings are rare in neurofibromas. Both may show homogeneous or inhomogeneous enhancement, but schwannomas may have a typical ring or target type of enhancement in which the central portion of the mass remains relatively hypointense after contrast administration. Chronic compression of the spinal cord may result in the formation of syringomyelia.

Intradural Metastases (Leptomeningeal metastases)

Intradural metastases represent metastatic spread of primary malignant tumors into the spinal canal. Tumors of the CNS including medulloblastoma, choroid plexus papilloma and carcinoma, ependymomas, and high-grade gliomas may produce "drop metastases." In addition, primary systemic malignancies; most commonly breast cancer, lung cancer and melanoma, may also present with dural metastasis. The lumbosacral region is the most common location. Gadolinium-enhanced MRI is the imaging modality of choice to assess leptomeningeal spread. These intradural metastatic lesions often appear as small, round, multifocal lesions that enhance and coat the surface of the cord. More diffuse pial enhancement is seen in lymphomatous metastases, breast and prostate metastases.

EXTRADURAL TUMORS

Extradural neoplasms are localized between the osseous structures and dura mater or within the osseous structures themselves.[39] They account for approximately two-thirds of the cases of spinal tumors.[4] They can be classified into primary vertebral osseous tumors, tumors of the epidural space, and extraspinal tumors invading the spinal canal through the intervertebral foramina.

Imaging is used to evaluate the extent of involvement and neural tube compression.[40] Both MR imaging and CT are used to image these lesions because MR imaging allows for superior soft-tissue resolution, whereas CT better depicts the calcified components of lesions and the degree of adjacent osseous involvement.[4]

Multiple Lesions

Metastatic Disease

Spinal metastases are the most common tumors of the spine;[41] develop in approximately 10% of all patients with cancer and are multiple in 90% of cases. In adults, the most common primary tumors are adenocarcinomas of lung, prostate and breast. In children, most vertebral metastases arise from neuroblastoma and Ewing's sarcoma. The most commonly affected regions are the thoracic and lumbar and least commonly, the cervical spine. The metastatic foci may be in the posterior elements or in the vertebral bodies. Symptomatic spinal metastases produce a characteristic clinical syndrome beginning with local back or neck pain. Pain is followed by weakness, numbness and sphincter dysfunction.[41]

Most spinal metastases are lytic. Densely sclerotic metastases are typical (but not pathognomonic) for prostrate and rare cancers such as carcinoid tumors. Although nuclear medicine studies are very sensitive, their specificity is low. Uptake of most tracers requires destruction of cortical bone and thus metastases limited to bone marrow may be missed. Because of this reason, MRI is the imaging method of choice in these patients. Not only does MRI provide information regarding involvement of the bone, but also regarding overt or impending compression of the bone. Metastases to spine generally present as T1-hypointense and T2-hyperintense lesions that replace the normal marrow **(Figs. 11A to D)**. After contrast is given, most metastases enhance. Occasionally, the entire spine is involved by the tumor and its distribution may be so homogenous as to cause the vertebrae to appear normal at first glance (this is particularly true of prostrate metastases). A clue that this is happening is the fact that intervertebral disks appear brighter than bone marrow on T1 images (this is the inverse of what is normal, where the disks are darker than the vertebral body bone marrow on T1 images). By the time of diagnosis, many vertebral metastases have epidural extension.

MRI may be helpful to differentiate between a neoplastic compression fracture and an osteoporotic fracture. In neoplastic compression fracture, there is complete replacement of fatty marrow with neoplastic cells which may also extend beyond the spine. On the other hand, osteoporotic compression fractures may only demonstrate a band of marrow replacement representing edema. There is gradual return to the normal fatty marrow

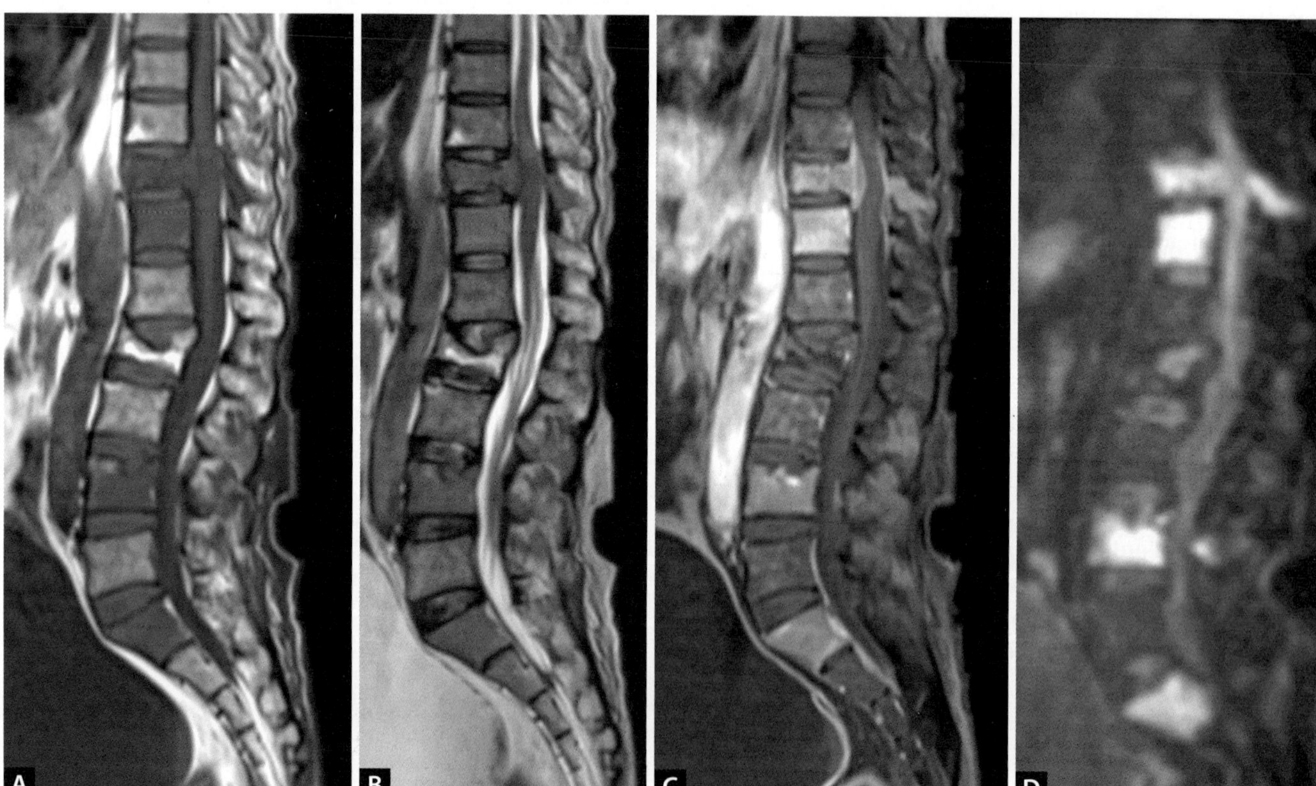

Figs. 11A to D: Spinal metastases: Sagittal T1WI (A), T2WI (B) post-gad fat sat T1WI (C) and diffusion-WI (D) show abnormal signal in T11, T12, L4 and S1 vertebral bodies with epidural soft tissue component at D11. These lesion are hypointense on T1 (A) and T2WI (B) and show restricted diffusion (D) and enhance following contrast administration (C). Note benign anterior wedging of L2 vertebrae without any enhancement or diffusion restriction.

on follow-up studies. The presence of multiple foci in the spine favors the diagnosis of metastatic disease. Diffusion weighted imaging may be helpful in differentiating benign osteoporotic vertebral body fractures (which have low signal intensity) from malignant ones (which have relatively high signal intensity).[42]

Multiple Myeloma

Multiple myeloma (MM) is a malignancy characterized by monoclonal proliferation of malignant plasma cells. Nearly always, the disease is systemic, but occasionally, it may be isolated (plasmacytoma). In most patients, plasmacytoma is the initial manifestation of the disease and MM develops in most of the cases 5 to 10 years after the initial diagnosis. MM is the most common primary neoplasm of spine with the majority occurring in the thoracic and lumbar spine. Most patients are men, 60 years of age or older. Plasmacytomas are expansile lytic masses that may extend into the epidural space; and may undergo pathological fracture.

On plain film or CT, they usually appear as focal lytic lesions, but often the disease may present innocuously, appearing only as diffuse osteopenia. The lesion may be sclerotic rather than lytic in case of POEMS (polyneuropathy, organomegaly, endocrinopathy, myeloma and skin changes) syndrome. Treated myeloma, after chemotherapy and/or radiation, may also exhibit sclerosis.[43]

MRI is superior to plain radiograph for both, focal and diffuse involvement. On MRI, five different infiltration patterns can be seen: (1) normal appearance of bone marrow despite minor microscopic plasma cell infiltration, (2) focal marrow involvement, (3) homogeneous diffuse marrow infiltration, (4) combined diffuse and focal marrow infiltration, and (5) "salt-and-pepper" pattern with inhomogeneous bone marrow with interposition of fat islands.[44] Typically marrow infiltrations are identified as hypointensities on T1WI, hyperintensities on STIR images and enhancement on gadolinium-enhanced images.[45] Diffuse involvement appears as homogeneous signal reduction on T1WI which enhances after contrast material administration. In general, however, MM is suspected whenever MR images depict an expansile focal mass; multiple focal masses in the axial skeleton; diffuse marrow involvement, particularly at known sites of normal hematopoiesis; or multiple compression fractures in a patient with no known primary malignancy.[45] These imaging features are suggestive but are not pathognomonic for MM and may also be seen in other marrow infiltrative disorders.

Recently, MRI has been used in clinical staging, guiding biopsies[45] and monitoring response to therapy in patients with multiple myeloma. In focal lesions, reduction of signal intensity on T2WI, lack of rim-like enhancement after contrast administration or even a normalization of bone marrow signal on T1 are signs of good response.[44] In diffuse lesions, a patchy reconversion to fatty marrow may be a sign of response to treatment.

Lymphoma

Spinal lymphoma occurs most often between the 5th and 7th decades of life. Most patients have underlying non-Hodgkin's lymphoma. Spinal involvement develops in approximately 2% of these patients and affects mostly the epidural space. Bone lesions are most frequent in the dorsal and lumbar spine and least frequent in the cervical spine. Bony involvement mostly results in osteolytic lesions, but patchy sclerosis and "ivory vertebrae" as well as mixed lytic and blastic lesions are also commonly seen.[46] Vertebral collapse may also occur.

On MRI, lymphoma appears as a nonspecific mass that is hyperintense on T1 images and hypointense or bright on T2 images. The T2 signal characteristics are related to the fact that lymphomas have a high nucleus-to-cytoplasm ratio. For similar reasons, lymphomas have restricted diffusion on DWI.[36] Lymphomas enhance intensely and may compromise the spinal canal, resulting in compression of the spinal cord. Radiation therapy can result in rapid reduction in the size and compressive effects of these lesions so early and accurate diagnosis is of particular importance. Paravertebral soft-tissue masses and gouge defects on the anterior borders of the vertebrae may be seen.

Vertebral Hemangiomas

Vertebral hemangiomas (VHs) are the most common primary bone tumor and are found in over 10% of population in autopsy studies. They are composed of thin-walled capillary-sized to cavernous blood vessels lined by endothelial cells infiltrating the medullary cavity between bone trabeculae. They are most commonly found in the fourth to sixth decades with slight female predominance. They may be solitary (70%) or multiple (30%). The most common locations are the thoracic, lumbar and cervical regions. Most of the hemangiomas arise in the body of the vertebra, but may also involve the pedicles and rarely, spinous processes. The majority of hemangiomas are asymptomatic, but occasionally, they may present as large and aggressive masses destroying a vertebra and producing pain and even compression of the spinal cord. Some hemangiomas enlarge and become symptomatic during pregnancy.

From a strict radiological point of view, VHs can be classified as typical, atypical, and aggressive (also called compressive).[47] The terms "typical" and "atypical" refer primarily to the MR imaging appearance, which is directly correlated with the ratio of fatty to vascular components and interstitial edema. The term aggressive refers to the presence of radiological features such as extension beyond the vertebral body, destruction of the cortex, and invasion of the epidural and paravertebral spaces.[47] Clinically asymptomatic VHs may show "typical" or "atypical" imaging findings, while symptomatic VHs more frequently appear "atypical" or "aggressive."

Typical Vertebral Hemangiomas

At radiography, typical VHs classically have a coarse, vertical, trabecular pattern, (which has been likened to corduroy) presumably a response to stress.[48] At CT, the thickened trabeculae are seen in cross section as small punctate areas of sclerosis, often called the 'polka-dot' appearance **(Fig. 12A)**. On sagittal and coronal reformatted CT images, classical vertical orientation of the thickened trabeculae is seen (the "corduroy" sign). **(Figs. 12B and C)**. The bony cortex is intact and no extraosseous extension is seen. On MRI, typical VHs appear as well-defined hyperintense lesions on both T1- and T2WI owing to the predominant fatty component and as slightly hyperintense lesions on FLAIR or STIR imaging because of their vascular component. Thickened vertical trabeculae appear as punctate and linear areas of iso- to hypointensity within the hyperintense lesion on T1WI. Variable enhancement is seen in postcontrast T1WI.

Atypical Vertebral Hemangiomas

Atypical VHs have less fatty and greater vascular content. Thus, they appear iso- to hypointense on T1WI and show very high signal intensity on T2W and fluid-sensitive images. Atypical VHs usually show varying degrees of enhancement following gadolinium administration, which is best appreciated on T1W fat-suppressed images. Like typical VHs, thickened vertical trabeculae on CT and MR images is a key feature for diagnosis, though this is more difficult to see in atypical VHs.

Aggressive Vertebral Hemangiomas

Aggressive VHs are more aggressive lesions that are usually made of less fat with more soft tissue hypervascular stroma. Plain radiograph may not detect abnormalities or may

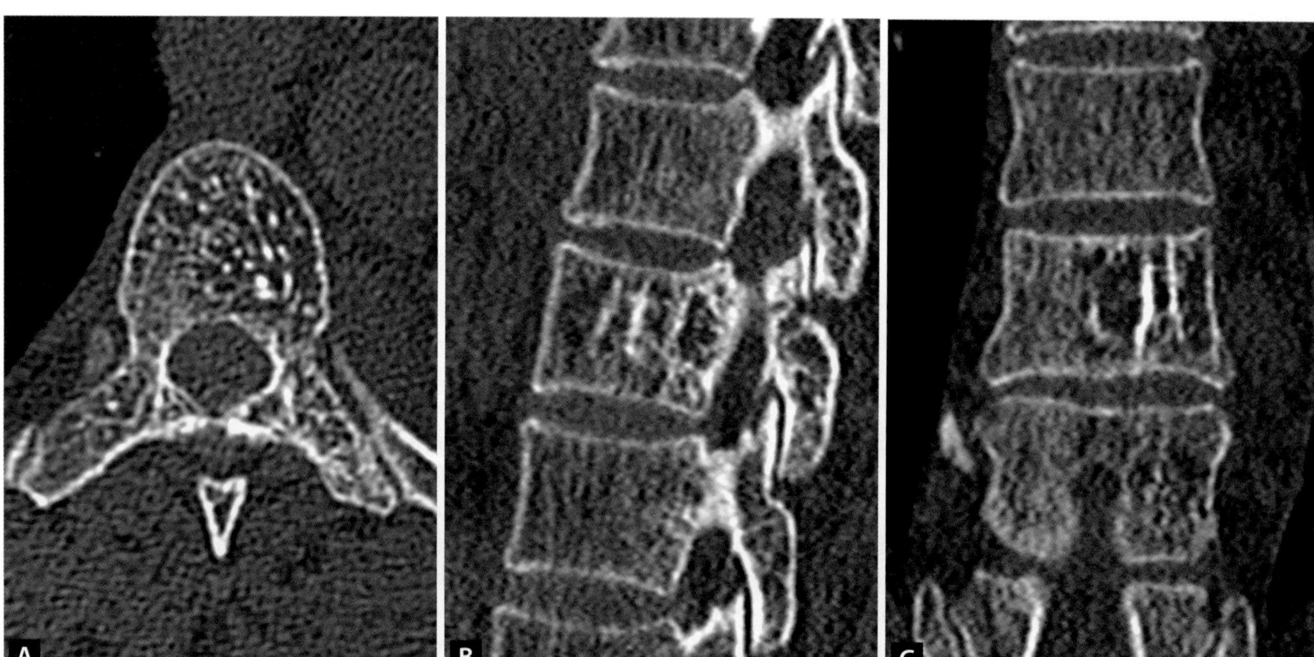

Figs. 12A to C: Hemangioma CT: (A) Axial CT of a L3 hemangioma with characteristic "honeycomb" appearance, also described as mottled appearance; Sagittal (B) and coronal (C) reconstructed images show sparse, vertically oriented thickened trabeculae that involve the vertebral body and posterior elements.

show nonspecific findings, such as osteoporosis, poorly defined or expanded cortex, vertebral collapse, pedicle erosion, or vertical trabecular pattern irregularities that are associated with lytic areas of varying size.[6,8] CT may show nonspecific findings such as ballooning[47] and lysis[49] of the cortex or extra-osseous soft tissue extension.[23,24] However, one must look for the typical "polka-dot" sign on axial CT images, even in the more aggressive/destructive lesions, because it can guide the correct diagnosis.

Aggressive VHs are difficult to diagnose by MR imaging as bone is not directly visualized and more aggressive lesions are usually made of less fat with more soft tissue hypervascular stroma. T1WI usually shows hypointense lesions. T2W and fluid-sensitive images usually show areas of very high intensity corresponding to the vascular components of aggressive VHs **(Figs. 13A to D)**.

Some imaging features that might suggest a diagnosis of aggressive VHs include: a maintained vertebral body height, a sharp margin with the normal marrow, intact cortex adjacent to a paraspinal mass, and enlarged paraspinal vessels.[50] The angiographic appearance of VHs is usually characteristic: dilatation of the arterioles of the vertebral body, multiple blood pools in the capillary phase, and intense opacification extending beyond the normal hemivertebral territory throughout the entire vertebral body.[48]

Solitary Lesions

Aneurysmal Bone Cyst

Aneurysmal bone cyst (ABC) accounts for lesser than 1% of all primary bone tumors. Approximately, 20% of all ABCs are located in the spine, particularly in the lower thoracic and lumbosacral regions, where the posterior elements are typically involved. The peak incidence is in the second decade of life with a slight female predominance. Patients complain of back pain and neurologic symptoms resulting from encroachment on the spinal canal.

ABCs may be primary (70%) or secondary. Secondary ABCs may be associated with GCT, osteoblastoma, chondroblastoma, metastases and osteosarcoma. Pathologically, ABCs consist of multiloculated blood-filled spaces, which are not lined by endothelium. Solid components are usually in septations and are composed of fibrous tissue, reactive bone and giant cells. In 5–7.5% of cases, the solid component is predominant.[51]

On plain radiographs, ABCs appear as marked expansile lesions causing bone remodelling. These lesions are centered in the posterior elements, with frequent extension into the vertebral body (75–90% of cases).[52,53] A thin, outer periosteal rim and septations may be seen. Similar to GCT and chordoma, spinal ABCs may also involve adjacent vertebral bodies, intervertebral disks, posterior ribs and paravertebral soft tissues.[54]

On CT scan, ABCs are eccentric, lytic, expansile, multiloculated lesions that resemble a "soap bubble" with a "blown-out" appearance **(Figs. 14A to C)**.[55] Cystic spaces with fluid-fluid levels can occasionally be detected on CT scan.[56] Relationship of the tumor with neural elements and fluid-fluid levels are better appreciated with MRI than CT. On MRI, the lobulated lesion is surrounded by a hypointense rim corresponding to an intact, thickened

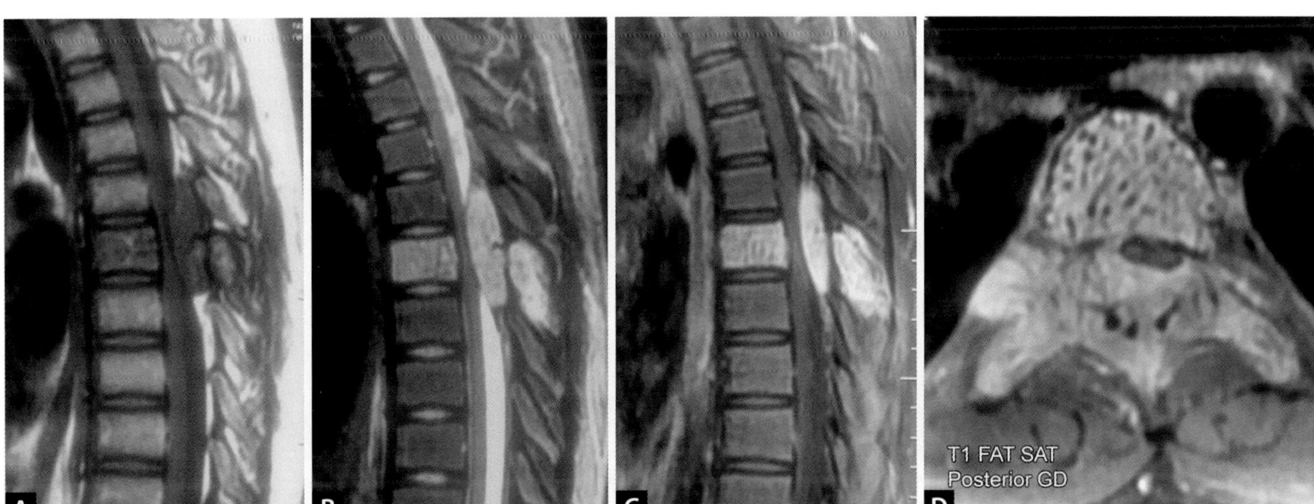

Figs. 13A to D: Hemangiomas aggressive: Sagittal T1WI (A) and T2WI (B) of the dorsal spine reveal D4 and D8 hemangiomas. The lesions are hypointense on T1WI and hyperintense on T2WI, suggesting aggressive hemangiomas. Axial T2WI (C) image shows right paravertebral and epidural soft tissue component, (D) compressing the spinal cord.

periosteal membrane **(Figs. 14A to C)**.[55] The cystic components vary in appearance on T1 and T2 scans, depending on the age of the blood products and debris within these cysts. Gadolinium contrast enhancement is seen in up to 96% of lesions.[57] and is usually seen within the rim and septations, rather than the cystic spaces.

The presence of fluid-fluid or hematocrit levels is suggestive, but not pathognomic of ABCs. I has also been reported in giant cell tumors, chondroblastomas, fractured simple cysts, fibrous dysplasia and malignant fibrous histiocytomas.[58] The presence of a solid component with diffuse contrast enhancement should raise suspicion for a secondary ABC, although it might also be encountered in the solid variant of ABC.[59]

Endovascular treatment with multiple embolic agents may be done as both, a preliminary procedure to lessen blood loss at surgery and as a stand-alone treatment.[52]

Giant Cell Tumor

Giant cell tumors (GCTs) of the spine are uncommon tumors and account for 3–7% of all GCTs. Spinal lesions occur during 2nd to 4th decades of life and are more frequent in women. Patients present with symptoms of pain (often radicular), weakness and sensory deficits.

Sacrum is the most common site of spinal GCTs.[60] Sacral GCTs are often eccentric and abut or extend across the sacroiliac joint,[35,44] in comparison to a more central location of sacral chordomas. Extra-sacral spinal GCTs are usually located in the vertebral body with or without extension to the posterior elements.[61] GCTs may involve the adjacent intervertebral disks and vertebrae.[62]

Pathologically, GCT is composed of abundant osteoclastic giant cells intermixed throughout a spindle cell stroma. Cystic areas and hemorrhage, with hemosiderin and prominent areas of fibrous tissue with high collagen content are often present.[63] Rarely, GCTs may metastasize and recur, especially with incomplete resection. Approximately 5–10% of GCTs are malignant.[54]

Typically, GCT appears as a lytic lesion with cortical expansion on a radiograph.[26,65] On CT scans, the tumor has soft-tissue density with well-circumscribed margins that may show a thin rim of sclerosis **(Figs. 15A and B)**. GCT shows heterogeneous signal intensity on both T1 and T2WI due to presence of necrosis, hemorrhage, or cystic spaces. Low T2 signal intensity due to presence of hemorrhagic and fibrotic content is often seen. Marrow edema is usually not seen in the absence of a pathological fracture. The lesion enhances after intravenous injection of contrast material.

At bone scintigraphy, GCT may reveal diffusely increased uptake of radionuclide. However, sacral GCTs commonly show the "doughnut" sign of central photopenia and increased peripheral activity. Angiography shows prominent vascularity of these tumors and is often reserved for preoperative embolization.

Osteoid Osteoma

Osteoid osteoma is a benign bone-forming tumor that is characterized by a small radiolucent nidus (usually < 2 cm

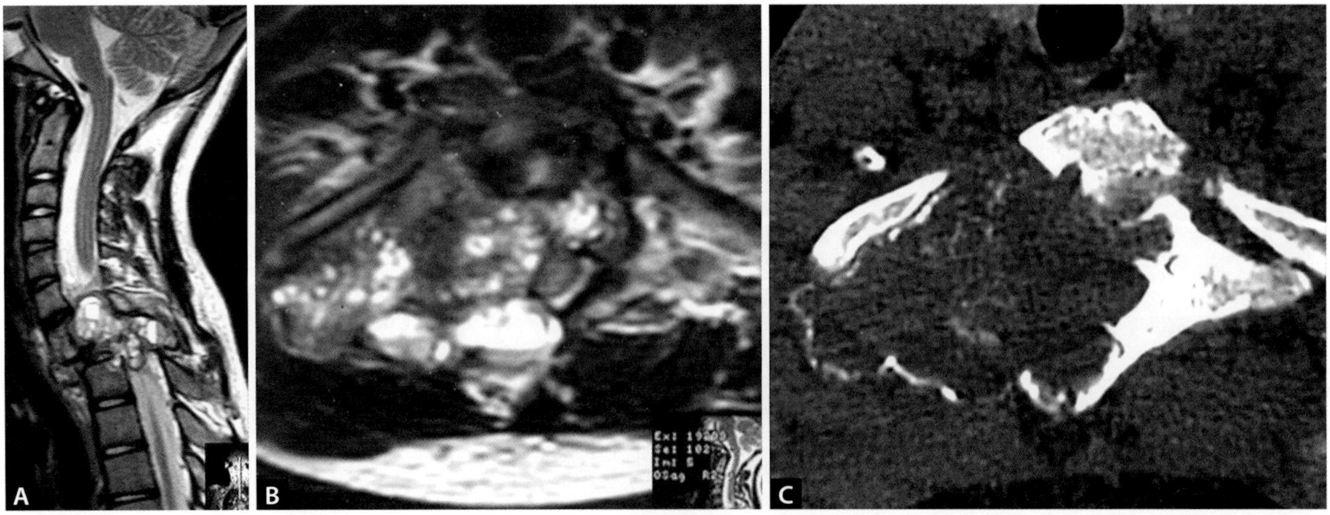

Figs. 14A to C: Aneurysmal bone cyst: Sagittal T2WI (A) and axial T2WI (B) of the cervicodorsal spine show and multicystic expansile mass involving the posterior arch, right pedicle and body of the D1 vertebra. The mass contains multiple septae with fluid-fluid levels. The spinal cord is displaced posteriorly and to the left; (C) CT scan shows the thin rim of bone marginating the mass.

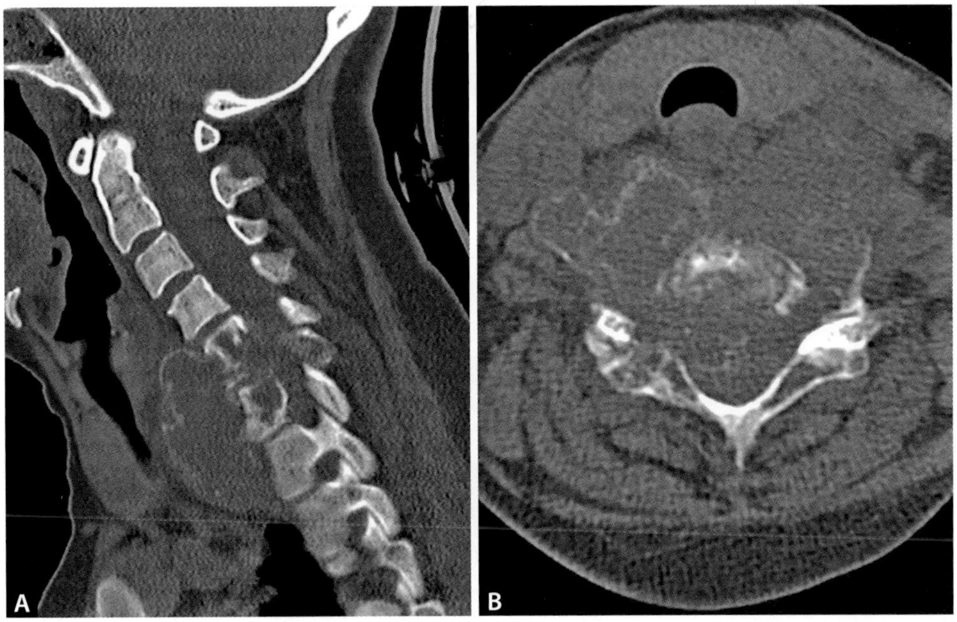

Figs. 15A and B: Giant cell tumor of C5 and C6: Sagittal (A) and axial (B) CT scans reveal an expansile lytic lesion centered in the vertebral body with posterior element extension.

in diameter). It involves the axial skeleton in 10% of cases.[48] Patients are usually affected between the ages of 10 and 20 years, with a male-to-female distribution of 1.5:2.[61,64] Clinical symptoms include painful scoliosis, focal or radicular pain, gait disturbance and muscle atrophy. Typically, the pain is worse at night and is relieved with aspirin.

The tumor involves the lumbar spine most commonly, followed by the cervical, thoracic and sacral regions.[65] The axial osteoid osteomas are most commonly present in the posterior elements of the vertebra (75%) and are rare in the vertebral body (7%).

Pathologically, the nidus of an osteoid osteoma is a small (<2 cm in diameter), round mass of pink to red tissue of osteoid and woven bone with interconnected trabeculae. The lesion is well circumscribed and may be surrounded by a variable degree of reactive cortical bone.

CT scan is an excellent imaging modality to detect an osteoid osteoma and define its exact location within the bone. CT shows the nidus as a round hypodense lesion surrounded by a hyperdense sclerotic ring **(Figs. 16A to C)**. Calcification within the nidus results in a target appearance of the lesion **(Figs. 16A to C)**. On MR imaging, nidus is generally of a low to iso signal intensity on T1WI, iso to high signal intensity on T2WI and enhances markedly; the surrounding osteosclerotic component results in a hypointense ring. Areas of calcification have low signal intensity on all pulse sequences. On MRI, a small nidus may be obscured by signal changes due to associated surrounding sclerosis, marrow edema and soft-tissue inflammation.[66] Radionuclide bone scans are extremely sensitive in the detection of osteoid osteomas.

Typically, management of spinal osteoid osteoma is complete surgical resection of the nidus. Percutaneous CT-guided removal and percutaneous ablation with a radiofrequency electrode, laser or alcohol are new methods of treatment.[67]

Osteoblastoma

It is classically believed that osteoblastomas differ from osteoid osteomas only in size (>2 cm in diameter). Osteoblastomas occur in young adults, with 90% of cases occurring in the 2nd and 3rd decades of life with a male predominance (2:1). Osteoblastomas present with dull localized pain and neurologic symptoms, including paresthesias, paraparesis and paraplegia.

Osteoblastomas of the spine represent 30–40% of all osteoblastomas and the lesions are equally distributed in the cervical, thoracic and lumbar segments.[68] These most frequently involve the posterior vertebral elements (55% of cases) with frequent extension into the vertebral body (42%).[61,64] Isolated vertebral body involvement in osteoblastoma is rare. Pathologically, the typical osteoblastoma is more than 2.0 cm in diameter. Histologic features resemble to those of osteoid osteoma

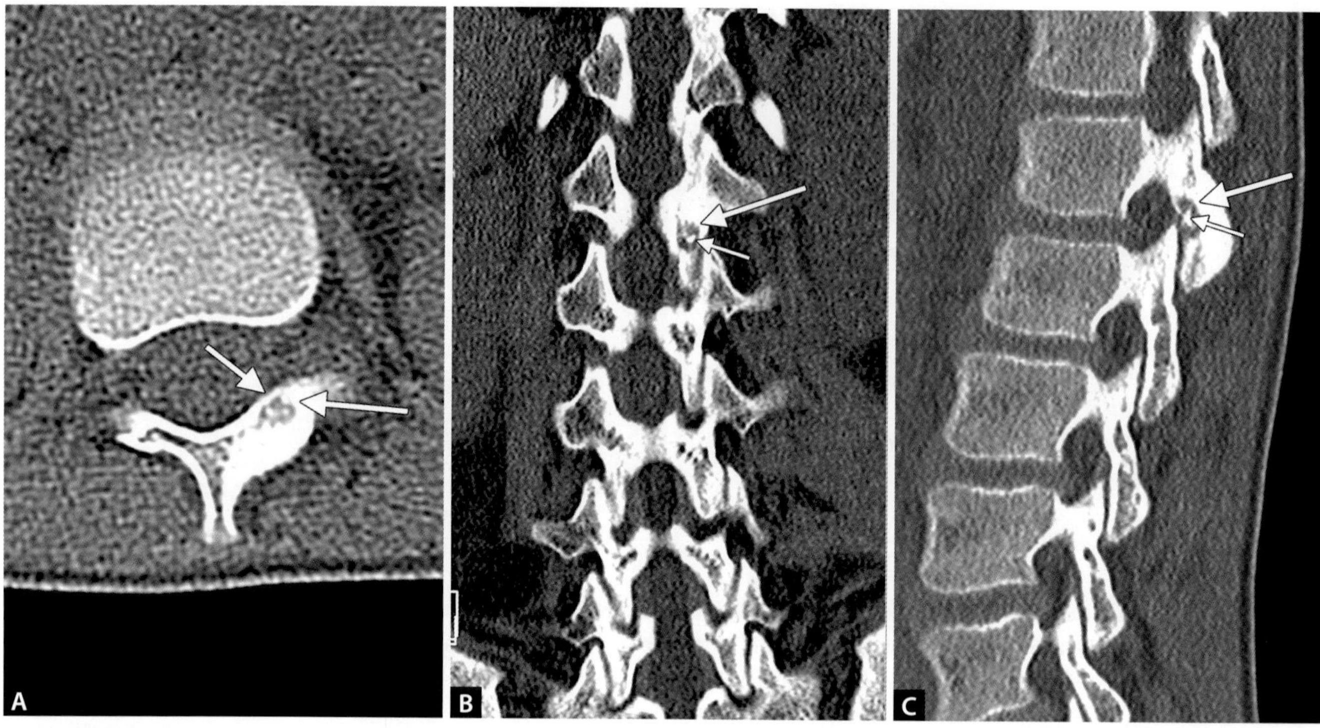

Figs. 16A to C: Osteoid osteoma in a 21-year-old man with low back pain: Axial (A), coronal reconstructed (B) and sagittal reconstructed (C) CT scans of lumbar spine show a focal lucency in the left L1 lamina (long arrows) with central mineralization (small arrows) and surrounding sclerosis typical of osteoid osteoma.

(interconnecting trabecular bone and fibrovascular stroma), but overall the microscopic pattern is not as well organized as that seen in osteoid osteomas.

Three radiographic patterns have been described with osteoblastoma.[68] In the first pattern, osteoblastoma may resemble osteoid osteoma but is usually larger (>2 cm in diameter). The second pattern appears as an expansile lesion with multiple small calcifications and a peripheral sclerotic rim. This is the most common appearance of spinal osteoblastomas **(Fig. 17)**.[69] The third pattern is the most aggressive pattern and appears as an expansile lesion with bone destruction, infiltration of surrounding soft tissue and intermixed matrix calcification. Interestingly, mineralization within an osteoblastoma may have the radiologic appearance (rings and arcs) of chondroid matrix.

At CT, the lesion shows areas of mineralization, expansile bone remodelling and sclerosis or a thin osseous shell about its margins. MR imaging appearance of osteoblastoma is generally nonspecific, with low-to-intermediate signal intensity seen on T1WI and intermediate-to-high signal intensity seen on T2WI.[68] MR imaging is sensitive to show relationship of the tumor with neural structures and surrounding soft tissues.[70]

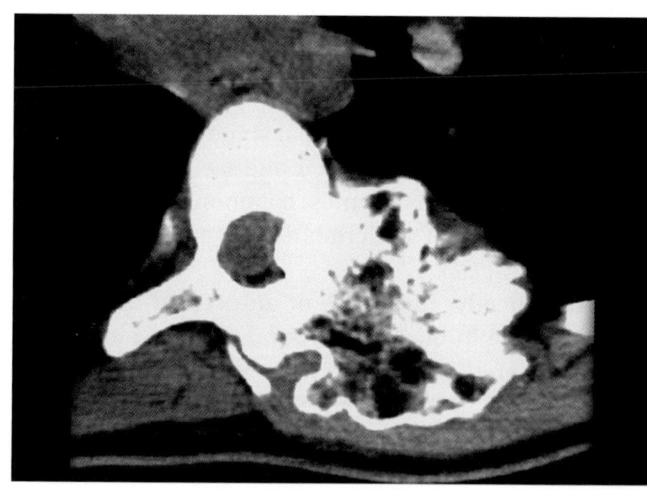

Fig. 17: Osteoblastoma: Axial CT of the dorsal spine reveals an expansile lesion of left pedicle and lamina of D6 vertebra with small foci of mineralized matrix.

Osteoblastomas show marked radionuclide uptake at bone scintigraphy.

Surgical resection is the treatment of choice for spinal osteoblastomas. The recurrence rate is 10–15% and early 50% for conventional and aggressive lesion respectively.[68,71]

Osteochondromas

Spinal osteochondromas are rare, accounting for only 1–4% of solitary exostoses and represent 4% of all solitary spinal tumors.[72] Generally, one spinal osteochondroma is present in 7–9% of patients with hereditary multiple exostoses.[73]

Spinal osteochondromas are often diagnosed during the 3rd and 4th decades of life when solitary and one decade earlier in patients with hereditary multiple exostoses.[72,73] Osteochondromas have a predilection for the cervical spine, particularly C2, though they can occur at all levels of the spine. Most commonly spinal osteochondromas arise from the posterior elements; some may arise from the vertebral body.

Osteochondromas have the composition of a normal bone (cortex and marrow space) with a cartilage cap from which growth occurs. Spinal osteochondromas may be sessile or pedunculated. The lesion is continuous with the marrow and cortex of the underlying bone.[72]

Thin-section CT is the best imaging modality to show pathognomonic marrow and cortical continuity of the lesion to the underlying bone. MR imaging usually shows yellow marrow centrally (T1 hyperintense and T2 isointense) with a low-signal-intensity cortex. The hyaline cartilage cap is often small and thin, with low to isointense signal intensity on T1WI and high signal intensity on T2WI. Marked cartilage cap thickening (>1.5 cm) should raise the suspicion of malignant transformation to chondrosarcoma in adults. Surgical excision of osteochondroma is usually curative.

Chordoma

Chordoma is a tumor arising from remnants of the primitive notochord and represents 2–4 % of malignant osseous neoplasms.[60] These tumors are almost always midline or paramedian in location. These tumors most commonly occur in the sacral regions (50%), followed by the skull base (35%) and the rest of the spine (15%).[60] Men are affected twice as frequently as women; the mean age of these patients is 50 years, with skull-base chordomas generally affecting a younger population, including children.[60]

Chordomas are slow-growing tumors that are commonly discovered as large masses. Enlarging chordomas tend to involve adjacent vertebral bodies and extend into the adjacent paraspinal tissues and epidural space.[74] Rarely, they can arise solely in the musculature of the perivertebral space.[74]

Pathologically, typical chordomas contain physaliphorous cells; and abundant intracellular and extracellular mucin. The chondroid or osteoid elements replace the mucinous matrix in atypical or dedifferentiated chordomas.[60]

On imaging, chordoma is seen as a destructive vertebral body lesion spanning several segments and sparing the disks with associated soft-tissue component.[75] It may have a "collar button" or "mushroom" appearance and a "dumb bell" shape. About 40% of chordomas are of the mobile spine and up to 90% of sacrococcygeal chordomas contain areas of amorphous calcifications.[55] Most chordomas are iso-or hypointense relative to muscle on T1WI. On T2WI, most chordomas have a high-signal intensity due to the presence of their signature physaliphorous cells (clear cells with intracytoplasmic vacuoles and abundant mucin) **(Figs. 18A to D)**.[60] The focal areas of hemorrhage, calcifications and high protein content of the myxoid and mucinous collections may account for the heterogeneous intratumoural T2 hypointensity and T1 hyperintensity.[55] The fibrous septa that divide the gelatinous components of the tumor appear as areas of low signal intensity on T2WI. T2-hypointense rim due to hemosiderin deposition has been reported in 72% of sacrococcygeal chordomas but is rare in spinal chordomas.[76] Most chordomas show moderate heterogeneous enhancement after gadolinium-injection.[75] Chordomas typically have a poor prognosis due to local recurrence following resection.

Chondrosarcoma

Chondrosarcoma is a malignant neoplasm that represents 10% of all primary bone tumors[77] and is second most common non-lymphoproliferative tumor of the spine. The most common age of presentation is in the fifth decade, with male predominance (M:F 2–4:1). The patient may present with pain, neurological symptoms and a palpable mass. The spine is affected in 3%–12% of cases.[61] Dorsal spine is the most common site, though it can occur at all levels of the spine. Chondrosarcoma may arise from the vertebral body (15% of cases), posterior element (40%), or both (45%).[55] Typically low grade, these neoplasms can arise *de novo* or secondarily from a pre-existing cartilage lesion such as an osteochondroma or an enchondroma.

Radiologically, these tumors appear as destructive lesions in the spine or as a paraspinal mass with calcification.[55] The characteristic chondroid matrix mineralization (rings and arcs) may be evident on radiographs, but are better evaluated with CT. Calcified matrix appears as areas of signal voids on MR imaging. Due to the high water content of hyaline cartilage, the non-mineralized portion of the tumor is hypodense

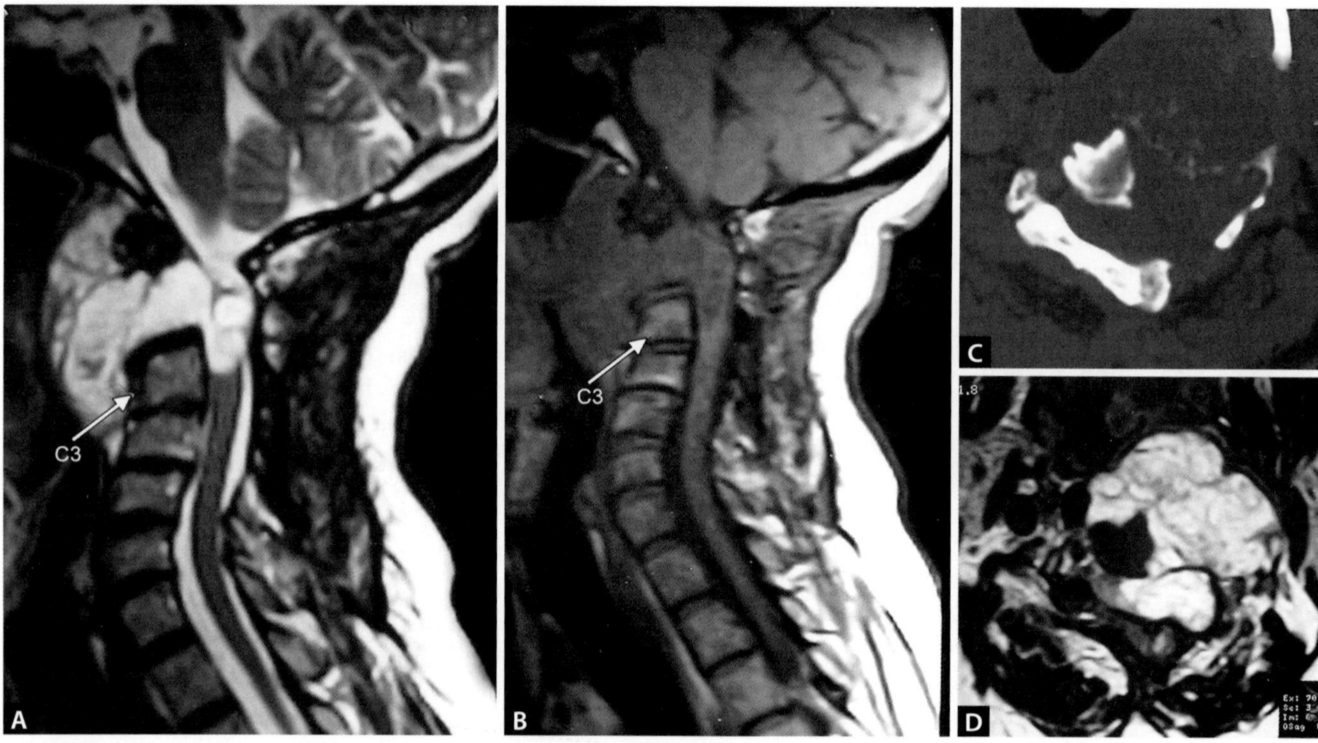

Figs. 18A to D: Chordoma: Sagittal T2WI (A), sagittal T1WI (B) and axial T2WI (C) show a mass lesion involving the body of C2 vertebra with a large prevertebral component. The mass is hypointense on T1 (B) and hyperintense on T2 (A and C). Axial CT scan (D) shows lytic destruction of the left half of the C2 vertebra.

on CT scans, low-to-intermediate signal intensity on T1WI and very high signal intensity on T2WI **(Figs. 19A to D)**.[78] Rings and arcs pattern of enhancement is seen at gadolinium-enhanced MR imaging; reflecting the lobulated growth pattern of these cartilaginous tumors. Transdiscal extension has been reported in 35% of cases[79] Chondrosarcoma arising from osteochondroma is seen as thickening of the peripheral cartilaginous cap of more than 1.5 cm. Surgical resection with adjuvant radiation therapy is the treatment of choice for spinal chondrosarcomas.

Fibrous Dysplasia

Fibrous dysplasia (FD) is a developmental anomaly wherein portions of the bone are replaced by fibrous connective tissue and poorly formed trabecular bone. FD affects primarily children and adolescents. FD may present in monostotic or polyostotic forms. Monostotic FD accounts for 80% of cases and tends to occur most often in the ribs, long bones, and skull. Involvement of the vertebral bodies is rare—only occurring in 2.5% of cases.[80,81] Spine involvement is more likely to present in the polyostotic form of the disease. Lumbar spine is most commonly involved in spinal FD. Vertebral body, with or without involvement of pedicles is the most common site of involvement.

Radiographically, spinal FD appears as a decrease in vertebral height. Classic plain radiographic appearance of a ground-glass matrix with definite sclerotic margins is not seen in spinal FD as opposed to FD occurring elsewhere in the body. However, on spine CT scans, "ground-glass" appearance can be seen and is the most common finding. In addition, a mildly expansile lesion with a "blown-out" cortical shell or a lytic lesion with a sclerotic rim and a decrease in body height can be seen. On MRI, FD shows variable characteristics, typically intermediate-to-low signal intensity on T1WI and variable signal intensity on T2WI. Benign FD lesions characteristically do not show cortical bone disruption or soft-tissue involvement; hypointense on T1W sequence and have fine well-circumscribed border between the lesion and the normal bone. Malignant transformation, though very rare, should be suspected when there is endosteal or cortical erosion; especially, if there is cortical destruction with associated soft-tissue. FD may be complicated by fractures.

Most lesions are metabolically active and hence show increased uptake on bone scans and increased metabolic activity with PET.

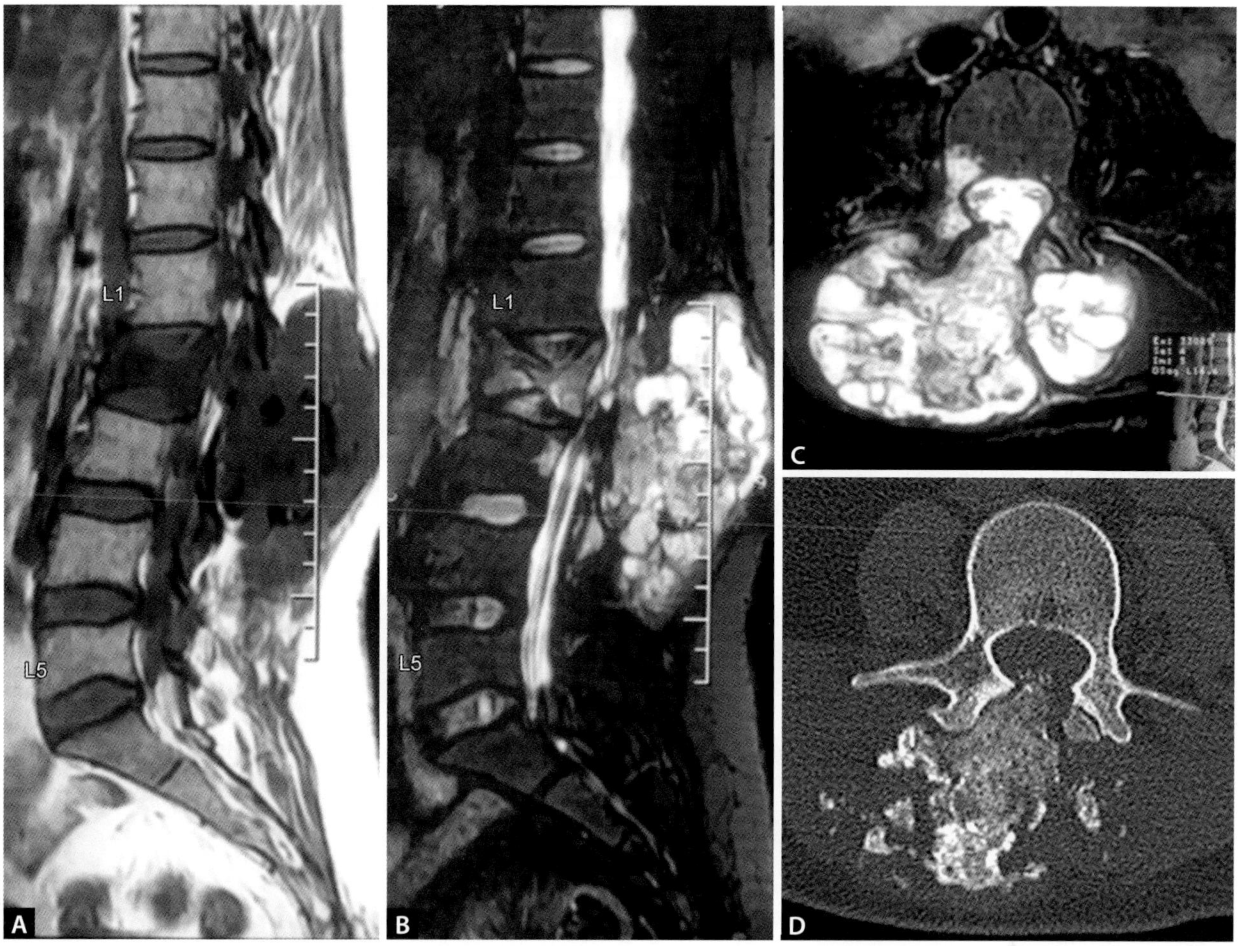

Figs. 19A to D: Chondrosarcoma: Sagittal T1WI (A), sagittal T2WI (B) and axial T2WI (C) show a mass lesion involving body and posterior elements of the L2 vertebra. The mass is hypointense on T1 (A) and hyperintense on T2 (B and C). Axial CT scan (D) shows ossification within the mass lesion.

EPIDURAL LESIONS

Angiolipoma

Spinal angiolipomas are rare lesions usually found in the epidural space of the thoracic spine.[82,83] Most patients present in their middle age with slowly progressive symptoms of spinal cord compression. Most of these lesions are found in adults and in the thoracic region. Spinal angiolipomas are typically located in the posterior and lateral aspects of the epidural space. However, infiltrating forms of tumor are generally located in the anterior epidural space.[82,83] On MRI, angiolipomas are predominantly hyperintense on T1WI and inhomogeneous owing to interspersed vascular elements **(Figs. 20A to D)**. A high vascular content is correlated with the presence of large hypointense regions on T1WI. These masses are hyperintense on T2WI.[83] The larger tumors may cause compression of the spinal cord. Intramedullary angiolipomas have rarely been described **(Figs. 21A to D)**.[83]

Epidural Lipomatosis

This entity, although not a tumor, may behave as one and result in compression of neural elements and thus is discussed here. The most common cause of epidural lipomatosis is prolonged treatment with steroids and rarely endogenous Cushing's syndrome.[84] Epidural lipomatosis may also be seen in morbidly obese patients. In this rare entity, there is hypertrophy of the normal epidural fat, particularly on the dorsal aspects of the thoracic spine and less commonly in the lumbar region. The most common symptom is back pain, but compression of the spinal cord may occur. If the fat grows at the level of neural foramina, radiculopathies may also occur.

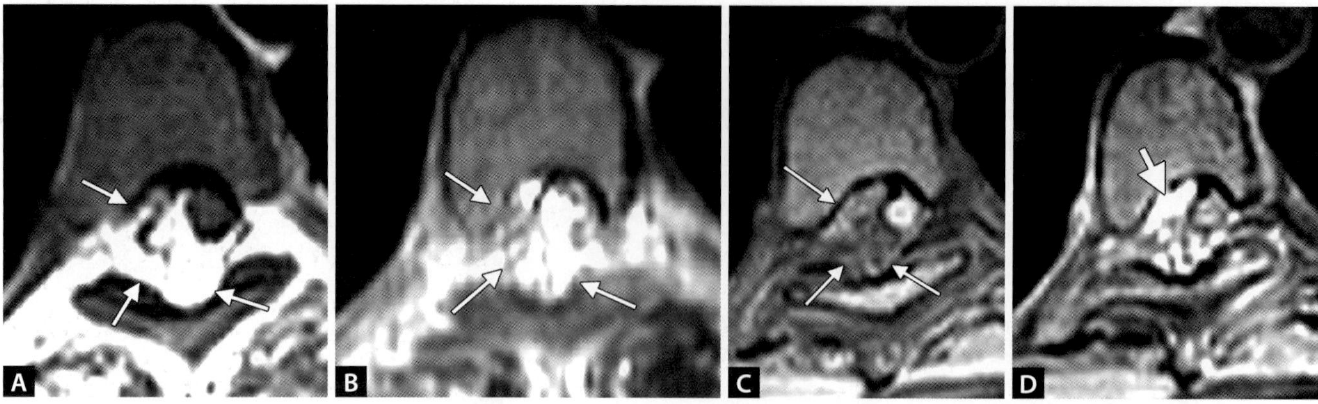

Figs. 20A to D: Extradural angiolipoma: Axial T1WI (A) and T2WI (B) show an extradural hyperintense mass (arrows in A and B) displacing the spinal cord anteriorly and to the left side. Axial T1-weighted fat-saturated image (C) showing diffuse, nearly homogeneous decrease in the signal intensity of the mass (arrows in C) suggestive of fatty tissue. Axial T1-weighted post-gadolinium fat-saturation image (D) showing enhancement of the extradural lesion (arrow in D).

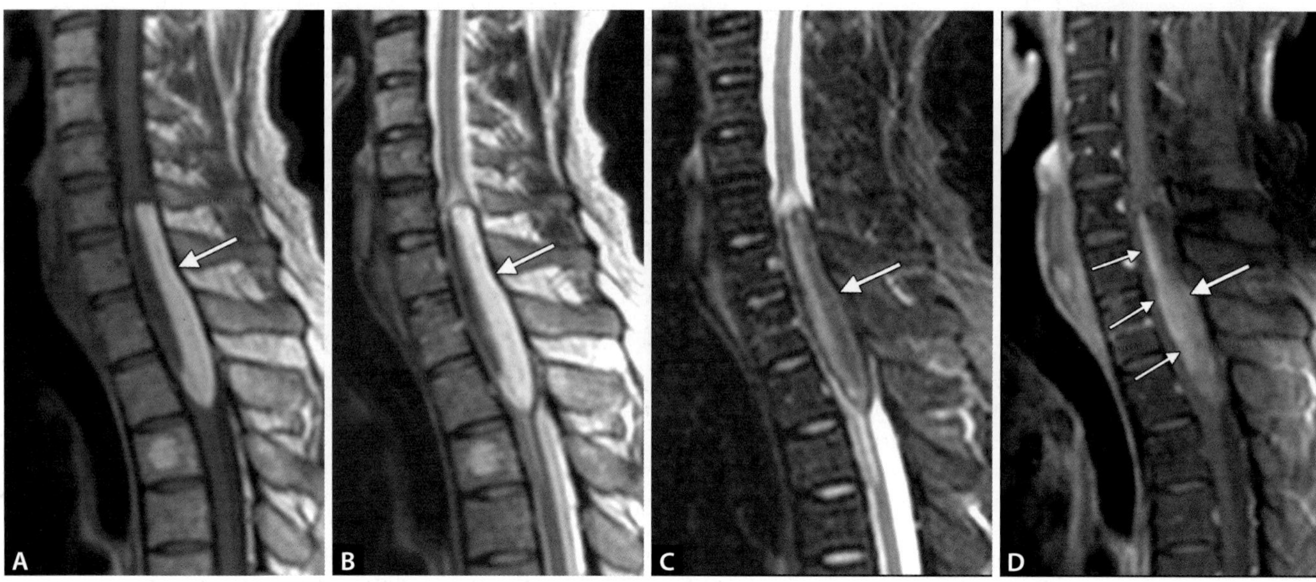

Figs. 21A to D: Intramedullary angiolipoma: Sagittal T1WI (A) and T2WI (B) showing the intramedullary angiolipoma. The dorsal component of the mass shows homogeneous high signal intensity, while the ventral component is heterogeneously hyperintense. No vascular flow voids are seen. Sagittal T1-fat-saturated image shows suppression of signal in the dorsal component (C and D).

The typical MRI appearance of epidural lipomatosis is that of T1 bright excessively thickened epidural fat (>5 to 6 mm) on the posterior aspect of the canal on sagittal images. The subarachnoid spaces are narrowed and the thoracic spinal cord appears thin. The superior and inferior aspects of the lipomatosis taper smoothly and usually extend at least six vertebral segments in length. On axial images, excessive fat is noted on the posterior aspect of the canal, extending laterally. This normal fat does not enhance after contrast administration. On CT, the abnormal fat is of low density and on myelography the fat may compress the canal and result in complete blockage of the passage of contrast. Similar findings are noted when epidural lipomatosis develops in the lumbar region.

CONCLUSION

It is important for the radiologist to be familiar with the imaging characteristics of spinal neoplasms. On the basis of patient's age, lesion location and radiologic appearance, a reasonable differential diagnosis can be arrived for most spinal tumors. A multimodality approach is very helpful to accurately characterize the lesion. It narrows down the differential diagnosis significantly. MR imaging is a particularly useful tool for evaluation of intramedullary neoplasms, whereas CT and MRI are complementary for the evaluation of extradural bony lesions.

REFERENCES

1. Moquin RR, Sandhu FA, Henderson FC. Cystic Intramedullary Neoplasms of the Spinal Cord. Seminars in Spine Surgery. 2006;18(3):168-74.
2. Smith AB, Soderlund KA, Rushing EJ, Smirniotopolous JG. Radiologic-pathologic correlation of pediatric and adolescent spinal neoplasms: Part 1, Intramedullary spinal neoplasms. Am J Roentgenol. 2012;198(1):34-43.
3. Sun B, Wang C, Wang J, Liu A. MRI features of intramedullary spinal cord ependymomas. J Neuroimaging. 2003;13 (4):346-51.
4. Koeller KK, Rosenblum RS, Morrison AL. Neoplasms of the spinal cord and filum terminale: radiologic-pathologic correlation. Radiographics. 2000;20(6):1721-49.
5. Kahan H, Sklar EM, Post MJ, Bruce JH. MR characteristics of histopathologic subtypes of spinal ependymoma. Am J Neuroradiol. 1996;17(1):143-50.
6. Nadkarni TD, Rekate HL. Pediatric intramedullary spinal cord tumors. Critical review of the literature. Childs Nerv Syst. 1999;15(1):17-28.
7. Choudhri AF, Whitehead MT, Klimo P, Jr, Montgomery BK, Boop FA. Diffusion tensor imaging to guide surgical planning in intramedullary spinal cord tumors in children. Neuroradiology. 2014;56(2):169-74.
8. Benesch M, Weber-Mzell D, Gerber NU, von Hoff K, Deinlein F, Krauss J, et al. Ependymoma of the spinal cord in children and adolescents: a retrospective series from the HIT database. J Neurosurg Pediatr. 2010;6(2):137-44.
9. Hallacq P, Labrousse F, Streichenberger N, Lisii D, Fischer G. Bifocal myxopapillary ependymoma of the terminal filum: the end of a spectrum? Journal of Neurosurgery: Spine. 2003;98(3):288-9.
10. Wippold FJ 2nd, Smirniotopoulos JG, Moran CJ, Suojanen JN, Vollmer DG. MR imaging of myxopapillary ependymoma: findings and value to determine extent of tumor and its relation to intraspinal structures. Am J Roentgenol. 1995;165(5):1263-7.
11. Jallo GI, Zagzag D, Epstein F. Intramedullary subependymoma of the spinal cord. Neurosurgery. 1996;38 (2):251-7.
12. Sarkar C, Mukhopadhyay S, Ralte AM, Sharma MC, Gupta A, Gaikwad S, et al. Intramedullary subependymoma of the spinal cord: a case report and review of literature. Clinical Neurology and Neurosurgery. 2003;106(1):63-8.
13. Hoeffel C, Boukobza M, Polivka M, Lot G, Guichard JP, Lafitte F, et al. MR manifestations of subependymomas. Am J Neuroradiol. 1995;16(10):2121-9.
14. Seo HS, Kim JH, Lee DH, Lee YH, Suh SI, Kim SY, et al. Nonenhancing intramedullary astrocytomas and other MR imaging features: a retrospective study and systematic review. Am J Neuroradiol. 2010;31(3):498-503.
15. Ducreux D, Fillard P, Facon D, Ozanne A, Lepeintre JF, Renoux J, et al. Diffusion tensor magnetic resonance imaging and fiber tracking in spinal cord lesions: current and future indications. Neuroimaging Clin N Am. 2007;17(1): 137-47.
16. Setzer M, Murtagh RD, Murtagh FR, Eleraky M, Jain S, Marquardt G, et al. Diffusion tensor imaging tractography in patients with intramedullary tumors: comparison with intraoperative findings and value for prediction of tumor resectability. J Neurosurg Spine. 2010;13(3):371-80.
17. Patel U, Pinto RS, Miller DC, Handler MS, Rorke LB, Epstein FJ, et al. MR of spinal cord ganglioglioma. Am J Neuroradiol. 1998;19(5):879-87.
18. Dudley RW, Torok MR, Gallegos DR, Mulcahy-Levy JM, Hoffman LM, Liu AK, et al. Pediatric low-grade ganglioglioma: epidemiology, treatments, and outcome analysis on 348 children from the surveillance, epidemiology, and end results database. Neurosurgery. 2015;76(3):313-9; discussion 9; quiz 9-20.
19. Lang FF, Epstein FJ, Ransohoff J, Allen JC, Wisoff J, Abbott IR, et al. Central nervous system gangliogliomas. Part 2: Clinical outcome. J Neurosurg. 1993;79(6):867-73.
20. Bambakidis NC, Robinson S, Cohen M, Cohen AR. Atypical teratoid/rhabdoid tumors of the central nervous system: clinical, radiographic and pathologic features. Pediatr Neurosurg. 2002;37(2):64-70.
21. Moeller KK, Coventry S, Jernigan S, Moriarty TM. Atypical teratoid/rhabdoid tumor of the spine. American Journal of Neuroradiology. 2007;28(3):593-5.
22. Niwa T, Aida N, Tanaka M, Okubo J, Sasano M, Shishikura A, et al. Diffusion-weighted imaging of an atypical teratoid/rhabdoid tumor of the cervical spine. Magn Reson Med Sci. 2009;8(3):135-8.
23. Rorke LB, Packer RJ, Biegel JA. Central nervous system atypical teratoid/rhabdoid tumors of infancy and childhood: definition of an entity. J Neurosurg. 1996;85(1):56-65.
24. Chu BC, Terae S, Hida K, Furukawa M, Abe S, Miyasaka K. MR findings in spinal hemangioblastoma: correlation with symptoms and with angiographic and surgical findings. Am J Neuroradiol. 2001;22(1):206-17.
25. Baker KB, Moran CJ, Wippold FJ, Smirniotopoulos JG, Rodriguez FJ, Meyers SP, et al. MR imaging of spinal hemangioblastoma. Am J Roentgenol. 2000;174(2): 377-82.
26. Faro SH, Turtz AR, Koenigsberg RA, Mohamed FB, Chen CY, Stein H. Paraganglioma of the cauda equina with associated intramedullary cyst: MR findings. Am J Neuroradiol. 1997;18(8):1588-90.
27. Shin JY, Lee SM, Hwang MY, Sohn CH, Suh SJ. MR findings of the spinal paraganglioma: report of three cases. J Korean Med Sci. 2001;16(4):522-6.
28. Lin YY, Lin CJ, Ho DM, Guo WY, Chang CY. Primary intramedullary spinal cord lymphoma. Spine J. 2012;12(6):527-8.
29. Flanagan EP, O'Neill BP, Porter AB, Lanzino G, Haberman TM, Keegan BM. Primary intramedullary spinal cord lymphoma. Neurology. 2011;77(8):784-91.

30. Koeller KK, Smirniotopoulos JG, Jones RV. Primary central nervous system lymphoma: radiologic-pathologic correlation. Radiographics. 1997;17(6):1497-526.
31. Kalaycı M, Çağavi F, Gül S, Yenidünya S, Açıkgöz B. Intramedullary spinal cord metastases: diagnosis and treatment—an illustrated review. Acta Neurochirurgica. 2004;146(12):1347-54.
32. Rykken JB, Diehn FE, Hunt CH, Schwartz KM, Eckel LJ, Wood CP, et al. Intramedullary spinal cord metastases: MRI and relevant clinical features from a 13-year institutional case series. Am J Neuroradiol. 2013;34(10):2043-9.
33. Rykken JB, Diehn FE, Hunt CH, Eckel LJ, Schwartz KM, Kaufmann TJ, et al. Rim and flame signs: postgadolinium MRI findings specific for non-CNS intramedullary spinal cord metastases. Am J Neuroradiol. 2013;34(4):908-15.
34. Yoshiura T, Shrier DA, Pilcher WH, Rubio A. Cervical spinal meningioma with unusual MR contrast enhancement. Am J Neuroradiol. 1998;19(6):1040-2.
35. Rossi A, Gandolfo C, Morana G, Tortori-Donati P. Tumors of the spine in children. Neuroimaging Clin N Am. 2007;17(1):17-35.
36. Van Goethem JWM, van den Hauwe L, Özsarlak Ö, De Schepper AMA, Parizel PM. Spinal tumors. Eur J Radiol. 2004;50(2):159-76.
37. Kyoshima K, Horiuchi T, Zenisaka H, Nakazato F. Thoracic dumbbell intra- and extramedullary schwannoma. Journal of Clinical Neuroscience. 2005;12(4):481-4.
38. Wilne S, Walker D. Spine and spinal cord tumours in children: a diagnostic and therapeutic challenge to healthcare systems. Arch Dis Child Educ Pract Ed. 2010;95(2): 47-54.
39. Pilavaki M, Chourmouzi D, Kiziridou A, Skordalaki A, Zarampoukas T, Drevelengas A. Imaging of peripheral nerve sheath tumors with pathologic correlation: Pictorial review. Eur J Radiol. 2004;52(3): 229-39.
40. Jaramillo D. Whole-body MR imaging, bone diffusion imaging: how and why? Pediatr Radiol. 2010;40(6):978-84.
41. Perrin RG, Laxton AW. Metastatic spine disease: epidemiology, pathophysiology, and evaluation of patients. Neurosurgery Clinics of North America. 2004;15(4):365.
42. Park SW, Lee JH, Ehara S, Park YB, Sung SO, Choi JA, et al. Single shot fast spin echo diffusion-weighted MR imaging of the spine—Is it useful in differentiating malignant metastatic tumor infiltration from benign fracture edema? Clinical Imaging. 2004;28(2):102-8.
43. Mulleman D, Gaxatte C, Guillerm G, Leroy X, Cotten A, Duquesnoy B, et al. Multiple myeloma presenting with widespread osteosclerotic lesions. Joint Bone Spine. 2004;71(1):79-83.
44. Baur-Melnyk A, Buhmann S, Durr HR, Reiser M. Role of MRI for the diagnosis and prognosis of multiple myeloma. European Journal of Radiology. 2005;55(1):56-63.
45. Angtuaco EJC, Fassas ABT, Walker R, Sethi R, Barlogie B. Multiple myeloma: Clinical review and diagnostic imaging. Radiology. 2004;231(1):11-23.
46. Guermazi A, Brice P, de Kerviler EE, Ferme C, Hennequin C, Meignin V, et al. Extranodal Hodgkin disease: spectrum of disease. Radiographics. 2001;21(1):161-79.
47. Cross JJ, Antoun NM, Laing RJ, Xuereb J. Imaging of compressive vertebral haemangiomas. Eur Radiol. 2000;10(6):997-1002.
48. Laredo JD, Reizine D, Bard M, Merland JJ. Vertebral hemangiomas: radiologic evaluation. Radiology. 1986;161 (1):183-9.
49. Gaston A, Nguyen JP, Djindjian M, Le Bras F, Gherardi R, Benhaiem N, et al. Vertebral haemangioma: CT and arteriographic features in three cases. J Neuroradiol. 1985; 12(1):21-33.
50. Friedman DP. Symptomatic vertebral hemangiomas: MR findings. Am J Roentgenol. 1996;167(2):359-64.
51. Sanerkin NG, Mott MG, Roylance J. An unusual intraosseous lesion with fibroblastic, osteoclastic, osteoblastic, aneurysmal and fibromyxoid elements. "Solid" variant of aneurysmal bone cyst. Cancer. 1983;51(12):2278-86.
52. Koci TM, Mehringer CM, Yamagata N, Chiang F. Aneurysmal bone cyst of the thoracic spine: evolution after particulate embolization. Am J Neuroradiol. 1995;16(4 Suppl): 857-60.
53. Kransdorf MJ, Sweet DE. Aneurysmal bone cyst: concept, controversy, clinical presentation, and imaging. Am J Roentgenol. 1995;164(3):573-80.
54. Diel J, Ortiz O, Losada RA, Price DB, Hayt MW, Katz DS. The sacrum: pathologic spectrum, multimodality imaging, and subspecialty approach. Radiographics. 2001;21(1):83-104.
55. Murphey MD, Andrews CL, Flemming DJ, Temple HT, Smith WS, Smirniotopoulos JG. From the archives of the AFIP. Primary tumors of the spine: radiologic pathologic correlation. Radiographics. 1996;16(5):1131-58.
56. Hudson TM. Fluid levels in aneurysmal bone cysts: a CT feature. Am J Roentgenol. 1984;142(5):1001-4.
57. Mahnken A, Nolte-Ernsting C, Wildberger J, Heussen N, Adam G, Wirtz D, et al. Aneurysmal bone cyst: value of MR imaging and conventional radiography. Eur Radiol. 2003;13(5):1118-24.
58. Tsai JC, Dalinka MK, Fallon MD, Zlatkin MB, Kressel HY. Fluid-fluid level: a nonspecific finding in tumors of bone and soft tissue. Radiology. 1990;175(3):779-82.
59. Suzuki M, Satoh T, Nishida J, Kato S, Toba T, Honda T, et al. Solid variant of aneurysmal bone cyst of the cervical spine. Spine. 2004;29(17):E376-E81.
60. Llauger J, Palmer J, Amores S, Bague S, Camins A. Primary tumors of the sacrum: diagnostic imaging. Am J Roentgenol. 2000;174(2):417-24.
61. Drevelegas A, Chourmouzi D, Boulogianni G, Sofroniadis I. Imaging of primary bone tumors of the spine. European Radiology. 2003;13(8):1859-71.
62. Schwimer SR, Bassett LW, Mancuso AA, Mirra JM, Dawson EG. Giant cell tumor of the cervicothoracic spine. Am J Roentgenol. 1981;136(1):63-7.
63. Aoki J, Tanikawa H, Ishii K, Seo GS, Karakida O, Sone S, et al. MR findings indicative of hemosiderin in giant-cell tumor

of bone: frequency, cause, and diagnostic significance. Am J Roentgenol. 1996;166(1):145-8.
64. Flemming DJ, Murphey MD, Carmichael BB, Bernard SA. Primary tumors of the spine. Semin Musculoskelet Radiol. 2000;4(3):299-320.
65. Tourniaire J, Bossard D, Gleize B, Tavernier T, Bochu M. Case report 801: osteoid osteoma of the coccyx. Skeletal Radiol. 1993;22(6):457-9.
66. Houang B, Grenier N, Greselle JF, Vital JM, Douws C, Broussin J, et al. Osteoid osteoma of the cervical spine. Misleading MR features about a case involving the uncinate process. Neuroradiology. 1990;31(6):549-51.
67. Kransdorf MJ, Stull MA, Gilkey FW, Moser RP Jr. Osteoid osteoma. Radiographics. 1991;11(4):671-96.
68. Kroon HM, Schurmans J. Osteoblastoma: clinical and radiologic findings in 98 new cases. Radiology. 1990;175(3):783-90.
69. Kumar R, Guinto FC, Jr., Madewell JE, David R, Shirkhoda A. Expansile bone lesions of the vertebra. Radiographics. 1988;8(4):749-69.
70. Crim JR, Mirra JM, Eckardt JJ, Seeger LL. Widespread inflammatory response to osteoblastoma: the flare phenomenon. Radiology. 1990;177(3):835-6.
71. Lucas DR, Unni KK, McLeod RA, O'Connor MI, Sim FH. Osteoblastoma: clinicopathologic study of 306 cases. Hum Pathol. 1994;25(2):117-34.
72. Albrecht S, Crutchfield JS, SeGall GK. On spinal osteochondromas. J Neurosurg. 1992;77(2):247-52.
73. Barros F TEP, Oliveira RP, Taricco MA, Gonzalez CH. Hereditary multiple exostoses and cervical ventral protuberance causing disphagia. Spine. 1995;20(14): 1640-2.
74. Wippold FJ, 2nd, Koeller KK, Smirniotopoulos JG. Clinical and imaging features of cervical chordoma. Am J Roentgenol. 1999;172(5):1423-6.
75. Smolders D, Wang X, Drevelengas A, Vanhoenacker F, De Schepper AM. Value of MRI in the diagnosis of non-clival, non-sacral chordoma. Skeletal Radiology. 2003;32(6):343-50.
76. Sung MS, Lee GK, Kang HS, Kwon ST, Park JG, Suh JS, et al. Sacrococcygeal chordoma: MR imaging in 30 patients. Skeletal Radiology. 2004;34(2):87-94.
77. Sundaresan N, Rosen G, Boriani S. Primary malignant tumors of the spine. Orthop Clin North Am. 2009;40(1): 21-36.
78. Mummaneni PV, Rosenberg WS. Spinal chondrosarcoma following adenocarcinoma of the breast: case report. Surg Neurol. 2000;53(6):580-2.
79. Shives TC, McLeod RA, Unni KK, Schray MF. Chondrosarcoma of the spine. J Bone Joint Surg Am. 1989;71 (8):1158-65.
80. Fitzpatrick KA, Taljanovic MS, Speer DP, Graham AR, Jacobson JA, Barnes GR, et al. Imaging Findings of Fibrous Dysplasia with Histopathologic and Intraoperative Correlation. American Journal of Roentgenology. 2004;182 (6):1389-98.
81. Park SK, Lee IS, Choi J-Y, Cho KH, Suh KJ, Lee JW, et al. CT and MRI of fibrous dysplasia of the spine. Br J Radiol 2012;85 (1015):996-1001.
82. Garg A, Gupta V, Gaikwad S, Deol P, Mishra NK, Sharma MC, et al. Spinal angiolipoma: report of three cases and review of MRI features. Australas Radiol. 2002;46(1): 84-90.
83. Samdani AF, Garonzik IM, Jallo G, Eberhart CG, Zahos P. Spinal angiolipoma: case report and review of the literature. Acta Neurochirurgica. 2004;146(3):299-302.
84. Bodelier AGL, Groeneveld W, van der Linden AN, Haak HR. Symptomatic epidural lipomatosis in ectopic Cushing's syndrome. European Journal of Endocrinology. 2004;151(6):765-9.

CHAPTER 34

Spinal Vascular Malformations

Shailesh B Gaikwad

INTRODUCTION

Vascular lesions of the spinal cord are heterogeneous group of disorders with wide spectrum ranging from lesions with simple angioarchitecture such as dural or pial arteriovenous fistula to complex arteriovenous malformations (AVM). Although they are relatively uncommon disorders, they are potentially curable causes of progressive myelopathy hence requiring comprehensive evaluation both clinically and radiologically. Diagnosis of spinal vascular malformations mainly rests on magnetic resonance imaging (MRI), while selective digital subtraction angiography (DSA) is needed for thorough understanding of the disease process, for characterization of its angioarchitecture and planning the therapeutic strategy.

Classification

Classification of vascular lesions of the spinal cord have been confusing in the literature, as there are multiple systems of classifications proposed, with overlapping criteria to classify these disorders.

Genetically spinal cord vascular malformations are classified as three broad categories.

1. Hereditary lesions caused by mutations in vascular germinal cells, e.g. malformations associated with hereditary hemorrhagic telangiectasia (HHT) **(Figs. 1A to E)**
2. Non-hereditary genetic lesions caused by somatic mutations which share metameric links, e.g. spinal AV metameric syndromes (Cobb, Klippel-Trenaunay, and Parkes-Weber syndromes)
3. Isolated sporadic lesions, that are not associated with any genetic links.

In 1993, Anson and Spetzler proposed morphologic classification of spinal cord vascular malformations into the four following morphologic categories, Type I to IV **(Table 1)**.

In 2006, Kim and Spetzler proposed a modified anatomic classification based on anatomic location and type of malformation **(Table 2)**.

In 2002, Spetzler suggested to include spinal artery aneurysms, and tumor and tumor like lesions such as cavernous malformations (cavernomas), hemangio-blastomas, which grossly complete the vascular lesions of spinal cord.

T Krings et al, proposed a simple classification scheme to classify vascular malformations of spine. It is based on a simple questionnaire, which is as follows:

1. Is there a shunt? If no—cavernoma
2. If there is a shunt, what is the feeding artery?
   a. If feeding artery is radiculomeningeal artery (RMA)—spinal dural arteriovenous fistula (SDAVF)
   b. If feeding artery is RMA, then what is the nidus architecture?
      i. Glomus type
      ii. Fistulous type—This is further subdivided into micro and macrofistulous form based on the shunt volume.

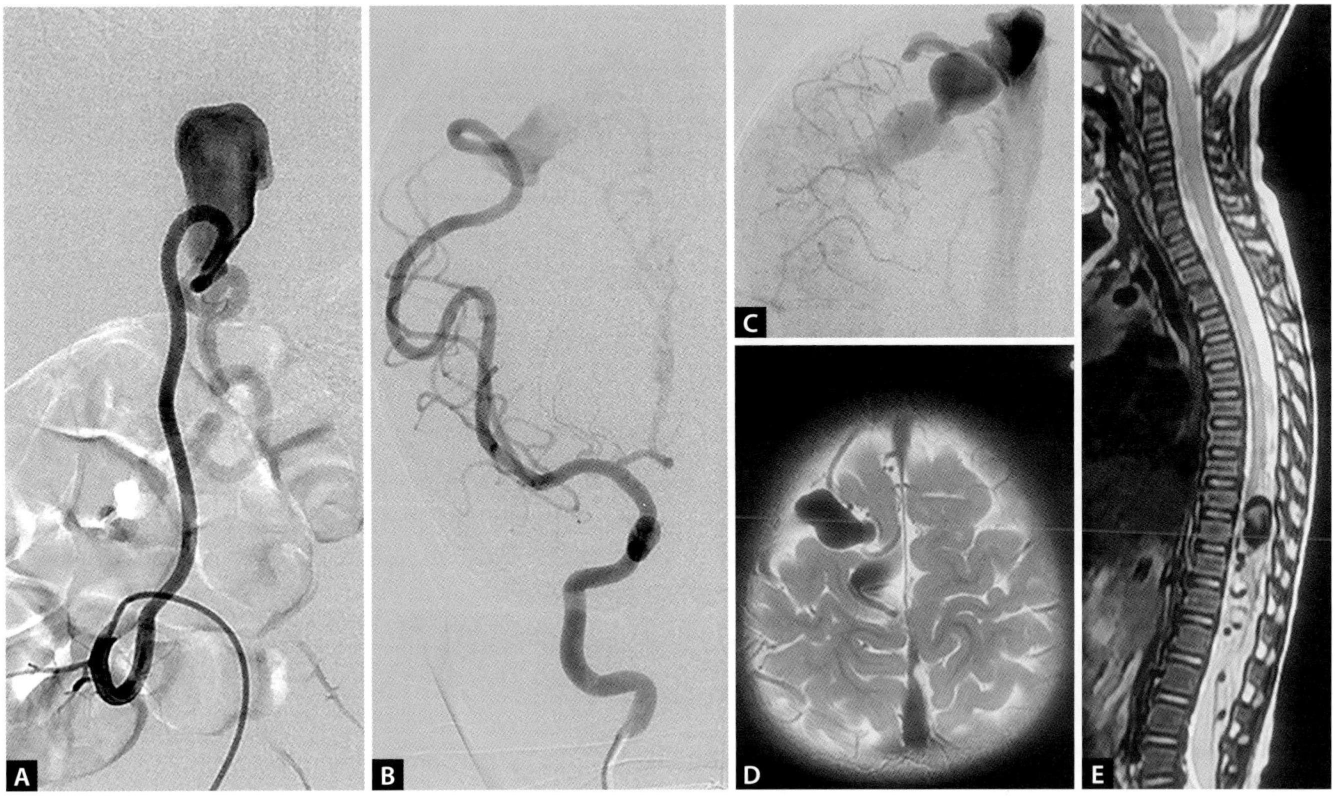

Figs. 1A to E: A 6-year-old boy with hemorrhagic telangiectasia (HHT) shows a spinal cord pial macrofistula (SCAVF) fed by radiculomedullary artery (A); Cerebral angiogram of the same child shows a pial AVF fed by right MCA branches with ectatic venous pouch (B and C). MR images showing right frontal and thoracic cord pial AVFs (D and E).

Table 1: Anson-Spetzler morphologic classification of spinal vascular malformations (1993).

Anson-Spetzler morphologic classification (1993)		*Description*
Type I	Spinal Dural AVF (SDAVF)	Radicular artery communicating directly with a dural vein
Type II	Glomus AVM	Intramedullary pial AVM fed by radiculomedullary or radiculopial arteries
Type III	Juvenile or metameric AVM	Complex juvenile metameric AVMs involving multiple compartments (extradural and intradural), along discrete somite levels
Type IV	Spinal cord AVF (SCAVF)	Pial AVF fed by radiculomedullary or radiculopial arteries

Table 2: Kim and Spetzler modified anatomic classification (2006).

Types		*Other descriptions*
Fistulae	Extradural	Osteodural or anterior epidural and posterior epidural fistulae belong to this group
	Intradural dorsal	Classic Type I lesions (SDAVF)
	Intradural ventral	Classic Type IV lesions (SCAVF)
AVM	Extradural-intradural	Classic Type III lesions (juvenile/ metameric AVM)
	Intradural	Classic Type II lesions (Glomus AVM)
	Conus	Conus AVMs

EXTRADURAL ARTERIOVENOUS FISTULAE (EPIDURAL FISTULAE)

The extradural arteriovenous fistulae, previously called as epidural fistulae, represent an abnormal connection between an artery and the epidural venous plexus (Batson's plexus). This produces engorgement of the epidural plexus and subsequent mass effect upon the spinal cord. Venous drainage can be confined to the epidural space or may reflux into the perimedullary veins. These occur commonly in the thoracic spine. Anatomically they can be further divided into anterior (osteodural) **(Fig. 2)** and posterior **(Fig. 3)** subgroups, depending upon the vein in which the

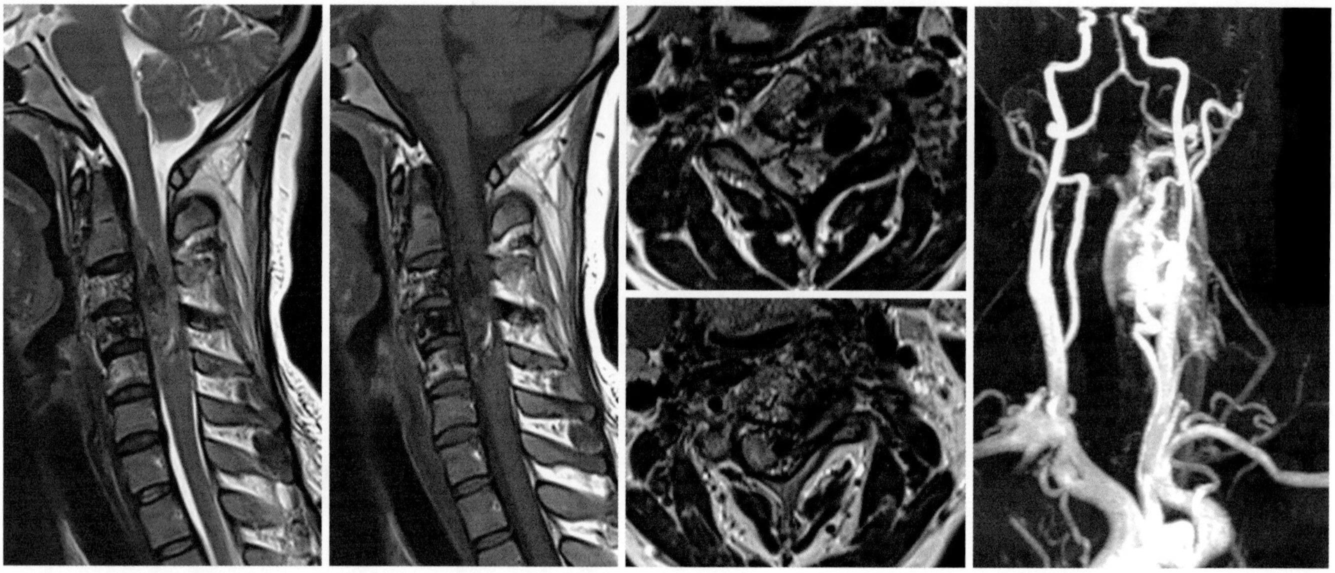

Fig. 2: Anterior epidural fistula: A 24-year-old female patient with paresthesia and quadriparesis. T1 and T2WI shows heterogeneous anterior extradural lesion with areas of hypointensity and hyperintensity s/o hemorrhages. Note extensive osteolysis involving vertebral bodies of C3 to C5. Axial images show extradural location of flow voids with mass effect over the cord. CE MRA images show the fistula fed by branches of left ascending and deep cervical artery.

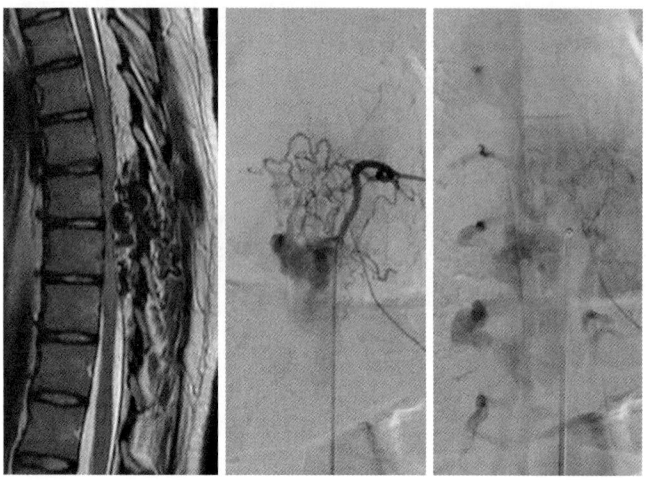

Fig. 3: Posterior epidural fistula: A 26-year-old male patient with paraparesis. T2WI shows multiple vascular flow voids in posterior epidural space, compressing the cord. Selective DSA shows the fistula fed by multiple small arterial feeders from the intercostal artery. Venous phase of the angiogram shows the venous drainage into azygos-hemiazygos system, and not into the intradural veins.

fistula is opening. Rangel-Castilla et al. proposed a subclassification system of extradural arteriovenous fistulae into three types: A, B1, and B2. Type A fistulae have at least one intradural draining vein, while type B have purely extradural drainage. Type B1 has mass effect on the thecal sac and cord, no mass effect is seen in type B2.

Clinically they present with progressive myelopathy, mainly secondary to mass effect over the cord by engorged epidural veins. Symptoms secondary to congestive myelopathy may be seen if the drainage is seen into the intradural veins. Patients may also present with radiculopathy due to mass effect over nerve roots. Hemorrhage is rare.

MRI examination reveals engorged epidural veins either anteriorly or posteriorly which may exert mass effect over the cord. Cord signal intensity changes may be present. Adjacent bones, especially vertebral bodies can show osteolysis. Selective DSA shows fistula draining into the epidural venous plexus. On very rare occasions an intradural draining vein may be seen.

These lesions are effectively treated by endovascular means, using liquid embolization agents mainly n-butyl cyanoacrylate (NBCA, glue) or Onyx. In cases were the fistula could not be approached by microcatheter, open surgery can be used. Incomplete occlusion of the fistula actively recruits new feeders, resulting in recurrence.

DORSAL INTRADURAL ARTERIOVENOUS FISTULA (SPINAL DURAL ARTERIOVENOUS FISTULA)

Dorsal intradural AVFs correspond to the classic Type I lesions in the Anson-Spetzler classification. They are the most common type of spinal AV fistula, making up about

70% of all spinal AV malformations. There is a male predominance (M:F - 5:1), and it is usually diagnosed in the 5th to 6th decades of life. They are mostly found in the thoracic and thoracolumbar regions (more than 80%).

SDAVFs are formed by an abnormal connection between one or more radiculomeningeal arteries and the venous outflow. The shunt is located intradurally at the level of the dural sleeve surrounding the nerve root and drains into perimedullary veins. They have slow flow and are grouped into 2 subtypes. Subtype A has a single feeding artery while Subtype B has multiple feeders. Unlike the other spinal vascular malformations, this type of AVF is acquired.

The pathogenesis of SDAVF was first described in 1926 by Foix and Alajouanine. They described a progressive subacute necrotizing myelopathy, now known as Foix-Alajouanine syndrome, and found vascular obstruction, spinal cord necrosis and tortuous and dilated vessels on the surface of the spinal cord. They proposed that spinal cord ischemia is secondary to venous congestion or hypertension, which is the hallmark of this disease. Venous hypertension results in decreased arteriovenous pressure gradient resulting in vascular slowing. This results in progressive venous congestion and edema of the cord parenchyma with progressive symptoms.

Early symptoms of SDAVF are often non-specific which leads to delay in diagnosis. Lower extremity weakness is the most common initial presenting symptom, seen in about half of the cases. Other symptoms seen at presentation, include gait disturbance, paresthesia, back pain and bladder/bowel or sexual dysfunction. Hemorrhage is rare.

MRI is the initial image modality used in the evaluation when SDAVF is suspected. MRI shows increased signal intensity in the cord on T2-weighted images, which corresponds to cord edema which usually spans multiple levels. Dorsal intradural flow voids may be present and are more evident on heavily T2-weighted images or contrast-enhanced T1-weighted images. Selective catheter angiography is the gold standard for diagnosis of SDAVF. It also provides an opportunity for possible endovascular treatment. It usually shows a small low-flow fistula fed by dorsal radiculomeningeal artery draining into intradural veins with venous congestion **(Figs. 4A to F)**.

Conventionally, surgery is used as the main modality of treatment. The target of surgical or endovascular treatment is the arterialized proximal part of the draining vein. After performing a hemi-laminectomy and opening the dura, corresponding dorsal radiculomeningeal artery is followed, as it heads towards the dorsal nerve root. The artery-vein connection is disrupted by either coagulation, ligation or clipping. Surgery is associated with very low morbidity (2%), with complete occlusion achieved in >98% of patients.

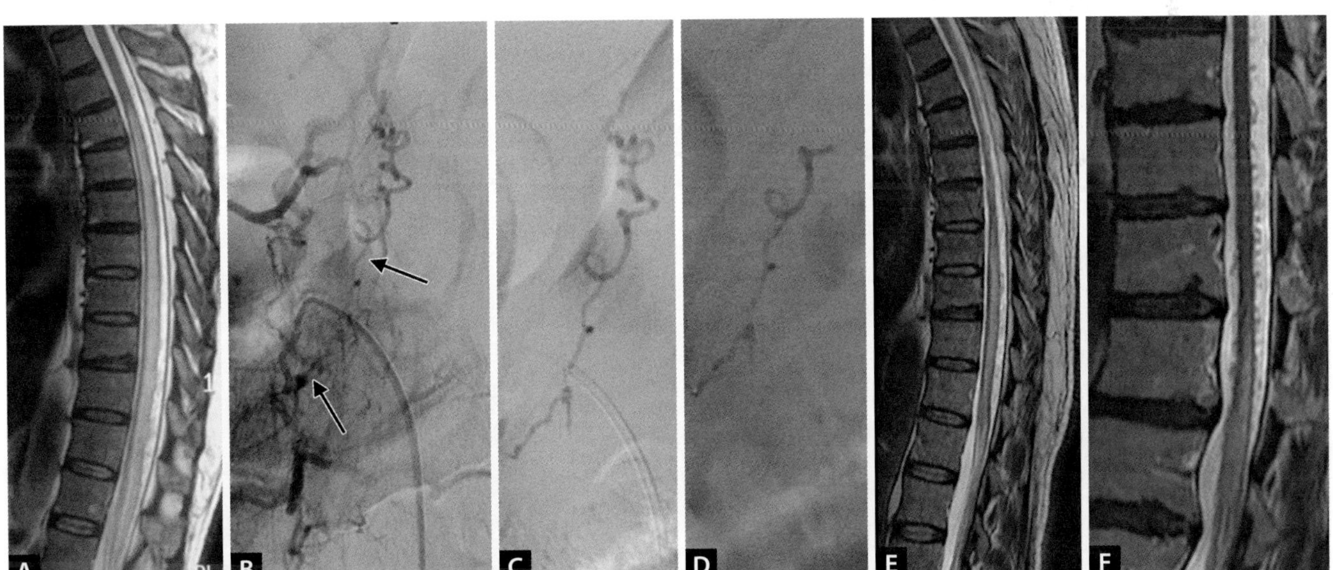

Figs. 4A to F: Dorsal intradural AVF (SDAVF): A 52-year-old male with slowly progressive paraparesis, bladder and bowel involvement. (A) Preprocedure MRI showing extensive spinal cord edema and vascular flow voids; (B) DSA and (C) microcatheter run showing fistula (black arrow, down) with draining vein (black arrow, up); (D) Glue cast; (E) Follow-up MRI showing reduction in spinal cord signal changes; (F) MRI of another patient with SDAVF shows spinal cord signal intensity changes and vascular flow voids dorsal to the cord in intradural location.

The recent advances in endovascular procedures have given an alternative to surgical treatment of SDAVFs. It is less invasive, and may be performed at the same time as the diagnostic spinal angiogram. Early endovascular procedures used polyvinyl alcohol particles (PVA), however, this had high recanalization rates. Recurrence is less with liquid embolization agents like NBCA and Onyx. Embolization is contraindicated in patients where a radiculomedullary artery arises from the same pedicle as the feeder. Endovascular attempts in such cases may result in spinal cord ischemia and grave neurological deficits. Due to the small size and tortuous anatomy of the arterial feeder, microcatheterization may fail, resulting in need for surgery.

Prognosis after treatment depends on the duration and severity of pretreatment symptoms. Motor symptoms improve better compared with sensory or bladder/bowel symptoms.

VENTRAL INTRADURAL AVF (SPINAL CORD AVF, SCAVF, PERIMEDULLARY AVF)

These lesions correspond to Classic Type IV lesions in the Anson-Spetzler classification **(Figs. 5A to F)**. They are also referred to as perimedullary AVFs or fistulous arteriovenous malformations and are extremely rare, compared with cord AVMs or SDAVFs. They occur in a younger population, commonly presenting in the first and second decade and has no sex predilection.

Ventral intradural AVFs originate from the anterior spinal artery. The fistulous communication lies outside the cord parenchyma and pia matter in the subarachnoid space, anterior to the cord in the midline. Blood flow through these AVFs is very fast and they may have flow-related aneurysms and venous pouches. In contrast to the dorsal types, ventral intradural AVFs are congenital lesions. They can be further subdivided into 3 distinct types based on feeding vessel size, shunt volume and drainage pattern.

1. *Type A:* Small with a single feeder and low shunt volume. The feeding artery and draining vein are not much dilated. Hemodynamic features are similar to dorsal intradural AVFs **(Fig. 6A)**.
2. *Type B:* These are of an intermediate size with a major feeder from anterior spinal artery as well as smaller feeders at the level of the fistula.
3. *Type C:* These are giant lesions with multiple large arterial feeders and massively dilated venous vascular channels and large shunt volumes. Hemodynamic features in this subtype is similar to intramedullary AVMs **(Fig. 6B)**.

SCAVFs were first described by Djindjian in 1977 and later classified as Type IV by Heros. There are no capillaries or nidus between the artery and the venous network.

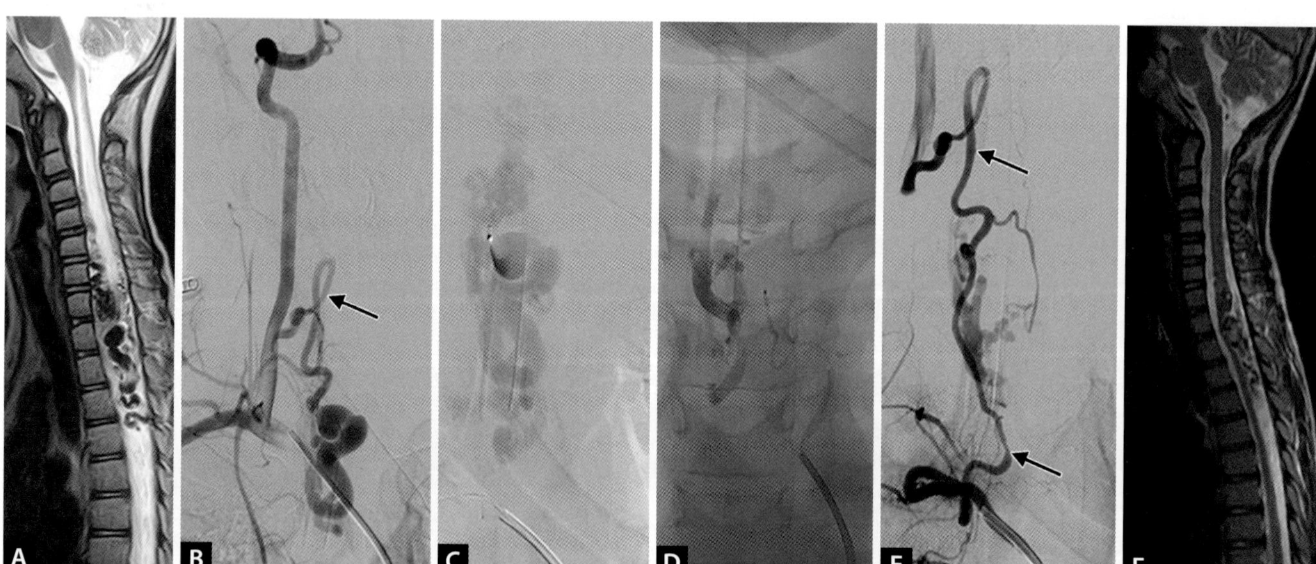

Figs. 5A to F: Ventral intradural AVF (SCAVF): A 7-year-old female with acute onset paraparesis. (A) MRI showing multiple dilated vascular flow voids with extensive cord edema; (B) DSA showing macrofistula fed by RMA (black arrow); (C) Microcatheter run; (D) Glue cast; (E) Check angiogram showing preservation of anterior spinal axis (black arrows); Follow-up MR (F) showing decrease in flow voids and resolution of edema.

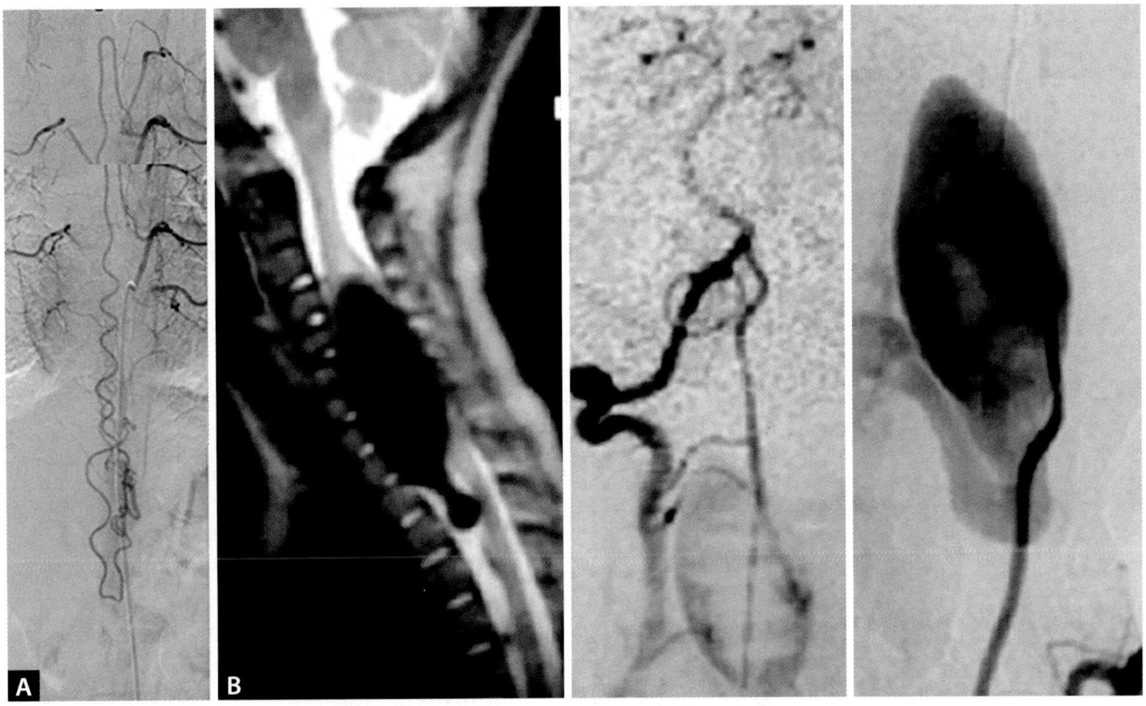

Figs. 6A and B: Spinal cord AV fistula (SCAVF): (A) Microfistula. A 8-year-old male with congestive myelopathy. DSA shows single hole fistula fed by radiculomedullary artery. Note the single arterial feeder directly communicating with vein with no intervening nidus. Note the absence of dilatation or ectasia in the venous side; (B) Macrofistula. A 2-year-old male with acute onset quadriparesis and respiratory distress. MRI shows large sac in the spinal canal; compressing the cord. DSA shows macrofistula with a large venous sac, fed by anterior spinal artery and RMA from left superior intercostal artery.

The pathology is similar to dorsal intradural AVFs with venous hypertension. However, the cause of the venous hypertension is due to vascular steal and mechanical compression, than from slow flow and venous congestion. Hemorrhage is more common and occurs in about 20–40% of patients.

Symptoms are produced by vascular steal, mechanical compression from engorged veins or by subarachnoid or intraparenchymal hemorrhage **(Figs. 7A to D)**. Symptoms are usually progressive in nature, with myelopathy the most common finding. Cases in which a patient present acutely or an acute exacerbation of baseline symptoms are usually a result of hemorrhage.

MR Imaging is often the initial image modality used to diagnose SCAVFs. T2 prolongation in the cord is seen with flow voids on the ventral aspect of the cord or thecal sac. Hemorrhage may be identified as T1 hyperintense signal.

Treatment depends on the subtype of the ventral intradural AVFs. Types A and B may be treated by surgical or endovascular means, while Type C lesions are almost always treated via endovascular route. Surgery is generally difficult since anterior or anterolateral approach is needed to reach the fistula.

Endovascular embolization with liquid embolic agent, especially NBCA with its rapid polymerization time is generally used to treat these fistulas. Care should be taken to preserve the anterior spinal axis while embolization. Outcome of the patient is generally good if the fistula is occluded and anterior spinal axis is preserved.

EXTRADURAL-INTRADURAL ARTERIOVENOUS MALFORMATIONS (JUVENILE/METAMERIC AVM)

Extradural-Intradural AVMs are rare and complex, and has been called type III, metameric, or juvenile AVM **(Figs. 8)**. They arise from single or multiple somites, having both intra and extradural components. They may also have soft tissue, bone or skin involvement, corresponding to the same metamer as that of the cord. Most often they are diffuse and do not have a nidus. They may also be a part of a syndromic complex such as the metameric angiomatosis (Cobb's syndrome), disseminated angiodysplasia (Osler-Weber-Rendu syndrome), Klippel-Trenaunay syndrome, or Parkes-Weber syndrome. This is a high-flow lesion with multiple feeding and draining vessels.

These type of lesions are commonly seen in adolescents and young adults who present with pain or progressive myelopathic symptoms from spinal cord compression, venous hypertension, or vascular steal. Intramedullary or subarachnoid hemorrhage could be the initial presenting symptom.

MRI is the modality of choice as it helps to find the extent of the AV malformation and the compartments involved. As the AVM is more extensive, the goal of the treatment should be to avoid morbidity and not complete radiological cure. Targeted approach is needed to specifically focus on selected problems like venous hypertension, obliterating a part of the AVM, which is causing mass effect or occluding the fistulous part of the AVM.

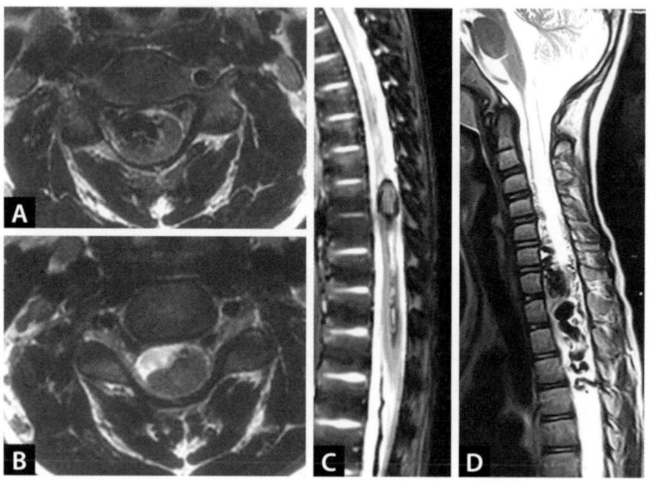

Figs. 7A to D: Causes of myelopathy in SCAVF: (A and B) Mass effect; (C) Hematomyelia; (D) Venous congestion.

INTRAMEDULLARY AVM (GLOMUS AVM)

A spinal intramedullary AVM consists of multiple abnormal vessels constituting a nidus with one or more feeding arteries and draining veins. These lesions were previously classified as type II (glomus) AVMs in the earlier classification by Anson and Spetzler **(Figs. 9A to F)**. The nidus may be intramedullary, intra and extramedullary or located in the conus. These lesions are mostly located in the cervicothoracic region. About 20–40% of spinal intramedullary AVMs are associated with aneurysms and their presence is related with increased risk of bleeding.

They are more simply classified as compact and diffuse forms (Spetzler). The compact forms were earlier classified as glomus type and the diffuse forms were classified as juvenile AVMs. The juvenile AVMs form a distinct subgroup in that they have an embryological basis for their location.

Patients usually present in the third decade of life. Hemorrhage is seen in up to half of the patients. The risk of

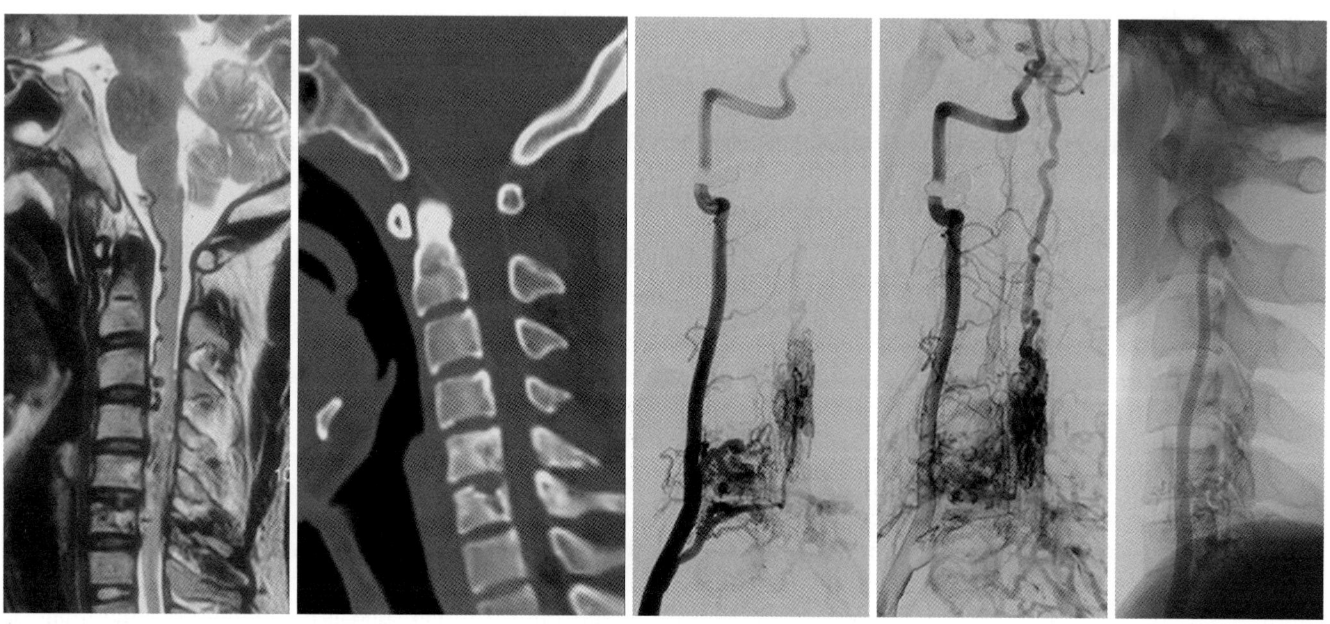
Fig. 8: Juvenile or metameric AVM: T2W sagittal images show osteodural lesions at C5 and C6 vertebral levels with few vascular flow voids within the cord and a prominent vascular channel anterior to cord. Sagittal CT images show osteolysis of C5 and C6 vertebral bodies. DSA images show an epidural fistula at the level of C5 and C6 vertebral bodies and a spinal cord intramedullary AVM at slightly higher level, corresponding to the same somite. Note the venous drainage into anterior spinal vein, which was seen as prominent vascular channel in T2W image.

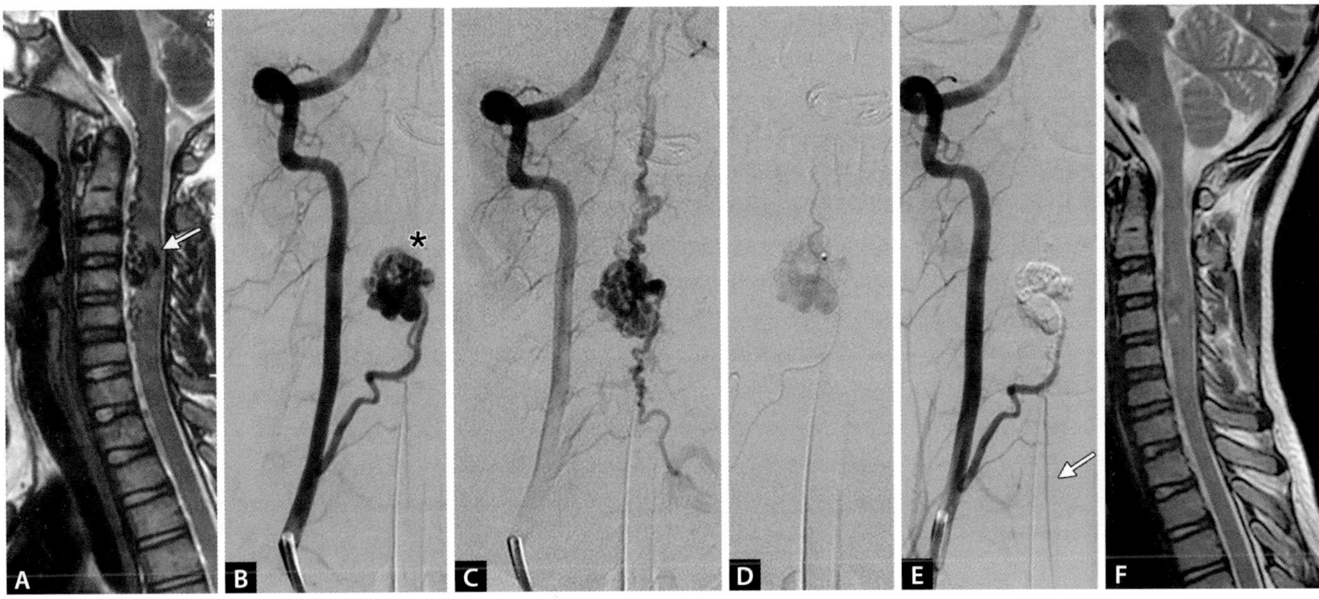

Figs. 9A to F: Intramedullary AVM: MRI of a 9-year-old child with acute onset quadriparesis shows cervical cord AVM (arrow, A). DSA showed glomus type of AVM fed by radiculomedullary artery arising from right vertebral artery (asterisk, B), draining into perimedullary veins (C). Microcatheter angiogram after super-selective catheterization shows visualization of only the nidus and draining vein (D). Embolization of the AVM nidus was done with n-butyl cyanoacrylate (glue). Check angiogram showed complete obliteration of AVM with preservation of anterior spinal axis (arrow, E). Follow-up MRI showed complete obliteration of AVM with non-visualization of flow voids (F).

re-bleeding in patients presenting with hemorrhage is 10% at one month and 40% at one year. No sex predilection is seen. Non-hemorrhagic manifestations include back pain, radicular pain, motor/sensory deficits, sexual disturbance, sphincter disturbances and bruit.

1. *Hemorrhage:* Half of the patients present with subarachnoid hemorrhage or acute medullary syndrome. These patients present with moderate to severe backache and sudden neurologic deficit.
2. *Venous hypertension:* The arterialized veins have dysplastic walls and are not capable of handling high blood pressure. This may either lead to rupture of vessels, or ischemia secondary to congestion. Symptoms may be positional with squatting or raising the leg above heart level causing exacerbation of symptoms.
3. *Venous thrombosis:* Thrombosis due to venous congestion is seen in low flow AVMs. It predisposes to ischemic damage of surrounding cord parenchyma and hemorrhage.
4. *Vascular steal:* Vascular steal is seen in high-flow AVMs. With limited ability to vasoconstrict, blood is sucked into the AVM and the surrounding normal tissue suffers ischemia.
5. *Mechanical compression:* The nidus and venous pouches can cause compression of the cord. Patient may present with combination of myelopathy or radiculopathy secondary to pressure effect of the AVM.

Magnetic resonance imaging (MRI) and magnetic resonance angiography (MRA) are the first choice of investigation although selective catheter angiography is the gold standard for definitive diagnosis and characterization of these lesions. MR features suggestive of vascular malformations include a serpentine pattern of flow voids and spinal cord signal changes due to venous congestion, myelomalacia, infarction and hemorrhage. MRA is increasingly being used for the diagnosis, localization and characterization of spinal AVMs. The limitations of MRA are difficulty in detecting multiple feeding vessels, low sensitivity for detection of spinal aneurysms, and inability to offer treatment in the same sitting.

Digital subtraction angiography is the gold standard for diagnosis of spinal AVM and characterization of its angioarchitecture. Segmental arteries should be individually catheterized on both sides to avoid missing silent lesions. The information to be sought on DSA includes location, feeding pedicle side and site, type of fistula and location of anterior spinal and posterior spinal arteries in relation to the AVM.

There are three modalities for treatment of spinal AVMs, which includes surgery, endovascular and stereotactic radiosurgery. In some cases, a combination of these

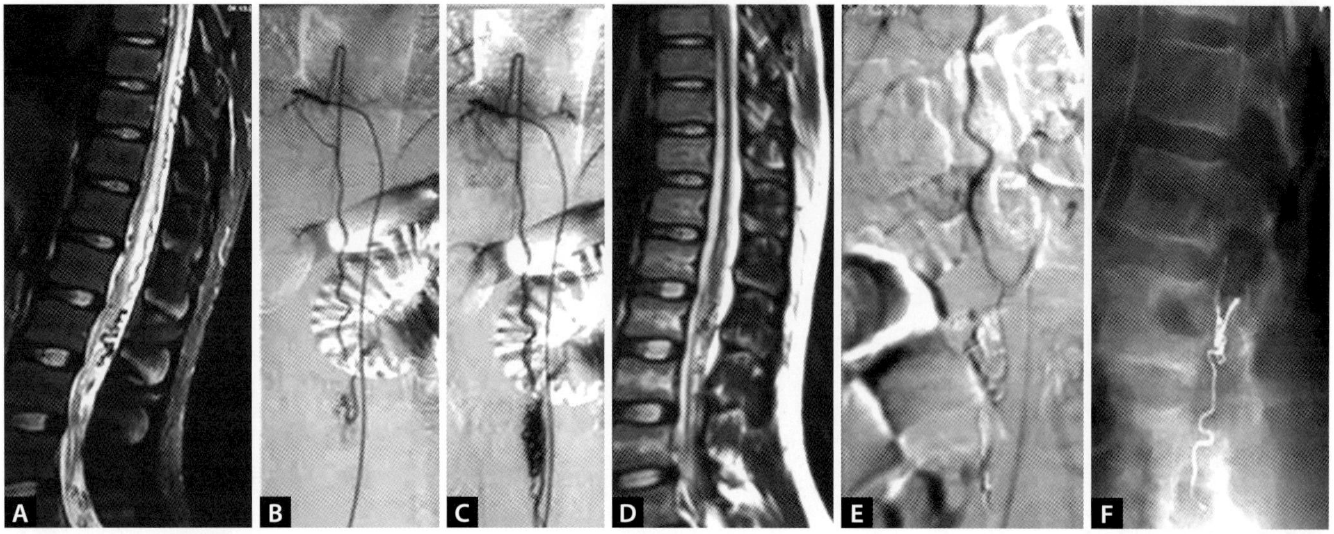

Figs. 10A to F: Spinal cord AVM (conus): (A) Sagittal T2W MRI showing the edematous swollen cord and multiple tortuous dilated vascular channels present both anteriorly and posteriorly; (B and C) RD9 injection, showing the enlarged radiculomedullary artery supplying the complex AVM through anterior spinal axis. Post-embolization imaging: (D) T2W sagittal MRI (done on second post-procedure day) showing complete resolution of the abnormal vascular flow voids and decrease in the bright signal and swelling of the cord; (E) Immediate post-embolization RD9 injection showing complete obliteration of the AVM with adequately filling anterior spinal axis; (F) Onyx cast.

treatment modalities may be tried. Although stereotactic radiosurgery is commonly used in cranial AVMs, its use in spinal AVM is only at the research level. Several articles have quoted the effectiveness of radiosurgery of spinal AVMs.

Endovascular therapy is used either primarily or to reduce the size and flow in the lesion before surgery. Super-selective catheterization of feeder arteries rather than the segmental artery helps in preventing ischemic damage to the normal parenchyma thus reducing the chance of neurological deficits. The most commonly used embolic materials for the embolization of spinal AVMs are NBCA and onyx. Factors that favor a successful endovascular occlusion include normal anterior spinal artery separate from the nidus, short distance between the arterial feeders and the nidus, and high flow through the AVM nidus. Occlusion of the nidus may lead to edema of the surrounding cord and neurological deterioration, which is usually a self-limiting condition and the patient recovers in a few weeks. Use of corticosteroids may be helpful in reducing the edema.

CONUS MEDULLARIS AVM

Conus AVMs are a subset of intramedullary AVMs and consists of lesions at the conus with multiple feeding arteries, multiple diffuse niduses and complex venous drainage. They have multiple direct AV shunts that derive from the anterior and posterior spinal arteries. Niduses are usually extramedullary and pial based. Because of the location of these lesions, patients may present with both upper and lower motor neuron symptoms **(Figs. 10A to F)**.

CAVERNOUS ANGIOMAS (CAVERNOMA) OF SPINAL CORD

Cavernomas are intramedullary vascular malformations which is made of dilated thin walled capillaries and sinusoids. There is generally no feeding artery or a draining vein. Cavernomas cause symptoms by acute cord hemorrhage or rarely subarachnoid hemorrhage. They can also present with progressive myelopathy due to repetitive hemorrhages or toxic degradation products of hemorrhage.

On MR imaging, hypointense hemosiderin rim is seen in T2WI and multi-echo gradient images, with a 'popcorn' hyperintense center. Subacute hemorrhage may be detected as T1 hyperintense signal. Usually no enhancement is seen. Cavernomas are angiographically occult **(Figs. 11A to E)**.

Asymptomatic lesions are followed up. Lesions that present with recurrent hemorrhages are best treated with microsurgical removal. As there is no definite feeding artery, endovascular treatment is not a treatment option for cavernoma.

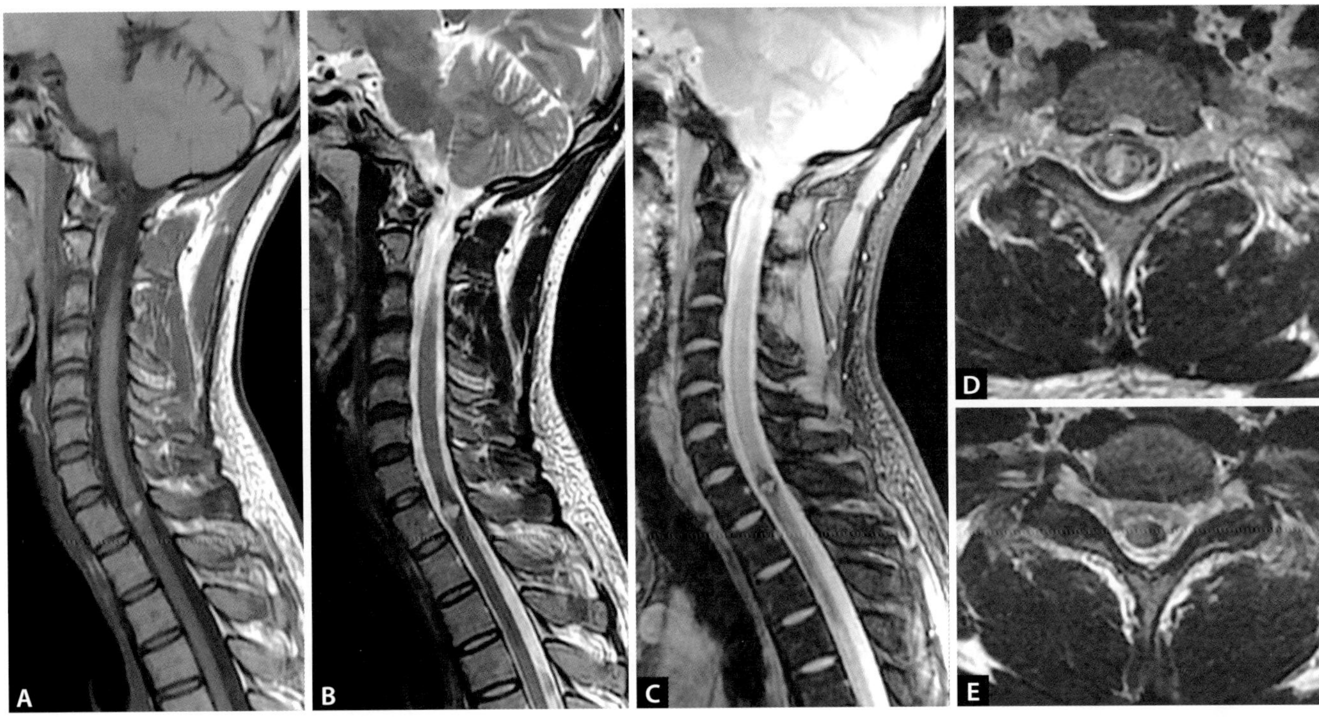

Figs. 11A to E: A 26-year-old male patient with acute onset neck pain and neurological deficits; T1 and T2WI (A and B) show a small focal hyperintense lesion in the cord with hypointense rim in T2WI and GRE (B and C); T2W axial images show hyperintense area of subacute bleed with cord expansion and hypointense area of chronic bleed (D and E).

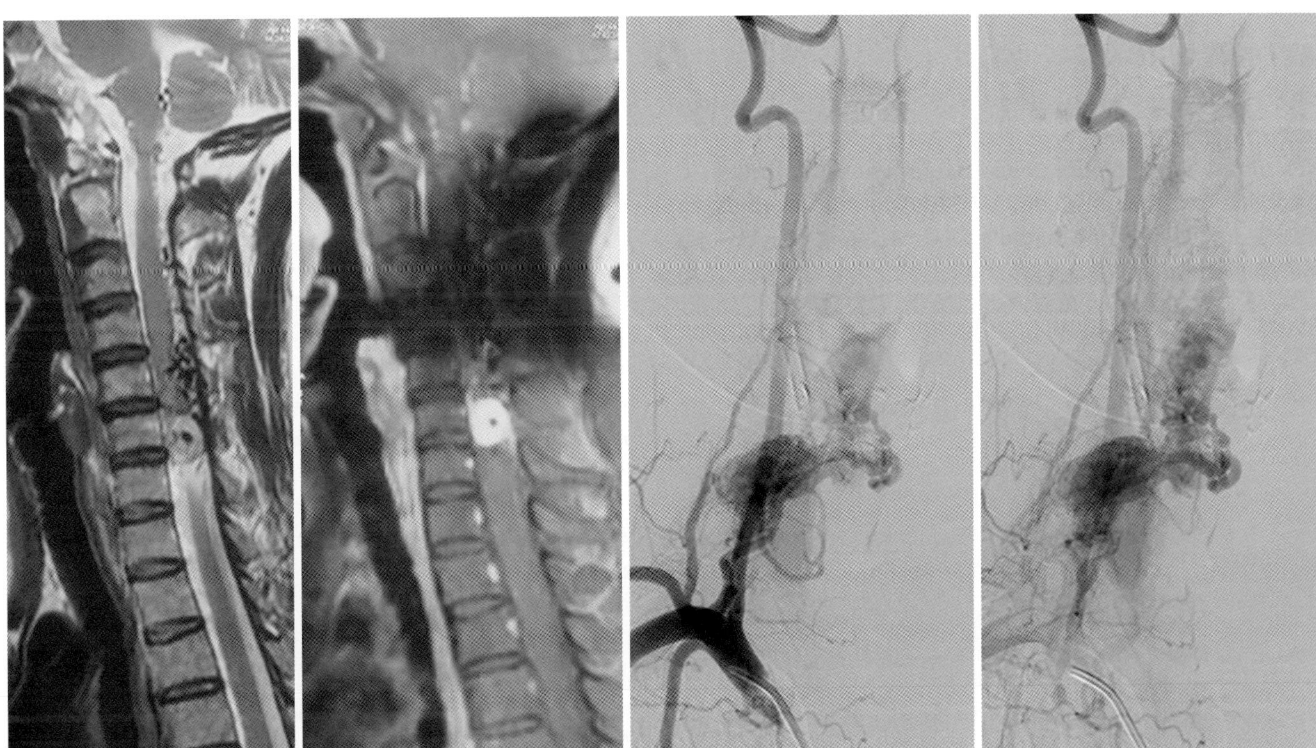

Fig. 12: Hemangioblastoma: Well-defined hyperintense lesion within the spinal canal in T2WI with intense enhancement is seen. Multiple vascular flow voids are seen, predominantly dorsal to cord. DSA shows tumor blush, fed by branches of ascending and deep cervical arteries with venous drainage into perimedullary veins.

OTHER LESIONS

Although not really vascular malformations, hemangioblastomas and spinal aneurysms are included under vascular lesions of spinal cord classification by Spetzler.

Spinal hemangioblastomas are highly vascular tumors with extensive arterial feeders and draining veins. With its high flow and steal phenomenon, they act like high flow spinal AVM or AVF, and may present with mass effect, venous hypertension, or ischemia secondary to steal. Symptoms of venous hypertension develop if hemangioblastomas drain into perimedullary veins. They appear as T2 hyperintense lesions with adjacent vascular flow voids representing arterial feeders and draining veins. Cystic components are commonly seen. After contrast administration, the solid components of the lesion show intense enhancement **(Fig. 12)**.

Spinal artery aneurysms are extremely rare when not associated with any high flow lesions like AVMs or SCAVFs. When associated with high flow lesions, management of the primary lesion would suffice to remodel and heal the walls of weakened aneurysm wall. In large aneurysms, especially when they have previously ruptures, it is safe to place one or two detachable coils in the aneurysmal sac to prevent re-rupture.

CONCLUSION

With a wide spectrum of disorders, along with their varied pathophysiology, it is essential to have a comprehensive idea about identification, classification and treatment of these disorders. It would help in early identification of the disease and avoids misdiagnosis, as it is one of the curable causes of progressive myelopathy.

ACKNOWLEDGMENT

The authors acknowledge and thank Dr Parthiban Bala, DM Resident in Department of Neuroimaging and Interventional Radiology, AIIMS, New Delhi, India, for active involvement and helping in writing the chapter.

SUGGESTED READING

1. da Costa L, Dehdashti AR, terBrugg E KG. Spinal cord vascular shunts: spinal cord vascular malformations and dural arteriovenous fistulas. Neurosurg Focus. 2009;26(1):E6.
2. Gonzalez LF, Spetzler RF. Treatment of Spinal Vascular Malformations.
3. Kim LJ, Spetzler RF. Classification and surgical management of spinal arteriovenous lesions: arteriovenous fistulae and arteriovenous malformations. Neurosurgery. 2006;59(suppl 5):S3-195-S3-201.
4. Krings T. Vascular malformations of the spine and spinal cord: anatomy, classification, treatment. Clin Neuroradiol. 2010;20(1):5-24.
5. Krings T, Geibprasert S. Spinal dural arteriovenous fistulas. Am J Neuroradiol. 2009;30(4):639-48.
6. Nachanakian A, El A, Abou G, Alayw M. In: Tjoumakaris S (Ed). Spinal Dural Arteriovenous Fistulas — Treatable Cause of Myelopathy. Arteriovenous Fistulas - Diagnosis and Management
7. Rodesch G, Hurth M, Alvarez H, Tadié M, Lasjaunias P. Classification of spinal cord arteriovenous shunts: proposal for a reappraisal—the Bicetre experience with 155 consecutive patients treated between 1981 and 1999. Neurosurgery. 2002;51(2):374-380.
8. Spetzler RF, Kondziolka D, Higashida RT, Kalani MYS, editors. Comprehensive management of arteriovenous malformation of the brain and spine. Cambridge: Cambridge University Press; 2015. 336 p. (Cambridge medicine).

CHAPTER 35

Imaging of Low Backache

Raju Sharma, Shivanand Gamanagatti, Devasenathipathy Kandasamy, Arun Kumar Gupta

IMAGING OF LOW BACK PAIN

Nearly half the adult population in India suffers from back pain, lasting at least 24 hours at sometime every year.[1] The impact of back pain on society is considerable and is associated with an enormous economic burden. Low back pain most commonly affects the 30–50 year age group, with the prevalence peaking during the sixth decade. Young people are more likely to have brief, acute episodes of back pain, whilst chronic pain tends to occur in older people. There is an equal sex distribution. This chapter summarizes the etiology, clinical presentation and radiological investigation of low back pain.

When to Image?

There are many causes of back pain with a complex inter-relationship between anatomical, pathological and psychological factors leading to the eventual clinical presentation. A careful history and physical examination remains the mainstay of initial assessment of back pain. Imaging is not necessary in most cases of back pain because of the high rate of spontaneous remission within 6–8 weeks.[2] Furthermore, the use of early imaging does not appear to alter management in most patients. There are, however, certain features or "red flags" that should suggest serious pathology and prompt early imaging.[3] It is increasingly recognized that plain radiographic evaluation of back pain in the absence of trauma is of limited value, as degenerative changes are very common and sinister pathology may easily be missed.

Indications of a more complicated status, often termed "red flags," include the following:[3]

- Recent significant trauma, or milder trauma, age >50 years
- Unexplained weight loss
- Unexplained fever
- Immunosuppression
- History of cancer
- Intravenous (IV) drug use
- Prolonged use of corticosteroids, osteoporosis
- Age >70 years
- Focal neurologic deficit with progressive or disabling symptoms
- Duration longer than 6 weeks

Four main clinical scenarios:[4]

1. Acute nonspecific back pain, which usually resolves spontaneously within 6–8 weeks. Imaging prior to six weeks does not improve outcome but does increase cost.
2. Chronic back pain without sinister features. This is a very common situation that is usually related to degenerative disease.
3. Back pain with sciatica: A condition usually caused by disk prolapse.
4. Possible serious pathology or cauda equina syndrome, this group encompasses various conditions such as tumor, infection and inflammatory disorders.

Of these conditions, the first two do not usually warrant imaging. In patients suffering from sciatica, the cause is usually a prolapsed disk, and those who have had a failed period of conservative therapy may require imaging. In patients with possible serious pathology, urgent imaging is indicated.

CONDITIONS CAUSING BACK PAIN

The physical causes of back pain can be divided into mechanical conditions such as disk disease and non-mechanical conditions, such as infection, inflammation or neoplasm **(Table 1)**.[4-6] There are also conditions which do not involve the spine, such as abdominal aortic aneurysms and urological conditions that may present with back pain. Due to the complexity of the bony, ligamentous, muscular and neural elements of the back, a specific anatomical diagnosis often cannot be made. Even when radiological investigations show an abnormality, the positive findings may not necessarily relate directly to the back pain. Close clinico-radiological correlation is therefore required.[4-6]

IMAGING MODALITIES

The purpose of diagnostic imaging is twofold: first is to provide accurate anatomic information and the second perhaps more important purpose is to affect the therapeutic decision-making process.

Radiographs

Radiographs are recommended when any of the above red flags are present. Lumbar radiographs may be sufficient for the initial evaluation of the following red flags, with further imaging indicated for treatment planning if findings are abnormal or inconclusive.[3,7]

- Recent significant trauma (at any age)
- Osteoporosis
- Age >70 years

Table 1: Causes of low back pain.

Mechanical (95%)	*Specific cause*
Acquired	Muscular injury Vertebral fracture Facet joint degeneration Disk degeneration Disk herniation Spinal stenosis Pars defects'
Congenital	Transitional vertebra Scoliosis Scheuermann's disease
Non-mechanical (5%)	Infection Neoplasm Spondyloarthropathy
Non-spinal cause	Abdominal aortic aneurysm, renal disease, pancreatitis, psychogenic

The initial evaluation of the LBP patient may also require further imaging if other red flags such as suspicion of cancer or infection are present.

Plain and contrast-enhanced MRI has the ability to demonstrate inflammatory, neoplastic, and most traumatic lesions as well as show anatomic detail not available on isotope studies. Gadolinium-enhanced MRI reliably shows the presence and extent of spinal infection, and is useful in assessing therapy.[7,8] MRI has therefore taken over the role of the isotope scan in many cases where the location of the lesion is known. The isotope scan remains invaluable when a survey of the entire skeleton is indicated (e.g. for metastatic disease).

Magnetic Resonance Imaging, Computed Tomography, Myelography and Myelography/CT

Uncomplicated acute LBP and/or radiculopathy (no red flags) do not warrant the use of any of these imaging studies. The early indiscriminate use of expensive imaging procedures should be avoided. The appropriate use of these imaging procedures is an important challenge. For example, LBP complicated by "red flags" suggesting infection or tumor may justify early use of CT or MRI even if radiographs are negative. The most common indication for the use of these imaging procedures, however, is the clinical setting of LBP complicated by radiating pain (radiculopathy, sciatica) or cauda equina syndrome (bilateral leg weakness, urinary retention, saddle anesthesia), usually due to herniated disk and/or canal stenosis.[3]

Magnetic Resonance Imaging

MRI of the lumbar spine has become the initial imaging modality of choice in complicated LBP, replacing myelography and CT in recent years. Although disk abnormalities are common on MRI in asymptomatic people, acute back pain with radiculopathy suggests the presence of demonstrable nerve root compression on MRI.

However, determining the cause of back pain is complicated as it is often multifactorial and anatomical abnormalities are common in the spine and may not necessarily translate into clinical symptoms. Thus, the use of MRI in nonspecific LBP should be avoided and it should be reserved for the investigation of severe or progressive neurological deficits or for those cases in which serious underlying pathology is suspected. However, it plays a vital role in planning surgical management in cases of radiculopathy and spinal stenosis.[3,7,8]

MRI is particularly efficacious for detecting "red flag" diagnoses, particularly using the short tau inversion recovery (STIR) and fat-saturated T2-weighted fast-spin-echo sequences. MR with contrast is useful for suspected infection and neoplasia. In postoperative patients, enhanced MRI allows distinction between disk and scar when tissue extends beyond the disk space.

MR Protocol for Imaging Patients with Backache[9]

Coils and patient position:

- Phased array spine coils should be used for all spine imaging. Patients are positioned supine in the magnet.

Image orientation:

- Sagittal and axial images are acquired in the lumbar region. In the axial imaging plane, stacked cuts are acquired that cover an entire block of the spine. Acquiring images angled only through the disks is considered inadequate because portions of the spinal canal are not imaged in the axial plane, and sequestered disk fragments and spondylolysis defects are often missed.
- Sagittal images alone are sometimes inadequate to detect a disk fragment that has migrated from the parent disk. Because sequestered disks are a cause of failed back surgery and persistent symptoms, it is important to identify them on MRI by obtaining stacked axial images in addition to sagittal images through the canal.
- In the unoperated lumbar spine, stacked axial images should be obtained from the middle of the L3 vertebral body to the middle of the S1 vertebral body.
- In the postoperative spine, stacked axial images (matched images before and after contrast administration) are obtained by centering at the level of the previous surgery.
- Axial images are often better than sagittal for detecting lesions in the neural foramina. Generally, axial and sagittal planes of imaging are complementary to each other.
- Coronal images may be useful to better define the anatomy in patients with scoliosis.

Pulse sequences and regions of interest:

- T1W and fast T2W images are the standard for sagittal imaging in any segment of the spine.
- Gradient-echo sagittal sequences are used when looking for blood in the cord after trauma to take advantage of the blooming effect.
- A fast STIR sagittal sequence also is useful in trauma patients when looking for ligamentous injury with changes of hemorrhage and edema.
- Gradient echo axial images are used to detect disk disease in the cervical spine, whereas fast T2W axial images are used in the thoracic and lumbar spine for the same indications.
- T1W and FSE T2W images are selected in the sagittal and axial planes for most indications. Slice thickness generally is 3 or 4 mm.
- The fields of view are as small as possible; larger ones are required for sagittal than for the axial imaging planes.
- Phase and frequency encoding gradients should be reversed for imaging the spine in the sagittal plane so that chemical shift artifacts at the diskovertebral interfaces do not obscure pathology in the vertebral body end plates or disks.
- For evaluation of the post-operative spine fast spin echo sequences are better than spin echo sequences and the latter are better than gradient echo sequences. The shortest possible echo time should be used. Increasing band width and decreasing voxel size are useful. The frequency encoding direction should be kept parallel to the long axis of the pedicle screw. Some vendors offer specific metal artifact reduction sequences (e.g. MAVRIK, SEMAC).[10]

Use of gadolinium-based contrast:

- Contrast medium is always used for postoperative spine imaging, suspected infection, tumor, intradural or nontraumatic cord lesions.
- If any abnormality is identified in the epidural space when evaluating for osseous metastases or cord compression, gadolinium is given to show these lesions better.

Standing MR Scanners are available in which the patient can be scanned in weight bearing position. This may sometimes reveal clinically significant pathology like lumbar spine instability, disc disease and spondylolisthesis not detected on the conventional supine MRI. Kinetic MRI can be done in flexion and extension position. It also overcomes the problem of claustrophobia and has some niche indications. However these open scanners use low field magnets and therefore images are of low signal to noise ratio.

COMPUTED TOMOGRAPHY

Computed tomography provides superior bone detail but is not quite as useful in depicting disk protrusions when compared with multiplanar MRI. With the added value associated with high-quality reformatted sagittal and coronal plane images, CT is useful for depicting spondylolysis, pseudoarthrosis, scoliosis, and for post-surgical evaluation of bone graft integrity, surgical fusion, and instrumentation.[3]

CT is useful in detecting tumors like osteoid osteoma. The advent of dual energy CT has further enhanced the role of this modality. Using three material decomposition algorithms virtual non-calcium (VNCa) images can be generated and they can detect marrow oedema and marrow infiltration before osteolytic lesions develop. This can be useful in trauma, spondylodiscitis and in marrow infiltrative disorders like myeloma and skeletal metastasis.[11]

CT is often used to evaluate post-operative spine. There are methods available for metal artifact reduction based on iterative algorithms which should be used to enhance image quality.

Myelography/CT

"Plain" myelography was the mainstay of lumbar herniated disk diagnosis for decades. It is now usually combined with post-myelography CT in problematic cases. The combined study is complementary to plain CT or MRI and occasionally more accurate in diagnosing disk herniation, but it suffers the disadvantage of requiring lumbar puncture and contrast injection.

Discography and CT Discography

When other studies fail to localize the cause of pain, discography may occasionally be helpful. Although the images often depict nonspecific aging or degenerative changes, the injection itself may reproduce the patient's pain, which may have diagnostic value.[12,13]

Isotope Bone Scan

The role of the isotope bone scan in patients with acute LBP has changed in recent years with the wide availability of MRI and especially contrast-enhanced MRI. The bone scan is a moderately sensitive test for detecting the presence of tumor, infection, or occult fractures of the vertebrae but is nonspecific. For spondylolysis or stress fracture in athletes, bone scintigraphy with single photon emission computed tomography (SPECT), followed by limited computed tomography (CT) if scintigraphy is positive, is more sensitive than MRI.

High-resolution isotope imaging, including SPECT, may localize the source of pain in patients with articular facet osteoarthritis prior to therapeutic facet injection.[14] Similar scans may be helpful in detecting and localizing the site of painful pseudoarthrosis in patients following lumbar spinal fusion.

TRANSITION VERTEBRA

In 1917, Mario Bertolotti, an Italian surgeon, was the first to put forward a possible relationship between low back pain and congenital anatomical abnormalities in the last lumbar vertebra, described as "sacral assimilation of the lumbar vertebrae".[15] The presence of a transverse mega-apophysis in a lumbar vertebra with transitional characteristics may be associated with low back pain. Four to seven percent of patients with low back pain have transitional vertebra. Motion between the transitional vertebra and the sacrum is reduced and asymmetrical, resulting in early degenerative changes within the "neoarticulation" or in the normal contralateral facet joint, which gives rise to facet pain. Biomechanical stress transferred to the upper mobile vertebral segment can accelerate the disk degeneration, another mechanism responsible for pain. Lumbosacral transitional disk has reduced height compared with normal lumbosacral intervertebral disks.

If a lumbosacral transitional vertebra (LSTV) is suspected on MRI, the decision of whether it represents a sacralized L5 or lumbarized S1 must be made. Many complimentary imaging findings have been described to identify the transition vertebra. The true nature of the lower vertebral segmentation can be established on conventional radiographs that include the thoraco-lumbar junction so that hypoplastic true ribs may be differentiated from large transverse processes, thus allowing correct identification of the L1 vertebral body. It has been recommended to use a whole spine localizer to count the number of vertebra from C2 with the assumption that there are 7 cervical and 12 thoracic segments which helps in assigning the LSTV.[16]

It has been proposed that the position of the right renal artery may be used to identify lumbar levels on sagittal MRI, because it usually lies closest to the L1-2 disk space and the aortic bifurcation lies at L4. The Iliolumbar ligament can be clearly identified on axial MRI as a single or double hypointense band extending from the transverse process of L5 to the posteromedial iliac crest that also helps in localisation of L5 vertebra. Bone marrow oedema may be seen in the transverse processes of LSTV but has a poor correlation with back pain. The L3 vertebra usually has the longest transverse process which can be used as an additional feature to correctly number the lumbar vertebrae. The identification of vertebral level and

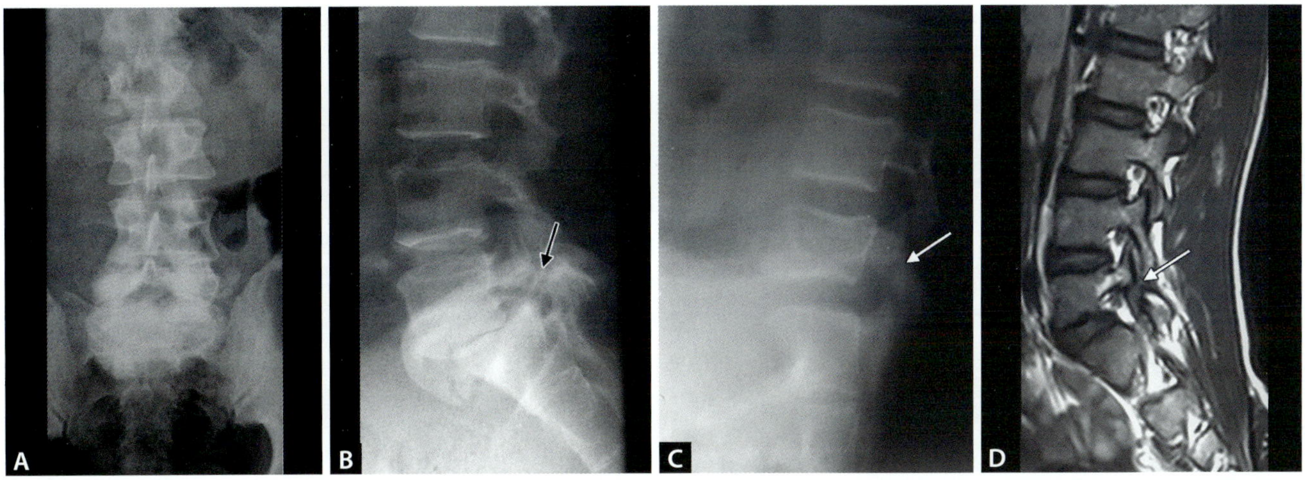

Figs. 1A to D: Anteroposterior (A) and lateral (B) radiographs of the lumbosacral spine showing break in the pars interarticularis (arrow) of L5 with grade II spondylolisthesis of L5 over S1. End plate sclerosis and osteophyte formation at L5-S1 levels are also noted. Lateral radiograph of a child (C) showing spondylolysis of L5 vertebra (arrow) and MRI T1 W sequence (D) showing the defect at pars inter-articularis.

transitional vertebra is also important in communicating the correct level of disk abnormalities to the operating surgeon.[16]

SPONDYLOLYSIS AND SPONDYLOLISTHESIS

Spondylolysis is defined as a defect in the pars interarticularis, which appears to be secondary to a stress fracture. A bilateral defect would result in spondylolisthesis (Forward slippage of a vertebra on the one below it) of varying degrees. Most common levels are L4-5 and L5-S1. The prevalence of spondylolysis is low in children and increases with age, there is a high incidence in adolescent athletes. The prevalence in general population is around 5% and commonly affects L5 (~90%) and L4 levels.[17] There is a genetic predisposition to spondylolisthesis, with 30% to 70% prevalence in other family members. Spondylolisthesis may be secondary to stress fracture of bilateral pars in young or may be due to degenerative disease in elders.[18,19]

Spondylolisthesis has been graded as follows, according to forward slippage of a vertebra on the one below it: Grade I (0–25%), II (25–50%), III (50–75%), Grade IV (75–100%).

Imaging

In spondylolysis the aim of imaging is: to detect lysis, distinguish acute and active lesions from chronic inactive non-union, assess bony healing in follow-up of acute lesions, detect listhesis and grade it, and identify spinal and neural foramina stenosis.[20,21]

Conventional radiography is often the first line imaging modality **(Figs. 1A to D)**, and techniques include routine anteroposterior (AP) lateral views and oblique views. Although chronic nonunion may be demonstrated, radiography is unreliable for detection of early and acute lesions. Oblique radiographs of the lumbosacral spine are more sensitive than frontal and lateral radiographs, which may miss 20% of unilateral pars defects.[22] Scotty dog with a collar around the neck is a typical sign described on oblique radiographs representing the break in pars. Bilateral spondylolysis with anterolisthesis of L5 over S1 may show the appearance of Napolean hat on frontal radiographs.

CT is probably the best method for demonstrating spondylolytic defects and may also be used for assessment of healing. Multiplanar reconstruction along the Pars has been utilized successfully for identifying defects, by demonstrating discontinuity in the bony ring of the posterior elements of the vertebra. It may simulate a facet joint giving rise to the "Extra facet sign". However, CT is limited in detection of other pathological processes, and it cannot reliably distinguish between active and inactive lesions.[20,21] Bone scan can be a useful technique to differentiate active stress reaction from inactive disease.

MRI may not depict the bony pars defects; however, it evaluates accurately the degree of slippage **(Figs. 2A to D)**, spinal stenosis, nerve roots, and the associated pathologic disk changes.

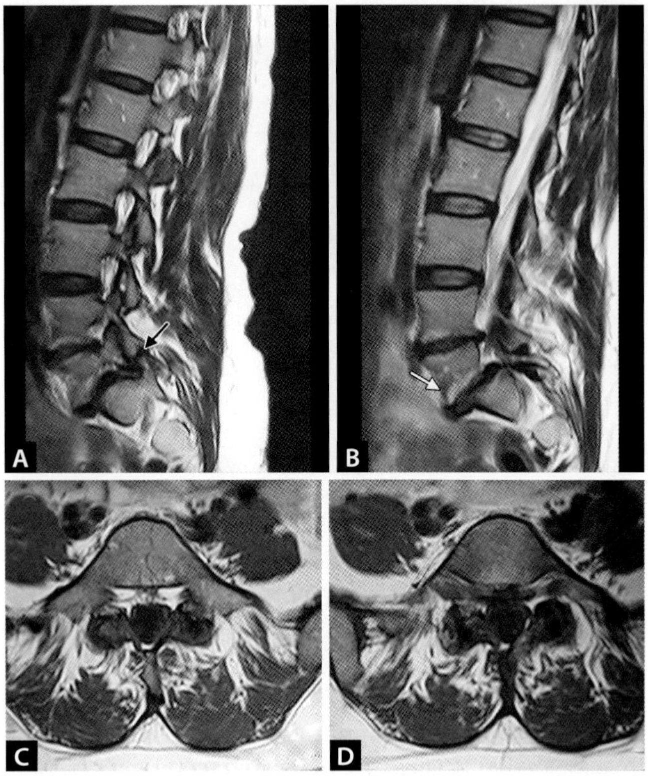

Figs. 2A to D: Sagittal T2W (A and B) and axial T1W (C and D) MR images showing spondylolysis seen at L5 (black arrow) with grade II spondylolisthesis (white arrow) of L5 over S1.

A new grading system has been described that utilizes both the morphological information of MRI combined with the presence or absence of marrow edema on fat-suppressed T2-W images. This distinguishes between stress reaction and active and inactive spondylolysis.[22,23]

Indications for surgery include worsening pain and progressive listhesis, significant neurologic findings and slippage of more than 50%. Healing is not a feature of developmental spondylolysis, and patients with chronic inactive lysis can usually return to normal physical activities.

Scheuermann's Disease

Scheuermann's disease, also known as juvenile kyphosis, is a disorder that presents with a rigid thoracic or thoracolumbar kyphosis.[24] Its incidence is estimated at 1 to 8%. Scheuermann disease affecting the lumbar region is more painful than the thoracic counterpart.

It was first described in 1920 by Scheuermann, who believed that the endplate irregularity and vertebral wedging was caused by avascular necrosis of the cartilage ring apophysis.[24] Although the etiology is still unknown, it is thought to be related to stress and repeated trauma. A recent study suggests that the presence of a gene defect in the COL9A3 gene is associated with Scheuermann disease and intervertebral disk degeneration.

Clinical Presentation

Adolescents typically present to medical attention because of cosmetic deformity; adults more commonly present because of increased pain.

Imaging and Diagnosis

The diagnosis of classical Scheuermann's disease is based on involvement of three contiguous thoracic vertebrae with 5° of wedging associated with end-plate irregularity, and a thoracic kyphosis greater than 40°. The diagnosis of lumbar Scheuermann's disease is based on varying degrees of end-plate irregularities and disk narrowing in the lumbar spine or thoracolumbar junction, but with no abnormal kyphosis.[24,25]

Radiographs may show vertebral endplate irregularities, anterior vertebral body wedging, Schmorl's nodes **(Figs. 3A and B)**, and relative narrowing of the disk spaces. MRI **(Figs. 3C and D)** has an important diagnostic role, particularly with severe and painful kyphosis. It demonstrates, with great detail, endplate irregularities, Schmorl's nodes, disk degeneration, disk space narrowing, and anterior wedging of the vertebral bodies. Assessment of vertebral canal is imperative, especially in case of severe kyphosis.[26]

When reporting on radiographs of the lumbar spine with a combination of features such as end-plate irregularity, disk narrowing and Schmorl's nodes, particularly at the thoracolumbar junction, which would usually be recorded as being indicative of Scheuermann's disease, radiologists should avoid the use of this term and report only the anatomical and pathological features seen. The radiological diagnosis of Scheuermann's disease should be restricted to those patients who demonstrate the above features associated with an increased kyphosis of the thoracic spine.[26]

DEGENERATIVE DISEASES OF LUMBAR SPINE

Degenerative Changes in the Anterior Elements

- Degenerative change of the nucleus pulposus
- Annular tears
- Disk herniation

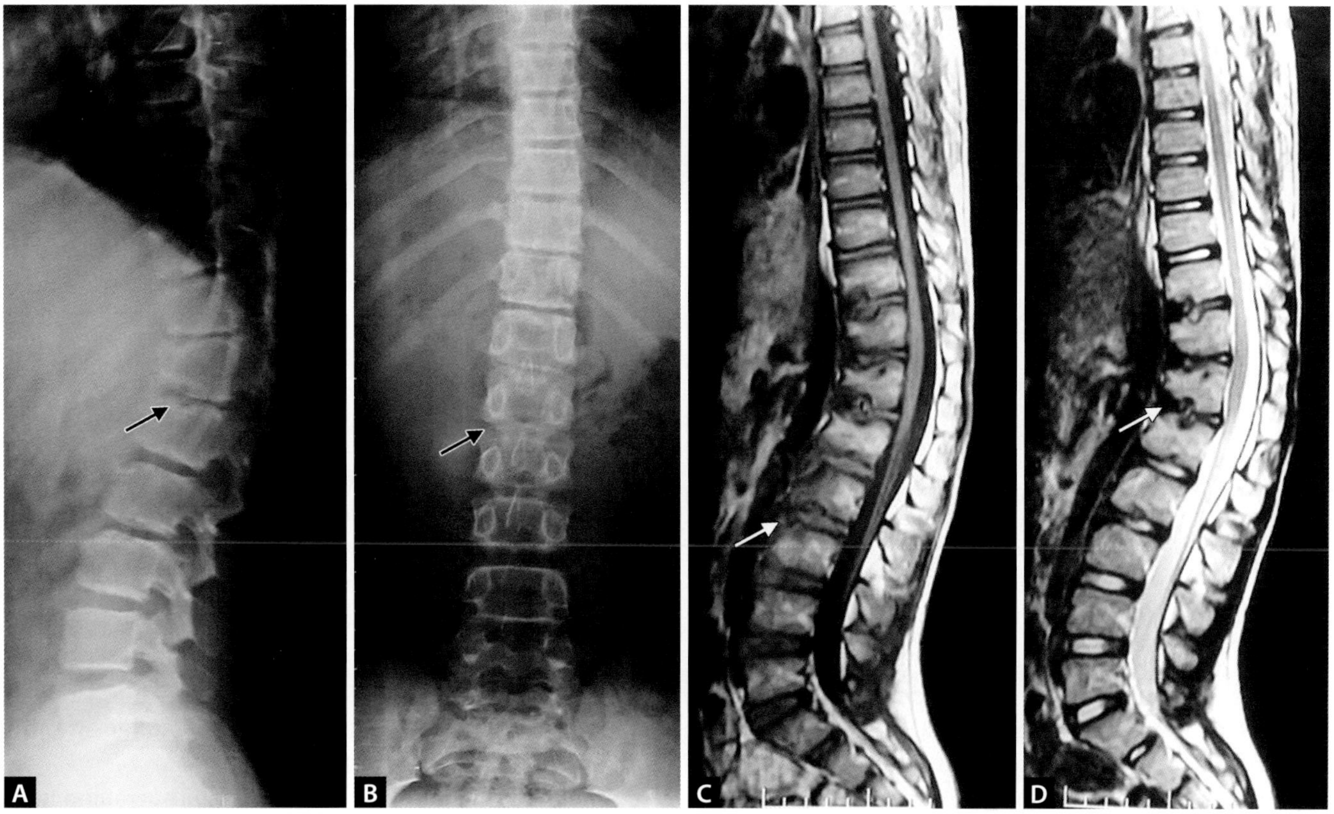

Figs. 3A to D: Scheuermann's disease: Anteroposterior (A) and lateral (B) radiographs of the dorsolumbar spine showing end-plate irregularities (black arrow) with decreased disk space at multiple levels and anterior wedging of lower dorsal and upper lumbar vertebral bodies. T1W (C) and T2W (D) MR images of the dorso-lumbar spine showing Schmorl's nodes (white arrow) at multiple levels in the lower thoracic and upper lumbar spine with kyphosis.

- Degenerative end plate changes
- Spondylosis deformans

Degenerative Changes in the Posterior Elements

Degenerative changes of the facet joints

Complications of Degenerative Spinal Disease

- Scoliosis and kyphosis
- Segmental instability
- Spinal stenosis
- Foraminal stenosis

Presentation

- Degenerative change may present with local back pain, radiculopathy, or myelopathy.
- Degenerative facet arthropathy, degenerative disk disease, degenerative end plate changes, and ligamentous injury are all possible pain generators in the setting of axial back pain.
- Narrowing of the spinal canal or neural foramina can result in myelopathy and radiculopathy, respectively.
- Segmental instability, kyphosis, and scoliosis malalignment that may occur secondary to degenerative disease.
- Imaging of patients who have suspected spine pathology characterizes the level and extent of degenerative changes that may be a source of symptoms.
- Significant morphological changes on imaging are often found in asymptomatic patients without any significant clinical symptomatology, which does not require further evaluation in terms of acquiring electrophysiologic data to determine the significance of anatomic findings seen on imaging studies.

DEGENERATIVE CHANGE OF THE NUCLEUS PULPOSUS

Normal Disk

Intervertebral disks consist of a central gelatinous nucleus pulposus composed of water and proteoglycans.

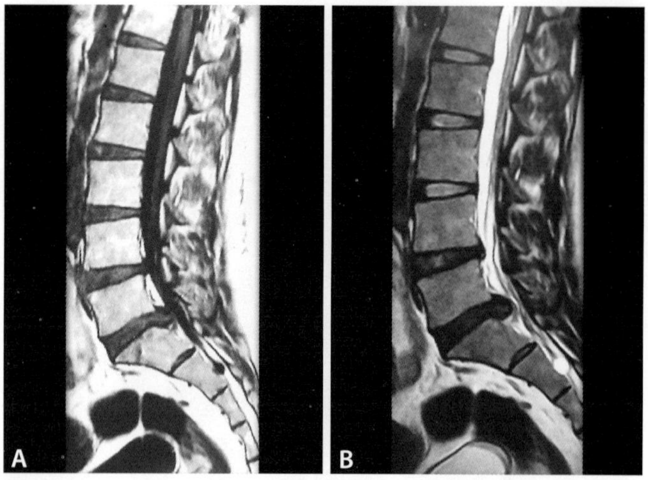

Figs. 4A and B: Sagittal T1W (A) and T2W (B) MR images showing normal signal in upper lumbar discs, loss of T2 hyperintensity suggesting dessication in L4 and L5 disks along with disk protrusion at these levels. Incidental perineural cyst is seen at S2 level.

The nucleus pulposus is surrounded by the annulus fibrosus. The inner portion of the annulus is composed of fibrocartilage, whereas the outer fibers are made of concentrically oriented lamellae of collagen fibers. The annulus is anchored to the adjacent vertebral bodies by Sharpey's fibers.

MR Appearance of Normal Disk

On MRI, the normal disk shows low signal intensity on T1W images, slightly lower signal than adjacent normal red marrow and very similar to muscle. T2W images show diffuse high signal intensity **(Figs. 4A and B)** throughout the disk except for the outer fibers of the annulus, which are homogeneously hypointense. Distinction between the nucleus pulposus and the inner annulus fibrosus is impossible by MRI.

Normal disks typically do not extend beyond the margins of the adjacent vertebral bodies; however, diffuse extension beyond the margins by 1–2 mm may occur in some histologically normal disks. The posterior margins of disks tend to be mildly concave in the upper lumbar spine, straight at the L4-5 level, and slightly convex at the lumbosacral junction.[27]

Abnormal Nucleus

With aging and degeneration, the intervertebral disks lose hydration, lose proteoglycans, and gain collagen as they become more fibrous. A horizontally oriented fibrous intranuclear cleft develops in the nucleus. MRI shows the intranuclear cleft as a horizontal, low signal intensity line that divides the disk into upper and lower halves on T2W sagittal images. Eventually, there is diffuse decreased signal intensity on T2W images **(Figs. 4A and B)** from the increased collagen content in the nucleus. The disk progressively loses height with increasing degrees of degeneration.[27] There is a five level grading system proposed by Pfirrmann et al which can be used to objectively evaluate the severity of disk degeneration on T2W spin echo images.[28,29]

Points to Remember

- The term "early degenerative changes" refers to accelerated age-related changes in the disk without evidence of structural failure
- A degenerated disk is a term reserved for those with structural failure combined with accelerated or advanced signs of aging
- Degenerative disk disease is best defined as symptomatic degenerative disk changes
- Many patients exhibit degenerative changes on MR without associated symptoms
- Intervertebral disk height at the lumbosacral junction is variable because of segmentation differences and a decreased disk height at this interspace is not necessarily pathologic.[27]

Annular Fissures

Annular fissure or tear represents a biomechanical failure of the annulus fibrosis and are usually associated with degenerative changes in the nucleus pulposus. The three basic types of annular tears are vertical, radial, and peripheral rim tears, of these radial tear is of practical interest.[30-32] Radial tears involve either part or the entire thickness of the annulus from the nucleus to the outer annular fibers. Radial tears run perpendicular to the long-axis of the annulus and occur more commonly in the posterior half of the disk, usually at L4-5 and L5-S1.[30-32] Radial tears may be source of pain either because the vascularized granulation tissue grows into the tear and causes painful stimulation of nerve endings or the chemical and mechanical irritation to the nociceptive fibers that normally exist in the annulus.

MR Appearance

- Show focal areas of high signal intensity on T2W images or on contrast enhanced T1W images.

- Radial tears may be seen on T2W sagittal images within the posterior annulus as globular or horizontal lines of high signal intensity.
- On axial images, radial tears may be seen as focal areas of high signal intensity that parallel the outer disk margin for a short distance.

Disk Herniation (Abnormalities in Disk Morphology)

It is a nonspecific term used to indicate disk that extends in some abnormal manner beyond the margin of vertebral body. Most surgeons dealing with spine disorders use a more standardized nomenclature that helps to distinguish what are likely to be clinically relevant lesions from lesions that probably are not. Standard nomenclatures used by the orthopedic surgeons include: *Diffuse disk bulge, Broad-based protrusion, Focal disk protrusion, Disk extrusion, and Sequestered disk.*[30-32]

Points to Remember

- A herniation is "focal" if it involves less than 25% of the disk circumference.
- A"broad-based" disk herniation involves between 25% and 50% of the disk circumference.
- Involvement of more than 50% of the circumference of the disk is defined as a "diffuse disk bulge."
- A "disk protrusion" **(Figs. 5A to D)** is defined as a herniation that demonstrates continuity with the adjacent disk. Herniated disk shows anteroposterior < mediolateral diameter.
- If the size of the disk fragment (in any plane) is greater than the width of the base (anteroposterior > mediolateral diameter), it is termed a "disk extrusion" **(Figs. 6A and B)**.
- A"sequestered disc" (free fragment) refers to a disk fragment that has lost all continuity with the parent disk **(Figs. 7A to D)**.

Method of Quantifying the Severity of Disk Disease

- Mild if the anterior epidural fat is not obliterated,
- Moderate if the epidural fat is obliterated and the thecal sac is being displaced, and
- Severe if the cord is being effaced or nerve roots displaced.

Diffusely bulging disk extends symmetrically and circumferentially by more than 2 mm beyond the margins of the adjacent vertebral bodies. This diagnosis is based on axial and sagittal images by comparing the size of the disk with the size of the adjacent vertebral bodies. A segment of

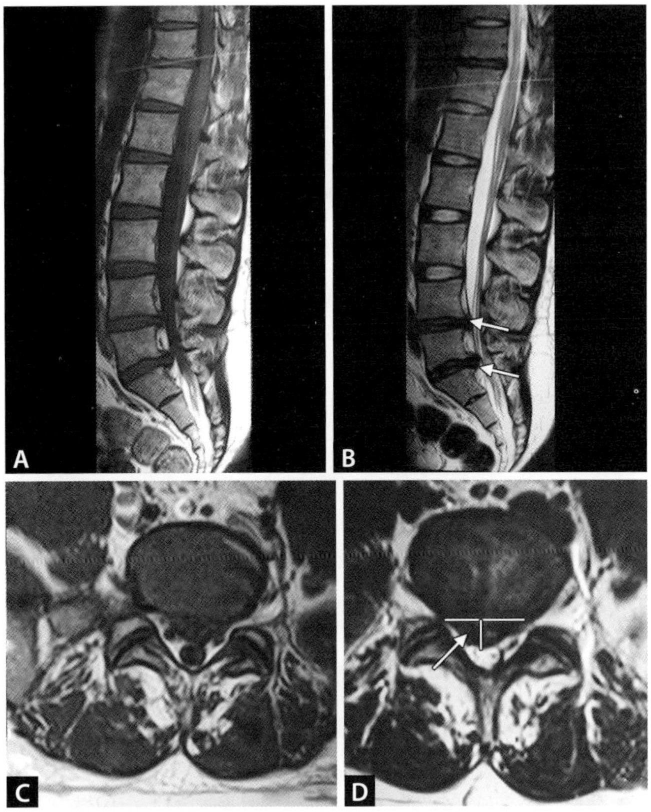

Figs. 5A to D: Disk protrusion: Sagittal T1W (A), T2W (B) and axial T1W (C), T2W (D) images showing disk dessication and protrusion at L4-L5 and L5-S1 levels (arrows). The herniated disk has a broad base which is more than its AP diameter, suggesting it is a protrusion. It is causing bilateral foraminal stenosis.

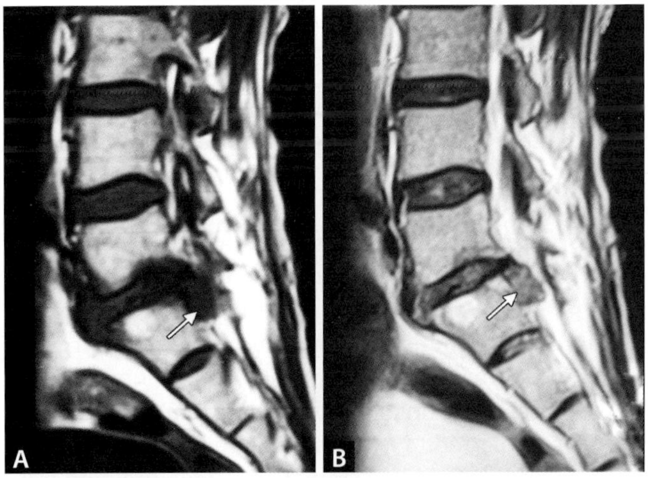

Figs. 6A and B: Sagittal T1W (A) and T2W (B) MR images showing disk extrusion at L5-S1 level with caudal migration.

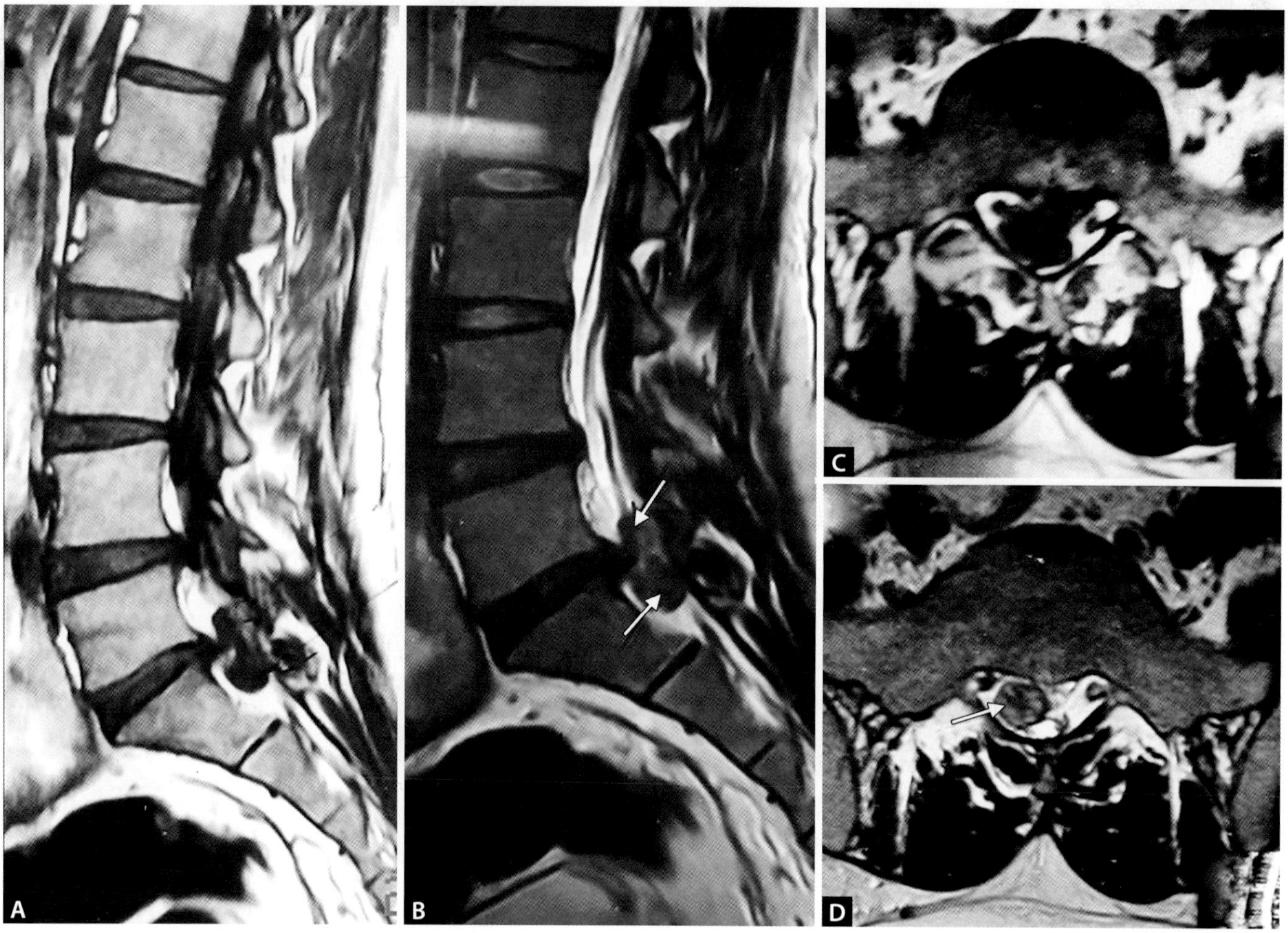

Figs. 7A to D: Sequestered disk: Sagittal T1W (A), T2W (B) and axial T1W (C), T2W (D) MR images showing a large herniated fragment of disk (arrow), which is mildly T2 hyperintense, located posterior to S1 vertebral body. This fragment has no attachment to parent disk.

disk tissue that projects beyond the margin of the vertebral body but that does not involve the entire circumference of the disk can be called either a focal bulge or a broad-based protrusion.

Disk protrusion is a focal, asymmetric extension of disk tissue beyond the vertebral body margin, usually into the spinal canal or neural foramen. The base (the mediolateral dimension along the posterior margin of the disk) is broader than any other dimension **(Figs. 5A to D)**. Some of the outer annular fibers remain intact, and hence it is referred to as a contained disk. The protruded disk does not extend in a cranial or caudal direction from the parent disk.

Extruded disk is a more pronounced version of a protrusion and often is responsible for symptoms. There is disruption of the outer fibers of the annulus, and the disk herniation usually is greater in its anteroposterior dimension than it is at its base (mediolateral dimension). The extruded disk may migrate up or down behind the adjacent vertebral bodies **(Figs. 6A and B)** but maintains continuity with the parent disk. These also may be referred to as non-contained disks. MRI shows the described contour abnormalities, and because of a significant inflammatory reaction that may occur in response to the extruded disk material, there may be high signal intensity on T2W and contrast-enhanced T1W images in or surrounding the disk. Lumbar disk extrusions that cause radiculopathy but are managed non-operatively have been shown to do well about 90% of the time. Spontaneous reduction in size of disk extrusions and protrusions that were managed conservatively has been well documented with imaging. The regression in disk size may not be the reason for reduction in pain. Much of the pain from extruded disks is probably from the inflammatory response to them rather than from compression of neural elements from the mass effect.

Sequestered disk, when extruded disk material loses its attachment to the parent disk, it is called a sequestered fragment or a free fragment **(Figs. 7A to D)**. These fragments may migrate in a cranial or caudal direction with equal frequency and generally remain within about 5 mm of the parent disk. They may be located between the posterior longitudinal ligament and the osseous spine or extend through the posterior ligament into the epidural space. They almost always remain in the anterior epidural space, but occasionally the fragment may migrate into the posterior epidural space. Rarely, the disk fragment can perforate through the thecal sac to reach the intradural space. It is extremely important to recognize these fragments because they may be overlooked at surgery. The fragment of disk material that migrates from the parent disk often shows peripheral or diffuse high signal intensity on T2W and contrast-enhanced T1W images, caused by the inflammatory reaction within or surrounding it. Otherwise, a low signal intensity mass resembling the signal of the parent disk is seen. Sequestrations are a contraindication to chymopapain, percutaneous diskectomy, and other limited disk procedures.

Location of Focal Disk Abnormalities

Most of the disk herniation in lower back occurs at L4-L5 or L5-S1 levels. While reporting a focal disk abnormality the size, contour, location and relationship to nerves or other important structures should be described. The location of a focal disk abnormality needs to be conveyed accurately so that the surgical approach can be planned properly and so that it can be determined whether symptoms correlate to the anatomic abnormality seen on MRI. Focal disk abnormalities that remain at the level of the parent disk should be described as being central, left or right paracentral, left or right foraminal, or left or right extraforaminal (also called lateral or far lateral).[30-32]

Significance of Disk Contour Abnormalities

Degenerative Disk Disease can Cause Following Consequences

- Neural compression
- Chemical irritation of nerves
- Osseous abnormalities
- Segmental instability
- Spinal stenosis
- Disk-related compressive myelopathy

Intraosseous Disk Herniations

Disk material not only projects into the spinal canal, but also may directly herniate into the adjacent vertebral bodies through the end plates which are known as a Schmorl's or cartilaginous nodes.

Presentation

These are usually asymptomatic; however traumatic Schmorl's nodes resulting from axial loading forces may be acutely painful. Multiple thoracic Schmorl's nodes can occur in very active teens from axial stresses and result in irregularity of several end plates, loss of disk height, and narrowing of the height of the affected anterior vertebral bodies from fractures, with a resultant kyphosis (Scheuermann's disease).[24,25] An inflammatory, foreign body-type response to intraosseous disk herniation may occur, with vascularization around the disk material and surrounding marrow edema, which may cause severe pain.

Points to Remember

Inflammatory Schmorl's nodes on MRI tend to have large, dome-shaped regions of marrow edema surrounding them; marrow edema is low signal on T1W and high signal on T2W and contrast-enhanced T1W images. A rim of contrast enhancement around the periphery of the Schmorl's node is seen in addition to the surrounding marrow edema. These can have an aggressive look, similar to infection or tumor, and careful evaluation is necessary to make the proper diagnosis.[30-32]

OSSEOUS DEGENERATIVE CHANGES

Vertebral Bodies

The vertebral bodies respond to degenerative changes in the adjacent intervertebral disks in two major ways: (1) formation of osteophytes and (2) marrow changes paralleling the end plates.

Osteophytes

Osteophytes are the excrescences of bone that occur on the upper or lower margins of vertebral bodies. They occur as disks degenerate and bulge, placing traction stresses on Sharpey's fibers, which attach the disks to the vertebral bodies. Osteophytes usually are located anteriorly in the lumbar and thoracic spine, but are commonly anterior or posterior in the cervical spine. MRI of most osteophytes shows low signal intensity cortical margins with fatty marrow that follow the signal of fat on all pulse sequences.

Endplates

The marrow in vertebral bodies adjacent to degenerated disks may change in response to the disk disease. Parallel bands of abnormal signal in the end plates have been divided into three types and are called Modic type 1, 2, or 3 changes. These marrow changes may be focal or diffuse along the end plate but tend to be linear and always parallel to the end plates.[31,32]

- *Type 1*: Decreased signal T1, increased signal T2 (inflammatory tissue)
- *Type 2*: Increased signal T1, follows fat on T2 (focal conversion to fat)
- *Type 3*: Decreased signal T1 and T2 (sclerosis)

Facet Joints

Normal facet joints: Are formed by the inferior articular process of the vertebra above articulating with the superior articular process of the lower vertebra. The articular surfaces are covered with hyaline cartilage. The osseous structures are enveloped in a joint capsule lined by synovium; these are true synovial joints. The anterior aspects of the facet joints and the laminae are covered by the ligamentum flavum.

Facet joint arthropathy: Degenerative changes of the facet joints manifest as cartilage fibrillation with joint space narrowing, subchondral sclerosis, subchondral cysts, and osteophyte formation that result in overgrowth or hypertrophy of the osseous portions of the joints. Synovial cysts may develop from degenerated spinal facet joints and project either anteriorly (through the ligamentum flavum) or posteriorly from the joints.[31,32]

Symptoms from degenerative changes of the facet joints may result from compression of adjacent neural structures (spinal stenosis) by overgrowth of the bone, inward buckling of the ligamentum flavum, protrusion of synovial cysts into the spinal canal, or the joints themselves being painful.

Imaging Findings

Most of the changes that occur in facet joint arthropathy are bony (sclerosis and joint space reduction) and they are better evaluated on CT scan compared to MRI which can underestimate the severity.[29,33] On the other hand MRI is superior in evaluating marrow edema and effusion.

MRI of degenerative facet joint disease is typical of degenerative changes in any joint (subchondral sclerosis is low signal intensity on all pulse sequences; Synovial cysts are low signal intensity on T1W and high signal intensity on T2W images).

The osteophytes and hypertrophic osseous changes create a rounded and enlarged appearance of the articular processes of the facets on axial images that may cause narrowing of the adjacent spinal canal, lateral recesses, or neural foramina.

Posterior Spinous Processes

Degenerative changes of the spinous processes and intervening interspinous soft tissues is called as kissing spine or Baastrup's disease. On CT scan the features are marginal sclerosis of involved spinous processes with faceted appearance, osteophytes and erosions **(Fig. 8)**. Ankylosis is a late feature. MRI may show marrow edema and hyperintense bursal fluid in the interspinous ligament region.

Spinal Stenosis

Spinal stenosis is narrowing of the central spinal canal, neural foramen, lateral recess, or any combination of these anatomic regions, by soft tissue or osseous structures that impinge on neural elements and may result in symptoms.[34]

Causes

- *Degenerative*:
  - Disk contour abnormalities (bulges, herniations)
  - Vertebral body osteophytes
  - Degenerative spondylolisthesis

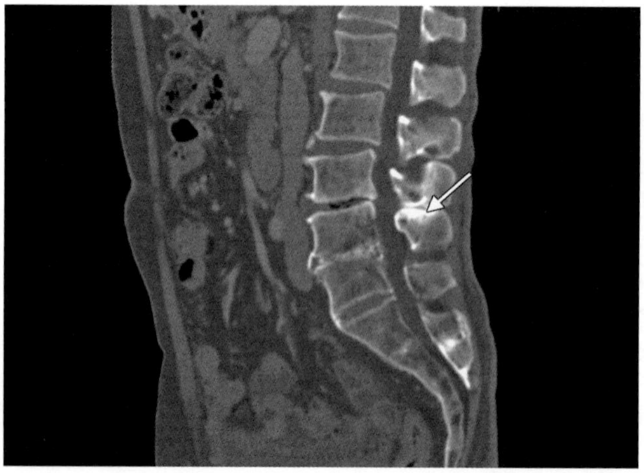

Fig. 8: CT scan of lumbosacral spine in sagittal plane showing reduction of interspinous space between L3-L4 level (arrow) and associated bone sclerosis suggestive of Baastrup's disease.

- Facet joint degeneration, osteophytes, synovial cysts
- Ligamentum flavum buckling

- *Congenital short pedicles*:
  - Usually requires superimposed degeneration to be symptomatic
- *Any mass arising from bone, disk, or within canal*:
  - Osseous tumor, fracture fragments
  - Spondylolysis, spondylolisthesis
  - Ossification of posterior longitudinal ligament
  - Epidural lipomatosis, hematoma, abscess, tumor, scarring

Symptoms from spinal stenosis are often nonspecific and include back pain, intermittent neurogenic claudication, extremity radiculopathy, pain with hyperextension relieved by flexion, and pain on standing relieved by lying down. The presence of imaging findings of spinal stenosis does not indicate that a patient has symptoms from the stenosis.

Types of Involvement

- Central canal
- Neural foramina
- Lateral recesses

Central Canal Stenosis

Central canal stenosis usually is the result of facet joint osteophytes and inward buckling of the ligamentum flavum posteriorly, with disk bulging anteriorly in the canal. Normally, the central canal and thecal sac are round or nearly round (a plump oval) structures on axial images; if they become flattened ovals or triangular in shape, it indicates central stenosis. Central stenosis can cause edema in the affected nerve roots, or, in the cervical spine, there may be abnormalities of the cord, probably myelomalacia from ischemia at the site of stenosis, which shows high signal intensity on T2W images.[34] Besides the encroachment by the osteophytes, disk bulge and hypertrophied ligamentum flavum, accordion shape of the cauda equina nerve roots is another feature which suggests significant canal stenosis. This appearance is best seen on T2 W sagittal images and it is because of the inability of the roots to slide smoothly during change in posture. There is a lot of variation regarding the imaging criteria used to diagnose canal stenosis. Despite various caveats, size criteria of 10 mm canal diameter is the widely used one. There is a four level grading method proposed by Schizas et al to grade the severity of canal stenosis.[35]

Lateral Recess Stenosis

Lateral recess stenosis usually is caused by hypertrophic degenerative changes of the facet joints, or less commonly by a disk fragment or postoperative fibrosis. Lateral recesses are located on the medial aspects of pedicles. Nerve roots lie in these recesses after leaving the thecal sac, but before entering the exiting neural foramina. There is a neural foramen bordering the upper and the lower margins of a lateral recess. If there is deformity in the shape of the recess, and the descending nerve is displaced or compressed, there is lateral recess stenosis. This space is best evaluated in the axial plane of imaging.

Neural Foramen Stenosis

Neural foramen stenosis occurs as a result of degenerative osteophytes of the facet joints or a foraminal disk protrusion **(Fig. 5D)**, extrusion, or sequestered fragment; a diffuse disk bulge; or postoperative fibrosis. Neurogenic tumors can occur in this location which can mimic a herniated disk **(Figs. 9A to C)**. MRI with contrast can be helpful in differentiating these two entities. Neurogenic tumors usually show iso to mild T2 hyperintensity and enhancement on post contrast images whereas herniated disk does not show any central enhancement.

Narrowing of the neural foramina can be evaluated on sagittal and axial images. On sagittal images, the normal neural foramen has the appearance of a vertical oval. If disk material extends into the foramen, the oval narrows inferiorly, creating a keyhole shape. Axial images may be more accurate for diagnosis because they show more of the extent of each foramen.[34]

Postoperative Changes

The imaging feature of postoperative spine depends on the type of surgery performed, interval after surgery and the basic disease itself. Generally, spine surgery is performed either for decompression or spine stabilization or both. Utility of radiographs are limited to check the positioning of implants and for most of the other indications CT or MRI is the modality of choice in post operative setting. The choice of sequences in MRI will depend on the presence of implant. Even MRI compatible implants cause significant local artifacts and hence the positioning and sequences are optimised to reduce artifacts. Recently, metal artifact reduction sequences have shown significant improvement in image quality.

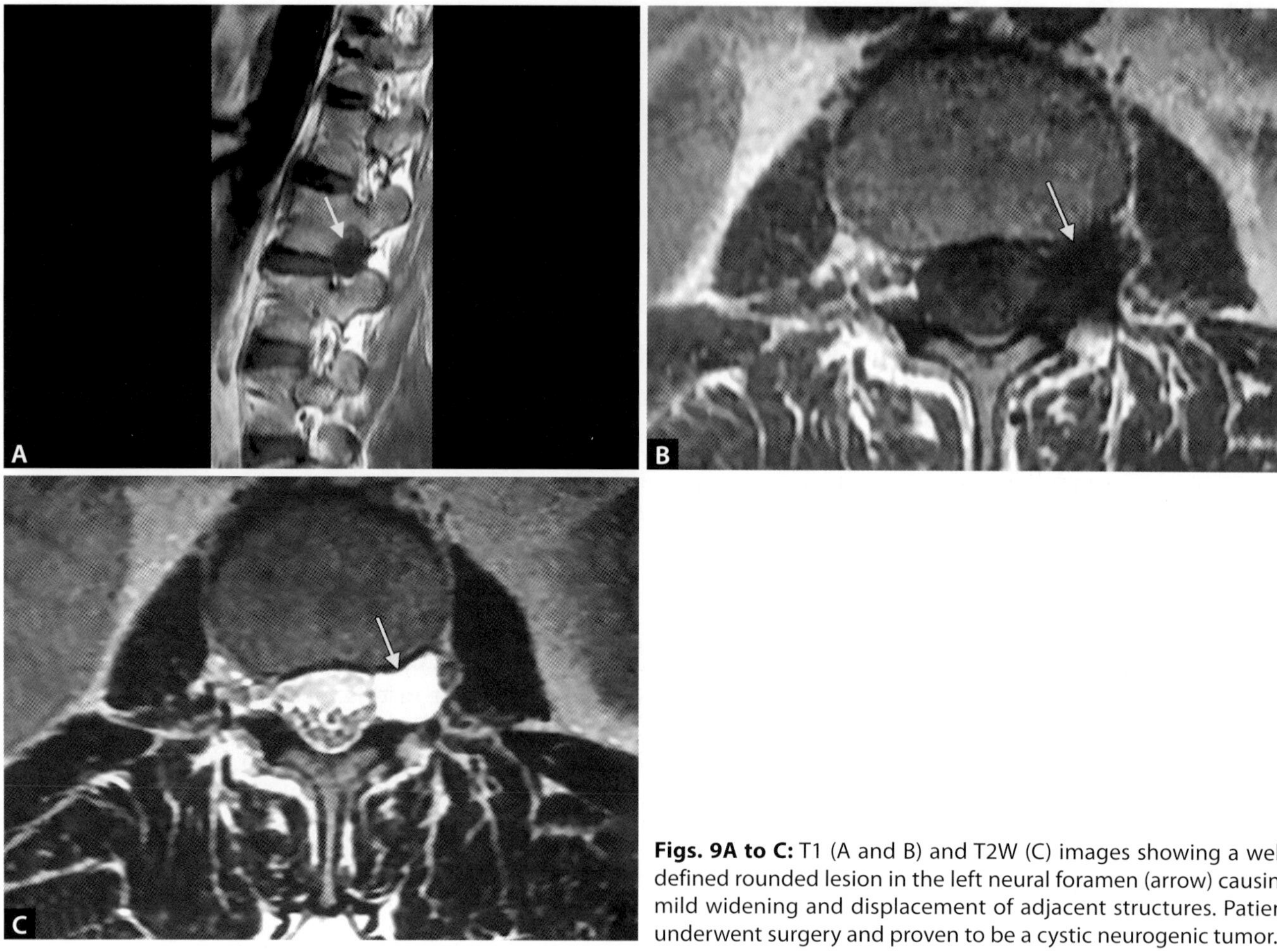

Figs. 9A to C: T1 (A and B) and T2W (C) images showing a well-defined rounded lesion in the left neural foramen (arrow) causing mild widening and displacement of adjacent structures. Patient underwent surgery and proven to be a cystic neurogenic tumor.

Failed Back Syndrome

Patients may have persistent, recurrent, or new and different symptoms after surgery of the spine. The reasons for these problems are many and varied. The most common reasons are recurrent or persistent disk extrusions, postoperative scarring, spondylodiscitis, arachnoiditis, nerve root damage (neuritis), and inadequate surgery.[36,37]

Distinguishing postoperative scarring (epidural fibrosis) from extruded disk material is one of the most important tasks for radiologists in evaluating postoperative MRI studies. All postoperative spine MRI studies should be done with contrast enhancement to distinguish between these two common causes of symptoms in postoperative patients. Scar tissue that is more than 6 months old enhances diffusely **(Figs. 10A to I)** and early after the intravenous administration of gadolinium (high signal intensity on T1W images). Disk material does not enhance until late, if at all, and usually enhances only peripherally. These rules do not work as well during the first 6 months after surgery, when asymptomatic fibrosis may show peripheral rather than diffuse contrast enhancement that is indistinguishable from an extruded disk. Extruded disk material may be an indication for another operation, whereas there is no benefit from reoperating on a patient with postoperative scarring.[36,37]

Other signs that may help distinguish postoperative scarring from a disk abnormality are that postoperative scarring often has irregular margins; it may not be contiguous with the adjacent disk; and, instead of producing a mass effect on the dural sac, it may cause retraction. Recurrent disk herniations, conversely, usually are contiguous with the disk, have sharp margins, and cause mass effect on the dural sac.[36,37]

Fluid collections in the operative site in the form of hematoma, seroma, pseudomeningocele and abscess, spondylodiskitis and arachnoiditis are the complications which can occur after surgery that can be diagnosed on imaging **(Figs. 11A and B)**.

Postoperative Imaging after Intervertebral Fusion and Instrumentation

Spinal instrumentations have been widely performed using various hardware primarily to maintain the alignment of spine. Interbody devices like mesh and cage are also used to promote fusion. Radiologists should be aware of the type of surgery performed and hardware used to identify the post-operative complications, identify the normal post-operative changes and evaluate the correct placement of implants. The common hardware related complications include implant malpositioning, migration, loosening, fracture and infection. The role of radiograph in this situation is limited and CT scan is a much better modality to show the position and alignment of implants precisely. Role of MRI is to evaluate the spinal cord and nerve roots and to detect infection. Pedicle screw is ideally placed in the center of pedicle parallel to the superior endplate of vertebra. The tip of pedicle screw should not breach the anterior cortex of the vertebral body or in contact with vascular structure. Interbody implants like cage is placed 2 mm from the posterior margin of vertebral body.[10]

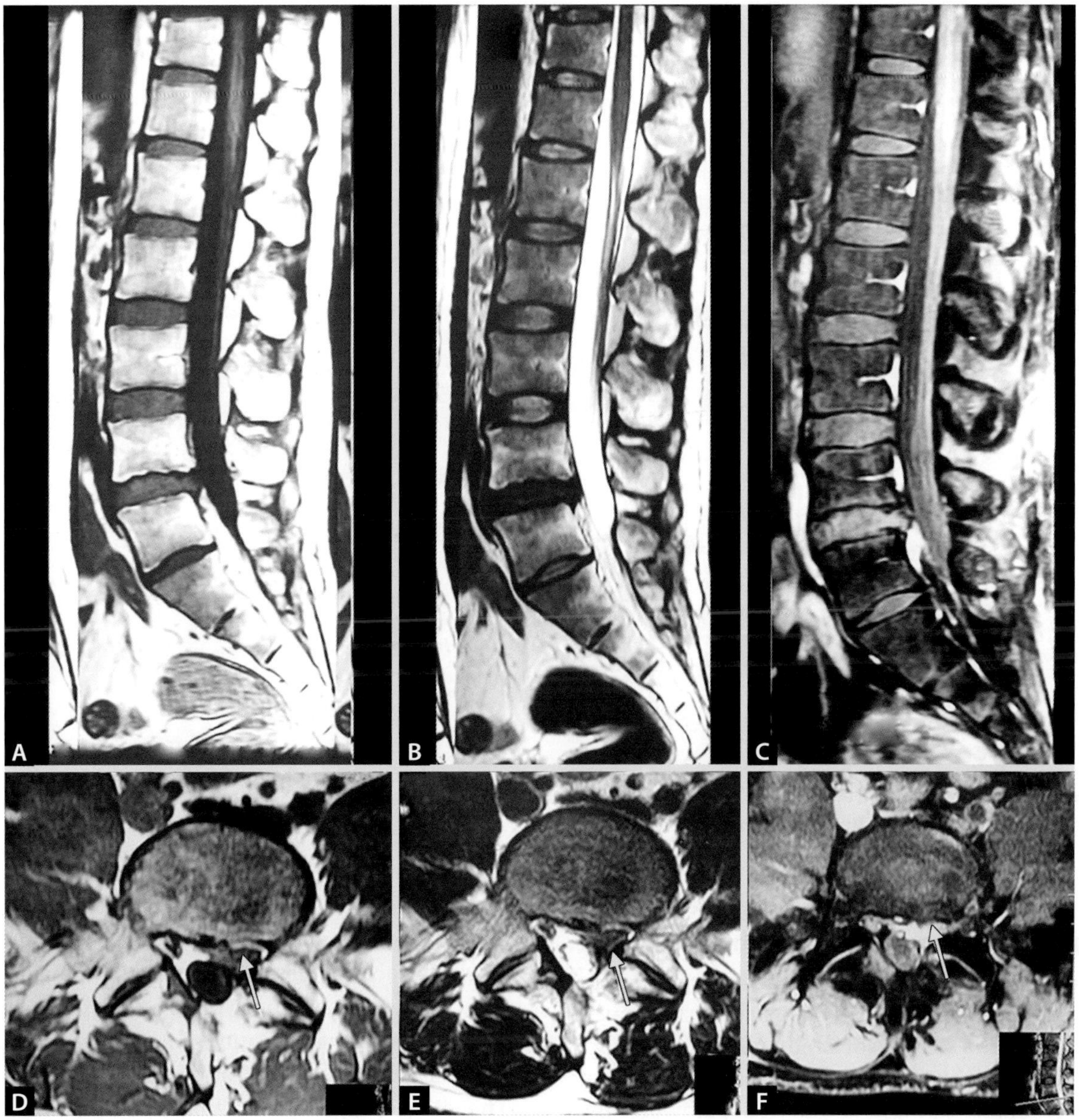

Figs. 10A to F

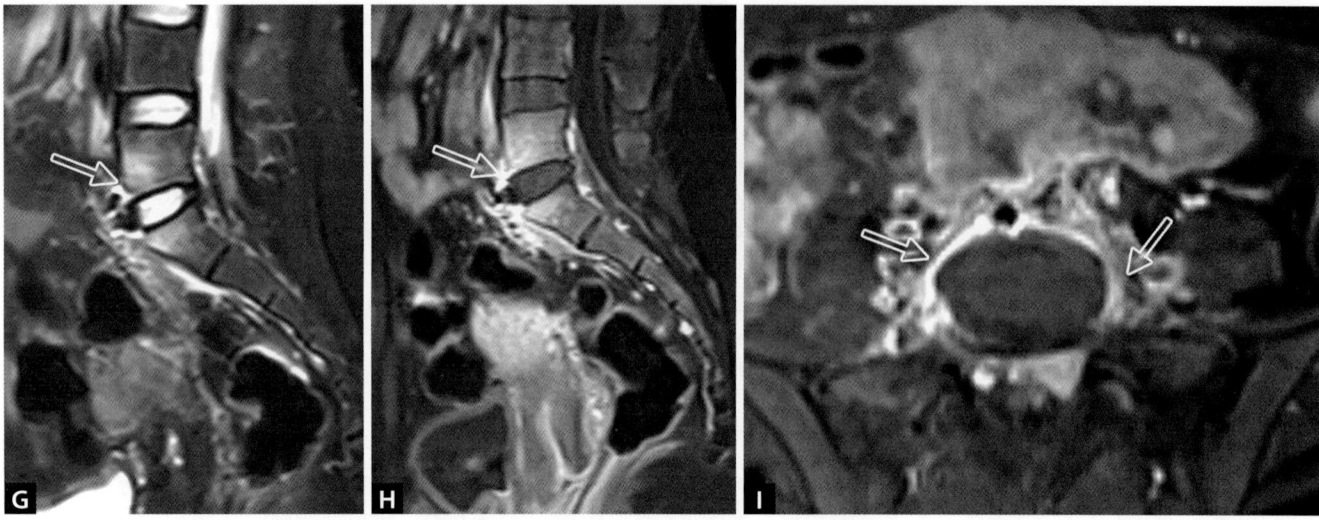

Figs. 10G to I

Figs. 10A to I: Failed back syndrome: Sagittal T1W (A), T2W (B) and fat-suppressed postgadolinium T1W (C) and axial T1W (D), T2W (E) and fat-suppressed T1W (F) MR images show an intermediate signal mass (arrow) in the left paracentral region of this patient, one year after left laminectomy. Contrast-enhanced images (C and F) show diffuse enhancement of the left paracentral mass, indicating this is scarring/ fibrosis, rather than a disk fragment. In another patient who underwent surgery in the lumbosacral region showing T2 hyperintensity (outlined arrow in G) in L5 and S1 marrow with associated soft tissue showing enhancement in postcontrast images (outlined arrow in H and I) suggestive of spondylodiscitis developing after surgery.

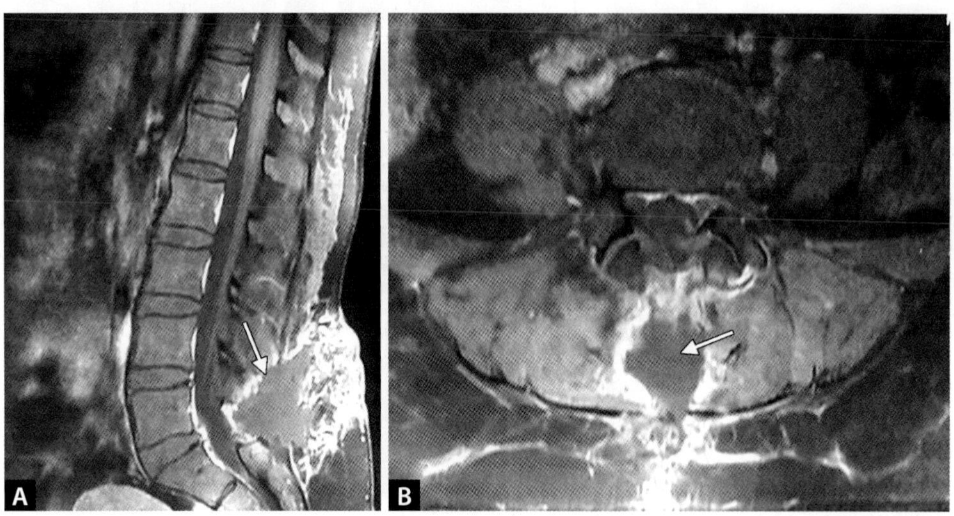

Figs. 11A and B: Post-contrast MRI images in sagittal (A) and axial (B) planes in a patient who underwent spinal decompression surgery showing a non-enhancing fluid collection posterior to spine (arrow) with irregular enhancing wall suggestive of abscess.

Seronegative Spondyloarthropathy

This group of disorders includes ankylosing spondylitis, Reiter's or reactive arthropathy, psoriatic arthropathy and spondyloarthropathy associated with inflammatory disease. They are characterized by rheumatoid factor negative inflammatory arthritis and enthesiopathy affecting the spine and sacroiliac joints. It presents in early to mid adulthood, more commonly in males with symptoms of low backache and stiffness which is worse in the morning. It has a strong association with HLA B27 haplotype. A detailed discussion of this entity is beyond the scope of this chapter and only the salient features are presented.

The disease first affects bilateral sacroiliac joints followed by the thoracolumbar junction and may

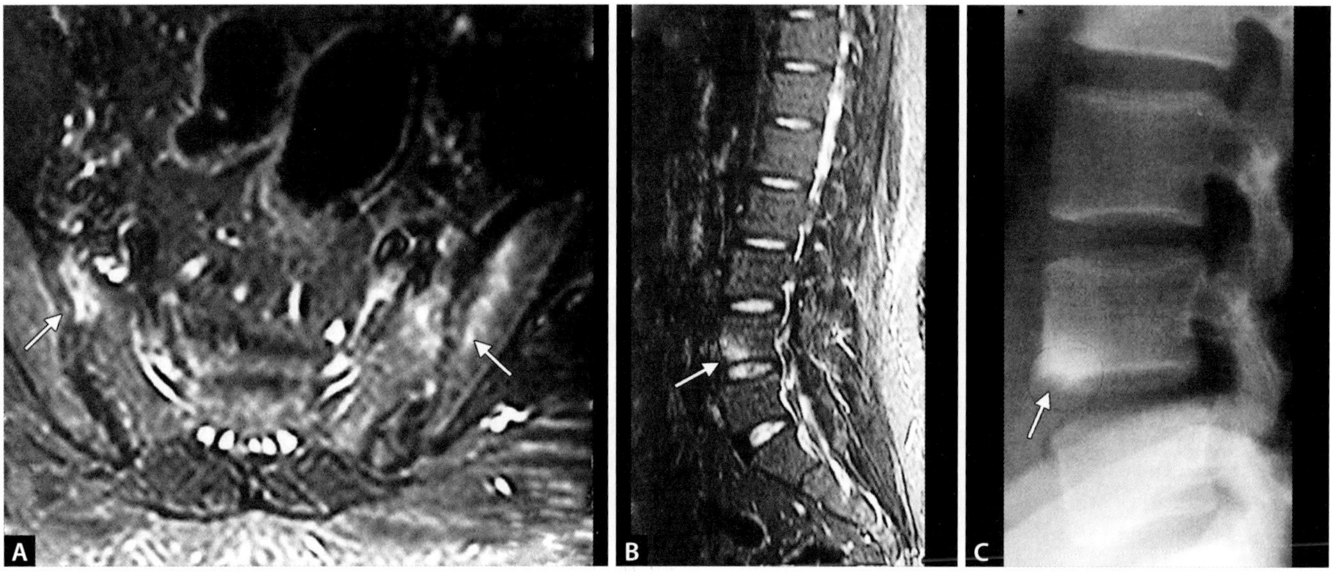

Figs. 12A to C: Ankylosing spondylitis: Axial STIR (A) image of bilateral sacroiliac joints and sagittal STIR (B) image of LS spine showing hyperintensity at articular margins of bilateral SI joints (arrows) and at anteroinferior margin of L4 vertebra typical appearance of early spondyloarthropathy. Lateral radiograph (C) of lumbar spine showing anterior corner erosions at the L4 vertebral body. The typical shiny corner sign (or Romanus lesion) is present (arrow).

eventually involve the entire spine. The erosive sacroilitis is best appreciated on a PA view of the pelvis and affects the lower third of the joint. The earliest sign is loss of definition of subchondral bone, and other features are small erosions, widening of joint space, sclerosis and eventually fusion of the joint.[38] Early manifestations of sacroilitis may be better evaluated by CT and MRI. Small erosions are well seen on CT and MRI in the early stage of disease shows T2 and STIR hyperintensity **(Figs. 12A to C)**.[39]

The vertebral bodies show squaring, corner erosions which undergo sclerotic repair. This leads to shiny corner sign or Romanus lesion **(Fig. 12C)**. Multilevel syndesmophytes give rise to a bamboo spine appearance. Facet joints are commonly involved and erosions progress to fusion.

Fractures and pseudoarthrosis may occur through the disk or endplate and are referred to as Anderson lesion **(Figs. 13A and B)**. This can mimic infectious spondylodiscitis and the differentiating feature is extension across the posterior elements.[39]

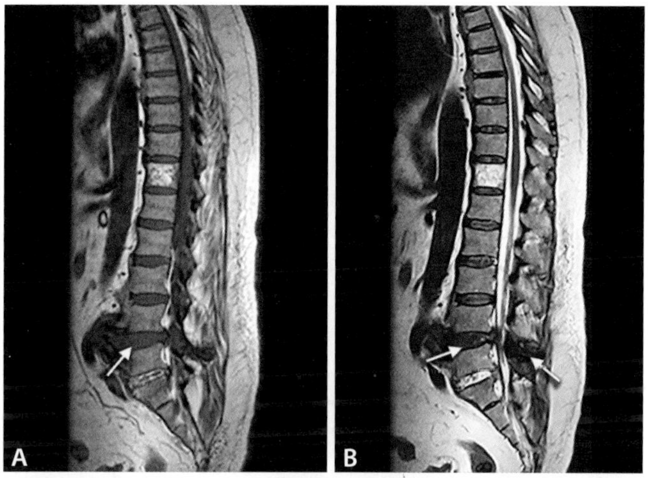

Figs. 13A and B: Sagittal T1W (A) and T2W (B) MR image of the thoracolumbar spine showing a fracture through the L5-S1disk which is extending across the posterior elements typical of Anderson lesion (white arrow). Incidental vertebral hemangioma of D12 vertebra is also seen (thick arrow).

INFECTIONS

Infections of the spine are a common cause of back pain in our country. Infection should be suspected in patients with severe back pain that does not improve with rest, that wakes them at night, and that is associated with a fever. Tuberculosis of the spine is common in India and needs to be kept in the list of differential diagnosis for a wide variety of spinal abnormalities. Conventional radiographs are the initial screening modality when infectious spondylitis is suspected. Compared to MRI and radionuclide scans, radiographs are relatively insensitive early in the course of infection. It takes weeks for destructive changes to become evident.[40] This initial imaging study, however, guides the next diagnostic step.

Tubercular Infection

The spine is the most common site of osseous tuberculous involvement, comprising in most series about 50% of cases. Patients present with long-standing and insidious onset of stiffness and local tenderness, with or without constitutional symptoms. The lower dorsal and upper lumbar vertebrae are most frequently affected; cervical and sacral involvement occurs uncommonly. The spread of tuberculosis to the spine is usually by hematogenous route, by perivertebral arterial or venous plexi, or rarely by extension from a paraspinal infection. It is often difficult to differentiate tubercular from pyogenic spondylytis both clinically and on imaging. There are four different patterns of involvement: paradiskal, central, subligamentous and posterior.[40]

Plain film evaluation of the tuberculous spondylodiskitis may demonstrate loss of vertebral height or disk interval, erosions, indistinct margins of end plates **(Figs. 14A and B)** paravertebral masses, and sequestrae. The infection usually begins in the anterior aspect of the vertebral body, adjacent to the vertebral endplate. Focal areas of erosion and osseous destruction in the anterior corners of the vertebral body are typical plain film findings. Involvement of the adjacent intervertebral disk or vertebral body results from penetration of the disk itself or spread of infection beneath the anterior or posterior longitudinal ligament. Contiguous vertebral involvement, destruction of the intervertebral disk and progressive vertebral body collapse result in the characteristic gibbus deformity of the spine commonly associated with spinal tuberculosis.[40] Paraspinal abscess formation may be detected on radiographs as fusiform paravertebral soft tissue masses.

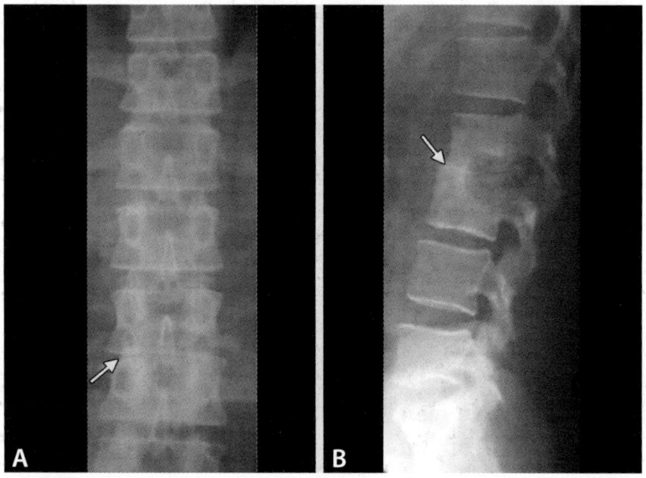

Figs. 14A and B: Tuberculosis: Anteroposterior and lateral plain radiographs (A and B) of lumbar spine showing reduced L2-3 disk space (arrow) with indistinct adjacent end plates and lytic lesion centered around the end plates suggestive of infective spondylitis.

Disk space narrowing may be quite subtle. Over 50% of the trabecular bone is lost before a lesion is conspicuous on plain film; this process may take up to 6 month. In the thoracic spine visualization of a paravertebral abscess requires an adequately penetrated view. In the lumbar spine asymmetry or bulging of the psoas shadow may be detected. Scalloping of the anterior vertebral contour (aneurysmal appearance) is more commonly seen with children. Plain film is limited in evaluation of the posterior arch, particularly in the thoracic spine. No specific or pathognomonic plain film signs distinguish tuberculous from pyogenic spinal infection, and correlation with the clinical picture is important.

Computed Tomography Features

Computed tomography (CT) is not a routinely used imaging modality in assessing the tuberculous spondylitis but it may be helpful in assessing the cortical breakdown, destruction of cancellous bone as well as spinal distortion in chronic cases. MDCT using thinnest collimation with multiplanar reconstruction in different planes, can be beneficial to assess the destruction of bone and gibbus/scoliosis deformity of the spine in chronic cases.

One of the major disadvantages of CT as compared to MRI, is difficulty in identifying the early marrow changes of the disease process within the bone. Another disadvantage of CT is its inability to identify subtle epidural soft tissue component due to beam hardening artifact.

However, CT is more sensitive in showing subtle soft tissue calcifications as compared to MRI. Computed tomography is useful for guiding percutaneous drainage of paravertebral abscesses, which are difficult to access under ultrasound guidance.

MR Features

Multiplanar capability and optimal tissue contrast make MR imaging the optimal modality for evaluation of spondylodiskitis.[41-43] The entire spine and canal can be visualized, including the posterior elements. MR imaging has higher sensitivity for early infiltrative disease including end plate changes and marrow infiltration than bone scan and plain films. MR imaging affords excellent definition of epidural, paravertebral, and intraosseous abscesses, and extent of cord compromise. Paravertebral abscesses may be large, and discharge through tracts well seen on multiple planes. The involved vertebrae show hypointense signal on T1-weighted images and heterogeneous increased signal on T2-weighted images. The intravenous administration of contrast improves definition of epidural abscesses and masses, and cord and nerve root compromise **(Figs. 15A to D)**. The abscesses show peripheral enhancement with central necrosis. Acute stage shows inhomogeneous enhancement in areas of marrow infiltration, and enhancing lesion borders. With tuberculous spondylodiskitis, the disk shows signal characteristics seen with pyogenic discitis in at least three quarters of cases, of bright signal on T2-weighted images, decreased signal on T1-weighted images, and enhancement of disk after contrast administration. Disk space preservation, normal signal intensity, and lack of enhancement have been reported in approximately 25% of cases.

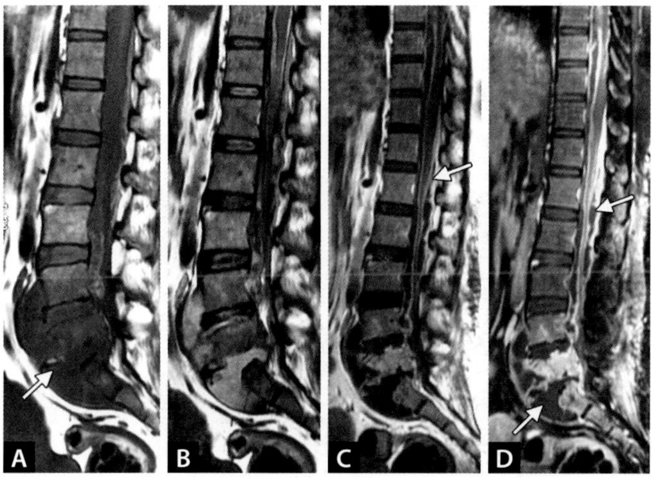

Figs. 15A to D: Tubercular spondylitis. Sagittal T1W (A), T2W (B) and postcontrast T1W (C and D) MR images showing destructive lesion involving the L5 vertebra, L5-S1 disk space and adjacent end plates associated with prevertebral soft tissue component which is showing peripheral rim enhancement suggestive of abscess. The abscess is extending into the spinal canal (extradural location) proximally till D12 level (arrow). Leptomeningeal enhancement is also seen.

In paradiscal variety MRI shows hypointense signal on T1W and high signal on T2W images in the end plate, narrowing of the disk, and large paraspinal and epidural abscesses. In the central type of lesion signal intensity abnormality is confined to the vertebral body and the disk space is preserved. The appearance can be indistinguishable from metastases or lymphoma.[41-45]

Uncommon Patterns

Infection limited to a single vertebral body in the form of osteitis may occur. It is detected late on plain radiographs and is better seen on MRI as a marrow signal abnormality **(Figs. 16A to G)**. Multiple vertebral levels may be involved in a non-contigous manner, manifested on plain radiographs as skip lesions of vertebral body destruction and collapse. The posterior elements of the spine are

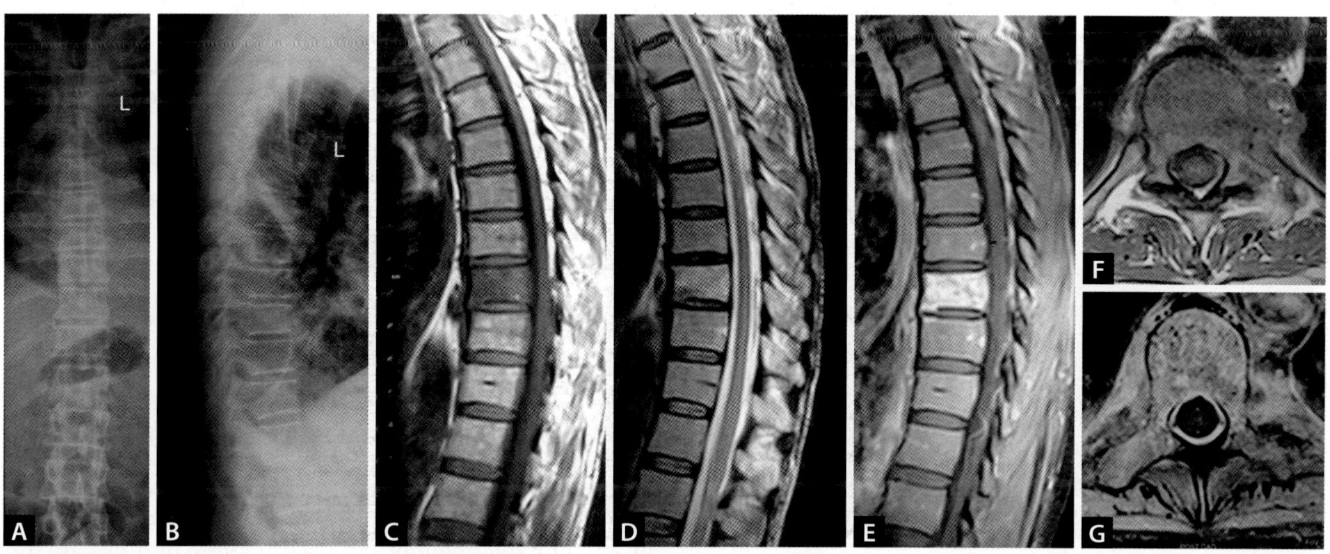

Figs. 16A to G: Central tuberculosis: Radiographs anteroposterior (A) and lateral view (B) of the dorso-lumbar spine are normal. Sagittal T1W (C) T2W (D) and postcontrast T1W (E) images and axial T1W (F) and postcontrast images (G) show T1 hypointensity, T2 hyperintensity and enhancement of the marrow of D6 vertebral body with small left paravertebral soft tissue. The height of the vertebra and adjacent disk space is maintained.

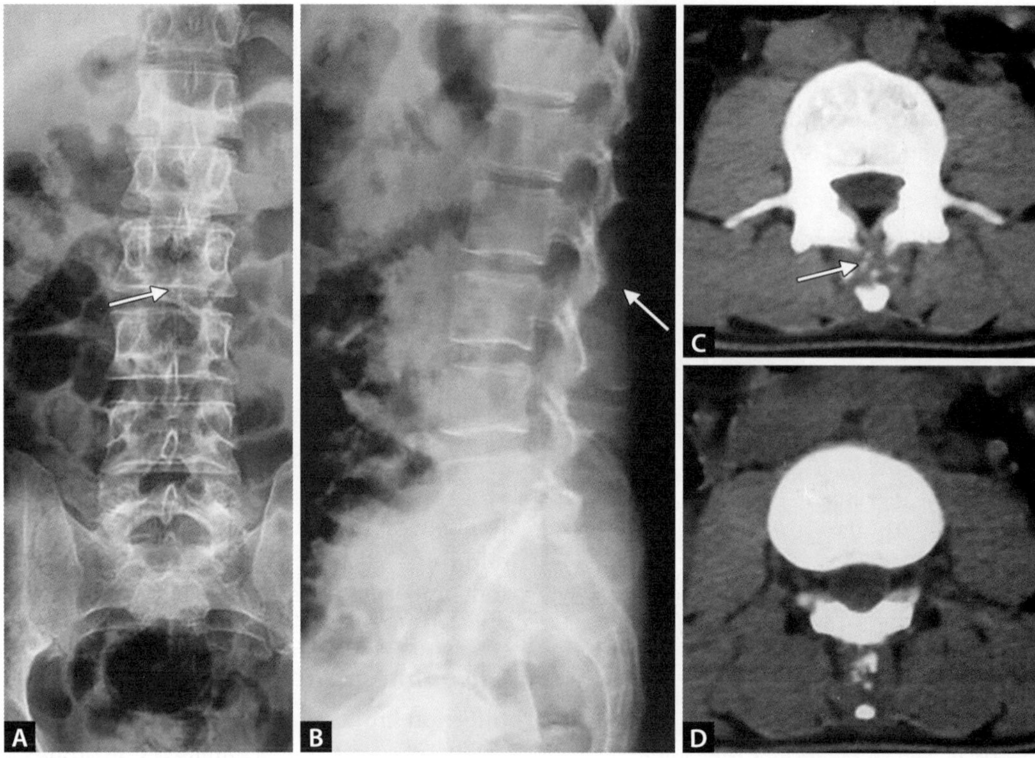

Figs. 17A to D: Posterior element TB: Anteroposterior (A) and lateral (B) radiographs of lumbar spine showing non-visualization of the spinous process of L2 vertebra. Axial CT sections (C and D) showing lytic destructive lesion involving the spinous process of L2 vertebra.

usually involved secondarily due to spread of infection from the vertebral body. However, isolated involvement of the posterior elements may occasionally occurs **(Figs. 17A to D)**.[43,44]

Response Assessment and Follow-up

There is an increasing move away from surgical intervention towards conservative therapy, percutaneous drainage of abscesses, or both. It is therefore critical to monitor treatment response. MR imaging is a valuable diagnostic tool not only for early diagnosis but is also used to effectively monitor treatment response. Particular emphasis should be placed on soft-tissue appearance in the early stages. Progressive reduction in gadolinium enhancement and the eventual loss of all enhancement are useful signs. Later on, fat deposition is a useful sign of healing. Gadolinium enhancement patterns vary and a reduction in gadolinium enhancement is a reliable sign, but an increase does not necessarily denote treatment failure.

Follow-up of patients with tuberculous spondylitis has to be based upon both clinical and radiological findings. Usually there is lag of 2 months for radiological improvement of a lesion to be seen on imaging, as compared to clinical improvement. It takes about 2–3 months to show a radiologically perceptible sclerosis (remineralization), following drug treatment.

MRI done at 2–3 months even in a responsive tuberculous spondylitis may show increased inflammatory response giving false impression of progression of disease. Thus, early MR imaging following the start of drug treatment may be unreliable. However, if MRI findings worsen at 5–6 months of treatment, one should suspect a therapeutically refractory case.

Also, if there is no clinical improvement or there is worsening of spinal abnormality or appearance of a new lesion or failure of healing of ulcer/sinus or dehiscence of wound after 4–5 months of surgery, one should think of either refractory or drug resistant tuberculosis. To label a case as multi-drug resistant tuberculosis, drug resistance has to be demonstrated on tissue sample.

Early healing: Reduction in amount or degree of gadolinium enhancement of soft tissue (These findings are the best indicators of early healing).

However, progression of bone or disk changes, either an alteration in signal intensity or increasing destruction, during early course of treatment do not indicate failed treatment.

Late healing: Signs of healed tubercular lesions on follow-up contrast enhanced MRI include complete disappearance of marrow edema, resolution of paravertebral collections and replacement of vertebral body marrow by fat, seen as increased signal on T1-weighted images.

These patients should be monitored for at least 2 years, following the completion of treatment regimen and follow-up MR is performed to show complete resolution of the lesion.

Role of FDG-PET Scan

Active tuberculosis shows increased uptake on FDG-PET scan, but this increased uptake is non-specific. It is also seen in neoplastic as well as other granulomatous diseases like brucellosis. FDG-PET may be requested in patients with equivocal MRI findings or for response evaluation when there are enhancing areas on MRI, after full clinical resolution of the symptoms and completion of ATT. In such situations, increased uptake on FDG PET supports presence of active infection. FDG PET also provides a quantitative measurement of the absolute fraction of the injected dose reaching a tissue called the Standard Uptake Value (SUV). SUV values are raised in cases of active tuberculosis.

Differential diagnosis

Uncommon infections: Brucellosis is a zoonotic infection, and the most common site of bone brucellosis is the spine. The imaging manifestations closely resemble tubercular spondylitis. Brucellar spondylitis has a predilection for the lower lumbar spine. Features reported in the literature include intact vertebral architecture inspite of diffuse vertebral osteomyelitis, marked T2 hyperintensity and enhancement of the intervertebral disk and facet joint involvement. Gibbus deformities are rare and paraspinal abscesses are smaller than those in tubercular spondylitis. This possibilty should be kept in mind when apparent tubercular spondylitis does not respond to treatment.[42]

Fungal spondylitis caused by organisms like Aspergillus may be seen in immunocompromised hosts and very rarely in immunocompetent patients. The imaging findings mimic pyogenic or tubercular spondylitis and diagnosis is made usually after tissue sampling. T2 hyperintensity in discs is typically lacking in this entity, a fact attribute to the paramagnetic and ferromagnetic elements in fungi.[45]

Non-infectious diseases that mimic spondylodiscitis: Non-infectious inflammatory diseases and degenerative disease may simulate spinal infection. *Discogenic vertebral body degeneration (Modic Type I)* may resemble infectious spondylitis because of the presence of bone marrow edema which has high signal intensity on T2W images. These marrow changes and the associated disk may also enhance on contrast-enhanced images. The lack of increased signal intensity of associated disk on T2W images and the absence of soft tissue abnormality distinguish degenerative changes from infectious spondylitis.[43,44]

Pseudoarthrosis secondary to spinal fracture *(Andersson lesion)* are not an uncommon complication of advanced ankylosing spondylitis. They commonly involve the disk space or juxtaarticular end plate. In pseudoarthrosis sub-chondral sclerosis and end plate erosion may be seen on radiographs that mimic infectious spondylitis. MRI can help in the differentiation by showing the extension of fracture line across the posterior elements.[43]

Occasionally *Schmorl's nodes* can also mimic infectious spondylodiscitis. The herniation of the disk into the vertebral endplate can incite marrow edema and vascularization which can result in vertebral end plate hyperintensity and enhancement. However, if the bone defect involves only one end plate and the disk does not show diffuse signal abnormality, Schmorl's node rather than spondylodiscitis should be suspected.

Neuropathic spine is seen in patients of diabetes, syringomyelia, syphilis, etc. It most often involves the thoracolumbar junction and lumbar spine. Destructive changes in the vertebral bodies lead to fracture, bone sclerosis, large osteophytes and decreased disk space. The disk space and surrounding marrow show lower T2 signal than in infectious spondylitis. Other distinguishing findings of this entity include facet involvement, osseous joint debris and joint disorganization.

In *neoplastic lesions,* the disk is usually preserved and disk height reduction is rare. The end plates are usually distinct. If posterior elements are involved, neoplastic lesions should be included in the differential.

Other infiltrative granulomatous lesions such as sarcoidosis may show signal intensity abnormalities similar to TB, but diskitis is usually not seen.

Pyogenic Infection

The vertebral infection generally begins adjacent to the endplate, it invades the subchondral bone and extends to the disk. The common causative organism is

Staphylococcus aureus. This pattern of hematogenous infection gives rise to the classic radiographic picture of infectious spondylitis: destructive changes of two adjacent vertebral bodies and the intervening disk. This is manifested on the radiograph as loss of height of the vertebral bodies and a narrowed disk space. Because of endplate destruction, the disk space may have an apparent increase in height, rather than narrowing. The destructive changes of metastatic tumor have a different pattern. Tumor tends to respect the endplates, extending into the surrounding soft tissues by cortical invasion.

The initial radiographs may be completely normal and the findings typically lag behind symptoms by two to three weeks. The earliest signs include blurring of endplates and decrease in the height of disk space followed by bone destruction in the adjacent vertebrae. Eventually sclerosis supervenes and is a manifestation of a reparative response. Radionuclide scan using Tc 99m has an accuracy as high as 90% in patients with more than two days of symptoms.[45-47]

TUMORS

A wide spectrum of tumors can affect the bony spine. Some of them like hemangiomas are common and discovered incidentally. The commonest malignant lesions in the spine are metastases and myeloma. Primary tumors are rare and radiographic and MR features can help to narrow the differential diagnosis.[48]

Benign Tumors

Hemangioma

They are benign vascular lesions, majority of which are asymptomatic and discovered incidentally. They have been reported in up to 10% of all individuals undergoing spinal imaging. Most spinal hemangiomas occur in thoracic spine and are usually confined to the vertebral bodies. They are usually asymptomatic and do not require clinical attention. However, rarely they are aggressive and can grow beyond the vertebral body and may compress the spinal cord or nerve roots.[48]

They show characteristic imaging findings. The radiographic appearance is of prominent vertical striations giving a corduroy cloth or honeycomb appearance. This translates into the polka dot appearance on CT. Thickened trabeculae are surrounded by hypodense fatty tissue. Typical hemangiomas appear hyperintense on both T1 and T2W sequences **(Figs. 18A and B)** and may enhance after contrast administration. The aggressive hemangiomas are hypointense on T1W and bright in T2W scans, may be associated with a paravertebral soft tissue **(Figs. 19A to F)** and resemble metastases or myeloma.[48,49]

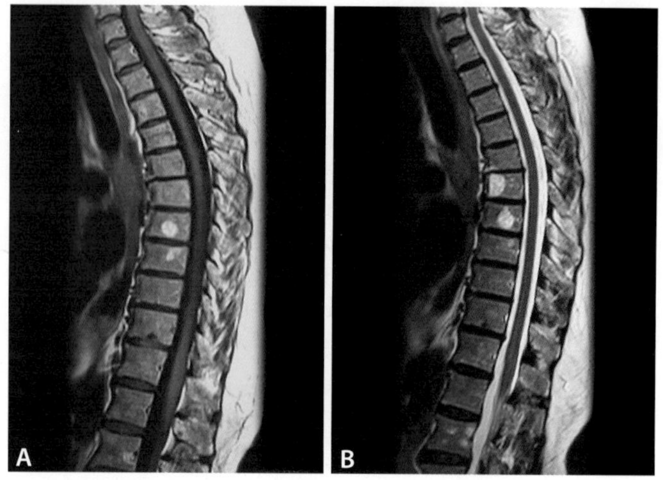

Figs. 18A and B: Sagittal T1W (A) and T2W (B) MR images showing lesions involving the vertebral bodies of two dorsal vertebra which are hyperintense on both T1W and T2W images suggestive of vertebral hemangioma.

Osteoid Osteoma

It is a relatively common benign osseous lesion. The peak incidence is in the second decade. It has a tendency to involve the posterior elements and occurs commonly in the pedicle. The lumbar spine is most commonly affected (59%) followed by cervical and thoracic spine.[50,51]

The histological hallmark is a nidus, which is smaller than 1.5 cm. Clinically, the spinal osteoid osteoma presents with a painful scoliosis. The pain is worse at night, and is relieved with aspirin. The lumbar spine radiographs may show scoliosis, concave to the side of the lesion. The central lucent nidus may be obscured by the reactive sclerosis. CT is the modality of choice for a careful search of a nidus **(Figs. 20A to C)**. The nidus is usually a subcentimeter lytic area with a sclerotic center surrounded by periosteal thickening. Occasionally, vascular channels leading to this lesion may be seen adjacent to the nidus. As with other nonaggressive osteoid lesions, MRI is not indicated. In fact, MR may be misleading, as the nidus is commonly not evident. If visible, it appears as a low signal focus with extensive adjacent marrow and soft tissue edema. The nidus is hypointense on T1W images and hypo to hyperintense on T2W images. Surrounding hyperintensity is reactive host response and involves a much larger area than the tumor. Severe reactive response may lead to a misdiagnosis of malignancy or infection.

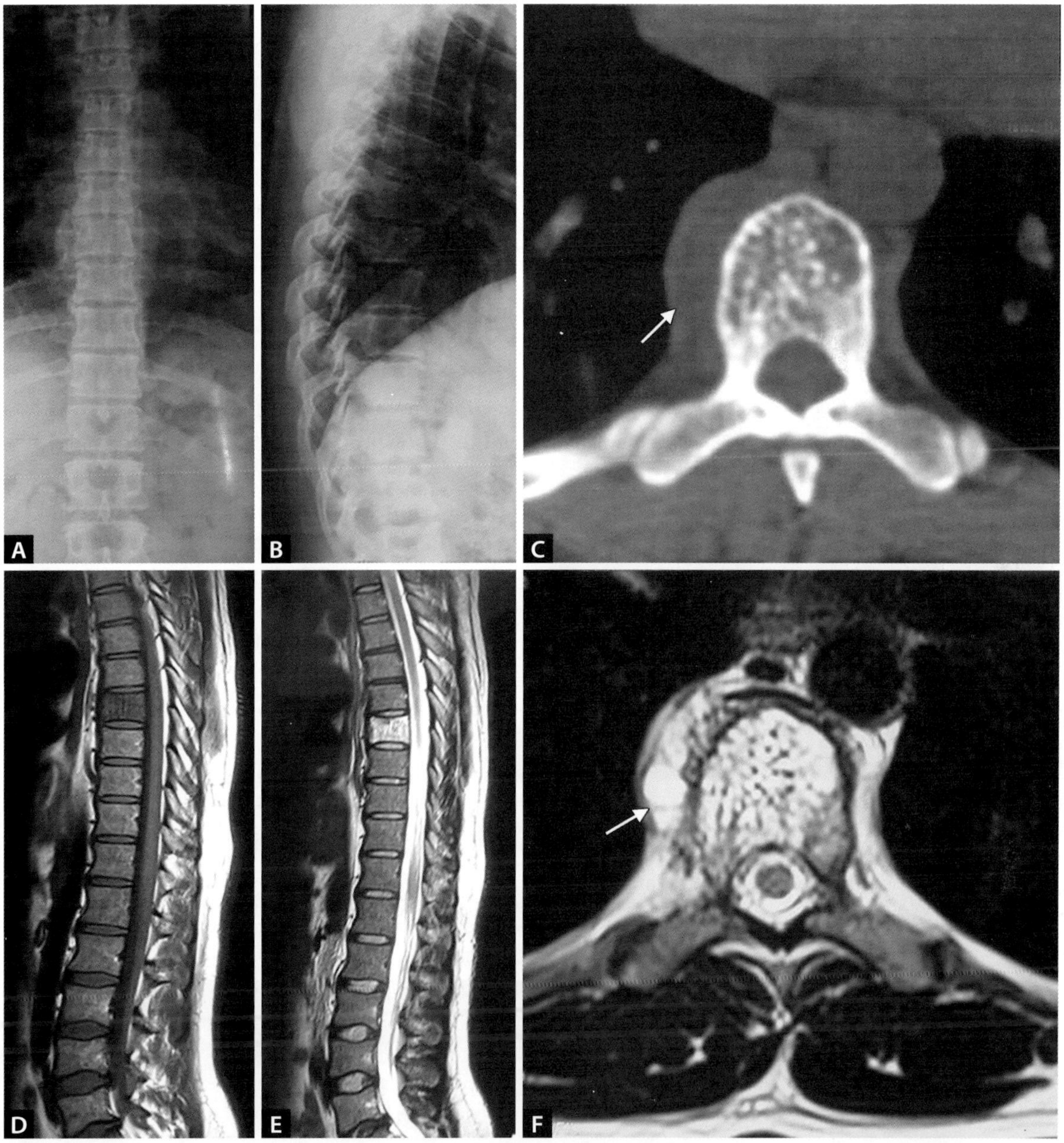

Figs. 19A to F: Aggressive hemangioma: Anteroposterior and lateral radiographs (A and B) of dorsolumbar spine show a small right paraspinal mass; Axial CT section (C) of D8 vertebra showing typical polka dot appearance involving the D8 vertebral body associated with right paravertebral soft tissue component (arrow); Sagittal T1W (D), T2W (E) and axial T2W (F) MR images showing lesion involving the vertebral body of D8 which is hypointense on T1W and brightly hyperintense on T2W associated with soft tissue component.

The lesion is positive on all three phases of a Tc-99m MDP bone scan. The differential diagnosis of osteoid osteoma in the spine includes osteoblastoma which is larger, unilateral absent pedicle, osteoblastic metastases, and stress fracture of pedicle. CT plays a valuable role in distinguishing these entities.[50,51]

The treatment is surgical or image guided percutaneous excision or RF ablation. The entire nidus has to be removed to prevent recurrence.

Osteoblastoma

Osteoblastomas are related to osteoid osteomas and by definition are larger than 1.5 cm in diameter. They are seen in patients in the first to third decades. Up to 40% osteoblastomas are found in the spine. They also have a tendency to involve the posterior elements.[48] Radiographs show a lytic, expansile lesion **(Fig. 21A)** in the posterior elements. CT is ideal to show the expansile lesion **(Fig. 21B)** with sclerotic border, which may have foci of calcification representing an osteoid matrix. MRI is usually not required except to show the relationship with the cord and nerve roots. It is T1 hypointense and shows intermediate to high signal on T2W images.[51] Secondary aneurysmal bone cyst may be seen within the lesion and they are T2 hyperintense **(Fig. 21C)** with fluid-fluid levels. Extensive peri-tumoral edema is common and may involve adjacent bones and soft tissues. The differential diagnosis includes osteoid osteoma, aneurysmal bone cyst, infection and metastases.

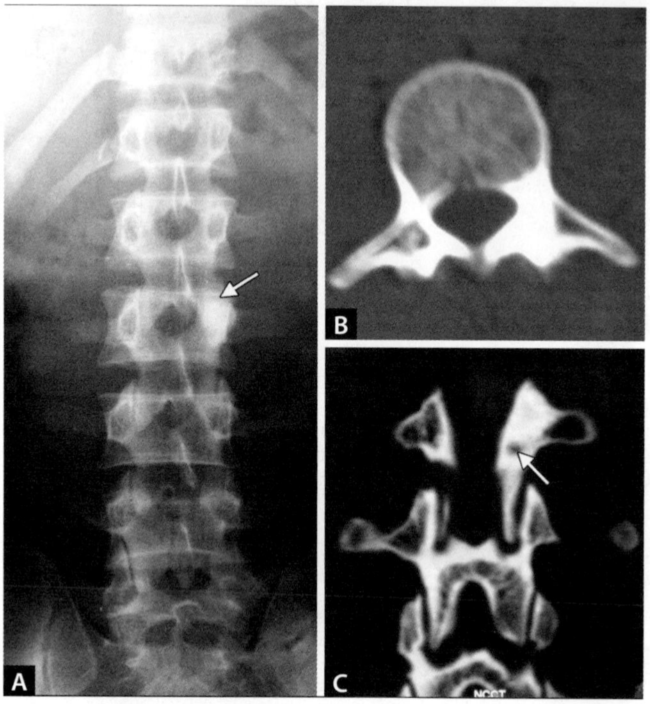

Figs. 20A to C: Osteoid osteoma: Anteroposterior radiograph of lumbar region (A) showing sclerotic left pedicle of L2 vertebra (arrow). Axial (B) and Coronal 3D reformatted CT (C) images showing sclerotic lesion involving left pedicle and lamina with small lucent nidus in the centre (arrow).

Aneurysmal Bone Cyst

They are benign lesions with blood filled cavities. They occur in the younger age group within the first two decades of life. The spine is a common location with the lumbar spine ranking second to the thoracic spine. Radiograph shows expansile lesion in the posterior elements **(Figs. 22A and B)** which often extends to involve the vertebral body. CT shows a lesion with balloon like expansion and thinned out cortex, with a non-sclerotic narrow zone of transition. Fluid-Fluid levels with sedimentation of blood products are a typical finding. It commonly extends into the epidural space and causes cord compression. MRI is ideal for showing the cystic spaces **(Figs. 22C and D)** within the lesion separated by septae. Fluid levels of varying signal intensities due to different stages of hemorrhage **(Fig. 22D)** are well seen on MRI.[48,50] On contrast administration only the periphery of the lesion and septae enhance.

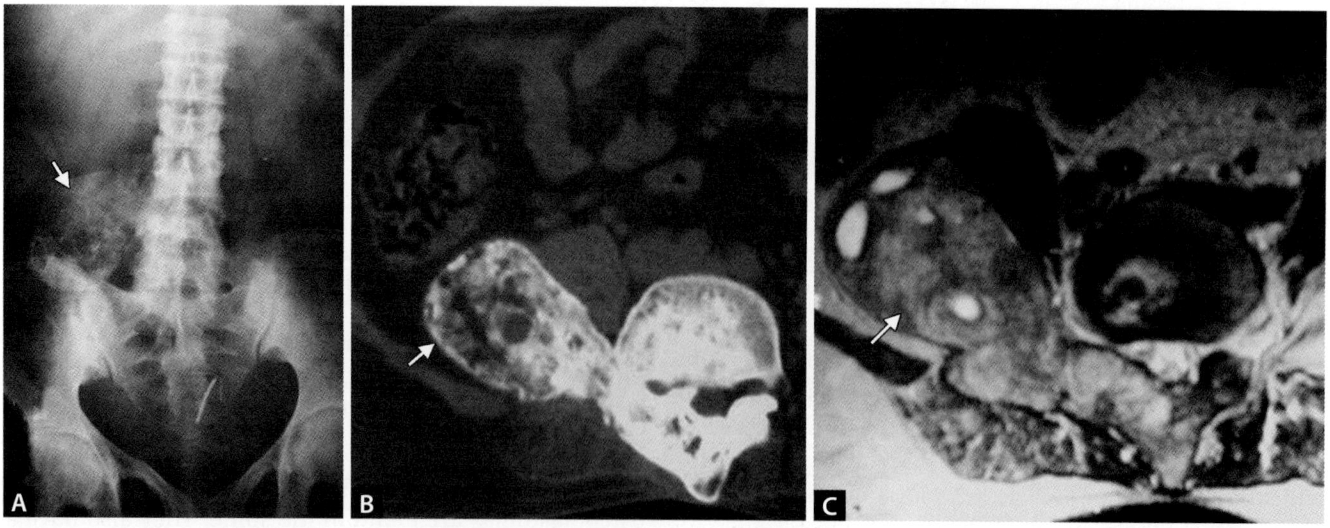

Figs. 21A to C: Osteoblastoma: Anteroposterior radiograph of KUB region (A) showing large expansile mixed lytic-sclerotic lesion arising from right transverse process of L4 vertebra (arrow); Axial CT (B) and axial T2W (C) MR images showing large expansile osseous lesion involving the right transverse process and lamina of L4 vertebra (arrow). Hyperintense foci are likely to be due to secondary aneurysmal bone cyst.

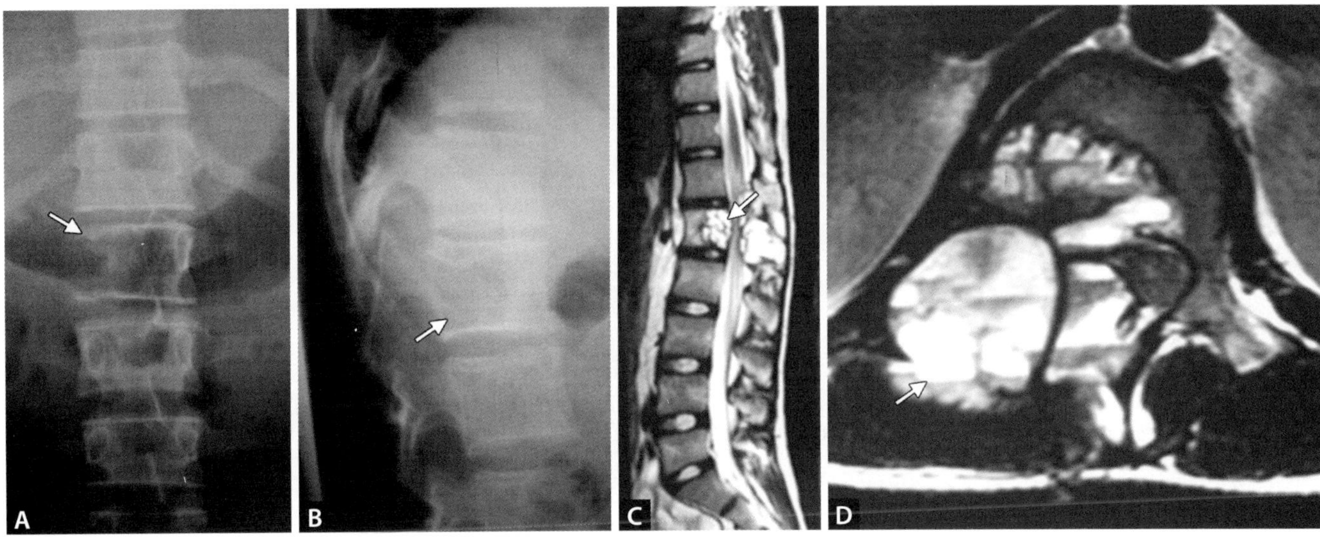

Figs. 22A to D: Aneurysmal bone cyst: Anteroposterior (A) and lateral (B) radiographs of lumbar spine showing a lytic destructive lesion involving the posterior vertebral body and right pedicle (arrow). Sagittal T2W (C) and Axial T2W (D) MR images showing hyperintense lesion in L1 posterior vertebral body, right pedicle and lamina with multiple blood fluid levels (arrow).

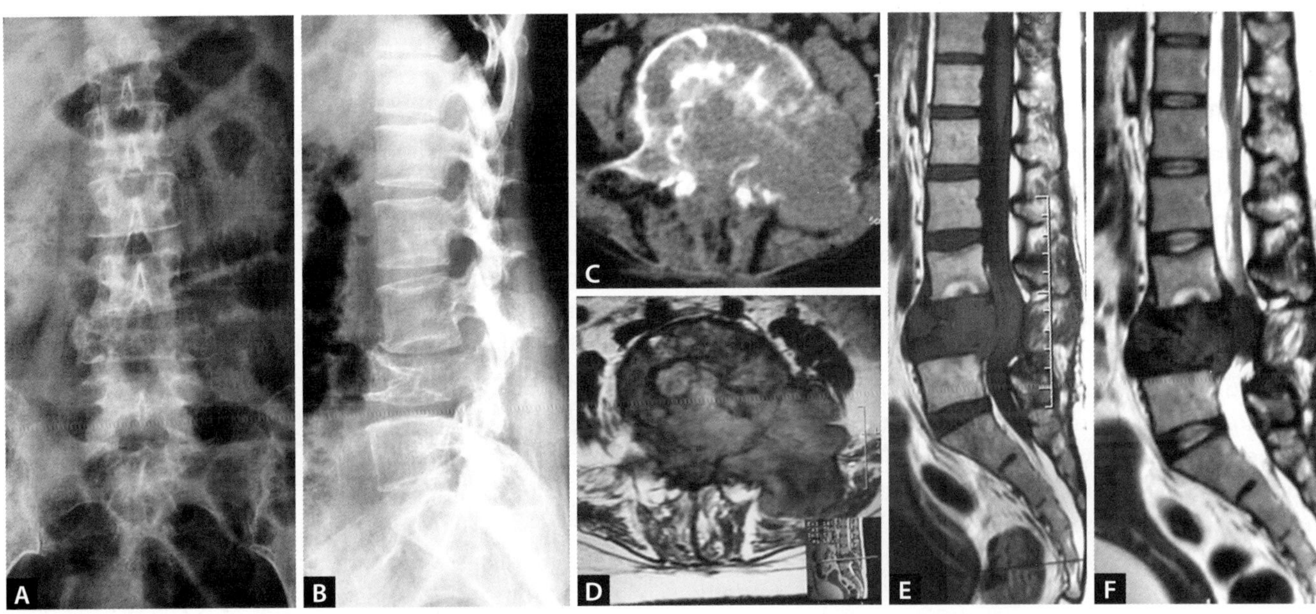

Figs. 23A to F: Giant Cell Tumor: Radiograph Anteroposterior (A) and lateral view (B) showing lytic expansile lesion in L4 vertebral body and pedicle with collapse; Axial CT image (C) shows an expansile lesion involving body, pedicle and left transverse process with soft tissue component; Axial T2W (D), Sagittal T1W (E), T2W (F) MR images show collapse L4 with posterior convexity which is hypointense on both T1 and T2W images, with an extradural intraspinal soft tissue component compressing the thecal sac.

Giant Cell Tumor

It is an aggressive but benign bone tumor composed of oesteoclastic giant cells. It occurs in mature skeleton commonly in the second to fourth decades. Spine is the fourth most common location for this lesion and majority of spinal GCTs occur in the sacrum.

Radiographs show an ill-defined expansile lytic lesion **(Figs. 23A and B)** with a narrow zone of transition and without a sclerotic border. Sacral lesions can be occult on radiography and may only be picked up on cross-sectional imaging. MRI is ideal for showing the extension into the spinal canal and cord compression. It shows a lesion which

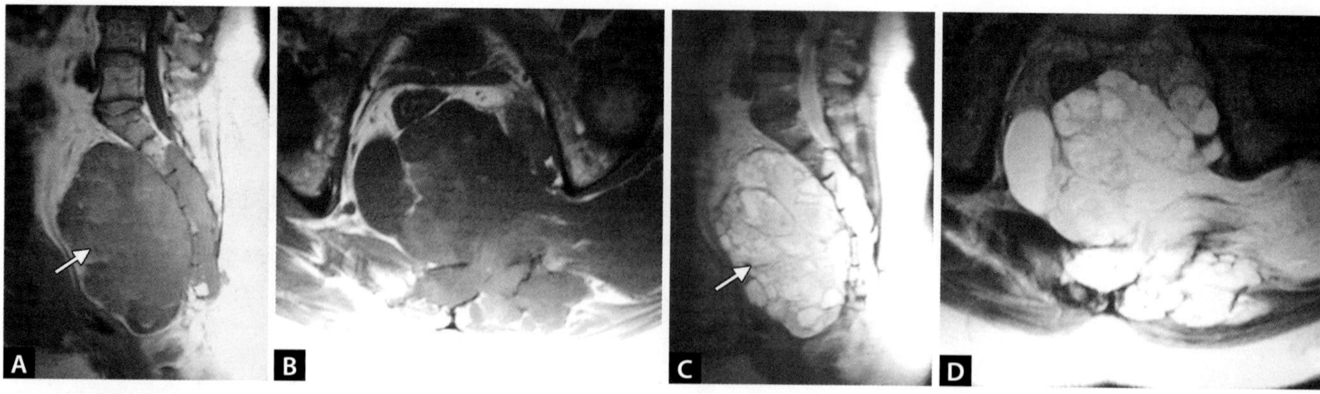

Figs. 24A to D: Sacral chordoma: T1W sagittal (A), axial (B), T2W sagittal (C) and axial (D) MR images showing altered signal intensity involving sacrum associated with large soft tissue component (arrow) which is hypointense on T1W and brightly hyperintense on T2W, extending into the sacral spinal canal.

is hypointense on T1 and intermediate to high signal on T2W images **(Figs. 23C to E)**. Secondary aneurysmal bone cysts are seen as T2 hyperintense foci within the lesion.[48] The differential diagnosis includes aneurysmal bone cyst, metastases, plasmacytoma and chordoma.

MALIGNANT TUMORS

Chordoma

Chordomas are relatively rare slow growing low grade malignant tumors. They arise from notochord remnants in the centers of the vertebral bodies. They are more common at the cranial and caudal ends of the spine, that is, clivus and sacrum, respectively, but may occur at any level, with 35% arising in the lumbosacral spine. Chordoma is always kept in the differential diagnosis when a midline lesion is seen involving the sacrum.[52] The clinical presentation depends on the location of the tumor. The tumors may present with nonspecific back pain, which may be accompanied with neurological symptoms. It commonly affects patients in the third to sixth decades, with no sex predominance. It appears as a lytic lesion on radiography and CT scanning with some amorphous calcification. MRI is the modality of choice for defining the extent of the tumor and its intraspinal extension. This tumor is hypointense on T1W and hyperintense on T2W sequence **(Figs. 24A to D)** with low signal septations.[50,52] Post-contrast images show mild to intense enhancement. These characteristics along with its midline location in an older patient are suggestive of this diagnosis. En bloc resection is the treatment of choice and radiotherapy may play a useful role.

Chondrosarcoma

It is a malignant tumor of connective tissue, characterized by formation of cartilage matrix by tumor cells. Most commonly affects dorsal spine followed by sacrum. Within the vertebra, body and posterior elements are equally affected. Typically they are of large size, at the time of presentation. On imaging, they appear as a lytic mass with chondroid matrix: higher-grade lesions tend to have larger areas without calcifications. CT scan helps in better delineation of extent of the lesion, bone destruction and calcification. MR helps in evaluating extent of tumor within bone and degree of extension into adjacent soft tissues.

Differential diagnoses include sacral chordoma. Chondrosarcomas arise off midline, from the sacroiliac joint space cartilage, and display heterogeneous signal intensity on T2-weighted MR images because they consist of both mineralized and nonmineralized chondroid matrix **(Figs. 25A to C)** Chondrosarcomas typically do not contain areas of hemorrhage, a fact that helps differentiate them from chordomas.

Metastases

Skeletal metastases are significantly more common than primary bone tumors. Spinal metastases are common because they occur in hematopoietic active bone marrow, which is predominantly located in the adult spine. Most spinal metastases are found in the thoracic and lumbar regions. They are frequently disseminated via the hematogenous route. Both venous dissemination and arterial dissemination may occur. Batson's plexus of veins, is a major source of spinal metastases, and it connects with venous plexuses inside the spinal canal. Pressure difference in these veins directs tumor cells from the pelvis (prostate) into the lumbar or thoracic vertebral bodies. They frequently invade the vertebral bodies or the pedicles. Metastases can also grow along nervous tissue

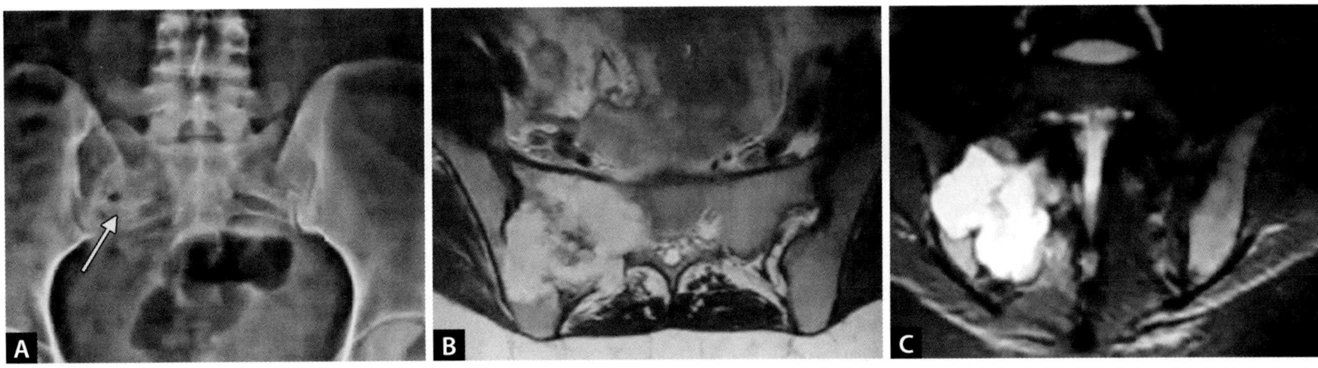

Figs. 25A to C: Sacral chondrosarcoma: Anteroposterior (A) radiograph of pelvis showing lytic destructive lesion with central calcification; Axial T2W (B), coronal T2W (C) with fat saturation MR images showing heterogeneous T2 bright lesion involving right half of the sacrum with contiguous extension across the sacroiliac joint.

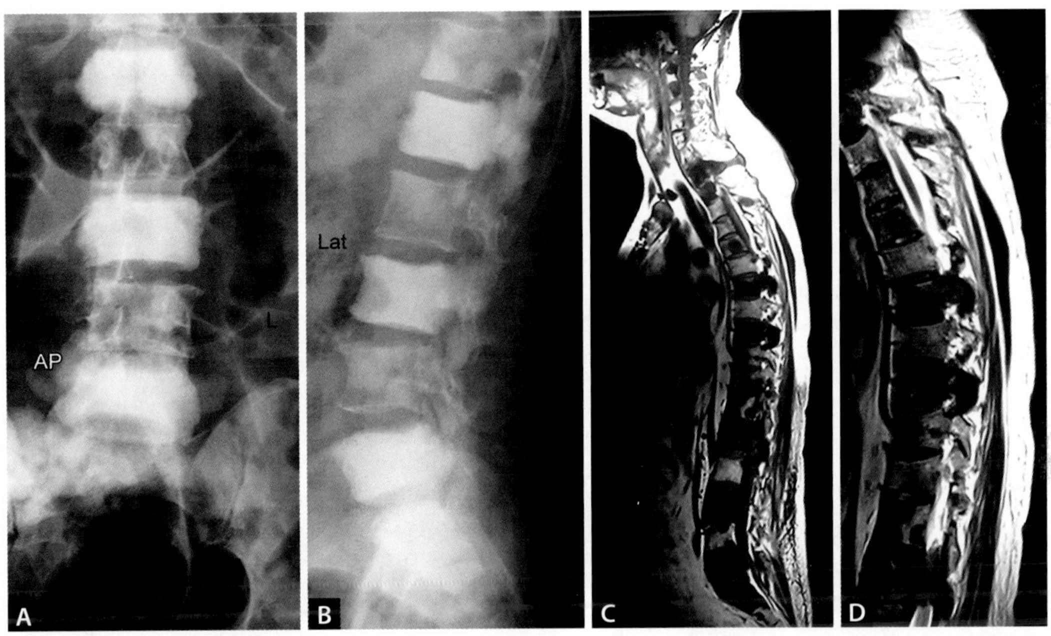

Figs. 26A to D: Sclerotic spinal metastases: Anteroposterior (A) and lateral (B) radiographs of lumbar spine showing dense sclerotic lesions involving multiple vertebrae; Sagittal T1W (C) and T2W (D) showing lesions hypointense on both T1 and T2 images involving both anterior and posterior elements.

and thus enter the epidural space inside the spinal canal. The most common sources of vertebral metastases are the breast, lungs, thyroid, kidney, and prostate.[48] As the metastatic lesions grow, they destroy the vertebral body, penetrate through cortical bone, invade the spinal canal, and compromise the neural elements. Cord compression and neurological deficits may also occur when vertebral bodies collapse due to bone destruction.

Radiographs have poor sensitivity for spinal metastases detection. Vertebral bodies can loose upwards of 50% of their density before it becomes detectable in plain films. The vertebral bodies may appear heterogeneous on plain films. This appearance is not specific and can be found in osteoporosis as well. The vertebral bodies' shape, texture, and cortices should be critically observed. Special attention should be paid to the posterior vertebral body wall. The metastatic deposit may be seen as a presence of a lytic or blastic vertebral lesion **(Figs. 26A to D)**. In some patients with metastatic prostate cancer the vertebral bodies may seem completely white. The pedicles should be inspected carefully. They are well seen in posteroanterior views and can be screened rather quickly. Absence, erosion, or sclerosis of a pedicle may indicate the presence of a bone metastasis at that location.

Bone scan is an efficient and inexpensive tool for detecting skeletal metastases which is sensitive but not specific. Multiplicity of lesions is well-evaluated. False positive scans may be seen in degenerative disease, fracture and infection. Areas of increased activity that may correspond to facet joints or disk spaces are more likely to be due to degenerative changes.

CT can also detect bony metastases and associated soft tissue mass in patients undergoing CT as a part of imaging work up to look for tumor or for staging of known malignancy. MDCT allows excellent sagittal and coronal MPRs **(Figs. 27A and B)** which when viewed on bone window can pick up vertebral metastases.

However, MRI is the most sensitive modality for picking up early vertebral metastases.[48,53] T1W and STIR sagittal sequences of the whole spine **(Figs. 28 to 30)** can be performed and are very sensitive for vertebral deposits and their impact on the spinal canal and the spinal cord. MRI is also very useful to differentiate osteoporotic vertebral collapse from neoplastic collapse. The features are summarized in **Table 2**.

PET-CT scan has emerged as an important tool to image the whole body for the evaluation of metastatic lesions. 18F FDG PET/CT scan performs better in the evaluation of lytic vertebral metastasis whereas 18F NaF PET/CT scan performs better in the evaluation of sclerotic or mixed lytic sclerotic lesions.

Osteoporotic Collapse versus Neoplastic Collapse

Osteoporotic collapse **(Figs. 31A and B)** is common in the elderly and in post-menopausal women. In the acute setting it may be difficult to distinguish it from malignant collapse, as the presence of edema gives rise to hypointense

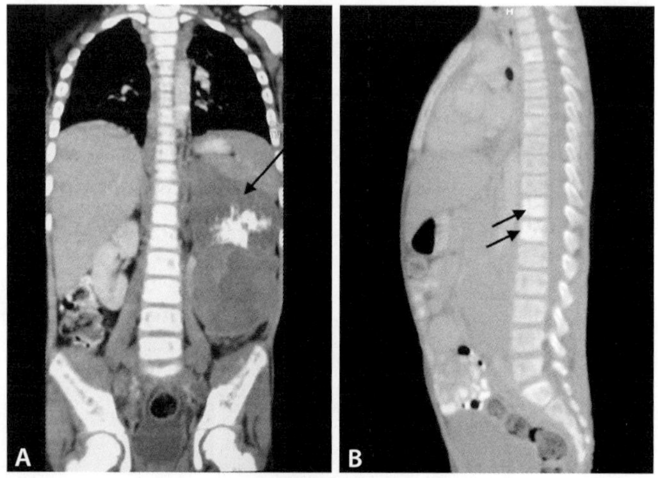

Figs. 27A and B: Neuroblastoma with vertebral metastases. Coronal and sagittal 3D reformatted CT images showing large soft tissue mass in left side of abdomen with dense coarse calcification (long arrow) in a child, associated with sclerotic lesions involving multiple vertebrae (small arrows).

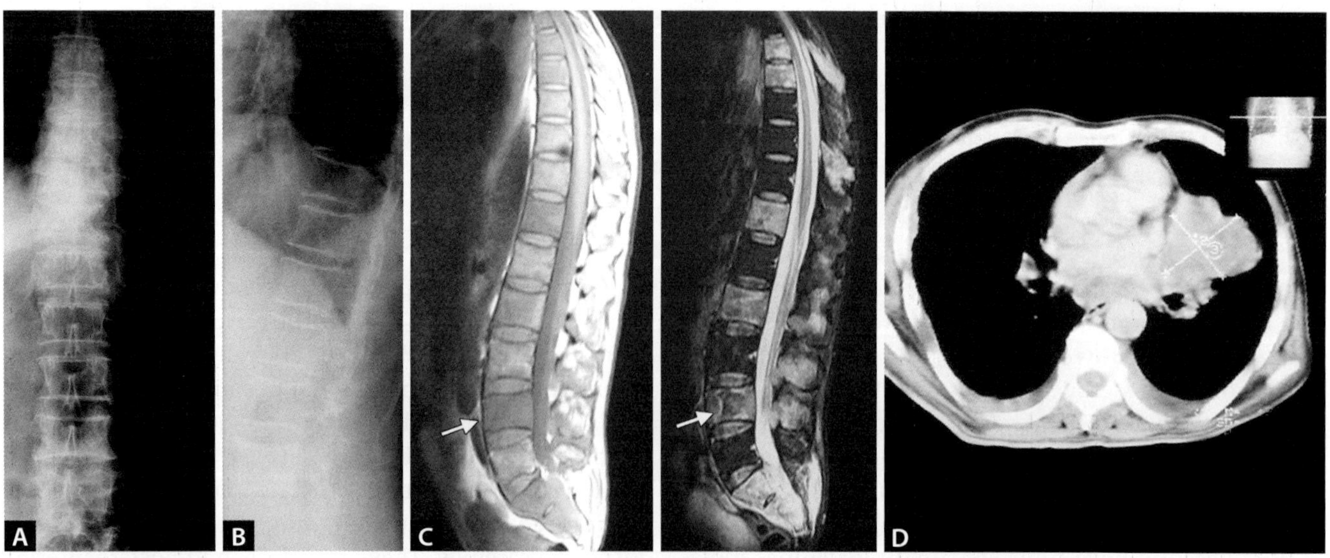

Figs. 28 A to D: Vertebral metastases from bronchogenic carcinoma: Anteroposterior (A) and lateral (B) radiographs of dorsolumbar spine show subtle lytic lesions involving pedicles. Sagittal T1W (B), STIR (C) MR images showing multiple lesions (hypointense on T1W and hyperintense on STIR) involving both anterior and posterior elements of vertebrae. Axial CT scan (D) showing large soft tissue mass in left hilar location with bilateral pleural effusion suggestive of carcinoma of lung.

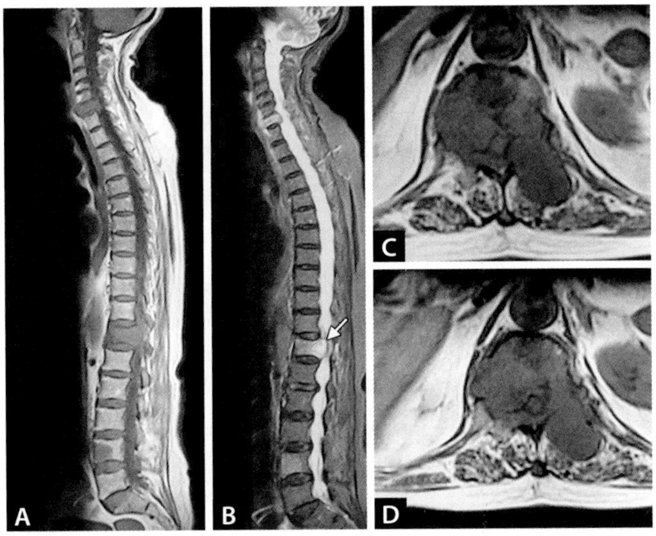

Figs. 29A to D: Spinal metastasis: Sagittal T1W (A), T2W (B) MR images showing altered signal intensity (hypointense on T1W and hyperintense on T2W) involving vertebral bodies of multiple vertebrae. Axial T1W (C) and T2W (D) MR images showing involvement of both anterior and posterior elements of vertebra associated with soft tissue component extending into the spinal canal causing spinal canal narrowing. Posterior vertebral margin of the involved vertebrae is showing convex border (arrow).

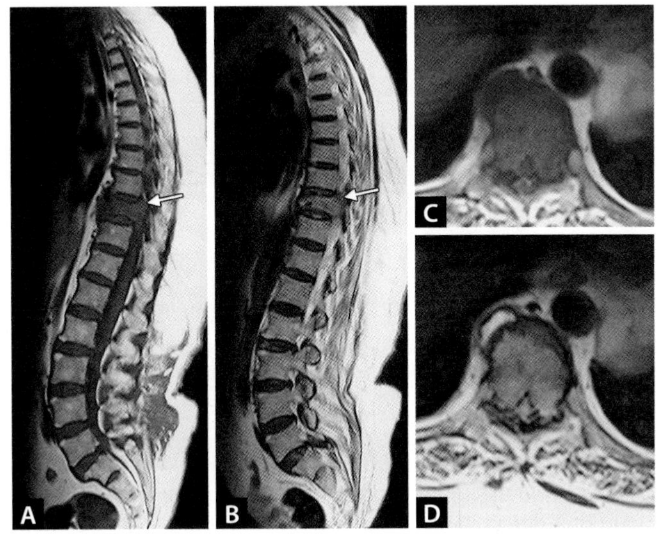

Figs. 30A to D: Sagittal T1W (A), T2W (B) MR images show a collapsed D10 vertebra with posterior convexity (arrow). The axial T1W (C) and T2W (D) images show involvement of body and pedicle with extradural soft tissue compressing the cord.

Table 2: Features of osteoporotic and neoplastic collapses.

Osteoporotic collapse	*Neoplastic collapse*
Anterior wedging, height relatively maintained posteriorly	Uniform collapse
Posterior margin flat	Posterior margin convex
Patchy abnormal signal, some fatty marrow present	Uniform replacement of fatty marrow by tumor giving uniform abnormal signal
Fracture line present	Fracture line absent
Absence of extraosseous Soft tissue	Presence of extraosseous soft tissue

signal on T1W images and hyperintense signal on T2W and STIR sequences. Majority of the times some fatty marrow signal is preserved, the posterior cortex remains concave and the pedicles are normal. The spectrum of findings are related to the age of the collapse and within three months of injury there is always some restoration of fatty marrow and a linear hypontense band may persist. In chronic fractures return to the fatty marrow signal occurs and at this stage there is no difficulty in distinguishing it from malignant collapse. Multiple lesions of different ages may occur confounding the problem further.[48,54]

Malignant collapse also shows T1 hypointensity and T2 hyperintensity and contrast enhancement.[55] Considering that up to one-third of vertebral collapse in patients with known malignancy are benign the diagnosis is difficult when there is a history of malignancy. The marrow replacement is usually complete, posterior cortex is convex, pedicles are commonly involved and associated soft tissue component may be present.

Recently diffusion weighted MRI has also been used for this distinction. Tumor infiltration will show restricted diffusion whereas osteoporotic collapse will not.

Occasionally central type of tuberculosis involving the vertebral body only without diskal or adjacent vertebral involvement may also mimic malignant collapse.

Multiple Myeloma

It is a plasma cell neoplasm of bone marrow and commonly involves the spine. The imaging appearance in spine is non-specific and mimics metastatic disease. The differential diagnosis is better made on radiographs which in myeloma show osteopenia and typical punched out lytic lesions in the skull vault **(Fig. 32A)**. Occasionally sclerotic lesions may be seen specially in the setting of POEMS syndrome (polyneuropathy, organomegaly, endocrinopathy, myeloma, sclerosis). Myeloma lesions are usually cold on bone scan. MRI is a sensitive screening tool but may be normal even in the presence of proven marrow infiltration. Focal T1 hypo- and T2 hyperintense

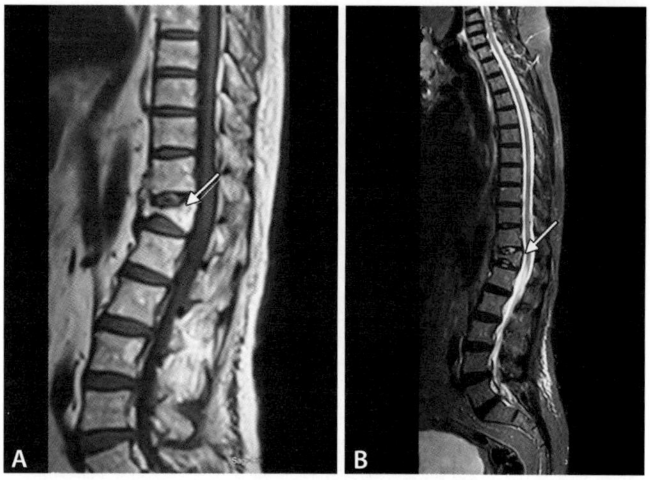

Figs. 31A and B: Sagittal T1W (A) and T2W (B) MR images showing near complete collapse with anterior wedging of D12 vertebra with preserved signal intensity (arrow) and straight posterior vertebral margin suggestive osteoporotic collapse.

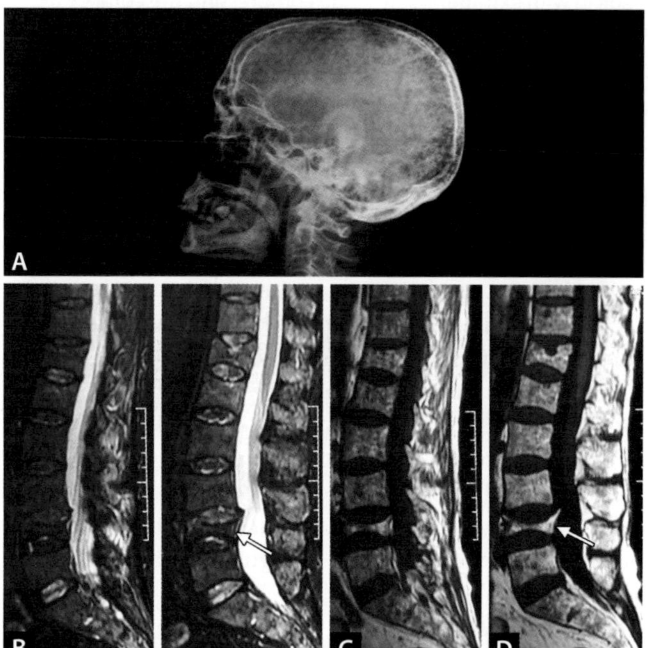

Figs. 32A to D: Multiple myeloma: Lateral radiograph of skull (A) showing multiple uniform sized punched out lytic lesions involving the entire calvarium. Sagittal T2W (B) and T1W (C and D) MR images showing patchy focal altered signal intensity involving multiple vertebrae associated with near complete collapse of L4 and partial collapse of D12 vertebrae. Posterior vertebral margin of the collapsed vertebra is straight (arrow) with preserved signal likely due to osteoporosis.

lesions of variable size **(Figs. 32B to D)** may be seen or there may homogeneously decreased signal may be seen on T1W images which can easily be overlooked. T2W images in the latter group will show hyperintense signal and enhancement will be seen on contrast administration.[48,56]

VNCa CT images may become useful in the future for detection of non-osteolytic infiltrative lesions of myeloma.

Lymphoma

Primary lymphoma of bone is a rare entity and spine is the fourth most common location for it. It is usually a Non-Hodgkin lymphoma with a peak incidence in fifth to seventh decade. Secondary lymphomas are far more common and up to 30% of systemic lymphomas have osseous involvement.

Lymphoma in the spine can present as an epidural mass, osseous involvement, lepto meningitis and as an intramedullary mass. In this discussion, we will confine ourselves to osseous lymphoma which is frequently associated with epidural soft tissue masses.

The radiographs show a nonspecific lytic lesion, but it may also be sclerotic. Bone scan shows increased uptake and 67 Gallium scintigraphy has been shown to have a high sensitivity and specificity.[53] MRI shows a lesion which is T1 hypointense and T2 iso to hyperintense, which enhances on contrast administration. The soft tissue mass may show T2 hypointensity due to hypercellularity.

Low backache is a very common clinical problem. Majority of patients do not require imaging. It is important to triage patients into chronic nonspecific pain versus those with more ominous pathology who would benefit with imaging. Plain radiographs and MRI play the most useful role and CT and scintigraphy are used as problem solving tools.

REFERENCES

1. Sharma SC, Singh R, Sharma AK, et al. Incidence of low back pain in workage adults in rural North India. Indian J Med Sci. 2003;57(4):145-7.
2. Gilbert FJ, Grant AM, Gillan MG, et al. Low back pain: influence of early MR imaging or CT on treatment and outcome—multicenter randomized trial. Radiology. 2004;231(2):343-51.
3. Davis PC, Wippold FJ, Brunberg JA, et al. ACR Appropriateness Criteria® on low back pain. J Am Coll Radiol. 2009;6(6):401-7.
4. Teh J, Imam A, Watts C. Imaging of back pain. Imaging. 2005;17(3):171-207.
5. Deyo RA, Weinstein JN. Low back pain. N Engl J Med. 2001;344(5):363-70.
6. Borenstein D. Epidemiology, etiology, diagnostic evaluation, and treatment of low back pain. Curr Opin Rheumatol. 1996;8(2):124-9.

7. Jarvik JG, Hollingworth W, Martin B, et al. Rapid magnetic resonance imaging vs radiographs for patients with low back pain: a randomized controlled trial. JAMA. 2003;289(21):2810-8.
8. McNally EG, Wilson DJ, Ostlere SJ. Limited magnetic resonance imaging in low back pain instead of plain radiographs: experience with first 1000 cases. Clin Radiol. 2001;56(11):922-5.
9. Singh K, Helms CA, Fiorella D, et al. Disc space-targeted angled axial MR images of the lumbar spine: a potential source of diagnostic error. Skeletal Radiol. 2007;36(12):1147-53.
10. Bellini M, Ferrara M, Grazzini I, et al. Neuroimaging of the Postoperative Spine. Magn Reson Imaging Clin. 2016;24(3):601-20.
11. Kellock TT, Nicolaou S, Kim SSY, et al. Detection of Bone Marrow Edema in Nondisplaced Hip Fractures: Utility of a Virtual Noncalcium Dual-Energy CT Application. Radiology. 2017;284(3):798-805.
12. Kim HG, Shin DA, Kim HI, et al. Clinical and radiological findings of discogenic low back pain confirmed by automated pressure-controlled discography. J Korean Neurosurg Soc. 2009;46(4):333.
13. Carragee EJ, Lincoln T, Parmar VS, et al. A gold standard evaluation of the "discogenic pain" diagnosis as determined by provocative discography. Spine. 2006; 31(18):2115-23.
14. Dolan AL, Ryan PJ, Arden NK, et al. The value of SPECT scans in identifying back pain likely to benefit from facet joint injection. Rheumatology. 1996;35(12):1269-73.
15. Elster AD. Bertolotti's syndrome revisited. Transitional vertebrae of the lumbar spine. Spine. 1989;14(12): 1373-7.
16. Konin GP, Walz DM. Lumbosacral transitional vertebrae: classification, imaging findings, and clinical relevance. Am J Neuroradiol. 2010;31(10):1778-86.
17. Syrmou E, Tsitsopoulos PP, Marinopoulos D, et al. Spondylolysis: a review and reappraisal. Hippokratia. 2010;14(1):17.
18. Beutler WJ, Fredrickson BE, Murtland A, et al. The natural history of spondylolysis and spondylolisthesis: 45-year follow-up evaluation. Spine. 2003;28(10):1027-35.
19. Fredrickson BE, Baker D, McHolick WJ, et al. The natural history of spondylolysis and spondylolisthesis. J Bone Joint Surg Am. 1984;66(5):699-707.
20. Campbell RSD, Grainger AJ, Hide IG, et al. Juvenile spondylolysis: a comparative analysis of CT, SPECT and MRI. Skeletal Radiol. 2005;34(2):63-73.
21. Harvey CJ, Richenberg JL, Saifuddin A, et al. The radiological investigation of lumbar spondylolysis. Clin Radiol. 1998;53(10):723-8.
22. Paajanen H, Tertti M. Association of incipient disc degeneration and instability in spondylolisthesis. Arch Orthop Trauma Surg. 1991;111(1):16-19.
23. Collier BD, Johnson RP, Carrera GF, et al. Painful spondylolysis or spondylolisthesis studied by radiography and single-photon emission computed tomography. Radiology. 1985;154(1):207-11.
24. Scheuermann HW. Kyphosis dorsalis juvenilis. Ugeskr Laeger. 1920;82:385.
25. Blumenthal SL, Roach J, Herring JA. Lumbar Scheuermann's. A clinical series and classification. Spine. 1987;12(9):929-32.
26. Summers BN, Singh JP, Manns RA. The radiological reporting of lumbar Scheuermann's disease: an unnecessary source of confusion amongst clinicians and patients. Br J Radiol. 2008;81(965):383-5.
27. Yu S, Haughton VM, Sether LA, et al. Criteria for classifying normal and degenerated lumbar intervertebral disks. Radiology. 1989;170(2):523-6.
28. Pfirrmann CW, Metzdorf A, Zanetti M, et al. Magnetic resonance classification of lumbar intervertebral disc degeneration. Spine. 2001;26(17):1873-8.
29. Clarençon F, Law-Ye B, Bienvenot P, et al. The degenerative spine. Magn Reson Imaging Clin. 2016;24(3):495-513.
30. Fardon DF, Milette PC. Nomenclature and classification of lumbar disc pathology: recommendations of the combined task forces of the North American Spine Society, American Society of Spine Radiology, and American Society of Neuroradiology. Spine. 2001;26(5):E93-E113.
31. Modic MT. Degenerative disc disease and back pain. Magn Reson Imaging Clin N Am. 1999;7(3):481-91.
32. Lee SH, Coleman PE, Hahn FJ. Magnetic resonance imaging of degenerative disk disease of the spine. Radiol Clin North Am. 1988;26(5):949-64.
33. Kalichman L, Hunter DJ. Lumbar facet joint osteoarthritis: a review. In: Seminars in arthritis and rheumatism. Elsevier; 2007. p. 69-80.
34. Modic MT, Masaryk T, Boumphrey F, et al. Lumbar herniated disk disease and canal stenosis: prospective evaluation by surface coil MR, CT, and myelography. Am J Roentgenol. 1986;147(4):757-65.
35. Schizas C, Theumann N, Burn A, et al. Qualitative grading of severity of lumbar spinal stenosis based on the morphology of the dural sac on magnetic resonance images. Spine. 2010;35(21):1919-24.
36. Ross JS, Masaryk TJ, Schrader M, et al. MR imaging of the postoperative lumbar spine: assessment with gadopentetate dimeglumine. Am J Neuroradiol. 1990;11(4):771-6.
37. Ross JS. Magnetic resonance assessment of the postoperative spine. Degenerative disc disease. Radiol Clin North Am. 1991;29(4):793-808.
38. Braun J, Bollow M, Sieper J. Radiologic diagnosis and pathology of the spondyloarthropathies. Rheum Dis Clin. 1998;24(4):697-735.
39. Vinson EN, Major NM. MR imaging of ankylosing spondylitis. In: Seminars in musculoskeletal radiology. Copyright\copyright 2002 by Thieme Medical Publishers, Inc., 333 Seventh Avenue, New York, NY 10001, USA. Tel.:+1 (212) 584-4662; 2003. p. 103-44.
40. Shanley DJ. Tuberculosis of the spine: imaging features. Am J Roentgenol. 1995;164(3):659-64.

41. Moorthy S, Prabhu NK. Spectrum of MR imaging findings in spinal tuberculosis. Am J Roentgenol. 2002;179(4):979-83.
42. Moore SL, Rafii M. Imaging of musculoskeletal and spinal tuberculosis. Radiol Clin. 2001;39(2):329-42.
43. Forrester DM. Infectious spondylitis. In: Seminars in Ultrasound, CT and MRI. Elsevier; 2004. p. 461-73.
44. Ledermann HP, Schweitzer ME, Morrison WB, et al. MR imaging findings in spinal infections: rules or myths? Radiology. 2003;228(2):506-14.
45. Thrush A, Enzmann D. MR imaging of infectious spondylitis. Am J Neuroradiol. 1990;11(6):1171-80.
46. Varma R, Lander P, Assaf A. Imaging of pyogenic infectious spondylodiskitis. Radiol Clin. 2001;39(2):203-13.
47. Carragee EJ. The clinical use of magnetic resonance imaging in pyogenic vertebral osteomyelitis. Spine. 1997;22(7):780-5.
48. Motamedi K, Ilaslan H, Seeger LL. Imaging of the lumbar spine neoplasms. In: Seminars in Ultrasound, CT and MRI. Elsevier; 2004. p. 474-89.
49. Baudrez V, Galant C, Berg BCV. Benign vertebral hemangioma: MR-histological correlation. Skeletal Radiol. 2001;30(8):442-6.
50. Flemming DJ, Murphey MD, Carmichael BB, et al. Primary tumors of the spine. In: Seminars in musculoskeletal radiology. Copyright\copyright 2000 by Thieme Medical Publishers, Inc., 333 Seventh Avenue, New York, NY 10001, USA. pp. 299-320.
51. Ozaki T, Liljenqvist U, Hillmann A, et al. Osteoid osteoma and osteoblastoma of the spine: experiences with 22 patients. Clin Orthop. 2002;397:394-402.
52. Diel J, Ortiz O, Losada RA, et al. The sacrum: pathologic spectrum, multimodality imaging, and subspecialty approach. Radiographics. 2001;21(1):83-104.
53. Nöbauer I, Uffmann M. Differential diagnosis of focal and diffuse neoplastic diseases of bone marrow in MRI. Eur J Radiol. 2005;55(1):2-32.
54. Uetani M, Hashmi R, Hayashi K. Malignant and benign compression fractures: differentiation and diagnostic pitfalls on MRI. Clin Radiol. 2004;59(2):124-31.
55. Tehranzadeh J, Tao C. Advances in MR imaging of vertebral collapse. In: Seminars in Ultrasound, CT and MRI. Elsevier; 2004. p. 440-60.
56. Angtuaco EJ, Fassas AB, Walker R, et al. Multiple myeloma: clinical review and diagnostic imaging. Radiology. 2004;231(1):11-23.

CHAPTER 36

Localization in Clinical Neurology

Manish Modi, Sudesh Prabhakar

LOCALIZATION IN CLINICAL NEUROLOGY

Localization, derived from Latin term locus, is the diagnostic exercise of determining from the signs or symptoms of the patient, what site of the nervous system has been affected by the disease process. Clinical localization has particular relevance to the adequate use of ancillary diagnostic procedures. Current techniques of imaging, electrodiagnosis and other laboratory studies have revolutionized the practice of neurology. However, their use must be integrated with findings of history and neurological examination.

Clinical Diagnosis and Lesion Localization

Clinical diagnosis in neurology requires several steps:

- Recognition of impaired function
- Identification of site of central nervous system (CNS) affected
- Definition of most likely etiology
- Use of ancillary procedures.

Recognition of impaired function depends on a good history and neurological examination. Abnormal neurological findings come in the form of abnormal behavior or cognition, impaired posture or gait, difficulty in movement of face or extremities, and finally the sensory disturbances, including pain.

Neuroanatomy is the key to localization. Neuroanatomy has two broad based aspects: (1) the morphology of the structure, and (2) its "functional representation". Functional representation refers to the function mediated by a given structure of the nervous system. Damage to a structure results in dysfunction in the realm mediated by this structure.

APPROACH TO NEUROLOGICAL DISORDER

Neurological localization and diagnosis is approached in each patient with the following six questions in mind:

1. Is there a disease in the nervous system?
2. At what level(s)?
3. What longitudinal system(s) is (are) involved?
4. Is the process—focal/multifocal/diffuse?
5. What is the lateralization right/left or bilateral?
6. What is the course acute/subacute/chronic? Then further queries like:
   a. Static versus progressive
   b. Relapsing/remitting or monophasic
   c. Onset sudden or insidious

Based on the anatomic-temporal profile, the neurological disorders are broadly grouped into:

- *Degenerative*: Progressive and tend to be chronic and diffuse.
- *Neoplastic*: Progressive, may be subacute or chronic, and tend to be focal or multifocal but may be diffuse (e.g. carcinomatous meningitis).
- *Vascular*: Acute and usually focal but may be diffuse (e.g. subarachnoid hemorrhage).
- *Inflammatory*: Subacute or chronic and tend to be progressive. They may be focal (e.g. abscess), diffuse (e.g. meningitis, encephalitis), or multifocal (e.g. autoimmune disease).

- *Demyelination*: Acute, focal, may be relapsing and remitting.
- *Toxic metabolic*: Diffuse and may have any time course.
- *Traumatic*: Processes are always acute, may be static and improving or progressive, and may be diffuse, focal, or multifocal.
- *Congenital*: Developmental diseases are chronic and typically diffuse, and may be static or progressive.

The present chapter will focus on few important symptoms and signs, which refer to a particular area of the neuraxis and help in clinical localization. The chapter is subdivided into disorders of cranial nerves, motor system, including gait and coordination, sensory system, and finally disorders of higher mental function.

DISORDERS OF CRANIAL NERVES

OLFACTORY NERVE (CRANIAL NERVE I)

Anosmia

Significant olfactory dysfunction has been described with Alzheimer's disease, Lewy body disease, Huntington's chorea, Parkinson's disease, spinocerebellar ataxia, multiplesclerosis. Tumors of sphenoid or frontal bone, pituitary tumors with suprasellar extension, nasopharyngeal carcinoma or giant anterior communicating artery aneurysm can also present with anosmia.

Foster-Kennedy syndrome noted with olfactory groove or sphenoid ridge mass and space occupying lesion of frontal lobe is characterized by:

- Ipsilateral anosmia
- Ipsilateral optic atrophy
- Contralateral papilledema.

Pseudo-Foster-Kennedy syndrome is noted when increased intracranial pressure of any cause occurs in patient who has previous unilateral optic atrophy. However, mostly pseudo-Foster-Kennedy syndrome is due to sequential anterior optic neuropathy or optic neuritis in which optic disk atrophies on the other side.

OPTIC NERVE (CRANIAL NERVE II)

Papilledema: Optic disk swelling, manifested by disk hyperemia, blurring of disk margin, loss of venous pulsations **(Fig. 1)** are usually secondary to raised intracranial pressure and can be manifestation of large number of pathological conditions **(Box 1)**.

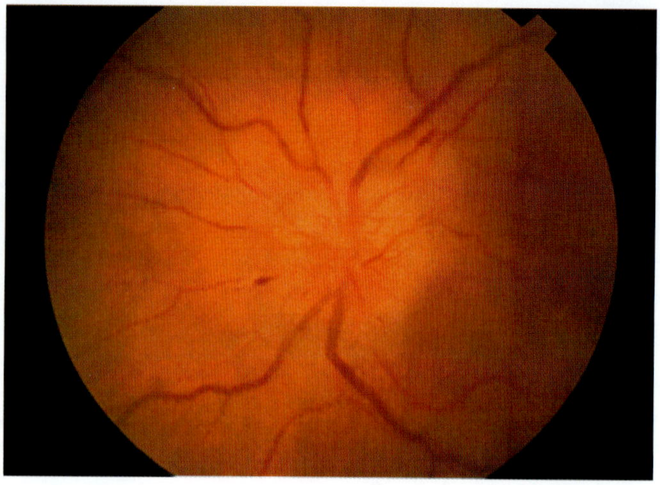

Fig. 1: Fundus photograph showing papilledema.

Box 1: Syndromes causing increased intracranial pressure and papilledema.

Primary causes
• Hydrocephalus • *Mass lesions*: Tumor, hemorrhage, large infarction, abscess • Meningitis/encephalitis • Subarachnoid hemorrhage • Trauma • High flow arteriovenous malformations with overloading venous return • Intracranial or extracranial venous obstruction • Pseudotumor cerebri syndrome

Visual Pathway Localization (Fig. 2)

Monocular visual loss is usually caused by lesions affecting retina or optic nerve.

Binocular visual loss is seen in lesions localized to or beyond optic chiasm.

Bitemporal field defects are most often due to a compressive mass lesion affecting the optic chiasm, such as pituitary tumor, suprasellar meningiomas, craniopharyngiomas and gliomas.

Binasal hemianopias are usually due to bilateral intraocular disease of retina or optic nerve. Rarely bilateral compression of lateral chiasma may result in binasal defect.

Homonymous hemianopia appears with lesions in the retrochiasmatic pathways, i.e. optic tract, lateral geniculate body, optic radiations or occipital lobe. A host of diseases like tumors, demyelination, trauma *arteriovenous malformation* (AVM), infections, surgery, etc. can lead to homonymous hemianopia.

Superior homonymous quadrantic defects ("pie in the sky" field defects) result from lesion of temporal loop (Meyer's loop) of optic radiation like space occupying lesion (tumor, abscess, hemorrhage), arteriovenous

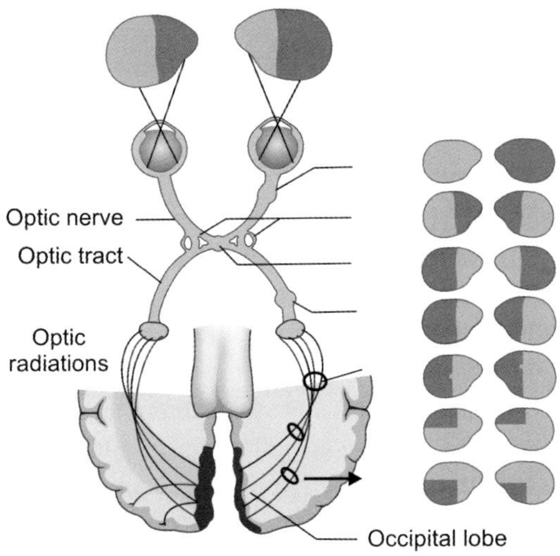

Fig. 2: Visual pathways and field defects.

malformation, infections, infarctions, demyelinating disease, trauma, etc.

Inferior quadrantic defects ("pie on the floor" field defects) occur due to involvement of optic radiations in the depth of parietal lobe.

OCULOMOTOR SYSTEM (CRANIAL NERVE III, IV, VI) (TABLE 1)

Supranuclear Lesions

Disturbance of conjugate gaze may be found in association with midbrain, pontine or cerebral lesions.

Destructive lesion of the motor eye field of the frontal lobe (area 8) causes paresis of the gaze to the opposite side, with deviation of eyes towards the side of the lesion, while an irritative lesion (or an epileptic focus) in this region causes strong, rapid involuntary conjugate deviation of the eye to the opposite side.

Table 1: Localization of lesions of ocular motor nerves.

Location	*Symptoms*	*Signs*
Extraocular muscle/ orbit	Eye swelling Monocular vision loss Dry eyes	• Periorbital edema • Conjunctival injection and chemosis • Proptosis • Eyelid retraction • Lagophthalmos (inability to close the eye completely) Lid lag (higher than normal lid position in downgaze) • Von Graefe's sign (dynamic slowing of lid descent during eye movement from upgaze into downgaze) • Optic neuropathy (from optic nerve compression)
Neuromuscular junction	• Fluctuating symptoms • Proximal muscle • Weakness • Shortness of breath • Swallowing difficulty • Worsening at night or with exercise	• Moment-to-moment or visit-to-visit variability • Fatigue of lids or eye elevation with prolonged upgaze • Cogan's lid twitch • Peek sign • Orbicularis oculi weakness • Ptosis and enhanced ptosis
Cranial nerve	Arm and leg weakness	Contralateral hemiparesis: pyramidal tract
Brainstem	• Clumsiness or imbalance • Facial numbness or tingling • Facial weakness	• *Ataxia:* Cerebella peduncle • *Ipsilateral facial sensory loss:* Trigeminal tracts and nuclei • *Upper and lower facial weakness:* Facial nerve fasciculus and nucleus
Cranial nerve Subarachnoid space	Stiff neck Vision loss Headache	• Kernig's and Brudzinski's signs • Papilledema
Cranial nerve	Facial numbness and tingling	Ipsilateral facial sensory loss in the first (V1) and second (V2) trigeminal distributions
Cavernous sinus cranial nerve	Facial numbness and tingling	• *Ipsilateral Horner's syndrome:* Sympathetic fibers • Ipsilateral facial sensory loss in the first (V1) trigeminal distribution
Orbital apex	Eye prominence	Proptosis
Supranuclear	• Arm and leg weakness • Clumsiness or imbalance • Facial numbness or tingling • Facial weakness	• *Contralateral hemiparesis:* Pyramidal tract • *Ataxia:* Cerebellar peduncle • *Ipsilateral facial sensory loss:* Trigeminal tracts and nuclei • *Upper and lower facial weakness:* Facial nerve fasciculus • *Ocular motility:* Saccades affected greater than smooth pursuit; vestibulo-ocular reflexes spared

Parinaud's syndrome is characterized by paralysis of conjugate upward gaze, impairment of convergence. It is seen in lesions at the level of superior colliculi (anterior quadrigeminal bodies), the foretectal region, or the posterior commissure and is found in tumor of pineal glands, encephalitis, multiple sclerosis vascular and other lesions.

Nuclear Lesions

Nuclear involvement of ocular nerves may result from vascular lesions (infarct or hemorrhage), inflammatory lesions, neoplasms, trauma, metabolic disorders, multiple sclerosis, and syringobulbia. There is usually associated involvement of medial longitudinal fasciculus, corticospinal tract, sensory pathways, cerebellar connections, other cranial nerve nuclei, sympathetic pathways, etc.

- *Weber's syndrome:* Caused by involvement of oculomotor nerve as it passes through the cerebral peduncles and produce ipsilateral third nerve paralysis with contralateral paresis of lower face, tongue and extremities.
- *Benedict's syndrome:* Caused by lesion of midbrain involving third nerve as it passes through the red nucleus. It is characterized by an ipsilateral oculomotor paralysis with contralateral ataxia, tremor and hyperkinesias of upper extremity.
- *Nothnagel's syndrome:* There is unilateral oculomotor paralysis combined with ipsilateral ataxia due to involvement of third nerve and brachium conjunctivum.
- *Millard-Gubler syndrome:* There is ipsilateral lateral rectus paralysis, ipsilateral facial paralysis with contralateral hemiplegia.
- *Raymond's syndrome:* Consists of an ipsilateral sixth nerve paralysis and contralateral hemiplegia.
- *Foville's syndrome:* Ipsilateral gaze paralysis, facial paralysis with contralateral hemiplegia. There is contralateral deviation of eyes and head.

Internuclear Ophthalmoplegia

Paralysis of adduction of the contralateral eye, together with variable paresis and monocular nystagmus of the abducting eye. Internuclear ophthalmoplegia (INO) is found in brainstem lesions and is seen with multiple sclerosis, vascular, neoplastic, inflammatory or degenerative lesions of the brainstem or compression of latter by neoplasms of the posterior fossa. There are usually symptoms and signs indicating involvement of neighboring centers and pathways.

Infranuclear Lesions

These may be caused by lesions within skull, middle cranial fossa, cavernous sinus, superior orbital fissure or orbit. Involvement in the skull may be produced by meningitis, trauma, subarachnoid hemorrhage, etc.

Cavernous sinus thrombosis consists of ipsilateral ptosis, chemosis, edema of eyelids and orbital tissue, paralysis of third, fourth, sixth cranial nerves, involvement of upper division of trigeminal nerve, and at times papilledema.

In *superior orbital fissure syndrome*, including Tolosa-Hunt syndrome, there is usually painful ophthalmoplegia with or without vision loss. It may also result from sphenoid sinusitis, skull fractures, etc.

Other Disorders of Oculomotor System

- *Nystagmus:* Involuntary oscillation or trembling of the eyeball. It can be congenital or acquired.
  - *Vestibular nystagmus* is caused by either irritation or destruction of semicircular canals, vestibular nerve or vestibular nuclei. It is a fine nystagmus, usually associated with vertigo.
  - *Cerebellar nystagmus* indicates that vestibulocerebellar pathways are affected, i.e. either the vermis or the inferior cerebellar peduncle, though can be seen in cerebellar hemispheric lesions. It is usually a coarse type of nystagmus.
  - Other *central nystagmus* is produced mainly by lesions affecting structures in the region of fourth ventricle or brainstem principally zone between oculomotor nuclei and vestibular nuclei.
  - *Downbeat nystagmus* is seen in brainstem lesions, especially in craniovertebral junction anomalies.
  - *Upbeat nystagmus* is usually caused by lesions of anterior vermis of the cerebellum though can be seen in any brainstem lesion.
  - *See-saw nystagmus,* in which one eye moves upward while the other moves down, is seen in patients with tumors of suprasellar region or anterior third ventricle.
- *Opsoclonus:* Coarse, irregular, nonrhythmic, agitated oscillations of eyes in both horizontal and vertical planes. These have been observed in encephalitis, cerebellar or brainstem disorders, comatose states, metabolic encephalopathies or as part of "paraneoplastic syndromes".
- *Ocular bobbing:* Coarse, synchronous, downward "bobbing" movements of eyes are observed in coma with pontine lesions and is of grave significance.

TRIGEMINAL NERVE (CRANIAL NERVE V)

The fifth nerve may be affected by lesions of brainstem or outside it at different level, by tumor of the cerebellopontine angle, tumors of base of skull, lesions within cavernous sinus, infections of petrous bone, orbital cellulitis, etc.

Trigeminal neuralgia (tic douloureux), characterized by sudden attacks of excruciating, lancinating pain, is usually caused by vascular pressure on the nerve outside the brainstem but can also be a presenting symptom of multiple sclerosis, syringobulbia, herpes zoster and cerebellopontine angle tumor.

FACIAL NERVE (CRANIAL NERVE VII)

Localization of Facial Nerve Lesions (Fig. 3)

Supranuclear Palsy

Supranuclear palsy is the paresis of lower part of the face with relative sparing of upper part. There are two varieties of central facial palsy: (1) Volitional and (2) *emotional* type.

In *volitional palsy*, the involvement is most marked on voluntary contraction (like baring teeth, etc.) while on involuntary contractions such as smiling, crying, etc. There is preservation of function with no evidence of paresis. This variety of volitional palsy is seen in lesions of cortical center in the lower-third of precentral convolution or pathways between this center and nucleus of facial nerve.

In *emotional ormimetic* type of facial palsy, the impairment is most marked on smiling or weeping, though the patient can voluntarily retract his mouth. This type of palsy is considered to be result of deep seated lesion in extrapyramidal, basal ganglia, thalamus, or hypothalamus or frontal lobe lesions anterior to precentral convolution.

Masked facies are seen in Parkinson's disease and other Parkinsonian syndromes. There is loss of associated movements like infrequent blinking and smiling.

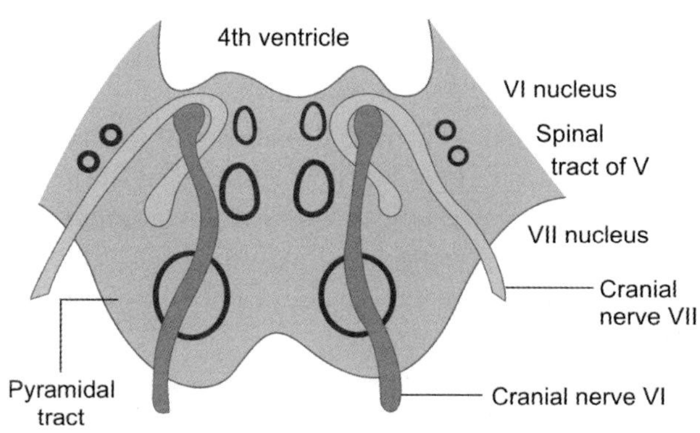

Fig. 3: Facial nerve course in pons.

Infranuclear Facial Nerve Palsy

It can occur in variety of conditions but the most common is *Bell's palsy*. In this condition, both upper and lower part of face is involved and patient is unable to close the eyes on the affected side. *Bell's phenomenon*, i.e. eyeball turns upward and cornea is hidden, when the patient attempts to close eyes on involved side.

VESTIBULOCOCHLEAR NERVE (CRANIAL NERVE VIII)

Vertigo is a sensation of movement and is often accompanied by feelings of unsteadiness and loss of balance. True organic or vestibular vertigo is usually rotator in type and has been described as *Objective*, if the external objects seem to be rotating around the individual, and as *Subjective*, if the individual himself is rotating. The presence of associated symptoms, like nausea, vomiting, staggering, deviation of eyes, disturbance of balance, tinnitus, hearing loss, effect of change of posture are important clues to localization.

In general, vertigo of *peripheral origin* is usually episodic in character, aggravated by change in posture, and accompanied by nystagmus, which that of *central origin* is more apt to be continuous, less clearly defined and may not be accompanied by nystagmus and there may be evidence of other CNS changes.

Deafness, tinnitus, and vertigo are important presenting symptoms of cerebellopontine angle neoplasms, usually a neurinoma or a neurofibroma.

Partial deafness may be an early symptom of a tumor of *glomus jugulare* (chemodectoma), later there may be tinnitus, vertigo, and involvement of other cranial nerves (facial, vagus and others).

GLOSSOPHARYNGEAL AND VAGUS NERVE (CRANIAL NERVE IX, X)

Lesions of these nerves lead to dysarthria and dysphagia, with associated nasal regurgitation of fluids and nasal intonation of voice. Examination reveals asymmetrical movement of uvula and impaired or absent gag reflex and palatal reflex.

Supranuclear involvement leads to pseudobulbar palsy with associated dysphagia and dysarthria. In this condition, the gag, palatal and jaw jerk reflexes are brisk.

Nuclear involvement occurs in a variety of vascular, demyelinating, neoplastic, degenerative conditions.

Wallenberg's syndrome (lateral medullary syndrome), caused by occlusion of posterior inferior cerebellar artery (PICA) or vertebral artery, leads to acute dysphagia, dysarthria, ipsilateral anesthesia of face, ipsilateral Horner's syndrome, ipsilateral cerebellar hypotonia and asynergy, with contralateral loss of pain and temperature sensation on limbs and trunk **(Fig. 4)**.

Infranuclear involvement may follow lesions at the base of skull, jugular foramen or along the course of vagus nerve.

Syndrome of Vernet, caused by lesion at the jugular foramen, is characterized by ipsilateral paralysis of ninth, tenth and eleventh nerves. It is usually of traumatic origin and follows basilar skull fracture; however, vascular or neoplastic lesions may also cause this syndrome.

Syndrome of Villaret is the result of lesion in the retropharyngeal space and results in paralysis of ninth-tenth, eleventh and twelfth nerve and Horner's syndrome.

Palatal Myoclonus

Palatal myoclonus is a rhythmic movement of palate and associated muscles, in frequency of 50–240/min. It probably results from brainstem lesion with interruption of connections between the inferior olivary body, dentate nucleus and red nucleus (*The triangle of Guillain and Mollaret*).

SPINAL ACCESSORY NERVE (CRANIAL NERVE XI)

The lesion of this nerve causes paralysis of sternocleidomastoid and trapezius muscles.

More commonly hyperkinetic manifestation with tonic or clonic spasm of the muscles is encountered. The muscle contraction of sternomastoid pulls head and occiput to one side and face to opposite side (*Torticollis*).

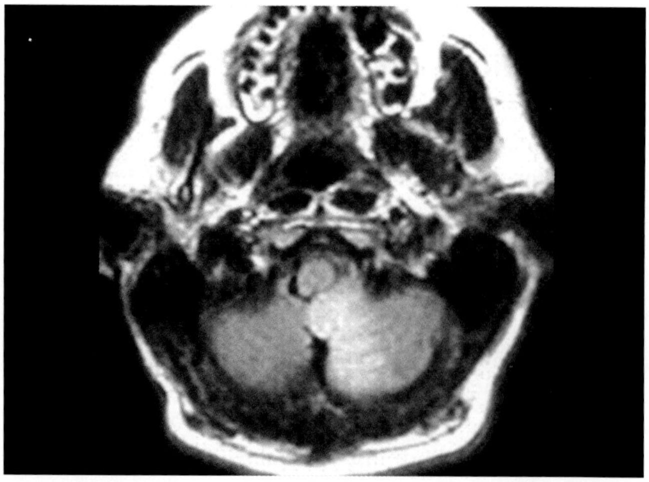

Fig. 4: Magnetic resonance imaging of the brain (T2WI) showing left lateral medullary syndrome.

There are many causes of torticollis: congenital, structural, traumatic and myogenic factors; Klippel-Feil syndrome, rickets, cervical arthritis, spina bifida, trauma, etc. Reflex torticollis may be secondary to vascular lesions, tumor, cervical lymph node metastasis, retrotonsillar abscess, etc. Disorders of extrapyramidal system, especially of the basal ganglia, are probably the most common causes of neurologic torticollis.

HYPOGLOSSAL NERVE (CRANIAL NERVE XII)

This nerve supplies the muscles of tongue. Lesions cause weakness and atrophy of the tongue muscles and may be seen in a variety of lesions in brainstem (neoplasm, vascular, granuloma, multiple sclerosis); within the skull (like meningitis, neoplasm), basilar invagination, Arnold-Chiari malformation; in the hypoglossal canal or in neck (trauma, tumor, vascular lesions).

DISORDERS OF MOTOR SYSTEM

Motor function is a complex process and involves many areas of the CNS, like cerebral cortex, basal ganglia, cerebellum, and reticular activating system in addition to the final common spinomuscular pathway. Lesions of any of the constituent portions of motor system lead to walking difficulty/weakness. The classical features of upper motor neuron lesion versus lower motor neuron are tabulated in **Table 2**.

The examination of motor system involves:

- Inspection for muscle bulk, wasting, fasciculation
- Power for objective weakness
- Tone for any increase or decrease in tone
- Tendon reflexes for any attenuated or exaggerated reflexes
- Coordination
- Gait *per se* can give important clue to the localization and diagnosis.

Muscle Bulk

Localized wasting or fasciculation in the weak limb indicates either radicular or anterior horn cell involvement, as well as plexus or nerve involvement. Focal wasting has great localizing value and can be seen in syringomyelia, cord tumors, spondylosis, motor neuron disease, etc.

Power Testing

It is done in individual group of muscles and is graded from Grade 0 (no contraction) to Grade V (normal power), as per Medical Research Council (MRC) grading.

Table 2: Upper motor neuron versus lower motor neuron signs.

Clinical test	*Upper motor neuron*	*Lower motor neuron*
Reflexes	Hyper-reflexia	Hyporeflexia
Muscle tone	Increased/spastic	Decreased/flaccid
Fasciculation	None	Present
Atrophy	None	Severe
Babinski sign	Present	Absent

Muscle Tone

It is the resistance to passive movement, when the patient is asked to relax. Tone is a reflex phenomenon and involves alpha motor and gamma efferent fibers. The tone is usually tested by supination-pronation of the forearm; flexion and extension of elbow and dorsiflexion and plantar flexion of wrist joint. In lower limbs, passive flexion and extension of hip, knee and ankle joint is done to assess the tone. Other soft signs of documenting abnormal tone are:

- *Pronator sign*: In the presence of hypotonia with cerebellar lesions, there is tendency of the hands to assume a position of pronation, when the arms are outstretched horizontally.
- *Pronator drift sign*: With eyes closed, the patient holds both arms outstretched in front of him. The elbows should be fully extended, the wrist extended and the hands open with palms up. In the presence of mild hemiparesis (there is mild increase in tone), there may be slow pronation of wrist, slight flexion of elbows and fingers, downward and lateral drift of the hand.

Various pathological conditions can cause either decrease (hypotonia) or increase in tone (hypertonia).

Hypotonia is usually seen in lesions involving spinomuscular level, proprioceptive pathways, cerebellar lesions and choreas.

Hypertonia is caused by interruption of impulses from supraspinal regions. Two types of hypertonia are observed clinically: (1) spasticity, and (2) rigidity.

Spasticity

This is seen with corticospinal lesions. There is *clasp knife* type of resistance, where there is elastic, spring like resistance to stretching at beginning of movement, which continues till certain point and then suddenly the muscle relaxes. Occasionally, spasticity is so marked that the examiner cannot passively move the extremity. The level of corticospinal tract affliction is generally based on associated symptoms and signs.

Extrapyramidal Rigidity

Lesions of extrapyramidal system produces either *lead pipe or cog wheel rigidity*. In this type of hypertonia, there is same degree of resistance in entire range of movement and is seen in both flexor and extensor groups. Often there is intermittent yielding of muscles to stretching.

Rigidity of this kind is seen in Parkinson's disease and other Parkinsonian syndromes. Parkinsonism is characterized by bradykinesia, tremor and rigidity. A large variety of Parkinsonian syndrome produce these symptoms and can be distinguished from Parkinson's disease by a variety of clinical and other diagnostic tests.

- *Idiopathic Parkinson's disease* is characterized by asymmetric onset rigidity, tremor and bradykinesia. Cognition is preserved till late stage and no gross dysautonomia is observed. Usually magnetic resonance imaging (MRI) of brain reveals age-related atrophic change.
- *Multisystem atrophy* is characterized by associated severe dysautonomia, affecting bowel, bladder and postural hypotension. MRI reveals cruciform hyperintensity in pons ("hot cross bun" sign) **(Fig. 5)**.
- *Progressive supranuclear palsy* is characterized by recurrent falls (usually backward), with predominant axial rigidity. There is severe upgaze and downgaze restriction and in later stages lateral gaze restriction is seen. MRI reveals atrophy of the rostral midbrain tegmentum, the pontine base, giving hummingbird appearance on midsagittal view.

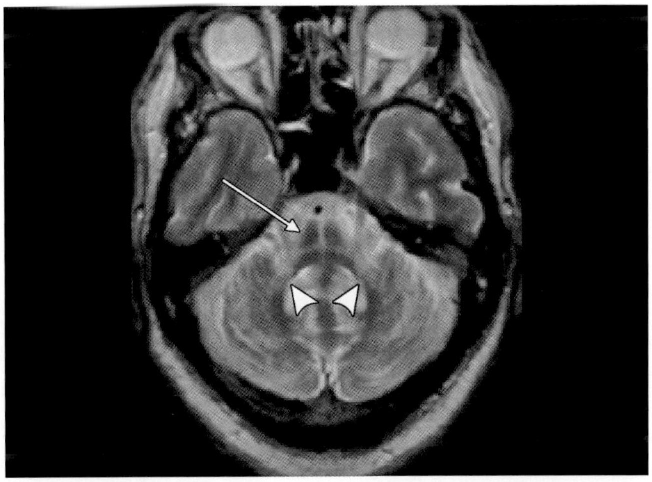

Fig. 5: Magnetic resonance imaging of the brain showing "hot cross bun" sign in *multiple-system atrophy* (MSA).

Reflexes

Reflex action requires a stimulus, a sensory pathway, a link with motor unit, motor neuron and finally, a contractile or other effector element. Any breach in this arc results in an absent reflex. Commonly used tendon reflexes are discussed below.

Biceps Jerk

Press forefinger gently on biceps tendon in antecubital fossa and then strike the finger with the hammer.

Normal result: Flexion of elbow with visible contraction of biceps muscle.

Segmental innervations: C5; Peripheral nerve: Musculocutaneous.

Supinator Jerk

Strike lower end of radius 5 cm above the wrist.

Normal result: Contraction of brachioradialis and flexion of elbow.

Segmental innervations: C5, C6; Peripheral nerve: Radial.

Triceps Jerk

Strike the triceps 5 cm above elbow, held in midflexed position.

Normal result: Extension of elbow and visible contraction of triceps.

Segmental innervations: C6, C7; Peripheral nerve: Radial.

Knee Jerk

Tap the patellar tendon in midflexed position of knee.

Normal result: Extension of knee and contraction of quadriceps.

Segmental innervations: L 3-4; Peripheral nerve: Femoral.

Ankle Jerk

Achilles tendon is struck after dorsiflexing the ankle.

Normal result: Plantar flexion of the foot and contraction of gastrocnemius.

Segmental innervations: S1; Peripheral nerve: Medial popliteal.

Hoffman Reflex

The terminal phalanx of the patient's middle finger is flicked downwards between examiner's finger and thumb. In hyper-reflexia, the tips of other fingers flex and the thumb flexes and adduct.

Abnormalities of Tendon Reflexes

- *Hyper-reflexia* is usually seen in pyramidal tract lesions but can also be seen in agitation, anxiety and fear.
- *Clonus* indicates marked degree of reflex excitability and usually means pyramidal system disease.
- *Absent reflex* indicates breach in a part of reflex arc either in sensory nerve, root or anterior horn cell, anterior root, peripheral nerve, etc. The other differences in upper versus lower motor neuron lesions are summarized in **Table 2**.
- *Inverted supinator reflex*: When supinator jerk is tested, there is no contraction of brachioradialis or biceps and only exaggerated finger flexion is seen. It indicates cord lesion at fourth or fifth cervical level, as in disk disease, syringomyelia, cervical neoplasm, etc.

Superficial Reflexes

Abdominal Reflexes

Lightly stroking the abdomen from without inwards in all four quadrants of abdomen.

Normal result: The muscles of the quadrant stimulated contract and umbilicus moves in that direction.

Segmental innervations: Upper abdominal, T9-10; midabdominal, T10-11; lower abdominal, T11-12.

The abdominal reflexes are usually absent in pyramidal tract lesions, though they may normally be absent in obese individuals and multiparous women.

Cremasteric Reflex

Inner part of thigh is stroked in downward and inward direction.

Normal result: The contraction of cremasteric muscle pulls up the scrotum and testicle on the side examined.

Segmental innervations: L1-2.

Anal Reflex

Lightly scratch the perianal skin.

Normal result: Contraction of external anal sphincter.

Segmental innervations: S4-5.

Plantar Reflex

Babinski sign: Extension of great toe with fanning of other toes on striking the outer aspects of foot with blunt key.

Other Important Reflexes

Grasp Reflex

Place first and second finger between the thumb and forefingers of patient's hand and try to draw them lightly away. If grasp reflex is present, the fingers will be held tightly by the patient's hand. It is due to bilateral corticospinal tract involvement, usually seen in neurodegenerative diseases like Alzheimer's disease, multi-infarct state, tumor or vascular accidents in the premotor cortex.

Forced Grasping Reflex

Lightly and repeatedly touching the side of palm results in hand following the stimulus and attempting to grasp it and is usually seen in widespread cerebral lesions. In advanced cases, patient may try to follow the movement of hand (*Groping reflex*).

Sucking Reflex

Touching the corner of mouth produces a sucking movement of the lips and is seen in widespread hemispheric lesions.

Glabellar Tap

Tapping at root of nose is accompanied by synchronous blinking and is commonly seen in Parkinson's disease.

Coordination

For proper coordination, both sensory and motor system should be intact. Various tests used to test coordination are:

Finger Nose Test

Each arm is drawn out to full abduction, with forefinger pointed. Patient is asked to alternatively touch the nose tip with his finger and the examiner's finger. In cerebellar disease, the finger moves to the nose in a wavering side to side or up and down fashion.

Heel-Knee Test

The patient is told to run heel down the front of shin to the top of the foot. In cerebellar disease, the heel overshoots the knee sideways and develops rotating oscillation as it approaches it.

Dysdiadochokinesis

There is failure to efficiently perform rapid alternating movements. Patient is asked to rotate hands rapidly at wrists, holding the forearms vertically, with elbows flexed. In cerebellar disease, the movements will be coarse, irregular and slow.

Past Pointing Test

Patient sits holding his arm forward, so that his fingers touch fingers of the examiner. Then he is asked to lower or raise the arm above head and bring it back to original position. In cerebellar disease, the arm on the side of lesion will deviate outwards towards the side of lesion.

Sensory System

The various modalities of sensation tested in clinical neurology are:

- Pain, light touch and temperature. These are *exteroceptive sensations* derived from sources outside the body.
- Sense of position, passive movement, vibration and deep pain. These are the *proprioceptive sensation* derived from the body itself.
- Stereognosis and graphesthesia are two point of discrimination. These are the cortical sensations.
- It is wise to move from area of impaired sensation to normal sensation, for the change is easier to detect.
- The common patterns of sensory loss with localizing value are:
  - *Total unilateral loss* of all forms of sensation is seen in extensive lesion of thalamus or internal capsule.
  - *Unilateral hyperalgesia* and hyperesthesia follows partial lesions of thalamus.
  - *Crossed hemisensory loss*, on face on one side and body on opposite side, is seen in lesions of medulla (lateral medullary syndrome).
  - *Bilateral loss of all sensations* below a definite level is seen in gross lesion of spinal cord.
  - *Suspended sensory loss*: Impairment of pain and temperature sensation over several segments with normal sensation above and below are seen in intrinsic lesion of the cord, like syringomyelia and intrinsic cord tumor.
  - *Saddle anesthesia*: Impairment of sensation over the lowest sacral segments is seen in cauda equina/conus medullaris lesion.
- Unilateral loss of pain and temperature below a definite level is seen in Brown-Sèquard syndrome of hemisection of cord, as in compression or demyelination.
- *Glove and stocking anesthesia* is seen in peripheral neuropathy.

- *Patchy areas* of sensory loss can be seen in a nerve or radicular distribution.
- *Romberg's sign*: The patient sways from the heels, when the eyes are closed, after making the patient stand with feet opposed. This is characteristic of proprioceptive deficiency (large fiber neuropathy or affliction of dorsal columns).

Gait

At the end of the clinical examination, the patient should be made to walk for few meters. Note the posture of the body while walking, the position and movements of the arms, legs, the distance between feet, the regularity of movement, the ability to maintain a straight course, the ease of turning and stopping. The various gaits of clinical significance are:

- *Dragging of feet*: The patient who drags one foot usually has an upper motor neuron lesion of that leg. In the presence of marked hemiparesis, he will throw the whole leg outwards from the hip, producing the movement called "*circumduction*". This is usually seen following hemiplegia of any cause.
- *Scissoring gait*: In bilateral upper motor neuron lesions, both feet drag, steps are slow and short, the gait is stiff legged. The feet tend to cross in "scissor" fashion, most commonly seen in spastic diplegia of childhood.
- *High stepping gait*: The patient raises the foot high to overcome a foot drop; the toe hits the ground first. This gait occurs in lumbosacral root, cauda equina lesions or peripheral nerve lesions causing anterior tibial muscle paralysis.
- *Stamping gait*: The heels tend to strike the floor first and result from loss of position sense, when the patient does not know where his foot is. The abnormality is increased in dark. This is seen in sensory neuropathies or disorders of posterior columns.
- *Shuffling gait*: Movement is a series of small, flat footed shuffles is commonly seen in extrapyramidal syndromes, particularly Parkinson's disease. The steps become quicker as the movement progresses (festination).
- *Gait apraxia*: The gait is irregular and hesitant with small stepped shuffling. The patient may lean backwards rather than forwards. This type of gait is seen in syndrome of normal pressure hydrocephalus (NPH) and can also be seen in multi-infarct states.
- *Ataxic gait*: The patient tends to reel and sway as if drunk and is seen in cerebellar diseases.
- *Waddling gait*: The pelvis is rotated through an abnormally large arc, accompanied by compensatory movements of upper trunk and associated with marked lordosis. This is usually seen in myopathies.
- *Hysterical gaits*: Bizarre gait, which varies from moment to moment and can be altered by suggestion.

DISORDERS OF HIGHER MENTAL FUNCTION

DISORDERS OF SPEECH

Two main types of speech defects are encountered in neurological disorders: (1) Dysarthria and (2) dysphasia (aphasia).

Dysarthria

When the articulation and enunciation of individual words and phrases is distorted, this is dysarthria. Articulation requires coordination of tongue, lips, palate, larynx and muscles of respiration and may be affected by lesions of upper and lower motor neuron, extrapyramidal and cerebellar systems. Various types of dysarthria are:

- *Spastic dysarthria*: This is caused by lesions of bilateral upper motor neuron. The tongue is small and spastic. The speech is slurred, as if the patient is talking from the back of the throat.
- *Rigid dysarthria*: Speech is monotonous, all inflections and accents disappear, and words run into one another. This is a result of extrapyramidal lesion.
- *Ataxic dysarthria*: Speech is irregular, slurred and drunken. The rhythm is jerky, sometimes explosive, staccato or scanning. This is a result of cerebellar disease.
- Weakness of facial, palatal, tongue muscles can also produce dysarthria. There is nasal intonation of speech in bulbar palsy.

Dysphasia

When the patient is failing to put into properly constructed words or phrases the thoughts he wishes to express, even if articulation is adequate, then it is called dysphasia (or aphasia). Evaluation of dysphasia includes assessment of spontaneous speech, comprehension, naming objects, repetition, reading, writing and calculation. Various types of dysphasias are:

- *Broca's aphasia*: Speech is nonfluent with preserved comprehension, poor repetition and naming ability. Usually seen in an infarct in the territory of anterior part of the left middle cerebral artery.

- *Wernicke's aphasia*: Speech is fluent with profoundly affected comprehension, impaired repetition. Naming is poor. The patient produces jumbled string of meaningless words and neologisms. Posterior left middle cerebral artery territory infarction is the most common cause with damage to the posterior third of superior temporal gyrus.
- *Transcortical aphasia*: There is retained repetition with fluent or nonfluent aphasia.
- *Echolalia*: Involuntary repetition of words and phrases spoken by someone else. The lesion lies in the temporo-parietal region.
- *Pure word deafness*: Patient cannot recognize the spoken word. This is due to a lesion in the middle of first temporal gyrus.
- *Pure word dumbness*: This is an apraxic speech defect with inability to articulate. The lesion may be widespread in the left hemisphere. Usually reading, writing, and copying are preserved.
- *Alexia*: Inability to understand written material. There is lesion in left occipital cortex and splenium of corpus callosum. There is associated right homonymous hemianopia and is seen in infarction of posterior cerebral artery.
- *Alexia with agraphia*: The patient cannot read or write spontaneously. The lesion lies in the left angular gyrus and is usually accompanied by nominal aphasia, acalculia, hemianopia and visual agnosia.
- *Agraphia*: Pure writing defect may occur in lesion that lies between angular gyrus and motor area.
- *Acalculia*: Inability to calculate may be seen in lesions of left angular gyrus.

APRAXIA

Inability to carry out well organized voluntary movement correctly despite the fact that motor, sensory, coordinative functions are not significantly impaired. Four types of apraxia are commonly recognized.

1. *Ideomotor apraxia*: Inability to imitate or mime an act involving use of objects. There is lesion between dominant parietal lobe and motor area.
2. *Ideational apraxia*: Carrying out a whole of complex act is defective though execution of different parts of complete act may be normal.
3. *Constructional apraxia*: Inability to make or copy simple designs. The lesion is in the angular gyrus of either hemisphere but when isolated, is usually from nondominant parietal lesions.
4. *Dressing apraxia*: The patient is unable to dress or undress himself in the absence of motor or sensory deficit. The lesion is usually in nondominant posterior parietal lobe lesions.

AGNOSIA

Failure to recognize some object or sound, when the sense by which it is normally recognized remains intact.

Visual Agnosia

The patient is unable to name or describe the use of the objects shown but is able to identify them, when he touches them. The site of lesion lies in second and third occipital gyri and the adjacent subcortical white matter in the dominant hemisphere.

The patient may be unable to find his way around an obstruction or find his way to a given point. This type of visual disorientation is seen in bilateral posteroinferior parietal lesions or in the nondominant hemispheric affliction.

Tactile Agnosia

The patient may be unable to recognize an object, by touching but is able to give its name on seeing. The patient with true tactile agnosia is able to describe its shape, size, texture. The site of lesion is in contralateral supramarginal gyrus or in corpus callosum.

Auditory Agnosia

The patient who is unable to recognize the sound, but can recognize the object on sight or touch, has auditory agnosia. The site of the lesion is in the posterior part of the temporal convolutions of the dominant hemisphere.

PARIETAL LOBE DYSFUNCTIONS

- *Right left disorientation*: Patient is unable to correctly point towards the right or left side of the body in parietal lobe lesion.
- *Autotopagnosia*: Patient is unable to identify any part of the body.
- *Finger agnosia*: Inability to pick out individual digit is termed finger agnosia.
- *Gerstmann syndrome*: It consists of finger agnosia, acalculia, right-left disorientation and agraphia without alexia and is found in lesions of the dominant hemisphere in the region of angular gyrus.
- *Anosognosia*: Complete lack of awareness of opposite half of the body is seen in lesions of parietal lobe of nondominant hemisphere.
- *Sensory inattention*: Bilateral stimulation by visual, auditory or tactile stimuli may result in inattention

in one of the fields, though can be appreciated when stimuli are given in individual fields. This phenomenon of inattention is commonly seen in parietal lobe lesion, usually after vascular accidents, or tumor of the contralateral hemisphere.

CONCLUSION

The importance of neurologic examination in the diagnosis of diseases of the nervous system cannot be overemphasized. Neurological examination is a time consuming and tiring exercise for both patient as well as physicians. However, a good history and proper examination can localize the disease process accurately and based on the temporal course of the disease a likely etiology can be postulated. This exercise helps in judicious use of ancillary investigations including radiology.

SUGGESTED READING

1. Brazis PW, Masdeu JC, Biller J. Localization in Clinical Neurology, 5th edition. Philadelphia, USA: Lippincott Williams & Wilkins. 2007.
2. Haerer AF. DeJong's The Neurologic Examination, 6th edition. Philadelphia, USA: Lippincott-Raven. 2005.
3. Hauser SL. Harrison's Neurology in Clinical Medicine. USA: McGraw Hill Professional. 2006.
4. Patten J. Neurological Differential Diagnosis, 2nd edition. New York, USA: Springer-Verlag. 2000.
5. Spillane J. Bickerstaff's Neurological Examination in Clinical Practice, 6th edition. USA: Wiley-Blackwell. 1996.

CHAPTER 37

Basic Neuropathology

Kirti Gupta, Rakesh Kumar Vasishta

REMOVAL OF THE BRAIN FROM SKULL

The most common method of removal of brain from the skull involves a reflection of the scalp followed by the removal of a generous cap of bone using a circumferential saw-cut. The left covering of the brain is called dura. This is the stage at which the superior longitudinal sinus can be tested in two ways: either by opening it or by simply running a fingertip along it and examining any motion of the surrounding blood. When the brain is suspended by the basilar artery, each side of the dura is incised and reflected medially, piercing through the bridging veins with knife or scissors. After dividing the anterior attachment of the falx, the dura is reflected backwards. The frontal lobes are lifted very gently from the base of the anterior cranial fossa, while trying to ensure that the olfactory bulbs remain attached to the brain. The optic nerves, internal carotid arteries (ICA), oculomotor nerves and pituitary stalk are cut neatly across close to the base, when they become visible. The tentorium is uncovered, first on one side then on other, by delicately lifting the temporal lobes; and the attachments of the tentorium to the petrous temporal bones are cut with a sharp knife. As a result of the piercing of the dura, the same cut will separate the roots of the trigeminal, facial and the auditory nerves. In the gap which shows up between the clivus and the pons, the visible abducents nerves are cut. The lower cranial nerves and the vertebral arteries, which are still holding the brainstem down are cut, either with a knife or with long-bladed scissors, without causing any damage to the lower brainstem. This can usually be carried out blind, but cutting as far as possible to each side. After the cutting of vertebral arteries, the lower brainstem and upper cervical cord become visible, thus making it possible to cut across with the knife. After this, a number of bridging veins remain, including the great vein of Galen, which performs the function of draining blood from the deeper cerebral gray matter into the straight sinus. Throughout the whole procedure, the brain should be held by the left hand very carefully, so that the tension and distortion remain at a minimum level. Once it is free, the brain should only be placed with its base upwards in a bucket of a suitable size containing buffered formalin, instead of a flat surface. It is gently suspended by a thread passing through the basilar artery and the ends of the thread are tied to the bucket handle.

REMOVAL OF VENOUS SINUS, CAVERNOUS SINUS AND MIDDLE EAR EXAMINATION

After removal of the brain all abnormalities in the dura at the base of the cranial cavity is noted and the patency of the principal venous sinuses (straight, lateral, sigmoid, superior longitudinal) is examined. A hammer and chisel are used for checking the internal carotid artery (ICA), the ear drums and middle ears. The chisel is applied to the base of the middle cranial fossa and a sharp hit with the hammer then displays the middle ear drum and ICA lying within the carotid canal, which can lead to the wall of the cavernous sinus. In the similar way, after removing the pituitary and the sphenoid sinus the frontal and ethmoidal sinuses are opened and demonstrated.

A vibrating saw is used for removing a square piece of sphenoid block for the cavernous sinus. The portion includes the area around the pituitary fossa containing the parts of ICA, optic tracts, cranial nerves—III, V, VI.

EXAMINATION OF THE BRAIN

After its removal, the brain is fixed in 20% buffered, neutral formalin for the duration of 10–14 days. The fixed brain is then weighed (usually the weight of brain is slightly higher than when unfixed). The normal brain weight ranges from 1,100 g to 1,600 g for males and 1,050–1,500 g for females.

Gross Features to be Noted

- *Meninges*:
  - For exudates
- *Gyri and sulci*:
  - For flattening and narrowing of sulci-cerebral edema
  - Narrowing and thinning of gyri—atrophy
- *Convexities/surface*:
  - *For exudates*:
    - Pyogenic meningitis
  - *Enlargement*:
    - Unilateral (space occupying lesion)
    - Bilateral (bilateral lesions, cerebral edema)
  - Atrophy of frontal lobes—senile atrophy
- *Base of brain*:
  - *Exudate*:
    - Tubercular meningitis
    - Mucoid—both at base and at convexities (cryptococcal meningitis)
  - *Circle of Willis*:
    - For aneurysm
    - For emboli—in case of stroke the most common sites being the bifurcation of an ICA and the origin of a branch of a middle cerebral artery (MCA)
    - Sites of atheromatous narrowing should be noted
  - Mammillary bodies and optic chiasm-atrophy (alcohol induced)
  - Uncal notching and tonsillar herniation
  - Atrophy of brainstem
  - Cerebellum—cerebellar atrophy
    - Ataxia, chronic debilitating illness.

Slicing of Brain

- *Coronal slicing*: Normally, the first incision separates the hindbrain (brainstem and cerebellum) from the cerebral hemispheres. This should be done with a clean transverse cut across the midbrain, just in front of the third nerve, at right angles to the long axis of the brainstem. The first cut passes through the optic chiasm or mammillary bodies, going through the anterior margin of the thalamus. The anterior part of the cerebrum is then placed to be cut surface down, between a pair of centimeter (or less) guides, and successive slices taken at centimeter intervals or less and laid out, posterior surface upward, with the right side on the right. The same procedure is repeated on the posterior part.
- In the cases which have undergone computerized tomography (CT) scans during their life are preferably sliced at the alternative-horizontal plane because that clearly shows the contrast between the actual and radiographic slices. Usually, the initial cut for horizontal slicing is at level of the upward end of the Sylvian fissure. The slices are spread out, upper surface upward, with right side facing right.
- *Hindbrain dissection*: After serving the midbrain, a clear observation of the occurrence of the trans-tentorial herniation becomes possible or not. It is visible in the following signs:
  - Excessive grooving of the parahippocampal gyrus, on one side or both, and
  - Lateral compression of the upper brainstem.

  There are two commonly practiced routines for slicing the hindbrain. The first, which is also the most commonly followed, involves cutting through the upper medulla at the level of the lateral apertures (foramina of Luschka) in a plane vertical to the long axis of the medulla, and continuing the cut through the cerebellum. This displays an extremely broad view of the *fourth ventricle*, the dentate nuclei, and the flocculi, uvula and nodulus of the cerebellum. Further cuts are made through the lower part of the specimen, using 5 mm guides or free-hand slices 3–4 mm apart, until it ends. On the other hand, if the interest is intended for the regional differences between areas of cerebellum, the alternate method can be applied. Oblique cuts are made to separate the cerebellum from the brainstem. These cuts pass through the cerebral peduncles ending in the fourth ventricle. These oblique cuts can then be made at right angles to the folia on the upper surface, and a midline cut will display the whole of cerebral vermis. The brainstem is sliced at 3–4 mm intervals as before.

Appearance of the Ventricles

The lateral ventricles may be larger or smaller than normal, or unequal.

Various points to note:

- Whether the ventricles contain blood
- Whether the capaciousness of the subarachnoid spaces between the cerebral sulci and in the basal cisterns is normal or abnormal. If it is more than normal, there is a presumption of cerebral atrophy; but if it is less, a block in the cerebrospinal fluid (CSF) pathway must be looked for
- Whether the dilation of the ventricles affects the ventricular system wholly or partially; and if it is partially affected, whether the difference can be accounted for by local atrophy or tissue destruction.

Choice of Blocks for Histology

There are no strict rules regarding the choice of blocks for embedding, except that at least some should be relevant to the probable diagnosis.

Five standards for brain:

1. The left frontal lobe to include the border zone between anterior and middle cerebral arteries
2. Hippocampus to include the Ammon's nucleus
3. Basal ganglia including globus pallidus, putamen, internal capsule, insular cortex
4. Pons
5. Cerebellum to include the dentate nucleus.

Pediatric Brain Examination

Special and intensive care is required for extracting infants' brains. The tissues of an infant's brain are not only softer and more friable, but the leptomeninges are also fragile. The risk involved in manipulating a soft brain can also be reduced by taking the brain out under water. The brain of an infant can easily be removed by cutting the sutures and reflecting the parietal and frontal bones outwards.

The maturity of the infant brain can be evaluated by weighing it, and by examining the state of development of the cerebral gyri and the extent and distribution of myelination. The same method is followed for slicing of pediatric brain as well as an adult brain.

Points to be noted:

- *Hemorrhages*: Subdural and subarachnoid hemorrhage **(Fig. 1D)**.
- *Congenital malformations*: Common
  - Anencephaly—failure of brain formation
  - Spina bifida occulta
  - Meningocele/meningomyelocele/encephalocele
  - Porencephaly
- Hydrocephalus (HC) characterized by dilated ventricular system **(Figs. 1A to D)**.
  - *Obstructive HC*: Secondary to obstruction within the ventricular system.
  - *Communicating HC*: Secondary to extraventricular obstruction or due to impaired absorption or overproduction of CSF.
  - *HC ex vacuo*: Secondary to primary cortical disease with cerebral atrophy
- Acquired perinatal lesions
- *Germinal matrix hemorrhage*: This is encountered in premature infants. These begin as hemorrhagic infarcts in the involuting subependymal matrix layer of the lateral ventricle. When extensive they produced massive—intraventricular hemorrhagic lesions **(Fig. 1C)**. Smaller lesions are resolved leaving subependymal matrix cysts.
- *Periventricular leukomalacia*: This is encountered more often in the premature infants and consists of focal areas of necrosis in the periventricular white matter. These necrotic foci may undergo mineralization.
  - *Kernicterus*: It refers to heavy bilirubin staining of deep gray nuclei with selective damage to some parts of brain in deeply jaundiced infants **(Fig. 1C)**.
  - *Hypoxia*: Dusky discoloration of central white matter **(Fig. 2)**.

INFECTIONS

While examining a neuropathological case with possibility of a central nervous system (CNS) infection the main aims to be established are:

- The root cause of the infection
- The route taken by the organism to reach nervous system
- The effects of the infection on the nervous system.

At autopsy, the following samples are taken:

- CSF samples for:
  - Microscopic examination
  - Culture and sensitivity
- Brain tissue for culture and sensitivity
- Crush smears for organisms, fungal hyphae
- Fresh tissue for PCR especially in case of:
  - Viral infections (1 cm^2 of tissue)
  - Cerebellum, hippocampus: Rabies

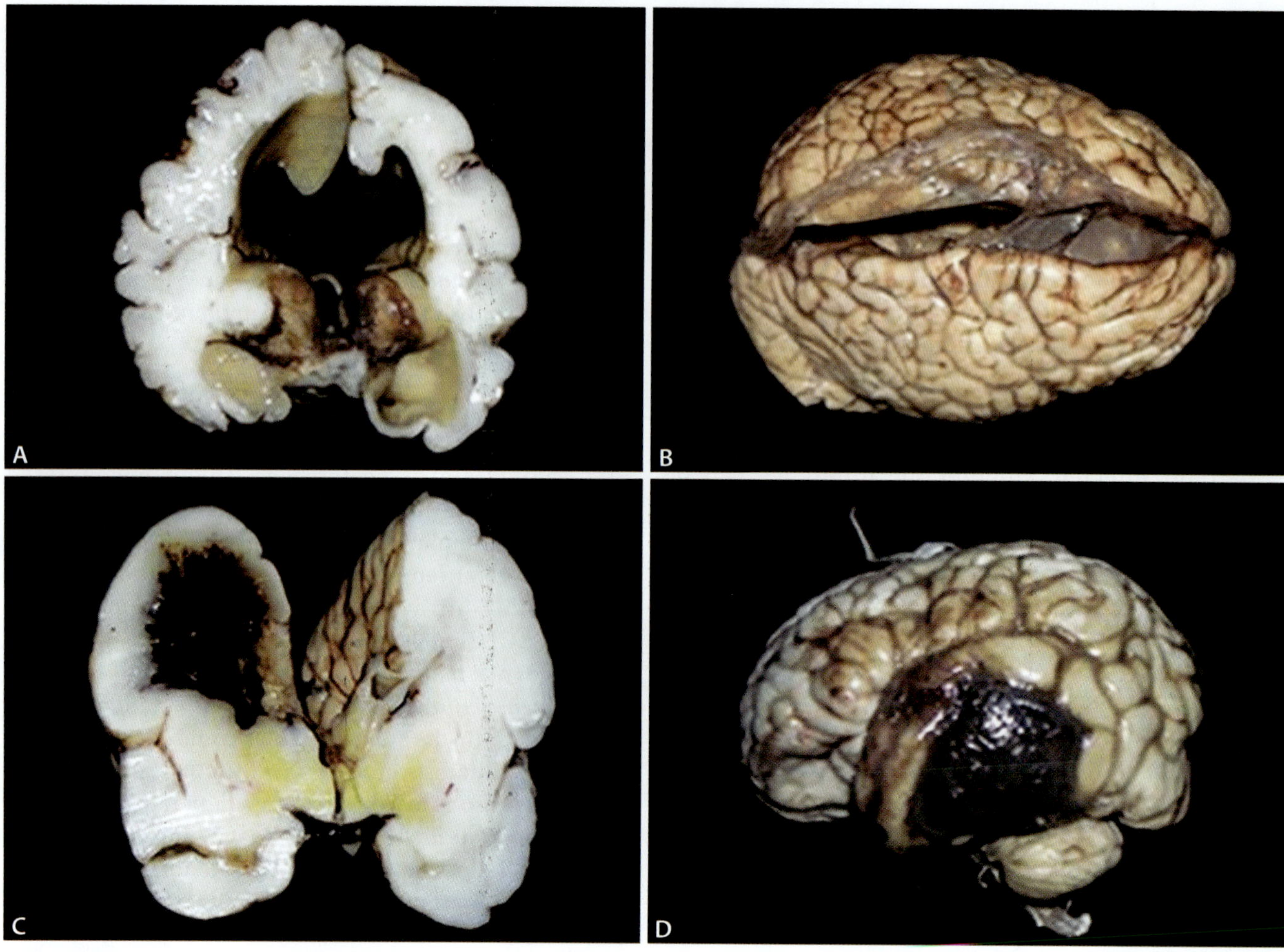

Figs. 1A to D: Hydrocephalus: (A) Dilated lateral ventricular system; (B) Superior view of the neonatal brain with hydrocephalus; (C) Intraventricular hemorrhage (left) with kernicterus (bilirubin staining of the thalamus); (D) Patch of subarachnoid hemorrhage over the left temporal lobe.

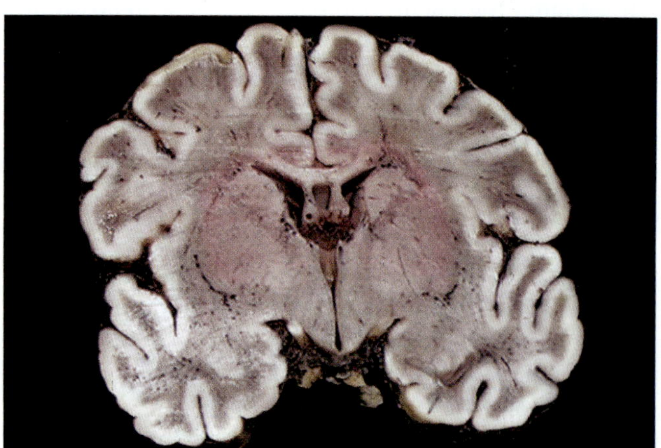

Fig. 2: Coronal slice of a neonatal brain showing marked hypoxic changes with dusky discoloration of the central white matter.

- Temporal lobe: Herpes simplex virus
- Portion of frontal cortex: Enteroviral encephalitis

Routes of Infection

- Hematogenous from established infection (e.g. osteomyelitis, septic arthritis, endocarditis, bronchiectasis)
- Spread from a nearby focus of infection (paranasal air sinuses, middle ears and bones of skull and spine)
- Penetrating injury.

The outcome is influenced by a number of factors including the virulence of the invading organism, the effectiveness of number of the defenses of the host and the pace of initiating the suitable antibiotic therapy. The CSF provides an excellent culture medium for many organisms to multiply at a rapid speed, it is because it is moderately removed from immune defenses. The low vascularity of

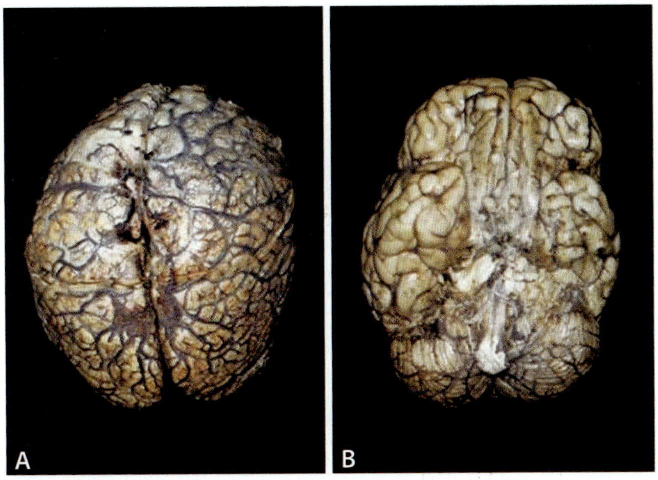

Figs. 3A and B: (A) Thick exudates over the surface of the convexities in a case of acute pyogenic meningitis; (B) Organized exudate at the base of the brain in a case of tubercular meningitis.

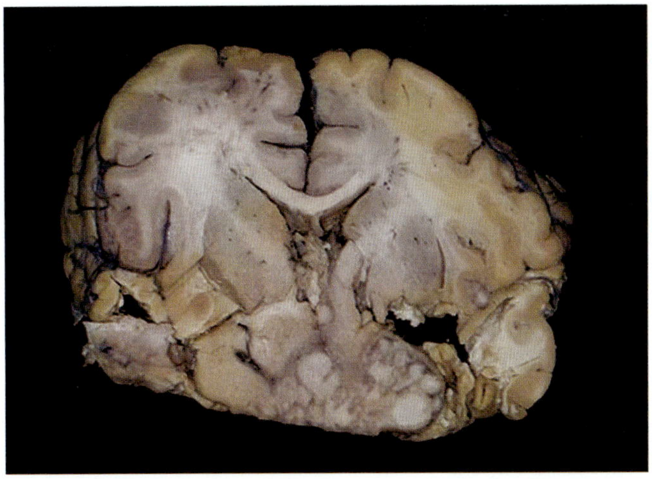

Fig. 4: Thick, organized exudates at the base of the brain with destruction of the bilateral basal ganglia, hippocampus, and optic chiasm in a case of tubercular meningitis.

the dura makes it difficult to remove organisms in the subdural space. Even antibiotics fail here due to poor penetration unless these are directly instilled.

Less virulent organisms, such as cryptococci and other fungi, and toxoplasmosis, are generally found in very young or elderly and debilitated patients because they have weak immunity, and may evoke little in the way of an inflammatory response.

Consequences of Infection

- Edema, acute, possibly fatal
- Sagittal sinus thrombosis with venous infarction
- Cerebral arterial infarction due to arteritis and HC.

Leptomeningitis

Acute Meningitis

A purulent exudate is readily evident in the subarachnoid space and it may be more marked over the vertex or at the base **(Figs. 3A and B)**. Acute inflammatory cells which are found in the superficial perivascular spaces surround the tiny penetrating vessels present on the walls of the cortex and the brainstem. Cortical and hippocampal neurons also show signs of acute hypoxic changes. The subarachnoid space and leptomeninges contain a neutrophil-rich infiltrate. Fibrin strands can also be frequently seen. Organisms may be demonstrated with the appropriate stains (Gram's, PAS), unless treatment with antibiotics during life has largely eradicated them. There may be adrenal or skin hemorrhages outside the CNS, along with evidence of more prevalent intravascular coagulation.

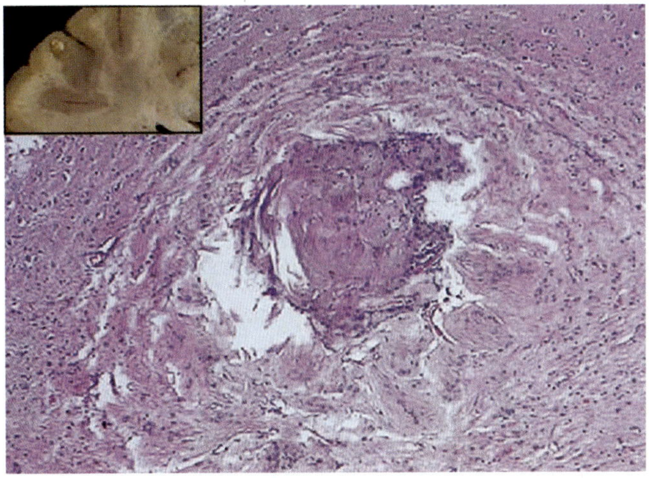

Fig. 5: Tuberculoma at the gray-white junction in the middle frontal gyrus. Microscopically shows a central necrotic focus with minimal inflammatory infiltrate.

Tubercular Meningitis (Figs. 3B to 6)

Thick exudates more at the base of the brain with opacity of meninges at the convexities. Microscopically, presence of epithelioid cell granulomas with Langhans' giant cells within the subarachnoid space is the characteristic feature. Meningeal vessels within the subarachnoid space may be entrapped producing arteritis leading to infarcts.

Tuberculomas may be single or multiple.

Sites of predilection— cerebellum, pontine tegmentum and paracentral lobule **(Fig. 5)**.

Round oval masses composed of necrotic, caseous center become cystic, fibrous and get calcified.

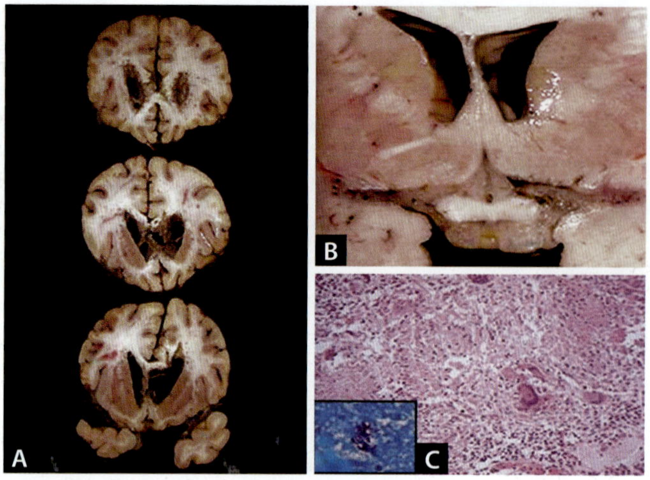

Figs. 6A to C: In a case of tubercular meningitis: (A) Ventriculitis with hydrocephalus; (B) Thick exudates at the base of the brain around the optic chiasm; (C) Epithelioid cell granuloma with acid fast tubercular bacilli (ZN stain, inset).

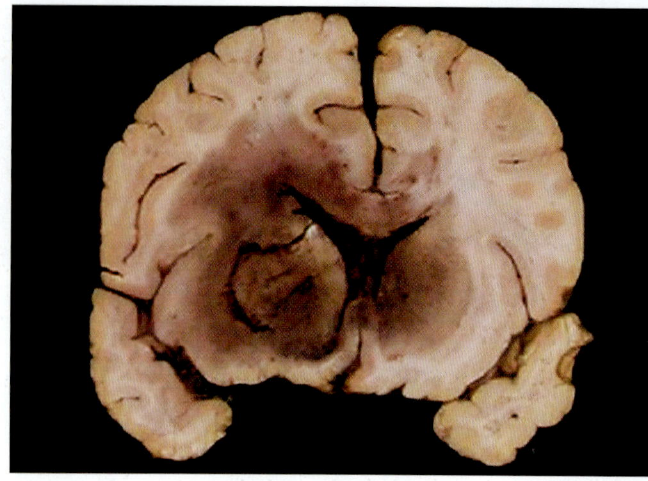

Fig. 7: In a case of fungal meningoencephalitis: Large areas of hemorrhagic necrosis involving the basal ganglia region, corpus callosum and central white matter.

Chronic Meningitis

Various organisms are responsible for causing chronic meningitis, which may be accompanied by granulomas or brain abscesses as well. When the inflammatory process in the subarachnoid space persists for duration more than a week or two, secondary effects also start developing in the brain.

- Hydrocephalus
- Multiple cerebral infarcts due to narrowing of, and thrombosis in, arteries affected by endarteritis obliterans, particularly common in fungal infections
- Collagenous thickening of leptomeninges, chiefly at the base
- *Cryptococcus* is liable to produce widened perivascular spaces, particularly in the basal ganglia
- Granulare pendymitis is invariably present in cases of chronic meningitis.

The organisms can themselves be identified with appropriate stains (Gram's for bacteria, Ziehl-Neelsen (ZN) for *Mycobacteria*), periodic acid-Schiff (PAS) and methenamine silver stains for fungi, Giemsa for protozoa).

Fungal Meningitis/Encephalitis

The more common fungi to involve the brain are:

- *Aspergillus*: Commonly in diabetics and produce large areas of hemorrhagic necrosis **(Fig. 7)**.
- *Zygomyces*: Commonly in diabetics and produce largeareas of hemorrhagic necrosis **(Figs. 8A and B)**.

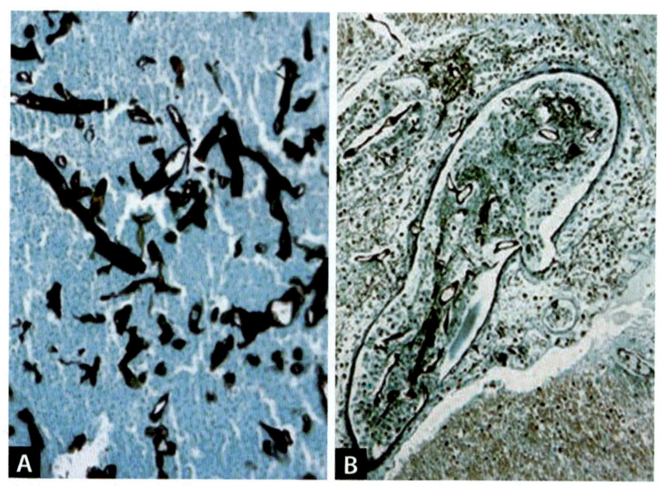

Figs. 8A and B: (A) Broad, aseptate hyphae of zygomycetes; (B) Fungal hyphae infiltrating the vessel wall with fibrinoid necrosis (Grocott's stain).

- *Candida: Usually in neonates produce large areas of hemorrhagic necrosis* ***(Fig. 9A)***.
- *Cryptococcus*: Produces meningitis with basal exudates and because of mucoid capsule gives a "slippery" feel to the brain **(Fig. 9B)**.

Subdural Empyema

It is from a focus of local osteomyelitis or paranasal sinus infection that the pus spreads in the subdural space. There may also be associated acute meningitis.

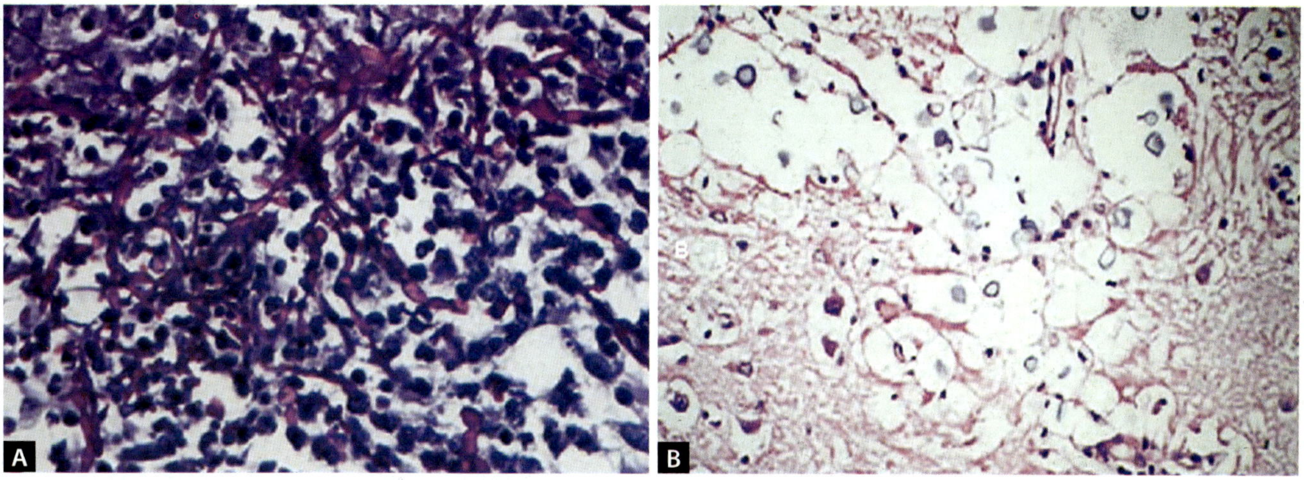

Figs. 9A and B: (A) Yeast and pseudohyphae of *Candida* in a neonatal case of fungal meningoencephalitis; (B) Cryptococci around the perivascular spaces.

Brain Abscess

Despite the probability of abscesses cropping up anywhere in the brain, these are most common in the white matter. Those with a local cause have particular sites of predilection. There may also be multiple, in which case they may be small and easily overlooked, especially when the organisms are blood-borne. At beginning, they consist of a small focus of liquefaction necrosis, or purulent encephalitis. Its expansion leads to the collection of pus in the center which forms a wall around it which composes of glial fibrils. If the abscess is situated near the ependymal surface, it may be incapable of to barring it from penetrating into the ventricle. Bacteria are the organisms most commonly responsible for the brain abscess are bacteria, but there can be involvement of other organisms as well, and these should be considered, particularly if bacterial cultures are not positive.

Purulent Encephalitis Associated with Subacute Bacterial Endocarditis

Septic emboli which arise from the infected heart valves occasionally become the cause of solitary or multiple brain abscesses. They may also block an artery and cause cerebral infarction, which eventually becomes an extension from the septic embolus. If numerous neutrophil polymorphs are found present in and around the edge of an infarct, it should raise the suspicion of the diagnosis, and immediately a Gram stain should be performed to find organisms. A *mycotic aneurysm is also another likely consequence of the presence of septic embolus in the cerebral artery.* It is caused by a local infection and weakening of the arterial wall. This in turn may crack, thus producing brain hemorrhage of the subarachnoid space.

Viral Encephalitis (Fig. 10)

Unlike bacteria and fungi, viruses depend for reproduction on the existence of suitable host cells. Aseptic meningitis due to viral infection is well recognized and relatively common, but generally self-limiting. Enterovirus infection is the most common cause of viral meningitis. Viral encephalitis and myelitis, due to infection of cells of the brain and spinal cord, tend to produce more severe disease, though the extent of the harm incurred is highly variable. The range of viruses pathogenic to nervous system is very wide. Some enter into the blood through bloodstream (e.g. arboviruses), whereas others take a neural route to the CNS after initial replication in extra neural tissues and uptake into peripheral nerves (e.g. rabies). HIV and arboviruses are the most widespread brain infections in the world so far.

Postmortem Examination in Cases of Suspected Viral Encephalitis

Cerebrospinal fluid and samples of serum should be collected for estimating the viral antibody titers. A rise in the serum antibody titer to a particular virus is not a sufficient evidence to declare a virus as the reason for encephalitis. However, with the comparison of antibody titers in CSF with those in serum it is possible to know if intrathecal synthesis of antibody to a specific virus has occurred or not. If it has, this is an indication of the existence of the virus within the CNS, despite the

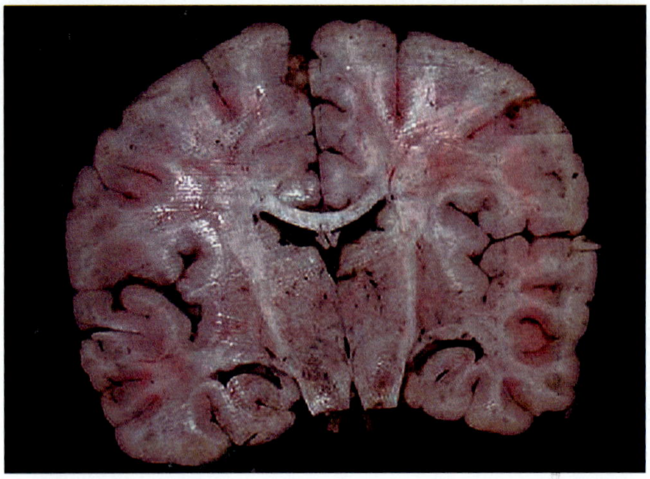

Fig. 10: A case of viral (Japanese B) encephalitis with softening and petechial hemorrhages in the thalami and the midbrain.

attempts to culture the virus being unsuccessful. In viral encephalitis there is usually also evidence of oligoclonal immunoglobulin in the CSF. Due to its characteristic of being sensitive and specific, the use of polymerase chain reaction (PCR) to detect specific viral nucleic acid in CSF or brain has become the chosen method for verifying the viral etiology of encephalitis.

Macroscopic Examination of the CNS and the Choice of Blocks for Microscopy

There is a possibility of some generalized swelling and congestion, perhaps with a few petechial hemorrhages on the pial surface. The meninges may be slightly blurred in the acute phase of herpes simplex encephalitis, there is swelling, hemorrhage and softening centered on one or both temporal lobes. If the patient survives until months or years later there is destruction and collapse of same regions. In chronic forms of encephalitis there is likely to be some degree of cerebral atrophy, granular discoloration of the white matter and fibrous thickening of the leptomeninges.

When preparing blocks for microscopy from cases of postmortem, samples should be taken both from areas which appear normal as well as from those which are obviously abnormal, and from transition zones in between. Samples from each major cerebral lobe, hippocampus, basal ganglia, thalamus and several levels of brainstem and cerebellum should be taken. It is necessary to have a wide sampling of the CNS because, although the *type* of damage caused by viral infections tends to be stereotyped, the location and distribution of the damage is often characteristic of particular viruses. The most reliable evidence about the cause of encephalitis appears from culture of a specific organism or detection of specific viral nucleic acid sequences by PCR, and from the use of immune-histological studies or in situ hybridization used to detect the presence of specific viral antigens or nucleic acid.

Pathological Features Common to Most Forms of Viral Encephalitis

- Death of cell with neuronophagia
- Perivascular lymphocytic collections
- Microglial nodules
- Inclusion bodies—which contain virus-coded material. Most characteristic are the RNA inclusions that form *Negri bodies*, cytoplasmic inclusions found in neurons in rabies. Round or oval, intranuclear, eosinophilic inclusion bodies, larger than nucleoli, and usually surrounded by a halo of clear nucleoplasm, are found in neurons and oligodendrocyte nuclei in subacute sclerosing panencephalitis (SSPE) and "immunosuppressive" measles encephalitis (Cowdry type A inclusions). They can sometimes be spotted in neurons in herpes simplex encephalitis.

NEUROVASCULAR DISEASES

These are those disorders attributable to pathologic structural and functional modifications of the blood vessels in the central, peripheral and autonomic nervous systems. This term is more encompassing and better than *stroke, or cerebrovascular disease*. Enormous importance should be imparted to the neurovascular diseases as these are the major cause of morbidity and are the third most common cause of death in this country.

Numerous causes can be attributed to the occurrence of a stroke and the following discussion is divided into hemorrhagic and ischemic. The *arterial infarcts* are generally ischemic and are characterized by the involvement of an area corresponding to a territory supplied by a major cerebral artery. The *venous infarcts* are hemorrhagic.

Arterial Infarcts or Territorial Infarcts

The arterial infarcts may be caused by thrombotic or embolic occlusion. The thrombotic infarcts are pale whereas embolic infarcts are hemorrhagic. The pale infarcts may also transform into hemorrhagic infarcts due to re-establishment of circulation.

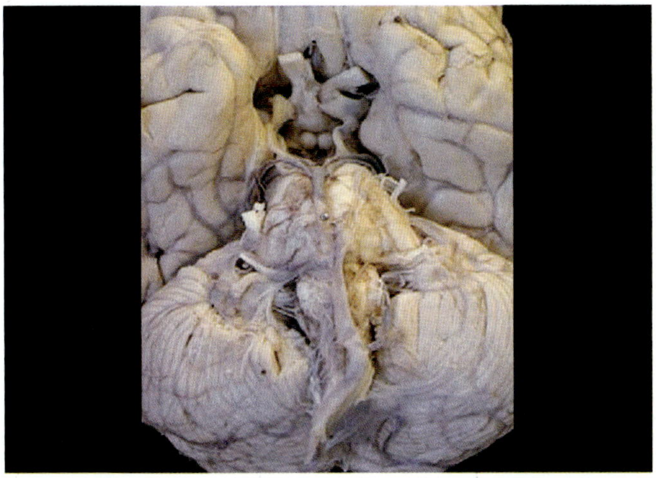

Fig. 11: Circle of Willis at the base of the brain.

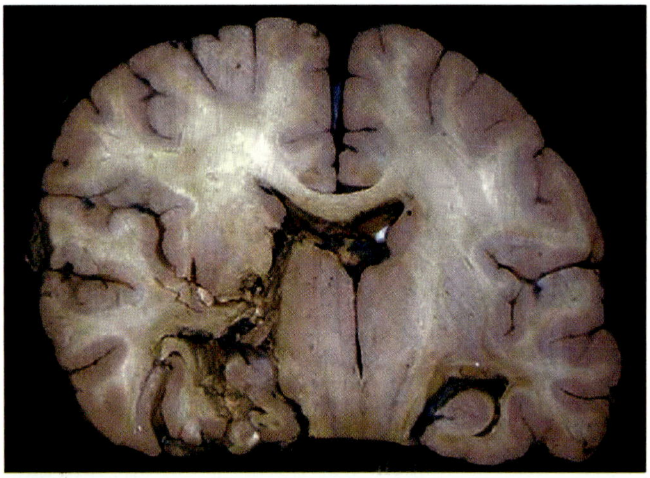

Fig. 12: Ischemic infarct in the region of MCA with softening and breaking down of the left cortical white matter (thalamus and hippocampus).
Abbreviation: MCA: Middle cerebral artery.

The three major branches coming of the circle of Willis **(Fig. 11)**, the anterior, middle and the posterior cerebral arteries, provide the vast majority of the arterial blood supply of the cerebral hemispheres. Territorial infarcts in the distribution of the *anterior cerebral artery* are extremely uncommon due to the adequacy of collateral flow through the circle of Willis. Most often these are the result of vasospasm related to rupture of a berry aneurysm on its proximal portion. Infarcts which involve the territory of the *posterior cerebral artery* are either embolic in nature, or are related to the effects of severe transtentorial herniation. Infarcts created by the *MCA* occlusion by embolic or thrombotic episodes manifest as massive strokes **(Fig. 12)**.

Embolic Infarcts

Since the total cerebral blood flow represents about 20% of the cardiac output, emboli are a relatively common cause of infarction. In several clinicopathological studies, embolic infarcts are said to be the most common cause of stroke. Such embolic infarcts may occur in virtually any location in the nervous system, but some locations are more typical. The embolic material rises up the cerebral vessels which bifurcate multiple times leading to the gradual narrowing of the lumina. The embolus finally settles in a vessel that is too small to enable its further travel. In situations with thromboembolism, the clot will rapidly break up into smaller fragments. Attempts to find the embolus by inspection or histologic investigation are mostly unsuccessful. Characteristically, thromboembolic infarcts are multiple and have the tendency of being peripheral in location and have a hemorrhagic appearance to some extent. Since emboli producing such lesions typically originate from either cardiac or carotid sources, they have a tendency of favoring the involvement of the cerebral hemispheres. There are innumerable possible sources for such emboli. In cases of chronic arterial fibrillation, mural thrombi in the auricular appendage of the left atrium may dislodge leading to the embolic infarction in the brain. Another common source of multiple cerebral emboli is from thrombi adherent to the endocardium following myocardial infarction with the formation of a left ventricular aneurysm. Carotid arteries are also a source of cerebral embolization. The carotid arteries, particularly in the region of the carotid bifurcation, are common sites for ulcerative atherosclerosis. Thrombi can form in the region of such lesions, and can embolize, as can fragments of atherosclerotic plaque. The cerebral artery at the center and its branches is the most common vessel to suffer embolic occlusion from an origin in the internal carotid artery. When emboli travel up the vertebrobasilar system, they can readily reach both posterior cerebral arteries, giving rise to bilateral infarcts in this distribution as a consequence of going either to the right or the left as they reach the top of the basilar artery.

Paradoxical embolization of the brain may occur in the situations in which natural filtering capacity of the capillary bed of the lungs has been bypassed, that is, in situations with right to left shunting of blood. Therefore, patients with patent foramen ovale, ventricular septal defects or pulmonary arteriovenous (AV) fistulae are at increased risk for cerebral embolization.

Cerebral Venous Infarcts (Fig. 13)

Thrombosis of one, or more, of major dural sinuses can give rise to the entity of cerebral venous infarcts. Within the system of venous drainage of the cerebral hemispheres, there are numerous interconnecting collateral channels, so one must achieve fairly extensive occlusion of a sinus and its associated major cortical veins, to cause a sufficient degree of interference in cerebral blood flow necessary to induce infarction of the tissues being drained. These causes include women who are taking oral contraceptives or who are postpartum, postoperative patients, hypercoagulable states associated with certain cancers, sickle cell disease, various forms of polycythemia, severe dehydration and cachexia. Local infection can also give rise to such occlusions with the formation of local thrombophlebitis. The resultant occlusion causes a hemorrhagic usually bilateral infarction within the area of drainage of the thrombosed veins.

Lacunar Infarcts

When the brain of elderly patients is being sliced, one commonly comes across small elongated, often multiple, cystic infarcts involving the thalamus, basal ganglia (especially the putamen and globus pallidus) and intervening internal capsule. These are called lacunes or lacunar infarcts and are usually bilateral and multiple. Advanced age, hypertension and diabetes influence the growth of such lesions. Lacunes stand for infarcts that are related to arteriosclerotic pathology in the lenticulostriate arteries arising from the proximal MCA. By definition, lacunes should not exceed 1 cm in their greatest dimension.

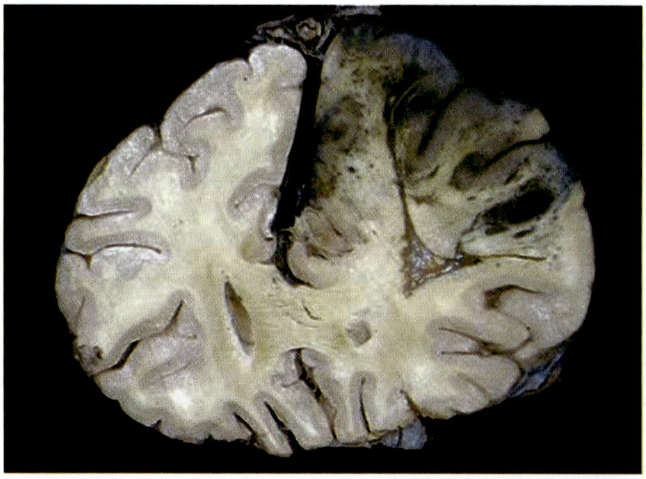

Fig. 13: Venous infarcts: Thrombosed superior sagittal sinus with hemorrhagic infarct involving the right frontal lobe with midline shift, edema and herniation of cingulated gyrus.

Practical Considerations

While evaluating a brain specimen suspected of having an ischemic lesion, the circle of Willis should be examined most carefully, along with its feeding and exiting vessels. Determine the extent and distribution of artherosclerotic lesions, possible occlusion, and for portions that are either incomplete or atretic. Understanding of ischemic stroke in the brain mostly involves a knowledge of the status of the carotid arteries, in particular, the relative patency. The practice of removing the carotid arteries has gone out of favor, leaving the prosector to guess as to what might or might not be present in these extremely important vessels.

Broad guidelines for autopsy on stroke patients:

- Look for extradural or subdural hemorrhage. If present, search for skull fractures.
- In case of SAH, examine circle of Willis and look for aneurysm, AVM, etc. in fresh state.
- Look at carotid siphon, cavernous sinus and dural venous sinuses and remove them if involved.
- Remove carotid arteries and vertebral arteries.
- Look for stenosis, atheroma, thrombosis (serial transverse sections), arterial dissection, etc. Gentle perfusion with water after removal and before cutting gives an idea of blockage.
- Size, site, anatomical location and nature of lesion whether arterial or venous infarct (usually hemorrhagic); single or multiple lesions. Infarcts-central or peripheral. Lesions—single or multiple.
- Observe edema, midline shift, ventricular size, herniation, secondary hemorrhages in pons, secondary infarction and whether hemorrhagic transformation of ischemic infarcts has occurred due to thrombolysis.
- For venous infarct sample the involved venous sinuses, infarcts with overlying thrombosed cortical veins, areas adjacent to look for vascular fibrin thrombi and their age, etc.

Intracranial Hemorrhage

Intracranial hemorrhage may occur as a result of head trauma or it may be spontaneous **(Flowchart 1)**.

The major causes of nontraumatic ICH are as follows:

- Hypertension—common sites are putamen, thalamus, lobar, cerebellum, pons **(Fig. 14)**
- AVM and aneurysms
- Cerebral amyloid angiopathy (CAA)
- Anticoagulant therapy
- Tumors
- Abuse of illicit with licit drugs.

Flowchart 1: Causes of intracranial hemorrhage.

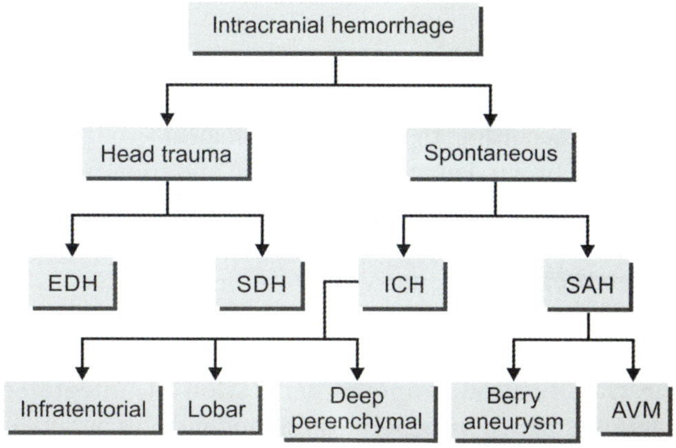

Abbreviations: AVM: Arteriovenous malformation; EDH: Extradural hemorrhage; ICH: Intracerebral hemorrhage; SDH: Subdural hemorrhage; SAH: Subarachnoid hemorrhage.

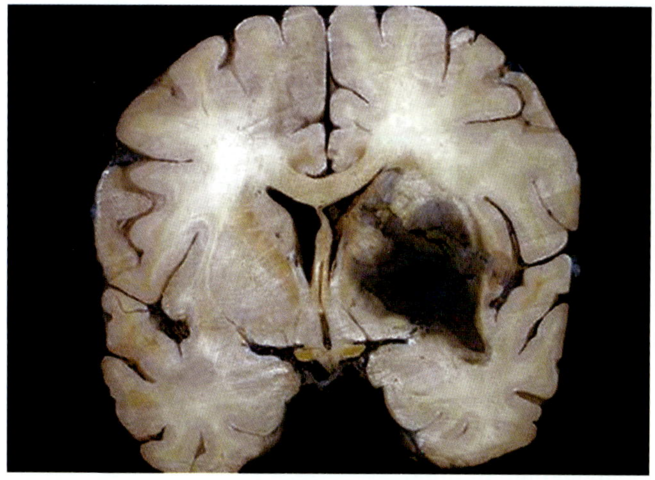

Fig. 14: Hypertensive bleed involving the right basal ganglia region.

Aneurysm

Subarachnoid hemorrhage is most commonly caused due to rupturing of berry aneurysm. With large aneurysm, a layered thrombus may be found partially filling the inner cavity. Berry aneurysms arise in a very particular geographic pattern of predilection, with approximately 70% of such lesions occurring within 1 cm of the anterior portion of the circle of Willis. Most common sites are the anterior communicating artery, the proximal anterior cerebral artery, the most distal extent of the internal carotid artery, the proximal MCA and the most rostral extent of the posterior extent of the posterior communicating artery.

Arteriovenous Malformations

Arteriovenous malformations may also be the underlying lesion leading to an intracerebral hemorrhage. Usually these represent developmental abnormalities in which arteries have direct communication with veins, without any intervention of a capillary bed. This subjects the veins associated with the malformation of arterial blood pressure directly. Greatly enlarged draining veins may be observed on the vertex lying over such a lesion. After cutting the brain, one can often see with the naked eye many irregular large vascular channel profiles within the hemorrhage. In some cases the arteriovenous malformation is so small that it can be completely eradicated by the hemorrhage. In such cases, identifying the underlying lesion may be quite difficult and require extensive histological sampling. The use of an elastic stain is helpful in visualizing the arterial vascular walls within the pool of blood clot.

Demyelinating Disease and Multiple Sclerosis

Gross Features

- Irregular gray patches on the normally whitish surface of the pons or on the cut surfaces of the upper cervical cord and optic nerves.
- When the brain is freshly incised, sharply demarcated gray or pinkish-gray firm patches (called plaques) can be found on the cut surfaces of cerebral hemispheres (especially subependymal region, angles of lateral ventricles, optic nerves) and spinal cord (mostly at cervical level).
- Chronic plaques are sharply demarcated with smooth edge.

Inherited Metabolic Diseases

In examining cases of inherited metabolic disease it is very important to reserve some fresh tissue for biochemical and genetic study before fixing the remainder of the tissue. Fresh tissue should be taken for electron microscopy.

TUMORS

Postmortem Examination of Brain with Tumor

When examining the CNS in cases with tumors, at the postmortem, the presence of midline shift, softening, necrosis and herniations, as a consequence of intracranial space occupying lesions should be noted. If the tumor caused epilepsy, the brain may show pathological changes associated with this condition, it is very crucial to examine the intracranial viscera very carefully, searching particularly for sources of metastatic deposits. There may also, rarely, be evidence of extracranial spread of primary CNS tumor to other sites.

General Guidelines

- Fresh tissue is snap frozen for rapid intraoperative diagnosis.
- Crush smears may also be prepared from fresh tissue for rapid diagnosis.
- Sampling of adjacent brain is essential to assess the margins and pattern of infiltration.
- Grading as proposed by WHO classification is followed which grades the tumor according to their malignant potential on a scale ranging from I for benign to IV for malignant tumors.
- *Common immunohistochemical stains*:
  - GFAP: Glial fibrillary acidic protein-astrocytic differentiation.
  - Synaptophysin, Neu N for neuronal differentiation.
  - NFP: Neurofilament protein-neuronal differentiation.
  - EMA (epithelial membrane antigen), cytokeratin.
  - Vimentin-mesenchymal marker
  - S-100: positive in choroid plexus tumors
  - CD20, CD3, CD45, CD68, MUM1, bcl2, bcl6-Lymphoid neoplasms
  - MAP-2 (microtubule associated protein)-Neuronal differentiation
  - CD 99: Peripheral PNET/Ewing's sarcoma
  - INI-1, Brg-1: Atypical teratoid rhabdoid tumors (AT/RT)
  - Ki-67: Marker of proliferative index
  - Markers for molecular subtyping/prognostication
  - IDH1 R132H, ATRX, p53: Primary glioblastoma versus secondary glioblastomas
  - H3K27 me3: Midline gliomas enriched for H3K27 trimethylation
  - BRAF V600E: Tumors enriched for *BRAF V600E* mutation
  - LIN 28: Positive in subset of central PNETs
  - YAP1, GAB1, beta-catenin: Molecular subgrouping of medulloblastoma
  - p53—to identify medulloblastoma enriched for *TP53* mutations

WHO Classification of CNS Tumors 2016 Update

For decades, the classification of brain tumors was based on the concept of histogenesis, i.e. the tumors could be classified according to their morphological similarities to the cell of origin. Large scale genomic and transcriptomic studies have significantly improved our understanding of biology and oncogenesis of brain tumors. The 2016 update breaks the century-old tradition of a histological classification and incorporates well-established molecular parameters into the classification of brain tumors. The classification proposes generation of 'integrated' diagnoses which incorporates phenotypic and genotypic classification **(Appendix J)**.

SUGGESTED READING

1. Banerjee AK. Postmortem Examination of the nervous system. Neurol India. 1997;45:120-5.
2. Chhang WH, Kak VK, Khosla VK, et al. Metastatic intracranial tumours : experience and review of literature. Neurol India. 1993;41(2):73-81.
3. Dastur DK, Lalitha VS, Udani PM, et al. The brain and meninges in tuberculous meningitis—gross pathology in 100 cases and pathogenesis. Neurol India. 1970;18(2):86-100.
4. Drlicek M, Bodenteich A, Urbanits S, et al. Immunohistochemical panel of antibodies in the diagnosis of brain metastases of the unknown primary. Pathol Res Pract. 2004; 200:727-34.
5. Gupta K, Salunke P. Molecular markers of glioma: an update on recent progress and perspectives. J Cancer Res Clin Oncol. 2012;138(12):1971-81.
6. Kleinschmidt-DeMasters BK. Central nervous system aspergillosis: a 20-year retrospective series. Hum Pathol. 2002;33(1):116-24.
7. Louis DN, Perry A, Reifenberger G, et al. The 2016 World Health Organization Classification of Tumors of the Central Nervous System: a summary. Acta Neuropathol. 2016; 131(6):803-20.
8. Murthy JM, Sundaram C, Prasad VS, et al. Aspergillosis of central nervous system: a study of 21 patients seen in a university hospital in south India. J Assoc Physicians India. 2000;48:677-81.
9. Salunke P, Aggarwal A, Gupta K, et al. Large demyelinating lesions: A neurosurgical perspective. Br J Neurosurg. 2012;26(4):490-8
10. Volpe JJ. Brain injury in the premature infant: Overview of clinical aspects, neuropathology, and pathogenesis. Semin Pediatr Neurol. 1998;5:135-51.

Appendices

APPENDIX A: HUNT-HESS GRADING OF SAH

Grade	*Description*
1	Asymptomatic, or mild headache and slight nuchal rigidity
2	Moderate-to-severe headache, nuchal rigidity, no neurological deficit
3	Drowsy, confused or mild focal deficit
4	Stupor, moderate-to-severe hemiparesis, early decerebrate rigidity or vegetative disturbances
5	Deep coma, decerebrate rigidity

Add one grade for serious systemic disease (e.g. HTN, DM, severe atherosclerosis, COPD) or severe vasospasm on arteriography.
Abbreviation: SAH: Subarachnoid hemorrhage.

APPENDIX B: GLASGOW COMA SCALE

Point	*Best eye*	*Best verbal*	*Best motor*
6	-	-	Obeys
5	-	Oriented	Localizes pain
4	Spontaneous	Confused	Withdraw to pain
3	To speech	Inappropriate	Flexor (decorticate)
2	To pain	Incomprehensible	Extensor (decerebrate)
1	None	None	None

APPENDIX C: WFNS SCALE

Grade	*GCS*	*Motor deficit*
I	15	Absent
II	14–13	Absent
III	14–13	Present
IV	12–7	Present/Absent
V	3–6	Present/Absent

Abbreviations: WFNS: World Federation of Neurological Surgeons; GCS: Glasgow Coma Scale.

APPENDIX D: COOPERATIVE ANEURYSM STUDY NEUROLOGICAL STATUS SCALES

Status	*Signs and symptoms*
Status 1	Symptom-free
Status 2	Minor symptoms
Status 3	Major neurologic deficit, but fully responsive
Status 4	Impaired state of alertness, but capable of protective or adaptive responses to noxious stimuli
Status 5	Poorly responsive, but with vital signs
Status 6	No response to shaking, nonadaptive response to stimuli, and progressive instability of vital signs

■ APPENDIX E: COGNARD CLASSIFICATION OF DURAL ARTERIOVENOUS SHUNTS

I	Venous drainage into dural venous sinus with antegrade flow
IIa	Venous drainage into dural venous sinus with retrograde flow
IIb	Venous drainage into dural venous sinus with antegrade flow and CVR
IIa and b	Venous drainage into dural venous sinus with retrograde flow and CVR
III	Venous drainage directly into subarachnoid veins (CVR only)
IV	Type III with venous ectasias of the draining subarachnoid veins

Abbreviation: CVR: Cortical venous reflux.

■ APPENDIX F: BORDEN CLASSIFICATION OF CRANIAL DURAL AVF

Type I	DAVFs drain into dural venous sinuses without pial reflux
Type II	DAVFs drain into venous sinuses, but show retrograde flow into a pial vein
Type III	DAVFs drain directly into a pial vein (or an isolated dural sinus segment) and are associated with significant venous hypertension

Each type is further characterized by the complexity of the architecture of the arteriovenous shunt into **Subtype A**, a simple fistula with a direct, single connection between the feeding artery and the draining vein or sinus, and **Subtype B**, a complex lesion with multiple fistulous connections.
Abbreviation: AVF: Arteriovenous fistula.

■ APPENDIX G: FISHER GRADE OF CEREBRAL VASOSPASM RISK IN SUBARACHNOID HEMORRHAGE

Grade	*Appearance of Blood on Head CT Scan*
1	No blood detected
2	Diffuse deposition or thin layer with all vertical layers (in interhemispheric fissure, insular cistern, ambient cistern) less than 1 mm thick
3	Localized clot and/or vertical layers 1 mm or more in thickness
4	Intracerebral or intraventricular clot with diffuse or no subarachnoid blood

■ APPENDIX H: MODIFIED FISHER CT SAH RATING SCALE

Grade 0	No SAH or IVH
Grade 1	Focal or diffuse, thin SAH, no IVH
Grade 2	Focal or diffuse, thin SAH, with IVH
Grade 3	Focal or diffuse, thick SAH, no IVH
Grade 4	Focal or diffuse, thick SAH, with IVH

Abbreviation: IVH: Intraventricular hemorrhage.

■ APPENDIX I: SPETZLER-MARTIN INTRACRANIAL AVM GRADING SCALE

	Score
Size	
0–3 cm	1
3.1–6.0 cm	2
>6 cm	3
Location	
Noneloquent brain area	0
Eloquent brain area*	1
Deep Venous Drainage	
Absent	0
Present	1

Score = sum of all categories, with lesions graded I to V based upon total sum (e.g. grade I = 1 point).
*Associated with significant neurologic impairment (e.g. language area, motor cortex, others).
From: Spetzler RF, Martin NA, J Neurosurg. 1986;65:476.
Abbreviation: AVM: Arteriovenous malformation.

APPENDIX J: WHO CLASSIFICATION OF TUMORS OF THE CENTRAL NERVOUS SYSTEM

Diffuse Astrocytic and Oligodendroglial Tumors	
Diffuse astrocytoma, IDH-mutant	9400/3
Gemistocytic astrocytoma, IDH-mutant	9411/3
Diffuse astrocytoma, IDH-wildtype	9400/3
Diffuse astrocytoma, NOS	9400/3
Anaplastic astrocytoma, IDH-mutant	9401/3
Anaplastic astrocytoma, IDH-wildtype	9401/3
Anaplastic astrocytoma, NOS	9401/3
Glioblastoma, IDH-wildtype	9440/3
Giant cell glioblastoma	9441/3
Gliosarcoma	9442/3
Epithelioid glioblastoma	9440/3
Glioblastoma, IDH-mutant	9445/3*
Glioblastoma, NOS	9440/3
Diffuse midline glioma, H3 K27M-mutant	9385/3*
Oligodendroglioma, IDH-mutant and 1 p/19q-codeleted	9450/3
Oligodendroglioma, NOS	9450/3
Anaplastic oligodendroglioma, IDH-mutant and 1 p/19q-codeleted	9451/3
Anaplastic oligodendroglioma, NOS	9451/3
Oligoastrocytoma, NOS	9382/3
Anaplastic oligoastrocytoma, NOS	9382/3
Other Astrocytic Tumors	
Pilocytic astrocytoma	9421/1
Pilomyxoid astrocytoma	9425/3
Subependymal giant cell astrocytoma	9384/1
Pleomorphic xanthoastrocytoma	9424/3
Anaplastic pleomorphic xanthoastrocytoma	9424/3
Ependymal Tumors	
Subependymoma	9383/1
Myxopapillary ependymoma	9394/1
Ependymoma	9391/3
Papillary ependymoma	9393/3
Clear cell ependymoma	9391/3
Tanycytic ependymoma	9391/3
Ependymoma, *RELA* fusion- positive	9396/3*
Anaplastic ependymoma	9392/3
Other Gliomas	
Chordoid glioma of the third ventricle	9444/1
Angiocentric glioma	9431/1
Astroblastoma	9430/3

Contd...

Contd...

Choroid Plexus Tumors	
Choroid plexus papilloma	9390/0
Atypical choroid plexus papilloma	9390/1
Choroid plexus carcinoma	9390/3
Neuronal and Mixed Neuronal-glial Tumors	
Dysembryoplastic neuroepithelial tumor	9413/0
Gangliocytoma	9492/0
Ganglioglioma	9505/1
Anaplastic ganglioglioma	9505/3
Dysplastic cerebellar gangliocytoma (Lhermitte-Duclos disease)	9493/0
Desmoplastic infantile astrocytoma and ganglioglioma	9412/1
Papillary glioneuronal tumor	9509/1
Rosette-forming glioneuronal tumor	9509/1
Diffuse leptomeningeal glioneuronal tumor	
Central neurocytoma	9506/1
Extraventricular neurocytoma	9506/1
Cerebellar liponeurocytoma	9506/1
Paraganglioma	8693/1
Tumors of the Pineal Region	
Pineocytoma	9361/1
Pineal parenchymal tumor of intermediate differentiation	9362/3
Pineoblastoma	9362/3
Papillary tumor of the pineal region	9395/3
Embryonal Tumors	
Medulloblastomas, genetically defined	
Medulloblastoma, WNT-activated	9475/3*
Medulloblastoma, SHH-activated and TP53-mutant	9476/3*
Medulloblastoma, SHH-activated and TP53-wildtype	9471/3
Medulloblastoma, non-WNT/non-SHH	9477/3'
Medulloblastoma, group 3	
Medulloblastoma, group 4	
Medulloblastomas, histologically defined	
Medulloblastoma, classic	9470/3
Medulloblastoma, desmoplastic/nodular	9471/3
Medulloblastoma with extensive nodularity	9471/3
Medulloblastoma, large cell/anaplastic	9474/3
Medulloblastoma, NOS	9470/3
Embryonal tumor with multilayered rosettes, CI9MC-altered	9478/3*
Embryonal tumor with multilayered rosettes, NOS	9478/3
Medulloepithelioma	9501/3
CNS neuroblastoma	9500/3
CNS ganglioneuroblastoma	9490/3

Contd...

Contd...

CNS embryonal tumor, NOS	9473/3
Atypical teratoid/rhabdoid tumor	9508/3
CNS embryonal tumor with rhabdoid features	9508/3
Tumors of the Cranial and Paraspinal Nerves	
Schwannoma	9560/0
Cellular schwannoma	9560/0
Plexiform schwannoma	9560/0
Melanotic schwannoma	9560/1
Neurofibroma	9540/0
Atypical neurofibroma	9540/0
Plexiform neurofibroma	9550/0
Perineuroma	9571/0
Hybrid nerve sheath tumors	
Malignant peripheral nerve sheath tumor	9540/3
Epithelioid MPNST	9540/3
MPNST with perineural differentiation	9540/3
Meningiomas	
Meningiomas	9530/3
Meningothelial meningioma	9531/3
Fibrous meningioma	9532/0
Transitional meningioma	9537/0
Psammomatous meningioma	9533/0
Angiomatous meningioma	9534/0
Microcystic meningioma	9530/0
Secretory meningioma	9530/0
Lymphoplasmacyte-rich meningioma	9530/0
Metaplastic meningioma	9530/0
Chordoid meningioma	9538/1
Clear cell meningioma	9538/1
Atypical meningioma	9539/1
Papillary meningioma	9538/3
Rhabdoid meningioma	9538/3
Anaplastic (malignant) meningioma	9530/3
Mesenchymal, Non-meningothelial Tumors	
Solitary fibrous tumor/hemangiopericytoma**	
Grade 1	8815/0
Grade 2	8815/1
Grade 3	8815/3
Hemangioblastoma	9161/1
Hemangioma	9120/0
Epithelioid hemangioendothelioma	9133/3
Angiosarcoma	9120/3
Kaposi sarcoma	9140/3

Contd...

Contd...

Ewing sarcoma/PNET	9364/3
Lipoma	8850/0
Angiolipoma	8861/0
Hibernoma	8880/0
Liposarcoma	8850/3
Desmoid-type fibromatosis	8821/1
Myofibroblastoma	8825/0
Inflammatory myofibroblastic tumor	8825/1
Benign fibrous histiocytoma	8830/0
Fibrosarcoma	8810/3
Undifferentiated pleomorphic sarcoma/malignant fibrous histiocytoma	8802/3
Leiomyoma	8890/0
Leiomyosarcoma	8890/3
Rhabdomyoma	8900/0
Rhabdomyosarcoma	8900/3
Chondroma	9220/0
Chondrosarcoma	9220/3
Osteoma	9180/0
Osteochondroma	9210/0
Osteosarcoma	9180/3
Melanocytic Tumors	
Meningeal melanocytosis	8728/0
Meningeal melanocytoma	8728/1
Meningeal melanoma	8720/3
Meningeal melanomatosis	8728/3
Lymphomas	
Diffuse large B-cell lymphoma of the CNS	9680/3
Immunodeficiency-associated CNS lymphomas AIDS-related diffuse large B-cell lymphoma EBV-positive diffuse large B-cell lymphoma, NOS Lymphomatoid granulomatosis	9766/1
Intravascular large B-cell lymphoma	9712/3
Low-grade B-cell lymphomas of the CNS	
T-cell and NK/T-cell lymphomas of the CNS	
Anaplastic large cell lymphoma, ALK-positive	9714/3
Anaplastic large cell lymphoma, ALK-negative	9702/3
MALT lymphoma of the dura	9699/3
Histiocytic Tumors	
Langerhans cell histiocytosis	9751/3
Erdheim-Chester disease	9750/1
Rosai-Dorfman disease	
Juvenile xanthogranuloma	
Histiocytic sarcoma	9755/3

Contd...

Contd...

Germ Cell Tumors	
Germinoma	9064/3
Embryonal carcinoma	9070/3
Yolk sac tumor	9071/3
Choriocarcinoma	9100/3
Teratoma	9080/1
Mature teratoma	9080/0
Immature teratoma	9080/3
Teratoma with malignant transformation	9084/3
Mixed germ cell tumor	9085/3
Tumors of the Sellar Region	
Craniopharyngioma	9350/1
Adamantinomatous craniopharyngioma	9351/1
Papillary craniopharyngioma	9352/1
Granular cell tumor of the sellar region	9582/0
Pituicytoma	9432/1
Spindle cell oncocytoma	8290/0
Metastatic Tumors	

The morphology codes are from the International Classification of Diseases for Oncology (ICD-O) [742A]. Behavior is coded/O for benign tumors; /1 for unspecified borderline, or uncertain behavior; /2 for carcinoma *in situ* and grade III intraepithelial neoplasia; and /3 for malignant tumors. The classification is modified from the previous WHO classification, taking into account changes in our understanding of these lesions.
*These new codes were approved by the IARC/WHO Committee for ICD-O.
Italics: Provisional tumor entities.
**Grading according to the 2013 WHO Classification of Tumors of Soft Tissue and Bone.

Abbreviations: NOS: Not-otherwise specified; MPNST: Malignant peripheral nerve sheath tumor; MALT: Mucosa-associated lymphoid tissue; CNS: Central nervous system; EBV: Epstein–Barr virus.

APPENDIX K: WHO GRADES OF SELECT CNS TUMORS

Diffuse Astrocytic and Oligodendroglial Tumors	
Diffuse astrocytoma, IOH-mutant	II
Anaplastic astrocyloma, IOH-mutant	III
Glioblastoma, IDH-wild type	IV
Glioblastoma, IDH-mutant	IV
Diffuse midline glioma, H3K27M-mutant	IV
Oligodendroglioma, IDH-mutant and 1p/19Q-codeleted	II
Anaplastic oligodendroglioma. IDH-mutant and 1p/19q-codeleted	III
Other Astrocytic Tumors	
Pilocytic astrocytoma	I
Subependymal giant cell astrocytoma	I
Pleomorphic xanthoastrocytoma	II
Anaplastic pleomorphic xanthoastrocytoma	III
Ependymal Tumors	
Subependymoma	I
Myxopapillary ependymoma	I
Ependymoma	II
Ependymoma, *RELA* fusion-positive	II or III
Anaplastic ependymoma	III
Other Gliomas	
Angiocentric glioma	I
Chordoid glioma of third ventricle	II

Contd...

Contd...

Choroid Plexus Tumors	
Choroid plexus papilloma	I
Atypical choroid plexus papilloma	II
Choroid plexus carcinoma	III
Neuronal and Mixed Neuronal-glial Tumors	
Dysembryoplastic neuroepithelial tumor	I
Gangliocytoma	I
Ganglioglioma	I
Anaplastic ganglioglioma	III
Dysplastic gangliocytoma of cerebellum (Lhermitte-Duclos)	I
Desmoplastic infantile astrocytoma and ganglioma	I
Papillary glioneuronal tumor	I
Rosette-forming glioneuronal tumor	I
Central neurocytoma	II
Extraventricular neurocytoma	II
Cerebellar liponeurocytoma	II
Tumors of the Pineal Region	
Pineocytoma	I
Pineal parenchymal tumor of intermediate differentiation	II or III
Pineoblastoma	IV
Papillary tumor of the pineal region	II or III
Embryonal Tumors	
Medulloblastoma (all subtypes)	IV
Embryonal tumor with multilayered rosettes, C 19MC-altered	IV
Medulloepithelioma	IV
CNS embryonal tumor, NOS	IV
Atypical teratoid/rhabdoid tumor	IV
CNS embryonal tumor with rhabdoid features	IV
Tumors of the Cranial and Paraspinal Nerves	
Schwannoma	I
Neurofibroma	I
Perineunrioma	I
Malignant peripheral nerve sheath tumor (MPNST)	II, III or IV
Meningiomas	
Meningioma	I
Atypical meningioma	II
Anaplastic (malignant) meningioma	III
Mesenchymal, Non-meningothelial Tumors	
Solitary fibrous tumor/hemangiopericytoma	I, II or III
Hemangioblastoma	I
Tumors of the Seller Region	
Craniopharyngioma	I
Granular cell tumor	I
Pituicytoma	I
Spindle cell oncocytoma	I

Source: Louis DN, Ohgaki H, Wiestler OD, Cavenee WK (2016) World Health Organization Histological Classification of Tumors of the Central Nervous System. International Agency for Research on Cancer, France.

APPENDIX L

National multiple Sclerosia society

2017 McDonald Criteria for the Diagnosis of Multiple Sclerosis

ECTRIMS EUROPEAN COMMITTEE FOR TREATMENT AND RESEARCH IN MULTIPLE SCLEROSIS

Diagnosis of MS requires elimination of more likely diagnoses and demonstration of dissemination of lesions in the CNS in space and time. See Lancet Neurology paper* for details.

CLINICAL PRESENTATION	ADDITIONAL DATA NEEDED TO MAKE MS DIAGNOSIS
...in a person with a typical attack/CIS at on onset	(see KEY below for definitions)
• ≥ 2 attacks and objective clinical evidence of ≥ 2 lesions • ≥ 2 attacks and objective clinical evidence of 1 lesion with historical evidence of prior attack involving lesion in different location	None. Dissemination in space (DIS) and dissemination in time (**DIT**) have been met.
• ≥ 2 attacks and objective clinical evidence of 1 lesions	**One** of these criteria: – **DIS:** additional clinical attack implication different CNS site – **DIS:** ≥1 symptomatic or asymptomatic MS-typical T2 lesions in ≥2 areas of CNS: periventricular, juxtacortical/cortical, intratentorial or spinal cord
• 1 attacks and objective clinical evidence of ≥2 lesions	**One** of these criteria: – **DIS:** additional clinical attack – **DIS:** simultaneous presence of both enhancing and non-enhancing symptomatic or asymptomatic MS-typical MRI lesions – **DIS:** new T2 or enhancing MRI lesion compared to baseline scan (without regard to limiting of baseline scan)

Colored text = revisions compared to previous McDonald criteria

KEV: **CIS:** clinically isolated syndrome **CNS:** central nervous system **CSF:** cerebrospinal fluid **DIS:** dissemination in space DIT: dissemination in time T2 lesion: hyperintense lesioin on T2-weighted MRI

*Thompson AJ, et al. Lancet Neurol 2017; online Dec 21,http://dx.doi.org/10.1016/S1474-4422(17)30470-2.

2017 McDonald Criteria for the Diagnosis of Multiple Sclerosis (continued)

CLINICAL PRESENTATION	ADDITIONAL DATA NEEDED TO MAKE MS DIAGNOSIS
...in a person with a typical attack/CIS at on onset	(see KEY below for definitions)
• 1 attacks and objective clinical evidence of 1 lesion	**One** of these criteria: – **DIS:** additional attack implicating different CNS site – **DIS:** ≥1 MS-typical symptomatic or asymptomatic MS-typical T2 lesions in ≥2 areas of CNS: periventricular, juxtacortical/cortical, intratentorial or spinal cord **AND** **One** of these criteria: – **DIS:** additional clinical attack – **DIS:** simultaneous presence of both enhancing and non-enhancing symptomatic or asymptomatic MS-typical MRI lesions – **DIT:** by new T2 or enhancing MRI lesion compared to baseline scan (without regard to limiting of baseline scan) – CSF-spcific (i.e. not in serum) oligoclonal bands
...in a person with a typical attack/CIS at on onset	
• 1 progression from onest	–**1** year of disability progression (retrospective or prospective) **AND** **Two** of these criteria: – ≥1 symptomatic or asymptomatic MS-typical T2 lesions (periventricular, juxtacortical/cortical or infratentorial) – ≥ 2 T2 spinal cord lesions – CSF-specific (i.e. not in serum) oligoclonal bands

The international panel on diagnosis of multiple sclerosis was convened under the auspices of the international advisory committee on clinical trials in MS, sponsored by the National MS society and the european committee for treatment and research in multiple sclerosis.

APPENDIX M: INTERNATIONAL LEAGUE AGAINST EPILEPSY (ILAE) CLASSIFICATION OF EPILEPSY

ILAE 2017 classification of seizure types expanded version[1]

Focal onset	Generalized onset	Unknown onset
Aware / Impaired awareness **Motor onset** • Automatisms • Atonic[2] • Clonic • Epileptic spasms[2] • Hyperkinetic • Myoclonic • Tonic **Non-motor onset** • Autonomic • Behavior arrest • Cognitive • Emotional • Sensory	**Motor** • Tonic-clonic • Clonic • Tonic • Myoclonic • Myoclonic-tonic-clonic • Myoclonic-atonic • Atonic • Epileptic spasms[2] **Non-motor (absence)** • Typical • Atypical • Myoclonic • Eyelid myoclonia	**Motor** • Tonic-clonic • Epileptic spasms **Non-motor** • Behavior arrest Unclassified[3]
Focal to bilateral tonic-clonic		

1 Definitions, other seizure types and descriptors are listed in the accompanying paper and glossary of terms.
2 These could be focal or generalized, with or without alteration of awareness
3 Due to inadequate information or inability to place in other categories

Source: Fisher et al. Instruction manual of the ILAE 2017 operational classification of seizure types. Epilepsia doi: 10.1111/epi.13671.

APPENDIX N: NIH STROKE SCALE

N I H
STROKE
SCALE

Patient Identification. ___ ___-___ ___ ___-___ ___ ___

Pt. Date of Birth ___ ___/___ ___/___ ___

Hospital ________________________(___ ___-___ ___)

Date of Exam ___ ___/___ ___/___ ___

Interval: [ ] Baseline [ ] 2 hours post treatment [ ] 24 hours post onset of symptoms ±20 minutes [ ] 7-10 days
[ ] 3 months [ ] Other ________________________________(___ ___)

Time: ___ ___:___ ___ [ ]am [ ]pm

Person Administering Scale ________________________________

Administer stroke scale items in the order listed. Record performance in each category after each subscale exam. Do not go back and change scores. Follow directions provided for each exam technique. Scores should reflect what the patient does, not what the clinician thinks the patient can do. The clinician should record answers while administering the exam and work quickly. Except where indicated, the patient should not be coached (i.e., repeated requests to patient to make a special effort).

Instructions	Scale Definition	Score
1a. Level of Consciousness: The investigator must choose a response if a full evaluation is prevented by such obstacles as an endotracheal tube, language barrier, orotracheal trauma/bandages. A 3 is scored only if the patient makes no movement (other than reflexive posturing) in response to noxious stimulation.	0 = **Alert**; keenly responsive. 1 = **Not alert**; but arousable by minor stimulation to obey, answer, or respond. 2 = **Not alert**; requires repeated stimulation to attend, or is obtunded and requires strong or painful stimulation to make movements (not stereotyped). 3 = Responds only with reflex motor or autonomic effects or totally unresponsive, flaccid, and areflexic.	______
1b. LOC Questions: The patient is asked the month and his/her age. The answer must be correct - there is no partial credit for being close. Aphasic and stuporous patients who do not comprehend the questions will score 2. Patients unable to speak because of endotracheal intubation, orotracheal trauma, severe dysarthria from any cause, language barrier, or any other problem not secondary to aphasia are given a 1. It is important that only the initial answer be graded and that the examiner not "help" the patient with verbal or non-verbal cues.	0 = **Answers** both questions correctly. 1 = **Answers** one question correctly. 2 = **Answers** neither question correctly.	______
1c. LOC Commands: The patient is asked to open and close the eyes and then to grip and release the non-paretic hand. Substitute another one step command if the hands cannot be used. Credit is given if an unequivocal attempt is made but not completed due to weakness. If the patient does not respond to command, the task should be demonstrated to him or her (pantomime), and the result scored (i.e., follows none, one or two commands). Patients with trauma, amputation, or other physical impediments should be given suitable one-step commands. Only the first attempt is scored.	0 = **Performs** both tasks correctly. 1 = **Performs** one task correctly. 2 = **Performs** neither task correctly.	______
2. Best Gaze: Only horizontal eye movements will be tested. Voluntary or reflexive (oculocephalic) eye movements will be scored, but caloric testing is not done. If the patient has a conjugate deviation of the eyes that can be overcome by voluntary or reflexive activity, the score will be 1. If a patient has an isolated peripheral nerve paresis (CN III, IV or VI), score a 1. Gaze is testable in all aphasic patients. Patients with ocular trauma, bandages, pre-existing blindness, or other disorder of visual acuity or fields should be tested with reflexive movements, and a choice made by the investigator. Establishing eye contact and then moving about the patient from side to side will occasionally clarify the presence of a partial gaze palsy.	0 = **Normal.** 1 = **Partial gaze palsy;** gaze is abnormal in one or both eyes, but forced deviation or total gaze paresis is not present. 2 = **Forced deviation,** or total gaze paresis not overcome by the oculocephalic maneuver.	______

Rev 10/1/2003

Contd...

NIH STROKE SCALE

Patient Identification. ___ ___-___ ___ ___-___ ___ ___

Pt. Date of Birth ___ ___/___ ___/___ ___

Hospital ______________________(___ ___-___ ___)

Date of Exam ___ ___/___ ___/___ ___

Interval: [ ] Baseline [ ] 2 hours post treatment [ ] 24 hours post onset of symptoms ±20 minutes [ ] 7-10 days
[ ] 3 months [ ] Other ______________________(___ ___)

Contd...

3. Visual: Visual fields (upper and lower quadrants) are tested by confrontation, using finger counting or visual threat, as appropriate. Patients may be encouraged, but if they look at the side of the moving fingers appropriately, this can be scored as normal. If there is unilateral blindness or enucleation, visual fields in the remaining eye are scored. Score 1 only if a clear-cut asymmetry, including quadrantanopia, is found. If patient is blind from any cause, score 3. Double simultaneous stimulation is performed at this point. If there is extinction, patient receives a 1, and the results are used to respond to item 11.	0 = **No visual loss.** 1 = **Partial hemianopia.** 2 = **Complete hemianopia.** 3 = **Bilateral hemianopia** (blind including cortical blindness).	____
4. Facial Palsy: Ask – or use pantomime to encourage – the patient to show teeth or raise eyebrows and close eyes. Score symmetry of grimace in response to noxious stimuli in the poorly responsive or non-comprehending patient. If facial trauma/bandages, orotracheal tube, tape or other physical barriers obscure the face, these should be removed to the extent possible.	0 = **Normal** symmetrical movements. 1 = **Minor paralysis** (flattened nasolabial fold, asymmetry on smiling). 2 = **Partial paralysis** (total or near-total paralysis of lower face). 3 = **Complete paralysis** of one or both sides (absence of facial movement in the upper and lower face).	____
5. Motor Arm: The limb is placed in the appropriate position: extend the arms (palms down) 90 degrees (if sitting) or 45 degrees (if supine). Drift is scored if the arm falls before 10 seconds. The aphasic patient is encouraged using urgency in the voice and pantomime, but not noxious stimulation. Each limb is tested in turn, beginning with the non-paretic arm. Only in the case of amputation or joint fusion at the shoulder, the examiner should record the score as untestable (UN), and clearly write the explanation for this choice.	0 = **No drift;** limb holds 90 (or 45) degrees for full 10 seconds. 1 = **Drift;** limb holds 90 (or 45) degrees, but drifts down before full 10 seconds; does not hit bed or other support. 2 = **Some effort against gravity;** limb cannot get to or maintain (if cued) 90 (or 45) degrees, drifts down to bed, but has some effort against gravity. 3 = **No effort against gravity;** limb falls. 4 = **No movement.** UN = **Amputation** or joint fusion, explain: ____________ **5a. Left Arm** **5b. Right Arm**	____ ____
6. Motor Leg: The limb is placed in the appropriate position: hold the leg at 30 degrees (always tested supine). Drift is scored if the leg falls before 5 seconds. The aphasic patient is encouraged using urgency in the voice and pantomime, but not noxious stimulation. Each limb is tested in turn, beginning with the non-paretic leg. Only in the case of amputation or joint fusion at the hip, the examiner should record the score as untestable (UN), and clearly write the explanation for this choice.	0 = **No drift;** leg holds 30-degree position for full 5 seconds. 1 = **Drift;** leg falls by the end of the 5-second period but does not hit bed. 2 = **Some effort against gravity;** leg falls to bed by 5 seconds, but has some effort against gravity. 3 = **No effort against gravity;** leg falls to bed immediately. 4 = **No movement.** UN = **Amputation** or joint fusion, explain: ____________ **6a. Left Leg** **6b. Right Leg**	____

Rev 10/1/2003

Contd...

NIH STROKE SCALE

Patient Identification. ___ ___-___ ___ ___-___ ___ ___

Pt. Date of Birth ___ ___/___ ___/___ ___

Hospital ____________________(___ ___-___ ___)

Date of Exam ___ ___/___ ___/___ ___

Interval: [ ] Baseline [ ] 2 hours post treatment [ ] 24 hours post onset of symptoms ±20 minutes [ ] 7-10 days [ ] 3 months [ ] Other ________________________(___ ___)

Contd...

7. Limb Ataxia: This item is aimed at finding evidence of a unilateral cerebellar lesion. Test with eyes open. In case of visual defect, ensure testing is done in intact visual field. The finger-nose-finger and heel-shin tests are performed on both sides, and ataxia is scored only if present out of proportion to weakness. Ataxia is absent in the patient who cannot understand or is paralyzed. Only in the case of amputation or joint fusion, the examiner should record the score as untestable (UN), and clearly write the explanation for this choice. In case of blindness, test by having the patient touch nose from extended arm position.	0 = **Absent.** 1 = **Present in one limb.** 2 = **Present in two limbs.** UN = **Amputation** or joint fusion, explain: __________	____
8. Sensory: Sensation or grimace to pinprick when tested, or withdrawal from noxious stimulus in the obtunded or aphasic patient. Only sensory loss attributed to stroke is scored as abnormal and the examiner should test as many body areas (arms [not hands], legs, trunk, face) as needed to accurately check for hemisensory loss. A score of 2, "severe or total sensory loss," should only be given when a severe or total loss of sensation can be clearly demonstrated. Stuporous and aphasic patients will, therefore, probably score 1 or 0. The patient with brainstem stroke who has bilateral loss of sensation is scored 2. If the patient does not respond and is quadriplegic, score 2. Patients in a coma (item 1a=3) are automatically given a 2 on this item.	0 = **Normal;** no sensory loss. 1 = **Mild-to-moderate sensory loss;** patient feels pinprick is less sharp or is dull on the affected side; or there is a loss of superficial pain with pinprick, but patient is aware of being touched. 2 = **Severe to total sensory loss;** patient is not aware of being touched in the face, arm, and leg.	____
9. Best Language: A great deal of information about comprehension will be obtained during the preceding sections of the examination. For this scale item, the patient is asked to describe what is happening in the attached picture, to name the items on the attached naming sheet and to read from the attached list of sentences. Comprehension is judged from responses here, as well as to all of the commands in the preceding general neurological exam. If visual loss interferes with the tests, ask the patient to identify objects placed in the hand, repeat, and produce speech. The intubated patient should be asked to write. The patient in a coma (item 1a=3) will automatically score 3 on this item. The examiner must choose a score for the patient with stupor or limited cooperation, but a score of 3 should be used only if the patient is mute and follows no one-step commands.	0 = **No aphasia;** normal. 1 = **Mild-to-moderate aphasia;** some obvious loss of fluency or facility of comprehension, without significant limitation on ideas expressed or form of expression. Reduction of speech and/or comprehension, however, makes conversation about provided materials difficult or impossible. For example, in conversation about provided materials, examiner can identify picture or naming card content from patient's response. 2 = **Severe aphasia;** all communication is through fragmentary expression; great need for inference, questioning, and guessing by the listener. Range of information that can be exchanged is limited; listener carries burden of communication. Examiner cannot identify materials provided from patient response. 3 = **Mute, global aphasia;** no usable speech or auditory comprehension.	____
10. Dysarthria: If patient is thought to be normal, an adequate sample of speech must be obtained by asking patient to read or repeat words from the attached list. If the patient has severe aphasia, the clarity of articulation of spontaneous speech can be rated. Only if the patient is intubated or has other physical barriers to producing speech, the examiner should record the score as untestable (UN), and clearly write an explanation for this choice. Do not tell the patient why he or she is being tested.	0 = **Normal.** 1 = **Mild-to-moderate dysarthria;** patient slurs at least some words and, at worst, can be understood with some difficulty. 2 = **Severe dysarthria;** patient's speech is so slurred as to be unintelligible in the absence of or out of proportion to any dysphasia, or is mute/anarthric. UN = **Intubated** or other physical barrier, explain:______________	____

Contd...

Rev 10/1/2003

NIH STROKE SCALE

Patient Identification. ___ ___-___ ___ ___-___ ___ ___

Pt. Date of Birth ___ ___/___ ___/___ ___

Hospital ________________________(___ ___-___ ___)

Date of Exam ___ ___/___ ___/___ ___

Interval: [ ] Baseline [ ] 2 hours post treatment [ ] 24 hours post onset of symptoms ±20 minutes [ ] 7-10 days
[ ] 3 months [ ] Other ________________________________(___ ___)

Contd...

11. Extinction and Inattention (formerly Neglect): Sufficient information to identify neglect may be obtained during the prior testing. If the patient has a severe visual loss preventing visual double simultaneous stimulation, and the cutaneous stimuli are normal, the score is normal. If the patient has aphasia but does appear to attend to both sides, the score is normal. The presence of visual spatial neglect or anosagnosia may also be taken as evidence of abnormality. Since the abnormality is scored only if present, the item is never untestable.	0 = **No abnormality.** 1 = **Visual, tactile, auditory, spatial, or personal inattention** or extinction to bilateral simultaneous stimulation in one of the sensory modalities. 2 = **Profound hemi-inattention or extinction to more than one modality;** does not recognize own hand or orients to only one side of space.	____

Rev 10/1/2003

APPENDIX O: MODIFIED RANKIN SCALE (MRS)

MODIFIED RANKIN SCALE (MRS)

Patient Name: ____________________

Rater Name: ____________________

Date: ____________________

Score	Description
0	No symptoms at all
1	No significant disability despite symptoms; able to carry out all usual duties and activities
2	Slight disability; unable to carry out all previous activities, but able to look after own affairs without assistance
3	Moderate disability; requiring some help, but able to walk without assistance
4	Moderately severe disability; unable to walk without assistance and unable to attend to own bodily needs without assistance
5	Severe disability; bedridden, incontinent and requiring constant nursing care and attention
6	Dead

TOTAL (0–6): ______

References

Rankin J. "Cerebral vascular accidents in patients over the age of 60." *Scott Med J* 1957;2:200-15

Bonita R, Beaglehole R. "Modification of Rankin Scale: Recovery of motor function after stroke." ***Stroke* 1988 Dec;19(12):1497-1500**

Van Swieten JC, Koudstaal PJ, Visser MC, Schouten HJ, van Gijn J. "Interobserver agreement for the assessment of handicap in stroke patients." ***Stroke* 1988;19(5):604-7**

Section 2

Recent Advances and Applied Physics in Imaging

CHAPTER 38

Ultrasound Instrumentation: Practical Applications

Kushaljit Singh Sodhi, Akshay Kumar Saxena, Mukesh Kumar Yadav

INTRODUCTION

Ultrasonography (USG) in the last few decades has undergone massive transformation and today occupies a crucial role in practice of most of the domains of medicine. Advances in ultrasound technology include enhanced spatial, vascular and contrast resolution, besides encompassing various therapeutic options. New transducers and emerging imaging paradigms allow real-time acquisition of large field of views and even three-dimensional volumetric data. In sonography, transducer, is the central component, which is responsible for both, generation of ultrasound beam and detection of returning echoes.[1] It is the changes in the generation of echo signals, it's reception, analysis and display that helps differentiate one scanner from another.[1] Its safety, portability, low cost and real-time application makes it one of the most widely used imaging modalities. This section provides a brief overview of practical aspects of ultrasound instrumentation.

MACHINE CONTROLS

In this section we shall briefly talk about some of the functions of the ultrasound machine which are most frequently put to use **(Figs. 1A and B)**. It is of course recommended that all sonologists must learn the various capabilities of their own equipment to optimize the quality of the image as well as the diagnosis.

- *Keyboard*: Various capabilities as provided by manufacturer
- *Transducer select*: To chose one of the many transducer probes attached to the transducer ports on the ultrasound machine

FREQUENCY OF TRANSDUCERS

Transducer frequency can vary from 2.0 MHz to 16.0 MHz and its selection is primarily based upon patient's body habitus and the region to be scanned.[2]

High-frequency Transducer

- Frequency range of 7.0–14.0 MHz
- Linear transducer mostly, sector transducer more suited for children
- Provides increased resolution of images, however, with reduced penetration
- Linear probes best for evaluation of superficial structures like, thyroid, scrotum, etc.

Medium-frequency Transducer

- Frequency range of 3.0–5.0 MHz
- Curvilinear or sector transducers
- Most commonly used probe for adult abdominal imaging.

Low-frequency Transducer

- Frequency of 2.0 MHz
- Transducer is sector type
- Provides increased depth of penetration but also results in loss of resolution

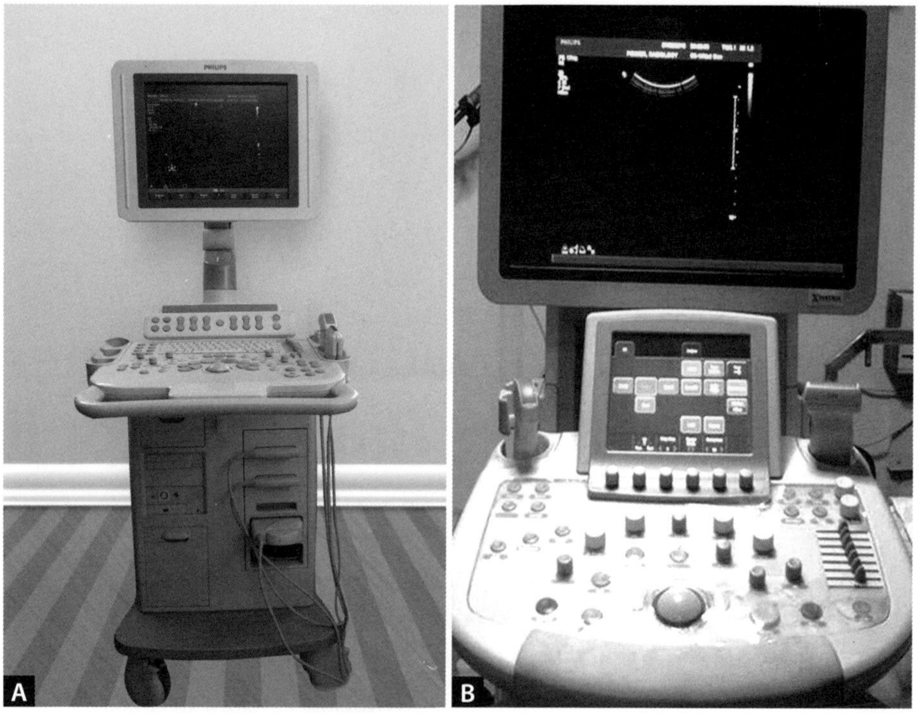

Figs. 1A and B: Modern ultrasound scanning unit with LCD screen.

- More suited for ultrasound studies of obese patients[2]
- *Overall gain control*: This is used for equal amplification of all signals received.
- *Time-gain compensation*: This is used to balance for attenuation of the ultrasound beam in the scanned tissue.[2] With time-gain compensation, a depth-dependent gain is applied to the echoes; with echoes that originate deeper in tissue (which are attenuated to a larger degree) have larger gain factors compared to those echoes which originate close to the transducer.[2,3] The signals from shallow structures are not amplified as much as those from deep structures. This process thus results in producing equally reflective structures to be displayed in B-mode image with the same brightness, regardless of their age. Time-gain compensation is controlled in most machines with a set of 6–10 gain knobs, each of which adjusts the receiver gain at a different depth.
- *Near and far gains*: These controls help in equalizing the differences in echoes received from various depths as they are displayed on the screen. When compensating for sound attenuation, the near to far gain controls (usually slide pods) should gradually be increased.[2,3]
- *Compression*: This is used to vary the amplitude range (dynamic range) of echoes which appear as shades of gray on the image. Most of the ultrasound machines apply logarithmic compression to the echo signals which emerge from the receiver; amount of compression is under the control of the operator.[2]

  Dynamic range is the ratio of the largest to smallest echo signals. It decreases as signals pass through imaging system as rejection and TGC remove many large and small signals.[3]
- *Depth*: This control is useful in adjusting the size of image so that the organs and adjacent structures or regions of interest can be equally clearly visible.
- *Focal point(s)*: This is a control which has one or more toggle buttons. This allows the operator to choose the level at which the ultrasound beam is focussed so as to enhance the resolution at a specific point or points. The placement of this control should be at the most posterior aspect of the organ or structure to be imaged.[2,3]
- *Postprocessing:* This can be used to change the appearance of echo signals, already stored in memory, on the image. Various postprocessing applications are available; each emphasizes different portions of the echo amplitudes stored in the image memory.
- Failure to properly adjust the gain control and/or improper placement of focal point during scanning might result in suboptimal image quality and misdiagnosis.

TYPES OF TRANSDUCERS

Ultrasound scanners automatically scan the ultrasound beam through transducers which consist of an array of many narrow piezoelectric elements.[3] Array may be made up of as many as 128–196 elements.[4]

Ultrasound transducers convert mechanical energy into electrical energy and produce images that can be displayed subsequently in a variety of formats. These can be of following types as shown in **Figures 2A to C**.

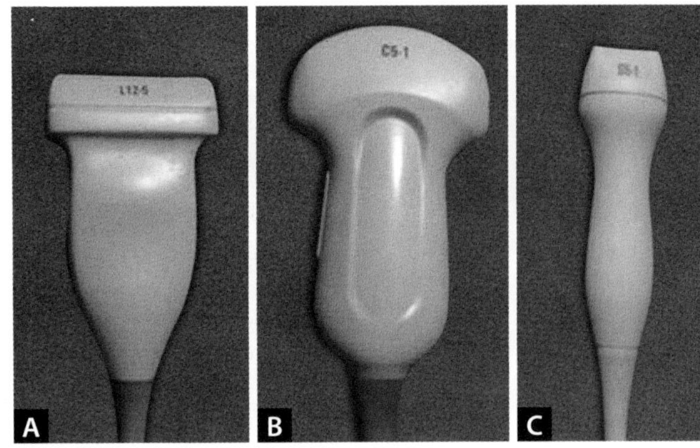

Figs. 2A to C: Photograph showing various types of transducers: Linear (A), curvilinear (B) and sector (C) array transducer.

Linear-array Transducer

Linear-array transducers are optimal for superficially placed structures, such as vessels, neck, testes. In this, final image is displayed as a rectangle. In a linear array, each time only a group of elements work together to transmit or receive.[2,5] The ultrasound beam is perpendicular to the transducer surface, centered over element subset and scans a rectangular area. Size of the field of view is equal in both the far field (area of penetration farthest away from transducer) and near field (area of penetration closest to transducer).[2]

Curvilinear-array Transducer

These are commonly used for routine abdominal and pelvic imaging. In curvilinear-array transducer, array of elements instead of a straight line (linear array) are arranged across a convex arc.[2,5] This fan like arrangement of elements result in a sector shaped imaging field. Compared to linear-array, curved array provides a wider image at large depths (field of view is wide in far field than near field) from a narrow scanning window.

Phased-array Transducer

In contrast to linear- and curved-arrays, all the elements work together in phased-array (all elements are used for each beam line).[5] Phase-array steer the beam by applying different delay on each element and it requires small acoustic window. Its main advantage is in providing a very broad imaged field at larger depths that too with a narrow transducer footprint. It is widely used in cardiac scanning as the transducer fits easily between the ribs (rib gap is a small acoustic window).

Doppler

The Doppler effect was first proposed by Christian Doppler, an Austrian physicist, in 1843.[6] According to this effect, if there is relative motion between an object and an observer (receiver), the frequency of sound wave perceived by the observer (receiver) is different from that emitted/reflected by the object.[5,6]

In diagnostic radiology, Doppler effect is utilized to detect blood flow in peripheral vessels (e.g. lower limb) as well as those supplying different organs (renal artery, portal vein, etc.). The information provided by a Doppler examination includes presence or absence of blood flow, direction of blood flow, type of blood flow (arterial high resistance/venous, presence and quantification of arterial stenosis, etc.[2] The difference in emitted frequency and received frequency is called the Doppler shift and is given by the equation:[6]

$$\Delta v = 2\, vS \cos\theta / V$$

where Δv = frequency change (Doppler shift)
v = frequency of original beam
S = velocity of blood
V = velocity of sound (1540 m/sec)
θ = angle between the direction of blood flow and sound beam

In clinical practice, three different Doppler techniques are utilized. Continuous wave Doppler is used for evaluation of peripheral vessels and the fetal heart. It provides information regarding the blood flow but lacks information regarding the depth from which the Doppler signal is coming from. Pulsed Doppler provides information regarding the presence, direction and depth from which the Doppler signal is coming from. Power Doppler is useful for the evaluation of slow flow.

The basic transducer for continuous wave Doppler contains an oscillator, two piezoelectric crystals and a demodulator **(Fig. 3A)**.[6] One of these crystals acts as the transmitter while the other acts as the receiver. Both of these crystals work continuously. The two crystals are inclined at an angle to each other. The purpose of inclining

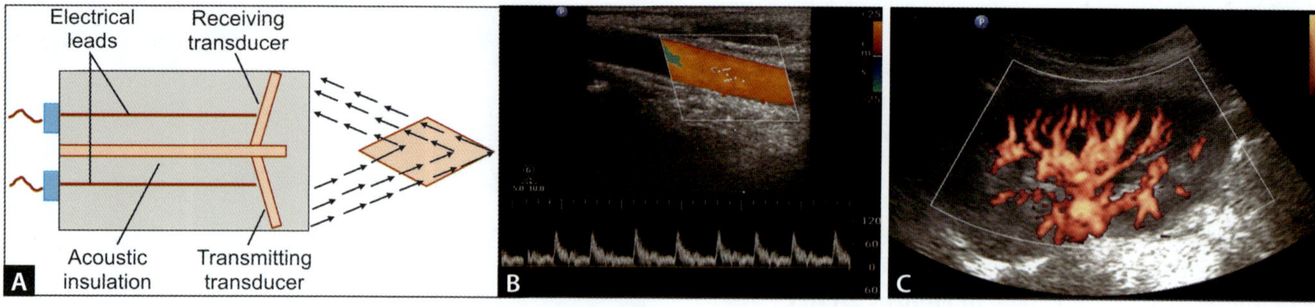

Figs. 3A to C: Components of a typical Doppler ultrasound transducer (A), color Doppler scan of common carotid artery (B) and power Doppler image showing normal Doppler signals in kidney (C).

the crystals is to cause overlap between the beam regions of the transmitter and receiver which in turn increases the sensitivity for detecting the returning signal (beam). The oscillator provides electrical voltage at the resonant frequency of the transducer which is converted into the transmitted ultrasound beam by the transmitter. The beam, after reflection, is received by the receiver piezoelectric crystal. The frequency of received beam is different from the transmitted frequency because of Doppler shift. The received signal is amplified and fed into the demodulator which also receives signal from the oscillator. The comparison of signals from the oscillator and received beam provides Doppler shift signal. The demodulator can also detect whether the received beam has frequency higher or lower than the transmitted frequency which provides information regarding the flow of blood towards or away from the transducer. It is important to note that apart from the moving blood, the moving vessel wall also generates Doppler shift. However, it has low frequency. The machines are equipped with circuits which filter off such low level frequencies and ensure that the signal from moving vessel wall does not hamper the evaluation of blood flow.[7-10]

The problem with continuous wave Doppler is that all the moving objects within the sonographic beam contribute to frequency shift. Thus, the observer cannot ascertain the depth from which the signal originates. This problem can be overcome by the use of pulsed Doppler. In this technique, very short bursts of the sound wave are repetitively emitted by the transducer. However, a new pulse is not emitted till such time the returning signal from the previous pulse is detected by the transducer. The receiver is designed to be turned on for a short period on at a specific moment. The time at which receiver is turned on (or gated on) provides the information regarding the depth at which the signal originated. The duration for which the receiver (or the gate) is turned on determines the axial length of the beam over which the signal is received. A combination of real-time imaging and pulsed Doppler is known as Duplex Doppler.

Although pulsed Doppler and duplex scanners provide information regarding the depth from which Doppler signal originates, it is limited to a very small region of the image. As a result, the sonologist needs to sample large number of areas to evaluate the entire vessel. This limitation is overcome in the color flow Doppler imaging. Recall that in pulsed (and duplex) Doppler, the depth from which Doppler signal is recorded is determined by the time lag (after emission of sound beam) after which the gate is opened to receive the signal.[8,9] Use of multiple gates, which open after different time lags, allows detection of depths of multiple Doppler signals. A modification of this principle is utilized in color flow imaging wherein electronically steered (phased array) transducers are used to detect signals at different depths of a real-time image. Thus, the signal can be detected from the vessels as well as surrounding tissues. The Doppler signal is assigned color proportionate to the strength of the Doppler signal. The superimposition of such colored information on the grayscale image generates the color flow image.

Pulsed Doppler does not provide information regarding the intensity (or power) of the Doppler signal. This information can be obtained in the power Doppler mode which displays the power (or intensity) of the Doppler signal, as it changes with time in every region within the chosen area. Higher intensity Doppler signals are imparted lighter hue of color. However, there is no information available regarding the velocity. The power Doppler has superior flow sensitivity as compared to conventional color Doppler and is used to evaluate the presence and characteristics of the flow in blood vessels that are poorly imaged with conventional color Doppler **(Figs. 3B and C)**.[10,11]

Tissue-harmonic Imaging

Tissue-harmonic imaging (THI) is a grayscale ultrasound mode that provides higher quality images than those of conventional sonography by using information from harmonics (which are generated by nonlinear wave propagation of ultrasound in tissue).[12-15] Harmonics are produced by the vibration of the tissues and are usually integral multiples of the transmitted frequency. In conventional grayscale sonography, the same frequency spectrum that is transmitted into the patient is subsequently received to produce the sonographic image. However, in THI, higher harmonic frequencies (multiples) generated by the propagation of the ultrasound beam through tissues are used in producing the image. Conventionally, only the second harmonic, or twice the fundamental frequency, is used for imaging. Tissue-harmonic imaging holds a great potential for improving the quality of image since it provides improved lateral resolution and signal to noise ratio and reduces the side lobe artifacts..[12,16]

The higher harmonic can also be used but it requires transducers with extremely wide bandwidth.[14] In THI, it is the reduced width of the ultrasound beam that improves lateral resolution (more harmonics are produced at the centre of a pulse than at the periphery). Increased lateral resolution improves the ability to resolve small anatomic structures and detail. Harmonic imaging is chiefly useful in obese patients because it reduces the deleterious effects of body wall. Intensity of harmonic waves generated is dependent upon the nonlinearity coefficient of the tissue insonated. Body tissues with a higher amount of fat have the highest nonlinearity coefficients, which increase the intensity of harmonic waves generated, thus improving the visibility of lesion in obese patients, whose body walls typically contain a high proportion of fat.[12,16,17]

Side lobe artifacts occur when the ultrasound beam hits an interface and is reflected back to the transducer, thus producing artifactual echoes. Reduction in side lobe artifacts improves the signal-to-noise ratio which results in an image which shows tissues as brighter whereas the cavities appear as darker. Harmonics are generated deep in relation to the body wall and because they are produced in tissues, they pass only once through the body wall, resulting in decreased artifacts from the body wall.[18-20]

Although better demonstration of cystic structures by THI has been emphasized, authors have now observed that THI provides additional information in both solid and cystic lesions[12,18] **(Figs. 4 and 5)**. Harmonic imaging increases diagnostic confidence in differentiating cystic from solid hepatic lesions, improves detection of the gallbladder and biliary calculi, improves the pancreatic definition and allows distinction between simple and complex renal cysts.

Another harmonic technique, known as 1.5 harmonic imaging has also been described.[21] This detects and visualizes signals that are a factor of 1.5 times higher than the fundamental center frequency of the transducer and are intermediate between the fundamental and the second harmonic frequency spectrum.[21,22] Obvious advantage is that this frequency range is nearly free of tissue echoes and only contains microbubbles echoes. Hence, it is featured with contrast improvement between tissue and microbubbles of 20dB or more compared to the second harmonic technique.

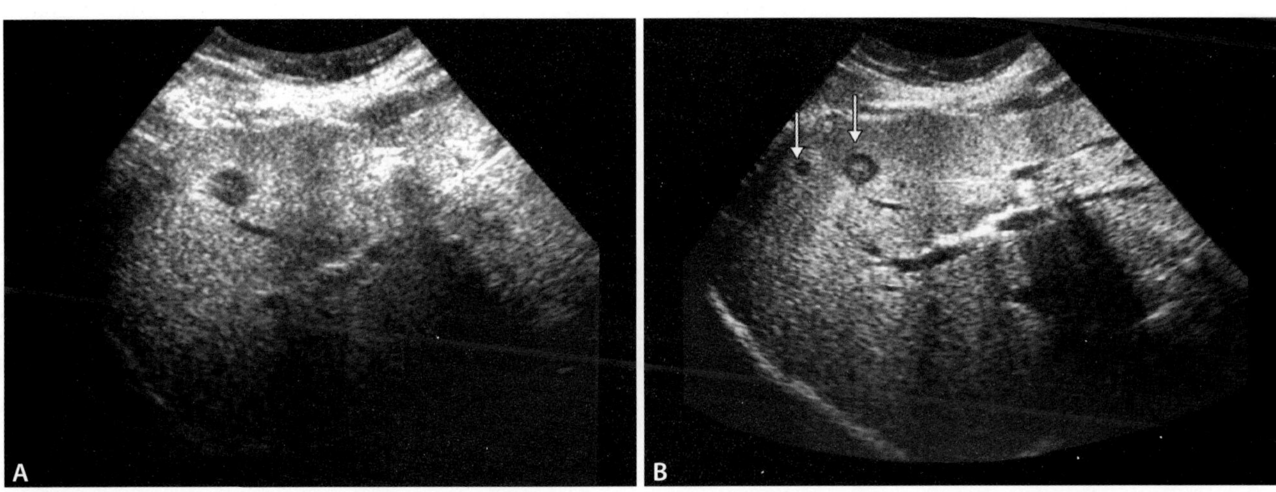

Figs. 4A and B: Comparison of conventional grayscale imaging (A) with THI (B) Tissue-harmonic imaging clearly demonstrates target lesions (indeterminate on conventional) in a metastatic liver disease. Also note that additional lesions are also detected with THI.

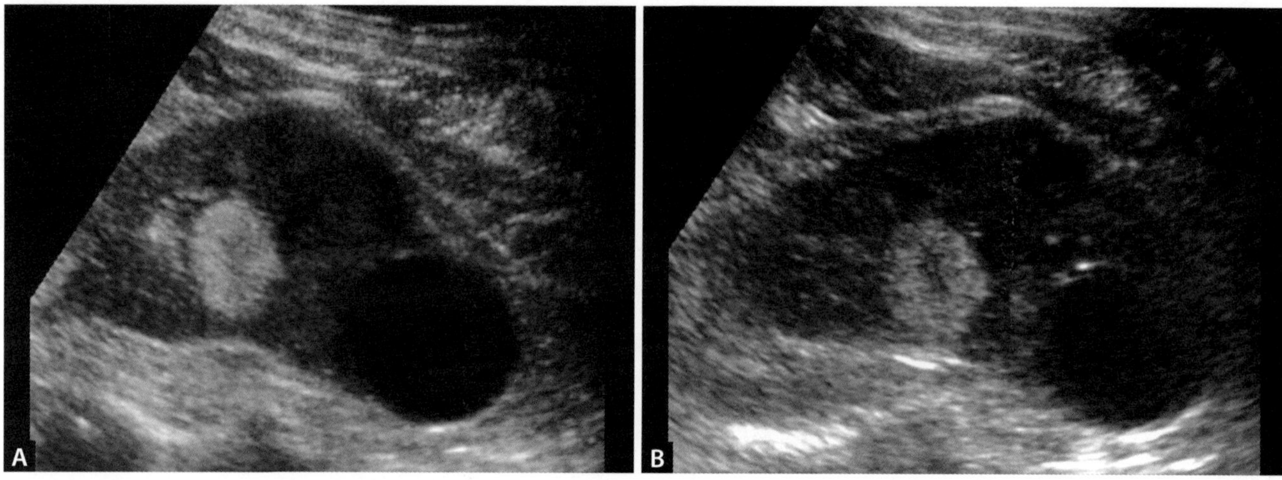

Figs. 5A and B: Tissue-harmonic imaging (A) demonstrates much better delineation of both cystic and solid lesions in this patient of renal angiomyolipomas, when compared to conventional grayscale imaging (B).

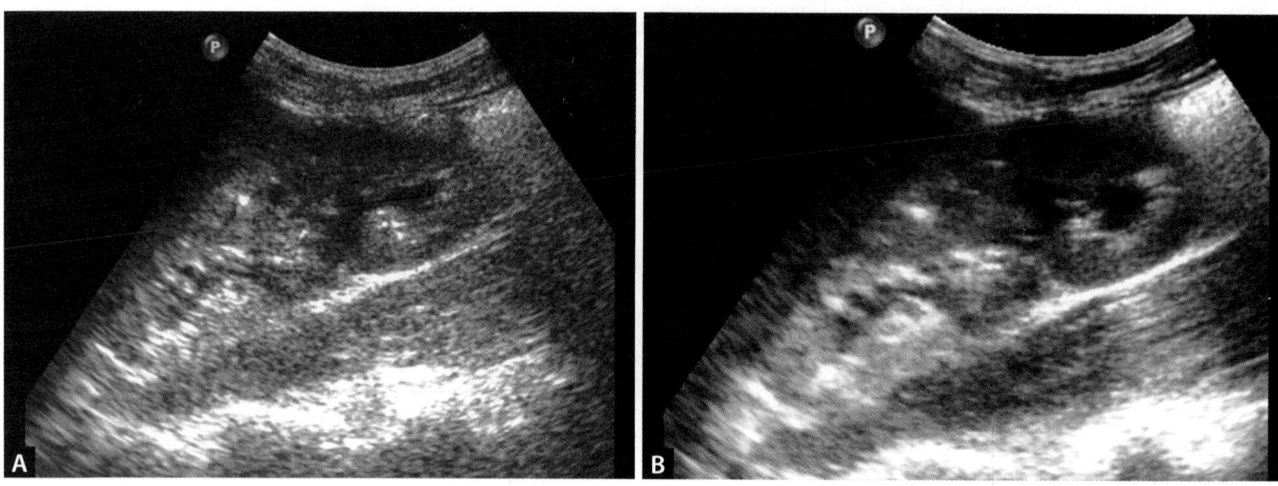

Figs. 6A and B: Spatial-compound imaging in a patient with nephrocalcinosis. Note medullary hyperechogenicity is not well appreciated on conventional grayscale mode (A), but is clearly demonstrated on compound imaging (B).

Spatial-compound Imaging

Spatial-compound imaging is a speckle reducing ultrasound technique, which uses electronic steering of ultrasound beams from a transducer array to obtain overlapping scans of a target object from different angles (same tissue is imaged many times by using parallel beams directed along different directions).[3,23] Resulting echoes from these multiple acquisitions are then averaged to produce a single compound image of improved quality due to reduction in image speckle. When compared to conventional B-mode imaging, in compound imaging, more time is required for acquisition of data (as here multiple ultrasound beams are used to evaluate same tissue) and frame rate is also reduced. Spatial-compound imaging demonstrates reduced level of speckle, noise, refraction, reduced shadowing and enhancement artifacts and improved contrast and margin definition[3,23,24] **(Figs. 6 and 7)**.

Application of spatial-compound imaging has been described in imaging of breast, peripheral vessels and musculoskeletal system. It can also be combined with other ultrasound applications, e.g. harmonic imaging.

EXTENDED FIELD OF VIEW

This technique available in most of the new scanners allows sonologists to visualize large anatomic regions in a single image. It can be performed on superficial structures with a linear array transducer or abdominal structures using a curvilinear probe, although most of its applications are in superficial structures.[3,23] Extended field of view imaging, also called panoramic imaging in some machines allows

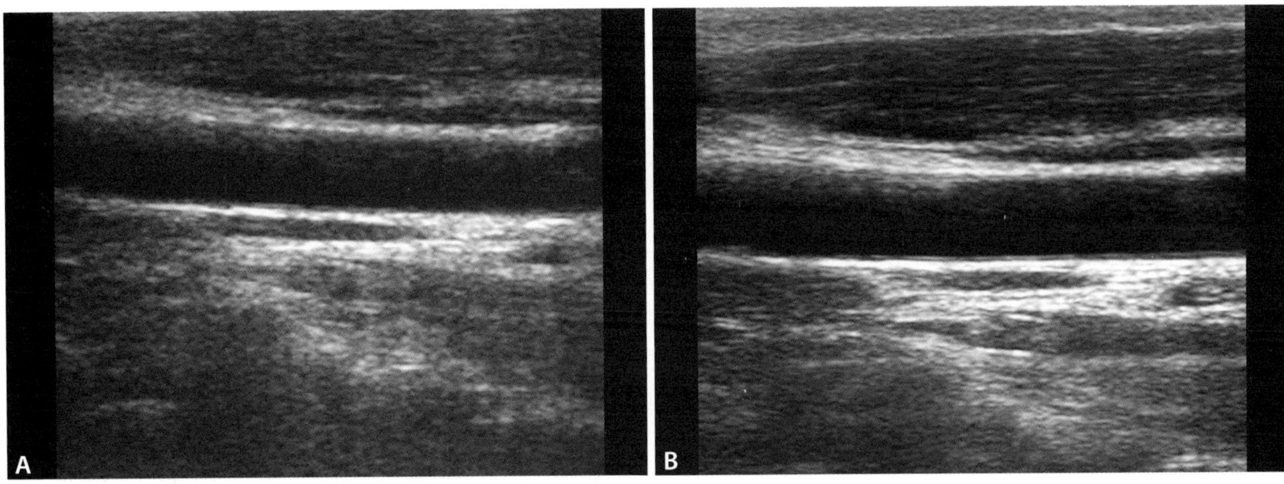

Figs. 7A and B: Spatial-compound imaging in carotid vessels helps clear depiction of intima-media thickness for accurate measurements. (A) refers to conventional grayscale while (B) refers to compound imaging.

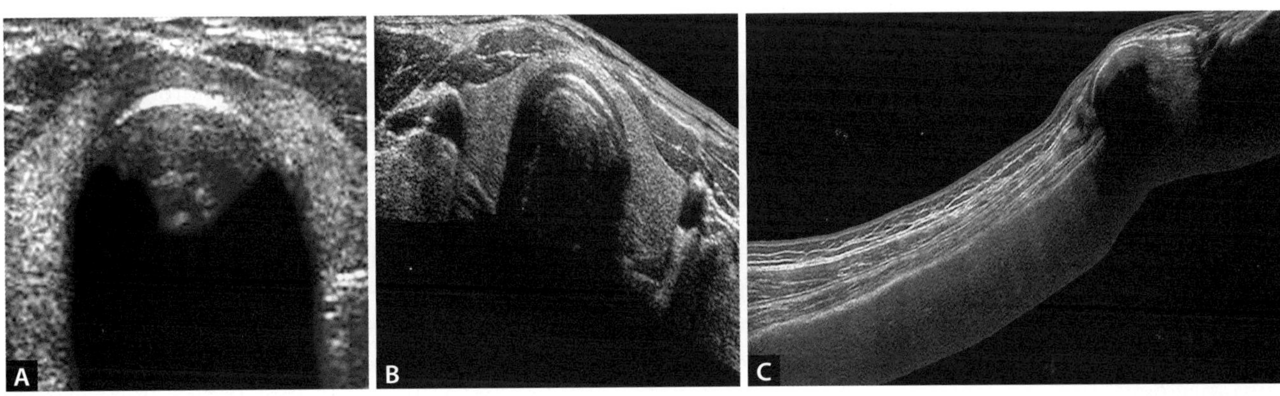

Figs. 8A to C: Extended field of view. Routine grayscale mode (A) is able to demonstrate only limited part of thyroid in a single image, while extended field of view mode (B) clearly demonstrates the composite image showing both lobes of thyroid, isthmus besides cervical vessels in a single image. Extended field of view (C) demonstrates quadriceps tendon, patella and patellar tendon in a single image.

easy measurements of large lesions/structures and exact delineation of anatomical relationships in a single image **(Figs. 8A to C)**. Transducer is initially moved laterally across the anatomic area of interest and multiple images are acquired from many transducer positions.[3] Images are registered with respect to each other. This registered data is subsequently combined to form one complete large field of view image.

Elastography

Imaging of tissue stiffness or elasticity is one of the rapidly evolving ultrasound based application. It is based on the fact that stiffness of tissue tends to alter with disease and can be imaged by measuring the tissue's distortion (strain) under an applied stress (compression from ultrasound transducer).[23] Images produced may be in grayscale, color or both. Although most of its initial application has been carried out in the breast, it is now increasingly being evaluated in diagnosis of complex cysts, liver cirrhosis, characterization of thyroid nodules and metastatic lymph nodes.[25]

3D and 4D Ultrasound

Three-dimensional USG or volume sonography is the imaging technology which involves acquiring a large number of data sets of 2D images from patient. After acquisition, this volumetric data can be qualitatively and quantitatively assessed with the use of many analysis tools, such as surface and volume rendering, multiplanar imaging and volume calculation techniques, etc. Hence similar to other cross-sectional imaging like computer tomography (CT) and magnetic resonance imaging (MRI), the volumetric data of this 3D ultrasound can also be 'postprocessed'. Because of volume imaging it is possible to display information in any orientation and any of the planes. If the 3D ultrasound is acquired and displayed over time, it is termed as 4D ultrasound, live 3D ultrasound or real-time 3D ultrasound.[26]

Currently there are two commonly used techniques to acquire 3D volumetric data—free-hand technique and automated technique. In the free-hand technique the examiner requires to manually move the probe within the region of interest. In the automated technique dedicated 3D probes (also called volume probes) have to be used. In this method, probe is held stationary and on activation the transducer elements within the probes automatically sweep through the 'volume box' which has been selected by the operator. The resultant images are digitally stored and can be 'processed' later in various display modes for analysis.[27]

It is perceived that the potential of 3D and 4D ultrasound has not been fully utilized till now. It is still being used as problem solving tool although it can be incorporated in routine day-to-day practice. There are numerous areas in which the use of 3D and 4D can be very useful **(Figs. 9A and B)**. Few of these are as follows:[26]

Gynecology

- For assessment of congenital anomalies of uterus[28,29]
- For evaluation of endometrial and uterine cavity (can also be done with saline infusion sonohysterography)
- For preprocedure localization of fibroids for planning myomectomy
- For evaluation of possible cornual ectopic pregnancies
- For exact delineation of intrauterine device location and type
- For imaging of adnexal lesions for better differentiation of ovarian lesions from tubal or uterine lesions
- Three-dimensional guidance for interventional procedures
- Evaluation and follow-up of patients of polycystic ovaries and tubal occlusion for infertility workup.

Obstetrics

- For evaluation of facial anomalies like cleft palate and cleft lip
- Evaluation of nasal bone, ears and cranial sutures
- Detection of central nervous system anomalies like corpus callosal agenesis and Dandy-Walker cyst
- For evaluation of ribs and intrathoracic masses
- For evaluation of spine, e.g. vertebral abnormalities, neural, tube defect,[30,31] diastematomyelia **(Figs. 9A and B)**, etc.
- For evaluation of extremities like club feet and skeletal dysplasia, etc.
- For evaluation of heart, placenta and umbilical cord
- For evaluation of multiple gestations for mapping of vasculature for twin transfusion syndrome
- Telemedicine and education
- Storing volumetric data for subsequent interpretation and review
- For quality control by way of central monitoring, e.g. procedures done at different peripheral sites and in multicenter research studies
- Teaching postprocessing techniques and standardized views to residents.

Studies have suggested that the mothers who are viewing the 3D images of the babies feel enhanced bonding with their fetus.[32]

With the use of 4D ultrasound many facial expressions, such as yawning, tongue protrusion, mouth opening, eye opening and blinking, etc. can also be studied in greater

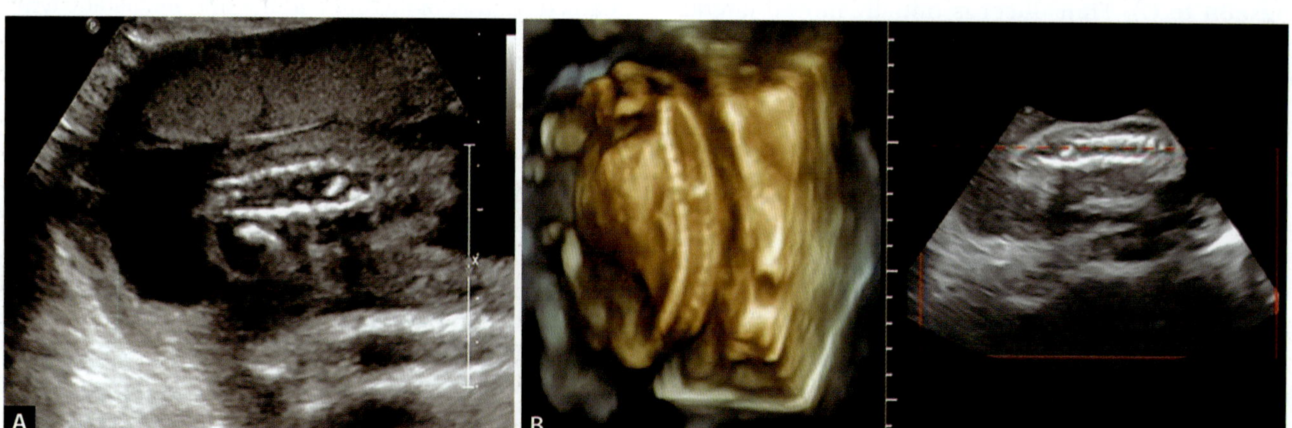

Figs. 9A and B: (A) Transabdominal sonographic coronal 2D image showing bony spur in a case of diastemeomyelia; (B) Corresponding 3D image showing the bony spur.

details.[33-35] Four-dimensional ultrasound has also been used in the evaluation of fetal heart.[36-38]

Three-dimensional images are very useful for demonstrating the abnormality to the referring physician as these images are better comprehended by those who are not tuned to understand grayscale format of 2D images. Similarly storage of 'volume' data allows us to reprocess the data in future for subsequent interpretation or reviews. These volume data can be sent to remote workstations for telemedicine and teaching purposes. It has also been shown in a few studies that acquisition of 3D data needs less time which can potentially increase patient through put and increase efficiency of the imaging department.[39]

Limitations

As 3D ultrasound information is dependent on reformation of acquired 2D ultrasound data, it is expected that the problems which affect the 2D ultrasound like motion, unfavorable body habitus, shadowing artifacts and suboptimal scanning techniques also result in poor quality 3D images.[27]

Fusion Imaging

Fusion imaging or hybrid imaging means combination of two imaging techniques. This can be in the form of fusion of two anatomical techniques like ultrasound with MRI or CT; or it can be fusion of anatomical technique (ultrasound, CT or MRI) with molecular imaging technique like SPECT or PET **(Figs. 10A to D)**. One example of fusion imaging is real-time virtual sonography (RVS).

To obtain virtual fusion images, an initial step is to transfer the previously acquired CT or MRI data to the ultrasound machine.[40] A point like magnetic positioning sensor unit is attached to the ultrasound probe to detect any change in position of probe during investigation. The transmitter of this sensor unit is placed onto the surface of patient. During examination ultrasound screen is seen as split images with virtual reconstructed CT/MR image on one side and currently acquired USG image on other side of the screen. An attempt is made to match these two images with each other. This is usually done by freezing the CT or MR section with some clearly visible anatomic landmark (e.g. portal vein bifurcation, superior most margin of kidney or the lesion itself, etc.) and identifying the same landmark by freehand USG.[41] Then these two images are matched. The real-time USG image can also be superimposed on the virtual reconstructed CT image with adjustable difference in the grayness **(Figs. 10A to D)**.

CLINICAL APPLICATIONS OF FUSION IMAGING

It has been observed that there are few lesions/tumors in liver which are isoechoic and hence not well appreciable on grayscale ultrasound. Similarly there are subgroups of patients who have been treated with either TACE or RFA and now there is recurrence in the vicinity of the primary tumor site. These lesions are also poorly localized on grayscale USG. Hence detection by USG or further biopsy/treatment by the local ablative therapies were difficult for such lesions. These lesions are usually clearly visible on contrast enhanced CT/MR. However, interventional treatment is usually easier to perform with USG guidance which also avoids radiation to the operator. The RVS combines the advantages of both imaging techniques.[42] In one way this technique provides real-time visualization of the needles in preprocedural CT scan images. The feasibility of RVS module has been proven in many studies.[43-45] The RVS module has been shown to be compatible with B mode, color Doppler mode as well as with harmonic imaging mode.[46] However, the data on accuracy and efficacy of this technique are still emerging.[47]

Limitations

Real-time virtual sonography cannot be used in those patients in whom CT/MRI are contraindicated (e.g. contrast allergy, renal failure, metallic implants, etc). Another limitation is that sometimes the best synchronization is not achievable hence limiting the utility.[46] It definitely prolongs the examination time and it is more expensive as it adds the cost of CT/MRI also.

Therapeutic Applications of Ultrasound

- Ultrasound guided aspirations, drainages and biopsies form the backbone of any interventional radiology unit. With the help of ultrasound, one can easily track the needle path and perform any such interventional procedure easily. Not only it is noninvasive, radiation free, portable modality, it also offers a real-time navigation facility to the interventionists.
- *High-intensity focused ultrasound (HIFU)*: High intensity focused ultrasound is rapidly emerging as a noninvasive method for tumor ablation. In this, high intensity ultrasonic waves are focused at a focal lesion with high accuracy, resulting in a lethal rise in the temperature at the desired target site, with resultant damage of the tumoral cells.[48] Simply put, tranducers help thermally ablate tumors without introducing

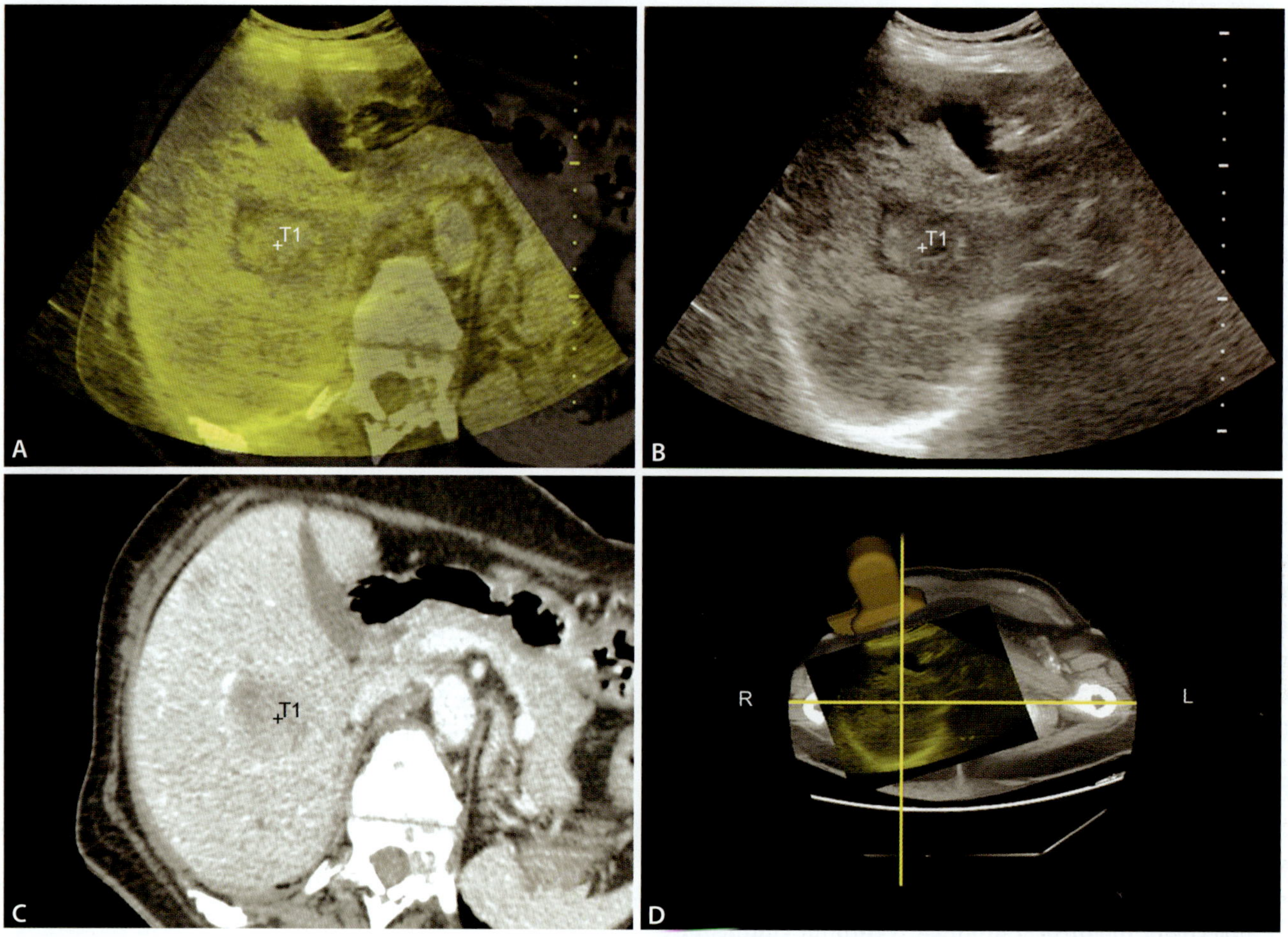

Figs. 10A to D: Application of fusion imaging on a patient with well-visualized lesion on both CT as well as on USG. Four split images seen on the screen. (A) Overlay image showing good matching of the lesions from sonographic and CT images; (B) Current sonographic image; (C) Previously acquired CT images feeded in ultrasound machine. On moving the ultrasound transducer, there will be automatic reformation of these feeded images corresponding to the axis of ultrasound transducer so that the same imaging plane is matched to the ultrasound image; (D) 3D view which is being displayed during the fusion workflow.

needles or wires into the tumor.[49] High intensity energy is absorbed and converted into heat at the focal lesion. This heat raises the temperature causing coagulative necrosis at the site.[50]

It is guided by real-time ultrasound imaging and can be run by one of several transducers with focal lengths varying from 90 to 160 mm. Although choice of transducer would depend upon depth of the target lesion, the most commonly used transducer is the one with a focal length of 135 mm and operating frequency of 0.8 MHz.[48,49] Presently, HIFU is being widely used for ablation of both benign and malignant tumors. It is most common applications worldwide are in the treatment of uterine fibroids, liver tumors and prostate cancer. Apart from these, it has also been used in the ablation of breast, bone, pancreas and soft tissue tumors.

Ultrasound-based Molecular Imaging and Oncotherapy

Ultrasound molecular imaging, which is based on the use of molecularly targeted contrast agents, combines the advantages of contrast enhanced ultrasound with the ability to characterize neoplastic processes at a molecular level.[51] Ultrasound molecular imaging has enormous potential applications, which can range from early cancer detection and tumor characterization to monitoring treatment response and guiding cancer therapies.[51,52] There is also potential role for ultrasound contrast agents in improved delivery of chemotherapeutic drugs and gene therapies across existing biological barriers. Most of the preclinical studies have used contrast micro-bubbles, which are emulsions (gas-liquid) of several micrometer in size, confined to intravascular space. Much smaller newer nanoparticles are currently being investigated for future application.

Ultrasound-image Artifacts

Image artifacts on ultrasound are commonly seen in day to day clinical ultrasound practice. Some artifacts are generated by the physical limitations of the modality while some arise secondary to improper scanning technique. Artifacts can interfere with image interpretation. Ultrasound artifacts can be understood with a basic appreciation of the physical properties of the ultrasound beam, the propagation of sound in matter and the assumptions of image processing.[53] Ultrasound artifacts often arise secondary to errors inherent to the ultrasound beam characteristics, the presence of multiple echo paths, velocity errors and attenuation errors. The beam width, side lobe, reverberation, comet tail, ring-down, mirror image, speed displacement, refraction, attenuation, shadowing and increased through-transmission artifacts are encountered on a routine basis in clinical practice.[53] An ability to recognize and then correct potentially correctable ultrasound artifacts is significant for patient care and improvement in the image quality.

Ultrasound artifacts can be grouped under the following:

- *Resolution-related artifacts includes*: Speckle in conventional ultrasound imaging results from the use of phase-sensitive transducer and occurs when structure in the object is on a scale too small to be resolved by the imaging system.[54] 'It is an interference phenomenon—small scatterers cause constructive and destructive phase interference at the receiving array. The ability of a speckle to mask small but perhaps diagnostically important image features makes it an undesirable property.'[55]

  Speckle pattern does not alter with time, so repeat imaging if obtained through same plane with same transducer position and orientation, will show the same speckle pattern. However, if we change the transducer orientation and position, the speckle pattern shall also change.
- *Attenuation-related artifacts include* attenuation, shadowing and enhancement attenuation. It occurs due to lack of transmission of sound through a mass lesion. It points to solid internal consistency of the lesion.[2]

  When an ultrasound beam encounters a focal object that attenuates the sound to a lesser or greater extent than in the surrounding tissue, the strength of the beam distal to this given structure will be either stronger or weaker than in the adjoining field. Thus, when the ultrasound beam encounters a strongly attenuating or highly reflective structure, the amplitude of the beam distal to this structure is diminished. The echoes returning from structures beyond the highly attenuating structure will also be diminished. In clinical practice, this is seen as a dark band known as a "shadow" deep to a highly attenuating structure (calculi) **(Fig. 11A)**.

  Similarly, when the ultrasound beam traverses a focal weakly attenuating structure within the imaging field, the amplitude of the beam beyond this structure is greater than the beam amplitude at the same depth in the rest of the field and thus echoes returning from structures deep to the focal weak attenuator will have

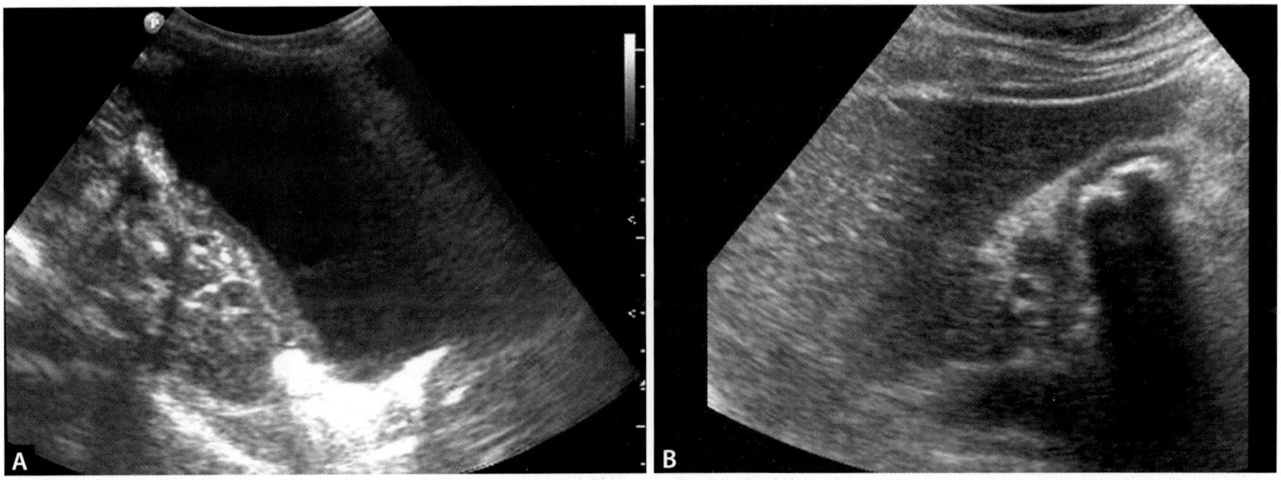

Figs. 11A and B: Ultrasound image artifact shadowing (A) and enhancement (B) in two different patients. (A) Demonstrates shadowing with gallbladder calculi; (B) Demonstrates enhancement from a large abdominal cystic lesion.

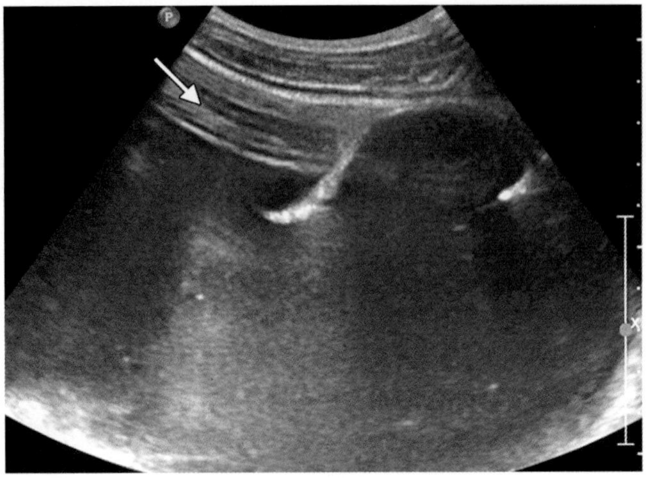

Fig. 12: Reverberation artifact (arrow) at anterior part of grossly hydronephritic kidney.

a higher amplitude and will be falsely displayed as increase in echogenicity or "enhancement", typically seen posterior to a cystic lesion (low attenuation lesion)[53-55] **(Fig. 11B)**.

- *Propagation-related (artifacts associated with multiple echoes)* ***(Fig. 12)***[56] includes reverberation, comet tail, ring down, sidelobe and mirror image artifacts.
  Reverberation: In the presence of two parallel highly reflective surfaces, the echoes produced from a primary ultrasound beam may be repeatedly reflected back and forth before returning to the transducer for detection. When this happens, multiple echoes are recorded and displayed. At imaging, this is seen as multiple equidistantly spaced linear reflections and is referred to as reverberation artifact.[53,56] Typically, it occurs when sound beam travels with minimal or no attenuation through a cystic (fluid) structure. These become weak as sound travels into the tissue deeper and can mimic solid component in a cystic structure (urinary bladder). This artifact can be resolved by simply changing the scanning angle.
  Comet tail artifact is also a form of reverberation. In this artifact, the two reflective interfaces and thus sequential echoes are closely spaced. The sequential echoes may be so close together on the display that individual signals remain unperceivable. It appears as a dense, tapering echoes distal to a structure which reflects strongly.[2] Classic examples include metallic objects which may produce such artifacts.
  Mirror image artifacts: are generated when a highly reflective interface is encountered by the primary beam. The reflected echoes then encounter the "back side" of a structure and are reflected back toward the reflective interface before being reflected to the transducer for detection.[53] The display shows a duplicated structure which is equidistant from but deep to the strongly reflective interface. In clinical imaging, this duplicated structure is commonly identified at the level of the diaphragm, where the pleural-air interface acts as the strong reflector.
- *Ultrasound beam characteristics related artifacts:*
  Beam width artifact: A highly reflective object located within the widened beam beyond transducer's margin may generate detectable echoes. Ultrasound display presumes echoes to be originating from within narrow imaging plane and displays them as such.[53] Its clinical application can be manifested as when anechoic structure (urinary bladder) shows peripheral echoes. This can be corrected and removed during scanning by adjusting the focal zone to the level of interest and by placing transducer at the center of the object. Side lobes are multiple beams of low amplitude ultrasound energy that project radially from the main beam axis and artifacts seen mainly with linear array transducers.[53] Similar to beam width artifact, this phenomenon is most likely to be recognized as extraneous echoes present within an expected anechoic structure, such as the bladder.[57]

REFERENCES

1. Rizzatto G. Ultrasound transducers. Eur J Radiol. 1998;27 (Suppl 2):S188-95.
2. Silkowski C. Ultrasound Nomenclature, Image Orientation and Basic Instrumentation. In: Abraham D, Silkowski C, Odwin C. Emergency Medicine Sonography. Jones and Bartlett Publishers; 2010. pp. 1-24.
3. Hangiandreou NJ. Radiographics AAPM/RSNA physics tutorial for residents. Topics in US: B-mode US: basic concepts and new technology. 2003;23(4):1019-33.
4. Thomenius KE. Instrumentation for B-mode imaging. In: Goldman LW, Fowlkes JB (Eds). Categorical course in diagnostic radiology physics: CT and US cross-sectional imaging. Oak Brook, Ill: Radiological Society of North America; 2000. pp. 9-20.
5. Zagzebski JA. Physics and Instrumentation in Doppler and B-mode ultrasonography. In: Zwiebel and Pellerito. Introduction to Vascular Ultrasonography, 5th edition. Elsevier Saunders; Philadelphia: Chapter 2. 2005. pp. 19-60.
6. Curry ST, Dowdey JE, Murry RC. Ultrasound. In: Christensen's Physics of Diagnostic Radiology, 4th edition. Lea & Febiger; 1990.pp. 323-70.
7. Kremkau F. Diagnostic ultrasound principles, Instrumentation and Exercises, 5th Edn. Orlando FL: Grune & Startton;1993.
8. Taylor KJW, Wells PNT, Burns PN. Clinical applications of doppler ultrasound. New York: Raven Press;1995.

9. Evans D. Doppler ultrasound physics instrumentation and clinical applications. New York: John Wiley and Sons; 1989.
10. Rubin JM, Bude RO,Carson PL, et al. Power Doppler US: A potentially useful alternative to mean frequency-based color doppler US. Radiology. 1994;190:853-6.
11. Martinoli C, Derchi LE, Rizzatto G, Solbiati L. Power Doppler sonography: general principles, clinical applications, and future prospects. Eur Radiol. 1998;8:1224-35.
12. Sodhi KS, Sidhu R, Gulati M, Saxena A, Suri S, Chawla Y. Role of tissue harmonic imaging in focal hepatic lesions: comparison with conventional sonography. J Gastroenterol Hepatol. 2005;20(10):1488-93.
13. Shapiro RS, Wagreich J, Parsons RB, Pasik AS, Yeh HC, Lao R. Tissue harmonic imaging sonography: evaluation of image quality compared with conventional sonography. AJR. 1998;171:1203-6.
14. Yucel C, Ozdemir H, Asik E, Oner Y, Isik S. Benefits of tissue harmonic imaging in the evaluation of abdominal and pelvic lesions. Abdom. Imaging. 2003;28:103-9.
15. Ward B, Baker AC, Humphrey VF. Nonlinear propagation applied to the improvement of resolution in diagnostic medical ultrasound. J Acoust Soc Am. 1997;101:143-54.
16. Rosenthal SJ, Jones PH, Wetzel LH. Phase inversion tissue harmonic sonographic imaging: a clinical utility study. AJR. 2001;176:1393-8.
17. Choudhry S, Gorman B, Charbonear JW, et al. Comparison of tissue harmonic imaging with conventional US in abdominal disease. Radiographics. 2000;20:1127-35.
18. Hann LE, Bach AM, Cramer LD, Siegel D, Yoo HH, Gaxia R. Hepatic sonography: comparison of tissue harmonic and standard sonography techniques. AJR. 1999;173:201-6.
19. Desser TS, Jeffrey RB. Tissue harmonic imaging techniques: physical principles and clinical applications. Semin. Ultrasound CT MR. 2001;22:1-10.
20. Lencioni R, Cioni D, Bartolozzi C. Tissue harmonic and contrast specific imaging: back to gray scale in ultrasound. Eur. Radiol. 2002;12:151-65.
21. Kollmann C. New sonographic techniques for harmonic imaging--underlying physical principles. Eur J Radiol. 2007;64(2):164-72. Epub 2007 Sep 17. Review.
22. Kawagishi T. Technical description of 1.5 harmonic imaging, an effective technique for contrast–enhanced ultrasound diagnosis. Medical review 2003-Cardiology special Issue. Cardiac imaging & Networking. Toshiba Medical systems.
23. Harvey CJ, Pilcher JM, Eckersley RJ, Blomley MJK, Cosgrove DO. Advances in Ultrasound. Clin Radiol. 2002;57;157-77.
24. Jespersen SK, Wilhjelm JE, Sillesen H. Multiangle compound imaging. Ultrason Imaging. 1998;20:81-102.
25. Garra BS. Elastography Current status, future prospects and making it work for you. Ultrasound Quarterly. 2011;27:177-86.
26. Benacerraf BR, Benson CB, Abuhamad AZ, et al. Three- and 4-dimensional ultrasound in obstetrics and gynecology: proceedings of the American Institute of Ultrasound in Medicine Consensus Conference. J Ultrasound Med. 2005; 24(12):1587-97.
27. Bega G, Lev-Toaff AS, O'Kane P, et al. Three-dimensional Ultrasonography in Gynecology Technical Aspects and Clinical Applications. J Ultrasound Med. 2003;22(11): 1249-69.
28. Raga F, Bonilla-Musoles F, Blanes J, et al. Congenital mullerian anomalies: diagnostic accuracy of three-dimensional ultrasound. Fertil Steril. 1996;65(3):523-8.
29. Wu MH, Hsu CC, Huang KE. Detection of congenital mullerian duct anomalies using three-dimensional ultrasound. J Clin Ultrasound. 1997;25(9):487-92.
30. Dyson RL, Pretorius DH, Budorick NE, et al. Three dimensional ultrasound in the evaluation of fetal anomalies. Ultrasound Obstet Gynecol. 2000;16(4): 321-8.
31. Lee W, Chaiworapongsa T, Romero R, et al. A diagnostic approach for the evaluation of spina bifida by three-dimensional ultrasonography. J Ultrasound Med. 2002;21(6):619-26.
32. Ji E, Pretorius D, Newton R, et al. Effects of ultrasound on maternal-fetal bonding: a comparison of two- and three-dimensional imaging. Ultrasound Obstet Gynecol. 2005; 25(5):473-7.
33. Kurjak A, Azumendi G, Vecek N, et al. Fetal hand movements and facial expression in normal pregnancy studied by four-dimensional sonography. J Perinat Med. 2003;31(6):496-508.
34. Kurjak A, Stanojevic M, Andonotopo W, et al. Behavioral pattern continuity from prenatal to postnatal life: a study by four-dimensional (4D) ultrasonography. J Perinat Med. 2004;32(4):346-53.
35. Kurjak A, Stanojevic M, Azumendi G, et al. The potential of four-dimensional (4D) Ultrasonography in the assessment of fetal awareness. J Perinat Med. 2005;33(1):46-53.
36. DeVore GR, Falkensammer P, Sklansky MS, et al. Spatio-temporal image correlation (STIC): new technology for evaluation of the fetal heart. Ultrasound Obstet Gynecol. 2003;22(4):380-7.
37. Viñals F, Poblete P, Giuliano A. Spatio-temporal image correlation (STIC): a new tool for the prenatal screening of congenital heart defects. Ultrasound Obstet Gynecol. 2003; 22(4):388-94.
38. Gonçalves LF, Lee W, Chaiworapongsa T, et al. Four dimensional ultrasonography of the fetal heart with spatiotemporal image correlation. Am J Obstet Gynecol. 2003;189(6):1792-802.
39. Benacerraf BR, Shipp TD, Bromley B. How sonographic tomography will change the face of obstetric sonography: a pilot study. J Ultrasound Med. 2005;24(3):371-8.
40. Real-time Virtual Sonography Unit. Instruction Manual. Hitachi Medical Corporation. 2004-2006.
41. Sandulescu L, Saftoiu A, Dumitrescu D, Ciurea T. The role of real-time contrast-enhanced and real-time virtual sonography in the assessment of malignant liver lesions. J Gastrointestin Liver Dis. 2009;18(1):103-8.
42. Sandulescu L, Dumitrescu D, Rogoveanu I, Saftoiu A. Hybrid ultrasound imaging techniques (fusion imaging). World J Gastroenterol. 2011;17(1):49-52.

43. Minami Y, Kudo M, Chung H, et al. Percutaneous radiofrequency ablation of sonographically unidentifiable liver tumors. Feasibility and usefulness of a novel guiding technique with an integrated system of computed tomography and sonographic images. Oncology. 2007;72(Suppl 1):111-6.
44. Minami Y, Chung H, Kudo M, et al. Radiofrequency ablation of hepatocellular carcinoma: value of virtual CT sonography with magnetic navigation. Am J Roentgenol. 2008;190(6): W335-41.
45. Kitada T, Murakami T, Kuzushita N, et al. Effectiveness of real-time virtual sonography guided radiofrequency ablation treatment for patients with hepatocellular carcinomas. Hepatol Res. 2008;38(6):565-71.
46. Sandulescu L, Saftoiu A, Dumitrescu D, Ciurea T. Real-time contrast-enhanced and real-time virtual sonography in the assessment of benign liver lesions. J Gastrointestin Liver Dis. 2008;17(4):475-8.
47. Krücker J, Xu S, Venkatesan A, et al. Clinical Utility of Real-time Fusion Guidance for Biopsy and Ablation. J Vasc Interv Radiol. 2011;22(4):515-24.
48. Shehata IA. Treatment with high intensity focused ultrasound: secrets revealed. Eur J Radiol. 2012;81(3):534-41.
49. Wu F, Wang ZB, Chen WZ, Zhu H, Bai J, Zou JZ, et al. Extracorporeal high intensity focused ultrasound ablation in the treatment of patients with large hepatocellular carcinoma. Ann Surg Oncol. 2004;11(12):1061-9.
50. Dubinsky TJ, Cuevas C, Dighe MK, Kolokythas O, Hwang JH. High-intensity focused ultrasound: current potential and oncologic applications. Am J Roentgenol. 2008;190(1):191-9.
51. Kaneko OF, Willmann JK. Ultrasound for molecular imaging and therapy in cancer. Quant Imaging Med Surg. 2012;2(2):87-97.
52. Kircher MF, Willmann JK. Molecular body imaging: MR imaging, CT, and US. Part II. Applications. Radiology. 2012;264(2):349-68.
53. Feldman MK, Katyal S, Blackwood MS. US artifacts. Radiographics. 2009;29(4):1179-89.
54. Burckhardt CB. Speckle in ultrasound B-Mode scans, IEEE Trans. Sonics Ultrasonics. 1978;SU-25:1-6.
55. Chen Y, Broschat SL , Flynn PJ. Phase Insensitive Homomorphic Image Processing for Speckle Reduction. Ultrasonic Imaging. 1996;18:122-39.
56. Bushberg JT, Seibert JA, Leidholdt EM, Boone JM. The essential physics of medical imaging, 2nd edition. Philadelphia, PA: Lippincott Williams & Wilkins; 2002. pp. 469-553.
57. Laing FC, Kurtz AB. The importance of ultrasonic side-lobe artifacts. Radiology. 1982;145(3):763-8.

CHAPTER 39

Image Optimization in Ultrasound

Rashmi Dixit

INTRODUCTION

Ultrasound imaging with its inherent flexibility, low cost and real time physiologic measurement capability with no known bioeffects, at intensities used in medical imaging, plays a vital role in diagnostics.

Image formation in ultrasound depends on the physical properties of ultrasound pulse formation, transmission and interaction with tissues. Acoustic energy undergoes essentially three different types of interactions in the tissues-reflection (specular and diffuse), refraction, and attenuation.

Diagnostic applications of ultrasound are based on detection and display of acoustic energy reflected from interfaces within the body. The amplitude of the reflected energy is used to generate ultrasound images while frequency shifts in backscattered ultrasound provide information relating to moving targets such as blood. Real-time, gray- scale, B-mode display, in which variations in display intensity or brightness are used to show signals of differing amplitude, is the mainstay of ultrasound imaging. Real-time ultrasound produces an impression of motion by generating a series of 2D images several times per second or frames per second.

The **quality of an ultrasound image**[1-3] depends on its spatial resolution, temporal resolution, contrast resolution and freedom from certain artifacts. Spatial resolution has three components: axial, lateral and elevational or azimuthal resolution. Axial resolution is the resolution along the axis of the ultrasound beam. It is also called longitudinal or depth resolution and depends on spatial pulse length, which is the product of wavelength and number of pulses, being equal to half the spatial pulse length. As frequency is increases the pulse length decreases permitting resolution of smaller details. Hence, axial resolution improves with increasing frequency (which reduces wavelength). Axial resolution at a frequency of 3.5 MHz is 0.5–1.0 mm. It does not change significantly with depth. Lateral resolution refers to the ability to distinguish two structures lying side by side. The width of the main beam defines the lateral resolution of the ultrasound image because objects can be resolved separately only if the beam is narrower than the distance between them. Hence in modern systems-transducers are focused to reduce beam width. Focal zone is the area where the beam is 3–4 wavelengths wide and the area where lateral resolution is highest, deteriorating rapidly beyond it. Lateral resolution with frequency of 3.5 MHz is approximately 2 mm. Focusing in the elevation plane is also possible with current technology.

Temporal resolution refers to the ability to locate the position of a particular moving structure in time. This increases as the frame rate increases. Contrast resolution is the ability to show very subtle difference in echo strength. Contrast resolution improves when a system can recognize and store a wide range of echo amplitudes.

New technical developments and remarkable improvement in image quality have marked several new applications for diagnostic ultrasound. The rise of state of the art, expensive equipment has greatly eased the sonologist's job. Nonetheless, it does not by itself guarantee, high-quality ultrasound images. Variables, many of which are under direct user control, must be managed to guarantee the production of quality studies. An accurate ultrasound diagnosis relies heavily on the experience and skill of the examiner and requires adjustment of the equipment settings from patient to patient and organ to organ. Hence, the image optimization is an essential prerequisite for diagnostic ultrasound imaging.

GRAYSCALE IMAGING

Basic Guidelines[2-5]

Patient should be positioned in such a way that the area of interest can be easily accessed and the patient is comfortable during the examination. Changing the patient position to better elucidate pathology is also important, e.g. an extended neck for thyroid examination, left lateral decubitus position for gallbladder calculi, etc.

A good acoustic window improves scanning accuracy and image quality. Solid organs like the liver or spleen or fluid filled structures, which do not attenuate the sound beam, e.g. full bladder or fluid filled stomach provide a good acoustic window to see deeper structures. Use of adequate amount of coupling gel is essential as air has high-acoustic impedance.

Factory Presets

The more complicated machine settings are saved as presets. Presets provide a useful starting point; however, these are settings which are optimized for patients of average body habitus and further optimization of the image by manual adjustments is invariably required in order to increase diagnostic confidence and avoid artifacts. A single touch image optimization is also available on some systems; however this only resets the parameters to the chosen preset.

Transducer Selection

Choosing the appropriate transducer both in terms of frequency as well as footprint is extremely important for a good examination. Higher frequencies provide a better resolution but are attenuated much more as attenuation is proportional to the fourth power of frequency. A trade off thus has to be made between the need for penetration and resolution.

While performing superficial scans as for the thyroid, musculoskeletal system or testicular examination a linear transducer with a high frequency (7–10 mHz or even 15–17 MHz) is suitable but for deeper structures a lower frequency, such as 2.5–3 MHz is used. Currently, many multifrequency and broad band width transducers are available. For intercostal scanning or scanning the neonatal brain transducers with a smaller footprint which fit into the small acoustic window are appropriate **(Figs. 1A and B)**. Sector transducers are thus useful to evaluate deeper structures through a small acoustic window, e.g. echocardiography. In sector scanning, however, resolution becomes poorer with increasing depth as the same echo lines are spread out over a wider area deeper in the tissue.

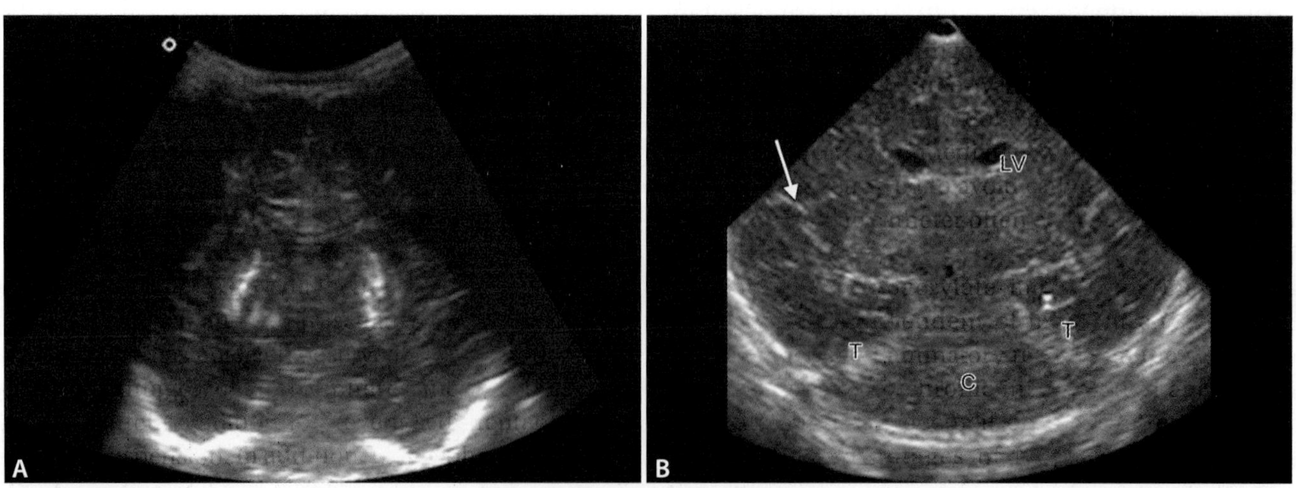

Figs. 1A and B: Cranial sonogram performed with a curvilinear array abdominal probe (A) shows shadowing obscuring the cerebral convexities on both sides due to mismatch between the large transducer footprint, acoustic window. The second scan (B) performed with a small footprint transducer shows good visualization of cerebral convexities. Arrow shows the sylvian fissure.
Abbreviations: T: Tentorium; C: Cerebellum.

Overall Gain

Overall gain amplifies all the returning echoes/signals uniformly. An excessively high gain can result in a washed out image and can obscure many details.

Time-gain Compensation

Time-gain compensation (TGC) is also referred to as distance-gain-compensation (DGC) or spatial-time compensation (STC). Signals that arrive later, i.e. from greater depths are amplified more than earlier signals to compensate for the attenuating effect of tissues. TGC controls permit the user to selectively amplify the signals from deeper structures or suppress signals from superficial tissues so that a smooth grayscale picture can be obtained **(Figs. 2A and B)**. Although most newer machines provide for some automatic TGC, manual adjustment by the user is one of the most important factors that may have a profound effect on image quality.

Depth Setting

This parameter selects the depth of the imaging field. If too much depth is selected the image will be small and the area of interest difficult to visualize, measurements may also be inaccurate. On the other hand of the depth setting is too shallow the complete region or organ is not visualized and pathology at a deeper levels may be completely missed **(Figs. 3A and B)**. Practically depth can be adjusted by starting at a higher depth, subsequently depths should be decreased so that the area of interest in at about three-fourth the depth of the screen. A small area should be available behind the area of interest of observe useful artifacts.

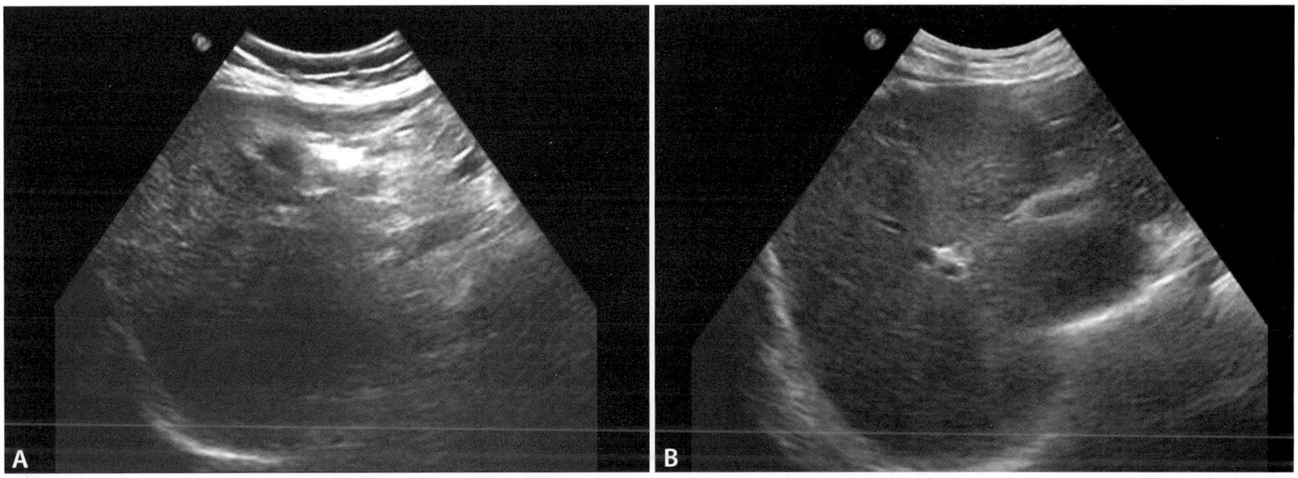

Figs. 2A and B: (A) Improper TGC setting resulting in a dark band over the deep aspect of the liver; (B) With the correct TGC setting the whole liver shows a uniform echopattern.

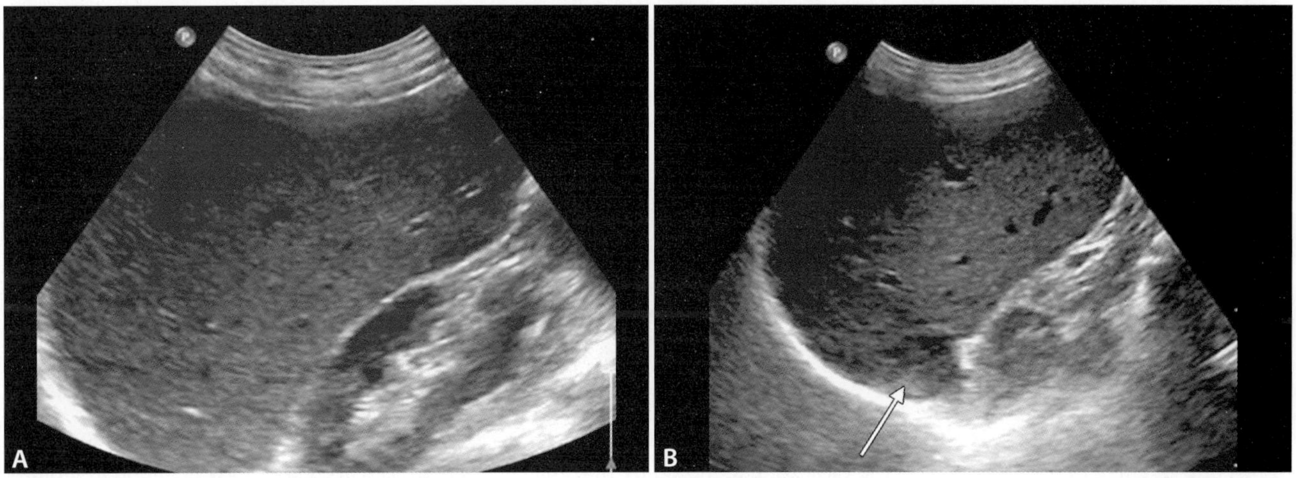

Figs. 3A and B: Improper depth setting in (A) results in nonvisualization of posterior most portion of liver with consequently missed metastatic focus, which is easily appreciated (arrow) with proper depth setting in (B).

Focal-zone Setting

To improve resolution diagnostic transducers are focused electronically. As already discussed, the resolution of ultrasound is best in the focal zone. The focal zone should thus be set over the area of interest. A significant difference in image resolution depending on the focal-zone setting is the hallmark of a well-focused beam **(Figs. 4A and B)**. Modern scanners allow the use of multiple focal zones; however, this may result in decreased frame rate and hence decreased temporal resolution.

Zoom

Zoom is used to magnify the area of interest. There are two types of zoom available. Read zoom is used to enlarge a frozen image whereas write zoom is used to enlarge the display magnification, when scanning is taking place.

In read-zoom-gray level values are read only from a small part of the computer memory and the pixels are enlarged while displaying, something like a magnifying glass. If the magnification factor is too large image matrix becomes obvious and renders the image to grainy.

In write zoom use is made of the fact that the echo samples are received fast enough for several samples to occur in each pixel. In this situation, the image scale can be enlarged to a point where only one sample occurs in each pixel. Each pixel, whose size remains unchanged, displays less tissue. Thus, there is magnification without loss of definition. If the scale is increased further, there is a larger space between scan lines so that further interpolation and smoothening may be required to maintain an acceptable image. More real-scan lines can be introduced using sophisticated signal processing so that definition is improved. One such option is referred to as high-density (HD) zoom. This magnifies the region of interest while increasing line density by redistributing and reformatting all scan lines for the defined region of interest.

Hence, one should always try to use the write zoom. Zoom is extremely useful for accurate measurement of small structures as the CBD.

Dynamic Range

Dynamic range is the ratio of the highest to the lowest amplitudes that can be displayed, expressed in decibels. Dynamic range adjustment changes the contrast. The widest dynamic range that permits best differentiation of subtle differences in echo intensity is preferred for the most applications. The narrower ranges increase the conspicuity of larger echo differences **(Figs. 5A and B)**.

ARTIFACTS IN B MODE IMAGING[3,5-7]

Artifact is a term used to describe any unwanted information generated in the process of image formation. Most artifacts interfere with image interpretation while some artifacts which contain diagnostic information are referred to as friendly artifacts.

A number of artifacts may occur during scanning. Understanding how and why a particular artifact occurs is imperative to eliminate it and avoid errors in diagnosis.

The ultrasound equipment relies on physical assump tions to assign location and intensity of each received echo. The assumptions are:

- The echo detected arose from within the main US beam

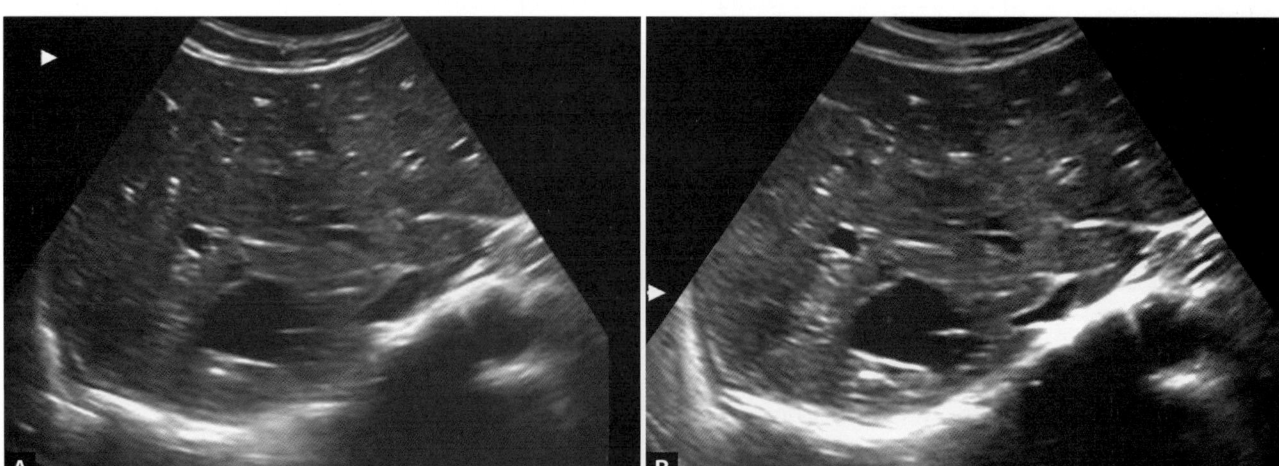

Figs. 4A and B: Effect of focal zone: In (A) the focal zone (denoted by the small arrowhead) is placed anteriorly resulting in a blurred appearance of the posteriorly placed hepatic cyst and diaphragm. These become more sharply defined with proper focal zone positioning over the area of interest (B).

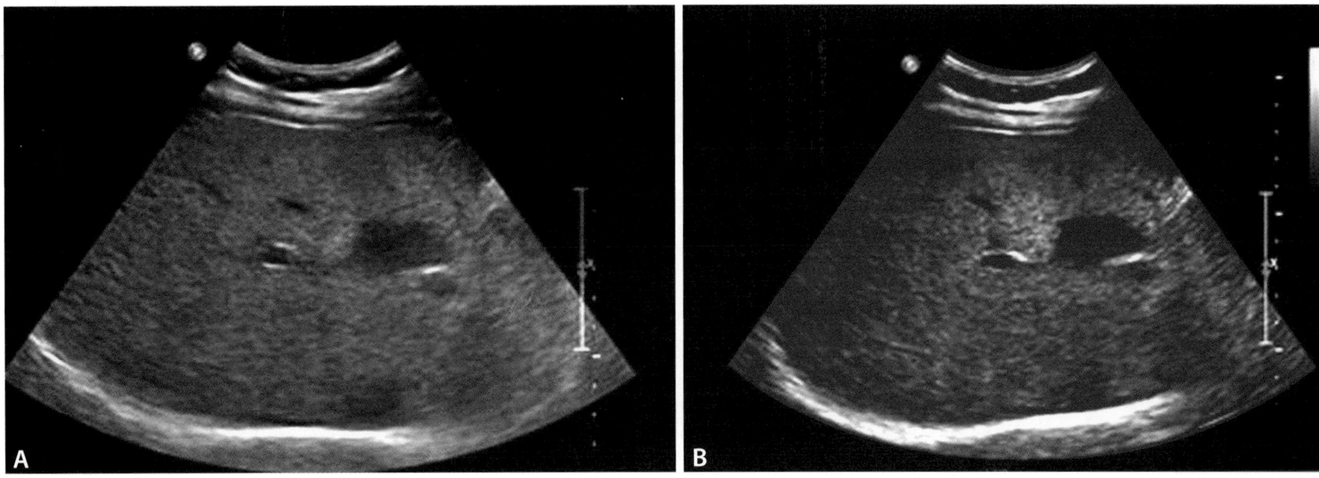

Figs. 5A and B: Images of the liver displayed at dynamic ranges of 70 and 36 dB are shown. The wide dynamic range (A) permits appreciation of subtle differences in echointensity between the diffusely fatty liver and a focal area of sparing. The narrow range (B) increases the conspicuity of larger echo differences with the area of focal sparing appearing darker and the diaphragm brighter than the wide dynamic range image.

- It has returned to the transducer after a single reflection
- The depth on an object is related only to the time taken by an ultrasound pulse to return as an echo to the transducer
- Sound travels at a constant speed and in a straight line in human tissue
- The acoustic energy in an ultrasound field is uniformly attenuated.

While examining patients using ultrasound these assumptions are often not maintained resulting in artifacts.

Beam-width Artifact

The real ultrasound beam is not of a uniformly narrow, laser-like configuration which would be optimal for image resolution. A typical ultrasound focused ultrasound beam exits the transducer at the same width as transducer and progressively narrows to a focus after which it spreads rapidly in the far field, where it may widen beyond the actual width of the transducer. A highly reflective object located within the widened beam beyond the edges of the transducer may generate detectable echoes. The system assumes that these echoes arose from within the imaging plane and displays them accordingly **(Fig. 6)**. The more intense the reflection the further off axis its echoes will be received.

During clinical scanning the artifact is recognized when a structure which should be anechoic has peripheral echoes. It is generally most obvious when a bony or gaseous structure lies adjacent to a fluid space **(Fig. 7)**.

This also means that a strong reflector will continue to give detectable echoes further from the central axis than a weak reflector. Hence, the resolution is better for weak reflectors than strong reflectors which tend to blur laterally and are therefore seen as cigar-shaped smears or streaks so that the width is exaggerated. It also results a general tendency to fill in small echo free regions, such as ducts producing slightly reduced measurements.

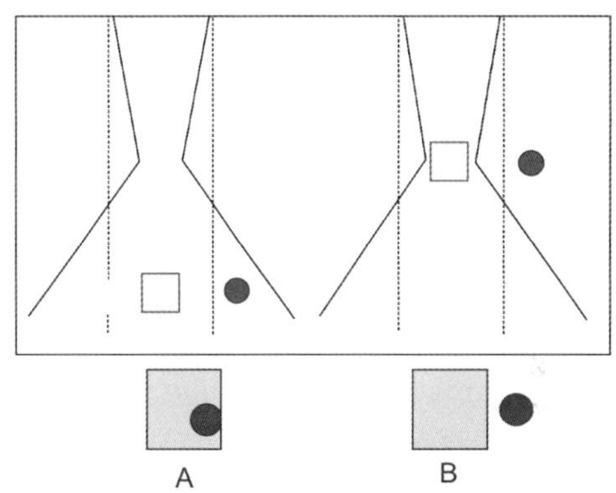

Fig. 6: Mechanism of beam-width artifact: Dotted lines represent the imaging plane. Echoes from the circle are assumed to arise from within the imaging plane in A and displayed within the square. This is rectified with proper focal-zone setting in B.

This can be rectified and image quality improved by adjusting the focal zone to the area of interest and placing the transducer over the center of the object of interest.

Slice-thickness Artifact

Beam-width artifacts also occur in the orthogonal plane, i.e. in the slice thickness or elevation plane. With circular transducers either simple disc or annular array types the beam is symmetrical in all planes but for linear and phased

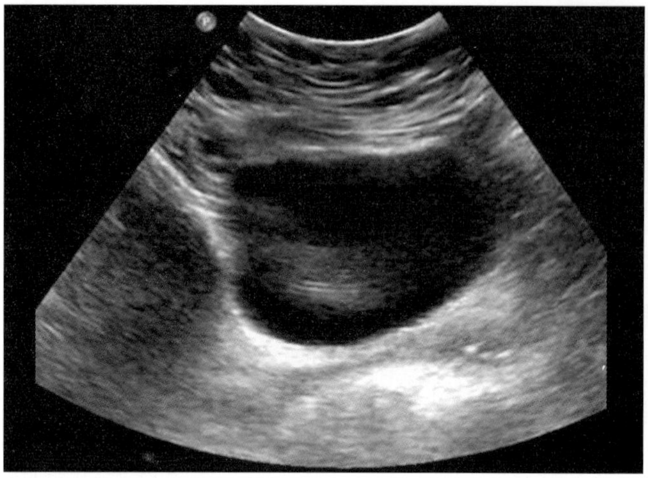

Fig. 7: Beam-width artifact: Strong echoes arising from a gas-filled bowel loop in the pelvis smear across the bladder.

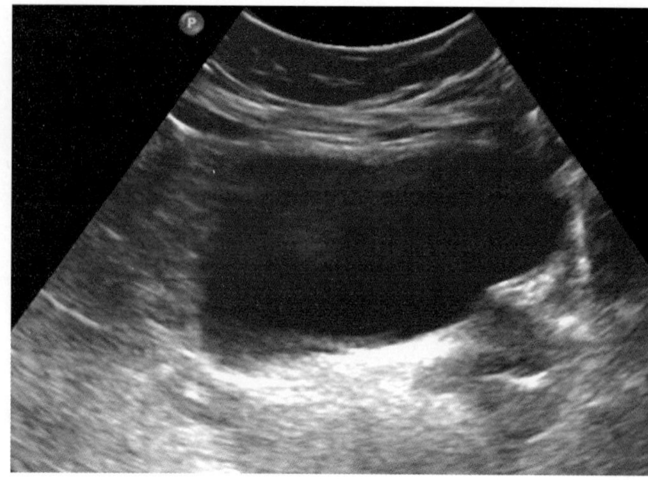

Fig. 8: Low-level echoes are seen in the bladder not from debris but due to slice-thickness artifact arising from gas present in the bowel in the adjacent planes.

array transducers the beam wider in the orthogonal plane resulting in information from adjacent planes being depicted in the image.

The beam width may be wider than a fluid collection. Some of the sound energy may hit structures outside the plane of intersection and may be projected into it to simulate a layer of sludge causing a simple fluid collection to appear complicated **(Fig. 8)**. Since the reflector which has caused the artifact is not visualized in the image it is more difficult to recognize them than the same artifact occuring in the scanned plane. However, with the latest 2D and X-matrix transducers, It is possible to focus the beam in the elevation plane a well-providing, a uniformly focused ultrasound beam.

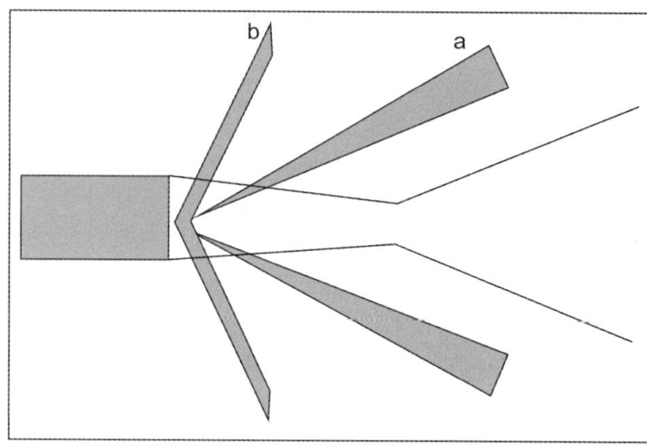

Fig. 9: Off-axis beams: Side lobes (a) and grating lobes (b).

Side-lobe and Grating-lobe Artifacts

These are low energy beams directed at angles away from the central line due to vibration of the edges of the transducer called side lobes and grating lobes. The latter occurs only in array transducers **(Fig. 9)**.

Strong reflectors present in the path of these low energy off-axis beams may generate echoes detectable by the transducer. These are displayed as having originated from within the main beam usually within an anechoic structure. They often have a convex shape and are also referred to as **Chinese hat artifacts**.

Artifacts Associated with Multiple Echoes

Reverberation Bands

A very important assumption in pulse-echo ultrasound imaging is that an echo returns to the transducer after a single reflection and that the depth is related to the time taken for the echo to return. If two highly reflective surfaces lie parallel to each other, the echoes generated may be reflected back and forth before they reach the transducer. The first echo returning after a single reflection is displayed in its proper position. The later echoes returning after multiple reflections are presumed to be arising deeper to the original structure (due to the delay) and are displayed as equally spaced linear reflections in a striped pattern called **reverberation artifact (Figs. 10 and 11)**. The deeper echoes are weaker than the superficial ones due to loss of sound energy due to attenuation by intervening tissues and incomplete reflection so that the bands become narrower and less intense with depth.

Since the distance between the reverberation bands depends on the distance between the reflectors if the reflectors are very closely spaced the sequential echoes

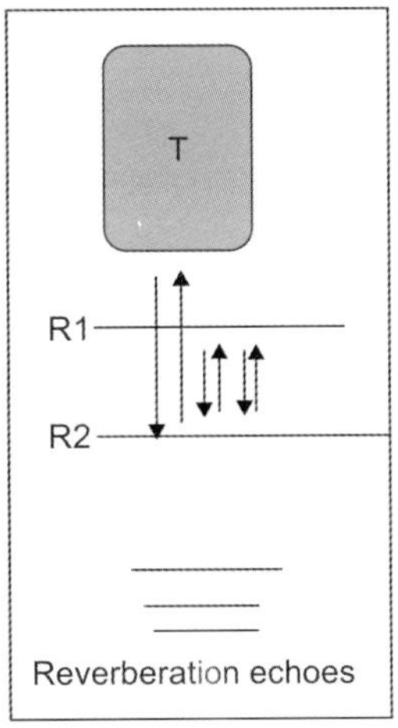

Fig. 10: Mechanism of reverberation artifact.
Abbreviations: T: Transducer; R1 and R2: Reflecting surfaces.

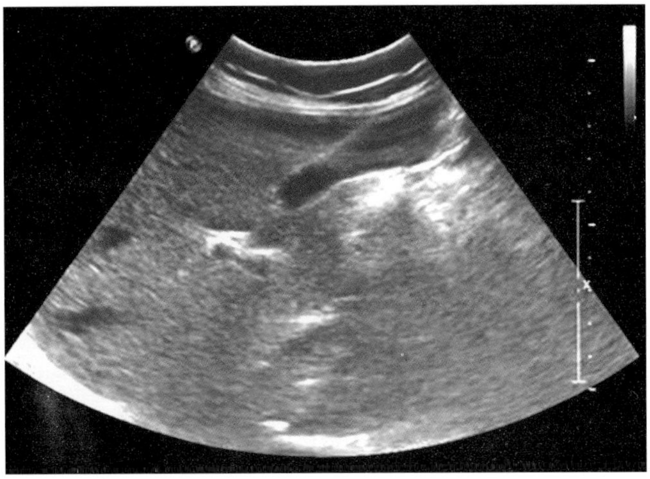

Fig. 11: Multiple equally spaced lines are seen within the gallbladder due to multiple reflections originating in the anterior abdominal wall.

may be so close that individual bands cannot be seen. The resulting artifact is triangular with a tapered shape resembling a comet with its bright tail hence referred to as a **comet-tail artifact**. This artifact is commonly seen deep to calcifications, surgical clips, IUCD and in adenomyosis of gallbladder. It is presumed that many small fluid spaces like the Aschoff–Rokitansky sinuses in the wall of the gallbladder in this condition cause repeated reflections from the walls of the fluid space producing reverberation or the comet tail artifact. The artifact is diagnostic of adenomyosis **(Fig. 12)**.

Another artifact the **ring-down** artifact was previously thought to bc a variant of comet-tail artifact because of the similar appearance of the two; however, this has a separate mechanism. The ultrasound energy is believed to cause vibrations within fluid trapped between air bubbles. These vibrations create a continuous sound wave that is transmitted back to the receiver. This is displayed as a line or series of parallel bands extending posterior to a gas collection.

Mirror-image Artifact

This artifact is also generated by a repeat echo. It is sometimes also referred to as a multipath artifact. The ultrasound beam encounters a highly reflective surface. The reflected echoes then encounter another reflective structure on their way back and are reflected back towards the reflective interface before being reflected to the transducer, where they are detected. The display shows a duplicated structure equidistant but deep to the strongly reflective interface. This artifact is commonly seen at the diaphragm with the air-pleural interface acting as a strong

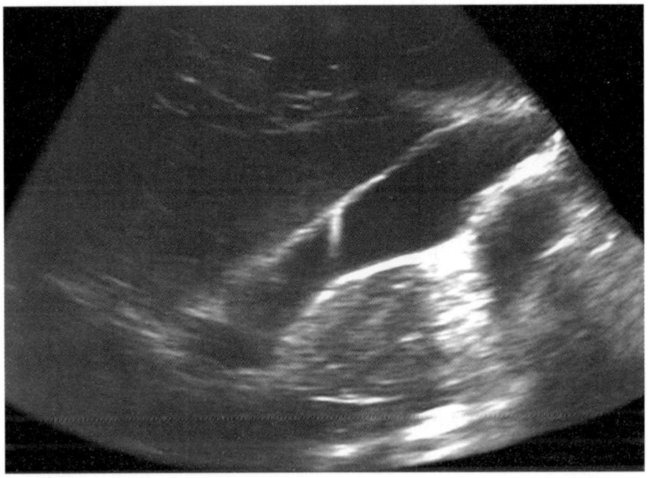

Fig. 12: Adenomyosis of the anterior wall of gallbladder producing a typical comet-tail artifact.

reflector. It is recognized as hepatic parenchyma seen in the expected position of the lung **(Fig. 13)**.

At this level, it does not cause any diagnostic problem, in fact may be useful, e.g. increased through transmission behind a peripheral cyst may be seen in the mirror image which would otherwise be obscured by the hyperechoeic reflection of air in the lung.

In some situations, this artifact can be confusing for example in the pelvis a repeat echo of the bladder or structures just behind it may appear as a deeper line apparently marking back of an echo poor mass. This in reality is a mirror image of the bladder. The clues that help to distinguish this pseudomass from the true mass are: the typical position, the back wall of the mass often lies behind the sacrum and hence is anatomically not possible, and

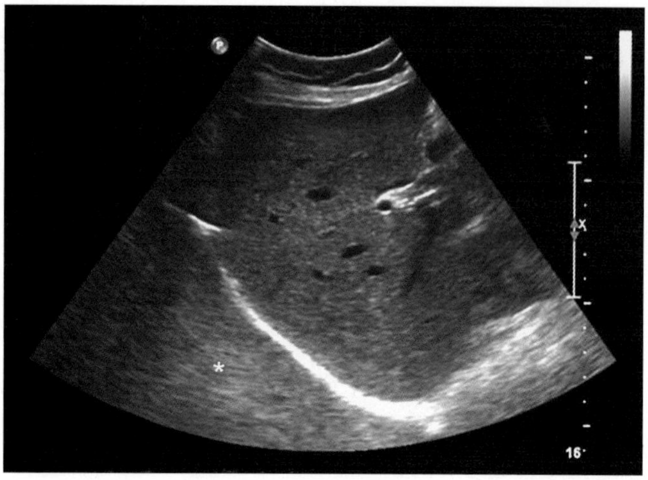

Fig. 13: Mirror reflection of the liver is seen above the diaphragm in this patient (asterix).

the poorly discerned or weak superior and inferior walls compared to strong anterior and posterior walls.

Artifacts Associated with Velocity Errors

An important assumption in ultrasound imaging is that the velocity of US in soft tissues is constant (1540 m/s). This is not absolutely true in clinical sonography; fat, for example, conducts sound about 15% slower than most other soft tissues do **(Table 1)**.

When sound travels through a tissue with a velocity significantly lower than the assumed constant of 1540 m/sec the returning echo takes longer to return to the transducer. Scanners use the amount of delay to calculate the depth of the echo (0.13 μs delay corresponding to ~1 cm depth on final image). The processor assumes that the delay is due to the increased distance traveled by the echo. The echoes are thus displayed deeper on the image than they actually are. This is called ***speed-displacement artifact*** or ***propagation- velocity artifact***. This geometric distortion does not affect the lateral dimension of the image as this is determined by the scanning action of the transducer rather than by the speed of sound. In clinical practice, this artifact is most commonly seen when an area of focal fat is encountered, e.g. areas of focal fat in the subdiaphragmatic region of the liver can result in a discontinuous appearance of the diaphragm because of fallacious posterior displacement of diaphragmatic segments behind the fatty change.

In most cases, velocity errors are too small to be clinically significant and may in fact provide diagnostic clues to the presence of fat within lesions. However, in ophthalmic measurement where great precision is

Table 1: Velocity of ultrasound in biologically important materials.[3]

Tissue type	*Velocity (m/s)*
Air	330
Fat	1450
Water	1480
Brain	1565
Muscle	1580
Liver	1600
Lens of eye	1650
Soft tissue average	1540

required the distortion caused by the significantly higher velocity in the lens can be important. The speed of sound in the lens of the eye is 1620 m/s (vs 1540 of average soft tissues) so regions of the retina imaged through the lens appear closer than the parts imaged through the sclera producing a shelf-like anterior distortion called **Baum's bumps** after sonologist who first described them.

Refractory Errors

Changes in velocity also produces refractory errors. When a nonperpendicular incident ultrasound beam encounters an interface between two materials with different speeds of sound, it changes direction. The degree of this change and the direction is dependent both on the angle of incidence and the difference in velocity between the two media. The scanner working on the assumption that the US beam travels in a straight line misplaces the echoes to the side of their true location. This situation may become important clinically during transabdominal pelvic scans due to refraction occurring deep to the junction of rectus abdominis muscle and midline fat. This can cause lateral stretching of pelvic structures and obstetric measurements made under these conditions may be erroneous. In more extreme cases, it may cause apparent duplication of structures Repositioning the transducer eliminates this artifact.

Attenuation Errors

As an ultrasound beam travels through the tissues, its energy gets attenuated due to combined effect of absorption, scattering and reflection. The greater distance the ultrasound beam travels through the body, the more the attenuation for a beam of similar energy. To compensate for this attenuation, ultrasound processing incorporates a compensatory amplification of echoes that take longer to return, i.e. arising in the deeper tissues. Attenuation also varies with different tissues depending on the attenuation coefficient which expresses the loss of ultrasound intensity per distance traveled **(Table 2)**.

Acoustic Shadowing

When the ultrasound beam encounters a tissue that attenuates sound to a greater extent than the majority of the tissue in the beam shadowing occurs. This is because the gain compensation is only set to an average value; hence, an inadequate correction will be applied to this region. Both it and tissues deeper to it are depicted as less reflective than they actually are. This is visible as a dark band called an acoustic or distal shadow **(Fig. 14)**. Shadowing can also be caused by an extremely efficient reflector such as gas bubble or calcification where 99% and 80% of the incident sound beam, respectively is reflected back. This is because very little of the sound energy penetrates to insonate deeper tissues and in addition any echoes from them would probably not cross the reflective layer on the return journey since they would be rereflected distally.

Edge Shadowing

Shadowing is also sometime seen deep to the edges of strongly curved surfaces, such as cyst walls, fetal skull and vessels. Fine dark lines can be seen extending distal to such edges and become even more striking in the case of a cyst due to the increased through transmission behind the cyst itself.

Two explanations have been offered for this: refraction of the ultrasound beam as it strikes a curved surface and **increased attenuation** at the edges because the ultrasound beam passing through the edge travels a larger distance through the cyst wall than that passing through the diameter of the cyst. Since the cyst wall is presumed to be more attenuating than the surrounding tissues, the beam is attenuated more resulting in shadowing. Although acoustic shadows have diagnostic significance and are useful for diagnosis of calcification or calculi, edge shadows do not have this diagnostic significance **(Figs. 15A and B)**. Edge shadows commonly occur in situations where shadowing erroneously suggests calcification, e.g. vessel walls in renal sinus or malignancy, Coopers ligaments in the breast. It is important to recognize them as artifactual and dismiss them.

Increased through Transmission or Distal Bright-up'

Attenuation errors also occur if a tissue attenuates less than its surrounding tissues (e.g. a full bladder or a simple cyst). In this situation the echoes from it and the tissues posterior to it are overcorrected appearing as a bright band often termed 'distal enhancement' but in view of the enhancing effect of ultrasound contrast agents it is better termed increased through transmission or distal bright up **(Fig. 16)**.

Table 2: Attenuation coefficients for selected tissues.[6]

Material	*Attenuation coefficient (dB/cm)*
Water	0.000
Soft tissue	0.3–0.8
Fat	0.5–1.8
Bone	13–26
Air	40

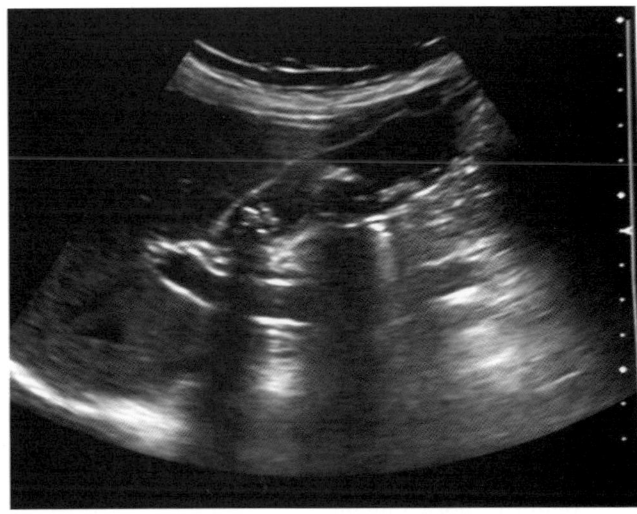

Fig. 14: Acoustic shadows: Seen as dark bands posterior to multiple gallbladder calculi.

Noise

All imaging systems are prone to two types of noise random and structured. Electrical components produce random low- level voltages which, when amplified, are seen as fluctuating moving grey spots on the image producing a snow storm appearance.

There are various other sources of'noise' within ultrasound images. Perhaps the most important is **speckle**. Speckle is an important source of image degradation and loss of contrast in ultrasound image. Small tissue reflectors approximately the size of wavelength of sound cause scattering of sound waves which are sent out almost uniformly in all directions. Constructive and destructive interference of these acoustic fields result in speckle. Most biologic tissues appear in US images as though they are

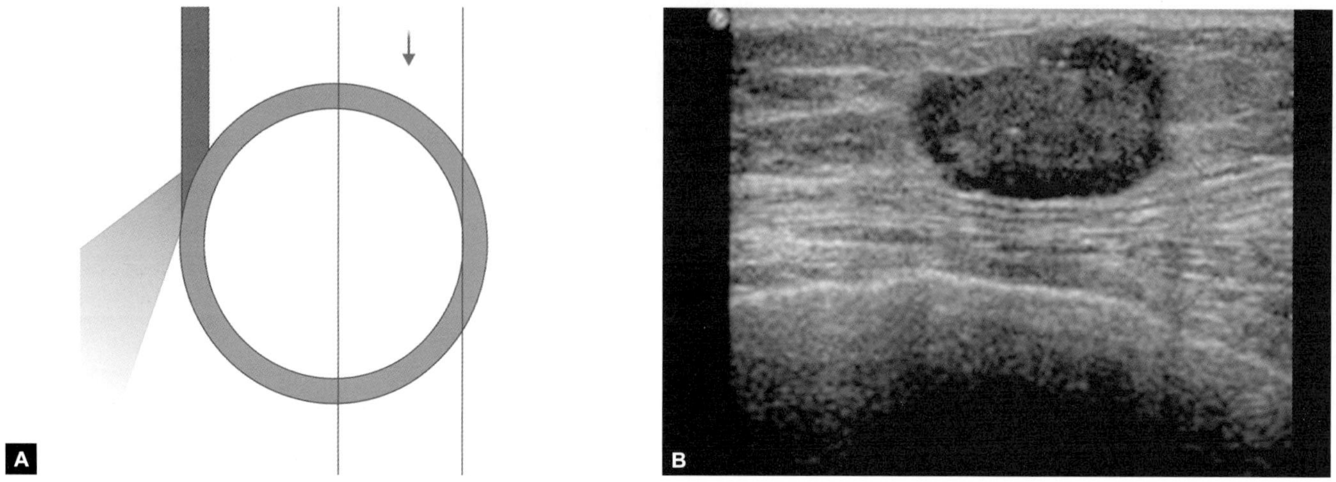

Figs. 15A and B: (A) Refractive and attenuation model to explain mechanism of edge shadowing; (B) Subtle edge shadowing seen along the edges of fibroadenoma breast.

filled with tiny scattering structures. Most of the visible signal in US images results from speckle interactions. The interference pattern also gives ultrasound images a characteristic grainy appearance reducing contrast and making identification of subtle features and abnormal tissue patterns more difficult.

Another problem is **clutter**, which arises from electrical interference or beamforming artifacts, reverberations, and other acoustic phenomena. Clutter consists of spurious echoes which can often be seen within structures of low echogenicity, such as a cysts, or within amniotic fluid, and which may be confused with 'real' targets as already discussed. Finally, another potential source of noise, especially in deep-lying regions, is thermal noise arising in the electronics of the transducer or beamformer. All these sources of noise affect the ability of the radiologist to recognize tissue anomalies by interfering with the pattern recognition process in the observer's brain. Various techniques, such as temporal smoothening (i.e. frame averaging or persistence) are used to reduce noise. The real information is reinforced while noise cancels out. In addition a number of special imaging modes are available on high end scanners to deal with these problems which are discussed later.

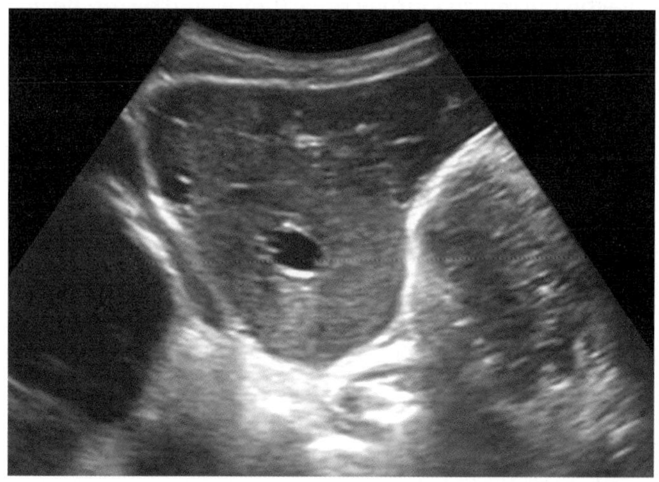

Fig. 16: A bright band is seen posterior to this hepatic cyst—Increased through transmission or distal bright-up.

SPECTRAL AND COLOR DOPPLER EXAMINATION

Basic Guidelines[7]

Gray-scale settings should always be optimized before color Doppler flow mapping is applied. Fine details, such as small plaques or intimal thickening may be washed over by color if the grayscale image is not evaluated first.

Of the various technical parameters that can be controlled the choice of the correct transducer or the correct transducer frequency is the most important like grayscale imaging. A trial of different transducer frequencies till the best compromise between penetration and signal strength is reached is usually required.

Knowledge of anatomic variants is very important while scanning for vascular especially venous disease; for example, failure to recognize duplication of common femoral vein can result in missing the diagnosis of deep venous thrombosis.

It is important to scan the entire length of vessel from its origin to termination when possible. If the ostium of a vessel is not evaluated, lesions at the ostia may be missed, e.g. atherosclerotic plaque commonly involve the origin of carotid and vertebral arteries. In such a situation, the elevated velocities may render evaluation of more distal stenotic lesions by velocity criteria alone difficult. Each vessel must also be examined in two planes, i.e. longitudinal and transverse to avoid missing partially occlusive eccentric thrombi, which may not be centered in the imaging plane in a longitudinal scan alone.

While scanning peripheral vessels, it is important not to mistake a collateral that runs parallel and close to the occluded vessels for the main vessel. Identification of the vein that accompanies the artery and familiarity with the normal orientation of the vessels can help in distinguishing a parallel collateral from the main vessel as the collateral usually runs quite separate from the vein. Use of a lower frequency transducer with a wide field of view which enables visualization of both the patent segments of the native vessel and the collateral is also useful. Another useful technique is to follow the vessel from its origin to be certain of its source.

Optimizing Color Doppler and Spectral Doppler Settings[7-11]

Color Box or Color Doppler Sampling Window

The color box is a user adjustable area within the ultrasound image in which all color Doppler information is displayed. The angle of incidence of the color box can changed by angling the color box to the 'right' or 'left' so called 'steering' or by angling the transducer. As the size width and depth of color box increases frame rate decreases, image resolution and quality are affected. Thus, the box should be as small and superficial as possible while still providing the necessary information. This will maximize the frame rate. The frame rate refers to the rate at which complete images are produced. Frame rate affects the temporal resolution. With grayscale imaging alone the frame rate can exceed 50 fps but the time required to produce color images is much longer. The frame rate in color imaging is dependent on several factors. The wider the color box more the scan lines required and longer it will take to acquire data to produce the image. Increasing the depth (or height) of the box alone will not produce any major change in the frame rate, increasing the imaging depth however will require a lower PRF (due to more time for the echo to travel to and fro) hence decreasing the frame rate.

Doppler or Color Gain

Gain refers to amplification of sampled information for purposes of improving the depiction of acquired data. It controls the amplitude of color display in color or power mode and the spectral display in pulsed Doppler mode. If flow is present and the gain is set too low it is possible that no flow will be depicted on the monitor; however, an excessively high gain setting produces noise obscuring true Doppler signal and filling in the spectral waveform resulting in falsely increased flow with little meaningful quantitative flow data.

For spectral Doppler the gain should be adjusted so that the tracing should be continuous and easy to visualize without any low level noise band above and below baseline.

For color imaging the color gain should be set as high as possible without displaying random color speckles. This is set by turning it up until noise (i.e. scattered isolated color pixels overwriting grayscale pixels) is encountered and then backing off until the noise just clears. The color should just reach the intimal surface of the vessel. A high color gain setting may cause bleeding of color or blooming into the wall or even outside the vessel lumen. This impairs visualization of plaques and partial thrombi **(Figs. 17A and B)**.

Velocity Scale

This is one of the most important parameters under user control during a Doppler examination. It determines the range of velocities that are depicted with either the color or spectral component. It is not synonymous with pulse repetition frequency (PRF) but PRF is related to the velocity scale setting so that increasing the velocity scale increases the PRF and vice versa. If the velocity setting is too low for the velocities being examined, the high velocity signals will not be displayed accurately and aliasing results. Aliasing is an incorrect and paradoxical display of the colors or spectral Doppler velocity. This is related to the fact Doppler and color flow utilize pulsed beams which are transmitted and received by the transducer. The number of such pulses sent determines the pulse repetition frequency. If the Doppler shift is higher than PRF/2 or the Nyquist limit then the display wraps around the scale and appears to change direction. For spectral Doppler the velocity peak is cutoff at the top of the scale and written from the lowest portion of the scale back toward the top. On the color Doppler image aliasing is seen as color change from red to yellow to light blue to dark blue. Color aliasing projects the color of reversed flow within central areas of higher

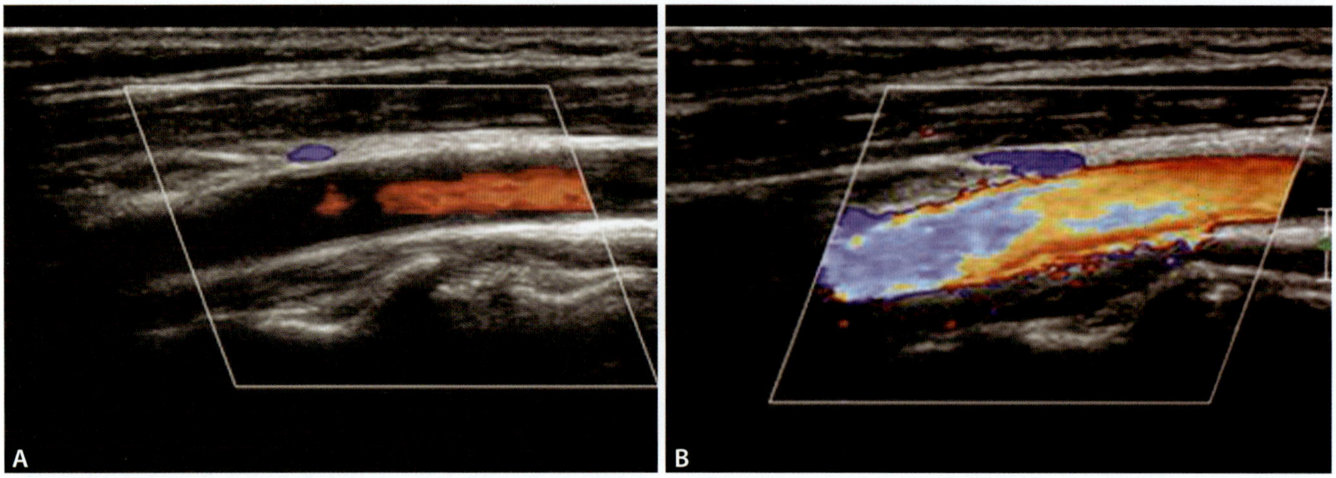

Figs. 17A and B: (A) Color Doppler images of the carotid with very-low-color gain showing incomplete color fill in the carotid; (B) Excessively high-color gain resulting in bleeding of color into the wall of the carotid and some noise in the surrounding tissues.

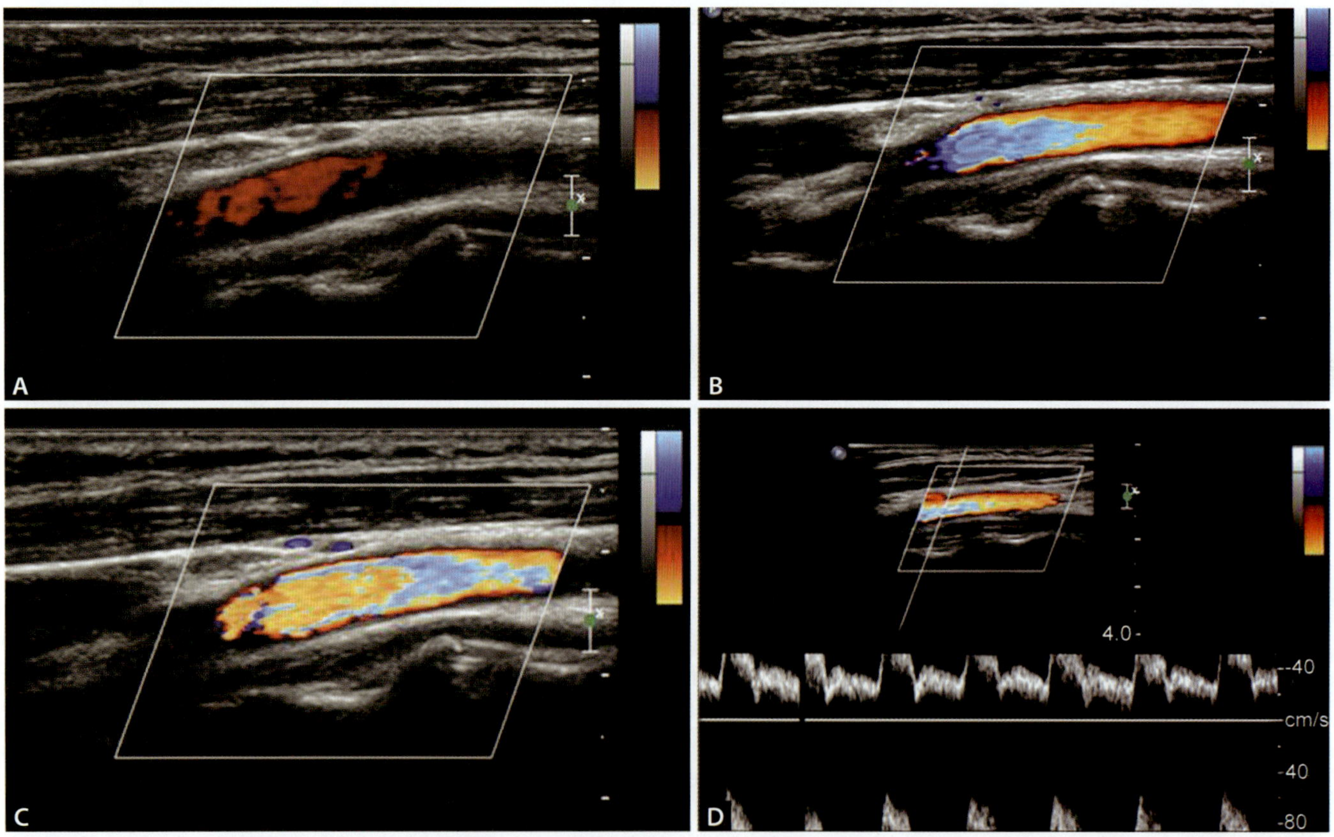

Figs. 18A to D: (A) At high PRF settings of 12000 Hz only minimal flow is seen in the carotid artery; (B) When the velocity scale is lowered to 4000 Hz complete wall-to-wall color fill is seen with an area of aliasing seen where the artery dips away from the transducer; (C) A very low PRF results in aliasing throughout the vessel; (D) Aliasing in spectral Doppler with the top of the peak being cut-off and written at the bottom.

laminar velocity. With aliasing no black stripe is seen from the low velocity filter between the reversed colors unlike flow reversal **(Figs. 18A to D)**. Higher velocities require a higher PRF for accurate sampling

Aliasing is one of the most important artifacts in Doppler and can be advantageously used to demonstrate high- or low-flow turbulence. It can be useful to quickly identify the higher velocity region within the vessel and readily place the sample volume for velocity measurement. However, if the color velocity scale is set much lower than the mean velocity of blood flow, aliasing occurs throughout the vessel lumen making it difficult to identify the high velocity turbulent jet associated with a significant stenosis. Tortuosity of a vessel can cause erroneously produce the appearance of aliasing.

The options available to reduce spectral aliasing are increasing the Doppler angle with resultant decrease Doppler shift, increasing velocity scale, changing the baseline setting or using a lower ultrasound frequency. Aliasing is not seen in power Doppler because it has no directional or velocity component.

Gate Size or Sample Volume Box

It is the user defined area from where the spectral Doppler information is obtained depicted as a pair of cross hairs within the 2D image. Although on the image it looks like a flat box, sample volume has a third dimension in and out of the plane of the image which may be up to a centimeter at times. Hence, signals may be displayed from unwanted areas of vessels or even unwanted vessels. Normally, the gate should cover approximately two thirds of the vessel lumen **(Figs. 19A and B)**. If the sample volume encompasses the entire vessel slower velocities from the vessel margins are included resulting in spectral broadening. However, if the gate is too small the Doppler signal may be missed. In addition, if the vessel is mobile as well the Doppler signal may be discontinuous with loss of diastolic signal in each cycle.

Increasing the Doppler gate is helpful when searching for trickle flow or trying to obtain a Doppler signal from behind a calcified plaque.

Sample Volume or Gate Position

The optimal position of a sample volume in a normal vessel is in the midposition parallel to the wall whereas in a diseased vessel there is some controversy whether the cursor should be angled parallel to the flow or parallel to the vessel wall. Whichever method is used the same technique must be used every time to allow reproducibility and standardization. If the sample volume is placed eccentrically too close to the vessel wall it will be degraded by signal from vessel wall motion and will also show artificial spectral broadening.

Angle Correction

In vascular applications optimal imaging of the vessel wall is obtained when the transducer is perpendicular to the vessel wall. However, this selection is not suitable for Doppler examination. In diagnostic Doppler imaging the Doppler equation is used to calculate the blood flow velocity, i.e.

$$\Delta f = (2f\,v/c)\,\cos\theta$$

where

Δf = Change in frequency

f = Original transmitted frequency

v = Velocity of blood flow

c = Speed of sound in tissue

θ = Angle of insonation.

Thus, the angle θ which is the angle between the direction of Doppler pulses and the direction of blood flow affects the frequency shift. At a Doppler angle of 0 the maximum Doppler shift is achieved as cosine of 0° equals is 1, conversely no Doppler shift will be recorded if the angle is 90° because cosine of 90° is 0. Ideally a

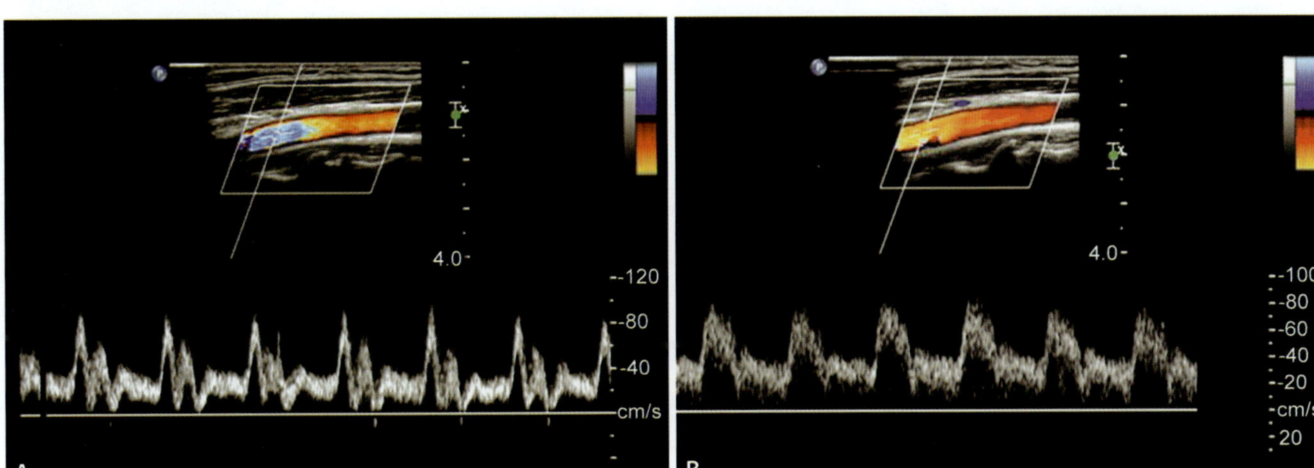

Figs. 19A and B: (A) A properly positioned sample volume in the center of the vessel covering almost 2/3rds of vessel lumen results in a spectral trace with a clear window; (B) An excessively large sample volume covering the entire vessel lumen results in inclusion of lower flow from the edges with consequent spectral widening.

small Doppler angle, i.e. less than 60° should be used approximately between 45° and 60° because within this range a linear relationship exists between Doppler shifts and velocity. The cosine of Doppler angle changes rapidly for angles more than 60°; hence, a small change in the angle is associated with a large change in the value of cos θ. Hence, a small error in estimation of Doppler angle will result in a large change in the estimated velocity producing unreliable results.

Color-write Priority

Color write priority is a setting closely related to color gain.

This selects a grayscale value above which all color information is suppressed. While larger vessels require a low setting of color-write priority, in small vessels that do no have resolvable anechoic lumen on grayscale color information can be suppressed by inappropriate color-write priority. In such a situation, color is not seen in the image even when the system has detected it. This is of particular importance in areas like the testis where the intratesticular vessels are small and Doppler is an important means of diagnosing torsion.

Baseline

The baseline is depicted on both the color bar and spectral waveform. It divides the color bar into positive and negative Doppler shifts. Baseline can be adjusted to emphasize certain aspects of flow, although the overall range of depicted velocities does not change, the depicted flow that is emphasized changes. Adjustment of baseline is one method to prevent aliasing.

Wall Filters

Wall filters selectively filter out all information below a defined frequency threshold. It eliminates the typically low-frequency–high-intensity noise that may arise from vessel wall motion. There are usually preset by the manufacturer as high, medium or low which can be applied separately to spectral, color and power imaging. The aim is to eliminate low frequency noise, but if it is set too high, it can result in the loss of signal from slow flow. In some arteries diastolic flow may be eliminated resulting in errors in calculation of Doppler indices, hence it should be kept as low as possible (typically in the range of 50–100 Hz). Filters can be applied separately to the color Doppler image or spectral Doppler depending on which scanning mode is active. On the color bar, the filter setting is indicated by a black band on both sides of the baseline. Increase in filter settings show up as widening of the black band. On spectral waveform a high wall filter wall results in loss of depicted spectral information immediately above baseline. Reducing the wall filter setting results in filling of spectral data towards the baseline.

Inversion of Flow

It is possible to electronically invert the direction of flow as depicted on both color flow and spectral waveform. This can result in red-blue color inversion on the color Doppler image and inversion of spectral waveform with spectral Doppler. Hence, flow direction in a vessel should never be presumed but carefully determined after comparing with the color bar. Misinterpretation of flow direction may erroneously suggest a malfunctioning TIPS or result in a missed flow reversal in an artery.

Directional Ambiguity

Directional ambiguity or indeterminate flow direction refers to a spectral Doppler tracing in which the waveform is displayed with nearly equal amplitude above and below the baseline in a mirror image pattern. Directional ambiguity can result when the interrogating beam intercepts the vessel at 90° (or close to 90°). If a Doppler signal is detected it is seen as a tracing both above and below the baseline. At higher gain settings directional ambiguity is worse. This can be corrected by changing the angle of interrogation.

This should be distinguished from true-bidirectional flow. In this case blood actually flows in two directions such as in the neck of a pseudoaneurysm. The clue here is that flow here is first in one direction and then in the other in the same cardiac cycle. It is never simultaneously symmetric above and below the baseline. Bidirectional flow can also be seen in the setting of high resistance organ flow such a torsion, venous thrombosis, etc. and is seen as diastolic reversal.

Slow Flow

If one is unable to visualize color flow in a vessel despite optimization of all Doppler parameters, the flow may be too slow for the color flow image to visualize. In such a situation use of power Doppler or spectral Doppler which are more sensitive to slow flow may help to detect flow. The power Doppler technique uses the intensity or power of the Doppler signal rather than the frequency shift. Strength of a Doppler signal that exceeds a particular threshold level is displayed, hence it is less angle dependent. It is also more sensitive as more extensive dynamic range can be used than with standard color Doppler imaging because noise that would overwhelm the color Doppler image can be assigned a uniform background color. The spectral wave form makes use of 256 pulse cycles per scan line and contains qualitative and quantitative diagnostic information for interpretation. The color map on the other hand contains only about 8 pulse cycles per scan line there by providing considerably less information than spectral Doppler. Also the color Doppler images display the mean frequency shift rather than the peak frequency shift.

Appropriate settings of the above mentioned Doppler parameters eliminate or greatly reduce Doppler artifacts related to machine settings. There are certain other artifacts, such as those due to anatomical factors or those unrelated to blood flow which one must be aware of to avoid misinterpreting the artifact as true flow.[7-12]

Anatomically Related Artifacts

Mirror-image artifacts

As already discussed in the section on grayscale imaging, reflection of ultrasound by an interface between zones of high and low acoustic impedance produces an image of an object on both sides, although it is located only on one side. A similar artifact can occur with color Doppler imaging most often in the supraclavicular region where mirror images of the subclavian artery or vein are caused by reflection from the pleura/lung causing apparent duplication of the vessel with the phantom vessel being projected deeper in the image. Carotid and brachial arteries may also show mirror images. Changing the scanning angle will cause the mirror artifact to disappear.

Artifacts Unrelated to Blood Flow

Pseudo flow

Pseudo-flow artifact is related to motion of fluid rather than blood flow within a vessel. The signal will appear as long as fluid motion continues. Pseudo flow may be caused by motion of ascites, amniotic fluid and urine from the ureteric orifice. It can mimic real blood flow on color or power Doppler. Spectral analysis reveals the presence of a Doppler signal but that which is atypical for a normal vessel. Some pseudo-flow artifacts, such as those seen at ureteral orifice are useful to identify the ureteric orifice and can be useful to exclude complete obstruction.

Twinkling artifact

This occurs behind a strongly reflecting granular interfaces such as urinary tract stones or parenchymal calcification.

Although primarily seen posterior to urinary calculi and parenchymal calcification it can also be seen behind any irregular highly reflective surface, biliary calculi, gallbladder adenomyosis and cholestrolosis Twinkling artifact is believed to be caused by a narrow band of intrinsic machine noise called phase (or clock) jitter. On a flat surface, system noise generates a narrow band of Doppler shift as a result of tiny clock errors. This is generally excluded by wall filters and not displayed. Rough surfaces increase the delays in measuring the signal and amplify the errors which increases the spectral bandwidth of this noise above the level of wall filter.

It is seen as rapidly fluctuating mixture of Doppler signals, i.e. red and blue pixels which imitate turbulent flow. On spectral Doppler analysis the tracing is absolutely flat suggestive of noise. The artifact is dependent on the color write priority and grayscale gain. As the color write priority decreases the twinkling artifact decreases. The key to the identification of twinkling artifact is that color is produced behind the calcification and concomitant Doppler spectral trace shows noise thus a calcified carotid plaque with twinkling can be differentiated from a potentially ulcerated plaque with flow in ulcer cavities. Also increasing the velocity scale eliminates flow signal but not twinkling **(Figs. 20A to C)**.

It is important to recognize this signal as artifactual in the gallbladder because it may simulate high velocity blood flow within a gallbladder mass suggesting the diagnosis of gallbladder carcinoma. On the other hand, the presence of twinkling artifact can be very useful for diagnosis of small stones that do not generate a strong echo. However, twinkling is not invariable. Authors suggest that calcium oxalate dihydrate and calcium phosphate calculi always produce twinkling artifact while calcium oxalate monohydrate and urate stones may lack a twinkling artifact.

Edge artifact

This is related to strong specular reflectors and is seen as steady color along the rim of calcified structures such as gall- stones or cortical bone. It is more commonly seen with power Doppler than color Doppler. The spectral Doppler tracing is characteristic being a straight line pattern equal above and below the baseline representing noise not true flow **(Figs. 21A and B)**.

Flash artifact

Flash artifact is a sudden burst of random color that fills the frame obscuring the grayscale image. It can be caused by tissue motion or transducer motion. It is most commonly seen in hypoechoic areas, such as cysts or fluids collection and in the left lobe of liver (due to cardiac pulsation). Power Doppler is more susceptible to flash artifact than color-flow Doppler because of the longer time required to build the image as more frames are averaged to create a power Doppler image than with standard color Doppler.

Flash artifact occurs due to a system setting that suppresses color pixels which would otherwise overwrite

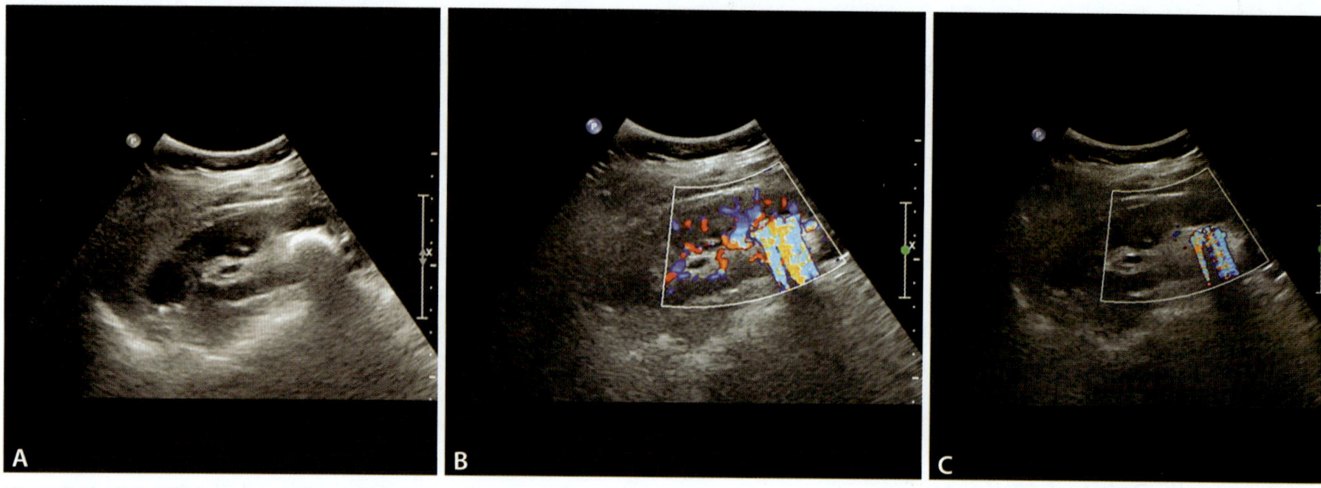

Figs. 20A to C: (A) The gray-scale image shows a large renal calculus with distal acoustic shadowing; (B) On application of color a mosaic of color is seen behind the calculus due to the twinkling artifact. Note the presence of flow in the intrarenal vessels as well; (C) On increasing the velocity scale, the intrarenal flow disappears but the twinkling artifact persists.

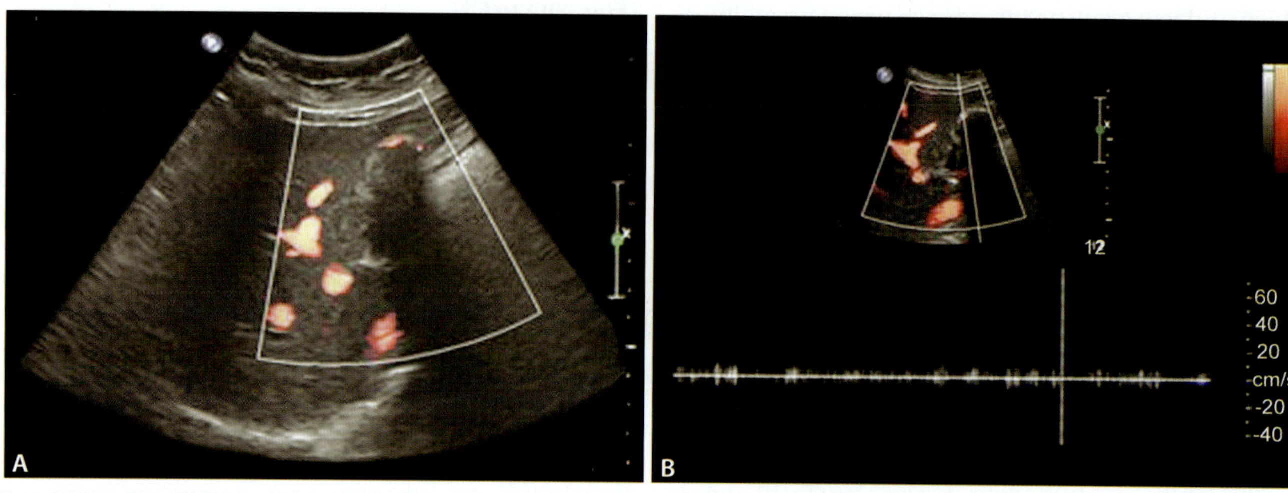

Figs. 21A and B: (A) Edge artifact: Power Doppler image showing steady color along the rim of a gallbladder calculus; (B) The spectral trace is characteristic of noise being a straight-line pattern above and below the baseline.

grayscale echoes or the color write priority. In the absence of grayscale echoes, color pixels take priority so that flow is seen in nearly stationary fluid. The artifact is transitory coinciding with transducer or patient motion such as respiration or cardiac pulsation and hence can be easily interpreted. In fact the flash artifact may at times be used to denote fluid nature of solid appearing material.

Perivascular or Color-bruit Artifact

This is a tissue motion artifact in which movement is generated within an organ rather than involving an entire organ or image. It is seen as a color mosaic in soft tissue (rather than a single homogeneous color) adjacent to vessels with turbulent flow and is thought to be caused by actual vascular tissue vibration. These artifacts are more common with low PRF as a result of increased sensitivity of the system but may also be caused by low wall filter setting.

This artifact is the imaging equivalent of an auditory bruit or palpable thrill. It varies with the cardiac cycle being most prominent in systole and least in diastole. It is commonly seen in association with anastamotic sites, stenotic arteries or arteriovenous fistulae and can be useful to detect their presence.

SPECIAL IMAGING MODES[1-3,10,13-16]

The modern imaging systems incorporate a number of special imaging modes involving advances in beamforming, ultrasound signal acquisition, and postprocessing to deal with inherent artifacts in ultrasound and improve image quality.

Tissue-harmonic Imaging

Difference in propagation velocity of ultrasound between tissues such as fat and other soft tissues, near the transducer results in phase aberrations that distort the ultrasound field producing noise and clutter. In addition, the focusing of the ultrasound beam depends on phase coherence of the sound waves at the focal zone and at the transducer surface during receive focusing. If the intervening tissue has heterogeneous velocities defocusing will occur because the waves no longer coincide precisely, degrading lateral resolution. Tissue harmonic imaging provides a means to reduce the effects of phase aberrations. The term harmonic refers to frequencies that are integral multiples of true frequency of the transmitted pulse which is called the fundamental frequency or first harmonic. The second harmonic has a frequency twice the fundamental.

Harmonics are generated due to the non-linear propagation of sound waves in the tissues. The wave velocity is higher for high pressure waves, i.e. compression than low pressure component, i.e. rarefaction. This causes increasing distortion of the ultrasound pulse as it travels through the tissue changing the wave pattern from a perfect sinusoidal shape to a sharper saw tooth shape. This generates waves of higher frequencies which are multiple of the fundamental frequency (2nd, 3rd, 4th, etc.) which are referred to as harmonics **(Fig. 22)**. The intensity decreases as the order of the harmonics increases. In addition, the higher-frequency harmonics are also attenuated more. Hence, current harmonic imaging is mostly performed using the second harmonic component (Work is in progress in order to utilize higher-order harmonics or the so called superharmonic imaging and frequencies lower than the transmitted frequency or subharmonic imaging for use with ultrasound contrast media). The final image is formed by the harmonic frequency bandwidth in the received signal after eliminating the transmitted frequency by frequency filtering, pulse inversion/phase cancellation or coded harmonics.

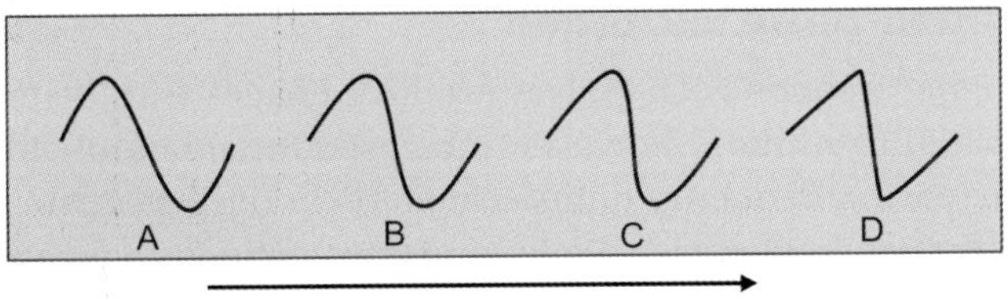

Fig. 22: Generation of harmonics: As the path length through the tissue increases the sinusoidal waveform (A). Changes to a more saw tooth pattern with higher frequency due to the compression wave traveling faster than the rarefaction wave (D).

The generation of harmonics requires interaction of transmitted pulse with the propagating tissues; hence, harmonic generation is not important near the transducer or skin surface and becomes important only some distance away from the transducer. Harmonic images therefore show good rejection of artifacts and clutter arising from the body wall and also reduce the defocusing effect of the body wall. Artifacts are also reduced in harmonic imaging as the amplitude of the harmonic waves is relatively small reducing detection of echoes from multiple scatters. In addition artifacts produced by the fundamental frequency and side lobes do not have sufficient energy to generate harmonic frequencies and are therefore filtered out during image formation. Penetration can be improved by using a low-fundamental transmitted pulse and imaging at the higher-harmonic frequency.

Other advantages include improved axial resolution due to shorter wavelength and better lateral resolution due to improved focusing with higher frequencies. Also because harmonics originate in regions of the ultrasound pulse with the greatest pressure amplitude, i.e. near the pulse center (as the amplitude at the periphery is too weak to generate harmonics) it results in a narrower beam producing images with superior lateral and elevational resolution. Harmonic images thus show less haze, noise, clutter and better cyst clearance **(Figs. 23A and B)**.

The technique is most useful in patients with thick complicated body wall structure or the so-called difficult patients for mid field imaging. At greater depths harmonic signals begin to decrease substantially relative to fundamental signal due to increased attenuation.

COMPOUND IMAGING

Compound imaging is the ability to aquire multiple frames from different frequencies, i.e. **frequency-compound imaging** or from different angles, i.e. **spatial-compound imaging**. Frequency compounding is the combination of multiple images detected from different frequency bands into a single image. This reduces noise and speckle as the appearance of speckle varies with frequency. This is possible with the use of broad band width transducers.

Spatial-compound Imaging

In spatial-compound imaging electronic steering of ultrasound beams from an array transducer is used to image the same tissue multiple times by using parallel

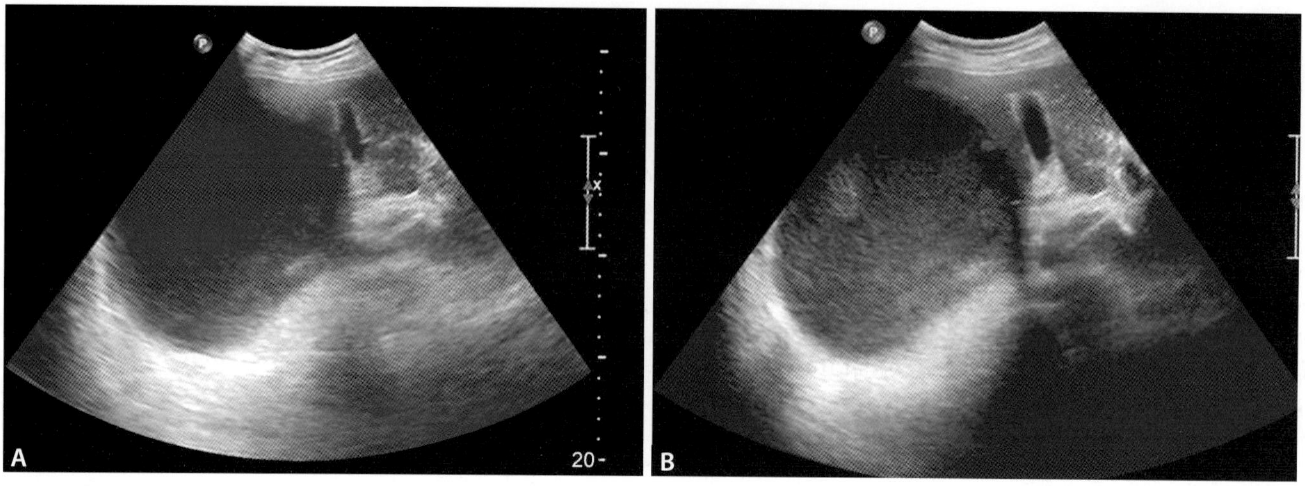

Figs. 23A and B: (A) A transverse scan of the liver in a relatively obese patient with a large-right-lobe abscess. Although the abscess is visualized in the image without harmonics; (B) The margins of the abscess, its internal echopattern and the diaphragm are much better appreciated in the harmonic-imaging mode.

beams oriented in different directions. Data from many such beam lines is acquired and averaged together into a single image. The appearance of speckle varies according to the beam line direction, averaging echoes from different directions tends to average and smooth speckle making the images look less grainy. Since speckle noise is random it cancels out during compounding while signal is reinforced.

Spatial compounding is also useful to image specular reflectors. Relatively large smooth surfaces reflect sound like a mirror with angle of incidence being equal to angle of reflection. Such specular reflectors include diaphragm, wall of urinary bladder, endometrial stripe, etc. Since the ultrasound beam is not dispersed like scatters, the signals are much stronger but are highly directional. Display of specular interfaces is therefore highly dependent on angle of insonation and specular reflectors return echoes to the transducer only if the sound beam is perpendicular to the interface. As the surface is titled away from 90° the signal intensity falls rapidly (as the sound beam is reflected away from the transducer). This results in poor margin definition and less distinct boundaries for cysts and other masses in conventional imaging where each scan line used to generate the image. It is of particular importance in sonography of the **musculoskeletal system** because of the anisotropic nature of muscles and tendons. The fibrillar pattern of a tendon is best appreciated when the ultrasound beam is perpendicular to the tendon and appears relatively echo-poor at oblique angles simulating tears or tendinosis. In spatial compound imaging since the image is generated from more than one angle of insonation the chances that at at least one of these is perpendicular to the specular reflector is greater, reducing anisotropic effects improving tissue plane definition and display of curved structures.

Spatial-compound images show reduced levels of speckle, noise, clutter and refractive shadows and improve contrast and margin definition. Enhancement and shadowing artifacts may be reduced which may be an advantage or potential drawback depending on the clinical situation **(Figs. 24A and B)**.

Another drawback is that because multiple US beams are used to image one tissue region instead of just one beam as in conventional B-mode imaging more time is required for data acquisition and processing so the compound frame rate is reduced compared to conventional B-mode imaging depending on the processing capabilities of the imaging system.

Spatial compounding can also be achieved by using a single transmit pulse and varying the crystals that receive. This typically maintains higher frame rates as less transmit pulses are used.

Coded-pulse Excitation

Higher frequency US pulses produce images with better spatial resolution, however, increased attenuation with increasing frequency limits evaluation of deep structures with high frequencies. Coded-pulse excitation is a means of overcoming this limitation providing good penetration at higher frequencies necessary for high-spatial resolution. This technique uses longer ultrasound pulses instead of the routinely used short ultrasound pulses. These longer

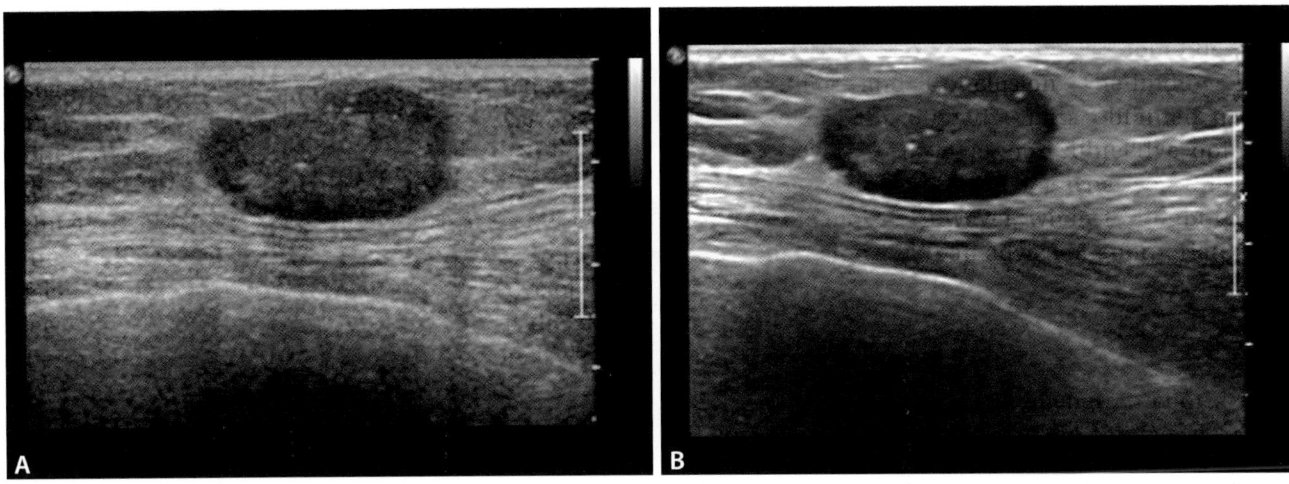

Figs. 24A and B: Fibroadenoma of the breast imaged without (A) and with spatial-compound imaging (B). The margins of the lesion, internal architecture and calcifications are better visualized. Note the reduced edge shadows.

pulses carry greater ultrasound energy, which increases the energy of echoes that return from the deeper tissues allowing use of higher frequencies. The coded pulses are produced with a very characteristic shape and the returning echoes also have a similar shape, which makes their identification from background noise easier **(Fig. 25)**. The returning echoes are then processed using a pulse-compression technique in which the location of the long characteristic pulse shapes are identified. These pulse shape locations may be determined with a tight-spatial tolerance and correspond to the location of structures from where they are reflected. Hence, the location of reflectors is identified with good spatial resolution. This produces an image with good echo signal and good spatial resolution at greater depths.

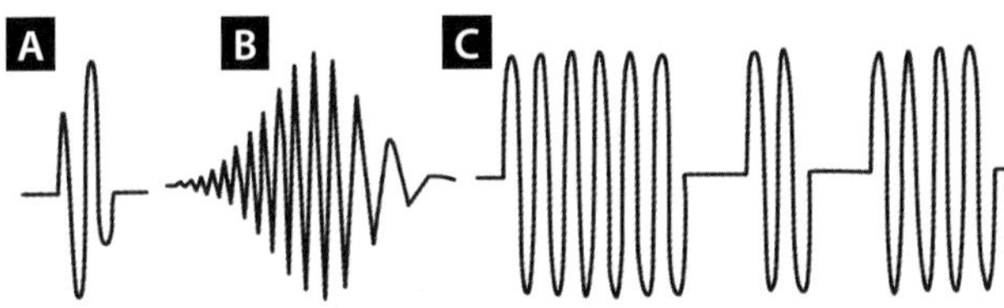

Fig. 25: (A) Normal pulse; (B) A chirp pulse; (C) A coded pulse.

Adaptive-image Processing

An adaptive-image processing algorithm is one that able to recognize the difference between real targets and artifacts, and to modify its processing accordingly. Multiresolution adaptive image processing algorithms to smooth speckle and enhance structural edges are now available (e.g. XRES Philips).

It involves an analysis phase (in which artifacts and targets are identified) and an enhancement phase (in which artifacts are suppressed and targets enhanced). The analysis phase takes into account multiple characteristics of the target, such as local statistical properties, textural and structural properties. The textural and structural information in particular is vital for identifying the strength and orientation of interfaces and thus allowing directional filtering of these targets in the enhancement phase. For example, smoothing is applied along an interface to improve continuity, while edge enhancement is applied in the perpendicular direction. In regions identified by the analysis phase as being homogeneous, smoothing is applied equally in all directions.

Photopic-ultrasound Imaging

This technique can be use to optimize image contrast. Gray levels are converted to monochromatic color value, allowing very subtle structural differences to be appreciated.

Extended Field of View Imaging

Early static B-mode scanners had a large field of view (FOV) which was lost with the introduction of real-time scanning. Extended-FOV imaging restores the capability of visualizing large anatomic regions in a single image.

The transducer is translated across the region of interest, during which multiple images are acquired from multiple transducer positions. Image features in regions of overlap between successive images are used to determine the exact position of the multiple images relative to each other by the scanner. The images are thus registered with respect to each other accounting for both translation and in plane rotation of the transducer. The registered image data is processed in a large image buffer and combined to form the large FOV image. It is a useful image presentation format

B-Mode Flow Imaging

B-mode flow imaging is a new method for flow imaging available in ultrasound. This technique shows blood flow with grayscale or B-mode imaging and is not a Doppler method. For B flow imaging digitally encoded wide band pulses are transmitted and reflected from moving blood cells. The returning echoes are decoded and filtered to increase sensitivity of moving scatterers and distinguish blood from tissue. Both the surrounding stationary tissue and flowing blood are shown in shades of gray.

As this is not a Doppler technique no velocity or frequency information is provided. It is a purely visual nonquantitative method. The major advantage is that it allows precise definition of the boundary between flowing blood and vessel wall. There is no problem of blooming or over amplification of flow signals as this is a non-Doppler technique. The technique does not degrade the spatial or temporal resolution of the grayscale image unlike color Doppler and is more accurate in showing the extent of plaque and surface irregularity of the plaque as compared to color Doppler or grayscale imaging alone in superficial vessels.

The technique is, however, most useful in superficial vessels as it relies on amplification of very weak echoes from red blood cells.

3D–4D Ultrasound

Although 3D–4D technology has been available in ultrasound for years it is mainly used in cardiology, obstetrics and gynecology. Uses in other areas are being gradually explored.

Among the primary approaches used for 3D data acquisition are the free hand scanning, mechanical devices integrated into the transducer and matrix array technology.

The 4D refers to real-time acquisition of 3D data set. Volume data is generally displayed using three primary methods, multiplanar images (3 slices orthogonal to each other) and rendered images that show entire structures throughout volume.

The 3D/4D ultrasound, provides the ability to acquire the entire volume at one time so that there is no risk of missing out details which were not included in the original scan. Organ volumes, especially of irregularly shaped organs may be more accurately measured using volume data, 3D data results in more reproducible measurements can thereby assist in monitoring therapy and allow better definition of fetal facial features, uterine congenital anomalies, etc.

CONCLUSION

With increasing technological advances, applications of ultrasound and Doppler have grown tremendously both for detection of pathology and physiology. Gaining maximum benefit from this complex technology requires a combination of skills, including knowledge of physical principles that empower ultrasound with its unique diagnostic unique capabilities. With this information the radiologist can gather maximum information from each examination while avoiding pitfalls and errors in diagnosis that may result from omission of information or misinterpretation of artifacts. Careful attention to technical parameters, appropriate use of special imaging features and diligence of examination technique will avoid day-to-day scanning pitfalls and result in studies with improved diagnostic accuracy.

REFERENCES

1. Hangiandreou NJ. B-mode US: basic concepts and new technology. Radiographics. 2003;23(4):1019-33. Review.
2. Merrit Christopher RB. Physics of ultrasound in Diagnostic ultrasound vol 1, 3rd edn. Rheumack Wilson SR Charboneau JW (Eds). Elsevier. 2005.pp.3-34.
3. Cosgrove D. Artefacts in B mode imaging in Abdominal and general ultrasound vol 1, 2nd edn. Meire H, Cosgrove D, Dewbury K, Farrant P (Eds). Churchill Livingstone; 2001. pp. 47-65.
4. Rubens DJ, Bhatt S, Nedelka S, Cullinan J. Doppler artifacts and pitfalls. Radiol Clin North Am. 2006;44(6): 805-35.
5. Farina Robrterto Saparano Amelia. Errors in ultrasonography in Errors in Radiology. Luigia Romano Antonio Pinto (Eds). Springer Verlag. 2012.pp.76-85.
6. Feldman MK, Katyal S, Blackwood MS. US artifacts. Radiographics. 2009;29(4):1179-89.
7. Acampara Ciro, Fabia Pinto, Magistris Giuseppe De Errors in color Doppler ultrasonography in Errors in Radiology. Springer Verlag; 2012.pp.86-103.
8. Tahmasebpour HR, Buckley AR, Cooperberg PL, Fix CH. Sono graphic examination of the carotid arteries. Radiographics. 2005;25(6):1561-75.
9. Kruskal JB, Newman PA, Sammons LG, Kane RA. Optimizing Doppler and color flow US: application to hepatic sonography. Radiographics. 2004;24(3):657-75.
10. Zagzebski James A. Physics in Doppler and B-mode ultrasound in Introduction to vascular sonography, 6th edn. Pellirito, Polak (Eds). Elsevier; 2012.pp.20-51.

11. Campbell SC, Cullinan JA, Rubens DJ. Slow flow or no flow? Color and power Doppler US pitfalls in the abdomen and pelvis. Radiographics. 2004;24(2):497-506.
12. Rahmouni A, Bargoin R, Herment A, Bargoin N, Vasile N. Color Doppler twinkling artifact in hyperechoic regions. Radiology. 1996;199(1):269-71.
13. Choudhry S, Gorman B, Charboneau JW, Tradup DJ, Beck RJ, Kofler JM, Groth DS. Comparison of tissue harmonic imaging with conventional US in abdominal disease. Radiographics. 2000;20(4):1127-35.
14. Rosenthal SJ, Jones PH, Wetzel LH. Phase inversion tissue harmonic sonographic imaging: a clinical utility study. Am J Roentgenol. 2001;176(6):1393-8.
15. Desser TS, Jeffrey RB. Tissue harmonic imaging techniques: physical principles and clinical applications. Semin Ultrasound CT MR. 2001;22(1):1-10.
16. Lin DC, Nazarian LN, O'Kane PL, McShane JM, Parker L, Merritt CR. Advantages of real-time spatial compound sonography of the musculoskeletal system versus conventional sonography. Am J Roentgenol. 2002;179(6):1629-31.

CHAPTER 40

Ultrasound Elastography: Principles and Application

Veenu Singla, Tulika Singh, Anindita Sinha

INTRODUCTION

Elastography is a noninvasive technique of imaging stiffness or elasticity of tissues by measuring movement or deformation of tissue in response to a small applied pressure. It is a method of "virtual palpation" of tissue or lesions, which has the potential to overcome the subjectivity associated with clinical palpation. It can also provide objective and quantitative measures of tissue stiffness.

BASIC PHYSICS

Some common terminologies like stress, strain, shear, elasticity, viscoelasticity and Hooke's law and Young's modulus are often used and a basic understanding of these is required to understand elastography.

Stress

Stress is defined as force per unit area. Unit of stress is Pascal or pounds per square inch (psi) (Pascal = Newton/m^2). Stress can be due to compression, which acts perpendicular to a surface and causes shortening of an object. Shear stress acts parallel to a surface and causes deformation.

In elastography, stress can be applied exogenously by transducer compression, vibrators or acoustic radiation force. Endogenous motion of vessels, cardiac or respiratory motion can also be utilized. Although endogenous sources overcome the shortcomings of exogenous source like attenuation (e.g. due to obesity or ascities), endogenous stress is difficult to quantify.[1]

Strain

When subjected to stress an object tends to undergo deformation of its original size and shape; the amount of deformation is known as strain. Longitudinal strain, like compression causes change in length of an object. Shear strain causes changes in angles of an object.

Strain is unitless, expressed as change in length per unit length of the object. So hard objects have lower strain values than softer objects. When compression is applied, lesions nearer the applied force undergo more displacement than objects lying in a deeper plane. This is similar to clinical difficulty in palpating deep seated lesions and is one of the factors which may influence efficacy of elastography.

Elasticity

The property of materials to return back to its original form after stress is removed, is known as elasticity. Elastic materials strain immediately when stressed and also return quickly back to their original position.

Viscosity

Viscosity is the measure of resistance of a fluid when it under-goes shear stress or tensile (compression or stretching) stress.

Viscoelasticity

This is the property of materials to exhibit both viscous and elastic properties. In viscoelastic material like soft tissue, there is a time delay between application of force and displacement. When stress is applied, the strain increases rapidly as free fluid in soft tissues is exuded. Then, the relationship of stress over strain becomes linear for small changes.

Poroelasticity

A material in which a solid matrix is permeated by an interconnecting network of fluid filled pores.

Tissue may be viscoelastic, poroelastic, anisotropic (e.g. muscle fibers or nerve fibers oriented in a particular direction) or contractile or a combination of these and disease conditions may modify their character.

Elastography techniques which can estimate visco/poroelasticity, give a more accurate estimate of tissue conditions than techniques where simple stress, strain or Young's modulus is measured, as here tissue is assumed to be a homogeneous and isotropic material.

Hooke's law states that stress is proportional to the strain within an object's elastic limit. Young's modulus (E) is the ratio of stress over strain and has the same unit as stress. Young's modulus measures the tissue's resistance to compression.

Hooke's law holds true for homogeneous isotropic solids. Softer tissues like fat undergo more deformation (strain) when stress (e.g. compression during palpation) is applied. Harder tissues like muscle and fibrous tissue resist strain and thus have a higher Young's modulus.[2-4]

Poisson's ratio: When exposed to stress, tissue may contract in one dimension (like width) while its length increases.

Poisson's ratio = lateral contraction per unit breadth/longitudinal extension per unit length.[5]

Poisson's ratio for normal soft tissue is 0.5.

Shear modulus: Shear modulus or modulus of rigidity (G) is the ratio between shear stress and shear strain.

Elasticity imaging can be based on imaging either strain, stress or Young's modulus, shear modulus or shear wave velocity imaging.

DEPICTION OF ELASTOGRAMS

Elastograms are generally viewed simultaneously with a sonogram to identify area of abnormality. This can be done with either grayscale depiction or a semitransparent color overlay of the elastogram over the sonogram.

On grayscale elastograms, stiffer lesions are darker and appear to increase in size when compared to sonograms. On color overlay images, blue and green depicts stiff areas and red to yellow denotes soft areas.

DIFFERENT ELASTOGRAPHY TECHNIQUES

Elastographic techniques vary depending upon:

- The method used for tissue excitement (either mechanical or ultrasonic force)
- By the response of tissue to compression, i.e. static or quasistatic, where a single compression is applied or dynamic system in which response to rapid compression or vibration is measured.

Compression Elastography

Compression elastography is calculating a strain profile in a direction perpendicular to the tissue surface in response to an externally applied force. This technique is most widely used in different ultrasound systems to evaluate the elastic properties of the tissues by analyzing the radiofrequency pulses generated by a structure in response to external compression.[6] Compression causes deformation of the tissue that varies as a function of the elastic coefficient. This principle is expressed by Young's modulus of elasticity.[7] RF waveform before and after compression are windowed and the signals in the same segment are compared to calculate the displacement. Around 97% of transmitted ultrasound waves are absorbed, only 3% of energy is scattered. Scattering occurs at the tissue boundaries, especially collagenous and fat surfaces.

Tracking of displacement of this scatter in real-time is the objective of strain imaging.[8] A simple approach to extract elasticity information from soft tissue involves acquiring maps of the tissues before and after the compression **(Fig. 1)**. Radiofrequency echo signals are typically the "map of tissue" used and tiny motion induces a change in the phase of radiofrequency echoes that can be tracked.[9] The amount of shift in the signal equals the amount of tissue displacement at the point in the image frame. This

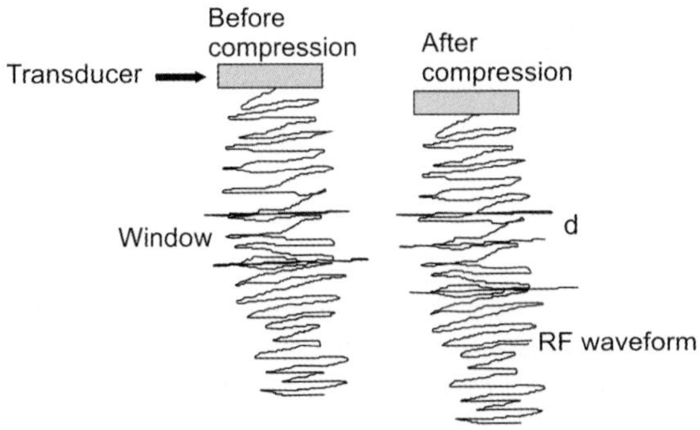

Fig. 1: The windowed segment of scattered RF waveform is cross-correlated with the waveform obtained pre- and postcompression. The amount of shift between the matching segments is equal to tissue displacement (d).

rate of change values is known as strain. Specialized software is used to calculate the relative difference in the tissue movement from one frame to another and then to estimate the tissue deformation.[10]

Three methods have been introduced for measuring tissue strain at elastography are spatial correlation method, phase shift tracking method and combined autocorrelation method. The spatial correlation method is 2D pattern matching algorithm to search for the position that maximizes the cross correlation between ROIs selected from two images. The phase shift tracking method is based on autocorrelation method and can be used rapidly and precisely to determine longitudinal tissue motion because of phase domain processing. This method fails when used for large displacement and it poorly compensates for lateral movement known as lateral slip.[11]

To overcome this problem, a method known as combined autocorrelation method is employed, which enables rapid and accurate detection of longitudinal displacement by using phase domain processing without aliasing.[12] Clinical implementation typically involves freehand scanning, which requires real-time implementation for instant feedback to the user to control the direction of deformation.[13] Hard or stiff materials tend to move as a whole with all points displacing with the same amount on compression, which results in zero or small rate of change of displacement called as zero or no strain. Softer tissue shows larger change in rate of displacement versus depth giving large strain values. The deformation measurement is mapped on elastogram on which stiffer areas are depicted as dark and elastic area lighter. This actually allows the differentiation of the lesion, which otherwise isoechoic on grayscale ultrasound image.[10] Free hand scanning is usually induced at a rate resulting in nearly completely elastic deformation making interpretation much easier than it otherwise. The most common clinical application is breast imaging. But any organ which can be clinically palpated has been scanned for elastography including breast, prostate, thyroid muscle and lymph node.

Limitations

The amount of tissue displacement and the rate of change in displacement vary with the amount of compression applied. Hence, the tissue strain is dependent on the amount of the compression applied and it does not quantify the intrinsic elastic property of the given tissue. This makes it operator dependent. It is a qualitative imaging of relative stiffness, so the actual strain value cannot be compared with the next imaging.[6] However, it can be used as semiquantitative elastography with evaluation of strain ratio, which is the ratio of strain between the lesion and adjoining normal tissue. Because it shows only changes in strain from one area to other in the same image, hence it is suitable for the detection and evaluation of the small focal lesion and not sensitive to the diffuse disease process that produces same stiffness all over in one image.

Acoustic Radiation Force Impulse

Principle and Technique

Acoustic radiation force impulse (ARFI) imaging is a technique where short duration acoustic forces known as pushing pulses are used to cause tissue displacements. No external or physiological (pulsation or respiration) compression is needed. The cessation of force causes tissue to return to its original position. Pushing pulses can be applied by the ultrasound transducer array (frequency of 2–7 MHz) to a volume of 2 mm^3 for 1 ms per pulse resulting in a displacement of 10–20 m. Pushing frequency is in the lower end of the transducer bandwidth, and the transmit voltage is at the upper end of the system capability. The pushing pulses are similar to those for power Doppler imaging; however, they are much longer in duration (200 cycles vs 10 cycles).

Measurement

Ultrasound pulses track these displacements by locating change in the peak along multiple tracking lines. The excitation can be performed in a sequential fashion by translating the tracking line along the tissue to assess the response. Parallel acquisition of push pulses and tracking displacements can also be done. Peak displacement, time taken to reach peak displacement and recovery time are utilized to characterize tissue response.

Tissue recoil also generates shear waves, which propagate away from the focal point of excitation. The speed of the shear waves is proportional to the tissue stiffness. Shear modulus can be calculated from the shear wave velocity **(Fig. 2)**. Mapping shear-wave velocity (cm/sec or m/sec) at multiple lateral points from the region of excitation can generate quantitative measurements of tissue stiffness.

Quantitative versus Qualitative

In lesion identification and monitoring ablation procedures, higher spatial resolution qualitative images are required. Quantitative analysis is required for diffuse stiffening associated with advanced liver fibrosis,

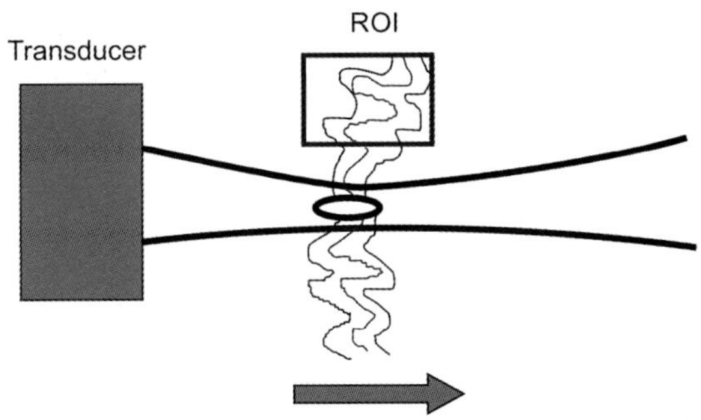

Fig. 2: Schematic diagram for shear wave sonography: Longitudinal acoustic pulse transmission causes tissue displacement. Shear waves propagate away perpendicular to transmitted pulse. Separate tracking pulses in the region of interest (ROI) track these shear waves. The stiffer the tissue, faster the shear-wave velocity.

differentiation of malignant and benign lesions based upon their absolute stiffness, and monitoring of disease progression and response to therapy.

Advantages

The ARFI images are found to be more homogeneous and have better contrast than surface displacement (compression) elastography. Deeper tissue, not accessible by superficial external compression elastography can be evaluated.

Disadvantages

Physiological (respiration, pulsation) and transducer motion can degrade image quality as 1-3 ms is required per tracking line pair. Lower ultrasound frequencies and motion compensation techniques like premonitory physiological motion and subtracting this expected motion have been applied to overcome these limitations.[5,14]

Tissues at a depth of more than 10 cm cannot be accurately assessed due to attenuation of the radiation force at greater depths.

Safety

Peak temperature increase for one pushing pulse from a single excitation is largest near the focal point. The typical temperature rise associated with an individual excitation ranges from 0.02°C to 0.2°C, varying primarily as a function of transmit frequency and pulse duration. The duration of pushing pulses and the frame rate is limited to keep within the standard diagnostic limits of mechanical and thermal index.[15]

Shear-wave Imaging

Principle and Technique

Shear waves are induced remotely within tissue when an impulsive acoustic radiation force of a focused ultrasound beam produced by the transducer interacts with tissue.

Shear waves propagate perpendicular to the axial displacement caused by the ultrasound pulse and attenuate about 10,000 times more rapidly than compression waves.[5] The high attenuation of shear waves enables mechanical oscillations to be induced within a very limited area of tissue. Deformations by the focused ultrasound radiation are generally very small (at submicron level). Sophisticated signal processing is required to detect such motion differences. A shear wave is created and tracked at lateral, spatially offset positions from the radiation force excitation by a parallel tracking method **(Fig. 2)**.[5,9]

Measurement

Velocity of shear waves (in cms^{-1}) can be measured and used to evaluate tissue stiffness by calculating the elastic Young's modulus according to the formula: $E = 3V^2$ (E—Young's modulus in kPa, V—shear wave velocity in cms^{-1}).

Qualitative versus Quantitative

This technique results in both qualitative color coded elastogram and also quantitative maps either of elasticity (in kPa) or of shear-wave velocity (in cms^{-1}).

Advantages

Lack of tissue compression makes it a more objective meas-urement, the direct assessment of elasticity and the quantita-tive measurements are provided.

Disadvantages

Assessment of superficial structures may be difficult, as a certain depth of ultrasound penetration is needed for shear waves to be produced.

Advances in Shear-wave Imaging

1. *Spatially modulated ultrasound radiation force (SMURF):* In this technique, a linear array transducer is used to acquire a reference scan at a specified position. Two pushing pulses are then transmitted and focused at the same depth laterally from the original position. This is followed by a series of scan lines, from which

the induced shear-wave peaks are estimated. This allows fast and accurate estimation of shear modulus with improved resolution.[16]

2. *Supersonic shear-wave imaging:* In supersonic shear-wave imaging, the focus of the radiation force from one location is changed to different depths (typically five) along the beam axis. Shear waves are created at multiple locations and these interfere constructively to create a conical shear wave front like a Mach cone of an aircraft traveling at supersonic speed.

   Imaging the shear-wave propagation requires an ultrafast scanner capable of 5000 frames per second. This is achieved by elimination of focusing of the pulses used for motion detection. One plane wave or a set of plane waves is transmitted with different angular direction to track the shear wave. B-mode data is also acquired in real time at about 50 frames per second.
   Measurement: Shear-wave propagation is measured and wave speeds are assessed to give viscoelastic moduli.[17]
3. *Axial shear-strain imaging:* Malignant lesions tend to be more tightly bound to surrounding tissue than benign lesions. Axial shear strain images as how tightly the lesion is fixed to the surrounding tissue. Loosely bound lesions have a thin band of color at the boundary whereas malignant lesions have a much thicker band. This simple depiction is much easier to interpret than elastography images.[18]

Harmonic-motion Imaging

Technique

Low frequency ultrasound (10–300 Hz) produces oscillations in tissue, which is measured at the center of vibration. Two separate focused ultrasound transducers are used. One transducer has a very large aperture, which is used to generate the radiation force. A small phased array transducer placed through a hole in the larger transducer detects motion.

Application

The same transducer, which generates the radiation force, can be utilized for creating thermal lesions. This allows real-time and simultaneous generation and monitoring of high-intensity focused ultrasound (HIFU) therapy. Tissue stiffening signifying successful ablation can be monitored and the treatment procedure can be performed in a time-efficient manner. Real-time monitoring of RF ablation of arrhythmogenic foci in the heart may help spare the surrounding healthy myocardium from ablation.[19]

Shear-dispersion Ultrasound Vibrometry

Technique

This involves creating a shear-wave by an external actuator or by acoustic radiation force. Multiple pushing pulses or excitation pulses are transmitted at a particular frequency and motion stimulated at harmonic frequencies is detected by ultrasound.

Measurement

Shear-wave speed dispersion is measured from the data generated at several frequencies. Dispersion of shear-wave gives a measurement of the viscoelastic properties of tissue.

Mechanical Imaging

Stress patterns of internal structures of tissue are measured by compressing the tissue by an ultrasound probe. Pressure sensors mounted on the contact surface of the probe detects the temporal and spatial changes in stress pattern, thus providing information about the different elastic properties (viscosity and porosity).

Measurement

Surface stress data is recorded, allowing 2D and 3D reconstruction of tissues on the basis of elasticity. Nonlinear elasticity imaging which is most sensitive to cancerous changes can be evaluated by mechanical imaging.[20]

Application

Detection of cancer and differentiating benign from malignant lesions.

ELASTOGRAPHY APPLICATIONS

Breast

As the breast cancer tissue is harder than the adjoining normal breast parenchyma, because of its desmoplastic reaction, the evaluation of breast masses to differentiate benign lesion from malignant was one of the initial application of the ultrasound elastography.[21] Initially elastograms were done by using a computer controlled device, which needed precise control of amount of compression which is typically very small (0.1–0.5 mm). It was slow and very few elastogram could be taken. It also needs postprocessing. Over a period of time, hand held compression with the ultrasound transducer was substituted with more recently developed real-time processing.[22]

The evaluation of hardness has the same principle of conventional clinical examination, i.e., palpation of any breast lump. Initial clinical work in this field appeared in 1997 and showed that cancer generally appeared stiffer (darker) than benign lesion and surrounding normal breast tissue.[23] Cancerous lesions almost invariably appeared larger on elastography. Other authors demonstrate the use of color maps to depict the tissue stiffness.[11] A proposed scoring system for the lesions on color maps is based upon elastographic properties of the tissue.

Elastosonographic Score (Fig. 3)

Score 1: Presence of even strain in the lesion (green)

Score 2: Prevalence of green with few, if any blue spots with inconstant locations

Score 3: Prevalently green but with central blue area

Score 4: Almost completely blue, with few green points, most of all in periphery.

Score 5: Completely blue, also with a peripheral glow around the nodule.

For elastography score when cut-off point is taken between 3 and 4 for the malignant lesion, it showed 86.5% sensitivity, 89.8% specificity and 88.3% accuracy in one study.[11] This gives information about local strain estimated at a given location in tissues, but it depends on surrounding mechanical properties and it is not quantitative **(Figs. 4 to 7)**.[24]

Recently, the methods of semiquantitative assessment of the breast lesions with strain ratio between the nodule and the adjoining normal breast tissue is used for the differentiation of benign versus malignant nodule have been developed.[25] With freehand compression, the influence of probe movement has certain limitation as the elasticity map obtained is highly dependent on the organ's compressibility limits under pressure and on the extent of tissue compression applied. This makes it operator dependent. To overcome this problem, the quantitative methods are developed with assessment of the shear module, which is overall tissue stiffness like shear wave elastography and supersonic shear imaging.

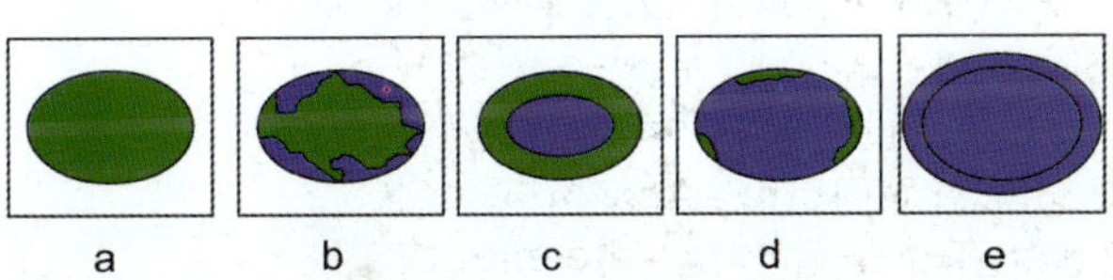

Fig. 3: Colored diagrams representing the general appearance of elasticity score breast nodule in Tsukuba scoring of 1(a), 2(b), 3(c), 4(d) and 5(e).

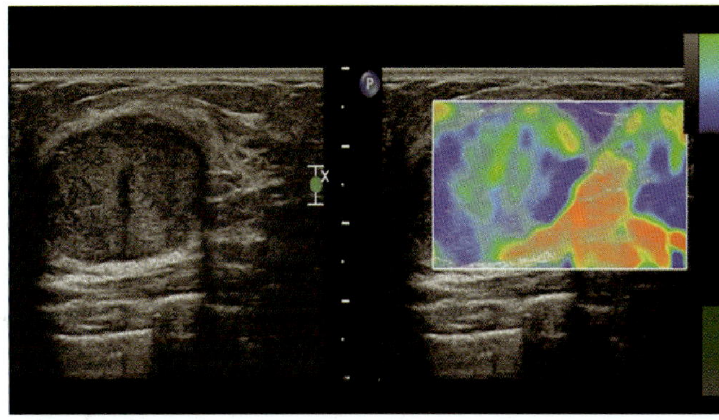

Fig. 4: Elastography image of fibroadenoma showing elastographic score 2 with few small blue areas of no strain in the periphery. B-mode image shows well-defined ovoid hypoechoic nodule with posterior acoustic enhancement.

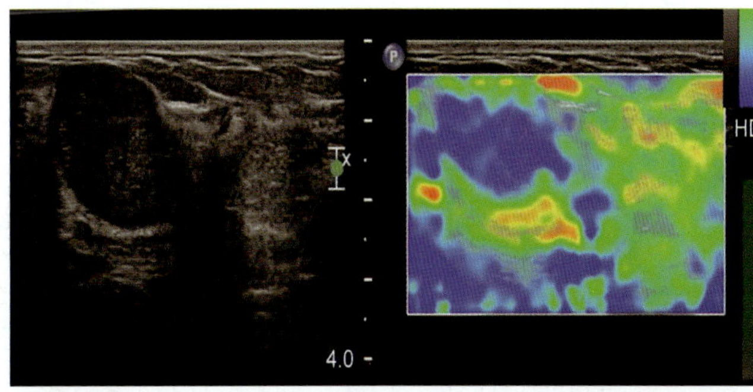

Fig. 5: Elastographic image of another fibroadenoma showing elastographic score 3 with more central blue areas of no strain.

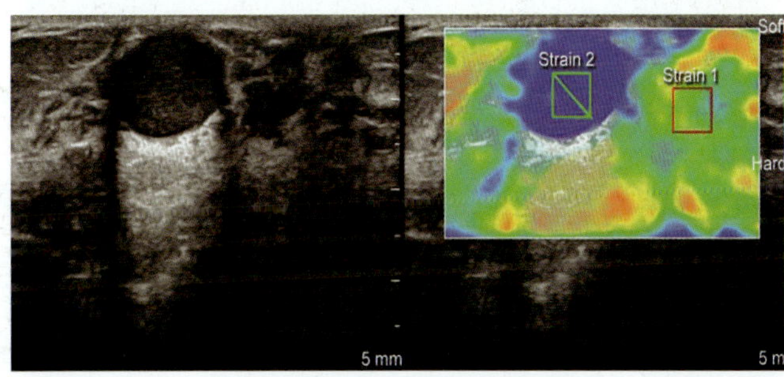

Fig. 6: Electrographic image IDC breast shows elastographic score 4 with complete lesion appearing blue with no strain. The picture also shows the strain ratio 4.4 between the lesion and the adjoining normal breast.

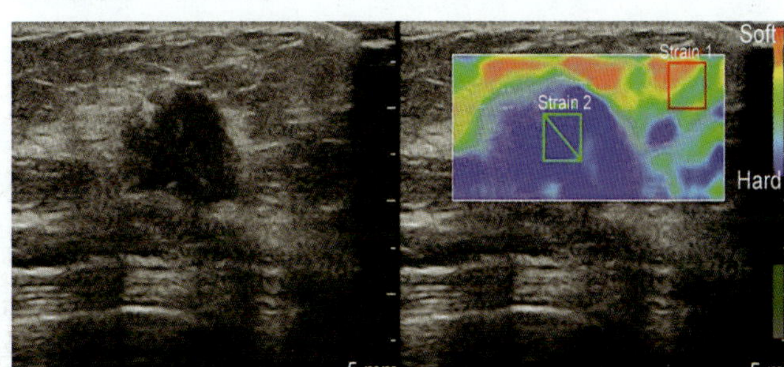

Fig. 7: Elastographic image of IDC breast shows elatsographic score 5 with blue area of no strain in the lesion and in the peripheral echogenic halo.

It combines two concepts. Instead of using mechanical external compression, the system itself remotely induces mechanical vibration by using acoustic radiation force created by a focused ultrasound beam. The displacement induced at the focus, generates a shear wave that conveys information linked to the local viscoelastic properties of the tissue, thus enabling a quantitative approach to elasticity values.[26]

The interpretation and measurement of elasticity is done in terms of the Young's modulus (in kilo Pascal, kPa). It is reported that mean elasticity values are significantly higher in malignant masses (153.3 kPa ± 58.1) than in benign masses (46.1 kPa ± 42.9) **(Fig. 8)**.[27]

Elastographic Appearances of the Breast Masses

Simple cyst versus complex cyst

Simple cyst is the most common type of breast lesion. It usually appears on conventional ultrasound as anechoic round or oval well-defined lesion with posterior acoustic enhancement, with imperceptible posterior wall. On elastography, it gives a target or bulls-eye appearance, with central bright area surrounded by a dark concentric rim.[28] Complex cyst with debris because of its internal contents can appear as a solid lesion on B-mode conventional ultrasound, and can be subjected to biopsy. Ultrasound elastography can help in revealing the cystic nature of the lesion with the typical target appearance.

Fibroadenoma: Represent most common type of solid breast lesion. Ultrasound typically shows fibroadenoma as well-circumscribed hypoechoic masses, which are wider than tall with long axis parallel to the chest wall. Sometimes, fibroadenoma can present as atypical shape like taller than wide.

In such cases, sonoelastography can help elucidate the benign nature of the lesion. Usually, it appears smaller than B-mode images in contrast to the malignant lesion,

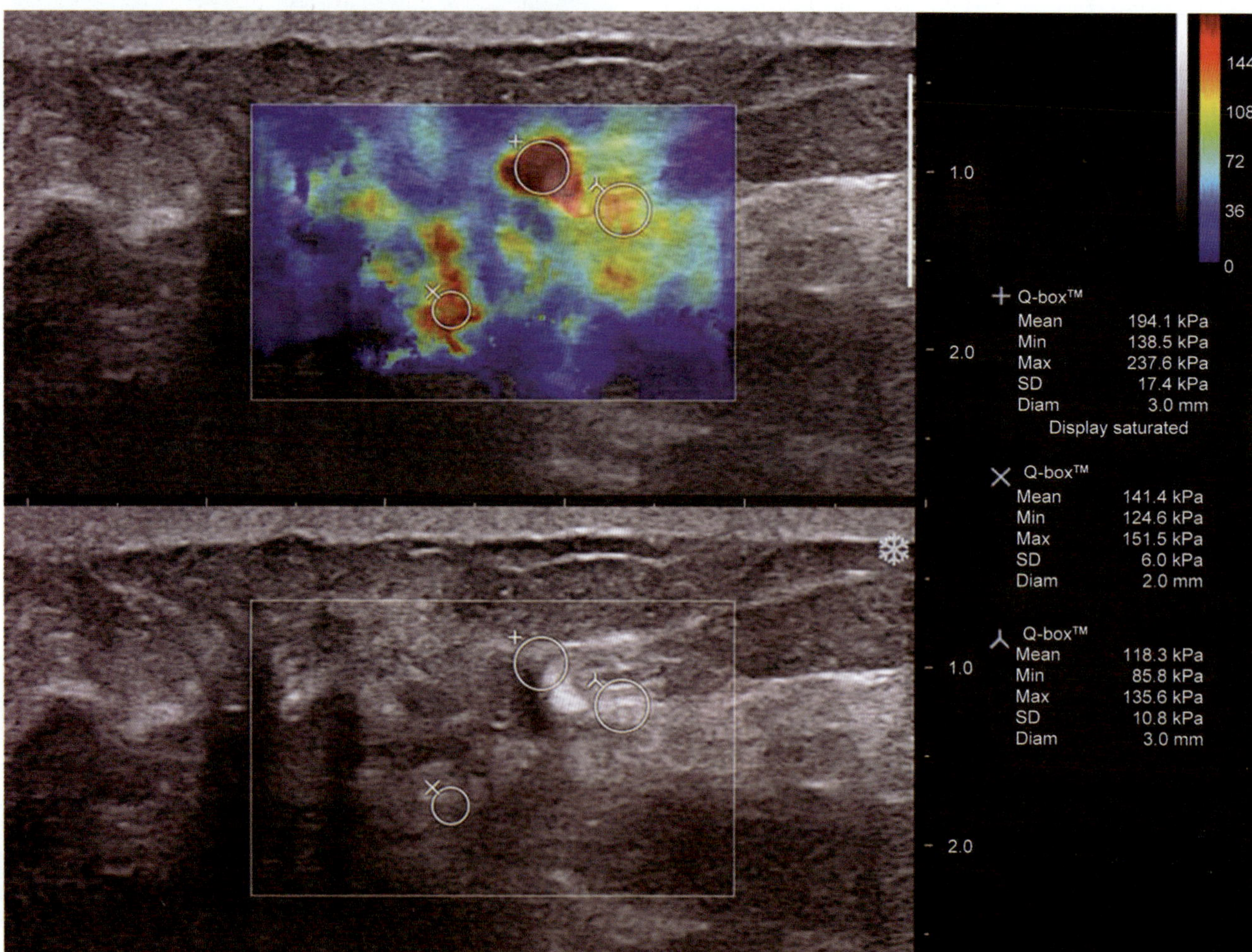

Fig. 8: Shear wave elastography image of malignant breast lesion showing red color in hard tissue with values above 130 kPa.

which show larger size on elastography because of its desmoplastic reaction in surrounding tissue. In one study as many as 73% of fibroadenoma could be differentiated from malignant on the basis of elastographic size and brightness criteria. Other methods to differentiate are quantitative and semiquantitative like calculating the strain ratio or assessment of overall stiffness as discussed earlier. Fibroadenoma larger than 2 cm and with calcification can give false positive for malignancy on elastography.[29]

Invasive ductal carcinomas: It is the most common invasive tumor of the breast. On B-mode ultrasound it appears as a hypoechoic spiculated or microlobulated mass, which is taller than wide with angular margins and a hyperechoic halo. On sonoelastography, invasive ductal carcinoma typically appears darker than normal tissue or benign lesion and it is slightly larger on the elastogram as compare to the B-mode ultrasound images.

Overall, ultrasound elastography is reported to have a sensitivity of greater than 95% and specificity of about 85% for differentiation between benign and malignant lesion using different qualitative and quantitative methods.[30] False negative elastogram can be seen in few well-defined benign looking masses, masses with tumor necrosis with acoustic enhancement can mimic cysts.

Liver

Diffuse Liver Diseases: Fibrosis, Cirrhosis, Acute Hepatitis, Nonalcoholic Fatty Liver Disease

In diffuse liver diseases, imaging modalities like B-mode ultrasound, CT and MRI have limited role in diagnosing liver fibrosis and early cirrhosis.

On ultrasound, hyperechoic nodular liver may be present with both liver fibrosis as well as fatty liver. A normal CT or MRI cannot rule out cirrhosis. Liver biopsy has been the reference method for diagnosing liver inflammation and fibrosis. However, it is an invasive procedure with accompanying risk and even life threatening complications and also prone to sampling errors as only a small volume of the liver is sampled. Interobserver variability is also high.

Elastography (by ultrasound or magnetic resonance) is a noninvasive modality for assessment of fibrosis and degree of fibrosis. It is painless, reproducible and repeatable and easy to perform, allowing monitoring of disease. Although MRI elastography is sensitive for evaluation of fibrosis, it has limited availability; is time consuming and costly and not suitable for screening patients for presence or degree of fibrosis.

Factors Influencing Liver Stiffness

1. Chronic liver parenchymal pathology may cause changes in liver stiffness by inducing fibrotic changes. On liver biopsy, fibrosis can be divided into four stages:[31]
   Stage 0 (normal): No fibrosis around portal triads
   Stage 1(portal fibrosis): Fibrosis surrounds the portal triads, but is limited to these areas
   Stage 2 (periportal fibrosis): Fibers begin to extend into the periportal space, but do not connect with other portal triads
   Stage 3 (septal fibrosis): Fibrous connective tissue links neighboring portal triads and begins to extend to the central veins. Shape of lobule is distorted
   Stage 4 (cirrhosis): Most portal triads are connected by fibrous tissue. Some portal triads and central veins are also connected.
2. Necro-inflammatory activity in the setting of acute hepatitis which causes hepatocyte swelling, edema and inflammatory infiltration may also increase liver stiffness. Patients with acute hepatitis (viral, autoimmune and drug-induced) may have a discrepancy between the liver stiffness measurement (LSM) and the fibrosis grade by biopsy.

   Liver stiffness may be in the cirrhotic range (above 12.5 kPa) whereas fibrosis staging by biopsy is not more than stage 2. Similar increase in stiffness measurement is found in patients with chronic viral hepatitis who have acute exacerbations associated with rise in alanine amino transferase.[32]
3. Congestive cardiac failure and extrahepatic cholestasis or congestive heart failure. Light meals also alter elasto graphy values.[33-35]

Ultrasound Elastography

Techniques for liver stiffness measurement

Transient elastography-Fibroscan™ apparatus (Echosens, Paris, France)—is a nonimaging modality which has been widely used for liver stiffness measurement **(Figs. 9A and B)**.

It uses a single cycle of low amplitude low frequency (50 Hz) vibration to induce a shear wave. The velocity of the shear wave is faster in dense fibrotic tissue.

Transient elastography probe has a 5 MHz ultrasound transducer probe mounted on the axis of a piston, which acts as a vibrator. The tip of the probe is placed in the intercostal space with the patient lying supine with abducted arms. Under control time motion (TM) and A-mode, the operator choses a liver portion within the right liver lobe at least

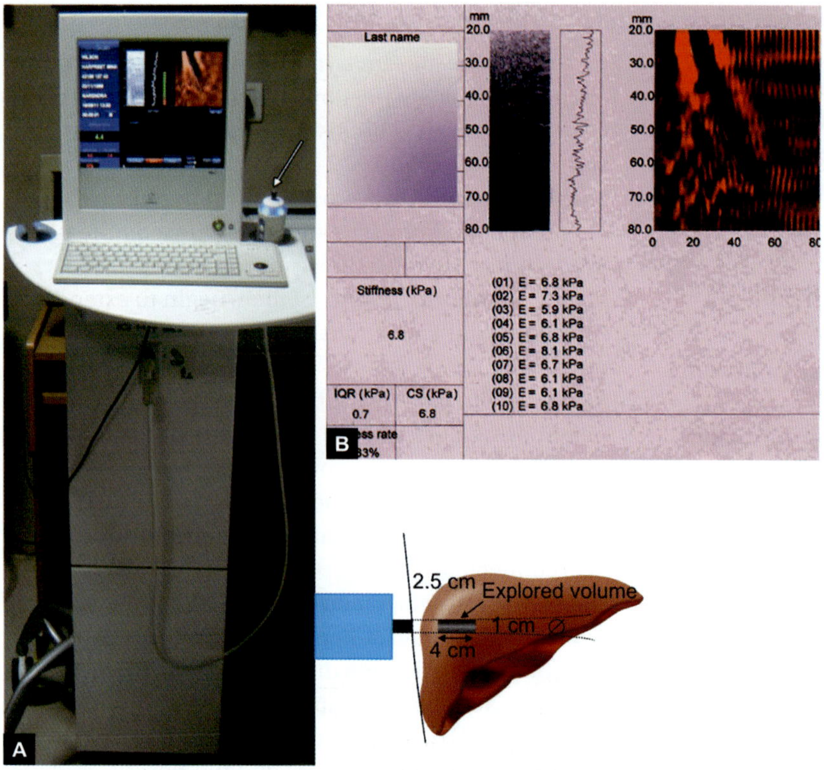

Figs. 9A and B: Image of the Fibroscan device (Echosens, Paris) for transient elastography: (A) The probe has a piston (arrow), which is placed in the right intercostal space. A single low frequency vibration is generated and shear wave elasticity in a cylinder of 1 cm × 4 cm of hepatic tissue is measured (inset). Measurements of 10 successful acquisitions in a normal liver (B) with a success rate of at least 60%, and with Interquartile Range (IQR-median of the middle 50% of the values) <30% of the median are taken. *Courtesy:* Dr Ajay Duseja, Associate Professor, Department of Hepatology, PGIMER, Chandigarh.

6 cm thick, free of large vascular structures and gallbladder. Stiffness is measured on a cylinder of hepatic tissue of 1 cm diameter and 2–4 cm length. The median value of 10 successful acquisitions, expressed in kilo-pascal (kPa), is taken as the liver stiffness. Measurements of 10 successful acquisitions with a success rate of at least 60%, and with Inter-quartile range (IQR- median of the middle 50% of the values) less than 30% of the median value are generally considered valid.

Values range from 2.5 to 75 kPa, with normal values around 5.5 kPa. Wide range of liver stiffness values are observed in patients with cirrhosis (13–75 kPa).[36] Transient elastography has excellent accuracy in diagnosing cirrhosis and significant degrees of fibrosis.

Comparison Between ARFI, Real-time Elastography and Transient Elastography for Liver Stiffness Measurement (Table 1)

Acoustic radial force imaging (ARFI) also has equal reliability in diagnosing liver fibrosis. ARFI is more sensitive for lesser degrees of fibrosis. Acute exacerbations of chronic liver disease have less influence on the liver stiffness by ARFI.[37,38]

Values for the liver stiffness measured with a transient elastography cannot be directly compared with ARFI or real- time (shear-wave) elastography since in the former a low frequency low amplitude pulse is given. This will lead to lower values when compared with real-time elastography.

The liver stiffness values with a transient elastography have a wide range (2.5–75 kPa), whereas ARFI values are in a very narrow range (0.5–4.4 m/s). This might make it difficult to differentiate normal form abnormal values with ARFI in a clinical setting, although values in healthy donors range between 0.85 and 1.25 m/sec.[36,39]

Post-treatment assessment

Elastography is also used for measuring liver stiffness changes in responders and relapsers undergoing antiviral treatment with interferon and ribavirin. Liver stiffness measurements show significant decrease in patients of viral hepatitis undergoing treatment with interferon and ribavirin. Relapse after treatment also leads to increase in stiffness.[40]

Assessment of portal hypertension/varices

Hepatic venous pressure gradient (HVPG) is the reference standard for measuring portal venous pressure (values > 6 mm Hg). However, it is an invasive procedure. Patients with cirrhosis and gastroesophageal varices have an HVPG of at least 10–12 mm Hg. Variceal hemorrhage, ascites or

Table 1: Comparison of different elastography techniques for liver diseases.

	Fibroscan (Transient elastography)	ARFI	Shear wave elastography
Imaging	Not possible	Yes	Yes
Assessment of focal lesions	Possible for large (>5 cm) and superficial lesions. Requires prior localization with B-mode imaging. No real-time image guidance	Yes	Yes Different areas within focal lesion can also be measured
Maximum depth of tissue for assessment	2.5–6.5 cm from skin	10 cm from skin	8 cm from skin
Maximum region of interest	1 cm × 5 cm	0.6 × 0.5 cm – 0.6 × 10 mm	Variable
Technique	Static–no images generated	Static images	Real-time 2D evaluation
Obesity	Difficult (better with XL probe)	Less difficult	Less difficult
Ascites	Difficult to impossible	Difficult assessment	Difficult assessment
Quantification	Yes	Possible	Yes
Range of values	Large	Small	Large

encephalopathy may develop when HVPG increases over a threshold value of 10–12 mm Hg.

Splenic elasticity has a close linear relationship with HVPG and can help predict the presence of esophageal varices in patients with chronic liver disease.

Values of splenic stiffness above 8.7 kPa correlates with HPVG above 6 mm Hg and values above 17.6–23 kPa correlate with severe portal hypertension (HVPG > 12 mm Hg). Splenic stiffness measurements show better and linear correlation with degree of portal hypertension than liver stiffness measurements. Combination of the liver stiffness with spleen diameter and platelet count, however, better correlates with degree of portal hypertension.[41]

Assessment of TIPSS

Splenic stiffness also decreases significantly with a functional TIPSS, whereas liver stiffness measurements do not show significant changes.[42]

Assessment of liver transplant

Repeated liver stiffness measurements (LSM) following transplant can discriminate between slow and rapid fibroses (fibrosis stage F2-F4 at 1-year). Liver transplant recipients with hepatitis C virus infection undergo rapid fibrosis within the first year. Serial measurements of elastography within the first year shows much higher LSM than non-HCV infected recipients (9.9, 9.5, 12.1 kPa vs 6.9, 7.5, 6.6 kPa).[43]

Assessment of nonalcoholic fatty liver disease

Nonalcoholic fatty liver disease (NAFLD) is a range of liver disorders with hepatic steatosis without alcohol consumption, viral, or drug-related etiologies. Histologically, it can be a simple accumulation of triglyceride droplets in hepatocytes or may progress to cellular injury and inflammation with resultant fibrosis and even cirrhosis and HCC.

Fibrosis and cirrhosis due to NAFLD can be detected by transient elastography or other routine elastographic techniques. A newer technique of controlled attenuation parameter (CAP) gives an estimate of the attenuation of ultrasound at 3.5 MHz and is expressed in decibel per meters (dB/m). CAP is evaluated using the same radiofrequency data and in the same region of interest that is used for transient elastography and is a nonimaging based modality which shows promise in assessing the degree of steatosis noninvasively.[44]

Advantages

Elastography is a noninvasive, painless and repeatable procedure.

- It can evaluate a much larger liver volume than liver biopsy
- It can be used for initial assessment, monitoring as well as diagnosis of complications (portal hypertension, esophageal varices)
- It can help in biopsy planning from stiffest regions to reduce sampling error
- Tumor ablation monitoring is also possible real-time with this procedure.

Limitations

Parenchymal thickness of less than 4 cm under the probe, presence of ascites, severe obesity, and the absence of an intercostal space sufficiently wide for probe, limit the usage of elastography. Male sex, body mass index more than 30, metabolic syndrome and acute viral hepatitis are all known to cause increased liver stiffness.[45]

Focal Liver Lesions

ARFI

Malignant and benign liver lesions appeared stiffer compared with the surrounding liver parenchyma on ARFI in a study by Shuang-Ming T et al. There were statistical differences between malignant and benign liver lesions. The median value of malignant and benign liver lesions were 3.14 m/sec (average value 3.16 ± 0.80 m/sec, range 1.17–4.45 m/sec) and 1.35 m/sec (average value 1.47 ± 0.53 m/sec, range 0.74–3.26 m/sec).

A cut-off value of 2.22 m/sec resulted in sensitivity, specificity, and accuracy for malignancy of 89.7%, 95.0%, and 92.2%, respectively.[46]

Compression ultrasonography

Onur MR et al. evaluated benign and malignant focal hepatic lesions, such as hemangiomas, focal nodular hyperplasia (FNH), nodular regenerative hyperplasia, adenomas, hepatocellular carcinomas (HCC), metastases, and cholangiocarcinomas. The strain ratio of liver parenchyma was compared with that of the focal lesion to give the strain index value. Mean strain index values of malignant liver lesions were significantly higher than that of benign lesions [The mean strain index value of malignant liver lesions ± SD (2.82 ± 1.82) was significantly higher than that of benign liver lesions (1.45 ± 1.28)]. Stiffness of hemangiomas vary depending on the amount of fibrotic septa dividing the vascular spaces. Strain index as well as mean values of hemangiomas on ARFI (1.5–2.3 m/sec) are significantly low.[47,48]

Shear wave

Shear-wave values (in kPa) can distinguish between FNH and adenoma. The FNH have a radial pattern of elasticity whereas adenomas and hemangiomas are homogeneous. Scars from radiofrequency ablation or healed abscesses have the highest stiffness values among benign lesions.

A significant difference was also found between HCCs and cholangiocarcinoma elasticity. Cholangiocarcinomas were the stiffest among malignant lesions (56.9 ± 25.6 kPa).

The HCC stiffness depends on the underlying liver, with lesions in cirrhotic livers appearing softer than lesions in normal or mildly cirrhotic livers. Metastasis stiffness also is highly variable and depends on the primary source. Carcinoid metastases are stiffer than colorectal metastases.[49]

Prostate

Prostate gland is one of the earliest organs for which elastography was proposed. Endorectal ultrasound continues to be most commonly used imaging modality for assessing the prostate. On B-mode ultrasound, most carcinoma prostate show varying echogenicity mostly being hypoechoic to few isoechoic or hyperechoic also. So the overall sensitivity is approximately 50%.[50]

Real-time endorectal elastography shows the sensitivity 68% with accuracy of about 76%.[51] Prostate cancers have a higher elastic modulus than that of surrounding normal prostate tissue.[13]

Eventually, the prostate cancer appears dark on elastogram more in the peripheral lesion. Sometimes, the malignant lesions which are very small or invisible on B-mode ultrasound images are prominent on elastogram as dark area of low strain **(Fig. 10)**.

Elastographic imaging of the prostate gland can be performed with manual compression strain imaging (two-dimensional) or with external vibration with Doppler imaging, which permits two- and three-dimensional imaging. Vibration elastography generates tissue displacement through the use of an independent external vibration source. Relative displacement is measured by using a variant of Doppler imaging that depicts differential motion of tissue types. This technique provides good correlation for tissues that have a large difference in stiffness.[52] Another role is for sonoelastographic guided prostate biopsies which increase the detection rate about three times than the routine endorectal ultrasound guided biopsies.[53]

Benign prostatic hyperplasia appears as heterogeneous hypoechoic area on endorectal B-mode ultrasound. Area with benign hyperplasia also show higher stiffness than that of normal prostate tissue but less than that of carcinoma prostate. However, it is difficult to differentiate between two and sometime it can give a false positive

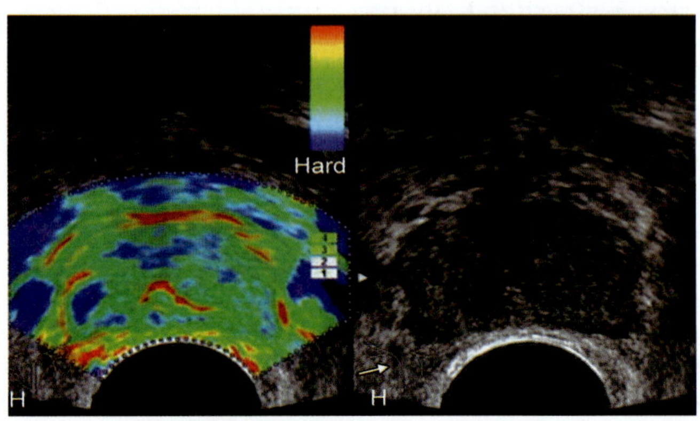

Fig. 10: Elastography image is showing hard nodule in the prostate in the right peripheral zone in blue color. Same nodule appeared hyperechoic on B-mode ultrasound image.

findings for the cancer prostate.[52] In a recent study, the ARFI was implemented to image excised human prostate.[53] The ARFI imaging is an elasticity imaging technique, which uses remotely generated, focused acoustic beam to excite tissue and generate the images of tissue displacement response.[54]

Various prostatic zonal structures and pathologies were demonstrated on ARFI imaging. The ARFI images are produced by evaluation of displacement within the ROE from multiple excitation and formation of an image from all location. The central zone (CZ), Ca prostate and atrophy show smaller displacement than the normal tissue in transitional zone (TZ) and peripheral zone (PZ). The stiffness ratio of Ca prostate to normal tissue calculated to be 2.2 with their shear moduli for Ca prostate, CZ and atrophy are from 8 to 10 kPa and for PZ and TZ/BPH are 4–5 kPa, respectively.[53]

More recently ARFI imaging is used for human prostate in vivo. Carcinoma prostate appears as bilaterally asymmetric stiff structures; benign prostatic hyperplasia (BPH) appears heterogeneous with a nodular texture, and the boundary of the transitional zone (TZ) forms a stiff rim separating the TZ from the peripheral zone (PZ). Compared with the matched B-mode images, ARFI images, in general portray prostate structures with higher contrast. The ARFI imaging holds promise for guidance of targeted prostate needle biopsies and therapy.[55]

Lymph Nodes

Elastography is also useful in differentiating reactive and metastatic axillary lymph nodes in carcinoma breast. As axillary lymph nodes status is the most important prognostic factor in carcinoma breast. The B-mode ultrasonography criteria for metastasis have based on the size, shape, hilum and the cortical thickening of lymph nodes.[56,57] For elastography, axillary lymph nodes also given on elasticity scoring system on the basis of color coding:

- Score 1: Absent or very small blue area
- Score 2: Small, scattered blue area, total blue area less than 45%
- Score 3: Large blue area, total blue area more than 45%
- Score 4: Blue area with or without a green rim.

Reported elasticity score of metastatic axillary lymph nodes (3.1 ± 0.7) is significantly higher than the score for reactive lymph nodes (2.2 ± 0.7; $p < 0.001$),[58] when the cut-off was taken between 2 and 3, the sensitivity and specificity was approximately 80%.

Similar kind of scoring done for cervical lymph nodes by Deng ke Teng et al. in which they found most benign lymph nodes showing elasticity score 1 or 2 and most of malignant node showing elasticity score 3 or 4 with sensitivity and specificity of 88.4% and 35.1%, respectively. They also calculated the strain ratio which showed strain ratio cut-off for malignant higher than 1.78 and for benign lower than 1.78 with sensitivity and specificity of 98.1% and 64.9%, respectively.[59]

Thyroid

Another area of potential usefulness is the evaluation of thyroid nodule because the ultrasound and nuclear medicine criteria for differentiating between benign versus malignant nodules are not reliable. A number of articles have shown the potential utility of nodular stiffness for characterizing it as malignant.[60,61] Similar to the breast and other nodular lesion, the malignant thyroid nodule is stiffer than the benign thyroid nodules. Mainly semiquantitative methods with compression elastography using strain index is utilized. It is calculated by dividing nodule strain value by the strain of adjacent normal thyroid tissue. Good quality elastography of thyroid is challenging because of the shape of neck with sloping contour, which can cause lateral movement of thyroid and the pulsation from the adjoining carotid artery. Even with these technical difficulties as more and more results are reported, it can be used to help in deciding which nodule to be biopsied when many nodules are present.[62] For the diffuse diseases of the thyroid quantitative or semiquantitative elastography is used. One study with shear wave velocity analysis shows increase stiffness in case of Hashimoto's thyroiditis.[63]

Gynecology

Cervical Elastography

Labor assessment

Cervical consistency and dilatation of internal os is assessed by palpation before induction of labor by prostaglandin or oxytocin. Cervical length measurement is done by ultrasound. Ripening of the internal os, which is not routinely evaluated during pregnancy by vaginal examination, can be assessed by transvaginal elastography. A soft internal os and harder external parts of the cervix are predictors of a favorable reaction to oxytocin during induction of labor. This can also help in deciding whether prostaglandins are required. Failed induction rates were higher in patients with increased stiffness of the internal os in a study by M Swiatkowska-Freund.[64]

Role

Elastography may play a role in predicting delivery, and in detecting patients with a high risk of preterm delivery.

Cervical Cancer

Transvaginal elastography has been evaluated for the diagnosis of cervical lesions. Malignant lesions are stiffer (blue on color coded maps), whereas benign lesions are of intermediate stiffness (green).

Significant differences in strain ratios have been noted between benign (polyp/fibroid/erosion/inflammation) and malignant lesions (Strain ratio was obtained by dividing the mean strain within the lesion by the mean strain from the parametrial tissue).

A cutoff value of strain ratio of 4.53 or higher has been suggested for confident diagnosis of malignancy. Elastography helps in the detection of endophytic cancers, which are more common in elderly women and are difficult to diagnose clinically or colposcopically. Depth of invasion of stroma can also be accurately assessed by elastography, helping in staging.[65] However, elastography is not helpful in the diagnosis of cervical intraepithelial neoplasia.[66]

Pitfalls

Transvaginal elastography of the cervix lacks a proper reference tissue where comparison studies are possible. Infiltration of parametrial tissue by tumor would give rise to errors in strain ratio measurement as parametrial tissue is taken as reference.

Normal cervix itself has heterogeneous elasticity. Moreover, the portion of the cervix nearest the transducer tip is prone to compression and even the mildest movement or pressure may result in erroneous impression of softening.[67]

Fibroids

Fibroids are often dense and the posterior acoustic shadowing poses difficulty in correct assessment of size and extent on ultrasound. Fibroids appear harder and have well demarcated borders on elastography. Color coded images in elastography can help in better delineation of fibroids and also in characterizing changes associated with treatments like embolization.[68]

Fibroids versus Adenomyosis

In adenomyosis and adenomyomas, which is often difficult to diagnose on B-mode ultrasound, elastographic color maps show a typical pattern of a soft lesion (green) with a central core which is even less stiffer (red). This pattern persists in both diffuse as well as focal varieties, though the margins are irregular in diffuse and well demarcated in the focal variety. Fibroids in comparison are stiffer and are depicted in blue on color maps.[69]

Endometrial Pathologies

Color-coded elastographic images and elasticity indices (where stiffer tissues are given lower scores) have shown that normal or atrophic endometrium has significantly lower scores than endometrial hyperplasia, cancer or polyps.[70]

Musculoskeletal

Compression ultrasonography has been the most commonly used technique for musculoskeletal applications. Strain of the region of interest is compared with the remaining tissue (usually fat) within the elastogram. The semiquantitative measurement method includes the ratio of the relative strains between the area of interest and a reference area. The ARFI and shear wave elasticity imaging are being increasingly used for musculoskeletal applications.

Appearance of Normal Tendons

Compression elastography: In healthy volunteers, the normal Achilles tendons were found to have two distinct elastography patterns. They were either homogeneously hard structures or in the majority they had considerable inhomogeneity with soft areas (longitudinal bands or spots), which did not correspond to any changes in B-mode or Doppler ultrasound.[71]

Shear wave

Shear wave elastography has also been used to measure mean elasticity values of muscles. For the gastrocnemius and masseter muscles, supraspinatus tendon, and Achilles tendon in both the longitudinal and transverse planes, shear wave elastographic values ranged from 11.1 ± 4.1 kPa (range 2–28 kPa), 10.4 ± 3.7 kPa (range 2–23 kPa), 31.2 ± 13 kPa (range 6–90 kPa), 74.4 ± 45.7 kPa (range 6–242 kPa), and 51.5 ± 25.1 kPa (range 10–111 kPa). The mean elasticity values for the muscles and tendons in the longitudinal plane were greater in men than in women, but the Achilles tendon in the transverse plane did not exhibit a significant difference between sexes. There was no significant correlation between age and elasticity for the muscles.[72]

Tendinopathy

Symptomatic tendons were found in compression elastography to contain marked softening in 57%, mild softening in 11% and no soft areas (hard structures) in 32% of cases.[73] The alterations in asymptomatic tendons were seen in the tendon mid-portion and were not always found to correspond to alterations in conventional ultrasound. Mild softening was not correlated with conventional ultrasound abnormalities, whereas marked softening was found mainly in cases with ultrasound evidence of disease. This could signify either a false positive finding or the increased sensitivity of elastography in early diagnosis.

Another study has found increasing stiffness in diseased tendons, probably reflecting the stage of the disease, with fibrosis being the predominant component.[74] Increased stiffness of extensor tendon has been noted in lateral epicondylitis, with elastography being more sensitive than conventional ultrasound.[75]

Normal muscle

Elastographic appearance of normal muscle needs further detailed investigation. Relaxed muscle gives an inhomogene-ous appearance of intermediate or increased stiffness (green/yellow or blue color, respectively) with scattered softer and harder areas especially at the periphery near boundaries.[71]

Exercise

Elastography has also shown increase in muscle hardness (changes in strain ratio) immediately after exercise which lasted from 30 minutes to 4 days.[76,77]

Rheumatological disorders

Soft tissue nodules: Elastography helps in differentiation of rheumatoid nodules and tophi; rheumatoid nodules were significantly less elastic than tophi and suggesting a possible role of this method for the investigation of soft tissue nodules.[78]

Synovitis

Inflammatory synovitis due to rheumatoid arth ritis was shown to be of intermediate stiffness, infectious synovitis (due to tuberculosis) was softer, whereas fatty villous proliferations (lipoma abrorescens) and pigmented villonodular synovitis were predominantly soft, as opposed to synovial sarcoma, which was hard.[79]

Skin

Elasticity of skin over the forearm in scleroderma patients have been evaluated with compression elastography leading to predominant blue areas (hard) as compared to green (intermediate) stiffness in controls.[80]

Soft tissue masses

Data on the elastographic appearance of soft tissue masses with histological confirmation is limited. A study revealed lipoma and low flow vascular malformations and thyroglossal cysts to be soft due to fat/liquid content. Neurogenic tumors and dermoid/sebaceous cysts were stiffer. Stiffness of abscesses varied from soft to intermediate, probably due to varying liquid and solid components.

Considerable overlap in elastography measurement was present. Elastography may be beneficial in cases of equivocal B-mode findings and for guiding aspiration or biopsy in abscesses or mixed solid/cystic lesions.[81]

Myofascial pain

Elastography has also been utilized in identifying active trigger points in myofascial pain, which is a major cause of nonarticular pain with motor and sensory symptoms. Measurements have shown increased hardness in trigger points as compared to normal areas. This helps in objective classification instead of the subjective clinical assessment of nodular hard areas in involved muscles.[82]

Inflammatory/dystrophic conditions

In inflammatory myositis, increased stiffness due to fibrosis and decrease in fatty infiltration has been documented using compression strain imaging. Elastography has shown correlation with serum markers in inflammatory myopathies and could help in disease monitoring.[83] Elastography may also be more sensitive in detecting dystrophic changes in muscle stiffness earlier than ultrasound and MRI.[84] In spasticity due to cerebral palsy, elastography has helped to establish site of botulinum toxin injection.[85]

Hyaline cartilage

Evaluation of elasticity of hyaline cartilage may help in evaluation prior to arthroscopy and in monitoring treatment.[86]

Standardization

Standardization is required, especially in musculoskeletal imaging. Differences in applied transducer pressure and ROI size can affect the elastic modulus even on shear wave imaging significantly. The larger the ROIs size, the higher the chance to include the muscle fascia, dense collagen fiber and bone. This leads to increase in the maximum value of elastic modulus, although mean values over large areas may remain the same. Increase in acquisition time may also lead to slippage of transducer from intended position.

Elastography on muscle and tendon should be performed with the lightest transducer pressure and a shorter acquisition time.[87] For the Achilles tendon, the suggested standard size for longitudinal scans is a depth of three times the tendon and about three-quarters of the screen, and for transverse scans the para-Tenon should be included.[88]

Role in musculoskeletal imaging

Elastography may be utilized for early diagnosis, staging and monitoring inflammatory, degenerative, myopathic or dystrophic conditions. It may also have a role in guiding interventions. However, clinical utility and validity of ultrasound elastography in musculoskeletal applications is still to be established by further studies involving larger number of patients.

OTHER APPLICATIONS

Renal Transplant Assessment

Supersonic shear-wave imaging, transient elastography and strain imaging have been utilized to diagnose chronic allograft injury. It can be used to monitor allograft stiffness, so that patients with serial increase can be subjected to a biopsy before renal function deteriorates, instead of all patients undergoing routine protocol biopsies. It can also monitor effect of treatment. However, subclinical rejection, infection or recurrence of underlying disease cannot be detected.[89]

Cardiovascular Applications

The two major areas of cardiovascular applications are strain imaging of the myocardium and of atheromatous plaque and the arterial wall.[90] Myocardial evaluation focuses on evaluation of localized areas of ischemia, infarction, and scarring. Arterial elasticity evaluation has focused on detection of vulnerable plaque and estimation of arterial wall compliance, as vulnerable plaques are known to be much softer than stable plaques. Elasticity estimation in these organs makes use of the normal movement of myocardium and vessel walls during the cardiac cycle rather than externally applied vibrations or pressure. Early work focused on intravascular ultrasound imaging of plaque,[91] but that method is invasive, and much of the current work is focused on external methods of plaque stiffness imaging.

Venous Thrombosis

The use of elasticity imaging for evaluation of venous thrombosis has also been reported.[92] This application is important because new thrombi are at a higher risk for embolization than are older more fibrotic thrombi. Because the stiffness of a thrombus increases with increasing age,[93] elasticity imaging may offer a way of gauging the age of thrombi, which can be difficult using grayscale sonography alone.

Skin and Soft Tissue

Elastography can visualize components of skin and soft tissue abscesses, including the abscess cavity and surrounding induration. A percentage of patients who fail therapy will progress to more invasive infections, either by local spread, such as deeper tissue infection or via systemic spread, such as bacteremia. While B-mode sonography can help differentiate the contents of an abscess cavity from the surrounding tissue, sonoelastography by measuring tissue stiffness can visualize the indurated tissue surrounding the abscess cavity. Asymmetry of the inflammatory changes surrounding abscess cavities has been reported to be associated with a higher rate of failure after standard therapy.[94] Also the size of the tissue indurations may predict progression to bacteremia or the time to resolution.[95]

Endoscopic Ultrasonography

Endoscopic ultrasonography (EUS) is one of the most recent advances in gastrointestinal endoscopy. The EUS with real time tissue elastography can be more useful than EUS with only a B-mode imaging ability. Real-time EUS elastography can be performed with the conventional EUS probes without any need for additional equipment that induces vibration or pressure. Elastographic imaging of the normal pancreas is characterized by a uniform, homogeneous green color distribution (representing intermediate stiffness) throughout the organ. A green-predominant pattern, either homogeneous or heterogeneous, excludes malignancy with a high accuracy. On the contrary, a blue-predominant pattern, either homogeneous or heterogeneous, favors the diagnosis of malignant tumor. On quantitative analysis, a healthy pancreas shows a mean elasticity value of 0.55%. A strain ratio higher than 15.41 or a mass elasticity value below 0.03% is 100% specific for malignancy.[96]

Limitations of EUS Elastography

The main pitfall of EUS elastography is the inability to control tissue compression by the EUS transducer. Use of EUS elastography is also hampered by the induction of motion artifacts due to respiratory or heart movements, which cannot be adequately eliminated or quantified. The presence of nearby structures with very low or high density and stiffness, such as the heart, major vessels or spine are also difficult to be excluded from the ROI analyzed. Selection of the ROI has to carefully include surrounding soft tissues only, since the methodology of elastography assumes computations relative to the average strain inside the ROI. An intrinsic limitation of qualitative elastography is the subjective interpretation of the elastographic pattern that may be associated with significant intra-and interobserver variability.

Pitfalls

Large lesions can be under assessed, with portions of the lesion lying out of the field of view. Moreover, painful lesions may be under-represented because of the increased discomfort related to elastography. Performing ultrasound elastography can be technically challenging in organs like the salivary glands in terms of achieving only longitudinal transducer compression, i.e. avoiding lateral or out-of beam movements, and achieving the correct amount of compression. In this respect, even slight nonaxial transducer movements detrimentally affect elastogram quality, observed as background noise, due to mistracking artifacts.

CONCLUSION

In conclusion, elastography has emerged as a useful adjunct tool for ultrasound diagnosis. Elastograms are images of tissue stiffness and may be in color, grayscale, or a combination of the two. In a typical elastogram, low strain areas denoting a stiff or hard material are given darker gray values, whereas high strain areas denoting very soft tissues are given lighter gray values. The rapidly advancing field of tissue elasticity imaging and estimation has already produced several applications. The goal in breast elastography is not necessarily to diagnose cancers but to confidently classify questionable lesions on the sonogram as definitely benign. This will help reduce the number of biopsies of a benign lesion.

Recent advances in elastography include quantification using strain ratios, ARFI and shear wave velocity estimation. These are useful not only for characterizing focal masses but also for diagnosing diffuse organ diseases, such as liver cirrhosis. Beyond breast mass evaluation, elastography is showing a greatest potential in the liver. Other promising applications include prostate cancer detection, atheromatous plaque and arterial wall evaluation, venous thrombus evaluation, graft rejection, and monitoring of tumor ablation therapy. Other modalities may be used for elasticity imaging, the most powerful being magnetic resonance elastography. Ultrasound, being less expensive and easier to use, will likely become the most widely used modality for clinical elasticity estimation and imaging.

REFERENCES

1. Palmeri ML, Nightingale KR. What challenges must be overcome before ultrasound elasticity imaging is ready for the clinic? Imaging Med. 2011;3:433-44.
2. Duck F. Physical properties of tissue, A Comprehensive Reference Book. NY; Academic Press:1990.
3. Sarvazyan A, Skovaroda AR, Emelianov SY, et al. Biophysical bases of elasticity imaging. Acoust Imaging. 1995;21: 223-40.
4. Sarvazyan A. Handbook of Elastic Properties of Solids, Liquids and Gases. Elastic properties of soft tissue. 2001. pp.107-27.
5. Peter NT Wells, Hai-Dong Liang. Medical ultrasound: imaging of soft tissue strain and elasticity. J R Soc Interface. 2011;8(64):1521-49. Published online 16 June 2011 doi: 10.1098/rsif.2011.0054.
6. Garra BS. Imaging and estimation of tissue elasticity by ultrasound. Ultrasound Q. 2007;23:255-68.
7. Fehrenbach J. Influence of Poisson's ratio on elastographic direct and inverse problems. Phys Med Biol. 2007;52:707-16.
8. Insana MF, Pellot-Barakat C, Sridhar M, Lindfors KK. Viscoelastic imaging of breast tumor microenvironment with ultrasound. J Mammary Gland Biol Neoplasia. 2004;9: 393-404.
9. Sarvazyan A, Hall TJ, Urban MW, et al. An overview of elastography-an emerging branch of medical imaging. Curr Med Imaging Rev. 2011;7:255-82.
10. Ginat DT, Destounis SV, Barr RG, et al. US elastography of breast and prostate lesion. Radiographics. 2009;29: 2007-16.
11. Itoh A, Ueno E, Tohno E, et al. Breast disease: clinical application of US elastography for diagnosis. Radiology. 2006;239(2):341-50.
12. Shiina T, Doyley MM, Bamber JC. Strain imaging using combined RF and envelope autocorrelation processing. In: Proceedings of the IEEE Ultrasonics Symposium. Savoy, Ill:Institute of Electrical and Electronics Engineers Ultrasonics, Ferroelectrics, and Frequency Control Digital Archive. 1996;2:1331-6.
13. Zhang M, Nigwekar P, Castaneda B, et al. Quantitative characterization of viscoelastic properties of human prostate correlated with histology. Ultrasound Med Biol. 2008;34:1033-42.
14. Kathy Nightingale. Acoustic Radiation Force Impulse (ARFI) Imaging: a Review. Curr Med Imaging Rev. 2011;7(4):328-39. doi:10.2174/157340511.
15. EE Drakonaki, GM Allen, DJ. Ultrasound elastography for musculoskeletal applications. Wilson. British Journal of Radiology. 2012;85:1435-45.
16. McAleavey SA, Menon M, Orszulak J. Shear-modulus estima tion by application of spatially-modulated impulsive acoustic radiation force. Ultrason. Imaging. 2007;29: 87-104.
17. Bercoff J, Tanter M, Fink M. Supersonic shear imaging: a new technique for soft tissue elasticity mapping. IEEE Trans Ultrason Ferro Electr Freq Control. 2004;51:396-409.
18. Thitai-Kumar A, Garra BS, Ophir J. Visualization of bonding at an inclusion boundary using axial-strain elastography: a feasibility study. Phys Med Biol. 2007;52(9):2615.
19. Maleke C, Konofagou EE. In vivo feasibility of real-time moni-toring of focused ultrasound surgery (FUS) using harmonic motion imaging (HMI). IEEE Trans Biomed Eng. 2010;57:7-11.

20. Krouskop TA, Wheeler TM, Kallel F, et al. Elastic moduli of breast and prostate tissues under compression. Ultrason Imaging. 1998;20:260-74.
21. Cespedes I, Ophir J, Ponnekanti H, et al. Elastography: elasticity imaging using ultrasound with application to muscle and breast in vivo. Ultrasound Imaging. 1993;15:73-88.
22. Hall TJ, Zhu Y, Spalding CS. In vivo real-time freehand palpation imaging. Ultrasound Med Biol. 2003;29:427-35.
23. Garra BS, Cespedes EI, Ophir J, et al. Elastography of breast lesions: initial clinical results. Radiology. 1997;202:79-86.
24. Burnside ES, Hall TJ, Sommer AM, et al. Differentiating benign from malignant solid breast masses with US strain imaging. Radiology. 2007;245(2):401-10.
25. Zhi H, Xiao X-Y, Yang H-Y, et al. Semi quantitating stiffness of breast solid lesions in ultrasonic elastography. Academic Radiology. 2008;15:1347-53.
26. Tanter M, Bercoff J, Athanasiou A, et al. Quantitative assessment of breast lesion viscoelasticity: initial clinical results using supersonic shear imaging. Ultrasound Med Biol. 2008;34(9): 1373-86.
27. Chang JM, et al. Clinical applications of shear wave elastography (SWE) in the diagnosis of benign and malignant breast diseases Breast Cancer Res Treat. 2011;29(1):89-97.
28. Booi RC, Carson PL, O'Donnell M, et al. Diagnosing cysts with correlation coefficient images from 2-dimensional freehand elastography. J Ultrasound Med. 2007; 26(9):1201-7.
29. Giuseppetti GM, Martegani A, Di Cioccio B, et al. Elastosonography in the diagnosis of the nodular breast lesions: preliminary report. Radiol Med. 2005;110(1-2):69-76.
30. Barr RG. Initial results of breast real-time elasticity imaging to characterize lesions [abstr]. Radiological Society of North America Scientific Assembly and Annual Meeting Program. Oak Brook: Radiological Society of North America; 2006. p. 644.
31. Carey E, Carey WD. Noninvasive tests for liver disease, fibrosis, and cirrhosis: Is liver biopsy obsolete? Cleaveland Clinic J Med. 2010;77:519-27.
32. Sagir A, Erhardt A, Schmitt M, et al. Transient elastography is unreliable for detection of cirrhosis in patients with acute liver damage. Hepatology. 2008;47:592-5.
33. Millonig G, Reimann FM, Friedrich S, et al. Extrahepatic cholestasis increases liver stiffness (FibroScan) irrespective of fibrosis. Hepatology. 2008;48:1718-23.
34. Millonig G, Friedrich S, Adolf S, et al. Liver stiffness is directly influenced by central venous pressure. J Hepatol. 2010;52:206-10.
35. Berzigotti A, de Gottardi A, Delgado MG, et al. Liver stiffness increases after a meal in patients with cirrhosis but its change does not correlate with the changes in HVPG (abstract). Hepatology. 2010;52:1074A.
36. Laurent Castera. Non-invasive assessment of liver fibrosis in chronic hepatitis C. Hepatol Int. 2011;5:625-34.
37. Sporea I, Bota S, Peck-Radosavljevic M, et al. Acoustic radiation force impulse elastography for fibrosis evaluation in patients with chronic hepatitis C: an international multicenter study. Eur J Radiol. 2012;81(12):4112-8. doi: 10.1016/j.ejrad. 2012.08.018. Epub 2012 Sep 20.
38. Rizzo L, Calvaruso V, Cacopardo B, Alessi N, Attanasio M, Petta S, et al. Comparison of transient elastography and acoustic radiation force impulse for noninvasive staging of liver fibrosis in patients with chronic hepatitis C. Am J Gastroenterol. 2011;106(12):2112-20. doi: 10.1038/ajg.2011.341. Epub 2011 Oct 4.
39. Son CY, Kim SU, Han WK, et al. Normal liver elasticity values using acoustic radiation force impulse imaging: a prospective study in healthy living liver and kidney donors. J Gastroenterol Hepatol. 2012;27(1):130-6. doi: 10.1111/j.1440-1746.2011.06814.x.
40. Martinez SM, Foucher J, Combis JM, et al. Longitudinal liver stiffness assessment in patients with chronic hepatitis C undergoing antiviral therapy PLoS One. 2012;7(10):e47715. doi: 10.1371/journal.pone.0047715. Epub 2012 Oct 17.
41. Laurent Castera, Massimo Pinzani, Jaime Bosch. Noninvasive evaluation of portal hypertension using transient elastography. J Hep. 2012;56 j:696-703.
42. Gao J, Ran HT, Ye XP, et al. The stiffness of the liver and spleen on ARFI Imaging pre- and post-TIPS placement: a preliminary observation. Clin Imaging. 2012;36(2):135-41.
43. Carrión JA, Torres F, Crespo G, et al. Liver stiffness identifies two different patterns of fibrosis progression in patients with hepatitis C virus recurrence after liver transplantation. Hepatology 2010;51(1):23-34. doi: 10.1002/hep.23240.
44. Sasso M, Beaugrand M, de Ledinghen V, et al. Controlled attenuation parameter (CAP): a novel VCTE™ guided ultrasonic attenuation measurement for the evaluation of hepatic steatosis: preliminary study and validation in a cohort of patients with chronic liver disease from various causes. Ultrasound Med Biol. 2010;36(11):1825-35. doi: 10.1016/j.ultrasmedbio. 2010. 07. 005. Epub 2010 Sep 27.
45. Roulot D, Czernichow S, Le Clésiau H, et al. Liver stiffness values in apparently healthy subjects: influence of gender and metabolic syndrome. J Hepatol. 2008;48:606-13.
46. Shuang-Ming T, Ping Z, Ying Q, et al. Usefulness of acoustic radiation force impulse imaging in the differential diagnosis of benign and malignant liver lesions. Acad Radiol. 2011;18(7):810-5. Epub 2011 Mar 21.
47. Onur MR, Poyraz AK, Ucak EE, et al. Semiquantitative strain elastography of liver masses. J Ultrasound Med. 2012;31(7):1061-7.
48. Gallotti A, D'Onofrio M, Romanini L, et al. Acoustic radiation force impulse (ARFI) ultrasound imaging of solid focal liver lesions. Eur J Radiol. 2012;81:451-5.
49. Aymeric Guibal, Camille Boularan, Matthew Bruce, et al. Evaluation of shear wave elastography for the characterization of focal liver lesions on ultrasound. Eur Radiol. DOI 10.1007/s00330-012-2692-y.
50. Kamoi K, Okihara K, Ochiai A, et al. The utility of transrectal real-time elastography in the diagnosis of prostate cancer. Ultrasound Med Biol. 2008;34(7):1025-32.

51. Akin O, Hricak H. Imaging of prostate cancer. Radiol Clin North Am. 2007;45(1):207-22.
52. Daniel T, Ginat, Stamatia V Destounis, et al. US Elastography of breast and prostate lesion. Radiographics. 2009;29:2007-16.
53. Zhai, et al. Characterizing the stiffness of human prostates using acoustic radiation force, ultrasound imaging. 2010;32(4):201-13.
54. Nightingale K, Palmeri M, Nightingale R, et al. On the feasibility of remote palpation using acoustic radiation force. JASA. 2001; 110:625-34.
55. Zhai, et al. Acoustic radiation force impulse imaging of Human Prostate: Initial in vivo demonstrations. Ultrasound Med Biol. 2012;38(1):50-61.
56. Choi YJ, Ko EY, Han BK, et al. High-resolution ultrasonographic features of axillary lymph node metastasis in patients with breast cancer. Breast. 2009;18:119- 122.
57. Bedi DG, Krishnamurthy R, Krishnamurthy S, et al. Cortical morphologic features of axillary lymph nodes as a predictor of metastasis in breast cancer: in vitro sonographic study. Am J Roentgenol. 2008;191:646-52.
58. Jae Jeong Choi, et al. Role sonographic elastography in the differential diagnosis of axillary lymph nodes in breast cancer. J Ultrasound Med. 2011;30:429-36.
59. Deng Ke Teng, et al. Value of US elastography in assessment of enlarged cervical lymph nodes. Asian Pacific J Cancer Prev. 13: 2081-5.
60. Hong Y, Liu X, Li Z, et al. Real-time ultrasound elastography in the differential diagnosis of benign and malignant thyroid nodules. J Ultrasound Med [serial online]. 2009;28(7):861-Y7.
61. Lyshchik A, Higashi T, Asato R, et al. Thyroid gland tumor diagnosis at US elastography. Radiology. 2005;237:202-11.
62. Dighe M, Kim J, Luo S, et al. Utility of the ultrasound elastographic systolic thyroid stiffness index in reducing fine-needle aspirations. J Ultrasound Med. 2010;29:565-74.
63. Bahn MM, Brennan MD, Bahn RS, et al. Development and application of magnetic resonance elastography of the normal and pathological thyroid gland in vivo. J Magn Reson Imaging. 2009;30:1151-4.
64. M Swiatkowska-Freund, K Preis. Elastography of the uterine cervix: implications for success of induction of labor. Ultrasound Obstet Gynecol. 2011;38:52-6.
65. Sun LT, Ning CP, Liu YJ, Wang ZZ, et al. Is transvaginal elastography useful in preoperative diagnosis of cervical cancer? Eur J Radiol. 2012;81(8):e888-92. doi: 10.1016/j.ejrad.2012.04.025. Epub 2012 Jun 18.
66. Thomas A, Kümmel S, Gemeinhardt O, et al. Real-time sonoelastography of the cervix: tissue elasticity of the normal and abnormal cervix. AcadRadiol. 2007;14(2): 193-200.
67. Molina FS, Gómez LF, Florido J, et al. Quantification of cervical elastography: a reproducibility study. Ultrasound in Obstetrics & Gynecology. 2012;39(6):685-9.
68. Ami O, Lamazou F, Mabille M, et al. Real-time transvaginal elasto sonography of uterine fibroids. Ultrasound Obstet Gynecol. 2009;34:486-8.
69. Tessarolo M, Bonino L, Camanni M, et al. Elastosonography: a possible new tool for diagnosis of adenomyosis? EurRadiol. 2011;21:1546-52. doi 10.1007/s00330-011-2064-z.
70. Preis K, Zielinska K, Swiatkowska-Freund M, et al. The role of elastography in the differential diagnosis of endometrial pathologies– preliminary report. GInekol Pol. 2011;82:494-7.
71. EE Drakonaki, GM Allen, DJ Wilson. Elastography for musculoskeletal applications. BJR. 2012;85:1435-45.
72. Arda K, Ciledag N, Aktas E, et al. Quantitative assessment of normal soft-tissue elasticity using shear-wave ultrasound elastography. AJR. 2011;197:532-6.
73. De Zordo T, Chem R, Smekal V, et al. Real-time sonoelastography: findings in patients with symptomatic Achilles tendons and comparison to healthy volunteers. Ultraschall Med. 2010;31:394-400.
74. De Sconfienza LM, Silvestri E, Cimmino MA. Sonoelastography in the evaluation of painful Achilles tendon in amateur athletes. Clin Exp Rheumatol. 2010;28:373-8.
75. De Zordo T, Lill SR, Fink C, et al. Real-time sonoelastography of lateral epicondylitis: comparison of findings between patients and healthy volunteers. Am J Roentgenol. 2009;193: 180-5.
76. Niitsu M, Michizaki A, Endo A, et al. Muscle hardness measurement by using ultrasound elastography: a feasibility study. Acta Radiol. 2011;52(1):99-105.
77. Yanagisawa O, Niitsu M, Kurihara T, et al. Evaluation of human muscle hardness after dynamic exercise with ultrasound real-time tissue elastography: a feasibility study. Clin Radiol. 2011;66(9):815-9.
78. Sconfienza LM, Silvestri E, Bartolini B, et al. Sonoelastography may help in the differential diagnosis between rheumatoid nodules and tophi. Clin Exp Rheumatol. 2010;28:144-5. Epub 2011 May 6. 80.
79. Lalitha P, Reddy MCh, Reddy KJ. Musculoskeletal applications of elastography: a pictorial essay of our initial experience. Korean J Radiol. 2011;12:365-75.
80. Iagnocco A, Kaloudi O, Perella C, et al. Ultrasound elastography assessment of skin involvement in systemic sclerosis: lights and shadows. Rheumatol. 2010;37(8): 1688-91. doi: 10.3899/jrheum.090974. Epub 2010 Jun 15.
81. Bhatia KS, Rasalkar DD, Lee YP, et al. Real-time qualitative ultrasound elastography of miscellaneous non-nodal neck masses: applications and limitations. Ultrasound Med Biol. 2010;36:1644-52.
82. Ballyns JJ, Shah JP, Hammond J, et al. Objective sonographic measures for characterizing myofascial trigger points associated with cervical pain. Ultrasound Med. 2011;30(10):1331-40.
83. Botar-Jid C, Damian L, Dudea SM, et al. The contribution of ultrasonography and sonoelastography in assessment of myositis. Med Ultrason. 2010;12:120-6.
84. Drakonaki EE, Allen GM. Magnetic resonance imaging, ultrasound and real-time ultrasound elastography of the

thigh muscles in congenital muscle dystrophy. Skeletal Radiol. 2010;39:391-6.
85. Vasilescu D, Dudea S, Botar-Jid C, et al. Sonoelastography contribution in cerebral palsy spasticity treatment assessment, preliminary report: a systematic review of the literature apropos of seven patients. Med Ultrason. 2010;12:306-10.
86. Zheng YP Mak, AFT Qin, L Ding CX. Ultrasound elastography of articular cartilage: a preliminary study. 20th Annual International Conference of the IEEE Engineering in Medicine and Biology Society; 1998.pp.1940-2.
87. Kot BCW, Zhang ZJ, Lee AWC, et al. (2012) Elastic modulus of muscle and tendon with shear wave ultrasound elastography: variations with different technical settings. PLoS ONE 7(8): e44348. doi:10.1371/journal.pone.0044348.
88. Klauser AS, Faschingbauer R, Jaschke WR. Is sonoelastography of value in assessing tendons? Semin Musculoskeletal Radiol. 2010;14:323-33.
89. Arndt R, Schmidt S, Loddenkemper C, et al. Noninvasive evaluation of renal allograft fibrosis by transient elastography—a pilot study. Transplant International. 2010;23:871-7.
90. Garra BS. Imaging and estimation of tissue elasticity by ultrasound. Ultrasound Q, 2007;23(4):255-68.
91. de Korte CL, Cespedes EI, van der Steen AFW, et al. Intravascular ultrasound elastography: assessment and imaging of elastic properties of diseased arteries and vulnerable plaque. Eur J Ultrasound. 1998;7:219-24.
92. Rubin JM, Xie H, Kim K, et al. Sonographic elasticity imaging of acute and chronic deep venous thrombosis in humans. J Ultrasound Med. 2006;25:1179-86.
93. Geier B, Barbera L, Muth-Werthmann D, et al. Ultrasound elastography for the age determination of venous thrombi. Evaluation in an animal model of venous thrombosis. Thromb Haemost. 2005;93:368-74.
94. Gaspari R, Blehar D, Briones J, et al. Sonoelastographic characteristics of abscess in duration associated with therapy failure. J Ultrasound Med. 2012;31(9):1405-11.
95. Gaspari R, Blehar D, Mendoza M, et al. Use of ultrasound elastography for skin and subcutaneous abscesses. J Ultrasound Med. 2009;28(7):855-60.
96. Lee TH, Cha S, Cho YD. EUS Elastography: advances in diagnostic EUS of the pancreas. Korean J Radiol. 2012; 13(S1):S12-S16.

CHAPTER 41

Computed Tomography Hardware: An Update

Ashu Seith Bhalla, Arun Deep Arora

INTRODUCTION

Since the first clinical use of computed tomography (CT) in 1972, its technology has made notable advances. The first CT scanner which was built by British engineer Hounsfield had a rotation time of about 300 seconds with a maximum image matrix of 80 × 80 pixels. It has been a long journey to the present day 256 to 320-slice scanners with rotation times of 0.33 seconds and an image matrix of 512 × 512 pixels. Several vendors today offer 256-slice spiral CT scanners and even 320 slice is now available. But the ever evolving technology has more in store: scanners with new detector materials for higher sensitivity, dual-source CT, dual-energy detectors and flat-panel detectors are further milestones of CT development.[1] The subject will be discussed under the following headings:

- Basic workflow of a CT scanner
- Determinants of an optimal image
- Advances in hardware
- *Special CT*: Cone-beam CT (CBCT)/volume CT, navigation systems.

BASIC WORKFLOW OF CT SCANNER

The CT scanner consists of three primary systems; including the gantry, the computer and the operating console. Each of these is made up of various subcomponents. The largest among these systems is the gantry assembly. It is made up of all the equipment related to the patient positioning, including patient support, the positioning couch, mechanical supports and the scanner housing. It also contains the heart of the CT scanner, the X-ray tube, as well as detectors arranged around the patient **(Fig. 1)**. Earlier versions of CT employed a pencil-like X-ray beam (with single detector) and the tube-detector movement was both linear and rotary, termed as the "rotate-translate" motion. In an attempt to shorten the scan time, a fan shaped beam with multiple detectors was adopted. The approach then shifted to "rotate-rotate" where multiple detectors are aligned as an arc and both detector arc and X-ray tube rotate around the patient. The quantum leap took place with the next level where the detectors formed a complete ring around the patient and only the X-ray tube rotates inside the detector ring, described as "rotate-fixed" motion.[2]

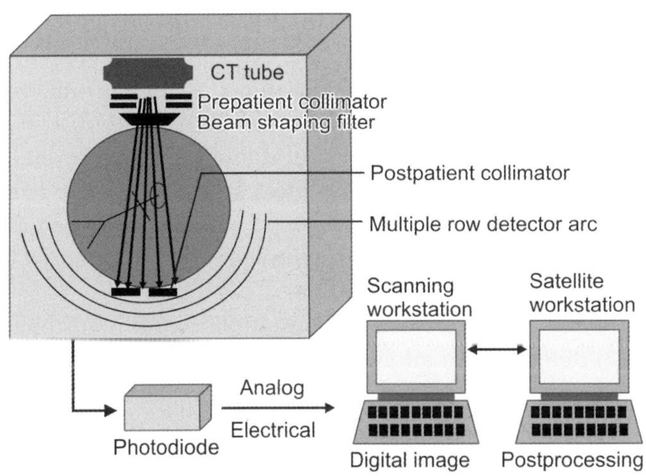

Fig. 1: Schematic diagram showing the basic components and workflow of a CT scanner.

DETERMINANTS OF AN OPTIMAL IMAGE

Determinants of an optimal image in CT as in any image acquisition system are:

- Spatial resolution
- Contrast resolution
- Temporal resolution.

Spatial Resolution

The key factors determining the spatial resolution are the detector size in the z-axis direction, reconstruction algorithms and patient motion. Spatial resolution is specified in the axial as well as z-axis plane. Scan plane is also called x-y plane and z-axis plane is also called out of plane **(Figs. 2A and B)**. The axial or x-y plane spatial resolution is dependent on the pixel size, which is a ratio of scan field of view (SFOV) and image reconstruction matrix. On the other hand, the number of rows in multidetector CT (MDCT) scanner and the detector size determines the out of plane (z-axis) resolution. The detector row width defines the minimum thickness of the reconstructed CT image and is influenced by the z-axis dimension of the individual detector element. For example, a detector row width of 0.6 mm allows a slice thickness of 0.6 mm. To achieve improved through-plane spatial resolution, some systems use an X-ray focal spot that alternates between two z-positions (i.e. z-flying focal spot) to acquire two overlapping slices for each detector row. This feature has been reported to improve z-plane spatial resolution to 0.4 mm[3].

Cone-beam CT uses a high-resolution two-dimensional (2D) detector and allows isotropic data acquisition and reconstruction leading to higher spatial resolution. These systems however, offer poor contrast resolution as shall be discussed subsequently in the chapter.

Temporal Resolution

The temporal resolution is determined by the gantry rotation time, acquisition mode, type of image reconstruction, and pitch. Gantry rotation time refers to the amount of time taken to complete one full rotation (360°) of the X-ray tube and detector around the patient. The recent advances in technology have brought considerable decrease in the gantry rotation time, almost as low as 330–370 msec. The lesser the gantry rotation time, the greater the temporal resolution achieved. Acquisition mode becomes especially important in cardiac CT where the dataset need be acquired at a very rapid speed to overcome the cardiac motion. It may be done through prospective ECG triggering wherein the data is acquired for only part of the complete gantry rotation, at a desired distance from the R-R peak in the cardiac cycle. This partial scanning reduces the radiation dose to the patient and achieves a temporal resolution in the range of 200–250 msec. The other mode of retrospective ECG gating in which data is acquired throughout the cardiac cycle and segmented reconstruction done from different cardiac cycles to increase temporal resolution to 80–250 msec. Multiple segment reconstruction, though increases the temporal resolution, but runs the risk of misregistration artifacts as the reconstruction data is selected from different heartbeat cycles. The pitch can be defined as the ratio of table increment per gantry rotation to the total X-ray beam width. The pitch factor plays a major role in improving both the temporal and spatial resolution but at

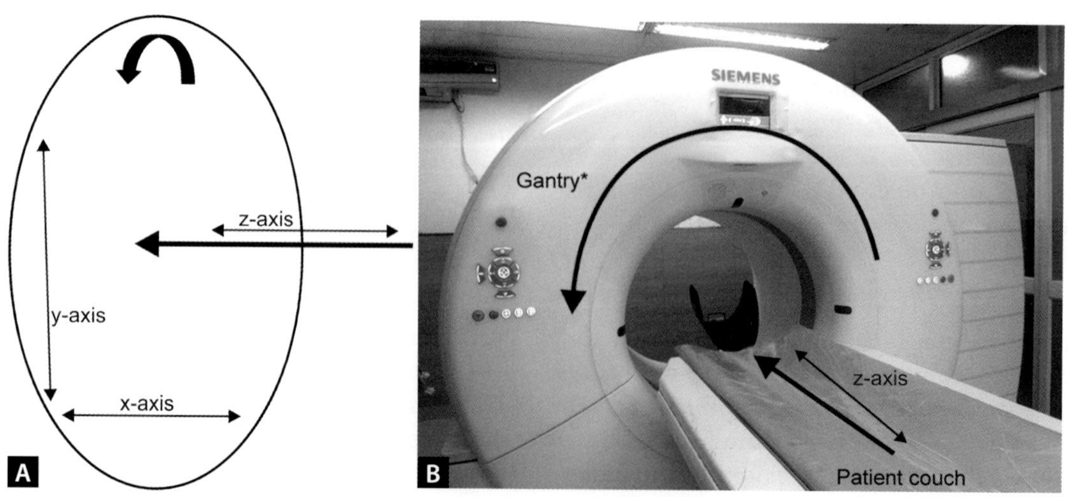

Figs. 2A and B: (A) Diagram showing the orientation of x, y and z-axis; (B) Photograph of a CT scanner. The gantry* houses the CT tube and the detector rows.

the same time has a dramatic effect on the overall radiation dose delivered during a spiral CT examination. Because radiation dose is inversely proportional to the pitch, the low-pitch protocols substantially increase radiation dose to patients.[3]

Another approach to increase the temporal resolution is to increase the number of X-ray sources (tubes) generating the X-rays. For a single-source scanner, the time required to collect all data needed for reconstruction of images (i.e. the acquisition time) is approximately one-half the gantry rotation time. The fastest single-source scanner currently available spins at 270 msec per rotation, for a nominal acquisition time and temporal resolution of 135 msec. For a dual-source scanner, the acquisition time is approximately one-fourth the gantry rotation time, because the two X-ray source/detector systems collect data in half the time needed for a single X-ray source/detector array. The fastest dual-source scanner currently available spins at 280 msec per rotation, for a nominal acquisition time of 70 msec.[3]

Contrast Resolution

Contrast resolution is the ability of a CT scanner to differentiate small attenuation differences on the CT image. It is crucial to remember that the linear attenuation coefficient is an absorption measurement and it is dependent on thickness of a material, density of a material, atomic number and photon energy. A change in kVp results in alteration of linear attenuation coefficient of the structure, even if the same structure is being imaged. Contrast resolution is limited by noise and with the increase of noise in an image, there is a decrease in the contrast resolution. Special filters called bow-tie filters absorb weaker energy photons, which reduce the probablility of scattered photons being detected by the CT detectors. An X-ray beam consists of polychromatic photons or photons having different energies. The bow-tie filters serve to absorb lower-energy photons primarily to "lessen" the effects from the polychromatic nature of an X-ray beam. A soft tissue, standard or smooth algorithm is used during the reconstruction process for enhancement of soft tissue and contrast resolution.[4]

ADVANCES IN HARDWARE

The newest technology offers significant advantages, but, current CT hardware releases are far from uniform across vendors, reflecting different approaches to image acquisition in the current era. No single CT scanner offers the full range of the newest features. This underscores the importance of understanding the properties and advancements of individual components of CT scanner.

Advances in CT Tube

Most modern commercial scanners use a hot-cathode, high-vacuum X-ray tube which is built with a liquid-cooled, copper-backed tungsten target. Lead can be found in various parts of the CT scanner system, which reduces the amount of excess radiation.

In conventional CT, the tube and detectors moves clock-wise and anti-clockwise 360° while in spiral/helical CT the tube and detector arrays continuously move with the table. The early CT scanners used the stationary anode X-ray tubes because the long scan times indicated that the instantaneous power level was low. Long scan times also allowed dissipation of heat. Shorter scan times in later versions of CT scanners required high-power X-ray tubes and use of oil-cooled rotating anodes for efficient thermal dissipation.

Several technical advances have been brought about in component design for achieving these power levels and dealing with the problems of target temperature, heat storage and heat dissipation. For example, the tube envelope, cathode assembly and anode assemblies including anode rotation and target design have been redesigned. A decrease in scan times has increased the anode heat capacity by as much as a factor of five, thus preventing the requirement for cooling delays during most clinical procedures, and tubes with capacities of 5–8 million heat units (MHU) are also available now. In addition, improvement in the rate of the heat dissipation (kilo-heat units per minute) has increased the heat storage capacity of modern X-ray tubes. The large heat capacities are achieved with thick graphite backing of target disks, anode diameters of 200 mm or more, improved high-temperature rotor bearings and metal housings with ceramic insulators among other factors.[5]

The working life of tubes used today ranges from 10,000 to 40,000 hours, with a marked improvement over the 1,000 hours typical of conventional CT tubes. Since many of the robust engineering changes led to an increase in the mass of the tube, a significant effort was also made towards reducing the mass to better withstand the increasing gantry rotational rates which were required by faster scan times.

With an increase in the gantry rotation speed, the stress on the gantry structure also increases, since rapid movement of heavy mechanical components inside the CT gantry makes it harder to achieve a further reduction in gantry rotation time. In fact, even a small incremental gain in the gantry rotation time requires great effort in the engineering design.[5]

A major landmark in development of CT tubes is the advent of directly cooled X-ray tube. It allows gantry rotation time below 0.4 seconds and allows virtually unlimited volume coverage at maximum scan speed without compromise on resolution and image quality. Direct anode cooling enables extremely high cooling rates and eliminates the need for anode heat storage capacity. The very compact design is robust. The anode and inner tube assembly are significantly smaller than in the conventional tubes. In conventional X-ray tubes, the entire anode including the bearings is encapsulated in a vacuum and the cooling fluid cannot reach it efficiently, which results in lower cooling rates. Robust X-ray tubes with higher heat storage capacity up to 8 MHU, allows scanning until the heat storage capacity is filled. Once overheated, even such state-of-the-art conventional X-ray tubes cool down to normal operation temperatures in 5–10 minutes.

The new directly cooled X-ray tubes provide direct cooling of the anode with all bearings being located outside the vacuum. Similar to a miniature electron beam CT, the electron beam in the tube is shaped and controlled by an electromagnetic field. The direct anode cooling enables unprecedented cooling rates of 4.7 MHU/min and eliminates the requirement for large heat storage capacities. In fact, the heat storage capacity of the new anode is close to 0 MHU. Even at maximum load, these tubes cool down within just 20 seconds which is much less than the time needed to begin the next scan or to position the next patient. With substantially higher tube lifetime even at much higher G-forces this revolutionary design is the key to increased gantry rotation speed and reduced life-cycle cost at the same time. A novel example of such a tube is Straton tube.[6]

X-ray tube with flying focus has a magnet system for deflecting and focusing the electron beam, whereby the magnet system including a carrier that is constructed as an iron yoke and that has four pole projections that are arranged around the axis of the electron beam offset from one another by 90 degree., on which two pairs of coils (z-coils and .phi.-coils) are arranged so as to be offset from one another by 90 degree. The individual coils of each pair supplied with a common high-frequency alternating current that deflects the electron beam in the .phi.- and z-directions, respectively, in a pulsed manner.[5]

Advances in Detectors

The detector array design in multiple-row detector CT varies with each manufacturer. The detectors are arranged in rows and columns. The number of active detector rows and the z-axis width of detectors in an array define the detector configuration. A detector design that is subdivided into equal elements, or portions, is called *uniform, matrix,* or *mosaic. Nonuniform* or Variable detectors use variable detector size in the orthogonal direction or along the z-axis (the longitudinal axis of the patient table). In combination with a physical postpatient collimator, signals from these detectors can be combined to form various values of image thickness in a manner that improves detector efficiency over that of uniform detectors. This improvement is a result of the smaller proportion of dead space due to the divisions (cell walls) between detector elements. *Hybrid detectors* has a number of narrow detector elements in the center of the detector and a different number of wider detectors (usually double the width of the narrow detectors) on both sides of the span of narrow detectors **(Figs. 3A to C)**. The number of narrow and wider detectors can vary among different vendors.[7]

Following the presentation of the first 4-slice CT scanner in 1998, all other manufacturers also offered scanners enabling acquisition of four simultaneous slices per rotation. The next step was the development of 16-slice CT scanners parallel to slimmed-down versions for the simultaneous acquisition of 6, 8, or 10 slices. And as the slice counts keep going up (128, 256 and even 320) the costs and clinical capabilities go up too.

In-plane spatial resolution is determined primarily by the number of X-ray projections available for reconstruction, the scan field of view and the image matrix. The highest in-plane spatial resolution of current MDCT scanners has been reported to be in the range of 0.23–0.4 mm.

During helical scanning, some overscanning in the longitudinal direction (z-overscan) is required to ensure that sufficient data are available for reconstruction. Dynamic or adaptive collimation is a hardware-based solution for collimating the X-ray beam such that extraneous radiation exposure is blocked by retractable collimator blades. Dynamic collimation has the greatest effect in reducing dose for shorter-scan lengths and higher-pitch values.

Z-overscanning can also occur during axial scanning. In this case, the amount of z-overscan depends on the planned scan length P and the total beam collimation. Adaptive collimation is a hardware solution offered on certain wide-detector array MDCT scanners. With this technique the detector collimation is automatically selected from a set of beam collimations in increments of 10 mm that are based on the planned scan length so as

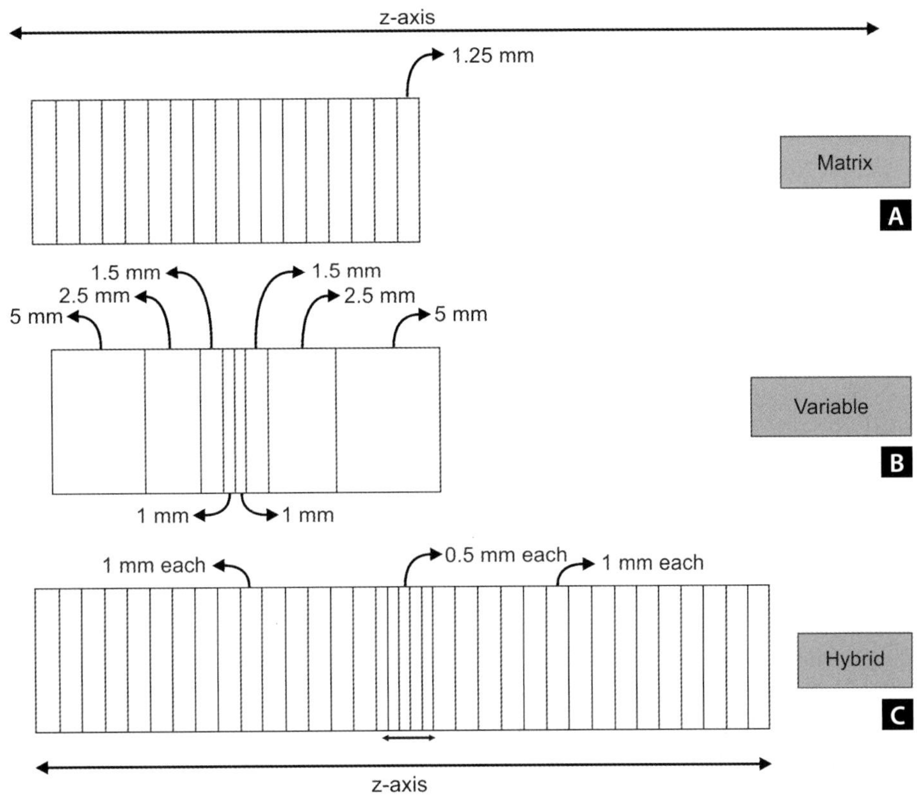

Figs. 3A to C: Diagram showing the basic design of matrix (A), variable (B) and the hybrid (C) detector. The measurements indicated in the diagram are relative and not to scale.

to minimize extraneous exposure. Adaptive collimation for axial scanning has the greatest effect in reducing dose with wide-detector array MDCT scanners because the portion of the total X-ray exposure in the axial scan mode attributed to z-overscanning increases with z-axis detector coverage.[1]

Dual energy may be principally achieved either by radiating the object with two different energy spectra from a single source through fast voltage switching or from multiple sources operating at different voltages, or by analyzing the energy spectrum on the detector side. A simple but effective solution lies in a double-layer detector design. The upper layer predominantly receives photons with lower energy and the lower layer receives photons with higher energy. Summing the signal from both detector layers returns the full signal as in a single layer detector, but separate readouts from both layers allow for simple spectral analysis of the X-ray beam.[1]

Most scanners use ceramic (solid-state) scintillation detectors coupled to photodiodes, which have improved spatial resolution and decreased noise compared with older xenon gas detector systems. Another milestone in CT technology lies in the development of new detector materials that exhibit higher sensitivity to radiation and allow faster sampling rates. There is a new scintillator that features a negligible afterglow in conjunction with a 100-fold faster reaction time, allowing for recording of 7000 views per second. Implementation of the new scintillator may be one of the prerequisites for single-source ultra-fast dual energy switching, promising almost simultaneous spatial and temporal registration and material decomposition without the limitation of a reduced FOV due to the second smaller detector in dual-source CT. They have very low afterglow, extremely low radiation damage and very good chemical durability, mechanical properties, uniformity and manufacturability. Approximately 50% fewer beam-hardening artifacts, metal artifact reduction and further improvements in contrast-to-noise ratio are some of the benefits resulting from the new scintillator. The new scintillator is configured to emit fluorescence when irradiated with X-rays and it has a primary decay time of only 30 nsec, making it 100 times faster than the conventional scintillator material. It has afterglow levels that reach only 25% of the levels of conventional scintillator material. The most advantageous feature of MDCT with garnet-based detectors is the improved spatial resolution (high-definition imaging at up to 230 mm resolution). An example of this is Gemstone, which is a newly developed transparent polycrystalline scintillator for CT from GE health care.[8,9]

Advances in Reconstruction

Conventionally, Filtered back projection method has been used for image reconstruction in single section CT, which involves processing of each ray sum immediately after it is obtained while the data acquisition continues for other ray sums. It attempts to project a uniform value of attenuation over the path of the ray such that the calculated attenuation over the path is proportional to the measured attenuation. The final image obtained is rather blurred as a result of the assumption that the beam attenuation occurs uniformly over the entire path of the ray. A technique to eliminate the blurring is the 'convolution operation' or 'filtering' which involves a 'filter function' or convolution 'kernel'. The filter or kernel may be chosen by the radiologist or automatically selected for a particular procedure. The most commonly used single-section spiral interpolation schemes are the 360° and 180° linear interpolation methods.[10]

Spiral CT requires an interpolation of the acquired measurement data in the longitudinal (through-plane) direction to estimate a complete CT data set at the desired plane of reconstruction. The 360° and 180° linear interpolation single-section spiral reconstruction approaches can be extended to multidetector row spiral scanning in a straightforward way but the cone angle of the measurement rays is not taken into account **(Fig. 4)**. Scanners that rely on 180° or 360° multidetector linear interpolation techniques and extensions thereof provide selected discrete pitch values to the user to provide optimized sampling schemes in the longitudinal direction and, hence, optimized image quality. Scanning at low pitch optimizes image quality and longitudinal resolution at a given collimation but at the expense of increased patient dose. To reduce patient dose, either milliampere settings should be reduced at low pitch values or high-pitch values should be chosen. A further refinement to spiral interpolation is the Z-filter approach, in which reconstruction is not restricted to the two rays closest to the image plane and is contributed by all rays within a selectable distance from the image plane. An example of z-filter technique is adaptive axial interpolation algorithm, which allows the system to trade off z-axis resolution with image noise. Unlike in single section spiral CT, patient dose is independent of spiral pitch.[11]

For CT scanners with 16 or more detector rows, modified reconstruction approaches that account for the cone-beam geometry of the measurement rays have been developed. In three-dimensional (3D) convolution back-projection technique for multisection spiral scanning, the reconstruction is based on sorting of raw data from individual detector channels. In the raw data space, which is typically four times as large as the image data space, the signals from the individual detector rows are computed in such a way that axial images in parallel orientation are directly obtained from the raw data.[1,11] Sorting of the raw data requires considerable processor power and more powerful computers. Direct 3D filtered back projection of raw data is superior to rebinning algorithms (mentioned later) in homogeneous distribution of image noise and uniform slice thickness in particular for scanners with larger cone angles. Iterative reconstruction techniques, based on back and forward projection promising significant noise reduction, have been proposed since the early times of CT technology. In single-slice spiral CT, the pitch factor did not affect image noise but higher-pitch factors resulted in thicker slices and increasingly blurred

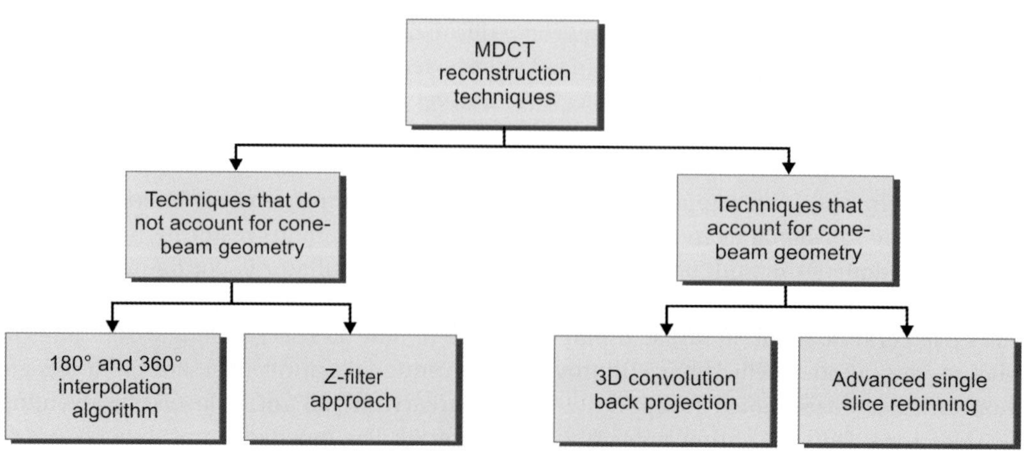

Fig. 4: Multidetector CT (MDCT) reconstruction techniques.

anatomy. Typical pitch factors used in spiral CT ranged between 1 and 2. In multislice spiral CT, the pitch factor does not affect the slice sensitivity profile of the reconstructed section but faster table feed (higher-pitch value) increases image noise because fewer photons are available for image reconstruction. This effect is compensated for on all scanners by automatically increasing the tube current (mA value) when a higher-pitch factor is selected. It is thus no longer possible to reduce the radiation dose by simply choosing a higher-pitch factor (which was possible on earlier spiral CT scanners). The image quality achieved with all currently available implementations of reconstruction algorithms may vary with the pitch factor. On most current scanners, optimal image quality is obtained when using pitch values slightly less than one because computation of supplementary projections obtained by overlapping scanning generally results in higher image quality.[1]

Rebinning Algorithms

Advanced single-slice rebinning (ASSR) and its variations are algorithms optimized for small cone angles. The algorithm reduces (3D) cone-beam data to tilted slices by minimizing the deviation of the reconstruction plane from the spiral. The image planes are no longer perpendicular to the patient axis; instead, they are tilted to match the spiral path of the focal spot generating pseudoaxial slices. In a final z-axis reformation step, the traditional transverse images are calculated by interpolating between the tilted original image planes. The ASSR algorithm operates efficiently and requires fairly little computing power to reconstruct images of clinically acceptable image quality. Representative examples for rebinning algorithms are the adaptive multiplanar reconstruction algorithm (AMPR) and the conjugate ray reconstruction (weighted hyperplane reconstruction).[1]

SPECIAL COMPUTED TOMOGRAPHY

Cone-beam CT/Volume CT

Cone-beam CT (CBCT) is an emerging CT variant which is designed to provide a compact, low-cost, low-radiation dose system that can be used to image high-contrast structures as in the head and neck. Cone-beam CT uses divergent X-rays forming a "cone" between the source and detector, unlike the "fan-beam" geometry in conventional CT **(Figs. 5A and B)**. In CBCT multiple images are acquired during a single rotation of the gantry around the patient head producing a volumetric data. On the other hand, conventional CT requires both rotation as well as z-axis translation of the gantry to be able to acquire 3D

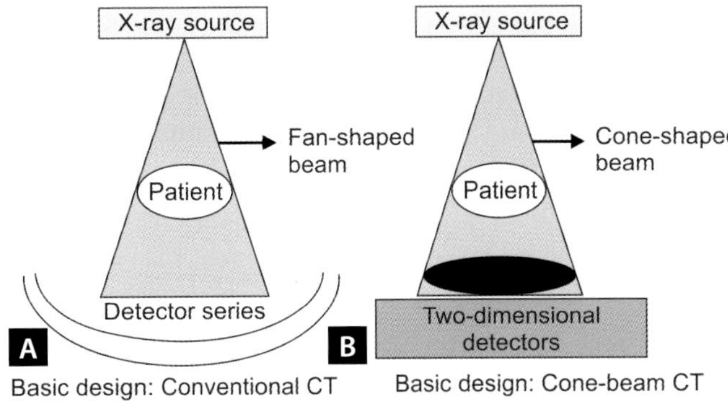

Figs. 5A and B: Schematic diagram showing basic design of a conventional CT (A) and cone-beam CT (B).

data. X-ray tubes of relatively low power requirements are employed. Recent versions of the system use flat panel detectors (FPDs) of the indirect-conversion type based on a cesium iodide (CsI) scintillator.[12] These digital flat panel CBCT systems can also be mounted on a C-arm for applications in interventional radiology suites.

Cone-beam CT thus produces an entire volumetric data set in a single gantry rotation as it utilizes a 2D detector system unlike the one-dimensional (1D) detector or series used in MDCT.[13,14] Depending on the variants of the system devised for various applications, several terms been used in literature to describe these new volumetric imaging techniques, such as cone-beam CT, C-arm CT, cone-beam volume CT, volume CT, angiographic CT and flat-panel CT.[13]

Cone-beam Geometry

Cone-beam CT uses a high-resolution 2D detector instead of a series of row of 1D detector elements as in MDCT.[13] Images obtained by CBCT have high-isotropic spatial resolution.[14] This is due to the isotropic nature acquisition and reconstruction in CBCT systems.[12] The volumetric data obtained in CBCT yield a dataset with isometric voxel size as small as 150 × 150 × 150 μm^3 at the isocenter, thus allowing high-quality multiplanar reconstructions.[12,15] Multidetector CT on the other hand produces individual sections which are subsequently stacked typically yielding spatial resolution of 500 × 500 μm^2 in-plane and 500–1000-μm in the z-axis.[12] Cone-beam CT however, suffers from poor contrast resolution due to higher scatter in cone-beam acquisition, a lower DQE of CBCT systems and reduced temporal resolution and dynamic range of the FPDs.[13] CBCT is thus suited for imaging of high-contrast structures. Higher scatter is a major limiting factor with the cone-beam vs conventional fan-beam geometry acquisition leading to image degradation. In order to counter this effect, several anti-scatter measures are employed, such as grids, software correction algorithms, beam-stop scatter mapping and alteration of object-to-detector distance (air-gap).[16] Cone-beam CT also suffers from limited anatomic coverage as it is based on acquisition of images during single gantry rotation.[13]

Flat-panel Detector

Cone-beam CT scanners use CsI scintillator detectors unlike the ceramic detectors used in MDCT. These suffer from a greater lag (afterglow) and hence scan times are much longer with CBCT relative to MDCT, thus reducing the temporal resolution of CBCT scanners. For instance, the current C-arm CBCT acquisitions take about 5 seconds.[13,15] In addition, CsI detectors also have a lower quantum efficiency reducing the dynamic range of the scanner.[13] The low-dynamic range also result in low-contrast resolution of these systems.

Reconstruction

Volumetric data thus acquired in CBCT as in MDCT can subsequently be manipulated and reconstructed with software to allow multiplanar as well as panoramic reconstructions.[12] The most commonly used reconstruction algorithm in CBCT systems is a modification of the filtered back-projection method called the Feldkamp algorithm.[15] Compared to MDCT, CBCT however takes longer times for acquisition as well as reconstruction of images despite the acquisition being done in a single rotation.

Radiation Dose

The other major advantage of CBCT is reduction of radiation dose relative to MDCT. Effective dose of commercial CBCT scanner has been estimated as 0.2 mSv Vs 1–2 mSv for MDCT head.[17,18] However, assessment of radiation dose during CBCT affords many challenges due to the altered beam geometry and underestimation of dose when using conventional methodology, such as ion-chamber inserts.[12,19] Also, conventional dosimetry metrics, such as the CTDIW cannot be directly applied to CBCT imaging. It is hence suggested that the difference in absorbed dose measurements may be insignificant when FOVs and image quality parameters between CBCT and MDCT are adjusted.[15,19]

Applications

Cone-beam CT provides a compact system wherein the scan can be performed with the patient sitting in an upright position. It has primarily found widespread applications in maxillofacial imaging including dental imaging, sinus and temporal bone imaging. It is most popular as an office based system for dental imaging. Cone-beam CT systems for maxillofacial imaging became available in 2001.[20] The compact design also makes the system significantly cheaper than MDCT. It also delivers a lower radiation dose than MDCT. Cone-beam CT has high spatial resolution but low-contrast resolution and limited anatomic coverage. It is not meant to be a substitute for MDCT which is distinctly superior in image quality but as a compact, inexpensive, low-dose system for applications. C-arm based CBCT systems are also used in interventional radiology suites.[13]

C-arm Based Cone-beam CT

The CBCT system is compact enough to allow it to be mounted on a C-arm. These systems allow projection radiography fluoroscopy, digital subtraction angiography, and volumetric CT applications through a single system. This has significant utility as it eliminates the need for transporting the patient to the CT room for procedures requiring guidance of cross-sectional imaging. Currently, all commercially available C-arm mounted CBCT systems employ digital flat-panel detectors.[13] Also, unlike MDCT as there is no z-axis translation and all acquisition occurs in a single rotation of the tube-detectors, it allows patient to remain stationary during the procedure.

Cone-beam CT has been employed for radiation therapy planning.[21] Cone-beam CT has also been used for surgical planning particularly in orthopedic, chest,abdominal, head and neck and neurosurgical procedures.[13,22]

Electron-beam tomography (EBT) is a specific form of computed tomography (CAT or CT) in which the X-ray tube is not mechanically spun in order to rotate the source of X-ray photons. In EBT, however, the X-ray tube itself is stationary and large and surrounds the imaging circle partially. Rather than moving the tube itself, electron beam focal point (and hence the X-ray source point) is swept electronically along a tungsten anode in the tube, tracing a large circular arc on its inner surface. This motion can be very fast. The heart always remains in motion and some important structures, such as arteries, move several times their diameter during each heartbeat. Thus, Rapid imaging is very useful to avoid the blurring of moving structures during the scan. It increasingly appears that the spiral CT designs, especially those with (b) 64 detector rows, (b) 3 × 360°/sec rotation speeds and designed for cardiac imaging, are largely replacing the EBT design from a commercial and medical perspective.

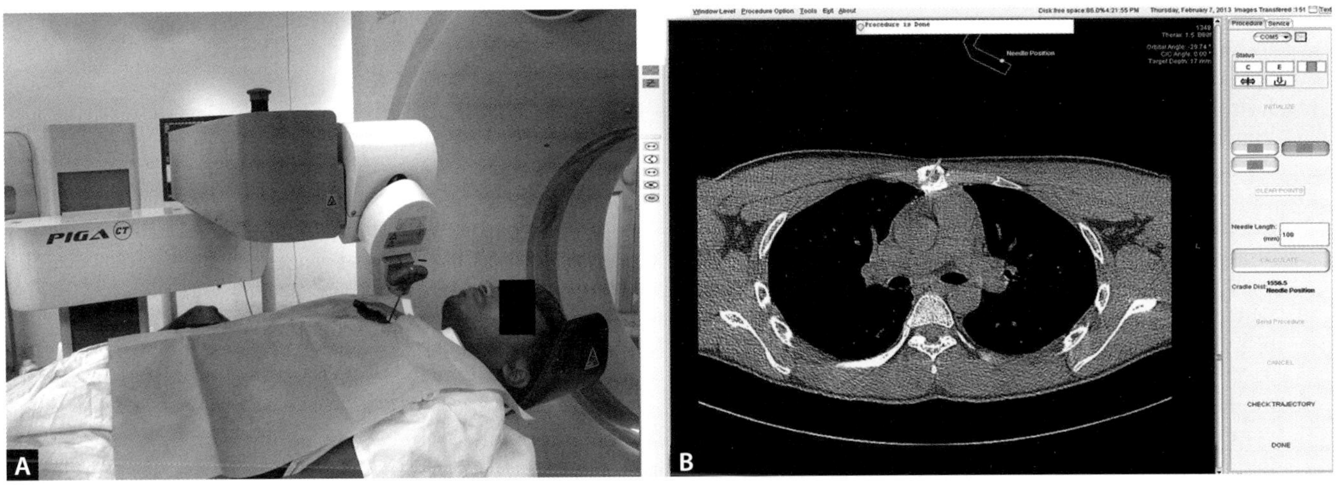

Figs. 6A and B: (A) Photograph showing sternal biopsy in a patient with the help of PIGA; (B) The planner image on the console projects the expected trajectory of the needle path.

Navigation Systems

Several navigation systems have recently become available to aid in CT guided interventions. One of the methods used for this purpose is electromagnetic tracking. These systems involve interaction with previously acquired images to provide real time spatial navigation information. This method does not involve continuous imaging of the patient. Combining electromagnetic tracking with preacquired imaging can be beneficial in guiding interventions, for instance in allowing real time targeting of lesions using previously acquired sequences in desired phase of enhancement.[23] Electromagnetic tracking also allows utilization of data from other imaging modalities. Similarly this technology is also being used to guide endoscopic and surgical procedures. Previously acquired CT images are loaded into proprietary software which reconstructs 3D images as desired. These are then used to mark target locations and plan path of intervention. Real time visualization of position of the endoscope is also then available in relation to these images. Navigation devices may also be based on optical tracking systems.[24]

Automated guiding systems for CT-guided biopsies are also available now. These typically involve the use of a robotic, electromechanical arm **(Figs. 6A and B)**. A computer interface receives the CT images and calculates coordinates on DICOM images and then guides needle placement through the arm.[25]

CONCLUSION

Computed tomography hardware thus is a rapidly evolving field, constantly introducing newer technologies for the user as the vendors continue to innovate.

REFERENCES

1. Rogalla P, Kloeters C, Hein PA, et al. CT Technology Overview: 64 –Slice and Beyond. Radiol Clin N Am. 2009;47:1-11.
2. Curry TS, Dowdey JE, Murry RC. Computed Tomography in Christensen's Physics of Diagnostic Radiology, 4th edition Philadelphia and London: Lea & Febiger; 1990. pp. 289-322.
3. Mahesh M, Cody DD. Physics of cardiac imaging with multiple-row detector CT. Radiographics. 2007;27(5):1495-509.
4. Reddinger W. www.e-radiography.net, [Place unknown] Out Source, Inc., 1998 [Updated 2013 January 1; cited 2013 March 08] Available from: www.e-radiography.net/mrict/CT_IQ.pdf
5. www.kau.edu.sa [cited 2013March 08] Available from: "X-Ray Tube in CT Scanner" www.kau.edu.sa/.
6. www.medical.siemens.com [cited 2013 March 08] Available from: www.medical.siemens.com/.../S_64-69_Science_Speed 4D.pdf
7. Cody DD, Mahesh M. Technologic Advances in Multidetector CT with a Focus on Cardiac Imaging. Radio Graphics. 2007;27: 1829-37.
8. www.gehealthcare.com [cited 2013 March 08]
9. Yanagawa M, Tomiyama N, Honda O, et al. Multidetector CT of the lung: image quality with garnet-based detectors. Radiology. 2010;255(3):944-54.
10. Miraldi F, Sims MS, Wiesen EJ. Imaging Principles in Computed Tomography in CT and MR Imaging of the Whole Body, 4th Edn. In: Haaga JR, Lanzieri CF, Gilkeson RC (Eds). United States of America: Mosby; 2003.pp.2-36.
11. Flohr TG, Schaller S, Stierstorfer K, et al. Multidetector row CT systems and image-reconstruction techniques. Radiology. 2005;235(3):756-73.
12. Miracle AC, Mukherji SK. Cone beam CT of the Head and Neck, Part 1: Physical Principles. AJNR. 2009;30:1088-95.
13. Orth RC, Wallace MJ, Kuo MD. For the Technology Assessment Committee of the Society of Interventional

Radiology. C-arm cone-beam CT: general principles and technical considerations for use in interventional radiology. J Vasc Interv Radiol. 2008;19:814-20.
14. Jaffray DA, Siewerdsen JH. Cone beam computed tomography with a flat-panel imager: initial performance characterization. Medical Physics. 2000;27:1311-23.
15. Gupta R, Grasruck M, Suess C, et al. Ultra-high resolution flat-panel volume CT: fundamental principles, design architecture and system characterization. Eur Radiol. 2006;16:1191-205. Epub 2006 Mar 10.
16. Endo M, Mori S, Tsunoo T, Miyazaki H. Magnitude and effects of X-ray scatter in a 256-slice CT scanner. Med Phys. 2006; 33:3359-68.
17. Bauhs JA, Vrieze TJ, Primak AN, et al. CT dosimetry: comparison of measurement techniques and devices. Radiographics. 2008;28:245-53.
18. Alspaugh J, Christodoulou E, Goodsitt M, et al. Dose and image quality of flat-panel detector volume computed tomography for sinus imaging. Med Phys. 2007;34:2634.
19. Fahrig R, Dixon R, Payne T, et al. Dose and image quality for a cone-beam C-arm CT system. Med Phys. 2006;33:4541-50.
20. Scarfe WC, Farman AG, Sukovic P. Clinical applications of cone-beam computed tomography in dental practice. J Can Dent Assoc. 2006;72:75-80.
21. Moore CJ, Am A, Marchant T, et al. Developments in and experience of kilovoltage X-ray cone beam image-guided radiotherapy.
22. Daly MJ, Siewerdsen JH, Moseley DJ, Jaffray DA, Irish JC. Intraoperative cone-beam CT for guidance of head and neck surgery: Assessment of dose and image quality using a C-arm prototype. Med Phys. 2006;33:3767-80.
23. Appelbaum L, Sosna J, Nissenbaum Y, Benshtein A, Goldberg SN. Electromagnetic navigation system for CT-guided biopsy of small lesions. AJR. 2011;196:1194-200.
24. Meier-Meitinger M, Nagel M, Kalender W, Bautz WA, Baum U. Computer-assisted navigation system for interventional CT-guided procedures: results of phantom and clinical studies. Rofo. 2008;180(4):310-7. [Article in German]
25. Chellathurai A, Kanhirat S, Chokkappan K, Swaminathan TS, Kulasekaran N. Technical note: CT-guided biopsy of lung masses using an automated guiding apparatus. Indian J Radiol Imaging. 2009;19(3):206-7.

CHAPTER 42

Dual-energy Computed Tomography

Arun Kumar Gupta, Manisha Jana

INTRODUCTION

Beginning from the single-slice sequential CT scanner and advancing towards multislice spiral CT with ultrafast true isotropic volume imaging, computed tomographic imaging technology has undergone significant changes in the last few decades. Conventional CT scanners, operating at a single energy, provide morphologic imaging only, with little material-specific information in body imaging. On the other hand, dual-energy CT utilizes the principle that different materials show different attenuation at varying energy levels, and this difference in attenuation can be used for tissue characterization. Since its inception, dual-energy CT scanning has undergone several technical modifications. This chapter describes the development, principle and applications of dual-energy CT.

HISTORICAL PERSPECTIVE

The concept of dual-energy CT existed from the very beginning of the history of computed tomographic imaging. In the early days, Sir Hounsfield proposed that "two pictures are taken of the same slice, one at 100 kV and the other at 140 kV... areas of high-atomic numbers can be enhanced... Tests carried out to date have shown that iodine (Z = 53) can be readily differentiated from calcium (Z = 20)".[1] Alvarez and Macovski[2] and Kalender et al.[3] also described the theoretical basis of dual-energy CT scanning in the late 1970s and early 1980s. The constraints in dual-energy imaging in early days were poor-spatial resolution, increased-radiation dose, slower-CT scanners leading to image misregistration, and significant noise in the lower-kilovoltage image.[4-8] With the advent of newer-multislice CT scanners having improved temporal resolution, dual-energy CT has finally become a reality in clinical applications. First commercially available dual-energy CT scanner came into use in 2006[8] (Somatom Definition, Siemens, Erlangen, Germany). It was dual-source dual-energy CT scanner (DS-DECT) having two X-ray tubes and two detector systems. Over the time, there have been newer modifications and advancements in the dual-energy scanners. In second generation of dual source dual-energy scanners, the dual-energy scan FOV was increased (from 26 to 33 cm); and the addition of a selective photon shield led to increased contrast to noise ratio and better and accurate material characterization. The DSDECT scanner was followed by the development of a single-detector, single-source DECT (SS-DECT) system with the capability for rapid alternation/fast switching between two kVp settings (Gemstone Spectral Imaging; GE Healthcare, Piscataway, NJ).[9] A SS-DECT scanner has a single ultrafast detector system with very-short afterglow and dual-energy scanning is made possible by rapid switching of the kVp settings of the tube. Currently available dual-energy CT scanners employ different technologies to obtain high and low-energy datasets:

- Dual-source dual-energy CT (DS-DECT)
- Single-source dual-energy CT (SS-DECT); and
- Single-source dual-energy scanner with dual-detector layers (under development with Philips, not commercially available).

PRINCIPLE

In clinical imaging, compton scatter and photoelectric effect are the two predominant interactions of matter with X-ray photons. The photoelectric effect occurs when an incident photon, having sufficient energy to overcome the K-shell binding energy of the electron in an atom, interacts with the atom to release the K-shell electron. The energy generated is released in the form of a photoelectron. The likelihood of photoelectric effect depends on the atomic number of the substance as well as the energy of the incident beam.[10] As the energy of the incident photon beam approaches the K-shell binding energy of an electron (which varies with the atomic number), the chances of photoelectric effect increases. K-edge refers to an increased photoelectric effect and a spike in attenuation at an incident energy level just greater than the K-shell binding energy.[7] The K-edge values of different materials are given in **Table 1**.

The principle of dual-energy CT imaging is based on the differential absorption of energy at variable kVp settings. For example, let us consider a substance (A) with K-edge at 60 kVp and another (B) at 130 kVp. If we image multiple combinations of A and/or B at 80 and 140 kVp, there will be differential attenuation at both these energy settings depending on the relative percentage of these substances. The object containing large amount of substance A will show higher attenuation at 80 kVp and lower attenuation at 140 kVp; whereas object containing larger amount of substance B will show higher attenuation at 140 kVp. In clinical applications, the constituents of soft tissues have a different K-edge (variable from 0.01 to 0.53), away from that of iodine (33.2) or calcium (4); hence iodine or calcium can be distinguished from soft tissues at dual energy imaging **(Fig. 1)**.

In diagnostic imaging, once the datasets at 80 kVp and 140 kVp are generated, the attenuation of the enhanced structures containing iodine (vessels, highly perfused organs) are more on a 80 kVp image than on a 140 kVp image. This difference in attenuation varies between different organs; for example, highly vascular organs and vessels have higher difference than muscles **(Figs. 2A to H)**. Postprocessing softwares use this information to generate a virtual noncontrast image, or to calculate the material composition within a specific region of interest.

DUAL-ENERGY RATIO

The material characterization on DECT largely depends on their dual-energy ratio. The dual-energy ratio is a material-specific parameter. It depends on the atomic number, not on the material density or concentration. For experimental derivation of dual-energy ratio of a given material X, the CT attenuations at any given kVp (for example, 140 kV) at different material concentrations are assessed and arranged along a graph (A). Similar graph (B) is made for different material concentrations at another kVp (for example 80 kVp). The dual-energy ratio of material X can be described as a ratio of the slope of the graph B to the slope of graph A.[12]

The difference between dual-energy ratio of different materials depends on several factors, for example:

1. Difference in the atomic number of the materials and
2. Spectral separation between X-ray spectra at the two energies. If the two incident X-ray beams have mean energies very close to each other, the difference in dual-energy ratios among various component materials (for example, iodine and soft tissue) will be less, and it will be difficult to differentiate them on imaging.

Table 1: Atomic number and k-edges of different substances and radiographic contrast agents[11]

Substance	*Atomic number*	*K-edge (keV)*
Hydrogen	1	0.01
Carbon	6	0.28
Nitrogen	7	0.40
Calcium	20	4
Iodine	53	33.2
Barium	56	37.45

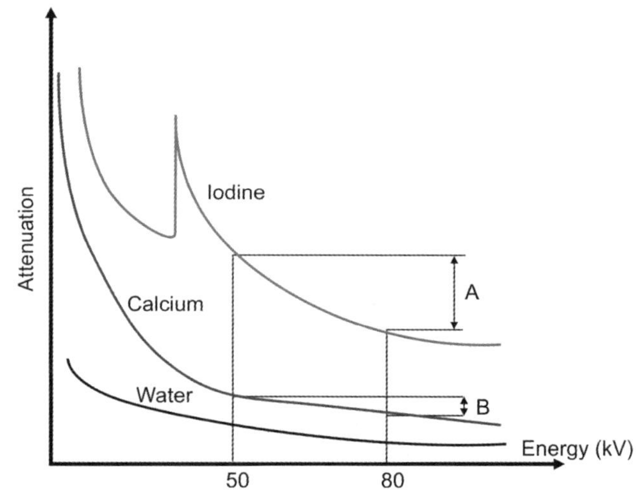

Fig. 1: Principle of dual-energy CT. Change in CT attenuation of substances at different energy levels of incident beam. Iodine (k-edge 33.2 keV), shows a peak attenuation at lower energies and a rapid decrease in attenuation at higher energies. When attenuation at 50 and 80 kVp are compared; iodine shows a greater decrease (A) in attenuation at higher energy than calcium (B). Water shows very minimal change in attenuation with changes in kV. This forms the basis of material characterization in dual-energy CT.

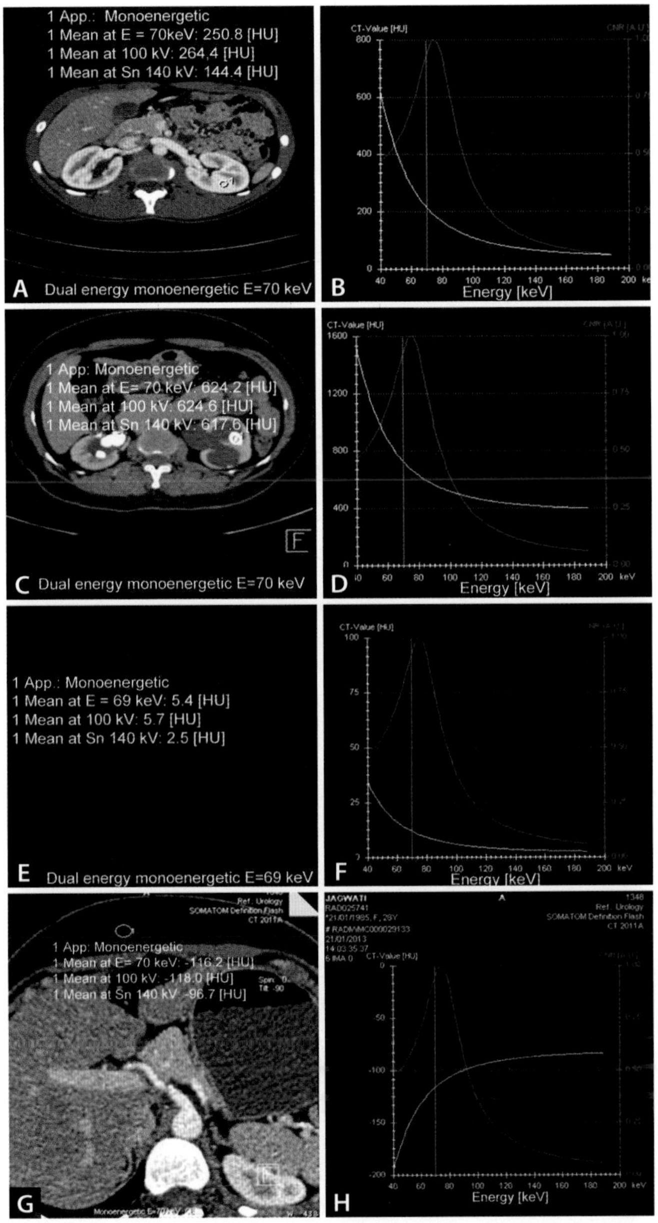

Figs. 2A to H: Different CT attenuation of tissues at different energy levels, based on their constituents. Highly vascular organs containing iodine on CECT shows higher attenuation at lower-energy images. For example, renal parenchyma shows an attenuation of 250.8 HU at 70 kV images and 144.4 HU on 140 kV images (A and B). Calcium shows very little variation in the attenuation values over a change of energy from 70 to 140 kV (C and D). Water also shows very little change in attenuation (E and F). Fat, to the contrary, shows a minimal increase in attenuation at higher energy images (G and H); –116.2 HU at 70 kV and –96.7 HU at 140 kV.

Spectral Separation and Selective-photon Shield

As a continuation of the previous discussion, for efficient dual-energy imaging the two incident X-ray beams should have sufficiently different energies. In reality, whenever X-ray is generated, it is emitted in the form of a continuous spectrum with photons having different energy levels (Bremsstrahlung) and a mean energy. The mean energy of an X-ray spectrum varies with the bombarding energy (kV). When two tubes with different kV are used, two spectra are generated with significant overlap between them (spectral overlap) **(Figs. 3A and B)**. As described earlier, the spectral overlap makes material characterization more difficult. Spectral overlap also reduces the dose efficiency as the 140 kVp spectrum contains significant percentage of low-energy photons also, which add to the patient dose. Spectral separation indicates a situation when there is minimal overlap between the different energy spectra, i.e. less spectral overlap.

Adequate spectral separation can be achieved by several methods:

1. Adding separate filtration to one or more tubes in DS-DECT.[13]
2. Adding split filtration to SS-DECT.[14]
3. Sandwich (dual) detectors.
4. Energy discriminating, photon counting detectors.

In DS-DECT, either one or both the tubes can have additional filtration. However, adding filters to the low-energy tube will further cut off the resultant kVp making it impossible to image a larger patient; hence, it is not practiced. Adding filtration to the higher-energy tube in the second-generation scanners using tin filters, termed selective photon shield, has led to improved spectral separation **(Figs. 3A and B)**.[12] Selective-photon shielding also improves the SNR efficiency and reduces dose to the patient. Tin is chosen as a filter component as it is inexpensive and easily available. The ideal thickness of filter varies between 0.5 and 0.8 mm.

Dual-source DECT

In the first-generation dual-source DECT scanner, X-rays are generated by two X-ray tubes, which are kept at 90 degrees angle to each other in the same gantry and operating at different kVp **(Fig. 4A)**. The average kVp of the higher-energy tube is 120–140 and that of the lower-energy tube is 80–100. The tube with larger kVp (tube A) has a larger detector of FOV 50 cm, and the lower energy tube (B) has a smaller FOV detector (26 cm). In the second-generation DS-DECT **(Fig. 4B)** scanner, the lower-energy tube (tube A) is paired with a detector with FOV of 50 cm while the higher-energy tube (tube B) is paired with a smaller detector with FOV of

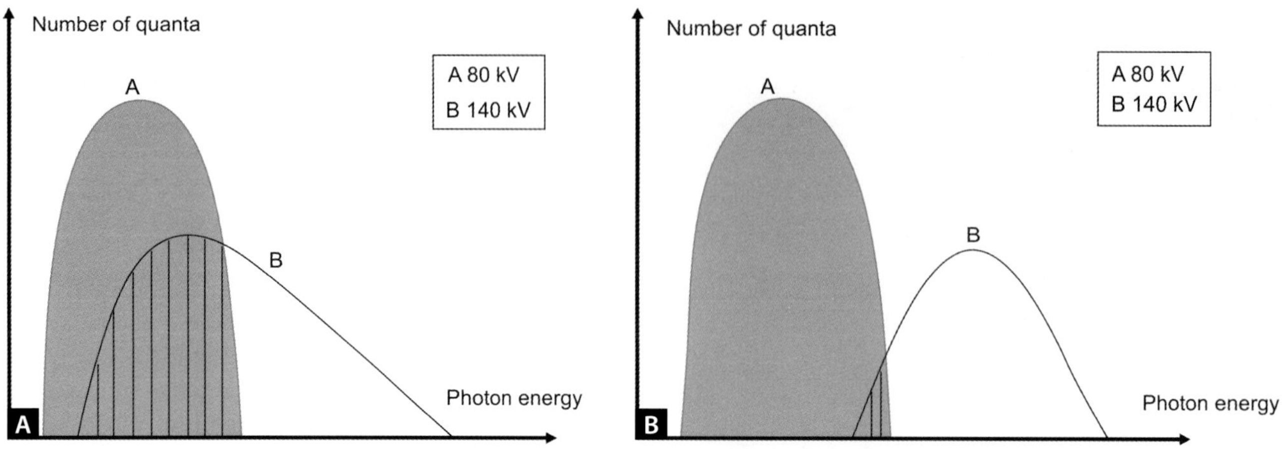

Figs. 3A and B: Spectral separation. When high- (140 kV) and low-energy X-rays (80 kV) are used, there is a significant energy overlap between them (shaded area A). Hence, generation of a true monoenergetic beam becomes difficult. After the use of a selective tin filter with the higher- energy tube in second-generation DS-DECT scanners (B), the lower-energy X-rays from 140 kV tube are filtered, thereby, reducing the overlap (shaded area B). This leads to better spectral separation, proper monoenergetic imaging and better material characterization.

33 cm. Higher-energy tube has a selective-proton shield made of tin filter. Two separate detector arrays lead to generation of two image datasets. Since both the tube kVp can be modified independently and additional selective-photon shield can be used in DS-DECT scanners, it results in better spectral separation. The temporal resolution of a DS-DECT is one- quarter of the rotation time (approximately 75 ms), as one X-ray tube acquires data during 90° of rotation.

However, the drawback of DS-DECT lies in term of temporal mis-registration, since the scans are not acquired simultaneously, but at a small time gap (although in ms). Another drawback is the limited dual-energy FOV (33 cm), which makes it difficult to image patients with larger body habitus.

Single-source DECT

Single-source DECT (SS-DECT) scanners use a single X-ray tube, which generates high- and low-energy X-ray spectra by rapid changing of the kVp settings (at an interval of 0.5 msec) in the same rotation **(Fig. 4C)**. Since the tube current cannot be changed so rapidly, in order to maximize the contrast to noise ratio, the exposure time ratio is changed between two acquisitions. For example, 65% exposure time is given for the 80 kVp beam and 35% for the 140 kVp beam.[15,16] The SS-DECT requires a very- fast detector and data-acquisition system with fast-sampling capability. The detector arrays used in SS-DECT are made of cerium-activated garnet (Gemstone Spectral Imaging; GE Healthcare, Piscataway, NJ).

The advantage of SS-DECT over DS-DECT includes:
1. Better temporal registration between two datasets, as the images from high and low-energy acquisition are acquired almost simultaneously.
2. Larger FOV of imaging (50 cm) and easier quantification of material density.

The disadvantage of SS-DECT includes a poorer spectral separation (hence less accurate material characterization compared to DS-DECT with selective photon shielding) as a selective-photon shield is not commercially available in such scanners (refer to previous paragraphs).

Dual-energy CT with Layered Detectors

This scanner contains a single X-ray source with hybrid detector for high and low energy imaging. The top layer captures low energy data and the bottom layer captures high- energy data; which are then used to reconstruct two separate image datasets.[17] Such scanners are under development with Philips, not yet commercially available. **Table 2** summarizes the comparison of DS-DECT and SS-DECT scanners.[18]

Processing of Data and Image Reconstruction in Dual-energy Imaging

The images generated from a DECT should have the combined morphologic data and material specific information. To obtain a material-specific image, the datasets can be processed in two ways:
1. Processing after the reconstruction of low- and high-energy images; which is also called 'image domain decomposition'. This method is used in DS-DECT

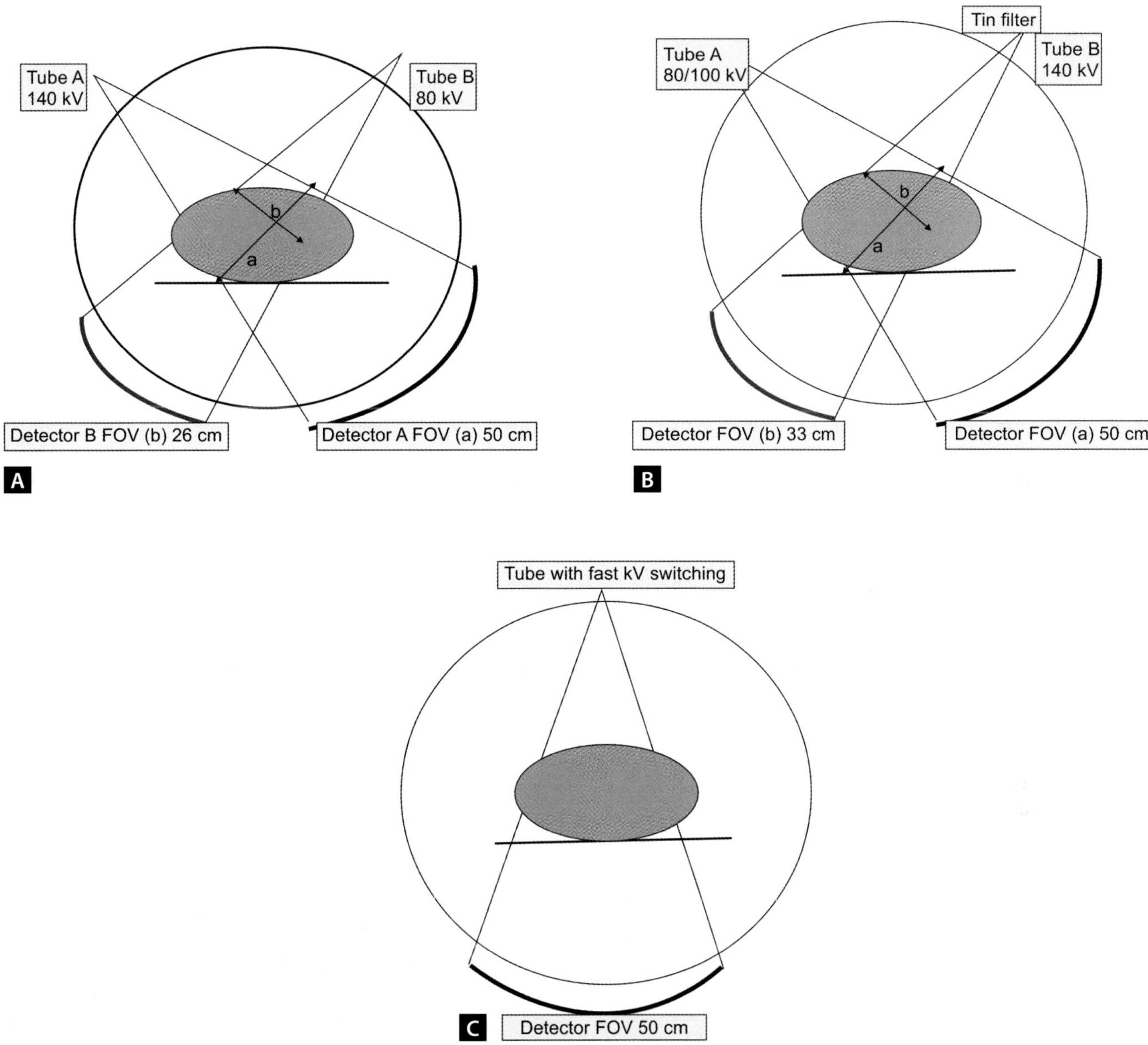

Figs. 4A to C: Dual-energy scanners—the first-generation DS-DECT scanners (A), the second-generation DS-DECT scanner (B) and SS-DECT scanner (C). In a first-generation DS-DECT scanner, two tubes are placed in the gantry at an angle of 90° to each other. Tube A has a higher kVp (140) and had a larger detector array of FOV 50 cm. The smaller-detector array (26 cm FOV) is paired against the lower-energy tube (80 KV). In a second-generation DS-DECT scanner, the smaller detector (FOV 33 cm) is paired with a higher-energy tube with a selective-photon shield. The SS-DECT scanner has a single tube and a detector array with 50 cm FOV. There is rapid switching of kVp in the tube.

scanners and dual (sandwich)-layer detector DECT scanners. In DS-DECT, images are generated by linear or non-linear sigmoidal blending of both (high and low energy) datasets.[19] In linear blending, a specific ratio of both high and low energy data are used. In sigmoidal blending, the pixels with higher attenuation are selected from the low energy datasets and the pixels with low noise are selected from high energy datasets. Material-specific images are obtained by calculating the difference in attenuation of varying materials between the low and high energy image datasets. For abdominal DS-DECT, a three-material decomposition (soft tissue, fat and iodine) process is commonly used to generate virtual noncontrast images. A color-coded overlay image (usually iodine overlay in abdominal imaging) is generated by assigning a color to the voxels containing the material and overlapping them on monochromatic images.[20,21]

Table 2: Comparison between single-source and dual-source dual-energy CT[17]

	Single-source-DECT	*Dual-source-DECT*
Tubes	Single X-ray tube with rapid switching of kVp	Two tubes operating at different kVp
Field of view (FOV)	Larger, 50 cm	FOV of dual energy acquisition 33 cm
Temporal and spatial registration	Good	Limited, as two separate image datasets are acquired
Spectral separation	Limited	Good, further improved by selective-photon shield (tin filter)
Data processing	Projection space dual-energy decomposition (more flexible)	Image domain decomposition (limited flexibility)
Noise on lower kVp images	Higher (as tube current can not be modulated while kVp is being altered)	Less (because of modulation of individual tube current)
Calculation of HU value on virtual NCCT image	Not possible	Possible
Prototype	Discovery CT 750 HD; GE healthcare	Somatom definition; Siemens

2. Processing before the images are reconstructed from high and low energy sinograms; also called 'projection-space decomposition'. It is a more robust processing which is preferred because of greater flexibility in material decomposition, and minimizing beam-hardening artifact.[9] In this method, after data acquisition, the 80 kVp images are not routinely reconstructed. The high- and low-energy datasets are calibrated and aligned in projection space to generate material density image and monochromatic images (providing energy-selective information). Material density image reconstruction in based on the theory of *basis material decomposition*; which proposes that the attenuation coefficients of any material can be computed as a weighted sum of the attenuation coefficients of two basis materials as long as the k-edge of the material is not within the evaluated energy range.[2,3] The two base materials should have highly different atomic number. The commonly selected dual energy basis material pairs are iodine and calcium, and iodine and water. Two separate sets of material density images are generated (iodine density and water density images, for example). The lesions containing iodine (for example, enhanced organs, vessels) will show higher attenuation on iodine-density images than on water density images. Monochromatic images are generated during the processing of material density images by calculating the linear attenuation coefficient (μ) of an object.[22]

Advantage of a monochromatic image generated from a DECT over a single-energy image at the same kVp includes the reduction of beam hardening artifacts and provides accurate CT numbers.

Image Display in DECT

Images generated in DECT can have two types of display:

1. *Material-density display* **(Figs. 5A and B)**: In DECT, the material-density display can be iodine-density display or water density display.
   - In an iodine-density display, the enhanced organs containing iodine appear bright whereas unenhanced areas remain dark. In abdominal imaging, iodine-density display has important role in the evaluation of a hyperdense cyst on CECT. Hemorrhagic/complicated cysts and often pose an imaging dilemma whenever incidentally detected on a CECT. On CECT images, they appear hyperdense and require an additional NCCT scan to rule out enhancement. On iodine-density display, they appear dark. Also, in the renal cysts, it can help reduce the problem of misdiagnosis of a cyst as a solid lesion due to 'pseudoenhancement', which refers to artifactual increase in CT numbers within a simple cyst on a single-energy CECT.[23]
   - The water-density display is equivalent to virtual unenhanced images. Water-density display can obviate the need of an additional NCCT image acquisition when a CT urographic image detects a calculus within the pelvicalyceal system; or for detection of calcification within an enhancing mass lesion.
2. *Monoenergetic image display* **(Fig. 6)**: The monoenergetic or pseudomonochromatic display are energy-specific display. Images are processed at any given kVp from the dual energy datasets, which resemble images physically acquired after scanning at that given kVp. Virtual monogengetic/

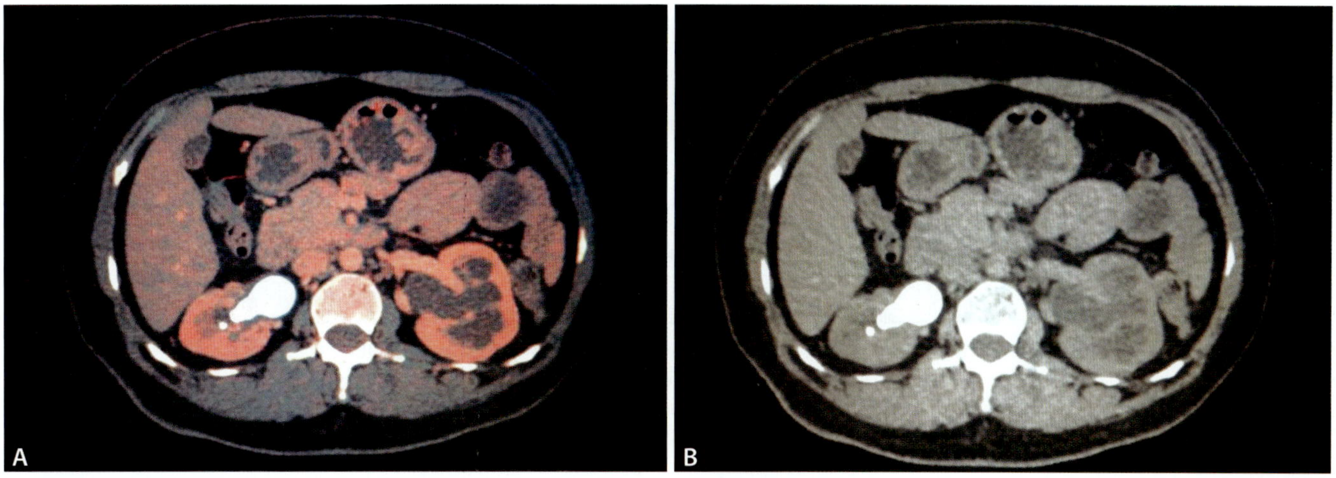

Figs. 5A and B: Material-density display. Iodine overlay map (A), created by overlapping the iodine-density images over monoenergetic image, highlight the organs containing iodine (colored red). The gradient of color varies according to the degree of enhancement of the organ. The water density display (B) is equivalent to virtual unenhanced image. Note that both calcium and iodine appear dense on a routine single-energy CT, but they can be differentiated on iodine map images as calcium will not be highlighted on a iodine map image (for example, the calculus in this image).

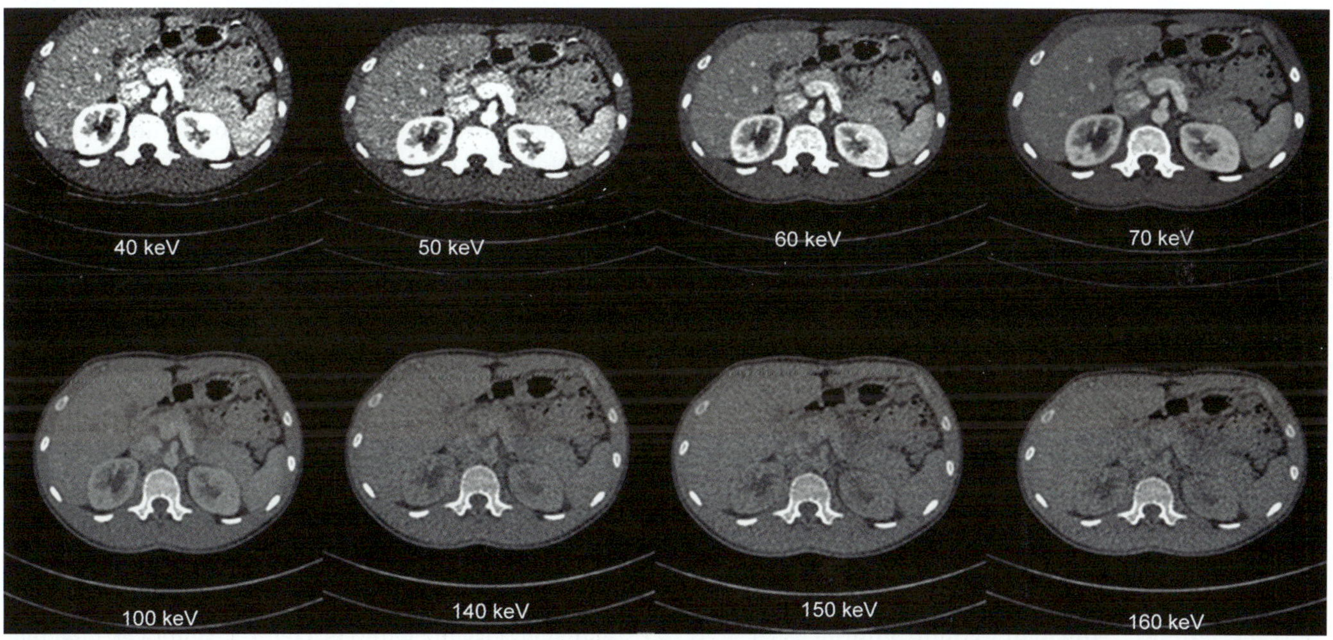

Fig. 6: Virtual monoenergetic images generated from a DS-DECT scanner. It is evident from the images that the attenuation of iodine and the image contrast are high at lower-energy images, although the images appear more noisy. As the kVp increases, the contrast difference between various tissues becomes negligible and the 160 keV image becomes identical to a noncontrast image.

pseudomonochromatic images at lower kVp show higher-image contrast and make small- enhancing lesions more conspicuous than routine display at 70 kVp. However, the images at lower kVp (for example 40 kV) have more noise and higher kVp images have less contrast. The optimum-image contrast to noise ratio is achieved at 70 kVp.

APPLICATIONS OF DECT

Applications in Abdomen

Renal Applications

1. *Renal calculi characterization* ***(Figs. 7A and B):*** On the basis of the dominant chemical component, urinary calculi can be divided into either uric

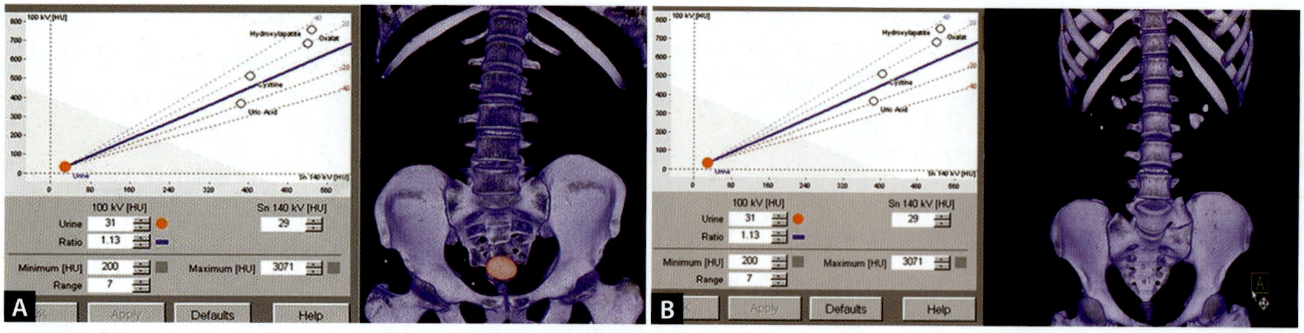

Figs. 7A and B: Renal calculi characterization by DECT. Images acquired at 100 and 140 kV in a DS-DECT scanner. A reference dual-energy ratio of 1.13 is taken to differentiate uric acid from nonuric acid calculi. The uric acid calculus (A) shows a dual energy ratio less than 1.13 and are colored red (arrow). The nonuric acid calculi show a dual-energy ratio above the reference line and are colored blue (B).

acid (UA) or nonuric acid calculi. Uric acid calculi are often associated with metabolic causes such as hyperuricemia or gout. These stones are lucent on radiograph but can be identified on CT. Nonuric acid calculi are further divided into calcium, cystine and struvite. Calcium calculi are the most common type and contains calcium oxalate monohydrate (COM), calcium oxalate dihydrate (COD), calcium phosphate and hydroxyapatite in a variable proportion. Struvite stones are composed of magnesium ammonium phosphate (triple phosphate) and are the major constituent of a stag horn calculus (calculus in pelvis with extension into at least two calyces). Cystine calculi are rare and associated with certain metabolic conditions, such as cystinuria. A calculus containing both uric acid as well as nonuric acid component is labeled as mixed calculus. Determining the composition of calculi has direct treatment implications. Uric acid stones can be treated medically whereas cystine and COM stones are resistant to extracorporeal shock-wave lithotripsy (ESWL) and percutaneous nephrolithotomy (PCNL) is preferred.[24]

Till now, single-energy NCCT has remained the usual standard investigation for evaluating urinary tract calculi. However, single-energy NCCT is unreliable for characterizing the type of calculi since calculi of different proportions of constituents can have overlapping CT attenuation values. When imaging is done on DECT scanners, the change in attenuation between high-and low-energy scans can be used to differentiate types of calculi.[25] UA calculi are composed of light elements whereas non-UA calculi are composed of heavy elements; hence, these two groups can be differentiated on imaging. On SS-DECT, calcium and uric acid material density images are generated, uric acid calculi are depicted on uric acid material density images and calcium containing calculi on calcium density images. DS-DECT has an added advantage of selective photon shield (tin filtration) in the 140 kVp tube for better spectral separation and more accurate composition analysis. In a DS-DECT scanner, keeping the reference dual-energy ratio at 1.13, the uric acid calculi are seen to lie below the reference line and non-UA calculi above it **(Figs. 7A and B)**. Several *ex vivo* studies have demonstrated the efficacy of DECT in characterizing stones, and also the advantage of additional tin filtration.[26-28]

2. *Renal cysts:* Detecting a simple cyst with water density is not an imaging challenge. Differentiating a complex/complicated renal cyst from a solid renal mass lesion is often difficult, and depends on the detection of enhancement in the lesion. Conventional single-energy CT will require two acquisitions, one NCCT and another CECT. Using dual energy CT, the additional acquisition of NCCT can be avoided as it is possible to generate virtual NCCT from the datasets. On iodine-density images, the enhancing solid mass will appear bright; whereas high density cysts will be dark, since they do not have any iodine in them.[29] In SS-DECT, it is not possible to calculate the HU value of the lesion, which is possible with DS-DECT.[30] Moreover, effective beam hardening reduction in DECT helps avoid the phenomenon of 'pseudoenhancement' (vide supra).
3. *Renal mass characterization and follow-up after ablation*: Calcification within an enhancing renal mass can be detected on a virtual NCCT image generated from a dual-energy dataset. After thermal ablation of solid renal masses, the imaging assessment should consist of multiphase scanning with and without contrast to detect enhancement in residual tumor tissue. While imaging on DECT scanners, one contrast-enhanced acquisition can generate virtual NCCT

scans, thus reducing the total dose to the patient. Iodine overlay maps help detect the enhancement in such masses.

Both DS-DECT and SS-DECT have a few technical limitations for the evaluation of renal masses. Firstly, virtual NCCT images have more image noise than real NCCT images. Second, because of the material decomposition algorithms used, calcification in renal lesions is less conspicuous on virtual unenhanced images than on real unenhanced images. Third, smaller amounts of fat in renal masses are difficult to detect on virtual NCCT images and can be measured only on conventional thin-section unenhanced CT images.

4. *CT urography*: CT urography is a routine imaging procedure in the evaluation of hematuria and multiple phase acquisitions (NCCT and delayed images) are performed for CT urography. On DECT imaging, virtual NCCT generated from the dual energy datasets can obviate the need for an additional NCCT acquisition and thus reduce the radiation dose. Takahashi et al.[31] reported that on virtual NCCT from excretory-phase CT urography performed with a DS-DECT scanner, the rate of detection of urinary tract stones was 100% for stones larger than 7 mm but decreased significantly (29%) for stones of 1–2 mm size.

Quality of the generated virtual NCCT images depends on iodine concentration within the pelvicalyceal systems, hence a highly concentrated iodinated contrast material within the PCS may lead to a 'rim artifact' at the margins and obscure small calculi. Incomplete subtraction of concentrated iodine can also be mistaken as calculi.[31]

Applications in Adrenal

Adrenal Adenoma

Adrenal adenomas are common imaging occurrences, and most of them are detected incidentally on abdominal CECT scans. Attenuation of less than 10 HU on NCCT image is virtually diagnostic of adrenal adenoma. When an incidental adrenal nodule is detected on single-energy CECT, it becomes essential to get a delayed scan or separate NCCT scan for characterization of the nodule. On a DE-CECT acquisition, virtual NCCT images generated from the dual energy datasets help eliminate the need of another NCCT scan.

The attenuation of adrenal adenoma at low and high kVp image depends on their lipid content. On several studies, there have been mixed reports related to the attenuation of adrenal adenoma on 80 and 140 kVp scans.[32,33]

Hepatic Mass Characterization

1. *Characterization of hepatic mass lesions:* Solid hepatic mass lesions are typically evaluated using a multiphase CECT. Like other organs, NCCT acquisition in liver also can be avoided by generating a virtual NCCT image from DECT acquisition in any one of the phases of multiphase CECT protocol. Secondly, hypervascular liver lesions are most conspicuous in arterial phase of examination, however detection of a hypervascular lesion on a delayed arterial phase becomes difficult. In such a scenario, on a DECT scan, the lesions can become more appreciable on a lower kVp image.[34,35] Monochromatic low kVp images and iodine-density display make detection of small hyperenhancing liver lesions easier. Non-enhancing lesions or cysts appear dark on iodine density maps **(Figs. 8A and B)**.
2. *Follow-up after hepatic tumor ablation or TACE*: After tumor ablation or embolization, detection of recurrence/ viable tumor depends on the demonstration of tumor mass enhancement, which in turn needs acquisition of both NCCT and a CECT scan in proper phase. With DECT, single CT acquisition can generate virtual non-contrast scans and iodine maps to detect enhancement; thereby avoiding excess radiation exposure.

   A word of caution needs to be remembered while imaging hepatocellular carcinoma after chemoembolization with lipiodol. Since lipiodol contains high concentration of iodine, iodine density display images shows the lipiodol accumulation as bright spot/hyperenhancement, which should not be diagnosed as recurrent or residual tumor.[36]
3. *Hepatic steatosis or iron deposition*: Hepatic focal fat deposition is often a diagnostic dilemma as it mimics solid tumor. Though there are several pointers like typical distribution and geographic nature of lesion and lack of mass effect on adjacent vasculature; sometimes, the diagnosis may be difficult on a single phase single energy CT. DECT can differentiate focal fat deposition from other hepatic mass lesion in the absence of iron deposition, which is a confounding factor.[11,37,38] Studies have described that attenuation values that are 9–13 HU lower at 80 kVp than at 140 kVp are suggestive of fat infiltration **(Figs. 9A to E)**.[37,38] Iron deposition in liver parenchyma will have higher attenuation at lower energy images.[11]

Application in Pancreas

Pancreatic neoplasms are usually hypovascular and their detection is based on the attenuation difference between

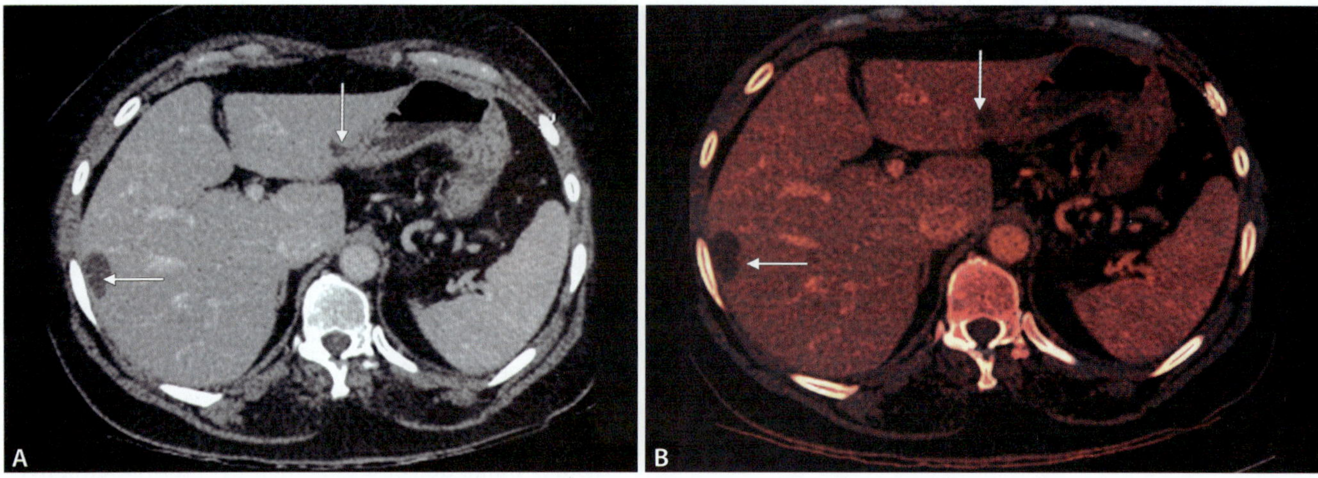

Figs. 8A and B: Simple hepatic cysts, imaging performed on a second generation DS-DECT scanner. Simulated monoenergetic image display at 70 kV generated from a dual-energy dataset (A) shows hypodense focal lesions in segment III and V (arrows). Iodine overlay maps (B) show them to be dark (not taking up iodine).

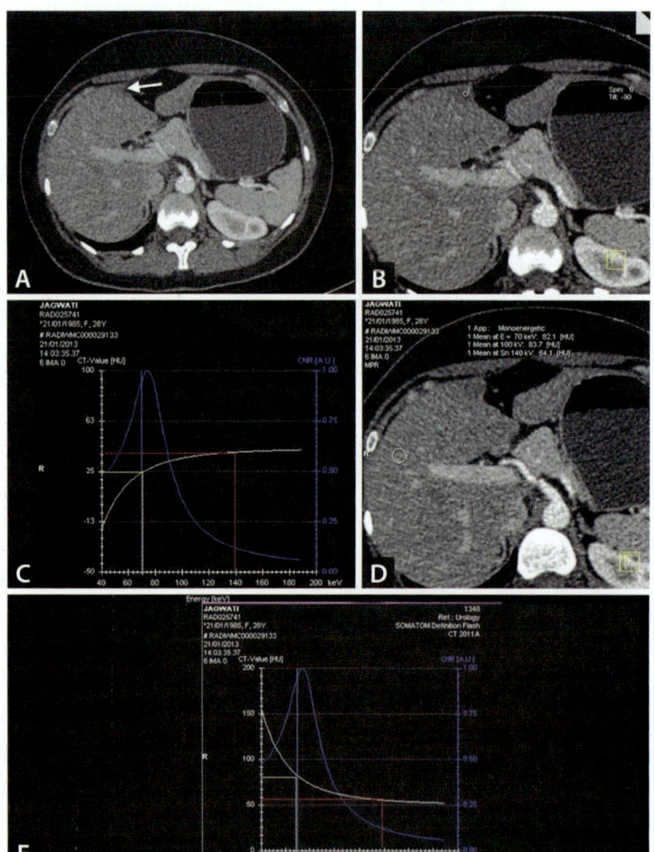

Figs. 9A to E: Focal hepatic steatosis. The area of focal fat deposition is seen as a hypodensity in segment 4b adjacent to the falciform ligament (arrow in A). Monoenergetic display (B) derived from a DS-DECT scanner (Somatom Definition Flash, Siemens) with tin filtration shows the increase in attenuation in higher kV images (attenuation of 23.8 at 70 kV, shown with a yellow line and 34.2 at 140 kV, shown with a red line) (C), which is suggestive of fatty change. In comparison, normal enhancing liver parenchyma shows a decrease in attenuation (D and E) in the higher energy images (attenuation of 82.1 at 70 kV and 64.1 at 140 kV images).

the normally enhancing pancreatic parenchyma and hypoenhancing mass lesion. Pancreatic parenchymal enhancement is best assessed in the pancreatic phase, 40–70 sec after injection of contrast material. However, significant percentage of pancreatic carcinomas are difficult to detect even on pancreatic phase images.[39] With DECT, the normally enhancing pancreatic parenchyma shows higher attenuation on monochromatic lower-energy display image and the iodine-density display. It has been seen that the attenuation difference between the lesion and normal pancreatic parenchyma (hence the lesion detection) increases with 80 kVp image than a single-energy routine 120 kVp scan.[40]

Another potential application of DECT in pancreatic imaging is the accurate identification of pancreatic necrosis; although the clinical importance is not yet established.[11]

Pulmonary Applications

1. *Pulmonary thromboembolism*: Pulmonary thromboembolism (PTE) imaging has undergone significant change in the past few years. Pulmonary CT angiography (CTA) has been accepted as the imaging modality of choice in case of suspected high-risk population. Pulmonary CTA can detect intraluminal thrombus in segmental arteries and smaller vessels also, but smaller clots/partial occlusion in subsegmental arteries can be missed on CTA. When imaging is done on a DECT scanner, smaller clots can be detected on an iodine overlay map visible as a perfusion defect. Compared to CTA and scintigraphy, dual-energy CT has a high sensitivity and specificity for perfusion mapping for the assessment of pulmonary embolism.[41,42] The perfusion defects in cases of pulmonary embolism are usually peripheral and wedge-shaped; although they can be absent in cases of very small nonoccluding thrombus in smaller vessels.

   For the generation of a proper iodine perfusion map of the lungs, the maximum and minimum value for material decomposition are usually kept at -600 and 960 HU. It excludes all the enhancing mediastinal structure and all central vessels in the lung parenchyma from the iodine perfusion map. Hence, the relatively less perfused area in case of thromboembolism can be easily visualized as perfusion defect **(Figs. 10A to I)**. For obtaining proper parenchymal enhancement, iodinated contrast agent should be injected at a proper rate (4–4.5 mL/sec), followed by 40 mL saline chase to reduce artifacts resulting from dense contrast in SVC/ brachiocephalic vein. Imaging should be done in both pulmonary and aortic phase. A threshold value of 20 HU mean iodine attenuation can be used to differentiate areas of lung parenchyma with negligible perfusion from those with demonstrable flow.

   Perfusion defects can also be seen from non-PTE causes; for example, in cases of aberrant pulmonary vascular supply,[43] or artefactual perfusion defects as in the lingual or right middle lobe (from cardiac pulsations), bilateral lower lobes near the diaphragm (from respiratory motion), in bilateral upper lobes (from streak artifacts in SVC or subclavian artery). Perfusion defects are also observed in parenchymal abnormalities, such as consolidation, atelectasis or emphysema **(Figs. 10A to I)**.[44,45]
2. *Xenon perfusion CT:* Xenon is a radiopaque gas with atomic number 54 and has photoelectric absorption characteristics similar to iodine.[46] During xenon ventilation CT, the patient usually inhales 30% xenon through a xenon gas inhalation system (Zetron V; Anzai Medical, Tokyo, Japan). Overlay maps are generated similar to iodine perfusion CT. DE xenon ventilation CT can be used to generate a ventilation map with areas of bronchial obstruction or atresia showing reduced ventilation.[47,48]
3. *Pulmonary nodule evaluation:* The degree of contrast enhancement on CECT is an important factor in differentiating a benign pulmonary nodule from a malignant one. DECT can generate virtual NCCT images and thereby quantify the enhancement. The differentiation of calcification from contrast enhancement is also possible on a single DE- CECT acquisition, thereby saving the additional radiation exposure of NCCT.

Musculoskeletal Applications

1. *Application in gout:* Gout is a disease resulting from intra-articular or soft-tissue uric acid crystal deposition leading to severe deforming arthropathy and gouty tophi formation. The causes may be multifactorial. Most often the diagnosis can be made on clinical and biochemical basis; however, the definitive diagnosis of gout requires microscopic analysis of fluid aspirated from the joint with the finding of negatively birefringent monosodium urate (MSU) crystals.[49] But few studies have described a rate of negative aspiration as high as 25% in acute attacks.[50]

   Plain radiography can show the arthropathy and corticated bone erosions in case of gouty soft tissue tophi. On DECT, the dual-energy ratio (vide supra) of uric acid varies significantly from that of calcium;

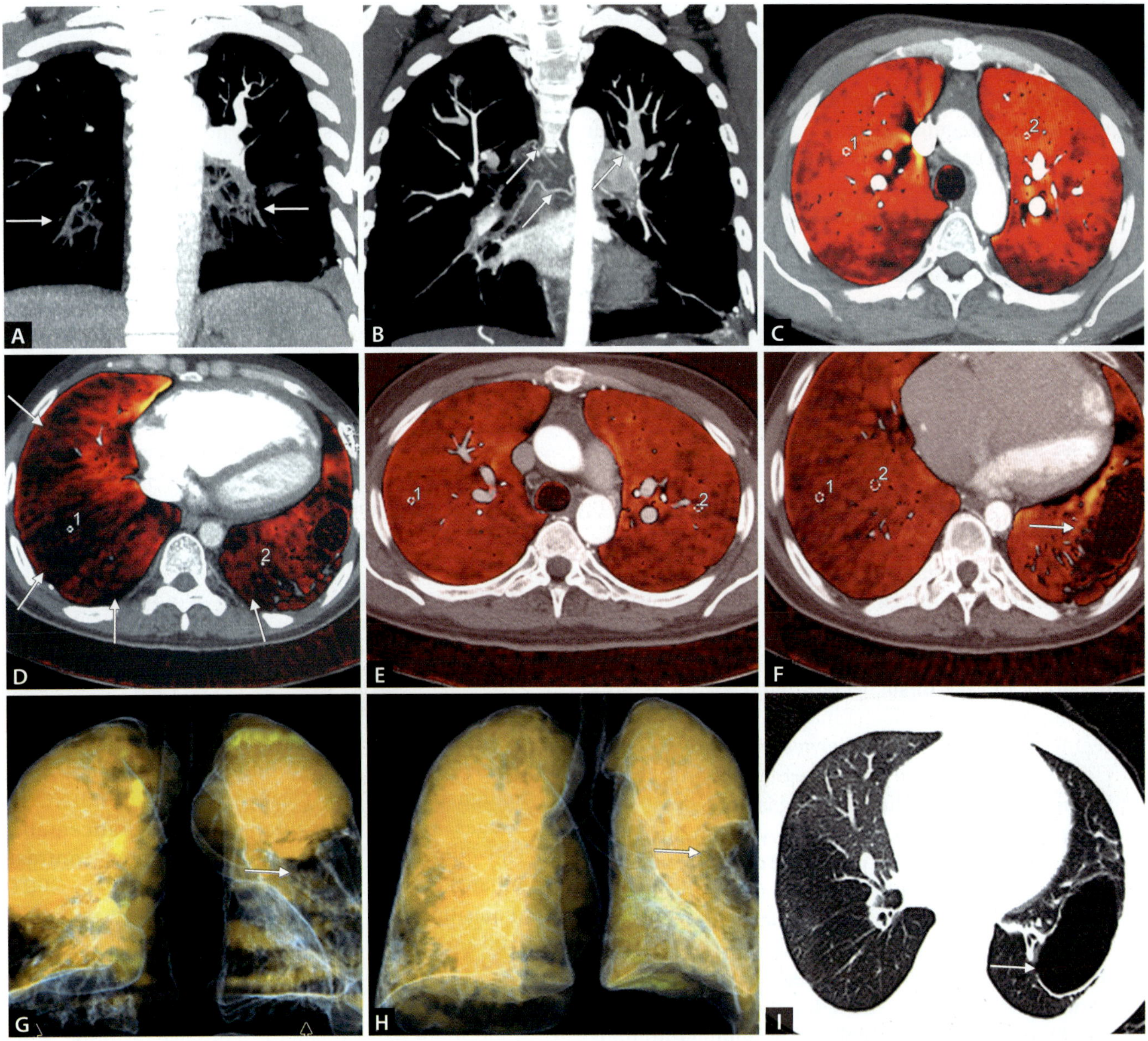

Figs. 10A to I: Dual-energy CT perfusion in chronic pulmonary thromboembolism. Coronal reformatted CTA image acquired at pulmonary phase (A) shows non-enhancement and attenuation in caliber of the lower lobe pulmonary arteries (arrows). Aortic phase image reveals hypertrophic bronchial arteries (small arrows in B). Iodine overlay maps generated from dual-energy CTA during pulmonary phase (C and D) reveal patchy areas of perfusion defect in the basal segments of both lower lobes (arrows in D). Iodine maps (E and F) generated from aortic phase images shows near complete perfusion (via bronchial collaterals) in the corresponding area. Volume-rendered images generated from iodine distribution maps in pulmonary phase (G) also shows the areas of perfusion defect (black arrow); whereas aortic phase image (H) shows near complete perfusion except a small area of non-perfusion (notched arrow) secondary to a large bulla. Lung window axial image (I) confirms the presence of the bulla (arrow).

hence, they can be easily differentiated. DS-DECT scans can generate material specific images and keeping the reference dual- energy ratio at 1.36, the uric acid crystals lie below the line and are differently color-coded (green), whereas the calcium deposits lie above the line **(Figs. 11A to D)**. The utility of DECT in gout diagnosis is twofold. First, it can diagnose gout in an easy, noninvasive and reproducible manner. Secondly, using automated volume software, the tophi volume can be quantitatively measured with less interobserver variability.[51,52]

2. *Metal artifact reduction:* Imaging of patients with metallic prosthesis remains a challenge. As the X-ray beam passes through metal prosthesis, the lower

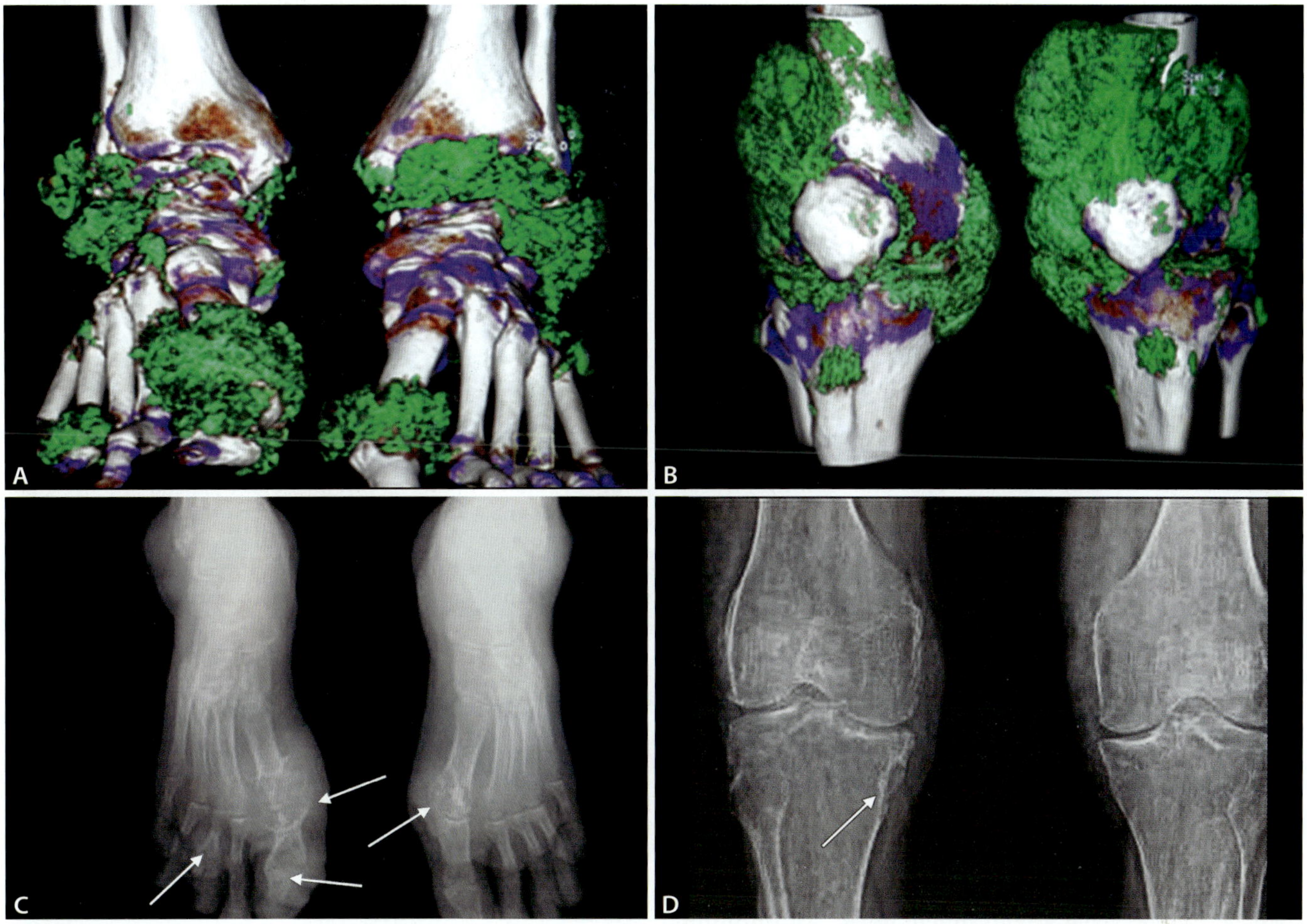

Figs. 11A to D: DECT in gout imaging. Scanning was performed at 80 and 140 kV in a patient with chronic gouty arthritis. Keeping a reference dual energy line at 1.36, MSU crystals are color-coded green. Color-coded volume-rendered imgaes of the ankle (A) and knee (B) reveal extensive MSU crystal deposition around the joints. Plain radiographs of the feet and knee reveals periarticular soft-tissue swellings and corticated erosions (arrows in C and D).

energy photons are absorbed and the character of the X-ray spectrum changes (it becomes 'harder', i.e. having higher energy photons only). This gives rise to the beam hardening artifacts around metallic prostheses which hamper the visualization of periprosthetic abnormalities. The usual modifications to reduce metal artifact in a single energy scanner include:

- Increasing the kVp,
- Increasing the mAs,
- Reducing slice collimation,
- Using a softer kernel for reconstruction, and
- Thicker slice reconstruction. Using DECT, monoenergentic reconstruction at a higher kVp has been shown in several studies to be more effective than routine single energy CT images at 120 kVp.[53,54]

3. *Other musculoskeletal applications:* Although evaluation of gout has remained the most widely used musculoskeletal application of DECT, there are several other applications, for example, detection of bone marrow edema[55] and evaluation of ligaments and tendons.[56-59]

Bone marrow edema is ideally best evaluated by MRI. Pache et al.[55] described high sensitivity and specificity of DECT imaging in the detection of post-traumatic bone marrow edema. Using a three material decomposition (water, fat and calcium), the virtual non-calcium subtracted images can be generated to detect marrow edema.

Tendons and ligaments are made up of collagen fibrils, which have a specific dual-energy ratio. In DECT, for material specific image generation a three material decomposition algorithm is used (collagen, fat and soft tissue). Several studies[56-59] have showed conflicting efficacy of DECT in the evaluation of tendons and ligaments. Thicker ligaments like anterior and posterior cruciate ligaments and patellar ligament can be adequately visualized, however visualization of thinner anatomical structures may not be appropriate.

Applications in Head and Neck

Like other parts of the body, DECT imaging in head and neck also has the advantage of generating a virtual NCCT image from the dual-energy dataset, without the need for an additional non-contrast scanning in order to quantify enhancement in a mass lesion. Iodine overlay maps can increase lesion conspicuity of head and neck masses. Recent study by Kuno et al.[60] has also demonstrated improved diagnostic performance and interobserver reproducibility by DECT imaging in laryngeal cartilage invasion in head and neck squamous cell carcinoma.

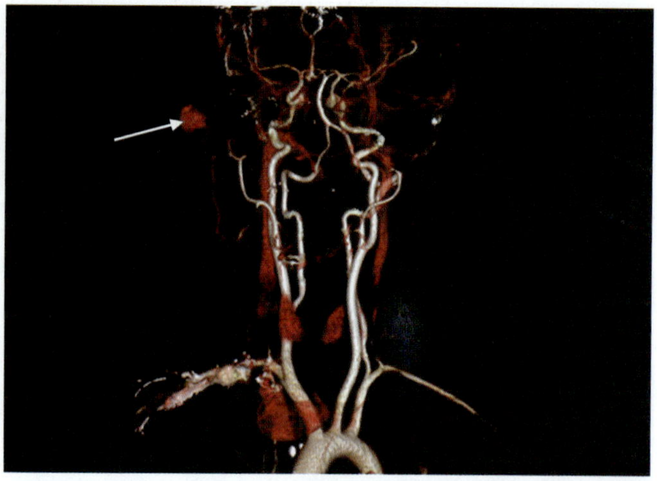

Fig. 12: Volume-rendered CTA image of the head and neck in a 10-year-old male with proliferative hemangioma (arrow) on the right side of face. The bone removal in dual energy CTA depends on material differentiation and leads to complete and quick bone subtraction compared to threshold-based bone subtraction.

Vascular Applications

Dual-energy CT angiography has been most widely used in aortic imaging. The advantages of DECT in aortic stent-graft imaging are multiple. First, virtual monoenergetic high kVp images in DECT are more effective in metal artifact reduction.[54] Secondly, the virtual monoenergetic low kVp images are more sensitive in detection of iodine (hence small endoleaks which are otherwise difficult to detect), though have a high image noise. An optimum monoenergetic image can be generated to balance the iodine density and the image noise. Third, the iodine overlay map can detect smaller endoleaks (differentiate between blood and contrast).[61] Fourth, DECT acquisition can help generate a virtual NCCT image which can detect intramural hematoma and has comparable image noise as that of a true NCCT image.[62] Fifth, the DE subtracted angiographic images are easier to generate and provide more complete bone removal. Finally, In endoleak detection, single-delayed DECT scanning followed by reconstruction of virtual NCCT and mono energetic low-kV images has very high sensitivity, specificity and positive predictive value (96–100%) compared with a conventional multiphase single energy CTA acquisition, thereby significantly reducing the patient dose (40–64%).[63,64]

In peripheral or neck angiography, the drawbacks of threshold based bone subtraction is that in cases of arteries lying close to bone, a part of the artery can be subtracted and may mimic stenosis or occlusion. Since the bone subtraction in DECT is based on material differentiation, it takes less time and yields more complete bone removal **(Fig. 12)**, which can reduce such artifacts.[65]

Unlike single energy CTA with threshold-based bone subtraction, DECT-CTA can remove calcified plaques also, with better visualization of vascular lumen. Compared to threshold-based bone removal, DECT bone subtraction are easier, quicker and more accurate in detection of vessel stenosis.[66]

Cardiac Applications

Coronary CT angiography in a multidetector row scanner has become an established imaging tool in the detection of significant coronary artery disease (CAD) in low-to-intermediate risk population.[67,68] However, the mere detection of an artery stenosis does not predict the hemodynamic significance of it, which can be predicted by myocardial perfusion imaging or wall motion abnormalities. Till now, myocardial perfusion studies have been performed using nuclear medicine studies (SPECT) and MRI. However, SPECT has poor spatial resolution and is not useful for coronary artery assessment. MRI can detect myocardial perfusion and cine-MRI can detect regional wall motion abnormality; but it is time-consuming and not useful for morphologic assessment of coronary artery disease.[69,70] With the use of DECT technology, material density (iodine) maps can be generated for the myocardium, reflecting the myocardial perfusion. Although termed 'perfusion', the map usually reflects the myocardial blood pool and is a static acquisition. A typical DECT cardiac perfusion study consists of the following phases—an initial calcium scoring followed by arterial phase scan, injection of IV adenosine and acquisition of

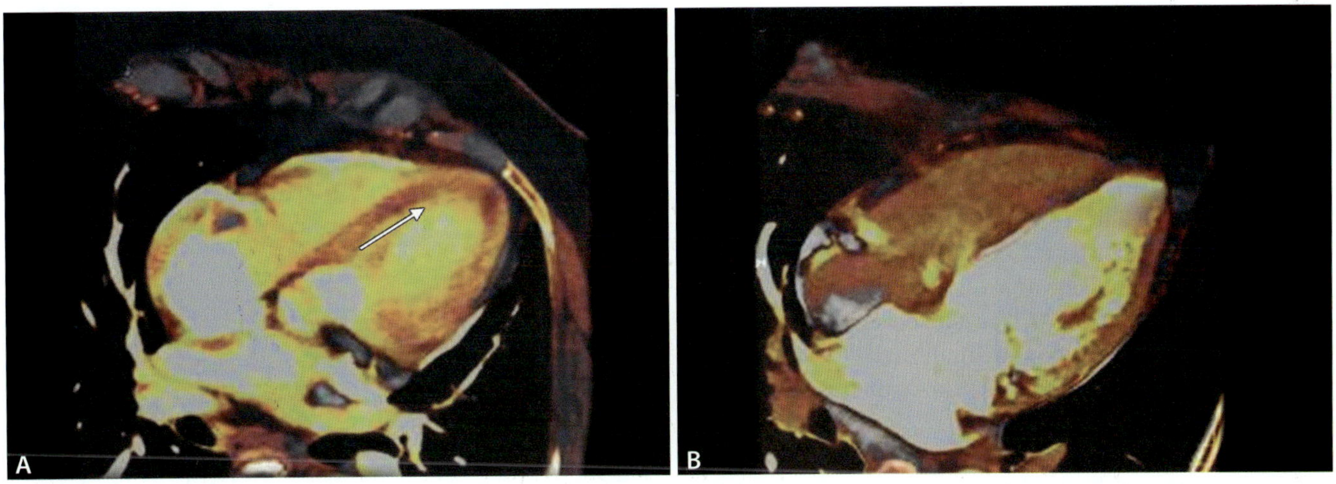

Figs. 13A and B: Stress myocardial perfusion imaging using DECT. A 52-year-old lady with effort intolerance. Iodine overlay maps at rest (A) shows perfusion defect (arrow) in the territory of the left anterior descending coronary artery (LAD) which is exaggerated on adenosine stress images (B); LAD territory ischemia.

stress images 3 minutes after IV adenosine (140 μg/min/kg) infusion, rest scanning 2 minutes after the stress scan when the heart rate returns to the baseline level. Finally, a delayed scan (5–10 min) is acquired. Monoenergetic low kV, high kV and iodine overlay maps are generated.[71] Normally perfused myocardium show uniform iodine distribution **(Figs. 13A and B)**. Myocardial infarcts are visualized as perfusion defects both at rest and under stress, whereas reversible ischemia shows perfusion defect only in stress images. Nonviable myocardium will show hyperenhancement on delayed scans.[72] DECT thus can combine the benefits of superior resolution morphologic imaging in CAD coupled with detection of its hemodynamic significance in the form of ischemia/infarction, which is unique to this modality.

Material differentiation based on dual-energy ratio has been tried in the characterization of plaques. Although differentiating a calcified from a noncalcified plaque is possible, but the differentiation of various types of non-calcified plaques have not been successful.[73]

Applications in Neuroimaging

As discussed for CTA elsewhere in the body, dual-energy CTA of intracranial vessels also has the similar advantage of easy and quick bone removal, especially with complex bony anatomy at the base of skull.[74] Other advantages of DECT scanning include avoidance of additional non-contrast scanning in certain circumstances. For example, In a patient with suspected subarachnoid hemorrhage, a preliminary NCCT scan can be avoided and direct dual-energy CTA can be performed to look for the etiology. The virtual NCCT images generated from the dual energy dataset helps detect hemorrhage and can save crucial time.[75]

Studies have described dual energy CTA to be the ideal tool for evaluating an acute intracranial hemorrhage. Apart from the ease of assessment of vascular cause of hemorrhage (vide supra); iodine overlay maps can be useful in differentiating tumor bleed from a simple hematoma.[76] Hemorrhage within a tumor will show hyperdensity on NCCT images and detection of any enhancing mass lesion in the background of hemorrhage can be an imaging challenge. Iodine overlay maps can detect the enhancing tumor tissue in the background of hematoma with greater accuracy; and also saves the patient from an additional radiation of NCCT scan.

DOSE CONSIDERATIONS

Although DECT scanning involves imaging with two different X-ray beams, the dose is not doubled in comparison to the single-energy scan. This is because the mAs are divided in the two sources; the higher-energy tube operates at a lower mAs and the lower-energy tube utilizes a relatively higher mAs. Till date, several experimental studies have been performed regarding dose comparisons of DECT scanning and single- energy scanning. Most of the experiments are based on DS-DECT scanners. Data are sparse regarding dose issues in SS-DECT. There has been various studies comparing dose of the single and dual energy scanners, but very few of them are performed with normalization of the contrast to noise ratio (CNR) or image quality.[77]

Schenzle et al.[77] performed a study on anthropomorphic phantom equipped with TLDs, with scanning performed at

140 and 80 kVp, 14 × 1.2 collimation in a first-generation DS-DECT scanner and in a second-generation DS-DECT scanner at 140 and 100 kVp settings with selective-photon shielding at 128 × 0.6 mm collimation. Dose comparison was done with a single-energy scan at 120 kV and 64 × 0.6 mm collimation at an equivalent dose index of 5.4 mGy x cm. The respective doses were 2.61 mSv (first-generation DS-DECT in dual-energy mode), 2.69 mSv (second-generation DS-DECT in dual-energy mode), 2.70 mSv (second-generation DS-DECT in single-energy mode). The image noise were also similar in all these three imaging techniques. Hence, there was no significant dose difference between the imaging techniques.

In coronary CTA, the dose received by DECT imaging has been assessed by Kerl et al.,[78] who compared the dose levels between DECT, first-generation DS-DECT in single- energy mode, and single-energy single source 16 slice MDCT. The investigators reported a lower dose, higher CNR and good diagnostic image quality in DECT than single-source MDCT. The increase in CNR was attributed to the low- kVp acquisition in DECT scanning by the investigators. Several other studies[78,79] regarding CT pulmonary angiography or CTA have shown that there is no significant increase in dose while scanning by DS-DECT scanning, compared to a single energy scanning. The added benefit of DECT scanning lies in the generation of virtual unenhanced scans, which can obviate the need of another NCCT scanning and reduce radiation dose. In renal imaging, the replacement of NCCT by virtual NCCT can result in a dose reduction of up to 35% in first-generation DECT and up to 50% in second-generation DECT.[80] Addition of tin filter in second-generation DS-DECT reduces the dose by eliminating lower-energy X-ray photons from the higher-energy spectrum.

Future trends in DECT imaging towards using a sandwich detector or an energy specific, photon counting detector can reduce the radiation dose further, retaining the benefits of material characterization on DECT.

Limitation

In spite of having significant advantages over single-energy CT in several applications, there are a few limitations of DECT **(Table 3)**. First, the FOV of the smaller detector is significantly less in DS-DECT (33 cm in second-generation DS-DECT) which leads to incomplete area coverage in obese patients. Second, the images generated from the lower-energy tube have inherently high noise. Finally, the large number of datasets generated leads to a problem in storage and archival. Pitfalls in organ-specific imaging have been discussed in their respective sections.

Table 3: Advantages and drawbacks of DECT

Advantages of DECT	*Disadvantages of DECT*
Material specific image can be generated. Characterization of renal calculi composition made possible	Increased radiation dose (which can be reduced using SPS)
Obviates the need for additional acquisition of NCCT images in many clinical indications, thereby reducing dose	Storage needs large capacity
Direct CT angiography—saves tedious post-processing and manual bone removal	Lower kVp image has inherent increased noise. Scanning may not be suitable in obese patients
Wider applications based on material characterization	Second detector in DS-DECT has smaller FOV, hence may not be beneficial in obese patients
Increased temporal resolution (helpful in cardiac CT)	

CONCLUSION

To conclude, dual-energy CT imaging adds another new dimension to conventional CT. the material-specific information gained by DECT scanning can be translated either to functional analysis of organs (for example, myocardial perfusion analysis), improvement in diagnostic confidence (noninvasive confirmation of clinical diagnosis in gout), aid in management decision-making (for example in renal calculi) or to easy image postprocessing and avoidance of unnecessary scanning.

ACKNOWLEDGMENTS

The authors sincerely acknowledge the contribution of Dr Gurpreet S Gulati for Figure 13 and Dr Ashu Seith Bhalla for Figure 10. The authors also sincerely acknowledge the contribution of Dr Sudeep Acharya and Dr Zohra Ahmad for Figures 7 and 11, respectively, from their MD thesis work at the Department of Radiodiagnosis, AIIMS, New Delhi, India.

REFERENCES

1. Computerized transverse axial scanning (tomography): Part 1. Description of system. GN Hounsfield, BJR. 1973;46: 1016-22.
2. Alvarez RE, Macovski A. Energy-selective reconstructions in X-ray computerised tomography. Phys Med Biol. 1976;21:733-44.
3. Kalender WA, Perman WH, Vetter JR, Klotz E. Evaluation of a prototype dual-energy computed tomographic apparatus. I. Phantom studies. Med Phys. 1986;13:334-9.
4. Rutherford RA, Pullan BR, Isherwood I. Measurement of effective atomic number and electron density using an EMI scanner. Neuroradiology. 1976;11(1):15-21.

5. Rutherford RA, Pullan BR, Isherwood I. X-ray energies for effective atomic number determination. Neuroradiology. 1976;11(1):23-8.
6. Millner MR, McDavid WD, Waggener RG, Dennis MJ, Payne WH, Sank VJ. Extraction of information from CT scans at different energies. Med Phys. 1979;6(1):70-1.
7. Chiro GD, Brooks RA, Kessler RM, et al. Tissue signatures with dual-energy computed tomography. Radiology. 1979;131(2):521-3.
8. Flohr TG, McCollough CH, Bruder H, et al. First performance evaluation of a dual-source CT (DSCT) system. Eur Radiol. 2006;16(2):256-68.
9. Zou YU, Silver MD. Analysis of fast kV-switching in dual energy CT using a pre-reconstruction decomposition technique. Proc SPIE 2008; 6913: Bellingham, Wash: International Society for Optical Engineering; 2008.
10. Curry TS III, Dowdey JE, Murry RC. Christensen's physics of diagnostic radiology, 4th edn. Philadelphia, Pa: Lea & Febiger. 1990.pp.61-9.
11. Coursey CA, Nelson RC, Boll DT, et al. Dual-energy multi-detector CT: how does it work, what can it tell us, and when can we use it in abdominopelvic imaging? Radio Graphics. 2010;30(4):1037-55.
12. Andrew N Primak, Juan Carlos Ramirez Giraldo, Christian D. Eusemann, Bernhard Schmidt, Birgit Kantor, Joel G. Fletcher, Cynthia H. McCollough. Dual-Source Dual-Energy CT With Additional Tin Filtration: Dose and Image Quality Evaluation in Phantoms and *In Vivo*. AJR. 2010;195:1164-74.
13. Kelcz F, Joseph PM, Hilal SK. Noise considerations in dual energy CT scanning. Med Phys. 1979;6:418-25.
14. Rutt B, Fenster A. Split-filter computed tomography: a simple technique for dual energy scanning. J Comput Assist Tomogr. 1980;4:501-9.
15. Chandra N, Langan DA. Gemstone detector: dual energy imaging via fast kVp switching. In: Johnson TRC, Fink C, Schönberg SO, Reiser MF, (Eds). Dual energy CT in clinical practice. Berlin, Germany: Springer-Verlag. 2011.pp.35-41.
16. Li B, Yadava G, Hsieh J, Chandra N, Kulpins MS. Head and body CTDIw of dual-energy X-ray CT with fast-kVp switching. In: Samei E, Pelc NJ, (Eds). Proceedings of SPIE: medical imaging. Bellingham, Wash: International Society for Optical Engineering; 2010. Vol 7622.
17. Vlassenbroek A. Dual layer CT. In: Johnson TRC, Fink C, Schönberg SO, Reiser MF (Eds). Dual energy CT in clinical practice. Berlin, Germany: Springer- Verlag. 2011;21-34.
18. Kaza RK, Platt JF, Cohan RH, Caoili EM, Al-Hawary MM, Wasnik A. Dual energy CT with single and dual source scanners: current applications in evaluating the genitourinary tract. Radiographics. 2012;32:353-69.
19. Fletcher JG, Takahashi N, Hartman R, et al. Dual-energy and dual-source CT: is there a role in the abdomen and pelvis? Radiol Clin North Am. 2009;47(1):41-57.
20. Johnson TR, Krauss B, Sedlmair M, et al. Material differentiation by dual energy CT: initial experience. Eur Radiol. 2007;17(6):1510-7.
21. Graser A, Johnson TR, Chandarana H, Macari M. Dual energy CT: preliminary observations and potential clinical applications in the abdomen. Eur Radiol. 2009;19(1):13-23.
22. Lehmann LA, Alvarez RE, Macovski A, et al. Generalized image combinations in dual kVp digital radiography. Med Phys. 1981;8(5):659-67.
23. Muller J, Vrtiska T, Schmidt B, et al. The impact of dual energy CT on pseudoenhancement of kidney lesions. In: Samei E, Pelc NJ, (Eds). Proceedings of SPIE: medical imaging 2010. Vol 7622. Bellingham, Wash: International Society for Optical Engineering; 2010.
24. Kambadakone AR, Eisner BH, Catalano OA, Sahani DV. New and evolving concepts in the imaging and management of urolithiasis: urologists' perspective. Radio Graphics. 2010; 30(3):603-23.
25. Eliahou R, Hidas G, Duvdevani M, Sosna J. Determination of renal stone composition with dual-energy computed tomography: an emerging application. Semin Ultrasound CT MR. 2010;31(4):315-20.
26. Joshi M, Langan DA, Sahani DS, et al. Effective atomic number accuracy for kidney stone characterization using spectral CT. In: Samei E, Pelc NJ, (Eds). Proceedings of SPIE: medical imaging 2010. Vol 7622. Bellingham, Wash: International Society for Optical Engineering, 2010.
27. Hidas G, Eliahou R, Duvdevani M, et al. Determination of renal stone composition with dual-energy CT: *in vivo* analysis and comparison with X-ray diffraction. Radiology. 2010;257(2):z394-401.
28. Vrtiska TJ, Takahashi N, Fletcher JG, Hartman RP, Yu L, Kawashima A. Genitourinary applications of dual-energy CT. AJR. 2010;194(6):1434-42.
29. Kaza RK, Caoili EM, Cohan RH, Platt JF. Distinguishing enhancing from nonenhancing renal lesions with fast kilovoltage-switching dual-energy CT. AJR. 2011;197(6):1375-81.
30. Mendonca PRS, Bhotika R, Maddah M, et al. Multi-material decomposition of spectral CT images. In: Samei E, Pelc NJ, (Eds). Proceedings of SPIE: medical imaging 2010. Vol 7622. Bellingham, Wash: International Society for Optical Engineering; 2010.
31. Takahashi N, Vrtiska TJ, Kawashima A, et al. Detectability of urinary stones on virtual nonenhanced images generated at pyelographic-phase dual-energy CT. Radiology. 2010;256(1):184-90.
32. Boland G, Jagtiani M, Kambadakone Ramesh A, Hahn P, Sahani D, Kalra M. Characterization of lipid poor adrenal adenomas: accuracy of dual energy CT (abstr). In: Radiological Society of North America scientific assembly and annual meeting program. Oak Brook, Ill: Radiological Society of North America; 2008.pp.390.
33. Gupta RT, Ho LM, Marin D, Boll DT, Barnhart HX, Nelson RC. Dual energy CT for characterization of adrenal nodules: initial experience. AJR. 2010;194(6):1479-83.
34. Marin D, Nelson RC, Samei E, et al. Hypervascular liver tumors: low tube voltage, high tube current multidetector CT during late hepatic arterial phase for detection—initial clinical experience. Radiology. 2009;251(3):771-9.
35. Schindera ST, Nelson RC, Mukundan S Jr, et al. Hypervascular liver tumors: low tube voltage, high tube current multi-detector row CT for enhanced detection—phantom study. Radiology. 2008;246(1):125-32.

36. Silva AC, Morse BG, Hara AK, Paden RG, Hongo N, Pavlicek W. Dual energy (Spectral) CT: applications in abdominal imaging. Radiographics. 2011;31:1031-46.
37. Raptopoulos V, Karellas A, Bernstein J, Reale FR, Constantinou C, Zawacki JK. Value of dual-energy CT in differentiating focal fatty infiltration of the liver from low-density masses. AJR. 1991;157(4):721-5.
38. Mendler MH, Bouillet P, Le Sidaner A, et al. Dual-energy CT in the diagnosis and quantification of fatty liver: limited clinical value in comparison to ultrasound scan and single-energy CT—with special reference to iron overload. J Hepatol. 1998;28(5):785-94.
39. Prokesch RW, Chow LC, Beaulieu CF, Bammer R, Jeffrey RB Jr. Isoattenuating pancreatic adenocarcinoma at multi-detector row CT: secondary signs. Radiology. 2002;224(3):764-8.
40. Spieler B, Macari M, Godoy M, et al. Dual source dual energy MDCT: comparison of 80 kVp and weighted average kVp data on pancreatic lesion conspicuity (abstr). In: Radiological Society of North America scientific assembly and annual meeting program. Oak Brook, Ill: Radiological Society of North America; 2008.p.522.
41. Fink C, Johnson TR, Michaely HJ, et al. Dual-energy CT angiography of the lung in patients with suspected pulmonary embolism: initial results. Rofo. 2008;180(10):879-83.
42. Thieme SF, Becker CR, Hacker M, Nikolaou K, Reiser MF, Johnson TR. Dual energy CT for the assessment of lung perfusion: correlation to scintigraphy. Eur J Radiol. 2008;68(3):369-74.
43. Boroto K, Remy-Jardin M, Flohr T, et al. Thoracic applications of dual-source CT technology. Eur J Radiol. 2008;68(3):375-84.
44. Pontana F, Faivre JB, Remy-Jardin M, et al. Lung perfusion with dual-energy multidetector-row CT (MDCT): feasibility for the evaluation of acute pulmonary embolism in 117 consecutive patients. Acad Radiol. 2008;15(12):1494-504.
45. Pansini V, Remy-Jardin M, Faivre JB, et al. Assessment of lobar perfusion in smokers according to the presence and severity of emphysema: preliminary experience with dual-energy CT angiography. Eur Radiol. 2009;19(12):2834-43.
46. Meyer JS, Hayman LA, Yamamoto M, Sakai F, Nakajima S. Local cerebral blood flow measured by CT after stable xenon inhalation. AJR. 1980;135(2):239-51.
47. Goo HW, Chae EJ, Seo JB, Hong SJ. Xenon ventilation CT using a dual-source dual-energy technique: dynamic ventilation abnormality in a child with bronchial atresia. Pediatr Radiol. 2008;38(10):1113-6.
48. Chae EJ, Seo JB, Goo HW, et al. Xenon ventilation CT with a dual-energy technique of dual-source CT: initial experience. Radiology. 2008;248(2):615-24.
49. Monu JU, Pope TL Jr. Gout: a clinical and radiologic review. Radiol Clin North Am. 2004;42:169-84.
50. Swan A, Amer H, Dieppe P. The value of synovial fluid assays in the diagnosis of joint disease: a literature survey. Ann Rheum Dis. 2002;61:493-8.
51. Choi HK, Burns LC, Shojania K, et al. Dual energy CT in gout: a prospective validation study. Ann Rheum Dis. 2012;71(9): 1466-71.
52. Dalbeth N, Aati O, Gao A, et al. Assessment of tophus size: a comparison between physical measurement methods and dual-energy computed tomography scanning. J Clin Rheumatol. 2012;18:23-7.
53. Bamberg F, Dierks A, Nikolaou K, Reiser MF, Becker CR, Johnson TR. Metal artifact reduction by dual energy computed tomography using monoenergetic extrapolation. Eur Radiol. 2011;21:1424-9.
54. Zhou C, Zhao YE, Luo S, et al. Monoenergetic imaging of dual-energy CT reduces artifacts from implanted metal orthopedic devices in patients with fractures. Acad Radiol. 2011;18:1252-7.
55. Pache G, Krauss B, Strohm P, et al. Dual-energy CT virtual noncalcium technique: detecting post-traumatic bone marrow lesions—feasibility study. Radiology. 2010;256:617-24.
56. Lohan DG, Motamedi K, Chow K, et al. Does dual-energy CT of lower extremity tendons incur penalties in patient radiation exposure or reduced multiplanar reconstruction image quality? AJR. 2008;191:1386-90.
57. Persson A, Jackowski C, Engström E, Zachrisson H. Advances of dual source, dual-energy imaging in postmortem CT. Eur J Radiol. 2008;68:446-55.
58. Deng K, Sun C, Liu C, Ma R. Initial experience with visualizing hand and foot tendons by dual energy computed tomography. Clin Imaging. 2009;33:384-9.
59. Sun C, Miao F, Wang XM, et al. An initial qualitative study of dual-energy CT in the knee ligaments. Surg Radiol Anat. 2008; 30:443-7.
60. Hirofumi Kuno, Hiroaki Onaya, Ryoko Iwata, et al. Evaluation of Cartilage Invasion by Laryngeal and Hypopharyngeal Squamous Cell Carcinoma with Dual-Energy CT. Radiology. 2012;265:488-96.
61. Ascenti G, Mazziotti S, Lamberto S, et al. Dualenergy CT for detection of endoleaks after endovascular abdominal aneurysm repair: usefulness of colored iodine overlay. AJR. 2011;196:1408-14.
62. Numburi UD, Schoenhagen P, Flamm SD, et al. Feasibility of dual-energy CT in the arterial phase: imaging after endovascular aortic repair. AJR. 2010;195:486-93.
63. Stolzmann P, Frauenfelder T, Pfammatter T, et al. Endoleaks after endovascular abdominal aortic aneurysm repair: detection with dual-energy dual- source CT. Radiology. 2008; 249:682-91.
64. Maturen KE, Kleaveland PA, Kaza RK, et al. Aortic endograft surveillance: use of fast-switch kVp dual-energy computed tomography with virtual noncontrast imaging. J Comput Assist Tomogr. 2011;35:742-6.
65. Yamamoto S, McWilliams J, Arellano C, et al. Dual-energy CT angiography of pelvic and lower extremity arteries: dual-energy bone subtraction versus manual bone subtraction. Clin Radiol. 2009;64:1088-96.
66. Brockmann C, Jochum S, Sadick M, et al. Dual energy CT angiography in peripheral arterial occlusive disease. Cardiovasc Intervent Radiol. 2009;32:630-7.

67. Mowatt G, Cummins E, Waugh N, et al. Systematic review of the clinical effectiveness and cost-effectiveness of 64-slice or higher computed tomography angiography as an alternative to invasive coronary angiography in the investigation of coronary artery disease. Health Technol Assess. 2008;12:iii–iv,ix–143.
68. Stolzmann P, Donati OF, Scheffel H. Low-dose CT coronary angiography for the prediction of myocardial ischaemia. Eur Radiol. 2010;20:56-64.
69. Gaemperli O, Schepis T, Valenta I, et al. Functionally relevant coronary artery disease: comparison of 64-section CT angiography with myocardial perfusion SPECT. Radiology. 2008;248:414-23.
70. Greenwood JP, Maredia N, Younger JF, et al. Cardiovascular magnetic resonance and single-photon emission computed tomography for diagnosis of coronary heart disease (CE-MARC): a prospective trial. Lancet. 2012;379:453-60.
71. Weininger M, Schoepf UJ, Ramachandra A, et al. Adenosine-stress dynamic real-time myocardial perfusion and adenosine-stress first-pass dual-energy myocardial perfusion CT for the assessment of acute chest pain: Initial results. Eur J Radiol. 2012;81(12):3703-10.
72. Arnoldi E, Lee YS, Ruzsics B, et al. CT detection of myocardial blood volume deficits: dual-energy CT compared with single-energy CT spectra. J Cardiovasc Comput Tomogr. 2011;5:421-9.
73. Henzler T, Porubsky S, Kayed H, et al. Attenuation-based characterization of coronary atherosclerotic plaque: comparison of dual source and dual energy CT with single-source CT and histopathology. Eur J Radiol. 2011;80:54-9.
74. Watanabe Y, Uotani K, Nakazawa T, et al. Dualenergy direct bone removal CT angiography for evaluation of intracranial aneurysm or stenosis: comparison with conventional digital subtraction angiography. Eur Radiol. 2009;19: 1019-24.
75. Postma AA, Hofman PA, Stadler AA, et al. Dual-energy CT of the brain and intracranial vessels. AJR. 2012;199(5 Suppl):S26-33.
76. Kim SJ, Lim HK, Lee HY, et al. Dual-energy CT in the evaluation of intracerebral hemorrhage of unknown origin: differentiation between tumor bleeding and pure hemorrhage. AJNR. 2012; 33:865-72.
77. Schenzle JC, Sommer WH, Neumaier K, et al. Dual energy CT of the chest: how about the dose? Invest Radiol 2010;45:347-53, Eur J Radiol. 2011;80:54-9.
78. Yuan R, Shuman WP, Earls JP, et al. Reduced iodine load at CT pulmonary angiography with dual-energy monochromatic imaging: comparison with standard CT pulmonary angiography—a prospective randomized trial. Radiology. 2012;262:290-7.
79. De Zordo T, von Lutterotti K, Dejaco C, et al. Comparison of image quality and radiation dose of different pulmonary CTA protocols on a 128-slice CT: high-pitch dual source CT, dual energy CT and conventional spiral CT. Eur Radiol. 2012;22:279-86.
80. Graser A, Johnson TR, Hecht EM, et al. Dual-energy CT in patients suspected of having renal masses: can virtual nonenhanced images replace true nonenhanced images? Radiology. 2009;252:433-40.

CHAPTER 43

Computed Tomography Perfusion Imaging

Veena Chowdhury

INTRODUCTION

Perfusion computed tomography (CT) allows functional evaluation of tissue vascularity. It measures the temporal changes in tissue density after intravenous injection of a contrast medium (CM) bolus using a series of dynamically acquired CT images. The greatest impact of perfusion CT has been on the assessment of patients who have had strokes, wherein the rapid scan timing and faster image processing have cemented its role as the modality of choice for evaluation of structural and functional status of cerebral vasculature.[1] In the field of oncology, perfusion CT has found applications in diagnosis, staging, prognostic evaluation and monitoring of response to therapies.[2,3] Although the role of ultrasound and magnetic resonance imaging have been explored for perfusion, there is a linear relationship between iodine concentration and density changes seen on CT expressed as Hounsefield units (HU), hence CT may be regarded as a preferred technique for perfusion imaging in general. Perfusion CT also has the potential to become the preferred technique for the assessment of tumor response to antiangiogenic drugs.[4,5]

PERFUSION COMPUTED TOMOGRAPHY TECHNIQUE: BASIC PRINCIPLE

The fundamental principle of perfusion CT is based on the temporal changes in tissue attenuation after intravenous administration of iodinated contrast medium. This enhancement of tissue depends on the tissue iodine concentration and is an indirect reflection of tissue vascularity and vascular physiology. After intravenous injection of the iodinated CM, the ensuing tissue enhancement can be divided into two phases based on the distribution in the intravascular or extravascular compartment. In the initial phase, the enhancement is mainly attributable to the distribution of contrast within the intravascular space and this phase lasts for approximately 40–60 seconds from the time of contrast injection. In the second phase, contrast passes from the intravascular to the extravascular compartment across the capillary basement membrane and tissue enhancement results from contrast distribution between the two compartments. In the first phase, the enhancement is determined to a great extent by the tissue blood flow (BF) and blood volume (BV) whereas in the second phase, it is influenced by the vascular permeability to the CM.[6] By obtaining a series of CT images in quick succession in the region of interest during these two phases, the temporal changes in tissue attenuation after injection of CM can be recorded. By applying appropriate mathematic modeling, tissue perfusion can be quantified. The various analytical methods vary from scanner to scanner and among the commercial vendors. Two most commonly used analytical methods are as follows:

1. *Compartmental analysis*: In this kinetic modeling technique, analysis can be undertaken using the single compartment or double compartment method.[4,6] The single compartment method assumes that the intravascular and extravascular spaces are a single compartment and calculates tissue perfusion based

on the conservation of the mass within the system. It estimates perfusion using the maximum slope of peak height of the tissue concentration curve normalized to the arterial input function.[7] Conversely, the double compartment method assumes that the intravascular and extravascular spaces are separate compartments and estimates capillary permeability and BV using a technique called Patlak analysis, which quantifies the passage of contrast from intravascular space into the extravascular space.

2. *Deconvolution analysis*: This CM kinetic modeling is based on the use of arterial and tissue time concentration curves to calculate the impulse residue function (IRF) for the tissue. The IRF is a theoretic tissue curve that is obtained from the direct arterial input, assuming that the concentration of contrast material in the tissue is linearly dependent on the input arterial concentration when the BF is constant.[6,7] After accounting for the flow correction, the height of this curve reflects the tissue perfusion and the area under the curve provides the relative BV estimation.[7] For the estimation of capillary permeability, a distributed parameter model is used, which is essentially an extended deconvolution method.

Compartmental and deconvolution modeling methods have been found to be generally comparable, with differences in their theoretic assumptions and their susceptibility to noise and motion.[8] Compartmental analysis is based on the assumption that bolus of CM has to be retained within the organ of interest at the time of measurement, which may result in underestimation of perfusion values in organs with rapid vascular transit or with a large bolus injection.[7] Deconvolution analysis, however, assumes that the shape of the IRF is a plateau with a single exponential washout. Although this assumption is believed to work for most organs, it might not be suitable for assessing perfusion in such organs as the spleen and kidney, which have complex microcirculations. Hence, it is preferable to use compartmental analysis for organs with the complex circulatory pathways. Deconvolution method is appropriate for measuring lower levels of perfusion (<20 mL/min/100 mL) because they are able to tolerate greater image noise attributable to the inclusion of the complete time series of images for calculation.[7] This is particularly beneficial for the accurate measurement of the lower perfusion values typically seen in tumors after treatment response. A potential drawback of including all the acquired images for the calculation is the possibility of image misregistration secondary to motion of the patient. Conversely, compartmental analysis effectively uses three images of perfusion measurement: the baseline image and the images immediately before and after the moment the maximal rate of contrast tissue enhancement is reached.[6,7] Hence, patient motion has relatively less impact in compartmental analysis. The mathematic modeling technique employed also has implications on the CT protocol used. The deconvolution method being less sensitive to noise, allows the use of lower tube current and permits scanning with higher temporal resolution for the dynamic cine acquisition. For the compartmental model, the presence of the image noise results in miscalculation of perfusion values; hence, a higher tube current with low image frequency is preferred for the dynamic study.

PERFUSION COMPUTED TOMOGRAPHY PROTOCOLS

A variety of the perfusion CT protocols have been proposed, and they typically depend upon the target organ, mathematic modeling technique, CT scan configuration and clinical objective. Nevertheless, a typical perfusion CT protocol consists of a baseline acquisition without contrast-enhancement, followed by a dynamic acquisition performed sequentially after intravenous injection of CM. The dynamic acquisition study includes a first pass study, delayed study, or both depending on the pertinent physiological parameters that need to be analyzed (**Table 1**).

Unenhanced CT Acquisition

The baseline unenhanced CT acquisition should provide wide coverage to include the organ of interest. This study basically serves as a localizer to select the appropriate tissue area to be included in the contrast-enhanced dynamic imaging range. Depending upon the scanner configuration, a 2 cm coverage area (for a 4 or 16 row CT scanner) or a 4 cm coverage area (for 64 row CT scanner) can be selected for dynamic scanning. Larger coverage area (8–16 cm) is now feasible with the availability of newer scanner with 128 to 320 rows of detectors.

Dynamic CT Acquisition

The first pass study for the perfusion measurements comprises images acquired in initial cine phase for a total of approximately 40–60 seconds. For the typical first pass study based on the deconvolution method, image acquisition is done every 1 second, whereas for the compartment method, image acquisition is done every 3–5 seconds.[9]

For obtaining permeability measurements, a second phase ranging from 2 to 10 minutes is supplemented after

Table 1: Terms commonly used in computed tomography perfusion.[6,7]

Perfusion parameters	*Definition*	*Marker (in oncology)*	*Units*
Blood flow (BF) or perfusion	Flow rate through vascuature in tissue region	• Tumor vascularity • Tumor grade	mL per 100 g/min
Blood volume (BV)	Volume of flowing blood within vasculature in tissue region	Tumor vascularity	mL per 100 g
Mean transit time (MTT)	Average time taken to travel from artery to vein	Perfusion pressure	Seconds
Permeability surface (PS) area product	Total flux from plasma to interstitial space	Immature leaky vessels	mL per 100 g/min
Time to peak (TTP)	Time from arrival of contrast in major arterial vessels to the peak enhancement	Perfusion pressure	Seconds
Peak enhancement intensity (PEI)	Maximum increase in tissue density after contrast injection	Tissue blood volume	HU

the first pass study. The second phase images are acquired every 10 seconds for 2 minutes after the first pass study for a deconvolution method-based study. For permeability measurements with compartment model, images are acquired every 10–20 seconds.[9]

Technique of CT Perfusion

- Step I involves acquisition of unenhanced CT images to cover the entire region of interest
- Step II involves selection of the slice for dynamic imaging. The selected slices should be chosen to cover the maximum tumor area. The total tumor coverage area is 2 cm for 16-MDCT and 4 cm for 64-MDCT and up to 9 cm for 128-MDCT scanner
- Step III involves contrast-enhanced dynamic image acquisition
- Step IV involves postprocessing of CT data to generate colored perfusion maps of blood flow (BF), blood volume (BV), mean transit time (MTT) and permeability surface area product. Time attenuation curves showing the enhancement characteristics of the artery and tumor during the first pass and delayed phase of perfusion CT acquisition can be obtained.

Contrast Medium

One of the important considerations for adequate assessment of tissue perfusion is the CM bolus used for the intravenous injection. As there is a linear relation between iodine concentration and tissue enhancement, a higher concentration of CM is preferred (iodine 370 mg/mL). A contrast bolus of 40–70 mL and an injection rate ranging from 3.5 to 10 mL/s are normally adequate for optimal perfusion analysis. The scan delay for the cine acquisition from the start of the CM injection is determined by the CM circulation time to the region of interest. Typically, for most body applications, a scan delay of 5–10 seconds is considered suitable (5–8 seconds for neck/chest/abdomen studies and 10–15 seconds for studies of the pelvis and extremities).

Acquisition Parameters

The selection of acquisition parameters for perfusion CT needs to be done judiciously in keeping with the body part scanned, modeling technique used and radiation exposure.[10,11] Use of lower tube voltage (kilovolt peak, kVp) and the tube current (milli-Ampere-second, mAs) is recommended to reduce the radiation exposure.

It is important to note that movement during data acquisition can lead to image misregistration and can cause errors in the measurements of perfusion values.[10] Hence, efforts should be made to minimize motion by appropriate approaches, such as breath holding instructions to the patients for chest and upper abdominal applications. Likewise, anterior abdominal wall motion can be restricted by the use of abdominal straps.[11] Use of motility inhibiting agents, such as hyoscine butylbromide or glucagon, is recommended to curtail bowel peristalsis during the perfusion examination of bowel. In addition, luminal distention with water or saline is encouraged for study of hollow viscera to enable optimal tumor delineation. This is particularly relevant in follow-up examinations after therapy, in which tumor conspicuity is often in question after successful treatment. Metallic stents, prostheses and surgical implants cause beam hardening artifacts and can negatively influence the perfusion measurements. Finally, selecting the region of interest is crucial, and areas with excessive tumor necrosis or those located along organs with motion (in chest examinations) and areas near metallic prostheses or stents should be avoided.[12]

COMPUTED TOMOGRAPHY PERFUSION IN ACUTE ISCHEMIC STROKE

A stroke, or cerebrovascular accident, is defined as an abrupt onset of a neurologic deficit that is attributable to a vascular cause. Stroke is one of the leading causes of mortality and disability worldwide. Atherosclerosis of the carotid arteries is by far the most common predisposing condition for stroke. Strokes are ischemic approximately 85% of the time with the rest being hemorrhagic.

The concept of an ischemic penumbra (tissue at risk) has been a major impetus for developing pharmacologic interventions in the treatment of acute stroke. The ischemic penumbra is defined as the part of the brain that is sandwiched between brain regions committed to die and those that receive enough blood to communicate and that the cells in the ischemic penumbra could survive if the blood flow is restored.[13] The penumbra phase generally begins when blood flow falls below 20 mL/100 g/min and electrical communication between neurons cease with infarction not occurring until blood flow falls below 10 or 12 mL/100 g/min.

The identification of potentially salvageable ischemic tissue in the hyperacute period is of critical importance because the tolerance of perfusion disturbances is related to its duration, which can determine the progression of ischemia from the core into the oligemic penumbral region. This has led to the development of several functional imaging techniques, such as brain perfusion imaging.

Perfusion CT imaging is a functional imaging modality to differentiate between the infarcted core and the ischemic penumbra. Perfusion CT provides absolute and relative information about brain perfusion parameters, namely cerebral blood flow (CBF), cerebral blood volume (CBV), mean transit time (MTT), and time to peak (TTP) **(Figs. 1A to D)**. CBF is the total volume of blood moving through a voxel in a given unit of time. CBV is a measure of the total volume of blood within a voxel which includes blood in both the tissues and blood vessels. MTT is the time elapsed between the arterial inflow and the venous outflow. TTP refers to the time elapsed from the start of the contrast material injection to the attainment of maximum attenuation within the selected region of the brain. Normally, the relationship between these aforementioned parameters is expressed by the 'central volume principle' which is expressed by the equation, $\mathrm{CBF} \times \mathrm{MTT} = \mathrm{CBV}$.[14]

The diagnosis of acute ischemic stroke on perfusion CT is done commonly by visual inspection of CBF, CBV, MTT and TTP maps generated in a dedicated postprocessing workstation.[15,16] Areas showing perfusion abnormalities in CBF, CBV and MTT maps represent the infarct core while areas having relatively preserved CBV and with prolonged MTT and reduced CBF represent the ischemic penumbra[17,18] **(Figs. 2A and B)**. The perfusion abnormalities in acute stroke are tabulated in **Table 2**.

The perfusion parameter that most accurately describes the tissue at risk of infarction in case of persistent arterial occlusion is the relative MTT more than 145%. The perfusion parameter that most accurately describes the infarct core is the absolute CBV with an optimal threshold at 2 mL/100 g.[19]

Wintermark M et al. have defined a widely accepted threshold of increase in the relative MTT of more than 145% as the most accurate parameter to define the ischemic penumbra with an absolute increase in MTT of more than 7 seconds as the next best criterion. MTT values more than 145% suggest ischemic penumbra while much higher values are seen in infarct core.

In infarct core, the MTT values are prolonged and the CBV is reduced while the ischemic penumbra is the area of mismatch between the MTT and CBV maps (MTT-CBV), i.e. the MTT is prolonged while CBV is normal or increased,

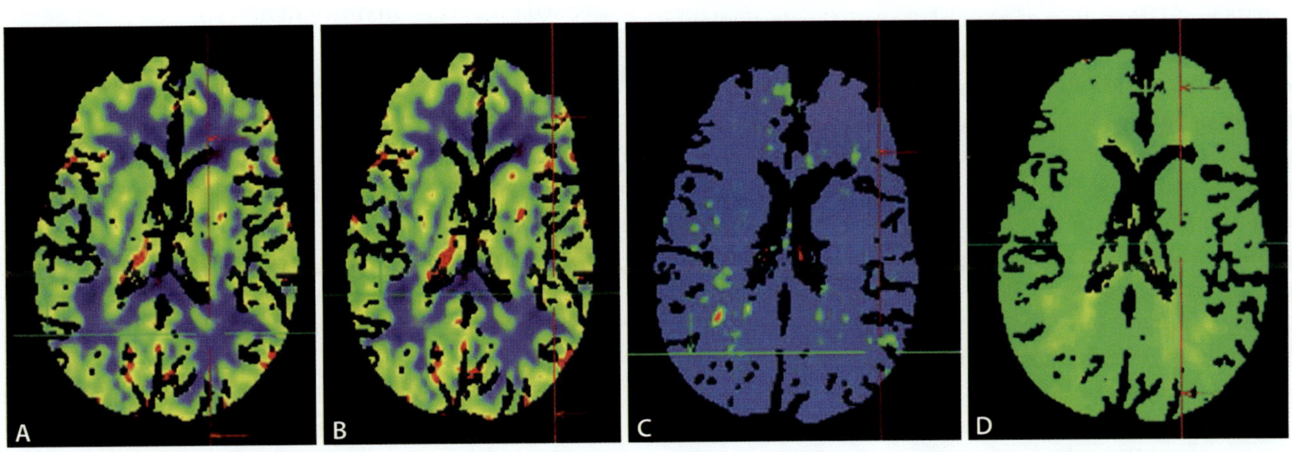

Figs. 1A to D: Normal cerebral perfusion CT maps representing cerebral blood flow (A), cerebral blood volume (B), mean transit time (C), and time to peak (D).

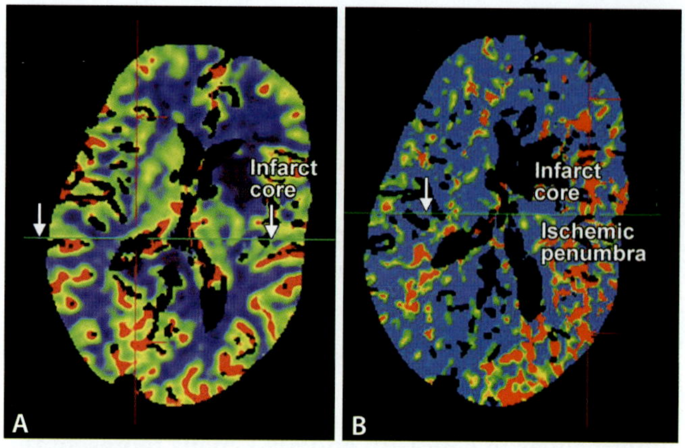

Figs. 2A and B: Perfusion CT maps representing CBV (A) and MTT (B) in a patient showing a central infarct core (CBV = 1.2 mL/100 mL) in the region of the left basal ganglia with a large surrounding ischemic penumbra (rMTT = 210%) revealing CBV-MTT mismatch (relatively preserved CBV with increase in MTT values)—Case of acute ischemic stroke.

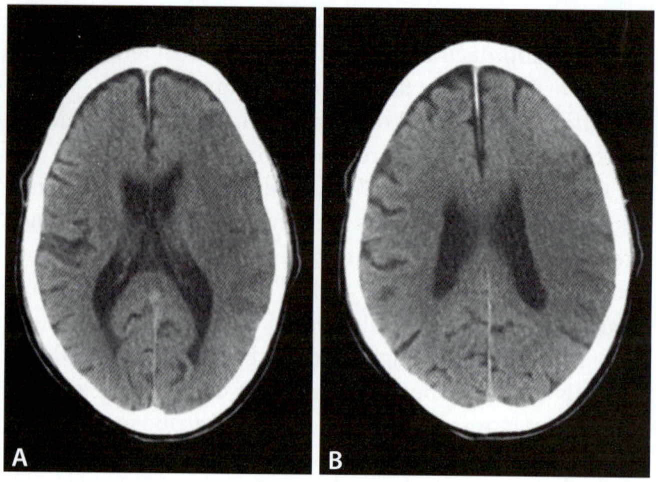

Figs. 3A and B: Noncontrast axial CT images reveal large areas of subtle loss of gray-white matter differentiation in the left frontoparietal region—Case of large hemispheric infarct.

Table 2: Perfusion abnormalities.[14]

Perfusion parameter	*Infarct core*	*Ischemic penumbra*
CBF	Reduced	Reduced
CBV	Reduced	Normal or increased
MTT	Prolonged	Prolonged
TTP	Prolonged	Prolonged

which can be depicted using automated summary maps **(Figs. 3 and 4)**.[20,21] A significant drawback of using CBF thresholds for ischemic penumbra is that differences in gray and white matter CBF values, and their respective ischemic thresholds (with ischemic gray matter CBF values being close to normal white matter CBF values), interfere with the use of CBF thresholds to define the penumbra.[22] Also, CBF values to define infarct core and penumbra vary widely within the literature.

The main limitation of most of the previously available multidetector row CT scanners in the evaluation of cerebral perfusion was the relatively narrow range of brain tissue covered primarily at the level of the basal ganglia resulting in the exclusion of a large volume of brain parenchyma including the superior cerebral hemispheres, posterior fossa and brainstem. However, the advent of modern CT scanners with increased number of detector rows, whole brain perfusion CT with substantially increased vertical scanning range is feasible which allows for complete and comprehensive evaluation of the entire areas of suspected ischemia/infarction.[23]

There are certain inherent advantages of CT perfusion imaging over MR perfusion imaging in that CT is very fast and much more widely available as compared to MRI thus reducing the imaging time. It is relatively less expensive. In addition, it is easily performed and MRI is much more limited by patient contraindications or intolerance.

There are multiple advantages of adding CT perfusion imaging to the routine stroke imaging protocol in an emergency setting which are as follows:[24-26]

1. It has been shown to increase diagnostic certainty for stroke detection.
2. It permits the estimation of amount of potentially salvageable tissue, hence guiding in patient management.
3. It allows the accurate prediction of the final infarct size and the evaluation of clinical prognosis for acute stroke patients at the time of emergency evaluation.
4. Thrombolytic therapy can be extended beyond the 3 hours window if the patients are carefully selected based on perfusion mismatch.

COMPUTED TOMOGRAPHY PERFUSION IN ONCOLOGY

There has been a gradual increase in the utility of perfusion CT in oncology, with a wide spectrum of clinical applications, including:

- Lesion characterization (differentiation between benign and malignant lesion)
- Identification of occult malignancies
- Vascularity
- Monitoring therapeutic response of various treatment regimens, including chemoradiation and antiangiogenic drugs.

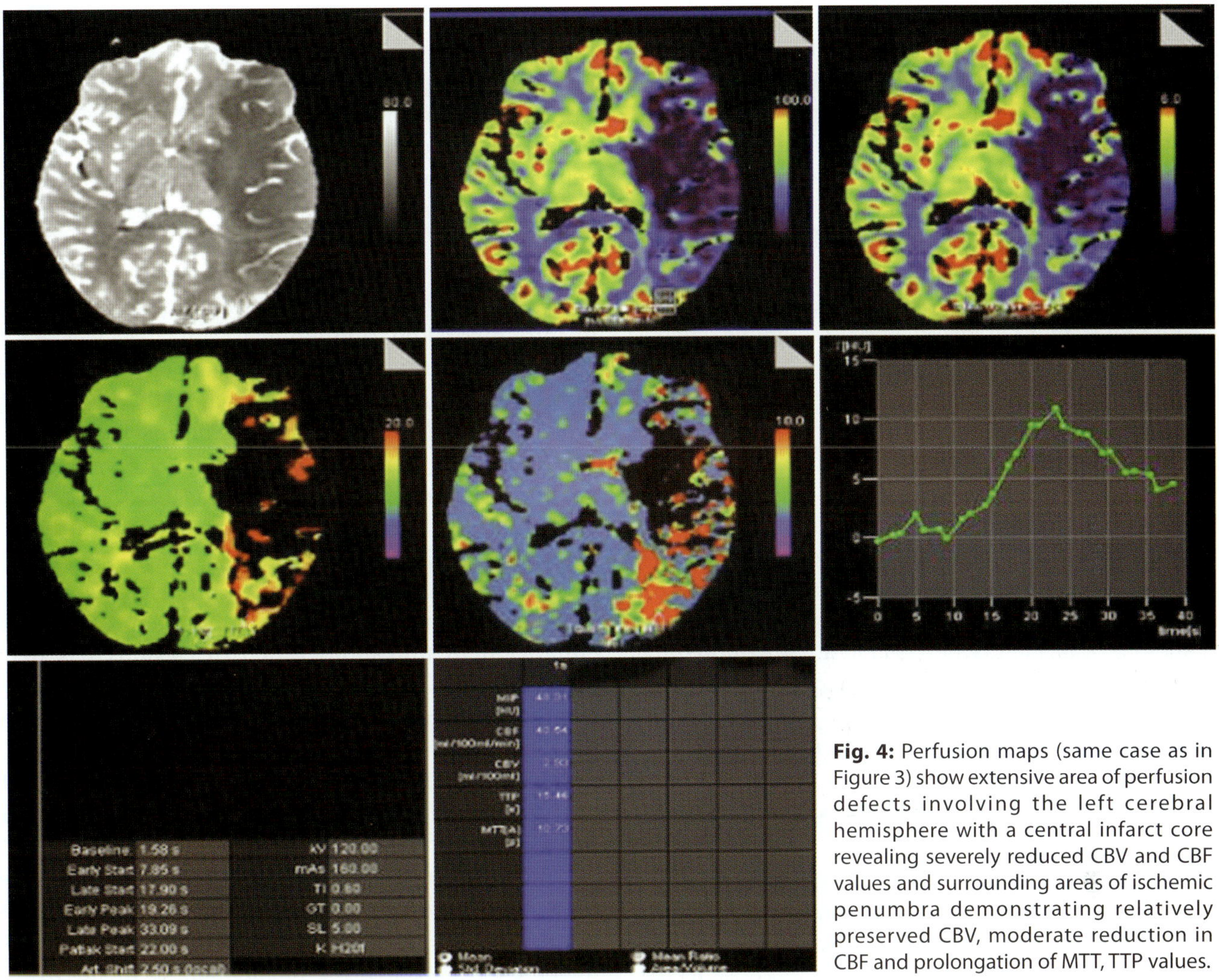

Fig. 4: Perfusion maps (same case as in Figure 3) show extensive area of perfusion defects involving the left cerebral hemisphere with a central infarct core revealing severely reduced CBV and CBF values and surrounding areas of ischemic penumbra demonstrating relatively preserved CBV, moderate reduction in CBF and prolongation of MTT, TTP values.

An emerging approach of cancer care is the individualized approach, in which the treatment strategies are targeted according to the tumor biology.[27] One of the key elements of tumor physiology that influences the aggressiveness of cancer and its response to treatment is tumor microvasculature (neoangiogenesis), and the presence of high vascularity usually suggests aggressive behavior and is associated with a poor outcome.[28,29] The tumor angiogenesis is defined as a process of developing new capillary blood vessels, resulting in vascularization of the tumor. This process, which is integral part to the growth and spread of tumor, consists of several dynamic processes mediated by the host growth factors, such as vascular endothelial growth factor, fibroblast growth factor, and platelet derived endothelial cell growth factor.[30,31] Perfusion CT displays and permits quantification of the abnormal vasculature within tumors, thus allowing assessment of tumor aggressiveness.

Development of newer antiangiogenic drugs has necessitated the use of functional imaging techniques, such as perfusion CT or dynamic contrast enhanced MR, to monitor their therapeutic effects, because conventional methods of monitoring response are not effective for these drugs.[32] Moreover, given that functional changes precede morphologic changes after treatment, techniques like perfusion CT allow earlier assessment of treatment effect than conventional methods, which rely on tumor size. Perfusion CT can measure vascular physiologic changes by virtue of changes in the contrast enhancement characteristics of tissues.[6] Accordingly, perfusion CT can be considered as surrogate (indirect) imaging biomarker for in vivo evaluation of response to antiangiogenic drugs. This is in contrast to microvessel density (MVD), which represents the actual tumor blood vessels (i.e. direct biomarker) that form the target of antiangiogenic drugs, and hence is considered the "gold standard" for quantifying and monitoring angiogenesis.[33] MVD has also been established as a prognostic indicator for many cancers. The most direct strategy for the measurement of MVD, and hence monitoring antiangiogenic therapy, would require periodic biopsies. There are several limitations in the routine use of microvessel density as biomarker, including:

- The requirement of invasive tissue sampling, such as biopsy
- The need for standardization
- The presence of random sampling errors
- The fact that such studies do not explore entire tumor volume, which can hamper evaluation because of heterogeneity of malignant tumors.[30] Indirect biomarkers like perfusion CT are hence used because of their observed benefits like noninvasiveness, they can be repeated frequently, and they dynamically reflect the microvasculatory function in a living individual. Several investigators have validated the utility of CT perfusion as a biomarker for measuring angiogenesis and monitoring response to treatment.[34]

HEPATIC COMPUTED TOMOGRAPHY PERFUSION[35-39]

The liver has a dual blood supply, the portal vein and the hepatic artery. Hepatic perfusion relies on the resolution of each component of its dual blood supply as contributions from each are altered in many diseases. Most disease processes affect blood flow regionally or globally or both. Perfusion CT can provide quantitative information about arterial and portal perfusion of liver lesions combined with a good anatomic detail **(Fig. 5)**.

Perfusion Parameters of Normal Liver

There are some disagreements in normal liver perfusion parameters from different sources due to different choices of computational model and people. However, they are all verged about 1/4 - 1/3 as the ratio of hepatic arterial perfusion/portal vein perfusion, in rough approximation of the blood supply from hepatic artery and portal vein **(Table 3)**.

CT Perfusion in Hepatocellular Carcinoma

Neovascularization, production of new blood vessels within the tumors, is an essential process for sustaining tumor growth. The spatial resolution of diagnostic imaging is insufficient to visualize tumor microvessels directly, however, functional imaging has the ability to evaluate neovascularization and help in the detection of tumors even before morphologic changes.[40] CTA and CTAP can be used to detect blood flow of hepatic artery and portal vein for HCC evaluation. Blood in the hepatic artery is increased and decreased in the PV while the blood volume is increased.[41]

The enhancement imaging features of HCC lesions have been correlated with tumor microvessel density and its intratumoral distribution characteristics **(Figs. 6A to C)**.[42] HAP is increased in the periphery and decreased in the center. The hepatic blood flow and HPI are higher in primary hepatic carcinoma than the normal liver.

Changes in perfusion parameters are valuable in qualitative and differential of primary HCC. CT perfusion can detect the abnormalities in liver perfusion before morphologic changes occur.

The peak enhancement value, contrast enhancement ratio, the pattern of time density curve and the gross enhancement morphology of HCC lesions has been correlated with tumor MVD and reflects the distributive features of tumor microvessels within the HCC lesions. Correlation has been found between the likelihood of intrahepatic metastasis of the HCC lesion with densely enhanced pseudocapsules and rich pseudocapsular tumor MVD.[42]

In HCC, CT perfusion has a role in making the differential diagnosis, evaluating tumor aggressiveness, monitoring therapeutic effects and determining the final patient outcome. HCC demonstrates higher BF, BV and PS and lower MTT measurements compared with the background liver **(Fig. 7)**.[43,44] There is also difference between CT perfusion values of well differentiated tumors and those of moderately and poorly differentiated tumors. Well differentiated HCCs demonstrate relatively higher BF, BV and PS and lower MTT measurements than do moderately and poorly differentiated HCCs. Tumor tissues with the highest malignant grade can be taken by biopsy under CT guidance, thus avoiding errors of grading occurring in selection of biopsy region.[45] The presence of cirrhosis and tumor thrombus in the portal vein does not significantly alter the perfusion values in HCC confirming that the blood supply of primary hepatic carcinoma is mainly provided by hepatic artery.[46]

Perfusion CT allows accurate quantification of changes in liver tumor perfusion during and after an embolization procedure, thus helping to optimize therapeutic outcome. CT perfusion is also able to assess changes in liver tumor perfusion in response to antiangiogenic treatment. HCCs

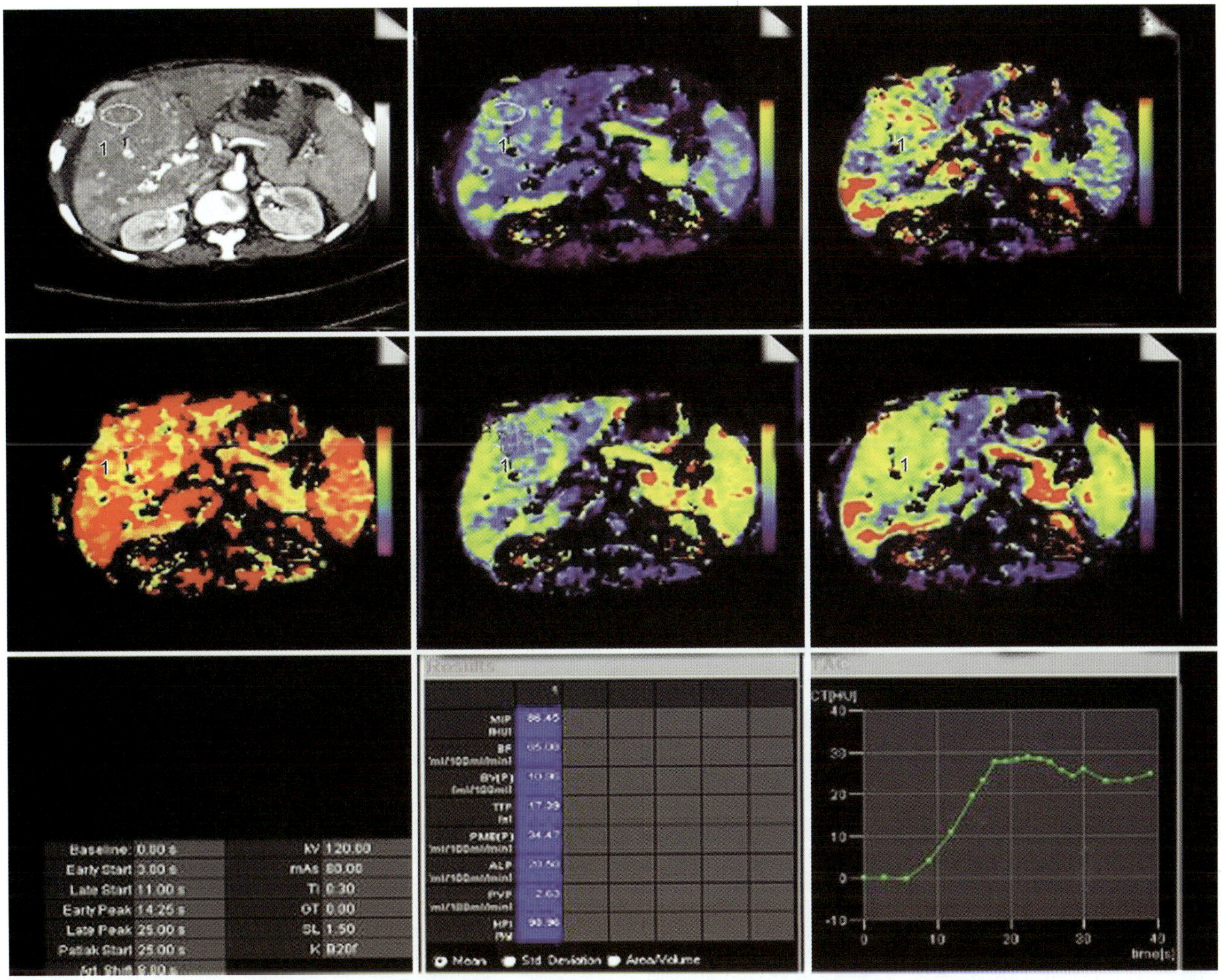

Fig. 5: Perfusion maps in normal liver parenchyma show blood flow of 85.0 mL/100 mL/min, blood volume of 10.5 mL/100 mL and time to peak of 17 seconds.

Table 3: Perfusion parameters of normal liver.

Sources	***HAP***	***PVP***	***HPI***	***HBF***	***HBV***	***MTT***
Miles et al.[35]	0.17	0.34	32%			
Blomley et al.[36]	0.19	0.93				
Weidekamm et al.[37]	0.2+/–0.08	1.02+/–0.35				
Zhou et al.[38]	0.17+/–0.08	0.9+/–0.04	16+/–16%	106.24+/–54.53	20.24+/–8.26	15.06+/–8.94
Hashimoto et al.[39]			18.4+/–5.6%	103.9+/-18	12.5+/–2.0	11.1+/–1.6

Abbreviations: HAP: Hepatic arterial perfusion (mL/min); PVP: Portal vein perfusion (mL/min); HPI: Hepatic perfusion index (%); HBF: Hepatic blood flow (mL/min/100 g); HBV: Hepatic blood volume (mL/100 g); MTT: Mean transit time (sec).

after bevacizumab treatment demonstrate reduction in perfusion values and the changes seen in MTT correlate with clinical outcome.[46] Earlier identification of tumor recurrence after various intervention procedures is also potentially possible with perfusion CT.

CT Perfusion in Metastatic Disease

Diagnosis of liver metastatic disease is very important for its staging, prognosis and treatment. Routine CT and MRI are insensitive to occult and early stage hepatic micrometastasis of tumors.[47] Although there may be no

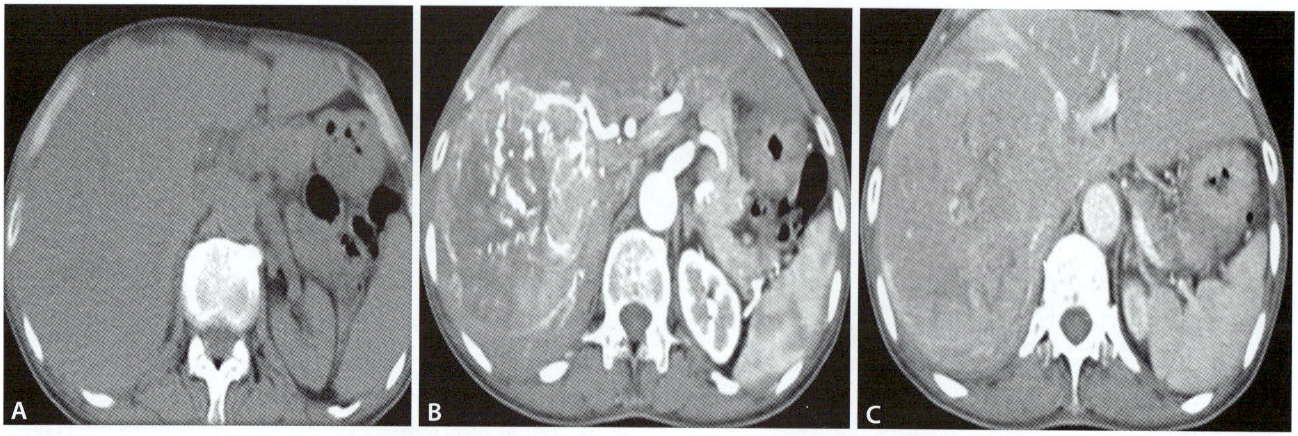

Figs. 6A to C: Triphasic study reveals a large iso- to hypodense lesion in right hepatic lobe on noncontrast scan (A). It shows intense enhancement in arterial phase (B), with relative washout in portal venous phase (C)—Case of hepatocellular carcinoma.

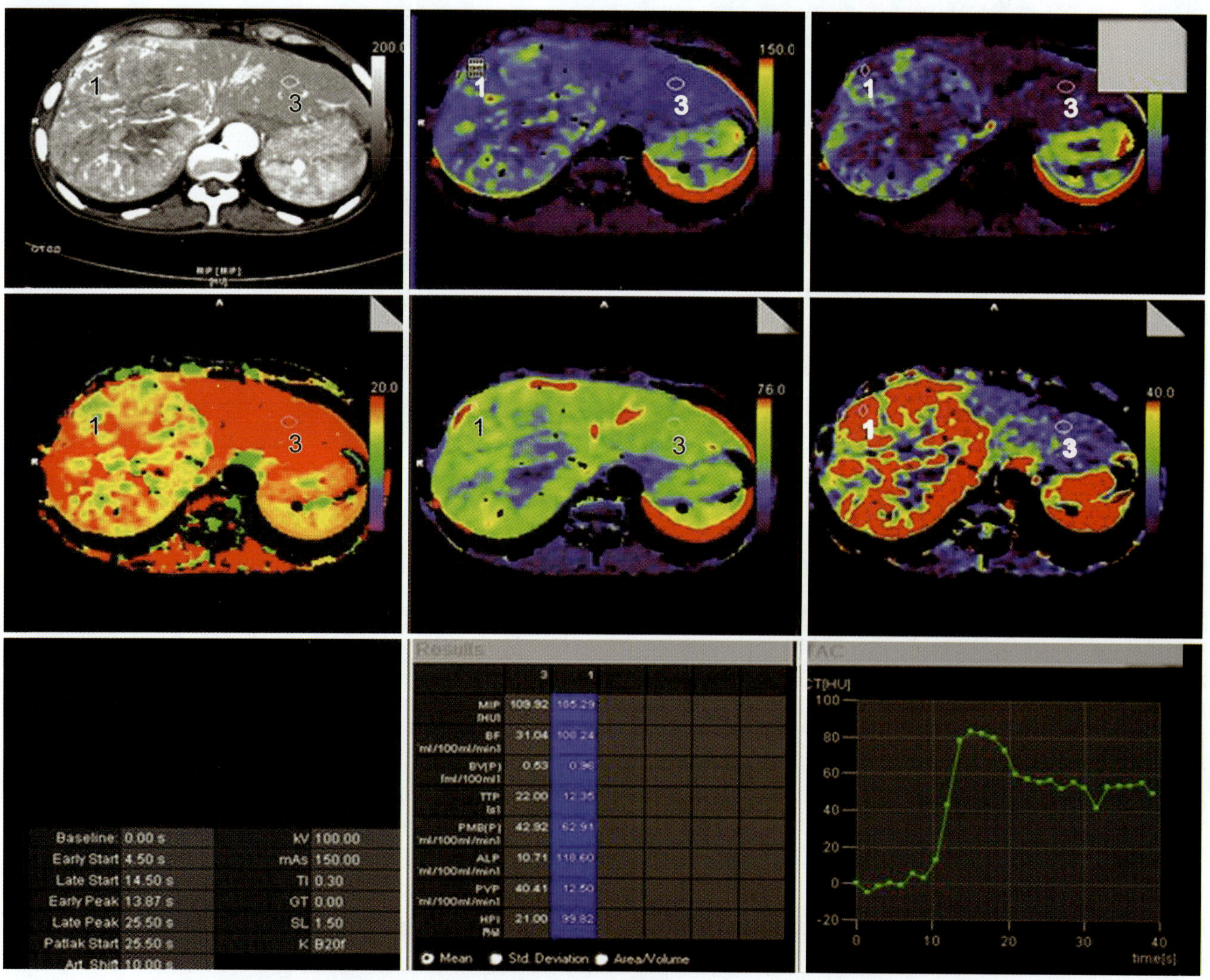

Fig. 7: Color maps (same case as in Figure 6) show increased ALP as indicated by red color, increased BF, BV as indicated by patchy areas of green color and decreased TTP shown by areas of yellow within the lesion in a case of hepatocellular carcinoma.

apparent abnormal morphology, CT perfusion can display changes in hemodynamics through its functional imaging. Improved detection and characterization of metastatic disease to the liver has profound implications for the prognosis and treatment of patients at risk.[47,48] The earlier diagnosis of the patients with micrometastatic disease may facilitate future use of targeted chemotherapeutic strategies and antiangiogenic therapies targeted against vascular endothelial growth factors. Exclusion of the presence of micrometastatic disease could obviate adjuvant chemotherapy in some patient groups.[49]

In a study conducted to assess changes in hepatic perfusion in patients of colorectal cancer with CT, arterial and portal perfusion were calculated from temporal changes in attenuation after intravenous administration of iodinated contrast material.[50] Arterial perfusion greater than 0.25 mL/min/mL (0.17 mL/min/mL for normal liver) was seen in 82% patients with overt metastasis versus 38% of the patients with no overt metastasis. Portal perfusion of 0.25 mL/min/mL or less (0.34 mL/min/mL for normal liver) was found in 46% patients with overt metastasis versus 19% of patients with no overt metastasis. Follow-up imaging showed progressive metastatic disease in 11% patients, all of whom had decreased portal perfusion. It was concluded that increased arterial perfusion was an indication of liver metastasis whereas reduced portal perfusion could indicate progressive disease[49,50] **(Figs. 8 and 9)**.

CT Perfusion in Focal Liver Lesions

Small liver lesions are also associated with changes in liver blood flow. Early detection of primary or metastatic hepatic focal lesions and characterization of other focal lesions may be possible on the basis of relative increase in hepatic arterial blood flow associated with these diseases. It has been suggested by some authors that differentiation between benign and malignant focal liver lesions is possible based on CT perfusion parameters.[51,52] Mean hepatic perfusion index (HPI) was less than 30% in all benign focal lesions and more than 30% in cases of malignant focal lesions **(Figs. 10 and 11)**.[53]

COMPUTED TOMOGRAPHY PERFUSION IN PANCREATIC NEOPLASMS

Pancreatic cancer remains one of the most difficult neoplasms to diagnose at an early stage. Despite recent advances in imaging including multidetector CT (MDCT), only 10–30% of patients with pancreatic cancer have resectable disease at diagnosis, therefore, long-term survival is extremely rare. Many researchers have been making every effort to find a method for early diagnosis, accurate staging and effective treatment of pancreatic cancer **(Figs. 12A to C)**.[54] In some clinical areas, difficulties can arise in differentiation of autoimmune pancreatitis (AIP) and chronic mass forming pancreatitis from pancreatic cancer. The differentiation between these entities is paramount in planning management for the patients. CT perfusion imaging allows noninvasive absolute quantification of pancreatic perfusion and adds to the precision of the differential diagnosis of pancreatic cancer and mass forming pancreatitis.[55]

All pancreatic adenocarcinomas and mass forming chronic pancreatitis exhibit a lower blood flow than controls. The low blood flow of mass forming chronic pancreatitis reflects the pancreatic fibrosis and necrosis that occurs in these cases.[56] The decrease of blood flow of pancreatic adenocarcinoma reflects that the blood perfusion in tumor areas is less than that of normal

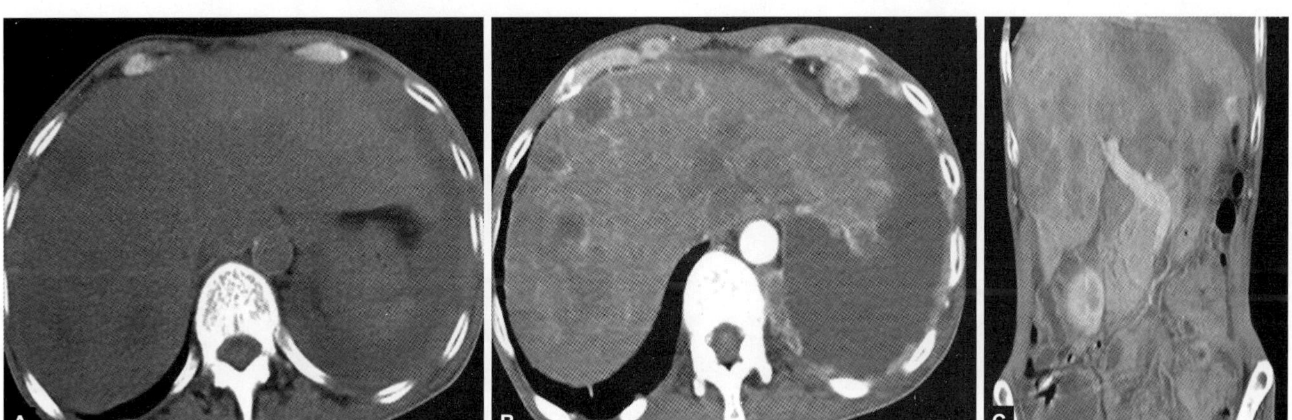

Figs. 8A to C: Triphasic CT reveals hypodense lesions in noncontrast scans (A), showing complete ring enhancement in arterial phase (B). Lesions appear hypodense on portal venous phase (C)—Case of metastatic adenocarcinoma.

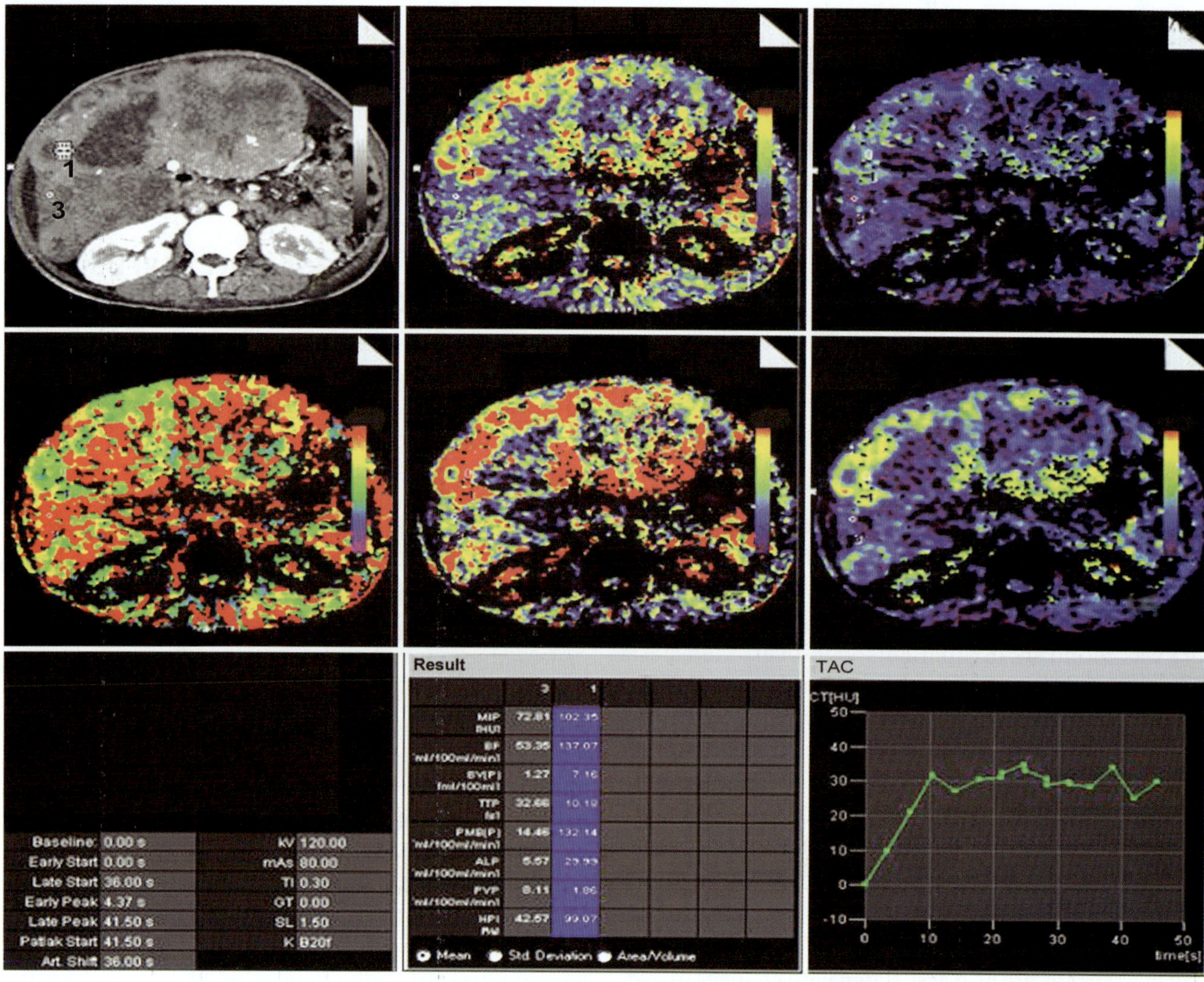

Fig. 9: Perfusion study (same case as in Figure 8) reveals focal areas of green and red color along anterior aspect of the largest lesion. Tumor reveals high blood flow, arterial liver perfusion and hepatic perfusion index with reduced portal vein perfusion.

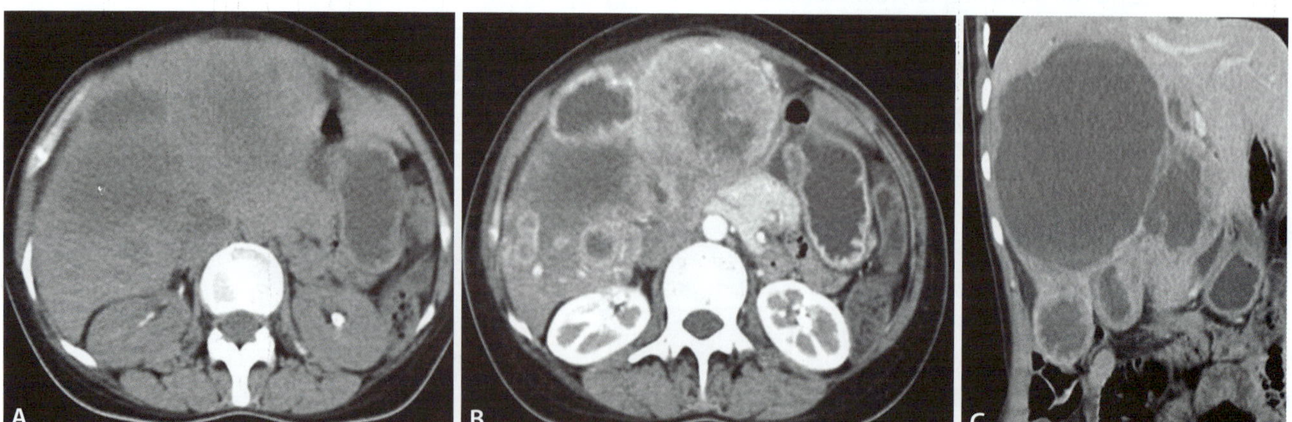

Figs. 10A to C: Triple phase study reveals multiple necrotic hypodense lesions with thick irregular walls and internal septations (A), which shows enhancement during arterial phase (B) and washout in portal venous phase; (C) Metastatic neuroendocrine tumor.

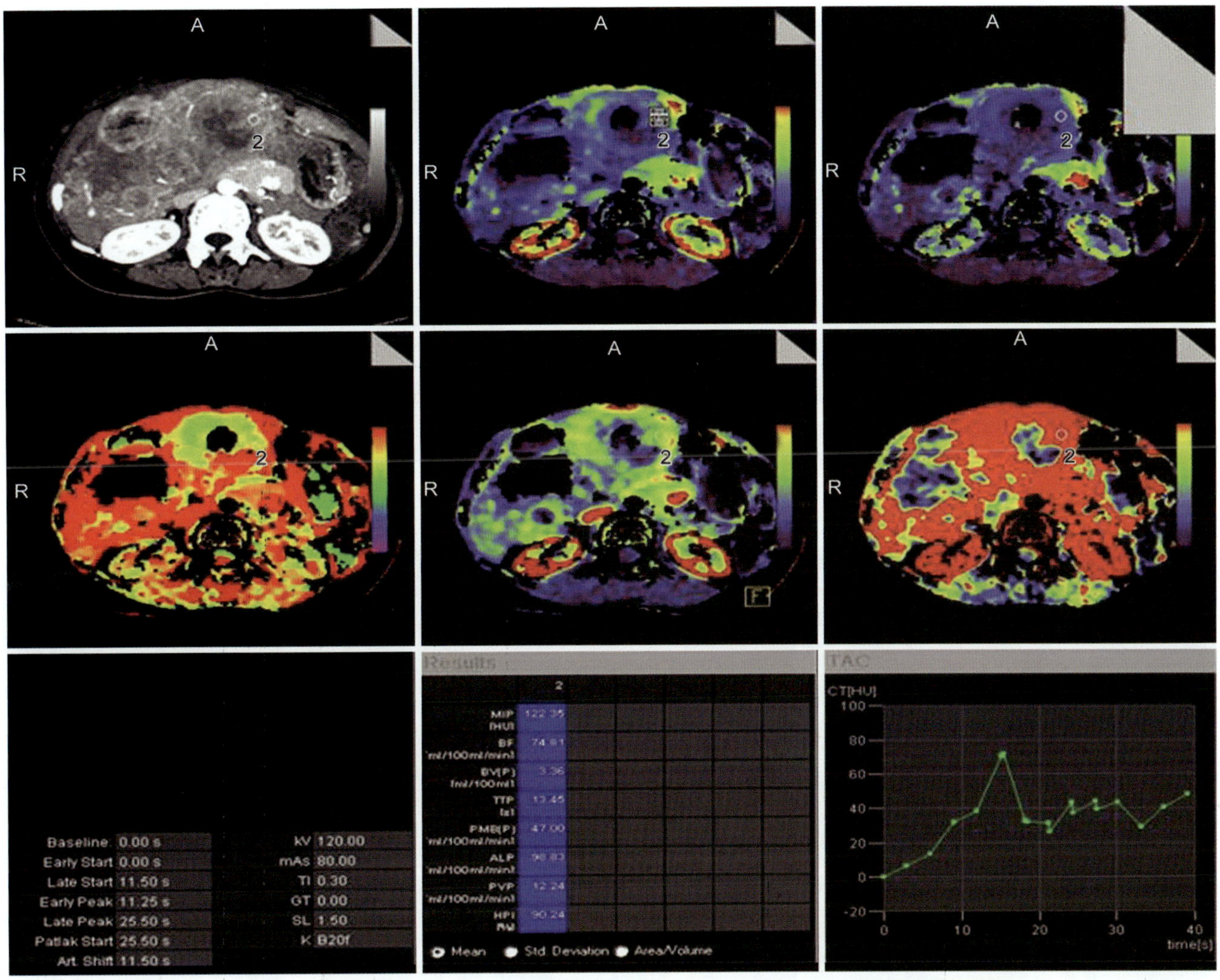

Fig. 11: Region of interest (ROI) placed over the edge of cavitatory lesion (same case as in Figure 10) show ALP 98 mL/100 mL/min and HPI of 90%, suggesting malignant etiology.

pancreas.[57] Decreased blood flow can be taken as the first characteristic of pancreatic adenocarcinoma and mass forming chronic pancreatitis. It has been seen in several studies that BF was 77% lower and BV was 65% lower in patients with pancreatic adenocarcinoma than in controls[58] **(Fig. 13)**. There was no significant difference noted in BF, BV, permeability, peak enhancement and TTP between pancreatic adenocarcinoma grade 1 and grade 2–3, and grade 4 and between grade 1 and grade 4. No significant difference between pancreatic adenocarcinoma stage I and stage II and III, between stage II and III and stage IV and between stage I and stage IV was found either, thereby indicating that the parameters cannot predict the grade and stage of pancreatic adenocarcinoma.[58]

The decrease in BV of pancreatic adenocarcinoma and mass forming chronic pancreatitis is related to the facts that the total number of vessels in pancreatic adenocarcinoma tissue and mass forming chronic pancreatitis is relatively less than normal and the number of regional capillaries is also less and this brings about the decreases in BV.[59] Decreased BV is the second characteristic of pancreatic adenocarcinoma and mass forming chronic pancreatitis.

The lower peak enhancement and the longer time to peak of pancreatic adenocarcinoma and mass forming chronic pancreatitis correspond to the decrease of BF and BV and reflect the lower enhancement on contrast CT imaging. This can be taken as third characteristic which can also be visualized on time density curves by lower and later peak of enhancement of pancreatic adenocarcinoma and mass forming chronic pancreatitis as compared to controls. Permeability was 559% higher in pancreatic cancer and 821% higher in mass forming

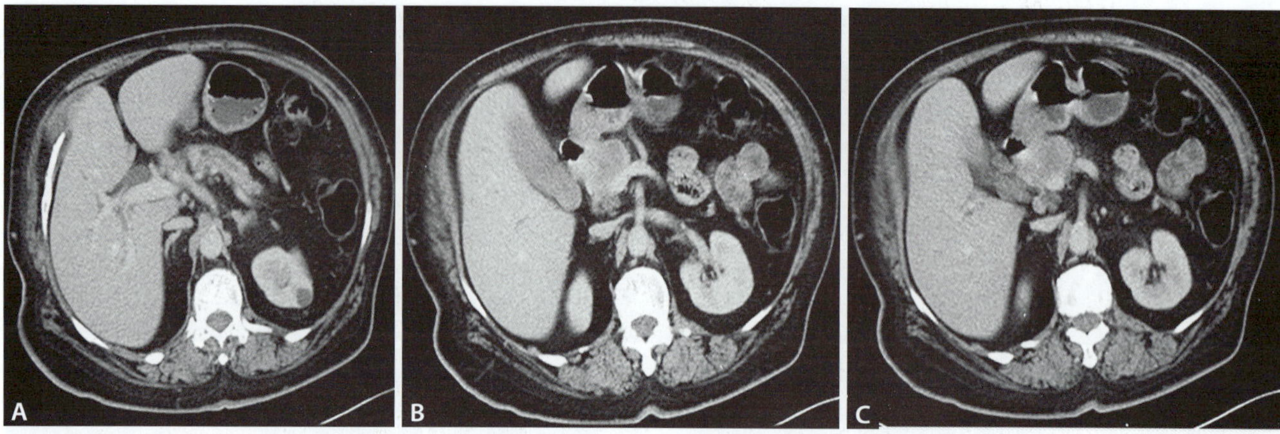

Figs. 12A to C: Cranial to caudal: Contrast-enhanced CT images show a hypodense mass lesion in the head of pancreas abutting the portal vein posteriorly and second part of duodenum medially, along with surrounding fat stranding. Upstream ductal dilatation and parenchymal atrophy is also seen—Case of pancreatic adenocarcinoma.

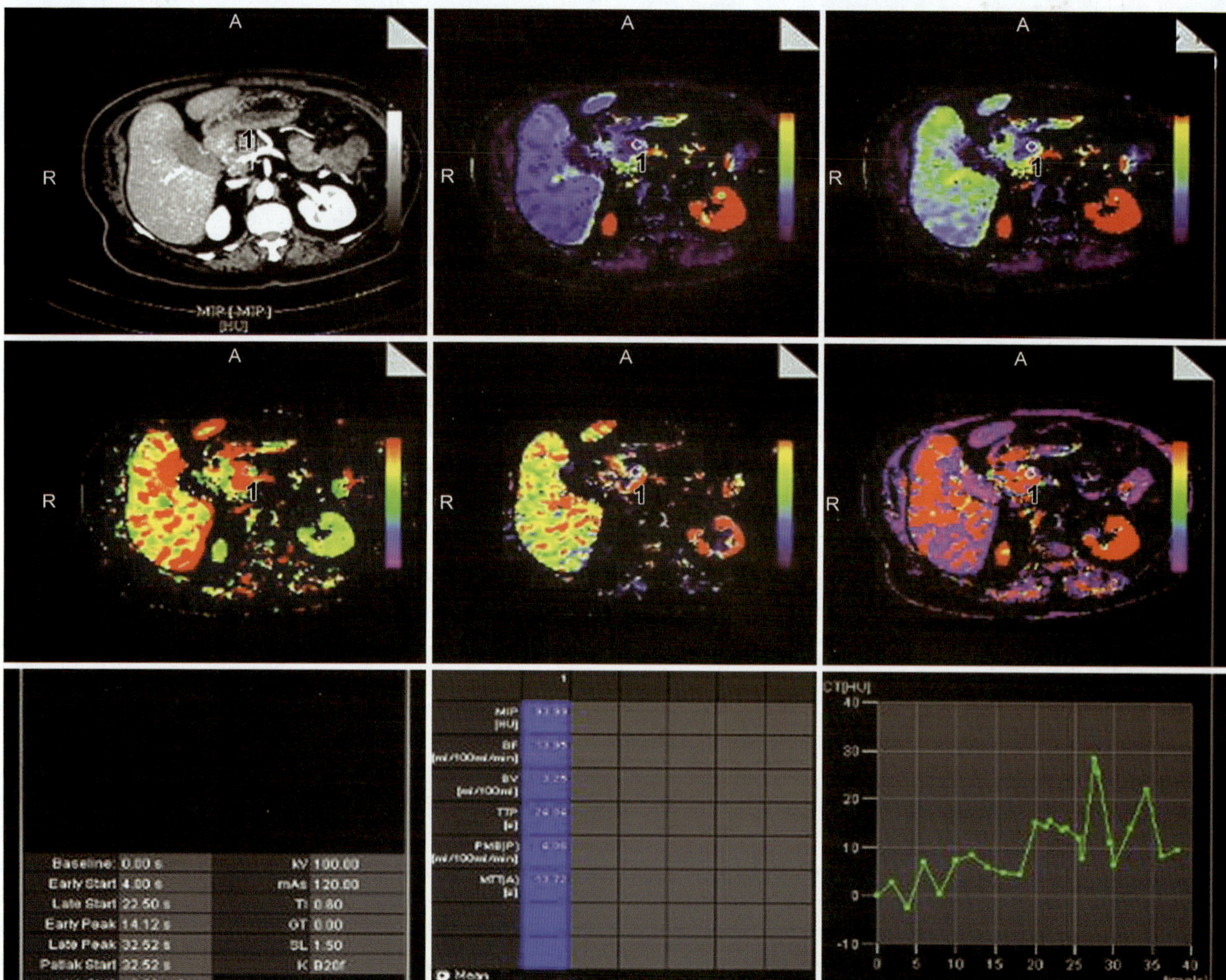

Fig. 13: Perfusion CT images with ROI at the pancreatic mass (same case as in Figure 12) reveal markedly reduced blood flow and blood volume within the lesion with increased permeability compared to normal controls.

chronic pancreatitis than controls.[58] The increase of permeability of pancreatic adenocarcinoma and mass forming chronic pancreatitis might be associated with a decrease in the integrity of vascular endothelium of tumorous and inflammatory vessel dilatation **(Figs. 14 and 15)**.[60]

Between adenocarcinoma and mass forming chronic pancreatitis, the BF, BV and peak enhancement are lower in patients with pancreatic adenocarcinoma than with mass forming chronic pancreatitis. Blood flow was 56% lower and blood volume was 53% lower in patients with pancreatic adenocarcinoma than with mass forming chronic pancreatitis.[58] The pancreatic adenocarcinoma is a hypovascular tumor and parenchyma of gland in patients with mass forming chronic pancreatitis appears less affected than that with pancreatic adenocarcinoma.[57] Malignant tumors with liver and lymph node metastasis have long MTT.

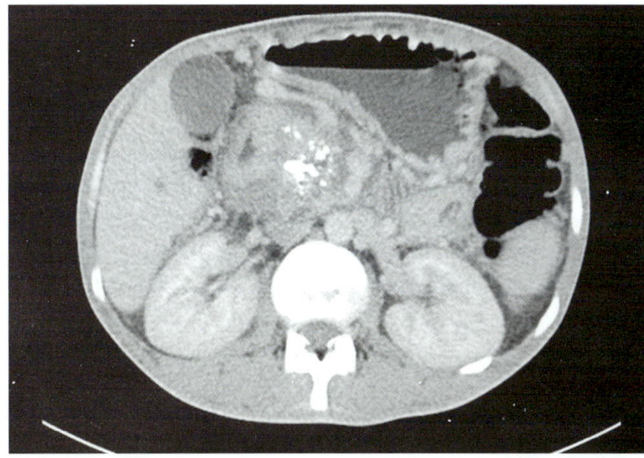

Fig. 14: Contrast-enhanced CT image shows a hypodense mass lesion with calcification in the head of pancreas abutting the portal vein posteriorly and second part of duodenum medially, along with surrounding fat stranding—Case of chronic calcific pancreatitis.

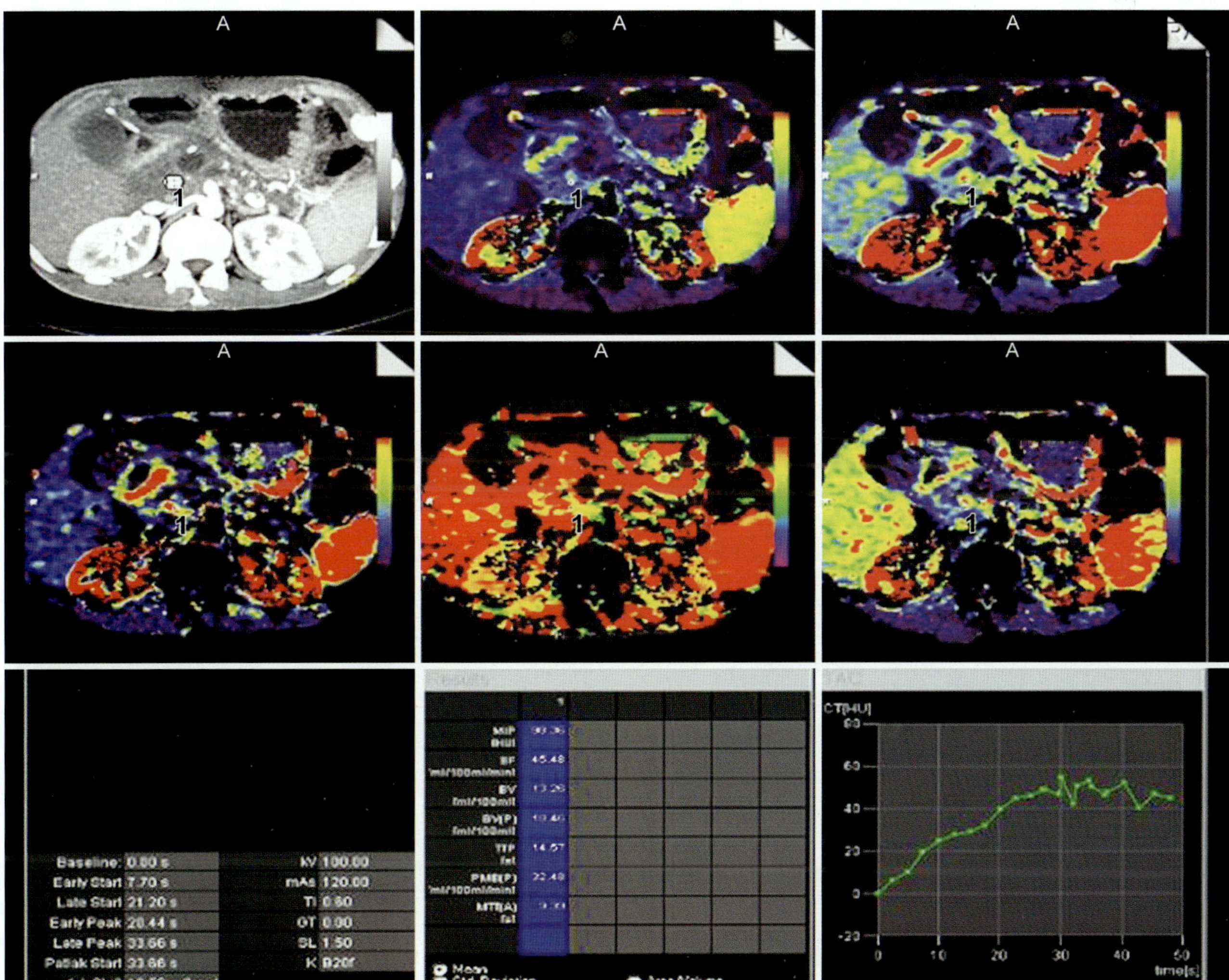

Fig. 15: Perfusion CT images with ROI within pancreatic head (same case as in Figure 14) reveal reduced blood flow and blood volume, and increased permeability in comparison to normal controls.

The comparison of perfusion parameters in patients with pancreatic adenocarcinoma, mass forming chronic pancreatitis and normal subjects (mean +/–SD) is given in **Table 4**.

Thus CT perfusion provides additional quantitative information on the function of microvasculature of tumor and carries the potential to evolve as a clinically valuable tool in pancreatic cancer. It has been noted that pancreatic tumors with high pretreatment volume transfer constant (K trans) between blood plasma and extravascular space indicate regular intratumoral flow and respond better to concurrent chemotherapy and radiotherapy (CCRT).[61] This might aid in the development of a tailored approach to therapy in these patients.

Substantially, high blood perfusion has been observed in hypervascular tumors, such as insulinomas compared with background pancreatic parenchyma **(Table 5)**.[62] Whereas conventional MDCT can depict tumor size, vascularity and presence of liver metastasis in pancreatic endocrine tumors, perfusion CT provides additional quantitative preoperative prognostic factors that could influence therapeutic treatment of patients. For example, in patients with small pancreatic tumors located in the head, where benefit of surgery has not been proved, favorable perfusion parameters could suggest follow-up rather than an aggressive approach.[63] It was seen in a study that blood flow was significantly higher in tumors measuring less than 2 cm in diameter, in those with a proliferation index of 29% or less and those without histological signs of microscopic vascular neoplastic involvement. A larger MTT was observed in tumors more than 2 cm in diameter and in those patients with lymph node or liver metastasis. Thus in contrast to most other tumors, the greater the vascularization, the lower is the grade in endocrine tumors of the pancreas.[62]

The pancreatic tumor perfusion measurements performed with CT were comparable to those performed with xenon CT, which is a more validated technique of CT perfusion.[64]

COMPUTED TOMOGRAPHY PERFUSION IN COLORECTAL CARCINOMA

Perfusion CT changes in colorectal cancer reflects its proangiogenic nature, since neovascularization is considered the initial triggering event in colorectal tumor growth and dissemination. Microvessel density progressively increases from normal colonic mucosa through adenoma to colorectal carcinoma.[65] Colorectal tumor size correlates significantly with microvessel density, and microvessel density counts from patients with lymph node metastasis, lymphatic vessel invasion, venous vessel invasion or relapse were significantly higher than those without.[66] Several investigators have validated the utility of CT perfusion as a biomarker for measuring angiogenesis. When compared with normal rectal mucosa, rectal cancer consistently showed higher blood flow and a shorter MTT **(Figs. 16 to 19 and Table 6)**.[67]

Given that functional changes precedes morphologic changes after treatment, techniques like perfusion CT allow earlier assessment of treatment effect than

Table 4: Comparison of perfusion parameters in patients with pancreatic adenocarcinoma, mass forming chronic pancreatitis and normal subjects (mean +/– SD).[58]

Parameters	*Pancreatic adenocarcinoma (n = 64)*	*Mass forming chronic pancreatitis (n = 15)*	*Controls (n = 33)*
Blood flow (mL/min/mL)	0.365+/–0.204	0.820+/–0.345	1.567+/–0.379
Blood volume (mL/mL)	0.089+/–0.042	0.191+/–0.088	0.258+/–0.041
Permeability (mL/mL/min)	0.956+/–0.556	1.336+/–0.582	0.145+/–0.088
Peak enhancement (HU)	30.858+/–15.860	42.166+/–23.109	57.000+/–13.382
Time to peak (sec)	47.047+/–6.124	36.133+/–7.726	24.858+/–2.881

Table 5: CT perfusion parameters in endocrine tumors and normal pancreas mean (median).[62]

Parameters	*Tumor*	*Normal pancreas*	*P value*
Blood flow (mL/100 g/min)	239.8 (183)	130.4 (94.4)	0.06
Blood volume (mL/100 g)	23.9 (21.8)	22.4 (23.3)	0.71
Mean transit time (sec)	10.9 (9.8)	14.9 (18.2)	0.28
Permeability surface area product (mL/100 g/min)	54.9 (55.3)	32.4 (16.5)	0.14

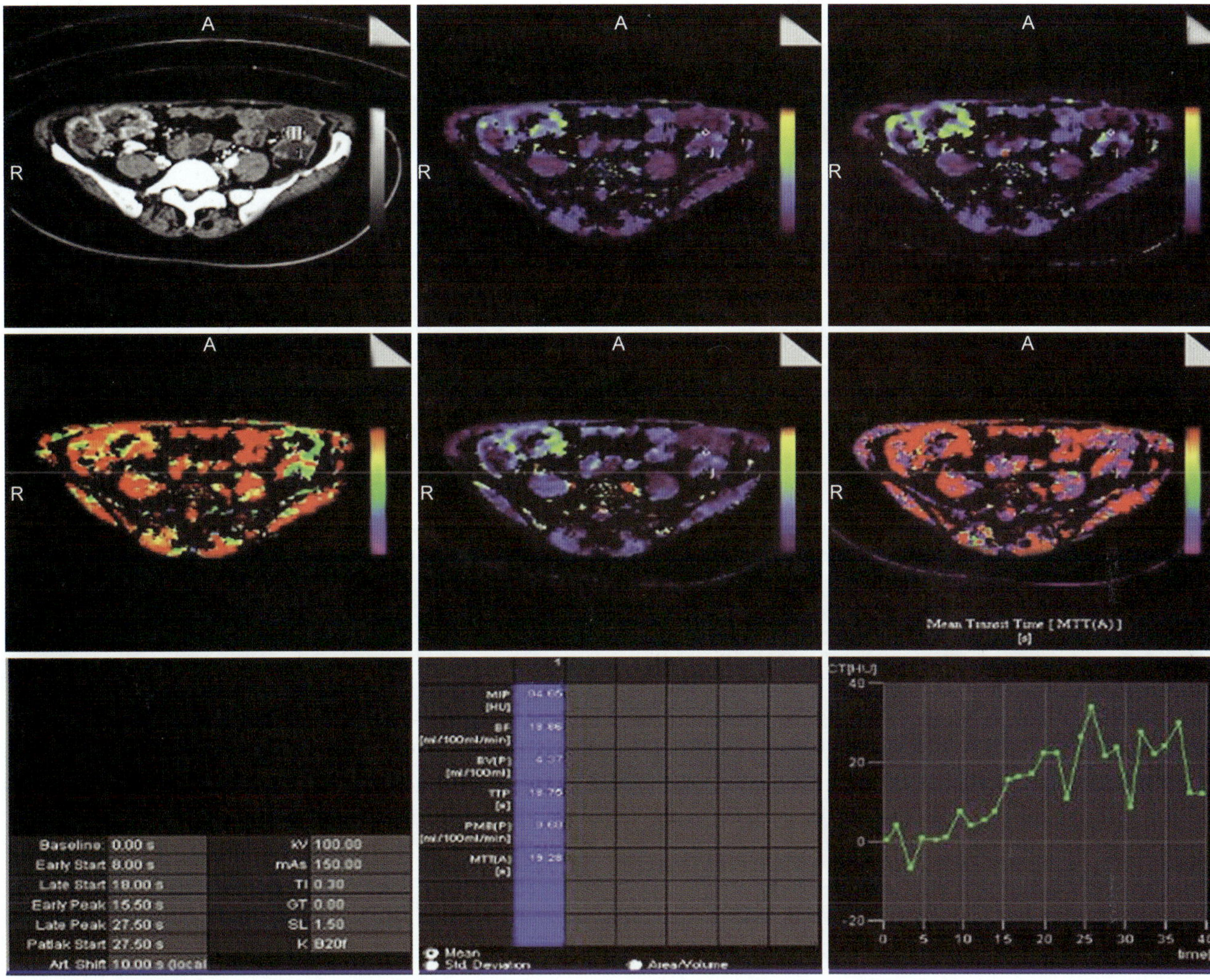

Fig. 16: CT perfusion maps from the normal appearing colon show blood flow of 18.8 mL/100 g/min, blood volume of 4.4 mL/100 g, permeability of 9.7 mL/100 g/min and mean transit time of 19.3 seconds.

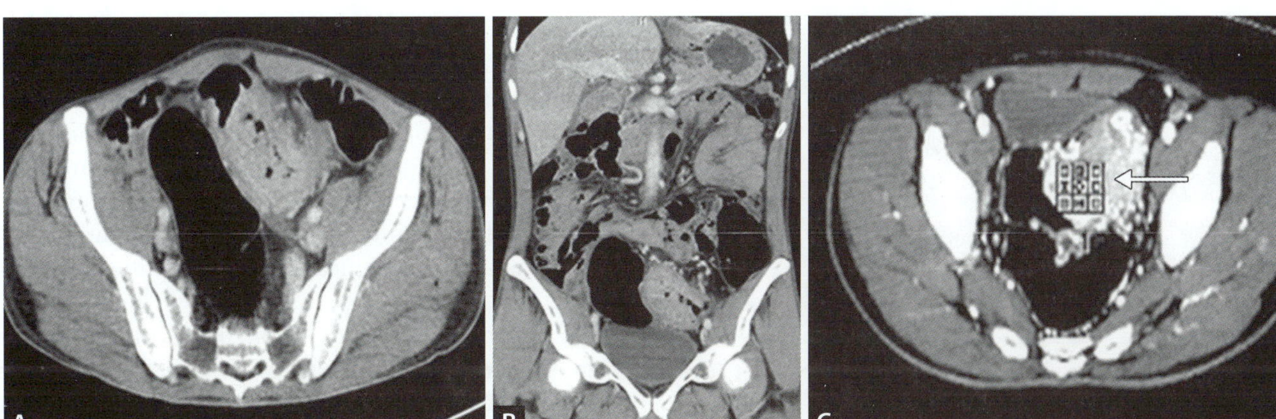

Figs. 17A to C: CECT axial (A) and coronal (B) images show asymmetric mural thickening in the sigmoid colon with heterogeneous enhancement and luminal narrowing. The maximum mural thickness was 2.7 cm. Minimal pericolonic fat stranding is noted. ROI placed over the enhancing part of the lesion is shown (arrow in C)—Case of moderately differentiated adenocarcinoma.

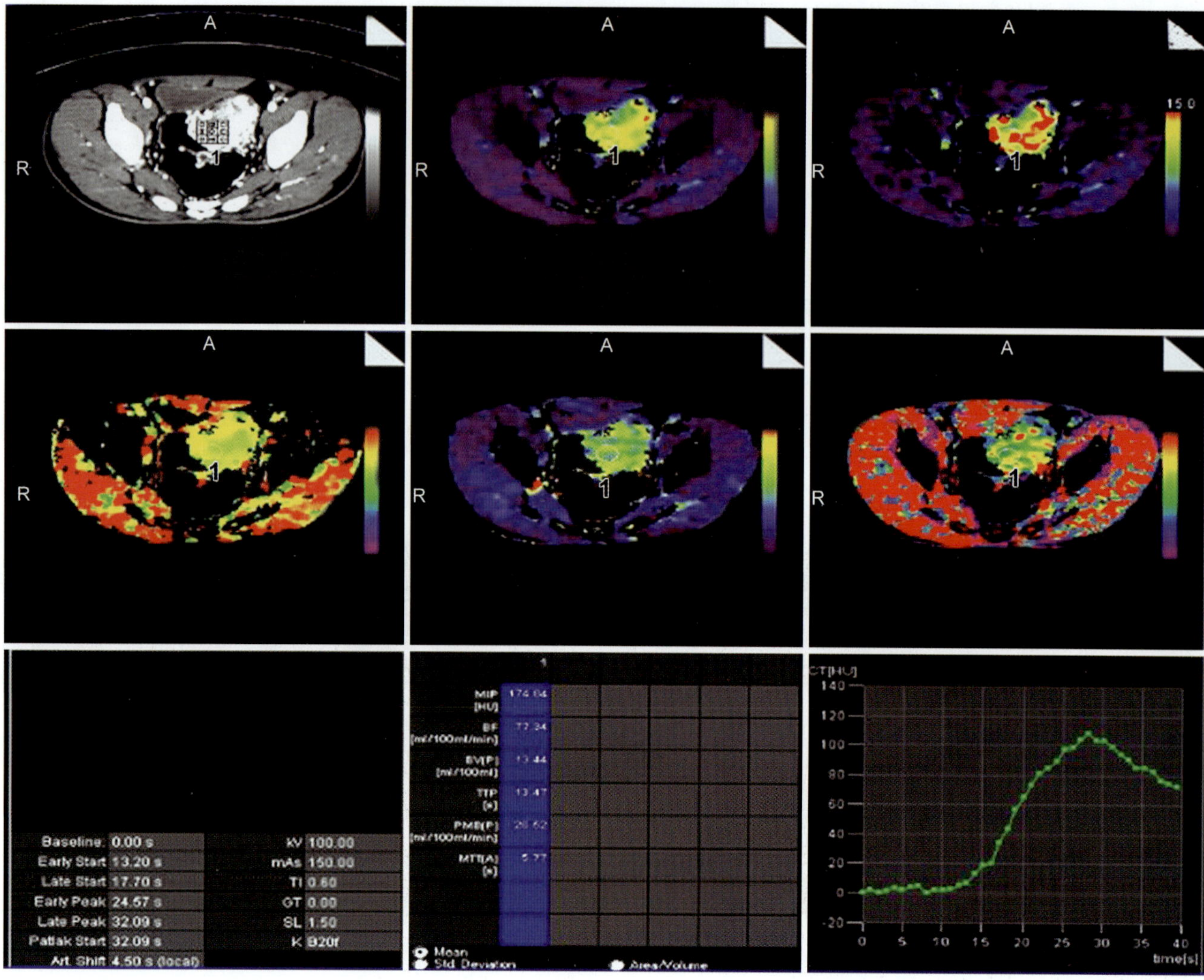

Fig. 18: Color maps (same case as in Figure 17) reveal very high blood flow of 77.3 mL/100 g/min, blood volume of 13.4 mL/100 g and permeability of 26.5 mL/100 g/min as coded by focal areas of green and red color (Note, scale on right side with red indicating highest value and violet lowest) suggesting malignant lesion.

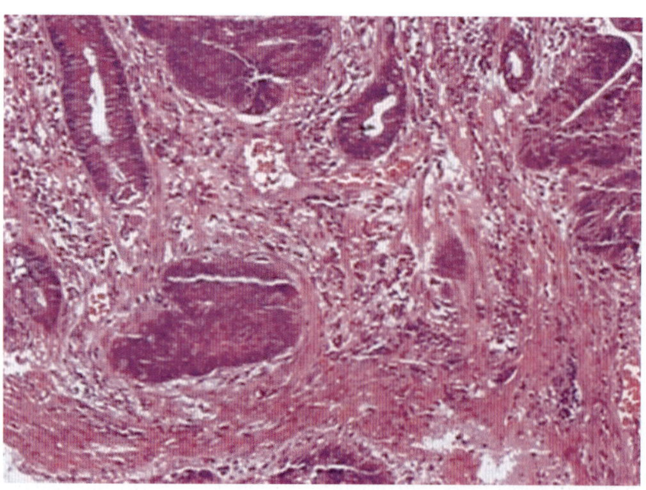

Fig. 19: Histopathological image of the case shown in Figure 17, showing moderately differentiated adenocarcinoma infiltrating the muscularis propria.

conventional method which rely on tumor size. The predominant application of perfusion CT in colorectal carcinoma is in assessing the response to radiotherapy and chemotherapy.[68,69] It has been seen there is significant fall in perfusion after two weeks of treatment with antiangiogenic drugs **(Table 7)**. After chemotherapy and radiotherapy, rectal carcinomas showed significant reduction in the blood flow and increase in MTT.[70]

Perfusion CT also has application in differential diagnosis of colonic lesions **(Figs. 20 and 21)**. The use of perfusion CT in characterization of colonic lesions was studied by Goh et al. in 2007 in which they have found that CT perfusion measurements can be used to differentiate between diverticulitis and colorectal carcinoma better than morphologic criteria.[71] Perfusion CT is able to differentiate colonic wall thickening attributed to diverticulitis from

Table 6: Perfusion values in rectal tumors and in normal rectum[70] (means+/–standard deviation).

Perfusion parameter	*Tumors*	*Normal rectum*	*P value*
Blood flow (mL/100 g/min)	60.33+/–29.13	31.02+/–15.55	0.02
Blood volume (mL/100 g)	3.78+/–1.01	3.38+/–1.59	0.25
Mean transit time (sec)	9.51+/–4.43	16.98+/–4.27	0.002
Permeability–surface area product (mL/100 g/min)	17.36+/–4.64	17.33+/–7.45	0.49

Table 7: Perfusion values in rectal cancer before and after therapy[70] (mean+/–standard deviation).

Perfusion parameter	*Before therapy*	*After therapy*	*P value*
Blood flow (mL/100 g/min)	62.57+/–26.50	23.36+/–13.18	0.001
Blood volume (mL/100 g)	3.58+/–1.18	2.83+/–1.09	0.10
Mean transit time (sec)	8.40+/–3.55	17.09+/–6.89	0.003
Permeability–surface area product (mL/100 g/min)	16.99+/–5.58	15.12+/–5.67	0.25

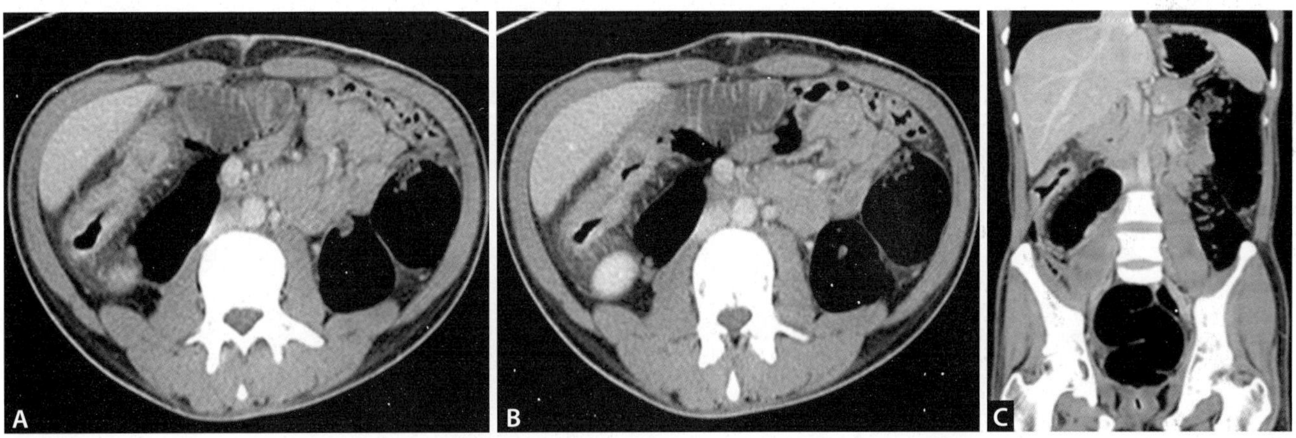

Figs. 20A to C: CECT axial (A and B) and coronal (C) images show circumferential mural thickening in the hepatic flexure and the ascending colon with luminal narrowing and an abrupt transition. The thickened bowel wall is homogeneously enhanced. This was misinterpreted as malignant lesion—Case of tuberculous colitis.

colorectal cancer based on the high perfusion values in colorectal cancer. Mean BV values of 6.0+/-1.2 mL/100 g and mean BF values of 80.1+/-31.5 mL/100 g/min are seen in colorectal carcinoma; while in diverticulitis, mean BV was 4.4+/-1.3 mL/100 g and mean BF was 52.0+/-27.3 mL/100 g/min.[71]

The association between poor prognosis and greater intensity of angiogenesis histologically is reflected in vivo by perfusion CT measurements **(Figs. 22A to C)**. Perfusion CT assessment of primary colorectal adenocarcinoma blood flow at staging can predict subsequent metastatic disease **(Figs. 23 and 24)**. The patients who had tumors with high blood flow and shorter mean transit time at baseline perfusion imaging showed a poor response to chemotherapy and radiotherapy.[72] High perfusion values in association with a poor response to chemotherapy and radiotherapy can be explained by large numbers of intratumoral arteriovenous shunts with a high perfusion rate and low exchange of oxygen.[70,73]

Quantitative measurements of blood flow using perfusion CT can be used for assessing clinicopathological features and prognosis in patients with colorectal cancer.[74] Well-differentiated tumors have higher blood flow than moderately differentiated tumors. Tumors with low blood flow show lymph node metastasis, vascular invasion, lymphatic invasion and distant metastasis.

Although histology is considered the gold standard for tumor grading, in heterogeneous tumors biopsies may be subjected to sampling error. Perfusion CT can assess tumor grade in vivo and can reduce the potential for sampling error by guiding biopsy to the tumor region most likely to be of the highest grade.

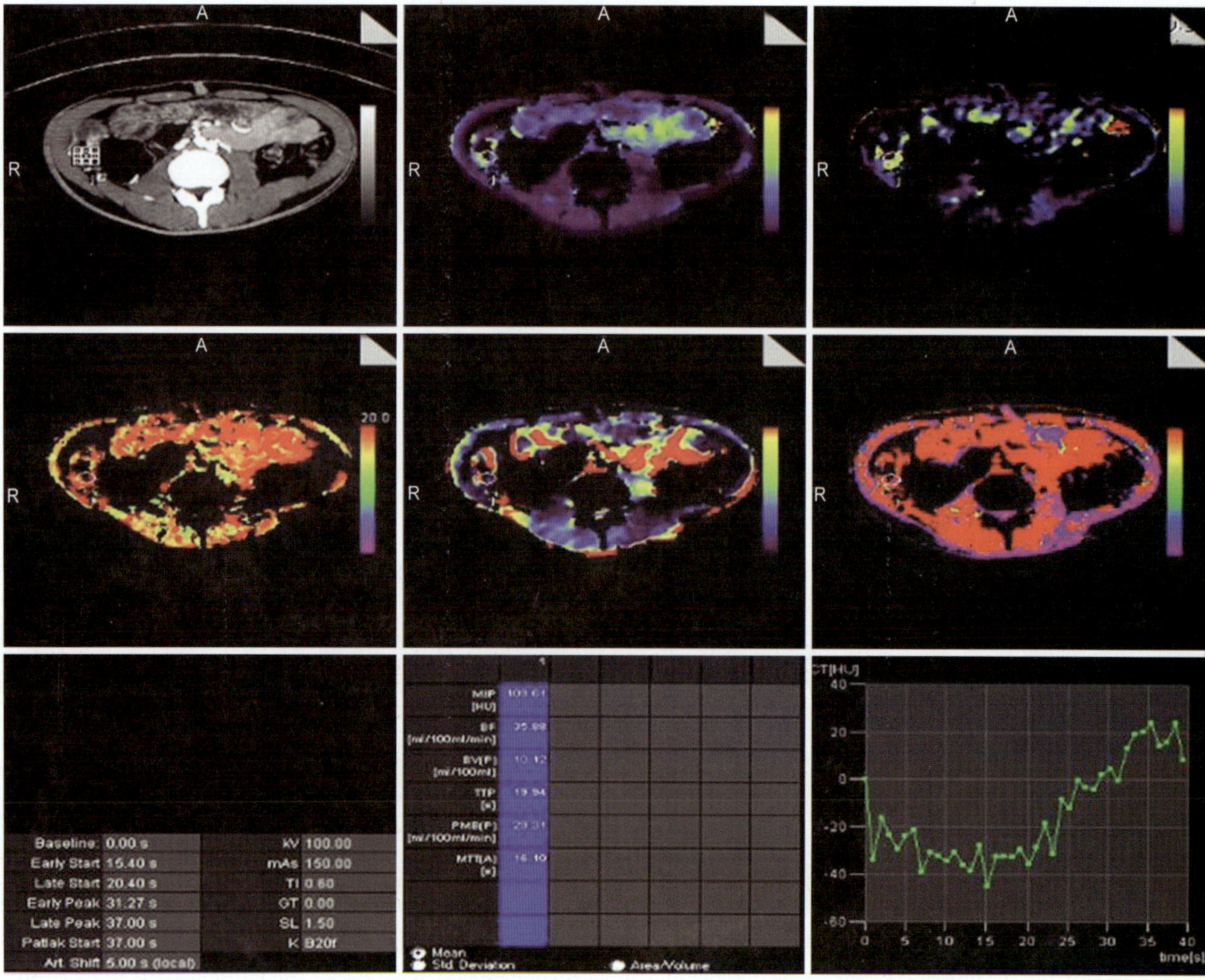

Fig. 21: CT perfusion study shows borderline values of BF 35.8 mL/100 g/min, BV 10.1 mL/100 g, PMB 20 mL/100 g/min and MTT of 16.1 seconds from the ROI drawn over the lesion. Histopathology revealed tuberculous colitis.

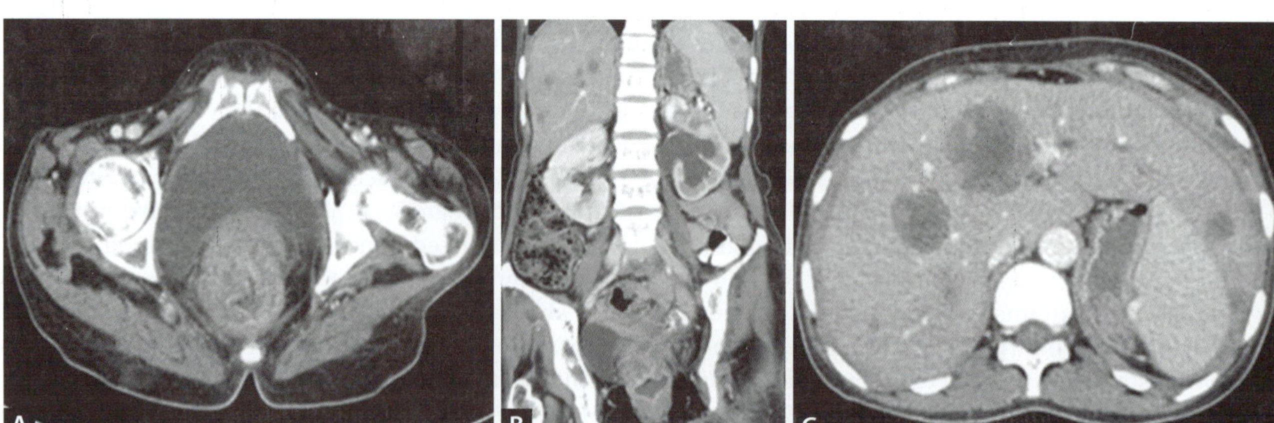

Figs. 22A to C: CECT axial (A) and coronal (B) images show irregular bowel wall thickening of the rectum and sigmoid colon with luminal narrowing and surrounding fat stranding. Heterogeneous enhancement is noted. Coronal MPR image (B) in addition shows left hydroureteronephrosis. CECT axial image through the liver (C) shows multiple round heterogeneously hypodense lesions of varying sizes in the right and left lobe of liver—Case of mucin secreting adenocarcinoma rectosigmoid with hepatic metastases.

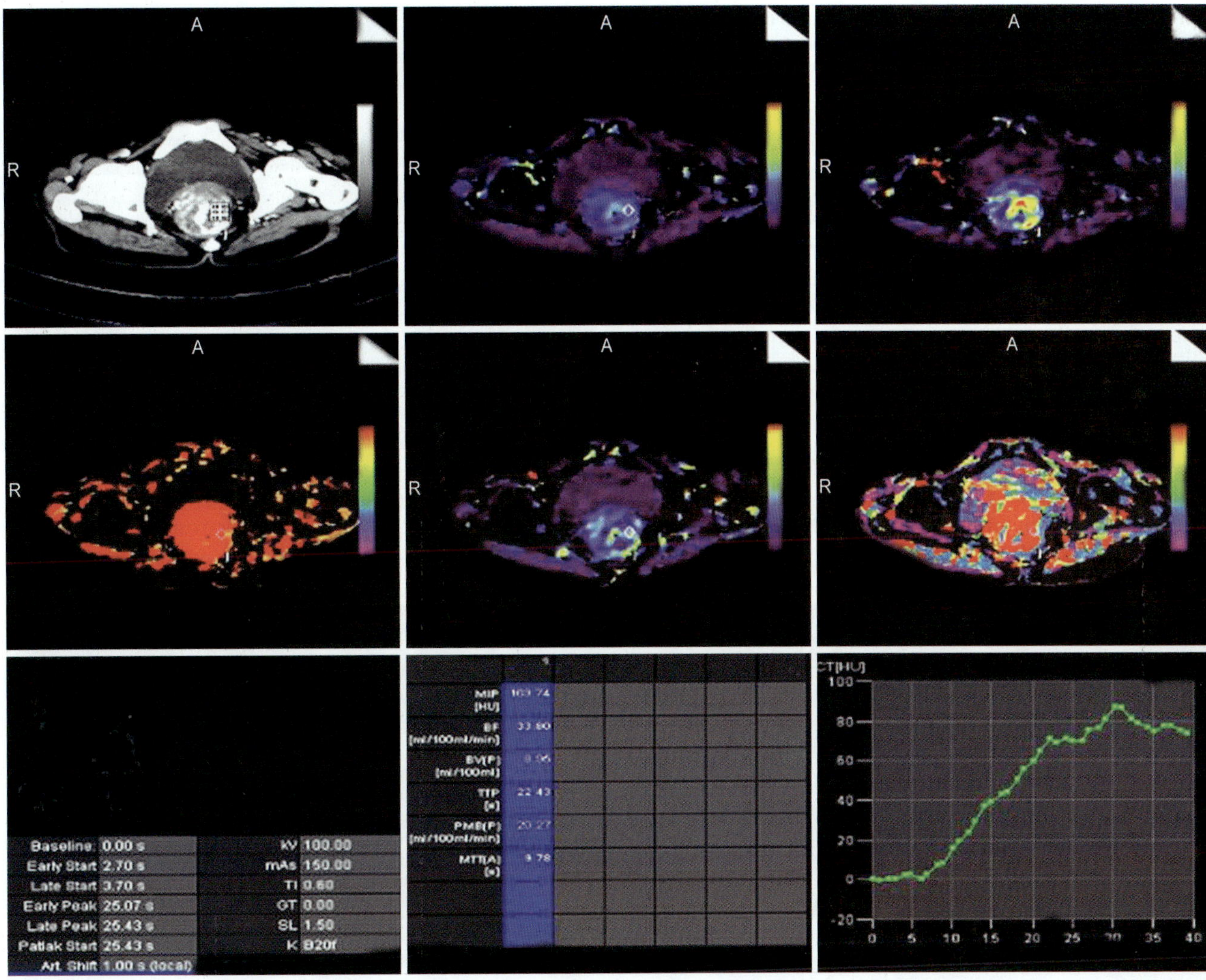

Figs. 23: Region of interest (ROI) placed over the lesion (same case as in Figure 22) shows high blood flow of 33.8 mL/100 g/min, blood volume of 9 mL/100 g, permeability of 20.3 mL/100 g/min and short MTT of 9.8 seconds suggesting malignant lesion.

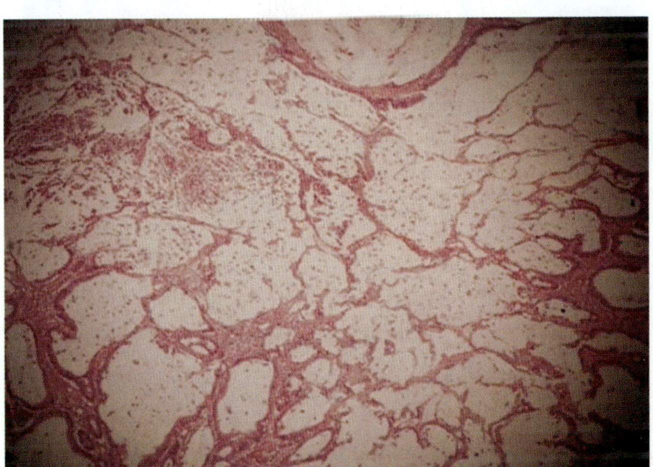

Fig. 24: Histopathological image of the case shown in Figure 20, shows extracellular mucin pool with intermingled atypical cells s/o mucin secreting adenocarcinoma.

COMPUTED TOMOGRAPHY PERFUSION IN PROSTATE CANCER

Though CT has been investigated to assess angiogenesis in malignant tumors of liver, lung, colon, rectum, pancreas, with the development of perfusion CT technique, the feasibility of the perfusion CT technique for evaluating prostate tumors has been shown only by a few studies. The reasons include:

1. Lack of contrast resolution makes identification of cancer on unenhanced CT scans impossible with the consequent inability to center the perfusion values on malignant areas.
2. Difficulty in morphologic differentiation between central and peripheral zone on CT images which do not allow identification of suspected malignant lesion.[75]

These problems have been overcome with the introduction of 64 and 128 MDCT scanner with larger volume coverage, enabling evaluation of the entire prostate. In a study published in 2012, substantial differences in mean values of BV, MTT and permeability surface area product parameters between prostate cancer, BPH, chronic prostatitis and healthy tissue have been found **(Figs. 25 and 26)**.[76]

The permeability surface area product and BV, which are respectively measures of capillary leak and functional vascular density, have been found to correlate with MVD in cancer fields **(Table 8)**. The BV, permeability surface area product reflects the main features of prostate cancer tumor vascularity which includes numerous and poorly formed vessels (high BV and MVD) with high permeability to macromolecules (high permeability surface area product), intermittent or unstable flow due to transient rises in already raised interstitial pressure (low BF value) and multiple arteriovenous shunts (low MTT values).

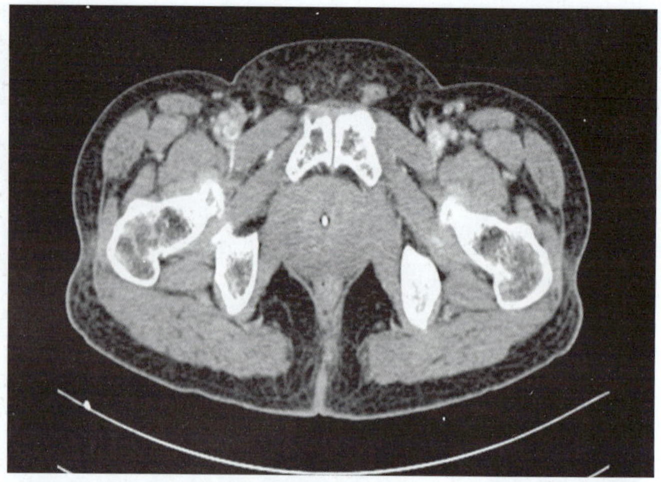

Fig. 25: Contrast-enhanced CT image shows a diffusely enlarged prostate with homogeneous enhancement and maintained fat planes. Note is made of Foley's catheter in situ—Case of benign prostatic hyperplasia.

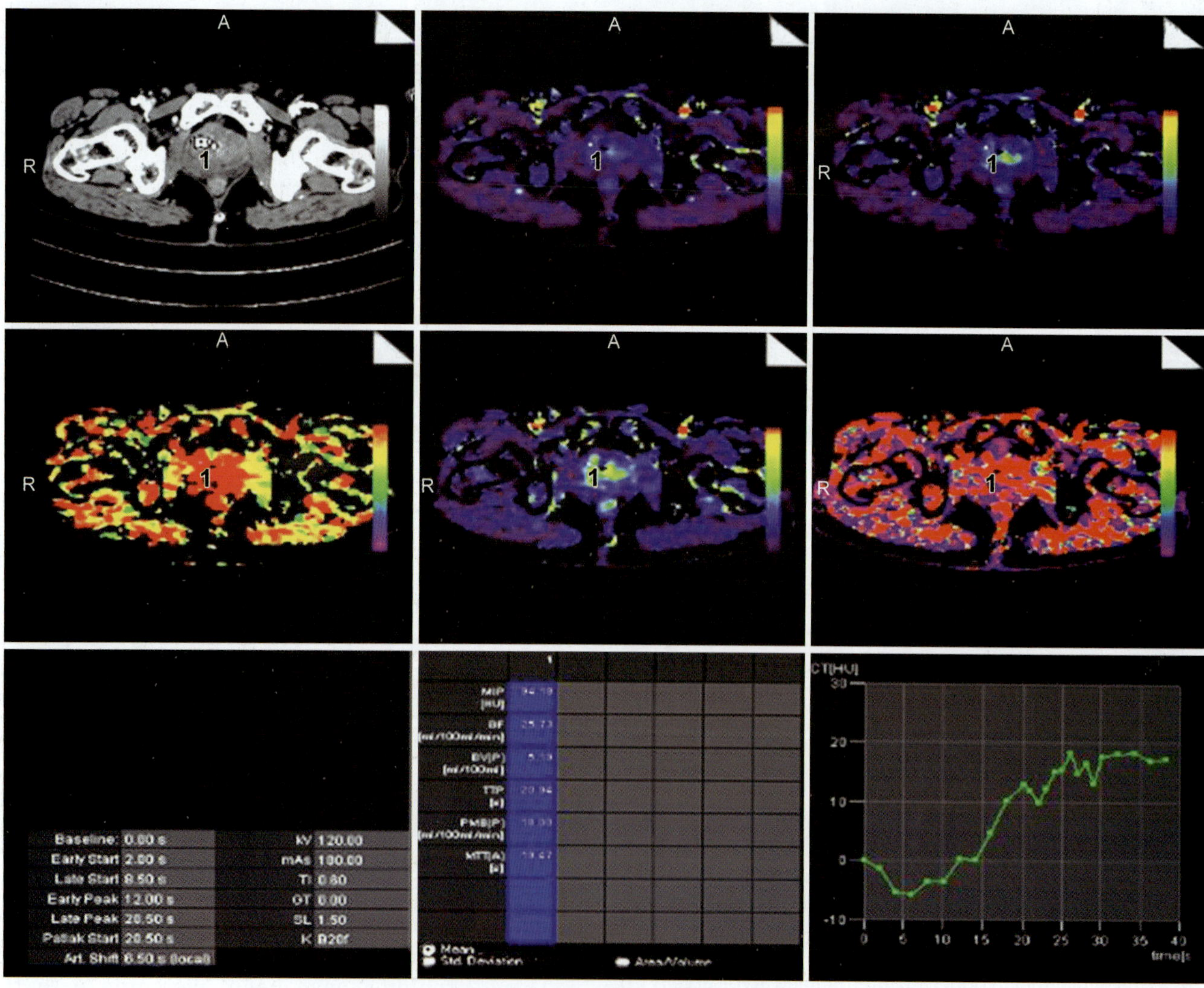

Fig. 26: CT perfusion maps in case of benign prostatic hypertrophy reveals prostatic perfusion values within normal limits.

Table 8: Perfusion CT parameters and histologic parameters in different prostatic tissues.[77]

Histologic diagnosis	*CT perfusion*				*Histology*	
	Blood flow	***Blood volume***	***Mean transit time***	***Permeability surface area product***	***Mean microvascular density***	***Mean vascular area***
Prostate cancer (n = 196)	18.36	8.45	19.19	26.34	70.78	0.0184
Benign prostatic hyperplasia (n = 461)	19.49	6.21	18.74	18.67	64.96	0.0171
Chronic prostatitis (n = 285)	19.67	4.94	16.24	18.08	54.91	0.0244
Healthy fields (n = 504)	20.32	5.44	16.37	19.93	60.51	0.0159

Thus quantitative assessment of microvessel density by CT perfusion may have a role in the detection of prostate cancer, metastasis, stage of disease and disease specific survival. It can accurately predict and localize tumor volume preoperatively and may be useful for selecting and guiding therapy for prostate cancer. It may provide baseline values (particularly BV and permeability surface area product) that may be well-suited for monitoring tumor response to radiation therapies or to antiangiogenic agents, such as bevacizumab, docetaxel and prednisone.[77] Perfusion CT data may also be used for targeted radiotherapy for tumor foci with minimal radiation to the surrounding tissue. It may also be used for future delineation of intraprostate subvolumes for intensity modulated radiation therapy which is difficult to do with parametric maps of DE-MRI. It may also have a role in the development of a 3D perfusion CT computer aided diagnosis (CAD) system for the detection of prostate cancer.

COMPUTED TOMOGRAPHY PERFUSION IN LYMPHOMA

Aggressive lymphomas are characterized by both a high metabolic turnover and a rather pronounced vascularity of tumor masses, whereas less aggressive lymphomas show a lower level metabolism and are generally considered to be less vascularized.[78] Metabolic activity is readily appreciated by ^{18}F-FDG PET imaging in these diseases, whereas vascular characteristics, such as perfusion and vessel wall permeability are detectable mainly by volume perfusion CT, dynamic contrast-enhanced (DCE) MRI, and DCE ultrasound. Contrast-enhanced volume perfusion CT measures changes in tissue density over time by using repeated CT scans of the volume being analyzed.

Subtypes of non-Hodgkin's lymphomas are characterized by a differing microscopic ultrastructure and a complex and variable vascularity, sometimes even within the same tumor lesion. These differences in histopathologic microarchitecture may lead to distinctive perfusion traits that may enable a differentiation between lymphoma entities.[79] Mean BF, BV and K^{trans} (transit constant) values have been found significantly higher in follicular lymphoma than in diffuse large cell lymphoma pointing towards distinct vascular properties due to differences in vascular microstructure and histopathologic lymphoma architecture. Mean BF values of 43.5+/−5.6 mL/100 mL/min and mean BV values of 9.5+/−2.3 mL/100mL are seen in follicular lymphoma while in diffuse large B cell lymphoma, the mean BF was 28.8+/−2.4 mL/100 mL/min and mean BV 4.6+/−0.5 mL/100 mL.[79] This is of particular relevance in patients with nonaggressive lymphomas, such as follicular lymphoma or chronic lymphocytic leukemia, which may show a transformation into high-grade lymphomas.[80] The use of perfusion imaging in lymphoma as a potential surrogate parameter of therapy response and early detection of transformation may allow tailoring treatment regimens accordingly.

Active lymphoma showed an increase in perfusion compared with inactive lymphoma and progression from inactive to active disease showed an increase in perfusion on serial evaluation.

COMPUTED TOMOGRAPHY PERFUSION IN BRAIN TUMORS

Brain tumors are an important cause of mortality and morbidity, hence, an early diagnosis and accurate characterization is necessary **(Fig. 27)**. Malignant brain tumors, of which gliomas are the most common primary neoplasm in adults and are very heterogeneous tumors. They are characterized by neovascularity and increased angiogenic activity resulting in higher proportion of immature and hyperpermeable vessels. High-grade gliomas can be highly invasive and extremely vascular tumors. Two of the most important factors in determining the malignancy of gliomas are their ability to infiltrate the brain parenchyma and to recruit or synthesize vascular networks for further growth (i.e. neoangiogenesis). Presently, brain tumor grading is based on the histopathological assessment of the tumor by stereotactic biopsy or cytoreductive surgery, which has inherent limitations due to sampling and its interpretation.

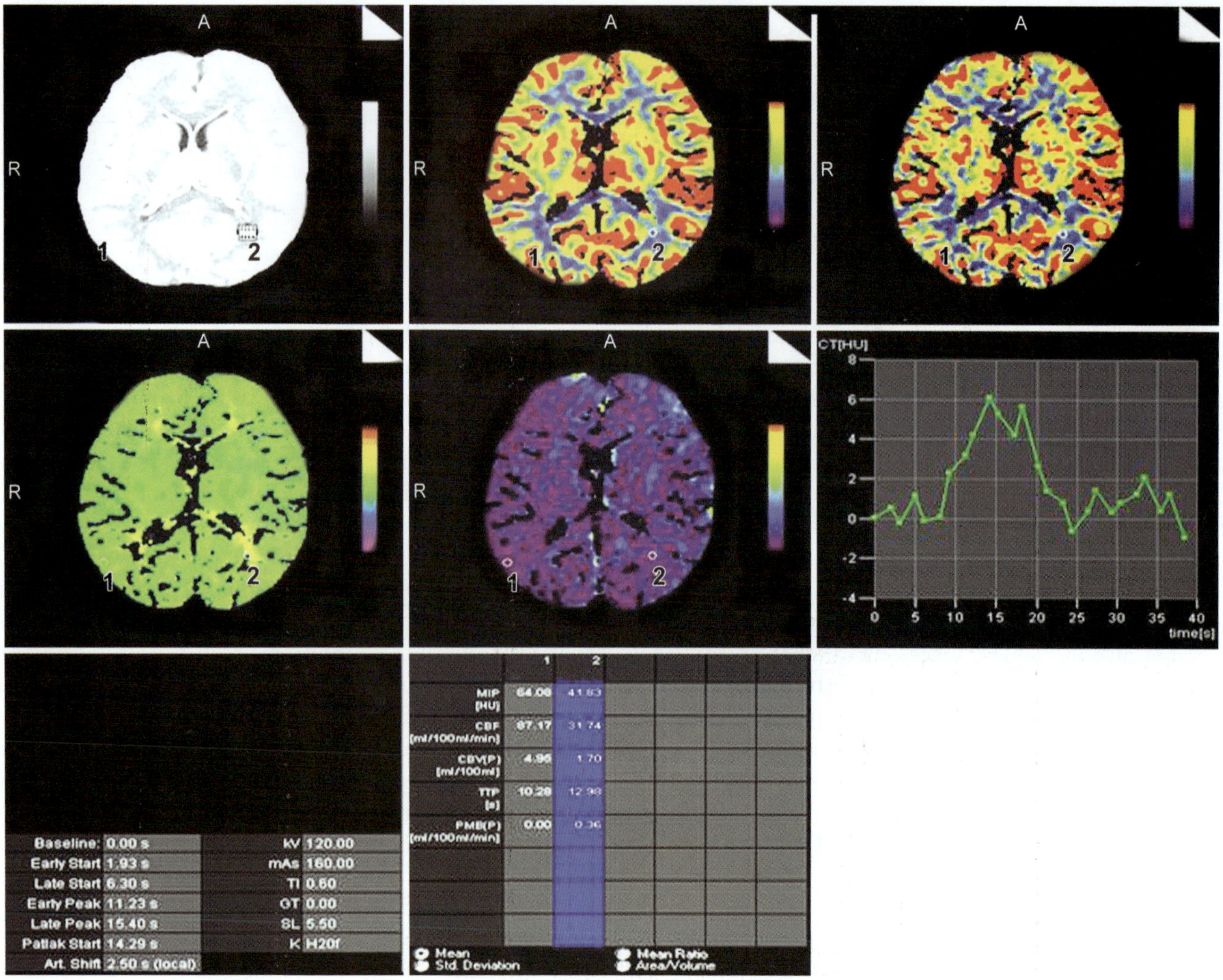

Fig. 27: Perfusion CT maps of normal cerebral parenchyma, i.e. CBF (top middle), CBV (top right), TTP (middle left), PMB (middle). Note the scale on the right side of the maps depicting the lowest values in violet and highest values in red. The normal gray matter and basal ganglia appear yellow to red on color coded maps of CBF and CBV while normal white matter appears blue. On PMB maps normal brain appears violet indicating intact blood brain barrier. Perfusion values through the normal white matter in this case (ROI 2) are CBF of 31.74, CBV of 1.70, TTP of 12.98 and PMB of 0.36. The graph indicates the time attenuation curve through the ROI.

Histologic evaluation of tumor angiogenesis by using various markers, such as microvascular density, microvascular cellular proliferation, and total vascular area is limited by this regional heterogeneity, and its confounding effect is worsened by its small size and limited number of samples obtained with surgical biopsy. These limitations can result in inaccurate classification and grading of gliomas due to sampling errors. Brain tumor angiogenesis is a continuously evolving process that can also be affected by various treatment modalities. Hence, there is a need for noninvasive in vivo clinical imaging tools that can study perfusion in the entire tumor which can be used to assess much larger volumes than small biopsy samples, and can probably guide biopsy and excision sites for better results.

Perfusion CT, which has also been used recently for glioma grading, provides a linear relationship between tissue attenuation and tissue concentration of a contrast agent, unlike perfusion MR imaging. Hence, it probably provides a more robust and less biased estimation of hemodynamic (tumor blood volume) and physiologic (tumor vascular leakiness) parameters. In addition, due to the wider availability, faster scanning times, and low cost compared with MR perfusion, perfusion CT is potentially well suited to study brain tumors and could potentially be useful as an easy clinical tool for quantitative estimates of perfusion parameters and their use as imaging biomarkers **(Figs. 28 and 29)**.[81]

In a perfusion CT study for cerebral neoplasms, grade IV tumors show highest mean CBF as well as the highest mean

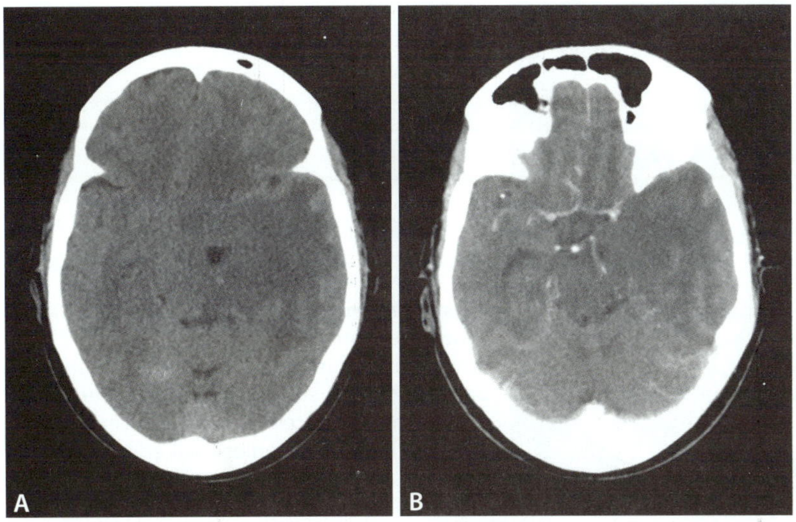

Figs. 28A and B: Axial noncontrast CT (A) and contrast-enhanced CT (B) scans show an ill-defined hypodense lesion in the left temporal region showing minimal enhancement with mass effect and rotation of the brain stem—Case of astrocytoma.

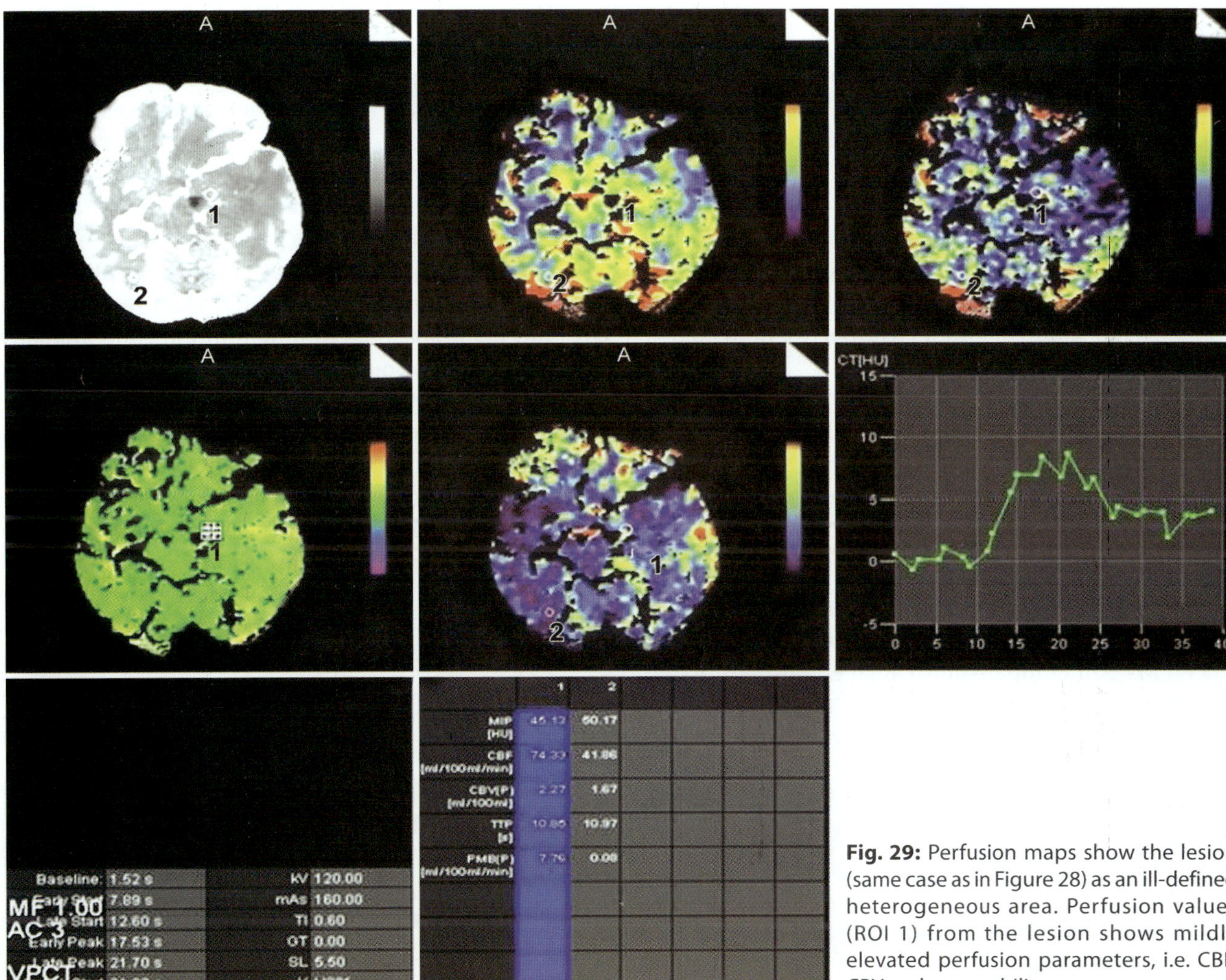

Fig. 29: Perfusion maps show the lesion (same case as in Figure 28) as an ill-defined heterogeneous area. Perfusion values (ROI 1) from the lesion shows mildly elevated perfusion parameters, i.e. CBF, CBV and permeability.

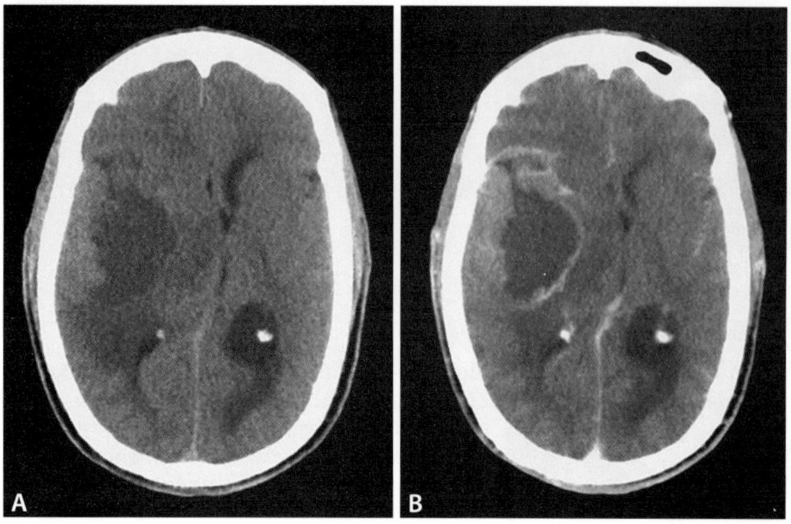

Figs. 30A and B: Axial noncontrast (A) and contrast-enhanced (B) CT scans showing a large heterogeneous mass lesion in the right temporoparietal region showing irregular peripheral enhancement and central nonenhancing necrotic areas with marked perilesional edema, midline shift and dilatation of contralateral ventricle—Case of glioblastoma multiforme.

CBV. Glioblastoma multiforme showed mean CBF value of 133.51, mean CBV value of 7.44 and mean permeability values of 15.15 **(Figs. 30 and 31)**. The normalized perfusion values observed in GBM were mean nCBF of 4.96, mean nCBV of 3.76 and mean nTTP of 0.85. Perfusion values were highest in GBM among astrocytomas. The correlation for CBF and CBV with tumor grade is better in astroglial tumors as compared to oligodendroglial tumors and is hypothesized to be due to the fine capillary network typically observed in oligodendrogliomas. Mean value of PMB was seen to show progressive increment with increasing grade of tumors irrespective of histologic subtype **(Figs. 32 and 33)**.

COMPUTED TOMOGRAPHY PERFUSION IN HEAD AND NECK TUMORS

Perfusion CT is being used in the evaluation of head and neck tumors **(Fig. 34)**. Benign tissues show lower BF and BV and longer MTT compared with malignant tissue **(Figs. 35 and 36)**.[64] It has been seen that squamous cell carcinoma shows substantially increased BF, BV, PS and reduced MTT in comparison to adjacent normal tissues **(Figs. 37 and 38)**.

It has been found that tumors with lower perfusion values showed a poor response to induction chemotherapy. This is attributed to the presence of tissue hypoxia within the tumor which hinders the treatment delivery and therapeutic effect of chemoradiation.

COMPUTED TOMOGRAPHY PERFUSION IN LUNG CANCER

Dynamic CT has been used for the characterization of solitary pulmonary nodules as benign or malignant based on the enhancement characteristics. Nodules with higher perfusion are more likely to be malignant. Multislice perfusion CT is also helpful to differentiate lung cancer from benign lung masses. BV, BF and PS were all found to be higher in malignant than benign masses. When BV more than or equal to 5 mL/100 mg was set as a diagnostic threshold, the sensitivity, specificity, positive-predictive value and negative-predictive value were 96%, 78%, 92%, 87%, respectively.[82]

Whole tumor perfusion analysis is technically feasible with 64 or higher detector row CT. High blood volume (BV) has been observed in lung tumoral zone indicative of the presence of numerous vessels.[83] Moreover, these areas also show a high capillary permeability, i.e. K^{trans}, a well known characteristic of tumoral vessels. Perfusion CT enables quantitative and qualitative assessment of lung tumor neovascularization. It is also a noninvasive tool for providing predictive and prognostic parameters in patients with lung cancer and for monitoring chemotherapy. Perfusion CT of pulmonary metastasis has potential in the assessment of early vascular changes that result from laser-induced thermotherapy (LITT) and predicting technical success immediately after treatment.[84] Tumors with perfusion measurements that do not change after therapy indicate progressive disease.

OTHER APPLICATIONS

Nephrology

Dynamic CT has been used to study the relative glomerular filtration rate and to determine the relative function of each kidney. The iodinated contrast agents used for CT are filtered at the glomerulus and not reabsorbed by the tubules. They can thus measure physiological indices, such as contrast

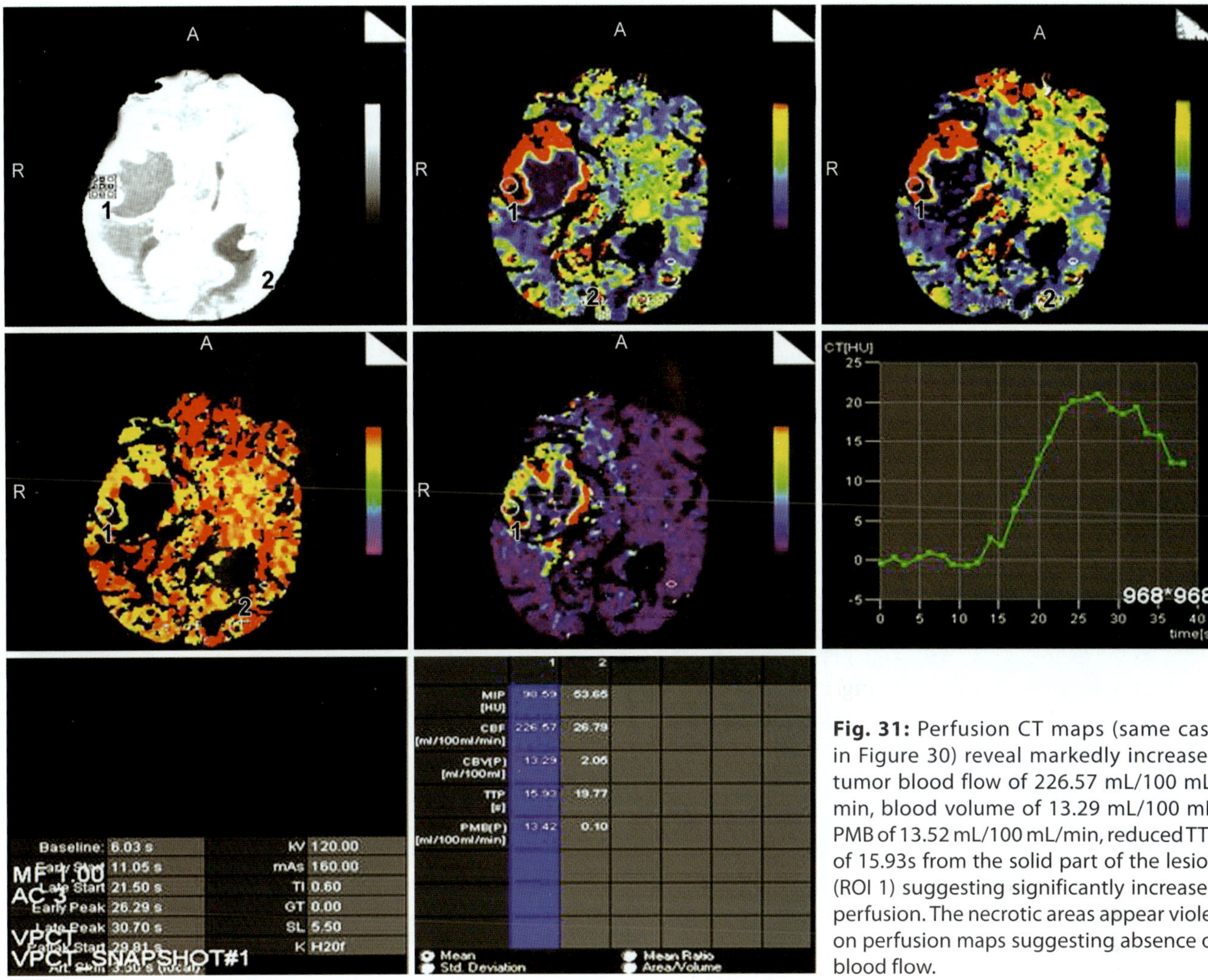

Fig. 31: Perfusion CT maps (same case in Figure 30) reveal markedly increased tumor blood flow of 226.57 mL/100 mL/min, blood volume of 13.29 mL/100 mL, PMB of 13.52 mL/100 mL/min, reduced TTP of 15.93s from the solid part of the lesion (ROI 1) suggesting significantly increased perfusion. The necrotic areas appear violet on perfusion maps suggesting absence of blood flow.

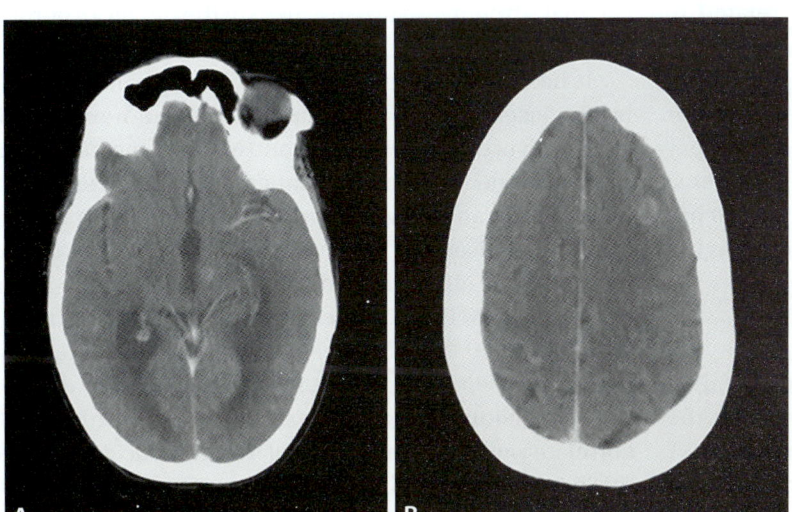

Figs. 32A and B: In a known case of carcinoma of breast axial contrast-enhanced scans show well-defined, small round lesions with moderate postcontrast enhancement in the left thalamus and left frontal region—Case of cerebral metastases.

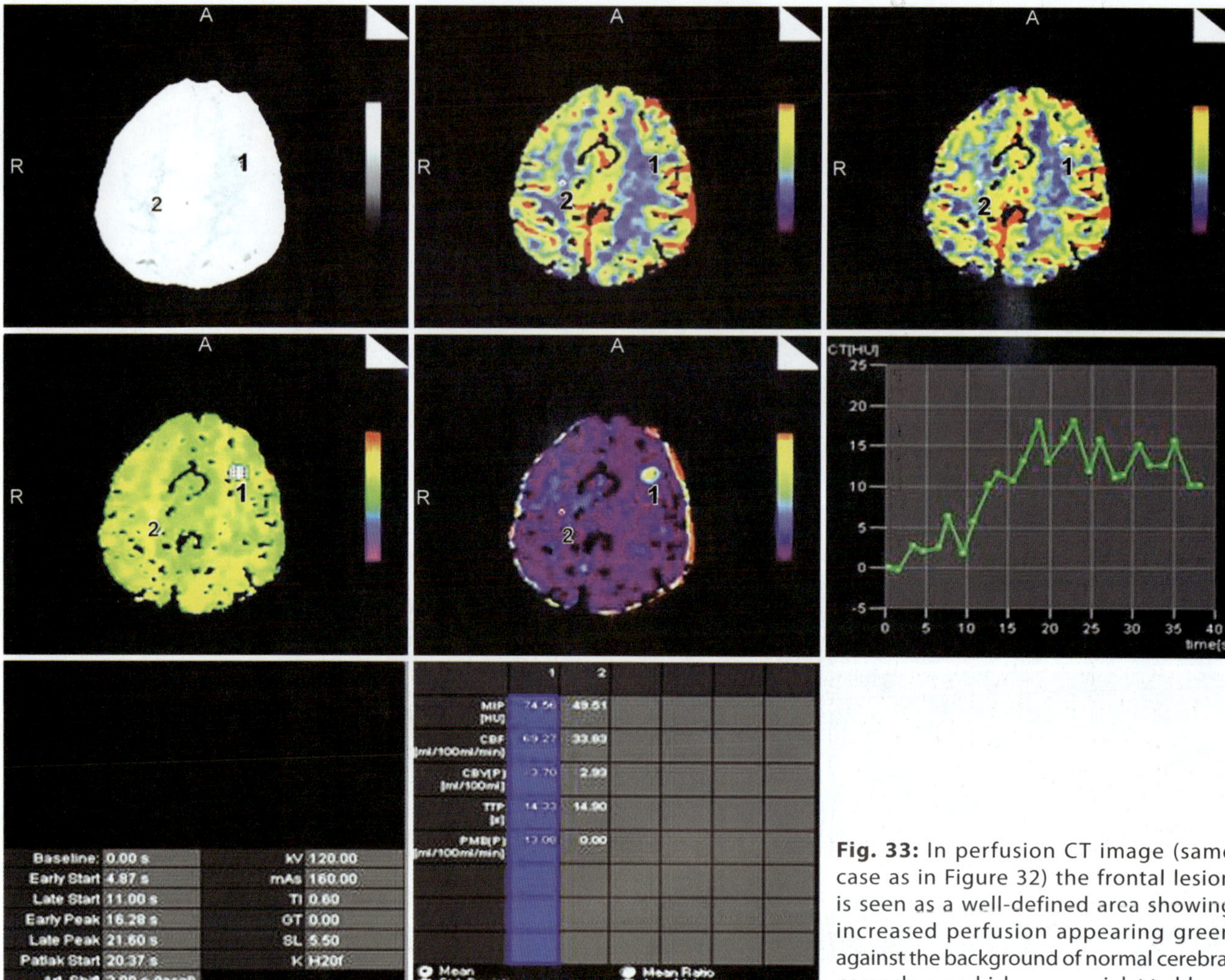

Fig. 33: In perfusion CT image (same case as in Figure 32) the frontal lesion is seen as a well-defined area showing increased perfusion appearing green against the background of normal cerebral parenchyma which appear violet to blue.

clearance per unit volume, which is closely related to glomerular filtration rate per unit renal volume of kidney. In normal kidneys clearance/volume averaged 0.49+/-0.11 mL/min/mL.[85] In patients with renovascular hypertension attributable to unilateral renal artery stenosis, perfusion CT was capable of distinguishing renal stenosis with and without preserved perfusion. It also has a role in the differentiation of rejection as compared to other causes of dysfunction in transplant kidneys.

Chronic Liver Diseases

Chronic liver diseases include chronic hepatitis, liver fibrosis and cirrhosis. Liver biopsy is considered the gold standard to assess the degree of liver cirrhosis. CT perfusion can show the pathological changes in the liver before cirrhosis, even at the early stage of fibrosis and it can make noninvasive assessment of the degree of chronic liver disease.

It has been reported that total liver perfusion (TLP) is decreased in patients with cirrhosis and noncirrhotic chronic liver disease while HPI and MTT are increased. The hepatic perfusion indices of patients without liver disease were significantly lower than that of those with child B and C liver disease. The best cut-off point to differentiate patients with cirrhosis from those without cirrhosis was considered a MTT of 22.6 second with both sensitivity and specificity of 81%.[86] It has been reported that hepatic blood flow decreases with the severity of chronic liver disease. The perfusion changes as estimated by perfusion CT correlate well with the severity of liver chronic disease and this has implications in the follow-up of patients who have chronic liver disease.

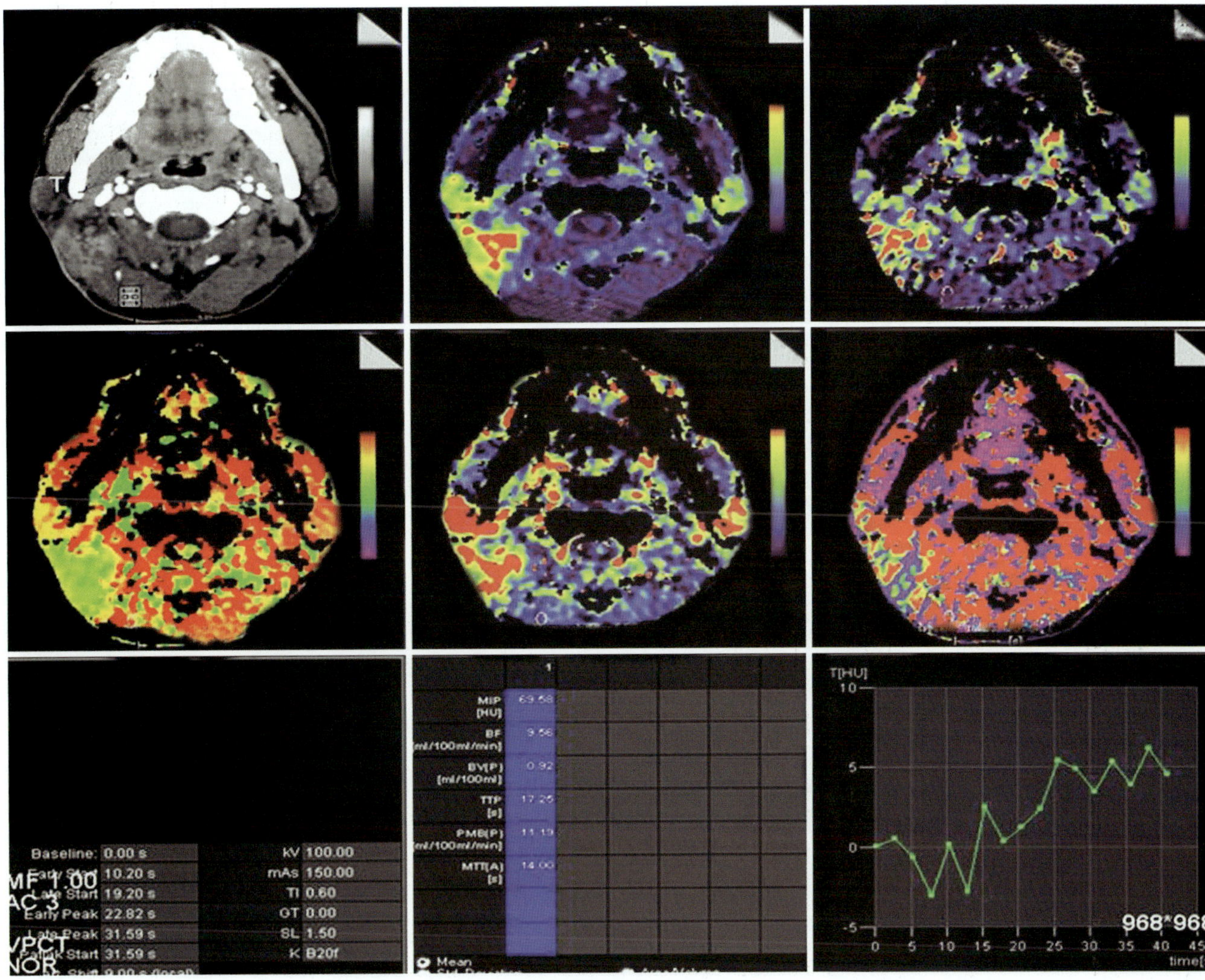

Fig. 34: Perfusion CT maps show color maps for blood flow (BF), blood volume (BV), mean transit time (MTT) and permeability (PMB) generated by software, in which every pixel is assigned a color that represents a numeric value for the perfusion parameter calculated for that voxel. High numeric values are represented by color shades of yellow and red, and low numeric values are represented by color shade of blue—Normal perfusion CT of neck.

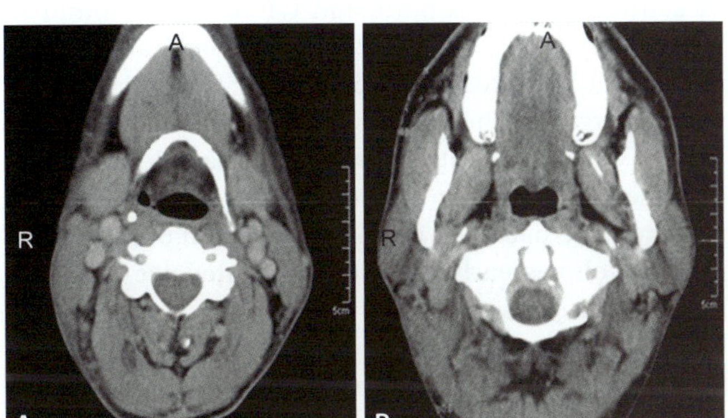

Figs. 35A and B: Axial contrast-enhanced CT scans at the level of hyoid bone (A) and at the level of atlas vertebra (B) show multiple hypodense lymph nodes along the jugular chain—Tubercular lymphadenitis.

CT Perfusion in Liver Transplantation

It is important to evaluate noninvasive liver perfusion after liver transplantation. CT perfusion can monitor the tendency of hemodynamic changes in portal vein and hepatic artery, contributing to the early diagnosis of blood vessel complications after transplantation.

Some studies showed changes in hepatic artery perfusion (HAP), while some in portal venous perfusion (PVP) and total liver perfusion (TLP). Authors hold that it is related to the selection of patients, and examination time after the transplantation, etc. Therefore, hemodynamic change after transplantation is dynamic process, and different patients have different hemodynamic characteristics.

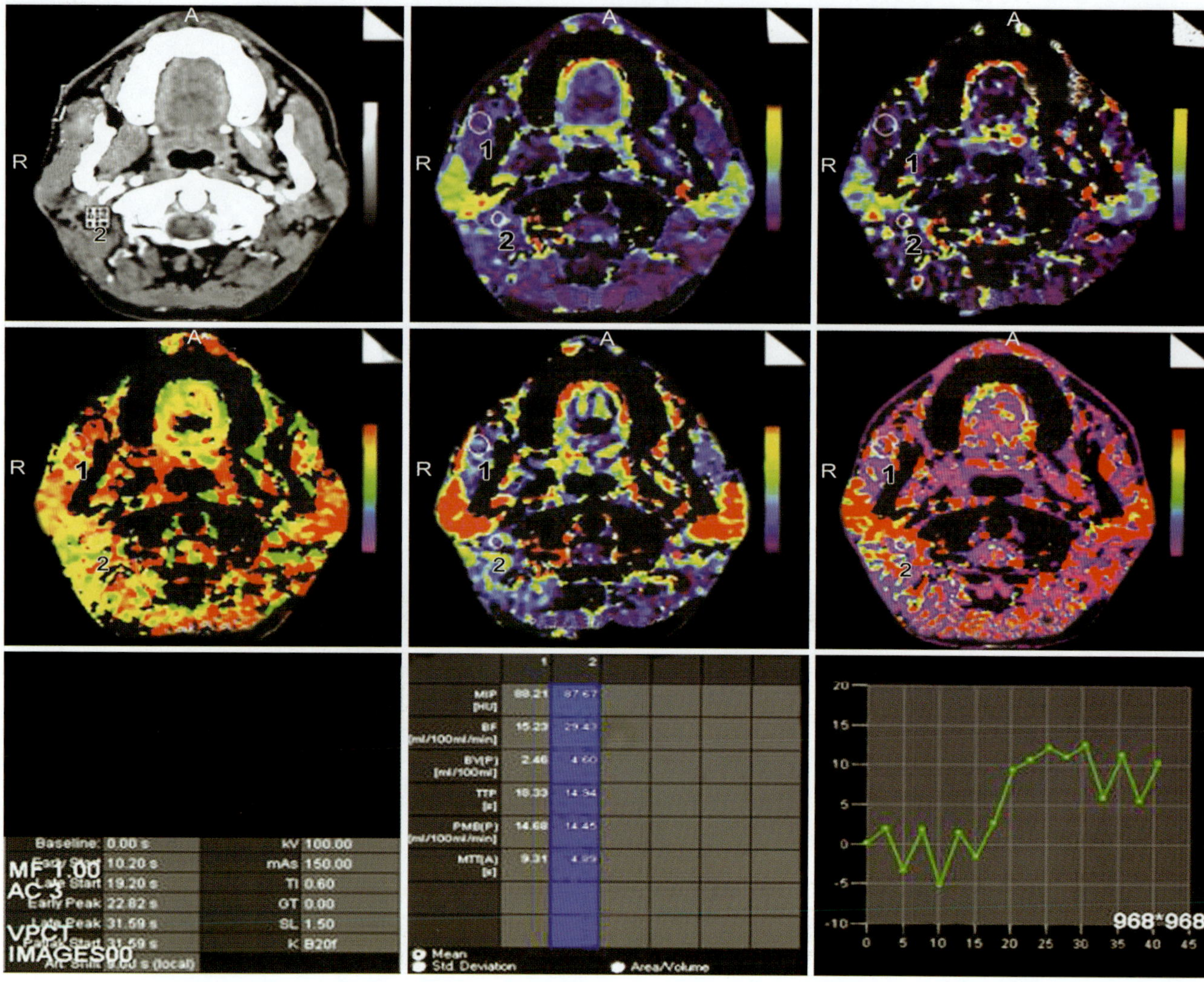

Fig. 36: Perfusion CT maps (same case as in Figure 35) show mildly elevated perfusion parameters from the enlarged cervical nodes (ROI 2).

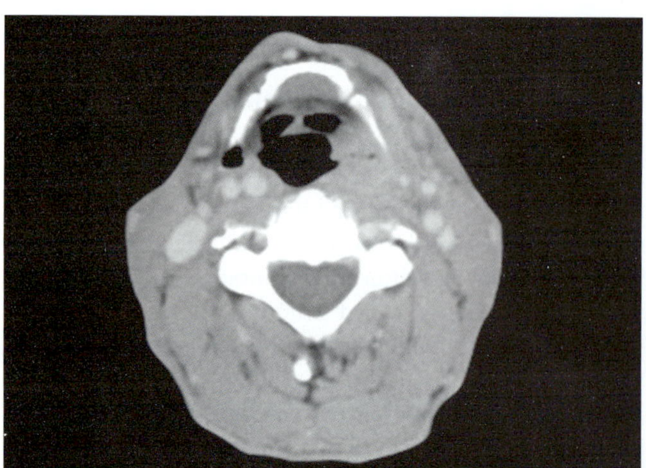

Fig. 37: Axial contrast-enhanced CT scan of the neck at the level of the hyoid bone shows an ill-defined heterogeneous enhancing mass lesion involving supraglottic larynx on the left side—Case of squamous cell carcinoma larynx (well-differentiated).

Acute Pancreatitis

In acute pancreatitis perfusion CT has been found to have a sensitivity and specificity of 100% and 95.3%, respectively in detection of pancreatic ischemia.[87] Areas with pancreatic ischemia showed a reduction in perfusion values. Compared with normal pancreas identification of these areas can help to predict the later development of pancreatic necrosis. The early detection of pancreatic necrosis allows early institution of intensive care and improves prognosis.

RADIATION ISSUES

A major concern of perfusion CT is the risk for exposure to ionizing radiation, especially in patients who require serial perfusion studies for monitoring treatment effects. Several techniques, including reduced tube current and tube potential can be employed to reduce radiation dose.

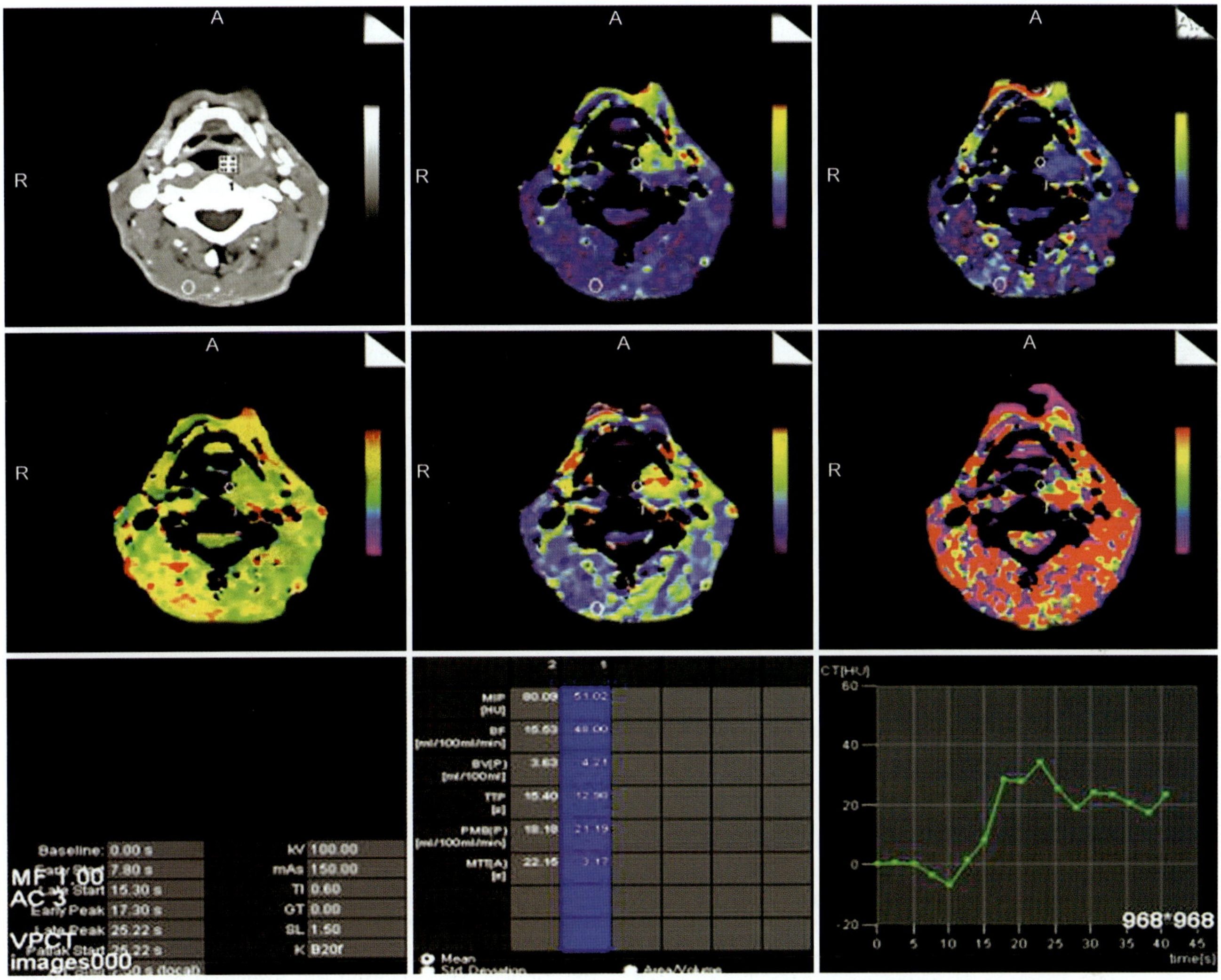

Fig. 38: On the perfusion CT maps, the lesion (same case as in Figure 37) stands out clearly. The perfusion values from the tumor (ROI 1) reveal markedly high tumor blood flow (48 mL/100 g/min), blood volume (4.21 mL/100 g), permeability (21.19 mL/100 g/min) and low mean transit time (3.17 sec).

Likewise, protocol modifications involving the use of higher temporal sampling rates, such as scanning every 2–3 seconds instead of 1 second during the first pass and limiting the scan duration of cine acquisition to 40–50 seconds, can substantially minimize the radiation exposure from each examination without compromising the data. Likewise, tailoring the perfusion CT protocol to the clinical objective or the relevant parameters can also diminish the radiation dose to the patient. For example, in clinical situations requiring tissue perfusion parameters like BF or MTT, it would be prudent to perform only the first pass study.[64]

■ CONCLUSION

Perfusion CT has achieved great strides as a functional technique since its inception and its scope in the clinical and research settings is increasing. With the advancement in perfusion software and the development of new generation scanners having a wider cine acquisition, it has allowed even single or multiple organ perfusions with the advantage of decreased radiation exposure and motion artifacts. Moreover, the integration of positron emission tomography (PET) CT systems with the prospect of combining perfusion measurements with PET data represents an exciting new innovative technology that has a wide range of clinical application as a single examination. Development of new contrast agents which remain longer in intravascular compartment may also overcome the complexities of physiological modeling. Thus perfusion CT which was primarily introduced as a research tool has emerged as a definitive functional technique not only in patients of stroke but also in oncology and other areas.

REFERENCES

1. Miles KA. Perfusion imaging with computed tomography: brain and beyond. Eu Radiol Suppl. 2006;16:M37-43.
2. Ma SH, Le HB, Jia BH et al. Peripheral pulmonary nodules: relationship between multislice spiral CT perfusion imaging and tumor angiogenesis and VEGF expression. BMC Cancer. 2008;8:186.
3. Perini R, Choe R, Yodh AG et al. Noninvasive assessment of tumor neovasculature: technique and clinical applications. Cancer Metastasis Rev. 2008;27:615-30.
4. Miles KA. Perfusion CT for the assessment of tumour vascularity: which protocol?. Br J Radiol. 2003;76:S36-42.
5. Harvey C, Dooher A, Morgan J et al. Imaging of tumour therapy responses by dynamic CT. Eur J Radiol. 1999;30:221-6.
6. Miles KA. Tumour angiogenesis and its relation to contrast enhancement on computed tomography: a review. Eur J Radiol. 1999;30:198-205.
7. Miles KA, Charnsangavej C, Lee FT et al. Application of CT in the investigation of angiogenesis in oncology. Acad Radiol. 2000;7:840-50.
8. Cao J, Yang A, Long XY, et al. CT hepatic volume measurement combined with CT perfusion imaging in evaluating the hepatic functional reserve. Zhong Nan Da Xue Xue Bao Yi Xue Ban. 2007;32:422-6.
9. Sahani DV, Kalva SP, Hamberg LM et al. Assessing tumor perfusion and treatment response in rectal cancer with multisection CT: initial observations. Radiology. 2005;234:785-92.
10. Goh V, Halligan S, Gartner L et al. Quantitative colorectal cancer perfusion measurement by multidetector row CT: does greater tumour coverage improve measurement reproducibility?. Br J Radiol. 2006;79:578-83.
11. Goh V, Halligan S, Hugill JA et al. Quantitative assessment of colorectal cancer perfusion using MDCT: inter and intraobserver agreement. Am J Roentgenol. 2005;185: 225-31.
12. Goh V, Halligan S, Hugill JA et al. Quantitative colorectal cancer perfusion measurement using dynamic contrast-enhanced multidetector row computed tomography: effect of acquisition time and implications for protocols. J Comput Assist Tomogr. 2005;29:59-63.
13. Koenig M, Kraus M, Theek C et al. Quantitative assessment of the ischemic brain by means of perfusion related parameters derived from perfusion CT. Stroke. 2001;32:431-7.
14. Hoeffner EG, Case I, Jain R et al. Cerebral perfusion CT: technique and clinical applications. Radiology. 2004;231:632-44.
15. Koenig M, Klotz E, Luka B et al. Perfusion CT of the brain: diagnostic approach for early detection of ischemic stroke. Radiology. 1998;209:85-93.
16. Mayer TE, Hamann GF, Baranczyk J et al. Dynamic CT perfusion imaging of acute stroke. Am J Neuroradiol. 2000;21:1441-9.
17. Klotz E, Koenig M. Perfusion measurements of the brain: using dynamic CT for the quantitative assessment of cerebral ischemia in acute stroke. Eur J Radiol. 1999;30:170-84.
18. Keith CJ, Griffiths M, Petersen B et al. Computed tomography perfusion imaging in acute stroke. Australas Radiol. 2002;46:221-30.
19. Wintermark M, Flanders AE, Velthuis B et al. Perfusion CT assessment of infarct core and penumbra: receiver operating characteristic curve analysis in 130 patients suspected of acute hemispheric stroke. Stroke. 2006;37:979-85.
20. Wintermark M. Brain perfusion CT in acute stroke patients. Eu Radiol Suppl. 2005;15:d28-31.
21. De Lucas EM, Sánchez E, Gutiérrez A et al. CT protocol for acute stroke: tips and tricks for general radiologists. Radiographics. 2008;28:1673-87.
22. Wintermark M, Reichhart M, Thiran JP et al. Prognostic accuracy of cerebral blood flow measurement by perfusion computed tomography, at the time of emergency room admission, in acute stroke patients. Ann Neurol. 2002 ;51:417-32.
23. Murayama K, Katada K, Nakane M et al. Whole brain perfusion CT performed with a prototype 256 detector row CT system: initial experience. Radiology. 2009;250:202-11.
24. Lui YW, Tang ER, Allmendinger AM et al. Evaluation of CT perfusion in the setting of cerebral ischemia: patterns and pitfalls. Am J Neuroradiol. 2010;31:1552-63.
25. Parsons MW. Perfusion CT: is it clinically useful?. Int J Stroke. 2008;3:41-50.
26. Allmendinger AM, Tang ER, Lui YW et al. Imaging of stroke: Part 1 perfusion CT-Overview of imaging technique, interpretation pearls, and common pitfalls. Am J Roentgenol. 2012;198:52-62.
27. Miles KA. Functional computed tomography in oncology. Eur J Cancer. 2002;38:2079-84.
28. Brawer MK, Deering RE, Brown M et al. Predictors of pathologic stage in prostatic carcinoma. The role of neovascularity. Cancer. 1994;73:678-87.
29. Fontanini G, Vignati S, Basolo F et al. Angiogenesis as a prognostic indicator of survival in non-small cell lung carcinoma: a prospective study. J Natl Cancer Inst. 1997;89:881-6.
30. Cuenod CA, Fournier L, Balvay D et al. Tumor angiogenesis: pathophysiology and implications for contrast-enhanced MRI and CT assessment. Abdom Imaging. 2006;31:188-93.
31. Phongkitkarun S, Kobayashi S, Kan Z et al. Quantification of angiogenesis by functional computed tomography in a matrigel model in rat. Acad Radiol. 2004;11:573-82.
32. Li WW. Tumor angiogenesis: molecular pathology, therapeutic targeting, and imaging. Acad Radiol. 2000;7:800-11.
33. Provenzale JM. Imaging of angiogenesis: clinical techniques and novel imaging methods. Am J Roentgenol. 2007;188:11-23.
34. Miles KA. Functional CT imaging in oncology. Eur Radiol. 2003;13:134-8.

35. Miles KA, Hayball MP, Dixon AK. Functional images of hepatic perfusion obtained with dynamic CT. Radiology. 1993;188:405-11.
36. Blomley MJ, Coulden R, Dawson P et al. Liver perfusion studied with ultrafast CT. J Comput Assist Tomogr. 1995;19:424-33.
37. Weidekamm C, Cejna M, Kramer L et al. Effects of TIPS on liver perfusion measured by dynamic CT. Am J Roentgenol. 2005;184:505-10.
38. Zhou Z, Huang H, Xu B. Clinic application with MSCT perfusion in liver tumor. Journal of Clinical Radiology. 2006;3:013.
39. Hashimoto K, Murakami T, Dono K et al. Assessment of the severity of liver disease and fibrotic change: the usefulness of hepatic CT perfusion imaging. Oncol Rep. 2006;16:677-83.
40. Komemushi A, Tanigawa N, Kojima H et al. CT perfusion of the liver during selective hepatic arteriography: pure arterial blood perfusion of liver tumor and parenchyma. Radiat Med. 2003;21:246-51.
41. Ippolito D, Sironi S, Pozzi M et al. Perfusion computed tomographic assessment of early hepatocellular carcinoma in cirrhotic liver disease: initial observations. J Comput Assist Tomogr. 2008;32:855-8.
42. Chen WX, Min PQ, Song B et al. Single-level dynamic spiral CT of hepatocellular carcinoma: correlation between imaging features and density of tumor microvessels. World J Gastroenterol. 2004;10:67-72.
43. Sahani DV, Holalkere NS, Mueller PR et al. Advanced hepatocellular carcinoma: CT perfusion of liver and tumor tissue—initial experience. Radiology. 2007;243:736-43.
44. Tsushima Y, Funabasama S, Aoki J et al. Quantitative perfusion map of malignant liver tumors, created from dynamic computed tomography data. Acad Radiol. 2004;11:215-23.
45. Zhong L, Wang WJ, Xu JR. Clinical application of hepatic CT perfusion. World J Gastroenterol. 2009;15:907-11.
46. Zhu AX, Holalkere NS, Muzikansky A et al. Early antiangiogenic activity of bevacizumab evaluated by computed tomography perfusion scan in patients with advanced hepatocellular carcinoma. The oncologist. 2008 ;13:120-5.
47. Cuenod CA, Leconte I, Siauve N et al. Early changes in liver perfusion caused by occult metastases in rats: detection with quantitative CT. Radiology. 2001 ;218:556-61.
48. Shi GF, Wang SJ, Wang Q et al. Effect of perfusion CT scan on hepatic hemodynamic changes in rats with liver micrometastases. Ai Zheng. 2006;25:849-54.
49. Leggett DA, Kelley BB, Bunce IH et al. Colorectal cancer: diagnostic potential of CT measurements of hepatic perfusion and implications for contrast enhancement protocols. Radiology. 1997;205:716-20.
50. Glover C, Douse P, Kane P et al. Accuracy of investigations for asymptomatic colorectal liver metastases. Dis Colon Rectum. 2002;45:476-84.
51. Wang JY, Wang SQ, Chen L et al. Application of CT perfusion imaging in discrimination of liver carcinoma and hemangioma. Linchuang Gandan Bing Zazhi. 2006;22:455-7.
52. Meijerink MR, van Waesberghe JH, van der Weide L et al. Total liver volume perfusion CT using 3D image fusion to improve detection and characterization of liver metastases. Eur Radiol. 2008;18:2345-54.
53. Perkins AC, Whalley DR, Ballantyne KC et al. Reliability of the hepatic perfusion index for the detection of liver metastases. Nucl Med Commun. 1987;8:982-9.
54. Schima W, Ba-Ssalamah A, Kölblinger C et al. Pancreatic adenocarcinoma. Eur Radiol. 2007;17:638-49.
55. Kandel S, Kloeters C, Meyer H et al. Whole organ perfusion of the pancreas using dynamic volume CT in patients with primary pancreas carcinoma: acquisition technique, post-processing and initial results. Eur Radiol. 2009 ;19:2641-6.
56. Takeda K, Mikami Y, Fukuyama S et al. Pancreatic ischemia associated with vasospasm in the early phase of human acute necrotizing pancreatitis. Pancreas. 2005;30:40-9.
57. Xu J, Liang Z, Hao S et al. Pancreatic adenocarcinoma: dynamic 64-slice helical CT with perfusion imaging. Abdom Imaging. 2009;34:759-66.
58. Lu N, Feng XY, Hao SJ et al. 64-slice CT perfusion imaging of pancreatic adenocarcinoma and mass-forming chronic pancreatitis. Acad Radiol. 2011;18:81-8.
59. Mirecka J, Libura J, Libura M et al. Morphological parameters of the angiogenic response in pancreatic ductal adenocarcinoma--correlation with histological grading and clinical data. Folia Histochem Cytobiol. 2001;39:335-40.
60. Von Dobschuetz E, Pahernik S, Hoffmann T et al. Dynamic intravital fluorescence microscopy—a novel method for the assessment of microvascular permeability in acute pancreatitis. Microvasc Res. 2004;67:55-63.
61. Park MS, Klotz E, Kim MJ et al. Perfusion CT: noninvasive surrogate marker for stratification of pancreatic cancer response to concurrent chemo and radiation therapy. Radiology. 2009;250:110-7.
62. d'Assignies G, Couvelard A, Bahrami S et al. Pancreatic endocrine tumors: tumor blood flow assessed with perfusion CT reflects angiogenesis and correlates with prognostic factors. Radiology. 2009;250:407-16.
63. Falconi M, Plöckinger U, Kwekkeboom DJ et al. Well differentiated pancreatic nonfunctioning tumors/ carcinoma. Neuroendocrinology. 2006;84:196-211.
64. Kambadakone AR, Sahani DV. Body perfusion CT: technique, clinical applications and advances. Radiol Clin North Am. 2009;47:161-78.
65. Li ZP, Meng QF, Sun CH et al. Tumor angiogenesis and dynamic CT in colorectal carcinoma: radiologic pathologic correlation. World J Gastroenterol. 2005;11:1287-91.
66. Takebayashi Y, Akiyama SI, Yamada K et al. Angiogenesis as an unfavorable prognostic factor in human colorectal carcinoma. Cancer. 1996;78:226-31.

67. Goh V, Bartram C, Halligan S. Effect of intravenous contrast agent volume on colorectal cancer vascular parameters as measured by perfusion computed tomography. Clin Radiol. 2009;64:368-72.
68. Willett CG, Boucher Y, Di Tomaso E et al. Direct evidence that the VEGF specific antibody bevacizumab has antivascular effects in human rectal cancer. Nat Med. 2004;10:145-7.
69. Bellomi M, Petralia G, Sonzogni A et al. CT perfusion for the monitoring of neoadjuvant chemotherapy and radiation therapy in rectal carcinoma: initial experience. Radiology. 2007;244:486-93.
70. Sahani DV, Kalva SP, Hamberg LM et al. Assessing tumor perfusion and treatment response in rectal cancer with multisection CT: initial observations. Radiology. 2005;234:785-92.
71. Goh V, Halligan S, Taylor SA et al. Differentiation between diverticulitis and colorectal cancer: quantitative CT perfusion measurements versus morphologic criteria—initial experience. Radiology. 2007;242:456-62.
72. Wu GY, Ghimire P. Perfusion computed tomography in colorectal cancer: protocols, clinical applications and emerging trends. World J Gastroenterol. 2009;15:3228-31.
73. Kerbel RS. Tumor angiogenesis. N Eng J Med. 2008;358:2039-49.
74. Goh V, Halligan S, Daley F et al. Colorectal tumor vascularity: quantitative assessment with multidetector CT—do tumor perfusion measurements reflect angiogenesis?. Radiology. 2008;249:510-7.
75. Ives EP, Burke MA, Edmonds PR et al. Quantitative computed tomography perfusion of prostate cancer: correlation with whole mount pathology. Clin Prostate Cancer. 2005;4:109-12.
76. Osimani M, Bellini D, Di Cristofano C et al. Perfusion MDCT of prostate cancer: correlation of perfusion CT parameters and immunohistochemical markers of angiogenesis. Am J Roentgenol. 2012 ;199:1042-8.
77. Harvey CJ, Blomley MJ, Dawson P et al. Functional CT imaging of the acute hyperemic response to radiation therapy of the prostate gland: early experience. J Comput Assist Tomogr. 2001;25:43-9.
78. Ruan J, Hajjar K, Rafii S et al. Angiogenesis and antiangiogenic therapy in non-Hodgkin's lymphoma. Ann Oncol. 2008;20:413-24.
79. Spira D, Adam P, Linder C et al. Perfusion and flow extraction product as potential discriminators in untreated Follicular and diffuse large B cell lymphomas using volume perfusion CT with attempt at histopathologic explanation. Am J Roentgenol. 2012;198:1239-46.
80. Nogai H, Dörken B, Lenz G. Pathogenesis of non-Hodgkin's lymphoma. J Clin Oncol. 2011;29:1803-11.
81. Jain R. Perfusion CT imaging of brain tumors: an overview. Am J Neuroradiol. 2011;32:1570-7.
82. Bai RJ, Han MJ, Wang LP et al. CT perfusion imaging in solitary pulmonary nodule. Chinese Journal of Medical Imaging Technology. 2004;6:019.
83. Tacelli N, Remy-Jardin M, Copin MC et al. Assessment of non-small cell lung cancer perfusion: pathologic CT correlation in 15 patients. Radiology. 2010;257:863-71.
84. Hegenscheid K, Behrendt N, Rosenberg C et al. Assessing early vascular changes and treatment response after laser-induced thermotherapy of pulmonary metastases with perfusion CT: initial experience. Am J Roentgenol. 2010;194:1116-23.
85. Tsushima Y. Functional CT of the kidney. Eur J Radiol. 1999;30:191-7.
86. Beers BE, Leconte I, Materne R et al. Hepatic perfusion parameters in chronic liver disease: dynamic CT measurements correlated with disease severity. Am J Roentgenol. 2001 ;176:667-73.
87. Bize PE, Platon A, Becker CD et al. Perfusion measurement in acute pancreatitis using dynamic perfusion MDCT. Am J Roentgenol. 2006;186:114-8.

CHAPTER 44

Magnetic Resonance Instrumentation: An Update

Anjali Prakash

INTRODUCTION

A magnetic resonance (MR) image represents the relative response of specific nuclei to absorbed radiofrequency energy. The Dutch physicist CJ Gorter[1] first proposed the NMR concept in 1936, which was furthered by the work of Block and Purcell. They were awarded the Nobel Prize for Physics in 1952. Between 1950s and 60s, it was used primarily as an analytical tool for chemists and physicists to determine the chemical structure, configuration and reactive processes. Modern clinical use started after Paul Lauterbur's[2] suggestion in 1973, that operator controlled magnetic field gradients could be used to encode position dependent information in the NMR signal. Magnetic resonance imaging (MRI) has been selected along with computed tomography (CT) as example of the benefits to society of basic research in physics. In 2003, Paul Lauterbur and Sir Peter Mansfield received the Nobel Prize in medicine for their discoveries concerning magnetic resonance imaging.

The main constituents of an MRI scanner is the **magnet subsystem** which produces a spatial and temporally constant magnetic field B_0, the **gradient subsystem** to produce varying magnetic field gradients for spatial encoding, **RF subsystem** to transmit and receive radiofrequency B_1 and the **computer and microprocessors** to specify and control the pulse sequence calculate, process, display, store and transfer the resultant clinical image. This includes an acquisition and control system, reconstruction system. There is viewing console for operator input of control parameters and display of imaging. In addition, magnetic and RF shielding is required. Patient table, hardware for physiological monitoring of patient (ECG and respiratory gating) and monitoring equipment is also needed **(Figs. 1 and 2)**.[3]

During imaging, patient is placed on the MRI table which brings the patient into strong magnetic field, such that the anatomy to be imaged is in the region of maximum uniformity of the field—isocenter. The B_0 field lines are aligned along the longest body axis—Z-axis. The other two short axes are X and Y-axis. A required scan is selected; the selected information is passed on to the gradient pulse generator that adjusts the amplitude and waveform of the three gradients. The gradient amplifier then increases the power required to drive the gradient coils to generate the gradient field strength required. RF transmission also starts with the host computer which sets the required B_1 field frequency on the frequency synthesizer. Using an amplitude modulator, the carrier frequency is modulated into apodisced fine pulses. The RF amplifier increases the power of the pulse from milliwatts to kilowatts, which is used to drive the RF transmit coil. The signal from the body is acquired with an RF receive coil which induces in it an alternating voltage of a few microvolts. After amplification by an RF amplifier (receiver), tuned to the resonant frequency, the amplitude or envelope of this signal is sampled, digitized and computer analyzed.

THE MAGNET

The magnet is the key component of the MR scanner. It determines the appearance, cost and capacity of the

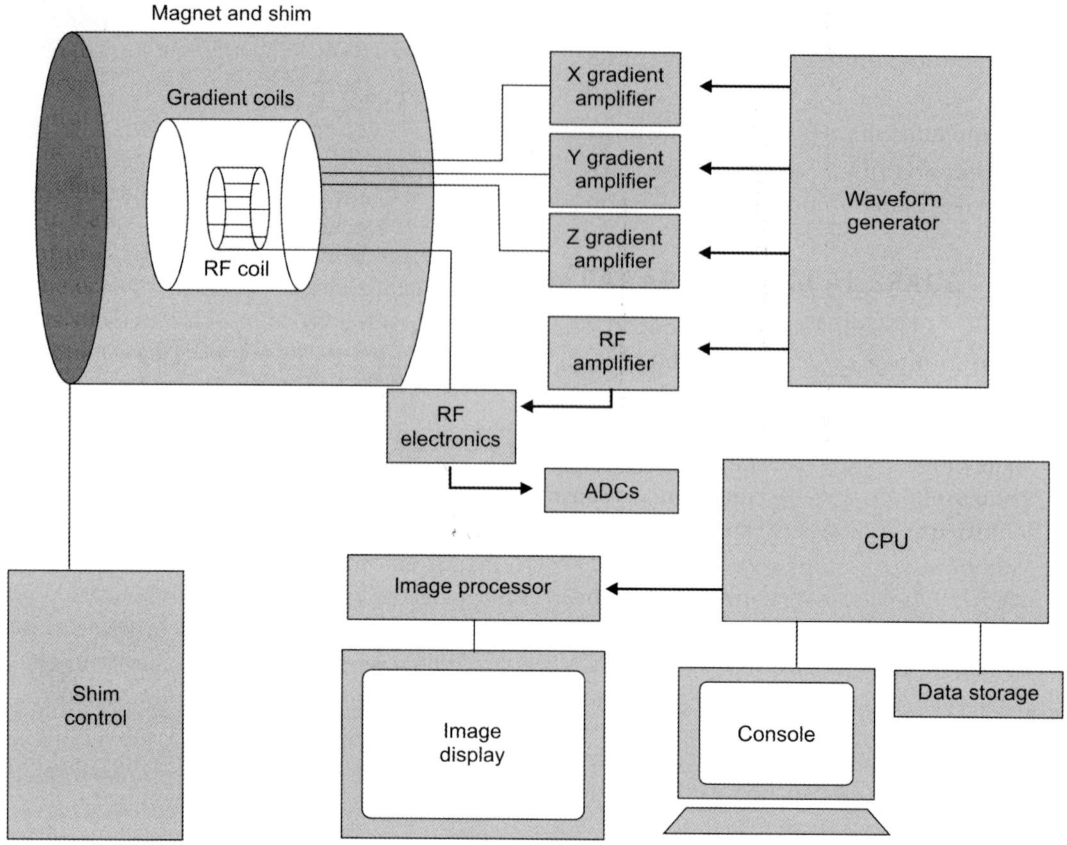

Fig. 1: Various hardware components of MRI scanner.

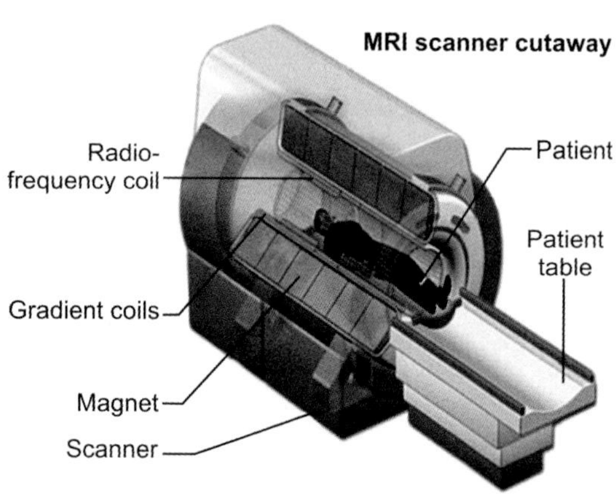

Fig. 2: Magnetic resonance imaging scanner indicating position of various coils.

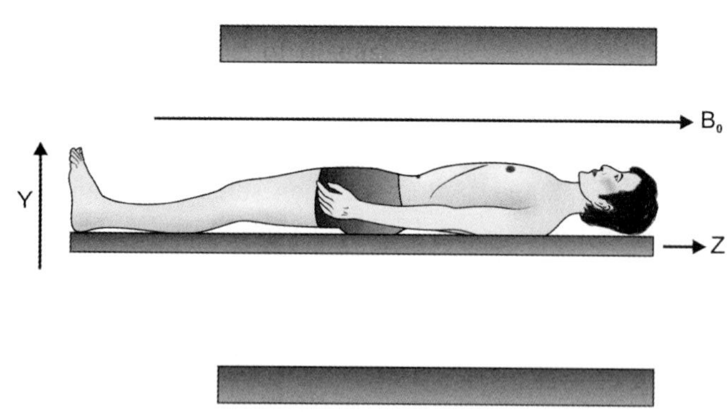

Fig. 3: Schematic depiction of the Z-axis along the main magnetic field B_0.

device. The **strength of the magnet** is measured in tesla (T), research systems with a magnetic strength of 9.4 T[4] are available for use in humans. There are three types of magnets used in MRI—permanent magnets, resistive magnets and superconducting magnets.

The main magnetic field needs to be very **uniform or homogeneous** in terms of its strength and direction unaffected by ambient temperature. It defines a direction in space that is conventionally referred to as Z-direction. The Z-component of the main field at the center of the magnet is designated as B_0, Z-axis usually runs along the cylindrical axis of the main magnet and in the direction from the patients head to feet **(Fig. 3)**. Any variation of this longitudinal field Bz from its central value B_0 has a

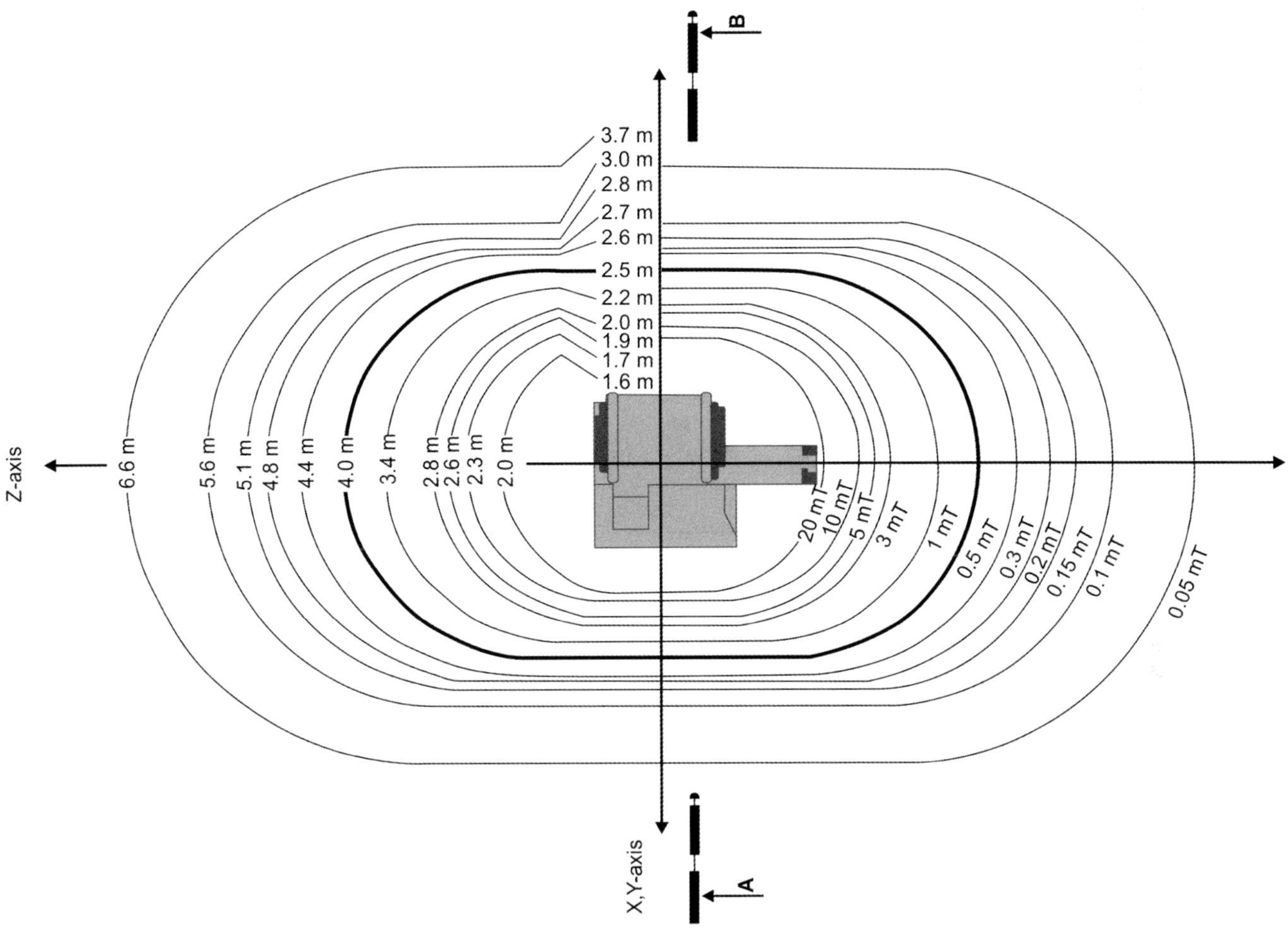

Fig. 4: Fringe field around the MR scanner. The 0.5 mT (5 Gauss) line is marked in bold.

significant effect on motions of spin system. Consequently, the design of the main field coils is chosen to minimize variations in the strength of the B_0 field over the desired region of imaging. The straightness of magnetic lines within the center needs to be perfect. Within a specified region called **diameter spherical volume (DSV)** the field is uniform with a typical magnetic flux variation of 5 ppm for imaging and 1 ppm for spectroscopy. A main magnet with DSV positioned at **magnet isocenter** is called a symmetric magnet. In an asymmetric (open-bore) magnet, DSV is shifted a certain distance away from the isocenter towards one end of the magnet. The magnet should have a bore size large enough to accommodate the patient. Open-bore magnet allows better patient access and helps claustrophobic patients.

The magnetic field lines form closed loops and crowd together within a solenoid but spread widely outside it as **'fringe' field**. This effect is reduced by an iron shroud weighing many tonnes or by additional shimming coils. The fringe fields are negligible in a permanent magnet, being concentrated in the iron yoke. Patients with pacemakers need to be kept away from areas where stray fields are greater than 0.5 mT (5 Gauss line). This defines the controlled area for safety purposes around MRI installations. Siting of the machine should be done away from steel girders and reinforced concrete, which may become manifested in the fringe field **(Fig. 4)**.

Permanent magnet: It consists of two opposing flat faced magnetized pole pieces fixed to an iron frame. The materials used are iron and alloys of aluminum, nickel and cobalt. Once magnetized, these maintain magnetization indefinitely without power input. Permanent magnets require no power input and cannot be shut down. They provide low strength (0.3 T or less), vertical fields.

Permanent magnets are very heavy up to 80–100 tonnes. Running costs are relatively less. Permanent magnet systems are used for claustrophobic patients, children, obese adults and interventional procedures. These are constructed as open access configuration unlike solenoid magnets.

A newer magnetic alloy of iron neodymium and boron has been described which are of lower weight, with higher strength. Other materials used are metallic alloy alnico, ceramic barium ferrite and rare earth alloy samarium cobalt ($SmCO_3$).[5]

Resistive magnet: This is a set of DC coils with copper or aluminum conductors, in which the magnetic field is generated by passage of electric current through a wire. It requires 50–100 KW of stable power supply to produce a homogeneous magnetic field. The heat produced is removed by cooling water pumped rapidly through the hollow coils. The vertical or horizontal magnetic field is limited by heating to 0.5 T and has significant fringe fields. It can be switched off at the end of day or in an emergency setting. It takes 15–30 minutes to reestablish the magnetic field. It is cheapest and smallest, weighing only 2 tonnes. Resistive magnets have a limited role, these days.

Hybrid magnets: Combine feature of more than one basic type. Magnet may include both a set of permanent magnet and a set of electric coils to achieve a stronger magnetic field.

PREPOLARIZED MRI

In 2001, a research team at Stanford University invented a new technique called prepolarized MRI/PMRI.[6] They demonstrated that two magnets can be used together, one strong, but not very uniform and the other very homogeneous, but not so strong. The magnet that is strong produces a strong magnetic field which varies in uniformity by as much as 40%. A second magnet produces a more precise magnetic field. These magnets can be ordinary copper wound magnets, lowering cost. As the magnetic field is "tuned" by the second magnet, a PMRI scan can be obtained adjacent to a metal implant.

Superconducting Magnet

Superconductivity is a property of materials, such that they lose electrical resistance at very low temperatures. Examples of such materials are some metals (Hg) and alloys—niobium/titanium, niobium/tin and vanadium/gallium. It takes many hours for the superconducting state to be reached and the current to build up. Then the coil is short-circuited and power source switched off. Once energized, the current continues in a loop as long as superconducting temperature is maintained. The current continues to flow, while using no power like permanent magnets, they require no external power source once it is energized.

A superconductive electromagnet is a DC solenoid about 1 m in diameter, commonly made of niobium–titanium alloy in a copper matrix **(Fig. 5)**. This becomes superconducting at 10° Kelvin and the magnet is operated at temperature maintained by a cryogen-liquid helium at 4°K (-269°C/-452°F). The length of the superconducting wire in the magnet is several miles long; this length of the wire has to be constructed without interruption of its superconducting properties. The magnet is immersed in a liquid-helium vessel called the cryostat—Dewar (at 4.2 K with ~1700 L of liquid helium) which is surrounded by liquid nitrogen at 77.4 K. This creates a temperature gradient from the magnet core to the surrounding room to minimize thermal energy losses and stabilizes the internal core temperature. The expensive liquid helium is replenished periodically as the cryogens boil off due to heat leaks. The coldhead is used for minimizing the helium boil-off and to recondense some helium vapor back into the liquid bath. The heat which reaches the cryo shields of the magnet is absorbed and passed via the coldhead to an external heat exchanger which is part of the refrigerator system. A rhythmical thud that is heard in the system while it is not acquiring images is due to the operation of helium refrigeration pump **(Fig. 6)**. The coldhead must be in permanent operation.

In newer designs, the liquid nitrogen has been replaced by a cryogenic refrigerator with the cooling lines going to the cold head in the liquid helium. This eliminates the need

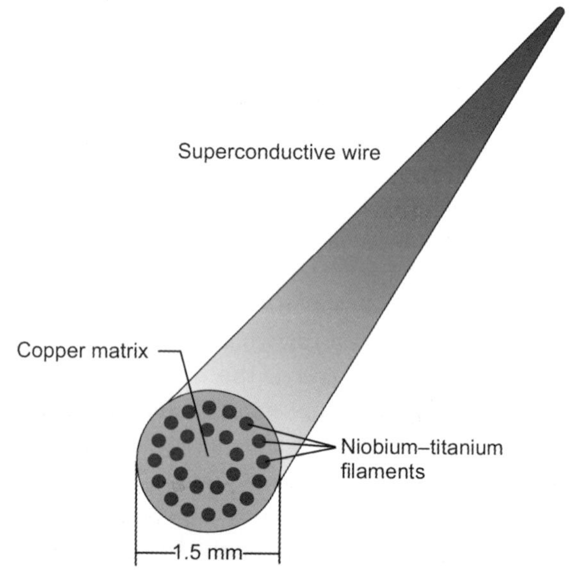

Fig. 5: Cut section of a superconductive wire made of Niobium-titanium alloy imbedded in copper matrix.

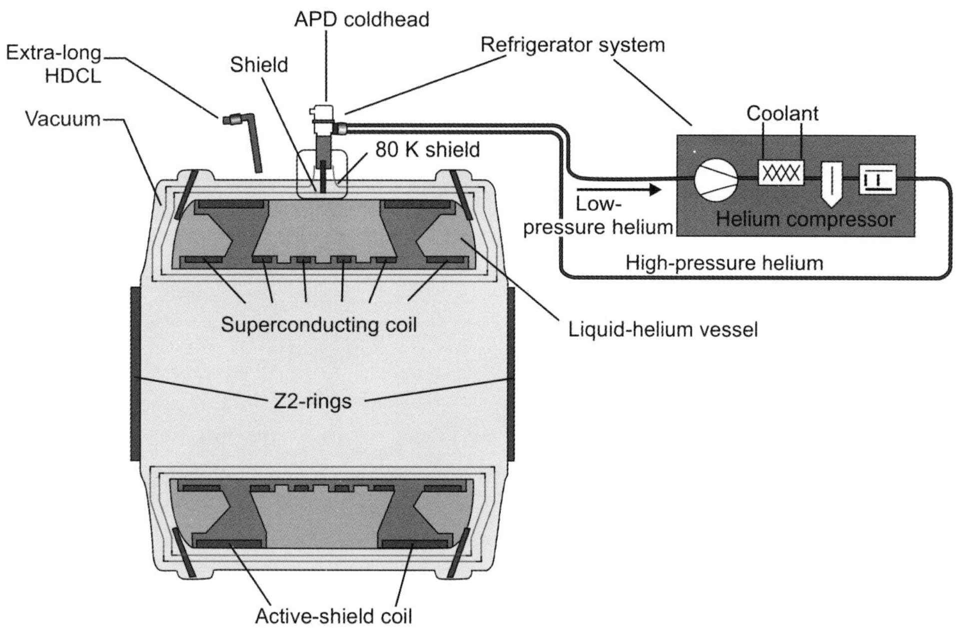

Fig. 6: The magnet assembly in a superconducting magnet is seated into an all welded stainless steel vessel filled with liquid helium.

to add liquid nitrogen and increases the hold time of liquid helium.[3,7-9]

The machine is correspondingly large and expensive. It has a tunnel configuration, which makes it claustrophobic to patients'. Typical performance specifications include a spatially uniform field, at the magnet center to be better than 10 ppm over a sphere of 40 cm and drift of the field to be less than 0.1 ppm. Ultralight magnet (magnet weight 6 tons) have been designed with nearly zero helium boil-off.

Quench

The magnet has to be kept at a temperature below the critical/transition temperature. If a small region of wire is heated to temperature above this, it begins to dissipate heat and there is increase in temperature. This leads to a process called quench wherein the stored energy in the magnetic field is converted into heat. This raises the temperature of the liquid helium above its boiling point and magnetic field collapses. Magnets sense the onset of a quench and activate heaters that spread energy deposition throughout the coils. If this were not to happen, deposition of energy at a point could melt wire locally and destroy it.[7,8]

After a quench, magnet itself is rarely damaged and may be recooled and energized. To minimize possibility of quench due to frictional heating, magnet is 'trained' at the time of manufacture by cycling magnetic fields above the planned level of operation. Quenches are also possible if the cryostat vacuum fails or cryogenic fluid is not refilled in time. The coolant level is hence logged daily.

Superconducting magnets are supplied with an emergency switch system that permits a deliberate quench in case of an emergency, like a person being trapped against or inside the magnet by a ferromagnetic object. The field decreases from initial value to nearly zero in one minute.

In a controlled quench, safety aspects need to be considered as helium gas is very cold and contact should be avoided. External venting channels should be clear. Helium may displace room oxygen and harm people.

MAGNET GEOMETRY

Tunnel systems: These have a tunnel bore with horizontal magnet field, best magnetic field homogeneity and are seen only with superconducting systems.

Wide-bore designs have superior homogeneity for large FOVs, while short-bore magnets provide relief from claustrophobia **(Fig. 7)**.

Open systems have a vertical magnetic field; can be permanent or superconducting magnet **(Fig. 8)**.

Specialty magnets are specially designed for a particular type of examination usually for musculoskeletal applications. These have a superconducting/resistive magnet. 70 Mt/m of power and a slew rate of 300 T/m is the available gradient strength with one vendor.[10] Dedicated RF coils (80–180 mm in diameter) are available for a range of anatomies. There is a chair/recliner so that the patient is seated comfortably **(Fig. 9)**.

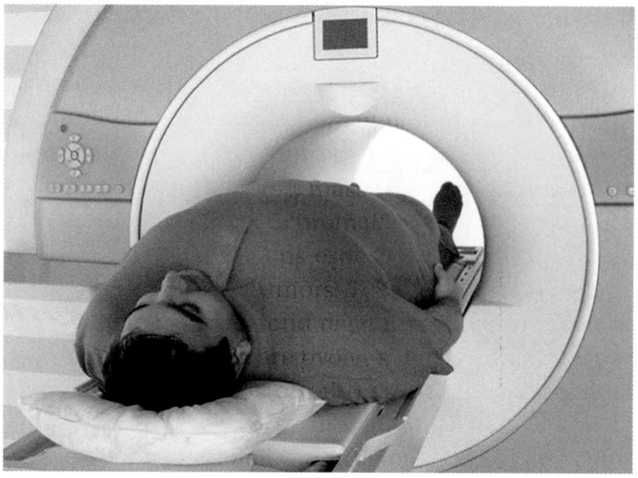

Fig. 7: Wide-bore (70 cm) tunnel magnet.

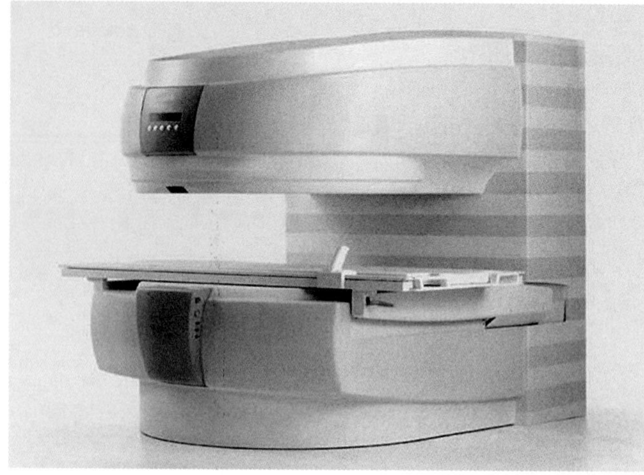

Fig. 8: Open low-field MRI with a permanent magnet.

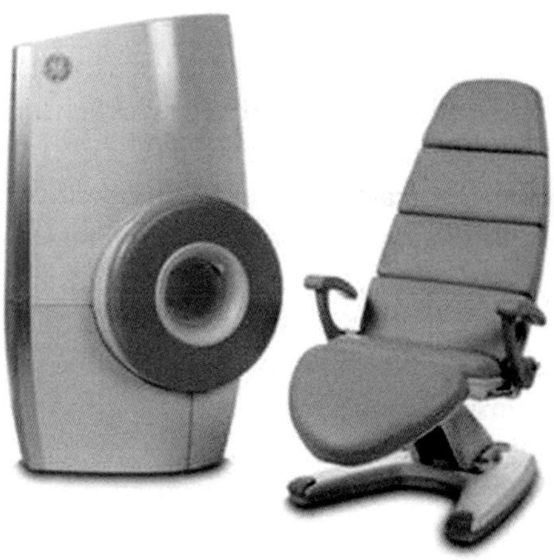

Fig. 9: Specialty magnet system used in musculoskeletal imaging.

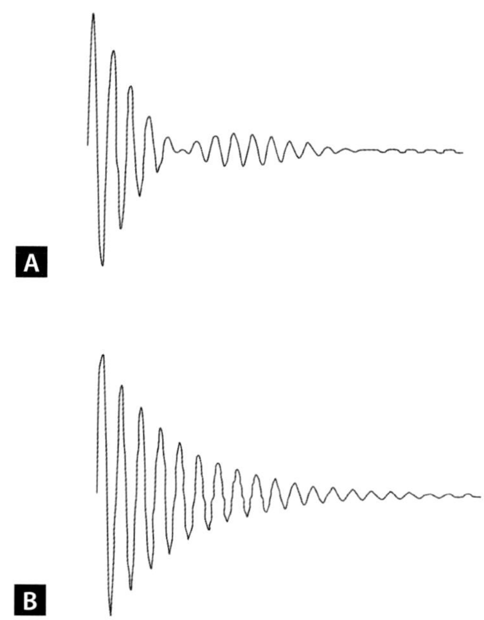

Figs. 10A and B: FID signal from a poorly shimmed sample (A) showing a complex decay envelope, while an exponentially decaying amplitude (B) indicates proper shim.

Shim Coils

The magnetic field must be stable and not affected by temperature. The homogeneity of a magnet is specified as the maximum deviation of the field in points per million (ppm) over a spherical volume of a given diameter (dsv). The uniformity should be in the range of 5 ppm.

Imperfections in manufacturing of the coils lead to harmonic error field. The process of 'shimming' is required to overcome these errors.

Two methods are available for shimming:

Passive shimming: It is achieved by placing small permanent magnets at strategic locations at time of installation within the bore of the magnet to counteract field in homogeneities.

Active shimming: A set of coils is used and current is passed through these 'shim coils'. This generates small magnetic fields gradients superimposed on the main magnetic field and remove the field nonuniformities. Field homogeneity is measured by examining an FID signal in the absence of field gradients. The FID from a poorly shimmed sample shows a complex decay envelope with many humps. Shim currents are adjusted to provide a large amplitude exponentially decaying FID indicating a homogeneous B_0 field **(Figs. 10A and B)**. Active shimming is computer optimized for each imaging volume.

The shim coils can be superconducting and located within the cryostat and maintained at low temperature.

Shim coils can also be a set of resistive shim coils, when they are placed in the room temperature bore of the magnet.

3 TESLA AND HIGHER-MAGNET STRENGTHS

Superconducting magnets operating at 1.5 T have been the standard, though in recent years 3 T systems have gained prominence. Research systems of 7 T/9.4 T have been installed at a few sites; whereas individual prototypes of higher strength have been introduced. There are many advantages and challenges with the higher-strength magnets.

The signal to noise ratio SNR is $\infty B_1.\sqrt{NEx}.Np/BW$, where B_1 is field strength, NEx is the number of excitations, Np is the number of phase encoding lines and BW is the receiver bandwidth. The SNR at 3 Tesla should be double to that at 1.5 T, however, in practice is slightly less than double.[11] Larger MR signal and improved SNR produce excellent images and many special applications like functional, diffusion weighted imaging and multinuclear spectroscopy are now possible.

The drawback of a higher field is increased T_1, necessitating a longer TR and longer imaging time. Chemical shift artifacts are increased at higher field strengths. It is harder to make the static magnetic field uniform. Inhomogenities in the magnetic field reduce T_2*, producing focal loss of signal at air soft tissue interfaces, near metallic clips. This susceptibility artifacts increases at 3 T. The artifact can be used to increase detection of hemorrhage, free intraperitoneal air-susceptibility weighted imaging. A higher magnetic field increases the specific absorption rate SAR-energy deposited by RF field. SAR is four times higher at 1.5 T. Use of parallel imaging decrease SAR, while maintaining SNR. Another artifact that can be seen at 3 T is Dielectric shading.[11,12] This is nonuniform RF distribution to the body caused by the fact that waves cannot uniformly penetrate the body due to tissue conductivity and shielding effects. This is more pronounced at 3.0 T since the RF wavelength at 3 T (~25 cm) approaches the size of the body. The effects of dielectric shading are manifested in MRI images as areas with different contrast and uniformity. A common method of compensating general image nonuniformity in conventional high-field imaging systems is to use a postprocessing normalization filter that derives an intensity correction function directly from the final image. These so-called "Bias Field Correction (BiFiC)" image filters[13] can produce a uniform image appearance.

Gradient System

Gradient coils spatially encode the position of protons by varying the magnetic field linearly across the imaging volume. The Larmor frequency will then vary as a function of position in the X, Y, Z-axis. The magnetic field gradient in the X, Y and Z directions required for an imaging study are produced by three sets of orthogonally positioned coils **(Fig. 11)**. The slice selection gradient and RF pulse define a slice, a second magnetic field gradient applied orthogonally to the slice selection gradient serves as a readout gradient or frequency encoding gradient. By repeated rotation and application of the readout gradient, spatial information in more than one direction can be obtained. A third gradient—the phase encoding gradient completes the spatial encoding of spins.

Each of the three sets of gradient coil has separate power supply and independent computer control which alter the slope of the magnetic field. These are switched off and on frequently to allow slice selection, frequency and phase encoding. All three coils are wound on a cylinder and situated in the warm bore of the magnet. These coils are connected to **gradient amplifiers** that control the rise time and maximum value of the gradients. The direction of the current (DC) passed through the coil determines the increase or decrease in the field strength relative to the center. Each gradient individually produces a field in a specific direction; a gradient field in any chosen direction can be generated by activating two or all three of the gradient coils. This makes it possible to select imaging planes in any of the directions.

Gradients are resistive electromagnets consisting of metallic coils driven by power amplifiers. Gradient coil wires are usually made of copper and are circular or rectangular in cross-section with a diameter of

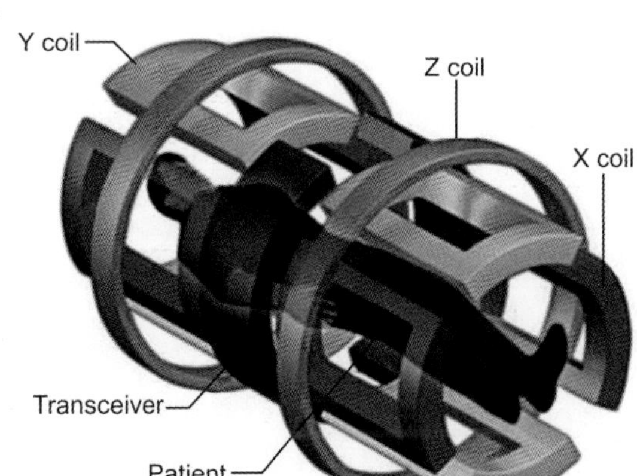

Fig. 11: Gradient magnets in the X, Y and Z direction.

~5 mm **(Figs. 12A and B)**. A **Maxwell coil** produces linear variation in field along Z-axis, in other axes it is done using a **Saddle–Golay coil**. The current necessary to generate a typical gradient field of ~40 mT/m is of the order of few hundred amperes. The peak power is an important design criterion of the gradient amplifier.

The slice select or Z-axis gradient field is switched on during the application of RF pulse. The steeper the gradient, thinner the slice. In the time of a few milliseconds, when MR signal is being received, current is passed through another set of gradient coils -XX coils. This alters the magnetic field gradient from side to side in the X direction. This is for frequency encoding, a steeper gradient is used for a smaller FOV.

The third set of coils (YY) coils for phase encoding are energized, immediately after the 90° pulse, but before it is inverted by the 180° pulse. This produces a gradient from front to back of the patient. Steeper gradients are required for finer phase matrices.

The maximum gradient amplitude that can be generated (in millitesla per meter) has a direct impact on the minimum slice thickness and FOV and thereby of the maximum spatial resolution that is available. The current in these coils are rapidly switched on and off (on a millisecond time scale between various levels). The time required to switch between two current levels or **slew rate** (time, rate of change of gradient length in T/m/s) is an important technical specification of the scanner capability. This sets the limit to the minimum TR and TE values that can be achieved and consequently the minimum acquisition time. A slew rate of a gradient system (in tesla per meters per second) is defined as the ratio of gradient strength divided by rise time. Slew rate depends on both the gradient coil (it takes more time to ramp up/down a large coil than a small coil) and on the performance of the gradient amplifier (it takes a lot of voltage to overcome the inductance of the coil) with significant influence on image quality. Slew rates up to 100–200T/m/sec while gradient strengths up to 40–50 mT/m is now available.

Another factor is **linearity of the gradient**. If the gradient falls off nonlinearly on either side of the magnet isocenter, then the image will be distorted at edges of FOV. Gradient performance is measured in **amplitude** (in millitesla per meter, mT/m) and **rise time** (in μ seconds).

Scan speed is dependent on the performance of the gradient system. Stronger gradients allow faster imaging and higher resolution. Applications, such as MR angiography, cardiac MR and diffusion tensor imaging require high- amplitude gradients (>20 mT/m) with a fast slew rate. Fast switching gradients can lead to induction of **eddy currents** due to the changing magnetic fields produced. These degrade imaging sequences by producing geometric distortion, blurred images and artifacts like ghosting **(Fig. 13)**. To overcome this, shielding of gradient coils is done, where a second coil surrounds the primary gradient coil and carries current in the opposite direction. These cancel the eddy currents but also reduce the overall strength of the gradient fields. These actively shielded gradients are increasingly used as rapid scan imaging protocols based on gradient echoes gained prominence.

Specialized gradient coils are being developed for a variety of clinical applications. In echoplanar imaging, the requirements of gradient strengths, rise times and

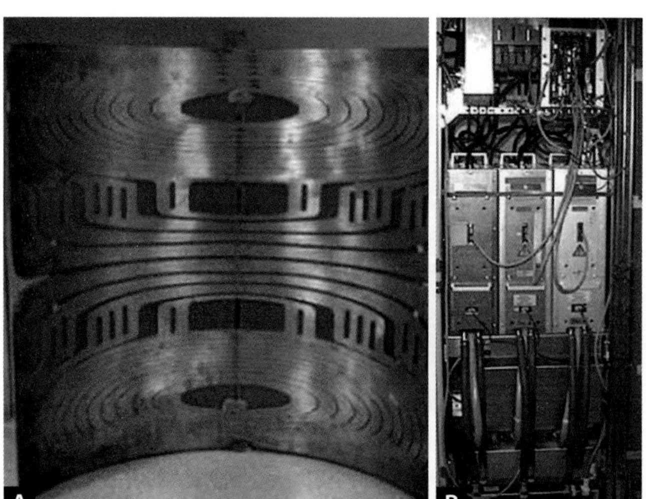

Figs. 12A and B: (A) Gradient coil; (B) Gradient amplifier.

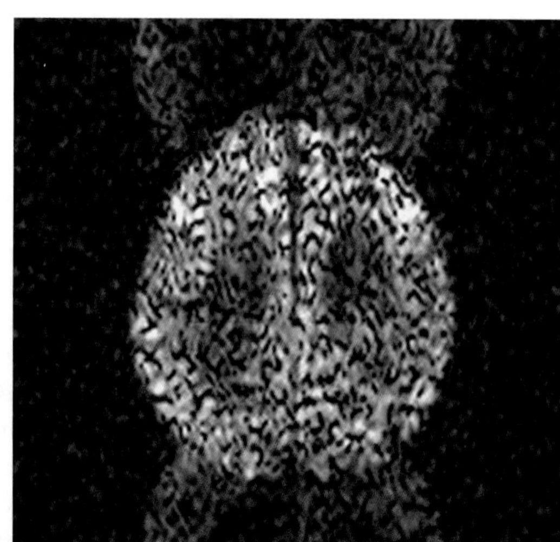

Fig. 13: *Eddy current* artifact—inhomogeneities in the gradient cause distortion in the image.

duty cycle have been increased as all the space is to be traversed in a single excitation. This requires each phase encoding projection to be acquired in less than 0.8 ms. Gradient coils required would have a maximum amplitude of 20 mT/m, minimum rise time of 0.1 ms (slew rate 200 T/m/s) and a duty cycle of 50–60%. This requires matching of gradient to power supplies that are capable of responding to the resonant mode at maximum amplitude and holding it at that level for a short period of time. Dual gradients' have been developed wherein there is a short, higher-performance central region provided by one of the segments of the gradient tube and another mode of operation with the standard full region gradient. Specifically, in head imaging a physically smaller gradient tube can be used which combines improved gradient performance with satisfactory physical stimulation.[14]

At time of switching interval, the resulting force on the gradient coils is longer, producing a loud bang. **Acoustic noise** is the signature complaint of most patients about MRI. As gradient strength is increasing, so is the noise. Improvements in mounting techniques, use of damping materials and advances in materials used, placing the gradient tube in a vacuum have all been used to decrease the acoustic noise.

One drawback of powerful gradients is **peripheral nerve stimulation**. There are standards that limit stimulation based on duration of the stimulus and the rate at which the magnetic field changes (db/dt). The shorter the stimulus the faster the magnetic field has to change to cause the stimulus. To decrease db/dt, gradient can be made shorter.

Powerful gradient amplifiers are sited in a room with restricted access adjacent to the magnet room.

Radiofrequency System

Radiofrequency system is required to transmit and receive signals at or near the Larmor frequency of the precessing spins. The frequency of the RF coil is defined by the Larmor equation. The Larmor frequency of protons being 63.8 MHz at 1.5 Tesla. MRI uses a Fourier transformation technique. This utilizes a brief burst of RF energy (lasting a few milliseconds) from a RF transmitter to excite the spins, followed by detection of the FID (free induction decay) signal that lasts 10–1000 ms. RF field B_1 is two vectors rotating in opposite directions in a plane transverse to B_0. At the Larmor frequency the vector rotating in the same direction as the precessing spins will interact strongly with the spins. RF coils work efficiently when physically aligned to receive signal that originate perpendicular to the main magnetic field B_0.

The RF subsystem consists of a **transmitter**, a **receiver coils**. The RF transmission system consists of RF synthesizer; amplifier and transmitter coil (usually built into the body of the scanner). RF transmitter generates a temporally stable basic frequency for the RF, delivers an appropriate waveform to amplifier which delivers an RF pulse of shape and flip angle to the coil and time the deliver of the pulses. This can be achieved by analog or digital process. The transmitter must display linearity, i.e. the output of the power amplifier should be directly proportional to the input power. This is achieved by a process called as envelope feedback. RF amplifier converts a low-level RF demand signal to a high-power level. RF source is combination of independent input signal and amplifiers. **RF coil** is a combination of coil elements arranged to produce an advantageous B_1 field distribution. **RF channel** denotes the number of connections to the RF coil. **Coil element** is an arrangement of electrical conductors for converting an electrical current into magnetic field.

RF receiver subsystem: The RF receiver consists of the coil, preamplifier and signal processing system.

The primary role of the receiver in an MRI scanner is to convert the analog coil signals into digital format. The design of a modern digital receiver is based on an analog-to-digital converter (ADC), which samples the analog MRI signal and converts it into digital format. Important characteristics of the ADC are its conversion bandwidth and resolution. The conversion bandwidth equals half the digitization rate. State-of-the-art ADCs allow conversion bandwidth of over 50 MHz at 14 bit resolution. Since frequencies are generally well above 50 MHz, usually an alias of the MRI signal is detected.

Prior to input into the ADC, the MRI scanners signal needs to be amplified and filtered. Amplification serves to match the voltage range of the MRI signal to the input range of the ADC, in order to engage its full dynamic range. Analog filtering serves to reduce noise and interference signals that alias into the ADC conversion band from outside the target band around the MRI scanner Larmor frequency. In addition, depending on Larmor frequency, down conversion might be required to bring the signal frequency to within the input band of the ADC. The choice of ADC digitization rate is to some extent dependent on the master clock of the MRI scanner exciter. To avoid phase errors between excitation and reception, the digitization clock of the ADC needs to be synchronized to the clock of the MRI scanner exciter frequency that is a multiple of the exciter clock. In addition, it is beneficial to avoid digitization frequencies that put the Larmor alias at around 0 Hz. After digitization, digital down-sampling is performed to reduce the amount of data. The output bandwidth and center frequency can be adjusted to match those of the MRI scanner signal bandwidth and (aliased) center frequency. An added advantage of down-sampling is the increase in dynamic range, which amounts to 1 bit for every factor of 4 of down-sampling.

RF coils can be **transmit and receive** or **transmit only/ receive only coils**. Receive only and transmit only coils must be electronically isolated. This means that when the transmitter is on, the receiver is open circuited to prevent the transmitting power from entering the receiving chain. During signal reception, the transmitting coil is open circuited to prevent mutual coupling. When the power amplifier is not active, its output is disconnected to avoid the output noise from interfering with the sensitive signal that is being received.

A wide range of RF coil designs are available in MRI. Ongoing developments in the RF system are one of the most profound changes in MRI system development. There are many types and geometries of the coil.

RF coils are classified into two types—**volume** and **surface coils**. Volume coils surround the imaged object and provide homogeneous transmission and reception over a large anatomic region. These are both transmit and receive coils (transcieve). Head and body coils are referred as volume coils **(Fig. 14)**. As the noise is nonlinearly proportional to the volume of tissue being imaged; the SNR of these is lower than the surface coils. Body coils are constructed on cylindrical coil forms—diameter of 50–60 cm and a length of 70–80 cm. These are large enough to surround the patient's chest and abdomen. Head coils are smaller, 40 cm long and 28 cm in diameter.

Surface coils are usually receiving coils with a limited area of sensitivity from which they receive signal. Surface coils fit closely over specific anatomic region. The sensitivity of the coil is related to the radius of the coil. As the coil size is increased, noise will also increase. These include circular coil configuration for orbits and TM joints, rectangular coils for lumbar spine or irregular shapes for shoulder, cervical spine. Surface coils are advantageous as they increase the SNR; however, the sensitivity is not uniform over its field of view. These need to be positioned carefully. Surface coils can be rigid or flexible in design. Flexible coils can be closely applied to the contour of the body, are more comfortable and however, are less durable due to higher wear and tear **(Fig. 15)**.

A large coil (body coil) is used as a transmitter and a smaller surface coil as a receiver combining the advantage of uniform excitation of a large coil and increased SNR of a smaller coil. However, if two separate coils are used, they need to be tuned to the same frequency. Coil decoupling is necessary to prevent current in one coil to excite current in the other.

For a solenoidal magnet the transmitter and receiver coils are **saddle shaped** and have the volume of the greatest B_1 field homogeneity along the linear portion of the coil, the ends being inhomogeneous **(Fig. 16)**. An alternate design called a **bird cage coil or resonator** has improved B_1 homogeneity and has higher sensitivity. These are volume coils consisting of two circular or elliptical conducting end rings joined by conducting

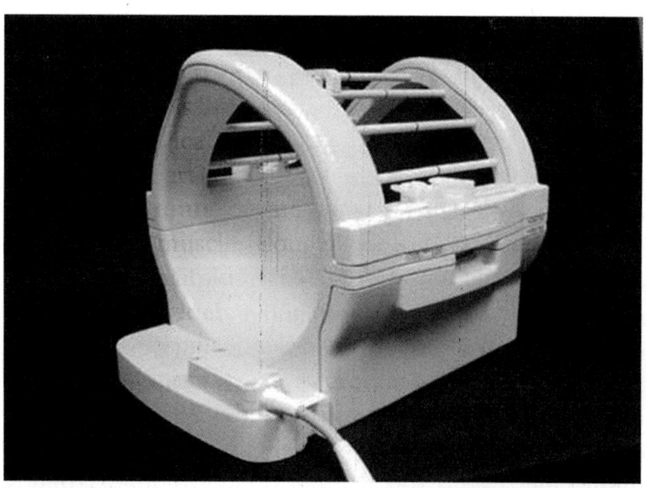

Fig. 14: Circularly polarized head coil, volume coil—both transmit and receive.

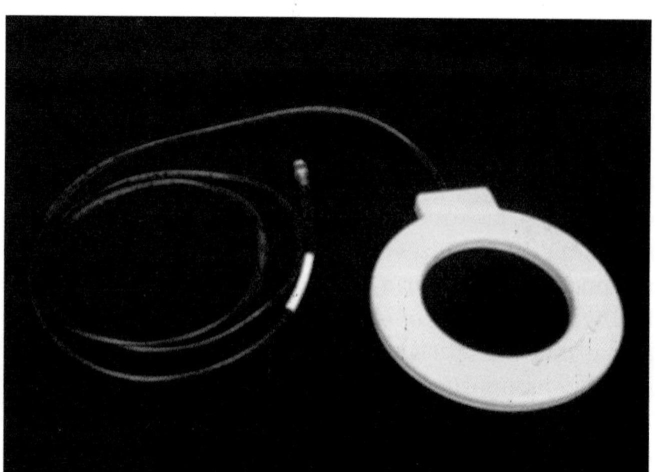

Fig. 15: Surface loop coil—receive only.

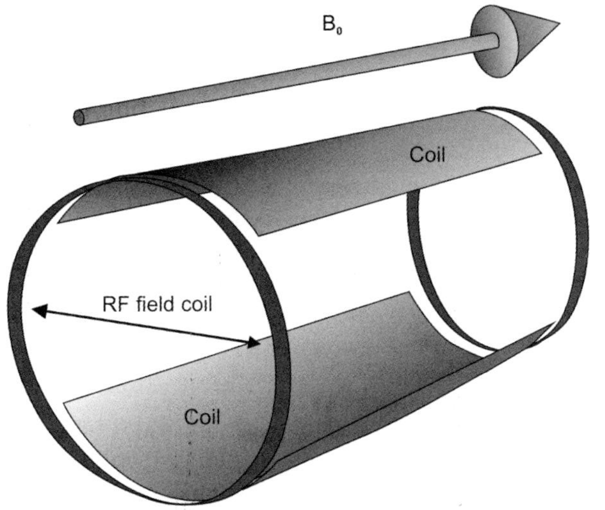

Fig. 16: Linearly polarized body coil comprising flat conductors configured in a hollow tube.

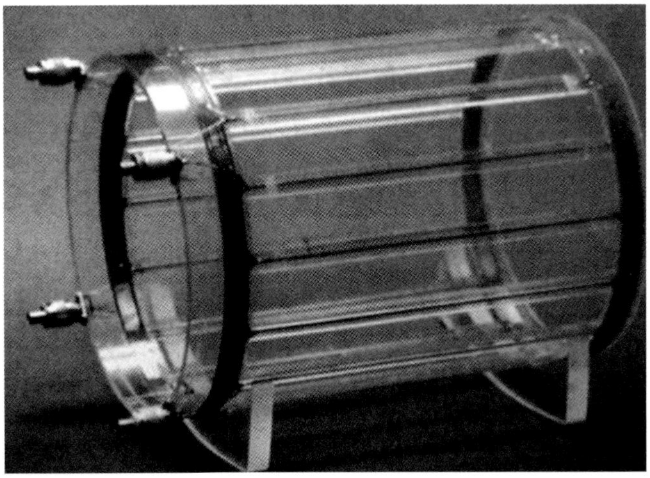

Fig. 17: Bird cage resonator.

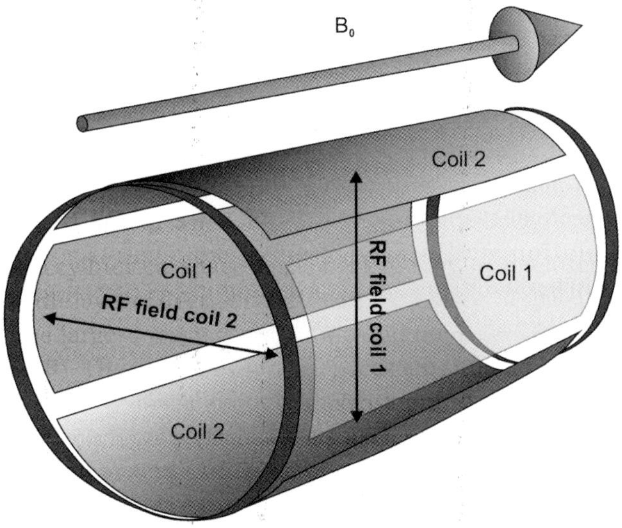

Fig. 18: Design of a circularly polarized body coil showing 2 RF fields with a phase shift.

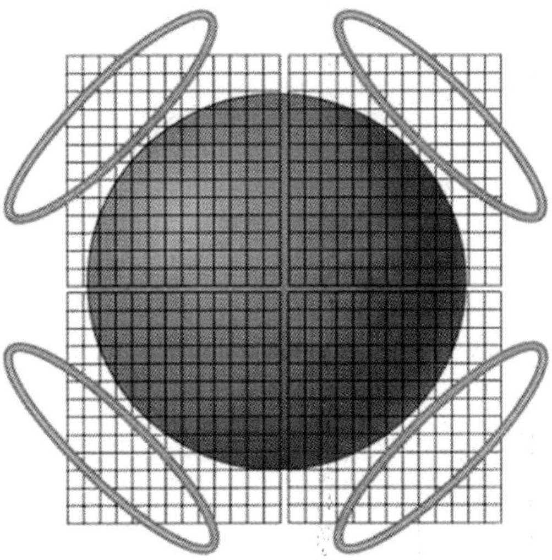

Fig. 19: Phased array coil—multiple coil elements, increasing SNR and FOV.

rings or legs **(Fig. 17)**. A common version uses 16 loops to span the cylinder. These coils provide a uniform RF field. **Quadrature reception** is applied with volume coils to improve SNR. Two pairs of coils (phase sensitive detectors) are used to detect signal that are out of phase. The signal of the two is combined to form a final image. A coil operating in this manner is called **"circularly polarized" (Fig. 18)**. This increases SNR by a factor of $\sqrt{2}$. It requires only half the power to generate; therefore less power is deposited in tissues. A circularly polarized birdcage resonator is called a quadrature coil and is the most frequently used RF coils in MRI today. Whole body sized birdcage coils are available. A related form of multimode resonator, referred to as TEM (transverse electromagnetic) resonator is also useful for head and neck imaging at higher field strengths. These are fitted just inside the gradient coil set. RF transmitting coils are also shielded to minimize power losses.[15-17]

Phased array coils: Arrays of surface coil are used to extend the effective FOV of the receiver coil while maintaining the improved SNR characteristics of a limited FOV of a single coil **(Fig. 19)**. The coils in array can be activated remotely as single receivers and cover a limited FOV in the region of interest. There is also another method where each coil in the phased array has a separate receiver channel. The signal is collected from all coils in the array simultaneously, data combined to give an image of a complete FOV, with a SNR equivalent to a single coil. As number of receiver channels increase, so does the cost.

The coils are electromagnetically decoupled from one another by selecting the overlap between neighboring coils, so that mutual inductances disappear. This is achieved by the use of low-impedance preamplifiers on the output of each individual coil or by physically overlapping the coil receiver elements. The hexagonal arrangement of coils and extent of overlap are chosen to minimize mutual inductances between coil elements. Noise is proportional to sensitivity volume of the coil, which is smaller for surface coil than for a volume coil.

Phased array coils have to be positioned perpendicular to the main magnetic field. Phased array coils require an individual hardware channel for each reception element demanding more computer processors. As the number of channels increase, the coil elements become smaller and penetration may be compromised. This may lead to inhomogeneous SNR, which would be maximum near the surface of the coil and less within the deeper parts. This has been overcome with the use of postprocessing algorithm to correct intensity variation.[18]

Transmit phased array coils: A current is produced on each element via special amplifiers. Precise control of the relative amplitude and phase of each element enables them to be mutually independent. With reduced pulse duration, higher SNR, improved field homogeneity and reduced SAR, parallel MRI can be used in the excitation phase as in transmit SENSE at higher field strengths.[7]

Hybrid coil: This is a transmit/receive coil. It consists of a localized dedicated transmitter coil whose size is just optimized for a target FOV and an independent set of receiver coils. As the transmitter coil is much smaller than the typical whole body transmitter coil, it requires less input power to generate the necessary B_1 with a potentially reduced SAR. Hybrid coils are thus useful for higher static magnet fields.

Most of the RF transmit and receive subsystem component, such as digital to analogue converters, analogue to digital converters, power amplifiers, frequency mixers are sited in the electronics/cabinet room.

Careful shielding of the MR scan room is required to prevent contamination of the weak signal arising from the patient with extraneous signal at the same frequency. These can be from broadcasting stations or operation of electronic equipment. MRI rooms have a shield called as **Faraday cage**, consisting of a conductive metal lining of copper or aluminum through which RF electromagnetic radiation will not pass. It keeps external electrical noise out and the generated RF signal within the examination room. Electronic filters are used to prevent noise from entering the scan room via wiring cables. Screened rooms possess wave guides/tubes fixed into the wall of the room, through which nonconductive tubing, such as fiber optical coil passes. The examination room door should be shut while acquiring data to enable the shield to work effectively. Machine should be away from lifts/elevators and power cables, which may cause RF interference, distorts the image and produce linear artifacts. A hardware and software system is provided which provides protection for the patient against the **heating effect of RF energy absorption** and RF hardware from excess transmitted RF energy or hardware failure in the RF transmit path. This takes into account various coil types, amount of transmitted power allowed for the body coil is much higher than that of a transmit receive head coil as the body coil is larger and can handle more power. Correct calibration of the MR system is essential.

MULTICHANNEL RF COILS AND PARALLEL IMAGING

Multichannel radiofrequency and parallel imaging technologies are hardware and software implementations, respectively, aimed at improving the coverage, signal resolution and speed of MRI examinations. With multichannel RF technology, the MRI signal used to form an image is collected by an array of separate detectors, or coil elements. Each element relays signal information along a separate channel to an image reconstruction computer. Such arrays of coil elements and receivers can improve imaging coverage and the ratio of signal-to-noise in the image. The connection to the system of a coil with more elements than the number of channels requires complex logic switches in the coil, number of elements in the array of detectors and receivers is an important factor in characterizing an MRI scanner. Parallel imaging technology uses complex software algorithms to reconstruct the signals from multiple channels in a way that can reduce imaging times and/or increase image resolution.

The concept of "multielement phased arrays receive coils" started around 1990; as a result MRI systems typically had up to 4 receive channels. Towards the end of the 1990s, with the introduction of parallel imaging, the technology related to MRI receiving architecture made enormous progress: over a period of 10 years, the number of receiving channels increased from the original 2–32. In the last decade, the move towards higher channel counts in coils has been at the forefront of MR development. This trend towards higher number of channels has resulted in an increased complexity of the MRI system with increased initial costs. Also upgrades to a higher number of channels are costly because a substantial expansion of the RF chain is required.

Acquisition time in MRI is proportional to the number of phase encoding steps. Increasing the distance between each phase encoding lines in k space by a factor of R, reduces the acquisition time by the same factor, while keeping the spatial resolution fixed. Acquisition time is reduced by a factor (R = acceleration factor), equivalent to the number of independent coil elements (4–32). In practice, only a time reduction of 2–3 is possible as SNR is inversely proportional to $\sqrt{R}$ and at higher R, SNR becomes unacceptably low. Decreasing the phase encoding lines decreases the FOV, resulting in aliasing or wraparound.

There are two techniques to remove or prevent aliasing:

1. ***Simultaneous acquisition of spatial harmonics (SMASH)***: The missing k space lines are restored prior to Fourier transformation.[19] Generalized autocalibrating partially parallel acquisition (GRAPPA) is a variant of SMASH in which a small number of additional lines of k space data are acquired during the acquisition, eliminating the need for a separate coil sensitivity.
2. ***SENSE***: ***Sensitivity encoding***[20]—data is first Fourier transformed, resulting in an aliased image. This is then by "unwrapped" by using the spatial information from the coil sensitivity profile.

SENSE is the most commonly used parallel imaging technique available with many vendors as ASSET (GE healthcare, Waukesha, Wis), SPEEDER (Toshiba medical systems, Tokyo, Japan), SENSE (Philips medical system, Cleveland, Ohio), Siemens (Erlangen, Germany) offers both SENSE and GRAPPA as a single package under the trade name iPAT.

Parallel imaging is useful in conditions where scan speed outweighs the need for a high SNR, e.g. cardiac imaging.

Multitransmit technology: Imaging in conventional MR scanners, uses a single source to transmit a signal to the patient. Multitransmit uses multiple RF sources, each source individually adapted to patients anatomy. This cancels out dielectric shading seen at 3.0 T. Multitransmit also reduces local specific absorption rate SAR. Interleaved sequences and saline bags are not required. Another advantage, as claimed by the vendor, of using multiple RF sources is increase in scanning speed by 40%.[21,22]

Total imaging matrix: Provided by one vendor,[23] the system contains up to 102 matrix coil elements integrated seamlessly with up to 32 independent RF channels. These provide high SNR associated with local coils for an FOV ranging from 5 to 196 cm. There is no requirement for patient/coil repositioning. This system provides a PAT factor up to 16. Tim46 ultrahigh density array up to 204 coil elements with 128 RF channels increase SNR considerably (**Fig. 20**).

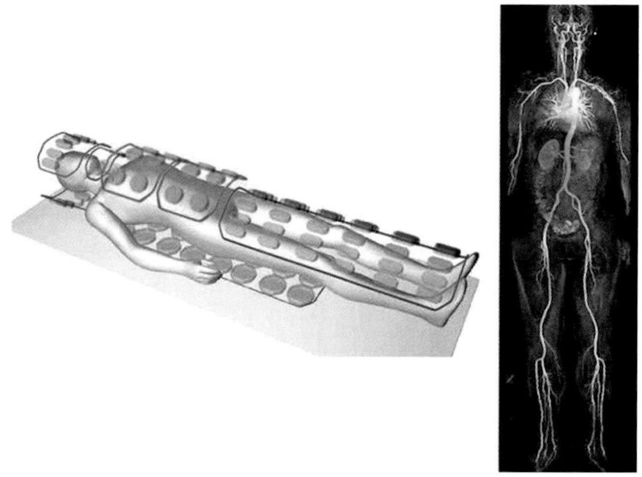

Fig. 20: Total Imaging Matrix®—102 coil elements with 32 channels providing whole body coverage of up to 205 cm.

Computer

The computer is the command center of the MRI system. It shapes and times the RF pulses, turns the gradients on and off, controls the RF receiver to collect data. After data collection, it is required for manipulation, storage, retrieval. A processor is required for computation.

Data Processing and Image Reconstruction

The two primary dedicated digital control systems are the pulse generator and the data acquisition system.

The pulse generator synchronizes the gradients and RF pulses after selection at operator console. Digital synchronization is provided for the receive channel analog to digital convertor, such that the detected signal correlate with the applied gradient and RF frequency. The **temporal positional accuracy and repeatability (TPAR)** is an important specification of the system.

Data is collected from one or more receiver channels. This may be in analog or preferable digital domain. **Digital broadband MR** is a new technology that samples the MR signal directly in the coil on the patient. The fiberoptic transmission of digital broadband data from the coil to the image reconstruction removes potential noise that is associated with analog RF. In conventional MR system, multiple analog coaxial cables are required (one per element/channel as digitization is performed away from the RF coil). In digital broadband system digitization is inside the RF receive coil, the number of RF channels is now determined by the coils, rather than the system. There is a single broadband fiberoptic cable that is independent of number of elements/channels in an RF coil. A gain of 40% in SNR is claimed. System also is channel independent. In a conventional system, 8 channels can receive coils up to 8 channels; to support a 16 channel coil an upgrade would be required. Digitization in the coil makes number of channels required redundant.

Data processing from multiple channels in the digital domain allows for correction of the inhomogeneous sensitivity of the coil and produces an acceptable image with a required FOV.

The required data acquisition rate increases with the number of channels being sampled. The sampling frequency needs to be twice the receiver bandwidth to meet the Nyquist criteria and prevent aliasing. To account from phase errors that may occur, a sample frequency of four times the bandwidth is used. Analog to digital converter are used. Digital data processing speeds are critical in higher field magnets with larger matrix size.

The complex MR signal is sampled and computer analyzed into a spectrum of component frequencies using a mathematical process called Fourier analysis. The data from every signal in a selected slice are stored in k space. This space is a spatial frequency domain in the computer where the signal spatial frequencies and their origin are stored. The number of lines filled in k space matches the number of encodings in the sequence.[7] The central part of k space is filled with data from shallow encoding gradients, low spatial frequencies, less details, but stronger signals. The upper and lower parts are filled with data from the steeper gradients, high spatial frequencies, better detail but low-signal intensity. k space has to be completely filled with the data from the imaging sequence before the signal is analyzed and processed into the image. The data once acquired, is stored in a large memory array after being filtered. The memory is very large and a cached disk system is used. Powerful reconstruction processors are used computer servers, are important components of MR hardware and have many forms, rackmount servers used in many systems. Image reconstruction algorithms are implemented to distribute computational load and save time. The sample frequency and the number of simultaneously acquired channels determine the maximum data rates through the system.

After the image is reconstructed, may be displaced for instantaneous viewing or stored in a database for review.

ADVANCED MR APPLICATIONS AND HARDWARE

Magnetic Resonance-High-Density Focussed Ultrasound (or MRgFUS)

A noninvasive method using high-density focused ultrasound and using MR for planning and temperature monitoring was first used in 2008 as an alternative to surgery for treatment of uterine fibroids. The clinical applications of this are increasing to include management of bone metastasis, prostate, etc.

A focusing transducer is used to transmit ultrasound energy into a small volume at the target locations inside the body. The ultrasound energy penetrates the intact skin and soft tissue to produce a well-defined region of coagulative necrosis by producing high temperature and only in the focused area. Three-dimensional MR provides the anatomical reference data for planning. MRI based temperature map acquired in real-time during ablation provides monitoring support. This is an outpatient procedure. Dedicated abdominopelvic coils designed for therapy applications are integrated within the table for positioning ease. The same system can be used for both therapy and diagnosis. This is exclusive to GE MR Systems[10] in collaboration with Insightec's Ex-ablate 2000 **(Fig. 21)**.

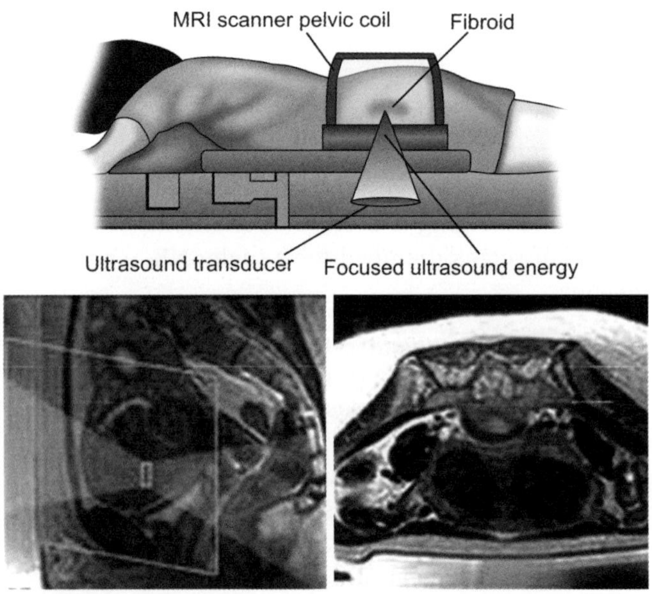

Fig. 21: Magnetic resonance-guided focused ultrasound—depicts the position of the patient, ultrasound transducer and the focused beam.

Magnetic Resonance Elastogram

This is an acquisition hardware and reconstruction application that produces images with contrast related to stiffness of soft tissue. Sound waves (40–200 Hz) are generated in the body by using an MRI compatible acoustic driver. These are then imaged by a special phase contrast MRI sequence. Finally the data generated is processed to generate elastograms—color coded anatomic images that depict the relative stiffness of tissue in the cross section of interest. The hardware component is compromised of an active sound wave generator and a passive transducer that produces vibrations in the subject to be scanned. The data is reconstructed in both magnitude and phase formats and the latter is used to produce strain wave and relative stiffness images. This technique is used to assess liver fibrosis.

MR Surgical Suite: Interventional MRI

Interventional MRI is the use of MR techniques for guidance of both diagnostic and minimally invasive therapeutic interventions. The magnet is of the 'open' type to allow access to the patient. There is video camera sensor array which detects the correct location and orientation of the hand held instrument. Use of new fast gradient echo pulse sequences allows continuous MR images (0.3–7 seconds per image). These are viewed through a high-resolution radiofrequency shielded monitor in the operating room. This modality is especially useful in areas of complex anatomy like skull base, retropharynx, etc.

Magnetic Resonance-Positron Emission Tomography

Fully integrated magnetic resonance-positron emission tomography (MR–PET) suite has been introduced. This has integrated cooling feature with specialized shielding to eliminate magnetic field interference in PET data processing. The detectors used in PET are MR compatible. This is dealt with in detail elsewhere in the book.

The MRI is now a widely used and well-developed modality. Intense technical development is continuing to increase its clinical applications including in the field of molecular imaging and to provide the necessary hardware for the same.

REFERENCES

1. Gorter CJ. Negative result of an attempt to detect nuclear spins. Physica. 1936;3:995-8.
2. Lauterbur PC. Image formation by induced local interactions: examples employing nuclear magnetic resonance. Nature. 1973;242:190-1.
3. Schneck JF, Kelley DAC, Marinelli L. Instrumentation: Magnets, coils and Hardware. In: Wolters Kluwer (Ed). Magnetic Resonance Imaging of the Brain and Spine Atlas SW, 4th edn. Lippincott Williams & Wilkins; 2009. pp.2-24.
4. Vaughan T, DelaBarre L, Synder C, et al. 9.4 T human MRI: preliminary results. Magn Med. 2006;56:1274-82.
5. Sagawa M, Fujimura S, Togawa N, et al. New material for permanent magnets on a base of Nd and Fe. J Appl Phys. 1984; 55:2083-7.
6. Scott Greig, Chronik Blaine, et al. A prepolarized MRI scanner.Proc Intl Soc Mag Med. 2001;9:610.
7. Allisy-Roberts P, Williams J. Farr's Physics For Medical Imaging, 2nd edn. Saunders Elsiever; Magnetic Resonance Imaging 189.
8. McRobbie DW, Moore EA, Graves MJ, Prince MR. MRI from picture to proton. Cambridge: Cambridge University Press. 2003.
9. Adam A, Dixon AK, Grainger RG, Allison DJ. Magnetic Resonance Imaging Basic Principles in Diagnostic Radiology. 2008;87-107.
10. GE Healthcare. GE MR Systems. [online] Available from *https://www.gehealthcare.com/en/global-gateway*. [Accessed December, 2018].
11. Akisk FM, Sandrasegaran K, Aisen AM, et al. Abdominal MR imaging at 3.0 T. Radiographics. 2007;27:1443-4.
12. Merkle EM, Dale BM. Abdominal MRI at 3.0 T: the basics revisited. Am J Roentgenol. 2006;186:1524-32.
13. Jellúš V, et al. New Modification of the Homomorphic Filter for Bias Field Correction. Proc ISMRM. 2005. p. 2247.
14. Turner R. Gradient coil design: a review of methods. Magn Reson Imag. 1993;11:903-20.
15. Walker KM, Tsuruda JS, Hadley JR, et al. Radiofrequency coil selection for MR imaging of the brain and skull base. Radiology. 2001;221:11-25.
16. Fujita H. New Horizons in MR Technology: RF coil designs and trends. Magn Reson Med Sci. 2007;6(1):29-42.
17. Schenck JF. Radiofrequency coils: types and characteristics. In: Bronskill MJ, Sprawls P (Eds). The Physics of MRI. Woodbury, NY: American Institute of Physics; 1993. pp.98-134.
18. Roemer PB, Edelstein WA, Hayes CE, et al. The NMR phased array. Magn Reson Med. 1990;16(2):192-225.
19. Sodickson DK, Manning WJ. Simultaneous aquistion of spatial harmonics (SMASH): fast imaging with radiofrequency coil arrays. Magn Reson Med. 1997;38: 591-603.
20. Prussmann KP, Weiger M, Scheidegger MB, et al. SENSE: Sensitivity encoding for fast MRI. Magn Reson Med. 1999; 42:952-62.
21. www. heathcare.philips.com/main/products/mri.
22. Harvey PR, et al. SAR behavior during whole-body multi-transmit RF shimming at 3.0 T. Proc. ISMRM. 2009;p. 4786.
23. Siemens. Medical solutions. [online] Available from *https://www.siemens.com/medical%20solutions*. [Accessed December, 2018].

CHAPTER 45

Image Optimization in Magnetic Resonance Imaging

Jyoti Kumar

INTRODUCTION

Optimizing image quality means finding a balance between the different aspects of image quality and image speed. For an image to be optimal for diagnosis, the anatomic and pathologic features within the image must be distinguishable from each other.

Ideally, an image should have a high signal-to-noise ratio (SNR), high-spatial resolution, excellent contrast, minimum artifacts and an acceptable scan time. Generally, there is a conflict amongst these criteria. Knowledge about various MR parameters within the user interface that can be modified by the radiologist helps find the most appropriate balance between image quality and scan time.

In this chapter, we shall discuss image optimization under these major headings:

- Signal-to-noise ratio
- Contrast-to-noise ratio (CNR)
- Spatial resolution
- Scan time
- Artifacts and their remedial measures.

SIGNAL-TO-NOISE RATIO

MR signal is the voltage received by the receiver coil from each voxel in a slice after it is stimulated by a radiofrequency pulse. This is recorded at time interval TE and at specific frequencies. Bright pixels in the image represent stronger signals, and darker pixels represent weaker signals in the image.

Noise is an unwanted occurrence in the MR image. Noise appears as a grainy random pattern superimposed on the MR image. This represents statistical fluctuations in signal intensity that is superimposed on the image and compromises image quality. It usually occurs at almost all frequencies at random times. The source of this noise is Brownian motion of charged particles throughout the body of the patient whereas signal comes from just the selected slice. The electronic noise of the receiver technology and the environment also contribute to the noise.

The SNR refers to the ratio of the amplitude of the MR signal to the amplitude of the background noise. A high SNR improves image quality. To increase the SNR, we need to increase the signal relative to the noise. The parameters which affect SNR are field strength, proton density, coil type and position, TR, TE, flip angle, number of signal averages, slice thickness and receiver bandwidth.

Field Strength

With higher field strength, more protons are aligned parallel to the main field (spin up nuclei) as fewer protons have energy which could be enough for opposing this increased field strength and lie antiparallel to the main field (spin down nuclei). The net magnetism of the patient (termed the net magnetization vector or NMV), displays the balance between the parallel and antiparallel magnetic moments. In high field strengths, NMV increases and therefore the signal increases.

Proton Density

The signal strength depends on the quantity of signal generating protons in the voxel (proton density). For example, pelvis contains structures with a high proton density, such as fat, bone and muscle, giving a high signal. On the other hand, chest contains air filled lungs and vessels with low proton density, and hence imaging of chest requires measures to boost SNR.

Coil Type and Position

Imaging of small anatomical regions, such as extremities (e.g. ankles, wrists), neck or the breasts require specialized surface coils to maximize both the SNR and spatial resolution. Large coverage is provided by the large coils, such as the body coil but it results in a lower SNR. A phased array coil combines the two advantages by using multiple small coils which provide good SNR and the data from these are combined to produce an image with good coverage.

Positioning of coils is also of great importance. To understand this, let us revise few basic principles of MR imaging. In an external magnetic field (B0), spin up and spin down nuclei are in a state of equilibrium. Excess spins generate constant magnetization in the longitudinal plane (Z-axis). Spins are also precesssing like a wobbling top and they are out of phase with each other. NMV is zero in the transverse plane. Application of RF pulse leads to two things: energy absorption and phase coherence. Hydrogen nuclei absorb energy. If the appropriate amount of energy is absorbed, the number of nuclei in the spin up position is equal to the number in the spin down position. Consequently, the longitudinal magnetization reduces to zero. Secondly, on application of an RF pulse, the spins move into phase with each other. When spin up and spin down nuclei are equal in number, the net effect is one of precession so that NMV now precesses in the transverse or XY plane. As the NMV has been moved through 90° from the direction of the main magnetic field or the Z-axis, it is called a 90° RF pulse. It is the magnetization in the transverse plane that is used to produce the signal. As the NMV rotates in the transverse plane, it passes across the receiver coil to induce a voltage in it. This voltage is the MR signal. The position of the coil is kept such that the transverse magnetization created in the XY plane remains perpendicular to the coil. In a superconducting system, this means positioning the coil either over, under, or to the right or left of the area to be examined. A coil positioned perpendicular to the table results in zero-signal generation.

Repetition Time

Repetition time (TR) is the time between the application of two RF pulses. It is measured in milliseconds (msec). When the RF pulse is removed, longitudinal magnetization recovers (T1 recovery) and transverse magnetization begins to decay (T2 decay). The T1 time of a tissue is inherent in nature and refers to the time it takes for the recovery of 63% of the longitudinal magnetization. The period of time in which this longitudinal recovery occurs is the time TR. The longer the TR, the greater is the recovery of longitudinal magnetization, which is now available to be flipped into the transverse plane on the application of the next excitation pulse. Hence, the SNR is improved with a long TR. A short TR reduces the SNR. Although a short TR is required for T1 weighting, reducing this parameter excessively may severely compromise the SNR.

Echo Time

Echo time (TE) refers to the time between an RF excitation pulse and collection of the signal. It is also measured in milliseconds (msec). The T2 decay time of a particular tissue is also inherent to the tissue. It is the time it requires for 63% of the transverse magnetization to be lost. The time period over which it occurs is the time between the excitation pulse and the MR signal or the TE. The TE determines the extent of T2 decay occurring in a particular tissue. At short TEs, very little transverse magnetization has dephased, so the signal amplitude and hence SNR is high. A long TE reduces the SNR. Although a long TE is required for T2 weighting, an excessive increase in this parameter may severely compromise the SNR.

Flip Angle

It is the angle through which NMV is moved as a result of RF excitation pulse. When a large flip angle is used, longitudinal magnetization is entirely converted into transverse magnetization resulting in maximum signal. On the other hand, small flip angles convert only a proportion of the longitudinal magnetization to transverse magnetization. A small flip angle is used in gradient echo imaging which results in a low SNR and hence measures may be needed to improve it.

Number of Signal Averages

Number of signal averages (NSA) determines the number of times frequencies in the signal are sampled with the same slope of phase encoding gradient. Multiple measurements of one slice are obtained and the results are averaged in a single image. Increasing the number of excitation (NEX) increases the signal collected. We need to remember that noise is also being increasingly sampled. As noise occurs randomly and at all frequencies, doubling the number of signal averages does not double the SNR but only increases the SNR by a square root of two. Also, when NEX is doubled the time required to obtain the scan is also doubled **(Figs. 1A and B)**.

Slice Thickness

When we obtain thicker slices, the voxel is enlarged and hence more proton spins contribute to the signal, thereby increasing the signal intensity. Noise remains the same because it is not just coming from the slice, but the patient's entire body and MR environment. Hence, SNR is directly proportional to the slice thickness. The drawback is that, increasing the slice thickness reduces the spatial resolution resulting in partial volume effects **(Figs. 2A and B)**.

Receiver Bandwidth

This is the range of frequencies sampled within the FOV during readout in the frequency encoding direction. It is measured in kilo Hertz (kHz). Reduction of the receiver bandwidth reduces the proportion of noise sampled relative to signal, hence effectively increasing the SNR.

The drawback here is that to reduce the bandwidth, the sampling time has to be increased to satisfy Nyquist theorem. This theorem states that the sampling rate must be at least double the frequency of the highest frequency

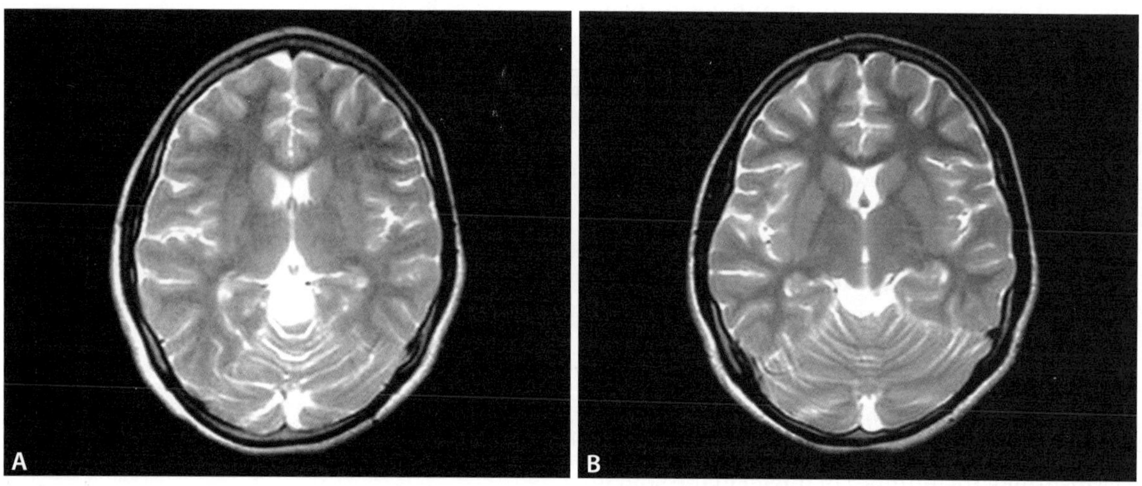

Figs. 1A and B: Image comparison: T2-weighted axial images of the brain acquired with one signal average on the left (A) and four signal averages on the right (B). The SNR of the image (B) was double than that of (A). Also, the scan time of (B) was four times than that of (A).

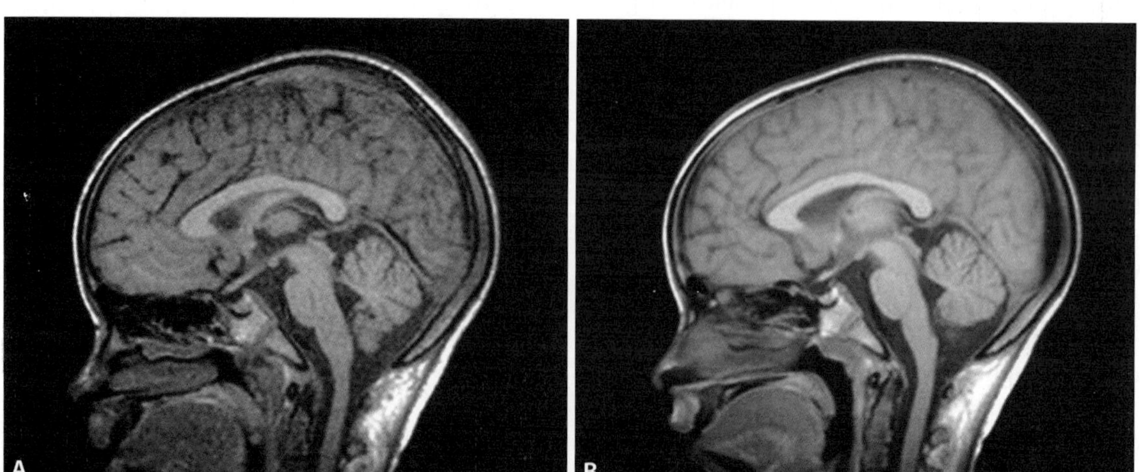

Figs. 2A and B: Image comparison—T1-weighted sagittal images of the brain: The image on the right (B) was acquired with double the slice thickness on the left (A). The SNR of the image (B) was double that of (A). However, this occurred at the expense of spatial resolution.

in the echo to accurately reflect all the frequencies in the signal. If receiver bandwidth is reduced keeping all parameters unchanged, then sampling time needs to be increased to be able to sample all frequencies accurately. As the echo is centered in the middle of the sampling window, TE need to be increased. Therefore, it is not suitable for T1 or proton density weighted imaging, where a low TE is used. Also, chemical shift artifact is increased when receiver bandwidth is decreased. Reduced receive bandwidths should be used when there is no requirement of a short TE (T2 weighting) and when fat is absent (example: brain, and any other examination when fat is suppressed).

CONTRAST-TO-NOISE RATIO

MR images would have no clinical value without satisfactory image contrast which is defined as the difference in signal strength between two tissues in the image. A high SNR does not guarantee easy differentiation of two structures in an image. The CNR is the most significant image quality factor because this allows for differentiation between anatomical tissues in the image and also in differentiation between pathological and normal tissue, hence aiding in final analysis of the image. Superior soft-tissue contrast is a major advantage of MR imaging versus alternative modalities, such as computed radiography.

Contrast in MR is a complex function of intrinsic characteristics of the structure, i.e. proton density, T1- and T2-relaxation times, magnetic susceptibility of the nuclei as well as programmable pulse-sequence parameters, e.g. TR, TE, flip angle, slice thickness, etc. For example, a longer TR permits more time for T1 relaxation and produces more signal from tissues with long T1 values. Longer TE, on the other hand, allows more time for T2 relaxation and produces more signal from tissues with long T2 values.

The factors that increase CNR are administration of a contrast agent, magnetization transfer constant, chemical suppression techniques and T2 weighting, where difference between pathology and anatomy is increased.

Administration of a Contrast Agent

A contrast agent like gadolinium shortens the T1 time of structures, especially of pathological lesions when they have a break in blood brain barrier. Enhancing tissue appears much brighter, hence boosting the CNR.

Magnetization Transfer Constant

In biological systems, protons usually exist in two pools. The 'free pool' consists of relatively mobile protons in free bulk water and some fat containing tissues. With standard MRI, this pool provides the bulk of the signal. The second pool or 'bound pool' consists of restricted protons bound in proteins, other large macromolecules, and cellular membranes. With conventional MRI, this pool does not contribute to MR signal due to very short T2.

Under normal MR conditions magnetization is exchanged from the 'free pool' to the 'bound pool' and vice versa, that results in a situation of equilibrium situation which is characteristic for that type of tissue.

When additional RF pulses are use to suppress bound protons, it results in no net magnetization of the 'bound pool.' A difference in magnetization between the pools is thereby created. The cross relaxation processes transfers the magnetization from the 'free pool' to the 'bound pool.' A new equilibrium is reached decreasing the SNR of a particular tissue. Hence the contrast with the surrounding tissue is accentuated. It is primarily used to suppress normal tissue.

Chemical Suppression

Signal is suppressed either from fat or water. For example, fat suppression techniques null fat and hence CNR between lesions and the surrounding normal tissues that contain fat is increased.

Echo-train Length

In fast-spin-echo (FSE) sequence, a train of 180° rephasing pulses are used. The number of these pulses and resultant echoes is called the echo train length or turbo factor. Since each echo has a different TE and data from each echo are used to produce one image, the contrast of FSE is unique. On T2 FSE, fat is hyperintense as this echo train reduces spin-spin interactions in fat, thereby increasing T2 decay time (J-coupling). Muscle appears darker because the echo train increases magnetization transfer effects that produce saturation.

Time from Inversion

The time from inversion (TI) is the primary factor that controls the contrast in Inversion Recovery (IR) sequences.

These are spin-echo-sequences that begin with a 180° pulse which flips the NMV by 180°. At time TI after the 180° inverting pulse, a 90° pulse is applied which is then followed by 180° pulse for rephasing spins that produces echo at time TE. If TI is long enough to let NMV pass through the transverse plane before the 90° pulse is applied, the contrast will depend on how much saturation this 90° pulse produces. Saturation is when NMV is pushed beyond the transverse plane by the 90° pulse and results in T1 weighting. TIs of 300 to 700 ms result in heavy T1 weighting. Certain specific TI values result in suppression of signal from specific tissues. For example, TI of 100–180 ms is used in STIR sequence. 90° pulse is here applied after this TI when NMV of fat is passing exactly through transverse plane. At this null point, there is no longitudinal magnetization of fat and hence no transverse magnetization results on application of 90° pulse, therefore resulting in no signal from fat. Similarly, TIs of 1700–2200 ms are used to null the signal from CSF on FLAIR imaging.

SPATIAL RESOLUTION

Spatial resolution is defined as the ability to distinguish between two points that are close to each other in the patient. The size of the voxel determines the spatial resolution. The imaging volume is divided into slices. Each slice displays an area of anatomy which is called the field of view (FOV). This FOV is divided into pixels. The size of the pixels is determined by the matrix. The FOV may be specified separately for the frequency encoding and phase encoding directions which may be the same in a square or isotropic FOV and different in an anisotropic or a rectangular FOV. Frequency and phase encoding gradients are applied to spatially locate the signal coming from each pixel in the FOV.

Voxel Volume, FOV, Matrix

Voxel volume is a product of pixel size and slice thickness. Therefore, slice thickness, FOV and matrix size determine voxel volume. The greater the voxel volume, more are the number of spins that contribute to MR signal, resulting in a higher SNR per voxel. However, when the voxels are larger, spatial resolution falls as the likelihood of two points close to one another in the patient, being in separate voxels decreases.

When FOV is decreased, pixel size and hence voxel volume decreases, thereby decreasing the SNR and increasing spatial resolution **(Figs. 3A and B)**. When small coils are used which boost local SNR, a small FOV may be used. However, a small FOV should be used with caution with a large coil as SNR will be severely compromised unless other measures like increasing NEX is used.

When the matrix is changed, the number of pixels that must fit into the FOV also changes. As the matrix increases, the dimension of each pixel decreases. This reduces the SNR but improves spatial resolution. In addition as the phase matrix increases, the scan time also increases **(Figs. 4A and B)**. However, if we increase the frequency matrix only, it increases the resolution but the scan time does not increase as only the phase matrix determines scan time. A rectangular FOV where the FOV is reduced in the phase direction reduces the scan time keeping the resolution same as that of square FOV. This is especially useful when anatomy of the area examined fits into a rectangle, as in sagittal image of pelvis.

Increasing the slice thickness increases the voxel volume, hence increasing SNR at the expense of spatial resolution **(*see* Figs. 2A and B)**.

SCAN TIME

The longer the examination time, the greater the discomfort to the patient resulting in increased chances of a bad image. Good immobilization is also vital, since a

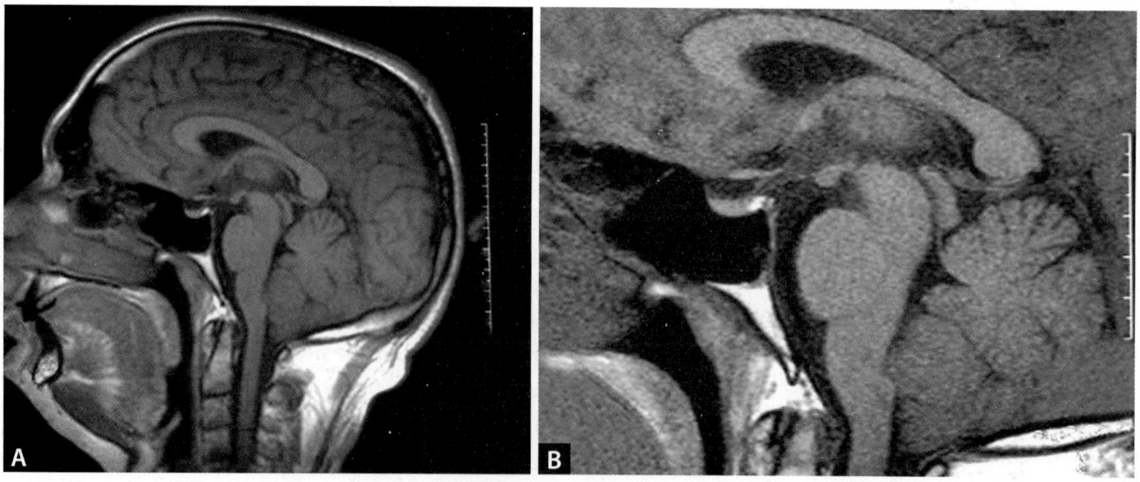

Figs. 3A and B: Image comparison—T1-weighted sagittal images of the brain: The image on the right (B) was acquired with reduced FOV and reduced pixel size compared with left (A). The spatial resolution of (B) was increased at the expense of reduced SNR.

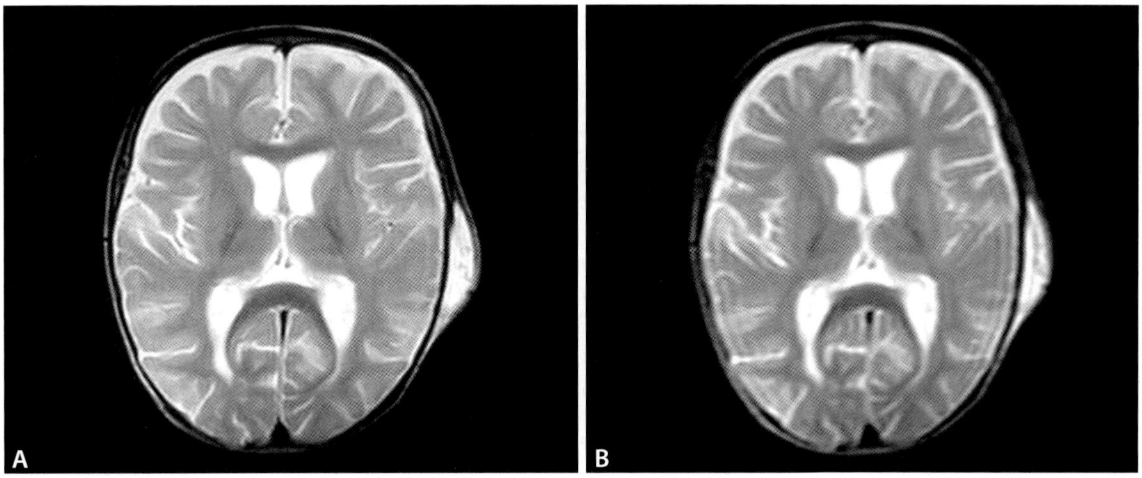

Figs. 4A and B: Image comparison—T2-weighted axial images of the brain: The image on the left (A) was acquired with increased matrix and hence, reduced pixel size compared with right (B). The spatial resolution of (A) was improved. As the phase matrix was increased, the scan time was also increased.

few minutes spent in making the patient comfortable can save us many minutes of wasted sequences. The scan time is determined by the following factors.

Scan time = TR × number of excitations × number of phase encodings

Repetition Time

The greater is the time between the application of two RF pulses, the greater is the scan time. When we reduce the repetition time (TR), we can reduce the scan time. However, reducing TR reduces SNR as already discussed. As less longitudinal magnetization recovers during each TR period, the next 90° pulse flips it to beyond the transverse plane. This is called saturation and increases T1 weighting. As there is less time to excite slices in this reduced TR, the number of slices that can be acquired in a single acquisition also decreases.

Number of Excitations

When the NEX or signal averages is increased, more and more measurements of one slice are being obtained to average the results. This increases the scan time (***see* Figs. 1A and B**). But when we reduce the NEX to reduce scan time, SNR falls because now, the number of times data is stored in k-space is reduced. Since averaging of noise is also less, there is also an accompanying increase in motion artifact.

Phase Matrix

Increasing the phase matrix increases scan time **(Figs. 4A and B)**. To understand this, we shall first discuss the basic physics behind MR gradients. Gradients are coils of wire which change the magnetic field strength of the magnet in a controlled manner when current is passed through them. They change the precessional frequency and phase of the spins. These are employed along three orthogonal axes, XYZ, to enable us to select a slice (slice-selection gradient), and to spatially locate the signal along the two dimensions of the image within a slice (frequency encoding and phase encoding gradient).

Frequency encoding gradient is switched on to locate signal along one axis of the image (usually the long axis) and produces a frequency shift. At a frequency matrix of 256, 256 different frequencies are mapped along the long axis of the image. Fourier transformation allows us to determine signal contribution of each frequency, enabling us to allocate this signal to the location of origin along one axis of the image. Fourier transformation is like a prism (which disperses white light into its spectra) that causes physical dispersion of the frequencies collected and assigns them to a structure in the image.

Phase-encoding gradient alters the phase of the nucleus, causing a phase shift. When this gradient is switched off, phase shift of spins remains. This phase shift is used to locate the signal along one dimension of the image (usually the short axis). For a phase resolution of 256, we have to generate 256 signals with different phase encodings for 256 different locations. The pulse sequence has to be repeated 256 times for a phase matrix of 256. Hence, the phase matrix is an important determinant of scan time. If we reduce the phase matrix to reduce scan time, the spatial resolution of the image falls.

Number of Slice Encodings in 3D Sequences

In three-dimensional fast scan sequences, scan time is depends upon the number of slice locations needed in the volume in addition to TR, NEX and number of phase encodings

Scan time = TR × number of excitations × number of phase encodings × slice encodings

ARTIFACTS

Artifacts are structures in the MR image that do not correspond to spatial distribution of tissue in the image plane. The cause of this signal misregistration is variable; artifacts are divided into three main types based on the cause:

1. Motion artifacts
2. Artifacts related to particular measurement technique or parameters used, e.g. chemical shift, wrap around and truncation artifacts.
3. External artifacts results from either a malfunction of the MR scanner or external interference.

Motion Artifacts (Phase Mismapping)

These may result from accidental patient movement, respiration, heart beat, blood flow, eye movements or swallowing motion. These signal misregistartions occur in the phase encoding direction. The tissue is excited at one location but is mapped to a different location during readout due to its motion. This occurs in the phase encoding direction rather than the frequency encoding or readout direction because the encoding of phase by the phase encoding gradient occurs before signal detection, whereas frequency encoding gradient, also called the readout gradient, is applied concurrently with signal detection. For example, if the abdominal wall is at one position during the application of phase encoding gradient, its phase shift value is allocated to it in accordance with this position. During readout, the abdominal wall moves to another position, but the system still allocates it according to its first position resulting in ghosting artifact. Also, patient motion normally is much slower than the faster sampling process along the frequency encoding direction (in order of milliseconds). On the other hand, sampling along phase encoding direction needs all phase encoding steps and is in the order of seconds. This is another reason why motion artifacts are appreciable more along phase encoding direction.

Ghosting and Smearing

While ghosting results from periodic motion, smearing is a result of aperiodic motion.

The periodic rise and fall of thorax/abdomen during breathing produces an artifact called ghosting **(Figs. 5A and B)**. If the respiration rate is constant, then during inspiration, the abdomen is in several equidistant phase encoding steps during the inspiration phase and it is in the expiration phase in the intervening steps. This periodic motion is seen a locally offset double or multiple structures in the phase encoding direction. These ghosts are offset by the true image by an amount that is proportional to the respiration rate. Structures rich in signal, for example subcutaneous fat, further increase ghosting artifact. In a strictly periodic motion, the localization of the ghost can

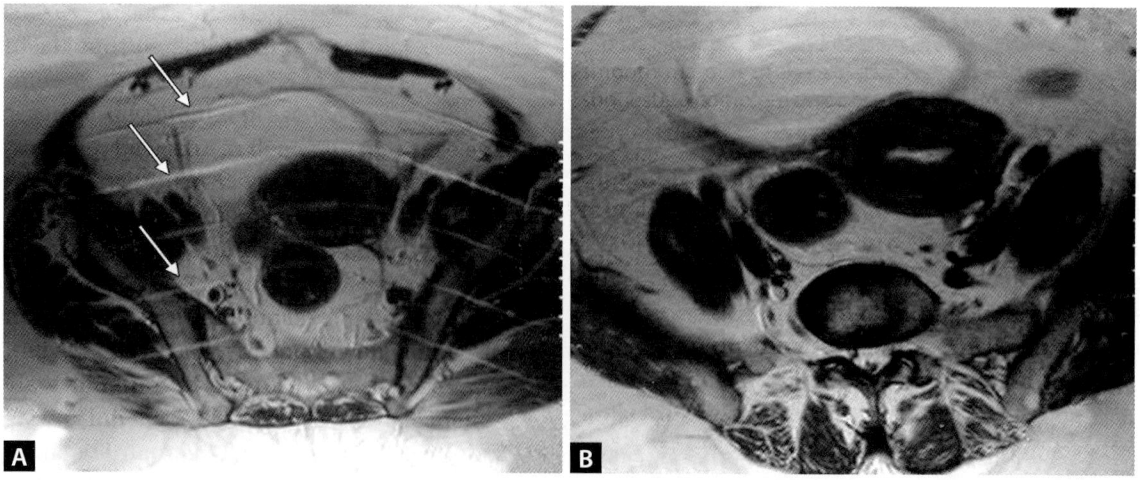

Figs. 5A and B: Ghosting artifact: T2-weighted image of the pelvis (A) shows marked ghosting artifact (arrows) due to periodic respiratory motion. This was reduced in (B) by increasing the number of signal averages and placing a spatial-presaturation pulse in the overlying subcutaneous fat. However, both these techniques contributed to an increase in scan time.

be predicted by a simple formula, describing the distance between the ghost image and the original structure.

Distance = TR × phase encoding steps × NEX × motion frequency

The higher the frequency of the motion, e.g. higher the breathing rate, the greater the distance between the original and the ghost artifact. We can increase the distance between the ghosts by increasing TR, phase matrix or NEX so that the first ghost lies outside the image,; however scan time is increased by all these methods. The brightness of the ghost depends upon the amplitude of motion; larger the pulsation, brighter the ghost.

Another type of artifact that may result from aperiodic motion like that of eyes is smearing **(Fig. 6)**. Peristalsis, which is a random movement, produces motion artifacts that result in generalized blurring of the image, which appears to be superimposed by a layer of noise.

Blood flow is a very common cause of motion artifacts in the image. Fast continuous flow compared to TR produces a continuous artifact throughout the FOV, resulting in blurring, as in spin echo images. In-plane flow, parallel to the slice plane produces a diffuse artifact seen in coronal images. Flow in aorta and IVC affects the entire image acquired in coronal plane as these great vessels extend through the entire image. CSF flow artifacts can also degrade the image of the spine on T2-weighted images. Periodic motion due to pulsatile through plane flow (flow perpendicular to the image plane) will be discussed later.

Remedy: Various methods are tried to decrease the severity of motion artifacts in the final image, depending upon whether signal from moving tissue is desired in the image or not. While spatial-presaturation pulse may be used in the former case, other remedial measures are required when signal from moving tissue is desired in the image.

Spatial-presaturation pulse: When signal from moving tissue is not desired, spatial presaturation pulse can be used to reduce these artifacts. These are used in spine examinations to suppress cardiac and abdominal motion artifacts **(Figs. 7A to C)**. These saturation pulses are applied at the beginning of the pulse sequence and hence reduce the number of imaging sections that can be obtained

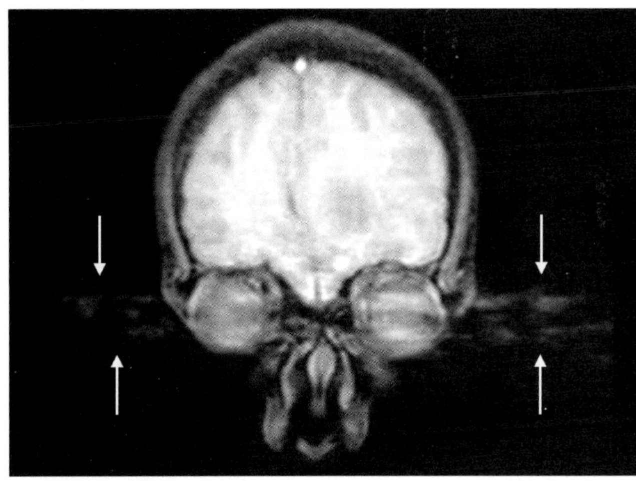

Fig. 6: Smearing artifact: T1-weighted coronal image of the brain shows smearing artifact (arrows) due to aperiodic motion of the eyes.

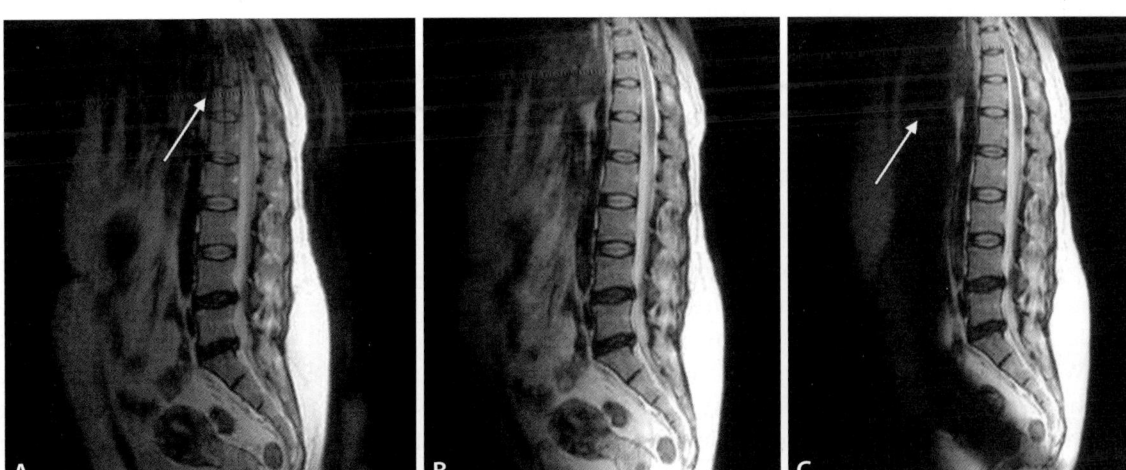

Figs. 7A to C: Motion artifact: T2-weighted sagittal images of the spine show marked motion artifacts degrading the image (A) (arrow) when the phase encoding direction was anterior to posterior. On changing the phase encoding direction to head to foot (B), the motion artifacts from the heart do not degrade the image. There is further improvement in image quality when a spatial-presaturation band (arrow) is used to suppress motion artifacts from the great vessels (C).

per TR in multislice acquisitions. They may also result in increased heat deposition when specific absorption rate (SAR) is already high.

When signal from moving tissue is desired in the image, other methods may be used. These include use of faster sequences, modification of acquisition parameters, physiological triggering and flow compensation.

Faster imaging: The most effective technique may be shortening of acquisition time to minimize motion artifacts. This has been achieved through the improvements in MR imaging hardware, which include faster and stronger gradients, multichannel coils, and higher magnetic field strengths.

There are various techniques to obtain faster sequences. Fast spin echo sequences use multiple 180° refocusing pulses and allow multiple echoes to be obtained within a given TR. The number of additional echoes obtained is called the echo train length (ETL). However, excessive ETLs may blur the image and increase some flow artifacts. Sequences such as half Fourier single-shot turbo spin echo (HASTE) allow rapid acquisition by filling only half of k-space. Parallel imaging technique also reduces the scan time and hence motion artifacts. This technique uses multichannel, multicoil technology, with each coil possessing a distinct known sensitivity profile over the field of view. At least 2 coil elements are aligned in the phase encoding direction. The phase encoding steps are reduced by a factor of X, known as the parallel imaging factor. Only one of every X lines of k space is filled up in the phase encoding direction. The other lines are inferred from the signal amplitude and known sensitivity profile of the coils used. Several data extrapolation algorithms like generalized autocalibrating partially parallel acquisition (GRAPPA) and sensitivity encoding (SENSE) are used before and after Fourier transformation, respectively. The major disadvantage is a decreased SNR. However, overall increase in SNR at 3T makes higher parallel imaging factors possible in clinical practice.

Radial k-space filling technique: Multi-shot radial acquisition technique (e.g. syngoBLADE, Siemens healthcare, Erlangen, Germany; PROPELLOR, GE healthcare. Milwaukee, Wis) fills the k-space radially instead of standard line by line rectilinear filling. With this technique, MR imaging datasets are acquired in multiple overlapping radial sections. A series of low resolution images is reconstructed from each radial section which is then combined to produce high resolution images. Because the phase encoding direction varies with each radial section, ghosting artifact from motion is not propagated in the phase encoding direction but dispersed through the radial sections. The main disadvantage it has is the low spatial resolution because the periphery of k space is less densely filled than its central region.

Modification of parameters: Parameters may be modified to alter the appearance of motion artifacts. Frequency and phase encoding direction can be swapped, which alters the position of the artifact **(Figs. 7A to C)**. These may now be relocated to image areas that do not affect image interpretation. For example, motion artifacts due to eye movement may obscure brain parenchyma if phase encoding direction is antero-posterior for an axial image. This may be overcome when phase encoding direction is made right to left and the artifact now lies outside the brain.

Increasing NEX is another method of reducing motion artifacts. Increasing the number of signal averages increases the signal from the tissue and the motion artifact signal is reduced relative to the tissue signal **(Figs. 5A and B)**.

Physiological triggering/gating: Physiological triggering synchronizes the data collection with a periodic signal produced by the patient, such as pulse or heartbeat allowing normal movement of tissue. Data collection may be synchronized with ECG signal using lead wires, pulse using pulse sensor on an extremity, respiration using pressure transducer on the patient or a navigator echo indicating diaphragmatic motion. ECG gating is used in cardiac evaluation where artifacts from cardiac motion need to be minimized. This may be prospective or retrospective gating. In the prospective method, the timing signal is first detected. The echo signal is collected at the same time following the time signal. Since the moving tissue is stable at this time, there is minimal misregistration of signal. This is typically used in static cardiac examinations. Prospective triggering also allows the rejection of arrhythmic beats, which can degrade MR image quality. In the retrospective method, the timing signal and the echo signal are first acquired together. The timing signal does not control data collection. These are analyzed only after the scan is complete and the data collection is gated to the timing signal. This method is commonly used in cine cardiac imaging where sequential images are produced according to their time point in the cardiac cycle to allow a dynamic evaluation of cardiac function. Further artifact suppression can be achieved while imaging the heart, if the acquisition is performed during breath holding. The disadvantages of a triggered study include a longer scan time and misregistration artifacts if the trigger signal is irregular, e.g. with an irregular heart rate.

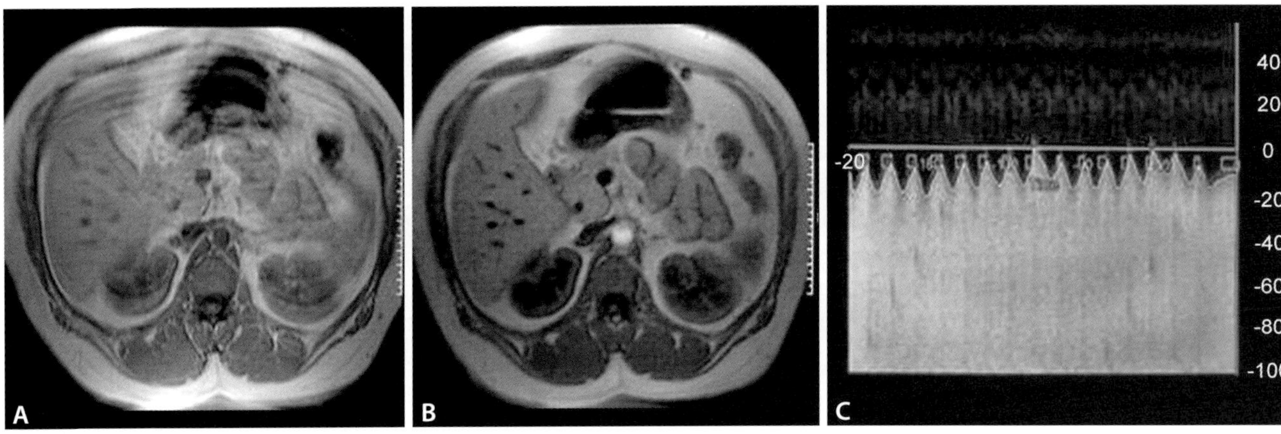

Figs. 8A to C: Motion artifact: Axial T1-weighted gradient echo image of the abdomen shows marked respiratory motion artifact resulting in blurring of the image (A). There is marked reduction in motion artifact (B), using a navigator echo pulse (C).

In contradistinction to cardiac gating, respiratory gating is not frequently used in clinical imaging. The method of breath holding is used to avoid respiration artifacts. In infants, children, and patients with respiratory and cognitive impairment, either short sequences are used or imaging examination is divided into multiple brief sequences if the patient can hold breath for a limited time. However, multiple breath holds require cooperation from the patient. In respiratory gating, bellows or a belt is encircled over the abdomen and the acquisition is timed to end expiration when there is minimum motion. The disadvantages include an increased acquisition time and an additional setup time. Respiratory compensation or phase reordering [respiratory ordered phase encoding (ROPE)] is another effective way to reduce respiratory artifacts. In this technique, phase encoding steps are ordered on the basis of the phase of the respiratory cycle. K-space lines are reordered such that the adjacent samples in the final data have minimal differences in the respiratory phase. This works well only with regular respiratory rate. Navigator echo is a commonly used method to suppress periodic motion artifacts from breathing; it uses an additional navigator pulse. This is most commonly used in abdominal imaging where a small one dimensional spatial encoding gradient is placed perpendicular to the diaphragm **(Figs. 8A to C)**. The imaging dataset is then corrected by the navigator echo so that only the data acquired at end expiration (when diaphragm is at peak) is used in reconstruction of final image.

Gradient moment rephasing: GRE flow compensation uses additional gradient pulses to correct for phase shifts of the moving protons. It is also known as gradient motion rephasing (GMR) or motion artifact suppression technique (MAST). Additional gradient pulses are used to eliminate the phase shifts in moving protons, bringing them back into phase with no effect on static spins. In most instances, correction is needed only for spins flowing with constant velocity (first order motion compensation). As additional gradient pulses are used, there is a modest increase in TE. In pulse sequences in which short TEs are desired, short duration high amplitude gradient pulses need to be used. This limits the minimum FOV for the sequence. Higher-order compensation can also be done for spins with either constant or varying acceleration, but this further increases the echo time.

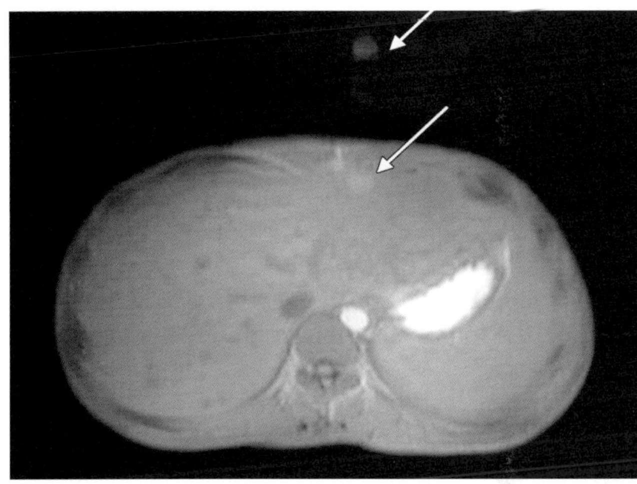

Fig. 9: Ghosting artifact from pulsatile aortic flow: Pulsatile through plane flow in the aorta is seen as ghost vessels at discrete points (arrows) on this T1-weighted axial gradient image.

Pulsatile Flow-related Artifacts

Periodic motion due to pulsatile through plane flow (flow perpendicular to the image plane) results in ghost vessels at discrete points, frequently seen in axial abdomen gradient echo images **(Fig. 9)**. The distance between the ghosts depends on the difference between the heart rate and TR. GRE images are more prone to these ghost artifacts than SE sequences. In spin-echo sequences, flowing blood usually appears dark. This is because after being exposed to the 90° excitation pulse in SE sequences, flowing blood moves out of the imaging section before the refocusing 180° pulse is applied, while the blood protons that move into the imaging section has not been exposed to the excitation pulse; hence, resulting in dark signal. In contrast, bright blood phenomenon is seen on GRE sequences.

Remedy

Saturation pulse: A common way to reduce the motion artifact due to through-plane flow is to apply a saturation band adjacent to the imaging section. The protons in this slab are saturated with the use of 90° RF pulse and then spoiled by strong gradients before image acquisition, hence resulting in no signal when spins flow into the imaging volume. When applied superior to the acquisition slab in the abdomen, it eliminates arterial pulsation artifact. When placed inferiorly, it eliminates artifacts from venous inflow in the iliac veins.

Advantage of pulsation artifacts: Pulsation artifacts from vascular lesions can help us reach the correct diagnosis, when in doubt. The vascular nature of the lesion is confirmed if we see associated pulsation artifacts.

Artifacts due to Measurement Technique/Parameters

Aliasing

Aliasing (wraparound artifact) occurs when the imaging FOV is smaller than the anatomy being imaged. This occurs mostly in the phase encoding direction. The tissue stimulated outside the sensitive volume of the coil contains higher or lower phase and frequency information. These are misinterpreted during Fourier transformation. This tissue is misrepresented in the image on the opposite side **(Figs. 10A and B)**. To explain this, let us recapitulate that the phase of the signal originating from inside the FOV has a range from 0 to 360°. Due to the circular nature of phase, a signal from outside the FOV with a phase of 400° (= 360° + 40°) is not distinguishable from a phase of 40° from inside the FOV and hence is misinterpreted within the FOV during Fourier transformation. Thus, the part of the body that lies beyond the borders of the FOV is wrapped inside to the other side of the image. This can mask anatomical structures in the FOV.

Wraparound is seldom encountered along the frequency encoding axis because the frequency encoding direction is typically oversampled within the system. In the new imaging systems, the digital receiver automatically filters out unwanted high frequencies or makes use of a high bandwidth in the frequency encoding direction. Aliasing can also be seen in the section direction in volume imaging. The sidelobes of the RF pulse that excites the entire volume of tissue can also produce a signal form outside this slab and information in the first section of the slab may be aliased in the last section of the 3D acquisition **(Fig. 11)**.

Remedy

Increase FOV: The wraparound can be eliminated by enlarging the phase FOV to accommodate the entire object. Increase in FOV increases the SNR but decreases the spatial resolution.

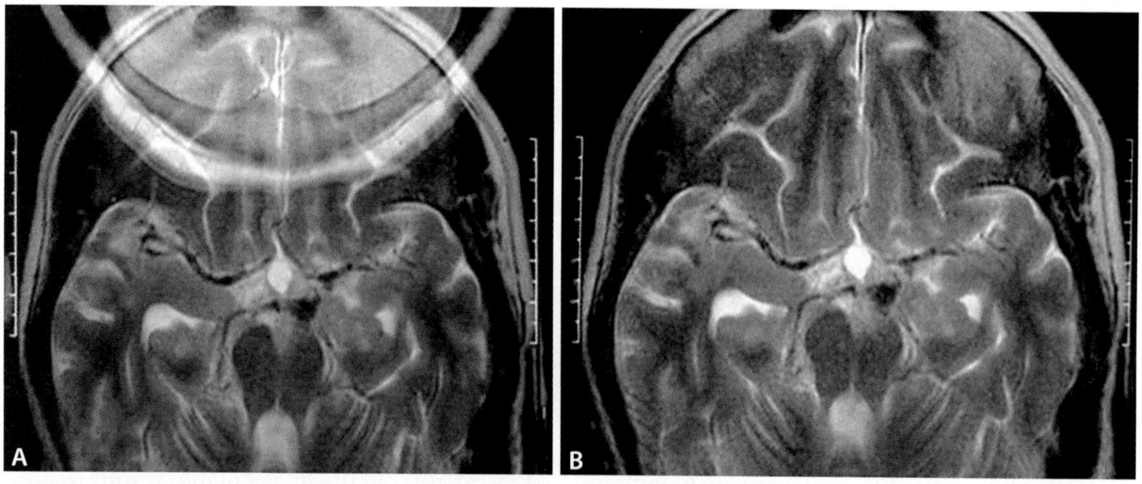

Figs. 10A and B: Aliasing artifact: T2-weighted axial images of the brain depict aliasing artifact when it was acquired with a reduced FOV smaller than the anatomy of the image. The tissue outside the FOV was misrepresented on the opposite side (A). This was overcome by oversampling in the phase encoding direction (B). However, there was no penalty in scan time as NEX was halved.

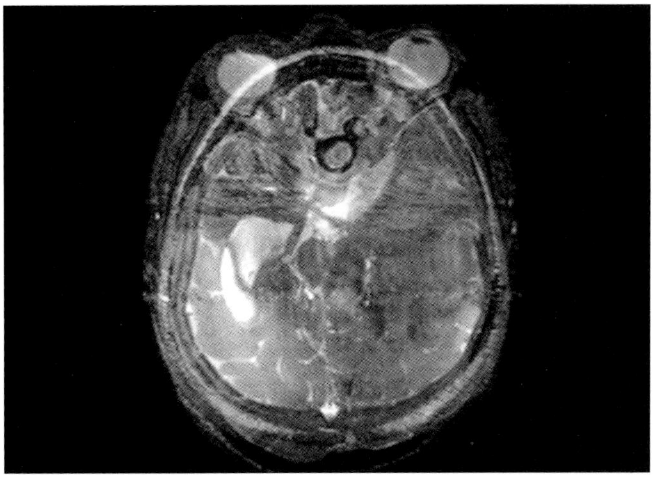

Fig. 11: Aliasing artifact in volume imaging: 3D constructive interference in steady state (CISS) GRE sequence shows overlap of information of the first and last sections of the sequence due to aliasing.

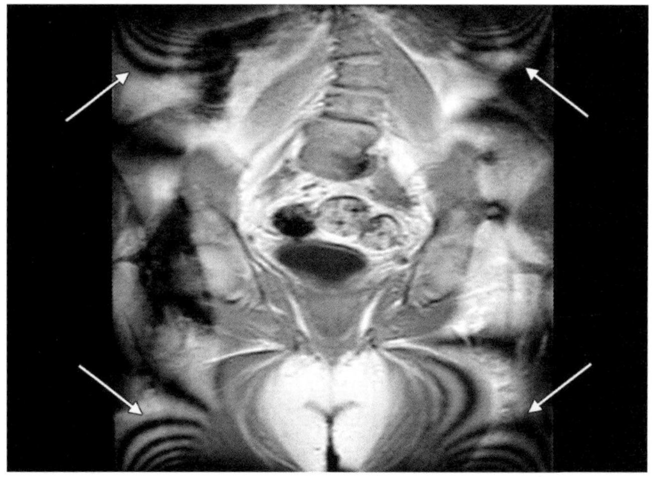

Fig. 12: Moiré artifact: T1-gradient coronal image of the abdomen in a heavy patient using a large FOV that is still smaller than the patient depicts the Moiré artifact. This is seen as stripes (arrows), and occurs as a result of a combination of aliasing and field inhomogeneities between the two edges. These are especially prominent at areas of susceptibility borders (e.g. air tissue interfaces).

Swapping the phase and frequency encoding direction: The phase encoding and frequency encoding directions may also be swapped if the phase encoding is not already along the shorter axis.

Oversampling/no phasewrap: Oversampling may be done in the phase encoding direction. This is done by increasing the sampling points; however, these are not used for image creation **(*see* Figs. 10A and B)**. The FOV is doubled in the phase direction along with doubling of the phase matrix to avoid any decrease in spatial resolution. Oversampling increases the scan time. Hence the NEX is usually halved to compensate for doubling of phase matrix. Usually, there is no penalty in scan time, SNR and spatial resolution. This may not be possible in fast scan techniques like those in abdominal imaging, when NEX is already minimum.

Saturation pulse/regional coils: Aliasing can also be minimized by suppressing signal from outside the region of interest using a presaturation pulse or with the use of regional coils to diminish the amount of signal received from outside the region of interest.

In 3D sequences, aliasing can be minimized by exciting only a limited part of the volume in the Z-direction by applying a Z-gradient pulse during the RF excitation.

Moiré /Fringe Artifact

In heavy patients, a special artifact may be seen in coronal imaging when a large field of view which is still smaller than the object is used. This results in aliasing superimposed on phase differences between the two edges. Over large fields of view, homogeneity of the field degrades at the edges, causing phase differences between the edges. Aliasing along with mismatched phases over the edges produces the moiré or fringe artifact **(Fig. 12)**. These are seen in gradient echo images. Use of spin-echo sequences eliminates these artifacts. Another measure that may be taken to reduce these artifacts is to ensure that the arms of the patient are by the side of his/her body while positioning so that they are within the FOV while imaging chest/abdomen.

Chemical-shift Artifacts

The chemical-shift phenomenon can be defined as the signal-intensity alterations that occur due to the inherent differences in the resonant frequencies of precessing protons. Clinically, the chemical-shift phenomenon is most evident between the signals of water and lipid. In water, hydrogen is linked to oxygen and in fat, it is linked to carbon. The protons hence have different chemical environments. When placed in an external magnetic field, these protons have slightly different precessional frequencies. Hydrogen in fat resonates at a lower frequency than water. Because fat and water protons have different precessional frequencies, these are allocated to different image pixels along the frequency encoding axis. Although this occurs throughout the image, this is most apparent at fat fluid interfaces, e.g. in imaging of fluid filled structures like bladder, orbits and kidneys which are surrounded by fat. When the chemical shift misregistration is greater than or equal to the size of an individual pixel, a dark or bright band of signal intensity will occur at the lipid-water interface in the frequency-encoding direction of the image. The dark bands appear because of the shifting of the lipid proton signals to a lower frequency, away from the actual lipid–water interface, which causes a signal void. The bright bands result from the overlapping of water signal with "shifted" lipid signal on the high-frequency side of the interface. Despite their presence, the bright bands may be more difficult to appreciate when an object with curved surface is being imaged.

The approximate chemical shift between lipid and water is 3.5 parts per million. At field strength of 1.5 T, protons from fat resonate at a point approximately 220 Hz downfield from water protons. This difference is directly proportional to magnetic field strength. The number of pixels involved in this shift is directly proportional to the field strength and frequency matrix but inversely related to the receiver bandwidth.

$$CSA = \Delta\omega \cdot N_{freq}/BW_{rec}$$

CSA = chemical sift artifact, $\Delta\omega$ = frequency difference between fat and water dependent on field strength, N_{freq} = frequency matrix, BW_{rec} = receiver bandwidth

In high-field-strength magnets, frequency difference between fat and water increases, resulting in greater CSA. However, higher SNR at this field strength allows higher bandwidth sampling rates, which diminishes these artifacts. Use of narrow receiver bandwidths and large matrix in the frequency encoding direction can accentuate these artifacts. These artifacts were commonly seen in T2-weighted images before the invention of TSE imaging as the former used low bandwidths to increase the low SNR inherent in T2-weighted sequences.

Remedy: To reduce these artifacts, various measures may be taken. The phase and frequency-encoding direction may be swapped. The frequency-encoding direction may be used along the axis where there is narrow fluid–fat interface or in a direction where this artifact does not hamper the primary area of interest. Suppression of fat or water signal by the use of STIR/chemical/spectral presaturation is another means of reducing this artifact.

Receiver bandwidth is another parameter that may be altered to reduce this artifact. Receiver bandwidth is the range of frequencies sampled within the FOV during readout in the frequency encoding direction. When this is increased, more frequencies are mapped across the same number of pixels. Consequently, there is a reduction in the chemical shift. However, when we increase the receiver bandwidth, signal to noise ratio of the image drops.

Advantage

Chemical shift along the frequency axis forms the basis of MR spectroscopic imaging.

Chemical Shift in Echoplanar Imaging

These artifacts also occur with echoplanar imaging, but in the phase-encoding direction. These are fast sequences where images are acquired in 50–80 ms. The receiver bandwidth is normally very large in the frequency encoding direction (greater than 100 kHz), hence chemical shift is not appreciable in this direction. However, the phase encoding occurs in a continuous fashion with a low bandwidth, resulting in pronounced chemical shift artifacts in this direction. Fat suppression techniques are necessarily used to minimize the artifact **(Figs. 13A and B)**.

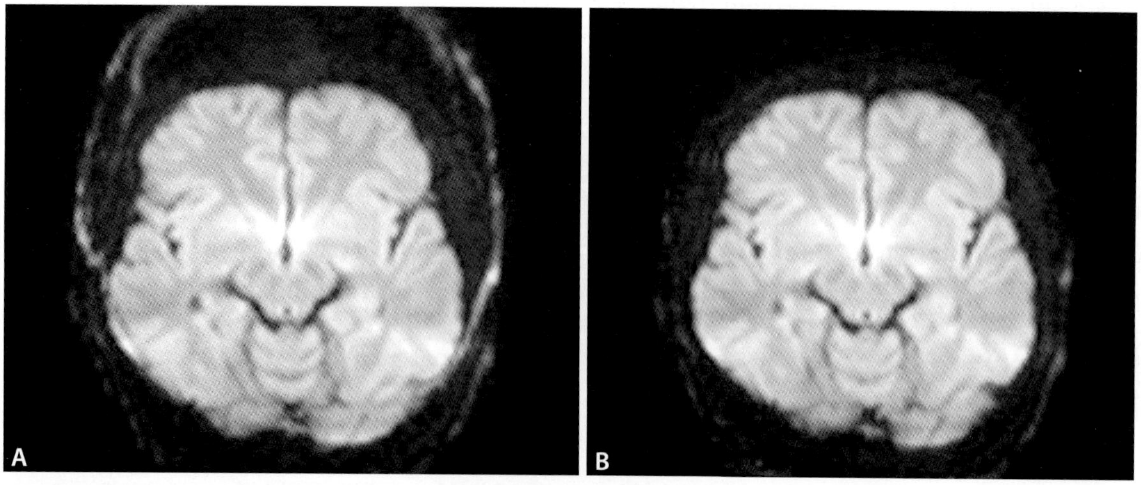

Figs. 13A and B: Chemical-shift artifact: (A) Echoplanar imaging depicts chemical shift artifact in phase encoding direction which is anterior to posterior; (B) Fat-suppression technique can be used to minimize the artifact.

Phase-cancellation Artifact

This is the second artifact induced by chemical-shift differences between fat and water protons. It can also be referred to as chemical-shift artifact of the second kind. These artifacts are observed in gradient-echo images and not in spin echo sequences which use a 180° refocusing pulse. This pulse redirects the fat and water proton spins back into phase with respect to one other by the time of readout (TE). The lack of a 180° refocusing radio-frequency pulse in gradient-echo sequences results in the cycling of fat and water proton signals in and out of phase with respect to each other over time. The time interval between fat and water being in phase is called the periodicity. This time, depends on the frequency shift and hence the field strength. At 1.5 T, the periodicity is 4.8 ms. This periodicity decreases at lower field strengths, hence the time at which fat and water protons are in phase with each other increases at low field strengths. At 1.5 T, fat and water signals precess in phase approximately every 4.8 msec; every 7.2 ms at 1.0 T; and every 36.7 msec at 0.2 T.

This periodicity is used to obtain in-phase and opposed-phase MR images. In in-phase images, fat and water have the same phase orientation. The signal contribution of fat and water protons therefore is additive in the final image. In opposed-phase images, the transverse magnetization of fat and water cancel each other. Hence, in voxels containing equal fat and water such as those at interfaces between fat and water based tissues, this signal cancellation results in a dark ring surrounding the tissue, also known as contour artifact **(Figs. 14A and B)**.

Advantage

Opposed-phase images are used to detect intracellular fat and can be used in assessment of fatty infiltration of liver, adrenal masses and in assessment of marrow infiltration.

Truncation Artifacts

Truncation or Gibbs artifacts are ripple like features that appear at regions of abrupt transition between high and low signal intensity structures, e.g. in T1 weighted images when high signal from fat at the edge of the region is still present at the end of data collection or in T2 weighted MR images of the spine at the interface of low signal intensity spinal cord with high signal intensity CSF. These are seen as stripes or rings in the image with alternating high and low signal intensity. These are also known as edge oscillations.

These artifacts are a result of insufficient digital sampling of the echo. Since there is a limited window period available for measurement of signal, there is interruption of this measurement at certain locations and data is truncated or omitted in k-space. Approximation errors in Fourier transformation of these signals lead to truncation artifacts. As Fourier transformation is better used for estimating gradual transitions, abrupt transitions at high contrast interfaces results in these artifacts.

These sharp borders which exist between areas of high contrast are represented by high spatial frequency data. The highest sampled frequency is inversely proportional to the size of the pixels. When we use a lower matrix, i.e. a bigger pixel size in the phase encoding direction, the higher frequencies are cut off, which leads to incorrect

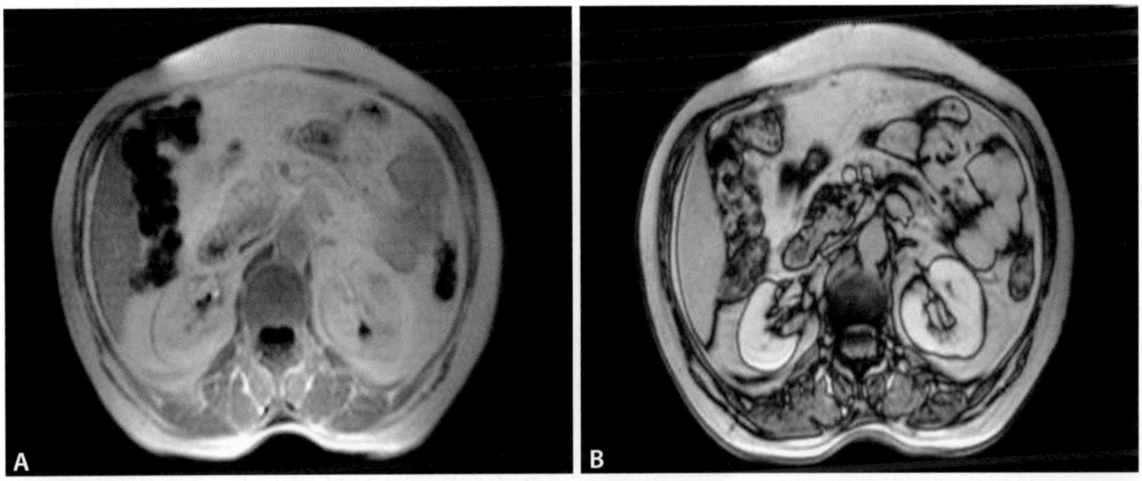

Figs. 14A and B: Phase-cancellation artifact: In (A) and opposed (B) phase-gradient echo MR images of the abdomen at TE 4.8 msec and TE 2.4 msec, respectively in a 1.5 T MR system show a dark rim surrounding the structures at fat water interfaces on the opposed phase images.

imaging of sharp edge lines. These artifacts can be seen in both phase and frequency encoding direction. However, they are usually seen in the phase encoding direction because usually a smaller phase matrix is used as compared to frequency matrix in order to reduce the acquisition time.

Remedy: These artifacts can be diminished by reducing the size of pixels, by increasing the acquisition matrix. However, this occurs at the expense of reduced SNR and increased acquisition time. Another method of reducing these artifacts is by applying various filters. Raw data filters may be used prior to Fourier transformation (e.g. Fermi, Gaussian, Hanning filters). These filters force the signal amplitude to zero at the end of data collection period. These improve the SNR of the image as high frequency noise is removed from the signal. However, excessive filtering may result in loss of sharpness of the image as this eliminates high frequencies responsible for edge definition, resulting in blurring. Image reconstruction of rectangular raw data matrices automatically uses a weak filter.

Magnetic Susceptibility Difference Artifacts

Magnetic susceptibility is a measure of spin polarization or magnetization induced by external magnetic field. The magnetic field contribution from the tissue may add to or subtract from the main magnetic field, depending upon whether the structure is paramagnetic or diamagnetic respectively. Differences in tissue susceptibility hence lead to magnetic-field inhomogeneities. Tissues, such as cortical bone or air filled organs, such as lungs and bowel have small magnetic susceptibility. Soft tissues, on the other hand, have more polarisable material and greater tissue susceptibility. At the interface between these regions with high and low magnetic susceptibility, significant distortion artifacts result due to local magnetic field gradients or field inhomogeneities. These result from enhanced dephasing of protons located at the boundaries of structures with a very different magnetic susceptibility. These artifacts are seen as areas of signal void. The second effect is that of strong distortion of the main magnetic field resulting in geometric distortion of anatomy **(Figs. 15A and B)**. The paranasal sinuses, the orbits, the lungs, heart, stomach and intestinal loops are the problematic areas. These are also observed in kidneys and bladder after administration of paramagnetic contrast agent which concentrates in these organs leading to significant signal loss.

These artifacts are more pronounced with gradient echo sequences **(Fig. 15A)** and EPI imaging **(Fig. 16A)**. In gradient echo imaging, signal amplitude is a function of T2*, in which proton dephasing from magnetic field inhomogeneities is an important factor that affects image contrast. On the other hand, spin-echo sequences use a refocusing 180° pulse which rephases the protons and hence minimizes these artifacts **(Fig. 15B)**. With EPI imaging, the entirety of k-space is filled by data from one RF pulse. This single-shot readout using gradient refocusing over a long period is predisposed to these artifacts. Generally, high bandwidth of this sequence in frequency encoding direction protects it from these distortions in this direction. However, low bandwidth in EPI sequence in the phase encoding direction affects distortions in this direction. Therefore, the phase encoding gradient is oriented along the axis of the susceptibility gradient (anteroposterior direction while imaging the

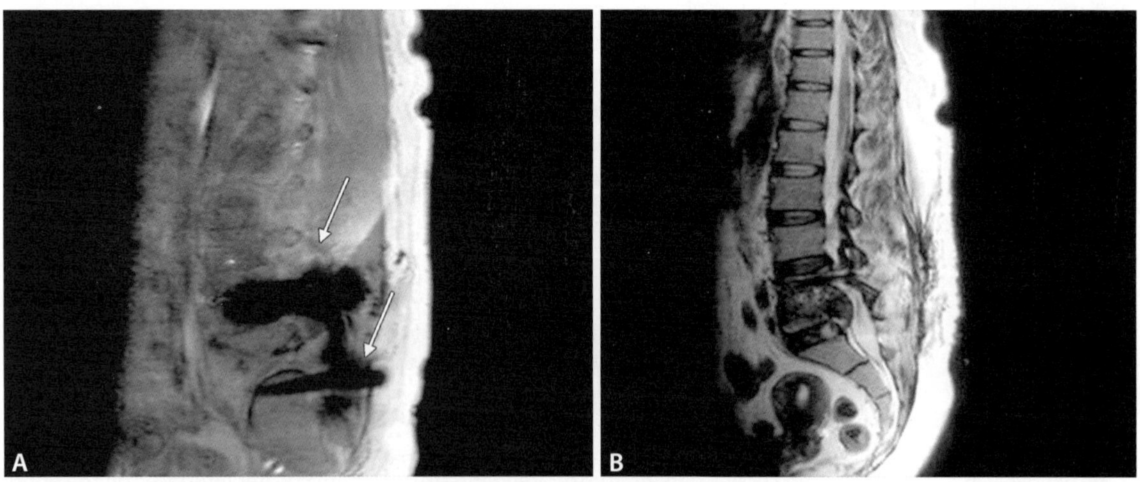

Figs. 15A and B: Magnetic-susceptibility artifact: Gradient-echo sagittal image of the spine shows magnetic susceptibility artifact due to a metal fixator, seen as areas of signal void and geometric distortion (arrows in A). Use of spin-echo sequence (B) minimizes the artifact.

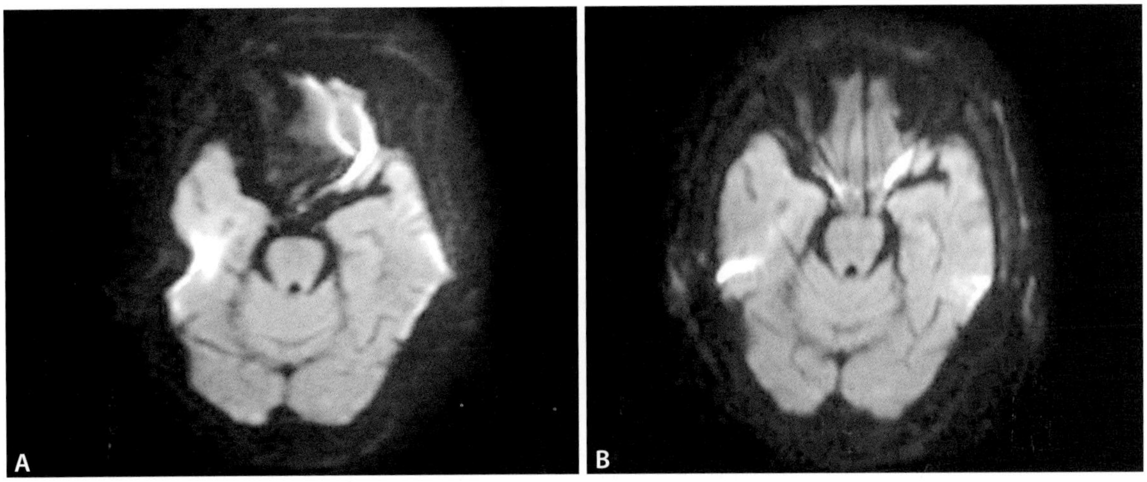

Figs. 16A and B: Magnetic-susceptibility artifact: Echoplanar imaging shows marked distortion when the phase-encoding gradient is from right to left (A). This is minimized by keeping the direction of the phase-encoding gradient from anterior to posterior, and hence, along the susceptibility gradient in brain (B).

brain) to reduce the distortion in EPI imaging **(Fig. 16B)**. The higher the field strength of the main magnetic field, the stronger are these artifacts. Also, these artifacts are more pronounced when sequences having long echo times are applied. The longer the TE, greater is the time available for dephasing of protons.

Remedy: Following remedies may be done to eliminate or reduce these artifacts. Spin echo sequences may be used which use a rephasing 180° pulse. TE may be reduced as longer the TE, greater is the time available for dephasing of protons. The best combination of spin echo and short TE is found in fast spin echo techniques rather than the conventional spin echo sequences. The voxel size may be reduced to reduce the local magnetic field inhomogeneities. Larger bandwidth sequences also reduce these artifacts. Although these susceptibility artifacts are more pronounced at higher field strengths, inherent improvement in SNR in 3T systems allows the use of higher bandwidth and parallel imaging to reduce these artifacts. These artifacts can be reduced in multishot EPI acquisitions, with parallel imaging and with radial k-space sampling technique.

Advantage

These artifacts can be of great advantage when hemorrhage is being investigated, as blood products become more apparent due to magnetic susceptibility or blooming artifacts. They are also used to our advantage as they form the basis of perfusion imaging, functional imaging of the brain, quantification of liver iron content and use of reticuloendothelial specific agents in liver imaging.

Section Cross Talk

In multisection two dimensional sequences, crosstalk artifact can result if there is no interslice gap. This is a result of imperfect shape of the RF slice profiles which should ideally be rectangular but are actually more curved shaped. Side lobes of RF pulses can excite part of adjacent sections. Hence these are excited twice by an RF pulse in the same TR, resulting in saturation and low-signal intensity. This is seen in all sections except the first and last slices.

This is not seen in three dimensional sequences as the whole volume of tissue is excited together and gradients are used to obtain sections within this volume.

Remedy: This can be overcome by using RF pulses with sharper section profiles, increasing the gap between sections, and/or imaging multiple sections in separate batches (interleaving).

Parallel-imaging Artifact

Parallel-imaging techniques such as GRAPPA and SENSE help us to reduce acquisition time by extrapolating data before and after Fourier transformation, respectively. However, we must take care to avoid very high acceleration factors as the noise level increases and SNR falls with use of high acceleration factor. This noise can be seen in the center of the image **(Figs. 17A and B)**. Also, if field of view is smaller than the object being imaged, increased noise can be seen in addition to aliasing artifact. This aliasing artifact may also be projected in the central portion of the image. This moves outwards as the parallel imaging factor is reduced.

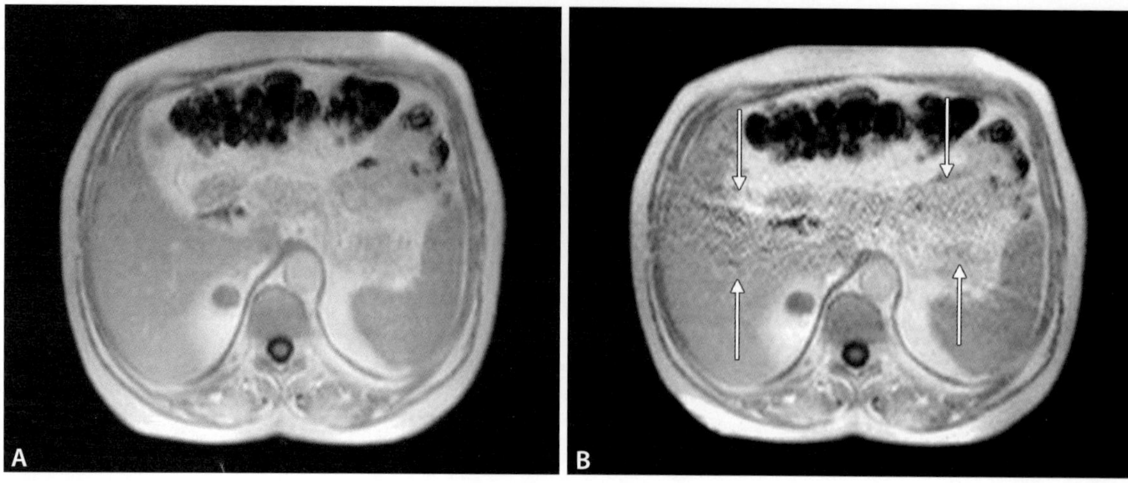

Figs. 17A and B: Parallel-imaging artifact: Axial T1-weighted gradient image acquired without parallel imaging (A) and axial T1-gradient image acquired with a parallel imaging factor of 2 (B) shows noise and reconstruction artifacts in the middle of the FOV in the latter image (arrows) which limit the diagnostic quality of the image.

External Artifacts

External artifacts are generated from sources other than the patient. These could be classified into two categories—those that are hardware related and those that are not. Improper calibration of gradients, RF transmitter and receiver system can lead to various distortions and incorrect spatial localization. The gradient system and RF transmitter system can sometimes malfunction and work in an unstable manner. This can result in amplitude and phase modulations resulting in ghosting or smearing artifacts and occur throughout the image field in the phase encoding direction. These may be indistinguishable from motion artifacts. These system related artifacts could be transient effects generated within one or more of the subsystems or could be a sign of degradation of some of the electronic components in the subsystem.

Artifacts Caused by Field Distortions

Distortions artifacts may be caused by main magnetic field inhomogeneities or nonlinearity of the gradient field or RF field inhomogeneities.

Main field inhomogeneities: Although most manufacturers very carefully construct MR systems with homogeneous magnetic fields, but some inhomogeneities still occur because of field falloff towards the magnet periphery. This is more pronounced in large bore or open MR systems. This is especially important in spectral-fat suppression sequences. If the magnetic field is not homogeneous, fat suppression pulse may not uniformly suppress the fat. This is mostly seen at the edges of an image with large FOV. To minimize the artifact, the anatomy should be centered within the magnet as much as possible and field homogeneity correction should be done just prior to the scan, with the patient inside the scanner.

Distortions in the main magnetic field may also result from ferromagnetic substances like zippers, metal clips on the patient's body/clothing **(*see* Figs. 15A and B)**. These result in magnetic susceptibility artifacts as described above, but these are more severe as metals have much higher magnetic susceptibility than body tissues. These can be minimized by using fast SE sequences using a high bandwidth and decreased echo time. However, care should be taken in these cases as metallic objects can result in more energy absorption and heating as compared to normal body tissues.

Gradient-field nonlinearity: Gradient-field nonlinearity is related to gradient falloff due to finite size of gradient coils. Gradient coil produces a varying magnetic field that is linear through the isocenter of the magnet but tapers towards the side of the magnet. This leads to distortion and loss in spatial resolution. In a large FOV image, gradient field distortion is seen as compression of the structures at the edge of the image **(Fig. 18A)**. As this is a predictable artifact, MR imaging software can correct these distortions before the final image is reconstructed. Postprocessing techniques can also correct the distortions but not the accompanying loss in spatial resolution **(Fig. 18B)**.

RF-field inhomogeneities: Inhomogeneities in RF pulse are not the cause of geometric distortions but can lead to non-uniformity in signal. These may be due to problems in RF construction or from dielectric (standing wave) effects. Dielectric effect is especially prominent at 3T

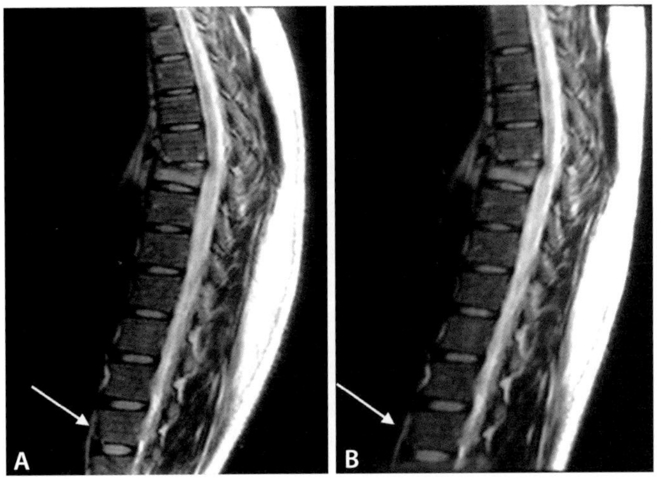

Figs. 18A and B: Field distortion due to gradient-field nonlinearity: Sagittal T2-weighted image of the thoracic spine shows geometric distortions resulting from gradient nonlinearity, with vertebral bodies appearing progressively smaller toward the inferior edge of the FOV (arrow in A). Distortion correction software was used to correct the distortion (arrow in B).

systems because high-frequency low-wavelength RF pulse is required to excite protons at this high-field strength because of increased Larmor frequency of protons. The wavelength of these RF pulses approximates the dimensions of the anatomic structure and standing waves may result. These waves manifest as bands of destructive and constructive interference, seen as dark and bright zones respectively. Dielectric pads may also be used to change the patient's apparent girth to reduce the effect.

RF field distortions can also lead to inhomogeneous fat suppression on STIR imaging. RF shimming can help reduce the artifact. Alternatively, spectral-fat saturation may be used instead of STIR sequence to suppress fat. STIR is a nonspecific technique of fat suppression, as signal is suppressed from all tissues with a T1 equal to that of fat. Spectral-fat saturation, in contradistinction, suppresses the fat signal only because it is based upon differentiation of resonant frequency of fat from water.

Spike (Herringbone) Artifact

Spikes are noise bursts of short duration that can occur randomly during data collection. These are a result of loose electrical connections that produce arcs or because of breakage of interconnections in an RF coil. These are more frequently encountered when gradients are applied at high-duty cycle, e.g. in echoplanar imaging. These produce bad data points or a spike of noise, in k-space. Fourier transformation of this spike of noise results in a specific 'crisscross' or 'herringbone' pattern seen as dark stripes overlaid on the image **(Fig. 19)**. Spike noise is usually transient but can become chronic if not attended to.

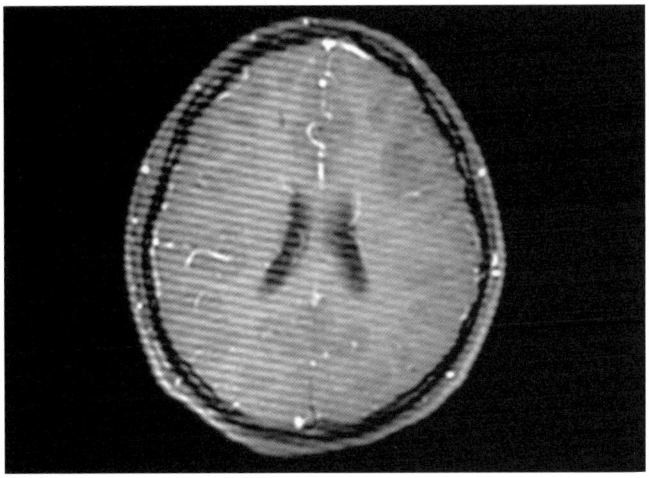

Fig. 19: Spike or herringbone artifact: Loss of data points in the process of acquisition due to a spike of noise can lead to a "crisscross" or "herringbone" pattern of artifact.

Advantage

This pattern of stripes produced by spiking can be utilized for tagging, which is a vital technique in cardiac imaging.

Zipper Artifact

Zipper artifact is an artifact that is caused by external interference resulting from external RF fields, as those caused by open doors, radios, mobile telephones, electronic controls, etc. These emit interfering electromagnetic signals that hamper MR image quality. Zipper artifact appears as a region of increased noise with a width of 1 or 2 pixels that extends perpendicular to the frequency encoding direction, throughout the image series.

Remedy: To prevent these artifacts, MR tomographs are installed in RF-sealed rooms, also known as Faraday cage. These sealed rooms not only protect the equipment from external RF interference but also shield the environment from RF fields generated by the tomograph. The door of the MR room should always be closed properly to prevent this interference. If any constructional changes take place after the installation of the MR tomograph, e.g. drilling holes for cables, it may lead to interference in RF shielding. In this case, the source of interference needs to be carefully looked for. Sometimes, electrical connections from any patient monitoring device which work on alternating current can also interfere with RF shielding. The persistence of the artifact even after the equipment is removed indicates compromise of the RF shield.

CONCLUSION

Clinical MR imaging is becoming more and more versatile and complex, making it difficult for the radiologist to grasp the physical principles underlining the changing technology. Nevertheless, knowledge of basic MR physics plays a key role in clinical imaging as its understanding can help us modify imaging protocols to obtain optimum image quality within acceptable scan time. Good-quality images enable us to reach the correct clinical diagnosis with greater confidence.

SUGGESTED READING

1. Brown MA, Semelka RC. Artifacts. In: MRI- Basic principles and applications, 3rd edn. New Jersey: Willey Liss Inc; 2003. pp. 113-40.
2. Brown MA, Semelka RC. Measurement parameters and image contrast. In: MRI- Basic principles and applications, 3rd edn. New Jersey: Willey Liss Inc; 2003. pp. 93-102.
3. Hood MN, Ho VB, Smirniotopoulas JG, Szumowski J. Chemical shift: the artifact and clinical tool revisited. Radiographics. 1999;19:357-71.
4. Mitchell DG, Cohen M. In: MRI principles, 2nd edn. Philadelphia, Pa: Saunders; 2004. p. 416.
5. Morelli JN, Runge VM, Ai F, Attenberger U, Vu L, Schmeets SH, Nitz WR, Kirsch JE. An image based approach to understanding the physics of MR artifacts. Radiographics. 2011;31:849-66.
6. Stadler A, Schima W, Ba-Ssalamah A, Kettenbach J, Eisenhuber E. Artifacts in body MR imaging: their appearance and how to eliminate them. Eur Radiol. 2007;17(5):1242-55.
7. Westbrook C. Artifacts. In: MRI at a glance, 1st Edition. Great Britain: Blackwell Science; 2002.pp.73-78.
8. Westbrook C. Image quality. In: MRI at a glance. 1st edn. Great Britain: Blackwell Science; 2002. pp. 64-72.
9. Yang RK, Rith CG, Ward RJ, deJesus JO, Mitchell DG. Optimising abdominal MNR imaging: approaches to common problems. Radiographics. 2010;30:185-99.
10. Zhuo F, Gullapaali RP. MR artifacts, safety and quality control. Radiographics. 2006;26:275-97.

CHAPTER 46

Diffusion-weighted Magnetic Resonance Imaging

Devasenathipathy Kandasamy, Raju Sharma

INTRODUCTION

Magnetic resonance imaging (MRI) imaging has become an important imaging tool in the current clinical practice mainly because of its excellent contrast resolution without the risk of any ionizing radiation. This has become even more relevant with the growing concern for radiation issues in computed tomography (CT) and other imaging modalities which utilize ionizing radiation. Diffusion-weighted imaging (DWI) is a promising technique which was originally described by Le Bihan 30 years back and because of the recent developments in MR hardware this has found a place in routine clinical MR protocols. The basic principle of DWI is based on the Brownian motion of water molecules which takes place in the body and it utilizes motion sensitizing gradients to study this motion.[1,2] It provides unique information at a microstructural and functional level which can be used to characterize cellular dense lesions and this has applications in oncology. Other reasons why this technique is appealing are that it can be performed rather quickly and does not require the use of exogenous contrast agents.

Diffusion can be assessed both qualitatively and quantitatively. It is quantified by the parameter called apparent diffusion coefficient (ADC) which is derived from the diffusion images. The ADC is a scalar quantity which has only magnitude without any directional information.[3] This chapter will focus on the basic principles of DWI and optimization of the technique and briefly review its clinical applications.

BASIC PRINCIPLE

Water molecules in the body undergo a random motion called "Brownian motion" which is as a result of body heat.[2] Theoretically, these constant random motions are uniform in all directions. But the diffusion in body tissues is restricted by various organelles, membranes and tissue planes. The intracellular diffusion is more hindered than the extracellular component because of the presence of cell membrane.[4] In case of malignant tumors the cells are densely packed with large nuclei and scanty cytoplasm which results in restriction of diffusion **(Fig. 1)**. On the other hand, benign cells are loosely packed with small nucleus and abundant cytoplasm that facilitates diffusion.[5] Because of the interaction of water molecule within biological tissues which can impede the actual diffusion the measured diffusion is termed as ADC which is expressed in mm^2/s. When the diffusion is not restricted in any particular direction it is called isotropic diffusion as seen in CSF space and cystic lesions. When the diffusion occurs preferentially in a particular direction it is called anisotropic diffusion which is usually seen in white matter of brain.[6] In white matter and peripheral nerves the water diffuses preferentially along the axon.

Diffusion-weighted imaging can generate images in which the contrast between the structures is based on the diffusion characteristics. There are various types of sequences with diffusion sensitising gradients incorporated within but the basis of all of them is the technique suggested by Stejskal and Tanner in 1965 and

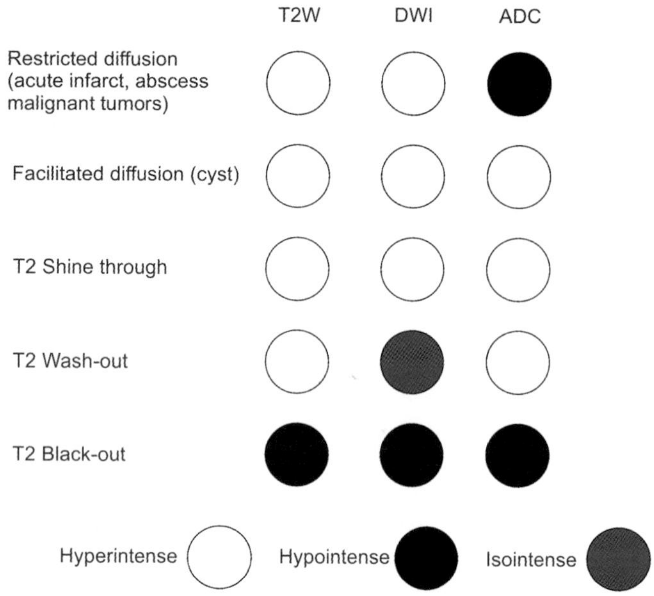

Fig. 1: Schematic representation of signal intensities on T2W, DW sequence and ADC map for disease entities and artifacts which are commonly encountered in day-to-day practice.

implemented by Le Bihan in 1986.[7,8] Their technique essentially involves adding two diffusion sensitizing gradient, one on either side of 180° refocusing pulse. These gradient lobes have the same magnitude but are opposite in direction. The first gradient lobe is called dephasing gradient which will dephase the spins of water molecules and the second is called the rephasing gradient which will rephase the spins to their original state. The 180° pulse will eliminate the dephasing due to the inhomogeneity of external magnetic field. This principle has been adopted with or without slight variation even in modern day sequences.[9] The idea behind this technique is that the water molecules whose diffusion is not restricted will get dephased by the first gradient lobe and during the process the molecules will move to another location in which the water molecules will be subjected to a different magnetic environment so that the rephasing pulse will not exactly rephase them to their original state. This will cause attenuation of signal from these water molecules as they are not exactly rephased to produce a strong echo. Whereas, water molecules whose diffusion is restricted will not move and they will be subjected to the same magnetic environment and the dephasing and rephasing gradients will exactly neutralize each other and their spins will be in phase to produce a strong echo. These diffusion gradients can be applied in any of the axis (x, y, z) or in any combination and it is called diffusion sensitizing direction. This diffusion gradient addition can be applied in spin echo or in steady state sequences as long as they have a long TE to accommodate them and this is the reason why the diffusion sequences are T2 weighted.

B VALUE

The magnitude, duration of diffusion gradient applied and the duration between the dephasing and rephasing lobe determines the sensitivity of the sequence to water diffusion which is described by a factor called diffusion weighting factor or b factor (s/mm^2). All the above factors are directly proportional to the b value. Usually, the magnitude is kept maximal and the other two are altered to get a desired b value. At least 2 b values are needed for the calculation of ADC and multiple b values are used for more accurate quantification.[2] When multiple b values are used the TE time which is maximum for highest b value is usually kept constant for all b values for better quantification.[6] The choice of b value is very important and depends on the hardware, region of study, type of sequence and the quantitative or qualitative nature of the study. The usual thumb rule is that b value is about inverse of the expected ADC value.[9] For example if the expected ADC value of a tissue is 1.2×10^{-3} then the approximate b value is 800. The SNR of the sequence is grossly affected by the b value selection. When the b value is increased, the SNR of the sequence reduces and at very high values the SNR becomes very low so as to make the quantification unreliable. At the same time low b value will not generate an image whose contrast characteristics are truly based on diffusivity of water molecules. So optimal b value is a balance between the SNR required for quantification and the diffusion contrast of the image. High b values (>1000) are used in imaging techniques like diffusion weighted whole body imaging with background body signal suppression (DWIBS) in which background signal suppression is important. Although multiple b values increase the accuracy of quantification of diffusion it also increase the acquisition time and associated artifacts. There are several approaches developed to circumvent these issues which are discussed later in the chapter.

APPARENT DIFFUSION COEFFICIENT AND EXPONENTIAL IMAGE

Apparent diffusion coefficient (ADC) image is a parametric map which is derived from the DW image and it is devoid of T2 shine through (vide infra). It needs images acquired at minimum of two b values to calculate ADC and in present day scanners the calculation of ADC map is automatic. The ADC value is dependent on the b value used where it is inversely proportional to the b values used even in the same patient. It is also dependent on the field strength of the scanner, gradient hardware and the type of image processing software used.[2] Since ADC map is the Gray Scale representation of pixel by pixel ADC values calculated from diffusion images, the artifacts associated with the diffusion sequences will also get reflected. In addition poor SNR in high b value images also adds to the deterioration of image quality. This is the reason for ADC map having poor image quality when compared to the diffusion image and in isolation it is not very useful for diagnostic purposes. Apparent diffusion coefficient values are usually inversely proportional to the degree of restriction. Area of restricted diffusion is seen as hyperintense on diffusion weighted images and hypointense on ADC and vice versa.

Another way to remove the T2 effect on the diffusion weighted image is generating an exponential image which is done by calculating the ratio of diffusion weighted image and b 0 image.[10] Contrary to ADC map, hyperintensity on the exponential image corresponds to hypointensity on ADC map and suggests diffusion restriction and vice versa.

DWI SEQUENCES AND OPTIMIZATION

Many sequences are altered to introduce the diffusion gradient pair for the development of DWI sequences. Some of the most commonly used sequences are discussed here.

Echo Planar Imaging

Although echo planar imaging (EPI) was initially proposed by Mansfield in 1978, it is the recent advancements in MR hardware and reconstruction software that made this sequence useful for clinical studies. It is an extremely fast technique which can fill the entire k space in single shot. It is robust and insensitive to motion artifacts which made it useful in DWI. After the initial excitation pulse, diffusion gradient pair, a series of fast gradient oscillations is applied for readout and the entire k-space is filled with a long echo train **(Fig. 2)**. This can be implemented as spin echo EPI or gradient echo EPI. Typically, separate acquisition is done for 3 orthogonal axes which are averaged into one final image. One of the disadvantages of EPI is significant phase shift gets accumulated between the water and fat protons and this leads to geometric distortion along the phase encoding direction.[6] As a result the fat signals can be offset by many pixels which will deteriorate the image quality, more so in higher field strengths. So, it is of paramount importance that all EPI sequences are done with fat suppression. There are various methods of fat suppression, such as water only excitation, chemical fat suppression, short-tau inversion recovery (STIR) and spectral selection attenuated inversion recovery (SPAIR) of which the latter two are inversion recovery sequences. SPAIR is a very good method of fat suppression for small FOV in which the fat suppression is uniform along with good SNR. For larger FOV, STIR is the best method to provide uniform suppression but at the cost of reduced SNR. Another disadvantage of EPI is that in longer echo train the water protons tend to show phase shift especially in the air-soft tissue and bone-soft tissue interfaces resulting in geometric distortion in the phase encoding direction.[9] This can be reduced by using parallel imaging and high-performance gradient coils which will shorten the echo train length, echo spacing and the readout time. Another problem with single shot EPI is limited spatial resolution in the order of 128 × 128 because of the rapid signal decay and limited SNR. These problems can also be reduced by splitting the acquisition into more than one excitation. This is a challenge if it has to be implemented in body imaging where motion is an important consideration. For body diffusion several approaches are followed which are discussed here. First approach is to perform a single shot acquisition with breath hold in which the disadvantages are the poor spatial resolution, limited number of b values, less number of averages and less anatomical coverage. Poor SNR can lead to unreliable ADC values. Second approach is acquisition across multiple excitations with respiratory/cardiac trigger. This overcomes the problems with single shot breath hold technique. However, triggers cannot totally rule out motion artifacts and the imaging time gets prolonged. Third approach is free breathing technique with multiple averages and can use multiple b values.[11] Regarding the choice of b values it is a balance between the accuracy

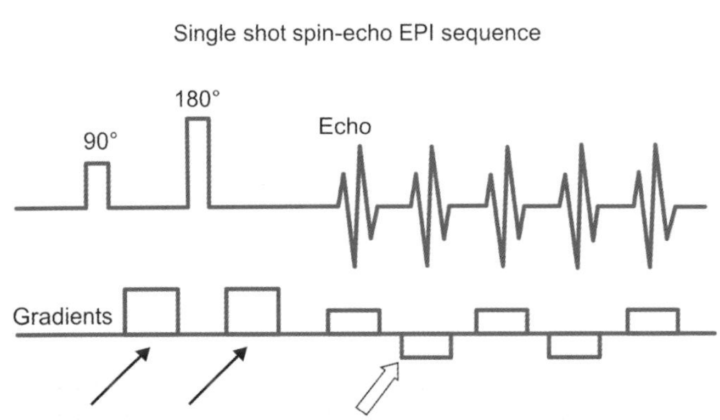

Fig. 2: Schematic representation of DW spin echo EPI sequence showing the motion probing gradients (arrows) used to detect the diffusion of water molecules and multiple gradient oscillations (outlined arrow) to generate echoes. In this single-shot sequence, the entire k space is filled in single excitation.

of quantification and contrast resolution in the diffusion image (vide supra).

Turbo Spin Echo Sequences or Half-Fourier-acquisition Single-shot Turbo-spin Echo

This is an alternative to DW-EPI sequence and it is also relatively insensitive to motion and can perform a single shot readout and the entire k-space is filled in single excitation. An important difference from EPI is that 180° refocusing pulse is applied during each readout so that the phase shift accumulation, because of long echo train, is avoided **(Fig. 3)**. This reduces the geometric distortion and susceptibility artifacts. Apart from this it has other disadvantages of single shot EPI sequence. Parallel imaging can improve the spatial resolution and reduction of geometric distortions. This sequence can also be segmented into multi-shot acquisition which has similar advantages as multi-shot EPI.

Steady-state Free-precession

Steady-state free-precession (SSFP) is also a fast sequence so it is relatively insensitive to motion. It is an atypical diffusion sequence in comparison to the above two with regard to the usage of diffusion sensitizing gradients. Here, both the dephasing and the rephasing gradients are not applied in the same repetition time (TR). They are applied in different TRs and not necessarily in the immediately following TRs. Consequently, it is almost impossible to quantitate the diffusion using this sequence. However, the contrast resolution is excellent so that it can be used for qualitative assessment of images. Recently, three-dimensional diffusion weighted sequences have also been developed.

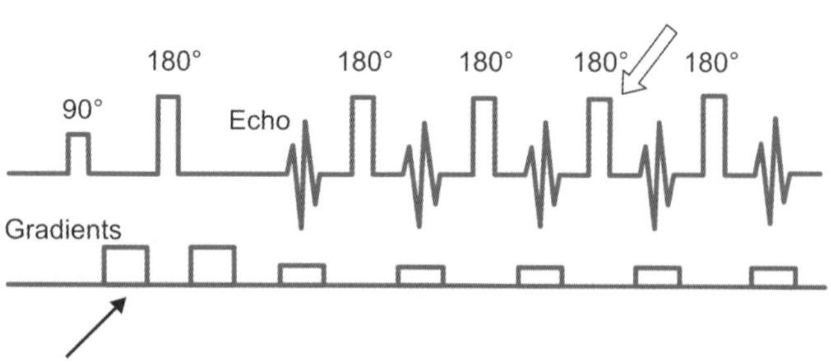

Fig. 3: Schematic representation of single shot fast spin echo sequence showing motion probing gradients (arrow) to detect the water diffusion. Multiple 180° refocusing pulses (outlined arrow) rather than gradient oscillations are used to generate echoes. In contrast to SE-EPI sequence, the use of refocusing pulses avoid the accumulation of phase shifts thereby reducing artifacts. This is also a fast sequence which is capable of acquiring the entire image in single excitation.

ARTIFACTS AND PITFALLS

There are many artifacts and pitfalls which are inherent to the technique itself, so it is very important for the radiologists and the technicians to be aware of those. In this chapter we will discuss few of the important ones which are relevant to clinical practice.

T2 Shine Through

This is one of the well-known phenomenon which can potentially lead to a wrong diagnosis when diffusion weighted images are interpreted in isolation. It is because DW sequence is based on a T2 weighted sequence and its effects are shown in the final image. It is very prominent in low b value images where the T2 effects predominate. For example, simple cysts in which diffusion is not restricted are seen as hyperintense structure on DW images. The ADC map or exponential images can help overcome this pitfall since both of them eliminate the T2 effect in the image and represent diffusion characteristics only **(Fig. 1)**. In the above example of simple cyst the ADC map will show hyperintensity because of unrestricted diffusion. At the same time when the lesion is hyperintense on T2 weighted images and hypointense on ADC, the hyperintensity in DW images will get accentuated.[6] When multiple b value images are available then the hyperintensity which is due to T2 effect decreases with increase in b value whereas the hyperintensity due to diffusion is retained.

T2 Washout

This phenomenon is seen when the T2 hyperintensity is balanced by the increase in ADC in the DW image.[12] This is usually seen in vasogenic edema in which there is increase in ADC because of increased diffusivity and that effect is balanced by the T2 hyperintensity. Thus in the DW image the lesion appears isointense. Again this effect can be circumvented by interpreting DW images along with ADC map in which the lesion appears hyperintense **(*see* Fig. 1)**.

T2 Blackout

This effect is noted when the T2 hypointensity is reflected on the DW image as hypointensity **(Fig. 1)**. It is usually seen in hematoma which is seen as T2 hypointensity because of susceptibility effect.[13,14]

Eddy Current Artifacts

Eddy current artifact is worth mentioning here because it is commonly associated with EPI sequences which is the most common sequence used for DWI. Eddy Currents are produced in the patient body and in the scanner hardware by rapidly changing magnetic gradients which are used in EPI sequence for sensing diffusion and readout. This can cause image distortion, spatial blurring and misregistration artifacts. This necessitates postprocessing of the data before ADC calculation to prevent quantification errors.[15] This artifact can also be reduced by using proper shielding in the hardware.

Susceptibility Artifacts

This is also commonly seen in EPI sequences at the bone-soft tissue or air–soft tissue interface like close to skull base, sinuses, mastoids, bowel and lung bases. This leads to accumulation of phase shifts which are more pronounced in the phase encoding direction. This gets even worse if the matrix size is increased because of prolonged readout time. This can be reduced by using DW-HASTE sequences in which the phase shifts are periodically corrected or by using multi-shot acquisition or by using parallel imaging so that the readout time is reduced.

Chemical-shift Artifacts

Usually in conventional spin echo sequences the effect of difference in precession frequency of water and fat protons are seen along the frequency encoding direction. Whereas in EPI sequences the artifact is seen along the phase encoding direction and it is very prominent again because of accumulation of phase shifts during longer readouts. This can be prevented by using effective fat suppression techniques (vide supra).

Motion Artifacts

Motion artifacts are due to gross patient movement or cardiac/respiratory/bowel motion. Although the currently available single shot techniques are fast enough to avoid motion artifacts, multi-shot techniques suffer from motion in body imaging. This can be reduced by using cardiac/respiratory triggered sequences, parallel imaging, propeller or high-amplitude gradients.[2]

Effect of Contrast Media

The gadolinium-based contrast media used for MR imaging can have an effect on the diffusion parameters especially in kidneys where they are concentrated by causing paramagnetic effects locally. Recent evidence suggests that the ADC values of kidneys can be significantly lower in the postcontrast image than the precontrast image. Similar effects were not found in the liver, pancreas and spleen.[16]

ADVANCED DW TECHNIQUES

Diffusion Tensor Imaging

There are newer techniques, such as diffusion tensor imaging (DTI) which have both magnitude and the directional information of diffusion also. The DTI is extensively studied in brain where it is used to show the white matter tracts. It uses the property of anisotropy of diffusion of water molecules. Because of the myelinated axons in the brain white matter, the diffusion is unhindered along the direction of the fiber which is called diffusion anisotropy. Diffusion information given by the DWI is a scalar quantity which lacks the directional component. To obtain the directional component gradient lobes are used in multiple directions and the resulting data is processed. As a result each voxel has the effective direction of diffusion which is called as Eigen vector and the value of diffusion in that direction is called as Eigen value. This information is used to reconstruct fiber tract network in the brain which is called as tractography. Although this tensor model holds good in many situations, it can be limited if there are crossing fibers with different direction of diffusion in a voxel. So there are newer approaches to overcome this limitation, such as high angular resolution diffusion imaging (HARDI) which can be used to study the complex diffusion process.

Whole Body Diffusion-weighted Imaging

There is evidence that whole body DWI along with anatomical images, such as T1 and T2 can be very useful for the evaluation of malignant tumors.[2,17] The DWIBS is a whole body diffusion technique which is done typically using DW-EPI sequence and STIR for fat suppression. It is a free breathing technique in which the scans are usually taken from the skull base till the level of mid-thigh. Acquisition is done in multiple stations using multiple thin slices and a large number of signals are collected and averaged. Typically, b value in the range of 1000 is used which will provide good background suppression. But, more than one b value can be used if quantification is needed at the expense of time. These multiple slices are fused and usually displayed in inverted gray scale with white background similar to PET images. It can be visualized as radial projections of MIP in coronal plane. Because of the high b value, body fat muscle and most of the organs gets suppressed which highlights the abnormal areas. However, normal structures with restricted diffusion, such as spleen, lymph nodes, uterus, ovary and testis can be seen. The MIP images should always be interpreted along with the source images because improper fat suppression can lead to pseudotumor appearance. One disadvantage of this technique is long acquisition time. It has been shown to perform as well as PET/CT in the evaluation of tumors, such as lymphoma and nonsmall cell lung cancer.[18] The DWIBS is a noninvasive technique without the use of radiation and has a huge potential in oncologic imaging.

DIFFUSION KURTOSIS IMAGING

Diffusion of water molecules in a homogeneous solution follows a Gaussian distribution whereas diffusion of water molecules in biological tissues actually follows a non-Gaussian distribution.[19] This difference in distribution is because of cellular microstructure (cell membranes and organelles) which alter the water diffusion.[14] It is especially true in the brain where diffusion is restricted by the myelinated axons. Quantification of non-Gaussian diffusion can be useful in characterization of intracellular structures. Kurtosis is a metric which quantifies the non-Gaussianity of any distribution. Generally, a large kurtosis signifies higher diffusional heterogeneity and tissue complexity. This principle has been studied in the brain imaging especially in ischemia with promising results.

Intravoxel Incoherent Motion

Intravoxel incoherent motion (IVIM) was initially described by Le Bihan in 1980s.[8,20] They described D* as pseudo-diffusion coefficient which is dependent on capillary perfusion. The IVIM is based on the fact that the diffusion imaging at low b values (b 0–100) will have the effect of both the tissue perfusion (pseudo-diffusion) and the true diffusion. In fact at low b values the pseudo-diffusion predominates. This effect gets reduced at high b values where the true diffusion predominates. This is one proposed reason for decrease in ADC values with increase in b value. In a normally perfused tissue at low b value the motion of water molecules because of blood perfusion in tortuous capillary network adds to the actual water diffusion. So acquiring images at increasing b values would enable us to quantify the perfusion in a tissue noninvasively. Since IVIM is very sensitive to motion and other sequence related artifacts it should be performed with single shot EPI sequence and high-performance hardware. The current model available in most of the commercial scanners for the calculation of ADC is based on monoexponential function, considering that the logarithm of relative signal intensity plotted against the b value is a straight line which is not true.[21] So ADC calculated with the monoexponential fit would have a component of microcapillary perfusion in addition to true diffusion especially with low b values. The IVIM model suggests that the relationship between the signal intensity and b value is not monoexponential rather biexponential. Based on the IVIM model there is evidence that shows that DWI is sensitive to tissue perfusion and this potential can be applied to obtain the tissue perfusion assessment in addition to diffusion measurement.[21–24]

Histogram Analysis of ADC

Usually ADC value is calculated by drawing region of interest (ROI) which will typically provide mean or median ADC value of the region. Recently attempts have been made to use histogram based analysis of ADC values. In this, the ADC values across a region can be represented as histograms, i.e. frequency of voxels having the ADC values.[25] This will provide better understanding of heterogeneity of the lesion. It generally, utilizes volumetric evaluation of the lesion so that all the voxels of the lesion from different slices are evaluated rather than a selected ROI. The ADC calculation by this method is reproducible because the entire lesion is analyzed and the errors in ROI placement are reduced. Histogram analysis can provide various useful metrics, such as percentiles, kurtosis and skewness of distribution of ADC values which will provide better insights into the pattern of distribution. Comparison of these metrics based on histogram analysis between the pre- and post-treatment imaging can evaluate the response to therapy.

CLINICAL APPLICATIONS OF DWI

Although initially DWI was established and successfully used in neuroimaging, recent developments in the sequence protocols and their optimization, hardware enhancements and improvements in software have made this technique a robust tool for body imaging also.

Brain

Diffusion weighted imaging has become a gold standard in imaging of stroke to identify the infarct core mainly because of its ability to detect the infarcted area within minutes after the onset of symptoms, much earlier than other MRI sequences and CT can show changes.[26] Diffusion weighted imaging is highly sensitive (81–100%) and specific (86–100%) in detecting the ischemic area within 12 hours of symptom onset.[14] It is also superior to FLAIR and T2-weighted sequences in detecting small area of infarct and has the ability to differentiate acute infarct from old lesions and nonspecific white matter changes **(Figs. 4A to C)**. Those areas which show diffusion abnormality usually progress to infarction unless early thrombolysis therapy is started. The area of diffusion abnormality also correlates well with the final clinical outcome thereby directing appropriate management for patients. The DWI and ADC parameters are used for the prediction of hemorrhagic transformation of infarct.[14] The diffusion imaging in brain is further enhanced by newer sophisticated techniques, such as DTI and diffusion kurtosis imaging (DKI) (vide supra). They give additional information regarding the microstructural status of the brain tissue which will help in better understanding of the disease process.[27] It also has an important role in brain tumor imaging as well. It helps in characterization of tumors and their response assessment to treatment. Solid gliomas which show low ADC values are associated with higher grade.[28] Similarly, medulloblastoma and rhabdoid tumors have been shown to have low ADC values compared to ependymoma and astrocytoma in posterior fossa.[27] The DTI also has a proven role in the preoperative assessment of brain tumors. Response of brain tumors after chemoradiation is assessed by DWI. Changes in ADC values in the first few weeks after the therapy are found to be noninvasive biomarkers for response to therapy and it can be used for prognostication also.[29,30]

Head and Neck

Diffusion weighted imaging has potential to differentiate pleomorphic adenoma from other benign and malignant lesions of parotid gland.[31] Because of the presence of glandular component and fluid these tumors show significantly higher ADC value than Warthin tumors which have hypercellular stroma.[31] It can differentiate sinonasal malignant lesions from benign lesions because in the former ADC is lower. The ADC values can also be used to characterize a tumor, for instance it can differentiate squamous cell carcinoma (SCC) from lymphoma. The lymphoma usually shows low ADC values compared to SCC because of the hypercellular nature.[32,33] The limitation of its use is that some malignant lesions like chondrosarcoma can have high ADC values.[31] Prediction of tumor grading can be done by ADC values as poorly differentiated solid lesions show low ADC values compared to well-differentiated lesions. By differentiating necrotic area from viable tumor it can also help identify areas from where biopsy can be performed.[31,34] In the assessment of tumor response to therapy one of the major limitations of PET is that it is sensitive to inflammatory changes also. The DWI has the potential to overcome this difficulty because the inflammatory lesions show high ADC values whereas tumor tissue would show low ADC values. So it can be used as a surrogate marker to assess the tumor response very early during therapy. Apparent diffusion coefficient values in SCC have been shown to significantly change even after the first week of treatment and the complete responders show higher increase in ADC when compared to partial responders.[35] There is a recent study which evaluated the role of DWI in the orbit and suggested that it may help differentiate pseudotumor from lymphoma and cellulitis

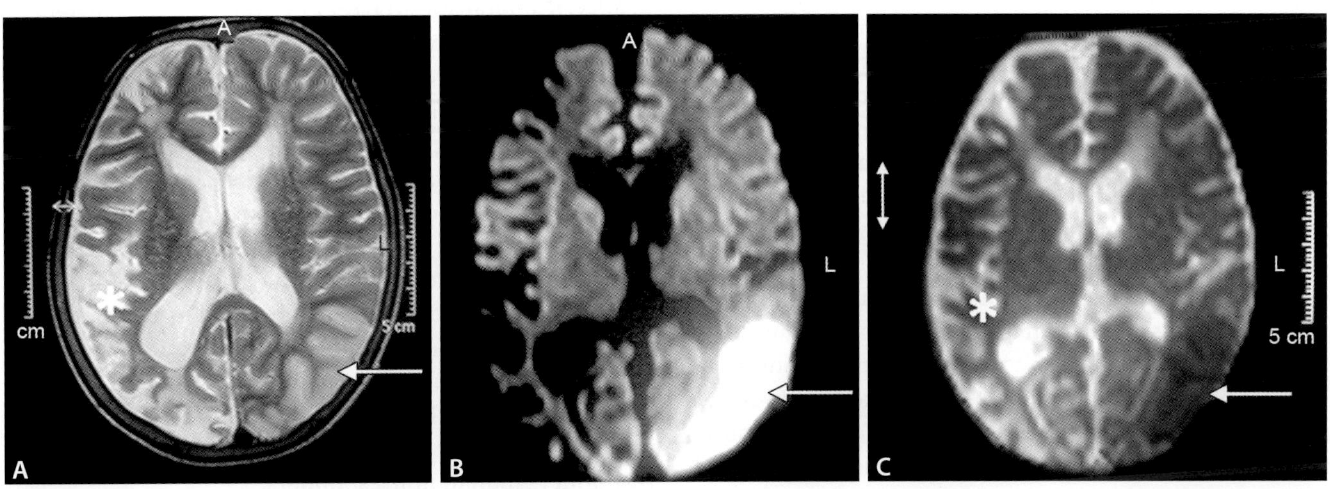

Figs. 4A to C: T2W axial image (A) of brain shows mild gyral hyperintensity (arrow) and swelling seen in the left parieto-occipital cortex. Multifocal areas of hyperintensities (*) seen in right cerebral hemisphere with associated volume loss suggestive of chronic infarct. DW-EPI sequence with b value of 1000 in axial plane (B) shows a brightly hyperintense area (arrow) which on ADC map (C) shows hypointensity (arrow). The above features are suggestive of acute infarct on the left side. Apparent diffusion coefficient map also shows multifocal hyperintensity in right cerebral hemisphere suggestive of facilitated diffusion. As depicted in this case, DWI along with ADC can be very useful for the chronological dating of infarcts.

which is again based on the fact that lymphoma shows low ADC compared to pseudotumor and cellulitis.[36] The DWI can reliably differentiate necrosis within a tumor from abscess formation. Abscess shows very low ADC because of the presence of macromolecules and increased viscosity.

Pediatric Applications

The use of ionizing radiation in children is a concern because of long-term effects, so DWI can be an alternate technique in this age group. The DWI does not involve the use of contrast media so it can be used whenever contrast-enhanced imaging is not possible because of deranged renal function. Experience of DWI in paediatric imaging is limited but promising. The ADC values can be used to detect malignant tumors, characterize them and assess the treatment response. Studies have been done in variety of pediatric tumors and they found that DWI performed better or similar to conventional MRI.[37,38]

Thorax

Diffusion weighted imaging in thorax needs faster sequences with high-performance gradients and parallel imaging techniques along with phased array coils. The low proton density in lung and magnetic field inhomogeneity makes quantitative DWI even more challenging. Usually, two b values are used and STIR is used for fat suppression especially if quantification is needed. It can be done in breath holding or free breathing with respiratory and cardiac triggers. Studies have used various methods, such as qualitative, semiquantitative and quantitative to differentiate malignant lesions from benign lesions.[4] In qualitative method the intensity of the lesion is compared with the intensity of spinal cord or chest wall muscle and the malignant lesions are usually hyperintense to spinal cord or chest wall muscles. In semiquantitative analysis, the ratio of the signal intensity of the lesion and the signal intensity of the reference structure is used to characterize the lesion. The quantitative analysis depends on the ADC measurement of the lesion itself.

Most of the work has been done in lung carcinoma. Studies have shown that the ADC of the malignant lesions is usually lower than the benign lesions and small cell carcinoma which has closely packed cells shows lower ADC when compared to nonsmall cell carcinoma although overlap may occur. At the same time small metastatic nodules, inflammatory nodules and fibrotic nodules cannot be reliably differentiated.[39] In case of collapsed lung it is very difficult on routine imaging to delineate the tumor boundary. Diffusion weighted imaging has been used successfully to delineate the tumor from the collapsed lung.[40] Diffusion weighted imaging has also been used to characterize the mediastinal nodes in patients with carcinoma lung.[41,42] The ADC values of malignant nodes were significantly lower than that of benign nodes. Another potential application of DWI is in the evaluation of tumor response after therapy.

Breast

Contrast-enhanced MRI of the breast is an established technique in the diagnosis of carcinoma breast with sensitivity of 89–100% and specificity of 72%.[18] Several studies have attempted to use DWI to differentiate malignant lesions from benign. There are no uniform b values or calculation methods used by the investigators which have resulted in different ADC cut-off values. Generally, the malignant lesions showed lower ADC values when compared with benign lesions **(Figs. 5A to D)**. But there is significant overlap between the two groups.[4] Lesions with fibrotic components, such as fibroadenoma and fibrocystic disease can result in low ADC values leading to diagnostic difficulty. Many optimizations were proposed including normalization of ADC of the lesion to the ADC of ipsilateral glandular parenchyma which would eliminate the ADC variations because of scanning parameters and effects of menstrual cycle.[43] This approach has been shown to improve the diagnostic accuracy. Efforts have been made to use DWI in addition to dynamic contrast-enhanced imaging and this has also been shown to improve diagnostic accuracy.[18] Diffusion weighted imaging has been used to grade the tumor, predict the histological type and to better evaluate the local extent of the tumor. Recently, many studies have been published regarding the role of DWI in the evaluation of response to treatment. Decrease in size of the lesion as response criteria is not an optimal parameter since it takes a long time to show a significant difference. Chemotherapeutic agents are toxic and they have various side effects which necessitates earlier assessment of response. Studies have shown that the increase in ADC value in comparison with the pretreatment value can be used as a noninvasive biomarker of disease response.[44,45] Using the change in ADC values, response can be evaluated as early as after the first cycle of chemotherapy and it has been found that the increase in ADC values was significantly more in responders than in nonresponders.

Liver

It is challenging to apply DWI in any abdominal organ mainly because of the respiratory motion and

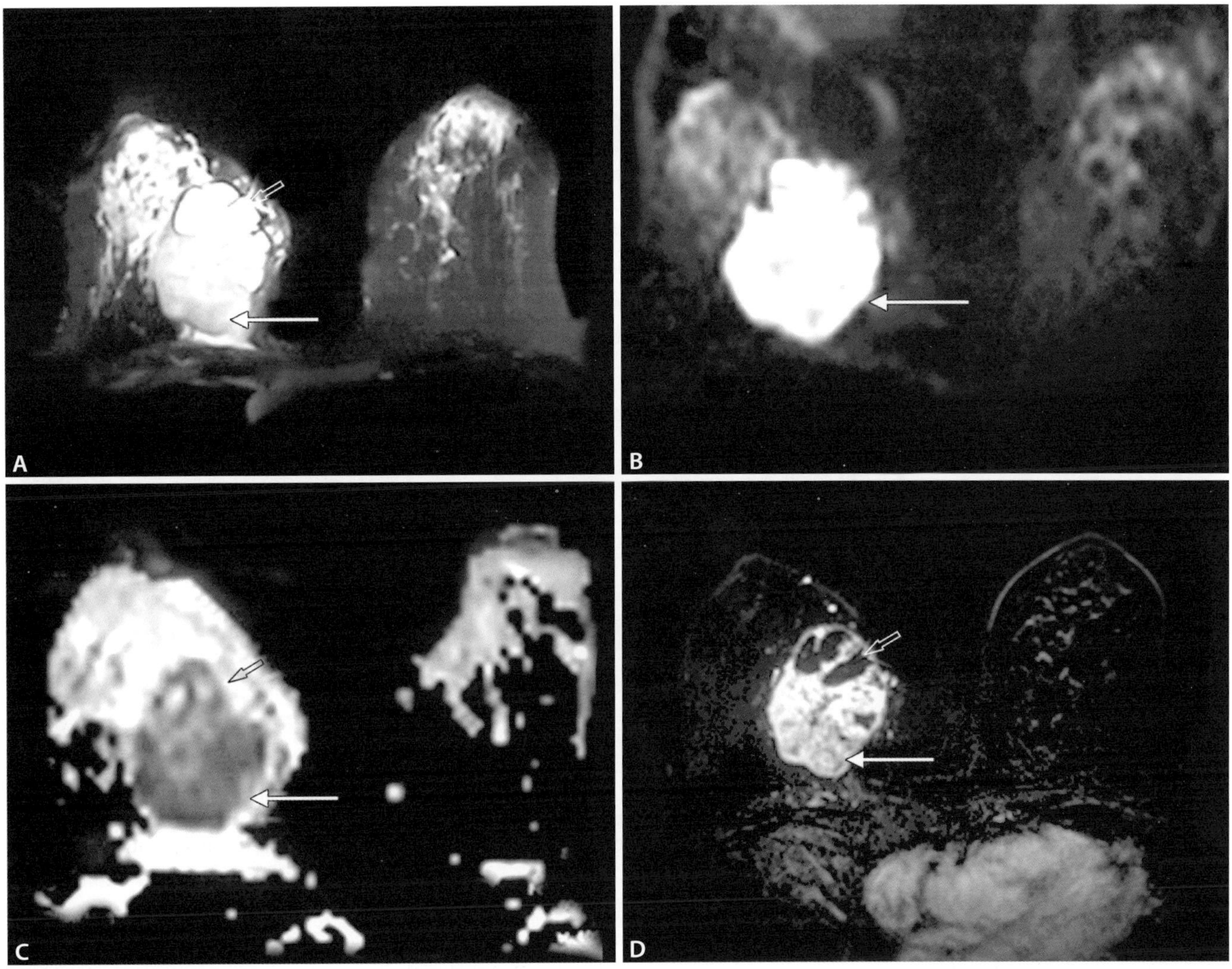

Figs. 5A to D: Axial T2W sequence of bilateral breasts (A) shows a hypointense mass lesion (arrow) in the right breast. It also shows areas of necrosis (outlined arrow) within. Diffusion-weighted sequence with b value of 1000 (B) shows a markedly hyperintense lesion (arrow) with good background suppression of other structures making the lesion more conspicuous. Apparent diffusion coefficient map (C) shows hypointensity (narrow) suggesting marked restriction of diffusion consistent with a highly cellular mass. Few areas show facilitated diffusion (outlined arrow) consistent with necrosis. These findings are also confirmed on subtracted postcontrast T1 fat suppressed image (D). Histopathology showed infiltrating ductal carcinoma.

susceptibility. The Liver is one of the most studied organs in abdomen using DWI. The Liver parenchyma shows relatively short T2 relaxation times, so the b values and the TE of the sequence should be optimized accordingly. Too high b value might cause unacceptable signal suppression which is because of long T2 time rather than diffusion characteristics itself. Usually, the recommended b values are 0, 100 and 500.[3] Presence of branching vessels within the liver parenchyma poses a difficulty in the detection of small focal lesions. In black blood DWI images, the vessels are suppressed so that the lesion detection is relatively easier especially on low b values. At the same time lesion characterization is better done on high b value images. To support this studies have shown that DWI is better than fat suppressed T2 weighted sequences.[46,47] Diffusion weighted imaging can be applied as a useful adjunct or can be used as a reasonable alternative to contrast enhanced images for the evaluation of the liver metastasis.[48,49] Hemangioma and simple cysts show significantly high ADC values that they can be reliably differentiated from hepatocellular carcinoma (HCC) and metastasis which show low ADC values **(Figs. 6 and 7)**. However, benign solid lesions like hepatic adenoma and focal nodular hyperplasia can have overlapping values

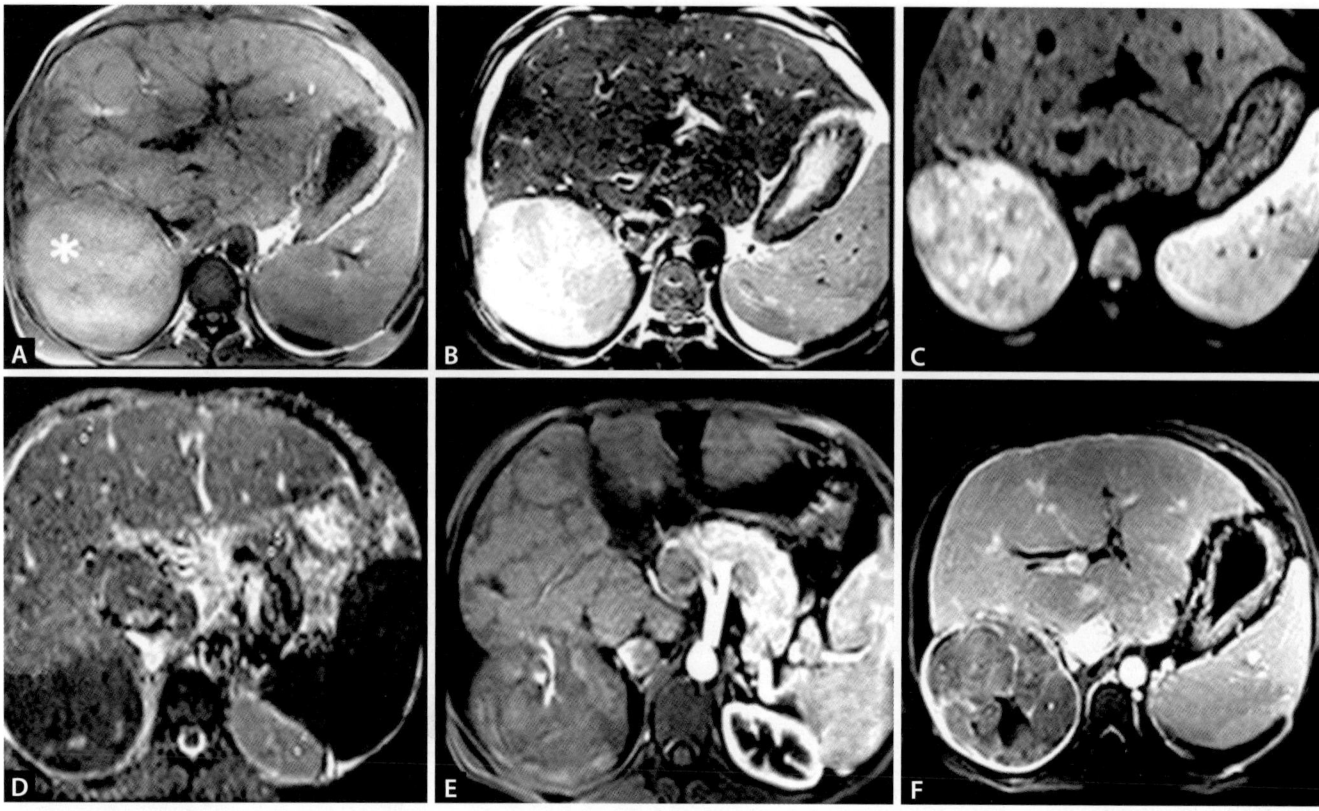

Figs. 6A to F: Axial T1W GRE sequence (A) shows an exophytic mildly hyperintense lesion (*) arising from the right lobe of liver. Rest of the liver is showing features of chronic liver disease. Lesion is markedly hyperintense on T2W sequence (B). Diffusion-weighted image with b value of 500 (C) shows the hyperintense lesion which on ADC map (D) shows marked diffusion restriction suggestive of hypercellular tumor. With these findings along with arterial enhancement in postcontrast T1W image (E) and capsule formation in delayed postcontrast image (F), diagnosis of hepatocellular carcinoma was made.

which cannot be reliably differentiated from malignant lesions.[3,18] Similarly, malignant lesions which are necrotic and mucinous tumors can have high ADC values and can mimic benign lesions on DWI. Diagnosis and detection of HCC and dysplastic nodules in a cirrhotic liver is very difficult based on ADC values because the diffusion is as it is restricted in cirrhotic liver as a result of fibrosis. As in other tumors, DWI has a role in the evaluation of tumor response and it has been shown to demonstrate significantly more ADC changes in responders than in nonresponders. In addition, the pre-treatment high ADC values have been correlated with poorer response to therapy. It is well known that ADC values are low in cirrhotic liver and a recent study showed that ADC values correlated well with US elastography and serum markers for moderate and severe fibrosis.[50]

Gallbladder and Biliary Ducts

There is emerging evidence that DWI can be helpful in differentiating malignant gallbladder lesions from benign. Malignant lesions tend to show high signal intensity on DWI and low ADC values compared to benign lesions.[51] It can distinguish adherent or tumefactive sludge from gallbladder malignancy. A recent study has shown that DWI performed better than conventional MRCP in the detection of extrahepatic cholangiocarcinoma.[52]

Pancreas

Apparent diffusion coefficient values of pancreas have been shown to vary with age of the patient and the location in pancreas. With increase in age pancreas undergoes atrophy, fatty replacement and fibrosis which is proposed to be a cause for change in ADC.[53,54] The ADC values of head and body of the pancreas is shown to be significantly more than the tail of pancreas.[54] Carcinoma of pancreas shows low ADC values compared to the rest of normal pancreas and the ADC values depend on the histological characteristics as well. However, there is overlap of ADC values of carcinoma pancreas with focal pancreatitis because of which their distinction is

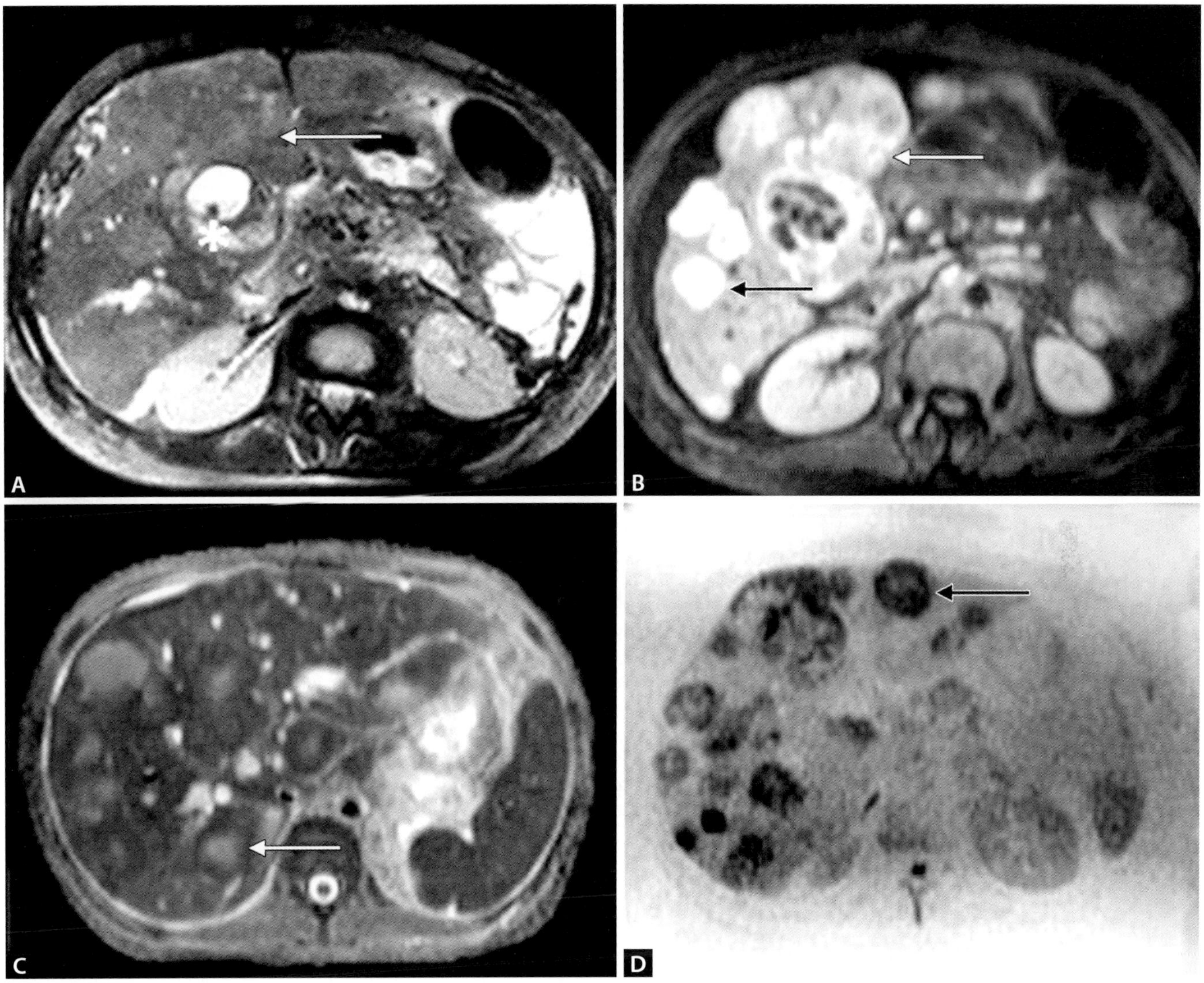

Figs. 7A to D: Axial T2W sequence (A) shows a mass lesion involving the gallbladder (*) with adjacent liver infiltration. Calculi were also noted in the gallbladder. Multiple subtle hyperintense lesions (arrow) in both lobes of liver are suggestive of metastases. Diffusion-weighted sequence with b value of 500 (B) shows these focal lesions (arrows) much better than the T2W sequence. Apparent diffusion coefficient map (C) also shows multiple focal lesions (arrow) which are showing restricted diffusion in the periphery of the lesion. Most lesions on ADC map show central hyperintensity suggestive of necrosis. Diffusion-weighted sequence with b value of 1000 displayed in inverted gray scale (D) shows multiple metastatic lesions (arrow) with very good background suppression which is comparable to positron emission tomography image.

difficult. Cystic lesions of pancreas, such as pseudocysts, simple cysts show a relatively high ADC values compared to pancreatic abscesses, hydatid cysts and cystic neoplasms.[55]

Kidneys and Adrenal

Diffusion weighted imaging has been successfully used in differentiating malignant renal lesions from benign lesions. Renal cysts show high ADC values than the normal parenchyma and other solid lesions **(Figs. 8A to E)**. Among the cysts, those with T1 hyperintensity show lower ADC than those which are T1 hypointense.[56] This has been attributed to the presence of blood or proteinaceous content which can alter diffusion and the same can be helpful in differentiating simple cysts from necrotic neoplasms. Recent studies have shown DWI can be helpful in characterization of renal malignant masses and ADC values can be used to predict the histological subtype of renal cell carcinoma.[57,58] Renal Abscesses and infected cysts show low ADC values than other cystic

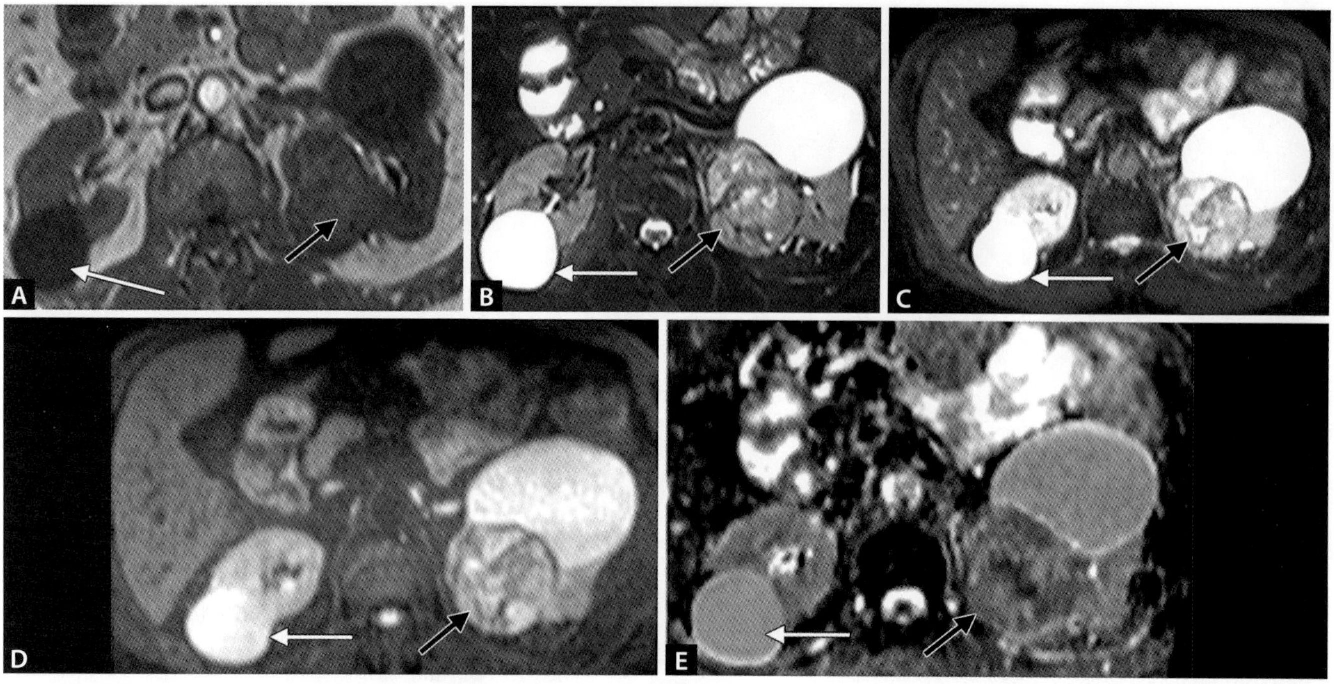

Figs. 8A to E: Axial T1W sequence of bilateral kidneys (A) shows hypointense exophytic lesions (arrow) in both the kidneys and an isointense lesion (outlined arrow) in the posterior cortex of left kidney. T2-weighted fat suppressed and DW sequence with b value of 0 (B and C) shows markedly hyperintense lesions (arrow) in both kidneys suggestive of simple cysts whereas the posterior cortex lesion in left kidney (outlined arrow) is isointense to kidney parenchyma. On DW sequence with b value of 500 (D) the simple cysts are loosing signal compared to b 0 image whereas the posterior cortex lesion is retaining signal suggestive of solid nature of the lesion. Apparent diffusion coefficient map (E) shows the cystic lesions as hyperintense to renal parenchyma which is consistent with simple cysts. The solid lesion in the left kidney (outlined arrow) is mildly hypointense to renal parenchyma which is consistent with a hypercellular solid tumor. Solid lesion in the left kidney was proven to be clear cell carcinoma

lesions.[59] According to recent studies, DWI is not useful in differentiating benign adrenal lesions from malignant lesions based on ADC values although cysts and to some extent pheochromocytoma showed higher ADC values.[60,61]

Prostate

Prostate is rich in glandular structures which facilitates free diffusion of water. Recent usage of high field strength, advancements in hardware and sequences have made DWI possible in the prostate with good SNR. The usage of endorectal coils have been shown to improve the image quality. Several studies have shown that prostate cancer is seen as hyperintense area in DWI and show hypointensity on corresponding ADC maps.[62] However, there is overlap of ADC values of prostate cancer with focal chronic prostatitis and benign prostatic hyperplasia.[2] There is a significant negative correlation found between the ADC values and the Gleason score which would help in management decisions. It is also found to be useful in locoregional staging and lymph nodal detection.[2] It can be used as a biomarker to assess response in patients who are treated with radiation. The ADC values have been shown to increase in response to therapy.[63]

Female Pelvis

Conventional MRI has an important role in detection and staging of female pelvic malignancies. Diffusion weighted imaging can be used as an adjunct to it to increase its diagnostic accuracy. Normal endometrium shows varying diffusion characteristics and ADC values during different phases of menstrual cycle. Lowest ADC values are seen at the end of the cycle.[4] This variation should be taken in to account while interpreting the DW images and ADC values. Endometrial carcinoma has been shown to have significantly low ADC value compared to the normal endometrium.[4,18,64] It can show the extent of myometrial invasion which is important in the management especially if contrast media cannot be used. It can differentiate endometrial carcinoma from other benign endometrial lesions, such as hyperplasia and polyp. Diffusion weighted imaging can detect the malignant nodes even though they are normal according to size criteria. Cervical carcinoma is a hypercellular tumor whose ADC values are less than the normal cervical stroma. It can clearly show the depth of invasion in cervix and can also be used for detection of involved nodes allowing to stage the disease more accurately.[65] Because of low ADC value of SCC, it can be differentiated from adenocarcinoma of cervix. However, there is no clear-cut cut-off value for ADC available in the literature mainly because of variations in the technique and hardware used. There are contradicting reports regarding the potential of DWI to differentiate malignant ovarian lesions from benign lesions.[66,67] However, it improves the detection of peritoneal deposits when combined with a conventional MRI sequences than the latter alone.[68]

CONCLUSION

Diffusion weighted imaging is an evolving technique that provides a new paradigm for tissue characterization. Its ability to provide both qualitative and quantitative insight in to complex diffusion mechanisms and changes at a cellular level with only a small time penalty have made this technique a valuable addition to clinical MR protocols. However, DW sequences must be interpreted in conjunction with other MR sequences to avoid the pitfalls of this technique.

REFERENCES

1. Bonekamp D, Jacobs MA, El-Khouli R, Stoianovici D, Macura KJ. Advancements in MR imaging of the prostate: from diagnosis to interventions. Radiographics. 2011;31(3):677-703.
2. Malayeri AA, El Khouli RH, Zaheer A, Jacobs MA, Corona-Villalobos CP, Kamel IR, Macura KJ. Principles and applications of diffusion-weighted imaging in cancer detection, staging, and treatment follow-up. Radiographics. 2011;31(6):1773-91.
3. Chandarana H, Taouli B. Diffusion and perfusion imaging of the liver. Europ Journ of Radiol. 2010;76(3):348-58.
4. Türkbey B, Aras Ö, Karabulut N, Turgut AT, Akpınar E, Alibek S, Pang Y, Ertürk \cS M., El Khouli RH, Bluemke DA. Diffusion-weighted MRI for detecting and monitoring cancer: a review of current applications in body imaging. Diagn Interv Radiol. 2012;18:46-59.
5. Herneth AM, Mayerhoefer M, Schernthaner R, Ba-Ssalamah A, Czerny C, Fruehwald-Pallamar J. Diffusion weighted imaging: lymph nodes. Eur J Radiol. 2010;76(3): 398-406.
6. De Figueiredo EH, Borgonovi AFNG, Doring TM. Basic concepts of MR imaging, diffusion MR imaging and diffusion tensor imaging. Magn Reson Imaging Clin N Am. 2011;19(1):1.
7. Stejskal EO, Tanner JE. Spin diffusion measurements: Spin echoes in the presence of a time-dependent field gradient. The J Chem Phys. 1965;42:288.
8. Le Bihan D, Breton E, Lallemand D, Grenier P, Cabanis E, Laval-Jeantet M. MR imaging of intravoxel incoherent motions: application to diffusion and perfusion in neurologic disorders. Radiology. 1986;161(2):401.
9. Dietrich O, Biffar A, Baur-Melnyk A, Reiser MF. Technical aspects of MR diffusion imaging of the body. Europ Journ Radiology. 2010;76(3):314-22.
10. Provenzale JM, Engelter ST, Petrella JR, Smith JS, MacFall JR. Use of MR exponential diffusion-weighted images to eradicate T2“ shine-through” effect. Amer Jour of Roentg. 1999;172(2): 537-9.
11. Koh DM, Thoeny HC. Diffusion-weighted MR Imaging: Applications in the Body. Springer. 2010.
12. Provenzale JM, Petrella JR, Jr LCHC, Wong JC, Engelter S, Barboriak DP. Quantitative Assessment of Diffusion Abnormalities in Posterior Reversible Encephalopathy Syndrome. AJNR. 2001;22(8):1455-61.
13. Hiwatashi A, Kinoshita T, Moritani T, Wang HZ, Shrier DA, Numaguchi Y, Ekholm SE, Westesson PL. Hypointensity on diffusion-weighted MRI of the brain related to T2 shortening and susceptibility effects. Amer Journ Roentg. 2003;181(6):1705-9.
14. Fung SH, Roccatagliata L, Gonzalez RG, Schaefer PW. MR diffusion imaging in ischemic stroke. Neuroimaging Clin N Am. 2011;21(2):345.
15. Haselgrove JC, Moore JR. Correction for distortion of echo-planar images used to calculate the apparent diffusion coefficient. Magn Resonan Med. 2005;36(6):960-4.
16. Wang CL, Chea YW, Boll DT, Samei E, Neville AM, Dale BM, Merkle EM. Effect of gadolinium chelate contrast agents on diffusion weighted MR imaging of the liver, spleen, pancreas and kidney at 3T. Europ Journ Radiol. 2011;80(2): e1-e7.
17. Takahara T, Imai Y, Yamashita T, Yasuda S, Nasu S, Van Cauteren M. Diffusion weighted whole body imaging with background body signal suppression (DWIBS): technical improvement using free breathing, STIR and high resolution 3D display. Matrix. 2004;160(160):160.
18. Bonekamp S, Corona-Villalobos CP, Kamel IR. Oncologic applications of diffusion-weighted MRI in the body. Journ Magn Resonan Imag. 2012;35(2):257-79.
19. Jensen JH, Helpern JA, Ramani A, Lu H, Kaczynski K. Diffusional kurtosis imaging: the quantification of non-Gaussian water diffusion by means of magnetic resonance imaging. Magn Reson Med. 2005;53(6):1432-40.
20. Le Bihan D, Breton E, Lallemand D. Perfusion in intravoxel incoherent motion MR imaging. Radiology. 1988;168:497-505.
21. Koh DM, Collins DJ, Orton MR. Intravoxel incoherent motion in body diffusion-weighted MRI: reality and challenges. Amer Journ Roentg. 2011;196(6):1351-61.
22. Wang Z, Su MY, Najafi A, Nalcioglu O. Effect of vasodilator hydralazine on tumor microvascular random flow and blood volume as measured by intravoxel incoherent motion (IVIM) weighted MRI in conjunction with Gd-DTPA-Albumin enhanced MRI. Magn resonan imag. 2001;19(8):1063-72.

23. Pickens III DR, Jolgren DL, Lorenz CH, Creasy JL, Price RR. Magnetic resonance perfusion/diffusion imaging of the excised dog kidney. Investigative radiology. 1992;27(4):287-92.
24. Lemke A, Laun FB, Simon D, Stieltjes B, Schad LR. An *in vivo* verification of the intravoxel incoherent motion effect in diffusion-weighted imaging of the abdomen. Magn Resonan in Med. 2010;64(6):1580-5.
25. Downey K, Riches SF, Morgan VA, Giles SL, Attygalle AD, Ind TE, Barton DPJ, Shepherd JH, deSouza NM. Relationship Between Imaging Biomarkers of Stage I Cervical Cancer and Poor-Prognosis Histologic Features: Quantitative Histogram Analysis of Diffusion-Weighted MR Images. AJR. 2013;200(2):314-20.
26. Hjort N, Christensen S, Solling C, Ashkanian M, Wu O, Røhl L, Gyldensted C, Andersen G, Ostergaard L. Ischemic injury detected by diffusion imaging 11 minutes after stroke. Ann Neurol. 2005;58(3):462-5.
27. Heiss WD, Raab P, Lanfermann H. Multimodality assessment of brain tumors and tumor recurrence. Journ of Nucl Med. 2011;52(10):1585-600.
28. Arvinda HR, Kesavadas C, Sarma PS, Thomas B, Radhakrishnan VV, Gupta AK, Kapilamoorthy TR, Nair S. Glioma grading: sensitivity, specificity, positive and negative predictive values of diffusion and perfusion imaging. Journ Neuro-oncolo. 2009;94(1):87-96.
29. Hamstra DA, Chenevert TL, Moffat BA, Johnson TD, Meyer CR, Mukherji SK, Quint DJ, Gebarski SS, Fan X, Tsien CI. Evaluation of the functional diffusion map as an early biomarker of time-to-progression and overall survival in high-grade glioma. Proc Natl Acad Sci USA. 2005;102(46):16759-64.
30. Hamstra DA, Galbán CJ, Meyer CR, Johnson TD, Sundgren PC, Tsien C, Lawrence TS, Junck L, Ross DJ, Rehemtulla A. Functional diffusion map as an early imaging biomarker for high-grade glioma: correlation with conventional radiologic response and overall survival. Journ Clini Oncol. 2008;26(20):3387-94.
31. Razek AAKA. Diffusion-weighted magnetic resonance imaging of head and neck. Journ Comp Assis Tomog. 2010;34(6):808.
32. Maeda M, Kato H, Sakuma H, Maier SE, Takeda K. Usefulness of the apparent diffusion coefficient in line scan diffusion-weighted imaging for distinguishing between squamous cell carcinomas and malignant lymphomas of the head and neck. Amer journ of Neuroradiol. 2005;26(5):1186-92.
33. Sumi M, Ichikawa Y, Nakamura T. Diagnostic ability of apparent diffusion coefficients for lymphomas and carcinomas in the pharynx. Europ Radiol. 2007;17(10):2631-7.
34. Razek AAKA, Megahed AS, Denewer A, Motamed A, Tawfik A, Nada N. Role of diffusion-weighted magnetic resonance imaging in differentiation between the viable and necrotic parts of head and neck tumors. Acta Radiologica. 2008;49(3):364-70.
35. Kim S, Loevner L, Quon H, Sherman E, Weinstein G, Kilger A, Poptani H. Diffusion-weighted magnetic resonance imaging for predicting and detecting early response to chemoradiation therapy of squamous cell carcinomas of the head and neck. Clinic Canc Resear. 2009;15(3):986-94.
36. Kapur R, Sepahdari AR, Mafee MF, Putterman AM, Aakalu V, Wendel LJA, Setabutr P. MR imaging of orbital inflammatory syndrome, orbital cellulitis, and orbital lymphoid lesions: the role of diffusion-weighted imaging. Amer Journ Neuroradiol. 2009;30(1):64–70.[cited 2012 Dec 23].
37. Uhl M, Altehoefer C, Kontny U, Il'yasov K, Büchert M, Langer M. MRI-diffusion imaging of neuroblastomas: first results and correlation to histology. Eur Radiol. 2002;12(9):2335-8.
38. Humphries PD, Sebire NJ, Siegel MJ, Olsen E. Tumors in pediatric patients at diffusion-weighted MR imaging: apparent diffusion coefficient and tumor cellularity. Radiology. 2007;245(3):848-54.
39. Satoh S, Kitazume Y, Ohdama S, Kimula Y, Taura S, Endo Y. Can malignant and benign pulmonary nodules be differentiated with diffusion-weighted MRI? Amer Journ Roentgenol. 2008;191(2):464-70.
40. Qi LP, Zhang XP, Tang L, Li J, Sun YS, Zhu GY. Using diffusion-weighted MR imaging for tumor detection in the collapsed lung: a preliminary study. Europ radiol. 2009;19(2):333-41.
41. Kosucu P, Tekinbas C, Erol M, Sari A, Kavgaci H, Öztuna F, Ersöz S. Mediastinal lymph nodes: Assessment with diffusion-weighted MR imaging. Journ Magn Reson Imag. 2009;30(2):292-7.
42. Nomori H, Mori T, Ikeda K, Kawanaka K, Shiraishi S, Katahira K, Yamashita Y. Diffusion-weighted magnetic resonance imaging can be used in place of positron emission tomography for N staging of non-small cell lung cancer with fewer false-positive results. Journ Thorac Cardiovasc Surg. 2008;135(4):816-22.
43. Khouli RHEI, Jacobs MA, Mezban SD, Huang P, Kamel IR, Macura KJ, Bluemke DA. Diffusion-weighted Imaging Improves the Diagnostic Accuracy of Conventional 3.0-T Breast MR Imaging. Radiology. 2010;256(1):64-73.
44. Sharma U, Danishad KKA, Seenu V, Jagannathan NR. Longitudinal study of the assessment by MRI and diffusion-weighted imaging of tumor response in patients with locally advanced breast cancer undergoing neoadjuvant chemotherapy. NMR in biomed. 2009;22(1):104-13.
45. Park SH, Moon WK, Cho N, Song IC, Chang JM, Park IA, Han W, Noh DY. Diffusion-weighted MR Imaging: Pretreatment Prediction of Response to Neoadjuvant Chemotherapy in Patients with Breast Cancer. Radiology. 2010;257(1):56-63.
46. Bruegel M, Gaa J, Waldt S, Woertler K, Holzapfel K, Kiefer B, Rummeny EJ. Diagnosis of hepatic metastasis: comparison of respiration-triggered diffusion-weighted echo-planar MRI and five T2-weighted turbo spin-echo sequences. Amer Journ Roent. 2008;191(5):1421-9.
47. Zech CJ, Herrmann KA, Dietrich O, Horger W, Reiser MF, Schoenberg SO. Black-blood diffusion-weighted EPI acquisition of the liver with parallel imaging: comparison with a standard T2-weighted sequence for detection of focal liver lesions. Investig Radiol. 2008;43(4):261-6.

48. Koh DM, Brown G, Riddell AM, Scurr E, Collins DJ, Allen SD, Chau I, Cunningham D, Desouza NM, Leach MO. Detection of colorectal hepatic metastases using MnDPDP MR imaging and diffusion-weighted imaging (DWI) alone and in combination. Europ Radiol. 2008;18(5):903-10.
49. Hardie AD, Naik M, Hecht EM, Chandarana H, Mannelli L, Babb JS, Taouli B. Diagnosis of liver metastases: value of diffusion-weighted MRI compared with gadolinium-enhanced MRI. Europ Radiol. 2010;20(6):1431-41.
50. Lewin M, Poujol-Robert A, Boëlle P-Y, Wendum D, Lasnier E, Viallon M, Guéchot J, Hoeffel C, Arrivé L, Tubiana J-M, Poupon R. Diffusion-weighted magnetic resonance imaging for the assessment of fibrosis in chronic hepatitis C. Hepatology. 2007; 46(3):658-65.
51. Sugita R, Yamazaki T, Furuta A, Itoh K, Fujita N, Takahashi S. High b-value diffusion-weighted MRI for detecting gallbladder carcinoma: preliminary study and results. Europ Radiol. 2009;19(7):1794-8.
52. Cui XY, Chen HW. Role of diffusion-weighted magnetic resonance imaging in the diagnosis of extrahepatic cholangiocarcinoma. World Journ Gastroenterol. 2010;16(25): 3196.
53. Ichikawa T, Haradome H, Hachiya J, Nitatori T, Araki T. Diffusion-weighted MR imaging with single-shot echo-planar imaging in the upper abdomen: preliminary clinical experience in 61 patients. Abdomin Imag. 1999;24(5):456-61.
54. Yoshikawa T, Kawamitsu H, Mitchell DG, Ohno Y, Ku Y, Seo Y, Fujii M, Sugimura K. ADC Measurement of abdominal organs and lesions using parallel imaging technique. AJR. 2006;187(6):1521-30.
55. Inan N, Arslan A, Akansel G, Anik Y, Demirci A. Diffusion-weighted imaging in the differential diagnosis of cystic lesions of the pancreas. Americ Journ Roentgenol. 2008;191(4):1115-21.
56. Zhang J, Tehrani YM, Wang L, Ishill NM, Schwartz LH, Hricak H. Renal Masses: Characterization with Diffusion-weighted MR Imaging- A Preliminary Experience. Radiology. 2008;247(2):458-64.
57. Goyal A, Sharma R, Bhalla AS, Gamanagatti S, Seth A, Iyer VK, Das P. Diffusion-weighted MRI in renal cell carcinoma: a surrogate marker for predicting nuclear grade and histological subtype. Acta Radiol. 2012;53(3):349-58.
58. Paudyal B, Paudyal P, Tsushima Y, Oriuchi N, Amanuma M, Miyazaki M, Taketomi-Takahashi A, Nakazato Y, Endo K. The role of the ADC value in the characterisation of renal carcinoma by diffusion-weighted MRI. British Journ Radiol. 2010;83(988):336-43.
59. Goyal A, Sharma R, Bhalla AS, Gamanagatti S, Seth A. Diffusion-weighted MRI in inflammatory renal lesions: all that glitters is not RCC. Eur Radiol. 2013;23(1):272-9.
60. Miller FH, Wang Y, McCarthy RJ, Yaghmai V, Merrick L, Larson A, Berggruen S, Casalino DD, Nikolaidis P. Utility of diffusion-weighted MRI in characterization of adrenal lesions. Americ Journ of Roentg. 2010;194(2):W179-85.
61. Tsushima Y, Takahashi-Taketomi A, Endo K. Diagnostic utility of diffusion-weighted MR imaging and apparent diffusion coefficient value for the diagnosis of adrenal tumors. Journ Magnet Reson Imag. 2009;29(1):112-7.
62. Gibbs P, Pickles MD, Turnbull LW. Diffusion imaging of the prostate at 3.0 Tesla. Investig Radiol. 2006;41(2):185-8.
63. Song I, Kim CK, Park BK, Park W. Assessment of response to radiotherapy for prostate cancer: value of diffusion-weighted MRI at 3T. Americ Journ Roentg. 2010;194(6):W477-82.
64. Fujii S, Matsusue E, Kigawa J, Sato S, Kanasaki Y, Nakanishi J, Sugihara S, Kaminou T, Terakawa N, Ogawa T. Diagnostic accuracy of the apparent diffusion coefficient in differentiating benign from malignant uterine endometrial cavity lesions: initial results. Europ Radiol. 2008;18(2):384-9.
65. Lin G, Ho KC, Wang JJ, Ng KK, Wai YY, Chen YT, Chang CJ, Ng SH, Lai CH, Yen TC. Detection of lymph node metastasis in cervical and uterine cancers by diffusion-weighted magnetic resonance imaging at 3T. Journ Magnet Reson Imag. 2008;28(1):128-35.
66. Moteki T, Ishizaka H. Diffusion-weighted EPI of cystic ovarian lesions: Evaluation of cystic contents using apparent diffusion coefficients. Journ Magnet Reson Imag. 2000;12(6):1014-9.
67. Nakayama T, Yoshimitsu K, Irie H, Aibe H, Tajima T, Nishie A, Asayama Y, Matake K, Kakihara D, Matsuura S. Diffusion-weighted echo planar MR imaging and ADC mapping in the differential diagnosis of ovarian cystic masses: Usefulness of detecting keratinoid substances in mature cystic teratomas. J Magn Reson Imaging. 2005;22(2):271-8.
68. Low RN, Sebrechts CP, Barone RM, Muller W. Diffusion-weighted MRI of peritoneal tumors: comparison with conventional MRI and surgical and histopathologic findings: a feasibility study. Amer Journ Roentg. 2009;193(2):461-70.

CHAPTER 47

Functional Magnetic Resonance: Perfusion and Dynamic Contrast-enhanced Magnetic Resonance Imaging

Niranjan Khandelwal, Sameer Vyas

PERFUSION MAGNETIC RESONANCE IMAGING

Perfusion can provide valuable information for detection, characterization and monitoring therapies in various disease processes like neoplasm, inflammations and ischemia.[1,2] It is also referred as capillary or tissue-specific blood flow, and is an established physiologic and pathophysiologic measure of the volume of blood flowing through the microvasculature of a mass of tissue in a certain period of time. It is a quantitative measure, which can be determined with many different experimental techniques and often expressed in mL/100 g/minute.[3] The values of perfusion should be comparable across measurement modalities and the theoretical equations are usually used for determining perfusion that can be translated from one measurement technique to another.

The perfusion can be noninvasive measured by the use of a tracer. Depending on the characteristics of these tracers, the blood flow measures can be divided into mainly three types, viz. diffusible tracers, intravascular tracers and microsphere type tracers.[4,5] The diffusible tracers can easily pass through blood vessel walls and include H_2O, or H_2O^{15} (used in positron emission tomography), and xenon (used in computed tomography-based perfusion measures). The intravascular tracers are those tracers which remain within the vessel walls and include iodinated contrast in CT and gadolinium and other contrast agents in magnetic resonance imaging (MRI). However, these agents are partially diffusible in most tissues of the body and separating perfusion from vessel permeability effects can be a challenge. The microsphere type tracers are slightly larger than capillaries, and hence, they get stuck within the microvasculature indefinitely. They are widely used for invasive animal studies and are considered too risky for human studies. Clinical agents, such as the single-photon emission computed tomography (SPECT) agent Tc-HMPAO mimic microspheres by remaining in the target tissue for a long time but they achieve this by diffusing into tissue and then undergoing a chemical transformation within the tissue that discourages diffusing back out.

As unusual nuclear species are readily detected in the body with MRI, perfusion imaging is possible with many different tracers, including fluorinated compounds, deuterated water, O^{17} and hyperpolarized gas, xenon.[5-7] The normal concentration of these tracer agents (nuclei) in tissue is almost zero and the only signal observed in clinical MRI is because of perfusion effects as the signal from these can be well separated from the water proton signal. These techniques are interesting and potentially promising, however these agents generally produce weak signals to noise ratio, have low spatial resolution, and lack the sensitivity of the proton MRI techniques, which is usually employed for clinical studies. Proton-based perfusion techniques using the strong signal from water protons in tissue have been found to be useful in the clinical setting and clinical research.

Perfusion imaging with the proton signal can be performed either by dynamic imaging following the bolus injection of an MR contrast agent or by labeling of the water in the inflowing arterial blood.[8-12] Contrast agent-based methods are commonly used as the effects of contrast agents in the vessels or tissue are quite strong. The bolus tracking technique is most widely used and it involves the injection of a bolus of magnetic contrast agent while repeatedly imaging.[13,14] It is usually performed using T2* (or T2) contrast where the signal change is due to the magnetic susceptibility of the contrast agent and is known as dynamic susceptibility contrast (DSC) MR perfusion or the T1 properties of the contrast agent, where the signal change is due to the T1-shortening effects of the contrast agent and is known as dynamic contrast enhancement (DCE) MR perfusion.[13-17] The DSC imaging is mostly employed in the brain whereas DCE-MR perfusion is usually employed outside the brain. By selectively affecting the MRI signal from water in the inflowing arterial blood, imaging without contrast agent is possible and is known as arterial spin labeling (ASL) technique. It produces a smaller signal change than the contrast agent methods but the lack of an injection and the use of diffusible water as the tracer make this approach an interesting alternative option.[11,15]

Magnetic-contrast Agents in Neural Tissues

MR-contrast agents (paramagnetic and superparamagnetic) are intravascular within normal brain tissue, as they are too large to cross the blood–brain barrier. The signal changes resulting from alterations to the intravascular signal are relatively small because the brain-blood volume is small (3–6%). However, the magnetic-contrast agents within the vasculature can have effects beyond the vessels as an intravascular-contrast agent and can affect tissue signal by altering the magnetic fields in the nearby tissue.[18-21] In addition, spins can move between small blood vessels in the microvasculature and the tissue.

Imaging Techniques and Methods

Three techniques are mainly used for performing MR perfusion imaging: dynamic susceptibility contrast-enhanced perfusion, dynamic contrast-enhanced perfusion and arterial-spin labeling.[1]

All these techniques involve repetitive serial imaging during the passage of blood that has been labeled with either contrast material or with an endogenous magnetic tracer label. In clinical studies, dynamic-susceptibility contrast-enhanced (DSC) MR perfusion is currently the most commonly used technique and it is very simple to perform in a clinical environment.

Dynamic-susceptibility Contrast-enhanced MR Perfusion

Principle: Dynamic-susceptibility contrast-enhanced MR perfusion (DSC-MRP) technique utilizes the T2* susceptibility effects of gadolinium, rather than the T1-shortening effects which are mostly associated with contrast-enhancement on conventional imaging.[22-26] It uses rapid measurements of MR signal change following the injection of a bolus of a paramagnetic MRI contrast agent.[1] The susceptibility effect is the shortening of T2 and T2* relaxation times, which leads to lower signal on T2- or T2*-weighted images. The signal loss which results from the passage of the contrast agent bolus on T2* weighted images helps in calculating the change occurring in the contrast concentration of each pixel. Contrast agent is treated as an intravascular marker and leakage into the interstitial space is either ignored or eliminated if possible. This data can be utilized to derive calculated estimates of cerebral blood volume (CBV), mean transit time (MTT) and cerebral blood flow (CBF).

Image acquisition: The patient should be positioned comfortably with sufficient cushioning to reduce movement and light restraining straps be used in the same manner as used for normal MRI. Data is acquired by applying a fast imaging technique, such as single or multishot echoplanar imaging (EPI) to produce a temporal resolution of approximately 2 seconds. The imaging sequence may be gradient echo which will maximize T2* weighting. Alternatively, a spin echo approach can also be used which minimizes the signal contribution from the large vessels. A series of at least five precontrast images should be collected prior to the passage of the bolus and many centers will collect for up to 1 minute to provide a large number of precontrast images to improve the estimation of the signal intensity baseline during analysis. A standard contrast dose (0.1 mmol/kg) is usually adequate, but a double dose of gadolinium (0.2 mmol/kg) may be used to improve the signal to noise ratio. The contrast is usually injected through an 18- or 20-gauge IV catheter at a high rate (3–7 mL/sec) using a power injector, to allow for a tight bolus of contrast material. After the injection, a saline flush of at least 25 mL (20–30 mL) should be delivered at the same rate to make sure that the bolus, which enters the central circulation is as coherent as possible. Alternatively, a careful manual injection technique can also be used. However, for manual techniques the injection should be given through a large cannula (at least 18 G). It should preferably be introduced into a large antecubital vein so that the resistance of the injection system is reduced. The injection should be given at an even rate and should be immediately followed by a chaser of the same amount of normal saline given at the same rate. Successive images of the region of interest (ROI) are then acquired during the first pass of contrast material.

Data analysis: The analysis of DSC-MRI is based on the assumption that the contrast agent remains within the vascular space throughout the examination acting as a blood pool marker.[25,26] This assumption does not stand true except within the brain where there is absence of contrast leakage because of the blood–brain barrier. The drop in T2* signal caused by the susceptibility effects of gadolinium is computed on a voxel-by-voxel basis and used for constructing a time-versus intensity curve. The degree of signal drop is then assumed to be proportional to the tissue concentration of gadolinium, so that relative concentration-time curves can be obtained (delta R2 curves) **(Figs. 1A to C)**.[26-31] Relative cerebral-blood volume (rCBV) can be obtained by calculating the area under the concentration-time curves, normalized to a contralateral, uninvolved region. "Relative" refers to the fact that an arterial input function is not used in the calculation of CBV, and therefore, precise quantification of cerebral blood volume is not performed. Repetition of this process on a voxel-by-voxel basis can be done to construct an rCBV map **(Fig. 2)**. The MTT is then estimated as some form of standardized measurement of the width of the curve, such as the width at half the maximum height (full width at half maximum; FWHM). The blood flow can then be calculated using the central volume theorem CBF = CBV/MTT.

The initial calculation of local-contrast concentration from the observed signal change a straightforward and contrast concentration is linearly related to the T2 rate changes ($\Delta R2$), which can be calculated for using the relationship:

$$\Delta R2 = -\ln [S(t)/S(0)]/TE$$

where,

S(0) is the base line signal intensity

S(t) is the pixel intensity at time t and TE is the echo time.

This allows transformation of signal-intensity time course data to contrast concentration time course data ***(see* Figs. 1A to C)**. In addition to these flow related parameters, maps can also be produced on the basis of time taken by the contrast to reach the voxel using the time of arrival or, more commonly the time-to-peak (TTP) concentration.

Problems with DSC MRI: There are several major problems/errors with the DSC MRP, therefore, numerous major modifications have been brought in the analysis approach as an attempt to produce more accurate quantitative estimates of blood flow.[26-43] Three main problems with the technique include:

1. Contrast recirculation
2. Contrast leakage
3. Bolus dispersion.

- ***Contrast recirculation:*** Analysis of the contrast bolus passage assumes that the bolus passes through the voxel and that the concentration of contrast then returns to zero. However, the contrast recirculates through the body and a second recirculation peak follows the first **(Fig. 3A)**. When the contrast continues to circulate, the bolus disperses and widens so that the second peak is lower and broader than the first and by the time of the third recirculation the intravascular contrast must

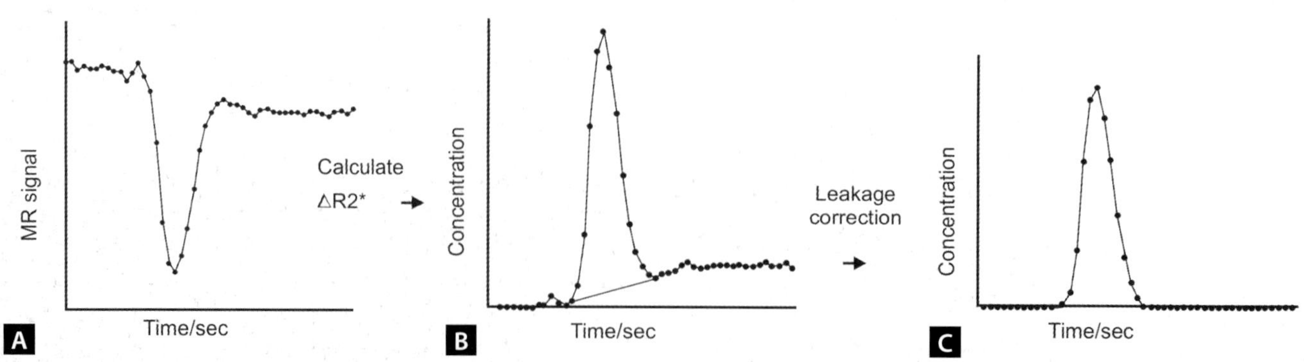

Figs. 1A to C: Figures show data analysis in DSC perfusion: (A) Time-versus MR signal intensity curve where signal intensity decreases during passage of contrast agent bolus and is measured through a series of MR images; (B) Tissue concentration versus time curve where change in the relaxation rate ($\Delta R2^*$) is calculated from signal intensity, and a baseline subtraction method is applied to measured data; (C) Corrected $\Delta R2^*$ curve after leakage correction.

have evenly mixed throughout the blood volume, thus causing a small constant baseline elevation in the contrast concentration. Errors in measurement of CBV are due to the presence of both first pass and recirculating contrast in the vessels during the latter part of the bolus passage. The error can be approached is by use of curve fitting technique, which also smoothes the data, effectively reducing noise and eliminates the contamination of the first pass bolus due to contrast agent recirculation.

- ***Contrast leakage and tissue enhancement:*** Leakage of contrast into the interstitial space causes signal changes, principally by relaxivity mechanisms. High permeability in regions of severe bloodbrain barrier breakdown (e.g. high-grade neoplasm) leads to extravasation of contrast material into the interstitium, which increases signal above baseline due to the T1-shortening effects of gadolinium (i.e. enhancement) **(Fig. 3B)**. Since, the algorithm for calculation of rCBV assumes a constant baseline, the area above baseline is interpreted by the algorithm as negative blood volume, and subtracted from the area below baseline caused by the drop in T2* signal. This leads to significant underestimation of rCBV. Imaging methods based on susceptibility allow the separation of these relaxivity and susceptibility based effects and produce images in which the effects of contrast leakage are either removed or reduced. The use of techniques with reduced T1 sensitivity, such as low flip angle gradient echo-based sequences and increase the repetition time (TR), or uses a dual echo technique or use pre-enhancement [preinject an additional small dose of gadolinium (0.05 mmol/kg) to presaturate the interstitium, effectively elevating the baseline before the dynamic acquisition], which effectively removes relaxivity effects. In addition, newer contrast materials, which can act as 'blood pool' agents

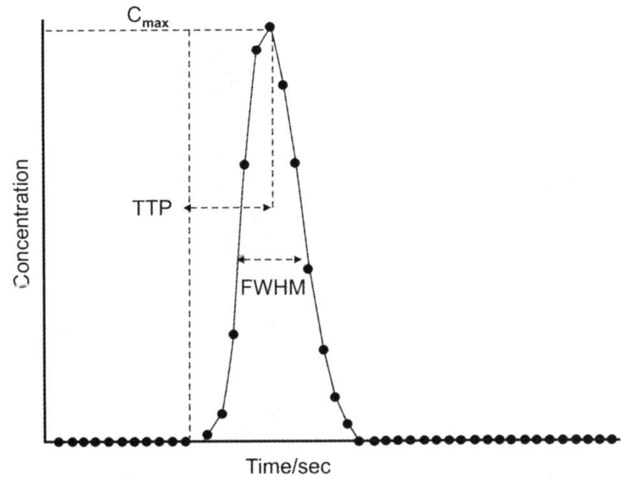

Fig. 2: Contrast (tissue concentration) versus time curve showing the different parameters. Area under curve represents cerebral blood volume, height of curve represents cerebral blood flow and area/height of curve represents mean transit time. C_{max}, peak height and, full width half maximum (FWHM), time-to-peak (TTP) concentration.

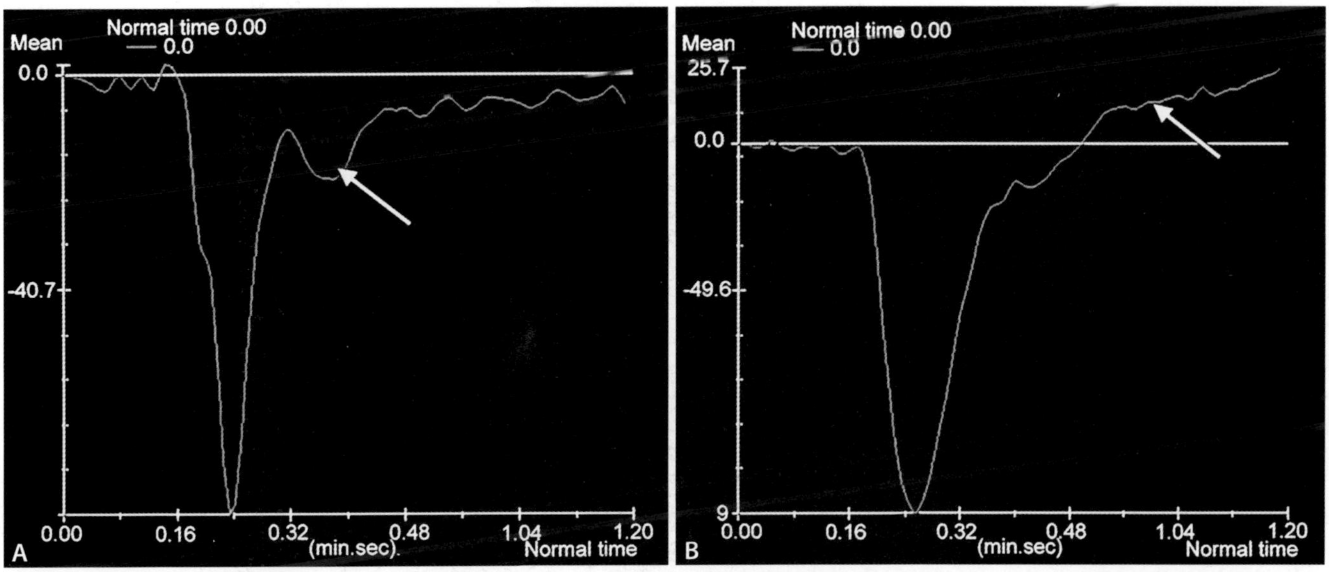

Figs. 3A and B: (A) Signal-intensity time curve showing marked signal-intensity decrease during arrival of the contrast agent, followed by partial recovery of the signal-intensity loss. A second decrease in signal intensity (arrow) is due to recirculation; (B) Signal-intensity time curve showing contrast leakage and signal above baseline due to the T1 shortening effects of gadolinium.

(such as gadobenate dimeglumine and monocrystalline iron oxide nanoparticles) may ameliorate this problem. The change which occurs in signal intensity due to T1 shortening is biexponential so that for any given sequence, there is a plateaux phase during which signal intensity remains relatively constant. The effect of this response curve is that pre-enhancement of tumors will reduce the relaxivity-based signal intensity responses to subsequent contrast doses. However, each approach offers a perfect solution and the choice of method must be based on individual analysis task to be undertaken.

- ***Bolus dispersion and the measurement of absolute CBF:*** To measure the absolute CBF it is assumed that the technique can produce quantitative measurements of CBV and MTT. However, the use of the area under the curve to estimate CBV results in relative measurement that allows comparison of CBV between tissues rather than producing an absolute measurement.[44-48] In addition, the measurement of CBF also requires accurate estimation of MTT (calculated from the width of the contrast bolus). The width of the contrast bolus is affected by the arterial input function (AIF), changes in bolus width (due to regional alterations in flow) and physical bolus broadening (due to dispersive effects).

MRI Sequence Type

Gradient-echo versus spin-echo: Both gradient-echo and spin-echo acquisitions can be used, but rapid spin-echo imaging capable of dynamic perfusion measurements is only practical with echoplanar systems. Theoretically, spin-echo produces signal changes which predominantly reflect the passage of contrast through the capillary bed and reflect the tumor physiology at the capillary level; however several studies have shown that in comparison to the benefit of using spin-echo images, there is more of compromise in terms of signal to noise ratio. Spin-echo techniques are selectively sensitive to small vessels that are less than 20 μ in diameter, whereas gradient-echo images incorporate signals from larger tumor vessels as well as the microvascularity. Gradient-echo techniques have shown a stronger correlation between tumor grade and blood volume.

Spatial coverage versus time resolution: The selection of the spatial coverage and time resolution usually happens as a compromise, in accordance with the particular application and tissue under study. The time resolution is limited by the transit time of the bolus through the tissue as for accurate quantification of DSC-MRP data, a proper characterization of the transient signal drop is required. Typically, a repetition time (TR) of 2 s or less is necessary for acquisition of the fast changes during the first pass. Therefore, the spatial coverage will be limited by the maximum number of slices that can be acquired within this TR. Echo planar imaging (EPI), segmented EPI, FLASH, etc. can be used.

2D versus 3D sequences: Both 2D and 3D sequences can be used. 2D sequences are usually preferable; however 3D sequence allows increased coverage, but typically, it occurs at the expense of an increased TR, or a decreased spatial resolution.

Single-echo versus dual-echo sequences: Dual-echo sequences provide a simple way to remove the relaxivity effects and allows the quantification of changes in R2* without assumption regarding the T1 behavior.[41,42] However, the sampling of two echoes increases sampling time and thus reducing the maximum number of slices that can be acquired (and therefore, coverage) in a given TR. when spatial coverage is important, single-echo sequences with a pre-dose of contrast may be used as the use of a pre-enhancement approach is proven effective.

Dynamic Contrast-enhanced MR Perfusion

Dynamic contrast-enhanced MR perfusion (DCE-MRP) provides insight into the nature of the tissue properties at the microvascular level by demonstrating the wash-in, plateau, and washout contrast kinetics of the tissue.[49-55] The DCE-MRP, which is also referred as 'permeability' MRI, is an entirely different approach to MR perfusion that mainly focuses at the evaluation of tumor permeability.[48-65] The main advantage of T1-based techniques is that tumor leakiness (enhancement) is used for data analysis rather than considering it as an artifact as in DSC-MRP. It has been established that quantification of contrast leakage can provide powerful indicators of the state of neovascular angiogenesis in pathologies, such as tumors and inflammatory tissue; and capillary leakage of contrast on MRI can provide an approach for monitoring the effects of the antiangiogenic drugs.

Principle: The T1-weighted technique measures the 'relaxivity effects' of the paramagnetic contrast material. The relaxivity effect of paramagnetic contrast material refers to the shortening of T1 relaxation time, leading to higher signal on T1-weighted images. The DCE-MRP is based on a two-compartmental (plasma space and extravascular-extracellular space) pharmacokinetic model **(Fig. 4)**.

Image acquisition: The patient should be positioned as used for normal MRI. The general steps in acquisition of DCE-MRP are perform baseline T1 mapping, acquire

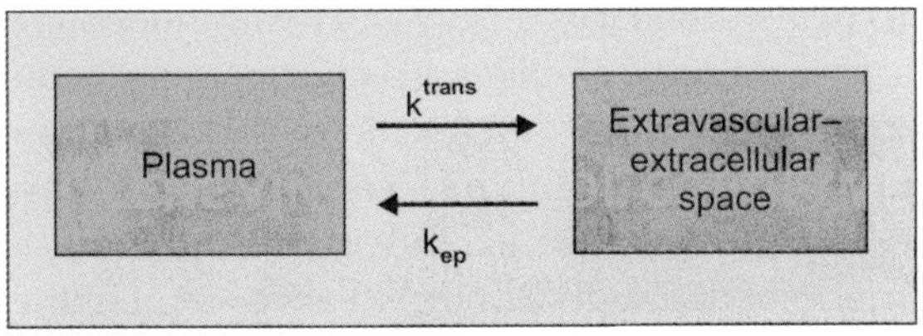

Fig. 4: Dynamic contrast-enhanced MR perfusion: Two-compartment model demonstrates the exchange of contrast between plasma and extravascular-extracellular space.

DCE-MRP images, convert signal intensity data to gadolinium concentration, determine the vascular input function, and perform pharmacokinetic modeling.[56,57] The dynamic-imaging sequence must include precontrast images for a sufficient period to allow accurate estimation of the extracellular space and of the contribution of renal excretion. The data is acquired by three-dimensional (3D) gradient echo sequence. A bolus injection technique as used for DSC-MRP is used. A lower dose of gadolinium is administered (typically a single dose of 0.1 mmol/kg) at a lower rate (2 mL/sec) and repetitive acquisitions are then made through the lesion at longer intervals, typically every 15–26 seconds. Imaging is carried out over a much longer period of time than with T2*-based techniques, to allow for the contrast to leak out into the extravascular space and come into equilibrium over several passes of the contrast bolus through the tumor bed.

Data analysis: Various techniques can be employed for quantification of the contrast-enhancement effect, which include simple measures of the rate of enhancement to complex pharmacokinetic analyses.[59-65]

Simple-analysis techniques: The quantification of enhancement can be done by directly comparing the signal-intensity curves from ROI. There are many measurements that allow this type of analysis and are designed to minimize the variation, which will occur among patients due to variations in contrast dose, injection and scanning techniques and scanner type. The simplest of these is a measurement of the time taken for the tumor tissue to attain 90% of its subsequent maximal enhancement (T90). Another parameter measures the maximum rate of change of enhancement [maximal intensity change per time interval ratio (MITR)]. Various curve shapes can also provide insight into the quantification and calculate a standardized slope of the enhancement curve. However, the enhancement curve is poorly reproducible and most of these methods which are based on signal intensity remain sensitive to variations between acquisition systems as the relationship between contrast concentration and signal intensity is non-linear.

Pharmacokinetic-analysis techniques: With pharmacokinetic modeling of DCE MRP data, several metrics are commonly derived: the transfer constant (k^{trans}), the fractional volume of the extravascular extracellular space (v_e), the rate constant (k_{ep}, $k_{ep} = k^{trans}/v_e$), and the fractional volume of the plasma space (v_p). These quantitative techniques are intended to calculate the biological features, such as endothelial permeability and the endothelial surface area, which are relatively independent of imaging approach (scanner type, scanning technique or individual patient variations). The most frequently used metric in DCE MRP is k^{trans}. It can have different interpretations depending on blood flow and permeability. In situations, in which there is very high permeability, the flux of gadolinium-based contrast agent is limited only by flow, and thus k^{trans} mainly reflects blood flow; whereas if there is very low permeability, the gadolinium-based contrast agent cannot leak easily into the extravascular–extracellular space, and thus k^{trans} mainly reflects permeability. The product of the endothelial permeability and endothelial surface area represents the transfer coefficient k^{trans} which controls the leakage of contrast from the vascular to the extravascular compartment. The leakage of contrast can be calculated by:

$$v_e \frac{dc_1}{dt} = k^{trans}(C_p - C_1)$$

where,

- v_e is the proportion of the voxel into which contrast can leak (contrast distribution space)
- C_1 is the concentration of contrast in the space
- C_p is the concentration of contrast in the blood.
- k^{trans} can be calculated if we accurately estimate the change in concentration of contrast in the bloodstream and in the tissue over time. The calculation of contrast concentration also requires knowledge of the initial T1 value of the tissues before contrast arrival which must therefore be measured before the dynamic imaging is performed and is usually measured by the use of gradient echo images with variable flip angles.

Problems with quantitative measurement of DCE MRI: The measurement of k^{trans} with pharmacokinetic analysis techniques have few disadvantages, which includes partial volume averaging effects, long acquisition time and flow dependency of k^{trans}.

Partial-volume averaging effects: The pharmacokinetic analysis technique is based on the assumption that the samples derived from voxels in blood vessels will represent changes in the blood concentration whereas voxels within the target tissue will represent leakage in the extravascular contrast. However, this assumption is not correct and voxels within the target tissue are actually likely to represent a mixture, some of which will have significant intravascular contrast content. This will result in overestimation of k^{trans} in these voxels which can be seen as areas of apparently high permeability in areas of normal brain. This problem can be approached by excluding any voxel which produces values over a certain threshold (1.2/min) as being vascular in origin or more complex pharmacokinetic models.

Long-acquisition time: Another major problem with permeability imaging is long acquisition time as the measurement takes a considerable period of time (at least 5 min). There is rarely any misregistration of data in brain perfusion and can be easily corrected by data coregistration. However, in other areas of the body which are affected by respiratory motion, there is significant misregistration and respiratory gating techniques distinctly limit the image acquisition strategy and the achievable temporal sampling rate. This can be approached by modifying the pharmacokinetic model and describing only the first passage of the contrast bolus. This technique also eliminates the problems with partial volume averaging described above and produces highly reproducible parametric maps of both k^{trans} and CBV.

Flow dependency of k^{trans}: The measurements of k^{trans} will be markedly affected by flow to the voxel as well as the permeability and surface area of the vascular endothelium. For measurements of k^{trans} it is assumed that for any given combination of intravascular and extravascular contrast concentrations the rate of contrast leakage will be proportional to the permeability and surface area of the vascular endothelium; however, it is true only where the supply of contrast to the vascular space is sufficiently high that the intravascular concentration will not be affected by the contrast leakage. There is limitation, in areas where there is contrast leakage and the blood flow is not adequate to replenish the contrast at an adequate rate; as a result plasma contrast concentration decreases and k^{trans} will reflect local blood flow.

Arterial-spin Labeling MR Imaging

Arterial-spin labeling (ASL) is an alternative technique of performing MR perfusion without the use of an intravenous contrast agent.[66-68] The ASL can be thought of as a natural extension of magnetic resonance angiography (MRA) and is also closely related to blood flow imaging with H_2O^{15}PET. Many recent studies show that ASL provides similar information to the DSC or DCE MRP, and even have more advantages as compared to these techniques, including better ASL flow maps in detecting regions of disturbed vascularity and being independent of tumor permeability, so that corrections are not required. Hitherto, limitations of ASL like long imaging times and decreased spatial resolution as compared with contrast-based techniques have excluded widespread clinical application of ASL, but with recent advancement the ASL may contribute significantly to the future of MR perfusion imaging.

Principle: ASL uses magnetically labeled blood as an endogenous contrast agent. In this technique, spatially selective excitation pulses or flow encoding gradient pulses are applied to inflowing blood to differentiate between static tissue and flowing blood. Time is allowed for the blood to move out of the vessels and into the perfused tissue, and then the signal change in tissue caused by the selective labeling of the arterial blood is measured which is closely related to the blood flow into that tissue. The arterial-spin labeling methods measure CBF by taking the difference of two sets of images: tag images, in which the longitudinal magnetization of arterial blood is inverted or saturated, and control images in which the magnetization of arterial blood is fully relaxed.[69,70] To remove the contribution of the static tissue to the tag image, a control image of the same slice is acquired in which inflowing blood is not tagged. The magnetization difference ($\Delta M = M_{contr} - M_{tag}$), i.e. difference of the control and tag images yields an image that is proportional to CBF. Tag and control images are typically acquired in a temporally interleaved fashion, and the running difference of the control and tag images is used to form a perfusion time series.

Image acquisition and labeling techniques: Different labeling techniques of ASL, that have been described or used for *in vivo* studies, are very similar and differ only in subtle aspects of implementation. However, they are broadly divided into spatially selective ASL and velocity-selective ASL.[71-79] In spatially selective ASL, a spatial separation between the imaged region and inflowing arterial blood is required to cause signal change in the image whereas in velocity-selective ASL, bipolar gradients are used to label flowing blood. Velocity-selective ASL, resemble phase contrast angiography, and can be used to label blood within the slice or slab and thus may permit labeling even closer to the capillary bed than spatially selective ASL. In most of the ASL techniques, magnetization is labeled along the main magnetic-field direction (Mz). The advantage of labeling Mz is that changes in Mz return back to the equilibrium on the time scale of T1. The magnetization can also be labeled along the transverse direction (Mx or My) but since the transverse magnetization decays with T2, typically 5–10 times faster than T1 decay, the signal produced would be much smaller.

Spatially selective ASL is by far the well-developed technique and most studies have been performed using this technique. It is similar to time-of-flight angiography. Inflowing blood may be tagged continuously or intermittently and can be broadly divided into continuous ASL and pulsed ASL **(Figs. 5A to C)**. Different pulsed labeling strategies differ from each other in primarily two issues. First is what inversions are applied to other tissue, including the imaged region, and secondly what is done to insure that the differences between the two RF preparations do not cause direct effects on the image which are independent of perfusion.

Pulsed ASL: In this technique, single perturbing pulse is applied to the spins outside the slice at a single-time point, and then time is given for the spins to enter the tissue **(Figs. 5B and C)**. Usually, an RF pulse is applied at a time approximately 1 second before imaging. An inversion RF pulse is usually used as it creates the largest change in the arterial magnetization and the time before imaging is referred to as TI, as in inversion recovery sequences. Two images are obtained, one with the region containing the inflowing artery inverted and one where it is not inverted. The signal change with pulsed techniques is smaller than with continuous techniques as the spins which enter the tissue later are perturbed earlier than in the continuous technique, there is additional T1 decay of the label and generally. However, this technique also have additional advantages including more traditional RF and gradient strategies, are less subject to certain types of systematic error, and can produce excellent images. Pulsed ASL methods include echo planar imaging and signal targeting with alternating radiofrequency (EPISTAR), flow-sensitive alternating inversion recovery (FAIR), signal targeting with alternating radio frequency (STAR), transfer insensitive labeling technique (TILT) (Gobay 1999) and proximal inversion with a control for off-resonance effect (PICORE) (Wong 1997).[80-84]

The EPISTAR technique is the simplest pulsed inversion strategy and was first proposed by Edelman et al. In this technique, a slab-selective inversion pulse is applied inferior to the imaged brain region to label arterial spins and a superior inversion slab is applied during the control image preparation. The superior inversion insures equal magnetization transfer effects from the two preparation pulses.

The FAIR is an alternative strategy to EPISTAR where a nonselective inversion pulse is applied for the labeling and a slab selective inversion containing the entire imaged region is applied for a control image. In this technique, the effect on inflowing spins inferior to the slice is the same as in EPISTAR, but the spins in the imaged slab are inverted in both cases, rather than left unaffected.

Because any slight difference in the flip angle of the two pulses will have a big effect upon the measured signal, special RF pulses with low sensitivity to variations in RF amplitude and very sharp slice profiles must be employed. There are number of variations of these basic labeling techniques and most of them may provide small improvements to the results but variations in implementation and methods of assessment overshadow these small differences.

Continuous ASL: In this technique, spins are continuously inverted at a specific location before they enter the tissue.

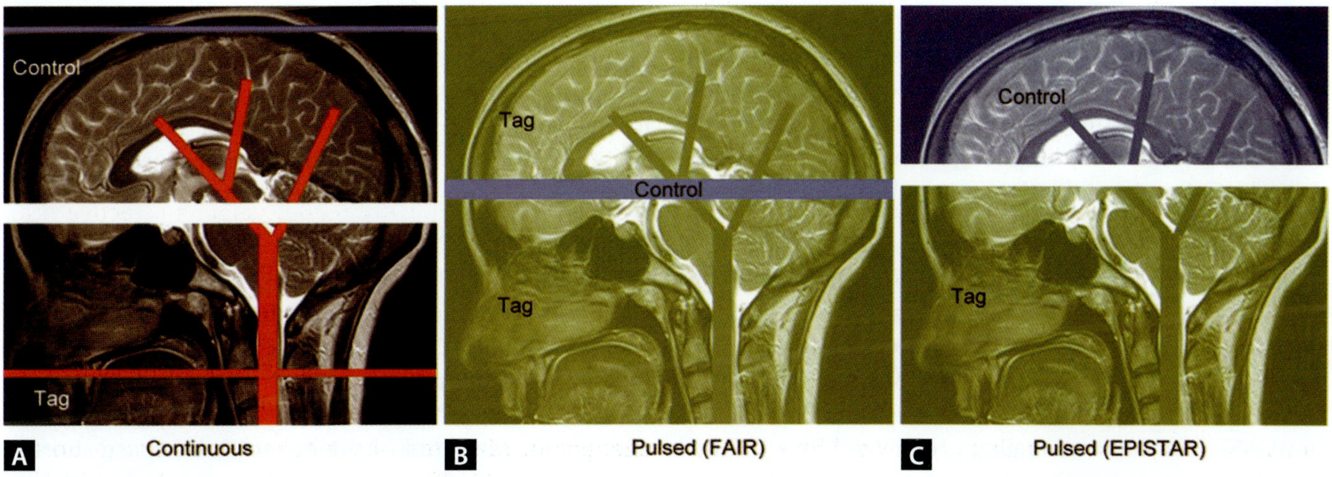

Figs. 5A to C: ASL techniques, schematic diagram illustrating arterial spin labeling strategies. (A) Continuous ASL (CASL) labels arterial spins as they flow through a labeling plane; (B and C) Pulsed ASL (PASL) labels arterial spins using a spatially selective labeling pulse.

Thus spins which enter the tissue first are labeled first and spins which enter later are labeled later. One can approximate continuous saturation of spins as they flow past a certain plane by applying a series of thin saturation pulses repeatedly, but trying the same strategy with inversion pulses is problematic; some spins may remain within the saturation slab for two or more inversions and get doubly inverted. Inversion pulse is considered highly desirable to use a continuous inversion technique as it provides a stronger signal change. Continuous ASL methods include Saturation, inversion (Williams 1992) with flow-driven adiabatic inversion pulse and labeling with 2nd coil. Continuous ASL (CASL) usually employs a special RF labeling scheme known as flow-driven adiabatic inversion. Flow-driven adiabatic inversion is a simple technique because it requires only turning on a constant gradient and RF **(*see* Fig. 5A)**. While the pulsed ASL experiment is essentially a decaying bolus experiment where the labeled blood transiently enters the tissue, the continuous ASL experiment can be operated as a steady-state experiment. If the labeling is left on for a long time, a balance between the inflow of newly labeled spins and the T1 decay of the labeled spins already in the tissue is reached. This makes quantification of perfusion relatively simple. As compared with pulsed ASL, the continuous ASL can achieve a signal approximately 2–3 times larger is generally more sensitive. The greatest disadvantage of the continuous labeling approach is the unusual RF requirements of the labeling. As in CASL (Flow-driven adiabatic inversion), weaker RF for an extended period of time is required, implementation may be difficult because many scanners are designed specifically for brief, widely spaced pulses of RF at high power.

Vessel-selective labeling: A recent approach has been introduced in which arterial water is labeled selectively on the basis of the blood velocity, termed velocity-selective ASL. The main difference between velocity-selective ASL and the other ASL techniques is that the arterial water is labeled everywhere, including the volume of interest, therefore minimizing the time for the blood to reach any region of interest.

Pseudo-continuous arterial spin labeling (pCASL): This is also known as pulsed continuous arterial spin labeling (pCASL). This is a newly proposed technique that has eased the technical restrictions of CASL and employs a train of discrete RF pulses that mimics continuous ASL.[85,86] In pCASL, continuous labeling is achieved by a train of rapidly repeating low tip RF pulses and alternating sign (bipolar) magnetic field gradients which is also suitable for MR systems that do not have continuous RF capabilities. Moreover, it has been shown that pCASL can achieve better compensation of adverse MT effects than CASL.

Data analysis (calculating blood flow from arterial-spin labeling measurements): The control and tag images ASL are acquired in an interleaved fashion and a perfusion time series is then formed from the running subtraction of the control and tag images.[87-90] Hence, the simple subtraction image obtained can be a good reflection of relative blood flow without any calculations. However, because differences in tissue T1 and other factors can lead to different sensitivity to blood flow across the image and quantitative measurements of blood flow can be useful for some purposes, it can be useful to convert the difference images into actual blood flow maps in physiologic units. This conversion requires some consideration of how inflow impacts tissue MR signal.

Problems with ASL: Despite its advantages, ASL imaging is limited by a large background signal and the motion artifacts. In addition, the small signal level of ASL reduces the signal-to-noise ratio of the ASL perfusion imaging. With recent advancement in MRI technology, good quality images can be obtained.

DYNAMIC CONTRAST-ENHANCED MRI

Dynamic contrast-enhancement techniques are well established for characterizing the benign or malignant lesions by providing functional information to the anatomically detailed morphological images as the malignant lesions usually show faster and higher levels of enhancement than normal tissue.[91] This enhancement pattern of the malignant lesions reflects increased vascularity (neoangiogenesis) and higher endothelial permeability to the contrast molecules than do normal or less aggressive malignant tissues. Nowadays, dynamic contrast-enhanced MRI (DCE-MRI) is modality of choice for the diagnosis and characterization of the tumors of the brain, breast, prostate, liver, cervix and musculoskeletal system.[92-95]

Principle: The DCE-MRI relies on fast MRI sequences obtained before, during and after the rapid intravenous (IV) administration of a gadolinium-based contrast agent.[64] IV-injected contrast agents pass from the arteries to the tissue microvasculature and extravasate within seconds to the extravascular–extracellular space. Contrast agents in vessels and in the extracellular space shorten local relaxation times, leading to increased signal on T1-weighted sequences. The ability to measure vessel leakiness is related to blood flow (i.e. it is difficult to identify leakiness if the flow is too low). Thus, the signal measured on DCE-MRI represents a combination of perfusion and permeability. The DCE-MRI is sensitive to alterations in vascular permeability, extracellular space and blood flow. The DCE-MRI enables the depiction of physiologic alterations as well as morphologic changes. It is an emerging imaging method to assess tumor angiogenesis and the clinical application of DCE-MRI for cancer is based on data showing that malignant lesions usually shows rapid, intense enhancement followed by a relatively rapid washout compared to normal healthy tissue.

Image acquisition: The acquisition of DCE-MRI is done by acquiring a minimum of three sections through the tumor and imaging volume that includes a region outside the tumor, such as an artery or muscle for normalization. Quantity of the injected contrast material is usually standardized according to the patient's body weight and preferentially should be injected at a constant rate with a power injector typically using 3D T1-weighted acquisition (spoiled gradient-echo sequences) to repeatedly image a volume of interest after the administration of a bolus of IV contrast agent. T1-weighted spoiled gradient-echo sequences provide high sensitivity to T1 changes, high signal-to-noise ratios (SNRs), adequate anatomic coverage, and rapid data acquisition. Serial image sets are obtained sequentially every 5 seconds (ranging from 2–15 seconds) for up to 5–10 minutes. The rapidity with which MRI must be acquired necessitates that larger voxels (i.e. lower matrix sizes) must be obtained to maintain adequate SNRs.

Data analysis: Signal intensity (SI) enhancement patterns on T1W images can be evaluated by different analysis techniques, viz. qualitative, semiquantitative and quantitative. The complexity and standardization of analytic technique is needed to be adjusted.

Qualitative: The qualitative or visual analysis is most readily accessible analytic but also the least standardized method. It is based on the general assumption that tumor vessels are leaky and more readily enhance after IV contrast material. It is expressed by a fast exchange of blood and contrast media between capillaries and tumor tissues. Thus, DCE-MRI patterns for malignant tumors are expected to show early rapid high enhancement after injection followed by a relatively rapid decline compared with a slower and continuously increasing signal for normal tissues during the first few minutes after contrast injection. The qualitative analysis shows higher accuracy and less interobserver variability but there is overlap of malignant and benign tissues, which is limiting the capabilities of this approach. Moreover, the qualitative approach is inherently subjective and therefore difficult to standardize among institutions, making multicenter trials less reliable.

Semiquantitative analysis: Semiquantitative analysis calculates various curve parameters and is also referred as curveology. It is also based on the assumption of early and intense enhancement and washout as a predictor of malignancy. Parameters are obtained to characterize the shape of the time-intensity curve, such as the time of first contrast uptake, time to peak, maximum slope, peak enhancement, and wash-in and washout curve shapes. There are three common dynamic curve types after initial uptake: type 1, persistent increase; type 2, plateau; and type 3, decline after initial upslope. Type 3 is considered to be indicator of malignancy. The semiquantitative approach is widely used and has the advantage of being simple to perform. It has limitations in terms of generalization across acquisition protocols, sequences, and all other factors contributing to the MR signal intensity, which in turn affect curve metrics, such as maximum enhancement and washout percentage.

Quantitative analysis: Quantitative analysis is most generalizable but most complex method. It depends on contrast concentration curves over time and pharmacokinetic models are applied to calculate permeability constants. Dynamic imaging data obtained with DCE-MRI can generate curves which are mathematically fit to compartment pharmacokinetic models. For functional analysis of tissue microcirculation, two-compartment model is considered for the kinetic parameters which demonstrates the exchange of contrast between plasma and extravascular space as proposed by Tofts et al. To describe tumor and tissue permeability, various kinetic parameters include, K^{trans} [transendothelial transport of contrast medium from vascular compartment to the tumor interstitium (washin)], k_{ep} [reverse transport parameter of contrast medium back into the vascular space (washout)], fpV (plasma volume fraction compared to whole tissue volume) and Ve [extravascular, extracellular volume fraction of the tumor; the fraction of tumor volume occupied by extravascular-extracellular space (EES)]. Physiologically, the value of k^{trans} is tissue dependent; k^{trans} will indicate the tissue perfusion per unit volume, if the contrast uptake of the tissue is flow limited; on the other hand, k^{trans} indicates the tissue permeability, if the uptake is permeability limited. In majority of tumors, k^{trans} indicates a combination of both flow and permeability properties of the tissue and high k^{trans} values usually reflect both high permeability and high perfusion. This is thus a fundamental limitation of DCE-MRI that the parameters it generates are inherently ambiguous with regard to their physiologic significance.

REFERENCES

1. Essig M, Shiroishi MS, Nguyen TB, Saake M, Provenzale JM, Enterline D, et al. Perfusion MRI: the five most frequently asked technical questions. Am J Roentgenol. 2013;200:24-34.
2. Hochberg AR, Young GS. Cerebral perfusion imaging. Semin Neurol. 2012;32:454-65.
3. Lammertsma AA, Cunningham VJ, Deiber MP, et al. Combination of dynamic and integral methods for generating reproducible functional CBF images. J Cereb Blood Flow Metab. 1990;10:675-86.
4. Axel L. Cerebral blood flow determination by rapid-sequence computed tomography. Radiology. 1980;137:676-86.
5. Yonas H, Darby JM, Marks EC, et al. CBF measured by Xe CT: approach to analysis and normal values. J Cereb Blood Flow Metab. 1991;11:716-25.
6. Detre JA, Eskey CJ, Koretsky AP. Measurement of cerebral blood flow in rat brain by F-19 NMR detection of trifluoromethane washout. Magn Reson Med. 1990;15:45-57.
7. Kim SG, Ackerman JJH. Quantification of regional blood flow by monitoring of exogenous tracer via nuclear magnetic resonance spectroscopy. Magn Reson Med. 1990;14:266-82.
8. Detre JA, Leigh JS, Williams DS, et al. Perfusion imaging. Magn Reson Med. 1992;23:37-45.
9. McGehee BE, Pollock JM, Maldjian JA. Brain perfusion imaging: How does it work and what should I use? J Magn Reson Imag. 2012;36:1257-72.
10. Ostergaard. Principles of cerebral perfusion imaging by bolus tracking. J Magn Reson Imag. 2005;22:710-7.
11. Wu, Ostergaard. Technical aspects of perfusion-weighted imaging. Neuroimaging Clin N Am. 2005;15:623-37.
12. Duyn, van Gelderen. Technological advances in MRI measurement of brain perfusion. J Magn Reson Imaging. 2005;22:751-3.
13. Rosen BR, Belliveau JW, Buchbinder BR, et al. Contrast agents and cerebral hemodynamics. Magn Reson Med. 1991;19:285-92.
14. Keston P, Murray AD, Jackson A. Cerebral perfusion imaging using contrast-enhanced MRI. Clin Radiol. 2003;58:505-13.
15. Williams DS, Detre JA, Leigh JS, et al. Magnetic resonance imaging of perfusion using spin inversion of arterial water. Proc Natl Acad Sci USA. 1992;89:212-6.
16. Calamante F, Thomas DL, Pell GS, et al. Measuring cerebral blood flow using magnetic resonance imaging techniques. J Cereb Blood Flow Metab. 1999;19:701-35.
17. Villringer A, Rosen BR, Belliveau JW, et al. Dynamic imaging with lanthanide chelates in normal brain: contrast due to magnetic susceptibility effects. Magn Reson Med. 1988;6:164-74.
18. Weisskoff RM, Zuo CS, Boxerman JL, et al. Microscopic susceptibility variation and transverse relaxation: theory and experiment. Magn Reson Med. 1994;31:601-10.
19. Yablonskiy DA, Haacke EM. Theory of NMR signal behavior in magnetically inhomogeneous tissues: the static dephasing regime. Magn Reson Med. 1994;32:749-63.
20. Kiselev VG, Posse S. Analytical model of susceptibility-induced MR signal dephasing: effect of diffusion in a microvascular network. Magn Reson Med. 1999;41:499-509.
21. Petrella JR, Provenzale JM. MR perfusion imaging of the brain: techniques and applications. Am J Roentgenol. 2000;175:207-19.
22. Aksoy FG, Lev MH. Dynamic contrast-enhanced brain perfusion imaging: technique and clinical applications. Semin Ultrasound CT MR. 2000;21:462-77.
23. Cha S. Perfusion MR imaging: basic principles and clinical applications. Magn Reson Imaging Clin N Am. 2003;11:403-13.
24. Covarrubias DJ, Rosen BR, Lev MH. Dynamic magnetic resonance perfusion imaging of brain tumors. Oncologist. 2004;9:528-37.
25. Chavhan GB, Babyn PS, Thomas B, Shroff MM, Haacke EM. Principles, techniques, and applications of T2*-based MR imaging and its special applications. Radiographics. 2009;29:1433-49.
26. Boxerman JL, Hamberg LM, Rosen BR, et al. MR contrast due to intravascular magnetic susceptibility perturbations. Magn Reson Med. 1995;34:555-66.
27. Fisel CR, Ackerman JL, Buxton RB, et al. MR contrast due to microscopically heterogeneous magnetic susceptibility: numerical simulations and applications to cerebral physiology. Magn Reson Med. 1991;17:336-47.
28. Rempp KA, Brix G, Wenz F, et al, Quantification of regional cerebral blood flow and volume with dynamic susceptibility contrast-enhanced MR imaging. Radiology. 1994;193:637-41.
29. Edelman RR, Mattle HP, Atkinson DJ, et al. Cerebral blood flow: assessment with dynamic contrast-enhanced T2-star-weighted MR imaging at 1.5 T. Radiology. 1990;176:211-20.
30. Levin JM, Kaufman MJ, Ross MH. Sequential dynamic susceptibility contrast MR experiments in human brain: residual contrast agent effect, steady-state, and hemodynamic perturbation. Magn Reson Med. 1995;34:655-63.
31. Barbier EL, Lamalle L, Decorps M. Methodology of brain perfusion imaging. J Magn Reson Imag. 2001;13:496-520.
32. Rosen BR, et al. Contrast agents and cerebral hemodynamics. Magn Reson Med. 1991;19:285-92.
33. Kassner A, Annesley DJ, Zhu XP, et al. Abnormalities of the contrast re-circulation phase in cerebral tumors demonstrated using dynamic susceptibility contrast-enhanced imaging: a possible marker of vascular tortuosity. J Magn Reson Imaging. 2000;11:103-13.
34. Heiland S, Benner T, Debus J, et al. Simultaneous assessment of cerebral hemodynamics and contrast agent uptake in lesions with disrupted blood–brain barrier. Magn Reson Imag. 1999;17:21-7.

35. Weisskoff RM, Chesler DA, Boxerman JL, et al. Pitfalls in MR measurement of tissue blood flow with intravascular tracers: which mean transit time. Magn Reson Med. 1993;29:553-9.
36. Akbudak E, Conturo TE. Arterial input functions from MR phase imaging. Magn Reson Med. 1996;36:809-15.
37. Duhamel G, Schlaug G, Alsop DC. Measurement of arterial input functions for dynamic susceptibility contrast magnetic resonance imaging using echoplanar images: comparison of physical simulations with *in vivo* results. Magn Reson Med. 2006;55:514-23.
38. van Osch MJ, van der Grond J, Bakker CJ. Partial volume effects on arterial input functions: shape and amplitude distortions and their correction. J Magn Reson Imaging. 2005;22:704-9.
39. Perman WH, Gado MH, Larson KB, et al. Simultaneous MR acquisition of arterial and brain signal time curves. Magn Reson Med. 1992;28:74-83.
40. Vonken EP, van Osch MJ, Bakker CJ, et al. Simultaneous quantitative cerebral perfusion and Gd-DTPA extravasation measurement with dual-echo dynamic susceptibility contrast MRI. Magn Reson Med. 2000;43:820-7.
41. Vonken E, van Osch M, Bakker C, et al. Measurement of cerebral perfusion with dual-echo multi-slice quantitative dynamic susceptibility contrast MRI. J Magn Reson Imag. 1999;10:109-17.
42. Ostergaard L, Weisskoff RM, Chesler DA, et al. High resolution measurement of cerebral blood flow using intravascular tracer bolus passages. Mathematical approach and statistical analysis. Magn Reson Med. 1996;36:715-25.
43. Liu HL, Pu T, Andrews T, et al. Cerebral blood flow measurement by dynamic contrast MRI using singular value decomposition with an adaptive threshold. Magn Reson Med. 1999;42:167-72.
44. Calamante F, Gadian DG, Connely A. Delay and dispersion effects in dynamic susceptibility contrast MRI: simulations using singular value decomposition. Magn Reson Med. 2000; 44:466-73.
45. Ostergaard L, Sorensen AG, Kwong KK, et al. High resolution measurement of cerebral blood flow using intravascular tracer bolus passages. Experimental comparison and preliminary results. Magn Reson Med. 1996;36:726-36.
46. Calamante F, Morup M, Hansen LK. Defining a local arterial input function for perfusion MRI using independent component analysis. Magn Reson Med. 2004;52:789-97.
47. Mouridsen K, Christensen S, Gydensted L, et al. Automatic selection of arterial input function using cluster analysis. Magn Reson Med. 2006;55:524-31.
48. Lorenz C, Benner T, Lopez CJ, et al. Effect of using local arterial input functions on cerebral blood flow estimation. J Magn Reson Imag. 2006;24:57-65.
49. Sourbron S, Ingrisch M, Siefert A, Reiser M, Herrmann K. Quantification of cerebral blood flow, cerebral blood volume, and blood-brain-barrier leakage with DCE-MRI. Magn Reson Med. 2009;62:205-17.
50. Tofts PS, Brix G, Buckley DL, et al. Estimating kinetic parameters from dynamic contrast-enhanced T1-weighted MRI of a diffusable tracer: standardized quantities and symbols. J Magn Reson Imaging. 1999;10:223-32.
51. Dean BL, Lee C, Kirsch JE, et al. Cerebral hemodynamics and cerebral blood volume: MR assessment using gadolinium contrast agents and T1-weighted turbo-FLASH imaging. AJNR. 1992;13:39-48.
52. Moody AR, Martel A, Kenton A, et al. Contrast-reduced imaging of tissue concentration and arterial level (CRITICAL) for assessment of cerebral hemodynamics in acute stroke by magnetic resonance. Invest Radiol. 2000;35:401-11.
53. Shin W, Cashen TA, Horowitz SW, et al. Quantitative CBV measurement from static T1 changes in tissue and correction for intravascular water exchange. Magn Reson Med. 2006;56:138-45.
54. Lu H, Law M, Johnson G, Ge Y, et al. Novel approach to the measurement of absolute cerebral blood volume using vascular-space-occupancy magnetic resonance imaging. Magn Reson Med. 2005;54:1403-11.
55. ME Raichle, JO Eichling, MG Straatmann, et al. Blood-brain barrier permeability of 11C-labeled alcohols and 15O-labeled water. Am J Physiol. 1976;230:543-52.
56. Edelman RR, Siewert B, Darby DG, et al. Qualitative mapping of cerebral blood flow and functional localization with echo-planar MR imaging and signal targeting with alternating radio frequency. Radiology. 1994;192:513-20.
57. Kwong KK, Chesler DA, Weisskoff RM, et al. MR perfusion studies with T1-weighted echo planar imaging. Magn Reson Med. 1995;34:878-87.
58. Paldino MJ, Barboriak DP. Fundamentals of quantitative dynamic contrast-enhanced MR imaging. Magn Reson Imaging Clin N Am. 2009;17:277-89.
59. Tofts PS, Brix G, Buckley DL, et al. Estimating kinetic parameters from dynamic contrast-enhanced T(1)-weighted MRI of a diffusable tracer: standardized quantities and symbols. J Magn Reson Imag. 1999;10:223-32.
60. Tofts PS, Kermode AG. Measurement of the blood-brain barrier permeability and leakage space using dynamic MR imaging. Fundamental concepts. Magn Reson Med. 1991;17:357-67.
61. Cron GO, Santyr G, Kelcz F. Accurate and rapid quantitative dynamic contrast-enhanced breast MR imaging using spoiled gradient-recalled echoes and bookend T(1) measurements. Magn Reson Med. 1999;42:746-53.
62. Cron GO, Kelcz F, Santyr GE. Improvement in breast lesion characterization with dynamic contrast-enhanced MRI using pharmacokinetic modeling and bookend T(1) measurements. Magn Reson Med. 2004;51:1066-70.
63. Nguyen TB, Cron GO, Mercier JF, et al. Diagnostic accuracy of dynamic contrast-enhanced MR imaging using a phase-derived vascular input function in the preoperative grading of gliomas. Am J Neuroradiol. 2012;33:1539-45.
64. Jackson A. Analysis of dynamic contrast enhanced MRI. Br J Radiol. 2004;77:S154-66.
65. Claussen C, Laniado M, Schorner W, et al. Gadolinium-DTPA in MR imaging of glioblastomas and intracranial metastases. AJNR. 1985;6:669-74.

66. Talagala SL, Ye FQ, Ledden PJ, Chesnick S. Whole-brain 3D perfusion MRI at 3.0 T using CASL with a separate labeling coil. Magn Reson Med. 2004;52:131-40.
67. Wang Z, Wang J, Connick TJ, Wetmore GS, Detre JA. Continuous ASL (CASL) perfusion MRI with an array coil and parallel imaging at 3T. Magn Reson Med. 2005;54: 732-7.
68. van Laar PJ, van der Grond J, Hendrikse J. Brain perfusion territory imaging: methods and clinical applications of selective arterial spin-labeling MR imaging. Radiology. 2008;246:354-64.
69. Buxton RB, Frank LR, Wong EC, et al. A general kinetic model for quantitative perfusion imaging with arterial spin labeling. Magn Reson Med. 1998;40:383-96.
70. Frank LR, Wong EC, Buxton RB. Slice profile effects in adiabatic inversion: application to multislice perfusion imaging. Magn Reson Med. 1997;38:558-64.
71. Golay X, Stuber M, Pruessmann KP, et al. Transfer insensitive labeling technique (TILT): application to multislice functional perfusion imaging. J Magn Reson Imaging. 1999;9:454-61.
72. Edelman RR, Chen G. EPISTAR MRI: multislice mapping of cerebral blood flow. Magn Reson Med. 1998;40: 800-5.
73. Kim SG. Quantification of relative cerebral blood flow change by flow-sensitive alternating inversion-recovery (FAIR) technique: application to functional mapping. Magn Reson Med. 1995;34:293-301.
74. Yongbi MN, Branch CA, Helpern JA. Perfusion imaging using FOCI RF pulses. Magn Reson Med. 1998;40: 938-43.
75. Dixon WT, Du LN, Faul DD, et al. Projection angiograms of blood labeled by adiabatic fast passage. Magn Reson Med. 1986;3:454-62.
76. Wong EC, Buxton RB, Frank LR. A theoretical and experimental comparison of continuous and pulsed arterial spin labeling techniques for quantitative perfusion imaging. Magn Reson Med. 1998;40:348-55.
77. Wong EC, Buxton RB, Frank LR. Quantitative imaging of perfusion using a single subtraction (QUIPSS and QUIPSS II). Magn Reson Med. 1998;39:702-8.
78. Herscovitch P, Raichle ME. What is the correct value for the brain–blood partition coefficient for water. J Cereb Blood Flow Metab. 1985;5:65-9.
79. Maccotta L, Detre JA, Alsop DC. The efficiency of adiabatic inversion for perfusion imaging by arterial spin labeling. NMR Biomed. 1997;10:216-21.
80. Siewert B, Bly BM, Schlaug G, et al. Comparison of the BOLD and EPISTAR technique for functional brain imaging by using signal detection theory. Magn Reson Med. 1996;36:249-55.
81. Garcia DM, Duhamel G, Alsop DC. Efficiency of inversion pulses for background suppressed arterial spin labeling. Magn Reson Med. 2005;54:366-72.
82. Zaharchuk G, Ledden PJ, Kwong KK, et al. Multislice perfusion and perfusion territory imaging in humans with separate label and image coils. Magn Reson Med. 1999;41:1093-8.
83. Alsop DC, Detre JA. Multisection cerebral blood flow MR imaging with continuous arterial spin labeling. Radiology. 1998;208:410-6.
84. Deibler AR, Pollock JM, Kraft RA, Tan H, Burdette JH, Maldjian JA. Arterial spin-labeling in routine clinical practice, part 1: technique and artifacts. AJNR. 2008;29:1228-34.
85. Järnum H, Steffensen EG, Knutsson L, et al. Perfusion MRI of brain tumours: a comparative study of pseudo-continuous arterial spin labelling and dynamic susceptibility contrast imaging. Neuroradiology. 2010;52:307-17.
86. Nezamzadeh M, Matson GB, Young K, Weiner MW, Schuff N. Improved pseudo-continuous arterial spin labeling for mapping brain perfusion. J Magn Reson Imaging. 2010;31:1419-27.
87. Golay X, Petersen ET, Hui F. Pulsed star labeling of arterial regions (PULSAR): a robust regional perfusion technique for high field imaging. Magn Reson Med. 2005;53:15-21.
88. Werner R, Norris DG, Alfke K, et al. Continuous artery-selective spin labeling (CASSL). Magn Reson Med. 2005;53:1006-12.
89. Warmuth C, Gunther M, Zimmer C. Quantification of blood flow in brain tumors: comparison of arterial spin labeling and dynamic susceptibility-weighted contrast-enhanced MR imaging. Radiology. 2003;228:523-32.
90. Gonzalez-At JB, Alsop DC, Detre JA. Cerebral perfusion and arterial transit time changes during task activation determined with continuous arterial spin labeling. Magn Reson Med. 2000;43:739-46.
91. Hayes C, Padhani AR, Leach MO. Assessing changes in tumour vascular function using dynamic contrast-enhanced magnetic resonance imaging. NMR Biomed. 2002:15;154-63.
92. El Khouli RH, Macura KJ, Jacobs MA, et al. Dynamic contrast-enhanced MRI of the breast: quantitative method for kinetic curve type assessment. AJR. 2009;193:W295-300.
93. Overview of Dynamic Contrast- Enhanced MRI in Prostate Cancer. AJR. 2012;198:1277-88.
94. Jackson AS, Reinsberg SA, Sohaib SA, et al. Dynamic contrast-enhanced MRI for prostate cancer localization. Br J Radiol. 2009;82:148-56.
95. Türkbey B, Thomasson D, Pang Y, et al. The role of dynamic contrast-enhanced MRI in cancer diagnosis and treatment. Diagn Interv Radiol. 2010;16:186-92.

CHAPTER 48

Magnetic Resonance Angiography

Ajay Kumar, Sameer Vyas, Naveen Kalra

HISTORY AND INTRODUCTION

The term angiography stands for the imaging depiction of vascular structures, and there are many ways to evaluate the vascular structures like Doppler, computed tomographic, catheter and magnetic resonance angiography (MRA). In last decade, MRA has been increasing in demand because of its physiological nature on the contrary to CTA and catheter angiography which involves catheterization, radiation and nephrotoxic iodinated contrast agents. However, there are many limitations, such as availability, cost, time consuming and high sensitivity to motion and flow related artifacts.

The first research meeting devoted to MRA was hosted by Roberto Passariello in L'Aquila, Italy in 1989. Those days three-dimensional phase-contrast MRA would take 19 hours from the time the patient entered the magnet until images could be seen; one hour to acquire the image and 18 hours of overnight image postprocessing. Computational capabilities of modern equipment have reduced the delay to a few seconds. Postprocessing now has taken a more central role in the communication of enormous amounts of data with less cumbersome two- or three-dimensional projections.

Many variations on the MRA theme have been presented over the ensuing 15 years. Dennis Parker developed the 3D multislab time-of-flight (TOF) MRA technique which remains in routine clinical use to this day. Pulse sequence design plays a major role in the continuing advancements in the field, most notably as a consequence of more sophisticated and novel k-space filling strategies. The work of Kent Yucel and Martin Prince at the Massachusetts General Hospital in1992 brought gadolinium-enhanced MR angiography to clinical utility. The first-pass dynamic contrast-enhanced MRA method provides robust and reproducible imaging results that have propelled the adoption of MRA into wider clinical use. This advance reliably produced images of sufficient quality to replace invasive catheter-based X-ray contrast angiography for most diagnostic purposes.

The advent of very high field clinical scanners operating at 3.0 tesla is now reinvigorating the earlier used noncontrast methods. 3.0 T MRA benefits from two key phenomena:

- The signal to noise of 3.0 T is twice that of the 1.5 T, offering the opportunity to either increase the spatial resolution or to shorten scan times by up to a factor of four
- The longer T1 of tissues at 3.0 T, ~20 to 40% higher than 1.5 T, provides better background suppression, additional inflow enhancement, and improved contrast-to-noise.

FLOW PHENOMENA

Flow phenomena in blood or cerebrospinal fluid (CSF) also influence the MR image contrast, in addition to inherent tissue factors like T1, T2 and proton density. Blood flow is complex and variable inside the body, so it is important to understand the various types of flow that are as follows:

- Laminar flow is flow where the particles move along in concentric sheets and laminae, i.e. different but consistent velocities across the vessel. It is seen in normal vessels

- Plug flow is flow where all fluid particles move forward in parallel lines with the same speed and has a characteristic blunt profile. It is seen in the descending thoracic aorta
- Turbulent flow is flow at different velocities which varies, i.e. velocities across the vessel changes and is seen at vascular bifurcations
- Vortex flow is flow after narrowing and is seen after stricture or stenosis. In it, the high velocities are seen at the center
- Stagnant flow is flow that nearly behaves like stationary tissue and is seen in occluded vessels and large aneurysms.

The moving spins (spins that move during acquisition of data) show different contrast characteristics from the stationary spins. The moving spins causes mismapping of the signal because of the flow phenomena and result in flow motion artifacts or phase ghosting. The flow phenomena is generally categorized into time of flight, entry slice phenomenon and intravoxel dephasing.

Outflow-related Signal Loss (Washout Effect, T2 Flow Void)

When images are obtained with a spin-echo (SE)-pulse sequence, the blood flowing at a high velocity perpendicular to the imaging plane produces a weaker signal than the surrounding stationary tissue. This phenomenon is caused by the washout of flowing spins from the slice during the imaging process. Spin-echo techniques are characterized by a sequence of slice-selective 90° and 180° radiofrequency (RF) pulses. Only those tissue components that are affected by both pulses can provide an MR signal. Moving material, such as blood in the vessels, flowing through the excited slice at a sufficiently high velocity, is affected by only one of these pulses, and therefore does not contribute to the MR signal. This is the so-called "flow void" **(Figs. 1A and B)**. The intensity of the vascular signal declines with decreasing slice thickness, increasing echo time (TE), and increasing flow velocity.

If the blood flow velocity is so high that all spins leave the slice between the 90° and 180° pulses ($v \geq s/(TE/2)$, then there will be no signal and the vessel will appear dark. Spins flowing within the imaging plane are not affected by this phenomenon. The washout effect is observed only for SE sequences and is most pronounced on T2- weighted imaging because of the long echo times used. With gradient-echo (GRE) techniques, the echo is refocused without a 180° pulse simply by reversing the imaging gradients. Since only one RF pulse is needed to form an echo, the washout effect does not occur. With standard SE sequences, the washout effect provides valuable and reliable information about blood flow. The absence of a

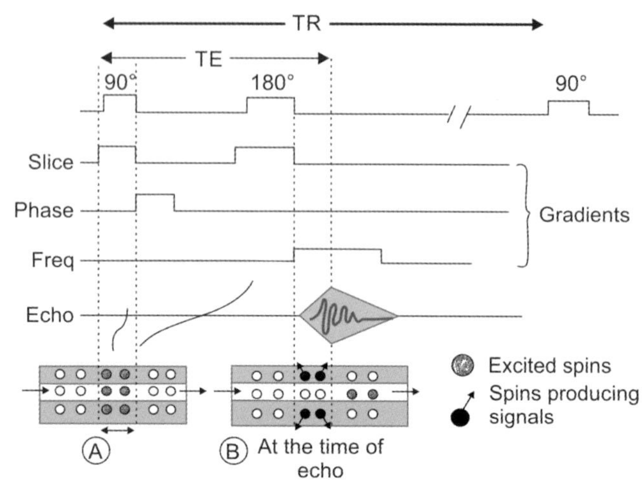

Fig. 1A: Spin-echo sequence depicting the "Flow void" phenomenon (A and B) represents the tissue sample with shaded area as stationary tissue (spins) and central nonshaded area as vessel having moving spins. (A) At the time of 90° excitation and 180° rephasing RF pulse for that particular selected slice location. (B) Same tissue with same slice location at the time of receiving signal or TE, now only stationary spins are giving signal in the selected slice, however, the moving spins have migrated out of selected slice with new nonexcited spins in that place giving no signals.

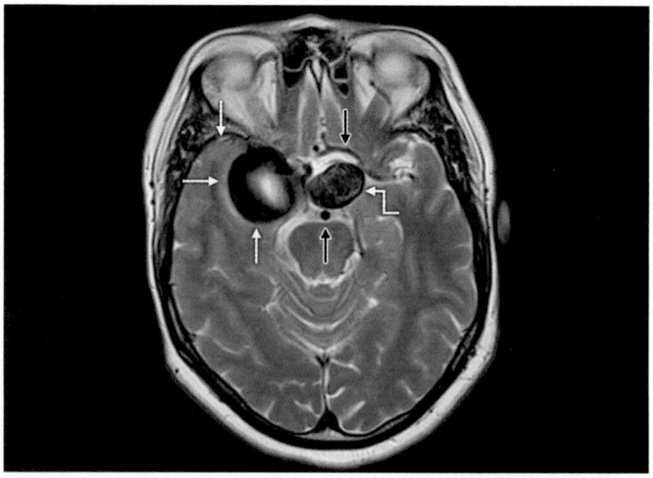

Fig. 1B: T2W axial image of the patient with bilateral ICA aneurysms shown to explain "Flow voids"—Normal arteries, i.e. left ACA and basilar arteries (black arrows) are seen hypointense due to flow void, left aneurysm (white elbow arrow) postcoiling shows heterogeneous hypointese signals due to partial thrombosis. Right patent aneurysm (white arrows) reveals flow voids at periphery due to high flow, however, central part giving bright signals due to relative stasis of blood.

flow void on T2-weighted imaging should be considered as indicative of very slow flow or even occlusion of the vessel. On the other hand, occlusion of the vessel can be excluded if a flow void is present.

Inflow-related Signal Enhancement (Inflow Effect)

The signal of blood flowing rapidly out of the measured slice is reduced with SE sequences, under these circumstances the opposite effect may occur: spins flowing into the slice may generate a higher signal than the surrounding tissue. This effect is referred to as "inflow enhancement". On T1-weighted imaging, contrast is generated by repeated RF pulses that are applied with a time interval (repetition time, TR) that is shorter than the T1 relaxation time of the tissue (typically TR < 700 msec). As a result, the tissue components are saturated unequally, depending on their individual T1 times. This is the basis of T1-weighted image contrast. Irrespective of flow effects, blood in the vessels would appear hypointense on a normal T1-weighted image due to its relatively long T1 time. The signal emitted by the tissue diminishes when the TR is reduced. With GRE sequences, repetition time shorter than 50 msec can be achieved. This allows the majority of nonmoving spins to become saturated, thus minimizing the background signal. Spins outside the excited slice (or volume) are not influenced by the RF pulses. Consequently, blood entering into the slice being imaged is fully relaxed, experiencing not more than a few excitations on its way through the slice. As a result, flowing blood gives rise to considerably higher signal intensity relative to that of the saturated spins in the stationary tissue. This effect is called "inflow enhancement" or "flow-related enhancement". The signal intensity of flowing blood increases with decreasing slice thickness, and increasing flow velocity.

If the blood flow velocity is so high that all vessel spins are replaced by unsaturated spins in the time interval TR, flow enhancement is maximal and the vessel appears bright on a gray or black background. Although the inflow effect occurs both with SE and GRE sequences, SE sequences are not practical for the TOF method because the competing washout effect tends to overbalance the inflow effect at higher flow velocities, leading to decreased flow signal. Consequently, flow-related enhancement using GRE sequences to produce bright-blood images is the basis of time-of-flight angiography.

Phase Effects

Phase effects concern the transverse component of the magnetization. They occur whenever spins are moving in the presence of magnetic field gradients, as are applied for spatial encoding of the MR signal. Magnetic field gradients provoke a change in the Larmor frequency depending on gradient strength and spin position. A gradient pulse of certain length and amplitude, therefore, induces a phase shift of the transverse magnetization, which can be compensated by a second gradient pulse with identical strength and duration but opposite sign. Thus for stationary spins the net phase shift is zero. In contrast, the same gradients applied on a flowing spin generate a non-zero phase shift. Since the spins change their position during the bipolar gradient application, the second gradient pulse is no longer able to completely compensate for the phase shifts induced by the first gradient. The remaining phase shift Φ is proportional to the velocity component v of the spins along the gradient direction. On standard MR imaging, this flow-induced phase shift causes a spatial misencoding of the signal leading to ghost artifacts that are typically found in the phase-encoding direction. Spins in a blood vessel are moving with different velocities. Often, a parabolic flow profile is found. Spins moving faster, experience a larger phase shift than those moving more slowly. If there is a velocity distribution inside a voxel, phase dispersion (intravoxel dephasing) occurs resulting in decreased signal in the blood vessel. The extent of spin-dephasing depends on the strength and time interval of the gradient pulses, as well as the distribution of spin velocities. When complex flow patterns are encountered, for example, in vessels with turbulent flow, there may be a very broad spectrum of velocities within a voxel, leading to total signal loss in the vessel.

Using additional gradient pulses of appropriate amplitude and duration, flow-induced phase shifts can be compensated, thus eliminating any signal loss. This technique is called "gradient motion rephasing (GMR)" or just "flow compensation".[1] However, GMR is normally restricted to first-order movements, i.e. spins that move at a constant velocity. Turbulent flow and effects of acceleration cannot be completely compensated by GMR. Optimal reduction of flow-induced phase effects can be achieved by combining GMR with as short a echo times (TE) as possible, in order to reduce the time available for spin dephasing. Short TE also diminish the impact of pulsatile blood flow and turbulence **(Fig. 2)**.

TIME-OF-FLIGHT ANGIOGRAPHY: TECHNIQUES

The contrast mechanism of time-of-flight (TOF) MRA is based on the inflow effect. Fully relaxed blood entering the measured volume behaves as an endogenous contrast

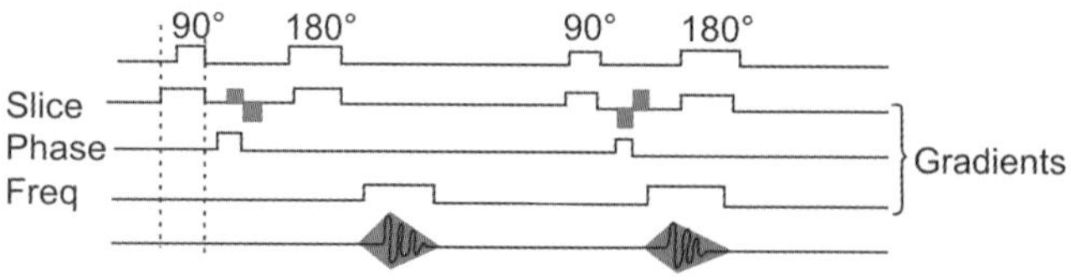

Fig. 2: Diagrammatic representation of phase-contrast MRA pulse sequence, note the velocity encoding gradient are in slice direction.

agent, by producing a bright signal. The bright depiction of flowing blood, however, requires the use of flow rephasing techniques (GMR) in order to overcome the effects of spin-dephasing due to transverse magnetization. TOF MRA using GRE sequences has several advantages: Firstly, GRE sequences are not affected by the washout phenomenon that diminishes the signal of fast flowing blood when using SE techniques. Secondly, GRE techniques permit the use of short repetition times (TR <40 msec), which are needed to efficiently saturate stationary tissue. Thirdly, TE can be kept short (TE < 5 msec), thus further reducing spin-dephasing.

Generally, it is advisable to apply in-phase echo times in order to avoid opposed-phase effects at the vessel walls that would impair the depiction of small vessels. Finally, GRE techniques are characterized by short acquisition times which are important when acquiring volume (3D) datasets. TOF techniques can be divided into three groups:

- Sequential 2D multislice method
- 3D single-slab method
- 3D multislab method.

With 2D techniques, the vessel is imaged by sequentially scanning multiple thin slices. This method has two advantages in comparison to the interleaved multislice technique: Firstly, very short TR times can be used which boost the inflow effect, and secondly, partially saturated blood is hindered from flowing from one slice to another. The method guarantees sufficient inflow enhancement even in vessels with a very slow flow and produces constant vessel-background contrast in the covered region, because each slice is an entry slice.[2] Problems arise with 2D TOF MRA if the vessels to be imaged do not flow in a perpendicular direction to the imaging plane. If the vessels run partly inside the slice (in-plane) or return to the slice in a looped form, then signal loss may occur due to the partial saturation of flow **(Figs. 3A and B)**. In order to achieve a sufficient signal-to-noise ratio, a slice thickness of at least 2–3 mm is necessary. However, this results in reduced spatial resolution and increased spin-dephasing due to the larger voxel size required. 2D slices do not have rectangular RF profiles and therefore, exhibit signal variations at the edges that can lead to step like artifacts in maximum intensity projection (MIP) reconstructions. However, this effect can be largely overcome by overlapping the slices. In vessels exhibiting very pulsatile flow, the extent of inflow enhancement varies during the heart cycle. The periodic change of inflow enhancement generates ghost images of the vessels. Saturation of blood spins can occur due to slow flow in the diastolic phase. The use of ECG triggered 2D TOF sequences may overcome many of these problems by confining data acquisition to the phase of maximum inflow. Thus blood signal is enhanced and ghost artifacts are eliminated. By synchronizing data acquisition with the heart cycle, the vessel is mapped in each slice with equal intensity. Unfortunately, a drawback of this approach is the prolonged acquisition time.

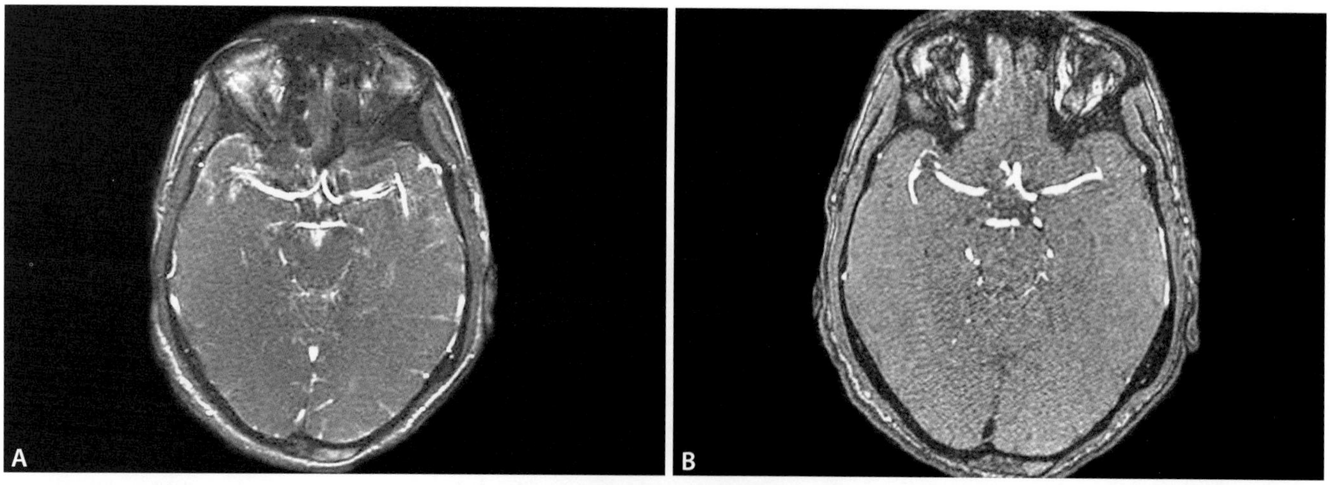

Figs. 3A and B: 2D TOF MRA (A) shows loss of flow-related signal in M1 segment of left middle cerebral artery (MCA) due to in-plane saturation; however, in same patient, MCA showing normal caliber and flow-related signal on 3D TOF MRA (B).

In 3D TOF MRA, the entire imaging volume, usually 30–60 mm thick, is excited simultaneously and then partitioned into thin slices by an additional phase encoding gradient along the slice-select direction.[3] 3D TOF MRA has the advantage of high spatial resolution together with high signal-to-noise ratio, thereby facilitating the improved depiction of particularly small vessel structures. The technique allows slices of less than 1 mm thickness and isotropic voxels to be acquired easily. One major problem of the 3D technique, however, is the progressive saturation that occurs when blood flowing through the volume is subjected to repeated RF pulses. As a result, the signal intensity decreases continuously in the direction of flow. The extent of saturation depends on the length of time in which the blood stays inside the volume. In slow flow vessels, signal begins to diminish when only a short distance has been covered. Conversely, in faster flowing blood the signal remains visible for a greater distance. Consequently, the maximum volume thickness should be kept as small as possible, matched to the size of the vessel region of interest. A reduction of saturation can also be achieved by increasing the TR. Larger vessel sections can be investigated by subdividing the volume of interest into several thin 3D slabs that are acquired sequentially **(Table 1)**.[4]

One such multislab technique which retains the advantages of 3D TOF yet has reduced saturation effects like 2D TOF, is called multiple overlapping thin slab acquisition (MOTSA). Generally, the chosen slab thickness has to be small enough to avoid saturation within the slabs. However, adjacent slabs must overlap by about 20–30% in order to compensate for signal attenuations arising at the slab edges due to nonrectangular excitation profiles. This results in compromised time efficiency and longer overall acquisition times. Frequently, 2D TOF MRA is favored for imaging veins because of the high sensitivity to slow flow. 3D TOF MRA, on the other hand, is more appropriate for fast arterial flow and for those cases in which high spatial resolution is required **(Figs. 4 and 5)**.

Important Points for Optimization of TOF Angiography[5-7]

- Orientation of slices or volume perpendicular to flow direction
- 2D for slow flow, 3D for fast flow
- 3D multislab for larger vessel sections
- Spatial presaturation to isolate arteries and veins
- Use of minimum TE reduces signal loss due to spin dephasing

Table 1: Comparison of 2D and 3D TOF

2D TOF	*3D TOF*
Less susceptible to saturation effect	More susceptible to saturation effect
Visualize slow as well as fast flow	Good for high flow
Low resolution and SNR	High resolution and SNR
Better for relatively larger FOVs	Smaller FOVs
Used mainly for cerebral venographies, abdominal and peripheral angiographies	Cerebral angiography

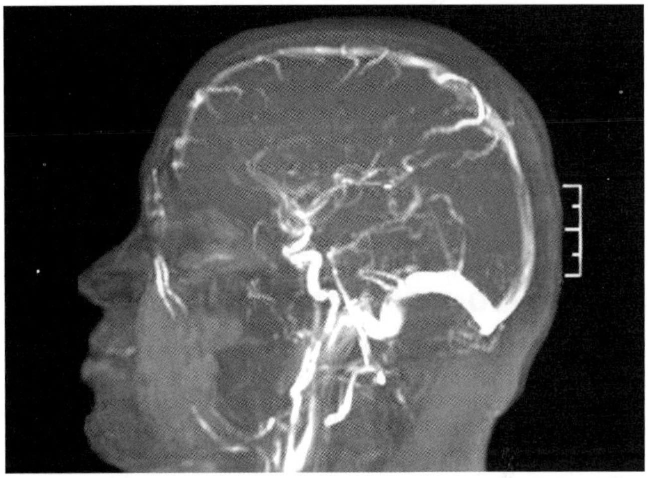

Fig. 4: 2D TOF MR venography reveals adequate visualization of cerebral venous system.

- TONE pulse reduces saturation effects in 3D TOF
- Magnetization transfer (MTC) and fat suppression improve vessel contrast.

Pitfalls with TOF MRA

- Methemoglobin in thrombosed vessels (cavernous: sinus thrombosis) may mimic blood flow (i.e. vessel patency)
- Work around—compare MIP with precontrast T1 images or use phase-contrast MRA
- Short T1 tissues (fat, bleeding, tissue that take up contrast) may simulate vessels
- Pulsation artifacts in CSF may simulate vessel lesions
- Signal loss occurring with turbulent or very slow flow causes overestimation of stenosis and artifacts in the depiction of aneurysms
- Signal loss due to susceptibility artifacts (coils, clips)
- Signal loss in case of in-plane flow (2D) or slow flow (3D)

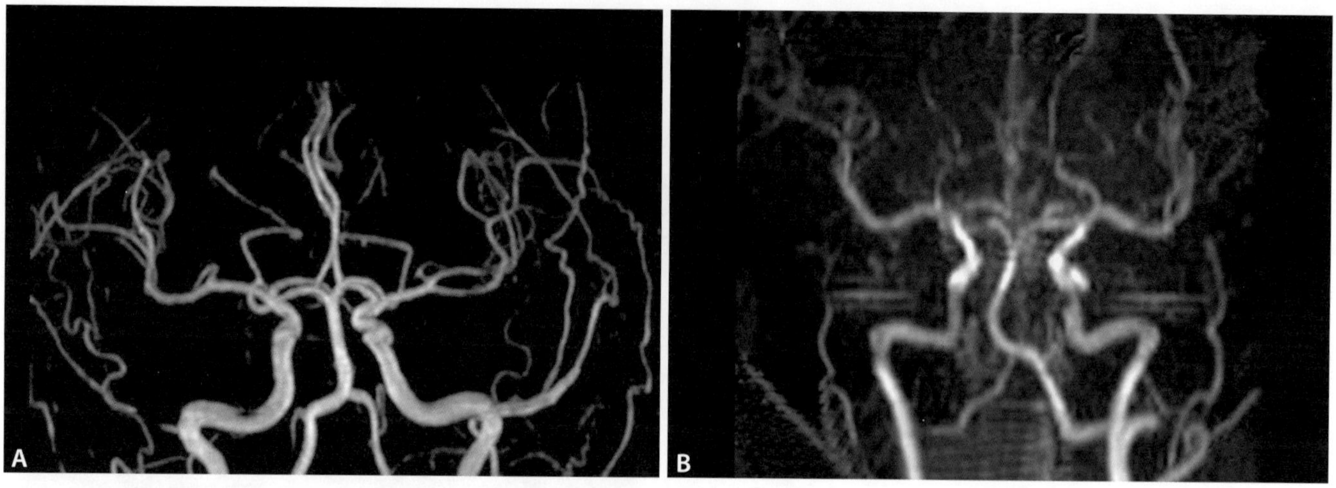

Figs. 5A and B: 3D TOF MRA (A) showing very good cerebral vascular anatomy with high spatial resolution and SNR in comparison to 2D TOF MRA (B) in same patient.

- Overlap of arteries and veins after contrast administration, particularly in intracranial MRA.

PHASE-CONTRAST ANGIOGRAPHY

Whereas phase effects are suppressed as fully as possible in TOF MRA, it is the flow-induced phase shift of the transverse magnetization that is employed to image blood vessels with phase-contrast techniques. There are two ways of using phase effects to selectively depict blood flow:

1. Magnitude contrast (rephased-dephased) method.
2. Phase-contrast method.

Today, magnitude contrast is only rarely used. Conversely, techniques that in a stricter sense are referred to as "phase contrast", have gained greater importance both as an imaging method and as an accurate approach to measuring blood flow velocity and direction.

Magnitude-contrast Technique

The concept of magnitude-contrast angiography is analogous to X-ray digital subtraction angiography (DSA). The basic idea is to acquire two datasets—one flow-rephased and one flow-dephased.[8] First, a flow-compensated measurement is performed using GMR in order to image flowing blood with high signal intensity. In the second acquisition, flow-sensitizing bipolar gradient pulses are applied specifically to induce velocity-dependent phase shifts of moving spins. If the flow-sensitizing gradient is strong enough, the spins within a voxel possessing different velocities may totally dephase resulting in dark vessel signal. Since stationary tissue appears the same in both acquisitions, subtraction of one dataset from the other results in the signal of the stationary tissue being cancelled leaving only the moving blood as visible. Interleaving the acquisition of both datasets can diminish the impact of motion artifacts on the subtraction process. The signal intensity in the subtracted image depends only on the velocity component along the flow-sensitizing gradient which is normally applied in the frequency-encoding direction. Therefore, the imaging volume should be oriented in such a way that the main flow direction in the vessel of interest is parallel to the read-out direction. Information about all three orthogonal flow directions can be obtained by repeating the flow-encoded acquisition with altered gradient orientations. As a result, a total of four acquisitions has to be performed (one rephased, three dephased), which impacts on the overall acquisition time. Although not in widespread use, magnitude contrast MRA can be considered applicable for imaging of peripheral vessels (arm, leg) since it allows larger sections of arteries to be visualized. If flow is unidirectional, a single pair of rephased and dephased acquisitions is sufficient, thereby reducing the overall acquisition time. Magnitude contrast MRA requires a spectrum of flow velocities within a voxel. Laminar flow with its parabolic flow profile is therefore, readily detected. The signal acquired is a direct result of the velocity distribution in each voxel, ensuring complete background suppression. The method is well adapted for depicting slow flow with good spatial resolution, covering larger sections of vessels. One disadvantage arises from the fact that this technique does not provide any information on flow direction or flow velocity.

Phase-contrast Technique

Similar to magnitude contrast, phase-contrast angiography is based on the acquisition of two datasets that differ in the phase of moving spins.[9,10] At first, a flow-rephased sequence (S1) is applied which defines the phase of transverse magnetization under conditions of total flow compensation. The second measurement (S2) is flow-sensitive, utilizing special flow-encoding gradients to provoke a measurable phase shift. Contrary to the magnitude contrast technique, the chosen gradient is weak enough to avoid complete phase dispersion arising from the velocity distribution of the spins. Complex subtraction of the two datasets S1 and S2 yields the phase difference Φ as well as the difference vector ΔS, both of which depend on the velocity component of the spins along the flow encoding gradient. There are two different approaches to utilizing flow-induced phase shifts to generate angiographic images. In the so-called phase map images, it is the phase difference Φ that is depicted as signal intensity. The sign of the phase shift encodes the flow direction. Nonmoving tissue appears as medium shade of gray while flowing blood is either brighter or darker, according to the direction of flow. As the intensity of each pixel is linearly proportional to flow velocity, phase images are particularly well suited for flow quantification and for identifying flow direction. In the second approach magnitude images, which reveal the length of the difference vector ΔS, are applied to anatomically image the vessels. However, while the brightness in each pixel is a measure of the local flow velocity, there is no information about the flow direction. The difference vector ΔS increases with rising spin velocity, reaching a maximum at $\Phi = 180°$. The corresponding critical velocity is called flow sensitivity or velocity encoding (VENC) and is determined by the strength of the bipolar flow-encoding gradients. The manufacturers of MR scanners provide a set of sequences adapted to different velocity ranges. In clinical practice, it is important to estimate the maximum flow velocity expected to occur in the vessel in advance in order to choose the phase-contrast sequence with an adequate VENC value. With phase contrast, only those velocities ranging between –VENC and +VENC, corresponding to phase shifts between –180° and +180°, can be uniquely detected. If the flow velocity exceeds the VENC value, there is an abrupt change of signal intensity in the phase image from bright to dark or vice versa. Blood flow that provokes a phase shift of 190° cannot be distinguished from oppositely directed flow that generates a phase shift of –170°. This ambiguity is called aliasing. In the magnitude image, maximum intensity is reached when the flow velocity equals the VENC value. At higher velocities, the signal intensity begins to decrease again. If the flow velocity in a voxel is exactly twice the VENC value, no signal emanates from the voxel, and the vessel appears to be interrupted. As an example, for a VENC value of 40 cm/sec spins flowing at a rate of 40 cm/sec provoke a phase shift of 180° yielding maximum signal intensity. Spins that flow at 60 cm/sec possess a phase shift higher than 180°. Therefore, on the magnitude image they appear less bright than the spins flowing at 40 cm/sec, but equally as bright as spins flowing at a rate of 20 cm/sec. Likewise, if there are spins flowing at a rate of 80 cm/sec, they will provide zero signal and appear as stationary spins. The phase-contrast method is sensitive only for the velocity component along the flow-encoding gradient. In order to obtain information on all flow directions, one dedicated flow-encoding gradient for each orthogonal direction of space is required. Thus a phase-contrast sequence comprises a total of four acquisitions: one flow-compensated measurement and three flow-encoded acquisitions in the X-, Y-, and Z-directions. Interleaving the four datasets can reduce artifacts caused by patient motion. Phase and magnitude images of the flow components in the three orthogonal directions are obtained by complex subtraction of flow-encoded and flow-compensated datasets. The three magnitude subtraction images can be added to obtain a sum magnitude image that depicts blood flow with bright signal regardless of flow direction **(Figs. 6 and 7)**.

Optimization

- Adapting flow sensitivity (VENC) to maximum flow velocity
- Encoding different flow velocities (multivenc) or different flow directions
- Contrast agent improves flow signal
- 2D acquisition provides one single projection within a short acquisition time
- 3D acquisition permits MIP postprocessing
- ECG triggering can be applied in cases of pulsatile flow
- Presaturation pulses can separate arteries and veins.

CONTRAST-ENHANCED MR ANGIOGRAPHY

Contrast-enhanced MR angiography (CE-MRA) has emerged as a technique of choice for vascular images. It relies on T1 shortening effects of Gd-chelate contrast in blood. This is different from the flow-based TOF and PC-MRA technique which uses the inherent motion of blood flow to generate vascular signal.[11]

Unlike 3D TOF MRA, it requires a gradient system with high slew rates for ultrafast aquisition and additive tools for proper timing of scan with regard to the bolus arrival.[12]

The basic sequence used for CE-MRA is ultra short TR/TE 3D spoiled gradient echo sequence. The TR is made as short as possible to speed up the image aquisition and

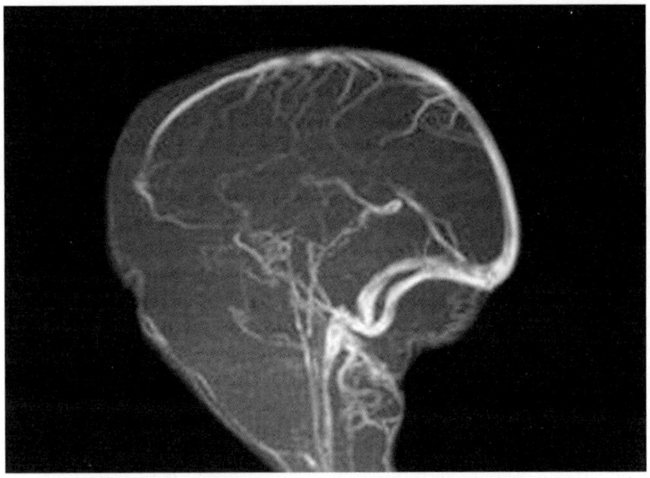

Fig. 6: Phase-contrast 3D MRV showing excellent cerebral venous system.

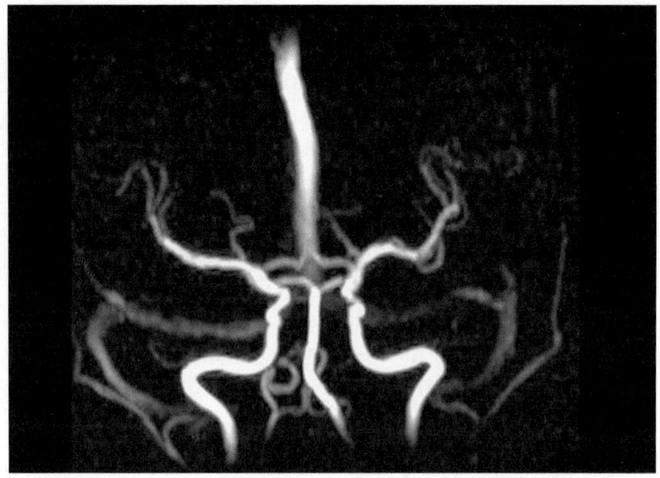

Fig. 7: Phase-contrast 3D MRA giving adequate depiction of arterial anatomy.

capture the first pass of contrast. The presence of Gd makes the blood immune to saturation, so the short TR tends to saturate only background tissue. In general, the highest flip angle achievable by the MRI machine is used. The TE is also made as short as possible—ideally approximately 1.0 msec, so as to limit any flow-induced dephasing effects.[13]

Different techniques are used to ensure optimal contrast of the arteries, e.g. bolus timing, automatic bolus detection, bolus tracking and care bolus, etc.[14]

The rate of injection affects the peak Gd concentration and thus the achievable arterial SNR. Generally, a faster injection rate will result in higher arterial SNR, but shorter bolus duration and earlier venous enhancement. Injection rates of 2 mL/sec are ideal for most CE-MRA applications, with little benefit shown for higher rates.[15]

For most CE-MRA examinations, a dose of 0.15–0.2 mmol/kg (typically 20–30 mL) is sufficient. If timing is good, lower doses (0.1 mmol/kg) have also been found to be adequate. In general, the use of a larger contrast agent dose has the benefit of prolonging the arterial phase and providing the operator with an additional buffer to compensate for errors in timing.[15,16]

One final consideration for contrast administration is that of saline flush. In practice, a large saline flush (at least 30 mL) should be used for all CE-MRA examinations. A large flush will ensure that the entire contrast dose is administered beyond the tubing and that the bolus will travel through the peripheral veins into the right heart, thus ensuring sufficient Gd concentrations are delivered to the more distal arteries. The use of a large flush increases the slope of the enhancement curve, increases the duration of the arterial phase of the bolus (up to 50%), and delays significant venous enhancement, all of which are preferable for arterial CE-MRA.[15,17]

The goal is to record the central region of k-space during the maximum enhancement of the artery. The center of k-space contains the lowest (spatial) frequency wave data, so it represents the major structures of the image and thus most of the gross image form and contrast; therefore, the center of k-space should be acquired during the time of highest contrast agent concentration.[18]

Also, a high rate of change of the contrast agent concentration during the acquisition of central k-space must be avoided to prevent ringing artifacts, arising in the fourier transform.[18] So, the enhancement is maximized by timing the contrast agent injection such that the period of maximum arterial concentration corresponds to the k-space acquisition.[14]

Special considerations with respect to timing must be undertaken with certain vascular problems, such as aneurysms: since the flow can be much slower through an aneurysm, more time must be allowed between the injection of contrast agent and the image acquisition.[18]

A high resolution with near isotropic voxels and minimal pulsatility and misregistration artifacts should be striven for. The postprocessing with the MIP enables different views of the 3D data set **(Figs. 8 to 11)**.

CE-MRA Advantages[14]

- The 3D MRA can be acquired in any plane, which means that greater vessel coverage can be obtained at high resolution with fewer slices (aorta, peripheral vessels)
- The possibility to perform a time resolved examination (similarly to conventional-catheter angiography)

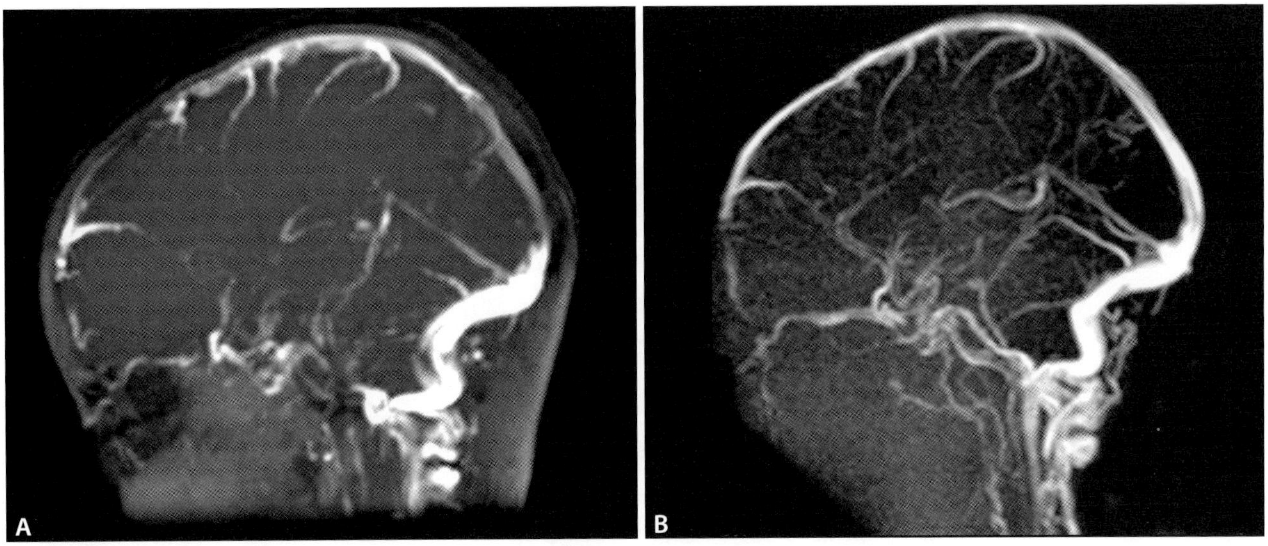

Figs. 8A and B: Phase-contrast 3D MRV showing better cerebral venous sinuses and smaller veins than 2D TOF MRV in same patient.

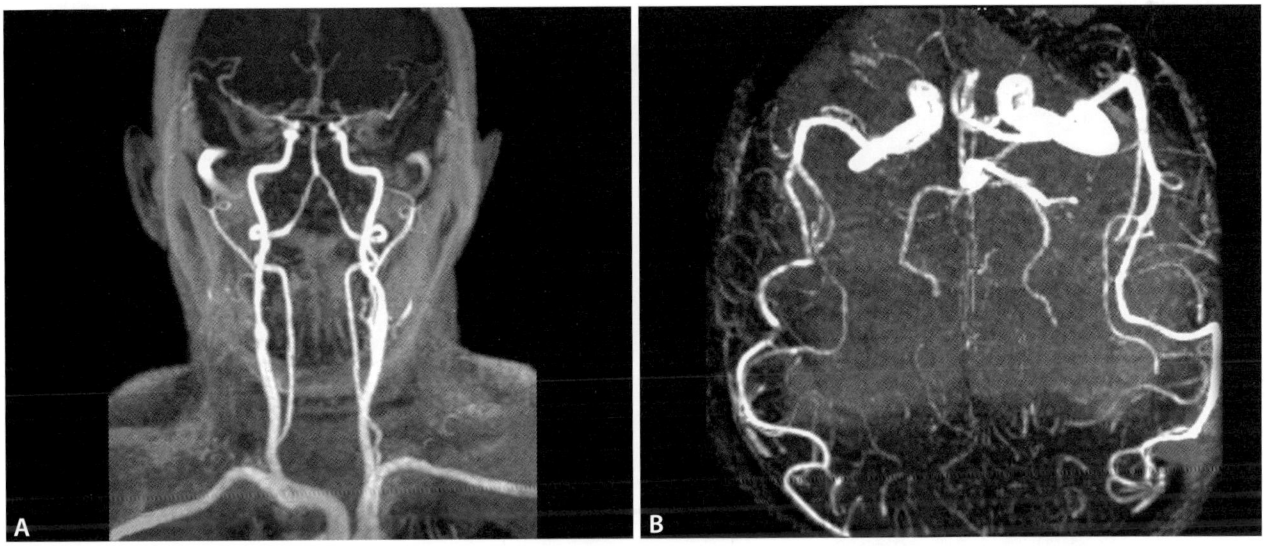

Figs. 9A and B: Contrast-enhanced MRA showing good neck and cerebral arterial anatomy.

- The CE-MRA reduces or eliminates most of the artifacts of time-of-flight angiography or phase-contrast angiography
- Minimal invasiveness with no associated risk of neurologic complications, reduced patient discomfort and inconvenience, greater cost savings
- No use of ionizing radiation; paramagnetic agents have a beneficial safety
- The CE-MRA does not prove to be better in evaluation of carotid artery atherosclerotic stenosis[19] however it appears to give better depiction of postcoiling larger residual/recurrent aneurysms[20]
- Other very important use of CE-MRA is that it differentiates between active and inactive disease in case of Takayasu arthritis by showing the intense enhancement of vessel wall.[21]

On the other hand, CE-MRA has some disadvantages. Due to the short arteriovenous transition time in the cerebral circulation, early enhancement of venous structures limits the time window for scan acquisition, and a trade-off is therefore, necessary between scan time, volume coverage and spatial resolution. Another disadvantage is the possibility of a false neck remnant in postcoiling patient with intracranial aneurysm, which may

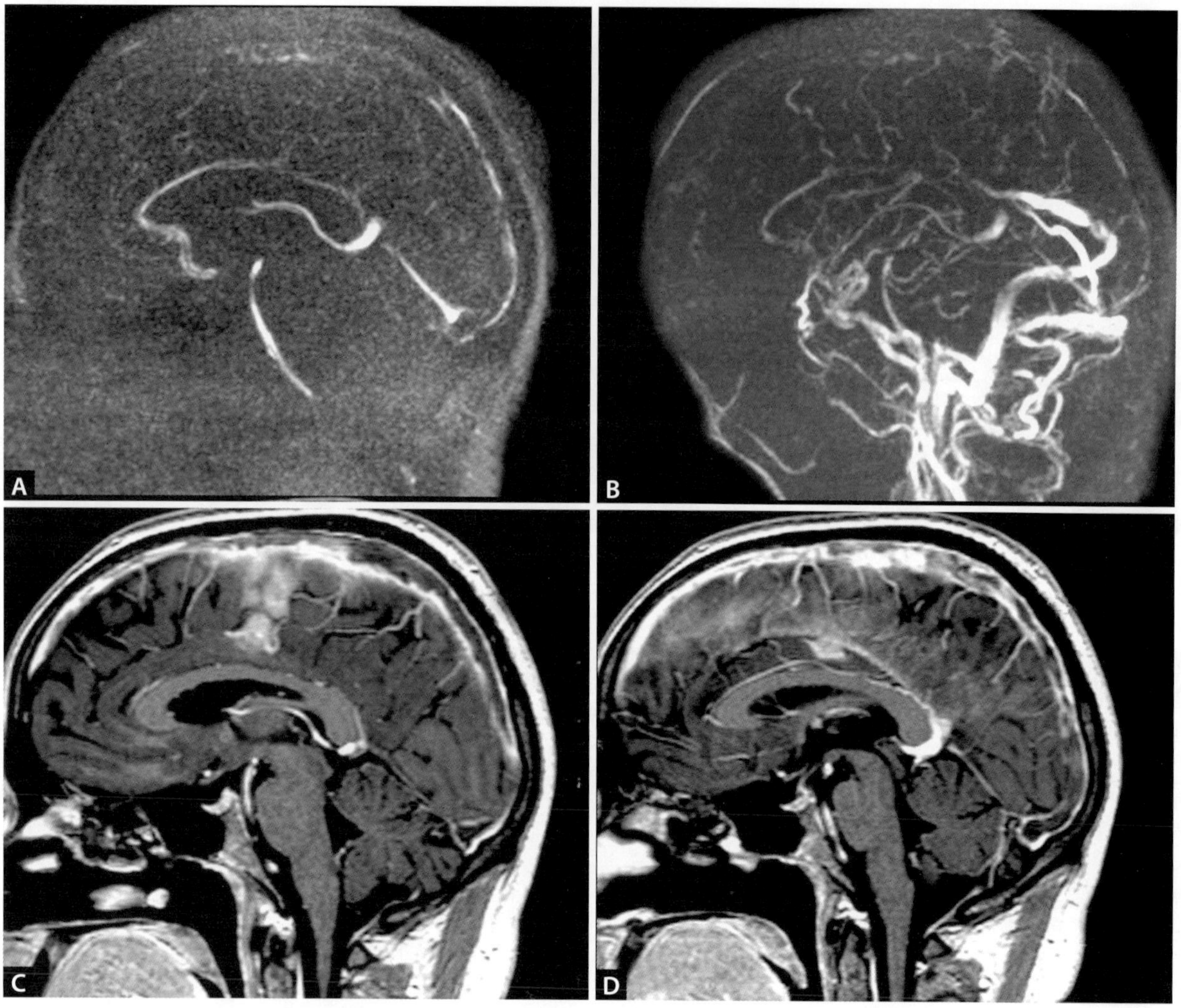

Figs. 10A to D: Case of superior sagittal venous sinus thrombosis showing nonvisualization of sinuses on PC 3D MRV (A and B); Postcontrast T1W (C and D) images confirm the filling defects in sinus.

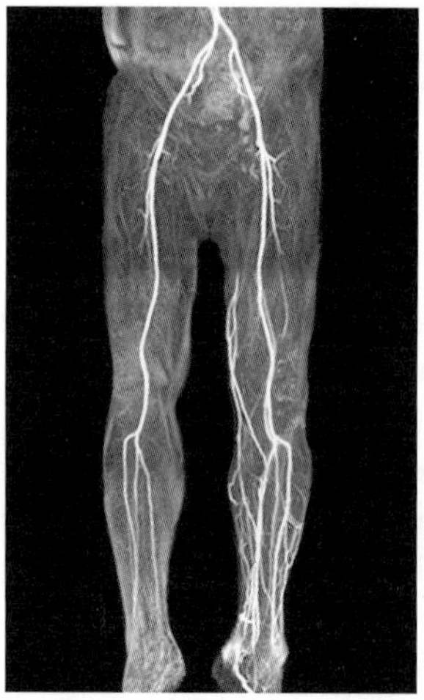

Fig. 11: CE-MRA bilateral lower limbs showing adequate visualization of lower limb arteries, early draining veins are seen on left side due to underlying vascular malformation.

be explained by the peripheral contrast enhancement of the organized thrombus or by the vasa vasorum within the aneurysm wall.[12,22]

Parallel Imaging[12]

Parallel acquisition techniques (PAT) have recently been developed and are now being increasingly used for vascular imaging. The PAT uses multichannel coil arrays to shorten the measurement time by reducing the number of phase encoding steps. The spatial information is instead extracted from the sensitivity profiles of the coil elements.

Numerous image acquisition algorithms have been described, including sensitivity encoding (SENSE), simultaneous acquisition of spatial (SMAS) harmonics, and generalized auto-calibrating partially parallel acquisitions (GRAPPA).

In intracranial 3D TOF imaging, PAT with an eight channel phased-array head coil has been used to save 43% of measurement time while maintaining the same image quality. However, it must be kept in mind that using PAT reduces the signal-to-noise ratio (SNR) by approximately the square root of the acceleration factor. The inherently high SNR of contrast-enhanced MRI makes PAT particularly suited for CEMRA.

In arterial CEMRA, PAT can be used to accelerate the acquisition (and hence avoid venous contamination), to increase spatial resolution and/or volume coverage, or to combine the two.[12]

Time Resolved/4D CE-MRA

Vascular malformation imaging work-up always needs a dynamic depiction of the disease. However, the conventional MRA, dynamic TOF, PC and CE-MRA lacks the ability in showing the different angiographic phases as early arterial, arterial and venous. At the same time, conventional angiography suffers from motion artifacts specially in unstable patients.

The time resolved CE-MRA includes combination of k-space segmentation into central, mid, and peripheral zones with sampling the central zones of the k-space at a more frequent rate.

Scan parameters used for rapid acquisition short TE of 0.9 ms and a short TR of 2.2 ms, fractional echo acquisition, 2.6 mm section thickness. MR contrast is injected at a rate of 2 mL/s to a total of 15 mL, followed by 30 mL of saline. Sagittal or coronal section are obtained with a FOV of about 28 × 22.4 cm, matrix of 192 × 192, NEX of 0.75, and flip angle of 20° at every 1.8–2.0 seconds. About 30 to 35 sections are acquired (**Figs. 12A to D**).[23]

Advantages of Time-resolved MRA

- Useful for unstable and moving patients[24]
- Better depiction of AVM feeders, nidus and venous drainages[25]
- Gives an idea about flow dynamics of AVM/AVF and aneurysms[24]
- Good for follow-up of postembolization or gamma surgery residual AVMS.[25]

Limitation

- High dose of contrast is required
- Time taking sequences
- Nonvessel selective on the contrary to catheter angiography.

FUTURE PERSPECTIVES

Presently, MRA techniques are well established tool for vascular imaging, however, still there is a need of decrease acquisition times, increase temporal and spatial resolution with more dynamic information. With advent of 3T MR scanner, these problems has been addressed in clinical imaging. Use of high fields such as 7T are in developing and research phase and the recent studies reveals that CEMRA at 7T demonstrates the feasibility and current constraints of ultra-high filed contrast-enhanced MRA relative to NC MRA.[26]

Also there are evidences of work under research reveals that TOF MRA at 7T have increase SNR and spatial restoration, especially for the assessment of brain AVM and high-grade gliomas. Other applications like arterial spin labeling are mentioned in other chapter on perfusion in this book.

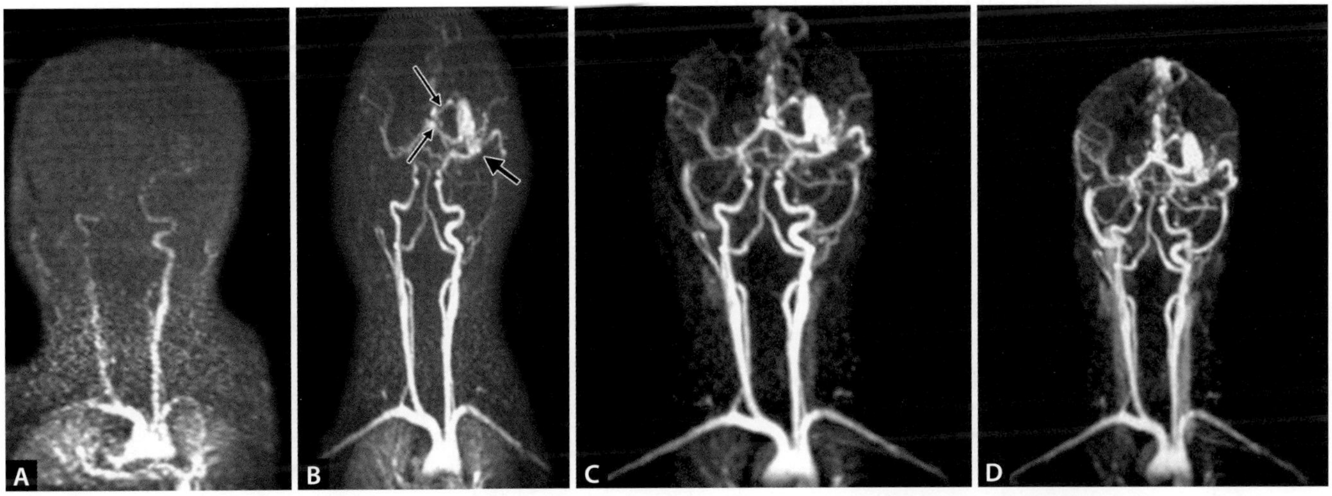

Figs. 12A to D: Time-resolved CE-MRA in a case of cerebral AVM demonstrating the AVM nidus, its feeders (thick arrow) and venous drainage (thin arrows) in a dynamic manner comparable to catheter angiography.

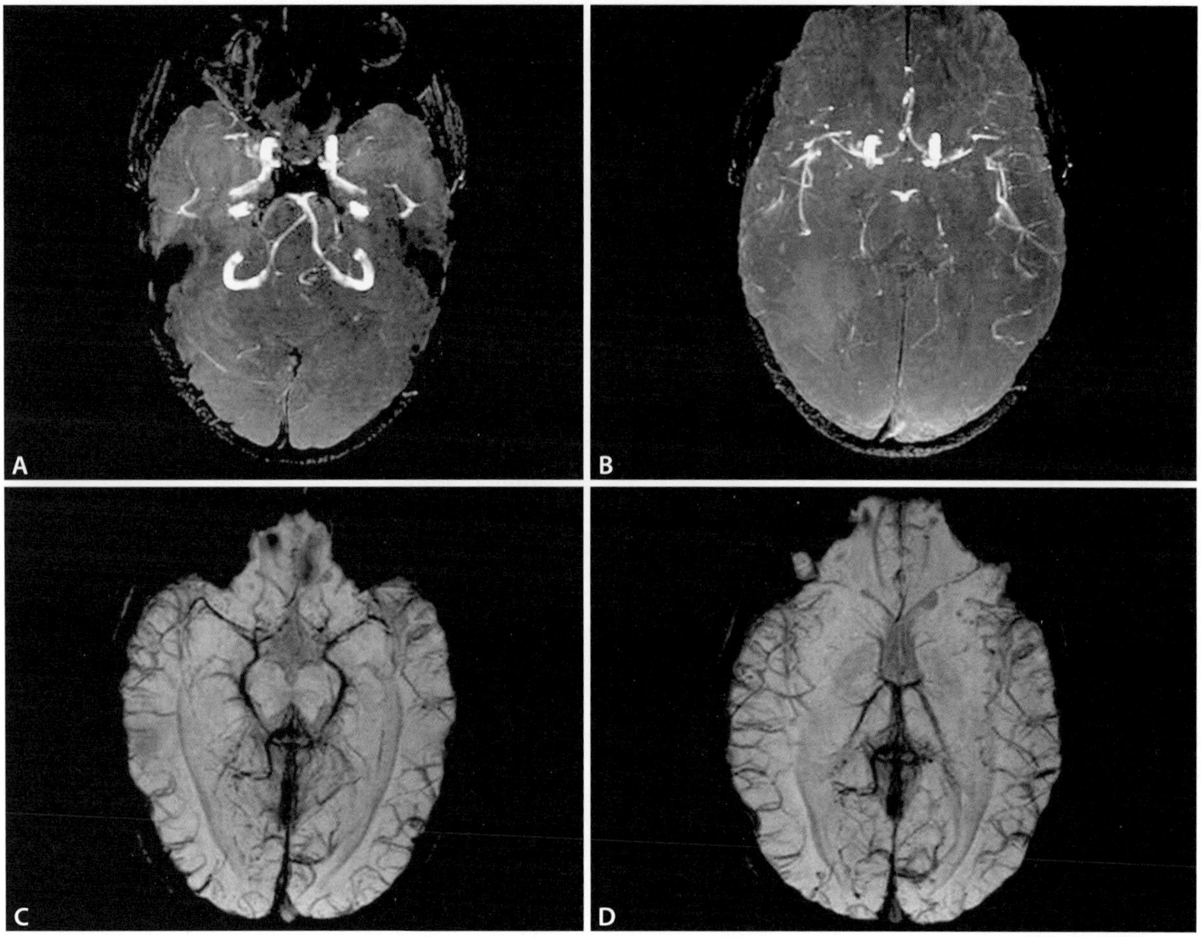

Figs. 13A to D: PC MRA application of SW imaging, images (A and B) are showing intracranial arterial anatomy due to TOF inflow effect and images (C and D) reveals the venous structures on SWI in same patient.

Newer techniques like SWI-MRA are also in developmental phase, it makes possible to image both artery as well as vein simultaneously and can be evaluated separately.[27] Veins are dark due to T2* effect with SWI processing, same time arteries are seen bright due to TOF inflow effect **(Figs. 13A to D)**. In addition, it can also provide the information about hemorrhage and calcification whether parenchymal or mural in case of atherosclerotic disease.

Lastly, there is lot more in future for MRA application due to advent of ultra-high field scanners and development of advance imaging sequences.

REFERENCES

1. Lenz G, Haacke E, Masaryk T, et al. Inplane vascular imaging: pulse sequence design and strategy. Radiology. 1988; 166:875-82.
2. Keller PJ, Drayer BP, Fram EK, et al. MR angiography with two-dimensional acquisition and three-dimensional display. Radiology. 1989;173:527-32.
3. Laub GA, Kaiser WA. MR angiography with gradient motion refocusing. J Comput Assist Tomogr. 1988;12:377-82.
4. Parker GL, Yuan C, Blatter DD. MR angiography by multiple thin slab 3D acquisitions. Magn Res Med. 1991;17:434-51.
5. Tkach J, Masaryk T, Ruggieri P, et al. Use of Tilted Optimized Nonsaturating Excitation. SMRM. 1992;2:3905.
6. Atkinson D, Brant-Zawadzki M, Gillan G, et al. Improved MR angiography: Magnetization transfer suppression with variable flip angles excitation and increased resolution. Radiology. 1994;190:890-4.
7. Edelman RR, Ahn SS, Chien D, et al. Improved time-of-flight MR angiography of the brain with magnetization transfer contrast. Radiology. 1992;184:395-9.
8. Axel L, Morton D. MR flow imaging by velocity compensated/ uncompensated difference images. J Comp Assist Tomogr. 1987;11:31-4.
9. Dumoulin CL, Hart HR. Magnetic Resonance Angiography. Radiology. 1986;161:717-20.
10. Dumoulin CL, Souza SP, Walker MF, et al. Three-dimensional phase contrast angiography. Magn Res Med. 1989;9:139-49.

11. Schneider G, et al. Magnetic resonance angiography: techniques, indications and practical applications. Springer-Verlag Italia, 2005.
12. Papke K, Brassel F. Modern cross-sectional imaging in the diagnosis of follow-up of intracranial aneurysms. Eur Radiol. 2006;16:2051-66.
13. Lohan DJ, et al. Contrast-enhanced MRA vs Nonenhanced MRA: Pros and Cons. Applied radiology, Journal of Practical medical imaging and Management. Supplement to May, 2007.
14. Contrast-enhanced Magnetic resonance angiography; *www.mr-tip.com.*
15. Kopka L, Vosshenrich R, Rodenwaldt J, et al. Differences in injection rates on contrast-enhanced breath-hold three-dimensional MR angiography. Am J Roentgenol. 1998; 170(2):345-8.
16. Lee VS, Rofsky NM, Krinsky GA, et al. Single dose breath-hold gadolinum-enhanced three-dimensional MR angiography of the renal arteries. Radiology. 1999;211:69-78.
17. Boos M, Scheffler K, Haselhorst R, et al. Arterial first pass gadolinium CM dynamics as a function of several intravenous saline flush and Gd volumes. J Magn Reson Imaging. 2001;13(4):568-76.
18. Bart E Muhs, Hence JM Verhagen, Matthew G Huddle, et al. Theory, technique, and practice of magnetic resonance angiography. Vascular. 2007;15(6):376-83.
19. LS Babiarz JM, Romero EK, Murphy B Brobeck. Contrast-enhanced MR Angiography is not more accurate than unenhanced 2D time-of-flight MR Angiography for determining >70% internal carotid artery stenosis. Am J Neuroradiol. 2009;30:761-8.
20. A TJ, Kaufmann J, Huston III HJ, Cloft J Mandrekar L. A prospective trial of 3T and 1.5T time-of-flightand contrastenhanced MR angiography in the follow-up of coiled intracranial aneurysms. Am J Neuroradiol. 2010;31:912-8.
21. Maurizio Papa, Francesco De Cobelli, Elena Baldissera. Takayasu Arthritis: Intravascular Contrast medium for MR Angiography in the evaluation of disease activity. AJR. 2012; 198:W279-W284.
22. Lubicz B, et al. Is digital substraction angiography still needed for the follow-up of intracranial aneurysms treated by embolization with detachable coils? Neuroradiology. 2008;50:841-8.
23. RI Farb R, Agid RA, Willinsky DM Johnstone. Cranial dural arteriovenous fistula: diagnosis and classification with time-resolved MR Angiography at 3T. Am J Neuroradiol. 2009; 30:1546-51.
24. Kristine A Blackham, Matthew A Passalacqua, Gurpreet S Sandhu. Applications of time-resolved MR Angiography. AJR. 2011;196:W613-20.
25. HK Lim, CG Choi, SM Kim. Detection of residual brain arteriovenous malformations after radio surgery: diagnostic accuracy of contrast-enhanced four-dimensional MR angiography at 3.0T. BJR. 2012;85:1064-9.
26. Umutlu L, Maderwald S, Kinner S. First- pass contrast-enhanced renal MRA at 7 Telsa: initial result. Eur Radiol. 2012 Oct (Epub ahead of print).
27. Samuel RS. Barnes, Mark Haacke. Susceptibility Weighted Imaging: Clinical angiographic applications. Magn Reson Imaging Clin N Am. 2009;17(1):47-61.

CHAPTER 49

Magnetic Resonance Imaging Pulse Sequences: An Evolution

Vivek Gupta, Niranjan Khandelwal

INTRODUCTION

Magnetic resonance sequences are continuously evolving, from simple sequences like conventional spin echo they have increased in number as well as complexity. However, the ultimate aim of every sequence is bring about better tissue contrast in least amount of time. Therefore, different sequences are designed to account for varied tissue characteristics. Also, with the tremendous improvement in computational powers now the sequences have become less time consuming and less prone to artifacts. It is a vast and complex topic but basic understanding of the sequences is essential to interpret the MR images they produced. **Table 1** gives an overview of the present generation of pulse sequences by various vendors.

MR sequence is a series of different RF pulses, which are applied at a particular time and in a specified way to obtain an image.

A pulse sequence diagram is a schematic diagram, which depicts various pulse or gradients that are applied over a period of time.

There are minimum of four horizontal lines, which depict the excitatory RF pulse, and three representing each gradient, i.e. phase gradient, frequency gradient and slice encoding gradient **(Fig. 1)**. Additional lines may be used to depict the generated echo and other pulse or gradients used.

BASIC TERMINOLOGIES

Image contrast is generated by variation of repetition time (TR) and echo time (TE) in any given sequence. TR is the time interval between application of an RF excitation pulse and start of the next RF pulse. TE is time between the initial RF pulse and the peak of the echo, which is produced. Both are usually in milliseconds. T1- and T2-weighting are other terms, which need to be understood. T1-weighted images would mean that though, image show all types of contrast but the T1 effect is more pronounced. T1 effect would mean that the TR and TE are both short and the difference between relaxation of longitudinal magnetization of fat and water can be detected. In T1-weighted images fat, blood products, slow moving blood and MR contrast would all be bright and tissues with fluid, mineral rich content like bone and air would be dark. T2-weighting is opposite of this. Here the TR and TE are both prolonged and thus the difference in T2 signal decay of fat and water can be detected. At short TE, this difference is not apparent. This makes high free water containing tissues bright of T2-weighted images. Another type of images are proton density images where TR is long and TE is short, thus the images are neither T1-weighted and nor T2-weighted but the image contrast produced is due to difference in proton density of the tissues, those having higher density of protons giving higher signal.

TYPES OF SEQUENCES

Spin echo sequences were the first sequences to be used for MR imaging. These were closely followed by gradient echo imaging. As more and more limitations of these classic sequences became apparent, they were modified to bring about better tissue contrast in less time. This was

Table 1: MR pulse sequences and their classification

	Technique	Sequences	Weighting	Features	Application
Spin-echo (SE) sequences					
1.	ConventionaL SE	SE	T1, T2 and proton density (PD)	Robust sequences. Less susceptible to T2* effects	Now replaced by fast SE sequences
2.	Fast SE (RARE)	TSE (Turbo SE) FSE (Fast SE)	T1, T2 and proton density (PD)	Faster Less susceptible to motion artifacts and T2* effects	High resolution neurological and orthopedic imaging. Single breath hold abdominal imaging
3.	HASTE	SS-FSE (single-shot fast-spin echo)	T- weighting	Faster	Used in MRCP
4.	Inversion recovery	IR, turbo IR, TIRM (turbo IR magnitude reconstruction), IR TSE	T1-weighting	High resolution imaging	For good contrast between white and gray matter
		FLAIR (fluid attenuated inversion recovery)	T2-weighting	Very useful in brain imaging	To suppress fluid and make adjacent lesions more prominent
		STIR (short T1 inversion recovery)	T1- and T2-weighted	Insensitive to susceptibility artifacts	To suppress fat signal
Gradient-echo (GRE) sequences					
A.	Coherent sequences				
1.	Postexcitation steady state sequences	FISP (fast imaging with steady-state precession), GRASS (gradient recalled acquisition in the steady state), FFE (fast field echo)	T1 and T2*	High SNR and T2* weighting, suitable to 3D imaging	Application in orthopedic imaging
2.	Pre-excitation steady-state refocused sequences	PSIF (reversed FISP), SSFP (steady state free precession)	T2-weighted	True T2 weighting achievable, lower SNR	CSF flow studies, inner ear imaging
3.	Fully refocused steady state sequences	True FISP, FIESTA (fast imaging employing steady state acquisition), Balanced FFE (fast field echo)	T1- and T2-weighting	Less sensitive to motion	Cardiac, fetal imaging Abdominal imaging
4.	Combination of A3 and A4	DESS (dual echo steady state)	T1- and T2-weighting		Orthopedic imaging
5.	Combination of A3 and A4	CISS (constructive interference in the steady state), FIESTA-C	T2-weighting	Less prone to banding artifacts in comparison the true FISP	Inner ear 3D imaging
B.	Incoherent/Spoiled sequences				
1a.	2D-spoiled GRE	FLASH (fast low angle shot), T1-FFE (T1 fast field echo), SPGR (spoiled gradient echo)	T1-weighted imaging	Fast imaging	MR angiography, In-out phase imaging
1b.	3D-spoiled GRE	VIBE (volumetric interpolated breath hold examination), THRIVE (T1-weighted high resolution isotropic volume examination)	T1-weighting	Isotropic imaging, high resolution, fast imaging	Body imaging
2.	Ultrafast GRE	Turbo FLASH, TFE (turbo field echo)	T1-weighted	Very fast imaging	To get rapid images like to track contrast arrival
3.	3D-ultrafast GRE	MP-RAGE (magnetization prepared rapid acquisition GE), 3D-TFE	T1-weighted	High resolution 3D sequence	Cerebral T1 3D imaging
4.	Echo planner imaging	EPI	T2* weighting	Ultrafast sequence	Diffusion, perfusion and functional MRI
Hybrid Sequences					
1.	Gradient/spin echo hybrid	Turbo GSE (gradient spin echo), GRASE (gradient echo and spin echo)	T2/T2* weighting	Fast imaging with low SAR	T2 weighting imaging of brain and orthopedic imaging

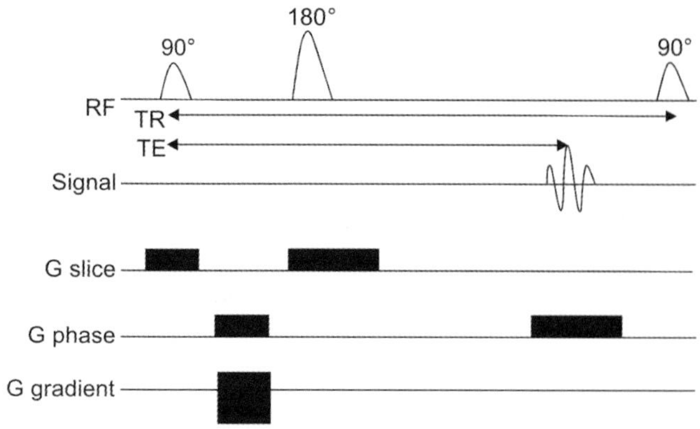

Fig. 1: Pulse sequence diagram of conventional spin echo sequence. Here a single180° RF pulse is applied after an initial 90° excitatory pulse. Since TR and TE are short, the image is T1-weighted.

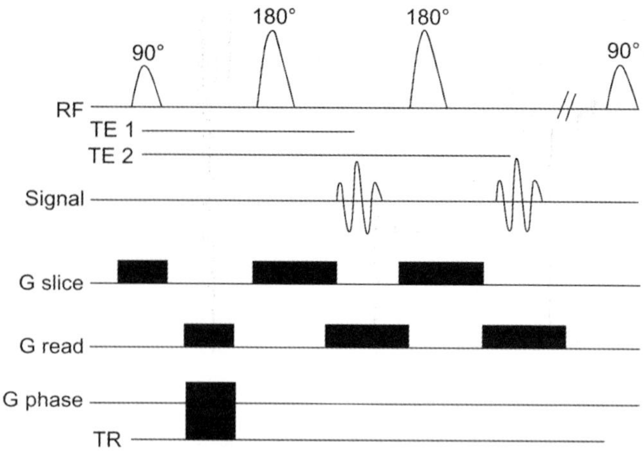

Fig. 2: Dual-echo-pulse sequence. Here first echo is proton-weighted as TE is short and second echo is T2-weighted as TE is prolonged. TR is prolonged.

followed by ultrafast sequences in both these groups. Finally, sequences with features of both of these were created to generate hybrid sequences.

Conventional Spin-echo Sequences

In a typical spin echo sequence, an initial 90° radio-frequency excitation pulse is followed by a 180° rephasing pulse which is then followed by an echo **(Fig. 1)**.

If there is only one 180° rephasing pulse, a T1-weighted image is produced since the resultant TR and TE are short. When two 180° pulse are used of results in two images. First image is proton density weighted, since here TR is long and TE is short and the second image is T2-weighted, as TR and TE are both prolonged **(Fig. 2)**.

Conventional spin echo sequences can be used in any part of the body with predictable tissue contrast characteristics. The major constrain in this sequence is the long acquisition times.

Parameters

Usually following parameters are applied:

- Single echo T1-weighting
  - *TR*: 300–500 ms
  - *TE*: 10–30 ms
- Dual echo T2-weighting
  - *TR*: 2000 ms
  - *TE1*: 20 ms
  - *TE2*: 80 ms.

Fast-spin-echo Sequences

This sequence was developed to overcome the limitation of conventional spin-echo sequence, it involves use of

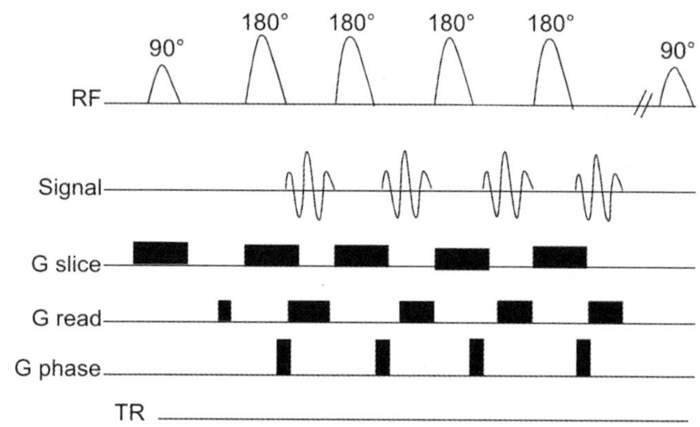

Fig. 3: Fast-spin-echo sequence. Here multiple 180° pulse are applied after an initial 90° pulse. The acquisition time is reduced as for a single 90° pulse multiple phase encoding steps take place.

multiple 180° rephasing pulses after the initial 90° RF pulse **(Fig. 3)**. This sequence reduces time by reducing the phase encoding steps (The scan time is dependent on TR, phase encoding steps and the number of signal averaging or the number of excitations).

Here each 180° rephasing pulse fills k-space by doing a phase encoding. Thus for a single excitatory RF pulse (90°) multiple 180° rephasing pulse are applied which in turn fills multiple lines in k-space, thereby filling the k-space faster and reducing the scan time. Typically 2,4,8,16 rephasing pulse are used and the time reduction achieved is inversely proportionate to them. The number of 180° pulse and the resultant echo is called "echo train length (ETL)". Rapid acquisition and relaxation enhancement (RARE) sequence employ this method (e.g. Turbo-SE and fast-SE sequences are examples of this technique).

Parameters

Usually following parameters are applied:

- Single echo T1-weighting
  - *TR*: 600 ms
  - *TE*: 17 ms
  - *ETL*: 4
- Single echo T2-weighting
  - *TR*: 4000–8000 ms
  - *TE*: 102 ms
  - *ETL*: 16
- Dual echo T2-weighting
  - *TR*: 2500-4500 ms
  - *TE1 effective*: 17 ms
  - *TE2 effective*: 102 ms
  - *ETL*: 8.

Half-fourier Acquisition Single-shot Turbo Spin Echo

Half-fourier acquisition single-shot turbo spin echo (HASTE) is another modification of fast spin echo where only half the lines of k-space are filled in a single shot (Single shot filling of k-space can also be done in RARE but filling of entire k-space will result in long acquisition time thus prone to significant T2 decay). For example, SS-FSE, FSE-ADA, FASE. Since k-space is symmetrical, rest half of k-space can be filled with interpolation.

Inversion Recovery Sequence

This is basically a spin echo sequence where an additional 180° inverting RF pulse is applied which inverts the net magnetizing vector (NMV) through 180°. After removal of pulse the NMV begins to recover, a 90° excitation pulse is applied at a time interval TI (inversion time) after the initial 180° inverting pulse. Following which, like in conventional spin echo sequences a 180° rephasing pulse is applied to produce an echo at a time TE **(Fig. 4)**.

This sequence can be both T1- and T2-weighted. If inversion time is sufficiently long to allow net magnetizing vector to pass through the transverse plane and then the 90° excitation pulse is applied, then the contrast is predominantly T1-weighted. Here TE is to be kept short. For T2-weighting the TE is prolonged so that T2 decay can occur and the resultant image is T2-weighted.

The TR, the interval between the two inverting 180° pulses should be kept long to allow for complete recovery of NMV to the longitudinal plane.

- *Short T1 inversion recovery (STIR):* This sequence is predominantly used to suppress fat to delineate the structures surrounded by fatty tissues. Here inversion time is kept low and 90° excitation pulse is applied when NMV of fat is crossing the transverse plane. At this point the longitudinal component of fat is zero so it does not contribute to any signal thus is suppressed.
- *Fluid attenuated inversion recovery (FLAIR) sequence:* This is commonly used sequence in brain to suppress the CSF signal. Here inversion time is kept long (as opposed to in STIR) and 90° excitation pulse is applied when NMV of water is crossing the transverse plane. This selectively suppresses the CSF/free fluid signal.

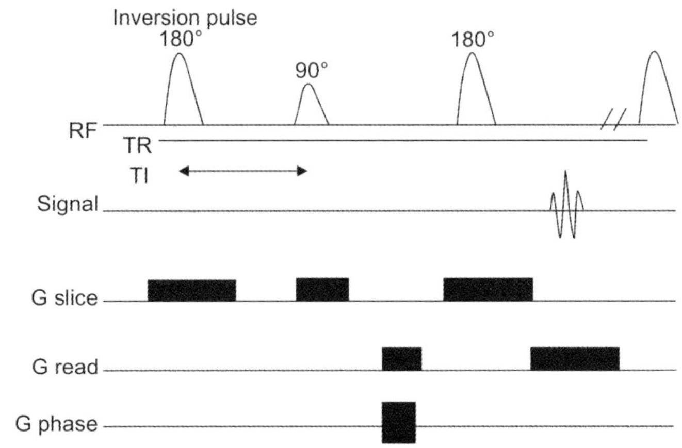

Fig. 4: A typical inversion recovery pulse diagram. A 180° inversion pulse is applied before 90° excitatory pulse to flip NMV by 180°. Inversion time (TI) is the time interval between the inversion pulse and initial excitatory pulse.

Parameters

- STIR
  - TI 100–180 ms
  - TE 70 ms + (for T2 weighting)
  - TR long
  - ETL-16
- FLAIR
  - *TI 1500*: 2200 ms
  - TE 70 ms + (for T2 weighting)
  - TR long
  - *ETL*: 12.

Gradient-echo Sequences

This is fundamentally different sequence when compared to spin echo sequence. In this type, an initial excitation pulse is applied with certain strength that it flips the NMV into transverse plane at an angle less than 90°. The angle to which it flips the NMV is called flip angle. After the pulse is withdrawn, the magnetic moments start to dephase due to presence of magnetic field inhomogeneities, which is called as T2* decay. A gradient pulse is then applied which dephase and then rephases the magnetic moments in the transverse component. This is followed by generation of signal called gradient echo **(Fig. 5)**. Since the rephasing by a gradient is not as effective as the RF pulse some nuclei, which are dephased (due to T2* effect) are not rephased and thus the resultant GRE image has some T2* effect.

Parameters

- T1-weighting
  - *TR*: <50 ms
  - *TE*: 5-10 ms
  - *Flip angle*: 60°–120°
- T2* weighting
  - *TR*: <500 ms
  - *TE*: 15–20 ms
  - *Flip angle*: <30°.

Steady State Sequences

When a RF pulse is applied the NMV is flipped into the transverse plane and it is the sum of both longitudinal and transverse magnetization. After the pulse is switched off, the transverse magnetization component begins to decrease as the magnetic moments move out of phase. If repeat excitation pulse is applied at a time shorter than T1 and T2 time of any tissue, then there will be a residual transverse magnetization. This accumulates over time if repeated pulse are applied and a state is reached when NMV remains constant. This is called "steady state". Two types of signals are produced once the steady state is achieved. First echo (S+) is due to free induction decay after the recent RF pulse of the NMV at short TE which contains both T1 and T2* weighting and the second signal (S–) is due to refocusing of the residual spin echo just before the next RF pulse is applied. This latter echo is predominantly T2-weighted.

Coherent-gradient-echo Sequence

In these sequences the residual transverse magnetization is utilized by applying a rephrasing gradient, which is similar to initial phase encoding gradient but is of opposite polarity. This rephases the residual magnetic moments and bring them in phase and then they contribute to signal during second excitation.

The sequences which sample the first echo are termed as postexcitation refocused steady state sequences **(Fig. 6)** and are mainly T2*-weighted (FISP, GRASS, FFE, FAST).

The sequences which sample the second spin echo are pre-excitation steady state refocused sequences **(Fig. 7)** and are mainly T2-weighted (PSIF, SSFP, T2-FFE).

The sequences which sample both the first (S+) and second (S–) echoes are fully refocused steady state sequences **(Fig. 8)** and are both T1- and T2-weighted (true FISP, FIESTA, balanced FFE).

CISS/FIESTA-C

Contstructive interface in steady state/fast imaging employing steady state acquisition

These are modified, fully refocused steady state sequences by different vendors. Since fully refocused steady state sequence like true-FISP is prone to 'banding artifacts', this aims to remove those. In this sequence, two true-FISP sequences are acquired one with alternating

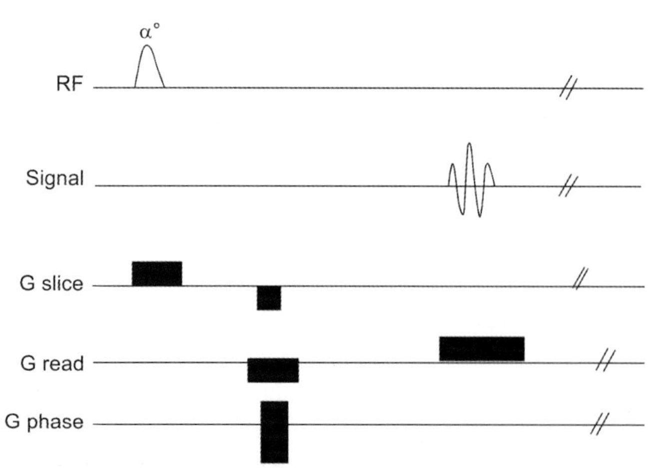

Fig. 5: Gradient-echo sequence. Here after an initial 90° pulse a gradient pulse is applied instead of 180° refocusing pulse as in spin echo sequence.

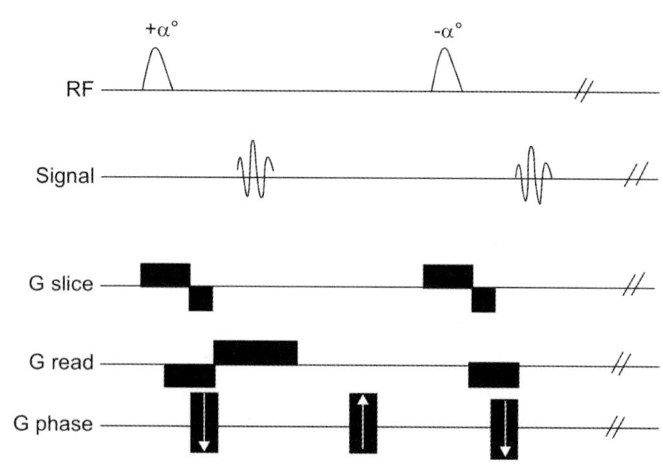

Fig. 6: Postexcitation refocused steady state sequence. Here the first echo after the recent RF pulse is sampled which is due to free induction decay and hence is predominantly T2*-weighted (short TE).

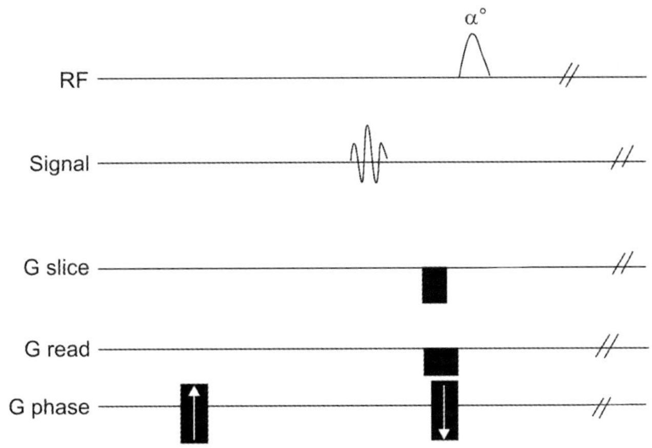

Fig. 7: Pre-excitation steady-state refocused sequence which is mainly T2-weighted as the second echo is sampled which is produced due to refocusing of the residual spin echo just before the application of next RF pulse (long TE).

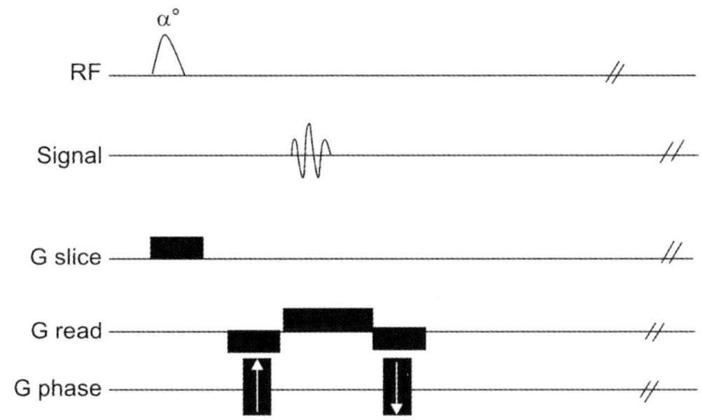

Fig. 8: Fully refocused steady-state sequence.

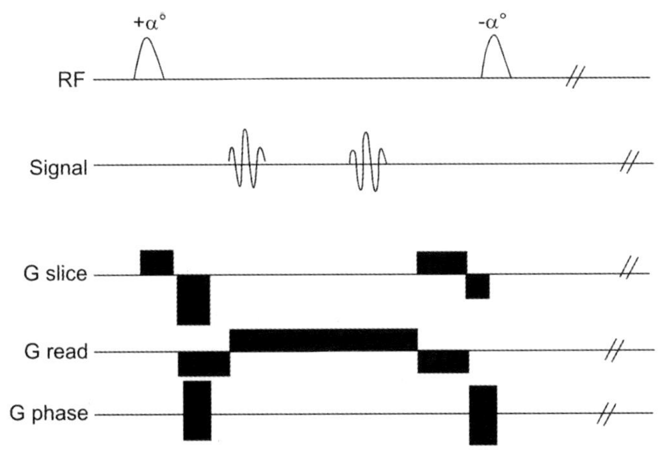

Fig. 9: Dual-echo-steady-state sequence.

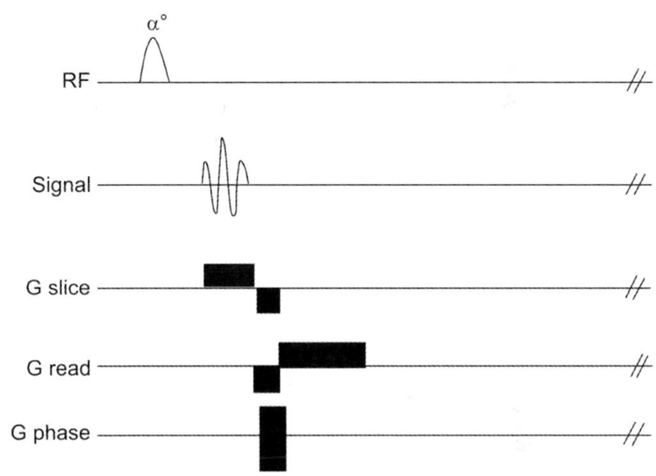

Fig. 10: Incoherent/spoiled gradient-echo sequences

phase RF pulse and second with nonalternating phase RF pulse. Combination of these two images displaces the banding artifacts. This results in high resolution 3D, T2-weighted image.

Dual-echo steady-state sequence

This is another variation of true-FISP. In true-FISP, being a balanced sequence S+ and S- signals are combined to form the image. In DESS, images are formed with FISP (S+) and reversed FISP (S-) and are then combined **(Fig. 9)**. FISP component provides the T1 component and PSIF signal provides the T2 component of the image.

Incoherent/spoiled gradient echo sequences

In these, the residual transverse magnetization is dephased by applying a gradient **(Fig. 10)**. Thus this does not contribute to signal. Since this is also a steady state sequence TR is short and flip angle is medium. The TE is kept very short so that T2* effect does not dominate and the resultant image is T1-weighted. (FLASH, SPGR, MPGR, T1-FFE).

Ultrafast Sequences

These are very fast sequences which employ multiple techniques to shorten the imaging time.

They can be discussed by the predominant weighting they employ.

T2-weighted Ultrafast Sequences*

Echo-planner imaging

This is one of the earliest ultrafast MR sequence where the time is reduced by filling all the lines of k-space in single echo train length. These echoes can be produced either by 180° rephrasing pulse or by gradients. Former is called spin echo EPI and the latter gradient EPI. Multiple echoes which are generated are phase encoded by different slope of gradient to fill separate k-space lines. The phase encoding gradient and the frequency encoding gradient are very rapidly turned on and off allowing rapid filling of k-space. EPI is now technique of choice for diffusion and perfusion imaging.

Diffusion-weighted imaging

For this either echo planer or fast gradient imaging is used. Two large gradients are applied after the excitation. If the protons are not moving, the first gradient dephases and the second rephrases the protons, thereby giving high signal. However, if the protons are moving they are not affected by one of the gradients. They are either dephased and not rephrased or opposite of this, thereby attenuating the signal as compared with stationary protons.

Perfusion-weighted imaging

It employs ultrafast T2 or T2* sequences. It employs use of intravenous gadolinium contrast bolus which decrease the T2 or T2* signal in and around the microvessels that perfuse the tissue. This attenuation is platted against time to generate cerebral blood volume, flow and mean transit time.

Perfusion imaging can also be carried out without contrast injection by tagging the spins with a inversion pulse before they enter the imaging volume. Single shot EPI sequence is commonly used for this imaging technique.

Ultrafast-gradient-echo Sequence

GE sequences, which acquire the images in less than one second are called ultrafast. This is achieved by first applying a magnetization preparation pulse before a GE sequence is applied. Typically, it is a 180° RF pulse. This increases the T1-weighting in the image and all lines of k-space are acquired after this. Images in this can be acquired in less than a second which is advantageous in tracking the arrival of contrast in a given area, typically used in bolus tracking MR angiography. For example, turbo FLASH, TFE, fast SPGR.

3D Ultrafast-gradient-echo Sequence

This is the 3D variant of above mentioned sequence. The difference in these two sequences is that it is a 3D sequence, the acquisition time is long. Thus a single preparatory magnetization pulse is not sufficient and instead multiple preparatory pulse are applied before filling a set of k-space lines. This sequence is applied to acquire very high resolution 3D T1-weighted images of the brain. For example, MP-RAGE, 3D TFE, 3D fast SPGR.

Hybrid Sequences

Gradient/Spin-echo Hybrid

This sequence employ combination of spin echo (RARE) and gradient echo (gradient EPI) for faster image generation. Like in RARE sequence multiple 180° refocusing pulses are applied after an initial 90° pulse to generate multiple echos. But in addition, multiple gradient echoes are generated by switching gradient after each 180° pulse. This sequence is generally employed to get high-resolution T2-weighted images.

SUGGESTED READING

1. Bitar R, Leung G, Perng R, et al. MR pulse sequences: what every radiologist wants to know but is afraid to ask. Radiographics. 2006;26(2):513-37.
2. Boyle GE, Ahern M, Cooke J, et al. An interactive taxonomy of MR imaging sequences. Radiographics. 2006;26(6):e24.
4. Chavhan GB, Babyn PS, Thomas B, et al. Principles, techniques, and applications of T2*-based MR imaging and its special applications. Radiographics. 2009;29(5):1433-49.
3. Chavhan GB, Babyn PS, Jankharia BG, et al. Steady-state MR imaging sequences: physics, classification, and clinical applications. Radiographics. 2008;28(4):1147-60.
5. Eugene Lin. Body MRI sequences: A conceptual framework. Applied radiology. 2012;41(1).
6. MRI at a Glance. Catherine Westbrook Hoboken, 2nd Edn. NJ: Wiley-Blackwell; 2010.
7. Pooley RA. AAPM/RSNA physics tutorial for residents: fundamental physics of MR imaging. Radiographics. 2005;25(4):1087-99.

CHAPTER 50

Digital Radiography: An Update

Alpana Manchanda

INTRODUCTION

Radiography is an art and science of recording images produced by X-rays on X-ray film. Till the past decade, the conventional film-screen system was the most widely used and accepted method of recording images, wherein the film acts as an image receptor, display medium and a source of permanent record. Though these films are relatively inexpensive and provide high image quality, they have many limitations.[1]

LIMITATIONS OF FILM SCREEN RADIOGRAPHY

- Radiographic film has a defined latitude (range of densities) that can be recorded simultaneously. This problem is particularly highlighted in chest radiography where 40% of lung area is obscured by heart, mediastinum and diaphragm. Mediastinum and retrocardiac portion of lung remain under penetrated when exposure is given for optimal lung details.
- Film-screen systems are intolerant to exposure errors, with under/over exposure leading to loss of radiographic contrast
- Films cannot be transmitted or duplicated without some loss of quality and this involve significant cost
- Acquisition, display and storage of image are nonseparable
- Another limitation of radiographic film is the noise inherent in these images. Both radiography and fluoroscopy use area beams, i.e. large rectangular beam of X-rays. The Compton scattered portion of the remnant X-ray beam increases with increasing field size. This increases the noise of the image
- Storage of conventional radiographs also poses a problem
- Film quality can deteriorate with time, especially if chemical processing is suboptimal
- Another important limitation of film screen imaging system is that the image cannot be manipulated before it is displayed and image quality is therefore not necessarily the same in all the images.

Image optimization is therefore essential to achieve good diagnostic images at the lowest possible dose.

Significant advancement in electronics and computer technology have resulted in film-screen radiography (FSR) systems being replaced by digital radiography (DR) systems which have become the standard technology in most departments. The process wherein digital detectors are used to capture information of an object is termed as digital radiography. There are many advantages of producing images in a digital format—in a format that can be stored and processed in a computer and displayed on a monitor.

ADVANTAGES OF DIGITAL RADIOGRAPHY[2,3]

- Digital images do not deteriorate physically or degrade chemically over time
- They allow a true reproduction of quality from copy to copy and from generation to generation

- Digital images are flexible, allowing a variety of manipulation such as magnification, cropping, edge enhancement, compression, etc.
- Digital detectors allow implementation of a fully digital picture archiving and communication system (PACS) in which images are stored digitally and available anytime.
- The images can be distributed electronically by web-based technology with no risk of losing clarity
- A higher patient through put is possible as compared to FSR system
- Increased dose efficiency and wide dynamic range of digital detectors with possible reduction of radiation exposure to the patient.

EVOLUTION OF DIGITAL RADIOGRAPHY

Digital-imaging system was installed in the 1970s until the microprocessor and semi conductor memory systems were developed in the 1980s and were designed to process the large amount of data generated from this system.[3] **Table 1** highlights the developments in digital radiography.

Table 1: Evolution of digital radiography.[3]

Year	Technique
1977	Introduction of digital subtraction angiography (DSA)
1980	DSA first put into clinical use
1980	Use of storage phosphor image plates
1987	Amorphous selenium-based image plates
1990	Charged-couple device (CCD) was introduced for direct capture of X-rays for digital image
1994	Selenium drum DR
1995	Amorphous silicon–cesium iodide (scintillator) flat-panel detector
1997	Gadolinium-based (scintillator) flat-panel detractor
2001	Gadolinium-based (scintillator) portable flat-panel detector
2001	Dynamic flat-panel detector fluoroscopy digital subtraction angiography
2007	Portable CR system

PHYSICS BEHIND DIGITAL RADIOGRAPHY

Digital imaging uses binary system in which information is interpreted as bits. A binary (base 2) digit can assume only one of two values, rather than one of ten as for decimal (base 10) system. The decimal representation of a binary number is calculated such that the digits are multiplied by power of 2 rather than power of 10.

Most digital systems handle individual pixels with eight-bit accuracy for displayed brightness. An individual pixel can therefore have any brightness value from 0 through 255 decibel, a total of 2^8 (256) possible brightness values. Most of the information in radiology is displayed as shades of black and white. The analog imaging system displays a smooth variation in brightness from completely dark to maximum brightness. In digital system the display would be more step like.

Thus, digital information is any information that is represented in discrete units, while analog information is one that is represented in continuous rather than discrete fashion **(Fig. 1)**.[4]

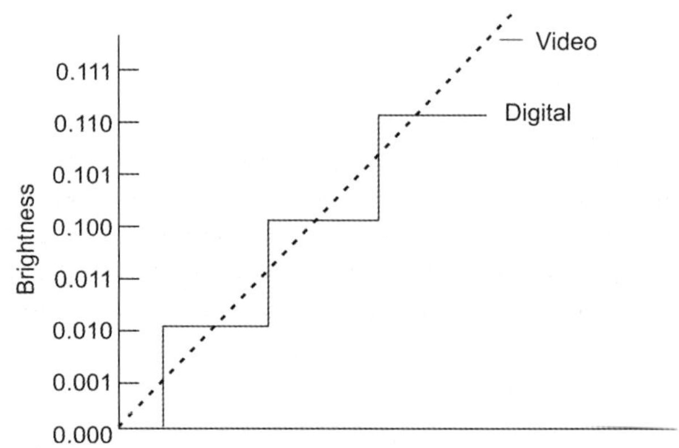

Fig. 1: Comparison of analog video voltage and digitized values.

In contrast to film screen radiography (FSR) in which the film serves as both detector and storage medium, digital detectors are used only to generate the digital image, which is then stored on a digital medium.

Digital imaging consist of four separate steps:

1. Image generation
2. Image processing
3. Image archiving
4. Presentation of the image.

PRINCIPLE OF DIGITAL RADIOGRAPHY

The digital detector is exposed to X-rays generated by a standard tube. The energy absorbed by the detector is transformed into electrical charges, which are then recorded, digitized and quantified into a gray scale. After sampling, postprocessing software is required for organizing the raw data into a clinically meaningful image.[3]

DIGITAL-RADIOGRAPHY SYSTEMS

Digital-radiography systems have evolved in recent years as advancements in FSR technology had almost reached the limit of further improvement.

In digital radiography, a digital detector replaces films and intensifying screens. There are two basic types of digital radiography systems depending upon the types of detectors used to capture the radiographic information.[3,5]

1. **Computed radiography (CR) system** use a storage phosphor image plate (photostimulable phosphor plate) enclosed in a light tight cassette. CR utilizes a two stage process with image capture and image readout done separately.
2. **Direct-digital radiography (DR)** uses detectors that have a combined image capture and image read out process. DR systems can be further divided to direct and indirect conversion groups, depending on the type of X-ray conversion used **(Flowchart 1)**.

Computed Radiography

Computed radiography (CR) systems use storage phosphor image plates with a separate image read out process. In CR systems, photostimulable crystals, i.e. photostimulable phosphor plates (PSP) is the detective layer in place of films and screens. These plates are coated with europium activated barium fluorohalide (Ba FX: Eu^{2+}), the halide being bromide, iodide or a combination of both. CR cassettes are used on conventional X-ray machines like normal cassettes and are available in similar sizes. Image generation in CR is a two step process.

When the storage phosphor image plates (IP) are exposed to X-rays, the X-ray energy is absorbed and temporarily stored by the crystals (detective layer of the plate) by bringing electrons to higher energy levels. X-ray energy can be stored for several hours depending on the specific physical properties of the phosphor crystals used. However, the readout process should start immediately after exposure because the amount of stored energy decreases over time.

In the readout process, the image plate/detective layer after exposure to X-rays is taken to a CR reader where it is scanned by a high-energy laser beam of a specific wavelength. The stored energy is set free as higher energy blue light having a wavelength different from that of the red laser light. This light is collected by photodiodes/photomultipliers and signal converted digitally into electrical signal by an analog-to-digital converter (ADC) then amplified, digitized and used to form an image **(Figs. 2 and 3)**.[5]

The imaging plate is ready for use again after exposure to white light.[5]

In a CR system, the patient information and cassette ID needs to be linked as there is no direct electrical connection between the CR reader and the cassette. A bar code reader or a chip embedded on the CR cassette is used for this purpose. The PSP imaging plates may be flexible or rigid, with the base in these plates being opaque or translucent. Different types of CR cassette designs and image readers are available, so all cassettes from the same vendor may not be compatible with all readers. Some of the CR plate readers can process one plate while holding multiple cassettes in a queue. This is known as "drop and go" which helps improve workflow.[5]

Some CR systems using PSP plates with translucent bases have a dual side readout. These systems use laser scanning from one side but capture light from both sides of the plate, increasing the DQE by 50–100% (DQE or detective quantum efficiency refers to the efficiency of a detector in converting incident X-ray energy into an image signal).

The spatial resolution of the CR images depends on:
- The laser spot size
- Photostimulable phosphor plate characteristics (packing density, thickness of the phosphor layer)
- Sampling rate of the emitted light.

Flowchart 1: Comparison of analog video voltage and digitized values.

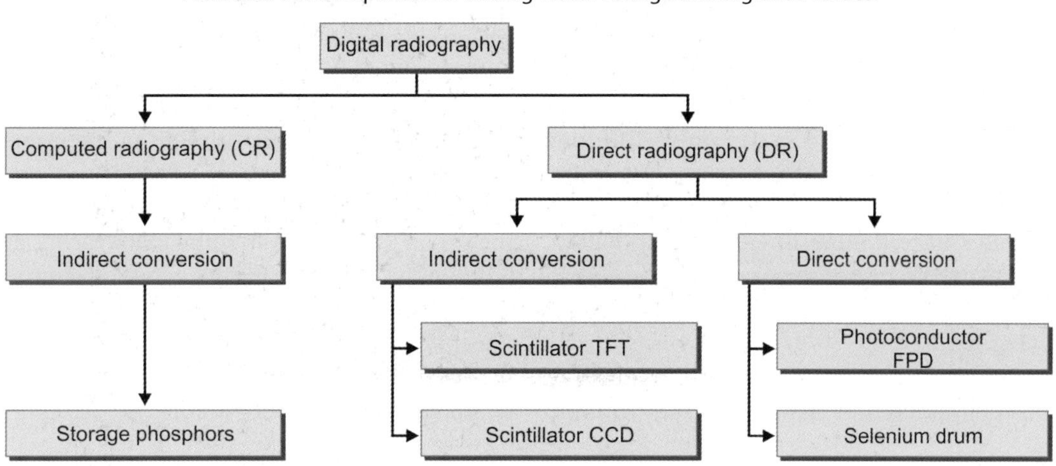

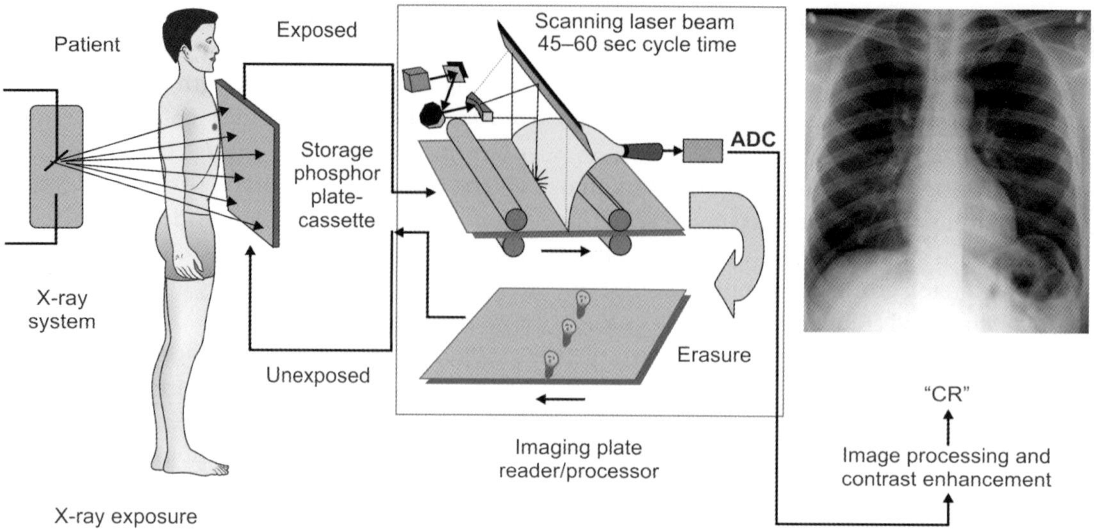

Fig. 2: Schematic representation of a CR imaging system, screen and scanner.

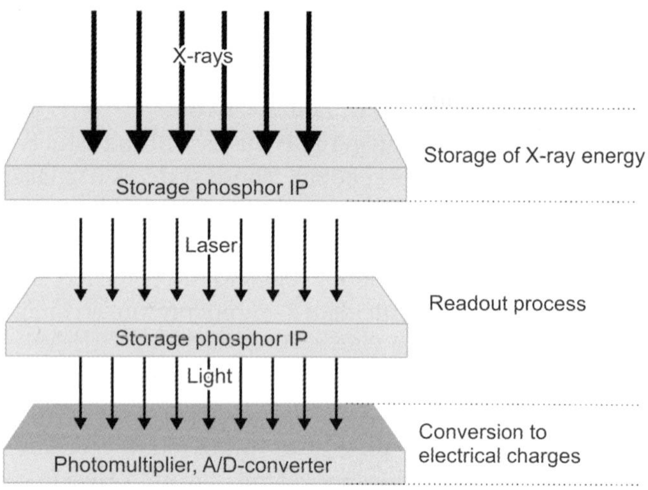

Fig. 3: Illustrates a CR system based on storage-phosphor image plates.

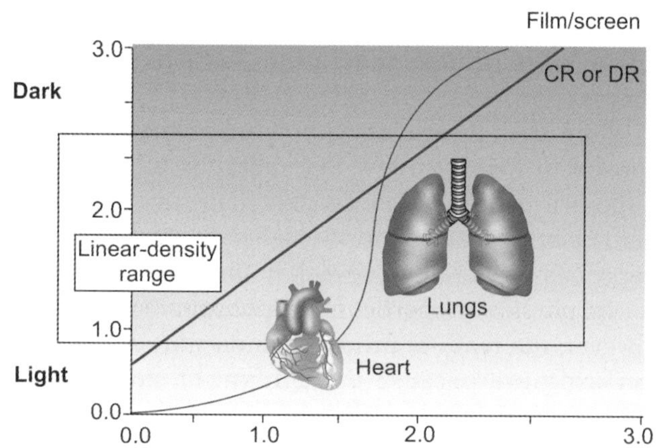

Fig. 4: Optical density versus radiation exposure response curves.

Diffusion of the scanning laser light and emitted light leads to some loss of spatial resolution.

The time taken for scanning a PSP plate varies from 40 to 90 seconds and depends on the plate size, resolution desired and dual/single side readout. Some newly introduced CR systems use line scanning techniques thereby reducing the image readout time to 20–30 seconds or even less.

Phosphor plates have a more linear, optical density versus radiation exposure response curve than the classic sigmoid-shaped curve of the conventional film-screen combination **(Fig. 4)**.

The CR technology thus gives a greater latitude of exposure which is useful under challenging radiographic circumstances, such as the intensive case unit. It allows structures of widely differing radiographic density to be well visualized on the same image, such as the area behind the cardiac silhouette and the lung vessels or the soft tissue of the neck or cervico thoracic junctions. This feature allows a reduction compared with FSR in the number of repeat images taken due to errors in selecting the correct exposure. The spatial resolution of CR is lower (i.e. 2½ line-pairs per mm) than that of conventional FSR which is approximately 5 line pairs per mm. But its superior contrast resolution more than compensates for its limited spatial resolution. Phosphor plates can be reused repeatedly for a thousand or more exposures. CR equipment is cheaper than direct DR equipment, especially for mobile radiographic units.[6]

Advantages of Storage Phosphor Systems

- Being cassette based, CR systems can easily be integrated into existing radiographic equipment
- Single CR systems can convert multiple radiography rooms to digital technology
- They have a wide dynamic range leading to reduced rates of failed X-ray exposure
- They are easy to use for bed side examinations and immobile patients
- CR cassettes can be placed in any position thereby enabling flexibility for positioning for difficult views
- Multiple cassette sizes are available
- In case of defect in the image plate, it can easily be replaced by the radiographer with no need for specialized equipment or service personnel.

Drawbacks of CR/Storage Phosphor Systems

- It is a time consuming technique
- Image reader takes time before the image can be displayed, with time taken being comparable to that required for film processing
- Spatial resolution is lower than that of film screen radiography
- Radiation dose required is same or more than film screen radiography.

Direct-digital Radiography

Digital-radiography (DR) or direct digital-radiography is a way of converting X-ray into electrical charges by means of a combined image capture and image readout process. DR systems are also called DDR or ddR systems by some vendors. DR systems can be further divided into direct and indirect conversion groups depending on the type of X-ray conversion used.[7]

- **Direct-conversion detectors** have an X-ray photoconductor, such as amorphous selenium that directly converts X-rays photons into an electric charge.
- **Indirect-conversion detectors** have a two-step process for X-ray detection
  - A scintillator is the primary material for X-ray interaction. When X-rays strike the scintillator the X-ray energy is converted to visible light
  - The visible light is then converted into an electric charge by means of photodetectors, such as amorphous silicon photodioide arrays or CCDs (charged-couple device).

In both direct- and indirect-conversion detectors, the electric charge pattern that remains after X-ray exposure is sensed by an electric-readout mechanism, and analog-to-digital conversion is performed to produce the digital image.

Direct Conversion

Direct-conversion type of detectors uses amorphous selenium as photoconductor that converts X-rays photons into electrical charges by setting electrons free. The photoconductor materials include amorphous selenium, lead iodide, thallium bromide and gadolinium compounds. The more commonly used element is selenium. All these elements have a high intrinsic spatial resolution. As a result, the pixel size, matrix and spatial resolution of direct conversion detectors are not limited by the detector material itself, but only by the recording and readout devices used.[3]

Selenium-based direct conversion DR systems are equipped with either (a) a selenium drum or (b) a flat panel detector.

Selenium Drum-based System of Direct Conversion

A rotating selenium drum with a positive electric surface charge is exposed to X-rays. During exposure, a charged pattern proportional to that of incident X-rays is generated on the drum surface and is recorded during rotation by an analog-to-digital converter **(Fig. 5A)**.

Several clinical studies have proved that selenium drum detectors provide good image quality that is superior to that provided by film-screen or CR system.[8] However, a limitation of selenium drum detectors is that they are dedicated thorax stand systems with no mobility at all.[3]

Large area, thin film transistor arrays

Thin-film transistor arrays (TFTs) are used as active electronic elements in both direct and indirect conversion, flat-panel detectors. Thin film transistor arrays are typically deposited onto a glass substrate in multiple layers, beginning with readout electronics at the lowest level and followed by charge collector arrays at higher levels. Then, depending on the type of detector being constructed, X-ray elements, light sensitive elements, or both, are deposited to form the top layer of TFT array. The whole assembly is encased in a protective enclosure with external casing for computer connection.[7]

Thin-film Transistor—Direct Conversion

Direct-conversion system-based on thin-film transistor arrays are constructed by adding an X-ray photoconductor as the top layer of the electronic thin-film transistor sandwich. Amorphous selenium is used as the photoconductor material because of its excellent X-ray

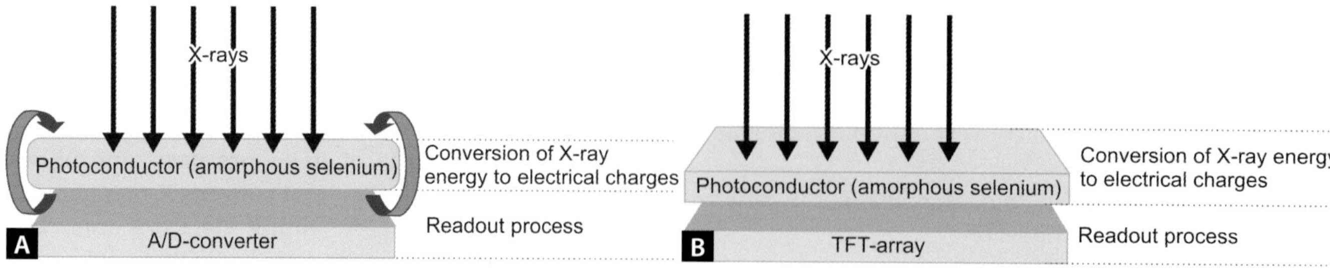

Figs. 5A and B: Direct-conversion DR system: (A) Selenium drum-based system; (B) Thin-film transistor.

detection properties and extremely high intrinsic spatial resolution.

It is sandwiched between two electrodes to which high voltage is applied. When this layer is exposed to X-rays, electrons and holes are produced, proportional to the amount of X-rays absorbed. The applied voltage separates the electrons and holes, so that the signal does not spread. The electronic charge is stored in capacitors and is read out sequentially. Thus, the X-rays are directly converted to electrical signal **(Fig. 5B)**. These detectors have very high spatial resolution, moderate X-ray absorption efficiency (DQE) and an excellent fill factor. The area of the detector that is sensitive to X-ray in relation to the total detector area is known as the "fill factor". Detectors with higher fill factors use absorbed radiation more efficiently.[5]

An advantage of amorphous selenium TFT array over selenium drum is that these detectors can be mounted on thorax stands and bucky tables. As selenium is used in its amorphous form, selenium plates can be made by means of evaporation relatively easily and inexpensively.[7]

Direct conversion of DR technology has mainly been derived from the use of selenium drums in photocopier machines and xeroradiography. Selenium has relatively low atomic number resulting in less X-ray absorption in general radiography KV range. The K-edge of selenium is more suited for the diagnostic KV range required in mammography. As a result, direct conversion FPDs are more popular in mammography than in routine radiography.[5]

Thin-film Transistor—Indirect Conversion

Indirect-conversion-based on thin-film transistor (TFT) arrays are constructed by adding amorphous silicon photodiode circuitry and a scintillator as the top layers of the thin-film transistor sandwich. These layers replace the X-ray photoconductor layer that is used in direct conversion devices.

Mechanism

When X-rays strike the scintillator, visible light is emitted proportional to the incident X-ray energy. Visible light

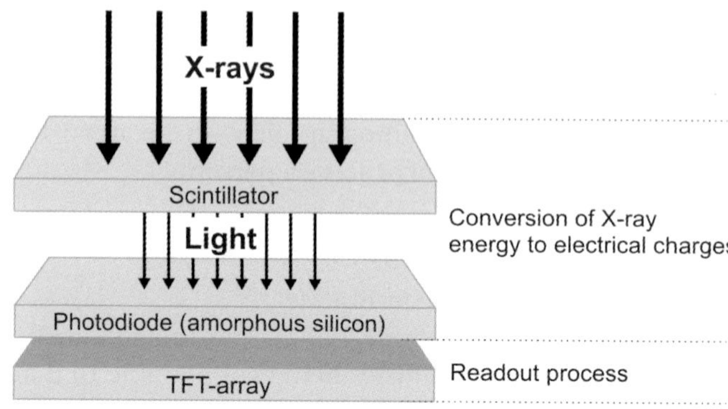

Fig. 6: Drawing illustrates an amorphous silicon-based indirect-conversion DR system.

photon are then converted into an electric change by the photodiode array, and the charge collected at each photodioide is converted into a digital value by using the underlying readout electronics **(Fig. 6)**.

TYPES OF SCINTILLATORS

The scintillators used in indirect conversion detectors can be either structured or unstructured **(Fig. 7)**.

Unstructured scintillator: With use of unstructured scintillator, the visible light emitted by the material can spread to adjacent pixels, thereby reducing spatial resolution.

Structured scintillators: To reduce the problem of scatter, some manufacturers now use a structured scintillator that consists of cesium iodide crystals that are grown on the detector. The crystalline structure consists of discrete and parallel 'needles' (5–10 μ wide) which channel most of the signal directly to the photodiode layer. As light spreading is greatly reduced in a structured scintillator, it maintains a good spatial resolution. Thicker layer of the material can be used in the detector. This increases the number of X-ray photon interactions and thus the available visible light.

Thallium-doped cesium iodide (CsI) is the most commonly used phosphor material. Another material that is used is gadolinium oxysulfide or Gadox (Gd_2O_2S).

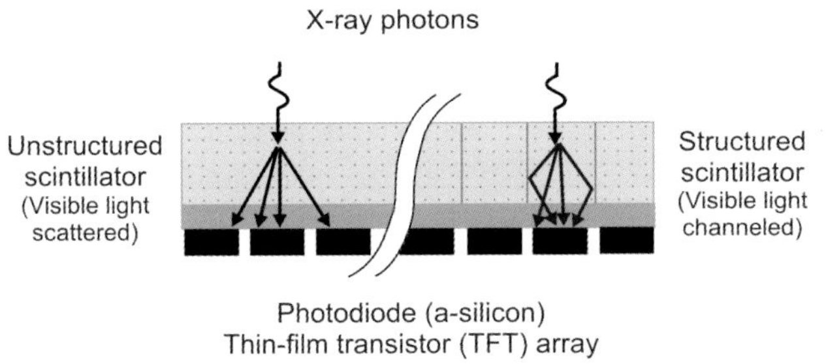

Fig. 7: Diagrammatic representation of indirect-conversion detectors—the X-ray scintillator can be structured or unstructured.

It has an amorphous structure that permits spread of light produced by X-ray absorption, resulting in poorer, spatial resolution. CsI- based detectors are more efficient in X-ray absorption than gadox detectors and have better DQE.[5]

The small size of the flat panel detectors is of advantage as it allows integration into existing bucky table or thorax stands. But as CsI-based flat-panel detectors are highly vulnerable to mechanical load because of their fragile nature, these detectors are to be handled with the utmost care. These systems cannot be used outside fixed installations and hence lack mobility. Portable flat panel detector systems make use of Gd_2O_2S-based scintillators as they are resistant to mechanical stress.[3]

Most flat panel detectors are available in large sizes of 43 × 43 cm, 41 × 41 cm, 43 × 35 cm, etc. Image generation with flat panel detectors is almost instant, with a time lapse less than 10 seconds. Also more number of patients can be imaged in the same amount of time than with other radiographic devices.[3]

Charged-coupled Devices

Charged-coupled devices (CCDs) is a light sensitive sensor for recording images that consists of an integrated circuit containing an array of linked or coupled capacitors. X-ray energy is converted into light by a scintillator, such as thallium doped cesium iodide. The amount of light emitted is then recorded by the CCD, and the light is converted into electrical charges. As the detector area cannot be larger than the CCD chip, it is necessary to combine several chips to create larger detector areas.[3]

Charged-coupled devices can be used for radiography as part of either (a) a lens coupled CCD system, or (b) a slot-scan CCD system.

The lens system is an array consisting of several CCD chips which form a detector area similar to that of a flat panel detector. Optical lenses are needed to reduce the area of the projected light to fit the CCD array **(Fig. 8)**. A drawback of the lens system is that it substantially reduces the number of photons that reach the CCD. This increases

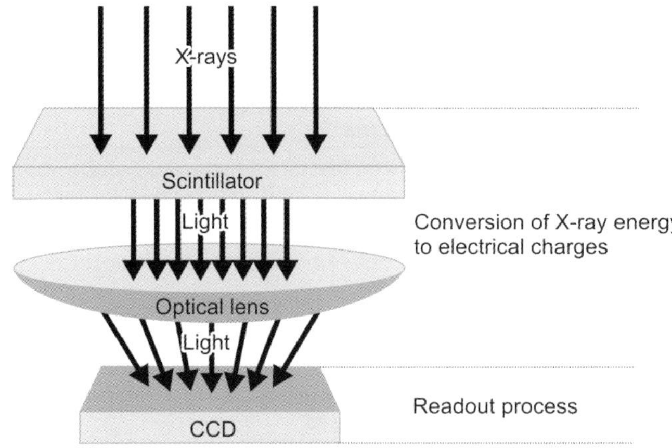

Fig. 8: Lens-coupled CCD-based indirect-conversion DR system.

the image noise (quantum mottle) and degrades image quality. In addition, optical coupling with lenses can introduce geometric distortion, optical scatter, and reduce spatial resolution.

Slot-scan CCD system—makes use of a special X-ray tube with a tungsten mode. The patient is scanned with a collimated fan-shaped beam, which is linked to a simultaneously moving CCD detector array having a matching detector. The combination of a small collimated beam and a concordant detector reduces the impact of scattered radiation in the images. The exposure time to the patient is about 20 m sec, and the readout time takes about 1.3 seconds.[3] Slot-scan CCD systems are dedicated to chest radiography, mammography or dental radiography.

The performance of lens-coupled CCD system has been found to be inferior to that of slot-scan system because of their technical principle, substantlally lower quantum efficiency, and lower signal-to-noise ratio (SNR).

Photon-counting Type DR System

Photon-counting type of DR system has construction similar to the slot scanning type, but uses a different type of detector. These systems use a multislit detector made of crystalline silicon (Si) as a scintillator. The principle is similar to the one used in direct type of flat panel detector. A voltage of about 100 volts is applied across the array of thin Si crystals (50 μm). The absorbed X-ray produce electrons and holes which is counted in a meter. The photon counting type of DR system produces images with a high SNR as the electrical pulse generated is much higher than the electronic noise. The images are of high contrast and detail resolution with no ghost image due to previous exposure residue. Presently, this technology is used for mammography.[9] In **Table 2**, differentiating features of direct and indirect types of flat panel digital detectors are enumerated.

Table 2: Main differentiating features of direct and indirect type of flat-panel digital detectors.[9]

S. No.	Direct-digital conversion	Indirect-digital conversion
1.	Direct conversion of X-rays to electrical signal X-rays ⟶ electrical signal	Indirect conversion of X-rays to electric signal X-rays ⟶ light ⟶ electrical signal
2.	Uses a photoconductor that directly converts the absorbed X-rays to electrical signal without any intermediate light production	Phosphor converts X-rays to light and photodiode array converts emitted light into electrical signals
3.	Detector material used—amorphous selenium (a-Se)	Phosphor used commonly—thallium-doped cesium iodide (CsI) or gadolinium oxysulfide (Gd_2O_2S)
4.	The signal does not spread as the applied high voltage separates the electrons and holes produced by absorbed X-rays	Light scatter reduces spatial resolution more with Gd_2O_2S as phosphor than CsI
5.	Resolution of the images is maintained as the thickness of the photoconductor is increased	With increasing phosphor thickness, poorer resolution images are obtained
6.	Fill factor ~ 100%	Moderate fill factor depending on pixel size
7.	Moderate DQE for KV used for conventional radiography, but high DQE for mammography KV range	High DQE for KV range used in conventional radiography

IMAGE PROCESSING

After exposure and readout, the raw imaging data needs to be processed for display on the computer. Image processing is one of the important features of digital radiography and greatly influences the way the image appears to the radiologist. Even though software products from several manufacturers use similar algorithm such as edge enhancement, noise reduction and contrast enhancement to alter the appearance of the image, the resulting image may differ considerably.[3]

Image processing is used to improve image quality by reducing noise, remove technical artifacts and optimize contrast for viewing. Spatial resolution cannot be influenced by the processing software as it is dependent on the technical variables of the detector (pixel size).

Noise limits the ability to see low contrast detail. In real time acquisition system such as fluoroscopy, noise can be reduced by adding the signal from successive frames to give a time averaged image. This is equivalent to increasing exposure time in radiography. Frame averaging is a useful technique provided that there is no movement between frames, otherwise the image will be blurred.

Noise may also be reduced by low-pass spatial filtering. In this technique, to the grayscale value stored in each pixel, a proportion of the value of the neighboring pixels and resultant value is averaged. The effect is to smooth the final image, but it blurs small details or edges.

Direct-radiography systems convert X-ray image information into electronic charges held by the TFT array. As indirect-conversion systems rely on light, substantial scatter occurs before the energy is converted to charge which reduces SNR.

Edge enhancement or high pass filtering has the opposite effect. Rather than display a weighted average value of neighboring pixels, a high pass filter adds in a proportion of the difference between the grayscale value of the pixel and that of its neighbor. The effect is to exaggerate the contrast at the boundary between structures, thus making the structures more visible.[10]

Image processing software is usually bundled with the detector and cannot be replaced by other software.

ASPECTS OF IMAGE QUALITY

Although the image in digital technique may appear as a conventional video or radiographic image, it is not. It is formed from individual image elements—pixels. With conventional imaging, X-rays form an image directly on the receptor. Efficient detection of the spatially dependent, attenuated transmitted beam is the first and most important task of an X-ray detector. With digital technique, X-rays form an electronic image on a radiation detector and are manipulated by a computer, temporarily stored in memory and displayed as a matrix of intensities, each having a dynamic range of values.

The major factors effecting digital image quality are mentioned here:

Pixels

The pixel is the foundation block of digital imaging. It is the smallest complete sample of an image. The two dimensional collection of pixels in the images is called the matrix, which is usually expressed in length (in pixels) by width (in pixels) Maximum achievable spatial resolution is defined by pixel size and spacing. Pixel size is a measure of resolution, wherein, smaller the pixel size (or larger the matrix), better the resolution.

Detector Size

The physical dimensions of the X-ray detector have an influence on the radiographic examinations performed. The detector should be sufficiently large to capture the desired anatomic views and sufficiently compact for all clinical applications.[7] Larger detector areas are needed for chest imaging than for imaging of the extremities.

Grayscale

Grayscale refers to shades of gray available for reproducing faithfully subtle differences in densities in an accurate manner. Grayscale images are different from black and white images. Unlike the latter, which have two colors (black, white), grayscale images have a number of shades of gray in between. More the number of shades available, superior is the display. The shades of gray that compose an image range from pure black at the weakest intensity to pure white at the strongest.

For routine visual display, 2^8 or 256 intensities (shades of gray) are recorded on a nonlinear scale. However, in medical imaging more shades of gray are required which allows 2^{16} or 65536 gray levels.

Spatial Resolution

It describes the ability to distinguish fine spatial detail and to differentiate objects in an image. In digital acquisition systems, resolution is governed by a term called spatial frequency. Resolution implies how frequently an object is sampled. As a rule of thumb:

- Increasing the sampling frequency helps increase resolution
- Images composed with a greater number of pixels have a higher spatial resolution. However, images with higher resolution require large file sizes.[2]

Increasing the radiation applied to the detector will not improve the maximum spatial resolution. In fact, scattering of X-ray and light photons with the detector influences the spatial resolution. Hence, spatial resolution for selenium-based direct conversion detectors is higher than for indirect conversion detectors. Structured scintillators are advantageous over unstructured scintillators.[3]

The image resolution in capturing devices is not synonymous with the image resolution of output devices, such as computer monitors or printers. In general, for capturing devices, the imaging resolution is expressed as ppi (pixel per inch) and for output devices as dpi (dots per inch).[3]

Spatial resolution in digital acquisition systems is expressed as pixel size, pixels/mm, or line pairs per millimeter (lp/mm). Line pairs per millimeter are a measure of resolution wherein pairs of lines are closely approximated. The unaided human is capable of distinguishing about 10–14 lp/mm. More the lines placed within a millimeter implies higher the resolution.

The spatial resolution of newer digital acquisition systems such as CR and DR are comparable to each other, but less than film-screen radiography.[2] It is possible to achieve a resolution of 5–10 pixel/mm in general purpose CR cassettes while a resolution of 20 pixel/mm is available in most CR systems approved for mammography.[5]

- *Detection of signal in a noisy background and noise reduction methods are*:
  - Flat fielding
  - Signal averaging
  - Anti-scatter grids
- *Dose reduction methods*:
  - High peak voltage
  - Added tube filtration
  - Detector technology
- Image processing, consistency and reproducibility are achievable by DR.

Contrast Resolution and Dynamic Range

Contrast resolution refers to the amount of grayscale differentiation that exists in an image. For digital image acquisition equipment, it means the number of shades of gray that a detector can capture. Digital detectors have high contrast resolution thus enabling thousands of shades of gray to be displayed. The superior contrast resolution of digital detectors more than compensates for the reduced spatial resolution.[2]

Dynamic image is the measure of the signal response of a detector that is exposed to X-rays. In a conventional film-scan combination, the dynamic range is S-shaped with a narrow exposure range for optimal film blackening, i.e. the film has a low tolerance for exposure at higher or lower than required, resulting in failed exposures or insufficient image quality **(Fig. 9)**.

In digital detectors, dynamic range is the range of X-ray exposure over which a meaningful image can be obtained. Digital detectors have a wide and linear-dynamic range. In contrast to film-screen system, the curve for digital detectors is less steep and covers a wider range. As a result, an optimal signal response will occur over a wider exposure range with digital detectors than with film-screen combinations. Another advantage of a wide-dynamic range is that differences between specific tissue

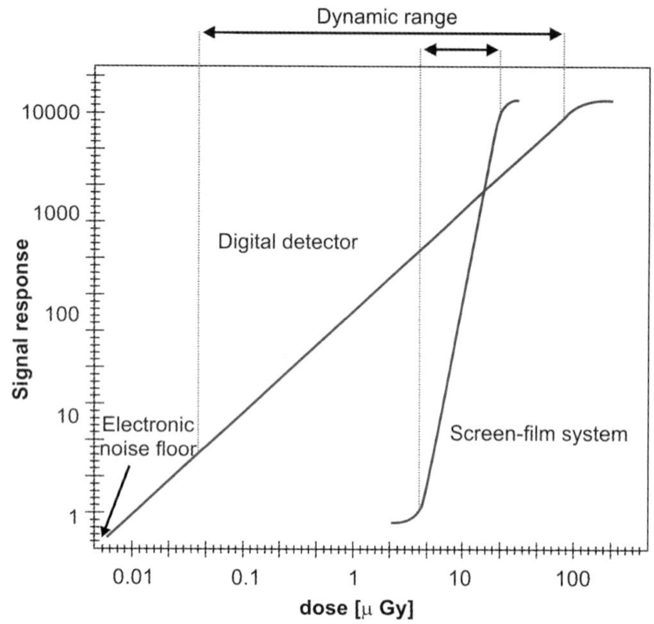

Fig. 9: Graph illustrates the dynamic range of screen-film combinations and digital detectors.

absorption (e.g. bone vs soft tissue) can be displayed in one image without the need for additional images.[3]

Modular Transfer Function

Objective methods can be used to determine detectors and X ray system performance (image quality) and efficiency (dose). Measurement include frequency dependent signal transfer via the MTF(f), noise power spectrum NPS(f) and signal transfer efficiency (input to output) via the DQE metric [DQE(f)]. Different detectors have different modulation transfer characteristics.

Modular transfer function (MTF) is the capacity of the detector to transfer the modulation of the input signal at a given spatial frequency to its output. At radiography, objects having different sizes and opacity are displayed with different gray scale values in an image. MTF has to do with the display of contrast and object size. It is responsible for converting contrast values of different sized objects (object contrast) into contrast intensity levels in the image (image contrast).[10]

The ratio of the output and input modulation is known as the modulation transfer function. MTF varies with spatial frequency. Generally reduces progressively from 100% at low spatial frequencies towards zero at higher frequencies.[10]

Detective-quantum Efficiency

Detective-quantum efficiency (DQE) is one of the important physical variables related to image quality in radiography and refers to the efficiency of a detector in converting incident X-ray energy into an image signal. It is calculated by comparing the signal to noise ratio at the detector output with that at the detector input as a function of spatial frequency. DQE depends on radiation exposure, spatial frequency, modulation transfer function, detector material and quality (voltage and current) of the radiation applied.[3]

An ideal situation is 100% quantum detection and conversion efficiency. Three types of materials are used and they are classified into three categories:

1. Unstructured scintillators (e.g. gadolinium oxysulfide and barium fluorobromide).
2. Structured phosphors (e.g. cesium iodide, cesium bromide).
3. Semiconductor direct detectors (e.g. amorphous selenium).

Digital systems with structured phosphors or semiconductors can achieve good spatial resolution. However indirect TFT technology based systems are more dose efficient.

Detectors with higher DQE will require less radiation dose than the detectors with lower DQE for similar image quality or SNR. Both MTF and DQE are depicted in the form of a graph as a function of frequency or spatial resolution in line pairs/mm^3 (lp/mm) **(Fig. 10)**. Both are higher at low resolution and decrease with increasing spatial resolution.[5]

An ideal detector should have a DQE of 1 which means that all the radiation energy is absorbed and converted into image formation. However, in practice, the DQE of digital detectors is limited to about 0.45 at spatial frequency of 0.5 cycles/mm^3. While the maximum reported DQE for

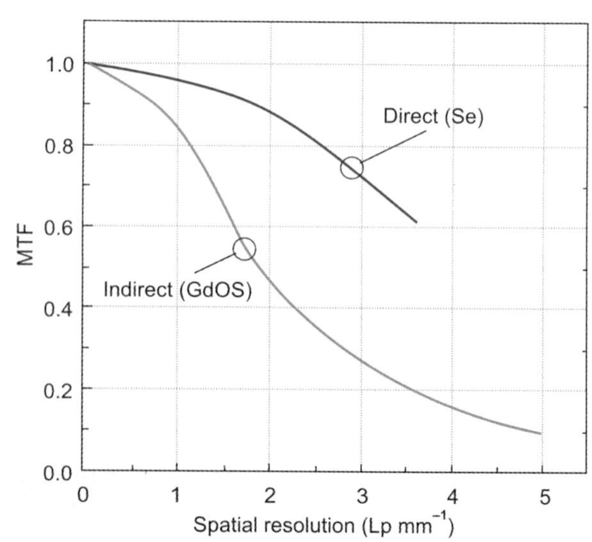

Fig. 10: MTF of direct- and indirect-digital systems.

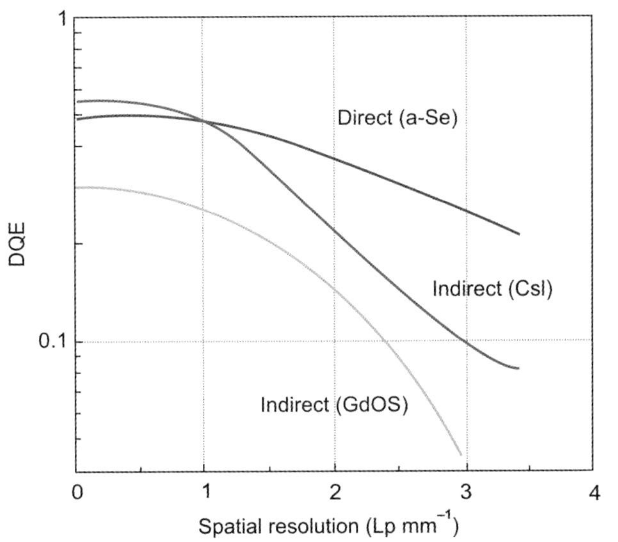

Fig. 11: DQE as a function of spatial frequency for 3 detector systems at 70 kVp.

film-screen and computed radiography are typically 0.15–0.25 under similar conditions **(Fig. 11)**.[11]

Over the years, various methods for measuring DQE have been established. In 1999 the IEC62220-1 standard was established to improve the comparability of DQE measurements of digital X-ray imaging devices. The exposure level is measured at the detector surface with calibrated radiation meters after removing all protective parts including antiscatter grid, the AEC chamber and other cover plates out of the beam. The IEC62220-1 standard will enable manufacturers to specify DQE values on the basis of an internationally accepted methodology. This helps users to compare detectors and imaging systems and to make optimal use of the detectors.[12]

Radiation Exposure

Digital detectors besides providing better image quality have the potential for substantially lowering the patient exposure. Efforts have been made to optimize both image quality and exposure in digital radiography. The most obvious way of minimizing patient exposure is to greatly reduce the number of failed exposures and requisite additional images.

In contrast to storage phosphor systems in which the possibility of exposure reduction is limited, DR systems offer a significantly higher potential for general exposure reduction because of their far superior quantum efficiency. Various studies have concluded that flat-panel detectors achieve the best results in high image quality at lower doses, followed by other DR systems, such as selenium drum and CCD-based systems.[3,13]

Use of CR for chest imaging leads to an increased in radiation dose, as storage phosphor plates are not suited for high kVp techniques. Moreover, storage phosphor plates are more sensitive to scatter, which makes the use of high ratio grids mandatory and so radiation exposure is increased.[13] Studies show that digital system optimization is an important parameter in reducing patient dose. Hence, technical requirements for digital systems should be set for achieving the same.[13]

Newer Applications in CR

Newer technological advances in CR have been introduced to overcome some of the limitations of CR system, such as cassette handing, long readout time of PSP plates, low DQE and poor resolution.

- *Automated CR systems:* Efficiency of CR systems has been recently improved by reducing the readout time and by removing the step of cassette handling. The readout time of PSP plate is reduced to less than 10 sec by line scan lasers and photodiode detectors in automated CR systems. In these systems, the image data acquisition is totally automatic as there is no cassette handling.
- *Newer structured phosphor for PSP plates:* Newer phosphors like cesium bromide having a structured needle-shaped configuration of crystals have been recently introduced which reduce light diffusion. They are also more efficient with an increased DQE.
- *Mobile CR systems:* To save labor, time and improve workflow of critically ill patients requiring bedside X-rays, portable, compact CR systems have been introduced in 2007. These systems have a mobile X-ray unit with an integrated CR reader which does away with the physical transport of the cassette to the CR reader, hence image is available in less than 25 seconds.[9]

Newer Applications in DR

A number of technological advancements have taken place in digital radiography in hardware as well as software applications **(Table 3)**.

- *Tomosynthesis:* In this technique multiple low dose exposures are given from various angles while the X-ray tube moves in an arc and the detector remains stationary. Multiple images with different focal zones can be created by addition of these low dose images after pixel shift. The images can be viewed singly or in a wire loop. An additional advantage of digital tomosynthesis compared to conventional tomography is that computer processing methods can be used to minimize the contribution of the blurred out of plane structures to the images deducted at each plane of

Table 3: List of select manufacturers of DR systems with details of their exposure indicator (EI).

Manufacturer	*EI name*	*EI symbol*	*Units*
Agfa	Log of median of histogram	1gM	Bels
Alara CR	Exposure indicator value	EIV	Mbels
Canon	Reached exposure value	REX	Unitless
Canon	EXP	EXP	Unitless
Carestream (formerly Kodak)	Exposure index	EI	Mbels
Fujifilm	S value	S	Unitless
GE	Uncompensated detector exposure	UD Exp	µGy air kerma
GE	Compensated detector exposure	CD Exp	µGy air kerma
GE	Detector exposure index	DEI	Unitless
Konica	Sensitivity number	S	Unitless
Philips	Exposure index	EI	Unitless
Siemens	Exposure index	EI	µGy air kerma

interest.[14] It is considered useful in chest, IVU studies and mammography.[9]

- *Dual-energy imaging:* Dual energy radiography methods are used to generate separate images of bone and soft tissue structures from two exposures made using different radiographic techniques, i.e. using high and low kilo voltage technique.[14] It is particularly useful in chest radiography where the interference of ribs is removed from lung tissue. Dual-energy techniques are most effective when both images are acquired simultaneously. Similar results are obtained with two exposures within a very short period of time. Though flat panel dual energy systems produce images with less noise, they are prone to artifacts from tissue motion occurring between the two exposures. Dual energy imaging is useful in chest radiography particularly in the evaluation of partially calcified nodules and pleural plaques.[9]
- *Computer-aided diagnosis (CAD):* They are important in early detection of cancer of the lung and breast. The suspicious areas are marked by the software for review by the radiologist. The main advantage of CAD is that it alerts the radiologist to avoid overlooking diagnostically significant findings.[9]
- *Automatic image stitching:* This feature is useful when precise measurements in lengthy anatomical regions like the spine or lower limb are required. With use of the largest flat panel DR plates, i.e. 43 × 43 cm, only a limited portion of the body can be imaged at a time. To overcome this problem of inability of studying the whole spine or entire lower limb, multiple sequential exposures at different patient positions are acquired in a patient who is absolutely still. Automatic stitching is then performed to reconstruct a larger composite image.
- *Mobile DR:* It consists of a 17 × 14 inch flat-panel detector connected by a cable to a mobile X-ray system having a monitor. The high cost and fragility of the FPDs hampers the use of mobile DR system. On comparison with FSR system, a mobile DR system is not affected by the availability, storage, transportation and disposal of films and chemicals.
- *Wireless FPDs:* A wireless portable DR system can transfer image data wirelessly to the DR system. It does not have any cables and does not interfere with surrounding machines. A 17 × 14 inch image is ready within 3 seconds and allows radiography of difficult regions of the body like the axilla or the TM joint. Also, with wireless FPDs, radiography of a limb with limited mobility (flexed/having contractures) is possible.
- *Fluoroscopy and radiography:* Real time digital imaging facilitates high quality radiography and fluoroscopy with up to 30 images/sec. The fluoroscopy feature is used in gastroenterology, urology and vascular applications.

Exposure Indicator for Digital Radiography

In contrast to FSR, where visual features, such as under/overexposure help in recognizing exposure errors, digital system lack in recognizing the same. As a result, the radiographer needs to monitor the exposure indicator (EI) associated with digital imaging system. Exposure indicators have been developed by most equipment manufacturers. The purpose of the EI is to allow the radiographer to know the level of exposure the receptor has received and thereby determine if the correct exposure technique for the image was used. It is important to note that EIs are not measures of radiation dose to the patient but records the level of exposure to the image receptor.

The exposure indicator varies among different manufactures, even having different names, symbols and units. **Table 3** shows a list of select manufactures and details regarding their EI as of 2011.[15]

ACR Practice Guideline for Digital Radiography

Radiographic examinations represent more than two-thirds of all radiologic examinations performed in both adults and children.[16] The Society for Pediatric Radiology in 2004 emphasized the need for ALARA Principle in digital imaging. The ACR developed a practice guideline of digital radiography in 2007 in "order to deliver optimal image quality at appropriate radiation doses so as to provide excellent safety and care for patients undergoing digital radiography examination".[15]

CONCLUSION

The future of radiography is digital and it is imperative that radiologists be familiar with the technical principles, criteria for image quality and radiation exposure issues with the various digital radiography systems that are currently available along with the technological advancements that are taking place.

REFERENCES

1. Selman J. The fundamentals of X-ray and radium physics, 8th Edn. Charles C Thomas; 1994.
2. Indrajit IK, Verma BS. Digital imaging in radiology practice: An introduction to few fundamental concepts. IJRI. 2007;17(4): 230-6.
3. Körner M, Weber CH, Wirth S, Pfeifer KJ, Reiser MF, Treitl M. Advances in digital radiography: physical principles and system overview. Radiographics. 2007;27(3):675-86.
4. Cury TS, Dowdey JE, Murry RC. Digital radiography in Christensen's Physics of Diagnostic Radiology, 4th Edn. Lea and Febiger; 1990.pp.392-431.
5. Verma BS, Indrajit IK. Advent of digital radiography: Part I. IJRI. 2008;18(2):113-6.
6. Strickland NH. Picture archiving and communication system and digital radiology. In Grainger & Allison Diagnostic Radiology. A textbook of Medical Imaging, 5th Edn, Vol. I: 3-30, 2008, Edited by Adam A, Dixon AK, Chruchill Livingstone.
7. Chotas HG, Dobbins JT 3rd, Ravin CE. Principles of digital radiography with large-area, electronically readable detectors: a review of the basics. Radiology. 1999;210(3):595-9.
8. Fischbach F, Freund T, Pech M, Werk M, Bassir C, Stoever B, et al. Comparison of indirect CsI/a:Si and direct a: Se digital radiography. An assessment of contrast and detail visualization. Acta Radiol. 2003;44(6):616-21.
9. Verma BS, Indrajit IK. Impact of computers in radiography: the advent of digital radiography, Part-2. IJRI. 2008;18(3):204-9.
10. Roberts PA, Williams J. Digital radiography in Farr's Physics for Medical Imaging (2nd edn), Saunders Elsevier. 2008;79:90.
11. Dowsett DJ, Kenny PA, Johnston RE. The digital image in The Physics of Diagnostic Imaging (2nd edn), International Thomson Publishing; 2006.pp.313-63.
12. Illers H, Buhr E, Hoeschen C. Measurement of the detective quantum efficiency (DQE) of digital X-ray detectors according to the novel standard IEC 62220-1. Radiat Prot Dosimetry. 2005;114(1-3):39-44.
13. Neofotistou V, Tsapaki V, Kottou S, Schreiner-Karoussou A, Vano E. Does digital imaging decrease patient dose? A pilot study and review of the literature. Radiat Prot Dosimetry. 2005;117(1-3):204-10.
14. Flynn M. Technical advances in CR and DR part 2. Available from. *http://www.imagingeconomics.com/issues/articles/2004-04_ 16.asp* (Last accessed on 2008 April 25th)
15. Herrmann TL, Fauber TL, Gill J, Hoffman C, et al. Best practices in Digital Radiography. White Paper (American Society of Radiologic Technologists); 2012.pp.1-26.
16. Harmon R. Realizing the full benefit of digital radiography. Imaging Economics 2001. Available from: *http://www.imagingeconomics.com/issues/articles/2001_12.20asp.*

CHAPTER 51

Digital Mammography

Smriti Hari, Chandrashekhara SH, Surabhi Vyas

INTRODUCTION

Mammography is one of the most technically challenging areas of radiography, requiring high spatial resolution, excellent soft tissue contrast and low-radiation dose. In thicker and denser breasts, wide image latitude is also needed. Reported sensitivities of screening mammography range from 45% to 85% with performance suffering as parenchymal density increases.[1] Several studies have shown improved detection of cancer with digital mammography in younger women who have dense breasts.[2,3]

Although the digital technique has many similarities to screen film and many of the requirements for an optimal image are the same, such as correct compression and positioning, the digital mammogram is constructed in a different way from screen-film images. Having an understanding of how the images are created and how different variables influence image quality is important to the radiologist for both diagnostic reasons and quality assurance purposes. New applications of digital mammography, such as digital breast tomosynthesis (DBT), stereo mammography and contrast-enhanced mammography are expected to further improve the diagnostic accuracy of mammography.

DIGITAL MAMMOGRAPHY

Although screen-film mammography (SFM) produce images of extremely high spatial resolution, the analog system can only function within a narrow dynamic range; markedly reducing the degree of object contrast that can be depicted in the image.

For this reason, digital platforms capable of mammographic imaging were developed. These digital systems have allowed the functions of image acquisition, display and archiving to be decoupled, thus allowing their individual optimization. The practical result of this implementation has been a significant increase in the dynamic range of contrast that can be captured in the mammographic image, potentially offsetting the effect of increasing breast density on the sensitivity of the examination. In digital mammography, the image is obtained in the same manner as in SFM, using a compression plate and an X-ray tube, with the screen-film cassette replaced by a digital detector.

BASIC PHYSICS OF DIGITAL MAMMOGRAPHY

Detectors

The first part of the digital imaging chain is the acquisition unit. From a technical point of view, the efficient use of the X-ray beam and the resultant quality of the image is dictated by the materials of the system and the method by which the X-ray beam information is recorded. There are several types of technology deployed in digital detectors.[4] Detectors are classified as either direct or indirect capture. In indirect capture, the energy from the X-ray beam is converted by an X-ray scintillator first into light and then into a digital signal. This is similar to how the image is produced with SFM. Charge couple devices (CCDs), photostimulable phosphors and amorphous silicon are types of indirect digital detectors currently in use. Direct capture units do not have this light conversion step; instead the substrate used is a photoconductive material that is able to directly convert the X-ray photons into an electrical charge. Amorphous selenium detectors are direct capture as are crystal silicon detectors that use photon counting technology. An ideal material for a mammography detector is selenium since it has high X-ray absorption efficiency, extremely high intrinsic resolution, low noise and a well-established manufacturing process.[5] With every alteration of the X-ray beam, noise is introduced into the images and information is lost; in theory then, direct capture units have the advantage of potentially using more of the primary beam than indirect systems.

Another approach to digital mammography is the computed radiography (CR) approach, which uses a photo-stimulable phosphor plate. The plate is used to absorb X-rays just as a screen-film cassette. However, rather than emitting light immediately after exposure through fluorescence, X-ray absorption prompts the electrons within the phosphor material to a higher energy level within the crystal. The image is then read out by placing the screen in a separate reader and scanned with a laser beam, electrons are released and higher-energy (blue) light is emitted in proportion to the X-ray exposure. The amount of blue light emitted is measured by an optical collecting system (photomultiplier tube). Currently, new detectors have size of 50 µm and read out from both sides. The major advantages of this technology are small detector-element size, ease of having multiple plate sizes and relatively low cost. Problems with this system include inefficient light collection and scatter of laser light in the phosphor material resulting in loss of spatial resolution and increased noise.

Spatial Resolution

All systems capture the exposure onto a digital matrix that is comprised of a grid of detector elements, or dels. The spatial resolution of a system is determined in large part by the size and spacing of the dels (dels are also called pixels and the distance between the center of 2 adjacent dels is called pixel pitch). The smallest structure that can be resolved by the detector turns out to be one that is twice the size of a del. This is called the Nyquist frequency of the detector.[6] So for a detector with a 70 µm pixel pitch, the smallest resolvable structure is 140 µm. In SFM, spatial resolution is defined by how many line pairs could be resolved per millimeter of film. Now, we must translate our understanding of spatial resolution to pixel pitch and dels. It so happens that half of the pixel pitch in millimeters is equal to the line pair resolution. So, for the same 70 µm detector, the line pair resolution would be 0.5×7 mm = 3.5 line pairs/mm. For comparison, screen-film systems have a requirement to have a minimum of 11 or 13 line pairs/mm depending on the orientation of the X-ray tube.

Pixel pitch is only part of the determination of spatial resolution as it is also dependent on the focal spot size, the spread of the signal in the detector and motion. Each of these variables is evaluated by its modulation transfer function (MTF). The MTF is the percentage of the signal strength entering the system relative to the signal coming out of the system, at varying frequencies and is a good measure of spatial resolution. In essence, the MTF simply describes how precisely any shape is transmitted through the system. Another way to think of MTF is that it describes how much of the original contrast is lost in the system for each exposure. Most systems have a nearly perfect MTF (of 1) for large shapes and a lower MTF as shapes become more fine. The MTF gives some but not all of the indication of system efficiency. The other important parameter is the detective quantum efficiency (DQE), which takes into account not only the spatial resolution (and thus considers pixel pitch and MTF) of a system but also the signal-to-noise ratio (SNR).[7] The DQE basically describes what percentage of the beam (or signal) produces an image versus how much is lost as noise in the system. Digital systems have higher DQEs than screen-film units and so direct-conversion systems offer the possibility of similar image quality at lower doses or improved image quality at the same dose as screen film.

Analog to Digital Units

Once the energy from the beam is captured in the detector, the signal is converted into an image. All detectors have a matrix into which the signal from the acquisition is stored. The matrix is divided into rows and columns of pixels (dels). As the X-ray energy is collected in the pixels, the information is stored as analog to digital units (ADUs). Essentially, each time an electron reaches a pixel, it is counted as an ADU. Therefore, the denser the patient tissue overlying anyone pixel, the lower the ADU count of that pixel. For each exposure, an ADU map is created on the matrix. This ADU map is converted into a gray scale image. The size of each pixel and the size of the matrix vary between equipment. As mentioned earlier, pixel pitch describes the distance from the center of one pixel to the center of the adjacent pixels. Currently available systems have pixel pitches of 50, 70 or 100 µm. Although there are detectable differences in the clinical images from these different pixel pitches, no study to date has definitively shown anyone of all the available units to be better for cancer detection than another.

Most systems have an automatic exposure control (AEC) that determines the optimal imaging parameters, such as kilovolt peak (kVp) and milliamps (mA). Unlike screen-film mammography where the AEC is used primarily to control image brightness, the AEC in digital mammography is used mainly to ensure that the radiation exposure is optimized for appropriate SNR.[8] This feature works by having a very low-dose fast test exposure given to the patient before the diagnostic exposure which generates a test ADU map that allows the system to evaluate one or more areas for determination of the correct exposure. The AEC uses this information along with the compressed breast thickness to determine the correct exposure parameters.

Processing Algorithms

To convert the digital signals captured during an exposure into a readable mammographic view, multiple types of processing algorithms are applied. The first category of processing is detector correction algorithms designed to remove any inhomogeneity's in the detector that may be perceived on the final image. Two examples are masking of dead pixels and flat-field calibration.

The second type of processing is used to generate a diagnostic image. These include thickness equalization (also called peripheral equalization) and contrast enhancement algorithms. Thickness equalization refers to a process whereby the areas of breast tissue containing high ADU counts, such as the subcutaneous fat and retroglandular fatty areas, are enhanced so that they can be easily seen at display. Contrast enhancement algorithms bring out the differences in ADU counts between adjacent pixels or groups of pixels by making those differences larger. This processing enhances calcifications and fine details like the spicules of a cancer and are meant to aid visibility because of the lower MTF of the systems for these high-frequency structures.

Dynamic Range

The bit depth of a system describes how many shades of gray are available for viewing. Most digital systems collect 12–14 bits of data, but through processing and transfer some of this information is lost and so at display, only 8–10 bits of data are available to the radiologist. This is the dynamic range of the image.

Comparison between Digital Mammograms and Film/Screen Mammograms

Screen-film cassettes used for mammography have a line-pair resolution of 18–21 lp/mm. Full-field digital mammography (FFDM) systems have spatial resolutions ranging from 5 to 10 lp/mm. In digital mammography systems, it is the size of the pixels that determines the spatial resolution. The pixel size for FFDM systems ranges between 50 and 100 microns. Reduction in the pixel size of any digital imaging system results in a rapid increase in the amount of data contained in the image, which increases system costs in terms of data storage, network bandwidth and display capabilities.[9]

The lower spatial resolution of FFDM systems compared to SFM is offset by the increased contrast resolution of FFDM systems. The contrast resolution of a system is described in terms of dynamic range. The limited dynamic range of screen film prevents visualization with equal clarity of all breast tissue regions from the chest wall to the skin line. As the digital system has greater dynamic range, it can record and differentiate subtle variations in contrast, that are not differentiated by screen film.

Unlike SFM, in which the image cannot be manipulated after exposure and processing, FFDM images can be optimized after image capture by image postprocessing and adjustment of image display. The window width and window level for all digital images viewed with soft copy display on review workstations can be adjusted, changing the contrast and brightness of the images, respectively, as well as digitally magnifying images.

Another important difference between SFM and FFDM is that screen-film images have a linear relationship between the logarithm of X-ray exposure and film optical density only in the central portion of the characteristic curve. In FFDM systems, there is a linear relationship between X-ray exposure and signal over the entire dynamic range of the detector. Thus, digital images do not suffer contrast loss in underexposed or overexposed areas of the mammogram and instead show similar contrast over the full dynamic range of the detector **(Fig. 1)**. Digital mammography also eliminates the variability and noise added by film processing.

In terms of breast dose, FFDM has a mean glandular dose lower than, or comparable to, the radiation dose of SFM. The average single-view mean glandular dose for FFDM is 1.86 mGy, 22% lower than the average SFM mean glandular dose of 2.37 mGy.[10]

A number of studies have evaluated the performance of digital mammography compared to SFM for screening

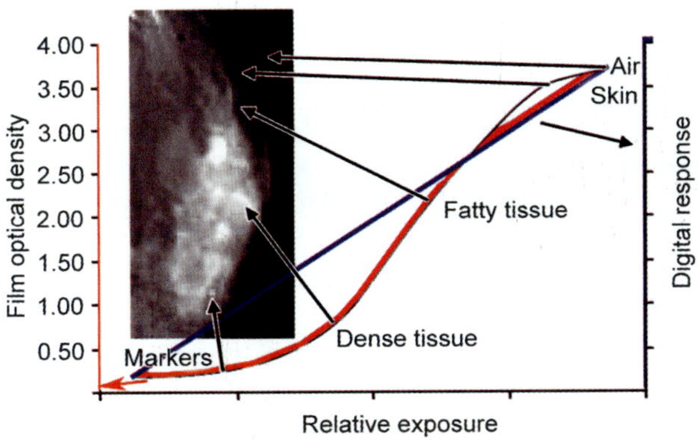

Fig. 1: Typical response curves for screen-film mammography (SFM) and digital mammography. Screen-film images have a linear relationship between the logarithm of X-ray exposure and film optical density only in the central portion of the characteristic curve. In FFDM systems, there is a linear relationship between X-ray exposure and signal over the entire dynamic range of the detector leading to visualization with equal clarity of all breast tissue regions from the chest wall to the skin line.

asymptomatic women for breast cancer. Early studies showed comparable or slightly worse results for FFDM compared to SFM.[11,12] Larger studies however, showed some benefits of FFDM compared to SFM. The American College of Radiology (ACR) Imaging Network Digital Mammographic Imaging Screening Trial (ACRINDMIST), which included nearly 50,000 women, showed no difference overall but found that FFDM was a better screening tool than SFM for women under age 50, for premenopausal and perimenopausal women and for women with denser breast tissue (BIRADS density categories 3 and 4).[13]

Storage of Digital Images

The FFDM systems present certain technical challenges related to the image size and the storage and archiving of digital images by computer systems. A digital image is a two-dimensional grid of picture elements (pixels), which is defined by its size and bit depth. The size of an image is calculated by multiplying its length in pixels to its width in pixels and the bit depth can be identified as the number of shades of gray that can be displayed. The demand for high spatial resolution in mammography requires higher digitization and smaller pixel size. Therefore, FFDM image size is dependent on the digital detector size, the number of pixels per image and the type of digitization. If the detected digital signals are digitized to 12 bits, it implies 212 or 4,096 signal values stored per pixel and 14-bit digitization yields 214 or 16,384 signal values stored per pixel. Whether the system provides 12- or 14-bit digitization, a digital detector of N pixels requires storage of 2N bytes. Generally, a typical screening mammography examination (two craniocaudal and two mediolateral oblique images) requires anywhere from 33 to more than 200 MB of computer storage space.

Display of Digital Images

Currently, various approaches are available for display of digital images. In the absence of soft-copy reading, digital images were printed on dry laser printers and read on high-luminance view boxes, similar to SFM images. This approach doesn't let the user benefit from the full range of advantages available on digital displays. Soft-copy display on high-resolution (5-megapixel) computer monitors allows easy manipulations of resolution, contrast and gray scale **(Fig. 2)**. Workstations need to be fast as mammography screening and diagnosis requires efficiency (i.e. ability to review old studies, magnification of areas of concern and comparison of both breasts and different views).

The workstation should be entirely compatible with PACS. Integrated multimodality workstation should be linked to the general archival system, so that different imaging modalities can be correlated to arrive at final diagnosis.

Artifacts

Artifacts in digital mammography can arise from a detector failure, a processing failure, corrupted calibration files, extraneous objects in-between the X-ray target and detector, or a failure of the components, such as the grid or the plate transporter in a CR unit. Aside from dust and debris on the surface of the detector or paddles, detector artifacts are the most commonly seen artifacts and include ghosting, dead pixels and flat-field inhomogeneities. Ghosting is the result of latent charge remaining in the detector from previous exposures and is specific to one of the weaknesses of using amorphous selenium direct detectors and photostimulable phosphor plates in CR imaging. Both substrates retain charge and need to be cleared. For the phosphor plates, the charge can generally be cleared by putting the plate through the cassette reader, which uses laser technology to clear it. For amorphous selenium, a flat field can be done and the detector recalibrated to overcome the ghosting or, in some instances, the detector must be replaced.

All digital detectors can have dead pixels. A few are of no clinical concern and they appear as bright white dots on the image. A row of dead pixels is seen as a straight thin white

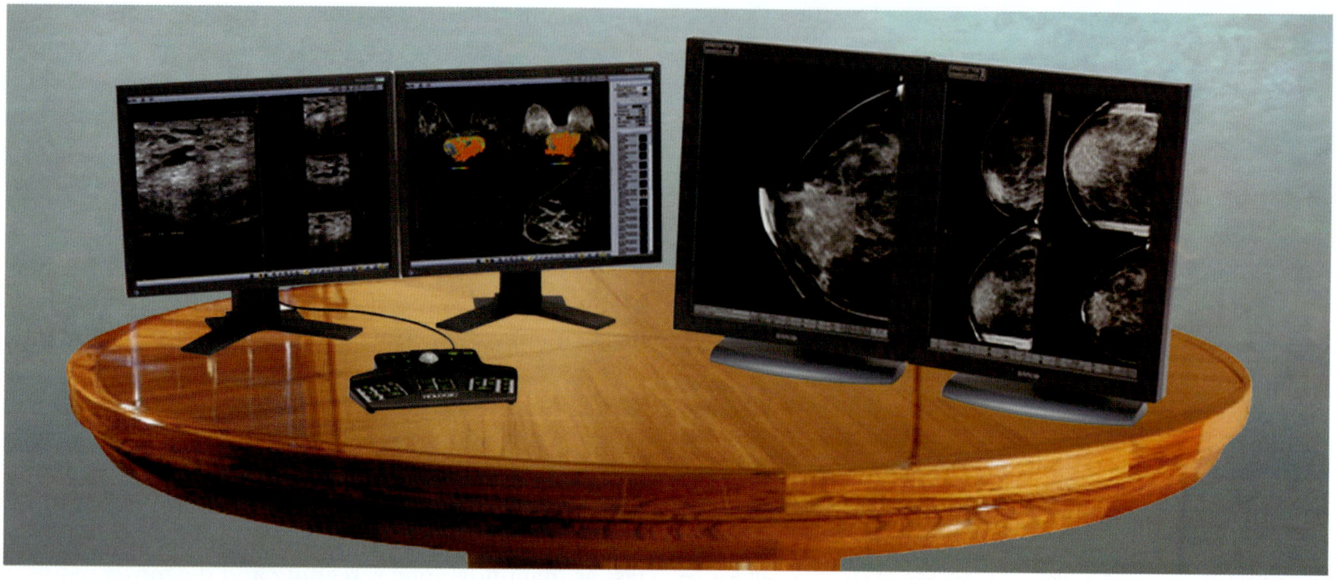

Fig. 2: Soft-copy display on high-resolution (5-megapixel) computer monitors allows easy manipulations of resolution, contrast and gray scale.

line. Many detectors are constructed as groups of arrays with associated amplifiers that are smaller than the matrix. These arrays are placed in the detector housing to create the matrix. Occasionally, 1 array may appear different than the adjacent ones and this background inhomogeneity can be visible to the radiologist.[14] If an exposure is done at high dose or a display has little dynamic range, these arrays are visible in the background of the image. A flat-field image using an acrylic slab will identify these and a flat-field recalibration will generally correct it.

Processing algorithms occasionally fail and this can create artifacts. Typically, these are seen as dark straight lines in the images. Occasionally, when the quality control technologist performs the unit calibration, the collimator is not properly aligned and this will produce either a dark or white vertical band at the chest wall side of the image. To eliminate this artifact, the system must have a flat-field recalibration after the collimator position is corrected.

Because mammography evaluates calcifications of 300 μm on average, detectors are built to have a maximal spatial resolution higher than that and the resultant mammographic images are large. For example, if a detector has a pixel pitch of 50 μm, the matrix can contain more than 20 million pixels. Mammography display monitors typically have only 5 million pixels and so the mammogram at full resolution will not fit in the field of view for display in most cases. As a result, the workstation has the requirement of intelligently displaying the mammograms with different sampling of the data so that the radiologist can perform the tasks of comparison to prior images and close inspection of the current study. Most workstations have the ability to create hanging or display protocols to accomplish this. There are only a few display modes used for all protocols and they are called fit to viewport, same size, true size, view actual pixels and magnification. The radiologist chooses the order of these modes when building a protocol.

Fit to viewport is the mode whereby adjacent pixels' ADUs are averaged together and displayed as 1 ADU to fit the image onto a portion of the monitor. Same size is a variation of fit to viewport whereby the workstation takes into account the different matrices from different manufacturers or different paddles (i.e. 100 μm vs 70 μm or small detector vs large detector from the same vendor) and scales all the images to look the same size to the radiologist. This allows for much more efficient evaluation of change over time. These modes are used for comparison of current and prior studies and comparison of right and left images. The workstation should readily display the functional pixel pitch of display and what percentage that resolution is compared with both true size and view actual pixels. True size is the mode that displays the true physical size of the breast and is useful when planning for surgery or stereotactic biopsy or when printing hard copy for comparison with screen-film mammography. The mode view actual pixels displays each acquired pixel on one display pixel. This is the mode that gives full-resolution images and is best for evaluation of calcifications and subtle mass margins. The mammogram is almost always bigger than the monitor in this mode so either manual panning of the image or some predetermined stepwise display of the image is needed to see the entire breast. Zooming the image with optical magnification at the workstation can be done but this is a mathematical up interpolation of data and does not provide more information to the image; it is just making the image larger for ease of viewing and at the same time introduces some noise to the image. Air gap magnification (using a magnification stand exactly like the technique used for SFM) allows a small portion of the breast to be sampled by the detector increasing spatial resolution, because more pixels in the detector are used to sample a smaller area of the breast. For this reason, magnification has been shown to be beneficial for evaluating calcifications with digital mammography and should still be used.[15]

APPLICATIONS OF DIGITAL MAMMOGRAPHY

The development of digital breast imaging does not constitute an end point but rather represents the beginning of a new era for mammography: an era in which the digital platform serves as the basis for development of innovative radiographic methods of imaging the breast, innovations that were not possible on the analog platform.

Computer-aided Detection and Diagnosis

Computer-aided detection (CADe) and computer-aided diagnosis (CADx) are computer software systems that are designed to review mammograms for bright clustered specks and converging lines, which represent microcalcifications and spiculated masses, respectively. These programs were developed to help radiologists search for signs of cancer against the complex background of dense breast tissue. The CAD marks potential abnormalities directly on the image displayed on the workstation **(Fig. 3)**. The radiologist interprets and analyzes the marked findings and each finding is dismissed as insignificant or further worked up. It thus decreases the chances of overlooking these abnormalities.[16] It acts as second opinion to the experienced radiologists and may help inexperienced radiologists.[17] The CADe refers to those algorithms that simply mark areas to be reviewed without providing any information regarding likelihood of malignancy. The CADx algorithms go a bit further and actually convey some additional information through variable sizing of marks and lesion metrics, such as likelihood of malignancy of similar lesions that were used to train the system. These marking methods are meant to be adjunctive to the radiologist's interpretation and not

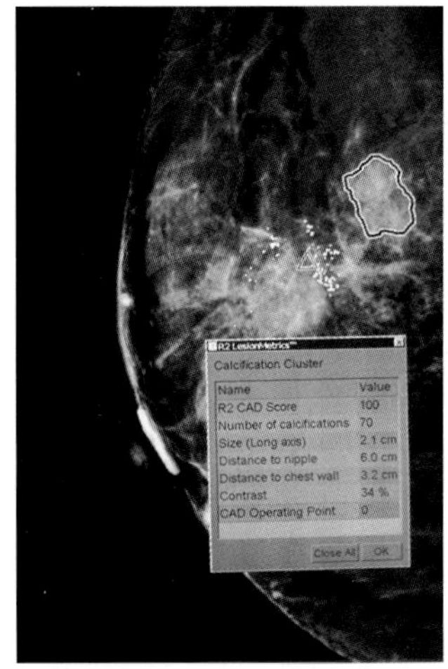

Fig. 3: Computer-aided detection marks potential abnormalities directly on the image displayed on the workstation.

intended to cause the radiologist to dismiss any lesion that was seen without the aid of the CAD marks.

Dual-energy Subtraction Mammography

The basic principle of dual-energy subtraction mammography is that if exposures are taken with both high- and low- operating potentials, using the same radiographic projection, some breast structures will exhibit greater absorption of low-energy compared with high-energy photons. Thus, assuming that there is no patient motion between exposures, one digital image can be electronically subtracted from the other causing most structures (those that do not exhibit differential absorption) to cancel out completely.[18] It takes advantage of the fact that the change in attenuation is greater for calcifications than for soft tissues when the kVp is altered from high energies to low energies. Dual energy mammography requires a modified mammographic machine that is capable of producing normal mammographic images and images obtained at higher energy (45–50 kV).

Contrast-enhanced Digital Mammography

The advantage of contrast-enhanced digital mammography is to obtain the functional contrast information attributed to the malignant neovascularity directly linked to anatomic information of high quality.[19] A precontrast image is obtained and then images are obtained following the intravenous administration of the contrast agent. By subtracting the two, only the contrast image remains, making the cancer more evident because of its nest of neovascularity.[19] Two main methods have been described for contrast-enhanced digital mammography;

serial examinations over time and dual energy imaging. Use of iodinated contrast material and modified digital mammography units are required for the technique. Before contrast injection, a noncontrast image is obtained. Next, series of images are taken after injecting the contrast. The enhanced images are subtracted from the baseline image leaving areas of enhancement visible with simultaneous construction of enhancement curves. The major problem with this study is the ability to image the breast in a single projection at a time. Therefore, dual energy methods have been developed to facilitate imaging of both breasts with a single contrast administration. After injecting the contrast, the patient is subjected to two pair of exposures, one at low kilovolts and other at high kilovolts. A subtraction image is produced that highlights areas of iodine concentration or enhancement. The mammographic image at low energy can be used as a routine gray scale mammographic interpretation. This technique does not allow for kinetic assessment of enhancement curves.

Digital Breast Tomosynthesis

Digital breast tomosynthesis has been developed to improve detection and characterization of breast lesions especially in women with dense breasts. In this technique, multiple projection images are reconstructed allowing visual review of thin breast sections offering the potential to unmask cancers obscured by normal tissue located below and above the lesion.

Technique

Conventional digital mammography exposes a compressed breast to ionizing radiation. The X-ray tube, the breast and the detector remain stationary. The image thus produced is a two-dimensional representation of three-dimensional space. In DBT, the X-ray tube is moved through a limited arc angle while the breast is compressed and a series of exposures are obtained **(Fig. 4)**. If there is a 45° arc of movement and an exposure is taken every 3°, there are 15 individual exposures. These projection image datasets are reconstructed through specific algorithms. The radiologist is presented with a series of slices (typically 1 mm thickness) through the entire breast that are read at a workstation similar to review of a computed tomography or magnetic resonance imaging study.

Several manufacturers have applied different methods to develop and perform tomosynthesis. Engineering constraints include total radiation dose, image time, patient motion, detector performance, detector motion and ability to image the entire breast. Manufacturers vary the arc of movement (typically 11–60°), the number of individual exposures, use of continuous or pulsed exposure, stability or movement of the detector, exposure parameters, total dose, effective size of pixels, X-ray source/filter source, single or binned pixels and patient position. The dataset can be reconstructed for the radiologist to read by displaying different thicknesses. For example, if a 60 cm compressed breast is reconstructed at 1 mm thickness, it will present 60 slices to be reviewed for the physician. If the images are reconstructed at 0.5 mm thicknesses, there will be 120 images to be reviewed. If the images are reconstructed at 10 mm thick slabs using maximum intensity projection (MIP) thick slices, there will be 6 images to review.

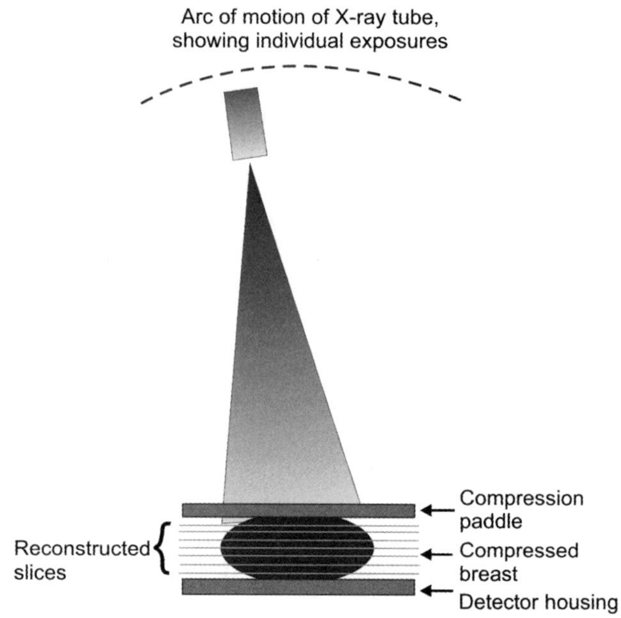

Fig. 4: Digital breast tomosynthesis: The X-ray tube moves through a narrow arch while the breast is in compression. A series of exposures results in multiple projection image datasets. Each exposure is a fraction of the dose of a conventional mammographic view. Projection image datasets are reconstructed into multiple thin-slice images (e.g. 1 mm thickness) for interpretation by the radiologist.

Radiation Dose

Digital breast tomosynthesis manufacturers and regulators impart a major consideration to the balance between dose and image quality. Since image quality has a tendency of being directly related to dose, compromises become necessary. All manufacturers have produced equipment with dosing parameters less than the current FDA limit of 300 mrad per exposure. The common conventional mammographic dose per view is 150–250 mrad.

Potential Benefits of Clinical Breast Imaging with Tomosynthesis

The potential benefits of DBT include improvement in screening sensitivity, improvement in lesion size at detection, improvement in characterization and decrease in recall rates. The DBT may be useful in both the screening and diagnostic evaluation. Neither has been proved in randomized controlled trials. In theory DBT, with thin section display, should allow superior detection of lesions that historically have been masked by overlying tissue **(Figs. 5A and B)**. The primary benefit of DBT is expected to be for noncalcified mammographic findings, such as masses, asymmetries and distortion.

Although many consider tomosynthesis to be a technique used for dense breast tissue, it may also have significant applications for those patients with nondense breasts by allowing detection of smaller lesions. The DBT also offers the possibility that characterization or specificity may be increased by better assessment of detected lesions and reduction in false-positive recalls. This is because the margin of a mass or character of an asymmetry may be better visualized. Malignant lesions may appear more malignant and benign lesions more benign. If these concepts are borne out, DBT may allow for improved sensitivity coupled with improved specificity. Diagnostic evaluation of potential masses and asymmetries found by screening mammography could also be a DBT function.

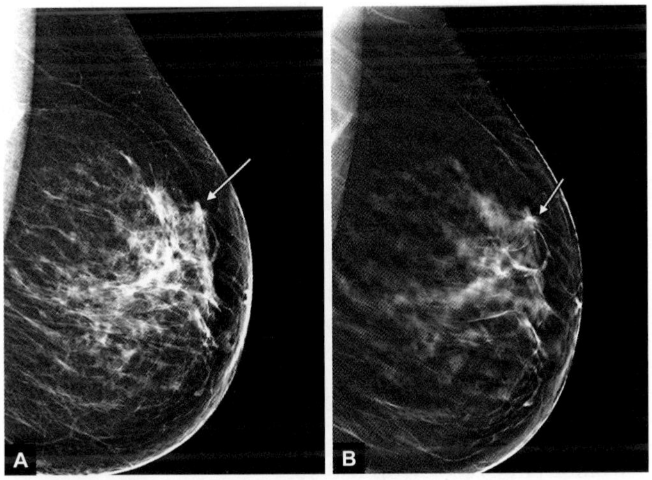

Figs. 5A and B: Conventional film screen MLO mammography view (A) of a patient with invasive ductal cancer. The cancer, although vaguely apparent on the conventional mammogram (arrow), is much better visualized on the 1 mm thick tomosynthesis image (B) (arrow). Note the clarity of the spicules and the separation from surrounding tissue.

Clinical Tomosynthesis Evaluations

Several early experimental clinical DBT studies for masses have generally shown good patient acceptance, physician preference for DBT images, improvement in sensitivity, improvement in characterization and often longer physician reading times.[20-22]

The literature is limited as regards the clinical microcalcification assessment by DBT for detection and characterization. While the in-plane resolution of DBT is good, out-of-plane resolution is poor. Because calcifications may be dispersed in three-dimensional space, viewing thin DBT images may make perception of calcification clusters difficult as only 1 or 2 may be visible on a slice. To overcome this issue, manufacturers have developed MIP images consisting of thick slices, such as 1–2 cm for reviewing calcifications.

Teleradiology Applications

Telemammography can become very effective with digital mammography, since it allows better access for the underserved and geographically remote populations to the latest in breast care. Electronic transfer of digital images to remote viewing sites can be accomplished almost as rapidly as between the display workstation and computer storage. Radiologists who work in several different hospitals can monitor and interpret examinations that are carried out in nearby, or distant locations. Mammography screening in mobile units can be improved, not only by eliminating the need to transport films from the site of examination to the site of interpretation, but also by permitting interpretation while patients are still available for repeat or additional examination. In addition, teleradiology can also be used to facilitate second opinion interpretation by providing rapid transfer of images to the second reader's display monitors.

Stereotactic Breast Biopsy

A full-field digital mammography detector can also be used for diagnostic and stereotactic-breast-biopsy imaging. This enables a multipurpose system ideal for both screening and follow-up imaging tasks.

Stereo Mammography

Acquisition of binary images, separated by a few degrees, allows the display of mammograms in a stereo fashion, to facilitate the visualization of the three-dimensional characteristics of mammographic features.[23] Computer display of stereo images requires either glass synchronized to display frame updates, or polarizing glasses. This technique has shown promise in improving three-dimensional depth discrimination in mammograms.

CONCLUSION

Full-field digital mammography offers the potential for significant advances in breast cancer diagnosis, including lower radiation dose with improved cancer detection rates. Transition from conventional film screen mammogram to digital mammogram is quite expensive but is compensated by numerous benefits. Radiologists face unique challenges when transitioning to digital mammography. The advanced applications and future developments available with digital mammography hold great promise for the improved early diagnosis and screening of breast cancer.

REFERENCES

1. Mandelson MT, Oestreicher N, Porter P. Breast density as a predictor of mammographic detection: comparison of interval- and screen-detected cancers. J Natl Cancer Inst. 2000;92:1081-7.
2. Pisano ED, Gatsonis C, Hendrik E. Diagnostic performance of digital versus film mammography for breast-cancer screening. N Engl J Med. 2005;353:1773-83.
3. Vinnicombe S, Pereira SP, McCormack VA, et al. Full-field digital versus screen-film mammography: comparison within the UK breast screening program and systematic review of published data. Radiology. 2009;251:347-58.
4. D'Orsi CJ, Newell MS. Digital mammography: clinical implementation and clinical trials. Semin Roentgenol. 2007;42:236-42.
5. Pisano ED, Yaffe YJ. Digital mammography. Radiology. 2005; 234:353-62.
6. Noel A, Thibault F. Digital detectors for mammography: the technical challenges. Eur Radiol. 2004;14:1990-8.
7. Samei E, Ranger NT, Mackenzie A, et al. Detector of system? Extending the concept of detective quantum efficiency to characterize the performance of digital radiographic imaging systems. Radiology. 2008;249:926-37.
8. Pisano ED, Yaffe MJ. Digital mammogarphy. Radiology. 2005;234:353-62.
9. Rowlands JA, Zhao W, Blevis IM, et al. Flat-panel digital radiology with amorphous selenium and active-matrix readout. Radiographics. 1997;17:753-60.
10. Hendrick RE, Pisano ED, Averbukh A, Moran C, Berns EA, Yaffe MJ, et al. Comparison of acquisition parameters and breast dose in digital mammography and screen-film mammography in the American College of Radiology Imaging Network Digital Mammographic Imaging Screening Trial. Am J Roentgenol. 2010;194(2):362-9.
11. Lewin JM, Hendrick RE, D'Orsi CJ, et al. Comparison of full-field digital mammography with screen-film mammography for cancer detection: results of 4,945 paired examinations. Radiology. 2001;218:873-80.
12. Skaane P, Young K, Skjennald A. Population-based mammography screening: comparison of screen-film and full-field digital mammography with soft-copy reading-Oslo I study. Radiology. 2003;229:877-84.
13. Pisano ED, Gatsonis C, Hendrick E, Yaffe M, Baum JK, Acharyya S, et al. Digital Mammographic Imaging Screening Trial (DMIST) Investigators Group. Diagnostic performance of digital versus film mammography for breast-cancer screening. N Engl J Med. 2005;353(17):1773-83.
14. Ayyala RS, Chorlton MA, Behrman RH, et al. Digital mammographic artifacts on full-field system: what are they and how do I fix them? Radiographics. 2008;28:1999-2008.
15. Kim MJ, Kim EK, Kwak JY. Characterization of microcalcification: can digital monitor zooming replace magnification mammography in full-field digital mammography? Eur Radiol. 2009;19:310-7.
16. Birdwell RL, Ikeda DM, O'Shaughnessy KF, et al. Mammographic characteristics of 115 missed cancers later detected with screening mammography and the potential utility of computer-aided detection. Radiology. 2001;219:192-202.
17. Karssemeijer N, Otten JD, Verbeek AL, et al. Computer-aided detection versus independent double reading of masses on mammograms. Radiology. 2003;227:192-200.
18. Lewin JM, Isaacs PK, Vance V, Larke FJ. Dual-energy contrast-enhanced digital subtraction mammography: feasibility. Radiology. 2003;229(1):261-8.
19. Jong RA, Yaffe MJ, Skarpathiotakis M, et al. Contrast-enhanced digital mammography: initial clinical experience. Radiology. 2003;228:842-50.
20. Poplack SP, Tosteson TD, Kogel CA, et al. Digital breast tomosynthesis: initial experience in 98 women with abnormal digital screening mammography. Am J Roentgenol. 2007;189: 616-23.
21. Andersson I, Ikeda D, Zackrisson S, et al. Breast tomosynthesis and digital mammography: a comparison of breast cancer visibility and BIRADS classification in a population of cancers with subtle mammographic findings. Eur Radiol. 2008;18:2817-25.
22. Gur D, Abrams GS, Chough DM, et al. Digital breast tomosynthesis: observer performance study. Am J Roentgenol. 2009;193:586-91.
23. Goodsitt MM, Chan HP, Hadjiiski L. Stereomammography: evaluation of depth perception using a virtual 3D cursor. Med Phys. 2000;27(6):1305-10.

CHAPTER 52

Fluoroscopy and Digital Subtraction Angiography

Deep Narayan Srivastava, Kumble S Madhusudhan

OVERVIEW

Fluoroscopy is an imaging technique which uses X-rays for real-time visualization of internal organs or structures of the body. A fluoroscope is used for the same which in its basic form consists of an X-ray source and a fluorescent screen between which patient is positioned. From its initial use in the early 20th century, the fluoroscope has undergone significant technological improvements with current fluoroscopic machines using larger sized flat-panel detector (FPD) with digital processing.[1] Digital subtraction angiography (DSA) is a fluoroscopic technique in which real-time subtraction of precontrast images is done for better visualization of contrast-filled structures.[2] Fluoroscopy is used in various diagnostic and therapeutic procedures, including assessment of dynamic processes, such as swallowing and cardiac function, provision of road map for positioning vascular or nonvascular catheters, evaluation of vessels using contrast in DSA and detection of gastrointestinal abnormalities in barium studies. For safe and efficient use of fluoroscopy, it is essential to have adequate knowledge of these equipments and newer developments. The chapter describes principles of fluoroscopy, early fluoroscopic equipments and newer advances in fluoroscopic imaging along with safety issues.

FLUOROSCOPY

The term fluorescence means emission of light by a substance when it is exposed to electromagnetic radiation. Fluoroscope consists of this substance in the fluorescent screen which is stimulated by X-rays. The fluorescent substance used in the initial days of fluoroscopy was barium platinocyanide which produced very dim images. Also, the substance was unstable. This substance was later replaced by cadmium tungstate and subsequently by zinc cadmium sulfide which though increased image brightness but still needed darkroom.[1] Fluorography means serial acquisition of higher-quality images for diagnosis and documentation.

In its early days, fluoroscopy was performed in a darkroom (darkroom fluoroscopy) as the light emitted by the fluorescent screen was dim. The radiologist had to adapt his/her eyes in the room for some time to enhance visualization. The image emitted by the screen was directly viewed by the examiner **(Figs. 1A and B)**. The

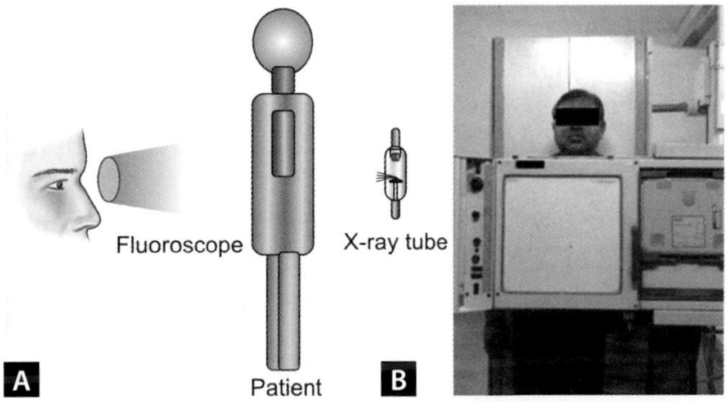

Figs. 1A and B: Darkroom fluoroscopy: (A) Shows early hand-held fluoroscope used in darkroom for direct visualization; (B) Is an improvised darkroom fluoroscope fixed to the table, but movable in all four directions. Here, X-ray tube is under the table.

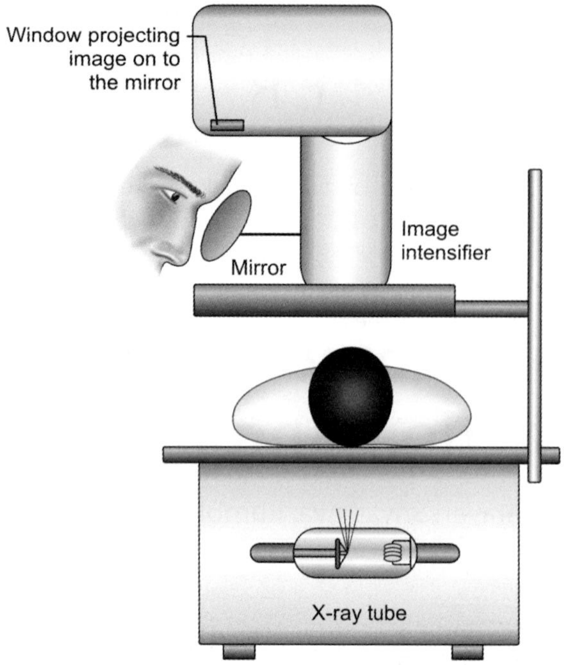

Fig. 2: First fluoroscopy machine with image intensifier. The image formed is intensified and reflected on to the mirror for visualization by the operator.

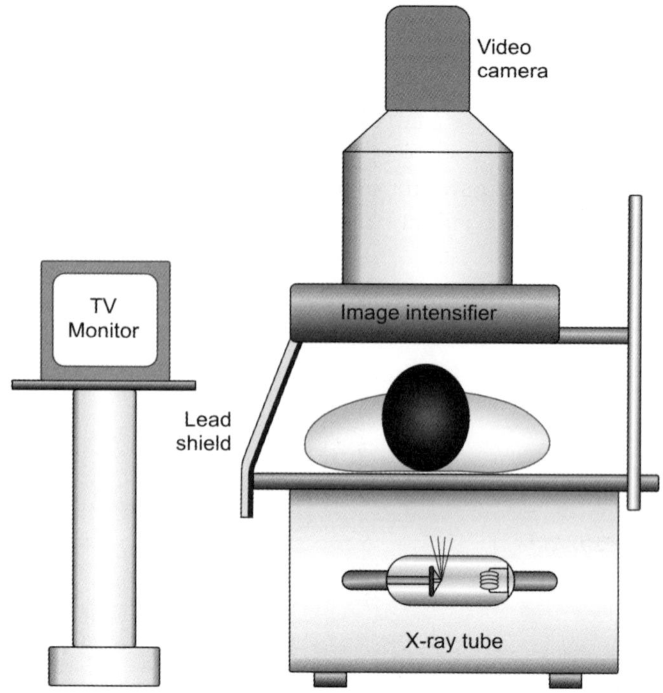

Fig. 3: Image intensifier fluoroscopy system with optical coupling system, video camera and television monitor display.

performance of the technique was mainly affected by the limitations of human eye at low light levels which reduced spatial and contrast resolution of the image viewed. This shortcoming was removed by image intensifier (II) which was introduced in 1953.[3] The II amplified the brightness of the light image for improved visualization. The major problem with the initial II was small viewing angle which needed the radiologist to move his/her position frequently as and when the II moved **(Fig. 2)**. This limitation was overcome with the development of video camera for image viewing and displaying it on monitor **(Fig. 3)**. Today, the II has larger size (40 cm) compared to the older ones (15 cm). With the development of digital technique, there is improvement in the performance of the imaging chain. The latest addition is the introduction of FPD which has replaced the II and video camera.

The main advantage of fluoroscopy over radiography is the use of low tube currents, in the range of 1–6 mA compared to 500–800 mA for routine radiography. Typical exposure rate of fluoroscopy for an average adult is in the range of 10–30 mGy/min (compared to a chest radiograph –0.3 mGy/30 msec or 600 mGy/min). But longer times may increase the risk of radiation injury. Hence, highly sensitive imaging receptors are needed to detect such low photon flux.

Components of Fluoroscopic System

The typical fluoroscopic imaging chain consists of a generator, X-ray tube, collimators and filters, grid, image intensifier and video camera system **(Fig. 4)**. The generator, X-ray tube, collimator and grid are similar to radiography system with few differences which are described here.

The generator used for fluoroscopy is similar to that used for radiography with an additional circuit for fluoroscopic procedure.[4] High-frequency generator with faster switching is preferred due to its best exposure reproducibility (beneficial for DSA).

The X-ray tube has two focal spots: small (0.3–0.6 mm) and large (1.0–1.2 mm). Small focal spot is used for fluoroscopy as it provides sharp images. For radiographic exposure, either of them can be used. The main additional feature in the tube used for fluoroscopy is high heat capacity (about 700 kHU) which is needed for prolonged X-ray exposure.[5] This is achieved by high-speed anode rotation (above 10000 rpm), oil heat exchanger and cooling fans in the housing assembly and grid-controlled exposures. Further, in the modern imaging system, the tube heat loading is constantly monitored which regulates exposure if there is tube overheating. Mobile C-arm systems incorporated with X-ray tubes having fixed anode contain single or dual focal spots (0.5 mm for fluoroscopy and 1.8 mm for radiography) and lower heat capacity (30–50 kHU). Modern C-arms have rotating anode for longer fluoroscopy procedures.

Collimators and filters are used to reduce unwanted radiation. One of the filters which needs special mention here is 'equalization filter'. It is used to reduce glare near the edges of the patient. They are partially radiolucent and made of lead-rubber or lead-acrylic material **(Figs. 5A and B)**. To attenuate low-energy X-rays (beam hardening), copper filters are preferred over aluminum as they are more effective in filtering low-energy X-rays. The grids used in fluoroscopy are of lower ratios (6:1–10:1) compared to that used for radiography (8:1–16:1) to limit increase in radiation dose. Some systems provide grids which can be removed when small part of the body is examined or small FOV is used and when II is positioned at a distance from the patient (for access for intervention or difficult anatomical part) which results in air gap. These modes produce less scatter and grid can be avoided to reduce patient radiation dose.

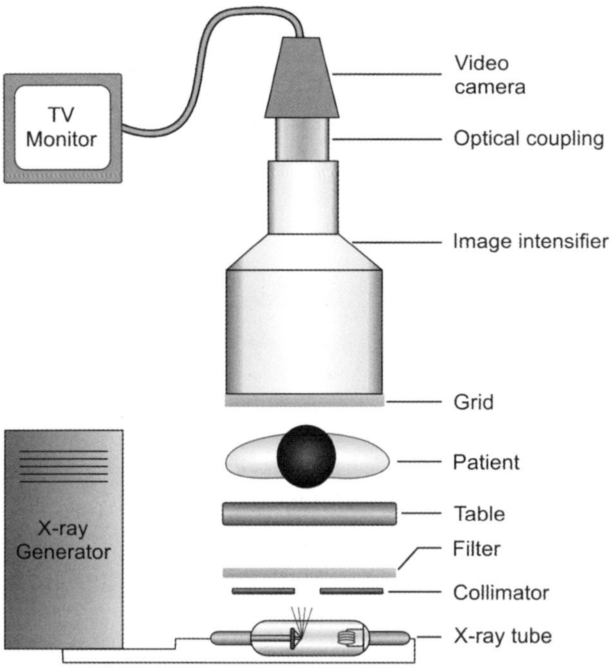

Fig. 4: Components of image intensifier fluoroscopy system.

Conventional continuous fluoroscopy involves continuous production of X-rays at low mA and images are acquired at 30 frames per second (fps). Pulsed fluoroscopy (PF) is a mode of operation in which X-rays are generated in pulses (2.5–30 fps) by two methods—generator controlled and tube controlled **(Fig. 6)**. In conventional generator controlled PF the current is supplied to the X-ray tube in short pulses lasting 3–10 milliseconds. However, due to the presence of long high-resistance cables between the generator and the tube the pulse has a bell shaped curve (slow rise to peak and fall to zero; **Fig. 7**). This increases the low-energy X-rays which results in reduced image quality and no significant decrease in radiation dose, a limitation overcome by grid-controlled PF. In grid-controlled PF, a negative charge is applied between cathode and anode of X-ray tube in a pulsatile manner which regulates incidence of electrons on anode **(Fig. 8)**. It produces uniform pulses without any low-energy photons **(Fig. 7)**. The advantages of pulsed fluoroscopy are improved temporal resolution (which reduces motion blur) and reduced radiation dose. The disadvantages include increase in noise perception,

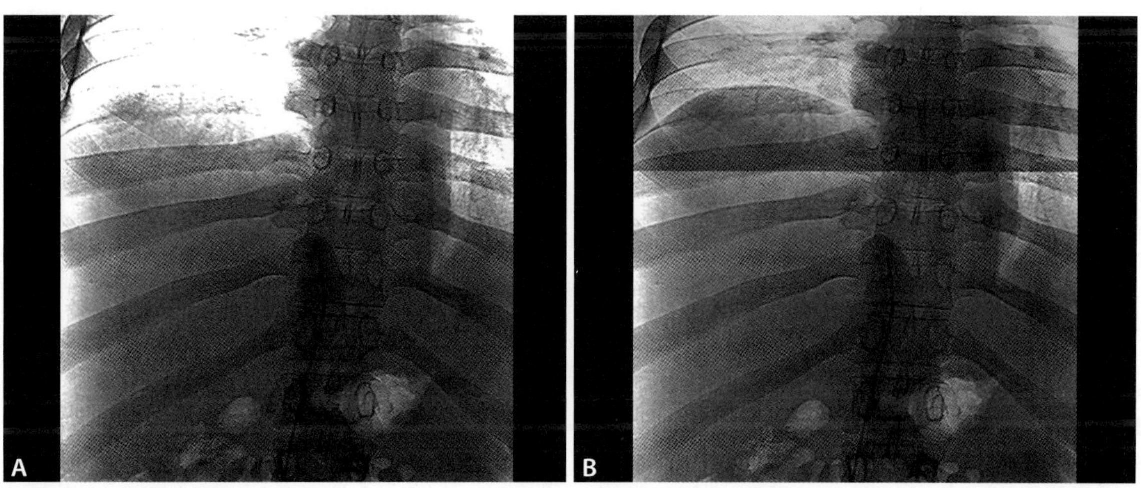

Figs. 5A and B: In a patient with inferior venacavogram, veiling glare is seen in the regions of lower lungs affecting the visualization of diaphragm and subdiaphragmatic regions (A). After placement of equilization filter, the glare is significantly reduced with better visualization of diaphragmatic outline (B).

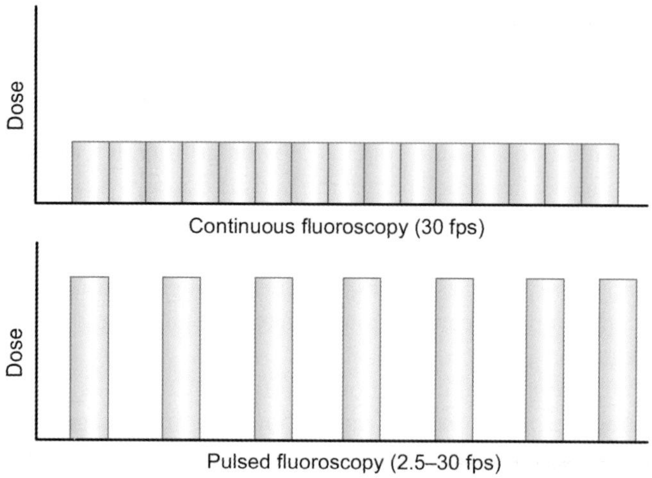

Fig. 6: Schematic diagram comparing continuous and pulsed fluoroscopy. Although there is increase in dose per pulse in the latter to maintain same image details, overall radiation dose is reduced.

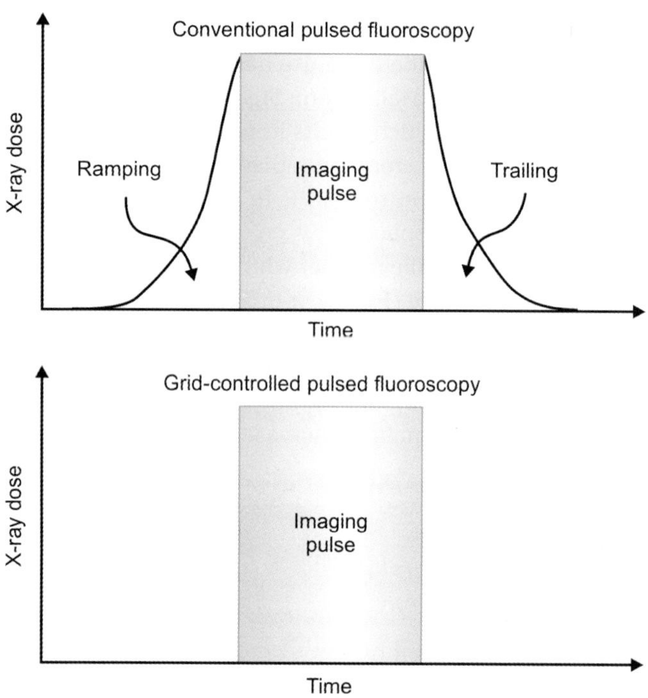

Fig. 7: The pulsing in conventional PF shows initial ramping and terminal trailing leading to generation of low-energy X-rays which increases radiation dose. Grid-controlled PF shows no such effect.

flicker effect and reduced visibility of fine catheters/ guidewires. The flicker effect may be reduced by interleaved image display where gap between two frames are filled by previous images from memory. The reduced radiation dose with pulsed fluoroscopy happens only when mAs remain constant. But often, vendors try to increase the mAs to compensate for increase in noise that occurs with reduced

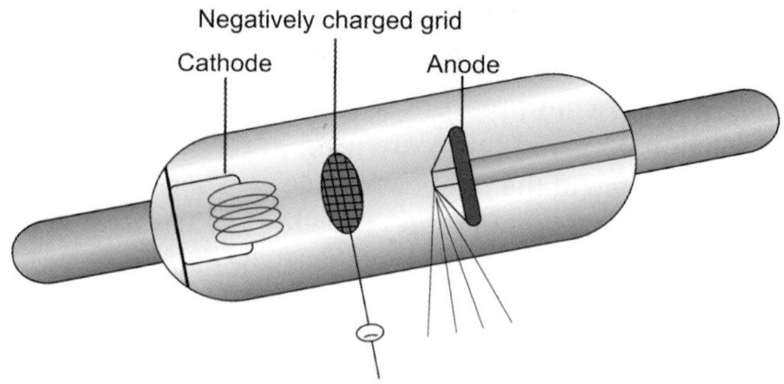

Fig. 8: Grid-controlled X-ray tube shows negatively charged grid between cathode and anode which can be switched on and off to control incidence of electrons on anode.

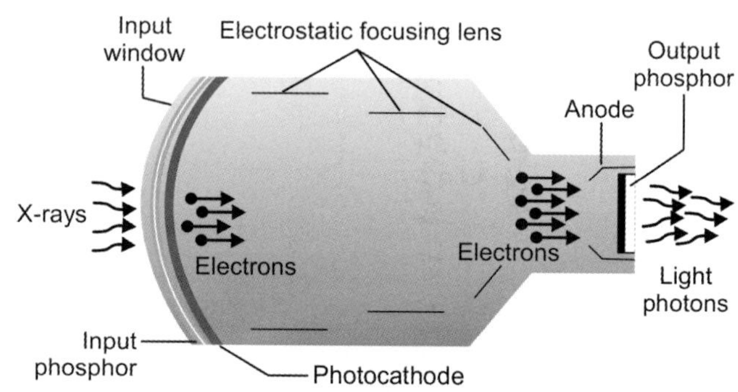

Fig. 9: Schematic diagram of image intensifier.

pulse rate. This may result in only modest decrease in radiation dose.

Image Intensifier

The main purpose of image intensifier is to amplify the brightness of the fluoroscopic image, thus obviating the need of dark adaptation by the radiologist. Two important functions of II are fluorescence (conversion of X-ray photons into visible light) and light signal amplification.[6] The basic elements that make an image intensifier are contained in a vacuum case and include input phosphor, photocathode, focusing lenses, anode and output phosphor **(Fig. 9)**. The vacuum case itself is covered by a protective metallic housing which is made of lead to absorb scatter radiation, mu-metal to protect electrostatic lenses from external magnetic forces and an outer aluminum shell. This aluminum shell also covers and protects the input window of the II.

Input Screen

This consists of input window, supporting layer (of aluminum), input phosphor and photocathode. Input window is a part of the vacuum case of II. It is convex in shape and is made of 1 mm thick aluminum. The convex shape reduces II to patient distance and increases field of view. The support layer for input phosphor and photocathode is thin enough to allow all the X-rays to pass through.

The main function of input phosphor is to convert X-ray photons into light photons. In modern equipments, input phosphor is made of cesium iodide–sodium (CsI:Na) **(Fig. 10)**. The advantages of CsI:Na over the previously used zinc cadmium sulfide (ZnCdS) are as follows:

- Cesium iodide-sodium has a mass attenuation coefficient which better matches with the radiation emitted from the patient than ZnCdS
- It has higher atomic number resulting in higher X-ray absorption
- It can be crystallized in needle form which reduces lateral scatter and improves spatial resolution
- Light emitted by CsI:Na has a range which matches with the sensitivity spectrum of the photocathode.

The thickness of the input phosphor is a trade-off between X-ray absorption efficiency (which increases with thickness) and spatial resolution (which decreases with increased thickness due to increased lateral scatter). The thickness in the presently used II is usually between 300 μ and 500 μ with efficiency of 60–70%.

The photocathode is adjacent to the input phosphor and is made of antimony cesium ($SbCs_3$) measuring about 20mminthickness.Itsproductionefficiencyisabout10–15%. A single X-ray photon of 60 keV incident on the screen is convertedintoabout2600lightphotonsofwhich1600reach photocathode, which converts these into approximately 200–300 photoelectrons.

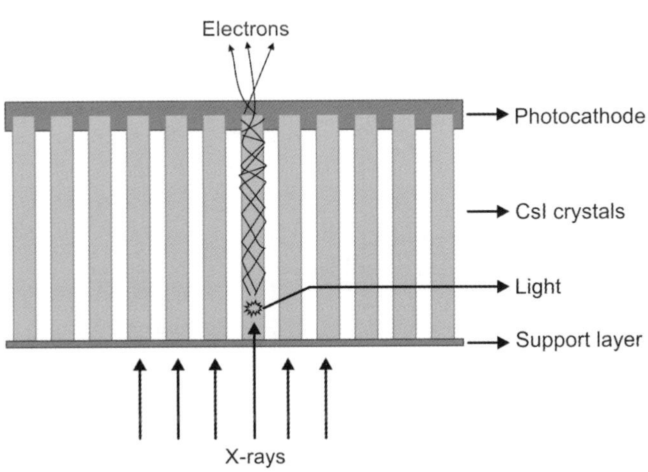

Fig. 10: Schematic diagram of input phosphor of image intensifier showing cesium iodide (CsI) crystals in needle form. This significantly reduces lateral scatter of light photons.

Electrostatic Lens

It consists of 3 sets of focusing electrodes which accelerate the photoelectrons to the anode. The voltage between input and output phosphor is about 25–35 keV. The electrodes increase the velocity and kinetic energy of the photoelectrons incident on output phosphor which increases the number of light photons generated per electron. The electrodes are sensitive to external electric and magnetic fields and are protected by efficient housing assembly.

Output Phosphor and Anode

The output phosphor is a fluorescent compound made of silver activated ZnCdS (ZnCdS:Ag, also called P20). It is in the form of a thin layer (4–8 μ) on the inner aspect of output window of vacuum chamber. About 2,000 photons are produced by the output phosphor for every 25 keV photoelectron. The anode is a thin layer of aluminum on the vacuum side of output phosphor surface.

Properties of Image Intensifier

The performance of an II is determined by various characteristics, including input size, spatial resolution, brightness gain, conversion factor, contrast ratio and magnification mode.[6] Larger input size provides larger viewing field but increases the cost. Larger sized II are useful in gastrointestinal and genitourinary investigations. The spatial resolution of II is about 4–6 line pairs/mm which increases with magnification.

Brightness gain is defined as the ratio of output luminance of II to that of a fluorescent screen when both are exposed to same level of radiation. This measurement is not reproducible. Hence, actual measurement is a function of two factors: minification gain and flux gain. Minification gain is the ratio of input area to output area of II. Flux gain is defined as number of photons generated by the output phosphor for every photon generated by input phosphor. Brightness gain is the product of minification gain and flux gain. It is usually in the range of 5,000–20,000.

Conversion factor is currently used by many manufacturers for evaluating the efficiency of II. It is defined as the ratio of output luminance level (Cd/m^2) of an II to its entrance exposure rate (μGy/sec). The typical values range from 25 to 30 Cd-sec/μGy-m^2. The output of an II reduces over time.

Contrast ratio is the ratio of brightness of the periphery to the center of the output window when the center of the II input window is completely blocked by appropriately thick lead disc. It is the measure of veiling glare. The typical values for modern II range from 10:1 to 30:1.

Magnification is performed by collimating to the region of interest thus reducing the field of view at input screen. This however, reduces minification gain. To compensate for this, there is increase in exposure at the input screen. Thus when magnification is increased, radiation dose to the patient is also increased.

Limitations of Image-intensifier System

Various drawbacks and artifacts of older II have lead to the development of better systems. However, knowledge of these is important to identify them and take adequate measures to their correction wherever possible.

The II system is bulky which results in some difficulty in positioning patients. The system includes a vacuum tube which is associated with risk of air leak. Air leak affects transmission of electrons and thus image quality. The dynamic range of II is lower compared to FPD. Magnification reduces FOV and thus increases radiation dose to maintain brightness.

Defocusing is an effect which occurs when electrons do not pass through in proper plane leading to image blurring. It results from alterations in voltage of electrostatic plates which occurs in older systems or by external magnetic field. This drawback also leads to *S distortion*, where effect of the external magnetic field is more on the outer beam of electrons than the central beam. Mu metal protects the plates from external effects, although not completely.

Lag is the delay that occurs after formation of an image by II before it is ready to transmit next image. This reduces the temporal resolution of the system. Older systems had a lag of 30–40 ms, but modern systems have a lag of about 1 ms.

As the input phosphor is convex and the output phosphor is flat, the outer electrons travel a longer path compared to the central ones. This results in two artifacts—vignetting and pin cushion distortion. *Vignetting* refers to increased brightness of the center of an image compared to its periphery due to higher concentration of electrons in the center than periphery. *Pin cushion* distortion refers to magnification and stretching of the periphery of an image.

Veiling glare or flare occurs due to scattering of light and defocusing of electrons within the II **(Fig. 5A)**. Here, areas of low density like lungs or external air partially occupying the FOV result in high electron flux leading to saturation of the phosphor. This results in difficult visualization of adjacent structures. Glare also occurs for a short time period when image intensifier is moved from a dense area to less dense area till automatic exposure control (AEC) adjusts the exposure. This can however, be significantly reduced by use of pulsed fluoroscopy.

Quality control should be done at regular basis to evaluate spatial and contrast resolution and radiation exposure. The resolution and brightness gain of II decrease over time and these need regular monitoring. Further details regarding quality control are described in a different chapter.

Optical Coupling and Video System

The II is optically coupled to a camera which converts light photons from II to voltage signal.[7] This signal is then transmitted to film camera or video camera for viewing. The system consists of an optical distributor and a video system.

Optical Distributor System

The main functions of optical distributor are as follows:

- Transmission of clear focused image from the output phosphor to all the cameras in the system
- Transmission of images of sufficient intensity/brightness to each camera and
- Transmission of brightness information to the AEC circuit of the X-ray generator. The system consists of a series of mirrors, lenses and camera apertures **(Fig. 11)**.

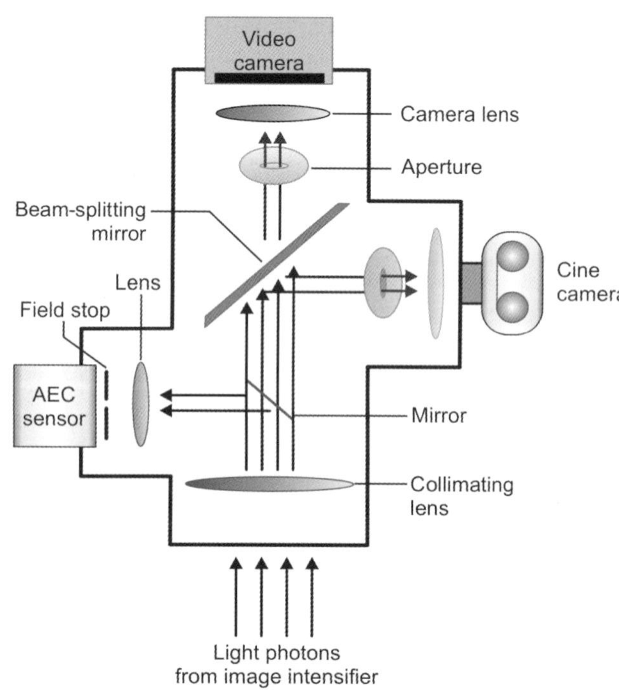

Fig. 11: Optical distributor system with its components.

Beam-splitting mirror is partially silvered and splits the light beam exiting the output phosphor through collimating lens into two, one reaching the film camera for recording and the other to video camera for viewing. There is an additional small mirror or prism between the collimating lens and beam-splitting mirror which transmits part of the light beam to AEC sensor. The AEC sensor uses a field stop between it and its lens to prevent the periphery of the light beam, which is not usually the area of interest, reaching the sensor to determine exposure.

Two types of lenses are present in the optical coupling system. The collimator lens is located at a distance from the output phosphor equal to the focal length of the lens. The light beam exiting the lens is collimated and parallel. Camera lens is present in each of the camera used in the system and is located at a distance equal to its focal length form the camera target.

The light beam reaching the camera lens is controlled by camera aperture or iris. The aperture determines the speed of the system which is a measure of total X-ray exposure needed to produce a proper image on camera. It is designated by f-number. Faster the speed, lesser is the X-ray exposure required. The apertures used can either be fixed or adjustable. Fixed apertures are usually used where detected X-ray exposure level is same across patients as in film cameras. But in video cameras, the X-ray exposure varies from low levels in fluoroscopy to high levels in angiography and thus need an adjustable aperture (motor-driven iris). Sometimes, additional neutral filter may be needed to prevent overexposure at high doses.

Every region in the light beam from the collimating lens contains information from all points of output phosphor. Hence, mirrors and apertures placed between two lenses are not visualized on the image.

Video System

This plays role in image display and recording and also provides input to the digital processor. It includes a camera head which converts light image into voltage signal and a camera control unit which process the voltage signal for display and digitization **(Fig. 12)**.

Two types of devices are used for signal generation, older vacuum tube sensor (pickup tube) and the modern charge-coupled device (CCD) sensor. The pickup tube contains a photoconductor which absorbs the light photons to generate electron-hole pairs within it. The electric field placed across the target causes the holes to move towards the inner surface of the target. The hole density, which is proportional to the light image

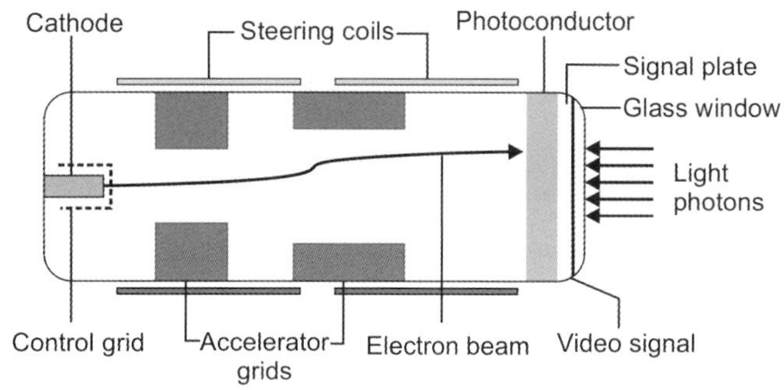

Fig. 12: Video camera pickup tube and its components.

intensity, is measured by focused electron beam and converted into voltage signal constituting the video output of the pickup tube. The photoconductor used include antimony trisulfide (SbS_3; Vidicon), lead oxide (Plumbicon) or a composite of amorphous selenium, arsenic and tellurium (Saticon). Plumbicon has very low lag time with good temporal resolution and hence used in cardiac angiography. Saticon has the advantage of linear response to light intensity. In CCD system, the target (Thallium-doped CsI) generates electron-hole pairs but the electrons accumulate in potential wells depending on the intensity of the light photons incident on it. The charge is then transferred to adjacent storage region where it is readout to generate an image. CCD is better than the pickup tube as it results in better dynamic range (12-bit depth), higher signal to noise ratio (SNR) and contrast resolution thus reduced patient dose. Its linear response is very useful in subtraction imaging. Further it is compact, robust, consumes less electricity, lacks maintenance and is not associated with lag phenomenon and geometric distortion. Currently, CCD cameras are available for both fluoroscopy and angiography systems.

Two operating properties of video system are lag and linearity. *Lag* refers to the time delay in the output of the video system in response to the changes in the input sensor of the video camera. CCD cameras have no lag. In pickup tubes, lag varies with high values seen in those using SbS_3 as target material. Lag is also higher in dark parts of the image than bright parts. Lag results in blurring of moving objects. One advantage of higher lag is significant reduction in image noise, which is high in CCD cameras. *Linearity* indicates relationship between light input and video signal output. A nonlinear response is desirable as smaller signals are better amplified.

The video signal output from the target (pickup tube or CCD) is converted into one-dimensional voltage signal which is displayed on the monitor by raster scanning

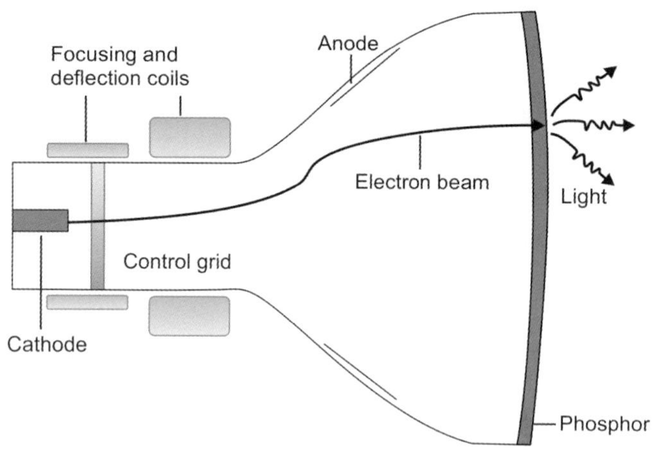

Fig. 13: Television picture tube and its operation.

(Fig. 13). Here, the voltage signal is scanned in a horizontal line from one end to the other, which is terminated by H-sync signal moving the scanning to next line. Once the whole screen is filled by horizontal lines, the V-sync signal shifts the scanning to the top of the image to restart scanning. H-sync and V-sync pulses produce dead time, equal to about 15% of the total horizontal period for the former and 7% of the total vertical period for the latter. The video scanning may be done in continuous manner (line 1, line 2, line 3, etc. in order) or interlaced manner (odd lines first followed by even lines). The standard scanning mode of a conventional video is 30 fps, 525 lines per frame and 2:1 interlaced video. Modern systems employ 60 fps and above and scan conversion for improved visualization. One has to note that this frame rate is different from the frame rate of X-ray generator.

The spatial resolution of fluoroscopic equipment is determined by the size of focal spot, the II, the digital system and the video system. The resolution of video system has two components: vertical resolution and horizontal resolution. Vertical resolution is determined by the number of horizontal lines on the screen and measured in terms of line pairs per mm. It is calculated by taking into account the size of II, magnification and number of lines of horizontal scanning. Older systems employed 525 lines per scan height but modern angiography system use 1049 lines. Horizontal resolution of video system is decided by the bandwidth of the system. A low-pass filter limits the bandwidth preventing too low or too high values thus ensuring that horizontal resolution matches vertical resolution. The bandwidth ranges from 4.5 MHz for 525 line system to 18 MHz for 1049 line system at 30 fps. Currently, many equipments use 1023-line raster line video system with liquid crystal display (LCD) monitor.

Digital Fluoroscopy

The initial fluoroscopic systems used cassettes for documentation of images. This resulted in high film usage, lag time between cassette changes and delay in viewing the spot films. Further, conventional fluoroscopic systems are associated with longer examination times, higher radiation doses, need for repetition of acquisitions due to non-availability of postprocessing, need for multitasking (turning on fluoroscopy, cassette changes, patient positioning) by radiologist and more staff. These problems are surmounted by the development of digital fluoroscopy which is easy to use, provides better image quality by postprocessing, reduced examination time and radiation dose.

The main principle behind digital fluoroscopy is conversion of analog video signal into digital data using an analog-to-digital convertor (ADC).[2] Other methods of digitization are use of CCD cameras and FPD. The fundamental theory of digital imaging included binary numbers, pixels and gray levels. Binary system uses two digits, i.e, 0 and 1, the values of which are determined by the number of digits (bits). A 2-bit number has 2^2 or 4 values (00, 01, 10, 11). A 3-bit number (000 to 111) can have 2^3 or 8 values, 4-bit number (0000 to 1111) 2^4 or 16 values, 8-bit number 2^8 or 256 values and so on. Each pixel in an image has a position, size and value. Pixel size is determined by field of view (FOV) and matrix size. Smaller the pixel size better is the resolution and sharper are the images. This can be done by increasing the matrix and/or reducing the FOV **(Figs. 14A to D)**. Pixel value is the gray level of the

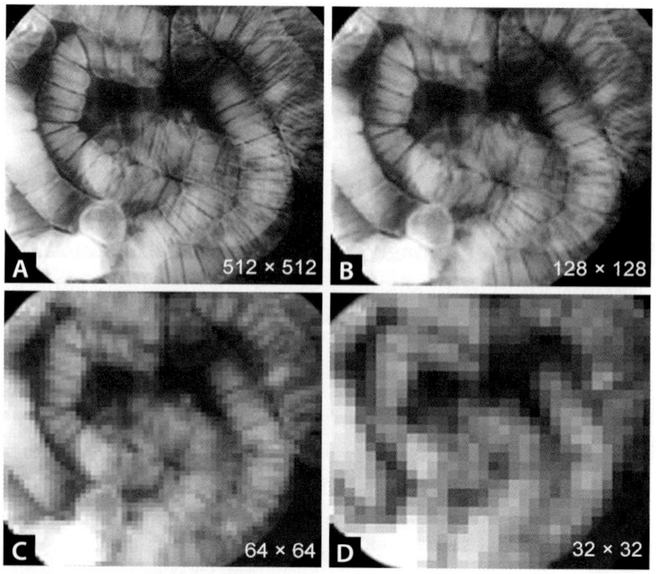

Figs. 14A to D: Spatial resolution of fluoroscopic image at various matrix sizes. Note the decrease in spatial resolution as matrix size is reduced.

image. The range of gray scale in an image depends on the bit depth of the system. Higher the bit depth, better is the contrast resolution **(Figs. 15A to C)**.

The ADC system collects the output signal of the video camera at regular intervals and converts it into binary values (0 and 1) for storage. The range of values depends on the bit depth of the ADC (e.g. an 8-bit ADC displays 2^8 or 256 values) and are expressed as varying gray scale intensity. The resolution of ADC system is determined by the resolution of the video camera which is about 1–2 lp/mm. The digital image thus formed can be stored for subsequent printing on film. Further the images can be processed to improve visualization.

The CCD cameras have substantially reduced the size of the bulky video system. As mentioned in previous section, the CCDs convert light signal from the scintillator into electrical charges which is readout and transmitted to the monitor. The CCDs have a resolution of 1.7 lp/mm. Flat-panel detectors (described later) used in some of the modern fluoroscopy systems do not need a video system.[8] They directly or indirectly convert X-ray photons incident on them into electronic signals which is displayed on the monitor. The electronic signal generated varies with the intensity of incident X-ray photons. With both these systems, ADC digitizes the signal for display and storage.

Postprocessing Techniques

Last image hold (LIH) is an important feature of digital fluoroscopy. The last image/frame of cine fluoroscopy at which imaging stops, is captured and continuously displayed on the monitor even after switching off the fluoroscopy. This image can be transferred to reference monitor and is used for guidance without additional radiation to the patient and medical staff. This is applicable for static objects. For areas which are in motion (e.g. cardiac imaging) *fluoroscopy loop* can be captured and made available for review when needed. Here, the last 150–300 frames or about 10 seconds of fluoroscopy can be saved.

Grayscale processing involves adjustment of brightness and contrast of the image. This is done by adjusting two values: window level and window width. Window level is the central value of the gray scale range of the image and window width is the range displayed on either sides of window level. For example, window level of 80 and window width of 50 means the central value of gray scale is 80 and 25 grayscale values can be visualized on either side of 80 (55–105) beyond which the image is either black or white. The level and width are adjusted depending on the region of interest with darker objects needing lower window level, brighter objects higher window level and soft tissues needing higher window width values.

Temporal frame averaging is a feature to reduce image noise. Here two or more images are averaged to form single image with less noise. The drawback of this property is image lag in dynamic fluoroscopic imaging, but may be useful for static images. *Edge enhancement* increases the sharpness of the image and may be used to make lesion more conspicuous.

Measurement of distance of objects can be done on digital image. This usually needs calibration by measuring known dimension of a reference object (e.g. catheter) in the field of view. The machine calculates this in terms of number of pixels and uses it as reference for distance measurements on the image. Other techniques which are available include black-white reversal, image flip (horizontal/vertical), electronic shutter and annotation.

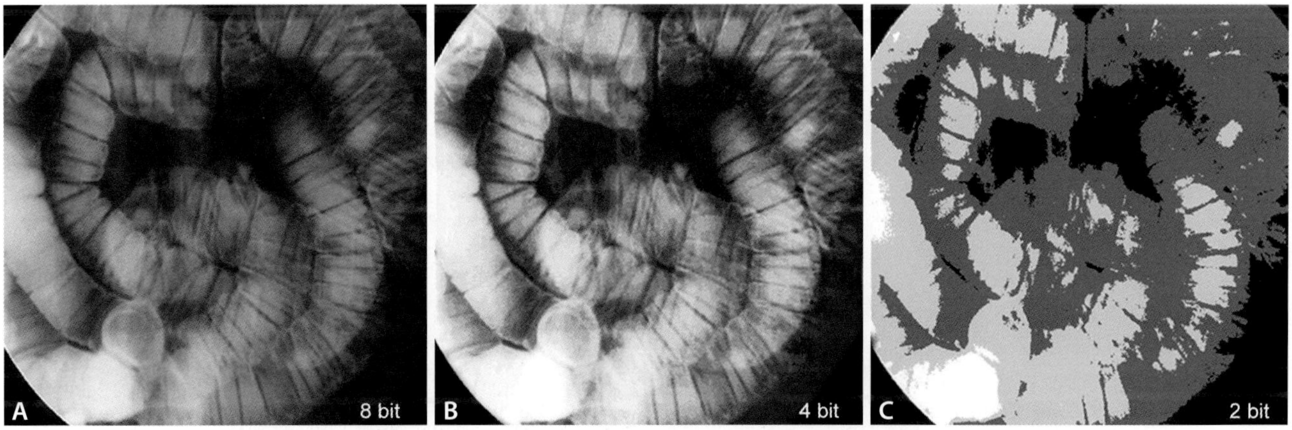

Figs. 15A to C: Contrast resolution of fluoroscopic image at various bit depths. Note the drastic fall in contrast resolution with reduction in bit depth (range of gray scale).

DIGITAL SUBTRACTION ANGIOGRAPHY

Digital subtraction angiography refers to a digital imaging technique for better visualization of contrast filled vessels.[9] This technique permits use of lower amount of contrast medium. Here, the precontrast image is digitally subtracted from postcontrast image to provide background suppression. This allows better visualization of low-contrast vessels, but at a cost of increase in noise. Usually the effect of noise is overcome by averaging two or more frames. Thus, this technique (subtraction) increases the noise which is countered by increased mA (compared to unsubtracted image).

Types of Subtraction

The types of subtraction techniques include mask mode, time interval, dual energy and hybrid subtractions.

Mask-mode subtraction is the most widely used process of DSA in which temporal subtraction is done **(Figs. 16A and B)**. It involves initial acquisition of a frame of region of interest which is used to stabilize the exposure factors. Then a second image is taken and stored as mask image. This mask image is subtracted from subsequently acquired images on pixel-by-pixel basis and show only contrast-filled structures. If any movement occurs after acquisition of mask image, misregistration occurs in the subtracted images. This can be overcome to some extent by pixel shifting.

Time interval difference subtraction is another mode of temporal subtraction where a consecutive previous frame is subtracted from current frame (e.g, frame 1 from frame 2, frame 2 from frame 3 and so on). This technique is very useful in cardiac imaging where there is rapid motion. The images obtained can then be stacked to provide a composite image without motion.

Dual energy subtraction is another technique in which the region of interest is exposed to higher kV (120–130 kV) and lower kV (70 kV) at very short interval (about 50 ms). Then, the higher kV image is subtracted from the lower kV image to produce an iodine and bone image (the soft tissue and gas shadows are eliminated). This technique has the advantage of elimination of motion artifacts. The limitations of this mode of subtraction include increased radiation dose, reduced opacity of contrast-opacified structures, reduced SNR and increased complexity of the equipment.

Hybrid subtraction is a combination of dual energy and temporal subtraction.

Techniques used in DSA

Road map is a technique in which static fluoroscopic image is subtracted from densely opacified vessel. Here, a short contrast run of the vessel is done under fluoroscopy to select the frame with maximum opacification of the vessel as the road map mask, which is stored in memory. Then subsequent live fluoroscopic image is subtracted from the road map mask for visualization of the vessel and the catheter/guide wire **(Figs. 17A and B)**. This technique is very useful in placement of catheters and guidewires in complex and small vessels. Motion after road map acquisition may affect subsequent intervention. Another similar technique is *fluoroscopy fade* in which a reference DSA image is overlaid on the real time fluoroscopic image. Dynamic 3D road mapping which is new development allows projection of 3D reconstructed vessel on live 2D fluoroscopic image.

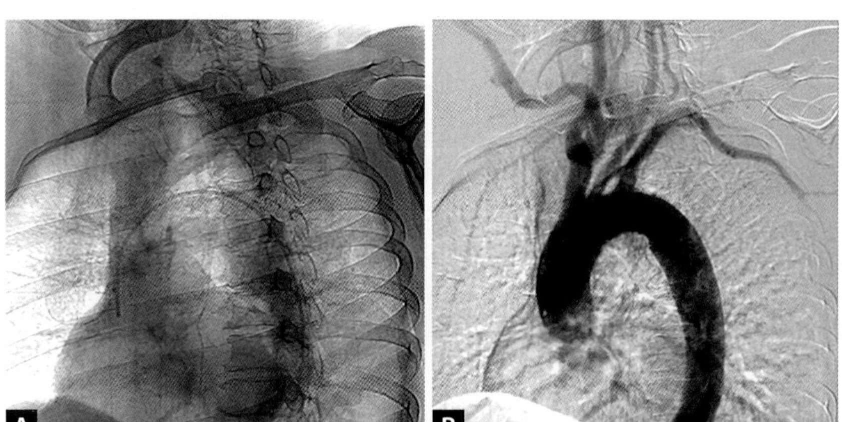

Figs. 16A and B: Mask-mode subtraction: (A) The initial image stored as mask; (B) Shows Subtracted aortogram depicting only vessels.

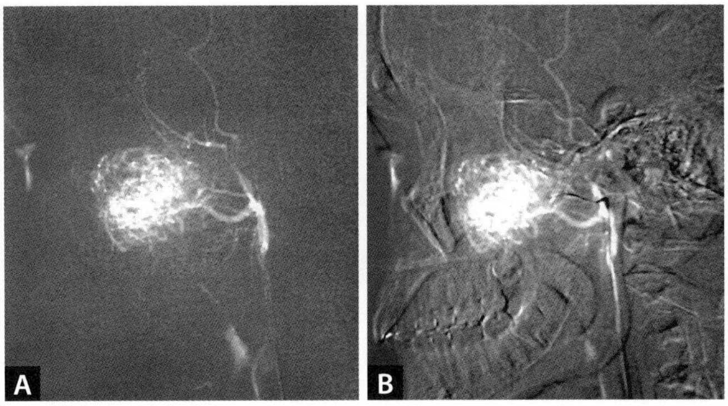

Figs. 17A and B: Road map in a case of preoperative embolization of nasopharyngeal angiofibroma. Subtracted fluoroscopic image with maximum contrast opacification is stored as mask image (A) and subsequent images are subtracted from mask image to visualize the guide-wire/catheter within the opacified vessel (B).

Peripheral DSA can be performed with single contrast injection using *stepping technique*. This is of two types. In stepping table technique, the table moves into three stations with X-ray tube and detector remaining fixed. In stepping gantry method, the tube-detector/II moves keeping the table fixed. In both methods, precontrast images are acquired at different stations and stored as mask image. Subsequently, matching postcontrast injection images are taken at same positions while chasing the bolus of contrast and subtracted from the corresponding mask image to produce clear image of peripheral arteries. The benefits of this technique are significantly reduced use of contrast and reduced examination time. The main disadvantage is increased chances of movement between precontrast and postcontrast images.

An important advancement in digital fluoroscopy is *rotational angiography* where the X-ray tube-detector system rotates through usually 90°–180° while acquiring continuous images.[10] Rotational angiography was available with II systems too. But with improvements in mechanical aspects of systems (rotation) and availability of faster detectors today they produce good quality images **(Figs. 18A and B)**. Mask images are initially acquired at 0.8°–2° gaps followed by postcontrast rotation and acquisition at same positions. Then DSA images are produced at each angle and reconstructed to produce 3D angiograms. The same technique without subtraction is used in some systems to provide axial images (volume or cone beam CT; **Fig. 18C**). The volume data acquired is reconstructed in different planes at a predetermined thickness. This helps in accurate planning of complicated interventions, but at the cost of higher radiation dose. Also, the images have very low contrast resolution due to higher proportion of scatter radiation (due to divergent beam or cone beam).

Postprocessing in DSA

Mask pixel shift is a software modification feature used when smaller patient motion occurs after the mask image is acquired. By shifting the pixels of the mask image, reregistering of the mask with postcontrast image is possible thus obviating motion artifacts **(Figs. 19A and B)**. This technique may be manual or automatic. *Remask* is a similar feature where another mask image is selected, which is temporally closer to the contrast image. This is useful when patient motion occurs prior to contrast image, but after initiation of the acquisition.

Image summation is a property in which two or more frames of a DSA acquisition are summed into a single image **(Figs. 20A to C)**. This is beneficial when rapid acquisition opacifies part of a vessel in each frame and summation adds up the frames to produce a single image showing the entire vessel. Stacking is a similar technique used in carbon dioxide angiography where the fragmented boluses of the gas are added to produce a complete picture of the opacified structure.

Land marking is a feature in which lesser intensity (10–20%, but is manually adjustable) of original image is added to the subtracted image **(Figs. 21A to C)**. This provides anatomical landmarks in subtracted images, useful in subsequent intervention.

Flat-panel Detector

Even after their availability in early 90s, the use of FPD in fluoroscopy was delayed due to the requirement of rapid recording and readout process. The first commercial unit was made available in 2001 intended for cardiac imaging.[11]

Flat-panel detector is the modern solid-state detector array which is used as image receptor.[8] The detector consists of an array of detector elements (DELs), the size of which range from 140 μm to 200 μm. Each DEL consists of photodiodes or capacitors and thin film transistors (made of hydrogenated amorphous silicon) depending on the type of conversion. The total size of the detector varies from 25 × 25 cm to 43 × 43 cm and thus each FPD may house 1.5–5 million individual DELs. This feature is responsible for the high cost of FPD. Thus they are mainly used in interventional angiography suites and rarely for diagnostic fluoroscopy. The X-rays passing through the patient are directly incident on the FPD and its DELs. This process generates an electronic signal either indirectly or directly **(Figs. 22A and B)**.

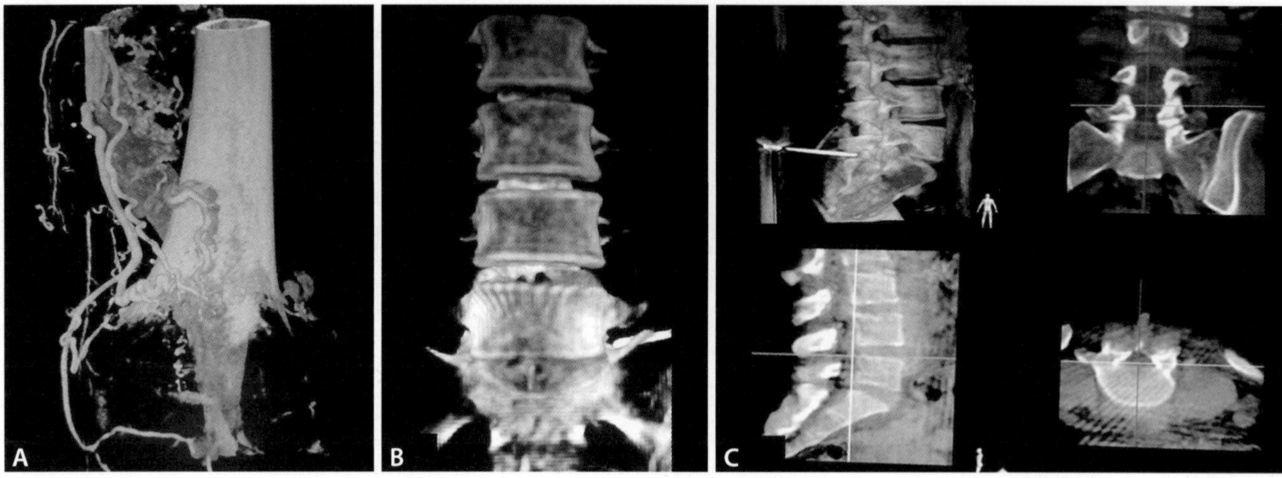

Figs. 18A to C: Three-dimensional rotational angiography image (A) acquired during contrast injection with rotation of the tube and detector in a case of arteriovenous fistula of lower limb; (B) shows lumbar spine during disc intervention. Note the images are of high contrast without soft-tissue visualization. Cone beam CT (C) is similar with the ability of multiplanar reconstructions.

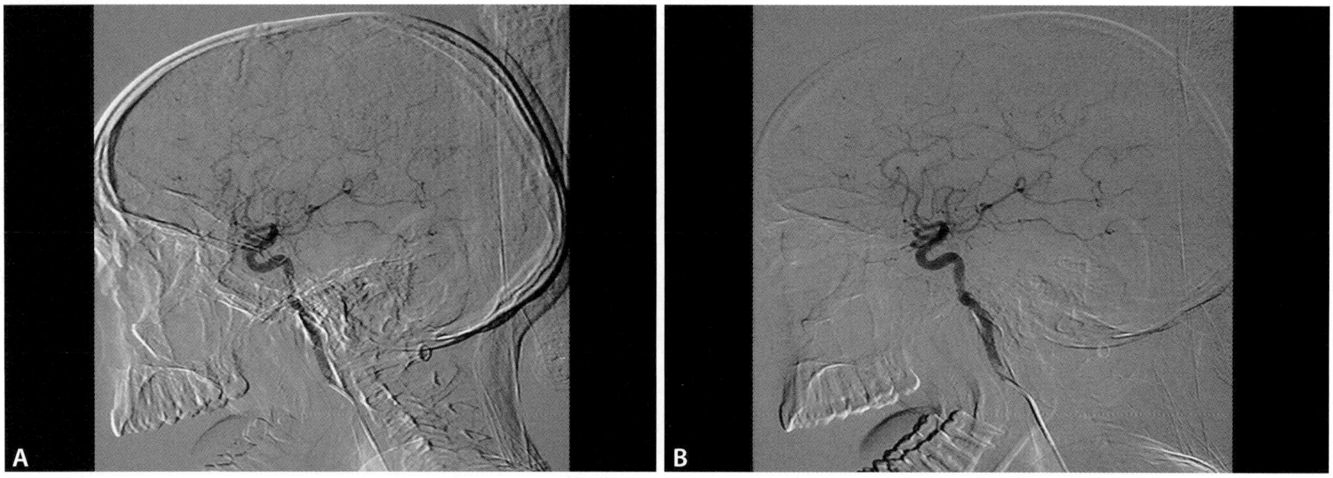

Figs. 19A and B: Motion after acquiring mask image results in misregistration and degradation of image quality (A) This can be partially overcome by pixel-shift technique (B).

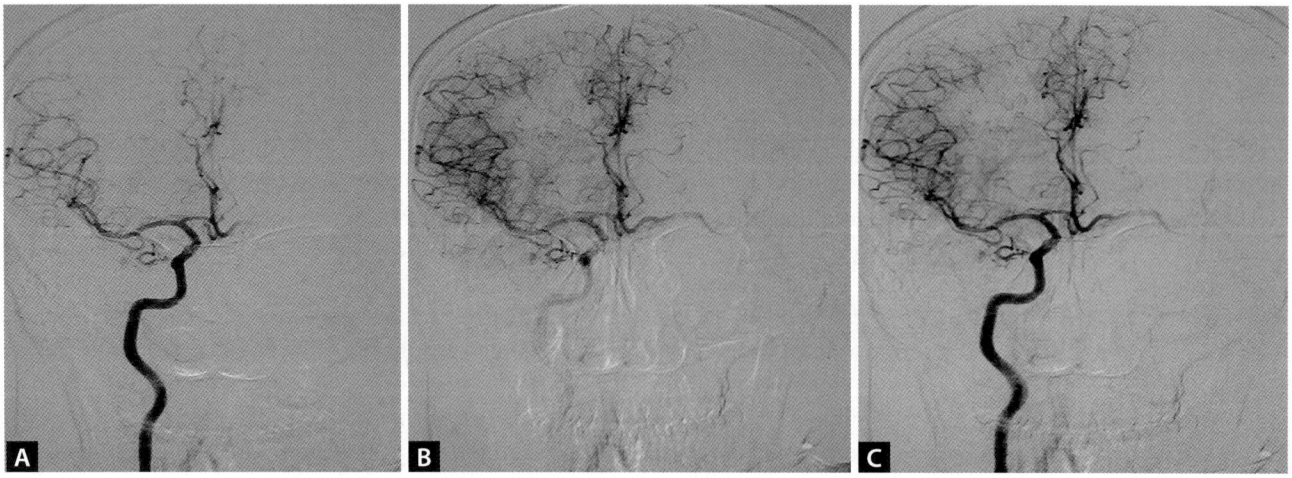

Figs. 20A to C: (A and B) Partial opacification of right internal carotid artery and its branches which can be overcome by summation technique (C) which adds the images to provide a composite image.

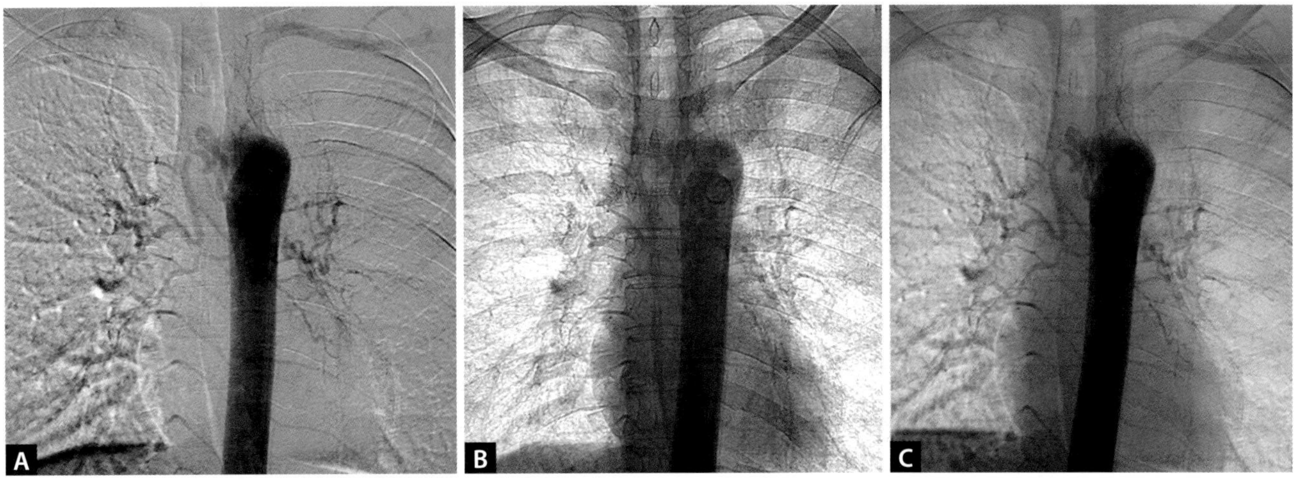

Figs. 21A to C: (A) Subtracted aortogram with bronchial and intercostal arteries without bony landmarks. Conventional image (B) although shows bones well, the arteries are not well seen. Land marking (C) shows both the arteries and bones.

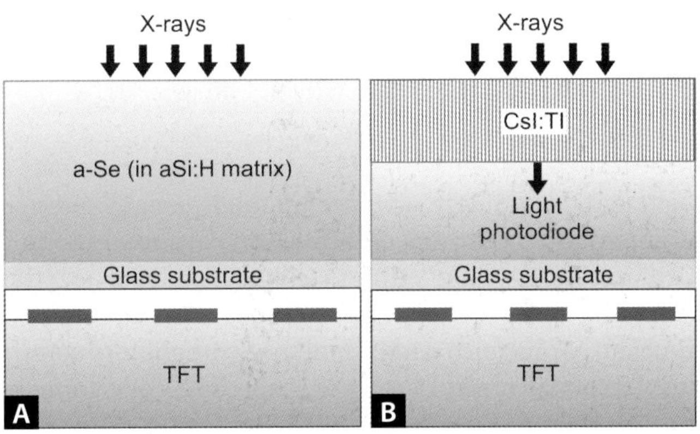

Figs. 22A and B: Basic structure of flat-panel detector, with direct conversion (A) and indirect conversion (B).

Indirect system FPDs consist of DELs which contain a scintillation layer made of thallium-activated cesium iodide (CsI:Tl). The CsI is arranged in the form of crystals which convert incident X-rays into light signal, intensity of which depends on the amount of incident X-ray flux. Cesium (Z = 55) and Iodine (Z = 53) have high atomic numbers and thus good X-ray absorption property. The arrangement of CsI is in the form of closely packed needle shaped crystals which reduces scatter and thus improves spatial resolution. Hence, thicker layers (550–650 µ) can be used which reduce patient dose. The DQE of CsI is in the range of 60–70%. The light signal from scintillator is then transmitted to the adjacent photodiode-transistor layer (contained in thin layer of hydrogenated amorphous silicon—aSi:H) which generates electronic signal depending on the light intensity. Majority of current systems (Siemens, Philips, GE) use this type of detector in combination with grid-controlled pulsed fluoroscopy.

Direct system FPDs directly convert incident X-rays into electric signal. These detectors are made of amorphous selenium (a-Se) in aSi:H matrix. Selenium has lower atomic number (Z = 34) and hence lower X-ray absorption efficiency. Thus, thicker layers (up to 1000 µ) are needed to avoid increase in radiation dose. Higher thickness results in partial loss of charge as it travels to the storage material. Also, increased noise aliasing is encountered with direct conversion. Higher voltages (~10 kV) which need to be applied across the detector may damage the TFT. Shimadzu and Toshiba manufacture direct-conversion fluoroscopic systems.

The process of image formation by FPDs is different from other methods. Here, each DEL is connected to a capacitor which is fully charged initially. During X-ray exposure, the capacitor discharges its stored charge, the amount of which depends on the intensity of the incident X-ray flux. Once exposure is over, the readout electronics measure the change in the charge of all the capacitors in the FPD to produce an image. Subsequently, a light is flashed to discharge the capacitors before fully charging them again. This process is repeated many times per second.

Advantages and Limitations of FPD Systems

The FPD is small, compact and reliable. Most of the artifacts associated with image-intensifier systems are not seen with FPD. As DELs are arranged in rows and columns S-distortions pin cushion artifacts are not encountered. The digital detector system ensures excellent uniformity which obviates vignetting. The fixed positions of DELs prevent defocusing effects. The detector directly produces an electronic signal and a television camera is not needed. The digital system reduces image noise. The FPD has larger dynamic range than II (14-bit vs 4–6-bit) and hence flare or veiling glare is usually not seen. The DQE (ratio of number of detected photons to number of incident photons) of FPD is better than II.

The limitations include increased cost of the detector and difficulty in manufacturing FPD not containing defective DELs. The data from such DELs are interpolated by software which results in some artifacts. The FPDs are temperature and mechanical shock sensitive, changes in which may damage the DELs.

The spatial resolution of FPD is about 2.5–3.4 lp/mm which is lower than that of II (4–6 lp/min; although the effective displayed resolution is 1–1.2 lp/mm). The resolution is limited by size of DELs (pitch) and by binning. Although reducing the size of DELs may improve spatial resolution, this happens at a cost of increase in radiation, as the effective readable surface area (which actually forms image or fill factor) is reduced. This increases image noise which is overcome by increasing radiation. Further with larger FOV, large numbers of elements are activated which substantially increases data transfer rates difficult to be handled by the system. To surmount this limitation, manufacturers carry out a process called *binning* for large FOVs where data from four DELs are grouped to form a single data (similar-to-single DEL). This reduces spatial resolution but also reduces noise. Further, magnification with FPD system also increases radiation dose to reduce noise, but to a lesser extent than that of II.

Another limitation of FPD system (and also II system) is 'ghosting'. This occurs because of persistence of previous image in the scintillation crystal as a ghost and thus affects image quality. Another reason for ghosting is recursive software filtration which adds previous frames of fluoroscopy to current frame. This results in image blurring/ghosting while scanning moving structures. However, this may be beneficial for static imaging as it reduces noise and improves SNR **(Table 1)**.

Table 1: Features of image intensifier and flat-panel detector systems.

Features	Image-intensifier system	Flat-panel detector system
Size	Large and bulky	Small and compact
Construction	In vacuum tube (risk of air leak)	Solid state
Cost	Cheaper	Expensive
Defocusing effect	Present	Absent
Pincushion effect	Present	Absent
S distortion	Present	Absent
Vignetting	Present	Absent
Veiling glare	Present	Absent
Resolution of II	About 5 lp/mm	2.5–3 lp/mm
Dynamic range	Lower (30:1)	Higher (14-bit)
Television system	Needed; Low resolution (1–1.2 lp/mm)	Not needed
Image noise	High	Low

Automatic Exposure Control

Regulation of radiation exposure to image detector is needed in fluoroscopy and image documentation.[12] Automatic exposure control frees the operator from adjusting kVp and mA to obtain optimal penetrated and bright image. A feedback signal is provided by an ionization chamber in case of spot films or photodiode in case of cameras. The signal is then stored in a capacitor until a predefined value is reached when the exposure is terminated. This principle is followed during recording of images. For fluoroscopy, the exposure is not terminated but continuously compared with a reference value and regulated accordingly. This technique is usually referred as automatic brightness control (ABC). Another method is to use the TV video output signal as feedback to X-ray generator. The exposure rate is adjusted by varying kVp, mAs and X-ray pulse width. Automatic brightness control has a response time of 1–1.5 sec. This can be overcome by the use of automatic gain control (AGC). In AGC, TV camera electronically increases the brightness of the image on the monitor when it is dim and noisy. This only maintains brightness and does not change radiation exposure. The lag time for AGC is in terms of milliseconds. Dynamic-density optimization (DDO) is a real time preprocessing algorithm which results in uniform grayscale distribution across the image in both fluoroscopy and DSA.

Recording Fluoroscopic Images

A number of techniques are available for recording and storing fluoroscopic images.[12] They are broadly classified into three types. They include direct-film recording, indirect recording and recording of motion.

Direct-film Recording

Here, as the name suggests, the images are directly exposed on photographic films located in front of II. Two types of devices do this type of image recording.

Spot-film devices use conventional screen-film cassettes for documenting images. The cassette is parked out of the way during routine fluoroscopy and during acquisition moves into the field. The images can be documented in different formats (from 1 to 6 images) on a single film, which has a resolution of about 7 lp/mm and speed of 400. The limitations include inability to use larger sized cassettes (14" × 17") and delay that occurs during acquisition for the cassette to move into the field.

Automatic-film changers are mounted on II and include a supply magazine containing unexposed films (up to 30 films), pair of high-speed screens, a receiving magazine which receives exposed films and a motor system for moving films (usually at a maximum rate of 4 films/second). The films have a resolution of 5 lp/mm and speed of 800 which reduces radiation dose. The disadvantages include use of only single film size, delay in documentation, motion blurring, film fogging and jamming and missed exposures.

Indirect Recording

These devices are placed behind the II and hence called indirect recording. This can be done by photofluorography and digital fluorography.

Photofluorography allows rapid filming up to an extent of 12 films per second. The photospot camera is side mounted and obtains image transmitted from beam-splitting mirror. The films used are roll films which are typically 105 mm wide. Thus the images here are minified. Although, the roll films have resolution of about 200 lp/mm, this is limited by the resolution of II (4–5 lp/mm). The advantages include reduced dose, cheaper films, less storage space and less delay in exposure. The limitations include poorer resolution and smaller sized images.

Digital fluorography uses CCD cameras or FPD where the images are digitally stored. The matrix may vary from 1 to 9 megapixels with resolution varying from 2.4 lp/mm to 3.4 lp/mm. This limitation in resolution is surmounted by the ability of postprocessing of the images. Other benefits include option of film less system, immediate viewing of images without delay and linear response which obviates over or under exposure.

Recording Motion

Motion recording is useful in visualization and reviewing of dynamic processes of the body. Cine camera and videotapes are used for this purpose.

Cine fluorography is regularly used for recording of movement of contrast in the vessels. It uses smaller (35 mm wide) and longer (120 m) film with acquisition capacity of 90 images/second. The frame rate of exposure can be adjusted as needed. Grid-controlled tubes are often used to turn X-ray exposure on and off quickly in synchrony with the camera shutter. Since II produces a circular image, exact framing is needed to fit this image on rectangular film. The effective resolution of the system is 16 lp/mm.

Videotape recording uses super VHS (S-video) technology with its electronic bandwidth matching with that of the TV. They however, produce half the resolution of cine fluorography.

Types of Fluoroscopic Equipment

Various configurations of fluoroscopic systems are available depending on the individual needs. Each system has its own advantages and disadvantages. The types of machines available are as follows:

Radiography–Fluoroscopy Unit with Under-couch Tube

This system has an under the table X-ray tube and collimator with image intensifier or detector above the table **(Figs. 23A and B)**. The II or detector with the tube can be adjusted by the operator to the field of interest. The advantage of this machine is reduced scatter radiation and thus reduced dose to the operator and patient. The disadvantages include need for an additional X-ray tube for radiography which adds to the cost and need for the presence of operator within the examination room for positioning and fluoroscopy (which exposes the operator to radiation) as remote control switches are not available with such systems. The II/ detector is fixed with a handle grip which allows effortless and smooth movement of the detector in all four directions; further it is integrated with fluoroscopic/acquisition button on it.

Radiography–Fluoroscopy Unit with Over-couch Tube

Here, the tube is located above the table at a distance, which is either fixed or adjustable to some extent depending on the vendor **(Figs. 24A and B)**. The detector is under the table. The benefits include available space for patient access, option for tube angulation, remote control operation (with some units) and ability to use the same tube for radiography. The remote control operation prevents primary beam irradiating the operator. The disadvantages are increased scatter radiation, need of additional lead protection devices (additional cost) and operator away from the patient.

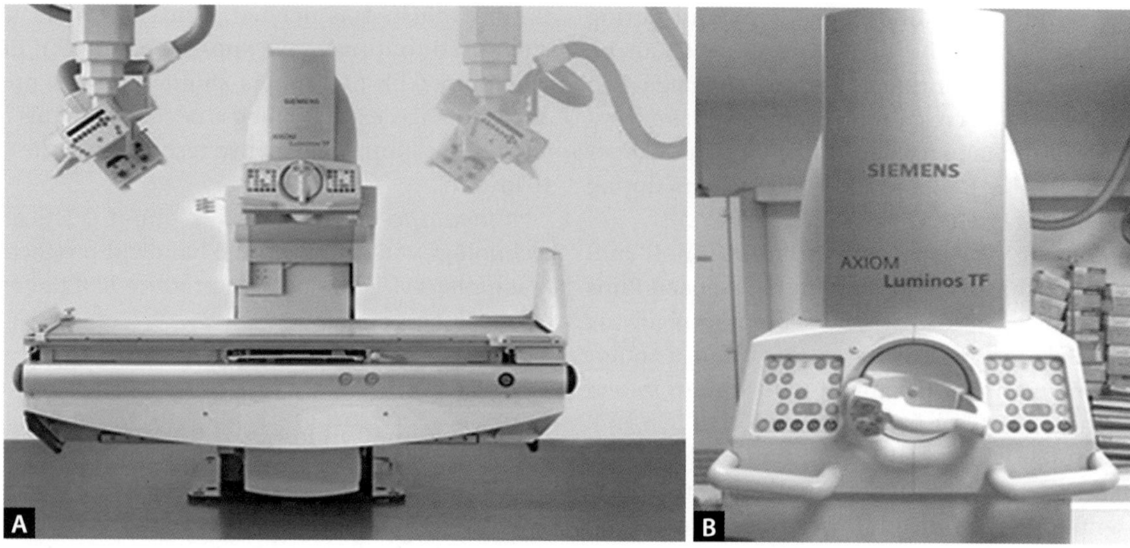

Figs. 23A and B: Radiography–fluoroscopy unit with under the couch X-ray tube (A). The second ceiling mounted X-ray tube is used for radiography. Close-up view of the image intensifier is seen with handle grip (B). (*Courtesy:* Siemens Medical Systems).

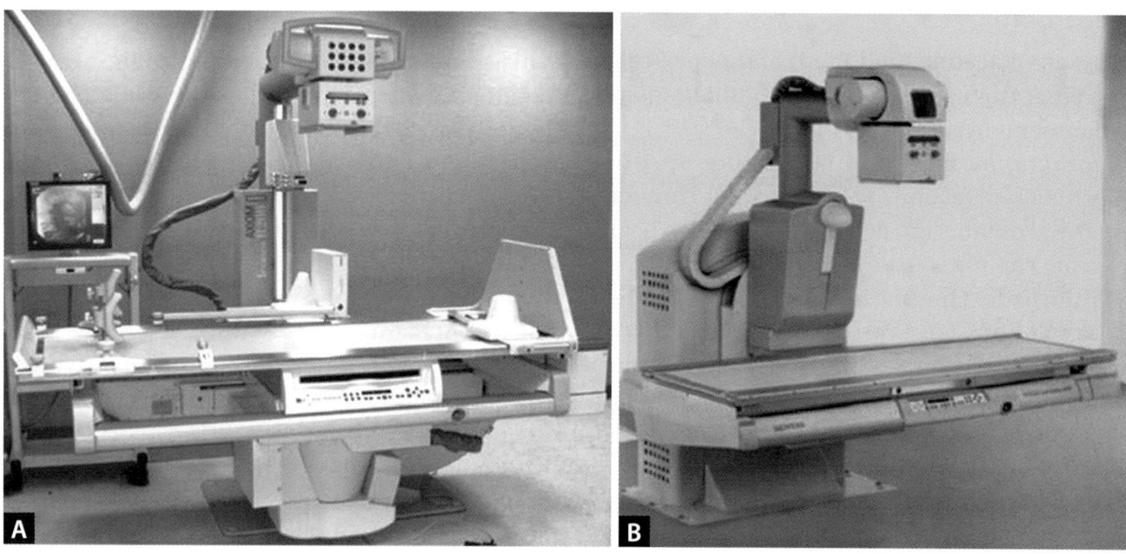

Figs. 24A and B: Radiography–fluoroscopy unit with over-couch X-ray tube and under the table image intensifier (A) and flat-panel detector (B). (*Courtesy:* Siemens Medical Systems)

Fixed C-arm Fluoroscopic System

This type of system is mainly used in angiography. This consists of a C-shaped apparatus with X-ray tube assembled at one end and II or detector at other end **(Figs. 25A and B)**. The shape allows for increased mobility of tube-detector assembly. The C-arm is either ceiling mounted or floor mounted. In addition, it includes a mobile floating table which is fixed to the floor at one end. Biplane C-arm system includes two C-arms, one ceiling mounted and the other floor mounted **(Fig. 26)**. This unit allows acquisition in two projections (e. g. AP and lateral) with single contrast injection.

Mobile C-arm System

This system is mainly used in operation theaters and wards to check the position of orthopedic implants, pacemakers or vascular implants **(Fig. 27)**. This system is cheaper and mostly uses image intensifiers, usually with CCD cameras. Due to the cost involved and need of proper care, FPD C-arm systems are slowly increasing in availability.

Factors Affecting Image Quality

The quality of fluoroscopic images is determined by a number of factors. The image quality is most importantly defined by spatial resolution and contrast resolution.

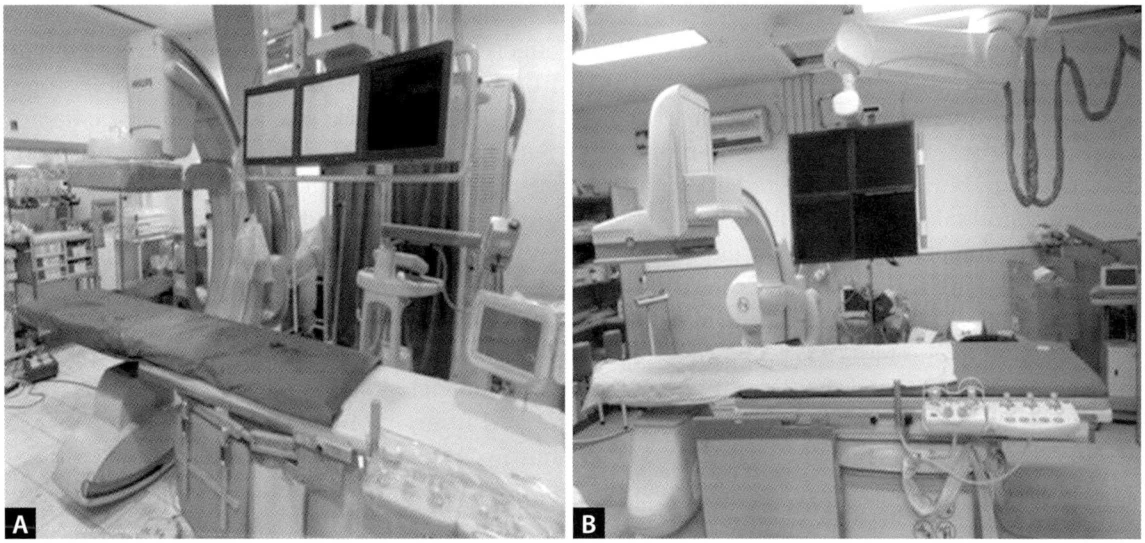

Figs. 25A and B: Fixed C-arm flat-panel detector fluoroscopy system used for angiography with the C-arm being ceiling mounted (A; *Courtesy:* Philips Medical Systems) or floor mounted (B; *Courtesy:* GE Medical System).

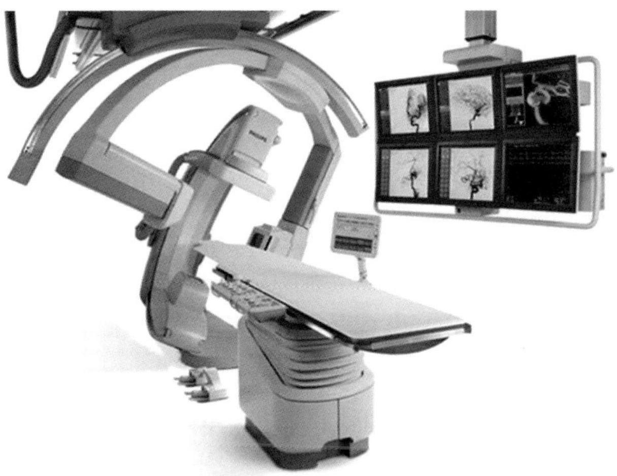

Fig. 26: Biplanar fixed C-arm system, with one arm ceiling mounted and the other floor mounted. (*Courtesy:* Philips Medical System).

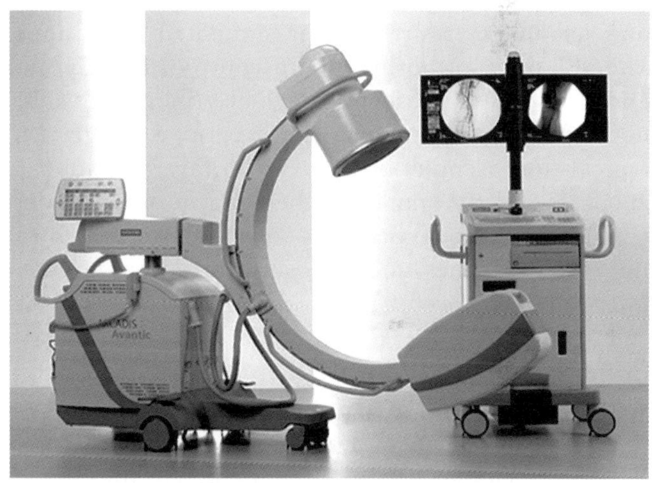

Fig. 27: Mobile C-arm fluoroscopy unit. (*Courtesy:* Siemens Medical Systems).

Spatial resolution of an image is determined by FOV, matrix, size and number of DELs, binning, video capability, focal spot size and mode of fluoroscopy (continuous vs pulsed). Contrast resolution is affected by scatter, glare, kVp, filtration, collimation, mA (which determines noise/SNR) and image processing techniques. Other factors include source-image receptor distance, patient-image receptor distance, ABC, aperture of optical-video system and conversion gain.

Evaluation of image quality is the most important part of quality control in fluoroscopy. Contrast resolution is evaluated using an aluminum step wedge with holes of different diameter, spatial resolution by line pair phantom, focal spot size by star phantom and temporal resolution by motor-driven rotating disc. These quality control tests should be carried out at regular intervals, typically annually, for optimal performance.

Radiation Safety in Fluoroscopy

From the initial days when fluoroscopy was introduced in medicine, there has been an increase in its utilization. In the past two to three decades, tremendous increase in its utilization in various diagnostic and interventional procedures has occurred which has increased the total fluoroscopy times greatly, sometimes even over one hour. Availability of newer intravascular devices has further added to its growth. All these together have increased radiation exposure to patients and to medical staff working with fluoroscopy. Most important of various radiation induced effects is skin burns caused by radiation. It has an insidious onset and take weeks to manifest in its full extent. The radiation induced skin injury is a deterministic (nonstochastic) effect with severity increasing with increase in exposure dose. The importance of skin injury in fluoroscopy is due to the fact that radiation dose is highest at skin entrance point and that skin in the region of interest suffers as the fluoroscopy time increases. The measurements which are typically used to measure radiation dose of a fluoroscopy system are receptor entrance exposure and skin entrance exposure rates.[13]

Receptor entrance exposure (REE) is defined as exposure at the entrance of image receptor required to produce a single image with grid removed. Skin entrance exposure (SEE) is the dose at entrance surface of a patient and usually measured under simulated conditions. The SEE limit for normal fluoroscopy is 100 mGy/min and high-dose fluoroscopy is 200 mGy/min. The values depend on kVp, patient thickness, grid, SID, etc. The typical fluoroscopic SEE rate for an average adult is about 10–30 mGy/min, but higher for acquisition modes. Usually, diagnostic procedures are associated with lower fluoroscopic times and exposure rates compared to interventional procedures.

Patient Dose Monitoring Methods

These methods are described in detail elsewhere. In short, they are of two types.

Direct methods use thermoluminescent dosimeters (TLD), photographic films and diodes or metal-oxide semiconductor field effect transistor (MOSFET) detectors. The TLD is the most accurate but due to smaller size cannot cover the entire field and may not correctly measure the peak dose field. Photographic films are inexpensive and useful in determining high-dose region and the dose. But the sizes available are limited. Both these methods are associated with time delay in reading out the measured doses. The MOSFET detectors provide dynamic measurement of skin dose and are accurate.[14] They have good linear response, low detection threshold and low error percentage (10%), but are detectable in the imaging field.

Indirect method most widely used is dose area product (DAP) meter. Since it is a product of dose and area, same values can be obtained with low dose exposed to larger area and higher dose exposed to smaller area. But the skin effect of these two modes is not the same as the latter results in more skin damage. The SEE can be computed from DAP reading if dose rate and field size data is available. But this is often difficult as both, dose rate and field size change dynamically during fluoroscopy. Still, DAP meters are widely used in modern systems for dose measurement. One new system is available which dynamically measures and displays an estimate of SEE and is called PEMNET (Patient Exposure Management Network). This records patient dose from all radiation related procedures (CT, cardiac, angiography, interventions) and is available for review from any workstation in the network. Currently however, there is no perfect dose monitoring system for fluoroscopy and interventional procedures.

Dose-reduction Techniques

Various dose reduction techniques include reduction of exposure time, improving collimation, reducing tube current, reducing spot exposures, using better detectors and reducing II/detector–patient distance.

Intermittent fluoroscopy is the most important due to the fact that the radiologist can control fluoroscopy time and can judiciously use it intermittently to reduce total patient and personnel dose. Last image hold (LIH) has been described above. Use of reference image, especially in DSA is helpful in significantly reducing radiation dose and contrast medium. Modern systems are available with electronic collimation which can be done on LIH without additional fluoroscopy.

Pulsed fluoroscopy provides substantial reduction in patient radiation exposure. Reducing the number of pulses increases image noise and this is overcome in many models by increasing mA which increases dose. Thus instead, there is only modest reduction in dose. The radiation dose of continuous fluoroscopy and pulsed fluoroscopy at 30 fps are similar. When the pulse rate is reduced from 30 to 15, 10, and 7.5 per second, the dose is approximately reduced by 22, 38 and 49% respectively.[15] No significant change in image quality is seen between continuous fluoroscopy and PF at 15 fps, 7.5 fps and 3.75 fps.[16] Further, at lower frame rates and magnified fields, instead of increasing exposure, the video camera aperture can be increased to maintain brightness. Automatic dose rate and image quality (ADRIQ) control modulates kVp, mAs, pulse width and filtration as per patient characteristics to produce lowest radiation with good image quality.[17]

The use of cumulative exposure timer, typically set at 5 minutes, alerts the operator of fluoroscopy time. Further, real time display of total exposure time, kVp, mAs and total dose also helps the radiologist to regulate patient radiation exposure.

Dose spreading is a method to reduce skin dose when lengthy interventional procedures are performed. Here, the tube-detector system is rotated about the region of interest as center to spread the skin dose to different area, so that single area is not overexposed. The quality of X-ray beam can be adjusted to remove low-energy X-rays (beam hardening). This can be done by increasing kVp (which reduces SEE) and use of metal filters like aluminum or copper (especially the latter as 0.1–0.3 mm of Cu reduces SEE by 30–50%).[18]

Magnification, either geometric or electronic results in increase in skin dose. Higher magnification may result in reduced spatial resolution due to focal spot blur if smaller focal spot is not used. High-dose fluoroscopy mode, available in few systems, is uncommonly used for very obese patients or thick body regions and results in high skin dose.

SUMMARY

Fluoroscopy is one of the basic X-ray techniques and is widely used for various diagnostic and interventional procedures. From the initial darkroom fluoroscopy considerable advancements have led to the development of image intensifiers, digital processing techniques and the present day FPD. Solid-state FPD systems produce better image with less artifacts and results in less radiation dose. Radiologists, as end users, should be aware of the basic structure and function of these equipments so that judicious adjustments are made on case to case basis. A constant note has to be made of the fluoroscopic time and radiation dose to the patient during each procedure. Adequate knowledge of methods of dose reduction during fluoroscopy and DSA is important to prevent radiation effects, especially on skin. Some recent technological developments like new detector technology based on crystalline silicon, emitter technology of X-ray tube, functional imaging protocols that provide physiological information of the lesion and patient and intravascular ultrasound with angiography are in the initial stages of research and may have potential to get established in the field of interventional radiology.

REFERENCES

1. Schueler BA. The AAPM/RSNA physics tutorial for residents: General overview of fluoroscopic imaging. Radiographics. 2000;20:1115-26.
2. Pooley RA, McKinney JM, Miller DA. The AAPM/RSNA physics tutorial for residents: Digital fluoroscopy. Radiographics. 2001; 21:521-34.
3. Krohmer JS. Radiography and fluoroscopy, 1920 to the present. Radiographics. 1989;9:1129-53.
4. Seibert JA. The AAPM/RSNA physics tutorial for residents: X-ray generators. Radiographics. 1997;17:1533-57.
5. Zink FE. The AAPM/RSNA physics tutorial for residents: X-ray tubes. Radiographics. 1997;17:1259-68.
6. Wang J, Blackburn TJ. The AAPM/RSNA physics tutorial for residents: X-ray image intensifiers for fluoroscopy. Radiographics. 2000;20:1471-7.
7. Van Lysel MS. The AAPM/RSNA physics tutorial for residents: Fluoroscopy: optical coupling and the video system. Radiographics. 2000;20:1769-86.
8. Nickoloff EL. The AAPM/RSNA physics tutorial for residents: Survey of modern fluoroscopy imaging: flat panel detectors versus image intensifiers and more. Radiographics. 2011; 31:591-602.
9. Curry TS III, Dowdey JE, Murry RC Jr. Christensen's Physics of Diagnostic Radiology, 4th Edn. Philadelphia, Pa: Lea & Febiger; 1990.
10. Orth RC, Wallace MJ, Kuo MD. Technology Assessment Committee of the Society of Interventional Radiology. C-arm cone-beam CT: general principles and technical considerations for use in interventional radiology. J Vasc Interv Radiol. 2008; 19:814-20.
11. Cowen AR, Davies AG, Sivananthan MU. The design and imaging characteristics of dynamic, solid-state, flat-panel X-ray image detectors for digital fluoroscopy and fluorography. Clin Radiol. 2008;63:1073-85.
12. Geise RA. The AAPM/RSNA physics tutorial for residents: Fluoroscopy: recording of fluoroscopic images and automatic exposure control. Radiographics. 2001;21:227-36.
13. Mahesh M. The AAPM/RSNA physics tutorial for residents: Fluoroscopy: patient radiation exposure issues. Radiographics. 2001;21:1033-45.
14. Miksys N, Gordon CL, Thomas K, Connolly B. Estimating effective dose to pediatric patients undergoing interventional radiology procedures using anthropomorphic phantoms and MOSFET dosimeters. Am J Roentgenol. 2010;194:1315-22.
15. Aufrichtig R, Xue P, Thomas CW, Gilmore GC, Wilson DL. Perceptual comparison of pulsed and continuous fluoroscopy. Med Phys. 1994;21:245-56.
16. Boland GWL, Murphy B, Arellano R, Niklason L, Mueller PR. Dose reduction in gastrointestinal and genitourinary fluoroscopy: use of grid-controlled pulsed fluoroscopy. Am J Roentgenol. 2000;175:1453-7.
17. Lin PJ. The operation logic of automatic dose control of fluoroscopy system in conjunction with spectral shaping filters. Med Phys. 2007;34:3169-72.
18. Nicholson R, Tuffee F, Uthappa MC. Skin sparing in interventional radiology: the effect of copper filtration. Br J Radiol. 2000;73:36-42.

CHAPTER 53

Tools in Interventional Radiology

Atin Kumar, Chandan Jyoti Das

INTRODUCTION

The common procedures performed in an interventional radiology set-up could be vascular as well as nonvascular. The need of hardware starts from the giving of local anesthesia or intravenous access till the suturing or plastering of the wound of the procedure in interventional radiology. Both the procedures have some common as well as specific needs. The common needs are like local anesthetic agent, blades, puncture needles and suturing agent. Some of the tools used to perform the interventional procedures are common for both vascular and nonvascular procedures, while some are specific to each type.

The various tools which constitute the armamentarium of an interventional radiologist are discussed in this chapter.

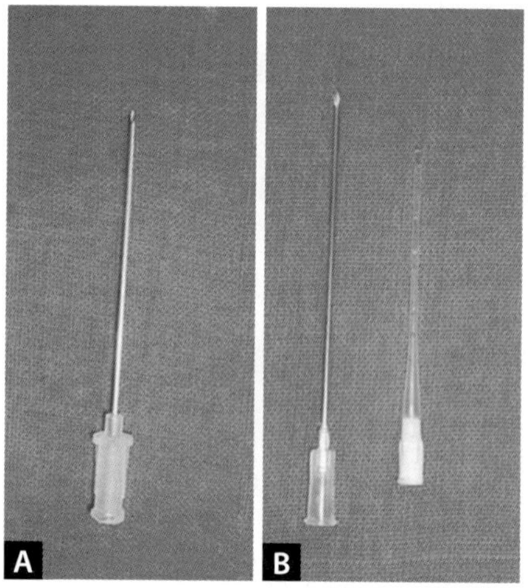

Figs. 1A and B: Puncture needles: (A) Single-piece needle; (B) Seldinger needle (Medicut).

PUNCTURE NEEDLES

Puncture needles are small-sized needles which are used to gain access to the vessel and are therefore also called as access needles. They are also used for nonvascular indications like gaining access to bile duct, pelvicalyceal system, abscess, etc. The typical access needle has a sharp, beveled distal edge for puncturing the artery **(Fig. 1A)**. The guidewire is introduced through its lumen into the vessel once blood comes out from the proximal end. Some access needles have an inner stylet which protrudes slightly out of the outer lumen needle. The tip of the inner stylet is sharp to puncture the artery but the tip of the outer needle is round and blunted to prevent vessel injury. Once the vessel is punctured, the stylet is removed to allow entry of guidewire.

The size of the access needle is measured in gauges. Higher-gauge number indicates smaller lumen diameter. The typical access needles are of size 18 G or 19 G.

The Seldinger needle (Medicut 18 G) is a double lumen type of access needle commonly used in vascular puncture in which the outer lumen is soft, pliable and nontraumatic cannula with a stylet with sharp and beveled edge within its lumen **(Fig. 1B)**. Once the vessel is entered, the inner stylet is removed and the soft cannula remains within the vessel through which the guidewire can be introduced. The commonly used intravenous cannula is almost similar and can be used for the same purpose. It is important to check the compatibility of the guidewire through the lumen of the access needle before the vessel is punctured. A 19 G needle accepts a 0.035 inch guidewire.

The vessel puncture can be single or double wall puncture. In the single wall technique, only the anterior wall of the artery is punctured by the advancing needle and when the tip is in the lumen (as evidenced by pulsatile backflow of blood), the guidewire is advanced within the lumen. The nonstylet access needles are preferred for this type of puncture whereas the needles with stylet are used for the double wall technique. In the double wall technique, the puncture needle is advanced through the vessel till it punctures the posterior wall also. Then the stylet is removed and the needle slowly withdrawn till the tip is within the lumen of the vessel. The double wall technique is comparatively easier. The single wall technique is preferred in cases of coagulopathy or when thrombolysis is planned to prevent excessive bleeding.

Another technique of vessel puncture is by micropuncture access set **(Fig. 2)**. In this, the needle used has a sharp beveled tip needle of very small diameter (usually 21 G) which is initially used to puncture the vessel. A compatible 0.018 inch guidewire is then introduced through the needle followed by removal of the needle. A coaxial dilator system with a 3 F inner dilator within a 4 F or 5 F outer dilator is then advanced over the guidewire. It is then followed by removal of the guidewire and the inner dilator to provide a large bore access within the lumen through which the normal 0.035 inch guidewire can be introduced. This technique is commonly used in situations where the access is difficult, e.g. antegrade femoral puncture, brachial artery punctures, pediatric patients, anatomically sensitive regions like jugular venous access and in conditions where thrombolysis is planned.

Seldinger technique is the systematic procedure of gaining access into the vessel. The vessel is first punctured with a needle which is followed by guidewire insertion through it. The needle is then removed over the wire and exchanged with a tapered catheter of appropriate size. This technique is also used in nonvascular procedures to gain access into biliary channels, pelvicalyceal system or into an abscess cavity.

DILATORS

Dilators are short stiff-tapered plastic catheters which are used to spread the soft tissues/fascia and the wall of the vessel so as to facilitate the subsequent passage of a catheter. Sequential use of increasing size dilators over a guidewire (preferably stiff guidewire) leads to an increase in the size of the initial percutaneous puncture. The dilators are also frequently used in nonvascular percutaneous procedures to dilate the track like in abscess drainage, percutaneous nephrostomy, percutaneous transhepatic biliary drainage, etc. **(Fig. 3)**.

The sizes of the dilators (and access needles) are measured in gauges. The size in inches equals 1/gauge. Hence, a 20 G needle measures 0.05 inches whereas a 25 G needle measures 0.04 inches. Smaller gauges indicate larger diameters.

SHEATHS

Introducer sheaths are small thin-walled catheters which are open at one end and are capped with a hemostatic

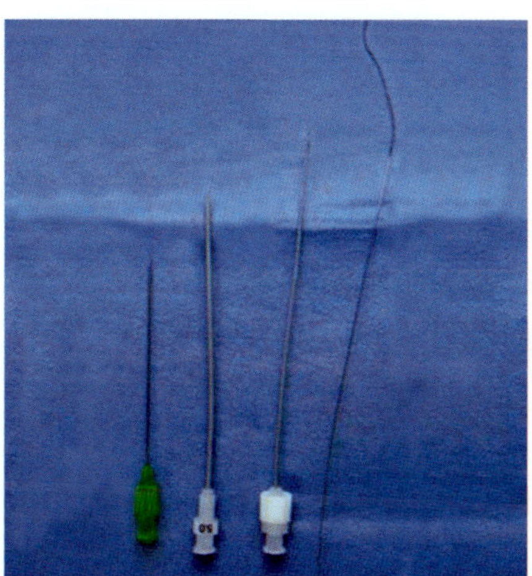

Fig. 2: Micropuncture access set: Consists of beveled tip needle, coaxial dilators and a 0.018 guidewire.

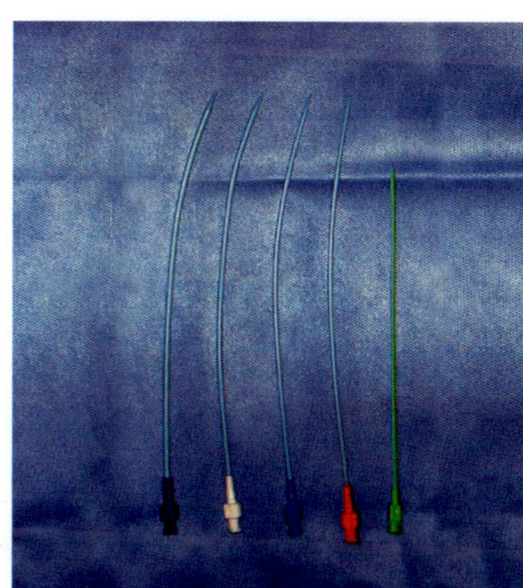

Fig. 3: Dilators of varying sizes (increasing from right to left). Each size is universally color coded.

valve or diaphragm at the other end. There is a short clear side arm which is used for flushing or injection of contrast. The distal end of the sheath is generally nontapered in contrast from normal catheters. The purpose of the sheath is to provide a continuous secured access within vessel lumen for multiple exchanges of various catheters and guidewires through a single puncture and access site. It is introduced as a coaxial system with a dilator within it to ensure smooth access. The introducer sheaths are also widely used for access in nonvascular interventions and drainage of fluid collections **(Fig. 4)**.

The sheaths being slightly stiffer, are also used to improve the pushability of a diagnostic catheter through them into tortuous vessels. Long length sheaths are also available which are mainly used for interventional procedures including nonvascular procedures. The use of crossover sheaths (across the aortic bifurcation) significantly enhances the selective catheterizations of contralateral iliac/femoral vessels and use of long sheaths can enable easy and direct advancement of catheters into selective distal main vessels.

The sheath sizes are described in French (F) and represents the maximum actual size in French of the catheter which can be introduced through its lumen. Hence, a 5 F sheath size means that a 5 F catheter can be introduced through it. Note that for sheaths the size represents the inner lumen diameter whereas for catheters and dilators, it represents the outer diameter. The sheaths are available in diameters 4–14 F with lengths ranging from 10 to 90 cm. There is a universal color coding system for the sizes of the sheaths. 4 F sheaths are of red color, 5 F gray, 6 F green and 7 F orange colored.

CATHETERS

The word catheter is derived from a latin word 'katheter' which means to push down. It is a hollow flexible tube that can be inserted into a body cavity, duct or vessel, thereby allowing drainage or injection of fluids, distending a passageway or providing access to surgical instruments. The process of inserting a catheter is catheterization.

Catheters are the backbone of an interventional radiological procedure. They come in various shapes, sizes and material types with each serving a specific function.

Parts of Catheter

A typical catheter consists of following parts **(Fig. 5)**:
- *Tip:* The distal tapered part
- *Shaft:* The long tubing
- *Hub:* The proximal part with a plastic funnel for ease of guidewire insertions and attachment of syringes for contrasts injections.

Materials

The catheters can be made of various materials including teflon (polytetrafluoroethylene or PTFE), polyethylene, polyurethane or nylon. The choice of the material decides the torque, stiffness, flexibility, thrombogenicity, burst pressure and the friction. Stiffness allows the pushing of the catheter while flexibility allows bending of the catheter to follow the curve of the vessel. High burst pressure measures the strength of the material and its ability to withstand the high injection rate without bursting. The ability of the catheter tip to rotate based on rotation of the catheter hub measures its torque ability. Mechanical

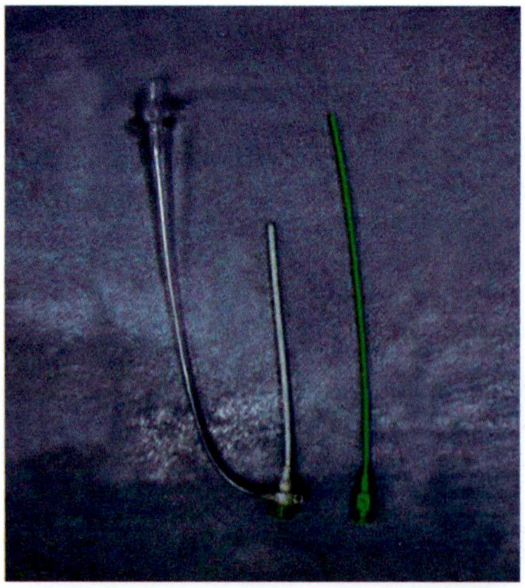

Fig. 4: Sheath: Size 6 F (green color).

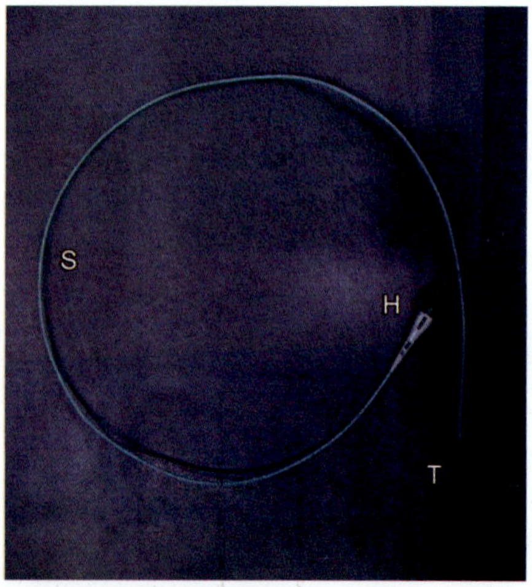

Fig. 5: Catheter parts: Hub (H), shaft (S) and tip (T).

braiding of the catheter wall by materials, such as nylon or stainless steel enhances the torque ability of the catheter and facilitates selective catheterization of vessels. Decreased friction of the catheter material on the luminal surface allows higher flow rates and on the outer surface enables easier advancement of the catheter with minimal buckling and wedging. Catheters can be coated by hydrophilic polymers to allow easier trackability, e.g. slip catheter (Cook). Impregnation of the catheter wall with barium sulfate, tungsten or lead salts is often done to increase the fluoroscopic visibility as the catheters are generally faintly radiopaque.

In general, PTFE or nylon catheters are stiffer with high tensile strength and burst pressure and hence are used for purpose of flush injections requiring high flow rates and pressures. In contrast, polyethylene catheters are less stiff and more flexible and hence are used for purpose of selective catheterizations.

Sizes

The catheters can be of varying diameter and lengths. The diameter of the catheter is conventionally measured in French size (F). (3 F = 1 mm = 0.038 inches). The catheter size in French refers to the outer diameter of the catheter. It is a factor in deciding the size of the catheter to be used based upon the size of the vessel to be catheterized. The general used intravascular catheters are commonly of size 4 F to 6 F. Catheters smaller than 4 F are not used for flush purpose but are required for pediatric use and for selective catheterization of tortuous or smaller vessels like intracerebral vessels. They are known as microcatheters and are usually of 2 F or 3 F size. Larger catheters of size 7 F to 9 F are used as guiding catheters and are mainly used to guide smaller catheters or devices within them to be used as a coaxial system. The guiding catheters are usually stiffer and firmer to allow passage of balloon catheters, PTCA wires and stent delivery system through them. Mild stiffness comes due to the wire-braided design. It should be noted that for guiding catheters the size in French refers to the inner diameter of the catheter (like the introducer sheaths) in contrast to standard use catheters and hence is determinant of the size of the standard catheter which can be coaxially passed through it. For example, a 6 F guiding catheter would be able to accommodate a 6F standard catheter.

The length of the catheter is the distance between the hub and the tip. It is conventionally measured in centimeters and usually varies between 60 and 110 cm for standard catheters. Smaller catheter lengths are required when the target vessel is close to the site of puncture (usually the femoral artery), such as contralateral iliac, renal or visceral arteries and in pediatric patients. Longer lengths measuring up to 260 cm are required for upper limb, calf, intracranial vessels selective catheterization. The microcatheters are usually of long length as they are to be used coaxially within another catheter and their tips must come out a reasonable distance out of the outer catheter.

Shapes and Holes

The shape of the catheter tip is the most essential element determining the type of use of the catheter. Depending upon the shape, the catheters are categorized as the following:

- *Simple straight/angled tip catheters:* These have a single curve or angle **(Fig. 6)**. The curve ranges from slightly curved (multipurpose) to more angled (hockeystick or picard) to completely circular (pigtail). These are either used as flush catheters (pigtail) or to catheterize arteries with angled origins to the direction of catheter like aortic arch branches (picard).
- *Complex curve catheters:* These have more than one curve and are usually used for selective catheterization of branches of the descending aorta. The curve closest to the tip is known as the primary curve while the farther curves are known as secondary curves or the tertiary curves. The primary curve helps to hook a target vessel at an angle while the secondary curve hits the back wall of the main vessel (the wall opposite to the origin of target vessel) and helps to push the

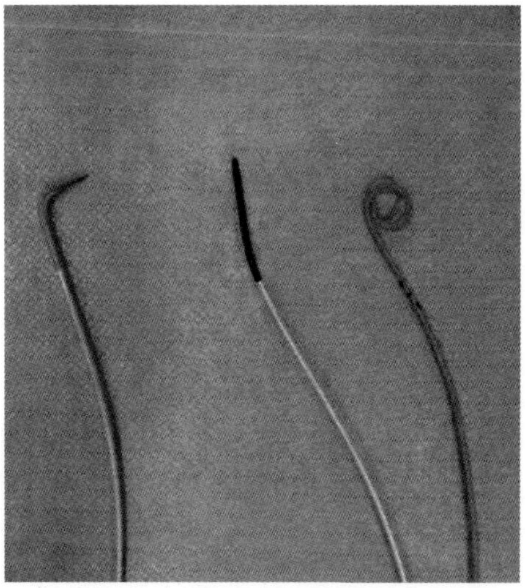

Fig. 6: Simple curve catheters: From left to right–picard, multipurpose and pigtail.

catheter further into the target vessel. These catheters are of two types:

- The primary and secondary curves are in the same direction, e.g. cobra, renal double curve, head hunter, etc. **(Figs. 7A to C)**. They are best used for selective catheterization of vessels which have origins angled caudally like the visceral arteries.
- The primary and secondary curves in opposite direction—reverse curve catheters, e.g. Simmons (1,2 and 3) catheters **(Fig. 7D)**. These are best used for selective catheterization of vessels which have steep obtuse angle like the left gastric artery or steep acute angled vessels (sometimes visceral arteries, left common carotid in atherosclerotic aortic arch). These catheters are straightened over a guidewire before advancing and their curves need to be reformed within the aorta after removal of guidewire. Several techniques have been described for the formation of these curves either in the arch or at aortic bifurcation. After hooking the target vessel by the tip of the catheter over a guidewire, these catheters are advanced into the vessel till the level of apex of secondary curve by partial withdrawal of the catheter at the groin (instead of pushing as done in all standard forward curve catheters). Only after this point the catheters can be further pushed into the vessel by advancing over a stiff guidewire. Due to their shape, they have increased chances of vessel wall injury while pulling out. Hence, these catheters should always be withdrawn after straightening over a guidewire under fluoroscopic monitoring.

Depending upon the position and number of holes, the catheters are divided into two types:

1. *End-hole catheter:* These are the standard diagnostic catheters which have a single hole at the tip of the catheter. The size of the hole is tapered to allow the maximum allowable sized guidewire to just pass through it snugly. These are used for selective catheterization. Pressure injector is not used with these catheters as it may cause plaque dislodgement and dissection.
2. *Side-hole catheters:* The side holes are usually multiple with an end hole. These catheters are used as flush catheters to obtain angiograms of large vessels. The side holes vary in number with typical pigtail flush catheter having 8–12 side holes. Though the size of an individual side hole is smaller than the size of the end hole (to prevent exiting of guidewire through this hole), the combined size of the side holes is larger than the end hole allowing much larger volume of contrast dispersal through these holes than the end hole. The multiple side hole catheters are preferred for flush injections as they cause uniform dispersal of contrast in the vessel. The side hole catheters are also used for thrombolysis as they result in uniform distribution of the thrombolytic agent within the thrombus. However, these catheters are not used for embolization as the embolising agents may either diffuse out through these holes resulting in nontarget embolization or may occlude the end hole at the tip due to lesser pressure delivered at the tip. The embolising coils may also get struck within the side holes.

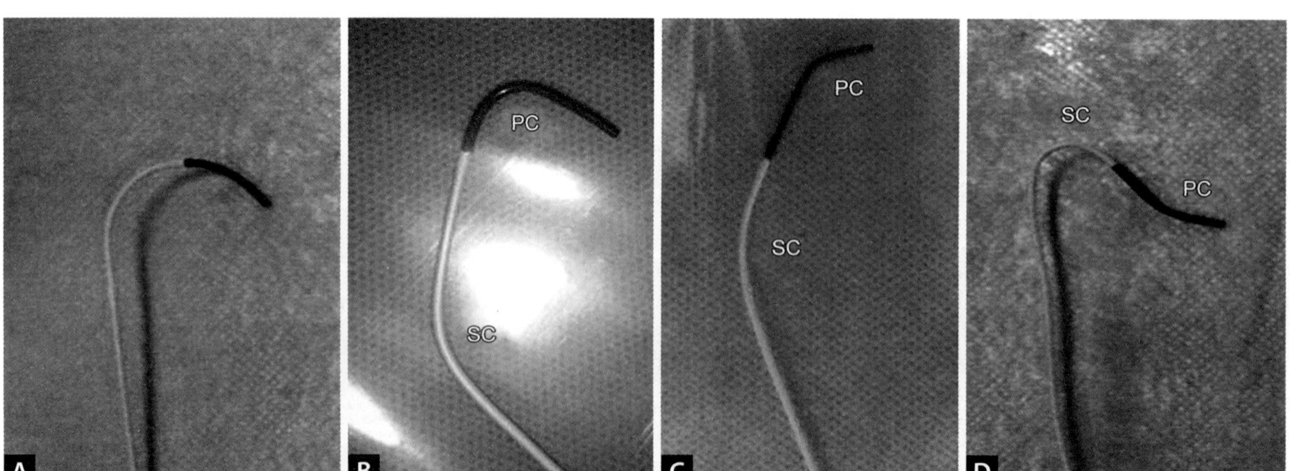

Figs. 7A to D: Complex curve catheters: (A) The primary and secondary curves are in same direction in cobra; (B) Renal double curve; (C) Head- hunter; (D) Catheters while in reverse curve catheters, they are in opposite direction as in Simmons catheter.

The commonly used catheters in clinical practice are:

- *Multipurpose* **(Fig. 6)**: It has straight tip. It can have end hole which is used for selective catheterization of small vessels or in pediatric patients. The side holes in multipurpose catheter is used for flush injections in smaller vessels which cannot accommodate the loop of pigtail catheter, e.g. iliac vessels.
- *Pigtail* **(Fig. 6)**: It is a multiple side hole and end hole catheter with a circular shape and is used for flush injections in large lumen vessels like aorta. The pigtail shape prevents direct intimal injury and ensures much less recoil of catheter after forceful injection of contrast through a pressure injector. It is also commonly used for drainage of collections as it gets secured within the cavity.
- *Picard* **(Fig. 6)**: It is an end hole catheter with tip angled at obtuse shape (100°). It is commonly used to selectively catheterize forward facing angled origin vessels like the arch vessels and bronchial arteries.
- *Cobra* **(Fig. 7A)**: It is an end hole catheter with a double curve shape and is commonly used for selective catheterization of visceral vessels. It is available in three different curve shapes C1, C2 and C3 with C2 being the most commonly used.
- *Renal double curve (RDC)* **(Fig. 7B)**: As the name suggests, it has two curves and is used for catheterization of renal vessels. The secondary curve rests against the aortic wall whereas the primary curve enters the vessel.
- *Head hunter* **(Fig. 7C)**: It has three curves. It is used for selective catheterization of the head and neck vessels.
- *Simmons* **(Fig. 7D)**: These are reverse curved catheters which are available in three curve shapes S1, S2 and S3 with increasing length of the curved segment. They are used to catheterize vessels with very acute or obtuse angled origin.
- *Slip catheter:* These are catheters with a special hydrophilic coating to increase their pushability within the vessel. They can be of various tip shapes from straight to curved.

Balloon Catheters

These are catheters with a balloon mounted on them close to their distal end. These are used for dilatation of a stenosed vessel, i.e. angioplasty. The balloons can be compliant, i.e. get stretched and increase their diameter on inflation beyond a certain pressure or noncompliant, i.e. do not get stretched beyond a maximum diameter. A noncompliant balloon provides greater dilating force than a similar compliant balloon.

The balloons are most commonly made of polyethylene terephthalate (PET) which is a relatively noncompliant polyster derivative. It appears like a very thin plastic. These balloons should not be used on calcified plaques or metal stents because of high chances of rupture.

Balloons are also be made of nylon derivatives which are relatively more compliant than PET. These are softer but more scratch resistant than a PET balloon. They are commonly used for mounting balloon expandable stents.

The balloons used in interventional radiological practice are of two types:

1. *Noncompliant, high-pressure balloons:* Mainly used for angioplasty. They are most often made of PET. These are used mainly in lower limb, renal, visceral and internal carotid arteries. The larger-sized balloons are used in aorta, veins or in valves. They may also be used for nonvascular applications like dilatation of esophagus, duodenum or colon.
2. *Compliant, low-pressure balloons:* Made of latex, silicone or polyurethane. They are used for temporary vascular occlusion, embolectomy or molding of stent grafts. The vascular occlusion by balloon may be required for the purpose of preventing reflux of embolic material proximally during embolization, or to minimize antegrade blood flow during embolization when alcohol is used as embolising material as in alcohol embolization of renal cell carcinomas or arteriovenous malformations. The embolectomy balloon catheters used for removing acute thrombi and clots from vessels are also compliant. The most commonly used is the Fogarty balloon catheter.

GUIDEWIRE

Medical guidewire is used to access the vascular, biliary and pelvicalyceal system for a variety of diagnostic and therapeutic medical procedures. The purpose of the guidewire is safe introduction and selective positioning of the catheter which is subsequently placed. An initial guidewire, or access wire, is first inserted through body passageways to a location where a medical procedure or treatment is to take place. In the next step, a catheter is advanced over the inserted guidewire, which enables the catheter to follow its predefined pathway to the point of treatment. Thereafter, other devices or fluids may be inserted via the catheter tubing, as needed. A guidewire is typically advanced beyond a stenosed area to allow balloon catheters and stents to treat the area.

The typical guidewires used in interventional radiology are constructed of a tightly wound fine outer wire of steel and a stiff inner "Mendrel" core wire. Addition of nitinol may be done to prevent kinking. Platinum and gold are added for better radiopacity. These wires are made in a variety of sizes and lengths but usually range from 0.010 to 0.038 inch in diameter and 50–300 cm in length. The outside of guidewire frequently has hydrophilic coating or Teflon coating to reduce friction and may be impregnated with heparin to reduce thrombogenicity. The hydrophilic coating works best when the wire is wet. The inner core provides the rigidity of the wire. The inner core wire is tapered towards the introduction end of the guidewire and ends at a variable distance from the tip. Varying the taper and the distance that the core extends towards the ends of guidewire allows one to vary tip flexibility and the transition zone length. Some wires have movable cores so that the flexibility of the tip can be changed at will. Most guidewires have a fine safety wire along the full length to prevent the outer wire coil from uncoiling and breaking off.

Flexible tip standard wires are generally used for routine percutaneous introduction of catheters. Tip flexibility allows the wires to buckle and avoid damaging the vessel. However, one must be aware that even a flexible guidewire may act as a sharp object when it first exits the tip of catheter. Exchange wires are long and allow enough length of the wire between the target site and external site so that a new catheter may be introduced without losing wire purchase internally.

Based on the stiffness of the guidewire, they may be classified as floppy, of normal stiffness (e.g. Terumo hydrophilic guidewire) or stiff/extra stiff (e.g. amplatz). The guidewires may also be classified as (1) steerable which have shaped tips with good torque control and hydrophilic coating and are used for negotiating stenosis, and (2) nonsteerable, which are stiffer wires allowing the positioning of the catheter but not used for crossing the stenosis.

Most guidewires are fragile and can be very expensive. Care should be taken to preserve their useful life as long as possible. Guidewires should be wiped with a saline soaked gauze or lint free pad after each introduction into the body. The build-up of blood clot, fibrin, or dried contrast can render the wire useless. It may also cause it to stick inside the catheters or cause emboli. The guidewires should be stored loosely coiled in a bowl of saline. The saline can be heparinised (5000 U/L) to help prevent thrombus formation.

Selection of Guidewires

Guidewires are a tactile-based surgical tool, which means that physicians take several factors into consideration when choosing their guidewire. Some wires have tapered cores at each ends allowing both ends to be used for introduction. Some guidewires are specially made to enhance their torquability which is the ability to translate rotational movement of the wire on the outset to the tip inside the patient. These wires can be steered into the desired location in the body.

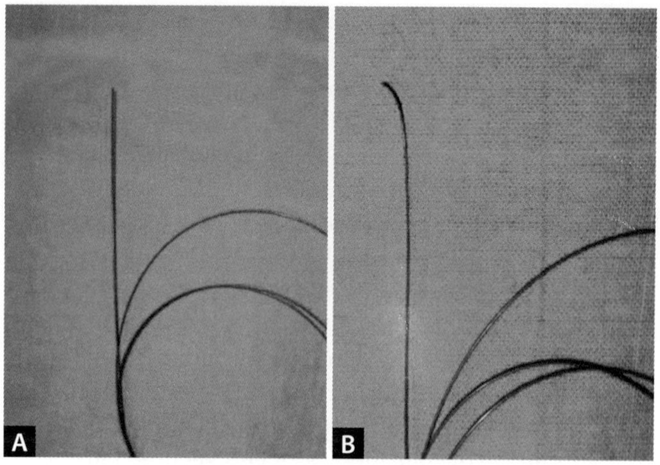

Figs. 8A and B: Guidewire: (A) Straight tip; (B) J-tip.

Based on the shape of the tip, the wires are of two types– J-tip or straight tip **(Figs. 8A and B)**. The J-tip wires are frequently used for hooking the ostium of various arteries. Straight tip guidewire is used to negotiate biliary obstruction during percutaneous biliary drainage (PTBD). The hard end of the guidewire may be used to push the coil inside the catheters from the cartage where it is lodged. The extra or superstiff guidewire are commonly used for inserting percutaneous drainage catheters or insertion of stents into biliary system.

FINE NEEDLE ASPIRATION CYTOLOGY AND BIOPSY NEEDLE

Biopsy or Fine needle aspiration cytology (FNAC) are procedures to obtain a sample of tissue from a tumor for pathological examination. The FNAC is a simple and fast procedure for cytological diagnosis. The core needle biopsy is more reliable than FNAC but requires thicker needle, longer processing time and is a little more invasive than FNAC. Needle biopsy may be used to take tissue or fluid samples from muscles, bones and organs, such as the liver or lungs.

The various types of needles that are commonly used for radiologic procedures are as follows:

- *Needle size:* Fine needles (20–25 Gauge) are ideal for cytology and can be safely introduced even through the bowel (except colon) with less chance of hemorrhage.

Larger needles (14–19 Gauge) have a better yield of tissue which can help in further subtyping. But it is more traumatic.
- Cutting edge of the needle could be end cutting (acute bevel/ninety degree bevel) or side cutting (cannula gap/ stylet gap).
- Spring loaded/automated side cutting needles are also available.

The selection of the size of needles usually depends on the procedure, size and location of the target. Small lesions at deeper location may require 20 G needle as it is stiffer than 22 G which can bend during insertion. However, 22 G needles will be optimum for FNAC of superficial lesions like thyroid or lesions located in the surface of liver. Whenever there is a need to transgress bowel (as in FNAC of pancreatic mass or mesenteric nodes) or a potential space (as in FNAC of lung mass through pleura) or in very hypervascular mass (as in kidney, thyroid), fine needles of 20–25 G need to be used for less complication. Thicker needles (14–19 G) should be used in suspected case of lymphoma as well as in equivocal fine needle aspirate in case of unknown primary. Longer needles like Chiba (20–25 G, Cook catheter, Bloomington, IN) are used whenever samples to be taken from a deeper location.

When a single needle technique is used, multiple punctures are required to obtain multiple samples. This can be more traumatic at times. Alternatively, a co-axial needle system can be used to obtain multiple samples using a single puncture. In this system, a thinner inner needle is inserted through a larger outer needle called an introducer. True-cut-type cutting needles powered by spring-activated handles can be used to obtain a bigger core of tissue, which is of particular importance in the diagnosis of benign lesions (as in benign lung nodules-granulomas/hamartomas) and in lymphoma.

STENT

A stent is a fine tubular structure open at both end that is usually placed into a tubular structure to keep its lumen open.

The procedure of placing a stent is called stenting. Commonly placement of stents is done in vascular, biliary and urinary system. Other reasons to use stents include keeping open a blockage in the airways. The general categories of stents are self-expanding (SE), balloon-expandable (BE), and stent-grafts (SGs).

SE stents **(Fig. 9A)** are composed of nitinol or elgiloy that are compressed into a delivery catheter that is unjacketed at the point of delivery. They are flexible but are prone for foreshortening. The example of SE stents are wallstent (Boston Scientific), SMART (Cordis Endovascular) and Zilver (Cook).

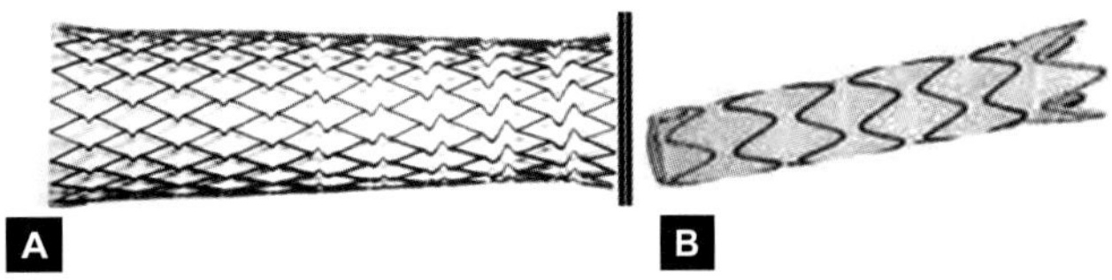

Figs. 9A and B: Stents: Self-expanding stent (A) and covered stent graft (B).

The BE stents are manufactured premounted on a balloon and deployed by dilating with a balloon with an inflator. The BE stents possess stronger radial force but have the potential for dislodgement from the balloon. The Palmaz (Cordis Endovascular) and Express (Boston Scientific) are examples of BE stents.

The stent-grafts (SGs) may SE or BE which are covered with synthetic material, such as Dacron or PTFE **(Fig. 9B)**. Potentially they can prevent the restenosis by their barrier effect but they are costly. Wall graft (Boston Scientific) is a self-expanding stent graft whereas iCast (Atrium Medical, Hudson) is a balloon-expandable stent graft used for aorto-iliac occlusion. These are used when the walls of the vessel need to be covered as in pseudoaneurysms and arterio-venous fistulas. The disadvantage of these stent-grafts in vascular use is that if there are branches arising from the segment of parent vessel in which graft is placed, they get blocked.

Commonly placement of stents is used in vascular, biliary and excretory system. Other reasons to use stents include keeping open a blockage in the airways.

Vascular Stent

The commonly performed vascular stenting is used for coronary, carotid, aorta and lower limb arteries. Vascular stenting is used after angioplasty to treat conditions that involve a narrowing or blockage of arteries or veins throughout the body, including:
- Narrowing of large arteries (aorta and its branches) due to atherosclerosis, or hardening of the arteries, a gradual process in which cholesterol and other fatty deposits, called plaques buildup on the artery walls.
- Peripheral artery disease (PAD), narrowing of the arteries in the legs or arms. In patients with PAD, angioplasty alone or angioplasty with stenting may be used to open up a blocked artery in the pelvis, leg or arm.
- Renal vascular hypertension, high blood pressure caused by a narrowing of the kidney arteries. Angioplasty with stenting is a commonly used method

to open one or both of the arteries that supply blood to the kidneys. Treating renal arterial narrowing is also performed in some patients to protect or improve the kidney function.

- Carotid artery stenosis, narrowing of the neck arteries supplying blood to the brain.
- Coronary artery disease, a narrowing of the coronary arteries that carry blood and oxygen to the heart muscle. An intraluminal coronary artery stent is a small, self-expanding, metal mesh tube that is placed inside a coronary artery after balloon angioplasty to prevent the artery from reclosure.
- Venous narrowings involving the central veins (in the chest, abdomen or pelvis). In some cases, stenting of the narrowed vein is also needed.
- Keeping artificial communication between hepatic vein and portal vein in TIPS.
- Narrowing in dialysis fistula or grafts. When there is decreased flow in the graft or fistula so that it is not adequate for dialysis, angioplasty is generally the first line of treatment. Stenting or stent-grafting may also be needed in some cases.

A drug-eluting stent is coated with a medicine that stops the growth of fibroblast further prevent the arteries from reclosing. It is like any other coronary artery or peripheral artery stents which is left permanently in the artery.

Biliary Stent

Biliary stents are usually placed to relieve a benign or malignant obstruction of the biliary tree. It may be plastic or metallic and the two most common methods that are used to place a biliary stent are endoscopic retrograde cholangiopancreatography (ERCP) and percutaneous transhepatic cholangiography. Biliary stenting is used to treat obstructions that occur in the bile ducts. There are a number of conditions, malignant or benign, that can cause strictures of the bile duct. Pancreatic cancer is the most common malignant cause, followed by cancers of the gallbladder, bile duct, liver, and large intestine. Noncancerous causes of bile duct stricture include injury to the bile ducts during cholecystectomy, gallstones, pancreatitis and primary sclerosing cholangitis.

An internal stent prevents the problems related to external drainage like, pericatheter leakage of bile. The disadvantage is the procedure of insertion which is invasive. Better patency rates are reported with metallic than with plastic stents in cases of malignant obstruction, though no effect on survival is noted. Plastic internal stents **(Fig. 10)** are cheapest but reportedly prone to migration. Various types of plastic stents in use include the Carey-Coons stent (Percuflex; Meditech/Boston Scientific) and silicone stents (Malecot; Cook, Inc).

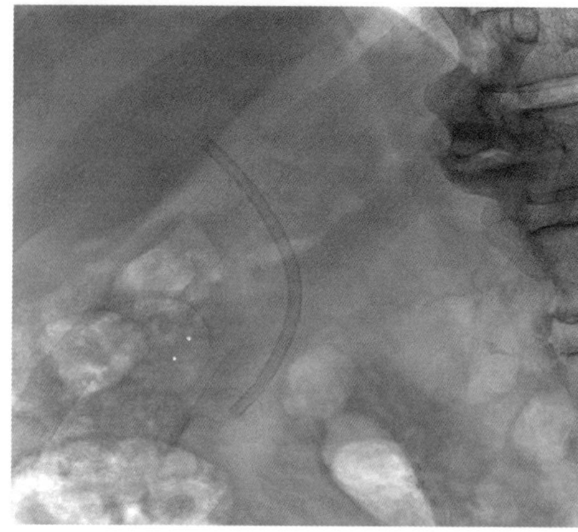

Fig. 10: Plastic stent seen within the common bile duct.

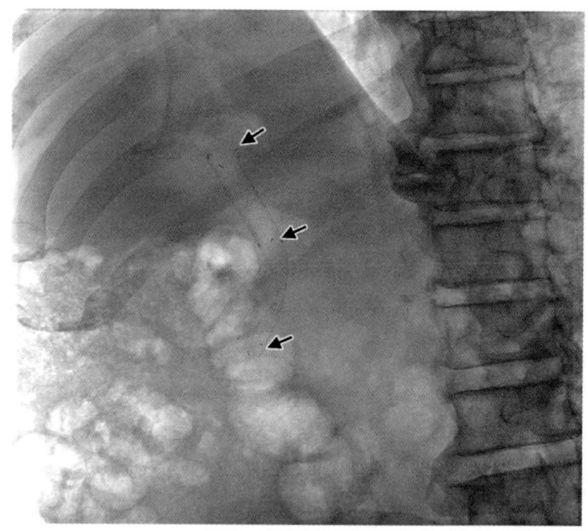

Fig. 11: Metallic stent inside the CBD—note the radiopaque markers (arrows) in the upper, mid and lower part of the stent.

Metallic stents **(Fig. 11)** are generally not used in the treatment of benign disease because studies have shown poor long-term patency rates. The Gianturco-Rosch Z stent (Cook, Inc), a metallic stent, has been used in benign strictures, but it should not be used for primary treatment. Limited applications may include the treatment of patients who are poor surgical candidates or of those in whom surgical treatment fails. Most postoperative strictures are treated surgically, though endoscopic and (less commonly) percutaneous placement of nonmetallic stents has increasingly been used in the past few years.

In cases of malignant obstruction, stents are placed as a palliative measure only if the tumor is unresectable. Various stents are approved for use in the biliary system, including self-expanding and balloon-mounted stents. Various self-expanding stents include the Wallstent (Boston Scientific; Natick, Mass), Luminex stent (Bard; Tempe, Ariz), and Smartstent (Cordis Endovascular; Miami, Fla).

Ureteral Stents

Ureteral stents **(Fig. 12)** are used to ensure the patency of a ureter. Ureteral stents are used to relieve ureteral obstruction, promote ureteral healing following surgery, and to assist with ureteral identification during pelvic surgery. This method is sometimes used as a temporary measure to prevent damage to a blocked kidney until a procedure to remove the stone can be performed. Indwelling times of 12 months or longer are indicated to hold open ureters which have been compressed by tumors in the neighborhood of the ureter or by tumors of the ureter itself. In many cases, these tumors are inoperable and the stents are used to ensure drainage of urine through the ureter. If drainage is compromised for longer periods, the kidney can be damaged. The main complications with ureteral stents are dislocation, infection, and blockage by encrustation. Recently, stents with coatings (e.g. heparin) have been approved to reduce infection, encrustation and, therefore, the frequency of stent replacement.

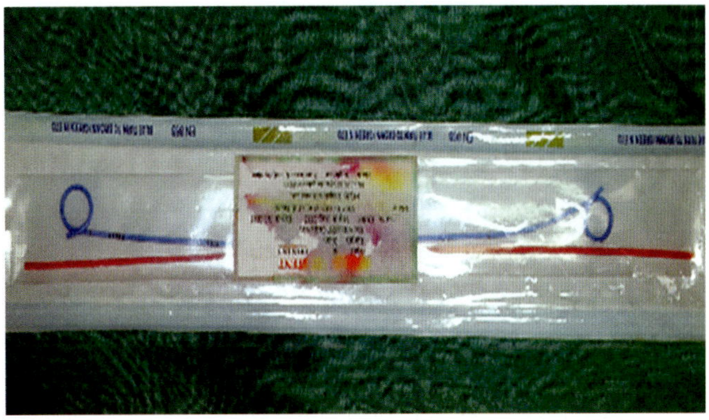

Fig. 12: Plastic double J ureteric stent with the pusher.

EMBOLIZING AGENTS

Embolizing agents are materials used to acutely stop blood flow in a vessel by mechanical occlusion. The clinical uses are to stop hemoptysis, hematuria, hematochezia, internal bleed or a pseudoaneurysm. Embolization may also be done as an adjunct to surgery or for palliation of malignant tumors. The embolising agents can be temporary or permanent. The embolization can be done in proximal vessel or in distal bed. Further, the embolization may or may not lead to organ/cellular death. Based on these requirements, the embolising agents are divided into four main categories:

- Permanent proximal occluders
- Permanent distal occluders
- Temporary proximal occluders
- Temporary distal occluders.

Permanent Proximal Occluders

- *Coils:* These are made of steel or platinum. They commonly have constituent thrombogenic polyester fibers. They are introduced within the vessel in straightened condition but form a spring shape when ejected out of the distal end of delivery catheter. They form a scaffolding upon which thrombus forms leading to permanent occlusion of the vessel. The coils come in various sizes depending upon the size of the wire used, the length of the coil and the diameter of the unconstrained coil. A typical example is 35-3-4. The 35 represents the diameter of the wire used to make the coil in inches which in turn determines the catheter lumen through which it will pass through. The 3 represents the length of straightened coil in centimeter which is chosen based on length of vessel available for deployment of coil and the 4 represents the diameter of the unconstrained coil loop in milimeter which is chosen based on diameter of the vessel in which the coil is to be deployed. Coils measuring .018 inches or less are termed microcoils and require microcatheters for their deployment. Nester coils are special fibred coils on a platinum strut which are soft and pliable. They conform to the target vessel anatomy when deployed and mainly used for filling-up space in large vessels or aneurysms as they bunch up within the lumen. The coils are of two types based on method of deployment: (1) pushable can be pushed out of the catheter by a guidewire or coil pushers, and (2) detachable are detached from the catheter tip *in vivo* by either mechanical pressure or electrolytically.
- *Amplatzer vascular plug* is a nitinol mesh device which is self-expandable occlusive agent. It is deployed by mechanical detachment and is used to occlude vessels ranging from 4 to 16 mm diameter.

The other less commonly used materials in this category are detachable balloons made of latex or silicon (used for treatment of caroticocavernous fistulas), small intestinal submucosa, suture material and bare angiographic wires.

Permanent Distal Occluders

- *Polyvinyl alcohol (PVA) particles* **(Fig. 13A)**: This is an inert plastic particle which comes in varying sizes from 100 to 1100 µm. It is available in small vials with each vial having particles of a range of sizes, e.g. 300–500 µm, 500–700 µm, etc. It is in fine dry coarse powder form which needs to be suspended in saline or contrast before it is injected through the catheter. The size of the particles to be injected is chosen based on the size of the distal vessel bed to be embolized. The particles go and form clumps within the vessels to permanently occlude it. If larger size particles are chosen they may cause clumping within the catheter or proximal vessel itself to lead to their occlusion. These are most commonly used in tumor bed embolizations (often preoperatively to decrease the vascularity), bronchial artery embolizations, uterine fibroid embolizations, etc. The end point is distal occlusion of the small arterioles without proximal vessel occlusion thereby, keeping the option of future repeat embolization of the same vascular territory. One vial of PVA particles costs approximately ₹ 5000. PVA is also available in the form of spherical PVA which makes it more compressible and therefore, facilitates the delivery. The typical examples are bead block made of hydrogel PVA or embospheres constituted from triacryl gelatin spherical hydrophilic spheres.
- *Sclerosants:* These are liquid agents which produce vascular occlusion by causing inflammation and thrombosis. Absolute alcohol and sodium tetradecyl sulfate (STS) are the two most commonly used sclerosants. Absolute alcohol, besides causing permanent vessel occlusion, also leads to cell death and tissue ablation. It is therefore, reserved for use where the end-organ cell death is acceptable, e.g. in renal cell carcinomas. It is a very painful procedure and thus is best performed under general anesthesia or liberal analgesia at least. The use of protective devices like proximal balloons is often required with the use of alcohol to prevent nontarget embolization. Sodium tetradecyl sulfate (STS) **(Fig. 13B)** is a relatively milder sclerosant which does not lead to cell death. A 3% concentration solution is used. It is mainly used for spermatic vein ablations, pelvic congestion syndrome and for venous vascular malformations.
- *Cyanoacrylates:* These are tissue adhesives. The most common used product is N-butyl cyanoacrylate (NBCA) or glue **(Fig. 13C)**. These are in the form of clear liquids at room temperature which get instantly polymerized when they come in contact with an ionic environment. Thus even a small amount of saline or blood leads to initiation of polymerization reaction of cyanoacrylates. For this reason when they are to be injected via the delivery catheter, the catheter should be flushed completely with a nonionic solution (most commonly used 20% dextrose) before and after each injection to prevent polymerization of the agent within the catheter. As soon as the agent ejects out of the distal catheter tip within the vessel, it comes in contact of blood (ionic) and gets polymerized to form a cast. Also, since the cyanoacrylates are radiolucent, they are delivered by mixing them with a radiopaque

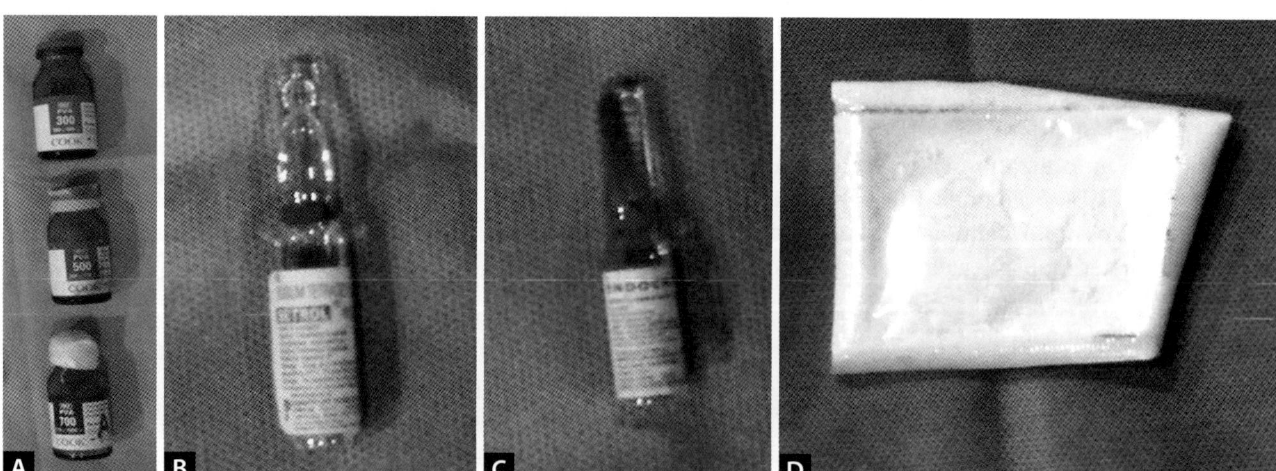

Figs. 13A to D: Embolizing agents: (A) PVA particles of various sizes; (B) Sodium tetradecyl sulfate; (C) N-butyl cyanoacrylate; (D) Gelfoam.

substance to make them visible under fluoroscopy. Ethiodol (brand name Lipiodol by Guerbet) is the most commonly used nonionic substance for the same. It is usually mixed in ratio of 1:1 to 5:1 to make 50–20% concentration of glue respectively. Higher the concentration of glue (lesser the amount of ethiodol added), the more proximal and earlier is the cast formation of glue when it comes in contact with blood at the distal end of catheter within the body. A lesser concentration leads to farther delivery of the embolic agent with a slightly delayed cast formation. The embolus which ultimately forms is larger than anticipated with the amount of cyanoacrylate as the substance draws blood elements within it. One vial of glue costs approximately ₹ 500.

- *Onyx:* It is a liquid embolic agent formed by combination of ethylene-vinyl alcohol copolymer, dimethyl sulfoxide and tantalum powder. It comes in the form of two vials, one containing the copolymer mixed with tantalum powder and the other containing dimethyl sulfoxide. These need to mixed and shaked in a shaker for 20 minutes immediately prior to injection for the agent to become ready for use. The onyx forms a cast as soon as it gets in contact with ionic material (like glue). The cast formation starts from outer surface to inner region. The major advantage of using onyx is much better control over the injection than glue but the deterrent is significantly higher in cost with one vial costing approximately ₹ 40,000.
- *Thrombin:* It is an enzyme which participates in the coagulation pathway and converts fibrinogen to fibrin. It is mainly used for hemostasis on surgically cut surfaces in the operation theater. Intravascularly, it has been used to induce thrombosis of pseudoaneurysms. Care is required to prevent its propagation into main vessel so as to prevent its occlusion.
- *Ethiodol:* It is manufactured under the brand name lipiodol. It is an inert oil-based contrast agent which is also used as embolising agent. The radiopaque properties of lipiodol help to make it visible during embolization procedure. Once injected into the vessel, the fat droplets get released and travel distally into smaller vessels till they cannot cross due to their size and then occlude the vessel. This level of distal embolization is at the level of small arterioles. It is commonly used mixed with glue for embolization. The radiopacity of lipiodol adds contrast to glue while the oil-based structure does not allow glue to solidify within the syringe/catheter till it comes in contact with ionic blood. Lipiodol is also used for embolization of hepatocellular carcinoma in combination with chemotherapeutic agents. It has affinity for the lesion and gets deposited in it even when injected nonselectively besides providing radiopacity to the mixture.

Temporary Proximal Occluders

- *Gelatin sponge:* It is most commonly used in the form of gelfoam **(Fig. 13D)**. It is available as a block which is cut into small pledgets and is made as a slurry mixed with contrast agent for intravascular injection. It leads to temporary mechanical occlusion of proximal vessels for a period of one week to few months. It is used in situations where preservation of blood flow is required in the long- term, e.g. to control bleeding from liver, spleen and in immediate preoperative embolization of tumors. Being inexpensive and easy to use, it is often used as a scaffold for combined embolization with coils.
- Autologous clot used for very short-term temporary embolization as it gets lysed within few hours. It may also be used in coagulopathic patients to control bleeding.
- Nondetachable occlusion balloon used in specific situations like before surgery to reduce intraoperative blood loss, for precise placement of embolic material or to reduce reflux of embolizing material into parent vessel.

Temporary Distal Occluders

- *Starch microspheres:* These are produced from vegetable sources like corn and potato. They are used for very short duration (few minutes) occlusion of distal small vessels, e.g. in procedures like intra-arterial chemotherapy.
- *Gelatin sponge powder:* It is also available in powder form. When delivered; it reaches distal circulation to block it temporarily.

SUGGESTED READING

1. Bakal CW. In: Mauro MA, Murphy K, Thomson K , Venbrux AC, Morgan R and Zollikofer CL (Eds). Image-guided Interventions. Philadelphia: Elseviers; 2008.
2. Gabelmann A, Hamid H, Brambs HJ, Rieber A. Metallic stents in benign biliary strictures: long-term effectiveness and interventional management of stent occlusion. Am J Roentgenol. 2001;177(4):813-7.
3. Kaufman JA. In Image-guided interventions, Mauro MA, Murphy K, Thomson K, Venbrux AC, Morgan R and Zollikofer CL (Eds). Philadelphia: Elseviers, 2008.

4. Klein JS, Solomon G, Stewart EA. Transthoracic needle biopsy with a coaxially placed 20-gauge automated cutting needle: results in 122 patients. Radiology. 1996;198:715-20.
5. Lopez RR Jr, Cosenza CA, Lois J, et al. Long-term results of metallic stents for benign biliary strictures. Arch Surg. 2001; 136(6):664-9.
6. Seldinger SI. Catheter placement of needles in percutaneous arteriography: a new technique. Acta Radiol. 1953;39:328-76.
7. Stavropoulos SW, Rajan D, Cope C. In: Baum S, Pentecost MJ (Eds). Abram's angiography: vascular and interventional radiology, 2nd edition. Philadelphia: Lipincott Williams & Wilkins; 2006.
8. Strauss KJ, Damiano MM and Kandarpa K. In: Kandarpa K, Aruny JE (Eds). Handbook of Interventional Radiological Procedures, 3rd edition. Philadelphia: Lipincott Williams & Wilkins; 2002.

CHAPTER 54

Magnetic Resonance Contrast Media

Anju Garg

INTRODUCTION

In the early days of magnetic resonance imaging, it was thought that the excellent soft tissue contrast would obviate the need for any type of contrast agent, making the procedure completely noninvasive. Contrast in MRI arises mainly from the heterogeneous distribution of tissue-relaxation times, and the lack of need for contrast materials is one of the major advantages of MR over other imaging techniques. However, it was noted that many important pathological conditions did not display specific enough changes in relaxation times to differentiate them from surrounding healthy tissue. Exogenous MR contrast agents were therefore developed shortly after the first commercial MR system became available in the 1980s. Presently exogenous contrast agents are frequently used in a significant proportion of MR examinations:

- To differentiate structures that are similar in appearance
- To provide additional specificity in describing regions of abnormal signal
- To specify or highlight spaces
- To depict tissue vascularity and perfusion.

BASIC PRINCIPLES OF MR CONTRAST AGENTS

Contrast agents for X-ray and CT show contrasting effects according to the electron-density difference, and they produce direct contrast effects on their positions. However, the contrast mechanism is more complicated for MRI, where the contrast enhancement occurs as a result of the interaction between the contrast agents and neighboring water protons, which can be affected by many intrinsic and extrinsic factors, such as proton density and MRI pulse sequences.

The basic principle of MRI is based on nuclear magnetic resonance (NMR) together with the relaxation of proton spins in a magnetic field. When the nuclei of protons, i.e the body's hydrogen atoms, are exposed to a strong magnetic field, their spins align either parallel or antiparallel to the magnetic field. During their alignment, the spins precess under a specified frequency, known as the Larmor frequency which is dependant on the strength of the magnetic field applied. When a 'resonance' frequency in the radiofrequency (RF) range is applied, the protons absorb energy and realign from a longitudinal to a perpendicular (or transverse) axis. After the disappearance of the RF pulse, the excited nuclei relax to their initial, lower-energy state. There are two different relaxation pathways. The first, called longitudinal or T1 relaxation, involves the decreased net magnetization recovering to the initial state. The second, called transverse or T2 relaxation, involves the induced magnetization on the perpendicular plane disappearing by the dephasing of spins.

MR contrast agents act by altering these relaxation times and this is measured as relaxivity. The relaxivity of an agent is proportional to the magnitude of its moment, its tumbling frequency in solution and its spin-relaxation time. Based on their relaxation processes, the contrast agents are classified as T1- and T2-contrast agents.

Molecules or ions with one or more unpaired electrons when placed in a magnetic field, generate a magnetic moment which aligns with the applied field. These ions or molecules are referred to as paramagnetic, superparamagnetic or ferromagnetic ions depending on their specific electronic configuration. The most commonly used MR contrast agents are a group of exogenous paramagnetic compounds of gadolinium, manganese and iron.

CLASSIFICATION OF MR CONTRAST AGENTS

MR contrast agents can be classified according to:

- Magnetic property of the agent
- Dominant effect of the agent on the signal intensity
- Biodistribution of the agent.

Magnetic Properties

This is the most common method used to classify the contrast agents into 2 main groups, namely paramagnetic and superparamagnetic.

Paramagnetic Contrast Agents

Paramagnetic materials have their own magnetic field and the local magnetic field of a paramagnetic agent reduces the T1- and T2-relaxation times of surrounding hydrogen nuclei, thus increasing signal on T1-weighted images. There are many paramagnetic metal ions that could potentially be used as MR contrast agents but the transition metal gadolinium (Gd^{3+}) is by far the most commonly used. This is due to a favorable combination of many (seven) unpaired electrons combined with a long electron spin-relaxation time which makes this metal a very efficient relaxation enhancing agent. Manganese, which has relaxation properties similar to gadolinium has also been used. All paramagnetic contrast agents are chelated with an appropriate ligand to minimize *in vivo* toxicity of free metallic ion.

Superparamagnetic Contrast Agents

Superparamagnetic agents behave in a manner similar to a paramagnetic substance. In clinical MRI, small or ultrasmall particles of superparamagnetic iron oxide are used as contrast agents. If the iron ions are magnetically ordered within the crystal, the net magnetic moment is so large that it greatly exceeds that of typical paramagnetic ions. This effect is referred to as superparamagnetism and is characterized by a large magnetic moment in the presence of an external magnetic field but no remnant magnetic moment when the field is zero. Superparamagnetic agents can also induce strong enhancement of the T1-relaxation rate of water (depending on size and composition of the particles), but their dominant effect is on T2/T2* relaxation due to the large magnetic moment of the nanoparticles.

Image Enhancement

The effect of the contrast agent on the signal intensity can either be positive (increase in signal or T1-enhancement) or negative (signal reduction or T2-enhancement). Almost all MR contrast agents will affect both T1- and T2-relaxation times and the distinction depends on many MR-specific parameters as well as contrast agent dose, e.g. gadolinium generally act as a positive enhancers on T1-weighted images but also have a weak T2-negative enhancing effect whereas iron oxide based contrast agents have a predominant T2 and T2* shortening effect and are negative agents.

Biodistribution

The biodistribution of a contrast agent describes how the agent is distributed *in vivo* after intravenous administration.

Extracellular-fluid Agents

Small-molecular weight (MW) paramagnetic agents are small enough to diffuse from the plasma into the interstitium and are thus distributed to the extracellular fluid. These agents are referred to as extracellular-fluid (ECF) agents. They are not taken up by cells and are therefore eliminated by renal excretion with a half-life determined by the glomerular filtration rate, e.g. gadolinium-based contrast agents.

Intravascular Agents

Intravascular agents are contrast agents with a MW large enough to prevent leakage from the vascular to the extravascular space. All iron oxide nanoparticles are intravascular agents, with a half-life in blood ranging from a few minutes to several hours. In blood, iron oxide agents with the appropriate composition can produce significant T1 shortening and several studies have investigated the use of nanoparticles for MR angiography. Other types of intravascular agents are based on macromolecular gadolinium compounds. Such agents are designed either by linking Gd^{3+} ions to a macromolecular polymer during synthesis or by making the Gd^{3+}-complex bind to plasma proteins after injection and thus forming macromolecules in blood.

Tissue-specific Agents

Tissue-specific agents are agents which have been specifically designed to accumulate in a given organ or tissue type. Intravascular iron oxides are taken up by the Kupffer cells of the liver, spleen and lymphatic system. Once taken up by the liver the nanoparticles will be accumulated into larger particulate clusters in the Kupffer cells and relaxation will be completely dominated by T2/T2* effects. Iron oxides can thus be said to be both intravascular agents as well as tissue specific agents. Mangafodipir trisodium and few gadolinium chelates also act as liver specific agents as they are taken up by hepatocytes.

Contrast agents have also been developed, and are in clinical testing, for targeting of atherosclerotic plaques as well as different types of tumor antibodies.

GADOLINIUM-BASED CONTRAST AGENTS

In the early 1980s, Copper (Cu^{2+}), Manganese (Mn^{2+}) and Gadolinium (Gd^{3+}) were recognized as paramagnetic ions capable of shortening the T_1 of water. After extensive testing of many paramagnetic chelates, the gadolinium diethlye triamine penta-acetic acid salt (Gd-DPTA) was singled out because of its high tolerability in animals and preserved good relaxation properties. Gadolinium-DTPA was first tested in humans in 1983 and in early 1988, the pharmaceutical product gadopentetate dimeglumine was launched as the first MR contrast medium.[1]

Gadolinium has an atomic number 64 and is one of a series of 17 chemically inert metals, the lanthanides. Gadolinium is named after the Finnish chemist Johan Gadolin.[2] It is a paramagnetic agent because of its seven unpaired electrons. This strong paramagnetic effect disturbs the relaxivity of nearby water protons resulting in a decrease of both T1- and T2-relaxation times. The reduction in the T1-relaxation time is greater at low gadolinium concentrations and this is seen as increased signal intensity on T1-weighted spin-echo or gradient-echo images.

Free Gd^{3+} ion is highly toxic *in vivo* because it competes with calcium. As gadolinium has a higher binding affinity for calcium-binding enzymes, it can displace calcium and thus alter all biological processes catalyzed by these enzymes. Free gadolinium also interferes with calcium channels to block physiological pathways that rely on Ca^{2+} influx, i.e. neural transmission and coagulation.[3] However, when it is bound (or chelated) to an organic ligand, gadolinium is generally regarded as safe for use as an MR contrast agent.

Currently there are nine Gadolinium-based contrast agents (GBCAs) approved for use in the United States and/or the European Union. Most available GBCAs are low molecular weight polyamino-carboxylate compounds **(Table 1)**.

They can broadly be classified into two categories based on their binding to serum proteins: (i) nonspecific-extracellular gadolinium chelates or agents which do not bind to serum proteins and (ii) high-relaxivity agents, which bind to serum proteins. The **nonspecific-extracellular GBCAs** include gadopentetate, gadoterate, gadodiamide, gadoteridol, gadobutrol, and gado-versatamide. They do not bind to any protein and their biodistribution and pharmacokinetics are essentially similar to iodinated water-soluble contrast media.

Table 1: Gadolinium-based contrast agents approved for clinical use.[6]

Generic name	*Trade name/ Manufacturer*	*T1-relaxivity (L/mmol/s at 1.5 T)*	*Molecular weight*	*Excretion*	*Protein binding*
Gadopentetate dimeglumine Gd-DTPA	Magnevist/Bayer	4.1	939.0	Renal	None
Gadoterate meglumine Gd-DOTA	Dotarem/Guerbert	3.6	558.6	Renal	None
Gadodiamide Gd-DTPA-BMA	Omniscan/GE	4.3	573.6	Renal	None
Gadoteridol Gd-HP-DO3A	ProHance/Bracco	4.1	558.7	Renal	None
Gadobutrol Gd-DO3A-butrol	Gadovist/Bayer	4.7	604.7	Renal	None
Gadoversetamide Gd-DTPA-BMEA	Optimark/Mallinckrodt	4.7	661.8	Renal	None
Gadobenate disodium Gd-BOPTA	MultiHance/Bracco	8.3	1058.2	96% renal, 4% hepatic	<5%
Gadoxetate disodium Gd-EOB-DTPA	Primovist, Eovist/Bayer	6.9	682.0	50% renal, 50% hepatic	<10%
Gadofosveset trisodium	Vasovist, Ablavar/Bayer	19	958.0	91% renal, 9% hepatic	>85%

After intravenous injection, they rapidly diffuse into the interstitial extravascular space. Reverse diffusion into the intravascular compartment also occurs and a state of equilibrium between diffusion in and out is usually reached within 2 hours. They are eliminated unchanged from the intravascular compartment by passive glomerular filtration and by 24 hours greater than 95% of the injected dose is excreted in urine with normal renal function. A very small amount (less than 0.1%) is eliminated via feces. Biological half-life is approximately 1.5 hours in patients with normal renal function.

Three basic phases of vascular and tissue enhancement occur following administration of GBCAs: arterial, blood pool and extracellular phases. Routine postcontrast images are acquired when the contrast has reached the extracellular interstitial space, i.e. approximately 2 minutes after injection. As the extracellular enhancement changes little over several minutes, fast scanning techniques are not essential for imaging. Interstitial enhancement is particularly conspicuous with suppression of the lipid signal intensity and T1W, fat suppressed images give the best contrast. However, if fat is nulled via inversion recovery with a short inversion time (STIR), enhancing tissue is also nulled because of its short T1 relaxation time. Therefore, the STIR technique is not recommended after administration of T1-shortening contrast agents.

Interstitial contrast agent is particularly prominent in tissues such as neoplasms and areas of inflammation. Fibrous tissue typically has a large interstitial space, therefore is much enhanced on extracellular phase images even though it is usually hypovascular. Many metastases also have large interstitial spaces and are hyperintense on extracellular phase images. Brain and testicular capillaries are not permeable to these contrast agents, unlike capillaries throughout the rest of the body. So, the enhancement of the brain is minimal, owing entirely to enhancement of the blood pool. Tumors and injured brain parenchyma enhance much more because of the enhancement of their interstitial space and so the depiction of brain lesions in postcontrast images is very high. In addition to diffusing across tissue capillary walls, GBCAs diffuse across glomerular walls into the renal tubules, within which they are concentrated as water is reabsorbed. This makes them highly effective for enhancing the kidneys and the urinary tract.

Arterial phase images are best acquired during the first pass of contrast agent through the arterial system, i.e. within 20 seconds of contrast administration. Early arterial images are best for depicting arteries, and later arterial phase images are better for depicting hypervascular tissues. Blood pool or the portal venous phase occurs at 60–90 seconds after contrast administration during which contrast is typically distributed throughout the body's vessels. Maximum liver parenchymal enhancement is also achieved during this phase. Dynamic imaging for detection and characterization of lesions in the liver and other organs can be performed, similar to CT, using nonspecific extracellular GBCAs.

The **high-relaxivity agents** include gadobenate, gadoxetate and gadofosveset. These agents bind to proteins and have a higher T1 relaxivity than the above mentioned gadolinium chelates **(Table 1)**. **Gadobenate and gadoxetate** act as nonspecific extracellular gadolinium chelates immediately after the bolus injection but later they are taken up by liver cells and so act as liver specific agents in the delayed phase. They are excreted through both, renal and hepatobiliary pathways. *Gadobenate dimeglumine* has a capacity for weak and transient protein bonding. Only 2 to 4% of the injected dose is taken up by liver cells and its delayed imaging time is 90–120 minutes. *Gadoxetate disodium* has the maximum biliary excretion (almost equal biliary and renal excretion) and has a convenient delayed imaging time of 10–20 minutes. It also results in a much more intense liver parenchymal enhancement than gadobenate. These two agents behave similarly to other gadolinium chelates during the initial phase and thus are helpful in assessing tumor enhancement and characterization. During the later phases, they selectively increase the signal intensity of the liver (via hepatocyte uptake), thus aiding in the detection of small tumors. This is dependent on the degree of differentiation of the tumor, as well-differentiated hepatocellular carcinoma may take up the contrast and become less conspicuous. However, these agents are best utilized for detection of metastases. In addition, because of biliary excretion during the delayed phase, the biliary ducts can be mapped well using T1-weighted images.

Gadofosevet has 80–90% binding to serum albumin. This high protein binding has 2 effects: firstly, it markedly increases the relaxivity (hence requiring lower doses and concentration) and secondly, it results in the agent being effectively confined to the vascular space. Due to its prolonged intravascular retention, it has been successfully used as a blood pool agent for MR angiography. The protein binding is reversible and gadofosevet is ultimately excreted unchanged by the kidneys through glomerular filtration.

As mentioned earlier, gadolinium must be chelated to reduce its toxicity. There are differences in the chemical structure of chelates used to bind the gadolinium ion—macrocyclic or linear. The chemical structure of a typical macrocyclic and a typical linear GBCA are depicted in **Figures 1A and B**. Gadolinium chelates can also be categorized into 4 classes based on their biochemical structure—macrocyclic or linear, and ionicity—ionic or nonionic as given below:

Linear, ionic—gadopentetate, gadobenate, gadoxetate and gadofosveset
Linear, nonionic—gadodiamide and gadoversetamide
Macrocyclic, ionic—gadoterate
Macrocyclic nonionic—gadoteridol and gadobutrol

The GBCAs vary with respect to osmolality and viscosity. Their osmolality ranges between 0.63 osmol/kg to 1.97 osmol/kg **(Table 2)**. *In vivo*, the the osmotic load of all the GBCAs is very low, compared to iodinated contrast media, because only a small amount of the contrast agent is required to produce a diagnostic MR examination. The nonionic agents tend to have lower osmolarity and are less viscous. Nonionic low-osmolar GBCAs also have lesser negative-isotropic effects, which is an important consideration for cardiac patients. Low viscosity GBCAs require less pressure to inject and can be administered using smaller-gauge needles or catheters.

The stability of an agent describes the affinity of the gadolinium atom for its compound and depends on its thermodynamic and conditional stability. The dissociation constants **(Table 2)** can be used to describe the stability of the linear GBCAs. The higher the dissociation constants, the greater the stability of the agent. Unlike the linear agents, the macrocyclic agents require a significant amount of energy to dissociate the gadolinium complexes. With these agents the kinetics of dissociation are described by the dissociation rate and the dissociation half-life. In general, the ionic agents are more stable than the nonionic ones.[4] When considering agents by class, the stability increases from nonionic linear to ionic linear to macrocyclic agents.[5,6]

Given the toxicity of the free metal ion, many agents are bound to excess chelate **(Table 2)**. The excess chelate is considered necessary because of the possibility for transmetallation with trace amounts of zinc in the

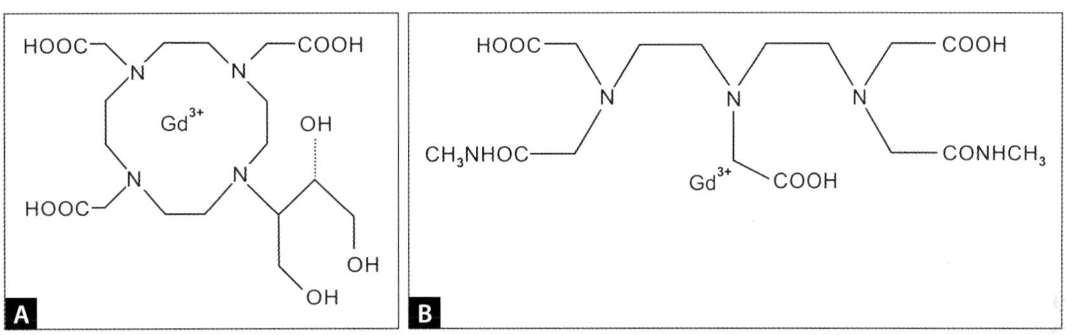

Figs. 1A and B: Chemical structure of gadolinium-based contrast agents: (A) Typical-macrocyclic agent—gadobutrol; (B) Typical-linear agent—gadodiamide.

Table 2: Physicochemical properties of gadolinium-based contrast agents.[7]

Generic name/ Trade name	*Osmolality (37°C, osmol/kg H_2O)*	*Viscosity (mPa at 37°C)*	*Thermodynamic stability constant*	*Conditional stability constant at pH 7.4*	*Metal chelates (mg/mL)*	*Excess chelates (mg/mL)*
Gadopentetate/Magnevist	1.96	2.9	22.1	18.1	469	0.4
Gadoterate meglumine/ Dotarem	1.35	2.0	25.8	18.8	278.3	0
Gadodiamide/Omniscan	0.79	1.4	16.9	14.9	287	12
Gadoteridol/Prohance	0.63	1.3	23.8	17.1	279.3	0.23
Gadobutrol/Gadovist	1.6	4.96	21.8	14.7	605	0.5
Gadoversetamide/Optimark	1.11	2.0	16.6	15.0	330.9	28.4
Gadobenate/Multihance	1.97	5.3	22.6	18.4	334	0
Gadoxetate/Primovist/Eovist	0.688	1.19	23.5	18.7	181.4	1
Gadofosveset/Vasovist	0.825	1.8	22.1	18.9	244	0.27

blood and a resulting release of free gadolinium ion. Accordingly, the least stable agents, gadodiamide and gadoversatamide, the two agents with the weakest thermodynamic stability constants, each have considerably larger amounts of excess chelate (12 mg/mL and 28.4 mg/mL, respectively) than the most stable agents, gadoterate and gadoteridol (0 and 0.23 mg/mL of excess chelate, respectively). The presence and quantity of excess chelate can be taken as an indirect marker of the instability of the contrast agent.[6,7]

Interaction between Extracellular Magnetic Resonance Contrast Agents with Clinical Tests

Extracellular magnetic resonance contrast agents may cause spurious hypocalcemia as they can interfere with the assay method of calcium measurement. Awareness of this effect on calcium measurements by some magnetic resonance contrast agents is important in order to avoid incorrect and potentially hazardous treatment. Caution should be exercised when using colorimetric assays for angiotensin-converting enzyme, calcium, iron, magnesium, total iron-binding capacity and zinc in serum samples of patients who have recently received gadolinium based contrast media. Therefore, biochemical assays are better performed before contrast media injection, or delayed for at least 24 hours afterwards or longer in patients with renal impairment.

Dose: Generally the recommended dose for clinical use is 0.1 mmoL/kg body weight, but up to 0.3 mmoL/kg body weight may be used, particularly for MRA. Smaller doses can be used for the high relaxivity agents.

Adverse Effects of GBCAs

Extracellular magnetic resonance contrast agents are well tolerated and have a low incidence of adverse effects. Mild adverse reactions, such as nausea, vomiting and urticaria occasionally occur after GBCA administration. Other uncommon adverse events include headache, taste disturbance, dizziness, and paraesthesia. While adverse reactions are rare in the general patient population, they are more common in patients with a history of asthma or allergy, and in patients injected at a faster rate.[3]

These types of adverse events are similar with all GBCAs, with no significant differences between agents. The incidence of mild adverse effects is less than 5%. Anaphylactoid reactions have been reported, but they are very infrequent. Life-threatening reactions are very rare with an incidence around 1:100000. Fatal reactions may occur, however, are extremely rare.[8,9]

Contrast-induced Nephropathy

Extracellular magnetic resonance agents are more nephrotoxic than iodinated contrast media in equimolar doses. However, as the dose of gadolinium-based contrast medium required for a diagnostic MRI examination is very small in comparison to doses of iodinated contrast media for CT and other radiographic examinations, nephrotoxicity due to these agents is uncommon even in patients with renal disease. In patients with marked reduction in renal function (particularly due to diabetes mellitus), contrast-induced nephropathy (CIN) may occur even at the standard doses of gadolinium based MR contrast agents.[10]

Gadolinium attenuates X-rays and hence its use for radiographic examinations instead of iodinated contrast media has been advocated in patients with history of serious adverse reactions to iodinated-contrast media and in patients who are to undergo imminent thyroid treatment with radioactive iodine, providing the renal function of these patients was normal. In patients with renal impairment, GBCAs should not be used in place of iodinated contrast media as they can induce nephrotoxicity at the doses required to produce adequate radiographic enhancement.[3]

Extravasation

Monitoring a patient for extravasation can be a challenge in MRI, especially when the patient is deep in the bore of the MR unit. An extravasation can occur at a distance from the injection site. Extravasation of GBCAs into the surrounding tissues can cause edema, inflammation and necrosis.[3] However, in most cases the effect is minimal with no long-term sequelae. Certain patient categories like infants, young children, unconscious and debilitated patients, patients with arterial insufficiency or compromised venous/lymphatic drainage are less able to tolerate extravasation. Low-osmolar, nonionic GBCAs reduce the risk of an extravasation because they tend to be lower viscosity, and because they are better tolerated, the severity is less following extravasation.[11]

Nephrogenic-systemic Fibrosis

Gadolinium-enhanced MRI was considered one of the safest imaging procedures. However, the concern of associated nephrogenic–systemic fibrosis (NSF) have forced the radiology community to rethink its imaging practices. The first case of NSF was described in 1997 as a skin disorder resembling scleromyxedema and termed as nephrogenic- fibrosing dermopathy.[12] Later, when systemic manifestations were identified, the nomenclature was changed to nephrogenic systemic fibrosis. NSF is characterized by scleroderma—like skin changes (swelling, skin induration, skin colored erythematous papules, woody skin) that mainly affect the limbs—lower limbs more than upper limbs and trunk. Fibrotic changes may also affect other organs such as muscles, heart, lungs, liver, kidneys and testes. The disease can be aggressive in some patients leading to severe physical deformity or even death.

The association of gadolinium with development of NSF was first described in 2006 by Grobner.[13] Since then, several studies have documented the presence of gadolinium in the tissues of patients with NSF and have supported the causative role of the contrast agent in the development of this condition.[14-16] The time between injection of GBCA and the onset of NSF symptoms occurs within days to months in the vast majority of patients; however, in rare cases, symptoms have appeared years after the last reported exposure.[6]

Although the exact mechanism of NSF is not yet established, it is known to occur exclusively in patients with decreased renal function (glomerular filtration rate <30 mL/min/1.73 m^2). The most widely held hypothesis is that because of the prolonged clearance time of GBCAs in renally impaired patients, gadolinium chelates have a propensity to undergo transmetallation, in which other cations in the body displace gadolinium from its chelate, releasing free gadolinium. This free gadolinium then binds with an anion, such as phosphate, and the resulting insoluble precipitate is deposited in various tissues. A fibrotic reaction ensues involving the activation of circulating fibrocytes. This theory is supported by the presence of gadolinium in affected tissues of NSF patients relative to unaffected states.[15]

Currently, there is no effective treatment for NSF. Trials with corticosteroid, photopheresis, plasmapheresis, thalidomide, methotrexate, etc. have not had much success. There is also no evidence that immediate hemodialysis protects against the development of NSF. Improving renal function seems to slow or arrest progression of this condition.

Risk Factors for Nephrogenic-systemic Fibrosis

Patient factors: The patients at highest risk for development of NSF are those on dialysis or with acute or chronic renal failure. It is estimated that patients with end-stage chronic kidney disease (CKD5, eGFR <15 mL/min/1.73 m^2) and severe CKD (CKD4, eGFR 15 to 29 mL/min/1.73 m^2) have a 1–7% chance of developing NSF after one or more exposures to at least some GBCAs. There has been only one published case report of a patient with eGFR values above 30 mL/min/1.73 m^2.[17]

It is not understood why some patients with severe CKD or acute kidney injury (AKI) develop NSF following exposure to GBCAs and others do not. One study described 30 patients who had an eGFR of under 30 mL/min/1.73 m^2 and who were exposed to high doses of gadodiamide (median dose of 90 mL and range of 40–200 mL). One of the 30 patients subsequently developed NSF, an observed incidence of about 3%.[18] So, it is postulated that gadolinium is necessary but not sufficient to trigger NSF. A number of possible cofactors have been postulated to play a role. These include metabolic acidosis or medications that predispose patients to acidosis, elevated iron, calcium, and/or phosphate levels, high-dose erythropoietin therapy, immunosuppression, vasculopathy, and infection, or other acute pro-inflammatory events.[19] However, none of these have been consistently confirmed as true cofactors. As a result, routine screening for them prior to GBCA administration is not recommended, although such screening may be performed on an optional basis. Hepatic disease in and of itself, in the absence of AKI or severe CKD, is not considered a risk factor for NSF.[20]

Contrast medium factors: NSF cases have been reported for almost all GBCAs. Although the majority of NSF cases involve the linear GBCAs—the most commonly reported agent being gadodiamide followed by gadopentetate and gadoversatamide—NSF has also been reported for gadoteridol, the macrocyclic formulation.[21] The stability of the binding of the gadolinium within the chelate has been found to be an important factor in pathogenesis of NSF (as discussed above), with macrocyclic chelates offering better protection and binding to gadolinium ion in comparison to the linear molecules. However, the American College of Radiology (ACR) Manual on Contrast Media states, "It must be emphasized that the frequency with which NSF has been associated with different GBCAs may reflect a combination of differences in toxicity, market share, number of years that the agent has been in use, and possible reporting bias. In addition reported frequency is also further confounded by the fact that some agents, particularly gadodiamide, may have been used disproportionately more frequently in patients receiving high doses of GBCAs for magnetic resonance angiography".[20]

The ACR has classified the GBCAs into three groups based on the reported prevalence of NSF with the various agents **(Table 3)**. There is limited data for Group III agents, although, to date, few, if any, unconfounded cases of NSF have been reported.[20]

Table 3: ACR classification of GBCAs based on reported prevalence of NSF.[20]

Group I: Agents associated with the greatest number of NSF cases • Gadodiamide (Omniscan®) • Gadopentetate dimeglumine (Magnevist) • Gadoversetamide (OptiMARK)
Group II: Agents associated with few, if any, unconfounded cases of NSF • Gadobenate dimeglumine (MultiHance) • Gadoteridol (ProHance) • Gadoteric acid (Dotarem) • Gadobutrol (Gadovist)
Group III: Agents which have only recently appeared on the market in the US • Gadofosveset (Ablavar) • Gadoxetate disodium (Eovist)

Besides the chelate stability, high doses of GBCAs, either as a single administration or cumulatively in multiple administrations over months to years, are also associated with higher incidence of NSF.

In spite of differences in the incidence of NSF, there is no evidence that any of the approved GBCAs are safe in the at-risk patient population. Conversely, in patients without renal disease, all gadolinium-based contrast agents seem to be safe.

Guidelines on GBCA Usage

The American College of Radiology (ACR), the Food and Drug Administration in the United States (FDA) and European Commision/European Medicines Agency (EC/EMA) have all given their recommendations on the use of GBCAs. The three groups use different words; however, there are only minor differences between their recommendations.[22] The ACR guidelines are given below:

The ACR recommends that, prior to an MRI using a GBCA, physicians should identify patients who have severe renal failure (GFR <30 mL/min/1.73 m^2) by questioning patients for a history of renal disease and should obtain an eGFR measurement within six weeks of the procedure in patients with (i) renal disease (including patients with a solitary kidney, renal transplant, or renal neoplasm), (ii) over the age of 60 years, and (iii) with hypertension, diabetes mellitus, or a history of severe liver disease. When a high-risk patient is identified, the ACR recommends considering alternative studies and informing these patients about the potential risks of GBCA-enhanced studies and should such studies be deemed necessary, using the lowest-possible dose of GBCA to obtain the necessary clinical information, and avoiding double or triple dose studies, if possible, and avoiding using those GBCAs that have been most frequently associated with NSF.

The ACR has specific recommendations for specific groups of patients: Patients with end-stage renal disease on chronic dialysis: If a contrast-enhanced cross-sectional imaging study is essential it would be reasonable to consider administering iodinated contrast media and performing a CT rather than an MRI. However, if a contrast-enhanced MR examination must be performed in a patient with end-stage renal disease on chronic dialysis, injection of group I agents **(*see* Table 3)** is contraindicated. Also, use of the lowest-possible dose needed to obtain a diagnostic study is recommended and is appropriate. The ACR also recommends that GBCA-enhanced MRI examinations be performed as closely before hemodialysis as is possible, as prompt postprocedural hemodialysis, although unproven to date, may reduce the likelihood that NSF will develop.

Chronic kidney disease stage IV or V (eGFR <30 mL/min/1.73 m^2) not on dialysis: The correct course of action in this patient group is problematic, as administration of iodinated-contrast media for CT may lead to further deterioration of renal function, while administration of GBCA for MRI could result in NSF. It is recommended that any GBCA be avoided in this patient group. However, if GBCA enhanced MRI is deemed essential, use of the lowest possible dose needed to obtain a diagnostic study is recommended Although there is no absolute proof that any GBCA is completely safe in this patient group, group I agents **(*see* Table 3)** have been contraindicated. Further, it may be prudent to avoid readministration of GBCA for several days to a week.

Chronic-kidney disease stage III with eGFR between 30 and 59 mL/min/1.73 m^2: NSF developing after GBCA administration to patients with eGFR > 30 mL/min/1.73 m^2 is exceedingly rare. However, eGFR determinations may fluctuate from one day to the next (with an eGFR level just above 30 on one day changing to an eGFR below 30 on another day). It is for this reason that the precautions described above for CKD4 and CKD5 patients are also recommended for inpatients with an eGFR < 40 mL min/1.73 m^2. In comparison, no special precautions are required in patients with an eGFR of 40 to 59 mL/min/1.73 m^2.

Chronic kidney disease stage I or stage II with eGFR >60 mL/min/1.73 m^2: There is no evidence of increased risk of NSF and all GBCAs can be safely administered using a dose of less than or equal to 0.1 mmol/kg.

Patients with acute kidney injury (AKI): Due to the temporal lag between eGFR (which is calculated using serum creatinine values) and actual glomerular filtration rates, it is not possible to determine whether a given patient has AKI based on a single eGFR determination. Accordingly, caution should be exercised in use of GBCA in patients with known or suspected AKI regardless of measured serum creatinine or calculated eGFR values. The GBCA should only be administered to these patients if absolutely necessary. When GBCA administration is required, agents associated with the greatest apparent NSF-associated risk (Group I agents) should be avoided and lowest possible dose used.

Patients on hemodialysis: There is no evidence supporting the use of hemodialysis in preventing or treating NSF in patients not already undergoing hemodialysis, but it may be useful to remove GBCAs in patients already on hemodialysis according to the EMA. The ACR recommends that enhanced MRI be done shortly before hemodialysis and if the patient is totally anuric, CT (using iodine based contrast material) should be considered.

GBCA Administration in Children[20]

To date, few pediatric cases of NSF have been reported, and no cases have been reported in children under the age of 6 years. Nevertheless, there is not enough data to demonstrate that NSF is less likely to occur in children than in adults with similarly significant renal disease. Therefore, it is prudent to follow the same guidelines for adult and pediatric patients as described above. It should be noted, however, that eGFR values in certain premature infants and neonates may be <30 mL/min/1.73 m^2 simply due to immature renal function (and not due to pathologic renal impairment). In these individuals, the ACR Committee believes that caution should still be used when administering GBCAs, although an eGFR value <30 mL/min/1.73 m^2 should not be considered an absolute contraindication to GBCA administration.

GBCAs during Pregnancy and Lactation[20]

It is known that GBCAs cross the human placenta and into the fetus when given in clinical dose ranges. No adequate and well-controlled terratogenic studies of the effects of these agents in pregnant women have been performed. A single cohort study of 26 women exposed to gadolinium chelates during the first trimester of pregnancy showed no evidence of teratogenesis or mutagenesis in their progeny.[23] Because it is unclear how gadolinium-based contrast agents will affect the fetus, these agents should be administered only with extreme caution. Each case should be reviewed carefully and gadolinium-based contrast agent administered only when there is a potential overwhelming benefit to the patient or fetus that outweighs the possible risk of exposure of the fetus to free gadolinium ions. The radiologist should confer with the referring physician and document the following in the radiology report or the patient's medical record:

- That information requested from the MR study cannot be acquired without the use of contrast or by using other imaging modalities.
- That the information needed affects the care of the patient and fetus during the pregnancy.
- That the referring physician is of the opinion that it is not prudent to wait to obtain this information until after the patient is no longer pregnant. It is recommended that the pregnant patient undergoing an MR examination provide informed consent to document that she understands the risk and benefits of the MR procedure to be performed, and the alternative diagnostic options available to her (if any), and that she wishes to proceed.[20]

Only tiny amounts of GBCAs given to a **lactating mother** reach the milk and only a minute proportion in absorbed from the baby's gut,[24] therefore the ACR recommends that they can be safely administered to a lactating mother. However, the EMA recommends discontinuation of breast feeding for at least 24 hours for all patients receiving high NSF risk GBCAs.

As healthcare providers have been restricting their use of GBCAs in patients at risk for NSF, the incidence of NSF has been dropping. This reduction reflects the changes that have been implemented in MR practice since the risks of NSF have widely publicized.[25]

MANGANESE-BASED CONTRAST AGENTS

Manganese (Mn^{2+}) like gadolinium (Gd^{3+}) is also a strongly paramagnetic substance due to the presence of five unpaired electrons in its structure. Its compound, Mangafodipir trisodium (MnDPDP, Teslascan) has a chemical similarity to vitamin B_6, and because of this, it is specifically taken up by hepatocytes. It increases the signal intensity of normal hepatic parenchyma thus giving a high lesion-to-liver contrast and providing improved detection, characterization and evaluation of liver lesions.[26] During the later phases, MnDPDP is excreted into bile and provides excellent biliary ductal detail aiding in the diagnosis of various biliary pathologies.[27] MnDPDP was also found to accumulate in the pancreatic parenchyma and has been clinically useful for the evaluation of pancreatic lesions.

Unlike the gadolinium agents, MnDPDP readily dissociates after injection to yield free manganese ions. The instability of the chelate *in vivo* raised concerns in the scientific literature about potential toxicity. Free manganese, in chronic exposure, accumulates in the brain and causes a parkinsonism-like syndrome. It can also have a depressive action on heart function. Moreover, evidence suggests that significant neurological risk is associated with manganese intoxication in subjects with chronic liver failure whose ability to eliminate manganese is reduced. Hence, MnDPDP has effectively been withdrawn from the market.[7]

Mn-based nanoparticles are currently under research for use as high performance contrast agents with reduced toxicity.

IRON OXIDE-BASED CONTRAST AGENTS

Superparamagnetic iron oxide particles were suggested as a potential liver specific MR contrast agents as early as 1980s. These agents contain a crystalline core of water insoluble iron oxide crystals, usually magnetite (Fe_3O_4) or maghemite (γ-Fe_2O_3) with a core diameter in the range of 4 to 10 nm. To prevent particle aggregation, these iron oxide crystals are coated by dextran or some other biodegradable polysachharide which makes the total size of the iron oxide particle substantially larger and also modifies their biological behavior.[28]

Each iron oxide crystal contains several thousand paramagnetic Fe ions (Fe^{2+} and Fe^{3+}). When these particles are subjected to an external magnetic field, they exhibit strong magnetization which can cause microscopic field inhomogeneity and activate the dephasing of protons. Thus, iron oxide nanoparticles shorten T2- and T2*-relaxation times of the neighboring regions, and produce a decreased signal intensity in T2- and T2*-weighted MR images.

Unlike low-molecular weight water soluble GBCAs, iron oxide agents do not leak into the interstitium and therefore, act as intravascular contrast agents or blood pool agents as long as the vessel endothelium is not altered by any pathological process. They are eliminated from blood by uptake into the reticuloendothelial system (RES) cells in liver, spleen, bone marrow and lymph nodes.[28]

The blood half-life and biological distribution of the nanoparticles are directly dependant on their size. They have been subdivided into two groups according to their mean-total diameter and the distribution of particle sizes of the iron oxide agent: (i) superparamagnetic iron oxide particles (SPIOs) and (ii) ultrasmall superparamagnetic iron oxide particles (USPIOs).

- *Superparamagnetic iron oxide (SPIOs) particles:* These are particles with aggregated iron oxide cores and a mean particle diameter greater than 50 nm. Two SPIOs have been developed clinically and approved for MR imaging:
  - *Fexumoxide* (also known as Feridex or AMI-25) with a particle size of 50–180 nm. It has a thin, incomplete dextran coating that causes individual particles to form polycrystalline aggregates. These aggregates behave in solutions or within cells as large particles. They are phagocytosed rapidly by reticuloendothelial cells and are cleared from the blood in an hour or less. It is administered as a slow I/V infusion over 30–60 minutes. Imaging is typically performed 1–4 hours after infusion. The liver appears darkest on T2* weighted and T2-weighted images in the first 24 hours after the infusion. Complete metabolism requires 14–28 days but the signal intensity of the liver typically returns to normal within 7–14 days. The most common complication of Feridex is acute severe low back pain, which may lead to discontinuation of the infusion in patients. This complication can be minimized with a slow infusion.[29]
  - *Ferucarbotran* (also known as Resovist or SH U 555 A) has a particle size of about 60 nm. The SPIO particles are coated with low molecular weight carboxydextran. Resovist is provided as a ready to use formulation and is administered as a rapid bolus and so is used with both dynamic and delayed imaging. The reported overall incidence of adverse events with Resovit was 7.1%, with vasodilation and parasthesias the common event reported.[7]

As mentioned before, these iron oxide contrast agents are phagocytosed by macrophages throughout the body. The SPIO agents are preferentially entrapped by the Kupffer cells in the liver and spleen and reduce the T2 relaxation time of these organs, thus the normal liver appears dark on T2 weighted images. Most liver tumors, whether benign or malignant, primary or metastatic, are deficient in Kupffer cells and do not exhibit SPIO particle uptake and appear relatively hyperintense after SPIO administration. However, well-differentiated tumors which have not lost all their Kupffer cells, will take up SPIO agents and exhibit reduced signal intensity.[27,29] Some, not all, focal nodular hyperplasias show SPIO uptake. Use of SPIO agents may help improve detection of HCC in cirrhotic patients. SPIO agents may also be used in combination with GBCAs to increase overall lesion detection.[29]

- *Ultrasmall superparamagnetic iron oxide (USPIOs) particles:* These are particles with non-aggregated (monodisperse) iron oxide cores with mean diameter less than 50 nm. As USPIOs are very small, they are extravasated from the blood vessels into interstitial spaces and transported to lymph nodes via the lymphatic channels. MR imaging is done 24–36 hours after contrast administration. The accumulation of the contrast within the normal nodes causes them to appear dark in T2 or T2* weighted while diseased nodes (e.g. metastatic nodes) do not show any change in signal intensity and appear uniformly or focally bright. When the hyperintense focus accounts for more than 30% of the nodal area, the node is considered metastatic. Harisinghani et al. reported the successful detection of lymph node metastases in patients with prostate cancer using USPIOs.[30] Sinerem and Combidex are two commercially available USPIO agents. USPIOs have also been tested as blood pool agents as they remain in the intravascular space for a long time.[31]

ORAL-CONTRAST AGENTS

Oral-contrast agents are required to delineate bowel pathology and distinguish bowel from other organs or mass lesions. The properties of an ideal oral contrast agent should be—little or no absorption by the stomach or intestines, complete excretion, no motion or susceptibility artifacts, uniform marking of the GI tract, good patient acceptance in terms of taste, volume to be ingested and timing of oral administration, be safe, and be of low cost.[32] A variety of oral contrast agents have been developed for improved delineation of the bowel in MR imaging studies. They can broadly be divided as:

- Low-signal intensity on all pulse sequences—low-low intensity (proton displacement or T2 shortening)
- High-signal intensity on all pulse sequences—high-high intensity (T1 shortening)
- Low-signal intensity on T1-weighted images and high-signal intensity on T2-weighted images—low-high intensity (water based)
- High-signal intensity on T1-weighted images and low-signal intensity on T2-weighted images—high-low intensity (T1 and T2 shortening)

The last two categories are also known as biphasic agents.

Low-low Intensity (Dark Lumen)

The signal intensity in bowel can be reduced by displacing the bowel contents with a material that contains no protons, such as air. Air can be administered by intubating the small bowel or rectum. However, due to patient discomfort and degradation of T_2*-weighted gradient-echo images and echoplanar images by susceptibility artefacts, air is not featured as an oral contrast agent.

Perfluorocarbons are agents which do not contain protons, but they have the same susceptibility as water and thus, do not cause artefacts. Perflubron, a perfluorocarbon formulation was the first oral MR contrast agent approved for clinical use. However, as it was very expensive, it was withdrawn from the market.[33]

SPIOs in high concentration can shorten T2 and T2* enough to eliminate signal from bowel even on so-called T1 weighted images. Their major disadvantage is the resulting distortion of the local magnetic field, which can exacerbate artefacts making fat-suppression particularly vulnerable. Currently, ferumoxsil – a silicon-coated SPIO is commercially available as GastroMARK (Mallinckrodt) or Lumirem (Guerbert) for use as an oral contrast agent. Side effects such as nausea and vomiting, flatulence and feeling of fullness have been reported in 15% of patients.[32]

Clays such as kaolin, attapulgite and helonite restrict the motion of water, thus shortening the T1- and T2-relaxation times. However, T1 weighted gradient echo images with a T_E of less than 3 msec have little T2-contrast and therefore depict clay in bowel contents as high-signal intensity owing to their short T1.[33]

High-high or Bright Lumen

Positive-contrast agents cause a reduction of T1 relaxation time; consequently they act on T1-weighted images by increasing the signal intensity of the bowel lumen (bright lumen). Positive-contrast agents are represented by paramagnetic materials, mainly gadolinium chelate solutions but also ferrous and manganese ions. Gadolinium chelate solution was among the first contrast agents proposed as an oral contrast for MRI. Gadolinium chelate dissolved in water at a concentration of approximately 1 mmol/L provides sufficient reduction of the T1-relaxation time of water to generate an increase in signal intensity on T1-weighted images. As the concentration is low it has no T2 effect, so it does not shorten the T2-relaxation time; consequently the signal intensity is also high on T2-weighted images. One of the first commercially available positive oral contrasts was gadopentetate dimeglumine solution (Magnevist Enteral–Schering AG).

Blueberry juice can be used as a positive agent due to its high content of manganese, a paramagnetic ion, which shortens the T1-relaxation time. Fat-containing food materials like milk, vegetable oil and icecream have an intrinsically short T1, thus providing high signal on T1-weighted MRI.[32]

High-low Intensity

Materials which shorten both T_1- and T_2-relaxation times enough that bowel contents have high signal intensity on T_1-weighted images and low signal intensity on T_2-weighted images. The major advantage is that the resulting signal intensity of bowel on all the pulse sequences is different from those of tumors and simple fluid collections, which tend to have low-signal intensity on T_1-weighted and high-signal intensity on T_2-weighted images. However, some T_2-weighted pulse segments (e.g. fast spin echo) may depict bowel more clearly if its contents have high signal intensity, so this form of contrast is not necessarily desirable for every application.

Examples of this type of contrast agent include clay, gadolinium chelates in high concentration and compounds of manganese. Manganese is present in high concentrations in some foods, such as bananas and blueberries.

Low-high Intensity

The least expensive, most widely available, and best understood oral contrast agent used for MRI is water which makes bowel as low-signal intensity on T1-weighted and high-signal intensity on T2-weighted images. It provides good small bowel distension, but its major limitation is intestinal absorbtion, which does not allow good distention of distal small bowel. For this reason, water is used in conjunction with different additives that reduce intestinal absorbtion, e.g. mannitol, sorbitrate, etc.

Dilute suspensions of $BaSO_4$ or dilute solutions of iodinated contrast material, such as those used in opacification of bowel for CT are very useful as low-high MR oral contrast agents.

Polyethylene glycol (PEG) is a strong hydrophilic molecule, which simulates the properties of water with regard to signal intensity with the added advantage of nonabsorbability. Using 600 mL of PEG, a good distension of bowel loops can be obtained with no significant side effects.[32] Low-high agents are also useful for delineating the pancreas; however, bowel may be difficult to distinguish from simple fluid collections and tumors; high bowel signal intensity can intensify motion artefacts.

The choice of a single agent presents advantages and disadvantages; thus the radiologist should choose the appropriate contrast agent according to clinical setting, MR experience, availability of agent and patient tolerance.

ONGOING RESEARCH AND FUTURE TRENDS

Currently most available MR contrast agents are useful in improving visibility and definition of pathology, but are not suitable for extended intravascular (blood pool) or tissue/organ specific imaging and do not allow molecular imaging. The iron oxide agents, although organ specific, are negative contrast agents and give a signal decreasing effect, which renders images of lower contrast than T1-contrasted agents. To overcome these limitations, there have been continuing efforts in searching for more specific contrast agents that can offer diagnosis with the accuracy approaching that otherwise only achievable with biopsy or histopathology. T1-nanoparticulate agents, target specific agents tumor specific, thrombus specific etc, smart agents like enzyme activated agents, chemical exchange saturation transfer (CEST And PARACEST) agents, fluorinated agents are some of the agents under research. The majority of these agents are in preclinical levels of research; however, successful *in vivo* imaging has been reported with many preclinical studies.[31,34-36]

CONCLUSION

At present, gadolinium chelates are the most widely used contrast agents in MR imaging and the only MR contrast agents available in India. They are easily available, have good tolerability and provide excellent lesion detection and characterization. The main concern with GBCAs is NSF, which is seen to occur only in patients with severe renal disease. The tissue-specific agents can be used for specific indications, depending on their availability.

REFERENCES

1. De Haen. Conception of the first magnetic resonance imaging contrast agents; a brief history. Top Mag Reson Imaging. 2001; 12:221-30.
2. Wastie ML, Latief KH. Gadolimium: named after Finland's most famous chemist. Br J Radiol. 2004;77:146-7.
3. Ersoy H, Rybicki FJ. Biochemical safety profiles of gadolinium-based extracellular contrast agents and nephrogenic systemic fibrosis. J Magn Reson Imaging. 2007;26:1190-7.
4. Kei PL, Chan LP. Gadolinium chelate-associated nephrogenic systemic fibrosis. Singapore Med J. 2008;49:181-5.
5. Schmitt-Willich H. Stability of linear and macrocyclic gadolinium based contrast agents. Br J Radiol. 2007;80(955): 581-2.
6. Juluru K, Vogel-Claussen J, Macura KJ. MR Imaging in Patients at risk for developing nephrogenic systemic fibrosis: protocols, practices, and imaging techniques to maximize patient safety. Radiographics. 2009;29:9-22.

7. ISMRM. Contrast Agents: Safety profile. [online] Available from *http://cds.ismrm.org/ismrm-2008/files/Syllabus-069.pdf.* [Accessed December, 2018].
8. Muroff LR. MRI contrast: current agents issues. Appl Radiol. 2001;30(Suppl):5-7.
9. Thomsen HS. Contrast media, safety issues and ESUR guidelines. Berlin Heidelberg New York, Springer, 2006.
10. Thomsen HS, Almen T, Morcos SK. The members of the contrast media safety committee of the European Society of Urogenital Radiology (ESUR): gadolinium-containing contrast media for radiographic examinations: A position paper. Eur Radiol. 2002;12:2600-5.
11. Bellin MF, Jakobsen JA, Tomassin I, et al. Contrast medium extravasation injury: guidelines for prevention and management. 2002;12:2807-12.
12. Cowper SE. Gadolinium—is it to blame? J Cutan Pathol. 2008;35:520-2.
13. Grobner T. Gadolinium—a specific trigger for the development of nephrogenic fibrosing dermopathy and nephrogenic systemic fibrosis? Nephrol Dial Transplant. 2006;21:1104-8.
14. Broome DR, Girguis MS, Baron PW, et al. Gadodiamide-associated nephrogenic systemic fibrosis: why radiologists should be concerned. AJR. 2007;188(2):586-92.
15. High WA, Ayers RA, Chandler J, et al. Gadolinium is detectable within the tissue of patients with nephrogenic systemic fibrosis. J Am Acad Dermatol. 2007;56(1):21-6.
16. Mackermann P, Skov L, Rossen K, et al. Nephrogenic systemic fibrosis: suspected causative role of gadodiamide used for contrast-enhanced MRI. J Am Soc Nephrol. 2006;17(9):2359-62.
17. Shibui K, Kataoka H, Sato N, Watanabe Y, Kohara M, Mochizuki T. A case of NSF attributable to contrast MRI repeated in a patient witrh stage 3 CKD at a renal function of eGFR >30 mL/min/1.73 m^2. Japanese Journal of Nephrology. 2009;51:676.
18. Bridges MD, St Amant BS, McNeil RB, Cernigliaro JG, Dwyer JP, Fitzpatrick PM. High-dose gadodiamide for catheter angiography and CT in patients with varying degrees of renal insufficiency: prevalence of subsequent nephrogenic systemic fibrosis and decline in renal function. Am J Roentgenol. 2009;192:1538-43.
19. Swaminatan S, Shah MV. New insights into nephrogenic systemic fibrosis. J Am Soc Nephrol. 2007;18:2636-43.
20. American College of Radiology. Manual on Contrast Media. Version 8 2012. Available at: *http://www.acr.org/~/media/ACR/Documents/PDF/QualitySafety/Resources/Contrast%20Manual/FullManual.pdf.*
21. Elmholdt TR, Jorgensen B, Ramsingh M, et al. Two cases of nephrogenic systemic fibrosis after exposure to the macrocyclic compound gadobutrol. NDT Plus Advance Access. Published online on March 19, 2010. Available at: *http://ndtplus.oxfordjournals.org/cgi/content/abstract/sfq028.*
22. Thomsen HS. Contrast-enhanced MRI in patients with impaired renal function: recent recommendations to minimize the risk of nephrogenic systemic fibrosis. Solutions in contrast imaging. 2010;1(2):1-8.
23. Webb JA, Thomsen HS, Morcos SK. The use of iodinated and gadolinium contrast media during pregnancy and lactation. Eur Radiol. 2005;15:1234-40.
24. Hylton NM. Suspension of breast-feeding following gado-pentetate dimeglumine administration. Radiology. 2000; 216:325-6.
25. Singer RM. A review of gadolinium-based contrast agents in magnetic resonance imaging. CE Web Source. 2014.
26. Rofsky NM, Earls JP. Mangafodipir trisodium injection (MnDPDP): a contrast agent for abdominal MR imaging. Magn Reson Imaging Clin N Am. 1996;4:73-85.
27. Kalva SP, Blake MA, Sahani DV. MR Contrast agents. Appl Radiol. 2006;35:18-27.
28. Wang YXJ, Hussain SM, Krestin GP. Superparamagnetic iron oxide agents;physicochemical characteristics and applications in NMR imaging. Eur Radiol. 2001;11: 2319-31.
29. Gandhi SN, Brown MA, Wong JG, et al. MR contrast agents for liver imaging: What, When, How. Radiographics. 2006;26: 1621-36.
30. Harsinghani MG, Barentsz J, Hahn PF, et al. Noninvasive detection of clinically occult lymph-node metastases in prostate cancer. N Engl J Med. 2003;348:2491-9.
31. Na HB, Song C, Hyeon T. Inorganic Nanopraticles for MRI Contrast Agents. Advanced Materials. 2009;21:2133-48.
32. Laghi A, Paolantonio P, Iafrate F, et al Oral contrast agents for magnetic resonance imaging of the bowel. Topics in Magnetic Reson Imaging. 2002;13:389-96.
33. Mitchell DG, Cohen MS. "Particulate and oral contrast agents" in MRI principles, 2nd Edition. Elseiver; 2004. pp.295-304.
34. Laurent S, Elst LV, Muller RN. Contrast Agents for MRI: recent Advances. eMagRes. Online John Wiley & Sons, Ltd, 2009.
35. Knight JC, Edwards PG, Paisey SJ. Fluorinated contrast agents for magnetic resonance imaging; a review of recent developments. RSC Advances. 2011;1:1415-25.
36. Vithanarachchi SM, Allen MJ. Strategies for target-specific contrast agents for magnetic resonance imaging. Cur Mol Imaging. 2012;1:12-25.

CHAPTER 55

Ultrasound Contrast Agents

Shashi Bala Paul, Manisha Jana

INTRODUCTION

Ultrasound imaging technology has evolved incessantly and come a long way since the time. It was first used in medical practice in 1942 by Dr Karl Theodore Dussik in Austria.[1] Ultrasound is the most widely used imaging modality owing to its characteristics of wide availability, simple to perform, lack of radiation, real-time scanning ability and above all the cost-effectiveness. With the development of the digital technologies, the last 60 years have witnessed the multifaceted evolution of diagnostic ultrasound with the emergence of innovative techniques like tissue harmonic imaging, color Doppler, power Doppler and the use of contrast agents for ultrasound imaging called contrast-enhanced ultrasound (CEUS).

Contrast-enhanced ultrasound has twin components, the ultrasound contrast agent (UCA) and the contrast-specific imaging modes. CEUS can detect the hemodynamics of the targeted organ and provide detailed information of the microvascularity and microperfusion observed by real-time scanning. Thus CEUS has exhibited the potential of overcoming the limitations of conventional B-mode ultrasound (US) and color (CD) or power Doppler (PD) ultrasound.[2]

Ultrasound contrast agents (UCAs) are microbubbles of gas with a protein, lipid or polymer shell. They are blood pool agents and remain confined to the intravascular space after intravenous injection as they are unable to pass through the vascular endothelium. Small microbubbles (1–10 μm) can pass through the lung capillaries and remain in circulation for a short-time and eventually get dissolved. The gas gets exhaled while the shell gets metabolized in the liver.[3,4] The UCAs, while in circulation, strongly increase the ultrasound backscatter and produce enhancement of echogenicity for the assessment of blood flow.[2] Contrast-enhanced Doppler imaging is possible because the low mechanical index (MI) amplifies the Doppler signals for better characterization of tumor vascularity. Low MI of 0.07 to 0.2 is needed for real-time evaluation of different phases of enhancement (arterial, venous and delayed) of the target organ subsequent to the intravenous administration of UCAs.[5] Detection of this flow requires the contrast-specific imaging modes like the pulse inversion or amplitude modulation technology which are now available in the ultrasound machines. These sequences take advantage of the nonlinear behavior of the microbubbles within the ultrasound field, bringing real-time perfusion imaging of the target organs into reach.

Contrast-enhanced ultrasound based parametric imaging (pCEUS) is used for quantitative assessment of the perfusion of the tumors. A dedicated software (Qontrast 4.00. Bracco, Milan, Italy) is used for generating perfusion maps of the tumor vascularity using the acquired data of tumoral enhancement obtained by continuous recording after the UCA injection. The time to peak (TTP), estimated perfusion (EP), peak intensity (PI) and area under the time-intensity curve (AUC) can be generated providing quantitative information on the tumor vascularity.[6]

EVOLUTION OF ULTRASOUND CONTRAST AGENTS

The first generation UCAs came into existence in the late 1960s **(Table 1)**.[2] These comprised of soluble gas and thus had a short life. Moreover, their large size prevented them from passing through the pulmonary circulation.[7] Thus they were used primarily for right heart imaging. Evaluation of the heart and great vessels by injecting agitated liquid via catheter was first undertaken by Gramiak et al.[8] The air bubbles within the solution greatly increased the returning echoes, but had a tendency to dissolve into the solution very quickly, resulting in short imaging window. Apart from the agitated saline, hydrogen peroxide, iodocyanine green dye, and iodinated contrast agents were also tried as ultrasound contrast media. In 1991, Echovist (Bayer Schering Pharma AG, Berlin, Germany), the first commercially available UCA, was introduced.[9] It was made of air bubbles coated with galactose and too had a very short life in the blood with minimal transpulmonary circulation limiting its clinical utility. Echovist was predominantly used for the evaluation of the cardiac shunt and the female genital tract.

Albunex (molecular biosystems Inc, San Diego, CA,1994) was the first FDA-approved contrast agent used clinically. It was composed of air-filled albumin microspheres suspended in 5% w/v human albumin solution.[10] In vitro, the linear relationship of Albunex concentration with scattered power was demonstrated by De Jong.[11] It had a mean size of approximately 3.5 µm. Although it was stable in albumin solution in vitro, it did not have significant recirculation (half life < 5 minutes) in vivo. It was used predominantly for the evaluation of cardiac shunts and valvular regurgitation with limited extracardiac applications. It is no longer manufactured.

In 1996, a relatively longer lasting UCA called Levovist came up. It contained air bubbles with a galactose/palmitic acid surfactant coating (Schering). Main indications for use were cardiac, intracranial and abdominal. However, the Levovist bubbles easily collapsed under ultrasound emission owing to its fragile properties, therefore, real-time images could not be obtained for a longer period.

By now, the need to develop more stable UCAs for prolonged window period for imaging was very evident. This formed the basis for the development of the second generation UCAs.

Second generation UCAs **(Table 2)** contain insoluble gases like sulphur hexafluoride (SF6) or perfluorocarbons and have a surface shell made of different substances like phospholipids, albumin or polymers providing better stabilization. Their smaller size enables a successful transpulmonary passage to reach the various target organs. After intravenous injection, due to their low solubility in water, better stabilization and strong harmonic response, prolonged visualization of dynamic enhancement of the organ can be observed on real-time ultrasound scanning.[7]

In 1998 and 2006, Optison (GE Healthcare) and Luminity (Bristol-Myers Squibb) made of octafluoropropane coated with albumin and lipid shell respectively, were introduced. The octafluoropropane gas has low-water solubility and is more stable providing longer imaging period. However, their sole indication for use has been cardiac.

In 2001, SonoVue (Sonovue, Bracco Milan. Italy) was introduced which contains sulfur hexafluoride stabilized by phospholipid shell. The second generation UCAs are pure blood pool agents as they are unable to destroy the vascular endothelium and thus remain exclusively intravascular resulting in prolonged enhancement of the vascular system. No extravasation into the interstitial fluid occurs. These pharmacokinetics are different from the contrast used in computed tomography (CT) and magnetic resonance imaging (MRI) which is rapidly cleared from the blood into the extracellular space.[2] These features make SonoVue an ideal ultrasound contrast agent for vascular phase imaging of different target organs and is being used widely with promising results.[2,12] SonoVue is the only contrast agent available in India.

The most recent second generation UCA is Sonazoid (Daiichi-Sankyo, Tokyo, Japan), which contains

Table 1: First generation ultrasound contrast agents.

UCAs	*Gas*	*Stabilization*
Agitated saline	Air	None
Echovist	Air	None
Levovist	Air	Palmitic acid*
Albunex	Air	Sonicated albumin*

*Have transpulmonary stability

Table 2: Second generation ultrasound contrast agents.

UCAs	*Gas*	*Stabilizing shell*
Optison	Octafluoropropane (approved in US and Europe)	Sonicated albumin
Luminity	Octafluoropropane perflutren	Lipids
Sonovue*	Sulfur hexafluoride (SF6)	Phospholipids
Sonazoid#	Perfluorobutane	Sonicated albumin

*The only available contrast in India
#Approved only in Japan

perflubutane and has a hard shell. Sonazoid differs from other agents in exhibiting the longest window period for imaging, the extended late phase. It has been successfully used in the evaluation of liver tumors. This UCA can depict the hemodynamics of the liver in the vascular and the postvascular phase also called the 'Kupffer phase'. This is because, the Kupffer cells of the liver phagocytose Sonazoid microbubbles and thus persist in the liver for long.[13] The experience with Sonazoid is limited to Japan only since it is available exclusively in that country.

Contrast-enhanced ultrasound is a promising modality and has many advantages over CT/MRI. It is a simple procedure which is easily available and requires few minutes to perform. It is free from ionizing radiation and can be safely used for repeated follow-up. No laboratory investigations for assessment of renal function are required prior to the study unlike that for CT/MRI as the UCAs are not nephrotoxic. Portability is another advantage. The CEUS machine with the contrast-specific modes can be carried anywhere in the hospital for performing bedside procedures on immobile patients.

TECHNIQUE OF CONTRAST-ENHANCED ULTRASOUND

A good US machine equipped with low MI contrast imaging mode is required. For intravenous use, the usual recommended dose of SonoVue is 2.4 mL. A higher dose is used for endoscopic contrast-enhanced ultrasound (CE-EUS) and when using high frequency transducers. For renal and pancreatic evaluation a low dose of 1.0 mL is used. For extravascular use, a few drops of SonoVue in 10–100 mL of saline may be sufficient.[14]

For intravenous use of UCAs, an access in the antecubital fossa using 20 gauge venflon with a three-way connector is obtained. The contrast material in the vial, e.g. (SonoVue) is prepared in the soluble form 5 minutes prior and shaken well to be properly dissolved for use. The target organ is visualized on the B-mode US and then keeping the lesion in focus the contrast-specific imaging mode is turned on. A simultaneous display of the tissue and contrast signals can be seen on the monitor as a dual window (option in some machines) which ensures the target lesion remains in the field of view throughout the study. The freshly prepared SonoVue is administered as an intravenous bolus followed by flushing with 10 mL of 0.9% normal saline. The enhancement characteristics of the target organ is observed on real-time by continuously scanning till the three vascular phases postinjection. The observation is recorded on the cine mode. Postprocedure, the patient is observed for about an hour for any adverse reaction if any due to the UCA.

SAFETY OF UCAs

Ultrasound contrast agents are well tolerated and are safe with few nonspecific side effects. The clearance of UCA is very fast and 80–90% of it gets eliminated through the lungs in 11 minutes.[15] Life threatening anaphylactoid complications are very rare (0.001%).[16] With its use in echocardiography, some fatal incidents have been reported in very ill patients. The use of UCAs mandate precautionary measures to be ready despite low incidence of side effects. Unlike other contrast agents used for CT or MRI, the UCAs are not nephrotoxic as they have no renal excretion. Hence, CEUS can be safely done in patients with compromised renal function.[17] Contraindications to the use of UCAs are cardiopulmonary disease, use prior to extracorporeal shock wave therapy, pregnancy, breast-feeding and severe coronary artery disease. Cautious use is recommended in neonates.

DIAGNOSTIC APPLICATIONS OF UCAs

A set of guidelines and recommendations for the use of CEUS were developed in early 2004 by the European Federation of Societies for Ultrasound in Medicine and Biology (EFSUMB).[18] These advocated its use for hepatic imaging and since then, CEUS has fully established itself for its use in a whole lot of applications in liver conditions.[14] Over period of time, various nonhepatic applications have also been developed with early encouraging results.[12]

Applications in Hepatic Imaging

Contrast-enhanced ultrasound is ideally suited for the evaluation of liver lesions. It is because of the fact that liver has a dual blood supply comprising of the hepatic artery and the portal vein which allows evaluation of the liver by real-time scanning in three vascular phases after the intravenous administration of the UCA. The continuous change in the intralesional hemodynamics depicted as the enhancement pattern of the liver nodule is observed in the arterial phase (AP) up to 30 seconds, portal venous phase (PP) from 31 to 120 seconds and the delayed phase (DP) from 120 to 180 seconds. Intermittent scanning is done in individual cases where the contrast is seen persisting in the late phase up to 5 minutes or so. If another mass needs to be studied in the same patient, then the same procedure is repeated with a fresh bolus of UCA after 10 minutes.

Detection of Focal Liver Lesions by CEUS

Traditionally, US has been the first imaging modality for the detection of focal liver lesion (FLL). However, its diagnostic accuracy for the detection and characterization of FLL is much lower than CT and MRI.[19,20] The sensitivity of US is low for early detection of hepatocellur carcinoma (HCC) in patients of chronic liver disease. US is unable to detect small nodules less than a cm, isoechoic nodules in a cirrhotic liver and lesions located in the subdiaphragmatic regions. Therefore, evaluation of vascularity of the suspicious liver nodules by CD and PD also have limitations like inability to detect slow flow, evaluate deep-seated vessels and frequently associated artifacts.[21,22]

With the use of CEUS, the diagnostic accuracy of FLL has improved from 27 to 42% of conventional US to 87–89% by CEUS.[23,24] Studies have also reported superiority of CEUS over CT in detection of FLL and a comparable accuracy of the two for the overall performance.[25,26]

Small malignant lesions are invariably seen as hypoenhancing nodules in the PP or LP of the mutiphasic imaging of CT/MRI. CEUS, by virtue of the use of the UCA, acquires similar ability to study the hemodynamics of the nodule in different vascular phases. Due to this fact, CEUS has led to improved detection of small lesions compared to conventional US and even in comparison to CT.[26,27]

Further, improved results have been shown with the use of a newly launched UCA called Sonazoid (only available in Japan). It has the additional advantage of Kupffer imaging which allows prolonged scanning up to 60 minutes resulting in better detection of malignant lesions in the postvascular phase.[27] CEUS with Sonazoid has shown a high sensitivity of 95% and specificity of 93% for detection of malignant lesions.

Characterization of FLL

Characterization of FLL should be done with the prior knowledge of the clinical history and any previous imaging. It is important to know whether the FLL is present in an underlying normal liver or a cirrhotic liver because the tumor types vary in the cirrhotic and noncirrhotic livers. CEUS is a useful modality for the characterization of FLL and can safely be considered as the first imaging modality for this purpose.[28,29] It has a high sensitivity of 98% and an accuracy of 93% in differentiating benign from malignant nodules.[30]

The enhancement pattern of the liver nodule is termed in relation to the adjacent liver parenchyma. The nodule is hyperenhancing if it enhances more, isoenhancing if it is similar to the liver parenchyma and hypoenhancing if it is less enhancing than the surrounding liver parenchyma. No enhancement refers to no change in enhancement subsequent to the contrast administration.

Confident and accurate characterization of the nodules requires eliciting their enhancement patterns in the different phases of CEUS. Late phase of CEUS is a vital part of the study helping in the characterization of the liver nodules. Benign liver lesions are iso- to hyperenhancing in the PP and LP, while the malignant lesions characteristically are hypoenhancing (show washout).[31] This occurs because, in the benign lesion the UCA is retained in the healthy liver due to slow flow through the sinusoids whereas, in the malignant lesions the UCA fail to retain due to lack of sinusoids resulting in hypoenhancement of the nodules (seen as dark defects).[32] This pattern occurs in 86–93% of benign and 78–98% of malignant liver nodules.[30,33,34]

CEUS Patterns of Benign Focal Liver Lesions (Table 3)

Hemangioma *is* the most common benign liver tumor with a prevalence of 1–20%.[35] CEUS has a sensitivity of 95% and specificity of 98% in diagnosing hemangioma.[36] The most common pattern of enhancement is the early peripheral nodular arterial enhancement with delayed centripetal fill-in which is similar to that seen on CT or MRI **(Figs. 1A to C)**. It is encountered in 52–88% of the cases. Sustained enhancement during the late phase has been reported in as high as 83–100% of cases.[33,34,37-39]

The high diagnostic accuracy of hemangioma on CEUS is comparable to that of MRI, which includes even small hemangiomas. If the typical features of enhancement are seen, further confirmation of the diagnosis by any other imaging is not required.[40] Atypical features occur in very small shunts (<15 mm), very large (more than 4 cm) hemangiomas which have arterioporto-venous shunts called high flow hemangiomas or shunt hemangiomas which are rapidly filling and the ones that have features of calcification, thrombosis or venoliths.[41] The chance of missing out on any rapidly enhancing hemangiomas (flash-filling) on CEUS is remote because of the advantage of continuous real-time scanning.

Focal nodular hyperplasia (FNH) is the second most common benign liver tumor with a prevalence of 0.9–3%.[42] It results from the proliferation of abnormally arranged non-neoplastic hepatocytes as a response to an area of vascular malformation or venous thrombosis. It is commonly associated with a central fibrous scar and anomalous arteries. It is important to differentiate FNH from other entities like hepatic adenoma or carcinoma (fibrolamellar type), because FNH is managed conservatively.

Being a hypervascular tumor, FNH shows homogeneous hyperenhancement in the arterial phase in nearly all the cases. In the portal and late phase, it is isoenhancing or slightly hyperenhancing, seen in about 87–100%. of the cases.[38,43,44]

The central scar occurs in 23–31% of cases and shows two types of enhancement the stellate vascularity and

Table 3: Enhancement patterns of benign focal liver lesions.

Focal liver lesion	***Arterial phase***	***Portal venous phase***	***Late phase***
Noncirrhotic liver			
Hemangioma Typical features Additional features (small lesion)	 Peripheral nodular enhancement Complete, rapid centripetal enhancement	 Partial/complete centripetal fill-in	 Complete enhancement Nonenhancing regions
Focal nodular hyperplasia Typical features Additional features	 Hyperenhancing from the center, complete, early Spoke wheel arteries, feeding artery	 Hyperenhancing Unenhanced central scar	 Iso/hyperenhancing Unenhanced central scar
Hepatocellular adenoma Typical features Additional features	 Hyperenhancing, complete Nonenhancing regions	 Isoenhancing Hyperenhancing Nonenhancing regions	 Isoenhancing Slightly hypoenhancing Nonenhancing regions
Focal fatty infiltration/sparing	Isoenhancing	Isoenhancing	Isoenhancing
Abscess Typical features Additional features	 Peripheral enhancement, no central enhancement Enhanced septa hyperenhanced liver segment	 Hyper-/isoenhancing rim, no central enhancement Hypoenhancing rim Enhanced septa hyperenhanced liver segment	 Hypoenhancing rim, no central enhancement
Simple cyst	Nonenhancing	Nonenhancing	Nonenhancing
Cirrhotic liver			
Regenerative nodule (± dysplastic)			
Typical features Additional features	Isoenhancing Hypoenhancing	Isoenhancing	Isoenhancing

In cirrhotic liver simple cysts, hemangiomas and abscesses may also be found and show the same enhancement pattern as in noncirrhotic livers. All other entities are rare findings in cirrhotic livers.
Source: https:*//www.thieme-connect.com/ejournals/pdf/10.1055/s-0032-1325499.pdf.*Guidelines and good clinical practice recommendations for CEUS in liver-update 2012. Accessed on Dec 25, 2012.

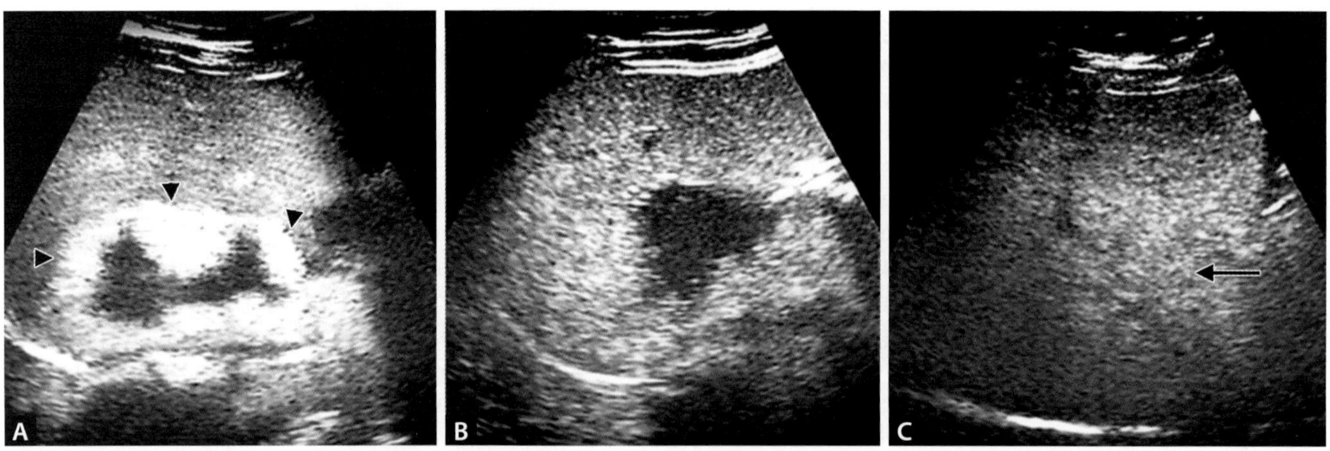

Figs. 1A to C: Hemangioma – Typical pattern: CEUS images of the FLL in segment VII showing peripheral nodular enhancement (arrow heads) in the AP at 23 seconds postcontrast injection (A) with progressive centripetal enhancement (B) becoming isoenhancing (arrow) in the LP at 240 seconds (C).

centrifugal filling. An anomalous artery courses in the scar in a linear and stellate fashion depicting a spoke wheel pattern, seen in 45–89% of the cases.[39,45,46]

Hepatocellular adenoma (HA) is a rare, benign liver tumor. It has a relatively nonspecific pattern of enhancement on CEUS. Being hypervascular, the ususal pattern is of hyperenhancement in the AP. Small HA shows homogeneous hyperenhancement while the larger ones are heterogeneously hyperenhancing due to the presence of intratumoral hemorrhage or necrosis. Very rarely, it may show iso- or hypoenhancement on the portal and late phases of enhancement and may thus mimic HCC posing a diagnostic dilemma. Even on histopathology, differentiation of HA from well-differentiated HCC is often challenging. Similar pattern may be depicted by hypervascular metastasis as well.[46]

Liver abscess: Pyogenic abscess is most frequently encountered abscess in the liver. The CEUS findings like the conventional US, vary with the stage of the abscess. The abscess usually shows areas of hyperenhancement.[47] Early abscess is generally solid and shows diffuse heterogeneous enhancement in the AP persisting in the PP and LP. A transient perilesional enhancement also occurs in the AP which in very few cases may show hypoenhancement in the PP.[47] If this rare finding is seen, this needs to be differentiated from a necrotic metastasis which appears as a punched out enhancement defect in the LP, while the abscess depicts an ill-defined area of hypoenhancement. As the abscess matures, it develops fluid within, which shows as an enhancing rim postcontrast injection. The internal septations enhance on CEUS leading to a honeycomb appearance.

Liver cysts always need to be diagnosed on conventional US where they are seen as thin-walled, anechoic well-defined areas with posterior enhancement. Cysts lack enhancement on any phase of CEUS.

Focal fatty change (Fatty infiltration of fatty sparing) may mimic masses on US. However, their location is typical adjacent to the falciform ligament, portal veins and gallbladder. They have geographical margins with no mass effect and vessels are seen traversing through the lesion.[48] If they are nodular or atypical in location, they may pose a diagnostic dilemma. After contrast enhancement, areas of focal fatty change show similar enhancement as the adjoining hepatic parenchyma in all the vascular phases.

CEUS Patterns of Malignant Focal Liver Lesions (Table 4)

CEUS has a sensitivity of 90% and specificity of 99% and an accuracy of 89% in diagnosing malignant lesions.[49] It is useful for detection of metastases, HCC in high-risk patients of cirrhosis, evaluate multistep carcinogenesis of HCC, serve as a guidance procedure for the biopsy or percutaneous ablative therapy and for assessment of therapeutic response to loco-regional treatment for HCC.

Metastases is the most frequent indication for performing US of the liver. The diagnosis can be simple when the patient has a known primary but very challenging, if no such history is available.

Conventional US has limitations in detection of metastases and its accuracy is significantly lower than CT/MRI.[50] Improved accuracy has been noted with the

Table 4: Enhancement patterns of malignant focal liver lesions.

Focal liver lesion	*Arterial phase*	*Portal venous phase*	*Late phase*
Noncirrhotic liver			
Metastasis:			
Typical features	Rim enhancement	Hypoenhancing	Hypo/nonenhancing
Additional features	Complete enhancement Hyperenhancement nonenhancing regions	Nonenhancing regions	Nonenhancing regions
HCC:			
Typical features	Hyperenhancing	Isoenhancing	Hypo/nonenhancing
Additional features	Nonenhancing regions	Nonenhancing regions	Nonenhancing regions
Cholangiocarcinoma:			
Typical	Rim-like hyperenhancement, central hypoenhancement	Hypoenhancing	Nonenhancing
Additional features	Nonenhancing regions Inhomogeneous/hyperenhancement	Nonenhancing regions	Nonenhancing regions
Cirrhotic liver			
HCC:			
Typical features	Hyperenhancing, complete nonenhancing areas (if large)	Isoenhancing	Hypoenhancing (slightly or moderately)
Additional features	Basket pattern, chaotic vessels Enhancing tumor thrombus Hypo/nonenhancing	Nonenhancing regions Nonenhancing	Isoenhancing Nonenhancing

Explanation: Other malignancies in cirrhosis have the same patterns as in noncirrhotic livers.
Source: https://www.thieme-connect.com/ejournals/pdf/10.1055/s-0032-1325499.pdf. Guidelines and good clinical practice recommendations for CEUS in liver-update 2012. Accessed on Dec 25, 2012.

use of CEUS.[51] Metastases show variable patterns of enhancement depending upon the vascularity of the primary tumor in the AP, while, they are typically rapidly hypoenhancing (within 20 secs) during the PP.[33,43]

More than 85% of the metastases show very short lasting peripheral rim enhancement, diffuse or mosaic enhancement followed by rapid washout.[33,38,43]

Rim enhancement with early washout is the hallmark of metastases. Hypervascular metastasis showing complete enhancement may be mistaken for HCC in which case other findings like clinical history, serum alpha-fetoprotein levels may come to rescue.

Hepatocellular carcinoma (HCC): HCC is the most common primary hepatic malignancy. More than 80% of HCC occur in patients with chronic liver disease of viral etiology.[52] The curative therapeutic options of HCC can be applicable only if the disease is diagnosed early. Hence, early detection and characterization of the nodule is imperative.

CEUS plays a pivotal role in evaluating the multistep carcinogenesis of HCC in cirrhosis. HCC is exclusively supplied by the abnormal arteries while the regenerative nodule (RN) and the dysplastic nodule (DN) contain normal hepatic arteries and portal veins. In the process of progression of DN towards malignancy, the abnormal arterial supply increases while the normal arterial and portal supply decreases.[5]

Regenerative nodule are small and seen on conventional US as either coarse and heterogeneous liver or as multiple, tiny, hypo- or hyperechoic nodules. On CEUS, most RN and DN do not show any enhancement (isoenhancing) in any phase. At times, they may show transient hypoenhancement in the AP. DN may have variable and inconsistent arterial and portal supplies or significant overlaps of vascular supply leading to problems in diagnosis on all modalities (CEUS, CT, MRI). Since CEUS has the advantage of continuous real-time scanning, it may pick up subtle transient patterns of enhancement in order to differentiate between HCC and DN.[5]

CEUS patterns of HCC: Typical HCC is supplied exclusively by the abnormal arteries. More than 90% of the HCCs are hyperenhancing in the AP, also termed arterialization. About one-third of the cases show a basket pattern (peripheral vascularity and penetrating the lesion).[38] On the late phase, 83–97% of HCCs show hypoenhancement, classically called washout **(Figs. 2A and B)**. This washout is generally slower and milder that than seen in metastases.

A good corelation of the enhancement pattern is seen with the histological differentiation of HCC. The more the differentiation of the lesion, more slowly is the washout of the nodule in the late phase. Moderately differentiated HCC shows typical pattern of arterial hyperenhancement and LP hypoenhancement. Atypical patterns are common with well-differentiated and poorly differentiated HCC.[53] Well differentiated HCC may or may not show hypoenhancement in the LP as they take long to washout **(Figs. 3A to C)**. In such cases, the observation on real-time scanning should be done for a longer duration. In a patient of cirrhosis, any nodule that is isoenhancing in the PP and LP should not be considered benign as about half of the well-differentiated HCCs do not show washout.[53,54]

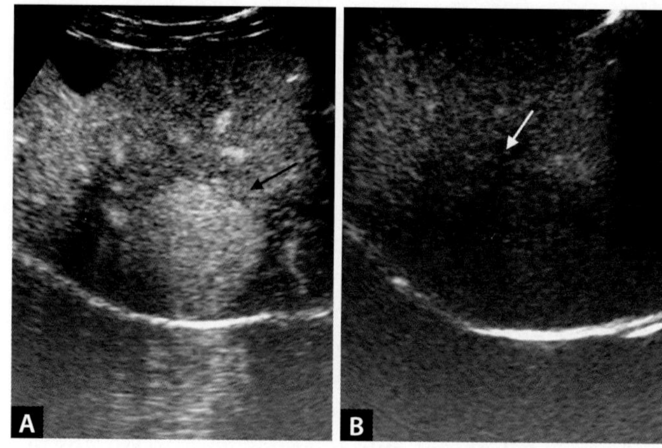

Figs. 2A and B: HCC-typical pattern: AP image of CEUS at 26 seconds showing hyperenhancement (arrow) of the FLL (A) with hypoenhancement (arrow) in the VP at 45 seconds (B).

CEUS can reliably differentiate between benign and malignant thrombus of the portal vein. Benign thrombus is generally avascular while the malignant one shows heterogeneous enhancement or irregular linear vessels following contrast injection.[55]

Intrahepatic cholangiocarcinoma (ICC): ICC typically depicts peripheral rim enhancement in the AP.[56,57] Hypoenhancement is seen in the PP and LP. This feature is in contrast to the findings of ICC seen on CT/MRI where, centripetal enhancement of the tumor occurs. This difference in pattern again is probably largely due to the fact that contrast agents of CT and MRI diffuse into the extracellular space leading to the enhancement of the tumor in the LP.

Guidance for Interventional Procedures

Ultrasound is the most commonly used modality for guiding procedures for tumor biopsy or percutaneous ablation. Conventional ultrasound fails to detect nodules that are isoechoic to liver parenchyma, with indistinct margins or infiltrative in nature. In some cases, the liver

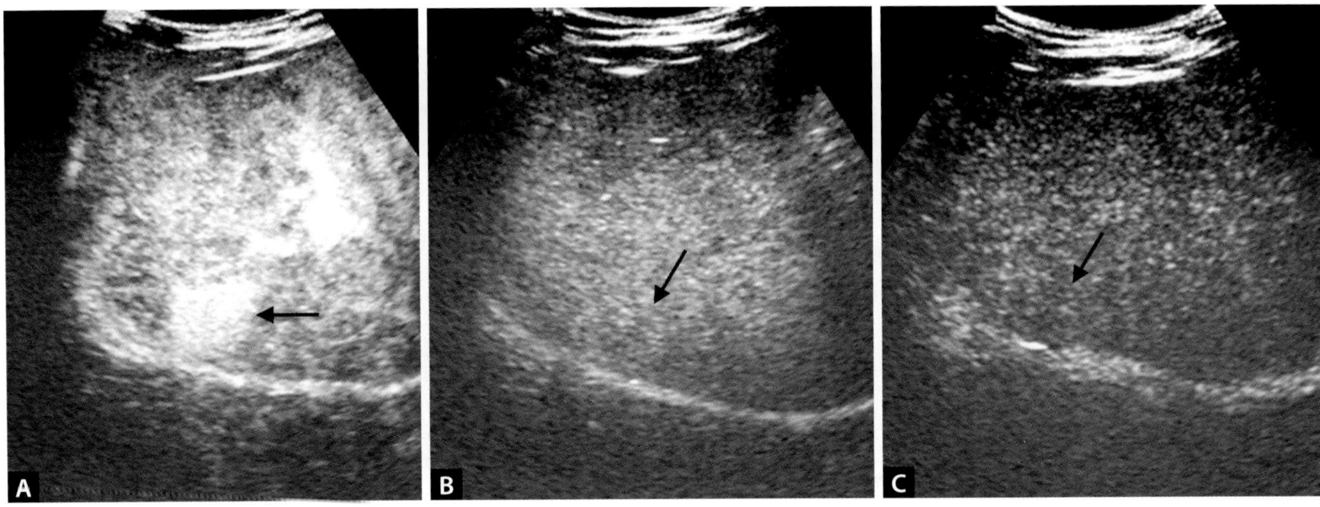

Figs. 3A to C: HCC- Atypical pattern: AP CEUS image of a known patient of cirrhosis with FLL showing homogeneous hyperenhancement (arrow) of the lesion at 30 seconds (A) with retained contrast appearing isoenhancing (arrows) in the VP and LP at 110 and 240 seconds respectively (B and C). Histopathology suggested well differentiated HCC.

nodule may not be seen at all and management of such nodules becomes problematic.

Since 2004, CEUS guidance has been used successfully for ablating the tumor that was not seen on conventional US.[58] CEUS plays a key role in the intervention of such cases. It improves the detectability of the nodules and aids in accurate guidance of the needle placement resulting in decreased number of treatment sessions for complete ablation.[59] Better local tumor outcome in terms of local tumor progression rate following CEUS-guided RFA has been reported in the range of 0–12% in the follow-up of 4.3–11 months.[60-62]

Many a times, the tumors with indistinct margins are seen larger in size on CEUS because the margins get well delineated and the extent of malignant infiltration can be reliably depicted following contrast injection.

Assessment of Treatment Response of Malignant Tumors and Plan Additional Treatment

Monitoring of response to locoregional therapy for HCC can be done with the use of CEUS. Locoregional therapy is the most commonly used treatment for HCC which comprises of transarterial chemoembolizaion (TACE) and percutaneous ablative therapies like radiofrequency ablation (RFA), ethanol (PEI) or acetic acid ablation (PAI) and microwave/laser ablation.

Percutaneous ablative therapies aim at producing coagulation necrosis of the tumor rendering it nonviable. The response to therapy is assessed by estimating the presence of the residual viable tumor tissue depicted by residual vascularity of the remaining tumor. Multiphasic CT/MRI have been the gold standard imaging modalities for assessment of treatment response of HCC.[36] However, these cross-sectional imaging modalities have their own limitations. Easy availability, costeffectiveness is a big issue. With CT, because of the association of ionizing radiation, and errors in contrast bolus timing, repeat scanning has its own risks which undermines its utility for follow-up use.

Contrast-enhanced ultrasound has the potential to overcome these shortcomings and can reliably differentiate between viable and nonviable tumor tissue following all types of percutaneous ablative therapy. This ability of CEUS is comparable with that of CT or MRI.[63] Postablation, the completely ablated tumor is seen as a hypoenhancing, well-defined area with margin of uniform thickness all around and no area of hyperenhancement within or in the periphery of the hypoenhancing defect **(Figs. 4A and B)**. Residual disease following ablation is often seen as an area of hyperenhancement in the AP at the margin or within the ablated tumor site, showing washout in PP and LP **(Figs. 5 and 6)**. CEUS can accurately detect the residual tissue post ablation. The assessment post-RFA can be done as early as immediately postablation and the results are comparable to CT performed at 24 hours.[63,64] CEUS can be safely used for repeated follow-up posttherapy as it is free from ionizing radiation and has a low risk of allergic and hypersensitivity reactions.

Transarterial chemoembrolization involves delivery of mixture of chemotherapeutic drugs with iodised oil (lipiodol) through the hepatic artery feeding the malignant liver tumor and subsequently embolizing the feeding

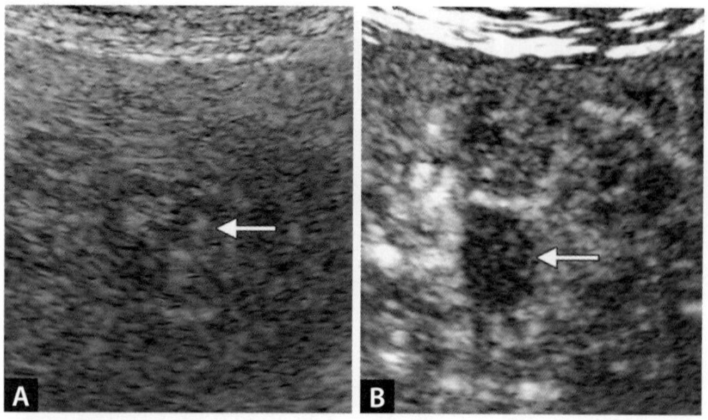

Figs. 4A and B: Post-RFA complete response of segment IV A HCC: Simultaneous US display images of tissue and contrast signal, showing a heteroechoic, ill-defined focal liver lesion [arrow (A)] which on CEUS shows a well-defined hypoenhancing ablative defect (arrow) with no hyperenhancing viable tissue within or at the margin on AP image of CEUS (B) suggesting complete response to ablation.

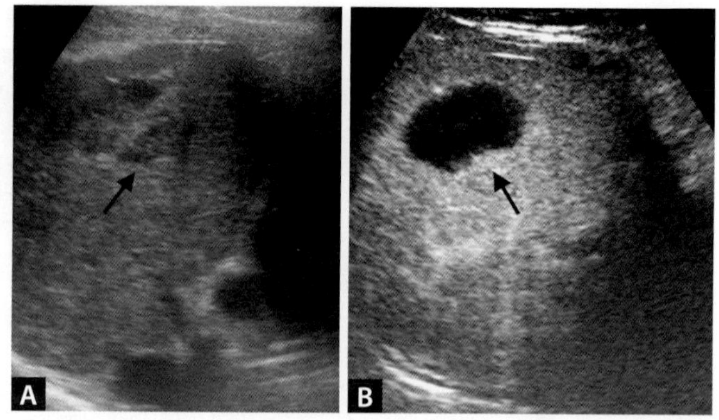

Figs. 5A and B: Residual disease Post RFA in a patient of cirrhosis with solitary HCC. On response assessment at one week post RFA, the US image showing a heterogeneous mass lesion in the liver with no clue of the viable or nonviable tumor tissue (A). On CEUS , the mass shows a focal area of hyperenhancement along the posteroinferior margin of the RFA defect (arrow) suggesting residual disease (B). A repeat RFA was planned subsequently.

artery temporarily. This results in devascularising the hypervascular HCC. Post-TACE assessment of response involves the depiction of residual viable, enhancing tumor. Multiphasic CT (MPCT) often has limitations in detecting the residual disease following TACE because the lipiodol used in TACE gets deposited in the viable as well as in the nonviable areas of the hepatic parenchyma and thus MPCT has to be undertaken after a minimum period of 4 weeks for proper assessment of response.[32] Moreover, the presence of deposited lipiodol in the tumor masks the status of viability of the tumor tissue in the adjoining hepatic parenchyma. MRI is considered the modality of choice in these cases. Diagnostic accuracy of CEUS in picking up residual disease in the lipiodol covered tumor is high as the UCAs particularly Sonazoid can demonstrate intranodular blood flow and produces prolonged sustained enhancement of the tumor tissue which can well depict the viable tumor despite the presence of lipiodol. CEUS has been found to be useful in detecting response as early as one week following TACE.[65] The viable disease would show up as areas of hyperenhancemnt in AP with washout in the PP and LP, while the nonviable tissue does not show any enhancement **(Figs. 7 and 8)**.

Parametric CEUS can additionally provide information by quantitative assessment of the perfusion of the residual tumor. The evaluation of the tumor vascularity can be done and perfusion maps illustrating contrast kinetics like TTP, PI and the AUC can be generated.[66] The PI in CEUS could reflect the microvessel density (MVD) in HCC. Therefore, quantification of CEUS seems to be helpful for assessment of tumor vascularity in HCC and provide

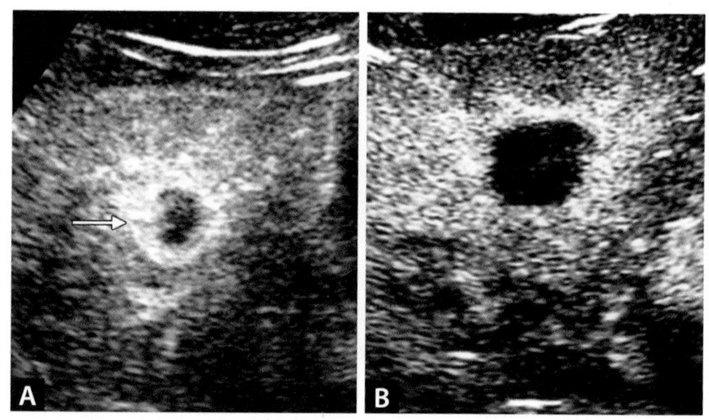

Figs. 6A and B: Post-PAI Residual disease: AP image of CEUS done at 4 weeks following PAI, depicting hyperenhancing area all along the margin and predominantly in the superolateral aspect (arrow) of the segment II/III HCC suggestive of residual disease (A). A repeat PAI was done and CEUS performed subsequently showing smooth margins of the ablative lesion with no enhancing tissue suggesting complete response (B).

quantitative assessment of the residual disease in the tumor posttherapy.

Monitoring response to antiangiogenic therapy for advanced HCC can also be done with CEUS and pCEUS. The antiangiogenic drugs induce necrosis of the tumor without eradicating the tumor. CEUS can reliably depict the absence of tumor vascularity following therapy indicating response to treatment.[67,68]

Hepatic Vein Transit Time Estimation

The arrival time of the UCA bolus in the hepatic artery and portal/hepatic vein can be measured and the calculation

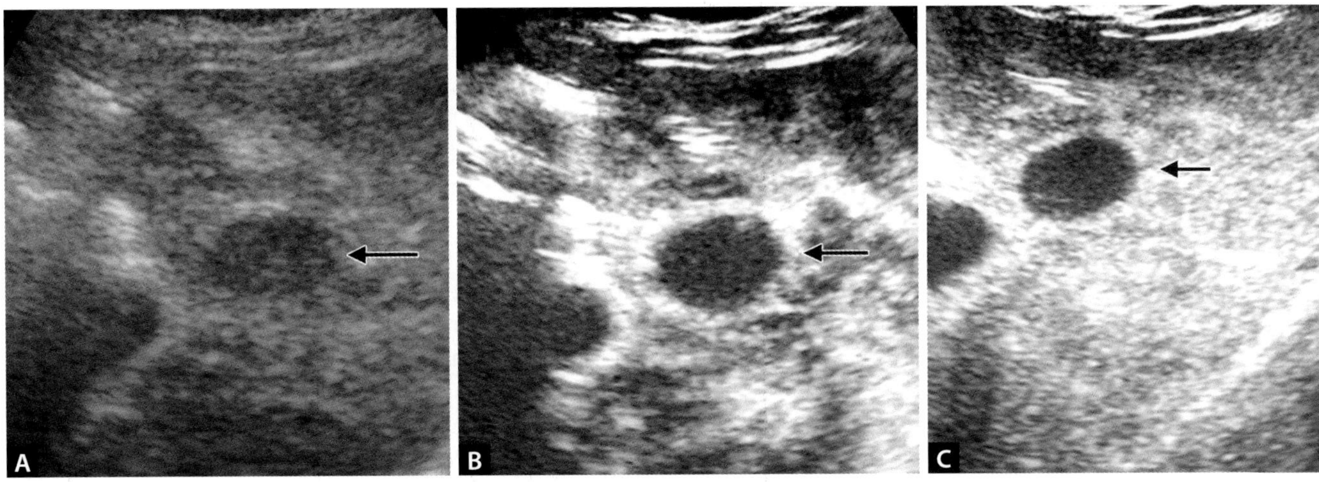

Figs. 7A to C: Post-TACE complete response—Segment II HCC post-TACE, seen as a well-defined hypoechoic lesion (arrow) with slightly hyperechoic margins on US (A). On CEUS, the mass is seen as a hypoenhancing lesion with uniform hyperenhancing margins (arrows) in the AP at 22 seconds and DP at 62 seconds suggesting complete response post-TACE (B and C, respectively).

of the transit times can be done. Shortening of the transit time is encountered in pathologies like liver cancer, cirrhosis and chronic hepatitis and this finding is quite nonspecific.[69,70]

CEUS has a number of limitations as well, despite having established itself as an important imaging tool for the evaluation of liver. Lesions located in the subdiaphragmatic areas are difficult to evaluate. Moreover, since CEUS has limited penetration, in patients of chronic liver disease, the deep-seated lesions may not be visualized due to steatosis and fibrosis of the liver. Small-sized metastases less than 5–10 mm can often be missed as they may be too small to be detected. CEUS is not useful for staging of malignancy because of the difficulty in examining the entire liver in the arterial phase. Moreover, one injection of UCA per nodule is required if the nodules are present in different segments of liver. This defeats its purpose of cost-effectiveness. CT/MRI needs to be resorted to in such a situation.

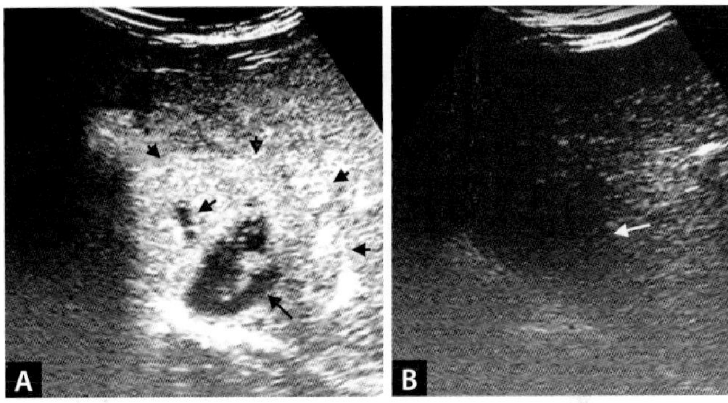

Figs. 8A and B: Residual disease post TACE: CEUS performed for a large segment VII HCC treated with TACE, showing , a large hyperenhancing tissue (arrowheads) with hypoenhancing necrotic areas (small arrow) within, in the AP (A) and showing uniform hypoenhancement (arrow) in the LP (B). Findings are suggestive of significant residual disease post-TACE. A repeat session of TACE was planned.

Liver Transplant

Contrast-enhanced ultrasound has also been tried in patients of liver transplant for evaluation of hepatic artery flow. Hepatic artery thrombosis is the most common vascular complication following transplant even though portal vein, hepatic vein and caval thrombosis can also occur but these conditions are relatively less common. Though Doppler is very useful in majority of the patients, however, at times due to postoperative edema, inaccessible hepatic arteries, it may fail to provide an answer. In such patients, CEUS has been tried with successful results.[31]

Applications in Pancreatic Imaging

The main utility of CEUS in pancreatic diseases lies in the characterization of pancreatic mass lesions and in the imaging of acute pancreatitis. After administration of UCAs, the pancreatic parenchyma shows early enhancement, immediately after aortic enhancement (10–30 sec). Maximal enhancement is reached at 60 seconds. After the arterial phase, a venous phase imaging should also be performed (30–100 seconds).[12,71,72] Once the pancreatic study is completed, delayed imaging of the liver should also be performed to rule out metastases, utilizing the same contrast agent.[73]

Detection of Focal Pancreatic Lesions

For pancreatic adenocarcinoms, the usual investigation modality is CECT. They are schirrhous tumors and commonly hypovascular compared to the normal pancreatic parenchyma. The detectability of small pancreatic mass lesions on CEUS is superior to US alone, comparable efficacy with that of EUS and more diagnostic accuracy than CT in the detection of tumors less than 2 cms.[71] Four patterns of enhancement of focal pancreatic lesions are seen: no enhancement (type I), vascularity less than adjacent pancreatic parenchyma (type II), vascularity equal to (type III) and more than the (type IV) adjacent pancreatic parenchyma. Pancreatic adenocarcinoma usually demonstrate type I and II patterns.[71]

Pancreatic neuroendocrine tumors can depict significant enhancement in the arterial phase of CEUS even when it may not show significant increased vascularity on Doppler imaging.[74,75]

Differentiation of Cystic Pancreatic Tumors from Pancreatic Pseudocyst

Common pancreatic cystic neoplasms include mucinous and serous cystic tumors, intraductal papillary mucinous tumors (IPMT). Mucinous cystic tumors are potentially malignant lesions. Imaging features include unilocular cystic lesions with internal septations and echogenic content. On CEUS, they show avid enhancement of the wall, internal septations and nodules.[76] Serous cystadenomas are usually microcystic lobulated masses, hypervascular and show enhancement of the internal septations. CEUS can differentiate a cystic pancreatic neoplasm from a pseudocyst by demonstrating the enhancement of septae, nodules and solid components in a tumor.[73] On the contrary, pancreatic pseudocysts are devoid of any contrast enhancement, even though the internal contents may appear echogenic on US.[76]

IPMT can be of the main duct type or branch duct type. In the main duct type, the main pancreatic duct is dilated and may show intraductal debris/clot. Branch duct type IPMT usually presents as a multiseptated cystic mass lesion in the head of pancreas. In IPMT, CEUS can differentiate a clot (which is avascular) from an enhancing nodule.

Detection of Pancreatic Necrosis in Acute Pancreatitis

The detection of necrosis at an early stage of development is of significant clinical importance as early treatment of necrosis (either percutaneous drainage or surgical debridement) can be planned to reduce morbidity and mortality. The routine diagnostic imaging modality in acute pancreatitis is CECT. CEUS can also be used as an alternative to CECT in the follow-up of acute pancreatitis.[77] After administration of UCAs, the necrotic pancreatic parenchyma remains unenhanced.[77]

Contrast-enhanced Endoscopic Ultrasound

Contrast-enhanced endoscopic ultrasound (CE-EUS) is a newer imaging modality which combines the benefit of superior resolution of EUS and assessment of enhancement characteristics (as in CEUS) in a single investigation.[78-82]

CE-EUS is useful for the differentiation of pancreatic ductal adenocarcinoma from focal pancreatitis and other focal lesions; and to differentiate cystic pancreatic tumor from pancreatic pseudocyst.[12] Since pancreatic adenocarcinomas tend to be fibrous in nature and have a tough capsule, they show less or no venous signals, owing to increased intratumoral pressure. On the contrary, focal pancreatitis shows both arterial and venous signals. CE-EUS increases the sensitivity of EUS (from 73.2% to 91.1%) in differentiation of pancreatic adenocarcinoma from focal pancreatitis.[83]

Applications in Renal Imaging

The main role of CEUS in renal lesions include the evaluation of a focal renal lesion,[84-87] differentiating a renal tumor from a pseudotumor,[88] and also in the evaluation of renal vascular lesions.[86,89] Other applications include guidance to radiofrequency ablation of renal tumors[90-93] and monitoring of renal abscesses in proven cases of urinary tract infection.[94] Kidneys are highly perfused organs and the microbubble contrast enhancement pattern of the kidneys follow a pattern similar to that seen on CECT. After administration of UCAs, the vascular pedicle of kidney enhances first, followed by the cortex and the medulla at the last. The tip of the renal medullary pyramid is the last to enhance. UCAs do not show excretion into the pelvicalyceal system.

CEUS is recommended for the following renal indications.[12]

Characterization of Renal Masses

Contrast-enhanced computed tomography (CECT) is the usual investigation for characterization and staging of renal mass lesions. However, on a single phase CECT, it becomes difficult to differentiate complicated hyperdense cyst and a solid enhancing mass lesion. Similarly, a hypodense nonenhancing solid mass lesion may be difficult to differentiate from a cystic lesion on CECT.

Since CEUS is more sensitive to detection of blood flow than CECT, it can differentiate a solid mass lesion from a cystic one with greater accuracy. It also scores over CECT in characterization of complex cystic renal masses as it can detect the septa and solid components in Bosniak grade 2–4 cysts with better sensitivity than CECT.[84-87]

Differentiation of Renal Tumors from Pseudotumors

Renal pseudotumors are proliferation of normal renal tissue which mimic tumor. US may fail to differentiate the two. After administration of UCAs, the enhancement of pseudotumors is similar to the normal renal parenchyma on all phases of enhancement.[88] On the contrary, the enhancement pattern of solid renal tumors differs from that of the normal renal parenchyma in at least one phase of enhancement. Although the differentiation of a benign from a malignant renal tumor cannot be done on the basis of enhancement characteristics, it is helpful in differentiating a "true" renal tumor from a pseudotumor.

Renal Vascular Lesions

Renal infarcts are better differentiated from ischemic areas on CEUS compared to unenhanced Doppler US/US as the infarcted area shows no enhancement whereas hypoperfused area retains its blood flow, although reduced.[86,89] CEUS also differentiates renal infarct from cortical necrosis, which shows preserved hilar vascularity.

Renal Tumor Ablation under CEUS Guidance

Like the use of CEUS guidance for liver tumors, renal tumors too can be ablated. CEUS can be used before the ablation procedure to increase tumor visibility. After the ablation procedure, CEUS performed 5–10 minutes later (once the gas and related artifacts disappear) can detect residual viable tumor seen as areas of enhancement whereas ablated regions appear nonenhancing.[90,91] Studies have demonstrated CEUS to be as accurate as CT and MRI in assessing adequacy of ablation treatment.[92,93]

Application in Abdominal Trauma

Contrast-enhanced computed tomography is the gold standard imaging modality in blunt abdominal trauma. The present role of CEUS in the abdominal trauma lies in the evaluation of intraabdominal solid organ injuries and triaging critically ill trauma patients without hampering with the resuscitation procedure in the emergency ward. Although bedside US has proven an effective modality to detect free intraperitoneal fluid, its utility is limited in detecting parenchymal injuries in solid abdominal organs.[95,96] Studies have shown that CEUS can detect intra-abdominal solid organ injuries (including liver, splenic, renal lesions) with higher sensitivity and specificity than US.[97,98]

The solid abdominal organs can be evaluated in a staged manner in two-part examination (one for the right hypochondrium, evaluating liver and right kidney) and another examination for the left hypochondrium for spleen and left kidney. Normal organs usually show homogeneous increased echogenicity in the parenchymal phase of the examination. A contusion is seen as a hypoechoic area within the enhancing parenchyma with ill defined borders; a laceration is a more well-defined linear nonenhancing area. In hypovolemic shock all the abdominal solid organs show reduced enhancement. Since UCAs are not excreted in the urine, they cannot be used to detect renal collecting system injury.

Applications in Breast Imaging

The main role of CEUS in breast is in the characterization of indeterminate breast masses. Mammography is the established screening modality in breast cancer, and US is widely employed for evaluation of palpable and imaging detected masses.[99] The utility of US can be limited in characterization of BI-RADS category 3 and 4 lesions, and role of different modalities like Doppler sonography and elastography has been evaluated in this group of patients.[100-102] Doppler sonography has shown limited utility in the characterization of breast lesions prior to the use of CEUS.

The advent of breast MRI led to an increase in sensitivity in cancer detection, although it had a low specificity.[103] The cancer detection on breast MRI was based upon both morphologic as well as contrast enhancement kinetics. The principle of use of CEUS in the detection of breast cancers depends on similar rationale of gaining superior resolution grayscale image, coupled with contrast imaging to assess neovascularity. Although one of the earliest applications of CEUS was in the evaluation of breast masses, unfortunately, till now it does not have any recommended role[12] as no specific pattern of enhancement or CEUS characteristics could be consistently detected as a marker of malignant mass lesion. The potential roles of CEUS in breast are discussed below.

Characterization of Breast Masses

Several studies have described difference in tumor vascularity between benign and malignant masses. The benign lesions (e.g. fibroadenoma) show smooth vessels at the periphery and less avid enhancement **(Figs. 9A**

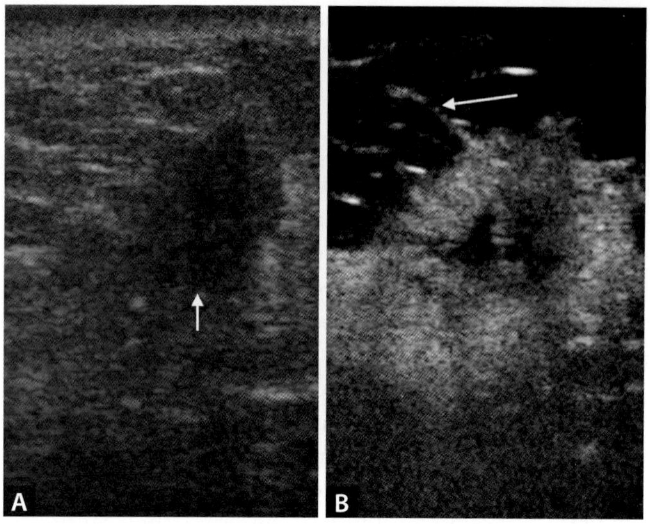

Figs. 9A and B: Benign breast mass (Fibroadenoma): Simultaneous US display image shows a well-defined smoothly marginated mass lesion without posterior acoustic shadowing (arrow) (A). CEUS image reveals minimal enhancement and peripheral branching vessels (arrow) (B).

and B), whereas the malignant masses appear spiculated **(Figs. 10A and B)**, have more tortuous vessels with irregular course, and have intervascular shunts.[104,105] Although several studies have shown malignant lesions to enhance earlier than benign lesions,[104] there is significant overlap between the two in other studies.[105]

Assessment of Tumor Response after Chemotherapy in Breast Cancer

Breast cancers which are not amenable for upfront surgery, usually undergo neoadjuvant treatment and the response to neoadjuvant chemotherapy can predict prognosis of the patient. Malignant tumors exhibit neovascularization, and the characterization and detection of tumor vessels can be useful for prediction of biologic activity of the tumor. After chemotherapy or hormone therapy, tumors tend to show reduced neoangiogenesis. Studies have shown CEUS to be more effective than Doppler US in the detection of tumor vascularity before and after treatment.[106]

Application in Prostatic Imaging

Till date, the evidence towards CEUS as a diagnostic modality in prostatic imaging is limited and described as a research tool.[12]

Prostatic adenocarcinoma is associated with neovascularity, but the detection of these microvessels is beyond the resolution of Doppler US. UCAs can increase the sensitivity of Doppler sonography. Prostatic

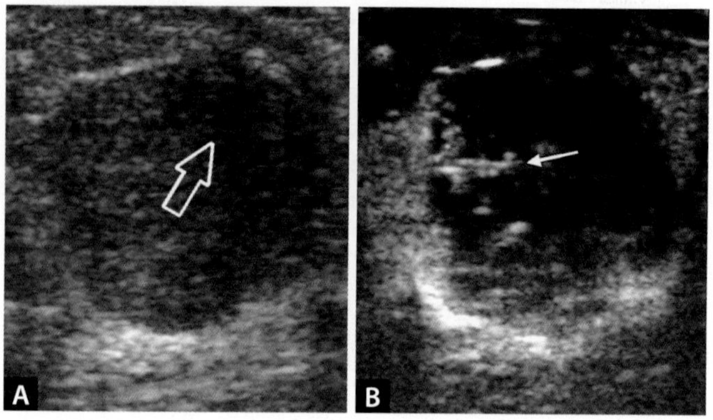

Figs. 10A and B: Invasive ductal carcinoma of breast: Simultaneous US display image (A) reveals an ill-defined hypoechoic mass lesion (block arrow) which is taller than wide. CEUS (B) demonstrates the spiculated margins of the mass and avid peripheral enhancement with central nonenhancing area. The ductal extension of tumor also shows avid enhancement (arrow).

adenocarcinoma tends to show early enhancement after administration of UCAs **(Figs. 11A and B)**. Several studies have compared the efficacy of CEUS guided targeted biopsy with systematic biopsy. It has been demonstrated that CEUS increased the detection rate of malignancy in the peripheral zone, but was not helpful in the central zone.[107,108] Some studies compared the yield of CEUS guided targeted biopsy with systematic biopsy and found a significantly increased detection rate on targeted biopsy,[109,110] although the detection of enhanced lesions lacked specificity or specific pattern of enhancement in adenocarcinomas.[111-113]

Miscellaneous Intravascular Applications

In the gastrointestinal tract, UCAs have been used in the disease activity evaluation in inflammatory bowel diseases[114-118] and clinical monitoring of Crohn's disease activity.[119] UCAs have also been used to differentiate between inflammatory and fibrotic strictures.[120] In spleen, UCAs can be used for lesion characterization,[121] to characterize suspected accessory spleen[122] and to confirm splenic infarction.[123] Tumor response assessment can be done in metastatic GIST using UCAs.[124,125]

While performing testicular sonography, use of UCAs have been recommended in the evaluation of a suspected segmental infarction (for better delineation of the infarct)[126], testicular trauma (for better detection of fracture line),[127] detecting areas of abscess formation in epididymo-orchitis.[128] and differentiating a neoplastic from a non-neoplastic focal lesion.[129]

Endometrial carcinoma is another frontier where the utility of CEUS has been explored where transvaginal CEUS can assess the depth of myometrial invasion, especially when the endometrial lining thin after biopsy.[130]

Application of CEUS in lung and pleural diseases is limited. In peripheral consolidations, CEUS can be used to differentiate embolic consolidation from an inflammatory etiology and to detect an area of abscess within a peripheral area of lung consolidation.[131-133] Vascular applications include carotid plaque characterization, differentiating a complete carotid occlusion from a tight stenosis, detection of dissection of carotid vessels and aorta,[134-137] characterization of suspected inflammatory abdominal aortic aneurysm, and detection, characterization and follow-up of endoleaks after abdominal aortic aneurysm repair.[138-140] For lymph node evaluation, it has been used for sentinel lymph node sampling in cancer patients, although not recommended in recent guidelines.[141]

Intracavitary Applications

Contrast-enhanced ultrasound has nonvascular applications as well. Assessment of the physiological cavities include voiding sonocystourethrogram or the evaluation of vesicoureteric reflux,[142] sono-hysterosalpingo-contrast sonography for tubal patency assessment,[143] CEUS-guided percutaneous cholangiography,[144] T-tube cholangiogram,[145] CEUS sialography for obstructive lesions of the salivary ducts,[146] CEUS guided nephrostomogram. Nonphysiologic cavities too can be evaluated by CEUS. Delineation of fistulae, abscesses and intraperitoneal collections and gastroesophageal reflux can be done successfully by different approaches.[147-149]

Upcoming Applications

Contrast-enhanced ultrasound is being tried in a big way for various novel applications. Some of the newer applications are worth mentioning in this chapter, such as assessment of transplanted kidneys,[150] perforator vessels in vascularized myocutaneous flaps, postoperative assessment of vascularity in myocutaneous flaps,[151-154] differentiation of an adherent GB sludge from a mass and detection of GB perforation in the setting of acute cholecystitis and for assessment of vascularity in uterine artery embolization for uterine fibroids.[155]

To conclude, the advent of UCAs have revolutionized the role of US in clinical practice. CEUS has emerged as a major player in hepatic imaging. It combines the advantage of superior spatial resolution of US with the real-time contrast kinetics assessment of focal liver lesions. While several nonhepatic applications are still in the experimental stage, but, the combination of new generations of UCAs and new ultrasound image sequences appears to be very promising. CEUS has the potential to become the most widely used imaging modality.

ACKNOWLEDGMENTS

The authors acknowledge the contribution of Dr Sanjay Sharma and Dr Vishal T for **Figures 11A and B**, from

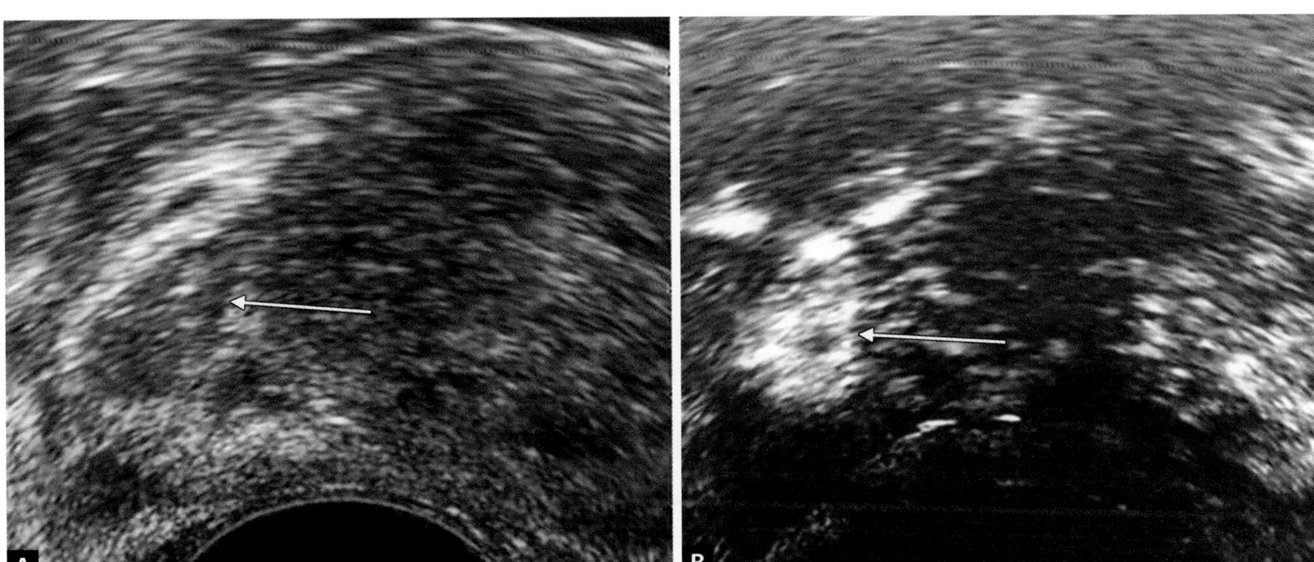

Figs. 11A and B: Transrectal sonography of adenocarcinoma of prostate: Simultaneous display US (A) shows hypoechoic mass lesion in the right half of the prostate (arrow); which shows increased enhancement compared to the rest of the gland after administration of UCAs (arrow in B).

the MD thesis work performed in the Department of Radiology, AIIMS (November 2009–November 2011).

REFERENCES

1. Shampo MA, Kyle RA. Karl Theodore Dussik- pioneer in ultrasound. Mayo Clinic Proceedings. 1995;70:1136.
2. Claudon M, Cosgrove D, Albrecht T, et al. Guidelines and good clinical practice recommendations for contrast-enhanced ultrasound (CEUS)—update 2008. Ultraschall Med. 2008;29:28-44.
3. Brannigan M, Burns PN, Wilson SR. Blood flow patterns in focal liver lesions at microbubble-enhanced US. Radiographics. 2004;24:921-35.
4. Cosgrove D, Blomley M. Liver tumors: evaluation with contrast-enhanced ultrasound. Abdom Imaging. 2004;29:446-54.
5. Kim TK, Lee KH, Khalili K, et al. Hepatocellular nodules in liver cirrhosis: contrast-enhanced ultrasound. Abdom Imaging. 2011;36:244-63.
6. Moschouris H, Malagari K, Marinis A, et al. Hepatocellular carcinoma treated with transarterial chemoembolization: Evaluation with parametric contrast-enhanced ultrasonography. World J Radiol. 2012;4:379-86.
7. Hui-Xiong Xu. Contrast-enhanced ultrasound: the evolving applications. World J Radiol. 2009;1:15-24.
8. Gramiak R, Shah PM. Echocardiography of the aortic root. Invest Radiol. 1968;3:356-66.
9. Nico de Jong, Marcia Emmer, Annemieke van Wamel, et al. Ultrasonic characterization of ultrasound contrast agents. Med Biol Eng Comput. 2009;47:861-73.
10. Christiansen C, Kryvi H, Sontum PC, et al. Physical and biochemical characterization of Albunex, a new ultrasound contrast agent consisting of air-filled albumin microspheres suspended in a solution of human albumin. Biotechnol Appl Biochem. 1994;19(Pt 3):307-20.
11. N de Jong, L Hoff. "Ultrasound scattering properties of Albunex microspheres". Ultrasonics. 1993;31:175-181.
12. Piscaglia F, Nolsoe C, Dietrich CF, et al. The EFSUMB guidelines and recommendations on the clinical practice of contrast enhanced ultrasound (CEUS): Update 2011 on nonhepatic applications. Ultraschall in Med. 2012;33:33-59.
13. Yanagisawa K, Moriyasu F, Miyahara T, et al. Phagocytosis of ultrasound contrast agent microbubbles by Kupffer cells. Ultrasound Med Bio. 2007;33:318-25.
14. Dietrich CF, Cui XW, Schreiber-Dietrich DG, et al. EFSUMB guidelines 2011: comments and illustrations. Ultraschall Med. 2012;33:S11-21.
15. Dietrich CF, Cui XW, Boozari B, et al. Contrast-enhanced ultrasound (CEUS) in the diagnostic algorithm of Hepatocellular and Cholangiocellular carcinoma, comments on the AASLD Guidelines. Ultrashall in Med. 2012;33:557-66.
16. Piscagalia F, Bolondi L. The safety of SonoVue in abdominal applications: retrospective analysis of 23188 investigations. Ultrasound Med Biol. 2006;32:1369-75.
17. Lencioni R, Piscaglia F, Bolondi L. Contrast-enhanced ultrasound in the diagnosis of hepatocellular carcinoma. Journal of Hepatology. 2008;48:848-57.
18. Albrecht T, Blomley M, Bolondi L, et al. Guidelines for the use of contrast agents in ultrasound. Ultraschall in Med. 2004;25:249-56.
19. Noone TC, Semelka RC, Chaney DM, et al. Abdominal imaging studies comparison of diagnostic accuracies resulting from ultrasound, computed tomography, and magnetic resonance imaging in the same individual. Magn Reson Imaging. 2004; 2219-24.
20. Wernecke K, Rummeny E, Bongartz G, et al. Detection of hepatic masses in patients with carcinoma comparative sensitivities of sonography, CT, and MR imaging. Am J Roentgenol. 1991;157:731-9.
21. Dietrich CF, Ignee A, Hocke M, et al. Pitfalls and artifacts using contrast-enhanced ultrasound. Z Gastroenterol. 2011;49:350-6.
22. Mitchell DG. Color Doppler imaging principles, limitations, and artifacts. Radiology. 1990;177:1-10.
23. Dai Y, Chen MH, Yin SS, et al. Focal liver lesions: can SonoVue-enhanced ultrasound be used to differentiate malignant from benign lesions? Invest Radiol. 2007;42:596-603.
24. Bartolotta TV, Taibbi A, Galia M, et al. Characterization of hypoechoic focal hepatic lesions in patients with fatty liver: diagnostic performance and confidence of contrast-enhanced ultrasound. Eur Radiol. 2007;17:650-61.
25. Hohmann J, Albrecht T, Hoffmann CW, et al. Ultrasonographic detection of focal liver lesions: increased sensitivity and specificity with microbubble contrast agents. Eur J Radiol. 2003;46:147-59.
26. Solbiati L, Tonolini M, Cova L, et al. The role of contrast-enhanced ultrasound in the detection of focal liver leasions. Eur Radiol. 2001;11:E15-E26.
27. Hatanaka K, Kudo M, Minami Y, et al. Sonazoid-enhanced ultrasonography for diagnosis of hepatic malignancies comparison with contrast-enhanced CT. Oncology. 2008;75 (Suppl) 1:42-7.
28. Xu HX, Liu GJ, Lu MD, et al. Characterization of small focal liver lesions using real-time contrast-enhanced sonography diagnostic performance analysis in 20 patients. J Ultrasound Med. 2006;25:349-61.
29. Sporea I, Badea R, Martie A, et al. Contrast-enhanced ultrasound for the evaluation of focal liver lesions in daily practice: a muticentric study. Medical Ultrasonography. 2012;14:95-100.
30. Nicolau C, Vilana R, Catalá V, et al. Importance of evaluating all vascular phases on contrast-enhanced sonography in the differentiation of benign from malignant focal liver lesions. Am J Roentgenol. 2006;186: 158-67.
31. Claudon M, Dietrich CF, Choi BI, et al. Guidelines and Good clinical practice recommendations for contrast-enhanced ultrasound (CEUS) in the liver—update 2012. Ultraschall Med. 2012 - PMID: 23129518.
32. Kono Y, Steinbach GC, Peterson T, et al. Mechanism of parenchymal enhancement of the liver with a microbubble-based US contrast medium; an intravital microscopy study in rats. Radiology 2002;224:253-7.
33. Von Herbay A, Vogt C, Willers R, et al. Real-time imaging with the sonographic contrast agent SonoVue

differentiation between benign and malignant hepatic lesions. J Ultrasound Med. 2004;23:1557-68.
34. Wilson SR, Burns PN. An algorithm for the diagnosis of focal liver masses using microbubble contrast-enhanced pulse-inversion sonography. Am J Roentgenol. 2006;186:1401-12.
35. Mergo PJ, Ros PR. Benign lesions of the liver. Radiol Clin North Am. 1998;36:319-31.
36. Xu HX. Contrast-enhanced ultrasound: the evolving applications. World J Radiol. 2009;1:15-24.
37. Ding H, Wang WP, Huang BJ, et al. Imaging of focal liver lesions low-mechanical-index real-time ultrasonography with SonoVue. J Ultrasound Med. 2005;24:285-97.
38. Leen E, Ceccotti P, Kalogeropoulou C, et al. Prospective multicenter trial evaluating a novel method of characterizing focal liver lesions using contrast-enhanced sonography. Am J Roentgenol. 2006;186:1551-9.
39. Morin SHX, Lim AKP, Cobbold JFL, et al. Use of second generation contrast-enhanced ultrasound in the assessment of focal liver lesions. WJG. 2007;13:5963-70.
40. Burns PN, Wilson SR. Focal liver masses enhancement patterns on contrast-enhanced images-concordance of US scans with CT scans and MR images. Radiology. 2007;242:162-74.
41. Dietrich CF, Mertens JC, Braden B, et al. Contrast-enhanced ultrasound of histologically proven liver hemangiomas. Hepatology. 2007;45:1139-45.
42. Nguyen BN, Flejou JF, Terris B, et al. Focal nodular hyperplasia of the liver a comprehensive pathologic study of 305 lesions and recognition of new histologic forms. Am J Surg Pathol. 1999;231441-54.
43. Quaia E, Calliada F, Bertolotto M, et al. Characterization of focal liver lesions with contrast-specific US modes and a sulfur hexafluoride-filled microbubble contrast agent diagnostic performance and confidence. Radiology. 2004;232420-30.
44. Shortell CK, Schwartz SI. Hepatic adenoma and focal nodular hyperplasia. Surg Gynecol Obstet. 1991;173426-31.
45. Kim TK, Jang HJ, Burns PN, et al. Focal nodular hyperplasia and hepatic adenoma differentiation with low-mechanical-index contrast-enhanced sonography. Am J Roentgenol. 2008;190:58-66.
46. Dietrich CF, Schuessler G, Trojan J, et al. Differentiation of focal nodular hyperplasia and hepatocellular adenoma by contrast-enhanced ultrasound. Br J Radiol. 2005; 78:704-7.
47. Catalano O, Sandomenico F, Raso MM, et al. Low mechanical index contrast-enhanced sonographic findings of pyogenic hepatic abscesses. Am J Roentgenol. 2004;182:447-50.
48. Kim TK, Jang HJ, Wilson SR. Benign liver masses: imaging with microbubble contrast agents. Ultrasound. Q 2006;22: 31-9.
49. Von Herbay A, Westendorff J, Gregor M. Contrast-enhanced ultrasound with SonoVue differentiation between benign and malignant focal liver lesions in 317 patients. J Clin Ultrasound. 2010;38:1-9.
50. Hagspiel KD, Neidl KF, Eichenberger AC, et al. Detection of liver metastasescomparison of superparamagnetic iron oxide-enhanced and unenhanced MR imaging at 1.5 T with dynamic CT, intraoperative US, and percutaneous US. Radiology. 1995;196:471-8.
51. Dietrich CF, Kratzer W, Strobe D, et al. Assessment of metastatic liver disease in patients with primary extra-hepatic tumors by contrast-enhanced sonography versus CT and MRI. World J Gastroenterol. 2006;121:699-705.
52. Pisani P, Parkin DM, Ferlay J. Estimates of the world-wide mortality from eighteen major cancers in 1985: implications for prevention and projections of future burden. Int J Cancer. 1993; 55: 891-3.
53. Jang HJ, Kim TK, Burns PN, et al. Enhancement patterns of hepatocellular carcinoma at contrast-enhanced US: comparison with histologic differentiation. Radiology. 2007;244:898-906.
54. Jang HJ, Yu H, Kim TK. Imaging of focal liver lesions. Semin Roentgenol. 2009;44:266-82.
55. Rossi S, Ghittoni G, Ravetta V, et al. Contrast-enhanced ultrasonography and spiral computed tomography in the detection and characterization of portal vein thrombosis complicating hepatocellular carcinoma. Eur Radiol. 2008;18:1749-56.
56. Chen LD, Xu HX, Xie XY, et al. Intrahepatic cholangio-carcinoma and hepatocellular carcinoma: differential diagnosis with contrast-enhanced ultrasound. Eur Radiol. 2010;20:743-53.
57. Vilana R, Forner A, Bianchi L, et al. Intrahepatic peripheral cholangiocarcinoma in cirrhosis patients may display a vascular pattern similar to hepatocellular carcinoma on contrast-enhanced ultrasound. Hepatology. 2010;51:2020-9.
58. Numata K, Isozaki T, Ozawa Y, et al. Percutaneous ablation therapy guided by contrast-enhanced sonography for patients with hepatocellular carcinoma. Am J Roentgenol. 2003;180:143-9.
59. Masuzaki R, Shiina S, Tateishi R, et al. Utility of contrast-enhanced ultrasonography with Sonazoid in radiofrequency ablation for hepatocellular carcinoma. J Gastroenterol Hepatol. 2011;26:759-64.
60. Maruyama H, Takahashi M, Ishibashi H, et al. Ultrasound-guided treatments under low acoustic power contrast harmonic imaging for hepatocellular carcinomas undetected by B-mode ultrasonography. Liver Int. 2009;29:708-14.
61. Minami Y, Kudo M, Hatanaka K, et al. Radiofrequency ablation-guided by contrast harmonic sonography using perfluorocarbon microbubbles (Sonazoid) for hepatic malignancies: an initial experience. Liver Int. 2010;30:759-64.
62. Miyamoto N, Hiramatsu K, Tsuchiya K, et al. Contrast-enhanced sonography-guided radiofrequency ablation for the local recurrence of previously treated hepatocellular carcinoma undetected by B-mode sonography. J Clin Ultrasound. 2010;38: 339-45.
63. Lu MD, Yu XL, Li AH, et al. Comparison of contrast-enhanced ultrasound and contrast enhanced CT or MRI in monitoring percutaneous thermal ablation procedure in patients with hepatocellular carcinoma: a multicenter study in China. Ultrasound Med Biol. 2007;33: 1736-49.
64. Meloni MF, Andreano A, Franza E, et al. Contrast-enhanced ultrasound: Should it play a role in immediate evaluation of

liver tumors following thermal ablation. European Journal of Radiology. 2012;81:e897-e902.
65. Xia YU, Kudo M, Minami Y, et al. Response evaluation of Transarterial chemoembolization in hepatocellular carcinomas: the usefulness of Sonazoid-enhanced harmonic sonography. Oncology. 2008;65:99-105.
66. Wang Z, Tang J, An L, et al. Contrast-enhanced ultrasonography for assessment of tumor vascularity in hepatocellular carcinoma. J Ultrasound Med. 2007;26:757-62.
67. Lassau N, Chami L, Chebil M, et al. Dynamic contrast-enhanced ultrasonography (DCE-US) and antiangiogenic treatments. Discov Med. 2011;11:18-24.
68. Lassau N, Koscielny S, Chami L, et al. Advanced hepatocellular carcinoma: early evaluation of response to Bevacizumab therapy at dynamic contrast-enhanced US with quantification-preliminary results. Radiology. 2010;b258:291-300.
69. Li N, Ding H, Fan P, et al. Intrahepatic transit time predicts liver fibrosis in patients with chronic hepatitis B: quantitative assessment with contrast-enhanced ultrasonography. Ultrasound Med Biol. 2010;36:1066-75.
70. Lim AK, Taylor-Robinson SD, Patel N, et al. Hepatic vein transit times using a microbubble agent can predict disease severity noninvasively in patients with hepatitis C. Gut. 2005;54:128-33.
71. Kitano M, Kudo M, Maekawa K, et al. Dynamic imaging of pancreatic diseases by contrast-enhanced coded phase inversion harmonic ultrasonography. Gut. 2004;53:854-9.
72. Badea R, Seicean A, Diaconu B, et al. Contrast-enhanced ultrasound of the pancreas—a method beyond its potential or a new diagnostic standard? Clinical Imaging J Gastrointestin Liver Dis June. 2009;18(2):237-42.
73. D'Onofrio M, Megibow AJ, Faccioli N, et al. Comparison of contrast-enhanced sonography and MRI in displaying anatomic features of cystic pancreatic masses. Am J Roentgenol. 2007;189:1435-42.
74. D'Onofrio M, Mansueto G, Falconi M, et al. Neuroendocrine pancreatic tumor: value of contrast-enhanced ultrasonography. Abdom Imaging. 2004;29:246-58.
75. Dietrich CF, Braden B, Hocke M, et al. Improved characterization of solitary solid pancreatic tumours using contrast-enhanced transabdominal ultrasound. J Cancer Res Clin Oncol. 2008;134: 635-43.
76. Rickes S, Wermke W. Differentiation of cystic pancreatic neoplasms and pseudocysts by conventional and echo-enhanced ultrasound. J Gastroenterol Hepatol. 2004;19:761-6.
77. Ripolles T, Martinez MJ, Lopez E, et al. Contrast-enhanced ultrasound in the staging of acute pancreatitis. Eur Radiol. 2010; 20:2518-23.
78. Becker D, Strobel D, Bernatik T, et al. Echo-enhanced color and power Doppler EUS for the discrimination between focal pancreatitis and pancreatic carcinoma. Gastrointest Endosc. 2001;53:784-9.
79. Bhutani MS, Hoffman BJ, van Velse A, et al. Contrast-enhanced endoscopic ultrasonography with galactose microparticles: SHU508 A (Levovist). Endoscopy. 1997;29:635-9.
80. Dietrich CF, Ignee A, Frey H. Contrast-enhanced endoscopic ultrasound with low mechanical index: a new technique. Z Gastroenterol. 2005;43:1219-23.
81. Dietrich CF. Contrast-enhanced low mechanical index endoscopic ultrasound (CELMI-EUS). Endoscopy; 2009;41 (Suppl 2):E43-E44.
82. Kitano M, Sakamoto H, Matsui U, et al. A novel perfusion imaging technique of the pancreas: contrast-enhanced harmonic EUS (with video). Gastrointest Endosc. 2008;67:141-50.
83. Hocke M, Schulze E, Gottschalk P, et al. Contrast-enhanced endoscopic ultrasound in discrimination between focal pancreatitis and pancreatic cancer. World J Gastroenterol. 2006;12(2):246-50.
84. Quaia E, Bertolotto M, Cioffi V, et al. Comparison of contrast-enhanced sonography with unenhanced sonography and contrast-enhanced CT in the diagnosis of malignancy in complex cystic renal masses. Am J Roentgenol. 2008;191:1239-49.
85. Clevert DA, Minaifar N, Weckbach S, et al. Multislice computed tomography versus contrast-enhanced ultrasound in evaluation of complex cystic renal masses using the Bosniak classification system. Clin Hemorheol Microcirc. 2008;39:171-8.
86. Park BK, Kim B, Kim SH, et al. Assessment of cystic renal masses based on Bosniak classification: comparison of CT and contrast-enhanced US. Eur J Radiol. 2007;61:310-4.
87. Ascenti G, Mazziotti S, Zimbaro G, et al. Complex cystic renal masses: characterization with contrast-enhanced US. Radiology. 2007;243:158-65.
88. Mazziotti S, Zimbaro F, Pandolfo A, et al. Usefulness of contrast-enhanced ultrasonography in the diagnosis of renal pseudotumors. Abdom Imaging. 2010;35:241-5.
89. Bertolotto M, Martegani A, Aiani L, et al. Value of contrast-enhanced ultrasonography for detecting renal infarcts proven by contrast-enhanced CT. A feasibility study. Eur Radiol. 2008; 18:376-83.
90. Wink MH, Lagerveld BW, Laguna MP, et al. Cryotherapy for renal-cell cancer: diagnosis, treatment, and contrast-enhanced ultrasonography for follow-up. J Endourol. 2006;20:456-8, discussion 458-9.
91. Johnson DB, Duchene DA, Taylor GD, et al. Contrast-enhanced ultrasound evaluation of radiofrequency ablation of the kidney: reliable imaging of the thermolesion. J Endourol. 2005;19:248-52.
92. Hoeffel C, Pousset M, Timsit MO, et al. Radiofrequency ablation of renal tumours: diagnostic accuracy of contrast-enhanced ultrasound for early detection of residual tumour. Eur Radiol. 2010;20:1812-21.
93. Meloni MF, Bertolotto M, Alberzoni C, et al. Follow-up after percutaneous radiofrequency ablation of renal cell carcinoma: contrast-enhanced sonography versus contrast-enhanced CT or MRI. Am J Roentgenol. 2008;191:1233-8.
94. Correas JM, Claudon M, Tranquart F, et al. The kidney: imaging with microbubble contrast agents. Ultrasound Q. 2006;22:53-66.
95. Paajanen H, Lahti P, Nordback I. Sensitivity of transabdominal ultrasonography in detection of intraperitoneal fluid in humans. Eur Radiol. 1999;9:1423-5.

96. Poletti PA, Kinkel K, Vermeulen B, et al. Blunt abdominal trauma: should US be used to detect both free fluid and organ injuries? Radiology. 2003;227:95-103.
97. Valentino M, Serra C, Zironi G, De Luca C, Pavlica P, Barozzi L. Blunt Abdominal Trauma: Emergency Contrast-enhanced sonography for detection of solid organ injuries. AJR. 2006; 186:1361-136.
98. Catalano O, Aiani L, Barozzi L, et al. CEUS in abdominal trauma: multicenter study. Abdom Imaging. 2009;34:225-34.
99. Del Cura JL, Elizagaray E, Zabala R, et al. The use of unenhanced Doppler sonography in the evaluation of solid breast lesions. Am J Roentgenol. 2005;184:1788-94.
100. Ozdemir A, Ozdemir H, Maral I, et al. Differential diagnosis of solid breast lesions: contribution of Doppler studies to mammography and gray scale imaging. J Ultrasound Med. 2001;20(10):1091-101.
101. Italian Society of Medical Radiology. Charta senologica. Diagnostic approach to breast diseases. Radiol Med. 2004;108:569-87.
102. Chapellier C, Balu-Maestro C, Bleuse A, et al. Ultrasonography of invasive lobular carcinoma of the breast: sonographic patterns and diagnostic value: report of 102 cases. Clin Imaging. 2000;24:333-6.
103. Baum F, Fischer U, Vosshenrich, et al. Classification of hypervascularized lesions in CE MR imaging of the breast. Eur Radiol. 2002;12:1087-92.
104. Kedar RP, Cosgrove D, McCready VR, et al. Microbubble contrast agent for color Doppler US: effect on breast masses—work in progress. Radiology. 1996;198:679-86.
105. Stuhrmann M, Aronius R, Schietzel M. Tumor vascularity of breast lesions: potentials and limits of contrast-enhanced Doppler sonography. Am J Roentgenol. 2000;175: 1585-9.
106. Vallone P, D'Angelo R, Filice S, et al. Color-Doppler using contrast medium in evaluating the response to neoadjuvant treatment in patients with locally advanced breast carcinoma. Anticancer Res. 2005;25:595-9.
107. Halpern EJ, McCue PA, Aksnes AK, et al. Contrast enhanced sonography of the prostate with Sonazoid: comparison with prostatectomy specimens in twelve patients. Radiology. 2002;222:361-6.
108. Halpern EJ, Ramey JR, Strup SE, et al. Detection of prostate cancer with contrast-enhanced sonography using intermittent harmonic imaging. Cancer. 2005;104:2372-83.
109. Mitterberger MJ, Aigner F, Horninger W, et al. Comparative efficiency of contrast-enhanced color Doppler ultrasound targeted versus systematic biopsy for prostate cancer detection. Eur Radiol. 2010;20:2791-6.
110. Wink M, Frauscher F, Cosgrove D, et al. Contrast-enhanced ultrasound and prostate cancer, a multicentre European research coordination project. Eur Urol. 2008;54:982-92.
111. Aigner F, Pallwein L, Mitterberger M, et al. Contrast-enhanced ultrasonography using cadence-contrast pulse sequencing technology for targeted biopsy of the prostate. BJU Int. 2009;103:458-63.
112. Sano F, Terao H, Kawahara T, et al. Contrast-enhanced ultrasonography of the prostate: various imaging findings that indicate prostate cancer. BJU Int. 2010;107:1404-10.
113. Strazdina A, Krumina G, Sperga M. The value and limitations of contrast-enhanced ultrasound in detection of prostate cancer. Anticancer Res. 2011;31:1421-6.
114. Robotti D, Cammarota T, Debani P, et al. Activity of Crohn disease: value of color-power-Doppler and contrast-enhanced ultrasonography. Abdom Imaging. 2004;29:648-52.
115. De Pascale A, Garofalo G, Perna M, et al. Contrast-enhanced ultrasonography in Crohn's disease. Radiol Med. 2006;111:539-50.
116. Serra C, Menozzi G, Labate AM, et al. Ultrasound assessment of vascularization of the thickened terminal ileum wall in Crohn's disease patients using a low-mechanical index real-time scanning technique with a second generation ultrasound contrast agent. Eur J Radiol. 2007;62: 114-21.
117. Migaleddu V, Scanu AM, Quaia E, et al. Contrast-enhanced ultrasonographic evaluation of inflammatory activity in Crohn's disease. Gastroenterology. 2009;137:43-52.
118. Girlich C, Schacherer D, Jung EM, et al. Comparison between a clinical activity index (Harvey-Bradshaw-Index), laboratory inflammation markers and quantitative assessment of bowel wall vascularization by contrast-enhanced ultrasound in Crohn's disease. Eur J Radiol 2011; epub DOI: 10.1016/j.ejrad.2011.02.054.
119. Guidi L, De Franco A, De Vitis I, et al. Contrast-enhanced ultrasonography with SonoVue after infliximab therapy in Crohn's disease. Eur Rev Med Pharmacol Sci. 2006;10:23-6.
120. Wilson SR, Burns PN. Microbubble-enhanced US in body imaging: what role? Radiology. 2010;257:24-39.
121. Yu X, Yu J, Liang P, et al. Real-time contrast-enhanced ultrasound in diagnosing of focal spleen lesions. Eur J Radiol 2011; epub DOI: 10.1016/ j.ejrad.2010.12.052.
122. Gorg C, Bert T. Second-generation sonographic contrast agent for differential diagnosis of perisplenic lesions. Am J Roentgenol. 2006;186:621-6.
123. Gorg C, Graef C, Bert T. Contrast-enhanced sonography for differential diagnosis of an inhomogeneous spleen of unknown cause in patients with pain in the left upper quadrant. J Ultrasound Med. 2006;25:729-34.
124. Lassau N, Lamuraglia M, Chami L, et al. Gastrointestinal stromal tumors treated with imatinib: monitoring response with contrast-enhanced sonography. Am J Roentgenol. 2006;187:1267-73.
125. Giorgi U, Aliberti C, Benea G, et al. Effect of angiosonography to monitor response during imatinib treatment in patients with metastatic gastrointestinal stromal tumors. Clin Cancer Res. 2005;11:6171-6.
126. Bertolotto M, Derchi LE, Sidhu PS, et al. Acute segmental testicular infarction at contrast-enhanced ultrasound: early features and changes during follow-up. Am J Roentgenol. 2011;196:834-41.
127. Valentino M, Bertolotto M, Derchi L, et al. Role of contrast enhanced ultrasound in acute scrotal diseases. Eur Radiol 2011; epub DOI: 10.1007/s00330-010-2039-5.
128. Moschouris H, Stamatiou K, Lampropoulou E, et al. Imaging of the acute scrotum: is there a place for contrast-enhanced ultrasonography? Int Braz J Urol. 2009;35:692-702, discussion 702-695.

129. Lock G, Schmidt C, Helmich F, et al. Early experience with contrast-enhanced ultrasound in the diagnosis of testicular masses: a feasibility study. Urology. 2011; 77:1049-53.
130. Liu ZZ, Jiang YX, Dai Q, et al. Imaging of endometrial carcinoma using contrast-enhanced sonography. J Ultrasound Med. 2011;30:1519-27.
131. Gorg C. Transcutaneous contrast-enhanced sonography of pleural based pulmonary lesions. Eur J Radiol. 2007;64:213-21.
132. Bertolini FA, Goerg C, Mathis G. Echo contrast ultrasound in subpleural consolidations. Echo contrast ultrasound in subpleural consolidations. 2008;18 (Suppl S395).
133. Gorg C, Bert T, Gorg K. Contrast-enhanced sonography for differential diagnosis of pleurisy and focal pleural lesions of unknown cause. Chest. 2005;128:3894-9.
134. Coli S, Magnoni M, Sangiorgi G, et al. Contrast-enhanced ultrasound imaging of intraplaque neovascularization in carotid arteries: correlation with histology and plaque echogenicity. J Am Coll Cardiol. 2008;52:223-30.
135. Giannoni MF, Vicenzini E, Citone M, et al. Contrast carotid ultrasound for the detection of unstable plaques with neoangiogenesis: a pilot study. Eur J Vasc Endovasc Surg. 2009;37:722-7.
136. Clevert DA, Horng A, Jung EM, et al. Contrast-enhanced ultrasound versus conventional ultrasound and MS-CT in the diagnosis of abdominal aortic dissection. Clin Hemorheol Microcirc. 2009;43:129-39.
137. Clevert DA, Sommer WH, Zengel P, et al. Imaging of carotid arterial diseases with contrast-enhanced ultrasound (CEUS). Eur J Radiol. 2011; epub DOI: 10.1016/j.ejrad.2010.12.103.
138. Clevert DA, Schick K, Chen MH, et al. Role of contrast-enhanced ultrasound in detection of abdominal aortic abnormalities in comparison with multislice computed tomography. Chin Med J (Engl). 2009;122:858-64.
139. Clevert DA, Minaifar N, Weckbach S, et al. Color duplex ultrasound and contrast-enhanced ultrasound in comparison to MS-CT in the detection of endoleak following endovascular aneurysm repair. Clin Hemorheol Microcirc. 2008;39:121-32.
140. Ten Bosch JA, Rouwet EV, Peters CT, et al. Contrast-enhanced ultrasound versus computed tomographic angiography for surveillance of endovascular abdominal aortic aneurysm repair. J Vasc Interv Radiol. 2010;21:638-43.
141. Sever AR, Mills P, Jones SE, et al. Preoperative sentinel node identification with ultrasound using microbubbles in patients with breast cancer. Am J Roentgenol. 2010;196:251-6.
142. Lebowitz RL, Olbing H, Parkkulainen KV, et al. International system of radiographic grading of vesicoureteric reflux. International Reflux Study in Children. Pediatr Radiol 1985; 15:105-9.
143. Lanzani C, Savasi V, Leone FP, et al. Two-dimensional HyCoSy with contrast tuned imaging technology and a second-generation contrast media for the assessment of tubal patency in an infertility program. Fertil Steril. 2009;92:1158-61.
144. Ignee A, Baum U, Schuessler G, et al. Contrast-enhanced ultrasound-guided percutaneous cholangiography and cholangiodrainage (CEUSPTCD). Endoscopy. 2009;41:725-6.
145. Mao R, Xu EJ, Li K, et al. Usefulness of contrast-enhanced ultrasound in the diagnosis of biliary leakage following T-tube removal. J Clin Ultrasound. 2009;38:38-40.
146. Zengel P, Berghaus A, Weiler C, et al. Intraductally applied contrast-enhanced ultrasound (IA-CEUS) for evaluating obstructive disease and secretory dysfunction of the salivary glands. Eur Radiol. 2011;21:1339-48.
147. Henrich W, Meckies J, Friedmann W. Demonstration of a recto-vaginal fistula with the ultrasound contrast medium Echovist. Ultrasound Obstet Gynecol. 2000;15:148-9.
148. Volkmer BG, Nesslauer T, Kufer R, et al. Diagnosis of vesico-intestinal fistulas by contrast medium enhanced 3-D ultrasound. Ultraschall in Med. 2001;22:81-6.
149. Chew SS, Yang JL, Newstead GL, et al. Anal fistula: Levovist-enhanced endoanal ultrasound: a pilot study. Dis Colon Rectum. 2003;46:377-84.
150. Lefevre F, Correas JM, Briancon S, et al. Contrast-enhanced sonography of the renal transplant using triggered pulse-inversion imaging: preliminary results. Ultrasound Med Biol. 2002;28:303-14.
151. Gardiner MD, Nanchahal J. Strategies to ensure success of microvascular free tissue transfer. J Plast Reconstr Aesthet Surg. 2010;63:e665-73.
152. Prantl L, Pfister K, Kubale R, et al. Value of high resolution ultrasound and contrast-enhanced US pulse inversion imaging for the evaluation of the vascular integrity of free-flap grafts. Clin Hemorheol Microcirc. 2007;36:203-16.
153. Prantl L, Schmitt S, Geis S, et al. Contrast harmonic ultrasound and indocyanine- green fluorescence video angiography for evaluation of dermal and subdermal microcirculation in free parascapular flaps. Clin Hemorheol Microcirc. 2008;38:105-18.
154. Prantl L, Schreml S, Walter M, et al. Evaluation of microcirculation of free flaps of the lower leg by contrast harmonic imaging (CHI) with time intensity curve (TIC) analysis. Clin Hemorheol Microcirc. 2008;39:343-50.
155. Marret H, Sauget S, Giraudeau B, et al. Contrast-enhanced sonography helps in discrimination of benign from malignant adnexal masses. J Ultrasound Med. 2004;23:1629–39, quiz 1641-2.

CHAPTER 56

Iodinated Contrast Media: An Update

Chandrashekhara SH, Sanjay Thulkar

INTRODUCTION

Iodinated contrast media (ICM) are widely used pharmaceutical agents in radiology and have become an integral part of many diagnostic imaging studies. Most commonly they are used intravenously, but for many diagnostic studies, they can also be used intra-arterially, intrathecally, orally and intra-abdominally. Although ICM are safe to use, adverse events do occur, which vary from mild physiological disturbances to life-threatening complications. The radiologists must recognize early and manage these adverse reactions, which are inherent in the use of contrast media.[1]

The ideal qualities of intravascular contrast agents are as follows:

- Water solubility
- Chemical and heat stability
- Biological inertness (nonantigenic)
- Low viscosity
- Lower or same osmolality as human serum
- Selective excretion (i.e. kidney)
- Safety
- Low cost
- Their formulations should be free of substances interfering with physiological homeostasis.[2-4]

HISTORY OF DEVELOPMENT OF IODINATED CONTRAST MEDIA

All the researches in the development of contrast media have proceeded with basic objectives (i.e. increased efficacy and reduced toxicity) which characterize all pharmaceutical research.

- In 1920s, the first radiographic contrast medium introduced for clinical practice was sodium iodide, which had limitations of high toxicity and poor radiographic contrast.[5]
- The first major breakthrough in the development of safer contrast media came, when iodine was bound to organic molecules, enabling significant reduction of iodine toxicity compared with sodium iodide (an inorganic salt). First organic salt, uroselectan (Iopax) was developed by Moses Swick, was readily excreted by kidneys and was surprisingly of relatively low toxicity. However, the major disadvantage of uroselecton was lesser efficacy in terms of contrast enhancement, as each molecule bound to only one iodine atom. Uroselectan-B (Neoiopax) [which is a bisodium salt with two iodine atoms and two particles in solution] quickly replaced uroselectan, providing slightly more iodine per molecule, lower toxicity and improved solubility.
- Diodrast (Iodopyracet), a di-iodinated N-pyridone compound was the dominant agent for excretory urography from early 1930s until acetrizoate was developed.
- In the 1950s, sodium and meglumine salts of tri-iodinated benzoic acid (acetrizoic acid), were introduced, which were of much lower toxicity but hyperosmolar (having osmolality five to eight times that of the blood). Acetrizoate (Urokon) provided adequate urograms at that time. In order to improve

efficacy and safety, various modifications of this tri-iodinated contrast medium, i.e. acetrizoic acid were done. It was postulated that the presence of a hydrogen atom on the tri-iodinated benzene ring gives a higher degree of protein binding than when the hydrogen atom has been substituted. It was also hypothesized that an increase in protein binding factor incited anaphylactic reactions.[6]

- Diatrizoate (Hypaque, Renografin) replaced acetrizoate (Urokon) in 1955–1956 as sodium and meglumine salts of diatrizoic acid proved safer and more diagnostically efficacious than earlier drugs. In diatrizoate, the unsubstituted hydrogen of acetrizoate has been exchanged for another acetamido unit, which caused increased biologic tolerance.[7]
- In the 1960s, majority of water soluble contrast media used were salts of iodinated fully substituted benzoic acid derivatives. These organic acids have 3 hydrogen atoms replaced by iodinated atoms and 3 hydrogen atoms replaced by simple side chains; for every 3 iodine atoms in solution, 2 particles are produced (one anion and one cation) in the ratio of 3:2. Subsequently, iothalamate (Conray) joined the market place in 1962, and the meglumine salt was first designed for urography.
- The next major development came in the 1970s with the introduction of low-osmolar contrast media (LOCM), which was achieved by converting tri-iodinated benzoic acid into a nonionic molecule by replacing the ionizing carboxylic acid (COOH) radical with hydrophilic structures that could be covalently bound to the benzene ring, i.e. an amide ($CONH_2$). This molecule does not dissociate in solution providing three atoms of iodine with only one active particle [ratio of 3:1] compared to a ratio of 1.5 [3 iodine atoms: 2 particles] seen with high-osmolar contrast medium. Dr Torsten was the first one to propose that nonionic molecules could reduce osmolality. Subsequently, Almen introduced the first ratio-three nonionic monomer, metrizamide in 1977.[8-10] Low-osmolar contrast media of this generation, which are now in widespread clinical use includes iohexol, ioversol, iopamidol and iobitridol.[11] Iohexol (Omnipaque) is the first nonionic contrast agent introduced, has the longest track record worldwide and is used for intravascular and intrathecal imaging studies. Iopamidol (Isovue) is used for intravascular and intrathecal imaging studies and ioversol (Optiray) used in intra-arterial and intravenous (IV) applications.
- In the 1980s nonionic-dimeric contrast media were introduced; two nonionic tri-iodinated benzoic rings were attached, giving iodine: particle ratio of 6:1, since there are 6 iodine atoms and only one active particle in each molecule.
- In 1980s and 1990s, there was an ongoing development of nonionic isotonic dimers. These agents are consequence of further applications of principles, such as eliminating ionicity, increasing hydrophilicity, lowering osmotoxicity and increasing the iodine atoms per molecule.

BASIC CHEMISTRY OF ICM

Tri-iodinated benzene ring is the basic constituent of all ICM **(Figs 1A to D)**. Benzene ring has 6 carbons numbered 1–6 clockwise. Carbon 1 attachment differentiates ionic from nonionic contrast media. At C1 in ionic contrast media, acidic group with sodium or meglumine is attached. At C1 in nonionic contrast media, amide group is attached.[12,13] Iodine atoms are attached at position 2, 4, 6 carbons. C3 and C5 have amide attachments to increase solubility and also to reduce protein binding. Iodine (atomic weight 127) provides excellent radioopacity because of higher atomic number and K-shell electron binding energy of 34 keV, which is lower than but close to mean energy used in diagnostic X-rays and thus maximizing the photoelectric effect.

TYPES OF ICM

Iodinated contrast media are divided based on their osmolality and ionicity. **High-osmolar contrast media (HOCM)** have more than 1400 mOsm/kg H_2O osmolality

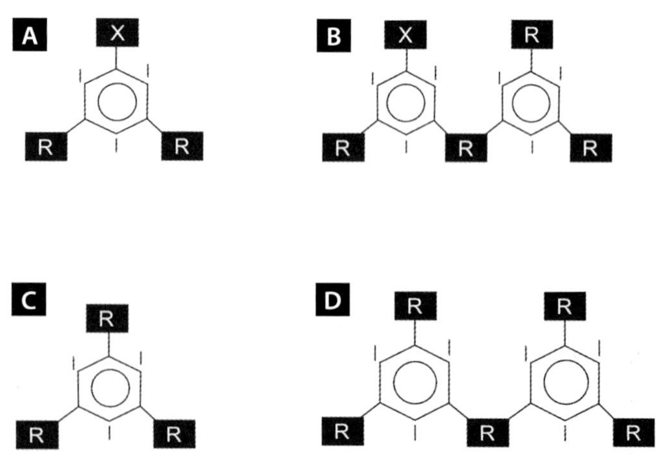

Figs. 1A to D: Types of iodinated contrast media. All ICM are based on tri-iodinated benzene ring. (A) Ionic monomer; (B) Ionic dimer; (C) Nonionic monomer; (D) Nonionic dimer (R-Hydrophilic, nonionizing side chains; X-Ionic moiety, $-COO^-$ and either sodium or meglumine cation).

(5–8 times the osmolarity of plasma) and most of them are ionic. **Low-osmolar contrast media** have 600–800 mOsm/kg H_2O (2–3 times the osmolarity of plasma) and consists of both ionic and nonionic contrast media. **Iso-osmolar contrasts** have osmolality of 290 mOsm/kg H_2O (same osmolarity as blood, plasma and cerebrospinal fluid) and only one product, which is nonionic is currently available.

Broadly, ICM are characterized as ionic or nonionic types. Ionic contrast medium breakdown into cations (positively charged particles) and anions (negatively charged particles) when enter solutions, such as blood.[11] This results in more molecules per kilogram of water with increase in osmolality. For every 3 iodine molecules present in an ionic contrast media, one cation and one anion are produced on entering a solution and thus described as 3:2 compounds. In contrast, nonionic contrast media does not dissolve into charged particles on entering a solution. For every 3 iodine molecules in a nonionic contrast media, one neutral molecule is produced and thus referred as 3:1 compounds.

Ionic and nonionic contrast media can be monomeric or dimeric types. Usually each benzene ring of ICM produces 3 iodine atoms. Monomer contains only one benzene ring. For delivering more iodine with each molecule of contrast, 2 benzene rings may be combined to produce a dimer, which would deliver 6 iodine atoms with each molecule.

The iodinated benzene ring contains ionizing carboxyl groups with a cation, usually sodium or meglumine.[2] Meglumine is the chosen organic cation since it has lower pharmacological activity in comparison to the sodium ion (and therefore better tolerance), but being a much larger ion, it increases viscosity. The carboxyl groups ionize in solution, making the agents water soluble. Since these compounds dissociate into ions in solution and contain only one iodinated benzene ring, these are described as **ionic monomeric agents**. Commonly used contrast material anions are diatrizoate and iothalamate. In a solution, ionic monomers break up into their anion and cation components, delivering 3 iodine atoms (3:2 ratio of iodine to osmolar particles). Thus, these have a relatively high osmolality (>1400 mOsm/kg at 50–76% by weight concentrations). Ionic monomer preparations, commonly available in India are meglumine iothalamate, sodium iothalamate, meglumine and sodium diatrizoate.

Nonionic monomers are the most widely used among lower-osmolality contrast agents. In nonionic monomers, the tri-iodinated benzene ring is made water soluble by adding five or six hydrophilic hydroxyl groups to organic side chains placed at 1, 3 and 5 positions. As there is no carboxyl group, these do not ionize in solution and a single molecule delivers 3 iodine atoms (3:1 ratio of iodine to osmolar particles). These have relatively low osmolality (600–800 mOsm/kg) at comparable iodine concentrations. Nonionic monomer preparations currently available in India are iohexol, iopromide, ioversol, iopamidol and iomeprol.

Ionic dimers are formed by joining two ionic monomers together and eliminating one of the carboxyl groups. These would deliver 2 ionic components per 6 iodine atoms (6:2 ratio of iodine to osmolar particles). These agents have concentration of 59% (320 mg iodine/mL) and a relatively low osmolality of 600 mOsm/kg at comparable iodine concentrations. Ioxaglate (Hexabrix) is the only ionic dimer currently available and is used widely for peripheral arteriography than for IV studies.

Nonionic dimers consist of two joined nonionic monomers. Single nonionic dimer delivers 6 iodine atoms (6:1 ratio of iodine to osmolar particles) and thus, are the most ideal contrast medium as they deliver the most iodine with the least effect on osmolality (approximately 290 mOsm/kg). At approximately 60% by weight concentration, these are iso-osmolar with plasma.[3] However, it results in higher viscosity and greater resistance to catheter injection.[14] Nonionic-dimer iodixanol (Visipaque) is currently available in India and has an osmolality of 290 mOsm/kg H_2O, same as blood.

In brief, there are four classes of ICM, i.e. high-osmolar ionic monomers, low-osmolar nonionic monomers, low osmolar ionic dimers and iso-osmolar nonionic dimers **(Table 1)**. These are available in various concentrations of iodine and have different physicochemical properties (osmolality, viscosity, hydrophilicity, ions content and pH). All ICM are distributed in the extracellular compartment and do not cross an intact blood–brain barrier and all are excreted via glomerular filtration.[3]

The iodine concentration of an individual contrast agent establishes the radioopacity of the contrast agent. The higher the iodine concentration, more the X-ray photons will be absorbed and thus particular contrast agent may be more radioopaque than the agent with comparative low iodine concentration. The iodine concentration affects the severity of an adverse reaction. The higher the iodine concentration, the more is the risk of an adverse reaction. Thus, more iodine ratio represents better opacification and fewer particles of contrast medium mean lower osmotoxic effect.[15]

ICM PHARMACOKINETICS

The salient pharmacokinetic properties of ICM are high-water solubility, low-lipid solubility, low-plasma protein binding and molecular weight ranging from 600 to 1650.

Table 1: Most commonly available iodinated contrast media.

Name of the contrast media	*Iodine/particle ratio*	*Iodine concentration (mg/kg)*	*Osmolality (mOsm/kg)*	*Viscosity (cPs at 37°C)*
• *Ionic monomer*:				
– Diatrizoate (Hypaque 50; GE Healthcare)	3/2(1.5)	300	1,550 (high)	5.2
– Metrizoate Isopaque (Coronar 370; Nycomed A/S)		370	2,100 (high)	2.34
• *Ionic dimer*:				
– Ioxaglate (Hexabrix; Guerbet lab.)	6/2(3.0)	320	580 (low)	7.5
• *Nonionic monomer*:				
– Iopamidol (Isovue-370; Bracco Diagnostics Inc.)	3/1(3.0)	370	796 (low)	3.0–9.4
– Iohexol (Omnipaque 350; GE Healthcare)		350	884 (low)	1.5–10.4
– Iomeprol (Iomeron-350,400; Bracco Intl.)		350	618 (low)	7.5
		400	726 (low)	12.6
• *Nonionic dimer*:				
– Iodixanol (Visipaque 320; GE Healthcare)	6/1(6.0)	320	290 (iso)	6.3–11.8

They are distributed only in the extracellular fluid and not metabolized. They are excreted mainly by glomerular filtration. Due to affinity for proteins and membrane bound receptors, ICM have minimal pharmacological action. Small size of the contrast molecules and high-water solubility permits free distribution of contrast across the vascular endothelium and thus between the intravascular extracellular space (blood pool) and extravascular extracellular compartment (interstitium).

There is no evidence of any substantial penetration of these contrast media molecules through the intact cell membrane or into the interior of the viable cells, except for the proximal tubular cells of the kidney. Theoretically, the differences in the molecular weight and size between the monomeric and dimeric contrast agents could lead to slightly-slower distribution rates into extracellular space for the larger dimers. This effect, however, appears to be quite small and is probably clinically insignificant. The effects of isotonic dimers on increased renal intratubular viscosity are yet to be fully assessed.[16,17]

When the contrast media molecules enter the systemic circulation, the molecules rapidly equilibrate across capillary membranes (except an intact blood-brain barrier) and are distributed throughout the intra- and extravascular extracellular space.[18] In the first phase of distribution, increase in the intravascular osmolality for the hypertonic agents, including the LOCM, causes a rapid fluid shift across capillary membranes toward the hypertonic (intravascular) compartment. As the contrast medium molecules pass through the capillary bed, rapid movement occurs through the capillary pores into the interstitial, extracellular space, as well as glomerular filtration into the renal tubules. Early vascular enhancement depends on the rate of iodine administration and blood flow; whereas parenchymal enhancement depends on the total iodine dose and volume of distribution. The main factors which influence the contrast enhancement include cardiac output and central blood volume, both of which have a correlation with the body weight.

All the current commercially available ICM are excreted in the kidney by glomerular filtration with no significant tubular excretion or resorption. Few older contrast media, such as iodopyracet (Diodrast) were excreted by means of both glomerular filtration and tubular secretion. Around 99% of the IV dose of contrast medium is eliminated through the kidney and instantaneous rate of removal is equal to the glomerular filtration rate times the plasma iodine concentration. Less than one percent is excreted through extrarenal routes that include hepatobiliary system, small and large intestines, sweat, tears and saliva. Vicarious excretion of contrast material occurs through extrarenal routes, in cases of renal insult or renal failure.

The half-life of ICM in patients with normal glomerular filtration rate is approximately 2 hours whereas in patients with severe renal dysfunction it can prolong to more than 30 hours depending on the extent of renal impairment.[10] Therefore, in patients with end-stage renal failure the plasma contrast medium concentration stays high for a fairly long span of time. In these patients, the extracellular concentration of iodine will reach the value given by the total iodine injected divided by the extracellular volume, which is approximately 200 mL per kilogram of body weight. The requirement of emergent dialysis after contrast administration has been debated in renal failure patients. The ICM are readily dialyzable as they are not protein bound and possess relatively low-molecular weights. It is believed that approximately one third of either HOCM or LOCM would have already been naturally eliminated through extrarenal routes before dialysis can be set up and begun.[11] The HOCM produces larger osmotic diuresis and so have lower urinary concentration than LOCM.

Basic Properties

The biocompatibility of iodine and its physical properties (k-edge at photon energy of 34 KeV) allow safe intravascular injection of large volumes at high concentration. All the other chemical elements in the molecules serve only to carry, or protect the iodine on the benzene ring. It is the iodine in the radiographic beam and the volume distribution of the contrast material that provide optional contrast enhancement for imaging.[19] The basic properties of ICM include osmolality, viscosity and ionicity.

Osmolality of intravascular contrast media refers to the number of particles in solution, per unit liquid, as compared to blood. Most of ICM have a greater osmolality than blood plasma. High-osmolality contrast media have osmolality approximately in the range 1400–1515 mOsm/kg, or about 5–8 times that of human blood. Low-osmolality contrast media have much lower osmolality ranging approximately 600–800 mOsm/kg, or roughly 2–3 times the osmolality of human blood.[18] Hyperosmolar contrast cause tissue damage and responsible for the sudden drawing of water from the cellular and interstitial spaces towards plasma, thereby producing local effects, such as heat and pain. Increased osmolality can cause systemic effects, such as vasodilatation, alteration to the permeability of vessel endothelium, hyperemia and osmotic diuresis. The HOCM cause strong osmotic diuretic effect. The lower osmotic effect of the LOCM, however, is not significant disadvantage because a higher iodine concentration is achieved in the urine. For urography and to some extent for CT scanning, some degree of osmotic diuresis is required. Nonionic-dimer contrast agent (Visipaque, GE Healthcare) has the osmolality 290 mOsm/kg or equal to that of blood and is referred to as an iso-osmolar contrast media. It has been suggested that iso-osmolar contrast media may offer some advantages, particularly in patients at risk of renal complications.

Viscosity is a physical property which is the thickness or friction of the fluid as it flows. The viscosity is related to the concentration, the size of the molecules in a specific contrast agent and the temperature of the contrast agent. This property will influence the injectability of intravascular agents through small bore needles and IV catheters. Contrast media with higher-viscosity values have to be injected at a comparatively slow rate. The other factors which influence contrast-media flow are iodine concentration, temperature of the contrast media, catheter inner diameter, catheter length and the number of catheter holes. A significant decrease can be brought in the viscosity of the contrast material if the liquid is heated to body temperature for injection. The concentration of iodine in the ICM affect its viscosity; the higher the concentration of iodine, the more will be the viscosity of the solution. The viscosity is largely controlled by the compositions of the side chains on the molecules. Meglumine side chain in the ICM helps achieve water solubility and biologic tolerance but also increases the viscosity. Ionic ICM have reduced viscosity and high hyperosmolality; Nonionic ICM have reduced viscosity and limited hyperosmolality; nonionic dimers have high viscosity and iso-osmolality. Viscosity also plays a role at the level of the nervous system, as a direct correlation has been observed between viscosity of the solution and magnitude of damage to the blood-brain barrier.[20] If associated with high-viscosity, isotonicity of radiopaque solutions also produces unwanted effects at renal level.

Ionicity refers to the ability of a molecule to break down into a positively-charged cation and a negatively-charged anion, resulting in more molecules per kilogram of water and thus increasing osmolality. This property is absent in non-ionic agents which makes them less osmolar. Ionic contrast agents are composed of molecules that will disassociate into ions when in solution. The molecules contained in nonionic contrast media do not dissociate. Although most nonionic contrast agents also have low osmolality, the two terms are not synonymous.

Pulmonary Effects of ICM

Pulmonary adverse effects of ICM include bronchospasm, increased pulmonary vascular resistance and pulmonary edema. Patients with history of asthma, pulmonary hypertension and incipient cardiac failure are at increased risk. It is recommended to use iso-osmolar contrast media and avoid large doses of contrast media to reduce the risk of pulmonary adverse effects.

Effects of ICM on Blood and Endothelium

It has been proved that all contrast media have anticoagulant properties, especially the ionic agents. The HOCM may induce thrombosis due to endothelial damage, particularly in phlebographic procedures. Low- or iso-osmolar contrast media should be used for diagnostic and interventional angiographic procedures. Meticulous angiographic techniques with advanced interventional devices reduce the thromboembolic complications.

General Policies for ICM Administration

There are certain policies, which everybody should follow in administering ICM. Only authorized persons, i.e. technologists and registered nurses should inject ICM under the supervision of radiologist. The dose and technique of ICM injection is decided under the guidance of radiologist. The ICM should be stored at less than 37°C for maximum period of one month. Multidose bottles of ICM should be discarded if not used within 8 hours after being opened. All multidose contrast containers/vials should be properly labelled along with the time they were opened. All ICM stock should be monitored by designated nursing and CT staff. All radiologists/technologists/nurses should personally inspect contrast containers/vials for integrity, signs of contamination and also check expiry date. All the expired contrast containers/vials should be timely disposed. Most of the adverse contrast reactions tend to occur either immediately or within 20 minutes postcontrast injection and hence, all the patients should be observed for sometime in the radiology department after ICM administration. All areas where contrast is given must be equipped with an emergency box containing supplies required for the treatment of contrast reactions.

Guidelines for Intravenous Administration of ICM

Intravenous injection via stable IV access is the most common parenteral route of contrast administration. Contrast is injected directly into the vein with a butterfly needle, an angiocatheter or through an established IV line. When the power injector is utilized, 22 G or large needle or cannula 1.25"–1.5" length is preferred for IV-contrast injection. It is advisable to obtain a good backflow of blood to test if the needle is adequately positioned in the vein. Adequate position of the cannula in the vein is checked again by saline flush into the vein before the contrast can be injected.

Care has to be taken when injecting ICM through existing access routes. Only power-injection rated peripherally inserted central catheters (PICC) or central lines are approved for power injection. Preexisting IV lines will be flushed with 10 mL of saline flush, to ensure patency, prior to contrast injection. The maximum flow rate and psi set for adult and pediatric injections are 5 mL/sec at <300 psi and 2 mL/sec at <300 psi respectively. The injection rate will depend on the specific catheter type, size and specific examination protocol.

Special care is to be taken whenever injecting contrast media via. any central line catheters. If not power rated, the contrast injection must be hand injection. Hand injection of contrast is acceptable if the examination does not require arterial phase of injection. The 5 rights for medication administration (i.e. right patient, right contrast/medication, right dose, right route and right time) should be strictly followed.

It is essential to know the serum creatinine levels and glomerular filtration rate (GFR) before injecting the contrast. Ideally, recent serum creatinine reports (done within 6 weeks) should be obtained. If there has been significant interval change in the patient's condition, a more recent serum creatinine report can be considered. If the serum creatinine level is >1.5 mg/dL in a diabetic patient, >2.0 mg/dL in a nondiabetic patient, or the GFR is <30 mL/min, the injection of ICM ideally should be avoided and alternate diagnostic test should be considered. The contrast may be given after discussion with the referring clinician/nephrologist considering risk-benefit ratio. This conversation must be properly documented. For patients with end-stage renal disease who are on chronic peritoneal dialysis, noncontrast study should be considered and contrast should only be given after discussion with the patient's nephrologist. Immediate dialysis is advised after the contrast study in the patients of significant renal compromise.

Dosage of Iodinated Contrast Media Administration

Dose of ICM is considered as potential risk factor for adverse contrast reactions and nephropathy. In practice, dose is only a concern in certain situations, such as patients undergoing catheter angiography and CT on the same day. In such circumstances, the clinical need for an optimal study should be duly regarded rather than strictly adhering to a relatively empiric maximum recommended dose. Regardless of the type of iodinated contrast agent, the lowest dose necessary to obtain adequate visualization should be used. It is advisable to discuss the relative risks and benefits with the patient and referring clinician. Standard dose of iodinated contrast administration is 1–2 mL/kg at concentration of 300 mg/mL. The maximum limit of contrast administration is typically 200 mL of an agent with a concentration of 320 mg/mL (a total of 64 grams of iodine). In general volumes of over 250–300 cc in a 24-hour period should be avoided. The maximum safe dose may also depend on the individual factor, such as a patient's level of hydration. It should be noted that specific circumstances may necessitate exceeding this 200 mL guideline. A radiologist is responsible for determining in what instances and to what extent, standard guidelines can be safely exceeded.

Adverse Reactions

Iodinated contrast agents are one of the safe and widely used medications. However, these agents are not completely devoid of risks and sometimes adverse side effects may occur. The LCOM generally cause less discomfort to the patient and lesser adverse reactions than do HOCM. Reactions are usually infrequent and range from 5 to 12% for HOCM and from 1 to 3% for LOCM.[21,22] The mild and moderate contrast reactions occur more frequently with HOCM (6–8%) than for LOCM (0.2%), but the incidence of severe reactions remains similar. Anaphylactic reactions are more common with HOCM, whereas cardiovascular decompensation is more common with LOCM. It is impossible to accurately predict which patients will have an adverse reaction. The drugs and equipment needed to treat acute contrast reactions must be readily available and all the radiology staff must be trained to treat quickly. Adverse reactions and their relationship to preexisting conditions and treatment are discussed in detail in the separate chapter. Since 1996, the Contrast Media Safety Committee has reviewed all the safety aspects of ICM and formulated the guidelines for the use and management of contrast reactions. European Society of Urogenital Radiology (ESUR) guidelines have been well received by the radiology community all over the world and are now standards for good practice at many institutions.[23]

In spite of taking all the precautions of the risk factors and selecting appropriate contrast media, it is not possible to opine confidently how the patient will ultimately react to contrast media. Hence, considering the medicolegal aspects, it is advisable that a proforma outlining the availability of various contrast media, their possible reactions and the cost should be made available to the patient. One must discuss directly with the patient/his relatives on these issues before planning a study and an informed consent signed by the patient and relative is mandatory.

ICM Interaction with Other Drugs and Clinical Tests

The ICM may interact with other drugs and interfere with biochemical assays. It is essential to know the patient's drug history and proper records of the ICM injection (time, dose, name and batch number) should also be kept. Drugs which require special attention include metformin, cyclosporine, cisplatin, aminoglycosides, nonsteroidal anti-inflammatory drugs, beta-blockers, interleukin-2 and hydralazine. Beta-blockers may impair the response to treatment of bronchospasm induced by contrast medium. The ICM should never be mixed with other drugs in the tubes or syringes. Biochemical analysis of blood or urine, collected within 24 hours of ICM injection should also be avoided. One of the pharmacodynamic effects of the ICM is the reduction of renal function, particularly in patients with preexisting renal dysfunction. This leads to the retention of drugs, which are excreted exclusively through the kidneys. The ICM injection has the tendency of interfering with some isotope studies, therefore it should be avoided for minimum 24 hours before isotope bone scanning and before labeling red blood cells for isotope studies. Patients undergoing the radioactive iodine therapy should not have received ICM for at least 2 months before treatment. Isotope imaging of the thyroid should be avoided for 2 months after ICM injection.[24]

Guidelines for Selective Use of LOCM

Few of the studies have suggested that the cost-effectiveness of low-osmolality agents is poor if they are used indiscriminately for the general population. The agents should be used selectively for patients at the highest risk for a reaction to a high-osmolality agent.[25] Various organizations, such as American College of Radiology or the American College of Cardiology have recommended the guidelines, which can serve as starting points for the establishment of institution's policies and procedures for the use of contrast media.

American College of Radiology (ACR) developed guidelines for the selective use of LOCM.[1] It recommends that LOCM be administered to the following:

- Patients having history of a previous adverse reaction to contrast material, except for a sensation of heat or flushing or a single episode of nausea or vomiting,
- Patients having history of asthma or allergy,
- Patients with history of cardiac dysfunction, including recent or potentially imminent cardiac decompensation, severe arrhythmias, unstable angina pectoris, recent myocardial infarction and pulmonary hypertension,
- Patients with generalized severe debilitation,
- Other circumstances, such as patients having sickle-cell disease, increased risk for aspiration, anxious patients, patients with whom communication cannot

be established to know about the risks and patients who request for the use of LOCM.

Many institutions use low-osmolality ICM agents in patients with preexisting renal insufficiency alone or accompanying diabetes.[26] Nowadays, most of the institutes use the LOCM in all or most of the patients, whenever contrast needs to be given.

It is not always possible to limit the use of LOCM to a selected group of patients. This is because some of the above mentioned guidelines can be interpreted differently by different individuals. Also, there is tendency for referring clinicians and radiologists to use the better tolerated nonionic agents increasingly to reduce patient discomfort or the likelihood of a reaction. There is also tendency for low-risk patients to choose nonionic agents when they are allowed specifically to select the type of contrast material that they are to receive.

It is also difficult to identify the patients, who are at risk for the administration of any contrast media. Estimations of patient risk are derived from a variety of sources and previous history. However, not all at risk patients are always readily identified. In emergency situations or when adequate assessment with steroid is not possible, all patients should be injected by LOCM. It is also essential to use minimum dose of contrast media for the given study and decrease waste of contrast material. The final decision on choice of contrast usage depend on public policy makers, organized medicine, individual physician and the patient.

Iso-osmolar Dimeric Contrast Media

Iso-osmolar dimeric nonionic contrast medium currently available is iodixanol, which is sold under the trade name Visipaque (GE Healthcare) in two main concentrations 270 mgI/mL, 320 mg/mL and hence the name Visipaque 270 or 320. It has osmolality of 290 mOsm/kg H_2O, similar to blood. Contrast-induced renal vasoconstriction and renal ischemia (major factor in the pathogenesis of contrast induced nephropathy) increases with increasing osmolality of the contrast agent. Isotonicity and lack of osmotoxicity of these contrast media result in better renal tolerance. Iodixanol is less likely to produce any incidence of adverse events as compared to other nondimeric contrast media because of its physical properties. Indeed, pharmacodynamic studies have indicated that iodixanol has fewer cardiovascular effects, causes less renal damage and is associated with similar or smaller changes to the blood-brain barrier and neurological function than the nondimeric nonionic contrast media. Iodixanol generally causes less frequent and less intense discomfort on injection. However, it is relatively expensive. It was believed that the use of low-osmolar contrast media is associated with a significantly lower incidence of contrast-induced nephropathy (CIN) compared with high-osmolar contrast media in patients with renal failure. Recently, the opinion regarding use of iso-osmolar dimeric contrast media in CIN has been divided among experts. Recent studies and clinical trials found no significant reduction in the risk of CIN with the use of iodixanol, as compared with LOCM.[27]

FUTURE OF ICM

The current nonionic dimers are highly viscous. High viscosity has been real problem in injection through thin catheters and occurrence of nephrotoxicity. In future, a low-viscous nonionic iso-osmolar dimer may find place in the market. New contrast media, including organ-specific agents are expected in near future.

CONCLUSION

Iodinated contrast media are most widely used and are quite safe to use. Reactions are usually mild at occurrence but may occasionally progress to life-threatening proportions. An in depth knowledge of contrast media, their adverse reactions, causes, predisposing factors, clinical features, management strategies, choice of agents and premedication regimens for high-risk patients, is essential to minimize the threats posed by these factors.

REFERENCES

1. American College of Radiology Manual on Contrast Media, 4th Edn. Reston, VA: American College of Radiology; 1998.
2. Katzberg RW. Acute reactions to urographic contrast medium: incidence, clinical characteristics, and relationship to history of hypersensitivity states—a commentary. AJR. 2008;190(6):1431-2.
3. Cohan RH, Ellis JH. Iodinated contrast material in uroradiology- choice of agent and management of complications. Rad Clin North Am. 1997;24(3):471-91.
4. Thomsen HS, Webb JAW. Contrast Media: Safety Issues and ESUR Guidelines, 2nd revised Edition. Springer publications; 2009.
5. McClennan BL, Preston M. Hickey memorial lecture. Ionic and nonionic iodinated contrast media: evolution and strategies for use. AJR. 1990;155(2):225-33.
6. Contrast media—a multifactorial approach. In: Carlo Del Favero-Intramed communications; 1997.
7. Lesser E, Farr RS, Fusjimagari T, et al. The significance of protein binding of contrast media in roentgen diagnosis. AJR. 1962;87:338-60.
8. Almen T. Contrast agent design: some aspects on the synthesis of water soluble contrast agents of low osmolality. J Theor Biol. 1969;24:216-26.

9. Almen T. Development of nonionic contrast media. Invest Radiol. 1985;20:52-9.
10. Almén T, Boijsen E, Lindell SE. Metrizamide in angiography I. Femoral angiography. Acta Radiol Diagn (Stockh). 1977;18(1): 33-8.
11. Katzberg RW. Urography into the 21st century: new contrast media, renal handling, imaging characteristics, and nephrotoxicity. Radiology. 1997;204(2):297-312.
12. Costa N. Understanding contrast media. J Infus Nurs. 2004;27: 302-12.
13. Bettmann MA, Morris TW. Recent advances in contrast agents. Radiol Clin North Am. 1986;24:347-57.
14. Peter Dawson. Adverse reactions to intravascular contrast agents. BMJ. 2006;333(7570):663-4.
15. Almen T. Visipaque- a step forward. A historical review. Acta Radiol Suppl. 1995;399:2-18.
16. Dobrato M, Powell CJ, Holtz E. Biochemical and morphological effects of contrast media on the kidney. Acta Radiol. 1995; 399:196-203.
17. Jokobson JA. Renal effects of iodixanol in healthy volunteers and patients with severe renal failure. Acta Radiol. 1995;36:196-203.
18. Rapport SI, Levitan H. Neurotoxicity of X-ray contrast media: relation to lipid solubility and blood-brain barrier permeability. Am J Roentgenol. 1974;122:186-94.
19. McClennan BL, Stolbery HO. Intravascular contrast media. Ionic versus nonionic: current status. Radiol Clin North Am. 1991;29(3):437-54.
20. Segal AJ. Optimizing urography. World J Urolol. 1998;16(1):3-8.
21. Singh J, Daftary A. Iodinated contrast media and their adverse reactions. J Nucl Med Technol. 2008;36:69-74.
22. Cochran ST, Bomyea K, Sayre JW. Trends in adverse events after IV administration of contrast media. AJR. 2001;176:1385-8.
23. Thomsen HS. European Society of Urogenital Radiology (ESUR) guidelines on the safe use of iodinated contrast media. Eur J Radiol. 2006;60:307-13.
24. Morcos SK, Thomsen HS, Exley CM. Members of contrast media safety committee of European society of urogenital radiology (ESUR). Contrast media: interaction with other drugs and clinical tests. Eur. Radiology. 2005;15:1463-8.
25. Ratko T. Technology assessment: low-osmolality contrast media. In: Oak Brook. UHC Technology Advancement Center, University Hospital Consortium,1993.
26. Cohan RH, Ellis JH, Dunnick NR. Use of low-osmolar agents and premedication to reduce the frequency of adverse reactions to radiographic contrast media: a survey to the society of uroradiology. Radiology. 1995;194: 357-64.
27. Heinrich MC, Häberle L, Müller V, Bautz W, Uder M. Nephrotoxicity of iso-osmolar iodixanol compared with nonionic low-osmolar contrast media: meta-analysis of randomized controlled trials. Radiology. 2009;250(1): 68-86.

CHAPTER 57

Contrast Reactions and its Management

Gaurav S Pradhan, Rajat Jain

INTRODUCTION

Iodinated contrast media are among the most commonly used contrast agent in the modern radiology practice. These contrast agents can be used almost anywhere in the body by whatever route, i.e. oral, intravenous, rectal, intra-arterial and intrathecal. It is important to remember that ionic contrast media should not be used intrathecally, as it can be life-threatening. Only nonionic contrast should be used for intrathecal administration and also for children with tracheoesophageal fistula.

The iodinated contrast agents are usually safe and adverse reactions are generally mild and self-limiting. Nonetheless, as any drug can cause side effects, contrast agents are no exception and severe or life-threatening reactions can occur.

Radiologists and other medical personnel involved in the use of contrast agents must be aware of risk factors for reaction to contrast media. They should be aware of and use strategies to minimize adverse events and be prepared to promptly identify and manage them.

For immediate reactors, the intradermal tests are the most sensitive, whereas delayed intradermal tests in combination with patch tests are needed for optimal sensitivity in non-immediate reactors. Contrast medium cross-reactivity is more common in the nonimmediate than in the immediate group. The datas suggest that at least 50% of hypersensitivity reactions to contrast media are caused by an immunologic mechanism. Skin testing appears to be a useful tool for diagnosis of contrast medium allergy and may play an important role in selection of a safe product in previous reactors.[1,2]

TYPES OF ADVERSE REACTION

Adverse reactions to contrast media are broadly divided into two main groups **(Flowchart 1)**:

1. Idiosyncratic anaphylactoid reactions
2. Nonidiosyncratic reactions.

IDIOSYNCRATIC ANAPHYLACTOID REACTIONS

Idiosyncratic anaphylactoid reactions (also described as allergy-like or anaphylactoid) are defined as unpredictable reactions which occur within 1 hour of contrast medium administration and which are unrelated to the amount of contrast medium above a certain level. They are the most dreaded and most serious complications as they occur without warning, cannot be reliably predicted and are not preventable in the present state of our knowledge.

Flowchart 1: Adverse reactions.

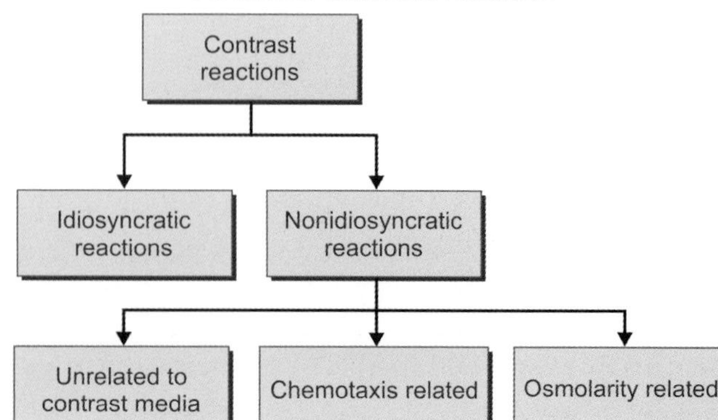

Mechanism of Idiosyncratic Anaphylactoid Reactions[1,3-7]

Idiosyncratic reactions vary greatly in severity and clinically may closely mimic true anaphylactic and allergic reactions, although there is no confirmatory evidence of a true antigen IGE antibody immunological reaction to contrast media. The mechanisms by which idiosyncratic reactions occur are not fully understood. However, they do appear to involve the release of active mediators, such as histamine, bradykinin, leukotrienes, prostaglandins and complement factors. Available evidence suggests that there are a variety of complex interactions between the complement, contact, coagulation and immune systems.[1,3-6]

- *Inhibition of enzymes:* Cholinesterase resulting in increased concentration of acetylcholine; may lead to vagal overstimulation, e.g. cardiovascular collapse, bradycardia, bronchospasm
- *Release of vasoactive substances:* Histamine, serotonin or bradykinin may result in vasomotor collapse
- *Activation of physiological cascade systems:* Complement activation system, the kinin system with bradykinin release, the coagulation system inducing intravascular coagulation and the fibrinolytic system causing lysis of fibrin and blood clots
- The immune system disturbances
- *Anxiety, apprehension and fear:* Activating a hypothalamic reaction resulting in cardiovascular and respiratory collapse and even death.

It is probable that many of these mechanisms are inter-related and that a self-perpetuating vicious circle is established, resulting in severe and perhaps fatal cardiovascular collapse.

Risk Factors for Acute Idiosyncratic Drug Reactions[8]

Risk factors for acute reactions
• Type of contrast agent • Previous adverse reaction to contrast medium • Asthmatics • Allergic and atopic patients • Patients on certain drugs like beta-adrenergic blockers • Patients with impaired cardiovascular and renal systems • Diabetics • Patients with various metabolic and hematological disorders • Thyrotoxic: goitrous patients • Feeble infants and aged patients • Patients with a severe general debility • Very nervous, anxious patients

- *Type of contrast agent:* More with high-osmolality contrast agent than with low/ iso-osmolar contrast agent
- *Previous adverse reaction to contrast medium:*
  - Most important patient factor predisposing to an acute idiosyncratic reaction
  - With ionic agents, the risk of a reaction in a patient who reacted previously has been stated to be 16–35%
  - When a patient who previously reacted to an ionic agent is given a nonionic agent, the risk of a repeat reaction is reduced to approximately 5%.
- *Asthmatics:* Katayama et al. described an 8.5 times increased risk with ionic agents and a 5.8 times increased risk with nonionic[8]
- *Allergic and atopic patients:*
  - A history of allergy to foods, drugs or other substances is associated with an increased risk of contrast medium reaction, usually by a lesser amount than with a history of asthma
  - Other conditions, such as hay fever, eczema, etc. are associated with an increased risk of reaction, but by a lesser amount than asthma.
- *Patients on certain drugs like beta-adrenergic blockers:*
  - Whether or not beta-blockers affect the incidence of idiosyncratic contrast medium reactions is controversial. It is, however, agreed that the use of beta-blockers can impair the response to treatment if a reaction does occur
  - Patients who are receiving or have received interleukin-2 are at increased risk of adverse events following iodinated contrast media.
- *Patients with impaired cardiovascular and renal systems:* A high sodium load caused by a large volume of HOCM containing sodium salts may exacerbate cardiac decompensation due to hypervolemia and myocardial depression
- Diabetics
- Patients with various metabolic and hematological disorders
- Thyrotoxic: goitrous patients
- Feeble infants and aged patients
- Patients with a severe general debility
- Very nervous, anxious patients.

Prevention of Acute Idiosyncratic Reactions[9-11]

If a patient has previous history of reaction to contrast media than, the possibility of obtaining the necessary diagnostic information from another test, not using iodinated contrast medium [e.g. ultrasonography, magnetic resonance imaging (MRI)], must be considered. If iodinated contrast medium is still considered necessary, the risk can be reduced by an appropriate choice of contrast medium and premedication. Patient should remain in the radiology department for at least 30 minutes as most severe reactions occur within the first 30 minutes after contrast medium injection. In high-risk subjects, monitoring for the first hour is recommended.[9,10]

- *Choice of contrast media:* The single most important method of reducing the risk of idiosyncratic contrast medium reactions is to use nonionic, low-osmolality agents, which are associated with a 4–5 times lower risk of reaction.[8,12-14] If there is prior documentation of contrast reaction from one contrast agent, then change to different low-osmolality contrast agent may be helpful[15,16]
- *Premedication:*[1,17-21] Most frequently, steroids with or without additional H_1 antihistamines have been recommended.
  - *Elective premedication:* Prednisone—50 mg by mouth at 13 hours, 7 hours and 1 hour before contrast media injection and diphenhydramine—50 mg intravenously, intramuscularly, or by mouth 1 hour before contrast medium.
    If the patient is unable to take oral medication, 200 mg of hydrocortisone intravenously may be substituted for oral prednisone
  - *Emergency premedication:* Hydrocortisone sodium 200 mg intravenously every 4 hours until contrast study required and diphenhydramine 50 mg IV, 1 hour prior to contrast injection
    - No use of steroids if given less than 4–6 hours before contrast administration
    - Diphenhydramine 50 mg IV (with no steroids) in very urgent scans.

Types and Management of Acute Idiosyncratic Reactions[1]

Guidelines from ACR Manual on Contrast Media Version 8; 2012[1]

Acute idiosyncratic reactions are usually characterized as mild, moderate or severe. Mild or minor reactions include nausea, mild vomiting, urticaria and itching. They usually do not require medical treatment other than reassurance and restoration of the patient's confidence. Vital signs should be obtained to detect hypotension that may be clinically silent while the patient is supine. Any patient with a mild allergy-like reaction should be observed at least for 20–30 minutes to ensure clinical stability or recovery. Treatment with an antihistamine may be given however, is not required most of the times.

Moderate reactions include more severe vomiting, marked urticaria, bronchospasm, facial or laryngeal edema, and vasovagal reactions. Moderate reactions require close patient monitoring until they resolve completely. Moderate adverse events are not immediately life-threatening, but often require medical treatment. The treatment depends on the type of reaction encountered.

- *Urticaria:*
  - Discontinue injection if not completed
  - No treatment needed in most cases
  - Give H_1-receptor blocker: diphenhydramine PO/IM/IV 25–50 mg.
    If severe or widely disseminated: give alpha-agonist adrenaline S/C (1:1,000) 0.1–0.3 mL (if no cardiac contraindications).
- *Facial or laryngeal edema:*
  - Give O_2 6–10 L/min (via mask)
  - Give alpha-agonist adrenaline SC or IM (1:1,000) 0.1–0.3 mL or, especially if hypotension evident, adrenaline (1:10,000) slowly IV 3 mL preferably under ECG control
  - Repeat as needed up to a maximum of 1 mg
  - If not responsive to therapy or if there is obvious acute laryngeal edema, seek appropriate assistance (e.g. cardiopulmonary arrest response team).
- *Bronchospasm:*
  - Give O_2 6–10 liters/min (via mask)
    Monitor: electrocardiogram, O_2 saturation (pulse oximeter) and blood pressure
  - Give beta-agonist inhalers (bronchiolar dilators, such as metaproterenol, terbutaline, or albuterol) 2–3 puffs; repeat as necessary. If unresponsive to inhalers, use SC, IM, or IV adrenaline
  - Give adrenaline SC or IM (1:1,000) 0.1–0.3 mL or, especially if hypotension evident, adrenaline (1:10,000) slowly IV 1–3 mL preferably under ECG control.

Repeat as needed up to a maximum of 1 mg.

Call for assistance (e.g. cardiopulmonary arrest response team) for severe bronchospasm or if O_2 saturation <88% persists.

Severe reactions include severe hypotension, hypertension, cardiac arrhythmias, cardiac arrest, convulsion and pulmonary edema.

- *Hypotension with tachycardia:*
  - Legs elevated (preferred) or Trendelenburg position
  - Monitor: Electrocardiogram, pulse oximeter, blood pressure
  - Give O_2 6–10 L/min (via mask)
  - Rapid intravenous administration of large volumes of Ringer's lactate or normal saline.

If poorly responsive: Adrenaline (1:10,000) slowly IV 1 mL.

Repeat as needed up to a maximum of 1 mg.

If still poorly responsive seek appropriate assistance (e.g. cardiopulmonary arrest response team).

- *Hypotension with bradycardia (vagal reaction):*
  - Secure airway: Give O_2 6–10 L/min (via mask)
  - Monitor vital signs
  - Legs elevated 60° or more (preferred) or Trendelenburg position
  - Secure IV access: Rapid administration of Ringer's lactate or normal saline
  - Give atropine 0.6–1 mg IV slowly, if patient does not respond quickly to steps 2–4
  - Repeat atropine up to a total dose of 0.04 mg/kg (2–3 mg) in adult
  - Ensure complete resolution of hypotension and bradycardia prior to discharge.
- *Hypertension, severe:*
  - Give O_2, 6–10 L/min (via mask)
  - Monitor: Electrocardiogram, pulse oximeter, blood pressure
  - Give nitroglycerine 0.4 mg tablet, sublingual (may repeat × 3); or, topical 2% ointment, apply 1-inch strip
  - If no response, consider labetalol 20 mg IV, then 20–80 mg IV every 10 minutes up to 300 mg
  - Transfer to intensive care unit or emergency department
  - For pheochromocytoma: Phentolamine 5 mg IV (may use labetalol if phentolamine is not available).
- *Seizures or convulsions*
  - Give O_2 6–10 L/min (via mask)
  - Consider diazepam 5 mg IV (or more, as appropriate) or midazolam 0.5–1 mg IV
  - If longer effect needed, obtain consultation; consider phenytoin infusion — 15–18 mg/kg at 50 mg/min
  - Careful monitoring of vital signs required, particularly of pO_2 because of risk to respiratory depression with benzodiazepine administration
  - Consider using cardiopulmonary arrest response team for intubation if needed.
- *Pulmonary edema:*
  - Give O_2, 6–10 L/min (via mask)
  - Elevate torso
  - Give diuretics: Furosemide 20–40 mg IV, slow push
  - Consider giving morphine (1–3 mg IV)
  - Transfer to intensive care unit or emergency department.

NONIDIOSYNCRATIC REACTIONS[22-25]

These are dose-related reactions and dependent on the physicochemical properties of the contrast medium, i.e. chemical composition, osmolality and concentration of contrast medium and also on the volume, speed and multiplicity of the injection.

- *Reactions unrelated to contrast media:* Pyrogenic (unsterile injection), vasovagal especially in anxious or psychosomatic patients, hypertensive attacks in patients with pheochromocytoma, excessive dehydration and hypoglycemia
- *Chemotoxic reactions:* As iodine is very firmly bound to the benzene rings, these side effects are probably due to toxicity to the contrast medium ion rather than to its iodine content. These include cardiac, neurological and renal toxicity as well as vascular manifestations
- *Hyperosmolar reactions:* Due to very high osmolality of these compounds predominantly HOCM, adverse reactions may occur when large volumes are injected into the circulation predominantly because of erythrocyte damage, endothelial damage, blood-brain barrier damage, vasodilatation, hypervolemia and cardiac decompression.

As these reactions are predominantly related to the hyperosmolality of the contrast media and depend on the dose, concentration and volume of contrast used, they can be significantly reduced by substituting LOCM for the very hypertonic HOCM.

Extravasation of Contrast[26-30]

It refers to the escape of contrast material from the vessel into which it is introduced, into the surrounding tissue or body cavity. It occurs with a frequency of about 0.1–0.9% of patients getting contrast injections, more commonly seen in patients having atherosclerotic peripheral vascular disease, diabetic vascular disease, Raynaud's disease, venous thrombosis, prior radiation therapy or extensive surgery, severely-ill or debilitated patients, injection through indwelling peripheral intravenous lines (>than 24 hours) and multiple punctures into the same vein.

Clinical Features

- *Mild:* Tissue edema, erythema, stinging, tenderness
- *Severe:* Compartment syndromes, skin ulceration and tissue necrosis.

Prevention is better than cure, and a good secured intravenous access reduces the incidence, along with extravasation detectors as present in some of the modern automatic pressure injectors prevents excess of contrast extravasation.

Contrast-extravasation Treatment

<20 mL extravasation	*>20 mL extravasation*	*>100 mL extravasation*
• Elevate the arm and observe	• Aspirate • Intermittent ice • Hyaluronidase (50–250 U) at local extravasation site	• Aspirate • Intermittent ice • Hyaluronidase (50–250 U) at local extravasation site • Immediate plastic consult if: – Blistering, – Altered perfusion, – Pain worsens after 2–4 hours – Change in sensation distally

Contrast-induced Nephropathy

Contrast-induced nephrotoxicity (CIN) is a sudden deterioration in renal function following the recent intravascular administration of iodinated contrast medium in the absence of another nephrotoxic event.

Diagnosis

There are no standard criteria for the diagnosis of CIN; criteria used in the past have included percent change in the baseline serum creatinine (an increase of variously 25–50%) and absolute elevation from baseline serum creatinine (e.g. an increase of variously 0.5–2.0 mg/dL). One of the most commonly used criteria has been an absolute increase of 0.5 mg/dL.

Acute Kidney Injury Network: Definition of Acute Kidney Injury[28,31]

The diagnosis of acute kidney injury is made according to the AKIN criteria if one of the following occurs within 48 hours after a nephrotoxic event (e.g. intravascular iodinated contrast medium exposure):

- Absolute serum creatinine increase of ≥0.3 mg/dL (≥26.4 μmol/L).
- A percentage increase in serum creatinine of ≥50% (1.5-fold above baseline).
- Urine output reduced to ≤0.5 mL/kg/hour for at least 6 hours.

Pathogenesis

The exact pathophysiology of CIN is not understood. Nephrotoxicity of contrast media is likely to be due to the following:

- Decreased renal perfusion due to renal vasoconstriction (low BP, peripheral vasodilatation)
- Glomerular injury manifests as proteinuria.
- Tubular injury due to osmolarity, chemotoxicity, ischemia.
- Contrast media precipitation of Tamm Horsfall protein that blocks tubules.
- Swelling of renal tubular cells causing obstruction.
- Both osmotic and chemotoxic mechanisms may be involved, and some investigations suggest agent-specific chemotoxicity.

Symptoms: Usually asymptomatic. Creatinine peaks in 3–5 days. In severe oliguric patients: peaks in 5–7 days.

Incidence:[32-38] The incidence of CIN in patients with normal renal function is <1% with intravenous and 2–7% with intra-arterial administration of contrast media. The incidence is higher (16%) in nonazotemic diabetic patients. The incidence may be as high as 33% in patients with preexistent azotemia. Incidence of 3–16% has been reported in patients undergoing percutaneous coronary interventions. Patients undergoing percutaneous coronary interventions (PCI) often have associated risk factors for developing CIN, such as diabetes mellitus, congestive heart failure and preexisting renal impairment.

Risk Factors for CIN

- Preexisting renal impairment (serum creatinine >1.3 mg/dL, GFR <60 mL/min)
- Dehydration
- CHF
- Use of nephrotoxic drugs (NSAID, aminoglycosides)
- Hypersensitivity disease (Multiple myeloma)
- Hypertension
- Hyperuricemia (as in active gout)
- Proteinuria (>0.5 gm/dL)
- DM
- Age >70 years.

Prevention of contrast induced nephropathy in high-risk patients[11,39-46]

- *Avoidance of iodinated contrast medium:* In high-risk patient it is best to avoid use of iodinated contrast media and the possibility of obtaining the necessary diagnostic information from another test, not using iodinated contrast medium (e.g. ultrasonography,

MRI), must be considered. In some clinical situations where the use of intravascular iodinated contrast medium may be necessary the lowest possible dose of contrast medium to obtain the necessary diagnostic information should be used[9-11]

- *Contrast media selection:* Increased osmotic overload on the diseased kidney is considered to be the major etiology of CIN. This can be significantly reduced by substituting LOCM for the very hypertonic HOCM[39]
- *Hydration:* Adequate hydration is considered to be the single most-effective way to prevent CIN. The ideal infusion rate and volume is unknown, but isotonic fluids are preferred (lactated Ringer's or 0.9% normal saline). One possible protocol would be 0.9% saline at 100 mL/hr, beginning 6–12 hours before and continuing 4–12 hours after intravascular iodinated contrast medium administration. Oral hydration has also been utilized, but with less demonstrated effectiveness. Pediatric infusion rates are variable and should be based on patient weight[40,41]
- *Sodium bicarbonate:* It has been found to be useful in prevention from CIN according to some studies[42,43]
- *N-acetylcysteine:* The role is controversial. There is evidence that it reduces serum creatinine in normal volunteers without changing cystatin-C (cystatin-C is reported to be a better marker of GFR than serum creatinine). This raises the possibility that *N*-acetylcysteine might be simply lowering serum creatinine without actually preventing renal injury. *N*-acetylcysteine should not be considered a substitute for appropriate preprocedural patient screening and adequate hydration[44,45]
- *Diuretics (Mannitol and furosemide):* There is no reported benefit and neither mannitol nor furosemide is recommended for CIN risk reduction[46]
- *Other agents:* The evidence for other theoretically renal-protective medications, such as theophylline, endothelin-1 and fenoldopam is even less convincing. Use of these agents to reduce the risk of CIN is not recommended.

Renal Dialysis Patients and the Use of Iodinated Contrast Medium[1]

Contrast agents are not protein-bound, have relatively low molecular weights and are readily cleared by dialysis. Unless an unusually large volume of contrast medium is administered or there is substantial underlying cardiac dysfunction, there is no need for urgent dialysis after intravascular iodinated contrast medium administration.

Patients with anuric end-stage chronic kidney disease can receive intravascular iodinated contrast medium without risk of further renal damage because their kidneys are no longer functioning.

Patients receiving dialysis are also at theoretical risk from the osmotic load imposed by intravascular iodinated contrast medium because they cannot clear the excess intravascular volume. This osmotic load can theoretically result in pulmonary edema and anasarca. Hence, contrast medium dosing should be as low as necessary to achieve a diagnostic result (as in all patients).

Recommendation of Contrast Agents Based on Serum Creatinine Level

Serum creatinine	*Recommendations*
<1.5 mg/dL	Can use either ionic or nonionic contrast
1.5–2 mg/dL	Use nonionic contrast
2–2.5 mg/dL	Use of nonionic only in extreme indications, but contraindicated in diabetics
>2.5 mg/dL	No contrast to be given

Contrast Administration and Pregnancy[1]

Diagnostic iodinated contrast media have been shown to cross the human placenta and enter the fetus when given in usual clinical doses.

While it is not possible to conclude that iodinated contrast media present a definite risk to the fetus, there is insufficient evidence to conclude that they pose no risk. Consequently, the Committee on Drugs and Contrast Media recommends the following:

- The radiologist should confer with the referring physician and document in the radiology report or the patient's medical record the following:
  - That the information requested cannot be acquired without contrast administration or via another image modality (e.g. ultrasonography).
  - That the information needed affects the care of the patient and fetus during the pregnancy.
  - That the referring physician is of the opinion that it is not prudent to wait to obtain this information until after the patient is no longer pregnant.
- It is recommended that pregnant patients undergoing a diagnostic imaging examination with ionizing radiation and iodinated contrast media provide informed consent to document that they understand the risk and benefits of the procedure to be performed and the alternative diagnostic options available to them (if any) and that they wish to proceed.

Contrast Administration and Lactation[1]

Less than 1% of contrast media are secreted in human milk and <1% of ingested contrast is absorbed by gut, thus it appears safe to continue breast-feeding after receiving such an agent. If the mother remains concerned about any potential ill effects to the infant, she may abstain from breast-feeding for 24 hours with active expression and discarding of breast milk from both breasts during that period. Expressed breast milk prior to contrast study may be used during this period.

Contrast Administration in Patients on Metformin[1]

Metformin, an oral biguanide hyperglycemic therapy for diabetes mellitus type 2, is primarily excreted unchanged by the kidneys, probably by both glomerular filtration and tubular excretion. The renal route eliminates approximately 90% of the absorbed drug within the first 24 hours. Metformin seems to cause increased lactic acid production by the intestines. Any factors that decrease metformin excretion or increase blood lactate levels are important risk factors for lactic acidosis. Renal insufficiency, then, is a major consideration. In patients with severe renal impairment, intravascular accumulation of the biguanide may occur after contrast media and this may precipitate biguanide lactic acidosis (vomiting, diarrhea, somnolence)—a potentially fatal complication.

Limiting the amount of contrast medium administered and hydrating the patient lessen the risk of contrast media-induced dysfunction; both of these measures should be considered in patients with known or incipient renal dysfunction.

Recommendations[1]

Category 1	*Category 2*	*Category 3*
Normal renal function with no known comorbidities No reason to discontinue metformin	Normal renal function with known co-morbidities +, then suspend metformin for 48 hours If the patient had normal renal function at baseline, was clinically stable and had no intercurrent risk factors for renal damage (e.g. treatment with aminoglycosides, major surgery, heart failure, sepsis, repeat administration of large amounts of contrast media), metformin can be restarted	Renal dysfunction then suspend metformin for 48 hours and restart only if repeat KFT is normal

Comorbidities for Lactic Acidosis with Use of Metformin

- Decreased metabolism of lactate
- Liver dysfunction
- Alcohol abuse
- Increased anaerobic metabolism
- Cardiac failure
- Myocardial or peripheral muscle ischemia
- Sepsis or severe infection.

Remember: Metformin + Chronic renal insufficiency + IV contrast = Lactic acidosis.

Contrast Administration and Interleukin-2 Therapy[47,11]

- Always ask the oncologist of possible IL-2 therapy
- Inform patient of possible risk involved
- Generally mild symptoms (12% patients), e.g. rash, flu-like symptoms, pruritus, hypotension, tachycardia, joint pain, but few may require hospitalization
- Steroids cannot be given (steroids counteracts intended IL-2 action)
- If previous history of reaction to contrast present , then do not give contrast until extremely necessary
- Monitor patient for 2 hours, if uneventful send patient home.

Contrast Administration and Thyroid Dysfunction[11]

- Manifest active hyperthyroidism is an absolute contraindication to radiographic contrast media administration
- Patients at risk: Graves' disease and multinodular goiter with thyroid autonomy (especially in elderly/ patients living on iodine deficient diet)
- Contrast may cause thyrotoxicosis (though rare)
- Patient becomes unfit for diagnostic thyroid scintigraphy, radioiodine treatment of thyroid malignancy for 2 months.

Prophylaxis of Contrast-induced Thyrotoxicosis

Elective contrast-enhanced studies: Sodium perchlorate 300 mg 3 times daily (start the day before and continue for 8–14 days).

Emergency contrast-enhanced studies: Sodium perchlorate 800 mg once daily (directly prior to examination, continue with 3 × 300 mg for 8–14 days).

Contrast Administration in Pheochromocytoma and Paraganglioma[11]

There is a theoretical risk of hypertensive crisis in patients of paragangliomas due to release of catecholamine however, studies have shown no elevation of catecholamine levels after the IV injection of nonionic contrast media. Direct injection of either type of contrast medium into the adrenal or renal artery is to be avoided, however, as this may cause a hypertensive crisis.[47,48]

Contrast and Drug Interaction[47]

- Drugs which enhance renal effect of contrast: NSAIDS, gentamicin, cisplatin, cyclosporine
- Drugs which enhance diuretic effect of contrast: acetazolamide, furosemide, spironolactone
- Drugs which enhance allergic reactions: β-blockers, IL-2, interferons and hydralazine (should be avoided until extremely necessary as it can provoke SLE like syndrome)
- Drugs which enhance negative inotropic effect of contrast: CCB, digoxin.

Delayed Adverse Events to Iodinated Contrast Media

These are uncommon reactions occurring from 30–60 minutes to up to one week following contrast material exposure, with the majority occurring between three hours and two days. The most frequent delayed adverse events following contrast media administration are allergic-like and cutaneous in nature.[49,50] They are more frequent in patients with previous history of reaction to contrast and in patients with asthma or other allergic disorders. Delayed cutaneous reactions commonly manifest as urticaria and/or a persistent rash which, may occasionally present with a maculopapular exanthem or generalized exanthematous pustulosis. Few cases resembling Stevens–Johnson syndrome, toxic epidermal necrolysis and cutaneous vasculitis have also been described.

A variety of noncutaneous sign and symptoms like nausea, vomiting, fever, drowsiness and headache have also been reported. Each of these is usually self-limited and does not require therapy.

Iodide "mumps" (iodine-related sialoadenopathy or salivary gland swelling) and a syndrome of acute polyarthropathy are two additional delayed contrast reactions that have been reported rarely after contrast media administration. These reactions appear to be more frequent in patients with renal dysfunction.[51,52]

Low-molecular nonionic contrast has been reported to cause fewer delayed skin reactions as compared to iso-osmolar contrast. Prophylaxis is not recommended for delayed adverse reactions.

Treatment

Most of these reactions are self-limiting and do not require any treatment, treatment is usually supportive, with antihistamines and/or corticosteroids used for cutaneous symptoms, antipyretics for fever, antiemetics for nausea and fluid resuscitation for hypotension. If manifestations are progressive or widespread, or if there are noteworthy associated symptoms, consultation with an allergist and/or dermatologist is an appropriate next step.[53]

Recommendations for the Departments Performing Contrast-related Investigations[54,55]

- The radiologist must always weigh the risk-benefit ratio for the possible advantages from the diagnostic procedure against the very small but ever-present risk of a severe adverse reaction (and even death) to the contrast medium
- In high-risk patient it is best to avoid use of iodinated contrast media and the possibility of obtaining the necessary diagnostic information from another test, not using iodinated contrast medium (e.g. ultrasonography, MRI), must be considered
- In the presence of risk factors, the referring clinician should be consulted and advised. The patient should also be informed, consulted and reassured. The discussion and result should be recorded in the patient's notes
- Although a routine test dose is generally not necessary, it is advisable to perform a small 1 mL test dose, either by IV or dermal testing in patients considered to be at increased risk of contrast reactions
- In high-risk patients premedication is strongly advised, especially in asthmatic and allergic patients according to the protocols
- Before administering the injection, the emergency trolley, alarm system and availability of experienced assistance must be confirmed
- An individual trained in recognizing and treating severe contrast reactions, including anaphylaxis, should be immediately available in the department
- Adequate hydration must be ensured in all patients receiving contrast media particularly if there is previous renal impairment and those patients receiving large

quantities of contrast media, in order to excrete the contrast media as completely and quickly as possible

- Nonionic, low or iso-osmolar agents are five to ten times safer than the high-osmolar ionic agents
- The smallest dose of contrast media that will give reliable, comprehensive diagnostic results should be used
- A patient should not be left alone or unsupervised in the first five minutes after an injection of the contrast agent
- Patient should remain in the premises for 15–30 minutes after the contrast administration as most of the contrast reactions occur during this period only
- All contrast reactions, with details of their nature, severity and the agent used, should be included in the radiological report and updated in the patient's hospital notes
- Radiographic contrast media like any drug are useful for the patient but not free from side effects and minor to severe life-threatening side effects can occur with their use and hence radiologists and other medical personal involved in the use of contrast agents should be aware of and use strategies to minimize adverse events and be prepared to promptly identify and manage them
- Reactions related to MR contrast media are covered in Chapter 54: Magnetic Resonance Contrast Media.

REFERENCES

1. ACR Committee on Drugs and Contrast Media; ACR Manual on Contrast Media. 2012;Version 8.
2. Brockow K, Romano A, Aberer W, Bircher AJ, Barbaud A, et al. Skin testing in patients with hypersensitivity reactions to iodinated contrast media—a European multicenter study. Allergy. 2009;64(2):234-41.
3. Nelson RC, Anderson Jr FA, Birnbawm BA, et al. Contrast medium extravasation detection accessory. Radiology. 1988; 209:837-43.
4. Dawson P, Cosgrove DO, Grainger RG. Textbook of Contrast Media. Oxford: ISIS Medical Media; 1999.
5. American College of Radiology: Manual on Contrast Media, 4th edition. Reston, Virginia, USA: American College of Radiology, 1999.
6. Thomsen HS, Muller RN, Mattrey RF. Trends in Contrast Media. Germany: Springer-Verlag; 1999.
7. European Society of Urogenital Radiology. 2003; Version 3.0.
8. Katayama H, Yamaguchi K, Kozuka T, Takashima T, Seez P, Matsuura K. Adverse reactions to ionic and nonionic contrast media. A report from the Japanese committee on the safety of contrast media. Radiology. 1990;175:621-8.
9. Hartman GW, Hattery RR, Witten DM, Williamson B. Mortality during excretory urography: Mayo Clinic experience. Am J Roentgenol. 1982;139:919-22.
10. Shehadi WH. Death following intravascular administration of contrast media. Acta Radiol Diagn. 1985;26:457-46.
11. Thompson HS, Webb JAW. Contrast media; Safety issues and ESUR Guidelines, 2nd revised edition. 2009.p.40-9.
12. Palmer FJ. The RACR survey of intravenous contrast media reactions: final report. Austr Radiol. 1988;32:426-8.
13. Wolf GL, Miskin MM, Roux SG, et al. Comparison of the rates of adverse drug reactions: ionic contrast agents, ionic agents combined with steroids and nonionic agents. Invest Radiol. 1991;26:404-10.
14. Bettman MA, Heeren T, Greenfield A, Gondey C. Adverse events with radiographic contrast agents: results of the SCVIR Contrast Agent Registry. Radiology. 1997;203:611-20.
15. Thomsen HS, Bush WH. Adverse effects of contrast media: incidence, prevention and management. Drug Safety. 1998; 19:313-24.
16. Dewachter P, Laroche D, Mouton-Fqaivre C, Clement O. Immediate and late adverse reactions to iodinated contrast media: a pharmacological point of view. Anti-Inflammatory Anti-Allergy Agents Med Chem. 2006;5:105-17.
17. Lasser EC, Berry CC, Talner LB, et al. Pretreatment with corticosteroids to alleviate reactions to intravenous contrast material. N Engl J Med. 1987;317:845-9.
18. Greenberger PA, Patterson R. The prevention of immediate generalized reactions to radiocontrast media in high-risk patients. J Allergy Clin Immunol. 1991;87:867-72.
19. Greenberger PA, Halwig JM, Patterson R, Wallemark CB. Emergency administration of radiocontrast media in high-risk patients. J Allergy Clin Immunol. 1986;77:630-4.
20. Grainger RG. Intravascular contrast media. The past, the present and the future. Br J Radiol. 1982;55:1-18.
21. Morris TW. X-ray contrast media. Where are we now and where are we going?. Radiology. 1993;188:11-6.
22. Aspelin P, Aubrey SG, Fransson SG, et al. Nephrotoxic effects in high-risk patients undergoing angiography. N Engl J Med. 2003;348:491-9.
23. Heinrich MC, Kuhlmann MK, Grgic A, et al. Cytotoxic effects of ionic high-osmolar, nonionic monomeric and nonionic iso-osmolar dimeric iodinated contrast media on renal tubular cells *in vitro*. Radiology. 2005;235:843-9.
24. Yoshikawa H. Late reactions to nonionic contrast media. Radiology. 1992;183:737-40.
25. Spring DB, Bettman MA, Barkan HE. Deaths related to iodinated contrast media reported spontaneously to US Food and Drug Administration 1978-1994: Effect of availability of low osmolality contrast media. Radiology. 1997;204:333-7.
26. IV extravasation management guidelines at children hospital; Westmead) practice guideline No: 0/C/12:8007-01:00.
27. http://radres.ucsd.edu/documents/CALL/Extravasation.pdf. ucsdmc policy/procedure-radiology Intravenous Contrast Media Guidelines-Adult.

28. Bellin MF, Jakobsen JA, Tomassin I, et al. Contrast medium extravasation injury: guidelines for prevention and management. Eur Radiol. 2002;12:2807-12.
29. Cohan RH, Ellis JH, Garner WL. Extravasation of radiographic contrast material: recognition, prevention, and treatment. Radiology. 1996;200:593-604.
30. Wang CL, Cohan RH, Ellis JH, Adusumilli S, Dunnick NR. Frequency, management, and outcome of extravasation of nonionic iodinated contrast medium in 69,657 intravenous injections. Radiology. 2007;243:80-7.
31. Mehta RL, Kellum JA, Shah SV, et al. Acute Kidney Injury Network: report of an initiative to improve outcomes in acute kidney injury. Crit Care. 2007;11:R31.
32. D'Elia JA, Gleason RE, Alday M, Malarick C, Godley K, Warram J, et al. Nephrotoxicity from angiographic contrast material: a prospective study. Am J Med. 1982;72:719-25.
33. Porter GA. Radiocontrast-induced nephropathy. Nephrol Dial Transplant. 1994;9(Suppl 4):146-56.
34. Barrett BJ, Parfrey PS, Vavasour HM, McDonald J, Kent G, Hefferton D, et al. Contrast nephropathy in patients with impaired renal function; high versus low osmolar media. Kidney Int. 1992;41:1274-9.
35. Lautin EM, Freeman NJ, Schoenfeld AH, Bakal EW, Haramati N, Friedman AC, et al. Radiocontrast associated renal dysfunction: Incidence and risk factors. Am J Roentgenol. 1991;157:49-58.
36. Rihal CS, Textor SC, Grill DE, Berger PB, Ting HH, Best PJ, et al. Incidence and prognostic importance of acute renal failure after percutaneous coronary intervention. Circulation. 2002; 105:2259-64.
37. McCullough PA, Wolyn R, Rocher LL, Levin RN, O'Neill WW. Acute renal failure after coronary intervention: Incidence, risk factors, and relationship to mortality. Am J Med. 1997;103:368-75.
38. Gruberg L, Mehran R, Dangas G, Mintz GS, Waksman R, Kent KM, et al. Acute renal failure requiring dialysis after percutaneous coronary interventions. Catheter Cardiovasc Interv. 2001;52:409-16.
39. Barrett BJ, Carlisle EJ. Meta-analysis of the relative nephrotoxicity of high- and low-osmolality iodinated contrast media. Radiology. 1993;188:171-8.
40. Weisbord SD, Palevsky PM. Prevention of contrast-induced nephropathy with volume expansion. Clin J Am Soc Nephrol. 2008;3:273-80.
41. Taylor AJ, Hotchkiss D, Morse RW, McCabe J. Preparation for Angiography in Renal Dysfunction: a randomized trial of inpatient vs outpatient hydration protocols for cardiac catheterization in mild-to-moderate renal dysfunction. Chest. 1998;114:1570-4.
42. Merten GJ, Burgess WP, Gray LV, et al. Prevention of contrast-induced nephropathy with sodium bicarbonate: a randomized controlled trial. JAMA. 2004;291:2328-34.
43. Navaneethan SD, Singh S, Appasamy S, Wing RE, Sehgal AR. Sodium bicarbonate therapy for prevention of contrast-induced nephropathy: a systematic review and meta-analysis. Am J Kidney Dis. 2009;53:617-27.
44. Stenstrom DA, Muldoon LL, Armijo-Medina H, et al. N-acetylcysteine use to prevent contrast medium-induced nephropathy: premature phase III trials. J Vasc Interv Radiol. 2008;19:309-18.
45. Vaitkus PT, Brar C. N-acetylcysteine in the prevention of contrast-induced nephropathy: publication bias perpetuated by meta-analyses. Am Heart J. 2007;153:275-80.
46. Solomon R, Werner C, Mann D, D'Elia J, Silva P. Effects of saline, mannitol, and furosemide to prevent acute decrease in renal function induced by radiocontrast agents. N Engl J Med. 1994;331:1416-20.
47. Morcos SK, Thomsen HS, Exley CM. Contrast media: interactions with other drugs and clinical tests. Eur Radiol. 2005;15:1463-8.
48. Katayama H, Yamaguchi K, Kozuka T, et al. Adverse reactions to ionic and nonionic contrast media. Radiology. 1990;175:621-8.
49. Meth MJ, Maibach HI. Current understanding of contrast media reactions and implications for clinical management. Drug Saf. 2006;29:133-41.
50. Christiansen C, Pichler WJ, Skotland T. Delayed allergy-like reactions to X-ray contrast media: mechanistic considerations. Eur Radiol. 2000;10:1965-75.
51. Berman HL, Delaney V. Iodide mumps due to low-osmolality contrast material. Am J Roentgenol. 1992;159:1099-100.
52. Gilgen-Anner Y, Heim M, Ledermann HP, Bircher AJ. Iodide mumps after contrast media imaging: a rare adverse effect to iodine. Ann Allergy Asthma Immunol. 2007;99:93-8.
53. Webb JA, Stacul F, Thomsen HS, Morcos SK. Late adverse reactions to intravascular iodinated contrast media. Eur Radiol. 2003;13:181-4.
54. Grainger RG, Thomsen HS, Morcos SK. Intravascular Contrast Media for Radiology, CT and MRI. In: Adam: Grainger & Allison's Diagnostic Radiology, 5th Edn.
55. Royal College of Radiologist. Standard for intravascular contrast agent administration to adult patients. Approved guidelines by board of faculty of clinical radiology, July 2011.

CHAPTER 58

Picture Archiving and Communication System and Radiology Information System

Shivanand Gamanagatti, Devasenathipathy Kandasamy, Arun Kumar Gupta

INTRODUCTION

Imaging informatics is a well-recognized subspecialty of radiology which deals with the flow of information from person to person or place to place.[1,2] It covers every aspect of radiologists and technicians day-to-day work in any digital radiology department. Modality, radiology information system (RIS) and picture archiving and communication system (PACS) form the important component for reliable running of the radiology service. The concept of PACS was envisioned in 1980s by the members of radiology community and since then it has grown into a robust entity. In the last decade, there have been numerous PACS installations worldwide. It greatly reduces the turn-around time which is the time interval between the acquisition and preparation of report. After the acquisition images are available instantaneously for the radiologists to report and the previous imaging studies can be prefetched for comparison. This increases the efficiency of the workflow in a department and deceases the manual filing and entries. Security issues are paramount regarding the patient data which is transferred across networks for various purposes. Security implementations are easier and robust in a digital environment than in analog environment because they provide application level security and tiered access to data. With digital environment, clinicians can place an order, it can be tracked and once the reports are ready they have access to both the image and report. This makes PACS and RIS more clinician friendly and helps them efficiently use their time also. RIS and PACS are considered to the heart of a digital radiology department and because of numerous advantages and improvements in computer technology it is set to become more popular and the standard of care in near future. Current industry standards and important aspects of PACS and RIS will be discussed in this chapter.

PICTURE ARCHIVING AND COMMUNICATION SYSTEM

Picture archiving and communication system (PACS) is an acronym for picture archiving and communication system:

- *Picture:* Referring to radiographic images and radiology reports.
- *Archiving:* Referring to the film file or film-jacket component of storing images.
- *Communications:* Referencing multiple viewers of images and reports at virtually unlimited viewing sites called workstations.
- *System:* Adopting the concept that a complex coordinated network makes it all possible.

The PACS is hardware and software that stores and manipulates digital information in the form of images and text data. It provides a modern radiology department with optimal storage of images and patient data files. It is also a digital centralized electronic storage system that provides easy access to images transmittable to any workstation on its network.[3]

There are several advantages claimed for PACS. These are as follows:
- The increased efficiency of acquisition, viewing and reporting of images
- Efficient data management, including fewer lost films
- Cost savings
- Space savings
- Environmental benefits
- Increased efficiency of retrieval of historical images

Potential disadvantages are as follows:
- High capital investment, and ongoing costs (training, specialist staff and equipment, and so on)
- The necessary infrastructure may not be available—PACS can place high demands on computer networks, and so it may be necessary to install a new network
- The technical skills required for the support of a PACS may be in short supply.

The PACS is an important aspect in the digital radiology department which handles the images generated by various digital modalities, and it is generally interfaced with RIS. PACS comprises of various components, such as acquisition modalities, workstations, network and storage. The size of the storage, network bandwidth and number of workstations vary among institutions with around 50 GB of data are generated in larger institutions. Apart from the components of PACS, well trained information technology team with in-depth knowledge is also a requirement for the smooth running. But there are some basic aspects of PACS which the radiologists should know will be discussed here.

Components and Architecture of PACS

Hurlen et al. (2008) defined the properties of a PACS, as a system that typically acquire, store, transmit, display, and process digital images.[4]

On the basis of this definition the basic components can be separated into the following:
- For acquiring and preprocessing of the images an image acquisition component is needed
- An archive server is composed of a database server or image manager, short-term and long-term storage, and a computer that controls the PACS workflow, known as a workflow manager
- Finally, to display the digital images, a viewing component is required, referred to as workstation.

Workflow

Workflow is a term simply means how a process is done, step by step. In radiology, the term *workflow* is used to describe how we complete an examination from order entry to transcribed report **(Flowchart 1)**.

Flowchart 1: Workflow in a typical radiology department.

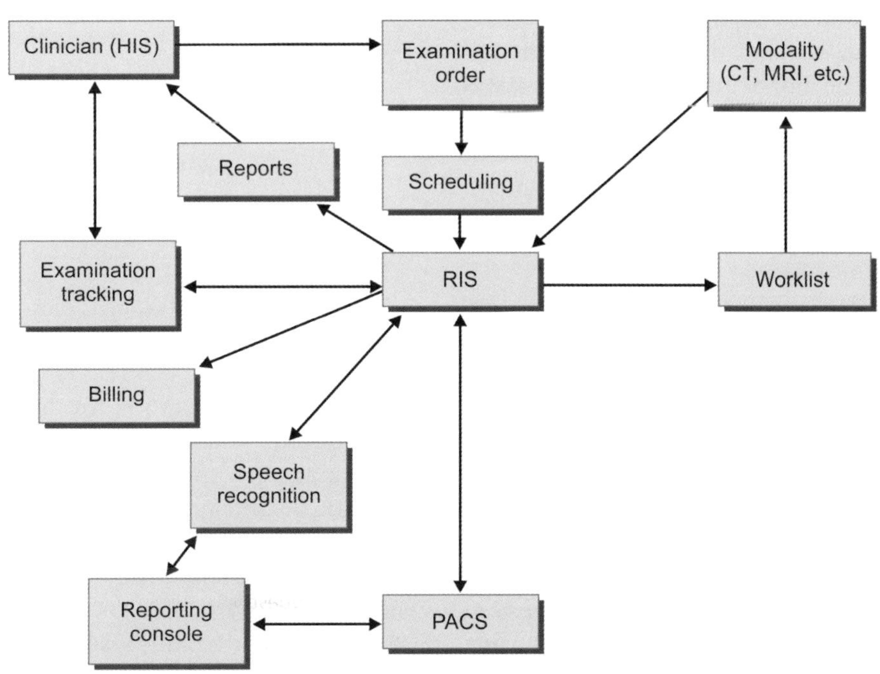

Abbreviations: HIS: Hospital information system; RIS: Radiology information system; PACS: Picture archiving and communication system.

Mini-PACS

A mini-PACS generally refers to a small-scale PACS, usually limited to one imaging modality or department. In a typical mini-PACS installation, one or more image acquisition devices of the same modality are connected to a local digital storage device, and one or two workstations are attached to the storage device, allowing retrieval and display of stored images.

A mini-PACS has some advantages and disadvantages over a full PACS. Advantages include the relatively low initial investment compared to a full PACS implementation, the possibility of a mini-PACS growing into a full PACS, and the chance for hospital staff to gain familiarity with PACS concepts. Disadvantages are centered on the fact that the benefits of a PACS are not fully realized—for example, if images need to be viewed outside the area covered by the mini-PACS, film still needs to be printed.

Teleradiology

Teleradiology can be defined as the ability to acquire a diagnostic image at one location and review it at a remote location, that remote location not being attached to the same local area network as the original image acquisition device. The basic components of a teleradiology system are the image acquisition and sending device, the network used to transfer the image data, and the receiving and viewing station.

Although there are many parallels between PACS and teleradiology, and in the equipment used to create PACS and teleradiology systems, there is a fundamental difference in the ultimate aim of the two systems: a PACS is designed to store image data and to transmit that data for display within an institution; a teleradiology system transmits image data to a remote location for diagnosis, but may or may not include an element of archive storage.

Acquisition

Image acquisition forms the entry point for PACS data, so any error at this point will affect the entire process. Digital modalities like CT, MRI and digital radiography (DR) can directly send the images to PACS. Even in fully digital radiology departments there is a requirement for digitization of films coming from outside hospitals for comparison. This is done by digitizers which scan the films using visible light or laser and they are converted into digital format. Usually the output of these digitizers is in DICOM format which can be transmitted to PACS using DICOM interface. In computed radiography (CR) the existing conventional X-ray machine can be used along with photostimulable phosphor plates to generate digital images.

Image Compression

Average radiology exam is (e.g: CT head) = 20 MB.

Types of Image Compression

- Lossless compression—JPEG : 2:1 = 10 MB/exam
- Lossy compression—Wavelet : 20:1 = 1 MB/exam
- *JPEG 2000*:
  - Combines lossless techniques and lossy wavelet
  - Standards based on wavelet compression
  - DICOM approval of advanced compression by 2000

There are two types of compression: (1) Lossy and (2) Lossless.

In lossy compression, the decompression of the image will not result in the original image. There will be an irreversible loss of image information during this process.

Using the lossless compression technique, which is a completely reversible process the original image can be obtained after decompression. This is the most preferred compression algorithm used in PACS.

Bits and Bytes

Single bits are rarely seen alone in computers. They are almost always bundled together into 8-bit collections, and these collections are called bytes. In medical imaging devices (CT, MR, US, CR, etc.), typically references 8-bit, 10-bit or 12-bit Grayscale images are encountered. This means each digital element of the image called a pixel, will be represented by 8-bit, 10-bit or 12-bit values.

- 1 bit = a light switch, ON or OFF, 0 or 1 (2 values)
- 1 byte = 8 bits '0000'0000' to '1111'1111' (256 values)
- 1 kilobyte (KB) = 1,000 bytes
- 1 megabyte (MB) = 1,000 KB
- 1 gigabyte (GB) = 1,000 MB
- 1 terabyte (TB) = 1,000 GB
- 1 petabyte (PB) = 1,000 TB

The word pixel stands for "picture element", and represents the smallest element in a digital image. A digital image is a two-dimensional array of pixels that represent an image. For example, if we talk about a 640 × 480 pixel image, it means that the image consists of 640 rows of pixels, with 480 pixels in each row. This would equate to a total of 307,200 total pixels (640 × 480 = 307,200), each having a separate grayscale or color intensity value **(Table 1)**. As we decrease grayscale resolution from 12-bits (2 bytes) to 8-bits (1 byte), we are

Table 1: Relationship between pixel size, bit depth and storage size.

		Storage size (bytes)			
Array size	*Total pixels*	*8-bit image (1 byte/pixel)*	*10,12 and 16-bit images (2 bytes/pixel)*	*24-bit image (3 bytes/pixel)*	*32-bit image (4 bytes/pixel)*
256 × 256	= 65536	**65536**	131072	196608	262144
512 × 512	= 262144	**262144**	**524288**	**786432**	1048576
1024 × 1024	= 1048576	**1048576**	**2097152**	**3145728**	4191304
2048 × 2048	= 4194304	4194304	**8388608**	12582912	16777216
2048 × 2560	= 5242880	5242880	**10485760**	15728640	20971520
4096 × 5120	= 20971520	20971520	**41943040**	62914560	83886080

Note: Dark shaded cells represent the most common resolution/bit depth configurations.

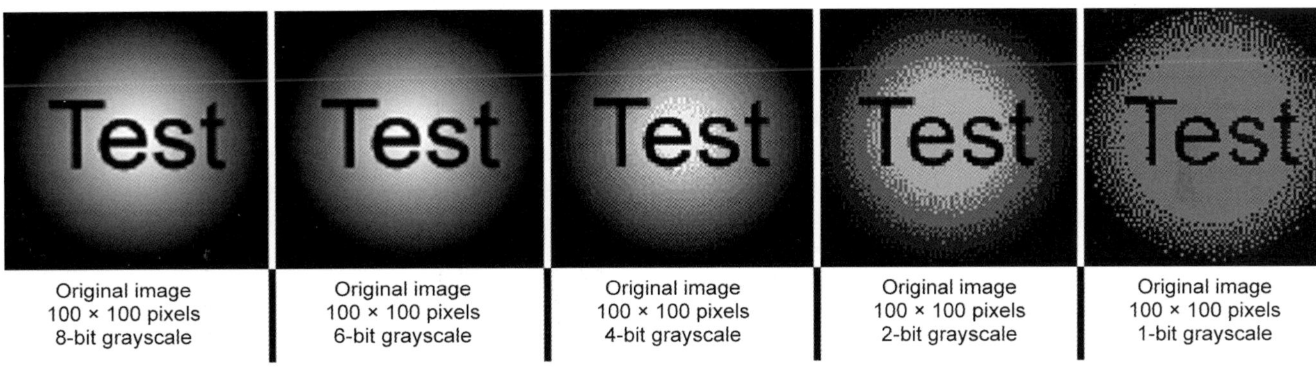

Fig. 1: Diagramatic representation on showing relationship between bit size and resolution of image.

decreasing the level of subtle details that we will capture from the film, but the file size that has to be transferred is half the size due to the storage of 1 byte of data per pixel instead of the 2 bytes required for the 12-bit image **(Fig. 1)**.[5]

Database Server

The main PACS server holds a database of all patient examination information. This database includes details of patient demographics, and the examinations the patient has had since the PACS was installed (and possibly earlier examinations, if digitized). It also contains the information necessary for the PACS to be able to find the images for those examinations, and to direct copies of the images to local storage as required (depending on the architecture of the system). The server also performs routine scheduled tasks required for system maintenance, and allows the system administrator to carry out manual tasks and system tuning as required. The regularly scheduled tasks can include daily and/or weekly backups, prefetching of historical images for review purposes, "flushing" of the online storage. Manual tasks can include management of user accounts, reconciling discrepancies within the database, and managing interfaces with external information systems.[5]

Storage

Data archive

Following acquisition, image data is likely to be stored on on-line, hard disk-based storage. The data may subsequently be saved on near-line or offline archive storage, which may be tape or disk based.

Archiving can be online, near-line or offline depending on the availability of data. Usually hard drive is used for online storage and data in online storage is readily available and it can be accessed almost immediately. Tapes and optical media which are loaded automatically by juke-box are called as near-line storage.[6] In near-line storage, data are available in less than a minute. In offline storage data are loaded manually and the loading time may vary. Some authors discourage the use of the term near-line.[2] This multi-tier system is used because the cost factor involved in online storage. But the cost of hard drives have been decreasing day by day so the use of offline storage should be reduced as far as possible mainly because of the manual intervention and the errors associated with it.

Another method is to store the data in a long-term archive in addition to PACS. In this case the data is stored permanently and available in long term archive even when the study is not available online. Availability of imaging data used in health care is very critical, so it is also sometimes recommended to store a copy of data in a different geographical location which is called as disaster recovery.

The amount of storage needed for a department should be calculated based on the number and types of imaging studies done and also the time duration for which they are kept in archive. Another consideration in choosing an appropriate storage is that it should be a robust and viable technology and should be upgradable in future. Any storage technology can fail so it is very important to have a failover mechanism especially in healthcare services. This is typically done by creating redundant copies so that even if a storage medium fails data can be recovered from another medium.

In order to calculate the archive storage requirements for a PACS, the data on the typical image sizes for each modality can be used. For each modality, multiply the typical image size by the average number of images per examination, and multiply this figure by the number of examinations performed in a year. This will give the annual storage requirements. This figure can be modified according to the amount of compression to be used on the data.

280,000 examinations = ~5.6 terabytes/year

Storage Hardware

The most common types of hardware used to provide storage solutions are those using magnetic and optical technologies. This can be further broken down into disk and tape technologies.

Disk-based storage

- *Redundant array of inexpensive disks:* The redundant array of inexpensive disks (RAID) was devised at the University of California in the late 1980s as a solution to the cost of large hard disks.

  The RAID is a popular technology employed in PACS and is exclusively used for online storage. Instead of using a single large hard disk to provide the required storage capacity, the RAID uses a number of smaller, cheaper disks to provide, in total, the same storage capacity. The RAID is a disk system that allows online access to the data and can provide fault tolerance and redundancy through the use of data striping and data mirroring. The functioning of this array of hard drives as a unit is controlled by the RAID controller. Since data is stored in multiple hard drives recovery of data possible when there is a failure
- *Data stripping:* This technique spreads the blocks of each file across multiple disks but provides no redundancy of the data. Each file is separated into fixed sized blocks, or stripe units, and striped across multiple disks in a "Round Robin" manner. However, the use of this striping provides no redundancy of the data. Round Robin is a scheduling algorithm in which processes are activated in a fixed cyclic order
- *Data mirroring:* A technique in which data are written to two duplicate disks simultaneously hence providing redundancy in the system. If one of the disk drives fails, the system can instantly switch to the other disk without any loss of data or service. The disadvantage of data mirroring is that there is no increase in speed of access with a higher cost and double the capacity being required. Disk mirroring is used commonly in online database systems, where it is critical that the data be accessible at all times
- *RAID levels:* There are number of different RAID "levels," each providing differing amounts of speed of access and fault tolerance. The most common are level 0, level 3, and level 5. The various levels are defined as:
  - *Level 0:* Provides data stripping. This improves data transfer performance but does not deliver fault tolerance or redundancy
  - *Level 1:* Provides disk mirroring. This data transfer is robot or carousel, to a reading/writing area; the time for this similar to a single disk and provides redundancy in the system
  - *Level 2:* Bits (rather than bytes or groups of bytes) are interleaved across multiple disks. Although this has high-transfer rates, it is rarely used
  - *Level 3:* Same as Level 0, but also reserves one dedicated disk for error correction data. It provides good performance and some level of fault tolerance
  - *Level 4:* Similar to Level 3, but manages disks independently rather than in unison. Not often used
  - *Level 5:* Provides data striping at the byte level and also stripe error correction information. This results in excellent performance and good fault tolerance
  - *Level 6:* Highest reliability, but not widely used. Similar to RAID 5, but does two different parity computations or the same computation on overlapping subsets of the data.

The access capability should be able to withstand disk failure and can have the facility to reconstruct the data from a failed disk.

- *Digital-versatile disk (DVD):* This is a form of storage media which uses a similar technology to CD-ROM. However it has a more efficient recording algorithm. Digital versatile disks (DVDs) come in several formats: they can be dual sided, and they can have multiple layers, which in turn allows for an increase in storage capacity. DVD has the ability to store large amounts of data, up to 4.7 GB per side for single-sided, single-layer disks.
- *Magneto-optical disk (MOD):* A type of disk that combines magnetic disk technologies with CD-ROM technologies. The Magneto optical disk (MOD) uses a laser to read the disk and a laser and magnet to write to the disk using the magneto-optical effect. A double-sided disk can store up to 9.1 GB of data.

Tape storage

There are many tape formats used for near-line and offline storage.

- *Advanced intelligent tape:* Advanced intelligent tape (AIT) comes in two formats, AIT-2 and AIT-3, which can store 50 and 100 GB respectively, with a data transfer rate of 12 MB/ sec for the AIT-3. The advantage of this technology over other tapes is the in-built chip in the tape housing, which holds indexing information of the data stored on the tape. This facilitates fast retrieval of data, since it is not necessary to read indexing information from the tape in order to locate the required data. This also allows for less wear and tear on the tape as limited searching through the tape is required to retrieve the data.
- *Jukebox:* The media used in archive storage are housed in a device known as a jukebox. A jukebox can contain one of many types of media (CD-ROM, tape or disks). The jukebox moves the media from its storage location, by means of a movement of disk to read is usually in the order of 10–30 seconds.

SAN versus NAS

Although the names sound similar, each storage technology is different.

NAS stands for **Network Attached Storage**

SAN stands for **Storage Area Network.**

Network attached storage unit

A network attached storage (NAS) is a unit that typically has multiple hard drives. The drives are then arranged in a RAID configuration to prevent against data loss due to hardware failure. Then, an operating is embedded in the NAS unit to perform all of the file operations, sharing, network communication, etc. Most NAS units are connected to your network via IP and can be managed through a web interface. The embedded-operating system allows the unit to create users, shares, permissions, and sometimes even act as a file transfer protocol (FTP) server to allow the access of files via the internet.

The NAS units offer better sharing capabilities between different operating system such as Windows and MAC due to the different file access methods in the embedded NAS operating system. NAS units also offer many additional features, such as automated backup, bit torrent downloading, file quotas, and print sharing.

Storage area network unit

The storage area network (SAN) units are also comprised of multiple disks configured in RAID to protect against data loss due to hardware failure. SAN units typically use higher end hard disks that spin between 10,000 RPM and 15,000 RPM for increased performance. SAN units do not have any type of embedded-operating system. SANs deal with data on the block level. This means that in order to utilize a SAN in your environment, it has to be attached to a host or multiple host machines. SANs connect to their host machine via a fiber channel. The host machine controls the file operations, sharing, permissions, etc. Typically, SANs are used in enterprise environments or in environments where fast input-output operations are required.

SAN units usually offer larger storage capacities due to the amount of physical hard drives they support. Also, data read and write speeds are faster in part due to the fiber channel link between the host server and the unit as well as the high end hard drive speeds.

Which is best NAS or SAN?

Choosing the right storage unit can be tricky. A NAS is a good choice if your organization is looking to create a centralized file storage system or your organization just needs some extra-file storage. If you are a larger enterprise and larger storage requirements as well as read write performance are necessary, then it may be wise to invest in a SAN over a NAS.

Workstation

It is the interactive component of PACS where the radiologists interpret and generate a report. It is the responsibility of radiologist to ensure the image quality which necessitates the radiologists to understand the basics of hardware. A typical workstation comprises display monitors, computer, local storage which is connected by network cables. The computer should have enough computing power in the order of 3 MHz or above, more and faster random-access memory (RAM) to do 3D rendering of large CT and MRI data sets.[1] In advanced workstation used for cardiac and vascular studies dedicated video graphics card is usually present to improve the performance.

Display Monitors

For radiologists basic knowledge of display monitors is very important. Cathode ray tube (CRT) monitors utilize older technology which has been used in televisions for decades and they are relatively cheaper. Liquid crystal display (LCD) is a newer technology which is relatively expensive. However, the LCD technology has been improved to match the quality of best CRT monitors and they are becoming cheaper. It is expected that in near future LCD monitors will replace CRT monitors. Compared to CRT the advantages of LCD monitors are:

- Thin and light weight
- Less power consumption
- Brightness of display
- Flat surface
- Aspect ratio is maintained.

One disadvantage of LCD monitor which is worth mentioning is that it has narrow viewing angle than CRT monitors.

Resolution

Spatial resolution of monitors is expressed in megapixels which is the number of million pixels. Very high-resolution monitors are expensive and they are slow to respond. So it is important to choose the resolution of monitors for the type of usage and workstation requirements.[2] For modalities like US, CT and MRI which have fixed matrix size can be viewed optimally in 2 megapixel monitors. Radiographs pose a problem because they have very high resolution which is usually more that the resolution of display monitors. One approach is to down sample the original image and it is displayed at a lower resolution in the monitor. Although finer details are lost in the process of down sampling it has been shown that resolution of more than 2–3 megapixels has no significant improvement in diagnostic accuracy.[7] Another approach is with lower resolution monitors the image can be zoomed and panned so that the finer details are visualized. Visualization of microcalcification is very critical in mammography and it demands for higher-resolution monitors. Monitors with 5 megapixel resolution are recommended for mammography interpretation.[2]

Color and Grayscale display

Most of the radiological images are in gray scale although Doppler, PET, nuclear medicine images used colors. Color LCD monitors are very good in displaying color images. The quality of display of grayscale monitor is superior to the corresponding color monitors because the images are blurred and less bright in color monitor. Color monitor is also expensive than the grayscale monitor which is also a reason for increasing usage of grayscale monitors in many radiology departments. Lower-resolution color monitors are used for viewing colored images whereas grayscale monitors are used to view high-resolution images. Typically, one low resolution color monitor and two high resolution gray scale monitors are used in workstations.

Radiologist Reading Stations

The radiologist reading station is used by a radiologist when making a primary diagnosis. The reading station has the highest quality hardware, including the best monitor. The computer hardware meet the needs of the PACS vendor, but it will usually be very robust, requiring little downtime. The keyboard and mouse can be customized. There are many different styles of mice available that can increase the efficiency of the software being used.

There is generally access to a nearby RIS, with a dictation system near or even connected to the PACS station. Many PACS have software that integrates the RIS and dictation system.

Physician Review Stations

The physician review workstations is a step-down model of the radiologist reading station. Many vendors use the same level of software but may eliminate some of the more advanced functions. One of the most important features on a physician review station is the ability to view current and previous reports along with images.

Network

Network is another important component which transmits data from one place to other. Four important factors to be considered while setting up a PACS network are: (1) performance or the speed of the network, (2) reliability, (3) upgradability, and (4) the cost involved. The workstations or computers used by radiologists to report are usually clients which are connected to a server. Clients get data from the server based on various queries. Typically there are many clients connected to a server by means of network cables. There are various equipment in a network, such as router, switch which are used to manage the network and use the bandwidth efficiently. This kind of connections between computers with in a hospital is called as local area network (LAN). This can be a wired network using cables or a wireless network. Usually wired network is preferred because of its performance, reliability and security reasons. When multiple LANs are connected it is called as wide area network (WAN). Performance of the network and the reliability depends on how it is managed which necessitates the requirement of trained personnel in the department. Network and error logs need to be checked on daily basis to ensure smooth running of network. Another technology which is virtual private network (VPN) is commonly used nowadays to view the images from anywhere in the world using the internet infrastructure. One of the problems in transmitting the images outside the hospital is lack of control and security over the transmitted data. Using this VPN protocol the internet infrastructure is tunnelled and used to reach the hospital LAN. This protocol ensures security of the transmitted data though the data is transmitted across various public networks. This also enables the radiologists to use all the facilities in the hospital LAN as if there are within the LAN. Users are given username and passwords and their privileges are set-up so that the data is secured in the network and it is not misused. Also, numerous network and PACS configurations are possible, such as certain information will be accessed by certain people.

It is very important to have a dedicated network for PACS and it should not be shared with other non-PACS network. This will ensure proper functioning and reduce congestion in the network. When many users are using the network simultaneously it will cause congestion and network will be slow to respond which can occur even in high bandwidth networks. To avoid this problem to some extent, there are techniques to compress the image which will reduce the network load.

System Architecture

System architecture can be defined as the hardware and software infrastructure of a computer system. In a PACS, the system architecture normally consists of acquisition devices, storage, display workstations, and an image management system. The following discussion outlines three common PACS architectures and takes a look at the flow of images after acquisition.

Client/Server-based Systems

In a client/server-based system, images are sent directly to the archive server after acquisition and are centrally located. The display workstation functions as a client of the archive server and accesses images based on a centralized worklist that is generated at the archive server. The healthcare worker at the display workstation chooses a name from the central list, and the archive server sends the image data to display station. Once the "client's session" is finished, the image data is flushed from its memory. Most systems allow basic image manipulation at the display workstation or "client," and the changes are saved on the archive server.

Advantages

Any examination sent to the PACS is available anywhere without other interventions. Only one person can open the study with the intent to read it. Others that open the study will receive a message that the study is open and being read. There is no need to pull or send historic images to a particular workstation because the old studies are available along with the new studies on the archive.

Disadvantages

The archive server is seen as a single point of failure. If the archive goes down, the entire system is down, and no image movement can take place. All newly acquired images must remain at the modality until the archive is up and can again receive the images.

The system is heavily network dependent. The images are flying back and forth between the archive and the workstations, and the network can become bogged down because of the large volume of data being moved. The archive server is handling many requests at once and can become bottlenecked because of the high volume of requests.

Distributed Systems

In a distributed or stand-alone system, the acquisition modalities send the images to a designated reading station and possibly to review stations, depending on where the order originated (i.e. ICU or ER). In some systems, the images are sent from the modality to the archive server, and the archive server distributes the images to the designated workstation. The reading station designations may be designed based on radiologist reading preferences. For example, MRI may be sent to one station and CT to another, or all cross-sectional neurological images may be sent to one station but all body imaging are sent to another. The designation is decided after extensive workflow observation. Moreover, in a distributed model, the workstations can query and retrieve images from the archive. All images are then stored locally and then are sent to the archive server after they have been read. These images remain on the local hard drive of the workstation until they are deleted either by a user or by system rules.

Advantages

If the archive server goes down, local reading at the workstations is not interrupted, other than not being able to get historic images. After the archive comes backup, the images that have been changed and signed off by the radiologist will be forwarded automatically to the archive to be saved. Because the images can be distributed to many locations at once, copies of an examination exist at various locations. Therefore, it is less likely that PACS data will be lost. The system is less dependent on the network for its speed. The user can be working on one examination while the workstation is pulling and getting the next examination ready to be read. The workstation can fetch historic images according to rules the user sets up.

Disadvantages

There is heavy reliance on the assumption that the distribution of images is being done correctly. If the distribution is wrong, the prefetching of historic examinations will not be correct either. Each workstation has a different worklist, and therefore only one person can be working on that list at a time. It can be inconvenient to read additional studies; the radiologist would have to move to another workstation to read the images designated for that workstation. The users must depend on the query-and-retrieve function when nonscheduled examinations arrive at the workstation to be read.

It is also possible for two radiologists to be reading the same examination and not knowing until they try to start dictation. The paper requisition is very important with this type of PACS.

Web-based Systems

A web-based system is very similar to a client/server system in how data flow. The significant difference is that both the images and the application software for the client display are held centrally. In a client/server system, the client still has application software locally loaded to the client, and only the images are held at the archive.

Advantages

The hardware at the client can be anything that will support an appropriate web browser. This allows for greater flexibility with hardware but can also be a disadvantage because image displays (monitors) may not be able to support diagnostic quality. The same application can be used on site and at home in teleradiology situations. Teleradiology is a term used to describe the reading of images outside the hospitals walls. It can be down the road at the radiologist's home or on the other side of the world during night-time hours.

Disadvantages

The system's functionality may be limited because the software is not installed locally. The bandwidth of the network connection limits the amount of data that can be transmitted for download, and some programs are too large to be transmitted over the network that is installed. As with client/server systems, the network is the biggest obstacle to performance.

Related Applications

Apart from RIS and PACS, radiologists also commonly use various applications and software which can make the interpretation of images easier, to do advanced postprocessing and generating reports in quicker and easier way. Some of the commonly used applications are discussed here.

Three-dimensional and advanced viewing

In the modern era of imaging thin high resolution images are routinely acquired and they are utilized in three-dimensional (3D) reconstructions. Many currently available commercial applications can provide a range of 3D reconstructions such as maximum intensity projection (MIP), surface shaded display (SSD) and volume rendering technique (VRT), etc. These techniques help the radiologists to make use of the fullest potential of the modality. Curved reconstructions and VRT used to be a time-consuming exercise but now these processes are automated by a click of a button. Other postprocessing techniques such as virtual bronchoscopy and colonoscopy can provide virtual endoluminal view. Modern workstations are also equipped with advanced postprocessing applications such as dual energy applications and computer-aided detection (CAD).

With the emerging technology of dual energy CT, various postprocessing applications are available to decompose the image based on the material density. In this way it is possible to generate iodine only image and virtual noncontrast scans. Spectral imaging is also possible in which the keV can be changed by the user and image is processed by the workstation according to the selected keV. This processing can be useful in studying the material characteristics over a range of photon energies. The clinical application of this technique is in differentiating hyperdensity because of bleed from contrast enhancement in postcontrast scans.

Computer-aided detection is a technique in which the computer will analyze the image to show the region of interest based on predefined rules. Those areas will be again analyzed by the radiologist to come to a conclusion. This method has been applied in mammography, lung nodule detection and polyp detection. Advanced segmentation algorithms are available nowadays which can be useful in determining the volume of tumor or any solid organ. This can be very useful in determining the response evaluation of tumors.

Speech recognition

Report generation is a time-consuming process if it involves typing of the report. Speech recognition software is aimed at reducing the time delay involved in typing a report. Various attempts were made since 1980s to device a robust speech recognition software.[6] But the earlier applications suffered many setbacks because of poor accuracy and inability to adapt to the accent of the radiologists. Various improvements have been made since then and the currently available speech recognition applications are robust enough to adapt itself to the accent of user and it has in-built spelling check which includes words used in radiology. In addition, it has seamless integration with the PACS software.

Industry Standards

Earlier, transmission of textual or image data across network used to be very difficult because the differences in the vendor, operating system and the application environment. To facilitate free flow of information across modalities and networks in health care industry standards have been developed. By this way, images and data from various vendors can be handled in an organized manner. Currently, Health Level 7 (HL7) is the industry standard for the transmission of textual information and digital imaging and communications in medicine (DICOM) is the industry standard for the image data and communication protocols. Vendors have quickly adopted these standards and because of their conformance to these standards it is possible to seamlessly transmit data across hospital information system (HIS), RIS and PACS and even between hospitals.

Health Level Seven International

Health Level Seven (HL7) is an international community of healthcare subject matter experts and information technology scientists collaborating to create standards for the exchange, management and integration of electronic health care information. HL7 standard was established in 1984 by a committee formed by the vendors and the users. It established the standard of exchange of electronic information in health care. It uses the highest level which is the application layer in open systems interconnection (OSI) model and it is independent of other lower layers. The information is exchanged as messages in HL7 format. Whenever there is an event such as admission, discharge or transfer, HIS sends a message containing key details RIS parses the message and updates its database. RIS can also send messages in HL7 format to PACS carrying key information. HL7 has been improved and updated thereafter in versions 2 and 3.

Digital imaging and communications in medicine (DICOM): It is a standard for handling, storing, printing, and transmitting information in medical imaging. It was also necessary to standardize the format of images and communication protocols used in imaging so as to facilitate flow of information across the hospital regardless of the vendors involved. A standard was developed together by American College of Radiology (ACR) and National Electrical Manufacturers Association (NEMA) to promote exchange of information among equipment from various vendors. This was aimed to integrate various equipment used in radiology, such as radiography machines, CT scanners, MRI, printers, digitizers, etc. with PACS. The first version was released in 1985 and it was called as ACR-NEMA version 1. Later in 1988, the second version namely ACR-NEMA 2.0 was also released with enhancements. In 1992, a newer version was released with major improvements, and it was named as DICOM 3.0.[6]

RADIOLOGY INFORMATION SYSTEM

In the modern digital radiology department radiology information system (RIS) forms the backbone which controls almost all aspects of radiology workflow. The RIS drives the workflow and transfer of information across the department. It deals with nonimage text-based computing functions, such as scheduling of an appointment, generation of worklist, order tracking, billing and reporting.[5] Scheduling can be done from RIS or the orders can come from HIS. RIS is responsible for collecting the patient demographic data and it will send it to the modality where it is needed in the form of worklist. The modality can use the worklist and proceed with the acquisition. In this way manual entry of patient data in the modality is avoided since manual data entry is the common cause of error. The accuracy of the patient data is very important so that the older imaging studies can be automatically prefetched from the archive and to enable correctness in the billing procedure. Pre-fetching of images can be done from the long term storage (LTS) or list of patients can be generated which is to be taken out manually from the record room. The scheduling can be done automatically by the software based on the set of rules or manually. Once the scheduling is done, the status of the examination can be tracked till the generation of the report.

After the scheduling, RIS will prepare the worklist and provide necessary data to the radiologist and technician who will perform the examination in the modality. This worklist can be either in paper format or electronic format. Besides the patient data and the clinical information it will also provide information regarding the patients ambulatory condition, sensitivity to drugs and contrast, etc. which is important in proper completion of the examination. Since the patient data are fetched electronically by the modality there is no scope for manual entry errors. Once the study is completed the images are sent to PACS and then RIS and PACS will interact to validate the available image information by matching with the order placed. Then RIS will generate a list of studies and will send it to appropriate specialty or radiologist in the department. The reports are then sent to the destined department and that is available for viewing and it will also update the billing department of the hospital. RIS archives the order, exam data and report. Thus, RIS controls the workflow in the radiology department.

REFERENCES

1. Branstetter BF 4th. Basics of imaging informatics. Part 1. Radiology. 2007;243(3):656-67.
2. Hersh WR. Medical informatics. JAMA: the journal of the American Medical Association. 2002;288(16):1955-8.
3. Dreyer KJ, Mehta A, Thrall JH (Eds). PACS—A Guide to the Digital Revolution, (New York: Springer-Verlag, 2002), ISBN 0-387-95291-8.
4. Hurlen P, Stbye T, Borthne A, Gulbrandsen P. Introducing PACS to the Late Majority. A Longitudinal Study. Journal of Digital Imaging Online. 2008.
5. Huang HK (Ed). PACS: Basic Principles and Applications (Wiley-Liss, New York, 1999), ISBN 0-471-25393-6.
6. Mildenberger P, Eichelberg M, Martin E. Introduction to the DICOM standard. European Radiology. 2002;12(4):920-7.
7. Simborg DW. The case for the HL7 standard. Comput Health. 1988;9(1):39-40.

CHAPTER 59

Evidence-based Radiology

Sanjay Sharma, Manisha Jana

INTRODUCTION

Evidence-based medicine (EBM) is defined as the integration of best research evidence with clinical expertise and patients' values and expectations.[1-3] Dr Guyatt and Dr Sackett, from the Evidence-based Medicine Working Group at McMaster University, Ontario, Canada, are the pioneers of EBM in modern clinical practice and first coined this term.[4] For proper understanding of EBM, all three of its basic constituents must be imbibed. Best research evidence implies clinically relevant research (which has been properly validated), in the field of diagnostic or therapeutic practice. Clinical expertise depends on the decision making ability and expertise in treatment, based on one's clinical knowledge, experience and skill.

This chapter includes the overview of evolution, types, components, strength and caveats of evidence-based practice (EBP) in our daily lives.

BACKGROUND

The practice of medicine has hitherto remained 'eminence based' that is, based on individual experience and expertise.[3] According to Frieldland,[5] the basic assumptions of this traditional medical practice are as follows:

- The measure of authority is proportional to the weight of individual experience
- Understanding pathophysiology forms the foundation for clinical practice
- Conventional medical training and common sense are enough to enable a physician to evaluate new tests and treatments
- Clinical experience and expertise in a given subject area are enough for the physician to develop clinical practice guidelines.

Traditional 'eminence-based practice' is more didactic, based on individual expertise and does not always take into consideration the existing best research evidence. This is where the proponents of EBP differ from traditional practice. The foundation of EBP rests upon the proper use of validated research evidence (e.g. meta-analysis, randomized controlled trials) to support one's clinical decision in diagnostic procedures, interventions and therapy. In no way it undermines the importance of individual knowledge or pathophysiology of disease.[6]

WHY EVIDENCE-BASED PRACTICE?

The growing awareness and practice of EBP worldwide can be explained by a few basic needs in healthcare services. Firstly, with the ever-increasing number of newer disease entities, the physician needs to be constantly updating himself about the diagnosis, prognosis and treatment of the disease.[7] In this respect the conventional textbooks as a resource often prove inadequate.[8] Also searching for the desired data from the deluge of available medical journals is practically impossible for a busy medical practitioner, owing to the lack of time.[9,10] Secondly, the improved clinical skills in an experienced professional very often coexists with a declining up-to-date knowledge.[11] This forms an increasing 'knowledge gap' among the practitioners. In clinical practice, the knowledge of healthcare workers forms the backbone of the clinical decision making. The 'knowledge gaps' appear when the healthcare provider's knowledge is insufficient to meet the need of the patient.[3,12] The gap can be in 'background knowledge', i.e. general information regarding a disease or treatment; or 'foreground knowledge' which pertains to the latest information regarding the disease condition, any new diagnostic test or intervention.[3] The 'background knowledge' is usually obtained from books and well established texts, e.g. radiological anatomy and procedures for radiologists. 'Background knowledge' gaps can be encountered in rare diseases or an uncommonly performed procedure.[3] 'Foreground knowledge' gaps are more common. Sources of this type of knowledge lie in latest published literature. It becomes important for a practicing physician to identify the knowledge gap and be aware about where to search for the required evidence.[13]

The rising costs of health care make it imperative to justify the decision for any specific diagnostic test or treatment. Moreover, the freely available internet, effective search engines (MEDLINE, Pubmed, Google scholar, etc) and development of systematic reviews of the existing evidences in health care, such as the 'Cochrane Collaboration' have made tracking any evidence easier,[14] further supporting the evidence, based approach towards medical decisions. Archie Cochrane, a British epidemiologist, highlighted in 1972 that most treatment decisions were not based on systematic review of clinical research but on random selection of existing evidence or 'expert opinion'.[15] Cochrane collaboration is a nonprofit organization consisting of volunteers all over the world who analyse the existing evidence and make the up-to-date evidence-based information available.[14] Another reason for growing popularity of EBP is the development of evidence-based journals (e.g. *Evidence-based Medicine*) which contain systematic reviews, meta-analyses and evidence-based guidelines.[16]

Forms of Evidence-based Practice

There are two forms of EBP, the 'top-down' and the 'bottom-up'.[3,17] The 'top-down' practice is usually carried out by experts working for a government, large centralized resource like Cochrane Collaboration or a professional body like American College of Radiology. However, what practitioners (clinician or radiologist) are more concerned in daily life is with the 'bottom-up' approach. 'Bottom-up' EBP starts from the practitioner who encounters a problem, asks an answerable question regarding the problem, searches for the best available evidence and applies it in his practice after critical appraisal. These two forms of EBP are not mutually exclusive, but complementary.[18] In the following sections of this chapter, we have elaborated the steps of 'bottom-up' EBP.

'Bottom-up' Evidence-based Practice

As described earlier, bottom-up EBP is more relevant to daily practice of a busy clinician or radiologist. The concept was started by David Sackett in 1996. These steps are listed in **Table 1**.

Step 1: Ask

The first step of 'bottom-up EBP' is asking a question, arising from either the background or foreground knowledge gap.

It is the foreground question that is usually needed to be answered to address the clinical problem. The foreground questions usually have four components, patient, intervention, comparator and outcome (PICO)[1,19] **(Table 2)**.

The questions in clinical practice can relate either to the etiology, risk factors, diagnosis or management of a certain entity. The radiologists in practice are more concerned with the diagnosis or management of a disease entity. While searching for the answers to a question, the practitioner should be aware of the kind of study to be looked for. For example, if a question relates to an etiology or risk factor, the ideal study design would be a randomized control trial (RCT), prospective cohort study or case-control study. The questions related to disease frequency can be best answered by a prospective cohort study or a cross-sectional study. For questions related to diagnostic procedures, a cross-sectional study with consecutive or random sampling may be ideal. A cohort/survival study will be ideal to answer a question related to the disease prognosis; and therapy/intervention related questions can be better answered by a RCT or cohort study.[3]

While searching for evidence, one should be aware about the hierarchy of evidence.[20,21] The study designs are graded by the levels of evidence. On top of the hierarchy, are

Table 1: Steps of bottom-up EBP[2,3].

Step	*Summary*	*Explanation*
1.	Ask	Asking an answerable question
2.	Search	Searching for the best available research evidence
3.	Appraise	Critical appraisal of the evidences for validity and impact assessment
4.	Apply	Application of the evidence in practice
5.	Evaluate	Evaluation of efficacy and effectiveness of first 4 steps

the systematic reviews of RCTs and cohort studies (Level 1a) which are considered the least-biased evidences. Level 1b includes RCTs and cohort studies with good validation and follow-up. Hitherto considered a superior evidence, an 'expert opinion' is downgraded at level 5. The levels of evidence are tabulated below **(Table 3)**.

In evidence-based radiology (EBR), when one searches for evidence, it must be valid and relevant. Since diagnostic imaging is not directly related to patient outcome and in view of the increasing cost of medical imaging, the technology assessment of an imaging tool has to be performed with assessment of some additional parameters.[22] The need for separate technology assessment also stems from the concern regarding risk of increased radiation exposure in the imaging modalities.[22] A conceptual framework of the technologic assessment was described by Thornbury,[23] McNeil, et al.[24] and later Fryback.[22,25] In short, the hierarchy of technical assessment deals with the following level:

- The technical efficacy
- Diagnostic accuracy (described by sensitivity, specificity, PPV, NPV)
- Diagnostic thinking efficacy (the pre- and post-test probability and likelihood ratios)
- Therapeutic efficacy (whether the imaging modality can change the treatment decision)
- Patient outcome efficacy (impact of the test on the patient)
- Societal efficacy (the cost-effectiveness).

The statistical terms used are explained later in this chapter.[22,25]

Step 2: Search

Once the question is formulated, the next step in EBP is searching for the best evidence. For this, the practitioner

Table 2: Components of a question (PICO), illustrated by an example[19].

Example: How effective is CT pulmonary angiography in the detection of pulmonary embolism compared to ventilation-perfusion scan, in patients with suspected pulmonary embolism?		
Component	***Explanation***	***Example***
Patient population/ clinical problem (P)	Patient's clinical situation or the problem of interest	Patients with suspected pulmonary embolism
Intervention (I)	Main intervention, which can be an exposure, diagnostic procedure or a treatment in question	Computed tomography (CT) pulmonary angiography
Comparator (C)	Exposure, diagnostic test or treatment to which the main intervention is compared	Ventilation-perfusion scan
Outcome (O)	Result/outcome of interest	The accuracy in the diagnosis of pulmonary embolism

Table 3: Levels/hierarchy of evidence[20,21].

Level of evidence	***Description***
1a	Systematic review (with homogeneity) of level 1 diagnostic studies or a clinical decision rule with 1b studies from different clinical centers
1b	Independent blind comparison of an appropriate spectrum of consecutive patients, all of whom have undergone both the diagnostic test and the reference standard
1c	Diagnostic finding for which specificity is so high that positive result rules in the diagnosis or for which sensitivity is so high that negative result rules out the diagnosis
2a	Systematic review (with homogeneity) of level 2 diagnostic studies
2b	Independent blind comparison but either in nonconsecutive patients or confined to a narrow spectrum of study patients (or both), all of whom have undergone both the diagnostic test and the reference standard; or a clinical decision rule not validated by means of a test set
3a	Systematic review (with homogeneity) of studies with a level of 3b and better
3b	Nonconsecutive study or independent blind comparison of an appropriate spectrum, but reference standard not applied to all study patients
4	Reference standard not applied independently or not applied blindly
5	Expert opinion without explicit critical appraisal or based on physiology, bench research, or "first principles"

needs to be aware of how and where to look for. As already described, the textbooks are a good source of background knowledge, but the foreground knowledge gap need latest evidences, which can not usually be found in textbooks, as they may be already outdated by the time they are published. The most up-to date resources for the best evidences are the electronic resources (journals, search engines, information systems).[3] The common electronic resources are listed in **Table 4**.

Radiologic electronic resources: Unfortunately, there are limited available electronic resources providing information regarding diagnostic imaging modalities. Evidence-based radiology website (http://*www.evidencebasedradiology.net*) was developed by the St Vincent's University hospital in Ireland and provides proper 5-step process of EBM. Critical appraisal worksheets and excel spread sheets can be downloaded to create graph of conditional probabilities.[26,27]

Step 3: Critically appraise

Once the proper evidences are available, one needs to assess them for validity and impact assessment. In routine practice, we tend to read an article without its proper critical appraisal. First step of critical appraisal of a primary research article (first-hand studies, such as RCT, experiments and survey) is the assessment of its validity, that is, whether the study is close to the truth and without bias.[28] The next step comprises of the impact assessment and applicability in one's own clinical practice.

- ***Validity assessment:*** The simple steps for validity assessment of a study are searching for answers to the following questions:[29]
  - What is the PICO of this study and whether they are relevant in one's own clinical scenario?
  - How well was the study performed?
  - Can the results be due to chance (bias)?

  Assessment of validity of a study by asking the PICO questions is done by following the steps described by an acronym **RAMMbo (Table 5)**. It also describes the processes to eliminate bias at each step. While critically appraising any study, the practitioner must try to get answers to all these questions, in order to decide if the results of the study are trustworthy. Additionally, while appraising the internal validity of a study describing any new diagnostic test, the following questions are to be answered[29]
  - Whether the test was evaluated on a group of patients similar to those on whom it is to be used in practice?
  - Whether there was an independent reference standard for proper blinded comparison?
  - Was the reference standard applied on all patients, independent of the test result?
  - Was the test validated on a separate, independent group of patients?

  In an ideal study, answers to all of the above questions should be 'yes'. After the internal validity and methodology assessment, if study comes out to be a proper blinded randomized study without bias, the results are to be assessed for their relevance. A statistically significant result is known by its p value. It is a measure of the probability that the result is purely by chance.[28,30] A p value of less

Table 4: Electronic resources for EBM[13].

Name	***Web Link***
McMaster University Health Information Research Unit: Evidence Based Health Informatics	http://*hiru.mcmaster.ca/hiru*
Pubmed: US National Library of Medicine and National Institutes of Health	http://*www.ncbi.nlm.nih.gov/sites/entrez*
Google Scholar	http://*scholar.google.com*
MD Consult	http://*www.mdconsult.com*
Cochrane Collaboration	http://*www.cochrane.org*
SUM Search	http://*sumsearch.uthscsa.edu*
American College of Physicians Journal Club	http://*www.acpjc.org*
British Medical Journal Evidence-based Medicine	http://*ebm.bmj.com*
BMJ Clinical Evidence	http://*clinicalevidence.bmj.com/ceweb*
National Library of Medicine	http://*www.nlm.nih.gov*
Center for Evidence-based Medicine at Oxford	http://*www.cebm.net*
Center for Evidence-based Radiology at the Brigham and Women's Hospital	http://*www.brighamandwomens.org/cebi/default.aspx*

Table 5: Assessment of validity of study in PICO format[29].

Questions	*Assessment*		*Possible error/bias*	*Ways to circumvent*
PICO	RAMMbo			
Patient (P)-population in the study	Assessing for fair recruitment **(R)**	R	Selection bias (the subjects are not representative of the population of interest), or Small study sample leading to imprecise results	Randomization or consecutive recruitment Increase the size of study population
Intervention (I)	How fairly were the subjects allocated **(A)** into groups?	A	Allocation bias (lack of proper matching of subjects in the two groups, e.g. age, sex, etc.)	Randomization
	Whether equal management and follow-up were done (fair **M**aintenance) in both (except for the index test/ intervention)?	M	Treatment bias	Equal management in both the groups apart from the index test or intervention
Comparator (C)	Same as above		Same as above	
Outcome (O)	Assessing for fair **M**easurement—valid and un**b**iased **o**utcome measurement	M	Measurement bias	Double blinding
		b o		

than 0.05 is considered statistically significant. Confidence intervals (CI) are an estimate of the range of values that are likely to include the real value. Usually they are described with 95% CI values.[28] Studies with larger samples tend to have narrower CI and are therefore more reliable.[31-33]

- ***Impact assessment:***
  - *Impact assessment of diagnostic literature:* After assessment for validity, the study should be evaluated for its impact or strength, usually found in the 'result section'. The important statistical parameters to be considered are sensitivity, specificity (with 95% CI), positive predictive value, negative predictive value, positive likelihood ratio, negative likelihood ratio and how these affect the pre- and post-test probability.[34] For understanding these parameters, let us start with a contingency table **(Table 6)**.

True-positive indicates the persons who are having the disease and are correctly detected positive by the test and true-negative indicates persons who do not have the disease and are correctly identified with the test. Sensitivity is a measure of how well a test can correctly identify the persons having a disease. Specificity is a measure of how well a test can detect the persons not having a disease. Sensitivity is closely related to a type II error/β (accepting a null hypothesis when it should have been rejected) and specificity is closely related to the type I error/a (rejecting a null hypothesis when it should have been accepted). Sensitivity and specificity, ideally, should be expressed with a 95% CI, which gives a better estimate of precision. For example, if a study states a range of sensitivity and specificity with 95% CI, it means that if the study is repeated 100 times, the values of sensitivity and specificity will lie within the given range 95% of the times.[31-33]

Table 6: A 2 × 2 contingency table describing outcome of a diagnostic test[27].

Test outcome	*Disease*	
	Present	*Absent*
Positive	True-positive (TP)	False-positive (FP)
Negative	False-negative (FN)	True-negative (TN)

Likelihood ratios (LR, positive and negative) reflect the discriminative power of a test.[35] Positive likelihood ratio (PLR) is the ratio of probability of a positive test result in a patient with disease to the probability of a positive test in a person without disease. Similarly, negative likelihood ratio (NLR) is the ratio of probability of a negative test in a person with disease to the probability of a negative test in a person without disease. A PLR>10 and NLR <0.1 is considered significant. A PLR of >10 is considered strongly positive, 2–5 moderately positive and 0.5–2 weekly positive. Similarly, NLR of <0.1 is considered strongly negative and 0.2–0.5 moderately or weakly negative.

Pretest probability is the likelihood that the person will have the disease in question even before the test is performed. It is usually decided by the prevalence of the disease and assessed by clinician without any mathematical analysis being involved **(Table 7)**. The pretest probability is important for interpreting the results of a diagnostic test, comparing more than one test or deciding whether it is worth doing the test at all.[34,36] Once the pretest probability and likely ratios are known, the post-test probability can be calculated. If LR>1, the post-test probability will be higher than the pretest probability. It is the post-test probability that the practitioner is more concerned about while treating a patient. The concern is whether the test has altered the disease probability

Table 7: Statistical jargon explained.

Term	*Mathematical expression/relationship*	*What does it imply for a diagnostic test?*
Sensitivity	TP/TP+FN	How well a test can identify patients with the disease?
Specificity	TN/ TN+FP	How well a test can identify the persons without the disease?
Positive predictive value	TP/TP+FP	
Negative predictive value	TN/TN+FN	
True-positive rate	TP/TP+FN	Equivalent to sensitivity
True-negative rate	TN/TN+FP	Equivalent to specificity
False-positive rate	FP/FP+TN or 1–specificity	
False-negative rate	FN/FN+TP or 1–sensitivity	
Power	1–false-negative rate or = sensitivity	Probability that the test will reject a false null hypothesis (i.e. it will not make a type II error) or The true-positive detection rate
Accuracy	TP+TN/TP+TN+FP+FN or True results/total population or Sensitivity × prevalence + (Specificity)/(1–prevalence), provided the prevalence is known	100% accuracy implies that the test will rightly detect all patients with or without the disease in a given population
Prevalence	TP+FN/ TP+FN+TN +FP	
Positive likelihood ratio (PLR)	Sensitivity/(1–specificity)	High PLR implies that if the test result is positive, there is a high chance that the disease will be present
Negative likelihood ratio (NLR)	(1–sensitivity)/specificity	Low NLR implies that if the test result is negative, there is a high chance that the disease will be absent
Pretest odds	Prevalence/(1–prevalence)	
Pretest probability	Patients with a disease/(patients with a disease+ patients without the disease)	Represents the likelihood of a disease in subject, prior to investigation. Usually determined by clinicians based on the likelihood of the patient having a disease. Zero percent pretest probability indicates that the patient in all probability will not have disease
Post-test odds	Pretest odds x likelihood ratio	Represents how confident a radiologist/physician is that the patient will have the suspected disease, after performing the test in question. It increases if the pretest probability is high
Post-test probability	Post-test odds/(post-test odds + 1)	
p value	Measurement of the probability that a result is purely by chance	Lower the p value, higher the probability that the observed result is statistically significant and not by chance

so that it now lies above the treatment threshold or below an exclusion threshold.[37] To calculate the post-test probability, one can multiply the pretest odds by the LR, or refer to the graph of conditional probability or Fagan's nomogram **(Fig. 1)**.[38-40] Further details of these tools are beyond the scope of this chapter.

For better understanding, let us consider a situation relevant to a practicing radiologist. When a clinician questions whether it is prudent to perform a CT pulmonary angiography (CTPA) in a patient with suspected pulmonary thromboembolism (PTE), the radiologist needs to know the pretest probability of PTE, i.e. what according to the clinician is the risk of PTE in the given patient. The pretest probability of 50% means that the clinician thinks there is a 50% chance that the patient may have PTE. Now after proper literature search, he finds that the PLR of CTPA is 10 and NLR is 0.02. Consulting the Fagan's nomogram, he finds that the positive post-test probability is around 90% and negative post-test probability of around 0.3%. This means the test can effectively rule in or rule out PTE, therefore, can be used.

- *Impact assessment for therapeutic literature:* Critical appraisal for a therapeutic literature for internal validity should be performed in similar ways as described before. For impact assessment of a therapeutic literature, the important statistical parameters are relative risk (RR), absolute risk reduction (ARR), relative risk reduction (RRR), absolute risk increase (ARI) or relative risk increase (RRI), number needed to treat (NNT) or number needed to harm (NNH) and odds ratio.[41]

For calculation of the above mentioned para meters, let us consider another contingency **Table 8**.

Relative risk means the risk of an event or developing a disease relative to exposure.[41] Mathematically, RR can be expressed as the ratio of risk in the treated/exposed group to the risk in the control group [(a/(a+b))/ (c/(c+d)]. A relative risk >1 implies increased risk in the exposed group. Absolute risk reduction is the difference in the event rate between treatment and control groups [(a/(a+b)) – (c/(c+d)]. Relative risk reduction is the difference in event rate between treatment and control groups, expressed as percentage (1-RR). Another important parameter is the number needed to treat (NNT) which is the inverse of ARR. A lower NNT means that only a small number of patients are needed to be treated to get a desirable benefit in at least some of them.[41-43]

Diagnostic systematic review and meta-analysis: Meta-analyses are statistical methods used to combine results from a number of different studies. A systematic review is a systematic assembly, critical appraisal and synthesis of all relevant studies on a specific topic.[44] Over the last few decades, as the number of available diagnostic and screening tests have increased significantly, the need of systematic analysis of all the available literature has also increased. Some of these studies may have inherent biases in their design whereas others may be well conducted. Since there is a plethora of evidence, a summary of all the available evidences should be deducted from them. Meta-analysis model aims at estimating the following: (a) the summary sensitivity and specificity and/or summary ROC curves and (b) common threats to the validity of the summary estimates.[45-48]

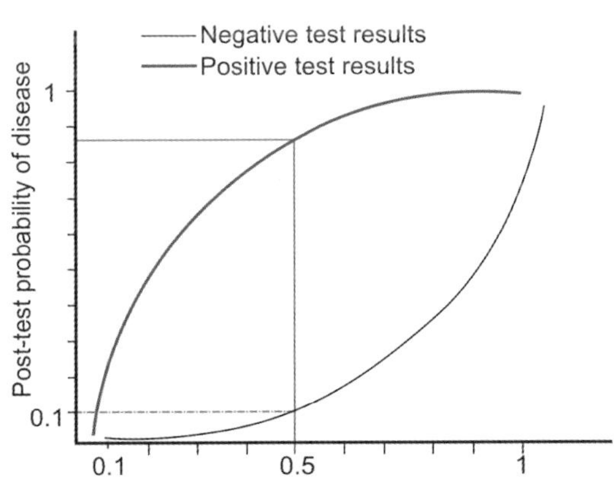

Fig. 1: Graph of conditional probability of a test showing high sensitivity and high specificity. Here, for a pretest probability of 0.5, the post-test probability of a negative diagnostic test outcome is 0.1 and post-test probability of a positive test result is 0.85 (85%), which means the test can successfully 'rule out' the diagnosis as well as 'rules in' (confirm) the diagnosis.

Table 8: A 2 × 2 contingency table describing a therapeutic test outcome[41].

Exposure	***Outcome of events***		
	Yes	No	Total
Yes	Events in experimental group (a) EE	b	(a+b) Subjects in experimental group ES
No	Events in control group (c) CE	d	(c+d) Subjects in control group CS

The steps involved in conducting a systematic review of a diagnostic test includes the following:

- Finding the evidence
- Assessing the study quality and applicability
- Summarizing the evidence qualitatively and quantitati vely (meta-analysis) and
- Clinical interpretation and application in developing a recommendation.[45] Steps 1 and 2 have been discussed earlier. Discussion on the meta-analytical integration of evidence and the analysis is beyond the scope of this chapter. In the integration of diagnostic data, two or more paired statistics are taken into consideration viz. sensitivity and specificity, PPV and NPV, etc. Summary estimate of sensitivity and specificity of various studies can be derived from various methods, summary ROC curves, Forrest Plot, etc.

While pooling data for meta-analysis, 'publication bias' should be kept in mind. It refers to the association of the publication probability of a study to its statistical significance. A study showing positive or good statistical significance is more likely to get published. There are several methods to estimate publication bias in a meta-analysis, e.g. Funnel plot. For the detailed understanding of Funnel plot the readers are requested to refer to more detailed treatise.[44]

In the clinical interpretation of evidence related to a diagnostic test, the important step is to determine the post-test probability, using the Fagan's nomogram or a graph of conditional probability, as described above.

Step 4: Apply

After proper critical appraisal of the available evidences, one should assess its applicability in the prevailing clinical context. This step can also be called 'external validation'.[49] Before applying the results in the individual patient, the following points should be considered.

- Whether the diagnostic test/treatment are feasible in your existing setup?
- Are there any other feasible alternatives?
- Are the patients in existing clinical scenario sufficiently similar to the subjects of the study?
- Whether the diagnostic test is changing the pretest probability?

  (Here one needs to calculate the LR of a study, which can be calculated from sensitivity and specificity, vide supra. If the PLR of a study is >10 or NLR <0.1, the test can significantly alter the pretest probability).
- Consider the pros and cons of the diagnostic/or therapeutic test

  (It is particularly important when the test or treatment under consideration has side effect or a risk, e.g. radiation exposure in diagnostic CT. In such cases, the risks associated with the test/treatment can be outweighed by the risk of the disease).[50]
- Must take into consideration the patient's opinion.

Step 5: Evaluate

The last step is to evaluate your results in clinical practice, after going through all the four previous steps. This can be performed by evaluating the efficiency in executing all the four steps, and taking initiative to improve them.

How does Evidence-based Radiology Differ from Evidence-based Medicine?

Since Radiology is a technology based subject, the practice of EBR differs from that of EBM in a few additional points under the step 'critical appraisal'. The additional five questions to be asked when assessing any imaging modality are as follows:[51]

- Has the imaging methodology been described in sufficient detail to allow to reproduce the study in your own department?
- Has the reference (gold standard) and the imaging test under evaluation been performed to the same standards of excellence?
- Have technology development within the same modality been adequately considered in the study design and discussion?
- Has the issue of radiation exposure been considered?
- How were the MRI/CT images reviewed, on hard copy images or on a monitor?

Limitations of Evidence-based Practice

While the proposers of EBP see it as a tool of paradigm shift in the clinical decision-making, the critics suggest that it should be considered as an additional tool in the existing practice, giving importance to the other alternate forms of clinical practice also. They criticize the 'bottom-up EBP' for being time-consuming and not practically feasible in daily clinical practice. While EBP necessitates the convergence of various modalities and enhances multimodality practice, it is often seen as unhelpful. Some also believe that it is unproven, threatens professional autonomy and narrows the research agenda.[52,17]

How can a radiologist practice EBR in his or her daily life?

- ***In justifying a new diagnostic test:*** When confronted to a question about performing a new diagnostic test in a patient, follow the previously stated five steps of EBP. It can help the radiologist in deciding whether the test is going to change the pretest probability so as to establish or exclude the diagnosis.

- ***While studying an article, critically appraising it*** (as described above) before applying its recommendations in your practice. Most radiology articles lack in proper statistical analysis and the information needed to assess validity is inadequate. Consolidated standards of reporting trials (CONSORT)[53] and the standards for reporting of diagnostic accuracy (STARD)[54] are two initiatives to improve the reporting of clinical trials and studies of diagnostic accuracy. While studying any article, the radiologist should test them using the STARD or CONSORT criteria. One can use the proper format for critical appraisal of a diagnostic literature (available at http://www.srs-mcmaster.ca). In this manner, knowing the strength and weakness of the existing literature can help the radiologist to plan a proper study in a specific field.
- ***Applying principles of EBR in academic activities*:** While presenting an article in a departmental Journal Club, a radiology resident could critically appraise it in the proper format, check for adequacy of the STARD criteria and summarize the strength and caveats of the article. This will help spread the practice of EBR among the fellow colleagues.

CONCLUSION

Evidence-based practice in radiology is a relatively new concept with its own advantages and limitations. Every radiologist should be aware of its concept and be able to apply it in their daily practice. In practice, clinical decision making remains a combination of 'expert opinion,' critical appraisal of the existing evidence and the judgment of the practitioner. A perfect balance between them can bring out the best patient care.

REFERENCES

1. Strauss SE, Rosenberg W, Glasziou P, et al. Introduction, in Evidence Based Medicine: How to Practice and Teach EBM 3rd edn. Churchill Livingstone, Edinburgh: Elsevier; 2005. pp.1-12.
2. Sackett DL, Rosenberg WM, Gray JA, et al. Evidence based medicine: what it is and what it isn't. BMJ. 1996;312:71-2.
3. Guyatt Kelly Am. Evidence based practice: an introduction and overview. Semin in Roentgenol. 2009;43:131-9.
4. Guyatt G, Cairns J, Churchill D, et al. Evidence-based medicine, a new approach to teaching the practice of medicine. J Am Med Assoc. 1992;268:2420-5.
5. Friedland D. Introduction, In evidence based medicine: a framework for clinical practice. Stamford Conn, Appleton and Lange; 1998.pp.2-3.
6. Woods BP. What's the evidence? Radiology. 1999;213: 635-7.
7. Currie LM, Graham M, Allen M, et al. Clinical information needs in context: an observational study of clinicians while using a clinical information system. AMIA Annu Symo Proc. 2003.pp.190-4.
8. Antman EM, Lau J, Kupelnick B, et al. A comparison of results of meta-analyses of randomized control trials and recommendations of clinical experts. Treatments for myocardial infarction. JAMA. 1992;268:240-8.
9. Haynes RB. Loose connections between peer-reviewed clinical journals and clinical practice. Ann Intern Med. 1990;113:724-8.
10. Sackett DL, Strauss SE. Finding and applying evidence during clinical rounds: the evidence cart. JAMA. 1998;280:1336-8.
11. Shuval K, Berkovits E, Netzer D, et al. Evaluating the impact of an evidence-based medicine educational intervention on primary care doctors' attitudes, knowledge and clinical behavior: a controlled trial and before and after study. J Eval Clin Pract. 2007;13:581-98.
12. Strauss SE, Richardson WS, Haynes RB. Our reactions to knowing and not knowing. In: Evidence Based Medicine: How to Practice and Teach EBM, 3rd edn., Edinburgh: Churchill Livingstone, Elsevier; 2005.pp.18-9.
13. Kelly Am. Evidence based radiology: step 2- searching the literature (search). Semin Roentgenol. 2009;43:147-52.
14. Cochrane Collaboration Website: available at http://*www.cochrane.org*.
15. Cochrane AL. Critical review, with particular reference to the medical profession. In: Medicines for the year 2000. London: Office of Health Economics; 1979.pp.1-11.
16. Evidence based medicine journal website. Available at http:// *ebm.bmj.com*.
17. Malone DE, Staunton M. Evidence-based practice in Radiology: step 5 (evaluate) - caveats and common questions. Radiology. 2007;243:319-28.
18. Van Beek EJ, Malone DE. Evidence-based practice in radiology education: why and how should we teach it? Radiology. 2007;243:633-40.
19. Glasziou P, Del Mar C, Salisbury J, et al. Formulate an answerable question. In: Evidence based practice workbook, 2nd edn. Boston: Blackwell Publishing; 2007. pp.21-34.
20. Levels of evidence. Oxford Centre for Evidence-Based Medicine Website. http://*www.cebm.net/levels_of_evidence.asp*.
21. Dodd JD. Evidence-based practice in Radiology: steps 3 and 4-Appraise and apply diagnostic radiology literature. Am J Radiol. 2007;242:342-54.
22. Fryback DG, Thornbury JR. The efficacy of diagnostic imaging. Med Decis Mak. 1991;11:88-94.
23. Thornbury JR, Fryback DG. Technology assessment—an American view. Eur J Radiol. 1992;14:147-56.
24. McNeil BJ, Adelstein SJ. Determining the value of diagnostic and screening tests. J Nucl Med. 1976;17:439-48.
25. Finberg HV. Evaluation of computed tomography: achievement and challenge. Am J Roentgenol. 1978;131: 1-4.

26. Center for evidence based radiology in Ireland. Available at http//*www.evidencebasedradiology.net/index.html.*
27. Maceneaney PM, Malone DE. The meaning of diagnostic test results: a spreadsheet for swift data analysis. Clin Radiol. 200;55:227-35.
28. Cronin P. Evidence-based Radiology: step 3- primary literature validity (critical appraisal). Semin Roentgenol. 2009;43:153-7.
29. Sackett DL, Strauss SE, Richardson WS, et al. Evidence Based Medicine: How to Practice and Teach EBM, 2nd edn. Churchill Livingstone, Edinburgh: Elsevier; 2000.
30. Guyatt G, Jaeschke R, Heddle N, et al. Basic Statistics for clinicians:1. Hypothesis testing. CMAJ. 1995;152:27-32.
31. Gardner MJ, Altman DG. Confidence intervals rather than p values: estimation rather than hypothesis testing. BMJ (Clin Res Ed). 1986;292:746-50.
32. Guyatt G, Jaeschke R, Heddle N, et al. Basic Statistics for clinicians: 2. Interpreting study results: confidence intervals. CMAJ. 1995;152:169-73.
33. Montori VM, Kleinbart J, Newman TB, et al. Tips for learners of evidence based medicine: 2. Measures of precision (Confidence intervals).CMAJ. 2004;171:611-5.
34. Cronin P. Evidence-based Radiology: step 3- critical appraisal of diagnostic literature. Semin Roentgenol. 2009;43:158-65.
35. Cronin P, Dwamena BA, Kelly AM, et al. Solitary pulmonary nodules and masses: A meta-analysis of the diagnostic utility of alternative diagnostic tests. Eur Radiol. 2008;18:1840-56.
36. McGinn T, Jervis R, Wisnivesky J, et al. Tips for teachers of evidence-based medicine. Clinical prediction rules (CPRs) and estimating pretest probability. J Gen Intern Med. 2008;23:1261-8.
37. Chang PJ. Bayesian analysis revisited: A radiologist's survival guide. Am J Roentgenol. 1988;152:721-7.
38. Sackett DL, Haynes RB, Guyatt GH, et al. The interpretation of diagnostic data. In: Clinical Epidemiology: A basic Science for clinical medicine, 2nd edn. Boston/Toronto/ London: Little, Brown; 1991.pp.92-3.
39. Fagan TJ. Nomogram for Bayes theorem. N Eng J Med. 1975;293:257.
40. Sackett DL, Richardson WS, Rosenberg W, et al. Is this evidence about a diagnostic test important? In Evidence based medicine, how to practice and teach EBM, 1st edn, Vol 127. Edinburgh: Churchill Livingstone; 1998.
41. Cronin P. Evidence-based Radiology: step 3- critical appraisal of therapeutic literature. Semin Roentgenol. 2009;43:166-9.
42. Jaeschke R, Guyatt G, Shannon H, et al. Basic statistics for clinicians. III. Assessing the effects of treatment: measures of association. Can Med Assoc J. 1995;152:351-7.
43. Barratt A, Wyer PC, Hatala R, et al. Tips for learners of evidence based medicine. I. relative risk reduction, absolute risk reduction and number needed to treat. Can Med Assoc J. 2004;171:353-8.
44. Sterne JAC, Harbord RM. Funnel plots in meta-analysis. The Stata Journal. 2004;4:127-41.
45. Dwamena BA. Evidence-based radiology: step 3- diagnostic systematic review and meta-analysis (critical appraisal). Semin Roentgenol. 2009;43:170-9.
46. Whiting P, Rutjes AWS, Reitsma JB, et al. The development of QUADAS: a tool for the quality assessment of studies of diagnostic accuracy included in systematic reviews. BMC Med Res Methodol. 2003;3:25.
47. Lijmer JG, Bossuyt PM, Heisterkamp SH. Exploring sources of heterogeneity in systematic reviews of diagnostic tests. Stat Med. 2002;21:1525-37.
48. Deeks JJ, Macaskill P, Irwig L. The performance of tests of publication bias and other size effects in systematic reviews of diagnostic test accuracy was assessed. J Clin Epidemiol. 2005; 58:882-93.
49. Cronin P. Evidence-based Radiology: step 4- Apply. Semin Roentgenol. 2009;43:180-1.
50. Del Mar C, Doust J, Glasziou P. Clinical Thinking: evidence, communication and decision making. London: BMJ Books. Blackwell Publishing Ltd; 2006.
51. Dodd JD, MacEnenaey PM, Malone DE. Evidence based radiology: how to quickly assess the validity and strength of publication in the diagnostic radiology literature. Eur Radiol. 2004;14:915-22.
52. Trinder L. A critical appraisal of evidence based practice. In: Trinder L, Reynolds S, (Eds). Evidence-based practice: a critical appraisal. Oxford, England: Blackwell Science; 2000. pp.212-41.
53. Moher D, Schulz KF, Altman D. The CONSORT statement: revised recommendations for improving the reports of parallel group randomized trials. JAMA. 2001;285:1987-91.
54. Bossuyt PM, Teitsma JB, Bruns DE, et al. Towards complete and accurate reporting of studies of diagnostic accuracy: the STARD initiative. BMJ. 2003;326:41-4.

CHAPTER 60

Radiation Hazards and Radiation Units

Pratik Kumar, Anil K Pandey

INTRODUCTION

Radiation can be defined as a packet of energy. The amount of energy the radiations can deposit in a given space varies with each type. It also differs in the power to penetrate. It may be ionizing and nonionizing. Nonionizing radiations do not affect at molecular levels. They may cause electrical shocks and burns. For example, prolonged exposure to microwaves radiation, which is nonionizing, may cause cataracts.

Ionizing radiations, such as X-rays have power to penetrate inside the body; therefore, they interact as well as provide information at the atomic level. X rays are directed towards the patient body and transmitted X-rays are used to form the image. Since X-rays are very small in size (in the unit of Angstrom), some of them can cross the body without interaction, some will interact with atoms and lose its energy completely, others will get scattered and come out from the body. Thus, the transmitted X-rays have energy from zero to a maximum value and when they fall on a two dimensional image receptor and deposit its energy, they create an image of the organ exposed.

X-ray (radiation) is extremely useful and becoming integral part of diagnosis and disease management. On the other hand, it ionizes the atoms and molecules when they pass through the body and creates biological damage.

In this chapter we are going to discuss the harmful effect of radiation on human body (radiation hazards), how to protect the patient, staff and public from radiation generated during the diagnostic and interventional procedures performed in radiology and units associated with measurement of radiation in these modalities.

RADIATION HAZARDS

Harmful effect of radiation on human body is called radiation hazards which can be created by direct and indirect mechanism of interaction of X-rays with human body.

Interaction of radiation with living things (human body cells) and nonliving things is different. All human beings are made of tiny structures called cells. The bigger a person is, the more number of cells he or she has. Children do not have as many cells as adults, but they have greater proportion of dividing cells. Chemical contents, physical shape and size of a living cell are continuously changing. A new cell is made when an existing cell grows and divides into two. The new cell is an exact copy of the old one. This change may be rapid or slow. In natural growth cycle of a cell, one step is linked with other as it is a continuous process, but for convenience these steps are named as different phase of growth cycle of the cell, such as M phase, G_1 phase, S phase and G_2 phase. The cells are most sensitive to radiation during Mitosis (i.e. M phase) and G_2 phase (i.e. Premitosis or RNA synthesis) and least sensitive during S phase (DNA synthesis).

First step of cell development is necessary to move on to the second step. In case of rapid development, the gap between the first step and second step is less, so the minimum time required to repair the damage created by the radiation, may not be available in case of rapid developing cells. In slow developing cell the time period to repair the break is available; therefore, slow developing cells are less sensitive to radiation in comparison to the fast/rapid developing cells. Similarly, any damage inflicted by radiation on the cell is expressed soon in case of rapidly developing cells as they progress fast through their cell-cycles.

DAMAGE TO DNA BY THE RADIATION

The X-ray energy used in the diagnostic radiology varies from 25 to 125 kVp. They deposit their energy in a very small volume and are sufficient to produce ionization inside the human body. Radiation creates damage to the DNA by direct and indirect mechanism. In the direct mechanism, the X-ray hits the DNA molecules directly. DNA molecule gets ionized resulting in damage. In indirect mechanism, water molecules absorb the X-ray energy and dissociates into H^+ and OH^-. OH free radical contains an unpaired electron in the outer shell and is highly reactive. It reacts with DNA and creates the damage. It is estimated that 60–70% of radiation-caused DNA damage is due to OH free radical.

THE EFFECT OF RADIATION

Chemical bonds hold DNA together. Loss of electrons causes chemical bond to change. Thymine, one of the four bases of DNA, is supposed to bind with adenine on its opposing strand. However, loss of electrons caused by radiation makes thymine bind with another thymine on the same strand. When DNA is replicated to make new cells, coding errors occur and mutations result. Mutations result in damaged chromosomes. Cells then reproduce abnormally, causing both defects and cancer.

The types of damage that can occur to DNA molecules are as follows:

- DNA single-strand breaks
- DNA double-strand breaks
- Sugar damage
- Base damage
- Local denaturation (separation of the two strands)
- DNA-DNA crosslinks
- DNA-protein crosslinks.

These damages can lead to:

- Slow down in the cell synthesization (copies of its own DNA) so that there is a delay in cell dividing into two cells
- Delay in repair mechanism that will delay the cell cycle progression (as the cell progresses towards next cell division)
- Delays in cell proliferation (increase in cell number) of a population of cells
- Death of the cell
- Mutation of the cell
- Cell transformation (changes in the cell which will make them to behave as a cancer cell).

Cell death have been given special names also as cell necrosis (death of a contiguous fields of cell, the content of the cell leaks out into the surrounding tissue and blood supply), cell lysis (the cell simply bursts open and releases its contents into the surrounding), apoptosis (or programmed cell death) which is under genetic control (specific gene must be present active or inactive) and it requires energy and when the cells die, DNA fragments of specific sizes and the content of the cells, are encapsulated in membranes as small vesicles.

The damages incurred by different kinds of tissue vary with the type of radiation to which the person is exposed and the means of exposure. Direct exposure to radiation can affect the whole body. The body attempts to repair the damage caused by the radiation. However, at times the damage is so severe and widespread that repair is impossible. For example, thyroid gland is one of the most radiation-sensitive parts of the body, especially in babies and children. Absorption of too much radioactive iodine can cause thyroid cancer to develop several years after the exposure.

Different types of cell aberration can occur depending on the position of the cell cycles at the time of exposure to ionizing radiation. Most common is formation of dicentric and ring which can be visualized under microscope after the exposure above 10–25 cGy. Visualization of the ring or dicentric aberration means cell death has occurred. Certain types of aberration and/or mutation in gene can cause cancer.

Mutation may occur even at low dose. There is no threshold of dose below which an ionizing radiation cannot induce mutation. However, at low doses and dose rates, the risk of mutation is very low and it is lower for low-dose rates at all doses. The relationship may be either linear or linear quadratic depending on type of radiation. X-rays follow linear-quadratic model, at low doses the relationship is linear with increase in dose, while at higher dose the relationship is square of the dose.

Stochastic and Nonstochastic (Deterministic) Effects

The effect of radiation can be broadly classified as stochastic and deterministic effect. Stochastic effects are observed at low doses and these effects have no threshold. At low-radiation dose the probability of occurrences of stochastic effect is low. As the dose increases the probability of occurrence of stochastic effect also increases. There is a linear relationship between absorbed dose and probability

Table 1: Radiation dose and its observable effects on humans.

Radiation dose	*Observable effects*
0–50 mSv	None (irrespective of acute or protracted exposure)
50–100 mSv	None, might not be existing or too small to detect (irrespective of acute or protracted exposure)
100–500 mSv	Slightly increased cancer risk. Decrease in blood counts at around 500 mSv
500–1 Sv	Some observable effect may be visible in acute exposure Increased cancer risk over longer duration Above 500 mSv some changes in blood cells occur but recovers quickly
1–2 Sv	Nausea and fatigue in acute exposure Increased cancer risks over longer duration
2–3 Sv	Nausea and vomiting within 24–48 hours, medical attention is required
3–5 Sv	Nausea, vomiting and diarrhea within hours, loss of hair and appetite occurs within a week, medical attention is must, half of the population exposed will die, if no medical attention is given
5 Sv–12 Sv	Death within a few days
Greater than 100 Sv	Death within a few hours

of effect. Examples of stochastic effects include hereditary effects and cancers. Cancer (which includes leukemia) and genetic effects follow linear nonthreshold dose-response relationship.

Deterministic effects start after the absorption of certain amount of dose. It has a threshold, once the absorbed dose crosses the threshold these effects appear in all exposed subjects and as the absorbed dose increases, the severity of the effect also increases. Examples of deterministic (also called nonstochastic) effects are various somatic effects including skin erythema, epilation, cataracts, impaired fertility, etc. The threshold for skin effect is above 2 Gy.

Radiation Doses and Expected Effect

The radiation dose to human body and its effect can be summarized in **Table 1**.

Radiation Effect on Embryo

All human beings start life as a single cell that divides over and over again and grows into babies inside their mothers' bodies.

Embryo is composed of relatively few cells and has high rates of cell division and cell differentiation. Rapidly developing cells have found to be more sensitive to the radiation. Since embryo/fetus has rapid developing cells, they are more sensitive to radiation than the adult.

Radiation produces no unique abnormalities.The effects vary with the amount of radiation dose, dose rate with which exposure has occurred and stage of development of the embryo/fetus. Many researchers follow the limit of 10 rad (100 mGy) to fetus in case of accidental exposure. Even in case of radiation dose to fetus in excess of 10 rad the risk incurred remains low for lower doses.

The effects of radiation on embryo/fetus are loss of pregnancy (embryonic, fetal or neonatal death), malformations and mental retardation. However, these occur at high doses generally not encountered in diagnostic radiology during normal investigations. Any decision for termination of pregnancy due to fetal exposure during radiological examination must be weighed against the information that the rate of spontaneous abnormality is quite high at 4–6% with respect to risk incurred due to fetal radiation exposure.

Ten-day Rule

It must be emphasized that both the ICRP and NCRP recommended application of the 10-day rule only to those studies that do not contribute to management of current disease. It, therefore, follows that studies which do contribute to diagnosis or treatment of current disease should be performed in fertile women without regard to stage of the menstrual cycle. It is suggested that all potential female patients due to radiological investigations should be inquired about her probable pregnancy. Missing menstrual period should be taken as pregnancy. If the patient does not think that she is pregnant (there is no missing period) the radiological investigation may be carried out. If it turns out that the patient is pregnant the radiologist/referring physician should weigh benefit and risk associated with the X-ray investigation and should obtain informed consent from the patient and her attendants for the further necessary action.

Protection of Patient, Staff and Public from Radiation

Radiation Risk

Radiation risk calculation are based on the type of radiation, amount of energy absorbed, and which part of the body these energies is deposited. For example, certain amount of radiation energy deposited to the wrist has really no effect, however, similar amount of energy deposited to blood forming organ may have an effect. One of worth-notable effect of low-dose radiation which we come across in diagnostic and therapeutic radiological investigations is probability of cancer induction. The probability of cancer induction is low at low dose but never zero theoretically and therefore calls for the optimisation of radiation doses for all radiological investigations. One should keep in mind that it is not possible to differentiate or detect the cancer caused by diagnostic X-rays from cancer caused by other factors, such as environmental, chemical or biological. The latency period of cancer induction may be in years or even in decade. This may be true for all carcinogens including radiation. This is especially true for low dose and low-dose rate radiation. If the low level of radiation exposure has occurred today, its effect as a cancer may be expressed after few years of exposure.

Radiation Protection Guidelines and LNT Model

In 1950s, the scientific group created the radiation protection guidelines. At that time no one really knew the effect of low dose of radiation. It was decided to assume that the relation between the radiation dose and its effects are linear and proportional. It was also decided that any dose, no matter how small, could bring an effect. This is called a linear no-threshold (LNT) model. Still this LNT model is in use to set radiation protection guidelines. Since this concept was easy to use and explain, most people presented this as a fact rather than saying that we do not know the effects of low doses of radiation or whether the low doses of radiation is safe. Effect of radiation at low doses is a controversial topic since it is difficult to get ideal epidemiological data. Cancer induction may be the only effect at low dose of radiation but there are also spontaneous incidences of cancer without radiation exposure (due to various other environmental carcinogens and biological factors). Such comparison demands similar control and study group in terms of life style, socioeconomic status, environment, age, sex, etc. except in radiation-exposure history. Obviously it is hard to meet this ideal situation. Ubiquitous background radiation is another confounding factor which exposes all people living on this planet all the time with on an average 2–3 mSv (milli Sievert) annual dose.

On the other hand, there are researchers and their preliminary experimental results which may indicate about the existence of beneficial effect of low-level radiation (called radiation hormesis) **(Fig. 1)**. At present it is thought prudent to consider low-level radiation having linear relationship with risk (without having any threshold of a minimum dose) which signifies that even low-level radiation entails some risk.

Every country has a regulatory authority to set the guidelines regarding radiation protection, make laws and to enforce them. These guidelines are based on LNT model and made in such a way that if followed properly, patient, staff and public all are protected. We must obey them.

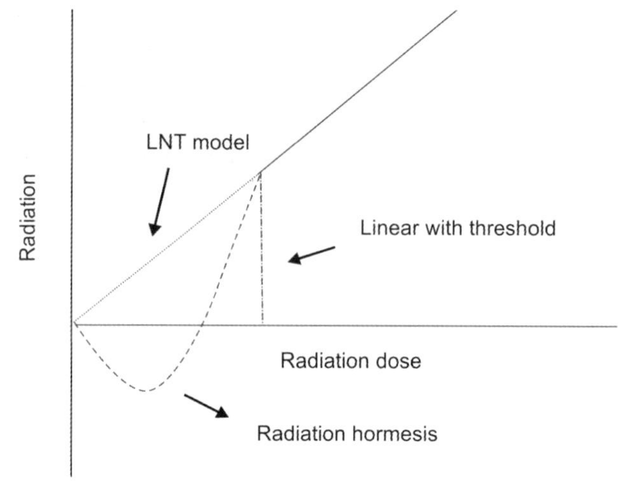

Fig. 1: Various hypotheses of low-level radiation dose and its effect.

Atomic Energy Regulatory Board (AERB), Mumbai is the competent authority to enforce radiation safety in practice in India.

The first principle of radiation protection for the patient is justification.

Justification

X-ray examination should be undertaken only when there is medical question which need to be answered, the amount of benefit which patient is going to receive in comparison to the risk associated with this X-ray examination is high and the information needed cannot be answered by any other investigation involving nonionizing radiation. In such condition, we say that X-ray examination is justified.

Some facts that can help in protecting staff patients and public from radiation

- X-rays are produced, emitted in isotropic direction; X-ray tube is shielded to protect patient and staff operating the machine.
- X-rays produced from the X-ray machine have a mixture of continuous spectrum starting from zero to maximum energy (equal to the kVp applied) and characteristic spectrum. If the spectrum is not filtered, the low-energy X-rays (also called soft X-rays) will be absorbed completely on superficial organs of the patient body and contribute to the patient dose; however, these X-rays will not contribute in the image formation. X-rays are passed through the filter to

remove these soft X-rays. Application of additional filter reduces the patient dose significantly.

- The X-rays emitted from the X-ray tube and directed towards the patient body are called primary X-rays. When these primary X-rays interact with the patient body, as a result of interaction scattered radiation are emitted in all direction.
- The energy of scattered radiation is almost equal to the primary radiation (a few keV less than the primary radiation). So it is most likely that the person standing in the room while X-rays are being energized will receive radiation exposure from the secondary radiation emitted from the patient body as a result of scattering.
- In case of over couch X-ray tube, the radiologist will receive maximum exposure to the face, because scattered X-rays from the patients are directed towards the face. In under couch X-ray tube, the scattered radiations are directed towards the legs. Therefore, lead rubber flaps can be used to protect legs. Goggles must be used to protect the eyes.
- The lead apron of 0.25–0.50 mm Pb equivalent is worn by the radiologist to protect them from the secondary scattered radiation. In the interventional procedures they have to wear it for a longer duration. Due to prolonged time period of wearing the lead apron, some orthopedic problems of spinal injury have been reported in the literature for the interventional radiologist. Therefore, it is important (for both the radiologist and patient's viewpoint) that interventional radiological procedures or radiation related procedures will only be adopted when there is no other option available. Now-a-days, vest-skirt type lead aprons are available which shifts weight of the skirt apron at the waist.
- Lead-free aprons incorporating tungsten, antimony and bismuth or barium, aluminum, tin, titanium, bismuth are available in the market. These aprons are environment friendly and recyclable as well. Lead is toxic and therefore, disposal of lead aprons need proper care. It is desirable to check the protection/attenuation efficiency offered by these new lead-free protection aprons before it is put to use. Lead free aprons may offer the weight which is 20–40% lesser than that of conventional lead apron.
- Radiation burns (Radiation hazards) are different than the burn by the fire and hence requires specific expertise and experience to treat such cases. Radiation burns have been reported in the literature during the interventional fluoroscopic examinations. This needs to be prevented.

Since X-rays have high-penetrating power, X-ray machines are needed to be installed in room having sufficient wall thickness such that outside the room the radiation penetrating through the wall must not exceed the limit set for public exposure. The entry of public or attendants is not allowed in the X-ray room while X-rays are being energized. There must be some warning signal displayed outside the X-ray room so that public must know that X-rays are being produced here. Public must know that X-rays beam is ON. The wooden door of the X-ray room must have sufficient lead shielding.

Cardinal principle of radiation protection is distance, time and shielding. The dose from the X-ray beam diminishes with the square of its distance from the source. This law is known as inverse square law. If the distance from the source is doubled, the dose reduces by ¼. So, one should maintain the maximum distance from the source to reduce dose. Radiation dose is directly proportional to the time duration spent with the source. It indicates to complete the job quickly (i.e. efficiency in job). By interposing shielding between the source and detector, the radiation dose decreases. One HVL (Half Value Layer) of a shielding material like lead, concrete or brick is the thickness of the material which when interspersed will attenuate the radiation to half.

General dose reduction measures that can be adopted to reduce patient doses are as follows:

- Increasing the distance between X-ray tube and patient helps reduce dose. Doubling the distance will make the dose one-fourth.
- Collimation at the target/patient's body reduces dose and improves image quality also due to lesser scattering.
- Compression of the body reduces the thickness of the body and hence volume of irradiation. Amount of scattering is directly proportional to the volume of irradiated tissue. Therefore, compression of body reduces the amount of scattering and improves image contrast. With reduced thickness lower-radiation dose is absorbed inside the body. That is why breast is compressed during mammography.
- Antiscatter grids are located between the patient and the image intensifier, or cassette or digital detector. Grids absorb most of the scatter radiation. Higher the grid ratio, better is the image quality but higher is the radiation dose to the patient. So, an optimum value of grid ratio needs to be selected. 8:1 for radiography and 5:1 for mammography is optimum. In radiography of children one may remove the grid since there is less scatter anyway due to smaller body volume of the

children. Removing grid will enable the radiographer to reduce the radiographic parameters and hence reduce the dose to the pediatric cases.

- With increase in kVp, penetrating power of X-ray beam increases. It will deposit less amount of energy inside the patient body during radiography and hence the patient dose will reduce. However, this will reduce the contrast in the image. In CT, higher kVp increases the patients' dose.
- X-ray beam contains both soft and hard X-rays. When X-ray beam is allowed to pass through the filter made of copper and aluminum the filter will attenuate the soft X-rays and allow the hard X-rays to pass through. Soft X-rays get absorbed on superficial organs and contribute to absorbed radiation dose and do not take part in the image formation. There is regulatory limit of minimum 2.5 mm aluminum total equivalent filtration to be present in X-ray beam in all radiography machines having 100 kVp or more.
- X-ray machines are available with automatic exposure timing control facility called automatic exposure control (AEC). These sensors monitors the transmitted X-ray from the patients, when amount of X-ray beam required for an optimum image quality is reached, it automatically turns off the X-ray beam falling on the patient body. In this way, it ensures that smallest amount of radiation have been administered to patient.
- Table top material should not absorb much radiation as the X-ray passes through it before reaching to patient/detector. However, it should be strong enough to carry the bulky patients. Carbon fiber has been proven to be the best material for X-ray system table top.
- Pulsed fluoroscopy reduces the dose to patients and staff significantly in interventional fluoroscopy. In pulse fluoroscopy the X-ray is emitted in pulses instead of continuous exposure. This effectively reduces the total time of emission of X-rays. Fifteen frames per second reduces radiation dose by about 25% while 7.5 frames per second may reduce the radiation dose to half. However, very-low frame rate may lead to choppy image especially during imaging of a moving organ. Modern technology uses digital refresh memory to digitize the last image and showing it in the gap time of two consecutive X-ray pulses unless next pulse refreshes the image. This reduces the flickering of the image on monitor when very-low frame-rate pulse fluoroscopy is operated.

We need to quantify the damage created by the ionizing radiation. Following radiation units are used in radiology.

RADIATION UNITS

When X-rays used in medical imaging interacts with any medium (human body or material like cassette, imaging plate, film, etc.), it transfers energy to the medium. This energy transfer is influenced by many factors. It is important to understand its nitty-gritty since risk to radiation has to be defined on the basis of the energy transfer pattern between interacting radiation and the medium it traverses through.

Fluence

X-ray may be thought of consisting of stream of energy packets (particles like) called X-ray photons. The stream of X-ray photons is called "X-ray Fluence" which is defined as number of X-ray photons passing through per unit area when the area is perpendicular to the direction of photon stream.

$$\text{Hence, X-ray fluence} = \frac{\text{Number of photons}}{\text{Area of cross section}}$$

Unit for fluence is cm^{-2}.

Flux

X-ray flux is defined as the X-ray fluence per unit time. In other words, number of X-ray photons passing through per unit area per unit time is called Flux. It may be seen that flux is nothing but fluence rate which is fluence per unit time.

$$\text{X-ray flux} = \frac{\text{Number of photons}}{\text{Area}} \cdot \frac{1}{\text{Time}}$$

In fluoroscopy the concept of flux is important since radiation is "on" for longer time.

Energy Fluence

It is defined as amount of energy passing through unit area. If we know the energy of each X-ray photon the energy fluence may be defined as:

Energy fluence = Fluence × Energy of each X-ray photon

Since X-ray photons from x-ray tube are polyenergetic, therefore mean energy of X-ray photons have to be considered while calculating energy fluence.

$$\text{Mean energy of X-ray photons} = \frac{\text{Total energy of photons}}{\text{Number of photons}}$$

Energy fluence

$$= \frac{\text{Number of photons}}{\text{Area}} \cdot \frac{\text{Total energy of photons}}{\text{Number of photons}}$$

$$= \frac{\text{Energy}}{\text{Area}}$$

The energy of X-ray photon is in terms of keV.

(The maximum energy of X-rays photons is the maximum potential applied across cathode-anode in X-ray tube by selecting tube voltage at control console in terms of kVp).

Energy fluence has unit keV per cm^2 which may be written as $keVcm^{-2}$.

Exposure

Exposure is defined as electrical charge produced by ionization created by the incident X-rays (radiation) in unit mass of air.

$$\text{Exposure} = \frac{\text{Amount of charge produced}}{\text{Irradiated mass of air}}$$

$$= \frac{\text{Charge}}{\text{Mass}}$$

$$= \frac{\text{Coloumb}}{\text{kg}} \text{ (SI unit)}$$

Traditional unit is roentgen (R) which is defined as 1 R = 2.58×10^{-4} coulomb/kg of air

Or, 3876 R = 1 coulomb/kg of air

The exposure rate is expressed in R/hr or mR/min.

R is valid for X-rays and gamma rays with energy up to 3 MeV. It is to note that the exposure and its unit R take care of the interaction of X-rays and gamma rays with air only.

Exposure is not applicable to electrons, beta or any charged particle. Exposure may be measured using ionization chamber. Since, there is not much difference between effective atomic number of air and soft tissue for the diagnostic range of energy, the absorbed dose to air or soft tissue may be regarded same. The concept of absorbed dose is for material.

Absorbed Dose

Absorbed dose indicates the amount of energy deposited by interacting ionization radiation (X-rays, gamma rays, electrons, beta, neutrons, alpha, protons, all radiation) with unit mass of matter.

$$\text{Absorbed dose} = \frac{\text{Amount of energy deposited}}{\text{Mass of matter}}$$

The unit of absorbed dose is joule per kilogram ($J\ kg^{-1}$) and a special name given to this in SI unit is gray.

1 gray (Gy) = 1 joule/kg

The traditional unit of absorbed dose is rad (radiation absorbed dose)

1 Gy = 100 rad

1 rad = 0.01 Gy = 0.01 Joule/kg

The conversion factor between "exposure" and "absorbed dose" is called roentgen to rad conversion factor (or F factor)

$$F = \frac{\text{Absorbed dose (rad)}}{\text{Roentgen (R)}}$$

F is defined as the absorbed dose in rad for a matter per roentgen exposure for a given energy. For diagnostic energy range the F factor is about 1 for soft tissue and it signifies that for keV range R and rad is approximately same. However, value of 'F' for bone in keV range of X-rays is about 4 and this shows that bone absorbs about 4 times more dose than soft tissue due to predominant photoelectric effect at lower energy which increases with substance of high atomic number (like bone with respect to soft tissue).

The relation between absorbed dose to air and exposure is as follows:

Dose to air (mGy) = 8.76 × Exposure (R)

1 R deposits 0.877 rad to dry air. This dose to air or air dose may also be equated with air kerma. The unit for air kerma is gray (Gy). Air kerma in air is the sum of kinetic energy of all charged particles generated when X-rays and gamma rays pass through unit mass of air.

Kerma

The ionizing radiation may be of two types, directly ionizing and indirectly ionizing. Directly ionizing radiations are those which carry charge with it (like alpha, electrons and beta). Directly ionizing radiation interacts with the electron of the atom of the medium through columbic forces. Indirectly ionizing radiation does not carry any charge and includes neutron, X-rays and gamma rays. The indirectly ionizing radiation deposits energy in the medium through two steps. In the first step, the interacting X-rays (or gamma and neutron) deliver/provides kinetic energy to the electrons of the medium through photoelectric, compton or pair production processes depending upon the energy of the incident X-rays. The electrons so produced are directly ionizing and in step two, they deposit their energy in the medium through the process of ionization and excitation. In some cases, where the range of such electrons is sufficiently high, some electrons may escape the medium.

The kerma stands for the kinetic energy released in the medium and is defined as total initial kinetic energy of all charge particles (electrons) released in the medium by the interacting X-ray (indirectly ionizing radiation) in a given mass. Kerma defines the above step one.

$$\text{Kerma (K)} = \frac{E_{tr}}{m}$$

E_{tr} = Sum of kinetic energy of electrons produced

m = Mass of the medium

Unit of kerma is joule/kg which is the unit for dose as well. SI unit for kerma is gray (Gy) and traditional unit is rad. Kerma is defined for X-ray, gamma ray and neutrons only.

The kerma may be considered made of two parts, collision part and radiative part. When the electrons are liberated by the incident X-ray on the medium of low atomic number (air, water, soft tissue) the majority of these electrons expend their energy during interaction with the orbital electrons of the atoms of the medium. A very small part of liberated electrons may interact with the nuclei of the atoms of the medium giving off Bremsstrahlung X-rays (radiative part). If the energy transferred by the incident X-rays to the liberated electrons in the medium is deposited locally and Bremsstrahlung loses (radiative lose) is negligible, the absorbed dose equals to kerma. For diagnostic energy range absorbed dose equals to kerma. At higher energy of incident X-rays and gamma rays radiative loss is not negligible.

The quantity "Exposure" indicates the amount of ionization in air due to radiation interaction while radiation dose (or called radiation absorbed dose) refers to the amount of radiation energy deposited to the medium (may be patient's body) with which the radiation (X-ray) has interacted. The term "radiation exposure" and "radiation dose" are many times used interchangeably especially in case of medical imaging where energy of X-rays used is in kilovoltage range. Generally "exposure" is measured using ionization chamber or any suitable measuring device while "Dose" is calculated from exposure and energy absorbed by X-rays per unit mass of the body.

Equivalent Dose

Equivalent dose may also be called radiation protection unit as it takes into account the potential of the radiation to cause biological damage. The ability to cause biological damage (effectiveness) varies with the type of radiation and is closely related with its ionizing capability. Various types of radiation has been assigned a "quality factor" which, though arbitrary chosen, may be linked with its relative biological effectiveness (RBE) related to linear energy transfer (LET) of radiation. The quality factor is called radiation weighing factor (W_R). W_R for X-rays, gamma rays, beta and electrons are 1, protons (>2 meV) has 5, neutrons (depending upon energy) has 5–20 and alpha particles W_R are 20.

Equivalent dose = Absorbed dose × W_R

The traditional unit for equivalent dose is rem and the SI unit is sievert (Sv). For X-rays $W_R = 1$ and hence, 1 mGy = 1 mSv.

Effective Dose

Radiosensitivity of various tissues is different. Therefore, radiation induced effect in different tissues are likely to be different even for similar equivalent dose for these tissues. Tissue have been assigned a tissue weighting factor (W_T) which represents the detriment (risk) of the radiation exposure to that tissue with respect to the uniform whole body radiation exposure. Bone marrow, colon, lung, breast, stomach each have been given W_T at 0.12, gonads at 0.08, bladder, liver esophagus and thyroid at 0.04, skin bone surface, brain and salivary glands have been given 0.01.

Effective dose = Σ Equivalent dose × W_T

Effective dose may be defined as sum of weighted radiation equivalent dose to various tissues/organs.

Effective dose has similar units as that of equivalent dose, i.e. traditional unit is rem and SI unit is sievert (Sv).

Radiation Dose Measurement in CT

The radiography is a projection imaging while CT scanner is a cross-sectional imaging. In the former, the radiation enters single body surface and maximum dose was delivered to the skin at the entrance. This measurement in case of radiography was called entrance skin dose (ESD). The ESD depends upon kV and mAs set on the control panel of the radiography machine. In contrast, radiation enters the body from all direction as X-ray tube revolves around the patient during exposure in CT scan. It makes the measurement of dose complex due to presence of significant amount of scatter dose and transmitted radiation when the X-ray tube is not directly over the point of measurement. Due to narrow collimation and requirement of good image, the mAs used in CT scanner are much higher than that in radiography. Computed tomography doses are measured in cylindrical phantom made of acrylic (or PMMA) with holes at center and periphery for placing ionization chambers **(Fig. 2)**. The body phantom has a diameter of 32 cm and head phantom has a diameter of 16 cm. Both phantoms have a length of 15 cm in Z-axis. The holes with diameter of 1 cm are made at 12, 3, 6 and 9'o clock positions and are provided with well-fitted acrylic plug to fill the gap (hole) when not in use (by ionization chamber).

Computed Tomography Dose Index

Computed tomography dose index (CTDI) was originally planned as an index of dose and not a real-patient dose. However, later CT dosimetry method for patient dosimetry

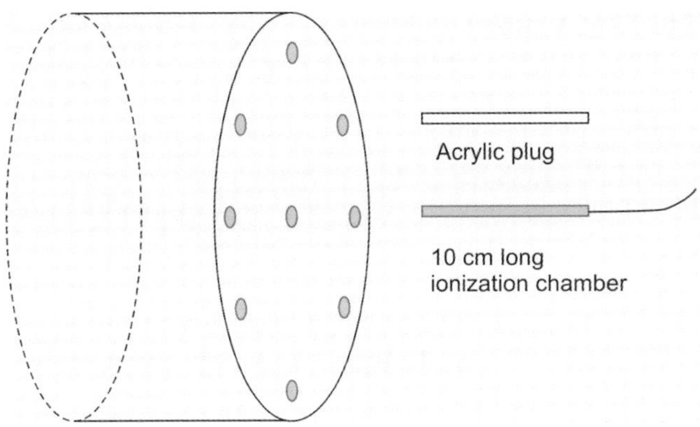

Fig. 2: Computed tomography dose index phantom with chamber.

was based upon CTDI. The $CTDI_{100}$ is a dose measured in a 100 mm long cylindrical ionization chamber when the chamber is placed in CT scanner at its isocenter. The ionization chamber is aligned (its long axis) with the axis of the patient couch (i.e. Z-axis). One single axial scan is performed at the center of the ionization chamber without movement of the table.

$$CTDI_{100} = \frac{1}{\text{Beam width}} \cdot \int_{l=-50\text{ mm}}^{l=+50\text{ mm}} D(z).dz$$

D(z) = radiation dose profile along Z-axis

The single axial scan at the center of the chamber with its beam width (i.e. in MDCT it is the product of number of channels and the size of the detector in channel) opened causes collection of charges created in ionization chamber, 50 mm on either side of its center due to scatter radiation along the Z-axis as well. Beam width may be denoted as NT where N is number of tomographic sections imaged or number of data channel used and T is the width of tomographic section along the Z-axis imaged by single data channel. For $CTDI_w$, the measurement of $CTDI_{100}$ is done at central and peripheral holes of the cylindrical acrylic (or PMMA) phantom.

$CTDI_w$ is a weighted measurement of $CTDI_{100}$

Computed tomography dose index depends upon the field of view (FOV). Doses at the periphery and center of the phantom (i.e. $CTDI_{100,\ center}$ and $CTDI_{100,\ periphery}$) are not equal. Computed tomography dose index at surface may be double of that at center. The average $CTDI_{100}$ which represents average dose to phantom has been termed as $CTDI_{weighted}$ or $CTDI_w$.

$$CTDI_w = 1/3\ CTDI_{100,\ center} + 2/3\ CTDI_{100,\ periphery}$$

In real work, we use CT scanner for series of slices or scans. These slices may be at gap, contiguous or overlapped.

$CTDI_{volume}$ describes the dose to phantom in CT scan with series of slices and abbreviated as $CTDI_{vol}$.

$$CTDI_{vol} = \frac{1}{\text{Pitch}} \cdot CTDI_{100}$$

Pitch is defined in helical or spiral CT scanning as distance travelled by patient table in gantry (mm) during a full rotation of X-ray tube around the patient or phantom for unit beam width (NT) in mm.

$$\text{Pitch} = \frac{\text{Table movement per axial scan (mm)}}{\text{Nominal beam width (NT) (mm)}}$$

$CTDI_{vol}$ represents the average radiation dose to phantom during scan and is reported on CT console for specific scan protocol. These values have been fed by the manufacturer after carrying out the measurement in phantom using specific scan protocol.

DLP is dose length product which is the product of $CTDI_{vol}$ and length of the CT scan.

$DLP = CTDI_{vol} \times$ scan length.

The unit for $CTDI_{vol}$ is mGy. It should be noted that $CTDI_{vol}$ though represents average radiation dose to phantom but may be substantially different for a phantom which has different size from the phantom used in measurement. $CTDI_{vol}$ is independent of the length of the scan, i.e. coverage of scan. However, DLP takes length of scan into account. AAPM report 204 provides conversion factor for $CTDI_{vol}$ for different sizes of phantom which is called size-specific dose estimates (SSDE). These factors may help us in arriving near the real doses involved in CT scan.

Radiation Dose Measurement in Fluoroscopy

In fluoroscopy the users may use direct or indirect method of assessment of radiation dose to patient and staff. Direct method utilizes some measurement devices to be put at the point of measurement (patient's skin, at some reference point, etc.) The measurement devices may be TLD, radiochromic film, MOSFET (Metal Oxide Semiconductor Field Effect Transistor) dosimeter, etc. Indirect method provides an estimate of radiation dose to patient by the direct measurement of some radiation-linked quantities (like, fluoroscopy time or dose–area product, i.e. DAP).

All fluoroscopy machines come equipped to measure the fluoroscopy X-ray "on" time. Fluoroscopy X-ray active time is also called "fluoroscopy time". This parameter is not good enough to provide the estimate of patient skin dose or staff dose.

Another indirect method to measure radiation dose to patient is DAP [or kerma–area product (KAP)]. Dose-area product or KAP meter is a large area, flat, transparent,

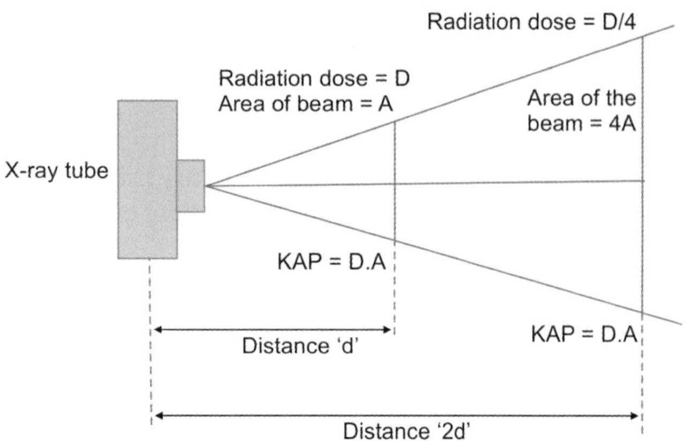

Fig. 3: Dose-area product is independent of distance.

ionization chamber that is fitted into the collimator of X-ray tube. The X-ray passes through it and KAP meter intercepts the whole beam (X-ray field). It gives the measurement as the product of kerma and the area of the radiation beam in the unit Gy.cm^2 or any of its derivative like mGy.cm^2, Gy.m^2, cGy.cm^2, etc. This quantity is independent of distance and can be measured anywhere in the beam. This is true since as we go away from X-ray source the X-ray dose decreases with square of the distance from source (inverse square law) but area of the beam increases due to divergence, again, with square of the distance. This results in the product of radiation dose (kerma) and the X-ray field (area of the beam) to remain constant throughout the X-ray beam and hence KAP can be measured anywhere in the X-ray beam **(Fig. 3)**. Kerma-area product represents the total energy incident on the patient and hence is considered a good indicator of stochastic risk of the radiation exposure. KAP values may be used to arrive at effective dose as the conversion factor is available in literature.

The KAP takes nonuniformity of the dose within the X-ray field into account like due to heel effect or due to utilization of any semitransparent shutter in any area of the field. It is easy to measure and all new fluoroscopy machines provide this data in real time. In some fluoroscopy machine, KAP may be calculated (rather measured) using generator and collimator settings. One should bear in mind that cumulative KAP reading does not indicate the risk of skin-exposure (skin burn) directly in the patient. Nonetheless, the scatter dose around the patient is largely proportional to KAP reading and hence may be a relative indicator of the radiation field around.

Nowadays, the fluoroscopic machines give cumulative doses at some reference point in terms of mGy which was designed to be an indicator of skin dose in the patient. The point of measurement of air kerma (calibrated free in air) has been defined at 15 cm from the isocenter of the isocentric machine (like c arm) towards the X-ray source. This point is intended to refer to the skin of the patient where radiation beam enters the patient. This reference point is called interventional reference point (IRP) and has been defined by International Electrotechnical Commission (IEC) standard 60601-2-43. However, one should keep in mind that cumulative dose at IEC reference point does not take into account back-scatter, table attenuation or in-field nonuniformity of dose. Also, actual skin may not be at IRP since the skin's position depends upon the position of the patient with respect to isocenter, patient thickness, angulations of beam, etc.

SUGGESTED READING

1. Bushberg JT, Seibert JA, Leidholt EM Jr, Boone JM. The essential Physics of Medical Imaging. Lippincott Williams & Wilkins; 2002.
2. IAEA. Radiation Protection of Patients. https://*rpop.iaea.org/ RPoP/RPoP/Content/index.htm.*
3. Khan FM. The Physics of Radiation Therapy. Lippincott Williams & Wilkins; 2009.

CHAPTER 61

Radiation Protection

Sapna Singh

In November 1895, Wilhelm Roentgen discovered X-rays. Roentgen was diligent in his investigation of the behavior of these new-found rays and he established their physical characteristics almost fully within a short period. It was, however, the tragedy of the radiation pioneers that drew attention to the fact that these X-rays were not only wonderful and useful in medicine, but harmful too. However, it took several years before radiation protection measures and the concept of a limit to the exposure dose for radiation workers was established.[1]

HISTORICAL PERSPECTIVE

Within few months of Roentgen's discovery, eye complaints and severe progressive dermatitis were reported. In 1896, one of Edison's assistants Clarence E Dally, involved in the production of X-ray tubes, who had been using his own hand to test their output, developed ulcerating carcinoma of his repeatedly exposed left hand. Delayed effects of radiation began to be documented only 20 years after their initial discovery, through individual case reports. The death of Professor Benjamin Brown in 1911 was also attributed to X-ray exposure causing visceral degeneration, as a result of his earlier experiments, of fluoroscoping his own abdomen continuously for a period of 2 hours during 1896. Germline mutation as a delayed effect of ionizing radiation was documented by Muller in 1927 and won him the Nobel Prize. In 1928, Murphy reported 14 cases of microcephaly and mental retardation in children of mothers who had received pelvic radiotherapy early in pregnancy. In 1929, Murphy and Goldstein documented 16 more patients with similar defects of microcephaly and mental retardation among children whose mothers had received pelvic radiotherapy early in pregnancy. In 1936, Percy Brown, a Radiologist historian, recorded case histories of adverse effects of radiation which occurred in people exposed from 1911 onwards. In 1940s and 1950s, it was a common practice to treat ankylosing spondylitis patients with radiation. It was a permanent cure and remained the treatment of choice for approximately 20 years, until it was discovered that some of the patients who had been cured by radiation are dying from leukemia. In 1942, Dunlap reported radiation induced leukemia in radiologists and other radiation workers.[2]

In 1947, the Atom Bomb Casualty Commission (ABCC) was established to undertake scientifically designed studies in Hiroshima and Nagasaki, to establish the radiation effects following the atomic bomb blasts in these two cities. This commission reported the incidence of genetic effects, mutations, cataracts, leukemias and other malignancies in the population exposed in these blasts. These studies also documented effects on unborn fetuses, including microcephaly and mental retardation. In 1956, Stewart et al. reported increased frequency of leukemia in children with history of radiation exposure during fetal life. In 1975, the ABCC was reorganized and renamed the RERF (Radiation effects and research foundation), funded equally by the United State of America and Japan. The RERF continues its work on genetics, cancer induction and other delayed effects of ionizing radiation.[2]

RADIATION UNITS

Conventional Units

These units are known as the "three Rs", the roentgen, rad (radiation absorbed dose), rem and curie. All of these are very practical units. However, they did not fit into the SI unit system that is being promoted for the sake of having one unified system of units for all physical quantities.

SI Units

The SI radiation units have been adopted by most organizations and publications. These are Gray (Gy), Sievert (Sv), Coulomb/kilogram (C/kg) and Becquerel. Different measurements of radiation are given in **Table 1**.

Table 1: Measurement of radiation.

	Exposure	*Absorbed dose*	*Dose equivalent*	*Radioactivity*
Common units	Roentgen (R)	Rad	Rem	Curie (Ci)
SI units	Coulomb/ kilogram (C/kg)	Gray (Gy)	Sievert (Sv)	Becquerel (Bq)

SPECIFIC QUANTITIES AND THEIR ASSOCIATED UNITS EXPOSURE

The unit of radiation exposure is the Roentgen (R). Roentgen is defined as an amount of X-rays or gamma rays that produces a specific amount of ionization in a unit of air under standard temperature and pressure. This quantity can be measured directly in the air chamber, it is 2.58×10^{-4} C/kg of air.[3]

Exposure is quantified by the unit of kerma. Kerma is an acronym for kinetic energy released in material. Kerma quantifies the amount of energy transferred to charged particles from ionizing photon radiation. The unit of kerma was the rad and now gray (Gy).

Absorbed Dose

Absorbed dose is defined as the quantity of radiation energy absorbed per unit mass of tissue.[4]

Units

The conventional unit for absorbed dose is the rad, which is equivalent to 100 ergs of absorbed energy per gram of tissue.

The SI unit is the gray (Gy), which is equivalent to the absorption of 1 Joule of radiation energy per kilogram of tissue.[4] The relationship between the two units is:

1 gray (Gy) = 100 rads[3]

10 mGy = 1 rad

For a specific type of tissue and photon energy spectrum, the absorbed dose is proportional to the exposure (R) delivered to the tissue.

BIOLOGICAL IMPACT

It is sometimes desirable to express the actual or relative biological impact of radiation. It is necessary to develop a distinction between the biological impact and the physical quantity of radiation because all types of radiation do not have the same potential for producing biological change. For example, one rad of one type of radiation might produce significantly more radiation damage than one rad of another type. In other words, the biological impact is determined by both the quantity of radiation and its ability to produce biological effects. The following two radiation quantities are associated with biological impact:

Dose Equivalent

Dose equivalent (H) is the quantity commonly used to express the biological impact of radiation on persons receiving occupational or environmental exposures. Personnel exposure in a clinical facility is often determined and recorded as a dose equivalent.

Dose equivalent is proportional to the absorbed dose (D) and the quality factor or weighting factor (W_R) for the radiation.[5] That is,

Dose equivalent (Sv) = Absorbed dose (Gy) × W_R[5]

The conventional unit for dose equivalent is the rem (roentgen equivalent man), and the Sl unit is the sievert (Sv).

Sievert is defined as the dose in gray multiplied by quality factor. When the quality factor is 1, the different relationships between dose equivalent (H) and absorbed dose (D) are dose equivalent values can be converted from one system of units to the other by:

1 Sv = 100 rem

Most radiations encountered in diagnostic procedures (X-ray, gamma, and beta) have quality factor values of 1. Therefore, the dose equivalent is numerically equal to the absorbed dose. Some radiation types consisting of large (relative to electrons) particles have weighting or quality factor values greater than 1. For example, alpha particles have a quality factor value of approximately 20 **(Table 2)**.[6]

Three quantities: Exposure, absorbed dose, and dose equivalent, although each expresses a different aspect of radiation, they all express radiation concentration. For the types of radiation used in diagnostic procedures,

Table 2: Radiation weighting factors.

S. No.	Type of radiation	Weighting/ Quality factor
1.	X, gamma or beta radiation	1
2.	Alpha particles and multiple charged particles	20
3.	Neutrons <10 keV	5
	10 keV to 100 keV	10
	>100 keV to 2 MeV	20
	>2 MeV to 20 MeV	10
	>20 MeV	5
4.	Protons	2

Table 3: Weighting factors for tissue.

Tissue	Weighting factor
Gonads	0.2
Active bone marrow, colon, lungs, stomach	0.12
Bladder, breast, esophagus, liver, thyroid	0.05
Bone surfaces, skin	0.01

Table 4: Typical effective doses from exposure to medical radiation.[8]

Diagnostic procedure	Typical effective dose (mSv)	Number of chest X-rays leading to comparable exposure
Chest (PA)	0.02	1
Extremities	0.01	0.5
Skull	0.07	3.5
Thoracic vertebrae	0.7	35
Lumbar vertebrae	1.3	65
Hip	0.3	15
Pelvis	0.7	35
Abdomen	1.0	50
Mammography (bilateral in 2 planes)	0.5	25
Intravenous pylography	2.5	125
Head CT	2.3	115
Chest CT	8	400
Abdomen or pelvis CT	10	500
Positron emission tomography	7.2	360

the factors that relate the three quantities have values of approximately 1 in soft tissue. Therefore, an exposure of 1 R produces an absorbed dose of approximately 1 rad, which in turn, produces a dose equivalent of 1 rem.

Effective Dose Equivalent (Effective Dose)

Irradiation from external environment affects the entire body, whereas medical diagnostic procedures generally affect only selected areas. To compare the risk assessment for all types of exposures, the concept of effective dose equivalent has been developed. It takes into account the specific organs and areas of the body that are exposed. The point is that all parts of the body and organs are not equally sensitive to the possible adverse effects of radiation, such as cancer induction and mutations.

For the purpose of determining effective dose, the different areas and organs have been assigned tissue weighting factor (w_T) values. For a specific organ or body area, the effective dose is: Effective Dose Equivalent (Sv) = Dose Equivalent (Sv) × w_T

If more than one area has been exposed, then the total body effective dose is just the sum of the effective doses for each exposed area. Also, by using effective dose it is possible to put the radiation received from diagnostic procedures into perspective with other exposures, especially natural background radiation.

The weighting factors for various tissues are discussed in **Table 3**:[5,7]

There is often a need to compare the amount of radiation received by patients for different types of X-ray procedures, for example, a chest radiograph and a CT scan. The effective dose is the most appropriate quantity for doing this.

Effective dose equivalent from a chest radiographic examination is 0.02 mSv, it means that the risk involved from a CXR is the same as the risk involved in exposing the entire body to an X-ray exposure of 0.02 mSv **(Table 4)**.[8]

This leads to the conclusion that a chest CT leads to 400 folds greater radiation exposure for the patient than conventional chest projection radiography.[9]

INTERACTION OF RADIATION WITH MATTER RADIATION TYPES AND SOURCES

Radiation can take several different forms and is simply a mechanism whereby energy is transmitted through space. Medical imaging modalities that involve ionizing radiation make use of electromagnetic waves located near one end of the electromagnetic spectrum. This spectrum consists of differing electromagnetic waves that are defined by their electromagnetic wavelength. At one end of the spectrum are the long-wavelength and relatively innocuous radio- and microwaves. As the electromagnetic wavelength decreases, radiation passes through the spectrum of visible light, after which the short-wavelength, high-energy X-rays, gamma rays, and cosmic rays are encountered. This energy has the capacity to be harmful to biologic tissue because it carries the potential to displace electrons from its energy level or shell around the nucleus. This can lead to ionization of the affected atom and explains why these forms of electromagnetic waves are termed "ionizing radiation". The effects of ionizing radiation on biologic tissues at the atomic and molecular level are concerning for several reasons. First, a displaced electron can cause damage to other cell components as it is ejected rapidly from its orbit. Second, the resulting highly chemically reactive ionized atom, or "free radical", can have deleterious effects on the cell of which it is a part. Third, the altered structure of the atom that occurs once an electron is lost may affect the function of the tissue involved; this result may be particularly grievous if the involved tissue is a chromosome within a radiosensitive cell, such as those found in the breast or ovary.

Humans are exposed to unavoidable forms of ionizing radiation each day. This type of radiation is classified as background radiation and is an unavoidable consequence of living. Background radiation originates from radon gas seeping out of the earth, natural radioactivity being emitted from rocks and other organic compounds in the ground, and cosmic rays that constantly rain down from space, among other sources. Although man-made radiation sources include airport security scanners, smoke detectors, television sets, and fluorescent lamp starters; medical imaging accounts for 95% of all exposure from man-made radiation sources. The reason for this rapid alteration in the proportions of exposure from man-made radiation sources over the past few years has been the phenomenal increase in the use of ionizing radiation in medical imaging.[10]

There are three major ways in which radiation is absorbed, especially X-rays and results in ionization: the photoelectric effect, the Compton effect and Pair production.

1. At low energies (30–100 kev), as in diagnostic radiology, the photoelectric effect is important. In this process, the incident photon interacts with an electron in one of the inner shells of an atom (typically K, L, or M). If the energy of the photon is greater than the binding energy of the electron, then the electron is expelled from the orbit with a kinetic energy that is equal to the energy of the incident photon minus the binding energy of the electron.[11] The photoelectric effect varies as a function of the cube of the atomic number of the material exposed (Z); this fact explains why bone is visualized much better than soft tissue on radiographs **(Fig. 1)**.

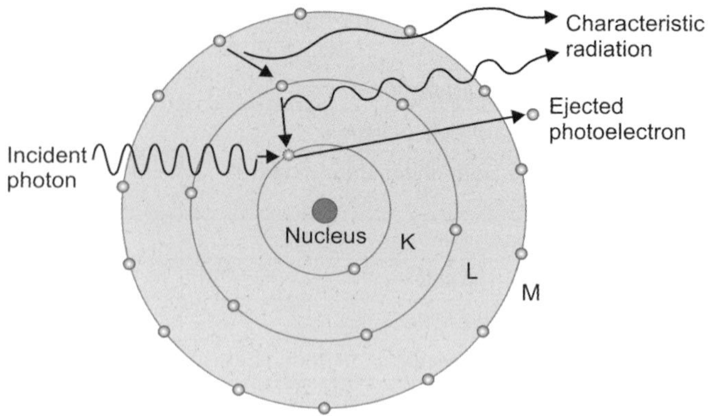

Fig. 1: Photoelectric effect.

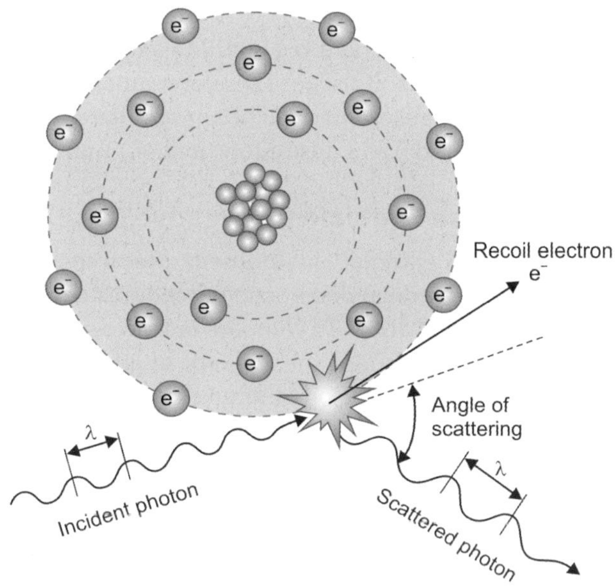

Fig. 2: Compton scattering.

2. At intermediate energies, as used in therapeutic radiology, the Compton effect dominates. In this process, the incident photon interacts with an electron in an orbital shell. Part of the incident photon energy appears as kinetic energy of electrons and the residual energy continues as a less energetic deflected photon **(Fig. 2)**.[11]
3. At energy levels above 1.02 MeV, the photons may be absorbed through pair production. In this process, both a positron and an electron are produced in the absorbing material. A positron has the same mass as an electron but has a positive instead of a negative charge. The positron travels a very short distance in the absorbing medium before it interacts with another electron. When that happens, the entire mass of both particles is converted to energy, with the emission of two photons in exactly opposite directions **(Fig. 3)**.

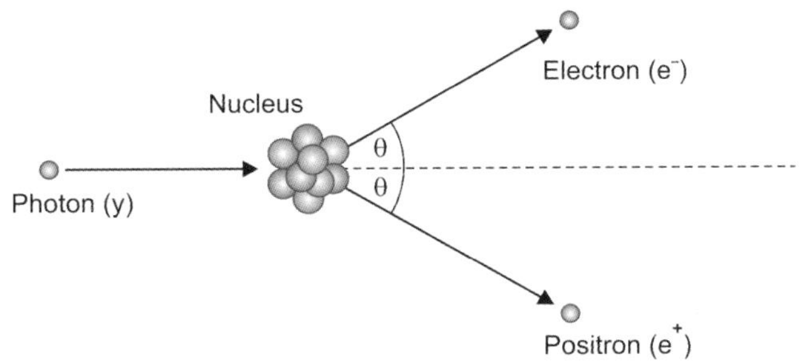

Fig. 3: Pair production.

BIOLOGICAL EFFECT OF RADIATION

- Critical target in cell-DNA
- Result from damage to DNA
- Radiation may be directly or indirectly acting **(Fig. 4)**.

Direct action: DNA directly gets ionized or excited, leading to biological damage.

Indirect action: Radiation interacts with other atom/ molecules (water) to produce free radicals which than dam-age DNA. Two-thirds of X-ray damage to DNA caused by hydroxyl radical.[12]

Absorption of radiation may result either in killing of cell or its modification by genetic change.

CLASSIFICATION OF RADIATION INJURY

Since the majority of radiation exposure is from man-made sources and that the majority of this exposure originates from medical imaging, it is important to understand the possible effects and risks of this radiation exposure for the human body. Radiation effects can be divided into two general types: deterministic effects and stochastic effects **(Table 5)**.

- Deterministic effects are the result of the excessive cell death that can occur following ionizing radiation exposures. These effects include skin erythema, epilation, necrosis, and lens cataract formation. Because these effects occur only after a critical mass of cells have died, they have a known radiation exposure threshold below which their occurrence can be avoided. Thus deterministic effects or certainity effects are directly related to a known dose of radiation and have a dose threshold and their severity is also dose-related.
- Stochastic radiation effects are random events which are not dose-related but their probability increases with an increase in radiation dose. Stochastic effects include carcinogenesis and hereditary effects. The possibility of a stochastic effect taking place supports the practice of exposures being kept as low as reasonably achievable (ALARA).

The effect of both are being summarized in **Table 6**.

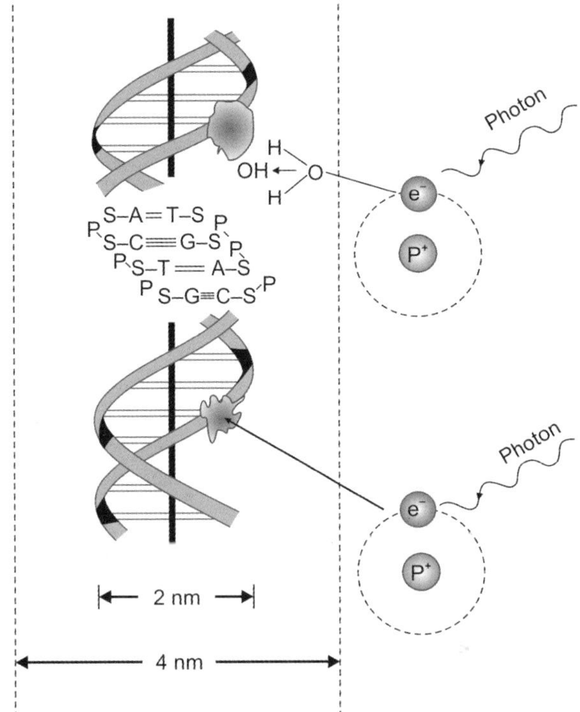

Fig. 4: Radiation may be directly/indirectly acting on the DNA of the cell.

Table 5: Types of radiation effects.

Type	*Effects*
Deterministic	Erythema, epilation, skin necrosis, cataract formation
Stochastic	Carcinogenesis, hereditary effects

Table 6: Radiation effects of deterministic and stochastic.

	Deterministic effects	*Stochastic effects*
1.	Cell killing	Cell modification
2.	Threshold described	No threshold for occurrence
3.	Severity is dose dependent	Severity is independent of dose
4.	Erythema, epilation, skin necrosis, cataract formation	Carcinogenesis, hereditary effects

Malignancies Associated with Radiation Exposure

Carcinogenesis is stochastic in nature.

Leukemia: Two types of adult leukemias are associated with radiation exposure. These are acute and chronic myeloid leukemias. Radiation exposure during childhood results in an increased incidence of acute lymphatic leukemia. The latency period of leukemia is a minimum of 2 years, peaks at 7–12 years and returns to zero at about 30 years.[13]

Other radiation-induced cancers: Malignancies of skin, lung, bone, blood dyscrasias and meningiomas have been described. Other malignancies known to be associated with radiation are osteosarcomas, breast carcinoma and thyroid carcinoma.[14]

Genetic Effects of Radiation

Genetic effects are stochastic by their nature.

- Radiation can either damage the DNA or affect the chromosome itself. Genetic effects on humans manifest as mutations leading to congenital defects in the offspring or causing malignancies.
- The genetic effects of radiation are evaluated on the basis of their mutational effects which is expressed as the "genetic doubling dose". Genetic doubling dose is an estimate of the amount of acute radiation which will double the spontaneous mutation rate or will cause an increase in the mutation rate which is equal to the number of spontaneous mutations which normally occur.
- The most common genetic effects, such as autosomal and X-linked changes and chromosomal alterations in an exposed population have been estimated to be occurring at 1×10^{-2} per Sv (0.01 mutations per Sv).[12,13]

Genetically significant dose (GSD): It is a genetic dose index. It is the gonad dose, that if received by every member of the population would be expected to produce the same total effect on the population as the sum of the individual dose as actually received. The GSD is therefore, a genetic dose index of the presumed genetic impact of radiation exposure on the total population due to radiation induced mutations on the reproduction of cells of this generation that can be translated as risk to the descendents.[15] The GSD is merely an attempt at estimating the dose received by the population gene pool[1] and an analysis of the GSD from diagnostic radiology can be used to estimate possible detriment from a specific practice.[15]

DETERMINISTIC EFFECTS AS DOCUMENTED FROM RADIATION ACCIDENTS

Acute Total-body Irradiation

The data regarding the acute effects of total-body irradiation on humans comes primarily from Japanese survivors of the atomic bomb. Marshall Islanders exposed to fallout radiation and victims of a few nuclear installation accidents, such as Chernobyl (in Ukraine).[16] Clinical manifestations depend on the total-body dose.

- At doses in excess of 100 Gy to the total body, death usually occurs within 24–48 hours from neurologic and cardiovascular failure. This is known as the cerebrovascular syndrome. Because cerebrovascular damage causes death very quickly, the failure of other systems do not have time to develop.
- At doses between 5 and 12 Gy, death may occur in a matter of days, as a result of the gastrointestinal syndrome. The symptoms during this period may include nausea, vomiting and prolonged diarrhea for several days, leading to dehydration, sepsis and death.
- At total-body doses between 2 and 8 Gy, death may occur several weeks after exposure and is due to effects on the bone marrow, which results in the hematopoietic syndrome. The full effect of radiation is not apparent until the mature hematopoietic cells are depleted. Death from the hematologic damage occurs at about 20–30 days after exposure and the risk of death continues over the next 30 days. Clinical symptoms during this period may include chills, fatigue and petechial hemorrhage. The threshold for this syndrome is 1 Gy.[16]
- *Mean lethal dose or LD 50:* The lethal dose 50 or LD 50 is a term borrowed from pharmacology and is defined as the dose of an agent that causes mortality in 50% of given population in a given time. For radiation, LD 50 has been estimated from the atomic bomb explosion at Hiroshima and Nagasaki and from accidental exposures. Based on this data and the observation that with medical support humans can survive a total-body dose of 4 Gy, estimates of LD 50 for humans is 3 to 4 Gy.[12]

Chronic Radiation Effects

These effects result from prolonged exposure of lower intensity or may appear as late effects in survivors of more acute exposures. These may be due to whole body or partial body irradiation.

- *Central nervous system:* Mild encephalopathy, focal neurological changes and transverse myelitis are known side effects of CNS irradiation. A unique late effect of cranial radiation combined with chemotherapy known as leukoencephalopathy, has been described as a necrotizing reaction and is usually noted 4–12 months.[16] Radiation necrosis occurs in 1–5% of patients after 55–60 Gy doses fractioned over 6 weeks, 75% of the cases occur within 3 years.[17]

- *Skin:* The changes include erythema, desquamation, thinning of epidermis, pigmentation and hair loss.
- *Heart and blood vessels:* Asymptomatic pericardial effusion, chronic constrictive pericarditis and pancarditis.
- *Lung:* Radiation pneumonitis develops in 3–6 weeks following exposures of more than 25 Gy. This can lead to permanent scarring.[17]
- *GIT:* Chronic phase of radiation enteropathy usually presents between 6 months and 5 years of exposure. The terminal ileum is the most commonly affected part. The changes include fibrosis, perforation, fistula formation, stenosis, etc.
- *Hematopoietic system:* Fatty replacement of marrow occurs above a threshold of 50 Gy.[17]
- *Eye:* Cataract has been recorded at 2 to 8 Gy of single exposure.[17]
- *Bladder:* Interstitial fibrosis, telangiectasia, ulceration and reduced capacity.

THE REGULATORY BODIES

There are several regulatory bodies at the International and National level.

The regulatory bodies lay down norms for protection against radiation and also recommend the dose limits for radiation workers and the general public. The ICRP or the International Commission for Radiation Protection is the international regulatory body. Each country has its national counterpart of the ICRP. In America, the counterpart is the NCRP or The National Commission for Radiological Protection and in India, it is the AERB or the Atomic Energy Regulatory Board.

- The International Commission of Radiation Protection (ICRP) was formed in 1928, on the recommendation of the first International Congress of Radiology in 1925. The commission consists of a chairman, a secretary and 12 members who are chosen from across the world based on their expertise. ICRU is the International Commission on Radiation Units and measurements.[18]
- The Indian regulatory board is the Atomic Energy Regulatory Board (AERB). It was constituted on November 15, 1983 by the President of India by exercising the powers conferred by Section 27 of the Atomic Energy Act, 1962 (33 of 1962) to carry out certain regulatory and safety functions under the Act. The Board consists of a full time chairman, an exofficio member, three part-time members and a secretary.[19]
- *Radiation safety Act in India:* Radiation safety in handling of radiation generating equipment is governed by section 17 of the Atomic Energy Act, 1962, and the Radiation Protection Rules (RPR), GSR - 1601, 1971 issued under the Act. The "Radiation Surveillance Procedures of Medical Applications of Radiation, GSR-388, 1989", issued under rule 15 specify general requirements for ensuring radiation protection in installation and handling of X-ray equipment.[19]

Role of AERB

According to AERB, safety code for medical diagnostic X-ray equipment and installations document, regulatory controls of AERB are as follows:[19]

- *Design certification:* Every medical diagnostic X-ray equipment shall meet the design safety specifications stipulated in the AERB Code. The manufacturer/vendor shall obtain design certification from the competent authority prior to manufacturing the X-ray equipment.
- *Type Approval/No Objection Certificate:* Prior to marketing the X-ray equipment, the manufacturer shall obtain a type approval certificate from the competent authority for indigenously made equipment. Only type-approved and NOC validated equipment shall be marketed and used in the country.
- *Approval of layout:* No X-ray unit shall be commissioned unless the layout of the proposed X-ray installation is approved by the competent authority.
- *Registration of X-ray equipment:* Acquisition of X-ray equipment, by purchase, transfer, gift, leasing or loan, shall be registered with the competent authority by the person acquiring the equipment. Registration shall be done only after the installation is approved from radiation safety viewpoint.
- *Commissioning of X-ray equipment:* No X-ray equipment shall be commissioned unless it is registered with the competent authority.
- *Inspection of X-ray installations:* The diagnostic X-ray installations shall be made available by the employer/owner for inspection, at all reasonable times, to the competent authority or its representative, to ensure compliance with the code.
- *Decommissioning of X-ray installations:* Decommissioning of X-ray equipment shall be registered with the competent authority immediately by the employer/owner of the equipment/installation.
- *Certification of RSO:* Any person accepting consultancy assignment to discharge the duties and functions of radiation safety officer (RSO) in diagnostic X-ray installations shall do so only after obtaining certification from the competent authority for the purpose. Such certification shall be granted on the basis of adequacy

of the person's qualifications, experience and testing/survey/dosimetry equipment available.

- *Certification of service engineers:* Only persons holding a valid certificate from the competent authority shall undertake servicing of X-ray equipment. Certification shall be granted on the basis of qualification, training, experience, and safety record of such person and availability of servicing facilities.
- *Penalties:* Any person who contravenes the provisions of the Radiation Protection Rules, 1971, elaborated in this Code, or any other terms or conditions of the license/ registration/certification granted to him/her by the competent authority, is punishable under sections 24, 25 and 26 of the Atomic Energy Act, 1962. The punishment may include fine, imprisonment or both, depending on the severity of the offence.

Radiation Protection Survey and Program (Flowchart 1)

The responsibility for establishing a radiation protection program rests with the hospital administration/owners of the X-ray facility. The administration is expected to appoint a Radiation safety committee (RSC), and a radiation safety officer (RSO). Every department should have an RSO. This officer should be an individual with extensive training and education in areas, such as radiation protection, radiation physics, radiation biology, instrumentation, dosimetry and shielding design. In India, AERB has specified duties of the RSO which include assisting the employer in meeting the relevant regulatory requirements applicable to his/her X-ray installation.[19] He/she shall implement all radiation surveillance measures, conduct periodic radiation protection surveys, maintain proper records of periodic quality assurance tests, and personnel doses, instruct all workers on relevant safety measures, educate and train new entrants, and take local measures, including issuance of clear administrative instructions in writing, to deal with radiation emergencies. The RSO should also ensure that all radiation measuring and monitoring instruments in his/her custody are properly calibrated and maintained in good condition.[19] The duties also include maintaining a record of all radiation surveys performed, deficiencies observed and remedial actions taken.

It is recommended that the RSC should comprise of a radiologist, a medical physicist, a nuclear medicine personnel, a senior nurse and an internist. It is the duty of RSC to perform a regular radiation protection survey. This survey has 5 phases which are as follows:[18]

1. *Investigation*: To obtain information regarding layout of the department, workload, personnel monitoring and records.
2. *Inspection*: Each diagnostic installation in the department is examined for its protection status with respect to its operating factors, control booth and availability of protection devices.
3. *Measurement*: Measurements are conducted on exposure factors. In addition, scattered radiation and patient dose measurements in radiography and fluoroscopy are performed.
4. *Evaluation*: The radiation protection status of the department is evaluated by examination of records, equipment working, status of protective clothing and the radiation doses obtained from phase-3.
5. *Recommendations*: A report is prepared on the protection status of the department and the problem areas if any identified, for which recommendations are made regarding corrective measures.[18]

Flowchart 1: Radiation protection program.

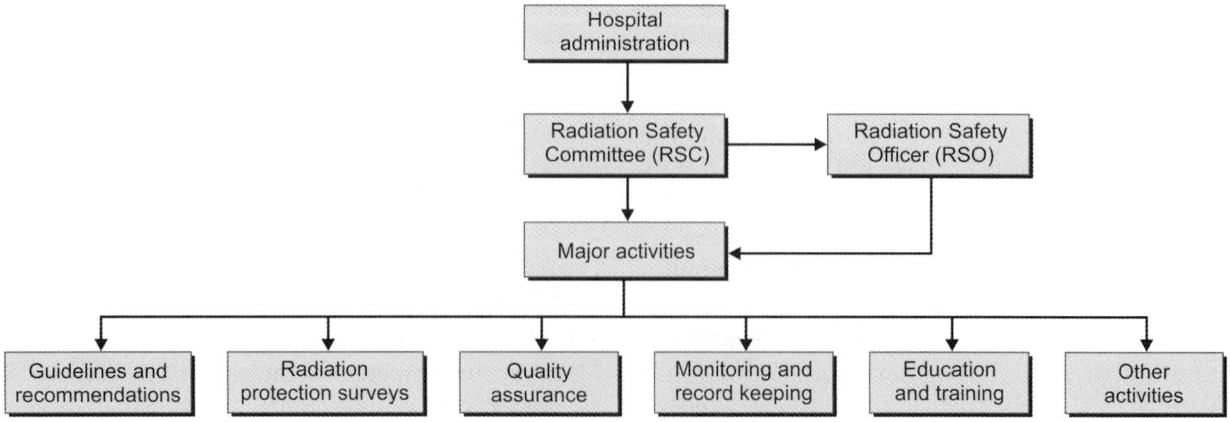

PROTECTION AGAINST RADIATION HAZARD PRINCIPLES OF RADIATION PROTECTION

The current radiation protection standards are based on three general principles, which are recommendations of the Inter-national Commission on Radiological Protection (ICRP). These include:[20]

1. *Justification:* No practice shall be adopted unless its introduction produces a net positive benefit.
2. *Optimization:* All exposures shall be kept as low as reasonably achievable, economic and social factors being taken into account.
3. *Dose limitation:* The dose equivalent to individuals shall not exceed the limits recommended for the appropriate circumstances.
   - *Justifiable use:* A practice that entails exposure to radiation should only be adopted, if it yields sufficient benefit to the exposed individuals or to society, to outweigh the radiation detriment it causes or could cause (i.e. the practice must be justified).[21] Internationally, in countries with regulatory bodies, it is recommended that all diagnostic practices should be justified. This involves the correct assessment of the clinical indications for the requested examination, knowledge of the expected yield from the examination and the way in which the results are expected to influence the diagnosis and subsequent medical management of the patient. The expected clinical benefit must be such that it will offset the radiation detriment. For example, benefit to risk ratio is high for CT brain in cerebrovascular hemorrhage and low in screening mammography in women below 35 years. However, since CT examinations are known to contribute a large dose of diagnostic radiation, it is recommended that CT referrals should be reviewed meticulously.[22]
     It has been reported that in a well-justified series of barium enema examinations, justification being determined by the degree of symptoms suffered, only 30% of the examinations will be positive. This may seem a low-return and indicate that too many people are subjected to the procedure. However, the conclusion drawn was that the examination is well-justified and that a negative finding is a positive result.[23]
   - *Optimization and ALARA:* Radiation sources and installations should be provided with the best available protection and safety measures under the prevailing circumstances, so that the magnitudes and likelihood of exposures and the numbers of individuals exposed be kept as low as reasonably achievable (ALARA), economic and social factors being taken into account.[24] In the United Kingdom (UK), this has for reasons of legal precedent been amended to read ALARP-As Low As Reasonably Practicable (ALARP).[25] Following the principle of ALARA or ALARP, the radiation protection worker is generally more structured and controlled than in the case of the patient where rules and regulations are more difficult to standardize.
   - *Dose limitation:* There is no absolute evidence of a threshold below which no damage occurs. Even the lowest doses may cause damage to the cells which might, later lead to malignancy or hereditary effects if the cells irradiated are germ cells in the gonads. Therefore, we have to assume that the probability of radiation induced cancer or serious hereditary defects are proportional to the radiation dose right down to the lowest levels.[26] This suggests that no radiation dose, however low, can be considered absolutely safe. Although this may be an overestimation of the true radiation effects at low-dose levels, it is preferable to hold the model and it is the basis for radiation protection standards today. Individual doses due to the combination of exposures from all relevant practices should not exceed specified dose limits for occupational and public exposure. Different dose limits are specified for the radiation workers as the expected benefit from the work they do while handling radiation will outweigh the small increase in risk (**Tables 7 and 8**).

- *Maximum permissible dose equivalent (MPD):* It may be defined as the maximum dose of ionizing radiation which an individual may accumulate over a long period of time with a negligible risk of significant body or genetic damage.
  - MPD = 5(N-1)R, where N is age in years more than 18 years and R is the exposure in Roentgens. The unit of MPD is rem
  - The newer recommendation is MPD = Age in years × 1 rem, i.e. the individual effective dose for a lifetime should not exceed the value of his/her age.

CARDINAL PRINCIPLE OF RADIATION PROTECTION

The triad of radiation protection measures is "time-distance-shielding", that is discussed below:

1. Keep the time of exposure to radiation as short as possible.

Table 7: Recommended dose limits for radiation workers and general public.[18,19]

	Occupational workers		Public	
	Limit	***Annual equivalents***	***Limit***	***Annual equivalents***
ICRP	20 mSv/yr over 5 years	20 mSv	1 mSv/yr over 5 years	1 mSv
NCRP	Cumulative dose = Age in yrs × 10 mSv	50 mSv	5 mSv for 5 years period	1 mSv
AERB	100 mSv for 5 years period	30 mSv	1 mSv/yr for 5 years	1 mSv

Abbreviations: ICRP, International Commission on Radiological; NCRP, National Council on Radiation Protection; AERB, Atomic Energy Regulatory Board.

Table 8: Recommendations for dose limits to eye and skin for occupational workers.[18,19]

Dose limits to skin, hands, feet (mSv/yr.)		***Dose limits to lens of eye (mSv/yr.)***
ICRP	500	150
NCRP	500	150
AERB	500	150

Abbreviations: ICRP, International Commission on Radiological; NCRP, National Council on Radiation Protection; AERB, Atomic Energy Regulatory Board.

2. Maintain as large a distance as possible between the radiation and the exposed person.
3. Insert shielding material between the radiation source and the exposed person.

Time

The exposure time is related to radiation exposure and exposure rate (exposure per unit time) as follows:

Exposure = Exposure rate × Time

The algebraic expressions simply imply that if the exposure time is kept short, then the resulting dose to the individual is small.[18]

Distance

The second radiation protection action relates to the distance between the source of radiation and the exposed individual. The exposure to the individual decreases inversely as the square of the distance. This is known as the inverse square law, which is stated mathematically as:

$$I \sim \frac{1}{d^2}$$

Where I is the intensity of radiation and d is the distance between the radiation source and the exposed individual. For example, when the distance is doubled the exposure is reduced by a factor of four.[4]

Shielding

The third radiation protection action relates to shielding. Shielding implies that certain materials (concrete, lead) will attenuate radiation (reduce its intensity) when they are placed between the source of radiation and the exposed individual.

- X-ray tube shielding
- Room shielding
  - X-ray equipment room shielding
  - Patient waiting room shielding
  - Control room shielding
- Personnel shielding
- Patient shielding.

Three types of radiations have to be considered in radiation protection which are as follows:

1. Useful beam is the radiation passing through the tube aperture, previously called the primary beam.
2. Leakage radiation includes all the radiation passing through the tube housing, other than the useful radiation.
3. Scattered radiation which has undergone a change in direction during passage through matter.

X-ray Tube Shielding (Source Shielding)

The X-ray tube housing is lined with thin sheets of lead because X-rays produced in the tube are scattered in all directions. This shielding is intended to protect both patients and personnel from leakage radiation. Manufacturers of X-ray devices are required to shield the tube housing so as to limit the leakage radiation exposure rate to less than 0.1 R hr^{-1} at 1 meter from the tube anode.[27] AERB recommends a maximum allowable leakage radiation from tube housing not greater than 1 mGy/hour/100 cm.[19]

Room Shielding (Structural Shielding)

- The lead-lined walls of radiology department are referred to as protective barriers because they are designed to protect individuals located outside the X-ray rooms from unwanted radiation.
- A 2-mm lead is equivalent to 25 mm layer of high quality barium plaster, 225 mm of solid brick, 150 mm of concrete or ½ brick thickness and ½ inch plaster.[11]

- A basic principle of permanent barriers is that joints and holes must be covered by the same or equivalent protective barrier as the wall.
  There are two types of protective barriers:
  - *Primary barrier:* It is one which is directly struck by the primary or the useful beam and whose atomic number and thickness is sufficient to reduce the exposure rate of the useful beam to the MPD.
  - *Secondary barrier:* It is one which is exposed to stray radiation either by leakage from X-ray tube or by scattered radiation from the patient.
- The shielding of X-ray room is influenced by the nature of occupancy of the adjoining area. In this respect, two types of areas have been identified.
  - *Control area:* It is defined as the area routinely occupied by radiation workers who are exposed to an occupational dose. For control area, the shielding should be such that it reduces exposure in that area to less than 26 mC/kg/week.
  - *Uncontrolled areas:* They are those areas which are not occupied by occupational workers. For these areas, the shielding should reduce the exposure rate to less than 2.6 mC/kg/week.

Exposure Calculations

Five factors must be considered for exposure calculations at any point:[28]

1. *Workload (W):* It is the quantity of X-rays generated per week.
   Workload = mAs/patient × patients/hour × hours/week = mAs/week.
2. *Exposure (E'):* Roentgen per mA.min at 1 meter. This is to convert the workload into Roentgens.
3. *Use factor (U):* It is the fraction of time that the beam is directed at a particular barrier.
4. *Occupancy factor (T):* Amount of time that the area will be occupied. T = 1 means that the area will be occupied by the same individuals throughout the full work day.
5. Distance (d).
   Weekly exposure at a point in question (E) can be calculated as
   $E = E' WUT/d^2$.[28]
   The value, thus calculated can be used to determine the thickness of the primary barrier.

- *Half-value layer (HVL):* It is the thickness of a specific substance that when introduced into the path of a beam of radiation, reduces the exposure rate by 50%.[28] For example, if the exposure at a point is 3.2 R/week and the permissible exposure is 0.1 R/week, the required number of HVLs calculated, which will reduce 3.2 R/week–0.1 R/week, is 5. If the HVL of the beam is 0.25 of lead, the barrier thickness would be 1.25 mm (0.25 × 5 = 1.25 mm) **(Table 9)**.
- In general, the primary protective barrier should consist of 1/16 inch lead extending 7 feet from the floor, when the X-ray tube is 5–7 feet from the wall. This barrier also takes care of the leakage radiation.
- A secondary protective barrier under the same operating conditions should consist of 1/32 inch of lead. This secondary barrier extends from the top of the primary barrier to the ceiling and should overlap the primary barrier at least 0.5 inches at the seam.[28]
- Patient waiting areas are provided outside the X-ray room. A suitable warning signal, such as red light and warning placard at a conspicuous place should be provided and kept 'ON' when the unit is in use to warn persons not connected with the particular examination from entering the room.[19]

Shielding of the X-ray Control Room

The control room of X-ray equipment is a secondary protective barrier which has two important aspects:

1. The walls and viewing window of the control booth, which should have lead equivalents of 1.5 mm.
2. The location of control booth, which should not be located where the primary beam falls directly, and the radiation should be scattered twice before entering the booth.

The AERB recommends the following shielding for the X-ray control room:[19] The control panel of diagnostic X-ray equipment operating at 125 kVp or above (as in CT) is installed in a separate room located outside but contiguous to the X-ray room and provided with appropriate shielding, direct viewing and oral communication facilities between the operator and the patient. In case of X-ray equipment operating up to 125 kVp, the control panel can be located in the X-ray room. AERB recommends that the distance between control panel and X-ray unit/chest stand should not be less than 3 m for general purpose fixed X-ray

Table 9: Tube potential and half-value layer (HVL) calculation.

	HVL[28]	
Tube potential (kVp)	***Lead (mm)***	***Concrete (inches)***
40	0.03	0.13
80	0.19	0.42
100	0.24	0.6
125	0.27	0.76
150	0.28	0.86

equipment. In mobile radiography, where there is no fixed protective control booth, the technologist should remain at least 2 m from the patient, the X-ray tube and the primary beam during exposure. In this respect, the ICRP as well as the NCRP recommends that the length of the exposure cord on mobile radiographic units should be at least 2 m long. The size of the CT room housing the gantry of the CT unit as recommended by AERB should not be less than 25 m^2.[19]

Personnel Shielding

Shielding of occupational workers can be achieved by following methods:

- Personnel should remain in the radiation environment only when necessary (step behind the control booth, or leave the room when practical).
- The distance between the personnel and the patient should be maximized when practical as the intensity of radiation decreases as the square of distance (inverse square law).
- Shielding apparel should be used as and when necessary which comprise of lead aprons, eye glasses with side shields, hand gloves and thyroid shields.

Lead aprons are shielding apparel recommended for use by radiation workers. These are classified as a secondary barrier to the effects of ionizing radiation. These aprons protect an individual only from secondary (scattered) radiation, not the primary beam.[29]

- The thickness of lead in the protective apparel determines the protection it provides. It is known that 0.25 mm lead thickness attenuates 66% of the beam at 75 kVp and 1 mm attenuates 99% of the beam at same kVp. It is recommended that for general purpose radiography, the minimum thickness of lead equivalent in the protective apparel should be 0.5 mm.[29] It is recommended that women radiation workers should wear a customized lead apron that reaches below midthigh level and wraps completely around the pelvis. This would eliminate an accidental exposure to a conceptus.[30]
- *Care of the lead apparel:* It is imperative that lead aprons are not abused, such as by dropping them on the floor, piling them in a heap or improperly draping them over the back of a chair.[31] Because all of these actions can cause internal fracturing of the lead, they may compromise the apron's protective ability. When not in use, all protective apparel should be hung on properly designed racks. Protective apparel also should be radiographed for defects such as internal cracks and tears at least once a year.
- *Gonad shield:* Gonad shields shall have a minimum lead equivalence of 0.5 mm.
- Other protective apparel includes eye glasses with side shields, thyroid shields and hand gloves. The minimum protective lead equivalents in hand gloves, gonadal shields and thyroid shields should be 0.5 mm.

Patient Shielding

Radiation protection of the patient involves both technical and medical decisions. The technical decisions relate to the choices of the appropriate equipment and to the technique. It is noted that the reduction in radiation dose by changes in the equipment will result in a more consistent reduction while reduction due to radiological technique need constant effort to maintain the benefit.[32]

Equipment

There are many radiation protection features and accessories on modern X-ray equipment. These include:

- *Beam filtration* causes lower energy photons to be absorbed by the filters and thus increase the mean energy of the beam and its penetration power and hence decrease the patient dose. Absorption primarily takes place with X-rays of less than 40 keV of energy and virtually all X-rays below 10 keV are absorbed.[33] These low energy X-rays contribute to patient dose without contributing to the image.

Total filtration should be indicated on the tube housing. The total permanent filtration in the tube should be not less than 1.5 mm Al **(Table 10)**.

For mammography, the AERB guideline states that the total filtration in the useful beam shall be not less than 0.03 mm of molybdenum for screen-film mammography for Mo-W alloy target type and 0.5 mm of aluminum for xeromammography for W-target X-ray tubes.[19]

- *Beam collimation:* During any radiographic procedure, the area of the patient exposed to the X-ray beam should be limited to the area of clinical interest. Tissues inside the primary beam receive doses that are orders of magnitude higher than doses received by tissue outside the primary beam. By using collimation

Table 10: Minimum total filtration for X-ray tubes.

Maximum-rated tube potential (kVp)	*Minimum total filtration (mm Al)*
Less than 70	1.5
70 to and including 100	2.0
Above 100	2.5

to expose only the area of clinical interest, one can substantially reduce unnecessary patient exposure.[34] Use of collimation has another important effect: by reducing the area of the X-ray beam, the amount of scattered radiation that reaches the image receptor is also decreased. The resulting images have better contrast.

- The table top should be one which allows a high beam transmission which increases the quantity of diagnostically important photons reaching the film. A carbon fiber material is generally used for a high transmission table top.
- *Image receptors:* The intensifying screen was designed to optimize absorption of the radiation by converting absorbed X-ray energy into visible light, which would be more readily absorbed by the film than the more energetic X-ray photons. The advent of fluorescent intensifying screens, which act as an image amplifier and their use with X-ray film, which is highly sensitive to the visible light photons, significantly reduce the absorbed dose to the patient while still maintaining the image quality. The intensification factor is the radiation exposure required without screens divided by the exposure required with screens to provide the same film blackening effect. This factor is dependent on the screen, the film and the exposure factors. One method of classifying screens is to put them into categories according to their relative light output or speed. In radiography, the speed of an image receptor is inversely related to the radiation exposure required to produce a certain amount of film blackening. Therefore, a fast screen (high-speed) requires less X-ray exposure than a slow screen (low-speed) to provide a given image density. Rare-earth screen film combinations, in use today, reduce the patient dose considerably without loss of diagnostic quality.[35] The image intensifier tubes, in use today, also have efficient input phosphors that play a role in reducing the dose to the patient.
- *Source to image receptor distance (SID):* The dose to the patient is reduced when the source-to-skin-distance (SSD) is increased and the SSD is related to the source-to-image-receptor distance (SID). Therefore, equipment with a larger SID will result in a lower dose to the patient.
  This is of importance both for standard radiography and for fluoroscopy. The recommended source-to-skin distance for an under couch fluoroscopic tube is a minimum of 30 cm and more when possible as the patient dose is very much higher when the tube is close to the table top.[32]
- *Antiscatter grids* reduce scattered radiation reaching the film thus improving the quality of the resulting radiograph and reducing chances of repeat exposures.[18,31]

Fluoroscopy X-ray equipment: According to the AERB safety code, the following have been recommended for fluoroscopy X-ray equipment.[19]

- *Fluoroscopy tube housing and filtration:* Every housing for medical diagnostic X-ray equipment shall be so constructed that leakage radiation through the protective tube housing in any direction, averaged over an area not larger than 100 cm^2 with no linear dimension greater than 20 cm, shall not exceed an air kerma of 1 mGy in one hour at a distance of 1.0 m from the X-ray target when the tube is operating at the maximum rated kVp and for the maximum rated current at that kVp. There shall be a distinctly visible mark on the tube housing to indicate the plane of focus.
- *Protective lead glass:* Protective lead glass covering of the fluorescent screen shall have a lead equivalent thickness of 2.0 mm for units operating up to 100 kVp. For units operating at higher kilovoltages the lead equivalence shall be increased at the rate of 0.01 mm per kVp.
- *Lead rubber flaps:* X-ray table and fluoroscopy screen shall be provided with means of adequate protection for the radiologist and other staff against scattered X-rays. Protective flaps having lead equivalence of not less than 0.5 mm and sufficient dimensions to protect the radiologist shall be so provided that they are suspended from the bottom of the screen such that the flaps overlap the fluoroscopic chair in vertical fluoroscopy, and from the edge of the screen, nearest to the radiologist, such that the flaps extend down to the table top in case of horizontal fluoroscopy. The 'bucky-slot' shall be provided with a cover of 0.5 mm lead equivalence on the radiologist's side.
- *Tube-screen alignment:* X-ray tube and fluoroscopic screen shall be rigidly coupled and aligned so that both move together synchronously and the X-ray beam axis passes through the center of the screen in all positions of the tube and screen.
- *Field limiting diaphragm:* Tube housing should be provided with a field-limiting diaphragm. Its control mechanism should be so mechanically restricted that even when the diaphragm is fully-opened and the screen is at the maximum distance from the table, there is still an unilluminated margin of at least 1 cm all along the edges of the screen. The diaphragm control

knobs shall be located on the frame of the fluorescent screen and provided with local shielding of at least 0.25 mm lead equivalence.

- *Focus-to-table top distance:* The focus-to-table top distance should be not less than 30 cm for fluoroscopy units.
- *Fluoroscopy timer:* The unit shall have a cumulative timer and its maximum range shall not exceed 5 minutes. There shall also be provision for an audible signal at the end of the preset time. Fluoroscopy units should have a built-in cumulative timer device and an audible warning system which rings after a preset fluoroscopy time has elapsed. This can be reset without canceling the recording of the total screening time and radiologists must be aware of the serious patient dose implications if the alarm is reset during the examination such that the screening time exceeds the preset time. The elapsed timer does not ensure safe operation but is of value as a training device for physicians learning the techniques of fluoroscopy and for all users as a means for monitoring the passage of exposure time.
- *Foot-switch and visual indicator:* A foot-operated pressure switch should be provided for conducting fluoroscopy examinations. There should be a visual indication on the control panel when the beam is "ON".
- *Table-top exposure:* The air kerma rate measured at table- top for the minimum focus-to-table top distance shall be as low as possible, and in any case shall not exceed 5 cGy per minutes.
- *Control panel:* Control panel should be provided with means to indicate control and exposure parameters including tube potential, exposure time and tube current/integral exposure in mAs. A clearly marked and identifiable indicator shall be provided at the control panel to show whether the X-ray beam is "ON" or "OFF".

Technique: The use of good radiographic technique and optimum film processing is important for the quality of the image but is also a critical factor in patient dose as repeat exposures to the patient give an additional radiation dose. It must be stressed that repeat images taken due to technical error must be kept to a minimum in order to reduce the patient dose from this unnecessary exposure.

- Optimum film processing helps to avoid repeat examinations.
- *Tube voltage and tube current:* The radiographer can alter the beam quality, that is the penetrating power of the beam, by adjusting the kVp and the beam quantity, which is the number of photons in the primary beam, by adjusting the mA. A higher kVp means that the electrons move faster in the tube current, which results in an increase in the quality of X-rays produced that in turn leads to a more penetrating primary beam. Doses will generally be lower at high kV because of the better penetration of the beam that leads to reduced scatter within the body. A compromise must be sought in order to use the highest kVp possible, so that the dose to the patient is at the lowest possible level, without reducing the image contrast to an unacceptable level. The NCRP recommends that the kVp and mA should be visible to the person doing the fluoroscopy at all times.[32]
- *Screening time and exposure factors:* Significant reduction in radiation dose to the patient can be made by conscious efforts of the practitioner to keep the screening time to a minimum. Intermittent fluoroscopy rather than continuous fluoroscopy is often adequate and should be followed. The screening mA and kV should be kept as low to give an adequate image. During fluoroscopy, the beam should be collimated the smallest that still shows. The magnification mode should be avoided as this increases the dose.

SAFETY OF RADIOGRAPHIC IMAGING DURING PREGNANCY

Ten-day rule: The greatest risk to the fetus of chromosomal abnormalities and subsequent mental retardation is between 8 and 15 weeks of pregnancy and examinations involving radiation to the fetus should be avoided during this period. For examinations in a female of reproductive age group, the radiograph should be carried out during the first 10 days of the menstrual cycle to avoid irradiating any possible pregnancy.

When a patient undergoes diagnostic procedures and subsequently finds she is pregnant, the immediate concern is about abnormalities in the developing fetus. Effects on the fetus may be both deterministic and stochastic. Deterministic effects result from the killing of the cells and there is a threshold dose. Examples are fetal death, gross malformations, mental retardation and growth retardation. Fetal malformations reported in the CNS are exencephaly, microcephaly, mental retardation, skull malformations and hydrocephalus. The ocular malformations reported with radiation are absence of eyes, microphthalmia, absence of lens and cataract. Skeletal malformations are stunting, cleft palate, club feet, deformed arms and spina bifida. Other malformations are genital malformations.[36] Animal data suggest that doses of 5–10 rad (50–100 mGy) received before embryonic implantation may result in prenatal death. Small head size (microcephaly) has been the primary anomaly reported, in children of the survivors of Hiroshima and Nagasaki, who

Table 11: Effects of prenatal exposure.

Gestational stage	Days after conception	Fetal dose		Observed effect
		Rad	mGy	
Perimplantation	0–14	5–10	50–100	Prenatal death
Major organogenesis	8–56	20–25	200–250	Most sensitive stage for growth retardation
	14–105			Small head size; most sensitive time for induction of childhood cancer
Rapid neuron development and migration	56–105	>10	>100	Small head size, seizures, decline in IQ points: 25 points/100 rad (1 Gy)
After organogenesis and rapid neuron development	105–term	>10	>100	Increased risk of childhood cancer
		>50	>500	Severe mental retardation observe at 16–25 wk

sustained in utero radiation exposure. The most sensitive period for this defect is 2–15 weeks after conception. In fetuses who received in utero exposure during the later half of this period, i.e. 8–15 weeks, severe mental retardation and intellectual deficits are also of concern at low doses as low as 10 rad (100 mGy).

Table 11 presents the effects of prenatal exposure as a function of gestational age.[4]

Radiation-induced childhood malignancy caused by in utero radiation exposure is also a concern. Data suggest that a fetus exposed in utero to 1 rad (10 mGy) during the first trimester would be 3.5 times more likely to develop childhood malignancy. In the unexposed population, the frequency of childhood cancer is one in 1500 or 0.07%. Because natural frequency is so low, 3.5 times that value is still quite low (3.5×0.07=0.25%), which leaves a high probability of 99.75% that the child exposed in utero will not develop childhood cancer.[37]

Table 12 gives the recommendation for continuing pregnancy after radiation exposure as a function of gestational age and dose.[37]

RECOMMENDED DOSE LIMITS TO PREGNANT WOMEN[18,19]

The recommendations of various authorities are as follows:

- *ICRP:* In pregnant females, a supplementary equivalent dose limit of 2 mSv applied to the surface of her lower abdomen for the remainder of her pregnancy, once pregnancy is established
- *NCRP:* Recommends dose limit 0.5 mSv per month for the embryo/fetus for occupational pregnant workers
- *AERB:* Recommends that once pregnancy is established, the dose equivalent to surface of pregnant woman's abdomen should not exceed 2 mSv for the remainder of the pregnancy.

Table 12: Fetal absorbed dose.

Gestational age	<5 rad (<50 mGy)	5–15 rad (50–150 mGy)	>15 rad (>150 mGy)
< 2 weeks	Recommended	Recommended	Recommended
2–8 weeks	Recommended	May consider termination (in presence of other risk factors)	May consider termination (in presence of other risk factors)
8–15 weeks	Recommended	May consider termination (in presence of other risk factors)	Higher risk conditions, but termination is not necessarily recommended
15 weeks to term	Recommended	Recommended	Recommended

RADIATION DETECTION AND MEASUREMENT

The instruments used to detect radiation are referred to as radiation detection devices. Instruments used to measure radiation are called radiation dosimeters.

Methods of Detection

There are several methods of detecting radiation, and they are based on physical and chemical effects produced by radiation exposure. These methods are:[31]

- Ionization
- Photographic effect
- Luminescence
- Scintillation.

Ionization

The ability of radiation to produce ionization in air is the basis for radiation detection by the ionization chamber. It consists of an electrode positioned in the middle of a cylinder that contains gas. When X-rays enter the chamber, they ionize the gas to form negative-ions (electrons) and positive-ions (positrons). The electrons are collected by the positively charged rod, while the positive-ions are attracted to the negatively-charged wall of the cylinder. The resulting small current from the chamber is subsequently amplified and measured. The strength of the current is proportional to the radiation intensity.

Photographic Effect

The photographic effect, which refers to the ability of radiation to blacken photographic films, is the basis of detectors that use film (e.g. film badge).

Luminescence

Luminescence describes the property by which certain materials emit light when stimulated by a physiological process, a chemical or electrical action, or by heat. When radiation strikes these materials, the electrons are raised to higher orbital levels. When they fall back to their original orbital level, light is emitted. The amount of light emitted is proportional to the radiation intensity. Lithium fluoride, for example, will emit light when stimulated by heat. This is the fundamental basis of thermo luminescence dosimeter (TLD), a method used to measure exposure to patients and personnel.

Scintillation

Scintillation refers to a flash of light. It is a property of certain crystals, such as sodium iodide and cesium iodide to absorb radiation and convert it to light. This light is then directed to a photomultiplier tube, which then converts the light into an electrical pulse. The size of the pulse is proportional to the light intensity, which is in turn proportional to the energy of the radiation.[18]

PERSONNEL DOSIMETRY

Personnel dosimetry refers to the monitoring of individuals who are exposed to radiation during the course of their work. Personnel dosimetry policies need to be in place for all occupationally-exposed individuals. The data from the dosimeter are reliable only when the dosimeters are properly worn, receive proper care, and are returned on time. Proper care includes not irradiating the dosimeter except during occupational exposure and ensuring proper environmental conditions. Monitoring is accomplished through the use of personnel dosimeters, such as the pocket dosimeter, the film badge or the thermoluminescent dosimeter. The radiation measurement is a time-integrated dose, i.e. the dose summed over a period of time, usually about 3 months. The dose is subsequently stated as an estimate of the effective dose equivalent to the whole body in mSv for the reporting period. Dosimeters used for personnel monitoring have dose measurement limit of 0.1–0.2 mSv (10–20 mrem).[18]

Pocket Dosimeter

The pocket dosimeter monitors dose to personnel. It consists of an ionization chamber with an eyepiece and a transparent scale, as well as a hollow charging-rod and a fixed and a movable fiber. When X-rays enter the dosimeter, ionization causes the fibers to lose their charges and, as a result, the movable fiber moves closer to the fixed fiber. The movable fiber provides an estimate of gamma or X-ray dose rate.

Film Badge Monitoring

- These badges use small double coated X-ray films sand-wiched between several filters to help detect radiation.
- Emulsion on one side is slow and that on the other side is fast.
- The film dosimeter is energy dependent, because silver and bromine have much higher atomic numbers than the tissue or air.

  To identify various components of incident radiation, film badge sandwiches the film between at least 6 pairs of filters **(Fig. 5)**.

  Six type of windows are:
  - Open window: Alpha rays
  - Plastic: Gray- beta rays
  - Cadmium: Yellow-slow neutrons
  - Thin copper: Green-diagnostic X-rays
  - Thick copper: Pink-gamma and therapeutic rays
  - Lead: Black-fast neutrons and gamma rays
- Radiation of a given energy is attenuated to a different extent by various type of absorbers. Therefore, the same quantity of radiation incident on the badge will produce a different degree of darkening under each filter.
- In India, film badges have been replaced by TLD badges.[31]

Thermoluminescent Dosimetry Monitoring

The limitations of the film badge are overcome by the thermoluminescent dosimeter (TLD). Thermoluminescence is the property of certain materials to emit light when they are stimulated by heat. Materials, such as lithium fluoride (LiF), lithium borate ($Li_2B_4O_7$),

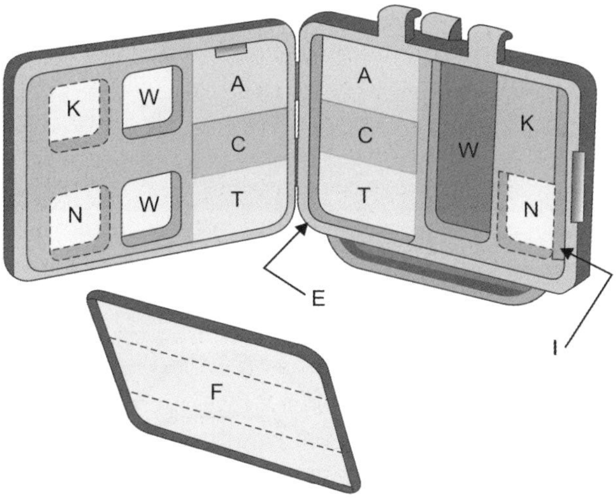

Fig. 5: A film badge.

calcium fluoride (CaF_2), and calcium sulfate ($CaSO_4$) have been used to make TLDs.

- When a LiF crystal is exposed to radiation, a few electrons become trapped in higher energy levels. For these electrons to return to their normal energy levels, the LiF crystal must be heated. As the electrons return to their stable state, light is emitted because of the energy difference between two orbital levels. The amount of light emitted is measured (by a photomultiplier tube) and it is proportional to the radiation dose.[28]
- The measurement of radiation from a TLD is a two-step procedure:
  - In step 1, the TLD is exposed to the radiation
  - In step 2, the LiF crystal is placed in a TLD analyzer, where it is exposed to heat. As the crystal is exposed to increasing temperatures, light is emitted. When the intensity of light is plotted as a function of the temperature, a glow curve results. The glow curve can be used to find out how much radiation energy is received by the crystal because the highest peak and the area under the curve are proportional to the energy of the radiation. These parameters can be measured and converted to dose.

Whereas the TLD can measure exposure to individuals as low as 1.3 μC/kg (5 mR) the pocket dosimeter can measure up to 50 μC/kg (200 mR). The film badge, however, cannot measure exposures less than 2.6 μC/ kg (10 mR). TLDs can withstand a certain degree of heat, humidity, and pressure; their crystals are reusable; and instantaneous readings are possible if the department has a TLD analyzer. The greatest disadvantage of a TLD is its cost.

Table 13: Advantages and disadvantages of electronic dosimeters.

Advantages	***Disadvantages***
Film badges	
Relatively cheap Permanent record of exposure Wide dose ranges (0.2–2000 mSv) Identifies type and energy of exposure Easy to identify individual dosimeters	Requires darkroom and wet processing Lower threshold for hard gamma radiation is 0.15 mSv is affected by heat, humidity and chemicals
TLD badges	
Chips can be reused Wide dose range (0.1–2000 mSv) Direct reading of personal dose Energy independent within ± 10% Compact: suitable for finger dosimetry	Requires high capital initially No permanent record (other than glow curves cannot distinguish radioactive contamination)
Electronic personal dosimeter	
Direct reading and cumulative record storage (up to16Sv) Flat response (20 keV to 10 MeV) can be 'zeroed' by user without deleting cumulative record Measures personal dose at depth and at the skin directly to 1 micro Sv audible warning at high-dose rates	Requires a filtered badge to provide energy discrimination High cost Linear response to dose is quite heavy Battery should be renewed every year

Electronic Dosimeters

- Direct reading electronic dosimeters based on Geiger-Muller tubes or single silicon diodes
- It can provide immediate dose readings and effective alarms when dose limit is exceeded
- The sensitivity is 50–200 times that of TLD badges
- The advantages and disadvantages can be tabulated as in **Table 13.**[11,28]

Wearing the Dosimeter

During Radiography

During radiography (when no protective lead apron is worn), the personnel dosimeter is worn at one of two regions:

1. On the trunk of the body at the level of the waist.
2. On the upper chest region at the level of the collar area outside the lead apron.

At these positions, the dosimeter readings represent an estimate of exposure at two different levels, i.e. the whole body exposure is estimated by the trunk level badge and exposures dose to internal organs like thyroid is measured by the collar level badge.

During Fluoroscopy

During fluoroscopy, a protective apron should always be worn. It is further recommended that ideally, two dosimeters should be worn by radiation personnel, one at the collar level outside the lead apron and the other at the level of trunk underneath the lead apron.

The one at the collar level gives an accurate estimate of the radiation dose to the unprotected regions of head and neck. The dosimeter worn underneath the lead apron at the trunk level provides an accurate estimate of the radiation to the protected organs. If only one dosimeter is worn, it must be worn at the collar outside the lead apron, because, the neck receives 10–20 times more radiation than the trunk which is protected by lead.

COMPUTED TOMOGRAPHY (RADIATION EXPOSURE AND DOSE MODULATIONS)

Radiation Dose Measures: CT Specific

Because of its geometry and usage, CT is a unique modality and therefore, has its own set of specific parameters for radiation dose. This modality is unique because the exposure is essentially continuous around the patient, rather than a projectional modality in which the exposure is taken from one or two source locations.[37]

Projectional radiographic exposures are taken from one source position and the entrance skin dose is much larger than the exit skin dose, creating a large radiation dose gradient across the patient **(Fig. 6)**.

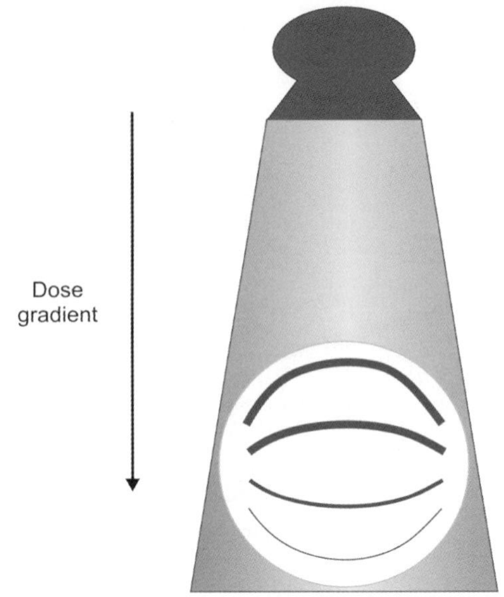

Fig. 6: Dose gradient resulting from a projectional radiographic exposure in which the source is stationary at one position. The thicker lines represent the entrance skin dose, which is much larger than the exit skin dose, represented by the thinner lines. This difference creates a linear difference through the patient.[37]

Conventional Radiographic Projections

In contrast, the tomographic exposure of CT scans with a full 360° rotation results in a radially symmetric radiation dose gradient within the patient.

CT Radiation Projections

However, there is a radial dose gradient which exists in computed tomography scanning **(Fig. 7)**.

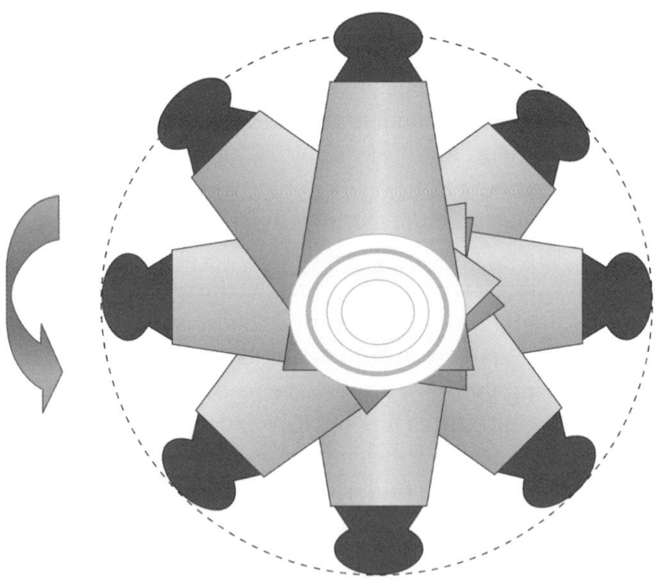

Fig. 7: Dose gradient resulting from a full 360° exposure from a CT scan. The thicker lines represent the entrance skin dose, which is much larger than the dose at the inner radius, represented by the thinner lines. This difference results in a radially symmetric radiation dose gradient within the patient.[37]

TYPICAL DOSE MEASUREMENTS

The radial dose gradient (the size of the difference from center to periphery) will be affected by several factors, including the size of the object, the X-ray beam spectrum, and the attenuation of the material or tissue **(Fig. 8)**.[37]

In addition to the variations within the scan plane, there are variations along the length of the patient or phantom. These can be characterized by the z-axis dose distribution or radiation profile **(Fig. 9)**. The radiation profile is not limited to the primary area being imaged, and there are tails to this distribution from the nonideal collimation of the X-ray source and from scatter of photons within the object being exposed. These contributions can add-up, creating additional absorbed dose in the primary area being imaged.

To account for the effects from multiple scans, several dose descriptors were developed.[37] These are as follows:

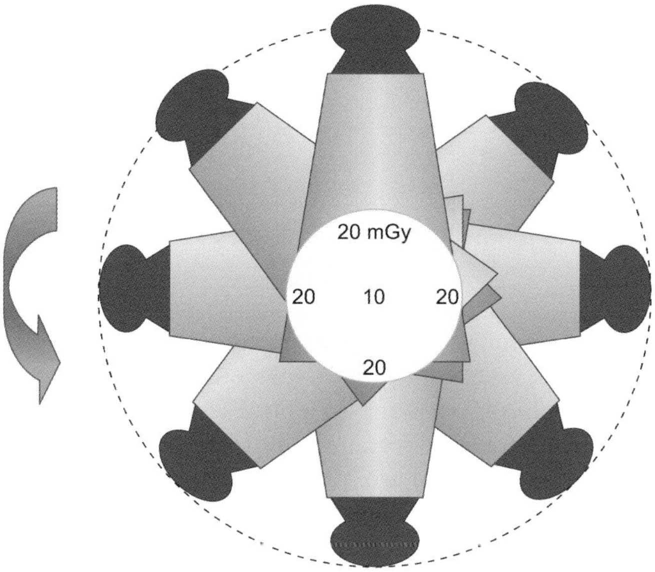

Fig. 8: Typical dose measurements in a 32 cm diameter (body) phantom from a single detector CT scan.[37]

- Multiple scan average dose (MSAD)
- Computed tomography dose index (CTDI)
- $CTDI_{100}$
- $CTDI_W$
- $CTDI_{vol}$
- Dose length product

Multiple Scan Average Dose

This is defined as the average dose resulting from a series of scans over an interval *I* in length.[38]

$$MSAD = (1/I)\int_{-\pi 2}^{\pi 2} D\ series(z)dz$$

where '*I*' is the interval of the scan length and '*D* series(*z*)' is the dose at position *z* parallel to the z (rotational)-axis resulting from the series of CT scans.

Computed Tomography Dose Index (CTDI)

It is defined as the radiation dose normalized to beam width measured from 14 contiguous sections.[39]

$$CTDI = (1/nT)\int_{-\pi}^{\pi} D\ single(z)dz$$

where *n* is the number of sections per scan, *T* is the width of the interval equal to the selected section thickness, and D single(*z*) is the dose at point *z* on any line parallel to the z (rotational) axis for a single axial scan.

However, to be measured according to the definition, only 14 sections could be measured and one had to measure the radiation dose profile—typically done with thermoluminescent dosimeters (TLDs) or film, neither of which was very convenient. Measurement of exposure could be done with pencil ionization chamber but its fixed

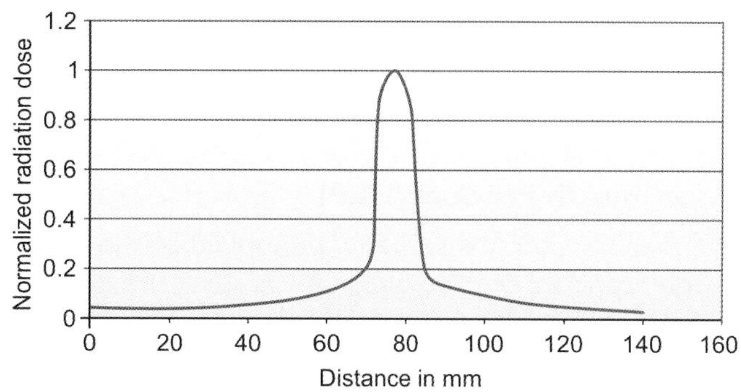

Fig. 9: Radiation profile of a full-rotation CT scan measured at isocenter. This profile is the distribution of radiation dose along the axis of the patient (the z-axis) and is known as D(z).

length of 100 mm meant that only 14 sections of 7 mm thickness could be measured with that chamber alone.

To overcome the limitations of CTDI with 14 sections, another radiation dose index—$CTDI_{100}$—was developed.

$CTDI_{100}$

This index relaxed the constraint on 14 sections and allowed calculation of the index for 100 mm along the length of an entire pencil ionization chamber.[38] This index can be measured and calculated for the center location as well as at least one of the peripheral positions.[40]

$$CTDI_{100} = (1/NT)\int_{-5\,cm}^{5\,cm} D\ series(z)dz$$

where '*N*' is the number of acquired sections per scan (also referred to as the number of data channels used during acquisition) and '*T*' is the nominal width of each acquired section.

$CTDI_W$

$CTDI_w$ was created to represent a dose index that provides a weighted average of the center and peripheral contributions to dose within the scan plane. This index is used to overcome the limitations of $CTDI_{100}$ and its dependency on position within the scan plane.

$$CTDI_w = (1/3)(CTDI_{100})_{center} + (2/3)(CTDI_{100})_{periphery}$$

$CTDI_{vol}$

One final CTDI descriptor takes into account the parameters that are related to a specific imaging protocol, the helical pitch or axial scan spacing, and is defined as $CTDI_{vol}$.

$$CTDI_{vol} = CTDI_w \times NT/I$$

where *N* is the number of acquired sections per scan and and *T* is the nominal width of each acquired section. The product of $N \times T$ is meant to reflect.

The total nominal width of the X-ray beam during acquisition and I is the table travel per rotation for a helical scan. Hence $NT/I = 1/\text{pitch}$

and $CTDI_{vol} = CTDI_w/\text{pitch}$.

Dose-length Product (DLP)

This value is simply the $CTDI_{vol}$ multiplied by the length of the scan (in centimeters) and is given in units of milligray-centimeters:

$$DLP = CTDI_{vol} \times \text{scan length}$$ [41]

This descriptor is used to obtain an estimate of effective dose.

The DLP values are easily converted to millisieverts by using conversion factors specific to the anatomic region imaged: the conversion factors listed by the American Association of Physicists in Medicine for the chest, abdomen, and pelvis are 0.014, 0.015, and 0.015.[42] These conversion factors are periodically updated, so care should be taken to apply the most recent ones **(Table 14)**.

Table 14: Effective radiation doses calculated from DLP values in a routine oncologic CT examination of the abdomen and pelvis.[43]

Region scanned	*DLP (mGy·cm)*	*Conversion factor*	*Effective dose (mSv)*
Abdomen and pelvis (portal venous phase)	681	0.015	10.2
Kidneys (delayed phase)	230	0.015	3.5
Bladder (delayed phase)	214	0.015	3.2

Techniques for Controlling Radiation Dose at CT

Multidetector CT protocols can be directly modified in a variety of ways. These include using an automated exposure control system or modifying individual acquisition parameters, such as the number of phases, section thickness, peak voltage (kVp setting), tube current–time product, and pitch.

USING AUTOMATED EXPOSURE CONTROL

Automated exposure control (AEC) systems are designed to reduce the radiation dose by dynamically altering the tube current as the X-ray tube rotates around the patient during multidetector CT scanning. The tube current is automatically modulated according to the attenuation level (i.e. the size) of the patient.[44] For smaller patients, i.e. the pediatric patients, the tube current is automatically decreased to adapt to the lower attenuation level. Conversely, the tube current is appropriately increased for larger patients. Use of AEC is an efficient way to tailor radiation dose to achieve a target image quality.

MODIFYING THE ACQUISITION PARAMETERS

Acquisition parameters, such as the number of scanning phases and the section thickness may be modified to achieve deeper dose reductions even when an automated exposure control system is used.

If CT angiography-venography protocol initially includes four scanning phases (precontrast), postcontrast arterial phase, postcontrast portal venous phase, and postcontrast delayed scanning), by decreasing the number of scanning phases to two (postcontrast arterial phase and slightly later portal venous phase), the radiation dose can be reduced by 50%.

The acquisition section thickness also has an important effect on image noise and, consequently, on the amount of radiation needed to meet the preset noise value. With regard to section thickness at 64-row multidetector CT, if the section thickness of 5 mm were decreased to 2.5 mm, Kanal et al. found, the noise index of 15.3 would have to be increased to 23.4 to keep the dose constant. Conversely, if the noise index were kept constant at 15.3, the relative dose with 2.5 mm thick sections would be approximately 2.3 times that with 5 mm thick sections.[45]

Reducing the Milliampere-seconds Value

The radiation dose is linear with milliampere seconds value, when all other factors are held constant, so the milliampere-seconds value is reduced by 50%, the radiation dose will be reduced by the same amount. However, this reduction will increase image noise by $1/\sqrt{(\text{mAs})}$, which means that a 50% reduction in the milliampere-seconds value results in a noise increase of 41%.

For example, detection of high-contrast objects in the lung may not require a low-noise imaging protocol and the reduction in milliampere-seconds may be well-tolerated. On the other hand, imaging low-contrast lesions in the liver does require a low-noise imaging protocol and the reduction in milliampere-seconds may limit the ability to detect these lesions.

Increasing Pitch

The radiation dose is inversely proportional to pitch. Increasing the pitch decreases the dose, increases the image noise, increases the effective section thickness, and reduces the scanning time.[46] The trade-off in increasing pitch is an increase in effective section thickness, which results in increased volume averaging, which in turn may reduce the image signal. The ability to use this type of dose reduction again depends on the clinical applications.

Varying the Milliampere-seconds Value by Patient Size

Computed tomography is an example of a digital modality in which the image quality continues to improve as the exposure increases. This is contrasted with analog projectional film, in which too high of an exposure results in an overexposed (too dark). However, the radiation dose to the smaller patient is potentially higher than is necessary to obtain a diagnostic image. Therefore, significant effort has recently been put into developing size- and weight-based imaging protocols. This has typically been in the form of a reduced milliampere-seconds value for reduced patient size and has led to the development of suggested technique charts for pediatric patients.

Optimum Tube Potential[47]

Use of an optimum tube potential may help improve image quality or reduce radiation dose particularly in pediatric CT examination. The main benefit of a lower tube potential is that it provides improved contrast enhancement, a characteristic that may compensate for the increase in noise that often occurs at lower tube potential and may allow radiation dose to be substantially reduced. The use of a lower tube potential should be carefully evaluated for each type of examination to achieve an optimum trade-off among contrast, noise, artifacts and scanning time.[47]

ITERATIVE RECONSTRUCTION

Computed tomography scanner vendors have been working to develop various image reconstruction techniques as alternatives to traditional filtered back projection for reducing image noise.

One such technique is iterative reconstruction, which is also known by the trade names iDose (Philips), iterative reconstruction in image space (IRIS; Siemens), adaptive iterative dose reduction (AIDR; Toshiba, Tochigi, Japan), and adaptive statistical iterative reconstructions (ASIR GE health care).[43] For example, the selection of "ASIR 30%" results in a combination of 70% filtered back projection data and 30% adaptive statistical iterative reconstruction data.

Ongoing development of iterative reconstruction techniques holds promise for achieving even lower levels of image noise, which will allow further reductions in radiation dose.

CONCLUSION

When used under properly controlled conditions, radiation is a safe and indispensable tool for medical diagnosis. Proper radiation safety management should ensure that radiologists and clinicians are knowledgeable about typical patient doses that are important in each type of radiologic examination and about the factors that affect these doses. This should ensure a judicious requisition for a radiological examination as well as help keep doses as low as possible while still creating optimum diagnostic quality images.

REFERENCES

1. Engel Hells P. Radiation protection in medical imaging. Radiography. 2006;12:153-60.
2. Millew RW. Delayed effects of external radiation exposure: a brief history. Radiation research. 1995;144:160-9.
3. Brateman L. Radiation safety considerations for diagnostic radiology personnel. Radiographics. 1999;19:1037-55.
4. Parry RA, Glaze SA, Archer BR. Typical patient radiation doses in diagnostic radiology. Radiographics. 1999;19: 1289-302.
5. International Commission on Radiological Protection. Recommendations of the ICRP. ICRP publication no. 26 Ann ICRP 1(3) Oxford, England Peragamon, 1977.
6. International Commission on Radiological Protection. Recommendations of the ICRP. ICRP publication no. 60 Ann ICRP 21(1-3) Oxford, England Peragamon, 1990.
7. National Council on Radiation Protection and Measurements. Limitation of exposure to ionizing radiation. NCRP report no 116, Bethesda Md:NCRP, 1993.
8. Strahlenschutzkommision: Orientierungshilfe fur radiologische und nuklearmedizinische. Untersuchungen Heft 30, Berlin H Hoffman 2006.
9. Shannoun F, Blettner M, et al. Radiation protection in diagnostic radiology. Dtsch Arztebl Int. 2008;105(3): 41-6.
10. Hricak H, Brenner DJ, Adelstein SJ, et al. Managing radiation dose in medical imaging: a multifaceted challenge. Radiology. 2011;258(3):889-905.
11. Selman Joseph. The Fundamentals of X-ray and Radium Physics, 7th Edn. Charles Thomas Publisher; 1985. pp.184-94.
12. Travis E. Bioeffects of radiation. In: Seeram E (Ed). Radiation Protection. Philadelphia; New York: Lippincott; 1997. pp. 73-81.
13. Sinclair WK. Radiation protection recommendations on dose limits: the role of the NCRP and the ICRP and future develop-ments. Int J Radiation Oncology Biol Phy. 1995;31(2): 387-92.
14. Schwenn MR, Brill AB. Childhood cancers 10 years after the Chernobyl accident. Curr Opin Pediatr. 1997;9(1):51-4.
15. Hall EJ. Radiobiology for the Radiologist, 4th edn, Philadelphia: JB Lippincott Company; 1994. pp. 419-52.

16. Cho LC, Glatstein E. Radition injury. In: Fauci AS, Braunwald E, Isselbacher KJ, et al (Eds). Harrison's Principles of Internal Medicine, 14th edn, New York: Hill; 1998. pp. 2259-504.
17. Rubin P, Constine LS, Williams JP. Late effects of cancer treatment: radiation and drug toxicity In: Perez CA, Brady LW (Eds). Principles and Practice of Radiation Oncology, 3rd Edn, Philadelphia, New York:Lippincott Raven; 1998. pp. 155-211.
18. Seeram E, Travis EC. Radiation protection. Philadelphia, New York: Lippincott; 1997.
19. AERB safety Code (Code no AERB/SE/MED-2), Mumbai; 2001; 1-20.
20. International Commission on Radiological Protection. Recommendations of the International Commission on Radiological Protection. ICRP publication. Oxford: Peragamon Press; 1991;60.
21. Shrimpton PC, Wall BF, Croft JR, Webb GAM. Medical exposure guidance on the 1990 recommendations of ICRP. Documents of NRPB. 1999;4(2):43-80.
22. Goldstone K, Yates SJ. Radiation issues governing radiation protection and patient doses in diagnostic imaging. In: Adam A, Dixon AK, Grainger RG, Allison DJ (Eds). Grainger and Allison's Diagnostic Radiology: A Textbook of Medical Imaging, 5th edn. New York: Churchill Livingstone; 2008. pp.159-71.
23. Burniston B. The barium enema—worthwhile examination? Radiography Today. 1993;59(675):4-12.
24. National Council on Radiation Protection and Measurements. Implementation of the principle of As Low As Reasonably Achievable (ALARA) for medical and dental personnel. NCRP report no 107, Bethesda, Md: NCRP, 1990.
25. Webb GAM. The requirement to keep radiation exposures as low as reasonably practicable (ALARP). London HMSO, National Radiological Protection Board (NRPB/P/B)1984.
26. Wall BF, Fisher S, Shrimpton PC, Rae S. Current levels of gonadal irradiation from a selection of routine X-ray examination in Great Britain Harwell: National Radiological Protection Board (NRPB – R 105)1980.
27. Simpkin DJ, Dixon RL. Secondary shielding barriers for diagnostic X-ray facilities: scatter and leakage revisited. Health Phys. 1998;74(3):350-65.
28. Christensen. Radiation protection. In: Curry TS, Dowdey JE, Murry RC (Eds). Christensen's Physics of Diagnostic Radiology, 4th edn. Philadelphia: London; 1990.
29. Shymko MJ. Minimizing occupational exposure. Radiologic Technology. 1998;70(1):89-90.
30. Wagner LK, Hayman LA. Pregnancy and women radiologists. Radiology. 1982;145:559-62.
31. Grover SB, Kumar J, Gupta A, et al. Protection against radiation hazards: regulatory bodies, safety norms, dose limits and protection devices. Indian J Radiol Imaging. 2002;12: 157-67.
32. National Council on Radiation Protection and Measurements. Medical X-ray, electron beam and gamma X-ray protection for energies up to 50 meV (equipment design, performance and use). Bethesda: NCRP publications (NCRP report no 102); 1989.
33. Sprawl P Jr. Physical Principles of Medical Imaging, 2nd Edn. Gaitherberg Md: Aspen; 1993.pp.165-7.
34. Graham DT, Cloke P. Principles of Radiological Physics, 4th edn. Edinburg:Churchill Livingstone; 2003. pp. 325-38.
35. Bushong SC. Radiological Science for Technologists, Physics Biology and Protection, 6th edn. St Louis year book; 1997. pp.442-7.
36. Steenvoorde P, Pauwels EKJ, Harding LK, et al. Diagnostic nuclear medicine and risk for the fetus. Eur J Nucl Med. 1998; 25:193-9.
37. McNitt Gray. Radiation dose in CT. Radiographics. 2002;22: 1541-53.
38. Jucius RA, Kambic GX. Radiation dosimetry in computed tomography. Appl Opt Instrum Eng Med. 1977;127:286-95.
39. Shope TB, Gange RM, Johnson GC. A method for describing the doses delivered by transmission. X-ray Computed Tomography Med Phys. 1991;8:488-95.
40. McCollough CM, Schueler BA. Calculation of effective dose. Med Phys. 2000;27:838-44.
41. Shrimpton PC, Edyvean S. CT scanner dosimetry. Br J Radiol. 1998;71:1-3.
42. American Association of Physicists in Medicine. The measurement, reporting and management of radiation dose in CT. Report no 96, College park Md: American Association of Physicists in Medicine, 2008.
43. Tamm EP, Rong XJ, Coly D, et al. CT radiation dose reduction: how to implement change without sacrificing diagnostic quality. Radiographics. 2011;31:1823-32.
44. Lee CH, Goo JM, Lee HJ, et al. Radiation dose modulation technique in multidetector CT era: from basics to practice. Radiographics. 2008;28:1451-9.
45. Kanal KM, Stewart BK, Kolokythas O, et al. Impact of operator selected image noise index and reconstruction slice thickness on patient radiation dose in 64 MDCT. AJR. 2007;189(1):219-25.
46. Primak AN, McCollough CH, Bruesewitz MR, et al. Relationship between noise, dose and pitch in cardiac multidetector row CT. Radiographics. 2006;26(6):1785-94.
47. Yu L, Bruesewitz M, Thomas KB, et al. Optimal tube potential for radiation dose reduction in Pediatric CT: principles, clinical implementations and pitfalls. Radiographics. 2011;31: 835-48.

CHAPTER 62

Planning a Modern Imaging Department

SC Bansal, Niranjan Khandelwal, Ajay Gulati

INTRODUCTION

During recent years, there has been increasing recognition that diagnostic imaging is an integral part of modern health care. Perhaps more than any other clinical service diagnostic imaging has been transformed by developments in information technology fueled by digital information technologies over the last thirty years. This has enabled earlier, more accurate diagnosis and more appropriate interventions for almost all major health conditions.

It is important to recognize that diagnostic imaging is not a technical service, but a clinical service that interprets information and requires the clinical expertise of imaging clinicians, who are increasingly making decisions about the management of patient care. There is increasing recognition of the need to place imaging early in care pathways to reduce the time to diagnosis and treatment and to improve efficiency and effectiveness.[1]

Most diagnostic imaging is carried out in clinical radiology departments, which deliver a range of services either within a hospital or as a stand-alone center. Apart from providing routine and specialized diagnostic services with various imaging techniques for indoor, outpatients and walk-in patients, the modern departments also provides therapeutic services like interventional radiology (minimally invasive treatments performed with imaging guidance). This acts as a big source of revenue generation for a hospital or a stand-alone center with high profitability.[2]

PLANNING AND ORGANIZATION

With rapid advancements in investigative technology, there is a continuous changing demand in the field of radiodiagnosis and imaging service resulting in an advanced and detailed systematic planning and organization for launching a modern imaging department. An understanding of what has changed—and what has not—is essential to developing safe, productive and comfortable imaging departments.

Launching a new diagnostic and therapeutic imaging center involves very specific requirements and roadmaps that have a direct impact on planning. The essential first step is to do a critical project analysis. Doing a cost-benefit analysis and determining if the return on the investment will be positive are important for a project's success. Good planning and communication with key staff members of the healthcare institution and the members of the design and construction team will help ensure successful implementation of any project. Analyzing the requirements for imaging equipment, space and personnel are other necessary steps. These are followed by scheduling and designing various aspects of the project.[3]

There are three horizontal levels of workflow (strategic, managerial and operational) in any organization, whether it is a government hospital or multinational corporate running a hospital. Planning must focus on the strategic level of decision making. The second level is the managerial or administrative level which focuses on daily issues such as employee attendance and productivity, patient backlogs, staff scheduling and reassignments. The operational level is where the work actually gets done in any organization **(Fig. 1)**.[4]

The major objectives of a radiology department include the following:

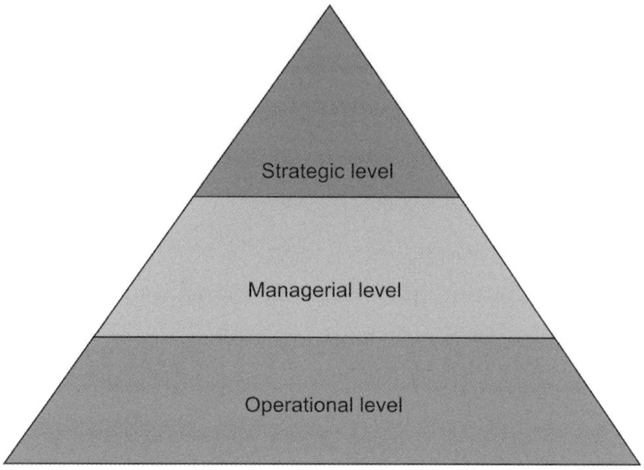

Fig. 1: Levels of radiological workflow.

- To provide comprehensive high quality imaging service
- Establishment and confirmation of clinical diagnosis
- Providing high quality therapeutic/interventional radiology
- Commitment to training and research.

Divisions of the Radiology Department

Radiology department generally has diagnostic as well as therapeutic sections.

The major components of radiology/imaging services are as follows:

- Radiography (X-ray machines/CR and DR System)
- Mammography
- Dual-energy X-ray absorptiometry (DEXA)
- Computed tomography (scan CT)
- Ultrasound and color Doppler
- Magnetic resonance imaging (MRI)
- Digital substraction angiography (DSA)
- Nuclear imaging systems.

To manage such large number of sophisticated machines whose rays/emissions are hazardous to healthcare calls for a critical planning taking in to consideration the safety aspect of patient, public and the department staff.[5]

LOCATION

The location of the department and the relative positions of the examination rooms have a considerable bearing upon the protection requirements. Aspects for planning are accessibility, convenience, privacy and traffic flow considerations, etc. i.e. that should be well connected. Accessibility towards OPD and emergency is a major point of consideration for this department. Central location on the ground floor with some space for future expansion is essential to allow upgradation and augmentation of services.[2] The location should be 10 meters away from the elevators due to their effect on the functioning of equipment in the department.[5]

The correct design of medical imaging facilities will reduce radiation and nonradiation hazards and contribute to the care and wellbeing of patients and staff. It is the general responsibility of the medical imaging service to ensure the optimum design of their facility and to ensure that there is no radiation risk to anyone working or waiting in any room adjoining the radiation zone. Therefore, strategic planning must be done to have a clear understanding of the operations in the department (staff movement, patient flow, material flow, technical procedures). Special attention to minor details related to operations can have significant impact on staff effectiveness and morale. Study of traffic patterns is the key to the efficiency of an imaging department. This study should be based on interactive discussions with the staff of the department and should consider the various activities like:[6]

- Movement of patients in and out of procedure rooms
- Activity sequence within procedure rooms
- Film processing and handling
- Image interpretation and reporting
- Filing.

LAYOUT

The layout of the department depends on the great extent the way the processes in the department are aligned and take place. Layout shall be prepared as per the AERB guidelines for layout and shielding of X-ray equipment. Planning should be done to create a safe, pleasant and efficient staff work environment. For a safe radiation environment, there are certain principles and considerations like "separation" of different functional areas helps control access:

- Public areas (waiting room, changing rooms, etc.)
- Staff areas (offices, reporting rooms, etc.)
- Work areas (radiation rooms, console rooms, labs, etc.)[2]

Corridors and doors leading to all patient areas and examination rooms should allow easy and safe movement of all patients, including handicapped or injured. Availability of toilet facilities is essential, particularly those suitable for handicapped patients. Also, the provision of safe storage facilities for patients' clothing and valuables during imaging is necessary.[6]

EQUIPMENT

The equipment used in this department are highly sophisti-cated and expensive. Major equipment are described below:

Conventional Radiography

The most important and easily performed imaging service in the front line of medical care is plain radiography. The X-ray unit must be able to perform all essential general radiographic examinations like chest, abdomen and extremities. Information is represented in the analog or continuous form rather than a discrete fashion. In conventional radiography, majority of the radiographic examinations have been carried out by projecting the beam through the patient allowing the transmitted beam to strike X-ray film or Intensifying screen to produce the latent image. Thelatent image can be made visible and permanent by processing the film with suitable chemicals **(Fig. 2)**.

Darkroom

When designing a darkroom, beside the operational considerations concerning the film development, the primary concern is the shielding of unexposed film from exposure to radiation (X-rays and daylight). The common location for a main darkroom is central in the imaging department. All construction provisions must be made to ensure that all potential openings to the outside are light tight (doors, ventilation, pass through, windows). Dry and wet areas should be separate from each other and chemicals must be stored safely.[6]

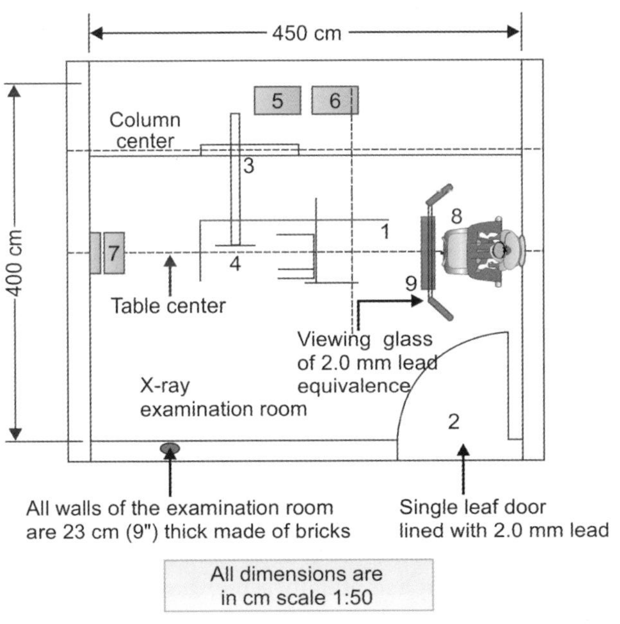

1. Examination table; 2. Spot film device; 3. Column stand; 4. X-ray tube head; 5 and 6. Unit electronics; 7. Chest stand; 8. Control unit; 9. MPB with lead glass viewing window of 1.7 mm lead equivalence

Fig. 2: Model Layout—X-ray installation.

Digital Radiography

Digital radiography is a form of X-ray imaging where digital X-ray sensors are used instead of radiography film. Digital radiography systems are replacing films in the modern departments. It is a representation of continuous analog information into digital form by the use of computer which processes the digital data to form an image. It not only has revolutionized communication between radiologists and clinicians, but also has improved image quality and allowed for further reduction of patient exposure. However, digital radiography also poses risks, such as unnoticed increase in patient dose and suboptimum image processing that may lead to suppression of diagnostic information. Advanced processing techniques, such as temporal subtraction, dual energy subtraction and computer-aided detection (CAD) will play an increasing role in the future and are all targeted to decrease the influence of distracting anatomic background structures and to ease the detection of focal and subtle lesions.[7]

The two most important objective performance measures to describe digital radiography systems with respect to dose requirements and detail resolution are the modulation transfer function (MTF) and the detector quantum efficiency (DQE).[8] DQE describes the efficiency of a detector to generate signal from X-ray quanta. MTF is a measure of image quality of an imaging system with respect to structural contrast and spatial resolution. Optimizing MTF and DQE simultaneously is a challenge: thicker detector material, for example, will improve absorption (thus, DQE), but generally also will induce more blur (deteriorate MTF).

The following sections discuss recent developments for the three main digital detector technologies: storage phosphors (computed radiography; CR), flat-panel detectors (digital radiography; DR) and charge-coupled device (CCD) detectors.

Storage Phosphor Radiography (Computed Radiography)

Computed radiography (CR) systems use storage-phosphor image plates having a detective layer of photostimulable crystals and separate image readout process.[9] A major advantage of CR systems is that they are cost effective way to getting digital images since they allow reutilization of existing X-ray equipment. CR cassettes utilize storage phosphors where electrons are trapped during exposure and subsequently extracted through a laser scanner.[10] Standard CR systems use a single laser beam and a detector screen covered with an amorphous (powder-based) detector material.

Dual-reading Computed Radiography Systems

Dual-reading CR systems are based on transparent detector material and employ light collection optics in the front and the back side of the detector. It improves quantum detection (DQE) and has only a minimum deteriorating effect on spatial resolution (MTF).[11]

Parallel Reading (Line Scanning)

Traditional CR scanners use principle of flying spot scanning for readout where a tightly focused laser beam stimulates the latent image in a moving storage phosphor plate one point at a time over the entire screen surface. Parallel reading employs a linear array of laser diodes (linear-line laser diode) that reads out all pixels in one line simultaneously, therefore speeding up the process tremendously. The dual side the reading and line scanning reading with columnar phosphors provide remarkable improvement compared to conventional CR systems and yield results comparable to most digital detectors for radiography.[10]

Needle-crystalline Computed Radiography Detectors

A new crystalline detector material (CsBr:Eu2+) for storage phosphor systems allows for creating a thicker detector layer (better DQE) without deteriorating spatial resolution (MTF). The principle is similar to that of indirect flat panel systems (CsI-photodiode/TFT detectors).

Flat-panel Direct Detector Systems

Two different DR technologies are available, both of which are based on TFT matrix arrays. Indirect conversion systems or opto-direct systems use a scintillator (e.g. cesium iodide, CsI or gadolinium oxysulphide, GOS or Gadox) layered on top of an array with light-sensitive photodiodes with thin-film transistors (TFTs). The scintillator converts radiation into light that is detected by the photodiode/TFT array. CsI-photodiode/TFT systems are widely used for chest radiography and provide better DQE than standard CR or Gadox-TFT systems **(Figs. 3 and 4)**.[12,13]

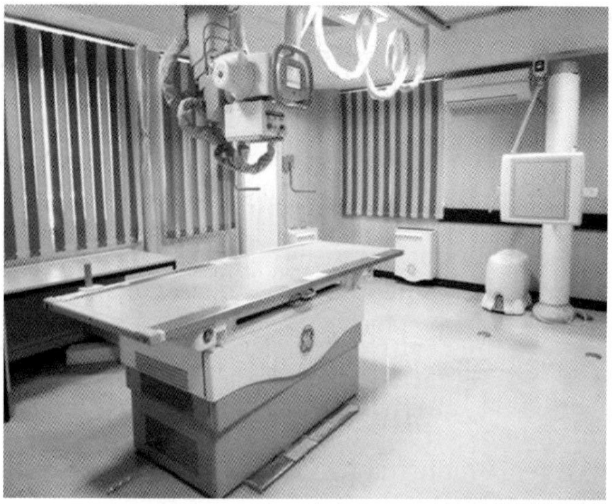

Fig. 3: Dual-reading flat panel X-ray unit.

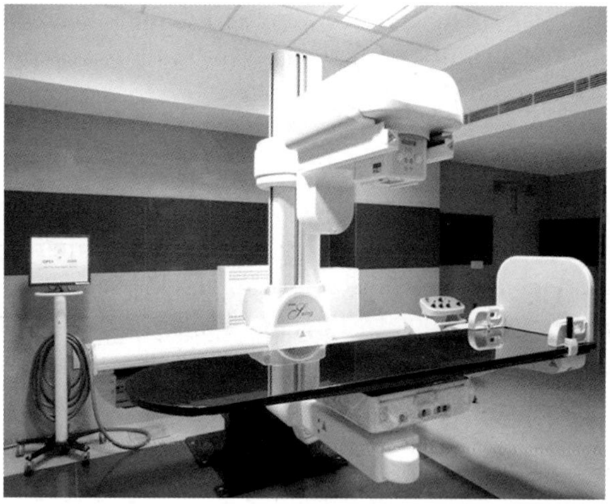

Fig. 4: Dual-reading and fluoroscopy unit (flat panel).

Direct conversion systems or electro-direct systems use a photo conducting layer (amorphous selenium, a-Se), in which the absorbed X-ray energy is directly converted into charge on top of a TFT array. These systems are excellent for the high spatial frequencies required for mammography, but because they absorb less X-ray energy, they suffer from a lower-dose efficiency (DQE), which makes them less suited for chest radiography.[12,14]

Charge-coupled Device Detector Technology

The light emitted by a scintillator screen has to be collimated to the CCD by optical coupling (demagnification), which can reduce dose efficiency and degrade image quality.[15] Recent improvements in coupling mechanism and use of larger CCD sensors have made these systems more attractive for chest radiography.[16]

Slot-scanning Charge-coupled Device Technology

No demagnification is required for slot-scanning CCD technology: a CsI scintillator is coupled to a linear array of CCDs that covers the whole slot that is used to scan the chest. The increased signal to noise yielded by scatter reduction effectively compensates for the 2.5 times lower intrinsic DQE of CCD technology.[17] The increased SNR can be used to improve image quality or to reduce patient dose.

The most advanced processing algorithms aim at analyzing images (CAD), selectively enhancing bones and soft tissues (dual-energy subtraction), and at visualizing change at follow-up (temporal subtraction).

Computer-aided Diagnosis

Computer-aided diagnosis (CAD) programs have the goal to aid the radiologist in detecting or differentiating various disease entities in the chest. Usually the system suggests a lesion or abnormal region that then has to be verified by the radiologist.

Dual-energy Subtraction

Dual-energy subtraction radiography involves taking a chest exposure at two different X-ray energies. By exploiting the difference in energy dependence of attenuation between bone and soft tissue, either bone or soft tissues can be eliminated by locally weighted subtraction of the two images. Dual-energy subtraction allows for differentiation of calcified and noncalcified lesions, improved detection of nodules and masses, especially in critical areas, and improved detection of rib lesions.[18,19]

Temporal Subtraction

Temporal subtraction is a processing technique based on the matching and subsequent subtraction of a follow-up radiograph and a baseline image.

Digital Tomosynthesis

Digital tomosynthesis is a medical imaging technique using a flat panel detector and tube rotation producing a series of slices at different depths. These projection images are subsequently shifted and added to bring objects in a given plane into focus, while other structures are spread across the image and are rendered with varying amounts of blur.[20] Most developments in tomosynthesis have been in breast imaging, but orthopedic, chest and urinary applications have also been used.[21]

X-ray equipment fall broadly into two groups portable/ mobile and fixed:

Portable radiography equipment means the X-ray unit is capable of being taken to the destination to be used. It is very simple to use and can be packed into carrying cases and so transported. Portable sets relatively have low mA setting, can be dismantled for transfer. The word "mobile" means that X-ray equipment is capable of being moved. It is mounted on the wheels and can be pushed by human power. It is larger and heavier than portable sets and need to be motorized or pushed between locations. It cannot be separated into smaller components and cannot be taken outside the hospital. Mobile sets have high MA value.

The digital mobile units are the ultimate solution to mobile X-ray imaging for digitalization in emergency rooms (ER), traumatology, intensive care units (ICU), in patient wards and pediatrics. These systems represents an evolutionary move in mobile diagnostic imaging equipment and include unique features in terms of operability, mobility and image quality.[22,23]

Wireless FPDs: Wireless portable DR system is now a reality. After exposure, it wirelessly transfer image data to the DR system. Alternatively the image data can be transferred to DR console via an Ethernet cable. It has no cables and does not interfere with surrounding machines, so it is easy to handle as a CR cassettes.[24] Typically a 17" × 14" image size is made available within 3 seconds **(Fig. 5)**.

Mobile Image Intensifiers Units

Mobile unit for fluoroscopy with an image intensifier is generally used in operating theater. This reduces the number of radiographs taken and saves the time during surgery.

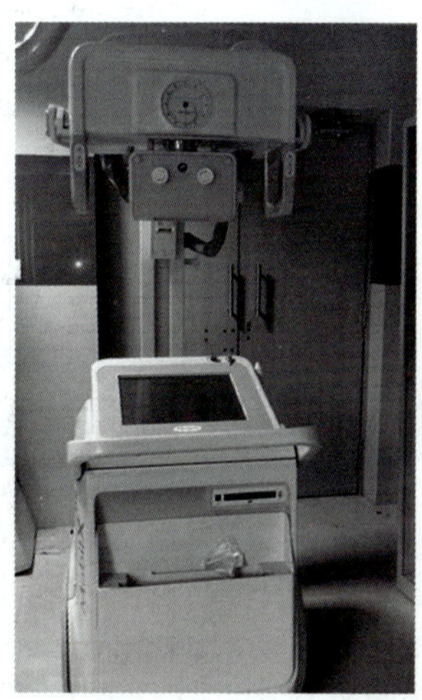

Fig. 5: Mobile digital radiography unit.

■ MAMMOGRAPHY

Mammography is a specific type of imaging using high precision X-ray machine which gives a reliable radiographic examination of the breast. The low dose X-ray study using mammography machine can aid in the early detection and diagnosis of breast diseases in women.[5] The use of mammography in breast cancer screening and treatment has represented a critical advance in the management of this disease. Current guidelines in India and by the American College of Radiology (ACR) recommended annual screening in women above the age of 40 years.

Screen film mammography SFM was traditionally considered the gold standard in mammography until recently, however full field digital mammography (FFDM) is now increasingly being recognized as an attractive alternative to SFM **(Fig. 6)**. The recent advances in mammography include digital mammography, computer-aided detection, breast tomosynthesis and performing stereotactic biopsy from indeterminate lesions.

Digital mammography, also called full-field digital mammography (FFDM), is a mammography system in which the X-ray film is replaced by solid-state detectors that convert X-rays into electrical signals. The electrical signals are used to produce images of the breast that can be seen on a computer screen or printed on special film similar to conventional mammograms.[25] FFDM has improved contrast resolution and greater ability to image dense breast tissue thereby increasing the diagnostic accuracy.

Computer-aided detection (CAD) systems use a digitized mammographic image and computer software then searches for abnormal areas of density, mass, or calcification that may indicate the presence of cancer. The CAD system highlights these areas on the images, alerting the radiologist to the need for further analysis and therefore improve the diagnostic capabilities.

Breast tomosynthesis, also called three-dimensional (3D) breast imaging, is a mammography system where the X-ray tube and imaging plate move in an arc during the exposure. It creates a series of thin slices through the breast that allow for improved detection of cancer and reduces the recall rates for additional imaging.[26]

Dual energy substraction mammography and contrast-enhanced digital mammography are also newer advanced techniques which help in improved lesion detection in difficult and indeterminate lesions.

Dual-energy X-ray Absorptiometry

Dual-energy X-ray absorptiometry (DEXA) is an imaging technology that uses a very low amount of X-ray energy to measure bone mineral density (BMD).

The technique relies on transmission measurements made at two photon energies to allow calcium and thereby bone mineral, be assessed. When soft-tissue absorption is subtracted out, the BMD can be determined from the absorption of each beam by bone. The first-generation of modern DEXA scanners used a pencil X-ray beam; later designs employ fan beams, cone beams and c-arm technology and thereby, allow more rapid and convenient scanning **(Fig. 7)**.[27,28]

Dual-energy X-ray absorptiometry is the most widely used and most thoroughly studied bone-density measurement technology.

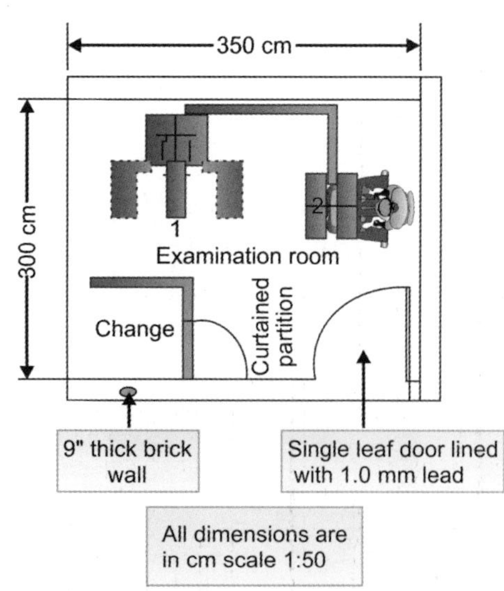

1. Mammography equipment, 2. Control unit with protective barrier of 1.5 mm lead equivalence
Fig. 6: Model layout—mammography installation.

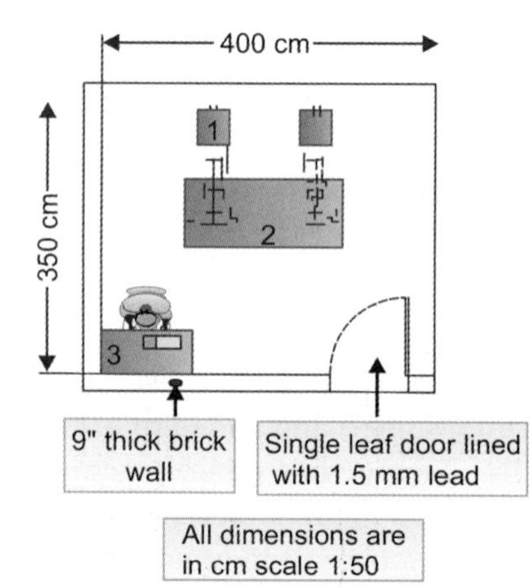

1. BMD equipment; 2. Examination table; 3. Evaluation unit
Fig. 7: Model layout—BMD installation.

The DEXA scan is the most accurate and reliable way to diagnose and follow osteoporosis and predicts the future risk of fracture. It contrasts to the nuclear bone scan, which is sensitive to certain metabolic diseases of bones in which bones are attempting to heal from infections, fractures, or tumors. DEXA scans can also be used to measure total body composition and fat content with a high degree of accuracy comparable to hydrostatic weighing with a few important caveats.[29] However, it has been suggested that, while very accurately measuring minerals and lean soft tissue (LST), DEXA may provide skewed results as a result of its method of indirectly calculating fat mass by subtracting it from the LST and/or body cell mass (BCM) that DEXA actually measures.

Sites central—lumbar spine, hip, whole body

Peripheral—forearm, calcaneous.

Whole body DEXA includes assessment of total Body Bone Mineral Content (calibrated against hydroxyapatite and consisting of about 80% cortical bone), total body lean mass (calibrated against saline and consisting of lean soft tissue), total body fat mass (calibrated against stearic acid and consisting of fatty soft tissue).[30]

COMPUTED TOMOGRAPHY

CT scan is a medical imaging modality which has become one of the most powerful tool for various diagnostic and therapeutic purposes in virtually all medical disciplines. The modern day CT systems generate volume of data that can be acquired by various techniques and protocols based on the clinical concern. CT is the workhorse imaging tool for the evaluation of chest, abdomen and pelvis. In a time sensitive situation particularly trauma, CT is generally the initial approach.

Innovations in image acquisition and reconstruction technologies have greatly expanded the range of CT applications available in the routine clinical setting. The modern day CT scanner (64 and 128 slice) can acquire sub-millimeter resolution images of entire body regions in a few seconds, allowing depiction of fine anatomical detail uncompromised by motion artifact **(Figs. 8A and B)**. With sophisticated visualization software, image data can be processed into multi-planar, volume-rendered, cine and other formats to better display anatomical abnormalities and facilitate newer applications such as dynamic CT, CT angiography, enterography, urography, tracheobronchography and cardiac CT. Newer applications including dual-energy material decomposition CT are furthering the transition of CT from a purely morphological to a combined anatomical, functional and metabolic imaging technique.[31]

Computed tomography angiography (CTA) enables the display of entire vascular system aided by injections of contrast medium. Several imaging post processing techniques are available enabling good display of the entire vascular system. The most widely used techniques are multiplanar reformation (MPR), thin-slab maximum intensity projection (MIP), shaded surface display (SSD) and volume rendering technique (VRT). Sophisticated segmentation algorithms, bone removal with thresh holding or subtraction algorithms and vessel analysis tools are also newer techniques which provide quality of vessel analysis comparable to DSA (conventional angiography). The clinical applications for these various image postprocessing methods include steno occlusive disease, aneurysms, vascular malformations.[32]

Virtual endoscopy (VE) is a recent development in postprocessing technique which is used to generate

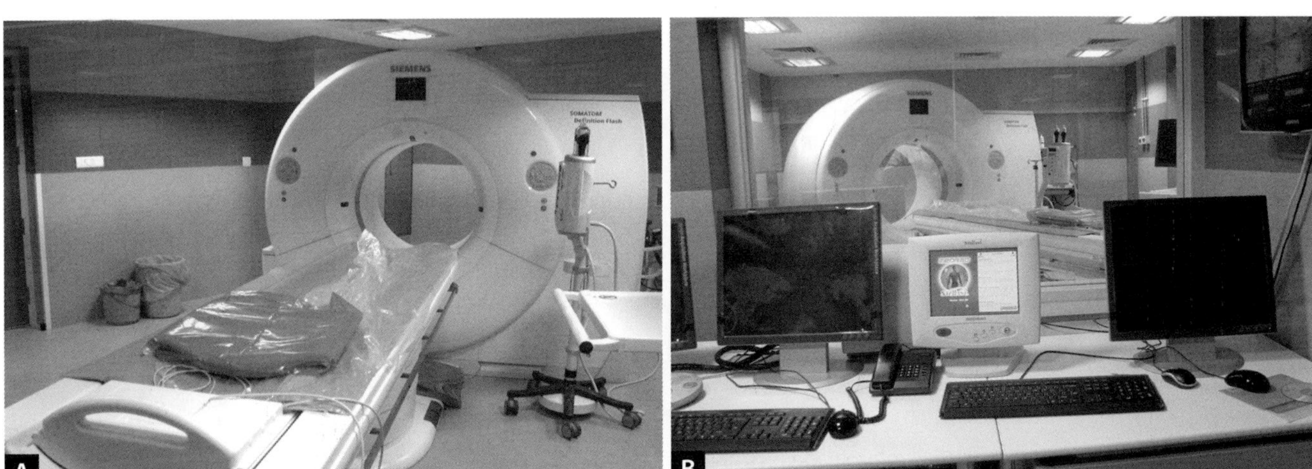

Figs. 8A and B: 128 slice dual source CT scanner.

virtual endoscopic views. This technique is used to obtain a perspective view of the display region mainly for anatomical cavities. These include, for example, the bronchial tree, large vessels, the colon and paranasal sinuses. VE is also used for areas not directly accessible for conventional endoscopy. The perspective volume rendering technique allows real-time fly through at high resolution mimicking the true endoscopy.

Installation of X-ray and CT scanner unit requires approval of AERB and need to conform to radiation protections measures **(Fig. 9)**. However, CT examination involves radiation exposure with potential risks and should be performed judiciously particularly in children who are more radio sensitive than adults.

ULTRASOUND

It is a noninvasive diagnostic medical modality that uses high frequency sound waves to visualize the internal structures of the body in real time. It has the important advantages of being widely available, low cost and does not use ionizing radiation. This modality has become one of the most preferred imaging for diagnostic, interventional, monitoring and follow-up of patients. It has a vital role in obstetrical imaging and is used both for assessing the fetal development and early diagnosis of many fetal anomalies.

Ultrasound is also useful for various guided interventions and can be performed on bed side in the triage of trauma patients. The quality of examination is however highly depen dent on the experience of the sonographer in addition to the patient body habitus. The advanced ultrasound system includes capable of harmonic imaging, color and power Doppler and 3D and 4D reconstructions **(Fig. 10)**. Technical advances like elastography and computer aided diagnosis have expanded the clinical applications especially in breast sonography.[33] Recently, therapeutic applications with high intensity focused ultrasound (HIFU) and micro-bubble assisted delivery of drugs and genes has shown great promise.[34]

Magnetic Resonance Imaging

Magnetic resonance imaging (MRI) is a medical imaging technique used in radiology which makes use of the property of nuclear magnetic resonance (NMR) to image nuclei of atoms inside the body. Unlike CT scans or traditional X-rays, MRI does not use ionizing radiation. MRI uses strong magnetic field to align atomic nuclei (usually hydrogen protons or any other nuclei with odd number of protons) within body tissues and various radio frequency pulses are put on and off repeatedly. The signal from human tissues are received by coils placed near the area of interest and fed to computer, which converts these signals into an image.

MRI provides excellent contrast between the different soft tissues of the body and can be used to image any part of the body. It is especially useful in musculoskeletal radiology and neuroradiology. It can detect or sometimes help in characterizing vital 'lesions' that might be missed or indeterminate on other imaging modalities.[35] The MRI provides excellent white and gray matter differentiation of nervous tissues. An advantage of MRI is its ability to produce images in axial, coronal, sagittal and multiple oblique planes with equal ease. MRI scans give the best

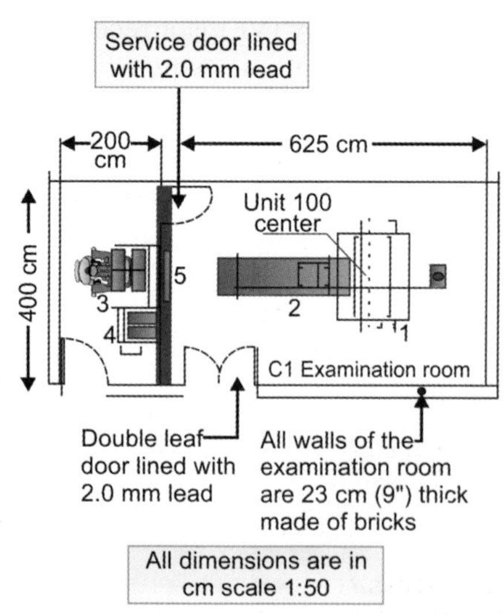

1. CT gantry; 2. Examination table; 3. Control unit; 4. Electronics; 5. Viewing glass 100 cm × 80 cm of 2.0 mm lead equivalence

Fig. 9: Model layout CT-scan installation.

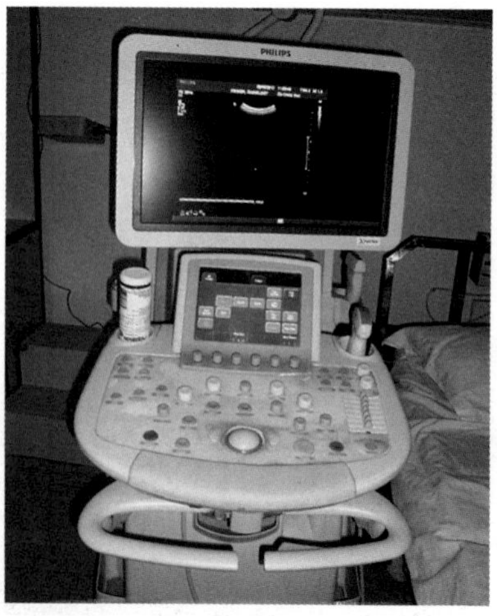

Fig. 10: Advanced ultrasound system.

soft-tissue contrast of all the imaging modalities. The advanced MR imaging techniques like perfusion imaging, diffusion-weighted imaging, and MR spectroscopy can improve the accuracy in diagnosis especially in the field of neuroimaging. With advances in scanning speed and spatial resolution and improvements in computer 3D algorithms and hardware, MRI has become an indispensable medical imaging technique in the current medical practice.

One disadvantage is the patient has to hold still for long periods of time in a noisy, cramped space while the imaging is performed. Claustrophobia severe enough to terminate the MRI exam is reported in up to 5% of patients. Recent improvements in magnet design, including stronger magnetic fields (3 tesla), shortening exam times, wider, shorter magnet bores and more open magnet designs, have brought some relief for claustrophobic patients **(Fig. 11)**. The modality is however contraindicated for patients with pacemakers, cochlear implants, some indwelling medication pumps, certain types of cerebral aneurysm clips and metallic prosthesis.[36]

Digital Subtraction Angiography

Digital subtraction angiography (DSA) is a type of fluoroscopy technique used in interventional radiology to clearly visualize blood vessels in a bony or dense soft tissue environment. Images are produced using contrast medium by subtracting a 'precontrast image' or the mask from later images, once the contrast medium has been injected.

Most cerebral angiography can be done with 3–5 frames per second (fps). Higher rates (e.g. 8–20 fps) are useful for imaging arteriovenous malformations and other high-flow lesions.[37] Not only anatomy but also function of blood flow can be studied using DSA, as X-ray images can be produced at a frame rate of up to 50 frames per second.[38] DSA is very successful in displaying the vascular system of the entire body and can be used both for diagnostic and therapeutic purposes.

While offering excellent spatial and temporal resolution as well as good contrast, single plane DSA suffers from its incapability of representing and displaying three-dimensional relationships. Such information can be introduced, if biplane angiography is applied **(Figs. 12 and 13)**. In biplane angiography, two X-ray devices generate images, which rotate around a common centre (called isocenter).

Planning and executing neuroradiological intervention is guided by biplane angiography because it provides fast information on the vascular system with high quality with 3D reconstructions. There has also been considerable progress in the development of catheters and embolization material. Using special microcatheters, the interventional neuroradiologist is able to reach almost every point in the brain by endovascular approach.

Three-dimensional (3D) reconstruction of the dataset acquired during rotational DSA represents the latest development in the neurovascular imaging armamentarium. This technique combines the anatomic resolution of DSA with the 3D visualization abilities previously offered only by CT or MR angiography, and hence provides more detailed information than does DSA alone. The adequate evaluation of 3D-DSA requires post processing by 3D reconstruction algorithms at an

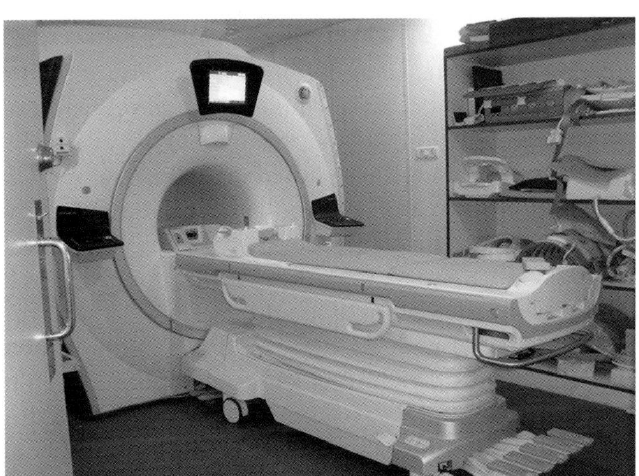

Fig. 11: Three tesla MRI system with coils.

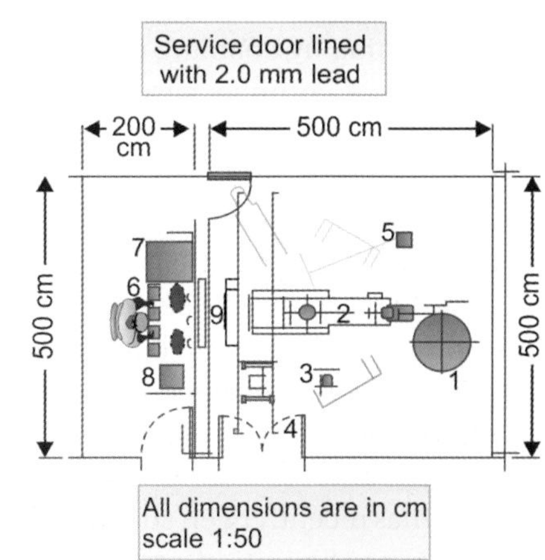

1. C-arm; 2. Examination table; 3. Monitor trolly; 4. Over head rails; 5. Fixed radiation shield; 6. Control unit; 7. Electronics; 8. Additional electronics; 9. Lead-glass viewing window 120 cm × 100 cm with 2.0 mm lead equivalence

Fig. 12: Model layout—Interventional radiology installation

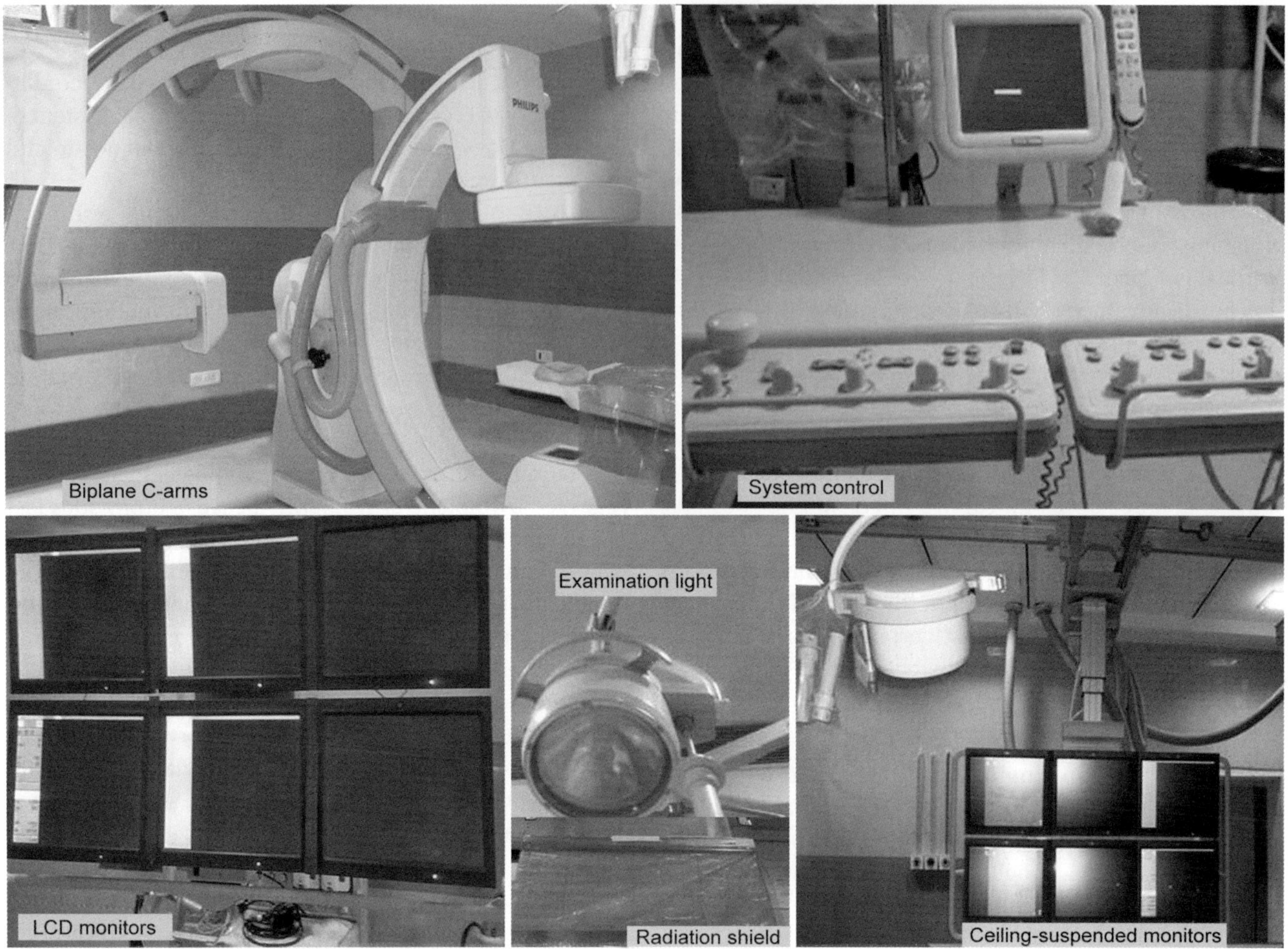

Fig. 13: Biplane DSA laboratory.

external workstation. 3D DSA has taken a prominent role in treatment planning by enabling exquisite detailed anatomic information of complex vascular lesions and also helps in choosing the most appropriate working projection for subsequent endovascular therapy. It provides precise vascular information in sophisticated tasks such as aneurysm volume measurement. Three-dimensional DSA is therefore essential for optimal diagnosis and endovascular management of cerebral aneurysms/arteriovenous malformations and can reduce the number of exposures.[39]

Digital flat-panel detector cone-beam computed tomography (CBCT) has recently been adapted for use with C-arm systems. This configuration provides projection radiography, fluoroscopy, digital subtraction angiography, and volumetric computed tomography (CT) capabilities in a single patient setup, within the interventional suite. Such capabilities allow the intervention list to perform intra procedural volumetric imaging without the need for patient transportation.[40]

Nuclear Imaging Systems

Nuclear medicine imaging noninvasively provides functional information at the molecular and cellular level by measuring the uptake and turnover of target-specific radiotracers in tissue. These functional processes include tissue blood flow and metabolism and by providing information on these processes, nuclear medicine imaging offers a broad array of tools for probing normal and disease-related states of tissue.

The principal imaging device is the gamma camera which detects the radiation emitted by the tracer in the body and displays it as an image. With computer processing, the information can be displayed as axial, coronal and sagittal images (SPECT images, single-photon emission computed tomography). SPECT has enabled the evaluation of disease processes based on functional and metabolic information. Positron emission tomography (PET) is also a nuclear medical imaging technique that produces a three-dimensional image or picture of functional processes in the body. The system detects pairs of gamma rays emitted indirectly by a positron-emitting radionuclide (tracer), which is introduced into the body on a biologically active molecule. If the biologically active molecule chosen for PET is FDG (fluorodeoxy glucose), the concentrations of tracer imaged then give tissue metabolic activity, in terms of regional glucose uptake. Use of this tracer to explore the possibility of cancer metastasis (i.e. spreading to other sites) is the most common type of PET scan in standard medical care (90% of current scans). However, on a minority basis, many other radiotracers are used in PET to image the tissue concentration of many other types of molecules of interest.

The addition of anatomic imaging provided by Integration of computed tomography (CT) to functional imaging of positron emission tomography (PET) and single photon emission computed tomography (SPECT) has further expanded the utility and accuracy of nuclear medicine imaging. By using combined-modality PET/CT and SPECT/ CT hybrid imaging, functional processes can be localized at anatomic sites or, in some instances, as yet unidentifiable structural alteration. These modalities have enhanced the accuracy of detection, determination of the extent and severity, and improved the ability to monitor patient's response to therapy in oncology patients.[41]

PICTURE ARCHIVING AND COMMUNICATION SYSTEMS

The development of electronic (filmless) department depends on the technological advances pertain to imaging and those arising from generally available computer technology. Picture archiving and communication systems (PACS) are computer systems dedicated to the storage, retrieval, distribution and communication of medical images from multiple modalities. Electronic images and reports are transmitted digitally via PACS; this eliminates the need to manually file, retrieve, or transport film jackets. The universal format for PACS image storage and transfer is digital imaging and communications in medicine (DICOM). Development of PACS has replaced the conventional analogue film, paper clinical request forms and reports with a format that has completely computerized electronic display. PACS offers several advantages to radiologists and radiology departments as they work to trim costs, improve patient care, increase throughput and efficiency and have a major added value is efficiency of data management. Access to electronic images helps foster collaboration and support seamless care for patients across the primary and secondary care sectors.

A modern PACS has (or should have) excellent capabilities for displaying new examinations in a user-friendly manner, perfecting and displaying pertinent prior examinations for comparison and providing access to prior reports. One would consider these features to represent baseline or core functionality for any modern PACS.[42]

The PACS architecture comprises of:

Centralized PACS-(hub and spoke, star topology)—single short-term storage unit to which every modality and every workstation is connected on a point to point basis.

Distributed PACS-composed of number of linked clusters, each with its own short-term storage unit and one or more image acquisition modalities and several diagnostic/review workstations. Short-term storage is provided by one or more random array of inexpensive disks (RAIDs). RAID is composed of magnetic hard disks which is linked to a server which is connected directly to the PACS workstations. Connection can be made at various bandwidths, the highest generally being gigabit ethernet **(Figs. 14A and B)**.

The major benefits of PACS result from digitization of data which allows easy comparison, simultaneous multilocation viewing, faster image retrieval, automatic chronological ordering and rapid database search.

Some of the disadvantages include the inherent costs and technological complexity which requires adequate trained hospital staff. A dedicated maintenance programme and a carefully devised plan to provide essential clinical services in require in case of PACS failure.[43,44]

There should be tight integration of the digital dictation stations to the PACS workstations. This eliminates keying errors on the part of the radiologists when logging in to read a particular case.

Digital reporting rooms: Incorporating image interpreta tion, PACS and radiology information systems are carefully designed for physical space demands, lighting and ergonomics. Lighting must be placed to avoid glare on the monitor. Individual work spaces must be designed to allow privacy and collaboration at the same time.

Hospital information system (HIS) stores demographic data of all the patients, e.g. patient name, identification number, date of birth and also records admission and discharge dates, outpatient appointments, clinicians responsible for patient care and so forth.

Radiology information system (RIS) can be a stand-alone computer platform, or may be a module of the HIS. It stores information specific to the radiology department

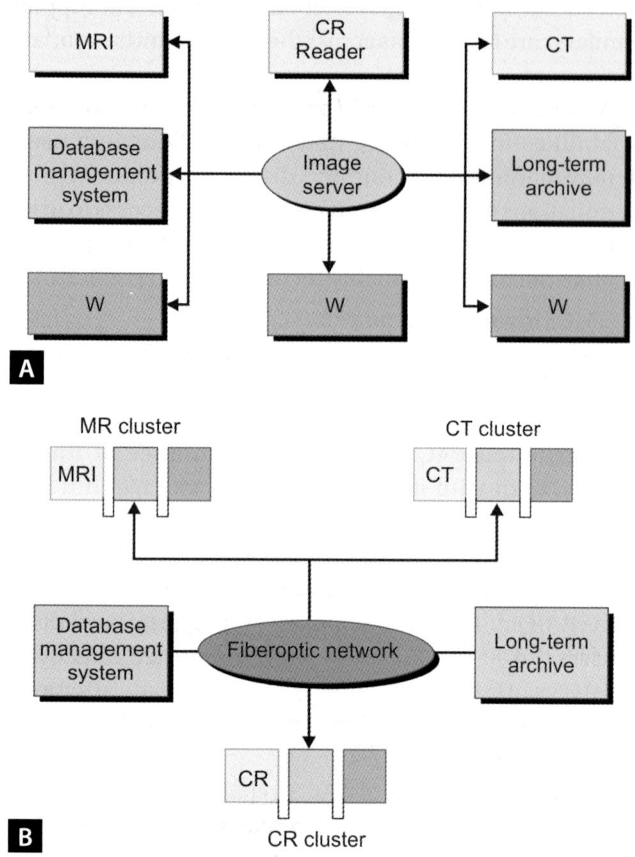

Figs. 14A and B: PACS architecture: (A) with workstation; (B) with networking.
Abbreviations: PACS: Picture archiving and communication system; MRI: Magnetic resonance imaging; CR: Computed radiography; CT: Computed tomography.

including radiological reports .Modern RIS will incorporate some DICOM features such as modality work list, modality performed procedure step, interpretation work list, and structured reporting.

Health level 7 is an internationally accepted standard for HIS and RIS systems. HIS-RIS-PACS integration should preferably be bidirectional. Input of demographic data is only once thereby minimizing human error. Any update to a patients demographic data or any scheduling is propagated to all systems HIS, RIS, or PACS automatically, hence providing advanced notice of events and allowing them to prepare.[45]

SAFETY STANDARDS AND QUALITY ASSURANCE

Safety standards and guidelines are an important aspect in early planning stages of a project. It is essential from the radiological safety view point, to exercise strict regulatory control over the safe use of ionizing radiation used in various diagnostic equipment. Statutory requirements for the safe operation of medical diagnostic equipment by hospitals, clinics and other medical institutions in India are given by atomic energy regulatory board, government of India.

Adopted safety guidelines should be referenced in planning standards or regulations. For ionizing radiation, shielding characteristics are based on the National Council on Radiation Protection and Measurements (NCRP) Report 147: Structural shielding design for medical X-ray imaging facilities. The information has been updated, including guidelines on new modalities.

Further, radiation protection devices **(Fig. 15A)** like lead flaps, radiation shield, thyroid shield, lead apron, lead goggles and lead gloves, etc. should have appropriate lead equivalent as per AERB guidelines. Further radiation warning signs **(Fig. 15B)** should be prominently displayed in front of the doors of all the radiation rooms in the radiology department.

Although the clinical use of X-rays is governed by optimization, justification and the as-low-as-reasonably-achievable (ALARA) principle, these are to supplemented by sound quality control (QC) practices. Imaging professionals should develop clearly defined guidelines that promote quality assurance in accordance with the latest technical knowledge of the equipment concerned. This professional approach will promote the due process of developing technical specifications, standards, and quality management.[46]

Digital images are created and processed with different parameters that must be continually assessed, different artifacts are possible from the digital processes, and complex computer systems can fail in subtle ways. Acceptance testing, regular calibration and proactive and consistent QC can prevent systematic errors that occur in digital acquisition or processing equipment and can contribute to overall department quality.[47]

TELERADIOLOGY

Teleradiology is the transmission of radiographic images from one location to another for interpretation by a radiologist. It is most often used to allow rapid interpretation of emergency room, ICU and other emergent examinations after hours of usual operation, at night and on weekends. The major advantage of teleradiology is the ability to utilize different time zones to provide real-time emergency radiology services around-the-clock. The disadvantages include higher costs, limited contact

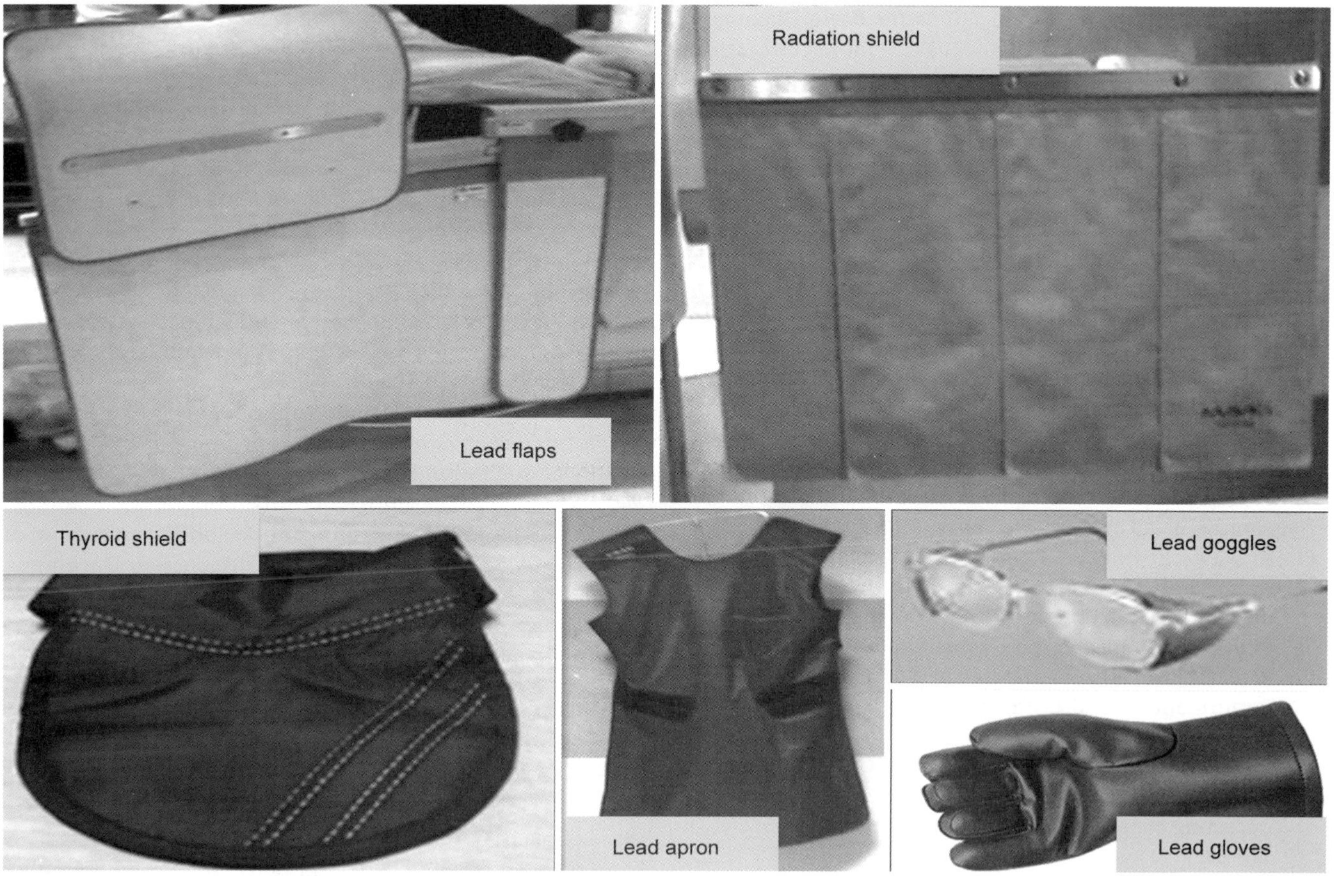

Fig. 15A: Radiation protection devices.

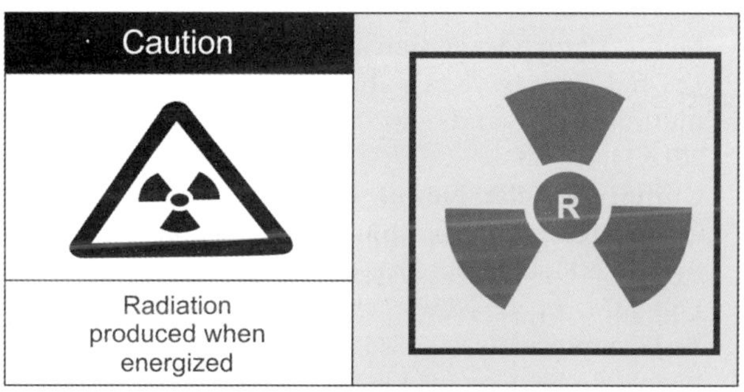

Fig. 15B: Radiation warning signs.

between the ordering physician and the radiologist, and the inability to cover for procedures requiring an onsite radiologist.

Successful planning of a modern imaging department depends on many things, and one of the most important factors relates to the amount of time and the quality of effort spent on strategic planning at the outset. Neglecting or skimping at this stage may lead to unforeseen problems that could ultimately derail the project. Fortunately, there are lessons that can be learned and applied from other healthcare organizations and even from the corporate world. Effectively utilizing planning as described in this article may help to steer a team in the right direction and ensure that underlying issues and the concerns of all facilities have been adequately addressed. Putting a high priority on strategic planning will relieve many of the headaches that can occur before, during and after the planning of a modern imaging department.

REFERENCES

1. Edwina H. The Future Delivery of Diagnostic Imaging Services in Wales. 2009.
2. Express Healthcare. Planning an Imaging Department. [online] Available from *http://www.expresshealthcare.in*. [Accessed December, 2018].
3. Woodford DA. Project planning in the diagnostic imaging department. Radiol Manage. 1997;19(3):35-9.
4. Evan Leepson. Strategic Planning for Radiology: Opening an Out-patient Diagnostic Imaging Center. Radiology management. 2003.
5. Singh H, Gayatri S. Radiology and Imaging Department. [online] Available from *http://www.drharisingh.com*. [Accessed December, 2018].

6. Salem D. Standard Specifications for Basic Diagnostic Radiology Departments. 2011. (*moh-gr.org/pdf/Standard%20 Specifications.pdf*)
7. Schaefor-Prokop C, Neitzal U, Venema HW, et al. Pigtail chest radiography: on and control of image quality update on modern technology dose containments. Eur Radio. 2008;18:1818-30.
8. Samei E. Performance of digital radiographic detectors: Quantification and assessment methods. Advances in digital radiography: RSNA: Categorical course in diagnostic Radiology Physics. 2003.pp.37-47.
9. Korner M, Weber CH, Wirth S, Pfeifer K, Reiser MF, Treitl M. Advances in digital radiography: physical principles and system overview. Radio Graphics. 2007;27:675-86.
10. Rivetti S, Lanconelli N, Bertolini M, Nitrosi A, Burani A, Acchiappati D. Comparison of different computed radiography systems: physical characterization and contrast detail analysis. Med Phys. 2010;37(2):440.
11. Arakawa S, Itoh W, Kohda K, et al. Novel computed radiography system with improved image quality by detection of emissions from both sides of an imaging plate. SPIE Medical Imaging, poster presentation. 1999.
12. Samei E, Flynn MJ. An experimental comparison of detector performance for direct and indirect digital radiography systems. Med Phys. 2003;30(4):608-22.
13. Metz S, Damoser P, Hollweck R, et al. Chest radiography with a digital flat-panel detector: experimental receiver operating characteristic analysis. Radiology. 2005;234(3):776-84.
14. Bacher K, Smeets P, Vereecken L, et al. Image quality and radiation dose in digital chest imaging: Comparison of an amorphous silicon and an amorphous selenium flat-panel system. AJR. 2006;187(3):630-7.
15. Bath M, Sund P, Mansson LG. Evaluation of the imaging properties of two generations of a CCD based system for digital chest radiography. Med Phys. 2002;29:2286-97.
16. Lawinski C, Mackenzie A, Cole H, et al. Digital detectors for general radiography: A comparative technical report. National Health Service report 05078. 2005. K-CARE website. *http/www. kcare.co.uk/publkications/abstracts/report05078.htm*
17. Samei E, Saunders RS, Lo JY, et al. Fundamental imaging characteristics of a slot scan digital chest radiographic system. Med Phys. 2004;31(9):2687-98.
18. MacMahon H. Improvement in detection of pulmonary nodu les: digital image processing and computer-aided diagnosis. Radiographics. 2000;20(4):1169-77.
19. Gilkeson RC, Sachs PB. Dual energy subtraction digital radio graphy: technical considerations, clinical applications, and imaging pitfalls (review). J Thorac Imag. 2006;21(4):303-13.
20. Dobbins JT, Godfrey DJ, McAdams HP. Chest tomosynthesis. Syllabus RSNA, Advances in digital radiography: RSNA categorical course in diagnostic radiology physics. 2003. pp. 211-7.
21. Brice J. Will new DR technologies offer alternative to CT? Part 2. *http://www.auntminnie.com/index.aspx?Sec=sup&Sub=xr a&Pag=dis&ItemId=90041*. Updated March 25, 2010. Accessed October 28, 2010.
22. MacMahon H, Yasillo NJ, Carlin M. Laser alignment system for high quality portable radiography Radiographics. 1992;12:111-20.
23. E-radiography. Mobile diagnostic imaging equipment. [online] Available from *www.e-radiography.com*. [Accessed December, 2018].
24. Lehnert T, Naguib NN, Ackermann H, Schomerus C, Jacobi V, Balzer JO, Vogl TJ. Novel, portable, cassette-sized, and wireless flat-panel digital radiography system: initial workflow results versus computed radiography. Am J Roentgenol. 2011;196(6):1368-71.
25. Radiology. Digital mammography. [online] Available from *http://www.radiologyinfo.org/en/info.cfm?pg=mammo*. [Accessed December, 2018].
26. Katherine A. Leslie. Digital Mammography: Planning, Implementation, and Integration [online] Available at *http://www.eradimaging.com*. [Accessed December, 2018].
27. Larkin A, et al. Commissioning and Quality Assurance of Dual Energy X-ray Absorptiometry (DEXA) systems, Rad. Prot. Dosim. 2008 (in press).
28. Sheahan NF, Dowling A, O'reilly G, Malone JF. Commissioning and quality assurance protocol for dual energy X-ray absorptiometry systems, Rad Prot Dosim. 2005;117:288-90.
29. Lohman TG, Harris M, Teixeira PJ, Weiss L. Assessing body composition and changes in body composition. Another look at dual-energy X-ray absorptiometry. Ann N Y Acad Sci. 2000;904:45-54.
30. Lorente Ramos, RM, Azpeitia Armán J, Arévalo Galeano N, Muñoz Hernández A, García Gómez JM, Gredilla Molinero J. Dual energy X-ray absorptimetry: Fundamentals, methodology, and clinical applications. Radiologia. 2012;54:410-23.
31. Guillerman RP. Newer CT applications and their alternatives: what is appropriate in children? Pediatr Radiol. 2011;41(Suppl 2):534-48.
32. Lell MM, et al. New techniques in CT angiography. Radiographics. 2006;26:S45-62.
33. Weinstein SP, Conant EF, Sehgal C. Technical advances in breast ultrasound imaging. Semin Ultrasound CT MR. 2006;27(4):273-83.
34. Harvey CJ, Pilcher JM, Eckersley RJ, Blomley MJ, Cosgrove DO. Advances in ultrasound. Clin Radiol. 2002;57(3):157-77.
35. Elsayes KM, et al. MRI characterization of 124 CT-indeterminate focal hepatic lesions: evaluation of clinical utility. HPB (Oxford). 2007;9(3):208-15.
36. Frank's Hospital Workshop. X-Ray. [online] Available from *http://www.frankshospitalworkshop.com/equipment/documents/X-ray/Radiology.pdf*. [Accessed December, 2018].
37. Harrigan MR, Deveikis JP. Biplanar DSA Diagnostic Cerebral Angiography. New York: Springer; 2013.

38. Toennies KD, Oishi S, Koster D, Schroth G. Accuracy of distance measurements in biplane angiography. Proceedings of Medical Imaging; Image Display: 1997;3031:19-30; SPIE San Diego: Yongmin K, editor.
39. JV Byrne, C Colominas, J Hipwell, et al. Assessment of a technique for 2D-3D registration of cerebral intra-arterial angiography. The British Journal of Radiology. 2004;77:123-8.
40. Orth RC, Wallace MJ, Michael D, Kuo MD. C-arm Cone-beam CT: general principles and technical considerations for use in interventional radiology. Vasc Interv Radiol. 2008;19:814-21.
41. Nuclear Medicine Imaging in Diagnosis and Treatment. National Research Council (US) and Institute of Medicine (US) Committee on State of the Science of Nuclear Medicine. Advan cing Nuclear Medicine through Innovation. Washington (DC): National Academies Press (US). 2007.
42. Ralston, Coleman RM, Beaulieu DM, Scrutchfield K, Perkins T. Progress toward paperless radiology in the digital environment: planning, implementation, and benefits. J Digit Imaging. 2004;17(2):134-43. Epu2004 Apr 19.
43. Samei E, Seibert JA, Andriole K, Badano A, Crawford J, Reiner B, et al. AAPM/RSNA tutorial on equipment selection: PACS equipment overview general guidelines for purchasing and acceptance testing of PACS equipment. Radiographics. 2004; 24:313-34.
44. Bryan S, Weatherburn GC, Watkins JR, Buxton MJ. The benefits of hospital-wide picture archiving and communication systems: a survey of clinical users of radiology services. Br J Radiol. 1999;72(857):469-78.
45. Dundas DD. Installation of a PACS system. The British Journal of Radiology. 2005;78:480-2.
46. Korir GK, Wambani JS, Korir IK. Establishing a quality assurance baseline for radiological protection of patients undergoing diagnostic radiology. SA Journal of Radiology. 2011.
47. Herrmann TL, Fauber TL, Gill J, et al. Best Practices in digital radiography. White paper Published by the American Society of Radiologic Technologists. 2012;84(1):88-9.

CHAPTER 63

Recent Advances in Positron Emission Tomography/Computed Tomography and Positron Emission Tomography/Magnetic Resonance

Rakesh Kumar, Anil Chauhan

INTRODUCTION

The last decade has witnessed a rapid advancement in the field of nuclear medicine. In this ever-expanding field, the onus goes to the advancement in instrumentation and radiotracers for clinical use, which is particularly evident in positron emission tomography/computed tomography (PET/CT) imaging. In this era of evidence-based medicine, the clinical indications for PET-CT has been increasing and expanding beyond oncology. Positron emission tomography/ magnetic resonance (PET/MR) imaging has been used in experimental setups for last 2 decades and recently has been introduced for clinical imaging in many centers.

The authors would discuss major recent advances in the clinical nuclear medicine related to PET/CT and PET/MR and their clinical applications. It is beyond the scope of this chapter to include the recent advances of the instrumentation and radiotracers.

POSITRON EMISSION TOMOGRAPHY/ COMPUTED TOMOGRAPHY

The PET is a functional diagnostic imaging technique, which can provide metabolic information for the underlying process that can either be normal physiological activity in the body or a pathological entity. There are many radiotracers that can be used for PET imaging, to provide information on glucose, amino acid and fatty acid metabolism, or target a particular receptor.

The PET alone is now universally replaced by PET/CT in routine clinical practice, as it had poor anatomical localization and early PET-only scanners had limited resolution of abnormal radiotracer accumulation in the body tissues. To overcome these two important limitations, combined PET/CT scanners were introduced in routine clinical practice after 2000. This widespread use of PET/CT was evidence based as PET/CT demonstrated higher specificity and sensitivity than either PET or CT alone for the management of various diseases especially in the field of oncology. Positron emission tomography/CT can provide the functional and morphological details of various pathological conditions in one procedure. Although many radiotracers are being used for PET-CT, ^{18}F-fluoro-2-deoxy-D-glucose (FDG) is the most commonly used radiotracer in PET/CT imaging. ^{18}F-fluoro-2-deoxy-D-glucose is an analog of glucose and the uptake is proportional to the metabolism of glucose by the pathological conditions. Most of these pathological conditions usually demonstrate high-glucose metabolism and show preferential uptake of FDG as compared to surrounding normal cells. After transport into tumor cell, FDG is phosphorylated by hexokinase into FDG-6-phosphate, which cannot continue through glycolysis because it is not a substrate for enzyme glucose-6-phosphate isomerase.[1,2] As a result, ^{18}F-FDG-6-phosphate is biochemically trapped within the cell. ^{18}F-FDG-PET is now an established standard in the initial staging, monitoring the response to the therapy and restaging after treatment of patients with various cancers as well as some nononcological conditions. In addition to qualitative image display, it is possible to quantify the FDG uptake value normalized to the injected dose and body weight/surface area, which is known as "standardized uptake value" (SUV). The SUV provides an approximate indicator that correlates with FDG metabolism in the tissue. A lesion with an SUV greater than 2.5 is considered to have a high probability of malignancy. However, that is not always true. Recently, a new quantitative parameter has been introduced which is described as tumor burden. This is a product of tumor volume and SUV. It has been reported to have higher accuracy than SUV alone in evaluating treatment response of solid tumors to chemotherapy.[3]

Clinical Applications of PET/CT

The PET/CT plays an important role in the management of cancer patients. It is primarily indicated for characterization of lesion equivocal on anatomical imaging, initial staging, treatment response evaluation, evaluation for recurrence, in detecting primary cancer in metastatic disease from unknown primary and to provide prognostic information for various cancers.

Diagnosis

The CT is the imaging modality of choice for detection and follow-up of lung nodules but has limited specificity especially in nodules less than 10 mm in size. Positron emission tomography/CT is increasingly being used to characterize small solitary pulmonary nodule (SPN), which are difficult to evaluate on CT. Positron emission tomography/CT provides additional functional information and is useful in differentiating benign lesions from malignant ones **(Figs. 1A and B)**. Two systematic reviews of the literature with meta-analysis reported sensitivity ranging from 96–97% and specificity of 78–86% using PET for detection of malignant SP.[4,5] It is important to note the limitations of PET-CT. ^{18}F-fluoro-2-deoxy-D-glucose PET/CT has low sensitivity in detecting low-grade tumors like bronchoalveolar carcinoma and bronchial carcinoid. Sarcoidosis and active granulomatous infection like tuberculosis and fungal infections (histoplasmosis or coccidioidomycosis) can be metabolically active and lead to false positive results.

Patients with cervical lymph-node metastasis from an unknown primary tumor present a big diagnostic dilemma from management perspective. FDG-PET can be a valuable tool in this subset of patients with an occult primary tumor in the head and neck region.[6] Positron emission tomography-CT is a valuable tool in these patients and can identify the primary tumor in approximately 30% patients.

Mammography is the widely used screening imaging technique for the detection of primary breast cancer but found to have lower sensitivity in women with radiographically dense breasts and in women with breast implants. Positron emission tomography/CT is useful in patients with dense breasts and patients with breast implants. Positron emission tomography/CT has also been found to be useful in detecting additional primary in contralateral breast in known breast cancer patients **(Figs. 2A and B)**. However, magnetic resonance imaging (MRI) remains the gold standard for this purpose in selected cases. Recently positron emission mammography (PEM) has been introduced for characterization of breast lesions and has shown encouraging results.[7] Patients with carcinoma-*in situ*, low-grade tumors, well-differentiated

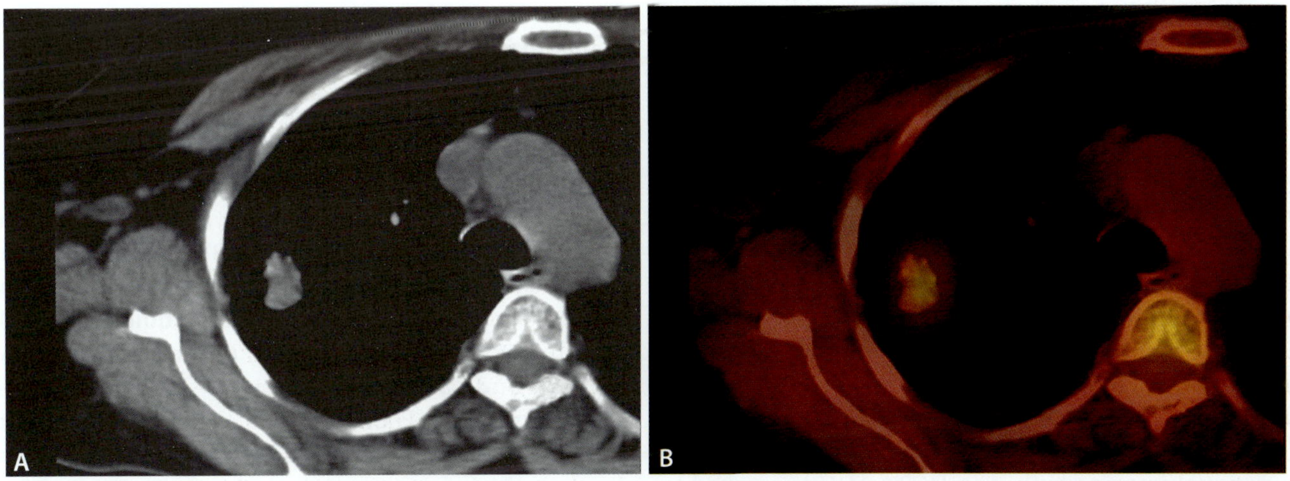

Figs. 1A and B: Chest CT of PET/CT shows solitary pulmonary nodule in right lung (A). Positron emission tomography/CT chest showing FDG uptake in the nodule suggestive of malignany (B). Fine needle aspiration cytology of nodule confirmed the diagnosis of malignancy (adenocarcinoma).

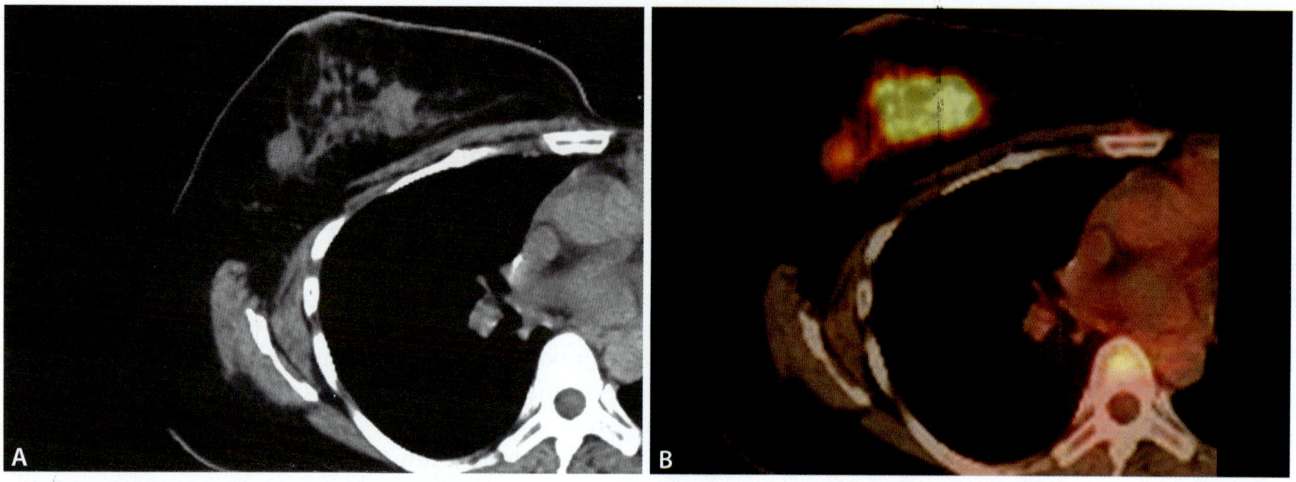

Figs. 2A and B: Computed tomography of PET/CT shows multiple nodules in right breast of patient who was treated for left breast cancer previously (A). Positron emission tomography/CT shows increased FDG uptake in all nodules suggestive of malignant nature of nodules (B) (additional primary in contralateral breast in known breast cancer patient).

ductal and lobular breast cancer usually have significantly lower SUVs and can be misinterpreted as benign lesions.

Till recently, the role of FDG-PET in bladder cancer was very limited due to urinary excretion of FDG. The detection of primary tumor and local visceral tumor recurrence is limited due to the presence of excreted FDG in the urinary tract, which often masks the pelvic lesion. An intervention, thus, to reduce the urinary radioactivity without altering the tumor uptake seems needed. In a recent study, we used diuretics administration as an intervention and demonstrated a sensitivity of 92% and specificity of 96% in patients with bladder carcinoma.[8] Diuretic administration significantly improved the detection of the primary tumor involving the bladder wall **(Figs. 3A to D)**.

Thymic tumors represent a broad spectrum of neoplastic pathologies with variable overlap in clinical and imaging presentation. Positron emission tomography/CT is useful in differentiating thymic hyperplasia from neoplasms, especially thymoma, carcinoma and lymphoma.[9] We have demonstrated that the difference between SUV max for thymic hyperplasia, thymoma and thymic carcinoma was statistically significant **(Figs. 4A and B)**.[10]

The FDG PET/CT has lower sensitivity and specificity for neuroendocrine tumors (NET). In addition to FDG, other positron-emitting radionuclides, such as somatostatin analog DOTA-D-Phe^{1}-Tyr^{3}-octreotide (DOTA-TOC), ^{11}C-Hydrox-yephedrine, ^{11}C-Epinephrine, ^{11}C-5-hydroxytryptophan and ^{18}F-DOPA, etc. are also used. Functional imaging with ^{68}Ga-DOTA-TOC is a valuable diagnostic tool in NETs as it targets the somatostatin receptors, which are molecular characteristics of most of these tumors. Our group demonstrated advantages of ^{68}Ga-DOTA-TOC over conventional FDG PET/CT in various NETs **(Figs. 5A to C)**.[11] ^{68}Ga-DOTATOC PET/CT emerged as the superior imaging technique with 100% sensitivity and PPV for detecting primary tumor, as compared to contrast-enhanced CT (CECT) that had a sensitivity of 83% in patients with NET. ^{68}Ga-DOTA-NOC PET-CT has been reported to be highly sensitive and specific for the detection of pheochromocytoma and paragangliomas as reported by Naswa et al. in 35 patients.[12] It seems better than ^{131}I MIBG scintigraphy for this purpose. Contrast-enhanced CT is a standard investigative procedure in the localization of gastrinomas. Small tumors are often missed and metastatic lesions may remain occult on CT. Naswa et al. demonstrated usefulness of ^{68}Ga-DOTANOC PET/CT in patients with gastrinoma with negative or equivocal results on CECT.[13]

In brain tumors, FDG PET/CT has limited application due to inherent high-glucose metabolism by brain parenchyma. FDG PET/CT may detect high-grade gliomas. FDG PET/CT has some role to play in patients with brain tumors treated by radiation therapy, where anatomical imaging modalities like CT and MRI can be limited in differentiating radiation necrosis from residual/recurrent tumor. New radiotracers like ^{11}C-methionine (^{11}C-MET), ^{11}C-tyrosine, ^{18}F-fluorotyrosine, ^{18}F-fluoroethyltyrosine (^{18}F-FET), 8-cyclopentyl-3-(3-^{18}F-fluoropropyl)-1-propylxanthine (^{18}F-CPFPX) and ^{18}F-fluoro-thymidine (^{18}F-FLT) have been studied as FDG has not much role due to its high normal uptake in brain. These nonFDG radiotracers however, are still experimental and not used in routine clinical practice.

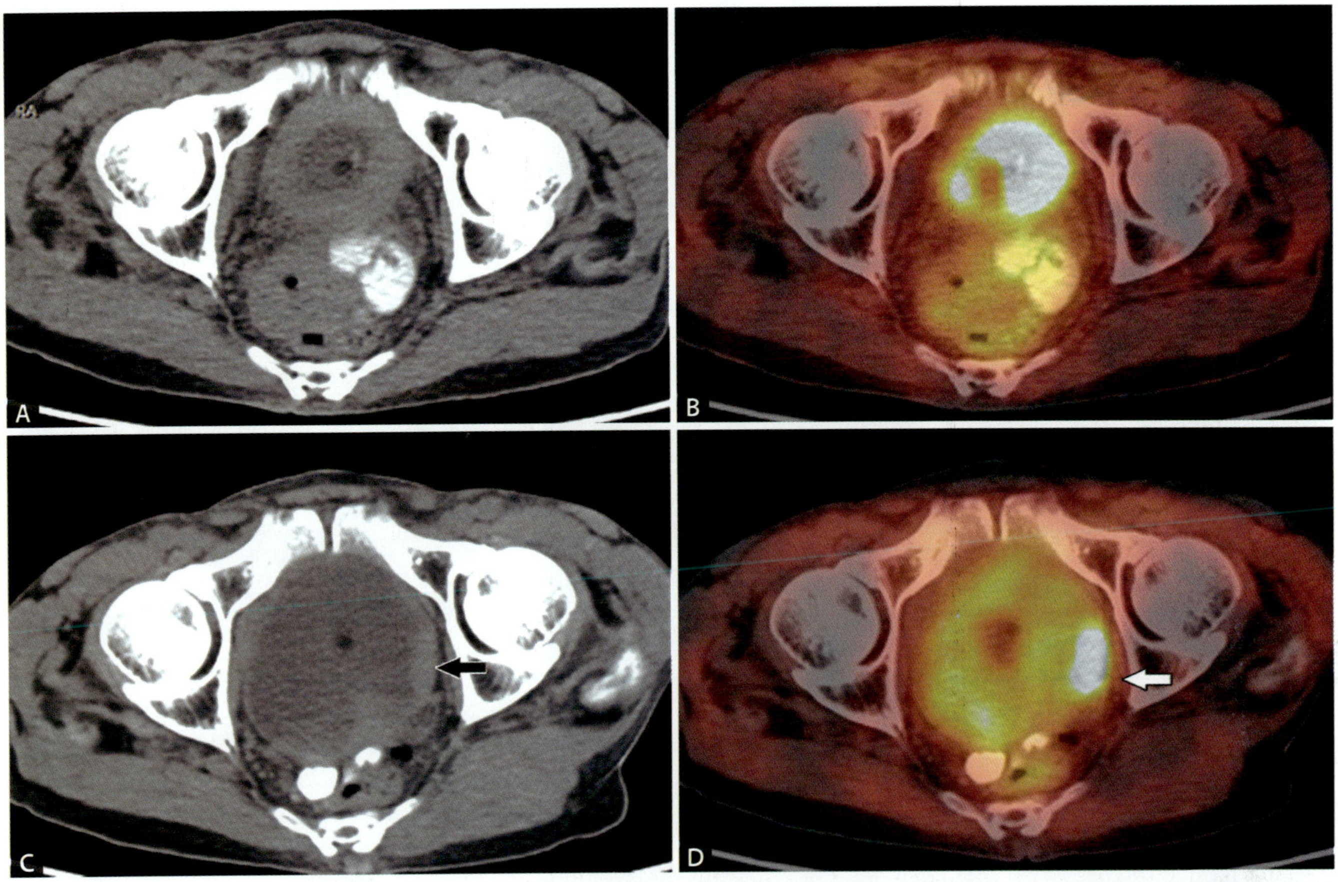

Figs. 3A to D: A 63-year-old man with carcinoma of the urinary bladder underwent staging PET/CT. Unenhanced axial CT image shows an diffuse tickening of urinary bladder wall with a catheter *in situ* (A). Corresponding axial PET/CT image shows a relative photon-deficient area in the region of the catheter bulb with urinary radioactivity occupying the remaining bladder cavity (B). Spot views of the urinary bladder were taken after diuretic administration which reveals the left lateral bladder wall thickening in a distended bladder on CT (C, black arrow), which shows intense uptake on axial PET/CT (D, white arrow) with a high target to background ratio after the residual bladder activity has been cleared.

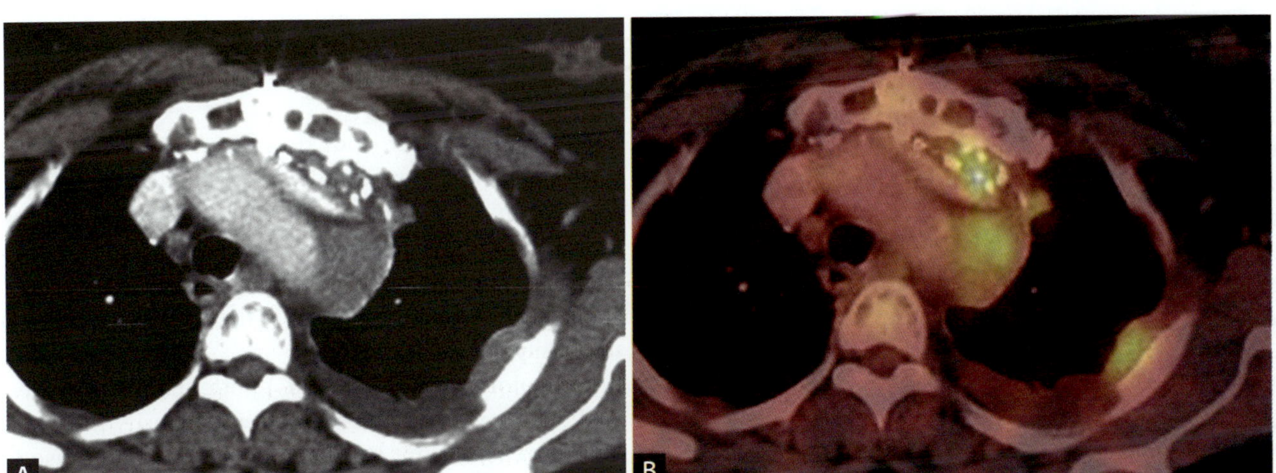

Figs. 4A and B: A 54-year-old man with thymic carcinoma underwent PET/CT. Contrast-enhanced CT axial image shows anterior mediastinal mass abutting arch of aorta with calcification. In addition there is left pleural thickening (A). Corresponding axial PET/CT image shows a intense uptake in the anterior medistinal mass seen on CT (B).

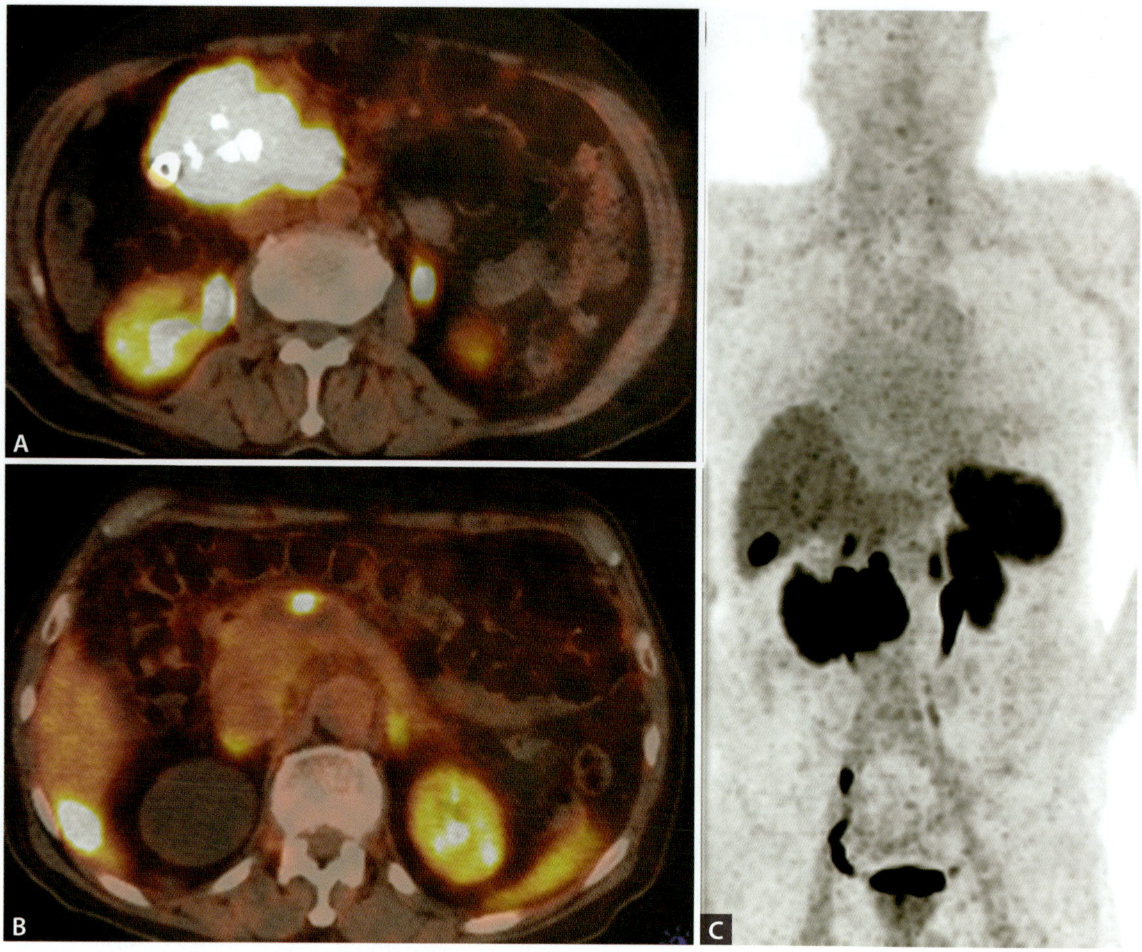

Figs. 5A to C: Transaxial ^{68}Ga-DOTATOC PET/CT images of abdomen (A) of a 42-year-old male patient presenting with pain abdomen showing intense tracer uptake in the pancreatic mass suggesting SSTR receptor expressing tumor. Also note a lesion in the liver showing increased ^{68}Ga-DOTATOC uptake suggesting metastasis (B). Projection image of whole body PET showing above described findings (C). A diagnosis of pancreatic NET was made. On histopathology the mass turned out to be a well-differentiated NET.

Initial Staging

The PET/CT has been found to play an important role in the initial staging of various tumors, which refers to assessing the extent of malignant neoplasms and in differentiating localized from disseminated disease.

For lung cancers, the FDG PET/CT has been primarily studied for nonsmall cell lung cancer (NSCLC) patients. In these patients regional and distant spread of the disease will change staging and guide the therapeutic approach **(Figs. 6A to E)**. Positron emission tomography/CT more accurately determines the T staging compared with either CT or PET alone. In one meta-analysis, PET/CT accurately predicted the T stage in patients with NSCLC in 82% of cases compared with 55% and 68% with PET alone and CT alone, respectively.[14] The additional advantages of PET/CT over CT are in differentiating central tumors from postobstructive atelectasis and detection of subtle areas of invasion.

In patients with Hodgkin's disease (HD) and Non-Hodgkin's lymphoma (NHL), PET/CT detects more lesions, which change the stage of the disease in almost 15% of patients when compared to conventional imaging like CT.[15] For histopathological examination of the lesion in HD and NHL, PET-CT can guide the biopsy from suitable and easily accessible site.

In colorectal cancer (CRC) patients, regional nodal or distant metastasis is present in majority of them at initial presentation. Computed tomography is used as initial investigation for staging but PET/CT is superior in detecting unexpected hepatic and extrahepatic metastases **(Figs. 7A to D)**. In a recent meta-analysis on the value of FDG PET/CT in preoperative staging of colorectal cancer

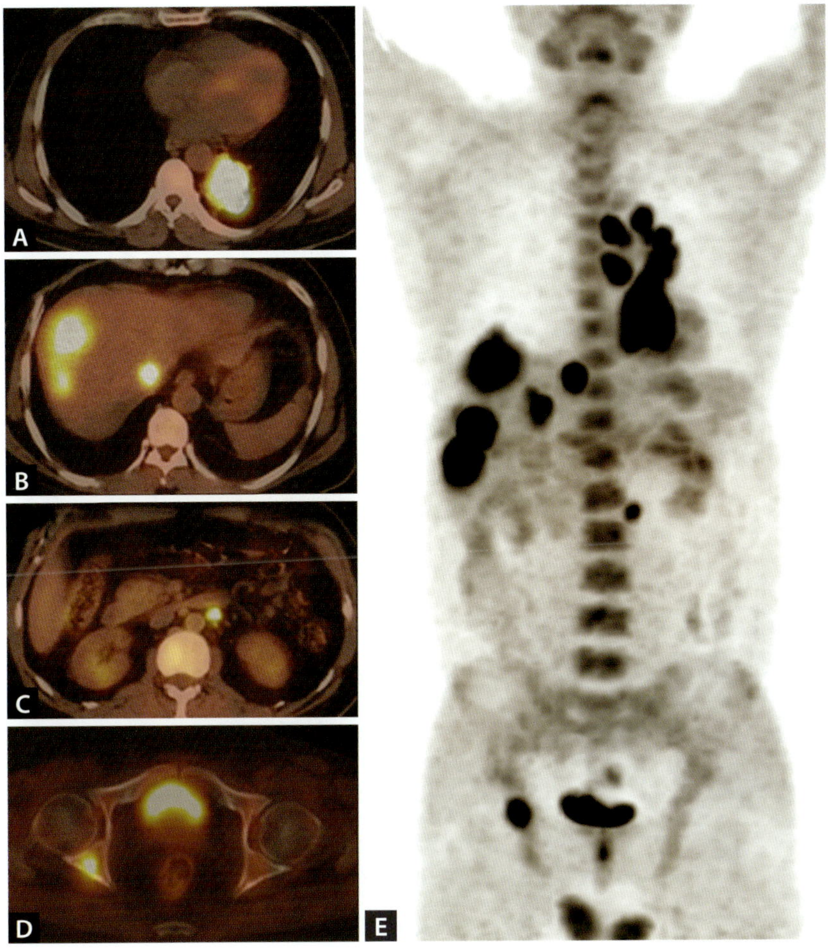

Figs. 6A to E: Transaxial [18]FDG PET/CT images of chest, abdomen and pelvis (A to D) of a 62-year-old male patient presenting with chest pain and hemoptysis, showing intense tracer uptake in the left lower-lung mass suggestive of malignant tumor (A). Also note multiple focal areas of increased FDG uptake in liver (B), left adrenal (C) and right acetabulum marrow (D) suggestive of metastatic disease. Projection image of whole body PET showing above described findings (E).

demonstrated a pooled sensitivity of 91%, and pooled specificity of 91%.[16] Mucinous adenocarcinoma is a subtype of CRC, which is less FDG avid and can produce false negative results in many cases.

Positron emission tomography/CT can be useful in initial staging evaluation of breast cancer as it can detect axillary node involvement, however, it is inferior in detecting lymph-node metastasis when compared to sentinel lymph-node biopsy. In selected patients who have high risk of nodal metastases, a clearly positive PET/CT carries a high-positive predictive value for nodal metastases. The advantage of PET/CT in initial staging in breast cancer is detection of internal mammary lymph node and distant metastasis **(Figs. 8A and B)**. ^{18}F-fluoro-2-deoxy-D-glucose PET/CT was found to be significantly more accurate for detecting axillary lymph-node and distant metastases in 106 women in a recently published study.[17] Management of 15 patients (14%) was altered based on the FDG PET/CT findings, including 3 patients with axillary lymph-node metastases, 5 patients with extra-axillary lymph-node metastases, 4 patients with distant metastases and 3 patients with synchronous malignancies.

Positron emission tomography/CT differentiates resectable and unresectable disease in esophageal and gastric cancers and helps in avoiding futile surgeries; however, the detection of regional nodal metastases is limited due to the small volume of disease in some lymph nodes and small size of the metastatic lymph nodes **(Figs. 9A to G)**. In a recent study authors from Australia have shown that PET/CT changed the stage group in 56 (40%) patients and changed management in 47 (34%) of 139 patients.[18] The authors concluded that PET/ CT provides incremental staging information compared with conventional imaging, changes management in one third of patients, and has powerful prognostic stratification in the primary staging of esophageal cancer. In a systematic review, Mazola et al. concluded that it appears reasonable to include FDG PET/CT in the diagnostic algorithm of patients with esophageal cancer in order to better define the optimal therapeutic approach.[19]

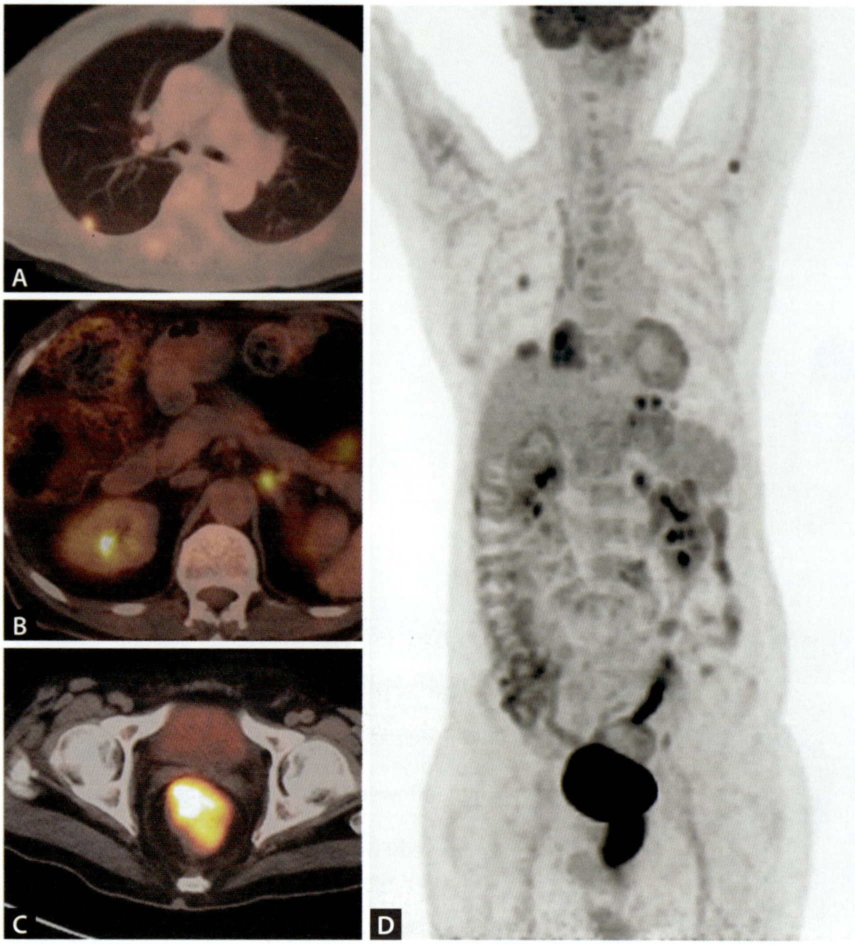

Figs. 7A to D: Transaxial ^{18}FDG PET/CT images of chest, abdomen and pelvis (A to C) of a 78-year-old male patient presenting with rectal mass, showing intense tracer uptake in the rectal mass suggestive of malignant primary tumor (C). Also note multiple focal areas of increased FDG uptake in the right lung (A) and left adrenal (B) suggestive of metastatic disease. Projection image of whole body PET showing above described findings (D).

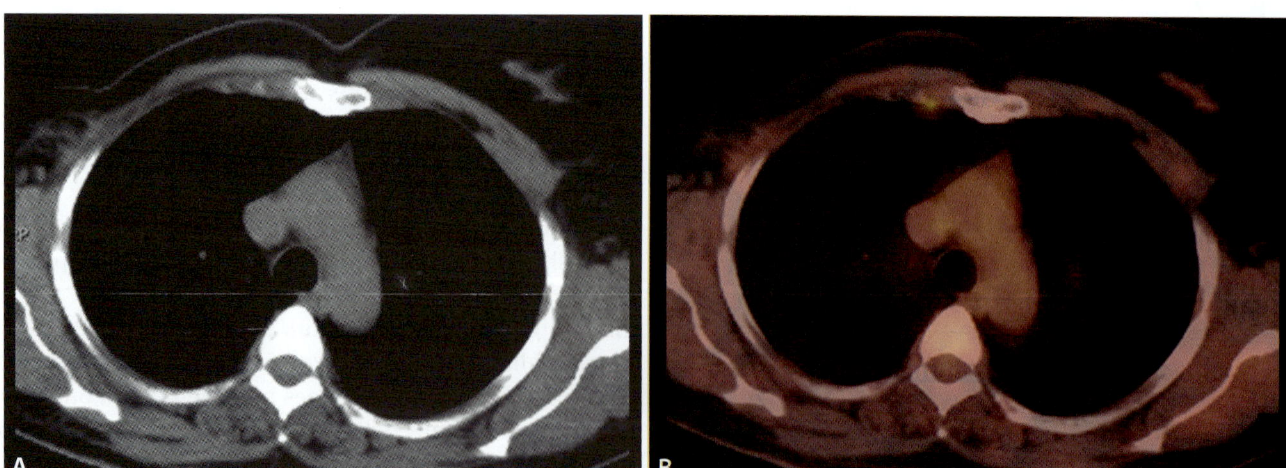

Figs. 8A and B: Chest CT of PET/CT shows no abnormality in a patient of right breast cancer (A). Positron emission tomography/CT chest showing FDG uptake in the subcentimeter right internal mammary suggestive of metastasis (B). Resolution of lymph node in postchemotherapy PET/CT confirmed the diagnosis of metastasis.

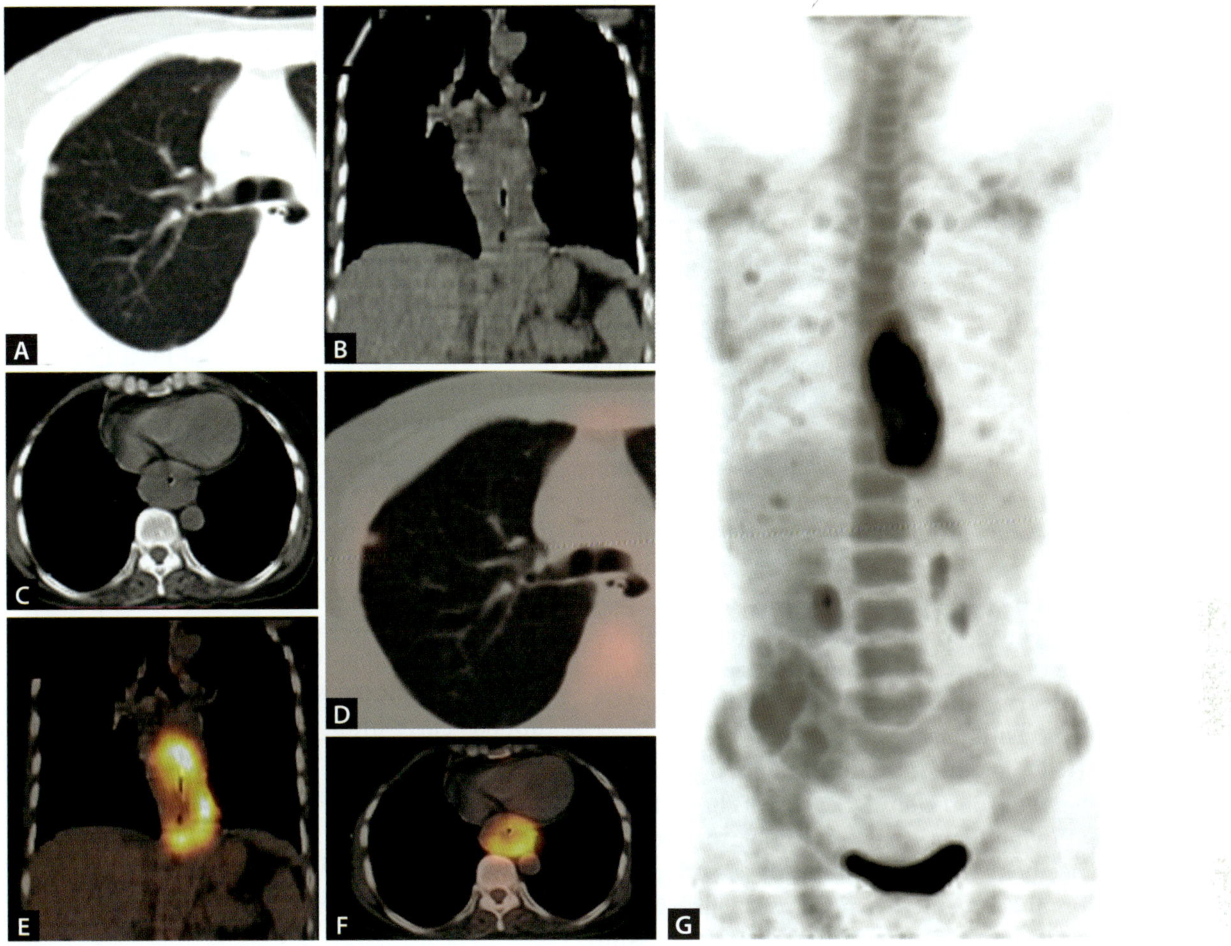

Figs. 9A to G: Chest CT of PET/CT show diffuse thickening of lower half of esophagus and right pulmonary nodule (A to C). Corresponding ^{18}FDG PET/CT images (D to F) show intense tracer uptake in the primary esophageal mass suggestive of malignant tumor and lung metastasis. Projection image of whole body PET showing above described findings (G).

The FDG PET/CT has a limited role in detecting soft-tissue metastasis to pelvic lymph nodes in patients with prostate cancer, owing to urinary excretion of FDG and low-glucose uptake by tumor cells (usually a well-differentiated neoplasm) in these patients. ^{11}C-choline PET/CT is more accurate than FDG PET-CT in patients with prostate cancer. In a systemic review and meta-analysis of ^{18}F-choline and ^{11}C-choline PET/ CT in the lymph-node staging of prostate cancer prior to surgery involving 10 studies and 441 patients, Evangelista et al. demonstrated pooled sensitivity of 49.2% and pooled specificity of 95%.[20] Another radiotracer ^{18}F-fluoro-5α-dihydrotestosterone (^{18}F-FDHT), a labeled analog of the major ligand for androgen receptor di-hydro-testosterone; has been used by some authors in limited number of patients. F18-Na-Fluoride PET/CT has high sensitivity for detecting bone metastases as compared to conventional bone scan due to high resolution of PET/CT scan.

The detection and staging of primary urothelial tumor and local visceral tumor recurrence is limited due to the presence of excreted FDG in the urinary tract, which often masks the pelvic lesion and probably the adjacent lymph-nodes. Diuretic administration significantly improved the detection of the primary tumor involving the bladder wall and regional lymph-nodes metastasis.[8] In a recent study, Divgi et al. studied the utility of iodine-124 ^{124}I-girentuximab PET/CT in 195 patients with renal masses and demonstrated higher sensitivity and specificity as compared to CECT.[21]

In NET, ^{68}Ga-DOTA-TOC PET/CT is superior to conventional imaging and FDG PET/CT for detecting occult metastasis. In our experience, we have found that

^{68}Ga-DOTA-TOC PET/CT is most sensitive and specific technique for initial staging of NET. Contrast-enhanced CT has been found to have higher accuracy as compared to FDG PET/CT but lower accuracy than ^{68}Ga-DOTA-TOC PET/CT.[11,12]

Treatment-response Evaluation

The PET/CT has emerged as a useful imaging modality that can evaluate the therapy response and differentiate respondersfromnonrespondersduringandaftercompletion of treatment. Since many of the chemotherapeutic drugs used for targeted therapy are cytostatic and not citocidal, conventional imaging like CT and MRI has limited value in evaluating the treatment response. The PET/CT being a metabolic imaging modality, can demonstrate the treatment response earlier by determining the glucose uptake by tumor, which decreases earlier than the size in solid tumors. The PET/CT performed after 1–2 cycles of chemotherapy can differentiate nonresponsive disease from adequate response better than conventional imaging modalities in various malignancies and can guide the treatment plan accordingly.

The PET-CT plays an important role in evaluation of treatment response soon after 1–2 cycles of chemotherapy in patients with lymphoma. It has been shown to have higher sensitivity, specificity and prognostic value when compared with CECT for mid-term therapy response **(Figs. 10A to J)**. Positron emission tomography-CT does not show any significant advantages over CECT when therapy evaluation is done after completion of treatment. In a recent study published by our group concluded though PET/CT depicts additional sites compared with contrast-enhanced CT and results in upstaging of disease. However, either PET/CT or contrast-enhanced CT may be used for response assessment and prognostication in stage III or IV nonlymphoblastic pediatric NHL.[22]

In breast cancer patients, PET/CT detects treatment-related metabolic changes much earlier than conventional imaging and clinical examination, once the chemotherapy has been initiated. There is strong correlation between the quantitative changes in SUV and overall clinical assessment of response of skeletal metastases to therapy and changes in tumor markers in breast cancer patients. We evaluated the role of FDG PET/CT for the assessment of response after two cycles of neoadjuvant chemotherapy (NACT) for breast cancer and concluded that FDG PET/CT can differentiate responders from nonresponders with high accuracy after two cycles of NACT in patients with locally advanced breast cancer (LABC).[23] ^{90}Y radioembolization [selective internal radiation therapy (SIRT)] has emerged as a valuable therapeutic option in unresectable, chemotherapy-refractory hepatic metastases from breast cancer. ^{18}F-fluoro-2-deoxy-D-glucose PET/CT appears to be useful for predicting survival in these patients.[24]

Neoadjuvant chemoradiation therapy may result in significant tumor regression in patients with gastrointestinal malignancies. Delta SUVmax (Absolute SUVmax change) and response index (RI, percent SUVmax change) are best predictive parameters in response evaluation of neoadjuvant chemotherapy. Hendlisz et al. assessed the predictive value of FDG PET/CT metabolic response after a single course of chemotherapy in patients with metastatic colorectal cancer and concluded that metabolic response measured by FDG-PET/CT after a single course of chemotherapy in metastatic CRC is able to identify patients who will not benefit from the treatment.[25] In patients with esophageal carcinoma, PET/ CT is more specific than CT and endoscopic USG for loco-regional lymph-node metastasis and response evaluation to neoadjuvant chemotherapy.

In bone tumors, PET/CT shows markedly reduced uptake early after the chemotherapy, while CT does not show definite change in tumor size. We studied 31 treatment naive osteosarcoma patients prospectively for treatment response by PET/CT scan after 3 cycles of neoadjuvant treatment and demonstrated that response can be predicted reliably by PET/CT scan early in disease course and PET/CT parameters correlate well with histologic necrosis.[26]

The CT scanning is the imaging modality of choice in gastrointestinal stromal tumors (GIST), which can locate a mass lesion, contiguous organ invasion and distant metastases. Since the introduction of Imatinib mesylate, PET/CT is being used widely in GIST. The PET/CT may show significant decrease in FDG uptake early after Imatinib therapy, while on conventional morphological imaging, tumor size may remain constant for a significant time and thereby, PET/CT accurately separates responders from non-responders in an early stage.

The PET-CT has shown promising results for assessment of treatment response from newer antiangiogenic agents (sunitinib and sorafenib) in patients with metastatic renal cell carcinoma, which might not show anatomical response, such as decreasing size on conventional imaging.

Restaging/Recurrence/Prognosis

Many of the cancers recur even after the successful initial therapy. The PET/CT is becoming standard of care in detecting the recurrence of various cancers and

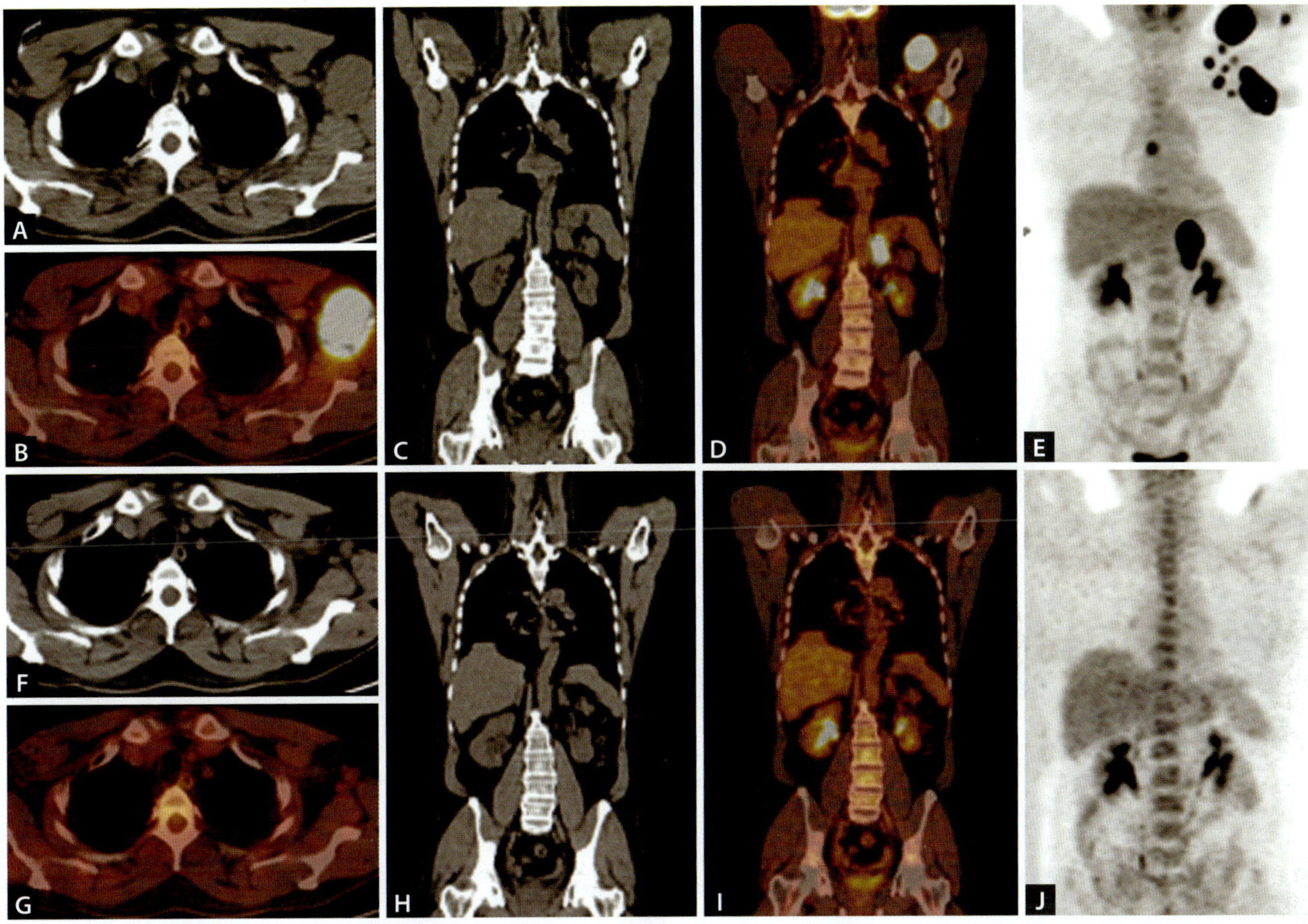

Figs. 10A to J: A 44-year-old man with NHL underwent baseline and postchemotherapy PET/CT for treatment response evaluation. In the baseline study (upper row), noncontrast CT of PET/CT shows enlarged left-axillary lymph nodes, left deltoid muscle deposit and left adrenal lesions (A and C). Corresponding ^{18}FDG PET/CT images (B and D) show intense tracer uptake in all lesion noted on CT. Projection image of whole body PET showing above described findings (E) PET/CT done after 2 cycles of chemotherapy (lower row) demonstrated resolution of all lesions, suggestion of complete remission (F to J).

in determining the prognosis. This is one of the most acceptable clinical indications of PET/CT in oncology. Positron emission tomography/CT has proven role in assessing the prognosis of colorectal cancer, NSCLC, pancreatic cancer, lymphoma **(Figs. 11A to D)**, cervical cancer, melanoma and other cancers.

In colorectal cancer, CT is frequently used to localize the site of possible recurrence, which has lower sensitivity and specificity. In a meta-analysis, comparing the diagnostic performance of PET, PET/CT, CT and MRI as whole-body imaging modalities for the detection of local and/or distant recurrent disease in CRC patients who have a (high) suspicion of recurrent disease, based on clinical findings or rise in carcinoembryonic antigen (CEA) level, demonstrated that whole-body PET and PET/CT are very accurate for the detection of local and/or distant recurrent disease in these patients **(Figs. 12A to F)**.[27] In another meta-analysis on colorectal liver metastases, FDG PET/CT had significantly higher sensitivity on a per-patient basis, compared with that of the CT, but not on a per-lesion basis. Sensitivity estimates for MR imaging with contrast were significantly superior to those for helical CT.[28]

The PET/CT has higher sensitivity and specificity compared to PET alone and diagnostic CECT for lesion detection in suspected recurrence in patients of gallbladder cancer. We have demonstrated a sensitivity of 97.6% and specificity of 90% in detecting gallbladder cancer recurrence using PET/CT in 62 PET-CT studies of 49 patients.[29]

In ovarian cancer, PET-CT has very important role in patients with rising tumor marker (CA-125) **(Figs. 13A to E)**. In a review by Son et al. PET/CT scan was found to

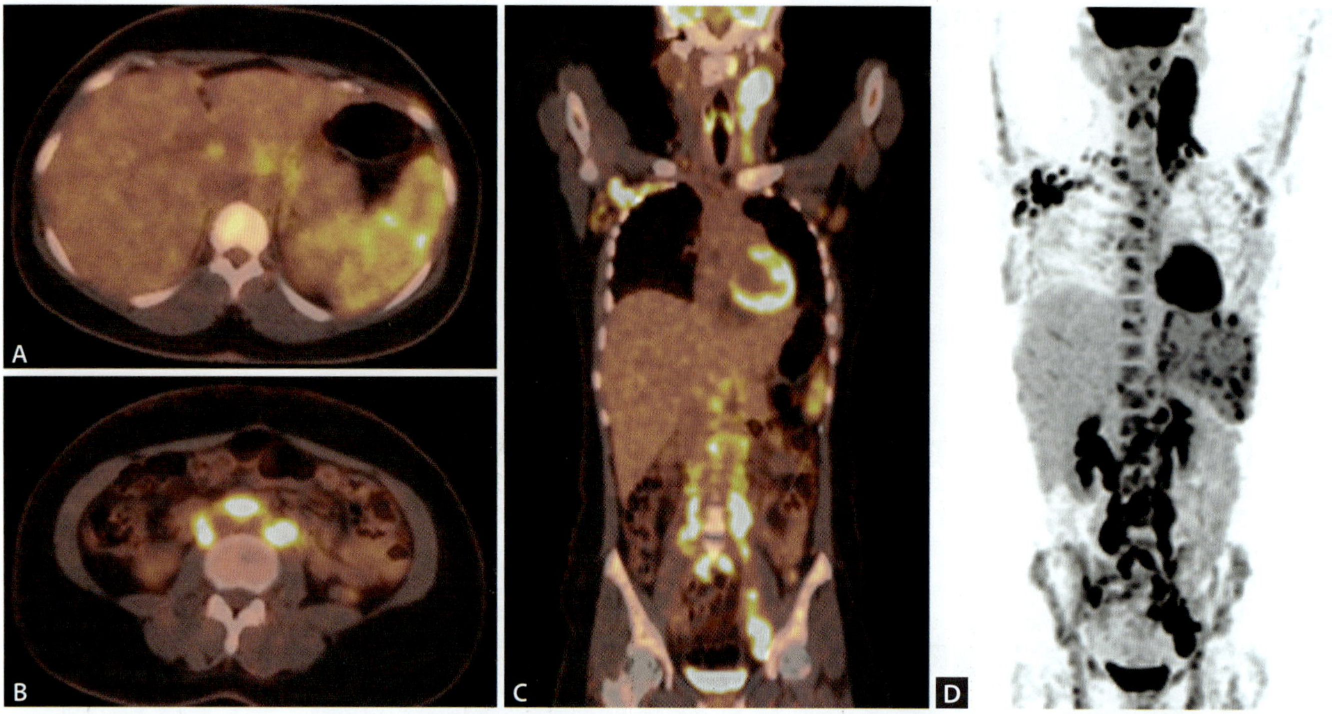

Figs. 11A to D: A 32-year-old man with NHL with complete remission after 6-cycles of chemotherapy presented with left cervical swelling and underwent PET/CT for restaging. Axial and coronal section of PET/CT shows splenic deposit, retroperitoneal, left pelvic, right axillary and left cervical lymph nodes (A to C). Projection image of whole body PET showing above described findings (D). These findings were suggestive of recurrent disease.

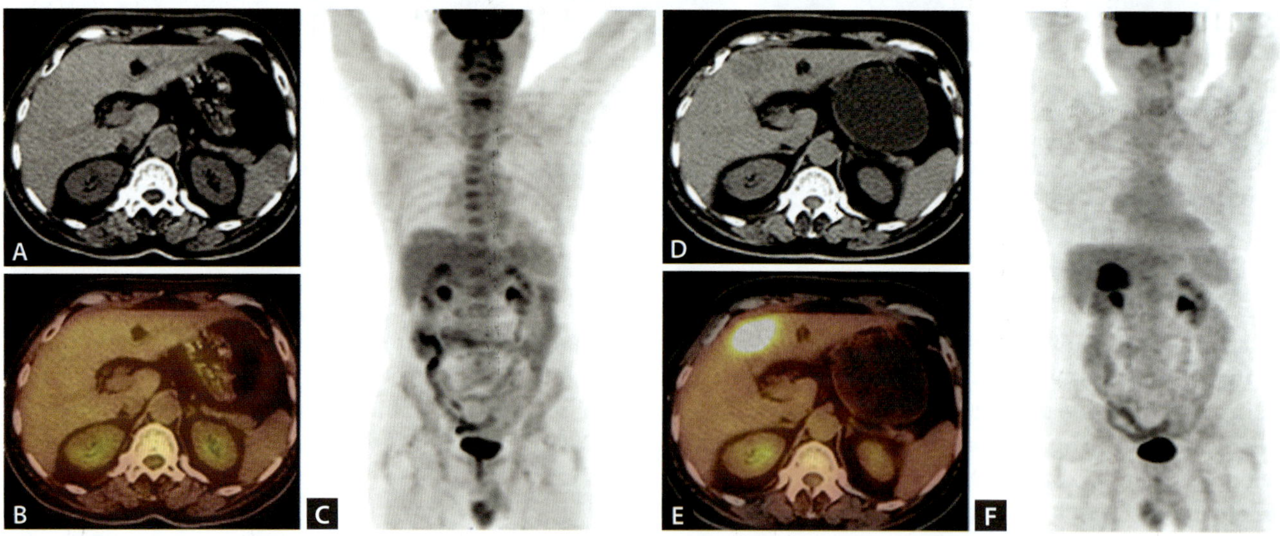

Figs. 12A to F: A 65-year-old man with a diagnosis of colorectal cancer who had normal PET/CT scan (right panel of images A to C) and CEA, 1-year back presented with recent rise in CEA levels, underwent PET/CT for restaging. Computed tomography of PET/CT shows hypodense liver lesion in segment IV (D). Positron emission tomography/CT shows increased FDG uptake in liver lesion suggestive of metastasis (E). Projection image of whole body PET showing above described findings (F). These findings were suggestive of recurrent disease.

be superior to CECT and MRI for detection of recurrent or residual ovarian cancer.[30] However, PET/CT may yield false-negative results in patients with small, necrotic, mucinous, cystic, or low-grade tumors. The PET/CT may be false-positive in the post-therapy setting, inflammatory and infectious processes. Despite these drawbacks, PET/CT is superior to CT and MR imaging for depiction of recurrent disease.

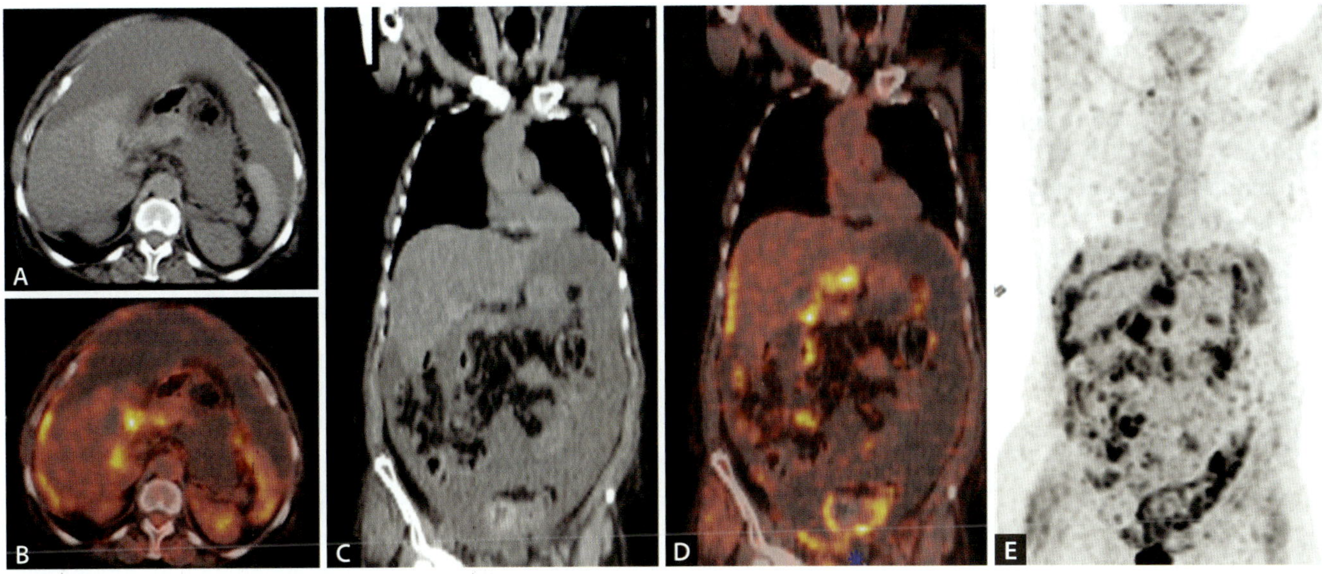

Figs. 13A to E: A 67-year-old woman with a diagnosis of ovarian cancer presented with recent rise in CA-125 levels and ascites, underwent PET/CT for restaging. Computed tomography of PET/CT shows ascites and peritoneal deposit (A and C). Positron emission tomography/CT shows increased FDG uptake in peritoneal deposit and ascites suggestive of metastasis (B and D). Projection image of whole body PET showing above described findings (E). These findings were suggestive of recurrent disease.

In NET, FDG PET/CT has no definite role except in evaluation of prognosis. A positive FDG PET/CT in patients with NET is suggestive of undifferentiated NET (WHO grade III) and poor prognosis.

Total lesion glycolysis (TLG), which combines volumetric and metabolic information from FDG PET/CT can provide a better evaluation of the prognosis. In 105 consecutive patients with NSCLC who underwent staging FDG PET/CT before any therapy, the 1-year PFS was 0.0% for patients with high whole-body TLG (>655) and 50.0% for those with low whole-body TLG (≤655).[31] This paragraph needs to be higher in hierarchy and another sentence about NSCLC needs to be included to talk in general and switch to more specific detail on TLG?

There are enough data in the literature on PET/CT regarding nononcology indications; however, there are no significant recent advances. Therefore, in this section, we have not discussed these as in nononcology indications of PET/CT.

POSITRON EMISSION TOMOGRAPHY/ MAGNETIC RESONANCE

The PET/CT has certain notable shortcomings, including the inability to perform simultaneous data acquisition leading to imaging artifacts and the significant radiation dose to the patient contributed by CT.[32,33] In addition, PET/CT has poor contrast among soft tissues and areas of complex anatomy, i.e. head and neck and pelvis. After 20 years of research work, an integrated PET/MR scanner (Siemens) which enables simultaneous acquisition of PET and MR imaging was launched in 2010 Munich, Germany.[34] There were many technical and practical hurdles before PET/MR was available for clinical imaging. Firstly, the photomultiplier (PMT)-based PET scanners do not work within or near the magnetic environment of an MR scanner. To overcome this, the developers used avalanche photo diode or silicon PMT- based PET detector systems.[35] Secondly, metallic objects, such as surface coils used to get best MR image quality interfere with the gamma rays from PET, causing unwanted attenuation. This can be achieved by modification of surface coils to reduce their metal content. Thirdly, MR data are not readily usable for attenuation correction like PET/CT.[36] Therefore, quantification of PET data was not possible. Various approaches to overcome this problem are currently under investigation.[37]

Clinical Applications of PET/MR

Oncology

Staging

Correct staging is very important for management of various cancers. Combined PET/MR imaging obtains concerted information about anatomy, cellularity and biological activity of the tumor. The sensitivity and specificity in oncology staging can be significantly improved using PET/

MR. There is relatively high-physiological FDG-activity in liver in PET/CT leading to masking of focal liver lesions with only slightly elevated FDG activity. Computed tomography also has intrinsically lower soft-tissue contrast compared with MRI in the liver. Lesion conspicuity was significantly better on the MRI component when compared with the CECT component.[38] That is why the most common indication of PET/MR is the detection and characterization of liver lesions (primary and metastatic) **(Figs. 14A to E)**. Positron emission tomography/MR is likely to be advantageous over PET/CT in the assessment of tumor invasion into adjacent structures in rectal, bladder, prostate and gynecological cancers.[39,40] Another indication requiring only regional extent imaging and expected advantages of PET/MRI is head and neck cancer due to its higher soft-tissue contrast. In these tumors, surrounding soft-tissue infiltration is important for local staging as well as surgical and radiotherapy planning.[39,40]

In addition, PET/MR will demonstrate improved accuracy in the assessment of spread to regional lymph nodes, especially in the pelvic, mediastinum and head-and-neck region **(Fig. 15)**.[41] It appears that combined PET/MR will enable a more thorough biological characterization of primary tumor and eventually metastases. Recently, Hirsch et al. reported PET/MR hybrid imaging in 15 children with multifocal malignant diseases and concluded that PET/MR is stable and reliable hybrid imaging modality, which generates a complementary diagnostic study of great additional value in pediatric cancer **(Figs. 16A to C)**.[42]

Overall, PET/MRI imaging has several advantages over PET/CT in many oncologic indications. Currently, the PET/ CT-MRI approach offers the highest flexibility to provide complete staging concepts.

Response evaluation

Accurate assessment of tumor response is essential in the management as well as in prognostication of cancer patients. Currently response is mainly evaluated by anatomical measures, known as the response evaluation criteria in solid tumors (RECIST) criteria. There are many limitations using these criteria in evaluating treatment response especially

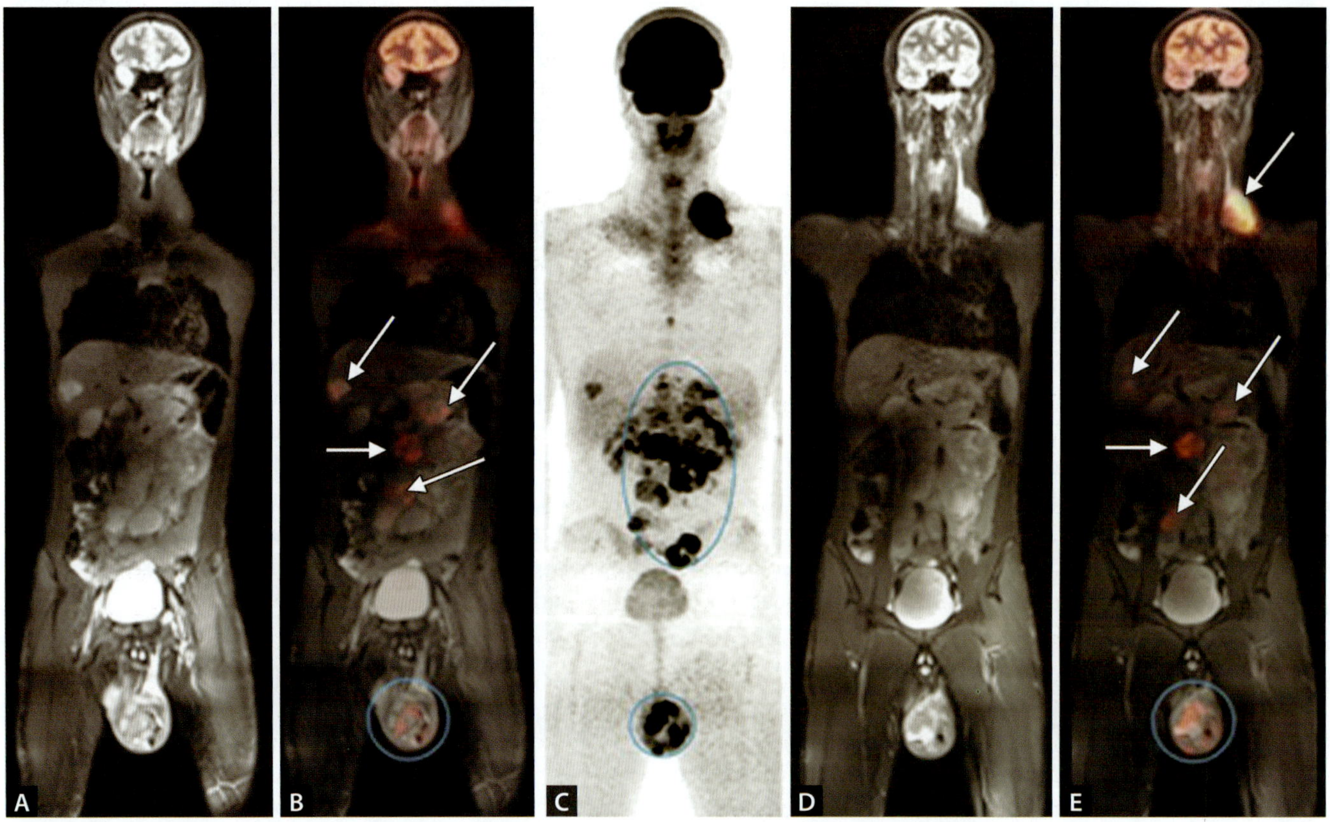

Figs. 14A to E: A 15-year-old boy with left testicular tumor with left retroperitoneal, supraclavicular and hepatic metastases (arrows). The primary tumor in the left testicle and the retroperitoneal metastasis exhibit a very inhomogeneous enhancement of the glucose metabolism with larger metabolically inactive areas showing no enhancement. This can only be explained in part by tumor necrosis. The liver metastasis shows significantly enhanced glucose uptake.

Source: Reproduced with permission from Franz Wolfgang Hirsch, Department of Pediatric Radiology, University of Leipzig, Liebigstr. 20a, 04103, Leipzig, Germany, hirw@medizin.uni-leipzig.de.

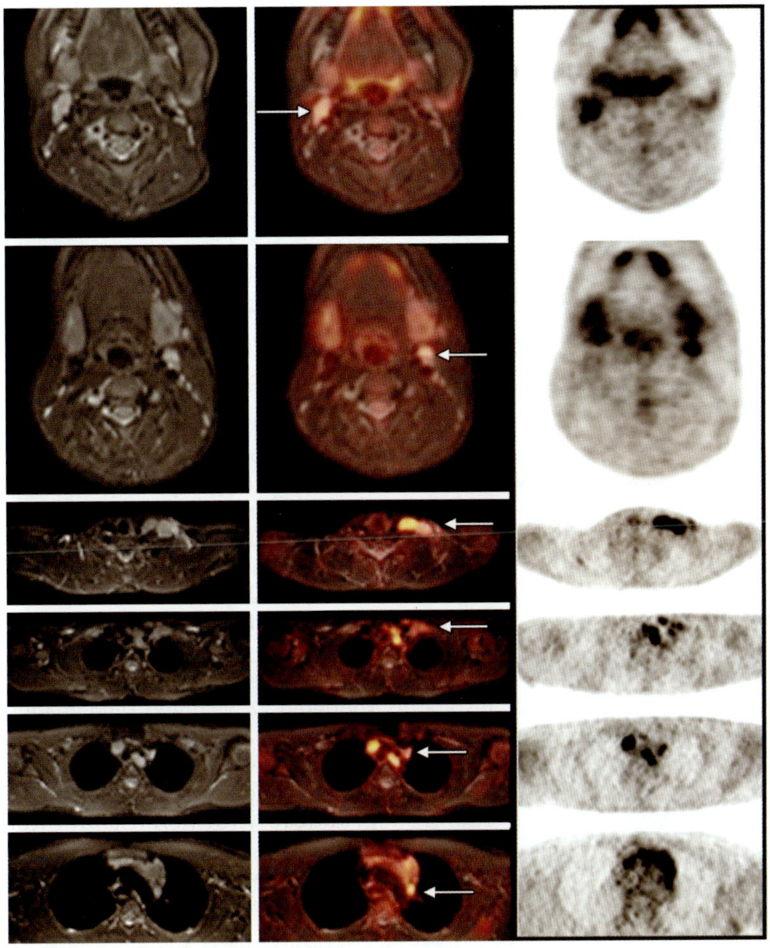

Fig. 15: A 13-year-old boy with Hodgkin disease stage II shows involvement of both sides of the submandibular, cervical and upper and middle mediastinum (arrows). Involvement of the submandibular lymph nodes (arrows) was not positively identified on MR criteria (size), but the PET image shows significantly enhanced FDG uptake. Arrows indicate positive PET/MR findings. *Source:* Reproduced with permission from Franz Wolfgang Hirsch, Department of Pediatric Radiology, University of Leipzig, Liebigstr. 20a, 04103, Leipzig, Germany, hirw@medizin.uni-leipzig.de.[41]

when patients are being treated with conventional cytoxic therapy or molecularly targeted agents, which can provide therapeutic benefit without significantly reducing the tumor size. The use of PET/CT, combining metabolic and anatomical information for therapy evaluation, has a huge potential impact on the quality of patient treatment as well as on the evaluation of new therapy regimes. Standardized criteria for response evaluation in solid tumors by PET/CT—PERCIST—was suggested in 2009[43] and the impact of PET in response evaluation in, e.g. lymphoma, is well established.[44] Similarly, diffusion-weighted MRI (DW-MRI) suggested that early changes in tumor-diffusion values correlate with response to therapy. Additionally, dynamic contrast-enhanced MRI can provide kinetics of tumor perfusion in pre- and post-treatment setting to assess the response to therapy. Therefore, the PET/ MR may provide unique advantages of both PET and MRI in exploring more specific changes in the tissue, making early therapy evaluation a safer endeavor.

Restaging

The FDG PET/CT can contribute in significant ways to the clinical management of patients particularly which have been previously treated by surgery or radiation and there is question of discrimination between post-treatment scar and recurrent tumor. However, in patients with brain tumors, metastatic liver disease and head neck cancer, PET/CT has limitations due to increased physiological FDG uptake and poor soft-tissue contrast. In these patients PET/MR will demonstrate improved accuracy in detecting recurrence. It has been demonstrated that CECT has high sensitivity for liver lesions, but generally MRI is still considered superior. However, there are only few studies evaluating CE PET/CT compared with MRI. A large meta-analysis did not find statistically significant differences in lesion detection.[45] Initial comparison of data acquired PET/CT-MRI system shows no difference in lesion detection when comparing CE PET/CT and non-CE MRI.[46]

Radiotherapy Treatment Planning

The best results of radiotherapy are obtained by the maximum radiation-dose delivery to target tissue and reducing dose to minimum to surrounding normal tissue. This can be obtained by the dose painting principle. Since

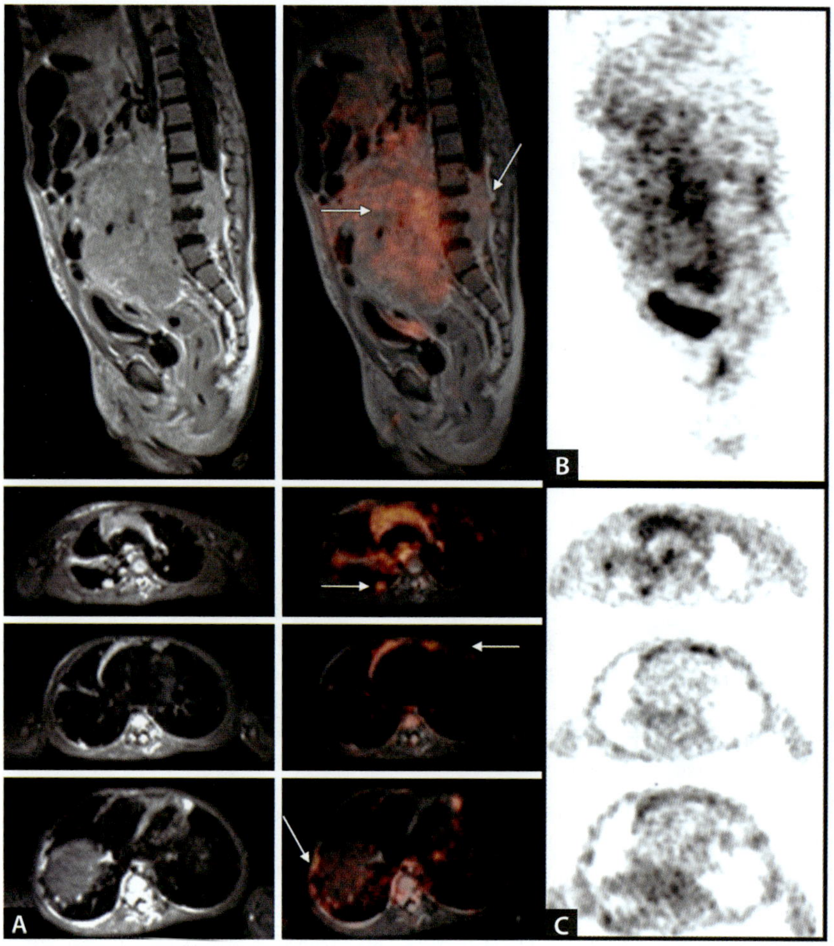

Figs. 16A to C: A 2-year-old boy with a large abdominal neuroblastoma that emanates from the sympathetic chain. Top row: the tumor (arrows) is growing into the spinal canal and involves the fourth and fifth lumbar vertebrae. The highly-differentiated tumor shows only slightly intense inhomogeneous FDG uptake. Lower row: transaxial slices show multiple (arrows) lung metastases and pleural metastases. The metastases are seen on the concordant respiratory-triggered T2-weighted TIRM images (A) and on the PET images (B and C); smaller metastases of 3–5 mm are clearly shown on the MR images. Arrows indicate positive PET/MR findings. *Source:* Reproduced with permission from Franz Wolfgang Hirsch, Department of Pediatric Radiology, University of Leipzig, Liebigstr. 20a, 04103, Leipzig, Germany, hirw@medizin.uni-leipzig.de.[42]

PET/MR has advantages of better tumor delineation because of high resolution of MR and metabolic status of tumor by PET, it can be used for better defining targeted radiotherapy of tumor and avoiding normal tissues. Another issue in radiotherapy is tumor hypoxia, which is a key mechanism leading to radiotherapy resistance. Therefore, imaging technique for hypoxia mapping which can be integrated with radiotherapy planning systems is always warranted.[47] Thorwarth et al. demonstrated feasiblility of dose painting using a dynamic ^{18}F-MISO-PET scan.[48]

Positron emission tomography based techniques using ^{64}Cu-ATSM, ^{18}F-MISO or ^{18}F-FAZA can image hypoxia by binding to intracellular macromolecules when pO_2<10 mm Hg.[49] Accumulation of most of PET tracers is flow-dependent while, MRI is thought to be most sensitive to perfusion-related hypoxia. By simultaneous PET/MR it will be possible to describe tissue hypoxia by PET hypoxia tracer together with blood-oxygen level dependent (BOLD) sequences, DW-MRI and/or DCE-MRI to distinguish between perfusion and diffusion as the most dominant cause of tumor hypoxia.[50,51]

Neurology

Anatomical imaging data is usually a prerequisite for processing and analysis of functional data in patients with neurological disorder. Till now this was achieved by software image fusion of structural and functional data. However, software image fusion has certain limitations, such as misregistration. Therefore an integrated PET/MR will be helpful in patients where visualized functional processes are time dependent in PET and MR. In functional neuropsychiatric examinations, MRI measuring the task-induced changes of the blood flow and oxygen consumption rates or the measurement of the arterial input function by MRI for its use in compartment modeling in quantitative PET studies are helpful.

In patients with Alzheimer's disease, PET/MR can be used for the early diagnosis, evaluation of disease progression and therapy response. In addition, morphologic images are essential to exclude other causes of dementia like multi-infarct dementia or normal-pressure hydrocephalus.[52,53]

Patients with refractory epilepsy despite medical treatment require surgery to resect the epileptogenic focus.[54] For success of surgical procedure structural and functional imaging data is of outmost importance. Therefore, these patients need to undergo a battery of imaging and non-imaging tests like morphologic MRI, functional MRI, PET and EEG for correct localization of epileptic focus. The PET/MR will be useful in such patients and data can be obtained using single imaging test in one day rather than multiple imaging tests on different days causing immense loss of time and money.

Cardiology

Myocardial perfusion imaging (MPI) using SPECT and SPECT/CT is well established technique for the management of coronary artery disease (CAD). Positron emission tomography still plays a limited role in daily clinical routine for MPI as there is lack of solid data to support a superior accuracy of PET over SPECT. The PET is the most reliable noninvasive tool for identification of myocardial viability in ischemic dysfunctional left ventricles and the only method validated in a prognostic interventional outcome study. However, it has not been used as there are competing radiation-free methods in the hands of cardiologists, such as echocardiography and MRI, which allow identification of viability. The PET/MR may be useful in evaluation of the vascular wall and the identification of plaques prone to rupture. It may help explore evolving and investigational fields of cardiovascular imaging, such as vulnerable plaque characterization, *in vivo* stem cell tracking and assessment of angiogenesis.

ACKNOWLEDGMENTS

We are highly thankful to Franz Wolfgang Hirsch for providing PET/MR **Figures 14 to 16**. These images were reproduced with permission from Franz Wolfgang Hirsch, Department of Pediatric Radiology, University of Leipzig, Liebigstr. 20a, 04103, Leipzig, Germany, hirw@medizin.uni-leipzig.de. Ref 42].

We thank Dr Suhas Singla and Dr Abhishek Kumar, Senior Resident, Nuclear Medicine, AIIMS for their help in selecting and getting other figures.

REFERENCES

1. Mochizuki T, Tsukamoto E, Kuge Y, et al. FDG uptake and glucose transporter subtype expressions in experimental tumor and inflammation models. J Nucl Med. 2001;42:1551-5.
2. McGowan KM, Long SD, Pekala PH. Glucose transporter gene expression: regulation of transcription and mRNA stability. Pharmacol Ther. 1995;66:465-505.
3. Sharma P, Gupta A, Patel C, Bakhshi S, Malhotra A, Kumar R. Pediatric lymphoma: metabolic tumor burden as a quantitative index for treatment response evaluation. Ann Nucl Med. 2012;26:58-66.
4. Gould MK, Maclean CC, Kuschner WG, et al. Accuracy of positron emission tomography for diagnosis of pulmonary nodules and mass lesions: a meta-analysis. JAMA. 2001;285:914-24.
5. Fischer BM, Mortensen J, Hojgaad L. Positron emission tomography in the diagnosis and staging of lung cancer: a systematic, quantitative review. Lancet Oncol. 2001;2:659-66.
6. Miller FR, Hussey D, Beeram M, Eng T, McGuff HS, Otto RA. Positron emission tomography in the management of unknown primary head and neck carcinoma. Arch Otolaryngol Head Neck Surg. 2005;131:626-9.
7. Berg WA, Madsen KS, Schilling K, et al. Comparative effectiveness of positron emission mammography and MRI in the contralateral breast of women with newly diagnosed breast cancer. Am J Roentgenol. 2012;198:219-32.
8. Nayak B, Dogra PN, Naswa N, Kumar R. Diuretic (18)F-FDG PET/CT imaging for detection and locoregional staging of urinary bladder cancer: prospective evaluation of a novel technique. Eur J Nucl Med Mol Imaging. 2012. [Epub ahead of print].
9. Gawande RS, Khurana A, Messing S, et al. Differentiation of normal thymus from anterior mediastinal lymphoma and lymphoma recurrence at pediatric PET/CT. Radiology. 2012;262:613-22.
10. Kumar A, Regmi SK, Dutta R, et al. Characterization of thymic masses using ^{18}F-FDG PET-CT. Ann Nucl Med. 2009;23:569-77.
11. Kumar R, Sharma P, Garg P, et al. Role of (68)Ga-DOTATOC PET-CT in the diagnosis and staging of pancreatic neuroendocrine tumors. Eur Radiol. 2011;21:2408-16.
12. Naswa N, Sharma P, Nazar AH, et al. Prospective evaluation of ^{68}Ga-DOTA-NOC PET-CT in pheochromocytoma and paraganglioma: preliminary results from a single centre study. Eur Radiol. 2012;22:710-9.
13. Naswa N, Sharma P, Soundararajan R, et al. Diagnostic performance of somatostatin receptor PET/CT using (68) Ga-DOTANOC in gastrinoma patients with negative or equivocal CT findings. Abdom Imaging. 2012. [Epub ahead of print].
14. De Wever W, Stroobants S, Coolen J, Verschakelen JA. Integrated PET/CT in the staging of non-small cell lung cancer: technical aspects and clinical integration. Eur Respir J. 2009;33:201-12.
15. El-Galaly TC, d'Amore F, Mylam KJ, et al. Routine bone marrow biopsy has little or no therapeutic consequence for positron emission tomography/computed

tomography-staged treatment-naive patients with Hodgkin lymphoma. J Clin Oncol. 2012;30:4508-14.
16. Brush J, Boyd K, Chappell F, et al. The value of FDG positron emission tomography/computerised tomography (PET/CT) in pre-operative staging of colorectal cancer: a systematic review and economic evaluation. Health Technol Assess. 2011;15:1-192.
17. Riegger C, Herrmann J, Nagarajah J, et al. Whole-body FDG PET/CT is more accurate than conventional imaging for staging primary breast cancer patients. Eur J Nucl Med Mol Imaging. 2012;39:852-63.
18. Barber TW, Duong CP, Leong T, et al. 18F-FDG PET/CT has a high impact on patient management and provides powerful prognostic stratification in the primary staging of esophageal cancer: a prospective study with mature survival data. J Nucl Med. 2012;53:864-71.
19. Marzola MC, De Manzoni G, Grassetto G, et al. Extended staging of oesophageal cancer using FDG-PET—a critical appraisal. Eur J Radiol. 2012;81:21-30.
20. Evangelista L, Guttilla A, Zattoni F, et al. Utility of choline positron emission tomography/computed tomography for lymph node involvement identification in intermediate-to high-risk prostate cancer: a systematic literature review and meta-analysis. Eur Urol. 2012. doi:pii: S0302-2838(12) 01107-4.
21. Divgi CR, Uzzo RG, Gatsonis C, et al. Positron emission tomography/computed tomography identification of clear cell renal cell carcinoma: results from the REDECT Trial. J Clin Oncol. 2013;31:187-94.
22. Bakhshi S, Radhakrishnan V, Sharma P, et al. Pediatric non-lymphoblastic non-Hodgkin lymphoma: baseline, interim, and posttreatment PET/CT versus contrast-enhanced CT for evaluation-a prospective study. Radiology. 2012;262:956-68.
23. Kumar A, Kumar R, Seenu V, et al. The role of ^{18}F-FDG PET/CT in evaluation of early response to neoadjuvant chemotherapy in patients with locally advanced breast cancer. Eur Radiol. 2009;19:1347-57.
24. Haug AR, Tiega Donfack BP, Trumm C, et al. ^{18}F-FDG PET/CT predicts survival after radioembolization of hepatic metastases from breast cancer. J Nucl Med. 2012;53:371-7.
25. Hendlisz A, Golfinopoulos V, Garcia C, et al. Serial FDG-PET/CT for early outcome prediction in patients with metastatic colorectal cancer undergoing chemotherapy. Ann Oncol. 2012;23:1687-93.
26. Bajpai J, Kumar R, Sreenivas V, et al. Prediction of chemotherapy response by PET-CT in osteosarcoma: correlation with histologic necrosis. J Pediatr Hematol Oncol. 2011;33:e271-8.
27. Maas M, Rutten IJ, Nelemans PJ, et al. What is the most accurate whole-body imaging modality for assessment of local and distant recurrent disease in colorectal cancer? A meta-analysis: Imaging for recurrent colorectal cancer. Eur J Nucl Med Mol Imaging. 2011;38:1560-71.
28. Bipat S, van Leeuwen MS, Comans EF, et al. Colorectal liver metastases: CT, MR imaging, and PET for diagnosis-meta-analysis. Radiology. 2005;237:123-31.
29. Kumar R, Sharma P, Kumari A, et al. Role of ^{18}F-FDG PET/CT in detecting recurrent gallbladder carcinoma. Clin Nucl Med. 2012;37:431-5.
30. Son H, Khan SM, Rahaman J, et al. Role of FDG PET/CT in staging of recurrent ovarian cancer. Radiographics. 2011;31:569-83.
31. Chen HH, Chiu NT, Su WC, et al. Prognostic value of whole-body total lesion glycolysis at pretreatment FDG PET/CT in non-small cell lung cancer. Radiology. 2012;264:559-66.
32. Chawla SC, Federman N, Zhang D, Nagata K, Nuthakki S, McNitt-Gray M, et al. Estimated cumulative radiation dose from PET/CT in children with malignancies: a 5-year retrospective review. Pediatr Radiol. 2010;40: 681-6.
33. Mattsson S, Söderberg M. Radiation dose management in CT, SPECT/CT and PET/CT techniques. Radiat Prot Dosimetry. 2011;147(1-2):13-21.
34. Delso G, Fürst S, Jakoby B, Ladebeck R, Ganter C, Nekolla SG, et al. Performance measurements of the Siemens mMR integrated whole-body PET/MR scanner. J Nucl Med. 2011;52:1914-22.
35. Pichler BJ, Judenhofer MS, Catana C, Walton JH, Kneilling M, Nutt RE, et al. Performance test of an LSO-APD detector in a 7-T MRI scanner for simultaneous PET/MRI. J Nucl Med. 2006;47:639-47.
36. Hofmann M, Pichler B, Schölkopf B, et al. Towards quantitative PET/MRI: a review of MR-based attenuation correction techniques. Eur J Nucl Med Mol Imaging. 2009;36(Suppl 1):S93-104.
37. Zaidi H, Ojha N, Morich M, Griesmer J, Hu Z, Maniawski P, et al. Design and performance evaluation of a whole-body Ingenuity TF PET-MRI system. Phys Med Biol. 2011;56:3091-106.
38. Assiri Y, Schmid D, Pietsch C, et al. Contrast-enhanced PET/CT vs. non-contrast enhanced PET/MRI in abdominal oncological lesions—Initial results. Annual Congress of the European Association of Nuclear Medicine, Milan, Italy, 2012.
39. Punwani S. Diffusion weighted imaging of female pelvis cancers: Concepts and clinical applications. Eur J Radiol. 2011;78:21-9.
40. Giannarini G, Petralia G, Thoeney HC. Potential and limitations of diffusion-weighted magnetic resonance imaging in kidney, prostate, and bladder cancer including pelvic lymph node staging: A critical analysis of the literature. Eur Urol. 2012;61:326-40.
41. Jansen JFA, Schöder H, Lee NY, et al. Tumor metabolism and perfusion in head and neck squamous cell carcinoma: pretreatment multimodality imaging with 1H magnetic resonance spectroscopy, dynamic contrast-enhanced MRI and [18F] FDG-PET. Int J Radiat Oncol Biol Phys. 2012;82:299-307.
42. Hirsch FW, Sattler B, Sorge I, et al. PET/MR in children. Initial clinical experience in paediatric oncology using an integrated PET/MR scanner. Pediatr Radiol. 2013 Jan 11. [Epub ahead of print]

43. Wahl RL, Jacene H, Kasamon Y, et al. From RECIST to PERCIST: Evolving Considerations for PET Response Criteria in Solid Tumors. J Nucl Med. 2009;50:122S-150.
44. Hutchings M, Loft A, Hansen M, et al. FDG-PET after two cycles of chemotherapy predicts treatment failure and progression-free survival in Hodgkin Lymphoma. Blood. 2006;107:52-9.
45. Niekel MC, Bipat S, Stoker J. Diagnostic imaging of colorectal liver metastases with CT, MR imaging, FDG PET, and/or FDG PET/CT: a meta-analysis of prospective studies including patients who have not previously undergone treatment. Radiology. 2010;257:674-84.
46. Crook DW, Mader C, Kuhn FP, et al. Diagnostic performance of PET/MR versus PET/CT in the abdomen. Presented at: European Congress of Radiology, Vienna, 2012.
47. Bentzen SM, Gregoire V. Molecular imaging-based dose-painting: a novel paradigm for radiation therapy prescription. Semin Radiat Oncol. 2011;21:101-10.
48. Thorwarth D, Eschmann SM, Paulsen F, et al. Hypoxia dose painting by numbers: a planning study. Int J Radiat Oncol Biol Phys. 2007;68:291-300.
49. Nehmeh SA, Lee NY, Schröder H, et al. Reproducibility of intratumor distribution of 18F-fluoromisonidazole in head and neck cancer. Int J Radiat Oncol Biol Phys. 2008;70:235-42.
50. Padhani AR, Krohn KA, Lewis JS, et al. Imaging oxygenation of human tumors. Eur Radiol. 2007;17:861-72.
51. Dirix P, Vandecaveye V, De Keyzer F, et al. Dose painting in radiotherapy for head and neck squamous cell carcinoma: value of repeated functional imaging with ^{18}F-FDG PET, ^{18}F-Fluoromisonidazole PET, diffusion-weighted MRI and dynam contrast-enhanced MRI. J Nucl Med. 2009;50: 1020-7.
52. Ossenkoppele R, Tolboom N, Foster-Dingley JC, et al. Longitudinal imaging of Alzheimer pathology using [11C] PIB, [18F]FDDNP and [18F]FDG PET. Eur J Nucl Med Mol Imaging. 2012;39:990-1000.
53. Kenny ER, Blamire AM, Firbank MJ, et al. Functional connectivity in cortical regions in dementia with Lewy bodies and Alzheimer's disease. Brain. 2012;135:569-81.
54. Duncan J. The current status of neuroimaging for epilepsy. Curr Opin Neurol. 2009;22:179-84.

CHAPTER 64

Common Drugs Used in an Imaging Department

Anupam Lal, Vivek Gupta, Manphool Singhal

INTRODUCTION

The beneficial or toxic effects of many plant and animal materials were known to us since the prehistoric times. Advances in chemistry and the further development of physiology in present time laid the foundation needed for understanding how drugs work at the organ and tissue levels. The last few decades have seen an exponential growth of information and understanding of the molecular basis for drug action. Better understanding of drug receptors and pharmacokinetics have led to modifying existing drugs for selective action or synthesizing newer drugs previously unknown to mankind.

The recent era has also witnessed a dramatic growth in the field of electronics and computerization, leading to development of faster and more precise medical imaging equipment that have made possible the minimally invasive image-guided interventional procedures. The interventional procedures continue to evolve and the list is ever increasing, that includes central venous catheter placements, tumor treatments (uterine fibroid therapy, radio- and chemoembolization of tumor, percutaneous radiofrequency and cryoablation), and procedures, such as angioplasty, abdominal aortic aneurysm stent-graft repair, vertebroplasty, kyphoplasty, and varicose vein therapies. There have also been advancements in standard biliary and urinary drainage procedures, percutaneous gastrointestinal feeding tube placement, and transjugular intrahepatic portosystemic shunts. These complicated procedures mandates use of drugs required for patient preparation, therapeutic applications and for preventing complications of the radiological interventions. The radiologists are no longer supervising only contrast administration and managing contrast reactions but also providing therapies for many diseases. The present imaging departments thus are equipped with modern anesthetic and life support machines and a large number of drugs that will be required in various interventional procedures. A thorough knowledge and understanding of these drugs is of paramount importance to the interventional radiologist for their judicious use and for preventing untoward reactions. A brief description of common drugs used in modern radiology department follows. The readers are encouraged to refer to standard textbooks of pharmacology for dosing and drug interactions in specific clinical scenario. Medications commonly used in radiology department can be divided into the following broad categories:

- Drugs used for patient preparation
- Drugs used for optimizing imaging evaluation
- Drugs affecting coagulation and antiplatelets
- Sclerosants and embolizing agents
- Drugs for transarterial chemoembolization (TACE).

DRUGS FOR PATIENT PREPARATION: SEDATIVES

Midazolam is the most commonly used short-acting benzodiazepine that possesses potent anxiolytic, amnestic, hypnotic, anticonvulsant, skeletal muscle relaxant, and sedative properties. Like all benzodiazepines it bind to specific $GABA_A$ receptor subunits at central nervous system (CNS) neuronal synapses facilitating GABA-mediated chloride ion channel opening and enhance membrane hyperpolarization. Midazolam is roughly 3–4 times more powerful and has twice the affinity for benzodiazepine receptors than diazepam and has more potent amnesic effects and also has a fast recovery time. Typical adult dose is 1–2.5 mg IV, and can be repeated every 5–10 minutes to a maximum dose of 10 mg. Midazolam has more potential than other benzodiazepines to cause respiratory depression and arrest hence should be administered slowly and extreme caution to be exercised in pediatric patients.

Intravenous midazolam is indicated for procedural sedation (often in combination with an opioid, such as fentanyl), for preprocedural sedation and for the induction of general anesthesia. Flumazenil, a benzodiazepine antagonist drug, can be used to treat an overdose of midazolam, as well as to reverse sedation. However, flumazenil can trigger seizures in mixed overdoses and in benzodiazepine-dependent individuals, so is not used in most cases.

Among the antihistaminics used for sedation, promethazine (Phenergan) 12.5–25 mg every 4 hourly or diphenhydramine (Benadryl) 25–50 mg are the most commonly employed.

Local Anesthetics

Local anesthetics (LA) effectively and reversibly block impulse conduction along nerve axons and other excitable membranes that use sodium channels as the primary means of action potential generation. Clinically, local anesthetics are used to block pain sensation from or sympathetic vasoconstrictor impulses to specific areas of the body. Newer local anesthetics were introduced with the goal of reducing local tissue irritation, minimizing systemic cardiac and CNS toxicity, and achieving a faster onset and longer duration of action.

They are broadly classified as follows:

- Aminoamides, e.g. lignocaine, bupivacaine, rapivacaine, etc.
- Aminoesters, e.g. procaine, benzocaine, cocaine, etc.

Lidocaine, is still a widely used local anesthetic, was synthesized in 1943 by Löfgren.

Methods of Administration

The choice of local anesthetic for infiltration, peripheral nerve blocks, and central neuraxis (spinal/epidural) blockade is usually based on the duration of action required. Procaine and chloroprocaine are short-acting; lidocaine, mepivacaine, and prilocaine have an intermediate duration of action; and tetracaine, bupivacaine, levobupivacaine, and ropivacaine are long-acting local anesthetics. The anesthetic effect of the agents with short and intermediate durations of action can be prolonged by increasing the dose or adding a vasoconstrictor agent (e.g. epinephrine or phenylephrine). The vasoconstrictor slows the removal of the local anesthetic from the injection site. In addition, it decreases the blood level and the probability of cardiovascular and CNS toxicity. The onset of local anesthesia can be accelerated by the addition of sodium bicarbonate (1–2 mL) to the local anesthetic solution. This maximizes the amount of drug in the more lipid-soluble (unionized) form. Repeated injections of local anesthetics can result in loss of effectiveness (i.e. tachyphylaxis) due to extracellular acidosis.

Infiltration Anesthesia

It is injecting the agent directly into the tissue without taking into consideration of course of cutaneous nerves. It is so superficial as to include only the skin. However deeper structures can also be included.

Others

- Surface anesthesia
- Nerve block
- Spinal anesthesia
- Epidural anesthesia
- Intravenous regional anesthesia.

Adverse Effects

CNS: Causes stimulation of CNS, producing restlessness and tremors that may proceed to clonic convulsions.

CVS: Usually due to inadvertent intravascular injection. Hypotension, due to arteriolar dilatation and cardiovascular collapse probably due to action on pacemaker or sudden onset ventricular fibrillation may occur.

Hypersensitivity: It is very rare and slightly more common with aminoesters. It can manifest either as allergic dermatitis or a typical asthmatic attack.

Sting Free LA

Addition of sodium bicarbonate reduced the stinging sensation related to the acidic nature of adrenaline containing LA.

- 2% lignocaine, 19 mL
- Adrenaline 1: 1000, 0.1 mL
- Normal saline, 20 mL
- Sodium bicarbonate (8.3%), 4 mL.

DRUGS USED FOR OPTIMIZING IMAGING EVALUATION: DIURETICS

Loop diuretics selectively inhibit NaCl reabsorption in the thick ascending limb of loop of Henle. Because of the large NaCl absorptive capacity of this segment and the fact that the diuretic action of these drugs is not limited by development of acidosis, as is the case with the carbonic anhydrase inhibitors, loop diuretics are the most efficacious diuretic agents currently available. Furosemide is the prototype of this group and is often used for optimizing urologic diagnostic procedures. The duration of effect for furosemide is usually 2–3 hours. Half-life depends on renal function. Reduction in the secretion of loop diuretics may result from simultaneous administration of agents such as NSAIDs or probenecid, which compete for weak acid secretion in the proximal tubule.

Uses

- *MRU*: Intravenous injection of low-dose furosemide (5–10 mg) and gadolinium (Gd) chelate is used for achieving a uniform distribution of the contrast material inside the entire urinary tract.
- *CTU*: Supplemental intravenous furosemide (10 mg) a vasodilator (an "inodilator") by selective inhibition of cAMP-may be used to optimize urinary collecting system opacification and distention.
- *IVU*: 10–20 mg lasix (1 mg/kg pediatric dose) is used to differentiate between complete or partial PUJO, PUJO and extrarenal pelvis at 4 hours of IVU study.

Contraindications

Furosemide, bumetanide, and torsemide may exhibit allergic cross-reactivity in patients who are sensitive to other sulfonamides, but this appears to be very rare. Overzealous use of any diuretic is dangerous in hepatic cirrhosis, borderline renal failure, or heart failure.

Vasodilators

They are used to treat angiographic and clinical vasospasm either alone or in combination with transluminal balloon angioplasty (TBA). Commonly used agents include papavarine, calcium channel blocker (nimodipine, verapamil, nicardipine) and milrinone.

Papaverine

Papaverine has been the most commonly used vasodilator for intra-arterial infusion therapy, a benzylisoquinoline alkaloid and a potent smooth muscle relaxant, is believed to act by the inhibition of phosphodiesterse activity in smooth muscle cells. It has been associated with seizures and elevations in intracranial pressure.

Dosage: 300 mg of papavarine diluted in 100 mL of normal saline forming a concentration of 0.3%. Approximately 2–4 mL of 0.3% papaverine solution injected as pulse spray. Papaverine should not be mixed with contrast agents or heparin because it may cause precipitation of crystals. Infusion of highly concentrated papaverine may have fewer vasodilatory effects and a higher risk of temporary deterioration, possibly because of emboli formed from papaverine precipitates.

Nimodipine

It is a dihydropyridine type of calcium channel blocker and specifically block L-type voltage-gated calcium channels. Dosage (intra-arterial)—Nimodipine diluted in a solution of NaCl 0.9% to obtain a 25% concentration.

Typical dose administered is 1–4 mg (5–20 mL) per vessel with the maximum rate of 2 mL/min. Intensive blood pressure monitoring is required during therapy as it can lead to hypotension.

Milrinone

Milrinone is a bypyridine methyl carbonitrile analog of amrinone. Its mechanism of action is similar to that of papaverine, which is a nonselective inhibitor of phosphodiesterase. Milrinone works as an inotropic drug and specific phosphodiesterase III in both cardiac and vascular smooth muscle. Parenteral milrinone delivered in large doses can cause systemic hypotension. Unlike Papavarine no significant elevation in intracranial pressure is seen.

Dosage: (Intra-arterial) Milrinone diluted in a solution of NaCl 0.9% to obtain a 25% concentration. Typical dose is infusion at a rate of 0.25 mg/min, with a total dose of 10–15 mg.

Recurrence of cerebral vasospasm, however, is common after vasodilator infusion, as these drugs have relatively short half-lives, therefore requiring additional infusion or TBA. At authors institute, Intra-arterial nimodipine is used and is reserved for patients with symptomatic vasospasm who have vessel diameter reduction between 25% and 50% of the initial diameter angiographically and in patients with distal vessel vasospasm not amenable to balloon angioplasty.

Patient Preparation in Suspected Pheochromocytoma

Older literature suggested premedication with oral alpha and beta-adrenergic blockade (phentolamine 5 mg and meto prolol 10 mg) for IV contrast medium usage in patients with pheochromocytoma, for preventing adrenergic crisis. It is to be remembered that beta blockade should never be used without alpha blockade in patients with pheochromocytoma. However recent studies indicate no need for routine prophylaxis when nonionic contrast media are employed.

Drugs for Cardiac Imaging

Cardiac CT

Cardiac CT (coronary angiography) is unique in that, the image quality is inversely proportional to motion artifacts and the best image quality is achieved at low heart rates <65 beats per minute (BPM). Thus, aggressive reduction of a patient's heart rate is advised before a scan for all patients with heart rates of more than 70 BPM especially when study is planned on 64-slice scanners, however with the availability of higher slice and dual-source CT scanners regulation of heart is not a concern but preferable. For regulation of heart rate to less than 65 BPM and make the rhythm regular the use of cardioselective (β1) β-blockers and newer drug ivadrabine is advocated.[1,2]

β-blockers

β-blockers reduce the heart rate by decreasing the frequency of the sinus node, slowing conduction in the atria and atrioventricular node, and by increasing the functional refractory period of the atrioventricular node. Various β-blockers in use are metoprolol, atenolol and esmolol, however metoprolol is the most preferred drug. Metoprolol can be given either oral or intravenous and protocols for its administration may vary from center to center. Intravenous yields higher (95%) bioavailability than oral (40%) administration due to high first-pass metabolism; hence, for faster reduction of heart rate intravenous administration is preferred. Its half-life is 3–4 hours. 50–100 mg oral metoprolol 1 hour before or intravenous metoprolol 5–20 mg immediately before the procedure can be employed. Intravenous administration should be slow over 1–2 minutes to be given in doses of 2.5–5 mg which can be repeated if required. In some centers oral metoprolol followed by intravenous metoprolol or esmolol is given. Esmolol being short acting (half-life—9 minutes) can be given as bolus doses for effective control of heart rate.[1,2]

Contraindications: Asthma and COPD patients, aortic stenosis, carotid stenosis, pulmonary embolism, atrioventricular block.

β-blockers causes significant reduction in ejection fraction, stroke volume and cardiac output therefore these agents should be avoided prior to imaging for evaluation of left ventricular functional analysis.[1]

Ivabradine

Ivabradine is a new drug which is pure heart rate lowering agent that acts by inhibiting ionic current in the pacemaker activity of sinoatrial node.[1] Results are better with higher heart rates. At present, it is available in oral form with dosage of 5–7.5 mg twice a day. It can be given as an alternative or adjunct to β-blockers.

Cardiac Stress MRI

The stress cardiac MRI is increasing being evaluated and now is clinical practice for the evaluation of inducible ischemia in patient with coronary artery disease and detection of myocardial viability. To invoke the cardiac stress during the MRI examination pharmacologic agents either positive inotrope (dobutamine or arbutamine) or vasodilator (dipyridamole or adenosine) are used.

Dobutamine

Dobutamine increases myocardial contractility and heart rate.[3] During the MRI (pre- and postdobutamine) the myocardial functions, contractility, perfusion and viability is assessed typically after injection of MRI contrast. It is given intravenously in the doses of 2.5–4.0 mg/kg/min. The side effects are chest discomfort and arrthymias. Its use should be terminated immediately once the signs of myocardial ischemia are detected by use of intravenous atropine in the doses of 0.3 mg increments every minute up to total dose of 1.5 mg.

Adenosine

Adenosine is a short acting (half-life less than 10 seconds) systemic arterial vasodilator. The intravenous dose is 140 μg/kg/min over 4–6 minutes (for a total dose of 0.84 mg/kg).

The common side effects include flushing, chest discomfort, anxiety, dyspnea and headache.[4]

DRUGS AFFECTING COAGULATION: PROCOAGULANTS

Thrombin

Thrombin is the product of the hemostatic response that converts fibrinogen to fibrin. It is also responsible for the aggregation of blood platelets in the formation of the "platelet plug" as well as the activation of factor VIII, factor V, factor XI, factor XIII and protein C. Percutaneous ultrasound-guided thrombin injection into the lumen of the pseudoaneurysm is a quick and valuable therapeutic alternative to endovascular management.[5,6] The technique has proven quick, safe, and comfortable for the patient, even in patients who have received anticoagulation and antiplatelet therapy. The most serious complication is distal arterial embolization, with a frequency of about 2%.

The initial thrombin was bovine in origin, and its use had been complicated by the formation of antibodies that cross react with human coagulation factors. This has been associated with life-threatening bleeding and in some circumstances anaphylaxis and death. Human thrombin, isolated from pooled plasma of donors, has been developed in an effort to minimize these risks, but its downside is the potential of transmitting blood-borne pathogens and limited availability. Recombinant thrombin has the advantage of being minimally antigenic and devoid of the risk of viral transmission. Human thrombin is more effective than bovine thrombin and thus the required dose for treating pseudoaneurysm is less. An injection of thrombin into the pseudoaneurysm is made through a thin 22 or 23 gauge needle and small boluses (0.1–0.3 mL) of the thrombin solution is given under ultrasound guidance till complete thrombosis of the aneurysm sac is achieved.[6] Thrombin is often used in conjunction with other hemostatic aids, including absorbable agents (like gelfoam, collagen, and cellulose), and with fibrinogen in fibrin glues. Fibrin glues contain thrombin and fibrinogen. When combined, the fibrinogen is activated by thrombin and converted into fibrin monomers. This forms an adhesive glue at the tissues applied. The fibrin monomers go on to interact with the patient's own factor XIII and calcium to convert the final product into a fibrin polymer that allows for platelet activation and aggregation with subsequent hemostasis. Fibrin glues come packaged with a dual chamber syringe that allows for the combination of the thrombin and fibrinogen after the plunger is depressed. The human thrombin is part of a commercial package sold as a fibrin sealant kit (500 U/mL or 1000 U/mL). Each packet contains a solution of human thrombin in calcium chloride and a fibrinogen concentrate with factor XIII and other proteins.

Anticoagulants

Intravascular procedures using indwelling catheters and sheaths would be impossible without inhibition of the coagulation cascade. These can be classified as follows:

- *Parenteral*
  - Heparin
    - Unfractionated heparin (UFH)
    - Low-molecular weight heparin, e.g. Enoxaparin, Dalteparin, Tcnzaparin
    - Heparinoids
    - Pentsaccharides—fondaparinux
  - Direct thrombin inhibitors (DTI)—hirudin, bivalirudin.
- *Oral*
  - Warfarin
  - Acenocaumarol
  - Phenindiones
  - Factor Xa inhibitors—rivaroxaban
  - Thrombin inhibitors, e.g. xemilgatron.

Heparin

Heparins in medical use are a heterogeneous population of linear polysaccharides belonging to the glycosaminoglycan family with molecular weight of 10,000–20,000. Heparin acts indirectly by activation of antithrombin (AT), leading primarily to the inactivation of clotting cascade factors Xa and thrombin (factor IIa). Thrombin is most sensitive to inhibition, and is 10 times more sensitive than factor Xa. Low dose of heparin prolong aPTT without significantly prolonging PT. High concentration of heparin prolong both aPTT and PT.

Injected IV, it acts instantaneously but after SC injection, anticoagulant effect develops after ~60 min. Heparin does not cross blood-brain barrier or placenta (the anticoagulant of choice during pregnancy). It is metabolized in liver and excreted in urine, so its half-life is longer in cirrhotics and renal failure patients. After IV injection of doses <100 U/kg, the averages half-life is 1 hr. Monitoring of heparin dosage during intervention procedures is guided by measuring activated clotting time (ACT) taken with 2 cc of whole blood. Normal range of ACT is 91–151 s, and it is to be taken every 1/2 hr.

Dosage of UFH for Optimal ACT Values in Endovascular Procedures[7-10]

- IV bolus of 3000 U, 5000 U, and 10,000 U, or ranging from 50 U/kg to 100 U/kg. A typical dose use in intervention procedures is 80U/kg bolus followed by 18 U/kg/hour
- Target ACT from 150–200 seconds to 350–400 seconds
- For low-risk procedures ACT—250–300 seconds
- For high-risk procedures, such as angioplasty and stent placement, ACT range of 300–350 seconds is recommended
- Goal of 400 sec for stent with filter device.

Bleeding due to overdose is the most serious complication of heparin therapy. Heparin-induced thrombocytopenia and osteoporosis (on long-term use) are the other adverse effects of heparin.

Heparin Antagonist: Protamine sulfate is a strongly basic low-molecular weight protein obtained from the sperm of salmon fish. It is used during hemorrhage in intervention procedure (AVM, aneurysm, vessel rupture). Given IV slowly it neutralizes heparin weight for weight, i.e. 1 mg is needed for every 100 U of heparin. In absence of heparin it itself has weak anticoagulant action. Being basic in nature it can release histamine in the body and can lead to hypersensitivity reactions.

Low-molecular Weight (LMW) Heparins: Low-molecular weight heparins (MW 3000–7000) have different anticoagulant profile; selectively inhibit factor Xa with little effect on factor IIa. Thrombocytopenia is less frequent. The major advantages are better SC availability with once daily sc administration. Dose is calculated on body weight basis. Since aPTT is not prolonged laboratory monitoring is not needed. They are mainly used in prevention and treatment of deep venous thrombosis.

Thrombolytics

Thrombolytic agents are used for the treatment of myocardial infarction, thromboembolic strokes, deep vein thrombosis and pulmonary embolism. They may also be used to clear blocked catheters that are used in long-term medical therapy.

Classification of Thrombolytics

1. *1st generation (Non fibrin-specific)*
   - Streptokinase
   - Urokinase
2. *2nd generation (Fibrin-specific)*
   - Prourokinase
   - Recombinant tissue plasminogen activator: Alteplase (Rt.-PA)
3. *3rd generation (Fibrin-specific)*
   - Reteplase (r- PA)
   - Tenecteplase (TNK-tPA)
   - Desmopletase.

Streptokinase: It is obtained from β hemolytic streptococci group C. It is inactive as such: combines with circulating plasminogen to form an activator complex which then cause limited proteolysis of other plasminogen molecules to plasmin. It has limited usefulness because many patients have preformed antistreptococcal antibodies and have potential for anaphylactic reaction. It is the least expensive of all the fibrinolytics.

Dosage: Bolus: 50,000U, Infusion: 5000U/hour for 12 hours.

Urokinase: It is an enzyme isolated from human urine and now prepared from cultured human kidney cells. It is non-antigenic.

Dosage: Bolus: 30,000–60,000U, Infusion: 4000U/hour for 2 hours, 2000U/hour for next 2 hours and 1000U/hour for next 8 hours.

Alteplase: It is produced by recombinant DNA technology. It is fibrin specific with little effect on circulating plasminogen. It has the drawback of lowering the levels of fibrinogen and plasminogen, leading to an increased risk of hemorrhagic complications. Presently, right-PA is the only agent approved by the FDA specifically for IV thrombolysis for ischemic stroke.

Dosage: It is available as 20–50 mg lyophilized powder, to be reconstituted.

- *Intravenous*: 0.9 mg/kg, 15%—Bolus, 85%—Infusion over a period of 30 minutes.
- *Bridging therapy*: 0.6 mg/kg IV (60 mg maximum over 30 minutes) followed by intra-arterially administration at the site of clot up to a total dose of 22 mg over two hours of infusion or until lysis of thrombus was obtained. 3rd generation agents offer the theoretical advantage of longer half-life and greater penetration into the thrombus matrix when compared to 2nd-generation agents. The half-life of alteplase is compared with that of other thrombolytic agents in **Table 1**. Retaplase is a genetically engineered, smaller derivative of recombinant right-PA that has increased potency and is faster acting than right-PA.

Dosage: Intra-arterial: 0.5 U/hour, Intravenous: 1 U/hour, maximum dose of 24 U in 24 hours.

Reversal of all thrombolytics can be done by administering fresh frozen plasma in the event of hemorrhagic complication.

Table 1: Half-life of thrombolytic agents.

Agent	*Half-life (min)*
Streptokinase	30–80
Urokinase	14–20
Prourokinase	20
Alteplase	3–5
Reteplase	15–18

Contraindications

Absolute

- Intracranial bleed
- Drug allergy.

Relative

- Surgery within 10 days
- Serious GI bleed within 3 months
- Hypertension with diastolic BP ≥110 mm Hg
- Active bleeding or hemorrhagic disorder
- Aortic dissection.

Adverse effects

- Bleeding complications at catheterization site, gastroin-testinal and cerebral hemorrhages may occur
- Rethrombosis can occur following thrombolysis and therefore anticoagulants such as heparin are usually co-administered, and continued after thrombolytic therapy.

Antiplatelets

These drugs decrease platelet aggregation and thrombus formation. They are effective in arterial circulation where anti-coagulants have little effect. Antiplatelets can be classified as:

- *Cyclooxygenase-1 (COX-1) inhibitor*: Aspirin
- *P2Y12 inhibitors (Thienopyridines)*: Ticlopidine, clopidogrel prasugrel
- *Phosphodiesterase inhibitors*: Dipyridamole, cilostazol
- *GPIIb/IIIa blockers*: Abciximab, eptifibatide, tirofiban.

Cyclooxygenase-1 Inhibitor

Aspirin induces a permanent functional defect in platelets, which can be detected clinically as a prolonged bleeding time. It primarily, acts by irreversible acetylation of COX-1, responsible for the formation of prostaglandin (PG) H_2, the precursor of thromboxane (TX) A_2.

The non-linear relationship between inactivation of platelet COX-1 and inhibition of TXA_2-dependent platelet function by low-dose aspirin has important implications: (i) a substantial reduction in platelet inhibition is associated with less than maximal inactivation of COX-1; (ii) recovery of platelet function is disproportionately rapid, occurring within 3–4 days upon drug withdrawal.

Moreover, inhibition of TXA2-dependent platelet function by aspirin leaves other platelet pathways [adenosine diphosphate (ADP)-P2Y12, thrombin-protease-activated receptor (PAR)-1] largely unaffected, thus providing a rationale for dual or triple antiplatelet therapy in high-risk settings.

Dosage: 50–325 mg oral.

Thienopyridines

Thienopyridines inhibit ADP dependent platelet function by irreversible modification of the platelet P2Y12 receptor through short-lived active metabolites, generated by liver cytochrome P-450 (CYP) isozymes. Recovery of platelet function after drug withdrawal occurs linearly over 7–8 days as a function of platelet turnover.

Genetic variation of the liver enzymes responsible for the metabolism of clopidogrel as well as drug–drug interactions [e.g. with proton pump inhibitors (PPIs)] are important determinants of the variable circulating levels of its active metabolite. These, in turn, are associated with variable inhibition of ADP-induced platelet aggregation and variable clinical response to clopidogrel treatment. It is used at a dosage of 75 mg for 3–5 days prior to the procedure followed by 75 mg maintains dose, post procedure for 3 months. In case of emergency scenario it can be used at the dosage of 450 to 600 mg 2 to 6 hours prior to the procedure. It is typically used in combination with aspirin.

Prasugrel is also a prodrug. It has more profound and less variable inhibition of platelet function observed when compared with clopidogrel. In contrast to clopidogrel, the lack of drug interaction potential and the apparent independence of CYP2C19 genetic variance result in a predictable antiplatelet response to prasugrel.

Antiplatelet agents such as aspirin and clopidogrel are cornerstones that have allowed and increased the use of minimally invasive treatment of cerebrovascular diseases and have reduced thromboembolic events.

Antiplatelet resistance

Drug resistance to antiplatelet agents has been a long-term problem, especially in known diabetic and hyper-cholesterolemia patient. These patients usually require a higher dose of these drugs for desired effect.

GPIIb/IIIa blockers

GPIIb/IIIa is an adhesive receptor (integrin) for fibrinogen and von Willebrand factor through which agonists like collagen, thrombin, TXA_2, ADP, etc. induce platelet aggregation. Thus antagonists prevent fibrinogen binding to activated GPIIb/ IIIa receptors and, thus, formation of fibrinogen bridges between platelets.

Abciximab, a non-competitive inhibitor of GPIIb/IIIa, is the humanized chimeric Fab-fragment of the monoclonal mouse antibody 7E3. Their effect on platelet aggregation is closely linked to plasma concentrations. Owing to their short plasma half-lives, continuous infusion is needed for sustained platelet inhibition.

Abciximab is used as a rescue agent in the management of thrombotic complications of intracranial and carotid angioplasty, intracranial aneurysm coiling. It has also been used in combination with fibrinolytic agents to enhance thrombolysis.

Dosage: Abciximab - 0.25 mg/kg IV bolus followed by 0.125 μg/kg/min continuous IV infusion for 12 hours.

For thrombosis associated with Aneurysmal coiling: Abciximab diluted with saline at concentration of 0.2 mg/mL. Injected intra arterially as bolus of 4–10 mg over a period of 10–20 minutes.

Phosphodiesterase Inhibitors

Cilostazol is a reversible type III phosphodiesterase inhibitor, with vasodilator and antiplatelet effects. It increases intra platelet CAMP, reduces cellular adenosine uptake, and inhibits vascular smooth muscle cell proliferation. Added to a standard combination of aspirin plus clopidogrel, cilostazol 100 mg bid has been found to potentiate inhibition of ADP-induced platelet aggregation when compared with aspirin and clopidogrel.

SCLEROSANTS AND EMBOLIC AGENTS

Historically, the first agent used for embolotherapy was auto logous blood clot. This was easily and quickly obtained and was inherently biocompatible. The drawback of autologous blood clot is that as the body's natural clot lysis dramatically limits the durability of occlusion; recanalization can recur within hours to days. The next agents developed were fascial strips harvested from dura and tensor fascia lata. Silk threads were also historically used as embolic agents, notably for intracranial vascular malformations. Today with the advent of modern liquid and particulates, silk, clot, and fascia are not used. Modern embolic agents are either temporary or permanent. Permanent agents are more common, and there are many applicable subsets, including liquid agents, particulates, coils, and detachable plugs and balloons.

GELATIN FOAM

Gelatin foam (Gelfoam, Upjohn, Kalamazoo, MI) has been used as an intravascular embolization agent for more than 30 years, with the first intravascular use in 1964 for cavernous carotid fistulas. Use of gelfoam is off-label for embolization, but its use is within the standard of care. Gelatin foam is a biologic substance made from purified skin gelatin. It is available in sterile sheets and as a powder comprised of 40–60 mm particles. Sheets can be cut into a variety of shapes.

Gelfoam cut into small 1–2 mm pieces can be mixed with dilute contrast and injected as pledgets, or be prepared as slurry.

Gelatin foam causes mechanical obstruction, slowing blood flow and hastening thrombus formation. In addition, it provides a scaffold for clot formation. Gelfoam embolization provides temporary vessel occlusion, allowing recanalization in a few weeks. The temporary nature of gelatin foam occlusion can be either an advantage or disadvantage depending on the clinical situation (e.g. temporary nature is advantageous in case of hemoptysis or trauma). Other advantages of gelfoam include low cost, versatility of use, and extensive clinical experience. However, it has been postulated that gelfoam can be associated with infection due to trapped air bubbles. Further, gelatin foam powder can potentially cause ischemia due to the small size (especially at sizes <70 mm) of the particles, allowing distal embolization.

POLYVINYL ALCOHOL

First introduced as an intravascular embolization agent in 1974 in the form of a sponge, current intravascular use of polyvinyl alcohol (PVA) is primarily in the form of particles.

The particles are made from a PVA foam sheet that is vacuum dried and rasped into particles. The particles are filtered with sieves and are available in sizes ranging from 100 mm to 1100 mm. Because of the method of preparation, PVA particles are slightly irregular in size. Particles are sorted by their ability to pass through a larger sieve, but not through a smaller sieve. Thus, oblong particles may have a long axis that is much longer than the stated size. One study evaluating actual size of PVA particles found that the majority were larger than the stated minimum size, with a few very small particles observed once the PVA particles were suspended in solution. Polyvinyl alcohol particles are irregular in shape, which promotes aggregation. They can be oblong, oval, irregular, sharp and angulated with small fragments after suspension.

Polyvinyl alcohol particles provide permanent occlusion by adherence to the vessel wall, causing stagnation of flow, in addition to lodging in the smallest vessel into which they will fit. The results are an inflammatory reaction and focal angio necrosis, with vessel fibrosis developing over time. Polyvinyl alcohol particles are biocompatible, and there is vast cumulative clinical experience with PVA particle embolization. The major disadvantage of PVA particles is their tendency to aggregate, occluding vessels more proximally than might be expected based on stated size. Particle clumping can also cause catheter occlusion, which is preventable by dilution of particles, proper suspension, and slow infusion. In addition, PVA particles can accumulate in the catheter hub and theoretically cause subsequent non target embolization when the catheter is flushed.

TRIS-ACRYL GELATIN MICROSPHERES

Use of tris-acryl gelatin microspheres was approved by the US Food and Drug Administration (FDA) in 2000 and gained specific approval for uterine fibroid embolization in December 2002. Embospheres are available in six size ranges: 40–120 mm, 100–300 mm, 300–500 mm, 500–700 mm, 700–900 mm, and 900–1200 mm. Embospheres are packaged in 20 mL prefilled syringes containing 2 mL of spheres in saline. Embosphere gold particles are colored for visibility. Tris-acryl gelatin microspheres are made from an acrylic polymer matrix impregnated and embedded with porcine gelatin. They are nonresorbable hydrophilic particles that are precisely calibrated by size. In addition, TAGM can be temporarily compressed by 20–30% of their initial diameter. Unlike PVA particles, TAGM are smooth and spherical in shape and fragmentation is not observed. Particle accumulation in the catheter hub, particle aggregation fragmentation, and catheter occlusion are uncommon with TAGM. In fact, larger TAGM may deform allowing delivery through a micro catheter with a lumen smaller than the maximum diameter of the sphere. By avoiding particle aggregation, Embospheres may penetrate into smaller vessels compared with PVA particles of the same size. Embospheres cause vascular occlusion by lodging in vessels and inciting a histological reaction similar to PVA particles when studied at 48 hours and 4 weeks. Embospheres are still identifiable in the tissue at 4 weeks, both intra- and extravascularly, and degeneration of the spheres has not been observed.

Disadvantages of Embospheres include the need for intermittent agitation to prevent sedimentation and maintain suspension. In addition, Embospheres are partly composed of porcine gelatin, which has allergic potential. Careful attention to sizing is necessary. The same size of Embosphere will penetrate more deeply compared with PVA and could cause unintended ischemia in some vascular beds such as the colon. The difference in effective particle size when using PVA particles versus Embospheres can be significant.

N-BUTYL-2 CYANOACRYLATE

N-butyl-2 cyanoacrylate (NBCA) is synthetic glue that was approved by the FDA in 2000 for cerebral AVM embolization. It is supplied as one or two 1 g tubes of NBCA, 10 mL of ethiodized oil, and 1 g of tantalum powder, which are mixed together immediately before use. It has been reported in the treatment of extracerebral and spinal tumors and spinal AVMs and AVFs. It has also been used for embolization of brain and spinal cord tumors, cerebral AVMS, and brain and spinal cord dural AVFs. N-butyl-2 cyanoacrylate is supplied as a free monomer, which is clear and free flowing. When exposed to an anionic environment, such as blood or water, polymerization occurs. Ethiodol is used as a vehicle and acts as a polymerization retardant. Tantalum powder is included to provide radiographic opacification, but also slows initiation of polymerization. Before use, adequate visualization should be confirmed with fluoroscopy. Polymerization of NBCA starts immediately on contact with anions, at a rate dependent on the concentration of the NBCA. Polymerization rate can be altered by varying the NBCA concentration with Ethiodol (Savage Laboratories, Melville, NY, USA) or glacial acetic acid.

To avoid unintended polymerization by premature contact with anions, catheter flushes should be performed with dextrose 5% (D5W) in water. In addition, cyanoacrylate can destroy polycarbonate, so polypropylene syringes should be used. N-butyl-2 cyanoacrylate embolization requires a special setup that includes attaching a syringe of NBCA and a syringe of D5W to the catheter via a three-way stopcock. Initial contrast injection is performed to determine the volume of glue injection required. Immediately after glue injection, the catheter tip is retracted to avoid catheter adherence to the vessel lumen. The catheter often occludes after one to two glue injections.

N-butyl-2 cyanoacrylate makes a permanent cast of the vessel, independent of inherent coagulation. It incites an acute inflammatory reaction in the vessel wall, which progresses to chronic inflammation and fibrosis. Recanalization can occur if only partial embolization is achieved. Advantages of NBCA are that it works instantly, completely occludes vessels, and is permanent. Disadvantages are that use of NBCA requires expertise. The catheter can become entrapped in the occluded vessel. Polymerization can spread distally or reflux proximally to the intended location. Finally, as part of embolization, catheter position must be abandoned.

ETHYLENE VINYL ALCOHOL COPOLYMER

Ethylene vinyl alcohol copolymer (EVOH) (Onyx, Micro Therapeutics, Inc. Irvine, CA) was first used as an embolic agent by Dr Taki in 1990 and was granted FDA approval in July 2005 as an embolic agent for cerebral AVM. It is a copolymer of ethylene vinyl alcohol prepared with dimethyl sulfoxide (DMSO) as solvent. Tantalum powder is added for opacity. On contact with blood, the DMSO diffuses away allowing polymerization of the EVOH, which forms a cast of blood vessels. In the United States, EVOH is available under the trade name Onyx, and comes prepared as Onyx 18 and Onyx 34, which differ in viscosity. Onyx 500 is available outside the United States and is indicated for the treatment of cerebral aneurysms. Lower concentration of Onyx results in a lower viscosity solution that can be injected into smaller vessels. Onyx comes packaged with a separate vial of DMSO, and special DMSO-compatible catheters must be used for the procedure. Once the catheter is placed in desired position, a small amount of DMSO is injected to fill the catheter dead space and to inhibit in-catheter Onyx polymerization. Once the catheter is in position, Onyx is delivered through the catheter under fluoroscopy. Histologic analysis of AVMs on a few patients embolized with Onyx demonstrated filling of the vessel lumen either partially or completely. Specimens resected 1 day post embolization showed with mild inflammation or angionecrosis. No specimen demonstrated extravasated Onyx. Others have reported successfully using Onyx alone or in combination with coils to treat peripheral vascular malformations.

Advantages of EVOH include that it is non-adhesive. This allows for longer injection times and the ability to temporarily suspend embolization and proceed with further angiography mid procedure if necessary. Although, there is a risk of embedding the catheter in Onyx if it refluxes around the catheter tip, the material is not adhesive and will not adhere to the catheter as does NBCA glue. Disadvantages of EVOH include the need for DMSO-compatible catheters and syringes. DMSO is toxic, and rapid injection of DMSO can cause vasospasm and necrosis. The safe injection rate is <0.3 mL injected longer than 40 seconds. The lowest toxic dose of Onyx in humans (that is, the maximum safe allowable dose) is 600 mg/kg.

ABSOLUTE ALCOHOL

Ethanol causes tissue infarction by inciting denaturation of proteins with resultant acute thrombosis and subsequent fibrosis. Use of absolute ethanol is generally limited to cases in which nontarget embolization is unlikely, such as in the kidney. It is generally used with flow control using balloons either in the arterial or venous portions or in some cases by using coils to slow the flow to acceptable levels. Venous outflow occlusion may be required if there is rapid systemic drainage of the lesion. Disadvantages of absolute alcohol embolization include difficulty to control placement, lack of opacity, and rapid dilution by vascular inflow. There are additional risks of damaging normal adjacent tissues including skin, mucosa, and nerves.

SODIUM TETRADECYL SULFATE

It is synthetic surface acting substance composed of sodium isobutyl ethyl octyl sulfate and 2% benzyl alcohol. It causes endothelial damage and intimal fibrosis. It is administered as a 3% solution, dose should not exceed 2 mL (usually used 0.1–1 mL).

Transarterial Chemoembolization

Chemoembolization is a palliative administration of anticancer drug directly into a tumor through its feeding blood supply, with concurrent or subsequent blockage of the feeding vessel by occlusive agents that are injected through the delivery catheter. This permits a higher concentration of drug to be in contact with the tumor for a longer period of time. Chemoembolization is most beneficial to patients whose disease is predominately limited to the liver.

Cancers that may be treated by chemoembolization include hepatocellular carcinoma and hepatic metastasis from colon, breast, carcinoid or other neuro endocrine tumors, islet cell tumors of the pancreas, ocular melanoma, sarcoma and other vascular primary tumors in the body. Chemoembolization with drug-eluting beads represents a new and clinically proven delivery device that can deposit a chemotherapeutic agent in the liver with minimal release into adjacent tissues.[11]

Lipiodol (iodized oil), an iodinated ethyl ester of poppy seed oil, was introduced as a drug carrier and an embolic agent in the early 1980s. When injected into the hepatic artery, Lipiodol selectively remains more in tumor nodules for several weeks to over a year due to a siphoning effect from hyper vascularization of the tumor vessels and an absence of Kupffer cells inside tumor tissues resulting in the embolic effects on smaller vessels. Lipiodol functions as a micro vessel embolic agent, as a carrier of chemotherapeutic agents and as an augmenter of antitumor effects of TACE by efflux into the portal veins. The anticancer drugs are vigorously mixed with the Lipiodol to prepare an emulsion, and when the emulsified Lipiodol and drug mixture is injected into a tumor supplying vessels, the anticancer drug is slowly released from lipiodol and remains in high concentrations within the tumor for a prolonged period. The stability of the emulsion could be more enhanced by adjusting the specific gravity of the contrast medium by adding a small amount of distilled water so it is close to the specific gravity of lipiodol.

Anticancer drugs used in conjunction with Lipiodol include doxorubicin, epirubicin, aclarubicin, 5-fluorouracil, mitomycin, cisplatin and SMANCS (styrene maleic acid neocarzinostatin). Several chemotherapeutic agents have been used with doxorubicin and cisplatin being the most common.

Doxorubicin (Adriamycin) is an anthracycline antibiotic, closely related to the natural product daunomycin, and like all anthracyclines, it works by intercalating DNA, with the most serious adverse effect being life-threatening heart damage. It is commonly used in the treatment of a wide range of cancers, including hematological malignancies, many types of carcinoma, and soft tissue sarcomas. Doxorubicin is photosensitive, and containers are often covered by an aluminum bag and/or brown wax paper to prevent light from affecting it. Doxorubicin is also available in liposome-encapsulated forms that forms a better emulsion with lipiodol.

Cisplatin was the first member of a class of platinum containing anti cancer drug, which now also includes carboplatin and oxaliplatin. These platinum complexes react in vivo, binding to and causing cross linking of DNA which ultimately triggers apoptosis. It is used to treat various types of cancers, including sarcomas, carcinomas (small cell lung cancer, ovarian cancer), lymphoma and germ-cell tumors. Usual dose for doxorubicin and cisplatin per session is 10–70 mg and 10–120 mg respectively. The criteria to determine the dosages of chemotherapeutic agents are variable and not standardized. Studies have failed to show significant differences in survival between the use of doxorubicin and other drugs, such as cisplatin or epirubicin, and to date, there is no evidence of the superiority of any single chemotherapeutic agent over other drugs or for monodrug chemotherapy versus combination chemotherapy.

REFERENCES

1. Pannu HK, Alvarez W Jr, Fishman EK. Beta-blockers for cardiac CT: A primer for the radiologist. AJR. 2006;186:S341-5.
2. Mahabadi AA, Achenbach S, Burgstahler C. Safety, efficacy, and indications of beta-adrenergic receptor blockade to reduce heart rate prior to coronary CT angiography. Radiology. 2010; 257:614-23.
3. Hundley WG, Hamilton CA, Thomas MS, et al. Utility of fast cine magnetic resonance imaging and display for the detection of myocardial ischemia in patients not well suited for second harmonic stress echocardiography. Circulation. 1999;100:1697-702.
4. Ranhosky A, Kempthorne-Rawson J. The safety of intravenous dipyridamole thallium myocardial perfusion imaging. Intra-venous dipyridamole thallium imaging study group. Circulation. 1990;81:1205-9.
5. Lew WK, Weaver FA. Clinical use of topical thrombin as a surgical hemostat. Biologics. 2008;2(4):593-9.
6. Victoria V, Reus M, Piñero A, Abellán D, Canteras M, de Rueda ME, Morales D, Parrilla P. Human Thrombin for Treatment of Pseudoaneurysms: Comparison of Bovine and Human Throm-bin Sonogram-Guided Injection. AJR. 2005;184(5):1665-71.
7. Schumacher HC, Meyers PM, Higashida RT, et al. Reporting standards for angioplasty and stent-assisted angioplasty for intracranial atherosclerosis. Stroke. 2009;40:e348-65.
8. Jiang WJ, Wang YJ, Du B, et al. Stenting of symptomatic M1 stenosis of middle cerebral artery: an initial experience of 40 patients. Stroke. 2004;35:1375-80.
9. Castellan L, Causin F, Danieli D, et al. Carotid stenting with filter protection: correlation of ACT values with angiographic and histopathologic findings. J Neuroradiol. 2003;30:103-8.
10. Qureshi AI, Luft AR, Sharma M, et al. Prevention and treatment of thromboembolic and ischemic complications associated with endovascular procedures. Part II. Clinical aspects and recom-mendations. Neurosurgery. 2000;46:1360-75, discussion 75-76.
11. Takayasu K. Transarterial chemoembolization for hepato-cellular carcinoma over three decades: current progress and perspective. Jpn J Clin Oncol. 2012;42(4):247-55.

CHAPTER 65

Molecular Imaging

Anish Bhattacharya, BR Mittal

INTRODUCTION

Molecular imaging is the characterization and measurement of the key biomolecules and molecularly based events using noninvasive medical imaging techniques. It helps in early detection, exact localization and determination of the extent of disease. In the era of personalized medicine, it helps physicians to personalize patient care by evaluating the response to specific therapy and thus selecting the therapy which is most effective in respect of the unique biological characteristics of the patient.

Molecular imaging has several advantages above anatomical imaging, because disease specific abnormal cellular activity occurs well before structural changes. Molecular imaging incorporates several modalities like optical imaging, nuclear imaging, ultrasound, magnetic resonance imaging, etc. **(Table 1)**. Nuclear medicine is a branch of molecular imaging, where the imaging agent is a radiotracer, a compound labeled with a radioisotope. The nonradioactive part of the tracer may be a pharmaceutical agent, an antibody, a protein fragment or even living cells. After its introduction into the body, the radiotracer accumulates in a specific target organ or attaches to specific cells. The imaging device (gamma camera/positron emission tomography (PET) scanner) detects the signal from the radioactive part of the tracer to show its distribution within the body.

The following pages of this chapter provide a brief overview of molecular imaging techniques used in nuclear medicine and their clinical applications.

MOLECULAR IMAGING PROBES IN NUCLEAR MEDICINE

Molecular imaging probes can be divided into four categories:[1]

1. Phenotypic probes are used in assessing general physiological features, such as metabolic changes secondary to pathology (F-18 FDG), cell proliferation (F-18 FLT), hypoxia (F-18 FMISO), angiogenesis, apoptosis and receptor study (Ga-68 DOTATATE).

Table 1: Molecular imaging modalities.

Modality	*Mechanism*	*Sensitivity range*	*Spatial resolution*	*Quantitative*
Ultrasound	High-frequency sound waves	~ 10 µM	~50 µm	+
MRI	Radiowaves	µM	~20 µm	++
SPECT	Gamma rays	nM	<1 mm (mSPECT)	+++
PET	Annihilation photons	nM	1 mm (mPET)	+++
Optical imaging	Visible NIR	pM	Several mm	No

2. Targeted probes are used to image specific biomolecules (e.g. signal transduction proteins or tumor-associated antigens) that are characteristic of a cell type.
3. Cell-tracking probes are used to localize and follow the movement of cells that may aid in the survival of the tumor (e.g. cancer cells, vascular endothelium, stromal cells).
4. Reporter gene probes are used in monitoring the actions of genes in biologic systems *in vivo*.

CLINICAL APPLICATIONS OF NUCLEAR MOLECULAR IMAGING

Oncology

Diagnosis and Staging

In the present time, the molecule that is most commonly used in PET is fluorine-18 fluorodeoxyglucose (F-18 FDG), a glucose analogue, developed to image glucose metabolism in the body. FDG is taken up in cells by glucose transporters. However, unlike glucose, subsequent conversion of FDG to FDG-6-monophosphate by the intracellular enzyme hexokinase traps the metabolite within the cells.[2]

Cancer cells usually have a higher rate of glucose utilization than normal cells (the Warburg effect) due to over-expression of glucose transporters and the transcription factor hypoxia inducible factor-1, which regulates genes involved in glycolysis.[3] The measurement of glucose metabolism as a surrogate marker of tumor activity has been utilized for a number of applications in cancer management, including cancer staging, recurrence detection, response assessment, prognostic evaluation and radiotherapy treatment planning. FDG is not specific for tumor cells, as any cells with increased metabolism will show increased FDG uptake. Furthermore, the low or variable glycolytic activity of some tumor types has a limiting effect on the utility of F-18 FDG PET in tumors, such as renal cell carcinoma, primary prostatic cancer and hepatocellular cancer. In addition, physiological uptake in the brain, nonspecific bowel uptake and urinary excretion of FDG also limit tumor detection.

Therefore, other PET tracers are emerging. FLT is a promising PET tracer for proliferation. It is taken up by proliferating cancer cells by thymidine kinase (TK-1) and trapped intracellularly.[4] Initial clinical studies have also demonstrated that FLT is more sensitive than FDG to image recurrent high-grade brain tumors, correlated better with Ki-67 values, and is a more powerful predictor of tumor progression and survival. There are studies emerging in support of F-18 FLT being useful in staging of nonsmall-cell lung cancer, high-grade brain tumors, etc.

F-18 fluoride bone scan is useful for detection of bony metastases in many cancers, such as breast cancer, prostate cancer, urinary bladder cancer. It has an advantage over conventional gamma camera bone scintigraphy due to better image resolution and the ability to provide 3-dimensional images. 18F-fluoro-dihydrotestosterone (FDHT), an antiandrogen receptor tracer, has shown promise in the detection of bone metastases in prostate cancer. Studies have shown that in many cases, bone metastases as well as lymph node involvement detected with FDHT-PET/CT were not detectable in either FDG-PET/CT or bone scan. This helps in accurate staging of prostate cancer. F-18 fluorocholine (FCH) has demonstrated promise in prostate cancer by detecting additional bony lesions and lymph nodes compared to FDG PET. C-11 choline PET/CT has high sensitivity and specificity for staging and restaging of prostate cancer.

Ga-68 DOTATATE and DOTANOC, being specific for somatostatin receptor expressing cells, are new tracers for imaging of neuroendocrine tumors. F-18 fluoro-dihydroxyphenylalanine (F-DOPA) is another tracer useful in diagnosis and staging of neuroendocrine tumors and low-grade brain tumors. Several other investigational tracers, like C-11 methionine for brain tumors and C-11 acetate for gliomas and prostate cancer, have been studied. All tumors do not behave in the same biological pattern in every individual. Thus these new tracers help in understanding the heterogeneity of tumor biology.

Assessment of Response to Treatment

In routine clinical practice, treatment response is usually evaluated with anatomical imaging modalities, with reduction in tumor size as a response guide. However, anatomical changes after treatment become evident much later than functional changes. Early identification of nonresponders may lead to alteration to more suitable therapy, thereby reducing the costs and side effects of ineffective therapy. Furthermore, with the introduction of cytostatic agents, which may not necessarily shrink the tumor, response evaluation is challenging with structural imaging. Thus molecular imaging has a great role in early response assessment to treatment. Recently, FDG-PET/CT has shown promising results in early response evaluation to treatment in many cancers like lymphomas,[5] lung cancer,[6] esophageal cancer,[7] etc. In malignant lymphomas, where after the completion of therapy, anatomical imaging often shows residual masses which could represent either persistent disease or fibrotic tissue, FDG-PET/CT has been accepted as the modality of choice for response evaluation **(Figs. 1A and B)**. Also, F-18 FLT-PET/CT has shown acceptable results in evaluation of response to cytostatic drugs in nonsmall-cell lung carcinoma.

Several studies have assessed the prognostic value of FDG-PET/CT. These studies in a variety of cancers, such as lymphomas,[8] lung cancer,[6] esophageal cancer,[7] etc. have demonstrated that early metabolic responders have a longer survival than nonresponders. Such a prognostic estimation by metabolic imaging could serve a guide for introducing modifications in therapy. It has been clearly demonstrated by several studies that persistent or increased focal FDG uptake in initially involved tumor sites in patients with Hodgkin's disease or non-Hodgkin's lymphoma is a strong predictor of residual or recurrent disease and is associated with a poor outcome.[9,10] In addition, residual FDG uptake after completion of treatment is associated with poor prognosis in other tumors, such as sarcomas,[11] esophageal,[12] lung,[13] head and neck[14] and cervical carcinomas.[15] Hypoxia imaging markers like F-MISO may be used in solid tumor for detection of radio-sensitivity of tumor cells to radiotherapy.

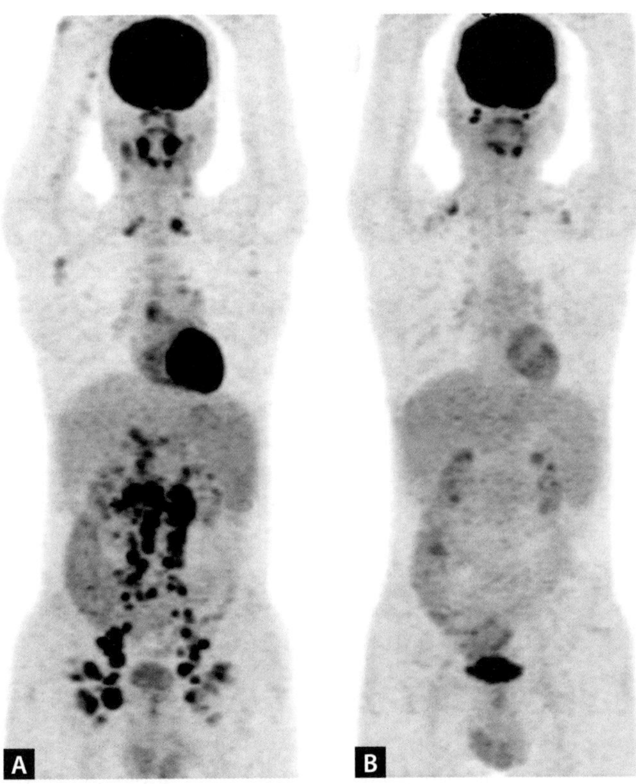

Figs. 1A and B: F-18 FDG PET maximum intensity projection (MIP) images in a patient with non-Hodgkin's lymphoma. (A) Pretreatment study showing involvement of lymph nodes both above and below the diaphragm; (B) Scan after 4 cycles of chemotherapy showing complete metabolic response in the involved lymph nodes.

Role in Drug Development

Metabolic imaging also serves as a pharmacodynamic endpoint in drug development, especially in studies with newer target-directed agents, where higher doses may not necessarily be better and an optimal therapeutic dose may exist. This will prevent an erroneous rejection of certain cytostatic agents, where a functional response may be observed in the absence of decrease in tumors size.

In addition, PET can provide information on in vivo normal tissue and tumor pharmacology, which has so far, relied on surrogate information obtained from body fluids. Understanding of both, the drug's pharmacokinetics and pharmacodynamics has the potential of rational modifications to drug development processes and hence save time. A number of PET tracers, such as [15O] H_2O and [18F] FDG have already been adopted as PET pharmacodynamic markers and are used in the evaluation of antineoplastic agents. PET may be useful in evaluation of a number of pharmacodynamic endpoints, which may either be a true endpoint or a validated surrogate endpoint. A pharmacodynamic relationship between dose and efficacy has been confirmed by PET studies. For example, in patients with metastases from colorectal cancer, labelled 5-FU PET has shown that higher 5-FU-tumor uptake (SUV), has association with longer survival.[16]

CENTRAL NERVOUS SYSTEM DISORDERS

Epilepsy

Single-photon emission computed tomography (SPECT) and positron emission tomography (PET) imaging are useful to detect brain disorders like stroke, Moya-Moya disease **(Fig. 2)**, dementia, epilepsy and movement disorders. Epilepsy is one of the common central nervous system disorders. Epilepsy is controlled by medication in around 70% of patients. In the rest of the patients who remain intractable to medical treatment, resection of the epileptogenic cortex may be considered. Nuclear medicine plays a crucial role in the presurgical assessment of patients with refractory epilepsy.

Ictal perfusion imaging with ^{99m}Tc-ethyl cysteinate dimer (ECD) or ^{99m}Tc-hexamethylpropyleneamine oxime (HMPAO) is commonly used to detect the seizure onset zone in a majority of the cases. However, ictal SPECT of the brain is only possible in some tertiary care centers. Interictal SPECT imaging is comparatively widely available, but is unreliable in determining the ictal onset zone. Interictal

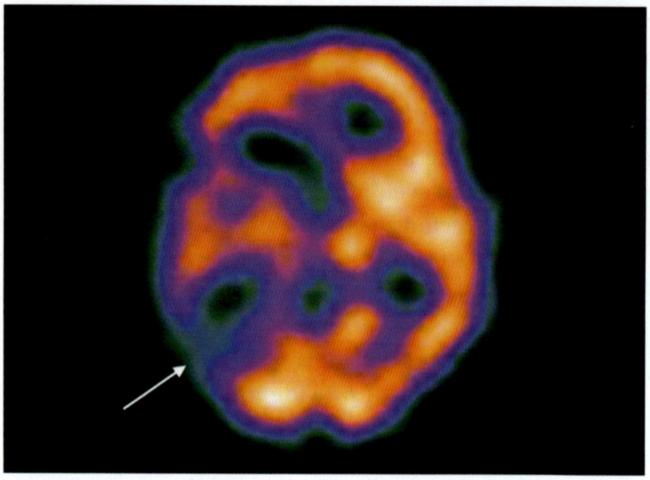

Fig. 2: Tc-99m ECD SPECT scan of the brain in a patient with Moya-Moya disease showing a focal perfusion defect in the right posterior parietal cortex.

FDG PET is more commonly used to detect a hypometabolic area in the brain, which usually encompasses but tends to be larger than the seizure onset zone. It has been shown that FDG PET is quite sensitive in detecting such sites, with 85–90% accuracy using modern techniques.[17]

In recent years, novel PET tracers have been developed to visualize specific receptor systems. In patients with epilepsy, changes in the γ-amino-butyric acid receptor (with 11C- or 18F-labeled flumazenil), opioid receptors (with 11C-carfentanil for μ-opioid peptide receptors; 11C-methylnaltrindole selective for δ-opioid peptide receptors), 5-HT_{1A} serotonin receptors (with 18F-FCWAY a selective 5-HT_{1A} receptor antagonist), nicotinic acetylcholine receptors and others may be detected with the newer PET tracers. However, its use is still limited in clinical practice.

Dementia

Fluorodeooxyglucose (FDG) PET measurements of cerebral glucose metabolism are well-validated in early diagnosis, differential diagnosis, and the evaluation of drug treatment for patients with dementia. Moreover, newer PET tracers **(Table 2)** have been developed to study the neuropathology and alterations of neurotransmitter systems underlying dementia, to advance our understanding of the pathophysiology of dementia, and to improve the accuracy of diagnosis. C-11 Pittsburgh compound B (PiB) appears most promising among all these new tracers, which has high-sensitivity in detecting amyloid pathology in vivo. It binds with high-affinity to neuritic Aβ plaques but not to diffuse plaques and neurofibrillary tangles.[18]

Table 2: PET tracers useful in evaluation of dementia.

Radionuclide tracer	*Molecular targets*
F-18 FDG	Glucose metabolism
C-11 Pittsburgh compound B (PiB)	Amyloid plaques
F-18 FDDNP	Tau-protein
C-11 PK11195	Microglial activation
F-18 DOPA	Dopaminergic neurons, dopa decarboxylation, and vesicular storage
F-18/C-11 altanserin	5HT2A receptors

Table 3: Potential PET radiotracer that can be used in investigations of movement disorders.

Radiotracers	*Molecular target*
F-18 DOPA	Dopaminergic neurons, dopa decarboxylation, and vesicular storage
F-18 FDG	Glucose metabolism
C-11 DTBZ	Type 2 vesicular monoamine transporters
F-18 CFT	Presynaptic dopamine transporters
C-11 raclopride	Postsynaptic dopamine D2 receptors

Movement Disorders

Positron emission tomography imaging with F-18 FDG has been extensively used for assessing local synaptic activity in the resting state in various movement disorders. Additionally, several new tracers **(Table 3)** have been developed which are useful for assessing of movement disorders and help enormously in the clinical management of patients. Among the compounds that have been explored, tracers that visualize the dopaminergic system have the highest potential for the assessment of movement disorders, for example, F-18-6-fluoro-L-dopa (F-DOPA).[19] Presynaptic dopamine transporters (DAT) SPECT tracers show high-sensitivity for detecting atypical Parkinsonian syndromes, for example, 123I- N-3-fluoropropyl-2b-carbomethoxy-3b-(4-iodophenyl) tropane (123I-FP-CIT).

CARDIOVASCULAR DISORDERS

Myocardial Viability

The hibernating myocardium in known coronary artery disease (CAD) patients represents a state of persistent left ventricular dysfunction in chronically decreased blood flow but preserved viability. Approximately 55–60% of the hibernating myocardium is expected to demonstrate functional improvement after intervention. In ischemic myocardium, normal free-fatty acid metabolism switches to glucose as the main source of energy. Increased F-18 FDG uptake is therefore, considered a marker of viability **(Figs. 3A and B)**. F-18 FDG PET is considered the "gold standard" for the detection of viable myocardium, with positive predictive value 74% and negative predictive value 87%.

Coronary Flow Reserve

The PET is the best noninvasive method for absolute quanti fication of myocardial blood flow (MBF) and quantification of coronary flow reserve (CFR). It is based on tracer kinetic models. O-15 water, N-13 ammonia and rubidium-82 are commonly used tracers. Clinical applications of absolute MBF quantification include preclinical diagnosis of CAD, accurate noninvasive diagnosis of multivessel disease, distinguishing the presence of collaterals and early hibernating myocardium is known as CAD and assessing response to therapy or intervention for CAD.

Atherosclerosis

Many tracers have been tried for imaging of atheroma, such as I-125 autologous human LDL, Tc-99m LDL, Tc-99m annexin V, FDG, etc. It has been seen that FDG is taken up in the atherosclerotic vessels. There is evidence that the uptake is mainly located in the intima and represents high metabolic activity in macrophages, which are in abundance in the atherosclerotic plaques. Another possibility is that the smooth muscles in the arterial wall are made visible due to the high use of glucose by this tissue.

INFECTIOUS AND INFLAMMATORY PROCESSES

Of the radiopharmaceuticals currently approved for imaging of infection/inflammation none is specifically for inflammation, and none can offer the option of directly distinguishing sterile from septic inflammation. Different mechanisms form the basis of accumulation of these agents in the inflamed tissues. Most radiolabeled agents have a tendency of accumulating at sites of infection if the local blood flow and the vascular permeability are increased. While scintigraphy with labeled activated leukocytes specifically depends on cellular migration to the site of inflammation, glucose uptake into inflamed tissue (as a result of increased metabolism) is another reliable mechanism to detect inflammation. Finally, Ga-67 binds to transferrin, with the complex being extravasated at sites of inflammation because of increased vascular permeability and then being transferred to locally present lactoferrin.[20]

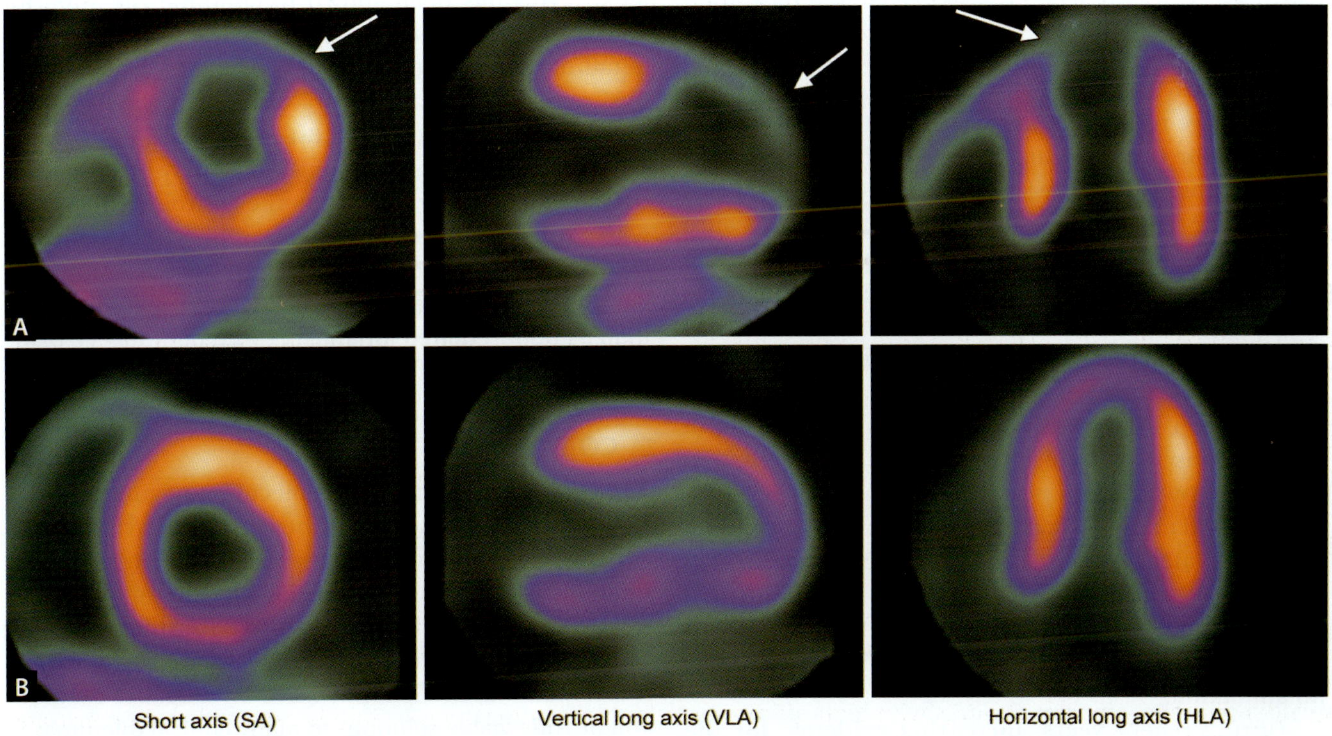

Figs. 3A and B: PET images using N-13 ammonia (A) and F-18 FDG (B) showing perfusion-metabolic mismatch. The perfusion defects in the anteroapical segment and apex (arrows) show good metabolic activity, indicating viable myocardium in these segments.

Ga-67 citrate is not used these days due to poor imaging characteristics, relatively high radiation exposure and prolonged imaging time (up to 72 hours). White blood cell scintigraphy comprises the isolation of autologous leukocytes, the ex-vivo labeling of these cells with either Tc-99m hexamethylpropylene amine oxime (HMPAO) or In-111 oxine and reinjection of the labeled cells into the patient. Radiolabeled autologous leukocytes are regarded as the most specific tracer for imaging of acute infection. However, the procedure requires handling of the patient's blood and meticulous attention to asepsis, in addition to imaging time of 24 hours.

Newer Agents for Imaging Infection/Inflammation

Several investigational radiopharmaceuticals, including radiolabeled nonspecific IgG, antigranulocyte antibodies, chemotactic peptides, interleukins (e.g. interleukin [IL]-1, IL-2, and IL-8), chemokines, and liposomes have been proposed as potential agents for imaging infection and inflammation. Four monoclonal antibodies, CEA-47, BW 250/183, IMMU-NN3, and MCA-480 have been examined for abscess/infection detection in humans. These agents have been investigated as potential replacements for radiolabeled leukocytes. Some of these have shown great promise in animal experiments. However, problems of cost, availability, immunological reactions and unforeseen adverse event reports, including two deaths and 15 life-threatening cardiopulmonary complications, have resulted in the suspension of their routine use.[21] The broad-spectrum antibiotic ciprofloxacin is a fluoroquinolone analog with specific binding to bacterial DNA gyrase that is present in all viable bacteria. Because of its specific binding to bacteria, it was hypothesized that Tc-99m labeled ciprofloxacin, a tracer designed to image microorganisms, may identify only the sites of infection and thus distinguish between sterile inflammation and infection. Localization, however, appears to be based primarily on extravasation and stasis at the sites of increased vascular permeability. It is rapidly cleared from circulation by the kidneys and shows no uptake in bone marrow, and minimal localization in liver and abdominal area. In clinical studies, Tc-99m labeled ciprofloxacin showed acceptable sensitivity and specificity in identifying a wide variety of infectious foci, but it does not appear to distinguish between infection and sterile inflammation.[22]

During recent years, increasing evidence for the application of 18F-FDG-PET in the evaluation of several infectious and aseptic inflammatory disorders has been published.[23,24] Although FDG-PET cannot reliably distinguish infection from noninfectious inflammation, it offers several practical advantages over conventional nuclear medicine techniques (white blood cell/bone marrow/bone imaging) including:

- Completion of the examination within a short period of time (1.5–2 hours)
- High-resolution tomographic images
- High target-to-background contrast ratios
- High sensitivity for chronic infections
- Minimal labor intensity
- High interobserver agreement
- Low-radiation dose (2–3 times lower than that of most conventional nuclear medicine techniques)
- Detection of infection in the axial skeleton; white blood cell (WBC) scanning in particular is of limited value in this setting.

The potential applications of FDG-PET imaging include evaluation of the complicated diabetic foot, painful joint prosthesis, fever of unknown origin (FUO), acquired immuno deficiency syndrome (AIDS)-related disorders, vascular graft infection and fistula, inflammatory bowel disease (IBD) and a variety of noninfectious inflammatory diseases.[21,25]

Recently, PET-CT imaging with F-18 FDG labeled leuko-cytes has been shown to combine the superior imaging characteristics of PET with the fine anatomical detail of CT and the specificity of leukocytes localizing to sites of acute inflammation.[26] In view of the negligible physiological uptake of F-18 FDG labeled cells in the intestine or urinary system, this tracer may be optimal to detect inflammatory foci within the gastrointestinal tract, with minimum confounding background physiological tracer activity.[27] The scanning procedure is completed within 2–3 hours after tracer injection, compared to more than 24 hour required for imaging with both In-111-oxine and Tc-99m HMPAO leukocytes.

CONCLUSION

The clinical applications of molecular imaging continue to grow, with the advent of newer radiotracers. While many new agents have shown great pomise in laboratory or animal studies, the cost, availability and safety of these tracers remain limitations in their routine use. With increasing applications of these techniques worldwide, it is hoped that these noninvasive investigative methods will provide viable solutions to many clinical dilemmas in future.

REFERENCES

1. Weissleder R, Pittet MJ. Imaging in the era of molecular oncology. Nature. 2008;452:580-9.
2. Buck AK, Herrmann K, Stargardt T, et al. Economic evaluation of PET and PET/CT in oncology: evidence and methodologic approaches. J Nucl Med. 2010;51:401-12.
3. Lu H, Forbes RA, Verma A. Hypoxia-inducible factor 1 activation by aerobic glycolysis implicates the Warburg effect in carcinogenesis. J Biol Chem. 2002;277:111-5.
4. Barthel H, Perumal M, Latigo J, et al. The uptake of 3'-deoxy-3'-[(18)F] fluorothymidine into L5178Y tumours in vivo is dependent on thymidine kinase 1 protein levels. Eur J Nucl Med Mol Imaging. 2005;32:257-63.
5. Juweid ME, Wiseman GA, Vose JM, et al. Response assessment of aggressive non-Hodgkin's lymphoma by integrated International Workshop Criteria and fluorine-18-fluorodeoxyglucose positron emission tomography. J Clin Oncol. 2005;23:4652-61.
6. Hoekstra CJ, Stroobants SG, Smit EF, et al. Prognostic relevance of response evaluation using [18F]-2-fluoro-2-deoxy-D-glucose positron emission tomography in patients with locally advanced nonsmall-cell lung cancer. J Clin Oncol. 2005;23:8362-70.
7. Weber WA, Ott K, Becker K, et al. Prediction of response to preoperative chemotherapy in adenocarcinomas of the esophagogastric junction by metabolic imaging. J Clin Oncol. 2001;19:3058-65.
8. Mikhaeel NG, Hutchings M, Fields PA, O'Doherty MJ, Timothy AR. FDG-PET after two to three cycles of chemotherapy predicts progression-free and overall survival in high-grade non-Hodgkin lymphoma. Ann Oncol. 2005;16:1514-23.
9. Cremerius U, Fabry U, Neuerburg J, et al. Prognostic significance of positron emission tomography using fluorine-18-fluorodeoxyglucose in patients treated for malignant lymphoma. Nuklearmedizin. 2001;40:23-30.
10. Spaepen K, Stroobants S, Dupont P, et al. Prognostic value of positron emission tomography (PET) with fluorine-18 fluorodeoxyglucose ([18F]FDG) after first-line chemotherapy in non-Hodgkin's lymphoma: is [18F]FDG-PET a valid alternative to conventional diagnostic methods? J Clin Oncol. 2001;19:414-9.
11. Schuetze SM, Rubin BP, Vernon C, et al. Use of positron emission tomography in localized extremity soft tissue sarcoma treated with neoadjuvant chemotherapy. Cancer. 2005;103:339-48.
12. Swisher SG, Erasmus J, Maish M, et al. 2-Fluoro-2-deoxy-glucose positron emission tomography imaging is predictive of pathologic response and survival after preoperative chemoradiation in patients with esophageal carcinoma. Cancer. 2004;101:1776-85.
13. MacManus MP, Hicks RJ, Matthews JP, et al. Positron emission tomography is superior to computed tomography scanning for response-assessment after radical radiotherapy or chemoradiotherapy in patients with nonsmall-cell lung cancer. J Clin Oncol. 2003;21:1285-92.
14. Kunkel M, Forster GJ, Reichert TE, et al. Radiation response noninvasively imaged by [18F]FDG-PET predicts local tumor control and survival in advanced oral squamous cell carcinoma. Oral Oncol. 2003;39:170-7.
15. Grigsby PW, Siegel BA, Dehdashti F, et al. Post-therapy [18F] fluorodeoxyglucose positron emission tomography in carcinoma of the cervix: response and outcome. J Clin Oncol. 2004;22:2167-71.
16. Moehler M, Dimitrakopoulou-Strauss A, Gutzler F, et al. 18F-labeled fluorouracil positron emission tomography and the prognoses of colorectal carcinoma patients with metastases to the liver treated with 5-fluorouracil. Cancer. 1998;83:245-53.
17. Newberg A, Alavi A, Reivich M. Determination of regional cerebral function with FDG-PET imaging in neuropsychiatric disorders. Semin Nucl Med. 2002;32:13-34.
18. Leinonen V, Alafuzoff I, Aalto S, et al. Assessment of beta-amyloid in a frontal cortical brain biopsy specimen and by positron emission tomography with carbon 11-labeled Pittsburgh compound B. Arch Neurol. 2008;65:1304-9.
19. Brooks DJ, Ibanez V, Sawle GV, et al. Differing patterns of striatal 18F-dopa uptake in Parkinson's disease, multiple system atrophy, and progressive supranuclear palsy. Ann Neurol. 1990;28:547-55.
20. Gotthardt M, Bleeker-Rovers CP, Boerman OC, et al. Imaging of inflammation by PET, conventional scintigraphy, and other imaging techniques. J Nucl Med. 2010;51:1937-49.
21. Basu S, Zhuang H, Torigian DA, et al. Functional imaging of inflammatory diseases using nuclear medicine techniques. Semin Nucl Med. 2009;39:124-45.
22. Goldsmith SJ, Vallabhajosula S. Clinically proven radiopharma ceuticals for infection imaging: mechanisms and applications. Semin Nucl Med. 2009;39:2-10.
23. Zhuang H, Yu JQ, Alavi A. Applications of fluorodeoxyglucose-PET imaging in the detection of infection and inflammation and other benign disorders. Radiol Clin North Am. 2005;43:121-34.
24. Zhuang H, Alavi A. 18-fluorodeoxyglucose positron emission tomographic imaging in the detection and monitoring of infection and inflammation. Semin Nucl Med. 2002;32:47-59.
25. Basu S, Chryssikos T, Moghadam-Kia S, et al. Positron emission tomography as a diagnostic tool in infection: present role and future possibilities. Semin Nucl Med. 2009;39:36-51.
26. Dumarey N, Egrise D, Blocklet D, et al. Imaging Infection with 18F-FDG-Labeled Leukocyte PET/CT: initial experience in 21 patients. J Nucl Med. 2006;47:625-32.
27. Bhattacharya A, Kochhar R, Sharma S, et al. Infection of pancreatic pseudocyst demonstrated on PET/CT using [18F] fluorodeoxyglucose-labeled autologous leukocytes. Clin Nucl Med. 2012;37:618-9.

CHAPTER 66

Ethical and Legal Issues in Radiology

Mandeep Kang, Manavjit Singh Sandhu

INTRODUCTION

With great power and the ability to handle human lives, comes great responsibility. The hippocratic oath makes us realize our duties and reiterates human expectations desired from us as medical professionals. We as true 'workers' try to achieve and maintain the greatest standards in treating 'OUR' patients. But being human, we falter at times, sometimes unknowingly and sometimes, though very rarely, knowingly. We have to realize the indubitable fact that in spite of doing the best we can as professionals, we are bound to be answerable for our actions even for the ones done for the betterment of patients. We cannot rest in the shade of the 'noble' medical profession. We have to be better equipped to prove at every step that the decisions we take are for the treatment of patient's infirmity. They say charity begins at home and the sooner we realize this, the better.

The two most significant changes in medicine in the past century were scientific development and the belief that no mistake, inadequacy and failure should be accepted as a normal part of life.

As we all live in a world governed by rules, laws and regulations which affect all citizens including doctors, we as radiologists, like all other doctors may be challenged legally on various grounds. Right from being accused by the police of committing a crime, facing claims of malpractice in a civil court to being charged with unprofessional conduct by medical boards and colleges, our community may be the subject of complaints registered by citizens through government agencies. In modern society, the dictum "If you provide a service, you may be used" is very true. The increasing accountability of service providers including doctors has lead to cessation of many specialized examinations by them because of high rates of such examinations landing up in court. An example is that many radiologists have given up interpreting mammograms especially in the West, where stricter laws hold them responsible for even minutest of shortcomings, e.g. delay in personal communication of results to the referring physicians.

The radiologists, as other medical professionals, have to be equipped to safeguard their privileges and be vigilant towards their duties and responsibilities. They should have knowledge of the ethical and legal issues that are bound to crop up during their day-to-day practice and be able to handle them with courage and self-belief. The following chapter highlights the various aspects, apart from the clinical/patient-oriented work, which one has to experience as a doctor with some suggestions regarding how to handle them.

ETHICAL ISSUES

The hippocratic oath teaches us to be ethically reasonable in our duties.[1] The moral principles or ethics as they are called are usually ingrained within us as individuals, however, there are circumstances when we may falter in the path to our duties and may inadvertently choose an unethical road which may bring our profession to disrepute. More often than not, this occurs as a result of our lack of awareness to certain regulations to be followed during practice. The various ethical issues are briefly discussed below.

DOCTOR-PATIENT RELATIONSHIP

Since time immemorial the doctor-patient relationship is one of sacred trust. A patient usually approaches a doctor with complete trust and faith to seek a solution to his/her pain and ailment. He assumes that the doctor has the requisite knowledge, skills and competence to treat the illness and thus confides in him. It thus becomes an unwritten agreement once the doctor begins on his job. The doctor cannot promise or guarantee a cure but should be empathetic and truthful towards the patient and his own-self, be it in diagnosis or treatment. If the doctor feels that a certain case requires special attention in which he is not competent enough, he should rightfully transfer the patient to the appropriate specialist.

The medical community must realize that the patient confides in them and thus confidentiality of the patient's information regarding the illness and disease should not be disclosed to anyone unless absolutely necessary. The radiologist should hand over the report to either the patient or the referring physician. All the investigations and procedures that are advised should be in the patient's interest and not be guided by other gains. The patient should be allowed to make informed decisions.

The doctor and all staff working under him/her should display utmost respect for the privacy and dignity of the patient. Their conduct and etiquette should be dignified and delicate. At the same time, the doctor must protect his own interests, e.g. performing a transvaginal ultrasound in the presence of a female attendant, to avoid embarrassing situations in case of any misunderstandings.

The doctor may be approached by patient's attendants at times who may try to influence him/her for any act of commission or omission that may not be in compliance with professional ethics or legal provisions, e.g. sex determination in a pregnant lady. In these cases, the doctor should remain vigilant, lest he/she may land in legal trouble. One should not easily succumb to any pressures or emotional blackmail and must not cross the ethical and legal boundaries.

RADIATION ISSUES

A radiologist must comply with legislation and appropriate measures to protect the health of patients and staff as he is the one who heads the gamut of various radiation-associated imaging procedures. He should ensure regular maintenance check of machines, adhere to badge monitoring requirements for staff and avoid excessive radiation exposure to patients in X-ray/CT examinations.[2] In all studies, he should adhere to the as low as reasonably achievable (ALARA) principle, especially in young patients who are most prone to the development of radiation-induced cancers in later life.

The radiologist heading a facility should ensure a detailed and documented procedure for protection of the patients and staff.

Patient Protection

The various measures that should be adopted are avoidance of unnecessary investigations, use of radiation protection devices and minimizing the radiation exposure times. In case of contrast-induced reactions in patients undergoing any radiological investigation, quick action must be taken by a concerned specialist. More practically, the radiologist himself/herself should be trained in the same.

Staff Protection

Radiation protection measures in the form of lead aprons, protective gloves, use of screens, personalized radiation dose monitoring equipment should be adhered to. The pregnant staff should be relocated in the radiation free zones for work.

The radiation records of the department personnel should be preserved during the working life of an individual until one attains the age of 75 years or at least 30 years after terminating work involving radiation exposure. The radiation records should be transferred to the next employer in case a worker changes jobs.

Public Protection

Appropriate signage should be displayed at appropriate places in the department which are under high-radiation exposure. The attendants should not be asked to accompany the patients for radiological investigations unless required and if so, with full protection. Periodic surveillance of radiation levels should be carried out in and around rooms housing the radiation equipment. A radiation safety officer having necessary qualifications should be appointed for the overview of radiation zones.

Pregnancy, whether in staff or public, requires special consideration as all such personnel should not be allowed to enter the radiation fields. It becomes the responsibility of the radiologist to perform radiation free imaging in such patients. Inadvertent use of radiation may be harmful to the developing fetus and may lead to litigations at a later date. Thus, all the investigations requiring ionizing radiation should be withheld unless there is definite beneficial effect on the patient's condition.

Protection During Interventions

Interventional radiology has emerged as a therapeutic sub-specialty of radiology and has picked up momentum over the last couple of decades as a minimally invasive treatment option. The risks involved in interventional procedures are more closely related to surgery than to diagnostic radiology. Thus, the duties of the radiologist performing interventions become stricter beginning right from when the patient comes for or is referred for some intervention till the time his/her condition improves for which he/she had been referred for initially. Just like any surgical procedure, the nature of the disease process and treatment options needs to be explained to the patient after which he can make an informed decision regarding the option chosen by him. A written informed consent should subsequently be taken before embarking on the procedure. It is the duty of an interventional radiologist's to perform the procedure to the best of his/her capability in keeping with international guidelines.[3,4] Moreover, he should regularly follow-up the patient on OPD basis.

LEGAL ISSUES

The physician community falls under constant surveillance due to the consumer-provider relationship that it shares with the patients. A thorough awareness of our expected responsibilities and understanding of the legalities associated with our profession will help us to provide our best to the patients without undergoing the stress of any repercussions. The specific aspects, where radiologists should be strategic are as follows:

Image Interpretation and Reporting

A radiologist is responsible for all aspects of a diagnostic examination. But it is his interpretation of the information obtained, embodied in the radiological report, that is the essential end product resulting from the contract between him and the patient. But the human eye and brain cannot match the extensive progress that radiology has seen in the recent past. In the words of Robinson:

"The performance of the human eye and brain has failed to keep pace with the enormous technical progress in the first full century of radiology. Errors and variations in interpretation now represent the weakest aspect of clinical imaging."

Alleged misdiagnoses account for majority of malpractice lawsuits (60–70%) against radiologists. Thus interpreting the obtained images forms the major component of a radiologist's job. A uniform approach may prevent inadvertent error in studying the images of the necessary examination.

First Study the Images

The clinical information should be withheld until after the images have been read because it can generate a framing bias and alter a radiologist's independent opinion. Also try not to refer to previous reports until you have formulated your own opinion.

Know How the Examination was Performed?

With such a wide range of imaging modalities available, the technical knowledge required has increased manifold. A radiologist should be well aware of the various technical aspects in various modalities like positioning, centering, etc. in radiography, pulse sequences in MRI, pitch in helical CT, Doppler effects in ultrasound, the physiology of contrast media, digital image evaluation and various artifacts involved in different imaging modalities.

How to Look (Detect the Abnormalities)?

It is the most important task requiring skills and practice. One should be adept at detecting the normal range of appearances. Patient data should be checked along with the dates of examinations before interpreting any examination. A pattern approach should be followed so that no region of the image is missed. Tuddenham studied the eye movements of experienced radiologists during film reporting and found an organized pattern of scanning, contrasting with the random scanning pattern of a beginner. Also try to think three-dimensionally!

When an Abnormality is Found?

It is the knowledge and experience that determine the probabilities that come to mind on viewing abnormal images. A detailed description of the abnormality is desirable for which following things should be kept in mind:

1. Determine the anatomy of each abnormality
2. Assess the radiopathology of each abnormality
3. Check any previous imaging investigations.

Reach a Conclusion

In reaching a conclusion to complete the interpretation, it is important to realize that "common diseases occur commonly" and it is reasonable to favor the most likely diagnosis. A radiologist should be in a sound position to suggest the most appropriate further investigation, if further diagnostic specificity is required. In formulating the report, it is helpful to clearly separate the objective findings from the subjective conclusion.

Interpretation of the imaging findings is followed by a written radiology report which has come to be regarded as factual, rather than the radiologist's subjective opinion in legal circles. The essence of report writing is the ability to describe things and express opinions concisely and precisely. An ideal radiology report is "most often right, though sometimes wrong, easy to read and not too long" as defined by a leading author.

When to Make the Report

The report should not be recorded until after the processes of interpretation and conclusion have been thought through as a thorough understanding of the case is essential for an accurate and precise report.

Giving the Report a Title

The title of the imaging should precisely include the region covered in the examination, e.g. a frontal view of the chest radiograph should be specified lest the examination is assumed to include both the frontal and lateral projections and may have a bearing on the future medicolegal consequence. It is also important to indicate the techniques used, especially in specialized CT and MR examinations where a particular technique or sequence can miss a particular finding, e.g. subarachnoid hemorrhage may be missed on a routine T1 and T2 image while it can be exquisitely demonstrated on a FLAIR or DWI sequence.

Proofread the Report

Before issue, the report should be checked by the reporting radiologist thoroughly, especially for typographical errors.

If an error is realized after dispatch of the report, a second report should be issued, replicating the first one with an addendum instead of an amended report.

General Format

The report can fall into two categories: those having a definite diagnosis and those in which a range of differential diagnoses are considered.

Definite diagnosis: Clearly mentioned in the final impression with utmost precision when in no doubt.

Indefinite diagnosis: When the diagnosis remains speculative, the format of the report should be divided into "Findings" and "Conclusion". The findings section should record the objective data obtained from the images. Never try to give your subjective opinion in the findings. Conclude by giving what you think is the possible diagnosis. However, when in doubt, give the differentials along with an advice of appropriate further investigations.

Length of the Report

In general, brevity is a virtue. Lengthy reports are not recommended because they tax the patience of referring physicians. It has been suggested that clinicians judge the confidence of the radiologist to be inversely proportional to the length of the report.

Negative Reporting

It is conventionally accepted that radiology reports record abnormalities and things not mentioned can be taken to be normal. In cases where the clinical information suggests an abnormal finding but the images appear normal, the report should report normality. There are cases where the borderline between normal and abnormal is uncertain. In such cases, it is reasonable to state "No definite abnormality seen".

Internal Architecture

Sentence construction, use of descriptive phrases and the order in which things are set out are all part of the report architecture. Such skills accumulate with experience though some guidelines may be helpful. A good report should have 'brevity, relevance and clarity'. The main objectives of the report should be to:

- Focus the reader's attention early
- Report the abnormalities as they are
- Use phrases and adjectives to qualify nouns
- Use familiar words
- Get the anatomical terms right
- Immediately communicate the findings to the referring physician when a life-threatening abnormality is detected
- Recommend further diagnostic investigations, if diagnosis is inconclusive.

Appropriate image interpretation and report writing form the major roles of a radiologist and thus should be as precise and accurate as possible. In spite of that there are occasions when the radiologist's report is put under scanner by the patient[5] and his/her physician. Most of these pertain to specific investigations and body systems like mammography for breast cancer, chest radiograph for lung cancer, etc.

LAWS/LEGAL ACTS APPLICABLE TO MEDICINE

PCPNDT Act

The Prenatal Diagnostic Techniques (Regulation and Prevention of Misuse) act (1994) and Preconception and Prenatal Diagnostic Techniques (Prohibition of Sex Selection) Rules, 1996.

The PNDT [(Prenatal Diagnostic Techniques (Regulation and Prevention of Misuse)] act came into existence in 1994[6] after the government realized that the cause of skewed sex ratio especially in parts of Northern India was the prenatal termination of female fetus. The advent and easy availability of ultrasound was being wrongly used for determining the sex of the fetus inside the mother's womb. As the girl child is unwelcome in many homes due to the traditional thinking, there was a high prevalence of "killing" the female child even before "she" was born. The census 2011[7] further reveals that the situation is far worse in respect of girl child population, particularly in the affluent areas of Punjab (893 girls to 1000 boys), Haryana (877), Chandigarh (817) and Delhi (866). To check and curb this malpractice, strict rules were formulated which banned the communication regarding the gender of the fetus by the sonologist to the patient/attendants.

In spite of the implementation of the PCPNDT act, the situation did not improve significantly as expected even after the amendment in the year 2002. An All India Conference of State Secretaries was thus called in 2005 in New Delhi where certain guidelines were revised and few new ones added. The ones pertaining to the radiologist community is that records of all diagnosis done by the ultrasound machines or other machines, as well as charts, forms, reports, consent letters, etc. used for the purpose of prenatal diagnosis should be maintained for at least two years. All new machines should have the facility of blocking any deletion from the memory unless authorized. A detailed overview of the guidelines can be had directly from the PCPNDT act or from a recent issue of the Indian Journal of Radiology and Imaging (IJRI 2012 Vol 22 Issue 2).

The act has been a blessing as there has been a constant though gradual increase in the female sex ratio. However, many doctors including the radiologists and gynecologists believed that the paperwork involved was too much which was eating into their occupation time. The laws were so strict that not completing the required data would invite strict action against them even if they had followed all the legal rules.

A study on Doctors' Perspective on PNDT act was conducted by Dhaduk et al.[8] A total of 26 obstetricians and 8 radiologists participated in the study. All the participants were given pretested and structured proforma to give their opinion on various aspects related to the PNDT act, viz difficulties faced, penalties for violation, punishment for violation, genuineness of information (Forms F and G), repercussions of the PNDT act, demand for gender determination, and suitable amendments in the PNDT act. Only 5.91% of the doctors felt that the PNDT act is the only tool for improving the gender ratio. As many as 79.41% of the doctors were of the opinion that the PNDT act is not the only tool to improve the gender ratio while 14.7% had no opinion. About a quarter (26.55%) of the doctors were of the view that penalties for violating the PNDT act are very heavy while three-quarters (73.45%) did not feel so. A total of 67.6% of the doctors were of the view that publicity through the media of court cases related to breaches of the PNDT act by doctors is beneficial for improving the gender ratio as it will act as a deterrent against flouting the provision of the PNDT act by doctors. A total of 32.41% of the doctors did not feel the same way.

On inquiring regarding completing forms F and G genuinely and completing it with true information, about half (55.9%) of the doctors stated that they completed these forms genuinely and with correct information; 2.9% stated that the information completed was absolutely false and 41.2% were not sure. With regard to the impact of the PNDT act on the future progress of the invention related to use of ultrasound technique in Medical Sciences; as many as 41.2% of doctors felt that the PNDT act can hamper the future course of medical invention, 44.1% of the doctors did not think so, and 14.7% of the doctors did not know. When asked about the demand from doctors for gender determination by patients in the outpatient department, 97.1% confirmed that there is such a demand from patients

Table 1: Different kinds of difficulties faced by doctors because of the PNDT Act.

Difficulties	*No. of respondents*	*%*
Excessive clerical work	29	85.29
Social difficulties	3	8.8
Hospital administrative difficulties	15	44.1
Police interference more than expected	10	29.4
No difficulties	6	17.6

or her family. Other difficulties faced by the doctors are given in **Table 1**.

The various State Governments have implemented the PNDT act in letter and spirit with all sincere efforts in order to check the declining sex ratio. An example of the actions taken is being quoted with respect to the state of Haryana. Haryana had been the first state where the first 3 court cases under this act were launched. It was also here that the first conviction took place under the PNDT act. Fourteen doctors/persons have been convicted in the State so far, under PNDT act with two convictions under MTP act. 1036 ultrasound clinics/ genetic clinics and 67 genetic counseling centers have been registered. 42 ultrasound machines have been registered in Govt sector while 115 ultrasound machines have been seized and sealed on account of being unregistered/other violations. 9,296 inspections of various ultrasound clinics have been conducted. Registration of 245 ultrasound centers has been suspended/cancelled. Four prosecutions were launched in the district courts by Faridabad in the month of Feb-March 2009. This is just an example of how the states across India are carrying on this work with zeal and the results have started showing up in the form of increase in the female ratios as observed in interim census across states.

The Indian Radiological and Imaging Association (IRIA) has also given support to this cause with active propagation of the theme of Save the Girl Child in form of sensitization of various individuals associated with it. It has started campaigns and is arranging various seminars to sensitize the member doctors to help in the government strategy of achieving the required goals of women empowerment and improving sex ratios.

A recent article[9] has shown that selective abortions of girls have increased tremendously in India, especially at homes where the first born child is a girl. The increasing sex-selection among the Asian communities in US and UK has forced the respective governments to introduce new legislation for curbing this act. The Prenatal Nondiscrimination Act (PRENDA) has recently been introduced in US which bans sex-selective abortions.

Consumer Protection Act (1986)

This Act was formulated by the Government of India in the year 1986 as an act to provide for better protection of the interests of consumers and for that purpose to make provision for the establishment of consumer councils and other authorities for the settlement of consumers' disputes and for matters connected therewith. Of the various service providers included in the act, doctor-patient relationship is also established as a consumer provider one. The doctor community is responsible for its actions and can be taken to task if an ill will can be proved against them. This may be harsh on us doctors as most of the times we try to alleviate the sufferings of 'our' patients with utmost care. We should not be delegated to the same level as other service providers like shopkeepers, etc., because our jobs are vastly different. Yet malpractice by certain unscrupulous elements in our community has made our whole profession answerable. Medical negligence constitutes a wide portal in the present judiciary which has seen many doctors being tried for their negligent acts. Many a times, doctors have been punished who have been bringing the medical profession to disrepute. Apart from the state judiciary which imposes sanctions on these individuals, the Medical Council of India also acts in coherence with the law agencies by debarring the practicing medical professionals from the state/national registers. These individuals can thereafter not practice medicine until and unless their names have been cleared of misdeeds.

The radiologists may become a part of various law suits due to a number of reasons. The following discussion enumerates the various aspects of duty required of us and how to be careful in the provision of these duties for the betterment of the patient without being held up by the consumer laws. A radiologist's role may primarily be as a defendant or as a witness.

Radiologist as a Defendant

In a Malpractice Claim

On receiving a court notice regarding a malpractice claim, the radiologist should act calmly and not be intimidated by the notice. One should do the following:

- Read the statement carefully to determine the exact nature of alleged malpractice
- Assemble all of the available documents you have including radiology reports, request forms and diagnostic images, if in your possession. Make copies and form a separate file
- Contact your insurer or medical defence lawyer without delay.

Duty of Care

A duty of care is intangible but generally accepted to be an obligation recognized by law to exercise diligence, care, knowledge, skill and caution in management. The duty may be different at different times for different patients. To further objectify the same, the Bolam principle is followed in many regions of the world and is most popular in Britain. It states that "a doctor is not negligent if he acts in accordance with a practice accepted at the time as proper by a responsible body of medical opinion." In spite of all linguistic endeavors regarding defining "duty of care", it is ultimately, for the judge to determine the breach of care which varies from case to case. Radiologists are required to provide the duty of care right from patient care to the interpretation of imaging findings.

Consent

The key elements of consent include:

- It must be voluntary
- It must be informed
- It must be given in writing by a person who has capacity to give it and should be witnessed preferably by a person unrelated to both the parties.

We as radiologists should personally obtain consent before carrying out an investigation even if it has been previously taken by the referring physician as he may not know precisely the risks involved in a particular investigation.

It is of more importance in case of invasive procedures like angiographies and radiological guided therapeutic procedures.[10] Any invasive procedure without informed consent is legally an assault—that is, the unlawful direct application of force to another individual. This is applicable in many countries across the world. No invasive procedure should be carried out without taking a written informed consent from the patient or nearest attendant.

Archiving and Ownership of Diagnostic Imaging Data

There are laws in many jurisdictions regarding retention of films in the public arena for a certain duration which may range from a minimum of 3 years up to 25 years of patient's age after which they may be destroyed without seeking patient's consent. Till this time, it is the responsibility of the concerned radiologist to preserve the imaging on which his/her reports are based. However, most patients and referring physicians opt to keep the films with them. The concept that the radiologist owns the images as 'tools of trade' is most important as the digital revolution portends a future of filmless radiology.[11] Until that is achieved, radiologists must record relevant hardcopy images on film, tape or disc. It is important that the images provided substantiate the dictated report.

Patient Referral

Although not a legal requirement, the importance of retaining referral information on each patient cannot be overstated from a medicolegal risk management point of view. Many a times the referral form by the physician is incomplete with respect to the clinical findings and provisional diagnosis. The information on the request form, often scanty, may be a telling factor in a radiologist's defence.

The second issue is whether a patient can self-refer himself/herself to a radiologist or has to be referred by a treating physician.[12] The patient can do a self-referral till the time it is not seen to transgress into the ethical and legal responsibilities of the radiologist.

Radiologist as a Witness

As Expert Witness

Radiologists are the expert witnesses allowed to give an opinion, and the basis for it, within their recognized field of specialized knowledge and experience. A radiologist may be required to give evidence-testimony in court for various reasons; as a defendant, or when the radiologist's report is relevant in other court actions. A summon is issued when a radiologist is required to provide evidence involving parties other than the radiologist. Refusal to attend court is not an option and failure to comply is a criminal offence.

Writing a Radiological Opinion

The document must show name, qualifications and address. The opinion should be honest, objective and based on the radiologist's experience and knowledge. Opinion should not be given on matters beyond one's limit of expertise.

Comments on Other Radiological Reports

As an expert, a radiologist may be required to be judgmental about reports by other professional colleagues. Without any bias, one should make his own opinion without belittling his fellow colleagues.

Appearing in Court

A good expert witness should understand his role and be well-prepared, objective, independent, and credible. One should be able to use simple, nontechnical language, explain technical terms to lay people, answer questions directly and clearly, use consistent body language and should dress like a professional.

Personal Communication by the Radiologists

Malpractice lawsuits alleging failure of communication of radiologic results are prevalent and becoming more so in the western world. One analysis of court transcripts disclosed that communication problems were present in more than 70% of depositions while another claims it to be a causative factor in as many as 80% of malpractice lawsuits. A survey categorizing causes of malpractice litigation involving radiologists released in 1997 by the Physician Insurers Association of America and the American College of Radiology (ACR) found that the number of medical malpractice claims alleging communication failure had grown to become the fourth most frequent primary allegation against radiologists. This survey also disclosed that in nearly 60% of malpractice lawsuits involving radiologists, the referring physician had not been directly contacted regarding urgent or significant unexpected findings, even though in 75% of these cases, the medical record had shown that a radiology report was issued in a timely manner. Thus, approximately 75% of claims against radiologists stems from various sorts of errors in communication.[13]

Malpractice litigation involving radiologic communi cation is moving to center stage in the legal arena. Traditionally, radiologists have considered themselves to be consultants or "doctors' doctors," in the sense that they initiated radiologic examination only on the request of a referring physician and then rendered a radiographic interpretation and transmitted it to the same physician. Most radiologists believed that their duty to communicate interpretations was fulfilled with the sending of the radiology report from the radiology department, destined to be received by the referring physician without being concerned that the report might not be received or noticed by that physician. Nowadays, due to easy and wide availability of radiologic techniques, we are receiving referrals for "screening" for various disorders with no apparent symptoms. In the traditional referral, the referring physician suspected an abnormality, actively awaited the radiologic results, and was likely to follow-up with the radiologist if a written report was not forthcoming in a timely fashion. In the case of screening investigation, however, the patient would have no clinical sign or symptom; it was likely that both the physician and patient expected the radiology report to reveal normal findings, and therefore, they might not actively seek the report—thus setting the stage for radiology reports to go astray without being noticed.

In the 1980s, the ACR issued its first Standard for Communication: Diagnostic Radiology. It stated: Some circumstances may require direct communication of unusual, unexpected, or urgent findings to the referring physician in advance of a formal written report. The timeliness of direct communication should be based upon the immediacy of the clinical situation.

Issue of Self-referral

The medicolegal responsibility of the radiologist when reporting X-ray films is the same whether they were ordered by a registered medical practitioner, a physician or the patient himself. He has a duty of care to interpret the films correctly, accurately and having taken account of all the information available. As radiological assessment nowadays involves complex imaging techniques, many of them being invasive involving considerable risks to the patient, the radiologist has to decide whether to agree to the request, having taken into consideration the source of the request, and whether the request is in the patient's best interest.[14] The radiologist would also have a duty to perform the test to the required standard, and without harm to the patient. If he agrees, he has a duty to ensure that the interpretation is correctly applied, having considered the individual patient and his clinical circumstances, even if the imaging has been done elsewhere.[15]

TELERADIOLOGY: WHO IS RESPONSIBLE?

Telemedicine has been defined by the World Medical Asso-ciation as "The practice of medicine over a distance, in which interventions, diagnostic and treatment decisions and recommendations are based on data, documents and other information transmitted through telecommunication systems."

The teleradiology system has evolved in a huge way over the last couple of decades. Safeguards aimed at limiting access to only those authorized to have access, and to prevent breach of patient confidentiality need to be in place. It is arguable whether there is a doctor-patient relationship in teleradiology between the remote radiologist, who acts more like a consultant, and the patient. However, it may be argued that a duty of care exists once the radiologist accepts a request to provide medical services.[16] The radiologist responsible for the report may be in breach, if it can be shown that he has not taken sufficient care when interpreting the films or in producing his report. Case law and legislation have yet to catch up with this rapidly developing area of healthcare. Recent reviews by Pattynama et al.[17] and Ross et al.[18] with relevance to the European system have generated apt questions and answers in this field of responsibility sharing. They have addressed some of these issues in their articles in the European Journal of Radiology.

The day we take the *Hippocratic oath* on the completion of our medical graduation, we promise ourselves the care, hard work, truth and just treatment that we would provide to all our patients. Although most of us strive to attain this at all cost, there may be times when we may falter either due to the governing circumstances or our inappropriate decisions. It is during this time that we are expected to stand for ourselves as practicing medical professionals and prove to the world our integrity. The awareness and knowledge of the medicolegal aspect of our practice is thus warranted. The brief review provided above may thus help in avoiding the legal hassles involved in providing appropriate care towards our patients. This review touches a few fronts where one can be challenged by patients, the duty that is often expected from us as professionals and some practical ways by which one can project one's work to the outer world without falling into legal conundrum in spite of giving our best for the community. Though a lot remains to be done in the Indian scenario with respect to the legal aspect of medicine, a thorough knowledge of medicine and laws is still essential for saving ourselves when the situation demands and to provide the best we can to our community and nation.

REFERENCES

1. Jhala CI, Jhala KN. The Hippocratic Oath: a comparative analysis of the ancient text's relevance to American and Indian modern medicine. Indian J Pathol Microbiol. 2012;55:279-82.
2. Lau LS, Pérez MR, Applegate KE, et al. Global quality imaging: emerging issues. J Am Coll Radio. 2011;8:508-12.
3. Zibners H. Legal Issues in Interventional Radiology: A private practitioner's perspective. Semin Intervent Radiol. 2001;18: 389-94.
4. Potchen EJ, JD, Hollstein BR. Information management and the legal aspects of interventional radiology. Semin Intervent Radiol. 2001;18:367-74.
5. Capaccio E, Podestà A, Morcaldi D, et al. How often do patients ask for the results of their radiological studies? Insights Imaging. 2010;1:83-5.
6. The Prenatal Diagnostic Techniques (Prohibition of Sex-Selection) Act, 1994. Act No. 57 of 1994 [20th September, 1994].
7. C Chandramouli (23 August 2011). Census of India 2011: A Story of Innovations. Press Information Bureau, Government of India.
8. Dhaduk KM, Parmar DV, Yadav BS, et al. A study on doctors' perspective on PNDT Act. Indian J Community Med. 2009; 34:160-1.
9. Jha P, Kesler MA, Kumar R, et al. Trends in selective abortions of girls in India: analysis of nationally representive birth histories from 1990 to 2005 and census data from 1991 to 2011. Lancet. 2011;377:1921-8.
10. Teoh MK. Medicolegal issues in radiology. SMA News. 2005;37:7-9.
11. Berlin R. Storing unread radiologic images in a PACs. Am J Roentgenol. 2011;196:W100.
12. Kilani RK, Paxton BE, Stinnett SS, et al. Self-referral in medical imaging: A meta-analysis of the literature. J Am Coll Radiol. 2011;8:469-76.
13. Berlin L. Communicating findings of radiologic examinations: whither goest the radiologist's duty? Am J Roentgenol. 2002;178:809-15.
14. Hutchinson M, Rowe E. Yet another flawed study of self-referral? Am J Roentgenol. 2012;199:W414.
15. Berlin L. Malpractice and ethical issues in radiology: limiting requests for outside radiographic interpretations. Am J Roentgenol. 2013;200:W92.
16. Ross P, Sepper R, Pohjonen H. Cross-border teleradiology-experience from two international teleradiology projects. Eur J Radiol. 2010;73:20-5.
17. Pattynama PMT. Legal aspects of cross-border teleradiology. Eur J Radiol. 2012;73:26-30.
18. Ross P, Pohjonen H. Images crossing borders: Image and workflow sharing on multiple levels. Insights Imaging. 2011;2: 141-8.

AIIMS-MAMC-PGI's
Comprehensive Textbook of
Diagnostic Radiology

AIIMS-MAMC-PGI's Comprehensive Textbook of

Diagnostic Radiology

SECOND EDITION

VOLUME 2

- **Gastrointestinal and Hepatobiliary Imaging**
- **Genitourinary Imaging**
- **Pediatric Imaging**

Editors

Arun Kumar Gupta MD FAMS
Professor and Head
Department of Radiodiagnosis
All India Institute of Medical Sciences
New Delhi, India

Anju Garg MD
Director Professor and Head
Department of Radiodiagnosis
Maulana Azad Medical College
New Delhi, India

Manavjit Singh Sandhu MD FICR
Professor and Head
Department of Radiodiagnosis
Postgraduate Institute of Medical Education and Research, Chandigarh, India

JAYPEE

JAYPEE BROTHERS MEDICAL PUBLISHERS
The Health Sciences Publisher
New Delhi | London | Panama

Jaypee Brothers Medical Publishers (P) Ltd.

Headquarters
Jaypee Brothers Medical Publishers (P) Ltd.
4838/24, Ansari Road, Daryaganj
New Delhi 110 002, India
Phone: +91-11-43574357
Fax: +91-11-43574314
Email: jaypee@jaypeebrothers.com

Overseas Offices
JP Medical Ltd.
83, Victoria Street, London
SW1H 0HW (UK)
Phone: +44 20 3170 8910
Fax: +44 (0)20 3008 6180
E-mail: info@jpmedpub.com

Jaypee-Highlights Medical Publishers Inc.
City of Knowledge, Bld. 235, 2nd Floor, Clayton
Panama City, Panama
Phone: +1 507-301-0496
Fax: +1 507-301-0499
E-mail: cservice@jphmedical.com

Jaypee Brothers Medical Publishers (P) Ltd.
Bhotahity, Kathmandu, Nepal
Phone: +977-9741283608
E-mail: kathmandu@jaypeebrothers.com

Website: www.jaypeebrothers.com
Website: www.jaypeedigital.com

Inquiries for bulk sales may be solicited at: jaypee@jaypeebrothers.com

AIIMS-MAMC-PGI's Comprehensive Textbook of Diagnostic Radiology (Volumes 1 to 3)

First Edition: 2016
Second Edition: **2019**

ISBN: 978-93-5270-704-1

Printed at: Replika Press Pvt. Ltd.

Dedicated to

THE SUPREME BEING

Who so mercifully helps us to accomplish gigantic tasks
so smoothly, effortlessly and so beautifully

Associate Editors

VOLUME 1

SECTION 1: Neuroradiology including Head and Neck Imaging

Paramjeet Singh MD
Professor
Department of Radiodiagnosis
Postgraduate Institute of Medical Education and Research
Chandigarh, India

Vivek Gupta MD DM
Professor
Department of Radiodiagnosis
Postgraduate Institute of Medical Education and Research
Chandigarh, India

Shailesh B Gaikwad MD
Professor and Head
Department of Neuroimaging and Interventional Neuroradiology
(CN Centre)
All India Institute of Medical Sciences
New Delhi, India

Ajay Garg MD
Professor
Department of Neuroimaging and Interventional Neuroradiology
(CN Centre)
All India Institute of Medical Sciences
New Delhi, India

SECTION 2: Recent Advances and Applied Physics in Imaging

Sanjay Sharma MD DNB MNAMS FRCR FICR
Professor
Department of Radiodiagnosis
Dr Rajendra Prasad Centre for
Ophthalmic Sciences
All India Institute of Medical Sciences
New Delhi, India

Ashu Seith Bhalla MD MAMS FICR
Professor
Department of Radiodiagnosis
All India Institute of Medical Sciences
New Delhi, India

Smriti Hari MD MAMS
Professor
Department of Radiodiagnosis
All India Institute of Medical Sciences
New Delhi, India

VOLUME 2

SECTION 3: Gastrointestinal and Hepatobiliary Imaging

Deep Narayan Srivastava MD MBA FAMS FICR
Professor
Department of Radiodiagnosis
All India Institute of Medical Sciences
New Delhi, India

Raju Sharma MD MAMS FICR
Professor
Department of Radiodiagnosis
All India Institute of Medical Sciences
New Delhi, India

SECTION 4: Genitourinary Imaging

Anupam Lal MD
Professor
Department of Radiodiagnosis
Postgraduate Institute of Medical Education and Research
Chandigarh, India

SECTION 5: Pediatric Imaging

Ashu Seith Bhalla MD MAMS FICR
Professor
Department of Radiodiagnosis
All India Institute of Medical Sciences
New Delhi, India

Sanjay Thulkar MD
Professor
Department of Radiodiagnosis
Dr BRA Institute—Rotary Cancer Hospital
All India Institute of Medical Sciences
New Delhi, India

VOLUME 3

SECTION 6: Chest and Cardiovascular Imaging

Sanjiv Sharma MD
Professor and Head
Department of Cardiac Radiology
Cardio-Thoracic Sciences Centre
All India Institute of Medical Sciences
New Delhi, India

Rashmi Dixit MD
Director Professor
Department of Radiodiagnosis
Maulana Azad Medical College
New Delhi, India

SECTION 7: Musculoskeletal and Breast Imaging

Anjali Prakash DMRD DNB MNAMS
Director Professor
Department of Radiodiagnosis
Maulana Azad Medical College
New Delhi, India

Contributors

Ajay Garg MD
Professor
Department of Neuroimaging and
Interventional Neuroradiology (CN Centre)
All India Institute of Medical Sciences
New Delhi, India

Ajay Gulati MD MAMS
Additional Professor
Department of Radiodiagnosis
Postgraduate Institute of Medical Education
and Research, Chandigarh, India

Ajay Kumar MD
Professor
Department of Radiodiagnosis and Imaging
Postgraduate Institute of Medical Education
and Research, Chandigarh, India

Akshay Kumar Saxena MD Dip NBE
Professor
Department of Radiodiagnosis
Postgraduate Institute of Medical Education
and Research, Chandigarh, India

Alpana Manchanda MD
Director Professor
Department of Radiodiagnosis
Maulana Azad Medical College
New Delhi, India

Amar Mukund MD
Associate Professor
Department of Radiodiagnosis
Institute of Liver and Biliary Sciences (ILBS)
New Delhi, India

Anil Chauhan
MBBS Board Certified in Radiology, USA
Fellow, Body Imaging
Department of Radiology
University of Texas MD Anderson
Cancer Center, Houston, USA

Anil K Pandey PhD
Assistant Professor (Medical Physics)
Department of Nuclear Medicine
All India Institute of Medical Sciences
New Delhi, India

Anindita Sinha MD
Additional Professor
Department of Radiodiagnosis
Postgraduate Institute of Medical Education
and Research, Chandigarh, India

Anish Bhattacharya DNB DRM MNAMS
Professor
Department of Nuclear Medicine
Postgraduate Institute of Medical Education
and Research, Chandigarh, India

Anjali Prakash DMRD DNB MNAMS
Director Professor
Department of Radiodiagnosis
Maulana Azad Medical College
New Delhi, India

Anju Garg MD
Director Professor and Head
Department of Radiodiagnosis
Maulana Azad Medical College
New Delhi, India

Ankur Gadodia MD DNB FRCR
Consultant
Goyal MRI and Diagnostic Centre
New Delhi, India

Ankur Goyal MD DNB MNAMS
Assistant Professor
Department of Radiodiagnosis
All India Institute of Medical Sciences
New Delhi, India

Anmol Bhatia MD
Assistant Professor
Department of Radiodiagnosis and Imaging
Postgraduate Institute of Medical Education
and Research, Chandigarh, India

Anuj Prabhakar DNB DM
Assistant Professor
Department of Neuroimaging and
Interventional Neuroradiology (CN Centre)
All India Institute of Medical Sciences
New Delhi, India

Anupam Lal MD
Professor
Department of Radiodiagnosis
Postgraduate Institute of Medical Education
and Research, Chandigarh, India

Arun Deep Arora MD
Former Senior Research Associate
Department of Radiodiagnosis
All India Institute of Medical Sciences
New Delhi, India

Arun Kumar Gupta MD FAMS
Professor and Head
Department of Radiodiagnosis
All India Institute of Medical Sciences
New Delhi, India

Arun Malhotra DRM PhD
Former Professor and Head
Department of Nuclear Medicine
All India Institute of Medical Sciences
New Delhi, India

Ashu Seith Bhalla MD MAMS FICR
Professor
Department of Radiodiagnosis
All India Institute of Medical Sciences
New Delhi, India

Atin Kumar MD DNB MNAMS
Professor
Department of Radiodiagnosis
Jai Prakash Narayan Apex Trauma Center
All India Institute of Medical Sciences
New Delhi, India

BR Mittal MD DRM DNB FICNM FAMS
Professor and Head
Department of Nuclear Medicine
Postgraduate Institute of Medical Education
and Research, Chandigarh, India

Chandan Jyoti Das MD DNB MNAMS
Associate Professor
Department of Radiodiagnosis
All India Institute of Medical Sciences
New Delhi, India

Chandrashekhara SH MD DNB MNAMS
Associate Professor
Department of Radiodiagnosis
Dr BRA Institute—Rotary Cancer Hospital
All India Institute of Medical Sciences
New Delhi, India

Chirag Kamal Ahuja MD DM
Assistant Professor
Department of Radiodiagnosis and Imaging
Postgraduate Institute of Medical Education
and Research, Chandigarh, India

Deep Narayan Srivastava MD MBA FAMS FICR
Professor
Department of Radiodiagnosis
All India Institute of Medical Sciences
New Delhi, India

Devasenathipathy Kandasamy MD DNB FRCR
Associate Professor
Department of Radiodiagnosis
All India Institute of Medical Sciences
New Delhi, India

Ekta Dhamija MD
Assistant Professor
Department of Radiodiagnosis
Dr BRA Institute—Rotary Cancer Hospital
All India Institute of Medical Sciences
New Delhi, India

Gaurav S Pradhan MBBS DMRD DNB
Director Professor
Department of Radiodiagnosis
Maulana Azad Medical College
New Delhi, India

Gurpreet Singh Gulati MD
Professor
Department of Cardiac Radiology
Cardio-Thoracic Sciences Centre
All India Institute of Medical Sciences
New Delhi, India

Hina Arif Mumtaz MD DNB
Former Senior Research Associate
Department of Radiodiagnosis
Postgraduate Institute of Medical Education
and Research, Chandigarh, India

Jyoti Kumar MD DNB MNAMS
Professor
Department of Radiodiagnosis
Maulana Azad Medical College
New Delhi, India

Kartik Ganga MD
Fellow
Department of Cardiovascular Radiology
and Endovascular Interventions
All India Institute of Medical Sciences
New Delhi, India

Kirti Gupta
MD Neuropathology Fellowship (St Jude, USA)
Professor
Department of Histopathology
Postgraduate Institute of Medical Education
and Research, Chandigarh, India

Kumble S Madhusudhan MD FRCR MAMS
Associate Professor
Department of Radiodiagnosis
All India Institute of Medical Sciences
New Delhi, India

Kushaljit Singh Sodhi MD MNAMS FICR
Professor
Department of Radiodiagnosis
Postgraduate Institute of Medical Education
and Research, Chandigarh, India

Kusum Joshi MD PhD
Professor and Former Head
Department of Histopathology
Postgraduate Institute of Medical Education
and Research, Chandigarh, India

Mahesh Prakash MD MAMS FICR
Professor
Department of Radiodiagnosis
Postgraduate Institute of Medical Education
and Research, Chandigarh, India

Manavjit Singh Sandhu MD FICR
Professor and Head
Department of Radiodiagnosis
Postgraduate Institute of Medical Education
and Research, Chandigarh, India

Mandeep Garg MD FRCR
Professor
Department of Radiodiagnosis
Postgraduate Institute of Medical Education
and Research, Chandigarh, India

Mandeep Kang MD DNB MAMS FICR
Professor
Department of Radiodiagnosis
Postgraduate Institute of Medical Education
and Research, Chandigarh, India

Manisha Jana MD DNB FRCR
Associate Professor
Department of Radiodiagnosis
All India Institute of Medical Sciences
New Delhi, India

Manish Modi MD DM
Professor
Department of Neurology
Postgraduate Institute of Medical Education
and Research, Chandigarh, India

Manphool Singhal MD DNB MNAMS
Additional Professor
Department of Radiodiagnosis
Postgraduate Institute of Medical Education
and Research, Chandigarh, India

Mukesh Kumar Yadav MD
Assistant Professor
Department of Radiodiagnosis
Dr BRA Institute—Rotary Cancer Hospital
All India Institute of Medical Sciences
New Delhi, India

Naveen Kalra MD MAMS FICR
Professor
Department of Radiodiagnosis
Postgraduate Institute of Medical Education
and Research, Chandigarh, India

Nidhi Prabhakar MD DNB
Assistant Professor
Department of Radiodiagnosis
Postgraduate Institute of Medical Education
and Research, Chandigarh, India

Niranjan Khandelwal MD Dip NBE FICR FAMS
Former Head
Department of Radiodiagnosis
Postgraduate Institute of Medical Education
and Research, Chandigarh, India

Pankaj Gupta MD DNB
Assistant Professor
Department of Radiodiagnosis and Imaging
Postgraduate Institute of Medical Education
and Research, Chandigarh, India

Paramjeet Singh MD
Professor
Department of Radiodiagnosis
Postgraduate Institute of Medical Education
and Research, Chandigarh, India

Pratik Kumar PhD Dip RP
Professor
Medical Physics Unit
Dr BRA Institute—Rotary Cancer Hospital
All India Institute of Medical Sciences
New Delhi, India

Priya Jagia MD DNB
Professor
Department of Cardiovascular Radiology
and Endovascular Interventions
All India Institute of Medical Sciences
New Delhi, India

Priyanka Naranje MD DNB MNAMS
Assistant Professor
Department of Radiodiagnosis
All India Institute of Medical Sciences
New Delhi, India

Punit Sharma MD
Former Senior Resident
Department of Nuclear Medicine
All India Institute of Medical Sciences
New Delhi, India

Radhika Batra MD DNB
Assistant Professor
Department of Radiodiagnosis
Maulana Azad Medical College
New Delhi, India

Radhika Srinivasan MD PhD
Professor
Department of Cytology and
Gynec-pathology
Postgraduate Institute of Medical Education
and Research, Chandigarh, India

Rajat Jain MD
Former Senior Resident
Department of Radiodiagnosis
Maulana Azad Medical College
New Delhi, India

Raju Sharma MD MAMS FICR
Professor
Department of Radiodiagnosis
All India Institute of Medical Sciences
New Delhi, India

Rakesh Kumar MD PhD
Professor
Department of Nuclear Medicine
All India Institute of Medical Sciences
New Delhi, India

Rakesh Kumar Vasishta MD FRCPath
Professor and Head
Department of Histopathology
Postgraduate Institute of Medical Education
and Research, Chandigarh, India

Rama Mohan Reddy MD (Nuclear Medicine)
Former Senior Resident
Department of Nuclear Medicine
All India Institute of Medical Sciences
New Delhi, India

Rashmi Dixit MD
Director Professor
Department of Radiodiagnosis
Maulana Azad Medical College
New Delhi, India

Sameer Vyas MD DM MAMS
Additional Professor
Department of Radiodiagnosis and Imaging
Postgraduate Institute of Medical Education
and Research, Chandigarh, India

Sanjay Sharma MD DNB MNAMS FRCR FICR
Professor
Department of Radiodiagnosis
Dr Rajendra Prasad Centre for
Ophthalmic Sciences
All India Institute of Medical Sciences
New Delhi, India

Sanjay Thulkar MD
Professor
Department of Radiodiagnosis
Dr BRA Institute—Rotary Cancer Hospital
All India Institute of Medical Sciences
New Delhi, India

Sanjeev Kumar MD
Assistant Professor
Department of Cardiovascular Radiology
and Endovascular Interventions
All India Institute of Medical Sciences
New Delhi, India

Sanjiv Sharma MD
Professor and Head
Department of Cardiac Radiology
Cardio-Thoracic Sciences Centre
All India Institute of Medical Sciences
New Delhi, India

Sapna Singh MD DNB MNAMS
Professor
Department of Radiodiagnosis
Maulana Azad Medical College
New Delhi, India

Satyam DNB MNAMS
Specialist
Department of Radiodiagnosis
Lok Nayak Hospital
New Delhi, India

SC Bansal MA MSc PhD
Former Lecturer
Department of Radiodiagnosis
Postgraduate Institute of Medical Education
and Research, Chandigarh, India

Shailesh B Gaikwad MD
Professor and Head
Department of Neuroimaging and
Interventional Neuroradiology (CN Centre)
All India Institute of Medical Sciences
New Delhi, India

Shamim Ahmed Shamim MD (Nuclear Medicine)
Assistant Professor
Department of Nuclear Medicine
All India Institute of Medical Sciences
New Delhi, India

Shashi Bala Paul PhD MAMS
Senior Scientist
Department of Radiodiagnosis
All India Institute of Medical Sciences
New Delhi, India

Shivanand Gamanagatti MD MAMS
Professor
Department of Radiodiagnosis
(Trauma Center Division)
All India Institute of Medical Sciences
New Delhi, India

Smita Manchanda MD DNB MNAMS
Assistant Professor
Department of Radiodiagnosis
All India Institute of Medical Sciences
New Delhi, India

Smriti Hari MD MAMS
Professor
Department of Radiodiagnosis
All India Institute of Medical Sciences
New Delhi, India

Subrat Kumar Acharya
DM FNASc FASc FNA JC Bose Fellow
Former Professor and Head
Department of Gastroenterology
All India Institute of Medical Sciences
New Delhi, India

Sudesh Prabhakar MD DM
Former Professor and Head
Department of Neurology
Postgraduate Institute of Medical Education
and Research, Chandigarh, India

Sudha Suri MD
Former Emeritus Professor
Department of Radiodiagnosis
Postgraduate Institute of Medical Education and Research, Chandigarh, India

(Late) Sumedha Pawa MBBS MD
Director Professor
Department of Radiodiagnosis
Maulana Azad Medical College
New Delhi, India

Surabhi Vyas MD DNB MNAMS
Associate Professor
Department of Radiodiagnosis
All India Institute of Medical Sciences
New Delhi, India

Swati Gupta MD DNB FRCR
Assistant Professor
Department of Radiodiagnosis
Maulana Azad Medical College
New Delhi, India

Tulika Singh MD
Additional Professor
Department of Radiodiagnosis
Postgraduate Institute of Medical Education and Research, Chandigarh, India

Ujjwal Gorsi MD
Assistant Professor
Department of Radiodiagnosis
Postgraduate Institute of Medical Education and Research, Chandigarh, India

Uma Debi MD
Assistant Professor
Department of Radiodiagnosis
Postgraduate Institute of Medical Education and Research, Chandigarh, India

Veena Chowdhury MBBS MD
Former Professor of Excellence
Department of Radiodiagnosis
Maulana Azad Medical College
New Delhi, India

Veenu Singla MD
Professor
Department of Radiodiagnosis
Postgraduate Institute of Medical Education and Research, Chandigarh, India

Vikas Bhatia MD DM
Assistant Professor
Department of Radiodiagnosis
Postgraduate Institute of Medical Education and Research, Chandigarh, India

Virendra Jain MD FRCR
Former Senior Resident
Department of Radiodiagnosis
Maulana Azad Medical College
New Delhi, India

Vivek Gupta MD DM
Professor
Department of Radiodiagnosis
Postgraduate Institute of Medical Education and Research, Chandigarh, India

Preface

In 1996, a unique venture was jointly initiated by the faculty of Radiodiagnosis, All India Institute of Medical Sciences (AIIMS), New Delhi; Maulana Azad Medical College (MAMC), New Delhi; and Postgraduate Institute of Medical Education and Research (PGIMER), Chandigarh, India, to organize continuing medical education (CME) programs based on a series of imaging courses. An integral part of this endeavour was publishing books covering all organ systems. The aim was to provide state-of-the-art knowledge for postgraduate students as well as the practicing radiologists along with establishing a uniform pattern of teaching in radiology across the country.

The first series of seven imaging courses was successfully completed in the year 2000. A second series of these courses was then initiated in the year 2002 and was completed in 2004. This was also highly successful. The third series of seven extremely popular and successful courses covering all the organ systems and advances in physics was started in 2008 and was completed in 2013. Currently, the fourth series is underway.

Every course in each of the series has resulted in publication of a book. These books have been very popular amongst residents as well as among practicing radiologists.

Considering the popularity of these books, the editors, along with publishers, M/s Jaypee Brothers Medical Publishers (P) Ltd, New Delhi, India, decided to combine the individual books into three volumes—*AIIMS-MAMC-PGI's Comprehensive Textbook of Diagnostic Radiology*.

In keeping pace with newer developments in the field of diagnostic radiology and in order to cater to the contemporary needs of users, the second edition of *AIIMS-MAMC-PGI's Comprehensive Textbook of Diagnostic Radiology* is now being presented after a gap of three years since the previous edition of this book. It is anticipated that with such a complete coverage of all the subjects, the users will not have to refer to any other book during their routine learning of diagnostic radiology.

We are sure that residents and radiologists will find these comprehensive three volumes easy to handle and very useful in day-to-day practice.

We are once again grateful to all the contributors from the three apex academic institutions of India, i.e. AIIMS, New Delhi; MAMC, New Delhi; and PGIMER, Chandigarh, India.

We are thankful to M/s Jaypee Brothers Medical Publishers (P) Ltd, for helping us to make our dream come true.

Arun Kumar Gupta
Anju Garg
Manavjit Singh Sandhu

Acknowledgments

We would like to put on record our deep appreciation and gratitude:

To Professors Manorama Berry, Sudha Suri and Veena Chowdhury (Past Editors) the three pioneers who in 1996 took a bold initiative and started a unique teaching course now popularly known as AIIMS-MAMC-PGI's imaging course. Up to 2013, three series of these courses have been completed and the fourth series was started at the end of 2016. This course series has become extremely popular and every course is followed by the publication of a book which too is highly appreciated and popular.

To Professors Sima Mukhopadhyay, Sushma Vashisht and Niranjan Khandelwal who have been the Editors of past series and who contributed to organizing the earlier courses in their capacity as Heads of Departments.

To all the Associate Editors of the different course books who put in immense effort to bring the books out on time.

To all the Authors who contributed chapters without whom we could not have collected such an outstanding content of teaching and academic material.

To our respective hospitals for giving us the privilege and unique opportunity to work, which enabled us to amass data from patients and document images of diverse diseases that provide the reader with a wide spectrum of knowledge.

Our sincere and grateful thanks to Shri Jitendar P Vij (Group Chairman), Mr Ankit Vij (Managing Director), Mr MS Mani (Group President), Ms Chetna Malhotra Vohra (Associate Director–Content Strategy), Ms Pooja Bhandari (Production Head), Ms Kritika Dua (Senior Development Editor) and other members of M/s Jaypee Brothers Medical Publishers (P) Ltd, New Delhi, India, for their untiring coordination efforts in the production of this book.

We are very proud indeed at the culmination of two decades of these course series, to compile and present them together in the form of these three volumes of *AIIMS-MAMC-PGI's Comprehensive Textbook of Diagnostic Radiology*.

Contents

VOLUME 1

NEUROradiology including head and neck imaging, recent advances and applied physics in imaging

SECTION 1: Neuroradiology including Head and Neck Imaging

VOLUME 2
GASTROINTESTINAL AND HEPATOBILIARY IMAGING, GENITOURINARY AND PEDIATRIC IMAGING

SECTION 3: Gastrointestinal and Hepatobiliary Imaging

SECTION 4: Genitourinary Imaging

SECTION 5: Pediatric Imaging

SECTION 7: Musculoskeletal and Breast Imaging

Section 3

Gastrointestinal and Hepatobiliary Imaging

CHAPTER 67

Imaging Techniques for Abdomen

Smriti Hari, Smita Manchanda

INTRODUCTION

The imaging techniques for evaluation of abdomen have evolved dramatically over the past few decades. Conventional radiographs and barium studies now have a limited role with the cross-sectional imaging modalities such as computed tomography (CT) and magnetic resonance imaging (MRI) being the mainstay of diagnosis. Ultrasound remains the first line investigation for suspected hepatobiliary and pancreatic pathologies. The recent advent of ultrasound contrast agents and elastography techniques has improved the diagnostic yield of ultrasound. The routine contrast-enhanced CT and MRI have been modified in the form of multiphase acquisition and enterography/colonography for an optimal delineation of hepatic/pancreatic and bowel pathologies respectively. There has been a significant advancement in the nuclear imaging studies with the advent of hybrid scanners like positron emission tomography (PET)-CT and PET-MRI that are capable of providing both anatomical and functional information.

CONVENTIONAL TECHNIQUES

Conventional radiographs of the abdomen are now limited to the emergency setting for the evaluation of suspected perforation and intestinal obstruction.

BARIUM STUDIES

Endoscopy is the investigation of choice for most esophageal pathologies with a complimentary role for barium studies. However, fluoroscopic barium studies **(Fig. 1)** are essential in the evaluation of motility disorders.

The stomach and duodenum are also best evaluated by endoscopy in cases of dyspepsia and abdominal pain. However, barium studies **(Fig. 2)** are required for assessing functional abnormalities like reflux and delayed emptying; submucosal masses and infiltrative processes. The barium/gastrografin oral contrast study is also the technique of choice for evaluation of early postoperative complications following gastric surgery.

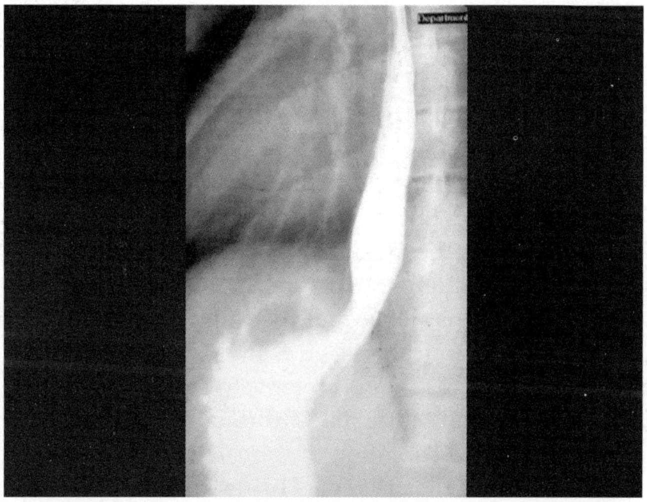

Fig. 1: The lower thoracic esophagus and gastroesophageal junction well seen in the distended state in a normal barium swallow.

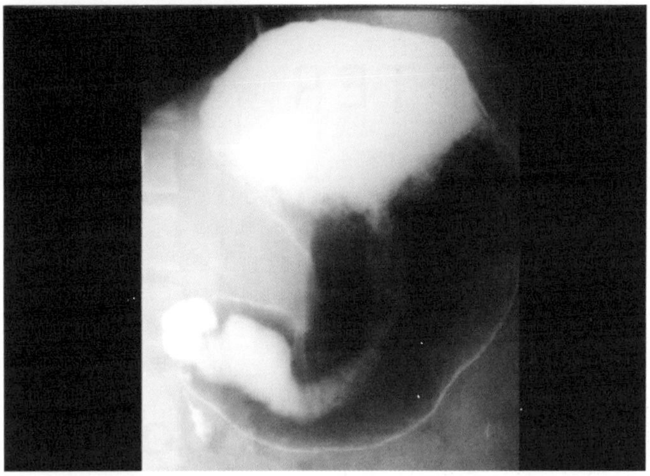

Fig. 2: Supine radiograph of double contrast barium swallow showing well-distended stomach and normal mucosal pattern.

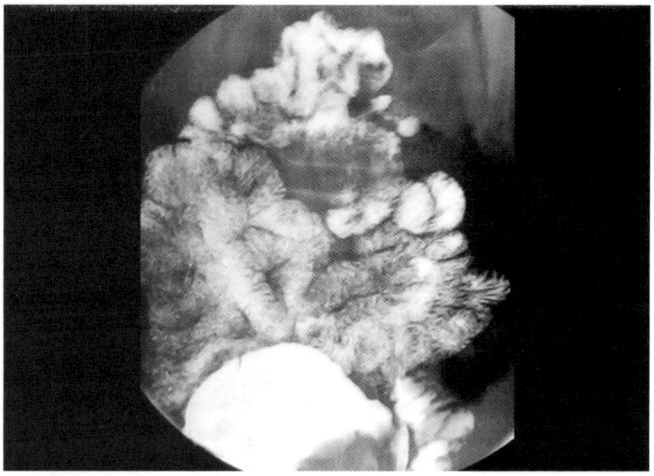

Fig. 3: Barium followthrough examination showing well-distended jejunal loops with normal villous pattern.

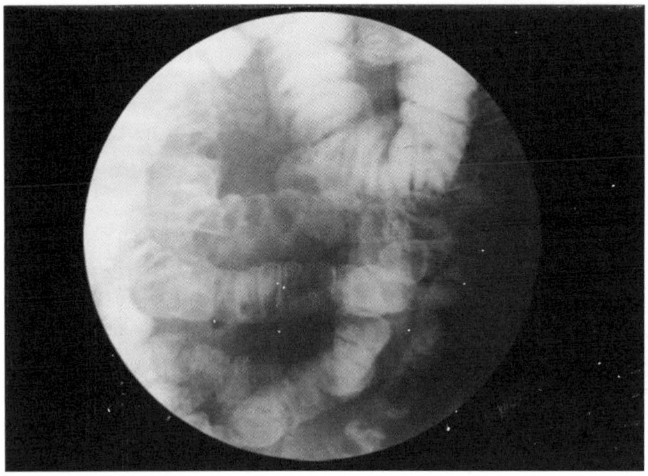

Fig. 4: Conventional small bowel enteroclysis showing normal distended jejunal and ileal loops in double contrast.

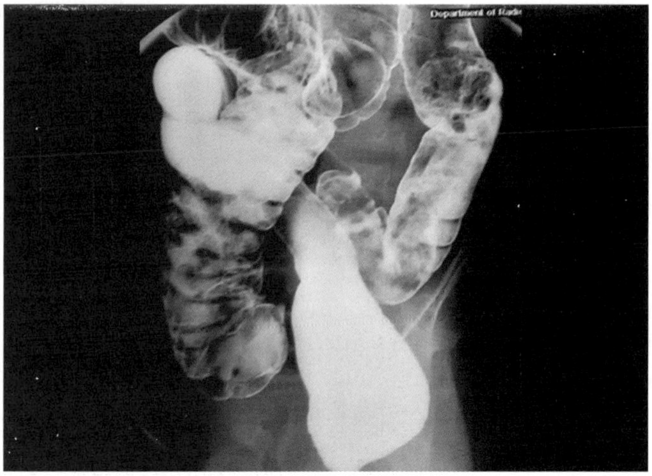

Fig. 5: Double contrast barium enema. Supine radiograph showing normal mucosal outline of the cecum, ascending colon, part of transverse colon and descending colon. The hepatic flexure and rectosigmoid colon are in a dependent position and hence seen in a barium-filled state.

For radiological evaluation of small bowel, both barium follow through **(Fig. 3)** and enteroclysis **(Fig. 4)**, are superior to CT/MRI examination in terms of demonstration of fine mucosal detail. The conventional enteroclysis has the advantages of shorter examination time, better distension of small bowel and better visualization of pathology but requires more radiologist time, greater technical skill, gives more radiation dose to patient and operator and is relatively uncomfortable for the patient. Small bowel follow through study is easy to perform, allows estimation of transit time and is more comfortable to the patient. However, complete and adequate distension of small bowel cannot be achieved in followthrough study.[1,2]

Colonoscopy is the investigation of choice for evaluation of colorectal diseases. However, barium enema **(Fig. 5)** is useful for delineating colonic caliber and configuration.[3] Also barium contrast enema is preferred in patients with question of large bowel obstruction, need for localization of colonic disease preoperatively or to assess the status of colon anastomosis.

Prior to undertaking any barium procedure, appropriate medical history along with results of previous investigations (including imaging and endoscopic procedures) should be obtained. **Table 1** highlights the indications, contraindications, brief technique along with special modifications of the commonly performed barium procedures.[4-7]

Table 1: Commonly performed barium procedures.

Procedure	Indications	Contraindications	Patient preparation	Examination technique	Modifications
Barium swallow	• Dysphagia • Odynophagia • Reflux disease • Atypical chest pain	• Recent esophageal surgery • Recent gastric surgery • Recent trauma • Uncooperative patient	• Nil orally for a minimum of 2 hours prior to the procedure • No smoking	• Low density (60–95% weight per volume [weight/volume]) barium suspension is used • Esophagus anatomy and motility is evaluated under fluoroscopy • Spot images taken to document normal (barium-filled and mucosal relief views) and abnormal findings • Gastroesophageal junction is documented along with evaluation for reflux • *Double contrast:* Performed using a high-density (210–250% weight/volume) barium suspension along with an effervescent agent	*Water-soluble contrast agent*: In cases, where leak or perforation is suspected *Iso-osmolar or low-osmolar contrast or dilute barium*: In cases, where aspiration or esophageal-tracheal or bronchial fistula is suspected
Barium meal upper GI	• Suspected reflux • Epigastric pain/ discomfort • Dyspepsia • Upper GI bleeding • Anemia • Weight loss	• Recent esophageal surgery • Recent gastric surgery • Recent trauma • Uncooperative patient	• Nil orally after midnight, a day prior • No smoking	• Fluoroscopic evaluation of esophagus, stomach and duodenum • *Double contrast*: Performed using a high-density (210–250% weight/volume) barium suspension along with an effervescent agent • Spot images to document normal and abnormal findings • Barium-filled and mucosal relief views of esophagus, stomach and duodenum • Overhead images for full anatomical delineation of stomach	*Water-soluble contrast agent*: In cases, where leak or perforation is suspected
Barium follow-through	• Suspected small bowel obstruction • Unexplained GI bleeding • Malabsorption • Suspected enteric fistula • Abdominal pain • Diarrhea	Uncooperative patient	Nil orally after midnight prior to the procedure	• 600 mL of 50% weight/volume barium suspension • Oral administration over one hour • Fluoroscopic evaluation after 30 minutes and regular overhead radiographs in prone position • Spot compression views of any focal abnormality • Compression of accessible loops • Ileocecal junction demonstration • Peroral pneumocolon, if required for better delineation of distensibility of cecum and ileocecal junction	*Water-soluble contrast agent*: Preferred, if there is suspicion of bowel leak or obstruction

Contd...

Contd...

Procedure	Indications	Contraindications	Patient preparation	Examination technique	Modifications
Enteroclysis	• Recurrent small bowel obstructions • Unexplained weight loss or gastrointestinal (GI) bleeding • Anemia • Malabsorption	• Inability to pass catheter • Patient intolerance for catheter	• Nil orally after midnight before the procedure • Laxative may be given on the day prior to the examination • Enteroclysis catheter placed under fluoroscopic guidance and nasal anesthetic spray • Tip-positioned several centimeters beyond the duodenojejunal flexure	• Single-contrast examination • Medium-density barium suspension given via the tube to maintain adequate small bowel distension • Double-contrast examination • High-density barium suspension followed by 0.5% solution of hydroxypropyl methylcellulose, volume of room air • Administered under fluoroscopic guidance, double-contrast mucosal coating and optimal distention of small bowel • Infusion rate controlled to avoid excessive peristalsis • Avoid reflux of large amounts of this fluid into stomach • *Technique*: External compression, rotation and palpation • Separate overlapping bowel loops • Spot compression views • Overhead large-format • Images of completely distended small bowel	
Barium enema	• Abdominal pain • Diarrhea/Constipation/ Change in bowel habits • Gastrointestinal bleeding • Anemia • Abdominal masses • Weight loss • Fever or sepsis • History of previous colon polyp or neoplasm • Familial inheritance pattern diseases involving the colon	• Unexplained pneumoperitoneum • Toxic colon • Uncooperative patient *Relative*: Rigid colonoscopy and biopsy	• Colon preparation to remove fecal matter and excess fluid • Dietary restriction • Hydration • Laxatives • Cleansing enemas	• Single-contrast enema • Low-density (15–25% weight/volume) barium suspension or water-soluble contrast • Spot compression views • Frontal views of entire filled colon • Lateral view of rectum • Angled-beam view of sigmoid colon • Postevacuation images • Double-contrast barium enema • Commercially available high-density (80% weight/volume or greater) barium suspension • Barium suspension and air introduced under fluoroscopic control • All segments of colon documented in double contrast • Overhead supine and prone radiographs of entire colon • Lateral view of rectum	*Water-soluble contrast*: • Immediate postoperative period • Suspected perforation • Bowel preparation not possible • Blind-ending colonic segments (e.g. Hartmann pouch) • May be therapeutic in cases of meconium ileus equivalent (cystic fibrosis)

Abbreviation: GI: Gastrointestinal.

ULTRASONOGRAPHY EVALUATION OF THE LIVER

Sonography is used as the initial imaging modality for suspected liver pathology.[8] It plays a vital role in the evaluation of focal liver lesions, screening for liver metastases in a patient with known malignancy, screening for hepatocellular carcinoma in the setting of hepatitis/cirrhosis, portal hypertension, surgical obstructive jaundice, hepatic veno-occlusive disease and preoperative work-up and postoperative follow-up of liver transplant patients. Sonography effectively differentiates a solid from a cystic lesion and provides significant information regarding the internal architecture of indeterminate lesions.

The addition of color Doppler flow imaging further helps in characterizing mass lesions and assessing patency of vessels.[9] Doppler is particularly helpful in liver transplants, Budd-Chiari syndrome and cirrhosis.

Technique

The liver is scanned in the supine or left decubitus position with a 3.5–5 MHz convex transducer in the transverse, sagittal and oblique planes, from a subcostal approach. The sub-costal approach may not suffice in all patients and intercostal scanning may have to be done with a small footprint transducer.[9] This is especially true in shrunken cirrhotic livers. An attempt is made to delineate the venous landmarks so that all the liver segments can be identified and scanned sequentially.

Sonographic Anatomy

Liver parenchyma is imaged as fine homogeneous mid-level echoes interrupted only by fissures and vessels. The liver echogenicity is usually greater but may be equal to renal echogenicity. Hepatic veins **(Fig. 6)** are well-defined tubular structures without significant marginal echoes, whereas portal veins have echogenic walls due to fibrous and fatty tissue **(Fig. 7)**. Bile ducts run parallel to portal vein branches, but their location in relation to veins is variable, and the axiom that ducts are always anterior to portal vein branches is not correct. The state of art electronically focused ultrasound equipment demonstrates normal intrahepatic biliary radicles quite well and a bile duct must be at least 40% of the size of its neighboring portal vein branch for it to be considered dilated. Therefore, the mere visualization of parallel channels in the liver parenchyma does not indicate biliary dilatation.[9]

The gallbladder is located in the interlobar fissure and is well evaluated by ultrasound. The wall of the gallbladder should not be thicker than 3 mm in the fasting state. The common duct lies anterior to the portal vein at the porta hepatis and should be measured at the place where the hepatic artery crosses perpendicularly between them. This level has been used because of the consistent acoustic window provided by the surrounding liver, which ensures reproducibility of the measurement. The common duct should not be wider than 6 mm at this point.

On Doppler examination, the normal hepatic vein trace reflects the transmitted right heart pressure changes leading to flow reversal during the right atrial contraction **(Fig. 8)**. The portal vein trace is continuously antegrade with a mean peak velocity of 15–22 cm/s. The portal venous flow shows slight undulation related to the cardiac cycle and respiration **(Fig. 9)**.

Intraoperative Ultrasonography

Intraoperative and laparoscopic ultrasonography (US) are very useful techniques that have had major impact on

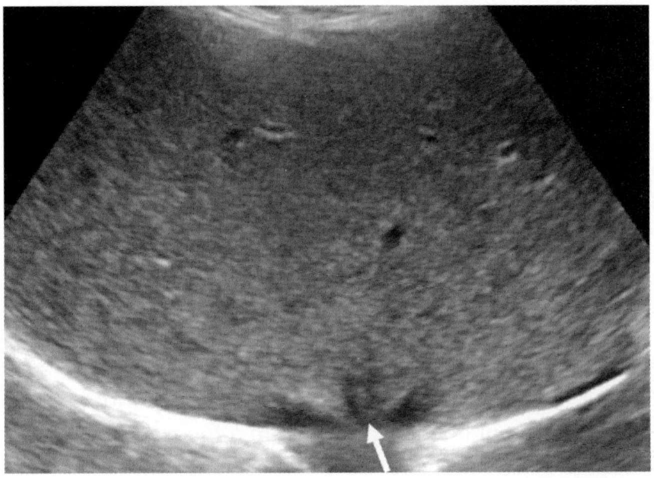

Fig. 6: Transverse US scan showing the three hepatic veins (arrow) joining the interior vena cava (IVC).

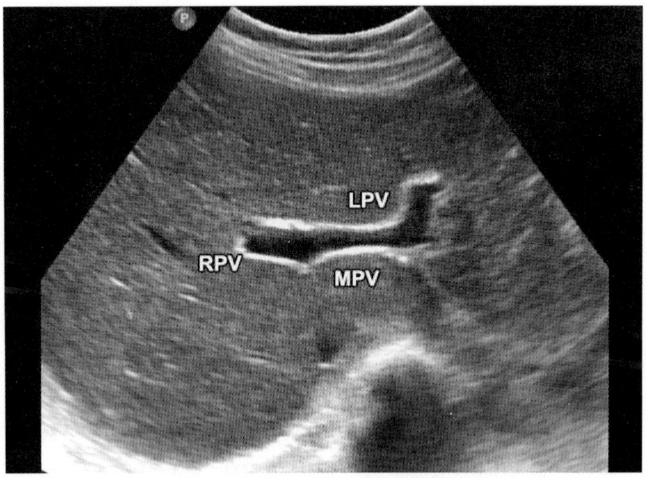

Fig. 7: Ultrasonography scan showing the bifurcation of main portal vein (MPV) into the right (RPV) and left portal veins (LPV).

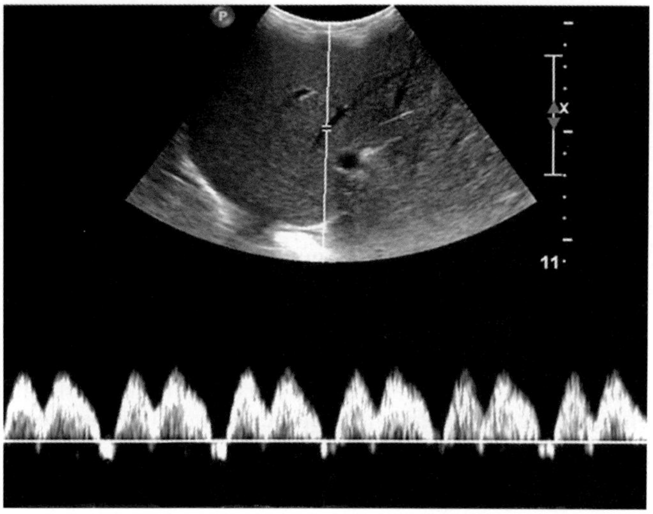

Fig. 8: Color Doppler flow imaging of hepatic vein showing normal triphasic flow pattern with a short phase of reversed flow.

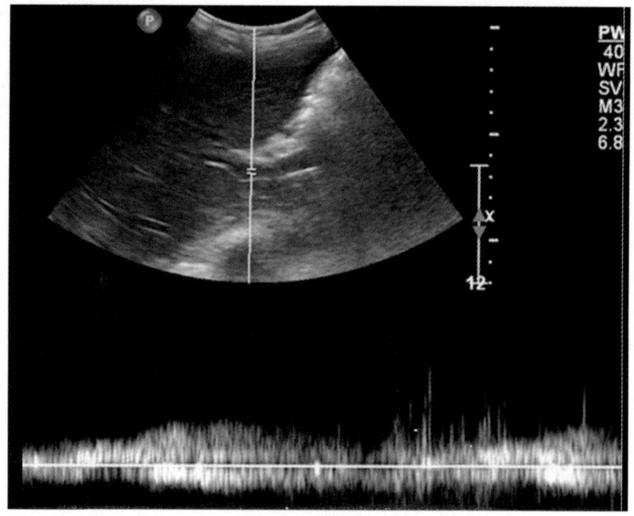

Fig. 9: Color Doppler flow imaging of portal vein showing continuous antegrade flow with minimal phasicity.

patient management. A 5–7 MHz T-shaped linear array probe is used for intraoperative scanning. The probe can be sterilized using ethylene oxide gas sterilization. The probe is applied directly to the liver surface and no gel or acoustic coupling agent is necessary. The liver is scanned from the dome to the caudal edge and from left to right in a sequential manner. Color Doppler can be coupled with the grayscale scan and is very useful to identify vascular landmarks and assess their patency.

Intraoperative ultrasonography (IOUS) provides useful real time information to the surgeon and can alter the surgical approach. Current applications for IOUS include tumor staging, metastases evaluation, tumor ablation processes, evaluation of patency of vessels, intrahepatic biliary disease, and in liver transplantation.[9]

Endosonography

The development of endoscopic US (EUS) has rendered the gastrointestinal tract amenable to high resolution US examination and histopathologic sampling when required in the same session. Higher frequency probes (6–10 MHz) are used during EUS and the echoendoscopes have biopsy channels for performing fine-needle aspiration (FNA).[10] It is useful for assessing the depth of tumor invasion and sampling of smaller lesions and adjacent lymph nodes. It is being used to stage esophageal and stomach malignancies in many centers.

Similarly, transrectal ultrasonography can be used for staging of colorectal carcinomas. Anal endosonography is useful in patients with injury to the external anal sphincter and presenting with fecal incontinence.

Endoscopic US is also used for the characterization of cystic lesions of the pancreas by identifying the ultrasound morphology and performing FNA with cyst aspiration.[10]

USG Elastography

Elastography is a recent development, which gives a measure of tissue stiffness.[11,12] Depending on the deforming force applied and the method used to study the resultant deformation, it can be classified as:

- Static elastography
- Impulse elastography
  - Unidimensional transient elastography (Fibroscan)
  - Acoustic radiation force impulse (ARFI) imaging mode elastography
  - Shear wave elastography.

Acoustic radiation force impulse (ARFI) elastography gives a quantitative measure of the shear wave speed (in m/s) induced by acoustic radiation through an external vibrator. The measurement area is a 1 × 0.5 cm rectangle placed on the B-mode ultrasound image. These measurements are taken in the right lobe of liver through the intercostal space. Its main use is in the assessment of liver fibrosis and hepatic masses. However, this technique is not real time, does not give standard deviation and the size of the measurement area cannot be changed.[11]

Shear wave elastography measures the speed of shear waves that are produced in the tissue perpendicular to the direction of displacement when a focused ultrasound beam provides an acoustic 'push'. The acquisition is real time with simultaneous display of the B-mode image and the corresponding shear wave elastography image (two- dimensional box with elastography color map). The speed of shear waves is used to calculate the elasticity in kilopascals (kPa and real time measurements can be made by placing the Q box over the region of interest **(Fig. 10)**. The system generates the maximum, minimum and mean values along with the standard deviation. The size and position of the Q-box can be altered and in addition, retrospective measurements can be made with this system.

USG Contrast Agents

Contrast-enhanced ultrasound (CEUS) uses microbubble-based contrast agents to improve the echogenicity of blood. It has major clinical applications in echocardiography, hepatology and vessel evaluation. It can be easily peformed after baseline ultrasound in the same sitting and provides functional vascular information without the use of ionic radiation.

The microbubbles have an average diameter of 1–4 µm and they oscillate at ultrasound frequencies of 1–15 MHz. These nonlinear oscillations generate echoes which are detected by the imaging system. With the availability of phase modulation and amplitude modulation techniques, the sensitivity of ultrasound equipment for microbubble detection has consistenly improved in the last decade.[13]

Examples of commonly used contrast agents include SonoVue (sulfur hexafluoride microbubble) and Levovist (microcrystalline suspension of galactose and palmitic acid). The contrast agent is available in the lyophilized powder form, which is to be mixed with 5 mL of 0.9% normal saline and injected as a rapid IV bolus followed by 5–10 mL of saline flush. USG scanning is started immediately and takes approximately 4–5 minutes. For the evaluation of liver lesions, real time imaging is performed through the arterial, portal venous and parenchymal phases **(Figs. 11A and B)**. Contrast is seen to pass through the hepatic artery and its branches with liver echogenecity increasing from the arterial to the portal phase. Lesion echogenecity is compared to the parenchyma at the same depth and their enhancement pattern is compared with that of the blood pool.[13,14]

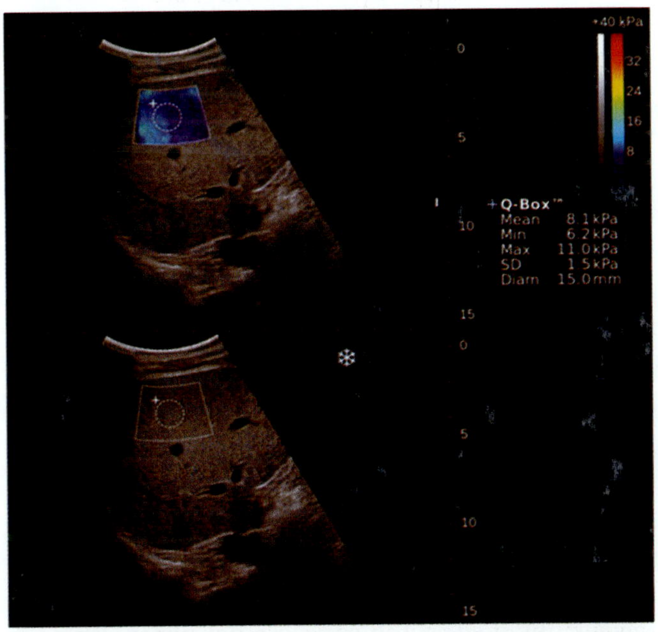

Fig. 10: Shear wave elastography of the liver seen as dual display. The color in the box corresponds to the velocity of the shear waves. The velocity is measured in kilopascals and is displayed in the vertical bar on the right.

USG Image Fusion and Navigation

The higher end ultrasound machines provide integrated image fusion and instrument navigation capabilities. The image navigation system provides real time guidance for soft tissue biopsy and ablation procedures in ultrasound combining the cross-sectional data available. Image fusion techniques makes it possible to target those lesions which are not well visualized on USG but are seen on another modality like CT or MRI. The CT/MRI images of the patient are added onto the ultrasound fusion system. The two-dimensional cross-sectional images are then transformed into dynamic, fused imaging maps that combine CT or MR imaging with live ultrasound.

CT EXAMINATION OF THE ABDOMEN AND PELVIS

For complete CT evaluation of abdomen and pelvis, images are acquired in the axial plane from the dome of diaphragm to below the ischial tuberosities in suspended respiration. The slice thickness is 5 mm or less. CT examination is optimized for each patient according to the relevant history and clinical indication. This includes determining the need for non-contrast scan and planning of the study as a single phase or multiphase study.[15]

Enteric contrast agent is used for better delineation of bowel loops and can be administered orally, via nasogastric tube, per rectally or in varying combinations. Positive contrast agents include dilute barium (1–2%) and water-soluble iodinated contrast material (2–3%). These help to differentiate intraluminal from extraluminal pathology and detect suspected leaks. However, bowel wall enhancement characteristics are difficult to interpret when positive contrast agents have been used. Similarly, they also interfere with the 3D reformatted angiographic

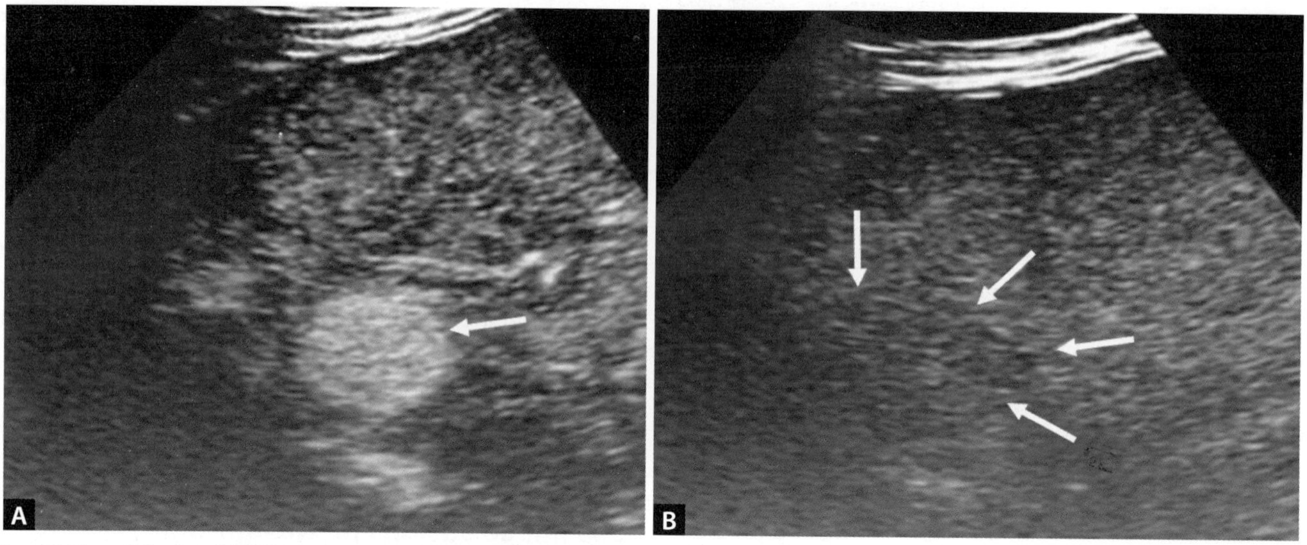

Figs. 11A and B: Small HCC in a 30-year-old man with chronic liver disease: (A) Arterial phase US image obtained 20 seconds after contrast material injection demonstrates diffuse homogeneous enhancement of the nodule (arrow); (B) Delayed phase US image obtained 192 seconds after injection shows washout (arrows).

images and should not be used in cases of suspected GI bleed.[15,16]

Neutral contrast material is more useful when bowel wall characteristics need to be evaluated and in vascular studies. These include water and agents with water density like mannitol, lactulose and methylcellulose. However, the evaluation of abscesses and hypodense collections becomes more challenging with use of neutral contrast agents.

Negative contrast agents like air and carbon dioxide are used routinely in CT colonography for optimal colonic distension.

When single-phase acquisition is planned, intravenous nonionic iodinated contrast (100 mL of 350 mg I/mL) is administered and images are acquired after 50–70 seconds. When evaluating CT abdomen, care should be taken to use different widow width and window level settings for viewing the visceral organs, the intra-abdominal fat, bony anatomy and lung bases as well. Multiphase acquisition is planned according to the area of interest as described below.[15]

CT Evaluation of Hepatic Pathology

Multiphase CT scanning should be performed for the evaluation of liver pathology.

Multidetector CT Evaluation

Typically a *triple phase CT* is performed in case of suspected liver lesion.

Non-contrast scan has a limited role, and is of use predominantly in patients treated with TACE or other ablative therapies. It can help to assess post-contrast enhancement in patients with siderotic nodules of increased attenuation. However, in order to keep the radiation dose low, most studies now do not recommend acquisition of the pre-contrast scan.[17,18]

Intravenous contrast is administered in a dose of 1.5–2 mL per kg body weight. The total iodine dose should be 525 mg iodine per kg or more; assuming iodine concentration of contrast to be 350 mg iodine per milliliter. Contrast should be administered at a flow rate of 3–4 mL/s using dual head mechanical injector and followed by saline flush. Most scanners now provide bolus-tracking software and passage of contrast through the descending aorta should be monitored to start the image acquisition.[19,20]

The images are acquired in the arterial, portal venous and delayed phases. The *early arterial phase* (about 10 seconds after the injection) is characterized by enhancement of the hepatic artery but not the portal vein. This phase is reserved for patients in whom CT angiography is required, such as potential transplant recipients, candidates for hepatic resection or cryoablation, or candidates for chemo-embolization.[21] CT angiography images can be created through three-dimensional reconstructions of the thin slice, isotropic images obtained in the early arterial phase. Water is preferred as the oral contrast agent for multiplanar CT angiography to allow optimal reconstructions from the 3D data sets. Maximum intensity projection, surface-shaded

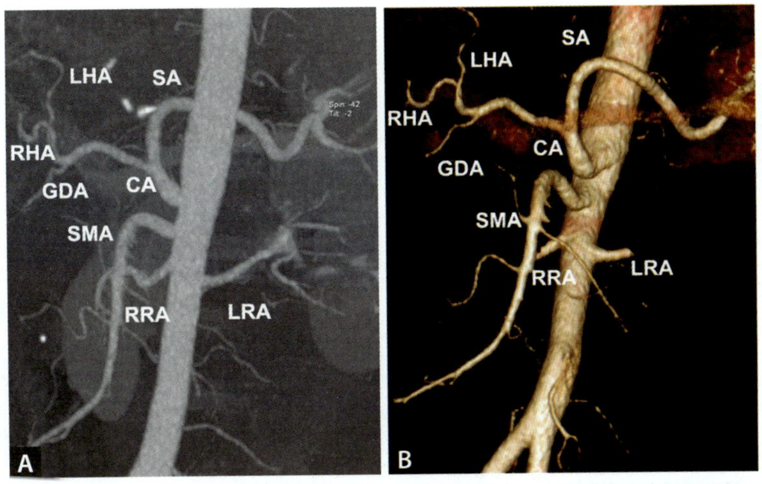

Figs. 12A and B: Coronal maximum intensity projection [MIP] (A) and volume rendered technique [VRT]; (B) reconstructed from the axial MDCT images obtained during early arterial phase of contrast enhancement demonstrates abdominal aorta and its branches. *Abbreviations*: CA: Celiac axis; SMA: Superior mesenteric artery; SA: Splenic artery; GDA: Gastroduodenal artery; RHA: Right hepatic artery; LHA: Left hepatic artery; RRA: Right renal artery; LRA: Left renal artery.

display, and volume-rendered techniques are used in the post-processing of CT angiography to depict vascular anatomy **(Figs. 12A and B)**.

The *late arterial phase,* which is acquired 20 seconds after contrast injection, is characterized by enhancement of hepatic artery, its branches and the portal vein.[22] This phase is critical for picking up hypervascular tumors. A combined CT angiogram/CT portogram can be obtained from the late arterial imaging phase and is used for delineation of the extrahepatic portal venous system in transplant cases and patients with pancreaticobiliary malignancy.[21] Venous compression, venous stenosis or thrombosis, and portal systemic venous collateral vessels can be displayed.

This is followed by the *portal venous* phase acquisition at 60–80 seconds after the start of injection of contrast. In this phase, there is peak parenchymal enhancement with optimal opacification of both the portal veins and the hepatic veins.[19,23]

The *delayed phase* is acquired to study the washout characteristics of liver lesions, capsular enhancement and to observe the delayed contrast enhancement of certain tumors like cholangiocarcinomas. This is acquired at 3–5 minutes post-contrast injection.[19]

The protocol has been summarized in **Table 2.** [19,23]

Table 2: Multidetector CT protocol (Hepatic evaluation).

Intravenous Contrast:
Iodinated contrast medium: Iodine concentration 350 mg/mL
- Volume: 1.5–2 mL/kg
- Flow rate: 3–4 mL/s
- Bolus tracking software
- Mechanical injector with saline flush

Oral contrast: 600 mL tap water
Image acquisition:
- *Non-contrast phase*:
  - Before the injection of contrast material
  - In patients treated with ablative therapies
- *Late arterial phase*:
  - 20 seconds after start of injection
- *Portal venous phase*:
  - 60–80 seconds after start of injection
- *Delayed phase*:
  - >120 seconds after start of injection (3–5 min)

Dual Energy CT Evaluation

Triple-phase CT on a dual energy CT scanner is performed similarly as described above for the multidetector CT. The main advantage is generation of virtual unenhanced images without adding to the radiation dose **(Figs. 13A to D)**. These help to detect the presence of calcification and fat within lesions. Few studies have reported that it is feasible to quantity iron deposition in the liver, with dual energy CT.[24]

VOLUME ESTIMATION

Volume estimation of the liver **(Fig. 14)** helps in accurate planning of hepatic resection by delineating the exact 3D anatomy of the liver.[21] Estimation of liver volume using three- dimensional techniques, when combined with clinical and laboratory evaluation of liver function, can aid in predicting postoperative liver failure in patients undergoing resection, assists in embolization procedures, and planning of staged hepatic resection for bilobar disease.[25]

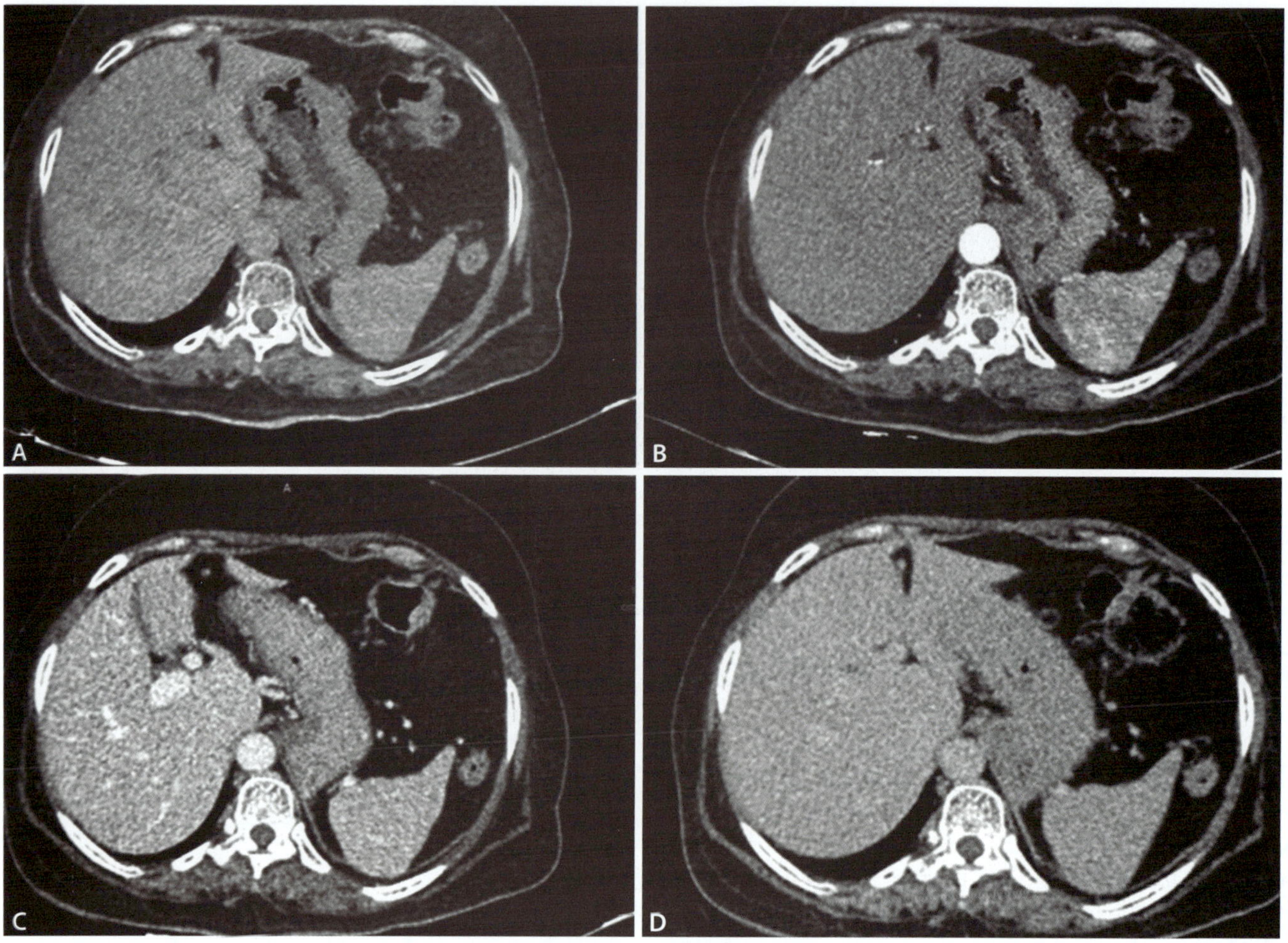

Figs. 13A to D: Multiphase CT acquisition for liver performed on a dual energy scanner. Virtual non-contrast (A); arterial (B); portal venous (C) and delayed (D) phase images reveal widening of the fissures in this known case of chronic liver disease. No focal lesion was detected.

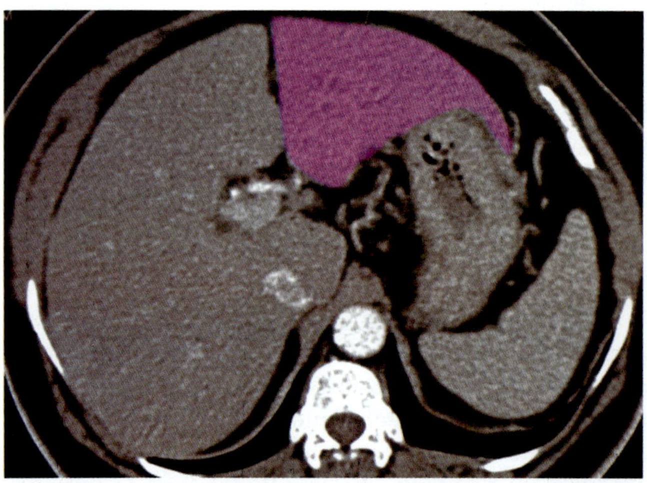

Fig. 14: CT volumetry in a patient planned for partial liver resection. Segments II and III are manually mapped out on contiguous axial slices and the volume is calculated using volumetric software.

MULTIDETECTOR COMPUTED TOMOGRAPHY EVALUATION OF PANCREATIC PATHOLOGY

For the evaluation of the pancreas, multiphase acquisition **(Figs. 15A and B)** is recommended.[26]

The precontrast images are followed by the arterial phase at 17–25 seconds after the start of contrast injection. This phase is recommended wherever optimal delineation of the arterial supply is required.

The peak parenchymal enhancement of the pancreas is seen at 35–50 seconds after the start of contrast injection. This pancreatic phase is best for peak tumor-parenchymal attenuation difference. Curved multiplanar reformat (MPR) can be obtained along the pancreatic duct for showing relationship of the duct with the tumor **(Table 3)**.

The portal venous phase is acquired 55–70 seconds after the start of contrast injection and is ideal for depiction

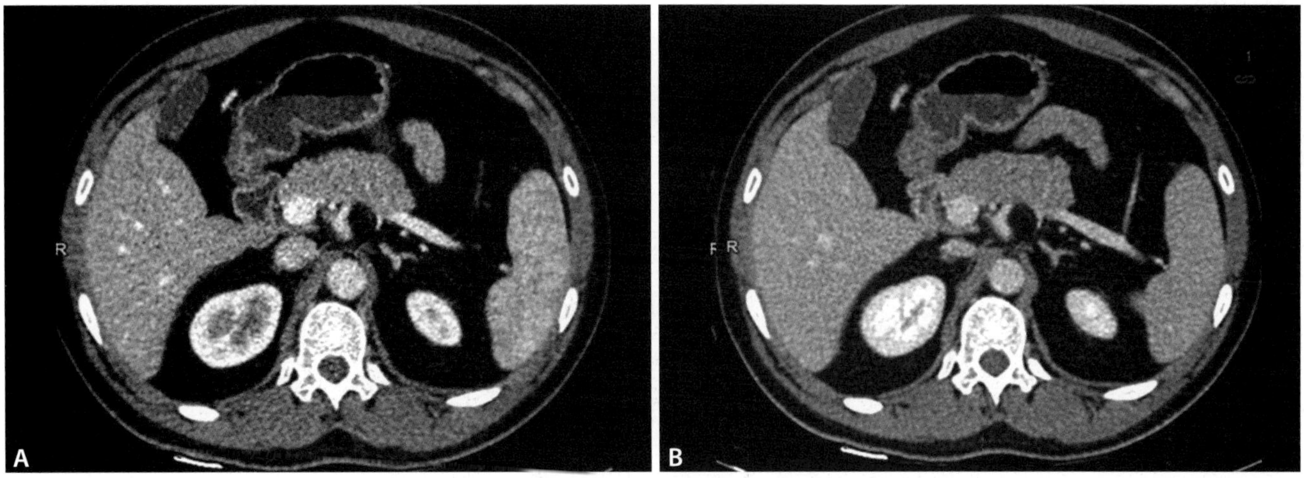

Figs. 15A and B: Multiphase CT acquisition for pancreas performed for suspicious lesion on USG. Pancreatic phase (A) is acquired at 35 seconds and portal venous phase (B) at 65 seconds after the injection of contrast medium. No focal lesion was detected.

Table 3: MDCT pancreatic protocol (Image acquisition).

- *Arterial phase*:
  - 17–25 seconds after start of injection
  - For angiography images and arterial supply delineation
- *Pancreatic phase*:
  - 35–50 seconds after start of injection
  - Peak tumor-parenchymal attenuation difference
- *Portal venous phase*:
  - 55–70 seconds after start of injection
  - Venous involvement and metastases

Table 4: CT enterography protocol.

- Nil orally
- Intestine cleansing: Polyethylene glycol lavage
- *Oral contrast*:
  - 300 mL 20% w/v mannitol mixed with 1.5 L water
  - 500 mL mixture given orally every 15 minutes
  - Remaining solution: On table oral administration
- Scan performed at 50 minutes
- *Intravenous contrast injection*:
  - 100–120 mL @ 3–4 mL/sec
  - Single phase/Multiphase acquisition

of venous involvement and liver metastases.[26,27] Minimum intensity projection (MinIP) images are used to delineate the anatomy of the pancreatic and biliary tree, which are seen as low-density structures.

BOWEL EVALUATION

CT Enteroclysis

Computed tomography (CT) enteroclysis involves the insertion of a nasojejunal tube under fluoroscopic guidance. The catheter tip is placed in the proximal jejunum and 1.5 L saline infused at 100 mL/min followed by on table infusion of 1.5 L saline with 100–120 mL intravenous contrast administration and single portal venous phase acquisition.[28] It has been replaced by CT enterography at most institutions.

CT Enterography

This is the preferred examination technique for the evaluation of small bowel pathology and is replacing traditional barium fluoroscopic studies, especially in cases of Crohn's disease.[29]

Neutral oral contrast agents are administered for optimal distension of small bowel. Bowel is prepared by prior fasting for 8 hours and intake of 50–100 mL of laxative diet solution (Polyethylene glycol lavage) one day prior to the study.[16] The neutral oral contrast agents used include water, mannitol, lactulose, methylcellulose, polyethylene glycol and 0.1% barium suspension. The CT attenuation of these agents is 0–30 HU and provides optimal contrast between bowel wall and lumen.[29]

The oral contrast should be consumed over 30–60 minutes. The protocol varies with institutions and a suggested protocol is given in **Table 4**.[16] Intravenous contrast is given (100–120 mL @ 3–4 mL/sec) and single-phase images are acquired between 50–70 seconds (either enteric or portal venous phase). However, in cases of obscure GI bleeding, both the arterial and portal venous phases must be acquired. Multiplanar reconstructions in the coronal plane **(Fig. 16)** better depict the anatomical relation of bowel loops and maximum intensity projection (MIP) images provide angiographic images for suspected GI bleed.[29]

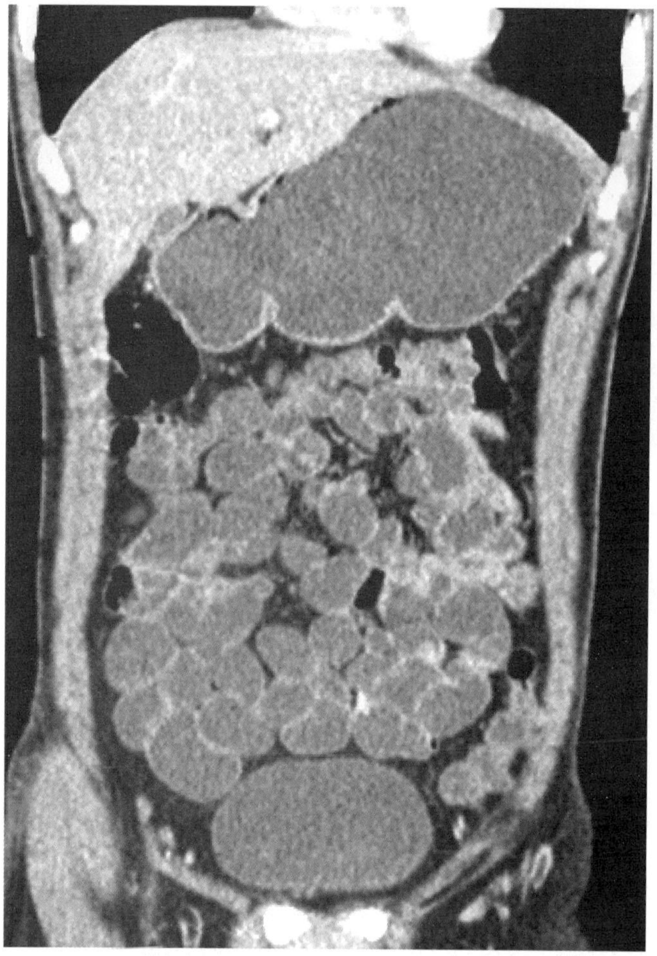

Fig. 16: CT enterography (coronal reformatted image) showing normal distension of the small bowel loops with no abnormal enhancement.

CT Colonography

CT colonography **(Table 5)**[16] is a minimally invasive procedure for evaluation of the large bowel. It can be used as a screening, surveillance or diagnostic modality depending on the patient profile. Colonic preparation is essential and consists of low fiber diet (for 1–3 days), hydration and 50–100 mL of laxative diet solution (Polyethylene glycol lavage), one day prior to the study. Fecal tagging is usually performed with oral administration of water-soluble iodinated contrast or dilute barium. This is done to incorporate positive contrast into residual fecal material and increase its CT density. The increased density helps to distinguish fecal material from polyps or malignancy.[30]

The patient should be asked to evacuate prior to the study. Soft and flexible rectal catheter is inserted and the colon is insufflated with carbon dioxide (mechanical) or room air (manual). CT scout film should be taken to check the adequacy of colonic distension. Low dose precontrast scan is acquired in the prone position, followed by intravenous contrast administration. Images are then acquired at 50–70 sec in the portal venous phase in the supine position. Optimal colonic distension is indicated by pencil thin colonic wall with thin haustral folds. Axial and coronal reconstructed images can be analyzed using CAD software, wherever available.[16,30]

Table 5: CT colonography protocol.

• *Patient preparation*: – Low fiber diet – Adequate hydration – Intestinal cleansing: Polyethylene glycol lavage • *Fecal tagging*: Oral administration of iodinated contrast or dilute barium • Evacuation prior to the study • *Colonic distension*: Carbon dioxide/Room air • *Scanning*: – Precontrast images; prone position – 100–120 mL intravenous contrast administration – Portal venous phase acquisition; supine position

MAGNETIC RESONANCE IMAGING

Magnetic resonance (MR) imaging is an excellent imaging modality because of its high contrast resolution, multiplanar capability, sensitivity to blood flow and lack of ionizing radiation. Technical advances in MR hardware and software have allowed the introduction of faster pulse sequences without the motion artifacts that previously posed limitations to abdominal MR imaging. The use of parallel imaging techniques with multi-channel phased array coils has significantly reduced the scan time. MRI of the abdomen **(Table 6)** is now an important modality for imaging the abdomen encompassing a variety of sequences, which are continuously being improvised.[31]

Higher field strengths are preferred (1.5 T or 3 T) for abdomen evaluation. The advantage of 3T imaging systems is increased signal-to-noise ratio, better delineation of post- contrast enhancement and reduced time for chemical shift sequences (echo times of in and opposed phase sequences is less compared with 1.5 T). At the same time, in comparison to 1.5 T, 3 T scanners have increased specific absorption rate (SAR) and suffer from greater magnetic field inhomogeneity making images more prone to susceptibility and chemical shift artifacts.[32,33]

Phased array surface coil is used for abdomen evaluation. T1- and T2-weighted imaging is performed using breath-hold or respiratory triggered sequences. The acquisition is usually multiplanar with slice

Table 6: MRI abdomen protocol.

• Fasting for 6 hours • Pelvic phased array surface coil • IV buscopan (1 mL~20 mg) • *Sequences*: – *T2WI*: Fat-suppressed; spin echo/hybrid sequence (axial, coronal) – Steady state fast field echo sequence: Axial – T1 in and opposed phase (Axial) – DWI (b value 0, 400, 800) – T2 (Multiecho) – *MRCP*: - Breath-hold rapid acquisition relaxation enhancement (RARE) or half-Fourier single-shot echo train spin-echo sequence (Thick slab acquisition) - 3D respiratory-triggered T2- weighted FSE technique	• *Postcontrast (Multiphase acquisition)*: – 2D or 3D T1-weighted sequences with fat suppression • *Pancreatic protocol*: – *Arterial phase*: 20 seconds after start of injection – *Portal Venous phase*: 45–65 seconds after start of injection – *Equilibrium phase*: 3–5 min after start of injection • *Hepatic Protocol:* – *Late arterial phase*: 20 seconds after start of injection – *Portal venous phase*: 60–80 seconds after start of injection – *Delayed phase*: >120 seconds after start of injection (3–5 min) – *Hepatobiliary phase*: Gadobenate dimeglumine (MultiHance): one hour postcontrast injection – *Gadoxetate (Eovist)*: 20 minutes postcontrast injection

thickness of 5-8 mm and interslice gap not more than 3 mm. Either spin-echo (TSE or FSE) or gradient echo sequences can be used for T1-weighted imaging, with at least one in and out-of-phase gradient T1 sequence. T2-weighted images include either spin-echo sequences (TSE or FSE) or hybrid gradient and spin-echo (GRASE) sequences. Fat suppression is required during T2 weighted imaging, and can be achieved by chemical selective fat saturation, short tau inversion recovery (STIR), or spectral presaturation inversion recovery (SPIR). 3D sequences (both T1 and T2) are also available and provide higher SNR with better fat suppression. Intravenous contrast (gadolinium chelates) is used depending on the study protocol. Post-contrast administration, 2D or 3D T1-weighted sequences with fat suppression are acquired.[31]

Heavily T2-weighted magnetic resonance cholangio-pancreatography (MRCP) sequences are used for evaluation of the biliary and pancreatic ductal system. The sequences used are breath-hold rapid acquisition relaxation enhancement (RARE) or half-Fourier single-shot echo train spin-echo sequence as a thick slab acquisition **(Fig. 17)** in multiple projections or as multiple thin (less than 5 mm) slices in coronal or axial plane. 3D respiratory-triggered T2- weighted FSE techniques with maximum intensity projection (MIP) reconstruction **(Fig. 18)** can also be used.[31]

Diffusion-weighted imaging for abdomen uses single-shot echo-planar sequences, breath-held or respiratory triggered. At least two b-values are used (b = 0 to 50 s/mm^2 and b = 500 to 1,000 s/mm^2) and ADC maps are generated for proper interpretation. DWI has short acquisition time and is now a part of the routine protocol. In patients with contraindications to MR contrast this sequence is particularly advantageous.[16,31]

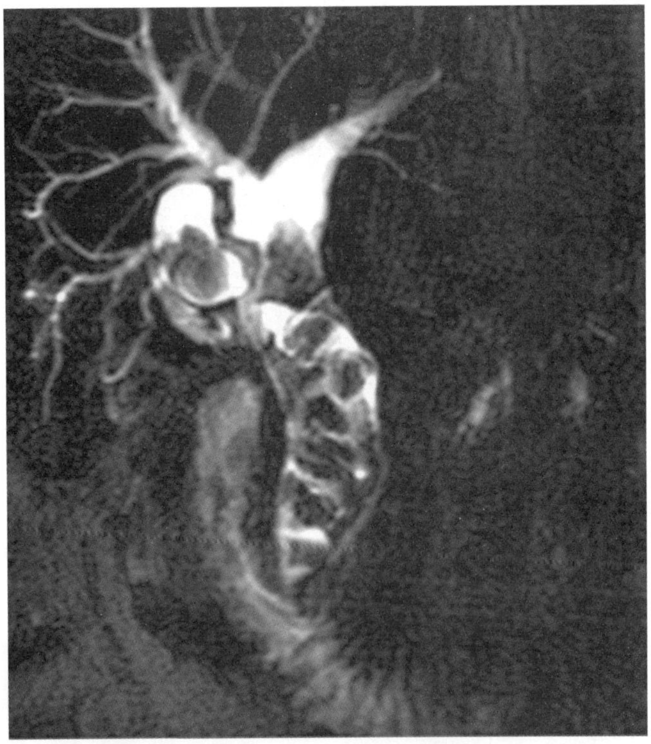

Fig. 17: Choledocholithiasis: Coronal thick slab projectional MRCP reveals multiple calculi in the common bile duct and right hepatic duct.

MRI of the Liver

MRI has evolved from a problem solving technique to first line investigative modality for liver lesions.

Pelvic-phased array surface coil is used with field of view including the entire liver. Acquisition is predominantly in the axial plane with additional coronal plane imaging to better depict the vascular anatomy and the hepatic dome.[34]

T1-weighted imaging is performed as in-phase and out-of-phase chemical shift gradient-recalled echo sequences prior to contrast administration. This is useful in evaluation of focal fat containing lesions and diffuse pathology like hepatic steatosis and iron overload.[35] In-phase (IP) and out-of-phase (OP) imaging is performed with a TE of 2.1 msec and 4.2 msec, respectively on 3T magnets. Both the images can be obtained in one TR by use of a double echo technique.[35]

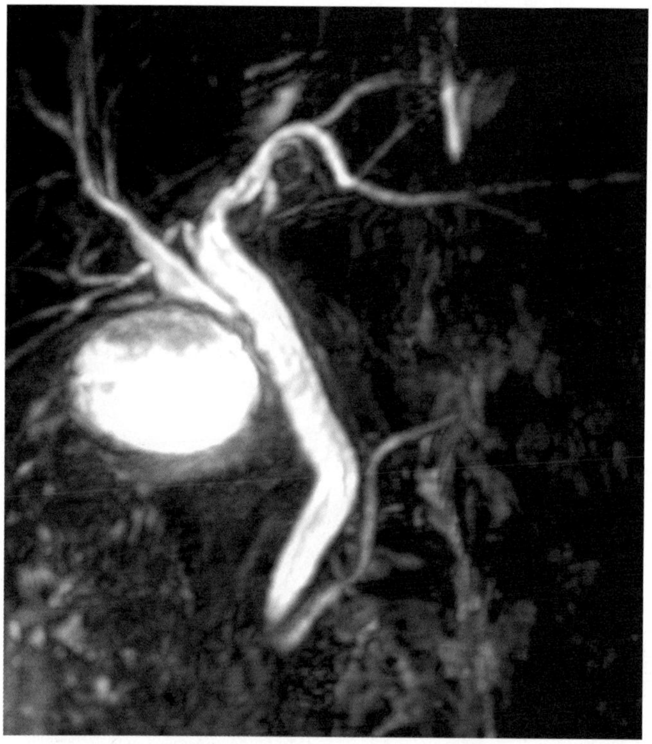

Fig. 18: MRCP (MIP) image showing normal intrahepatic biliary radicles, common bile duct and pancreatic duct in a case of carcinoma gallbladder.

T2-weighted images are acquired in the axial and coronal planes using a breath-hold or non-breath-hold technique. These include the accelerated fast spin-echo or single-shot accelerated fast spin-echo (half-Fourier single-shot turbo spin-echo (HASTE) or single shot fast spin-echo (SSFSE)) sequences. Respiratory compensation or respiratory triggering is employed whenever non-breath-hold sequences are used. An echo train length (ETL) of 16–20 provides optimal T2-weighted images in short scan time.[35] Echo-train spin echo sequences acquired as contiguous thin 2D sections or as a thick 3D volume slab, also form the basis for MR cholangiography.

The TE of T2-weighted images is usually around 80-90 msec and longer TE (150–250 msec) T2W imaging can be used to differentiate between cysts and solid lesions.

The liver parenchyma appears homogeneous on both T1 and T2-weighted images. The liver shows moderate signal intensity on T1W images, similar to the pancreas but brighter than spleen and kidneys **(Figs. 19A and B)**. On T2W images **(Fig. 20)**, the liver appears dark and has signal intensity less than that of spleen.

Post-contrast administration, dynamic fat-suppressed MR imaging **(Figs. 21A to D)** is performed using a 2-D or 3-D technique. Contrast is administered at a dose of 0.1 mmol/kg at a rate of 2 mL/s and followed by saline flush.[36] Pre-contrast scan is followed by the acquisition of scans in the late arterial (20 seconds after administration of contrast), portal venous (60–80 seconds) and delayed (2–5 minutes) phases. The bolus timing technique (includes automated bolus detection system or fluoroscopic

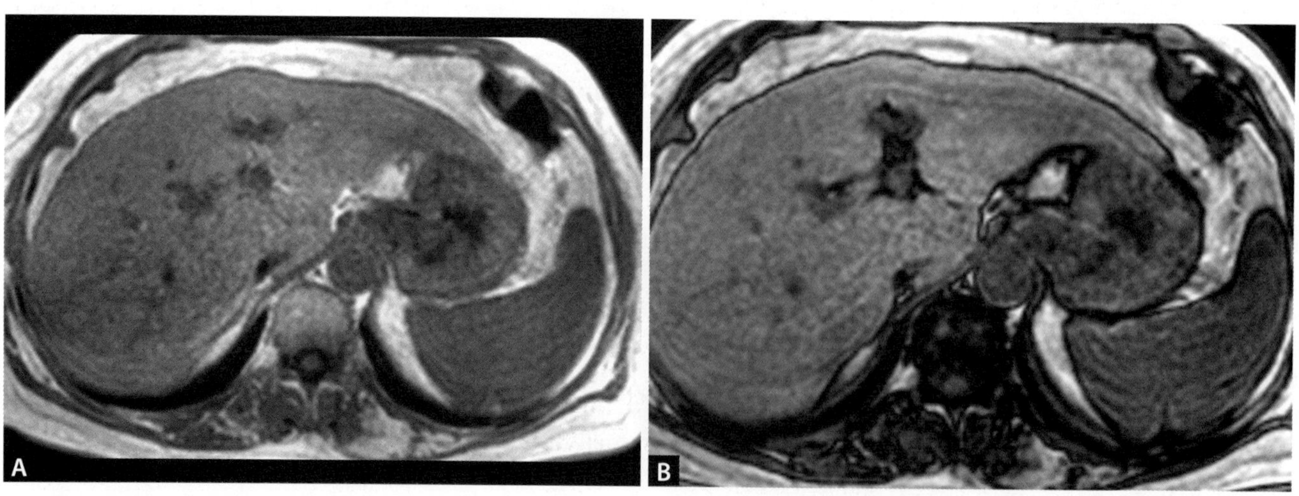

Figs. 19A and B: T1-weighted imaging for the liver. In-phase (A) and out-of-phase (B) chemical shift gradient-recalled echo sequences are performed prior to contrast administration. Liver shows homogeneous moderate signal intensity, greater than that of the spleen.

triggering) or acquisition of multiple repeated arterial-phase datasets is used for planning the arterial phase.

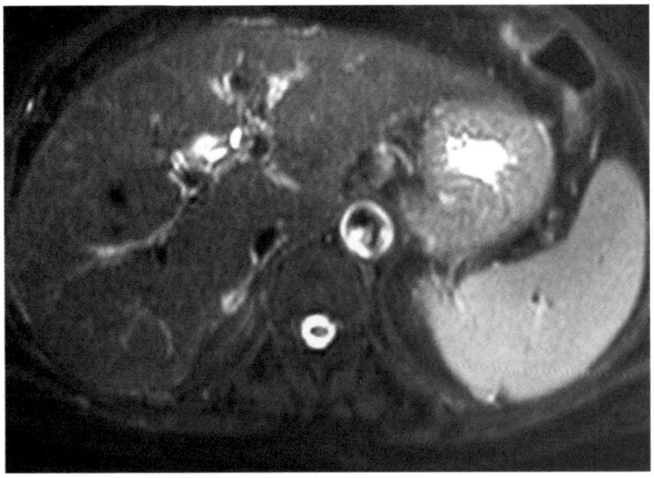

Fig. 20: Axial T2 WI fat-suppressed sequence reveals homogeneous signal intensity of the liver. Note the signal intensity of liver is less than that of spleen.

Additional delayed images (more than 5 minutes) may be required in cases of hemangiomas, vascular malformations, or cholangiocarcinomas.[37,38] Subtracted images (subtraction of the pre-contrast scan from the postcontrast scan) should be generated in cases of T1 hyperintense lesions.

The use of hepatobiliary specific MR contrast agents is recommended for liver imaging. When gadobenate dimeglumine (Multihance) is used, one hour delayed scan is performed. However, with the use of gadoxetate (Eovist), hepatobiliary phase is obtained at 20 minutes post-contrast injection. This phase is used to document retention of contrast in lesions like focal nodular hyperplasia and to better delineate the biliary anatomy. However, it is important to obtain MRCP images (T2-weighted imaging of biliary tree) before biliary excretion of contrast, as the enhanced bile is not visualized on the MRCP images. For optimal time utilization, T2-weighted and diffusion-weighted images can be obtained after the injection of gadoxetate disodium.[34]

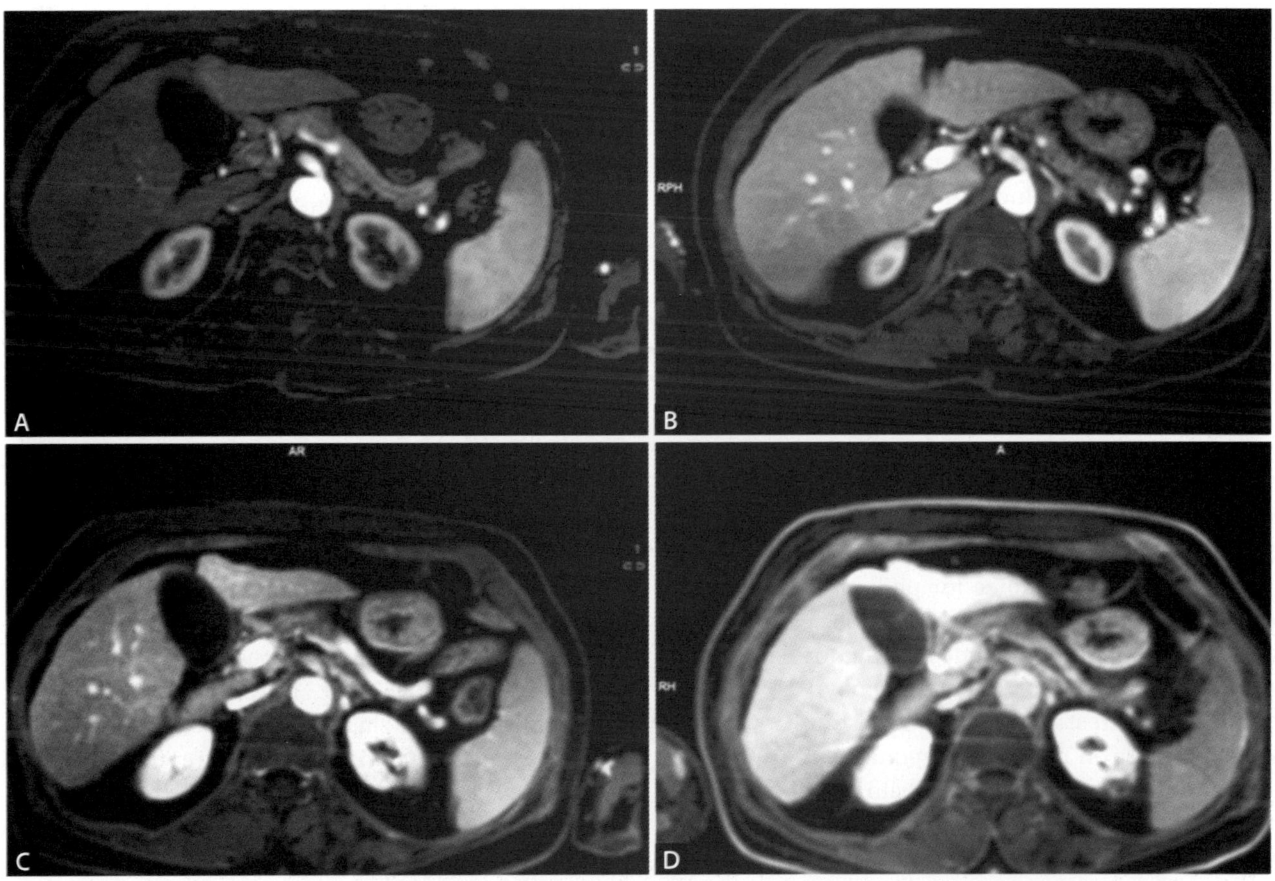

Figs. 21A to D: Multiphase MRI liver: Postcontrast (Gadobenate dimeglumine/Multihance) administration, T1-weighted fat-suppressed gradient echo images are obtained at 20 seconds [late arterial phase] (A); 65 seconds [portal venous phase] (B); 180 seconds [delayed phase] (C) and 1 hour [hepatobiliary phase] (D) in a patient of chronic liver disease. No focal lesion was detected.

Diffusion-weighted images are obtained using echo-planar imaging (EPI) with breath held, free breathing, or respiratory-gated techniques. Imaging time can be reduced with the use of parallel imaging. DWI is performed with at least two b-values (b=20–50 s/mm^2 and b=400 to 1000 s/mm^2). The use of ADC maps and calculation of ADC values is recommended to identify T2 shine through effect, which can be a confounding factor in the interpretation of DW images. DWI is useful in characterization of focal liver lesions, liver fibrosis and screening of the entire abdomen for additional lesions. It is of particular use in patients with contraindications to MR contrast medium. However, it is important to view the DWI images in conjunction with the other sequences and amalgamate, its findings with the morphology and enhancement characteristics for increased accuracy of diagnosis.[34]

MRI of Pancreatic Pathology

For the evaluation of pancreatic pathology, T1-weighted images are acquired as dual-echo GRE images in the axial plane and T2-weighted images as turbo spin-echo sequences in the axial and coronal plane. MRCP sequences using both 2D and 3D fast SE techniques are used to delineate the pancreaticobiliary anatomy. Intravenous gadolinium-based contrast medium is injected at a dose of 0.1 mmol/kg of body weight and dynamic scanning is performed. This includes the acquisition of arterial (20 sec after injection of contrast medium), portal venous (45–65 seconds) and equilibrium phase (3–5 min) images. Some authors recommend a coronal plane (parallel to the bifurcation of the portal vein) T1 GRE acquisition two minutes after the injection of contrast medium.[26,39]

MAGNETIC RESONANCE ENTEROGRAPHY

This is a noninvasive technique for the evaluation of small bowel pathology. Since there is no radiation exposure, it is the modality of choice for pediatric patients and monitoring of patients of inflammatory bowel disease.

Patient preparation includes fasting for 6 hours and intestinal cleansing as for CT enterography.

Biphasic contrast agents (hyperintense on T2-weighted and hypointense on T1-weighted sequences) are preferred as they provide maximal contrast with bowel wall on the post-contrast sequences. These include agents like water, mannitol, locust bean gum, low-dose barium, manganese compounds, and polyethylene glycol. The protocol varies with institutions and a suggested protocol is given in

Table 7: MR enterography protocol.

- Fasting for 6 hours
- *Oral contrast*:
  - 300 mL of 20% mannitol mixed with 1.5 L of water
  - Administered in divided aliquots over 1 hour
- *Intravenous contrast*:
  - 0.1 mmol/kg of gadolinium-based agent
  - Single phase acquisition at 50 sec (enteric phase)
- IV buscopan (1 mL~20 mg): after acquisition of cine BTFE
- *Sequences*:
  - *Steady state fast field echo (Cine)*: Coronal
  - *Steady state fast field echo*: Axial
  - *T2W FS*: Axial, coronal
  - *T1W Non FS*: Axial
  - *DWI (b VALUE 0, 400, 800)*: Axial
  - Post-contrast T1W FS: Axial, coronal

Table 7. Some centers advocate prone position as it decreases respiratory excursion and enables better separation of bowel loops.[16,40]

Images are acquired in both the axial and coronal planes **(Figs. 22A and B)**. T2W imaging can be performed as spin-echo sequence (TSE or FSE), gradient-echo (GRE) sequence, or a hybrid gradient and spin-echo (GRASE) sequence. Single shot technique is more useful as it is relatively insensitive to motion. Fat-suppressed sequences are preferred for the evaluation of active inflammation. T1 imaging can be performed as spin echo or gradient echo sequences with T1W 3D gradient-echo sequence having the advantage of short scan time allowing image acquisition within a single breath-hold.

"Cine imaging" of the bowel is real time, dynamic imaging of a predefined region of interest by employing a heavily T2W coronal slab or a single-shot steady-state free precession sequence. This is useful for the identification of fibrotic strictures.[40]

NUCLEAR IMAGING

Neuroendocrine tumors (NET) such as carcinoids and pancreatic NET express somatostatin receptors (SSTR) at the cell membrane.[41] Functional imaging uses the affinity of somatostatin receptor analogs for tissues, which express SSTR. There are six main subtypes of SSTR (1–5 including 2A and 2B) with SSTR-2 and SSTR-5 being the most commonly expressed in NET.

Octreotide scintigraphy (using octreotide labeled with indium 111) is the standard functional imaging modality for NET's. It is combined with single photon emission computed tomography for improved spatial resolution. It is also used to evaluate the response to treatment and for metastatic work-up of NET.[42] This technique has

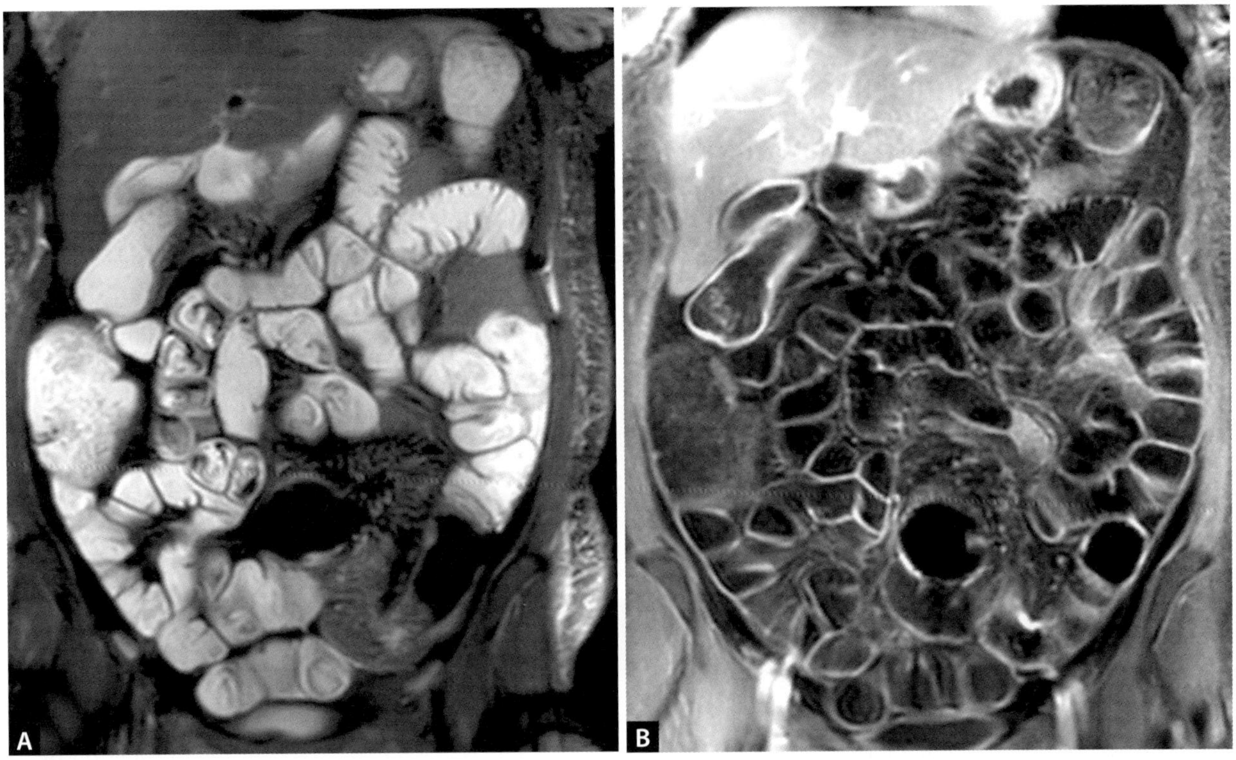

Figs. 22A and B: MR enterography: Coronal T2-weighted fat-suppressed fast spin echo (A) and post-gadolinium coronal T1 fat-suppressed gradient echo (B) acquisition shows good bowel distension and no abnormal enhancement.

greater sensitivity for carcinoids and gastrinomas than insulinomas.[42]

Iodine 123 (^{123}I) MIBG scintigraphy: This technique uses Metaiodobenzyl guanidine, which is a norepinephrine analog and binds to the norepinephrine transporter in NET.

PET/CT: Newer analogs labeled with gallium-68 are now used in combination with PET-CT imaging. However, they have more affinity to the SSTR-2 receptors than to the SSTR-3 and SSTR-5 receptors. Compared with octreotide scintigraphy, PET/CT requires less time and has a higher spatial resolution. In addition, the production of 68Ga-DOTA peptides is relatively less costly as it does not require a cyclotron.

Three types of ^{68}Ga-DOTA-peptide analogs are available:

1. ^{68}Ga-DOTA-Phe^{1}-Tyr^{3}-Octreotide (TOC)
2. ^{68}Ga-DOTA-NaI^{3}-Octreotide (NOC)
3. ^{68}Ga-DOTA-Tyr^{3}-Octreotate (TATE)

Out of these, DOTA-NOC has good affinity for SSTR-3 in addition to SSTR-2 and SSTR-5 receptors and is preferred as a broad-spectrum agent.[43]

^{68}Ga-DOTANOC PET enterography is useful for delineation of small bowel carcinoids.[16]

^{18}F FDG is also used as a glucose analog in FDG-PET (can be combined with CTE/CTC for evaluation of bowel neoplasms and inflammatory bowel disease) and ^{18}F DOPA is used as a catecholamine analog for DOPA PET in the evaluation of NET.[16,44]

ANGIOGRAPHY

Conventional hepatic/mesenteric angiography is now seldom used for diagnostic purpose as CT and MR imaging can generate high quality angiographic images in a non-invasive manner. The use of catheter angiography is now restricted to vascular interventions.

Technique

Coagulation profile and serum creatinine should be available prior to the procedure. The femoral artery is the preferred approach and Seldinger technique is used for the puncture. Angiography of the liver is performed by selective injections of the celiac axis and superior mesenteric artery (SMA) or one or more of their branches.

A 5-French right angle or reverse curve catheter such as Cobra is commonly used. The volume of contrast used is about 20–30 cc injected at a rate of 5–6 cc per second. The portal venous system is visualized by injecting the splenic artery or SMA coupled with prolonged filming.

Anatomy

The celiac axis **(Fig. 23)** is the first major branch of the abdominal aorta and it gives rise to three major branches (the common hepatic, left gastric, and splenic arteries). The common hepatic artery gives rise to the gastroduodenal artery after which it becomes the proper hepatic artery. The proper hepatic artery divides into the right and left hepatic arteries, which further divide to supply the corresponding segments. The main branches of the gastroduodenal artery are the retroduodenal, superior pancreaticoduodenal and right gastroepiploic arteries. The splenic artery gives rise to short gastric branches and the left gastroepiploic artery. The superior mesenteric artery (SMA) arises approximately 1 cm caudad to the celiac trunk and supplies the small bowel through the inferior pancreaticoduodenal, jejunal, and ileal arteries. The right colon is supplied by the ileocolic, right colic and middle colic artery branches of the superior mesenteric artery forming an arcade (marginal artery of Drummond), which anastomoses with the branches of the inferior mesenteric artery (IMA). The branches of the IMA include left colic artery, sigmoidal artery, rectosigmoid artery and superior rectal artery.[45]

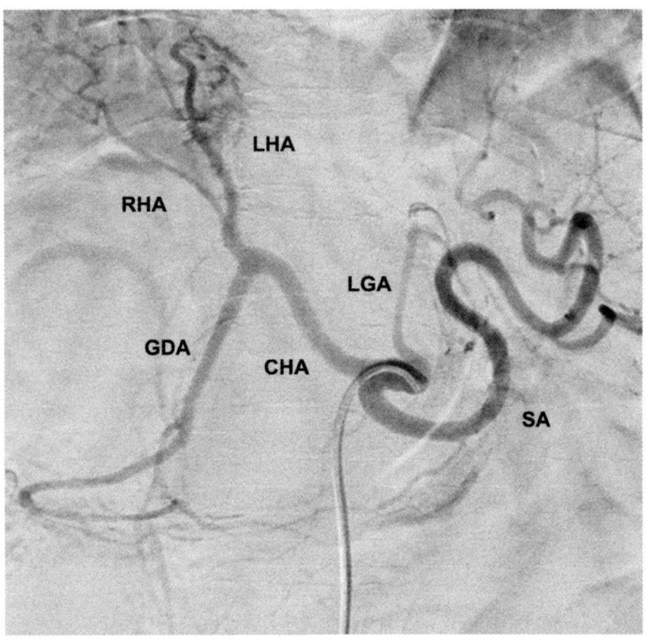

Fig. 23: Intra-arterial digital subtraction angiography (DSA) showing selective celiac axis injection, splenic artery (SA), left gastric artery (LGA), common hepatic artery (CHA), gastroduodenal artery (GDA), right hepatic artery (RHA) and left hepatic artery (LHA).

CONCLUSION

The imaging techniques for abdomen have evolved considerably in the past few years. Conventional radiographs and barium studies now have limited role in the evaluation of GI pathology. Recent advances in ultrasound like endosonography, elastography and contrast studies have significantly improved the diagnostic yield of a noninvasive and radiation free modality like ultrasound. Cross-sectional modalities such as CT and MRI remain the mainstay in the diagnosis and follow-up of most abdominal pathologies. A judicious use of the currently available imaging modalities is required for appropriate diagnosis and treatment of various abdominal diseases.

REFERENCES

1. Maglinte DDT, Sandrasegaran K, Chiorean M, Dewitt J, McHenry L, Lappas JC. Radiologic investigations complement and add diagnostic information to capsule endoscopy of small-bowel diseases. AJR. 2007;189:306-12.
2. Maglinte DDT. Capsule imaging and the role of radiology in the investigation of diseases of the small bowel. Radiology 2005; 236:763-7.
3. Halligan S, Robinson PJA. The large bowel: In: David Sutton (Ed). Textbook of Radiology and Imaging, 7th edn. Churchill Livingstone.
4. American College of Radiology. ACR practice parameter for the performance of esophagrams and upper gastrointestinal examinations in adults. *http://www.acr.org/~/media/5223A3FBC92E40378DF6E55FB8E6134B.pdf.* Accessed on September 07, 2016.
5. American College of Radiology. ACR practice parameter for the performance of a barium small bowel examination in adults. *http://www.acr.org/~/media/9408bdfc3c234e4287bd8610faafe3f1.pdf.* Accessed on September 07, 2016.
6. American College of Radiology. ACR–SAR practice parameter for the performance of an enteroclysis examination in adults. *http://www.acr.org/~/media/0CEECEA90E154EB99FC6562F1311E7E4.pdf.* Accessed on September 07, 2016.
7. American College of Radiology. ACR practice parameter for the performance of fluoroscopic contrast enema examination in adults. *http://www.acr.org/~/media/ACR/Documents/PGTS/guidelines/Fluoroscopic_Contrast_Enema.pdf.* Accessed on September 07, 2016.
8. Kono Y, Mattrey RF. Ultrasound of the liver. The Radiologic Clinics of North America. 2005;43(5):815-26.
9. Gazelle GS, Saini S, Mueller PR, (Eds). Hepatobiliary and Pancreatic Radiology: Imaging and Intervention. New York, NY, USA: Thieme Medical Publishers, 1998.

10. Kusera JN, Kucera S, Perrin SD, Caracciolo JT, Schmulewitz N, Kedar RP. Cystic lesions of the pancreas: Radiologic endosonographic correlation. Radiographics. 2012; 32:E283-E301.
11. Frulio N, Trillaud H. Ultrasound elastography in liver. Diagn Interv Imaging. 2013;94:515-34.
12. Ferraioli G, Parekh P, Levitov AB, Filice C. Shear wave elastography for evaluation of liver fibrosis. J Ultrasound Med. 2014;33:197-203.
13. Unnikrishnan S, Klibanov AL. Microbubbles as ultrasound contrast agents for molecular imaging: Preparation and application. AJR. 2012;199:292-9.
14. Catalano O, Nunziata A, Lobianco R, Siani A. Real-time harmonic contrast material-specific us of focal liver lesions. Radiographics. 2005;25:333-49.
15. American College of Radiology. ACR–SPR practice parameter for the performance of computed tomography (CT) of the abdomen and computed tomography (CT) of the pelvis. *http://www.acr.org/~/media/ACR/Documents/PGTS/guidelines/CT_Abdomen_Pelvis.pdf.* Accessed on September 07, 2016.
16. Das CJ, Manchanda S, Panda A, Gupta AK, Sharma A. Recent advances in imaging of small and large bowel. PET Clin. 2016; 11:21-37.
17. Iannaccone R, Laghi A, Catalano C, et al. Hepatocellular carcinoma: role of unenhanced and delayed phase multi-detector row helical CT in patients with cirrhosis. Radiology 2005;234(2):460-7.
18. Doyle DJ, O'Malley ME, Jang HJ, Jhaveri K. Value of the unenhanced phase for detection of hepatocellular carcinomas 3 cm or less when performing multiphase computed tomography in patients with cirrhosis. J Comput Assist Tomogr. 2007;31(1):86-92.
19. Choi JY, Lee JM, Sirlin CB. CT and MR imaging diagnosis and staging of hepatocellular carcinoma: Part I. Development, growth, and spread: key pathologic and imaging aspects. Radiology. 2014;272:635-54.
20. McEvoy SH, McCarthy CJ, Lavelle LP, Moran DE, Cantwell CP, Skehan SJ. Hepatocellular carcinoma: Illustrated guide to systematic radiologic diagnosis and staging according to guidelines of the American association for the study of liver diseases. Radiographics. 2013;33:1653-68.
21. Oto A, Tam EP, Szklaruk J. Multidetector row CT of the liver. The Radiologic Clinics of North America. 2005;43(5):827-48.
22. Kim MJ, Choi JY, Lim JS, et al. Optimal scan window for detection of hypervascular hepatocellular carcinomas during MDCT examination. Am J Roentgenol. 2006;187(1):198-206.
23. Laghi A, Iannaccone R, Rossi P, Carbone I, Ferrari R, Mangiapane F. Hepatocellular carcinoma: Detection with triple-phase multi-detector row helical CT in patients with chronic hepatitis. Radiology. 2003;226:543-9.
24. Coursey CA, Nelson RC, Boll DT, Paulson EK, Ho LM, Neville AM. Dual-energy multidetector CT: How does it work, what can it tell us, and when can we use it in abdominopelvic imaging? Radiographics. 2010;30:1037-55.
25. Wigmore SJ, Redhead DN, Yan XJ, et al. Virtual hepatic resection using three-dimensional reconstruction of helical computed tomography angioportograms. Ann Surg. 2001;233: 221-6.
26. Lee ES, Lee JM. Imaging diagnosis of pancreatic cancer: A state-of-the-art review. World J Gastroenterol. 2014;20:7864-77.
27. Chaudhary V, Bano S. Imaging of the pancreas: Recent advances. Indian J Endocrinol Metab. 2011;15:S25-32.
28. Manchanda SD, Prasad A, Sachdev N, De P, Abbas SZ, Baruah BP. Multidetector computed tomography (MDCT) evaluation of small bowel obstruction: pictorial review. Trop Gastroenterol. 2010;31:249-59.
29. American College of Radiology. ACR–SAR–SPR practice parameter for the performance of computed tomography (CT) enterography. *http://www.acr.org/~/media/99D260410DF44A3BA01F1AB716DE8F2F.pdf.* Accessed on September 07, 2016.
30. American College of Radiology. ACR–SAR–SCBT-MR practice parameter for the performance of computed tomography (CT) colonography in adults. *http://www.acr.org/~/media/A81531ACA92F45058A83B5281E8FE826.pdf.* Accessed on September 07, 2016.
31. American College of Radiology. ACR–SAR–SPR practice parameter for the performance of magnetic resonance imaging (MRI) of the abdomen (excluding the liver). *http://www.acr.org/~/media/8f5bc61adb114c5b9e46fe6914461d25.pdf.* Accessed on September 07, 2016.
32. Soher BJ, Dale BM, Merkle EM. A review of MR physics: 3T versus 1.5T. Magn Reson Imaging Clin N Am. 2007;15(3):277-90.
33. Leyendecker JR, Childs DD. Kidneys and MR urography. Magn Reson Imaging Clin N Am. 2007;15(3):373-82.
34. American College of Radiology. ACR–SAR–SPR practice parameter for the performance of magnetic resonance imaging (MRI) of the liver. *http://www.acr.org/~/media/6B520D299C0B4B018A90BE21A79D4F72.pdf.* Accessed on September 07, 2016.
35. Maniam S, Szklaruk J. Magnetic resonance imaging: Review of imaging techniques and overview of liver imaging. World J Radiol. 2010;2:309-22.
36. Arif-Tiwari H, Kalb B, Chundru S, Sharma P, Costello J, Guessner RW, Martin DR. MRI of hepatocellular carcinoma: an update of current practices. Diagn Interv Radiol. 2014;20:209-21.
37. Runge VM. A comparison of two MR hepatobiliary gadolinium chelates: Gd-BOPTA and Gd-EOB-DTPA. J Comput Assist Tomogr. 1998;22(4):643-50.
38. Soyer P, Bluemke DA, Reichle R, et al. Imaging of intrahepatic cholangiocarcinoma: 2. Hilar cholangiocarcinoma. Am J Roentgenol. 1995;165(6):1433-6.
39. Sandrasegaran K, Lin C, Akisik FM, Tann M. State-of-the-art pancreatic MRI. AJR. 2010;195:42-53.
40. American College of Radiology. ACR–SAR–SPR practice parameter for the performance of magnetic resonance (MR) enterography. *http://www.acr.org/~/media/99F8*

D0F593E64860AA3B1EC6CA1C758D.pdf. Accessed on September 07, 2016.

41. Woodbridge LR, Murtagh BM, Yu DFQC, Planche KL. Midgut neuroendocrine tumors: Imaging assessment for surgical resection. Radiographics. 2014;34:413-26.
42. Virgolini I, Traub-Weidinger T, Decristoforo C. Nuclear medicine in the detection and management of pancreatic islet-cell tumours. Best Pract Res Clin Endocrinol Metab. 2005;19:213-27.
43. Sharma P, Singh H, Bal C, Kumar R. PET/CT imaging of neuroendocrine tumors with 68Gallium-labeled somatostatin analogues: An overview and single institutional experience from India. Indian J Nucl Med. 2014;29:2-12.
44. Sahani DV, Bonaffini PA, Castillo CFD, Blake MA. Gastroenteropancreatic neuroendocrine tumors: Role of imaging in diagnosis and management. Radiology. 2013;266:38-61.
45. Stallard DJ, Tu RK, Gould MJ, Pozniak MA, Pettersen JC. Minor vascular anatomy of the abdomen and pelvis: A CT atlas. RadloGraphlcs. 1994;14:493-513.

CHAPTER 68

Imaging a Patient with Dysphagia

Alpana Manchanda, Jyoti Kumar, Gaurav S Pradhan

INTRODUCTION

Dysphagia is a common manifestation of many of the disorders affecting the esophagus. It is a nondescriptive term that literally means 'difficulty in swallowing'. It is defined as the subjective awareness of difficulty in swallowing or perception of obstruction of a solid or liquid bolus as it passes from the mouth to the stomach.[1] Dysphagia is considered to be clinically significant when such symptoms occur a minimum of several times a month. Dysphagia can result from functional or structural abnormalities of the oral cavity, pharynx, esophagus or gastric cardia. It may be further classified as oropharyngeal or esophageal (substernal), depending on the anatomic site of involvement. It is of utmost importance to differentiate between the two as their etiology, radiologic evaluation and management may vary greatly.[1]

EPIDEMIOLOGY

It effects nearly 22% of patients in the primary care setting; with two-thirds of the patients with dysphagia being more than sixty-five years of age.[2]

The diagnosis of dysphagia is important because of its associated morbidity and mortality. The elderly are at the highest risk of subsequent complications of dysphagia such as dehydration, weight loss, airway obstruction; the most dangerous being aspiration, which can be silent in up to 55% of patients.[2]

PHYSIOLOGY OF SWALLOWING

Swallowing is a complex activity which occurs in a coordinated manner to transport the ingested material from the mouth to the stomach. Normal swallowing is divided into oral, pharyngeal and esophageal stages and involves both voluntary and involuntary neuromuscular contractions starting from the mouth to the stomach.[2]

Oropharyngeal Stage

This stage is initiated by the contractions of the tongue and striated muscles of mastication which mix the food bolus with saliva and propel it from the oral cavity into the oropharynx. Once the food has left the oral cavity, swallowing is no longer under voluntary control. The bolus then activates the oropharyngeal sensory receptors which initiate the deglutition reflex which is a centrally-mediated wave of inhibition which precedes the peristaltic contraction. It not only propels the food through the pharynx and esophagus, but also prevents its aspiration (i.e. entry into the airway) and nasal regurgitation (retrograde flow into the nose). This is achieved in the following sequence of events—elevation of the soft palate which closes the nasopharynx, closure of the laryngeal vestibule which is critical for airway protection. This occurs as a result of upward and anterior movement of the larynx by the suprahyoid muscles. The epiglottis moves downwards to cover the airway. Finally the upper esophageal sphincter (UES) including the cricopharyngeus muscle relaxes due to which the bolus enters the cervical esophagus. The pharynx is cleared of the bolus by the sequential contraction of the pharyngeal constrictor muscles. The deglutition reflex lasts for approximately one second.[3]

Primary esophageal peristalsis is induced by a swallow at the pharyngesophageal junction. Caudad progression of a bolus is achieved by deglutitive inhibition.

Secondary peristalsis is induced by esophageal distension and initiates around the level of the aortic arch. It is a propulsive wave that occurs to clear the esophagus of any retained bolus.

Tertiary contractions are nonpropulsive and cause a variable degree of narrowing of the lumen. Between swallows, the esophagus is collapsed and the upper and lower esophageal sphincters are closed.

Esophageal Stage

The esophageal stage of swallowing begins once the bolus passes through the upper esophageal sphincter. In this phase, the peristaltic contractions of the smooth muscle of the thoracic esophagus propels the food towards the lower esophageal sphincter (LES) and stomach. The LES relaxes as soon as the swallow is initiated, which persists until the food bolus is propelled into the stomach.[3]

PATHOGENESIS OF DYSPHAGIA

The normal passage of the ingested bolus through the pharynx and esophagus depends on the size of the ingested bolus, size of the lumen, the force of peristalsis, deglutitive inhibition along with normal relaxation of the upper and lower esophageal sphincter during swallowing. When there is mechanical or structural cause to the dysphagia it is called *mechanical dysphagia*.

In contrast, *motor dysphagia* occurs due to weak peristaltic contractions or impaired deglutitive inhibition, causing nonperistaltic contractions and impaired relaxation of sphincters.[4]

Clinical Presentation

Dysphagia is a very nondescriptive term that can result from any problem from the proximal oral cavity to the proximal stomach.

A carefully taken history helps a physician to identify 80–85% of the causes of dysphagia. Specific questions such as the onset, duration, severity of dysphagia and any associated symptoms may help in narrowing the differential diagnosis to a specific diagnosis or to an anatomic or a pathophysiologic-related diagnosis.[5]

It is important to know if dysphagia is present during swallowing or at all times. Dysphagia which occurs during swallowing at all times without any organic cause is suggestive of globus hystericus. Dysphagia that occurs only for solids is likely due to a mechanical obstruction, while dysphagia for both solids and liquids is more likely to indicate a motility disorder.

Symptoms such as delayed or absence of swallow initiation, postswallow cough, nasopharyngeal regurgitation, repeated swallows to clear the bolus are indicative of oropharyngeal dysphagia.[6]

Abnormality of the oral phase of swallowing results in food dribbling from the mouth, difficulty in drinking or chewing, or difficulty in initiating a swallow. Soft palate insufficiency results in a nasal quality of voice or nasal regurgitation. Coughing or choking during swallowing indicates laryngeal penetration. Patients with pharyngeal dysphagia typically complain of a "lump in the throat" or of food "sticking in the throat" during swallowing. It may be caused by a functional abnormality such as cricopharyngeal dysmotility, amyotrophic lateral sclerosis or by a morphologic abnormality such as Zenker's diverticulum or pharyngeal tumor.[7]

A sensation of blockage at the level of the suprasternal notch or thoracic inlet raises the possibility of a cervical esophageal web, tumor or of extrinsic compression of the cervical or upper thoracic esophagus by an enlarged thyroid, mediastinal lymphadenopathy, or other mass lesion.[7] Substernal localization of dysphagia is usually due to a structural disorder such as reflux esophagitis, peptic stricture or Schatzki ring or motility disorder of the esophagus such as achalasia. A distal lesion (even carcinoma of the gastric fundus) may refer dysphagia proximally as far as the pharynx. The patient may complain of odynophagia (pain on swallowing) or chest pain. These symptoms may be due to esophageal spasm or other motor disorders, but may also be caused by infectious esophagitis, gastroesophageal reflux disease and ulcerated pharyngeal or esophageal tumors.

The duration and progression of symptoms also provide a clue to the etiology. Chronic and stable symptoms are suggestive of benign conditions such as peptic strictures, Schatzki's ring, while rapidly progressive symptoms associated with weight loss is suggestive of a malignant etiology. The timing of regurgitation in relation to swallowing or meals is also indicative of the underlying cause for example, regurgitation in between meals is suggestive of an underlying Zenker's diverticulum, while immediately after swallowing suggests esophageal retention of food.[6] (**Table 1**, lists the associated symptoms with possible etiologies of dysphagia).[4,5]

Dysphagia is also more common in patients with a history of gastresophageal reflux disease (GERD) than in those without GERD.[1]

Patients who develop dysphagia after a long history of reflux symptoms and those with poor control of symptoms may develop complications such as peptic stricture, Barrett's esophagus and even esophageal adenocarcinoma.[6] In young patients with history of atopy who present with dysphagia or obstruction to food bolus,

Table 1: Symptoms associated with possible etiologies of dysphagia.[4,5]

Symptoms	*Possible diagnoses*
Progressive dysphagia	Neuromuscular dysphagia
Sudden dysphagia	Obstructive dysphagia
Episodic dysphagia to solids	Lower esophageal ring
Difficulty in initiating swallow	Oropharyngeal dysphagia
Food sticks after swallow	Esophageal dysphagia
• Cough/choking-before, during or after swallow • In early phase of swallowing • In late phase of swallowing	• Indicative of aspiration • Neuromuscular dysphagia • Obstructive dysphagia
Weight loss: • In the elderly • With regurgitation	 • Carcinoma • Achalasia
Progressive symptoms: • Heartburn • Intermittent symptoms of dysphagia • Odynophagia	 • Peptic stricture, scleroderma • Rings and webs, diffuse esophageal spasm • *Esophagitis*: – Postradiation – Infectious – Pill induced
Chest pain with dysphagia	DES and related motor disorders
Worsening of pain by: • Solid food only • Solids and liquids	 • Obstructive dysphagia • Neuromuscular dysphagia
Regurgitation of old food	Zenker's diverticulum
Weakness and dysphagia	Stroke, muscular dystrophies, myasthenia gravis
Halitosis and dysphagia	Zenker's diverticulum
Dysphagia relieved with repeated swallows	Achalasia

eosinophilic esophagitis must be suspected and ruled out by endoscopic biopsy.

CAUSES OF DYSPHAGIA

These can be divided into two broad groups—mechanical and motor, involving oropharynx and esophagus **(Tables 2A to D)**.[4]

IMAGING TECHNIQUES IN THE EVALUATION OF DYSPHAGIA

As the anatomic structures and causes responsible for oropharyngeal and esophageal dysphagia are different, the approach to their evaluation also differ.[6]

Oropharyngeal dysphagia is evaluated by:
- Plain film
- Barium swallow
- Modified barium swallow/Videofluoroscopic Swallowing Study (VFSS)
- Nasopharyngeal-endoscopy
- Pharyngomanometry
- Cross-sectional studies (CT/MRI)

Esophageal dysphagia is evaluated by:
- Barium swallow
- Upper GI endoscopy
- Esophageal manometry
- Scintigraphy
- Cross-sectional studies (CT/MRI)
- Endoscopic ultrasound
- Intraesophageal pH measurement.

Even though there has been a decrease in the number of gastrointestinal fluoroscopic procedures, the number of contrast swallow studies have shown to increase.[9]

Barium studies and endoscopy are complementary investigations, but barium swallow is a useful first-line investigation for dysphagia. Its wide availability, non-invasiveness and it being a relatively inexpensive investigation are some of its advantages. It allows real-time continuous viewing of the bolus during transit from the oropharynx to the stomach and allows a good qualitative and functional assessment of the esophagus including the upper and lower esophageal sphincters.

A barium swallow may demonstrate an anatomical abnormality such as a stricture or mass lesion. It entails exposure to ionizing radiation and has poor sensitivity for subtle abnormalities, yet it is found to be more sensitive than esophagoscopy in detecting esophageal webs and rings.[6]

Examination Technique

Preparation: The pharynx, esophagus and stomach should be as free of fluid and secretions as possible to permit optimal mucosal coating during the barium study. The patient is instructed to fast overnight before the examination. The patient should avoid smoking or chewing gum as these activities may stimulate salivary and/or gastric secretions and impair mucosal coating.[7]

Plain Films

Although scout films are not obtained routinely, frontal and lateral plain films of the neck and chest may be helpful in cases of suspected foreign body, abscess, or fistula formation, and in the postoperative patient. The plain film may show fluid levels in the esophagus in a patient with

Tables 2A to D: Causes of dysphagia.

A: Mechanical oropharyngeal dysphagia
• Zenker's diverticulum • Cricopharyngeal bar or stenosis • Cervical (mucosal) Web-Plummer-Vinson syndrome • Retropharyngeal abscess • Oropharyngeal tumor • Head and neck surgery • Stricture-caustic, postradiation

B: Motor oropharyngeal dysphagia[6,8]	
1. Central nervous system	• Stroke • Parkinson's disease • Brainstem tumors • Alzheimer's disease • Drugs (Phenothiazines, benzodiazepines)
2. Degenerative diseases	• Amyotrophic lateral sclerosis • Huntington's chorea • Multiple sclerosis
3. Peripheral nervous system	• Spinal muscular atrophy • Guillain-Barré syndrome • Postpolio syndrome • Drugs (Botulinum toxin, cytotoxics)
4. Myogenic	• Myasthenia gravis • Dermatomyositis, polymyositis • Thyrotoxic myopathy • Drugs (amidarone, alcohol, cholesterol lowering drug)

C: Mechanical esophageal dysphagia	
1. *Intrinsic narrowing*	
i. Inflammatory/infective esophagitis	• Viral • Bacterial • Fungal • Caustic, chemical, thermal injury
ii. Webs and rings	• Congenital esophageal stenosis • Lower esophageal mucosal ring (Schatzki's ring)
iii. Benign strictures	• GERD and Barrett's esophagus • Peptic stricture • Caustic injury • Pill induced • Inflammatory (Candida, mucocutaneous lesions) • Postoperative or anastomotic • Postradiation
iv. Malignant stricture	
v. Foreign body	
2. *Extrinsic narrowing*	• Substernal thyroid • Posterior mediastinal mass • Vascular compression (aberrant right subclavian artery, right sided aorta, aortic aneurysm) • Enlarged vertebral osteophytes

Contd...

Contd...

D: Motor esophageal dysphagia[4]	
1. *Diseases of smooth muscles*	
i. Weak muscle contraction or LES tone	• Idiopathic • Scleroderma and related collagen vascular disease • Myotonic dystrophy • Metabolic neuromyopathy (amyloid/alcohol/diabetes) • Drugs (anticholinergics, smooth muscle relaxants)
ii. Enhanced muscle contraction	• Hypertensive peristalsis (nutcracker esophagus) • Hypercontracting lower esophageal sphincter (LES)
2. *Disorders of inhibitory innervation*	
i. Diffuse esophageal spasm (DES)	
ii. Achalasia	Primary, secondary (Chagas disease, carcinoma, lymphoma leading to pseudo-achalasia)
iii. Contractile (muscular/ lower esophageal ring)	

achalasia. In major esophageal dilatation, the esophagus expands to the right, producing a mediastinal edge that runs from the neck to the diaphragm with a single indentation produced by the azygos vein.

Barium Studies

Examination of the pharynx and esophagus requires a dynamic evaluation of motility as well as double-contrast spot films to detect morphologic abnormalities. Cineradiography or videofluoroscopy should be used to study swallowing dynamics. The recordings may be reviewed later to analyse tongue movement, soft palate evaluation, epiglottic tilt, laryngeal closure, cricopharyngeal opening and pharyngeal peristalsis.

The routine barium examination of the esophagus should be a biphasic study combining upright double contrast and prone single contrast technique. In the double contrast phase, the aim is to achieve adequate gaseous distension of the lumen with a thin layer of high density barium coating the mucosa. Gaseous distension is improved by the patient swallowing effervescent agents. The patient is also instructed to swallow rapidly the high density barium. Rapid drinking causes air swallowing and thus, esophageal distension. In addition, it interrupts the esophageal peristalsis, thus resulting in esophageal hypotonia.

The effervescent agent may be omitted in patients with suspected esophageal infections or obstructing lesions (because it is painful and may cause artefacts).

Prone views of the upper esophagus best shows esophageal webs and indentations by aortic arch anomalies. Barium-filled views of the distal esophagus are important for the detection of hiatal hernias, strictures, webs or rings as these may not be visible in the erect double contrast phase. Next, the patient is turned to the right and gastroesophageal junction is monitored fluoroscopically to elicit spontaneous gastresophageal reflux. The cardia is best shown in double contrast with the patient in the recumbent right lateral position.

Provocative testing in an attempt to reproduce symptoms may be useful in a patient with solid food dysphagia who has a normal study with liquid barium. A barium impregnated solid bolus may hold up at a subtle stricture or induce spasm not seen with liquid bolus.

A tube esophagogram may be performed if there is marked aspiration or penetration.

Evaluation of a patient presenting with dysphagia includes detailed evaluation of the pharynx, esophagus, gastroesophageal junction and the cardia using double-contrast and single-contrast barium examinations.[7]

Evaluation of Pharynx

The patient is positioned erect in the right lateral position with the fluoroscopy table being vertical and asked to swallow approximately 10 mL of 250% w/v of barium sulfate (high density) suspension. A cine recording of the oral and pharyngeal phases of swallowing is done both in full-field lateral views as well as collimated views of the pharynx. In addition to this, two lateral spot films are obtained during phonation (patient is asked to say "eeeeeee...") and during suspended respiration respectively.[10]

The patient's position is then changed to a frontal position and the head tilted backwards till the mandible is superimposed over the occiput. In this position, cine recording of two additional swallows is done. Two frontal spot films are obtained during Valsalva maneuvere and during suspended respiration respectively **(Figs. 1A and B)**.

Evaluation of the Esophagus, Gastroesophageal Junction and Cardia

The patient is positioned erect in the left posterior oblique position with the fluoroscopy table being vertical and asked to swallow effervescent granules with approximately 10 mL of water. The patient is then asked to rapidly swallow a mouthful of 250% w/v of barium sulfate suspension.

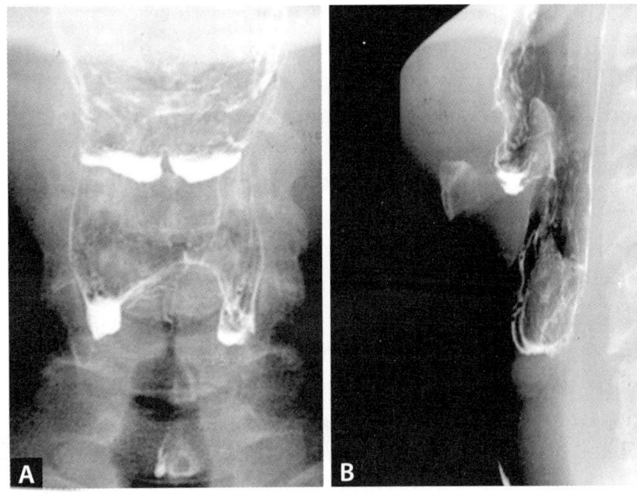

Figs. 1A and B: Spot views of the normal pharynx: (A) Frontal view shows normal smooth mucosal outline of the paired valleculae, pyriform sinuses and lateral walls of the hypopharynx; (B) Lateral view shows normal smooth mucosal outline of superimposed bilateral valleculae and pyriform sinuses.

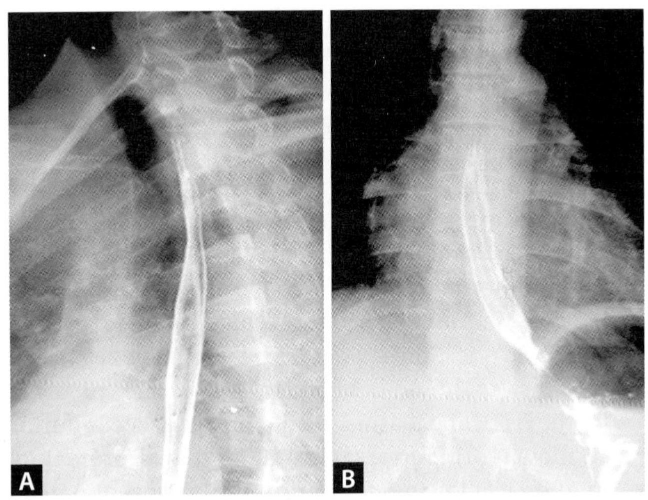

Figs. 2A and B: (A) Normal appearance of mid; and (B) Lower dorsal esophagus and gastroesophageal junction on Barium Swallow Study.

Spot films of the proximal and distal esophagus are obtained. In order to get proper double contrast views, the spot exposures should be timed with periods of optimal distension and coating **(Figs. 2A and B)**.

The fluoroscopy table is then made horizontal and the patient is asked to lie down in the right lateral position and spot films of the double contrast views of gastric cardia and fundus are obtained.

The patient is then turned prone in a right anterior oblique position and asked to swallow 100% w/v suspension of barium sulfate. Fluoroscopic examination of esophageal motility is done, along with spot exposures to obtain single contrast views of proximal and distal esophagus. In case of any abnormal esophageal motility detected, cine recording of additional swallows can also be done.

The patient is then asked to turn to his left side and then on to his back. The gastroesophageal junction is focused and monitored fluoroscopically as the patient is asked to slowly turn towards his right side in order to look for any spontaneous gastroesophageal reflux. If no spontaneous reflux is seen, then straight leg raising maneuver or Valsalva maneuver can be done to increase intra-abdominal pressure and gastroesophageal reflux is looked for.

Thus, there are several important principles in the evaluation of patients with dysphagia:[11]

- Radiographic evaluation of patients with dysphagia must include all structures involved in swallowing.
- If possible, the examination should be biphasic.
- Every patient should be examined in both the erect and recumbent positions.
- Each patient with dysphagia is different. Although there is a routine or basic examination, studies of patients with swallowing problems lend themselves to tailoring. Each examination is subtly altered on the basis of a short patient history taken by the radiologist. The routine examination is also modified by the clinical condition of the patient. The sicker the patient, less routine and more tailored the examination should be. The examination should be focused on answering a specific question such as "does the patient aspirate". The answer should not be just "yes" or "no" but "yes, for the following reasons". Aspiration may occur during swallowing due to a failure of laryngeal protection or after swallowing, for example, pharyngeal paresis may result in progressive retention of liquid in the pyriform sinuses and subsequent overflow aspiration, or gastroesophageal reflux may produce aspiration from esophagopharyngeal regurgitation of the refluxed material. Aspiration may also occur before swallowing if there is premature leakage from the mouth when the larynx is open and unprotected. The other important observation is whether the patient coughs during aspiration. With loss of sensory feedback, aspiration may be silent and not suspected clinically.

The Tailored Examination[7]

Recommended Approach

Patients with pharyngeal dysphagia or other symptoms localized to the pharynx, neck or suprasternal notch should undergo a careful radiologic examination of the pharynx with videofluoroscopic recordings and double contrast spot films. If the patient aspirates a substantial amount of barium, the examination should be terminated. If marked swallowing dysfunction occurs, particularly in stroke patients, a detailed study of the esophagus is unwarranted. However, patients with pharyngeal carcinoma have a significantly increased risk of synchronous esophageal carcinoma. Therefore, a double contrast examination of the esophagus should be performed in these cases. A normal pharyngeal study should always be followed by a careful examination of the esophagus and cardia to rule out more distal abnormalities causing referred dysphagia to the pharynx.

Conversely, patients with substernal dysphagia, odynophagia, reflux symptoms, or nonspecific chest pain should first undergo a detailed radiologic examination of the esophagus and cardia. Some esophageal disorders such as achalasia and gastroesophageal reflux disease may be associated with pharyngeal or cricopharyngeal dysfunction. However, pharyngeal abnormalities virtually never cause referred dysphagia below the level of the thoracic inlet, so a limited pharyngeal study may be performed in patients with substernal symptoms.

Videofluoroscopic Swallowing Study

It is also known as modified barium swallow and is the standard of reference for evaluating the swallowing mechanism. Videofluoroscopic swallowing study (VFSS) is a dynamic fluoroscopic study performed with high frame rate image capture and is useful for evaluating the motility of oropharynx and hypopharynx. The study is often performed in conjunction with a swallowing therapist and provides information about swallowing function in response to therapeutic measures and necessary dietary requirements. The images can be reviewed later with referring physicians, speech language pathologist, patients and their family members to explain the management recommendations.[3] VFSS provides real time visualization of the oropharyngeal and esophageal structures, movement and coordination of swallowing. The study best detects aspiration during swallow. Even though VFSS is a gold standard for dysphagia, it can be normal in patients with early or slowly progressive disease. Hence, if patient discomfort persists inspite of normal VFSS, they should be followed up.

Nasopharyngoscopy

It is also known as fiberoptic endoscopic swallowing study. This technique allows direct visualization of lingual, pharyngeal and epiglottic movements during swallowing and also assesses the presence of any pharyngeal retention of fluids after swallowing.[6]

Pharyngeal/Esophageal Manometry

Manometry is the most sensitive and accurate technique to assess esophageal motility and diagnose esophageal motility disorders. The study entails positioning a pressure sensing catheter within the esophagus. Test swallows are given to the patient following which esophageal contractility is observed. The upper and lower esophageal sphincters appear as zones of high pressure that relax on swallowing while the intersphincteric esophagus shows peristaltic contractions.[12]

With advancements in technology, the conventional manometry has been replaced by high resolution manometry (HRM) with substantial improvement in its recording power and fidelity. Pressure measurement of 1 cm or less can be measured along the entire esophagus thereby providing detailed mapping of esophageal motor function including upper and lower esophageal sphincters.

The traditional line plot in manometry has further largely been replaced by the topographical or contour or color plot which aids in more rapid interpretation of results. The combination of HRM with topography, also called high-resolution esophageal pressure topography allows more precise measurement of esophageal pressures **(Fig. 3)**. It has been shown to have higher sensitivity (72%) for achalasia as compared to conventional manometry (56%).[6]

Manometry is thus the "gold standard" test in diagnosing achalasia and esophageal spasm due to its high sensitivity in detecting pressure changes and its good correlation with bolus transit in these conditions.

Upper Gastrointestinal Endoscopy

Upper GI endoscopy not only provides direct visualization of the esophagus but also the oropharynx stomach and duodenum. It is the preferred investigation in patients with a history suggestive of mechanical obstruction and is useful in identifying intraluminal mass lesion, strictures, inflammatory disorders such as reflux disease, eosinophilic esophagitis and pill-induced ulceration.[6]

Endoscopes also have an instrumentation channel through which biopsy forceps, sclerotherapy catheters or balloon dilators can be passed and various therapeutic procedures can be performed simultaneously. Some of the advantages of endoscopy over contrast radiographic studies are:[12]

- Increased sensitivity for detection of mucosal lesions.

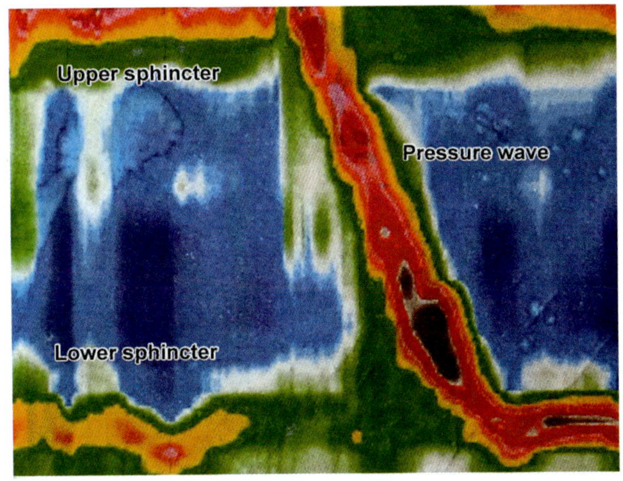

Fig. 3: Color plot depicting pressure waves of a normal swallow by esophageal manometry, also called high-resolution esophageal pressure topography.

- Increased sensitivity in the detection of Barrett's metaplasia which is mainly identified by its abnormal color.
- Obtaining biopsy specimen of suspected abnormalities for histopathological evaluation.
- The ability to effectively dilate strictures, which may be peptic, anastamotic or radiation induced or esophageal web or Schatzki's ring is a therapeutic capability of this technique. Endoscopic-guided pneumatic dilatation and botulinum toxin injection at the LES are some of the therapeutic alternatives which can be performed in patients of achalasia who are not suitable for surgical myotomy.[6]

Though upper GI endoscopy has relatively low sensitivity and specificity in the evaluation of underlying motility disorder it can suggest underlying achalasia in the presence of a dilated esophagus with features of reduced contractions which occlude its lumen and a tight LES. In the setting of achalasia, endoscopy provides direct visualization of the gastresophageal junction and gastric cardia to detect any underlying carcinoma causing pseudoachalasia.

Esophageal Scintigraphy

Scintigraphy is a screening test used to detect an abnormality in the esophageal transit time. It involves the ingestion of a liquid or solid bolus labeled with a radionuclide such as ^{99m}Tc-DTPA. The radionuclide movement is recorded by a gamma camera which measures the esophageal bolus time and clearance. The investigation is not used much even though it has been reported to have a high sensitivity and specificity in detecting esophageal motor abnormalities.[6] Handling of radioactive material and radiation exposure, poor anatomical definition compared with barium swallow and a lack of well-defined diagnostic criteria are some of the reasons why scintigraphy is rarely used in the investigation of dysphagia.

Intraesophageal pH Monitoring

This investigation is done in the setting of suspected gastroesophageal reflux disease (GERD). It can be performed in either of the two ways—a wireless pH—sensitive transmitter is anchored to the esophageal mucosa or a wire electrode is passed transnasally with the tip in the distal esophagus and an ambulatory 24–48 hours esophageal pH recording is done. The outcome is expressed as percentage and a pH value of less than 4 is indicative of recent acid reflux with values more than 5% indicative of GERD. Intraluminal impedance monitoring can be added to pH monitoring to detect reflux irrespective of whether it is acidic or not thereby increasing the sensitivity of the study.[12]

Endoscopic Ultrasound

Endoscopic ultrasound (EUS) combines an endoscope with an ultrasound transducer to create a transmural image of the tissue surrounding the endoscope tip. Its most important advantage in its greater resolution attributable to the proximity of the ultrasound transducer to the tissue being examined. There are two types of endoscopic probes-side viewing for imaging and at the tip for interventional purposes. The main esophageal application of endoscopic ultrasound are in the staging of esophageal cancer, in the evaluation of dysplasia in Barrett's esophagus and in the assessment of submucosal tumors.

Cross-sectional Imaging Studies

Imaging of the esophagus is challenging because the esophagus is a long tube, and poorly distensible, with a close relationship to many vital organs.[13]

Pharynx

Although the mucosal detail of the pharynx is studied best with barium contrast, the extraluminal anatomy is demonstrated in detail by CT, MRI and sonography. Axial techniques are therefore most useful as an adjunct to barium studies, particularly for tumor staging and the delineation of central and peripheral nervous system lesions producing pharyngeal dysfunction.

Esophagus

Although there is no absolute size of normal wall thickness, some authors define that the thickness should not exceed 3 mm in a well distended esophagus. Also, an eccentric thickening of the wall is suggestive of an underlying pathology.[6] Although, with increasing age, the esophageal caliber may increase, an anteroposterior (AP) diameter more than 10 mm and a transverse diameter greater than 24 mm are considered abnormal. Air may be seen in the esophagus in around 65% of normal population. However, an air-fluid level, fluid filled lumen or a lumen caliber more than 10 mm usually indicate obstruction or severe dysmotility.

Proper distension of the esophagus and stomach (by oral administration of effervescent granules and water) and optimally timed administration of intravenous contrast material are required to detect and characterize disease. Preoperative staging of esophageal carcinoma appears to be the main indication for MDCT. CT provides considerable information on the intramural and extramural extent of esophageal malignancy and is also an indispensable part of the planning for radiation therapy. CT and MRI have been used to stage esophageal carcinoma, because these techniques can reveal extraesophageal extension into adjacent mediastinal structures, including the trachea, bronchi, aorta, and pericardium, and can detect lymphadenopathy in the mediastinum. For assessing unresectability, CT and MR have comparable accuracy when using criteria such as tracheobronchial invasion and aortic invasion. However, CT appears more sensitive for detecting lymphadenopathy, particularly in the mediastinum.[14]

Though MR imaging is not routinely performed for esophageal pathology, the normal esophagus is well visualized in its entire length except the mid part which may be difficult to visualize as it is flattened behind the left atrium. On T1W images, the normal esophagus appears as a low signal intensity (SI) structure contrasted by high signal intensity of periesophageal fat. On T2W images, it appears as low signal intensity in contrast to high signal intensity of internal contents. Postcontrast MR images reveal moderate enhancement of the muscle layer of the esophagus. Use of phase array surface coils can provide high resolution MR images of individual layers of the esophageal wall. On high resolution T2W images the esophagus is seen as intermediate SI mucosa surrounded by high SI submucosa and low SI muscularis propria.[15]

FUNCTIONAL OROPHARYNGEAL ABNORMALITIES

Functional neuromuscular disorders (enlisted in **Table 2B**) can lead to the following pathophysiologic conditions with oropharyngeal dysphagia:

Laryngeal Penetration

During fluoroscopy, when the contrast material enters the laryngeal vestibule but does not pass below the level of the glottis through the true vocal cords, it is indicative of laryngeal vestibular penetration. In healthy people, spontaneous clearing of the contrast occurs from the laryngeal vestibule which is known as transient penetration or high penetration. It can arise from poor oral control of the bolus or from delayed initiation of the pharyngeal swallow.[3]

Aspiration

The term aspiration is used to describe the passage of foreign material including food and liquid through the true vocal cords into the trachea. Prevention of aspiration requires superior and anterior elevation of the larynx, closure of larynx and epiglottic tilt. These mechanisms can be evaluated at videofluoroscopy.[3] Aspiration can occur before, during or after swallow and is the most threatening symptom of oropharyngeal dysphagia.

Once aspiration has occurred, the immediate expected reflex is a cough due to excitation of recurrent laryngeal nerve receptors. In patients with dysphagia who present with aspiration, the cough response may be immediate, delayed or absent. The cough may also not be effective in throwing out material back into the hypopharynx. The severity of aspiration is determined subjectively by:

- The amount of material aspirated, i.e. minimal, moderate or severe.
- Quantification of the depth of aspiration.
- Response in terms of coughing.

The standard measure of severity of aspiration is the "8 point penetration aspiration scale" which includes both the depth of airway invasion (above or below the true vocal cords) and whether the material is ejected back into the hypopharynx or not. Silent aspiration is represented by a score of 8 in which material is aspirated below the true vocal cords without any overt clinical signs.

Postswallow Residue in the Pharynx

Following a swallow, the bolus may collect and remain in the valleculae and pyriform sinuses. This may be due to weak propulsion of bolus or inadequate opening of the upper esophageal sphincter. The residue in the pharynx may lead to secondary postswallow aspiration.

Cricopharyngeal Bar or Prominent Cricopharyngeus Muscle

The posterior indentation at approximately C5-C6 level by cricopharyngeus muscle normally effaces as a bolus passes through. Mild persistent indentation may be normal but more obvious prominence may be seen in patients with gastroesophageal reflux or functional or mechanical esophageal obstruction. It is postulated that acid reflux leads to edema, spasm and or hypertrophy of cricopharyngeus. On a contrast study on the lateral view it is seen as a smooth posterior bar-like or band-like protrusion into the lumen of the barium column at the junction of the hypopharynx and cervical (C5-C6 level) esophagus **(Fig. 4A)**. Cricopharyngeal bar may be seen in 5–10% of patients who are asymptomatic.

Extrinsic pharyngeal indentation caused by a cervical osteophyte may simulate cricopharyngeal prominence. Osteophytic impressions are fixed in position in relation to the spine, whereas cricopharyngeal indentations move with the pharynx and esophagus during swallowing.

STRUCTURAL OROPHARYNGEAL ABNORMALITIES

Postcricoid Webs

Webs are thin mucosal folds that are located in the anterior wall of the lower hypopharynx and proximal few centimeters of the esophagus. They typically present with dysphagia to solids but deglutitive aspiration may occur due to their proximal location.[8] They have been reported to be twice as common in women than men and more easily appreciated on barium swallow than on endoscopy[8] wherein they are seen as eccentric but occasionally circumferential 1–2 mm wide shelflike filling defect **(Fig. 4B)**. Characteristic "jet effect" may be seen on contrast swallow when a large bolus passes through a web. They arise on the anterior wall and never on the posterior

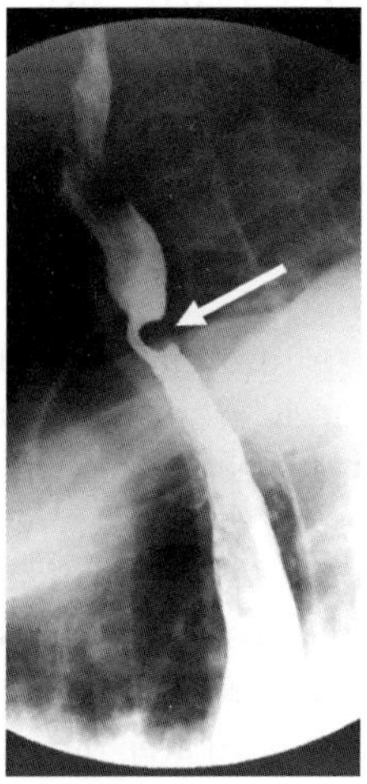

Fig. 4A: Prominence of the criocopharyngeus muscle seen as posterior indentation (arrow) on barium swallow study with mild proximal dilatation

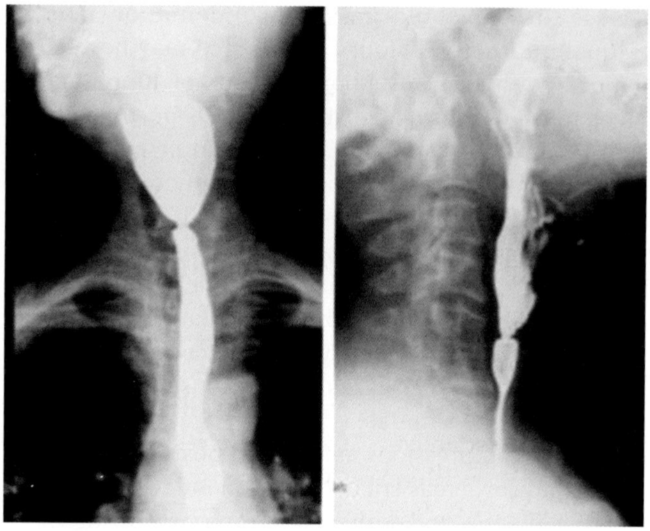

Fig. 4B: Barium swallow shows well-defined localized circumferential narrowing seen at the level of C5-C6 with minimal proximal dilatation—cricopharyngeal web.

wall and are best seen on the lateral projection. As rapid peristalsis allows cervical webs to be visualized only for fraction of a second, cineradiography is required to demonstrate them. Differentiation must be made between webs and the submucosal venous plexus which is a normal structure on anterior wall and causes an impression that is effaced as the bolus distends the lumen.

Cervical webs have been linked to underlying conditions such as GERD, epidermolysis bullosa and possibly associated with iron deficiency anemia (Plummer-Vinson Syndrome).

Pharyngeal Diverticula and Pouches

Several types of diverticula may be seen on oropharyngeal and upper gastrointestinal barium studies such as pharyngeal diverticula and pouches, Zenker's diverticulum and Killian-Jamieson diverticulum. Zenker's diverticulum has been found to be the most common of them and frequently implicated in pharyngeal dysphagia. This develops secondary to fibrosis and loss of compliance of the cricopharyngeus muscle.[8] It occurs as a result of increase in intraluminal pressure associated with distal obstruction in the form of a stenotic cricopharyngeus muscle (upper esophageal sphincter). Zenker's diverticulum is a false diverticula which involves herniation of the mucosa and submucosa through the muscular layer of esophagus. It is a pouch that develops as an area of anatomic weakness in the posterior hypopharyngeal wall between the horizontal and oblique fibers of the cricopharyngeus muscle. It is seen on the lateral view as a bulge or true sac extending posteriorly from the posterior hypopharyngeal wall just above the cricopharyngeal impression. On the frontal view a Zenker's diverticulum is seen as a barium-filled sac below the arcuate lines of the pyriform sinuses. This area is known as the triangle of Killian or Killian dehiscence. The mouth of the Zenker's diverticulum is present immediately above the cricopharyngeal muscle. Imaging in three projections are required for confirmation and assessment of the severity of a Zenker's diverticulum, i.e. anteroposterior, lateral and oblique. In contrast, the Killian-Jamieson diverticula originates below the cricopharyngeus muscle.

Small Zenker's diverticulae are usually asymptomatic. Dysphagia occurs as the diverticulum fills preferentially with food and obstructs the lumen of the esophagus. There is regurgitation of pouch contents and often, aspiration as its overflows. Recurrent chest infection are hence common.

The treatment of choice for Zenker's diverticulum is cricopharyngeal myotomy, either alone or combination with pouch resection. In the elderly with significant comorbidity, cricopharyngeal dilatation can provide symptomatic relief and can be performed as an alternative treatment.

Oropharyngeal Tumors and their Surgery

Tumors of the head and neck such as those arising from the tongue, palate, pharynx, tonsil and glottis may present with dysphagia. The surgical resection of these cancers can cause complications such as anastomotic leak, vascular injury and cranial nerve damage which can result in dysphagia. The effect of head and neck cancer surgery on swallowing can vary markedly from person to person and depends on many factors such as the extent of surgical resection, whether flap reconstruction is required, the nature of component structures removed, i.e. cartilaginous, muscular or bony or whether surgery has resulted in damage to neural innervations.

In those undergoing surgery for oral cancer, the extent of tongue resection is the most important factor which determines the severity of dysphagia. This is because tongue base motion is very important in generating pharyngeal propulsive forces. Also, following laryngeal surgery the degree of preservation of tongue base motion is an important prediction of recovery of swallow function.[8]

The majority of malignant pharyngeal tumors are squamous cell carcinomas. Small tumors may be seen as a nodular mucosal surface en face or as an irregular contour. Radiographic findings in large, advanced tumors include intraluminal mass, mucosal irregularity and asymmetric distensibility. An intraluminal mass may be seen as an abnormal luminal contour, abnormally located extra-barium-coated lines, a focal area of increased radiodensity, or a filling defect in the barium pool. Mucosal irregularity is recognized by abnormal barium collections due to ulceration or by a nonuniform nodular surface pattern. Asymmetric distensibility may be due to an infiltrating tumor or extrinsic mass **(Figs. 5A and B)**. The value of double-contrast pharyngography in patients with a known carcinoma is to determine the size, extent and inferior limit of the pharyngeal tumor and the degree of functional impairment. Pharyngoesophagograms are also useful for detecting separate co-existing carcinomas of the pharynx and esophagus. Extraluminal extent of the tumor (e.g. invasion of the pre-epiglottic space or cartilage destruction) and lymphadenopathy are best assessed by CT and MR imaging. **(Figs. 6A to C)**.

Postradiation Stricture

Radiotherapy for malignancies of oral and pharyngeal region is known to cause severe nerve and muscle damage. Chemotherapy and radiotherapy both are known to produce esophageal strictures leading to dysphagia with a lower risk of development of strictures at doses less than 60 Gy.

Video fluoroscopy or contrast swallow study can depict the pharyngeal or esophageal strictures developing secondary to radiotherapy for a laryngeal malignancy. The stricture may vary from short, smooth to complete obliteration of the lumen.[3]

It is important to take a history of radiotherapy for an oral or neck surgery in the past as radiation-induced dysphagia is known to manifest clinically more than 10 years post-treatment.[8]

Retropharyngeal Abscess

Retropharyngeal abscess may occur secondary to tonsillar infection, suppurative lymphadenopathy, spread of tubercular infection from the prevertebral space to the retropharyngeal space or from perforating injury of the pharynx or esophagus. It is more often seen in small children who may present with fever, neck stiffness and dysphagia. On lateral plain radiograph of the neck, findings are an increase in the retropharyngeal space, reversal of cervical lordosis and anterior displacement of the airway. The abscess may contain air and an air-fluid level may be seen. On CT, the abscess appears as an area of low attenuation with peripheral rim enhancement and on MR it is seen as high signal intensity on T2-weighted images **(Fig. 7)**.

Pharyngeal Foreign Bodies

A lateral radiograph of the neck taken at soft tissue exposure may show a radiopaque foreign body, but many impacted fish or chicken bones are poorly opaque. Evidence of perforation should be sought, including extraluminal gas and widening of the prevertebral soft tissues. A contrast swallow is performed with a small volume of low density

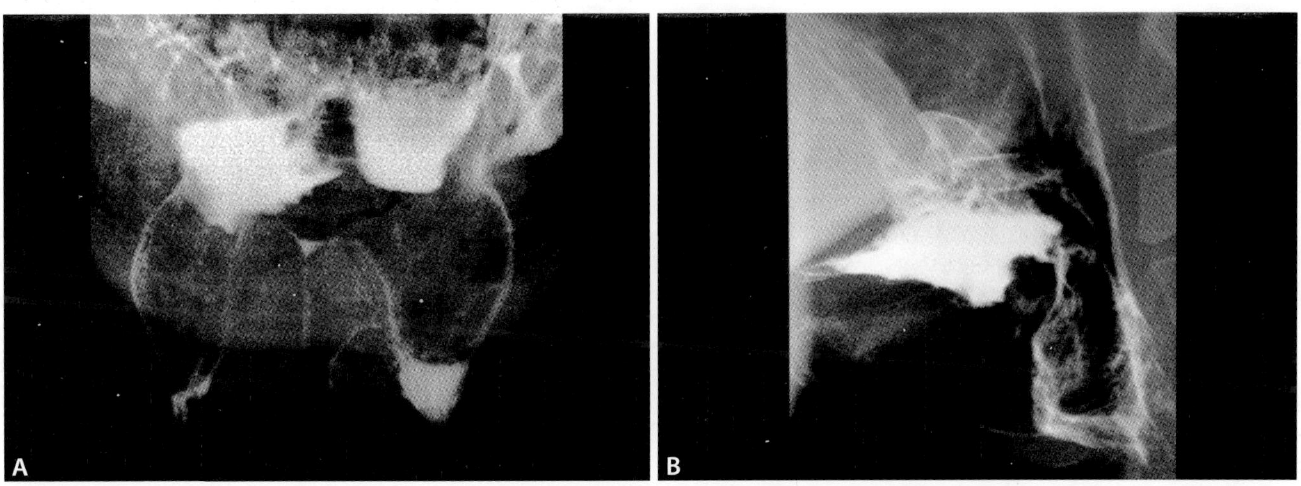

Figs. 5A and B: Contrast swallow: (A) Frontal; (B) Lateral spot views of the hypopharynx showing expansion and mucosal irregularity of the right vallecula by a malignant mass. The left vallecula and pyriform sinus appear normal—malignant right vallecular mass (SCC).

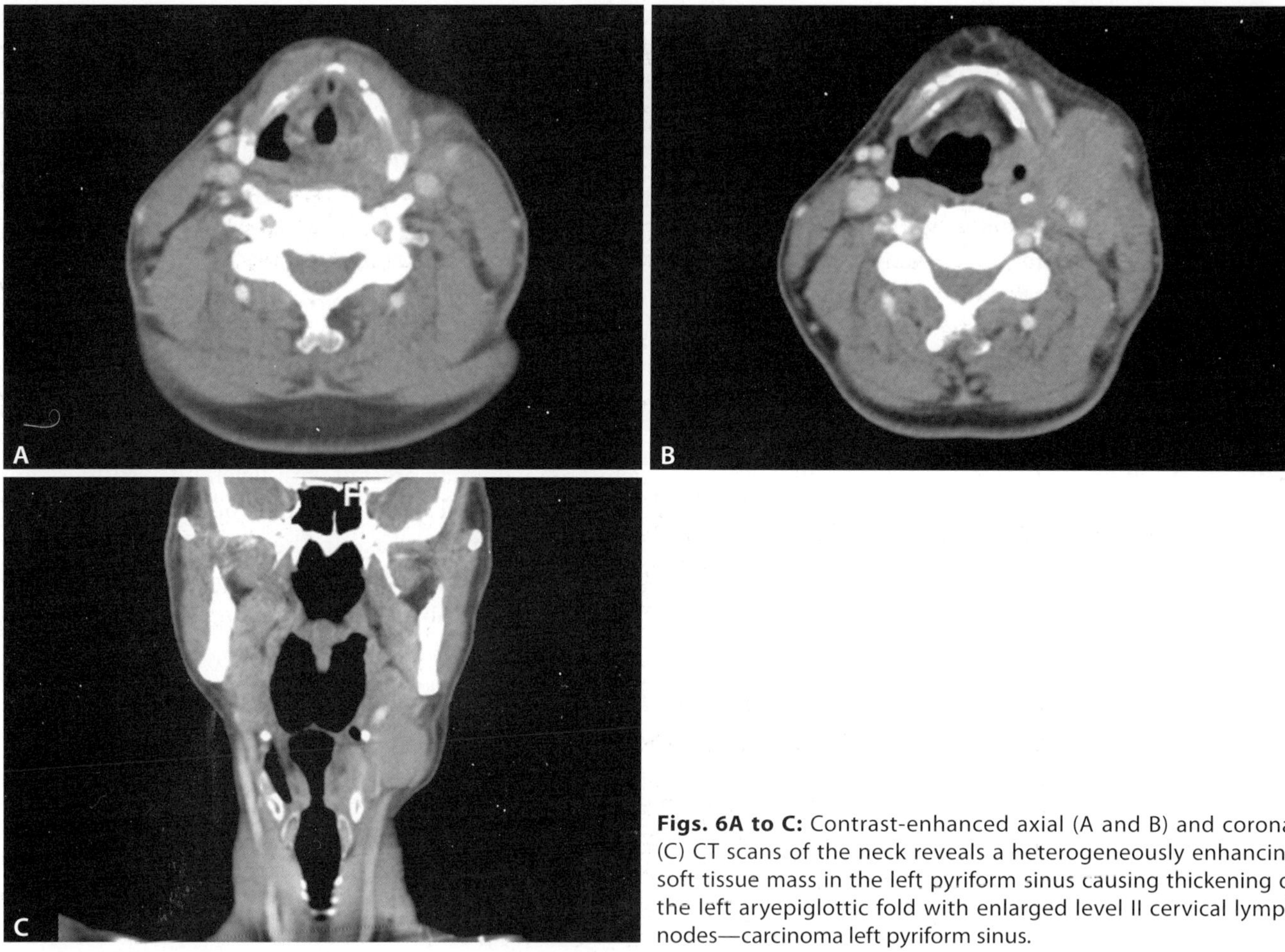

Figs. 6A to C: Contrast-enhanced axial (A and B) and coronal (C) CT scans of the neck reveals a heterogeneously enhancing soft tissue mass in the left pyriform sinus causing thickening of the left aryepiglottic fold with enlarged level II cervical lymph nodes—carcinoma left pyriform sinus.

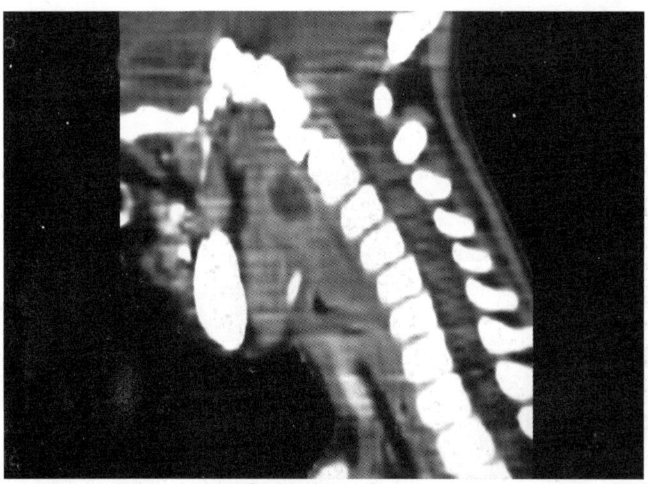

Fig. 7: Sagittal MPR image of CECT neck of a child with neck pain, fever and dysphagia shows a rim enhancing hypodense lesion in the retropharyngeal region causing compression of the oropharyngeal airway—retropharyngeal abscess.

barium, or water-soluble nonionic contrast if perforation is suspected. CT is an excellent investigation in localizing and identifying a foreign body, detecting complications such as perforation, collection or abscess formation and depicting involvement of adjacent structures.

ESOPHAGEAL MOTILITY DISORDERS

These disorders are those which are attributable to esophageal neuromuscular function and are commonly associated with dysphagia, chest pain or heart burn. The dysphagia is slowly progressive and occurs to both liquid and solid foods. The esophageal motility can be easily assessed at fluoroscopy with the patient in the prone right anterior oblique (RAO) position. Two to five individual swallows should be observed at fluoroscopy as the bolus passes. It is important to remember that in patients suspected of having an esophageal motility disorder, individual swallow should be evaluated, as a second or double swallow would interfere with primary peristalsis and limit evaluation of esophageal motility.

Specific motility disorders consist of diffuse esophageal spasm (DES), achalasia and scleroderma. However, the motility disorders may not fall into any of these categories and may occur in association with GERD.

PRIMARY MOTILITY DISORDER

Nonspecific Esophageal Motility Disorder

Motility abnormalities that do not meet the criteria of specific motility disorders fall into this broad category. Manometrically, abnormal peristalsis is seen in 20% of such cases. Peristalsis may be intermittently absent or of low amplitude. Lower esophageal sphincter dysfunction (incomplete relaxation) and frequent spontaneous or repetitive contractions are also detected. Radiologically a nonspecific disturbance of primary peristalsis and tertiary contractions are seen in 40–50% of cases **(Fig. 8)**.

Diffuse Esophageal Spasm

Clinical Presentation

Diffuse esophageal spasm is manifested by episodes of dysphagia and chest pain occurring due to abnormal esophageal contractions with normal lower esophageal sphincter (LES) relaxation on deglutition. Esophageal chest pain may closely mimic pain of angina. Features which suggest a pain of esophageal origin are it being unrelated to exertion, pain of prolonged duration which interrupts sleep, its relation to meals, relief with antacids and being accompanied by heartburn, dysphagia or regurgitation. All these presenting features also show overlap with cardiac pain. Both chest pain and dysphagia are also characteristic of peptic or infectious esophagitis. Hence, only after the more common entities mentioned above are excluded, that a diagnosis of diffuse esophageal spasm (DES) should be considered.[12]

Imaging Features

DES is characterized by the absence of primary peristalsis with simultaneous, spontaneous, repetitive, nonperistaltic uncoordinated esophageal contractions on manometry. The LES usually functions normally, although high resting pressures and incomplete relaxation may occur. It occurs in patients over 50 years of age and may be intermittent and noted mostly in the distal two-thirds of esophagus. Radiographically, there is loss of primary peristalsis in the distal esophagus. Nonperistaltic tertiary contractions are usually repetitive and simultaneous and may produce a corkscrew or rosary bead appearance **(Fig. 9)**. The findings are similar to those seen in nonspecific esophageal motility disorder. The clinical picture helps to distinguish the two conditions, because diffuse esophageal spasm is associated with chest pain. The esophagus is not usually dilated and the LES functions normally.

The radiological appearance of diffuse esophageal spasm is also known as pseudodiverticula or curling phenomena which can also be found with spastic achalasia.

Treatment

Various trials/treatment options for DES have been reported such as use of nitrates, calcium channel blockers, anxiolytics, with varying response. Surgery in the form of long myotomy or esophagectomy is generally not done.

Achalasia

Achalasia is an uncommon motility disorder of the esophagus characterized by a loss of primary esophageal

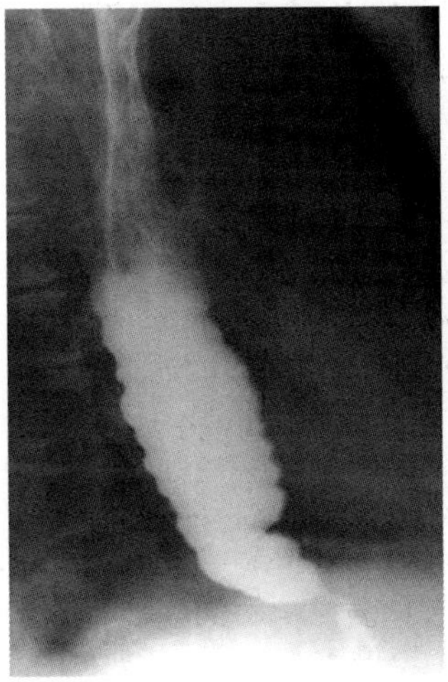

Fig. 8: Nonspecific esophageal motility disorder.

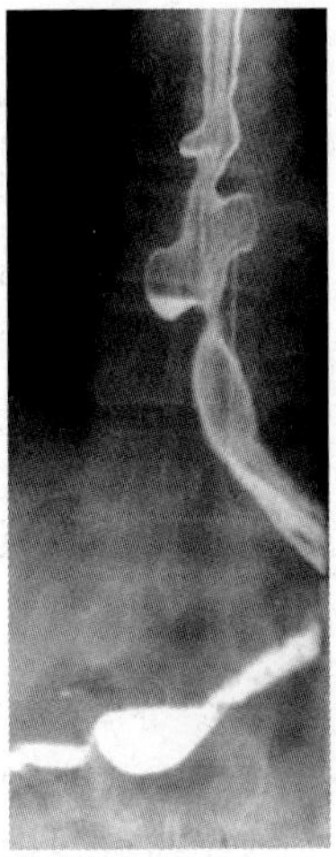

Fig. 9: 'Corkscrew' esophagus—nonpropulsive segmental contractions producing multiple areas of pronounced luminal narrowing with areas of sacculations.

peristalsis, incomplete relaxation of the lower esophageal sphincter in response to deglutition, increased resting LES pressure, and increased intraesophageal pressure.

All these lead to esophageal dilatation or megaesophagus. Of all the conditions associated with esophageal dilatation like achalasia, inflammatory narrowing, progressive systemic sclerosis (PSS) and carcinoma; achalasia causes the most severe generalized dilatation.[16]

Clinical Presentation

Achalasia can present at any age but is the most common in the 30–50 year age group. Dysphagia is usually worse with liquids than with solids, may initially be intermittent and eventually is persistent. It is diagnosed manometrically as esophageal aperistalsis and LES dysfunction, primary incomplete relaxation and elevated resting pressure. Esophageal dilatation is mild in the early stages, which may make radiographic diagnosis difficult.

Although the pathogenesis of achalasia is not known the most accepted theory is related to the paucity or absence of ganglion cells in the Auerbach's plexus in the distal esophageal wall.

Imaging Features

Plain chest radiographs are frequently sufficient for the diagnosis of achalasia. The esophagus is dilated with large amounts of retained food and fluid which may become markedly tortuous and present as a widened mediastinum mainly on the right side, adjacent to the cardiac shadow, often with an air-fluid level. Aspiration of the retained food from the dilated esophagus frequently leads to episodes of pneumonia. On an erect radiograph, air bubble of the gastric fundus is small or absent **(Figs. 10A and B)**.

Barium swallow with the patient erect demonstrates a variable degree of dilatation of the esophagus above a beak-like narrowing at the lower esophageal sphincter **(Figs. 11A and B)**. The sphincter opens intermittently under the force of the hydrostatic pressure of the barium column above it to allow bolus passage. A gradual, tapered, smooth, conical narrowing of the distal esophageal segment extending for 1–3 cm in length is known as bird's beak appearance and is the hallmark of achalasia. With the patient in erect position, sequential radiography can show small spurts of barium entering the stomach through the narrowed distal segment. The distal two-thirds of the esophagus, which contains smooth muscle is aperistaltic. Secondary stasis esophagitis is common. Esophageal carcinoma may develop which may be seen in 2–7% of patients with long standing achalasia. The carcinoma may develop in the mid esophagus secondary to stasis and irritation of esophagus. Whenever there is a worsening of symptoms in patients of achalasia, possibility of superimposed esophageal carcinoma is to be ruled out.[14]

It is essential that the patient with achalasia is examined in the recumbent position because in the erect position, gravity can simulate the effect of peristalsis and hide subtle abnormalities. Evaluation in the upright position is also necessary for the barium column to provide adequate hydrostatic pressure to force even small amounts of contrast into the stomach. In patients

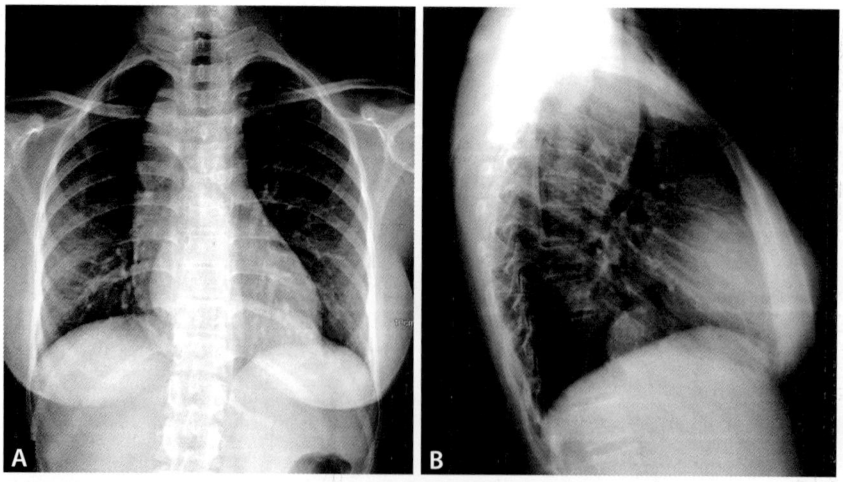

Figs. 10A and B: Chest (PA) erect (A) in a 21-year-old female with achalasia reveals a mediastinal shadow extending from the neck to the diaphragm on the right side due to markedly dilated esophagus. There is absence of air in the fundus of the stomach. Chest lateral (B) shows anterior displacement of the trachea by the dilated esophagus.

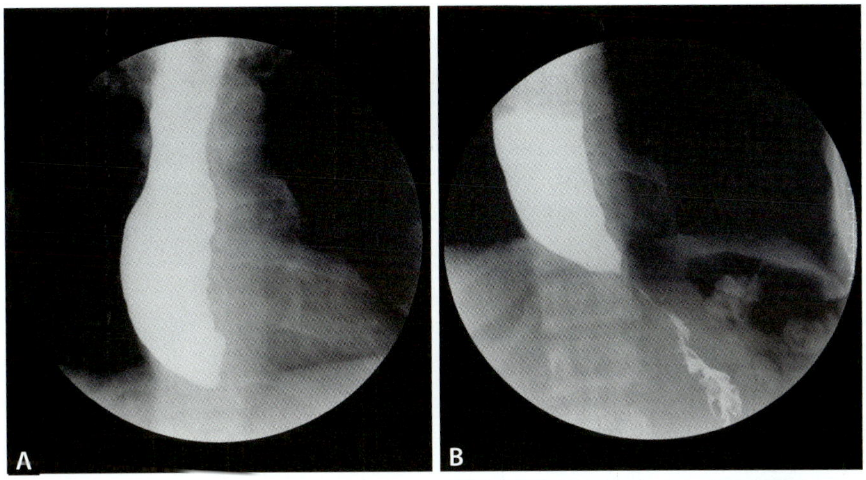

Figs. 11A and B: Barium swallow depicts: (A) A moderately dilated esophagus, (B) with a smooth conical narrowing of the distal esophagus: "Bird's beak" appearance-achalasia.

of achalasia, complete emptying of the esophagus does not occur even in the erect position. This is an important point to remember to differentiate from scleroderma radiologically, where emptying is usually normal in the erect position.[17]

Achalasia is diagnosed on barium swallow studies or esophageal manometry while the role of endoscopy is only in ruling out pseudoachalasia. Manometry is the most sensitive test in diagnosing achalasia as it identifies early disease before esophageal dilatation and food retention **(Fig. 12)**.[12] High resolution manometry identifies three subtypes of achalasia on the basis of pattern of pressurization in the aperistaltic esophagus: (1) Classic achalasia, (2) achalasia with compression and (3) spastic achalasia. All are characterized by impaired relaxation of the lower esophageal sphincter (LES) with absent peristalsis.

CT features of achalasia have been described by Rabuschka and colleagues[18] which consist of a moderate dilatation of the esophagus with a mean diameter of 4.5 cm at the carinal level, but having a normal wall thickness. They found that a normal wall thickness to be the most important feature that differentiates patients of achalasia from other esophageal diseases **(Figs. 13A to C)**. CT is routinely not indicated for the diagnosis of achalasia, but may be useful in confirming the diagnosis and detecting its complications. It may also suggest the presence of other diseases or superimposed benign or malignant processes.[16] The other causes of narrowing of the lower esophageal sphincter (LES) that may mimic achalasia are intrinsic or extrinsic neoplasm, peptic stricture and complications of scleroderma.

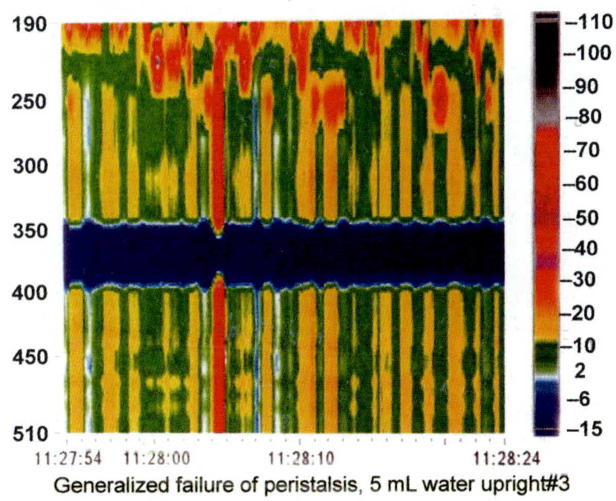

Fig. 12: Esophageal manometry in the patient with achalasia reveals absent esophageal peristalsis with incomplete relaxation of LES with high basal pressure.

Secondary achalasia refers to carcinoma of the gastric cardia or metastases involving the gastroesophageal junction resulting in a radiographic picture simulating achalasia. It is related to destruction of the intramural myenteric plexus. Secondary achalasia should be considered in older patients if symptoms are acute or if the tapered gastroesophageal junction shows mucosal nodularity or mass effect. Repeating the esophagogram after patient inhales amylnitrate may help to distinguish this entity from achalasia. This smooth muscle relaxant relaxes the lower esophageal sphincter in achalasia while in secondary achalasia the LES remains rigid and unchanged.

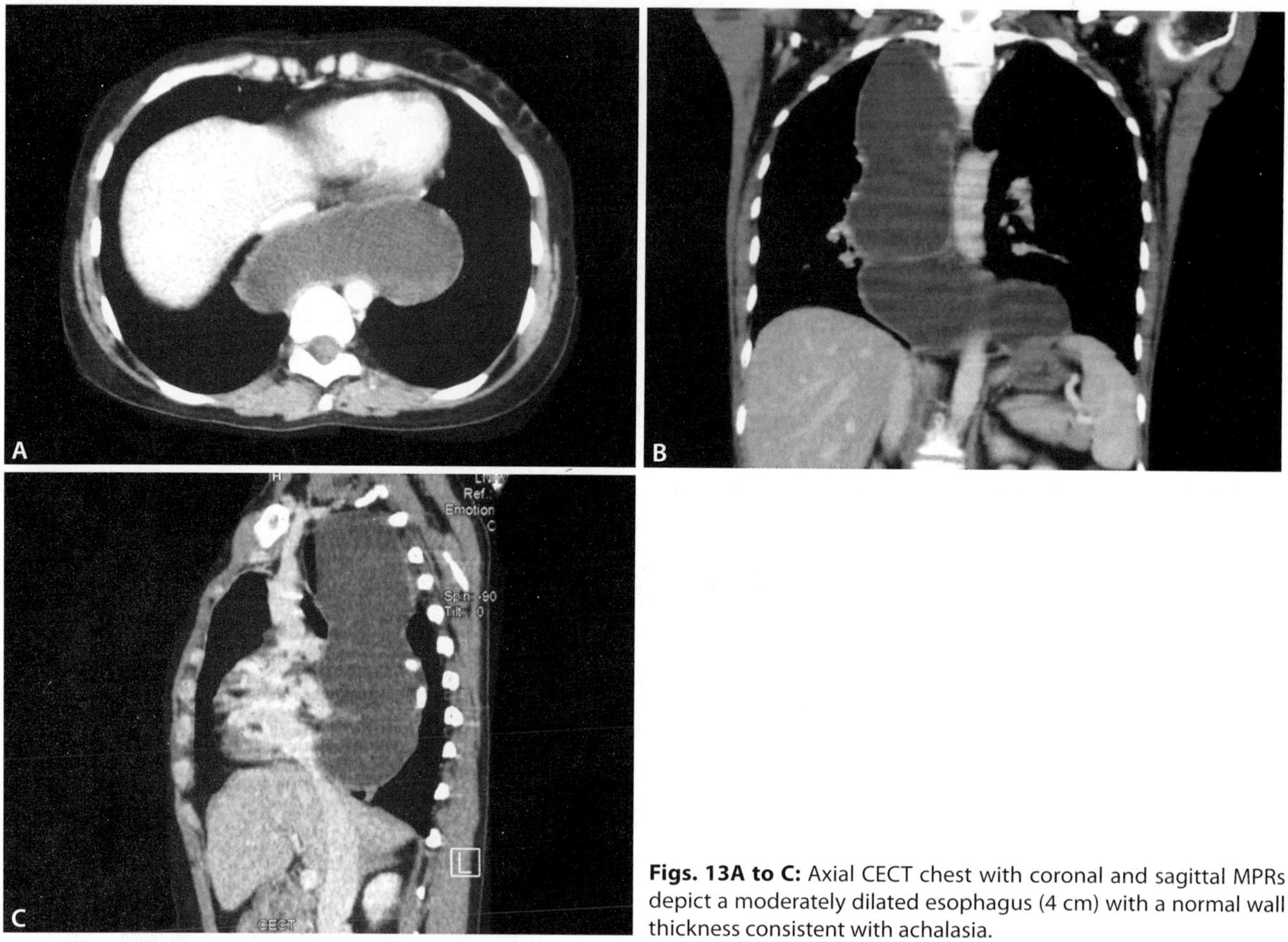

Figs. 13A to C: Axial CECT chest with coronal and sagittal MPRs depict a moderately dilated esophagus (4 cm) with a normal wall thickness consistent with achalasia.

Treatment

Achalasia cannot be prevented or reversed. Therapy is directed at reducing lower esophageal sphincter pressure, so that gravity and esophageal pressurization promote esophageal emptying. Peristalsis is rarely known to return. LES pressure can be reduced by pharmacological therapy, forceful dilatation or surgical myotomy. Pharmacological therapy in the form of nitrates or calcium channel blockers are used as temporary therapies and are administered before eating. Botulinum toxin injected under endoscopic guidance into the LES inhibits acetylcholine release from the nerve endings and is known to improve dysphagia in about 66% of cases for at least six months.[12]

The most reliable therapies for achalasia are pneumatic dilatation and Heller's myotomy. Pneumatic dilatation is an endoscopic technique which uses a noncompliant, cylindrical balloon dilator positioned across the LES and inflated to a diameter of 3–4 cm. The reported accuracy of this technique ranges from 32–98%. Esophageal perforation is the major complication which can occur rarely. Heller's myotomy is the most effective surgical procedure for achalasia. It is performed laparoscopically, usually in conjunction with partial Nissen's fundoplication, with good to excellent results being reported in 62–100% of cases. The surgery involves incising the circular muscle fibers down to the mucosa and allowing the mucosa to protrude through.

In patients with advanced achalasia who fail to respond to the above surgical measures, esophageal resection with gastric pull up or interposition of a segment of transverse colon may be the only option other than a feeding gastrostomy.

SECONDARY MOTILITY DISORDER

Scleroderma

Scleroderma results from atrophy or degeneration of smooth muscle in the lower half to two-thirds of the esophagus with subsequent replacement of esophageal musculature by fibrosis. Neural elements and ganglion cells are normal. The upper third of the esophagus is composed of the striated muscles which is usually not effected by scleroderma. Hence, on a barium swallow a normal peristaltic wave may be seen in this region. In the distal two-thirds esophageal region as the disease progresses, mild uncoordinated tertiary contractions seen early in scleroderma may disappear. As the LES tone is severely decreased in scleroderma, drinking in the erect position allows the bolus to the propelled down the esophagus by the striated muscles i.e. pharyngeal constrictors and carried by gravity into the stomach. Due to the incompetent lower esophageal sphincter , there is reflux of acid secretions into the distal esophagus leading to peptic esophagitis and stricture formation, resulting in heartburn and severe dysphagia. Distal esophageal peristalsis is absent or diminished which contributes to the severity of reflux esophagitis **(Figs. 14A and B)**.

STRUCTURAL ESOPHAGEAL DYSPHAGIA

Esophagitis

Numerous etiologic factors may cause esophagitis. The most common cause is gastroesophageal reflux.

Gastroesophageal Reflux Disease and Barrett's Esophagus

Patients with gastroesophageal reflux disease usually complain of a variety of symptoms like heartburn, regurgitation, substernal pain and also dysphagia in some cases. On double-contrast esophagography, early changes of reflux esophagitis may be recognized as a fine mucosal nodularity or granular appearance of the mucosa in the distal third or half of the thoracic esophagus, occurring due to the presence of mucosal edema and inflammation during the early stages of reflux esophagitis. As the disease progresses, double-contrast esophagography may demonstrate shallow ulcers and erosions, thickened longitudinal folds, inflammatory polyps and scarring. Reflux esophagitis may be recognized also on mucosal relief views as lobulation or nodularity of slightly thickened longitudinal folds. Superficial ulceration occurs with increasing severity, seen as tiny, punctate, linear or irregular collection of barium associated with mounds of edema and fold thickening and distortion. The changes of reflux esophagitis involve a continuous area in the distal esophagus extending proximally from the gastroesophageal junction. Sparing of distal esophagus indicates another cause for the radiographic abnormalities.[19]

A stricture may develop with chronic gastroesophageal reflux disease, which is a smooth, tapered and concentric narrowing in the distal esophagus. Occasionally, the benign stricture is asymmetric due to scarring. Sacculations may form with severe scarring. Esophageal dysmotility and dilatation of the esophagus due to atony may also be seen in gastroesophageal reflux disease.

Barrett's esophagus represents acquired progressive columnar metaplasia of the squamous epithelium in the distal esophagus. It is a premalignant condition. It occurs in about 10% of patients with long-standing gastroesophageal reflux and reflux esophagitis. Most strictures of Barrett's esophagus appear as peptic-type distal esophageal stricture. However, a more specific but less common finding is a mid to upper esophageal stricture, often associated with a sliding hiatal hernia or gastroesophageal

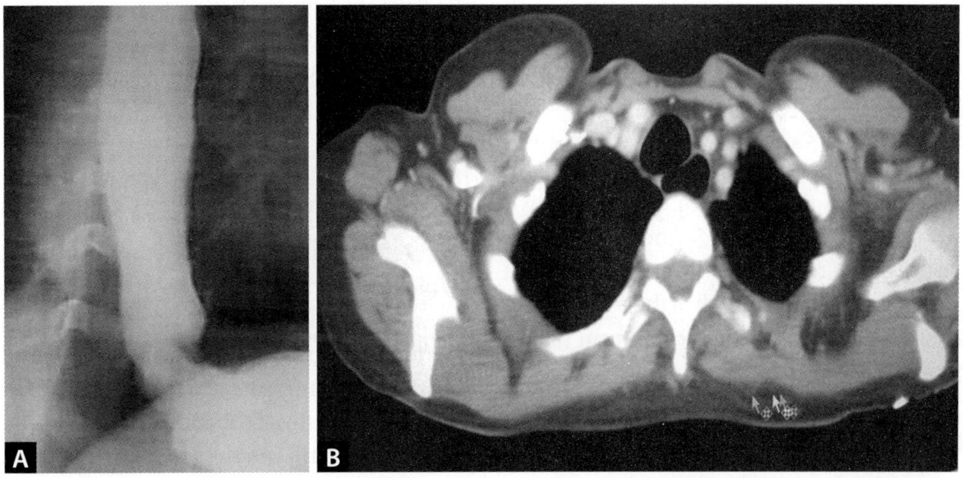

Figs. 14A and B: (A) Barium swallow spot film of lower dorsal esophagus showing dilated esophagus with patulous lower esophageal sphincter; (B) CT chest in the same patient shows dilated esophagus in a patient of scleroderma.

reflux. If Barrett's esophagus is suspected, patient should be kept under endoscopic surveillance with endoscopic biopsy performed as it carries a 100 fold increased risk of adenocarcinoma.[20]

Lower Esophageal Ring (Schatzki Ring)

A Schatzki ring is a thin, smooth, concentric, symmetric mucosal ring-like narrowing of the distal esophagus which marks the junction between the esophageal and gastric mucosa. The ring is constantly present and it does not change its position. However, Schatzki's ring is only seen on contrast swallow studies when the esophagus above and below it is dilated more than the width of the ring.It may be the result of gastresophageal reflux disease. These usually cause dysphagia when less than 13 mm in diameter but are usually asymptomatic when greater than 20 mm in diameter. [17]

The lower esophageal ring has been considered to be a transverse mucosal fold of non inflammatory origin. On barium studies it needs to be differentiated from a variant of ring-like peptic stricture with which it bears a resemblance. However, the ringlike peptic stricture is more asymmetric with tapered borders and generally longer than (greater than 4 mm) a Schatzki ring.[21]

Congenital Esophageal Stenosis

It is a rare condition which produces smooth fusiform narrowing of the esophageal lumen with varying degree of obstruction and proximal dilatation. Severe stenosis occurs in newborns and infants and usually requires surgery. However, a milder form of narrowing may go on till adulthood as patients adapt themselves to their eating habits to compensate for the stenosis. Its diagnosis can be made if a long concentric narrowing is seen in a patient with a long history of dysphagia often associated with recurrent food impaction with no other risk factors for developing esophageal stenosis.[17] On barium swallow the stenotic segment, usually in the mid-esophagus, may show mild narrowing with distinctive ring-like indentations ('ringed esophagus') in the region of the stricture. There are two schools of thought for this appearance. Some believe that the ring like indentations represent tracheobronchial remnants or cartilaginous rings in the wall of the esophagus. While others believe that it is an acquired condition which occurs secondary to gastroesophageal reflux disease.[21]

INFECTIOUS ESOPHAGITIS

Involvement of the esophagus by infective organisms such as *Candida* species, Herpes virus and cytomegalovirus (CMV) have become relatively common with the increase in use of immunosuppressive drugs for organ transplant as well as chronic inflammatory diseases, chemotherapy and acquired immunodeficiency syndrome (AIDS). In AIDS patients, infectious esophagitis is common when the CD4 count falls to < 100. CMV esophagitis occurs only in immunocompromised patients, especially transplant patients.

Regardless of the cause of the infectious agents, odynophagia (painful deglutition) is a characteristic symptom of infectious esophagitis with dysphagia, chest pain and hemorrhage also being common. Odynophagia is uncommon with reflux esophagitis, hence its presence should always raise the suspicion of an alternative etiology.[12]

On CT scan, esophagitis appears as a long segment, uniform, circumferential esophageal wall thickening, often with a 'target sign'. The thickening is as a result of edema, infiltration by inflammatory cells and muscular spasm. The mediastinal fat plane is preserved in esophagitis while esophageal carcinoma usually shows asymmetrical wall thickening with extension into mediastinum. Berkovick and associates found 55% of patients with esophagitis showed an esophageal wall thickness of more than 5 mm with 17% of patients depicting a target sign.[22]

Candida Esophagitis

Candida albicans is the most common cause of infectious esophagitis. It usually occurs opportunistically in immunocompromised patients. *Candida* is normally present in the throat but can become pathogenic and produce esophagitis in the compromised host and is thought to result from downward spread of the fungus from the oropharynx to the esophagus. *Candida* esophagitis can also result from local esophageal stasis caused by severe esophageal motility disorders such as achalasia and scleroderma. Symptoms range from asymptomatic to severe dysphagia.

Imaging Features

Since it is a mucosal disease, it can be identified on double contrast barium examination. In the diagnosis of *Candida* esophagitis, double contrast esophagography shows a sensitivity of about 90%. The findings include discrete, linear, or irregular plaque like filling defects with intervening normal mucosa **(Fig. 15)**. These plaques are oriented longitudinally within the esophagus and may slough off resulting in ulcerations scattered on a background of plaques. In advanced disease, there may be coalescent plaques, which have been likened to a

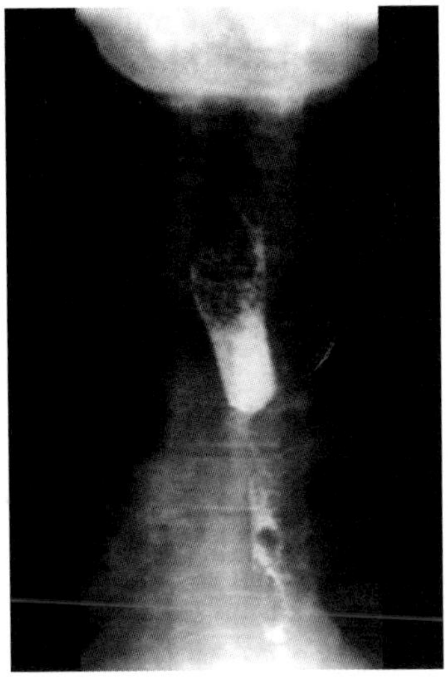

Fig. 15: *Candida* esophagitis: Esophagogram shows a shaggy contour with irregular plaque-like filling defects, seen above a stricture.

"cobblestone" or "snakeskin" appearance that correspond to the distinctive white plaques seen at endoscopy. Patients with AIDS may get a severe form of this disease, resulting in a grossly irregular or shaggy appearance secondary to extensive plaques and pseudomembranes that trap barium between them.

A newly described sign associated with esophageal candidiasis is the "foamy" esophagus seen on double contrast barium swallow study in the immunocompromised and in 25% of patients of esophageal stasis such as scleroderma, achalasia. It is characterized by the presence of multiple tiny, smooth, round lucencies (bubbles) of around 1–3 mm size that are intermingled with the barium suspension along the top of the barium column on upright views producing a layer of foam. The layer of foam may have a length ranging from 3 to 16 cm in the barium column. The pathophysiologic basis of the "foamy esophagus" is uncertain, but has been postulated to be produced directly by the fungal organisms that colonise the esophagus. These round lucencies in the foamy esophagus are bubbles, hence mobile and are usually distinguished radiographically from retained food or debris in the esophagus or diffuse nodularity of the esophageal mucosa. Undissolved effervescent granules used in a double contrast swallow may mimic the round lucencies seen in *Candida* esophagitis and hence should not be used in the initial swallows when candidial involvement is suspected.[22]

The CT findings of *Candida* esophagitis, though nonspecific and commonly seen in various kinds of esophagitis, are circumferential esophageal wall thickening of more than 5 mm, with relatively long segmental involvement. Enhanced scans may also depict the target sign (circumferential wall thickening and enhancing internal mucosa).[23]

Viral Esophagitis

Herpes esophagitis manifests usually as multiple discrete superficial ulcers separated by normal mucosa. The ulcers may be punctate, linear or stellate and are surrounded by radiolucent halos due to edema. In the appropriate clinical setting, the presence of small, discrete ulcers without plaques should be highly suggestive of herpes esophagitis, because ulceration in candidiasis almost always occurs against a background of diffuse plaque formation. When cytomegalovirus and HIV infect the esophagus, large, shallow ulcers up to several centimeters in size are seen in the mid- and sometimes the distal esophagus. The ulcer is usually solitary, ovoid in shape and longitudinal in orientation with smooth margins and often surrounded by a thin radiolucent rim of edematous mucosa. Since the treatment of CMV and HIV esophagitis differs widely, endoscopy with biopsies and cultures is required to differentiate the two infections.[19]

Tuberculosis

Tuberculous involvement of the esophagus is rare. When present, it is usually secondary to current or previous tuberculous infection in other sites. The esophagus may become infected as a result of direct extension from adjacent mediastinal or hilar lymph nodes, vertebral bodies, aortic aneurysms, tuberculous pharyngitis or laryngitis, or by inoculation of swallowed sputum, hematogenous or lymphatic spread.[24]

Tuberculous lesions can occur in any segment of the esophagus. However, they are most common in the middle third, just proximal to the tracheal bifurcation, because of its proximity to the mediastinal lymph nodes around the bifurcation of the trachea.[25] The changes in the esophagus may result from pressure, adhesions or actual involvement of mucosal surface.[24] The most common feature is extrinsic compression of the esophagus, usually by a mass of lymph nodes **(Fig. 16)**. Although the esophageal mucosa is often intact in such cases, the adventitia is usually implicated and this may produce classical traction diverticulum. When the disease process involves the esophageal mucosa, a tumorous lesion or an ulcer may result. Sinus or fistula as a result of rupture of caseous lymph nodes may also occur. Tracheoesophageal or bronchoesophageal fistula and

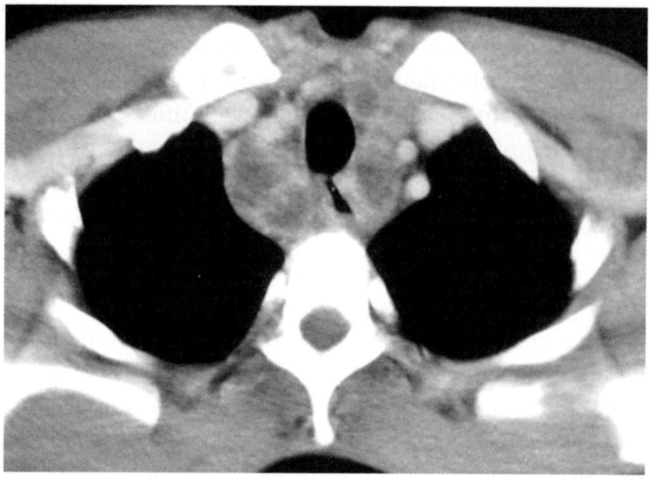

Fig. 16: CECT chest mediastinal window showing multiple variable sized rim enhancing necrotic mediastinal lymph nodes in bilateral paratracheal regions causing extrinsic compression of the esophagus—tuberculosis.

subsequent aspiration pneumonia or lung abscess may occur. A constricting lesion or kinking of the esophagus may be seen as a result of fibrosis.[25]

CT of the chest enables complete evaluation of the caseous mediastinal lymph nodes which surround and displace the esophagus and also depicts any fistulous tract extending from the esophagus to the nodal mass. The presence of amorphous gas in enlarged mediastinal lymph nodes in patients with tubercular lymphadenitis is suggestive of an esophageal nodal fistula.[12]

INFLAMMATORY ESOPHAGITIS

Corrosive/Caustic Esophagitis

Caustic ingestion can cause severe injury to the esophagus and stomach. The severity and extent of damage depends on the type, concentration, volume, physical form (solid or liquid) of the agent and duration of contact with the mucosa. Ingestion is usually accidental in children less than five years of age and intentional in adults. The most common cause is ingestion of a strong alkali (sodium or potassium hydroxide) present in drain cleaners, disc batteries, etc. The term 'lye' refers to substances which contain sodium or potassium hydroxide. Highly concentrated acids such as hydrochloric, sulfuric acid are contained in toilet cleaners, anti-rust compounds. Button batteries are highly concentrated alkaline solution which when lodged in the esophagus can cause burns within four hours and perforation within six hours.

The conventional school of thought is that acids preferentially damage the stomach as they are somewhat neutralized by the alkaline pH of the esophagus and alkalis injure the esophagus and spare the stomach. But extensive esophageal damage and perforation have been known to occur after acid ingestion.

Pathogenesis

Alkali ingestion results in a penetrating injury called liquifactive necrosis which spreads rapidly within seconds through the mucosa and wall of the esophagus resulting in esophageal perforation, mediastinitis and even death. This is most likely to occur with liquid preparations that coat larger mucosal surfaces. While solid lye preparation or alkaline batteries induce a more localized injury to the esophagus. The liquefactive necrosis usually lasts for 3–4 days with vascular thrombosis, mucosal inflammation, resulting in focal or extensive sloughing or ulceration. The esophageal wall becomes thinner in the next few weeks because of sloughing and development of granulation tissue and fibrosis. It takes 1–3 months for re-epithelialization be complete.

The likelihood of a stricture to develop depends on the depth of damage and the degree of collagen deposition.

Acid-induced injury produces a superficial coagulation necrosis that forms a protective layer over the mucosa. Being less viscous than alkaline solutions, they tend to pass quickly into the stomach. Patients of corrosive ingestion may complain of oropharyngeal, retrosternal or epigastric pain, odynophagia or dysphagia. Severe and persistent retrosternal or back pain may be indicative of esophageal perforation with mediastinitis.

Diagnosis and Staging

An upper GI endoscopy should be performed during the first 24 hours after caustic corrosive ingestion to assess the damage, establish the prognosis and guide further treatment. Endoscopy is contraindicated in a hemodynamically unstable patient, if there is severe respiratory distress or there is evidence of perforation.

An endoscopic grading system for corrosive esophageal injury has been developed for predicting clinical outcome, with grades 1 and 2A having an excellent prognosis while at the other end, grade 3B carrying a risk of early mortality in 65% cases. Patients with grades 2B and 3A are known to develop strictures in 70–100% cases.

Esophageal or gastric perforation can occur anytime during the first two weeks of ingestion. Water soluble contrast swallow should be performed to rule out the same. CT has been regarded more useful than endoscopy in assessing transmural damage and extent of necrosis and detecting perforation.

Sequelae of corrosive/caustic injury: Around one-third of patients of esophageal injury, mainly, those with grades 2B or 3 injuries, develop esophageal strictures. Dysphagia occurring due to stricture formation is generally seen two months after the corrosive injury. Barium swallow helps in evaluating the sequelae but is not able to differentiate if it is due to acid/ alkali ingestion. Strictures secondary to corrosive injury are usually long, smooth and mostly involve the middle and distal esophagus **(Figs. 17A to C)**. But variable appearances of caustic/corrosive strictures have been described. They can be short, long or multiple with a smooth outline with nodular defects or scalloping due to focal areas of submucosal fibrosis. It is important to perform a contrast study up to the pylorus to rule out concomitant gastric injury which can occur from 20% to 62.5% cases in the form of antral ulceration, pyloric stenosis or frank gastric outlet obstruction.

Treatment

Esophageal strictures are treated by esophageal dilatations which should be performed 3–6 weeks after the initial injury because of the associated high incidence of perforation if attempted early. The goal is to dilate the esophageal lumen to 15 mm and to completely relieve dysphagia. Long and eccentric strictures may be managed by endoscopic dilatation under fluoroscopic guidance so as to minimize the risk of perforation.

There is an increased risk for the development of esophageal squamous cell carcinoma (SCC) in patients of caustic/corrosive ingestion. This risk is substantially higher in victims of chronic lye ingestion as compared to the general population.[21] The latent period is generally in decades. Hence, these patients should be followed up periodically to rule out the same, with endoscopic surveillance for cancer recommended for 15–20 years after ingestion.

Drug-induced or Pill Esophagitis

Drug-induced esophagitis is caused most commonly by ingesting antibiotics, such as tetracycline and doxycycline which cause only superficial ulceration. Other medications include potassium chloride, quinidine, ferrous sulfate and anti-inflammatory drugs. They generally get lodged in the esophagus at sites of extrinsic compression. These drugs may result in severe esophagitis and strictures may develop.

Clinical Presentation

When such drugs dissolve in the esophagus, they cause mucosal injury by creating an acid pH or by a direct

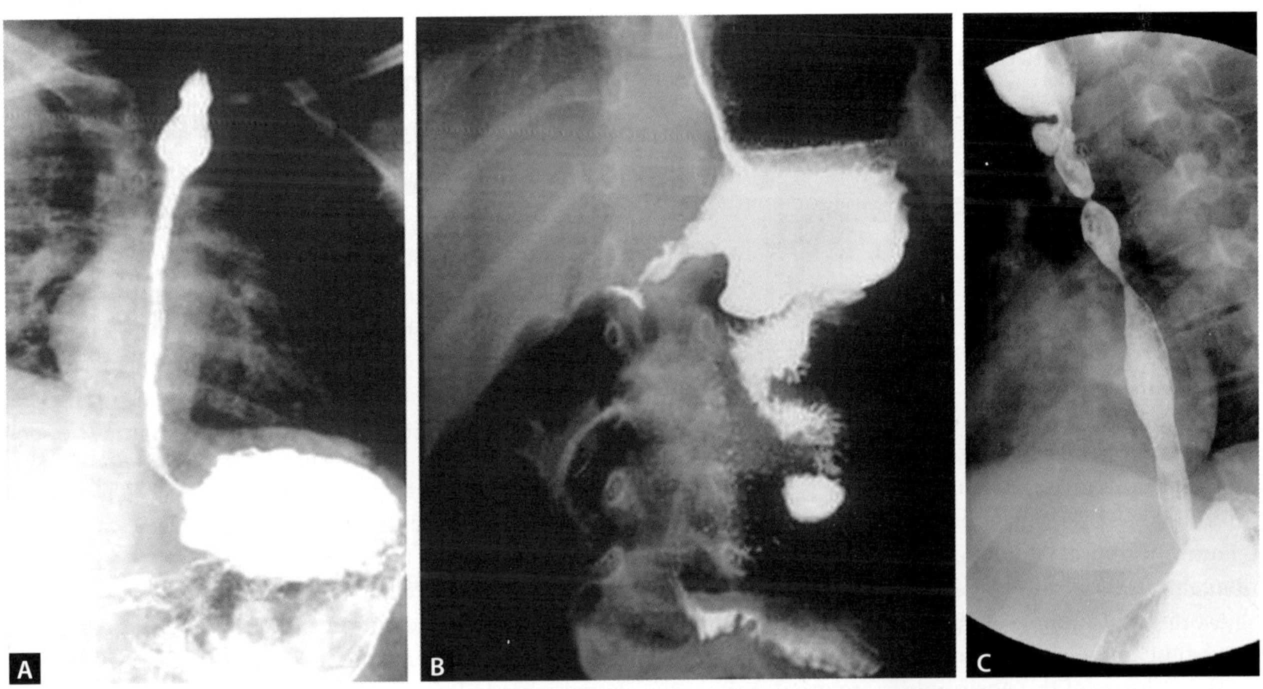

Figs. 17A to C: (A) Barium swallow showing a long stricture with nodular defects due to focal areas of submucosal fibrosis in a case of Caustic esophagitis; (B) The stomach shows narrowing of distal body and antrum with mucosal irregularity; Corrosive strictures in another patient showing (C) multiple, short, smooth strictures with proximal dilatation with diverticulum formation.

irritant effect in the epithelium. Hold up of tablets in the esophagus is favored by swallowing pills while lying down, taking them without water, abnormal esophageal motility, and cardiomegaly. Symptoms are usually sudden in onset and consist of chest pain, odynophagia or dysphagia. The pain of drug/pill-induced esophagitis characteristically develops over a period of hours or will awaken the patient from sleep. A history of ingesting the pill obviates the need for any diagnostic testing. Endoscopy when performed, reveals localized ulceration or inflammation.

Drug-induced esophagitis usually involves the proximal or middle esophagus. A typical location is the aortic arch level, where tablets are delayed because of the aortic indentation on the esophagus and the low contractile force of peristalsis.

Imaging Features

The radiographic findings consist of luminal irregularity, frank ulceration and luminal narrowing. The ulcers are usually ovoid, occasionally linear and clustered circumferentially. A repeat study 7–10 days after withdrawal of the offending agent will show healing of ulcers. CT chest may sometimes show esophageal thickening consistent with transmural inflammation. The condition usually resolves within days to weeks, but symptoms may persist for months. In severe cases, stricture may develop, which may required dilatation.[19]

Eosinophilic Esophagitis

Eosinophilic esophagitis is an increasingly common inflammatory condition characterized pathologically by eosinophilic infiltration of the esophagus that is thought to occur as an inflammatory response to food allergens in susceptible individuals.

Clinical Presentation

The condition should be strongly considered in children and adults with long standing dysphagia and recurrent food impaction. Majority of the patients present with an atopic history of food allergy, asthmas eczema, allergic rhinitis or peripheral eosinophilia.

The diagnosis of eosinophilic esophagitis (EoE) is based on a combination of typical esophageal symptoms and esophageal mucosal biopsies demonstrating infiltration of the esophageal squamous epithelium with eosinophils. It can also be seen with gastroesophageal reflux disease (GERD). However, if the eosinophils are greater than 20 eosinophils per high power field on endoscopic biopsy, a diagnosis of eosinophilic esophagitis should be made.[26]

Imaging Features

Eosinophilic esophagitis may cause segmental or diffuse esophageal strictures that can be diagnosed with esophagoscopy. Strictures may occur most often in the upper to mid thoracic esophagus. It may be associated with distinctive ring-like indentation known as "ringed esophagus". An esophagus with a small caliber may instead be seen in this condition. The "small caliber esophagus" is a radiographic sign that has been described in 2010 by White, Levine et al at barium esophagography and is defined as an esophagus with a caliber of less than 20 mm. The involved segment of esophagus is long with variable length of narrowing having a mean length of 15.4 cm with smooth contours and tapered margins.[26]

Endoscopy needs to be performed for a definitive diagnosis.

Treatment

Treatment includes dietary modification, proton pump inhibitors, steroid therapy, dilatation of strictures. Esophageal dilatation must be cautiously performed in patients with strictures because of increased risk of esophageal mural disruption and perforation.[1,12]

Intramural Pseudodiverticulosis

It is an unusual condition in which inflammation leads to dilatation of the ducts of the deep mucous glands. Intramural pseudodiverticulosis may occur as a consequence of scarring and is associated with strictures in 90% of patients.

Imaging Features

Radiologically, they appear as tiny, flask-shaped outpouchings of contrast material, 1–4 mm in size arranged in clusters or longitudinal rows **(Fig. 18)**. Often the neck of the pseudodiverticula are not opacified and they appear to be separated from the esophageal lumen by 1 or 2 mm and appear to float outside the esophagus. The condition may be segmental or diffuse, and may be seen in association with a peptic stricture in the lower esophagus.

ESOPHAGEAL NEOPLASMS

Benign Esophageal Neoplasms

Benign tumors comprise 20% of esophageal tumors. The most common benign intramural neoplasm of the esophagus is leiomyoma. Others such as hemangioma, schwannoma, neurofibroma and glomus tumor are very rare.

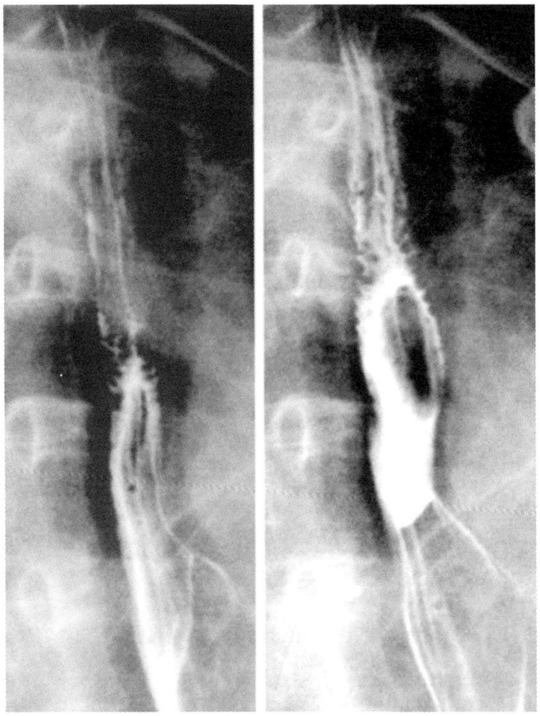

Fig. 18: Intramural pseudodiverticulosis: Tiny, flask-shaped outpouchings arranged in longitudinal rows produced by barium entering dilated esophageal glands, seen in the thoracic esophagus.

Mucosal-based benign tumors of the esophagus are squamous papilloma and adenoma.

Leiomyoma

They are neoplasms of mature smooth muscle cells and account for more than 50% of all benign esophageal neoplasms.[14] Leiomyomas are also the most common mesenchymal tumors of the esophagus in contrast to the rest of the gastrointestinal tract, where gastrointestinal stromal tumors (GISTs) are more common.

Clinical Features

They occur mostly in adults, being twice more common in males than females. However, rarely they may also be seen in children. Most patients are asymptomatic, but dysphagia and pain may develop depending on the size of the lesion and how much the esophageal lumen is getting compromised. Those effected generally have symptoms of more than two years duration[27] and dysphagia to solids is the predominant symptom. On immunohistochemistry, esophageal leio-myomas can be distinguished from GISTs as leiomyomas are negative for CD117 and CD34.

Esophageal leiomyomas mostly involve the mid (60%) and lower (30%) third of the esophagus, where smooth muscle is present.[27] They may arise from the muscularis mucosa or muscularis propria layers of the esophageal wall. Majority of the leiomyomas (97%) are intramural with 10% of them showing circumferential growth pattern. These tumors are mostly solitary with a size of <3 cm. Multiple leiomyomas (leiomyomatosis) can be familial and often associated with Alport syndrome in children. Esophageal leiomyomatosis can occur on its own or be associated with leiomyomas of the tracheobronchial tree and genital tract in the pediatric age group.

Imaging Features

On double contrast barium studies, esophageal leiomyomas appears as smoothly marginated filling defect that forms an obtuse angle with the adjacent esophageal wall. This appearance is characteristic of a submucosal mass.[27] On cross-sectional imaging, it appears as a smoothly marginated exophytic intraluminal mass or as an eccentric esophageal wall thickening **(Figs. 19A and B)**. It shows soft tissue homogeneous attenuation which may occasionally contain calcification. Leiomyomas are iso to hypodense to muscle on non-contrast CT and slightly hyperintense on T2W MR imaging. They show homogeneous enhancement on contrast imaging without any necrosis.[14]

Endoscopic ultrasound (EUS) has a diagnostic accuracy of 89% in the diagnosis of esophageal leiomyomas as it is able to depict which layer of the esophageal wall is involved.[6] On EUS, leiomyoma is seen as homogeneous hypoechoic mass in the muscularis mucosa, submucosa or muscularis propria. On PET-CT, leiomyomas do not usually show avid uptake as these tumors have a low mitotic rate.[27]

Differential diagnosis of esophageal leiomyomas includes duplication cysts, gastrointestinal stromal tumors, lymphoma and hematogenous metastases. Duplication cysts usually manifest in childhood and appear as cysts on all imaging modalities. Calcification is a feature of leiomyomas, but may be seen in GISTs. Small GISTs may mimic leiomyomas as they too appear as homogeneous intramural masses. However, small leiomyomas are relatively more common. Large GISTs may be differentiated on the basis of necrosis or cyst formation in them. Esophageal lymphoma and metastatic disease generally occur in a setting of contiguous invasion or widespread disease.[27]

Treatment

Treatment for esophageal leiomyomas consists of removal in the form of endoscopic resection or surgical enucleation

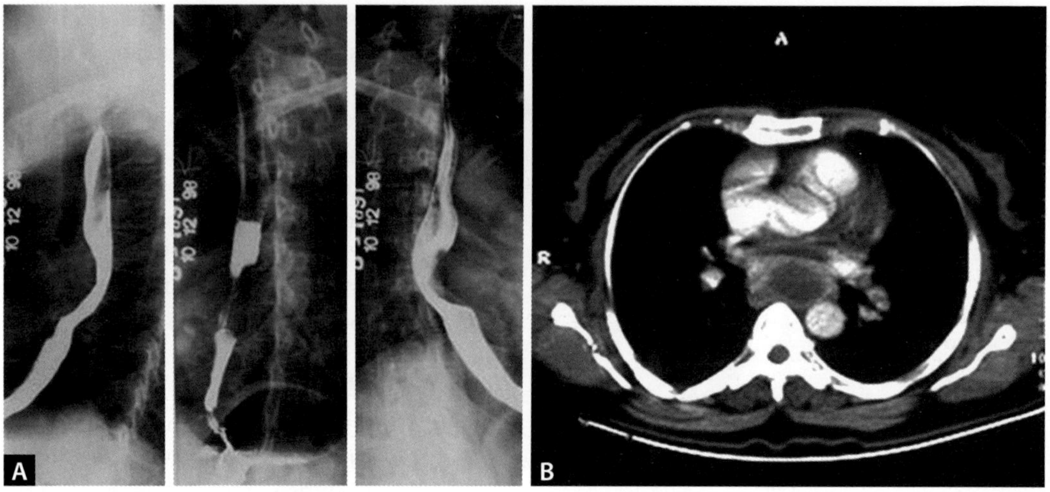

Figs. 19A and B: (A) Leiomyoma in the distal thoracic esophagus seen as a semilunar mass with intact mucosa, narrowing the barium column and widening the esophageal diameter; (B) CECT shows smooth hypodense mass seen indenting the esophageal lumen with intact fat planes around esophagus—leiomyoma.

or conservative follow-up. These lesions have a benign course and usually do not recur after surgery.

Gastrointestinal Stromal Tumors

Esophageal gastrointestinal stromal tumors (GISTs) are uncommon mesenchymal tumors as compared to leiomyomas of the esophagus. Esophageal GIST, similar to other gastrointestinal stromal tumors in the gastrointestinal tract, are positive for C-KIT (a cell surface transmembrane tyrosine kinase also known as CD117) and CD34. These tumors have a malignant potential and have overlapping imaging features with esophageal leiomyomas. Hence, it is important for the radiologist to be familiar with the clinicopathologic and imaging features of these tumors for appropriate patient management.

Clinicopathological Features

Esophageal GISTs are more commonly encountered than previously thought. They occur more often in the lower dorsal esophagus, the site for abundant intrinsic distribution of the gastrointestinal stromal tumor progenitor cells, the interstitial cells of Cajal. The patients generally present late with symptoms of dysphagia because of their submucosal, exophytic location and are usually large at presentation. Patients may also have pain and cough due to the mass effect exerted by the tumor on adjacent mediastinal structures.

Imaging Features

On barium studies GIST appears as a submucosal smoothly marginated mass. Ulceration may be seen in large GISTs on endoscopy or barium swallow study, while it is not a feature of esophageal leiomyomas.

On CT, esophageal GISTs appear as large, heterogeneous intramural soft tissue masses that are isoattenuating to muscles and show moderate postcontrast enhancement. Cystic areas are common in tumor larger than 4.5 cm while calcification is rare. Gastrointestinal stromal tumors show uniform FDG uptake on PET Scan.[28]

Treatment

Treatment consists of surgery alone or along with adjuvant imatinib (tyrosine kinase inhibitor) or radiation therapy. The table below **(Table 3)** lists the differentiating features between esophageal GIST and esophageal leiomyomas.[28]

Fibrovascular Polyp

Fibrovascular polyp is a rare, benign, tumor-like lesion of the esophagus composed of loose or dense fibrous tissue, adipose tissue and vascular structure. The polyp is covered by normal squamous epithelium. The components of fibrovascular polyp may vary from lesion to lesion and in different parts of the same lesion.

A fibrovascular polyp usually arises in the cervical esophagus near the level of the cricopharyngeus. It probably originates in the loose submuscular tissue of the cervical esophagus and gradually elongates over many years as it is dragged into the middle or distal third of the esophagus by esophageal peristalsis, until the intraluminal portion of the tumor becomes massive in size. Occasionally, it may even prolapse through the cardia into the gastric fundus.[29]

Table 3: Differences between esophageal GISTs and leiomyomas.

	Esophageal GISTs	*Esophageal leiomyomas*
1. Tumor size	Larger (~5–6 cm)	Smaller (< 3 cm)
2. Location	More frequently in distal esophagus	Mid (40%) and distal (50%) esophagus both locations
3. Barium swallow	Appears as smooth, submucosal nonobstructive filling defect	Appears as smooth, submucosal nonobstructive filling defect
4. CT scan	More heterogeneous attenuation	More homogeneous density
5. CECT	Moderately enhancing mass	Shows minimal to no enhancement
6. Ulceration	May be present. Seen on endoscopy or barium swallow study	No ulceration seen. Mucosa is normal
7. Calcification	Rare	Uncommon. Diffuse popcorn type
8. PET scan	FDG-avid tumor	Mild FDG uptake
9. Treatment	Surgical resection because of malignant potential/ adjuvant therapy or radiation	Resection/conservative follow-up if asymptomatic

Clinical Features

Fibrovascular polyp generally occur in elderly with slowly progressive dysphagia over years. Other symptoms include vomiting, weight loss, respiratory difficulty likely due to compression of the adjacent trachea by the distended esophagus. Very rarely fibrovascular polyp with a long stalk may regurgitate into the pharynx or mouth, resulting in sudden death from laryngeal occlusion.[14]

Imaging Features

On plain chest frontal radiographs, fibrovascular polyps may be detected as a right sided superior mediastinal mass and on a lateral view may cause compression and anterior bowing of the trachea. It can be differentiated from achalasia due to lack of distension of the distal esophagus.

On barium swallow studies it typically appears as a smooth, expansile, sausage-shaped intraluminal mass that arises in the cervical esophagus and extends to the middle or distal third of the esophagus. It can show a lobulated appearance which if marked, can mimic a malignant neoplasm radiographically. The CT appearance can vary depending on the amount of fat and fibrovascular tissue in the lesion. If fat is the predominant tissue, the presence of an intraluminal esophageal mass with fat attenuation in it is considered a typical sign of a fibrovascular polyp. When oral contrast surrounds the mass on CT, it may help in determining the intraluminal location of the lesion.

MR further aids in characterizing the composition of a fibrovascular polyp. Fat within the mass, mucoid secretion and nonacute blood depict a high signal intensity on T1W images while soft tissue and muscle within the tumor appear as low signal intensity on T2W images.[14]

Treatment

Fibrovascular polyps do not usually undergo malignant degeneration. But still these lesions warrant a removal because of the progressive and debilitating nature of the symptoms. Also, because of the known risk of asphyxiation and sudden death due to the gigantic sizes it can grow to in the esophagus, it is imperative to surgically remove these tumors.

MALIGNANT ESOPHAGEAL NEOPLASMS

Majority (~80%) of the esophageal neoplasms are malignant. More than 90% of these are squamous cell carcinomas or adenocarcinomas which are epithelial neoplasms.

Esophageal Carcinoma: Squamous Cell Carcinoma and Adenocarcinoma

Both squamous cell carcinoma and adenocarcinoma are very aggressive malignant epithelial neoplasms which disseminate early because of lack of serosa in the esophagus. The non- epithelial malignant neoplasms are rare in comparison and include sarcomas, particularly leiomyosarcoma. Lymphoma, malignant melanoma and metastasis also involve the esophagus rarely.

Clinical Presentation

Histologically, the most common esophageal cancer is squamous cell carcinoma (SCC) in 90% cases. However, in recent years there has been a marked increase in the prevalence of esophageal *adenocarcinoma* due to increasing weight gain and obesity and it has been recently found to be the most predominant type of esophageal carcinoma with Barrett's esophagus seen in many of these patients.[1,14] Barrett's esophagus is the most important risk factor which is implicated in the development of esophageal adenocarcinoma. It is a premalignant condition where the normal stratified squamous epithelium of the esophagus is replaced by columnar epithelium secondary to chronic gastroesophageal reflux and reflux esophagitis. These patients may present with symptoms secondary to underlying gastroesophageal reflux disease (GERD). However, most patients have advanced malignancy at the time of presentation with symptoms of dysphagia, odynophagia, rapidly progressive weight loss being similar to that seen in patients with advanced squamous cell carcinoma. Esophageal adenocarcinoma is seen predominantly in males in the seventh decade. Most of them involve the distal third of the esophagus with consequent invasion of the stomach by direct extension across the gastroesophageal junction.

Major risk factors of *squamous cell carcinoma* are tobacco and alcohol intake with other predisposing factors being achalasia, lye strictures, Plummer-Vinson syndrome, coeliac disease and tylosis. Patients with achalasia have a much higher risk of developing esophageal cancer which is 9–28 times that of a person without achalasia. The secondary cancers developing in achalasia patients usually present late in the disease course and have a poor prognosis. They may appear as large, bulky mass within a markedly dilated esophagus. Squamous cell carcinoma is more common in males than females with peak age group of involvement being 60–74 years.[14,27] They are most commonly located in the middle third of esophagus, followed by the lower third and then the upper third. Patients present with progressive dysphagia and by the time dysphagia develops, the esophageal lumen is more than 50% compromised and two-thirds of the circumference of the esophageal wall is invaded by the tumor. Ulceration in the tumor can produce odynophagia and patients may have chest pain unrelated to swallowing if the tumor has invaded the mediastinum.[16]

Independent of staging, the prognosis of esophageal adenocarcinoma is better than SCC, with a 5-year survival rate after resection being 42% compared to 30% for SCC.[27]

Imaging Features

On barium contrast studies, esophageal adenocarcinoma may be indistinguishable from SCC on the basis of morphological findings. Advanced esophageal carcinoma present with a variety of morphologic abnormalities. They may appear as annular apple-core lesion with overhanging margins **(Fig. 20)**, irregular narrowed segment, smooth tapering stricture, bulky endophytic mass **(Fig. 21)**, large ulceration, varicoid infiltrate **(Fig. 22)**, or diffuse nodularity **(Fig. 23)**. Varicoid carcinomas are those in which submucosal spread of tumor produces thickened, tortuous, longitudinal defects that mimic the appearance of varices. Varicoid tumors have a fixed configuration, whereas varices change in size and shape at fluoroscopy. In some cases, esophageal carcinoma spreads submucosally via the lymphatics and reappears at another site in the esophagus **(Figs. 24A and B)**. These satellite metastases may appear as polypoid, plaque-like, or ulcerated lesions separated from the primary tumor by normal mucosa.[19] Tumor also spreads subdiaphragmatically to the proximal stomach via submucosal lymphatics. Fistulization may occur spontaneously, or after radiotherapy.

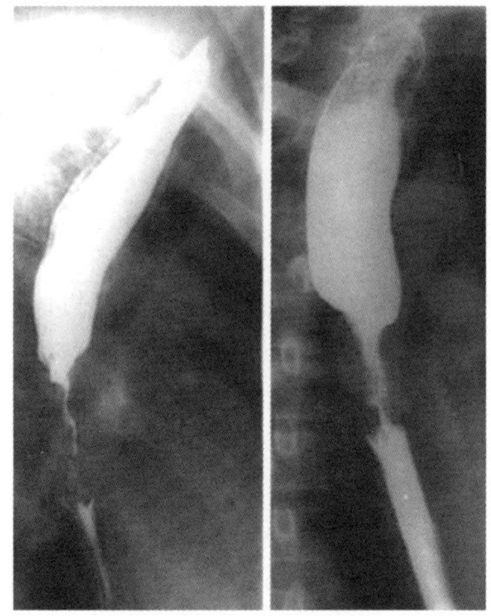

Fig. 20: Annular carcinoma in midportion of esophagus with circumferential infiltration and overhanging margins.

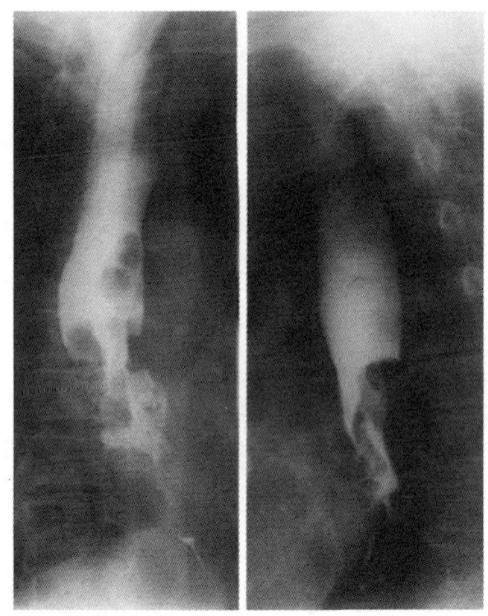

Fig. 21: Polypoidal filling defects with shouldering and irregular narrowing of lumen-carcinoma involving the mid and lower esophagus.

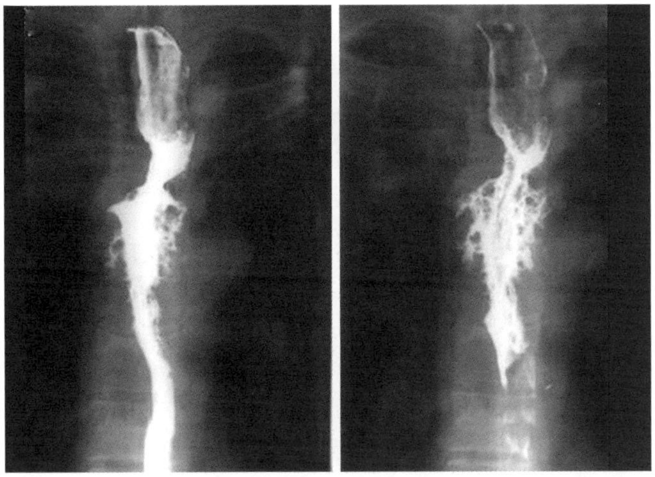

Fig. 22: Spot film of the esophagus at the level of aortic arch shows irregularity and nodularity of the mucosa with lymphatic infiltration-varicoid appearance in squamous cell carcinoma.

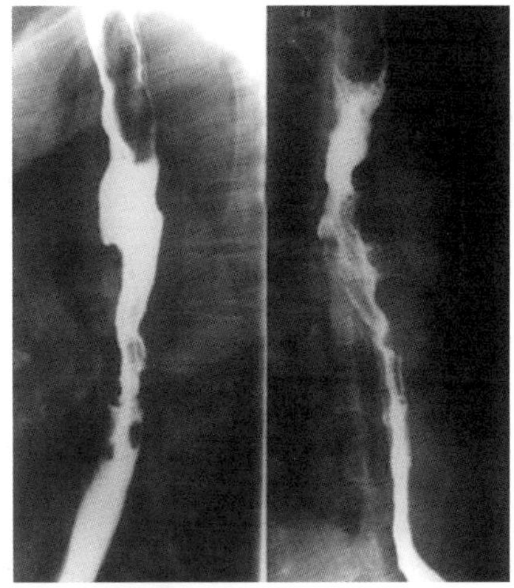

Fig. 23: Carcinoma involving mid esophagus with narrowing of lumen and diffuse nodular filling defects

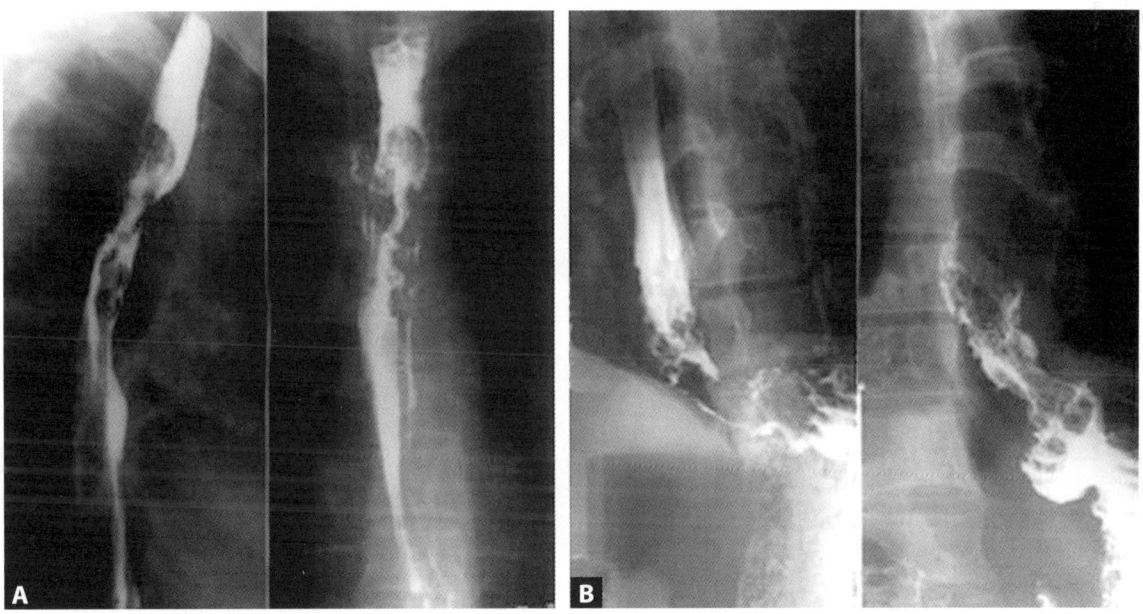

Figs. 24A and B: Carcinoma involving upper and mid esophagus in a circumferential manner. Another lesion is seen just above the esophagogastric junction—multicentric carcinoma.

On CT scans, esophageal carcinoma appears as a mass or wall thickening of soft tissue attenuation **(Figs. 25A to C)**. A recent study on dynamic CECT has shown that the optimal phase in depicting esophageal carcinoma in the late arterial phase as it best depicts the tumor enhancement and the attenuation difference between the tumor and the normal esophageal wall compared to early arterial and venous phases.[30]

On MR imaging the mass appears isointense to the residual esophageal wall on T1W images and intermediate or high signal intensity on T2W images. CT and MRI are both used for staging esophageal carcinoma and are both considered comparable for assessing resectibility in terms of mediastinal invasion, lymph node involvement and distant metastasis.[27] However, in routine clinical situations, CT is recommended.[14]

LEIOMYOSARCOMA

Leiomyosarcoma of the esophagus are rare, low grade malignant lesions accounting for less than 1% of all

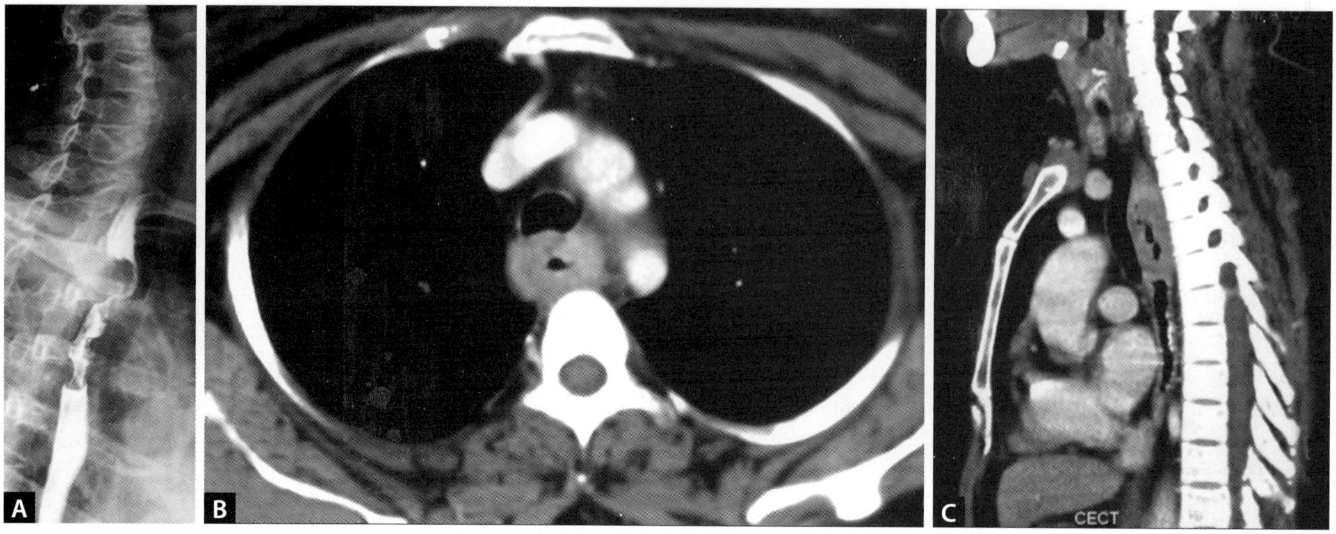

Figs. 25A to C: Barium swallow study (A) showing irregular area of luminal narrowing, ulceration with polypoid filling defect and shouldering involving upper dorsal esophagus; (B and C) axial and sagittal CECT reveals homogeneously enhancing circumferential mural thickening of the upper dorsal esophagus (D2-D5 level) with indentation of the trachea anteriorly. The periesophageal triangular fat pad is preserved: Carcinoma esophagus.

esophagal malignant neoplasms. They are characterised by slow growth and late metastasis, hence have a better prognosis than squamous cell carcinoma.

Leiomyosarcoma are seen in middle aged or older adults. Most of them are thought to arise de novo rather than from pre-existing leiomyomas.[30] They are usually located in the middle and distal thirds of the esophegas as the esophagus here is lined by smooth muscle. Leiomyosarcoma generally spread by direct extention into the mediastrinum or by hematogenous metastases.

Clinical Presentation

Patients present clinically with slowly progressive dysphagia and weight loss. But if tumor has a significant exophytic growth pattern without encroachment on the esophagus, dysphagia can be minimal or absent. GI bleeding can occur if the tumor ulcerates.

Imaging Features

Leiomyosarcoma may sometimes be detected on plain chest radiographs when they show a large exophytic component extending into the mediastinum. Two types of growth patterns have been described—polypoid or infiltrating. The typical appearance on barium studies is a submucosal mass that tends to be larger and more lobulated than benign leiomyoma and may sometimes contain areas of ulceration, cavitation or calcification **(Fig. 26)**.[31]

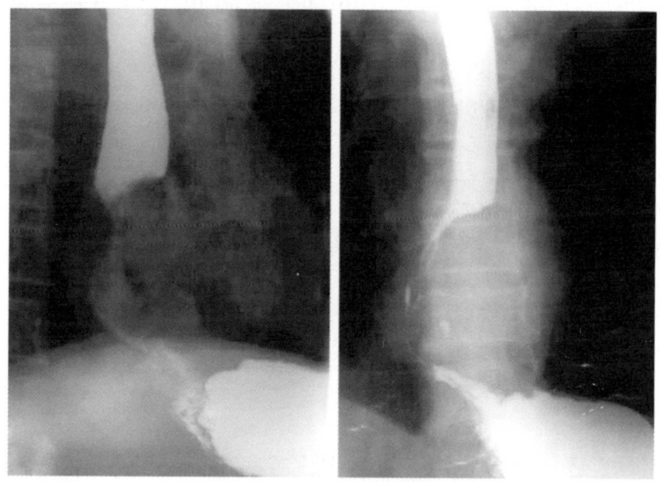

Fig. 26: Barium swallow shows a smooth extrinsic impression on the distal esophagus with a large exophytic component suggestive of an intramural mass—leiomyosarcoma.

On CT, leiomyosarcomas of the esophagus are seen as thickening of the esophageal wall with a large soft tissue exophytic component showing central areas of low attenuation due to necrosis and extraluminal air due to ulceration. An infiltrating type of lesion may be indistinguishable from an infiltrative esophageal cancer.[14] On MR imaging the tumor may appear as a mass that is isointense to skeletal muscle on T1-weighted images and hyperintense on T2-weighted images.

Early treatment is essential as leiomyosarcomas have a better prognosis than squamous cell carcinoma.

LYMPHOMA

Esophageal lymphomas are very rare, accounting for less than 1% of all gastrointestinal lymphomas. Esophageal involvement usually occurs secondary to contiguous spread of lymphoma from the gastric fundus or direct invasion by adjacent lymphomatous lymph nodes. Primary lymphoma has been reported in patients of AIDS.[27]

Clinical Presentation

Patients may present with dysphagia but often these tumors may not produce symptoms and have known to be discovered at autopsy with widespread disease.[14]

Imaging Features

Lymphomas most often occur in the distal esophagus with variable appearance on imaging. On barium studies, they are commonly seen as irregular narrowing of the distal esophagus due to direct spread of the tumor from the proximal stomach. They may also appear as multiple submucosal nodules, polypoid or ulcerated lesions, enlarged folds or rarely as aneurysmal dilatation of the esophagus.[27]

On cross-sectional imaging, lymphomas can cause concentric or asymmetric thickening of the esophageal wall with or without mediastinal lymphadenopathy. A helpful point to remember is that an intact fat plane between the esophageal tumor and adjacent structures goes in favor of an esophageal lymphoma **(Figs. 27A to C)**.[27]

On EUS, the tumor most commonly appears as homogeneously hypoechoic transmural thickening. On PET scan it mostly demonstrates avid FDG uptake.

Treatment

Esophageal lymphomas are treated by a combination of chemotherapy and radiotherapy which have been found to be as effective as surgery.

SPINDLE CELL CARCINOMA

These tumors of the esophagus have both carcinomatous and sarcomatous components and are currently considered as a variant of squamous cell carcinoma.

Imaging Features

Majority of the spindle cell tumors are located in the middle and distal esophagus and are characterized by intraluminal growth rather than esophageal wall invasion.[27] On esophagography it seen as a large polypoid intraluminal mass which mainly expands the esophagus without causing obstruction. The CT appearance is of a large intraluminal mass without proximal dilatation or localized wall thickening. On MR imaging, these tumors show greater enhancement than the esophageal wall.

The differential diagnosis of spindle cell carcinoma includes leiomyosarcoma, fibrovascular polyp, primary malignant melanoma and squamous cell carcinoma. Fibrovascular polyp also appear as polypoid intraluminal masses. This can be differentiated from spindle cell carcinoma as they have a very smooth contour and arise from the cervical esophagus while spindle cell carcinoma are more lobulated and arise from mid dorsal esophagus.

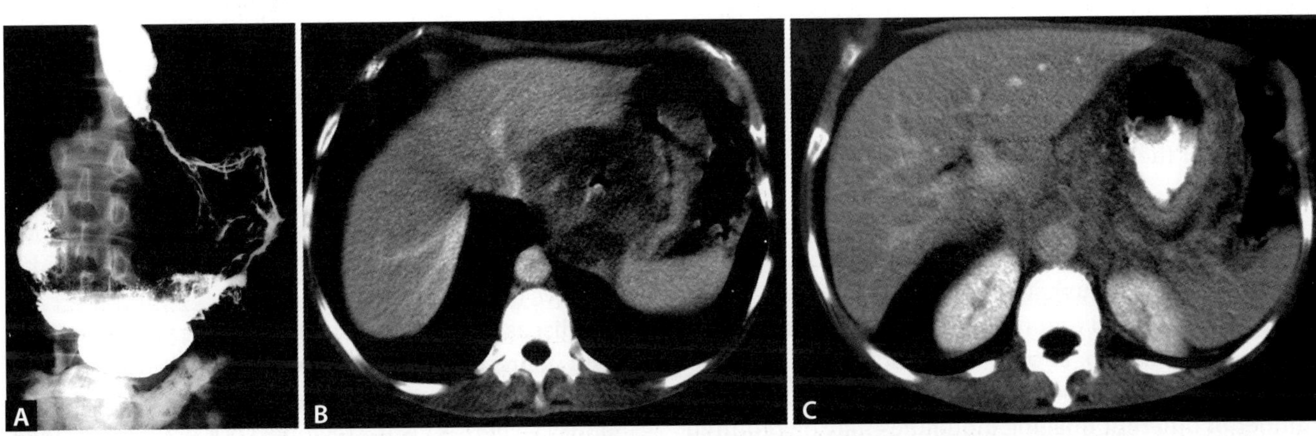

Figs. 27A to C: Barium swallow study (A) shows smoothly tapered narrowing of lower end esophagus with contiguous involvement of the proximal stomach. On CECT (B and C), there is bulky circumferential mass in the distal esophagus with diffuse infiltration into the stomach with preservation of fat planes: Primary esophageal lymphoma of lower end esophagus with contiguous involvement of proximal stomach.

PRIMARY MALIGNANT MELANOMA

These are very rare tumors of the esophagus which arise from malignant degeneration of the pre-existing melanocytes in the esophageal mucosa.

Imaging Features

On barium studies, primary malignant melanoma of the esophagus appear as polypoid intraluminal masses which expand the esophagus without causing significant obstruction. CT scan appearance is of a large intraluminal mass, surrounded by a rim of intraluminal air or contrast. They are not usually associated with lymphadenopathy.

SMALL CELL CARCINOMA

Small cell carcinoma is the most common histologic subtype of neuroendocrine carcinoma. It is a rare but aggressive malignant tumor of the esophagus which metastasizes early and resembles its counterpart in the lung.[27] The tumor usually expands the lumen of the esophagus.

Imaging Features

On contrast swallow it appears as a smoothly marginated, polypoid or fungating mass with ulceration. On CT, it shows irregular eccentric esophageal wall thickening and extensive lymph node metastasis to the mediastinum, supraclavicular region and abdomen. As spindle cell carcinoma is associated with extensive and distant metastasis, CT examination should include both the thorax and the abdomen.

STAGING OF ESOPHAGEAL CANCER

Staging of esophageal cancer is by the TNM classification which has been proposed by the American Joint Committee on Cancer (AJCC) has been revised in 2009 **(Table 4)**. It is the most widely accepted staging system for esophageal cancer and applies to all histologic types of carcinomas regardless of the pathologic type and longitudinal extent of tumor.

Accurate preoperative staging of esophageal cancer is difficult due to its proximity to other structures (aorta, trachea, left bronchus). The malignant nodes are also usually not enlarged and may arise some distance away from the tumor. Also, at time of diagnosis, unsuspected metastases may be present in 30% of cases. Hence, a number of different imaging modalities may be required for accurate staging such as endoscopy, CT, EUS and PET-CT. The multidisciplinary approach is crucial for planning appropriate treatment in patients of esophageal cancer.[32]

Table 4: Seventh edition (2009) of TNM staging system for esophageal cancer.

Category	*TNM Staging*
Tumor	Tis: High-grade dysplasia T1: Invasion of lamina propria, muscularis mucosae, or submucosa T2: Invasion of muscularis propria T3: Invasion of adventitia T4: Invasion of adjacent structures T4a: Resectable (pleura, pericardium, or diaphragm) T4b: Unresectable (aorta, vertebral body, or trachea)
Node	N0: Absent N1: 1–2 regional LNs N2: 3–6 regional LNs N3: ≥7 regional LNs
Metastasis	M0: Absent M1: Present

Initial diagnosis is usually with endoscopy as histological confirmation with biopsy is possible. A good quality double contrast swallow study can detect even early tumors. On a contrast swallow, if the appearance is of a symmetrical smooth narrowing, with gradual tapering to a normal caliber it is indicative of a benign stricture and malignancy can be ruled out safely. On the other hand, if a stricture shows ulceration, irregular mucosa, shouldering and shelf-like margins at fluoroscopy, it can be considered to be malignant at imaging.

Most of the patients undergo a CT scan at initial evaluation for staging. Even though CT is less sensitive than EUS and PET-CT, it is relatively specific for detecting locally advanced or metastatic disease. If these findings are picked up on CT, patient need not undergo further investigation for staging.

The introduction of the seventh edition of the TNM classification in 2009 has resulted in number of changes in the staging of esophageal cancer.[32] The changes which have been incorporated are:

- Tumors of the gastroesophageal junction (GEJ) have been reclassified as lower esophageal tumors if their epicenter is within 5 cm of the GEJ and they extend to involve the esophagus.
- T4 disease has been subdivided into resectable (T4a) and nonresectable (T4b) disease.
- Positive nodal disease has been subdivided into N1, N2 and N3 where N1 is 1–2 regional LN's, N2 is 3–6 regional LN's and N3 is ≥7 regional lymph nodes **(Fig. 28)**.

The spread of esophageal cancer to nodes occurs because of the longitudinal nature of lymphatic drainage. Hence, the revised manual defines regional

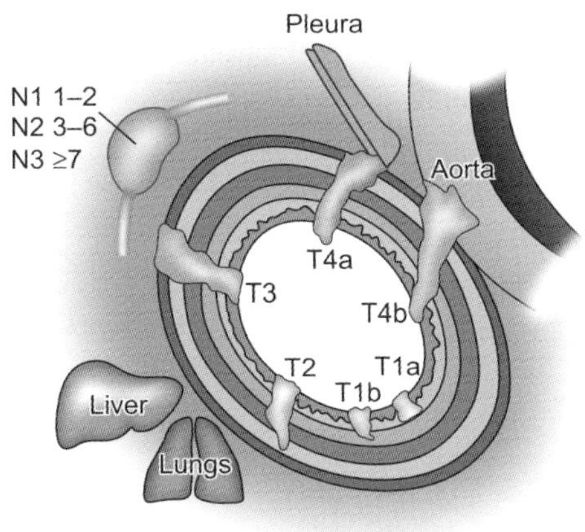

Fig. 28: Drawing illustrating the revised TNM staging system for esophageal cancer (seventh edition).

lymph nodes which includes any paraesophageal lymph node from the cervical nodes to the coeliac nodes.

- Cervical or coeliac axis lymph node involvement are not classified as metastasis (i.e. M1a or M1b) any longer and have been reclassified in regional nodes.

Hence, the new N classification is similar to that used in staging of cancer stomach where N describes the number of cancer positive nodes.[33]

CT for Esophageal Cancer

Role of CT in local or T staging of esophageal malignancy is limited as it is not able to delineate the individual layers of the esophageal wall. Hence, CT is only used for distinguishing T1-T3 stage from T4 stage (i.e. invasion to other structures). Signs of T4 disease are:

- Tumor having an arc of contact of more than 90° with aorta;
- Loss of the triangular fat which is normally seen between the esophagus, aorta and vertebral column; and
- Nodular protrusion of the tumor into the airways.

CT and MR both detect macroscopic periesophageal fat invasion by the tumor with accuracy ranging from 88% to 100%. However, microscopic invasion of the same is not discernible on cross-sectional imaging. Periesophageal fat invasion on CT appears as strand like areas of soft tissue attenuation in the periesophageal fat plane **(Figs. 29A to D)**. On MR imaging, it appears as focal loss of bright signal of fat with periesophageal invasion having ill-defined, irregular margins. Though periesophageal fat infiltration adversely effects prognosis, it is not a contraindication to en-bloc resection of the tumor.[14]

While assessing mediastinal involvement on CT or MRI, accurate assessment of the tracheobronchial tree and aorta (T4 disease) is important as their invasion is a contraindication to surgical resection. The features of tracheobronchial invasion are displacement or indentation of the posterior wall of the trachea or the bronchus by the tumor mass as well as evidence of direct extension of the tumor into the lumen of the airway **(Figs. 30A to D)**. The reported overall accuracy of tracheobronchial tree invasion which has been described ranges from 88% to 97%. It is important to remember that an absent intervening fat plane can also be seen in normal persons and does not always suggest tumor invasion.

Picus et al. in 1983 defined the criteria for aortic invasion on CT which has an accuracy of more than 90%. Aortic invasion is diagnosed when the area of contact between the esophageal cancer and aorta is an arc of more than 90°. When area of contact is less than 45°; aortic invasion is considered to be absent while an area of contact of 45°–90° is considered indeterminate.[34]

The presence of pleural, pericardial diaphragmatic or gastric invasion are not considered contraindications to surgery as the involved area can be removed with the tumor at the time of surgery.

CT is relatively insensitive in nodal staging of esophageal cancer as majority of the malignant nodes are not enlarged (i.e. appear less than 1 cm in short-axis diameter). Also, benign inflammatory nodes may be larger than the cut-off criteria nodes may not be detectable if inseparable from the primary tumor and it may not be possible to accurately measure the number of lymph node metastasis if they are matted. The periesophageal, subcarinal, left gastric and coeliac regions are the common sites of nodal involvement by an esophageal cancer. The supraclavicular and retroperitoneal abdominal lymph nodes are the most frequently involved nonregional lymph nodes, i.e. metastatic nodes. The liver, lungs, bones and adrenal glands are the sites for distant metastasis.

Endoscopic Ultrasound for Esophageal Cancer

Endoscopic ultrasound (EUS) is the modality of choice for assessing the depth of penetration of the primary tumor through the esophageal wall. It is superior to CT/MRI and PET-CT for locoregional or T-staging of the tumor as the individual layer from which the tumor arises is well-visualized. In advanced tumor, if the stricture is too tight the EUS probe may not be negotiable. This indicates that the stage to be almost T3 or T4. Hence, a combination of CT and EUS should usually be performed for initial staging of patients with esophageal cancer.

For nodal disease, EUS has a higher sensitivity than PET or CT, but a lower specificity. *For evaluation of metastatic*

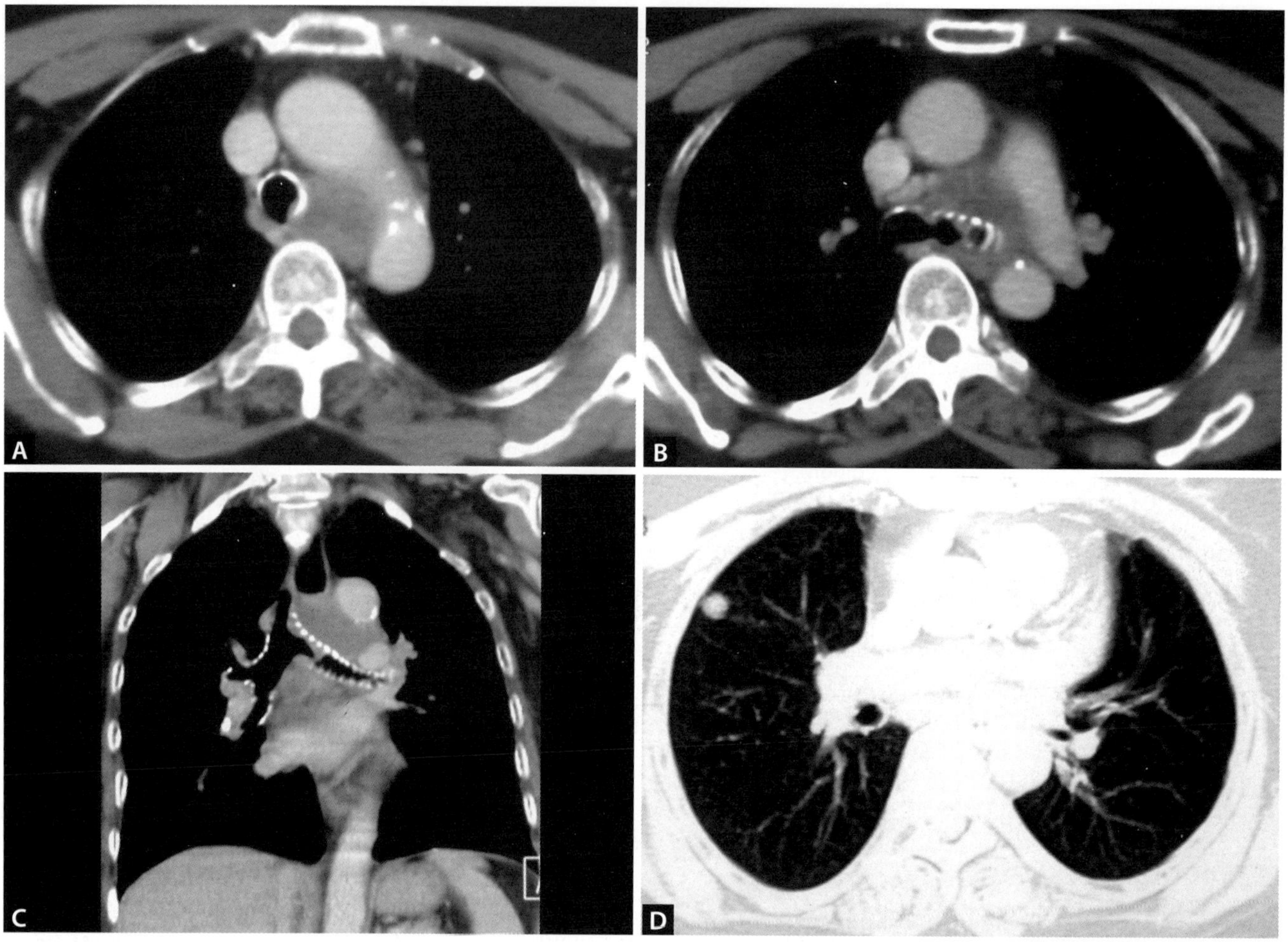

Figs. 29A to D: Contrast-enhanced CT chest in axial (A and B) and coronal planes reveals circumferential thickening of the esophagus with complete narrowing of its lumen with proximal dilatation at the level of carina (C). It is closely abutting the adjacent carinal wall, left pulmonary artery and descending aorta. (D) CT chest depicts a well-defined nodular opacity in the right upper lobe suggestive of a metastatic nodule. Carcinoma Esophagus—Stage IV.

disease, EUS does not have whole body coverage, hence it is to be used along with cross-sectional imaging for identifying the same.

PET-CT for Esophageal Cancer

PET-CT is the technique of choice for identifying metastases to nonregional lymph nodes and other tissues such as liver and skeletal muscle. It should be considered in all patients prior to radical treatment as it has the ability to correctly upstage up to 20% of patients. Even though most esophageal carcinomas appear FDG avid at PET-CT, the investigation has some limitations.[33]

- PET-CT has reduced spatial and contrast resolution which limits the entire anatomic extent of the primary mass to be evaluated.
- Not possible to assess the depth of local tumor invasion in most cases.
- May not be possible to detect early stage carcinoma on PET-CT.
- It has limited role in assessing spread to locoregional lymph node.

However, for T or local staging, PET is not the investigation of choice. If a tumor is not detected on PET-CT, it is likely to be T2 or less in 70% of cases.[32]

In the Seventh edition of the TNM staging system, the biologic activity of the tumor, i.e. histologic grade, is a new cancer characteristic that has been introduced where it is categorized as G1 (well differentiated), G2 (moderately differentiated) and G3 (poorly differentiated). While the stage groupings in the Sixth edition were according to the anatomic T, N, and M classification only, the new

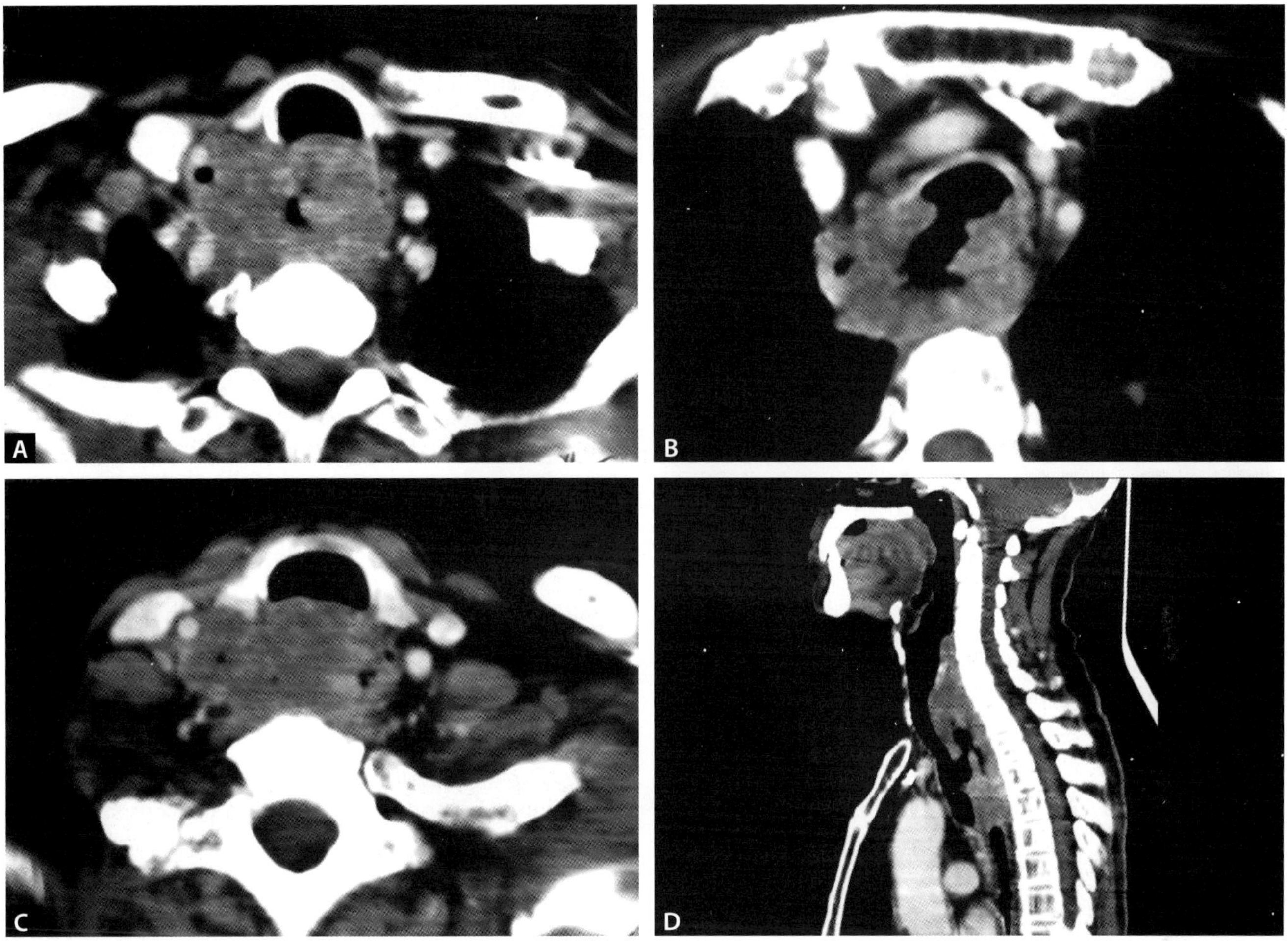

Figs. 30A to D: Axial (A to C) and sagittal (D) CECT reveals long segment asymmetric mass like mural thickening (~ 2.2 cm) of cervical, upper and mid thoracic esophagus (C6–D5 level) with infiltration and fistulous communication with posterior wall of trachea (B and D). There is partial encasement with loss of fat planes with right subclavian and proximal common carotid arteries (A and C): Squamous cell carcinoma (SCC) with tracheo-esophageal fistula.

stage groupings in the Seventh edition have been made according to the anatomic T, N, and M classification as well as nonanatomic cancer characteristics such as histopathologic cell type (SCC or adenocarcinoma), histologic grade (G1, G2 or G3) and cancer location (cervical, upper, mid or lower thoracic esophagus). These stage groupings have been introduced as they have been found to be consistent with data driven analysis and correspond to risk adjusted curves.[33] **Tables 5 and 6** give the stage groupings for esophageal adenocarcinoma and squamous cell carcinoma respectively.

Table 5: Stage groupings for adenocarcinoma.

	Stage				
	N0				
TM Category	***Grade 1-G2***	***G3***	***N1***	***N2***	***N3***
T1M0	IA	IB	IIB	IIIA	IIIC
T2M0	IB	IIA	IIB	IIIA	IIIC
T3M0	IIB	IIB	IIIA	IIIB	IIIC
T4M0			IIIC	IIIC	IIIC
T4a	IIIA	IIIA			
T4b	IIIC	IIIC			
Any T, M1	IV	IV	IV	IV	IV

Abbreviation: G: Histologic grade.

Treatment

A primary tumor that is T1 or T2, i.e. confined to the esophageal wall is potentially curable by esophagectomy. However, most of the patients present with locally advanced disease and 20–30% have distant metastasis at the time of presentation. Those with periesophageal involvement

Table 6: Stage groupings for squamous cell carcinoma.

Stage					
	N0				
TM Category	***G1***	***G2-G3***	***N1***	***N2***	***N3***
T1M0	IA	IB	IIB	IIIA	IIIC
T2M0			IIB	IIIA	IIIC
LE	IB	IA			
UME	IIA	IIB			
T3M0			IIIA	IIIB	IIIC
LE	IB	IIA			
UME	IIA	IIB			
T4M0			IIIC	IIIC	IIIC
T4a	IIIA	IIIA			
T4b	IIIC	IIIC			
Any T, M1	IV	IV	IV	IV	IV

Abbreviations: G: Histologic grade; LE: Lower esophagus; UME: Upper and middle esophagus.

(T3 stage) are treated with combined therapy in the form of neoadjuvant chemotherapy and radiotherapy followed by esophagectomy. T4 tumors are treated with definitive chemoradiotherapy, while patients with distant metastasis undergo palliative therapy.

EXTRINSIC NARROWING

Foreign Bodies

Foreign body ingestion is most commonly seen in children, those with psychiatric disorders, prisoners. In children, coins are the most frequently ingested foreign bodies. Bones from fish and chicken are the second most common foreign body in both children and adults. Most frequently they get lodged in the hypopharynx or cervical esophagus and may be difficult to visualize endoscopically. Patients with history of foreign body ingestion and impaction may present with symptoms such as dysphagia, odynophagia, foreign body sensation or food refusal. They are initially evaluated with plain radiographs of the neck, chest and abdomen. Barium studies are generally discouraged as they may hinder with attempts at endoscopic examination and retrieval later on. CT may be useful in select cases for definitive diagnosis or localization, prior to endoscopy or when perforation or another complication is suspected **(Figs. 31A to E)**.

Smooth foreign bodies, such as coins, buttons, dental crowns generally pass through the esophagus but may lodge in areas of normal anatomic narrowing at the thoracic inlet, aortic arch, or diaphragmatic hiatus. Sharp objects may arrest at any esophageal level. Metallic or dense foreign bodies are recognized on plain films of the neck or chest. Flat objects such as coins are oriented in the coronal plane of the esophagus in contrast to the sagittal plane orientation in the trachea. Obstructing foreign bodies may cause a gas-fluid level in the esophagus or tracheal displacement. Water-soluble contrast is indicated for the initial swallow to exclude perforation. Barium may be used for subsequent swallows. Cotton balls or marshmallows soaked in barium may be useful to demonstrate a small, hard-to detect foreign body. 80% of foreign bodies pass through the gastrointestinal tract spontaneously. If the diameter of the foreign body is too large to pass through the areas of esophageal narrowing, it lodges frequently at one of the three abovementioned areas of esophageal narrowing. Endoscopic removal of the obstructing foreign body may be required in such cases.

On plain frontal radiographs, coins can be differentiated from button batteries by their radiographic densities. While coins show homogeneous radiodensity, the ingested battery shows a central area of decreased density with a rim of increased density.[36]

A simple coin can be allowed to pass through the esophagus without worrying for any corrosive esophageal injury. However, button batteries need to be removed immediately by endoscopy, so as to prevent substantial damage to the esophagus. Due to its electrochemical properties, they can cause local cell death and mucosal necrosis. Complications secondary to ingestion of a button battery may range from local erosion to esophageal perforation to tracheoesophageal fistula. Fatal aortoesophageal fistulas have also been reported.

One must remember that proper history of the patient is very important as chronic impaction of a foreign body in the esophagus may produce features of erosion, fistula formation and inflammatory reaction which may be similar to findings produced by a malignant process.[37]

Vascular Ring

Vascular ring is an aortic arch anomaly in which the trachea and esophagus are surrounded by vascular structures. The most common aortic arch anomaly is the left aortic arch with an aberrant right subclavian artery which occurs in 1 in 200 individuals.[38] The aberrant right subclavian artery arises from the diverticulum of Kommerell which is a persistence of the embryologic right aortic arch. In most cases, the aberrant right subclavian artery crosses posterior to the esophagus **(Figs. 32A to C)**. Patients are symptomatic at extremes of age with children usually presenting with tracheal obstruction or dysphagia. While in adults, aneurysms of aberrant subclavian artery or a

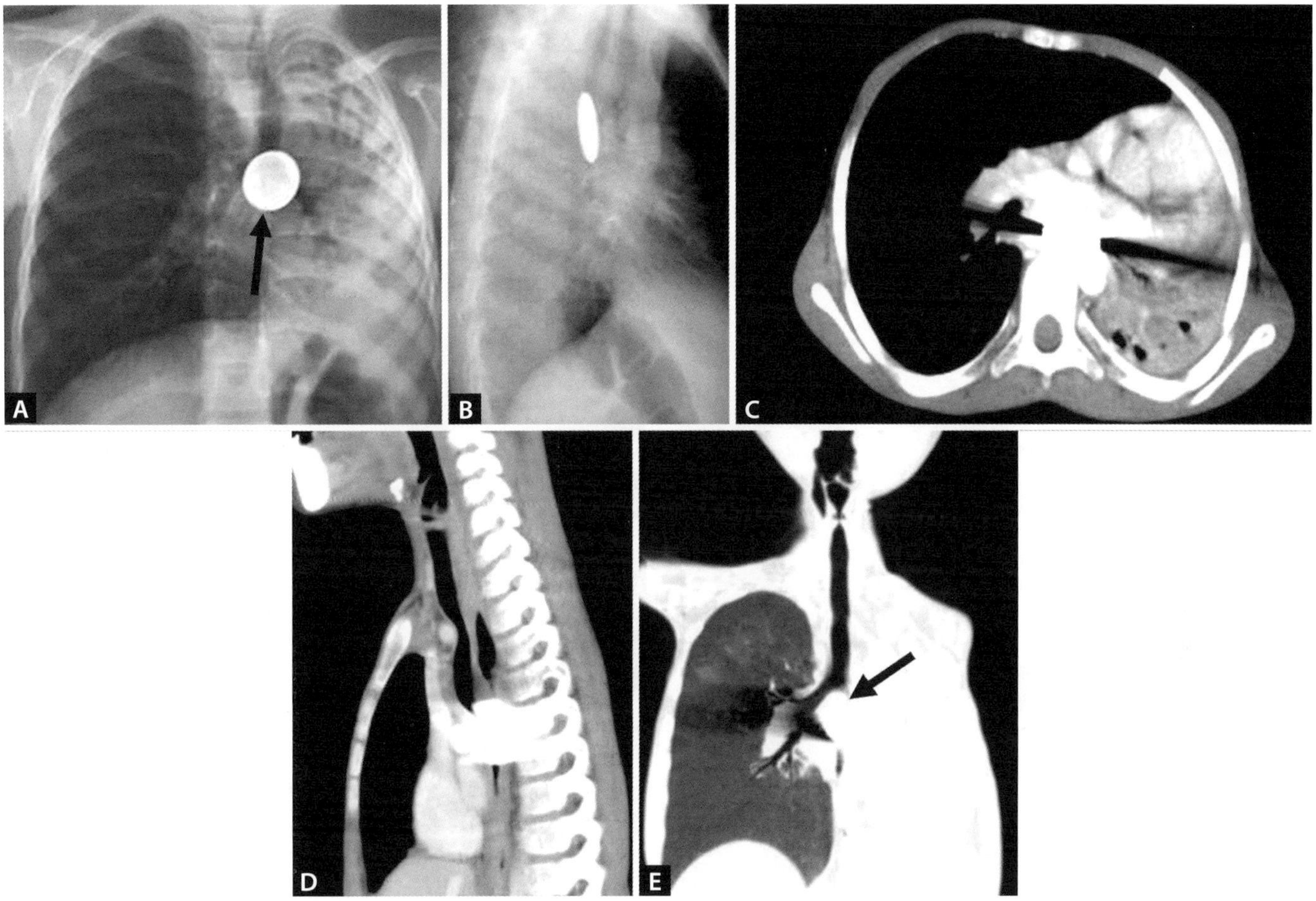

Figs. 31A to E: Impacted esophageal foreign body compressing airway: Frontal (A) and lateral (B) radiographs of chest reveal a well defined round radiopaque foreign body in the esophagus at the level of carina in the coronal plane on frontal X-ray (arrow in A) with associated volume loss of left lung. Contrast-enhanced axial (C) and sagittal MPR (D) images show a hyperdense foreign body giving streak artefacts impacted within the esophagus. (E) Coronal minimum intensity projection (MinIP) image shows near complete occlusion of left main bronchus (arrow) by the impacted esophageal foreign body with collapse of left lung.

prominent diverticulum of Kommerell can occur resulting in dysphagia, classically known as 'dysphagia Lusoria'.[36]

Enlarged Thyroid Gland

Mass effect due to enlarged thyroid gland is most often seen at the level of cervical esophagus. When the enlarged thyroid extends into the superior mediastinum it can result in a mass effect on the upper thoracic esophagus at esophagography. High resolution ultrasonography of the neck can confirm thyroid disease and CT neck apart from confirming helps in determining its extent **(Figs. 33A to C)**.

Enlarged Cervical Osteophytes

Cervical osteophytes are seen in around 20–30% of the elderly who may have neck stiffness and localized or radiating pain. However, large osteophytes have been known to cause dysphagia, odynophagia and globus symptoms. Dysphagia has also been found in patients of diffuse skeletal hyperostosis. The large osteophytes may impinge and mechanically compress the pharynx or upper esophagus causing obstruction **(Fig. 34)**. Another factor that can lead to dysphagia is the impaired tilting of the epiglottis over the laryngeal inlet by the mid cervical (C3-C4) osteophytes.

Retention of food and aspiration has been more often seen in patients with increased osteophytic size (>10 mm) that impinge on the pharynx than those without enlarged osteophytes.[39]

Cervical osteophyte-induced dysphagia is treated depending on the nature and severity of the disease. Sedation, anti-inflammatory drugs, muscle relaxants and

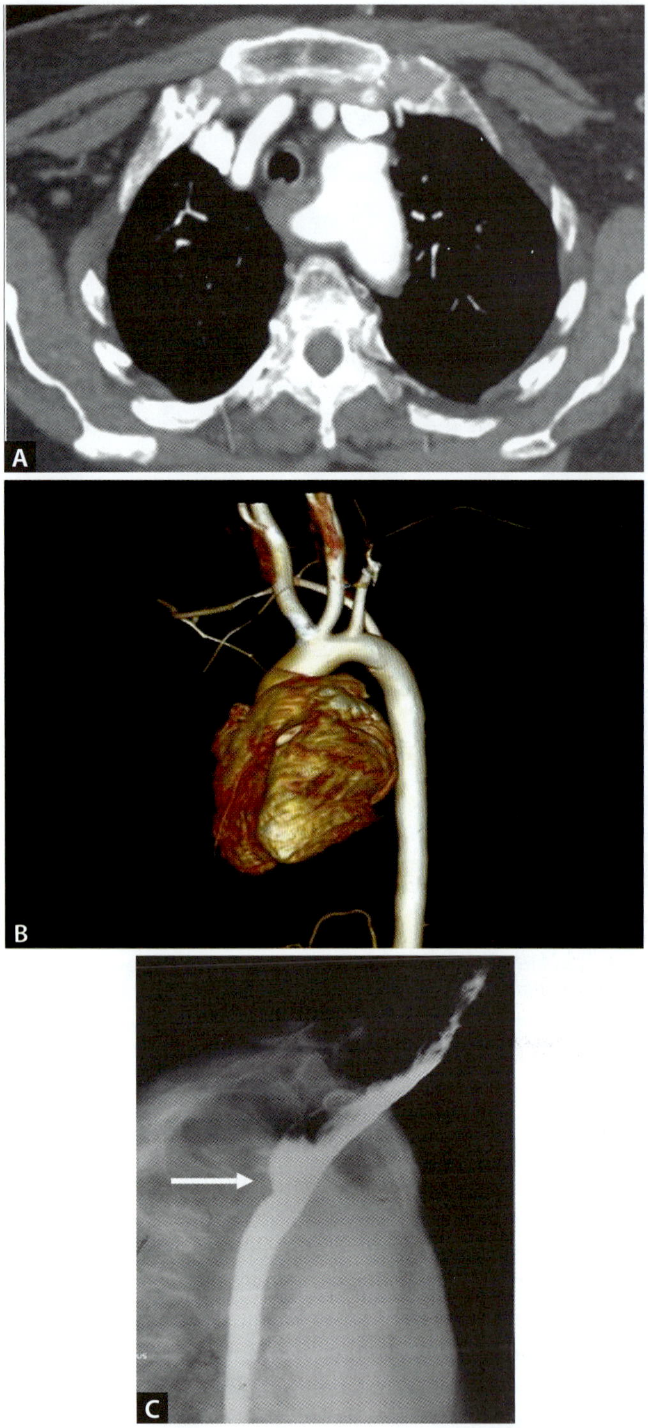

Figs. 32A to C: (A) Axial CECT image shows left aortic arch with aberrant origin of the right subclavian artery coursing behind the esophagus; (B) VRT image depicts the aberrant origin of the right subclavian artery behind the origin of the great vessels; (C) barium swallow study shows oblique indentation (arrow) on the upper esophagus-dysphagia lusoria.

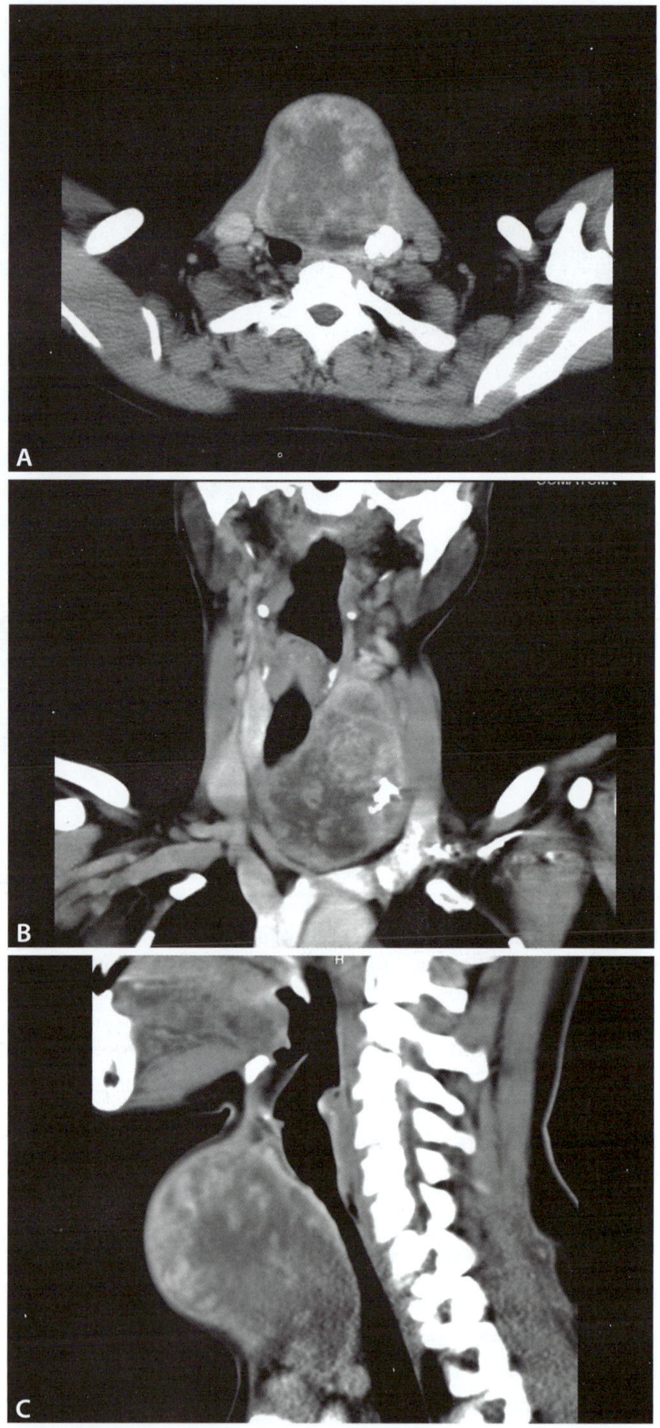

Figs. 33A to C: CECT neck reveals a heterogeneous mass of 5.7 × 7.4 cm predominantly involving the left lobe and isthmus of thyroid with hypodense nonenhancing areas and foci of calcification. The mass is extending to the suprasternal region causing marked tracheal deviation to the right with mild esophageal indentation—colloid goiter.

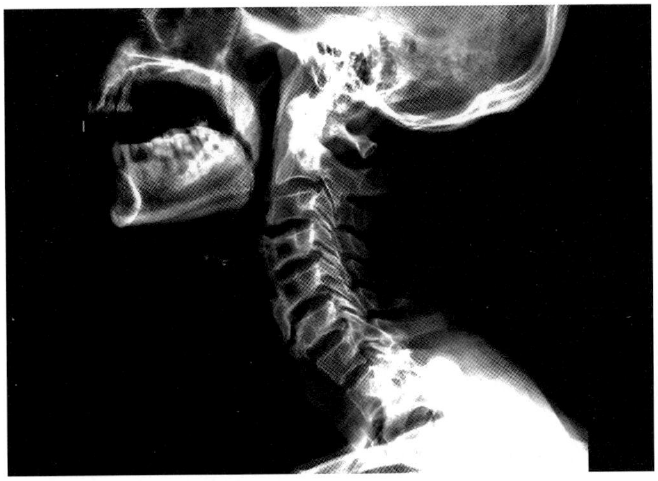

Fig. 34: X-ray lateral view cervical spine reveals enlarged osteophytes of C5, C6 vertebrae impinging on the esophagus.

appropriate soft diet are known to provide substantial relief. Surgical excision of large osteophytosis is reserved for patients with severe symptoms or those whose conservative treatment fails.

CONCLUSION

Dysphagia is a common problem and is generally due to an obstruction which may be either mechanical or functional. Patient demographics and symptomatology have an important role in determining the likely cause (i.e. oropharyngeal or esophageal) in around 85% of patients which helps in guiding subsequent investigation and management **(Flowchart 1)**. Knowledge of the radiological evaluation and imaging spectrum of the possible causes of dysphagia is essential for treatment planning.

Flowchart 1: Algorithmic approach to a patient with dysphagia.

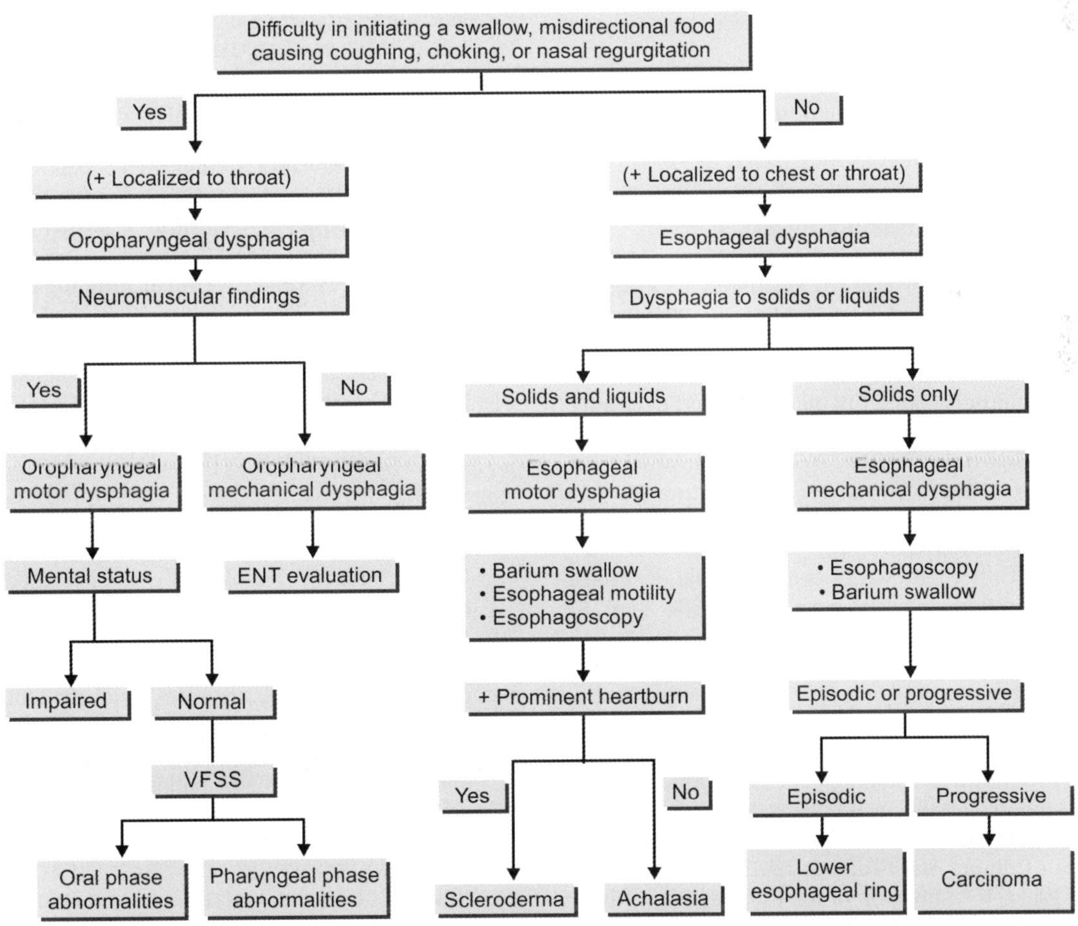

Abbreviations: VFSS: Videofluoroscopic Swallowing Study; ENT: Ear, nose and throat.

REFERENCES

1. Carucci LR, Turner MA. Dysphagia revisited: Common and Unusual causes. Radiographics. 2015;35:105-22.
2. Dodds WJ, Stewart ET, Logemann JA. Physiology and radiology of the normal oral and pharyngeal phases of swallowing. AJR. 1990;154:953-63.
3. Jaffer NM, Ng E, Au FW, Steele CM. Fluoroscopic evaluation of oropharyngeal dysphagia: anatomic, technical, and common etiologic factors. AJR. 2015;204:49-58.
4. Goyal RK. Alteration in gastrointestinal function. Dysphagia. In: Fanci AS, Kasper DL, Longo DL, et al (Eds). Harrison's Principles of Internal Medicine, 17th edition. McGraw Hill (Medical); 2008. pp. 237-42.
5. Spieker MR. Evaluating dysphagia. Am Fam Physician. 2000;61(12):3639-48.
6. Kuo P, Holloway RH, Nguyen NQ. Current and future techniques in the evaluation of dysphagia. Journal of Gastroenterology and Hepatology. 2012;27:873-81.
7. Levine MS, Rubesin SE. Radiologic Investigation of dysphagia. AJR. 1990;154:1157-63.
8. Cook IJ. Oropharyngeal dysphagia. Gastroenterol Clin N Am. 2009;38:411-31.
9. DiSantis DJ. Gastrointestinal fluoroscopy: what are we still doing? AJR; 2008.pp.1480-2.
10. Tao TY, Menias CO, Herman TE, McAlister WH, Balfe DM. Easier to swallow: Pictorial review of structural findings of the pharynx at barium pharyngography. Radiographics. 2013;33:E189-E208.
11. Jones B, Donner MW. Examination of the patient with Dysphagia. Radiology. 1988;167:319-26.
12. Kahrilas PJ, Hirano I. Disease of the esophagus. In: longo DL, Kasper DL, Jameson JL, et al (Eds). Harrison's Principles of Internal Medicine, 18th edition. McGraw Hill. 2012;292: 2427-37.
13. Ba-Salamah A, Zacheri J, Noebauer-Huhmann IM, et al. Dedicated multi-detector CT of the esophagus Spectrum of diseases. Abdom Imaging; 2007. p. 26.
14. Ha, HK, Park SH, Lee SS, Kim AY. Gastrointestinal tract–Esophagus In: Hagga JR, Dogra VS, Forsting M, et al (Eds). CT and MRI of the Whole Body, 5th edition. Mosby (Elsevier); 2009:30(2):1213-371.
15. Riddell AM, Hillier J, Brown G, et al. Potential of surface-coil MRI for staging of esophageal cancer. AJR. 2006;187: 1280-7.
16. Jang KM, Lee KS, Lee SJ, et al. The spectrum of benign esophageal lesions: imaging findings. Korean J Radiol. 2002;3:199-210.
17. Eisenberg RL, Esophagus (Section-1). In: Eisenberg RL (Ed). Gastrointestinal Radiology. A Pattern Approach, 4th edition. Lippincolt Williams & Wilkins; 2003. pp. 3-150.
18. Rabushka LS, Fishman EK, Kuhlman JE. CT evaluation of achalasia. J Comput Assist Tomogr. 1991;15(3):434-9.
19. Pawa S, Prakash A. Imaging of the esophagus. In: Gupta AK, Chowdhury V, Khandelwal (Eds). AIIMS-MAMC-PGI's Comprehensive Textbook of Diagnostic Radiology. 1st edition. The Health Sciences Publisher (Jaypee); 2016;70(2):1139-57.
20. Leslie P, Carding PN, Wilson JA. Investigation and management of chronic dysphagia. BMJ. 2003;326:453-6.
21. Luedtke P, Levine MS, Rubesin SE, Weinstein DS, Larfer I. Radiologic diagnosis of benign esophageal strictures: a pattern approach. Radiographics. 2003;23(4):897-909.
22. Sam JW, Levine MS, Rubesin SE, Laufer I. The "foamy" esophagus: A radiographic sign of Candida esophagitis. AJR. 2000;174:999-1002.
23. Berkovich GY, Levine MS, Miller WT. CT findings in patients with esophagitis. Am J Roentgenol. 2000;175(5):1431-4.
24. Rosario MT, Raso CL, Comer GM. Esophageal tuberculosis. Dig Dis Sci. 1989;34:1281-4.
25. Nagi B, Lal A, Kochhar R, et al. Imaging of esophageal tuberculosis. Acta Radiologica. 2003;44:329-33.
26. White SB, Levine MS, Rubesin SE, Spencer GS, Katzka DA, Laufer I. The small-caliber esophagus: radiographic sign of idiopathic eosinophilic esophagitis. Radiology. 2010;256: 127-34.
27. Lewis RB, Mehrotra AK, Rodriguez P, Levine MS. From the radiologic pathology archives: Esophageal neoplasms: radiologic-pathologic correlation. Radiographics. 2013;33: 1083-108.
28. Winant AJ, Gollub MJ, Shia J, Antonescu C, Bains MS, Levine MS. Imaging and clinicopathologic features of esophageal gastrointestinal stromal tumors. AJR. 2014;203:306-14.
29. Levine MS, Buck JL, Pantongrag-Brown L, Buetow PC, Hallman JR, Sobin LH. Fibrovascular polyps of the esophagus: clinical, radiographic, and pathologic findings in 16 patients. AJR. 1996;166:781-7.
30. Umeoka S, Koyama T, Togashi K, Saga T, Watanabe G, Shimada Y, Imamura M. Esophageal Cancer: Evaluation with triple-phase dynamic CT-initial experience. Radiology. 2006;239(3):777-83.
31. Levine MS. Esophageal cancer radiologic diagnosis. In: Gore RM (Ed.). The Radiologic Clinics of North America. 1997;35:265-94.
32. Godfrey EM, Freeman AH. The esophagus. In: Adam A, Dixon AK, Gillard JH, Schaefer-Prokop CM (Eds.). Grainger and Allison's Diagnostic Radiology (A textbook of Medical Imaging), 6th edition. 2015;26(1):610-26.
33. Hong SJ, Kim TJ, Nam KB, et al. New TNM staging system for esophageal cancer: What chest radiologists need to know. Radiographics. 2014;34:1722-40.
34. Picus D, Balfe DM, Koehler RE, et al. Computed tomography in the staging of esophageal carcinoma. Radiology. 1983;146:433-8.
35. Bruzzi JF, Munden RF, Truong MT, et al. PET/CT of esophageal cancer: its role in clinical management. Radiographics. 2007;27:1635-52.
36. Hryhorczuk AL, Lee EY, Eisenberg RL. Esophageal abnormalities in pediatric patients. AJR. 2013;201:W519-32.
37. Young CA, Menias CO, Bhalla S, Prasad SR. CT features of esophageal emergencies. Radiographics. 2008;28(6):1541-53.
38. Gilkeson RC, Kolodny S. Thoracic Aorta in Hagga JR, Dogra VS, Forsting M, et al. (Eds). CT and MRI of the Whole Body, 5th edition. Mosby (Elsevier). 2009;1:1091-132.
39. Strasser G, Schima W, Schober E, et al. Cervical osteophytes impinging on the pharynx: importance of size and concurrent disorders for development of aspiration. AJR. 2000;174:449-53.

CHAPTER 69

Tumors of Stomach and Duodenum

Gaurav S Pradhan, Rashmi Dixit, Jyoti Kumar, Virendra Jain

INTRODUCTION

Stomach and duodenum can be involved by a wide variety of benign as well as malignant tumors. Benign tumors of the stomach and duodenum, though of more infrequent occurrence than malignant tumors, are sufficiently common to warrant attention.

Benign tumors of the stomach and duodenum are uncommon, with an incidence of 0.4% in autopsy series and 3–5% in upper endoscopic series, most of them performed for unrelated reasons. Over the recent years, the incidence of these lesions is rising due to a higher level of suspicion exhibited by clinicians, and the availability and wide application of diagnostic tools, such as gastrointestinal endoscopy. Most patients with benign stomach and duodenal tumors remain asymptomatic for long periods of time. Symptoms may be vague like abdominal pain or may manifest on account of large size of tumor, obstruction and bleeding. Patients with tumors at specific sites like at GE junction, ampulla of vater may present with dysphagia and jaundice respectively. Some benign polyps can have malignant potential while others may co-exist with a malignant lesion. So, proper evaluation, periodic surveillance and timely treatment hold the key to correct management.

Malignant tumors of the stomach and duodenum include adenocarcinoma, lymphoma, carcinoids and gastrointestinal stromal tumors. Most common among these are carcinoma of the stomach and lymphoma, other tumors are comparatively uncommon. Stomach and duodenum can also be secondarily involved by other malignancies, either by contiguous extension from tumors of the adjacent organs or by hematogenous dissemination. They often produce no specific symptoms when they are superficial and potentially surgically curable, although up to 50% of patients may have nonspecific gastrointestinal complaints such as dyspepsia. The lack of early pathognomic symptoms often delays the diagnosis. Consequently, 80–90% of patients present with locally advanced or metastatic tumors that have poor rates of resectability. High index of clinical suspicion especially in patients with risk factors for gastric malignancy, requires thorough evaluation and due surveillance, so as to pick up the disease at a very early stage.

Endoscopy is the modality of choice for evaluation of upper gastrointestinal tract, not just because mucosal detail is well appreciated but also because simultaneous biopsy of suspicious lesions can be performed. Amongst imaging modalities, barium meal upper gastrointestinal examination remains unsurpassed in the depiction of mucosal detail compared to other imaging modalities such as multislice computed tomography, virtual gastroscopy. This aided by fluoroscopic evaluation of peristaltic activity greatly improves diagnostic accuracy. On the other hand, cross-sectional modalities like CT and MRI are superior to barium examinations in depiction of wall of the viscera as well as extraluminal disease. FDG-PET scanning is useful in the staging and postoperative assessment of various malignancies.

GASTRIC POLYPS

Gastric polyps are classified histologically into three types:

- Epithelial polyps
- Hamartomatous polyps
- Mesenchymal polyps.

Epithelial Polyps

These are the most common type of gastric polyps and they are further divided in three types mainly—*fundic gland polyps (FGPs), hyperplastic polyps, and adenomatous polyps.* The incidence has increased in recent years due to increased number of endoscopic examinations. The prevalence and the type of the polyps also depend on the risk factors in the population under consideration. Hyperplastic and adenomatous polyps are encountered more often in an *H. pylori*-infected territory while fundic gland polyps are seen with increased proton pump inhibitor (PPI) usage.[1] They are usually asymptomatic, however, large polyps often become pedunculated and may erode surface epithelium, which may result in chronic blood loss and iron-deficiency anemia. Rarely they present with gastric outlet obstruction due to prolapsed large polyp into antropyloric region. The clinical importance of these polyps is because of the variable malignant potential and their co-occurrence with other risk factors for gastric malignancy. For these reasons polyps need to be biopsied or resected wherever possible, along with multiple biopsies from surrounding flat gastric mucosa.[2]

On barium images, these lesions are seen as ring shadow enface and small surface nodules forming acute angle on in profile view with the gastric wall. On CT they appear as single or multiple small uniform masses which shows enhancement on contrast enhanced images.

Fundic Gland Polyps

Fundic gland polyps (FGPs) are one of the most common polyps found in the stomach seen on upper GI endoscopy.[3] Sporadic FGPs are sessile polyps and are distributed exclusively in the body and fundus[4] of the stomach with the lesions varying from 1 mm to 8 mm in size, most commonly noted in middle-aged women.[5] Hypergastrinemia associated with a gastrinoma, Zollinger-Ellison syndrome, or long-term therapy with PPIs has been shown to be associated with fundic gland polyps. Few studies also conclude that sporadic FGPs are not associated with atrophic gastritis and have low prevalence of *Helicobacter pylori* infection.[6]

About 30–100% of patients with FAP have been reported to have gastric polyps.[4] Majority (95%) are FGPs while only remaining 5% are actually adenomatous polyps and arise from a mutation in the *APC* gene.[7]

Dysplasia is not common and usually of low grade. The risk factors for dysplasia include large polyp size, and presence of antral gastritis.[8] Polyps associated with PPI use have virtually no malignant potential.[1] As per current guidelines[4] polypectomy is not required for sporadic FGPs because of their low malignant potential. Biopsy is usually indicated at the initial endoscopy to rule out dysplasia or adenocarcinoma. FGPs >1 cm in size are resected assuming sampling error from forceps biopsy alone.[5]

Hyperplastic Polyps

These are the second most common gastric polyps after FGPs and typically occur in the sixth and seventh decades. These polyps are usually sessile or pedunculated, usually less than 2 cm.[4] The polyps are small and are usually multiple and are randomly distributed anywhere in the stomach, although antrum is the typical site.

These are the most common polyps and have a strong tendency to occur in the setting of inflammatory disorders such as chronic gastritis, *H. pylori* gastritis, pernicious anemia, gastric surgical site, bile reflux disease and chemical gastritis.[9,10] In most cases, in addition to polyp biopsy it is also advised to biopsy background flat mucosa to identify etiologic factors if any. 80% of the hyperplastic polyps have been seen to regress after treatment of *H. pylori* infection.[11] They appear as radiolucent filling defects if present on dependent posterior wall or as ring shadows with white rim of barium, if present on nondependent anterior wall. They are found most frequently in the antrum. They are usually smooth, dome-shaped, and measure between 0.5 cm and 1.5 cm in diameter, although they may be much larger. Large hyperplastic polyps often become pedunculated and may present with gastric outlet obstruction because the polyp may obstruct or prolapse through the pylorus.

Like FGPs, hyperplastic polyps also seem to have low neoplastic potential but they have a tendency to have synchronous cancers in the adjacent gastric mucosa especially if associated with chronic gastritis.[12]

Because of low risk of dysplasia and synchronous cancers there is confusion regarding the management of hyperplastic polyps. Recommendations of size criteria for polypectomy range from >2 cm as per few authors and >0.5 cm as per others.[13] Because of more risk of adenocarcinoma in the surrounding nonpolypoid flat tissue as compared to polyps per se, multiple biopsies from the flat uninvolved mucosa is recommended.[4]

Adenomatous Polyps

Adenomatous polyps are the precursor for gastric cancer and are divided into tubular, villous and tubulovillous distinctions histologically. These polyps are usually solitary and seen in the antrum, however can be seen anywhere in the stomach. They are commonly seen as sessile or flat lesions but the pedunculated form may be seen uncommonly. They are also seen in various polyposis syndromes like FAP, Gardner's syndrome,Turcot syndrome. These lesions are usually seen in relation to atrophic gastritis and in the background of intestinal metaplasia. *H. pylori* infection has not been seen associated with them. They vary in size from millimeters to centimeters[5] and larger size >2 cm and villous histology increases the risk of neoplasia (28–40%).[14]

They are premalignant with high-grade dysplastic changes and are currently redefined as noninvasive intraepithelial neoplasia (NiN).[15] It is hence recommended to remove the adenoma with further examination of entire gastric mucosa and biopsy if necessary.

Hamartomatous Polyps

These are mucosal polyps which can arise from any of the 3 embryonic layers and are composed of disorganized tissue in situ. These polyps are seen sporadically, though occasionally they occur as part of a syndrome such as Peutz-Jeghers syndrome, juvenile polyposis, etc. Although hamartomatous means non-neoplastic, they can coexist with adenomatous polyps.[16]

Peutz-Jeghers syndrome is an autosomal dominant hereditary disorder which characteristically has multiple hamartomatous polyps along the entire gastrointestinal system and mucocutaneous hyperpigmentation at the lips.[17] Gastric polyps are seen in 15–30% of the cases. Gastric syndromic polyps are however often indistinguishable from nonspecific gastric hyperplastic polyps and hence endoscopic, pathologic and clinical correlation is required for proper diagnosis.

Juvenile polyps and juvenile polyposis syndrome: These are mucosal tumors that consist of excess lamina propria and dilated cystic glands and hence are occasionally called inflammatory polyps or retention cysts due to these distended glands, inflammatory cells and edema.

These lesions are typically solitary pedunculated polyps and range from 3 mm to 20 mm in size. However, when multiple, a syndrome of juvenile polyposis should be considered.

The different subtypes are difficult to differentiate radiologically. These polyps if small are well circumscribed with smooth, nodular surface if seen en face and are seen to form acute angle with the gastric wall when viewed in profile on barium studies. Larger polyps have a lobulated surface and areas of erosion or ulceration mimicking malignant growth.[18]

Mesenchymal Polyps

These are polyps which arise from mesenchymal tissue and are usually beneath the surface epithelium and hence impart a nodular rather than polypoidal appearance. These include inflammatory fibroid polyps, gastrointestinal stromal tumors, leiomyomas and will be discussed in the later section of the chapter.

MALIGNANT GASTRIC NEOPLASMS

Malignant tumors of stomach and duodenum include adenocarcinomas, lymphoma, gastrointestinal stromal tumors and carcinoid with the most common malignancy being adenocarcinomas comprising 90–95% of all malignant gastric tumors.[1] Gastric malignancy is the second most common malignancy after lung cancer, in the world with incidence in males being twice as common as compared to females. Carcinoma of stomach is significantly more prevalent in Eastern Asia (Japan, Korea, China) and hence most of the early diagnostic techniques and management plans have been developed in Japan. The disease is picked up late especially in western world due to lack of mass screening programmes and vague symptoms like loss of appetite, loss of weight and epigastric pain or discomfort.

GASTRIC ADENOCARCINOMAS

Peak age of incidence for gastric cancers is between 50 and 70 years. It is equally distributed in the antrum, body and the fundus-cardiac region of the stomach with only 10% being diffusely infiltrative. The incidence of more aggressive carcinomas around the gastroesophageal junction has increased over the last two decades.[19] Though a marked reduction has been observed in the incidence of gastric carcinoma in North America and Western Europe in the last 50 years, 5-year survival rates are less than 20%, as most patients present late and are unsuitable for curative, radical surgery. There is an increased recognition of the association with *Helicobacter pylori* infection believed to increase the risk by 3-6 fold.[20] Other associated risk factors include inherited genetic component, pernicious anemia, adenomas, atrophic gastritis, patients having "A" blood group and those who have undergone gastrectomy. A number of dietary factors like salted, smoked and pickled food and food rich in nitrates also predispose a person for gastric cancer.[21]

Screening methods with variable success rates like-endoscopy, *H. pylori* antibody and serum pepsinogen testing are used at various places.[22]

Pathophysiology

Gastric carcinomas are classified according to cell types with adenocarcinoma being most common. Gastric adenocarcinomas are divided into 2 types. Type 1 adenocarcinomas are intestinal tumors and have well-formed glandular structures. This form of gastric carcinoma is more likely to involve the distal stomach and occur in patients with atrophic gastritis. It has a strong environmental association. Type 2 adenocarcinoma is a diffuse type, though cardia is commonly involved. Gastric wall infiltration is more pronounced in this type and patients have worse prognosis than type 1 tumors.

EARLY GASTRIC CANCER

The need for early gastric cancer (EGC) to be recognized as a separate entity originated in Japan, as there is high prevalence of gastric malignancy in the region and early detection and definitive treatment hold the key to successful outcome. These lesions are confined to the mucosa or submucosa irrespective of the nodal metastasis[23] (T1, any N) and are classified into 3 types as per Japanese system (elevated, superficial, shallow):[24]

1. *Type I:* Elevated lesions in gastric wall, protruding more than 5 mm into the lumen
2. *Type II:* Superficial lesions that are elevated (IIa, <5 mm), flat (IIb), or depressed (IIc)
3. *Type III:* Excavated, irregular ulcers with nodular, clubbed mucosal folds.

Limited literature is available for role of double-contrast barium upper GI examination in early gastric cancers.[25,26] With the widespread use of endoscopy, multiple endoscopic biopsies of suspicious lesions are considered the diagnostic procedure of choice for early gastric cancer. Recent advances of CT like multiplanar reformatting (MPR), surface shaded display, virtual gastroscopy, and dynamic contrast imaging have significantly improved the detection rate of type 1 EGC. On CT EGC lesions are commonly seen as focal enhancing thickening of the inner layer with visible low-attenuation outer layer and maintained perigastric fat planes. However, lesions without thickening or enhancement are likely to be missed.[1]

ADVANCED GASTRIC CANCER

Advanced gastric cancer (AGC) is the most commonly diagnosed form of gastric cancer seen in western world, defined as involvement of muscularis propria and beyond. The gross morphology of advanced lesions on imaging can be either polypoid, infiltrative or ulcerative with considerable overlap among them. The polypoidal lesions can have acute angle with gastric wall suggesting epithelial nature of the lesion.[1] Advanced gastric cancers are usually larger than 3 cm and most symptomatic patients present in this stage. Borrmann classified the advanced gastric cancers morphologically into 4 types.[27] Type 1 are polypoidal lesions, Type 2 are ulcerative, Type 3 are ulceroinfiltrative and Type 4 infiltrating linitis plastica type lesions.

Staging of Gastric Cancer

Tumor, node and metastasis (TNM) staging by the AJCC/UICC is the most commonly used staging system for gastric cancer. Two modifications have been made in their 7th edition *Tumor Staging Manual*. Firstly tumors arising at the gastroesophageal junction or gastric tumors which are crossing it but arising in the stomach <5 cm from GE junction are staged using the TNM system for esophageal cancer. Secondly, the stomach T categories **(Tables 1 and 2)** [28] have been harmonized with the T categories of the rest of gastrointestinal tract.[29]

The T stage, representing the extent of penetration through the gastric wall, is categorized in the **Table 1**.

Table 1: T-category (Gastric cancer).

- TX primary tumor cannot be assessed
- T0 no evidence of primary tumor
- *Tis carcinoma in situ*: Intraepithelial tumor without invasion of the lamina propria
- T1 tumor invades lamina propria, muscularis mucosae or submucosa
- T1a tumor invades lamina propria or muscularis mucosae
- T1b tumor invades submucosa
- T2 tumor invades muscularis propria
- T3 tumor penetrates subserosal connective tissue without invasion of visceral peritoneum or adjacent structures.
  T3 tumors also include those extending into the gastrocolic or gastrohepatic ligaments, or into the greater or lesser omentum, without perforation of the visceral peritoneum covering these structures
- T4 tumor invades serosa (visceral peritoneum) or adjacent structures
- T4a tumor invades serosa (visceral peritoneum)
- T4b tumor invades adjacent structures such as spleen, transverse colon, liver, diaphragm, pancreas, abdominal wall, adrenal gland, kidney, small intestine and retroperitoneum

Table 2: TNM staging of gastric cancer.[28]

Stage of gastric cancer	*TNM grades*
0	Tis, No, Mo
1A	T1, N0, M0
1B	T1, N1, M0, T2, N0, M0
2A	T1, N2, M0, T2, N1, M0, T3, N0, M0
2B	T1, N3, M0, T2, N2, M0, T3, N1, M0, T4a, N0, M0
3A	T2, N3, M0, T3, N2, M0, T4a, N1, M0
3B	T3, N3, M0, T4a, N2, M0, T4b, N0 or N1, M0
3C	T4a, N3, M0, T4b, N2 or N3, M0
4	Any T, any N, M1

N Staging

In the TNM staging system, the N category is defined on the basis of number of metastatic lymph nodes involved. As opposed to TNM staging the anatomical nodal stations are used in the Japanese system (JCGC 13th edn).[1]

The N stage, representing the number and site of draining lymph nodes involved, is categorized as follows:

- NX-Regional lymph nodes cannot be evaluated
- N0-No lymph nodes involved
- N1-Metastases in 1-2 regional lymph nodes
- N2-Metastases in 3-6 regional lymph nodes
- N3-Metastases in >7 regional lymph nodes
- N3a-7-15 regional lymph nodes
- N3b-16 or more regional lymph nodes.

Lymph node involvement and their localization are of paramount importance in deciding the surgical management. Lymph node metastases occur in approximately 80% of patients with gastric cancer. The frequency is related to the size and depth of the tumor with local perigastric nodes being involved first, followed by the regional (celiac, hepatic, left gastric, splenic) and distant (left supraclavicular and axillary) nodes. A wide range of values for accuracy have been reported on CT/MRI which vary with the threshold values of the size, margin, architecture and enhancement pattern. It is recommended to report all visible lymph nodes regardless of their size and to leave it to the histopathology for accurate N staging.[1] CT depicts 75% of nodes larger than 5 mm in diameter, but it does not depict tumor in normal-sized nodes. CT is not useful in distinguishing between enlarged nodes due to reactive changes and those due to tumor. The local nodes (N1) are located in the prepyloric region and in the gastrocolic and gastrohepatic ligaments. These nodes are removed by performing the standard gastrectomy procedure. The regional nodes (N2), located in the porta hepatis, hepatoduodenal ligament and peripancreatic region, are not routinely removed during gastrectomy procedure. So their detection is more important.

Recently it has been suggested that EUS and MDCT are comparable for both T and N staging and considered complementary techniques for loco regional staging.[30,31]

M Staging

The M stage, representing the presence of metastases, is categorized as follows:

- M0—No distant metastases
- M1—Distant metastases.

As the portal vein drains the stomach, the liver is the most common site for hematogenous metastases. Less common sites are the lungs, adrenal glands and kidneys. Bony and cerebral metastases are uncommon.

Intraperitoneal and omental metastases are common in advanced gastric cancer. They consist of nodules, localized fluid collections, irregular thickening and stranding of the mesentery and omentum. Ascites and small-bowel obstruction may also occur.

Imaging Features of Advanced Gastric Cancer

Upper GI endoscopy is the preferred technique for detection of gastric cancer which is also useful in obtaining histological confirmation of suspicious gastric lesions. Many cancers are picked up at asymptomatic level by this technique. However, due to limitation of evaluation of gastric wall and locoregional spread its role is limited.

Barium UGI Features

Malignant gastric ulcer is the most common presentation of gastric cancer on upper GI barium studies, hence it is important to differentiate benign from malignant ulcers **(Figs. 1A to C)**. Malignant ulcers are usually nonprojecting, with ulcer brim being wide and thick with central ulceration (Carman-Kirklin meniscus sign), distorted irregular radiating folds stopping well short of ulcer brim.[7] As opposed to malignant ulcers, a typical benign ulcer shows projecting ulcer **(Fig. 2A)** with an ulcer collar or mound with symmetrical radiating folds reaching up to brim of the ulcer **(Fig. 2B)**. There is also undermining of gastric mucosa noted in benign ulcers which is seen as a filling defect/lucent line rimming the ulcer crater on double contrast barium meal (DCBM) known as Hampton's line (Pathognomonic) **(Fig. 2C)**. Barium meal fluoroscopic procedures help

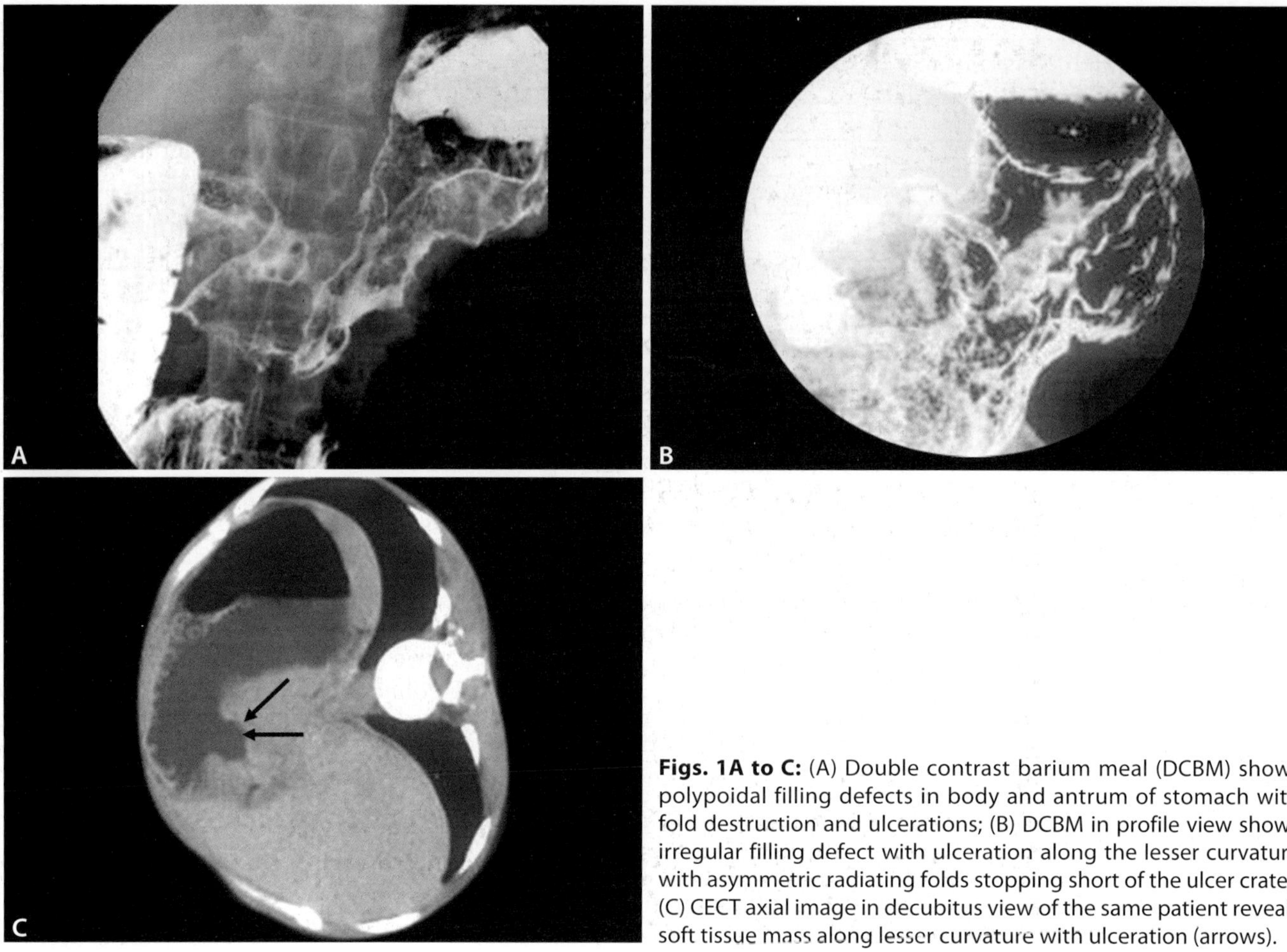

Figs. 1A to C: (A) Double contrast barium meal (DCBM) shows polypoidal filling defects in body and antrum of stomach with fold destruction and ulcerations; (B) DCBM in profile view shows irregular filling defect with ulceration along the lesser curvature with asymmetric radiating folds stopping short of the ulcer crater; (C) CECT axial image in decubitus view of the same patient reveals soft tissue mass along lesser curvature with ulceration (arrows).

in differentiating benign and malignant lesions and in evaluating response to treatment. However, the ease of direct visualization and choice of guided biopsy makes endoscopy a routine procedure of choice.[32]

Polypoid carcinomas are lobulated masses that protrude into the lumen. They may contain one or more areas of ulceration **(Fig. 3A)**. With ulcerated carcinomas, an irregular crater is located in a rind of malignant tissue. On profile view, these lesions are seen to be intraluminal as opposed to benign projecting ulcers, and on enface view, nodular distorted mucosal folds are seen converging to the edge of the ulcer **(Fig. 3B)**.

Infiltrative cancers on the other hand can have non-scirrhous or scirrhous (desmoplastic) histology. Non-scirrhous lesions have stomach wall thickening as well as rugal fold thickening in the form of nodularity or spiculation of the mucosa **(Fig. 4A)**. On the contrary aggressive scirrhous lesions exhibit wall thickening with loss of mucosal folds. If diffuse, scirrhous lesions are called linitis plastica. They cause narrowing of the stomach with a rigid structure (leather bottle stomach) and are better appreciated on fluoroscopic imaging than endoscopy **(Fig. 4B)**.[18]

In the lesions of the cardia, as distal esophagus is often involved, submucosal spread of tumors may result in pseudoachalasia or secondary achalasia with tapered, beaklike narrowing of the distal esophagus along with infiltration of the gastric cardia **(Figs. 5A to C)**.

CT Features of Gastric Cancer

Computed tomography (CT) has become an indispensable tool for diagnostic evaluation of the stomach because of its superiority to barium studies over depiction of gastric wall as well as extra luminal disease. CT is used preoperatively, primarily to determine the stage and extragastric spread of a gastric carcinoma. MDCT with thin collimation [1.25 mm sections reformatted at 1 mm intervals] is performed using water as oral contrast agent. Water is preferred as an oral contrast agent over positive oral contrast medium, as enhancing gastric wall and subtle abnormalities can be

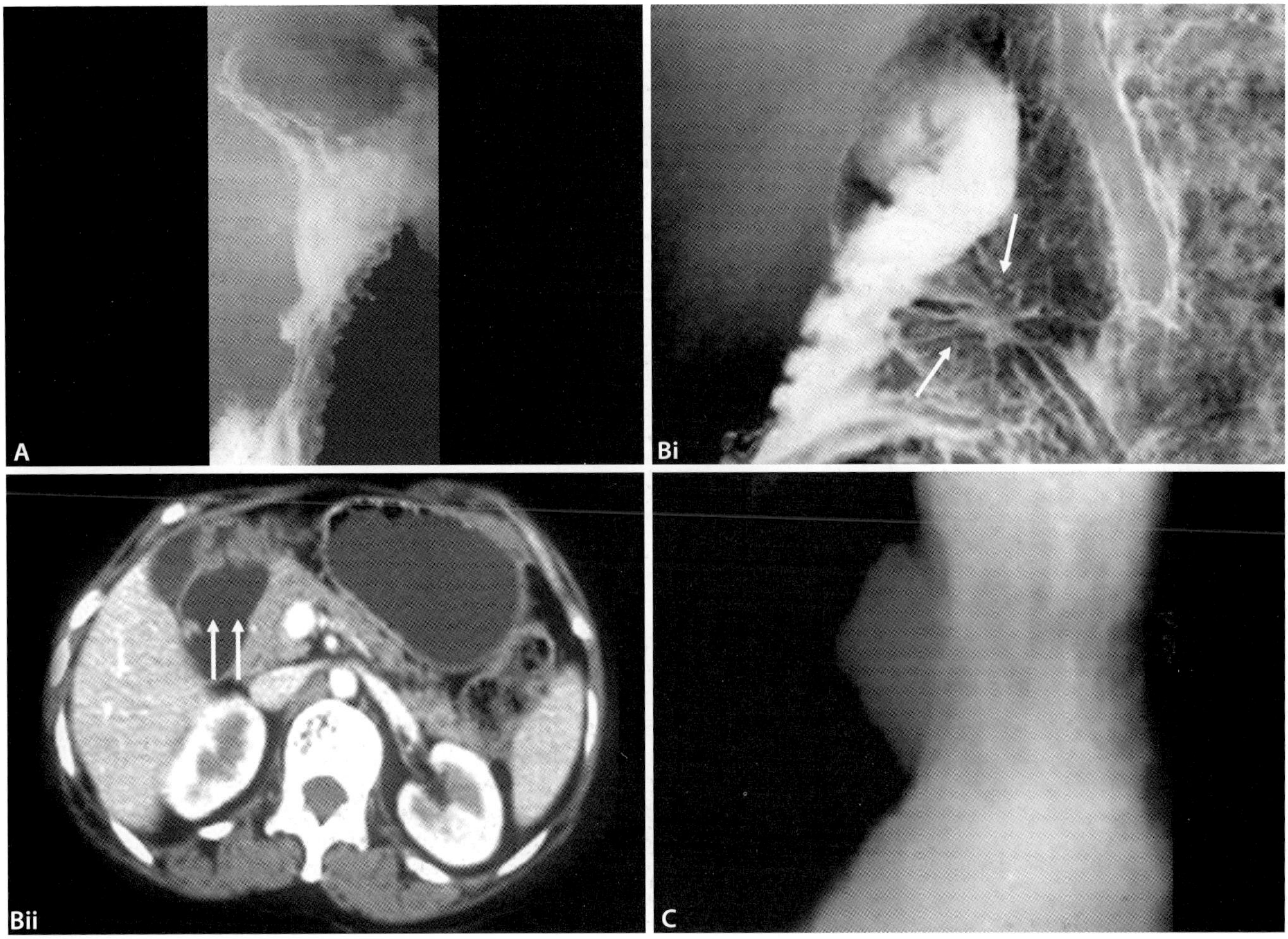

Figs. 2A to C: (A) Barium-filled crater seen projecting beyond the line of gastric contour on profile view; (Bi and ii) Double contrast barium meal study en face view showing a contrast-filled benign gastric ulcer along the anterior wall of stomach with the gastric folds seen reaching up to the ulcer margin. CECT of the same patient reveals mild gastric wall thickening in the antrum with ulceration; (C) Thin radiolucent line (Hampton's line) rimming the mouth of ulcer crater on profile view.

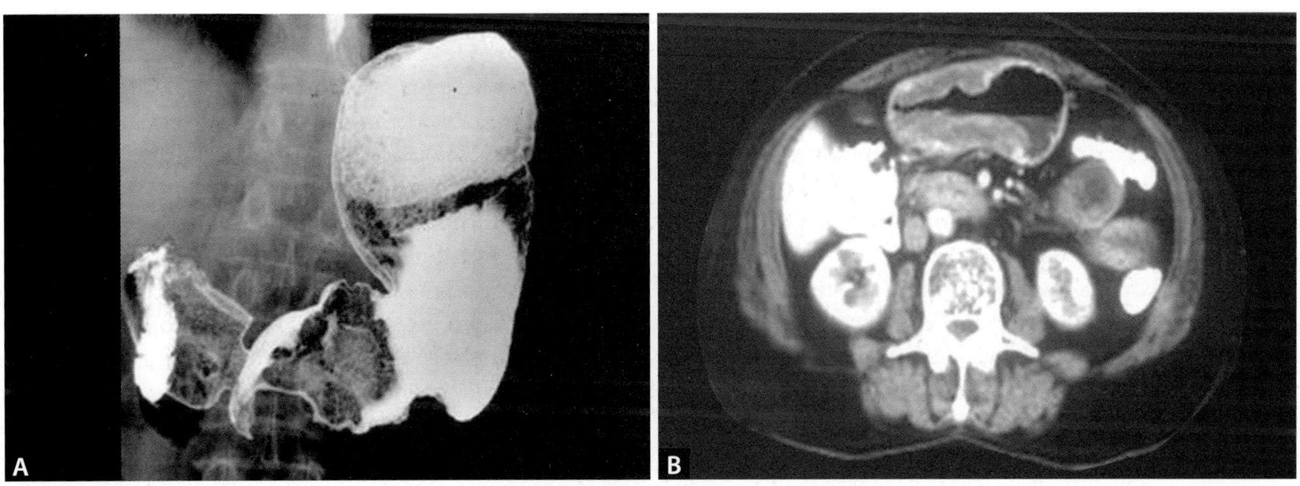

Figs. 3A and B: (A) Irregular polypoidal filling defect noted along greater and lesser curvature of the stomach distally on DCBM study with narrow string like pyloric canal and shouldering proximally. Visualized duodenum shows normal mucosal outline; (B) Heterogeneously enhancing polypoidal mural thickening noted in the gastric antrum on CECT. There is no perigastric extension noted.

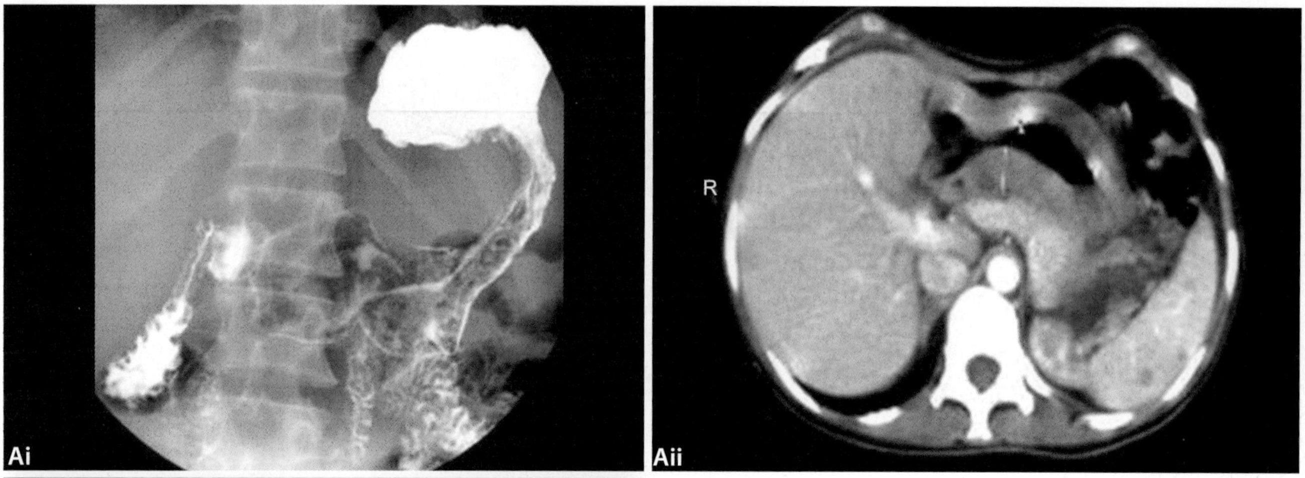

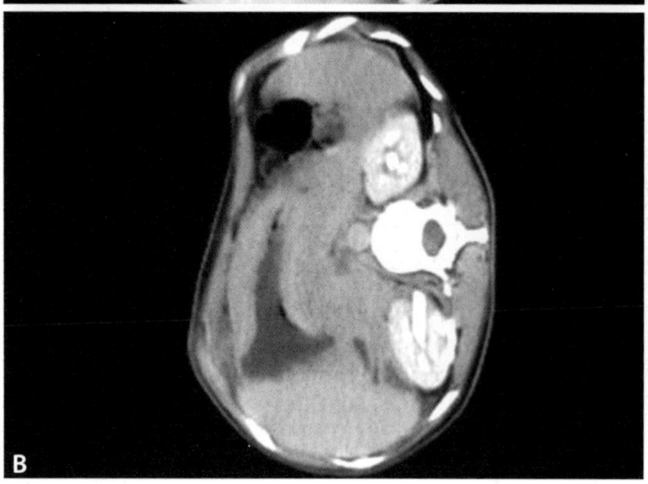

Figs. 4A and B: (A) DCBM reveals markedly reduced distensibility of body and antrum of stomach in a case of adenocarcinoma (Scirrhous type); (B) CECT of the same patient reveals diffuse circumferential mural thickening (~2 cm) in the region of body and antrum of stomach, in supine and decubitus position.

well visualized and because it does not interfere with 3D imaging and CT angiography. Normal gastric wall is about 5–10 mm. In gastritis, the thickness is usually less than 10 mm while in carcinoma it is usually more than 10 mm. In lymphoma, gastric wall thickness is more than 20 mm. We also need to evaluate thickening on parameters like eccentric or circumferential lesion, focal or diffuse and whether the thickening shows enhancement. Stomach wall may however appear thickened if poorly distended and if obliquely oriented in the scan plane, like the GE junction and cardia which can be taken care of by adequate gastric distension (hydro-CT) or by changing patient position. Combination of unenhanced MDCT with air distension of stomach and dual phase contrast enhanced MDCT with water distension also improves the detection and T staging of the primary tumor. In addition, biphasic evaluation with early arterial phase is used to assess enhancement of the gastric wall while the portal venous phase is used to assess the liver parenchyma for metastases because they are mostly hypovascular **(Fig. 6)**.

CT scans may show focal wall thickening, ulcerations, polypoidal mass with or without ulceration or diffuse wall thickening. Mucinous carcinomas have low attenuation (high mucin content) and occasionally may contain calcification **(Figs. 7A and B)**. Transpyloric extension of antral lesion is seen in both carcinoma and lymphoma. Although more common in lymphoma, statistically carcinoma is more common overall hence it is not a reliable finding to differentiate the two. Usually there is focal wall thickening with mucosal irregularity or ulceration, which may show marked contrast enhancement (typically scirrhous carcinomas). Tumor invasion of the perigastric (T3) fat is seen as soft-tissue stranding and further extension involves adjacent structures (T4). AGC can also involve diaphragm, adrenal glands, peritoneal cavity and abdominal wall. Gastric carcinoma can metastasize to ovaries. These metastases are usually bilateral and are known as Krukenberg tumors **(Fig. 8)**.

Direct extension of the tumor into adjacent structures is relatively common. The pancreas is invaded via the

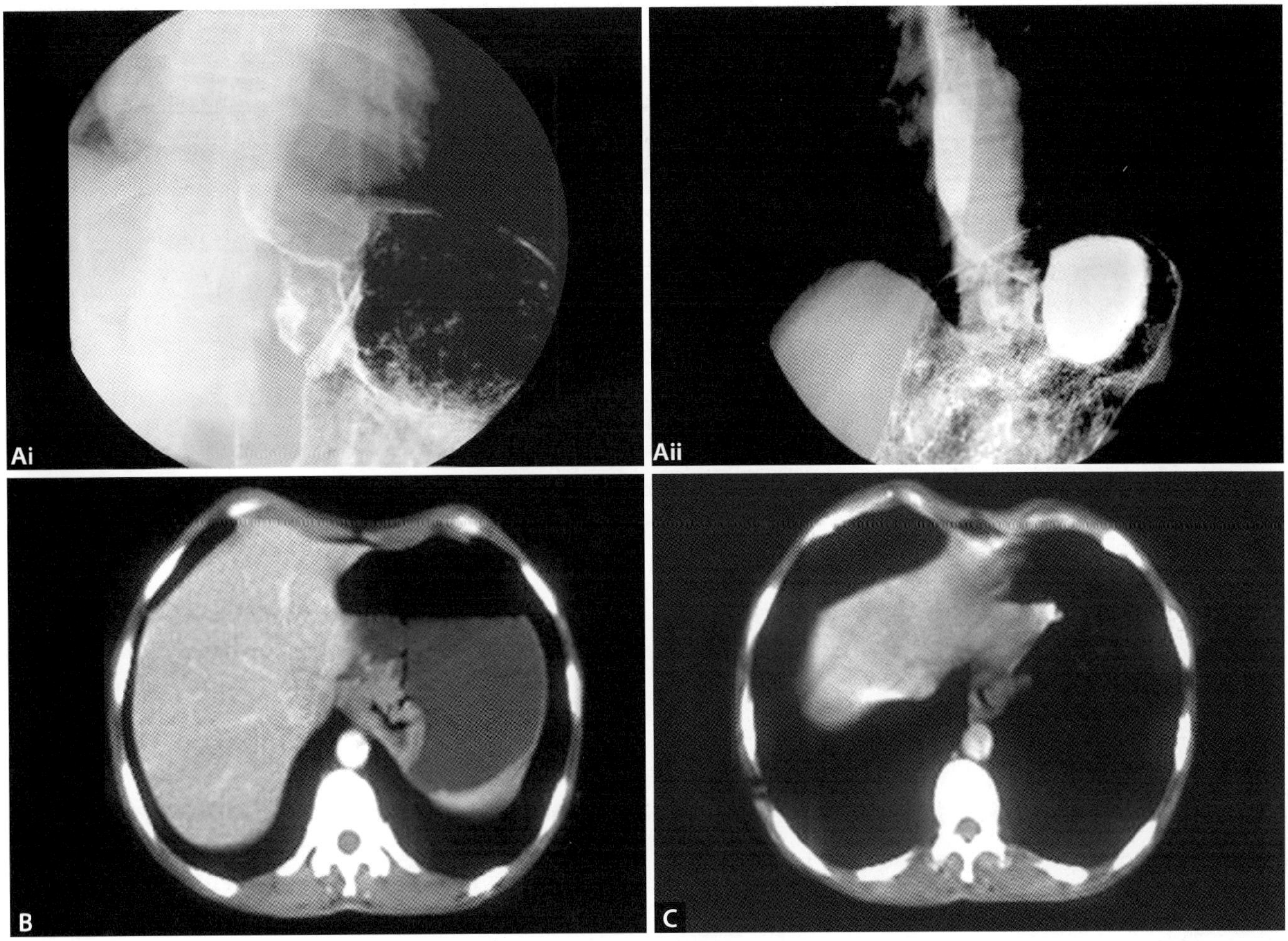

Figs. 5A to C: (A) Beak-like narrowing of GE junction with mass at gastric cardia with pooling of barium suggests ulceration on DCBM; (B and C) Axial CECT sections of the same patient reveal heterogeneously enhancing soft tissue mass at GE junction with ulceration in a patient of adenocarcinoma.

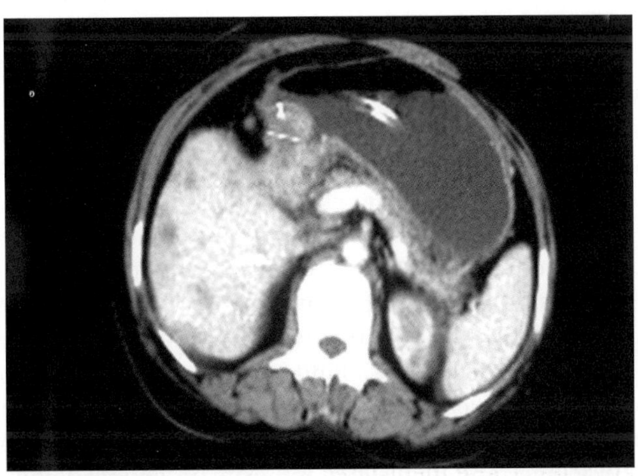

Fig. 6: CECT abdomen shows circumferential mural thickening of antropyloric region in a patient of adenocarcinoma with multiple non-enhancing hypodense lesions in the liver symptoms of metastasis.

lesser sac **(Figs. 9A and B)**, the transverse colon, via the gastrocolic ligament and the liver via the gastrohepatic ligament. Longitudinal spread to the distal esophagus occurs in as many as 60% of patients with carcinoma of the cardia. However, the duodenum is involved in only 5–20% of antral carcinomas[1] **(Fig. 9C)**. Left gastric nodes are consistently involved in most gastric cancers. The regional nodes (N2), located in the porta hepatis, hepatoduodenal ligament and peripancreatic region, are not removed by the routine gastrectomy procedure. So their detection is more important **(Figs. 10A and B)**.

Limitations of CT Scanning

Carcinoma in the region of the cardia is often missed on CT due to normal soft tissue thickening due to reflections of phrenicoesophageal ligaments and attachment of gastrohepatic ligament along lesser curvature. In

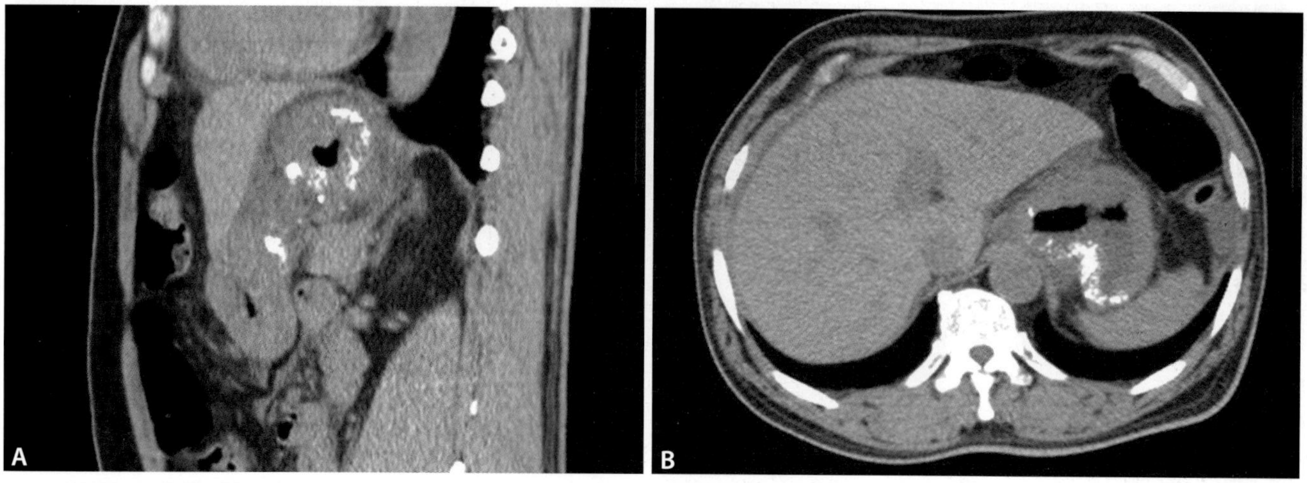

Figs. 7A and B: Noncontrast axial and sagittal scans of a patient with mucinous cystadenocarcinoma reveal diffuse thickening of the gastric wall with punctuate foci of calcification.

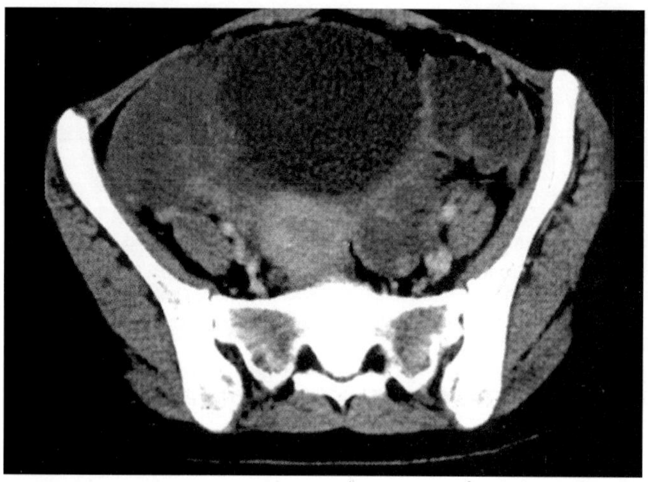

Fig. 8: In a postoperative case of carcinoma stomach, axial contrast-enhanced images reveals multicystic masses in bilateral adnexa suggests Krukenberg tumor in a postoperated case of recurrent gastric carcinoma.

double-contrast studies or on CT done after proper distension, normal anatomic landmarks are obliterated and replaced fallaciously by a plaque-like lesion. Moreover, loss of fat plane between the gastric wall and the left lobe of the liver may be seen.

On CT, T2 and T3 lesions may be difficult to distinguish. For AGC, the differentiation between serosal (T4A) versus the adjacent organ invasion (T4B) is more practical for surgeons for the planning of management. Focal change in the CT attenuation within the adjacent organs is required to make a diagnosis of adjacent organ invasion (T4b), not simply loss of intervening fat plane,[1] as loss of a fat plane between the tumor and pancreas may be due to an inflammatory reaction. In emaciated patients, loss of fat planes may simulate direct organ invasion and it is difficult to differentiate between T3 and T4 stage. CT may be inaccurate in assessing nodal involvement as small nodes may contain tumor, and large nodes may result from inflammatory causes. Further perigastric nodes may not be delineated, if the stomach is not well distended. CT may also fail to depict tiny omental and peritoneal deposits.

Inspite of inherent limitations, CT remains the staging modality of choice because it can help identify the primary tumor, assess for local spread, and detect nodal involvement and distant metastases.

Magnetic Resonance Imaging

Magnetic resonance imaging (MRI) provides better soft tissue resolution than CT and the fast-imaging technique is superior to CT in detecting serosal invasion. It is however, comparable to CT for T and N staging.[33] Since MRI is time consuming, costly and limited by motion artifacts it is not routinely used for diagnostic evaluation. Limited data is however, available for MRI of gastric lesions. The lesions show intermediate signal on T1W images compared to the surrounding normal mucosa and muscularis propria. Similar to CT, signal alteration on MR in adjacent organ implies involvement by tumor, rather than just loss of fat plane. Low signal intensity on T2W images and high signal intensity on opposed phase images are also noted.[34] MRI may be slightly better than CT for few T1 and T2 lesions but with similar results for T3-4 lesions, nodal and distant metastasis assessment. So

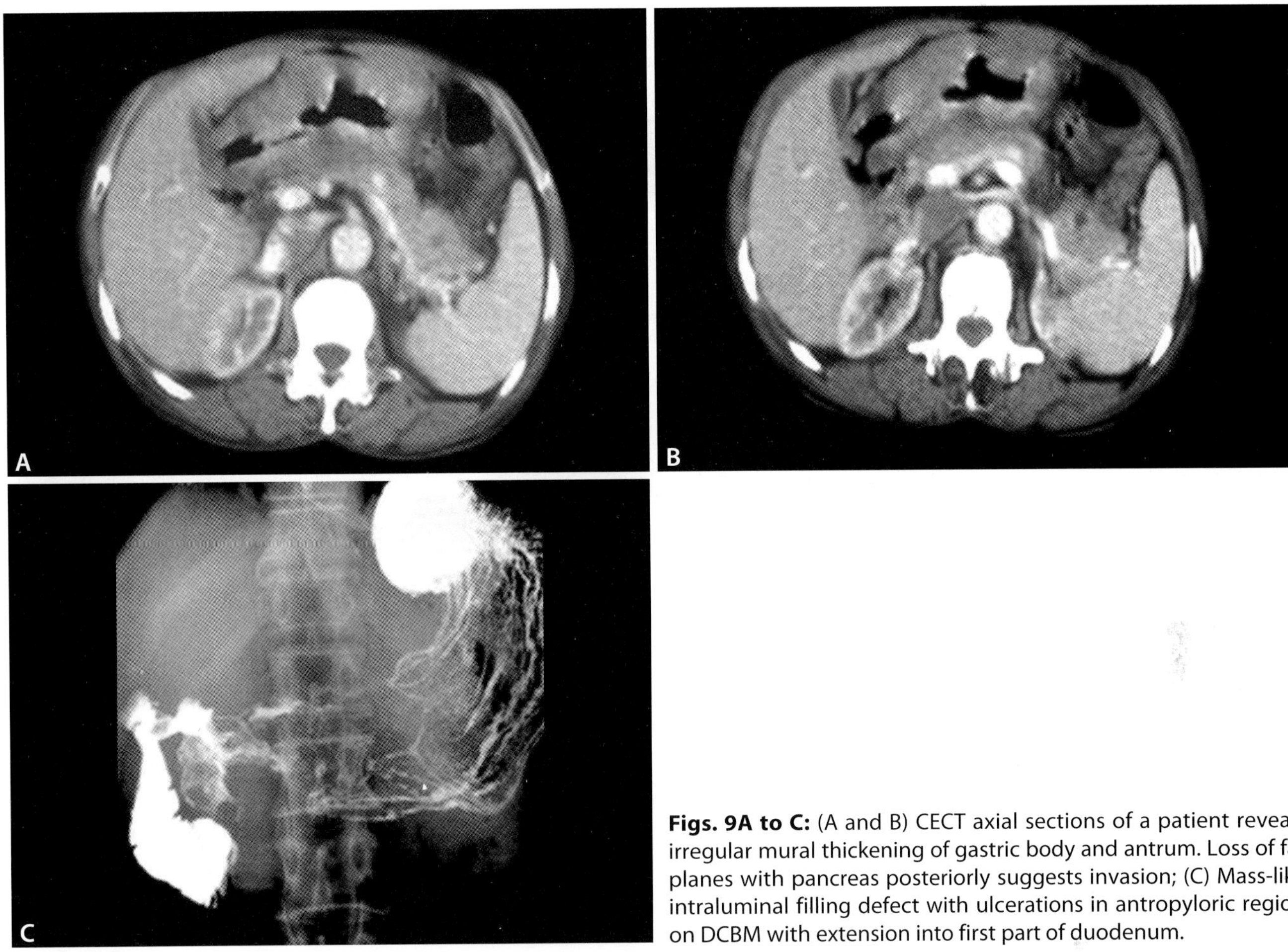

Figs. 9A to C: (A and B) CECT axial sections of a patient reveals irregular mural thickening of gastric body and antrum. Loss of fat planes with pancreas posteriorly suggests invasion; (C) Mass-like intraluminal filling defect with ulcerations in antropyloric region on DCBM with extension into first part of duodenum.

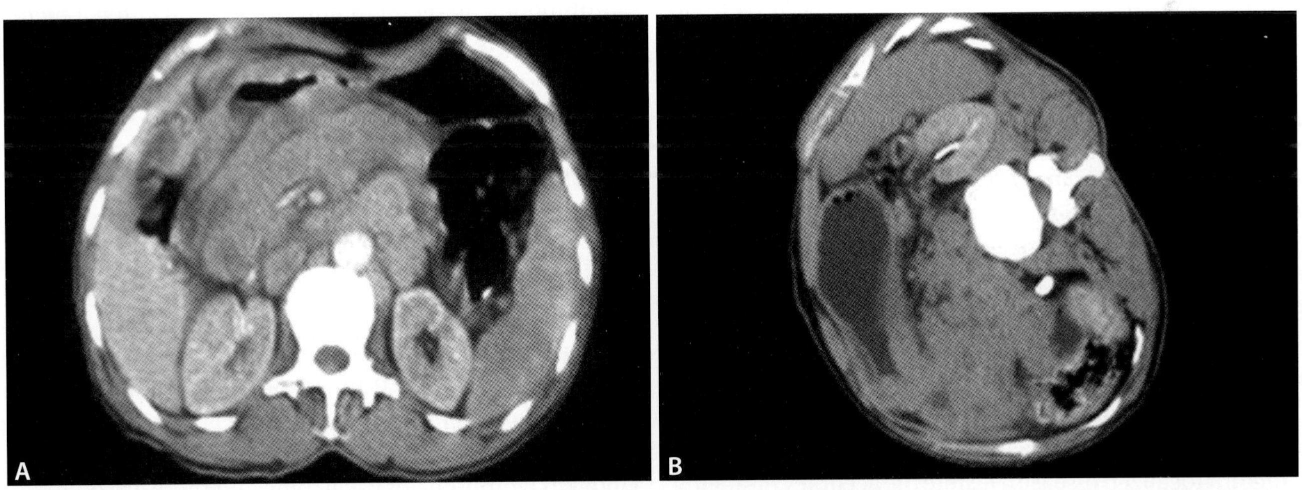

Figs. 10A and B: Supine and right lateral decubitus CECT scan showing mural thickening with heterogeneous enhancement in antropyloric region with multiple enhancing coeliac axis and aortocaval region lymph nodes (N1, N2).

now-a-days, MRI is predominantly used in patients where CT is contraindicated, like drug allergy and where there are concerns of radiation exposure.

Endoscopic Ultrasonography

The role of endoscopic ultrasonography (EUS) is to assess the depth of local invasion and the presence or absence of perigastric nodes. Unlike CT and MRI, EUS can depict stomach wall as 5 layered structure. This has improved the accuracy of local staging of gastric carcinomas on EUS as compared to CT and MRI. A gastric tumor is demonstrated as a hypoechoic mass with varying mural invasion. On endoscopic ultrasonography in T1 tumors, wall thickening is limited to the mucosa and submucosa. However, its depth may be overestimated because of the inflammatory response around the tumor, or underestimated because of microscopic spread.[35] Regarding N staging, involved nodes are rounder and more hypoechoic than normal nodes. EUS-guided FNAC can be done for lymph nodes although it is not a routine practice. Also EUS has limited role if there are long strictures, ulcerations and larger size lesions. It cannot evaluate distant metastasis and it is an invasive technique requiring lot of patient preparation and work-up.

Nuclear Imaging

FDG-PET depicts the primary tumor, but involved perigastric lymph nodes are not identified separately from the primary tumor because of poor spatial resolution. Mucinous, poorly differentiated adenocarcinomas and peritoneal metastasis can also be missed on FDG-PET on account of poor uptake. Superior spatial resolution of PET-CT makes it preferable over FDG-PET alone in detection of lymph nodes, metastasis and to evaluate therapeutic response. Diagnostic laparoscopy is highly sensitive for identifying peritoneal metastases and combined with laparoscopic ultrasound, peritoneal biopsy and ascitic cytology unnecessary surgeries can be avoided.[36]

Treatment and Prognosis

Gastric malignancy is an aggressive neoplasm with a 5-year survival rate of less than 20%, prognosis being correlated to the stage of the tumor at presentation. Surgical resection of the primary tumor and regional lymph nodes, if possible is the most definitive therapy. The important prognostic factors influencing survival in resectable gastric cancer are depth of invasion and the presence or absence of nodal metastases. Therefore, accurate staging of gastric cancer is essential because surgical resection is the treatment of choice for localized disease. Despite the accuracy of staging by CT a localized disease may be found unresectable and decision to proceed further is usually taken at laparotomy. Tumors within 5 cm of GE junction are treated with distal esophagectomy and partial gastrectomy combined with gastrojejunostomy. Localized tumors many a times are treated with neo-adjuvant chemotherapy to improve the chances of complete resection of tumor. Palliative surgery is sometimes indicated in advanced cancers to relieve obstruction at GE junction by placing stents.

CT also helps in detecting postoperative complications like afferent loop syndrome, anastomotic leaks and pancreatitis.

Differential Diagnosis

The differential diagnosis includes:

Gastric lymphoma in which the stomach remains pliable, despite large tumor bulk. Further, gastric lymphoma is associated with bulky lymphadenopathy extending below the renal hila, in contrast to adenocarcinoma.

GIST can also mimic the polypoidal form of adenocarcinoma, however GISTs are primarily exophytic and are usually not associated with lymphadenopathy.

Type III carcinoids are aggressive hypervascular masses with features of lymphatic and hematogenous invasion and can therefore mimic adenocarcinoma. So careful review is needed on CT scan to look for perigastric nodal or liver metastasis, which is uncommon in carcinoid tumors.

Metastasis present as multiple small submucosal masses which on having central ulceration give rise to "target or bull's eye" appearance. This can mimic malignant ulcer of adenocarcinoma.

In chronic gastritis, the gastric wall is thick and enhancing and can mimic adenocarcinoma, but the thickness is usually less than 10 mm. Further, there is no lymph node enlargement and the general clinical picture is of a relatively well preserved patient, as opposed to a cachectic patient suffering from malignant process.

Gastric Lymphoma

Gastric lymphoma constitutes 1–5% of the gastric malignancies. Lymphoma may involve GIT as primary malignancy or more commonly as a part of systemic illness and is considered the most common extranodal site for lymphoma. Gastric involvement is seen in about 50% cases and is the most common extranodal site of lymphoma overall.[35] Primary GIT lymphoma does not involve liver or spleen and is confined to stomach and the regional lymph nodes. Majority of lymphomas are non-Hodgkin lymphoma of B-cell type and there are only a few case reports of Hodgkin disease involving gastrointestinal system in literature.[37]

Primary gastrointestinal lymphomas usually affect one site. There are five diagnostic criteria, which have been described by Dawson[38] to make the diagnosis of a primary gastrointestinal lymphoma:

1. No palpable superficial lymph nodes.
2. No adenopathy on chest radiograph
3. Normal values of white cells in blood count.
4. Involvement of GI tract predominantly with involvement of drainage lymph nodes only if at all on laparotomy.
5. No lesions in the liver and spleen.

Patients frequently present with abdominal pain associated occasionally with malabsorption, abdominal mass and weight loss.

Modified TNM staging by European Gastrointestinal Lymphoma Study Group and Luguano staging[39] are two most commonly used staging protocols used for primary gastrointestinal lymphoma.

Most of lymphomas arise from mucosa associated lymphoid tissue (MALT) and have good prognosis as they remain localized for a long time. It is usually a low grade MALT lymphoma, however it can transform into intermediate or higher grade if not treated timely.[40] MALT lymphomas are now referred to as extranodal marginal zone B cell lymphoma (ENMZL), as they arise from the marginal zone of lymph node. Chronic *Heliobacter pylori* infection is associated with MALT lymphomas, and many low grade MALT lymphomas undergo regression with treatment of *H. pylori* infection. They may be low grade or high grade. Low grade lymphomas tend to spread superficially, accompanied occasionally by ulceration and manifest as small nodules with minimal mucosal thickening. Tumors <5 cm with <5 mitoses per high power field suggest low grade lymphoma. On the other hand, high grade lymphomas are usually large tumors, often >5 cms in size, polypoidal and associated with marked rugal fold thickening and have >5 mitoses per high power field. There is commonly necrosis within the tumor which may give rise to septated appearance and excavation may lead to communication with rest of the gastrointestinal tract or peritoneal cavity. Occurrence of hemorrhage may produce fluid-fluid level within the tumor. Direct invasion of adjacent organs or distant, omental and peritoneal metastasis may also occur.

T-cell lymphomas associated with enteropathy, Burkitt's lymphoma, etc are rare. Other risk factors for gastric lymphoma include inflammatory bowel disease, coeliac disease, HIV infection and immunosuppression after solid organ transplant.[41]

Diagnostic Imaging

Lymphoma can be focal or diffuse and involve any portion of the stomach. Though early lymphoma is confined to the mucosa and submucosa, gastric lymphomas are usually advanced at presentation and may mimic the appearances of gastric carcinoma.

Barium study and CT scan form the mainstay of diagnostic workup and radiographic findings of lymphoma parallel their gross morphological subtypes on both the techniques. The most common appearance is that of an infiltrating lesion with diffuse mural and fold thickening.

The CT reveals preservation of the perigastric fat planes even with a massive tumor. This favours the diagnosis of lymphoma over adenocarcinoma. Adenocarcinoma and lymphoma both are associated with lymphadenopathy, however bulky lymph nodes extending below the renal hila favor the diagnosis of lymphoma.[42] CT is also a better technique to diagnose complications like perforation, obstruction and fistulization. Moreover despite extensive infiltrative lesions stomach remains pliable and gastric outlet obstruction is uncommon in contrast to gastric adenocarcinoma.

The type of involvement can be infiltrative, ulcerative, polypoidal, nodular or a combination of above.

- *Infiltrative form*: Infiltration can be local or diffuse. It is associated with thick, nodular folds which are not effaced after hypotonic agent adminstration. Distensibility of stomach is maintained which helps in differentiation from linitis plastica due to adenocarcinoma. These patients are therefore less prone to develop gastric outlet obstruction[43] **(Figs. 11 and 12)**. Differential diagnosis includes Menetrier's disease, hypertrophic, lymphocytic and eosinophilic gastritis.

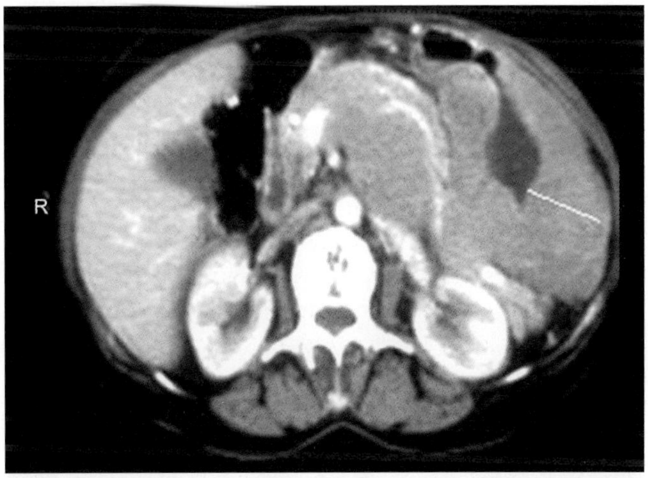

Fig. 11: Marked enhancing wall thickening (5 cm) noted in another patient of gastric lymphoma on CECT with multiple enlarged retroperitoneal nodes reaching up to renal hilum.
Courtesy: Dr Vinod G Maller, MAMC, New Delhi.

- *Ulcerative form*: Presence of ulcer accompanied by a polypoidal mass, absence of areae gastricae and associated rugal fold thickening are pointers of ulcerative form of lymphomatous involvement.
- *Polypoidal form*: There can be an intraluminal mass which may be lobulated or may present as submucosal mass. It may be associated with ulceration.
- *Nodular form*: These present as multiple submucosal masses. These often ulcerate giving "target or bull's eye" appearance.
- Extension to involve duodenum may be seen in about 40% cases **(Figs. 13A to C)**. Esophageal involvement is less common and seen in about 10% cases.[1]

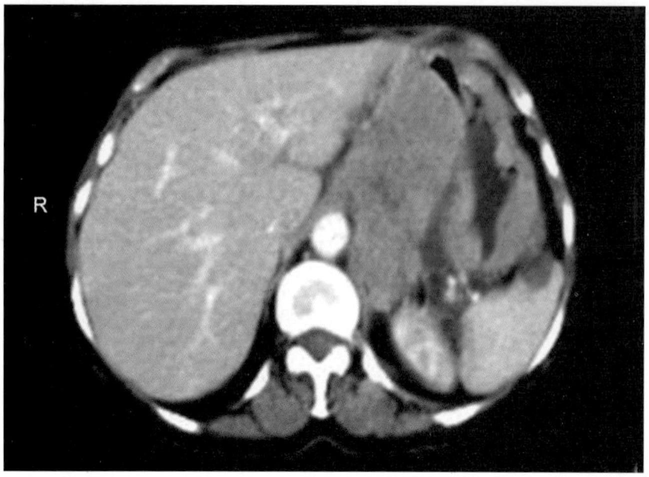

Fig. 12: Thick nodular folds in the region of gastric body along with enlarged lymph nodes noted in gastrohepatic ligament and paraaortic region. Note is also made of hypodense lesion in spleen. *Courtesy:* Dr Vinod G Maller, MAMC, New Delhi.

The MRI is useful in evaluating bowel wall thickening along with organ and lymph node involvement. Lymphomatous masses are hypointense on T1 and hyperintense on T2 weighted images as they have high free water content. MR is helpful in evaluating treatment due to reduction in signal intensity on T2 as a result of reduced cellular and water content.

In the detection of low-grade and MALT lymphomas cross sectional imaging may be limited; which can be best overcome by staging EUS which accurately assesses

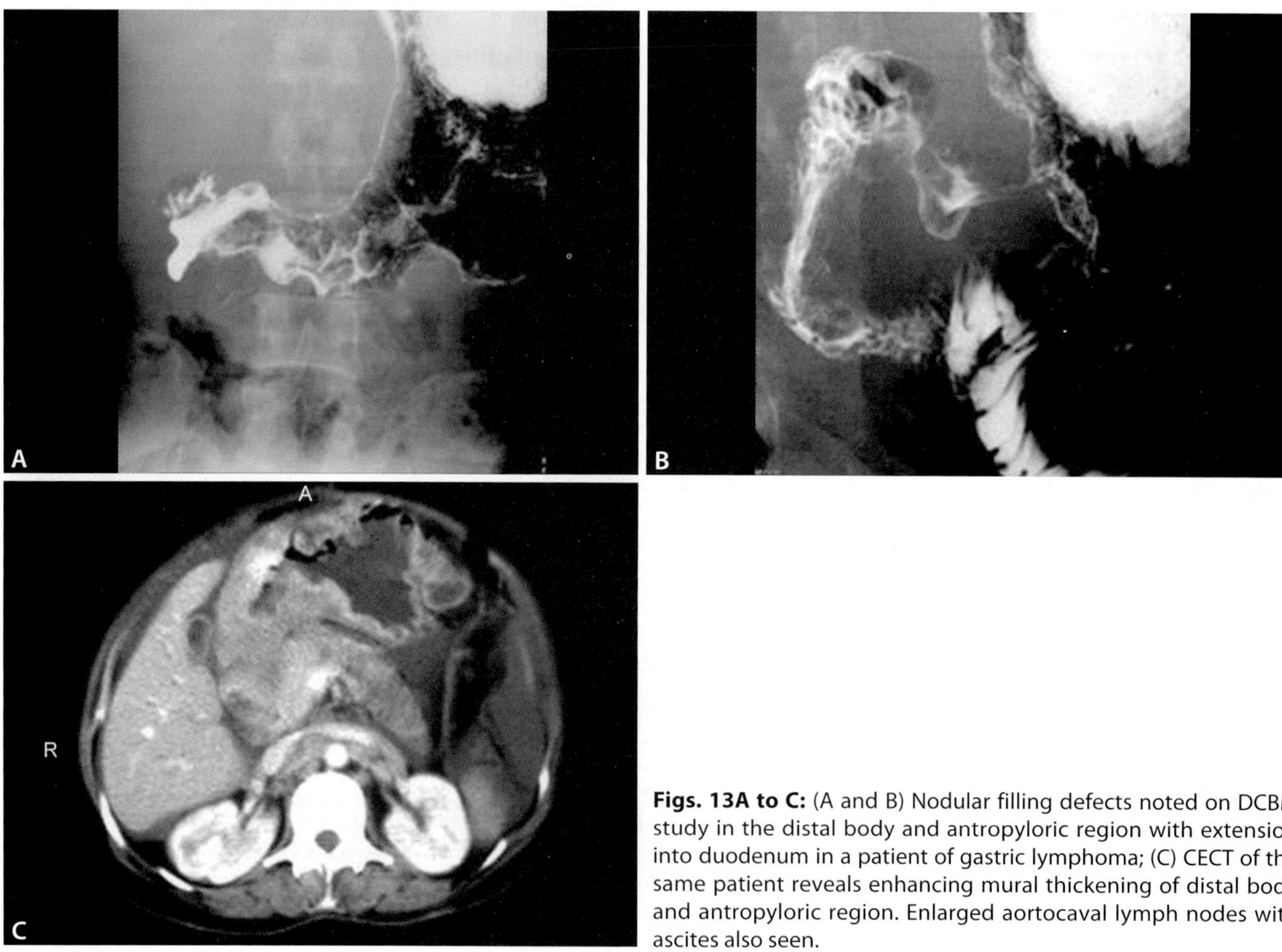

Figs. 13A to C: (A and B) Nodular filling defects noted on DCBM study in the distal body and antropyloric region with extension into duodenum in a patient of gastric lymphoma; (C) CECT of the same patient reveals enhancing mural thickening of distal body and antropyloric region. Enlarged aortocaval lymph nodes with ascites also seen.

the intramural infiltration, local node involvement, and response to therapy.[44]

Radionuclide imaging using FDG PET/PET-CT is helpful in evaluating lymph nodes as involved nodes show increased uptake, however its role is limited due to unpredictability and variability of degree of uptake in different subtypes.[45] FDG-PET is also found helpful in predicting the treatment response.

Metastatic Disease

Common tumors that metastasize to stomach include breast, malignant melanoma, lung, lymphoma and Kaposki sarcoma. These present as multiple small submucosal masses which on having central ulceration give rise to "target or bull's eye" appearance **(Figs. 14A and B)**. Differential diagnosis includes neurofibromas, pancreatic rest cells and leiomyomas.

Gastric and Duodenal Carcinoids

Gastrointestinal carcinoids are well differentiated endocrine neoplasms arising from specialized endocrine cells that populate the mucosa and submucosa of the gastrointestinal system. Hence theoretically they can be seen arising from any part of the gastrointestinal system and produce clinical symptoms depending on the type of the hormone they are secreting. Carcinoids arise most commonly from the distal ileum from enterochromaffin cells which produce serotonin. Usually they present as lymph nodal or liver metastasis.

Carcinoids of the stomach, duodenum or colon are however a relatively rare entity. Majority of the gastric carcinoids arise from gastric body and fundus from oxyntic cells.[46]

Gastric carcinoids are primarily divided into three types depending on their clinical, imaging and pathological differences by Bordi et al.[47]

Type I: Most common (74%), female predominance at an older age, usually associated with autoimmune chronic atrophic gastritis and usually encountered during endoscopy performed usually for dyspepsia or anemia. Achlorhydria, pernicious anemia or gastric G-cell hyperplasia may be seen.

They are usually small (<1 cm) and seen as multiple smoothly marginated mucosal and submucosal masses in the body and fundus of stomach showing enhancement on CECT.

Type II: Usually associated with Zollinger-Ellison syndrome in patients of multiple endocrine neoplasia (MEN type-I). They usually present as recurrent nonhealing gastric or duodenal ulcers with marked mucosal fold and rugal thickening, abdominal pain, bleeding or diarrhea due to hypergastrinemia by gastrin producing neoplasms **(Fig. 15)**. They have a more marked propensity to metastasize than type I carcinoids.

They are also usually multiple but of variable size unlike type I carcinoids and can show ulceration. Smaller masses like in type-I can be missed on CECT **(Fig. 16)**.

Type III: Type III ECL-cell carcinoids represent 10–15% of the gastric carcinoids which usually does not have any associated hypergastrinemia or atrophic gastritis and usually present with signs and symptoms of aggressive

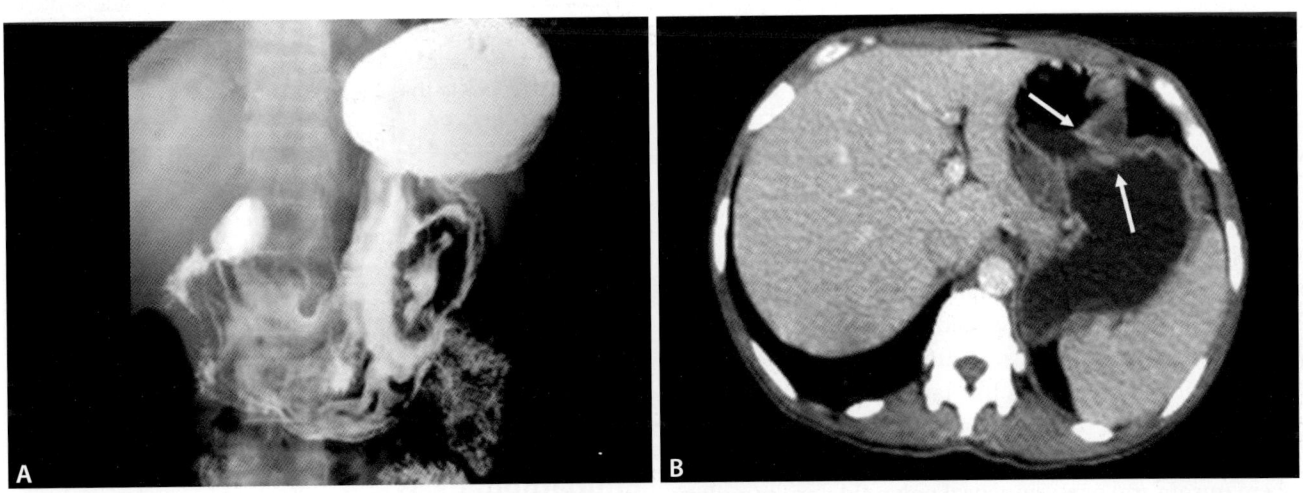

Figs. 14A and B: (A) Target/Bull's eye lesion—DCBM reveals a large filling defect in body of stomach with central pooling of barium; (B) CECT shows focal thickening of stomach wall in the region of body with central ulceration in a patient of submucosal metastasis from melanoma.

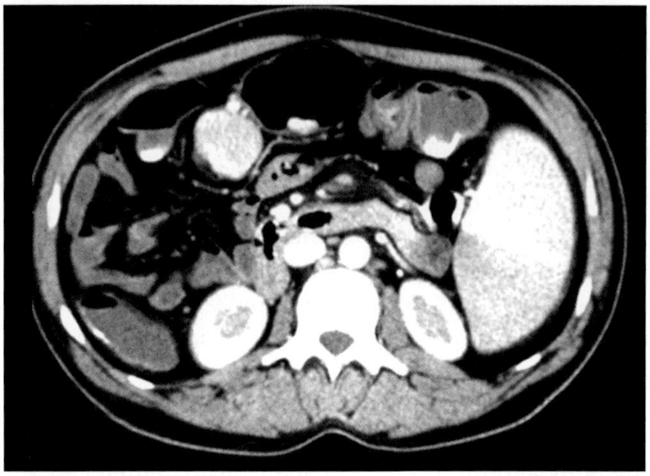

Fig. 15: A patient of gastrinoma showing heterogeneously enhancing mass lesion in relation to 2nd part of duodenum with intensely enhancing multiple nodular masses in the body and antrum region of stomach suggestive of multiple carcinoids.

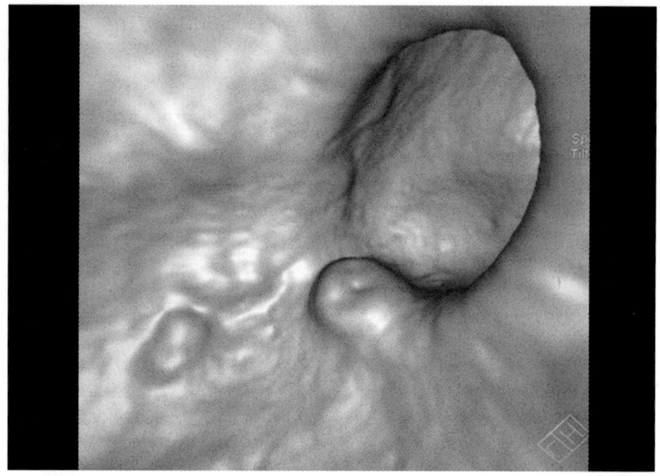

Fig. 16: Virtual gastroscopy of the same patient reveals multiple variable sized submucosal masses in the body and antrum of stomach with few of them showing central ulcerations.

mass like anorexia, weight loss, bleeding or pain abdomen.

It usually presents as large aggressive hypervascular solitary mass with exophytic component in the gastric fundus and body with features of lymphatic and hematogenous invasion on histopathology. So it needs a careful review on CT scan, to look for perigastric nodal or liver metastasis[46,47] **(Fig. 17)**.

The differentials for gastric carcinoids include other multifocal polypoidal masses like multiple hyperplastic polyps, adenomatous polyps in familial adenomatous polyposis syndrome, hamartomatous polyps in Peutz-Jeghers syndrome and juvenile polyposis for type I and II gastric carcinoids. Type III carcinoids can mimic adenocarcinoma, lymphoma, and gastrointestinal stromal tumors.

Majority of duodenal carcinoids are G cell type and they are also rare like gastric carcinoids. Patients with MEN 1 usually develop G cell carcinoids in 90% of the patients while D cell type usually associated with Neurofibromatosis type 1 (NF-1).

Gastrinomas usually present with abdominal pain, bleeding, recurrent nonhealing ulcers and diarrhea while somatostatin producing carcinoids are almost exclusively present around ampulla of Vater and hence present with obstructive symptoms like jaundice, pancreatitis or hemorrhage.

Duodenal carcinoids are usually small, homogeneous, 1–2 cm intramural or submucosal polypoid periampullary nodules which can show focal ulcerations. After adenocarcinoma, carcinoids are the second most common malignant tumors of the duodenum and may have similar syndromic associations as that of gastric carcinoid. Most of the tumors are small, however larger tumors (>1.5 cm in size) present with metastasis at the time of presentation.[48]

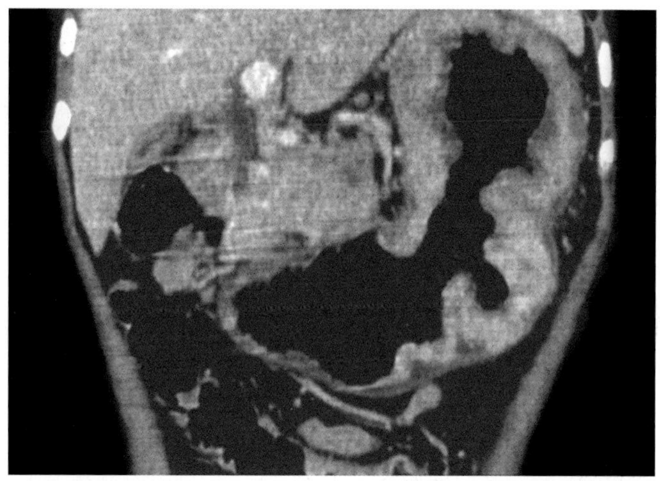

Fig. 17: Gastric carcinoid (Type-III)—CECT coronal reformat of another patient reveals diffuse mural thickening with irregular polypoidal lesions in the fundus and body of the stomach. There is a large heterogeneously enhancing mass lesion seen in the region of head of the pancreas.
Courtesy: Dr Prashant Nagpal, MAMC, New Delhi.

GASTROINTESTINAL STROMAL TUMOR

Etiopathogenesis

Gastrointestinal stromal tumor (GIST) is the most common mesenchymal neoplasm that can be found throughout the gastrointestinal tract with 60–70% of the tumors affecting the stomach.[49] Before the immunohistochemical tests were available, they used to be considered leiomyoma but the uniqueness of tumor being c-KIT (CD 117) positive helps to differentiate GIST from other neoplasms. 5% cases of GIST however do not show CD 117 immunoreactivity and rather harbor mutations for platelet derived growth factor receptor-alpha (PDGFR- alpha).[50]

They arise from pacemaker interstitial cells of Cajal normally present in myenetric plexus, which are responsible for peristalsis.[51] Because they arise from the deep muscularis propria, GISTs frequently have an exophytic or intramural pattern of growth. Endoluminal tumors although less common if present have features of intramural masses like smoothly circumscribed masses forming obtuse or right angles with the gastric wall.[52] Pressure necrosis can cause focal mucosal ulcerations in lesions larger than 2 cm which appears as "bull's eye" lesion on DCBM study.

Clinical Features

Clinical manifestations of the GIST depend on their size and location. Small lesions are discovered incidentally. Ulcerated lesions usually present with bleed in form of hematemesis, melena or iron deficiency anemia.[53] Larger masses usually present with abdominal pain and early satiety. However, because of predominantly exophytic nature of tumors, many of these patients remain asymptomatic until the tumors become quite large.[52]

Imaging Features

The typical CT appearance of small tumors are often of homogeneous density and that of large tumors is heterogeneously enhancing lobulated hypervascular exophytic mass with mucosal ulceration, central necrosis, hemorrhage, cavitation and areas of cystic degeneration[51] **(Figs. 18A to C)**. Ulcerations and fistulizations can be manifested as air and oral contrast

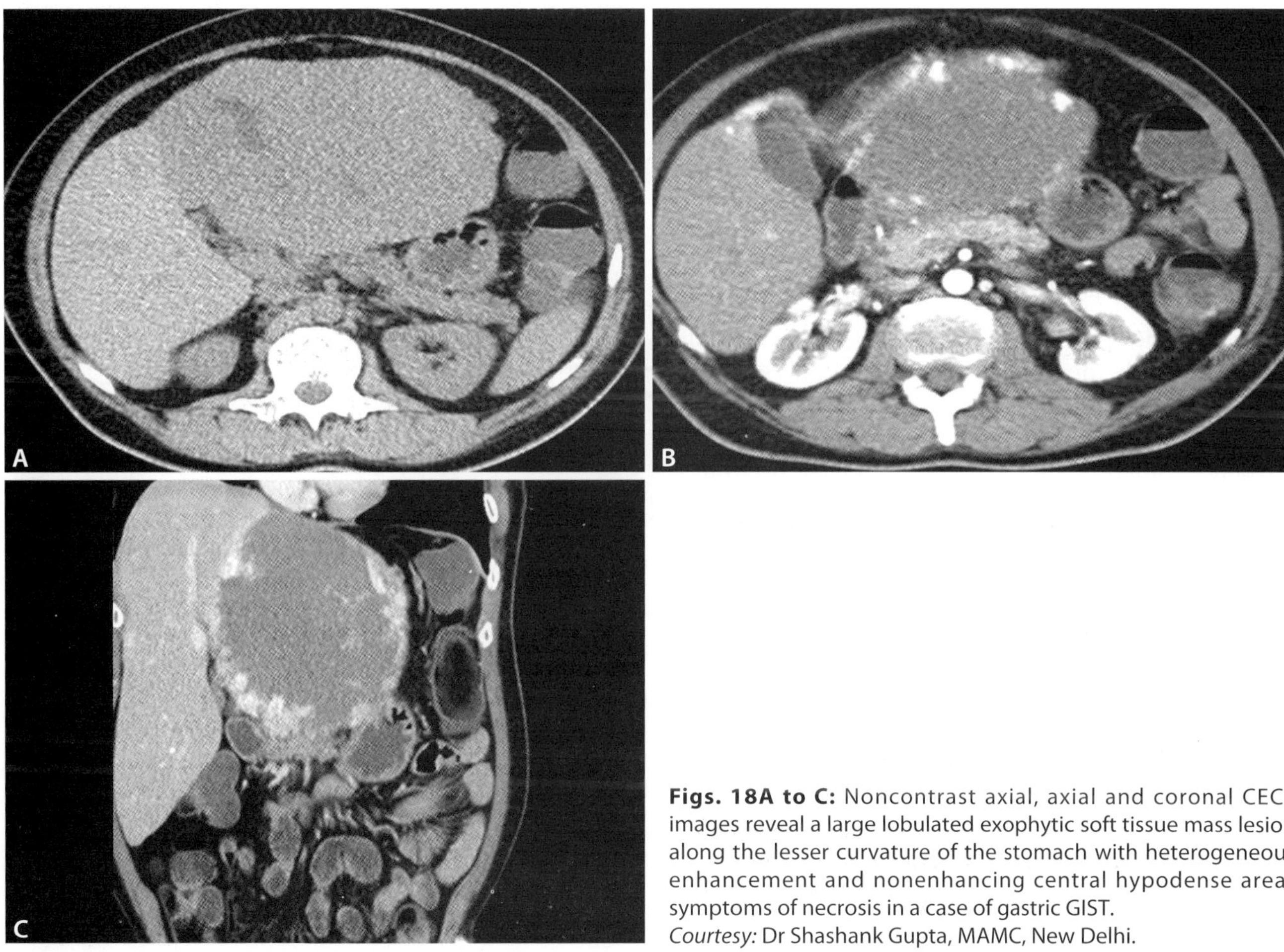

Figs. 18A to C: Noncontrast axial, axial and coronal CECT images reveal a large lobulated exophytic soft tissue mass lesion along the lesser curvature of the stomach with heterogeneous enhancement and nonenhancing central hypodense areas symptoms of necrosis in a case of gastric GIST.
Courtesy: Dr Shashank Gupta, MAMC, New Delhi.

within the lesion. 5–10% of the cases can show calcification. Size >5 cm, necrosis, mesenteric or contiguous organ infiltration and metastasis favors diagnosis of malignant GIST.[54,55] Rarely clumps of calcification can be seen. Nearly half of the patients present with metastasis in the advanced stages when the tumor has invaded the adjacent organs like colon, diaphragm and pancreas with deposits predominantly seen in liver and peritoneum. Nodal metastasis is infrequent in GISTs.[56]

Differential diagnosis for GISTs can be neural tumors like schwannomas, true leiomyomas and small type 3 solitary carcinoid tumors. Immunoreactivity to c-KIT or DOG1 however can confirm the diagnosis.[57] Other tumors showing intramural growth like gastric adenocarcinoma or lymphoma can mimic a GIST. However, lymphadenopathy is rare for GISTs. Submucosal metastases to the stomach from melanoma or breast cancer can manifest as bull's-eye lesions, they can be single, however usually they are multiple.[52]

The GISTs smaller than 2 cm are generally considered benign with a very low risk of recurrence. However, no GIST can truly be labeled benign.[58] A definitive diagnosis is particularly important because advanced GIST can now be treated with a new tyrosine kinase inhibitor imatinib with a remarkable response and a prolonged survival.[59,60]

On CT, GISTs typically become homogeneous and hypoattenuating from heterogeneously hyperattenuating appearence, with disappearance of enhancing tumor nodules and tumor vessels in the early post-treatment period by Imatinib. There is development of myxoid degeneration and occasional areas of hemorrhage and necrosis can be seen within the healing tumor which can paradoxically increase the size of tumor. However with overall reduction in tumor enhancement this does not indicate tumor progression. The term *cystic change* is usually avoided while under treatment by Imatinib. Development of a nodule within the treated tumor is unique to GISTs and indicates recurrence regardless of changes in tumor size.[61]

Duodenal GIST

In institutional review of GIST, about 20% of GIST's occurred in duodenum as compared to rest of the gastrointestinal tract. They were larger than their gastric counterparts, with the majority occurring in 2nd part of duodenum. Association of duodenal GIST's with neurofibromatosis has also been noted.

Duodenal GIST often present with bleeding and, occasionally pain.[62] Similar to gastric lesions these lesions are seen as large heterogeneously enhancing, exophytic masses with central ulceration and filling of central cavity by oral contrast on CECT **(Figs. 19A to C)**.

In addition to medical treatment as described for gastric GIST's, surgical resection options include pancreaticoduodenectomy and segmental duodenectomy with preservation of pylorus.

Gastric Lipomas (Table 3)

Gastric lipomas are solitary submucosal lesions usually detected incidentally in asymptomatic patients. They are composed of mature fat cells surrounded by fibrous capsule.[63] Small tumors are asymptomatic although, larger tumors can present with abdominal pain and bleeding due to ulceration of overlying mucosa. Infrequently they can develop into pedunculated lesions which can intermittently prolapse through pylorus and cause obstruction.[61]

The most common location of gastric lipomas is gastric antrum. They appear as smooth submucosal masses on fluoroscopy, however can show central ulceration. They also can change size and shape with peristalsis being soft tissue lesions.[61] On CT they appear as solitary, submucosal, well demarcated lesion with homogeneous fat attenuation. Occasionally linear strands of soft tissue at the base or mild adjacent gastric wall thickening may be present.[47] On CT images, attenuation values of –70 to –120 HU are diagnostic of a lipoma.[63] Rarely, they can present with complications like ulceration, intussusceptions and hemorrhage.[64] So, they can present as masses of soft tissue attenuation rather than fatty attenuation.

Liposarcoma/Leiomyoma/Leiomyosarcoma

Liposarcoma originates in undifferentiated mesenchymal cells within the submucosal and muscularis of stomach wall. There is predominately exophytic growth and as a result, delay in diagnosis. Four forms of liposarcoma are differentiated, myxoid, round cell and pleomorphic variety. Necrosis, hemorrhage, fatty or cystic areas may occur within the mass depending on various types.

Leiomyomas and leiomyosarcomas are well circumscribed intramural tumors and predominate in the region of gastric cardia. The true leiomyomas are rare benign tumor of stomach and are negative for c-KIT and strongly and diffusely positive for desmin and smooth muscle actin.

Leiomyomas appear on CT as homogeneous, low attenuation masses with an endoluminal growth pattern.[65-67] They too can have central ulceration if >2

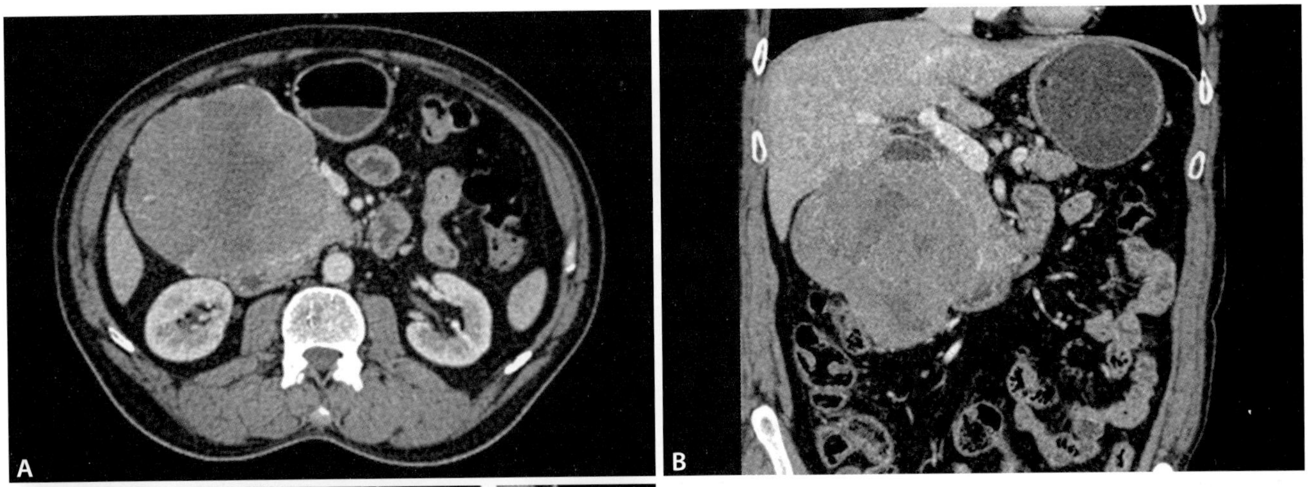

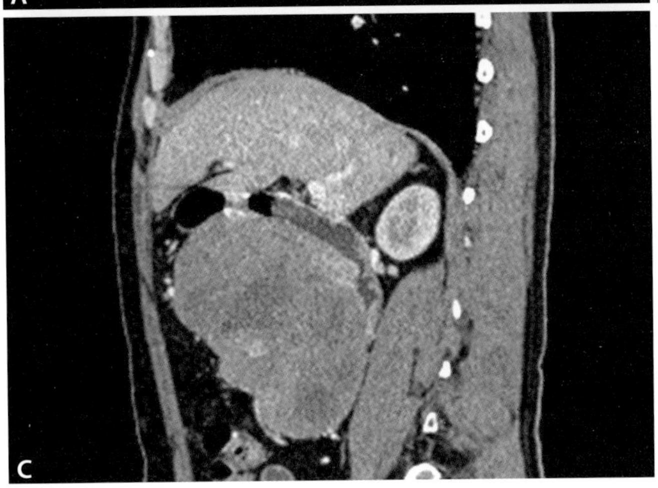

Figs. 19A to C: Axial, coronal and sagittal CECT images reveal a large lobulated exophytic heterogeneously enhancing soft tissue mass lesion along the 2nd part of duodenum (anterior aspect) with non-enhancing central necrotic hypodense areas in a case of duodenal GIST.
Courtesy: Dr Surabhi Gupta, MAMC and GB Pant Hospital, New Delhi.

Table 3: Other rare tumors and focal gastric lesions mimicking tumor.

Rare tumors	***Other focal gastric lesions mimicking tumor***
Gastric lipoma	Inflammatory pseudotumor/ myofibroblastic tumor
Leiomyoma/leiomyosarcoma/ liposarcoma	Ectopic pancreatic rests/ myoepithelial hamartoma
Neurogenic tumors	Gastric duplication cyst
Glomus tumor	
Hemangioma	
Plasmacytoma	

cm in size and hence includes GISTs and schwannomas as differentials.However, the malignant nature of leiomyosarcoma, is not easily distinguished by gross appearance and needs invasion and metastasis for the diagnosis **(Figs. 20A to C)**. Histological evaluation can only establish the final diagnosis in isolated cases. Sarcomas present mostly with bleeding due to hypervascular nature of tumor and central necrosis or massive mucosal erosion of the tumor and with partial obstruction if large. Endoscopically, the tumors appear as a smooth, submucosal mass over which the mucosal folds are stretched and effaced. Leiomyosarcomas can undergo hematogenous spread to the liver and lungs.[48]

Neurogenic Tumors of Stomach

These are benign submucosal neoplasms and comprise 4% of all benign gastric neoplasms and are nerve sheath tumors in origin (schwannoma).[68] They are believed to arise within the myenetric plexus in the muscularis propria. They are slow growing exophytic tumors which are mostly asymptomatic and because of this indolent growth these are usually discovered incidentally by cross sectional imaging or on endoscopy.[69] Carney's triad is associated with gastric neurogenic tumors along with pulmonary chondromas and extra adrenal paragangliomas.

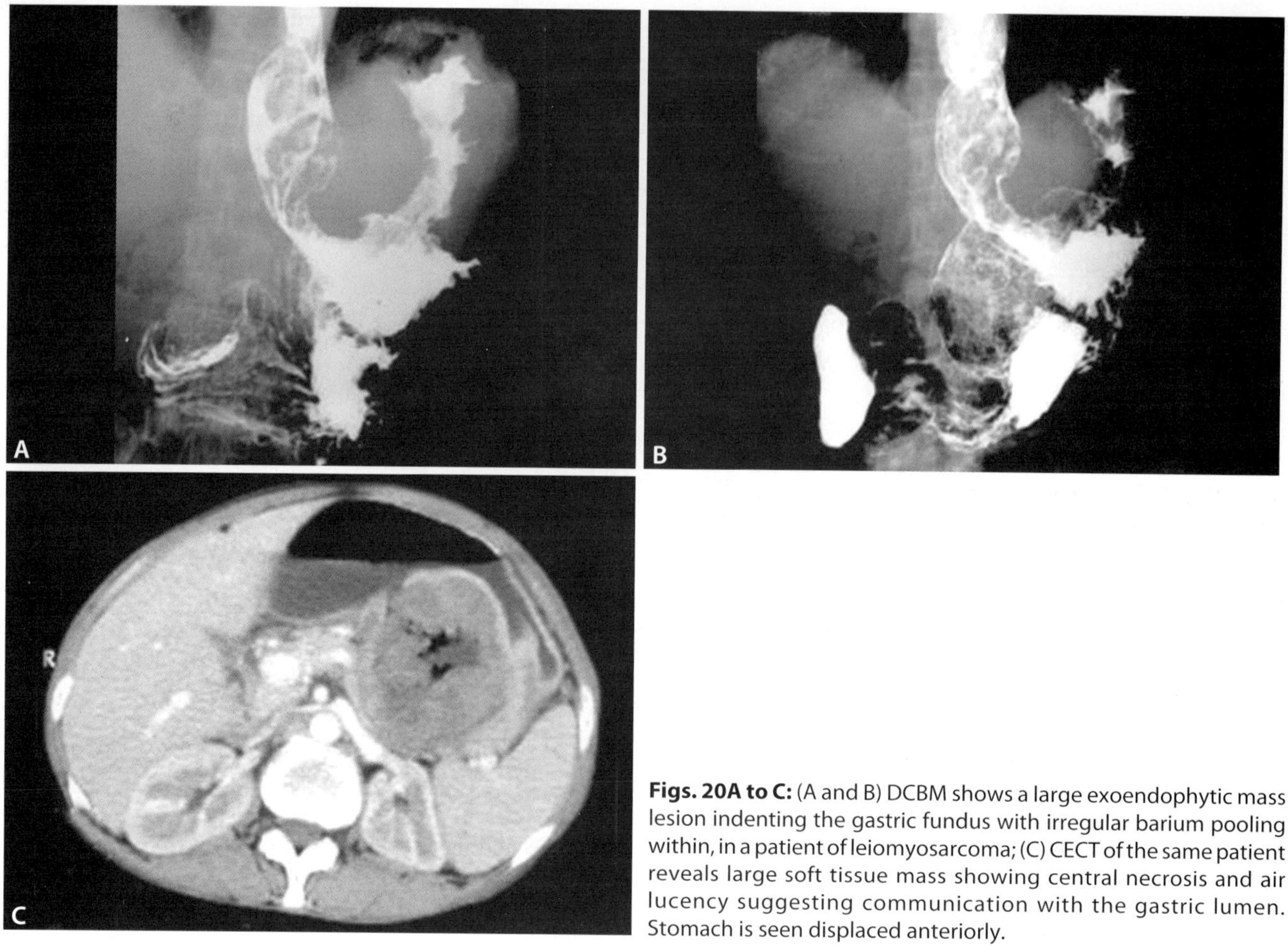

Figs. 20A to C: (A and B) DCBM shows a large exoendophytic mass lesion indenting the gastric fundus with irregular barium pooling within, in a patient of leiomyosarcoma; (C) CECT of the same patient reveals large soft tissue mass showing central necrosis and air lucency suggesting communication with the gastric lumen. Stomach is seen displaced anteriorly.

Schwannomas arising mostly in the gastric body can have an exophytic or intramural growth, may be asymptomatic or present with pain, bleeding or obstruction if large.[70]

Neural tumors in the stomach usually appear on CT scans as submucosal masses (with or without ulceration) that are indistinguishable from other mesenchymal tumors. Gastric schwannomas are usually homogeneous, low attenuation masses. Hemorrhage, ulceration, calcification and cystic changes are rare unlike in schwannomas at other places which commonly shows cystic changes which help them in distinguishing from more heterogeneous GISTs. Contrast enhancement is variable. They usually show minimal to no significant enhancement on arterial phase but show delayed enhancement on equilibrium phase.[52]

Glomus Tumor

Neuromyoarterial receptors or glomus bodies are composed of modified smooth muscle cells and account for 2% of benign gastric tumors and arise nearly in all cases in muscularis propria.[71]

Their clinical presentation varies from asymptomatic nature of disease to various features like pain, hematemesis or melena.

They usually present in gastric antrum as hypervascular lesions.[66,71] These tumors are also soft tumors like lipomas on barium studies and can change in size and shape. However, strong arterial enhancement with persistence on delayed films differentiate from lipomas on CT.[1] The differentials for gastric glomus tumors include GIST, carcinoids, lipomas, metastasis, ectopic pancreas and sometimes due to specific peripheral nodular pattern of enhancement with delayed filling-in, hemangioma becomes a differential.[66,71]

Hemangioma

Another solitary vascular gastric tumor which comprises less than 2% of benign gastric lesions.[72] It is a debate whether these are true neoplasms or congenital malformations and are found to be associated with number of syndromes such as Klippel-Trénaunay syndrome, Maffucci syndrome, blue rubber-bleb nevus syndrome, or Osler-Rendu-Weber disease.

They are mostly seen in children and gradually involute with age. However, with the possibility of massive GI bleed they are usually resected.

They are seen as intramural masses on fluoroscopy and show avid enhancement on CT scan. Phleboliths, if seen in the lesion are considered pathognomonic.

Plasmacytoma

About 10% of extramedullary plasmacytomas occur in the gastrointestinal tract with primary gastric plasmacytoma accounting for five percent of them.

The diagnosis is established by absence of any visceral involvement elsewhere, apart from stomach. In addition there is no serum M protein and bone marrow infiltration. Four forms of primary gastric plasmacytoma include nodular, infiltrative, ulcerative and polypoidal variety. There is poor enhancement of the wall of stomach and diagnosis is established with immunohistological diagnosis of deep gastric tissue biopsy.

Other Focal Gastric Lesions Mimicking Tumor

A number of conditions can mimic the neoplastic processes in the stomach and hence their importance cannot be ignored given the implications for management.

Inflammatory Pseudotumor/Myofibroblastic Tumor

The term inflammatory myofibroblastic tumor or pseudotumor denotes a pseudosarcomatous inflammatory lesion that contains spindle cells, myofibroblasts, plasma cells, lymphocytes and histiocytes which can frequently be a benign lesion or have a more aggressive behavior with propensity of local recurrence and a low rate of metastasis. The pathogenesis of IMT remains unclear, although various allergic, immunologic, and infectious mechanisms have been postulated. The myofibroblastic tumor cells often show reactivity for anaplastic lymphoma kinase (ALK). ALK-negative IMFTs have been associated with older patient age at presentation and can manifest with distant metastases.[73] In most cases IMT features mimic malignancy on upper flexible endoscopy and radiological imaging. For that reason, most IMT cases require surgical exploration and complete resection to obtain an accurate microscopic diagnosis.

It is seen mostly in children or young adults. It occurs in the soft tissue of children and young adults and lungs are the most commonly affected site. It is rare in abdomen, but when present, it is seen along terminal ileum or greater curvature of stomach.[74]

On CT, IMFTs appear as enhancing, aggressive intramural masses,[75] which can invade through the gastric wall into the peritoneal cavity or nearby organs. They can also have ulcerations and calcifications at occasions.[76] GIST, solitary fibrous tumor and schwannomas hence make the differentials because of similar appearences on CT imaging.

Ectopic Pancreatic Rests/Myoepithelial Hamartoma

This is also known as heterotopic, accessory, or aberrant pancreas and is defined as pancreatic tissue lacking anatomic and vascular continuity with the main body of the gland.

These lesions are most commonly found incidentally in asymptomatic patients mainly along the greater curvature of prepyloric region of stomach and duodenum. Some patients present with abdominal pain, gastrointestinal bleeding, and obstruction due to complications like pancreatitis, pseudocyst, insulinoma, and pancreatic cancer.[77]

Ectopic pancreas may manifest as a submucosal mass in the stomach or duodenum and may easily be misinterpreted as another submucosal tumor such as gastrointestinal stromal tumor (GIST) or leiomyoma. They can appear as well defined submucosal masses on either single or double contrast barium studies and can even have central umbilication and rarely barium may even be seen to enter into rudimentary ductal system. However, the typical location (prepyloric antrum and duodenum), endoluminal growth pattern, ill-defined border, prominent enhancement of overlying mucosa, and a long diameter/short diameter ratio of greater than 1.4 are considered significant CT features for differentiating ectopic pancreas from other tumors.[78]

Magnetic resonance imaging (MRI) is diagnostic, as ectopic pancreas follows pancreatic signal and enhancement pattern on all sequences.[79] Usually these lesions are flat (LD/SD > 1.4), however they can acquire ovoid form and protrude endoluminally after intra glandular cyst formation. Small cystic areas within the mass represent dilated anomalous ducts.[47]

Gastric Duplication Cyst

Duplication of the alimentary tract is a rare congenital anomaly with the gastric duplication cysts (GDCs) being rarest, representing only 4% of all alimentary tract duplications. The common age of presentation being the first decade with approximately 67% manifest within the first year of life.[80] Classically, barium studies show an intramural filling defect indenting the gastric contour. Typical NCCT appearance is a spheric to ovoid nonenhancing cystic lesion in close approximation to greater curvature. Occasionally marginal calcifications may be present. Contrast-enhanced CT scan typically demonstrates a thick-walled cystic lesion with enhancement of the inner lining. EUS can further add to the diagnosis by demonstrating an echogenic internal mucosal layer and a hypoechoic intermediate muscular layer making the diagnosis of GDC highly likely.

The essential criteria for diagnosis of a gastric duplication cyst includes—contiguity of the cyst wall with that of the stomach; smooth muscles in the cyst wall, which is continuous with the muscle of the stomach; and lining of the cyst wall by either gastric epithelium or any other type of gut mucosa.[81]

Majority of gastric duplications are cystic (80%) and do not communicate with lumen of the stomach. Few of them are tubular and may show some communication. It is defined as tubular when the lumen is contiguous with the stomach lumen and cystic when the lumen is not contiguous.

Because most of the duplication cysts occur along the greater curvature of the stomach, they can potentially compress the adjacent organs such as pancreas, kidney, spleen, and adrenal gland and hence lesions arising from these organs become the differential diagnosis of duplication cysts.

As with the native gastric mucosa, the cyst lining may undergo erosions, ulceration, bleeding and regenerative changes. In noncommunicating cysts pressure necrosis of the mucosa may be seen due to increased fluid production. These changes may lead to bleeding into the cyst or perforation into the peritoneal cavity. Duplication cysts have the potential for neoplastic transformation especially by production of onco-fetal antigens which raises the problem of a precancerous condition in long standing cases.

DUODENAL FOCAL LESIONS

Introduction

Prevalence of small bowel malignancies are 50 times less common than colonic neoplasms, duodenal involvement is seen in approximately 20% of these neoplasms. Their peak incidence is between the sixth and eight decade of life with nearly equal frequency of symptomatic benign and malignant duodenal tumors and a near equal sex distribution. It is speculated that protective factors might play role in the low incidence of these tumors as compared to adenocarcinoma of the colon and stomach like secretory immunoglobulins, rapid transit with lack of bacteria, small intestinal hydroxylases that could neutralize potential carcinogens and alkalinity can prevent formation of potential carcinogen. Benign tumors abound in duodenal cap, there being almost equal preponderance of benign and malignant tumors in second part, while malignant tumors predominate in the remaining part of duodenum.[82]

Symptoms can vary from obstructive jaundice due to obstruction of the ampulla, partial duodenal obstruction, or from bleeding due to ulceration with resultant hematemesis or melaena. Patients may occasionally also present with pancreatitis, intussusception, and symptoms due to the effects of hormone production in case of neuroendocrine tumors.

Flexure defect pseudotumor is a normal finding that occurs due to bunching of mucosal folds at the apex of the duodenal bulb where there is sudden change in the direction of duodenum. Annular pancreas, a relative common congenital abnormality may be confused with annular carcinoma. A prominent notch like defect in the lateral wall of the second part of duodenum causing eccentric narrowing without any accompanying ulceration is quite suggestive of annular pancreas and intact mucosa on endoscopy and CT can also help differentiate it.[48]

Double contrast barium meal and in selected cases, hypotonic duodenography are helpful modalities in fluoroscopic diagnostic evaluation of duodenal pathologies.

Carcinoid, leiomyoma and leiomyosarcomas have already been discussed.

BENIGN DUODENAL TUMORS

Adenomas

Most common benign tumors in the duodenum are adenomas and are of three main types including adenomatous polyps, Brunner's gland adenomas, or villous adenomas. Villous adenomas are discussed under malignant tumors due to high rate of their malignant transformation. They can present with anemia due to chronic blood loss or intermittent jaundice/pancreatitis due to blockage of ampula of vater.

Adenomatous Polyps

These polyps of duodenum are sessile, nodular, or pedunculated and usually <1 cm in diameter. They are commonly associated with familial polyposis coli, Peutz and Jegher's syndrome Gardner's syndrome and have potential to transform into villous adenomas and adenocarcinomas. Surveillance is required and it is recommended to do periodic upper gastrointestinal endoscopies with numerous biopsies. The polyps which are considered suspicious like large lesions, ulcerated or bleeding lesions, lesions with white or firm areas, and lesions found to have tubulovillous components are better removed and radical treatment is performed only if an invasive carcinoma is detected.

Brunner's gland adenomas: These adenomas present as pedunculated polyps, circumscribed nodular hyperplasia or diffuse nodular hyperplasia and have very low malignant potential. Brunner's gland adenoma is usually single and presents as filling defect. Histologically they resemble Brunner's gland and produce mucus. Treatment includes endoscopic or local open resection.[48]

Lipomas

These are smooth submucosal masses which have a characteristic yellow appearance on endoscopy. Most remain fairly small, but some may become pedunculated, cause pain and bleeding due to mucosal erosion and obstruction especially intussusception in younger patients. They can change shape due to palpation, peristalsis and gravity.[82] Local excision is usually sufficient for symptomatic lesions **(Fig. 21)**.

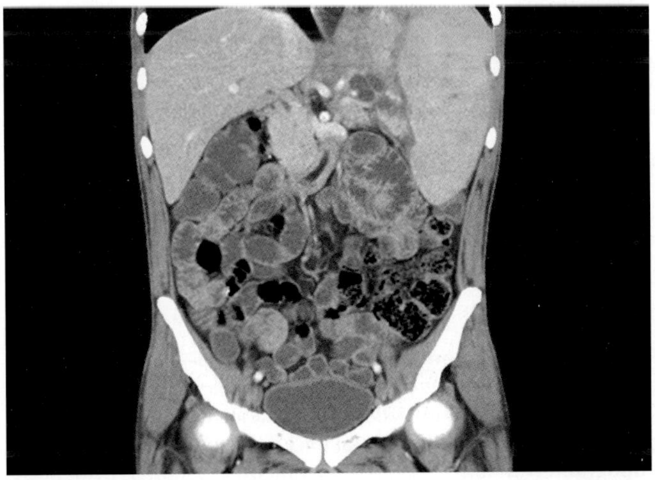

Fig. 21: Coronal CECT reveals a well-defined nonenhancing, submucosal hypodense lesion of fat attenuation seen along the 3rd part of duodenum extending along 4th part up to the DJ flexure suggestive of lipoma.

Other Benign Tumors

Other benign duodenal masses include hemangiomas and lymphangiomas which are well circumscribed submucosal masses, and are composed of predominantly blood vessels or lymphatic vessels, respectively and can be multifocal. Emergency laparotomy may be required if bleeding from hemangiomas is massive. Other multifocal lesions are neurofibromas and schwannomas which are poorly circumscribed lesions with wavy, fibrillary elements, identical to lesions seen at other places. These lesions mostly present with bleeding and excision of all symptomatic lesions is advocated.

Malignant Duodenal Tumors

The common malignant lesions are adenocarcinoma, lymphoma, villous adenoma, GIST and carcinoid tumors. Associated malignancies are most often other adenocarcinomas of the intestinal tract, bladder carcinoma, and lymphomas. Squamous cell carcinoma of the duodenum is very rare and may arise in congenital anomalies such as duplications and diverticula. Most of the squamous cell carcinomas of the duodenum are metastatic tumors from other solid organs such as cervix or lung.[82] Close monitoring of all patients with duodenal tumors is therefore warranted.

Adenocarcinoma

Duodenum is most common site and accounts for 50% carcinomas of the small bowel overall however, primary adenocarcinomas of the duodenum is a rare entity and account for only 0.5% of all GI malignancies. *Perivaterian carcinoma* is a term that includes malignancies in and around ampulla, inclusive of malignancies of duodenum, ampulla, pancreas and distal common bile duct.

Adenocarcinomas can be ulcerating, infiltrating to polypoid and virtually all are mucin producing. The most common site is periampullary region, and approximately 20% of duodenal adenocarcinomas arise in villous adenomas. Rarely, they arise in a duodenal diverticulum or in patients with nontropical sprue.

Duodenoscopy is considered a more sensitive diagnostic procedure than barium studies or hypotonic duodenography as it detects small lesions that may otherwise be missed. An upper gastrointestinal series should however be performed to rule out synchronous small bowel lesions. Computed tomography is the preferred investigation to assess extraluminal spread, involvement of lymph nodes and distant metastasis. The lesion can be stenosing, polypoidal or ulceroinfiltrative and mostly present as nodular heterogeneously enhancing circumferential mural thickening **(Figs. 22A to C)**. If it involves ampulla, it causes dilatation of both main pancreatic duct and common bile duct giving "double duct sign".

The treatment of choice for adenocarcinoma of the duodenum is pancreatico-duodenectomy. Small tumors in the fourth portion of the duodenum only are however treated with distal duodenectomy and duodenojejunostomy.

Lymphoma

Although primary lymphoma of the duodenum is rare, the duodenum may be involved in systemic lymphoma, more so in AIDS patients.[82] Only 5% of all lymphomas are primary intestinal lymphoma and less than 10% of these are located in the duodenum. The only way to establish the diagnosis of primary lymphoma is to exclude the presence of the disease in other organs. Similar to gastric lymphoma most duodenal lymphomas are non-Hodgkin's lymphomas of B-cell origin. Only a few reports exist of Hodgkin's lymphomas or T-cell lymphomas. Involvement of the mesentery and the draining lymph nodes is common.

Lymphomas are difficult to distinguish from carcinoma preoperatively, though they tend to be larger than carcinomas. Often endoscopic biopsies are nondiagnostic as lymphomas arise in the submucosa. There may duodenal fold thickening, polypoidal masses and multiple nodules in patients of lymphoma. In advanced disease, however, perforation and multiple lesions are more common in lymphomas than in adenocarcinomas of the small bowel.

Lymphomas cause symptoms similar to those of duodenal and pancreatic carcinomas, and their appearance on computed tomography may be confused with pancreatic cancer. Histological cell type and grade help in deciding further management. Primary lymphoma of the duodenum is curable by surgery in only 40% of patients and unresectable cases of lymphoma requires radiotherapy and chemotherapy. Surgery in such cases is

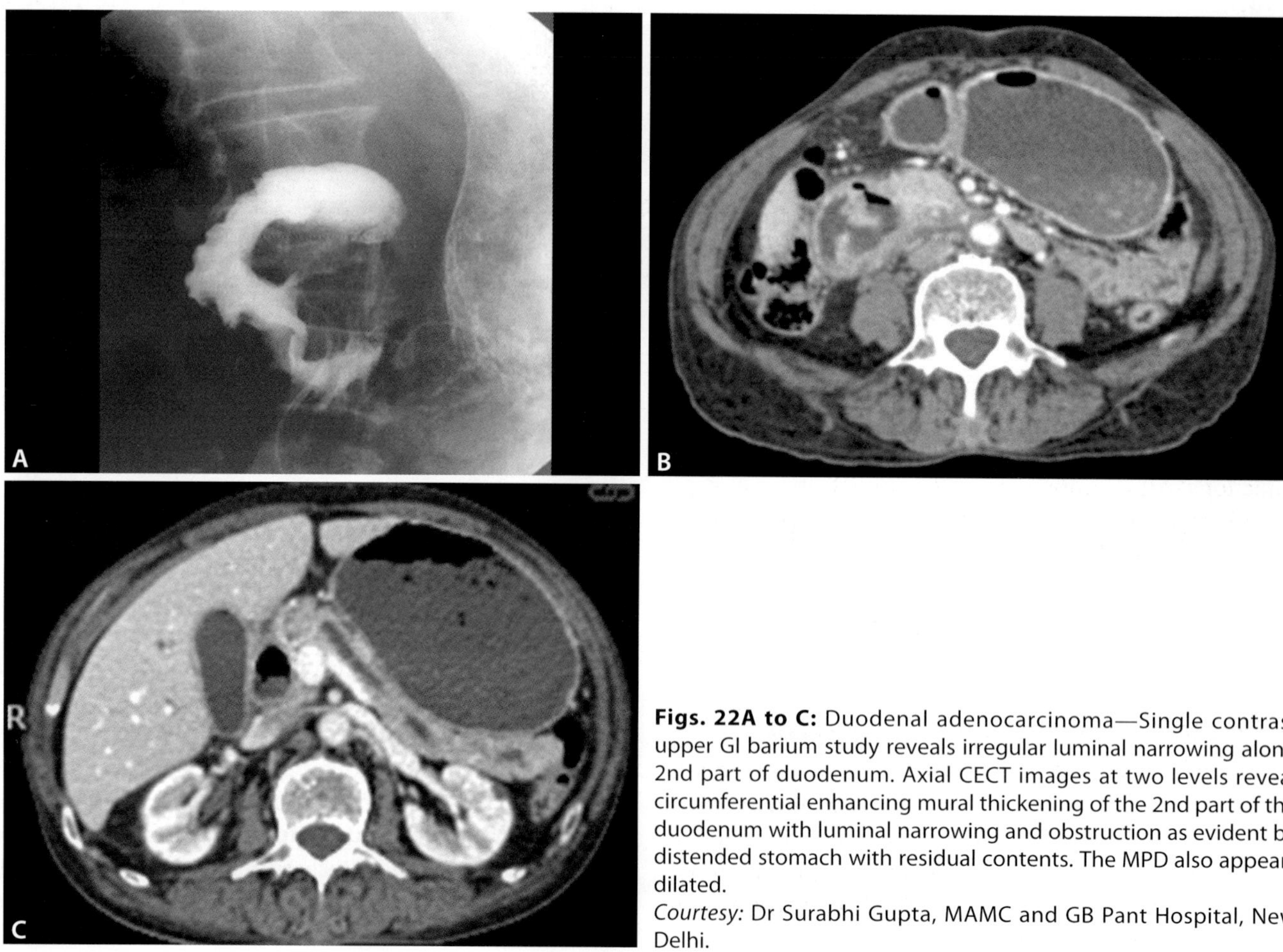

Figs. 22A to C: Duodenal adenocarcinoma—Single contrast upper GI barium study reveals irregular luminal narrowing along 2nd part of duodenum. Axial CECT images at two levels reveal circumferential enhancing mural thickening of the 2nd part of the duodenum with luminal narrowing and obstruction as evident by distended stomach with residual contents. The MPD also appears dilated.

Courtesy: Dr Surabhi Gupta, MAMC and GB Pant Hospital, New Delhi.

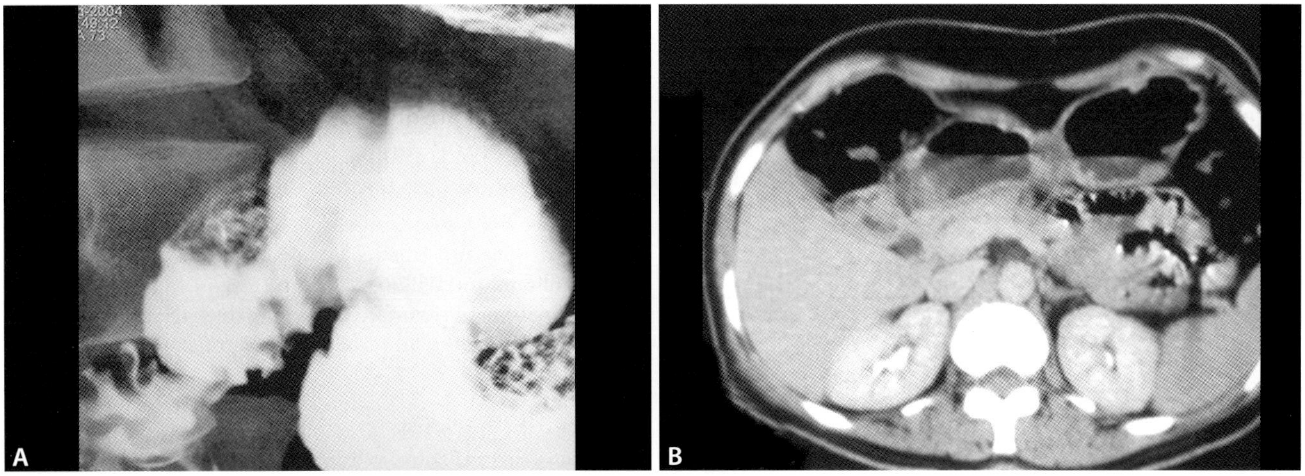

Figs. 23A and B: Villous adenoma: Polypoidal filling defect along lateral wall of duodenal bulb characteristic 'cauliflower' or 'soap-bubble' appearance on barium studies, caused by the trapping of barium in the crevices between the multiple frond-like projections of the tumor. CECT axial section reveals heterogeneously enhancing polypoidal mass lesion in first part of duodenum with nonenhancing fluid-filled hypodense linear areas symptoms of crevices between fronds with tracking of fluid in it.

being used only to treat complications such has bleeding from high-grade lesions.

Villous Adenoma

Majority of the villous adenomas are located around ampulla and become symptomatic much earlier than other duodenal tumors due to obstructive jaundice. Approximately 40–50% of villous adenomas of the duodenum harbor adenocarcinomas, irrespective of the size of the tumor. Definite diagnosis of the villous adenomas is made by examination of entire tumor histologically after complete removal as 50% of the lesions are missed on endoscopic biopsy alone. Villous adenomas exhibit a characteristic 'cauliflower'or 'soap bubble' appearance on barium studies, caused by the trapping of barium in the crevices between the multiple frond-like projections of the tumor[1] **(Figs. 23A and B)**.

Endoscopic resection is possible if the tumor is small and pedunculated. In all other cases duodenotomy is required. Since there is high incidence of co-existent malignancy, pancreaticoduodenectomy is the treatment of choice.

Secondary Involvement and Metastasis

Secondary involvement of duodenum by malignant process in adjacent viscera, like pancreas is fairly common and it is often not possible to distinguish a primary tumor of duodenum from a tumor of pancreas involving duodenum.[82]

Metastases to the duodenum can also occur and can present as filling defect with central ulceration and necrosis leading to classical "bull's eye" or "target" appearance. They are seen with metastasis from malignant melanoma **(Fig. 24)** and in patients with Kaposi's sarcoma.

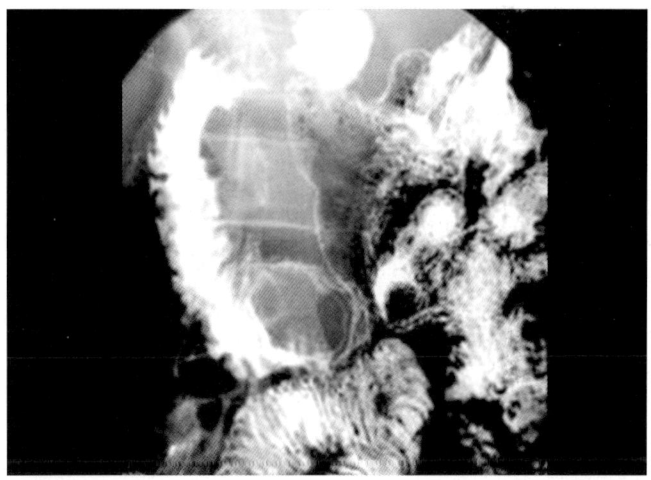

Fig. 24: Single contrast barium study showing large submucosal filling defect on enface view in the 3rd part of duodenum in a complaint of malignant melanoma symptoms of metastasis.

CONCLUSION

We should be aware of the advantages, pitfalls and limitations of the various imaging modalities in the diagnostic workup. Our aim should be to ensure early and accurate diagnosis of the tumors involving stomach and duodenum by judiciously using the various imaging modalities and techniques available and also ensure periodic surveillance for patients at risk.

REFERENCES

1. Grainger and Allison's Diagnostic Radiology—A Textbook of Medical Imaging, 5th edition, Churchill Livingstone; 2007.
2. Carmack SW, Genta RM, Graham DY, et al. Management of gastric polyps: a pathology based guide for gastroenterologists. Nat Rev Gastroenterol Hepatol. 2009;(6):331-41.
3. Stolte M, Sticht T, Eidt S, Ebert D, Finkenzeller G. Frequency, location, and age and sex distribution of various types of gastric polyp. Endoscopy. 1994;26(8):659-65.
4. Goddard AF, Badreldin R, Pritchard DM, Walker MM, Warren B. The management of gastric polyps. Gut. 2010;59(9):1270-6.
5. Chandrasekhara V, Ginsberg GG. Endoscopic management of gastrointestinal stromal tumors. Curr Gastroenterol Rep. 2011;13(6):532-9.
6. Shand AG, Taylor AC, Banerjee M, et al. Gastric fundic gland polyps in south-east Scotland: absence of adenomatous polyposis coli gene mutations and a strikingly low prevalence of *Helicobacter pylori* infection. J Gastroenterol Hepatol. 2002;17(11):1161-4.
7. el-Zimaity HM, Jackson FW, Graham DY. Fundic gland polyps developing during omeprazole therapy. Am J Gastroenterol. 1997;92(10):1858-60.
8. Bianchi LK, Burke CA, Bennett AE, Lopez R, Hasson H, Church JM. Fundic gland polyp dysplasia is common in familial adenomatous polyposis. Clin Gastroenterol Hepatol. 2008;6(2):180-5.
9. Abraham SC, Singh VK, Yardley JH, Wu TT. Hyperplastic polyps of the stomach: associations with histologic patterns of gastritis and gastric atrophy. Am J Surg Pathol. 2001;25(4):500-7.
10. Ohkusa T, Miwa H, Hojo M, et al. Endoscopic, histological and serologic findings of gastric hyperplastic polyps after eradication of *Helicobacter pylori*: comparison between responder and non-responder cases. Digestion. 2003;68(2-3):57-62.
11. Ljubicic N, Banic M, Kujundzic M, et al. The effect of eradicating *Helicobacter pylori* infection on the course of adenomatous and hyperplastic gastric polyps. Eur J Gastroenterol Hepatol. 1999;11(7):727-30.
12. Dirschmid K, Platz-Baudin C, Stolte M. Why is the hyperplastic polyp a marker for the precancerous condition of the gastric mucosa? Virchows Arch. 2006;448(1):80-4.
13. Ginsberg GG, Al-Kawas FH, Fleischer DE, Reilly HF, Benjamin SB. Gastric polyps: relationship of size and histology to cancer risk. Am J Gastroenterol. 1996;91(4): 714-7.
14. Schmitz JM, Stolte M. Gastric polyps as precancerous lesions. Gastrointest Endosc Clin N Am. 1997;7(1):29-46.
15. Rugge M, Nitti D, Farinati F, et al. Non-invasive neoplasia of the stomach. Eur J Gastroenterol Hepatol. 2005;17: 1191-6.
16. Calva D, Howe JR. Hamartomatous polyposis syndromes. Surg Clin North Am. 2008;88(4):779-817.
17. Beggs AD, Latchford AR, Vasen HF, et al. Peutz-Jeghers syndrome: a systematic review and recommendations for management. Gut. 2010;59(7):975-86.
18. Rubesin SE, Levine MS, Laufer I. Double-contrast upper gastrointestinal radiography: a pattern approach for disease of the stomach. Radiology. 2008;246:33-48.
19. Pisters PWT, Keslen DP, Tepper JE. Cancer of the stomach. In: Devita VT, Lawrence TS, Rosenberg SA (Eds), Cancer: principals and practice of oncology, 8th edition, Lippincott, Williams and Wilkins. 2008.pp.1043-79.
20. Parsonnet J, Friedman GD, Vandersteen DP, et al. *Heliobacter pylori* infection and the risk of gastric carcinoma. N Engl J Med. 1991;325:1127-31.
21. Ramon JM, Sera L, Cerdo C, et al. Dietary factors and gastric cancer risk: A case control study in Spain. Cancer. 1993;71:1731-5.
22. Hamashima C, Shibuya D, Yamazaki H, et al. The Japanese guidelines for gastric cancer screening. Jpn J Clin Oncol. 2008; 38:259.
23. Maruyama M, Baba Y. Diagnosis of the invasive depth of gastric cancer. Abdom Imaging. 1994;19:532-6.
24. Japanese Gastric Cancer Association. Japanese classification of gastric carcinoma—2nd English edition. Gastric Cancer. 1998. pp.10-24.
25. Low VH, Levine MS, Rubesin SE, et al. Diagnosis of gastric carcinoma: sensitivity of double-contrast barium studies. Am J Roentgenol. 1994;162:329-34.
26. Levine MS, Rubesin SE, Laufer I. Barium studies in modern radiology: do they have a role? Radiology. 2009;250:18-22.
27. Gore RM, Levine MS, Gahremani GG, et al. Gastric cancer: Radiologic diagnosis. Radiol Clin N Am. 1997;35:311-29.
28. Furukawa K, Miyahara R, Itoh A, et al. Diagnosis of the invasion depth of the gastric cancer using MDCT with virtual gastroscopy: comparison with staging with endoscopic ultrasound. Am J Roentgenol. 2011;197:867-75.
29. Washington K. Editorial: 7th edition of the AJCC Cancer Staging Manual: Stomach. Ann Surg Oncol. 2010;17:3077-9.
30. Kwee RM, Kwee TC. Imaging in local staging of gastric cancer: a systematic review. J Clin Oncol. 2007;25:2107-16.
31. Hwang SW, Lee DH, Lee SH, et al. Preoperative staging of gastric cancer by endoscopic ultrasonography and multidetector row computed tomography. J Gastroenterol Hepatol. 2010;25: 512-18.
32. Pradhan Gaurav S. Benign lesions of stomach and small intestine. AIIMS-MAMC-PGI's Comprehensive Textbook of Diagnostic Radiology, Jaypee Brothers Medical Publishers. 2016.pp.1158-72.
33. Edelman Robert R, Hesselink John R, Zlatkin Michael B, Crees John S. Clinical Magnetic Resonance Imaging Vol-3, 3rd edition. 2006.pp.2684-721.
34. Kim Il Young. MR imaging of gastric carcinoma. In: Ismaili N (Ed). Management of Gastric Cancer. InTech. 2011. pp. 19-36.
35. Ghai S, Pattison J, Ghai S, O'Malley ME, Khalili K, Stephens. Primary Gastrointestinal Lymphoma: Spectrum of Imaging Findings with Pathologic Correlation. Radiographics. 2007; 27:1371-88.

36. Lim JS, Kim MJ, Yun MJ, et al. Comparison of CT and 18F FDG-PET for detecting peritoneal metastases on the preoperative evaluation of gastric carcinoma. Korean J Radiol. 2006;7:249-56.
37. Isaacson PG. Gastrointestinal lymphomas of T and B-cell types. Mod Pathol. 1999;12:151-8.
38. Dawson IM, Cornes JS, Morson BC. Primary malignant tumors of the intestinal tract. Br J Surg. 1961;49:80-9.
39. Rohatiner A, d'Amore F, Coiffier B, et al. Report on a workshop convened to discuss the pathological and staging classifications of gastrointestinal tract lymphoma. Ann Oncol. 1994;5:397-400.
40. Yoo CC, Levine MS, Furth EE, et al. Gastric mucosa-associated lymphoid tissue lymphoma: radiographic findings in six patients. Radiology. 1998;208:239-43.
41. Parsonnet J, Hansen S, Rodriguez L, et al. Recent developments in our understanding of gastric lymphoma. Am J Surg Pathol. 1996;20(Suppl I):S1-7.
42. Miller FH, Kochman ML, Talamonti MS, Ghahremani GG, Gore RM. Gastric cancer: radiologic staging. Radiol Clin North Am. 1997;35:331-49.
43. Ciftci AO, Tanyel FC, Kotiloglu E, Hicsonmez A. Gastric lymphoma causing gastric outlet obstruction. J Pediatr Surg. 1996;31:1424-6.
44. Guglielmi G, Schiavon F, Cammarota T (Eds). Radiologia geriatrica, Springer; 2006.
45. Radan L, Fischer D, Bar-shalom R, et al. FDG avidity and PET/CT patterns in primary gastric lymphoma. Eur J Nucl Med Mol Imaging. 2008;35:1428-4330.
46. Levy AD, Sobin LH. Gastrointestinal Carcinoids: Imaging Features with Clinicopathologic Comparison. Radio Graphics. 2007;27:237-57.
47. Virmani V, Khandelwal A, Sethi V, Hill MF, Fasih N, Kielar A. Neoplastic stomach lesions and their mimickers: spectrum of imaging manifestations. Cancer Imaging. 2012;12:269-78.
48. Chappuis CW, Divincenti FC, Cohn I Jr. Villous tumors of the duodenum. Ann Surg. 1989;209:593-9.
49. Gong J, Kang W, Zhu J, Xu J. CT and MR imaging of gastrointestinal stromal tumor of stomach: a pictorial review. Quant Imaging Med Surg. 2012;2(4):274-9.
50. Heinrich MC, Corless CL, Duensing A, et al. PDGFRA activating mutations in gastrointestinal stromal tumors. Science. 2003;299(5607):708-10.
51. Lee NK, Kim S, Kim GH, et al. Hypervascular subepithelial gastrointestinal masses: CT-pathologic correlation. Radiographics. 2010;30:1915-34.
52. Kang HC, Menias CO, Gaballah AH, Shroff S, Taggart MW, Garg N, Elsayes KM. Beyond the GIST: Mesenchymal Tumors of the Stomach. Radiographics. 2013;33:1673-90.
53. Levy AD, Remotti HE, Thompson WM, Sobin LH, Miettinen M. Gastrointestinal stromal tumors: radiologic features with pathologic correlation. Radiographics. 2003;23(2): 283-304.
54. Salamah AB, Prokop M, Uffmann M, Pokieser P, Teleky B, Lechner G. Dedicated Multidetector CT of the Stomach: Spectrum of Diseases. Radiographics. 2003;23:625-44.
55. Kim H-C, Lee JM, Kim KW, et al. Gastrointestinal stromal tumors of the stomach: CT findings and prediction of malignancy. AJR. 2004;183:893-8.
56. DeMatteo RP, Lewis JJ, Leung D, Mudan SS, Woodruff JM, Brennan MF. Two hundred gastrointestinal stromal tumors: recurrence patterns and prognostic factors for survival. Ann Surg. 2000;231(1):51-8.
57. Espinosa I, Lee CH, Kim MK, et al. A novel monoclonal antibody against DOG1 is a sensitive and specific marker for gastrointestinal stromal tumors. Am J Surg Pathol. 2008;32(2):210-8.
58. Demetri GD, Benjamin R, Blanke CD, et al. NCCN task force report: optimal management of patients with gastrointestinal stromal tumors (GIST)—expansion and update of NCCN clinical practice guidelines. J Natl Compr Cancer Netw. 2004;2:S1–S26.
59. Joensuu H, Roberts PJ, Sarlomo-Rikala M, et al. Effect of the tyrosine kinase inhibitor STI571 in a patient with a metastatic gastrointestinal stromal tumor. N Engl J Med. 2001;344:1052-6.
60. Blanke C, Joensuu G, Demetri M, et al. Longterm follow up of advanced gastrointestinal stromal tumor (GIST) patients treated with imatinib mesylate (abstr). In: Proceedings of the 2004 Gastrointestinal Cancers Symposium: Current Status and Future Directions for Prevention and Management. Alexandria, Va: American Society of Clinical Oncology. 2004;43.
61. Hong X, Choi H, Loyer EM, Benjamin RS, Trent JC, Charnsangavej C. Gastrointestinal Stromal Tumor: Role of CT in Diagnosis and in Response Evaluation and Surveillance after Treatment with Imatinib. Radiographics. 2006;26:481-95.
62. Jayaraman MV, Mayo-Smith WW, Movson JS, Dupuy DE, Wallach MT. CT of the Duodenum: An Overlooked Segment Gets Its Due. Radiographics. 2001;21:S147-60.
63. Thompson WM, Kende AI, Levy AD. Imaging characteristics of gastric lipomas in 16 adult and pediatric patients. Am J Roentgenol. 2003;181(4):981-5.
64. Ferrozzi F, Tognini G, Bova D, et al. Lipomatous tumors of the stomach: CT findings and differential diagnosis. J Comput Assist Tomogr. 2000;24:854-8.
65. Miettinen M, Lasota J. Gastrointestinal stromal tumors: definition, clinical, histological, immunohistochemical, and molecular genetic features and differential diagnosis. Virchows Arch. 2001;438(1):1-12.
66. Hur BY, Kim SH, Choi JY, et al. Gastroduodenal glomus tumors: differentiation from other subepithelial lesions based on dynamic contrast-enhanced CT findings. Am J Roentgenol. 2011;197(6):1351-9.
67. Lee MJ, Lim JS, Kwon JE, et al. Gastric true leiomyoma: computed tomographic findings and pathological correlation. J Comput Assist Tomogr. 2007;31(2):204-8.
68. Park SO, Han JK, Kirn TK, et al. Unusual gastric tumors: radiologic pathologic correlation. Radiographics. 1999;19: 1435-46.
69. Raber MH, CMPZ des Plantes, Vink R, Vink R, Klaase JM. "Gastric schwannoma presenting as an incidentaloma on

CT-scan and MRI," Gastroenterology Research. 2010;3(6): 276-80.
70. Hong HS, Ha HK, Won HJ, et al. Gastric schwannomas: radiological features with endoscopic and pathological correlation. Clin Radiol. 2008;63(5):536-42.
71. Miettinen M, Paal E, Lasota J, Sobin LH. Gastrointestinal glomus tumors: a clinicopathologic, immunohistochemical, and molecular genetic study of 32 cases. Am J Surg Pathol. 2002;26(3):301-11.
72. Levy AD, Abbott RM, Rohrmann CA Jr, Frazier AA, Kende A. Gastrointestinal hemangiomas: imaging findings with pathologic correlation in pediatric and adult patients. Am J Roentgenol. 2001;177(5):1073-81.
73. Coffin CM, Hornick JL, Fletcher CD. Inflammatory myofibroblastic tumor: comparison of clinicopathologic, histologic, and immunohistochemical features including ALK expression in atypical and aggressive cases. Am J Surg Pathol. 2007;31(4):509-20.
74. Bjelovic M, Micev M, Spica B, Babic T, Gunjic D, Djuric A, Pesko P. Primary inflammatory myofibroblastic tumor of the stomach in an adult woman: a case report and review of the literature. World Journal of Surgical Oncology. 2013;11:35.
75. Karnak I, Senocak ME, Ciftci AO, et al. Inflammatory myofibroblastic tumor in children: diagnosis and treatment. J Pediatr Surg. 2001;36(6):908-12.
76. Narla LD, Newman B, Spottswood SS, et al. Inflammatory pseudotumor. Radiographics. 2003;23:719-29.
77. Grendell JH, Ermak TH. Anatomy, histology, embryology, and developmental anomalies of the pancreas. In: Sleisenger and Fordtran's gastrointestinal and liver disease. Philadelphia, PA: Saunders. 1998.pp.761-71.
78. Kim JY, Lee JM, Kim KW, Park HS, Choi Y, Kim SH, Kim MA, Lee JY, Han JK, Choi BI. Ectopic Pancreas: CT Findings with Emphasis on Differentiation from Small Gastrointestinal Stromal Tumor and Leiomyoma. Radiology: 2009;252(1).
79. Okuhata Y, Maebayashi T, Furuhashi S, et al. Characteristics of ectopic pancreas in dynamic gadolinium-enhanced MRI. Abdom Imaging. 2008;35:85-7.
80. Singh JP, Rajdeo H, Bhuta K, Savino JA. Gastric Duplication Cyst: Two Case Reports and Review of the Literature. Hindawi Publishing Corporation Case Reports in Surgery. 2013, Article ID 605059, 4 pages.
81. Horne G, Ming-Lum C, Kirkpatrick AW, Parker RL. "High-grade neuroendocrine carcinoma arising in a gastric duplication cyst: a case report with literature review." International Journal of Surgical Pathology. 2007;(15)2:187-91.
82. Winfield RD1, Hochwald SN, Vogel SB, Hemming AW, Liu C, Cance WG, Grobmyer SR. Presentation and management of gastrointestinal stromal tumors of the duodenum. Am Surg. 2006;72(8):719-22; discussion 722-3.

CHAPTER 70

Small Bowel Tumors

Rashmi Dixit, Gaurav S Pradhan, Anju Garg

INTRODUCTION

Tumors of the small bowel both benign and malignant are quite uncommon, this despite the fact the small bowel constitutes about 75% of the total length of the gastrointestinal tract and 90% of its mucosal surface. It also lies between two areas of high cancer risk, i.e. the colon and the stomach yet only about 3–5% of all GI tumors and less than 2% of all gastrointestinal malignancies arise in the small bowel.[1-3] However with advances in endoscopy and imaging an increasing number of small bowel tumors are being diagnosed.

About 40 different histologic types of tumors have been described in the small bowel. Although over 2/3 of lesions found at autopsy are benign, most symptomatic lesions and those detected at surgery tend to be malignant.[1] The major tumors are listed in **Table 1**.

Table 1: Small bowel tumors and polyps.

1. Epithelial Adenoma Carcinoma Neuroendocrine tumors/carcinoid Mixed carcinoid-adenocarcinoma Others
2. Nonepithelial/mesenchymal Lipoma Leiomyoma Hemangioma/lymphangioma Gastrointestinal stromal tumors (GIST) Leiomyosarcoma Kaposi's sarcoma Others
3. Lymphoid tissue Lymphomas
4. Neurogenic Neurofibroma Schwannoma
5. Secondary tumors/metastasis
6. Polyps

SMALL BOWEL CARCINOGENESIS–PATHOGENESIS

The exact reason for the low incidence of malignancy in the small intestine is not certain but several theories have been proposed including liquid contents of the small bowel causing less mucosal irritation, relatively rapid transit, lower bacterial load in small bowel and high levels of IgA due to increased lymphoid tissue.[1,4]

Certain syndromes or conditions are associated with increased incidence of specific histologic types of small intestine tumors, e.g. Peutz-Jeghers syndrome, familial adenomatous polyposis, Lynch syndrome and Gardner's syndrome predispose to adenoma and adenocarcinoma and von Recklinghausen's disease or neurofibromatosis to gastrointestinal stromal tumors. Gardner's syndrome also predisposes to multiple desmoid tumors.[1,4]

DIAGNOSTIC TECHNIQUES

The clinical presentation of most small bowel tumors is non-specific. The diagnosis is further challenged by lack of easy endoscopic access and relative rarity of disease leading to low index of suspicion. The various techniques available to evaluate the small intestine tumors are—conventional small bowel follow through examination, conventional enteroclysis, ultrasound, CT and MR (including CT and MR enterography and enteroclysis) and endoscopic techniques like capsule endoscopy, push enteroscopy.

Early diagnosis of small bowel tumors is challenging and currently there are no definite guidelines as to which technique should be used first, but it would be reasonable to use noninvasive imaging before more invasive and expensive endoscopic techniques are used.

Barium meal follow through may show some abnormal pattern in up to 83% cases of small bowel tumors however, direct evidence of presence of tumor is seen in only 30–44% cases. Enteroclysis has a sensitivity of 90–95% for the detection of small bowel tumors, but the technique is invasive and provides little information on mural and extramural extent of tumor.[5,6] With the advent of high end multiple detector computed tomography (MDCT) scanners and widespread use of CT enterography, conventional enteroclysis is rarely performed these days.

Ultrasound examination is generally not used for the primary diagnosis of small bowel tumors, however, because it is often the first investigation performed in nonspecific abdominal complaints it may detect a bowel mass especially when this is large. Malignant mass may be seen as asymmetric wall thickening, 'target lesion' or occasionally as a large exophytic mass where the organ of origin may not be clear like in gastrointestinal stromal tumors. Increased vascularity may be seen within the lesion on colour Doppler. Contrast enhanced ultrasound has also been used in bowel masses especially for follow-up of treated gastrointestinal stromal tumors. Associated findings such as nodal involvement and ascites can also be seen.[7]

Conventional CT has sensitivity of around 80% for small bowel tumors, however, CT/MR enterography have sensitivity of 85–95%.[4,8,9] CT enterography is generally the current standard practice given the excellent sensitivity to detect even small tumors due to superior tumor to background contrast enhancement owing to the use of neutral oral contrast. Due to its higher cost, lower spatial resolution as compared to CT and artifacts due to bowel motion MR enteroclysis/enterography is generally not used as a first line investigation unless radiation dose due to repeat examinations is a concern. However, MR of the gastrointestinal tract is gaining clinical acceptance. Cine sequences or MR fluoroscopy may also be performed during the exam allowing functional evaluation of small bowel as well. In some studies, MR enteroclysis was found to be more sensitive than CT enteroclysis in patients with Crohn's disease.[1,4]

Ultrasound and CT may also be used to guide percutaneous biopsy or needle aspiration .

18F-FDG-PET/CT may be useful in patients with adenocarcinoma, lymphomas and sarcomas mainly for staging. PET-CT with octreotide analogs is useful in detection and staging of carcinoids.[4]

Hybrid PET-MRI is a promising new technique that has very limited availability as yet but appears to hold promise for evaluation of gastrointestinal malignancy. It combines the high contrast and spatial resolution of MR with the high sensitivity of PET and allows use of multiple sequences for combined functional and anatomical evaluation. This may allow for improved staging and restaging of disease status after treatment.[10]

Capsule endoscopy is a relatively new technique used by gastroenterologists, that can screen the entire small bowel. Capsule endoscopy may detect lesions not detected on standard push endoscopy and imaging. It has higher sensitivity to detect tumors and polyps than push enteroscopy which evaluates only the first 120 cm of the small bowel beyond the ligament of Treitz. However, some lesions may be missed due to poor bowel preparation, orientation of camera away from lesion and rapid or delayed small bowel transit. It is also not very accurate in exact localization and size estimation and is contraindicated in patients with bowel stricture, intestinal obstruction, swallowing and motility disorders.[4,5]

Balloon enteroscopy allows evaluation of the entire small bowel. Double balloon enteroscopy (DBE) has a sensitivity of about 86% in detecting small bowel tumors which is comparable with capsule endoscopy. The decision to use single or double balloon enteroscopy is the investigator's choice, as no definite advantage of single balloon enteroscopy has been demonstrated. Capsule endoscopy is less invasive and is generally preferred as the initial exam although the two can be complementary as abnormal areas can generally not be biopsied on capsule endoscopy. All endoscopic methods are limited in the evaluation submucosal and mural lesions.[4,5]

BENIGN TUMORS AND POLYPS

Adenoma

Adenomas represent the most common benign tumor of the small intestine. Histologically, these can be tubular, villous or tubulovillous. Although adenomas are benign they are considered premalignant. Large size and villous component are associated with an increased risk of malignant transformation. They may occur as a pedunculated polyp or sessile polypoid lesion, usually 2–3 cm in size.

On barium studies, when seen in profile, they are seen as smooth or lobulated lesions forming acute angles with the bowel wall. In pedunculated lesions the pedicle can also be visualized. Sometimes the surface may appear granular due to barium trapping in the interstices. They may act as a lead point for intussusception.[11,12]

Adenomas are difficult to appreciate on routine CT or MR but may be seen on CT/MR enteroclysis or enterography. On CT enteroclysis they are seen as well-defined soft tissue lesions with moderate enhancement on post-contrast images and a clear fat plane around the lesion **(Figs. 1A and B)**.[13,14] On MR enteroclysis adenomas are seen as homogeneously enhancing intraluminal masses on fat saturated postcontrast T1W images, while on T2W images they appear as low signal intensity intraluminal masses. Generally there is no proximal dilatation.[15,16]

Inflammatory fibroid polyps also known as Vanek's tumors are an important differential diagnosis which are predominantly located in the ileum and represent rare non-neoplastic pseudotumorous submucosal lesions of uncertain etiology. They can be sessile or pedunculated polypoid lesions. Histologically, IFPs consist of mass of loose fibrous connective tissue, with presence of inflammatory infiltrate consisting of large number eosinophils. On CT a well-defined, smooth, homogeneous, low attenuation, nonenhancing or hypoenhancing polypoid mass is seen **(Figs. 2A to C)**.[17]

Multiple adenomas can be found in the hereditary polyposis syndromes. A major risk factor is familial adenomatous polyposis (FAP) where 80% patients develop duodenal adenomas. Patients frequently develop jejunal and ileal polyps also.[4]

Treatment includes endoscopic resection for pedunculated tumors and surgical removal of large sessile tumors.[1,4]

Lipoma

Lipomas account for 15–20% of all small intestinal neoplasms. The small bowel is the most common site in the gastrointestinal (GI) tract after the colon and within the small bowel ileum is the most common location. The vast majority of these are submucosal tumors that are composed of mature adipose tissue. About 5–10%, may be subserosal. Small lesions are mostly asymptomatic whereas larger lesions may produce intussusception, rarely surface ulceration may occur leading to gastrointestinal bleed.[13,16,18]

They can be sessile or pedunculated producing a sharply marginated ovoid or spherical polypoid defect on barium studies which may change shape with compression or on different views due to pliability. Sometimes the low density of fat may be apparent. Usually they are solitary but occasionally may be multiple. On CT lipomas are seen as a low density fat attenuation masses (between -60 to -120 HU) in the wall of the small intestine **(Figs. 3A to C)**. No contrast enhancement or nonfatty elements are seen, however, sometimes few linear strands of soft tissue attenuation may be seen at the base corresponding to prominent fibrovascular septae on histopathology. Such tumors may at times show surface

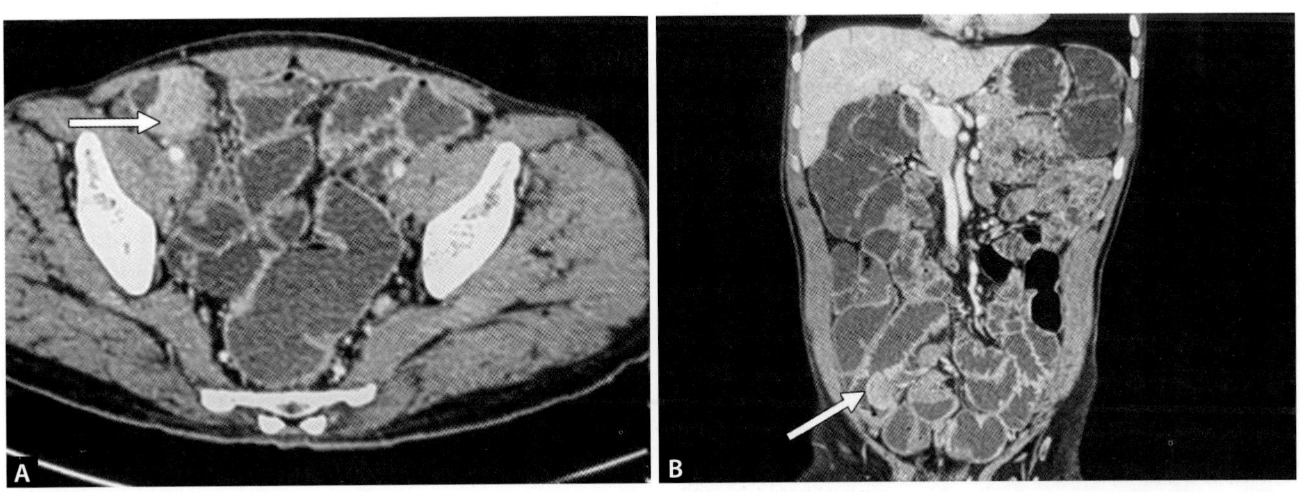

Figs. 1A and B: *Small bowel adenoma*: Axial (A) and coronal (B) CT enteroclysis images reveal a sessile polypoid moderately enhancing mass lesion in the ileum (arrows) with normal surrounding fat planes suggestive of an adenoma.

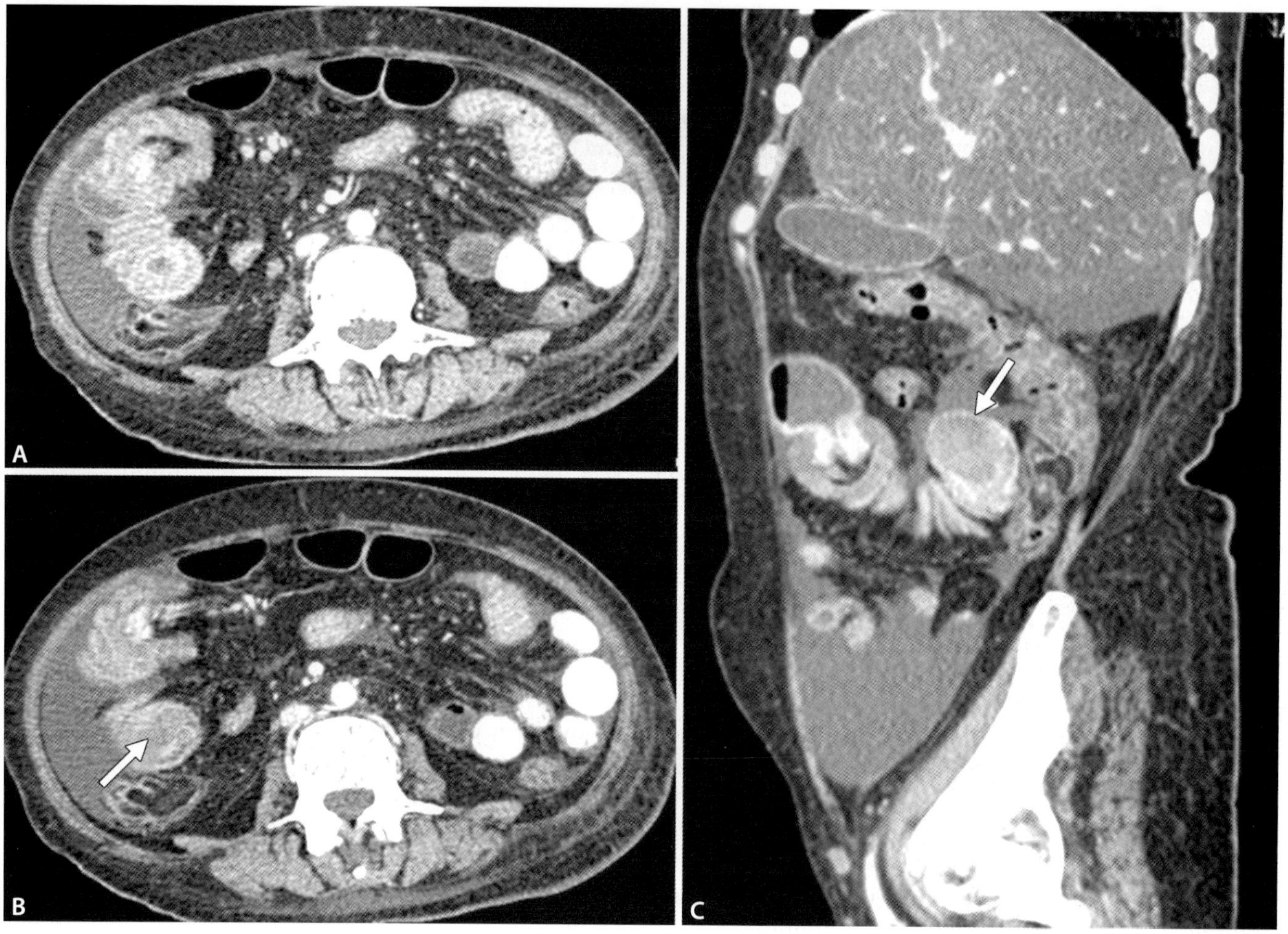

Figs. 2A to C: *Inflammatory fibroid polyp*: Axial (A and B) and sagittal (C) images show free fluid in the right paracolic region and telescoping of proximal ileum into a distal ileal loop along with a sleeve of mesenteric fat and vessels consistent with ileo-ileal intussusception. A well-defined poorly enhancing hypodense polyp is seen at the apex (arrows in B and C) which was proven to be an inflammatory fibroid polyp on histopathological examination.

ulceration and must not be mistaken for liposarcoma—the septae being presumably enlarged due to inflammation associated with the ulcer.[18] On MR enterography they are seen as well-circumscribed masses which are bright on T1W, match the signal on intra-abdominal fat on T2W images with signal suppression on fat saturated images and do not show contrast enhancement.[16]

Leiomyoma

True leiomyomas of the small intestine are extremely rare most lesions previously diagnosed as leiomyomas may actually represent gastrointestinal stromal tumors (GIST). They can be seen as round or crescentic predominantly submucosal masses showing homogeneous enhancement on CT or MR. They are virtually impossible to distinguish from small gastrointestinal stromal tumors on imaging. Occasionally intraluminal polyp or extraluminal masses may be seen.[1,13]

Hemangioma

Small bowel hemangiomas are rare most often situated in the jejunal submucosa and can be sessile, pedunculated or infilterative. Most lesions represent venous malformations rather than true tumors (hemangioma). Some cases can occur in association of syndromes like blue rubber bleb nevus and Klippel Trenaunay syndrome. In contrast to most other benign tumors most are symptomatic and commonly produce manifest or occult gastrointestinal bleed. Other symptoms include pain, obstruction due to intussusception and rarely perforation.[1,13]

On enteroclysis they may produce a nodular, pliable submucosal filling defect.[11] On contrast enhanced CT

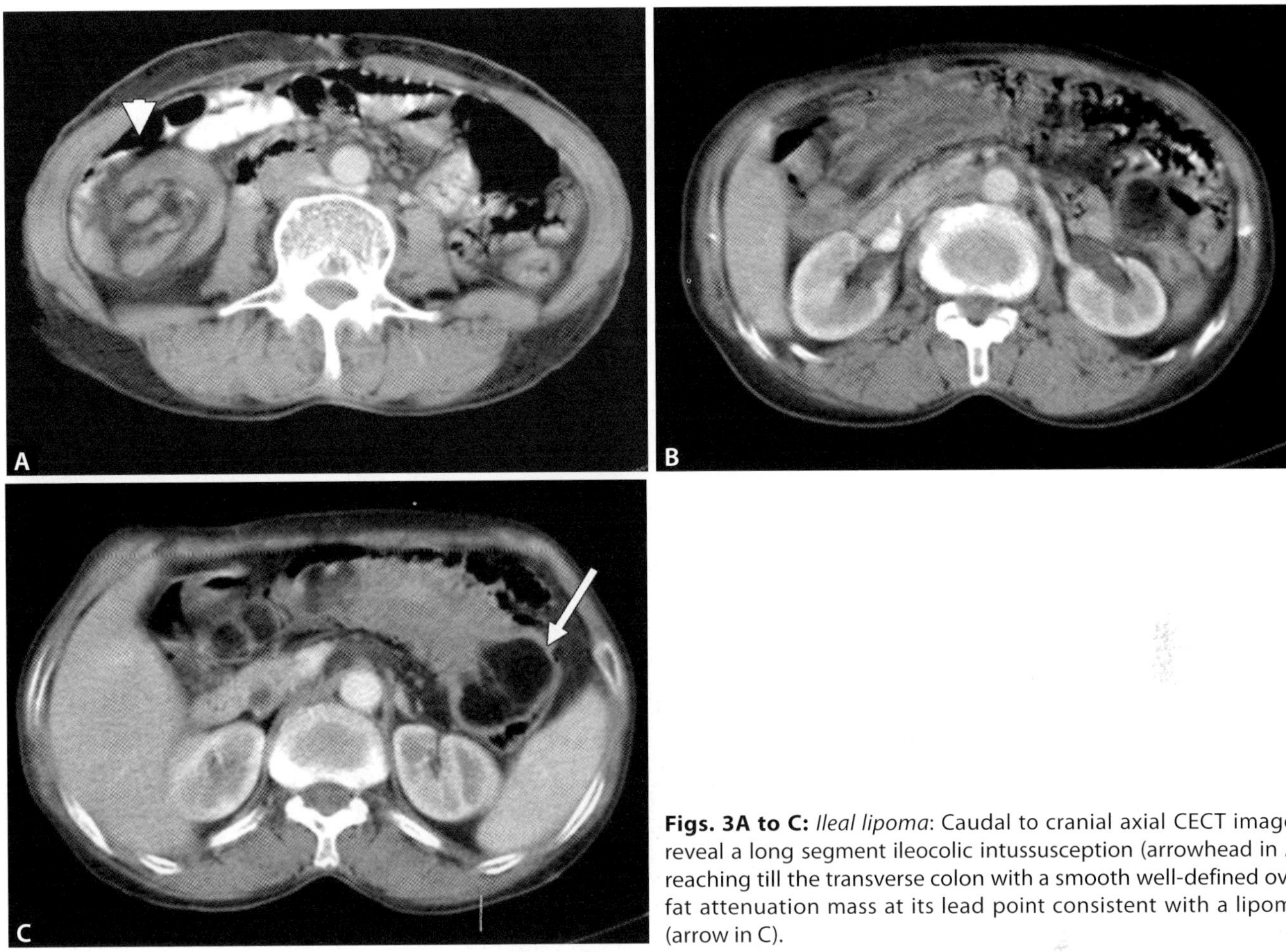

Figs. 3A to C: *Ileal lipoma*: Caudal to cranial axial CECT images reveal a long segment ileocolic intussusception (arrowhead in A) reaching till the transverse colon with a smooth well-defined oval fat attenuation mass at its lead point consistent with a lipoma (arrow in C).

enterography they can be seen as intensely enhancing lesion with or without phleboliths. Progressive enhancement may be seen with multiphase CT.[19,20] On MR they are T1 hypointense, markedly hyperintense on T2W images with no loss of signal on fat saturated images. Nodular enhancement has been reported in the arterial phase and homogeneous enhancement in the delayed phase.[16]

Neurogenic Tumor

Neurogenic tumors are relatively rare arising from the intramural neural plexus. Most often these are nonplexiform neurofibromas occurring as well-defined subserosal masses on the antimesenteric border, difficult to detect on contrast examinations. They can be multiple especially in patients with neurofibromatosis. Occasionally they are submucosal when it is difficult to distinguish them from other submucoasl masses on imaging. Schwannomas usually occur as solitary masses. Plexiform neurofibromas can also involve the small bowel.[13]

POLYPOSIS SYNDROMES INVOLVING THE SMALL BOWEL

Although a number of polyposis syndromes can involve the small intestine the important ones are; Peutz-Jeghers syndrome; familial adenomatous polyposis generalized juvenile polyposis; and Cronkhite-Canada syndrome. These disorders are characterized by the presence of multiple polyps affecting all or parts of the gastrointestinal tract. They are distinguished by the way they can be inherited, location, associated extraintestinal symptoms and the microscopic appearance of the polyps.

Peutz-Jeghers Syndrome

Peutz-Jeghers syndrome (PJS) is a rare autosomal dominant syndrome but has incomplete penetrance.[1,11] It is associated with mutation of STK II tumor suppression gene resulting in hamartomas throughout the gastrointestinal tract. The characteristic feature of PJS polyp is the smooth muscle core arising from muscularis mucosae extending into the polyp. The polyps are most common in the small bowel and less so in the stomach and colon. They tend to be multiple and vary in size and shape. These can be sessile or pedunculated and produce intraluminal filling defects.[1,11,21]

The polyps, being firm are especially prone to intussusception and may cause bleeding as well **(Figs. 4A to D)**. Although the polyps of PJS, being hamartomatous, are benign, the syndrome is associated with a definitely increased risk of small bowel adenocarcinoma. It is not clear whether this arises from the polyp or from coexisting adenomas. PJS is associated with 10–18 fold increase in gastrointestinal cancers.[1,11]

In patients presenting with multiple polyps the presence of multiple cororectal polyps and duodenal polyps (adenomas) favors the diagnosis of familial adenomatous polyposis (FAP) while the presence of small number of large polyps in the distal duodenum and jejunum favors PJS.[1,11] Other associated findings which help to clinch the diagnosis of PJS include pigmented lesions on the buccal mucosa, lips and on the skin especially hands and feet.[1,21]

Management of these polyps may be done by enteroscopic clearance. Intestinal resection is limited to the necessary minimum when required. The primary aim of polyp removal is to present intussusception.[1]

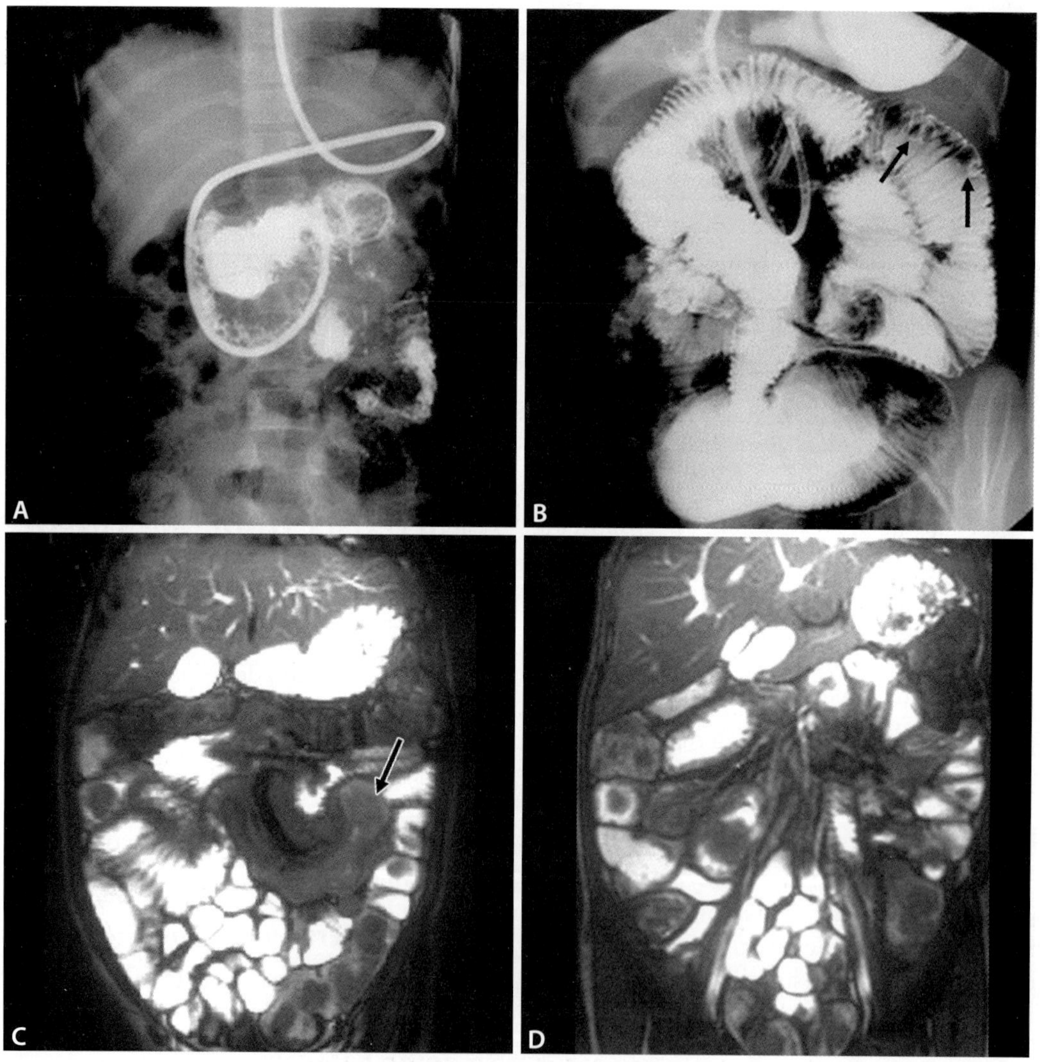

Figs. 4A to D: *Peutz–Jegher's syndrome*: Barium enteroclysis (A and B) in a patient with mucocutaneous pigmentation demonstrates multiple round to oval filling defects in the jejunum with jejuno-jejunal intussusception producing a coiled spring appearance in A. Coronal T2W (C and D) MR enteroclysis images of the same patient reveal multiple round to oval T2 iso to hypointense polyps in the jejunum. Jejuno-jejunal intussusception due to a polyp acting as a lead point is also well seen (arrow in C).

Cowden's Disease[4,21]

Cowden's disease consists of gastric, small bowel and colonic hamartomas and facial trichilemmomas.

Familial Adenomatous Polyposis[1,4,21]

Familial adenomatous polyposis is an inherited, autosomal dominant syndrome characterized by the presence of multiple adenomatous polyps in the colon 80% of patients can also have adenomas involving the small intestine most common in the duodenum. Extra-intestinal manifestation of familial adenomatous polyposis (FAP) include osteomas of mandible, long bones and skull, thyroid malignancy, adrenal adenoma/carcinoma, CNS tumors (particularly medulloblastoma) and desmoid tumors.

Turcot's syndrome and Gardner's syndrome are also associated with multiple adenomatous small bowel polyps.

Cronkhite-Canada Syndrome[21]

It is characterized by several intestinal polyps of the inflammatory type, hyperpigmentation, dystrophy of nails, alopecia and diarrhea. The onset is usually after 40 years. The polyps are most commonly found in the small intestine and are generally not considered premalignant. The patient's main problem is usually malabsorption and protein loss.

Juvenile Polyposis[22]

Juvenile polyps are most often seen within first 10 years of life. The term juvenile however refers to the histology of the lesion and not the age of onset. Solitary lesions occur in the colon commonly presenting with bleeding per rectum. Juvenile polyposis is an autosomal dominant condition with multiple, i.e. more than 5 polyps throughout the colon (juvenile polyposis coli) but polyps can occur anywhere in the GI tract (generalized juvenile polyposis) usually presenting in adolescence or late childhood. The familial variety may be associated with an increased risk of GI cancer most often colonic.

MALIGNANT TUMORS

Adenocarcinoma

Adenocarcinoma of the small intestine is less common in Asia and developing countries than the western world where it accounts for 30–50% of small bowel malignancies. It occurs usually in the 6th–7th decade and is slightly commoner in males than females.[1,23]

The duodenum and proximal jejunum are the most sites for adenocarcinoma, the jejunum accounting for about 30% cases of adenocarcinoma small bowel (generally within 30 cm of ligament of Treitz) and the duodenum for 50%. Ileal involvement is seen only in 20% cases and is commoner in patients with Crohn's disease.[1,14,24]

Etiopathogenesis

Risk factors and geographical distribution for adenocarcinoma of the small bowel are considered to be similar to colonic carcinoma. An increased risk of small bowel adenocarcinoma has been reported in colorectal cancer survivors. It is believed that an adenoma carcinoma sequence occurs in the small bowel as well. The presence of adenoma whether single or multiple is considered the most important risk factor for development of small bowel cancer. Syndromes such as familial adenomatous polyposis, Peutz Jeghers syndrome, Lynch syndrome, Cowden's disease, Gardner's syndrome[1,24,25] and inflammatory disorders like Crohn's disease and celiac disease also predispose to development of adenocarcinoma. Some studies have shown an association with alcohol consumption, high animal fat intake, consumption of red meat and salt cured or smoked meat. Some urological procedures like ileal conduit of ileocystoplasty also increase the risk of adenocarcinoma.[1,24,25] No risk factor may be evident in most cases.

Clinical Presentation

Small bowel adenocarcinomas tend to become symptomatic later than the lesions located in the duodenum. The clinical features are nonspecific and include nausea, vomiting, pain abdomen, small bowel obstruction, weight loss and gastrointestinal bleed which may be occult. The nonspecific nature of clinical symptoms and uncommon nature of disease results in diagnostic delay.[1,26] Misinterpretation of radiological studies can also cause diagnostic delay.[1,26] As a result most lesions are already metastatic by the time they are diagnosed. Small intestinal mucosa, unlike the large bowel, contains lymphatics which extend till the luminal surface and invasion of mucosal tumors into these lymphatics may be responsible for early tendency to metastases.[1] A significant proportion of patients may present acutely with obstruction, massive gastrointestinal bleed or perforation.[1,24,26]

Imaging Features

On barium studies adenocarcinoma produces a short segment circumferential narrowing with mucosal irregularity and ulceration. The lesions tend to have overhanging margins—the so called "apple core" lesion **(Figs. 5A to D)**. These strictures have a fixed unchanging character on compression and with advanced lesions bowel obstruction is common.[11,26]

Differential diagnosis of small bowel strictures on barium include infective or inflammatory disorders like tuberculosis and Crohn's disease. These strictures do not have overhanging margins. In the case of Crohn's disease, associated adenocarcinomas of the terminal ileum, the tumor may resemble an inflammatory exacerbation of a fibrous stricture making the diagnosis difficult. It is unusual for lymphoma or gastrointestinal stromal tumors (GIST) to produce strictures, when they occur they tend to involve longer segment and are more pliable on fluoroscopy than adenocarcinoma. Occasionally small bowel metastases may produce lesions indistinguishable from adenocarcinoma.[11,26]

On CT/MR enteroclysis or enterography a small lesion may be seen as a polypoid mass which is indistinguishable from other benign tumors or polyps. Larger lesions may produce a discrete polypoidal mass or moderate wall thickening resulting in short segment annular narrowing with abrupt overhanging edges. Annular lesions are more common in the distal small bowel while polypoid lesions are more common in the duodenum. The high grade stenosis may result in proximal small bowel obstruction.[4,14,24] On T2W MR images, the mass may show a heterogeneous signal. Moderate post-contrast enhancement which is heterogeneous may be seen on CT or MR.[27] Marked diffusion restriction has been also reported on DW-MRI.[28] Occasionally, the lesions can be large and bulky mimicking lymphoma or gastrointestinal stromal tumors,[26-28] but bowel obstruction is unusual in lymphoma or gastrointestinal stromal tumors (GIST). The features

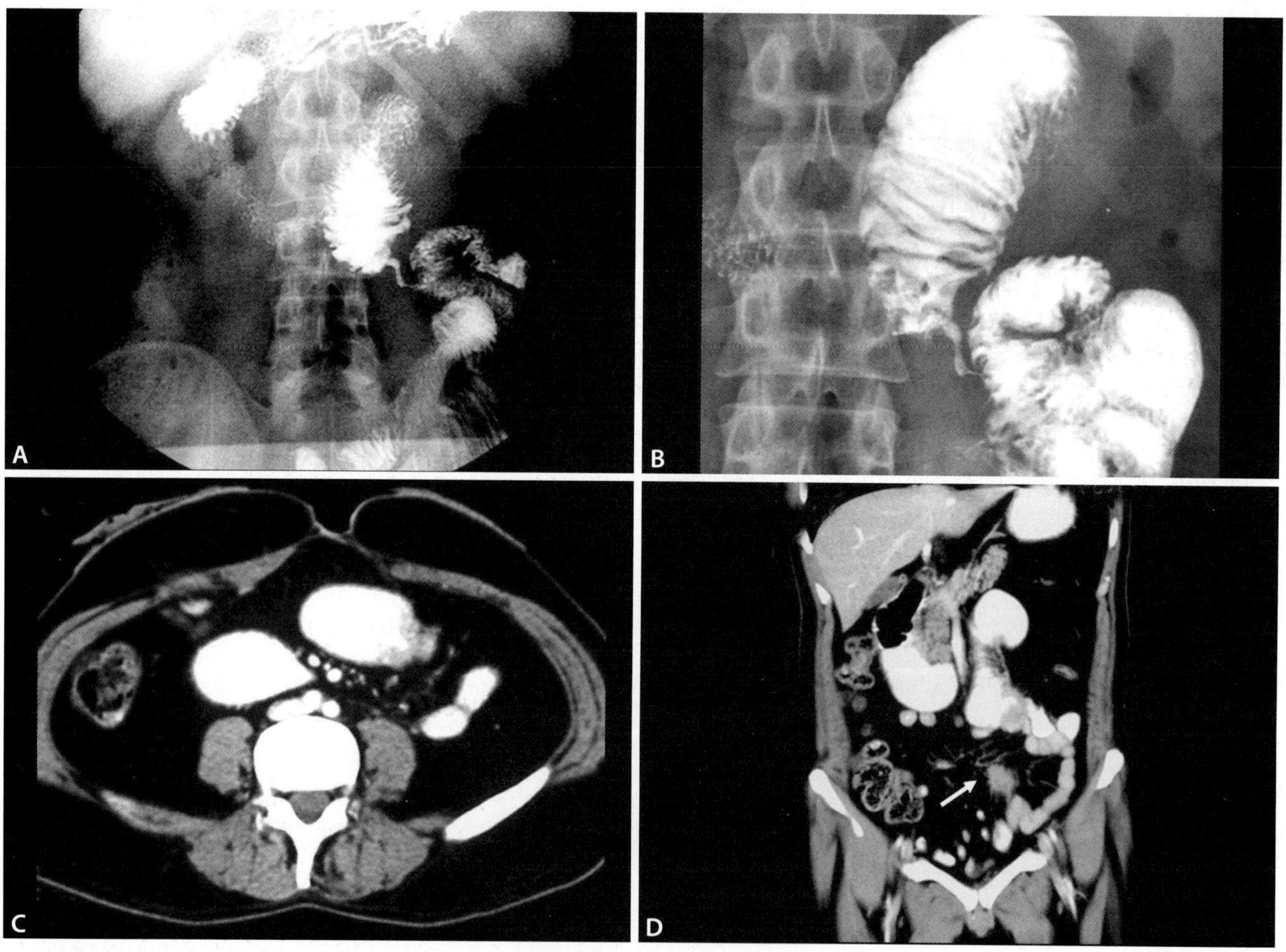

Figs. 5A to D: *Adenocarcinoma jejunum*: Barium meal follow through examination (A and B) showing a short segment tight stricture in the proximal jejunum with shouldering and mucosal irregularity—better appreciated on the magnified image (B). Axial and coronal CECT images (C and D) of the same patient depict homogeneously enhancing moderate wall thickening causing significant luminal narrowing with abrupt overhanging edges. Mesenteric lymphadenopathy is noted (arrow in D). Perivisceral fat appears normal.

favoring an adenocarcinoma include a short segment, solitary, stricturing lesion more common in the proximal small bowel with infiltration of perivisceral fat **(Figs. 6A to D)**.[16,26,27] The tumors are also FDG-avid and can be seen as increased activity on PET-CT.[29]

With advanced lesions invasion of mesentery and adjacent organs may occur. Retroperitoneal and mesenteric lymphadenopathy, hepatic and peritoneal metastases are the other findings that may be seen on cross sectional imaging.[26-28] DW-MR has been shown to be useful for detection of even small peritoneal metastases seen as nodular or linear areas of high signal on DW imaging which may be more easily seen with background suppression.[30,31] DW imaging has been reported to have high diagnostic accuracy especially when it is used in conjunction with oral and intravenous contrast enhanced MR.[30,32]

The key imaging findings are summarized in **Table 2**.

Staging and Prognosis

Once the diagnosis of small bowel adenocarcinoma is established a staging thoraco-abdominopelvic

Table 2: Adenocarcinoma small bowel: key imaging findings.

• *Site:* Duodenum, proximal jejunum
• *Barium:* Short segment stricture with shouldered margins
• *CT/MR*: Focal moderate wall thickening with overhanging margins
• Polypoid mass
• Heterogeneous moderate enhancement
• Associated findings
• Perilesional fat infiltration
• Lymphadenopathy
• Small bowel obstruction common

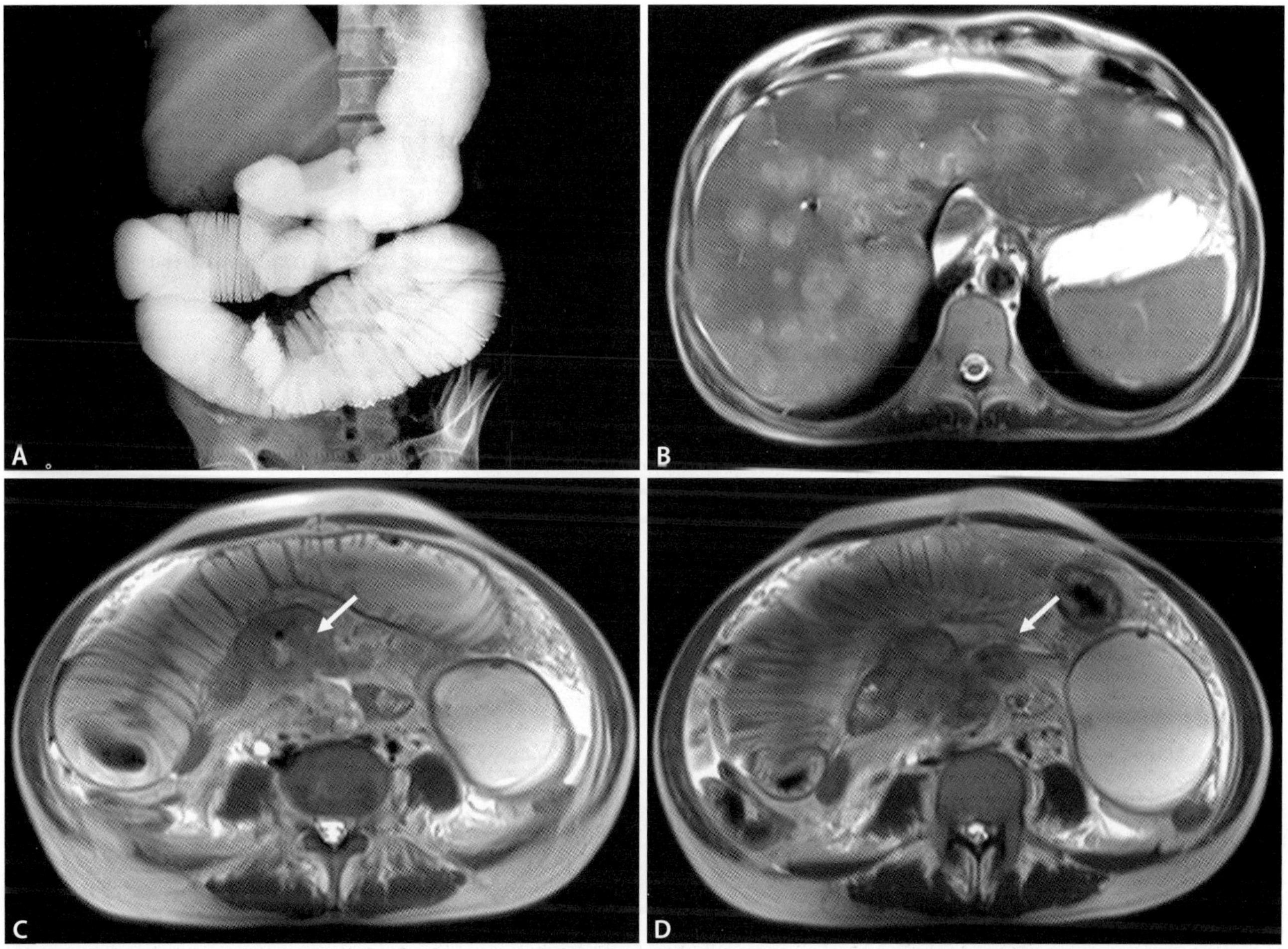

Figs. 6A to D: *Adenocarcinoma jejunum with hepatic metastases*: Barium meal follow through (A) reveals abrupt irregular narrowing of the jejunum producing complete obstruction and proximal dilatation. Cranial to caudal axial T2W MR images. (B to D) Images depict moderatecircumferential mural thickening of the jejunum in the same region with resultant marked luminal compromise (arrow in C) and adjacent lymphadenopathy (arrow in D). Multiple hepatic metastases and ascites are also noted.

CT to search for metastasis is recommended. Upper gastrointestinal endoscopy and colonoscopy may also be done to look for predisposing genetic disease such as polyposis syndromes.Baseline plasma carcinoembryonic antigen (CEA) and carbohydrate antigen (CA) 19.9 should be done in advanced disease as the levels of these tumor markers have prognostic significance. Since most patients have advanced disease by the time diagnosis is made the prognosis is generally poor. Ileal or jejunal lesions have a slightly better prognosis than duodenal lesions.[1,24]

TNM staging system[33] is used to stage adenocarcinoma small intestine given in **Table 3**.

Treatment

Though surgical resection is the primary and the only potentially curative treatment option, very few cases are resectable at the time of diagnosis. Complete resection of the primary tumor with locoregional lymph node dissection is essential. The main prognostic factor for localized small bowel adenocarcinoma is lymph node invasion. Also, the number of positive lymph nodes have prognostic value in stage III disease, patients with more than 3 lymph nodes having a worse prognosis than those with only one or two positive lymph nodes.[24]

If following surgery the disease is found to be stage 0 or 1 no adjuvant treatment is recommended. For stage 2 disease with pT4 tumor or stage III disease adjuvant treatment is recommended. No standard adjuvant regimen has been defined to date due to lack of randomized controlled trials. Generally a chemotherapy regimen similar to that for colorectal cancer[34] is followed. Patients with advanced disease may be treated by chemotherapy or radiotherapy for palliation. Radiotherapy being mainly used for duodenal lesions. Stenting of the bowel strictures can also be done as a palliative measure.[24]

Carcinoid Tumors or Neuroendocrine Tumors

Carcinoid tumors were originally described by Langhans and Lubarsch[35,36] but Oberndorfer in 1907 was the first to use the term carcinoid or 'Karzinoide' meaning 'carcinoma like.'[37] This is because these tumors displayed less aggressive growth than seen with most other gastrointestinal carcinomas.[38] The current preferred nomenclature for these tumors is neuroendocrine tumors (NET) NETs are relatively rare neoplasms arising from Amine Precursor Uptake and Decarboxylation (APUD) cells of the diffuse endocrine system.[39] These cells have a number of antigens that are common with nerve elements (neuroendocrine markers) hence the term neuroendocrine is used for these cell types and tumors.[40,41] There are several types of diffuse endocrine cells in the gastrointestinal tract such as Gastrin or G cells, D cell (somatostatin producing cell), enterochromaffin or EC cell, etc. They represent largest number of neuroendocrine cells in the body, therefore, the gastrointestinal tract is the most common site of NETs accounting for 60–70% cases.[39]

Small bowel carcinoids are generally sporadic. Those associated with MEN—I are mostly foregut carcinoids while patients with NF1 typically have periampullary carcinoids.[42,43]

Etiopathogenesis

The incidence of carcinoids as reported in the western literature has increased over the last two decades. The distribution of tumors along the GI tract has also changed.

Table 3: TNM staging of small bowel adenocarcinoma.

T Stage		
Tis	Tumor limited to epithelium or carcinoma *in situ*.	
T1	Tumor invades lamina propria submucosa or muscularis mucosa	
T2	Tumor extends into the muscularis propria	
T3	Tumor invades 2 cm or less into subserosa or into non-peritonealized perimuscular tissue (mysentery or retroperitoneum) surrounding the small bowel	
T4	Tumor invades into adjacent organs or extends through visceral peritoneum	
N Stage		
N0	No lymph node involvement	
N1	Metastases in one to three regional lymph nodes	
N2	Metastases in four or more regional lymph nodes	
M Stage		
M0	No distant metastases	
M1	Distant metastases present	
Stage 0	TisN0M0 (Carcinoma *in situ*)	Stage 3 N1 with any T M0
Stage 1	T1/T2N0 M0	Stage 4 Any T and N, M1
Stage 2	T3/T4 N0 nodes M0	

The appendix is no longer considered most common site and the small bowel or the rectum are more commonly involved.[39]

Small bowel carcinoids account for 26–30% of all gastrointestinal carcinoids. Ileum is the most common site, the usual location being within 60 cm of ileocecal valve.[39,44] They occur most frequently between the fifth to seventh decades and some studies report a slightly higher incidence in males for small bowel carcinoids, others report equal incidence in males and females. Rarely NETs can arise in a Meckel's diverticulum.[41,45]

Majority of the jejunal and ileal carcinoids arise from the enterochromaffin (EC) cell type of endocrine cells in the crypts of Lieberkuhn also called Kulchitsky cell. Carcinoids are submucosal tumors which may produce intramural masses or protrude into the lumen forming polypoid nodules with occasional focal ulceration of the overlying mucosa. These nodules can cause intussusception. The primary intestinal tumors are usually small—generally not more than 3.5 cm but have already invaded the muscularis propria at the time of diagnosis in most cases. These infiltrative tumor cells extend through the muscularis propria forming tumor masses in the subserosa of the intestine extending into the adjacent mesentery. Local release of serotonin and other substances as well as the pattern of growth described above results in desmoplasia, which is most marked in the submucosa and adjacent mesentery. In addition mesenteric vessels close to the tumor as well as those far away may be thickened with focal occlusions or stenosis due to the vasoactive substances released or vascular invasion.[45]

Conventional argentaffin and argyrophil silver staining techniques can be used to identify the tumor cells as EC cells. More recently immunohistochemical markers for serotonin, substance P and other tachykinins have been used. These tumors are also strongly positive for general endocrine markers such as chromogranin A, neuron specific enolase and synaptophysin.[41,45]

Many pathologic classification systems have been proposed for carcinoid/NET. Based on their location and embryologic origin they were traditionally classified as foregut, midgut and hindgut[39,45] to emphasize clinicopathologic difference between these groups. However, this did not explain the heterogeneity in their biologic behavior following which a WHO classification was developed in 2000 and then modified in 2010. According to this system carcinoids are categorized under the generic term of neuroendocrine tumors (NET Gr I).[45] This is given in **Table 4**. This classification has clinical implications. Intermediate and high grade

Table 4: World Health Organization 2010 classification of neuroendocrine tumors (NETs).

NET type	*Tumor classification*
NET, grade I	Well-differentiated, low-grade, mitotic count <2 per HPF, Ki-67, index <3%
NET, grade II	Well-differentiated, intermediate-grade mitotic count 2–20 per HPF, Ki-67, index 3–20%
NET, grade III, small cell	Poorly differentiated, high-grade, mitotic count >20 per HPF, Ki-67 >20%, small cell features
NET, grade III, large cell	Poorly differentiated, high-grade, mitotic count >20 per HPF, Ki-67 >20% large cell features

Note: HPF, high power field; Ki-67 index refers to the % of cells which are +ve for Ki-67–a marker for cell proliferation.

NETs are more likely to develop metastases so a shorter follow-up of 3 months is required for them than the usual follow-up at 6 months. Metastatic deposits from these tumors occur in lymph nodes, mesentery and liver and may become very large obscuring the primary tumor.[39,45]

Small bowel carcinoids are multiple in 30–40% of patients. A second primary malignancy (synchronous/metachronous) may present in gastrointestinal NET's. This is most frequent in the small intestinal NETs occurring in about 29% cases. Gastrointestinal adenocarcinomas are the most commonly associated malignancy others being prostate, breast, bronchus and bladder malignancies.[39]

Clinical Features

Most patients are asymptomatic because of the slow growing nature of these tumors. Symptoms may be related to the primary tumor, mesenteric involvement or metastatic disease. A long history of crampy abdominal pain, weight loss, fatigue or diarrhea and small bowel obstruction and very rarely obscure GI bleed may be seen.[45]

Carcinoid syndrome is seen in about 10% of all patients with gastrointestinal carcinoids and in around 17% of those with small bowel carcinoids. This occurs when vasoactive substance such as serotonin, kallikrein, bradykinin and prostaglandins produced by the tumor enter systemic circulation without metabolic degradation, which normally occurs in the liver. Patients with ileal carcinoids who have extensive hepatic metastases are most likely to develop carcinoid syndrome. The classic carcinoid syndrome consists of cutaneous flushing, diarrhea, abdominal pain, wheezing due to bronchospasm, palpitations and low blood pressure. This can be precipitated by alcohol, cheese, chocolate, exercise or emotional stress.[39,45] About 75% of patients with carcinoid syndrome develop carcinoid heart syndrome, i.e. right-sided valvular fibrosis and fibrosis of right cardiac chambers. Inactivation of the bioactive peptides in the lungs is thought to be responsible for left sided sparing.[39,45]

Laboratory tests that are useful in establishing the diagnosis of small bowel NETs/carcinoid include urinary 5 hydroxyindoleacetic acid (5-HIAA) a serotonin breakdown product which is elevated in 75% of midgut carcinoids and serum chromogranin A which is elevated in 80–90% of all gastrointestinal carcinoids (foregut, midgut and hindgut). The latter is also used to assess response to therapy.[39,45] In patients who have clinical features of carcinoid syndrome echocardiography is indicated to detect carcinoid heart disease which is an independent poor prognostic factor.[46]

Imaging

The imaging findings depend on primary tumor size, extent of mesenteric involvement and lymph node or hepatic metastases.

On barium studies/enteroclysis small carcinoids are generally not seen. When seen they produce mucosal elevations or rounded nodules with smooth overlying mucosa or surface ulceration producing a barium filled crater the so called 'bull's eye' or target appearance usually in the ileum. In the later stages, with bowel wall and mesenteric fibrosis,tethering and thickening of mucosal folds, rigidity, kinking, sharp angulations and narrowing of bowel loops is seen.[26]

While conventional abdominal CT has very low sensitivity for detection of small (<2 cm) lesions, multiphase helical CT with neural oral contrast, i.e. CT enterography or enteroclysis improve detection of smaller lesions because of improved tumor to background contrast.[47,48] The scan acquisition must be done earlier than usual, i.e. in the late arterial phase.[47,48] Some studies have reported that CT enteroclysis has a sensitivity of 100% for detection of small bowel carcinoids.Small ileal NETs may be seen as solitary or multiple hyperenhancing polyps, plaque like lesions or carpet lesions.[39,49]

Transmural extension of the tumor and associated mesenteric involvement and fibrosis are well seen on CT. About 50–75% cases of midgut carcinoids with median size of 3 cm have mesenteric masses more than 1.5 cm in size.[50,51] Transmural extension is seen on CT as concentric mural thickening with a focal soft tissue tumor mass adjacent to it. Deposits of carcinoid in the mesentery produce enlarged lymph nodes or masses which are commonly spiculated and produce mesenteric retraction. The soft tissue stranding or spiculation represents fibrosis rather than tumor infiltration and increases as the degree of fibrosis increases on histology. These masses may be much larger than the primary tumor and completely obscure it. Fine stippled or bulky and dense calcification may be seen in 40–70% of the mesenteric masses.[45,50] Histologically, this occurs in areas of mature fibrous scarring. The exact site of origin of mesenteric masses is not certain but they are usually thought to arise within the mesenteric fat or nodal tissue of small bowel mesentery.[52]

Mesenteric fibrosis angulates and kinks the involved intestine producing 'hair pin' bends—well appreciated on both axial images and multiplanar reconstructions **(Figs. 7A to E)**. It can also produce a 'spoke wheel' or 'sunburst' pattern of radiating mesenteric vessels.[45] 3D-CTA is a very useful technique to delineate full extent of the mesenteric mass and associated vascular involvement before surgical planning. Occasionally signs of bowel ischemia may also be seen due to vascular involvement. Rarely, diffuse mesenteric or peritoneal disease can occur producing miliary peritoneal implants, large masses, mesenteric caking or ascites.[45,53]

On MR enterography or enteroclysis carcinoids may be seen as solitary or multiple nodular masses or nodular fold thickening appearing isointense to muscle on T1W images and iso to mildly hyperintense on T2W images with intense contrast enhancement. The mesenteric mass itself is isointense on both T1W and T2W images due to fibrosis, mesenteric extension resulting in stretching, fixing and angulation of small bowel loops. Calcification though not as well seen as on CT may be seen as signal voids.[16,54]

Nuclear medicine studies in gastrointestinal NETs help in staging the disease, detect additional sites of involvement before surgery and detect unknown primary in patients presenting with metastases. Somatostatin receptor scintigraphy (SRS) is performed using radiolabelled synthetic somatostatin analogue ^{111}I octreotide because NET's express somatostatin receptors especially subtypes II and V. Overall sensitivity of somatostatin receptor scintigraphy (SRS) in detecting tumor burden both primary and metastatic for gastroenteropancreatic (GEP) NETs is 80–90% however, the sensitivity in detecting occult primary in a patient presenting with metastatic disease is disappointingly low at 2–23%.[39] Some recent studies suggest that with the availability of DOTANOC-PET for comparison the sensitivity of SRS is substantially lower than that reported in earlier studies.[39,55]

PET-CT using tracers like ^{68}Ga labeled DOTATOC/ DOTANOC which are octreotide derivatives and ^{11}C-5-hydroxytryptophan have higher sensitivity for tumor burden than SRS ranging from 93% to 97% while its sensitivity

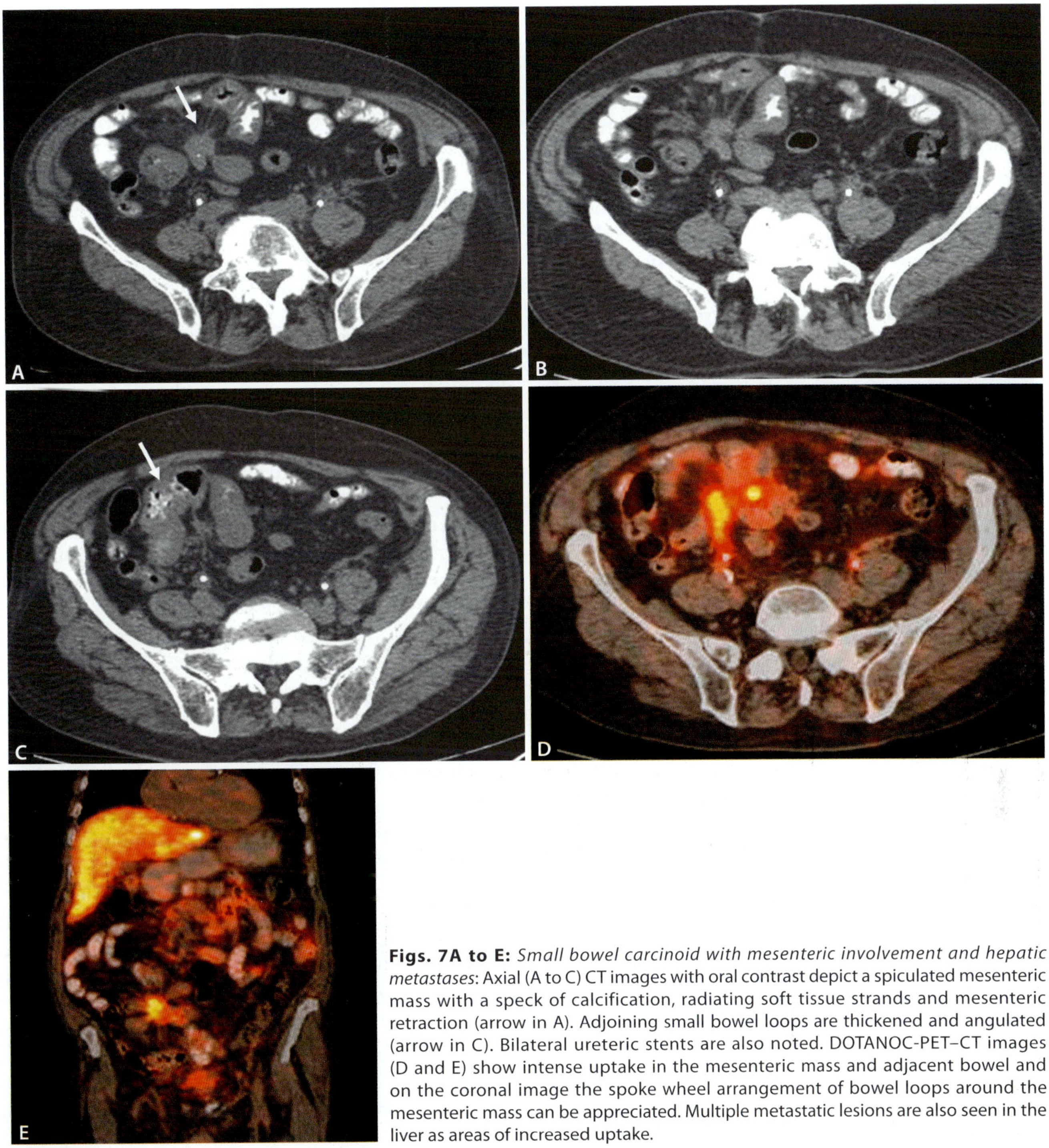

Figs. 7A to E: *Small bowel carcinoid with mesenteric involvement and hepatic metastases*: Axial (A to C) CT images with oral contrast depict a spiculated mesenteric mass with a speck of calcification, radiating soft tissue strands and mesenteric retraction (arrow in A). Adjoining small bowel loops are thickened and angulated (arrow in C). Bilateral ureteric stents are also noted. DOTANOC-PET–CT images (D and E) show intense uptake in the mesenteric mass and adjacent bowel and on the coronal image the spoke wheel arrangement of bowel loops around the mesenteric mass can be appreciated. Multiple metastatic lesions are also seen in the liver as areas of increased uptake.

for localizing unknown primary is around 59% **(Figs. 7A to E)**.[45,56]

^{18}F-FDG PET/CT is not useful in diagnosing typical low grade NET's because of the low glycolytic rate but has a role in prognostication of poorly differentiated NET's (WHO grade 3 and 4). The tumors that are ^{18}F-FDG PET/CT avid have a poorer prognosis and more rapid disease progression than those with negative uptake.[57-59] These poorly differentiated tumors do not express somatostatin receptors. Thus, there is an inverse relationship in which DOTANOC PET/CT and FDG PET/CT findings are inversely related at either end of the NETs differentiation spectrum.[55]

Imaging of Metastatic Lesions

In the case of midgut carcinoids, metastases are more common as the tumor size increases with the reported incidences being over 70% with a tumor size exceeding 2 cm.[54] In the vast majority of cases the primary tumor is usually so small that it may not be apparent on imaging and secondary findings are more common. Hepatic metastases are the most frequent finding followed by tumor induced fibrosis causing kinking of small bowel mesentery.[54] Liver metastases are seen in about 40% of ileal lesions at initial presentation. On ultrasound, liver metastases may be hyperechoic. Contrast enhanced ultrasound may help in improving sensitivity of ultrasound from 68% to 99%. Since the metastases are generally hypervascular they are best seen on arterial phase imaging on CT or MR. Occasionally they can be necrotic and may calcify. MR has reportedly a higher sensitivity of 95.2% for detection of liver metastases than CT, USG or SRS.[54] In one study PET-CT using ^{68}Ga labeled DOTATOC/NOC was superior to all conventional imaging techniques like CT/MR for detection of osseous and nodal metastases but was not found to be significantly superior for detection of hepatic metastases.[45,54,55]

Retroperitoneal or mesenteric lymphadenopathy has been reported in 20–30% of midgut carcinoids.[54] In these patients with retroperitoneal lymphadenopathy, retroperitoneal fibrosis may occur resulting in ureteric obstruction at times.[54] Other less common sites of metastases include bones, lungs, peritoneal cavity and ovary.[39]

Differential Diagnosis

The differential diagnosis of small primary tumors includes gastrointestinal stromal tumor (GIST), adenoma or leiomyoma. Other lesions that need to be distinguished from carcinoid include lymphoma, adenocarcinoma, metastases, GIST and Kaposi's sarcoma. Presence of fibrosis and angulation of bowel loops is characteristic of carcinoid, however it may occur with mesenteric extension of adenocarcinoma or metastases. DOTANOC-PET-CT can be extremely useful when the diagnosis is not clear.

The mesenteric mass of carcinoid tumor may mimic sclerosing mesenteritis and it may be very difficult to distinguish these conditions preoperatively. The soft tissue mass in sclerosing mesenteritis may envelop the mesenteric vessels with collateral vessel formation however, the fat around the mesenteric vessels is preserved, the so called "fat ring sign" unlike in carcinoid.[16]

Table 5 summarizes the important imaging findings in carcinoid tumors.

Table 5: Carcinoid/NET key imaging findings.

• Site-distal ileum
• Intensely enhancing polypoid mass/ bowel wall thickening
• Mesenteric mass with calcification and desmoplasia (spiculation)
• Mesenteric retraction
• Angulated or hair pin small bowel loops
• DOTANOC-PET avid

Future Directions[16]

Cytogenetic studies may help to understand the malignant potential of carcinoids better. Some studies have shown that if the metastatic tumor is positive for transcription factor CDX-2 then the primary is likely to be in the midgut. In addition, if it is negative for other transcription factors including pancreatic and duodenum homebox factor (PDX-1) neuroendocrine secretory protein-55 (NESP-55) and thyroid transcription factor (TTF-1) the primary tumor is most likely located in the ileum. In such a patient it may be appropriate to plan a CT enterography while a pancreatic CT protocol may be more useful in pancreatic NETs.

Treatment and Prognosis

Treatment depends on the extent of disease, symptomatology and receptor status. Localized small bowel NET's are treated surgically by removing the involved bowel and affected nodes. The entire bowel must be examined at surgery to rule out multiple lesions. Prophylactic cholecystectomy is recommended when treatment with somatostatin analogues is planned as these drugs cause impairment of gallbladder function with gallstones formation and cholecystitis. Even in patients with unresectable disease debulking may be carried out for symptomatic relief.

A multidisciplinary approach is required in patients with metastases. DOTANOC/DOTATOC–PET should be done if treatment with somatostatin analogues (octreotide/lanreotide/vapreotide) is planned to determine receptor status. Somatostatin analogue injections help to provide symptomatic relief in patients with carcinoid syndrome. They are also thought to inhibit the growth of tumors, hence have an important role in the treatment of carcinoid tumors with positive receptor status.

For limited liver metastases complete resection should ideally be done with curative intent. The various treatment options for extensive hepatic metastases include radiofrequency ablation (RFA), arterial embolization, chemotherapy, peptide receptor radionuclide therapy with ^{111}In, ^{90}Y or ^{177}Lu labeled octreotide analogues (DOTANOC-PET is useful in these patients to identify receptor status). Tyrosine kinase inhibitors and VEGF monoclonal antibodies are also being evaluated.[39]

Although carcinoids have a much less aggressive growth pattern than adenocarcinoma, the 5 years survival rate for small bowel carcinoids is about 54%. If complete surgical resection can be performed the survival rate improves greatly approaching 75%. The five years survival rate for patients with liver metastases in patients with few liver metastases (<5) is similar to those without metastasis and much better than in those with extensive hepatic metastases. In patients with distant metastases 5 years survival rate is below 20%.[47,54]

GASTROINTESTINAL STROMAL TUMORS

Gastrointestinal stromal tumors (GIST) are the most common nonepithelial or mesenchymal tumor of the gastrointestinal tract. The term was first used by Mazur and Clark.[60,61] Prior to 1983, these tumors were variably referred to as smooth muscle tumors; leiomyomas, leiomyosarcomas and leiomyoblastomas. However, they are distinct from true smooth muscle or neural tumors and are thought to arise from interstitial cells of Cajal. In 95% of patients, these tumors express KIT protein - CD117 a tyrosine kinase receptor which is the most important criterion for diagnosing GIST. Most GISTs are CD34 positive also. Immunoreactivity to KIT helps to differentiate gastrointestinal stromal tumors from true smooth muscle tumors.[60-62]

There is a small percentage of patients in whom the tumor does not show KIT mutation, instead mutations in the related tyrosine kinase platelet derived growth factor receptor alpha (PDGFR - α) are seen. A minority of gastrointestinal stromal tumors (GIST) have no KIT or PDG-FR and are known as 'wild type' GIST. The tumors seen in patients with neurofibromatosis are generally of the 'wild type' and have a low malignant potential.[63]

Clinical Features

The clinical presentation is extremely variable and depends on the size and location of tumors. Small gastrointestinal stromal tumors (GIST) may be discovered incidentally during radiological evaluation or surgery for another condition. Nausea, vomiting, abdominal pain, distension, palpable abdominal mass and feeling of satiety may occur with large masses.[64] Gastrointestinal bleeding from mucosal ulceration is a common manifestation of symptomatic gastrointestinal stromal tumors (GIST). This may be in the form of hematemesis melena or anemia due to occult bleed.[64]

Etiopathogenesis

The exact prevalence of gastrointestinal stromal tumors is difficult to ascertain however, it is estimated that there are about 5000–10,000 new cases every year.[62] Most patients are over 50 years at the time of diagnosis and there is no definite sex predilection. Ethnicity, race, occupation or geographic location have no association with gastrointestinal stromal tumors.

An increased incidence of GIST has been reported in patient with neurofibromatosis type 1 (NF1). Generally these patients have multiple small intestinal GISTs. Gastrointestinal stromal tumors are a probable feature of Carney's triad consisting of epithelioid leiomyosarcoma with paraganglioma and pulmonary chondroma. These do not necessarily occur at the same time. Other syndromes associated with GIST include Carney–Stratakis syndrome characterized by gastrointestinal stromal tumors (GIST) and paraganglioma and marked by germline mutations of succinate dehydrogenase (SDH) subunits A, B, C and D.[63,64]

Gastrointestinal stromal tumors (GIST) can arise all along the gastrointestinal tract, the stomach being the most frequent site followed by the small intestine. Any part of the small intestine can be involved. The esophagus is the only site in the gastrointestinal tract where leiomyomas are commoner than GIST accounting for 75% of mesenchymal esophageal tumors. Rarely, they can arise primarily in the omentum, mesentery and retroperitoneum.[64]

These tumors are well-circumscribed masses without a true capsule, size varying from few mm to over 30 cm. On gross pathology, cut surface is pink, tan or gray in color. Larger lesions can show focal areas of hemorrhage cystic degeneration and necrosis. GISTs arise from the outer muscular layer or muscularis propria of the gastrointestinal tract and tend to grow exophytically producing large masses arising from the intestinal wall and projecting into the abdominal cavity. Mucosal ulceration may be seen in a significant number of lesions as a component of the tumor extends to the mucosal surface.[64,65]

Histologically, these can be spindle cell, epithelioid or mixed cell types and on immunohistochemistry they express CD117 a transmembrane receptor for a growth factor called stem cell factor expressed on hematopoietic stem cells, myenteric plexus of adult gastrointestinal tract, etc. No gastrointestinal stromal tumor (GIST) can be unequivocally labeled benign although lesions less than 2 cm in size have a very low risk of recurrence and are mostly considered benign. Small bowel GISTs in general have a more aggressive course than gastric tumors hence the size threshold for estimating risk of metastases or recurrence may be smaller for small intestinal GISTs. Metastases tend to occur to the liver and peritoneum but do not involve the lymph nodes.[65,66]

Pediatric gastrointestinal stromal tumors (GIST) are extremely rare but constitute a distinct subset of GISTs which is associated with female predominance, lack of KIT/ PDGFRA mutations, mainly gastric lesions which tend to be multicentric with lymph node metastases.[63]

IMAGING APPEARANCES

Although plain radiographs have no role in the diagnosis of gastrointestinal stromal tumors they may reveal a soft tissue haze due to the mass. Rarely irregular gas collections may be seen when the masses are cavitating with presence of air in the cavity.[65]

Ultrasound can detect large masses which appear heterogeneous due to areas of necrosis however, it may be difficult to identify the exact organ of origin **(Fig. 8)**.[65]

On barium studies, due to a large extraluminal component these masses exhibit mass effect on the affected segment of intestine. A cavity or fistula communicating with the intestinal lumen hence filling with barium may be seen and rarely aneurysmal dilatation can be seen **(Figs. 9A to C)**. Small lesions may produce submucosal masses indistinguishable from other benign submucosal lesions, sometimes mucosal irregularity due to ulceration can be seen.[64]

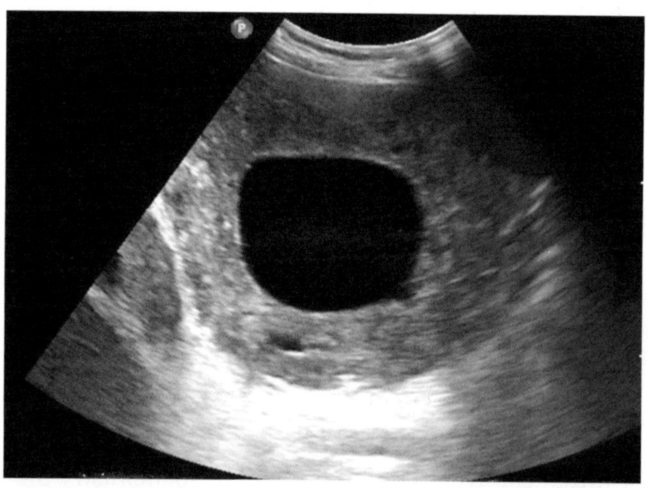

Fig. 8: *Gastrointestinal stromal tumor*: Grayscale ultrasound image reveals a large heterogeneous mass with a central area cavitation in a patient with GIST.

The CT is the mainstay for diagnosis and staging. The entire tumor including the mural, extramural and luminal component is well delineated on CT. In many cases the bulk of the tumor is extraserosal making its difficult to determine its origin from small bowel. The appearances are variable depending on the size and aggressiveness of the tumor, most lesions tend to be heterogeneous due to necrosis, hemorrhage or cystic degeneration and show inhomogeneous patchy enhancement following contrast administration **(Figs. 10A to C)**. Homogeneous attenuation is less commonly seen.[60,62,64,65] Calcification is rarely seen. Vascular supply is well-demonstrated on CTA using MIP or curved planar reconstructions. Usually the tumors displace adjacent organs but with advanced disease direct invasion of adjacent structures may be seen. Rarely the tumors may appear predominantly cystic and may be misdiagnosed as pseudocysts. Small GIST's usually produce homogeneous, submucosal or endoluminal polypoid masses.[60,62,64,65]

According to some reports nearly 50% of patients with gastrointestinal stromal tumors present with metastasis. Liver and peritoneal metastases are the most common occurring due to hematogeneous spread and peritoneal seeding respectively **(Figs. 11A and B)**. Less common sites of metastasis include lung, pleura and soft tissue. Lymph node metastases are distinctly uncommon.[60]

MR is indicated for evaluation of liver lesions indeterminate at CT, when CT is contraindicated and for surgical planning of rectal gastrointestinal stromal tumors. The MR appearances depend on the size, degree of necrosis and hemorrhage. The most common appearance is an exophytic bulky mass. Sometimes a protruding intraluminal mass or bidirectional growth pattern relative to the intestinal wall may be seen. The solid areas of the tumor are low signal on T1W images, high signal on T2W images and show enhancement after contrast administration. Areas of hemorrhage show variable signal intensity depending on the age of hemorrhage. Mesenteric masses in the case of gastrointestinal stromal tumors (GIST) tend to be smooth, without any spiculation.[16] DWI may reveal restricted diffusion with low ADC values **(Figs. 12A to F)**.[67]

^{18}F-FDG-PET/CT is also a highly sensitive technique for detection and staging of gastrointestinal stromal tumors but a small number of lesions are not FDG avid.[60]

The imaging findings are summarized in **Table 6**.

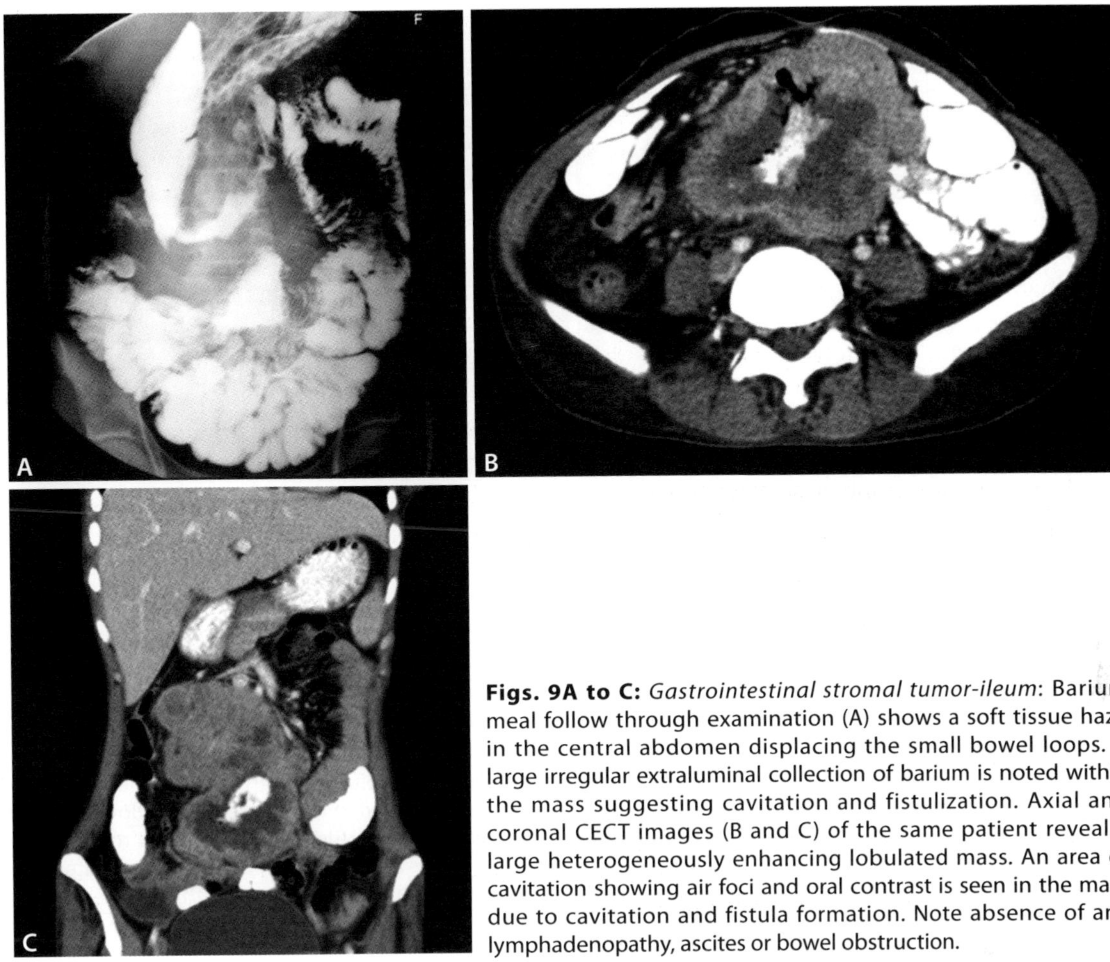

Figs. 9A to C: *Gastrointestinal stromal tumor-ileum*: Barium meal follow through examination (A) shows a soft tissue haze in the central abdomen displacing the small bowel loops. A large irregular extraluminal collection of barium is noted within the mass suggesting cavitation and fistulization. Axial and coronal CECT images (B and C) of the same patient reveal a large heterogeneously enhancing lobulated mass. An area of cavitation showing air foci and oral contrast is seen in the mass due to cavitation and fistula formation. Note absence of any lymphadenopathy, ascites or bowel obstruction.

STAGING AND PROGNOSIS

Contrast-enhanced computed tomography (CECT) of the abdomen and pelvis is the imaging technique of choice for staging and follow-up. FDG-PET-CT/MRI is especially useful when early detection of tumor response to molecular targeted therapy is to be done. A TNM staging system for gastrointestinal stromal tumors (GIST) has been developed by AJCC in the 7th edition of the TNM staging system, however, it has several limitations and is generally not used.[63]

Several criteria have been proposed to prognosticate gastrointestinal stromal tumors. The term benign and malignant are not applied any longer since all gastrointestinal stromal tumors have some potential to behave in a malignant fashion.[63] Risk of recurrence is dependent on tumor size, mitotic index and site (i.e. location in gastrointestinal tract). Nongastric location is associated with poorer prognosis than gastric lesions. Some authors have stratified tumors into risk categories. Tumors less than 2 cm in size with a mitotic count < 5/50 HPF are categorized as very low-risk; and tumors >5 cm with a mitotic count of >5/50 HPF, tumors greater than 10 cm and any mitotic rate, while tumors of any size with a mitotic rate >10/50 HPF are classified as high-risk. Between these two lie low-risk and intermediate risk categories. Presence of rupture whether spontaneous or iatrogenic and male sex are independent adverse prognostic features.[63,68]

Treatment

Management of gastrointestinal stromal tumors requires a multidisciplinary approach. Tumors 2 cm or more in size should be surgically resected. The management of lesions that are <2 cm in size and discovered incidentally is controversial. The recommended standard treatment for localized tumors is complete surgical resection with clear margins with no lymph node dissection of clinically negative nodes. Although smaller tumors may be laparoscopically resected (if expertise is available)

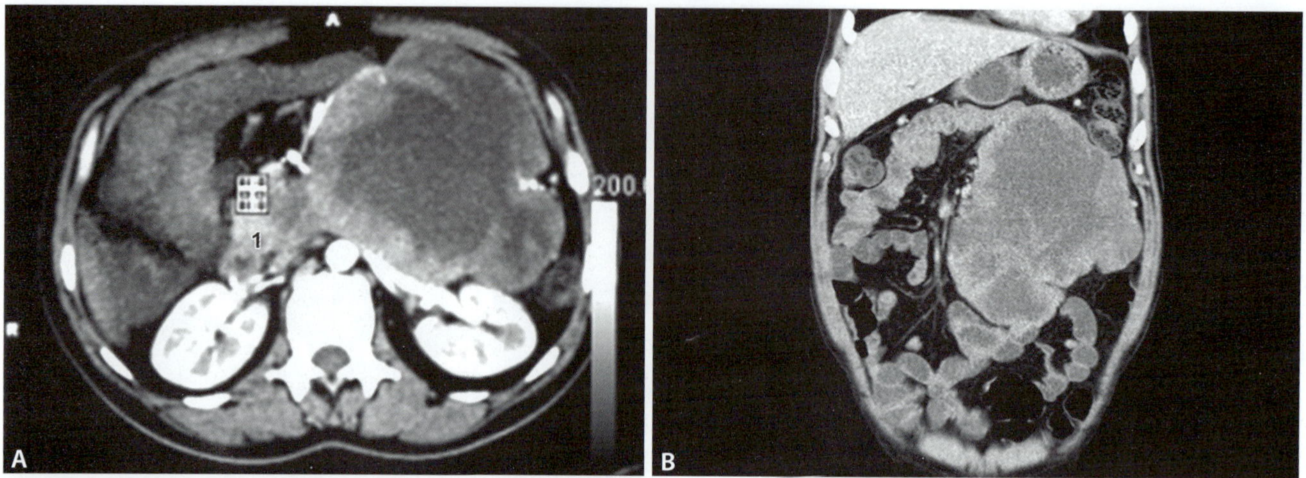

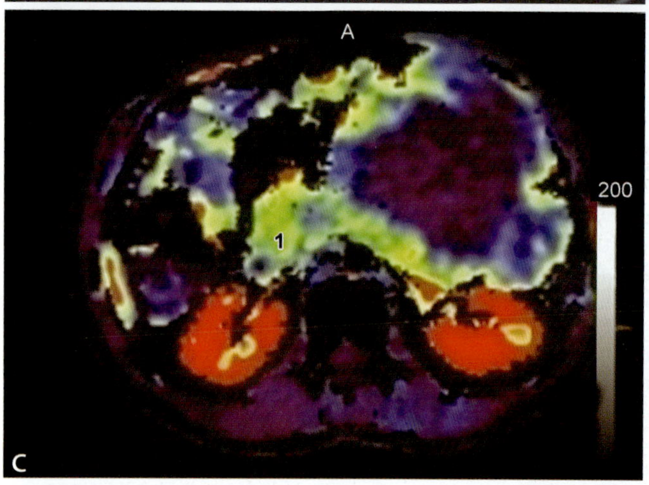

Figs. 10A to C: *Gastrointestinal stromal tumor-jejunum*: Axial and coronal (A and B) CECT images depict a large mass in close proximity to the jejunum with heterogeneous predominantly peripheral enhancement. Increased blood flow to this area is also confirmed on the perfusion CT blood flow map (C) seen as blue and green areas at the periphery. Note the lobulated but relatively smooth outer margin of the lesion with no evidence of mesenteric fat stranding or lymphadenopathy. On surgery a large jejunal GIST was resected.

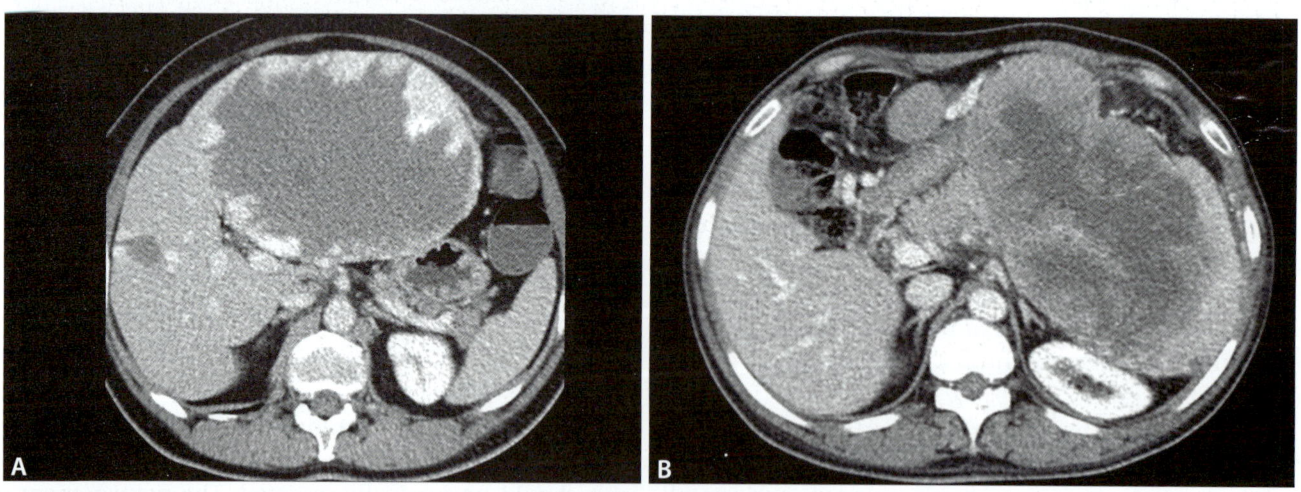

Figs. 11A and B: *GIST with hepatic metastases*: Metastasis to the left lobe liver in a patient with gastrointestinal stromal tumor (GIST) shows hypodense mass with multiple peripheral solid enhancing nodules on CECT. Also note the smaller lesion in the right lobe showing a similar appearance.

following the principles of oncologic surgery it is not recommended for large tumors due to higher risk of tumor rupture which has a very high-risk of recurrence. If the risk of relapse is substantial patient is put on adjuvant imatinib, a tyrosine kinase inhibitor (TKI) adjuvant treatment, close monitoring of treatment response is carried out during the

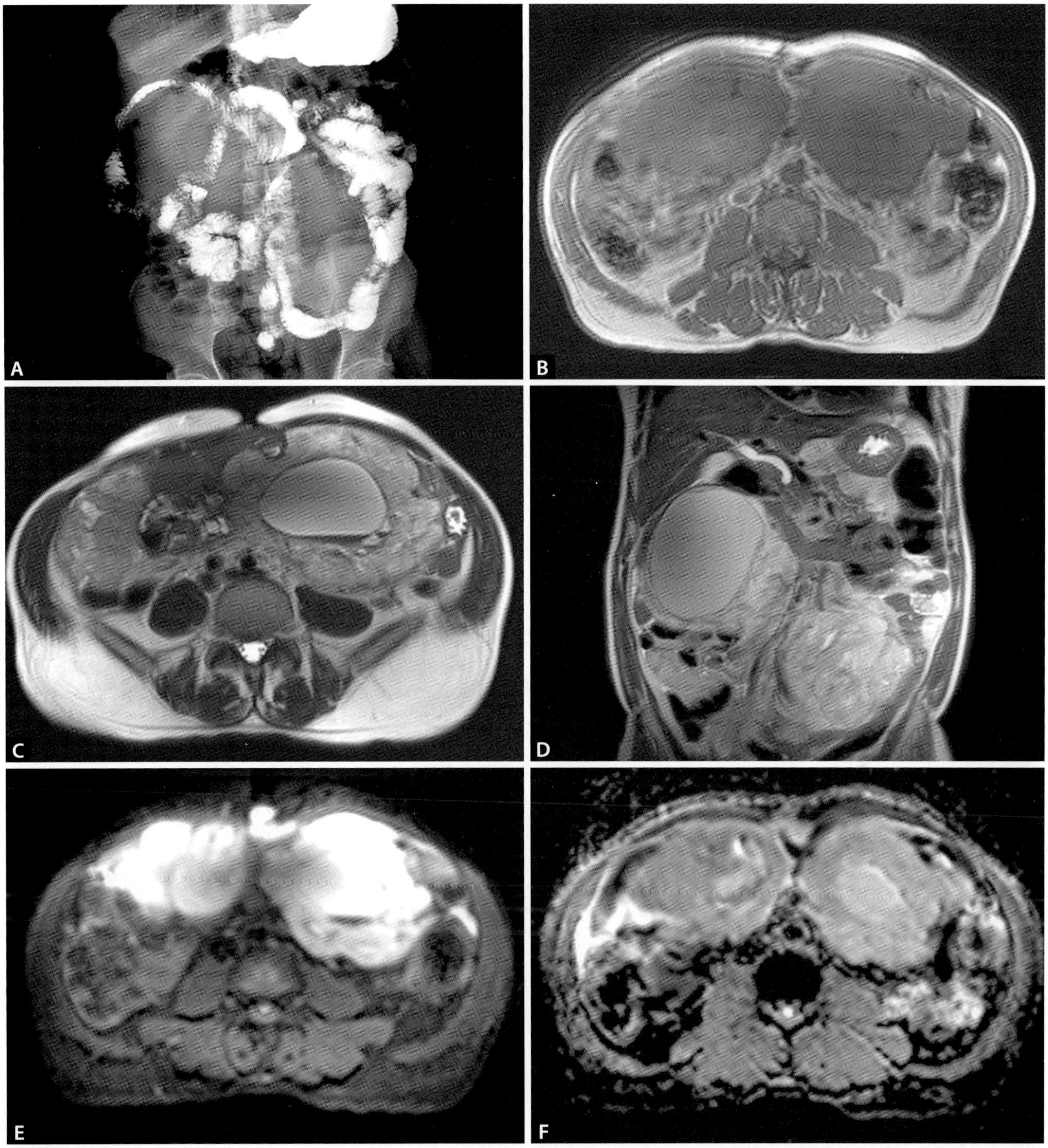

Figs. 12A to F: *Gastrointestinal stromal tumor*: Barium meal follow through examination (A) reveals evidence of extrinsic compression and displacement of small bowel loop around soft tissue masses. T1W (B); and T2W axial and coronal (C and D) MR images reveal T1W iso and T2W heterogeneously hyperintense masses in the mesentery in close proximity to the small bowel loops. A central area of cystic degeneration with fluid-fluid levels is seen in one of the lesions. (B) On DWI and ADC maps (E and F); there is evidence of restricted diffusion in the peripheral solid component appearing bright on DWI and dark on ADC maps. Note absence of lymphadenopathy or small bowel obstruction.

Table 6: GIST key imaging findings.

• Site–stomach followed by small bowel
• Bulky exophytic heterogeneous mass
• Moderate heterogeneous enhancement
• Smooth lobulated outline
• Internal gas, cavitation and fistulization
• Lymphadenopathy distinctly uncommon
• Usually no obstruction

treatment. Some authors recommend mutational analysis before adjuvant therapy since some subtypes may not be sensitive to TKI.[63]

Imatinib is also the standard treatment for inoperable and metastatic lesions. In case of confirmed nonresponse and disease progression or rarely intolerance to imatinib a second line TKI sunitinib may be used. Other drugs being tried include Regorafenib, sorafenib etc.[63]

RESPONSE EVALUATION AND SURVEILLANCE

Response evaluation to treatment is generally done on CT especially when ^{18}F-FDG-PET-CT/MR is not available and is generally done at 3 months. Traditional response evaluation criteria in solid tumors (RECIST) criteria based assessment of tumor response are insensitive in evaluating response to TKI as decrease in tumor size may take several months. Good response to imatinib is seen as lesions becoming homogeneous, hypoattenuating or hypodense, disappearance of enhancing nodules and tumor vessels. These changes represent a favorable effect even in the absence of anatomic decrease in size. Consistent similar signal changes on MR should also be considered as tumor response.[63] Choi et al proposed CT response criteria which take into account both the tumor size and density.[69] A complete disappearance of lesion with no new lesions is considered complete response while a 10% decrease in diameter or 15% decrease in density with no new lesions is required for partial response.

A paradoxical increase in tumor size may occur during treatment this does not imply tumor progression in the absence of enhancing nodules. It may be caused by myxoid degeneration or hemorrhage. Hemorrhage may also produce an increase in tumor attenuation complicating the CT based assessment further. Sometimes intratumoral hemorrhage may be significant, producing possible decrease in hemoglobin levels in the first 4–8 weeks of imatinib therapy.[60] At times even the appearance of new lesions in the liver may be due to their becoming more apparent with decrease in density rather than true lesions.[60,63] Imatinib therapy may result in fluid retention which is the most common side effect. This may be seen as ascites, pleural effusion, pericardial effusion or subcutaneous edema **(Figs. 13A and B)**. Hence, the presence of these on CT should not interpreted as new peritoneal disease.

Role of CT in early response evaluation is also being investigated, some studies reporting that decrease in attenuation of the tumor is seen within a month in most patients who respond to imatinib, in fact, it may be seen as early as 5 days after treatment. FDG-PET/MRI is extremely sensitive to detect early tumor response. A good response in the form of marked decrease in FDG uptake may be seen within 24 hours after a single dose. This may be very useful to identify early nonresponders. Even in patients showing a paradoxical increase in size on conventional CT due to hemorrhage or myxoid degeneration FDG-PET/CT can show no increase in metabolic activity resolving the dilemma.[60,63]

Other techniques that have been used include contrast enhanced ultrasound, perfusion CT and DW-MRI. On contrast enhanced ultrasound tumor response is seen as decreased tumor contrast uptake as early as day 5 or 7. Perfusion CT, has also been used to both prognosticate response to treatment and monitor treatment response with decrease in perfusion parameters such as blood flow and blood volume occurring with good response.[70,71] Using DW-MR some authors have reported that ADC values correlate closely with SUV parameters derived from PET-CT.

Surveillance is required for all cases as recurrence occurs in most patients even after complete resection, median time to recurrence being approximately 2 years. Generally recurrent disease first occurs in the liver or peritoneum. Criteria for progression include development of new lesions, increase in tumor size with new or enhancing nodules development of new lesions at previous site of disease and finally development enhancing nodules in hypoattenuating treated tumor even without increase in tumor size which is a typical pattern of progression seen in GIST **(Figs. 14A and B)**.[63]

LYMPHOMA

Gastrointestinal tract is the most common site for extranodal non-Hodgkin's lymphoma (NHL) since the lymphoid tissue occurring in the mucosa, lamina propria and submucosa forms the largest collection of lymphocytes compared to any other immune organ in the body. Most GI

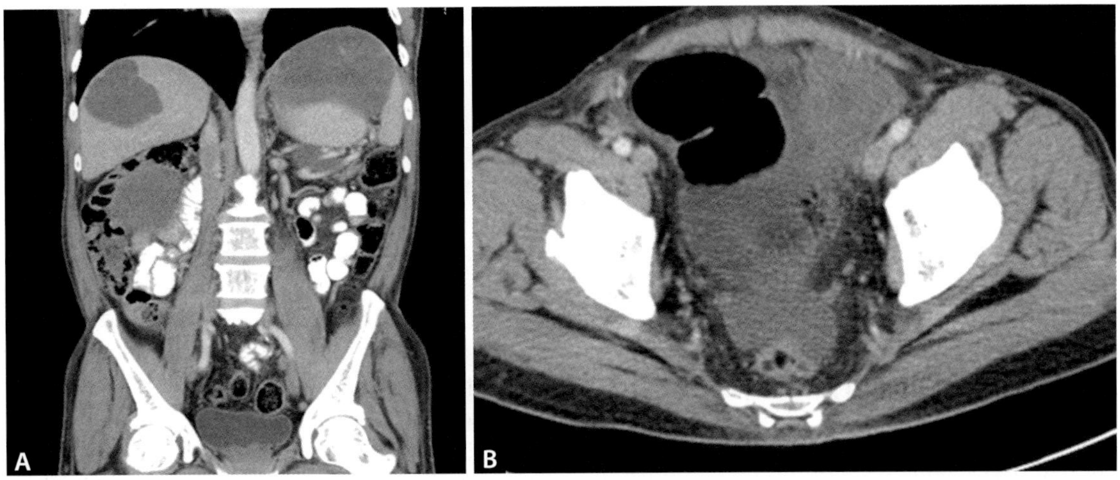

Figs. 13A and B: *GIST on imatinib therapy*: Coronal and axial CECT images of a patient with hepatic and peritoneal metastases from gastrointestinal stromal tumor (GIST) on imatinib reveal markedly hypodense lesions with no enhancing nodules consistent with a favorable response. Note the presence of free fluid in the pelvis due to fluid retention.

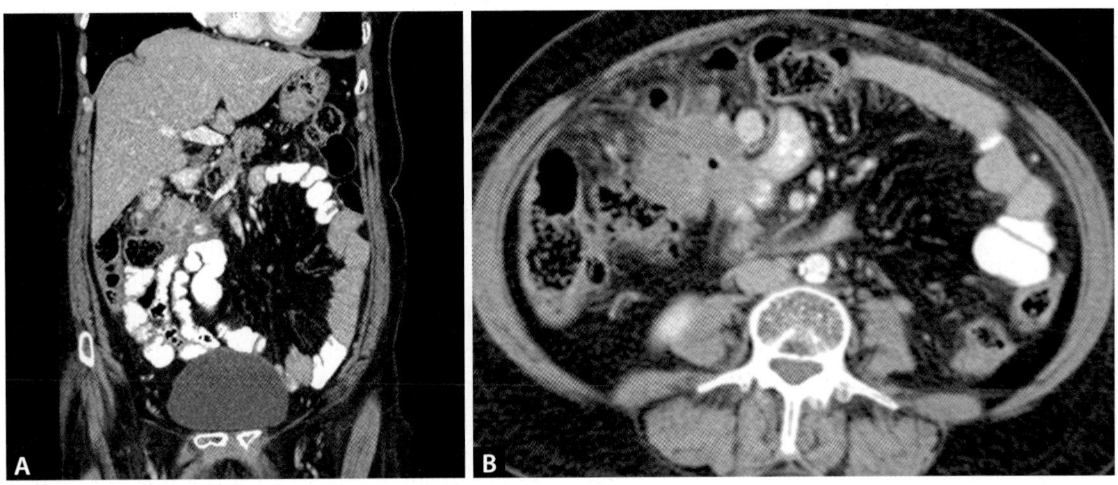

Figs. 14A and B: *Recurrent jejunal gastrointestinal stromal tumor*: Coronal and axial CECT images of an operated case of jejunal gastrointestinal stromal tumor showing a heterogeneously enhancing recurrent mass with irregular and spiculated margins at the site of previous disease involving the jejunum and adjacent transverse colon.

tract lymphoid tissue is referred to as mucosa associated lymphoid tissue.[72-74]

Involvement of the gastrointestinal tract can be primary or secondary to generalized disease. Primary gastrointestinal non-Hodgkin's lymphoma constitutes 10–15% of all non Hodgkin's lymphomas and 30–40% of extranodal lymphomas. These generally involve only a single site. The criteria described by Dawson et al.[75] are used to define primary gastrointestinal disease. These are:

- Predominant involvement of gastrointestinal tract with lymph node involvement restricted to primary drainage area.
- No palpable lymph nodes.
- No liver or spleen involvement.
- Normal chest radiograph, i.e. no mediastinal lymphadenopathy.
- Normal peripheral white blood cell count.

Although this definition was developed before the availability of cross sectional imaging, it is still applicable.[72] Some authors however advocate a more liberal definition of primary gastrointestinal lymphoma as lymphomas that predominantly involve the gastrointestinal tract presenting with gastrointestinal symptoms notwithstanding the presence or absence of lymph node involvement.[76,77]

Secondary gastrointestinal tract involvement in generalized disease is much more frequent since lymphomas commonly arise in retroperitoneal and mesenteric lymph nodes. At autopsy gastrointestinal involvement has been reported in up to 50% cases although this may not be clinically evident.[75]

The primary form when diagnosed sufficiently early has a much better progress than systemic lymphoma with gastrointestinal involvement. However, in advanced cases it may be difficult to distinguish between primary and secondary involvement clinically, radiologically and even pathologically.[78]

ETIOPATHOGENESIS AND CLASSIFICATION

The incidence of non-Hodgkin's lymphoma is reportedly increasing due to increasing incidence of HIV infection and a variety of environmental factors.[78] Risk factors that have been identified in the pathogenesis of small bowel lymphoma include HIV infection, celiac disease, inflammatory bowel disease and immunosuppression after solid organ transplantation. The risk of lymphoma is 45–100 times in patients who have received allograft or marrow transplants. These tumors are commonly associated with Ebstein-Barr virus (EBV) infection and referred to as EBV related post-transplant lymphoproliferative disorder.[78] Gastrointestinal tract involvement is seen in one-fourth to one-third of patients with AIDS and involvement of stomach, small and large bowel has been reported with an almost equal frequency.[72,78]

Peak incidence is in the 6th decade of life with a slight male predilection of 3:2, a small peak is also noted around 10 years. Although uncommon in childhood, lymphomas constitute the most common gastrointestinal tumor in children.[78] Small bowel involvement represents about 1/3rd of the cases of gastrointestinal lymphoma and is the second most common site after the stomach. It is a common malignant tumor of the small bowel constituting about 20% of all malignant lesions. The distal ileum is the most common site likely due to the abundant lymphoid follicles in this region.[72,76,78]

The recent WHO classification of lymphomas has categorized lymphomas into two major types - B-cell lineage (including Hodgkin's lymphoma) and T-cell or NK (Natural Killer) cell lineage.[72] The various types under these two categories that may involve the small bowel are given in **Table 7**.

Most small bowel lymphomas like other gastrointestinal lymphomas are of the B-cell lineage. Although any histological subtype can occur diffuse large B-cell lymphoma (DLBCL) is the most common type of gastrointestinal lymphoma in adults. Extranodal marginal zone B-cell lymphoma (ENMZL), so named because it arises from the marginal zone of Peyer's patches, is found predominantly in the stomach but does occur in the small and large intestine also. ENMZL was previously referred to marginal zone lymphoma of mucosa associated lymphoid tissue (MALT lymphoma).[76] Immunoproliferative small intestinal disease (IPSID) also known as alpha chain disease is a subtype of extranodal marginal zone B-cell lymphoma found in the small bowel. It is thought to occur as a result of combination of genetic risk factors and chronic infection by *Campylobacter jejuni*. It affects young adults with almost equal sex incidence and is associated with poor socioeconomic status. Patients may show alpha heavy chain immunoglobulins in the serum. Infiltration of the bowel wall by plasma cells leads to protein losing enteropathy. It can transform to high grade Mediterranean lymphoma. This condition is common in the middle east, far east and Mediterranean region.[78] Mantle cell lymphoma (MCL) produces multiple lymphomatous polyposis first described by Cornes in 1961.[79] Burkitt's lymphoma is a highly aggressive B-cell lymphoma.[78]

T-cell lymphomas of the small bowel represent about 10–20% of primary intestinal lymphomas. Though a variety of T-cell lymphomas may involve the small

Table 7: Classification of small bowel/gastrointestinal lymphoma and clinical behavior.

B-cell	*Clinical behavior prognosis*	*T-cell/NK cell*	*Clinical behavior prognosis*
Diffuse large B-cell lymphoma (DLBCL)	Aggressive curable	Enteropathy associated T-cell lymphoma (EATL)	Poor prognosis due to abdominal complications
Extranodal marginal zone B-cell lymphoma (ENMZL)	Localized curable	Type I and II (EATL)	
Mantle cell lymphoma (MCL)	Moderately aggressive incurable		
Follicular lymphoma	Indolent to moderately aggressive incurable		
Burkitt lymphoma	Aggressive curable		
Hodgkin's lymphoma	Potentially curable		

bowel most of these are enteropathy associated T-cell lymphomas (EATL) occurring in refractory celiac disease.[72] A Swedish study has shown a 6.6 times higher risk of non-Hodgkin's lymphoma in patients with celiac disease, majority being primary gastrointestinal tract lymphomas of the T-cell type. These usually manifest over 60 years and are commoner in men. Besides non-Hodgkin's lymphoma, celiac disease is also a risk factor for small bowel adenocarcinoma, esophageal carcinoma and melanoma.[73]

WHO has classified enteropathy associated T-cell lymphoma or EATL as type I which is strongly associated with celiac disease and accounts for 80–90% of cases of EATL. Type II EATL is also referred to as monomorphic CD56+ve intestinal lymphoma which is not related to celiac disease although enteropathy like changes may be found on histology. Type I generally involves the jejunum and proximal ileum as the jejunum is the site where most villous damage and inflammation occur.[72,73,80]

Clinical Presentation

Clinical features of small bowel lymphoma are nonspecific. Patients may present with malaise, pain abdomen, weight loss, fever, lump abdomen, chronic diarrhea and occasionally gastrointestinal bleed and small bowel perforation.[72]

Imaging

Conventional small bowel follow through series or enteroclysis are rarely performed these days but are useful to show small polypoid lesions. On ultrasound, these tumors produce hypoechoic circumferential or asymmetric bowel wall thickening. Aneurysmal dilatation or intussusception may also be appreciated **(Figs. 15A and B)**.[78]

The CT is useful both for initial diagnosis, staging and in the follow-up after surgery or chemotherapy. CT enterography is more useful in lower grades of lymphoma where the wall thickening may be subtle. MR and MR enteroclysis provide similar information.[81]

Traditionally described radiological patterns[72,73,81] that are evident on barium studies and a well performed CT or CT/MR enterography are:

- Infiltrating form
- Polypoid form/multiple nodules
- Endoexoenteric form with excavation and fistulization
- Mesenteric invasive form.

Infiltrative Form

Circumferential infiltration of the bowel wall by lymphoma causes bowel wall thickening and subsequently distortion or effacement of folds. On barium studies submucosal infiltration by tumor causes loss or effacement of mucosal folds to produce a smooth featureless appearance. The bowel lumen is generally not narrowed, in fact it may be dilated, referred to as 'aneurysmal dilatation'. This implies a localized nonobstructive dilatation of bowel lumen with diameter more than 4 cm in areas of bowel wall thickening and is seen in about 31% of small bowel lymphoma. The underlying cause is the loss of bowel wall tone due to infiltration of submucosal myenteric plexus and muscularis propria by tumor **(Figs. 16A to C)**.[72,81]

On CT or MR there is marked homogeneous circumferential thickening of bowel wall with diameter greater

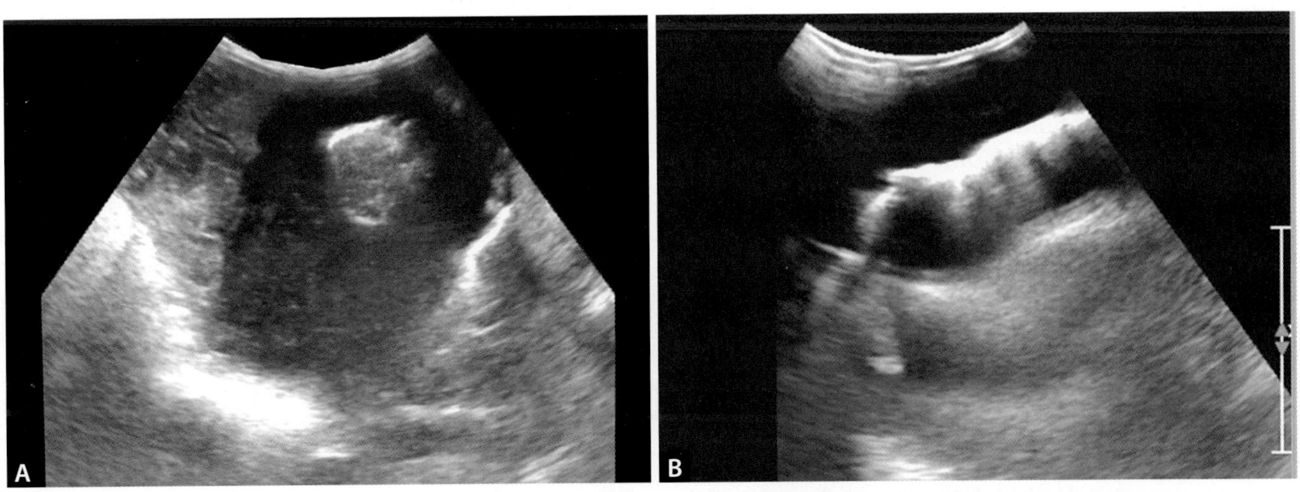

Figs. 15A and B: *Lymphoma small bowel*: Transverse and longitudinal ultrasound images reveal marked homogeneously hypoechoic bowel wall thickening with the dilated hyperechoic lumen in the center.

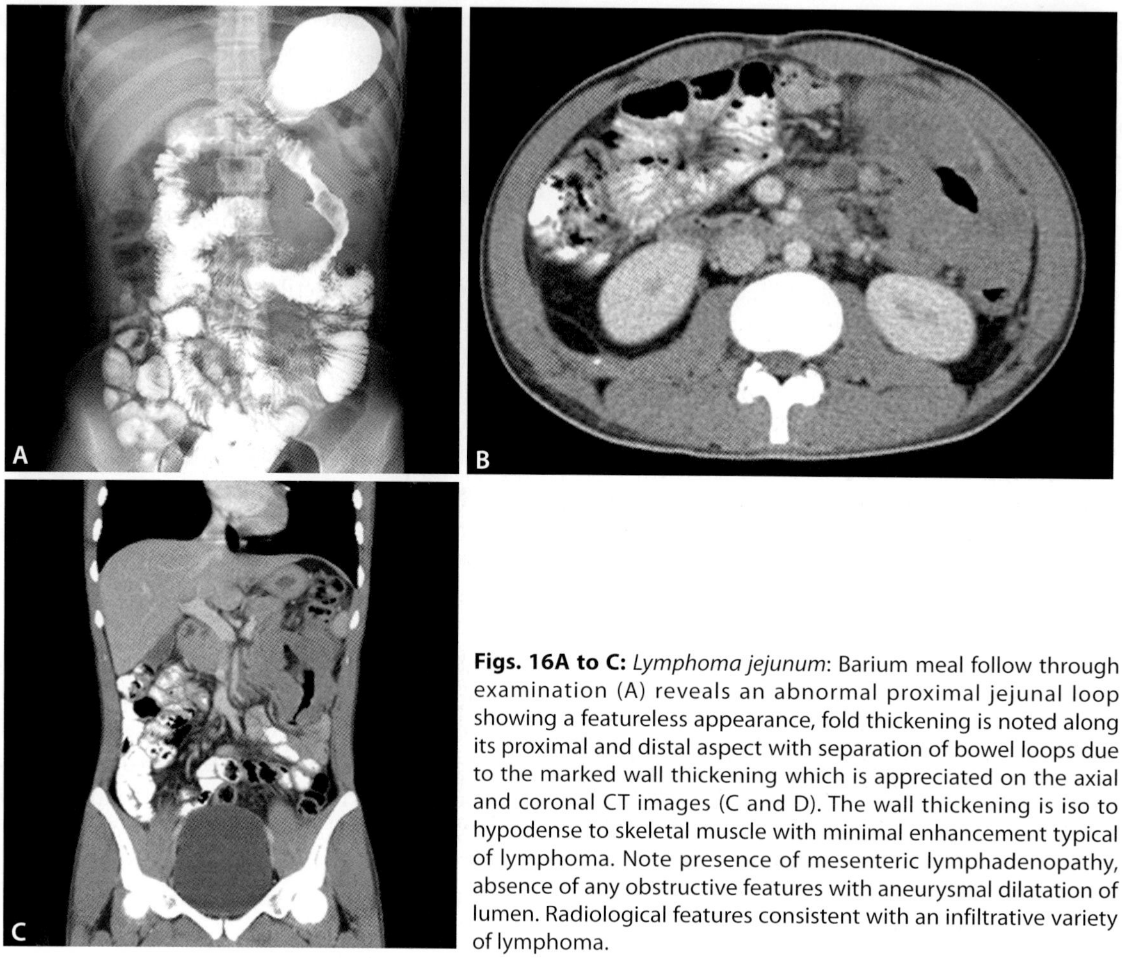

Figs. 16A to C: *Lymphoma jejunum*: Barium meal follow through examination (A) reveals an abnormal proximal jejunal loop showing a featureless appearance, fold thickening is noted along its proximal and distal aspect with separation of bowel loops due to the marked wall thickening which is appreciated on the axial and coronal CT images (C and D). The wall thickening is iso to hypodense to skeletal muscle with minimal enhancement typical of lymphoma. Note presence of mesenteric lymphadenopathy, absence of any obstructive features with aneurysmal dilatation of lumen. Radiological features consistent with an infiltrative variety of lymphoma.

than 2 cm, generally involving a long segment of bowel. The mural thickening results in separation of bowel loops which can also be appreciated on barium studies. The bowel wall attenuation is lower than or equal to muscle attenuation on CT **(Figs. 17A and B)**. On MR the wall tends to be iso on T1W and mildly hyperintense on T2W. These lesions tend to show homogeneous enhancement which is generally less than that in other malignant tumors.[15,16] One study has reported lower ADC values in small bowel lymphoma compared with adenocarcinoma.[67,82]

This variety of lymphoma can generally be distinguished easily from carcinoma. The longer length of involvement, lack of luminal narrowing or the presence of aneurysmal dilatation, absence of obstructive features and a smooth mural contour with bulky mesenteric adenopathy favor the diagnosis of lymphoma. Obstruction is less common than with other tumors because non-Hodgkin's lymphoma does not evoke a desmoplastic reaction. Although aneurysmal dilatation is considered a characteristic feature of lymphoma it can be seen with gastrointestinal stromal tumors, metastatic disease and rarely adenocarcinoma.[72,73]

Polypoid Form

This form produces multiple or solitary polypoid filling defects ranging from few mm to 4 cm on small bowel barium examination. A polypoid lesion that is large enough may produce a homogeneous solid nodule protruding into the lumen on CT or MR without wall thickening or lymphadenopathy.[78] Generally the polypoid nature of nodules may not be apparent on CT and the only findings that may be seen are nonobstructive wall thickening and a mass lesion. The polypoid lesions may act as a lead point for intussusception.[73] This pattern is generally produced by mantle cell lymphoma but may also be produced by ENMZL and follicular lymphoma. The differential diagnosis of multiple/solitary polypoid lesions include intestinal polyposis syndromes, gastrointestinal

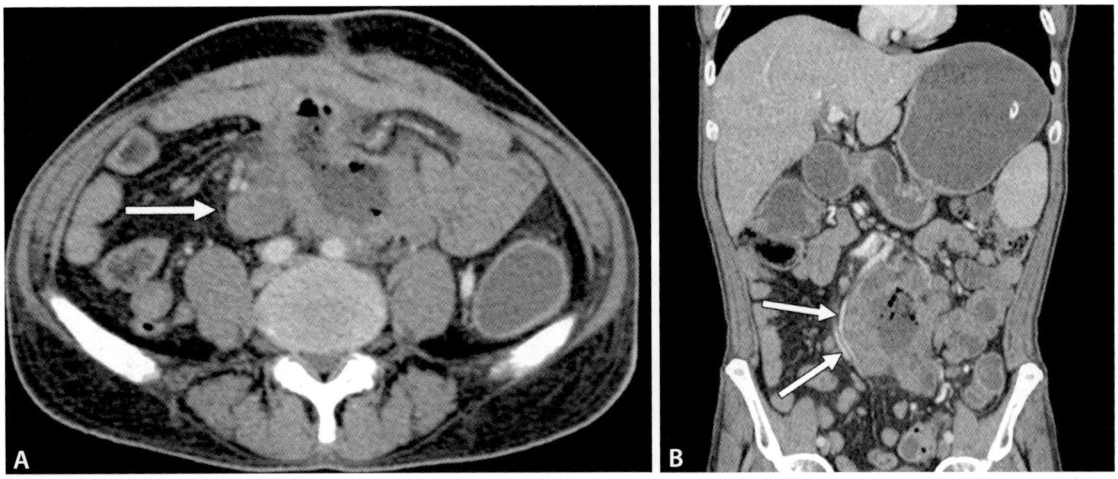

Figs. 17A and B: *Lymphoma ileum*: Axial and coronal CECT images reveal hypodense mildly enhancing wall thickening involving the ileum with aneurysmal dilatation of the lumen of the involved segment. Adjacent lymphadenopathy is also noted (arrow in A). The mesenteric vessels (arrows in B) are displaced by the mass but not encased or narrowed.

stromal tumors, lipomas, adenomas or metastases. The inherited polyposis syndromes are much more commonly responsible for multiple gastrointestinal polyps than mantle cell lymphoma. A positive family history (though not always present), presentation during childhood or early adulthood and characteristic extraintestinal findings may help to establish the diagnosis of polyposis syndromes.[72]

Metastases are generally larger, more randomly distributed and may produce submucosal masses, 'bull's eye' or target lesions with central ulceration with pooling of contrast.[73]

Endoexoenteric Form

This form is associated with bowel wall thickening, a large lymphomatous mass showing exocentric growth and deep ulceration. There may be formation of sinus tracts to mesentery with resultant sterile abscesses or fistulization to other abdominal viscera.[73] Barium studies may show a large barium filled cavity along the mesenteric border of the affected bowel. CT reveals gross wall thickening, large cavitating mass with extraluminal contrast extending into the cavity which commonly shows fluid and debris.[73,83] Similar findings may be found with cavitating gastrointestinal stromal tumors and occasionally metastatic melanoma.[73]

Mesenteric Invasive Form

It is believed that this variety occurs due to direct extension of disease from affected mesenteric nodes. This produces bowel wall thickening with tethered and angulated folds contiguous with bulky mesenteric nodes. This is the variety most commonly associated with obstruction. On CT/MR a 'sandwich appearance' may be seen with mesenteric vessels forming the middle of the sandwich and surrounding conglomerate nodal/intestinal masses forming the outer layers **(Figs. 18A to C)**.[72,83]

Table 8 summarizes the most common imaging appearances of lymphoma.

Radiological Appearances of Some Specific Lymphoma Types

Hodgkin's lymphoma rarely involves the bowel with only isolated case reports being available. This may produce a stenotic mass as it produces fibrosis unlike NHL.[72]

T-cell lymphoma on barium studies, especially enteroclysis, may depict thickened nodular folds with ulceration and stricture formation usually in the jejunum but it can be multifocal. On CT/MR there may be only mild to moderate wall thickening which is better appreciated on CT/MR enteroclysis **(Figs. 19A and B)**. Associated lymphadenopathy and infiltration of mesenteric fat may also be seen. Perforation is much more common in this variety of lymphoma and is believed to be due to angiocentric growth of lymphoid cells with infiltration of vessel walls producing vascular occlusion and ischemic necrosis. It has been reported that perforation may be present in 16%–33% of patient with type I and type II EATL respectively.[73] Laparotomy may be required in as many as 50% patients for complications such as hemorrhage, perforation or obstruction.[72] This variety of lymphoma needs to be distnguished from other complications of celiac disease such as chronic jejunoileitis (CJI) and

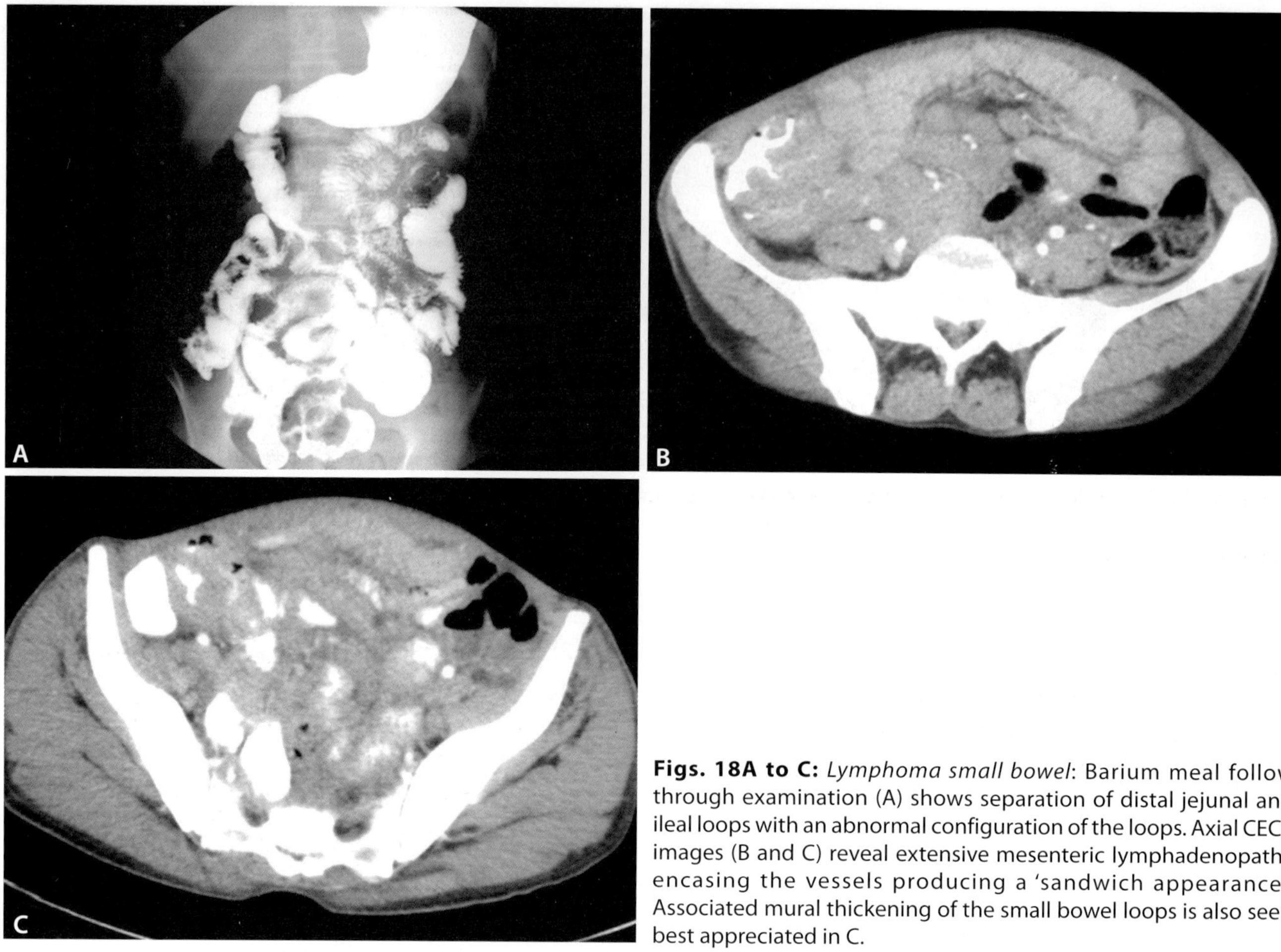

Figs. 18A to C: *Lymphoma small bowel*: Barium meal follow through examination (A) shows separation of distal jejunal and ileal loops with an abnormal configuration of the loops. Axial CECT images (B and C) reveal extensive mesenteric lymphadenopathy encasing the vessels producing a 'sandwich appearance'. Associated mural thickening of the small bowel loops is also seen best appreciated in C.

Table 8: Lymphoma key imaging findings.

• *Site*: Terminal ileum
• Long segment involvement
• *Barium*: Fold thickening/featureless appearance, aneurysmal dilatation
• *CT/MR*: Marked homogeneous hypodense/hypoattenuating wall thickening
• Minimal enhancement
• Smooth mural contour
• Associated findings
• Bulky adenopathy
• Bowel obstruction distinctly uncommon

refractory celiac disease (RCD). CJI is a rare complication difficult to distinguish and considered by some to represent a low grade enteropathy-associated T-cell lymphoma. Findings of effacement of jejunal folds, small bowel wall thickening, intussusception, infiltration of mesenteric fat, lymphadenopathy and splenic atrophy have been reported on CT and MR in refractory celiac disease (RCD). FDG PET has an important role in distinguishing between RCD and EATL as 86–100% of EATL lymphomas show increased uptake. The 5 year survival for T-cell lymphomas at 25% is much worse than the 75% survival rate for B-cell lymphomas.[72,73]

Burkitt's Lymphoma

The endemic variety of Burkitt's lymphoma is associated with Ebstein-Barr virus (EBV) infection and commonly involves the head and neck region. Other variants include sporadic variety and that associated with HIV infection (the immunodeficiency associated variant). It is a very rapidly growing tumor, commonly occurring in children and usually affects the terminal ileum or ileo-cecal region in sporadic cases. Less commonly it may involve the stomach or colon peak age of occurrence is 11 years. The genetic defects identified include translocation and deregulation of *c-Myc* gene on chromosome 8. On histology a typical 'starry-sky appearance' is seen due to

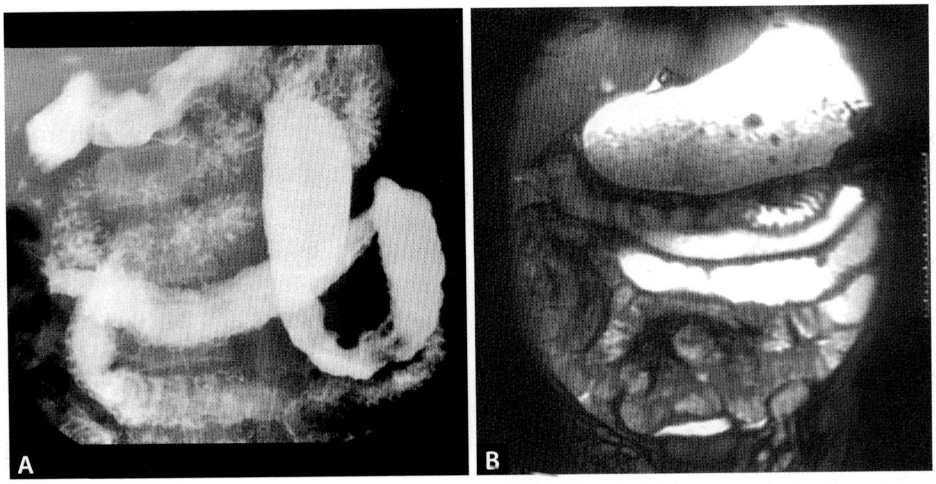

Figs. 19A and B: *T-cell lymphoma jejunum*: Barium enteroclysis (A) reveals nodular fold thickening in the jejunum with dilated featureless segment of jejunum in a patient with symptoms of malabsorption. Coronal T2W MR enteroclysis image (B) shows only mild wall thickening of the involved segments.

macrophage containing cellular debris lying scattered within dense sheets of lymphoid cells.[76,77]

Barium studies may show markedly thickened valvulae conniventes while grossly thickened bowel wall due to infiltration by tumor is seen on CT. There may be associated aneurysmal dilatation and intussusception with the thickened walls serving as the lead point. Diffuse lymphadenopathy, infiltration of the mesentery and peritoneum with peritoneal carcinomatosis may be seen. These tumors show high FDG uptake on initial scans due to their rapidly proliferating nature which reverts to normal following treatment **(Figs. 20A to F)**.

Endemic Burkitt's lymphoma is very chemosensitive and 5 years survival rates exceed 90% in children with localized disease. Sporadic and immunodeficiency associated Burkitt's are less sensitive to chemotherapy but 50–70% overall survival rate may be seen in adults after intensive chemotherapy.

Although radiological features of lymphoma are not specific to various pathogical types some radiologic pathologic correlation does exist[76] and is summarized in **Table 9**.

STAGING AND PROGNOSTICATION

Staging and response assessment systems in lymphoma have evolved over time owing to the introduction of radiation therapy, CT and FDG-PET/CT. 18F-FDG-PET/CT along with a CECT has been recommended as a staging tool for all FDG avid lymphomas. For the non-FDG avid varieties a CECT is recommended. It is also an excellent tool to evaluate response after treatment before morphological changes become apparent.[84]

Lymphomas comprise an extremely heterogeneous group of tumors hence their metabolic activity and glucose uptake is variable with low grade NHLs showing lower glucose uptake than aggressive lesions. Low grade follicular lymphomas and indolent extranodal marginal zone B-cell lymphoma (ENMZL) may show very low FDG uptake making it difficult to detect primary lesions. On the other hand diffuse large B-cell lymphoma (DLBCL), MCL, EATL, Burkitt's lymphoma and Hodgkin's disease are FDG avid. However, studies suggest that most low grade lymphomas can also be accurately staged with PET/CT.[84,85]

In some studies SUVmax (standard value uptake) varied greatly (between 3.2 and 43) among different lymphoma types. Aggressive lymphomas have a SUV max three times than that of indolent lymphoma on an average. A cut-off value of SUVmax at 10 reportedly had 71% sensitivity and 81% specificity in differentiating aggressive and indolent lymphomas.[84,85]

New tracers like 18F fluorothymidine being evaluated for PET-CT may be useful to distinguish between high grade and low grade lymphoma and early response assessment.[81,83] Their uptake is dependent on cell proliferation rather than glucose metabolism. However, high physiological tracer uptake in the abdomen limits the usefulness of these tracers for imaging of abdominal and pelvic lymphomas.

Whole body of diffusion-weighted MRI (WB-DWMRI) has also been evaluated as a tool to stage and follow-up gastrointestinal lymphoma with reports suggesting

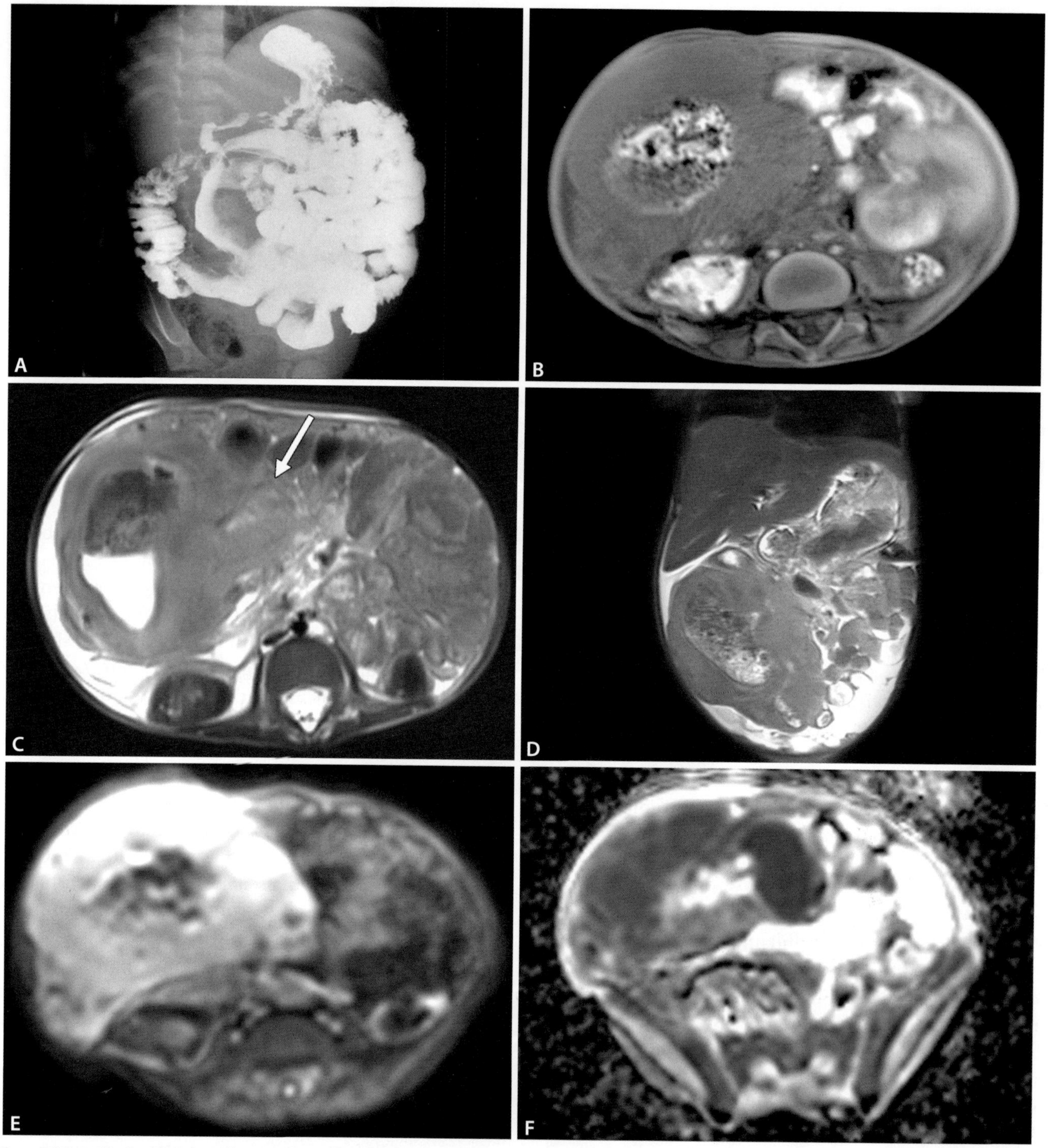

Figs. 20A to F: *Burkitt's lymphoma*: Barium meal follow through examination (A) of an 11-year-old boy presenting with a rapidly enlarging abdominal lump reveals long-segment effacement of mucosal folds resulting in a smooth featureless appearance of the distal ileum along with luminal dilatation. The presence of a significant extraluminal component is suggested by the surrounding soft tissue haze and displacement of bowel loops. T1W axial (B), T2W axial and coronal (C and D) depict marked wall thickening of the terminal ileum appearing hypointense on T1W images, mildly hyperintense on T2W images with evidence of diffusion restriction seen as bright signal on the DWI (E) and hypointense signal on ADC (F). Note the presence of ascites and adjacent lymphadenopathy (arrow in C).

Table 9: Correlation of radiologic findings with pathology in small bowel lymphoma.

Radiologic findings	*Likely lymphoma type*	*Therapeutic options*
1. Marked homogeneous nonobstructive bowel wall thickening, aneurysmal dilatation and bulky lymph nodes Site-distal ileum FDG-PET avid	DLBCL	Chemotherapy R-CHOP
2. *Barium*: Multiple small polyps *CT*: Polyps/nonobstructive bowel wall thickening and lymph nodes Site-distal ileum, colon and rectum Curvilinear areas of FDG-PET uptake	MCL Occasionally, ENMZL (more often in stomach/ colon) MCL	R-CHOP R-Hyper CVAD Consider stem cell transplant
3. Circumferential/asymmetric wall thickening polypoid mass FDG-PET avidity variable	ENMZL	*H. pylori* +ve–antibiotics *H. pylori* –ve/resistant–chemotherapy
4. Nodular fold thickening Site-proximal jejunum, entire small bowel in young adult males from middle east	IPSID	Tetracycline based antibiotic Unresponsive to antibiotics CHOP
5. Tiny polyps/fold thickening in jejunum FDG PET—unreliable	Follicular lymphoma	Wait and watch Chemotherapy—fludarabine based
6. Bulky terminal ileal/ileo-caecal disease in a child, rapidly progressive Strongly FDG-PET avid.	Burkitt's lymphoma	Chemotherapy—Magrath regimen*, hyper-CVAD
7. Barium nodular fold thickening, ulceration *CT*: Long segment eccentric circumferential mild wall thickening perforation in up to 50%. Associated features of celiac disease. Site-proximal jejunum FDG-PET avid.	EATL	Anthracycline containing Combination chemotherapy—CHOP

Abbreviations: CHOP: Cyclophosphamide, doxorubicin, vincristine, prednisone; R: Rituximab; Hyper-CVAD: Cyclophosphamide, vincristine, doxorubicin, dexamethasone methotrexate, cytarabine; DLBCL: Diffuse large B-cell lymphoma; ENMZL: Extranodal marginal zone B-cell lymphoma; IPSID: Immunoproliferative small intestinal disease; EATL: Enteropathy associated T-cell lymphoma.
*Magrath regimen, cyclophosphamide, doxorubicin, vincristine, methotrexate, ifosfamide, etoposide, cytarabine.

comparable diagnostic value as FDG PET-CT.[82,86] In a study comparing DW-MRI and PET-CT, DW-MRI was found to be only slightly inferior to FDG PET/CT for staging FDG avid lymphomas but for lymphomas with variable FDG avidity such as MALT lymphoma, DWI was superior to both 18FFDG-PET/CT and CECT (93.5% vs 64.5% sensitivity).[82,86] Thus WB-DW-MRI appears to be a promising tool for nodal and bone marrow of staging lymphomas. PET-MR Protocols are also being evaluated for lymphoma staging.[10]

A number of staging systems are available for GI lymphoma. The Mushoff modification of the Ann Arbor staging[87] is often used, however it suffers from the limitation that it does not address certain features specific to gastrointestinal lymphoma such as diffuse and incurable infiltration of the gastrointestinal tract.

An alternative staging system was first proposed by Blackledge and later modified by the international workshop in Lugano, Switzerland in 1994.[88] Lugano staging is a modification of the original Ann Arbor staging designed for the staging of primary GI lymphomas **(Table 10)**.

Table 10: Lugano classification for GI lymphoma.

• *Stage I*: Tumor confined to gastrointestinal tract, single primary or multiple noncontiguous lesions
• *Stage II*: Tumor extends into the abdominal cavity from primary gastrointestinal site
• *Stage II1*: Local nodal involvement
• *Stage II2*: Distant nodal involvement
• *Stage IIE*: Penetration of serosa to involve adjacent organ or tissue
• *Stage III*: no stage III in this system
• *Stage IV*: Disseminated extranodal involvement or gastrointestinal tract lesion with supradiaphragmatic nodal involvement (CME lymphoma—12).
• Specify site of involvement, e.g. IIE pancreas. If both nodal and adjacent organ involvement—both subscript 1 or 2 and E is used, e.g. II2E (pancreas)

The Paris staging system[89] proposed by European Gastrointestinal Lymphoma Study (EGILS) Group in 2003 has become increasingly accepted. This is summarized in **Table 11**. The major advantage of this staging system is its

Table 11: Paris staging system for primary gastrointestinal lymphomas (TNMB).

Stage	*Gastrointestinal lymphomas*
TX	Lymphoma extent not specified
T0	No evidence of lymphoma
T1	Lymphoma confined to the mucosa/submucosa
T1m	Lymphoma confined to the mucosa
T1sm	Lymphoma confined to the submucosa
T2	Lymphoma infiltrates muscularis propria or subserosa
T3	Lymphoma penetrates serosa (visceral peritoneum) without invasion of adjacent structures
T4	Lymphoma invades adjacent structures or organs
NX	Involvement of lymph nodes not assessed
N0	No evidence of lymph nodes involvement
N1	Involvement of regional lymph nodes
N2	Involvement of intra-abdominal lymph nodes beyond the regional area
N3	Spread to extra-abdominal lymph nodes
MX	Dissemination of lymphoma not assessed
M0	No evidence of extranodal dissemination
M1	Non-continuous involvement of separate site in gastrointestinal tract (e.g. stomach and rectum)
M2	Non-continuous involvement of other tissues (e.g. peritoneum, pleura) or organs (e.g. tonsils, parotid gland, ocular, adnexa, lung, liver, spleen, kidney, breast, etc.)
BX	Involvement of bone marrow not assessed
B0	No evidence of bone marrow involvement
B1	Lymphomatous infiltration of bone marrow
TNM	*Clinical staging:* Status of tumor, node, metastasis, bone marrow
$_{P}$TNMB	*Histopathological staging*: Status of tumor, node metastasis, bone marrow
pN	The histopathological examination will ordinarily include six or more lymph nodes

ability to record the depth of tumor infiltration, specific lymphoma spread and extent of nodal involvement.

The prognosis of NHL is better than that adenocarcinoma as it remains confined to the bowel wall for a long time and because more effective chemotherapy is available. The adverse risk factors for GI lymphoma include advanced stage, involvement of para-aortic nodes, large tumor bulk, serosal penetration, and intestinal rather than gastric origin. Other poor prognostic factors include advanced age of patient and higher grade of lymphoma.[78,81]

Treatment

Treatment[83] usually consists of a combination of chemotherapy, surgery and radiotherapy and is summarized in **Table 8**.

B-cell Lymphoma

Anthracycline based chemotherapy is the mainstay in the treatment of intestinal DLBCL. Primary surgery may be required at times to establish the diagnosis, reduce tumor bulk, to manage complications from perforation, obstruction and for staging. Radiotherapy may be used when there is bulky residual disease or only partial resection has been possible.

Immunoproliferative small intestinal disease (IPSID) is initially treated with tetracycline and metronidazole. A wait and watch policy may be adopted for lower grades of lymphoma like follicular lymphoma.

T-cell Lymphoma

Owing to its rarity the treatment of primary T-cell lymphoma is not well-defined. A gluten free diet helps to reduce the risk of lymphoma in celiac disease. Primary surgery along with chemotherapy is generally recommended due to the risk of perforation, hemorrhage and obstruction. However, following surgery initiation of chemotherapy is usually delayed because of postoperative infection and the difficulty in healing due to malnutrition.

Kaposi's Sarcoma

Kaposi's sarcoma is a tumor commonly associated with AIDS. It is a low grade systemic vascular neoplasm involving skin in the form of pigmented cutaneous lesions, internal organs and lymph nodes. In AIDS associated Kaposi' sarcoma early involvement of intestine and lymph nodes is seen. Lesions of Kaposi's sarcoma tend to be multiple and are generally seen as elevated submucosal nodules in the jejunum and ileum. Small bowel folds may be diffusely thickened. The lesions generally show mild heterogeneous enhancement. Associated retroperitoneal and mesenteric lymphadenopathy is common. Differentiation from lymphoma may be very difficult although Kaposi's sarcoma is more focal and nodular.[15,16]

Leiomyosarcoma

True leiomyosarcomas of the small bowel arise from the smooth muscle of the small bowel wall or blood vessels and are very rare accounting for less than 15% of primary intestinal malignant tumors. Usually these are solitary being situated in the jejunum and ileum and most commonly in Meckel's diverticuclum. The growth pattern is mainly slow extraluminal growth resulting in late presentation. Usually tumors exceed 5 cm in size at presentation.[14,16]

On barium studies a predominantly extrinsic lesion with barium filled cavitation may be seen. On CT/MR they produce large heterogeneous masses with area of necrosis and cystic degeneration with rim enhancement. There can be associated cavitation or fistulization **(Figs. 21A to C)**. Liver and peritoneal metastasis may also be seen which tend to be large with peripheral rim enhancement due to central necrosis. On imaging these cannot be distinguished from GIST.[1,14,16]

Metastatic Neoplasms

Secondary metastatic involvement of the small bowel is commoner than primary and may account for nearly half of all small bowel tumors.[1] The major pathways for metastatic spread are hematogenous, direct extension, intraperitoneal seeding and lymphatic.[1] Tumors from the stomach, colon, ovary and uterus spread to the small bowel either by direct invasion or intraperitoneal spread while hematogenous metastases are seen in carcinoma breast, lung and melanoma.

The extraintestinal malignancy with the greatest propensity to metastasize to the bowel is melanoma. Small bowel is the most frequent site involved in the gastrointestinal tract owing to its rich blood supply. The vasa recti form a rich submucosal plexus on the antimesenteric border of the small bowel hence hematogenous metastatic deposits occur on the antimesentric border. Hematogeneous metastasis may produce solitary or multiple submucosal nodules on barium studies with or without central ulceration—'the bulls eye' appearance. On CT or MR these produce a short segment wall thickening or focal mass with contrast enhancement and at times may mimic primary neoplasm **(Figs. 22A to D)**.[1,14,16,28]

Intraperitoneal metastases most commonly arise from the colon or ovary. Transperitoneal seedling follows the circulatory pathway of peritoneal fluid. This fluid after flowing over the mesenteric recesses settles at the termination of small bowel mesentery in the ileo cecal region. Therefore transperitoneal metastases occur at the mesenteric border. They produce small contrast enhancing nodules along the serosal surface with disease progression they can encase the small bowel and cause obstruction. Gadolinium enhanced fat saturated MR has been shown to be more sensitive than CT to detect small tumor nodules **(Figs. 23A and B)**.[1,30,32]

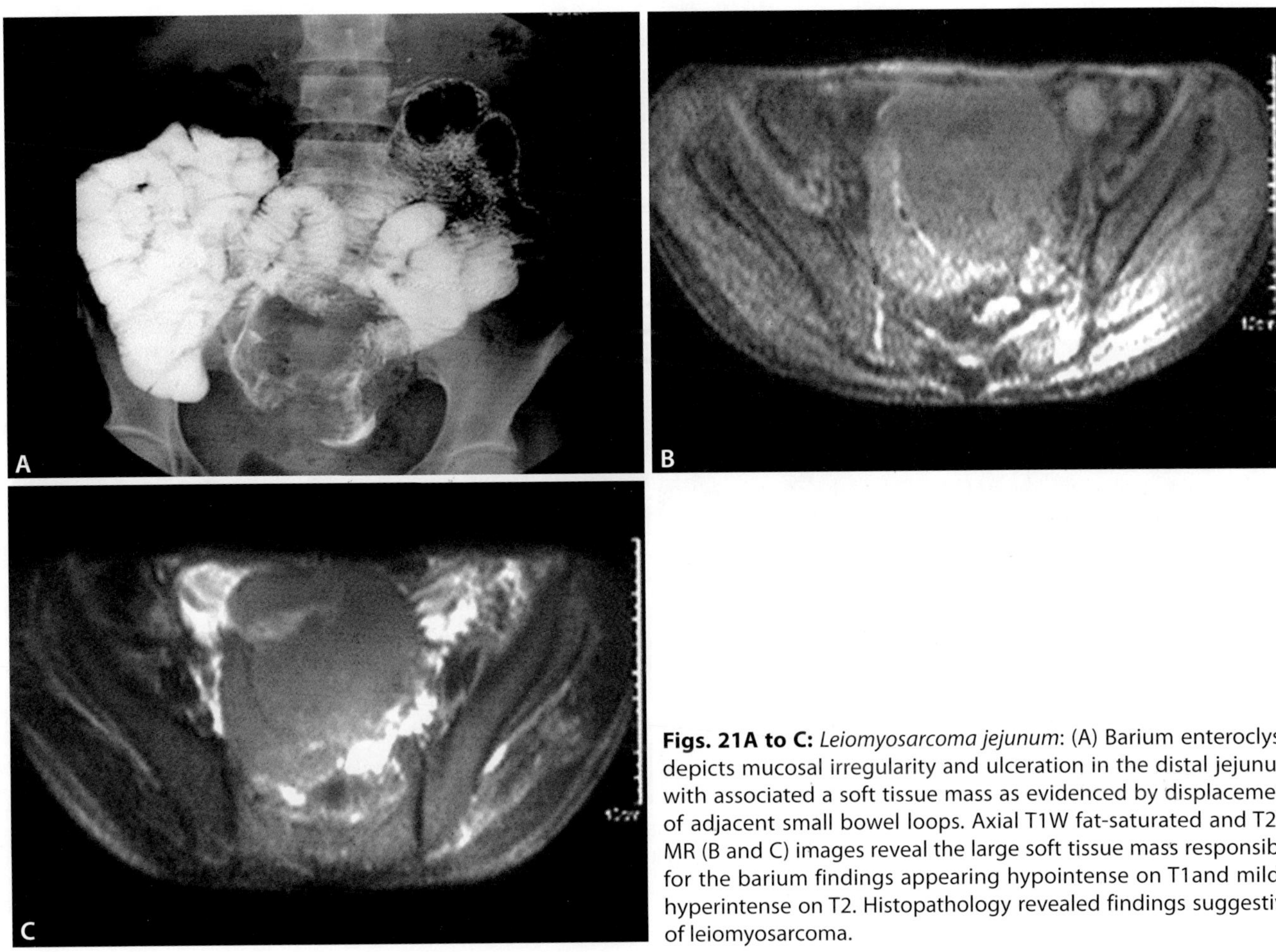

Figs. 21A to C: *Leiomyosarcoma jejunum*: (A) Barium enteroclysis depicts mucosal irregularity and ulceration in the distal jejunum with associated a soft tissue mass as evidenced by displacement of adjacent small bowel loops. Axial T1W fat-saturated and T2W MR (B and C) images reveal the large soft tissue mass responsible for the barium findings appearing hypointense on T1and mildly hyperintense on T2. Histopathology revealed findings suggestive of leiomyosarcoma.

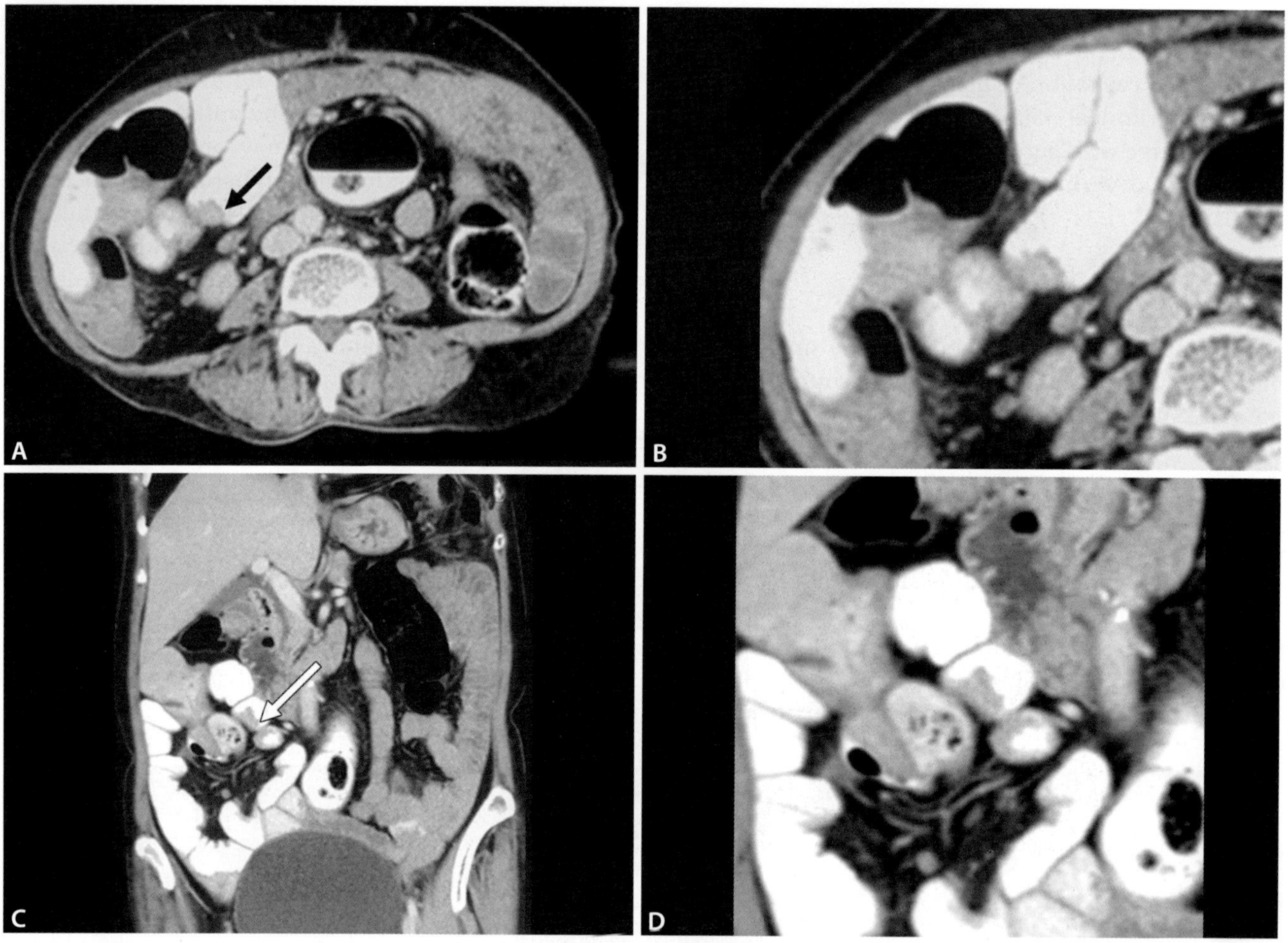

Figs. 22A to D: *Metastases small bowel*: Axial and coronal CECT images (A to D) in a patient of melanoma with hematogenous metastases reveals a focal polypoid intraluminal mass and wall thickening in the jejunum better seen on the magnified images (B and D) with mild dilatation of the loops.

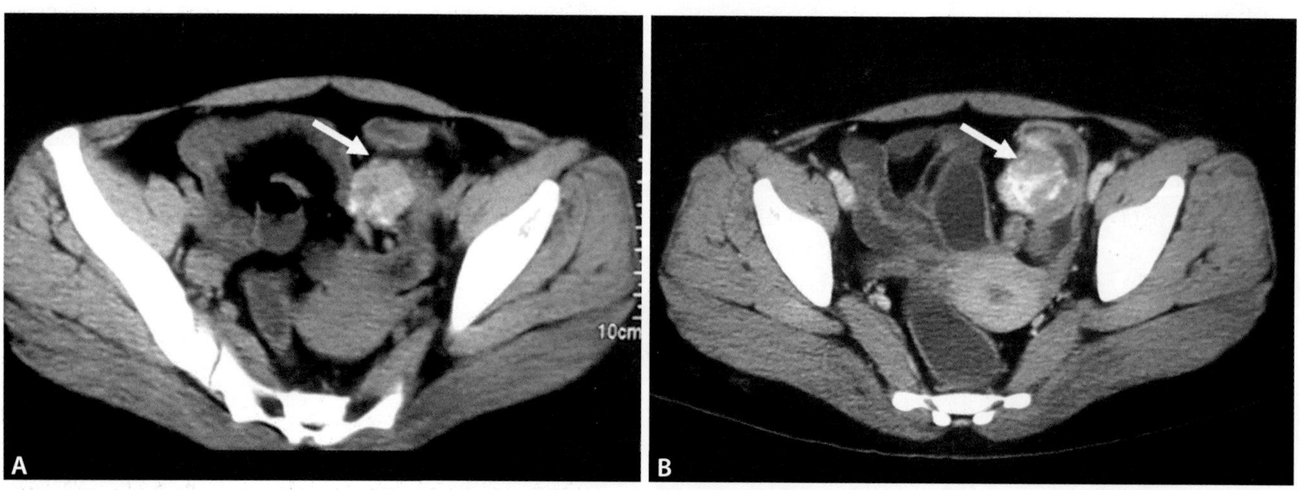

Figs. 23A and B: *Metastases small bowel*: Axial NCCT and CECT images show a serosal deposit on an ileal loop in the pelvis showing calcification and heterogeneous enhancement (arrows) in an operated case of adenocarcinoma ascending colon.

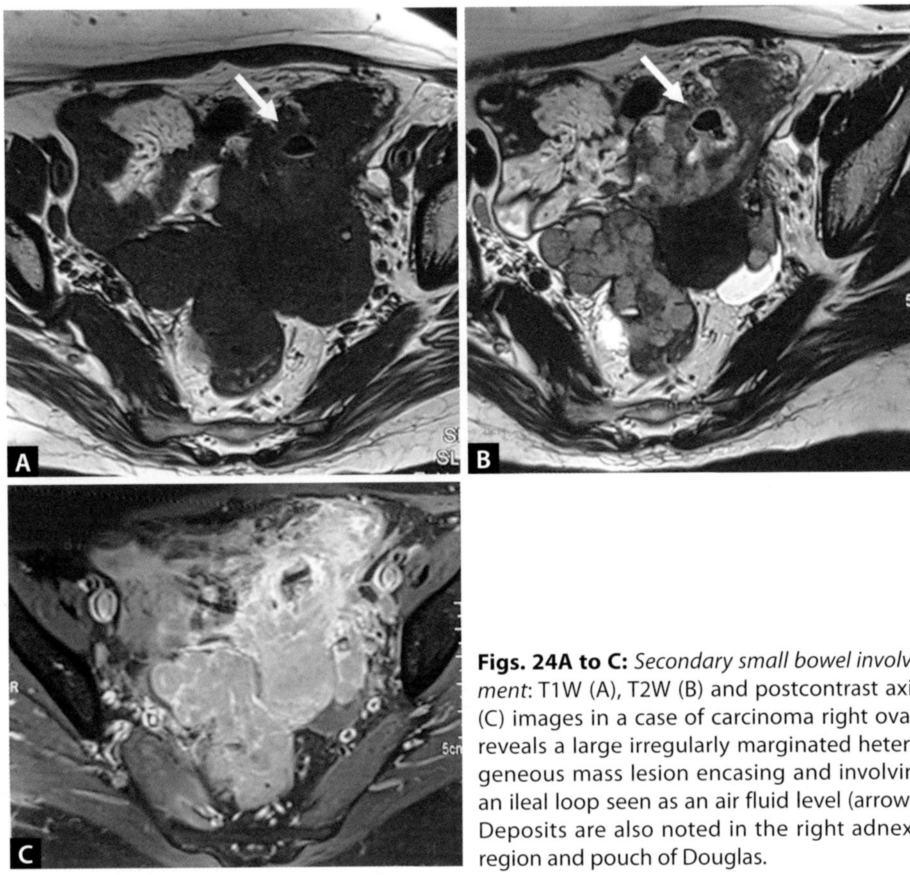

Figs. 24A to C: *Secondary small bowel involvement*: T1W (A), T2W (B) and postcontrast axial (C) images in a case of carcinoma right ovary reveals a large irregularly marginated heterogeneous mass lesion encasing and involving an ileal loop seen as an air fluid level (arrows). Deposits are also noted in the right adnexal region and pouch of Douglas.

Infiltration from advanced colonic, ovarian, pancreatic or biliary neoplasms can also involve the small bowel **(Figs. 24A to C)**.

CONCLUSION

Small bowel tumors are rare neoplasms, this combined with the nonspecific presentation and the relative difficulty in the evaluation of the small bowel makes early diagnosis of these lesions difficult. Despite advances in endoscopy, the radiologist continues to play a key role in their diagnosis. The imaging features of various small bowel tumors may overlap with each other, however, recognition of certain characteristic features on imaging studies may help to narrow the differential. The radiologist therefore needs to be fully conversant with the imaging features of small bowel tumors and consider these as a differential diagnosis in the appropriate clinical and radiologic context to avoid delay in diagnosis.

REFERENCES

1. Xynopoulos D, Mihas AA, Paraskevas E, Dimitroulopoulos D, Heuman DM, Mihas AA. Small bowel tumors. Annals of Gastroenterology. 2002;15(1):18-35.
2. Martin RG. Malignant tumors of the small intestine. Surg Clin N Am. 1986;66:779-85.
3. Neugut AI, Jacobson JS, Suh S, Mukherjee R, Arber N. The epidemiology of cancer of the small bowel. Cancer Epidemiol Biomarkers Prev. 1999;7:243-51.
4. Pourmand K, Itzkowitz SH. Small bowel neoplasms and polyps current gastroenterology reports. 2016;18:23. doi 10.1007s11894.016.0497.xfghg
5. Hara AK, Leighton JA, Sharma VK, Height RI, Fleischer DE. Imaging of small bowel disease: comparison of capsule endoscopy, standard endoscopy, barium examination and CT. Radiographics. 2005;25:697-718.
6. Nolan DJ, Traill ZC. The current role of barium examination of the small intestine. Clin Radiol. 1997;52:809-20.
7. Wale A, Pilcher J. Current role of ultrasound in small bowel imaging: seminars in ultrasound CT and MRI. 2016;37(5):482-97.
8. Pilleul F, Penigaud M, Milot L, et al. Possible small-bowel neoplasms: contrast-enhanced and water-enhanced multidetector CT enteroclysis. Radiology. 2006;241(3):796.
9. Pappalardo G, Gualdi G, Nunziale A, et al. Impact of magnetic resonance in the preoperative staging and the surgical planning for treating small bowel neoplasms. Surg Today. 2013;43(6):613.
10. Goh V, Prezzi D, Mallia A, Bashir U, Stirling JJ, John J, Charles-Edwards G, MacKewn J, Cook G. Positron

Emission Tomography/Magnentic Resonance Imaging of Gastrointestinal Cancers: Seminars in Ultrasound CT and MRI. 2016;37(4):352-7.
11. Levine MS, Rubesin SE, Laufer I. Pattern approach for diseases of mesenteric small bowel on barium studies. Radiology. 2008;249:2.
12. Rubesin SE. Simplified approach to differential diagnosis of small bowel abnormalities. Radiol Clin North Am. 2003;41: 343-64.
13. Lappas JC, Maglinte DD, Sandrasegaran K. Benign tumors of the small-bowel. Gore R, Levine M (Eds). Textbook of gastrointestinal radiology, 3rd edition. Philadelphia, PA: Saunders Elsevier; 2008. pp. 845-51.
14. Sailer J, Zacherl J, Schimaa W. MDCT of small bowel tumors. Cancer Imaging. 2007;7(1):224-33.
15. Masselli G, Polettini E, Casciani E, Bertini L, Vecchioli A, Gualdi G. Small-bowel neoplasm: prospective evaluation of MR enteroclysis. Radiology. 2009;251:743-50.
16. Masselli G, Colaiacomo MC, Marcelli G, et al. MRI of the small-bowel: how to differentiate primary neoplasms and mimickers. The British Journal of Radiology. 2012;85(1014):824-37.
17. CY Lee, MK Yuen. Inflammatory fibroid polyps causing intussusception in adult patients: Two case reports and review of literature focusing on radiological features. Hong Kong J Radiol. 2014;17:271-6.
18. Thompson WM. Imaging and Findings of Lipomas of the Gastrointestinal Tract American Journal of Roentgenology. 2005;184:1163-71.
19. Corsi A, Ingegnoli A, Abelli P, et al. Imaging of a small bowel cavernous hemangioma: report of a case with emphasis on the use of computed tomography and enteroclysis. Acta Biomed. 2007;78(2):139-43.
20. Huprich JE, Barlow JM, Hansel SL, et al. Multiphase CT enterography evaluation of small-bowel vascular lesions. American Journal of Roentgenology. 2013;201:65-72.
21. Buck JL, Harned RK. Polyposis syndromes. In: Gore RM, Levine MS (Eds). Textbook of gastrointestinal radiology, 2nd edition. Philadelphia, Pa: Saunders, 2000. pp. 1075-88.
22. Durno CA. Colonic polyps in children and adolescents. Can J Gastroenterol. 2007;21(4):233-9.
23. Brucher BL, Roder JD, Fink U, Stein HJ, Busch R, Siewert JR. Prognostic factors in resected primary small bowel tumors. Dig Surg. 1998;15:42-51.
24. Aparicio T, Zaanan A, Svrcek M, et al. Small bowel adenocarcinoma: epidemiology, risk factors, diagnosis and treatment. Dig Liver Dis. 2014;46:97-104.
25. Negri E, Bosetti C, La Vecchia C, Fioretti F, Conti E, Franceschi S. Risk factors for adenocarcinoma of the small intestine. Cancer. 1999;82:171-4.
26. Maglinte DD, Lappas JC, Sandrasegaran Malignant. Tumors of the small bowel. In: Gore R, Levine M (Eds). Textbook of gastrointestinal radiology, 3rd edition. Saunders Elsevier, Philadelphia, PA; 2008. pp. 853-69.
27. Masselli G, Gualdi G. Evaluation of small bowel tumors: MR enteroclysis. Abdm Imaging. 2010;35:23-30.
28. Faggian A, Fracella MR, D'Alesio G, Alabiso ME, Berritto D, Feragalli B, Miele V, Iasiello F, Grassi R. Small-Bowel Neoplasms: Role of MRI Enteroclysis: Gastroenterology Research and Practice Volume 2016, Article ID 9686815, 6 pages.
29. Cronin CG, Scott J, Kambadakone A, Catalano OA, Sahani D, Blake MA, McDermott S. Utility of positron emission tomography/CT in the evaluation of small bowel pathology. Br J Radiol. 2012;85(1017):1211-21.
30. Sinha R, Rajiah P, Ramachandran I, Sanders S, Murphy PD. Diffusion-weighted MR imaging of the gastrointestinal tract: technique, indications, and imaging findings. Radiographics. 2013;33(3):655-76.
31. Kyriazi S, Collins DJ, Morgan VA, Giles SL, deSouza NM. Diffusion-weighted imaging of peritoneal disease for non-invasive staging of advanced ovarian cancer. Radiographics. 2010;30(5):1269-85.
32. Low RN, Sebrechts CP, Barone RM, Muller W. Diffusion-weighted MRI of peritoneal tumors: comparison with conventional MRI and surgical and histopathologic findings—a feasibility study. AJR. 2009;193(2): 461-70.
33. Sobin LH, Gospodarowicz MK, Wittekind C. TNM classification of malignant tumors, 7th edition. Wiley Blackwell; 2009. pp. 153-9.
34. Cunningham D, Atkin W, Lenz HJ, et al. Colorectal cancer. Lancet. 2010;375(9719):1030-47.
35. Langhans T. Ubereinendrusenpolypimileum. Virchow Archiv Pathol Anatom Phys Klin Med. 1867;38:559-60.
36. Lubarsch O. Ueber den primaren krebs des ileum nebst bemerkungen uber das gleichzeitige vorkommen von krebs and tuberculose. Virchow Archiv Pathol Anatom Phys Klin Med. 1888;111:280-317.
37. Oberndorfer S. Karzinoide tumoren des dunndarms. Frankf Z Pathol. 1907;9:425-9.
38. Yao JC, Hassan M, Phan A, et al. One hundred years after "carcinoid": epidemiology of and prognostic factors for neuroendocrine tumors in 35,825 cases in the United States. J Clin Oncol. 2008;26:3063-72.
39. Ganeshan D, Bhosale P, Yang T, Kundra V. Imaging features of carcinoid tumor of gastrointestinal tract. Am J Roentgenol. 2013;201(4):773-86.
40. Rindi G, Bordi C. Highlights of the biology of endocrine tumors of the gut and pancreas. Endocr Relat Cancer. 2003;10: 427-36.
41. Chang S, Choi D, Jin Lee S, Jae Lee W, Park M, Sang Won Kim, Da Keun Lee, Kee-Taek Jang. Neuroendocrine neoplasms of the gastrointestinal tract: classification, pathologic basis, and imaging features. Radiographics. 2007;27:1667-79.
42. Williams GT. Endocrine tumors of the gastrointestinal tract-selected topics. Histopathology. 2007;50(1):30-41.
43. Duh QY, Hybarger CP, Geist R, et al. Carcinoids associated with multiple endocrine neoplasia syndromes. Am J Surg. 1987;154(1):142-8.
44. Karatzas G, Kouraklis G, Karayiannakis A, et al. Ampullary carcinoid and jejunal stromal tumor associated with von

Recklinghausen's disease presenting as gastrointestinal bleeding and jaundice. Eur J Surg Oncol. 2000;26(4):428-9.
45. Levy AD, Sobin LH. Gastrointestinal Carcinoids: Imaging Features with Clinicopathologic Comparison. Radiographics. 2007;27:237-57.
46. Moller JE, Connolly HM, Rubin J, et al. Factors associated with progression of carcinoid heart disease. N Engl J Med. 2003;348:1005-15.
47. Kamaoui I, De-Luca V, Ficarelli S, Mennesson N, Lombard-Bohas C, Pilleul F. Value of CT enteroclysis in suspected small-bowel carcinoid tumors. AJR. 2010;194:629-33.
48. Horton KM, Kamel I, Hofmann L, Fishman EK. Carcinoid tumors of the small bowel: a multitechnique imaging approach. AJR. 2004;182:559-67.
49. Paulsen SR, Huprich JE, Fletcher JG, et al. CT enterography as a diagnostic tool in evaluating small bowel disorders: review of clinical experience with over 700 cases. Radiographics. 2006;26:641-57, discussion 657-62.
50. Woodard PK, Feldman JM, Paine SS, Baker ME. Midgut carcinoid tumors: CT findings and biochemical profiles. J Comput Assist Tomogr. 1995;19:400-5.
51. Bader TR, Semelka RC, Chiu VC, et al. MRI of carcinoid tumors: spectrum of appearances in the gastrointestinal tract and liver. J Magn Reson Imaging. 2001;14:261-9.
52. Pantongrag-Brown L, Buetow PC, Carr NJ, et al. Calcification and fibrosis in mesenteric carcinoid tumor: CT findings and pathologic correlation. Am J Roentgenol. 1995;164:387-91.
53. Maglinte DDT, Herlinger H. Small bowel neoplasms. In: Herlinger H, Maglinte DDT, Birnbaum BA (Eds). Clinical imaging of the small intestine, 2nd edition. New York, NY: Springer; 1999. pp. 377-438.
54. Reznek RH. CT/MRI of neuroendocrine tumors. Cancer Imaging. 2006;6(Spec No A):S163-77. doi:10.1102/1470-7330.2006.9037.
55. Hofman MS1, Lau WF, Hicks RJ. Somatostatin receptor imaging with 68Ga DOTATATE PET/CT: clinical utility, normal patterns, pearls, and pitfalls in interpretation Radiographics. 2015;35(2):500-16. doi: 10.1148/rg.352140164.
56. Pelage JP, Soyer P, Boudiaf M, et al. Carcinoid tumors of the abdomen: CT features. Abdom Imaging. 1999;24(3):240-5.
57. Adams S, Baum R, Rink T, Schumm-Drager PM, Usadel KH, Hor G. Limited value of fluorine-18 fluorodeoxyglucose positron emission tomography for the imaging of neuroendocrine tumors. Eur J Nucl Med. 1998;25:79-83.
58. Binderup T, Knigge U, Loft A, et al. Functional imaging of neuroendocrine tumors: a head-tohead comparison of somatostatin receptor scintigraphy, 123I-MIBG scintigraphy, and 18F-FDG PET. J Nucl Med. 2010;51:704-12.
59. Zalom ML, Waxman AD, Yu R, Lee J, Ih G, Wolin EM. Metabolic and receptor imaging in patients with neuroendocrine tumors: comparison of fludeoxyglucose-positron emission tomography and computed tomography with indium in 111 pentetreotide. Endocr Pract. 2009;15: 521-7.
60. Hong X, Choi H, Loyer EM, Benjamin RS, Trent JC, Charnsangavej C. Gastrointestinal stromal tumor: Role of CT in diagnosis and in response evaluation and surveillance after treatment with Imatinib. Radiographics. 2006;26:481-95.
61. Mazur MT, Clark HB. Gastric stromal tumors: reappraisal of histogenesis. Am J Surg Pathol. 1983;7:507-19.
62. Sripathi S, Rajagopal KV, Srivastava RK, Ayachit A. CT features, mimics and atypical presentations of gastrointestinal stromal tumor (GIST). The Indian Journal of Radiology and Imaging 2011;21.3:176-81.
63. The ESMO/European Sarcoma Network Working Group Gastrointestinal Stromal Tumors: ESMO Clinical Practice Guidelines Ann Oncol. 2014;25 (Suppl 3):iii21-iii26.
64. Levy D, Remotti HE, Thompson WM, Sobin LH, Miettinen M. Gastrointestinal stromal tumors: radiologic features with pathologic correlation. Radiographics. 2003;23(2): 283-304.
65. King DM. The radiology of gastrointestinal stromal tumors. Cancer imaging. 2005(5):150-6.
66. GJ, Badran M, Al-Muderis O, et al. Malignant gastrointestinal stromal tumor:distribution, imaging features and pattern of metastatic spread. Radiology. 2003;226:527-32.
67. Afifi AH, Ela AM, Albanna A. Feasibility of diffusion weighted MRI in evaluation of different small bowel pathology. Ejrnm. 2015;46:459-69.
68. Fletcher CD, Berman JJ, Corless C, et al. Diagnosis of gastrointestinal stromal tumors: a consensus approach. Int J Surg Pathol. 2002;10:81-9. [PubMed].
69. Choi H, Charnsangavej C, de Castro Faria S, et al. CT evaluation of the response of gastrointestinal stromal tumors after imatinib mesylate treatment: a quantitative analysis correlated with FDG PET findings. Am J Roentgenol. 2004;183:1619-28.
70. Schlemmer M, Sourbron SP, Schinwald N, Nikolaou K, Becker CR, Reiser MF, Berger F. Perfusion patterns of metastatic gastrointestinal stromal tumor lesions under specific molecular therapy. Eur J Radiol. 2011;77:312-8.
71. Lassau N, Lamuraglia M, Chami L, et al. Gastrointestinal stromal tumors treated with imatinib: monitoring response with contrast-enhanced sonography. Am J Roentgenol. 2006;187:1267-73.
72. Gollub MJ. Imaging of gastrointestinal lymphoma: Radiol Clin N Am. 2008;46:287-312.
73. Lewis RB, Mehrotra AK, Rodríguez P, Manning MA, Levine MS. From the radiologic pathology archives: gastrointestinal lymphoma: Radiologic and Pathologic Findings: Radiographics. 2014;34:1934-53.
74. Levine MS, Rubesin SE, Pantongrag-Brown L, Buck JL, Herlinger H. Non-Hodgkin's lymphoma of the gastrointestinal tract: radiographic findings. AJR. 1997;168(1):165-72.
75. Dawson I, Cornes J, Morson B. Primary malignant lymphoid tumors of the intestinal tract. Report of 37 cases with a study of factors influencing prognosis. Br J Surg. 1961;49:80-9.
76. Manning MA, Somwaru AS, Mehrotra AK, Levine MS. Gastrointestinal lymphoma: radiologic-pathologic correlation. Radiol Clin North Am. 2016:54(4):765-84.

77. Krol AD, le Cessie S, Snijder S, et al. Primary extranodal non-Hodgkin's lymphoma: the impact of alternative definitions tested in the comprehensive centre west population-based NHL registry. Ann Oncol. 2003;55(1):1-16.
78. Ghai S, Pattison J, Ghai S, O'Malley ME, Khalili K, Stephens S. Primary gastrointestinal lymphoma: spectrum of imaging findings with pathologic correlation. Radiographics. 2007;27:1371-88.
79. Cornes JS. Multiple lymphomatous polyposis of the gastrointestinal tract. Cancer. 1961;14:249-57.
80. Catassi C, Bearzi I, Holmes GKT. Association of celiac disease and intestinal lymphomas and other cancers. Gastroenterology. 2005;128:S79-86.
81. Lo Re G, Federica V, Midiri F, et al. Radiological features of gastrointestinal lymphoma. Gastroenterology Research and Practice. 2016;2016:2498143. doi:10.1155/2016/2498143.
82. Mayerhoefer ME, Karanikas G, Kletter K, Prosch H, Kiesewetter B, Skrabs C, et al. Evaluation of diffusion-weighted MRI for pretherapeutic assessment and staging of lymphoma: results of a prospective study in 140 Patients. Clin Cancer Res. 2014;20(11): 2984-93.
83. Ghimire P, Wu GY, Zhu L. Primary gastrointestinal lymphoma. World J Gastroenterol. 2011;17(6):697-707.
84. Allen-Auerbach M, de Vos S, Czernin J. The impact of fluorodeoxyglucose-positron emission tomography in primary staging and patient management in lymphoma patients. Radiol Clin N Am. 2008;46:199-211.
85. Schoder H, Noy A, Gonen M, et al. Intensity of 18 flurodeoxyglucose uptake in positron emission tomography distinguishes between indolent and aggressive non-Hodgkin's lymphoma. J Clin Oncol. 2005;23(21):4643-51.
86. Stecco A, Buemi F, Quagliozzi M, Lombardi M, Santagostino A, Saccheti GM, et al. Staging of primary abdominal lymphoma: comparison of whole-body MRI with diffusion-weighted imaging and 18F-FDG-PET/CT. Gastroenterology research and practice, vol. 2015, article ID 104794, 8 pages, 2015. doi:10.1155/2015/104794.
87. Musshoff K. [Clinical staging classification of non-Hodgkin's lymphomas] Strahlentherapie. 1977;153(4):218-21.
88. Rohatiner A, d'Amore F, Coiffier B, et al. Report on a workshop convened to discuss the pathological and staging classifications of gastrointestinal tract lymphomas. Ann Oncol. 1994;5(5)397-400.
89. Ruskone-Fourmestraux A, Dragosics B, Morgner A, et al. Paris staging system for primary gastrointestinal lymphomas. Gut. 2003:52(6)912-3.

CHAPTER 71

Colorectal Tumors

Naveen Kalra, Mandeep Kang, Mahesh Prakash

INTRODUCTION

Colorectal tumors can be broadly classified as epithelial lesions, which include adenoma and adenocarcinoma; and nonepithelial or mesenchymal lesions, which include lipoma, leiomyoma, gastrointestinal stromal tumor (GIST), leiomyosarcoma and Kaposi's sarcoma. Other tumors are lymphoma, metastases and non-neoplastic benign polyps like hyperplastic and hamartomatous polyps. In this chapter, all these lesions will be discussed with particular focus on colorectal cancer.

EPIDEMIOLOGY

Colorectal cancer is the third most common cancer overall in both men and women. It is also the second leading cause of cancer deaths following lung cancer.[1] In men, it is the third most common cancer after lung and prostate cancer; and in women, it is the third most common cancer after lung and breast cancer.[2] The prevalence of colon cancer varies throughout the globe. While the incidence is high in North America, Europe and New Zealand, it is low in South America, Africa and Asia.[3] The reported incidence of colon cancer from eight population registries in India is 0.7–3.7/100,000 in men; and 0.4–3/100,000 in women with a higher incidence of rectal cancer (1.6–5.5/100,000 in men, 0–2.8/100,000 in women).[4] Colon cancer is more common in economically affluent populations, who have Western lifestyle practices like high intake of dietary fat, low intake of dietary fiber and sedentary lifestyle.[5] Minority (5.4%) of colorectal cancers occur in patients younger than 40 years.[5] The incidence of colorectal cancer rises after the age of 40 years with 90% of these cancers occur in persons more than 50 years old.[6] The median age at the time of diagnosis of colon and rectal cancer has been reported to be 71 years and 69 years respectively. Approximately, one half of the colon cancers occur in the rectum and sigmoid colon and these can be seen with the flexible sigmoidoscope.[7] There has been an increase in the right-sided lesions as opposed to the left-sided lesions. Distal lesions are more commonly found in men than in women.

RISK FACTORS

There are several risk factors, which are associated with the development of colorectal cancer. Primarily, these include dietary factors, hereditary factors, inflammatory bowel disease and other miscellaneous causes.

High-calorie, low-fiber diet rich in animal fats, including beef consumption is an important risk factor for the colon carcinogenesis. Excess intake of fat results in an increase in the level of fatty acids and free bile acids in the feces. This irritates the colonic mucosa and epithelial reparative proliferation ensues.[8] High fiber intake decreases exposure to the carcinogens by decreasing the fecal transit time. It also results in decreased bacterial-mediated conversion of primary to secondary bile acids by lowering the pH of the stool.[9]

There is an inverse relationship between the intake of calcium and of antioxidants such as vitamins A, C, E, selenium and colon cancer.[10] On the other hand, there is a direct relationship between alcohol consumption, smoking, hypergastrinemia in pernicious anemia patients, increased growth hormone level in patients with acromegaly and increased parathyroid hormone in patients with parathyroid adenomas, and the incidence of colorectal cancer.

Prior cholecystectomy has been reported to increase the risk of developing right-sided colon cancer in women by 1.5 times.[11] This is due to the deposition of potential carcinogens like bile salts and neutral sterols in the proximal colon while the distal colon is spared on account of their absorption proximally into the enterohepatic circulation. Prior ureterosigmoidostomy following cystectomy is also a potential risk factor for the development of adenocarcinoma at the site of anastomosis.

Occupational and environmental risk factors include exposure to asbestos, oils, printing materials, halogens, metal fumes, organic solvents, paint and dyes.

Radiation-induced colorectal cancers arise in rectum and sigmoid colon of patients with carcinoma of cervix, bladder and prostate. The latent period for such cancers is longer than 10 years with 3000 rad threshold value.[12] 1.5–9% of patients with colorectal cancer have been found to have a second synchronous cancer[13] and 5–8% subsequently develop a metachronous cancer.[14,15] The time interval between initial and metachronous cancer varies but the majority arises within 5 to 7 years of the index cancer.

Hereditary factors have been a subject of interest for colorectal cancer. Heredity has been shown to play a role in 5–6% of all colorectal cancers.[3] Familial adenomatous polyposis (FAP) is an autosomal dominant syndrome and is the result of germline mutation of the adenomatous polyposis coli gene. If a prophylactic colectomy is not performed in a patient with FAP, colorectal cancer always develops in these patients. Turcot's syndrome is a variant of FAP and in these patients, the extracolonic lesion is a brain tumor such as medulloblastoma.

In juvenile polyposis coli, there is a high incidence of colorectal neoplasia (dysplasia and adenocarcinoma) found in up to 20% patients at a relatively younger age (37 years).[10] Screening should be performed periodically in patients with Cronkhite-Canada syndrome, in which there are multiple juvenile polyps throughout the gastrointestinal tract except the esopahgus. These can undergo adenomatous and carcinomatous degeneration.

Hereditary nonpolyposis colorectal cancer or Lynch syndrome accounts for 4–6% of all colorectal cancers. In Lynch syndrome I, colorectal cancer is inherited as an autosomal dominant susceptibility with more metachronous and synchronous lesions. In Lynch syndrome II, there is an increased incidence of adenocarcinoma of endometrium, ovary and other organs in addition to colorectal cancer. The precursor lesion in Lynch-related colon cancer is a discrete proximal colonic adenoma. Right-sided colon cancer occurring at young age is the hallmark of Lynch syndrome. Colon cancers associated with Lynch syndrome have a better prognosis than other colorectal cancer varieties.[10]

Colon cancer in ulcerative colitis is uncommon, occurs in patients with pancolitis and constitutes about 1% of colorectal cancers. Patients with left-sided disease are at less risk. The risk begins to increase after 7–10 years of colitis. Actual risk of developing colorectal cancer is 0.5–2% after the initial 10 years of disease, 6.6% after 26 years, 11.4% after 32 years. Disease activity as such does not increase the risk of long-term colorectal cancer and lack of activity does not have a protective effect. The mean age of presentation in these patients is 40–45 years.[10]

The risk of developing adenocarcinoma of large and small bowel has been estimated to be 4 to 20 times more than that of general population in Crohn's disease. Most cancers develop in inflamed segments and in segments having strictures and fistulae. Excluded colon and rectum as well as bypassed small bowel segments are at particular risk. Multifocal carcinomas may be seen and are discovered late as they cannot be distinguished from benign strictures.[10]

PATHOGENESIS

Most colorectal cancers arise in adenomatous polyps.[16] Adenomas more than 1 cm in size have a higher risk of malignant transformation. The transition from benign adenoma to cancer usually takes 7–10 years. This adenoma-carcinoma sequence suggests that colon cancer is preventable if polypoid lesions larger than 1 cm are found and removed. This stresses the importance of screening programs for colon cancer.

In patients with inflammatory bowel disease, carcinoma evolves through a sequence of inflammation, dysplasia followed by carcinoma.

The malignant potential of an adenomatous polyp has four major determinants. These include size, presence of a stalk, villous architecture and degree of cellular atypia and dysplasia. Polyps less than 5 mm have little or no risk of malignant transformation, those between 1 and 2 cm carry a 5% risk and those which are more than 2 cm carry a 50% risk of harboring malignancy.[10] Sessile polyps are at higher risk for malignancy (>50%) than pedunculated polyps. In case a pedunculated polyp turns malignant, the invasion of the colonic wall by the cancer is rare if the length of the stalk is more than 2 cm. Adenomatous polyps are of three types— tubular, villous and tubulovillous. Malignant transformation is more likely with villous adenomas than with tubular adenomas.[17] This is because villous adenomas are usually sessile and penetration of the muscularis mucosa is more likely in a sessile polyp. Polyps with a greater degree of cellular atypia and dysplasia are more likely to become malignant.

CLINICAL FEATURES

Colorectal cancer is a slow-growing tumor. Therefore, symptoms may be absent or minimal at initial presentation. Symptomatic colorectal cancers usually present with evidence of bleeding. This may be in the form of occult blood in the stool, passage of frank blood per rectum or development of iron deficiency anemia. The symptoms depend upon the size and location of the tumor. Right-sided colon cancers usually grow to a large size before symptoms develop. This is because the right colon is more capacious and the contents are relatively fluid in consistency. Anemia and disordered bowel function are earlier findings in right-sided colon cancer. On the other hand, sigmoid cancers present, early as sigmoid colon is the narrowest portion of the large bowel and the cancer results in the obstruction to the passage of solid fecal matter early. These patients present with colicky, crampy abdominal pain that is relieved by a bowel movement. Left-sided colon cancers usually present with per-rectal bleeding or intestinal obstruction.

A feeling of incomplete bowel evacuation, persistent constipation or diarrhea and change in stool caliber should arouse suspicion of colorectal carcinoma in patients older than 40 years. Weight loss and anemia are seen in 50% of patients with colorectal carcinoma.

Patients with colorectal carcinoma usually have a normal physical examination. Sometimes, there may be a palpable mass or signs of intestinal obstruction. Palpable supraclavicular nodes may be seen with left-sided colon cancer and hepatomegaly may be present due to metastases. Among the laboratory investigations measurement of carcinoembryonic antigen (CEA) levels is a useful test. CEA is an antigen shed from the surface of tumor cells. Although not specific, CEA is a sensitive marker for colorectal cancer. The levels of serum CEA correlate with cancer stage and tumor size. Elevated preoperative CEA level predicts shorter disease-free survival.

PATHOLOGY

The gross morphology of the colorectal adenocarcinoma is related to its location. Large, polypoidal bulky masses overgrowing their vascular supply are seen in the cecum and ascending colon. They may also undergo necrosis. Tumors in the transverse and descending colon are ulcerated and infiltrative and have a large intramural component. Thus they are more invasive in nature. Tumors in the more distal colon and rectum are also infiltrative and have an annular constricting or 'napkin-ring' appearance. These tumors are the most biologically aggressive. In patients with inflammatory bowel disease, colon cancers are scirrhous, plaque-like or finely nodular.[18]

Malignancies of the large bowel are predominantly adenocarcinoma. Mucinous/colloid carcinomas are seen in the setting of inflammatory bowel disease and hereditary non-polyposis-related carcinoma in early age. They constitute 10 to 15% of the cancers with large lakes of mucin in which there is a scattered collection of tumor cells with signet ring cells. As the mucin is secreted within the interstitium of the gut wall, it dissects the wall, helps in the extension of the malignancy and worsens the prognosis. Calcification may occur in these tumors. Tumors that arise at the anorectal junction include squamous cell carcinoma, transitional cell carcinoma, cloacogenic carcinoma and melanocarcinoma.[10] They comprise less than 5% of malignant large bowel tumors. Primary lymphomas, carcinoid tumors and leiomyosarcomas comprise less than 0.1% of all large bowel tumors.[19] In addition, lymphoma, leiomyosarcoma and cancers of the breast, ovaries, prostate, lung and stomach can metastasize to the colon.

ROUTE OF SPREAD

There are five methods of tumor spread after the tumor has become invasive:

1. *Direct extension*: Direct invasion may occur along the tissue layers which provide the path of least resistance. As peritoneum represents a relative barrier, direct spread to neighboring intra-peritoneal organs is rare. After invading the visceral peritoneum, the tumor can spread to stomach, greater omentum, spleen, small bowel, another portion of the colon, uterus, bladder, fallopian tubes and ovaries. Retroperitoneal tumor may involve kidneys, pancreas, ureters and posterior truncal musculature. Rectal carcinoma after breaching fascia of Waldeyer may invade sacral plexus, sacrum and coccyx.[20] It may also invade internal iliac vessels and obturator musculature posterolaterally, and prostate, seminal vesicles, bladder, vagina and cervix anteriorly after compromising the fascia of Denonvillier's.
2. *Lymphatic spread*: Lymphatic spread occurs after the invasion of muscularis through submucosal lymphatics. Intramural spread of colorectal malignancy occurs to submucosal, muscular and subserosal lymphatics.

The first sites of involvement are usually the epiploic and paracolic lymph nodes. The intermediate lymph nodes (along vascular branches) and principal lymph nodes (at origins of colonic blood vessels) generally show involvement later in the course of the disease. The prognosis worsens when multiple lymph nodes are involved.

3. *Hematogenous metastases*: There exists the potential for hematogenous metastasis if colorectal malignancy invades the rich capillary network of lamina propria. The most common route is through branches of portal vein. Thus liver is the most commonly involved organ. Distal rectum drains through tributaries of internal iliac vein, which finally drain into the inferior vena cava. Batson's vertebral venous plexus is another path of hematogenous spread. In 20–40% colorectal carcinoma patients, liver is the sole site of metastases. Metastases to the lung are seen in 20% of patients. In 4% of patients, the lungs are the sole site of metastases. Other sites are less common and include adrenal glands, bone, kidney, pancreas, spleen and central nervous system.
4. *Peritoneal seeding*: Intraperitoneal seeding may occur during operation because of breach in serosa. The anterior wall of rectosigmoid junction is the site of metastatic seedling. Eventually, both the parietal and visceral peritoneal surfaces will be involved leading to malignant ascities.
5. *Intraluminal implantation*: Intraluminal tumor spillage at surgery is a likely source of implantation metastases and anastomotic recurrence.[21] Anastomotic recurrences may also be due to incomplete tumor excision or a metachronous tumor.

STAGING

Staging of colorectal cancer has evolved over many years. In 1932, Dr Cuthbert E Dukes, a London-based pathologist, in a study of 215 patients with rectal cancers, found direct relationship between survival and depth of tumor penetration into the intestinal wall and lymph node metastasis.[22] The Astler and Coller modification of the Dukes classification is commonly employed to stage colonic neoplasm.

In this method, the staging is as follows:

A Tumor limited to the mucosa

B1 Tumor extending into, but not through, the muscularis propria

B2 Tumor penetrating the bowel wall, but without any lymph node involvement

C Tumor with regional lymph node involvement. This is divided into C1, in which the primary tumor is within the bowel wall and C2, in which the primary tumor has spread beyond the bowel wall.

Turnball introduced an additional staging category in 1967 as stage D further divided into stage D1, which included fixed cancers that had invaded adjacent organs and stage D2, in which distant metastases had occurred. Currently the American Joint Committee on Cancer (AJCC) and International Union against Cancer (UICC) have recommended staging by TNM classification.[23] Local tumor staging or T staging depends on the depth of tumor penetration into the bowel wall. The extent of mural invasion is important, as it has shown to influence prognosis independent of lymph node involvement.

Primary Tumor (T)

TX: Primary tumor cannot be assessed
T0: No evidence of primary tumor
Tis: Carcinoma in situ
T1: Tumor invades submucosa
T2: Tumor invades muscularis propria
T3: Tumor extending through the muscularis propria into subserosa or non-peritonealized pericolic or perirectal tissue
T4: Tumor directly invades other organs or structures (T4a) or perforates the visceral peritoneum (T4b).

Regional Lymph Node (N)

NX: Regional lymph nodes cannot be assessed
N0: No regional lymph node metastasis
N1: Metastasis in 1–3 pericolic or perirectal lymph nodes
N2: Metastasis in 4 or more pericolic or perirectal lymph nodes.

Distant Metastasis (M)

MX: Presence of distant metastasis cannot be assessed
M0: No distant metastasis
M1: Distant metastasis.

Stage Grouping

Stage 0	Tis	N0	M0
Stage I	T1	N0	M0
	T2	N0	M0
Stage II	T3	N0	M0
	T4	N0	M0
Stage IIIA	Any T	N1	M0
	Any T	N2	M0
Stage IV	Any T	Any N	M1

ROLE OF RADIOLOGY

Radiology plays an important role in screening for colorectal cancer. The purpose of doing imaging studies in patients with colorectal cancer is to provide the surgeon and the oncologist comprehensive and accurate assessment of the primary tumor, local and distant spread of the disease, synchronous lesions and to detect clinically occult complications. Radiology has a critical role after treatment of colorectal carcinoma in the detection of recurrent or residual disease, local and distant metastases and metachronous cancers.[24]

Screening for Colorectal Cancer

The American Cancer Society has recommended that one of the following five testing schedules should be adopted, beginning at 50 years of age:[25]

1. Yearly fecal occult blood test (FOBT) or fecal immunochemical test (FIT)
2. Flexible sigmoidoscopy every 5 years
3. Yearly FOBT or FIT, plus flexible sigmoidoscopy every 5 years
4. Double contrast barium enema every 5 years
5. Colonoscopy every 10 years.

Fecal occult blood test (FOBT) is the most widely available and least expensive screening test for colorectal cancer. Colorectal cancers bleed intermittently and the blood that is lost into the stool is broken down into hematin. Hematin reacts with guaiac and the commonly used hemoccult test is based on the guaiac reaction. False-positive reactions are caused by ingestion of meat, certain vegetables and aspirin. False-negative results occur as cancers only bleed intermittently. Moreover, it is thought that a polyp must be over 2 cm in size before it bleeds regularly. The sensitivity for detection of colon cancer is lower than 50% and nearly 90% of polyps are undetected by FOBT.[26]

Flexible sigmoidoscopy visually inspects the rectum and distal sigmoid colon. Therefore approximately only half of the colorectal cancers can be detected by flexible fibreoptic sigmoidoscopy alone. Though it is a safe and well-tolerated procedure and does not require sedation, it is relatively expensive and has the potential for transmission of disease by contaminated instruments.

Double-contrast barium enema (DCBE) is a widely available, inexpensive and simple test. However, in a study comparing DCBE to colonoscopy, it was found that the sensitivity of DCBE for polyps less than 0.5 cm was only 32%, for polyps 0.6 to 1 cm, was 53% and for polyps greater than 1 cm was 48%.[27]

Colonoscopy can directly visualize most colon cancers. The National Polyp Study and the Italian Mutlicenter Study showed reduction in the incidence of colorectal cancer among patients who had adenomas detected and subsequently removed on colonoscopy.[28,29] Colonoscopy is regarded as the gold standard for determining sensitivities of other examinations of the colon. However in a review of tandem or back-to-back colonoscopies, an average of 21% of adenomas were missed.[30] 26% of these adenomas were 1–5 mm and 2% of them were 10 mm or more in size. There are blind spots in the colon behind folds and around flexures. Colonoscopy also has the risk of perforation or hemorrhage in 1:500 examinations and a fatality rate of 1:5000 examinations. The completion rate of colonoscopy ranges from 55% to 95%.

Virtual colonoscopy is a novel noninvasive technique wherein a three-dimensional endoluminal image is generated after processing data acquired by multidetector helical CT using specialized computer software. In the American College of Radiology Imaging Network (ACRIN) study conducted at 15 study centers on 2600 asymptomatic participants, it was found that CT colonography has a 90% sensitivity and 86% specificity for detection of polyps measuring 10 mm or more in diameter.[31] Thus virtual colonoscopy performs well in detecting lesions larger than 1 cm which are actually clinically significant lesions. The entire colon is also evaluated by virtual colonoscopy. However, patients found to have significant lesions must undergo optical colonoscopy. The reported rate of complications with this technique is relatively small (0.08%).

Double-contrast barium enema and virtual colonoscopy will be discussed in detail in subsequent sections.

DIAGNOSTIC METHODS

Imaging modalities available are plain abdominal radiographs, barium enema, ultrasound including endoluminal and Doppler ultrasound, computed tomography/CT colonography, MRI/MR colonography and angiography.

Plain Radiographs

These are usually not very informative except for depicting complications of advanced colorectal malignancy like obstruction and perforation. Dilatation of colon and small bowel in cases of obstruction, thumb printing suggestive of ischemic colitis proximal to an obstructing lesion and free intra-peritoneal air in cases of perforation and pericolonic abscess formation may be detected on plain films. There may be a fistula with gallbladder or urinary bladder. Calcification of carcinomatous lesion or hepatic metastases may be evident. When advanced, bony invasion is easily diagnosed by identifying destruction of bone and presence of associated soft tissue mass. Lung metastases may also be seen on chest skiagram.

Barium Enema

The major advantage of barium enema is its ability to examine the entire colon. It is reasonably accurate, minimally invasive and requires no sedation. Complications related to the investigation are rare. DCBE has a 20% better sensitivity than single-contrast barium enema for detecting adenomatous polyps less than 1 cm in size.[32] However, this difference in the sensitivity of the two types of barium enema is not there when we consider the detection of colorectal carcinoma. The reported sensitivity of barium enema is in the range of 90–95% for the detection of significant (1 cm) size polyps and cancer.[33] The most important prerequisite for an accurate radiological examination is thorough bowel preparation with selection of an appropriate technique, strict quality control during the study and careful interpretation of the radiographs. The most effective regimen is combination of dietary manipulation, oral catheters and cleansing enema. About 10–40% of colonic carcinomas can be missed on initial barium enemas due to poor colon preparation.[34,35] Presence of fecal matter can mimic or mask polyps and cancers and account for the most common reason for false-positive findings on barium enema. The single contrast barium enema is simpler in concept than the double contrast study, but requires meticulous technique. The selection of the type of barium enema to be performed depends on the indication for the examination, sensitivity for detecting specific diseases and the age and physical condition of the patient.

The DCBE gives better information of mucosa with better detection of smaller lesions. It is the ideal technique in patients who are older than 40 years, who have a personal or family history of colonic polyps, cancer or inflammatory bowel disease, and a positive FOBT. Other indications are patients with previous ovarian, breast or cervical carcinoma and with prior pelvic irradiation.

Single-contrast barium enema is simpler and does not require rigorous maneuvers. Therefore, it is indicated in patients who are more than 70 years old, debilitated or uncooperative patients and in those patients where barium study is indicated for exclusion of obstruction or diverticulitis. Young patients with low likelihood of colon disease may also be candidates for single contrast study. Manual or mechanical compression of the colon during fluoroscopy and spot radiographs of the various segments are critical in detecting small polypoid lesions. Technique protocols should be followed, the adequacy of colon cleansing assessed, careful fluoroscopy performed, poor quality films repeated and additional films of questionable lesions should be obtained when needed.

Meticulous interpretation of the barium enema films is needed to avoid diagnostic errors due to presence of stool, air bubbles and diverticulae, or confusion of normal anatomic structures for an abnormality. False-negative errors are caused by perceptive lapses, technical problems, interpretive mistakes, or a combination of these factors. Perceptive errors can be reduced by close scrutiny, second review or retrospective review of the films especially for diagnosing colonic polyps and sigmoid colon malignancies. Accuracy of DCBE for evaluation of colorectal polyps is dependent on the location of the lesion and the size of the colonic polyps. As stated earlier, the sensitivity of DCBE is poor for polyps under 5 mm, improving for polyps 5–9 mm and is best for diagnosing polyps over 1 cm.

Complications of barium enema are uncommon. The rates of perforation for barium enema are documented at 1:25,00 to 1:12,500 and for mortality at 1:50,000.[36,37] Subsequent to a biopsy performed through a rigid scope, enema should be deferred for 2 weeks due to risk of perforation. Enema need not be postponed if biopsy is performed through a flexible sigmoidscope or colonoscope as the depth of biopsy does not extend beyond the muscularis mucosa. Recent endoscopic polypectomy precludes enema for 2–3 weeks. Barium and latex sensitivity, barium impaction, transient bacteremia, dehydration and inadvertent placement of the enema tip into vaginal vault are other complications which may also be encountered. Despite the risk of transient bacteremia, there is presently no recommendation to give prophylactic antibiotics.

Colorectal malignancies have a broad spectrum of morphological appearances on imaging. The mucosal surface can be seen en face, either in the barium pool or in air contrast. The normal mucosal surface is smooth. An abnormal mucosal surface may have a granular, finely nodular or ulcerated surface. Early carcinoma is usually seen as a sessile polypoid mass. The radiologic detection of early carcinoma is primarily an exercise in the detection of small polyps. There are two common types of colonic polyps, hyperplastic and adenomatous. Hyperplastic polyps have no malignant potential. Small polypoidal carcinomas may have a smooth outline and be radiographically indistinguishable from benign tumors **(Figs. 1 and 2)**. Barium

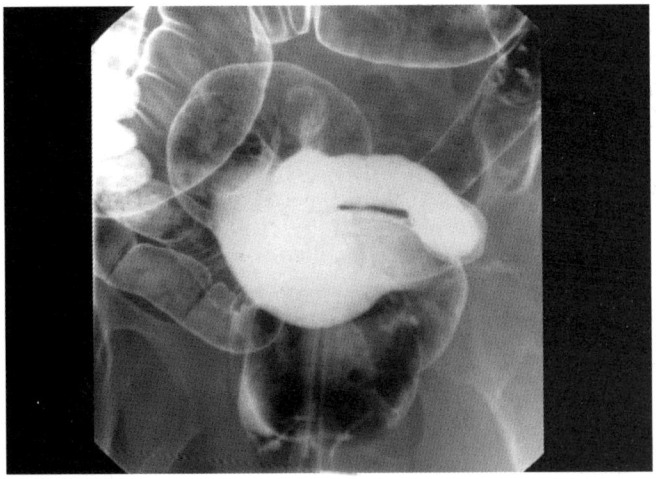

Fig. 1: Double-contrast barium enema DCBE shows a solitary, small, smooth polypoid lesion in the sigmoid colon which was malignant on histopathology.

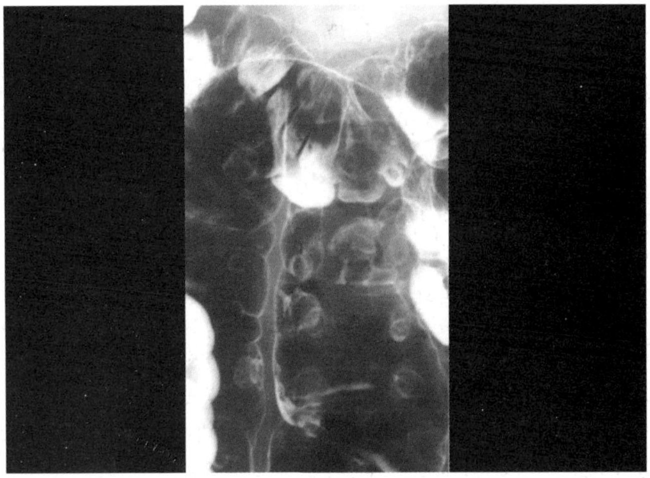

Fig. 2: DCBE in a patient with familial adenomatous polyposis showing multiple polyps in the colon.

enema cannot determine accurately, whether polypoid lesions in the size range of 0.5–3 cm are benign or malignant. Whenever, possible polyps more than 1 cm in size are found, they must be removed by colonoscopic polypectomy followed by histological examination.

Pedunculated polyps are best demonstrated on erect or lateral decubitus views of the colon. Those arising from the nondependent wall of the colon give the appearance of 'Mexican hat' sign,[38] where the central ring represents the stalk and the outer ring represents the head of polyps. In these cases, a change in position of patients shows the stalk in profile and confirms the diagnosis.

Sessile polyps may vary in appearance from a small, smooth polypoidal lesion to a bulky, lobulated mass forming acute angles with the adjacent colonic wall. When viewed en face, they appear as filling defects in the thin barium pool if they arise from dependent wall and etched in white if present on the nondependent surface. However, they may be missed if too much of high-density barium is present in the lumen, obscuring the lesion. When viewed in oblique projections, sessile polyps manifest as 'Bowler hat' sign,[39] with the dome representing the head of polyps and brim representing base of the polyp. Although the 'Bowler hat' sign can be produced by a diverticulum, the direction of the dome helps to distinguish a polyp from a diverticulum. When the dome points away from the axis of the bowel, the lesion is a diverticulum; and when it points towards the lumen of the bowel, it is a polyp.

Certain criteria have been described to assess the risk of malignancy of polyps based on their imaging features which include sessile versus pedunculated appearance, size of the polyp, number of polyps, basal indentation and surface contour. 1 cm is the threshold size for increased cancer risk of a polyp. In case of pedunculated polyps a stalk length >2 cm is not associated with malignant invasion into the adjacent wall. Smooth basal indentation is related to geometric factors and can be present in both benign and malignant lesions. Presence of basal irregularity is most predictive of malignant lesion when it is broad and irregular in larger polyps. The smooth surface contour is unreliable in distinguishing benign from malignant polyps. Lesions that have an irregular, 'soap bubbly' surface generally have villous elements and are likely to have malignant degeneration in at least 50% of lesions.[40,41] The majority of colonic adenomas are tubular adenomas. They have varying degrees of villous change which increases as the polyp increases in size. At the other end of the spectrum are villous adenomas which have a frond-like surface. There may be a transition from tubular adenoma to tubulovillous adenoma to villous adenoma. The risk of malignancy is related to the proportion of villous change in an adenoma. As the barium gets caught in the frond-like protrusions which go hand in hand with the villous change, the surface of the polyp assumes a 'soap bubbly' or a 'lacy' pattern. The term 'carpet lesion' has also been used to describe a flat lobulated lesion that manifests due to an alteration in surface texture of the bowel. These are again tubular adenomas with varying degrees of villous change.

Once a polyp is detected, there is a 3.5% risk of synchronous cancer and a 20% chance of an additional polyp.[42] Therefore, the remainder of the colon should be examined meticulously.

Advanced colorectal cancers have various morphological types. These include polypoidal, annular, scirrhous and flat lesions. The polypoidal lesions protrude into the lumen and have an irregular outline **(Figs. 3A to D)**. They may cause bowel obstruction or intussusception. Annular cancers are short in length with abrupt transition between normal and tumor mucosa **(Figs. 4 and 5)**. The mucosa is destroyed and there may be heaped up edges or ulceration. A focal area of spasm may cause confusion on DCBE but the mucosal folds remain intact within the area of the spasm. The differential diagnosis of annular colonic narrowing includes adhesions, inflammation, diverticulitis, endometriosis, radiation changes, metastatic disease and primary adenocarcinoma. Semiannular or 'saddle' tumor involves only a portion of the wall and results in asymmetry of bowel lumen. En face, these tumors produce overlapping lines with an abnormal orientation on double-contrast studies. Scirrhous tumor causes marked mural thickening and smooth strictures with submucosal and muscular invasion. Flat lesions are uncommon and usually occur in patients with long-standing ulcerative colitis. They can just result in abnormal lines on DCBE.

Problem Areas in Barium Studies

- *Distal rectum*: The catheter tip in the rectum can itself obscure plaque like or polypoidal lesions. Large internal hemorrhoids may mimic carcinoma, which appear on DCBE as thickened lobulated folds extending 3 cm or less from the anal verge or as cluster of small submucosal nodules in the rectum. However, low-lying rectal cancers that spread through the submucosa mimic hemorrhoids, but asymmetry of lesion and extent of rectal involvement suggests the diagnosis.

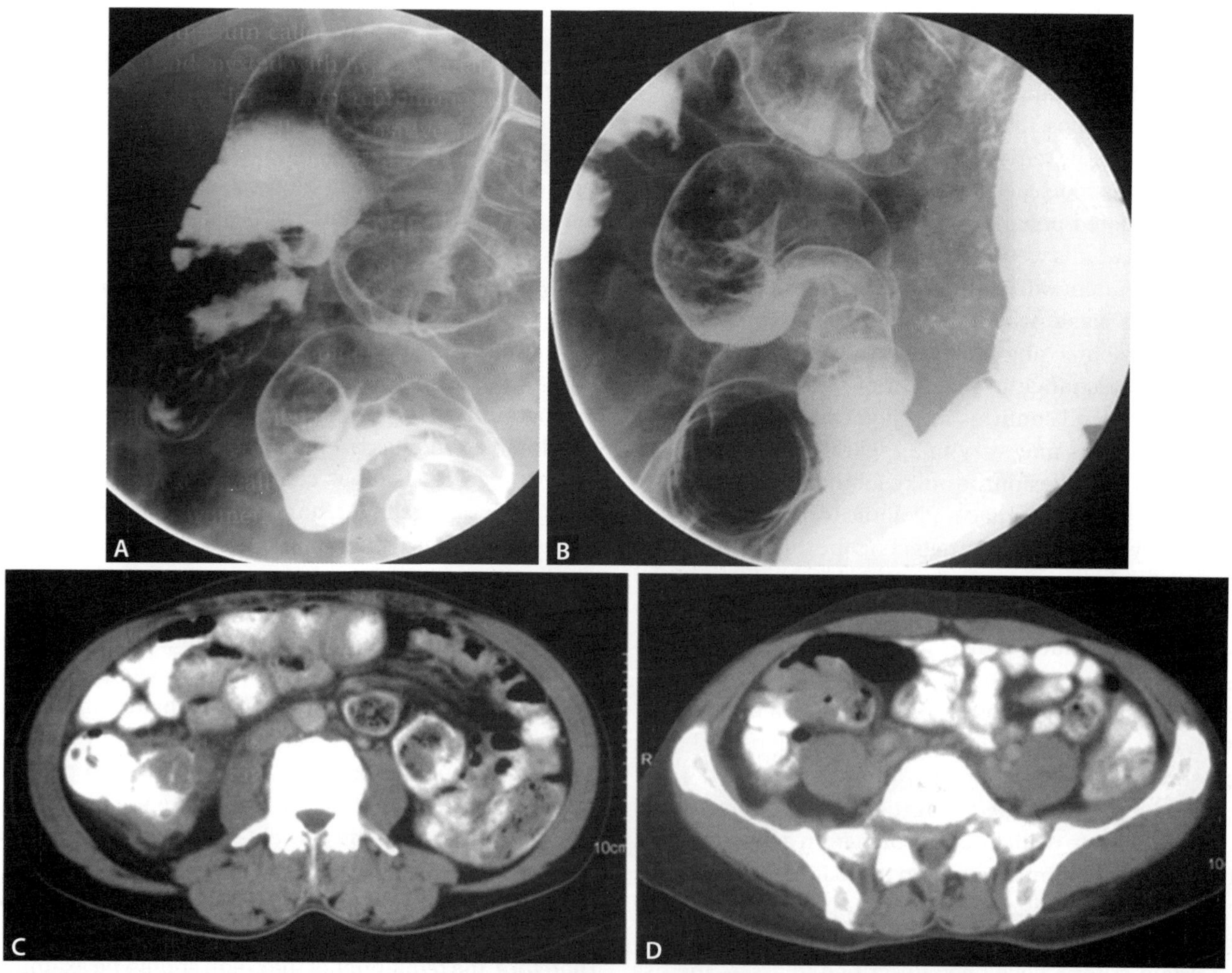

Figs. 3A to D: DCBE showing synchronous cancers in the ascending colon (A) and sigmoid colon (B). There is a short segment stricture in the ascending colon with a polypoidal component protruding into the colon. The sigmoid colon also shows a segment of narrowing. Axial CECT sections in the same patient showing circumferential mural thickening with a polypoidal component in the ascending colon (C). A similar lesion is also seen in the sigmoid colon with presence of ulcerations (D).

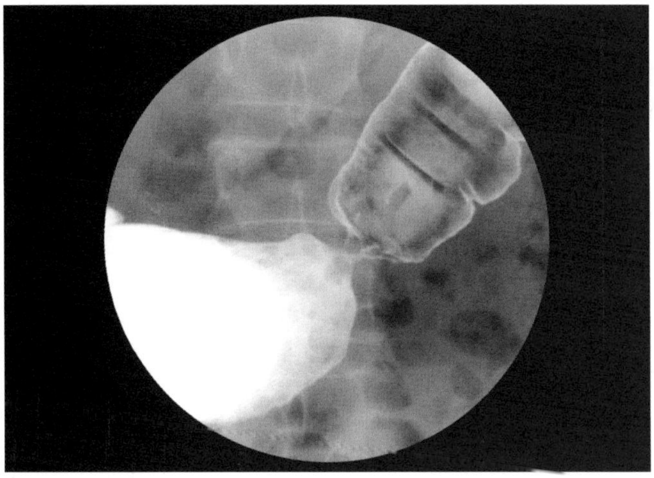

Fig. 4: DCBE showing a short annular stricture in the transverse colon with mucosal irregularity in a patient with colon cancer.

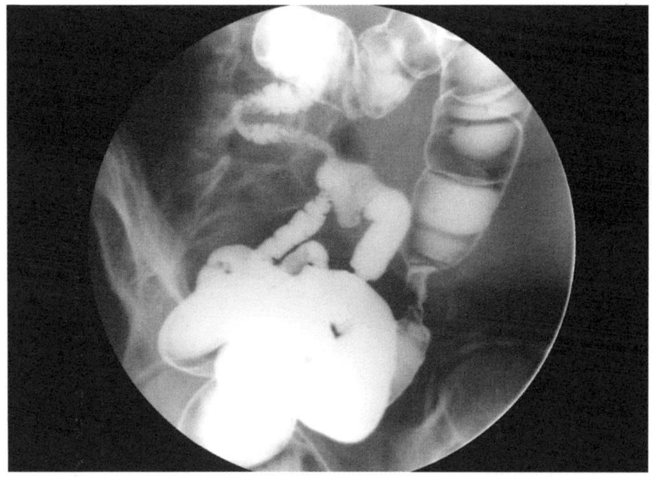

Fig. 5: Barium enema showing a stricture with mucosal irregularity in the descending colon in a patient with metachronous cancer. The patient had previous history of right hemicolectomy and ileo-transverse anastomosis for carcinoma of ascending colon.
Courtesy: Professor B Nagi, Department of Gastroenterology, PGIMER, Chandigarh, India.

- *Ileocecal valve*: Tumors arising in this area have subtle findings which include widening, splaying, straightening or asymmetric lobulation of the valve. These may be missed on initial observation.
- The presence of diverticulosis may obscure lesions. In patients who have equivocal lesions in the sigmoid colon, a 'sigmoid flush' may be performed at the end by introducing a small amount of low-density barium into the rectum to demonstrate polypoidal lesions as filling defects in the thin barium pool.[43] Common errors in barium interpretation can be due to:
  - Failure to detect small filling defects in a pool of barium.
  - Insufficient distension or overdistension.
  - Incomplete cleansing prior to the study.
  - Poor adherence of barium resulting in poor mucosal coating.
  - Failure to detect a synchronous lesion in presence of one lesion. Satisfaction or distraction by finding one lesion may result in overlooking a synchronous lesion.
  - Lesions may be obscured by haustral folds or overlying bowel loops.
  - Perceptive errors, because of extraneous material such as feces, anatomic variation such as redundant bowel loops or presence of diverticulae.

As most colorectal carcinomas are slow-growing, it is assumed that if a carcinoma is found within 3 years of a previous normal barium enema study, the tumor was missed on the previous examination.[33,44,45]

Ultrasound

The appearance of bowel on ultrasound depends not only upon the structures of the individual segment but more importantly upon its content and degree of distension. The bowel may be collapsed, containing only a small amount of mucus (the mucus pattern), or may contain fluid or gas. The mucus pattern is the classical target appearance. Large bowel tends to produce a more complex pattern, because it contains small amount of fluid and gas even in the fasting state. Sometimes, the colonic contents are reflective with distal shadows due to suspended fecal material. In case of colorectal malignancy, bowel wall thickening may be visualized by ultrasound resulting in a target or 'pseudokidney' configuration **(Figs. 6A to C)**. Normal bowel wall thickness in the non-distended state is 5 mm, reducing to about 3 mm when bowel is distended. When the bowel wall is thickened, the mucus pattern changes to a thickened, sometimes irregular 'halo' of bowel wall, with highly reflective irregular center giving a 'pseudokidney' sign.[45] This sign is nonspecific but strongly suggests bowel pathology. The site of the involved bowel must be inferred from the position of the lesion in the abdomen. In inflammatory processes of bowel wall the multiple layers are retained with a large segment of involvement. However, in neoplastic process a short segment involvement with obliteration of bowel wall layers is seen. The exception is lymphoma in which the wall layers are preserved. The diagnostic accuracy of transabdominal ultrasound is improved by retrograde instillation of fluid into the colon. This procedure known as sono-colonography, enables an accurate evaluation of the colonic lumen, colonic wall and also of the surrounding connective tissue. According to a study done by Bernd[46]

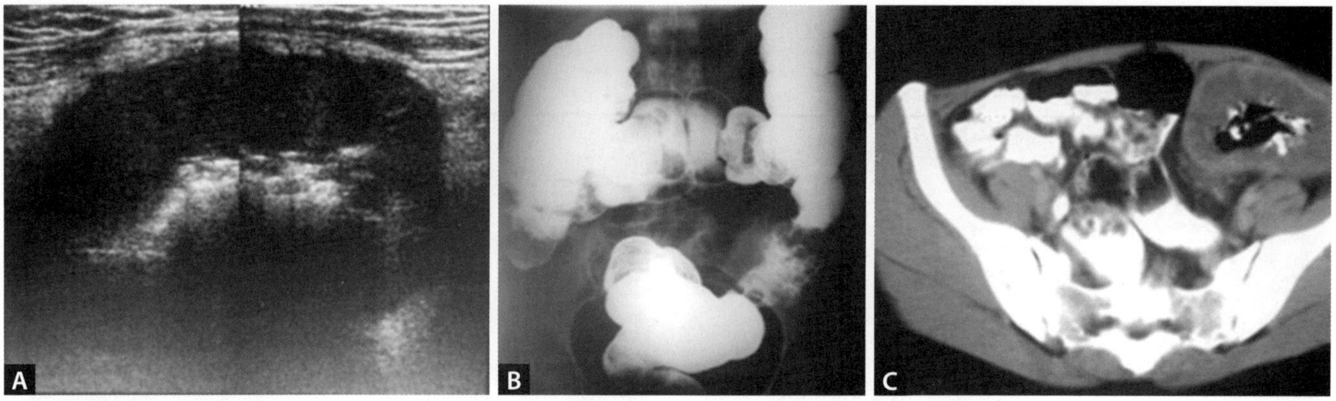

Figs. 6A to C: (A) Ultrasound of the lump in the left iliac fossa shows thickened bowel wall with highly reflective center consistent with 'pseudokidney sign; (B) Barium enema in the same patient shows a mass-like lesion with deep ulcerations in the region of descending colon; (C) Axial CECT section shows concentric mural thickening with ulcerations in the same segment.

the sensitivity of the technique in the detection of colonic carcinomas was 94% and the specificity was 100%. Ultrasound (US) screening of abdomen helps to find out liver metastasis and retroperitoneal lymphadenopathy. Fine needle aspiration and core biopsy is also possible using US guidance. It is particularly valuable in patients where confirmatory studies are either technically difficult or the findings are nonspecific.

Endorectal ultrasound (ERU): Evaluation of rectum with an endosonic probe was first done by Wilde and Reed in 1956.[45] The procedure is performed with an endorectally placed, rotating, high frequency transducer. If possible, the transducer should be passed proximal to the visualized tumor for complete assessment of mural involvement. The five layers of the rectal wall can be demonstrated as layers of alternating echogenicity with high-frequency transducers allowing an assessment of the depth of invasion of rectal tumors. The innermost ring is hyperechoic and represents the interface of the probe and the mucosa. The second ring is hypoechoic and is due to the muscularis mucosa. The third ring is hyperechoic and represents the submucosa. The fourth ring is again hypoechoic and is formed by the muscularis propria. The fifth ring is hyperechoic and is due to the perirectal fat or in areas of peritoneal reflection by the serosa and fat. Rectal carcinoma is seen as a hypoechoic mass with irregular borders interrupting the normal five-layer wall pattern. The accuracy of ERU in staging of colorectal carcinoma varies from 64% to 93%. Most of the errors are due to overestimates of the depth of invasion possibly as a result of co-existing inflammation. Tumor confined to the muscularis mucosa can be differentiated from tumor extending into the perirectal fat with invasion of adjacent structures and metastatic involvement of the perirectal lymph nodes **(Figs. 7A and B)**.

ERU may also help in differentiating benign villous adenomas from those with focal areas of invasive carcinoma. Glaser et al.[47] reported that benign villous adenoma appears hyperechoic and areas of invasive carcinoma appear hypoechoic. The presence of invasive carcinoma within a villous adenoma is determined by the involvement of the muscularis propria.[48] ERU can detect perirectal lymph nodes as small as 5 mm in size cannot be used to predict nodal involvement by malignancy. In fact, studies evaluating nodal metastasis based on the size of the lymph nodes have shown rather low accuracy rates. Nodal echo texture and morphology are the most often used criteria. Nodes which have sharply demarcated borders and an inhomogeneous hypoechoic pattern are more likely to be malignant unlike nodes with indistinct borders and a hyperechoic pattern. Limitation of ERU is in evaluating lymph nodes outside mesorectal fascia, lateral lymph nodes, distant metastasis, stenosing rectal carcinomas and tumors near the anal verge, which are difficult to visualize and may be missed. Other limitations of ERU include the inability to assess depth of penetration beyond the colonic wall as well as possible overestimation of tumor size in patients with extensive peritumoral inflammation or with preoperative radiation. Failure of the technique occurs in up to 15% of all rectal carcinomas.[45]

Transrectal US can distinguish three stages of disease based on TNM classification:

1. T1 tumor confined to mucosa and submucosa which does not interrupt the middle echogenic ring.
2. T2 tumor confined to rectal wall in which the outermost echogenic interface is intact.

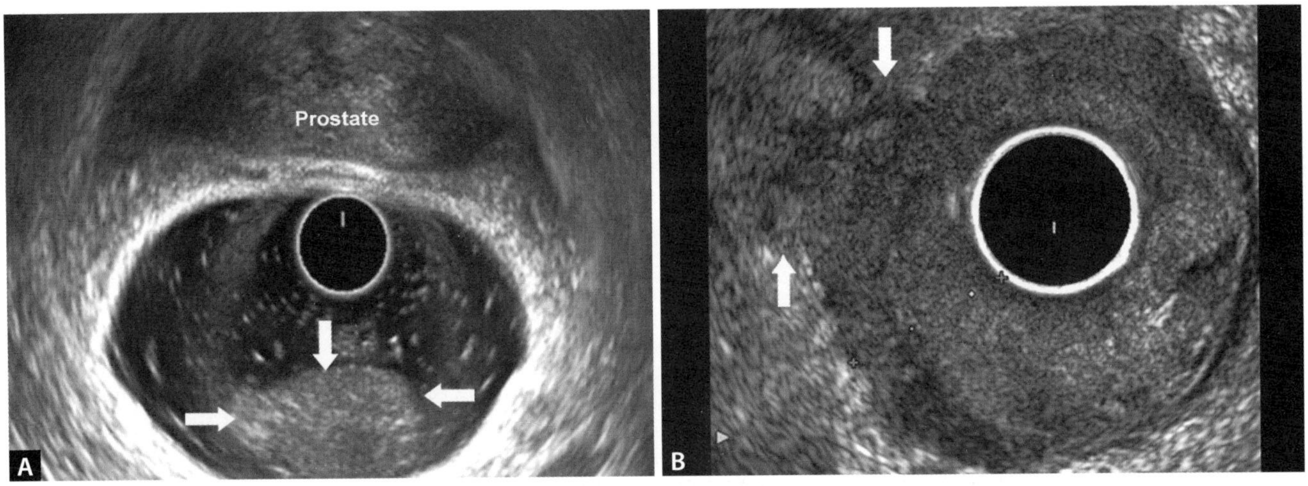

Figs. 7A and B: (A) EUS with radial echoendoscope shows polypoidal lesion (white arrows) with muscularis propria seen intact all around suggestive of T1 lesion; (B) EUS with radial echoendoscope shows involvement of all layers of rectum with infiltration of serosa and adjacent perirectal tissue (arrows) suggestive of T4 lesion.
Courtesy: Dr Surinder Rana, Department of Gastroenterology, PGIMER, Chandigarh, India.

3. T3 tumor which penetrates the perirectal fat and leads to disruption of outermost echogenic ring.

Doppler US may complement the US imaging by showing increased color flow, increased diastolic flow within tumor with low resistance waveform, as tumor vessels lack smooth muscle layer, thus offering little resistance **(Figs. 8A to E)**. A cut-off value of peak systolic velocity (PSV) greater than 25 cm/s is used to differentiate T3 and T4 tumors from T1 and T2 tumors and a PSV of more than 20 cm/s in lymph nodes is classified as malignant.

Computed Tomography

The primary aim of computerized tomography in imaging colorectal carcinoma is for preoperative staging, in assessing the postoperative complications and for the detection of tumor recurrence. It is estimated that up to 25% of patients with colorectal cancer have metastates at the time of diagnosis.[49] Therefore, staging technique should include both the primary colorectal neoplasm and sites of potential metastases.

Barium studies and colonoscopy/sigmoidoscopy provide excellent visualization of the mucosa. However, they cannot determine the depth of mural invasion by the tumor or the extent of metastatic involvement. Preoperative staging helps to assess tumor extent accurately to individualize therapy, assess risk of disease recurrence, and determine prognosis. CT and MRI have become the primary means for radiologic staging of colorectal carcinoma because of their ability to demonstrate the extent of wall invasion, extraluminal tumor spread, lymph node and distant metastasis. Complications of primary colonic malignancies such as obstruction, perforation and fistula formation can also be readily visualized with CT.

The accuracy of CT for colonic evaluation can be improved with several additional techniques including adequate cleansing of colon, administration of IV smooth muscle relaxants, distension of the colon with either air, carbon dioxide (CT colonography) or water and by having thin sections through the areas of tumor **(Fig. 9)**. A rectal enema may be given to delineate the descending colon and rectosigmoid region.

The normal wall thickening in a well-distended colonic segment is 3 mm, 3–6 mm is considered indeterminate, measurement greater than 6 mm is considered abnormal. Both the mucosal margin and outer colonic margin should be smooth and delineated by air/water-soluble contrast or pericolonic fat respectively. The rectum, rectosigmoid region, ascending and descending segments of the colon are relatively fixed structures and were, therefore, easily evaluated by conventional CT. Tumors in the flexures and transverse colon were less readily examined by conventional CT because bowel peristalsis and excursion of the diaphragm made these parts more difficult to evaluate. This has been overcome by the advent of fast helical CT scanners.

The primary bowel tumor is identified on CT as focal or circumferential wall thickening (>6 mm) with contour distortion or more frequently as a discrete mass. Occasionally, an intraluminal polypoid mass without wall thickening is seen. CT cannot depict the various layers of the bowel wall and cannot distinguish T1 from T2 stage.

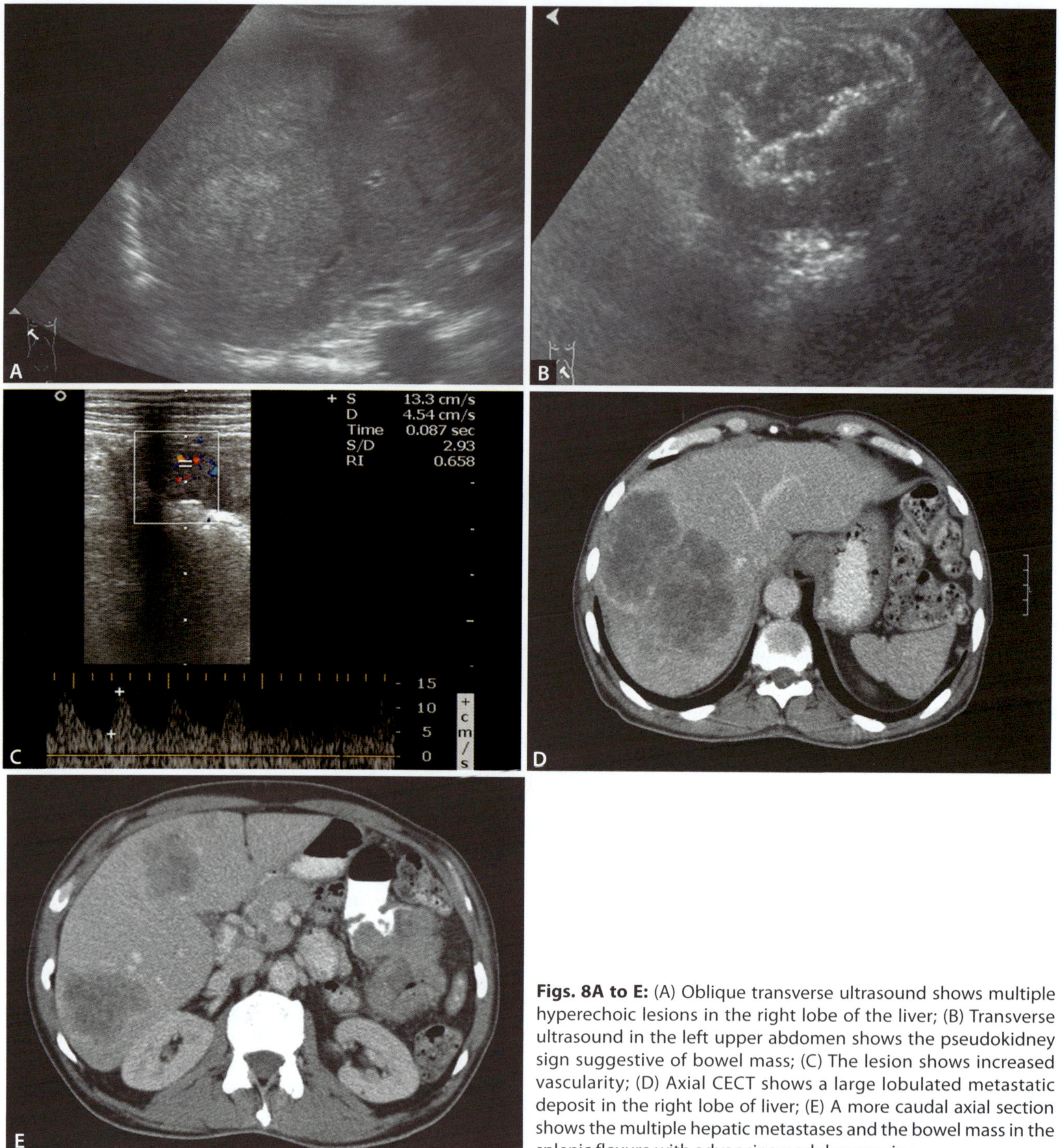

Figs. 8A to E: (A) Oblique transverse ultrasound shows multiple hyperechoic lesions in the right lobe of the liver; (B) Transverse ultrasound in the left upper abdomen shows the pseudokidney sign suggestive of bowel mass; (C) The lesion shows increased vascularity; (D) Axial CECT shows a large lobulated metastatic deposit in the right lobe of liver; (E) A more caudal axial section shows the multiple hepatic metastases and the bowel mass in the splenic flexure with advancing nodular margins.

Sometimes, contrast-enhanced CT scan with rectal contrast can demonstrate a typical 'napkin ring' lesion of annular contricting malignancy and plaque-like lesion. Large masses may undergo central necrosis and appear as a soft tissue mass with central low attenuation. Mucinous primary adenocarcinoma may rarely contain calcification, however, this occurs more often in hepatic metastasis than in the primary tumor. Rectal and sigmoid cancers may appear as asymmetric nodular wall thickening that narrows the lumen. This appearance may mimic diverticulitis, especially if the tumor involvement of the wall has resulted in infiltration of the pericolic fat. However, presence of fluid

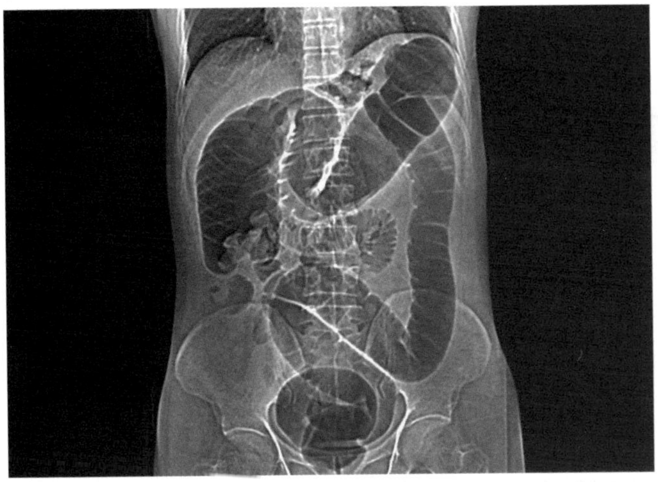

Fig. 9: Tomogram obtained before acquiring data for CT colonography shows the polypoidal mass lesion in the cecum. The rest of the colon is well distended with air.

in the root of the sigmoid mesentery and engorgement of adjacent sigmoid mesenteric vasculature favors the diagnosis of diverticulitis and presence of pericolic lymph nodes raises the suspicion of colon cancer. Pericolic lymph node adjacent to a segment of thickened colonic wall are seen much more frequently in cases of colon cancer than with diverticulitis. Thickening can occasionally appear symmetric and involve the entire circumference of the bowel wall. In such cases, it is difficult to differentiate malignant from benign causes of wall thickening, including inflammation and mural edema.

The pericolonic and perirectal fat appear uniformly hypodense without soft tissue stranding on CT. Thickening of the perirectal fascia produces the 'halo sign' which can be seen with extension of tumor into perirectal fat. Invasion beyond the bowel wall should be suspected whenever a focal mass deforms the contour of the outer colonic wall with an advancing nodular margin with or without pericolonic soft tissue stranding **(Figs. 10 and 11)**. Extracolonic tumor spread is also suggested by the loss of fat planes between the large bowel and the surrounding muscles like levator ani, obturator internus, piriform, coccygeus and gluteus. Unfortunately, the loss of fat plane is a nonspecific sign in cross-sectional imaging and can also be seen with cachexia and lymphatic or vascular congestion, this interpretation must be made with caution.[50] However, invasion is definite when a tumor mass is seen to extend directly into the adjacent muscle with obliteration of fat planes with enlargement of the individual muscle. Occasionally an enhancing intramuscular mass is seen.

Spread to contiguous organs in the pelvis should also be interpreted with caution and diagnosed only if a major portion of the viscera is enveloped or if an obvious mass involves an adjacent organ **(Figs. 12A and B)**. Primary or recurrent colonic cancers can invade the small and large bowel, the seminal vesicles, sciatic nerve, prostate, bladder, uterus and ovaries and also cause hydronephrosis by obstructing the ureters. Fistula between tumor and adjoining viscera such as bladder can be demonstrated by either direct visualization of fistulous tract on CECT or demonstration of air within the bladder. Fistulation into uterovaginal areas, ischiorectal fossa and small bowel can occur. Colonic cancers can destroy the adjacent bone. Minor invasion of bone can present as cortical destruction. In advanced cases, soft tissue mass with destruction of bones of sacrum, coccyx and ilium can be seen.

Regional lymph nodes are the most common metastatic site of colorectal carcinoma. CT cannot distinguish benign from malignant lymphadenopathy. Metastatic foci may be found in normal-sized lymph nodes (<1 cm). Likewise reactive inflammatory lymph nodes are frequently larger than 1 cm resulting in false-positive assessment of nodal disease. Only lymphangiography or guided biopsy can give a definite diagnosis. Any nonenhancing mass in the perirectal fat should be considered to be malignant lymphadenopathy irrespective of the size as hyperplastic lymph nodes do not occur in this region.

Sites of distant metastasis generally include the liver, lung, adrenals, peritoneum, kidneys and bone marrow. The liver is the most common site of extranodal metastasis. On noncontrast CT scans, hepatic metastases are typically discrete, hypodense lesions of variable size, although foci of calcification can be seen within metastatic mucinous adenocarcinoma. Following a bolus IV injection of iodinated contrast, deposits often show early peripheral enhancement or become uniformly hyperdense, go through an isodense phase and finally show washout of contrast. Scanning early in the dynamic phase to maximize liver-lesion contrast is critical to increase the lesion conspicuity.

Peritoneal carcinomatosis which is the result of spread of tumor over peritoneal surface, is usually well demonstrated by CT and appears as enhancing linear or nodular peritoneal thickening and is associated with ascites. In patients with disseminated disease, careful analysis of chest CT may reveal metastatic nodules. In women with an advanced stage of colon carcinoma, masses in the ovaries may be detected (Krukenberg's tumor).

CT scan is quite accurate in staging patients with advanced disease. Pitfalls occur in interpretation of

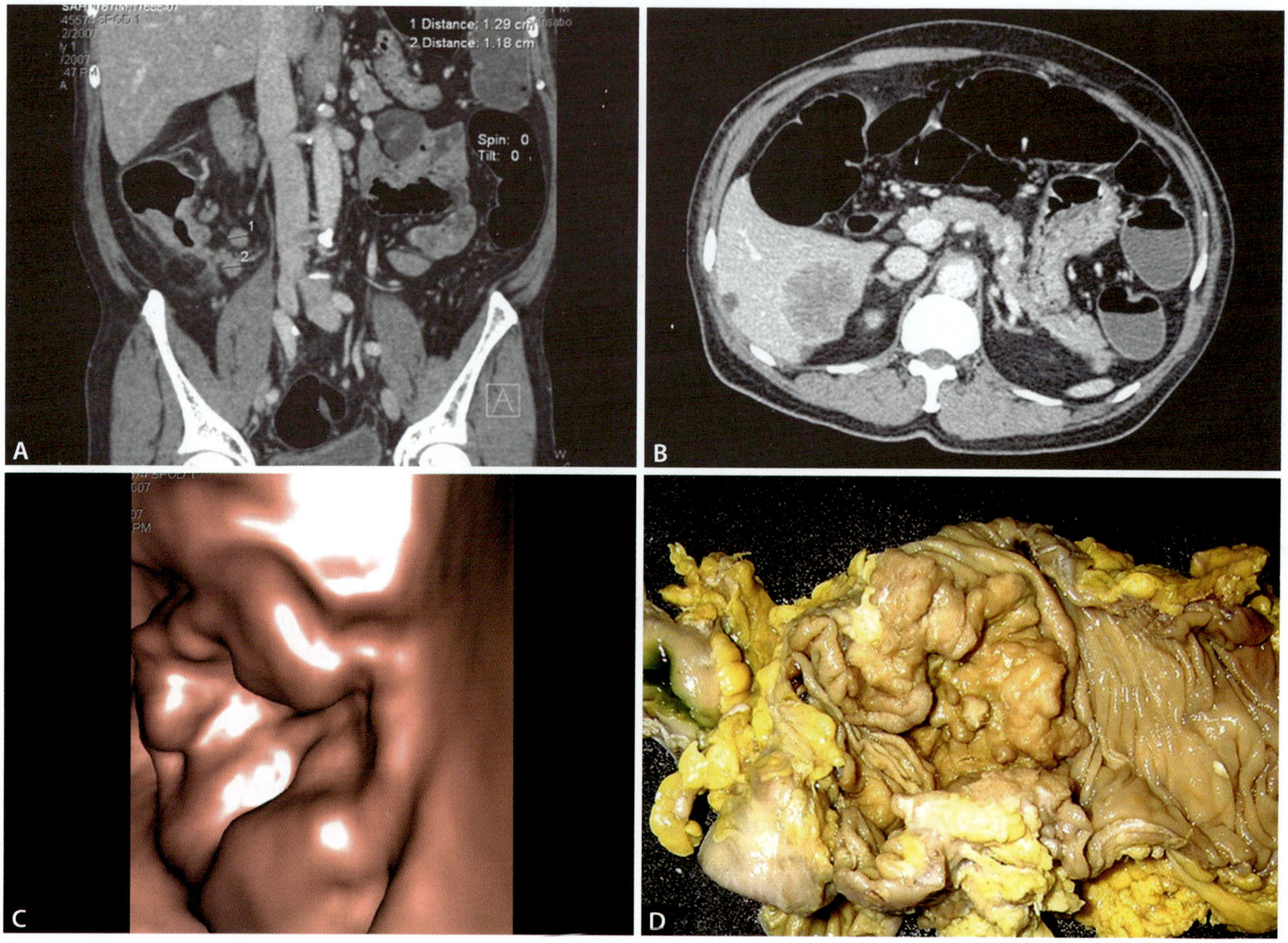

Figs. 10A to D: (A) Coronal MPR image shows concentric mural thickening with a polypoidal component in the cecum. Pericolonic stranding and multiple enlarged pericolonic lymph nodes are also seen; (B) Axial CECT section of the upper abdomen shows hypodense lesions in segment VI of liver suggestive of metastases; (C) CT colonoscopy endoluminal image shows the intraluminal irregular polypoidal growth; (D) Gross photograph of the ulceroproliferative growth involving the cecum which appears to be infiltrating up to the serosal fat.
Courtesy: Professor JD Wig, Department of General Surgery, PGIMER, Chandigarh, India.

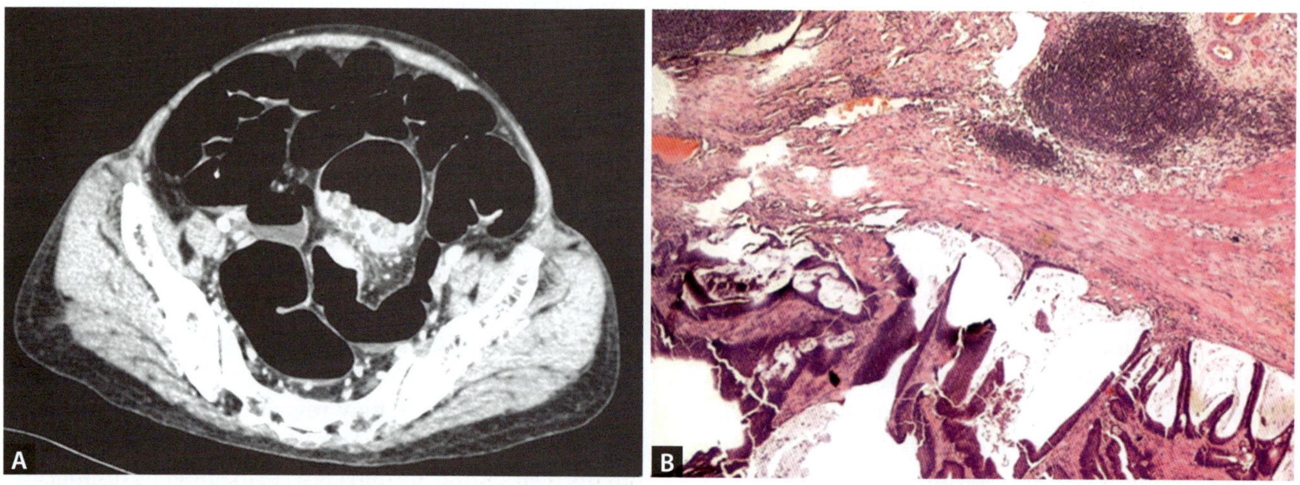

Figs. 11A and B: (A) CE-CTC image shows heterogeneously enhancing rectosigmoid growth with pericolonic stranding, CT Stage: T3; (B) Representative microphotograph of this T3 tumor showing infiltration through the muscularis propria into the subserosa consistent with stage T3. (H & E, × 250).
Courtesy: Professor K Vaiphei, Department of Histopathology, PGIMER, Chandigarh, India.

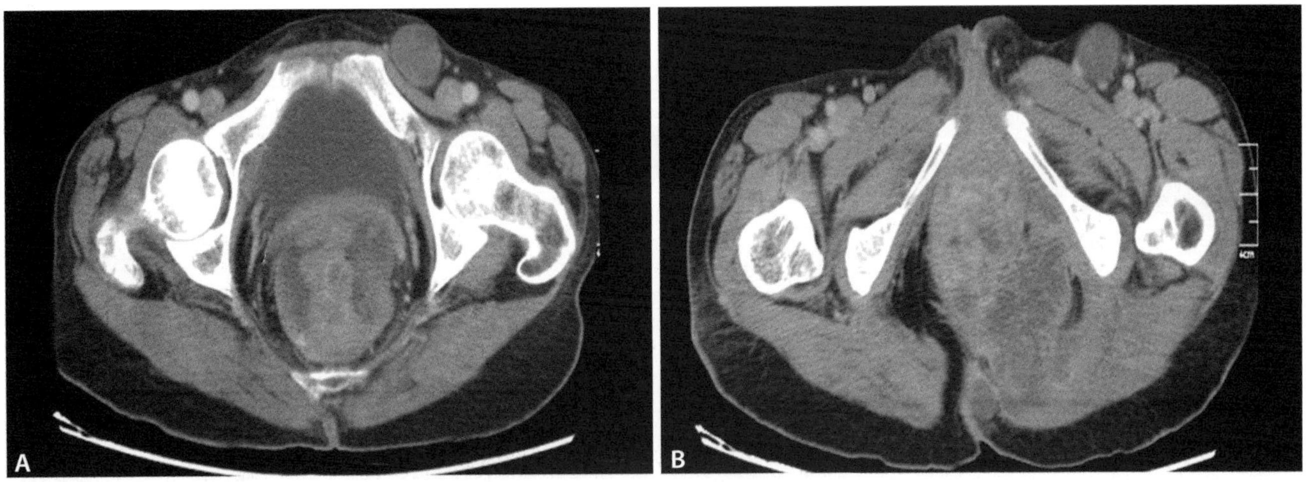

Figs. 12A and B: Axial CECT sections show a large heterogeneous mass in the rectum obliterating the lumen. The planes of the mass with the vagina, lateral pelvic wall and gluteal muscles on the left side are lost consistently with invasion. A large left inguinal lymph node is also seen.

scans in patients with less advanced tumors. Perforation/ulceration of colonic cancer can result in an inflammatory mass or abscess which obscures the underlying cancer. CT scan obtained after surgery or radiation therapy can demonstrate edema or hemorrhage of the pelvic structures simulating residual/recurrent disease.

CT staging is based on the combination of numerous findings like thickness of the colon wall, presence or absence of tumor spread to adjacent organs and presence or absence of metastases. Earlier studies have shown low accuracy (41–64%) for staging with conventional CT owing to low sensitivity of local tumor extent (53–77%) and of lymph node metastases (22–73%).[51] Recent studies have shown MDCT to be very useful in preoperative staging for colon cancer with accuracy of 4-slice CT being 83% for T-staging and 85% for N-staging.[52,53] In a study conducted at our Institute which was presented at the World Cancer Congress of UICC in 2008, the diagnostic accuracy for T-staging was 92.3% and for N-staging was 42.3%.[54] The lower specificity for lymph node metastases accounted for the lower accuracy of N-staging in this study **(Figs. 13A to D)**.

Computed Tomography Colonography

Computed tomography colonography (CTC) is an innovative technique that entails CT examination of the entire colon and computerized processing of the raw data acquired after colon cleansing and colonic distension. It was in 1994 that Vining and Gelfand from Bowman Gray University introduced CT colonography and exhibited the first CT colonography fly-through video at the annual meeting of the Society of Gastrointestinal Radiologists.[55]

The accepted indications for CT colonography are as follows:

- Incomplete colonoscopy due to an occlusive mass or stricture preventing examination of the proximal colon.
- Incomplete colonoscopy due to colonic tortuosity, adhesions, severe diverticular disease or patient intolerance of colonoscopy.
- Inability to perform colonoscopy due to requirement for anticoagulant therapy or risks of sedation.
- Patients who adamantly refuse to undergo colonoscopy but have a strong indication for diagnostic colonoscopy.

CT colonography is under analysis as a screening tool for colorectal cancer as it is relatively safe and has greater patient acceptance as compared with other available screening methods.

The contraindication for CT colonography are allergy to contrast, suspected colonic perforation, acute colonic infection (acute diverticulitis, severe infective colitis), acute lower GI bleeding, complete colonic obstruction, very recent colonic surgery (<1 week), medically unstable patients and refusal to undergo colonic preparation.

The technique involves colonic cleansing, colonic distension, image acquisition and post-processing of acquired data. For 'wet preparation' polyethylene glycol is used; while for 'dry preparation,' phospho-soda is used. Adequate colonic distension is critical for increasing polyp conspicuity. This can be achieved by using room air or carbon dioxide. Colonic perforation is rarely seen (0.59–0.08%).[56] Advanced age and underlying colonic pathology are the risk factors for colonic perforation. Air can be administered easily, is available at no cost but is

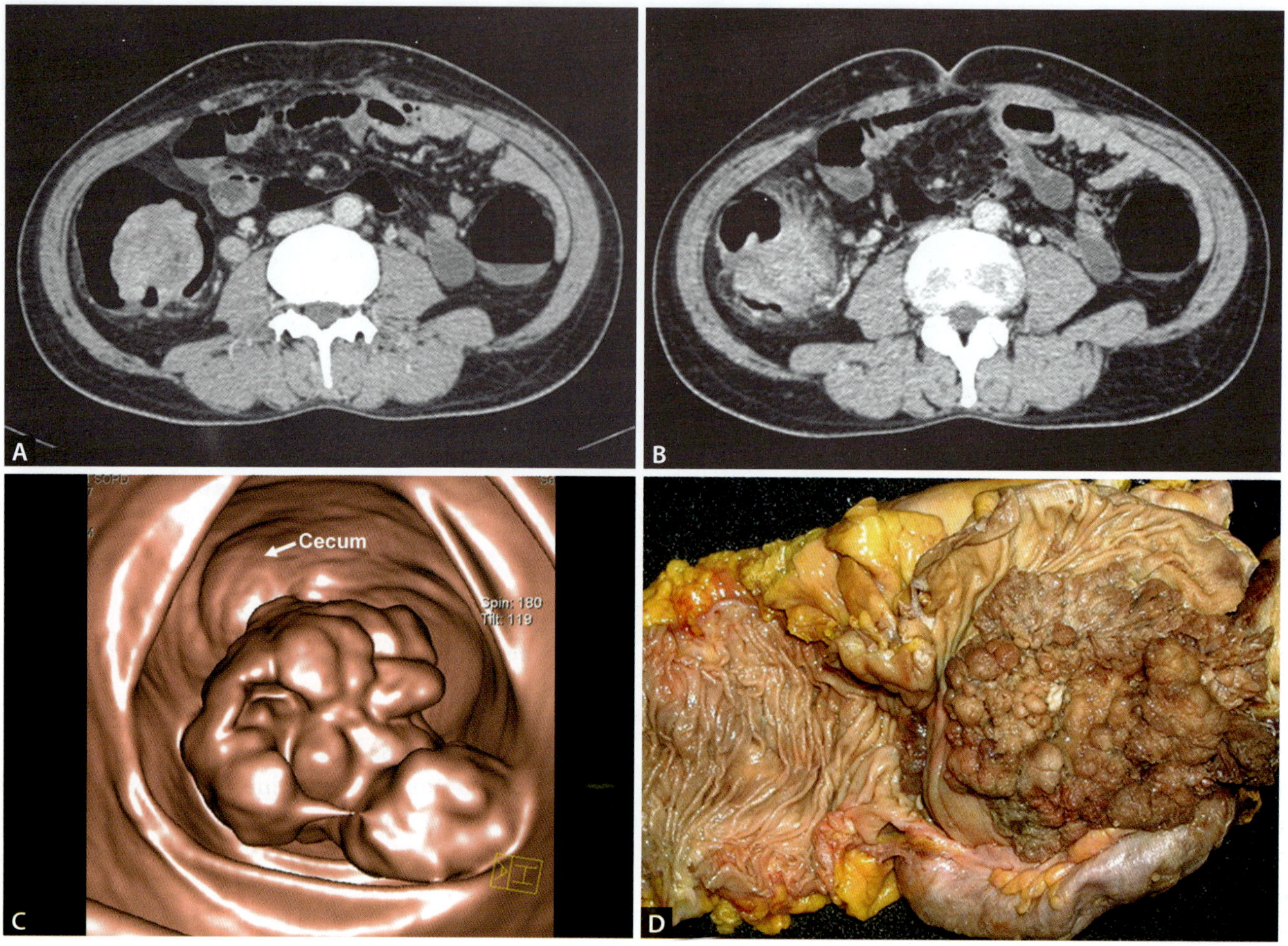

Figs. 13A to D: (A and B) Axial CE-CTC images show presence of polypoidal cecal growth with classical pericolonic stranding and lymph nodes—CT Stage: T3N2M0. Surgical Stage: T3N2M0. Histological stage: T3N0M0; (C) CT colonographic image of the same patient showing a polypoidal intraluminal cecal mass; (D) Gross photograph showing a proliferative tumor almost completely filling up the cecal lumen. *Courtesy:* Professor JD Wig, Department of General Surgery, PGIMER, Chandigarh, India.

less well tolerated than carbon dioxide as it is not absorbed by the colonic mucosa. Carbon dioxide, on the other hand, is gradually absorbed by the colonic wall, resulting in diminished discomfort to the patient **(Fig. 14)**. Image acquisition is done after colonic insufflation in supine and prone positions on a helical CT scanner using low-dose technique. The radiation dose is about half of the dose of a barium enema.[56] Intravenous contrast improves detection of medium-sized polyps (6–9 mm) especially in a suboptimally prepared colon.[57] After acquiring supine and prone scans, various software packages are used to display images in both 2D and 3D (endoluminal) views.

There are various mimickers of polyps which are potential pitfalls of CT colonography. These include adherent fecal matter, lipomas, inverted appendiceal stump, prominent ileocecal valve, inverted diverticulum

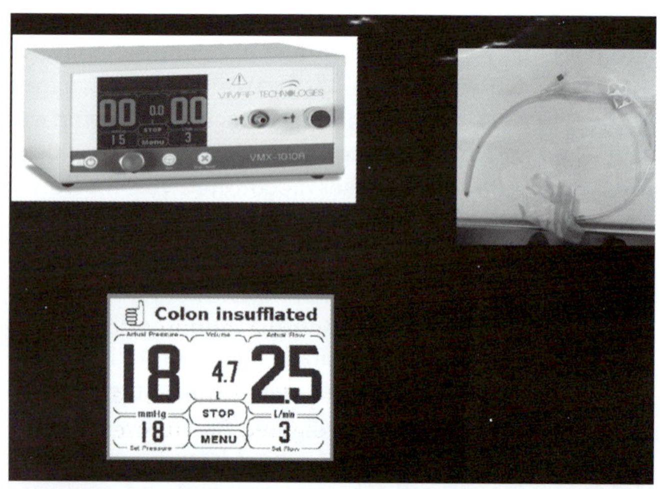

Fig. 14: CO_2 insufflation pump, insufflation tube catheter and the final message on the pump when the colon is completely insufflated.

and bulbous colonic folds. While some of these are due to technical errors on account of inadequate colon preparation or distension, others are due to perceptive errors.

In the first published study from India the sensitivity and specificity of CT colonography have been reported to be 65% and 77% respectively for lesions 1–5 mm; 97% and 83% respectively for lesions 6–9 mm; and 100% and 100% respectively for lesions 10 mm or larger.[58] CT colonography scores over optical colonoscopy as it provides information about extracolonic findings. The incidence of significant extracolonic findings ranges from 6.8% to 21%.[56] A reporting system for CT colonography has been devised by the Working Group on Virtual Colonoscopy and has been termed 'C-RADS' or CT colonography reporting and data system.[59] The aim of this reporting system is to achieve standardization of reporting. The advances in CT colonography include fluid and fecal tagging to achieve 'prepless' studies by digital bowel cleansing using subtraction techniques. Computer-aided detection (CAD) software and novel 3D views that slice open and flatten the colonic wall are being developed.

Magnetic Resonance Imaging

Magnetic resonance imaging (MRI) can be used to detect and stage rectosigmoid tumors more accurately than tumors in the rest of the colon. This increased accuracy is due to the fixed position of the rectosigmoid colon in relation to the pelvis. Many refinements have been described including MRI using an endorectal coil, addition of IV gadolinium chelate and the use of oral and rectal contrast agents to achieve bowel distension. High-performance gradient, faster pulse sequences, and high-resolution MRI are now routinely available, producing additional improvement in MRI quality.

Presently, MRI using thin sections and phased-array coils can distinguish tumors localized to mucosa and submucosa (T1) and those that infiltrate the entire colonic wall (T2) with a reasonable accuracy (65–85%).[60] Detection of tumor improves if proper colon cleansing and adequate distension can be obtained with administration of air, water or supraparamagnetic contrast medium. Imaging in prone position helps to decrease motion artifacts with better depiction of rectal tumors.

The different layers comprising the bowel wall on gadolinium-enhanced T1-weighted fat-suppressed spin echo images are the high-signal intensity mucosa, low-signal intensity muscularis mucosa and lamina propria, high-signal intensity submucosa and low-signal intensity muscularis propria.

In T1W SE images, rectosigmoid tumors are seen as wall thickening with signal intensity similar to or higher than skeletal muscles (long T1). Perirectal fat has short T1 and hence appears bright on T1WI and rectal air has no signal, thus these tumors are very well delineated on T1W images and their extension beyond the colonic wall is well visualized. If polyps or tumor contain a large amount of mucin, signal intensity can be higher on T1WI.

Gadolinium enhancement makes lesions more conspicuous **(Figs. 15A to C)**. On gadolinium-enhanced spoiled gradient-echo (SGE) MR images with oral and rectal contrast, the lesion is depicted as an enhancing soft tissue mass or as mural thickening.

On T2W images, the lesion is hyperintense to the muscle, but as fat is also hyperintense, contrast between the tumor and perirectal fat is not adequate and hence T2W images are not as useful as T1W images for diagnosing extracolonic extension. T2W images provide good contrast between tumor tissue and surrounding pelvic wall muscles as tumor is hyperintense and muscle hypointense on T2WI.

Studies have shown that T2WI is superior to T1WI for evaluating the extent of tumor in relation to the rectal wall layers and the mesorectal fascia.[61,62] T2WI can demonstrate the mesorectal fascia better than T1WI. This has assumed importance since the introduction of total mesorectal excision (TME) for rectal cancer. In this, the entire mesorectal compartment is removed, which includes rectum, surrounding mesorectal fat with the perirectal lymph nodes and a thin fascia that envelopes the two former structures and is known as mesorectal fascia. The recurrence rate of cancer after TME is reported to be less than 10%.[63] MRI technique and image quality play a prominent role in T-staging and accuracy is dependent on obtaining high-resolution images (0.5 cm voxel size) perpendicular to the plane of the tumor.

For evaluation of cancers involving the anal sphincter, images in the coronal plane are particularly useful. Routine MR imaging cannot recognize tumor foci in normal-sized lymph nodes. A T1W SE sequence with fat suppression, readily demonstrates lymph nodes. Depicting tumor in normal-sized lymph nodes may require the use of additional contrast agent directed at imaging nodal metastasis. Invasion of adjacent organs is best seen on transverse or coronal MR images. Neither CT nor MRI can detect microinvasion.

Liver and adrenal metastases are as well demonstrated on MR as on helical CT. All extrahepatic anatomic sites must be evaluated carefully to assess for possible metastatic tumor. Peritoneal carcinomatosis is difficult to detect on

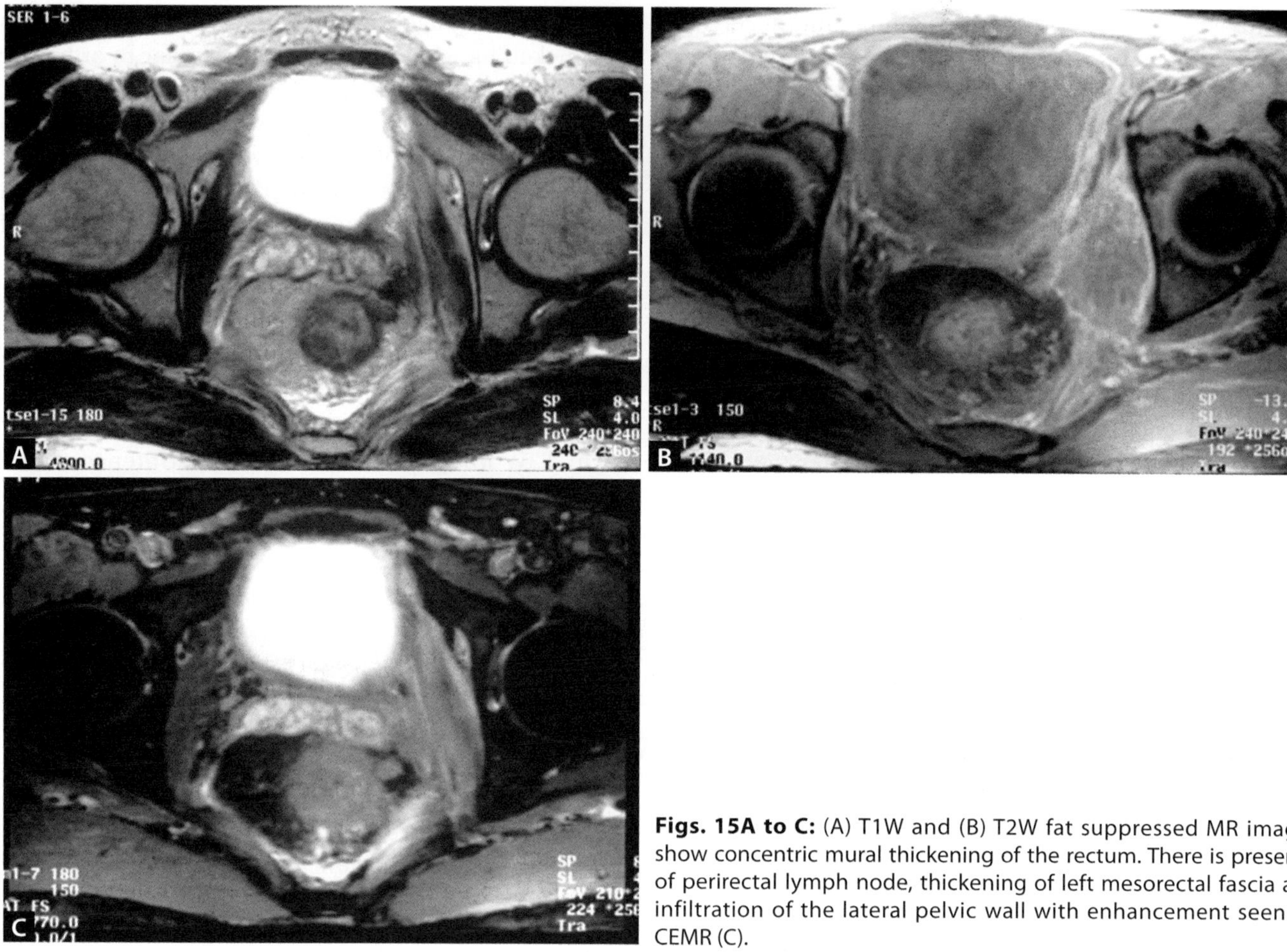

Figs. 15A to C: (A) T1W and (B) T2W fat suppressed MR images show concentric mural thickening of the rectum. There is presence of perirectal lymph node, thickening of left mesorectal fascia and infiltration of the lateral pelvic wall with enhancement seen on CEMR (C).

MR images. Fat-suppressed, gadolinium-enhanced SGE MR images are most useful for extrahepatic imaging. Peritoneal deposits enhance slowly with gadolinium and are most conspicuous on delayed images obtained after 5 minutes delay. Surface implants on the liver may be detected by T2 WI without IV contrast material. The ability of MRI to depict subtle osseous metastases is an advantage compared with helical CT. MR imaging is superior to CT at distinguishing between fibrosis and recurrent cancer and could eliminate the need for biopsies.

More advanced MR technique includes the use of an endorectal surface coil which has the potential to allow differentiation of the bowel wall layers and thus permits more accurate 'T'-stage determination. Comparison of endorectal MR (ERMRI), ERUS and 3D-ERUS have shown an overall similar accuracy for depicting the transmural extent of the rectal cancer, 91%, 84% and 88% respectively.[64] In a comparison of ERUS, ERMRI and CT in rectal cancer, Kim et al.[65] have shown comparable accuracies of 81% for both ERUS and ERMRI for depth of tumor penetration which was superior to CT (65%).

Endorectal MRI does have some limitations. This technique cannot be performed in patients with severely stenotic infiltrating lesions. It is a rigid device with a small radial area of acceptable signal to noise imaging. It cannot adequately assess the mesorectal fascia and the circumferential resection margin (CRM).

Magnetic Resonance Colonography

Magnetic resonance (MR) colonography is based on the acquisition of MR datasets of the abdomen which optimizes visualization of the large bowel. Data is acquired during single breath-hold scans. The bowel is distended per rectally with water, barium, room air or CO_2. Spasmolytics are given intravenously before rectal filling. Patient preparation involves use of cathartics and enemas. 2D and/or 3D fast imaging with steady-state precession (FISP) is a useful sequence for MR colonography. 3D TIW images are also acquired before and after administration of gadolinium intravenously. A T1W 2D FLASH (fast low-angle shot) sequence is also acquired in the axial plane for evaluation of adjacent abdominal organs. Axial, MPR and 'fly through' images are analyzed in both antegrade and retrograde directions. MR colonography has been reported to have 100% sensitivity for lesions larger than 10 mm and 89% for lesions 5–10 mm in size.[66] However, it has very limited accuracy for detecting lesions smaller than 5 mm.

The advantage of MR colonography over CT colonography is lack of ionizing radiation and superior soft tissue contrast. The disadvantages are lower spatial resolution, high susceptibility to motion artifacts, longer examination time and limited availability.

Arteriography

Arteriography has a limited value in colonic cancers. Its application is restricted to the investigation of patients with acute bleeding of apparent colonic origin with therapeutic embolization. The bleeding site may be demonstrated in patients with chronic low-grade blood loss. Arteriography with chemoembolization or radiofrequency ablation is also used for treating metastatic liver deposits in patients with colonic malignancies, who are not surgical candidates.

Immunoscintigraphy

Labeled anticarcinoembryonic antigen (CEA) monoclonal antibodies (MoAbs) have been used as *in-vivo* tumor localizing agents. Primary adenocarcinoma of colon and metastatic foci are seen as areas of increased radioactivity (hot spots). Depending on the size of tumor necrosis, liver metastases may appear as areas of intense, absent or intermediate uptake. The reported sensitivity of monoclonal antibody staging of colorectal cancer is 65–86% with specificity for detection of primary tumor, local recurrence and distant metastasis varying from 77% to 92%.[67]

Positron Emission Tomography

Fluorine 18-labeled deoxyglucose (^{18}FDG) is used, and there is a remarkably close correlation between tumor grade and glucose utilization. This method can be used for detection of distant, residual or recurrent disease **(Figs. 16 and 17)**. Malignant tissue demonstrates more rapid uptake with accumulation compared with normal tissue. Time activity curves of glucose utilization are generated for region of interest and pathologic areas are compared with surrounding normal tissue by generating a differential absorption ratio. Limitations of PET are decreased sensitivity in detecting colon lesion ≤10 mm in diameter and decreased tracer uptake by mucinous tumors. Nonspecific PET findings can result in negative impact on patient care in up to 9% patients.[68]

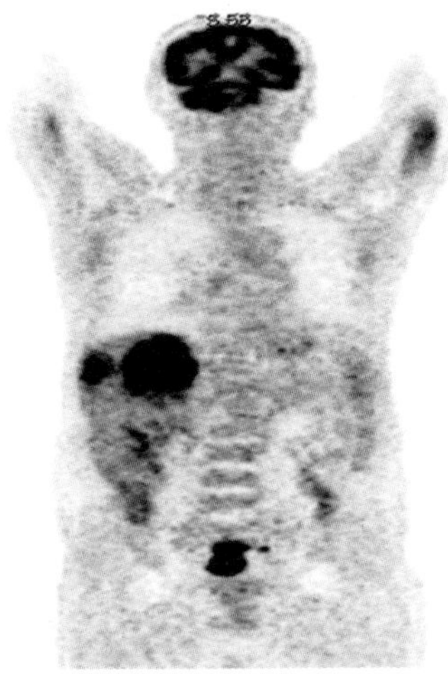

Fig. 16: Coronal PET image showing tracer avid rectal cancer with locoregional lymph node and liver metastases.
Courtesy: Professor BR Mittal, Department of Nuclear Medicine, PGIMER, Chandigarh, India.

RECENT ADVANCES

These include PET/CT colonography and CT perfusion imaging for colorectal tumors. PET/CT colonography involves the combination of 18F-FDG PET with CT colonography. It provides both anatomic and functional information. It has been used both for staging of colon cancer and for screening purposes.[69,70] The standard uptake value of malignant tumors has been reported to be between 4 and 20 with a mean of 9.[70]

Tumor perfusion of rectal cancer has been measured with first pass perfusion CT. Rectal cancers show higher blood flow (BF) and shorter mean transit time (MTT) compared with those of normal rectum. After chemotherapy and radiotherapy, responders show significant reduction in BF and increase in MTT.[71,72] Significant difference in baseline BF and MTT is seen between responders and nonresponders.

ACR RECOMMENDATIONS FOR COLORECTAL CANCER STAGING

The latest recommendations of the American College of Radiology (ACR) are based on the concept that for colon cancer, the role of imaging for locoregional staging (T and N stage) is of questionable utility. This is due to the fact that

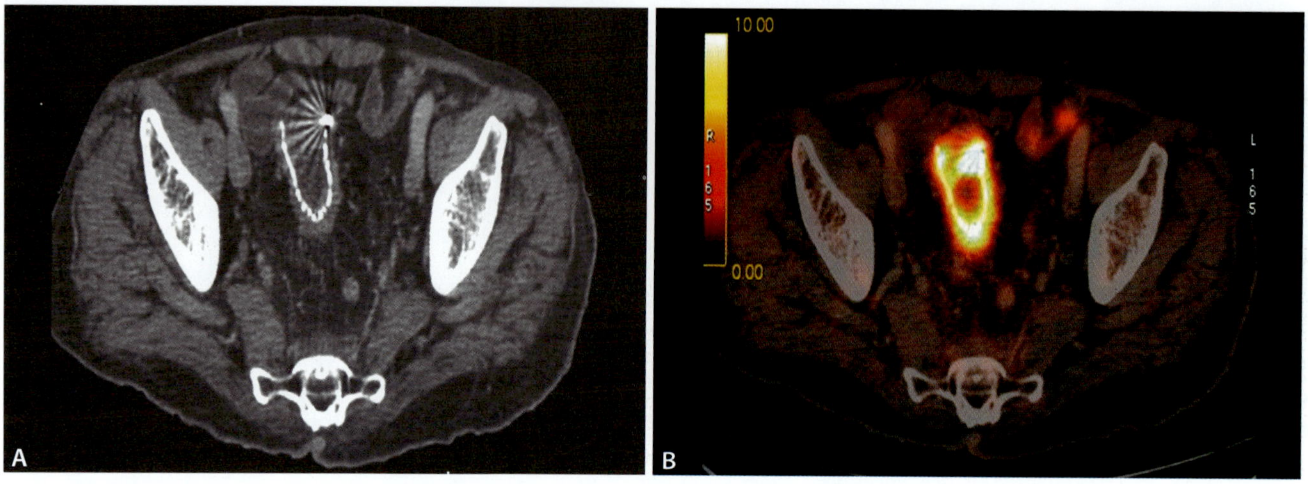

Figs. 17A and B: Axial CT (A) and PET-CT fusion image (B) in a patient postchemoradiation and postcolonic stent showing recurrent rectosigmoid thickening and locoregional lymph node. The bowel wall thickening showed more tracer uptake than the lymph node.
Courtesy: Professor BR Mittal, Department of Nuclear Medicine, PGIMER, Chandigarh, India.

neoadjuvant therapy has not shown any survival advantage over surgery alone and the standard surgical approach is radical resection. On the other hand for rectal cancer, the surgical options are more varied and are dependent on the involvement or sparing of the sphincter, circumferential resection margin and peritoneal reflection. Neoadjuvant chemotherapy and radiation, in addition to surgical resection have been found to decrease local recurrence and improve survival. Hence there is a need for accurate preoperative staging of rectal cancer.

As per the ACR appropriateness criteria of 2016, MRI pelvis without and with IV contrast is most appropriate for locoregional staging of rectal cancer. CECT of the chest, abdomen and pelvis is most appropriate for the staging for distal metastases of colorectal cancer. The sensitivity and specificity of MRI for assessment of circumferential resection margin range from 94% to 100% and 85% to 88% respectively.[73,74] Locoregional staging is not routinely required for colon cancer. The most common sites of metastatic involvement are liver and lungs. Accurate depiction of number, size and distribution is the primary goal of colon cancer staging. Multiphase CECT or contrast-enhanced MRI with optimization of technique are best suited for diagnosing liver metastases. MRI is more accurate in the setting of fatty liver and following neoadjuvant therapy. The use of chest CT, through controversial, is widely done along with CT or MRI of abdomen and pelvis. Only one quarter of pulmonary lesions found on CT are finally proven to be metastases. The routine use of PET-CT is not indicated for colorectal cancer.

OTHER EPITHELIAL TUMORS OF COLON

Squamous cell carcinomas are rare except in the rectum. Radiographic appearance is similar to adenocarcinoma and differentiation from other tumors is possible only by biopsy.

Cloacogenic carcinomas arise from transitional cloacogenic remnants of the anorectal junction. Radiographically the lesions are plaque-like and have a smooth or finely irregular surface. In profile, the borders form a tapered obtuse angle with the bowel wall. Ulceration is usually present. Since the lesions lie in the distal rectal areas, the catheter tip may completely obscure the lesion.

Carcinoid tumors present as submucosal lesions. The most common sites of colonic carcinoids are the rectum and cecum. They are seen as round, well-circumscribed masses **(Figs. 18A and B)**. Invasion of the bowel wall by tumor mass produces intense desmoplastic reaction and proliferation of fibrous tissue, resulting in contraction and kinking of the large bowel. Carcinoid tumors located in cecum and ascending colon are indistinguishable from adenocarcinoma on imaging.

NONEPITHELIAL TUMORS OF COLON

Mesodermal sarcomas of the large bowel are uncommon. They have a predilection for the rectal region. The lesions are usually rounded and lobulated but may be pedunculated. The tumors may grow extramurally and when the overlying mucosa ulcerates, necrosis and cystic cavitations can develop. Kaposi's sarcoma can involve any

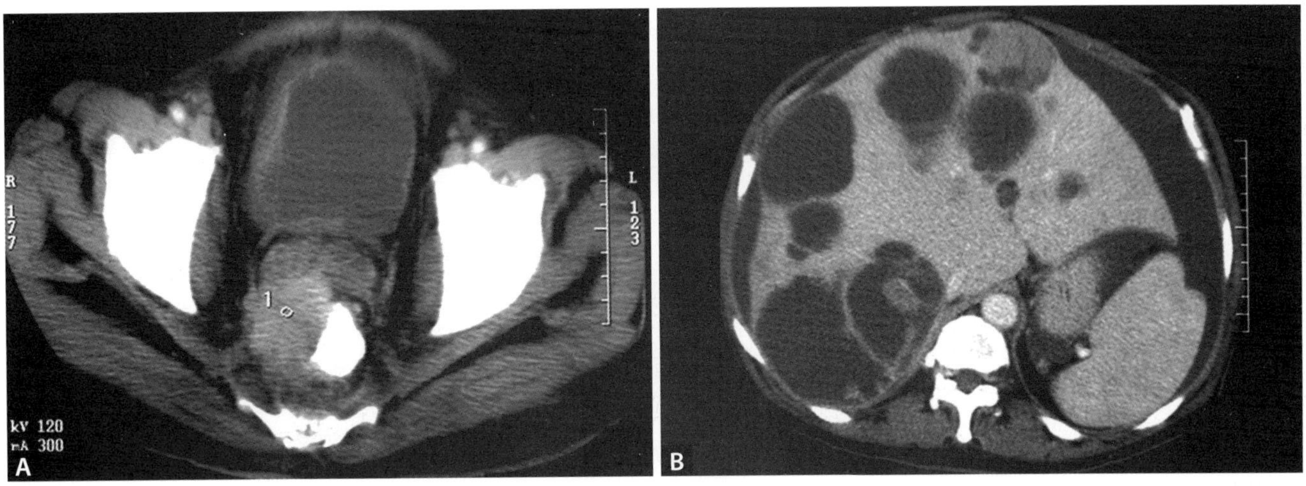

Figs. 18A and B: Axial CECT section shows a well-defined mass lesion along the right lateral wall of the rectum (A) with multiple cystic focal lesions in the liver (B) some of which are showing solid component in a patient with biopsy-proven carcinoid.

part of the gastrointestinal tract and presents as typical extramucosal mass or masses. On imaging, Kaposi's sarcoma is seen as a flat or plaque-like lesion, a small polypoid nodule or a polypoid submucosal lesion with or without umbilication.

Gastrointestinal stromal tumors (GISTs) arise from the interstitial cells of Cajal and express CD34. Only 1% of all GI tumors are of stromal origin and these are least commonly located in the colon. Small tumors are seen as sessile or pedunculated polyps. Large tumors may be seen as cavitating masses with a large extraluminal component or as submucosal masses with or without central ulceration **(Fig. 19)**. These lesions may mimic colonic lymphoma or carcinoma.

Colonic lipomas are uncommon benign tumors. Most lipomas are found in the right colon. About two thirds of these tumors are pedunculated. On barium enema, they are seen as smooth sessile or polypoidal lesions with a pedicle. Some of these lipomas may be lead points of intussusceptions. When this occurs, the lipomas may ulcerate and undergo fat necrosis resulting in CT attenuation more than fat. They are then confused with an intussuscepting carcinoma **(Figs. 20A to C)**.

Lymphoma of the colon is rare. The colon is the third most common primary site of lymphoma involving the gastrointestinal tract after stomach and the small bowel. As a primary lesion, lymphoma accounts for only 0.5% of all malignant tumors. Secondary involvement by lymphoma is usually multicentric **(Figs. 21A and B)**. The radiographic pattern may be localized or diffuse. In the localized form, the lesion is seen either as a polypoid mass that protrudes into the colonic lumen or as a constricting lesion that simulates an annular carcinoma. In the diffuse form, multiple small nodular lesions are seen. The defects are submucosal in origin with intact overlying mucosa. When lymphoma involves the mesentery, large masses may cause extensive compression on the colon.

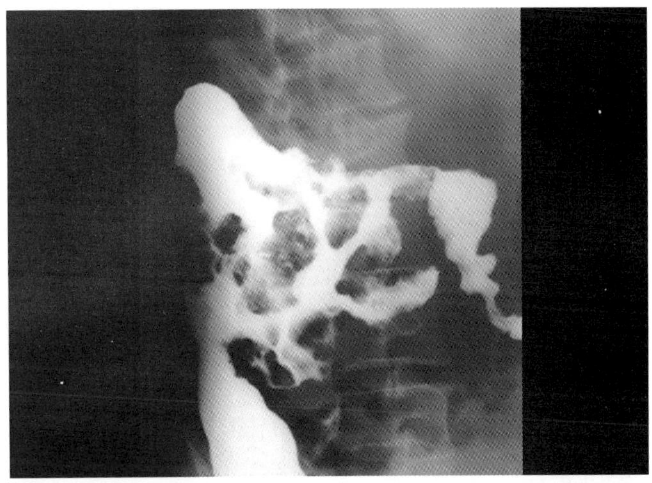

Fig. 19: Barium enema shows a large cavitatory mass lesion in the hepatic flexure with presence of deep ulcerations in a patient with leiomyosarcoma.

Courtesy: Professor B Nagi, Department of Gastroenterology, PGIMER, Chandigarh, India.

SECONDARY TUMORS OF COLON

Tumors that commonly metastasize to colon include stomach, breast, pancreas and gynecologic pelvic malignancies. Infiltration of the colon by secondary

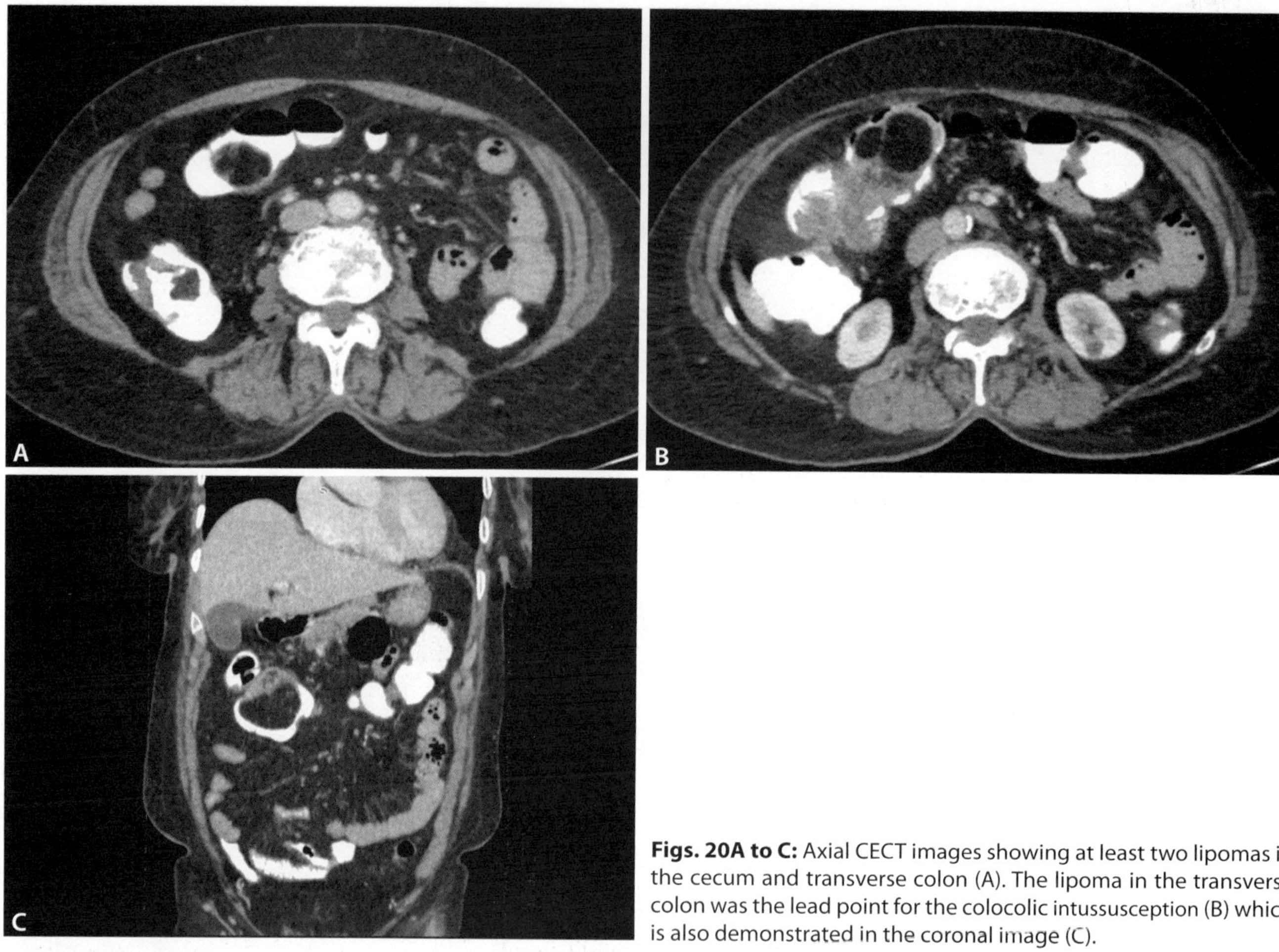

Figs. 20A to C: Axial CECT images showing at least two lipomas in the cecum and transverse colon (A). The lipoma in the transverse colon was the lead point for the colocolic intussusception (B) which is also demonstrated in the coronal image (C).

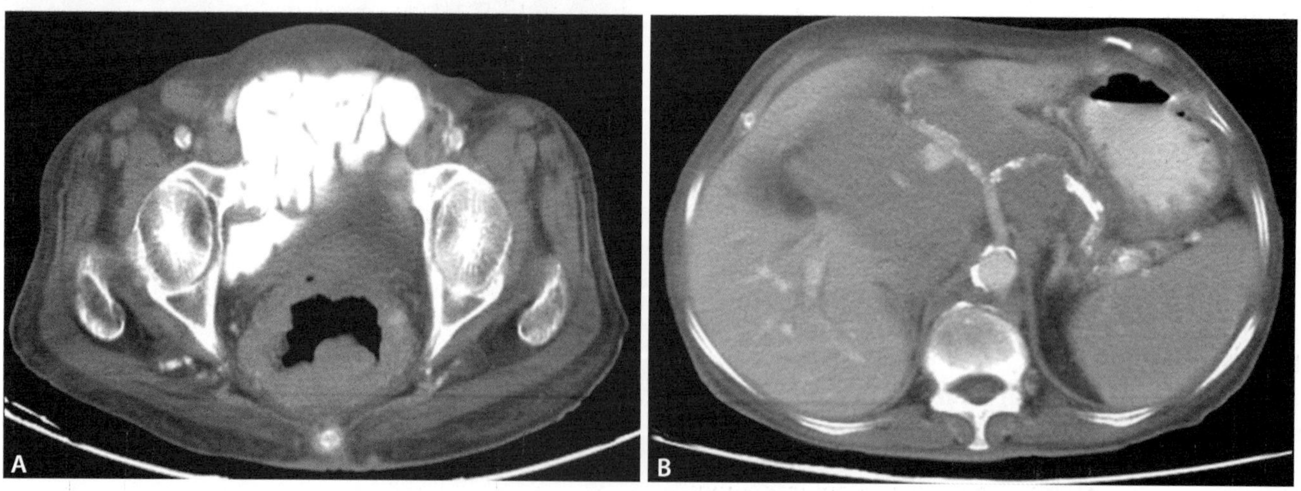

Figs. 21A and B: Axial CECT sections show concentric nodular mural thickening of the rectum (A) with conglomerate lymph nodal mass encasing the celiac trunk (B) in a patient with disseminated lymphoma.

tumors produces thickening of the colonic wall and mucosal folds. The classic radiographic appearances include indentations, spiculation, angulation, narrowing, displacement and fixation. Lymphogenous spread of tumors to the colon is characterized by the involvement of long segments, variable narrowing and loss of haustral markings. When metastases occur by the hematogenous route, as in melanoma, lesions present as smoothly marginated submucosal masses.

POSTOPERATIVE COLON AND RECURRENT CANCER

The radiologist should be aware of the various surgical techniques and postoperative anatomy for assessing the therapeutic response and for diagnosing tumor recurrence. In addition to the usual surgical resections like right hemicolectomy, extended right hemicolectomy, transverse colectomy, left hemicolectomy, sigmoid colectomy, the radiologist should be across more complex procedures such as Hartmann's procedure, anterior resection and abdominoperineal excision of rectum (APER).

Hartmann's procedure may be done for carcinoma of the sigmoid colon. It entails resection of the sigmoid and formation of the left-sided end colostomy. The rectum and distal sigmoid are closed off to form a rectal stump or Hartmann's pouch which is reattached to the colon within 3–6 months of the primary surgery. In anterior resection, the sigmoid and part of or the entire rectum, is resected. If the entire rectum is removed, that is, a low anterior resection is done, then a coloanal anastomosis is made. In case the entire rectum is not removed, a colorectal anastomosis is made. A temporary defunctioning stoma is usually made in cases of anterior resection. APER involves resection of the anus, rectum and part of the distal sigmoid colon through incisions made in the abdomen and perineum. This procedure is done for cancer of the distal third of rectum or anal canal and for salvage of the anal cancer that does not respond to chemoradiation.

T2-weighted MRI has been recommended for local restaging. Diffusion-weighted MRI adds to the response evaluation after chemoradiation **(Figs. 22A to E)**.[75,76] However, characterization of metastatic lymph nodes is challenging. Dynamic CEMR and perfusion CT assess the residual or recurrent tumor by showing contrast enhancement. The role of PET-CT is controversial. There are studies which show that irradiated rectal mucosa may show increased FDG uptake resulting in false-positive data.[77,78] Therefore, FDG PET is not recommended within the first four weeks after completion of chemoradiation.

POLYPOSIS SYNDROMES

Familial Adenomatous Polyposis Syndrome

It is the most common of the polyposis syndromes. Familial adenomatous polyposis syndrome (FAPS) is an autosomal-dominant disease and affects males and females equally. It is predominantly associated with development of adenomas in the colon which are small (80% are <5 mm in size) and sessile. Rectal sparing may be seen. Colonic carcinomas develop at around 40 years. The most common symptom is rectal bleeding and diarrhea. Treatment of choice is total colectomy with mucosal proectectomy and ileoanal anastomosis. Barium enema shows innumerable small sessile filling defects which carpet the entire colon. Extracolonic manifestations include fundal gastric polyps, premalignant gastric adenomas in the distal stomach and adenomas in the jejunum and ileum. Extraintestinal manifestations include sebaceous cysts, osteomas, fibrous tumors like desmoid, mesenteric fibromatosis and dental abnormalities (part of Gardner syndrome) and dental abnormalities. Congenital pigmented lesions of the retina are seen in >90% of patients with FAPS and may occur even before the colonic polyposis develops **(Fig. 23)**.[79] Several other tumors like medulloblastoma, meningioma, intracranial epidermoid cyst, papillary thyroid carcinoma and pancreatic carcinoma have been reported in patients with FAPS.

Peutz-Jeghers Syndrome

Peutz-Jeghers syndrome (PJS) is an autosomal dominant hereditary disease in which there are gastrointestinal hamartomas, mucocutaneous pigmentation and tumors outside the GI tract. Hamartomas is a non-neoplastic tumor composed of normal tissue elements. The hamartomatous polyps in PJS have a smooth muscle core from the muscularis mucosae, which is covered by the mucosa. The polyps may be the lead points of small bowel intussusceptions. The polyps are found in the jejunum, ileum, duodenum, colon and stomach in this order. They may be pedunculated or sessile. Pedunculated polyps are seen in the small bowel or colon while sessile polyps are seen in the stomach. The PJS polyps occur in clusters and not as carpet lesion.[80] Extraintestinal tumors include those of the pancreas, breast, ovary and uterus (adenoma malignum).

Cowden Disease (Multiple Hamartoma Syndrome)

Cowden disease is an autostomal dominant disease in which there are mucocutaneous lesions, thyroid gland abnormalities, breast cancer, GI tract hamartomatous polyps and abnormalities of the CNS. Facial trichilemmomas are pathognomic of Cowden disease.

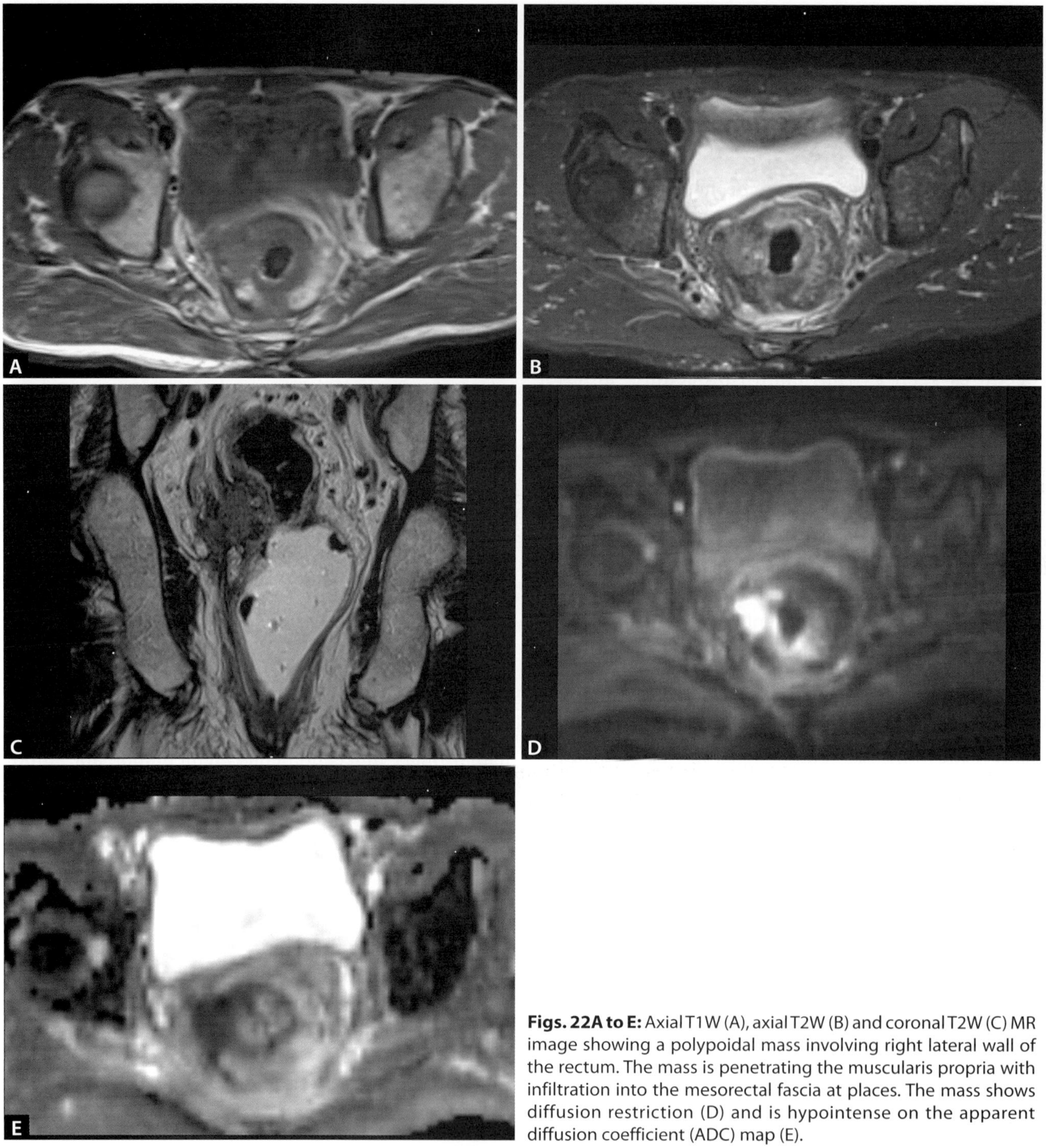

Figs. 22A to E: Axial T1W (A), axial T2W (B) and coronal T2W (C) MR image showing a polypoidal mass involving right lateral wall of the rectum. The mass is penetrating the muscularis propria with infiltration into the mesorectal fascia at places. The mass shows diffusion restriction (D) and is hypointense on the apparent diffusion coefficient (ADC) map (E).

Hamartomatous polyps are seen as multiple, small, sessile lesions with segmental or diffuse distribution. They are seen in rectosigmoid colon, stomach, duodenum, small bowel and esophagus in this order. Hyperplastic and adenomatous polyps may also be present.

Juvenile Polyposis

This is seen in the second decade of life. It is characterized by more than five juvenile polyps in the colon or rectum. The polyps can be seen throughout the GI tract as clusters. Juvenile polyps tend to be large lesions more than 1 cm in

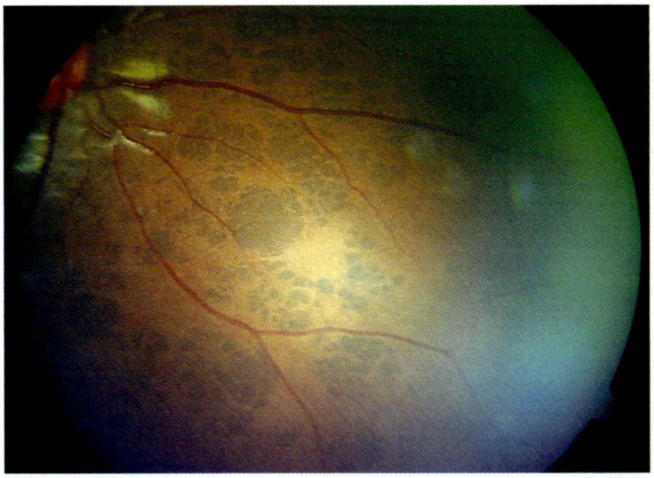

Fig. 23: Fundus picture showing sectoral hypertrophy of retinal pigment epithelium resembling animal footprints or pug marks. *Courtesy:* Dr Subina Narang, Department of Ophthalmology, GMCH, Chandigarh, India.

diameter. There can be sessile or pedunculated. Polyps are seen in the colon, stomach, small bowel and duodenum in this order.

Cronkhite-Canada Syndrome

Unlike the polyposis syndrome, Cronkhite-Canada syndrome (CCS) is not a familial disease. It is related to mental and physical stress. The lesions are predominantly inflammatory polyps.[81] Adenomatous, hyperplastic and hamartomatous polyps have also been reported. Polyps are seen as small, sessile or less commonly pedunculated lesions. They are seen in the stomach, small bowel and colon in this order. Ectodermal abnormalities of the hair, skin and nails occur after the onset of GI symptoms.

CONCLUSION

Colorectal cancer is a unique malignancy as it represents a preventable disease. The adenoma-carcinoma sequence reiterates the need for screening for polyps which are precursors of colorectal cancer. Screening is of immense importance in countries which have high prevalence of colorectal cancer. Though this malignancy has a low prevalence in the Indian subcontinent, it is expected to increase as more people are adopting Western lifestyle and dietary habits.

Imaging plays a key role in the screening program as well as for detection and staging of colorectal cancer. For screening purpose, the radiological options include CT colonography. The high sensitivity of CT colonography for detecting clinically significant polyps >1 cm has been possible due to the spectacular advances in CT technology.

Endoscopic sonography, CT and MRI are the primary cross-sectional techniques used for staging of colorectal cancer. Of these modalities, MRI is preferred for the locoregional staging of rectal cancer and CECT is preferred for the staging of colorectal metastases.

REFERENCES

1. Jemal A, Siegel R, Ward E, et al. Cancer statistics, 2007. CA Cancer J Clin. 2007;57:43-66.
2. Seidman H, Mushinski MH, Gelb SK, et al. Probability of eventually developing and dying of cancers: United States, 1995. CA Cancer J Clin. 1985;35:36-56.
3. Theoni RF, Laufer I. Polyps and carcinoma of the colon. In: Gore RM, Levine MS (Eds): WB Saunders, Philadelphia. Textbook of Gastrointestinal Radiology; 2008.pp.1121-66.
4. Mohandas KM, Desai DC. Epidemiology of digestive tract cancers in India. Ind J Gastroenterol. 1999;18:118-21.
5. Potter JD, Slattery ML, Bostick RM, et al. Colon cancer: A review of the epidemiology. Epidemiol Rev. 1993;15: 499-545.
6. Fleshner B, Slater G, Aufses AH. Age and sex distribution of patients with colorectal cancer. Dis Colon Rectum. 1989; 32:107-11.
7. Bond JH. Colonic tumors. Endoscopy. 1998;30:150-7.
8. Kritchevsky D. Colorectal cancer—the role of dietary fat and caloric restriction. Mutat Res. 1993;290:63-70.
9. Heilbrum LK, Nomura A, Hankin JH, et al. Diet and colorectal cancer with special reference to fiber intake. Int J Cancer. 1989;44:1-6.
10. Gore RM. Colorectal cancer: Clinical and pathologic features. Radiologic Clinics of North America. 1997;35:403-29.
11. McFaralane MJ, Welch KE. Gallstones, cholecystectomy and colorectal cancer. Am J Gastroenterol. 1992;87:1120-4.
12. Wilson RE, Donohue JH. Neoplasia of the colorectum. In: Phillips SF, Pemberton JH, Shorter RG (Eds). Raven Press, New York. The large intestine: Physiology, pathophysiology and disease; 1991. pp. 521-47.
13. Fenlon HM, McAneny DB, Nunes DP, et al. Occlusive colon carcinoma: Virtual colonoscopy in the preoperative evaluation of the proximal colon. Radiology. 1999;210:423-8.
14. Bulow S, Svendsen LB, Mellemgaard A. Metachronous colorectal carcinoma. Br J Surg. 1990;77:502-5.
15. Cali RL, Pitsch RM, Thorson AG, et al. Cumulative incidence of metachronous colorectal cancer. Dis Colon Rectum. 1993;36:388-93.
16. Lane N, Fenglio CM. The adenoma-carcinoma sequence in the stomach and colon: I. Observation on the adenoma as precursor to ordinary large bowel carcinoma. Gastrointest Radiol. 1976;1:111-19.
17. Cooper HS, Deppisch LM, Gourley WK, et al. Endoscopically removed malignant colorectal polyps: Clinicopathologic correlations. Gastroenterology. 1995;108:1657-65.

18. Lev R, Lee M. Colorectal carcinoma: Pathology. In: Rustgi AK (Ed). Gastrointestinal cancers: Biology, diagnosis, and therapy. Lippincott-Raven: Philadelphia; 1995. pp. 379-98.
19. Dodd GD. Malignancies. In: Alimentary tract radiology. Margulis AR, Burhenne HJ (Eds), 4th edn. The CV Mosby Company; 1989. pp. 1051-92.
20. Gore RM, Meyers MA. Pathways of abdominal and pelvic disease spread. In: Gore RM, Levine MS, Laufer I (Eds). Textbook of Gastrointestinal Radiology. WB Saunders: Philadelphia; 1994. pp. 2352-66.
21. Turnbull RB. The no-touch isolation technique of resection. JAMA. 1975;231:1181-5.
22. Johnson RD, Geisinger KR. Colorectal adenocarcinoma: Staging and histopathology. Seminars in Roentgenology. 1996;31:94-102.
23. Berlin JW, Gore RM, Yaghmai V, et al. Staging of colorectal cancer. Seminars in Roentgenology. 2000;35:370-84.
24. Silva AC, Hara AK, Leighton JA, et al. CT colonography with intravenous contrast material: varied appearance of colorectal carcinoma. Radiographics. 2005;25:1321-34.
25. Mandel JS. Screening for colorectal cancer. Gastroenterol Clin N Am. 2008;37:97-115.
26. Pamela M, McMahon G, Scott G. The case for colorectal screening. Seminars in Roentgenology. 2000;35:325-32.
27. Winawer SJ, Stewart ET, Zauber AG, et al. A comparison of colonoscopy and double-contrast barium enema for surveillance after polypectomy. National Polyp Work Group. N Engl J Med. 2000;342:1766-72.
28. Winawer SJ, Zauber AG, Ho MN, et al. Prevention of colorectal cancer by colonoscopic polypectomy. N Eng J Med. 1993;329:1977-81.
29. Citarda F, Tomaselli G, Capocaccia R, et al. Efficacy in standard clinical practice of colonoscopic polypectomy in reducing colorectal cancer incidence. Gut. 2001;48:812-15.
30. Van Rijn JC, Reitsma JB, Stoker J, et al. Polyp miss rate determined by tandem colonoscopy: a systemic review. Am J Gastroenterol. 2006;101:343-50.
31. Johnson CD, Chen MH, Toledano AY, et al. Accuracy of CT colonoscopy for detection of large adenomas and cancers. N Engl J Med. 2008;359:1207-17.
32. Gelfand DW. Colorectal cancer: Screening strategies. Radiology Clinics of North America. 1997;35:431-8.
33. Brady AP, Stevenson GW, Stevenson I. Colorectal cancer overlooked at barium enema examination and colonoscopy: A continuing perceptual problem. Radiology. 1994;192:373-8.
34. Ott DJ, Gelfand DW. How to improve the efficacy of the barium enema examination. AJR. 1993;160:491-5.
35. Ott DJ, Gelfand DW, Ramquist NA, et al. Causes of error in gastrointestinal radiology: II Barium enema examination. Gastrointest Radiol. 1980;5:99-105.
36. Gelfand DW, Ott DJ. Cost-effective screening for colorectal cancer. The radiologist's view. Primary Care and Cancer. 1992;12:11-3.
37. Stevenson GW. Normal anatomy and technique of examination of the colon: Barium, CT and MRI. In: Freeny PC, Stevenson GW (Eds): Margulis and Burhenne's Alimentary Tract Radiology. Mosby and Company, St Louis; 1994.p.692.
38. Laufer I, Kressel HY. Principles of double contrast diagnosis. In: Laufer I, Levine MS (Eds). Double-contrast gastrointestinal radiology. WB Saunders, Philadelphia; 1992.pp.9-54.
39. Youker JE, Welin S. Differentiation of true polypoid tumors of the colon from extraneous material: A new Roentgen sign. Radiology. 1985;84:610-5.
40. Boetow PC, Buck JL, Carr NJ, et al. Colorectal adeno carcinoma: Radiologic-pathologic correlation. Radiographics. 1995;15:127-46.
41. Delamarre J, Descombes P, Marti R, et al. Villous tumors of the colon and rectum: Double-contrast study of 47 cases. Gastrointest Radiol. 1980;5:69-73.
42. Bond JH. Polyp guideline: Diagnosis, treatment, and surveillance for patients with nonfamilal colorectal polyps. Ann Intern Med. 1993;119:836-43.
43. Lappas JC, Maglinte DDT, Kopecky KK, et al. Diverticular disease: Imaging with post-double contrast sigmoid flush. Radiology. 1988;168:35-7.
44. Kelvin FM, Gardiner R, Vas W, et al. Colorectal carcinoma missed on double contrast barium enema study: A problem in perception. Am J Roentgenol. 1981;137:307-13.
45. Dubbins PA. The small bowel and colon. In: Abdominal and general ultrasound. Cosgrove D, Meire H, Dewbury K (Eds). Churchill Livingstone. 1993;2:765-76.
46. Bernd L. Diagnosis of large bowel tumors by colonic sonography. The Lancet. 1990;20:144-6.
47. Glaser F, Schalg P, Harfarth C. Endorectal Ultrasonography for the assessment of invasion of rectal tumors and lymph node involvement. Br J Surg. 1990;77:883-7.
48. Hulsmans FH, Tio TL, Mathus-Vliegen EMH, et al. Colorectal villous adenoma: Transrectal US in screening for invasive malignancy. Radiology. 1992;185:193-6.
49. Scharling ES, Wolfman NT, Bechtold RE. Computed tomography evaluation of colorectal carcinoma. Seminars in Roentgenology. 1996;31:142-53.
50. Kalra N, Suri S, Gupta R, et al. MDCT in the staging of gallbladder carcinoma. Am J Roentgenol. 2006;186:758-66.
51. Regina GH, Beets T, Beets GL. Rectal cancer: Review with emphasis on MR imaging. Radiology. 2004;232:335-46.
52. Filippone A, Ambrosini R, Fuschi M, et al. Preoperative T and N staging of colorectal cancer. Accuracy of contrast-enhanced multidetector row CT colonography—Initial experience. Radiology. 2004;231:83-90.
53. Chung DJ, Huh KC, Choi WJ, et al. CT colonography using 16-MDCT in the evaluation of colorectal cancer. Am J Roentgenol. 2005;184:98-103.
54. Narayanan S, Kalra N, Bhatia A, et al. Staging of colorectal cancer using contrast-enhanced multidetector computed tomographic colonography. Singapore Med J. 2014;55:660-6.
55. Vining DJ, Gelfand DW. Non-invasive colonoscopy using helical CT scanning, 3D reconstruction and virtual reality. Presented in the syllabus of the 23rd annual meeting.

Society of Gastrointestinal Radiologists. Maui (Hawaii); 1994.
56. Summerton S, Little E, Cappell MS. CT colonography: Current status and future promise. Gastroenterol Clin N Am. 2008;37: 161-89.
57. Bhatia A, Saxena AK, Kalra N, et al. Intravenous contrast enhanced computed tomography colonoscopy in children with suspected colonic polyps. Eur J Radiol. 2013;82:905-12.
58. Kalra N, Suri S, Bhasin DK, et al. Comparison of multidetector computed tomographic colonography and conventional colonoscopy for detection of colorectal polyps and cancer. Ind J Gastroenterol. 2006;25:229-32.
59. Zallis ME, Barish MA, Choi JR, et al. CT colonography reporting and data system: A consensus proposal. Radiology. 2005;236:3-9.
60. Brown G, Radcliffe AG, Newcombe RG, et al. Preoperative assessment of prognostic factors in rectal cancer using high-resolution magnetic resonance imaging. Br J Surg. 2003;90: 355-64.
61. Beets-Tan RG, Beets GL, Vliegen RF, et al. Accuracy of magnetic resonance imaging in prediction of tumor-free resection margin in rectal cancer surgery. Lancet. 2001;357:497-504.
62. Brown G, Kirkham A, Williams GT, et al. High-resolution MRI of the anatomy important in total mesorectal excision of the rectum. Am J Roentgenol. 2004;182:431-9.
63. Heald RJ, Ryall RD. Recurrence and survival after total mesorectal excision for rectal cancer. Lancet. 1986;1:1479-82.
64. Hunerbein M, Pegios W, Rau B, et al. Prospective comparison of endorectal ultrasound, three-dimensional endorectal ultrasound and endorectal MRI in the preoperative evaluation of rectal tumors. Preliminary results. Surg Endosc. 2000;14: 1005-09.
65. Kim NK, Kim MJ, Yan SH, et al. Comparative study of transrectal ultrasonography, pelvic computerized tomography and magnetic resonance imaging in preoperative staging of rectal cancer. Dis Colon Rectum. 1999;42:770-5.
66. Ajay W, Pelster G, Treichel U, et al. Dark lumen magnetic resonance colonography: Comparsion with conventional colonoscopy for the detection of colorectal pathology. Gut. 2003;52:1738-43.
67. Britton KE, Granowska M. The diagnostic role of radiolabelled antibodies. In: Murrary IPS, EII PJ (Eds). Nuclear medicine in clinical diagnosis and treatment. Churchill Livingstone: Edinburgh; 1998. pp. 871-92.
68. Ramos E, Valls C, Martinez, et al. Preoperative staging of patients with liver metastases of colorectal carcinoma. Does PET/CT really add something to multidetector CT? Ann Surg Oncol. 2011;18:2654-61.
69. Kinner S, Antoch G, Bockisch A, et al. Whole-body PET/ CT colonography: a possible new concept for colorectal cancer staging. Abdom Imaging. 2007;32:606-12.
70. Gollub MJ, Akhurst T, Markowitz AJ, et al. Combined CT colonography and 18F-FDG PET of colon polyps: potential technique for selective detection of cancer and precancerous lesions. Am J Roentgenol. 2007;188:130-8.
71. Sahani DV, Kalva SP, Hamberg LM, et al. Assessing tumor perfusion and treatment response in rectal cancer with multi-section CT: initial observations. Radiology. 2005;234:785-92.
72. Bellomi M, Petralia G, Sonzogni A, et al. CT perfusion for the monitoring of neoadjuvant chemotherapy and radiation therapy in rectal carcinoma: initial experience. Radiology. 2007;244:486-93.
73. Purkayastha S, Tekkis PP, Athanasiou T, et al. Diagnostic precision of magnetic resonance imaging for preoperative prediction of the circumferential margin involvement in patients with rectal cancer. Colorectal Dis. 2007;9:402-11.
74. Videhult P, Smedh K, Lundin P, Kraaz W. Magnetic resonance imaging for preoperative staging of rectal cancer in clinical practice: high accuracy in predicting circumferential margin with clinical benefit. Colorectal Dis. 2007;9:412-7.
75. Sun Ys, Zhang XP, Tang L, et al. Locally advanced rectal carcinoma treated with preoperative chemotherapy and radiation therapy: preliminary analysis of diffusion-weighted MR imaging for early detection of tumor histopathologic downstaging. Radiology. 2010;254:170-8.
76. Hein Pa, Kremser C, Judmaier W, et al. Diffusion-weighed magnetic resonance imaging for monitoring diffusion changes in rectal carcinoma during combined preoperative chemoradiation: preliminary results of a prospective study. Eur J Radiol. 2003;45:214-22.
77. Konski A, Li T, Sigurdson E, et al. Use of molecular imaging to predict clinical outcome in patients with rectal cancer after preoperative chemotherapy and radiation. Int J Radiat Oncol Biol Phys. 2009;74:55-9.
78. Kalff V, Ware R, Heriot A, et al. Radiation changes do not interfere with postchemoradiation restaging of patients with rectal cancer by FDG PET/CT before curative surgical therapy. Int Radiol Oncol Biol Phys. 2009;74:60-6.
79. Iwamma T, Mishima Y, Okamoto N, et al. Association of congenital hypertrophy of the retinal pigment epithelium with familial adenomatous polyposis. Br J Surg. 1990;77:273-6.
80. Schumacher V, Vogel T, Leube B, et al. STK11 genotyping and cancer risk in Peutz Jeghers syndrome. J Med Genet. 2005;42:428-35.
81. Burke AP, Sobin LH. The pathology of Cronkhite-Canada syndrome polyps. Am J Surg Pathol. 1989;13:940-6.

CHAPTER 72

Ulceroconstrictive Diseases of the Gut

Devasenathipathy Kandasamy, Manisha Jana, Arun Kumar Gupta

INTRODUCTION

Imaging in ulceroconstrictive lesions of the gut has seen a paradigm change over the last few decades. While earlier conventional imaging studies relied predominantly on the luminal distension and opacification of the bowel lumen using positive oral contrast; newer modalities such as CT and MRI are capable of providing information on both intraluminal, as well as extrinsic abnormalities. CT enterography (CTE) and MR enterography (MRE) are unique imaging techniques having the combined advantages of both CT/MRI and enterography.

Plain Radiograph

The role of plain radiographs has diminished to a great extent because of the wider availability of cross-sectional modalities. They are useful only in a patient with acute or subacute intestinal obstruction, when they are often the first line modality. An erect abdominal radiograph can provide valuable information regarding the level and severity of bowel obstruction, and presence of pneumoperitoneum, although erect chest radiograph is the best method to detect the latter. Enteroliths can be seen sometimes proximal to the site of obstruction and presence of calcified lymph nodes can point towards the diagnosis of tuberculosis (TB). The drawback of this study is that it is often not helpful in detecting the etiology of obstruction. It plays no role in purely ulcerative disease entities.

Barium Studies

Barium meal follow through (BMFT) was the most widely used imaging technique for the evaluation small bowel until a few years ago. Constrictive lesions of the small bowel presenting as small bowel obstruction remain a challenge in diagnosis; as large part of the small bowel is not accessible by endoscopy. With the advent of better modalities such as multidetector computed tomography (MDCT) and MRI, the importance of BMFT has declined. BMFT, along with colonic evaluation by barium enema, can give valuable information regarding both small and large bowel obstructive lesions.[1] It is the best imaging technique to evaluate the mucosal details of small and large bowel. There are many classical signs described for TB and Crohn's disease (CD) on barium studies and they are good in demonstrating bowel narrowing, dilatation, mucosal ulcerations, kinking and clumping of bowel loops and fistulae **(Figs. 1 and 2)**. They are one of the few imaging techniques which are capable of studying the bowel motility which is an important parameter in bowel imaging. The evaluation of lesions in the ileum and cecum can be further enhanced by peroral pneumocolon (i.e. insufflation of air through the rectum).[2] Peroral pneumocolon can also provide valuable information regarding colonic pathologies.

Single contrast BMFT is usually performed with barium suspension having 66% w/v barium. With the technological advances in the field of fluoroscopic techniques, coupled

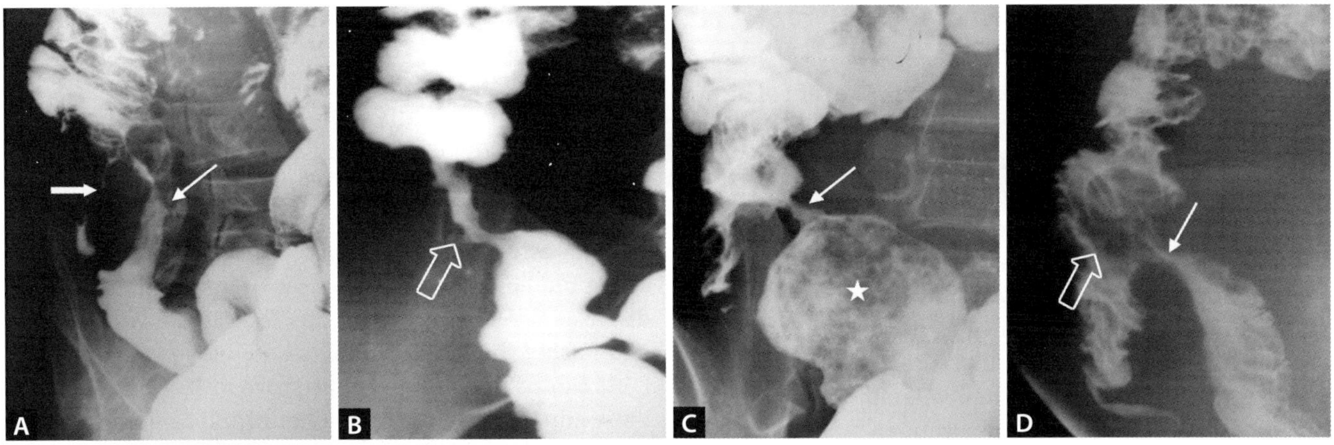

Figs. 1A to D: Ileocecal TB on barium studies: Barium meal follow through (BMFT) image (A) shows narrowing and mild mucosal irregularity (thin arrow) in the terminal ileum (string sign) with associated contracted cecum (thick arrow). BMFT image (B) of another patient shows narrowing of terminal ileum which is emptying directly into ascending colon (outlined arrow) with nonvisualization of cecum (Stierlin's sign). BMFT image (C) in a different patient shows fibrotic stricture in the terminal ileum (thin arrow) with proximal dilatation (star) and contracted cecum. BMFT image (D) of another patient shows mild gaping (thin arrow) and filling defect (outlined arrow) in the region of ileocecal valve (Fleischner's sign) due to edema of the valve.

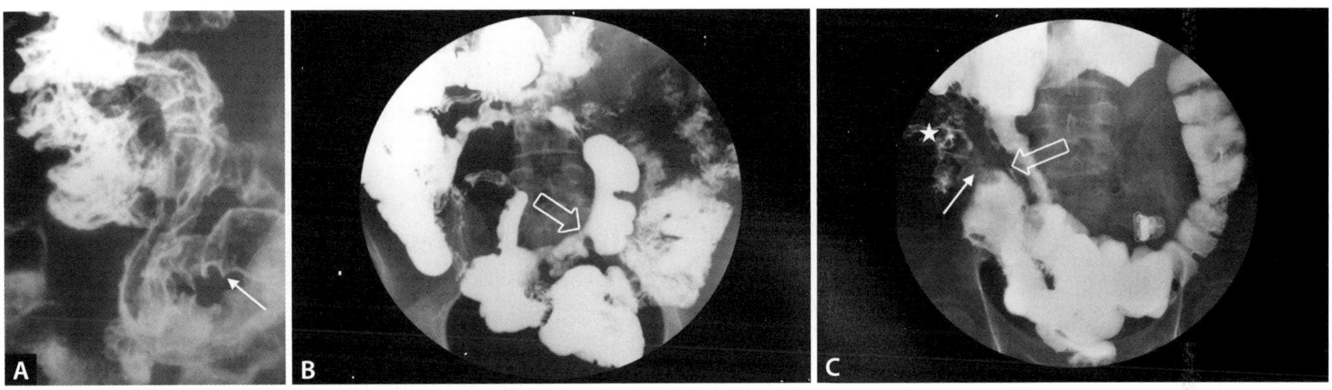

Figs. 2A to C: CD involving the small bowel: BMFT (A) showing mucosal irregularity in the terminal ileum and rose thorn ulcers (thin arrow). BMFT in another patient with CD (B) showing multiple strictures in distal ileum, shortening of mesenteric border and pseudosacculations in the antimesenteric border (outlined arrow). BMFT image (C) in a patient with CD showing narrowing of terminal ileum (thin arrow) with proximal dilatation, irregularity and narrowing of cecum (star). In one of the ileal loop there is a thin longitudinal extraluminal barium (outlined arrow) seen paralleling the bowel loop (double tracking) which is due to the presence of deep fissures in the bowel wall in CD.

with their wide availability and low radiation burden; most often the procedure is performed under fluoroscopic guidance nowadays. The major drawback in the evaluation of intestinal strictures by BMFT is the differentiation of a true stricture from a transient peristaltic contraction. In order to alleviate this drawback, enteroclysis (small bowel enema) came into practice; wherein the small bowel lumen is distended through a nasojejunal tube and using diluted barium. Enteroclysis yielded superior mucosal details compared to BMFT. Also, as the distension of bowel lumen was controlled and the luminal distension was visualized in real-time; this technique was superior to BMFT in the detection of subtle intestinal strictures. However, this technique entails ionizing radiation to the patient and the yield is also poor when compared with CTE or MRE. Hence, barium studies should be used only if CT or MR enterography is not available.

Single contrast barium enema and double contrast barium enema (DCBE) are two other important barium studies. While single contrast BE is adequate for delineating the strictures in the large bowel; DCBE is preferable in cases of suspected mucosal lesions such as in ulcerative colitis. However, colonoscopy is the primary modality of choice in the evaluation of patients with ulcerative colitis and imaging is not commonly performed for their evaluation.

CECT and CT Enteroclysis/CT Enterography

Contrast-enhanced CT (CECT) is the workhorse of imaging in suspected intestinal strictures. With the advent of newer generation fast MDCT scanners, CT can provide crucial information regarding mural/extraluminal findings in bowel pathology. CT enteroclysis combines the benefits of the two imaging modalities; good luminal distension similar to a conventional enteroclysis and visualization of extraluminal/transmural pathologies similar to CECT.[3] CT enterography (CTE) is a newer imaging technique wherein the luminal distension of small bowel is achieved without a nasojejunal tube; hence ameliorating patient discomfort arising from intubation. In this procedure either diluted mannitol/polyethylene glycol solution (PEG) is used as neutral oral contrast agent to distend the bowel loops. There are various protocols described for CTE in literature aimed at adequate bowel distension during scanning. The protocol given below is followed in our institute **(Table 1)**. CTE has been found to be a very sensitive tool in the diagnosis of inflammatory small bowel diseases; comparable to the capsule endoscopy.[4–6] Another important role of CTE is to rule out any strictures in the small bowel; prior to a capsule endoscopy; in order to avoid capsule impaction/retention.[6] Usage of ionizing radiation is an important drawback of CTE which limits its utility in follow up imaging. Radiation dose of a standard CTE study is around 15 mSv compared to 3-8 mSv for BMFT.[7,8] Radiation dose can be minimized by optimizing the scan parameters and using new techniques such as iterative reconstruction methods.

MRI/MR Enterography

Although CECT can provide a lot of diagnostic information in intestinal strictures; it comes with a high radiation burden; more so in patients of inflammatory bowel diseases who need repeated imaging.[9] MRI has the advantage of superior soft tissue contrast resolution; multiplanar imaging capability and lack of any ionizing radiation. MRI has the unique advantage of evaluating multiple paradigms such as T1 and T2 characteristics, diffusion restriction and pattern of contrast enhancement. In addition, new ultrafast sequences (True FISP – Cine MR) have made the real time evaluation of the small bowel possible; which is crucial for differentiating a stricture from a peristaltic contraction. MR enterography (MRE) has all the inherent advantages of CT enterography; with the additional benefit of being able to differentiate a fibrotic stricture from an active one. Diffusion weighted MRI (DWI) is also being increasingly used in cases of inflammatory bowel diseases.[10–13] The active lesions tend to show restriction of diffusion (hyperintense signal on high b value images). DWI can be an effective alternative to IV Gadolinium in the evaluation of lesion activity in inflammatory bowel diseases in patients in whom Gadolinium based contrast is contraindicated. Commonly used intraluminal contrast in MRE is diluted Mannitol, which can act as biphasic contrast agent. On the T2W images, it causes high signal intensity within the lumen and the bowel wall is seen as hypointense structure. On postcontrast T1W images, it serves as a 'negative' contrast agent and helps in better delineation of the wall enhancement against a dark lumen. The formulation of oral contrast and the timing of giving aliquots for MRE is the same as CTE protocol **(Table 1)**.

Table 1: CT Enterography protocol.

Preparation	***6 hours fasting***
Oral contrast	Water + Mannitol (300 mL of 20% mannitol in 1500 mL water)
Technique	450 mL at 60 min prior to scanning 450 mL at 40 min prior to scanning 225 mL at 20 min prior to scanning 225 mL at 10 min prior to scanning 250–300 mL on table just before scanning (plain water)

Ultrasonography and Contrast-enhanced Ultrasonography

Ultrasound (US) has limited role in the initial evaluation of intestinal obstruction; owing to gaseous abdominal distension which makes ultrasonographic visualization of bowel loops difficult. However, in cases of abdominal tuberculosis or inflammatory bowel diseases where the disease has been localized by other imaging modalities (such as CT or MRI); ultrasound is a useful tool for follow up evaluation. CT is associated with radiation burden, and MRI evaluation in children often needs sedation or general anesthesia. High-resolution US is an emerging technique to evaluate bowel disorders and it is very sensitive in detecting bowel wall abnormalities in the terminal ileum and ileocecal junction region. The spatial resolution of high resolution US is better than CTE or MRE and it can show wall thickening, dilated segment of bowel loop and bowel motility in real time. Increase in bowel and mesenteric vascularity can be detected on Doppler which is considered as a marker for disease activity in CD. Wide availability, repeatability and lack of radiation have made US an attractive technique in the evaluation of ulceroconstrictive bowel diseases. US is very sensitive to detect abnormalities in terminal ileum however for the evaluation of proximal small bowel loops the accuracy falls. Various studies across the globe have described a sonographic sensitivity and specificity for the diagnosis of CD ranging from 75 to 94% and 67 to 100%, respectively.[14,15]

Contrast enhanced ultrasonography (CEUS) is a recent advancement which has been evaluated and recommended in the evaluation of disease activity in inflammatory bowel diseases, distinguishing fibrous from inflammatory strictures, abscesses, and fistula.[16,17] It utilizes a special contrast agent such as sulfur hexafluoride microbubbles which is given intravenously to look for areas of abnormal enhancement. It can be used even in patients with renal impairment as the mode of excretion is via breath. Lack of expertise, limited availability of hardware and software for CEUS and contrast agent are the current limitations. The cine loops of CEUS can be processed using software and various quantifiable perfusion parameters can be obtained by placing region of interest (ROI) markers.

ABDOMINAL TUBERCULOSIS

Tuberculosis (TB) is one of the leading causes of death killing around 1.5 million people worldwide in 2014 and India constitutes 23% of all TB cases which is the highest in the world.[18] Abdominal TB constitutes about 17% of all inpatients admitted with the diagnosis of TB[19] Intestine is the sixth most common of all the extrapulmonary sites involved by TB.[20] TB is caused by *Mycobacterium tuberculosis* and abdominal TB generally includes involvement of gastrointestinal tract, lymph nodes, peritoneum and solid visceral organs of abdomen.

Gastrointestinal Tuberculosis

Gastrointestinal TB (GI TB) can present either with symptoms related to bowel like abdominal pain, vomiting, diarrhea and abdominal distension or systemic symptoms like fever, loss of appetite and weight.[21] The above symptoms of GI TB are not specific and can be seen in patients with CD. The role of imaging in differentiating GI TB and CD will be dealt later in this chapter. Apart from diagnosis, imaging is also useful in guiding FNAC or biopsy in patients where the diagnosis is uncertain on imaging alone. TB can involve any part of the gastrointestinal tract, but ileocecal region is most commonly involved (50–90%).[22,23] The other less commonly involved areas are ascending colon, jejunum, rest of the colon, rectum, duodenum, anal canal, esophagus and stomach in that order.[24,25]

Small Bowel Tuberculosis

Ileocecal region is by far the most common site for small bowel TB. There are various reasons hypothesized for this predilection which are as follows:

- Physiological stasis leading to longer contact
- Closer contact with tubercle bacilli
- Ileum is rich in lymphoid tissue
- Relatively neutral pH promoting bacterial growth.

Ileocecal TB has three morphological types—**ulcerative** (60%), **hypertrophic** (10%) and **ulcerohypertrophic** (30%). Ulcerative type is more common in immunocompromised individuals and hypertrophic type is more common in immunocompetent individuals. The ulcerohypertrophic form can closely mimic malignancy because of its morphology. The caseation necrosis occurring in the submucosal lymphoid tissue causes mucosal ulcerations whereas extensive inflammation and fibrosis in reaction to the bacilli leads to thickening in the hypertrophic type.

Before the advent of new cross-sectional techniques such as CTE and MRE, barium studies used to be the imaging modality of choice in suspected patients with ITB because of its unsurpassed ability to show the mucosal abnormalities. There are various signs on barium studies described in the different stages of ITB **(Fig. 1)**. Spasm, hypermotility, mucosal edema, edema of the ileocecal valve are the earliest signs of ileocecal TB. Fleischner or inverted umbrella sign which is due to the thickening of ileocecal valve with narrowing of terminal ileum is considered to be characteristic for ileocecal TB.[26] Stierlin's sign is due to rapid emptying of barium into cecum because of mucosal irritability **(Fig. 1)**. As the disease progresses there will be fibrosis and shortening of the involved bowel segment and napkin ring stenosis. This is called as string sign showing persistent narrowing of barium column in the area of stenosis **(Fig. 1)**. Cecum is pulled out of the right iliac fossa which is often referred to as pulled up cecum **(Figs. 3A to C)**. This also leads to contraction of cecum which can appear conical on imaging. Because of the cranial migration of cecum there is alteration in the angle between the terminal ileum and colon. The terminal ileum may appear hanging down and stretched from the contracted cecum which is called goose-neck deformity.

High resolution US can also show changes of GI TB in the form of abnormal wall thickening (>3 mm in distended state and >5 mm in collapsed state), inflammation in the surrounding mesentery and enlarged lymph nodes which may have calcification and necrosis. Bowel wall thickening is a nonspecific finding which can be seen in Crohn's disease, lymphoma, amoebiasis and carcinoma. However, TB commonly affects ileocecal junction and often the cecum is pulled up because of fibrosis. USG is optimal for the evaluation of ileocecal region wall thickening. However, USG is not sensitive to detect abnormalities in more proximal small bowel loops because of its inability to evaluate the entire length of bowel.

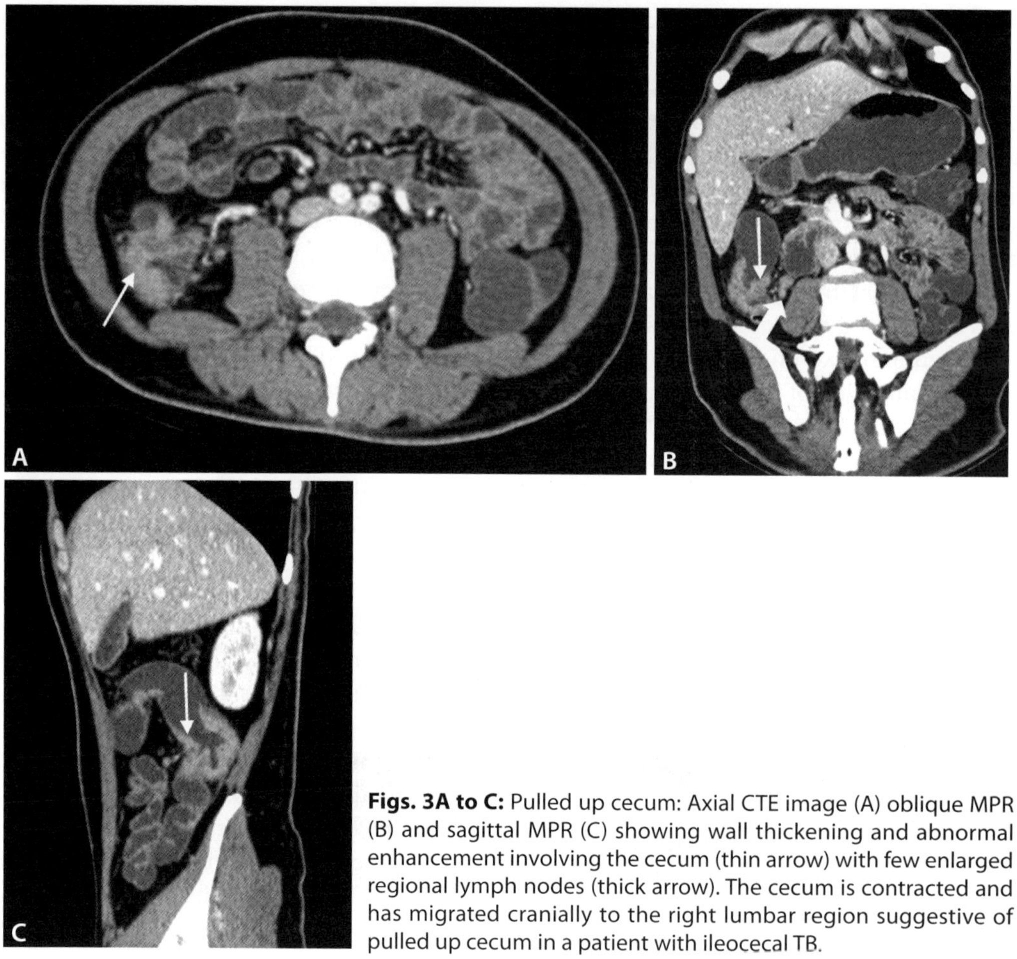

Figs. 3A to C: Pulled up cecum: Axial CTE image (A) oblique MPR (B) and sagittal MPR (C) showing wall thickening and abnormal enhancement involving the cecum (thin arrow) with few enlarged regional lymph nodes (thick arrow). The cecum is contracted and has migrated cranially to the right lumbar region suggestive of pulled up cecum in a patient with ileocecal TB.

Contrast-enhanced CT is better than USG to detect and characterize small bowel TB which can show the bowel wall thickening, mesenteric changes and adenopathy **(Fig. 4)**. The necrosis in the nodes is better detected on CECT. Though it is not sensitive for detecting early mucosal changes, it can comprehensively evaluate most of the other features of abdominal TB such as peritoneal and solid organ involvement. CTE is a relatively new technique which is considered superior to conventional CECT in the evaluation of mucosal abnormalities and in the detection of subtle wall thickening and narrowing of lumen. In the early stage CTE may show nonspecific inflammatory changes in the form of stratified wall thickening in distal ileum, ileocecal junction and cecum which can later progress to more severe homogeneous wall thickening and narrowing leading to obstruction **(Figs. 5 and 6)**. It can also show clumping of bowel loops, adhesions, mesenteric changes and occasionally

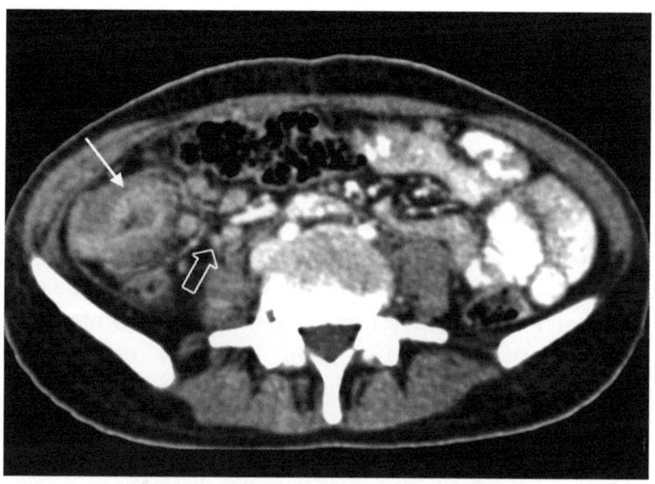

Fig. 4: Ileocecal TB: Axial CECT image showing circumferential wall thickening involving the cecum (thin arrow) with surrounding fat stranding and enlarged lymph nodes (outlined arrow). The above features are suggestive of TB.

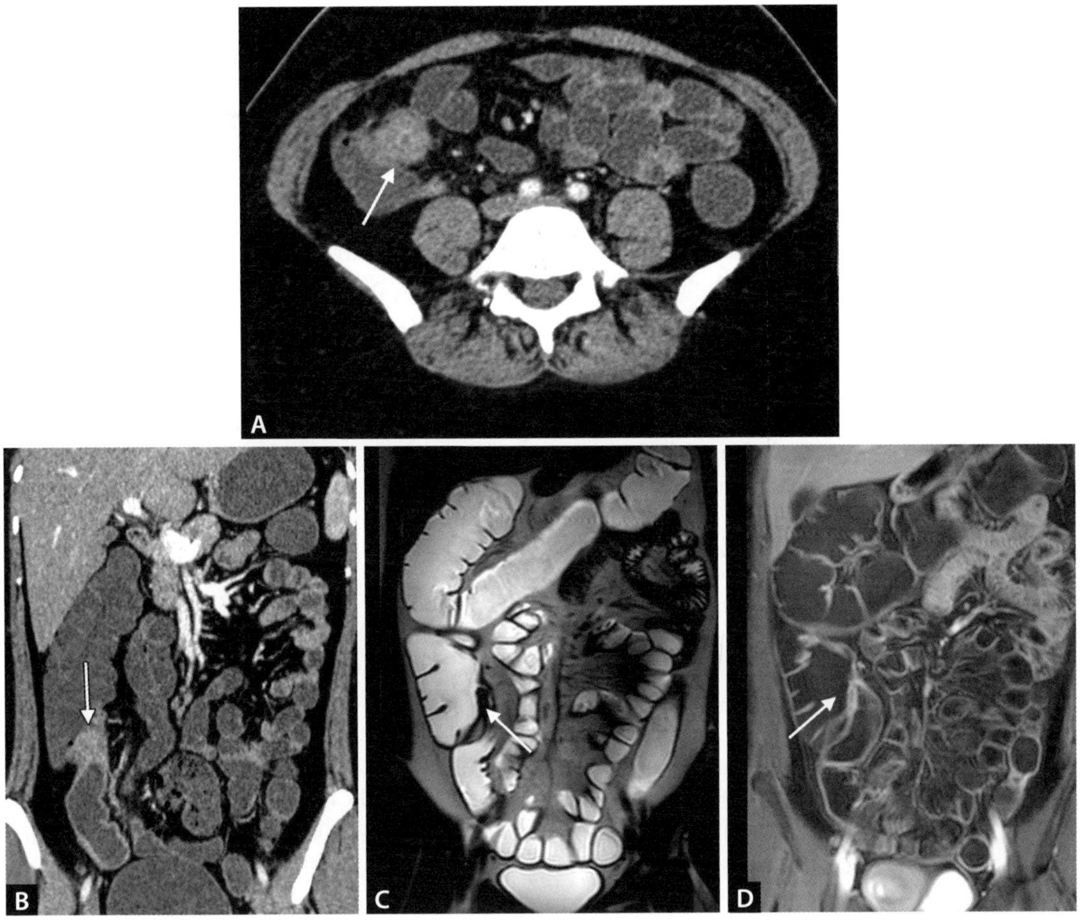

Figs. 5A to D: Fibrotic stricture in TB: CTE images (A and B) and MRE images (C and D) showing circumferential wall thickening involving the terminal ileum and ileocecal junction (thin arrow) causing mild proximal obstruction. The wall thickening is hypointense on T2-weighted image (C) and showing homogeneous enhancement on postcontrast image (D) suggestive of fibrosis.

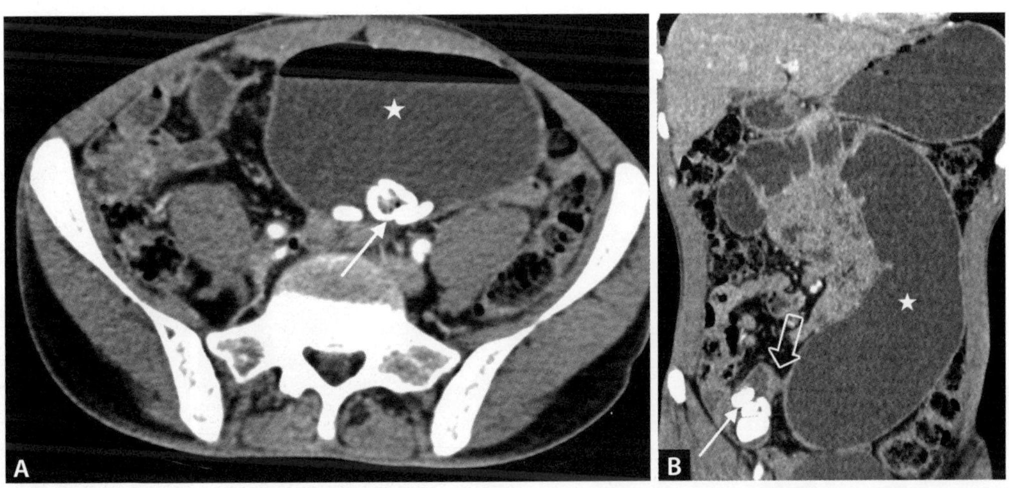

Figs. 6A and B: Small bowel obstruction with enteroliths: Axial CECT image (A) and coronal MPR (B) show a short segment ileal stricture (outlined arrow). There is marked proximal dilatation of small bowel with air-fluid level (star) suggestive of small bowel obstruction. Also noted is presence of multiple enteroliths (thin arrow).

cocoon formation in which varying length of bowel loop is encapsulated by a thick fibrotic membrane **(Figs. 7A to C)**. Because of superior contrast resolution MRI or MRE can also be used to show the features of GI TB. Sometimes the inflammatory changes in the bowel wall and in the surrounding mesentery are better seen on MRI as compared to CT and the tubercular lesions are usually hypointense on T1W images and hyperintense on T2W images **(Figs. 8A to D)**. MRE may show wall thickening, lymphadenopathy, ascites, peritoneal thickening and other associated extraluminal findings. It also shows good correlation with barium meal follow through studies in detecting wall thickening and has the advantage of being a radiation free one-stop shop technique.[27] Most of these findings are common to both GI TB and CD which makes the diagnosis difficult. There are imaging features which can help in this differentiation to a certain extent and are discussed later in this chapter.

Colonic and Anorectal TB

Colon is the second most common site of involvement in GI TB and isolated colonic involvement occurs in about 9% of patients.[28] Cecum is the commonest site followed by ascending colon. Colonic involvement usually presents with chronic pain in abdomen, rectal bleeding and alterations in bowel habit. On imaging colonic involvement presents as short or long segment thickening of the wall, ulcerations which are usually circumferential, and strictures with or without proximal dilatation. Occasionally, it can present with inflammatory polyps, bowel perforation or fistula formation. There may be other sites of involvement in the abdomen which can support the diagnosis. Barium enema can show the early mucosal abnormalities, ulcerations, spasm and stricture. Strictured area is seen as smooth narrowing producing an hour glass configuration as opposed to carcinoma colon which produces an apple core configuration. Colonic TB can closely resemble CD, ulcerative colitis, colonic carcinoma and amebic colitis.

Rarely, TB can involve the rectum and anal canal which can present as proctitis, strictures, fistula, ischiorectal fossa abscess, perianal fissures and warty growths. These findings are not specific for TB because they can occur in CD as well. Circumferential wall thickening because of tuberculous involvement can resemble carcinoma rectum. In doubtful cases, sampling should be done to confirm the diagnosis.

Duodenal Tuberculosis

It constitutes only about 2% of all GI TB and duodenum can be involved either by an extrinsic or intrinsic process.[29] Duodenum may be compressed or involved secondarily due to adjacent lymphadenopathy in which case barium studies can show widening of C-loop of duodenum and smooth narrowing. Primary involvement can manifest either as ulcerative or hyperplastic form which can be seen on barium studies as ulcers, polyps, fistula formation and narrowing of lumen. CT may show thickening of the duodenal wall commonly involving the second and the third part, which may be associated with stricture and proximal dilatation **(Figs. 9A to C)**.[30] Duodenal TB can mimic CD, lymphoma and carcinoma and it is usually difficult to differentiate them. Biopsy is confirmatory for the diagnosis.

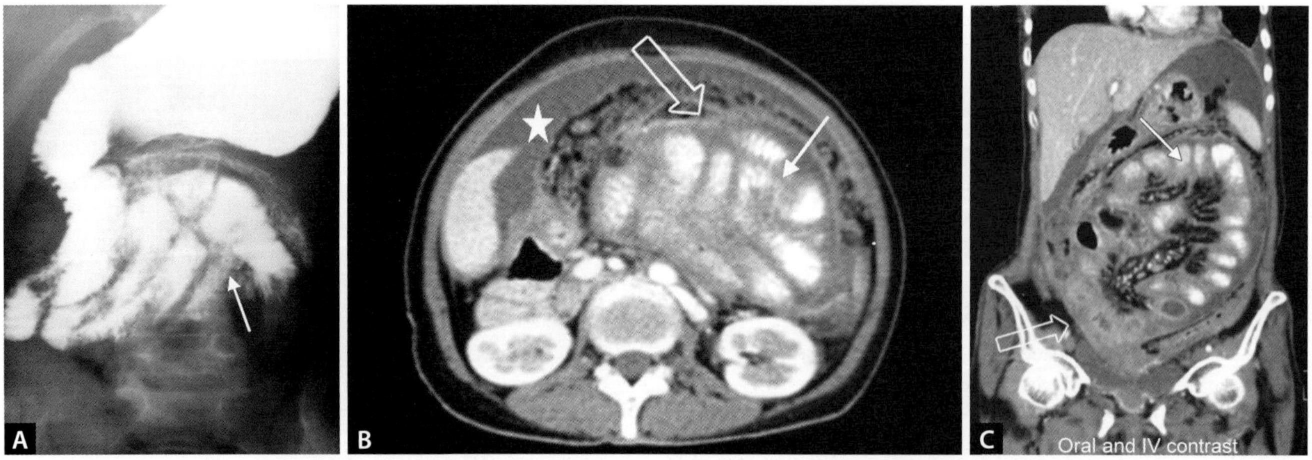

Figs. 7A to C: Sclerosing encapsulating peritonitis: Barium meal follow through (BMFT) (A) showing clumping and fixed position of the dilated small bowel loops (thin arrow) in the central abdomen. Axial CECT (B) and coronal MPR (C) image showing clumped dilated proximal jejunal loops which are encapsulated by a thick membrane (outlined arrow) all around suggestive of sclerosing encapsulating peritonitis (cocoon formation). There is associated loculated ascites (star) seen.

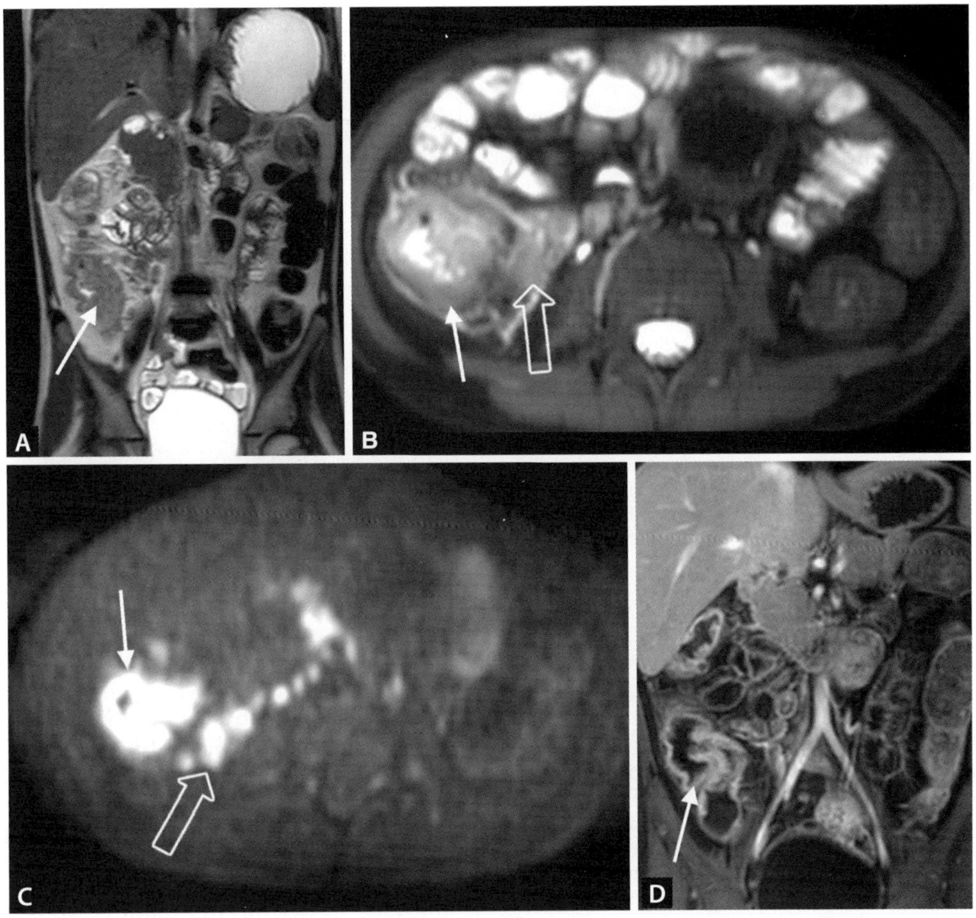

Figs. 8A to D: Ileocecal TB: MRE T2-weighted images (A and B) showing wall thickening which is hyperintense involving the ileocecal region (thin arrow) with enlarged regional lymph nodes (outlined arrow). The wall thickening shows diffusion restriction on diffusion weighted b-800 image (C) and hyperenhancement on post-gadolinium image (D) suggestive of active disease.

Gastric Tuberculosis

Stomach involvement by TB is exceedingly rare because of lack of lymphoid tissue in stomach, acidic environment and rapid emptying of gastric contents. Usually, spread of infection is via the hematogenous route or secondary to adjacent involved lymph nodes. Symptoms are very nonspecific like epigastric discomfort, vomiting and weight loss which can be seen in other diseases. Imaging features are usually nonspecific and depend on the nature of involvement. They are usually focal and commonly involve the antropyloric region of stomach. Ulcerative type can present with ulcer which can be seen on barium studies as a benign ulcer whereas the hypertrophic type can present with gross wall thickening which can mimic carcinoma or lymphoma. Stricture due to fibrosis can also be seen in the antropyloric region which can mimic CD. Occasionally, the entire stomach may be involved showing diffuse wall thickening and contracted stomach giving an appearance of linitis plastica. Diagnosis is usually confirmed on biopsy since the imaging features are not conclusive.

Esophageal Tuberculosis

Esophageal TB is a rare entity and it is usually secondary to adjacent mediastinal or pulmonary involvement. Tuberculous involvement of adjacent lymph node or vertebral body can spread to esophagus which is the commonest mode of spread.[29] Patients usually present with odynophagia, hematemesis and chest pain. Because of the close proximity with the lymph nodes, middle third of esophagus is the commonly involved site. Barium studies can show subtle findings such as ulcerations and mucosal irregularity. In advanced stages it may show stricture, traction diverticulum and sinus formation. Occasionally, there can be fistulous communication with the tracheobronchial tree. CT scan is more reliable in showing

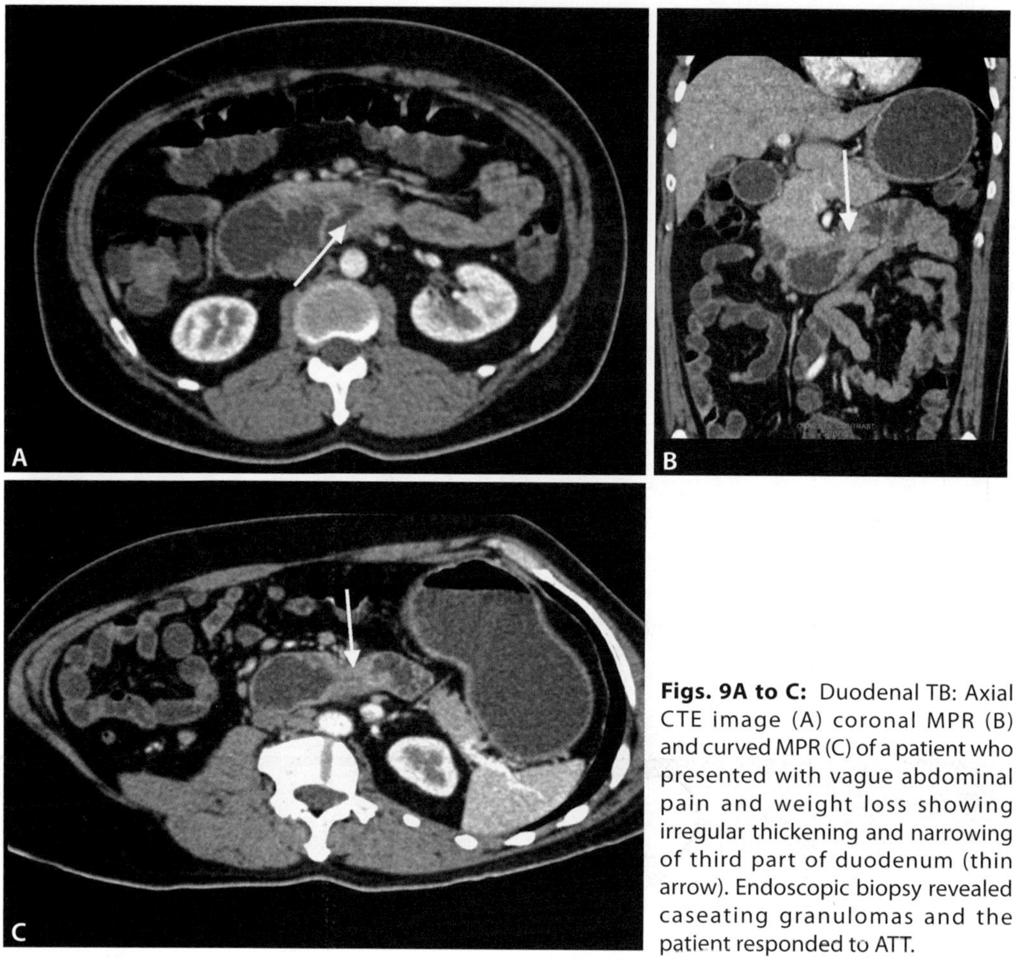

Figs. 9A to C: Duodenal TB: Axial CTE image (A) coronal MPR (B) and curved MPR (C) of a patient who presented with vague abdominal pain and weight loss showing irregular thickening and narrowing of third part of duodenum (thin arrow). Endoscopic biopsy revealed caseating granulomas and the patient responded to ATT.

the extraluminal findings and associated mediastinal and lung disease. It can closely mimic carcinoma esophagus because of which endoscopic sampling is necessary in almost all cases.

Extraintestinal Tuberculosis of Abdomen

Extraintestinal manifestation of TB can often be seen as associated findings in patients with GI TB. The salient features of extraintestinal TB will be covered briefly in this chapter.

Peritoneal Tuberculosis

Peritoneum is the most common location in the abdomen for involvement by TB, however, isolated involvement is relatively rare.[31] Most of the times it occurs in association with other sites of involvement. Involvement of peritoneum, mesentery and omentum are grouped under peritoneal TB. Spread of infection is either from rupture of involved lymph nodes or direct extension across the bowel wall. Peritoneal involvement manifests as thickening of the peritoneum (2–6 mm) with or without associated nodules. On USG the peritoneal thickening is seen as hypoechoic lesions and on CECT it is seen as smooth or nodular peritoneal thickening and enhancement. Contrast MRI may show the same features better mainly because of its superior contrast resolution and diffusion weighted MRI can also delineate this well. Ascites which can be either free or loculated is also a manifestation of peritoneal TB which can be seen in around 30–100% of patients.[32] USG is very sensitive in detecting ascites and also characterizing its nature. It is superior to CT in showing the septations and debris within the fluid. Usually high density ascites is seen in TB, but the density of ascites can range from water attenuation to high attenuation, depending on the amount of fibrin content and cellular debris.[33] Apart from characterizing ascites, imaging can also help in guiding aspiration of ascitic fluid for biochemical analysis. Tuberculous ascites usually shows low serum ascites albumin gradient (SAAG <1.1 g/dL) and elevated levels of adenosine deaminase (ADA) and lymphocytes. There are three types of peritoneal involvement based on the amount of ascites and associated features **(Figs. 10A to C)**:

1. Wet type—most common type, gross free or loculated ascites.
2. Fibrotic-fixed type—less common, with matted bowel loops, mesenteric masses and loculated ascites.
3. Dry-plastic type—rare, nodular dense fibrotic reaction of peritoneum.

Sclerosing encapsulating peritonitis (SEP) or cocoon is another manifestation of peritoneal TB in which a part or entire bowel loops or abdominal viscera is encapsulated by a fibrocollagenous membrane.[34] Barium studies may show clumping of bowel loops with or without obstructive features and CT scan show the membrane itself as a thick enhancing structure around the bowel loops **(Fig. 7)**. The other causes of SEP are chronic ambulatory peritoneal dialysis, ventriculoperitoneal shunts, sarcoidosis, gastrointestinal malignancies, etc.

Mesentery is frequently involved by TB and the appearance on imaging may be mild fat stranding, thickening, nodularity, diffuse infiltration or abscess formation.[31] Like mesentery, omental involvement may also show various imaging features. It may show a smudged, nodular thickening or caking of which smudged appearance is the most common type of involvement in TB **(Figs. 10A to C)**. Omental caking is a nonspecific finding and can be seen more commonly in peritoneal carcinomatosis.[31] CT scan is the preferred modality to evaluate the omental involvement and recently diffusion weighted MRI is also being evaluated in omental pathologies.[35]

Lymph Nodal TB

Mesenteric, omental, peripancreatic, periportal and upper retroperitoneal lymph nodes are commonly involved in TB **(Figs. 11 and 12)**. It is because these nodes are the regional draining sites for small bowel

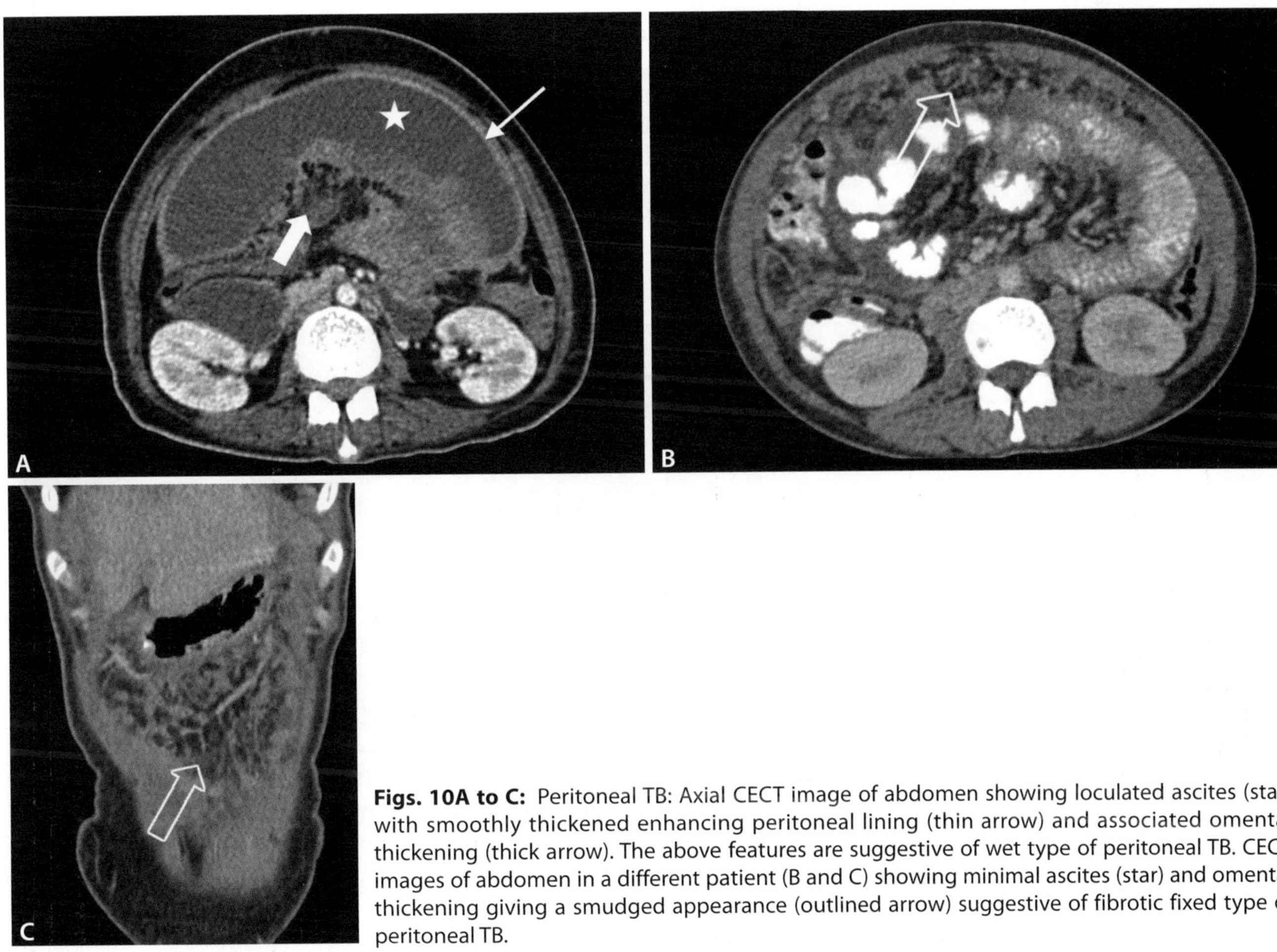

Figs. 10A to C: Peritoneal TB: Axial CECT image of abdomen showing loculated ascites (star) with smoothly thickened enhancing peritoneal lining (thin arrow) and associated omental thickening (thick arrow). The above features are suggestive of wet type of peritoneal TB. CECT images of abdomen in a different patient (B and C) showing minimal ascites (star) and omental thickening giving a smudged appearance (outlined arrow) suggestive of fibrotic fixed type of peritoneal TB.

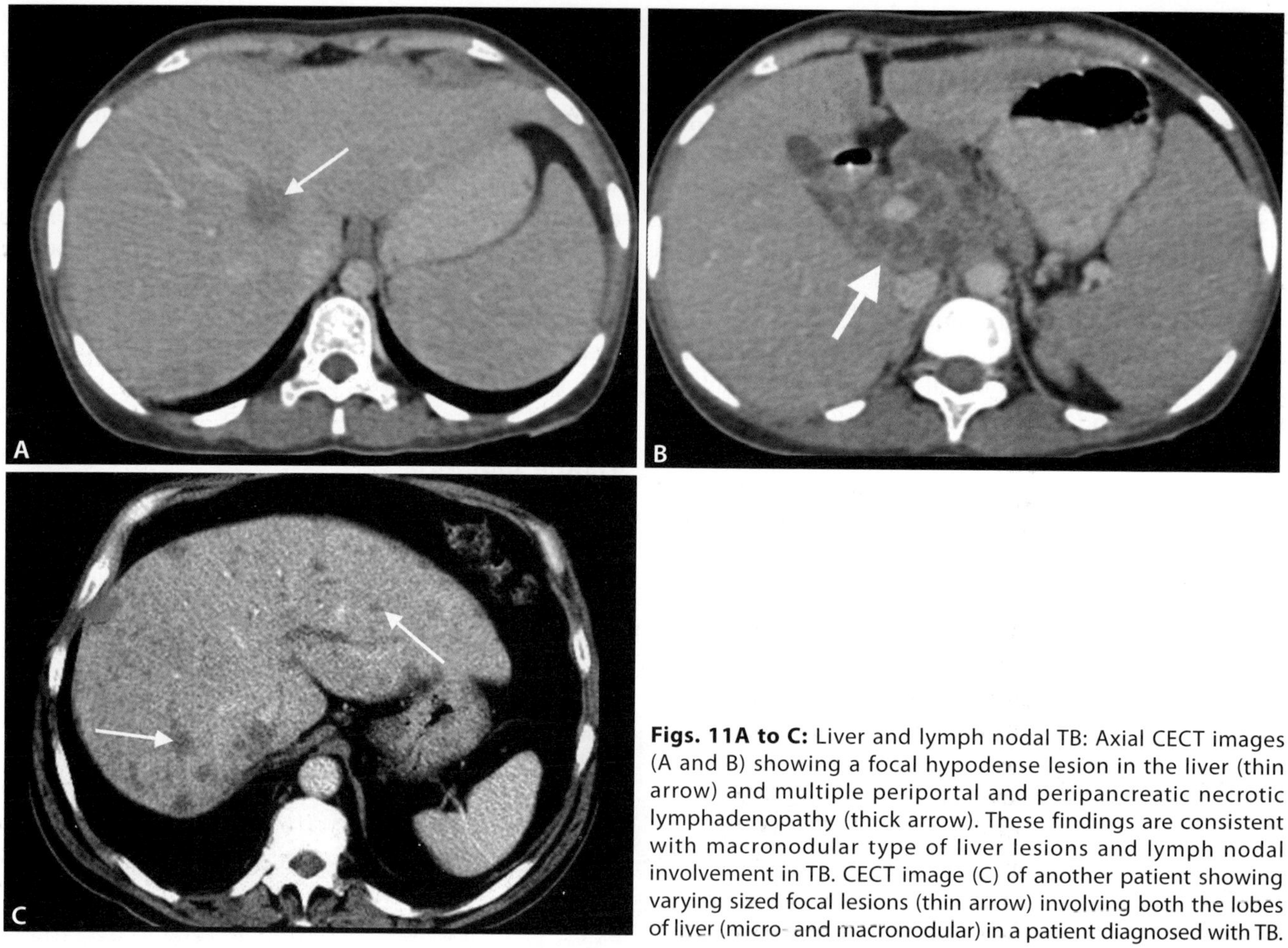

Figs. 11A to C: Liver and lymph nodal TB: Axial CECT images (A and B) showing a focal hypodense lesion in the liver (thin arrow) and multiple periportal and peripancreatic necrotic lymphadenopathy (thick arrow). These findings are consistent with macronodular type of liver lesions and lymph nodal involvement in TB. CECT image (C) of another patient showing varying sized focal lesions (thin arrow) involving both the lobes of liver (micro- and macronodular) in a patient diagnosed with TB.

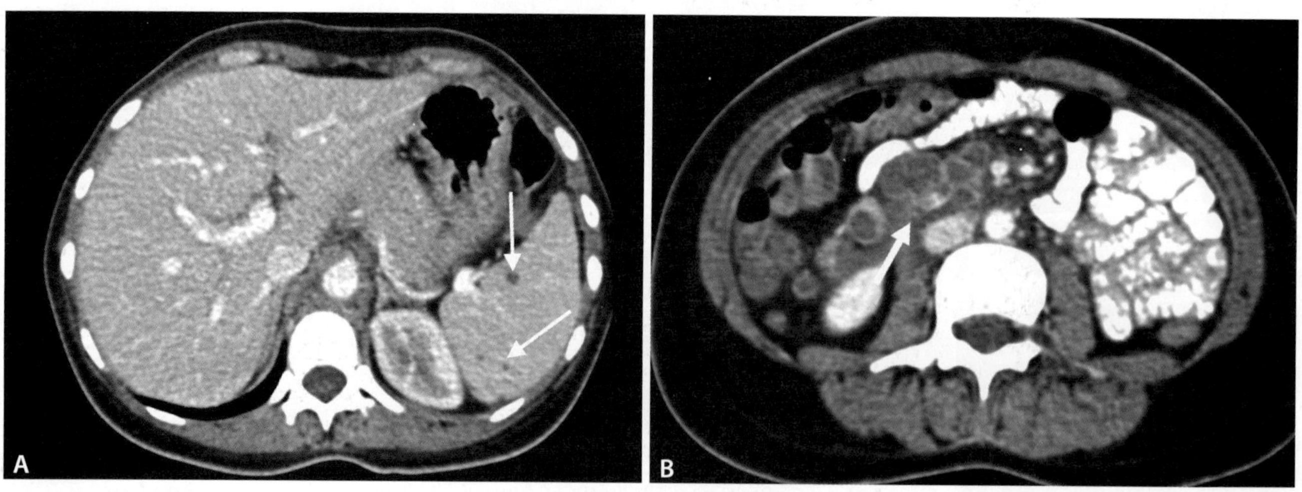

Figs. 12A and B: Splenic and lymph nodal TB: Axial CECT images of abdomen showing multiple hypodense lesions in the spleen (thin arrows) and multiple enlarged mesenteric lymph nodes which are showing peripheral enhancement and central necrosis (thick arrow). This patient responded to ATT confirming the diagnosis.

loops and proximal colon which are the common areas of involvement by TB.[33,36] The appearance of lymph node on imaging may vary depending on the stage of the disease. Enlarged lymph node with peripheral enhancement and central necrosis is the commonest type of appearance and is relatively specific for TB **(Figs. 11 and 12)**. However, central necrosis can be seen in malignancies, aggressive lymphoma and Whipple's disease.[36,37] Other less common appearances are homogeneous, heterogeneous or non-enhancement of the involved node. The nodes in TB tend to be matted and conglomerated because of periadenitis. Multiple normal-sized lymph nodes can also be a manifestation of TB, however not specific to TB. During the healing process the nodes can become smaller in size and become calcified. Enlargement of nodes, necrosis and calcification can be seen on both USG and CECT scan of which CT scan can provide a comprehensive evaluation of disease. Both can be used to guide sampling from the abnormal lymph nodes when imaging features are not conclusive. Enlarged nodes are seen as T1 hypointense and T2 hyperintense lesions on MRI. Necrosis and liquefaction in the center are seen as T2 hyperintensity within the node.

Visceral Solid Organ TB

Visceral organs such as liver, spleen and pancreas can be involved by TB and the usual route of spread is hematogenous.

Hepatosplenic TB

Hepatosplenic TB usually occurs as a part of military TB and it is found in 80–100% of patients with miliary TB according to an autopsy series.[30] However, diagnosis on antemortem imaging is quite unusual. Hepatosplenic TB can manifest as micronodular or macronodular type **(Fig. 11)**. In micronodular type the lesions are tiny and often they are less than the resolving ability of routine imaging. Diffuse enlargement of liver and spleen may be the only manifestation of this type. Sometimes, with high resolution USG images these micronodular lesions can be visualized as hypoechoic lesions. In this regard, USG is superior to CT scan. Other differential diagnoses for this type are sarcoidosis, metastasis, fungal infection and lymphoma. In the macronodular type, lesions are usually 1-3 cm in size and they are seen as hypoechoic lesions on USG and hypoenhancing lesions on CECT **(Figs. 11 and 12)**. These nodular lesions are hypointense on T1W scans and hyperintense on T2W scans. DWI can also help in detecting these lesions as they show restriction of diffusion. To start with these lesions may be solid and as the disease progresses they become liquefied and the imaging appearance changes accordingly. They get calcified during the healing phase and in patients with compromised immunity the lesions can progress in size and can become an abscess.

Pancreatic TB

Pancreatic TB is very rare and only few cases are reported in literature. It is thought to be because of the pancreatic juice which provides protection against the tubercle bacilli.[39] The most common site of involvement is the head of pancreas. There are three types of patterns described which are diffuse, focal and multifocal. Lesions can be seen as heterogeneously hypoechoic on USG and heterogeneously hypodense mass lesion on CT scan. Calcification can also be seen in some lesions which can be used to differentiate from pancreatic carcinoma. There may be enlarged lymph nodes with necrosis seen in the vicinity of the pancreas. None of these features are diagnostic for TB and it is usually difficult to differentiate tuberculous lesion from carcinoma pancreas or other inflammatory mass lesions. Most often the diagnosis is apparent only after sampling or after surgical resection. However, recently there have been efforts to differentiate these lesions using CT pancreatic perfusion.[39] There is limited role of MRI in these patients and it can be used to differentiate it from cystic neoplasms of pancreas.

INFLAMMATORY BOWEL DISEASE

Inflammatory bowel disease comprises a group of bowel disorders characterized by idiopathic chronic inflammation of bowel. It includes mainly Crohn's disease and ulcerative colitis. Majority of the times based on the clinical and imaging features it is possible to classify these disorders into one of these two entities. However, in a small subset it is not possible to categorize them accurately and they are grouped as indeterminate colitis or inflammatory bowel disease unclassified. There is another entity called microscopic colitis which is distinctly different from Crohn's disease and ulcerative colitis and can present with chronic watery diarrhea.[40] Microscopic colitis which includes collagenous colitis and lymphocytic colitis usually has normal appearance on colonoscopy and imaging. Inflammation can only be seen on microscopy and hence the name microscopic colitis.

Crohn's Disease

Earlier Crohn's disease (CD) was considered to be a disease of the west and thought to be uncommon in India. Only few cases were reported in the past from India and this was due to the fact that the clinical and imaging features of CD closely resemble TB which is endemic here. Diagnosing CD with reasonable certainty was difficult under those circumstances. However, in the recent years with the improvement in sanitation standards coupled with better understanding of disease and advancements in the field of imaging have led to increase in the detection of CD.[41] The true incidence of CD in India is still not clear because of sparse data availability.

Crohn's disease is a transmural granulomatous inflammatory process of the bowel wall characterized by waxing and waning course and discontinuous involvement of the bowel, which can be complicated by fistulae and abscesses. It can affect any part of the GI tract, from the oral cavity to the anus, often involving multiple discontinuous segments. Small intestine involvement is seen in 70% of cases, most commonly at the terminal ileum and colonic involvement can be seen in up to 50% of which exclusive colonic involvement is seen in 15–20% of patients.[42] Patients present with pain abdomen, diarrhea, low grade fever and easy fatigability. Fecal calprotectin is a reliable marker of bowel inflammation but is nonspecific as far as the etiology of inflammation is concerned and can be elevated in GI TB also.

Imaging is an integral part of the evaluation for CD and it provides vital luminal and extraluminal information. Often imaging can differentiate active inflammatory CD from fibrostenotic CD which is in fact one of the main purposes of imaging in these patients apart from diagnosis and evaluating the extent of disease and its complications. The above differentiation is of paramount importance because the management for these two stages is very different. Active CD is managed by medical treatment whereas fibrostenotic CD may need surgical management.

Many attempts have been made to standardize the classification and scoring of severity of the disease. Montreal classification is one of these which is widely used in clinical practice and research to describe the disease phenotype in CD **(Table 2)**.[43] It describes the type, extent and behavior of disease and studies have proven the reliability of the classification.[44–46] Crohn's Disease Activity Index (CDAI) is another widely used tool for scoring the disease severity which can be used to prognosticate CD and is useful in the follow-up of these patients.[47,48] Score of less than 150 is considered as remission of disease and score of more than 450 is considered as severe disease.

Table 2: Montreal classification of Crohn's disease.

Age at diagnosis (A)	
A1	16 years or younger
A2	17–40 years
A3	More than 40 years
Location (L)	
L1	Terminal ileum
L2	Colon
L3	Ileocolon
L4	Upper GI
Behavior (B) p-modifier for perianal disease, added as suffix to B	
B1	Nonstricturing, nonpenetrating
B2	Stricturing
B3	Penetrating

Imaging Features of Crohn's Disease

Imaging features of CD vary with the stage of disease process and the associated complications. Broadly, on imaging CD can be classified into four morphological subtypes:[49]

1. Active inflammatory subtype
2. Fibrostenotic subtype
3. Fistulising or perforating subtype
4. Reparative or regenerative subtype.

Double contrast barium enteroclysis was the imaging modality of choice before the emergence of cross sectional modalities like CTE and MRE. It is the best modality to show the aphthous ulcers seen in the active phase of disease as punctate collection of barium with surrounding radiolucent halo due to mucosal edema. When the disease progresses, the ulcers coalesce and form deep linear ulceration separating out the edematous mucosa **(Fig. 2)**. This is seen on barium studies as cobble-stoning. Later, the mesenteric border shortens due to fibrosis with formation of pseudosacculation along the antimesenteric border **(Fig. 2)**. Stenosis of the bowel loop with or without proximal dilatation and complications like bowel fistulization or contained perforation can also be seen on barium studies. In spite of the ability of double contrast barium to show the mucosal changes in great detail, the extraluminal changes of CD are not well evaluated for which the cross sectional modalities are better. In current practice barium studies are not routinely done for the diagnosis or follow up of CD. It may be done for few niche indications such as demonstration of aphthous ulcers, cobble-stoning of mucosa and fistula formation.[50] Ideal imaging modality for the evaluation of CD is CTE or MRE and the diagnostic performance of both the modalities are comparable for the detection of CD.[51–53] The choice between the two techniques depends largely on the local availability of equipment and expertise and few other clinical considerations. The radiation hazard involved in CTE and ability of MRE in differentiating active and fibrotic disease tilts the balance towards MRE in appropriate clinical scenario. When CD is suspected in a child or patient is being evaluated for response to treatment or follow-up imaging or there is suspicion of fistula, MRE is better than CTE. However, when CD is suspected in an elderly patient or clinical suspicion of CD is low or a diagnosis other than CD is suspected, CTE may be preferred over MRE because it is faster, reliable, relatively resistant to artifacts and gives consistent image quality.

Thickening of Bowel Wall

Bowel wall thickening is the most common finding in patients with CD **(Figs. 13 and 14)**. It is usually symmetrical and circumferential, most commonly involving the terminal ileum and the ileocecal junction. Often in CD, the degree of involvement of ileum is more than that of cecum.[54] Thickening of bowel wall is a nonspecific finding which can occur in both active inflammatory and fibrostenotic disease. In a distended bowel, wall thickness of more than 3 mm is abnormal. Single shot FSE or postcontrast sequence on MRE are the optimal sequences to look for wall thickening. This finding has high sensitivity and specificity in the range of 83–91% and 86–100%, respectively.[55] Wall thickening may reduce during the remission phase but, usually there will be some residual thickening compared to the normal segment. One pitfall of this finding is that bowel wall may apparently look thick when the bowel is collapsed. One should be careful not to label collapsed bowel loop as wall thickening.

Submucosal Edema

Submucosal edema leads to wall thickening and is usually seen as hypodense area on CTE and hyperintense area on T2 weighted sequence with or without fat suppression **(Figs. 13 to 15)**. Submucosal edema is a sign of active disease.

Bowel Wall Contrast Enhancement

Contrast enhancement of the involved segment can occur both in active inflammatory disease and in fibrostenotic phase. It is considered to be the earliest and the most sensitive sign for active CD.[56] It has been shown to correlate with the level of inflammation on histopathology. At the same time absence of abnormal enhancement almost excludes disease activity in CD.[57] Potential pitfalls in contrast enhancement are that the normal jejunal enhancement is more than ileal enhancement and collapsed bowel loops can show apparently increased enhancement. One should be aware of these pitfalls to avoid misinterpretation. There are three types of enhancement patterns described in CD–stratified, mucosal and homogeneous enhancement. Of the above types stratified bowel wall enhancement (target like) is specific for active inflammatory phase **(Figs. 13 and 15)**. Homogeneous enhancement is nonspecific and can be seen in both active and fibrotic phases **(Figs. 16 and 17)**. It is also known that often fibrosis and active inflammation can coexist and can present as varying features on imaging

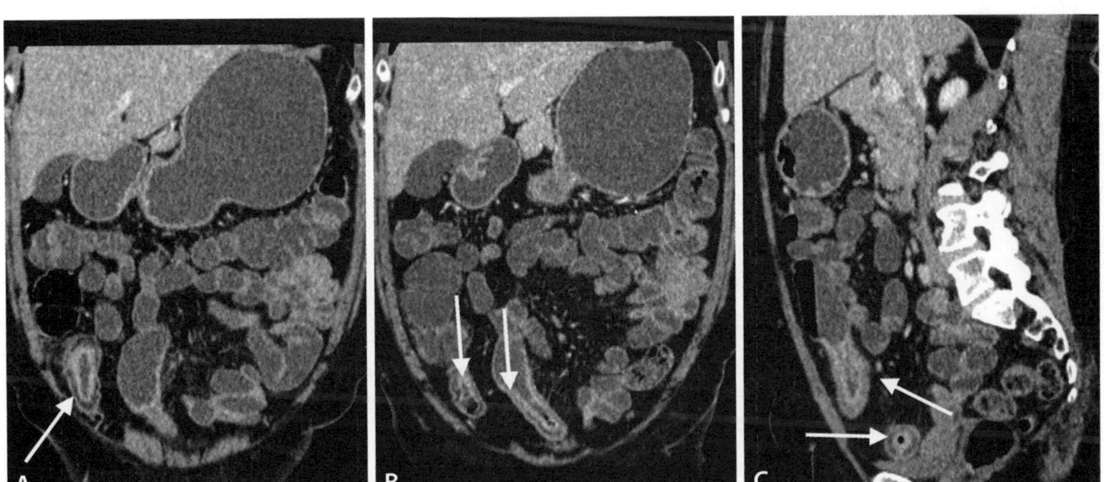

Figs. 13A to C: Stratified wall enhancement in active CD: Coronal CTE images (A and B) and sagittal MPR (C) showing thickening and stratified wall enhancement involving the ileal loops (thin arrow) which is a sign of active inflammatory stage of CD.

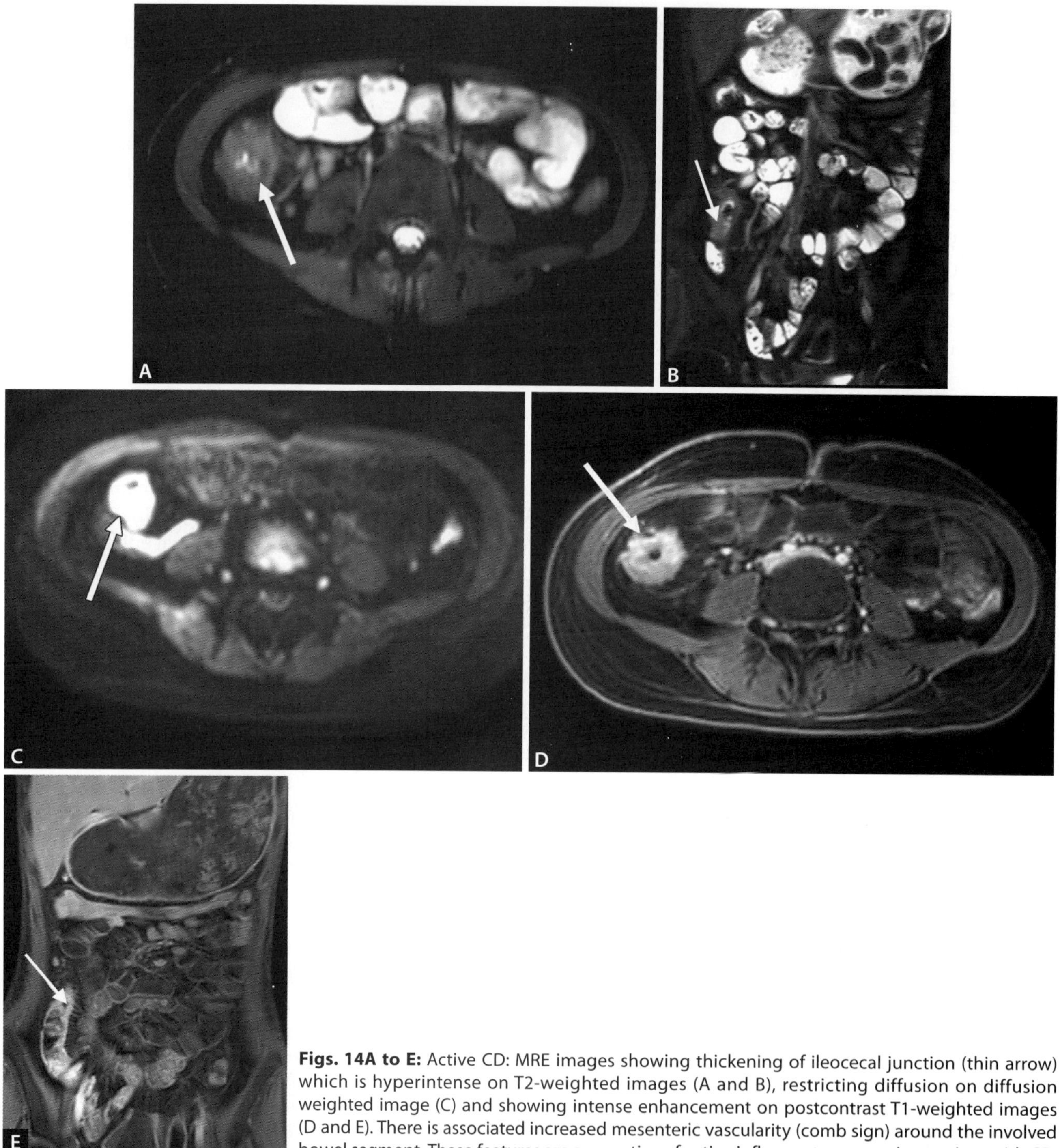

Figs. 14A to E: Active CD: MRE images showing thickening of ileocecal junction (thin arrow) which is hyperintense on T2-weighted images (A and B), restricting diffusion on diffusion weighted image (C) and showing intense enhancement on postcontrast T1-weighted images (D and E). There is associated increased mesenteric vascularity (comb sign) around the involved bowel segment. These features are suggestive of active inflammatory stage in a patient with CD.

(Figs. 18A to C). One promising alternative for contrast enhancement is diffusion weighted imaging in which the hyperintensity on trace images corresponds with active inflammation **(Fig. 14)**.[58] This technique is useful in patients where contrast cannot be administered for reasons like deranged renal parameters.

Submucosal Fat Infiltration

In patients with chronic inflammation there can be fat deposition in the submucosa which can appear markedly hypodense on CTE and loses signal on fat saturated sequences on MRE.[59,60] Although it is a nonspecific sign, the presence of submucosal fat infiltration in CD suggests chronicity.

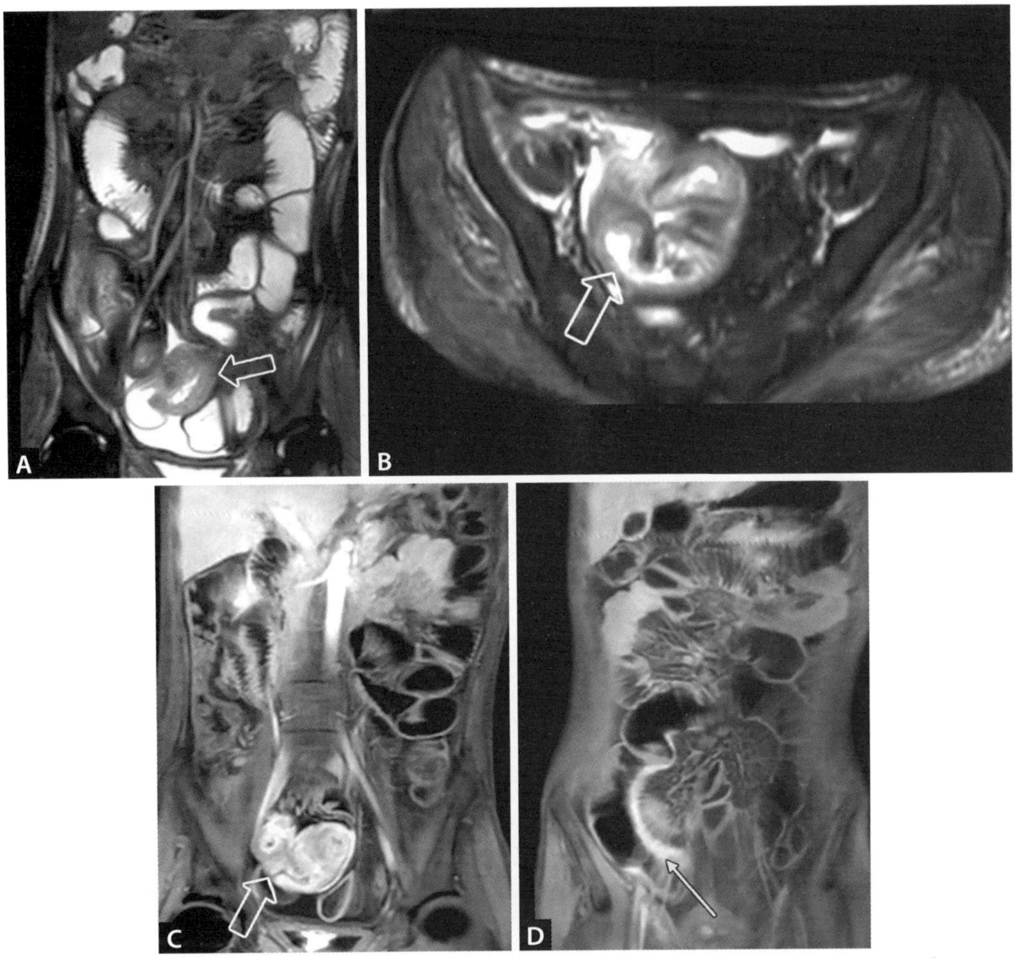

Figs. 15A to D: Active CD: Coronal MRE (A) and axial T2-weighted images (B) showing segmental wall thickening of a pelvic ileal loop (outlined arrow) which is showing T2 hyperintensity (A and B). Coronal postcontrast images (C and D) show stratified mural enhancement, asymmetrical wall thickening involving the mesenteric border of terminal ileum with intense enhancement (thin arrow). These findings are typical for active inflammatory stage of CD.

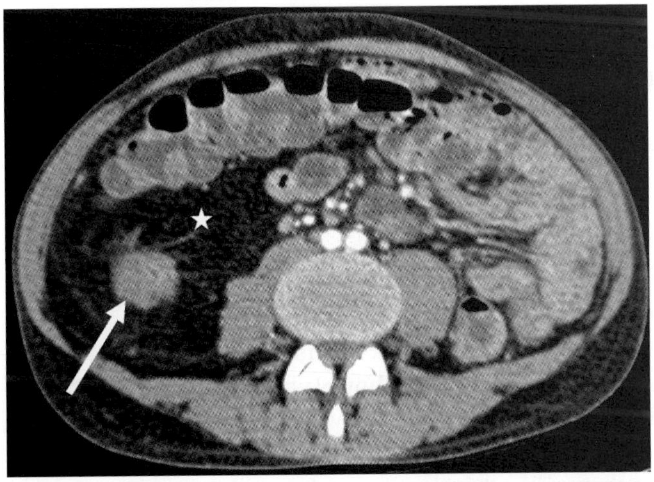

Fig. 16: Fat proliferation: Axial CTE image showing thickening of ascending colon (thin arrow) with surrounding fat proliferation (star). Minimal enhancement of the involved segment coupled with fat proliferation is suggestive of chronic fibrotic stage of CD.

Fibrosis

Recognising fibrosis on imaging is crucial for the management of CD because those patients are often considered for surgery as they are unlikely to benefit from medical therapy.[61] Fibrosis is a result of chronic inflammation which has a nonspecific appearance on CTE. MRE has an edge over CTE in this regard as fibrosis manifests as hypointensity on both T1 and T2-weighted images and shows progressive homogeneous enhancement in delayed phase **(Figs. 16 to 18)**.

Skip Lesions

This is defined as multifocal areas of involvement with normal healthy bowel in between. It is considered as an important sign to differentiate CD from other infective processes like TB but is not very specific.

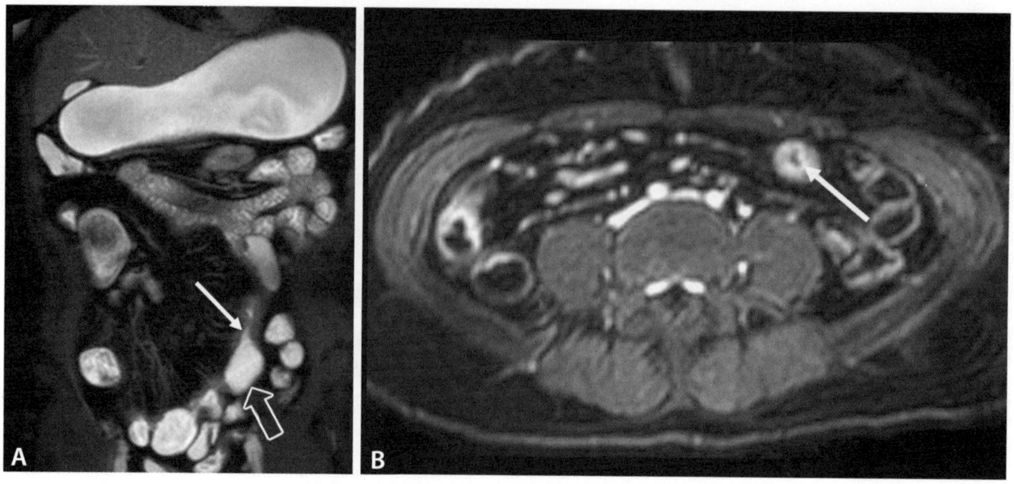

Figs. 17A and B: Pseudosacculations in fibrotic CD: Coronal T2-weighted image (A) of MRE study showing wall thickening and multiple segments of luminal narrowing involving the ileal loops (thin arrow). There are multiple pseudosacculations seen in the antimesenteric border (outlined arrow). Axial postcontrast T1 weighted image (B) shows homogeneous wall enhancement of the involved loop. The above imaging features are characteristic of fibrostenotic stage of CD.

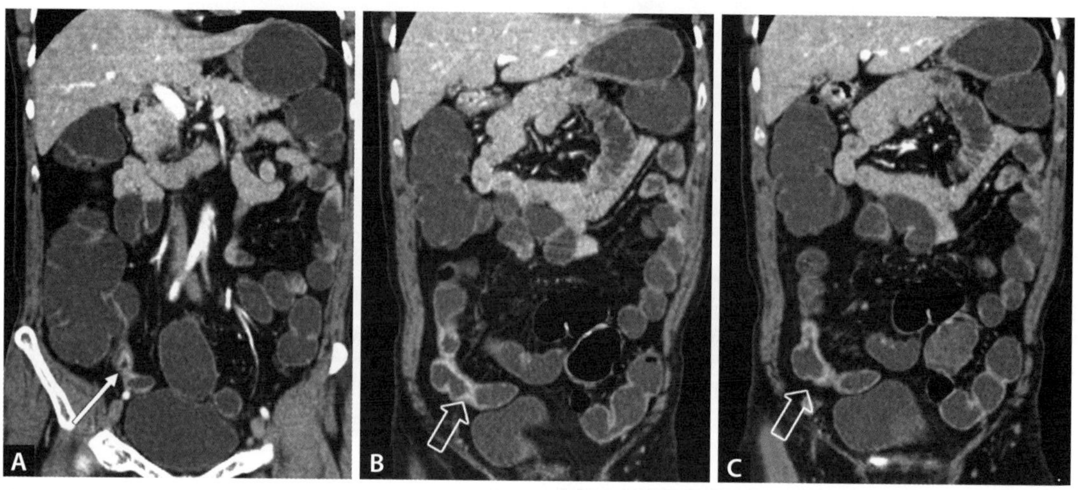

Figs. 18A to C: Coexisting active and chronic CD: Coronal CTE images (A to C) showing hyperenhancement with mural stratification (thin arrow) and pseudosacculation involving the antimesenteric border of distal ileum (outlined arrow). Mural stratification is a sign of active inflammatory stage whereas pseudosacculation is a sign of chronic CD.

Stenosis of Bowel Wall

Bowel wall narrowing in CD can be because of active inflammation leading to spasm or due to chronic fibrostenosing disease. This differentiation can sometimes be difficult based on imaging because of overlapping features. Presence of stratified enhancement, wall edema and ulcerations favor active inflammation whereas prestenotic dilated bowel loop indicate a chronic process.

Comb Sign

Comb sign is a manifestation of prominent vasa recta due to increase in vascularity in the mesentery. It is regarded as one of the specific signs of active inflammation **(Figs. 14 and 19)**. This is best seen on TruFISP (BTFE) and postcontrast sequences.

Mesenteric Edema

It is due to inflammation and resultant edema in the mesentery secondary to bowel wall inflammation. It is also considered as a sign of active inflammation. It is seen as increased attenuation on CTE (mesenteric fat stranding) and increased intensity on fat saturated T2-weighted sequences. In severe cases minimal free fluid can also be seen.

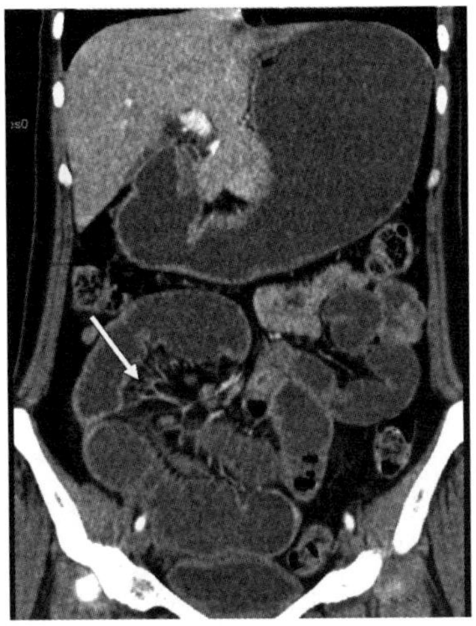

Fig. 19: Comb sign in active CD: Coronal CTE image showing a segment of dilated ileal loop with increased mesenteric vascularity (comb sign) (thin arrow) in a patient with CD. Presence of comb sign is a marker of active inflammatory stage of CD.

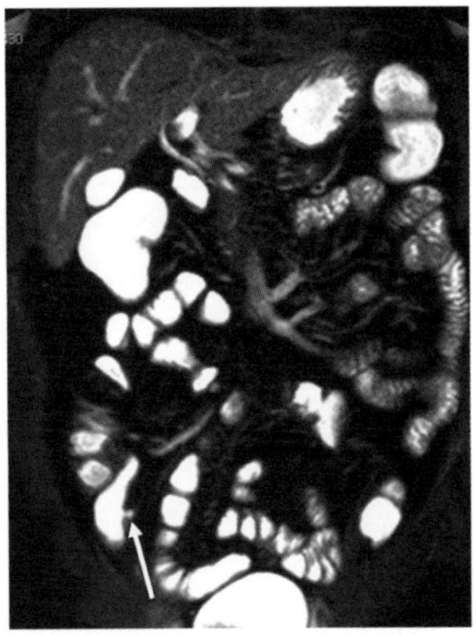

Fig. 20: Deep ulcer on CD: T2-weighted coronal image of MRE showing hyperintense outpouching (thin arrow) in the distal ileal loop suggestive of deep ulceration in a patient with CD.

Ulcerations

Ulcerations which are considered as a sign of active disease are sometimes seen on imaging especially on MRE when the loops are adequately distended **(Fig. 20)**. It may be seen as irregularity of the wall or thin linear hyperintensity extending into the wall. In a recent study, using high resolution MRE images, the sensitivity in detecting the mucosal features has been found to be in the range of 69–99% for superficial ulcers and 94–99% for deep ulcers.[62]

Abnormal Motility

Abnormal bowel motility is a known feature of active CD and sometimes it can be the early sign of disease. It can be classified into different patterns as follows:[63]

- Paralysis—when the involved segment does not show peristalsis
- Hypomotility—when the involved segment shows decreased motility
- Hypermotility—when the involved segment shows increased motility
- Intraluminal pendular movement—inefficient to and fro movement of bowel content.

The movement of the involved bowel loop is compared with the surrounding normal loops for any abnormality. If there is any abnormal movement of a segment, it has to be carefully studied in the other sequences on MRE to confirm the abnormality. Cine MR imaging which can be done as a part of MRE is the best way to evaluate bowel movement and it is found to increase the detection rate of lesions compared to standard MRE sequences.[63]

Abscesses, Sinuses and Fistulas

Abscesses, sinuses and fistulae developing in a patient with CD are considered as major complications and are also a sign of active disease. Abscesses are seen as hypodense lesion on CTE and hyperintense on T2-weighted sequences on MRE with the wall showing postcontrast enhancement. Sinuses and fistulae are seen as linear enhancing structures beyond the confines of bowel loop on CTE and MRE. In CD, there can be blind sinuses extending from the bowel wall, enteroenteric, enterocolonic, enterovesical, enterocutaneous or perianal fistula. A stellate configuration of bowel loops (star sign) which are adherent to each other is suggestive of enteroenteric fistula **(Fig. 21)**. The diagnosis of this entity has a bearing on management and may be an indication for initiating treatment with Infliximab. The sensitivity and specificity of CTE and MRE in detecting sinuses and fistulas is around 83% and 100% respectively.[60] However, MRE performs better in the diagnosis and evaluation of the extent of perianal fistulae in relation to the internal and external sphincters **(Figs. 22A to D)**.[64,65]

Pseudodiverticulum Formation

This sign is a result of asymmetrical fibrosis and shortening of the mesenteric border leading to apparent sacculations along the antimesenteric border. It is usually seen in chronic CD and associated with other features of chronic disease **(Figs. 2, 17 and 18)**.

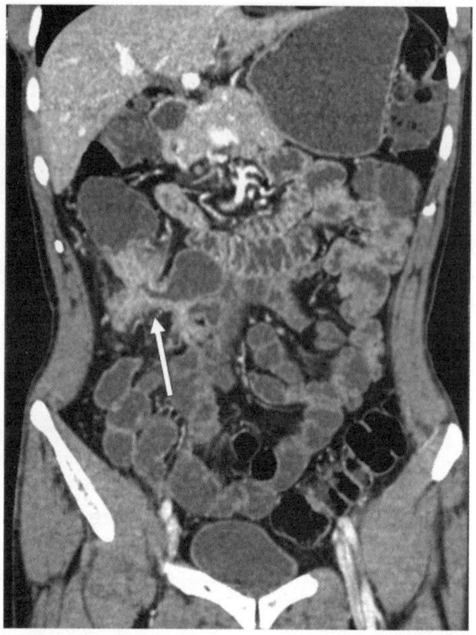

Fig. 21: Fistulizing stage of CD: Coronal CTE image showing abnormal thickening, distorted stellate configuration and communication between the small bowel loop and the ascending colon (thin arrow) suggestive of enterocolic fistula.

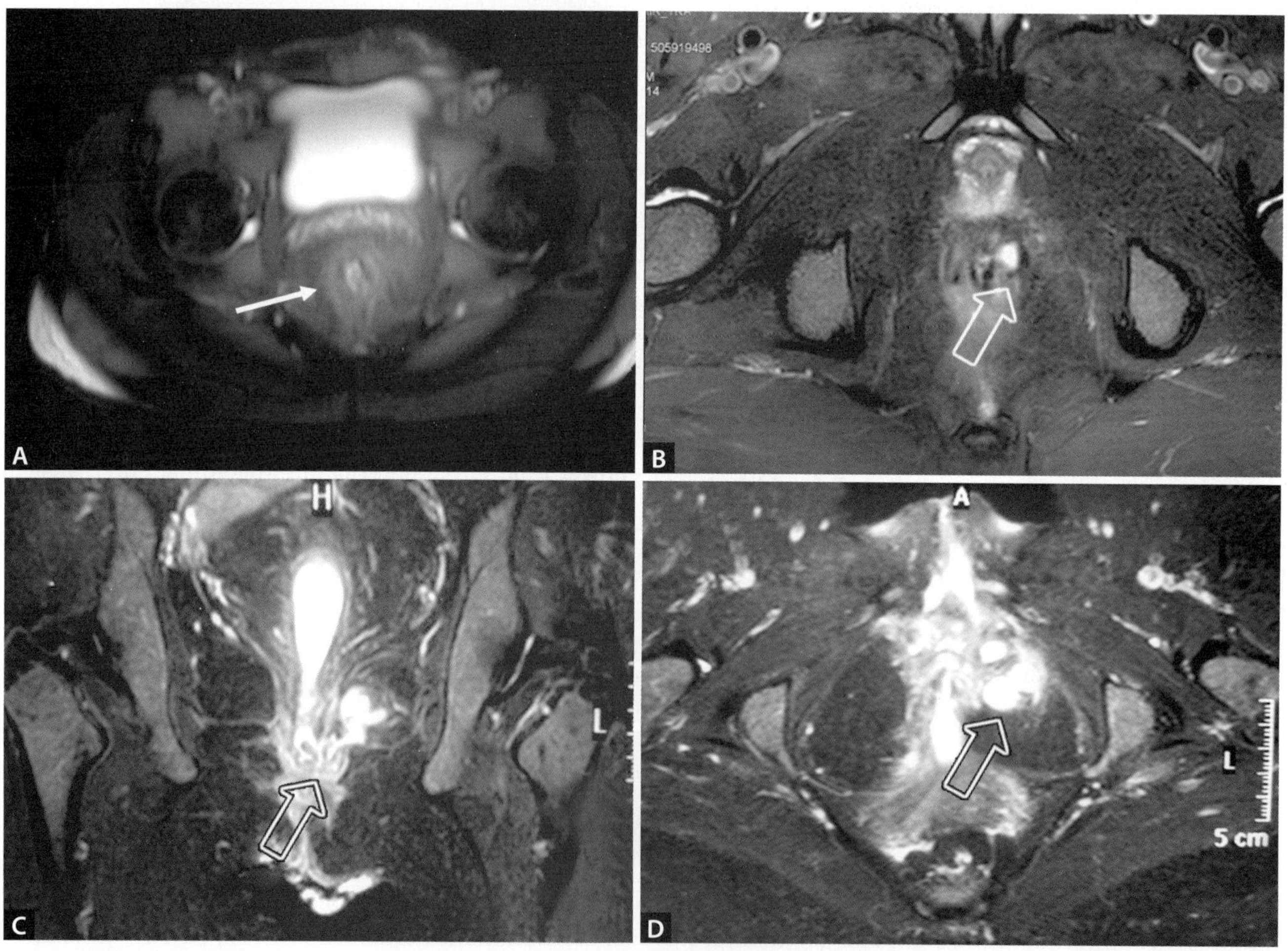

Figs. 22A to D: Perianal fistulas: T2-weighted MR images (A and B) of a patient with rectal involvement by CD (thin arrow) showing a small fistulous tract (outlined arrow) arising from the anal canal. T2-weighted images (C and D) of a different patient showing more complex fistulous tract and collections (outlined arrow) in left ischioanal fossa. Presence of fistula or sinus tract is a marker of active inflammatory stage in CD.

Fibrofatty Proliferation

It is seen in long standing CD as a result of chronic inflammation in bowel loops. It is seen as increased fat surrounding the involved bowel loops on all imaging modalities **(Fig. 16)**. This is a nonspecific finding and may be seen in any cause of chronic inflammation.

Reactive Lymphadenopathy

In India, enlarged regional lymph nodes with bowel wall thickening occur more commonly in TB. However, enlarged lymph nodes can occur in patients with CD also. However, lymph nodes in CD are usually less than 1cm in size. Mesenteric lymphadenopathy in CD is a nonspecific finding which can occur in both active and inactive disease. There is some evidence that the increased degree of nodal enhancement favors active disease in CD.[66]

Most of the features of CD described above are almost similar on CTE and MRE. Abnormalities such as submucosal edema, submucosal fat infiltration and fibrosis may appear as nonspecific hypoattenuation on CTE whereas they are more accurately characterized on MRE. The imaging features and their significance in differentiating active from fibrotic disease are listed in **Table 3**.

Imaging Features to Differentiate Intestinal TB from CD

Intestinal TB and CD have many features in common and their differentiation is difficult. This poses a greater problem in countries like India where TB is common and endemic. There is no single test which can reliably differentiate intestinal TB from CD. Hence a combination of clinical, endoscopic, imaging, histopathology and biochemical features should be used. Sometimes follow-up imaging and even a trial of anti-tuberculous therapy may be required to differentiate between them. Imaging is an important tool which is used routinely and the common imaging features used to differentiate both the entities are summarized in the **Table 4**.

Ulcerative Colitis

Ulcerative colitis (UC) is a characterized by superficial inflammation involving the colon. The colonic involvement in UC is symmetric and contiguous. Rectum is involved in almost all cases with varying length of proximal colonic involvement sometimes involving the entire colon (pancolitis).[67] Occasionally, terminal ileum can be affected and becomes edematous and dilated when the entire colon is involved and is called backwash ileitis. UC is well evaluated with colonoscopy and imaging is seldom used.

The earliest finding of UC on imaging is seen on double contrast barium enema (DCBE) as diffuse granular appearance of the mucosa because of inflammation and edema. This leads to thickening of wall and haustral folds. As the disease progresses to the submucosa, collar button ulcers develop. Collar button ulcers are not specific for UC because they can occur in other inflammatory diseases. In chronic disease, the colon shows narrowing and shortening and loses its haustral folds appearing featureless which is referred as lead pipe sign **(Figs. 23A and B)**.[68] When the mucosa gets denuded, residual mucosal mounds can develop into inflammatory pseudopolyps. Severe cases can be associated with backwash ileitis which may be seen as fixed and patulous ileocecal valve with dilated terminal ileum and granular appearance of mucosa. Because of chronic inflammation there may be increased presacral fat. One of the dreaded complication of UC is toxic megacolon which manifests as colonic dilatation more than 6 cm, thinning of wall and loss of haustrations. Plain radiography is usually diagnostic and barium studies are generally contraindicated because of the risk of perforation.

CT scan show the extraluminal changes of UC such as localized perforation, abscess, etc. CT is not sensitive in showing the early mucosal changes of UC. Inflamed bowel shows thickening and may show mural stratification. In chronic stage there may be narrowing of colon, alteration of haustral pattern and submucosal fat infiltration which can also be seen on CT. Narrowing of colon is usually because of benign strictures, however if there is asymmetry or

Table 3: Imaging features to differentiate active inflammatory from fibrostenotic disease in CD.

Active disease	*Fibrotic stage*	*Nonspecific*
• Submucosal edema • Early hyperenhancement • Stratified enhancement of wall • Comb sign • Mesenteric edema • Ulcerations • Abnormal motility • Abscesses, sinuses and fistulas	• Late progressive and homogeneous wall enhancement • Submucosal fatty infiltration • Fibrosis • Pseudodiverticulum • Fibrofatty proliferation	• Bowel wall thickening • Skip lesions • Bowel stenosis • Reactive lymphadenopathy

Table 4: Imaging features to differentiate GI TB and CD.

Imaging features	***Intestinal TB***	***CD***
Site of involvement	Cecum more than ileum	Ileum more than cecum
Length of involvement	Shorter segment	Longer segment
Multiple site involvement	Uncommon	Common
Skip lesions	Rare	Common
Type of wall enhancement	Homogeneous	Stratified
Mural stratification of wall	Rare	Common
Perianal fistula	Uncommon	Common
Mesenteric abscess	Very rare	Relatively common
Bowel fistulas	Rare	Relatively common
Strictures	Concentric	Eccentric with sacculations
Enteroliths	More common	Less common
Increased mesenteric vascularity	Uncommon	Common
Fibrofatty proliferation	Uncommon	Common
Mesenteric nodes	Large and necrotic	Small and homogeneous
Omental involvement	Often seen	Rare
Ascites	Frequent	Uncommon
Solid organ involvement	Relatively common	Very rare

Source: Modified and reproduced with permission from Sharma R, et al. Intestinal tuberculosis versus Crohn's disease: Clinical and radiological recommendations. Indian J Radiol Imaging. 2016;26(2):161-72.

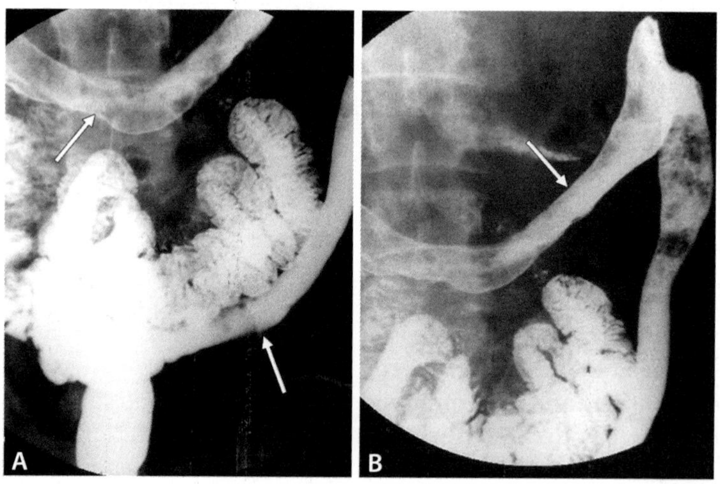

Figs. 23A and B: Lead pipe sign in chronic UC. Barium study images (A and B) of a patient with ulcerative colitis showing diffuse luminal narrowing and loss of haustrations (thin arrow) involving the entire colon without any skip areas. This featureless appearance of colon in chronic UC is known as lead pipe sign.

eccentric thickening with focal loss of mural stratification, malignancy developing in UC should be suspected. The overall risk of developing malignancy in UC is 3.7% and in CD is around 2.9%.[69,70] Pericolonic fat proliferation is much better seen on CT scan rather than on conventional modalities.[67,68] Pericolonic fatty proliferation or creeping fat around the colon occurs more frequently in CD as compared to UC.[71,72] MRI is not routinely used for the evaluation of UC but it can show most of the features which are seen on CT scan. USG is an emerging technique for bowel evaluation which can show bowel wall thickening and mural stratification.

MISCELLANEOUS DISEASES

This category includes radiation enteritis, NSAID enteropathy, eosinophilic enteritis, etc. which will be discussed in brief.

Radiation Enteritis

Radiation enteritis occurs as a result of toxic effects of radiation (usually more than 3000cGy) to the bowel wall and to the vasculature. Radiation effects can be acute, subacute or chronic depending on the time of onset of manifestations after radiation therapy. Acute stage occurs within 2 months whereas subacute and chronic stages occur after 2 months and 12 months respectively. In the acute phase, imaging may show spasm and edema of the involved bowel loops which can mimic other inflammatory conditions.[73] However, in radiation enteritis the involvement is limited to the irradiated area **(Fig. 24)**. In chronic stage there may be wall thickening, narrowing, ulceration and fat proliferation around the bowel. History of radiation and the area of involvement is the key to differentiate from other inflammatory diseases.

NSAIDs Enteropathy

Nonsteroidal anti-inflammatory drugs (NSAID) are one of the commonly prescribed drugs worldwide. They cause alterations in the protective mechanism of gut by affecting prostaglandin synthesis. It can affect the esophagus, stomach and small bowel and cause local complications. In esophagus and stomach it can cause multiple tiny mucosal erosions which may be seen on barium studies as focal collection of barium with surrounding halo due to edema around.[74,75] In the small bowel it can cause focal ulcers with associated wall edema in the acute phase. When the disease progress to chronic phase it can lead to ulcer and circumferential stricture which are typically thin and membrane like (mucosal diaphragm). They can cause bowel obstruction and lead to proximal bowel dilatation. Mucosal diaphragms are not specific to NSAID enteropathy because they can occur in other inflammatory diseases like CD.[74]

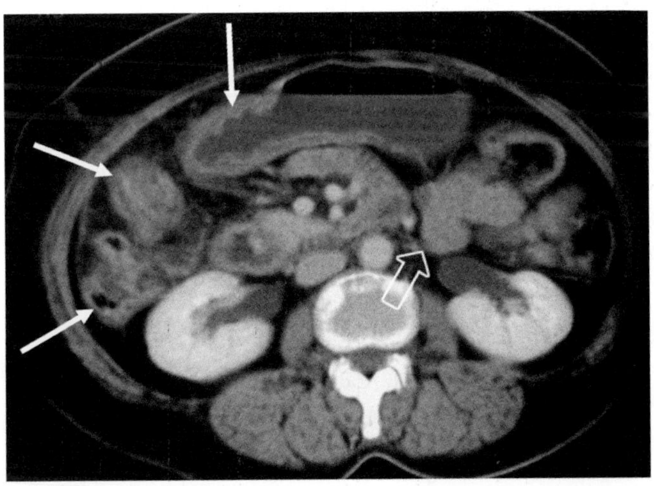

Fig. 24: Acute radiation enteritis. Axial CECT image of a patient who received radiotherapy for carcinoma gallbladder showing thickening of bowel loops with mural stratification and surrounding fat stranding (thin arrow) which are confined to the irradiated area. The bowel loops outside the irradiated area (outlined arrow) appear normal. These features are typical for acute radiation enteritis.

Eosinophilic Gastroenteritis

Eosinophilic gastroenteritis is a relatively uncommon entity which is characterized by patchy or diffuse infiltration of eosinophils in the bowel wall.[76] Majority of these patients have peripheral eosinophilia. Clinical features are nonspecific such as pain abdomen, vomiting or diarrhea. Gastric antrum is the most common site of involvement, however, it can also affect the duodenum and small bowel. It leads to mucosal fold thickening and submucosal infiltration which can be visualized on barium studies and CT scan. As the clinical and imaging features are nonspecific, the index of suspicion should be high to diagnose this condition and presence of peripheral eosinophilia is an important indicator.

CONCLUSION

In India where TB is endemic, it is often difficult to differentiate intestinal TB from CD only on the basis of clinical features. Imaging is an integral part of management of these patients and it can help in differentiating these two entities. A judicious combination of clinical, imaging, endoscopic and histological features should be used. Imaging also has an important role in the follow-up of these patients to look for complications and response to therapy. Hence, it is imperative for the radiologist to be aware of the imaging features so as to correctly diagnose these diseases and to avoid mismanagement.

REFERENCES

1. Maglinte DDT, Kelvin FM, O'Connor K, Lappas JC, Chernish SM. Current status of small bowel radiography. Abdom Imaging. 1996;21(3):247-57.
2. Nijhawan S, Kumpawat S, Mallikarjun P, Bansal RP, Singla D, Ashdhir P, et al. Barium meal follow through with pneumocolon: Screening test for chronic bowel pain. World J Gastroenterol WJG. 2008;14(43):6694.

3. Bender GN, Timmons JH, Williard WC, Carter J. Computed tomographic enteroclysis: one methodology. Invest Radiol. 1996;31(1):43-9.
4. Paulsen SR, Huprich JE, Fletcher JG, Booya F, Young BM, Fidler JL, et al. CT enterography as a diagnostic tool in evaluating small bowel disorders: review of clinical experience with over 700 cases. Radiographics. 2006;26(3):641-57.
5. Solem CA, Loftus EV, Fletcher JG, Baron TH, Gostout CJ, Petersen BT, et al. Small-bowel imaging in Crohn's disease: a prospective, blinded, 4-way comparison trial. Gastrointest Endosc. 2008;68(2):255-66.
6. Ha AS, Levine MS, Rubesin SE, Laufer I, Herlinger H. Radiographic Examination of the Small Bowel: Survey of Practice Patterns in the United States. Radiology. 2004;231(2):407-12.
7. Ilangovan R, Burling D, George A, Gupta A, Marshall M, Taylor SA. CT enterography: review of technique and practical tips. Br J Radiol. 2012;85(1015):876-86.
8. Mettler FA, Huda W, Yoshizumi TT, Mahesh M. Effective doses in radiology and diagnostic nuclear medicine: A catalog. Radiology. 2008;248(1):254-63.
9. Makanyanga JC, Taylor SA. Current and future role of MR enterography in the management of Crohn disease. Am J Roentgenol. 2013;201(1):56-64.
10. Kiryu S, Dodanuki K, Takao H, Watanabe M, Inoue Y, Takazoe M, et al. Free-breathing diffusion-weighted imaging for the assessment of inflammatory activity in Crohn's disease. J Magn Reson Imaging. 2009;29(4): 880-86.
11. Oto A, Zhu F, Kulkarni K, Karczmar GS, Turner JR, Rubin D. Evaluation of diffusion-weighted MR imaging for detection of bowel inflammation in patients with Crohn's disease. Acad Radiol. 2009;16(5):597-603.
12. Oto A, Kayhan A, Williams JT, Fan X, Yun L, Arkani S, et al. Active Crohn's disease in the small bowel: evaluation by diffusion-weighted imaging and quantitative dynamic contrast-enhanced MR imaging. J Magn Reson Imaging. 2011;33(3):615-24.
13. Oussalah A, Laurent V, Bruot O, Bressenot A, Bigard MA, Régent D, et al. Diffusion-weighted magnetic resonance without bowel preparation for detecting colonic inflammation in inflammatory bowel disease. Gut. 2010;59(8):1056-65.
14. Chiorean L, Schreiber-Dietrich D, Braden B, Cui XW, Buchhorn R, Chang JM, et al. Ultrasonographic imaging of inflammatory bowel disease in pediatric patients. World J Gastroenterol. 2015;21(17):5231-41.
15. Levine A, Koletzko S, Turner D, Escher JC, Cucchiara S, De Ridder L, et al. ESPGHAN revised porto criteria for the diagnosis of inflammatory bowel disease in children and adolescents. J Pediatr Gastroenterol Nutr. 2014;58(6):795-806.
16. Dietrich CF, Cui XW, Schreiber-Dietrich DG, Ignee A. EFSUMB guidelines 2011: comments and illustrations. Ultraschall Med-Eur J Ultrasound. 2012;33(S 01):S11–S21.
17. Dietrich CF. Comments and illustrations regarding the guidelines and good clinical practice recommendations for contrast-enhanced ultrasound (CEUS)–update 2008. Ultraschall Med-Eur J Ultrasound. 2008;29(S 04):188-202.
18. WHO | Global tuberculosis report 2015 [Internet]. WHO. [cited 2015 Nov 6]. Available from: *http://www.who.int/tb/publications/global_report/en/*.
19. Sircar S, Taneja VA, Kansra U. Epidemiology and clinical presentation of abdominal tuberculosis: a retrospective study. J Indian Med Assoc. 1996;94(9):342-4.
20. Marshall JB. Tuberculosis of the gastrointestinal tract and peritoneum. Am J Gastroenterol. 1993;88(7):989-99.
21. Sood R. Diagnosis of abdominal tuberculosis: role of imaging. J Indian Acad Clin Med. 2001;2(3):169-77.
22. Sharma MP, Bhatia V. Abdominal tuberculosis. Indian J Med Res. 2004;120(4):305-15.
23. Balthazar EJ, Gordon R, Hulnick D. Ileocecal tuberculosis: CT and radiologic evaluation. AJR. 1990;154(3):499-503.
24. Gulati MS, Sarma D, Paul SB. CT appearances in abdominal tuberculosis. A pictorial essay. Clin Imaging. 1999;23(1):51-9.
25. Ramesh J, Banait GS, Ormerod LP. Abdominal tuberculosis in a district general hospital: a retrospective review of 86 cases. QJM Mon J Assoc Physicians. 2008;101(3):189-95.
26. Carrera GF, Young S, Lewicki AM. Intestinal tuberculosis. Abdom Imaging. 1976;1(1):147-55.
27. Krishna S, Kalra N, Singh P, Kochhar R, Gupta R, Singh R, et al. Small-bowel tuberculosis: A comparative study of MR enterography and small-bowel follow-through. Am J Roentgenol. 2016;207(3):571-7.
28. Thoeni RF, Margulis AR. Gastrointestinal tuberculosis. In: Seminars in roentgenology [Internet]. Elsevier; 1979 [cited 2015 Sep 2]. p. 283-94. Available from: http://www.sciencedirect.com/science/article/pii/0037198X79900257.
29. Chong VH, Lim KS. Gastrointestinal tuberculosis. Singapore Med J. 2009;50(6):638-45; quiz 646.
30. Chavhan GE, Ramakantan R. Duodenal tuberculosis: radiological features on barium studies and their clinical correlation in 28 cases. J Postgrad Med. 2003;49(3):214-7.
31. da Rocha EL, Pedrassa BC, Bormann RL, Kierszenbaum ML, Torres LR, D'Ippolito G. Abdominal tuberculosis: a radiological review with emphasis on computed tomography and magnetic resonance imaging findings. Radiol Bras. 2015;48(3):181-91.
32. Akhan O, Pringot J. Imaging of abdominal tuberculosis. Eur Radiol. 2002;12(2):312-23.
33. Leder RA, Low VH. Tuberculosis of the abdomen. Radiol Clin North Am. 1995;33(4):691-705.
34. Jayant M, Kaushik R. Abdominal cocoon in a young man. World J Emerg Med. 2014;5(3):234-6.
35. Foti PV, Attinà G, Spadola S, Caltabiano R, Farina R, Palmucci S, et al. MR imaging of ovarian masses: classification and differential diagnosis. Insights Imaging. 2015;7(1):21-41.
36. Yang ZG, Min PQ, Sone S, He ZY, Liao ZY, Zhou XP, et al. Tuberculosis versus lymphomas in the abdominal lymph nodes: evaluation with contrast-enhanced CT. Am J Roentgenol. 1999;172(3):619-23.
37. Li DK, Rennie CS. Case Report Abdominal Computed Tomography in Whipple's Disease. J Comput Assist Tomogr. 1981;5(2):249-52.

38. Brauner M, Buffard MD, Jeantils V, Legrand I, Gotheil C. Sonography and computed tomography of macroscopic tuberculosis of the liver. J Clin Ultrasound. 1989;17(8):563-8.
39. Yadav AK, Nadrajah J, Kandasamy D, Sharma R, Gamanagatti S, Garg PK. Volume perfusion computed tomography as an aid to diagnosis of pancreatic tuberculosis. Trop Gastroenterol. 2015;35(4):264-6.
40. Bohr J, Wickbom A, Hegedus A, Nyhlin N, Hultgren Hörnquist E, Tysk C. Diagnosis and management of microscopic colitis: current perspectives. Clin Exp Gastroenterol. 2014;7:273-84.
41. Makharia GK. Rising incidence and prevalence of Crohn's disease in Asia: Is it apparent or real? J Gastroenterol Hepatol. 2006;21(6):929-31.
42. Yacoub JH, Oto A. New magnetic resonance imaging modalities for Crohn disease. Magn Reson Imaging Clin N Am. 2014;22(1):35-50.
43. Silverberg MS, Satsangi J, Ahmad T, Arnott IDR, Bernstein CN, Brant SR, et al. Toward an integrated clinical, molecular and serological classification of inflammatory bowel disease: report of a Working Party of the 2005 Montreal World Congress of Gastroenterology. Can J Gastroenterol J Can Gastroenterol. 2005;19 Suppl A:5A–36A.
44. Spekhorst LM, Visschedijk MC, Alberts R, Festen EA, van der Wouden E-J, Dijkstra G, et al. Performance of the Montreal classification for inflammatory bowel diseases. World J Gastroenterol WJG. 2014;20(41):15374-81.
45. Dassopoulos T, Nguyen GC, Bitton A, Bromfield GP, Schumm LP, Wu Y, et al. Assessment of reliability and validity of IBD phenotyping within the National Institutes of Diabetes and Digestive and Kidney Diseases (NIDDK) IBD Genetics Consortium (IBDGC). Inflamm Bowel Dis. 2007;13(8):975-83.
46. Krishnaprasad K, Andrews JM, Lawrance IC, Florin T, Gearry RB, Leong RWL, et al. Interobserver agreement for Crohn's disease sub-phenotypes using the Montreal Classification: How good are we? A multicenter Australasian study. J Crohns Colitis. 2012;6(3):287-93.
47. Best WR, Becktel JM, Singleton JW, Kern F. Development of a Crohn's disease activity index. National Cooperative Crohn's Disease Study. Gastroenterology. 1976;70(3):439-44.
48. Peyrin-Biroulet L, Panés J, Sandborn WJ, Vermeire S, Danese S, Feagan BG, et al. Defining disease severity in inflammatory bowel diseases: Current and future directions. Clin Gastroenterol Hepatol. 2016;14(3):348-54.e17.
49. Maglinte DD, Gourtsoyiannis N, Rex D, Howard TJ, Kelvin FM. Classification of small bowel Crohn's subtypes based on multimodality imaging. Radiol Clin North Am. 2003;41(2):285-303.
50. Marshak RH. Granulomatous Disease of the Intestinal Tract (Crohn's Disease): Annual Oration in Honor of Benjamin H. Orndoff, MD, 1881-1971. Radiology. 1975;114(1):3-22.
51. Grand DJ, Beland MD, Machan JT, Mayo-Smith WW. Detection of Crohn's disease: comparison of CT and MR enterography without anti-peristaltic agents performed on the same day. Eur J Radiol. 2012;81(8):1735-41.
52. Lee SS, Kim AY, Yang SK, Chung JW, Kim SY, Park SH, et al. Crohn Disease of the Small Bowel: Comparison of CT Enterography, MR Enterography, and Small-Bowel Follow-Through as Diagnostic Techniques. Radiology. 2009;251(3):751-61.
53. Siddiki HA, Fidler JL, Fletcher JG, Burton SS, Huprich JE, Hough DM, et al. Prospective comparison of state-of-the-art MR enterography and CT enterography in small-bowel Crohn's disease. Am J Roentgenol. 2009;193(1):113-21.
54. Sharma R, Madhusudhan KS, Ahuja V. Intestinal tuberculosis versus crohn's disease: Clinical and radiological recommendations. Indian J Radiol Imaging. 2016;26(2):161-72.
55. Constantino CPL, Rodrigues RS, Neto JAO, Marchiori E, Araujo ALE, de Mello Perez R, et al. Computed Tomography and Magnetic Resonance Enterography Findings in Crohn's Disease: What Does the Clinician Need to Know From the Radiologist? Can Assoc Radiol J. 2014;65(1):42-51.
56. Fidler JL, Guimaraes L, Einstein DM. MR Imaging of the Small Bowel. Radiographics. 2009;29(6):1811-25.
57. Lawrance IC. Correlation of MRI-determined small bowel Crohn's disease categories with medical response and surgical pathology. World J Gastroenterol. 2009;15(27):3367.
58. Buisson A, Joubert A, Montoriol PF, Ines DD, Hordonneau C, Pereira B, et al. Diffusion-weighted magnetic resonance imaging for detecting and assessing ileal inflammation in Crohn's disease. Aliment Pharmacol Ther. 2013;37(5):537-45.
59. Elsayes KM, Al-Hawary MM, Jagdish J, Ganesh HS, Platt JF. CT Enterography: Principles, Trends, and Interpretation of Findings 1. Radiographics. 2010;30(7):1955-70.
60. Sinha R, Verma R, Verma S, Rajesh A. MR enterography of Crohn disease: part 2, imaging and pathologic findings. Am J Roentgenol. 2011;197(1):80-85.
61. Van Assche G, Dignass A, Panes J, Beaugerie L, Karagiannis J, Allez M, et al. The second European evidence-based Consensus on the diagnosis and management of Crohn's disease: Definitions and diagnosis. J Crohns Colitis. 2010;4(1):7-27.
62. Sinha R, Murphy P, Sanders S, Ramachandran I, Hawker P, Rawat S, et al. Diagnostic accuracy of high-resolution MR enterography in Crohn's disease: comparison with surgical and pathological specimen. Clin Radiol. 2013;68(9):917-27.
63. Froehlich JM, Waldherr C, Stoupis C, Erturk SM, Patak MA. MR motility imaging in Crohn's disease improves lesion detection compared with standard MR imaging. Eur Radiol. 2010;20(8):1945-51.
64. Haggett PJ, Moore NR, Shearman JD, Travis SP, Jewell DP, Mortensen NJ. Pelvic and perineal complications of Crohn's disease: assessment using magnetic resonance imaging. Gut. 1995;36(3):407-10.
65. Halligan S, Buchanan G. MR imaging of fistula-in-ano. Eur J Radiol. 2003;47(2):98-107.
66. Gourtsoyianni S, Papanikolaou N, Amanakis E, Bourikas L, Roussomoustakaki M, Grammatikakis J, et al. Crohn's disease lymphadenopathy: MR imaging findings. Eur J Radiol. 2009;69(3):425-8.

67. Roggeveen MJ, Tismenetsky M, Shapiro R. Best cases from the AFIP: Ulcerative colitis. Radiogr Rev Publ Radiol Soc N Am Inc. 2006;26(3):947-51.
68. Gore RM, Balthazar EJ, Ghahremani GG, Miller FH. CT features of ulcerative colitis and Crohn's disease. AJR. 1996;167(1):3-15.
69. Eaden JA, Abrams KR, Mayberry JF. The risk of colorectal cancer in ulcerative colitis: a meta-analysis. Gut. 2001;48(4):526-35.
70. Canavan C, Abrams KR, Mayberry J. Meta-analysis: colorectal and small bowel cancer risk in patients with Crohn's disease. Aliment Pharmacol Ther. 2006;23(8):1097-104.
71. Deepak P, Bruining DH. Radiographical evaluation of ulcerative colitis. Gastroenterol Rep. 2014;2(3):169-77.
72. Parente F, Greco S, Molteni M, Anderloni A, Bianchi Porro G. Imaging inflammatory bowel disease using bowel ultrasound. Eur J Gastroenterol Hepatol. 2005;17(3): 283-91.
73. Addley HC, Vargas HA, Moyle PL, Crawford R, Sala E. Pelvic imaging following chemotherapy and radiation therapy for gynecologic malignancies. Radiogr Rev Publ Radiol Soc N Am Inc. 2010;30(7):1843-56.
74. McGettigan MJ, Menias CO, Gao ZJ, Mellnick VM, Hara AK. Imaging of Drug-induced Complications in the Gastrointestinal System. Radiogr Rev Publ Radiol Soc N Am Inc. 2016;36(1):71-87.
75. Frye JM, Hansel SL, Dolan SG, Fidler JL, Song LMWK, Barlow JM, et al. NSAID enteropathy: appearance at CT and MR enterography in the age of multimodality imaging and treatment. Abdom Imaging. 2015;40(5):1011-25.
76. Baig MA, Qadir A, Rasheed J. A review of eosinophilic gastroenteritis. J Natl Med Assoc. 2006;98(10):1616-9.

CHAPTER 73

Imaging of Ischemic Bowel Disease

Ajay Gulati, Naveen Kalra, Mandeep Kang

INTRODUCTION

Ischemic bowel disease occurs due to impaired arterial supply and/or venous drainage of splanchnic circulation, resulting in ischemic injury and altered bowel metabolism. Ischemic bowel disease present as complex spectrum of disorders with variable imaging manifestations depending upon time of onset, duration, severity of ischemic injury; the segment and length of bowel affected; vessels affected and status of collateral blood flow circuits. Ischemia may be acute or chronic; may be arterial or venous in origin. Ischemia may involve the small bowel, large bowel or both segments resulting in *mesenteric ischemia*, *colonic ischemia* and *ischemic enterocolitis* respectively. Variability in the above factors not only affects the clinical scenario, but also influences the management options, outcome and prognosis.

Bowel ischemia has numerous causes and variable presentations. Frequently patients complain of nonspecific symptoms. Classic triad of *abdominal pain, pyrexia and frank blood in stool* history is elicited only in less than one-third of the patients. Majority of the patients present with vague clinical symptoms including diarrhea, vomiting and abdominal discomfort.[1] Laboratory work up is often non-specific and time consuming. In the present modern era with advancements in imaging techniques, radiologists play a pivotal role in evaluation of bowel ischemia *by making an accurate diagnosis, and helping in treatment planning along with vital prognostic information*, as they are able to characterize and delineate the disease process.

ANATOMY OF SPLANCHNIC CIRCULATION

Relevant abdominal vascular anatomy knowledge is essential to understand and evaluate bowel ischemia; knowing the normal vascular pattern and its common anatomic variants is helpful in angiogram assessment and appropriate endovascular treatment planning. Splanchnic circulation consists of arterial supply and their collateral system; and venous drainage alternatively called as portal venous system.

Arterial Supply

Three major trunks arising anteriorly from abdominal aorta, namely *celiac axis, superior mesenteric artery, and inferior mesenteric artery* provide arterial supply to intra-abdominal viscera.

Celiac Axis

Celiac axis arises from aorta at T12 vertebral level, supply foregut derivatives such as liver, pancreas, spleen and bowel from stomach to 2nd part of duodenum by branching into *common hepatic artery, left gastric artery and splenic artery*. The common hepatic artery gives off gastroduodenal artery, right gastroepiploic artery and anterior superior pancreaticoduodenal artery branches. The splenic artery branches into left gastroepiploic artery and pancreatic artery **(Fig. 1)**.

Superior Mesenteric Artery

Superior mesenteric artery (SMA) arises from abdominal aorta at L1 vertebral level, supply midgut derivatives, from

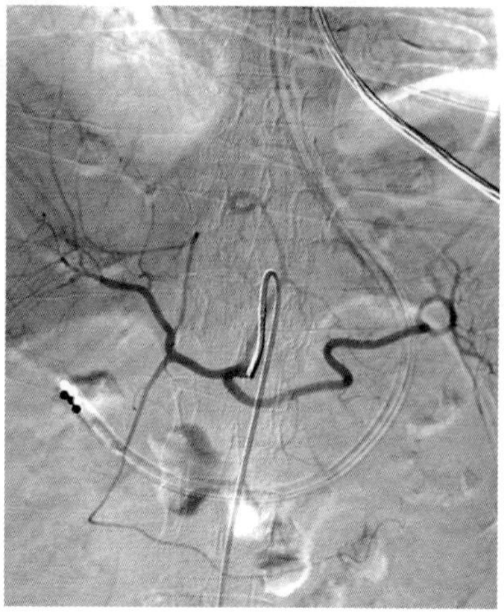

Fig. 1: Digital subtraction angiography (DSA) run of celiac axis trunk with its branches.

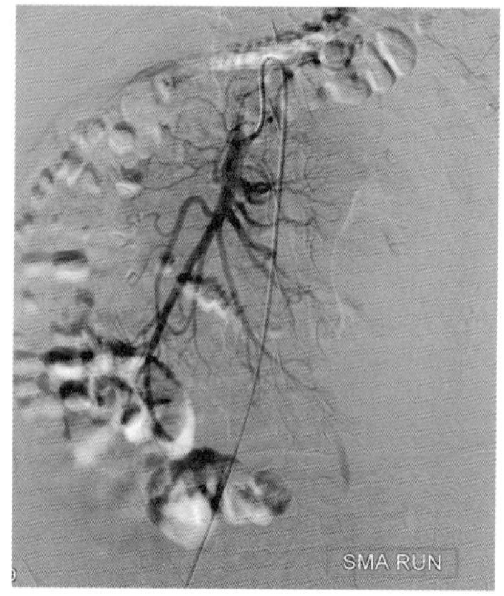

Fig. 2: DSA run showing superior mesenteric artery (SMA) and its branches.

2nd part of duodenum till middle third of transeverse colon. Anterior and posterior inferior pancreaticoduodenal arteries, middle colic artery, right colic artery, ileocolic artery and numerous jejunal and ileal arteries arise from superior mesenteric artery. All these branches contribute to form multiple vascular arcades, from which straight vessels perforate bowel wall **(Fig. 2)**.

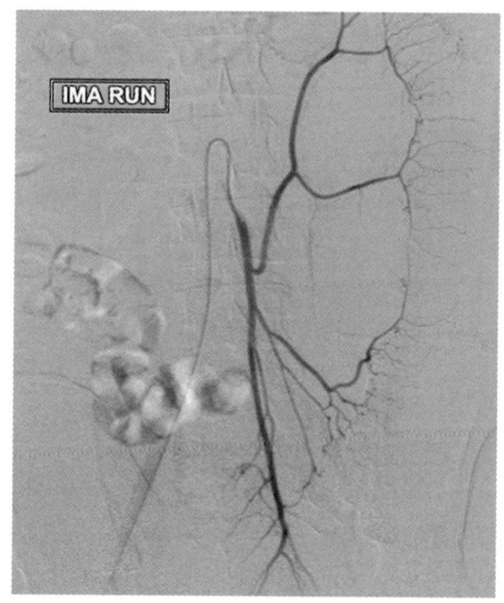

Fig. 3: DSA run showing inferior mesenteric artery (IMA) and its branches.

Inferior Mesenteric Artery

Inferior mesenteric artery (IMA) originates from anterior abdominal aorta at L3/L4 vertebral body level. Supply hindgut derivatives from distal third of transverse colon till proximal rectum, by left colic artery, sigmoidal arteries and superior rectal artery which are branched off from inferior mesenteric artery; distal rectum is supplied by hypogastric artery, which is a branch of internal iliac artery **(Fig. 3)**.

Collateral System

Abundant collateralization is seen between major mesenteric arterial trunks and the branches of mesenteric vascular arcades. These extensive collateral vessels are more conspicuous in the stomach, duodenum and rectum thereby accounting for inherent resistance to ischemia in these areas. The important collateral circuits:

- Pancreaticoduodenal arcade connecting celiac axis to superior mesenteric artery
- Marginal artery of Drummond
- Central anastomotic artery
- Arc of Riolan (aka the 'meandering mesenteric artery') are the potential conduits connecting superior mesenteric artery to inferior mesenteric artery **(Figs. 4A and B)**. Meandering artery connecting proximal middle colic artery of SMA with proximal left colic artery of IMA, may be visualized angiographically in presence of superior or inferior mesenteric artery occlusive pathology; hence it is essential to determine direction of blood flow within the meandering artery before dissecting any of the major mesenteric arteries.[1,2]

Portal Venous System

The small and large intestine is drained by superior and inferior mesenteric veins. Inferior mesenteric vein form common channel with splenic vein and join superior mesenteric vein (SMV) to form portal vein.

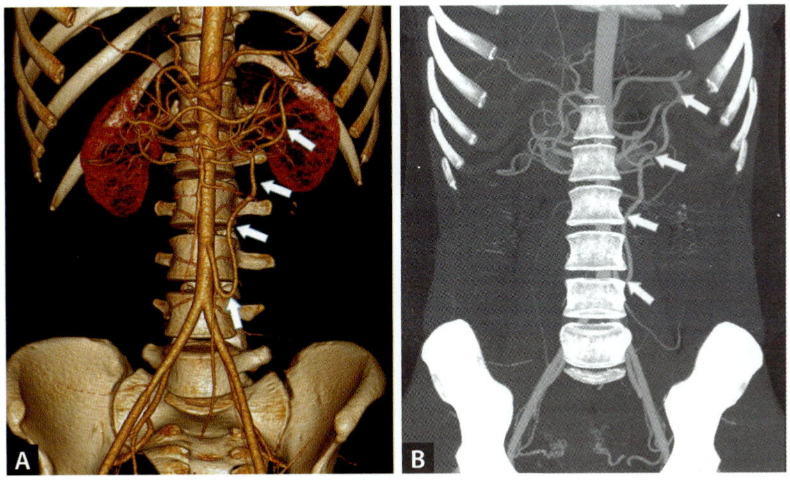

Figs. 4A and B: Coronal CT images (volume rendered and MIP) showing proximal superior mesenteric artery obstruction with arc of Riolan (arrows) reconstituting distal superior mesenteric artery (SMA) and its branches.

ETIOLOGY

Ischemic bowel disease is classified based on the time of presentation, anatomic segment of bowel involved and etiopathogenesis of disease **(Table 1)**.

PATHOPHYSIOLOGY OF ISCHEMIC BOWEL DISEASE

Ischemic injury deprives nutrition and oxygen supply necessary for cellular metabolism and their intactness. Collateral vessels are recruited after major vessel occlusion due to arterial pressure drop distal to the occlusion and provide alternate pathway to maintain the viability of the bowel. However, after critical period of time, persistence of ischemia causes development of vasoconstriction in the obstructed bed, elevating the arterial pressure and hampering the collateral flow. Arterial obstruction cause vasospasm with subsequent loss of cellular integrity, whereas venous ischemia causes blood column stasis with edema and subsequently reduced arterial blood flow causing mucosal cellular detachment. The common outcome in both these conditions is intestinal necrosis and peritonitis in its natural course. Persistent hypoxia or reperfusion injury plays a central role in setting and propagation of ischemic injury through oxidant free radical damage. It is essential to understand, differentiate and define the nature of vascular obstructive pathology radiologically, as the prognosis significantly differs with a mortality rate of 89% in the arterial occlusion and 11% in the venous obstruction.[4]

Understanding the ischemic pathology is important as the radiological findings correlate with extent of disease process as shown in **Table 2**.[4] The acute bowel ischemia

Table 1: Bowel ischemia types and etiology.[3]

A. Mesenteric ischemia	
1. *Acute*:	
i. Occlusive (80%) Occlusive arterial Occlusive venous (10–15%)	Thromboembolism Dissection/transection Closed loop obstruction Thrombophilia and hypercoagulable states Hypotension and shock
ii. Nonocclusive (20–30%)	Drugs (ergots/cocaine) Atherosclerotic disease
2. Chronic	Arterial hyperplasia Vasculitides
B. Colonic ischemia	Nonocclusive causes such as hypotension and vasculitides Occlusive causes
C. Ischemic enterocolitis	Vasculitides Latrogenic/traumatic vascular injury

Table 2: Radiopathological correlation of CT findings in ischemic bowel disease.

Pathologic events	***CT imaging correlation***
• Early vasodiltation • Vasoconstriction	• Wall hyperdensity (in both arterial and venous phase) • Absence/reduced bowel wall enhancement
Increased vascular permeability	• Bowel wall thickening • Bowel luminal dilatation
Mucosal cellular necrosis and microflora proliferation	• Pneumatoses intestinalis • Mesenteric/portal venous gas
Transmural bowel necrosis and bowel perforation	• Pneumoperitoneum • Retropneumoperitoneum • Ascites

evolves over time and includes 3 stages based on the extent of bowel wall involved; further superinfection of the involved segment facilitates necrosis and perforation.[1] The first radiological change seen on CT is secondary to vasodilatation, which is manifested as diffuse wall hyperdensity on both arterial and venous phases. This implies that ischemia has yet not progressed to advanced stage and is possibly reversible, if treated expediently. If ischemia persists and is severe enough, leads to vasoconstriction thereby hampering the collateral flow, which manifests as reduced bowel wall enhancement. Persistence of ischemia leads to necrosis of the bowel wall causing proliferation and migration of microbial flora into the bowel wall resulting in pneumatoses intestinalis, air in mesenteric and portal veins and their branches. Subsequently advanced cases result in bowel perforation causing pneumoperitoneum, retropneumoperitoneum and ascites.[4]

Stage 1	*Stage 2*	*Stage 3*
• Reversible • Pathology limited to mucosa only	Pathology extends to submucosa and muscularis propria	• Transmural involvement • Highest mortality

ACUTE MESENTERIC ISCHEMIA

Acute mesenteric ischemia is an abdominal emergency accounting for 5% of hospital admissions, which may be potentially life-threatening if not treated expediently. The reported mortality rate is high ranging ~60–80%, representing the extreme sensitivity of the small intestine to reduced blood supply.[5] Acute mesenteric ischemia results from occlusive and nonocclusive vascular pathology, and is further sub-classified into arterial, venous or both categories depending upon the vascular structure involved. Understanding the pattern of bowel changes aids in accurate diagnosis and planning appropriate treatment.

Superior Mesenteric Artery Thromboembolism

The superior mesenteric artery is the most predisposed arterial trunk involved by the thromboembolic events due to anatomic factors including wide caliber and narrow take off angle at its origin. Most commonly embolus lodges in initial ~3 to 8 cm from its origin **(Figs. 5A to C)**. Embolic event related ischemic patient generally present acutely, whereas it is not uncommon for thrombotic patients to present subacutely due to antecedent partially occluding atherosclerotic plaques causing collateral development. This group of patients may present as mesenteric angina and chronic mesenteric ischemia, or may present acutely due to superimposed thrombus in background of atherosclerotic disease causing ambient radiological features. Thromboembolic events are usually seen with pre-existing cardiovascular comorbidities such as atrial fibrillation, myocardial infarction, complicated atherosclerotic plaques, mycotic aneurysm, vasculitis and arterial dissection.[6]

Venous Mesenteric Ischemia

Less commonly venous occlusion cause mesenteric ischemia accounting for ~10% of bowel ischemia. Venous occlusive ischemic disease is seen in relatively younger patents with mortality rate of ~10–40%.[5] Closed loop obstruction is the most common cause for venous bowel ischemia **(Figs. 6A and B)**. Venous thrombosis may also

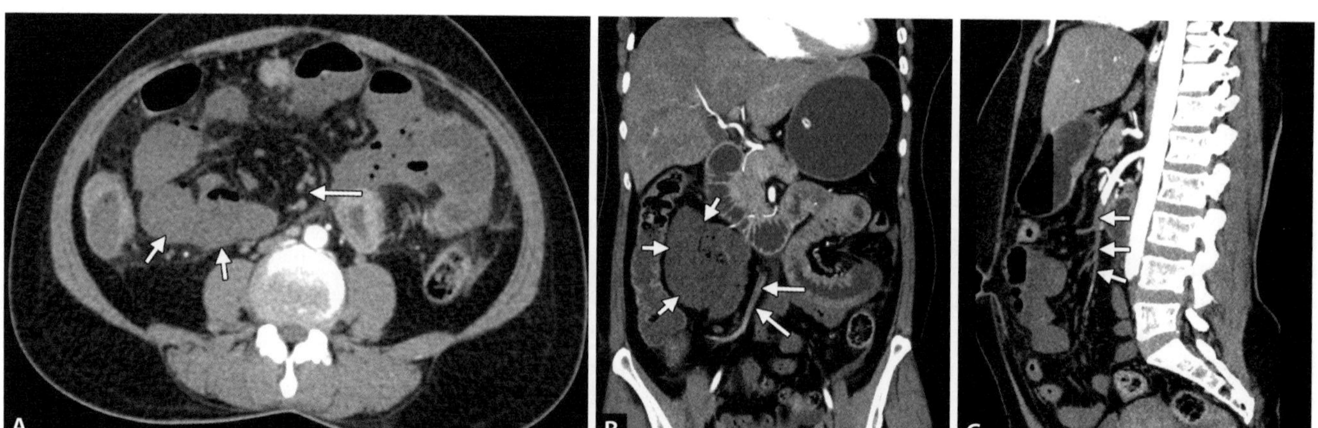

Figs. 5A to C: Axial, coronal, sagittal reconstructed CT images showing complete occlusion of the superior mesenteric artery (long arrows) with nonenhancing proximal small bowel loops in the right side of abdomen (short arrows).

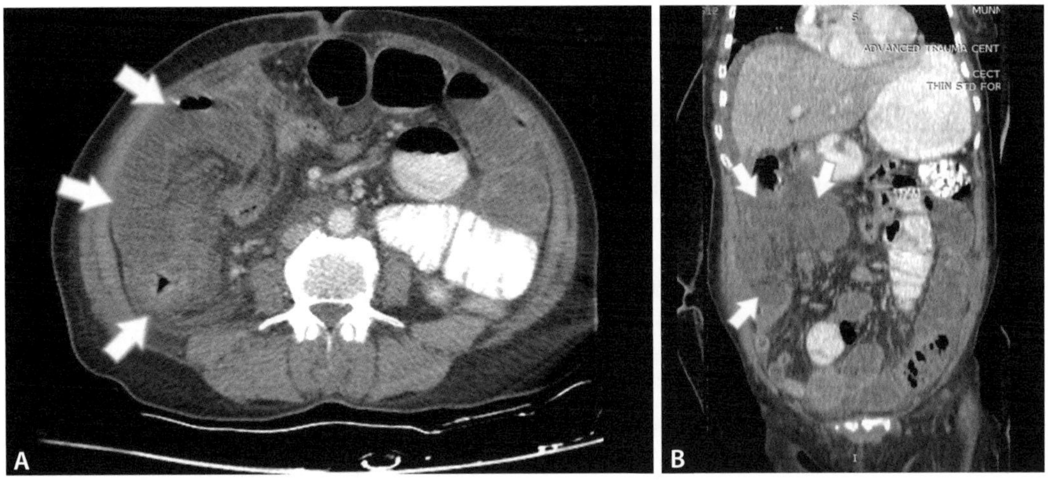

Figs. 6A and B: Venous ischemia secondary to closed loop (arrows) obstruction in the right upper quadrant with engorgement of vessels and fluid in the mesentery with thickened bowel wall.

be seen in patients with hyper coagulable hematological disorders, vasculitides, and less frequently in pregnancy, OCP consumption and underlying inflammatory conditions like SLE.[1]

Nonocclusive Mesenteric Ischemia

Nonocclusive mesenteric ischemia is seen commonly with patients admitted in critical care units and is multifactorial in cause, constituting 20–30% of ischemic disease. Due to its uncertain etiology and compromised host status mortality rate is generally high ranging 30–90%. Systemic hypotension provoke autoregulation and homeostasis, preserving cardiac and brain blood supply along with associated splanchnic vasoconstriction. Shock bowel injury generally seen with hypotensive and low cardiac output states. Any form of shock, renal failure with overly dialysis, drugs such as cocaine, amphetamines and ergotamines are attributed to causal role in nonischemic mesenteric ischemia.[1]

Imaging Modalities

Acute mesenteric ischemia patients generally present with vague clinical features and it is challenging to accurately diagnose this condition early, as it is utmost important to manage the condition timely, since the delay in the management will reflect in worse prognosis and higher mortality rates.

Plain radiographs may be the initial investigation preferred in patients presenting with acute abdomen. The findings are generally nonspecific and may demonstrate dilated bowel loops, thumb printing in early ischemic phase and may show pneumatoses, portal venous gas and

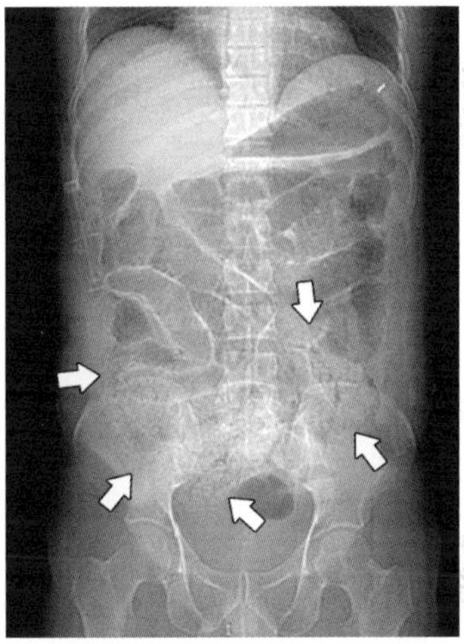

Fig. 7: Abdominal radiograph showing dilated bowel loops with pneumatosis intestinalis (arrows).

pneumoperitoneum in advanced ischemic stage.[4] The sensitivity is significantly low and normal radiograph does not exclude ischemic bowel disease **(Fig. 7)**.[7]

Ultrasonography is the another common modality employed for evaluation of patients presenting with acute abdomen and its role is mainly to exclude other potential causes of acute abdomen. The diagnostic yield in patients with mesenteric ischemia is more often suboptimal due to gaseous distension of bowel loops causing technical difficulty in evaluation of mesenteric vasculature.[4]

In the present modern era with significant technological advancements, MDCT is the investigation of choice for evaluating patients with suspected ischemic bowel disease. It has nearly replaced conventional angiography for diagnostic purposes and aids in making the correct diagnosis, as well as excluding other alternative pathologies.[3] In patients with ischemia CT examination can help in understanding pathophysiology to accurately diagnose and to characterize arterial versus venous occlusive disease, grade the severity of the disease, help in planning accurate treatment and also provide vital prognostic information. Comprehensive assessment of the bowel wall, mesenteric vasculature and surrounding mesentery is essential for the overall estimation of the severity and extent of the disease.[8]

Technical Aspects

The study protocol consists of biphasic CT abdomen with an arterial phase (35–40 sec) performed for evaluating the arterial stenosis and occlusions, and venous phase (65–70 sec) for assessing the mesenteric venous system and various abdominal viscera for changes of ischemia. Nonenhanced CT has been shown to be of benefit in some studies in literature as it can better evaluate the submucosal hemorrhage, hyperdense clots and also provide baseline attenuation of the bowel.[1,4] However, this is controversial subject as it adds to the radiation burden and timeliness and therefore remains contentious issue.

Pearl: Biphasic protocol with both arterial and venous phases is the standard imaging protocol in all patients with suspected mesenteric ischemia and arterial phase should not to be excluded from the examination in order to achieve dose reduction.

The role of oral contrast is again controversial in literature and preference is individualistic. In patients presenting acutely CT is obtained only with IV contrast, to expedite the study, although these cases may be technically difficult to evaluate due to inadequate distension of the bowel loops. In patients presenting with more subacute features, neutral oral contrast is generally preferred by most radiologists as it is helps in better assessment of the bowel wall and also improves the assessment of vascular tree by various post processing techniques.[1] Present generation MDCT scanners allow volumetric data acquisition which can be further postprocessed by various dedicated computer softwares on work stations. MPR and 3D reconstructions help in better anatomical and vascular evaluation, and increase the confidence of the radiologist in making an accurate diagnosis.[4] Masking the bowel enhancement pattern and interference with 3D reconstruction is a major drawback of administration of positive oral contrast agents and is therefore not generally recommended.[1]

The administration with IV contrast material CT examination may reveal dilated and thickened bowel loops associated with ascites and mesenteric edema in initial stages of acute mesenteric ischemia, whereas pneumatoses, pneumoperitoneum and portal and mesenteric venous gas signify advanced ischemic stage **(Figs. 8A and B)**. CTA and its dedicated reconstruction techniques such as MIP (maximum intensity projection), tissue transition projections (TTP) and vessel probe (VP) are more specific and often demonstrate arterial occlusions as filling defect within the vessel lumen with/without associated collateral formation **(Figs. 9A and B)**[4]. Similarly venous thrombosis is identified as central filling defect with mural rim enhancement.[9]

CT features of nonocclusive mesenteric ischemia are overlapping with other inflammatory or infectious conditions involving the bowel, which makes it challenging to diagnose this condition. CT findings may be variable from focal mucosal damage in watershed areas

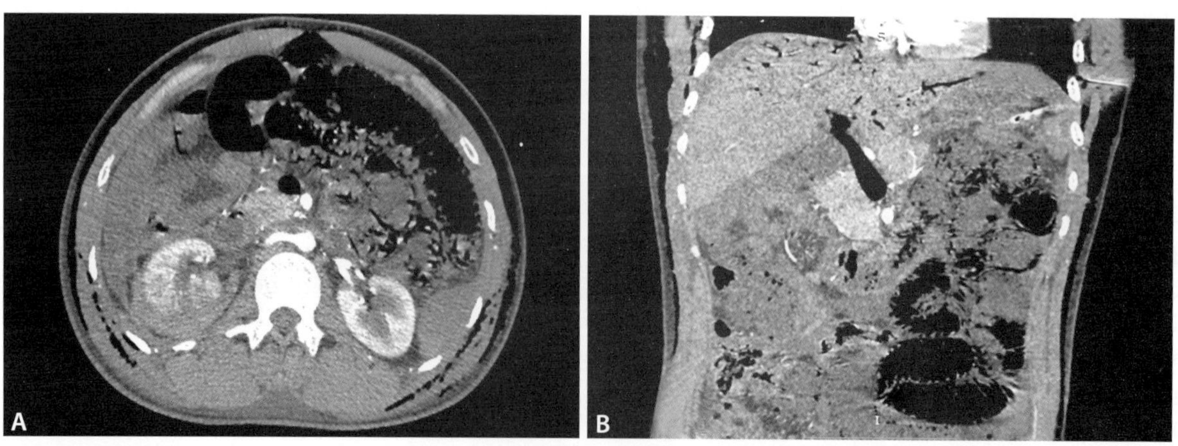

Figs. 8A and B: *Patient of blunt trauma abdomen*: Axial and coronal reconstructed CT images showing extensive pneumatosis, air in the mesenteric/portal venous branches and hemoperitoneum. Note is made of right renal contusion with perinephric hematoma.

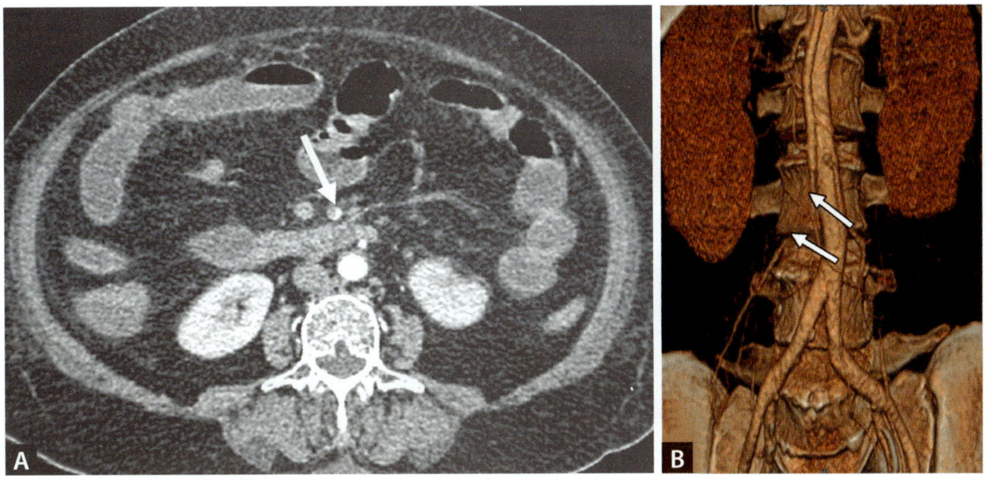

Figs. 9A and B: Axial, and volume rendered (VR) CT images showing occlusion of the branch of superior mesenteric artery (long arrows).

Table 3: Clinical and CT features of mesenteric ischemia.[1]

Features	***Arterial occlusive ischemia***	***Venous occlusive ischemia***	***Nonocclusive mesenteric ischemia***
Time of onset	Acute, chronic, acute on chronic	Acute or chronic	Acute or chronic
Predisposing conditions	Atrial fibrillation, recent myocardial infarction, atherosclerosis, aortic dissection, vasculitis, drugs like ergotamine and cocaine	Closed loop bowel obstruction and strangulation, hypercoagulable disorders, portal hypertension, pregnancy, malignancy, oral contraceptive pills (OCP)	Hypotension and shock, vasculitis, vasoconstricting drugs
Bowel wall status	May be thin in acute state or may be thickened with associated inflammation and edema	Edematous, markedly thickened bowel wall	Thickened bowel wall
Bowel wall enhancement	Depending on state of reperfusion, may nonenhance before reperfusion and may hyperenhance in reperfused state	Target sign with significant mucosal hyperenhancement **(Figs. 10A and B)**	Reduced enhancement
Mesenteric vasculature	Arterial stenosis/occlusion, aneurysm, dissection	Venous thrombosis	Nonspecific, with pruning of distal mesenteric vascular branches
Mesentery	Mesenteric fat stranding and free fluid in advanced stages	Significant mesenteric fat stranding and free fluid in early stages	Variable

to the damage of entire bowel. Small bowel loops generally show mural thickening with hyperenhancement.[1] Usually there is normal appearing colon. Ancillary features like reduced caliber of inferior vena cava and abdominal aorta may be identified along with intraperitoneal fluid in hypoperfusion conditions.[13] Appropriate and confident diagnosis of nonocclusive mesenteric ischemia is possible by angiography, which may show narrowing of origins of SMA branches, irregularity and spasm of mesenteric arcades **(Figs. 11A to C)**.

Regardless of the etiology, CT imaging features represent obstructive state traits and are based on pathophysiologic state of the disease. Few pattern of traits may aid in differentiating occlusive and non occlusive causes **(Table 3)**. Arterial occlusion generally causes paper thin bowel wall and hypoattenuation; whereas venous occlusive disease result in markedly thickened oedematous bowel wall, early mesenteric fat stranding and marked luminal dilatation seen even in the early stages **(Figs. 12A and B)**. Similar changes are however seen in advanced cases of arterial ischemia progressed to transmural necrosis **(Table 4)**. Distinguishing CT imaging features of arterial and venous ischemia are enumerated in **Table 4**.[1,10]

Dual energy CT with iodine overlay technique may be useful in detecting subtle bowel wall enhancement to

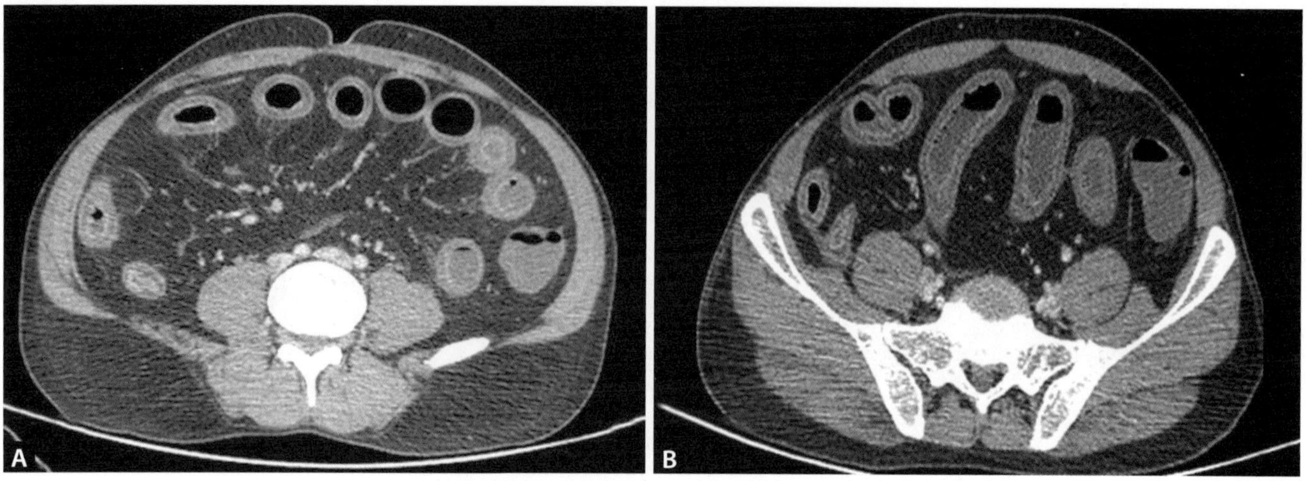

Figs. 10A and B: Axial CT images showing characteristic target sign with mucosal and serosal hyperenhancement in a patient of venous ischemia.

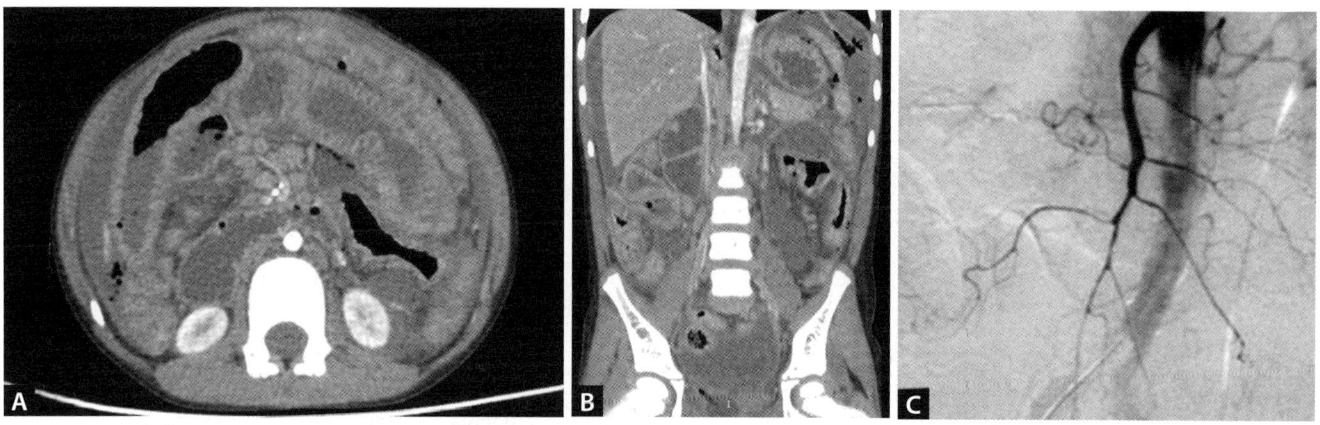

Figs. 11A to C: Patient of cardiogenic shock, CT Axial (A) and coronal (B) section showing reduced caliber of abdominal aorta with chinked IVC and showing diffuse concentric mural thickening involving bowel loops with ascites. DSA (C) SMA run showing reduced caliber and paucity of the distal branches with pruning.

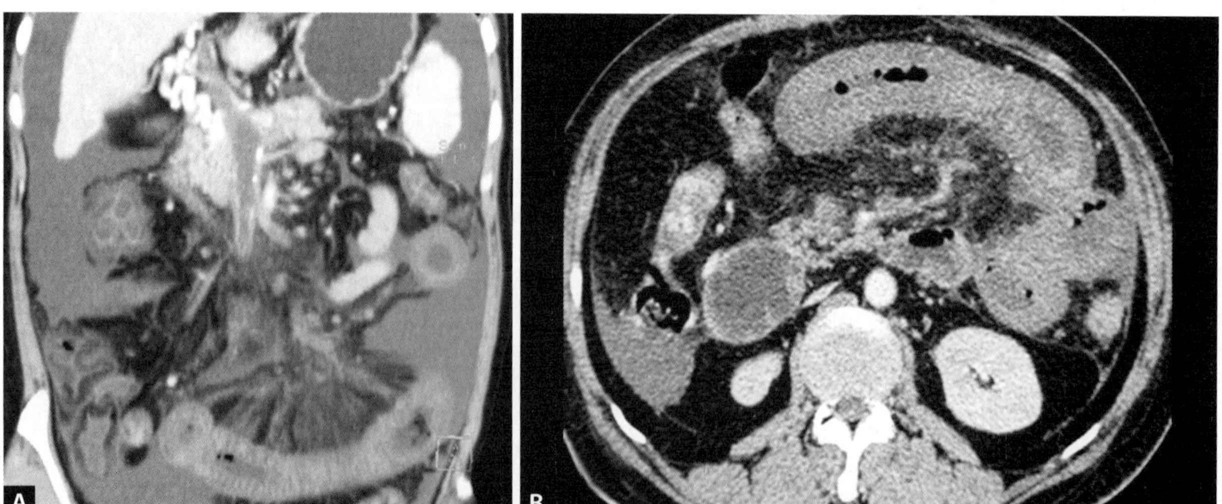

Figs. 12A and B: (A) Coronal CT image showing splenoportal thrombosis with thickened bowel loops and engorgement of mesenteric vessels suggestive of early venous ischemia; (B) Another patient of venous ischemia showing markedly thickened bowel wall with mesenteric changes.

Table 4: CT imaging features to differentiate arterial and venous occlusive ischemia.[10]

Arterial occlusion	*Venous occlusion*
Superior mesenteric artery (SMA) thrombosis	Superior mesenteric vein (SMV) thrombosis
No/subtle bowel wall enhancement	Hypo/Hyperdense bowel wall
Thinned out bowel wall	Significantly thickened bowel wall
Mucosal nonenhancement	Mucosal hyperenhacement
Bowel dilatation after transmural infarction	Dilated bowel lumen without infarction
Late mesenteric stranding, hemorrhage or edema	Marked early mesenteric fat stranding and hemorrhage

Note: Advanced cases of both arterial and venous ischemia show similar imaging manifestations such as air in mesenteric and portal venous system, pneumoperitoneum and retropneumoperitoneum.

Table 5: ACR appropriateness criteria for imaging acute ischemic bowel disease.[15]

Radiologic modality	*Rating*	*Remarks*
CTA abdomen with IV contrast	9	• Fast • Noninvasive • Evaluates other causes
Arteriography abdomen	8	Diagnosis and treatment in single procedure
X-ray abdomen	7	Initial tool to evaluate acute abdomen
MRA abdomen without and with IV contrast	7	• Time consuming • Limited benefits in distal thromboembolism and NOMI
US abdomen	6	• Better for venous occlusion • Assess other causes of abdominal pain
MRA abdomen without IV contrast	3	Lower sensitivity and specificity

Rating scale: 7, 8, 9 usually appropriate; 4, 5, 6 may be appropriate; 1, 2, 3 usually not appropriate.

differentiate ischemia from infective/inflammatory bowel wall thickening.[11]

Conventional angiography (DSA) is the gold standard for the evaluation and treatment of arterial thromboembolism. Acute mesenteric thromboembolism is visualized as filling defect, occluding the arterial lumen with/without collateral channels. Assessment of the distal vascular occlusion and catheter directed intervention may be performed in suitably selected patients. Angiography is also suitable for cases in which diagnosis is uncertain on CT; however, angiography is mainly performed with an intent of therapeutic purposes for performing interventions like thrombolysis, aspiration of thrombus or vasodilatory medication administration in patients where diagnosis has already been made on CT.[12]

MR is another advanced modality which has been employed in patients with mesenteric ischemia, its role in cases of acute mesenteric ischemia is generally not advocated due to long imaging duration and critical status of the patients.[13] Patients with subacute/chronic features may be assessed by gadolinium enhanced MRA which can provide accurate assessment of the mesenteric vasculature comparable to CT evaluation. Experimental studies have shown that MR techniques may be able to differentiate between acutely ischemic and infarcted segments based on signal changes on T2 weighted images and postcontrast gadolinium images.[14]

American college of radiology (ACR) has formulated rating system for various radiological modalities aiding in systematic, appropriate and timely evaluation of suspected ischemia in various clinical conditions **(Table 5)**.

Treatment of Acute Mesenteric Ischemia

Immediately prompt treatment is instituted after established diagnosis of acute mesenteric ischemia and treatment aims at revascularization of the mesenteric vessels to prevent further bowel ischemia. Early medical supportive management include fluid resuscitation, naso gastric/orogastric tube decompression, and anticoagulation. Broad spectrum antibiotics must be administered and care must be taken to avoid vasoconstrictive drug administration especially in nonocclusive mesenteric ischemic patients. The emphasis of treatment has shifted from surgical approach to endovascular therapy in recent years.

In the presence of peritoneal signs, emergency laparotomy recommended, immediate surgical embolectomy or bypass with resection of nonviable bowel is essential and intraoperatively meticulous bowel assessment for its viability is necessary. A second look laparotomy may be required after emergency surgery owing to vasospasm of normal vascular tree, inadequate resection of ischemic segment, doubtful perfusion of bowel segments or the condition of the patient fails to stabilize.[16]

Catheter guided therapies are performed on patients without frank imaging and clinical features suggestive of gangrene/bowel necrosis; these may be in the form of aspiration embolectomy or catheter thrombolysis using rt-PA or urokinase. If atherosclerotic changes are noted in in the vessel wall, this procedure can be electively followed by a percutaneous transluminal angioplasty with or without stenting. PTA with stent placement is more effective in immediate and long-term vessel patency than PTA alone as stents offered additional structural support to the vessel wall leading to lesser repeat interventions.[17] Endovascular techniques have led to a decrease in surgery related complications including decreased amount of bowel resected leading to lower incidence of short bowel syndrome, lesser incidence of systemic complications and reduced mortality.[18]

Acute nonocclusive mesenteric ischemia can be treated in the same sitting in which diagnostic catheter angiography is done for confirmation of diagnosis. The typical treatment consists of administration of intra-arterial vasodilators like papaverine, nitroglycerin or glucagon. Intravenous high dose prostaglandin E1 is equally effective in management if transarterial catheterization is not feasible. However, these vasodilator drugs can lead to systemic hypotension which must be taken care during the procedure.[18]

The mainstay of treatment of venous mesenteric ischemia is systemic anticoagulation. Long-term maintenance therapy on anticoagulants has a higher chance of recanalization of occluded veins and lower incidence of recurrence. One of its complications can be bleeding in the gangrenous bowel, however this should not prevent or delay in administration of the systemic anticoagulant and bleeding has to be managed if it occurs. Transhepatic or transjugular cannulation of the SMV and thrombolysis with or without thrombectomy needs to be considered in acute or subacute venous occlusion depending on the severity of the condition to prevent bowel infarction. Adjunct transjugular intrahepatic portosystemic shunt (TIPS) can be created to improve the outflow of the venous system.[18]

CHRONIC MESENTERIC ISCHEMIA

Chronic mesenteric ischemia is an uncommon condition which generally affects elderly population often with widespread atherosclerosis. The diagnosis is often late in its course as atleast two of the three major mesenteric vascular trunks, should have significant luminal narrowing before developing symptoms **(Figs. 13A and B)**.[19] Central clue for making the diagnosis of chronic mesenteric ischemia is not only the presence of significant vascular stenosis, but also prominent and tortuous collateral conduits between the mesenteric trunks which maintain the bowel viability. Frequently patients with this condition will be elderly, fragile, females who experience postprandial abdominal pain, develop fear of food and often avoid meals resulting in chronic weight loss.[20,21] Widespread atherosclerosis of the abdominal vasculature is the most frequent cause of chronic mesenteric ischemia, other less common conditions like vasculitis, radiation vasculopathy and fibromuscular dysplasia also cause chronic mesenteric ischemia **(Figs. 14A and B)**.[19,22]

Imaging Modalities

Noninvasive imaging modalities such as US, CTA, MRI/MRA are employed for the evaluation.[12] Angiography has its role in further evaluation of equivocal diagnosis or if endovascular treatment is contemplated.[12] According to ACR appropriateness criteria for evaluation of chronic mesenteric ischemia, the preference of the imaging modalities is discussed in the **Table 6**.

CT and CT angiography is the primary diagnostic tool as it allows accurate diagnosis and excludes other alternative causes of the clinical condition. CTA allows confident depiction of vascular tree with occlusions/stenosis and collateral channel formation. Mesenteric vasculature is better demonstrated by 3D imaging techniques and other post-processing tools available in the modern work stations.

Duplex USG is another promising modality which has an important role in nonacute presentations. Sonography alongwith color and spectral Doppler correlation can detect hemodynamically significant stenosis in proximal CA and SMA **(Figs. 15A to D)**. Peak systolic velocity of >275 cm/s and >200 cm/s in SMA and celiac trunk respectively, are reliable indicators of 70% or more stenosis in the fasting state.[9,23] Comparison of pre- and postprandial peak systolic velocity may also suggest vascular occlusion.

MRA also been shown to have comparable accuracy to CTA for evaluation of stenosis in the mesenteric vessels. Noncontrast sequences (time of flight and phase

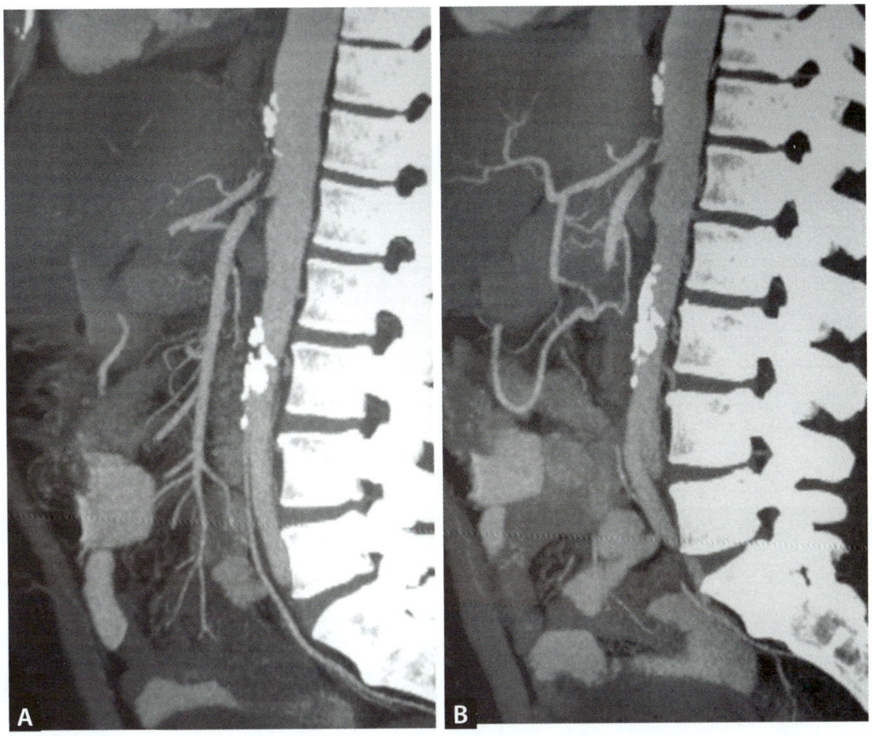

Figs. 13A and B: Patient of chronic mesenteric ischemia: Sagittal reconstructed CT images showing atherosclerotic changes with hemodynamically significant stenosis in the proximal celiac trunk and SMA.

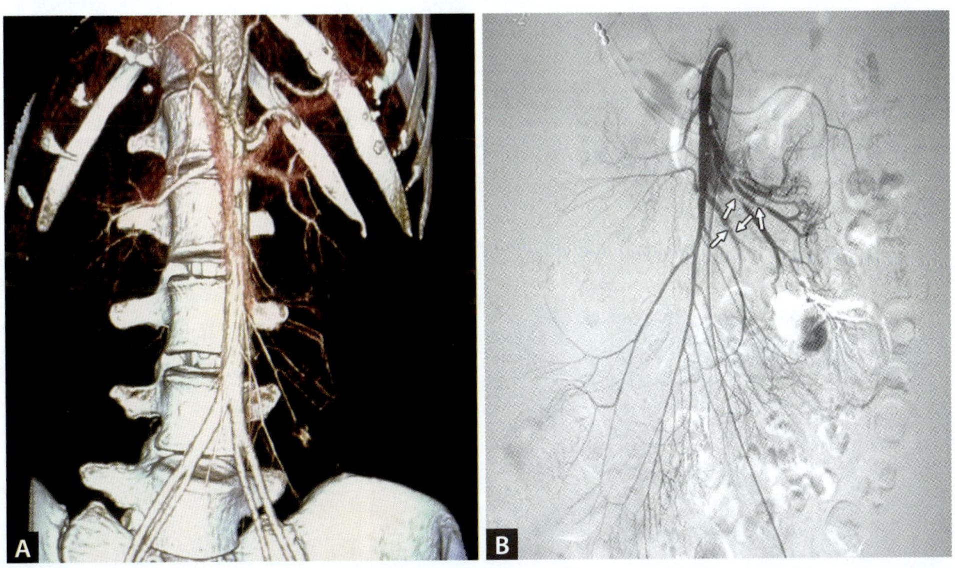

Figs. 14A and B: Patient of vasculitis with mesenteric angina: Volume rendered CT image showing subtle irregularity in the branches of SMA. DSA SMA run confirming the irregularities and multifocal narrowings in the branches of SMA.

contrast) can be employed in patients with renal function derangement in addition to the benefit of no radiation exposure. In chronic mesenteric ischemia, insufficient collateral channels may fail to meet the metabolic demands of bowel with decreased blood oxygenation in superior mesenteric vein or other mesenteric veins. This deranged physiology can also be assessed through MR perfusion techniques coupled with food challenge. Cine contrast phase imaging and MR oximetry can evaluate superior mesenteric vein flow and blood oxygenation respectively.[24]

Table 6: ACR appropriateness criteria to evaluate chronic mesenteric ischemia.[15]

Radiologic modality	*Rating*	*Remarks*
CTA abdomen with IV contrast	9	• Fast • Noninvasive • Evaluate other etiology
Arteriography abdomen	7	Diagnosis and treatment in single procedure
US abdomen	7	• Better for venous occlusive cause • Evaluate other causes
MRA abdomen without and with IV contrast	7	• Time consuming • Limited role in distal thromboembolism and NOMI
X-ray abdomen	3	Normal study does not exclude ischemia
MRA abdomen without IV contrast	3	Lower sensitivity and specificity

Rating scale: 7, 8, 9 usually appropriate; 4, 5, 6 may be appropriate; 1, 2, 3 usually not appropriate.

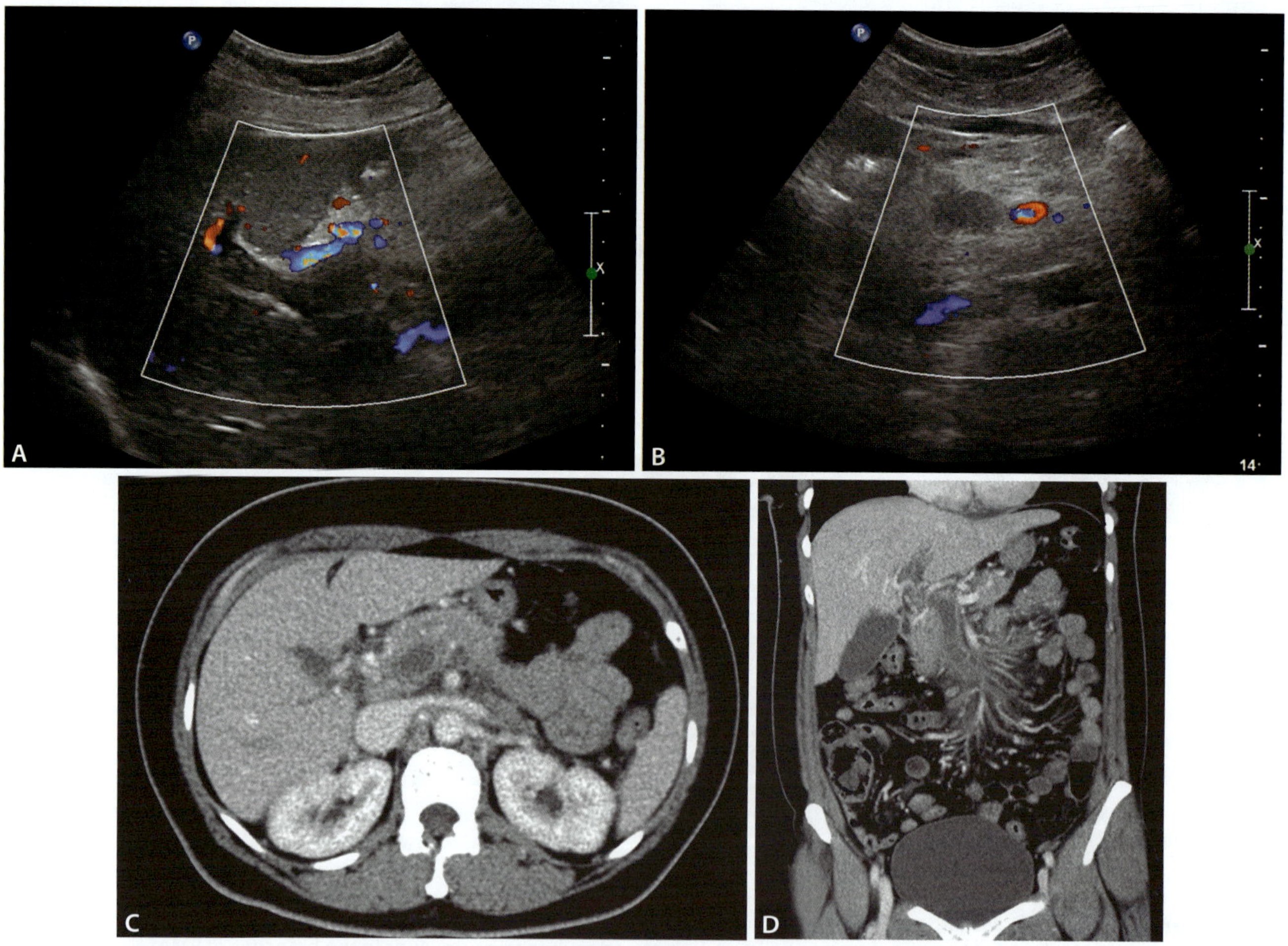

Figs. 15A to D: Doppler ultrasound images (A and B) showing dilated SMV and portal vein with no color filling suggestive of thrombosis; (C and D) Axial and coronal images confirming SMV and portal venous thrombosis.

Decrease in superior mesenteric venous flow in phase contrast imaging and reduction in superior mesenteric venous blood oxygenation level with resultant T2 value reduction after food challenge is noted with symptomatic chronic mesenteric ischemic patients.[24] However, lengthy acquisition time and inability to accurately evaluate the narrower caliber vessels such as IMA and other smaller branches are limitations in practice.

Treatment

Considering the individual patient anatomical factors and comorbities; life style changes surgery or endovascular treatment is advised, for relief of symptoms and to halt progression of chronic mesenteric ischemia into more acute events.[12,25,26] Angioplasty and stenting of the affected vascular segment are the endovascular procedures performed on affected vessels with high initial technical success rates of >90%. However, recurrent stenosis is not uncommon and reintervention is recommended **(Figs. 16A to F)**.[26-29] Endarterectomy, vascular bypass and arterial re implantation are the surgically available options for treating chronic mesenteric ischemia.[25] Revascularization of single vessel (usually SMA) is sufficient with long-term patency rate of 70-93%, despite multi vessel involvement.[25]

COLONIC ISCHEMIA

Colonic ischemia is the most common form of intestinal ischemia, usually seen in 7th decade of life, and second most frequent cause of lower gastrointestinal bleeding.[30] Underlying pathophysiologic changes are due to altered circulation, failing in meeting colonic metabolic demands. Most commonly vascular compromise results from non-occlusive etiology such as hypoperfusion states, vasculitis and other vasculopathy. Only 25% of patients are attributed to vascular occlusion.[31]

Vascular compromise can cause evolution of pathophysiologic changes in colon, may be seen sequentially as mucosal/submucosal damage, reversible colitis, ulcerative changes, stricture formation and gangrenous changes.[13,31] Patients usually present with mild lower abdominal pain

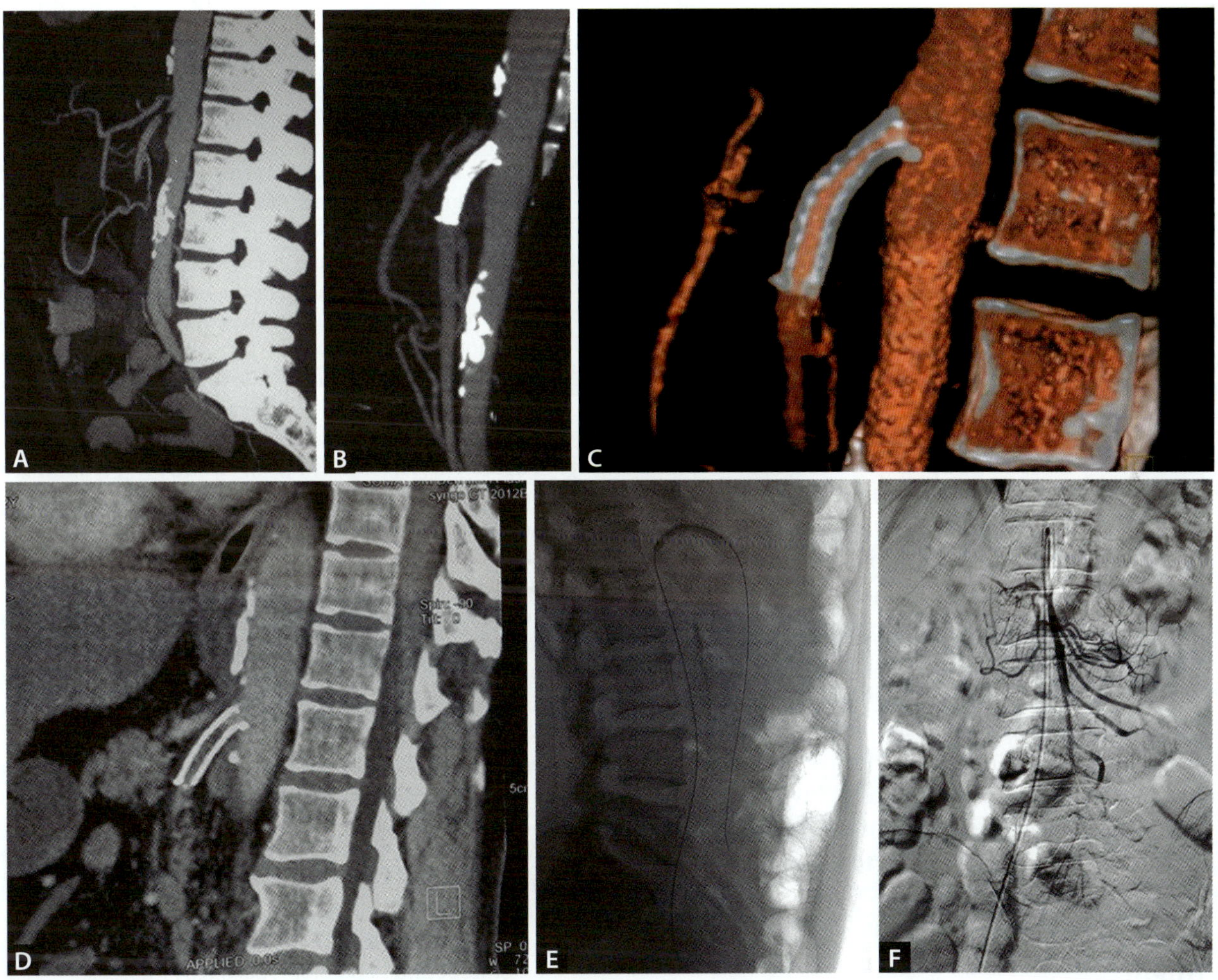

Figs. 16A to F: (A) Patient of chronic mesenteric ischemia with short segment stenosis involving proximal celiac trunk and SMA; (B and C) Metallic stenting performed in proximal SMA with good distal opacification; (D) Relapse of symptoms with CT repeated after 7 months showed in stent thrombosis with poor distal flow; (E and F) Reintervention with balloon dilatation performed across the stent with restored flow in the distal SMA and relief of symptoms.
Image Courtesy: Dr Vivek Gupta and Anupam Lal, Department of Radiodiagnosis, PGIMER, Chandigarh, India.

and bloody diarrhea.[32] Water shed areas of colon such as Sudecks point and Griffith points in splenic flexure and sigmoid colon are more prone for ischemic changes.[33]

Diagnosis

Radiographic changes depends upon the underlying pathophysiology and severity of bowel necrosis. Plain abdominal radiographic features can vary from normal study to very severe damage resulting in pneumo/retropneumo-peritoneum. Other features such as nonspecific ileus, thumb printing, transverse ridging and a haustration may be observed, occasionally pneumatosis or portal venous gas may be identified due to transmural bowel necrosis.[34,35]

Barium examination features vary with stage and degree of ischemic damage, serial changes in the barium study characteristics is the hallmark feature of colonic ischemia.[36-38] Features observed on barium studies may include thumb printing (most common), transverse ridging, spasm, ulceration, intramural barium and stricture formation.[34] Ultrasonography also demonstrates non specific bowel wall thickening and diminished color flow in involved bowel segment.[23]

CECT has become the gold standard investigation for diagnosing ischemic colitis which usually involves a specific segment of colon.[32] This is in contrary to the infective/inflammatory etiology which may be patchy or diffuse and is generally nonsegmental colonic involvement. Most common bowel segment affected is left colon;[32] CT features of ischemia include target/double halo sign, shaggy irregular contours, pneumatosis intestinalis, portal venous gas, peritoneal fluid, or pneumoperitoneum.[32] Limitations of CT evaluation is lack of specificity and difficult assessment of the bowel wall thickening secondary to inadequate bowel distension.[32] Also in colonic ischemia, initial imaging features cannot be utilised for definite prognostication.

Colonoscopic evaluation is the most sensitive diagnostic tool for colonic ischemia evaluation, and specific location and patchy segmental involvement may help in diagnosis. Favier classification is widely utilised by clinicians to make the diagnosis, to ascertain prognosis and to decide surgical intervention.[39,40]

Treatment

Correction of hypovolemia and treating primary cause is primary goal. Medical management consists of gastric rest, fluid and electrolyte management, administration of broad spectrum antibiotics and prophylaxis against venous thromboembolism. Resection of ischemic bowel with/without bowel anastomosis and/or cholecystectomy is the surgical management available for suitable patients.[32]

ACKNOWLEDGMENTS

Dr Muniraju M and Dr Akash Bansal, Department of Radiodiagnosis.

REFERENCES

1. Dhatt HS, Behr SC, Miracle A, Wang ZJ, Yeh BM, et al. Radiological evaluation of bowel ischemia. Radiol clin N Am. 2015;53:1241-54.
2. Gourley EJ, Gering SA. The meandering mesenteric artery: a historic review and surgical implications. Dis Colon Rectum. 2005;48(5):996-1000.
3. Upponi S, Harvey JJ, Uberoi R, Ganeshan A, et al. The role of radiology in the diagnosis and treatment of mesenteric ischemia. Postgrad med J. 2013;89:165-72.
4. Moschetta M, Telegrafo M, Rella L, Ianora AAS, Angelelli G, et al. Multidetector CT features of acute intestinal ischemia and their prognostic correlation. World J radiol. 2014;6(5):130-8.
5. Brandt LJ, Fuerstadt P. Intestestinal ischemia. Textbook of Sleisenger and Fordtran's Gastrointestinal and Liver Disease, 10th edition; volume 2:2076-2101.
6. Sandstorm CK, Ingraham CR, Monroe EJ, et al. Beyond decreased bowel enhancement: acute abnormalities of the mesenteric and portal vasculature. Abdominal Imaging. 2015;40(8):2977-92.
7. Oldenburg WA, Lau LL, Rodenberg TJ, et al. Acute mesenteric ischemia: a clinical review. Arch Intern Med. 2004;164:1054-62.
8. Furukawa A, Kanasaki S, Kono N, Wakamiya M, Tanaka T, Takahashi M, Murata K, et al. CT diagnosis of acute mesenteric ischemia from various causes. AJR. 2009;192:408-16.
9. Bradbury MS, Kavanagh PV, Bechtold RE, et al. Mesenteric venous thrombosis: diagnosis and noninvasive imaging. Radiographics. 2002;22(3):527-41.
10. Raman SP, Fishman EK, et al. Computed tomography angiography of the small bowel and mesentery. Radiol Clin N Am. 2016;54:87-100.
11. Fulwadhva UP, Wortman JR, Sodickson AD, et al. Use of dual energy CT and iodine maps in evaluation of bowel disease. Radigraphics. 2016;36:393-406.
12. Walker TG, Kalva SP, et al. Mesenteric ischemia. Semin Intervent Radiol. 2009;26:175-83.
13. Gore RM, Thakrar KH, Mehta UK, Berlin J, Yaghmai V, Newmark GM, et al. Clinical imaging, clinical gastro enterology and hepatology. 2008;6:849-58.
14. Wilkerson DK, Mezrich R, Drake C, Sebok D, Zatina MA. Magnetic resonance imaging of acute occlusive intestinal ischaemia. J Vasc Surg. 1990;11:567-71.
15. Oliva BI, Devarpanah AH, et al. ACR Appropriateness Criteria®—Imaging of Mesenteric Ischemia, 2012.

16. Klar E, Rahmanian PB, Bucker A, Hauenstein K, Jauch KW, Luther B. Acute mesenteric ischemia: a vascular emergency. Deutsches Arzteblatt International. 2012;109(14):249-56.
17. Landis MS, Rajan DK, Simons ME, Hayeems EB, Kachura JR, Sniderman KW. Percutaneous management of chronic mesenteric ischemia: outcomes after intervention. Journal of Vascular and Interventional Radiology. JVIR. 2005;16(10):1319-25.
18. Nicholas Fidelman AFA, Brooks D Cash, et al. ACR Appropriateness Criteria®—Radiologic Management of Mesenteric Ischemia, 2014.
19. Hohenwalter EJ, Heib RA, Patel PJ, et al. Chronic mesenteric ischemia: diagnosis and treatment. Semin Intervent Radiol. 2009;26:345-51.
20. Ujiki M, Kibbe MR. Mesenteric ischemia. Perspect Vasc Surg Endovasc Ther. 2005;17:309-18.
21. Kougias P, El Sayed HF, Zhou W, Lin PH. Management of chronic mesenteric ischemia. The role of endovascular therapy. J Endovasc Ther. 2007;14:395-405.
22. Sreenarasimhaiah J. Chronic mesenteric ischemia. Best Pract Res Clin Gastroenterol. 2005;19:283-95.
23. Reginelli A, Genovese EA, et al. Intestinal ischemia: US-CT findings correlations. Critical ultrasound journal. 2013;5:1-11.
24. Chow LC, Chan FP, Li KCP. A comprehensive approach to MR imaging of mesenteric ischemia. Abdom Imaging. 2002;27(5):507-16.
25. Schaefer PJ, Schaefer FKW, Mueller-Huelsbeck S, Jahnke T. Chronic mesenteric ischemia: stenting of mesenteric arteries.Abdom Imaging. 2007;32(3):304-9.
26. Atkins MD, Kwolek CJ, LaMuraglia GM, Brewster DC,Chung TK, Cambria RP. Surgical revascularization versus endovascular therapy for chronic mesenteric ischemia: acomparative experience. J Vasc Surg. 2007;45(6):1162-71.
27. Sharafuddin MJ, Olson CH, Sun S, Kresowik TF, Corson JD. Endovascular treatment of celiac and mesenteric arteries stenoses: applications and results. J Vasc Surg. 2003;38(4):692-8.
28. Matsumoto AH, Angle JF, Spinosa DJ, et al. Percutaneous transluminal angioplasty and stenting in the treatment of chronic mesenteric ischemia: results and longterm follow-up. J Am Coll Surg. 2002;194(Suppl 1):S22-31.
29. Sarac TP, Altinel O, Kashyap V, et al. Endovascular treatment of stenotic and occluded visceral arteries for chronic mesenteric ischemia. J Vasc Surg. 2008;47(3):485-91.
30. Paterno F, Longo WE. The etiology and pathogenesis of vascular disorders of the intestine. Radiol Clin North Am. 2008;46(5):877-85.
31. Balthazar EJ, Yen BC, Gordon RB. Ischemic colitis. Radiology. 1999;211:381-8.
32. Moszkowicz D, Mariani A, Trisallet C, et al. Ischemic colitis: the ABCs of diagnosis and surgical management. J Visc Surg. 2013;150(1):19-28.
33. Rogers AI, David S, et al. Intestinal blood flow and diseases of vascular impairment. In: Haubrich WS, Schaffner F, Berk JE (Eds). Gastroenterology, 5th edn, Philadelphia, Pa: Saunders. 1995. pp. 1212-34.
34. Parfitt JR, Driman DK. Pathological effects of drugs on the gastrointestinal tract: a review. Hum Pathol. 2007;38:527-36.
35. Wittenberg J, Athanasoulis CA, Williams LF, et al. Ischemic colitis: radiology and pathophysiology. AJR. 1975;123:287-300.
36. Gore RM, Calenoff L, Rogers LF. Roentgenographic manifestations of ischemic colitis. JAMA. 1979;241:1171-3.
37. Iida M, Matsui T, Fuchigami T, et al. Ischemic colitis: serial changes in double contrast barium enema examinations. Radiology. 1986;159:337-41.
38. Greenberg HM, Goldberg HI, Axel L. Colonic"urticaria" pattern due to early ischemia. Gastrointest Radiol. 1981;6:145-9.
39. Favier C, Bonneau HP, Tran Minh V, Devic J. Endoscopic diagnosis of regressive ischemic colitis. Endoscopic, histologic and arteriographic correlations. Nouv Presse Med. 1976;5:77-9.
40. Beppu K, Osada T, Nagahara A, et al. Relationship between endoscopic findings and clinical severity in ischemic colitis. Intern Med. 2011;50:2263-7.

CHAPTER 74

Gastrointestinal Hemorrhage: Imaging and Intervention

Deep Narayan Srivastava, Kumble S Madhusudhan, Shivanand Gamanagatti

INTRODUCTION

Gastrointestinal hemorrhage (GIH) is defined when bleeding occurs into any part of gastrointestinal tract (GIT), from esophagus to anal canal. It is a manifestation of various pathologies and is a serious symptom. It is associated with high morbidity and mortality, reaching up to 40% in severe cases.[1] The GIH may be acute or chronic/recurrent. Management of GIH involves multidisciplinary approach. The radiologist's role is in identifying the source and cause of bleeding and managing them with radiological interventions wherever needed.

CLASSIFICATION

The GIH may be upper (when the source of bleeding is proximal to ligament of Treitz) or lower, when the source is distal to it **(Box 1)**. Patients of upper gastrointestinal hemorrhage (UGIH) present with hematemesis (vomiting of blood) or melena (black tarry stools). For melena to occur (i.e. for stools to turn black) at least 60 mL of bleeding is needed and sufficient time should be available for blood to undergo degeneration by gastric and intestinal enzymes.[2] In lower gastrointestinal hemorrhage (LGIH), patients present with hematochezia, which is fresh blood in stools. However, this categorization is not absolute and may mislead the clinician.[3] Blood in gastrointestinal tract, due to cathartic properties, may rapidly reach the rectum and bleeding UGI source may present as hematochezia. Sometimes, due to slow colonic transit and bleeding rate, right colonic bleeding may present as melena. Occasionally, nasogastric tube may not show blood in cases of UGIH. Thus, evaluation of GIH should include both upper and lower GIT, till a source is identified.

Box 1: Classification of GIH.

Upper GIH	• Proximal to ligament of Treitz • From esophagus, stomach and duodenum
Lower GIH	• Distal to ligament of Treitz • From jejunum, ileum and colon (including rectum and anal canal)

Box 2: Types of GIH.

Overt GIH	Hemorrhage is grossly visible
Occult GIH	Hemorrhage is microscopic (positive on stool occult blood test)
Obscure GIH	Hemorrhage is not detectable on UGIE or colonoscopy

Overt GIH is when bleeding can be visualized by the patient or by the clinician **(Box 2)**. Occult GIH is when bleeding is not macroscopic and there is positive stool occult blood test. Obscure GIH is a condition when patient has bleeding but UGIE and colonoscopy are negative. Obscure GIH may be occult or overt.[4]

Clinical Presentation

The patients of GIH present with hematemesis, melena or hematochezia.[5] Tachycardia and hypotension is seen when acute blood loss is greater than 500 mL.[3] Severe/massive GIH occurs when at least 15% of blood volume is lost and patients present with shock. Patients with chronic or recurrent GIH present with anemia. Patients may be asymptomatic for hemorrhage less than 100 mL/day.

Etiology

Various etiologies are identified which can cause GIH.[6] These have been listed in **Table 1**. One can see from the table, that most of the lesions do not need imaging for making a diagnosis. The source of bleeding may be arterial, venous or capillary. Thus appropriate investigation must be chosen depending on the suspicion.

Evaluation

Endoscopy is the initial diagnostic procedure performed in all cases of suspected GIH **(Box 3)**.[7] This includes upper gastrointestinal endoscopy (UGIE) for UGIH and colonoscopy for LGIH. The advantage of performing endoscopy in patients of GIH is in detection of the lesion responsible for bleeding and in managing them endoscopically wherever required. In addition, sampling of the lesion can be done wherever necessary. Various endoscopic treatment options include injection of epinephrine or alcohol, thermal ablations like electrocoagulation or laser therapy and mechanical placement of clips or bands. The sensitivity and specificity of UGIE in evaluation of UGIH are 92–98% and 30–100% respectively.[8] Colonoscopy has a variable accuracy of 45–90%.[9] There are few limitations of endoscopy. Performing an endoscopy in a sick patient is difficult and may take time. Blood in the GIT may obscure the bleeding source and therapy may be impossible. In colonoscopy, bowel preparation needed for proper visualization may not be possible in acute setting. Despite these drawbacks, it is still the first line of investigation as most of the lesions responsible of GIH may not be seen on imaging.

Wireless capsule endoscopy is useful in patients where the source is not identified on other endoscopic techniques. It is a noninvasive technique and is useful in patient with occult or chronic GIH, with a diagnostic yield of about 63%.[10] Since the study takes long time (patient preparation, capsule transit time and download of data), it is mainly used in chronic an intermittent GIH and not in acute GIH. Its major risk is retention of capsule proximal to an intestinal stricture which needs surgical treatment. Double balloon enteroscopy can help in visualizing up to distal small bowel with diagnostic yield of 40–80%.

IMAGING MODALITIES

Various imaging modalities are available in the workup of patients presenting with GIH. These have been described here. It is important for the radiologist to choose the right type of investigation depending on the clinical presentation and suspicion.

Table 1: Etiology of GIH.

Upper GI bleed	*Lower GI bleed*
Peptic ulcer disease	Angiodysplasia
Varices	Diverticular disease
Gastritis/esophagitis/duodenitis	Neoplasms
Neoplasms	Colitis
Iatrogenic/postoperative	Iatrogenic/postoperative
Hepato-bilio-pancreatica	Hemorrhoids

Box 3: Routine investigations in GIH.

Clinical:
- Endoscopy/colonoscopy
- Enteroscopy/capsule endoscopy

Imaging:
- CT angiography/CT enterography
- Radionuclide scan
- Digital subtraction angiography

Box 4: Indications for imaging in GIH.

- Acute GIH when arterial source is identified on endoscopy
- Normal findings on endoscopy
- Hemobilia/hemosuccus pancreaticus on endoscopy
- Chronic/recurrent GIH
- Endoscopy not possible/difficult/failed
- Obscure or occult GIH

Indications

As described above, imaging is not needed in most patients presenting with GIH. The timing of imaging is also crucial in improving detection rates as bleeding is usually intermittent. Endoscopic diagnosis and management is sufficient. Also, in about 75% patients of UGIH and 80% patients of LGIH, the bleeding stops spontaneously and imaging may not detect any lesion. Thus about 20–25% patients of GIH require imaging.[3] Further, imaging may not identify a lesion in about 14% cases of UGIH and 20% of LGIH.[8] Thus, it is important to carefully define the indications for imaging in patients of GIH **(Box 4)**.

Radionuclide Studies

Radionuclide studies play role in the evaluation of patients with GIH with minimal risk and invasiveness to the patient.[11] The major indication is in cases where bleeding slow or intermittent as scanning can be done for longer periods. It is not useful in patients with massive continuous bleeding. It has variable accuracy and sometimes proximal or distal movement of the radionuclide between imaging sessions impair precise localization of the actual bleeding site.

The common radionuclides employed in patients with GIH are as follows:

^{99m}*Tc sulfur colloid:* It is cleared from the blood pool by the reticuloendothelial system. The half-life of the tracer in the blood pool is approximately 2.5–3 min. If active bleeding is occurring during this short time, the tracer extravasates into the bowel which can be identified on subsequent imaging. Although sulfur colloid scintigraphy can detect bleeding rates as low as 0.1 mL/min, this is possible only when there is active bleeding at the time of scan. In addition, isotope study can be repeated as often as required. The drawback is that bleeding into the hepatic or splenic flexures of the colon and UGIH will be obscured because of the overlap by normal accumulation of the tracer in liver and spleen.

^{99m}*Tc-labeled red blood cell (RBC):* These labeled RBCs in circulation extravasate during bleeding and can be detected. They have longer half-life in circulation. The advantage is that images can be obtained up to 2 hours after the initial injection and hence is especially useful for evaluating intermittent GIH. The major limitation is that activity seen in the lower GIT, when it may have occurred from more proximal segments of small bowel and sources of bleeding may be missed if frequent views are not obtained. This has a sensitivity and specificity of 93% and 95% respectively for bleeding rates > 0.04 mL/min.[12]

^{99m}*Tc-pertechnetate:* It is used in cases where bleeding from Meckel's diverticulum is suspected. This tracer accumulates in ectopic gastric mucosa present in the diverticulum and helps in identifying the source of GIH.

Computed Tomography

Computed tomography (CT) scan is the corner stone in the evaluation of GIH.[13] It is easily available, has high spatial resolution and can detect bleeding as low as 0.3 mL/min. Faster scans are possible with multidetector CT. The timing of CT scan is important due to intermittent nature of GIH and should be done as soon as GIH is clinically diagnosed.[14] Signs of GIH on CT scan include direct sign like extravasation of contrast into bowel lumen (jet like or swirling; **Figs. 1A to C**) and indirect signs like pseudoaneurysm **(Figs. 2A to D)**, vascular malformation or tumors.

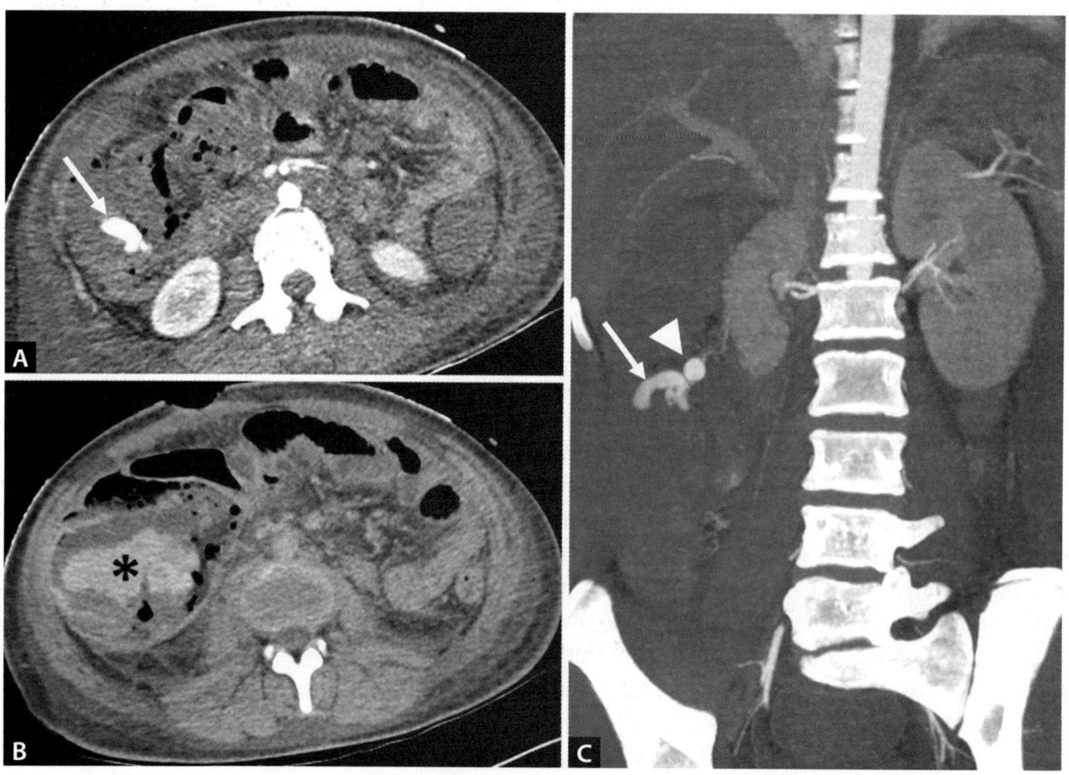

Figs. 1A to C: GIH presenting after ileal resection: Axial contrast-enhanced CT images in arterial phase (A) showing contrast extravasation into the ascending colon (arrow) from right colic artery with increase in extravasation in the venous phase (asterisk in B). Maximum intensity projection coronal image in arterial phase (C) also shows the pseudoaneurysm (arrowhead) with active extravasation of contrast (arrow).

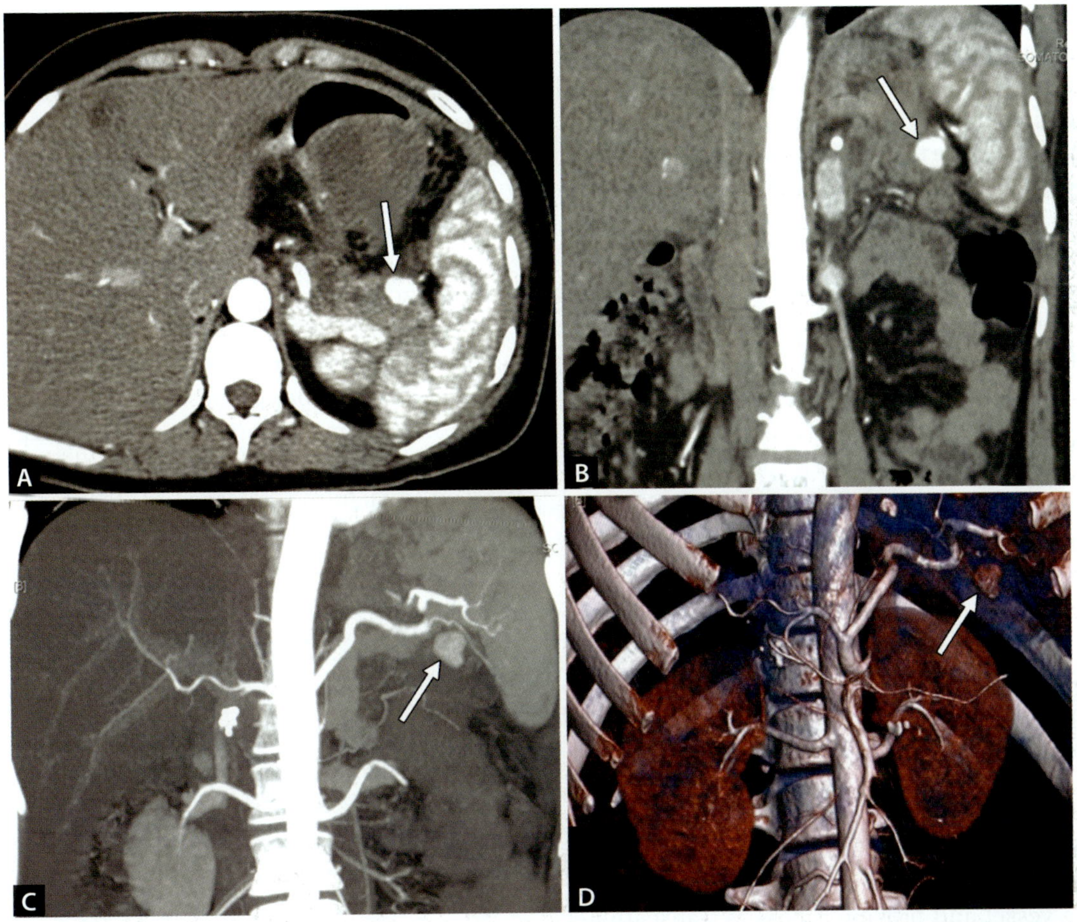

Figs. 2A to D: Chronic pancreatitis with GIH: Axial (A) and coronal (B) CT angiography images showing a pseudoaneurysm (arrow) arising from a branch of distal splenic artery. Coronal maximum intensity projection image (C) and 3D volume-rendered image (D) showing the pseudoaneurysm (arrow) and the source artery.

CT protocol: This typically involves performing an arterial and a venous phases. Iodinated contrast material is injected at the rate of 4 mL/sec. Oral contrast is usually not necessary. Arterial phase [CT angiography—(CTA)] is done at about 25–30 seconds after injection of contrast. This should be a late arterial phase to help detect small lesions and source of bleeding. Automatic bolus triggering is used for this with region of interest in abdominal aorta and trigger attenuation of 150 HU. Time delay after triggering should be about 10–15 sec. This is followed by venous phase (60–70 sec). In cases of UGIH, arterial phase should include area from dome of diaphragm to iliac crest and venous phase, the entire abdomen, including pelvis. For LGIH, the entire abdomen from dome of diaphragm to symphysis pubis should be scanned in both phases. When a small bowel source is suspected, CT enterography should be performed with neutral oral contrast and both arterial and venous phases should be acquired. Plain scans may be done and it may show acute hematoma in the bowel lumen.

The sensitivity, specificity and accuracy of CT angiography in the detection and localization of GIH are 90.9%, 99% and 97.6% respectively.[15] In addition to routine baseline images, reviewing the coronal reconstruction, maximum intensity projections (MIP) and volume rendered images are useful in identifying the source of bleeding and the feeding artery if any **(Figs. 2A to D)**. Low kV acquisition (100 kV) may be done for improved contrast resolution. Wide window settings will help in reducing the beam hardening artifacts due to high iodine concentration. With the advent of CTA for diagnosis of source of GIH, the role of conventional angiography has been largely limited to endovascular interventions. The advantages of performing CTA prior to digital subtraction angiography (DSA) are many. These include:

- CTA helps to plan DSA by identifying the source artery and anatomical variations.
- This decreases number of DSA exposures

- CTA information allows faster catheterization of bleeding vessels
- It decreases the amount of contrast material used during angiography
- It reduces procedure time and radiation exposure

Dual energy CTA is a recent addition and helps in reducing radiation dose due to its capability of generating virtual non-contrast images. In a recent study by Sun et al, it was shown that dual energy CTA with virtual noncontrast images and iodine maps is an accurate screening method in patients with active GIH with lower radiation dose.[16]

Angiography

Angiography plays a significant role in the management of patients with acute GIH by localizing the actual site of active bleeding and transcatheter embolization of the bleeding artery.[17] The role of angiography in the diagnosis of cause of GIH has diminished because of wider availability of endoscopy and CT angiography. However, it remains a valuable tool in patients with recurrent or continued GIH in whom source has eluded all other investigations. Angiography is beneficial in patients who fail to respond to conservative or invasive endoscopic management. It is also valuable in patients who are unstable and are bleeding massively. Angiography in these situations can locate the bleeding vessel and provide access to transcatheter management either to obviate surgery or to stabilize the patient before surgery.[2]

Angiography is especially important in whom bleeding has continued after blind laparotomy.[18] In acute GIH, angiography detects the site if bleeding exceeds 0.5 mL/min (blood loss exceeds four units within 24 hours). If bleeding is intermittent and the patient is stable, other less invasive examinations can be used and emergency angiography is not required. Evaluation of recurrent hemorrhage may be time consuming and expensive if bleeding is intermittent. Provocative pharmacoangiography and carbon dioxide angiography may be useful in select situations.

Technical Details

The renal function should be normal because angiography requires large amount of contrast medium. If renal function is deranged, alternative contrast media like carbon dioxide can be used for angiography.

A flush aortogram may be done initially, but often it is avoided and direct selective and superselective arteriography is done. In flush aortogram, the tip of pigtail catheter tip is placed above the level of celiac axis and a total of about 40 mL of iodinated contrast agent is injected using a mechanical injector at the rate of 18–22 mL/sec. This is followed by selective and superselective studies using various visceral angiographic catheters. Flush aortograms are important, particularly in cases of suspected aortoenteric fistula. If a major splanchnic artery cannot be catheterized or identified, a lateral aortography is used to accurately demonstrate and catheterize major aortic branches.

In mesenteric studies, the flow rate for contrast injection should be approximately 10 mL/sec for the celiac, 8 mL/sec for the superior mesenteric artery and 3 mL/sec for the inferior mesenteric artery. The imaging must be rapid during the arterial phase (2–3 frames/sec) and reduced to (1 frame/2–5 second) for the capillary and venous phases. Imaging should be carried out up to at least 30 seconds, to identify slow extravasation, suspected venous occlusion and vascular malformations. The suspected bleeding artery should be catheterized first if there is prior CTA information. If not, then all major branches of celiac artery (gastroduodenal, hepatic and left gastric) and then superior mesenteric (middle colic, right colic, ileocolic, major jejunal/ileal branches) and inferior mesenteric arteries (left colic and superior rectal) are sequentially catheterized. Microcatheters (2.5–2.8F) should be used wherever possible for catheterizing smaller or tortuous arteries. The more selective the catheter is placed, the higher the probability that active bleeding will be recognized. The rate of blood loss must be at least 5–6 mL/min for it to be detected on the midstream flush aortogram. However, selective arteriography may reveal bleeding sources with rate of bleeding as low as 0.5 mL/min. DSA of mesenteric arteries may sometimes be suboptimal due to bowel gas and peristalsis. Such motion artifacts may be misinterpreted as contrast extravasation and hence antispasmodic drugs are sometimes used to reduce bowel peristalsis. The sensitivity of DSA is 63–90% and 40– 86% for UGIH and LGIH respectively and specificity is 100% and positive findings are seen in about 24–78% patients of GIH.[19]

In approximately 70% of patients with gastric mucosal hemorrhage, bleeding occurs from left gastric artery (LGA). Hence, it is essential that LGA be well opacified during selective angiography. The celiac axis angiogram would not suffice if the tip of the catheter is distal to the origin of the LGA, or if the LGA originates from the aorta. In bleeding duodenal ulcers, contrast extravasation is most commonly noted from the supraduodenal branch of gastroduodenal artery. In variceal bleeding, contrast extravasation is rarely demonstrated as contrast medium gets diluted by the time it reaches the bleeding veins. The purpose of angiography in variceal bleeding is very limited.

Angiographic Findings in GIH

- *Extravasation of contrast:* It is seen as a puddling or staining that persists beyond the capillary and venous phases.
- Delayed films may show opacified intestinal folds due to luminal extravasation of contrast medium.
- If the lumen of the gastrointestinal tract is filled with clotted blood, a 'pseudovein' appearance is often seen as the extravasated contrast flows through the clot to the most dependent part. However, unlike the venous phase, it persists for a much longer time.
- Other findings include pseudoaneurysm **(Fig. 3)**, arteriovenous fistula, abnormal blush, neovascularity or hyperemia.
- Because bleeding may be intermittent, and spasm may preclude opacification of the target vessel, repeat injection or repeat angiography may be required to show the bleeding vessel **(Figs. 4A to C)**.

Provocative angiography may be done in patients of GIH when no cause is found on routine imaging.[20] Here, heparin, tissue plasminogen activator (tPA) and vasodilator (tolazoline) are injected through the catheter into the artery. This is followed by DSA to demonstrate any bleeding source. This technique increases blood flow into the vessel, relieves vasospasm and lyses any small clot, and thus improves detection of bleeding lesion. Provocative angiography has been shown to identify a cause in up to 33% patients of GIH with normal routine DSA.[21]

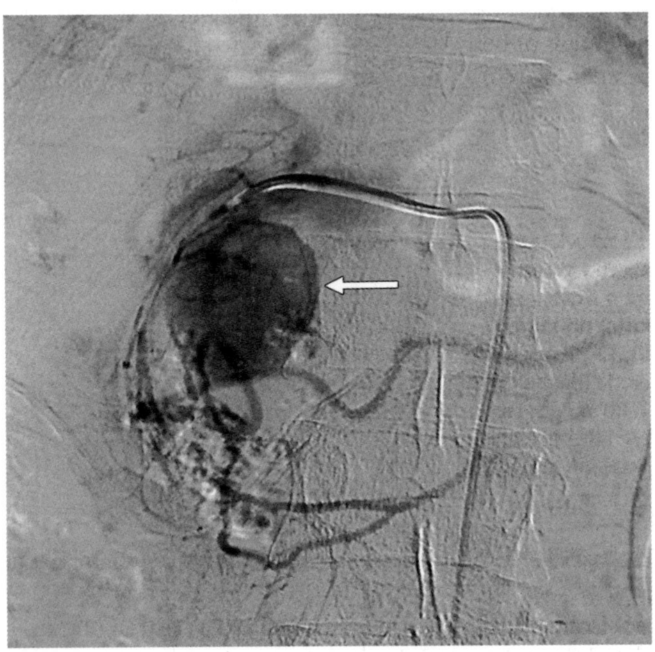

Fig. 3: DSA of gastroduodenal artery showing a large pseudoaneurysm (arrow) in a case of pancreatitis presenting with hematemesis.

Carbon dioxide angiography is useful in patients of renal failure and patients allergic to iodinated contrast agents. Carbon dioxide (CO_2) is an inert gas and easily dissolves in blood and is excreted by lungs.[22] It has low viscosity and has been suggested to be better in the evaluation of GIH.[23] It may be used in cases with high clinical suspicion and normal routine DSA.

Ultrasonography

Ultrasonography (USG) has limited role in the evaluation of patients with GIH. It specific situations like large superficial aneurysm/pseudoaneurysm and vascular abnormalities in solid organs (liver) color Doppler USG helps in detecting the lesion and may also guide if percutaneous intervention is needed. In addition, contrast enhanced USG assists in evaluating thickened segments of small bowel in patients with inflammatory bowel disease presenting with GIH.

Magnetic Resonance Imaging

Magnetic resonance angiography (MRA) has currently no role in the evaluation of acute GIH. Longer scan times, lower spatial resolution and need for breath hold limits its use in acute situations. However, in patients with chronic or recurrent GIH, MR enterography is useful in the evaluation of small bowel abnormalities such as inflammatory bowel disease, tumors, mesenteric ischemia and vasculitis.

RADIOLOGICAL INTERVENTIONS IN GASTROINTESTINAL HEMORRHAGE

After the bleeding site has been localized on imaging, minimally invasive angiographic procedures should be performed wherever possible to control the hemorrhage. This helps to avoid an emergency surgery in a patient with acute GIH. Endoscopic techniques like coagulation and mucosal injection of sclerosing agent controls bleeding in cases of ulcer and varices **(Box 5)**.

Radiological approaches used in the treatment of GIH include endovascular and percutaneous techniques.[24] Endovascular approach should be initially used in these patients as control is better and complications are fewer.

Endovascular Approach

Endovascular embolization has been used for lesions of the stomach, colon and small bowel. It is especially useful

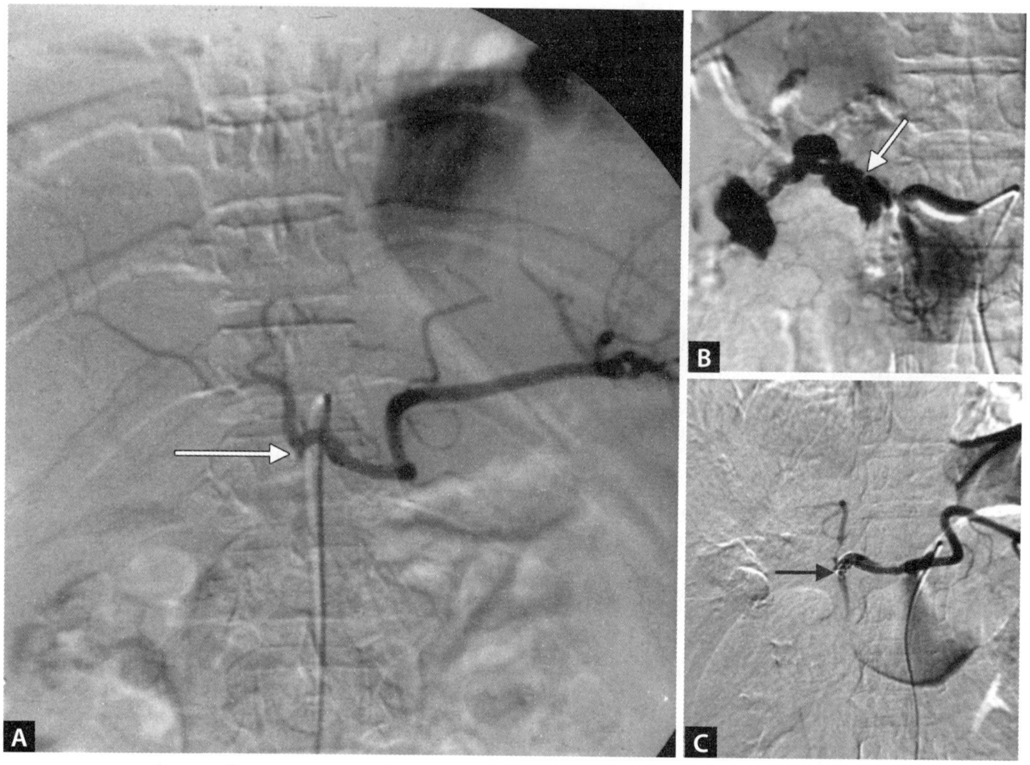

Figs. 4A to C: (A) Celiac artery angiogram in a case of GIH is showing spasm of gastroduodenal artery (arrow); (B) Hepatic artery angiogram showing extravasation of contrast in subhepatic area (arrow), and (C) Celiac artey angiogram after steel coil embolization not showing extravasation of contrast (arrow).

Box 5: Management of GIH.

Endoscopic • Coagulation • Sclerosant injection • EUS-guided thrombin/glue injection
Radiological *Endovascular* • Embolization–coils, glue, plug, gelfoam • Stents—stent graft, stent-assisted coiling • Balloon remodeling *Percutaneous—thrombin or glue injection*

in the treatment of bleeding pancreatic or hepatic artery pseudoaneurysms.[25] Here the target artery is catheterized superselectively and embolic agents are injected into the lesion or feeding artery to exclude the lesion from the circulation and thus control hemorrhage. The methods of endovascular treatment of pseudoaneurysm used include sandwich technique, proximal embolization, sac filling, stent assisted coiling, balloon remodeling and stent graft placement. The advantages are as follows:

- Control of bleeding is immediate
- Risk of visceral ischemia is minimal if embolization is superselective and collaterals are preserved.

Percutaneous Approach

This technique is used when endovascular approach fails or is not possible and in cases where the lesion is superficial and surrounded by solid parenchyma (e.g. intrahepatic pseudoaneurysm).[24] This is performed by direct puncture of the pseudoaneurysm by a thin needle (22G) under USG guidance followed by injection of embolic agent. The risks include rupture and non-target embolization.

Embolic Materials

Various embolic materials are available which are used in the management of GIH. These include permanent occluding agents like coils/microcoils, polyvinyl alcohol particles, n-butyl cyanoacrylate (nBCA or glue) and vascular plugs.[24,26] Temporary embolizing agents include gelatin sponge and autologous blood clot. Wherever a lesion is identified, permanent embolic agent should be used to avoid recurrence. Temporary agents may be used for per-operative and empirical (when bleeding source is not identified) embolization. The embolization in conjunction with vasopressin infusion is not recommended. The major risks of bowel embolization are ischemia and stricture formation, but these risks must be weighed against the high mortality rate of emergency surgery. Minimum amount of embolic material should be used to stop hemorrhage and should be injected as selectively as possible to avoid complications.

SPECIFIC SITUATIONS IN GASTROINTESTINAL HEMORRHAGES

Upper gastrointestinal hemorrhage (UGIH) can be differentiated from lower gastrointestinal hemorrhage (LGIH) by localizing the source of bleeding either proximal or distal to the ligament of Treitz. UGIH is 10 times more common than LGHI. Before imaging, a distinction must be made between UGIH and LGIH based on clinical findings.

Upper Gastrointestinal Hemorrhage

As described in **Table 1**, common causes (peptic ulcer disease, gastritis and varices) of UGIH account for up to 90% of all cases. Other less common causes include neoplasms of esophagus, stomach and duodenum, aortoenteric fistula, pancreatitis, hemobilia, arteriovenous malformations **(Figs. 5A to C)**, splanchnic arterial aneurysms and rarely mesenteric venous thrombosis and hepatobiliary and pancreatic tumors.[27,28] Acute UGIH due to penetration of a hepatic or left gastric artery aneurysm into the duodenal bulb **(Figs. 6A to D)** or stomach **(Figs. 7A to D)** is rare but has been reported.[29] Rarely primary blood dyscrasias, vasculitis, connective tissue disorders, hamartoma, jejunoileitis and uremia may also produce significant bleeding.[30]

Hemobilia

The causes are hepatic trauma, neoplasms, abscesses, hepatic artery aneurysm, laparoscopic and postoperative or interventional procedures of the liver **(Figs. 8 to 11)**. The presentation is characteristic, i.e. biliary colic, obstructive jaundice and UGIH. The diagnosis is made either on endoscopy by the appearance of blood from the ampulla of Vater or by diagnostic hepatic arteriography. The rupture of hepatic arterial branches and hepatic arterial aneurysms can be treated by angioembolization or surgical ligation of hepatic artery.[31]

Pancreatitis and Upper Gastrointestinal Hemorrhage

In pancreatitis a pseudocyst is frequently recognized on imaging, but a pseudoaneurysm is noted in less than 10% of cases. Intracystic hemorrhage has been reported in 6–10% of cases and this is due to extension of pancreatic inflammation to the nearby splenic artery. The pancreatic pseudocysts may present with the following five patterns of hemorrhage:[32]

1. Hemorrhage within the pseudocyst presenting with intermittent severe abdominal pain due to elevated intracystic pressure.
2. Gastrointestinal bleeding caused by fistula formation near the digestive tract.
3. Rupture into the peritoneum.
4. Hemorrhage caused by fistula formation with the bile duct.
5. Hemorrhage into the duodenum via the pancreatic duct (hemosuccus pancreaticus).

Celiac and superior mesenteric angiography should be done and selective arterial embolization may control the hemorrhage **(Figs. 12 and 13)**.

Lower Gastrointestinal Hemorrhage

Patients with lower gastrointestinal bleeding are usually older than those with gastric or duodenal lesions.

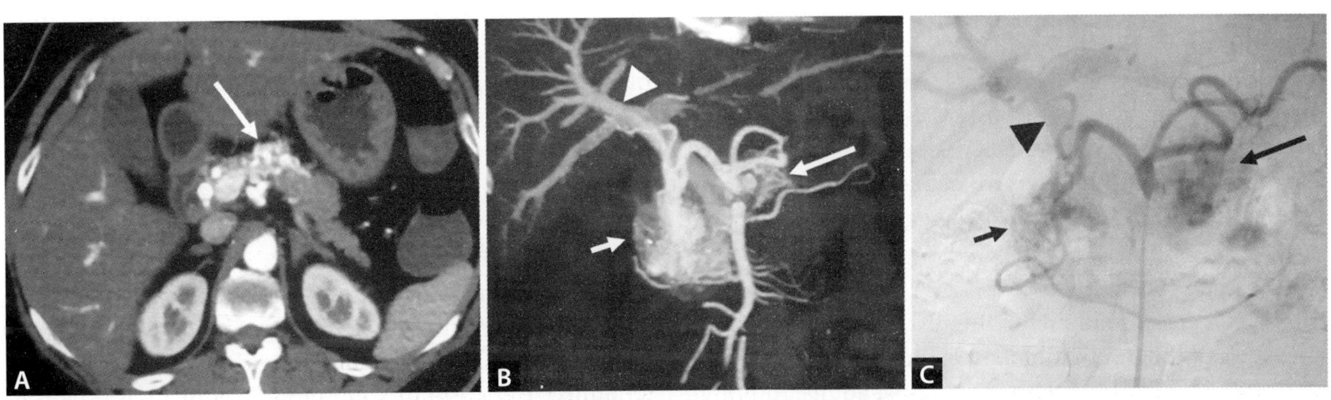

Figs. 5A to C: Pancreatic AVM. (A) Axial CT image in arterial phase showing cluster of vessels in the body of pancreas (arrow); (B) Coronal MIP image in arterial phase showing bunch of vessels at two locations, head (short arrow) and body (long arrow) region of pancreas with early filling of portal vein (arrowhead); (C) DSA of celiac artery showing the same two nidus, in head (short arrow) and body (long arrow) with arteriovenous shunting and opacification of portal vein (arrowhead). This was embolized preoperatively using PVA particles.

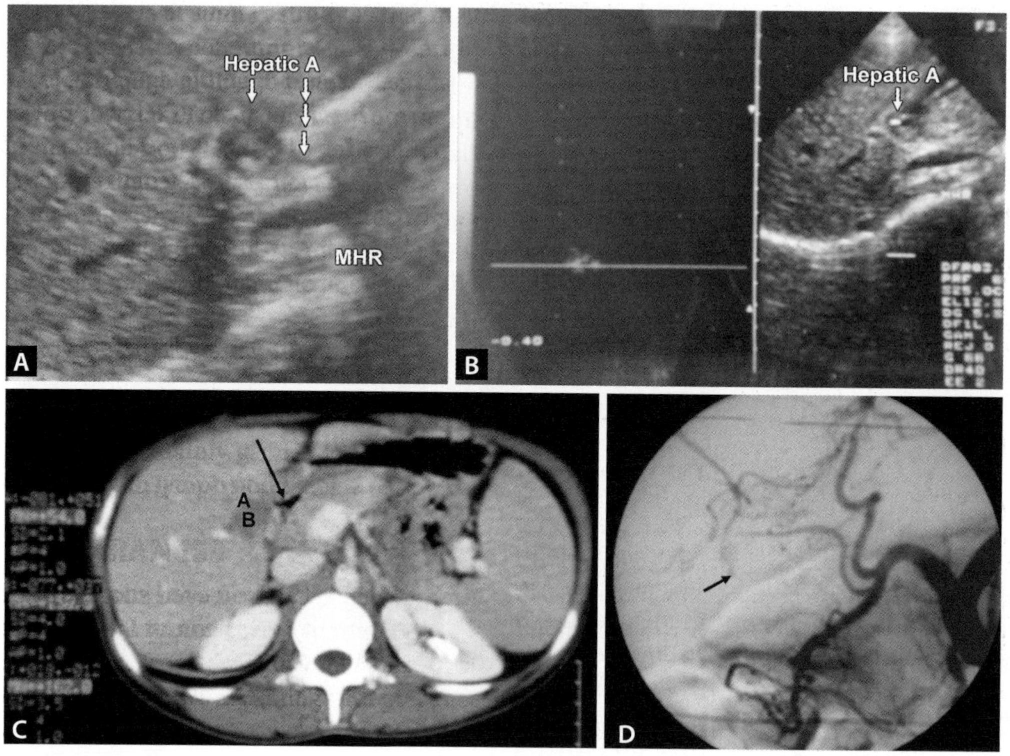

Figs. 6A to D: (A) Abdominal sonography showing a round, cystic mass at the porta; (B) Doppler sonography showing absence of signal in the echogenic area of the lesion; (C) Contrast-enhancing CT showing a low-attenuating area with an enhanced center lateral to second part at the duodenum (arrow). Selective celiac artery angiogram (D) is showing the aneurysm (arrow). At surgery, the partially thrombosed aneurysm was communicating to duodenal bulb

Causes of LGIH in India are nonspecific ulcers (30%), enteric ulcers (15%), tuberculosis (6%), neoplasms (6%) and others (31%). In western literature the causes are diverticular (33%), colitis and ulcers (22%), neoplasms (20%), angiodysplasia and others (25%). Some of the causes of the LGIH are discussed below.

Colonic Diverticula

They are mostly seen in the left sided colon. Bleeding is typically abrupt in onset, massive and painless, and does not recur in 60% of patients. Active diverticular bleeding can be demonstrated either by direct endoscopic visualization or by filling of the bleeding diverticulum with contrast medium at the time of angiography.

Meckel's Diverticulum

It is a congenital anomaly of the distal ileum, present in about 2% of the population and is an important cause of acute hemorrhage in children and young adults. Although only about 15% of these diverticula contain gastric mucosa, half the lesions, which cause acute bleeding, contain gastric mucosa. The acid secretions from gastric mucosa result in peptic ulceration, most often in the ileal mucosa adjacent to the gastric mucosa and may lead to gastrointestinal bleeding.[33] ^{99m}Tc-pertechnetate radionuclide scans can detect these bleeding diverticula. Identifying normal Meckel's diverticulum is difficult on CT scan. It may show nodular enhancing mucosa in a tubular structure. Angiography can show the vessel supplying the area of abnormally increased contrast medium accumulation in the distal ileum. Vitelline artery is a separate branch of the superior mesenteric artery, which is specific to Meckel's diverticulum, but in 80% of diverticula this vessel is involuted and is replaced by a distal ileal branch **(Figs. 14A to E)**.[34]

Angiodysplasia

It is a mucosal telangiectasia, often multiple, usually involving the cecum or ascending colon. These lesions are often multiple and represent dilated pre-existing vascular structures (mucosal or submucosal venules). It is caused mainly by intermittent obstruction of venous outflow, but ischemia or toxic effects of bowel contents also have their role in its pathogenesis.

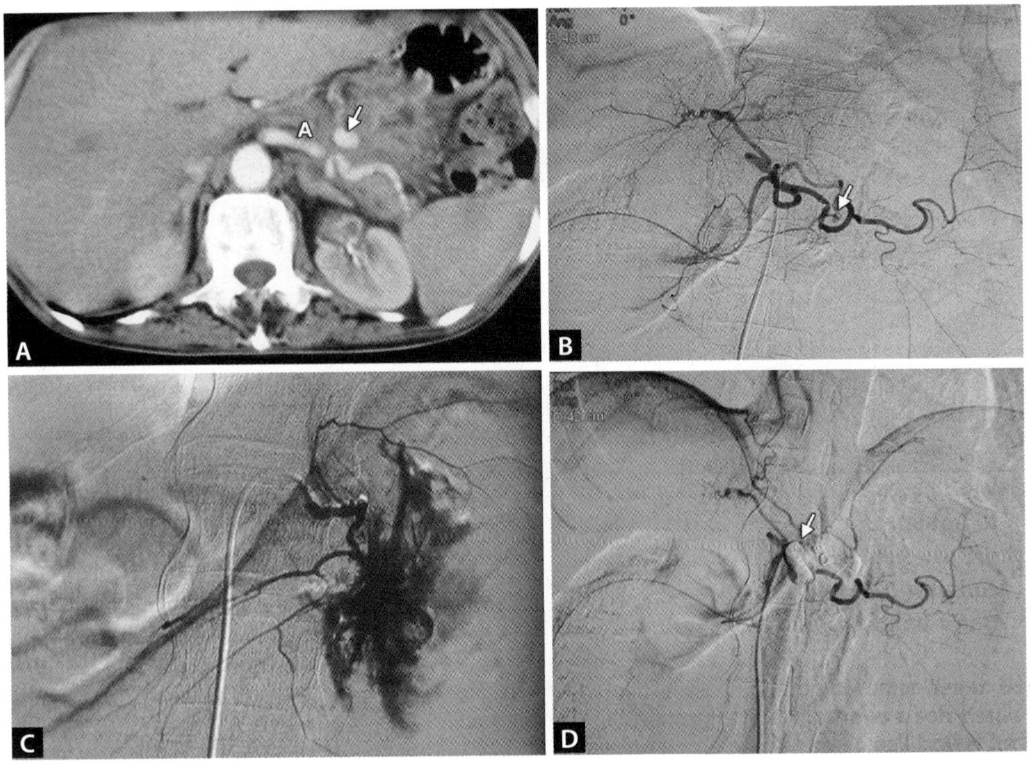

Figs. 7A to D: Contrast-enhanced arterial phase CT (A) and celiac artery angiogram (B) of a case of massive gastrointestinal hemorrhage is showing an enhancing aneurysm posterior to stomach (arrows). Selective left gastric artery angiogram (C) is showing leakage of contrast into stomach due to aneurysmogastric fistula. The left gastric artery was embolized (arrow) with steel coils (D) and partial gastrectomy was done later.

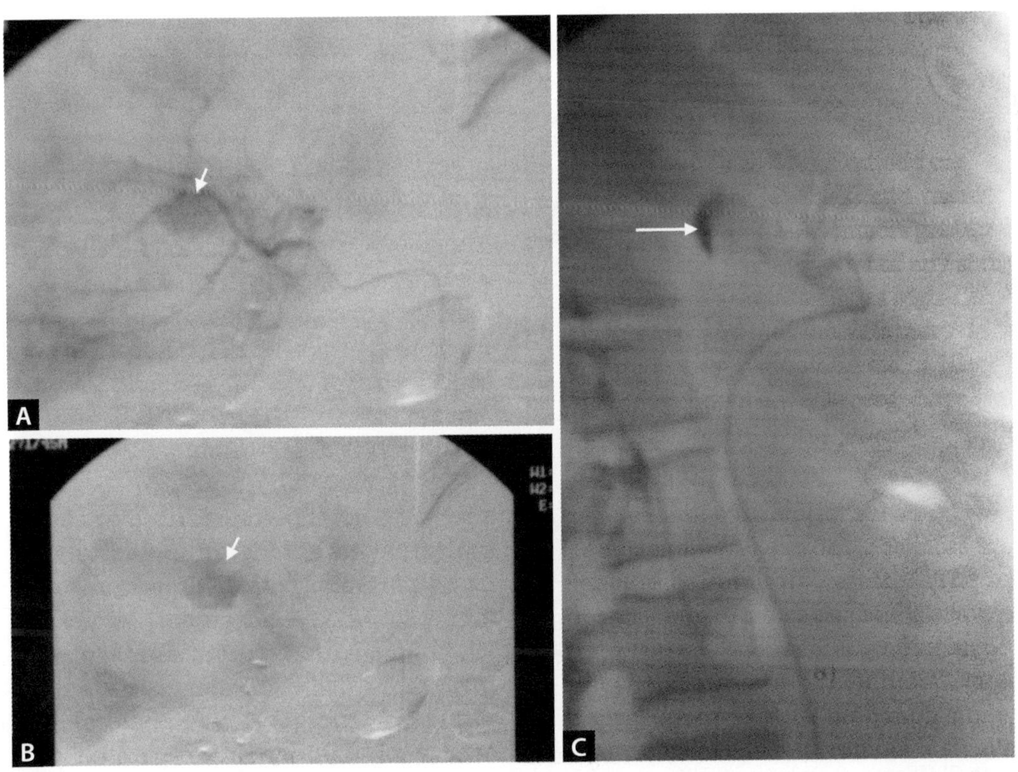

Figs. 8A to C: (A and B) Hepatic artery angiogram in a postoperative patient of road traffic accident showing extravasation of the contrast in the right lobe of liver (arrows); and (C) Lateral film showing pooling of contrast in a cavity (arrow).

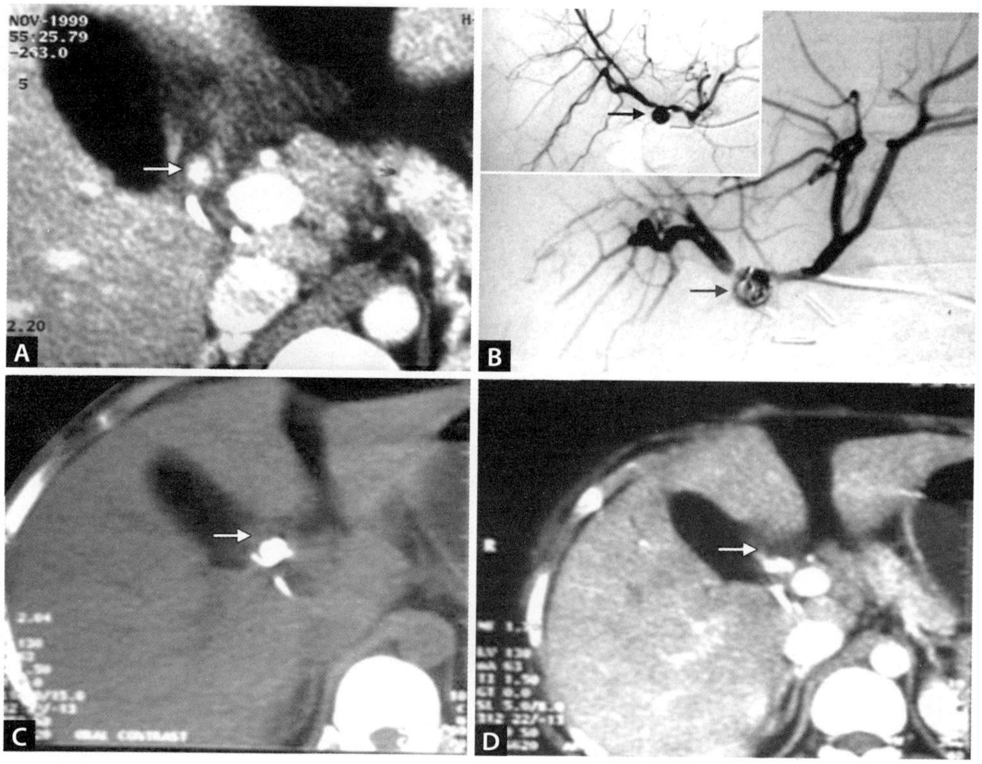

Figs. 9A to D: A 42-year-old woman with hemobilia following open cholecystectomy done two months ago shows right hepatic artery aneurysm (arrow) on CT (A) and hepatic angiography (B, inset). It was embolized using steel coils (B, arrow). Four months following embolization the noncontrast enhanced CT (C) shows aneurysm packed with coils (arrow). There is no enhancement of aneurysm on contrast-enhanced CT (D).

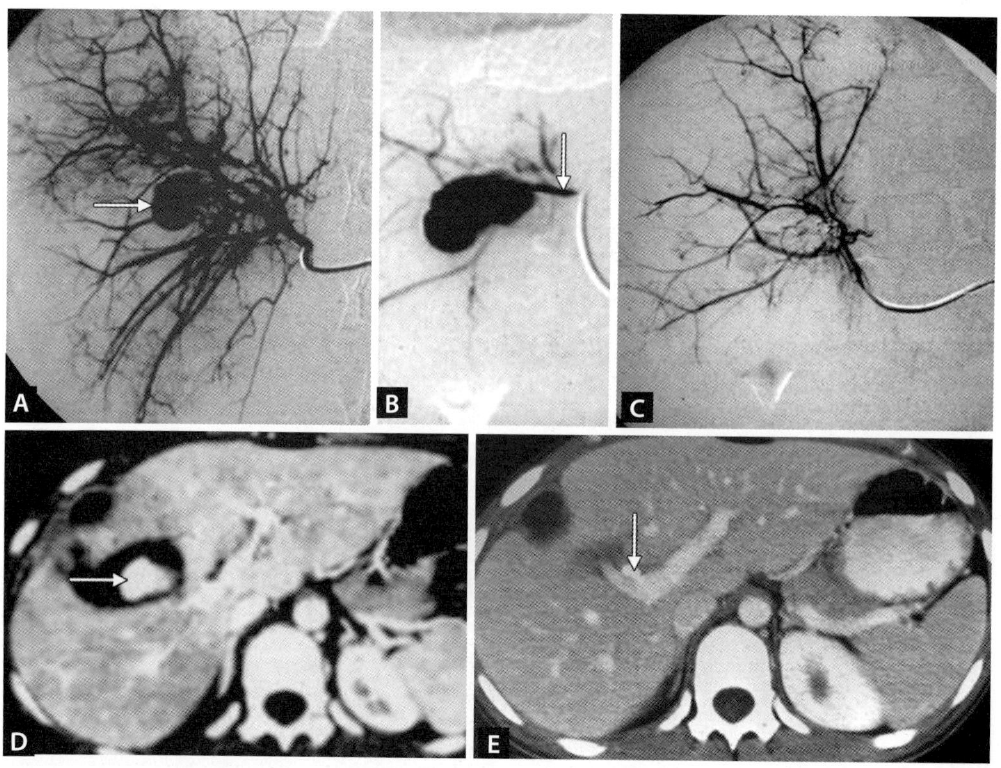

Figs. 10A to E: (A to C) Hepatic angiogram of a 28-years-old male a road traffic accident victim with a large pseudoaneurysm (arrow) filling by middle hepatic artery (arrowhead) was embolized with steel coil; (D and E) The aneurysm (arrow) and steel coil (arrowhead) are seen on pre- and postembolization three months CT.

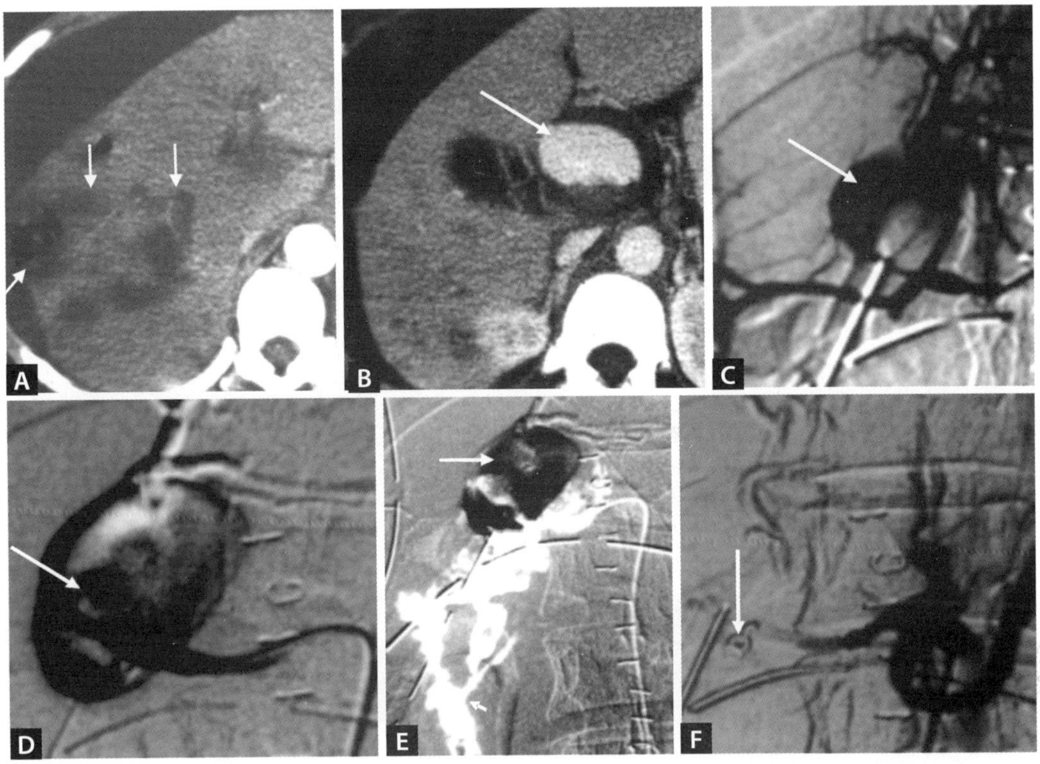

Figs. 11A to F: (A to D) A 35-year-old male with liver abscess (arrows) on treatment developed a large hepatic artery aneurysm (arrow); (E) There is simultaneous opacification of duodenum (arrows) due to communication of aneurysm to duodenum; (F) The hepatic artery was embolized using steel coils (arrow).

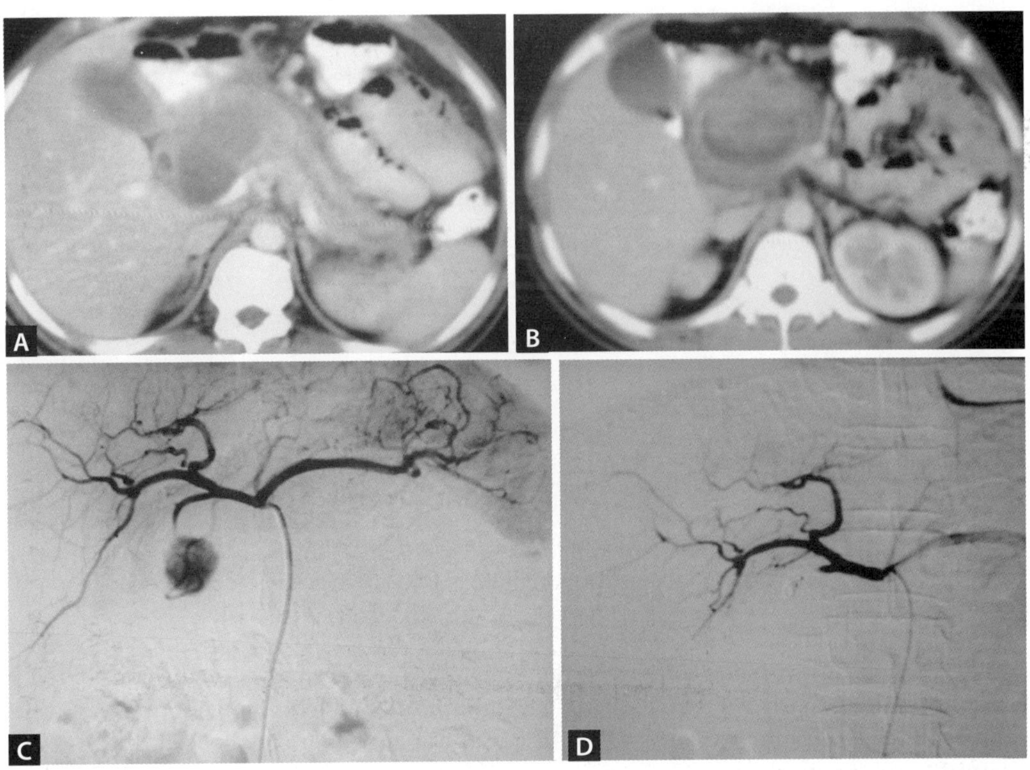

Figs. 12A to D: Contrast-enhanced CT (A and B) of a case of acute pancreatitis is showing a large pseudocyst with bleed and peripancreatic inflammation in head of pancreas. The pancreatic duct is dilated. Celiac artery angiogram (C) is showing an aneurysm of gastroduodenal artery. The artery was embolized with steel coils (D). Superior mesenteric angiogram was normal.

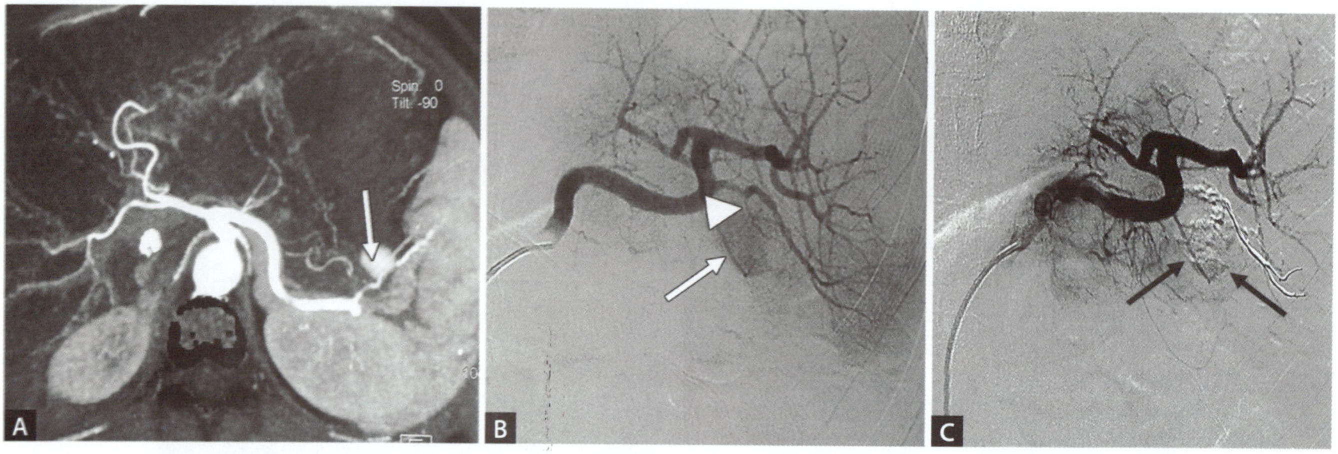

Figs. 13A to C: Splenic artery pseudoaneurysm: (A) MIP-CT image in arterial phase showing a contrast-filled outpouching (arrow) in the distal splenic artery; (B) DSA of splenic artery shows the pseudoaneurysm (arrow) arising from distal branch of splenic artery (arrowhead); (C) DSA after embolization with combination of coils and glue shows complete obliteration of the pseudoaneurysm (arrows).

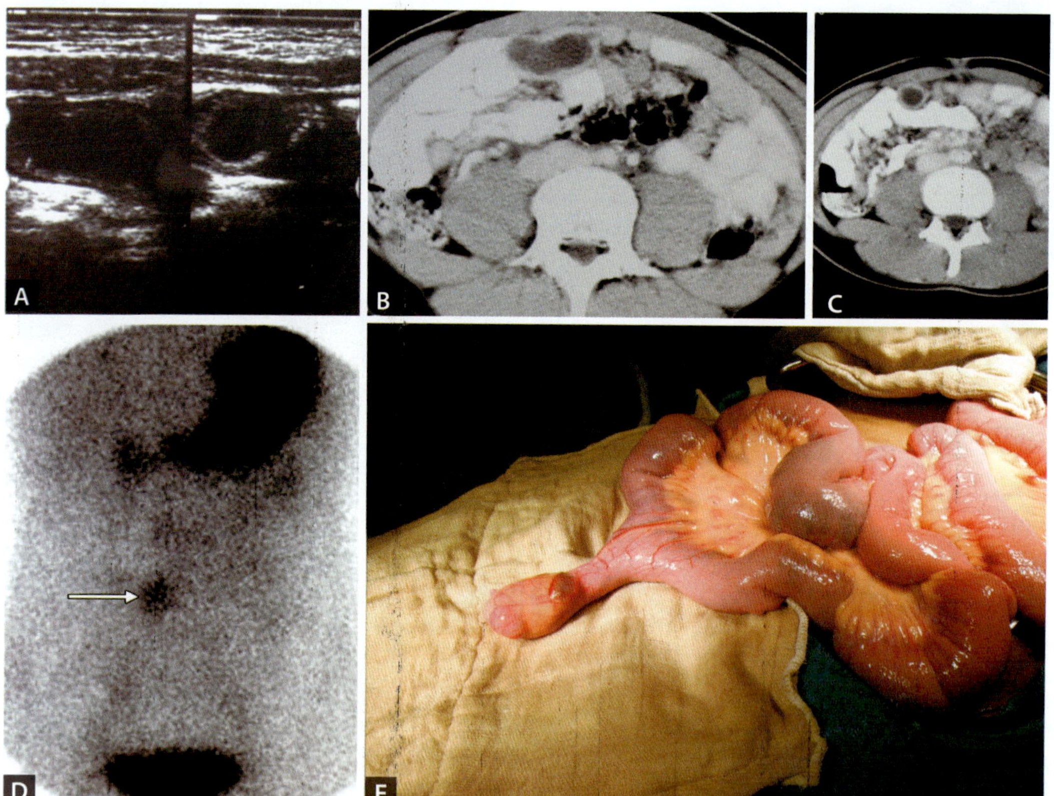

Figs. 14A to E: USG (A) showing a tubular, noncompressible, thick-walled blind ending structure in right paraumbilical region. On CECT (B and C) it was fluid filled with enhancing wall and showed active uptake of tracer (arrow) on ^{99m}Tc pertechnetate scan (D). The diagnosis of Meckel's diverticulum was confirmed at surgery (E).

On angiography it is seen as a vascular tuft appearing in the arterial phase with an early opacification of a draining vein, and delayed emptying of a dilated and tortuous intramural vein. To diagnose bleeding from angiodysplasia, actual extravasation of contrast must be demonstrated. If extravasation is not detected, carcinoma or some other lesion should be considered, because about one-third of all elderly patients may have angiodysplasia without any history of bleeding. After angiographic diagnosis of the lesion, catheter may be left in place for arterial injection of methylene blue for intraoperative localization of the lesion. Treatment of incidentally found angioectasias is not indicated in patients with no history of LGIH.

Hemangioma and Arteriovenous Malformation

Gastrointestinal tract hemangioma and AVM are rare but can cause significant morbidity **(Figs. 5 and 15)**. The clinical presentation may be acute, recurrent or chronic. MR imaging is sometimes useful in the evaluation of extent of the colonic lesion.[35]

Tumors

These can bleed spontaneously, but such blood loss is more likely to be chronic and intermittent rather than massive. On angiography some tumors like leiomyomas and leiomyosarcomas, adenoma and Kaposi's sarcoma are hypervascular and typically have an intense capillary stain **(Figs. 16A and B)**.

Inflammatory Bowel Diseases and Small Bowel or Colonic Ulcers

These produce nonspecific angiographic findings such as dilated arteries, mucosal outlining and sometimes pooling of contrast. Radiologic intervention is rarely needed.

Others

Mesenteric varices are rare and bleeding from these sites is unusual. The common location of these is in the rectosigmoid area. The most common cause of these varices is portal hypertension. Rarely these may be secondary to portal vein obstruction, congenital hepatic fibrosis (CHF), splenic vein thrombosis secondary to pancreatitis and splenorenal shunt block.[36] On angiography these can be demonstrated on delayed phase.

Ischemic colitis can be of occlusive or nonocclusive etiology. The occlusive causes are iatrogenic interruption of inferior mesenteric artery during aortic surgery, embolism, thrombosis, aneurysm of abdominal aorta, amyloidosis and vasculitis **(Figs. 17A and B)**.[37] Nonocclusive causes include low flow states due to cardiac dysfunction and hypovolemia. In the majority of patients, it is mild or transient. On barium enema, the hallmark of ischemic colitis is thumbprinting caused by submucosal hemorrhage and edema.

The rupture of arteriosclerotic aortic aneurysms into the small intestine (aortoenteric fistula) is almost always fatal. Rupture usually occurs after an arterial reconstructive surgery with fistula formation between synthetic graft

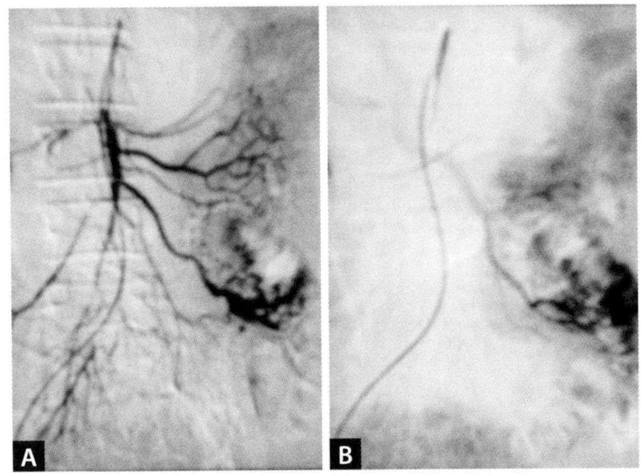

Figs. 15A and B: Superior mesenteric artery angiogram: (A) Early; (B) Delayed phase showing pooling of contrast in jejunal arteriovenous malformation.

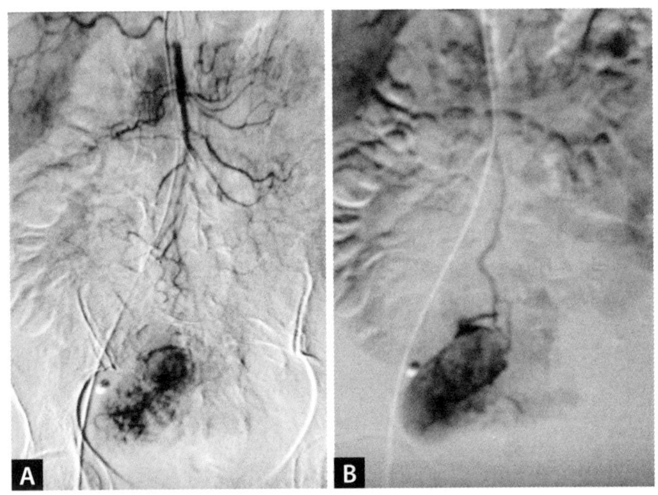

Figs. 16A and B: Superior mesenteric artery angiogram: (A) Early; (B) Delayed phase showing tumor vascularity in a case of ileal adenoma.

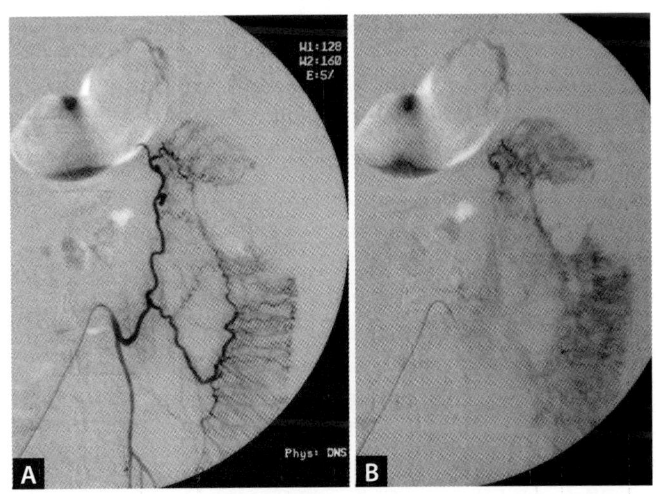

Figs. 17A and B: Inferior mesenteric artery angiogram: (A) Early; (B) Delayed phase showing avascular segment of descending colon.

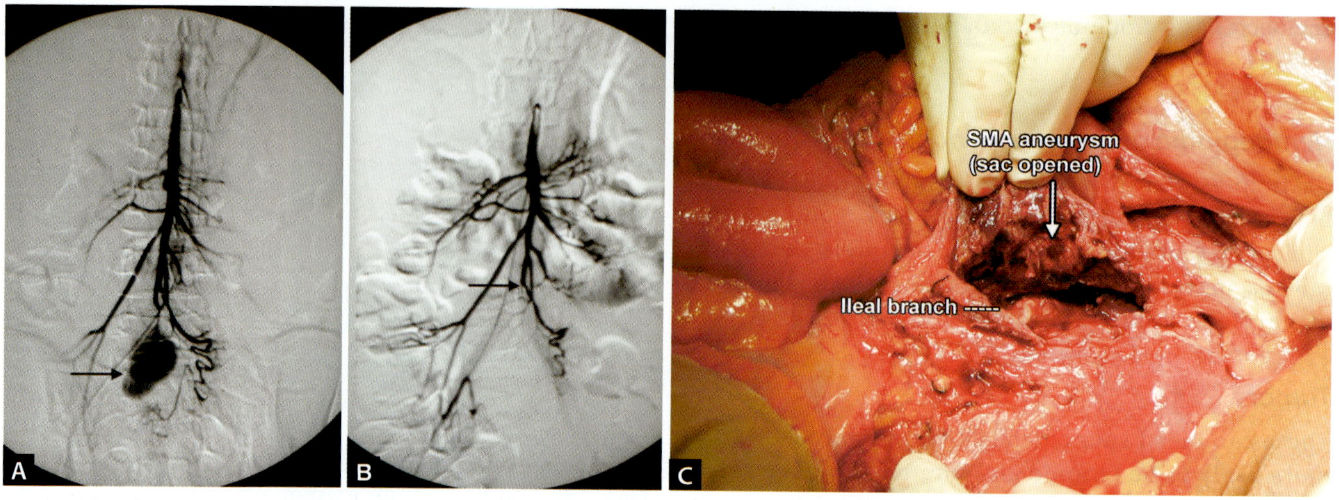

Figs. 18A to C: Superior mesenteric artery (SMA) angiogram (A) is showing a large aneurysm (arrow). The aneurysm was embolized (arrow) with steel coils (B) and later on surgically removed (C).

and bowel lumen. A small bleed may precede a sudden massive hemorrhage from an aortoenteric fistula. It is often difficult to diagnose it angiographically and on CT angiography, but observation of a nipple-like projection or a pseudoaneurysm in the presence of a vascular graft is presumptive evidence of a fistula. Mycotic aneurysm of mesenteric vessels are rare and are usually managed by surgery **(Figs. 18A to C)**.

Acute portal hypertension may also result in severe variceal bleeding which may not be controlled by endoscopy. Emergency transjugular intrahepatic portosystemic stent shunt (TIPSS) may be needed to save the patient. Bleeding fundal varices in patients with cirrhosis is difficult to manage by endoscopy and require an interventional procedure called balloon-occluded retrograde transvenous obliteration (BRTO) of varices. These procedures have been described elsewhere in the textbook.

CONCLUSION

GIH is a common clinical problem and needs a unified systemic approach by the physician, surgeon and radiologist with special expertise in vascular interventions. CT angiography should be the investigation of choice when endoscopy fails to diagnose the cause. DSA should be restricted to situations where interventions are required. In spite of many modern diagnostic techniques, quite often the cause of GIH remains undiagnosed.

REFERENCES

1. Kennedy DW, Laing CJ, Tseng LH, Rosenblum DI, Tamarkin SW. Detection of active gastrointestinal hemorrhage with CT angiography: a 4(1/2)-year retrospective review. J Vasc Interv Radiol. 2010;21:848-55.
2. Huprich JE, Alexander JA, Mullan BP, Stanson AW. Gastrointestinal hemorrhage. In: Gore RM, Levine MS (eds.) Gastrointestinal Radiology, 4th edition. WB Saunders, Philadelphia; 2015.pp.2271-81.
3. Laing CJ, Tobias T, Rosenblum DI, Banker WL, Tseng L, Tamarkin SW. Acute gastrointestinal bleeding: Emerging role of multidetector CT angiography and review of current imaging techniques. Radiographics. 2007;27:1055-70.
4. Kim BSM, Li BT, Engel A, Samra JS, Clarke S, Norton ID, Li AE. Diagnosis of gastrointestinal bleeding: A practical guide for clinicians. World J Gastrointest Pathophysiol. 2014;5:467-78.
5. Whelan CT, Chen C, Kaboli P, Siddique J, Prochaska M, Meltzer DO. Upper versus lower gastrointestinal bleeding: a direct comparison of clinical presentation, outcomes, and resource utilization. J Hosp Med. 2010;5:141-7.
6. Lee EW, Laberge JM. Differential diagnosis of gastrointestinal bleeding. Tech Vasc Interv Radiol. 2005;7:112-22.
7. Manning-Dimmitt LL, Dimmitt SG, Wilson GR. Diagnosis of gastrointestinal bleeding in adults. Am Fam Physician. 2005; 71:1339-46.
8. Jaskolka JD, Binkhamis S, Prabhudesai V, Chawla TP. Acute gastrointestinal hemorrhage: radiologic diagnosis and management. Can Assoc Radiol J. 2013;64:90-100.
9. Strate LL. Lower GI bleeding: epidemiology and diagnosis. Gastroenterol Clin North Am. 2005;34:643-64.
10. Triester SL, Leighton JA, Leontiadis GI, Fleischer DE, Hara AK, Heigh RI, et al. A meta-analysis of the yield of capsule endoscopy compared to other diagnostic modalities in patients with obscure gastrointestinal bleeding. Am J Gastroenterol. 2005;100:2407-18.
11. Mellinger JD, Bittner JG, Edwards MA, Bates W, Williams HT. Imaging of gastrointestinal bleeding. Surg Clin North Am. 2011;91:93-108.

12. Zuckier LS. Acute gastrointestinal bleeding. Semin Nucl Med. 2003;33(4):297-311.
13. Kim J, Kim YH, Lee KH, Lee YJ, Park JH. Diagnostic performance of CT angiography I patients visiting emergency department with overt gastrointestinal bleeding. Korean J Radiol. 2015;16:541-9.
14. Lee SM, Kim TO, Park HY, et al. Role of multi-detector row computed tomography for localisation of acute lower gastrointestinal bleeding. Korean J Gastroenterol. 2008;51: 298-304.
15. Yoon W, Jeong YY, Shin SS, et al. Acute massive gastrointestinal bleeding: detection and localization with arterial phase multi-detector row helical CT. Radiology. 2006;239(1):160-7.
16. Sun H, Hou XY, Xue HD, Li XG, Jin ZY, Qian JM, et al. Dual-source dual-energy CT angiography with virtual non-enhanced images and iodine map for active gastrointestinal bleeding: image quality, radiation dose and diagnostic performance. Eur J Radiol. 2015;84(5):884-91.
17. Srivastava DN, Sharma S, Pal S, Thulkar S, Seith A, Bandhu S, et al. Transcatheter arterial embolisation in the management of hemobilia. Abdominal Imaging. 2006;31(4):439-48.
18. Jaeckle T, Stuber G, Hoffmann MH, Jeltsch M, Schmitz BL, Aschoff AJ. Detection and localization of acute upper and lower gastrointestinal (GI) bleeding with arterial phase multidetector row helical CT. Eur Radiol. 2008;18:1406-13.
19. Abbas SM, Bissett IP, Holden A, et al. Clinical variables associated with positive angiographic localisation of lower gastrointestinal bleeding. ANZ J Surg. 2005;75:953-7.
20. Kim CY, Suhocki PV, Miller MJ Jr, Khan M, Janus G, Smith TP. Provocative mesenteric angiography for lower gastrointestinal hemorrhage: results from a single-institution study. J Vasc Interv Radiol. 2010;21(4):477-83.
21. Ryan JM, Key SM, Dumbleton SA, Smith TP. Nonlocalized lower gastrointestinal bleeding: provocative bleeding studies with intra-arterial tPA, heparin, and tolazoline. J Vasc Interv Radiol. 2001;12(11):1273-7.
22. Madhusudhan KS, Sharma S, Srivastava DN, Thulkar S, Mehta SN, Prasad G, et al. Comparison of intra-arterial digital subtraction angiography using carbon dioxide by 'home made' delivery system and conventional iodinated contrast media in the evaluation of peripheral arterial occlusive disease of the lower limbs. J Med Imaging Radiat Oncol. 2009;53(1):40-9.
23. Cho KJ. Carbon dioxide angiography: Scientific principles and practice. Vasc Specialist Int. 2015;31(3):67-80.
24. Madhusudhan KS, Venkatesh HA, Gamanagatti S, Garg P, Srivastava DN. Interventional radiology in the management of visceral artery pseudoaneurysms: A Review of Techniques and Embolic Materials. Korean J Radiol. 2016;17(3):351-63.
25. Srivastava DN, Gandhi D, Julka PK, Tandon RK. Gastrointestinal hemorrhage in hepatocellular carcinoma: management with transhepatic arterioembolization. Abd Imaging. 2000; 25:380-4.
26. Madhusudhan KS, Gamanagatti S, Garg P, Shalimar, Dash NR, Pal S, et al. Endovascular embolization of visceral artery pseudoaneurysms using modified injection technique with N-butyl cyanoacrylate glue. J Vasc Interv Radiol. 2015;26(11):1718-25.
27. Srivastava DN, Sharma S, Yadav S, et al. Pedunculated hepatic hemangioma with arterioportal shunt treated with angioembolisation and surgery. Australas Radiol. 1998;42:151-3.
28. Falodia S, Garg PK, Bhatia V, Ramachandran V, Dash MR, Srivastava DN. EUS diagnosis of a left gastric artery pseudoaneurysm and aneurysmogastric fistula seen with a massive GI hemorrhage. Gastrointestinal Endoscopy. 2008; 68(2):389-91.
29. Gandhi D, Srivastava DN, Choudhary VP, Pande GK, Datta Gupta S. Haemangiolymphangiomatous hamartoma of jejunum: an unusual cause of massive gastrointestinal hemorrhage. Trop Gastroenterol. 2001;22(2):95-7.
30. Chandrasekhar W, Srivastava DN, Mathur M, Bhatnagar V. Angiographic and immunologic studies in acute necrotizing jejunoileitis. J Trop Pediatr. 2002;48(2):88-92.
31. Ibrahim AS, Allangawi MH, Al-Muzrakchi AM. Massive bleeding from an arteriovenous malformation in the gastric fundus following gastric biopsy treated by embolisation. Int J Clin Pract. 2003;57:354-5.
32. Rao RCK, Kumar A, Berry M. Pseudoaneurysm of anomalous right hepatic artery as a cause of hemosuccus pancreaticus. Gastrointest Radiology. 1987;12:313-4.
33. Choi SY, Hong SS, Park HJ, Lee HK, Shin HC, Choi GC. The many faces of Meckel's diverticulum and its complications. J Med Imaging Radiat Oncol. 2016.
34. Bree RL, Reuter SR. Angiographic demonstration of a bleeding Meckel's diverticulum. Radiology. 1973;108:287-8.
35. Kandpal H, Sharma R, Srivastava DN, Sahni P, Vashisht S. Diffuse cavernous hemangioma of colon: magnetic resonance imaging features. Report of two cases. Australas Radiol. 2007; 51:147-51.
36. Srivastava DN, Yadav S, et al. Emergency percutaneous occlusion of surgical portosystemic shunt using steel coils and balloon catheter. Am J Roentgenol. 1999;172:1453-4.
37. Srivastava DN, Gulati MS, Tandon RK. Colonic infarction in acute pancreatitis: an unusual cause of gastrointestinal hemorrhage. Am J Gastroenterol. 1998;93(7);1186-7.

CHAPTER 75

Imaging of Appendix

Anju Garg, Sapna Singh

INTRODUCTION

The vermiform appendix is present only in humans, certain anthropoid apes and the wombat. Morphologically, it is the undeveloped distal end of the large cecum found in many lower animals. It usually arises from the posteromedial wall of the cecum about 2.5–4 cm below the ileocecal valve **(Fig. 1)**.[1] Although the relationship of the base of the appendix to the cecum is essentially constant, the remainder of the appendix is free, which accounts for its variable location in the abdominal cavity. If the cecum occupies a relatively normal position, the retrocecal position of the appendix is the most frequent. More than 50% of the appendices are retrocecal or retrocolic in position as judged from both operative and postmortem reports. The next most frequent position is pelvic and rarer situations are preileal, postileal, splenic and pericolic **(Fig. 2)**. A recent imaging based study showed that only in 4% cases is the appendix located at the classic McBurney point[2] (junction of the lateral and middle third of the line between the anterior superior iliac spine and the umbilicus).

The appendix is invested with a mesentery called the "mesoappendix". The wall of the appendix is composed of the mucosa, submucosa, muscularis and serosa, similar to the rest of the intestine. There is a 'valve' at its orifice in the cecum which probably does not function in life. At postmortem examination total occlusion of the lumen of the appendix is seen in 3–4% cases, whereas almost total/partial obliteration is found in an additional 25%. In persons greater than 60 years of age, the lumen is obliterated in more than 50% cases and may represent a etrogressive normal change with age.[3]

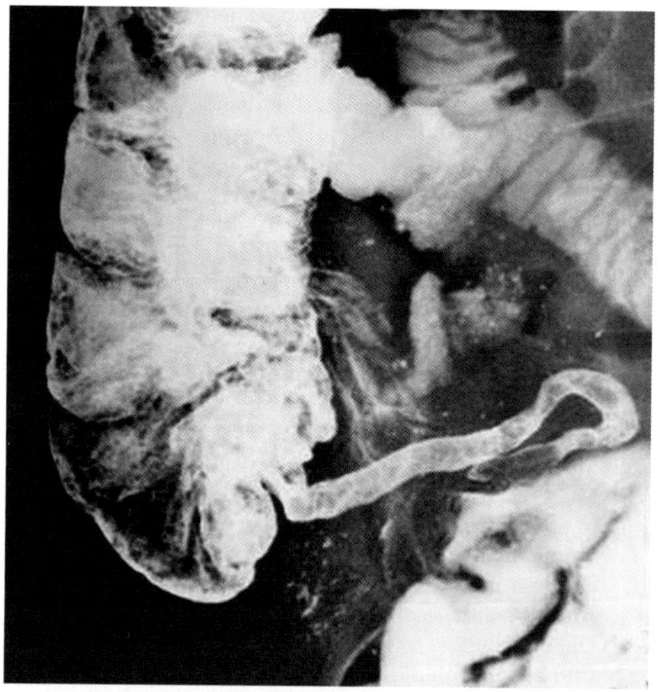

Fig. 1: Barium meal follow through study shows the origin of the appendix from the cecum below the ileocecal valve. A well-defined intraluminal filling defect is seen at its distal end due to a fecalith.

NORMAL IMAGING APPEARANCE

On plain films a normal appendix cannot be visualized. A calcified appendicolith may sometimes be detected, incidentally, as a laminated density of variable size (0.5–6 cm) in the right lower quadrant **(Fig. 3)**. It may occur in unusual locations when the appendix is in an abnormal position.

The normal appendix fills with barium in 80–90% of barium studies and is seen as a thin, tubular structure with a convex, rounded tip. There may be filling defects seen within the barium filled appendix which can be due to noncalcified fecaliths, air bubbles, or mucus **(*see* Fig. 1)**. The presence of air bubbles within the lumen may be a normal finding specially in the subhepatic, vertically directed appendix.

Occasionally the appendix may not fill immediately at the time of a barium examination but may be seen to contain barium in delayed films. In approximately 10% of cases the normal appendix may not fill at all. In some cases barium may be persistently retained in the appendix for a period of weeks or months after the barium examination **(Figs. 4A and B)**. Retention of barium can rarely predispose to the development of acute appendicitis.[4,5]

Sonography: In 1986, Puylaert[6] described a specific technique of graded compression applied with a high frequency transducer (> 5 MHz) for examination of the appendix. Using this technique the fat and bowel

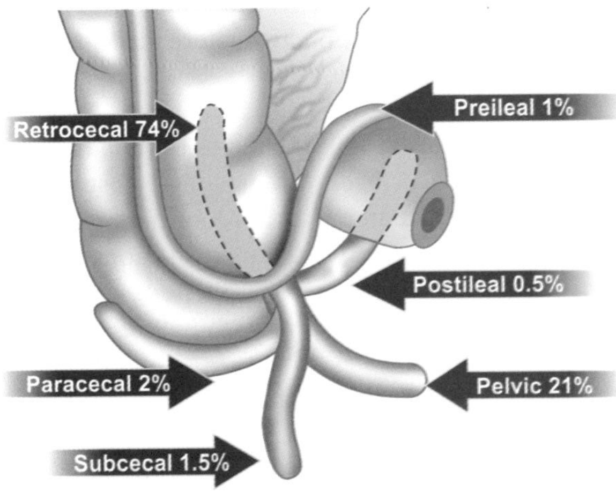

Fig. 2: The variable positions of the appendix.

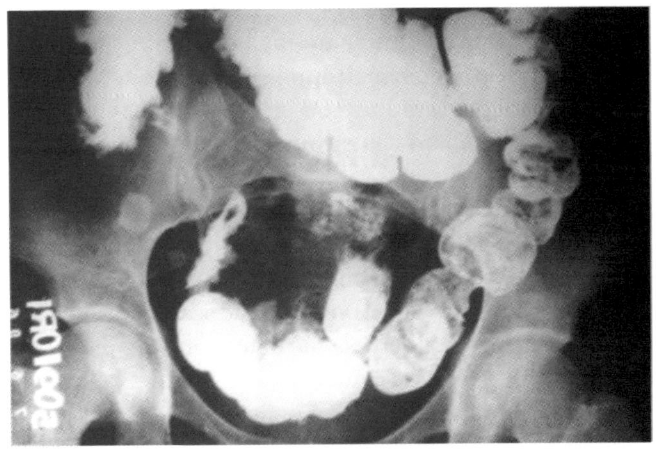

Fig. 3: Two appendicoliths can be seen in a noncontrast filled appendix on a barium study.

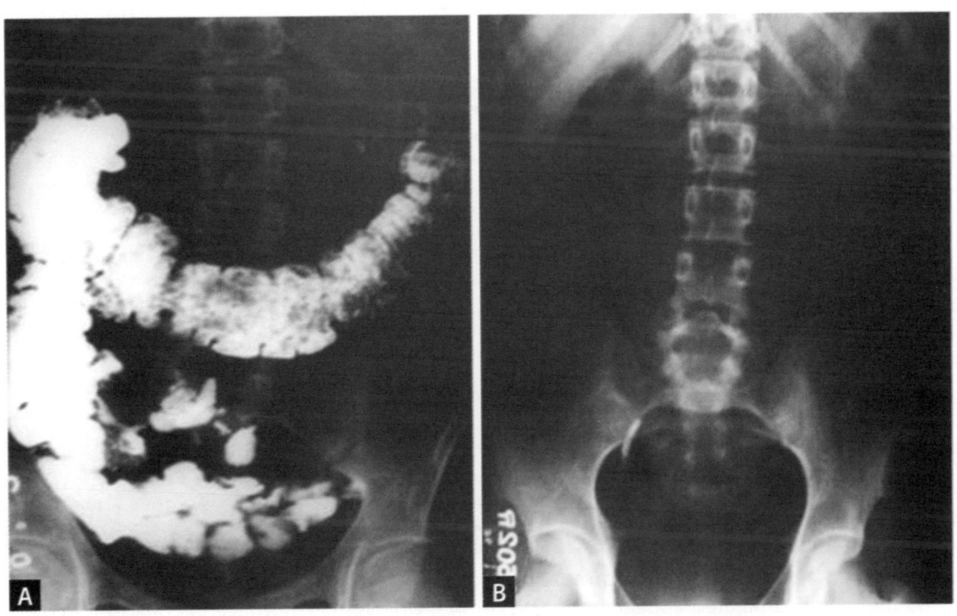

Figs. 4A and B: (A) Barium study showing a normally filling appendix; (B) Plain radiography done one month later shows retention of barium within the appendix.

are displaced or compressed. This eliminates artefacts from bowel contents and reduces the distance from the transducer to the appendix, allowing the use of a high frequency probe with better image quality.

The normal appendix, when identified, is seen as a compressible, tubular, blind ended structure, of double layer wall thickness < 6 mm, with or without echogenic intraluminal material (gas or feces) with no evidence of peristalsis.[7] The typical lamellated appearance may be seen even in the normal appendix representing (from outer to inner) the echogenic outer serosa, the hypoechoic muscular layer, the echogenic submucosa, followed by the hypoechoic muscularis mucosae and the innermost echogenic mucosal lining[8] **(Figs. 5A and B)**.

During computed tomography (CT) of the abdomen visualization of a normal appendix depends in great measure on the amount of intraperitoneal fat, the adequate opacification of terminal ileal loops and cecum, the type and quality of CT examination, and the diligence of the examiner. The normal appendix can be identified in 67–100% of adults who undergo dedicated thin-section helical CT scan.[9-11] Although the normal appendix may be seen in most cases even on unenhanced scans, intravenous and oral contrast do increase the detection rate.

Depending on its orientation, the appendix appears as a small tubular or ring-like density in the right lower abdomen which is either collapsed or can be fluid or air filled and has a thin wall with a sharp outer contour **(Figs. 6A to C)**. It is enveloped by the homogeneous fat density of normal mesenteric structures and may be located in the pelvis or posterior to the right colon in the retrocecal position. The diameter of the appendix has been seen to range from 3 mm to 10 mm which overlap the values used to diagnose appendicitis.[12] Appendicoliths may be seen in asymptomatic individuals presenting as ring like or homogeneous calcific densities associated with a normal looking appendix. The presence of air, fecal matter, or calcifications in the appendix has no immediate clinical implications without the expected inflammatory changes indicative of appendicitis.

ACUTE APPENDICITIS

Acute appendicitis is the most common cause of acute abdominal pain requiring surgery. Early diagnosis is crucial to the success of therapy, which consists of surgical removal of the inflamed appendix before it perforates.

Pathophysiology

The pathogenesis of acute appendicitis is thought to relate to obstruction of its orifice.[13,14] Mechanical obstruction by fecalith or solid fecal material in the cecum is demonstrated in one-third of the cases. Occasionally tumors, parasites, foreign bodies, etc. may be incriminated. However, no obstruction is demonstrated in up to half of the patients with appendicitis.

Fecaliths, which result from the inspissation of fecal material and inorganic salts within the appendiceal lumen, are the most common cause of obstruction and are present in 11–52% of patients with acute appendicitis.[15,16] True appendiceal calculi (hard, noncrushable, calcified stones) are less common than appendiceal fecaliths (hard but crushable concretions) but have been shown to be

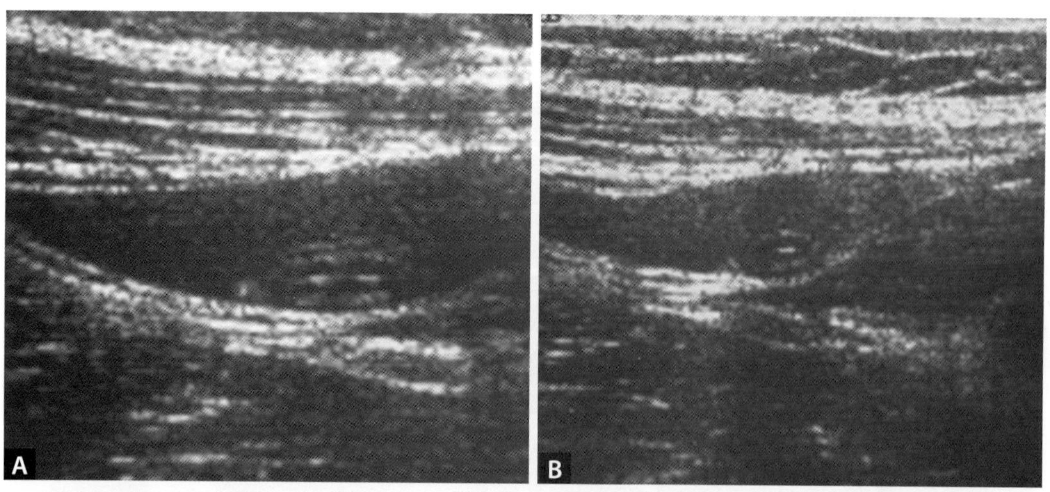

Figs. 5A and B: Sonographic visualization of the normal appendix in a case of ascites—longitudinal and transverse scans. The appendiceal wall shows the typical laminated appearance—the central hyperechoic interface of collapsed lumen, surrounded by the inner hypoechoic mucosa, echogenic muscularis propria bounded by the thin echogenic serosa. The total AP thickness of the appendix measured 3.8 mm.

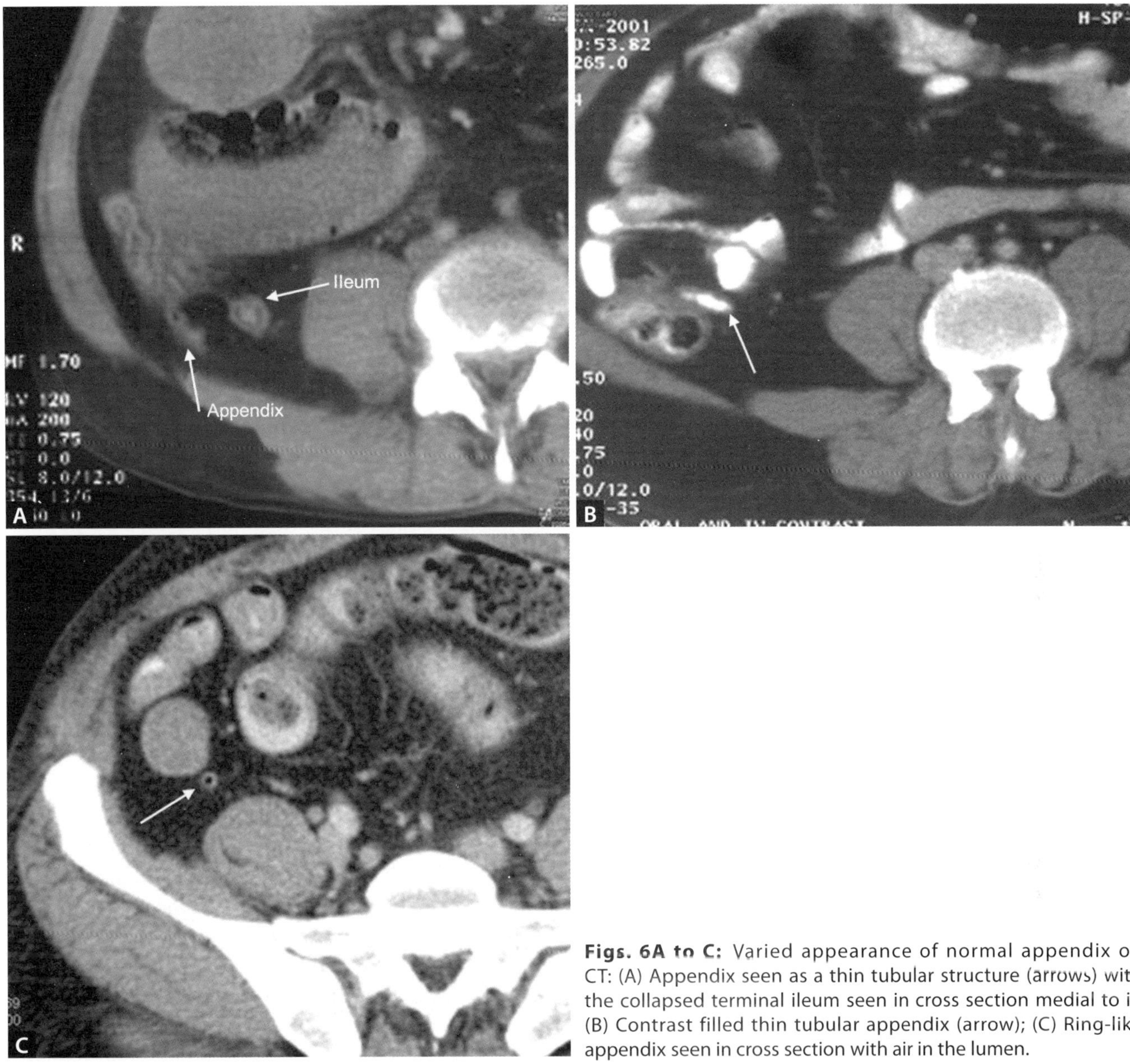

Figs. 6A to C: Varied appearance of normal appendix on CT: (A) Appendix seen as a thin tubular structure (arrows) with the collapsed terminal ileum seen in cross section medial to it; (B) Contrast filled thin tubular appendix (arrow); (C) Ring-like appendix seen in cross section with air in the lumen.

associated more commonly with perforating appendicitis and periappendiceal abscess.[15]

A relation between viral infection and appendicitis has also been described. Viral infection can cause lymphoid hyperplasia or lymph node enlargement which in turn can obstruct the appendiceal lumen. Another theory is that viral infections can cause mucosal ulceration leading to bacterial invasion of appendiceal wall and subsequent appendicitis.[16,17]

As the secretions distend the obstructed appendix, the intraluminal pressure rises, eventually leading to ischemia, mucosal ulceration and invasion of the wall by intestinal bacteria. The inflammation commences as a catarrhal appendicitis with congestion of the mucous membrane and variable reaction in the submucosal, muscular and peritoneal layers. It progresses rapidly, specially in the presence of a fecalith and the infected, necrotic wall becomes gangrenous which may perforate within 24–48 hours.[18]

Rupture of the appendix with spillage of pus into the peritoneal cavity results in localized or generalized peritonitis. In most cases, the spill of pus is limited, being walled off by omentum, mesentery, bowel loops and adhesions. If this protective measure is successful an "appendicular mass" is formed which may be a phlegmon or, in cases of circumscribed pus collection, an appendiceal abscess. The abscess may be intraperitoneal or retroperitoneal. It is most often located in the proximity of the appendix, so that the inflammatory mass usually lies adjacent to the cecum and terminal ileum. Depending on the position of the appendix, this may be in the right iliac fossa or in the pelvis. When the appendix is abnormally located or is unusually long, the abscess can be anywhere in the abdomen. Abscesses have been described in the left lower quadrant, the right flank, the anterior abdominal wall, the lesser sac, and in the subhepatic and subdiaphragmatic spaces.

Clinical Picture

Acute appendicitis typically presents with diffuse abdominal pain, anorexia, nausea and vomiting with subsequent migration of pain to the right iliac quadrant. However, this typical presentation is seen in only 50-60% of patients. The cardinal signs of appendicitis are localized abdominal tenderness, muscle guarding, pain on percussion and rebound tenderness. Laboratory abnormalities include leukocytosis and an elevated C-reactive protein. The differential diagnosis of appendicitis includes a long list of common gastrointestinal and genitourinary disorders[19] **(Table 1)**.

Imaging

Conventional Radiography

Plain abdominal radiographs are not indicated for clinically suspected appendicitis. Although they may be abnormal in approximately 50% of patients with acute appendicitis, they are not specific. The presence of calcified fecaliths (appendicoliths) is the single most important sign of appendicitis. Not only is their detection on the plain abdominal radiograph strong evidence of acute appendicitis, but their presence suggests perforation early in the course of the disease. Localized ileus, air-fluid level in cecum, cecal wall thickening and small bowel obstruction are other findings that can be seen on plain films.[20,21] Generalized paralytic ileus may occur in cases of perforated appendicitis but pneumoperitoneum is rare.

Table 1: Differential diagnosis of appendicitis.

- Acute mesenteric adenitis
- Acute gastroenteritis
- Crohn's disease
- Meckel's diverticulitis
- Diverticulitis
- Perforated peptic ulcer
- Intussusception
- Urinary tract infection
- Ureteral stone
- Ruptured Graafian follicle
- Epiploic appendagitis
- Endometriosis
- Ovarian torsion
- Ruptured ectopic pregnancy
- Pelvic inflammatory disease
- Ruptured hemorrhagic ovarian cyst
- Henoch-Schonlein purpura

Ultrasonography

Ultrasonography is a widely available and inexpensive modality with the potential for highly accurate imaging in the patient suspected to have acute appendicitis.[22] In experienced hands US has reported sensitivities of 75–90%, specificities of 86–100%, accuracies of 87–96%, positive predictive values of 91–94% and negative predictive values of 89–97% for the diagnosis of acute appendicitis.[7,23-25]

Ultrasonography technique: Puylaert's technique of using graded compression ultrasonography[6] is the most popular method of examination. It has a number of advantages. Firstly, it allows normal and gas filled loops of gut to be displaced from the field of view or compressed between the layers of musculature of the anterior and posterior abdominal wall. In contrast, abnormal loops of gut, or the obstructed appendix will be noncompressible and well seen on the grade dcompression image. This technique also allows for a successful examination of the patient who may have peritoneal irritation and sensitivity, as the compression is slow and gentle. Thirdly, the patient is able to provide input as to the point of maximal tenderness, which is often useful in focussing the examination in the correct area.[26] When a patient can self localize the site of maximal tenderness, there is a significant sonographic finding at this site in 94% of cases.[27]

Several additional maneuver have been shown to facilitate visualization of the appendix, e.g. applying pressure posteriorly to improve the degree of compression[28] or applying forceful upward sweeps with the transducer to displace the cecum and appendix upwards specially when the appendix is low lying or pelvic.[29] Turning the patient into the left lateral decubitus position is helpful in visualizing the retrocecal appendix.

Although high frequency linear probes are in wide use in patients suspected to have acute appendicitis, it has been reported that curvilinear probes work equally well and provide a slightly larger field of view and greater penetration. Transducers with a variable short focal zone and a frequency of 5-9 MHz have been recommended.[30] The use of harmonic imaging has also been shown to falicitate visualization of the appendix and the relevant surrounding structures.[31]

Sonographic findings: The inflamed appendix is seen as a blind ending, lamellated, a peristaltic tubular structure which is fixed, noncompressible and appears round on transverse sections. Traditionally appendicitis was diagnosed when its transverse diameter exceeded 6 mm. The threshold of 6 mm has a reported sensitivity of 98%,[32] however, sonographic studies of normal individuals show that up to 23% of normal patients have appendicular sizes > 6 mm.[33] Thus, the diameter of the appendix should be correlated with the associated findings, along with the clinical picture before a diagnosis of appendicitis is considered.

In early acute appendicitis-catarrhal stage-five layers can be identified **(Figs. 7A and B)**:

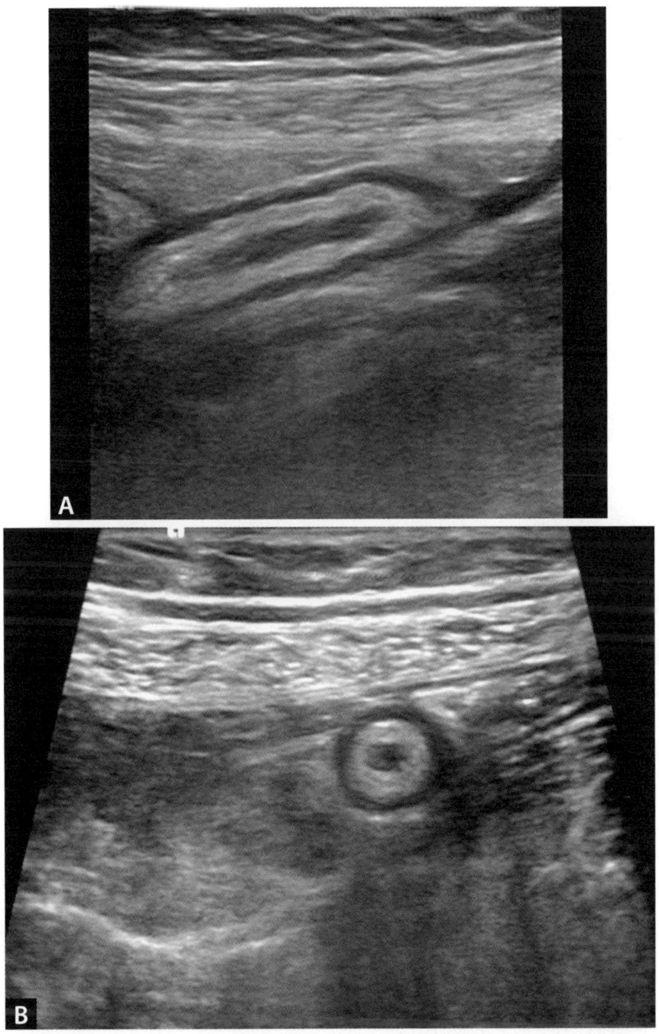

Figs. 7A and B: Acute appendicitis: (A) Oblique sonogram of right iliac fossa shows a blind-ending, tubular, layered, noncompressible inflamed appendix (maximal diameter 11 mm) which appears round on cross section; (B) Inflammatory changes can be seen as diffuse hyperechogenicity of the surrounding fat.

- A central, thin hyperechoic line representing the collapsed lumen and mucosal lining
- Hypoechoic layer (2–3 mm) representing the edematous lamina propria and muscularis mucosa
- Hyperechoic submucosa (2–3 mm)
- Hypoechoic muscular layer (2–3 mm)
- Outer most thin hyperechoic line representing the serosa.

In the later suppurative stages, the lumen of the appendix gets distended with pus/fluid **(Fig. 8)** and there may be an increase in the thickness of the submucosa and muscular layer in the range of 3–6 mm.

Appendicoliths are seen as bright, echogenic foci with clean distal acoustic shadowing **(Figs. 9A and B)**. Their identification within the appendix or in the adjacent perienteric soft tissue after perforation is highly associated with a positive diagnosis. Failure to see an appendicolith is noncontributory. Inflammatory change in the adjacent fat appears bright and noncompressible and is a sonographic clue to the presence of appendicitis in doubtful cases. Enlarged mesenteric lymph nodes may be identified.

An asymmetric thickening of the appendiceal wall suggests impending perforation **(Figs. 10A and B)**, whereas a focal/circumferential lack of visualization of the echogenic submucosa indicates perforation of the inflamed appendix. The lumen may or may not be distended.

An appendiceal mass is seen as a complex paracecal mass of mixed echogenicity and thickened paracecal fat. Phlegmonous change manifests as hypoechoic zones with poor margination within the inflamed fat **(Fig. 11)**.

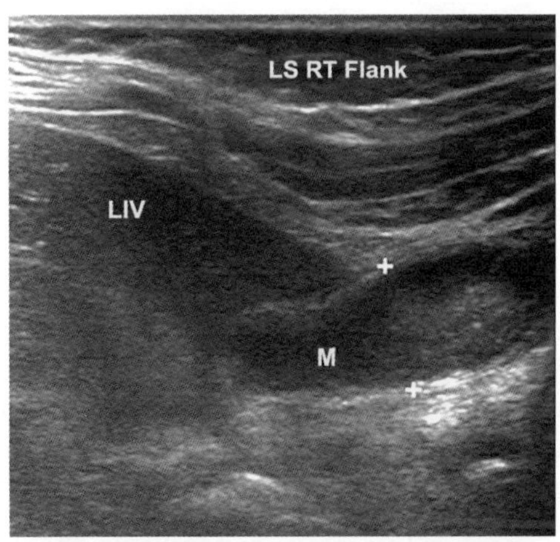

Fig. 8: Suppurative appendicitis in a subhepatic location. Longitudinal sonogram (LS) of right flank, in a 5-year-old boy, shows a markedly distended appendiceal lumen (++) with a fluid-debris level, just inferior to the liver (LIV).

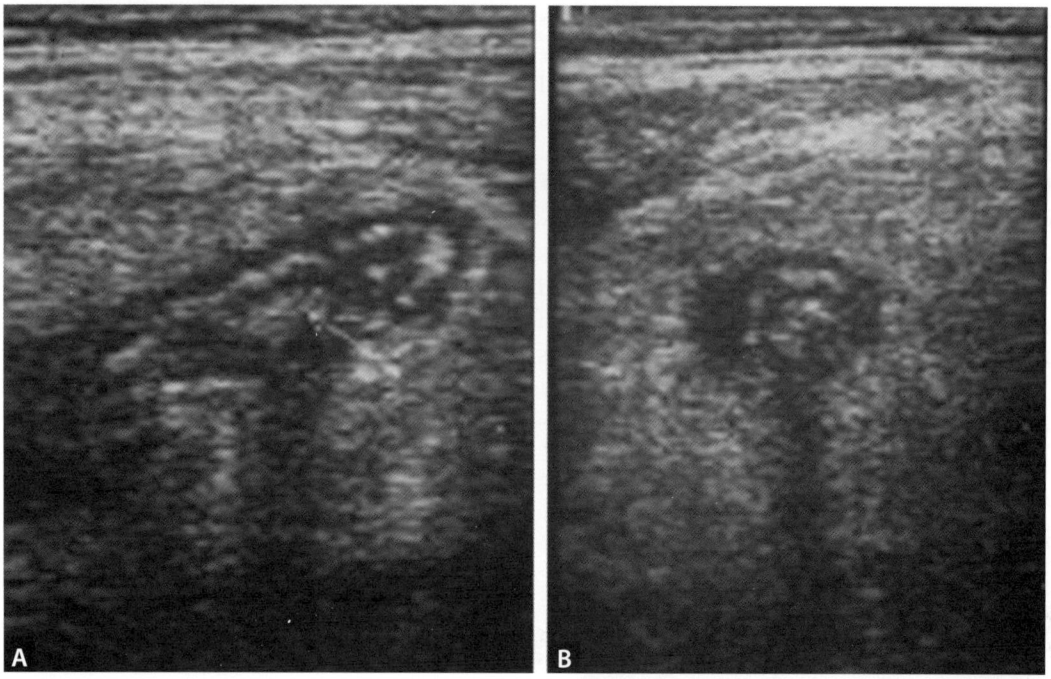

Figs. 9A and B: Acute appendicitis with appendicolith: (A) Longitudinal and (B) transverse sonographic images show an inflamed appendix with an appendicolith seen as an echogenic focus with distal shadowing within the lumen.

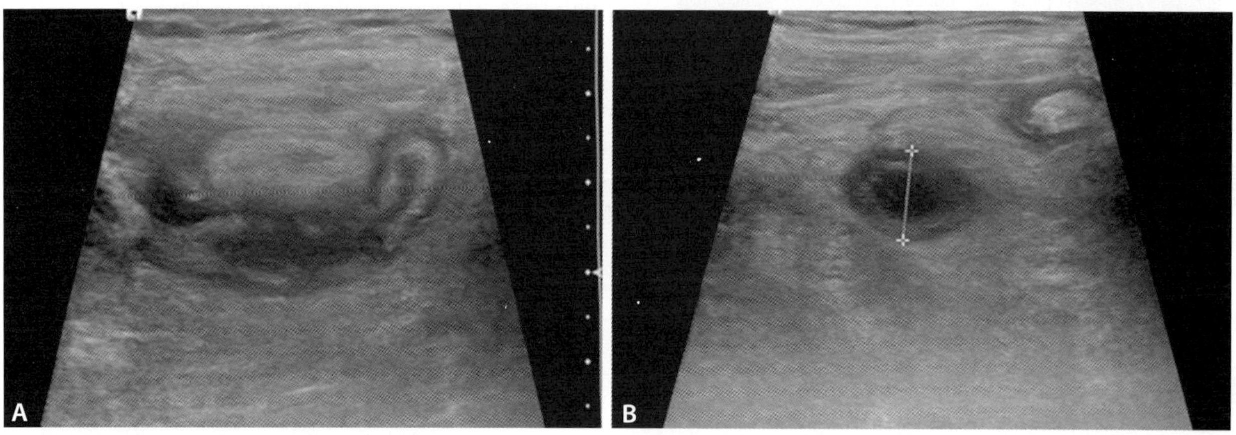

Figs. 10A and B: Acute suppurative appendicitis: (A) Longitudinal and (B) transverse sonographic images show a dilated appendix measuring 12 mm in diameter with a pus filled lumen and surrounding hyperechoic inflamed fat. The irregularly thickened echogenic submucosa suggests impending perforation.

Liquefaction and abscess formation will manifest as an actual fluid component. Gas bubbles within a collection suggest either perforation or gas forming organisms. Sympathetic thickening of the adjacent terminal ileum and ascending colon can often be seen.[30]

Doppler imaging: In cases of appendicitis, the presence of hyperemia in the appendiceal wall and adjacent mesoappendix **(Figs. 12A and B)** is a sensitive indicator of inflammation and can be well demonstrated on color Doppler.[34] The contribution of Doppler US is most evident in cases of equivocal grayscale US examination in which it is uncertain as to whether the imaged appendix is inflamed or normal.[35] When gangrenous changes supervene, color Doppler sonography may show decreased or no perfusion.

Pitfalls in Sonographic Diagnosis

Although ultrasound is highly specific for diagnosis of acute appendicitis, it requires considerable expertise.

The most important cause for a false negative result is overlooking of the appendix. Peritonism may prevent graded compression in patients with perforation, or the dilated, air filled loops of a dynamic ileus can hide the appendix from view. Other causes are obesity, focal appendicitis of appendiceal tip, a gas filled appendix and a retrocecal position of the appendix. The appendix may be relatively thickened in cases of perforated peptic ulcer or sigmoid diverticulitis and a false positive diagnosis is possible. In some cases the terminal ileum or a dilated fallopian tube may be misinterpreted as the inflamed appendix. The appendicular diameter in children with cystic fibrosis may be more than 6 mm.

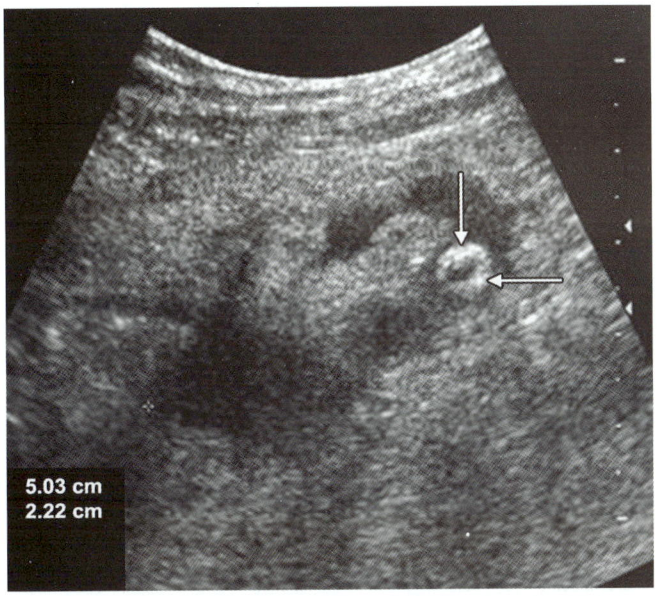

Fig. 11: Appendiceal mass: Sonography shows an ill-defined fluid collection and hyperechoic inflamed fat in the right iliac fossa with a small ring-shaped structure within it—the appendiceal remnant (arrows).

Computed Tomography

Computed tomography is a highly accurate and effective cross-sectional imaging technique for diagnosing and staging acute appendicitis. CT is readily available, operator independent and relatively easy to perform. It has reported sensitivities of 90–100%, specificities of 91–99%, accuracies of 94–98%, positive predictive values of 92–98% and negative predictive values of 95–100% for diagnosis of acute appendicitis.[30]

Computed tomography technique: Appendiceal CT protocols differ considerably with regard to the anatomic area to be included in the scan and to the use of intravenously, orally and rectally administered contrast material. The most popular and conservative approach is to perform helical CT scanning of the entire abdomen and pelvis with intravenous and oral contrast material. The main advantage of this technique is its ability to establish alternative or concurrent diagnoses. Scanning the entire abdomen also allows easy visualization of appendices in the nonstandard positions, including the right upper quadrant. The disadvantage of this technique is the time taken for the oral contrast to reach the cecum, which is essential for best results.

To overcome this drawback, simultaneous administration of rectal contrast has been recommended.[36] Not only does it shorten the delay of diagnosis, but the excellent visualization of the large bowel is helpful in identifying the appendix in difficult cases, in distinguishing

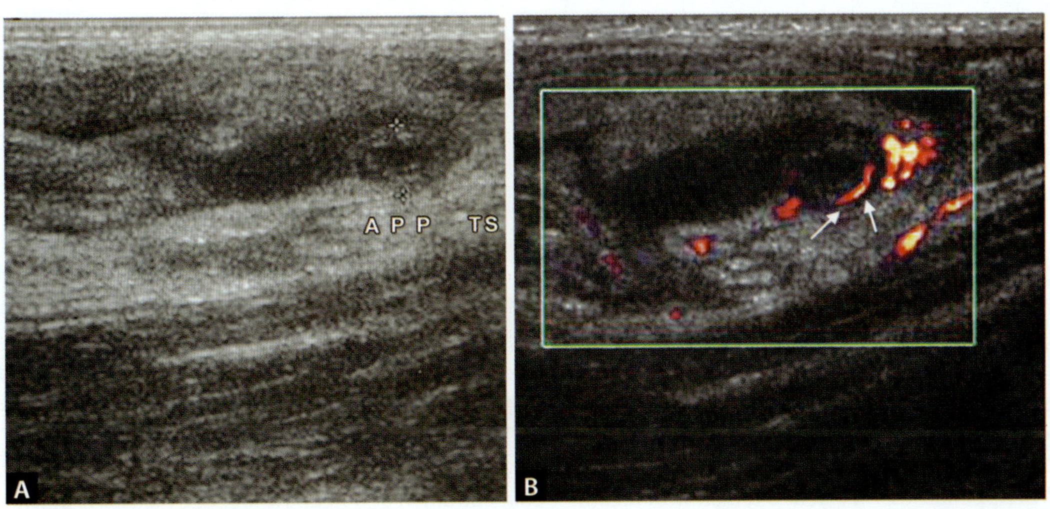

Figs. 12A and B: Color Doppler in acute appendicitis. Doppler demonstrates focally increased flow in the appendiceal wall and in the adjacent inflamed fat.

bowel pathology from appendicitis and in distinguishing pelvic organs from bowel loops.

Rao et al. advocated a focussed appendiceal CT technique in which a limited helical CT study of the right lower quadrant is performed after the rapid administration of colonic contrast material.[10] This technique has proved to be as accurate as those techniques in which intravenous and oral contrast material are administered, while allowing scanning to be completed within 15 minutes in the majority of patients examined. It also reduces the radiation dose to approximately one-third that received in a full abdomen and pelvis examination. A limitation of this scanning method is that a minority of patients will require additional scanning of the proximal abdomen or of the distal pelvis to identify disease not included in the scanning field of view.

The fastest CT protocol has been promoted by Lane et al.[37,38] who have advocated use of nonenhanced helical CT of entire abdomen and pelvis. This examination may be performed in less than 10 minutes, does not expose the patient to the potential risks associated with iodinated contrast agents, requires no bowel preparation and represents the most cost effective imaging alternative to ultrasound. This procedure is most effective in patients with large body habitus, as diagnostic accuracy may be compromised in patients with little abdominal and intrapelvic fat.

CT findings in acute appendicitis: A definitive CT diagnosis of acute appendicitis can be made if an abnormal appendix is identified or if a calcified appendicolith is seen in association with pericecal inflammation.[39,40] The inflamed appendix is seen as an enlarged, fluid filled, tubular structure associated with inflammatory stranding in the surrounding fat. Circumferential and symmetric wall thickening is nearly always present and is best demonstrated on images obtained with intravenous contrast enhancement **(Figs. 13A and B)**. The thickened wall usually enhances homogeneously, although mural stratification in the form of a target sign **(Fig. 14)** may be noted. Traditionally, the threshold diameter of 6 mm was used for diagnosis of appendicitis. However, it has been suggested that this may be too low, as studies in healthy adults have shown that the normal range of appendiceal size varies between 3 mm and 10 mm.[41] When the appendix diameter measures between 6 mm and 10 mm associated secondary changes such as fat stranding or cecal thickening should be present for a definitive diagnosis of appendicitis on CT. In the absence of secondary changes, a luminal diameter of 9 mm has been advocated as the threshold size for appendicitis.[42]

Linear fat stranding, local fascial thickening, and subtle clouding of the mesentery **(Fig. 15)** are characteristic findings of periappendiceal inflammation in nonperforated appendicitis; they may also be seen with microperforation. Other important findings include cecal apical thickening and the "arrowhead sign" **(Fig. 16)**. The latter finding occurs when cecal contrast material funnels symmetrically at the cecal apex to the point of appendiceal occlusion due to focal inflammatory thickening.[43] Another rare sign is the "cecal bar sign", which is seen when the inflamed cecal wall is interposed between cecal contents

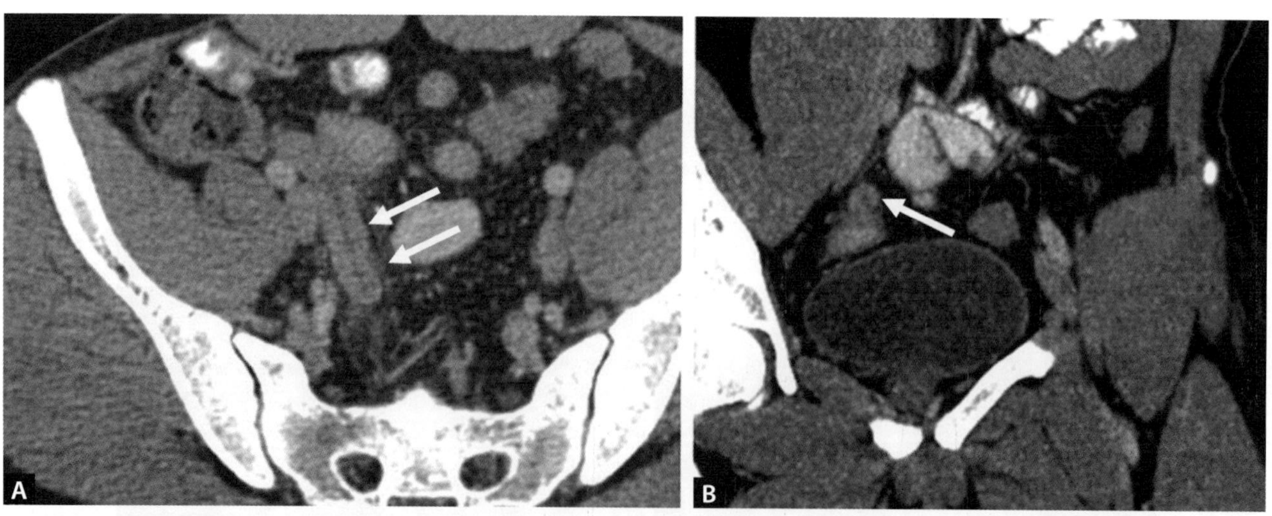

Figs. 13A and B: Appendicitis: A 27-year-old man with recurrent pain abdomen and negative US. CECT axial (A) shows the thickened, tubular, blind ending inflamed appendix (arrows) with subtle inflammatory stranding in the surrounding fat. The coronal oblique reformat (B) shows the inflamed appendix in cross section as a thickened ring (arrow). It measured 11 mm in diameter.

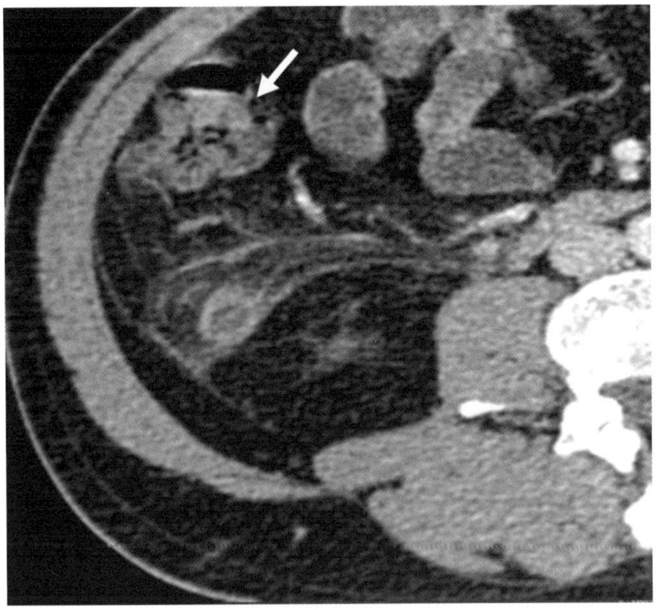

Fig. 14: Retrocecal appendicitis: CECT axial section shows the inflamed appendix as thickened, enhancing ringtarget sign—with marked surrounding inflammatory streaking. This was not seen on ultrasound as it was obscured by the cecum (arrow).

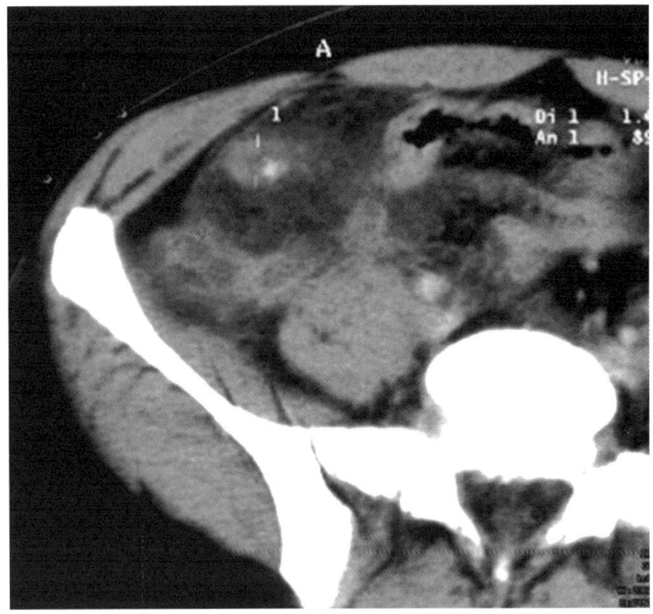

Fig. 15: Acute appendicitis: Axial CT section shows the appendix as a thick walled fluid filled structure (measuring 1.4 cm) with a small hyperdense focus within it—an appendicolith. Hazy, ill-defined, linear and streaky densities are seen in the adjacent mesentery due to severe peri-appendiceal inflammation.

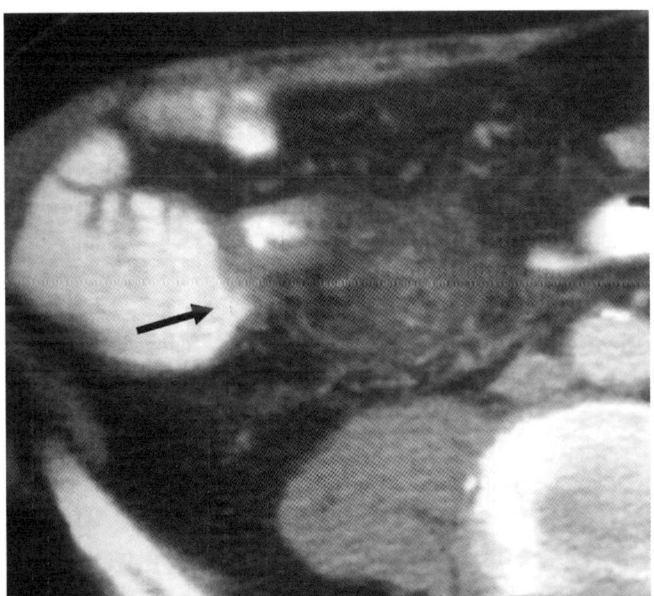

Fig. 16: Cecal arrowhead sign on CT: The focally thickened wall of the cecum seems to "funnel" the contrast material (arrow) towards the origin of the inflamed appendix.

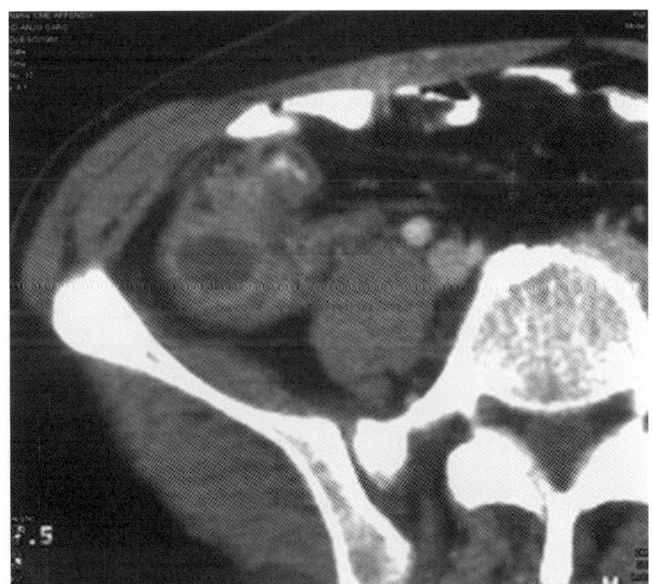

Fig. 17: CT of appendiceal abscess seen as a soft-tissue density mass with a central area of decreased attenuation in the right iliac fossa.

and a proximal obstructing appendicolith. Both, the arrowhead sign and the cecal bar sign can be seen only if positive contrast is present in the cecum.

Perforated appendicitis is usually accompanied by pericecal phlegmonor abscess formation **(Fig. 17)**. Associated findings include extraluminal air, marked ileocecal thickening, localized lymphadenopathy, peritonitis, and small-bowel obstruction. Contrast enhanced CT may be useful in cases of perforation by demonstrating the remains of a fragmented appendix. If the abnormal appendix is not seen, a specific diagnosis of appendicitis can be made by identifying an appendicolith with a periappendiceal abscess or phlegmon. Appendicolith detection rates for helical CT are approximately twice those for conventional CT.[9,10,37]

Although a pericecal phlegmon or abscess is strongly suggestive of appendicitis, these are nonspecific findings that may be seen with other disease entities. If substantial inflammation is present within the right lower quadrant, it may be difficult to differentiate primary appendicitis with secondary inflammation of the cecum and terminal ileum from ileocolitis with secondary inflammation of the appendix.

The creation of multiplanar reformatted images increases the confidence in identifying both the normal and the inflamed appendix.[44] Some of the factors that cause difficulty in the diagnosis of appendicitis at axial CT can be overcome with MPR. Coronal MPR image can help clinicians and radiologists since it is analogus to a conventional abdominal radiograph. Oblique (coronal and sagittal) and curved MPRs along the axis of the appendix can show the entire length of the appendix often with an obstructing appendicolith between collapsed and inflamed segment **(Figs. 18A and B)**

The CT findings of recurrent and chronic appendicitis are identical to those of acute appendicitis.[44] Distal appendicitis is diagnosed when CT reveals appendicitis that involves the distal, "upstream" aspect of the appendix, with a normal appearance of the proximal appendix and cecal apex. An obstructing pendicolith often is identified at the transition point between the normal and abnormal appendiceal segments. The proximal appendix in these cases may be collapsed or partially filled with contrast material or with air.

Pitfalls in CT diagnosis: The paucity of intra-abdominal fat represents the most common reason for a false negative diagnosis. This can be overcome by good opacification of small bowel loops with oral contrast which allows their differentiation from a distended appendix. Abnormal enhancement of the appendiceal mucosa seen with intravenous contrast may also help in establishing the diagnosis of appendicitis in these cases. Other causes for false negative diagnosis may be the atypical presentations, e.g. tip appendicitis or stump appendicitis or atypical location of the appendix, e.g. in the inguinal or femoral canal.

Magnetic Resonance Imaging

Magnetic resonance imaging (MRI) is not routinely advocated in cases of suspected appendicitis. It can be useful in cases where sonography is nondiagnostic or equivocal and is an alternative modality for evaluation of pregnant and pediatric patients in whom exposure to radiation is a concern.

On MRI, the normal appendix is best seen on T2W images as a blind, tubular structure with a diameter of less than 7 mm, and a wall thickness less than 2 mm.[45] The inflamed appendix is also is best visualized on

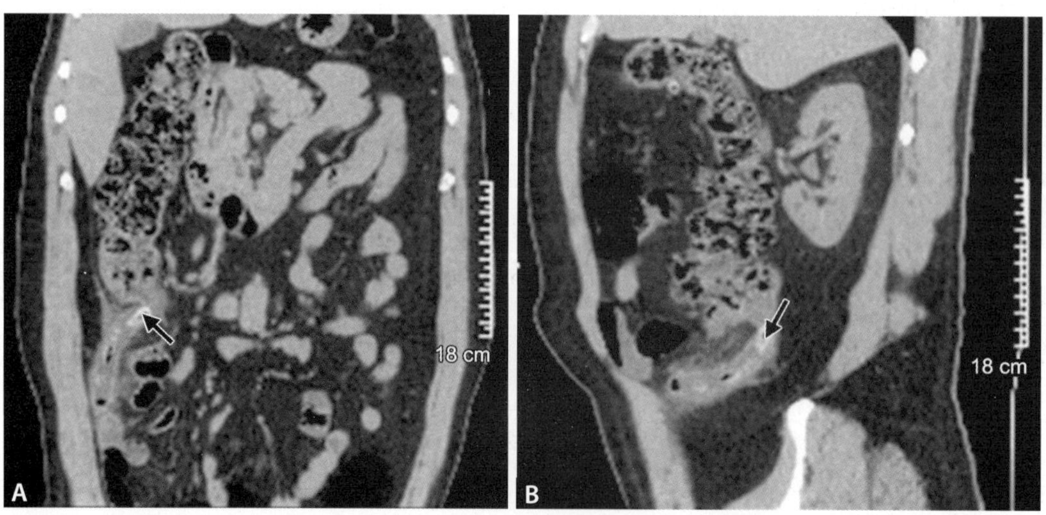

Figs. 18A and B: Coronal oblique and sagittal oblique reformats in another patient show the entire length of an enlarged, enhancing appendix arising from the cecum with an appendicolith (arrows) and few air lucencies within the lumen.

T2W sequences in the axial and coronal planes. T2W images are superior to T1W images because of better visualization of the bright signal intensity of inflammatory change associated with acute appendicitis.[46] The fat suppressed sequence in the axial plane shows the location of inflammation and free fluid collections better than other sequences although spatial resolution is less as compared with T1W and T2W sequences. On fat saturated, gadolinium enhanced T1W images enhancement of the wall of the inflamed appendix is well seen.[47]

On T2W imaging, the thickened appendiceal wall is seen as a slightly hyperintense ring with a markedly hyperintense center representing intraluminal fluid **(Figs. 19 and 20)**. The cutoff threshold of the appendix is the same as for CT. Periappendiceal inflammation gives a marked hyperintense signal. Appendicoliths are difficult to demonstrate on MRI as they are seen as intraluminal structures without signal intensity on all sequences.

Diffusion weighted MR imaging and ADC quantification have also been found to be effective in detecting an inflamed appendix. The average ADC values in patients with non-perforated appendix have been found to be lower than normal control groups (1.01 × 10-3 mm^2/s vs 1.85 × 10-3 mm^2/s). ADC values were also found to be lower in cases of perforation as compared to nonperforated appendicitis (0.79 × 10-3 mm^2/s vs 1.11 × 10-3 mm^2/s). Thus, ADC values can be of help in the diagnosis of acute appendicitis and its complications.[48]

MR has the advantage of good visualization of the abnormal appendix and adjacent inflammatory process, the ability to identify appendicitis in atypical locations, operator independence and lacks exposure to iodinated contrast media. However, its drawbacks are long scan time, high cost, limited availability, inability to visualize an appendicolith, and limitations related to claustrophobia and metal artefacts.

WHICH MODALITY AND WHEN?

In almost 80% of the cases, acute appendicitis presents with typical findings and no imaging is required. In the rest of the patients, who are usually young, old or pregnant the clinical picture may be obscure and diagnosis is sometimes impossible until laparotomy. It is in this group of patients that imaging plays an important role and cross sectional imaging has a distinct advantage over clinical assessment.

A large number of studies have been performed to assess the comparative accuracy of US, CT and MRI in the diagnosis of acute appendicitis. Doria, et al performed a meta analysis of the studies published between 1986 and 2004.[48] CT had a pooled sensitivity and specificity of 94% and 95% respectively in children and 94% and 94% respectively in adults. Ultrasound had a pooled sensitivity and specificity of 88% and 94% respectively in children and 83% and 93% respectively in adults. Also, studies which compared US

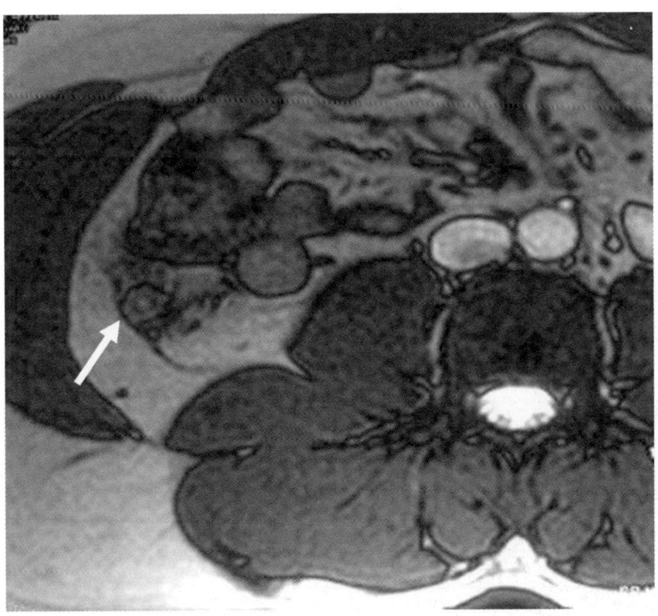

Fig. 19: MR-T2 weighted axial image showing a thickened, inflamed appendix in cross-section (arrow).

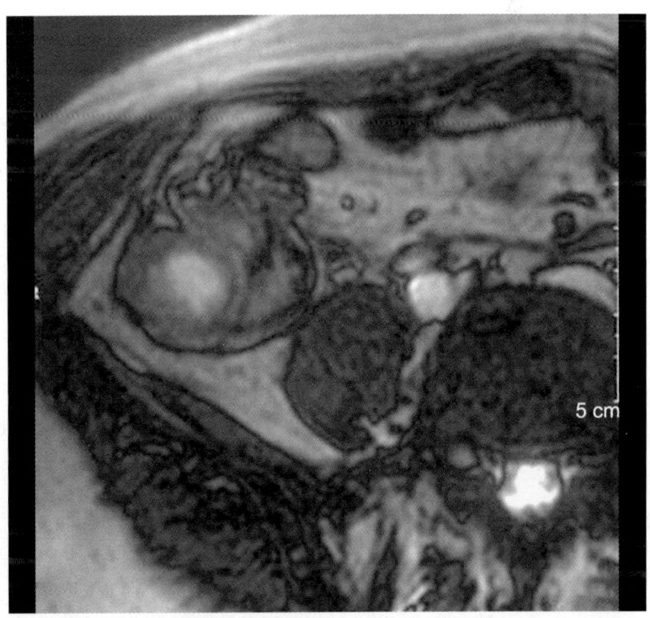

Fig. 20: MR-T2 weighted axial image in a case of appendiceal abscess shows a hyperintense fluid collection with a thick wall of lesser intensity.

and CT directly confirmed that CT was more sensitive than ultrasound.

Gaitini D[49] reviewed studies which were performed between 2006 and 2011 comparing graded compression US and CT performance and using surgery or clinical follow- up as the standard reference. Her results are presented in **Table 2**. It was found that the sensitivity of US and CT ranged between 74–88% and 91–100% respectively, whereas the specificity ranged between 83–97% and 90–100% respectively, with higher US sensitivity in children than in adults. Pedrosa et al[50] compared the role of US and MRI in 148 pregnant patients suspected of appendicitis and found that US had a low sensitivity (36%) but excellent specificity (99%), whereas sensitivity and specificity of MRI was 100% and 93% respectively.

Although CT seems to have an advantage over ultrasound in detection of acute appendicitis, US is substantially less expensive than CT and does not use ionizing radiation. It is also more universally available in our country. However, it is operator dependent and a small but finite number of false negative results occur regardless of expertise **(Table 3)**. Nevertheless, it is still recommended as the initial imaging modality specially in children, followed by CT only if sonographic diagnosis is uncertain. This approach seems to have excellent accuracy with reported sensitivity of 94 to 99% and specificity of 94 to 95%.[57-61]

Computed tomography, being the best modality for showing the extent of inflammatory process, should be used in patients with a high likelihood of perforation. This includes elderly, immunosuppressed patients and those with prolonged clinical symptoms (>72 hours duration) or a high fever and marked leukocytosis. CT is also the preferred modality for obese patients, patients with right lower quadrant masses and in those with persistent pain but a negative ultrasound.

Ultrasound is also the initial imaging modality in pregnant women with suspected appendicitis. However, several factors may limit its usefulness; the appendix may be displaced and adequate graded compression may be

Table 2: US and CT performance for the diagnosis of acute appendicitis.

Publication	*No. of patients*	*US sensitivity %*	*CT sensitivity %*	*US specificity %*	*CT specificity %*
Van Randen A 2008[51]	671	79	91	83	90
Doria AS 2007[52]	4341 A 9356 C	83 88	94 94	93 94	94 95
Poortman P 2009[53]	151 A	77	100	86	100
Gaitini D 2008[54]	420 A	74	100	97	99
Cuschieri J 2008[55]	3045 A	83	92		
Wan MJ 2009[56]	9356 C	88	97	94	94

Abbreviations: A: Adults, C: Children.
Source: Adapted from Gaitini D. Imaging acute appendicitis: state of Art. Journal of Clinical Imaging Science. 2011;3:1-9.

Table 3: Comparison of US, CT and MRI in imaging of acute appendicitis.

Feature	*US*	*CT*	*MRI*
Availability	High	Intermediate	Low
Oral contrast medium	No	Yes	No
Intravenous contrast medium	No	Yes (generally)	No
Sedation/general anesthesia	No	Yes (children)	Yes (children and claustrophobia)
Cost	Low	Intermediate	High
Speed	High	Low (contrast media ingestion)	Low
Operator dependence	High	Intermediate	Intermediate
Radiation exposure	No	Yes	No
Sensitivity	Intermediate	High	High
Specificity	High	High	High

Source: Adapted from Gaitini D. Imaging acute appendicitis: state of Art. Journal of Clinical Imaging Science. 2011;3:1-9.

difficult in the presence of the gravid uterus. In these cases MRI has emerged as a useful second line modality and has a reported high accuracy and low failure rate.[46,50]

TUBERCULOSIS OF THE APPENDIX

Primary involvement of the appendix by tuberculosis in which there is no detectable focus elsewhere is extremely rare. The appendix is more commonly involved secondary to ileocecal tuberculosis. Secondary involvement is also uncommon owing to the minimal contact of appendix with intestinal contents. Secondary involvement has been further classified as those secondary to:

- Local extension of ileocecal tuberculosis.
- Retrograde lymphatic spread from distant lesion in the cecum or ascending colon.
- Appendicular serositis/periappendicitis or peritoneal tuberculosis.

Majority of the patients present with symptoms of the associated intestinal lesion rather than acute appendicitis.

Radiological investigations do not establish the diagnosis which is always established by histopathology. Appendicectomy is advocated in all cases of appendicular tuberculosis as antitubercular drugs alone cannot control recurrent attacks of appendicitis. Antitubercular drugs are given with surgery to control local complications like sinus formation.[62]

MUCOCELE OF APPENDIX

Mucocele of the appendix is a descriptive term for an abnormal sterile, mucus accumulation distending the appendiceal lumen, regardless of the underlying cause. A precursor to the formation of a mucocele is obstruction of the appendiceal lumen which can occur due to fecalith, foreign body, carcinoid tumor, adhesions, endometriosis and mucinous cystadenoma or cystadenocarcinoma.[63] Mucoceles associated with primary mucinous cystadenoma or mucinous cystadenocarcinoma, are also termed malignant mucoceles.

There is formation of a globular or reniform smooth walled, broad based mass invaginating the cecum, with frequent calcification in the wall or substance of the mass. It may be asymptomatic or patients may present with vague abdominal pain—acute or chronic, and rarely intermittent colicky pain caused by intussusception of the mucocele into the cecum.

Plain films may show a soft tissue mass, with or without rim calcification. Barium studies will show nonfilling of the appendix with a globular, smooth, broad based filling defect that invaginates into the cecum.[64] The cecum may be displaced laterally and/or cephalad depending on the size of the mucocele. Ultrasound demonstrates a cystic mass extrinsic to the solid viscera in the right lower quadrant, which may show internal echoes, layering or polypoid excrescences **(Figs. 21A and B)**. Peripheral rim calcification may be seen in some cases.[65,66] On computed tomography a round, sharply defined mass with or without calcification or septation is seen. Attenuation values range from near water density to soft tissue density (0–40 H) similar to the attenuation values seen in mucinous ascites and other proteinaceous fluids[67] **(Figs. 21C and D)**.

Myxoglobulosis is a rare variant of mucocele in which the appendix is filled with clusters of pearly white mucus balls intermixed with mucus.[68] These mucus balls may calcify to form spherules 1–10 mm in diameter which can be seen on plain films. Unlike appendiceal calculi, the calcified spherules in myxoglobulosis are usually annular and non- laminated, shift within the mucocele and can layer in the upright position.

The treatment of mucocele is at variance with acute appendicitis as many surgeons do not advocate laparoscopic appendicectomy in these cases. In fact, some believe that it is contraindicated because rupture of the mucocele with subsequent spillage of mucus into the peritoneal cavity can lead to pseudomyxoma peritonei which has a poor prognosis. If a neoplastic cause of mucocele is identified, right hemicolectomy rather than laparoscopic appendicectomy is advocated. Also the chances of failure of the laparoscopic procedure are higher with higher luminal diameters. It is thus important to differentiate between acute appendicitis with associated mucocele from acute appendicitis without mucocele. The CT findings that favor the diagnosis of a co-existing mucocele include a luminal diameter greater than 13 mm, cystic dilatation of the appendix and mural calcification. If these findings are visualized in a patient, the surgeon should be made aware of a co-existing mucocele since the surgical management is different.[69]

PRIMARY APPENDICEAL INTUSSUSCEPTION

This may present as an acute surgical emergency without time for preoperative diagnostic studies, or as a subacute recurring condition. Primary appendiceal intussusception (PAI) can also be asymptomatic and may be noted only during a barium enema examination **(Figs. 22A to F)**. It produces an oval, round, or finger like filling defect projecting from the medial wall of the cecum along with nonvisualization of the appendix.[70]

The radiographic pattern of PAI must be differentiated from mural and intramural cecal defects due to other

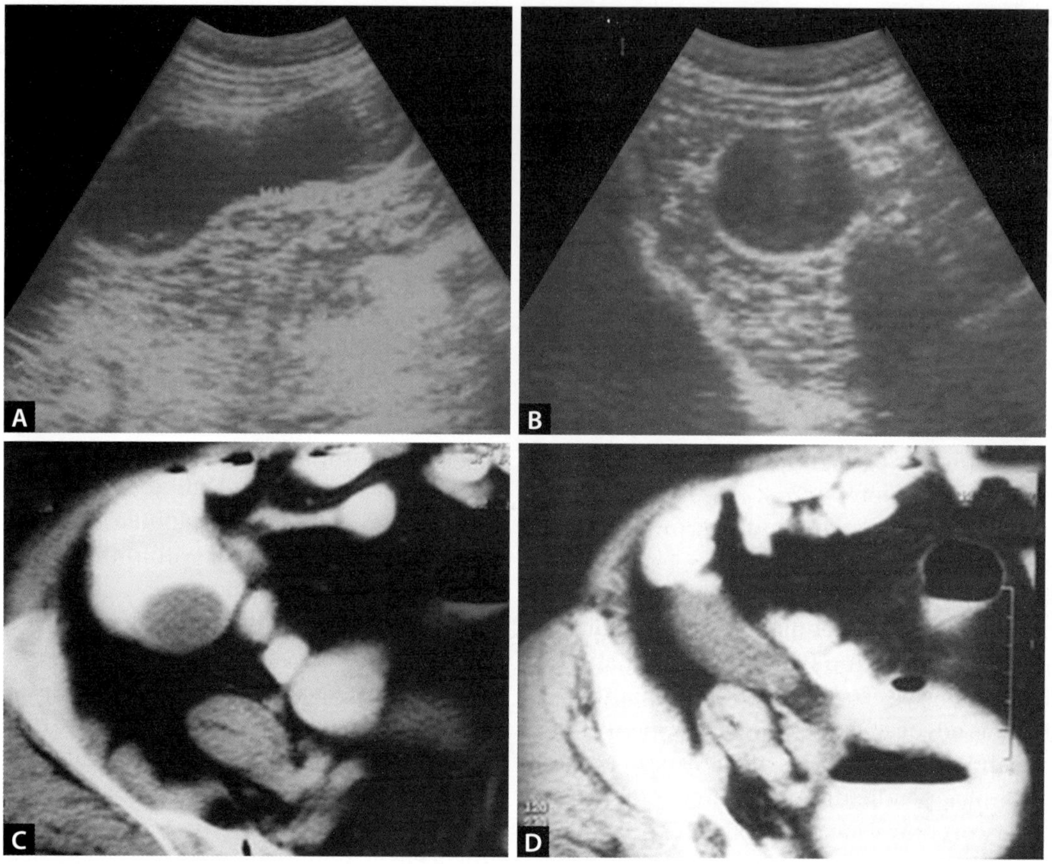

Figs. 21A to D: Mucocele of the appendix: (A and B) Axial and longitudinal views on sonography show a well-defined, thin walled, tubular, fluid-filled mass in the right iliac fossa; (C and D) Axial CECT scans show the mucocele invaginating into base of cecum.

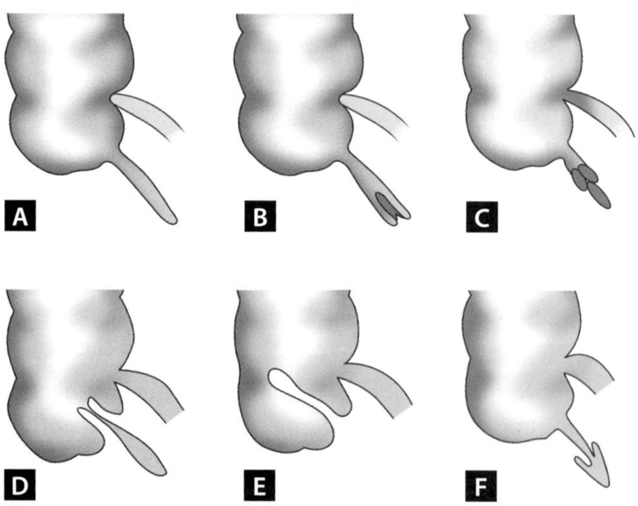

Figs. 22A to F: Types of simple primary appendiceal intussusception: (A) The normal appearance; (B, C and F) Variations of the appendicoappendiceal intussusceptions; (D) Incomplete appendiceal intussusception into the cecum (E) Complete appendiceal intussusception into the cecum. Only types D and E are visualized radiographically.

causes like benign and malignant tumors of the cecum, inverted appendiceal stumps, appendiceal tumors or abscesses. Such a differentiation may be greatly aided if a specific attempt is made to fill and visualize the appendix by appropriate pressure over the cecum during the barium enema examination. Should the defect remain constant and homolateral to the ileocecal valve on two examinations, definite differentiation cannot be made between irreducible intussusception, appendiceal and cecal masses.

POSTOPERATIVE APPENDICEAL DEFECTS

Postoperative defects in the cecum following appendicectomy may be secondary to inversion of the appendiceal stump, ligation of the stump without inversion or complete resection of the appendix.[70]

The inverted appendiceal stump produces a filling defect in the tip of the cecum at the base of the appendix on barium enema examination which varies widely in size from several millimeters to 3 cm. The inverted stump is particularly prominent for several weeks after surgery owing to persistent edema and inflammation. The surface may be smooth, lobulated or irregular, so that differentiation from a mucosal lesion of the cecum is often difficult, if not impossible.

The importance of recognizing the defect lies in differentiating an inverted appendiceal stump from a significant lesion. The inverted stump rarely causes symptoms, although cases of ulceration and intussusception have been reported.

TUMORS OF THE APPENDIX

Primary appendiceal neoplasms are uncommon, being found in approximately 0.5–1% of appendicectomy specimens at pathological evaluation.[71] Approximately 30–50% of all appendiceal neoplasms will manifest clinically with signs and symptoms of acute appendicitis. Other clinical manifestations include an asymptomatic palpable mass, incidental imaging findings, intussusception, GI bleeding, ureteral obstruction or hematuria or increasing abdominal girth from pseudomyxoma peritonei.

Although rare, a variety of primary neoplasms can arise from the appendix **(Table 4)**. Collins reported an incidence of carcinoid 0.5%, adenocarcinoma 0.08% and benign tumors 4.3%.[3] Benign tumors are rarely picked up preoperatively because of their small size. The diagnosis is usually an incidental finding at surgery.

Carcinoids (a neuroendocrine tumor) are the most common and represent up to 60% of all appendiceal neoplasms. They are commonly seen in young adults. Over 70% of these tumors are found in the distal third of the appendix and are <1 cm in size.[72,73] Most carcinoids are discovered in appendices removed incidentally at surgery for another procedure or because of acute appendicitis. Appendiceal carcinoids arise from subepithelial neuroendocrine cells.

Table 4: Primary neoplasms of the appendix.[58]

- *Adenoma or adenocarcinoma (epithelial)*:
  - Mucinous
  - Nonmucinous (colonic type)
- *Carcinoid tumor*:
  - Classic
  - Tubular
  - Goblet cell
- Lymphoma
- *Other tumors (rare)*:
  - Ganglioneuroma
  - Pheochromocytoma
  - Mesenchymal tumors
  - Kaposi sarcoma

Histologically, there are three types: classic type, tubular type and goblet-cell variety. Goblet-cell carcinoids are more aggressive and may represent a distinct subset of tumors with a malignant potential that is intermediate between carcinoids and adenocarcinomas.[74]

Computed tomography may not detect these tumors because of their small size. It may only show features of appendicitis. However, a larger tumor may be seen as a soft-tissue mass in the appendix with or without calcification.

Mucinous cystadenomas and cystadenocarcinomas commonly present as mucoceles in case they cause luminal obstruction, or pseudomyxoma peritonei in case of rupture of mucocele or direct tumor extension into the peritoneal cavity.

On imaging it is rarely possible to see the tumor as it is generally very small. Features of mucocele (described above) or pseudomyxoma peritonei may be seen. Pseudomyxoma peritonei is a diffuse intraperitoneal accumulation of gelatinous ascites. Some investigators posit that nearly all true cases of pseudomyxoma peritonei are appendiceal in origin and that associated ovarian lesions usually represent metastatic disease, although this is controversial.[75,76] Ultrasound shows multiple solid appearing intraperitoneal masses displacing the bowel posteriorly, or a multiseptated ascites. Scalloping of the surface of the liver and spleen is a pathognomonic feature. Computed tomography shows characteristic low attenuation (<20 HU) masses throughout the peritoneal space displacing the bowel loops centrally and scalloping the surfaces of the liver and spleen **(Figs. 23A and B)**. MRI additionally enables differentiation between mucinous and fluid ascites on T2W images. Synchronous metastatic ovarian tumors may be seen in almost 10% of cases.

The *colonic (nonmucinous) adenocarcinomas* are much rare than the mucinous adenocarcinomas. These tend not to form mucoceles, rather they manifest clinically with appendicitis, related to malignant luminal obstruction.[72] At CT, a focal soft tissue mass that involves the appendix but does not show a mucocele formation is most characteristic.

Lymphoma of the appendix is mostly of the non-Hodgkin's variety. The appendix becomes massively enlarged but typically maintains its vermiform appearance. On US, diffuse hypoechoic mural thickening with a soft tissue attenuation on CT can be seen. Aneurysmal dilatation of the appendiceal lumen has also been described.[77]

Other neoplasms: Other rare neoplasms of the appendix can be the *neuroendocrine tumors* of the appendix

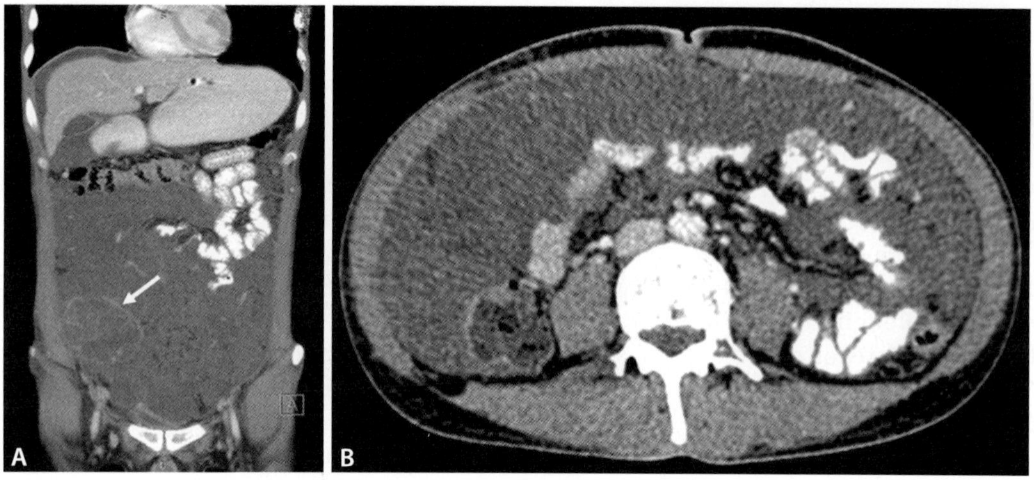

Figs. 23A and B: Pseudomyxoma peritonei from mucinous adenocarcinoma of the appendix manifesting as increasing abdominal girth in a 48-year-old man. Coronal (A) and axial (B) contrast-enhanced CT scans show a multiloculated mass in the right iliac fossa (arrow in A) with displacement and distortion of the bowel caused by diffuse intraperitoneal locules of pseudomyxoma peritonei which appear quite solid looking.

including ganglioneuromas and paragangliomas. Diffuse ganglioneuromatosis has been described and is associated with neurofibromatosis type 1. Mesenchymal tumors of the appendix are rare and are generally benign. Leiomyomas, leiomyosarcomas and gastrointestinal stromal tumors may all arise from the appendiceal smooth muscle. Neurofibromas and schwannomas also rarely arise in the appendix. Kaposi sarcoma can occur in patients with acquired immunodeficiency syndrome (AIDS) and needs to be differentiated from AIDS-related lymphoma which may be difficult on imaging.[72]

REFERENCES

1. Buschard K, Kjaeldfaard A. Investigation and analysis of the position, fixation, length and embryology of the vermiform appendix. Acta Chir Scand. 1973;139:293-8.
2. Oto A, Ernst RD, Mileski WJ, et al. Localisation of appendix with MDCT and inference of findings on choice of appendecectomy incision. AJR. 2006;186:987-90.
3. Collins DC. 71,000 human appendix specimens. A final report summarising 40 years' study. Am J Proctocol. 1963;14:265.
4. Totty WG, Koehler RE, Cheung LY. Significance of retained barium in the appendix. AJR. 1980;135:753.
5. Vukmer GJ, Trummer MJ. Barium appendicitis. Arch Surg. 1965;91:630.
6. Puylaert JB. Acute appendicitis: US evaluation using graded compression. Radiology. 1986;158:355-60.
7. Abu-Yousef MM, Bleichaer JJ, Maher JW, et al. High resolution sonography of acute appendicitis. AJR. 1987;149:53-8.
8. Rioux M. Sonographic detection of normal and abnormal appendix. AJR. 1992;158:733-78.
9. Rao PM, Rhea JT, Novelline RA, et al. Helical CT technique for the diagnosis of appendicitis: prospective evaluation of a focussed appendix CT examination. Radiology. 1997;202:139-44.
10. Rao PM, Rhea JT, Novelline RA, et al. Helical CT combined with contrast material administered only through the colon for imaging of suspected appendicitis. AJR. 1997;169:1275-80.
11. Stillman CA, Katz DS, Lane MJ. The normal appendix: evaluation with unenhanced helical CT (abstr) AJR. 1999;172(Suppl):58.
12. Karabulut N, Boyaci N, Yagci B, et al. Computed tomography evaluation of the normal appendix: comparison of low-dose and standard dose unenhanced helical computed tomography. JCAT. 2007;31:732-40.
13. Wangensteen OH, Denins C. Experimental proof of the obstructive origin of appendicitis in man. Ann Surg. 1939;110:629-47.
14. Pieper R, Kager L, Tidefelt U. Obstruction of the appendix vermiformis causing acute appendicitis: an experimental study in the rabbit. Acta Chir Scand. 1982;148:63-72.
15. Nitecki S, Karmeli R, Sarr MG. Appendiceal calculi and faecoliths as indicators for appendicectomy. Surg Gyn Obstet. 1990;171:185-8.
16. Alder AC, Tomly TB, Wayne A. Association of viral infection and appendicitis. Arch Surg. 2010;145(1):63-71.
17. Shaw RE. Appendix calculi and acute appendicitis. Br J Surg. 1965;52:451-59.
18. Trimaur-Dahl J. Roentgen examinations in acute abdominal diseases. Springfield, IL, Charles C Thomas, 1960.
19. Thompson JP, Selvaraj D, Nicola R. Mimickers of acute appendicitis. J Am Osteopath Coll Radiol. 2014;3(4): 10-21.
20. Soter CS. The contribution of the radiologist to the diagnosis of acute appendicitis. Semin Roentgen. 1973;8:375.

21. Graham AD, Johnson HF. The incidence of radio-graphic findings in acute appendicitis compared to 200 normal abdomens. Milit Med. 1966;131:272.
22. Jeffrey RB Jr, Laing FC, Townsend RR. Acute appendicitis: sonographic criteria based on 250 cases. Radiology. 1988;167: 327-29.
23. Jeffrey RB Jr, Laing FC, Lewis FR. Acute appendicitis: high-resolution real time US findings. Radiology. 1987;168:11-4.
24. Puylaert JBCM, Rutgers PH, Laosang RI, et al. A prospective study of ultrasonography in the diagnosis of appendicitis. N Engl J Med. 1987;317:666-9.
25. Sivit CJ, Newman KD, Boenning DA, et al. Appendicitis: usefulness of US in diagnosis in a paediatric population. Radiology. 1992;185:549-52.
26. Chesbrough RM, Burhard TK, Balsara EN, et al. Selflocalisation in US of appendicitis: an addition to graded compression. Radiology. 1993;187:349-51.
27. Chesbrough RM, Burkhard TK, Balsara ZN, et al. Selflocalization in US of appendicitis: an addition to graded compression. Radiology. 1993;187:349-51.
28. Lee JH, Jeong YK, Hwang JC, et al. Graded compression sonography with adjuvant use of a posterior manual compression technique in the sonographic diagnosis of acute appendicitis. Am J Roentgenol. 2002;78:863-8.
29. Lee JH, Jeong YK, Park KB, et al. Operator-dependent techniques for graded compression sonography to detect the appendix and diagnose acute appendicitis. Am J Roentgenol. 2005;184:91-7.
30. Birnbaum BA, Wilson SR. Appendicitis at the Millenium. Radiology. 2000;215:337-48.
31. Rompel O, Huelsse B, Bodenschatz K, et al. Harmonic US imaging of appendicitis in children. Pediatr Radiol. 2006;36(12):1257-64.
32. Kessler N, Cyteval C, Gallix B, et al. Appendicitis: evaluation of sensitivity, specificity, and predictive values of US, Doppler US, and laboratory findings. Radiology. 2004;230:472-8.
33. Rettenbacher T, Hollerweger A, Macheiner P, et al. Outer diameter of the vermiform appendix as a sign of acute appendicitis: evaluation at US. Radiology. 2001;218: 757-62.
34. Quillin SP, Siegel MJ. Appendicitis: efficacy of colour Doppler sonography. Radiology. 1994;191:557-60.
35. Lim HK, Lee WJ, Kim TH, et al. Appendicitis: usefulness of colour Doppler US. Radiology. 1996;201:221-25.
36. O'Malley ME, Halpert E, Mueller PR, et al. Helical CT protocols for the abdomen and pelvis: a survey. Am J Roentgenol. 2000;175:109-13.
37. Lane MJ, Katz DS, Ross BA, et al. Unenhanced helical CT for suspected acute appendicitis. AJR. 1997;168:405-09.
38. Lane MJ, Liu DM, Huynh MD. Unenhanced helical CT for suspected acute appendicitis: experience in 300 consecutive patients (abstr) AJR. 1999;172(suppl):114.
39. Birnbaum BA, Balthazar EJ. CT of appendicitis and diverticulitis. Radiol Clin North Am. 1994;32:885-98.
40. Balthazar EJ, Megibow AJ, Siegel SE, et al. Appendicitis: prospective evaluation with high resolution CT. Radiology. 1991;180:21-4.
41. Tamburrini S, Brunetti A, Brown M, et al. CT appearance of normal appendix in adults. Eur Radiol. 2005;15:2096-103.
42. Daly CP, Cohan RH, Francis IR, et al. Incidence of acute appendicitis in patients with equivocal CT findings. Am J Roentgenol. 2005;184:1813-20.
43. Rao PM, Wittenberg J, McDowell RK, et al. Appendicitis: use of arrow head sign for diagnosis at CT. Radiology. 1977;202:363-6.
44. Kim HC, Dal MY, Jin W, et al. Added diagnostic value of multiplanar reformation of multidetector CT data in patients with suspected appendicitis. Radiographics. 2008;28(2): 393-406.
45. Singh A, Danrad R, Blake MA, et al. MR imaging of the acute abdomen and pelvis: acute appendicitis and beyond. Radiographics. 2007;27:1419-31.
46. Rao PM, Rhea JT, Novelline RA, et al. The computed tomography appearance of recurrent and chronic appendicitis. Am J Emerg Med. 1998;16:26-33.
47. Hoerman M, Paya K, Eibenberger K, et al. MR imaging in children with non-penetrated acute appendicitis: value of unenhanced MR imaging in sonography selected cases. AJR. 1998;171:467-70.
48. Karul M, Berliner C, Keller S, et al. Imaging of appendicitis in adults. Fortsche Rontgenstr. 2014;186:551-8.
49. Giatini D. Imaging acute appendicitis: state of Art. Journal of Clinical Imaging Science. 2011;3:1-9.
50. Pedrosa I, Lafornara M, Pandharipande PV, Goldsmith JD, Rofsky NM. Pregnant patients suspected of having acute appendicitis: effect of MR imaging on negative laparotomy rate and appendiceal perforation rate. Radiology. 2009;250:749-57.
51. Van Randen A, Bipat S, Zwinderman AH, Ubbink DT, Stoker J, Boermeester MA. Acute appendicitis: meta-analysis of diagnostic performance of CT and graded compression US related to prevalence of disease. Radiology. 2008;249:97-106.
52. Doria AS, Moineddin R, Kellenberger CJ, Epelman M, Beyene J, Schuh S, et al. US or CT for diagnosis of appendicitis in children and adults? A meta-analysis. Radiology. 2006;241:83-94.
53. Poortman P, Oostvogel HJ, Bosma E, Lohle PN, Cuesta MA, de Lange-de Klerk ES, et al. Improving diagnosis of acute appendicitis: results of a diagnostic pathway with standard use of ultrasonography followed by selective use of CT. J Am Coll Surg. 2009;208:434-41.
54. Gaitini D, Beck-Razi N, Mor-Yosef D, Fischer D, Ben Itzhak O, Krausz MM, et al. Diagnosing acute appendicitis in adults: accuracy of color Doppler sonography and MDCT compared with surgery and clinical follow-up. Am J Roentenol. 2008;190:1300-6.
55. Cuschieri J, Florence M, Flum DR, Jurkovich GJ, Lin P, Steele SR, et al. The SCOAP Collaborative. Negative appendectomy and imaging accuracy in the Washington

State surgical care and outcomes assessment program. Ann Surg. 2008;248:557-63.

56. Wan MJ, Krahn M, Ungar WJ, Caku E, Sung L, Medina LS, et al. Acute appendicitis in young children: cost-effectiveness of US versus CT in diagnosis-a Markov decision analytic model. Radiology. 2009;250:378-86.
57. Inceseu L, Coskun A, Seleuk MB, et al. Acute appendicitis: MR imaging and sonographic correlation. AJR. 1997;168: 669-74.
58. Doria AS, Moineddin R, Kellenberger CJ, et al. US or CT for diagnosis of appendicitis in children and adults? A meta-analysis. Radiology. 2006;241:83-94.
59. Rybkin AV, Thoeni RF. Current concepts in imaging of appendicitis. Radiol Clin North Am. 2007;45:411-22.
60. Smink DS, Finkelstein JS, Garcia-Pena BM, et al. Diagnosis of acute appendicitis in children using a clinical practice guideline. J Pediatr Surg. 2004;35:392-5.
61. Hernandez JA, Swischuk LE, Angel CA, et al. Imaging of acute appendicitis. US as the primary imaging modality. Pediatr Radiol. 2005;35:392-5.
62. Singh MK, Arunabh, Kapoor VK. Tuberculosis of the appendix-a report of 17 cases and a suggested aetiopathological classification. Postgrad Med J. 1987; 63(774):855-7.
63. Higa E, Rosai J, Pizzimbono CA, et al. Mucosal hyperplasia, mucinous cystadenoma and mucinous cystadenocarcinoma of the appendix. A re-evaluation of appendiceal "mucocele". Cancer. 1973;6:1525-41.
64. Marohak RH, Gerson A. Mucocele of the appendix. Am J Digest Dis. 1960;5:49.
65. Dachman AH, Lichtenstein JE, Friedman AC. Mucocele of the appendix and pseudomyxoma peritonei. AJR. 1985;144:923-9.
66. Kim SH, Lim HK, Lee WJ, et al. Mucocele of the appendix: ultrasonographic and CT findings. Abdominal Imaging. 1998;23:292-6.
67. Madwed D, Mindelzun R, Jeffrey RB Jr. Mucocele of the appendix: imaging findings. AJR. 1992;159:69-72.
68. Lubin J, Berle S. Myxoglobulosis of the appendix. Arch Pathol. 1972;94:533.
69. Bennett GL, Tanpitukpongse TP, Macari M, et al. CT diagnosis of mucocele of the appendix in patients with acute appendicitis. Am J Roentgenol. 2009;192(3): W103-10.
70. Berk RN. Radiology of the appendix. In: Taveras JM, Ferucci JT (Eds). Radiology-Diagnosis—Intervention. Philadelphia: JB Lippincott Co. 1986;4(41).
71. Connor SJ, Hanna GB, Frizelle FA. Appendiceal tumors: retrospective clinicopathologic analysis of appendiceal tumors from 7,970 appendicectomies. Dis Colon Rectum. 1998;41:75-80.
72. In't Hof KH, van der Wal HC, Kazemier G, Lange JF. Carcinoid tumour of the appendix: an analysis of 1,485 consecutive emergency appendectomies. J Gastrointest Surg. 2008;12:1436-8.
73. Moertel CG, Weiland LH, Nagomey DM, et al. Carcinoid tumor of the appendix: treatment and prognosis. N Eng J Med. 1987;317:1699-1701.
74. Pickhardt PJ, Levy AD, Rohrmann CA, et al. Primary neoplasms of the appendix: radiologic spectrum of disease with pathologic correlation. Radiographics. 2003;23: 645-62.
75. Carr NJ, Sobin LH. Unusual tumors of the appendix and pseudomyxoma peritoei. Semin Diagn Pathol. 1996;13:314-25.
76. Hinson FL, Ambrose NS. Pseudomyxoma peritonei. Br J Surg. 1998;85:1332-9.
77. Pickhardt PJ, Levy AD, Rohrmann CA, et al. Non-Hodgkin lymphoma of the appendix: clinical and CT findings with pathological correlation. AJR. 2002;78(5)1123-7.

CHAPTER 76

Diffuse Liver Diseases

Surabhi Vyas, Ashu Seith Bhalla, Arun Kumar Gupta

INTRODUCTION

Diffuse liver diseases encompass a wide spectrum of entities of diverse etiology. Diagnosis based on imaging alone is generally more difficult than in focal liver lesions, as their effect on normal liver architecture may be minimal. However, imaging can help in assessing the severity and extent of the diffuse liver diseases and to demonstrate sequela such as portal hypertension and neoplasia. The following conditions are included under the term diffuse liver diseases:

- Hepatic steatosis
- Hepatitis—viral, alcoholic, radiation induced
- Hemochromatosis and hemosiderosis
- Amyloidosis
- Wilson's disease
- Granulomatous diseases
- Cirrhosis.

HEPATIC STEATOSIS (FATTY LIVER)

Hepatic steatosis or fatty liver is a benign condition resulting from an excessive accumulation of triglycerides in the form of small or large vacuoles (micro/macrovesicular types) within the hepatocytes. Excess fat deposition in the liver may result from excess synthesis, decreased utilization, impaired release of hepatic lipoproteins and excess mobilization from fatty tissue.

The common causes are alcoholism, diabetes mellitus and obesity. One-third of asymptomatic alcoholic patients and up to 50% of patients with diabetes mellitus develop fatty liver.[1] Malnutrition, chronic illnesses, ileal bypass, drugs and toxins, total parenteral nutrition, inflammatory bowel disease, severe hepatitis, steroid intake, acquired immune deficiency syndrome and congestive heart failure can also result in fatty liver.

With increasing prevalence of obesity, hepatic steatosis has become a major source of liver dysfunction even though in most cases fatty liver is asymptomatic with normal liver function tests. Radiologist is frequently the first to suggest the diagnosis. Mild hepatomegaly with or without vague right upper abdominal pain can be present in symptomatic patients. In acute fatty liver associated with pregnancy or alcoholic binge, patients may present with jaundice, acute hepatic failure or even encephalopathy.

NAFLD-NASH Continuum

In contrast to the alcohol-induced fatty liver, the nonalcoholic fatty liver disease encompasses a spectrum of disorders ranging from nonalcoholic fatty liver (NAFL) in which the hepatic enzymes are either normal or minimally increased and histologically there is no evidence of hepatocyte damage. On the other end of the spectrum is nonalcoholic steatohepatitis (NASH) which is characterized by deranged liver enzymes with or without jaundice. Histologically there is evidence of scarring and fibrosis.[1] It is similar to alcoholic liver disease in clinical and biochemical features. The exact etiology of NASH is unknown, however it is seen more commonly in patients with certain medical conditions like diabetes, obesity, hyperlipidemias and insulin resistance, which together are often called metabolic syndrome.[2,3]

Ultrasonography

Ultrasonography (USG) reveals hepatomegaly, increased parenchymal echogenicity with impaired visualization of the normally echogenic walls of intrahepatic portal venous branches. There is increased attenuation and poor penetration of the sound beam resulting in poor visualization of the deeper portion of liver, the diaphragm, hepatic and portal veins **(Fig. 1)**. Echogenicity of the liver can be compared with that of adjacent kidney. The degree of echogenicity is roughly proportional to the degree of steatosis and tends to parallel biochemical and clinical dysfunction. Focal fat infiltration may produce single or multiple hyperechoic lesions, while areas of focal fat sparing appear hypoechoic in an otherwise hyperechoic liver. In the presence of fatty liver, hepatic hemangiomas may appear hypoechoic necessitating MR or CT for their differentiation **(Figs. 2A to C)**. Hepatic steatosis and fibrosis often coexist and produce similar US findings. On the basis of ultrasound findings, fatty liver may be graded qualitatively as:

Mild: Increased echogenicity with maintained differentiation of intrahepatic vessels, portal vein braches and diaphragm.

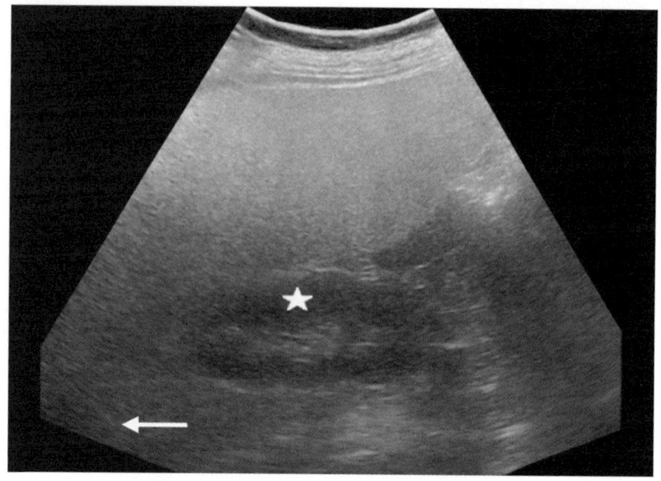

Fig. 1: Fatty liver: Increased echogenicity of the liver seen on ultrasound as compared to that of renal cortex (star). Note the poor depiction of diaphragm (arrow).

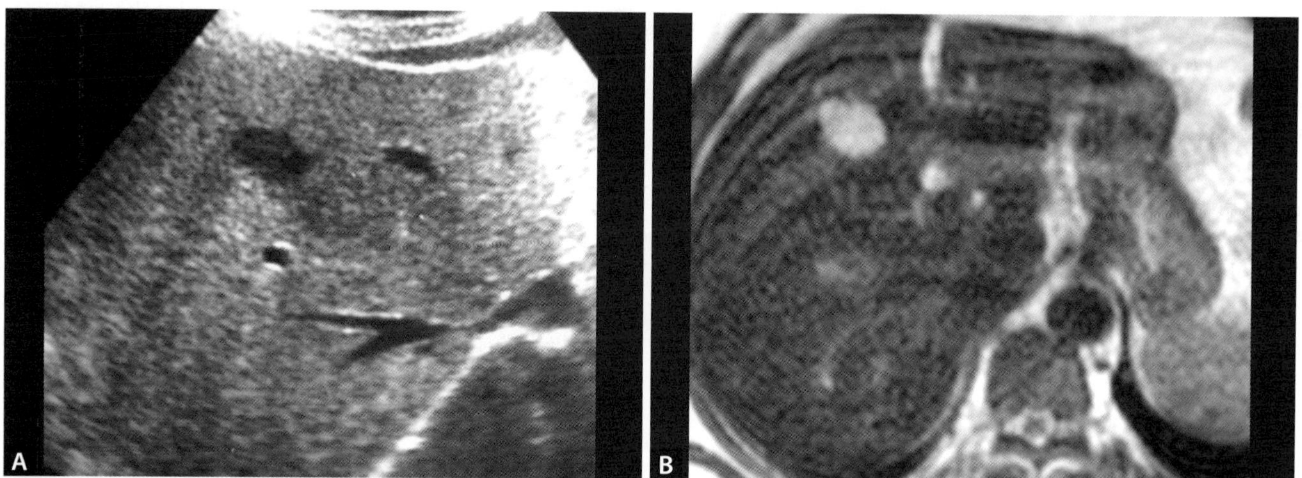

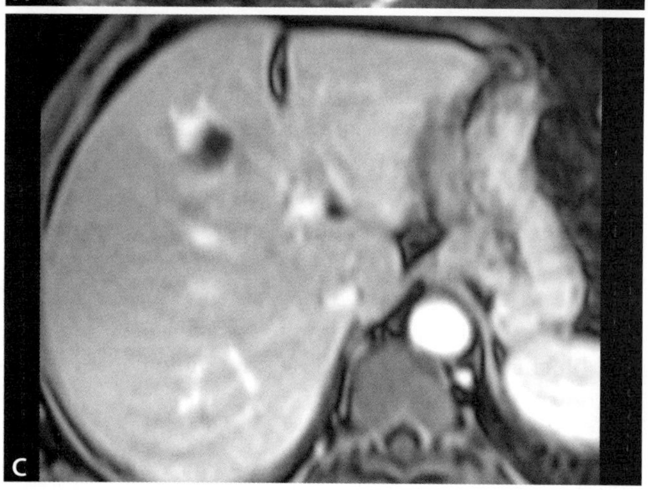

Figs. 2A to C: Fatty liver with hypoechoic hemangioma: (A) Transverse US of the liver shows a small hypoechoic focal lesion against a background of diffusely increased echogenicity of fatty liver (B) The lesion is hyperintense on T2W image, with (C) typical peripheral nodular enhancement, suggestive of hemangioma.

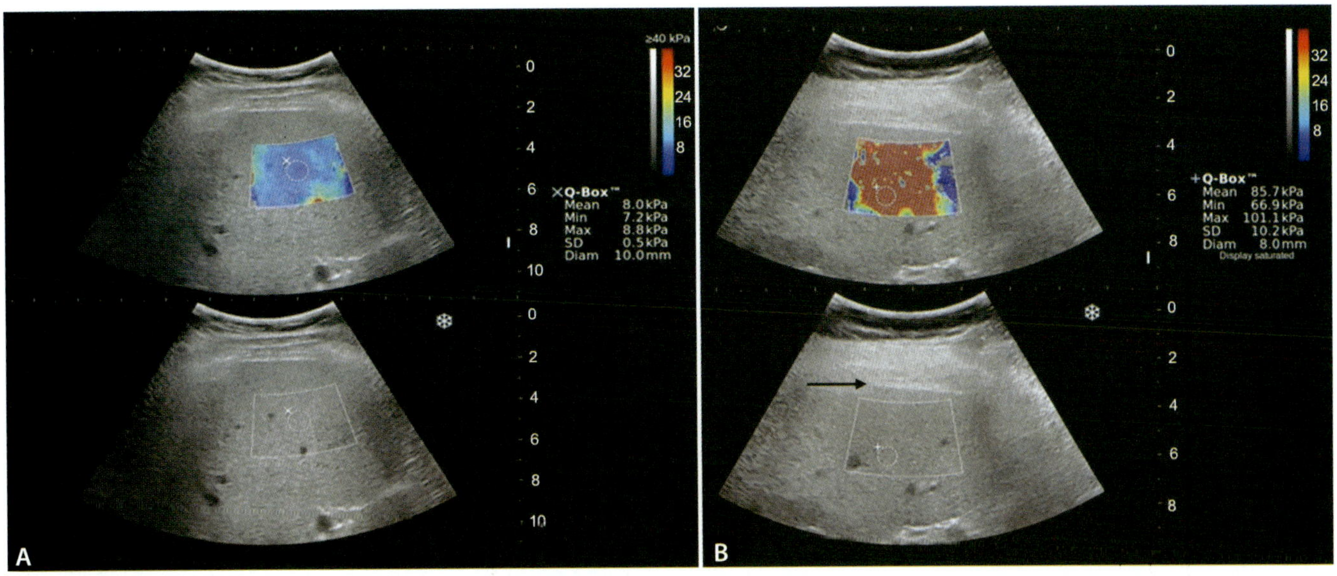

Figs. 3A and B: Shear wave elastography of liver showing a mean stiffness of 8 kPa, in case of mild fatty change (A), a higher value of 85.7 kPa in case of chronic liver disease (B). Also noted is irregularity of the hepatic surface in (B).

Moderate: Partially impaired demarcation of the portal vein and branches, diaphragm.

Severe: Markedly impaired demarcation of the portal vein branches and diaphragmatic contour.[4]

Quantitative assessment can be done by sonographic hepatorenal index (SHRI). In this method, a parasagittal image of the right lobe segment VI of liver and the right kidney is acquired. Region of interest (ROI) is placed on the liver parenchyma and renal cortex avoiding the vessels, renal pyramid and renal medulla. A numerical value based on the brightness/echogenicity in the selected pixel is assigned, and the ratio between the values of hepatic ROI to renal ROI is calculated to provide the SHRI.[5]

Ultrasound elastography is a noninvasive technique that assess the hardness of the target organ. The liver may show increased hardness in a variety of parenchymal disorders like parenchymal infiltrative disorders, cirrhosis, chronic inflammatory diseases and in congestive cardiac failure **(Figs. 3A and B)**. However, the liver stiffness may not increase in steatosis.

Computed Tomography

There exists an excellent correlation between the computed tomography (CT) attenuation of liver and the amount of fat deposition as determined on liver biopsy specimens.[6] Fatty liver is seen as reduced attenuation of the liver parenchyma **(Fig. 4)** Normal liver attenuation on unenhanced scans is 8–10 HU more than the spleen due to its glycogen content.[6] This relationship is reversed in fatty liver. A threshold CT attenuation value of 45 hounsfield units (HU) has been shown to be highly specific for moderate to severe steatosis.[7] The attenuation is often reduced below that of the normal portal vein and IVC so that these structures stand out prominently simulating contrast-enhanced image of the liver.[8] Unlike unenhanced scans, contrast enhanced CT is less reliable in the diagnosis of fatty liver.

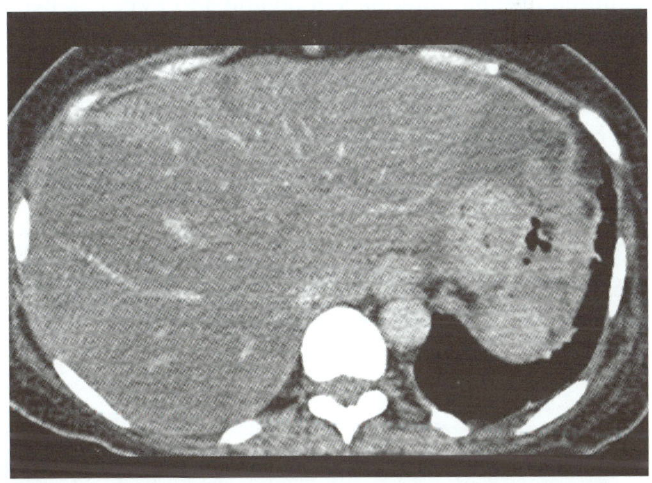

Fig. 4: Fatty liver: Axial CT image in a case of pancreatitis showing diffuse decrease in liver attenuation suggestive of fatty infiltration.

Liver attenuation index (LAI) can also be calculated as mean liver attenuation–mean splenic attenuation to provide a numeric value. CT-LAI of more than 5 implies low probability of hepatic steatosis, whereas a value between minus 10 and 5 signifies moderate to severe fatty change. A value less than or equal to 0 correlates well with significant hepatic steatosis.[9] Another numeric value that can be used is hepatic-to-splenic attenuation ratio which if less than 0.8 or 1 is highly specific (specificity, 100%) for the diagnosis of moderate to severe (>30%) macrovesicular steatosis.[10]

Decreased attenuation in fatty liver can hamper the detection of hypodense liver lesions like abscesses or neoplasms. A confident CT diagnosis of focal fat infiltration can be made when it is lobar, segmental or wedge shaped. In such cases, the area of decreased attenuation typically extends to the liver capsule, without causing contour bulge and typically has a straight margin. However, MRI may be required for confident differentiation of nodular areas of fat deposition or fat sparing from focal mass lesions.

Dual energy CT (DECT) has a role in calculation of the hepatic fat (hepatic fat fraction-HFF), where various material decomposition algorithms allow creation of fat specific and virtual noncontrast images from the images acquired at tube potentials of 80 and 140 kVP. The liver attenuation is reduced at low energy level and increases at higher energy levels in hepatosteatosis. It has been reported that an increase in attenuation by more than 10 HU on higher kVP suggests fatty infiltration greater than 25% **(Figs. 5A to C)**.[11]

Magnetic Resonance Imaging

There are two magnetic resonance (MR) techniques used for hepatic fat estimation—MRI and MR spectroscopy (MRS). Both make use of the difference in the water and fat proton resonance frequencies to measure signal due to fat fraction (SFF i.e. signal fat fraction or proton density fat fraction (PDFF).

MRS is a direct method of estimating signal fat fraction, and since the resonance frequencies of both protons are different, so are their peaks on the spectral tracing. Usually a single voxel technique is employed. Multivoxel MR technique is limited by shimming and the inability to acquire a relatively longer sequence in single breath hold leading to breathing artifacts. Once the peaks of water and fat are identified, the areas under the peak can be quantified **(Fig. 6A)**.

Magnetic resonance imaging (MRI) based techniques for signal fat fraction estimation include chemical fat suppression, and chemical shift-based imaging. In the former, two sets of images are acquired, with and without fat suppression. However, the problem of inadequate fat suppression may preclude adequate signal suppression and thus the latter is preferred.

Chemical shift imaging is based on acquiring images at two echo times (TEs). Here fat suppression pulse is not employed. Loss of signal on the opposed phase image when compared with the in-phase image readily identifies excess fat containing areas in the liver **(Figs. 6B and C)**. With the in and opposed images, liver signal fat fraction (FF) may be calculated (proportion of the fat signal divided by the total (water + fat) signal, FF = fat signal/(fat signal + water signal). On a 1.5T scanner signals from fat and water are in phase every 4.6 ms, out of phase at 2.3 ms and at their multiples. At 3T, the signals are in phase at 2.3 ms and out of phase at 1.15 ms and their multiples thereafter.

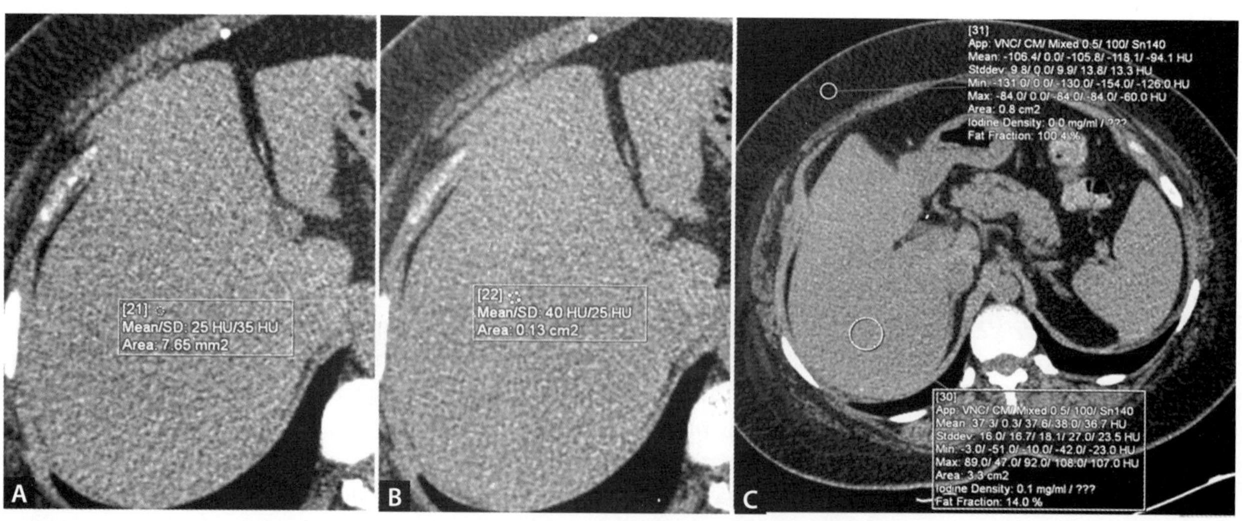

Figs. 5A to C: DECT hepatic steatosis at low keV (A) and higher keV (B) showing an increase in attenuation by more than 10 HU; (C) Liver fat fraction of 14% suggestive of steatosis. Note the fat fraction of subcutaneous fat is 100%.

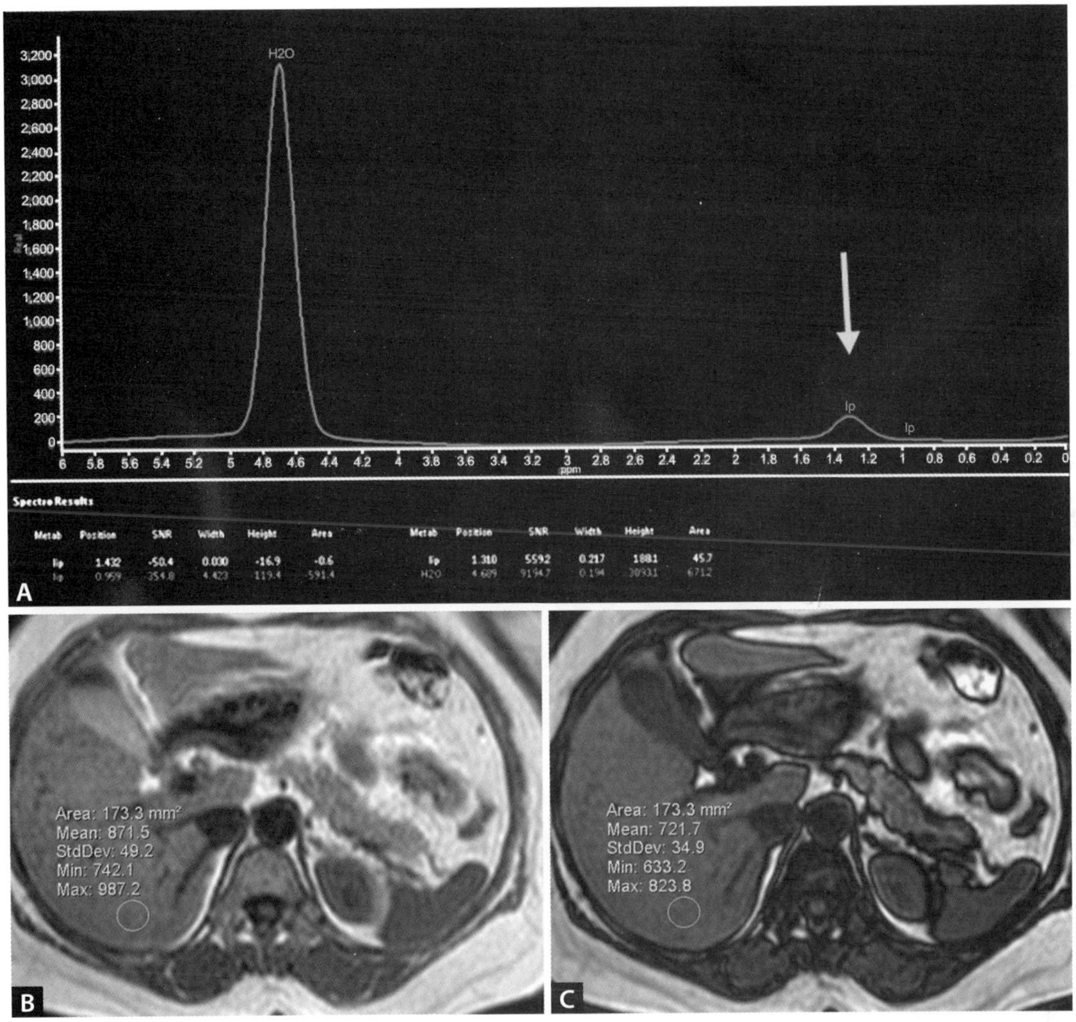

Figs. 6A to C: MRS spectrum in a case of fatty liver (A) showing a lipid peak at 1.3 ppm. Chemical shift MRI of fatty liver shows signal drop of liver parenchyma in the opposed-phase image (C) from in-phase image (B) due to steatosis.

Chemical shift MR imaging is the investigation of choice in cases with focal nodular or multifocal fat deposition/ sparing that may be confused with liver metastases on US or CT.

Although fatty infiltration may demonstrate increased signal intensity of liver on T1- and T2-weighted spin echo images this increase in signal may not be apparent even with massive fat deposition in liver.[12] Advanced MRI techniques based on 3D gradient echo imaging, are under evaluation for calculation of proton density fat fraction (PDFF), which allows quantitative evaluation of liver fat without the inherent limitations of the conventional chemical shift imaging which affect image quality such as choice of imaging parameters, field strength and coexisting biological factors like fibrosis, cirrhosis and iron overload.[13]

Contrast-enhanced MRI (CEMRI) using gadoxetic acid has been shown to have potential in differentiating simple steatosis from NASH, as the mean liver enhancement is found to be lower in NASH compared with simple steatosis likely due to increased hepatocyte volume reducing the sinusoidal space, and thereby the contrast uptake.[14] Similar observations have been seen by using USPIO, where poor hepatic uptake of USPIO has been seen in patients NASH than in simple steatosis.[15]

On cross-sectional imaging fat deposition is most often diffuse. Focal fat deposition and focal fat sparing are less common patterns that typically occur adjacent to the falciform ligament, fissure for ligamentum venosum, porta hepatis, gallbladder fossa and in the subcapsular portions of the liver. Their characteristic locations, geographic/ wedge shape configuration with angulated margins, lack

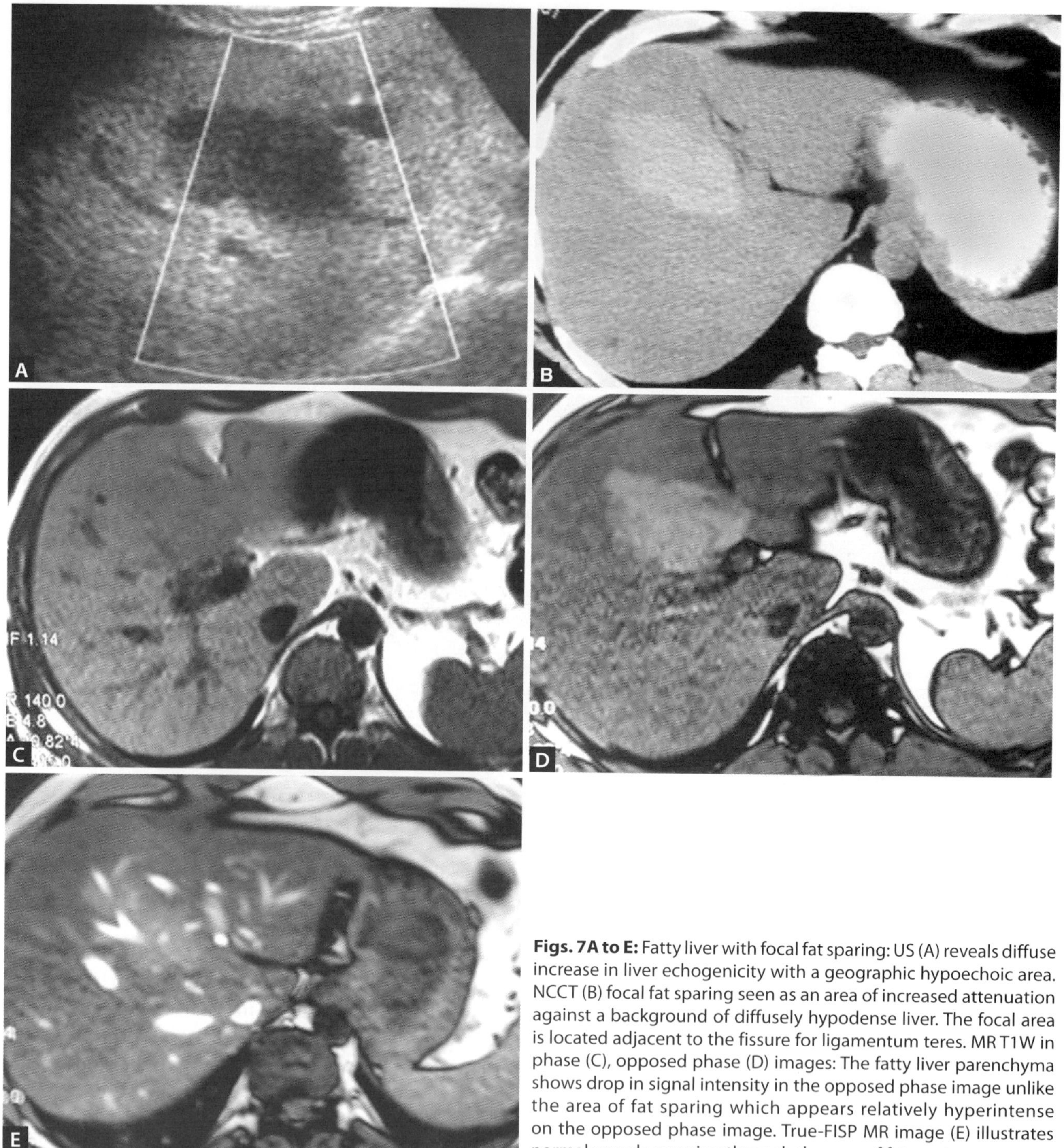

Figs. 7A to E: Fatty liver with focal fat sparing: US (A) reveals diffuse increase in liver echogenicity with a geographic hypoechoic area. NCCT (B) focal fat sparing seen as an area of increased attenuation against a background of diffusely hypodense liver. The focal area is located adjacent to the fissure for ligamentum teres. MR T1W in phase (C), opposed phase (D) images: The fatty liver parenchyma shows drop in signal intensity in the opposed phase image unlike the area of fat sparing which appears relatively hyperintense on the opposed phase image. True-FISP MR image (E) illustrates normal vessels coursing through the area of fat sparing.

of mass effect, presence of normal blood vessels coursing through them and enhancement similar to normal liver help differentiate these from true lesions. When multifocal or nodular these may however, simulate true masses and may require chemical shift MRI for their confirmation **(Figs. 7A to E)**.

VIRAL HEPATITIS

Hepatitis is diffuse inflammation of the liver that can be divided into acute and chronic forms. The latter is in turn, subdivided into persistent and chronic active categories. Imaging is relatively nonspecific but can help to exclude biliary obstruction in acute hepatitis. In chronic hepatitis, imaging is useful in monitoring the progression of the disease, development of portal venous hypertension and complications such as hepatocellular carcinoma.

USG

In acute viral hepatitis, liver and spleen are frequently enlarged. Severe acute hepatitis may result in diffusely decreased parenchymal echogenicity against which the portal vein branches appear brighter than normal.[1] This pattern is seen in up to 60% of patients with acute viral hepatitis and is best appreciated in thin patients.[16] Gallbladder wall thickening or contraction or both, are other nonspecific findings seen in patients with hepatitis. Paradoxical response of gallbladder to fatty food may be seen as dilatation of gall bladder. Severe chronic hepatitis causes coarsening of parenchymal echotexture and increased echogenicity resulting in poor visualization of portal venous branches. This finding, however, is nonspecific and is also seen in fatty infiltration and cirrhosis. Periportal lymphadenopathy may be seen in hepatitis.

CT

CT attenuation of liver is generally not altered in hepatitis unless fatty infiltration is present. Hepatomegaly, gallbladder wall thickening, and periportal hypodensity can be seen in acute hepatitis and periportal lymphadenopathy is commonly seen in chronic active hepatitis.

MRI

On MRI, the edematous liver in acute hepatitis may appear heterogeneous especially on T2-weighted images and early post contrast images. Periportal T2 hyperintense signal can also be seen. Likewise heterogeneous contrast enhancement and T2 hyperintensity signify severe ongoing inflammation in chronic hepatitis, while absence of patchy enhancement suggests low inflammatory reaction.[17] Progressive enhancement in the delayed phase suggests the presence of liver fibrosis in patients with chronic hepatitis.[18]

ALCOHOLIC HEPATITIS

Alcoholic liver disease manifests as three distinct but overlapping entities: fatty liver, alcoholic hepatitis and cirrhosis. Unlike acute viral hepatitis, liver echogenicity is increased in acute alcoholic hepatitis due to presence of concomitant fatty infiltration.

RADIATION HEPATITIS

In acute radiation hepatitis, CT shows a sharply defined, hypodense area in the liver corresponding to the radiation ports. This represents edema or fatty infiltration of the involved area. Clinically, onset is 2–6 weeks after therapy and is generally seen in patients receiving dose of more than 35 gray to the liver. The CT changes may be seen several weeks after the initiation of the therapy and resolve by 3–5 months. Radiation hepatitis on MR imaging is seen as geographic areas of edema on T1- and T2-weighted images.[19]

HEMOCHROMATOSIS AND HEMOSIDEROSIS

Hepatic iron overload can be divided into parenchymal iron deposition (hemochromatosis) and reticuloendothelial iron deposition (hemosiderosis). In hemosiderosis, the excess iron (body iron stores 10–20 g) is derived from red blood cells typically due to repeated blood transfusions or hemolytic anemia. Because such iron is deposited primarily in the reticuloendothelial system (liver, spleen, lymph nodes, bone marrow) organ function is generally preserved.

Hemochromatosis on the other hand is a more severe form of iron accumulation (body iron stores up to 50–60 g) that adversely affects organ function. Hemochromatosis may be primary or secondary. Primary hemochromatosis is an autosomal recessive metabolic disorder of excessive iron absorption in duodenum/jejunum. The causes of secondary hemochromatosis include excess iron intake, anemia due to ineffective erythropoiesis requiring multiple blood transfusions, congenital transferrin deficiency, portocaval shunts and alcoholic cirrhosis.

The excess iron in hemochromatosis is stored as ferritin and hemosiderin in various organs including liver, pancreas, myocardium, joints, endocrine glands like pituitary and skin, in decreasing order of severity. Sometimes iron is deposited in spleen and kidneys. Brain and nervous tissues are spared. A fibrous tissue reaction is found wherever iron is deposited. Iron deposits are greatest in liver and pancreas where they can contain 50–100 times the normal amount of iron. The liver is the first organ to be damaged in hemochromatosis resulting in hepatomegaly in 95% symptomatic patients. Fibrosis is maximal in periportal areas resulting in micronodular pigment cirrhosis. Fatty change is unusual. Iron-induced interstitial fibrosis in the pancreas affects endocrine functions to a greater extent than exocrine functions. Skin hyperpigmentation and diabetes mellitus results in so called *bronze diabetes* in these patients. Splenomegaly is present in approximately 50% cases, arthropathy of small joints of the hand with or without evidence of chondrocalcinosis on radiographs occurs in 20–50% and cardiac involvement is the presenting complaint in 15% cases. Diminished sexual activity, loss of body hair and testicular atrophy can be seen due to decreased production of gonadotropins.

Primary hemochromatosis usually presents in fourth to sixth decade of life. It is ten times more frequent in males. Women are generally spared due to iron loss with menstruation and pregnancy. The disease responds favorably to treatment that includes venesection/removal of blood and iron chelators. However, once cirrhosis sets in, it is irreversible and is complicated by development of hepatocellular carcinoma in about one-third of patients despite adequate therapy.[20] Early diagnosis and treatment of hemochromatosis is therefore of vital importance.

USG

Ultrasonography (USG) only depicts nonspecific changes of cirrhosis in patients with hemochromatosis and therefore has no role in the diagnosis.

CT

Unenhanced CT shows an overall homogeneous increase in density of hepatic parenchyma. While normal liver attenuation is between 45 and 65 HU, in hemochromatosis this ranges from 70 to 135 HU. The intrahepatic vessels stand out against the background of hyperdense liver. A CT value of 70 HU or more on unenhanced scan is very sensitive and fairly specific indicator of severe iron overload **(Fig. 8)**,[12] although amiodarone treatment and glycogen storage disease can result in similar increased attenuation.

CT also demonstrates increased density in spleen, pancreas, adrenal and lymph nodes. The increased background liver attenuation in hemochromatosis may hamper detection of hepatocellular carcinoma in the postcontrast images but facilitates tumor detection in unenhanced scans.

Dual energy CT has a proven role in estimation of liver iron content (LIC). It is based on three material decomposition of iodine, water and iron, to provide virtual iron content (VIC) as well as providing a virtual nonenhanced image by commercially available postprocessing softwares.[21]

MRI

MR imaging is the most sensitive and specific imaging modality for demonstration of hepatic iron overload and also for follow-up of patients under treatment.[17] Gradient echo sequences are more sensitive than spin echo sequences. On MRI, hemochromatosis is characterized by dramatic loss of T1 and T2 signal of the liver (90%) and pancreas (20%) **(Fig. 9)**. A liver/paraspinal muscle (L/M) signal ratio below 0.6 on spin echo T2-weighted images is suggestive of severe iron overload. It correlates well with the amount of iron present in the liver.[12] Iron estimation can also be done by in and opposed phase imaging where contrary to what is seen in fatty infiltration, iron deposition results in loss of signal in the in phase image which conventionally is acquired at a longer TE than the opposed phase image **(Figs. 10A to C)**.

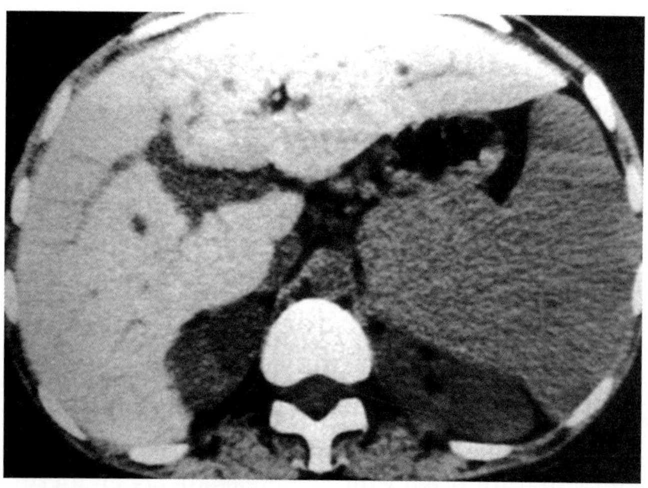

Fig. 8: Primary hemochromatosis: Unenhanced CT shows markedly increased attenuation of the liver parenchyma.

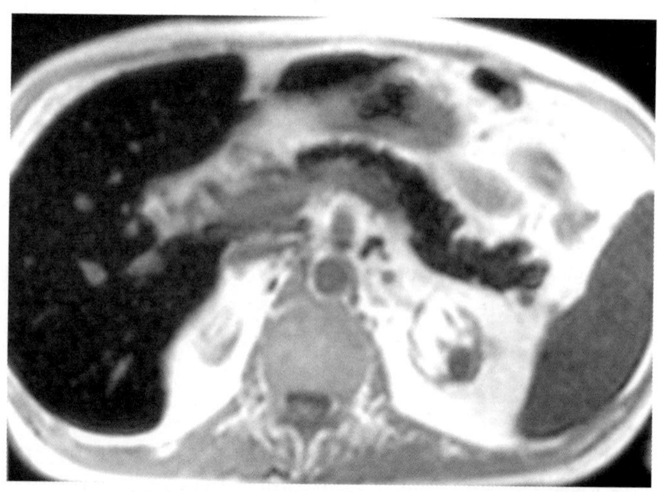

Fig. 9: Primary hemochromatosis: FSE T2W image reveals markedly hypointense signal of the liver and pancreas, while the spleen shows normal signal intensity.

Another method of iron estimation is based on T2 relaxometry. This technique is based on spin-echo and gradient-echo sequences. MR images are acquired at progressively longer echo times (TE), and the rate of signal decay is mathematically estimated. This generates a cross-sectional map of T2 (in spin echo) or T2* (in gradient echo) relaxation rates. Once the T2 or T2* value is calculated, the liver iron concentration (LIC) in mg of elemental iron/g of liver tissue by dry weight can be estimated by validated calibration curves.[22] Liver iron content can also be calculated by signal intensity ratio (SIR) between the liver and the paraspinal muscles from a set of multiple GRE sequences with fixed TR, different TE and flip angles for 1.5 T scanners using an online calculator developed by University of Rennes.[23]

Iron overload coexisting with fat deposition may present a diagnostic challenge and requires careful evaluation in all sequences. In fat deposition, there is loss of signal on opposed phase images, whereas in iron deposition there is low signal on 'in phase' images. Moreover, in presence of focal fatty sparing or focal fatty change on a background of iron overload (pseudolesion) may require enhancement pattern characterization.

Decreased signal intensity in hemochromatosis is also demonstrated in pancreas and myocardium, and only occasionally in spleen. In transfusional siderosis, the signal intensity of both spleen and liver is diminished while the signal of pancreas remains unchanged as it is devoid of reticuloendothelial cells **(Figs. 11A and B)** his feature helps to differentiate transfusional siderosis from hemochromatosis.

AMYLOIDOSIS

Amyloidosis is a rare condition characterized by the deposition of an extracellular fibrillar protein in the organs. It may be primary or secondary. Primary amyloidosis is due to deposition of amyloid light chain protein (AL). It may occur without pre-existing disease or may be seen as a complication of multiple myeloma. Secondary amyloidosis is due to the deposition of amyloid A protein

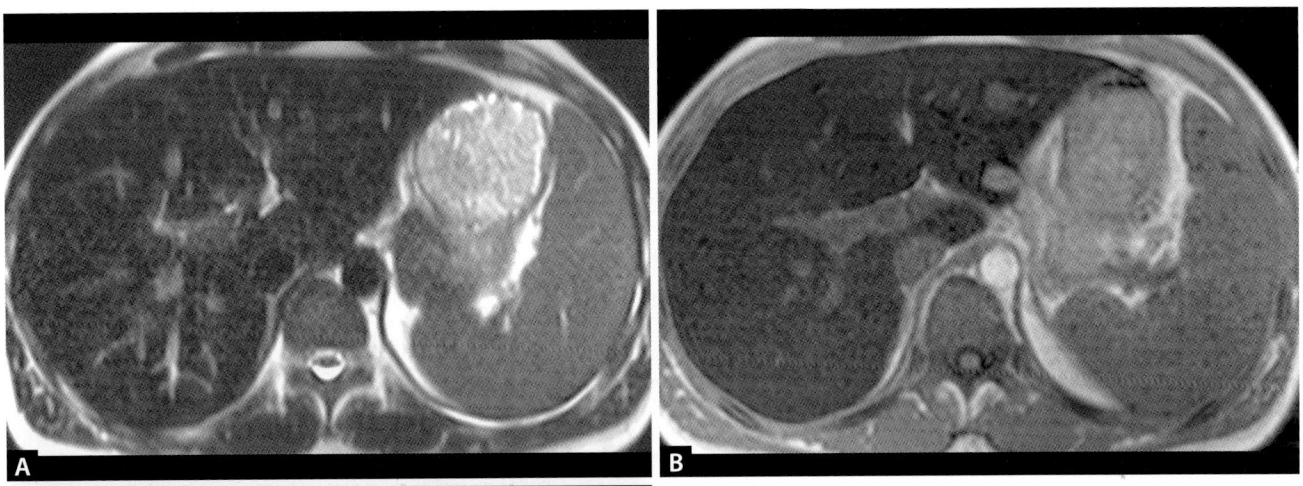

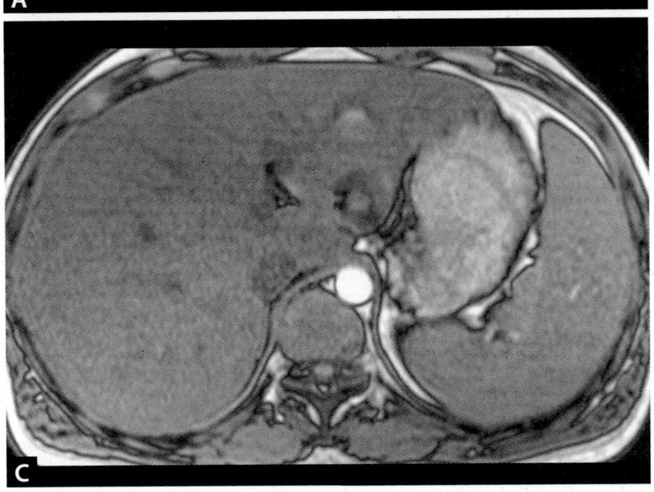

Figs. 10A to C: Hemosiderosis secondary to repeated blood transfusions: MRI HASTE T2W image (A) showing reduced signal intensity of liver. Spoiled GRE T1W in phase image (B) and opposed phase image (C) show increase in signal intensity of the liver parenchyma in the opposed phase image due to iron deposition. There are numerous similar hypointense foci in the spleen also

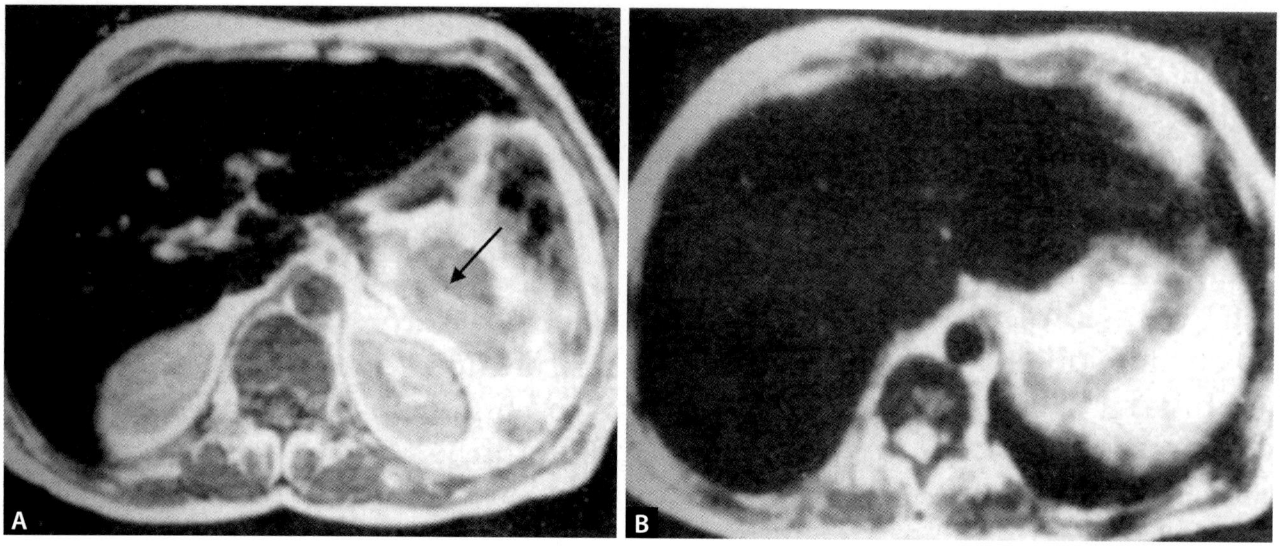

Figs. 11A and B: Hemosiderosis: Almost no signal intensity is seen on T1-weighted (A) and T2-weighted axial MR images (B). Normal signal intensity of the pancreas (↑) helps in differentiation from hemochromatosis. Spleen is not seen because of previous splenectomy in this patient.

(AA) and is seen with chronic infections, rheumatoid arthritis, ulcerative colitis, Crohn's disease, malignant tumors and Hodgkin's lymphoma. Clinically, there is smooth, non-tender hepatomegaly. Hepatic function is usually preserved despite massive amyloid deposition.

Ultrasound is usually normal except for presence of hepatomegaly. Rarely US reveals a heterogeneous echotexture due to nonuniform deposition. Increased liver stiffness is seen on ultrasound elastography which may be due to the protein deposition.[24]

On unenhanced CT scans amyloid deposition results in hepatomegaly and generalized decreased attenuation. On contrast-enhanced scans, focal areas of decreased enhancement corresponding to nonuniform involvement may be seen. The involved areas may show contrast enhancement in the delayed phase. Concomitant decrease in splenic enhancement may help differentiate amyloid deposition from fatty liver in appropriate settings. MR imaging has little role in the assessment of hepatic amyloidosis as there is no significant change in the T2 signal of involved liver.[25] MRI elastography also reveals increased tissue stiffness.

WILSON'S DISEASE

Wilson's disease or hepatolenticular degeneration is a rare, inherited autosomal recessive disorder of copper metabolism characterized by impaired biliary excretion of copper. Initially the excess copper accumulates in the liver. Subsequently copper deposition occurs in the basal ganglia, renal tubules, cornea, bones, joints and parathyroid glands. The spectrum of liver injury in Wilson's disease is nonspecific and includes fatty infiltration, acute hepatitis, chronic active hepatitis, cirrhosis or massive liver necrosis. Development of HCC is extremely rare.

Most patients present in childhood or adolescence with liver disease before the onset of neurologic manifestations. They may have progressive jaundice, ascites or even fulminant hepatitis. Patients presenting after the age of 20 years can present with a clinical picture simulating chronic active hepatitis or with neurological symptoms like Parkinson like movement disorder and psychiatric disturbance. The Kayser-Fleischer ring is a characteristic corneal pigment that is invariably present. Early recognition is important as treatment with penicillamine and zinc can prevent toxic deposition of copper in the liver and brain. Imaging findings of cirrhosis, fatty liver are nonspecific **(Figs. 12A and B)**. Fatty infiltration and excess copper can cancel each other out in advanced Wilson's disease, so that a high CT density is usually not seen. Skeletal changes are seen in over 85% patients with Wilson's disease.[26] These include osteomalacia, chondrocalcinosis, premature osteoarthritis, anterior wedging of dorsal vertebrae, Schmorl's nodes, osteochondritis dissecans and a periosteal reaction at the trochanters.

On MRI, copper deposition has no ferromagnetic effect on the liver signal intensity as it exists intracellularly in bound form. The changes on MRI are similar to those of cirrhotic liver disease with contour abnormalities

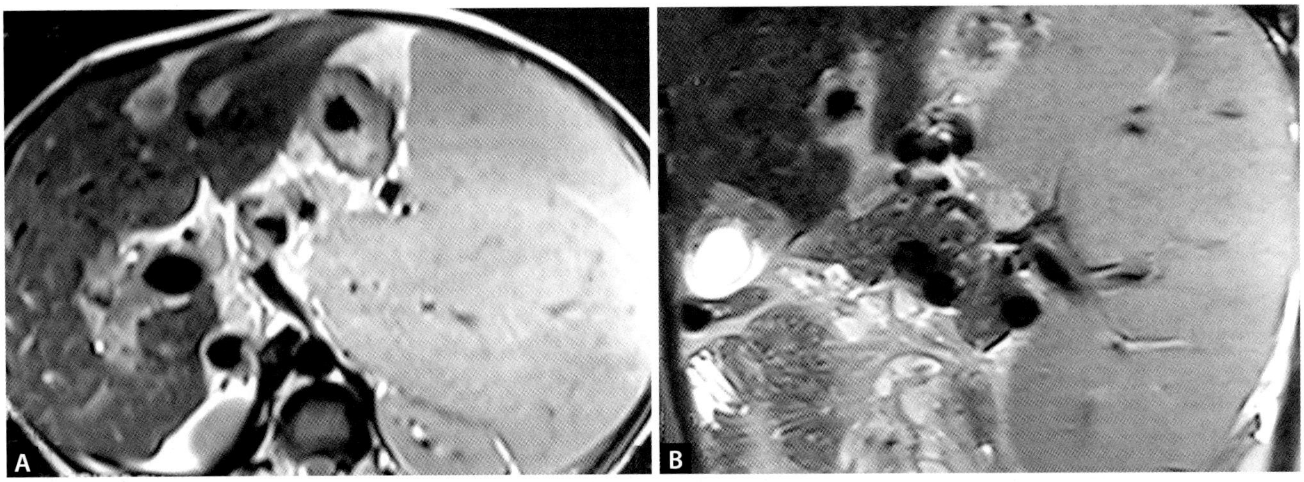

Figs. 12A and B: Wilson's disease: Axial (A) and coronal (B) TSE T2W image of a 15-year-old boy showing non-specific changes of liver cirrhosis with a shrunken liver and massive splenomegaly.

and regenerative nodules. A honeycomb pattern consisting of multiple low-intensity nodules surrounded by hyperintense septa on T2-weighted images may be seen. However, this finding is not specific to Wilson's disease.[27] Due to copper deposition T1 hyperintense and T2 hypointense nodules may be seen on MRI which may show resolution with chelation therapy.[28]

GRANULOMATOUS DISEASES

Granulomatous diseases denote the presence of a focal inflammatory process with the histological features of granuloma. The causes include various viral, bacterial, fungal and parasitic infections, sarcoidosis, granulomatosis with polyangitis (Wegener's), and toxic reaction to drugs and chemicals. Biochemical abnormalities in the form of elevated alkaline phosphatase (ALP) and gamma glutamyl transpeptidase (GGT) is frequently seen in various diffuse infiltrative diseases and alcoholic/viral chronic liver diseases.

Tuberculosis: Miliary tuberculosis is the most common form of hepatic tuberculosis. Usually it is not accompanied by radiological abnormalities because of its diffuse micronodular nature. Macronodular tuberculomas are uncommon and may be solitary or multiple. These are hypoechoic on ultrasound. CT scan shows hypodense masses with or without rim enhancement **(Fig. 13)**. Tubercular cholangitis and tubercular pyelophlebitis result from rupture of tubercular nodes/abscess and spread of caseous material into bile ducts and portal vein respectively. Both these conditions are rare. Multiple small intrahepatic calcifications with no associated masses seen on ultrasound and CT represent old healed granulomas.[12]

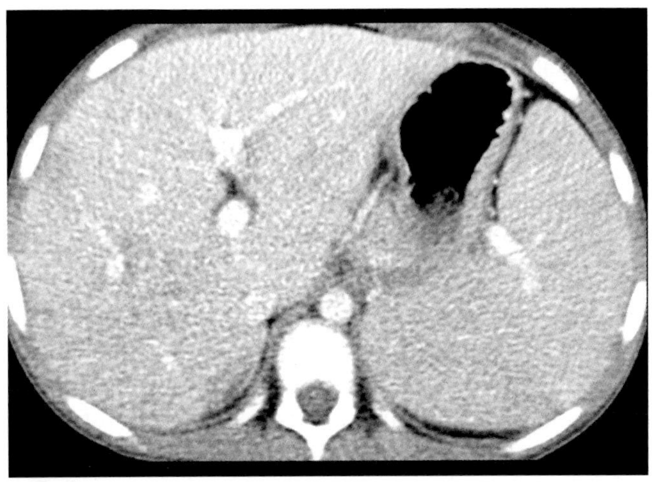

Fig. 13: Granulomatous disease: Contrast-enhanced CT of a young adult with disseminated tuberculosis reveals hepatosplenomegaly and ill-defined hypodense lesions in the right lobe of liver.

Sarcoidosis: Liver involvement occurs in 24–79% patients of sarcoidosis.[29] Clinically apparent liver disease is however rare. On imaging small (<2 mm) noncaseating granulomas are seen diffusely in the liver. Cross sectional imaging most frequently reveals hepatomegaly, often with associated splenomegaly. Less commonly granulomas are seen as nodular lesions 0.5–2 cm in size in the liver and spleen. These nodular lesions appear hypoechoic on US, hypodense on CT and hypointense on both T1- and T2-weighted MR images. Upper abdominal adenopathy is frequently associated in these patients. Occasionally, these nodes enlarge sufficiently to cause biliary obstruction at porta hepatis.

Schistosomiasis: It is a common parasitic infestation with high prevalence in endemic areas such as Africa, South America, Middle East, China and Japan. The adult worms release ova in portal and mesenteric veins, which embolize to the liver. The host reacts to the ova with a granulomatous inflammation, which is then replaced by fibrous tissue, leading to periportal fibrosis and portal hypertension. On ultrasound, periportal fibrosis is seen in the form of thick, echogenic bands replacing the normal portal venous walls, which radiate from porta hepatis to the periphery of the liver. These bands are seen as tubular, round or oval structures depending on the plane of the section. There may be evidence of portal hypertension. On unenhanced CT, the bands of periportal fibrosis are hypodense and they enhance markedly after contrast administration. They produce round, linear or branching patterns depending on the plane in which they are sectioned. The portal vein may not enhance, if it is thrombosed. Hepatic calcification, if seen, is fairly characteristic and has been termed as 'turtle back'.[30] It occurs within the capsule and hepatic parenchyma, perpendicular to the capsule looking like a septum. Sometimes the calcifications may be dense enough to be seen on the plain films.

Liver fluke or Fasciola hepatica: It is a trematode that infests cattle. Humans are accidental hosts. There is an acute phase of hepatic invasion that lasts for 1–3 months and a chronic phase of persistent adult flukes in the biliary tree. In hepatic fascioliasis, CT shows peripheral small, hypodense, serpentine or nodular lesions whose visibility is improved on dynamic or delayed enhanced CT. The tortuous peripheral channels correspond to the migratory tracts.[31]

There are many other causes of granulomatous infections, which include brucellosis, leptospirosis, syphilis, leishmaniasis, actinomycosis, aspergillosis and cryptococcosis. These are not associated with any specific radiological features.

CIRRHOSIS

Cirrhosis is a chronic disease of the liver, which is characterized by fibrosis, and nodular regeneration of the liver in response to hepatocellular necrosis. The etiology is diverse which includes viral hepatitis, alcoholism, prolonged cholestasis, hepatic venous outflow tract obstruction, malnutrition, cryptogenic cirrhosis, metabolic causes like hemochromatosis and Wilson's disease, various toxins and therapeutic agents. Cirrhosis is conventionally considered as an irreversibly scarred, end stage disease of the liver. Although the causes are many, the end result is same.[32] The response of the liver to the necrosis is limited, the most important being collapse of hepatic lobules, formation of diffuse fibrous septa and nodular re-growth of liver cells. The initiating hepatocyte injury leads to inflammation, structural collapse and fibrogenesis. The resulting fibrosis causes circulatory disturbances, portal hypertension and intrahepatic cholestasis. A vicious cycle is set-up whereby further hepatocyte injury occurs leading to progression of the disease. Morphologically cirrhosis is classified into micronodular and macronodular varieties. *Micronodular* disease is characterized by thick, regular septa, small regenerating nodules of uniform size, and involvement of every lobule. It may represent impaired capacity of re-growth as in alcoholism or malnutrition. *Macronodular* variety is characterized by septa and nodules of various sizes and presence of normal liver in between larger nodules.[32] There are many histological grading systems for categorizing hepatic fibrosis, *METAVIR* being the most common. It is a five point scoring system:

1. F0—no fibrosis
2. F1—portal fibrosis without septa
3. F2—few septa
4. F3—numerous septa without cirrhosis
5. F4—cirrhosis.[2]

A *regenerative nodule* is defined as a hepatocellular nodule containing one or more portal tracts located in a liver that is otherwise abnormal due to either cirrhosis or other severe disease. These nodules are present in all cirrhotic livers, and cirrhosis is classified on the basis of size of these on pathologic specimen as micronodular (less than equal to 3 mm), macronodular (more than 3 mm) or mixed. A *dysplastic nodule* is defined as a nodule of hepatocytes of at least 1 mm in diameter, with dysplasia of low or high grade but no histological criteria for malignancy. Dysplastic nodules are found in 15–25% of cirrhotic livers. Steatosis (fatty infiltration) can occur in either form, and either form may result in an enlarged or shrunken liver. *Focal confluent fibrosis* (or confluent hepatic fibrosis) refers to mass like fibrosis in advanced cirrhosis, associated with volume loss seen as retraction of overlying hepatic capsule or total shrinkage of segment or lobe.

Clinically, Child's classification is used to determine short-term prognosis. It takes into account jaundice, ascites, encephalopathy, serum albumin and nutrition status. In the Child-Pugh modification prothrombin time is used instead of nutritional status as a parameter. The total score classifies patients into grade A, B or C, with increasing severity of disease.[32] Complications of cirrhosis include portal hypertension, variceal bleeding, spontaneous bacterial peritonitis, coagulopathies, hepatic encephalopathy, hepatorenal syndrome and hepatocellular carcinoma (HCC). Risk of development of HCC in cirrhotic liver is approximately 3% per year. Although, cirrhosis of any etiology may lead to HCC, the risk is particularly high in cirrhosis which occurs secondary to viral hepatitis. Imaging studies play an important role in screening for HCC in cirrhotic patients.

USG

Liver is either enlarged or normal in size in the early stage of cirrhosis. A small shrunken liver is seen in advanced cases. Criteria for sonographic diagnosis include heterogeneously increased parenchymal echogenicity, decreased beam penetration through liver and poor depiction of diaphragm and intrahepatic portal venous walls. These features are common to both fatty infiltration and fibrosis and there is poor interobserver agreement on interpreting these finding. Echogenicity largely depends on gain settings; however, it can be compared with that of adjacent organs in cases of doubt. Normally, echogenicity of liver and renal cortex are almost equal or that of kidney is slightly lower than liver. In case the kidneys are diseased, comparison may be made with that of splenic echogenicity also as spleen has higher echogenicity than normal liver.

Morphological changes in cirrhosis include relative hypertrophy of the caudate lobe and segments 2, 3 of the left lobe and atrophy of the right hepatic lobe and segment 4 of left lobe. Sonographically, a right/left lobe ratio of sagittal diameters in midclavicular line and midline respectively of 1.3 or less can differentiate cirrhosis from normal liver with 93% accuracy, while a ratio of 1.4 or more excludes cirrhosis.[33] In advanced case of cirrhosis, accentuation of fissures, contour indentations, nodularity and regenerating nodules are seen. Regenerating nodules vary in size from 2 mm to 2 cm. These may be visible on US as hypoechoic nodules with echogenic border and are difficult to differentiate from small HCC on US. US scanning with a high frequency probe can depict a nodular liver contour even in early cirrhosis.[34] Atrophy of the liver, along with heterogeneous echotexture and poor beam penetration, however, limits the sonographic detection of small focal lesions in advanced cirrhotic liver. Sonography has a poor sensitivity in detection of HCC; it detects only 14% of lesions smaller than 2 cm and its sensitivity for detecting HCC during screening of cirrhotic patients is only 50%.[1,35]

Doppler evaluation is valuable as it provides hemodynamic information. Portal hypertension can be seen in the form of enlarged portal vein, diminution or reversal of portal venous flow and presence of portosystemic collaterals. Hepatic venous evaluation by Doppler is also helpful. Normal hepatic venous waveform is triphasic with a short phase of reversed flow. The fibrosis and decreased compliance of liver parenchyma leads to decreased amplitude of the phasic variations with loss of reversed flow. Alternatively, there may be a completely flat waveform. These features may be seen even in early stages of cirrhosis.[36] As the liver atrophies in end stage cirrhosis, hepatic veins may become attenuated and difficult to visualize. This can cause difficulties when the diagnosis of hepatic venous occlusion is being considered.[8]

The cirrhotic liver can be assessed noninvasively by three *ultrasound elastography* techniques, the transient elastography (fibroscan), acoustic radiation force impulse (ARFI) and shear wave elastography. The hepatic fibrosis correlates with the stiffness values generated on elastography such that value less than 6–7 kPa indicate no or mild fibrosis (F0-F1 METAVIR) and a value more than 12 kPa suggests cirrhosis (F3-F4 METAVIR) **(Fig. 3B)**.[3]

Contrast enhanced ultrasound using microbubble contrast agent has a role in characterizing focal liver lesions in cirrhotic liver and in screening of cirrhosis patients for hepatocellular carcinomas. It is a useful adjunct to CECT or CEMRI with the benefit of a real time contrast visualization without renal excretion of the contrast. Both dysplastic nodules and hepatocellular carcinomas show arterial phase hyperenhancement on CEUS, similar to CT and MRI.[37]

CT

Fatty liver is the most common CT feature of early cirrhosis. Morphological changes in advanced cirrhosis include an overall decrease in liver volume accompanied by atrophy of the right lobe and hypertrophy of left and caudate lobes. The dual arterial supply and shorter intrahepatic course of vessels supplying the caudate lobe along with the fact that caudate vein drains directly into the inferior vena cava permits better oxygenation and relative preservation of its function resulting in compensatory hypertrophy.[37] On the other hand it is postulated that alcohol and other toxins in the portal vein stream preferentially to the right hepatic lobe. Caudate lobe to right lobe size ratio has been proposed as an objective means of diagnosing cirrhosis. Three lines are drawn: Line 1 is parasagittal through the right lateral wall of main portal vein just caudal to its bifurcation, line 2 is parallel to line 1 through the medial margin of caudate lobe, and line 3 is perpendicular to these lines drawn midway between portal vein and IVC. The distances are measured on line 3. The distance between right abdominal wall and line 1 is right lobe size and distance between line 1 and line 2 is caudate lobe size **(Fig. 14)**. If the caudate lobe to right lobe ratio exceeds 0.65, cirrhosis is likely and it is definitive if it exceeds 0.73.[38] The hepatic fissure, gallbladder fossa and porta hepatis are widened due to parenchymal atrophy **(Fig. 15)**. These morphological changes are by and large similar irrespective of the underlying etiology of cirrhosis. However, patients with biliary cirrhosis and sclerosing cholangitis tend to have marked caudate lobe hypertrophy and often have atrophy of lateral segments of the left hepatic lobe in addition to atrophy of right lobe.

Cirrhotic liver often appears heterogeneous on both unenhanced and enhanced CT scans due to underlying fibrosis, iron accumulation, regeneration and altered portal venous flow.[8] Regenerating nodules and atrophy cause nodularity of liver contour. Ancillary CT features in cirrhosis include ascites, splenomegaly, enlargement of the hepatic artery, and evidence of porto-systemic collaterals, pericaval fat collection that may appear intraluminal on axial CT scans and increased attenuation of the mesenteric/retroperitoneal fat.

Regenerating nodules are usually less than 5 mm and are infrequently demonstrated on noncontrast CT, however may appear hyperdense if they contain iron (Siderotic nodules). These do not show arterial phase enhancement and remain isodense to minimally hypodense to the remaining parenchyma on portal venous phase.

Dysplastic nodules on the other hand measure 5–10 mm in size and show arterial phase enhancement due to progressive recruitment of hepatic arterial supply. The high grade dyplastic nodules may show portal venous washout similar to that of hepatocellular carcinomas.

Focal confluent fibrosis that is seen in 30% of patients with advanced cirrhosis can also simulate tumor appearing hypodense on unenhanced CT and isodense to slightly hypodense in contrast-enhanced CT. However, typical associated features including wedge-shaped lesion radiating from the porta hepatis, characteristic location in the anterior segments of right lobe and segment 4, delayed enhancement and focal retraction of the overlying liver capsule can help differentiate these from tumor. Similar to hepatitis, patients with cirrhosis can have enlarged upper abdominal lymph nodes and this finding is particularly common in patients with biliary cirrhosis and sclerosing cholangitis. Pseudocirrhosis results from distortion of the hepatic parenchyma due to treated multiple metastatic lesions, usually from breast carcinoma and can simulate changes of cirrhosis. Similar appearance may also result from pseudomyxoma peritonei or ovarian metastasis due to surface scalloping.

MRI

MR imaging can often detect cirrhosis at an earlier stage than US or CT.[1] In early cirrhosis, MRI demonstrates fine strands of fibrosis, which are seen as lace like hypointense

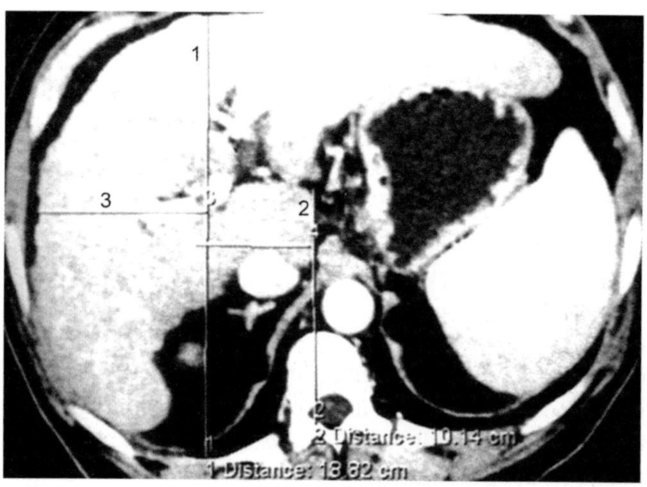

Fig. 14: CT scan shows method of measurements of right and caudate lobes. The diameters of right and caudate lobes are measured on line 3 as shown.

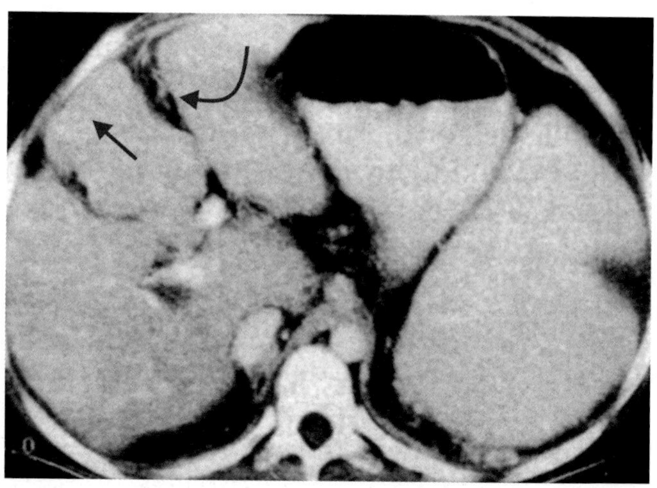

Fig. 15: Cirrhosis: Atrophy of the right lobe and hypertrophy of the caudate lobe with splenomegaly is seen on CT. Widened hepatic fissure (curved arrow), porta and nodularity of the contour of the liver (straight arrow) are also seen.

fine network on heavily T2-weighted images. Out of phase spoiled gradient echo images are very sensitive in this regard. These fine fibrotic strands show progressive enhancement following intravenous gadolinium. Enlargement of hilar periportal space, which is a space anterior to right branch of portal vein, is considered as an early manifestation of cirrhosis. It is caused by atrophy of segment 4. Early detection of cirrhosis by MRI is of clinical importance as these patients may benefit from newer treatment options now available.[22] As cirrhosis progresses, MRI demonstrates all features which are seen on CT, including contour nodularity, relative right lobe atrophy and left/caudate lobe hypertrophy, splanchnic vessels enlargement, hepatic arterial enlargement, collaterals, splenomegaly and ascites. Expansion and widening of interlobar fissure is also seen.

Abnormal hepatic periportal intensity, which is seen as hyperintense rings or track marks surrounding the portal vein branches on T2-weighted images, can be seen in cirrhosis. It is a nonspecific finding and also seen in many biliary or hepatocellular diseases. Gamna Gandy bodies in spleen are seen as multiple, small, low intensity spots on gradient echo images. These represent hemosiderin deposits in collagen bundles and may be the result of small hemorrhages and can be seen in portal hypertension due to other causes like EHPVO.

MR imaging is the modality of choice for characterizing nodules in cirrhotic liver and can demonstrate regenerating nodules with greater sensitivity than any other modality. While only approximately 25% of regenerating nodules are seen on CT mainly due to their iron content, MR can demonstrate 50% regenerative nodules **(Figs. 16A and B)**.[1] Dysplastic nodules (previously called adenomatous hyperplastic nodules) represent premalignant intermediary phase in pathway of hepatocellular carcinogenesis **(Figs. 17A to D)**. The MRI appearance of regenerative and dysplastic nodules on various MRI sequences and enhancement phases is summarized in **Table 1**.

Focal confluent fibrosis has T1 and T2 signal similar to HCC, i.e. hypointense on T1 and hyperintense on T2-weighted images. It may show arterial phase enhancement, however persistent enhancement in delayed phase helps in differentiation from hepatocellular carcinoma. Moreover, as with CT, characteristic location and associated capsular retraction also helps in differentiation. MR imaging is useful in differentiating viral from alcoholic cirrhosis. Larger caudate lobe volume, presence of a notch in the outline of right posterior segment of liver and smaller size of regenerating nodules favors the diagnosis of alcoholic cirrhosis over virus induced cirrhosis.[39]

MR elastography (MRE) has a role in noninvasive evaluation, staging and follow-up of hepatic fibrosis. It is based on modified phase contrast sequence where a mechanical propagation wave is produced in soft tissues usually of frequency 60 MHz. The propagation of the wave in the tissue creates an elastogram using complex algorithms. In various studies MR elastography has shown good agreement with ultrasound elastography, liver biopsy and other biochemical markers of hepatic fibrosis.[40,41] The advantages of MR elastography over ultrasound elastography include ability to evaluate the entire liver and eliminating the sampling error of USE.

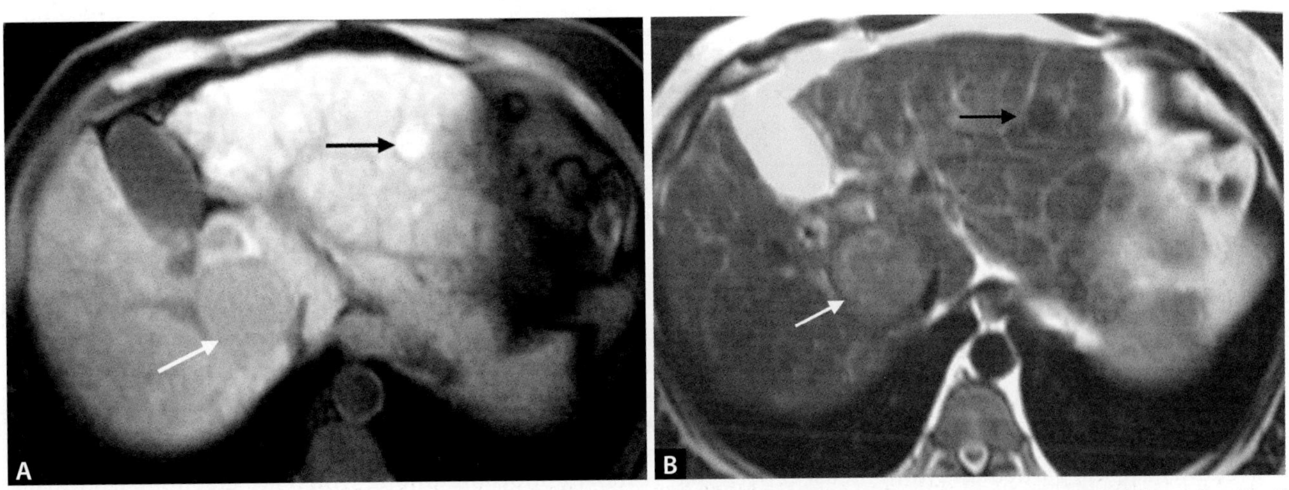

Figs. 16A and B: Cirrhosis with regenerative nodule and HCC: Axial T1W (A) and T2W (B) MR images shows a well-defined focal lesion in segment VIII of liver (white arrow) which is hypointense on T1 and hyperintense on T2W images suggestive of HCC. A regenerative nodule is also seen in segment II (black arrow) which appears hyperintense on T1 and hypointense on T2W images.

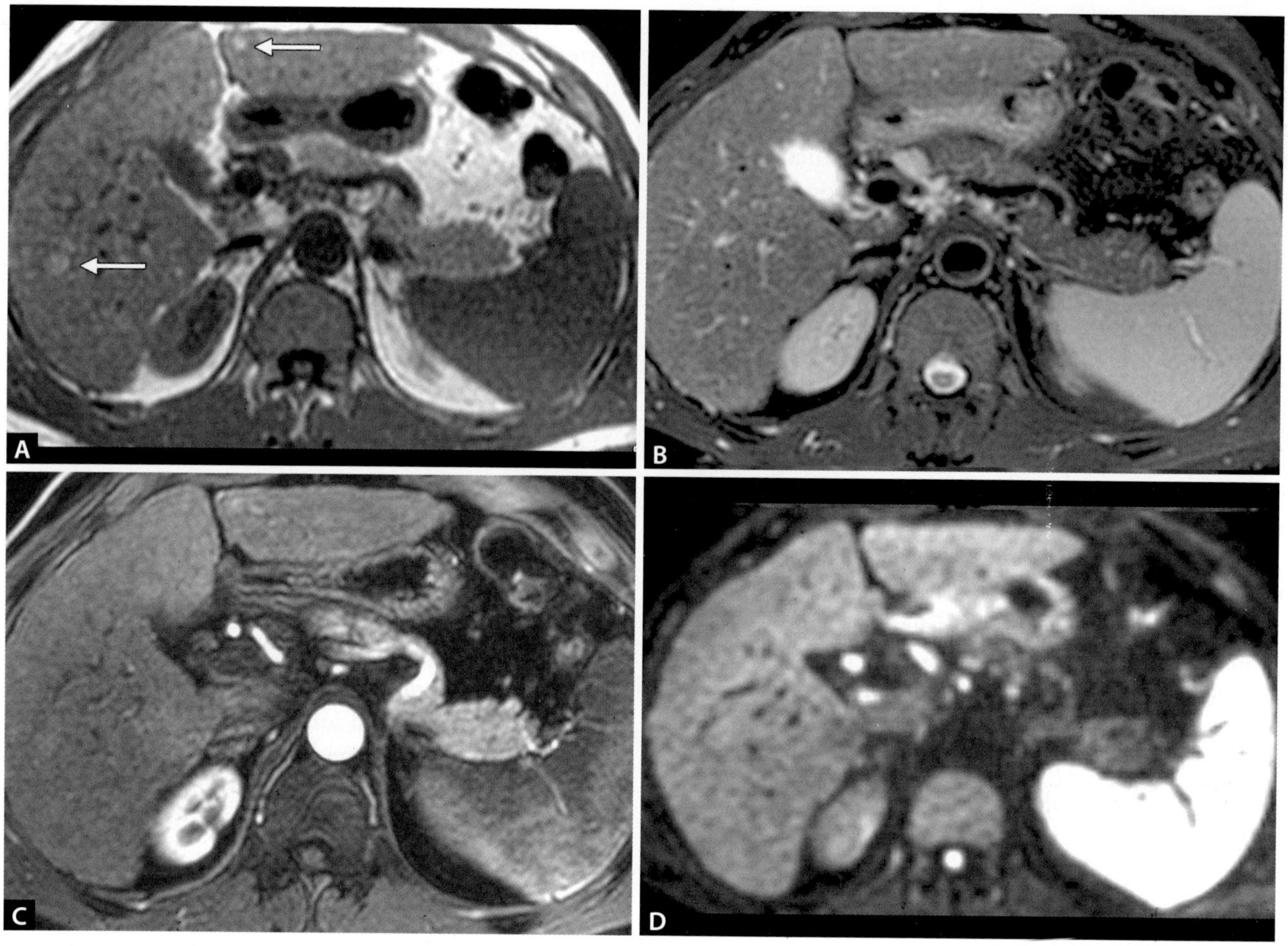

Figs. 17A to D: MRI findings of dysplastic nodules: In a patient of viral hepatitis related chronic liver disease showing irregular liver surface with multiple nodules (arrows) appearing hyperintense on T1W (A), isointense on T2W (B), with no arterial phase enhancement (C). Diffusion-weighted image (D) shows no areas of restricted diffusion.

Table 1: MRI features of nodules in liver cirrhosis.

	T1W	*T2W*	*Arterial phase*	*Venous/Delayed phase*
Regenerating nodule	Hyperintense	Iso- to hypointense	Isointense to liver	Isointense
Siderotic nodule	Hypointense	Hypointense	Isointense to hypointense	Iso- to hypointense
Low-grade dysplastic nodule	Iso- to hyperintense	Isohypointense	Isointense to liver	No washout
High-grade dysplastic nodule	Iso- to hyperintense	Isohypointense	Hyperenhancing	No washout

Moreover, MRE is unaffected by obesity and presence of ascites, which are known confounders in US elastography.

MALIGNANT DIFFUSE LIVER DISEASES

Occasionally, a malignant process may diffusely involve the liver. Metastases, particularly from breast cancer, may give rise to diffusely increased heterogeneous echotexture on ultrasound. Hepatocellular carcinoma, lymphoma and leukemia can also be seen as diffusely altered echotexture of the liver. Diagnosis is difficult in such situations and may require biopsy in the appropriate clinical context.[6]

CONCLUSION

Diffuse liver diseases may result from a variety of causes, most important among which are alcoholic liver disease and viral hepatitis due to their wide prevalence, and complications like cirrhosis and hepatocellular carcinoma. Imaging plays an important role in diagnosis as well as management of diffuse liver diseases. Multiphase contrast enhanced CT remains the workhorse modality however MRI with its superior contrast resolution and higher sensitivity for lesion detection and characterization is the modality of choice in indeterminate lesions on CT. New modalities such as ultrasound elastography, contrast-enhanced ultrasound and MRI elastography have further enhanced the imaging evaluation of diffuse liver diseases.

REFERENCES

1. Gore RM. Diffuse Liver disease. In Gore RM, Levine MS (Eds): Textbook of Gastrointestinal Radiology, 3rd edn. Saunders Elsevier: Philadelphia; 2008.pp.1685-729.
2. The French METAVIR Cooperative Study Group Intraobserver and interobserver variations in liver biopsy interpretation in patients with chronic hepatitis C. Hepatology. 1994;20:15-20.
3. Ziol M, Handra-Luca A, Kettaneh A, et al. Noninvasive assessment of liver fibrosis by measurement of stiffness in patients with chronic hepatitis C. Hepatology. 2005;41:48-54.
4. Skoczylas K, Pawełas A. Ultrasound imaging of the liver and bile ducts–expectations of a clinician. Journal of Ultrasonography. 2015;15:292-30.
5. Borges VF, Diniz AL, Cotrim HP, Rocha HL, Andrade NB. Sonographic hepatorenal ratio: a noninvasive method to diagnose nonalcoholic steatosis. J Clin Ultrasound. 2013;41: 18-25.
6. Park SH, Kim PN, Kim KW, et al. Macrovesicular hepatic steatosis in living liver donors: Use of CT for quantitative and qualitative assessment. Radiology. 2006;239:105-12.
7. Pickhardt PJ, Park SH, Hahn L, Lee SG, Bae KT, Yu ES. Specificity of unenhanced CT for non-invasive diagnosis of hepatic steatosis: implications for the investigation of the natural history of incidental steatosis. Eur Radiol. 2012;22:1075-82.
8. Lomas DJ. The liver. In: Grainger RG, Allison D, Adam A, Dixon AK (Eds): Diagnostic Radiology, 4th edn. Churchill Livingstone: London; 2001.pp.1237-76.
9. Lee SW, Park SH, Kim KW, et al. Unenhanced CT for assessment of macrovesicular hepatic steatosis in living liver donors: comparison of visual grading with liver attenuation index. Radiology. 2007;244:479-85.
10. Boyce C, Pickhardt P, Kim DH, et al. Hepatic steatosis (fatty liver disease) in asymptomatic adults identified by unenhanced low-dose CT. AJR. 2010;194(3):623-8.
11. Singh D, Das CJ, Baruah MP. Imaging of non alcoholic fatty liver disease: A road less travelled. Indian J Endocrinol Metab. 2013;17:990-5.
12. Venbrux AC, Freidman AC. Diffuse hepatocellular diseases. In: Friedman AC, Aachman AH (Eds). Radiology of the Liver, Biliary Tract and Pancreas. Mosby year book: St Louis; 1994.pp.49-167.
13. Reeder SB, Cruite I, Hamilton G, Sirlin CB. Quantitative assessment of liver fat with magnetic resonance imaging and spectroscopy. J Magn Reson Imaging. 2011;34(4):729-49.
14. Bastati N, Feier D, Wibmer A, et al. Noninvasive differentiation of simple steatosis and steatohepatitis by using gadoxetic acid–enhanced MR imaging in patients with nonalcoholic fatty liver disease: a proof-of-concept study. Radiology. 2014;271(3):739-47.
15. Smits LP, Coolen BF, Panno MD, et al. Noninvasive Differentiation between Hepatic Steatosis and Steatohepatitis with MR Imaging Enhanced with USPIOs in Patients with Nonalcoholic Fatty Liver Disease: A Proof-of-Concept Study. Radiology. 2016;278(3):782-91.
16. Tchelepi H, Ralls PW, Radin R, Grant E. Sonography of diffuse liver disease. J Ultrasound Med. 2002;21:1023-32.
17. Danet IM, Semelka RC, Braga L. MR imaging of diffuse liver disease. Radiol Clin North Am. 2003;41:67-87.
18. Martin DR, Semelka RC. Magnetic resonance imaging of the liver: review of techniques and approach to common diseases. Semin Ultrasound CT MR. 2005;26:116-3.
19. Semelka RC, Braga L. Armao D. Liver. In: Semelka RC (Ed). Abdominal Pelvic MRI. New York, Wiley-Liss; 2002. pp.33-318.
20. Kauffman JM, Grace ND. Hemochromatosis. In Weinstein WM, Hawkey CJ, Bosch J (Eds). Clinical Gastroenterology and Hepatology. Philadelphia, Elsevier-Mosby; 2005. pp.659-64.
21. Luo XF, Xie XQ, Cheng S, et al. Dual-Energy CT for patients suspected of having liver iron overload: can virtual iron content imaging accurately quantify liver iron content? Radiology. 2015;277(1):95-103.
22. Gandon Y, Olivie´ D, Guyader D, et al. Non-invasive assessment of hepatic iron stores by MRI. Lancet. 2004;363:357-62.
23. Online Gandon Y. Iron and liver. Available at: *www.radio.univ-rennes1.fr*
24. Lanzi A, Gianstefani A, Mirarchi MG, et al. Liver AL amyloidosis as a possible cause of high liver stiffness values. Eur J Gastroenterol Hepatol. 2010;22:895-7.
25. Srinivasan S, Tan YQ, Teh HS, Lee PJ, Khoo RN. Primary hepatic amyloidosis presenting as nodular masses on the background of diffuse infiltration and extreme liver stiffness on MR elastography. J Gastrointest Liver Dis. 2014;23:437-40.
26. Gitlin JD. Wilson's disease. In: Zakim D, Boyer TD (Eds). Hepatology: A Textbook of Liver Disease. Philadelphia, Saunders; 2003.pp.1273-88.
27. Vargas O, Faraoun SA, Dautry R, et al. MR imaging features of liver involvement by Wilson disease in adult patients. Radiol Med. 2016;121(7):546-56.
28. Hope TA, Ohliger MA, Qayyum A. MR imaging of diffuse liver disease: from technique to diagnosis. Radiol Clin North Am. 2014;52(4):709-24.
29. Karagiannidis A, Karavalaki M, Koulaouzidis A. Hepatic sarcoidosis. Ann Hepatol. 2006;5:251-6.
30. Fataar S, Bassiony H, Satyanatus P. CT of hepatic schistosomiasis. AJR. 1985;145:63-6.
31. Serrano MAP, Vega A, Oretega E, et al. CT of hepatic fascioliasis. J Comput Assist Tomogr. 1987;11:269-7.

32. Sherlock S, Dooley J. Hepatic cirrhosis. In: Sherlock S, Dooley J (Eds). Diseases of the Liver and Biliary System, 11th edn. Blackwell Science: Oxford; 2002.pp.365-8.
33. Goyal AK, Pokhrana DS, Sharma SK. Ultrasonic diagnosis of cirrhosis-reference to quantitative measurement of hepatic dimensions. Gastro Radio. 1990;15:32-3.
34. DeLeio A, Cestari C, Lomazz A, et al. Cirrhosis with sonographic study of the liver. Radiology. 1989;172:389-9.
35. Liu WC, Lim JH, Park CK, et al. Poor sensitivity of sonography in detection of hepatocellular carcinoma in advanced liver cirrhosis. Eur Radiol. 2003;13:1693-9.
36. Kemla A, Mural O, Umit C, et al. Hepatic vein Doppler waveform changes in early (child Pugh A) chronic parenchymal liver diseases. J Clin Ultrasound. 1997;25:15-1.
37. Giorgio A, Montesarchio L, Gatti P. Contrast-enhanced ultrasound: a simple and effective tool in defining a rapid diagnostic work-up for small nodules detected in cirrhotic patients during surveillance. J Gastrointestin Liver Dis. 2016;25(2):205-11.
38. Giorgio A, Amoroso P, Lettieri G, et al. Value of caudate to right lobe ratio in diagnosis with US. Radiology. 1986;161:443-4.
39. Okazaki H, Ito K, Fujita T, Koike S, Takano K. Matsunaga N. Discrimination of alcoholic from virus-induced cirrhosis on MR imaging. AJR. 2000;175:1677-8.
40. Kim D, Kim WR, Talwalkar JA, et al. Advanced fibrosis in nonalcoholic fatty liver disease: noninvasive assessment with MR Elastography. Radiology. 2013;268:411-9.
41. Singh S, Venkatesh SK, Wang Z, et al. Diagnostic performance of magnetic resonance elastography in staging liver fibrosis: a systematic review and meta-analysis of individual participant data. Clin Gastroenterol Hepatol. 2015;13:440-51.

CHAPTER 77

Clinical Aspects of Liver Cirrhosis: A Perspective for the Radiologist

Shashi Bala Paul, Shivanand Gamanagatti, Arun Kumar Gupta, Subrat Kumar Acharya

INTRODUCTION

Cirrhosis is characterized by the formation of regenerative nodules leading to architectural distortion, advanced fibrosis, scarring in response to chronic liver injury and resulting in end stage liver disease.[1] Diagnosis of cirrhosis is histological and imaging has a limited role in determining the presence of cirrhosis. On the contrary, it plays a vital role in diagnosing advanced changes of cirrhosis and its sequelae, particularly, portal hypertension and hepatocellular carcinoma (HCC). Imaging modalities are also widely used for screening of this "at risk" population and for therapeutic procedures for complicated cirrhosis. It is therefore, imperative for the radiologists to be familiar with the clinical presentation, natural course and imaging features of cirrhosis.

EPIDEMIOLOGY

Precise prevalence of cirrhosis worldwide is difficult to ascertain and is unknown. It is estimated to be 0.15% in the United States and a similar burden has been reported from Europe.[1] In contrast, higher figures are observed in Asia and Africa due to the high prevalence of chronic viral infections of hepatitis B or C. Last three decades have seen the emergence of a new entity termed nonalcoholic fatty liver disease (NAFLD), the spectrum of which ranges from simple steatosis to nonalcoholic steatohepatitis (NASH). The later can progress from hepatic fibrosis to cirrhosis and hepatocellular carcinoma.[2]

Nonalcoholic steatohepatitis (NASH) affects about 5–7% of the general population and 30-40% of the patients with raised liver enzymes. It has become the most common cause of liver dysfunction in the developed and developing countries.[2] NAFLD/NASH has an association with metabolic syndrome comprising of truncal obesity, type 2 diabetes mellitus, dyslipidemia, hypertension and insulin resistance.

In India, the exact burden of cirrhosis is not known. Hepatitis B virus (HBV) infection has intermediate endemicity with nearly 4% of the population being chronic HBV carriers.[3] Frequency of hepatitis C virus (HCV) infections is just about 0.87% in the community[4] while the prevalence of NAFLD varies from 8% to 25%.[5] There has been an alarming increase in the prevalence of diabetes and obesity globally. In India too, obesity is rampant amongst the adolescents and about 90% of the obese have NAFLD. The prevalence of type 2 diabetes is around 10%, the highest in India.[6]

It is likely that cirrhosis prevalence could be an underestimate due to the fact that the compensated cirrhotics invariably lack overt symptomatology and remain undetected. Moreover, undiagnosed cirrhosis may be encountered in countries where problems of NASH and hepatitis C exist. It has been estimated that about 20% of the patients with hepatitis C and 10% of NASH patients could progress to cirrhosis. Up to 1% of the population could have cirrhosis diagnosed only on histology.[1]

CAUSES AND RISK FACTORS OF CIRRHOSIS

Multiple causes of cirrhosis are known **(Table 1)**.[7] These can invariably be identified by the patient's history combined with serological and histological investigations. In North America, approximately 75% of patients with cirrhosis are chronic alcoholics. Viral hepatitis and other identifiable causes are seen in about 15% of patients; the remaining 10% of cases are of idiopathic (cryptogenic) cirrhosis. In Asia and Africa, cirrhosis is associated predominantly with chronic viral hepatitis.[8]

In India, viral hepatitis is the dominant cause of chronic liver disease and 50% is due to HBV while 20% by HCV infection.[3,9] Identification of the etiology helps in predicting complications and aids therapeutic management. Regular (moderate) alcohol consumption, older age (>50 years) are important risk factors for developing cirrhosis in viral hepatitis, whereas, truncal obesity, older age, insulin resistance or type 2 diabetes, hypertension and hyperlipidemia are responsible for NASH.[1]

Table 1: Main causes of cirrhosis.[7]

Etiology	*Examples*
Infectious	• Hepatitis B, C, D • Schistosomiasis • Syphilis • HIV (sclerosing cholangitis)
Metabolic/ inherited	• Non alcoholic steatohepatitis (NASH) in association with the metabolic syndrome • Wilson's disease • Hemochromatosis • Alpha-1 antitrypsin deficiency • Glycogen storage disease • Cystic fibrosis • Tyrosinemia • Galactosemia • Fructose intolerance • Byler's disease • Mucopolysaccharidosis • Abetalipoproteinemia • Prophyria • Wolman's disease
Biliary disease	• Extrahepatic obstruction • Intrahepatic obstruction
Immunological	• Autoimmune hepatitis • Primary biliary cirrhosis • Primary sclerosing cholangitis
Vascular	• Veno-occlusive disease • Budd-Chiari syndrome • Cardiac failure • Hereditary hemorrhagic telangiectasia
Drugs and toxins	• Alcohol • Amiodarone • Dantrolene • Halothane • Isoniazid • Methotrexate • Methyldopa • Aflatoxin • Diclofenac • Hypervitaminosis A
Miscellaneous	• Indian childhood • Malnutrition • Sarcoidosis • Ischemia • Graft versus host disease

NATURAL HISTORY AND PROGNOSIS

The natural history of cirrhosis is related to its underlying etiology and the treatment. Cirrhotics tend to remain compensated for years before the features of decompensation set in and once that happens, the mortality (without transplant) is as high as 85% in 5 years. The decompensation rates for hepatitis C and B are 4% and 10% yearly, respectively. Rapid decompensation generally develops in alcoholic cirrhosis if alcohol use is not discontinued. Mortality of cirrhotics with HCC is on the rise in most developed countries in contrast to the decreasing mortality trend of cirrhotics without HCC.[10]

PATHOLOGY

Histopathological changes of cirrhosis consists of inflammation, steatosis and progression to fibrosis which results in architectural distortion and development of a spectrum of nodules ranging from benign regenerating nodules to HCC.[11]

The nodular lesions are classified as regenerative, dysplastic or neoplastic according to the international nomenclature of hepatocellular nodules proposed in 1994.[12] Regenerative nodules represent a region of hepatic parenchyma that enlarges in response to necrosis and is surrounded by fibrous septa. The regenerative nodules are classified as micronodular (<3 mm), macronodular (>3 mm), or mixed forms. Macronodules rarely exceed 20 mm in size. When regenerative nodules contain iron, they are called siderotic nodules. Dysplastic nodules are classified as low or high grade on the basis of a spectrum of pathologic changes that include HCC. One such change is the appearance of a new vascular supply to the nodule, which becomes the dominant blood supply in large dysplastic nodules and small HCC.[13]

In the past, cirrhosis was labelled as an irreversible process of liver damage but recent studies have shown the reversal of cirrhosis by treating the underlying etiology at an early stage.[14]

TYPES OF CIRRHOSIS

Morphologically, cirrhosis is classified into micronodular, macronodular and mixed forms. Micronodular form is seen in cirrhosis due to chronic alcoholism, hepatitis C and biliary cirrhosis, and is characterized by the presence of regenerative nodules of relatively uniform and small size. Macronodular cirrhosis is a feature of chronic hepatitis B where the nodules are larger, coarser, and more variable in size. Mixed cirrhosis is a combination of both micronodular and macronodular forms in equal proportions.

CLINICAL PRESENTATION

Patients of cirrhosis present in either compensated or decompensated state. Compensated cirrhotics are often indolent and the disease may progress insidiously. Cirrhosis may be detected incidentally on routine clinical examination, biochemical screening, during abdominal surgery for some other ailment or on autopsy. About 30–40% of the cases of cirrhosis may be asymptomatic.[15] In the remaining, diagnosis is suspected when nonspecific symptoms like low-grade fever, general deterioration, anorexia, anemia, and weight loss appears.

Decompensated cirrhotics have clinical manifestations like jaundice, edema, coagulopathy, metabolic disturbances, gastroesophageal varices, ascites, spontaneous bacterial peritonitis, splenomegaly and hepatic encephalopathy **(Table 2)**.[16]

Table 2: Clinical features of cirrhosis.[16]

	Description	*Cause*
Jaundice	Icterus	Compromised hepatocyte excretory function, occurs when serum bilirubin >20 mg/L
Spider angiomata	Central arteriole with tiney radiating vessels, mainly on trunk and face	Raised estradiol, decreased estradiol degradation in liver
Nodular liver	Irregular, hard surface on palpation	Fibrosis, irregular regeneration
Splenomegaly	Enlarge on palpation or in ultrasound	Portal hypertension, splenic congestion
Ascites	Proteinaceous fluid in abdominal cavity, clinically detected when >1.5 L	Portal hypertension
Caput medusae	Prominent veins radiating from umbilicus	Portal hypertension, reopening of umbilical vein that shunt blood from portal vein
Cruveilhier-Baumgarten syndrome	Epigastric vascular murmur	Shunts from portal vein to umbilical vein branches, can be present without Caput medusae
Palmar erythema	Erythema sparing central portion of the palm	Increased estradiol, decreased estradiol degradation in liver
White nails	Horizontal white bands or proximal white nail plate	Hypoalbuminemia
Hypertrophic osteoarthropathy/finger clubbing	Painful proliferative osteoarthropathy of long bones	Hypoxemia due to right-to-left shunting, portopulmonary hypertension
Dupuytren's contracture	Fibrosis and contraction of palmar fascia	Enhanced oxidative stress, increased inosine (alcohol exposure or diabetes)
Gynecomastia, loss of male hair pattern	Benign proliferation of glandular male breast tissue	Enhanced conversion of androstenedione to estrone and estradiol, reduced estradiol degradation in liver
Hypogonadism	Mainly in alcoholic cirrhosis and hemochromatosis	Direct toxic effect of alcohol or iron
Flapping tremor (asterixis)	Asynchronous flapping motions of dorsiflexed hands	Hepatic encephalopathy, disinhibition of motor neurons
Fetor hepaticus	Sweet, pungent smell	Volatile dimethylsulfide, especially in portosystemic shunting and liver failure
Anorexia, fatigue, weight loss, muscle wasting	Occurs in >50% of patients with cirrhosis	Catabolic metabolism by diseased liver, secondary to anorexia
Type-2 diabetes	Occurs in 15–30% of patients with cirrhosis	Disturbed glucose use or decreased insulin removal by the liver

SEVERITY OF CIRRHOSIS

Grading of severity is on the basis of the Child Pugh Turcotte (CPT) classification[17] which takes into account the findings of serum bilirubin, serum albumin, prothrombin time, presence of ascites and encephalopathy **(Table 3)**. Estimated child's score categorizes the severity of cirrhosis into CPT class A, B and C on the score of 6 and less, 7–9 and more than 10, respectively. CPT class also predicts the development of complications and response to treatment. The 1-year survival rates of CPT class A, B and C patients are 100%, 80% and 45% respectively.[18] The model for end stage liver disease (MELD)[19] has been developed which is based on parameters of serum creatinine, bilirubin and international normalized ratio (INR) and does not include features of portal hypertension. It provides better prediction of severity and short-term mortality.

Table 3: Child-Pugh classification for grading the child's score.[17]

Clinical and biochemical measurements	***Points for increasing abnormality***		
	1	***2***	***3***
Encephalopathy (grade)	None	I and II	III and IV
Ascites	–	Mild	Moderate
Bilirubin (mg/dL)	1–2	>2–3	>3
Albumin (g/dL)	>3.5	2.8–3.5	<2.8
Prothrombin time (seconds prolonged)	1–4	>4–6	>6
Total score	5–6 = Child's A	7–9 = Child's B	10 or more Child's C

DIAGNOSIS OF CIRRHOSIS

Liver biopsy is needed to confirm cirrhosis in patients with compensated liver function in whom the ultrasound (US) is usually normal. On the other hand, if clear signs of cirrhosis are present, like small, shrunken liver, ascites or coagulopathy, biopsy confirmation is not necessary.[1] Liver biopsy is the gold standard for diagnosing cirrhosis due to its ability to grade inflammation, steatosis and stage fibrosis. It also aids in establishing the etiology of cirrhosis in about 20% of the patients of unknown etiology. Degree of fibrosis is used as a quantitative measure and various staging methods are available. METAVIR scoring, a commonly used method, grades fibrosis from F0–F4 where the later denotes cirrhosis **(Table 4)**.[20]

Table 4: METAVIR scoring.[20]

METAVIR fibrosis score		***METAVIR activity score***	
No fibrosis	F0	No activity	A0
Portal fibrosis without septa	F1	Mild activity	A1
Portal fibrosis with few septa	F2	Moderate activity	A2
Portal fibrosis with numerous septa without cirrhosis	F3	Severe activity	A3
Cirrhosis	F4		

Liver biopsy has a number of limitations as well. The procedure is invasive and associated with a significant level of morbidity and mortality. The biopsy sample represents 1/50,000 of the liver tissue and at times the sample may not be a representative of the overall disease as the disease has a nonhomogeneous pattern. The specimen smaller than 2 cm is almost always difficult to interpret. Additionally, there may be an inter or intraobserver variability. Thus, the sensitivity of liver biopsy is lower than 80% in detecting cirrhosis particularly in the macronodular type.[21]

The technique of obtaining liver biopsy varies from blind to image guided transabdominal approach, transjugular, and laparoscopic, open approach at surgery or autopsy. Use of ultrasound guidance aids in accurate targeting, reduce complication rate and improve the quality of samples.[22,23] The percutaneous route of liver biopsy is most commonly employed and in patients with increased risk of hemorrhage, a transjugular route is preferable.

Aspirin and other antiplatelet drugs are withheld one week before the scheduled procedure. Mild sedation is given prior and using local anesthesia, a 14/18 gauge needle is introduced under aseptic conditions into the last intercostal space as low and lateral, to avoid injury to the gallbladder and vascular structures. Biopsy is performed in sustained expiration to avoid penetrating the pleural space.

Contraindications to percutaneous liver biopsy are- an uncooperative patient, coagulopathy, massive ascites or generalized dilatation of the intrahepatic bile ducts which has an associated risk for choleperitoneum. Only 2–35% require hospitalization because of complications, of which pain and hypotension are the predominant causes. About 60% of the complications are encountered within 2 hours while 96% occur within 24 hours of the procedure. The mortality due to severe bleeding is extremely rare. In patients with moderate coagulopathy, the percutaneous liver biopsy can be performed with a prior transfusion of fresh plasma or platelets.

Short of biopsy, diagnosis of cirrhosis is formulated on the basis of clinical, biochemical, hematological, endoscopic and radiological findings. Clinical evaluation includes detailed history and physical examination. Presence of diabetes mellitus or hypertension is recorded. Investigations included complete blood count, liver function tests, blood sugar levels, lipid profile and serum alphafetoprotein. Viral markers for hepatitis B include HBsAg, total anti-HBc, HBeAg and HBVDNA while those for hepatitis C are anti-HCV and HCV RNA. Autoimmune markers are done, if the markers of hepatitis B and C are found negative. Radiological work-up comprises of an abdominal ultrasonography (US), multiphasic CT (MPCT) or MRI.

ENDOSCOPY

Endoscopy is routinely performed to look for the presence of esophageal varices. The size, extent and the appearance of varices is of immense relevance clinically. Grading of varices is done as the risk of bleeding increases with the size[24] and associated mucosal abnormalities.[25] The stomach and duodenum are also evaluated for features of gastropathy due to portal hypertension and associated ulcers are also looked for.

IMAGING IN CIRRHOSIS

Role of imaging in evaluation of cirrhosis is primarily for characterizing the morphologic manifestations of the disease, detection and quantitation of complications like ascites, portal hypertension, hepatic vein and portal vein thrombosis and detection of HCC. It is important to highlight that normal imaging findings do not exclude compensated cirrhosis. At the same time, in some patients with clinically unsuspected disease, the morphologic characteristics of the disease may be detected incidentally as part of screening strategies.

US is the most commonly used as it is widely available and inexpensive. Even though its role in determining the presence of cirrhosis is limited, it is often the first imaging modality. In the early stages of cirrhosis, liver appears normal in the majority of cases and often it is the advanced changes which are detected. These are, coarse, heterogeneous echo pattern of the liver, hypertrophied lateral segment of right lobe and caudate lobe, atrophy of medial segment of left lobe and the right lobe, liver surface nodularity, deep widened fissures, anteriorly placed gallbladder and shrunken size of the liver. **(Figs. 1 and 2)**.

US is useful for detecting the complications of cirrhosis[26,27] It is the first imaging modality for suspected HCC, although its sensitivity and specificity is less than that of CT and MRI. Doppler US (DU) and Color Doppler are useful in the evaluation of vascular structures by virtue of their ability for prompt differentiation between vascular and nonvascular structures. DU is the technique for differentiating benign from malignant thrombus, evaluating portal or hepatic venous system and confirming suspected portal hypertension **(Figs. 3A to D)**.

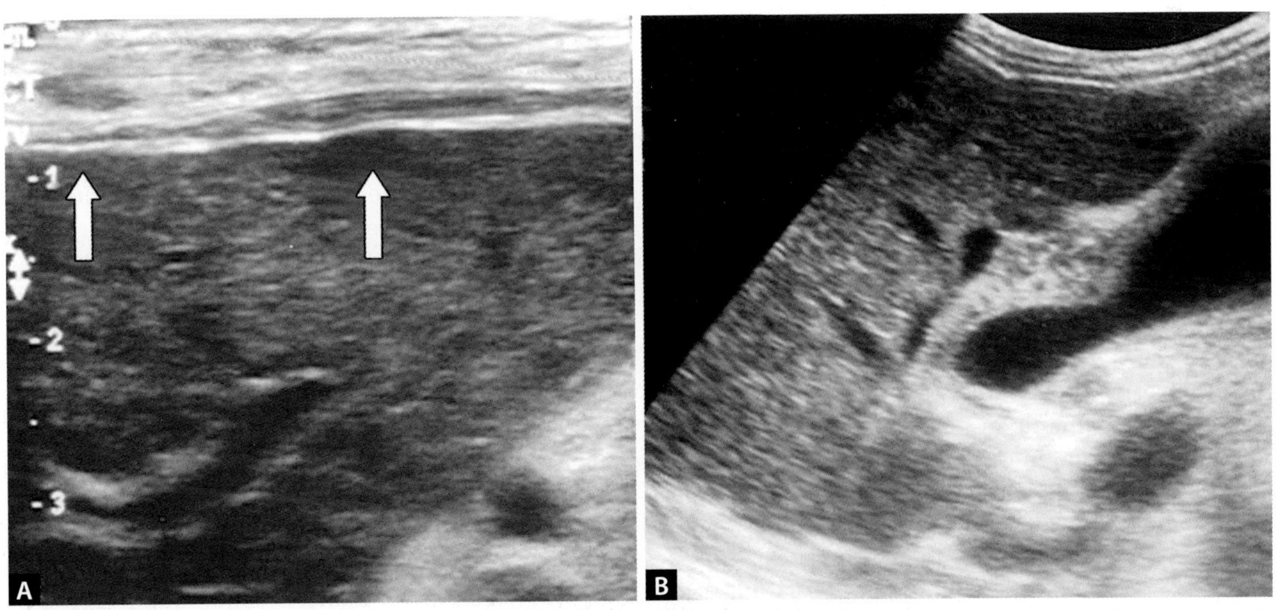

Figs. 1A and B: Changes of cirrhosis on US: (A) High frequency US depicting early changes of cirrhosis in the form of wavy and nodular outline of the surface of the liver; (B) In addition, the liver has coarsened echotexture. It is particularly useful to look for nodularity of the liver adjacent to the gallbladder.

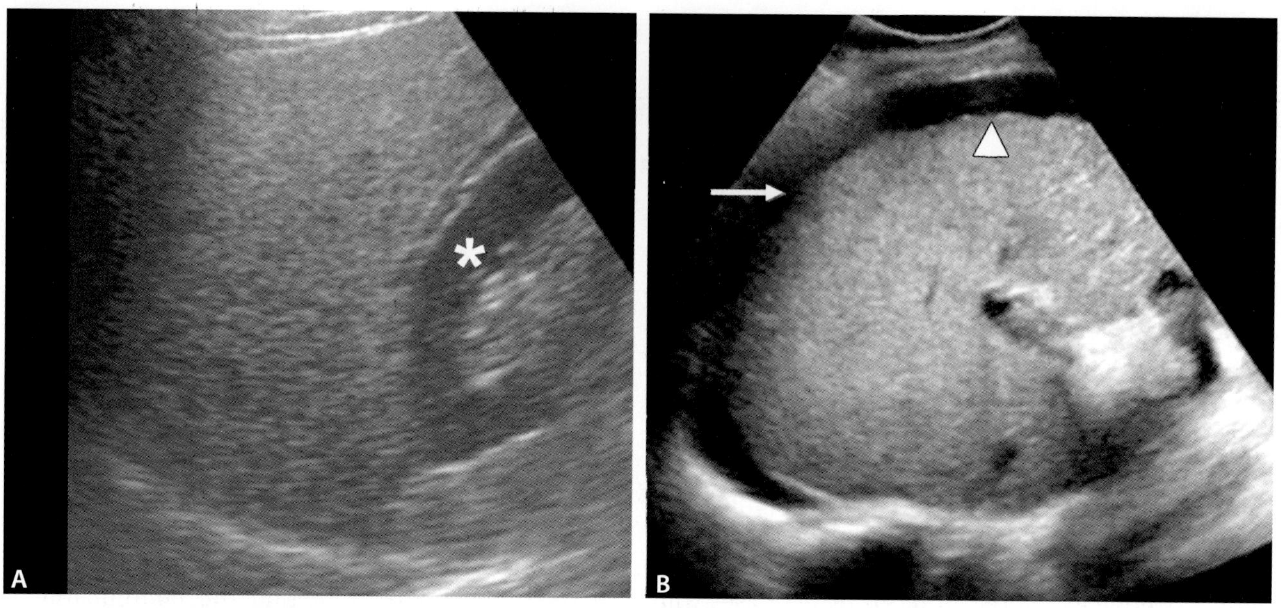

Figs. 2A and B: Late changes of cirrhosis on US: (A) Sagittal US image of the right lobe of liver showing increased echogenicity which is more than the right renal cortex (asterisk); (B) Small shrunken liver with surface nodularity (arrowhead) which is better appreciated due to the presence of ascites (arrow).

Conventional CT and MRI are used to define the severity of cirrhosis. Findings in cirrhosis are variable. Early parenchymal changes in cirrhosis may be subtle and may not be detected. However, the early findings of enlarged hilar periportal space with increased fat in the porta hepatitis may be seen on MRI. Morphological changes of advanced cirrhosis as seen on ultrasound are better seen on CT and MRI **(Figs. 4A and B)**. The regenerative nodules occurring in cirrhosis are difficult to detect on CT. Multiphasic MRI is the reference modality for detection and characterization of the small liver nodules in a cirrhotic liver, particularly early HCC **(Figs. 5A and B)** Moreover, specific MR sequences allow accurate detection of hepatic iron and fat content in hemochromatosis and liver steatosis as well.[28,29]

Since the emergence of the new concept of reversibility of changes of cirrhosis following treatment, the focus on accurate assessment of the grades of fibrosis in chronic liver disease has increased. The gold standard of biopsy being an invasive procedure, is unsuitable for repeated evaluation of therapeutic response. The last decade has seen the development of various noninvasive techniques for grading liver fibrosis. These are elastography techniques like transient elastography (Fibroscan), acoustic radiation force impulse (ARFI) quantification and 2D shear wave elastography (SWE) providing information regarding liver fibrosis by measuring the tissue stiffness.[30,31]

Transient elastography is one of the earliest and extensively used technique. It can reliably differentiate between significant fibrosis and mild fibrosis and also predict the occurrence of HCC on the basis of liver stiffness measurement.[32,33] With further refinements, ultrasound and MRI based elastography (MRE) techniques have been introduced with promising results. A meta-analysis on MRE has shown a sensitivity, specificity, AUROC of 92%, 96% and 0.98 respectively for differentiating advanced fibrosis and cirrhosis (more than F3) from less advanced fibrosis.[34] However, magnetic resonance elastography (MRE) has constraints of limited availability and high cost.

Ultrasound-based shear wave elastography (SWE) has gained immense popularity due to the easy availability and high diagnostic accuracy. It uses the combined information of the real time conventional ultrasound with both qualitative and quantitative liver stiffness assessment. Qualitative SWE refers to the display of various colors (vendor specific) corresponding to levels of tissue hardness in the small box placed at multiple sites in the liver. Similarly, the quantitative assessment is done by measuring the mean, maximum, minimum, standard deviation values of the shear wave speed in kilopascals or meters per second to provide the level of tissue stiffness interpreted as severity of fibrosis **(Figs. 6A and B)**. SWE estimates obtained from the right upper lobe show the best correlation with liver fibrosis severity on Metavir score on biopsy.[35] Recent meta-analysis containing 13 articles on SWE by Jiang T et al.[31] have reaffirmed the utility of SWE in estimating fibrosis. The pooled sensitivity and specificity for diagnosing advanced fibrosis (>F3) has been depicted

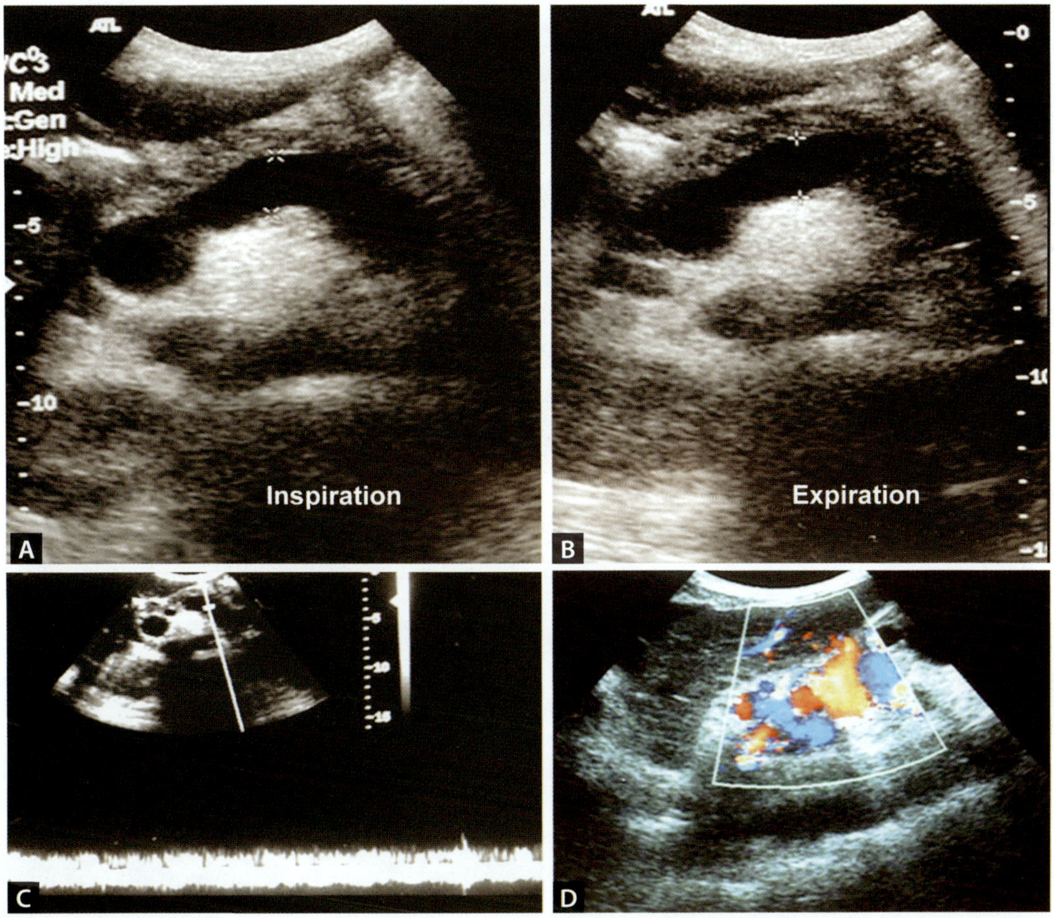

Figs. 3A to D: Cirrhosis with portal hypertension: (A and B) US of a known cirrhotic patient showing no appreciable change in size of the splenic vein during inspiration or expiration suggesting presence of portal hypertension; (C) Doppler of the same patient depicting dilated portal vein with continuous waveform without respiratory variation; (D) Color Doppler image of a different patient showing multiple gastric and perigastric collaterals with nodular left lobe of the liver.

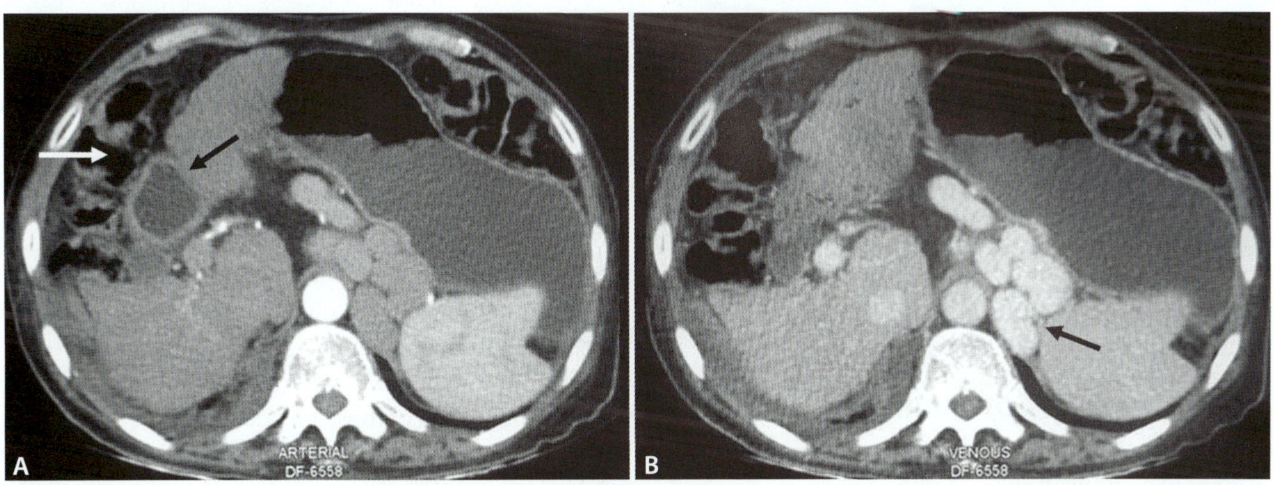

Figs. 4A and B: Cirrhosis with portal hypertension on multiphasic CT Liver: (A) Axial section arterial phase MPCT image showing a small, shrunken liver with deep widened fissures. There is atrophy of the right lobe and medial segment of left lobe with an enlarged caudate lobe. Colonic loop is interposed between the liver and the lateral abdominal wall (white arrow) and the gallbladder is placed anteriorly (black arrow); (B) Large, multiple perigastric and perisplenic collaterals are seen in the venous phase MPCT image (arrow).

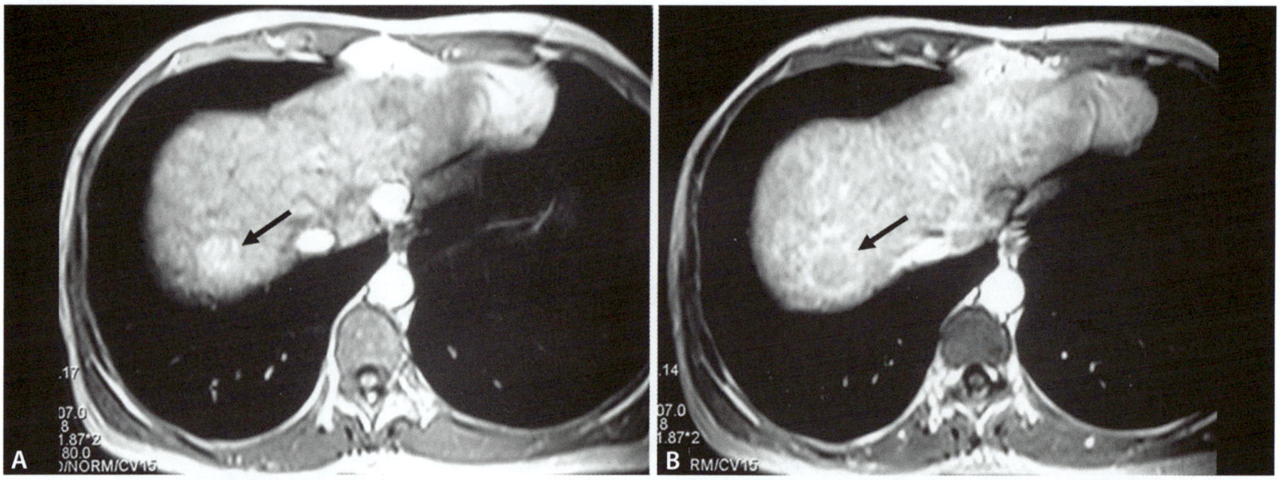

Figs. 5A and B: Characterizing nodules on multiphasic MRI liver: Axial arterial phase MRI image showing a cirrhotic liver with multiple variable sized nonenhancing (isointense) regenerating nodules and a solitary enhancing nodule (arrow, A) with wash out in the delayed phase (arrow, B) suggestive of HCC.

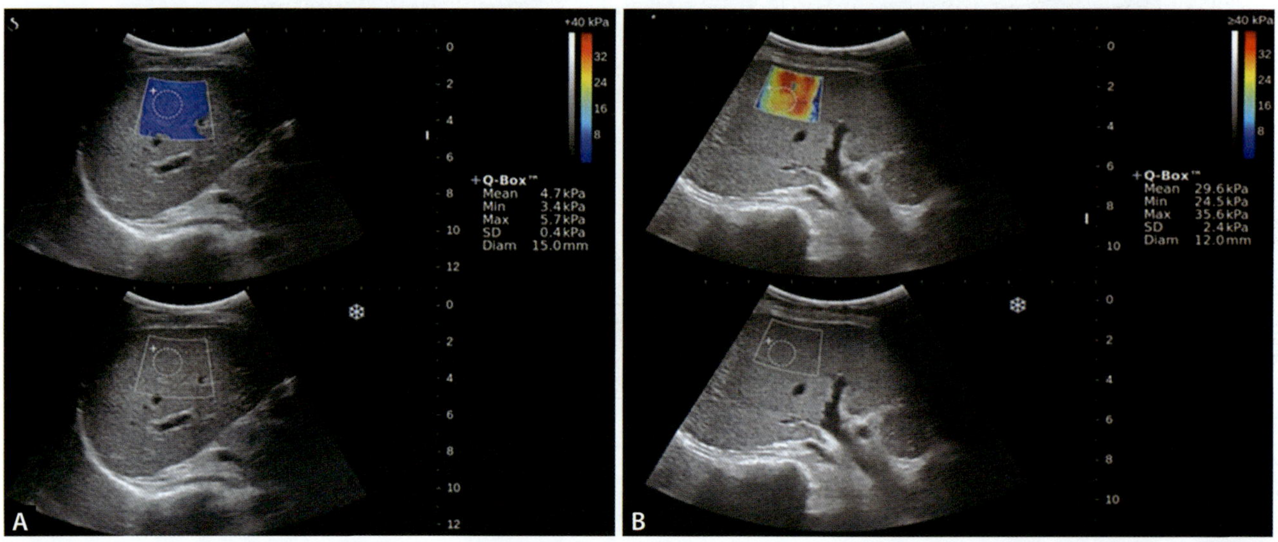

Figs. 6A and B: Estimation of liver fibrosis by SWE: (A) Simultaneous display of qualitative and quantitative SWE (a) and B mode US (b) of a chronic HBV patient—showing normal liver echogenecity (b) and depicting uniform deep blue color in the box with a mean stiffness value of 4.7 kPa. (a). The corresponding Metavir histological grade was F0 indicating absence of fibrosis; (B) Similar evaluation of another patient of chronic HCV showing an echogenic liver (b), and having colors of yellow, orange and red, with a mean elasticity of 29.6 kPa (a). The Metavir grade was F4, suggesting cirrhosis.

as 0.89 ($p = 0.56$, 95% CI, 0.86–0.92, $I2 = 0\%$), 0.86 ($p < 0.001$, 95% CI, 0.82–0.90, $I2 = 75.73\%$) respectively.

COMPLICATIONS OF CIRRHOSIS

Recent advances have focused on prevention and treatment of complications of cirrhosis.

Major clinical challenges are the sequelae of portal hypertension which include ascites, hypersplenism, renal dysfunction (hepatorenal syndrome) and gastrointestinal hemorrhage. The latter occurs more frequently and is most dramatic. Prospective studies have shown that as large as 90% of patients of cirrhosis develop esophageal varices and a third of these bleed.[25]

More recently, there has been an increasing understanding of cirrhosis *per se* on the myocardial effects resulting in cirrhotic cardiomyopathy. Sepsis is known to occur in 30–40% of hospital admissions due to cirrhosis[36] and this leads to 30% excess mortality independent of the severity of the liver disease. Hematological, endocrine, pulmonary and cardiac complications are also encountered. Gallstones and peptic ulcer are more common in these patients. However, it is the development of HCC that is the most severe and fatal complication.

CIRRHOSIS AND HEPATOCELLULAR CARCINOMA

More than 80% of the HCCs arises in the cirrhotic liver. It is the fifth most common neoplasm in the world, and the third most common cause of cancer-related deaths.[37] Incidence of HCC ranges from 5 to 15 patients per 100,000 in Europe and United States, and between 27 and 36 patients per 100,000 in Asian countries in India, the estimated incidence is 1.6 % per year.[38] It affects 5% of the asymptomatic cirrhotics and 15–20% of patients with acute decompensation in both low and high incidence areas.[37] In a study on screening symptomatic patients of cirrhosis at the tertiary care hospital in India, 35.5% of cirrhotics were found to have coexistent HCC at their first presentation to the hospital.[39]

Since, by and large, it is only the patients of cirrhosis who develop HCC, it would be prudent to screen the patients of cirrhosis for the presence of HCC at diagnosis and keep them under surveillance for early detection of HCC so that they are amenable to curative therapy. The patient of cirrhosis is a potential candidate for screening as it fits with the generic criteria enunciated for cancer screening.[40] This criteria states that the disease must be common with substantial morbidity and mortality, a clear cut 'at risk' population be identifiable (e.g. cirrhosis), the screening tests must have a low morbidity, high sensitivity and specificity, there must be an established treatment therapy, and the screening program must be cost effective. Surveillance of cirrhosis patients can potentially lead to diagnosis of HCC at an early stage when the tumor might be amenable to resection, liver transplantation or percutaneous ablation. Hence, it is imperative to screen these patients and treat this fatal disease at early stages.

The population at risk for HCC is relatively easy to identify. If HCC is detected on screening, it should always be followed by therapy. Longitudinal studies on patients with cirrhosis of different etiologies have shown that male patients, older age and having sustained high serum alanine aminotransferase (ALT) levels are at an increased risk and have rapid development of HCC.[10,41]

Sherman and Colombo reviewed the guidelines pertaining to the screening strategies at length.[42] The American Association for the Study of Liver Diseases (AASLD) and the European Association for the Study of the Liver (EASL) suggested screening for all patients of cirrhosis irrespective of etiology. The ideal target population defined was all carriers of HBV, Asian men older than 40 years and females more than 50 years, African/North American Blacks older than 20 years and family history of HCC. It was also suggested by The Asian Pacific Association for the study of Liver (APASL) to extend the screening to patients with NAFLD and hepatitis C with bridging fibrosis, respectively.[43] The EASL-EORTC guidelines[44] later laid down a more stringent criteria for surveillance in 2012 recommending screening for Child-Pugh stage A and B, Child-Pugh stage C awaiting liver transplantation, noncirrhotic HBV carriers with active hepatitis or family history of HCC. The benefit of screening has been documented in an US-based mass screening study in Taiwan.[45] More than 90% of all incident HCC cases could be diagnosed and a 31% reduction in the age and sex adjusted mortality ratio in the screened population was documented in comparison to unscreened population at similar risk.

Screening Tests

US and Alpha Feto Protein (AFP) have been the screening tests used in most surveillance programs and in addition CT has been used in special situations. US and AFP are simple screening tests, easily available and safe. However, both have associated limitations as well.

AFP has been used as a marker of HCC for many years. However, only 60–70% of patients of HCC in USA and Europe and 80–90% of patients in Asia have elevated serum AFP.[46] AFP is reported to have a sensitivity of 39–65%, a specificity of 76–94% and a positive predictive value (PPV) of 9–50% in diagnosing HCC.[47-50]

As patients with clinically overt disease often have high levels of AFP, the conventional diagnostic level of AFP in HCC is >400 ng/mL.[51] AFP levels could also be elevated in the presence of chronic viral hepatitis with reactivation but without HCC. On the other hand, 'normal' serum levels of AFP (<20 ng/mL) is not an uncommon occurrence in association with small HCCs.[52] A correlation between the level of AFP and the size of HCC masses has also been observed, larger the mass, higher the serum AFP level.[39] A high cut-off value of AFP (>400 ng/mL) has no place if AFP is to be used as a screening test to detect early, small HCCs that invariably produce lower levels of AFP. Lower AFP cut-off levels of 20 ng/mL also show a low sensitivity of 41–65% and specificity of 80–94%.[47-50]

Role of AFP as a screening test has been studied at length and no utility of a single cut-off value in screening was found.[39] Accordingly, serum AFP estimation is no longer recommended due to its poor sensitivity and specificity.[1] However, AFP more than 400 ng/mL has been used for characterizing the liver mass as malignant and because of this fact, it was included in the diagnostic criteria for HCC by the European Association for the Study of the Liver (EASL).[53]

With the revision of the various guidelines for diagnosing HCC, importance of noninvasive modality of imaging has been increased while that of invasive biopsy has decreased. Reduced AFP cut-off level to more than 200 ng/mL was suggested subsequently by the AASLD guidelines in 2005[54] and later the AFP marker has been excluded as a surveillance or a diagnostic tool in the revised EASL guidelines of 2012[44] **(Flowchart 1)**.

Ultrasound is invariably the first screening test used for detection of HCC **(Figs. 7A to C)**. It is noninvasive, radiation free, less expensive and easily available. Imaging of a cirrhotic liver poses a real challenge to the radiologist. In advanced cirrhosis, liver is shrunken and therefore the sonographic window is usually limited. Additionally, the hepatic echotexture is heterogeneous due to the presence of fibrosis, fatty infiltration, parenchymal necrosis and myriads of micro- and macronodular cirrhotic regenerative nodules. Detection of HCC in such a background liver becomes a difficult task. Sensitivity of US for detecting HCC in patients of cirrhosis is low and ranges from 27% to 94% and specificity from 90% to 98%.[49,55,56]

Detection of HCC is directly proportional to its size, as the size increases, the sensitivity increases. For detection of less than 2 cm and more than 2 cm nodules, US sensitivity is 31.6% and 78.6% respectively while that of CT is 59% and 94.7% respectively. Hence, CT fares better than US in lesion detection and also has an additional advantage of better delineation of the extent of disease.[57]

Contrast-enhanced ultrasound (CEUS) is a recent addition to the imaging tools for evaluation of liver. By the use of ultrasound contrast agents (UCA), CEUS is able to overcome the limitation of lesion characterization by conventional US. Currently, second generation contrast agents are used and SonoVue (Bracco, Milan,

Flowchart 1: Diagnostic algorithm and recall policy of European Association for the Study the Liver (EASL) 2012 guideline.[44]

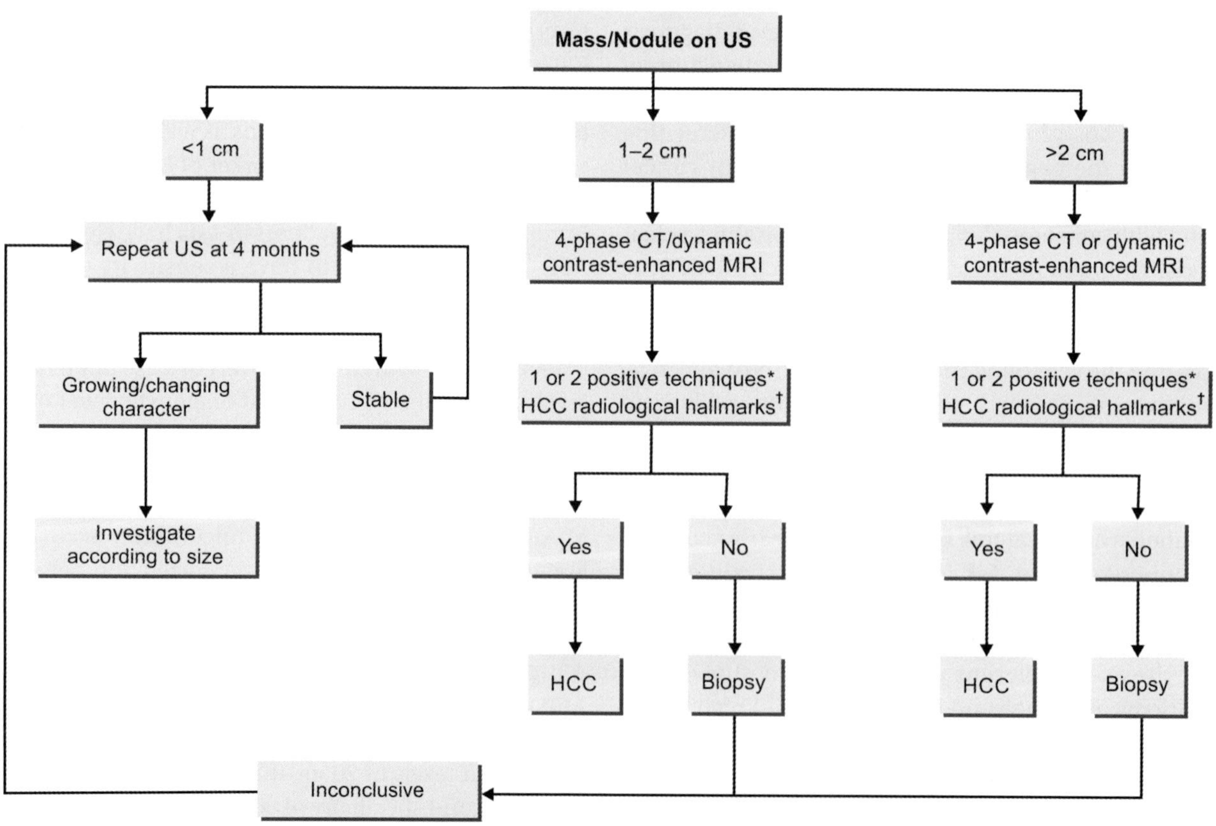

* One imaging technique only recommended in centers of excellence with high-end radiological equipment.
† Hepatocellular carcinoma (HCC) radiological hallmark: Arterial hypervascularity and venous/late phase washout.
Source: Adopted from European Association for the Study of the Liver.

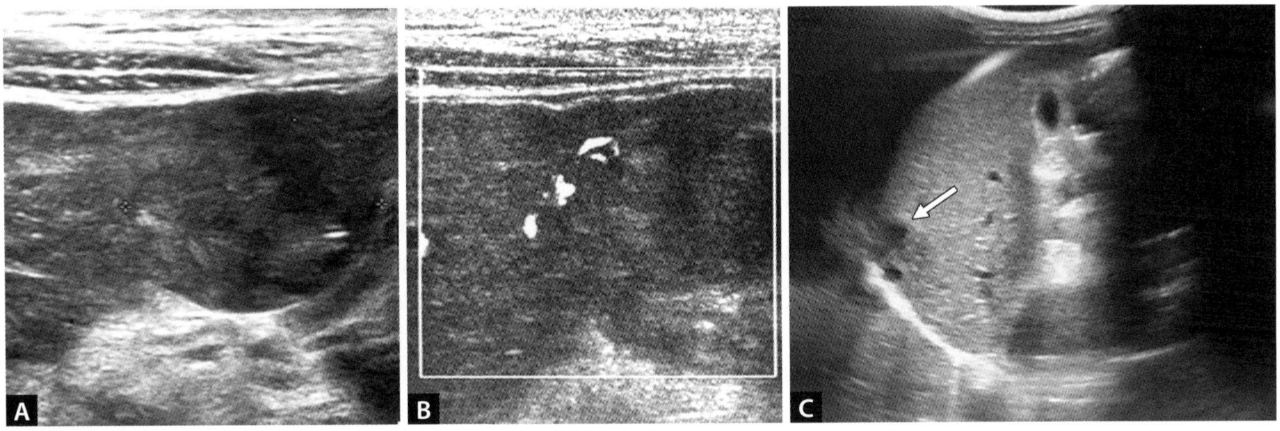

Figs. 7A to C: HCC detection on screening US: (A) High frequency screening US image of a patient with HCV cirrhosis, showing a 2.5 cm heterogeneously hypoecholc lesion in the left lobe of liver; (B) On power Doppler, a tortuous feeding artery is seen supplying the tumor; (C) US image of a decompensated HBV cirrhotic patient, showing a shrunken, echogenic liver with a small heteroechoic mass in the subdiaphragmatic location (arrow) suggestive of HCC in a cirrhotic liver.

Italy) is the only contrast agent available in India. It contains insoluble gases like sulfur hexafluoride (SF6) or perfluorocarbons and has a surface shell made of different substances like phospholipids, albumin or polymers providing better stabilization. Being blood pool agents, the UCA remains exclusively in the intravascular compartment providing detailed information of the intranodular hemodynamics on real time US and aiding in detection and characterization of the liver lesion. CEUS is now recommended by the World and the European Federation of Ultrasound as the first line imaging modality for liver lesions.[58] HCC exhibits typical enhancement patterns on CEUS quite similar to that seen on multiphasic CT/MRI. More than 90% of HCC are hyperenhancing in AP (arterialization) and 83–97% show washout (hypoenhancement) on DP **(Figs. 8A and B)**. CEUS has a sensitivity of 100%, specificity of 95.6%, PPV of 66.7% and NPV of 100% in diagnosing HCC when compared to either histopathology or CT/MRI.[59] In a multicentric study[60] CEUS was 30.2% more sensitive in diagnosing malignancy, 16.1% more specific in excluding malignancy with an overall accuracy of 22.9% compared to CT and/or dynamic MRI. When comparing the three modalities with histology, CEUS has a higher sensitivity (95.5%) and specificity (75%) in comparison to CT (72.2% and 37.5% respectively) and MRI (81.8% and 42.9% respectively). Since the comprehensive evaluation of the entire hepatic parenchyma cannot be done in a short span of arterial phase of CEUS, this modality has not found place in the screening protocols for HCC.

Contrast-enhanced MRI is the reference modality for evaluation of the patients of cirrhosis as it can accurately characterize different stages of the cirrhotic nodules developing during hepatocarcinogenesis ranging from the benign regenerative nodules to dysplastic nodules and early HCC. MRI performs better than CT in the detection of nodules less than 2 cm.[61] However, MRI has a major disadvantage in terms of limited availability and high cost which is a limitation for its wide use in a developing country.

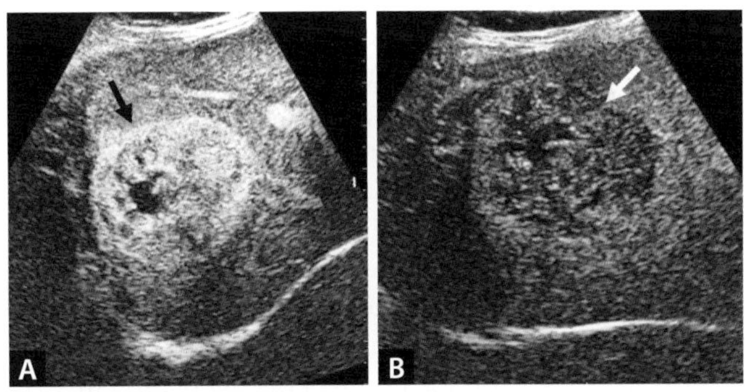

Figs. 8A and B: Typical pattern of HCC on CEUS: (A) Arterial phase CEUS image at 26 sec showing a large intensely enhancing mass in segment 7 mass of the liver with a small area of necrosis within (arrow); (B) The mass is showing hypoenhancement (wash out) in the delayed phase at 284 sec (arrow).

Surveillance Intervals

The optimal screening interval for HCC surveillance should depend on the information of the growth rate of HCC and the related premalignant lesions. According to studies on tumor growth, the reasonable interval is between 3 and 12 months.[62,63] Six months' surveillance interval allows most tumors to experience at least one doubling between surveillance intervals and allows ample opportunity to detect most tumors before they grow to more than 5 cm in diameter. Clearly, additional prospective studies are needed to validate this surveillance interval. Determination of this screening interval would have a direct implication on the stage of HCC detected and the cost effectiveness of the program.

Diagnosis of HCC and Protocol for HCC Surveillance

Earlier, the EASL protocol of 2000 was widely practiced world over.[53] It endorsed surveillance based on US and serum AFP every 6 months. In nodules smaller than 1cm, a 3 monthly follow-up was recommended. For larger nodules of 1–2 cm, HCC diagnosis required positive cytopathology. However, fine-needle biopsy has a false-negative rate of 30–40%.[64] It is important to note that a negative biopsy result, therefore, does not rule out malignancy. Further, a noninvasive diagnostic criteria was suggested for tumors larger than 2 cm which consisted of concomitant finding of two imaging techniques (CT, MRI) showing arterial hypervascularization, or by one positive imaging technique, showing hypervascularization associated with AFP level higher than 400 ug/L.[53]

The diagnostic criteria and recall policy for surveillance was later revised in 2012 by EASL[44] and the guidelines eliminated the role of AFP, recommended 4 monthly US for less than 1 cm nodule and introduced CT or MRI imaging even for nodules between 1–2 cm size. Thus greater emphasis has been attached to the imaging modalities subsequently and the role of biopsy has been reduced to situations where atypical imaging findings are encountered **(*see* Flowchart 1)**.

Typical imaging appearance of HCC is the presence of arterial phase enhancement followed by wash out in the venous or delayed phase of multiphasic CT/MRI. Larger tumors may also have small nonenhancing areas of necrosis in addition whereas the smaller tumors invariably are homogeneously enhancing in the arterial phase **(Figs. 9A and B)**.

Cost Effectiveness

The cost effectiveness of screening patients of cirrhosis depends on the incidence of HCC, efficacy of therapy and the age of the patient. In India, using the protocol of US and AFP six monthly and a yearly CT, the cost effectiveness of screening program from the patient perspective was ₹ 126,345 (US$ 2,808) for each HCC detected for local patients and ₹ 448,440 (US$ 9,965) for the outstation patients.[65] This cost per HCC case detected by the HCC surveillance program is exorbitant for low/middle income countries like India. Hence, measures for reducing cost need to be looked into.

TREATMENT OF CIRRHOSIS

Treatment is aimed at delaying the progression of disease and preventing the onset of complications. Delaying progression of compensated cirrhosis to decompensated status is important. A multifaceted approach is required for the management of these patients which includes treatment of the presenting signs and symptoms and the underlying cause of cirrhosis. Compensated cirrhotics need surveillance for developing HCC, screening for the presence of esophageal varices by upper GI endoscopy. Treatment of the etiology of cirrhosis is important. Specific therapy for hepatitis B or C infections, abstinence from alcohol to prevent progression to hepatic fibrogenesis and decompensation. Life style changes, weight loss,

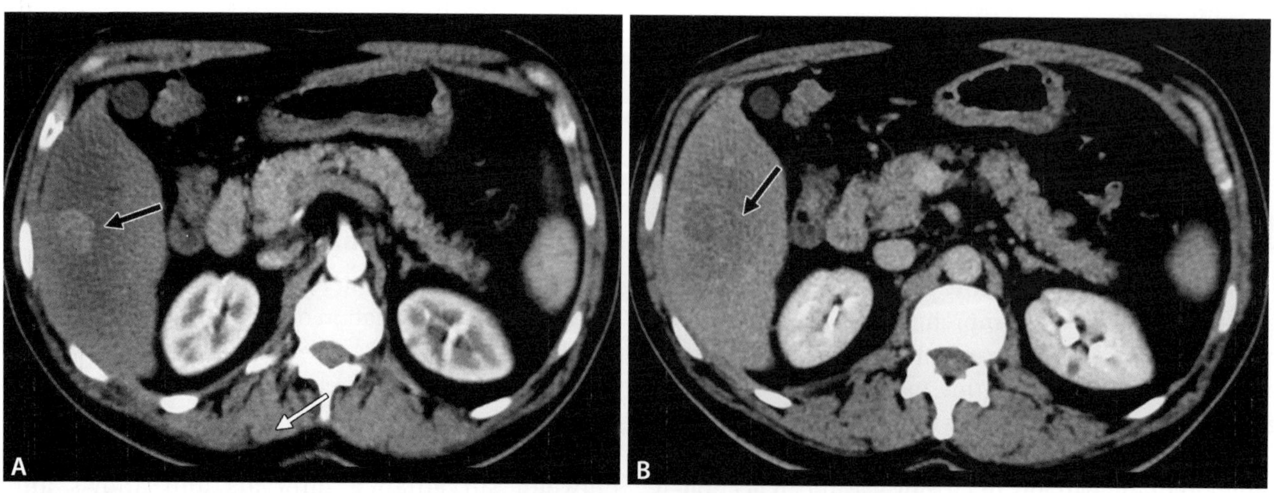

Figs. 9A and B: Typical pattern of HCC on multiphasic CT: (A) Arterial phase MPCT image depicting a small homogeneously enhancing mass in segment 6 of the liver (arrow,) with wash out in the delayed phase; (B) Liver has nodular margins suggesting presence of cirrhosis.

control of blood sugar levels in cases of diabetes are important in cases of NAFLD/NASH. Immunization for HAV, HBV, pneumococcal pneumonia and influenza are recommended. Protein calorie malnutrition needs redressal by encouraging small, frequent high protein meals. Some cases complain of fatigue, muscle cramps, sexual dysfunction which affect the performance status and quality of life. In them, a work up for anemia and thyroid function needs to be done.[66] Liver transplantation is recommended as an ultimate therapy for end stage liver disease. Survival rates following transplant at 1, 5 and 8 years are 83%, 70% and 61% respectively.[67]

TREATMENT OF COMPLICATIONS

Portal hypertension and its complications are managed with various radiological intervention procedures apart from surgery. Transjugular intrahepatic portosystemic shunt (TIPS) is indicated for control of active bleed refractory to sclerotherapy, intractable ascites, and an alternative to shunt surgery in high-risk patients and in cirrhosis due to hepatic venous outflow tract obstruction (HVOTO). Depending upon the site and extent of the venous block in HVOTO, various radiological procedure like angioplasty or stenting can be done to relieve obstruction.[68] Splenic artery embolization is considered these days for cases of hypersplenism since surgical splenectomy is associated with risk of morbidity.

HCC is the terminal, fatal complication of liver cirrhosis. Treatment of HCC is based on the Barcelona Clinic Liver Cancer (BCLC) staging classification **(Flowchart 2)** which links the stage of the disease with recommended treatment.[69]

Curative options of surgical resection and liver transplant are considered for BCLC stage 0 and stage A patients. A 5-year survival after resection can exceed 50% and in stage BCLC 0 (80–90%). The recurrence rate varies from 27% to 73%.

Liver transplant is considered in cases that fulfill the Milan criteria. Best results are seen within Milans criteria, where 4–5 years survival is seen in about 70–75%.[70] Locoregional therapies are the most widely used treatment option for HCC as most patients are not found suitable for

Flowchart 2: Barcelona Clinic Liver Cancer (BCLC) staging classification and treatment schedule.[69]

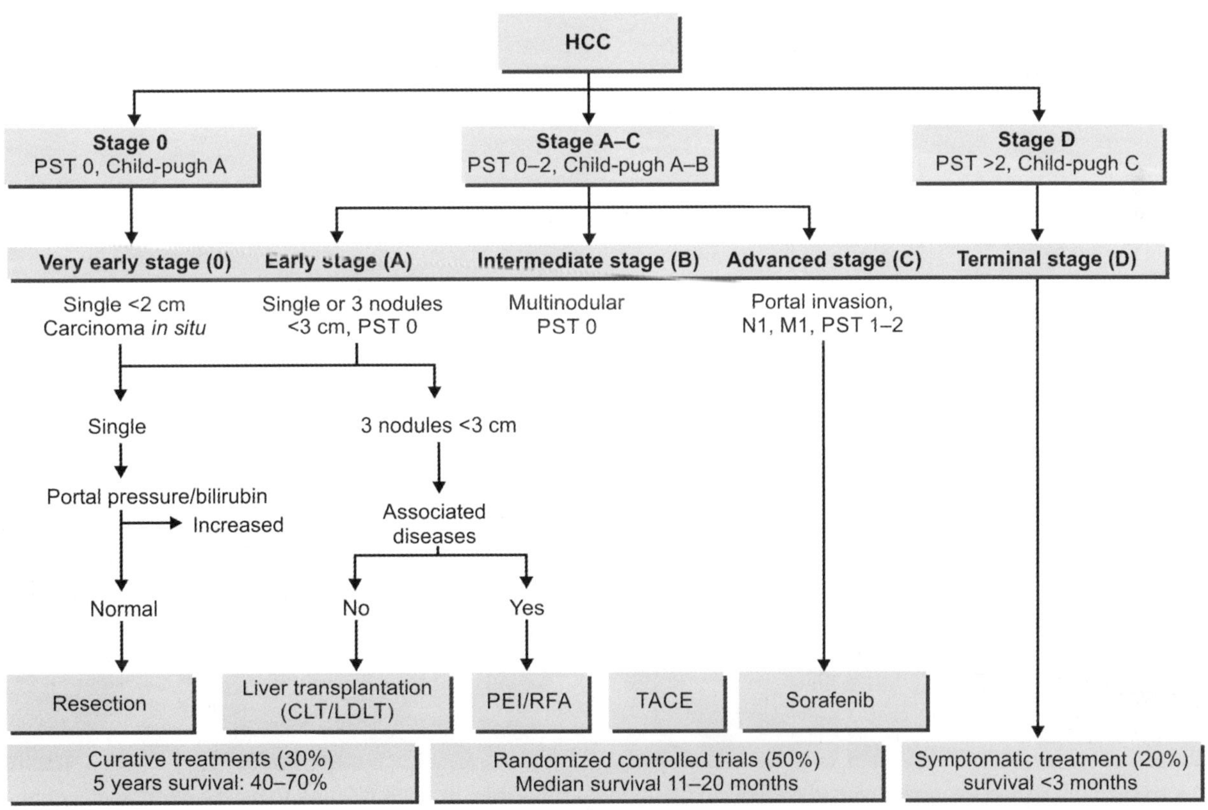

Abbreviations: PEI: Percutaneous ethanol injection; CLT: Cadaver liver transplant; LDLT: Living donor liver transplant; M: Metastases; N: Nodal stage; HCC: Hepatocellular carcinoma; PST: Performance status; RFA: Radiofrequency ablation; TACE: Transarterial chemoembolization.

surgery. Ablative procedures like radiofrequency ablation (RFA) or chemical ablation with ethanol (PEI) or acetic acid ablation (PAI) **(Figs. 10A to C)** have become the alternative to surgery. Outcome of RFA is almost at par with surgery (5-year survival rates of 40–70%) in selected candidates.[71] Due to such good outcome, certain centers have made RFA as the first line of therapy for BCLC A stage HCC and the cumulative survival rates of 95.2%, 69.5% and 58% at 1, 3 and 5 years respectively have been documented.[72] For BCLC stage B, palliative option of chemoembolization (TACE) is offered. Two meta-analyses of the randomized controlled trials have confirmed the beneficial effects of prolonged survival post-TACE. Initial tumor burden is an important predictor of survival.[73,74]

Radioembolization using yttrium-90 microspheres or oral chemotherapy using targeted anticancer agents are recommended for BCLC C stage where portal vein is thrombosed. Limited availability and high cost is the biggest limitation. However, studies have shown that patients with Child-Pugh A disease, regardless of portal vein thrombosis, have derived maximum benefit, whereas those with Child-Pugh B and portal vein thrombosis have had poor outcomes.[75] Rhenium too has been used in such patients with good results.[76] Sorafenib, an inhibitor of Raf kinase and tyrosine kinase activity of vascular endothelial growth factor, has been used to improve survival compared to patients undergoing supportive care.[77] The current trend is to resort to the multi-modality approach that is, combining regional and local therapies. This approach has been shown to produce better results than using single therapy alone.[78,79] Combinations tried are, TACE with RFA, TACE with PEI, TACE with PAI, or TACE with oral chemotherapy (Sorafenib) **(Figs. 11A to C)**. In advanced disease of BCLC D, the main stay of treatment is supportive therapy. However, oral chemotherapy too has been tried with little benefit.

CONCLUSION

Role of a radiologist is vital for patients of liver cirrhosis. Careful screening, early diagnosis, detection of life

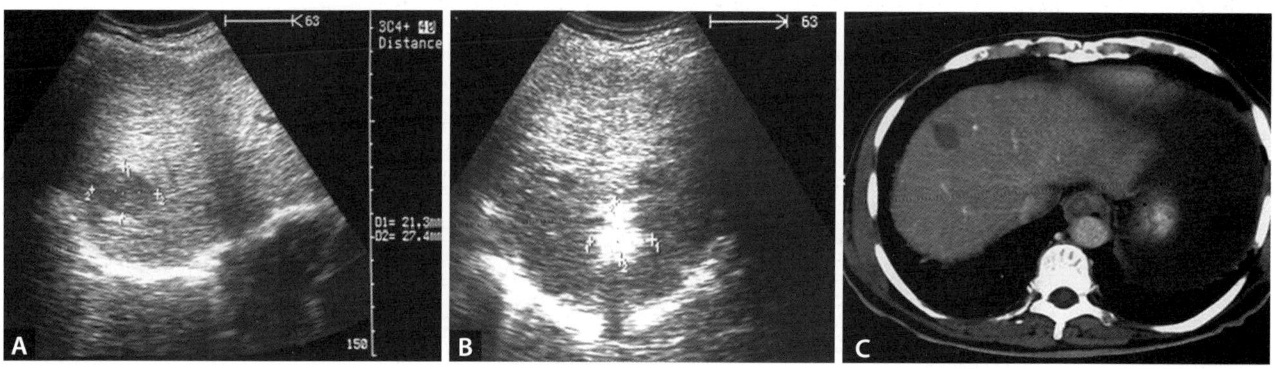

Figs. 10A to C: HCC treated with PAI: (A) US image of a patient of HBV cirrhosis showing a 2.5 cm hypoechoic lesion in the right lobe of the cirrhotic liver; (B) On subjecting to PAI, the lesion is completely hyperechoic on US immediately following PAI; (C) Follow-up CT at one year later shows that the ablative area has slightly reduced in size, is sharply demarcated with no residual or recurrent disease on the venous phase.

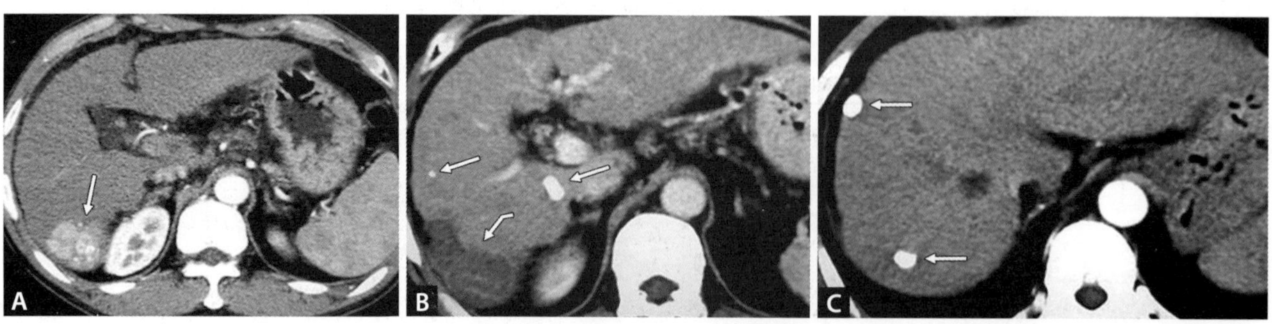

Figs. 11A to C: Combination treatment with RFA followed by TACE: (A) HBV cirrhosis patient found to have a small, solitary enhancing mass in segment 7 of liver on arterial phase CT, which was treated with RFA. At 18 months, multiple fresh lesions along with recurrence at the margin of the defect was noted and TACE was done; (B and C) Post TACE-CT images show all lesions covered with lipiodol (straight arrows and curved arrow respectively).

threatening complications and management by safe image- guided interventions has a significant impact on the outcome of the disease. Hence, understanding of the clinical profile, presentation, natural history and complications of this end stage liver disease is crucial for prolonging survival.

REFERENCES

1. Schuppan D, Afdhal NH. Liver cirrhosis. The Lancet. 2008;371:838-51.
2. Review Team, LaBrecque DR, Abbas Z, et al. World Gastroenterology Organisation global guidelines: nonalcoholic fatty liver disease and nonalcoholic steatohepatitis. J Clin Gastroenterol. 2014;48:467-73.
3. Tandon BN, Acharya SK, Tandon A. Epidemiology of hepatitis B virus infection in India. Gut. 1996;38:S 56-9.
4. Chowdhury A, Santra A, Chaudhuri S, et al. Hepatitis C virus infection in the general population: a community-based study in West Bengal, India. Hepatology. 2003;37:802-9.
5. Duseja A, Singh SP, Saraswat VA, et al. Non-alcoholic Fatty Liver Disease and Metabolic Syndrome - Position Paper of the Indian National Association for the Study of the Liver, Endocrine Society of India, Indian College of Cardiology and Indian Society of Gastroenterology. J Clin Exp Hepatol. 2015;5: 51-68.
6. Williams CD, Stengel J, Asike MI, et al. Prevalence of nonalcoholic fatty liver disease and nonalcoholic steatohepatitis among a largely middle-aged population utilizing ultrasound and liver biopsy: a prospective study. Gastroenterology. 2011;140:124-31.
7. Guha IN, Iredale JP. Clinical aspects and diagnostic aspects of cirrhosis. Textbook of Hepatology: From Basic Science to Clinical Practice, 3rd edition. 2008;1:604-19.
8. Brown JJ, Naylor MJ, Yagan N. Imaging of hepatic cirrhosis. Radiology. 1997;202:1-16.
9. Panigrahi AK, Panda SK, Dixit RK, et al. Magnitude of hepatitis C virus infection in India: prevalence in healthy blood donors, acute and chronic liver diseases. J Med Virol. 1997;51:167-74.
10. Fattovich G, Stroffolini T, Zagni I, Donato F. Hepatocellular carcinoma in cirrhosis: Incidence and risk factors. Gastroenterology. 2004;127:S35-50.
11. Popper H. Pathological aspects of cirrhosis: A review. Am J Pathol. 1977;87:228-64.
12. International working party: Terminology of nodular hepatocellular lesions. Hepatology. 1995;22:983-93.
13. Kamel IR, Bluemke DA. Imaging evaluation of hepatocellular carcinoma. J Vasc Interven Radiol. 2002;13:S173-83.
14. Benyon RC, Iredale JP. Is liver fibrosis reversible? Gut. 2000;46:443-6.
15. Conn HO, Atterbury CE. Cirrhosis. Diseases of the liver. In: Schiff L, Schiff ER (Eds). Philadelphia; Lippincort. 1987. pp. 725-864.
16. Chung RT, Podolsky. Cirrhosis and its complications. In: Braunwald E, Hauser SL, Fauci AS, Longo DL, Kasper DL, Jameson JL (Eds). Harison's Principles of Internal Medicine. New York; 2001.pp.1754-61.
17. Pugh RN, Murray-Lyon IM, Dawson JL, et al. Transection of esophagus for bleeding esophageal varices. Br J Surg. 1973;60:646-9.
18. Infante-Rivard C, Esnaola S, Villeneuve JP. Clinical and statistical validity of conventional prognostic factors in predicting short-term survival among cirrhotics. Hepatology. 1987;7:660-4.
19. Wiesner R, Edwards E, Freeman R, et al. Model for end-stage liver disease (MELD) and allocation of donor livers. Gastroenterology. 2003;124:91-6.
20. Bedossa P, Poynard T. An algorithm for the grading of activity in chronic hepatitis C. The METAVIR Cooperative Study Group. Hepatology. 1996;24:289.
21. Gaiani S, Gramantieri L, Venturoli N, et al. What is the criterion for differentiating chronic hepatitis from compensated cirrhosis? A prospective study comparing ultrasonography and percutaneous liver biopsy. J Hepatology. 1997;27: 979-85.
22. Caturelli E, Giacobbe A, Facciorusso D, et al. Percutaneous biopsy in diffuse liver disease: Increasing diagnostic yield and decreasing complication rate by routine ultrasound assessment of puncture site. Am J Gastroenterol. 1996;91:1318-21.
23. Farrel RJ, Smidy PF, Pilkington RM, et al. Guided versus blind liver biopsy for chronic hepatitis C: Clinical benefits and costs. J Hepatol. 1999;30:580-87.
24. Lebrec D, et al. Portal hypertension, size of esophageal varices, and risk of gastrointestinal bleeding in alcoholic cirrhosis. Gastroenterology. 1980;79:1139-44.
25. North Italian Endoscopic Club for the Study and Treatment of Esophageal varices. Prediction of the first variceal haemorrhage in patients with cirrhosis of the liver and esophageal varices. A prospective multicenter study. New England Journal of Medicine. 1988;39:319:983-9.
26. Larcos G, Sorokopud H, Berry G, et al. Sonographic screening for hepatocellular carcinoma in patients with chronic hepatitis or cirrhosis: An evaluation. 1998;171:433-5.
27. Zweilbel WJ. Sonographic diagnosis of diffuse liver disease. Semin Ultrasound CT MRI. 1995;16:8-15.
28. Bonkovsky HL, Rubin RB, Cable EE, et al. Hepatic iron concentration: Noninvasive estimation by means of MR imaging techniques. Radiology. 1999;212:227-34.
29. Qayyum A, Goh JS, Kakar S, et al. Accuracy of liver fat quantification at MR imaging: comparison of out-of-phase gradient-echo and fat-saturated fast spin-echo techniques: initial experience. Radiology. 2005;237:507-11.
30. Ultrasound Shear Wave Elastography for Liver Disease. In: Piscaglia F, et al. A Critical Appraisal of the Many Actors on the Stage. Ultraschall in Med. 2016;37:1-5.
31. Jiang T, Tian G, Zhao Q, Kong D, Cheng C, Zhong L, Li L. Diagnostic accuracy of 2D-shear wave elastography for liver fibrosis severity: a meta-analysis. PLoS One. 2016; 11:e0157219.
32. Jung KS, Kim SU, Ahn SH, Park YN, Kim DY, Park JY, Chon CY, Choi EH, Han KH. Risk assessment of hepatitis

B virus-related hepatocellular carcinoma development using liver stiffness measurement (FibroScan). Hepatology. 2011;53:885-94.
33. Wong GL, Chan HL, Wong CK, Leung C, Chan CY, Ho PP, Chung VC, Chan ZC, Tse YK, Chim AM, Lau TK, Wong VW. Liver stiffness-based optimization of hepatocellular carcinoma risk score in patients with chronic hepatitis B. J Hepatol. 2014;60:339-45.
34. Wang QB, Zhu H, Liu HL, Zhang B. Performance of magnetic resonance elastography and diffusion-weighted imaging for the staging of hepatic fibrosis: a meta-analysis. Hepatology. 2012;56:239-47.
35. Samir AE, Dhyani M, Vij A, et al. Shear-wave elastography for the estimation of liver fibrosis in chronic liver disease: determining accuracy and ideal site for measurement. Radiology. 2015;274(3):888-96.
36. Caly WR, Strauss E. A prospective study of bacterial infections in patients of cirrhosis. J Hepatol. 1993;18:353-8.
37. Llovet JM, Burroughs A, Bruix J. Hepatocelluar carcinoma. Lancet. 2003;362:1907-17.
38. Paul SB, Gulati MS, Sreenivas V, et al. Incidence of hepatocellular carcinoma among patients of cirrhosis of liver: an experience from a tertiary care centre in northern India. Indian J Gastroenterol. 2007;26,274-8.
39. Paul SB, Gulati MS, Sreenivas V, et al. Evaluating patients with cirrhosis for hepatocellular carcinoma: value of clinical symptomatology, Imaging and Alpha-fetoprotein. Oncology. 2007;72:117-23.
40. Prorok PC. Epidemiologic approach for cancer screening. Problems in design and analysis of trials. Am J Pediatr Hematol Oncol. 1992;14:117-28.
41. Benvegnu L, Fattovich G, Noventa F, et al. Concurrent hepatitis B and C virus infection and risk of hepatocellular carcinoma in cirrhosis. A prospective study. Cancer. 1994;74:2442-8.
42. Sherman M, Colombo M. Hepatocellular carcinoma screening and diagnosis. Semin Liver Dis. 2014;34:389-97.
43. Omata M, Lesmana LA, Tateishi R, Chen PJ, Lin SM, Yoshida H, et al. Asian Pacific Association for the Study of the Liver consensus recommendations on hepatocellular carcinoma. Hepatol Int. 2010;4:439-74.
44. European Association for Study of Liver; European Organisation for Research and Treatment of Cancer. EASL-EORTC clinical practice guidelines: management of hepatocellular carcinoma. Eur J Cancer. 2012;48:599-641.
45. Yeh YP, Hu TH, Cho PY, Chen HH, Yen AM, Chen SL, et al. Evaluation of abdominal ultrasonography mass screening for hepatocellular carcinoma in Taiwan. Hepatology. 2014;59:1840-49.
46. Matsumoto Y, Suzuki T, Asadi T, et al. Clinical classification of hepatoma in Japan according to serial changes in serum alpha fetoprotein levels. Cancer. 1982;49:354-6.
47. Sherman M, Peltekian KM, Lee C. Screening for hepatocellular carcinoma in chronic carriers of hepatitis B virus: incidence and prevalence of hepatocellular carcinoma in a North American urban population. Hepatology. 1995;22:432-8.
48. Trevisani F, D'Intino PE, Morselli-Labate AM, et al. Serum alpha-fetoprotein for diagnosis of hepatocellular carcinoma in patients with chronic liver disease: influence of HBsAg and anti-HCV status. J Hepatol. 2001;34:570-5.
49. Gambarin-Gelwan M, Wolf DC, Shapiro R, Schwartz ME, Min AD. Sensitivity of commonly available screening tests in detecting hepatocellular carcinoma in cirrhotic patients undergoing liver transplantation. Am J Gastroenterol. 2000;95: 1535-8.
50. Cedrone A, Covino M, Caturelli E, et al. Utility of alpha-fetoprotein (AFP) in the screening of patients with virus-related chronic liver disease: does different viral etiology influence AFP levels in hepatocellular carcinoma? A study in 350 western patients. Hepatogastroenterology. 2000;47:1654-8.
51. Daniele B, Bencivenga A, Megna AS, Tinessa V. Alpha fetoprotein and ultrasonography screening for hepato-celluar carcinoma. Gastroenterology. 2004;127:S108-12.
52. Johnson J. Tumor marker in the diagnosis and management of patients with hepatocullular carcinoma. Recent results in Cancer Research. 1986;100:68.
53. Bruix J, Sherman M, Llovet JM, et al. EASL panel of experts on HCC. Clinical management of hepatocellular carcinoma. Conclusion of the Barcelona 2000 EASL conference. European Association for the Study of Liver. J Hepatol. 2001;35:421-30.
54. Bruix J, Sherman M. Practice Guidelines Committee, American Associationfor the Study of Liver Diseases. Management of hepatocellular carcinoma. Hepatology. 2005;42:1208-36.
55. Bennett SL, Krinsky GA, Abitbol RJ, Kim SY, Theise ND, Teperman LW. Sonographic detection of hepatocellular carcinoma and dysplastic nodules in cirrhosis: correlation of pretransplantation sonography and liver explant pathology in 200 patients. Am J Roentgenol. 2002;179: 75-80.
56. Liu WC, Lim JH, Park CK, et al. Poor sensitivity of sonography is detection of hepatocellular carcinoma in advanced liver cirrhois: accuracy of pretransplantations sonography in 118 patients. Eur Radiol. 2003;13:1693-8.
57. Rao ARW, Chui AKK, Shi LW, et al. Sensitivity of radiological investigations in diagnosing hepatocellular carcinoma in cirrhotic liver. Transplantation Proceedings. 2003;35:348-9.
58. Claudon M, Dietrich CF, Choi BI, Cosgrove DO, Kudo M, Nolsøe CP, et al. Guidelines and good clinical practice recommendations for contrast enhanced ultrasound (CEUS) in the liver--update 2012: a WFUMB-EFSUMB initiative in cooperation with representatives of AFSUMB, AIUM, ASUM, FLAUS and ICUS. Ultraschall Med Stuttg Ger 1980. 2013;34:11-29.
59. Thakur S, Jhobta A, Dhiman DS, Sood RG, Chauhan A, Thakur CS. Role of contrast enhanced ultrasound in characterization of focal liver lesions. Egypt J Radiol Nucl Med. 2014;45:7-17.
60. Trillaud H, Bruel JM, Valette PJ, Vilgrain V, Schmutz G, Oyen R, et al. Characterization of focal liver lesions with Sono Vue (R) enhanced sonography: International multicenter-study

in comparison to CT and MRI. World J Gastroenterol. 2009;15:3748–56.
61. Burrel M, Llovet JM, Ayuso C, et al. MRI angiography is superior to helical CT for detection of HCC prior to liver transplantation: an explant correlation. Hepatology. 2003;38:1034-42.
62. Sheu J, Sung J, Chen D, et al. Growth rates of asymptomatic hepatocellular carcinoma and its clinical implications. Gastroenterology. 1985;89:259-66.
63. Barbara L, Benzi G, Gaiani S, et al. Natural history of small untreated hepatocellular carcinoma in cirrhosis: A multivariate analysis of prognostic factors of tumor growth rate and patient survival. Hepatology. 1992;16:132-6.
64. Durand F, Regimbeau JM, Belghiti J, et al. Assessment of the benefits and risk of percutaneous biopsy before surgical resection of hepatocellular carcinoma. J Hepatol. 2001;35:254-8.
65. Paul SB, Gulati MS, Sreenivas V, Madan K, Gupta AK, Mukhopadhyay S, Acharya SK. Economic evaluation of HCC surveillance program in India. Hepatol Int. 2008;2: 231-6.
66. Kamath PS, Shah VH. Overview of Cirrhosis, Sleisenger and Fordtran's Gastrointestinal and Liver Disease: Pathophysiology/Diagnosis/Management, 10th edn. PA: Elsevier Saunders. 2016;2:1254-60.
67. Roberts MS, Angus DC, Bryce CL, Valenta Z, Weissfeld L. Survival after liver transplantation in the United States: a disease-specific analysis of the UNOS database. Liver Transpl. 2004;204;10:886-97.
68. Mukund A, Gamanagatti S, Acharya SK. Radiological interventions in HVOTO: Practical tips Tropical Gastroenterology. 2011;32:4-140.
69. Llovet JM, Di Bisceglie AM, Bruix J, Kramer BS, Lencioni R, Zhu AX, et al. Panel of Experts in HCC-Design Clinical Trials. Design and endpoints of clinical trials in hepatocellular carcinoma. J Natl Cancer Inst. 2008;100:698-711.
70. Mazzaferro V, Bhoori S, Sposito C, Bongini M, Langer M, et al. Milan criteria in liver transplantation for hepatocellular carcinoma: an evidence-based analysis of 15 years of experience liver transplantation. 2011;17: S44-S57.
71. Lencioni R, Cioni D, Crocetti L, et al. Early-stage hepatocellular carcinoma in patients with cirrhosis: long-term results of percutaneous image-guided radiofrequency ablation. Radiology. 2005;234:961-7.
72. Choi D, Lim HK, Rhim H, Kim YS, Lee WJ, Paik SW et al. Percutaneous Radiofrequency ablation for early stage hepatocellular carcinoma as a first line treatment: long term results and prognostic factors in a large single-institution series. Eur Radiol. 2007;17:684-92.
73. Camma C, Schepis F, Orlando A, et al. Transarterial chemoembolization for unresectable hepatocellular carcinoma: meta-analysis of randomized controlled trials. Radiology. 2002;224:47–54.
74. Paul SB, Gamanagatti S, Sreenivas V, et al. Trans-arterial chemoembolization (TACE) in patients with unresectable hepatocellular carcinoma: experience from a tertiary care centre in India. Indian J Radiol Imaging. 2011;21:113-20.
75. Salem R, Lewandowski RJ, Mulcahy MF, et al. Radioembolization for hepatocellular carcinoma using Yttrium-90 microspheres: a comprehensive report of long-term outcomes. Gastroenterology. 2010;138:52–64.
76. Kumar A, Srivastava DN, Chau TTM, et al. Inoperable hepatocellular carcinoma: transarterial 188 Re HDD-Labeled iodized oil for treatment—Prospective multicenter trial. Radiology. 2007;243:509-19.
77. Llovet JM, Ricci S, Mazzaferro V, et al. SHARP Investigators Study Group. Sorafenib in advanced hepatocellular carcinoma. N Engl J Med. 2008;359:378-90.
78. Yamakado K, Nakatsuka A, Ohmori S, et al. Radiofrequency ablation combined with chemoembolization in hepatocellular carcinoma treatment response based on tumor size and morphology. J Vasc Interv Radiol. 2002:13:1225-32.
79. Kurokohchi K, Watanabe S, Masaki T, et al. Combined use of percutaneous ethanol injection and radiofrequency ablation for the effective treatment of hepatocellular carcinoma. Int J Oncol. 2002;21:841-6.

CHAPTER 78

Benign Focal Lesions of Liver

Sapna Singh, Anjali Prakash

INTRODUCTION

A focal liver lesion is defined as a discrete abnormality arising within the liver. Owing to the advances in imaging, focal liver lesions are being increasingly detected. There has been an increase in the detection of focal lesions in the millimeter range. Characterization of these multitude of lesions detected becomes important as the diagnosis of the lesion as benign rather than malignant greatly alleviates patient's anxiety. State of the art multi detector computed tomography (CT) (MDCT) with its excellent spatial resolution and 3T magnetic resonance imaging (MRI) allows for a near isotropic imaging.[1,2] The lesions are usually categorized on the basis of their morphology, vascularity, enhancement patterns and specific functional characteristics.

Benign focal lesions of the liver can be classified as developmental, neoplastic, inflammatory and miscellaneous. The benign hepatic tumors can be broadly classified according to the cell of origin as:

Pathologic classification of benign liver tumors (Based on cell of origin)[3]
Hepatocyte
• Hepatocellular adenoma • Hepatocellular hyperplasia • Focal nodular hyperplasia • Macroregenerative nodules • Nodular regenerative hyperplasia
Bile duct epithelium (Cholangiocellular)
• Hepatic cysts • Simple hepatic cysts • Polycystic liver disease/congenital hepatic fibrosis • Biliary cystadenoma • Bile duct adenoma
Mesenchymal cells
• Mesenchymal hamartoma • Hemangioma • Infantile hemangioendothelioma • Lymphangioma • Lipoma/angiomyolipoma/myelolipoma • Leiomyoma • Fibroma
Heterotopic cells

Mesenchymal hamartoma and infantile hemangioendothelioma are benign liver tumors seen in the pediatric population. Abscess, hydatid disease and tuberculosis constitute the infective group while fatty infiltration, peliosis hepatis and inflammatory pseudotumor can be grouped as miscellaneous.

HEPATIC CYSTS

Hepatic cysts are benign developmental lesions showing no communication with the biliary tree. Seen in 5–14% of the general population, a definite female preponderance (female: male ratio of 5:2) is seen.[3]

Pathology

Hepatic cysts are also called bile duct cysts and are believed to originate from hamartomatous tissue.[4] Hepatic cyst is a solitary unilocular cyst with a lining composed of a single primary layer of cuboidal bile duct epithelium. Its wall is usually less than 1mm thick and is composed of fibrous tissue.

Clinical Features

These are usually asymptomatic and discovered incidentally at routine imaging. Large hepatic cysts can cause compression of adjacent intrahepatic ducts and may rarely be symptomatic.[4]

Imaging Features

On ultrasonography, a simple hepatic cyst is seen as a well-defined anechoic lesion with thin imperceptible walls. There is enhanced through transmission like cystic lesions elsewhere[5] **(Figs. 1 and 2)**. Thin septations may be present. Thick septations, calcifications, nodules and debris are not seen in a simple hepatic cyst but may be seen in a complicated cyst. Ultrasound is almost 100% accurate in the diagnosis of simple hepatic cysts.[5]

Computed Tomography

On CT, a simple hepatic cyst is seen as a well-defined, round to oval, intrahepatic lesion with water attenuation (10–15 HU).[6] It has a homogeneous appearance with absence of any internal structures **(Fig. 3)**. The wall is thin and shows no evidence of contrast enhancement. Internal debris and contrast enhancement may however be seen in a cyst complicated by hemorrhage or infection.

Magnetic Resonance Imaging

On MRI, simple hepatic cysts are seen as well-defined homogeneous lesions with fluid signal intensity, hypointense on T1W and markedly hyperintense on T2W images[7] **(Figs. 4A and B)**. An increase in the signal intensity with increase in T2 weighting helps to differentiate these cysts from metastatic disease. A high signal on both T1 and T2- weighted images with a fluid level may be seen in the event of an intracystic hemorrhage. On diffusion weighted imaging (DWI), there is no restricted diffusion. These cysts show a decrease in signal intensity with increasing b values and are strongly hyperintense on apparent diffusion coefficient (ADC) sequence.

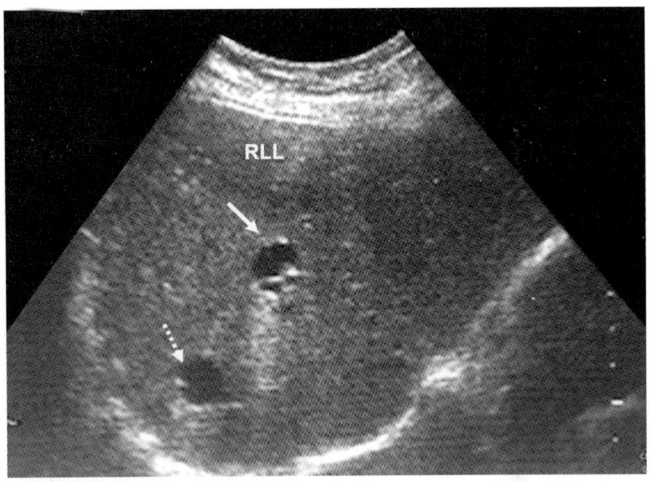

Fig. 1: Conventional US showing hypoechoic lesions in the right lobe of liver (RLL) with posterior acoustic enhancement and enhanced through transmission—simple liver cysts.

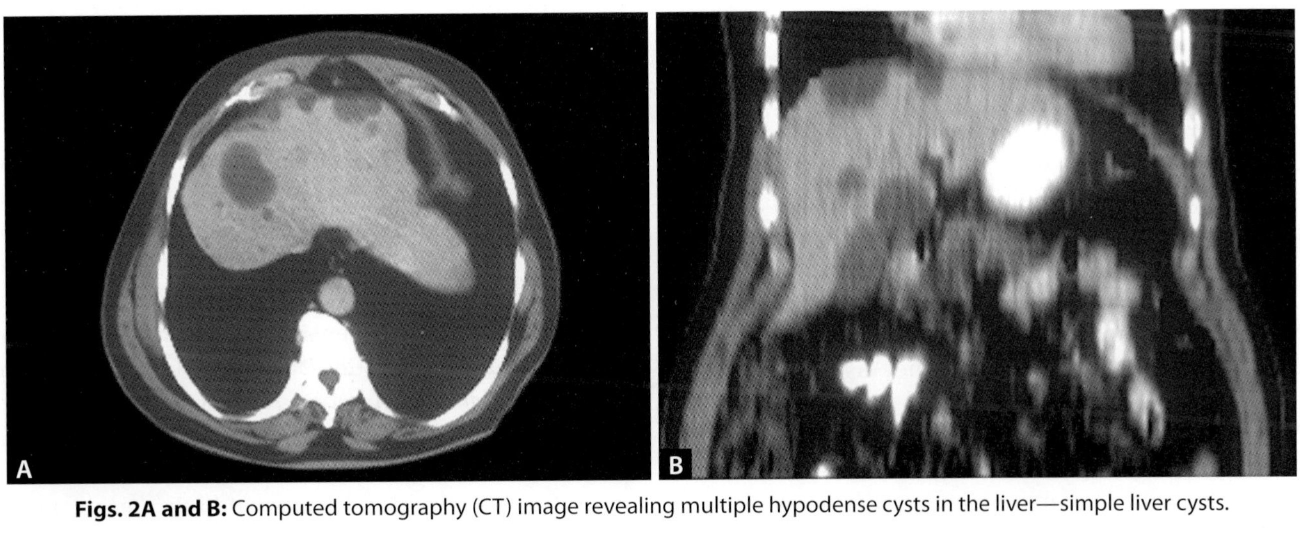

Figs. 2A and B: Computed tomography (CT) image revealing multiple hypodense cysts in the liver—simple liver cysts.

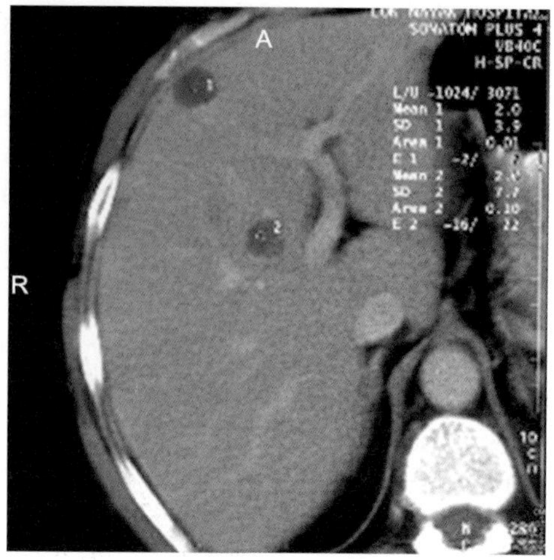

Fig. 3: Computed tomography (CT) image revealing small hypodense lesions in the liver having water attenuation—multiple simple liver cysts.

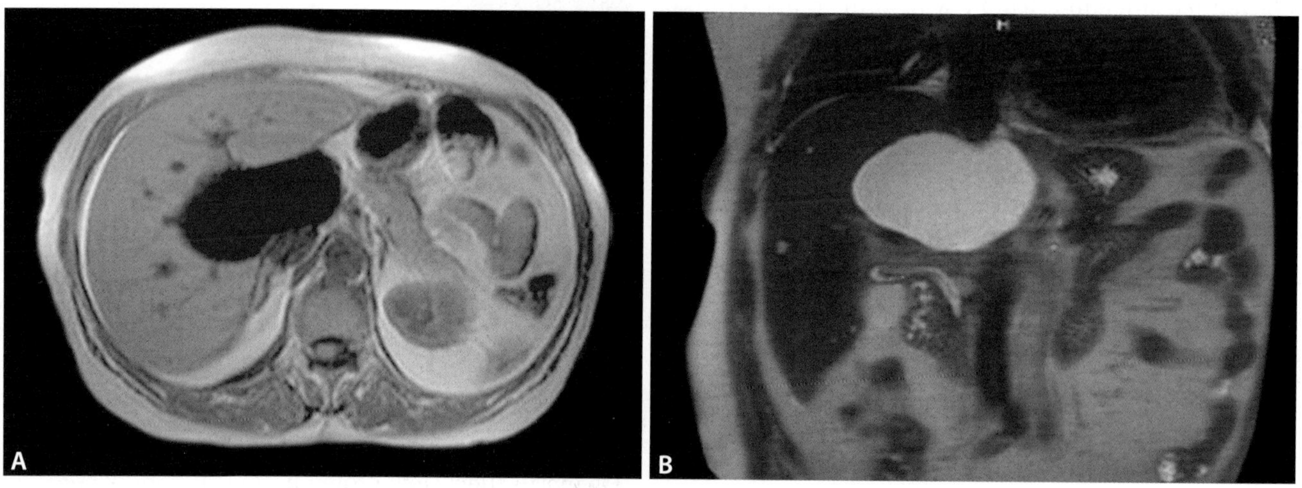

Figs. 4A and B: (A) T1W MR image showing a hepatic cyst as a homogeneous sharply marginated hypointense lesion; (B) T2W image reveals the cysts to be markedly hyperintense. Few smaller cysts are also seen in the periphery of the right lobe.

POLYCYSTIC LIVER DISEASE

When more than 10 cysts are present in the liver parenchyma, a polycystic disease should be considered. About 70% of patients with polycystic liver disease have autosomal dominant polycystic kidney disease while liver involvement occurs in 30–40% of patients with polycystic kidney disease.[8] Von Meyenberg's complexes and increased fibrous tissue are increasingly seen in the liver which surrounds the cysts in polycystic liver and autosomal dominant polycystic kidney disease.

CILIATED HEPATIC FOREGUT CYST

These cysts are congenital in origin and very rare. These are histologically similar to bronchogenic and esophageal duplication cysts.[9] They are usually solitary, seen more commonly in the medial segment of left lobe at the antero-superior margin or intersegmentally causing a bulge on the outer contour of the liver. A subcapsular location is characteristic. Most of these cysts are asymptomatic and discovered incidentally. Rarely, obstructive jaundice and portal hypertension due to mass effect on the biliary system or portal vein may occur. They are usually unilocular and smaller than 3 cm. On T1-weighted imaging, these cysts have a variable signal intensity, depending on serous or mucinous content while on T2-weighted images, these are homogeneously hyperintense. No restricted diffusion or contrast enhancement is seen.[9] Very rarely, a malignant transformation may occur. An irregular wall thickness or solid component developing within the lesion should be viewed with suspicion. Owing to the risk of malignant transformation, though rare, a complete surgical excision is recommended.

PERIBILIARY CYST

The peribiliary cysts represent cystic dilatation of the glands in the bile duct walls. These are associated with cirrhosis, specifically with portal hypertension. On imaging, these cysts are seen as anechoic structures along the portal tracts and may be mistaken for a dilated bile duct. Presence of thin septa within the cysts helps to differentiate these cysts from dilated bile duct.[9] CT shows hypoattenuating structures and MR reveals the cystic nature of the lesions on T2W images.

BILIARY DUCT HAMARTOMAS

It is also called Von-Meyenberg's complexes. Bile duct hamartomas are cystic lesions typically less than 1.5 cm in diameter diffusely scattered throughout the liver parenchyma.[10]

Pathology

They do not communicate with the biliary tree and are believed to originate from the embryonic bile ducts that fail to involute. They are considered a part of the spectrum of fibropolycystic liver disease that also includes congenital hepatic fibrosis, autosomal dominant polycystic liver disease and Caroli's disease. Histologically, they consist of focally disordered collections of bile ducts surrounded by abundant fibrous stroma.

Clinical Features

Usually asymptomatic and discovered incidentally at imaging.

Imaging Features

The CT and MR demonstrate the cystic nature of the lesions hypointense on T1 and markedly hyperintense on T2W images. They are seen as multiple cyst like hepatic nodules diffusely scattered in both lobes of the liver and typically measuring 0.5–1.5 cm in diameter and usually showing no enhancement. Very rarely, thin rim enhancement corresponding to the compressed liver parenchyma is seen. At MR cholangiography, no communication with the biliary tree is seen. No enhancement is seen with the liver specific contrast agents as they lack communication with the biliary tree.

On DWI, biliary hamartomas show no evidence of restricted diffusion and behave as simple hepatic cysts, showing signal intensity loss with increasing 'b' values and appearing hyperintense on ADC sequences.

Differential Diagnosis

Bile duct hamartomas need to be differentiated from multiple simple cysts. Simple hepatic cysts have a regular outline while bile duct hamartomas exhibit irregular outline. Hamartomas are typically less than 1.5 cm in diameter and occur without any renal involvement.

BILIARY CYSTADENOMA

Biliary cystadenomas are rare tumors of biliary origin. They are multilocular cystic lesions with the majority (85%) being intrahepatic.[11] They occur predominantly in middle aged women, are usually large in size (1.5–35 cm), and well-defined, multiloculated solitary masses occurring predominantly in the right lobe. Multifocality is rarely seen.

Pathology

Biliary cystadenomas are thought to be premalignant lesions.[11] On pathology, lesions are subdivided on the presence or absence of ovarian stroma which is useful in prognostication. Histologically, they are similar to mucinous cystic neoplasm of the pancreas. Gross features include a multilocular appearance and a fibrous capsule while on microscopy a single layer of mucin secreting cells is seen to line the cyst wall.

Clinical Features

Owing to their slow growing nature, they present with non-specific symptoms such as abdominal pain. Jaundice may occur due to associated biliary obstruction. They may be completely asymptomatic and discovered incidentally.

Imaging Features

USG and CT

Biliary cystadenoma appears as a well-defined solitary multi-loculated cystic mass with thin septations. The septations may show fine calcifications and show enhancement on administration of intravenous contrast. The fluid within the tumor is usually mucinous in nature but may be proteinaceous, hemorrhagic, gelatinous or purulent due to infection.

Coarse calcifications, polypoid excrescences, nodular projections, thick septations are seen in biliary cystadenocarcinomas rather than cystadenomas. Rarely, these tumors may communicate with the biliary tree and secrete mucinous material into the ducts.

MR Imaging

The lesions show fluid signal, hypointense on T1W and hyperintense on T2W images. A variable signal intensity is seen in the presence of hemorrhage and infection **(Figs. 5A and B)**. MR imaging can better demonstrate the relationship of the mass to the bile ducts or any intraductal tumoral extension.

Differential Diagnosis

A complex benign cyst, echinococcal cyst, cystic metastases, hematoma, undifferentiated sarcoma all constitute a differential diagnosis to these lesions. A percutaneous biopsy may be needed at times for a definite diagnosis. Resection of these lesions is usually complete and recurrence is rare.

HEMANGIOMA

Hemangioma is the most common benign neoplasm of the liver and is usually discovered incidentally. On routine cross sectional imaging studies, the reported incidence is 0.4% to 20%.[12] Hemangiomas range in size from a few millimeters to several centimeters; lesions larger than 10 cm are called giant hemangiomas. These are frequently located in a subcapsular location or in the vicinity of intrahepatic vessels though they may be located anywhere within the hepatic parenchyma. These are found more commonly in the right lobe and may rarely be pedunculated.

Pathology

On gross inspection, hemangiomas typically appear as soft reddish or bluish purple lesions. These are mesodermal in origin and are composed of blood filled cavernous vascular spaces lined by a single layer of endothelial cells supported by thin fibrous stroma. Depending on the size of the vascular spaces, hemangiomas are classified into two major types, the cavernous hemangioma and the capillary type, with cavernous type having large vascular spaces.[12] Thrombosis, fibrosis, calcification or ossification of the thrombus may occur due to slow blood flow within the spaces leading to involution. Involution is more common in lesions larger than 3 cm. Sclerosed hemangiomas represent the end stage of hemangioma involution and have obliterated and fibrosed vascular spaces. A hormonal influence has also been proposed in the etiopathogenesis as some hemangiomas enlarge during pregnancy while involution has been reported with corticosteroids.

Clinical Features

Hemangiomas occur most commonly in the 4th and 5th decades of life and are more common in women.[13] Majority of the cases are asymptomatic and are discovered incidentally.[14] Rarely, patients may present with abdominal pain owing to the compression on adjacent organs caused by large hemangiomas. A very rare complication of hemangiomas is the Kasabach-Merritt syndrome in which patients present with fever, leukocytosis, thrombocytopenia and consumptive coagulopathy. Hemorrhage is seen very rarely and is the reason for a prophylactic resection.

Imaging Features

USG: A very distinctive imaging pattern is seen in lesions <2 cm in diameter. Sonography shows a well-circumscribed homogeneously hyperechoic lesion

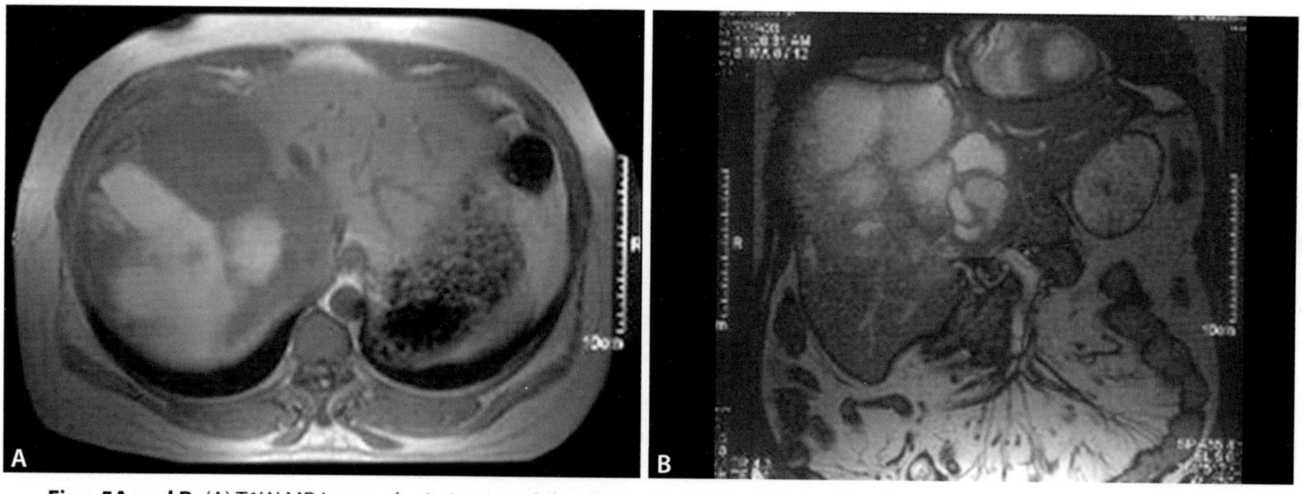

Figs. 5A and B: (A) T1W MR image depicting a multilocular cystic mass with variable signal due to the presence of fluid and hemorrhage/protein content; (B) T2W image showing the lesion to be high signal—biliary cystadenoma.

usually in a subcapsular location or in the vicinity of intrahepatic vessels **(Figs. 6 and 7)**. The echogenicity of hemangioma has been attributed to the interfaces between multiple vascular spaces. Larger lesions show a more heterogenous appearance owing to degeneration and fibrous replacement. On contrast US, a peripheral pooling or puddling of contrast expanding in a centripetal pattern followed by a complete fill in is seen.[15]

CT: On noncontrast scans, hemangiomas appear as low density lesions with well-defined lobulated margins. Following contrast administration, most hemangiomas show a characteristic peripheral nodular enhancement followed by a centripetal fill in and become isoattenuating with the liver parenchyma on delayed scans **(Figs. 8A to C)**. The initial peripheral nodular enhancement seen in hemangiomas in the arterial phase is isodense with the aorta, a finding which is 100% specific in differentiating hemangiomas from metastases. A peripheral centripetal fill in, coupled with delayed filling and persistence of enhancement constitute the diagnostic triad of hemangiomas by single level dynamic CT.[16,17] Though smaller lesions may show the characteristic imaging triad, larger lesions and giant hemangiomas exhibit nonenhancing areas corresponding to scar tissue, cystic degeneration or myxoid changes. Similarly, sclerosed hemangiomas may not show the characteristic imaging pattern. Capsular retraction, volume loss, geographic margins and nodular areas of internal enhancement suggest the diagnosis of a sclerosed hemangioma.

MRI: On MRI, these are seen as well-defined lesions hypointense on T1 and markedly hyperintense on T2-weighted images. Hemangiomas show a characteristic increase in hyperintensity with increasing TE values which

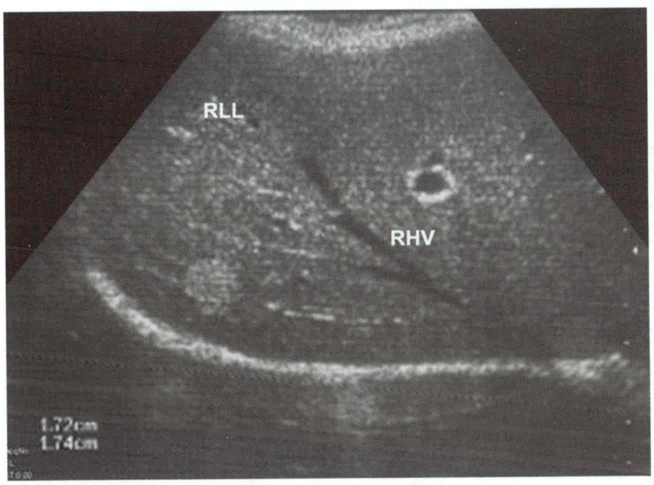

Fig. 6: US shows a well-circumscribed homogeneous hyperechoic lesion in the posterior segment of the right lobe of the liver—hemangioma.

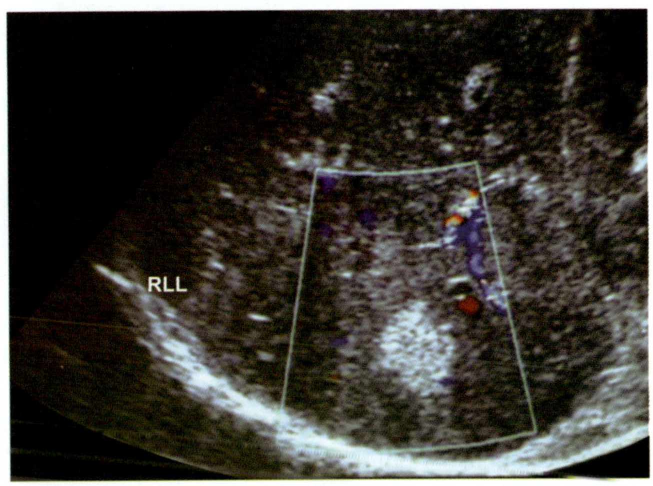

Fig. 7: Color flow imaging showing lack of internal vascularity in a hemangioma.

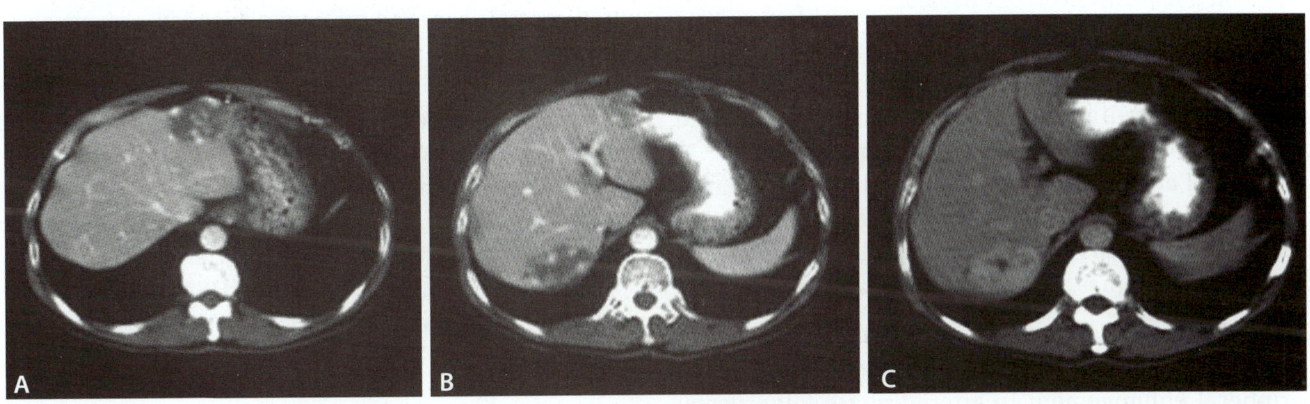

Figs. 8A to C: (A and B) Early phase CT (within 30 seconds) showing peripheral nodular enhancement in the hemangiomas; (C) Delayed phase enhancement 20 minutes later show complete fill in the hemangioma with a central fibrous scar seen in the larger one.

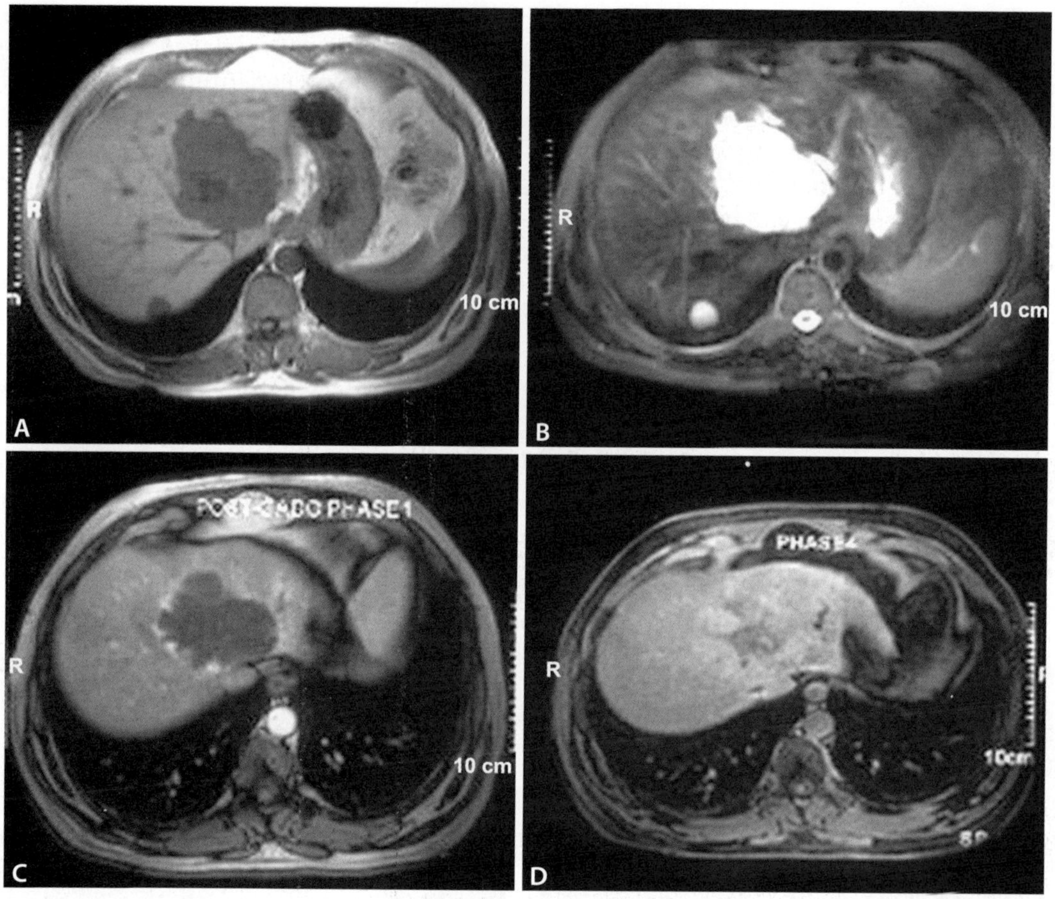

Figs. 9A to D: (A) T1 weighted MR image shows a well-demarcated lobulated hypointense lesion in the liver; (B) T2-weighted image reveals the lesion to be markedly hyperintense "light bulb appearance;" (C) Post-gadolinium image obtained within one minute of contrast administration shows peripheral enhancement within the lesion; (D) Delayed phase image shows centripetal fill in with a central scar-giant cavernous hemangioma.

has been called the "light bulb appearance" **(Figs. 9A to D)**.

On administration of Gadolinium, three enhancement patterns have been described with reported specificities of 100% and diagnostic accuracy of 95%.[12]

Type 1: A uniform, fast and intense enhancement of the hemangioma in the arterial phase remaining hyperintense to the surrounding liver parenchyma on delayed post-contrast images constitutes a type 1 pattern.[18] A perilesional enhancement reflecting high flow in efferent perilesional veins is seen. This pattern is usually seen in small hemangiomas (<1.5 cm) also called "small flash filling" hemangiomas.

Type 2: Medium size hemangiomas (1.5–5 cm) usually show a type 2 pattern characterized by typical nodular peripheral enhancement in arterial phase followed by centripetal fill in seen on the portal venous phase (70s) and a complete homogeneous fill in on delayed image (3–5 minutes).

Type 3: Giant hemangiomas show a type 3 pattern in which there is a failure to completely fill in and no enhancement of the central scar even on very delayed images up to 15 minutes **(Figs. 10A to F)**.[19,20]

Hemangiomas need to be differentiated from hypervascular metastases which are T2 hyperintense and arterially enhanced. Metastases usually demonstrate a target pattern of enhancement rather than a discontinuous rim seen in hemangiomas. The arterial enhancing rim in metastasis shows a washout in the portal venous phase.

With hepatocyte specific agents (HSA), hemangiomas show a hypointense appearance during the hepatocyte phase owing to the lack of hepatocytes within the lesion.[21] Since hemangiomas lack Kupffer cells, one would expect no signal drop with superparamagnetic iron oxide (SPIO)

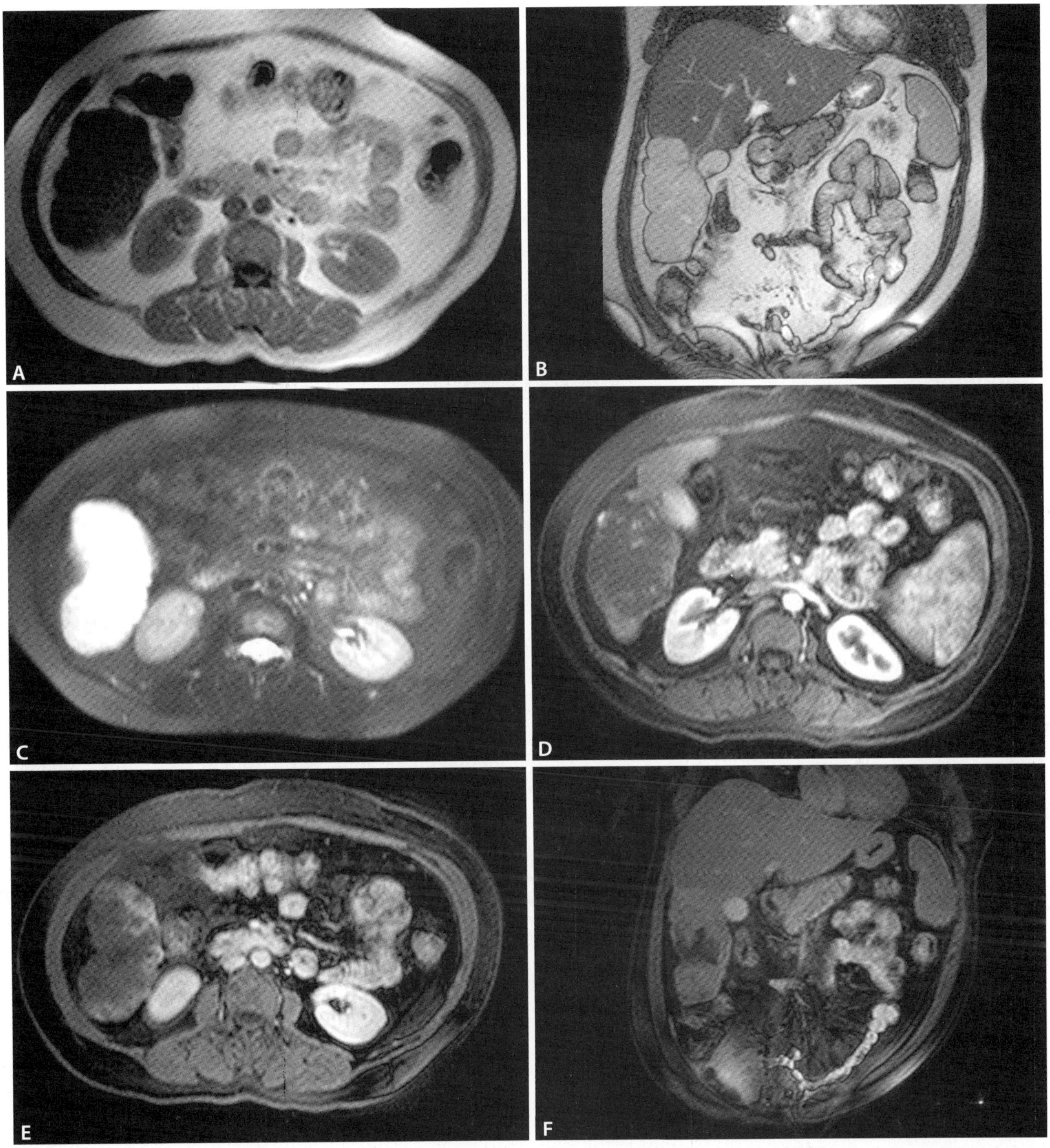

Figs. 10A to F: (A) T1W MR image showing an exophytic hepatic lesion hypointense on T1; (B) T2W image shows the lesion to be markedly hyperintense; (C) Marked hyperintensity seen with increasing TE value "light bulb appearance; (D and E) Postcontrast images showing the lesion with incomplete fill in; (F) No enhancement of the central scar seen even on delayed images—exophytic giant cavernous hemangioma

agents (ferucarbotran, ferumoxide) on a T2W image but a delayed drop in signal intensity (10–40 minutes) is seen owing to the blood pool phase of these agents. This blood pooling effect of SPIO is also seen in sclerosed or hyalinized type of hemangiomas. This finding helps to differentiate a hemangioma from metastases, as metastases do not show a drop in signal intensity as the blood pooling effect in metastases is negligible. On DWI, hemangiomas show a very high signal on ADC maps and a decrease in signal with increasing b values.[22] This pulse sequence along with contrast-enhanced MR can help in the differentiation between hemangiomas and cystic metastases.

FOCAL NODULAR HYPERPLASIA

It is the second most common benign liver tumor after hemangiomas, usually smaller than 5 cm with a mean diameter of 3 cm. When it involves an entire lobe, it is known as lobar focal nodular hyperplasia (FNH).[2]

Pathogenesis

A vascular etiology has been postulated as a congenital vascular malformation has been proposed to trigger hepatocyte hyperplasia. It has been suggested that hepatocyte hyperplasia occurs secondary to an increased arterial flow. This theory of pathogenesis is supported by the fact that FNH has been found in association with cavernous hemangiomas, vascular malformations elsewhere and with brain neoplasms.[12] As FNH is more common in women in 3rd–5th decade, a hormonal activity has also been proposed. Estrogens have been found to cause an increase in the size of the nodules (trophic effect). A regression in the size has been seen following the withdrawal of oral contraceptives suggesting a link between FNH and oral contraceptives (OCs).

Pathology

Focal nodular hyperplasia (FNH) is a well-circumscribed, nonencapsulated solitary lesion characterized by a stellate central scar. Histologically, it is composed of hepatocytes, bile duct elements, Kupffer cells and fibrous tissue. However, in FNH, the biliary elements are not connected with the normal biliary tree. FNH is classified into classic and nonclassic types. The classic form is the solid type containing the central scar. Malformed vessels and a nodular architecture are features of the classic type. Histologically, there are cellular areas of hepatic proliferation along with fibrosis. The nonclassic type is further subdivided as the (i) telangiectatic type (ii) FNH with cytologic atypia (iii) mixed hyperplastic and adenomatous FNH. A nodular architecture may be absent in the nonclassic form but it always shows bile duct proliferation. Of these, the telangiectatic variety is characterized by dilated blood filled spaces. In this type of FNH, the arteries are abnormal with a hypertrophic muscular layer and drain directly into the adjacent sinusoids. Necrosis and hemorrhage are common in this form. The other subtype contains areas of large cell dysplasia while the adenomatous form simulates an adenoma. Multiple lesions along with other lesions such as liver hemangiomas, meningiomas, astrocytomas, dysplastic systemic arteries and portal vein atresia constitutes the *multiple FNH syndrome*.[12]

Clinical Features

The FNH is more common in women in 3rd to 5th decade, though they occur at any age and in both males and females. Less than one third of the patients are symptomatic. Symptoms occur only when the lesions are very large in size and cause abdominal pain due to the expansion of Glisson's capsule or mass effect. Most of the lesions are asymptomatic and discovered incidentally on routine imaging.

Imaging Features

USG: FNH are usually seen as isoechoic homogeneous lesions usually identified only by the mass effect they exert **(Figs. 11A to C)**. Displacement of hepatic vessels may be the only identifiable abnormality. A hypoechoic halo seen around the lesion is due to the compressed liver parenchyma. Rarely they may be heterogeneous; a central scar may also be seen in larger lesions. When seen the central scar is usually hyperechoic. A stellate or spoke wheel pattern is seen corresponding to arteries running into radiating fibrous septa from the central scar on color Doppler. Spectral analysis reveals arterial waveform with a good diastolic flow and low resistive index. A continuous waveform from a draining vein may also be identified. On contrast-enhanced ultrosonography (CEUS), the lesion shows enhancement in the arterial phase and is isoechoic to the liver in the portal venous phase and beyond. On delayed imaging there is accumulation of contrast within the central scar.[23]

CT: FNH has been called a "stealth lesion" as it is not visualized on a noncontrast CT. It is a hypervascular lesion supplied by an enlarged anomalous hepatic artery and its drainage is always into the hepatic veins. The lesion shows intense enhancement in the arterial phase with a washout in the venous phase where it becomes isodense to the liver parenchyma. The central scar remains hypodense in the arterial or venous phases and shows accumulation of contrast only on the delayed images. The intratumoral vascularization of FNH is well demonstrated by 3D CT angiography which shows an arterial vessel leading directly into the lesion, lack of portal venous supply and presence of hepatic venous drainage.[24]

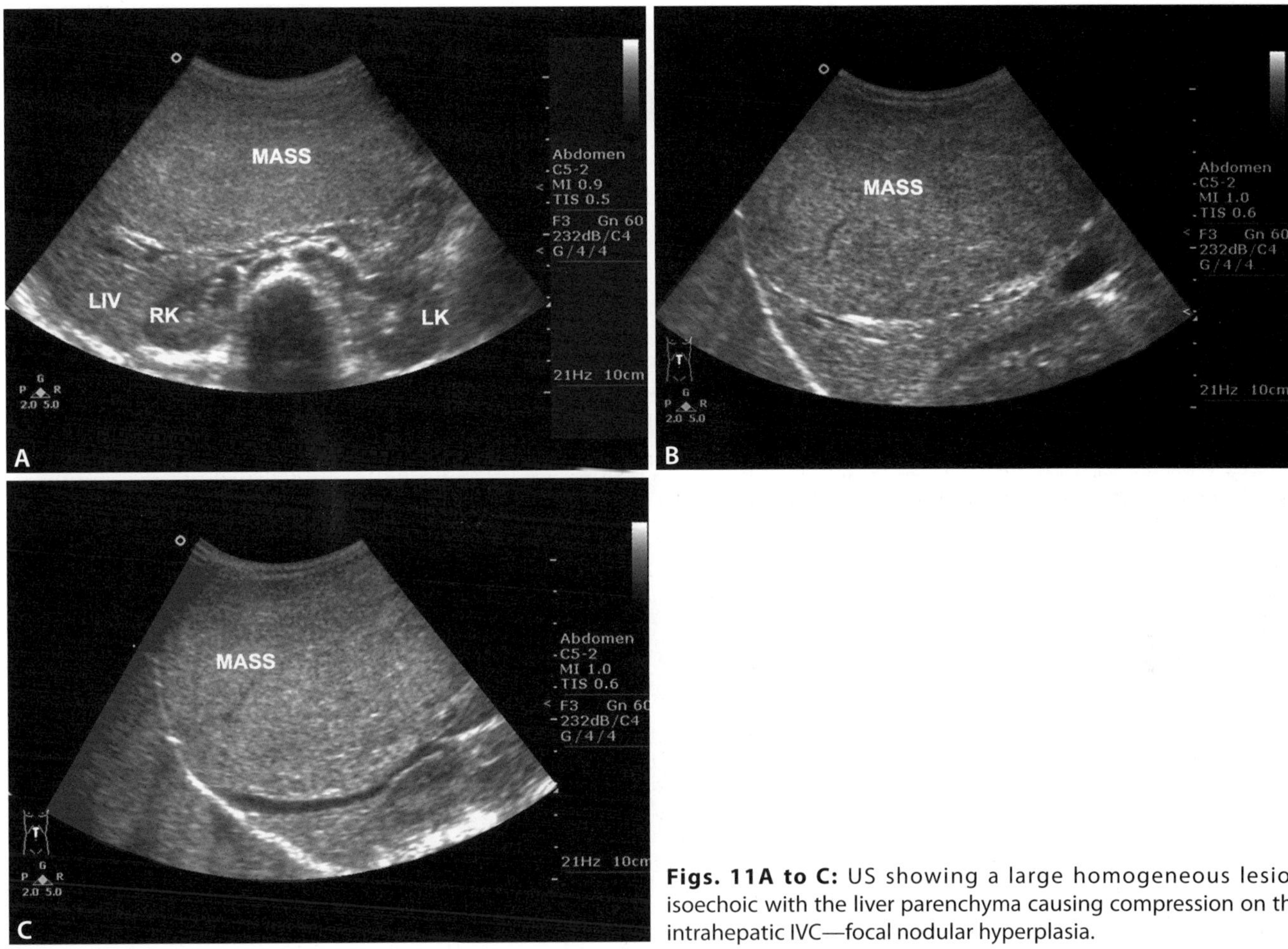

Figs. 11A to C: US showing a large homogeneous lesion isoechoic with the liver parenchyma causing compression on the intrahepatic IVC—focal nodular hyperplasia.

MRI: FNH shows a hypointense signal on T1W images and is hyperintense on T2W images. The central stellate radiating scar has a hyperintense signal on the T2W images owing to its vascular and myxoid tissue component. This is in contrast to the central scar seen in fibrolamellar hepatocellular carcinoma (HCC) which shows a low signal on both T1 and T2-weighted images owing to its fibrous nature.[25] A rapid enhancement in the arterial phase followed by a washout with the lesion becoming isointense in the venous phase is observed on administration of gadolinium. The central scar shows a delayed and persistent accumulation of contrast **(Figs. 12A to E)**.[26]

As a well-formed canalicular system is deficient in FNH, FNH shows a prolonged and excessive accumulation of Gd-BOPTA while adenomas show a hypointense appearance on delayed images owing to lack of bile ducts.[27,28] Other hepatocyte specific contrast agents like gadoxetate disodium can also be used. FNH contains Kupffer cells while adenomas do not. SPIO is a contrast agent that undergoes phagocytosis by the Kupffer cells. Hence in FNH there is a pronounced uptake of SPIO which shows a marked drop in signal intensity on T2W images while in adenomas a poor uptake of SPIO is seen due to lack of Kupffer cells.[29] SPIO also helps in differentiating between FNH and fibrolamellar HCC as the fibrolamellar carcinoma lacks Kupffer cells and shows no uptake of SPIO.

On DWI, FNH show a restricted diffusion with reported ADC values between 1 and 1.40 × $10^{-3}mm^2/s$ cm/s. However, these ADC values may also be seen in adenomas and malignant lesions.[22]

Differentiation between FNH and hepatocellular adenoma: FNH is usually managed conservatively while adenomas require resection due to their propensity for hemorrhage and hence the need for differentiation between FNH and adenomas.[2,3] A T1 isointensity, a homogeneous appearance, presence of central scar, a pronounced

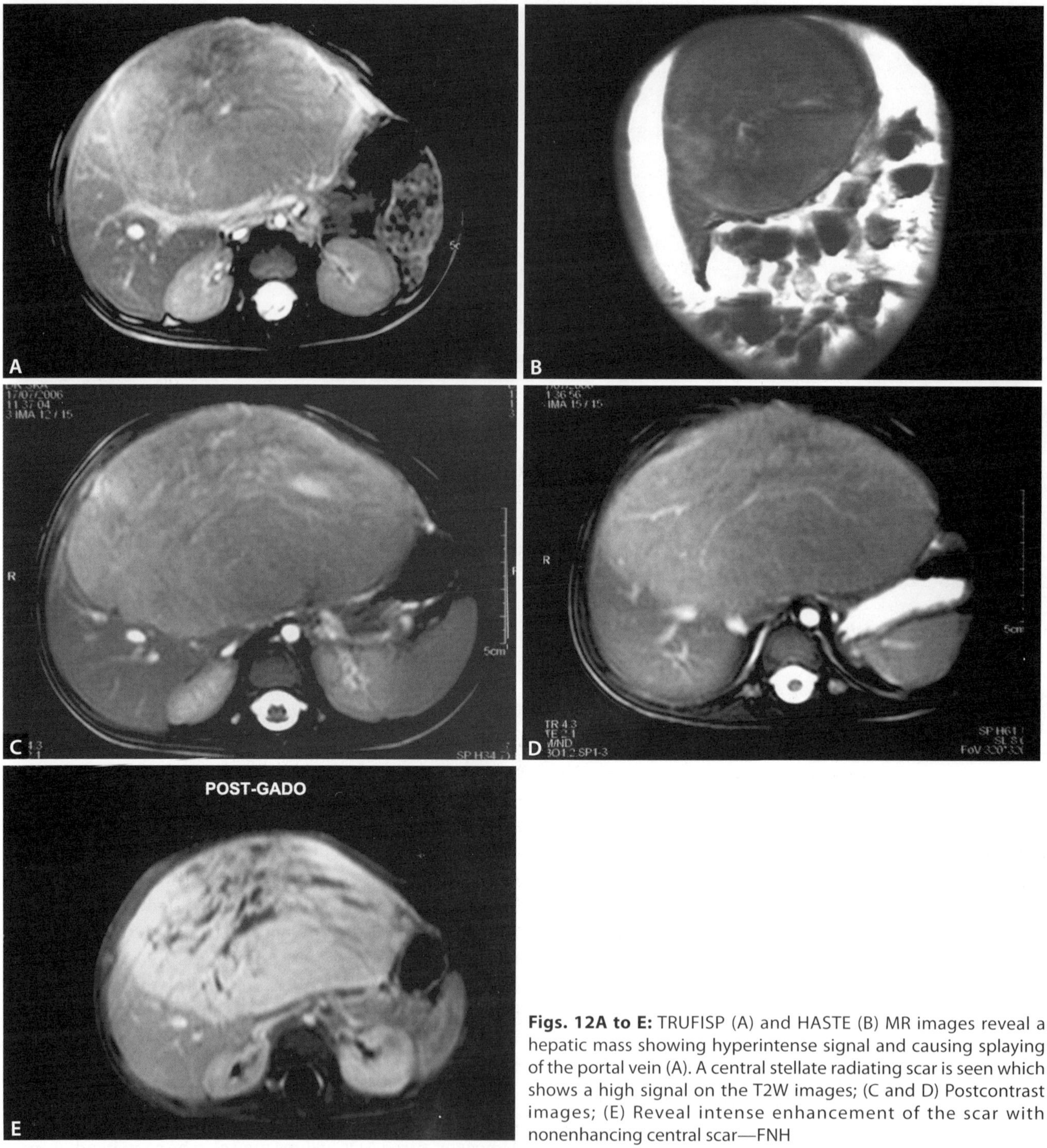

Figs. 12A to E: TRUFISP (A) and HASTE (B) MR images reveal a hepatic mass showing hyperintense signal and causing splaying of the portal vein (A). A central stellate radiating scar is seen which shows a high signal on the T2W images; (C and D) Postcontrast images; (E) Reveal intense enhancement of the scar with nonenhancing central scar—FNH

persistent hyperintensity with Gd-BOPTA, a marked uptake of SPIO are features suggestive of FNH while T1 hyperintensity, heterogeneity of the lesion, low uptake of SPIO and absence of enhancement with Gd-BOPTA are features of adenomas.

Differentiation between FNH and fibrolamellar carcinoma: A large size (>10 cm), tumor heterogeneity, a large scar (>2 cm), lymphadenopathy, invasion of adjacent vessels, calcification and metastases favors a diagnosis of fibrolamellar HCC.

	Focal nodular hyperplasia (FNH)	Hepatocellular adenoma (HA)	Fibrolamellar carcinoma
T1	Isointense	Hyperintense	Heterogeneously hypointense
Homogeneity	Homogeneous	Heterogeneous	Heterogeneous with central stellate calcification
Central scar	Present but < 2 cm, T2 hyperintense, rarely shows calcification	Absent	Large central scar > 2 cm, T2 hypointense, calcification common
Uptake of hepatocyte specific agents (HSA)	A pronounced persistent hyperintensity with HSA	Absence of enhancement	Absence of enhancement
SPIO	Pronounced uptake	Low uptake	No uptake
Invasion of adjacent organs	Absent	Absent	Present
Lymphade-nopathy	Absent	Absent	Present
Metastases	Absent	Absent	Present

HEPATOCELLULAR ADENOMA/ HEPATIC ADENOMA

Hepatocellular adenoma is an uncommon solid primary liver tumor. It is usually large in size (>10 cm) and is solitary. Hepatocellular adenomatosis is a rare condition in which multiple (>10) adenomas occur involving both lobes of liver.[30]

Pathogenesis

Although the exact pathogenesis is unknown, it is postulated that the development of adenomas, their number and size shows a definite relationship with the use of oral contraceptives in women and that of anabolic steroids in men. The dose and duration of intake also has a role with the annual incidence of adenoma reported to be 1 per million in women who have never been on oral contraceptives as compared to 30–40 per million in women on long term use.[31] Other associations include type I glycogen storage disease and Von-Gierke's disease where the possible mechanisms include glycogen/ insulin imbalance and glycogen overload.[31]

Abnormalities of the hepatic vasculature like absence or occlusion of the portal vein or porto-hepatic venous shunts have also been proposed in the etiopathogenesis particularly in patients with adenomatosis where the adenomas are non-steroid dependent, more prone to hemorrhage and malignant degeneration and are progressive in size. A genetic alteration has also been suggested with mutation of the HNF-1α gene and a β-catenin mutation found in patients with adenomas.

Pathology

Histologically, adenomas consist of atypical hepatocytes with areas of bile stasis, necrosis or hemorrhage. The hepatocytes are typically arranged in cords. Adenoma cells are larger than normal hepatocytes owing to their glycogen and lipid content. Intracellular and intercellular lipid present in the tumor accounts for its yellow appearance on cut section and the presence of fat is useful in its diagnosis on imaging studies. Adenomas lack Kupffer cells and bile ductules.[31] *The notable absence of bile ducts is a key distinguishing feature between adenomas and FNH on histology.* The tumor lacks portal tracts and terminal hepatic veins which accounts for its propensity to hemorrhage. Owing to the lack of a portal venous supply, adenomas are perfused directly from peripheral arterial feeding vessels. The feeding arteries and the extensive sinusoids make adenomas a hypervascular lesion. The high arterial pressure coupled with a poor support from the connective tissue makes these tumors prone to hemorrhage which may spread into the liver or the peritoneal cavity due to the lack of a true tumor capsule.

Different subtypes of HCAs have been described, 50% of adenomas are classified into a *inflammatory subtype* characterized by inflammatory infiltrates, sinusoidal dilatation and thick walled arteries.[32] The inflammatory subtype was earlier called the telangiectatic variety. The second most common subtype (30–35%) is the HNF-1α inactivated type. HNF-1α subtypes are also called *steatotic adenomas* because of their diffuse lipid content.[12] The β-catenin mutated subtype accounts for 10–15% of cases, is usually seen in men and is associated with anabolic steroids. This subtype also carries the risk of malignant transformation.[32] The reported incidence of malignant transformation in adenomas is 7%.[12]

Clinical Features

Most are asymptomatic and discovered incidentally on routine imaging. Some may present with a right upper quadrant fullness, usually seen in larger lesions. The classical clinical presentation is however acute abdominal pain caused by spontaneous hemorrhage or rupture leading to hypotension and even death in some cases.

Imaging Features

USG: Adenomas are echogenic masses, the echogenicity being attributed to the fat and glycogen content. They may have a heterogeneous appearance due to areas of hemorrhage and fibrosis. One third of the lesions may show a pseudocapsule, seen as a hypoechoic peripheral rim on USG. Color Doppler US may reveal intratumoral arteries which is a helpful differentiating feature from FNH. On CEUS, perilesional arteries are seen as intense enhancement around the lesion, rapid intense enhancement followed by an isoechogenicity due to wash out is highly diagnostic of an adenoma.[33]

CT: On noncontrast scans, adenomas are seen as isodense or hypodense lesions **(Figs. 13A to D)** due to presence of fat and glycogen within.[34] They may be heterogeneous due to intratumoral hemorrhage. On contrast administration, an early and rapid enhancement is seen during the arterial phase with the lesion becoming isodense on the portal venous phase. The enhancement does not persist owing to an arteriovenous shunting. A pseudocapsule may be seen in the larger lesions as a hypodense rim on the noncontrast scans and a hyperdense rim on the equilibrium phase[35] **(Figs. 14A to F)**.

MRI: Adenomas are usually T1 isointense or hyperintense lesions due to the presence of fat or glycogen content. On administration of gadolinium, these lesions exhibit an intense enhancement in the arterial phase followed by an isointensity in the venous phase. The lack of uptake of hepatospecific MR contrast like Gd-BOPTA, MnDPDP and SPIO helps to differentiate an adenoma from FNH which shows a pronounced uptake.[36] It is important to differentiate an adenoma from a hepatocellular carcinoma since both may contain intralesional fat (up to 40% HCC) and both show arterial hyperenhancement. The clinical history including patient demographics, any risk factors for HCC as well as a cirrhotic liver background help in the differentiation.[37]

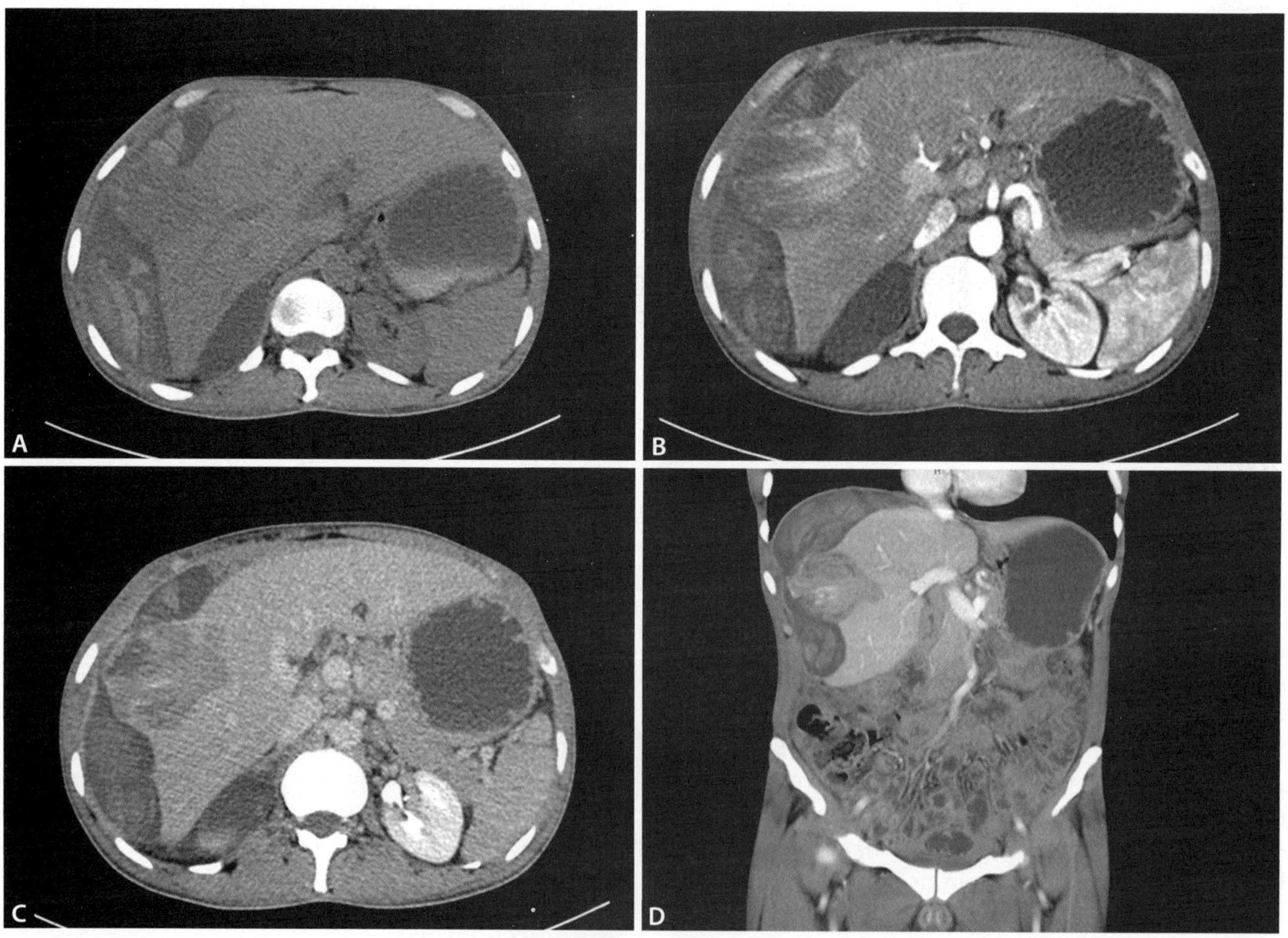

Figs. 13A to D: Noncontrast CT (A) shows a heterogeneous lesion in the liver with an exophytic component with evidence of subcapsular and subhepatic bleed. On contrast administration, an early and rapid enhancement in the arterial phase; (B) with the lesion becoming isodense in the portal venous phase; (C and D) is seen. Hepatocellular adenoma with hemorrhage.

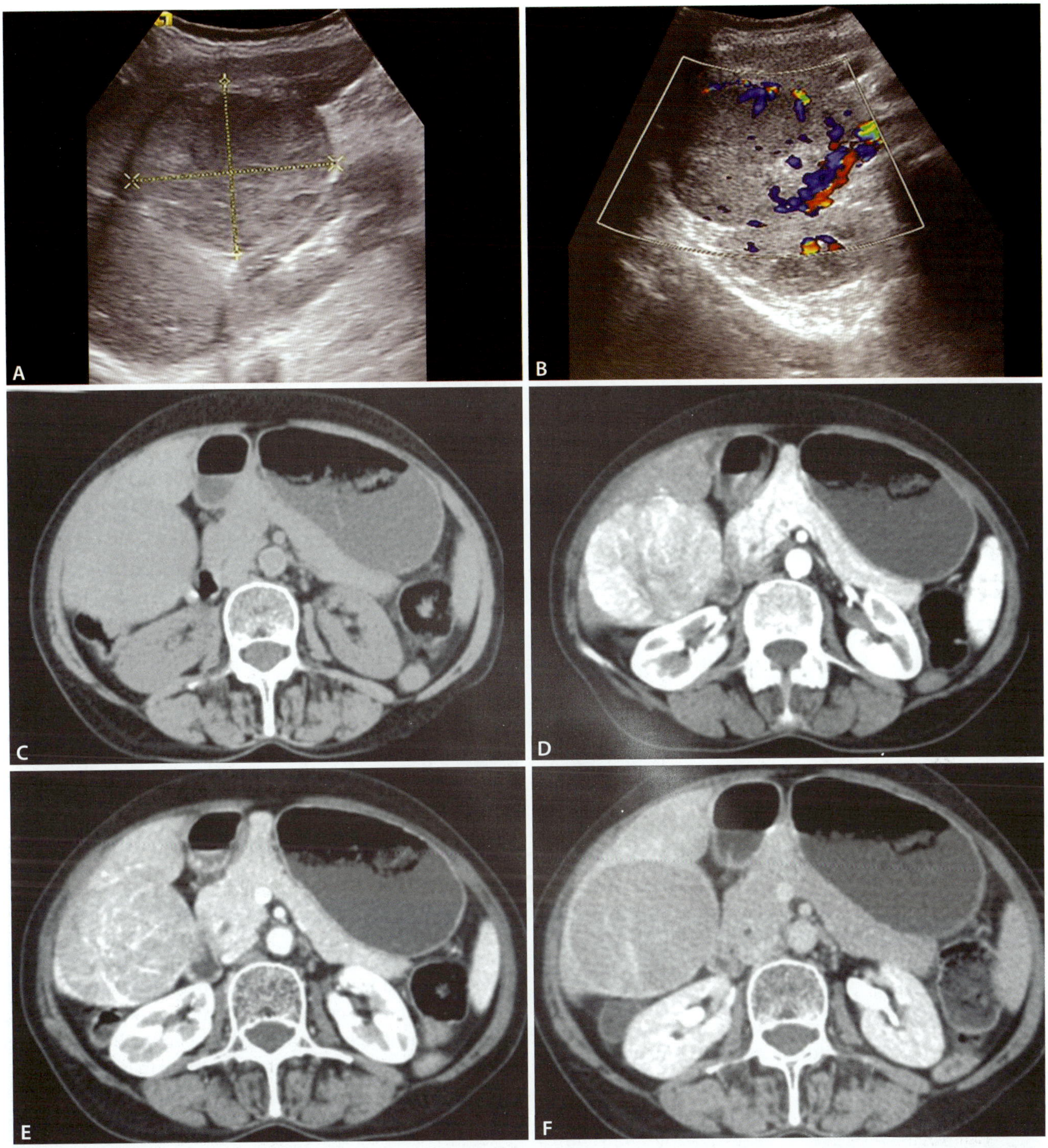

Figs. 14A to F: US showing a well-defined predominantly echogenic mass in the liver: with evidence of perilesional vascularity on color Doppler (A); NCCT scan (B); the mass to be isodense with the liver parenchyma, intensely enhancing in the arterial phase (C); becoming isodense in the portal venous phase (D); and hypodense in the equilibrium phase (E); Pseudocapsule can be seen in the delayed image as a hyperdense rim (F)—hepatocellular adenoma.

Since the HNF-1α inactivated subtype has the lowest risk of malignant transformation while the β-catenin mutated subtype has the highest risk, an attempt has been made by investigators to differentiate the subtypes on the basis of MR imaging.[12,32] Diffuse intralesional fat detected on chemical shift imaging (CSI) is characteristic of the HNF-1α inactivated subtype while marked T2 hyperintensity and strong arterial phase enhancement that persists on delayed images is highly suggestive of the inflammatory subtype. A characteristic "atoll sign" corresponding to a peripheral rim of hyperintensity and a central area of isointensity is seen in inflammatory hepatocellular adenomas (HCAs) resembling a coral atoll.[32] Scars and poorly defined T2 hyperintense areas suggest β-catenin mutated subtype.

Adenomas show a restricted pattern of diffusion though it may be seen in malignant lesions and FNH as well.[38] Management strategy for adenomas includes a lesion characterization by MRI as (i) steatotic (ii) heterogeneous (iii) nonsteatotic. If the patient is on oral contraceptives or anabolic steroids, a discontinuation of these followed by repeat imaging at 3–6 months is recommended.[32] If the adenomas are seen to regress, a follow-up is indicated, while in the growing lesions further evaluation is warranted. Surgical resection is recommended for large lesions (>5 cm) and those found in association with glycogen storage disease owing to an increased risk of malignant transformation.

NODULAR REGENERATIVE HYPERPLASIA

Nodular regenerative hyperplasia (NRH) is a condition characterized by multiple nodules replacing the hepatic parenchyma without the formation of fibrous septa within the nodules. The absence of fibrosis differentiates this condition from the regenerating nodules of cirrhosis.

Pathogenesis

The causes of NRH are varied. Various myeloproliferative disorders, rheumatologic disorders, steroids and anti-neoplastic drugs have been implicated as the causative factors. Association with portal hypertension is also seen.[39]

Clinical Features

The mean age of occurrence is around 50 years with no gender predilection. Children may be affected by this disorder when associated with congenital absence of the portal vein.

Imaging Features

US: In most cases NRH is not seen on ultrasound, the lesions being isoechoic with the adjacent liver parenchyma.[40] At times, isoechoic or hypoechoic nodules are seen. Color Doppler demonstrates arterial supply within the nodules.

CT: The CT appearance of NRH may range from that of a normal liver to focal hypoattenuating nodules ranging from 0.1 to 3 cm. The nodules enhance homogeneously after administration of contrast.

MRI: The lesions are typically isointense to the liver parenchyma on T1-weighted image while on a T2-weighted image the nodules appear iso or hypointense. The nodules show enhancement in the arterial phase. On the portal venous and equilibrium phases of contrast-enhanced dynamic MR imaging the lesions remain iso to slightly hyperintense.

On administration of Gd BOPTA, the lesions remain hyperintense owing to an abnormal biliary drainage. The presence of abundant Kupffer cells within the nodules accounts for a significant uptake of SPIO.

ADENOMATOUS HYPERPLASTIC NODULE

Adenomatous hyperplastic nodules (AHN) are benign but premalignant lesions usually seen in cirrhotic livers. They are also known as dysplastic nodules or macroregenerative nodules. They appear hyperintense on T1-weighted images and hypointense on T2W images. Dysplastic nodules that accumulate iron have a greater malignant potential owing to the tumor enhancing effects of iron.[41] Hepatocellular carcinoma (HCC) are hyperintense on T2W images, a finding that differentiates a dysplastic nodule from HCC. HCC are supplied by hepatic artery whereas dysplastic nodules have portal venous supply.[42]

The presence of "nodule within nodule appearance" consisting of a hyperintense nodule developing within a hypointense dysplastic nodule on T2W images is highly suspicious for the development of malignancy within the nodule.

PEDIATRIC LIVER TUMORS

Mesenchymal Hamartoma

Mesenchymal hamartoma is a benign cystic developmental lesion seen in the pediatric population. It is the second most common benign liver tumor occurring in the pediatric age group. Usually seen in children under the age of 2 years, it occurs twice as often in boys than girls.

Pathology

Mesenchymal hamartoma is a well-defined large encapsulated or pedunculated tumor.[43] It consists of gelatinous mesenchymal tissue with cyst formation and remnants of normal hepatic parenchyma and hence have a mixed solid cystic appearance in majority of the cases. They may have a predominantly cystic appearance if the cystic component predominates and solid appearance if the mesenchymal component predominates.

Clinical Features

Patients typically present with a gradually progressive enlarging abdominal distention. They may eventually develop vomiting, diarrhea or constipation as the mass enlarges. Respiratory distress may occur due to a mass effect on the diaphragm.

Imaging Features

USG: Usually seen as a well-circumscribed multilocular solid cystic lesion **(Figs. 15A and B)**. The cystic spaces are separated by echogenic septae.[44] The lesion may rarely have a solid appearance if the mesenchymal component predominates.

CT: It is seen as a multi-septated mass of water attenuation. The thin internal septations may show contrast enhancement. No calcification or hemorrhage is seen in these lesions **(Figs. 16A and B)**.

MRI: On MRI, the cystic component of the lesion is markedly hyperintense on T2W images while the mesenchymal (stromal) component is hypointense on both T1W images and T2W images **(Figs. 17A to C)**.[45,46]

INFANTILE HEPATIC HEMANGIOMA

Formerly, known as infantile hemangioendothelioma, infantile hepatic hemangioma is the most common benign hepatic tumor occurring in infants with females affected more commonly than males.[47]

Pathogenesis

Three subtypes of infantile hepatic hemangiomas have been described, the focal, multifocal and the diffuse types.

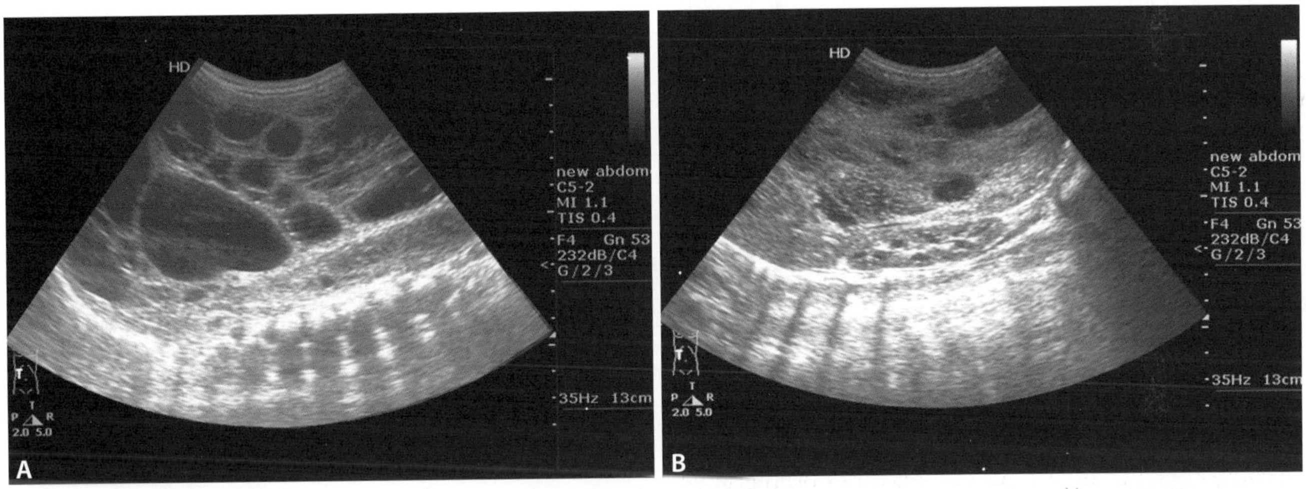

Figs. 15A and B: US shows a mixed solid cystic lesion within the liver in an infant—mesenchymal hamartoma.

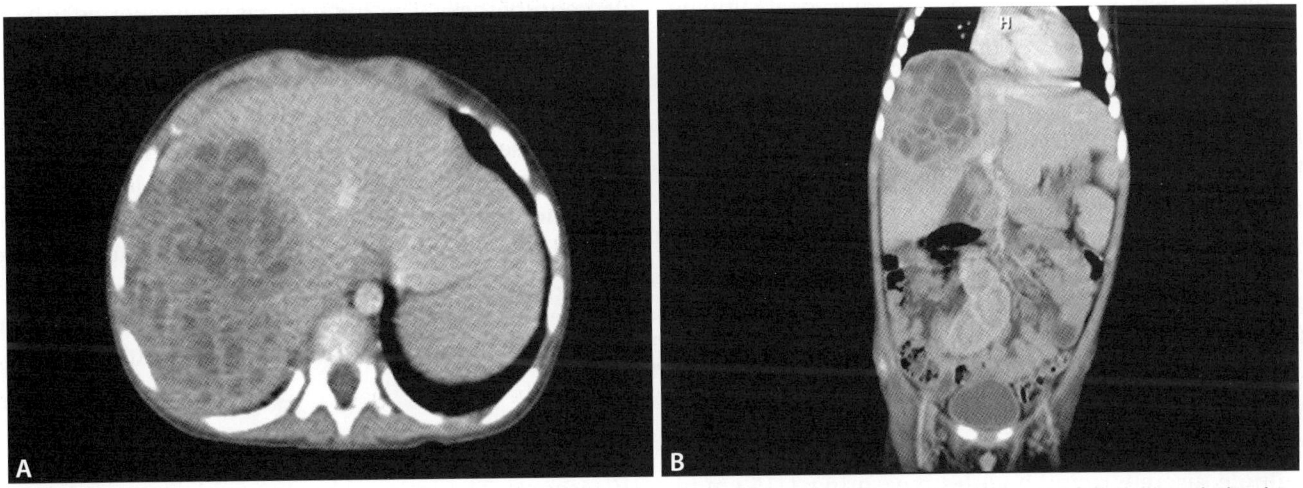

Figs. 16A and B: CT axial (A) and coronal (B) scans showing a multiseptated mass of water attenuation within the liver with the thin internal septations showing enhancement—mesenchymal hamartoma.

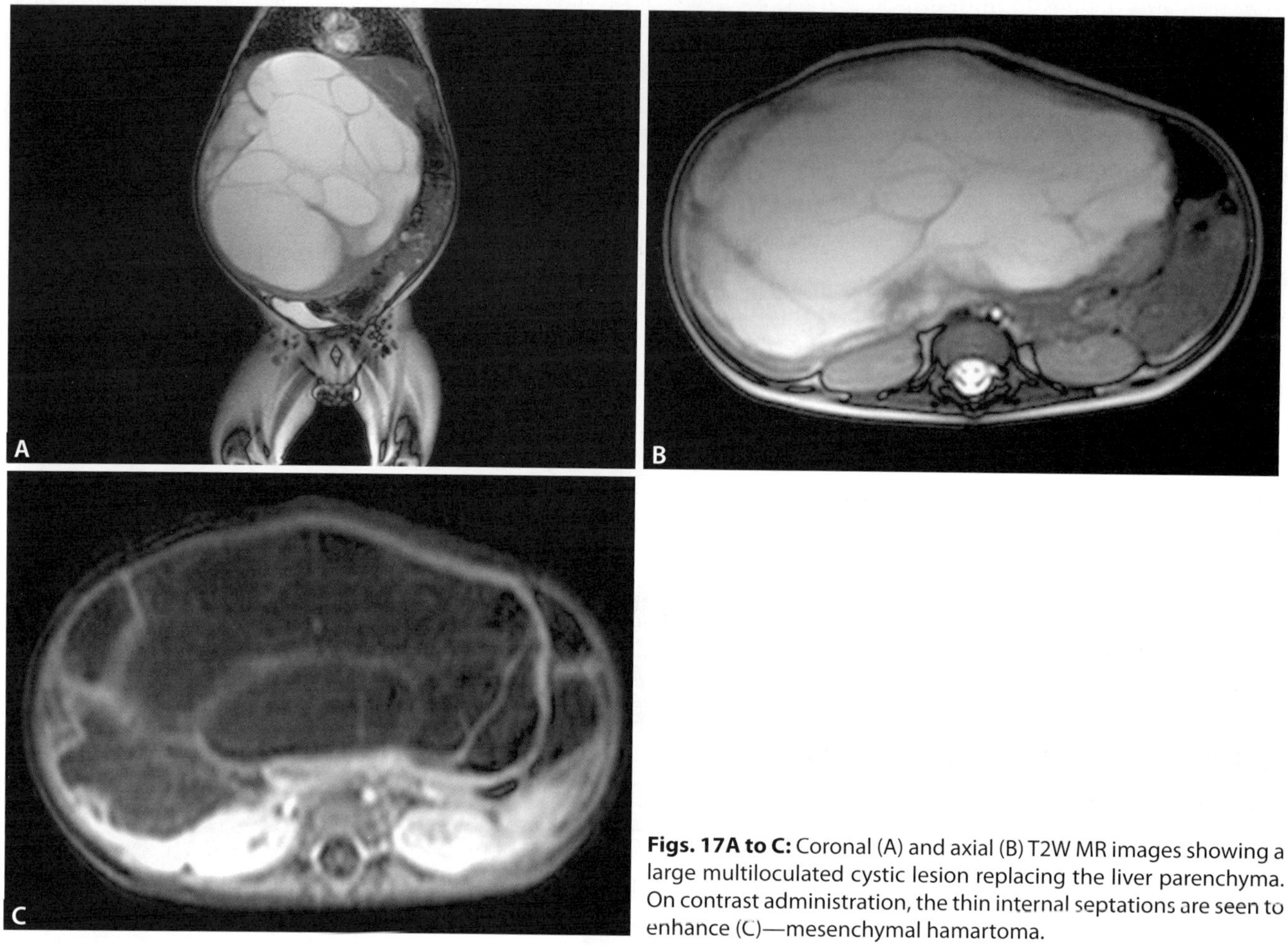

Figs. 17A to C: Coronal (A) and axial (B) T2W MR images showing a large multiloculated cystic lesion replacing the liver parenchyma. On contrast administration, the thin internal septations are seen to enhance (C)—mesenchymal hamartoma.

While the focal subtype is thought to be the hepatic form of rapidly involuting congenital hemangioma (RICH), the multifocal subtype is thought to be the hepatic form of simple cutaneous hemangioma. The multifocal subtype is often associated with multiple cutaneous hemangiomas in the same patient. Histopathologic antibody staining of endothelial cells in RICH is negative for glucose transporter protein 1 (GLUT 1) while it is positive in the multifocal variety similar to the cutaneous infantile hemangioma. The diffuse subtype is characterized by almost complete replacement of the hepatic parenchyma by infantile hemangiomas. These patients present with a large palpable abdominal mass and high output failure due to arteriovenous shunting.

Pathology

On gross examination, the tumor is composed of multiple discrete round nodules measuring 2–15 cm in diameter. Microscopically, two histological types have been described—the type 1 has vascular spaces lined by endothelial cells and supported by reticular fibers. Type 2 has larger, irregular spaces lined by immature pleomorphic cells. The 2nd type has been reported to have some malignant potential.

Clinical Features

90% of these lesions occur during the first 6 months of life. Affected infants may present with a palpable abdominal mass and bruit. Arteriovenous shunting occurring within the lesion may cause congestive heart failure in these infants. Occasionally, spontaneous rupture may lead to a massive hemoperitoneum or rarely thrombocytopenia due to platelet sequestration (Kasabach-Merritt syndrome) may occur.

Imaging Features

Ultrasound: The lesions show variable echogenicity, it may be highly echogenic, hypoechoic or anechoic with echogenic septa. Like hemangiomas, the increased echogenicity is attributable to the multiple interfaces that exist between the vascular spaces. A narrowing of the abdominal aorta below the origin of the coeliac axis, a dilated coeliac axis and common hepatic artery and prominent draining hepatic veins forms a characteristic imaging finding of infantile hepatic hemangiomas seen on color Doppler. These vascular abnormalities do not occur in a malignant hepatic tumor.[48]

CT: Noncontrast scans show the liver to be enlarged with multiple hypodense lesions within. Calcification may be seen in 40% cases. Contrast enhancement reveals a peripheral and centripetal enhancement followed by a prolonged and persistent enhancement on delayed scans similar to that seen in hemangiomas **(Figs. 18A to C)**. CT angiography depicts the dilated coeliac axis artery and narrowing of the aorta below its origin.

MRI: The lesions are typically hypointense on T1W images and hyperintense on T2W images with the contrast enhancement pattern similar to hemangiomas.[49]

UNUSUAL BENIGN TUMORS OF THE LIVER

Lipomatous Tumors

These include lipomas, angiomyolipomas and myelolipomas depending on fat, myeloid and vascular tissue component.[50]

Pathology

On gross examination, lipomas are solitary, well circumscribed masses containing variable amount of adipose, smooth muscle tissue and thick-walled blood vessels. The presence of prominent hematopoietic tissue makes it a myelolipomas or angiomyolipoma.

Clinical Features

Angiomyolipomas are rare benign tumors of the liver. They usually do not cause any symptoms and are solitary. Rarely, patients may present with abdominal pain owing to bleeding within these tumors. Multiple liver angiomyolipomas which are progressive and symptomatic occur in association with Bourneville-Pringle syndrome.

Imaging Features

USG: This lipomatous tumors are highly echogenic on US owing to their fat content. Differentiation from hepatic hemangioma is difficult although a mixed hyper hypoechoic pattern may be seen at times.

CT: Fat attenuation values (–20 to –115 HU are) typically seen on the noncontrast scans with a variable enhancement seen on contrast administration depending on the vascular component within **(Fig. 19)**.[50]

MRI: These tumors are seen to have a high signal on both T1- and T2-weighted images owing to the fat content. On the fat suppressed sequences, signal suppression with a hypointense appearance is seen. A signal drop seen on the opposed phase images during chemical shift imaging (CSI) suggests the presence of both macroscopic and microscopic fat.

LEIOMYOMAS

Leiomyomas are extremely rare benign hepatic tumors. They arise from the smooth muscles as solitary, well-circumscribed masses. An association has been seen

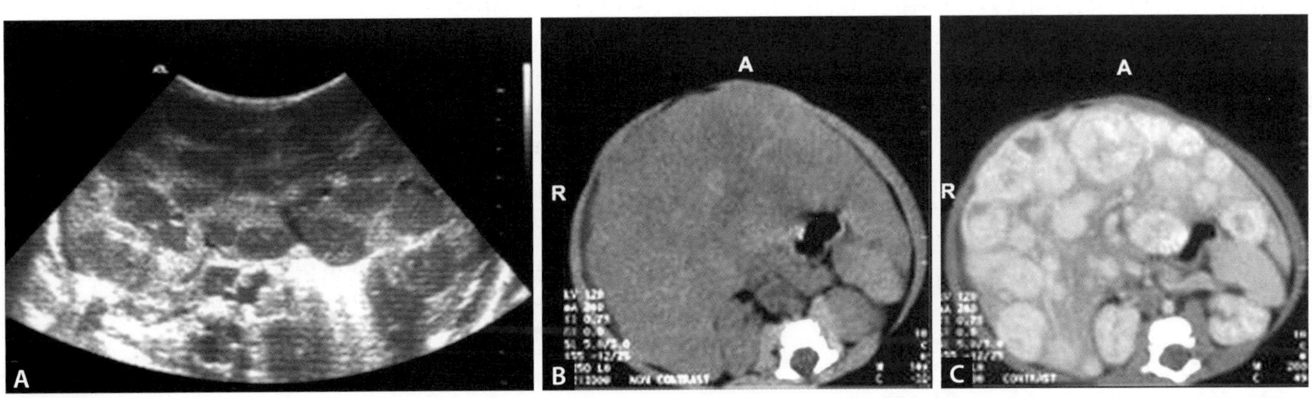

Figs. 18A to C: (A) US scan shows multiple hypoechoic lesions within the liver; (B) Noncontrast CT scan showing the liver to be enlarged with multiple hypodense lesions within; (C) Contrast-enhanced CT reveals peripheral and centripetal enhancement of the lesions—infantile hepatic hemangioma.

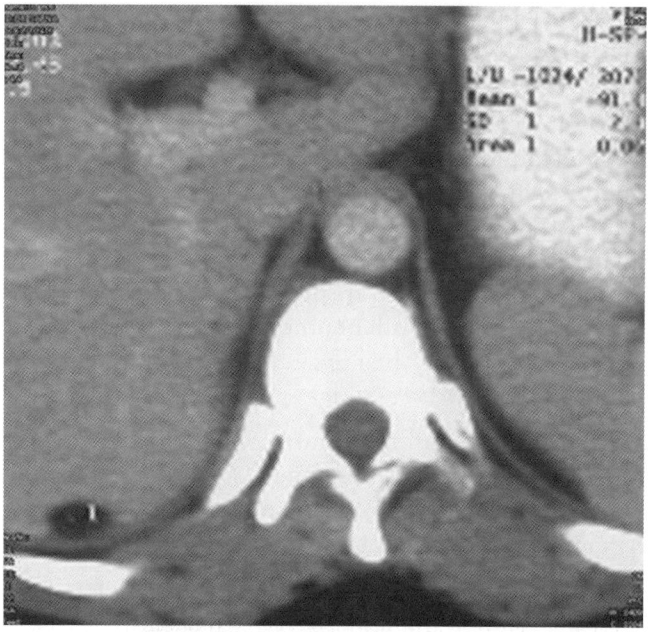

Fig. 19: CT image shows a small hypoattenuating lesion with fat attenuation value within the right lobe of liver—lipoma.

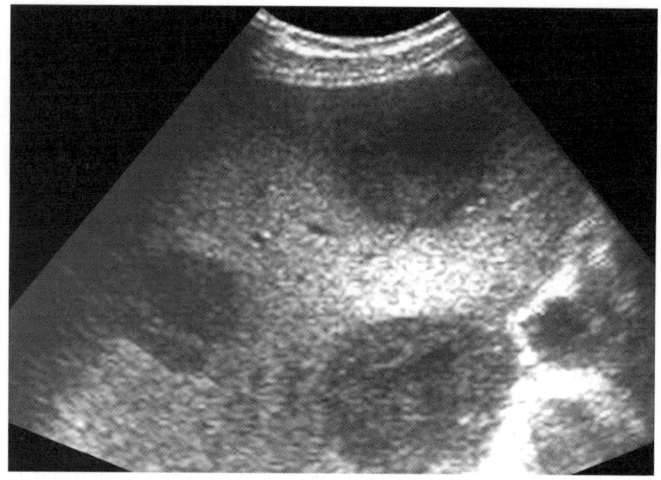

Fig. 20: US scan showing three lesions in the liver with well-defined walls and echoes within giving a solid appearance—pyogenic liver abscesses.

between HIV infection and leiomyomas as these have been reported in adults and children infected with the virus.

Imaging Features

USG: Leiomyomas appear as solid, hypoechoic masses with internal echoes.

CT: These appear as low attenuation masses on noncontrast scans with two distinct patterns of enhancement seen on contrast administration, a peripheral rim enhancement and a delayed homogeneous enhancement.

MRI: Leiomyomas are seen to have a hypointense signal on T1, a hyperintense signal on T2WI with an enhancement pattern similar to that seen on CT on contrast administration.

Paraganglioma

Paragangliomas are rare tumors of neural crest origin. Though usually seen along the sympathetic chain, these may very rarely be seen in the liver.[31] On imaging these are seen as well circumscribed lesions with intense contrast enhancement. Cystic areas and calcification may be seen.

INFECTIVE LESIONS

Bacterial (Pyogenic) Liver Abscess

A liver abscess may develop from several routes. The most common route is the biliary route owing to cholangitis secondary to obstructive biliopathy. Other routes include phlebitis of the portal or superior mesenteric vein secondary to appendicitis, diverticulitis, pancreatitis and other gastrointestinal infections. A direct extension from contiguous organs, arterial septicemia secondary to osteomyelitis, endocarditis, pneumonitis, a post-traumatic or an iatrogenic cause may also be the source of a liver abscess. A cryptogenic abscess may develop in patients with diabetes mellitus with no apparent source of infection. While abscesses of biliary origin are often multiple involving both lobes, abscess from the portal vein are often solitary and in 65% cases occur in the right lobe. *Staphylococcus* is the most common causative organism in children while *Escherichia coli* is the most common in adults.[51]

Clinical Features

The clinical symptoms include fever, pain in the right upper quadrant, nausea and vomiting and malaise. A tender hepatomegaly is seen with leukocytosis being the most common laboratory abnormality.

Imaging Features

Plain film findings: Elevation of the right hemidiaphragm, hepatomegaly, right pleural effusion and atelectasis may be seen in case of a large abscess.

USG: US can detect hepatic abscesses as small as 1.5 cm with a sensitivity of about 90%. They appear as well-defined lesions with thick, irregular walls **(Fig. 20)**. They are variable in echogenicity and are seen as anechoic in 50%, hyperechoic in 25% or hypoechoic in 25% cases.[52] Early lesions are hyperechoic and have well defined margins. Debris, septations, fluid-fluid level, air fluid level may also be seen. Echogenic foci with posterior reverberation artefacts are seen with gas producing organisms.

CT: On CT scans, abscesses are seen as low attenuation lesions with a characteristic peripheral rim enhancement **(Figs. 21A and B)**.[53] On administration of IV contrast, "double target sign" corresponding to perilesional edema and "cluster sign" representing coalescence of smaller lesions (<2 cm) to form a large abscess are characteristic features **(Figs. 22 and 23)**.[54] An air fluid level which is a specific sign of an abscess is seen in less than 20% of cases and may indicate an enteric communication.

MRI: These are seen as well-defined rounded lesions hypointense on T1W images, hyperintense on T2W images with intense peripheral rim enhancement on administration of contrast **(Figs. 24A and B)**. Peripheral edema seen as a high signal on T2W images is seen in only one third of the cases.[55] Diffusion weighted imaging of pyogenic abscesses shows a restricted pattern owing to the high cellularity and viscosity of pus.

AMOEBIC ABSCESS

Caused by the protozoan *Entamoeba histolytica*, amoebic liver abscess is the most common extraintestinal manifestation of amoebiasis. The organism may reach the liver from the colon, through the portal vein, via lymphatics or by direct extension.[56]

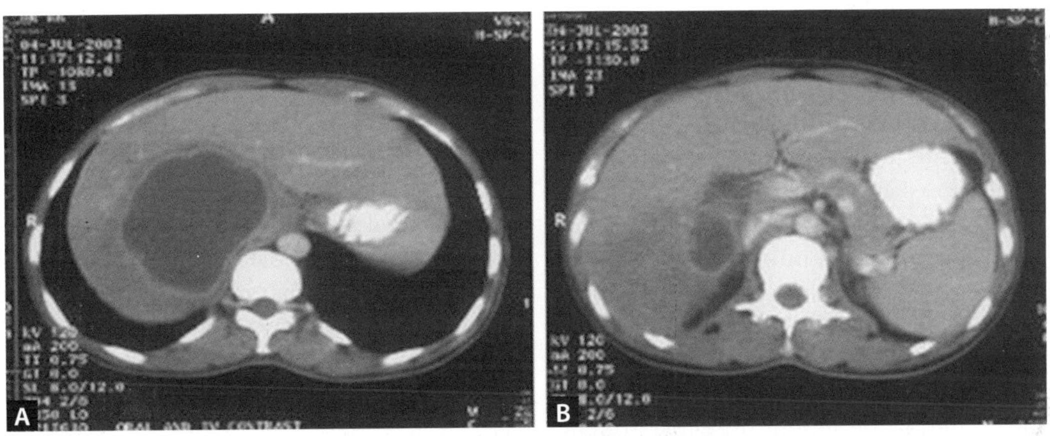

Figs. 21A and B: Contrast-enhanced CT showing irregular hypodense lesions in the liver with enhancing rim—pyogenic liver abscesses.

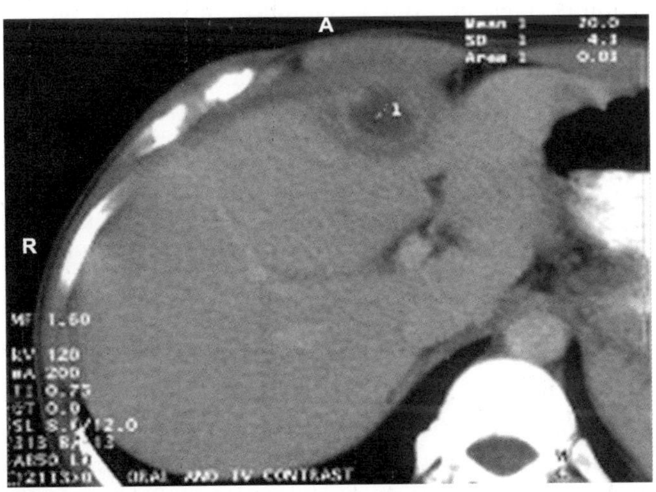

Fig. 22: Contrast-enhanced CT showing a hypodense lesion with perilesional edema giving a 'double target sign'—pyogenic liver abscess.

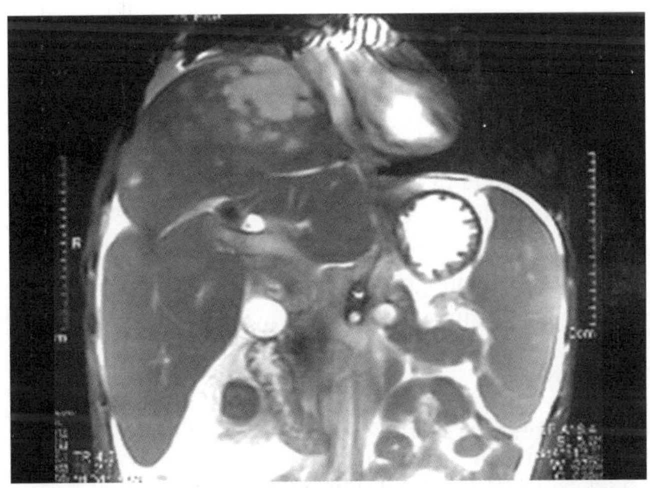

Fig. 23: MR image showing multiple small abscesses coalescing into a single cavity—"the cluster sign"—pyogenic liver abscesses.

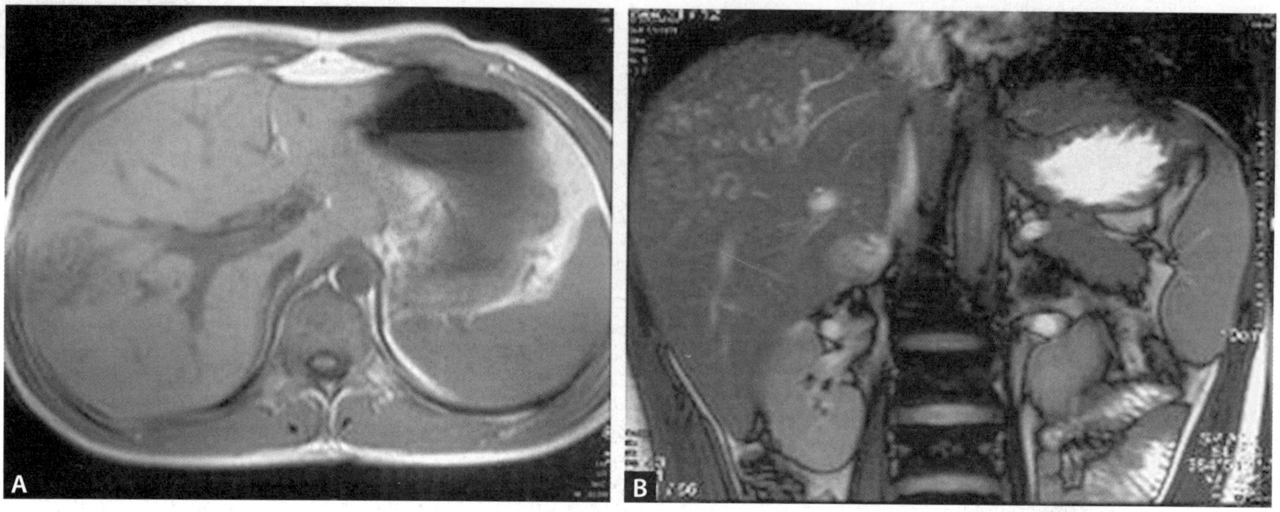

Figs. 24A and B: (A) T1 weighted MR image showing an ill-defined area hypointense in signal in the right lobe of liver; (B) T2-weighted image showing the area to have a high signal with multiple small lesions clustering together liver abscess.

Pathology

The cavitary amoebic abscess occurs as the liver parenchyma is frankly destroyed. Initially, the lesion contains necrotic tissue including the viable organism. As the lesion becomes larger, central cavitation is apparent and the active organism lies in the necrotic tissue lining the cavity. Surrounding this layer is an inflammatory zone of hepatic parenchyma invaded by the organisms. Centrally, the cavity is often filled by a thick fluid that resembles "anchovy paste". Frequently solitary, the abscess is most commonly located in the right lobe being related to the venous drainage from the usually infected right colon, via the superior mesenteric vein to the portal vein preferentially flowing into the right lobe of liver.

Imaging Features

Ultrasound

Amoebic abscess is seen as a round to oval solitary lesion in the right lobe of liver, with fine low level echoes and usually in continuity with the diaphragm **(Figs. 25A and B)**. A round or oval shape and a hypoechoic appearance with fine echoes are sonographic findings that favor an amoebic over a pyogenic liver abscess.[57]

CT Scans

Amoebic abscess appears as a low attenuation lesion with evidence of rim enhancement on contrast administration. Lesions in the early stage of development have a solid appearance with older lesions being cystic in appearance.[58] A target appearance due to an outer rim of lower attenuation surrounding the enhancing rim may be seen.

Magnetic Resonance Imaging

The abscess cavity is seen to have a low signal on T1 and a high signal on T2W images. The central cavity is often surrounded by a rim of high signal intensity corresponding to hyperemic reactive zone. On contrast administration, this reactive zone shows evidence of enhancement.

Complications

The most common complication of a liver abscess is rupture through the diaphragm resulting in pleuropulmonary amoebiasis occurring in 20–35% of patients **(Figs. 26A to C)**. Complications include pleural effusions, empyema, consolidation, lung abscess and very rarely hepatobronchial fistula.[59] Rupture into the peritoneal cavity is another complication **(Figs. 27A and B)**. Rarely, abscesses located in the left lobe may rupture into the pericardial cavity which is a serious life-threatening complication leading to cardiac tamponade or shock **(Figs. 28A to D)**. A rare complication is rupture of abscess into the biliary tree.

FUNGAL HEPATIC ABSCESSES

Fungal hepatic abscesses are uncommon. Immunocompromised states like HIV, chemotherapy, lymphoma, etc. are considered to be the predisposing factors. Liver is involved secondary to hematogenous spread of mycotic infection in other organs, most commonly in the lungs. *Candida* is the most common causative organism.

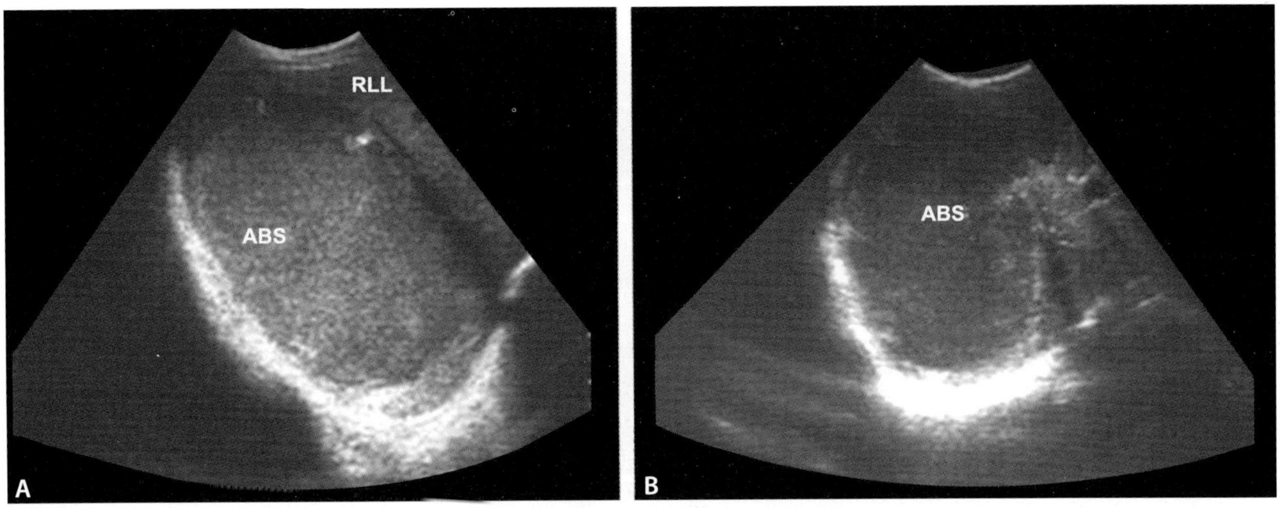

Figs. 25A and B: US showing a round hypoechoic lesion with low internal echoes within with absence of a well-defined abscess wall—amoebic liver abscess.

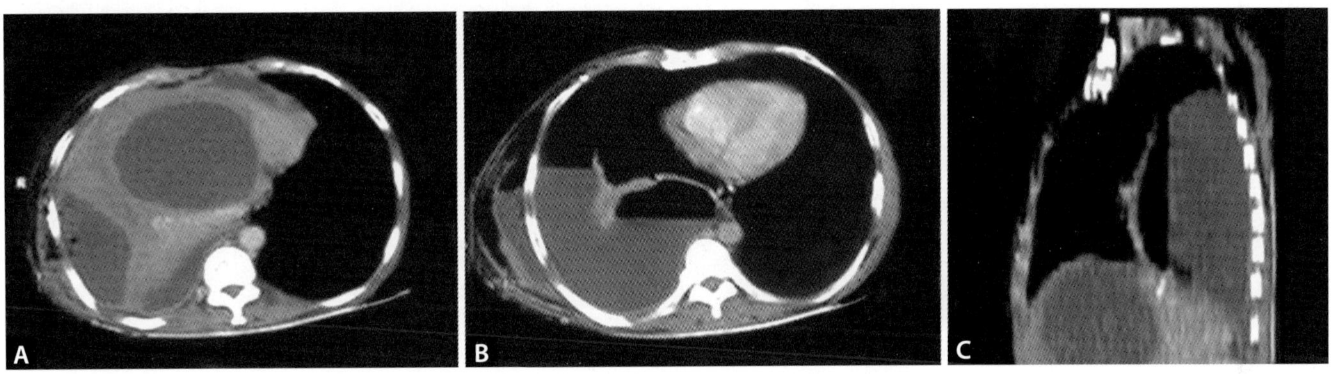

Figs. 26A to C: (A) Contrast-enhanced CT showing two abscesses in the liver with one of (A to C) lesions showing air loculi and indistinct margins; (B) A large hydropneumothorax is seen in the right pleural cavity; (C) Multiplanar reconstruction showing the communication between the abscess and the right hydropneumothorax—ruptured liver abscess.

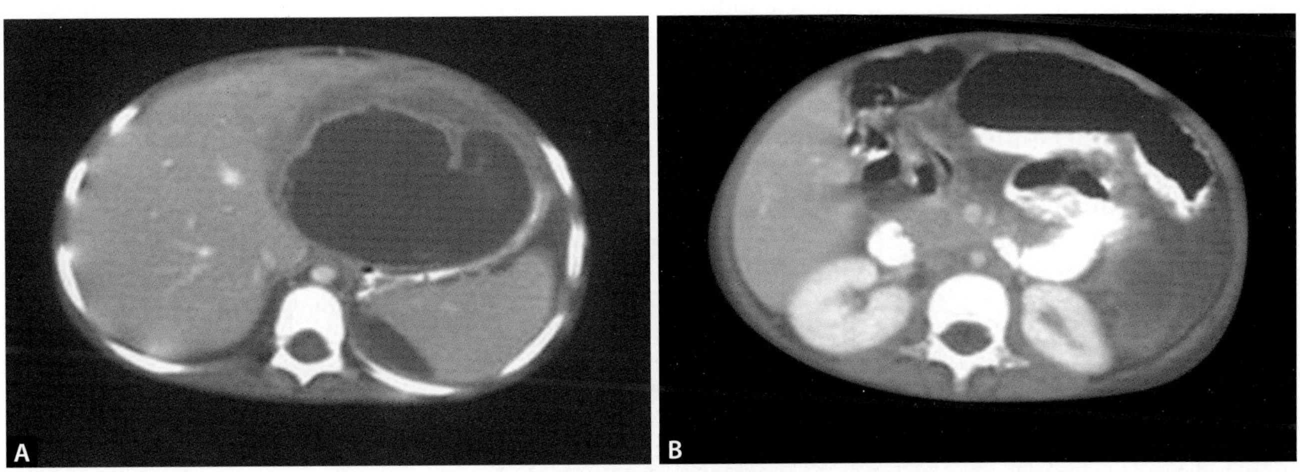

Figs. 27A and B: (A) Contrast-enhanced CT showing a large hypodense lesion with enhancing (A and B) rim in the left lobe of liver. Perilesional edema is noted. Fluid seen in the perihepatic and perisplenic region; (B) Fluid seen in the peritoneal cavity—intraperitoneal rupture of abscess.

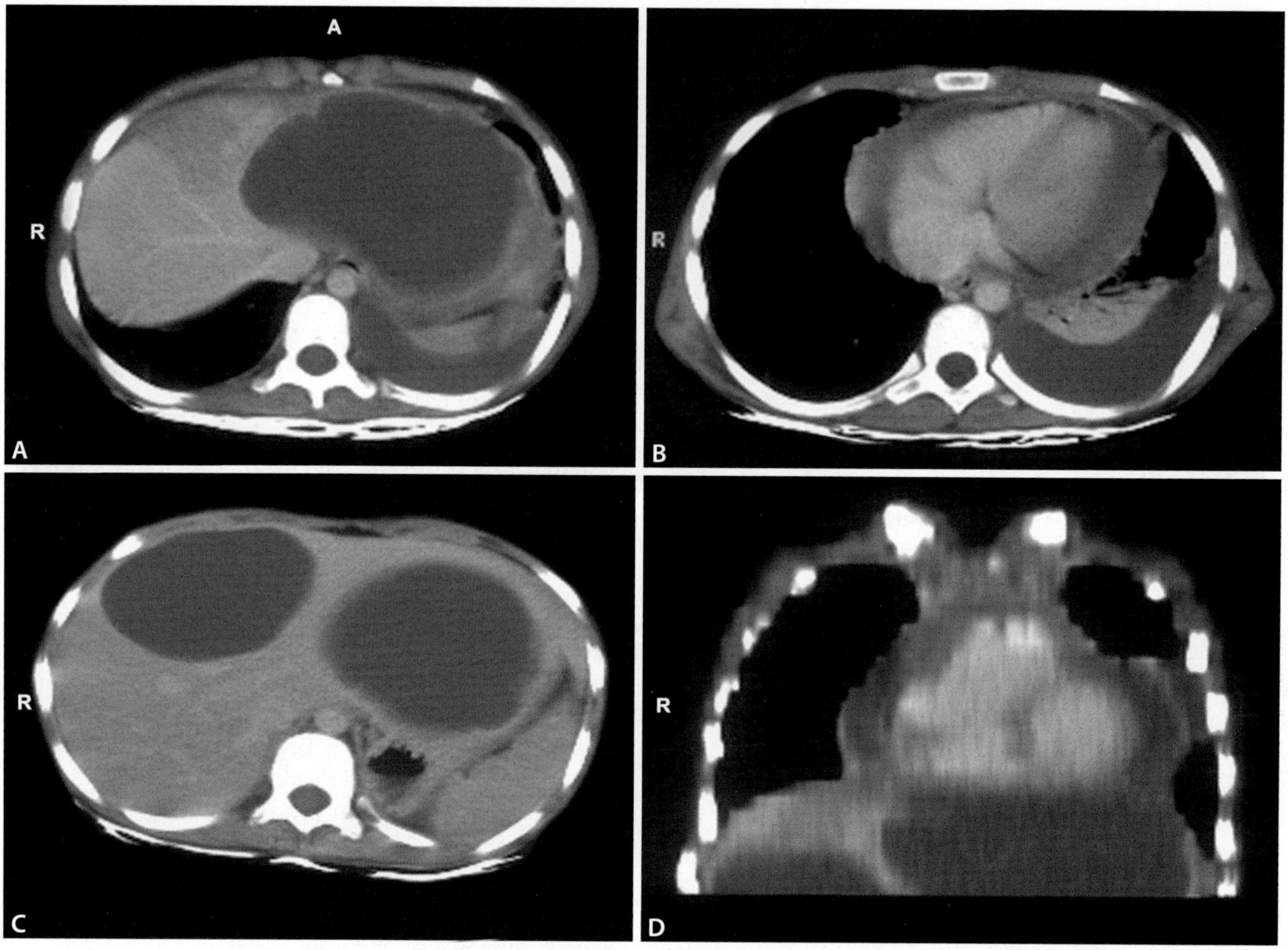

Figs. 28A to D: Contrast-enhanced CT sections reveal large abscesses in the liver with rupture of the left lobe abscess into the pericardium with pericardial and left pleural effusion—pericardial rupture of liver abscess.

Imaging Features

Sonographically, four major patterns of hepatic candidiasis are seen: (i) "wheel within a wheel", in which a peripheral zone surrounds an inner echogenic wheel (ii) "bull's eye", or target lesion in which a hypoechoic rim surrounds a hyperechoic center (iii) a "uniformly hypoechoic" appearance and (iv) "uniformly echogenic".

On CT scan, the most common pattern is multiple small, rounded hypoattenuating areas. Multiple punctate foci of increased attenuation due to calcification can be seen on NCCT.[60]

On MR, these lesions show increased signal intensity on T2-weighted images and STIR sequences.

HYDATID DISEASE

Hydatid disease is caused by the *Echinococcus granulosus*. Hydatid disease involves the liver in approximately 75% of cases with the right lobe more frequently involved.

Structure of Hydatid Cyst

The hydatid cyst is a trilaminated structure consisting of the pericyst, the ectocyst and the endocyst respectively. The pericyst is the outermost protective layer and comprises of modified host cells. The ectocyst allows passage of nutrients while the endocyst forms the true layer of the cyst, also known as the inner germinal layer. Daughter vesicles (brood capsules) that resemble a bunch of grapes arise from the inner germinal layer. Since the vesicles contain scolices, when they rupture the scolices pass to the cyst fluid forming a white sediment known as hydatid sand.[61]

Clinical Features

Classical symptoms of hydatid disease include abdominal pain and hepatomegaly. The majority may be asymptomatic and are discovered incidentally.

Imaging Features

Plain Film

Calcification is seen in 20–30% of hepatic hydatids, is usually seen in a curvilinear or a ring like pattern where the pericyst calcifies. Calcification of the pericyst, however, does not signify the death of the parasite which is usually represented by a dense complete calcification of the cyst.

Ultrasound

The sonographic patterns vary depending on the stage of evolution and maturity.

A well-defined anechoic cyst **(Fig. 29)** or a cyst with hydatid sand may be seen. The hydatid sand is seen as multiple echogenic foci within the cyst in a dependent position. Detachment of the endocyst from the pericyst may be either partial or complete. A partial detachment may produce a localized split in the cyst. Membranes are seen as serpentine, linear structures within the cyst giving rise to the "floating membranes" sign **(Fig. 30)**. An 'US water lily sign' is similar to the radiographic water lily sign seen in case of pulmonary hydatids.[62,63] A characteristic "honeycomb" pattern of cysts enclosed within cyst is seen in case of multiple daughter cysts from the germinal layer **(Fig. 31)**. The multiple septa seen represent the walls of the daughter cysts. A hydatid matrix of mixed echogenicity containing scolices, hydatid sand, membranes of broken daughter vesicles may be seen. Partial or complete calcification of the cyst wall may occur and may be seen as hyperechoic contour with acoustic shadowing. Hydatid cysts may become diffusely hyperechoic once infected and lose their characteristic sonographic appearance.

USG has been used to monitor the response to medical treatment. A reduction in the size, membrane detachment, mural calcification and increased echogenicity all indicate a favourable response to the treatment.

CT: On CT scans hydatid cysts have a density of near water attenuation. Daughter cysts when present give the lesions a multilocular appearance or a honeycomb appearance with the multiple septa representing the walls of daughter cyst.[64] The fluid in the daughter cysts has a lower attenuation than that of the fluid in the mother cyst. On contrast administration, the cyst wall does not show enhancement. Only the internal septae enhance **(Fig. 32)**.

Detachment of the laminated membrane from the pericyst can be visualized as linear areas of increased attenuation or the membranes may be free floating within the cyst **(Fig. 33)**. Calcification in the cyst wall is also easily detected by CT scan **(Figs. 34A and B)**.

MRI: Hydatid cysts appear as hypointense on T1W images and hyperintense on T2W images. The hydatid fluid and sand have a high signal on T2W images.[65] A characteristic imaging finding on MRI is the presence of a low signal intensity rim on both T1- and T2W-images surrounding the cyst as the pericyst is rich in collagen. The internal architecture or the honeycomb pattern is also well seen on MRI **(Figs. 35A and B)**.[66] Floating membranes are seen as linear low signal intensity structures within the cyst. Degenerated cysts decrease in size and appear heterogeneous, solid or pseudotumor like.

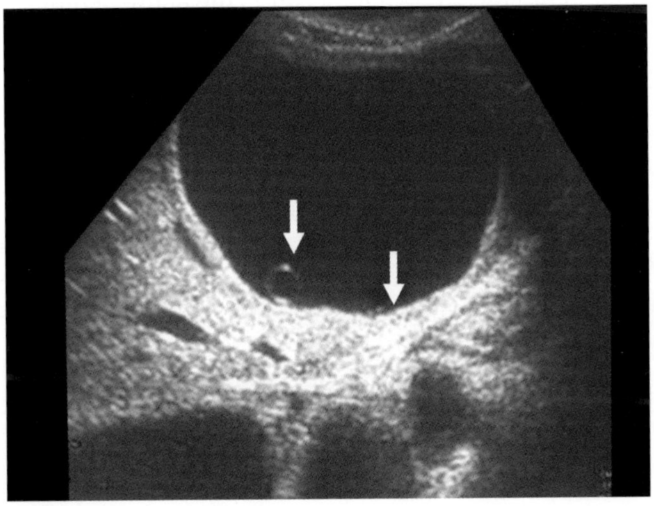

Fig. 29: US scan showing a well-defined anechoic cyst with a small cyst within—hydatid cyst.

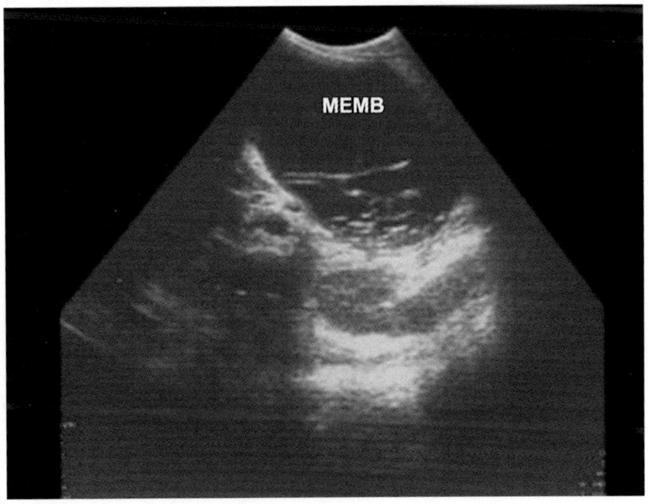

Fig. 30: US scan showing membranes as serpentine linear structures floating within a hydatid cyst.

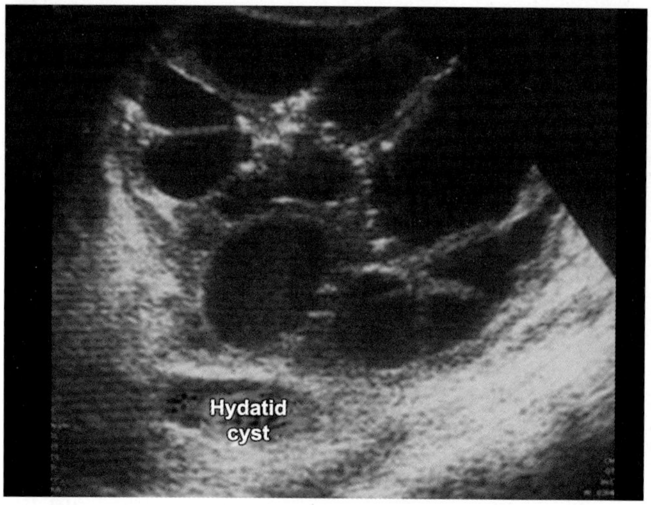

Fig. 31: US scan showing a characteristic appearance of cysts enclosed within a cyst giving rise to honeycomb pattern seen in a hydatid cyst.

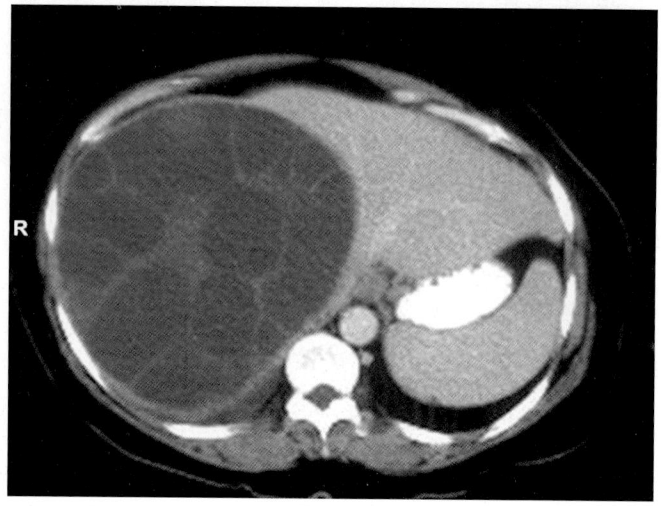

Fig. 32: CT scan showing the honeycomb pattern in a hydatid cyst with the multiple septae representing the walls of daughter cysts.

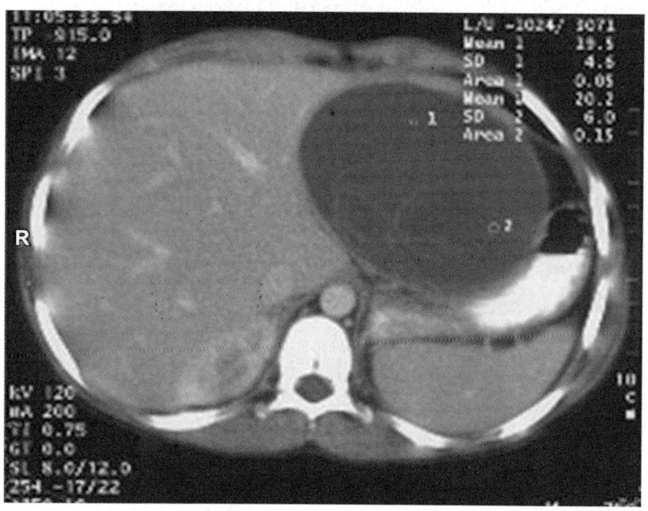

Fig. 33: Contrast-enhanced CT scan (CECT) showing detachment of the laminated membrane from the pericyst seen as linear areas of increased attenuation within the hydatid cyst.

COMPLICATIONS OF HYDATID CYSTS

Intrahepatic Complications

These include cyst rupture and infection. In direct cyst rupture there is free spillage of the hydatid material into the peritoneal, pleural or visceral cavity. A direct cyst rupture can occur when both the pericyst and endocyst rupture in contrast to a contained rupture where only the endocyst ruptures and the pericyst remains intact. A passage of cyst contents into the biliary tree constitutes a communicating rupture.[67] On MR imaging rupture will be seen as interruption of the low signal intensity rim of the cyst wall and extension of the contents through the defect.

Infection in the hydatid cyst can occur only when both the pericyst and endocyst rupture. Findings suggestive of an infection include a solid appearance, mixed pattern consisting of solid and fluid contents or air or air fluid levels within.

Peritoneal Seeding/Peritoneal Hydatidosis

Peritoneal seeding usually occurs secondary to hepatic hydatid disease through isolated cases of primary peritoneal echinococcosis can occur. The peritoneal cavity may be involved in 13% of the cases. Cysts are usually multiple, of varying sizes and may be located anywhere in the peritoneal cavity **(Figs. 36A to C)**.[68] An encapsulated multiloculated mass may be seen when the peritoneal hydatid disease grows and occupies the entire peritoneal cavity **(Figs. 37A to C)**.

Biliary Communication

The direct sign of rupture into the biliary tree is the visualization of the communication between the cyst wall and biliary radicles or the passage of hydatid cyst material into the biliary tree **(Figs. 38A to D)**. US can demonstrate echogenic linear filling structures without posterior acoustic shadow whereas CT can demonstrate high attenuation material in the biliary radicles or common bile duct. An air-fluid level or fat-fluid level are the indirect signs of a biliary communication.[69]

Other Complications

Hydatid cysts may grow exophytically to involve the bare area of the liver and the gastro hepatic ligament.

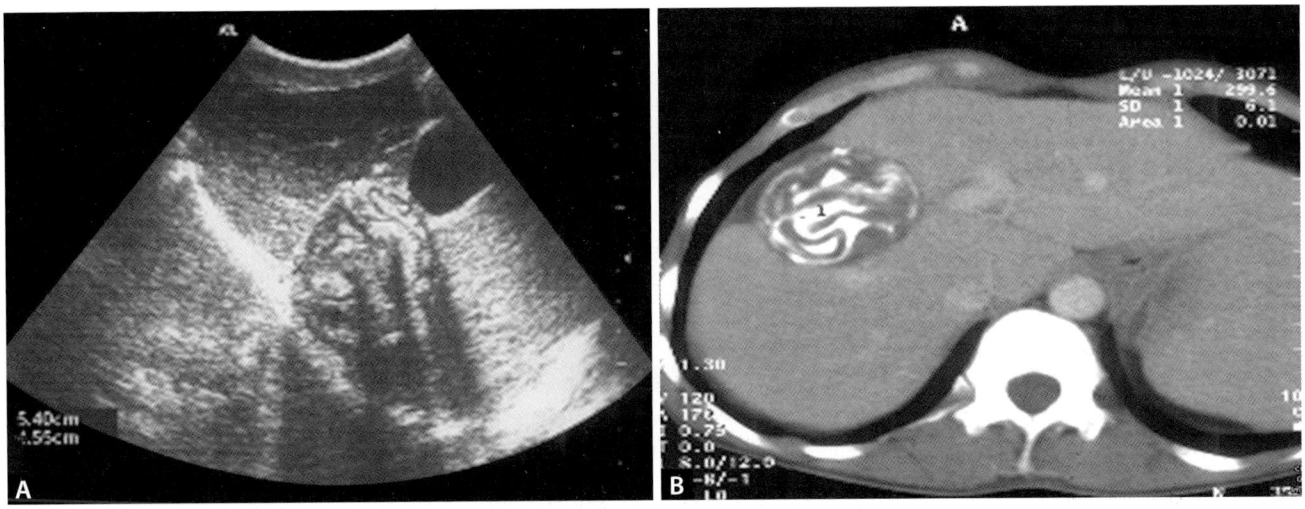

Figs. 34A and B: US (A) showing dense acoustic shadowing representing calcification in a hydatid cyst. CT (B) showing lamellar calcification in the membranes of the hydatid—calcified hydatid.

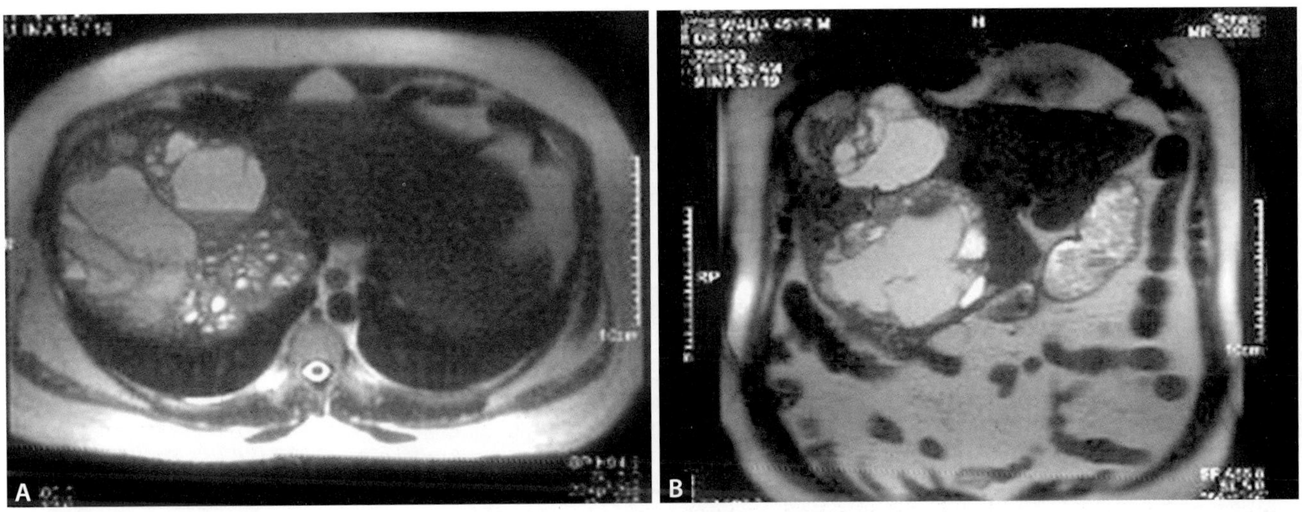

Figs. 35A and B: Axial (A) and coronal (B) MR images showing hepatic hydatids with multiple daughter cysts within appearing hyperintense on the T2-weighted images.

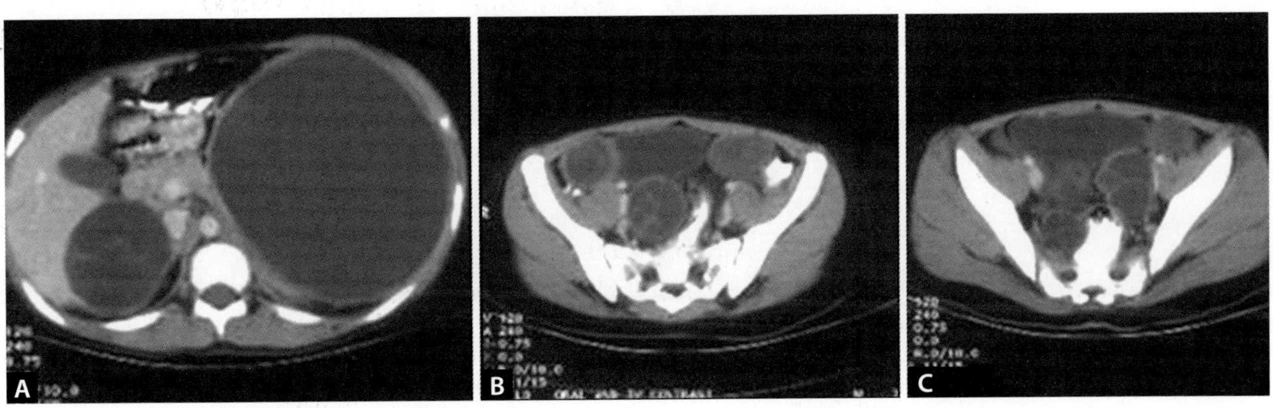

Figs. 36A to C: (A) CT scan showing hydatid cysts in the liver and spleen; (B and C) Multiple cysts of varying sizes seen in the peritoneal cavity—peritoneal seeding of hydatid cysts.

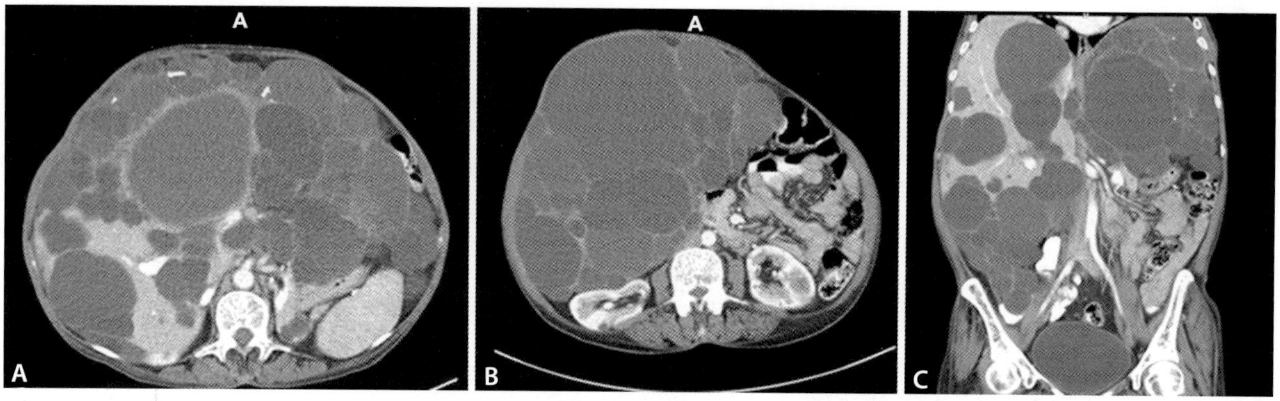

Figs. 37A to C: Contrast-enhanced CT scans revealing a multiloculated mass occupying the entire peritoneal cavity in addition to hydatid cysts within the liver—peritoneal hydatidosis.

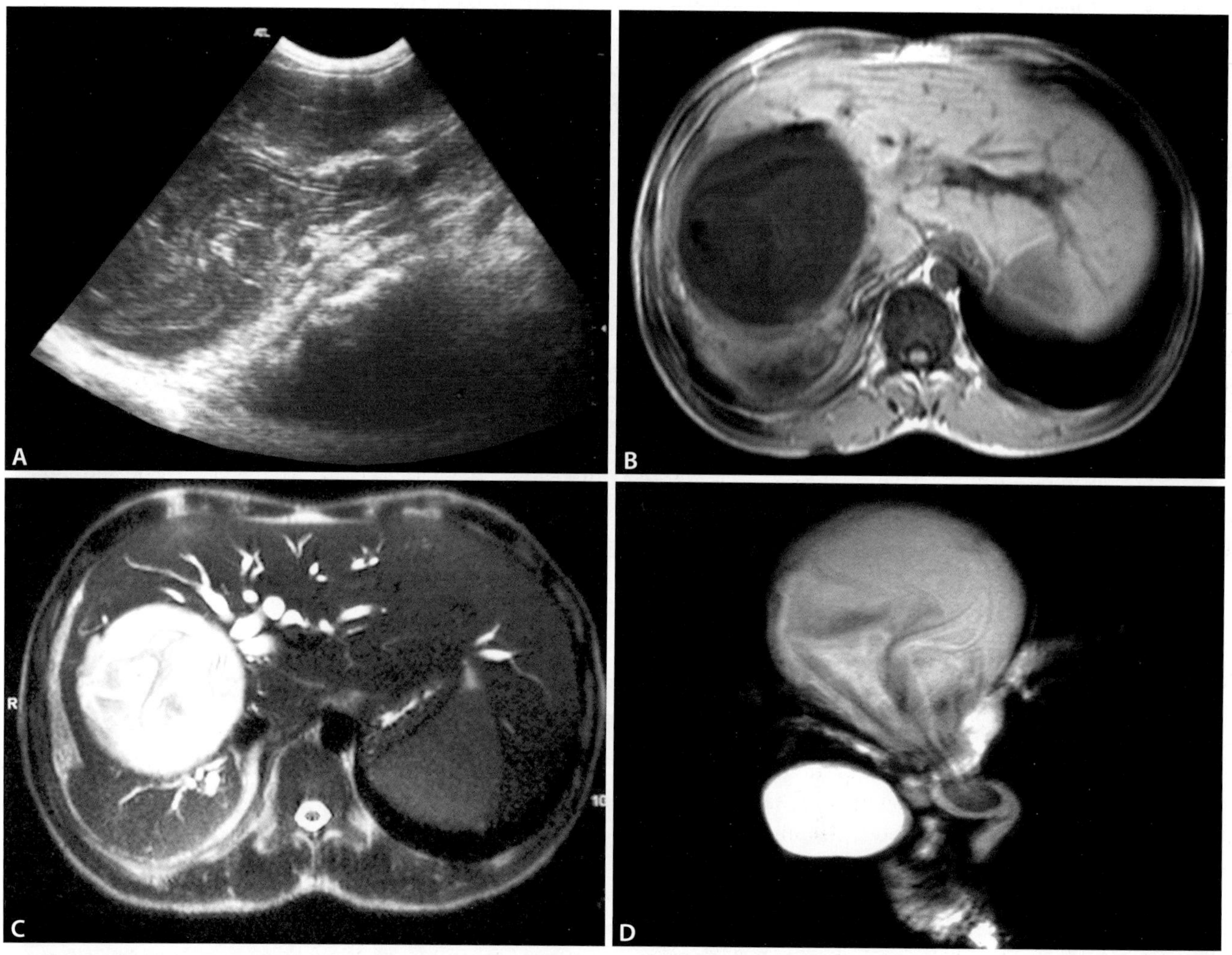

Figs. 38A to D: US (A) showing echogenic linear structures within the common bile duct. T1W (B) MR image showing the hydatid cyst as hypointense and T2W image (C) showing it as a hyperintense lesion with multiple linear low signal structures within s/o membranes. Passage of the cyst contents into the bile duct well depicted on the MRCP image—hydatid cyst with rupture into common bile duct.

Transdiaphragmatic thoracic involvement may be seen as pleural effusion, pulmonary lesion or chronic bronchial fistulas. Sagittal and coronal MR imaging is best to demonstrate the diaphragmatic defect and the migration of the hydatid cyst through it.[70] Perforation into the hollow viscera is an extremely rare complication seen in only 0.5% of cases. Patients may present with hydatidemesia or hydatidorrhea. Imaging may reveal an air-fluid level or orally administered contrast material inside the hollow viscus.[71] A portal cavernoma formation due to compression of the portal vein with secondary thrombosis is a rare complication. It is usually caused by hydatid cysts located in the caudate lobe.[72] Involvement of the abdominal wall may occur due to a direct communication between the cyst and the abdominal wall. An hour glass configuration may be seen due to the cysts passing through a small orifice.

HEPATIC ALVEOLAR ECHINOCOCCOSIS

The causative organism is *Echinococcus multilocularis*. It has a tendency to produce multilocular cysts anywhere in the organ or tissue with the liver being the most common site. Histologically, these cysts resemble alveoli rather than true cysts unlike hydatid cysts. These are usually 1–10 mm in diameter but may grow as large as 15–20 cm. They are usually solitary, multilocular or confluent.[73] The echinococcal cysts involve large regions of the hepatic parenchyma with an affinity for the porta hepatis with resultant portal hypertension and bile duct stenosis. Irregular margins, cystic and solid components and an in homogeneous enhancement pattern characterize the imaging appearances. Calcification begins in a scattered manner initially but eventually these become large calcified masses.

HEPATIC TUBERCULOSIS

Tuberculosis is a major cause of mortality and morbidity in the tropical countries and its incidence is increasing with the emergence of HIV and AIDS. Hepatic tuberculosis accounts for <1% of all tubercular infections,[74] being uncommon due to the low oxygen tension in the liver. The most common route of spread to the liver is hematogenous secondary to a tubercular focus elsewhere in the body resulting in a miliary pattern. Spread can also occur via the portal vein in cases of involvement of the gastrointestinal tract or via the lymphatic route in case of rupture of tuberculous lymph node along the portal tract.

Pathology

The histological hallmark of the disease is granuloma formation. Both caseating and noncaseating granulomas are seen. Presence of caseating epithelioid granuloma on histopathology is diagnostic of the disease.

Clinical Features

The disease may present at any age but is more common in young adults. Patients may present with high grade fever, weight loss, anorexia and upper abdominal pain. Rarely, patients may present with jaundice owing to biliary obstruction caused by periportal adenopathy.

Imaging Features

The disease can be classified into three forms: The parenchymal, serohepatic and tubercular cholangitis. The parenchymal form can be further subdivided as the micronodular and the macronodular pattern.[75]

Micronodular Form

This is the most common form of hepatic tuberculosis and usually occurs secondary to hematogenous dissemination.[76] A concomitant involvement of the lung may or may not be seen. The miliary hepatic lesions are randomly distributed throughout the hepatic parenchyma, are usually small in size and multiple. These may be at times, too small to be resolved by sonography and hepatomegaly may be the only imaging finding seen. A diffuse hypoechoic pattern of the liver parenchyma may be seen on sonography as the lesions are hypoechoic to the adjacent parenchyma.

On CT, the micronodular pattern is seen as micro-abscesses having a central hypodensity with peripheral rim enhancement on administration of contrast. This imaging appearance may mimic metastases, leukemic infiltration, lymphoma or fungal infections. Chronic lesions may calcify and the lesions may be seen as multiple echogenic foci with distal acoustic shadow on sonography or as multiple calcific foci on CT.

Macronodular Form

The macronodular form is less common than the micronodular variety.[77] Tubercular macronodules are also called pseudotumoral TB, tuberculomas or tubercular abscesses. These macronodules form as a result of conglomeration of miliary granulomas and may be seen as solitary or multiple complex hepatic masses. When solitary, the macronodular form may mimic a primary neoplastic lesion or other infective lesions. A "cluster sign" representing coalescence of multiple micronodular lesions into a macronodular lesion seen as a multiloculated cystic mass or a "target sign" representing a focus of calcification or enhancement in the center surrounded by low attenuation edema is highly suggestive but not pathognomonic of tubercular involvement.[78] At times, image guided biopsy is required for a definite histological diagnosis.[77]

Serohepatic Tuberculosis

This rare variety gives rise to a "frosted liver" owing to a predominant involvement of the subserosal plane of the liver. Imaging reveals multiple peripherally located conglomerated hypodense lesions with an overlying thickened enhancing capsule simulating sugar coating.[75] There may be associated bulky necrotic gastrohepatic and retroperitoneal adenopathy.

Tubercular Cholangitis

This can occur due to primary involvement of the biliary tree due to an extrinsic compression by periportal lymph nodes. Findings may vary from bile duct thickening, biliary dilatation and strictures with resultant obstructive biliopathy.[79]

HEPATIC SARCOIDOSIS

Liver involvement may be seen in 40–70% of patients with systemic sarcoidosis. The lesions are usually too small to be resolved by sonography and sarcoidosis may be seen as non-specific diffuse parenchymal heterogeneity, an increased parenchymal echogenicity or coarsening of the liver echotexture. CT and MRI will show the lesions as having a low attenuation with no enhancement seen on the post-contrast images.[74]

HEPATIC SCHISTOSOMIASIS

It is a serious parasitic infection of the humans usually having a chronic and insidious course. Hepatic involvement can occur due to *Schistosoma japonicum*, *Schistosoma mansoni* or *Schistosoma haematobium* infection. Patients may present with hematemesis due to portal hypertension or hematuria due to involvement of the urinary tract. Plain X-ray of the abdomen may show splenomegaly. Sonography may show periportal echogenicity due to fibrosis. Splenomegaly, collaterals and free fluid, i.e. features of portal hypertension can be seen. CT—A capsular or peripheral hepatic calcification is seen which is considered to be a hallmark of *Schistosoma japonicum* infection. Periportal areas of fibrosis may be seen as low density areas within the porta. Pseudoseptations within the liver, bands of calcification and liver notching are also characteristic imaging findings. MRI may show features of portal hypertension and low signal area within the porta due to fibrosis. Patients with schistosomiasis may develop hepatocellular carcinoma.

MISCELLANEOUS LESIONS

Fatty Infiltration

Fatty infiltration of the liver is a common occurrence resulting from increased deposition of triglyceride in hepatocytes. This arises from a variety of nutritional disturbances or toxic insults to the liver. These include obesity, nutritional deficiencies, diabetes mellitus, pregnancy, steroids, hepatotoxic drugs and alcoholism. The development of fatty infiltration is a dynamic process and changes may be seen in a few weeks of an insult and may regress within days. Most characteristically, the fatty involvement is uniform or geographic in distribution. However, occasionally it may be nodular or multifocal when it is indistinguishable from other focal hepatic lesions. Features suggesting the true nature of the process are sharp angular boundaries to the lesions and no evidence of displacement or effacement of venous structures. Chemical shift imaging on MRI will show focal fatty infiltration as an area of signal drop on the opposed phase images as compared to the in phase images.

Another well-recognized variant is focal sparing of small areas of normal liver in a more generalized fatty infiltration. The spared area appears as an echo-poor focal mass. A characteristic location for the spared area is the quadrate lobe anterior to the portal vein bifurcation or related to the gallbladder bed. The shape of the spared area or pseudomass is typically ovoid. Its location has led to the suggestion that the sparing relates to alteration of blood flow in this area.

Hematoma

The most common causes of hematoma are surgery and trauma. Hepatic lacerations, rib fractures and free fluid favor the diagnosis of a post-traumatic hematoma while iatrogenic hematoma usually occurs along a surgical plane. An intra or perihepatic hematoma can also occur due to bleeding in a hepatocellular adenoma. The CT appearance of a hematoma depends on the age of the blood products. While acute and subacute hematomas have a higher attenuation value due to aggregated fibrin components, a chronic hematoma has a fluid attenuation. On MRI subacute hematomas show a hyperintense signal on both T1- and T2-weighted images.[80] Gradient echo images are very sensitive for the detection of blood products.

Biloma

A rupture of the biliary system can produce bilomas. These can occur spontaneously, owing to trauma or following surgery. They can occur in an intrahepatic or perihepatic location. Pseudocapsule formation occurs due to the intense inflammatory reaction induced due to bile extravasation. On imaging bilomas appear as well defined cystic lesions within the porta. No septations or calcification are usually seen **(Figs. 39A to C)**. Clinical history, the location and imaging appearance helps in establishing the diagnosis.

Peliosis Hepatis

Peliosis hepatis is a benign vascular lesion characterized by sinusoidal dilatation and blood filled hepatic spaces. In 50% of cases, no cause can be found. In the remaining, the causative factors range from toxins (arsenic, PVC), drugs (steroids, oral contraceptives) to infections (*Bartonella*, tuberculous bacillus) and malignancies (HCC), renal and cardiac transplantation and diabetes.[80] A variable echogenicity with internal vascularity is seen on ultrasound. On noncontrast CT scans, a hypoattenuating area with an early brisk enhancement is noted on the postcontrast scans. Peliosis hepatis on MR is seen to be typically hypointense on T1 and hyperintense on T2W images.

Inflammatory Pseudotumor

Inflammatory pseudotumor (IPT) is a benign lesion consisting of inflammatory cells and fibrosis.[80] These may occur at all ages, they are more common in the young. Though the exact etiopathogenesis is unknown, it is postulated that they may occur secondary to an inciting hepatic infection. At US, inflammatory pseudotumors may appear as heterogeneous hyperechoic lesions with increased through transmission. These are seen as large hypoattenuating lesions on noncontrast CT. Contrast-enhanced CT reveals central hypodensity with thick peripheral hyperdensity **(Figs. 40A and B)**. The

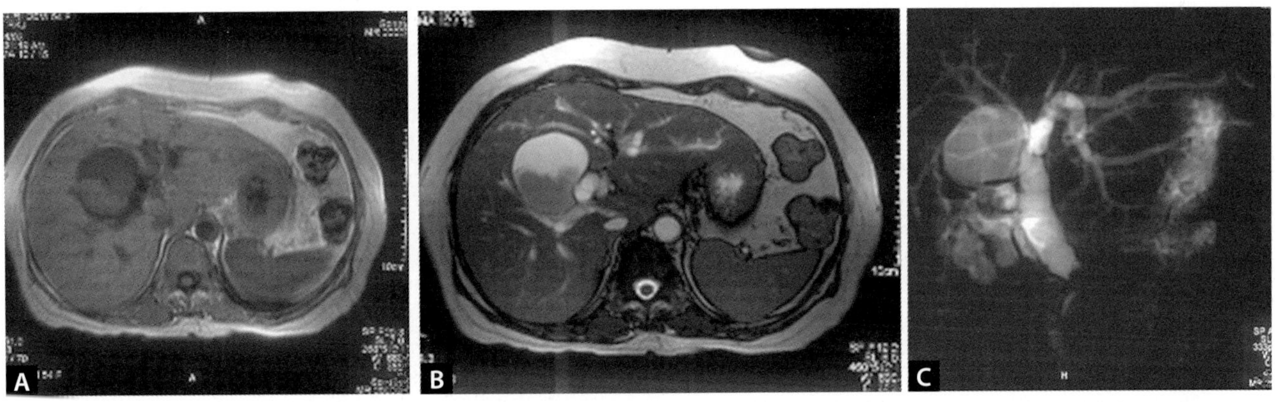

Figs. 39A to C: (A) MR image in a postcholecystectomy patient showing a well-defined hypointense lesion in the gallbladder fossa s/o biloma; (B) T2-weighted MR images shows a hyperintense signal in the cyst with a fluid-fluid level (due to Inspissated bile/sludge); (C) MRCP image depicting the biloma.

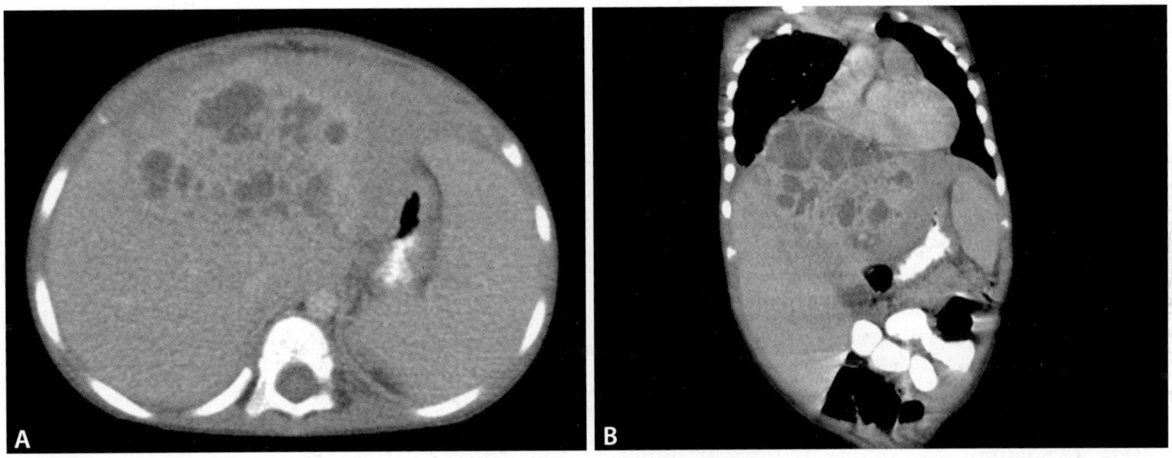

Figs. 40A and B: Contrast-enhanced CT reveals a mass with central hypodensity and thick peripheral hyperdensity in a child—inflammatory pseudotumor.

appearance may mimic a necrotic malignant mass. The hypodense center corresponds to inflammatory infiltrates while the hyperdense periphery corresponds to fibroblastic proliferation. The lesions are typically hypointense on T1W and hyperintense on T2W images.Contrast MRI reveals intense enhancement of the lesions with rapid washout and periportal involvement. It is difficult to differentiate this condition from a primary or metastatic neoplasm and biopsy may be required.[80]

CONCLUSION

There are myriad benign hepatic lesions; however the majority often display fairly specific imaging characteristics which allow a confident diagnosis. Atypical manifestations and the less familiar rarer benign tumors may pose a diagnostic challenge. An accurate patient history and relevant clinical data are important. Advances in imaging techniques such as diffusion-weighted magnetic resonance (DWMR) imaging, chemical shift imaging and the use of hepatocyte specific MR contrast agents allow a better understanding of the lesion itself and allow for an improved lesion diagnosis.

REFERENCES

1. Ata Soy C, Akyar S. Multidetector CT contributions in liver imaging. Eur Radiol. 2004;52:2-17.
2. Winterer JT, Kotter E, Ghanem M. Detection and characterization of bengin focal liver lesions with multislice CT. Eur Radiol. 2006;16:2427-43.
3. Ros PR. Focal liver masses other than metastases. In categorical course on gastrointestinal radiology. Oak Brook III, RSNA Publications; 1999.
4. Van Sonnenberg E, Wroblicka JT, D'Agostino HB, et al. Symptomatic hepatic cysts: Percutaneous drainage and sclerosis. Radiology. 1994;190:387-92.
5. Dewbury KC. Benign focal liver lesions. In: Meire H, Cosgrove D, Dewbery K, et al (Eds). Abdominal and General Ultrasound (2nd edn) Churchill Livingstone; 2001.
6. Blumke DA, Fishman EK. Spiral CT of liver tumors. In: Fishman EK, Jeffrey RB (Eds). Spiral CT Principles, Techniques and Clinical Application (2nd edn) Lippincott Raven, 1998.
7. Mathieu D, Vilgrain V, Mahfouz A, et al. Benign liver tumors. Mag Reson Imaging Clin N Am. 1997;5:255-88.
8. Vachha B, Sun M, RM, Siewert B, et al. Cystic lesions of the liver. AJR. 2011;196:W355-66.
9. Borhani AA, Wiant A, Heller MT. Cystic Hepatic Lesions: A review and an algorithmic approach. AJR. 2014;203:1192-1204.
10. Oto A, Tamm EP, Szklaruk J. Multidetector Row CT of the Liver Radiol Clin N Am. 2005;43:827-48.
11. Palacois E, Shannon M, Solomon C, et al. Biliary cystadenoma: Ultrasound, CT and MRI. Gastrointest Radiol. 1990;15:313-16.
12. Ba Ssalamah A, Baroud S, Bastati N, et al. MR Imaging of Benign Focal Liver Lesions. Mag Reson Imaging Clin N Am. 2010;18:403-19.
13. Matos AP, Velloni F, Ramalho, et al. Focal Liver lesions. Practical magnetic resonance imaging approach. World J Hepatol. 2015;16:1987-2008.
14. Birnbaum BA. Benign tumors of the liver: Hepatic haemangiomas. In: Margulis Burhennes (Eds) Alimentary Tract Radiology (5th edn), 1994.
15. Brannigan M, Burns PN, Wilson SR. Blood flow patterns in focal liver lesions at Microbubble enhanced US. Radiographics. 2004;24:921-35.
16. Powers C, Ros PR. Hepatic mass lesions. In: Haaga JR, Kanzieri CF, Gilkeson RC (Eds). CT and MR Imaging of the Whole Body (4th edn) Mosby, 2003.
17. Hanfusa K, Ohashi I, Himenso Y, et al. Hepatic haemangioma: Findings with two phase CT. Radiology. 1995;196:465.
18. Yu JS, Kim MJ, Kim KW, et al. Hepatic cavernous haemangioma: Sonographic pattern and speed of contrast enhancement on multiphase Dynamic MR Imaging AJR. 1998;71:1021-5.
19. Counbaras M, Weudum D, Cholley LM, et al. CT and MR Imaging features of pathologically proven Atypical Giant Haemangiomas of the liver. AJR. 2002;179: 1457-63.
20. Danet IM, Semelka RC, Braga L, et al. Giant haemangioma of the liver: MR imaging characteristics in 24 patients. Magnetic Resonance Imaging. 2003;21:95-101.
21. Francisco FAF, Araújo ALE, Neto, et al. Hepatobiliary contrast agents: differential diagnosis of focal hepatic lesions, pitfalls and other indications. Radio Bras. 2014;47(5):301-9.
22. El-Badrawy A, Ashmallah GA, Tawfik Am, et al. Diffusion weight MR imaging of benign hepatic focal lesions. Open Journal of Radiology. 2014;4:136-43.
23. Kim TK, Jang HJ, Burns PN, Lavallee JM, Wilson SR. Focal Nodular hyperplasia and hepatic adenoma: differentiation with low mechanical index contrast enhanced sonography. Am J Roentgenol. 2008;190:58-66.
24. Brancatelli G, Federle MP, Katyal S, et al. Haemodynamic characterization of focal nodular Hyperplasia using three dimensional volume rendered multidetector CT angiography. AJR. 2002;179:81-5.
25. Macky MD, Frazer C, deBoer WB. Magnetic resonance features of focal nodular hyperplasia of the liver. Australasian Radiology. 1999;43:315-20.
26. Elsayes KM, Narra VR, Yin, et al. Focal hepatic lesions. Diagnostic value of enhancement pattern approach with contrast enhanced 3D gradient echo MR imaging. Radiographics. 2005;25:1299-1320.
27. Grazioli L, Morana G, Federle M, et al. Focal nodular hyperplasia: Morphologic and functional information from MR Imaging with Gadobenate Dimeglumine. Radiology. 2001;221: 731-9.
28. Ba Ssalamah A, Schima W, Schmook MT, et al. Atypical focal nodular hyperplasia of the liver: Imaging features

of nonspecific and liver specific MR contrast agents. AJR. 2002;179:1447-56.
29. Beets Tan RGH, Van Engelshoven JMA, Greve JWM. Hepatic adenoma and focal nodular hyperplasia: MR findings with superparamagnetic iron oxide enhanced MRI. Clin Imaging. 1998;22:211-5.
30. Grazioli L, Federle MP, Ichikawa T, et al. Liver adenomatosis: Clinical, histopathologic, and imaging findings in 15 patients. Radiology. 2000;216:395-402.
31. Anderson SW, Kruskal JB, Kane RA, et al. Benign hepatic tumors and iatrogenic pseudotumors. Radiographics. 2009;29:211-99.
32. Cogley JR, Miller FH. MR Imaging of Benign Focal Liver Lesions. Radiol Clin N Am. *http//dx.doi.org/*10, 1016/ j. cl 2014.
33. Catalano O, Nunziata A, LobiancoR, Siani A. Real time harmonic contrast material specific US of focal liver lesions. Radiographics. 2005;25:333-49.
34. Horton KM, Blumke DA, Hruban RH, et al. CT and MR imaging of benign hepatic and biliary tumors. Radiographics. 1999; 19:431-51.
35. Tajima T, Honda H, Kuroiwa T, et al. Radiologic features of intrahepatic bile duct Adenoma: A look at the surface of the liver. J Comput Assist Tomography. 1999;23(5): 690-5.
36. King LJ, Burkill GJC, Scurr ED, et al. Mn DPDP enhanced magnetic resonance imaging of focal liver lesions. Clinical Radiology. 2002;57:1047-57.
37. Bartolozzi C, Cioni D, Donati F, et al. Focal liver lesions: MR imaging—Pathologic correlation. Eur Radiol. 2001;11:1374-88.
38. Caraiani C, Chiorean L, Fenesan DI, et al. Diffusion weighted magnetic resonance imaging for the classification of Liver Lesions as Benign or Malignant. J Gastrointest. Liver Dis. 2015;24:309-17.
39. Rha SE, Lee MG, Lee YS, et al. Nodular regenerative hyperplasia of the liver in Budd-Chiari Syndrome: CT and MR features. Abdom Imaging. 2000;25:255-8.
40. Quglia A, Tibballs J, Grasso A, et al. Focal nodular hyperplasia like areas in cirrhosis. Histopathology. 2003;42:14-21.
41. Krinsky GA, Lee VS, Nguyen MT, et al. Siderotic nodules at MR Imaging: Regenerative or Dysplastic J Comput Assist Tomography. 2000;24:773-6.
42. Bris FE, Bao Do AK, et al. Classification of hypervascular liver lesions based on hepatic artery and portal vein blood supply coefficients calculated from triphasic CT scans. Journal of Digital Imaging. 2015;28:213-33.
43. Ros PR, Goodman ZD, Ishak KG, et al. Mesenchymal hamartoma of the liver: Radiologic pathologic correlation. Radiology. 1986;158:619-24.
44. Ishak KG, Kabin L. Benign tumors of the liver. Med Clin North Am. 1975;59:995-1013.
45. Stanley P, Hall TR, Woolley MM, et al. Mesenchymal hamartomas of the liver in childhood: sonographic and CT findings. AJR. 1986;147:1035-9.
46. O'Neil J, Ros PR. Knowing hepatic pathology aids MRI of liver tumors. Diagn Imaging. 1989;11:58-65.
47. Ros PR, Rasmussew JF, Li KCP. Radiology of malignant and benign liver tumors. Curr Probl Diagn Radiol. 1989;18:95-155.
48. Srivastava DN, Mahajan A, Berry M, et al. Colour Doppler flow imaging of focal hepatic lesions. Australasian Radiology. 2000;44:285-9.
49. Keslar PJ, Buck JL, Selky DM. Infantile haemangioendothelioma of the liver revisited. Radiographics. 1993;13:657-70.
50. Prasad SR, Wang H, Rosas H, et al. Fat containing lesions of the liver: radiologic—pathologic correlation. Radiographics. 2005;25:321-31.
51. Brandborg LL, Goldman IS. Bacterial and miscellaneous infections of the liver. In: Zakim D, Boyer TD (Eds). Hepathology Philadelphia, WB Saunders, 1990.
52. Adeyiga AO, Lee EY, Eisenberg RL. Focal Hepatic Masses in Pediatric Patients. AJR. 2012;199:W422-40.
53. Halvovsen RA, Korobkin M, Foster WL, et al. The variable CT appearance of hepatic abscesses. AJR. 1984;141:941-6.
54. Jeffrey RB, Tolentino CS, Chang FC, et al. CT of small pyogenic hepatic abscesses: The cluster sign. AJR. 1988;151:487-9.
55. Balci NC, Semelhar RC, Noone TC, et al. Pyogenic hepatic abscesses: MRI findings on T1 and T2 weighted and serial Gadolinuim Enhanced Gradient Echo Images. J Magn Reson Imaging. 1999;9:285-90.
56. Gupta RK. Amoebic liver abscess. a report of 1000 cases. Int Surg. 1984;69:261-4.
57. Philips RL. Computed tomography and ultrasound in the diagnosis and treatment of liver abscesses. Australasian Radiology. 1994;38:165-69.
58. Radin DR, Ralls PW, Colletti PM, et al. CT of amoebic liver abscess. AJR. 1988;150:1297-1301.
59. Juimo AG, Gervez F, Angwafo FF. Extraintestinal amoebiasis. Radiology. 1992;182:181.
60. Shirkhoda A. CT findings in hepatosplenic and renal candidiasis. J Comput Assist Tomogr. 1987;11:795-8.
61. Beggs I. The radiology of hydatid disease. AJR. 1985;145:639-48.
62. Marti-Bonmati L, Menor Serrano F. Complications of hepatic hydatid cysts: Ultrasound, computed tomography and magnetic resonance diagnosis. Gastrointest Radiol. 1990;15: 119-25.
63. Von Sinner WN. New diagnostic sign in hydatid disease: Radiography, ultrasound, CT and MRI correlated to pathology. Eur J Radiol. 1990;12:150-9.
64. Pedroza I, Saiz A, Arrazola J, et al. Hydatid disease; Radiologic and pathologic features and complications. Radiographics. 2000;20:795-817.
65. Davolio SA, Canossi GC, Nicoli FA, et al. Hydatid disease: MR imaging study. Radiology. 1990;175:701-6.
66. Agildere AM, Aytekin C, Coskun M, et al. MRI of hydatid disease of the Liver: A variety of sequences J. Comput Assist Tomography. 1998;22(5):718-24.
67. De Diego J, Lecumberri FJ, Franquet T, et al. Computed tomography in hepatic echinococcosis. AJR. 1982;139:699-702.

68. Karavias DD, Vagianos CE, Kakkos SK, et al. Peritoneal echinococcosis. World J Surg. 1996;20:337-40.
69. Mendez JV, Arrazola J, Lopej J, et al. Fat–fluid level in hepatic hydatid cyst: A new sign of rupture into the biliary tree? AJR. 1996;167:91-4.
70. Gomez R, Moreno E, Loinaz C, et al. Diaphragmatic or transdiaphragmatic thoracic involvement in hepatic hydatid disease surgical trends and classification. World J Surg. 1995;19: 714-9.
71. Jain R, Sawhney S, Berry M. Hydatid disease: CT demonstration and follow-up of a cystogastric fistula. AJR. 1992;158:212.
72. Gil–Egea MJ, Alameda F, Girvent M, et al. Hydatid cyst in the hepatic hilum causing a cavernous transformation in the portal vein. Gastroenterol Hepatol. 1998;21:227-9.
73. Choji K, Fujita N, Chen M, et al. Alveolar hydatid disease of the liver: Computed tomography and transabdominal ultrasound with histopathological correlation. Clin Radiology. 1992;46: 97-103.
74. Chong V. Hepatobiliary tuberculosis: a review of presentations and outcomes. South Med J. 2008;101: 356-61.
75. Yu RS, Zhang SZ, Wu JJ, et al. Imaging diagnosis of 12 patients with hepatic tuberculosis. World J Gastroenterol. 2004;10(11): 1639-42.
76. Tatco UR, Margarita AM, Santos M, et al. The many faces of Hepatic tuberculosis. WFPITB Corner. 2015; 2:1-6.
77. Kakkar C, Polnaya AM, Koteshwara P, et al. Hepatic tuberculosis: a multimodality imaging review. Insights Imaging. 2015; 6:647-58.
78. Burrill J, William CJ, Bain G, et al. Tuberculosis: A Radiologic Review. Radiographics. 2007;27:1255-73.
79. Chong VH, Lim KS. Hepatobiliary tuberculosis. Singap Med J. 2010;51:744-51.
80. Alobaidi M, Shirkhoda A. Benign Focal Liver Lesions: Discrimination from malignant mimickers. Curr Probl Diagn Radiol. 2004;33:239-53.

CHAPTER 79

Malignant Focal Lesions of Liver

Raju Sharma, Kumble S Madhusudhan

INTRODUCTION

Imaging of the liver has undergone a paradigm shift during the last decade due to significant advances in technology and new contrast agents. This has led to greater understanding and better management of many diseases which affect the liver. The advent of ultrasound and MR elastography, dual energy CT and new MRI sequences and contrast agents (e.g. Gadoxetic acid) have increased the sensitivity for detection and accuracy for characterization of liver lesions.[1,2] Clinical information continues to be of paramount importance as it helps to tailor the imaging technique and narrows the differential diagnosis.

Malignant focal lesions of the liver are classified according to WHO as follows:[3]

- *Primary*:
  - *Hepatocellular tumors*:
    - Hepatocellular carcinoma (HCC)
    - Hepatocellular carcinoma, fibrolamellar
    - Hepatoblastoma, epithelial variants
    - Undifferentiated carcinoma
  - *Malignancies of mixed origin*:
    - Hepatoblastoma, mixed epithelial-mesenchymal
    - Combined hepatocellular-cholangiocarcinoma
  - *Bile duct lesions*:
    - Intrahepatic cholangiocarcinoma
    - Intraductal papillary neoplasm with invasive carcinoma
    - Mucinous cystic neoplasm
  - *Malignant mesenchymal tumors*:
    - Epithelioid hemangioendothelioma (EHE)
    - Angiosarcoma
- *Secondary*:
  - Metastatic deposits
  - Lymphoma.

Metastasis to the liver from an extrahepatic malignancy is by far the most common cause of a malignant hepatic neoplasm. Hepatic metastases are particularly common from primary malignancies of the gastrointestinal tract, breast and lung.

IMAGING TECHNIQUES AND ADVANCES

The imaging techniques used in the evaluation of focal liver lesions include ultrasonography (USG), computed tomography (CT), magnetic resonance imaging (MRI) and positron emission tomography (PET). Although ultrasonography is the initial imaging modality, most of the patients need further characterization by either multiphase contrast-enhanced CT or MRI. PET-CT is used in staging of the disease in case of liver metastases and lymphoma but not for the characterization of liver lesions. Recent advances in imaging techniques and contrast agents have further improved the accuracy of imaging in characterization of liver lesions.[4]

Elastography is a technique to assess the stiffness of tissues. Here either an external or an internal force is applied and the displacements of the tissue are subsequently measured. Various ultrasound elastography (USE) techniques are available including transient elastography (TE; fibroscan), acoustic radiation force impulse (ARFI) and 2D shear wave elastography (SWE).[5] TE and SWE give results directly in kilopascals whereas ARFI gives it in m/s (speed). Color coding is also done for different areas with different stiffness. USE may help in differentiation of benign from malignant focal liver lesions. Contrast-enhanced USG (CEUS) is a valuable technique for detection and characterization of focal liver lesions. Sulfur hexafluoride (Sonovue) is the widely used USG contrast agent. After contrast injection, dynamic imaging is done to assess the contrast flow characteristics within the lesion. Its limitations include operator dependence, difficulty in evaluating deeper lesions, lack of complete 3-dimensional information and difficulty in evaluating multiple lesions. It is also used to guide biopsies of liver lesions and in assessment of completeness of ablation of liver tumors immediately after the procedure. Other upcoming applications are quantitative perfusion imaging and molecular imaging. In the former, a time-intensity curve is generated and is useful in lesion characterization and assessment of treatment response of liver tumors. A recent addition is liver specific contrast agent—perflubutane (Sonazoid) which is taken up by Kupffer cells and normal liver shows uniform enhancement in Kupffer phase (15–120 min after injection). Focal liver lesions not containing Kupffer cells are seen as hypoechoic area in this phase. Thus, this helps in lesion detection and characterization.

Perfusion computed tomography (PCT) is a technique in which microvasculature of the tissue can be assessed after injection of intravenous contrast.[6] Improvement in the technology has resulted in larger coverage, reduced motion artifacts and radiation dose. This technique evaluates the vascularity of various tumors in liver and assists in making a diagnosis. It is also useful assessing response of tumors to chemotherapy and evaluating recurrence.

Dual energy computed tomography (DECT) is a recent addition to the existing imaging modalities.[7] In this technique, scan is done both at low energy (100 kVp) and high energy (140 kVp). The data obtained is then used in generation of iodine maps, virtual noncontrast images and material decomposition. Low kV images help in improving liver lesion detection by increasing the contrast to noise ratio. Iodine maps are useful in depiction of tumor vascularity in the liver based on iodine maps and iodine ratio and thus helps in differentiation of hepatic cystic/necrotic tumors from simple cysts and in assessing treatment response of tumors.[8]

MR elastography (MRE) is a technique similar to USE which uses shear waves to assess tissue stiffness.[4] Although, elastography is shown have role in differentiation of benign from malignant tumors, it is especially useful in differentiation of hepatic adenoma (softer) from focal nodular hyperplasia (stiffer) and hepatocellular carcinoma (softer) from cholangiocarcinoma (stiffer). They may also have a role in assessment of tumor response to chemotherapy. Liver specific MR contrast agents—Gadobenate dimeglumine and Gadoxetic acid are taken up by normal hepatocytes and excreted into the biliary tree in the hepatobiliary phase (60–90 min for gadobenate and 15–20 minutes for gadoxetic acid). Lesions not containing normal hepatocytes are seen as hypointense area. Thus, both these agents, in addition to initial dynamic contrast enhanced imaging, can be used in late phase imaging to improve lesion detection and characterization. Proton MR spectroscopy is also helpful in evaluation of focal liver lesions.[9] Studies have shown that malignant liver lesions show elevated choline compared to normal liver or benign lesions. Hepatocellular carcinomas after chemoembolization show reduction in choline on magnetic resonance spectroscopy and this may assist in evaluation of response. There is research still going on to improve the results by faster sequences, better hardware and faster processing.

PRIMARY MALIGNANT FOCAL LESIONS HEPATOCELLULAR CARCINOMA

Hepotocellular carcinoma (HCC) is the most common primary malignant neoplasm of the liver worldwide. The incidence varies, being more common in Africa and the far east. Etiology also varies among different population groups and the risk factors include hepatitis B and C infection, alcoholic cirrhosis, primary hemochromatosis, nonalcoholic fatty liver disease and exposure to carcinogens like aflatoxin. About 80% of cases of HCC arise in cirrhotic liver.[10] The 5-year cumulative HCC risk is 21% in hemochromatosis, 10% in hepatitis B virus infection, 8% in alcoholic cirrhosis and 5% in biliary cirrhosis.[11] Presence of multiple factors significantly increases the risk of HCC.[2] Any patient with chronic liver disease is at risk for the development of HCC with an annual incidence of 2–8%.[12,13] It is important to note that in patients with cirrhosis, in addition to HCC, there is an increased risk of development of intrahepatic cholangiocarcinoma.[14]

The HCCs which occur in cirrhotic liver are thought to arise in a stepwise fashion from a regenerating nodule which develops into a low grade dysplastic nodule, high grade dysplastic nodule which finally develops a focus of HCC to form early HCC and then progressed HCC.[15] The development of HCCs in liver without background cirrhosis is called *'de novo hepatocarcinogenesis'*.[16] Pathologically HCC may occur in three different forms: solitary, multifocal, or diffuse. In Asia, HCC usually presents as a well defined mass, either solitary or multifocal, associated with cirrhosis secondary to hepatitis B. In the west it usually presents as a diffusely infiltrating mass and has an association with alcoholic cirrhosis. Neo-vascularity is an important pathological characteristic of HCC. Capsule is seen in 65–82% of the lesions and encapsulated lesions have a better prognosis.[17]

Hepatocellular carcinoma frequently invades the portal vein (in about 40% cases) and less often the inferior vena cava and hepatic veins (15%).[2] Biliary invasion is uncommon. With various curative therapies now available (liver transplantation, hepatic resection, percutaneous ablative techniques, chemotherapy, immunotherapy), 5-year-survival rate is about 40–75%.[2]

The implementation of the screening programs has resulted in detection of HCC at an earlier stage **(Flowchart 1)**. Imaging is crucial for the diagnosis of HCC and biopsy is no longer performed.[18] The American Association for the Study of Liver Diseases (AASLD) recommends that if a mass >1 cm shows typical imaging features (arterial phase enhancement and washout in venous phase) on one modality [either Contrast-enhanced computed tomography (CECT) or Contrast-enhanced magnetic resonance (CEMR)] a diagnosis of HCC can be made. For lesions <1 cm, follow-up with USG should be done every 3 months to see if they progress or are stable.[18] Follow-up imaging is a must in all patients after treatment as recurrence rates are as high as 70% and most occur in the initial 3 years. This is done at 3-monthly intervals. Similar guidelines have also been suggested by National Comprehensive Cancer Network.[19]

Clinical Presentation

The clinical signs and symptoms are often obscured by the debilitating effects of cirrhosis. Upper abdominal pain, malaise, fever, weight loss, palpable mass and rapid deterioration of liver function in patients with long standing cirrhosis are possible indicators.

Alfa-fetoprotein (AFP) is a useful serum marker and is elevated in 50–70% cases. Serum levels more than 20 ng/mL are abnormal and levels above 1000 ng/mL are strongly suggestive of HCC.

Flowchart 1: Diagnostic algorithm for suspected focal lesion in patients with chronic liver disease.

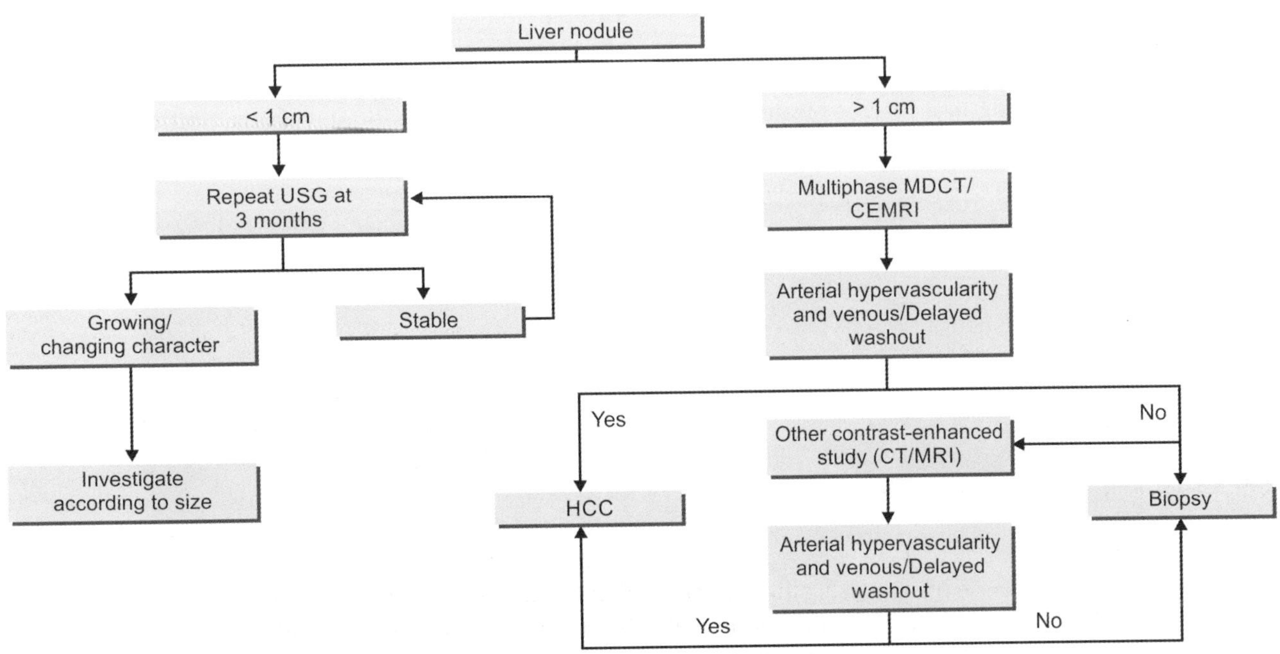

Abbreviations: MDCT: Multidetector-row computed tomography; CEMRI: Contrast-enhanced magnetic resonance imaging; USG: Ultrasonography
Source: Reproduced from AASLD Practice Guidelines 2010

Imaging in HCC

Imaging in HCC is a challenge as early diagnosis is critical for successful treatment. Lesions larger than 2 cm usually do not pose a diagnostic problem. However, nodules smaller than 2 cm often have nonspecific imaging features and create difficulties in diagnosis.[20] MRI scores over CT in detection of small HCCs in cirrhotic liver. The sensitivity of MRI and CT for detection of HCC is 81% and 68%, respectively. In addition differentiation of regenerative and dysplastic nodules from HCC, in cirrhosis, is vital for proper management.

Ultrasonography

Sonography being inexpensive and widely available is frequently used as the initial modality in the work-up of focal hepatic lesions. Recent advances in ultrasonography (USG) like liver specific ultrasound contrast agents and sonoelastography have increased its importance. The sensitivity of USG for detection of HCC ranges between 75% and 94% in various studies. However, sensitivity of USG for detection of HCC in the end stage cirrhotic liver is only about 50%, though the specificity has been reported to be as high as 98%. Most countries recommend a combination of USG and AFP every 6 months for HCC screening in high-risk patients.[18] Thus, any sonographically detected lesion in a cirrhotic liver should be evaluated according to the guidelines by American Association for Study of Liver Diseases.[18]

HCC has variable morphological presentations. Tumors can be solitary **(Fig. 1A)**, multifocal or diffusely infiltrating. The most common finding is a discrete lesion, either solitary or multiple. These lesions are usually hypoechoic, but are sometimes isoechoic and detected chiefly by virtue of a thin hypoechoic halo which corresponds to the tumor capsule. Encapsulated HCCs are more commonly seen in the Asian and Japanese population as compared to the west. Twenty-five percent of HCCs are echogenic.

The echo pattern has been shown to correlate with tumor morphology. Solid tumors without necrosis are hypoechoic whereas hyperechoic appearance is attributable to fatty metamorphosis, fibrosis, or sinusoidal dilatation **(Fig. 1B)**. The majority of small HCCs (<2 cm) are hypoechoic, whereas the larger HCCs are hyperechoic or of heterogeneous echo texture.

A less common pattern of HCC is diffuse parenchymal involvement with disorganization of the normal echo pattern. Multiple areas of decreased and increased echogenicity are present throughout the distorted liver without any distinct masses.

HCC has a propensity to invade the portal vein, hepatic vein or both, and this is depicted as echoes either partially or completely filling the lumen. Color Doppler flow imaging is a useful adjunct for detection of vascular invasion. The presence of arterial waveform within the thrombus indicates that it is neoplastic rather than bland thrombus. This distinction is vital because it has been shown that the presence of malignant portal vein thrombosis is the worst prognostic factor in predicting recurrence of HCC following surgical resection or liver transplantation. Color Doppler may also demonstrate intralesional vascularity in the form of a tangle of vessels within the tumor indicating hypervascularity and arteriovenous shunting. A basket pattern of intralesional vessels, indicating internal

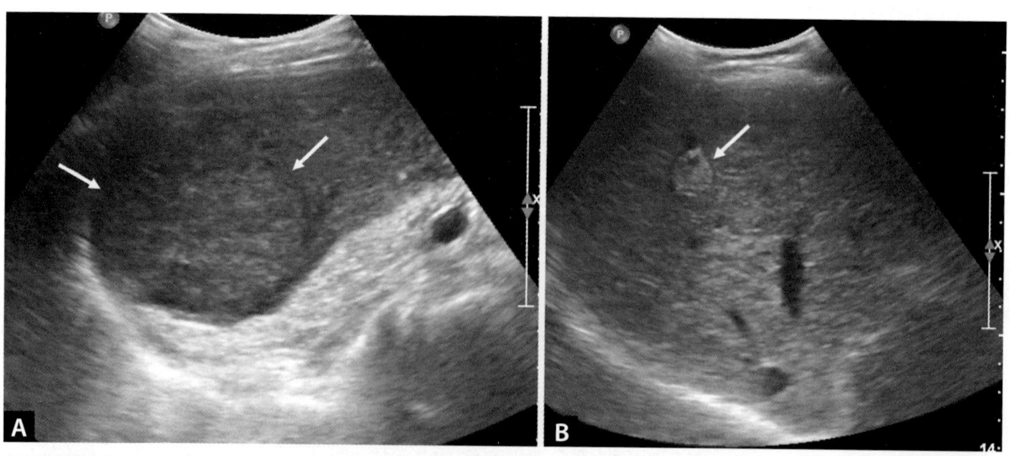

Figs. 1A and B: Sonographic appearance of hepatocellular carcinoma. (A) USG showing an isohyperechoic mass in the right lobe of liver (arrows) with normal background liver; (B) USG in a different patient with cirrhotic liver showing heterogeneous echotexture of parenchyma with an echogenic lesion (arrow) suggestive of HCC.

vascularity and shunting, may be seen in up to 15% of cases.[21] However, there is a lot of overlap in Doppler patterns. Contrast-enhanced USG with sonovue (Bracco, Milano, Italy) shows early hyperperfusion of HCC with washout in portal venous phase.[22] Liver specific USG contrast agent (Sonazoid; GE healthcare, Norway) has been developed but it is currently not available in India. It is a perflubutane based microbubble and provides both dynamic and liver specific images.[23]

Computed Tomography

The advent of helical CT made it possible to perform multi-phasic examination of the liver in the arterial and portal venous phase with the same bolus of contrast. This has had a major impact on the detection and characterization of hypervascular lesions like HCC. Multidetector computed tomography (MDCT) has allowed faster scanning of liver, thus reducing respiration artifacts and has increased the spatial resolution substantially, leading to improvement in the characterization of smaller lesions. Also, with MDCT, good quality multiplanar reconstructions and CT angiographic images can be obtained. The latter enables proper planning of surgical resection or transplantation.

The liver receives 75–80% of its blood supply from the portal vein and 20–25% from the hepatic artery. On the other hand, most liver tumors receive the majority of their blood supply from the hepatic artery. HCCs have a rich arterial supply and are better visualized on the arterial phase. It has been reported that up to 11% of lesions may be seen only on the arterial phase as they become isodense on the portal venous phase. In addition, arterial phase imaging is useful in demonstrating arterialportal shunting (early enhancement of intrahepatic portal venous branches) and enhancement of portal venous thrombus confirming it to be tumor thrombus.[1,15]

The CT features are variable depending on the size, vascularity and growth pattern. The multiphasic CT scan includes a noncontrast phase, followed by arterial, venous and delayed phases. Late arterial phase should be done as HCC shows enhancement in this phase. On unenhanced CT, most HCCs present as solitary or multiple low attenuating lesions. Areas of fat density may be seen. In a fatty liver, HCC may be seen as a hyperdense lesion. On arterial phase images the hypervascular tumor shows intense enhancement throughout the tumor **(Figs. 2A to C)**. The lesions are frequently encapsulated and the capsule is seen as a hypodense rim. Larger tumors are often heterogeneous due to necrosis and hemorrhage **(Figs. 3A to C)**. Arterial phase may demonstrate the presence of arterioportal shunting **(Fig. 4)**. During the portal venous phase there is rapid washout and the lesion becomes isodense to hypodense to normal liver **(Figs. 2B and 3B)**. On delayed phase, images the capsule and fibrous septa may show prolonged enhancement **(Fig. 3C)**. Contrast washout has very high specificity (96%) for the diagnosis of HCC.[24] Dual energy CT generates iodine maps which helps in detecting subtle lesions **(Figs. 5A and B)**. Vascular invasion is common with HCC. Portal vein invasion is due to portal venous drainage of HCC. A tumor thrombus in portal vein is diagnosed if the main portal vein has a diameter of ≥ 23 mm (bland thrombus rarely causes portal vein dilatation) and the thrombus shows enhancement (typically called "threads and streaks") in arterial phase **(Figs. 6A and B)**. HCCs may also extend into the hepatic veins or IVC **(Figs. 7A to C)**. HCCs may occasionally rupture and may lead to hemoperitoneum. A ruptured HCC is hypodense on arterial phase images showing only peripheral rim enhancement with focal discontinuity ('enucleation sign').[2]

Imaging accuracy is often more limited in the cirrhotic liver due to architectural distortion, presence of regenerating nodules and hemodynamic alterations. Therefore, the detection of HCC in a cirrhotic liver may require several complementary imaging techniques. Since the imaging appearance of HCC can be variable it is said that any mass in a cirrhotic liver that does not fulfill criteria for a cyst or hemangioma should be considered an HCC until proved otherwise.

Magnetic Resonance Imaging

Magnetic resonance imaging (MRI) with its superior contrast resolution and multiple paradigms for lesion characterization is superior to CT for the evaluation of HCC in a cirrhotic liver. The MR appearance depends on the type of disease (solitary, multifocal or diffuse), the degree of fibrosis, amount of fat as well as on the presence of necrosis and hemorrhage.

Usually, HCC is hypointense on T1W images and mildly hyperintense on T2W images **(Figs. 8A to E and 9A to E)**. The presence of fat or hemorrhage may result in increased signal intensity on T1W images **(Fig. 8A)**. Encapsulated lesions have a hypointense rim on T1W images and a single or a double layered hypointense rim on T2W images. Fast gradient echo sequences allow the liver to be imaged in a breath hold and multi-phasic dynamic gadolinium-enhanced MR imaging has been shown to improve detection of HCC and is superior to dual phase CT. MRI frequently demonstrates HCCs,

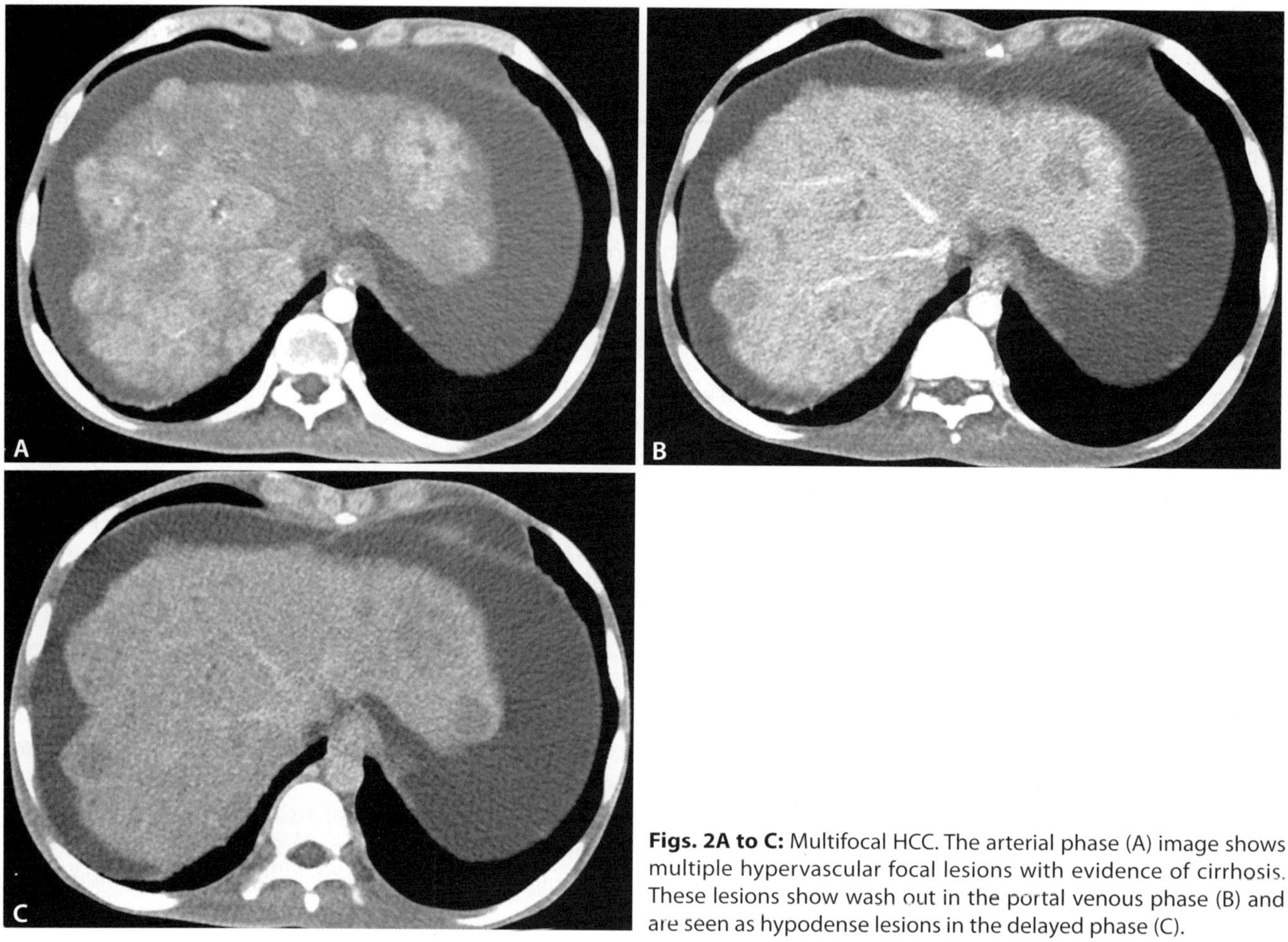

Figs. 2A to C: Multifocal HCC. The arterial phase (A) image shows multiple hypervascular focal lesions with evidence of cirrhosis. These lesions show wash out in the portal venous phase (B) and are seen as hypodense lesions in the delayed phase (C).

particularly tumors smaller than 1.5 cm, better than CT images. HCC is typically seen as a hypervascular mass with rapid washout. Tumors larger than 2 cm enhance in a heterogeneous fashion.[15]

The most sensitive sequence for detecting small HCC is the postgadolinium arterial phase on which small tumors enhance intensely. However, this feature is not specific as severely dysplastic nodules will also enhance. A more specific feature is washout of tumor below the signal of liver in venous or delayed phase with late enhancement of the capsule.[15] The arterial phase also allows distinction from metastatic disease because HCCs typically demonstrate enhancing stroma through the entire tumor whereas metastases have peripheral enhancement. However, metastases from hypervascular primaries (neuroendocrine tumors, renal cell carcinoma) may show similar enhancement and may pose diagnostic problem. The degree of vascularity in HCC may vary with the majority being hypervascular but some are hypovascular.

Diffuse infiltration with HCC may be subtle or simulate the appearance of chronic hepatitis or scarring. It may present as extensive hepatic parenchymal involvement with mottled punctate high intensity on T2W images and mottled enhancement on arterial phase images. Diffuse HCC is very frequently associated with portal vein thrombosis. MRI is useful in differentiation of tumor from bland portal vein thrombus. The hyperintense signal on T2W sequence is highly suggestive of tumor thrombus.[15] Other features favoring malignant thrombus include dilatation of the vein and contrast enhancement.

Liver specific MR contrast agents currently available include gadobenate dimeglumine and gadoxetic acid. Gadobenate dimeglumine (Gd-BOPTA) has the advantage of being both intravascular and hepatobiliary contrast agent.[15] Although it is mainly excreted by the kidneys, about 5% is excreted in the biliary tree, which is prominently seen 60–120 minutes after intravenous injection. Gadobenate, is available in India and should

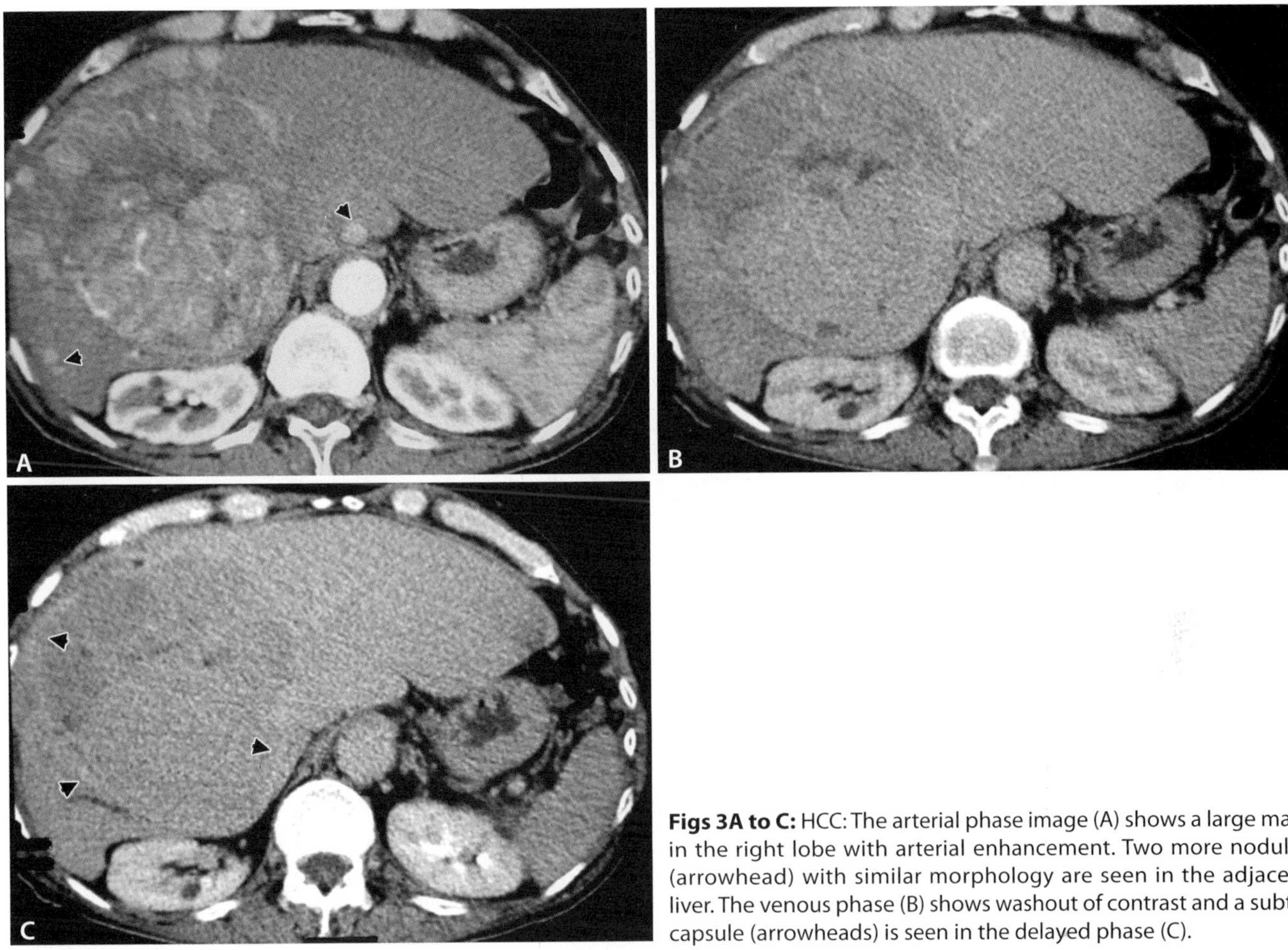

Figs 3A to C: HCC: The arterial phase image (A) shows a large mass in the right lobe with arterial enhancement. Two more nodules (arrowhead) with similar morphology are seen in the adjacent liver. The venous phase (B) shows washout of contrast and a subtle capsule (arrowheads) is seen in the delayed phase (C).

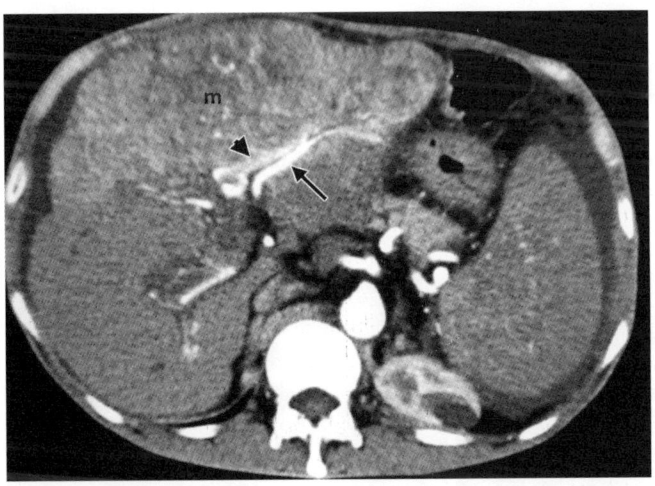

Fig. 4: Arterioportal shunt: The arterial phase CT image shows a large enhancing lesion (m) in the segments 3 and 4 of liver with contrast in the left hepatic artery (arrow) and left branch of portal vein (arrowhead) suggesting arterioportal shunting.

be routinely used as a contrast agent for dynamic CEMR with an additional delayed scan taken at 1–2 hours after injection. Another liver specific contrast agent is Gadoxetic acid (Gd-EOB), which has about 50% hepatic excretion.[25] With this agent the hepatobiliary phase can be acquired at 15–20 min after contrast injection. Both these agents are taken up by functioning hepatocytes through organic anionic transport polypeptide (OATP) receptors and excreted into biliary canaliculi. Thus, lesion which do not contain hepatocytes are seen as hypointense areas compared to the enhancing normal liver parenchyma on hepatobiliary phase **(Figs. 10A to F)**. This hepatobiliary phase thus improves detection of the lesions. However, well-differentiated HCCs may also show uptake of the agent **(Fig. 9E)**.

Diffusion-weighted imaging (DWI) is increasingly being used in abdomen. The typical b-values used are 0, 400 and 800 s/mm^2. DWI has an important role in differentiation of benign from malignant liver lesions and improves the accuracy of contrast-enhanced MRI in detection of HCC with only a minimal time penalty.[26,27] HCCs show restriction of diffusion and this sequence

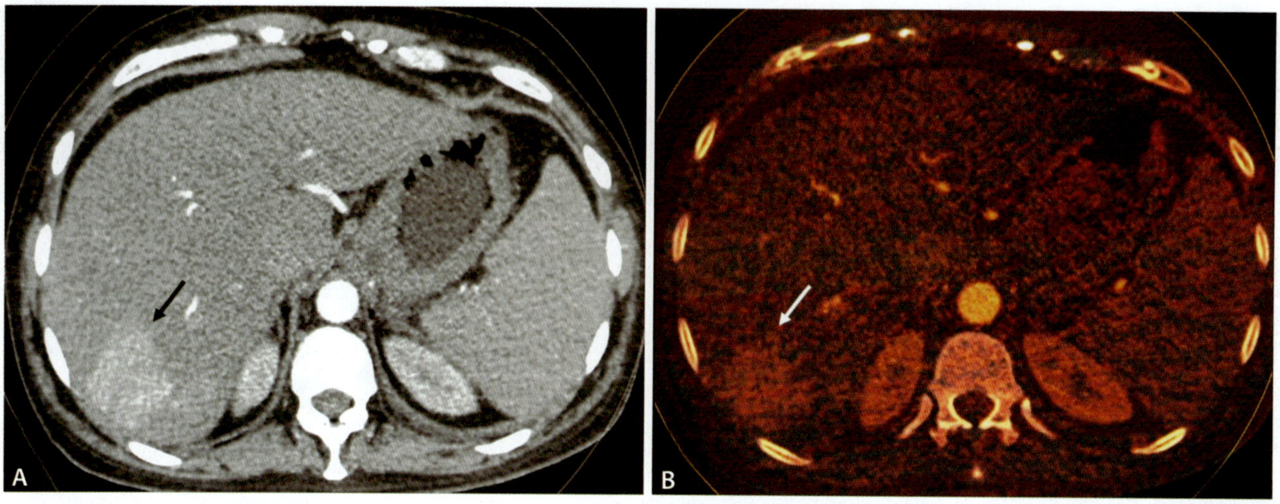

Figs. 5A and B: Dual energy CT appearance of HCC. (A) Axial CT scan in arterial phase showing enhancing lesion in segment 7 of liver (arrow); (B) Iodine map generated from dual energy CT data makes it easy to appreciate iodine uptake in the lesion (arrow).

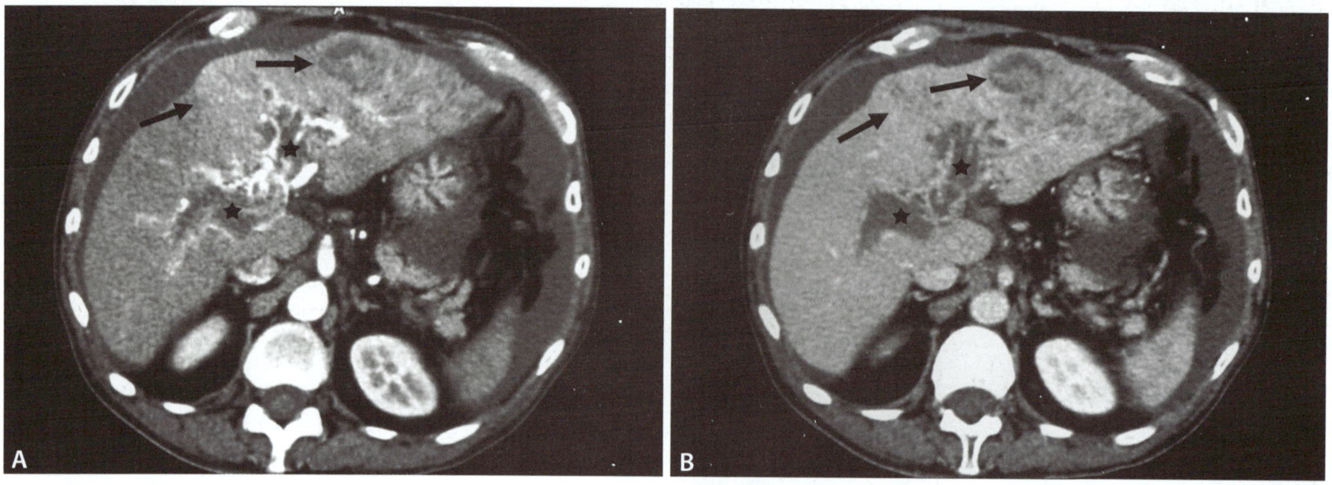

Figs. 6A and B: Portal vein thrombus: The arterial phase CT image (A) shows two enhancing lesions (arrows) in segments 3 and 4 of liver with arterioportal shunting. The portal vein in the venous phase image; (B) shows a large filling defect (stars) with 'thread and streak' pattern of enhancement suggestive of tumor thrombus.

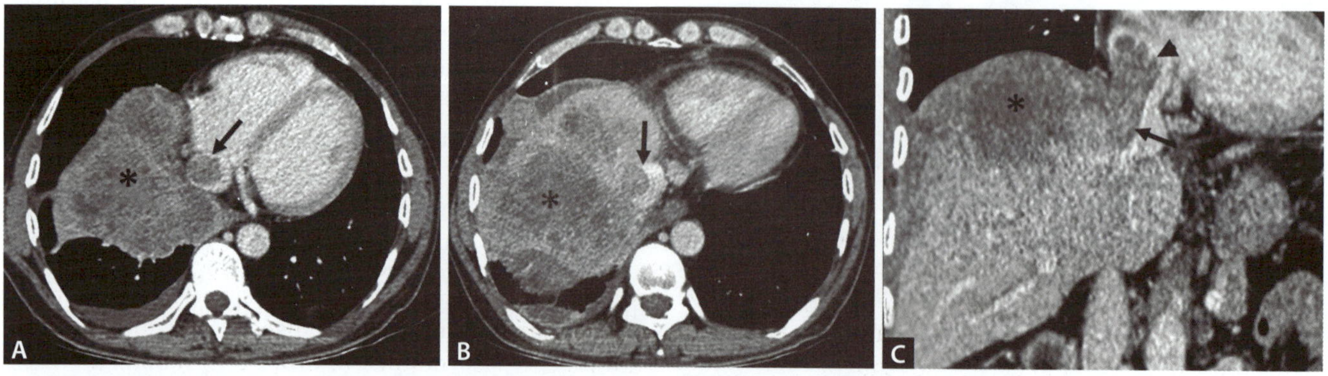

Figs. 7A to C: HCC with inferior vena cava extension. Axial (A and B) and coronal (C) contrast-enhanced CT scans in venous phase showing large mass in the liver (asterisk) with extension into the inferior vena cava (arrow) and right atrium (arrowhead in C).

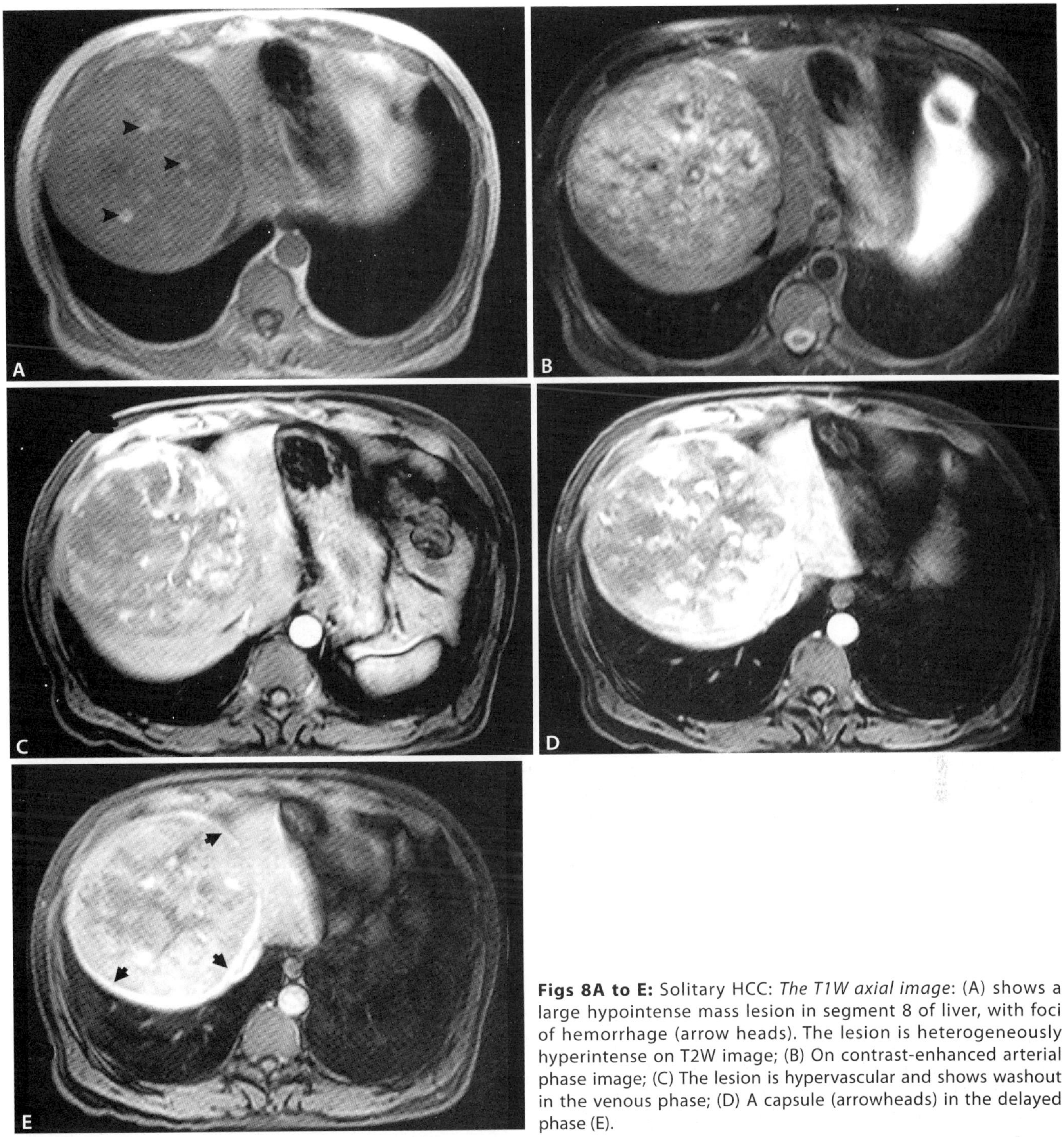

Figs 8A to E: Solitary HCC: *The T1W axial image*: (A) shows a large hypointense mass lesion in segment 8 of liver, with foci of hemorrhage (arrow heads). The lesion is heterogeneously hyperintense on T2W image; (B) On contrast-enhanced arterial phase image; (C) The lesion is hypervascular and shows washout in the venous phase; (D) A capsule (arrowheads) in the delayed phase (E).

may help in distinguishing it from other benign arterially enhancing lesions **(Figs. 9A to E)**.[28]

Various staging systems are available for HCC. The Barcelona Clinic Liver Cancer (BCLC) staging is the widely accepted one and it takes into consideration hepatic function (by Child-Pugh score), patient's performance status and tumor staging (tumor size and number and portal vein thrombosis) for disease classification.[29] In addition it also defines appropriate management for different disease stages. This is shown in **Flowchart 2**.

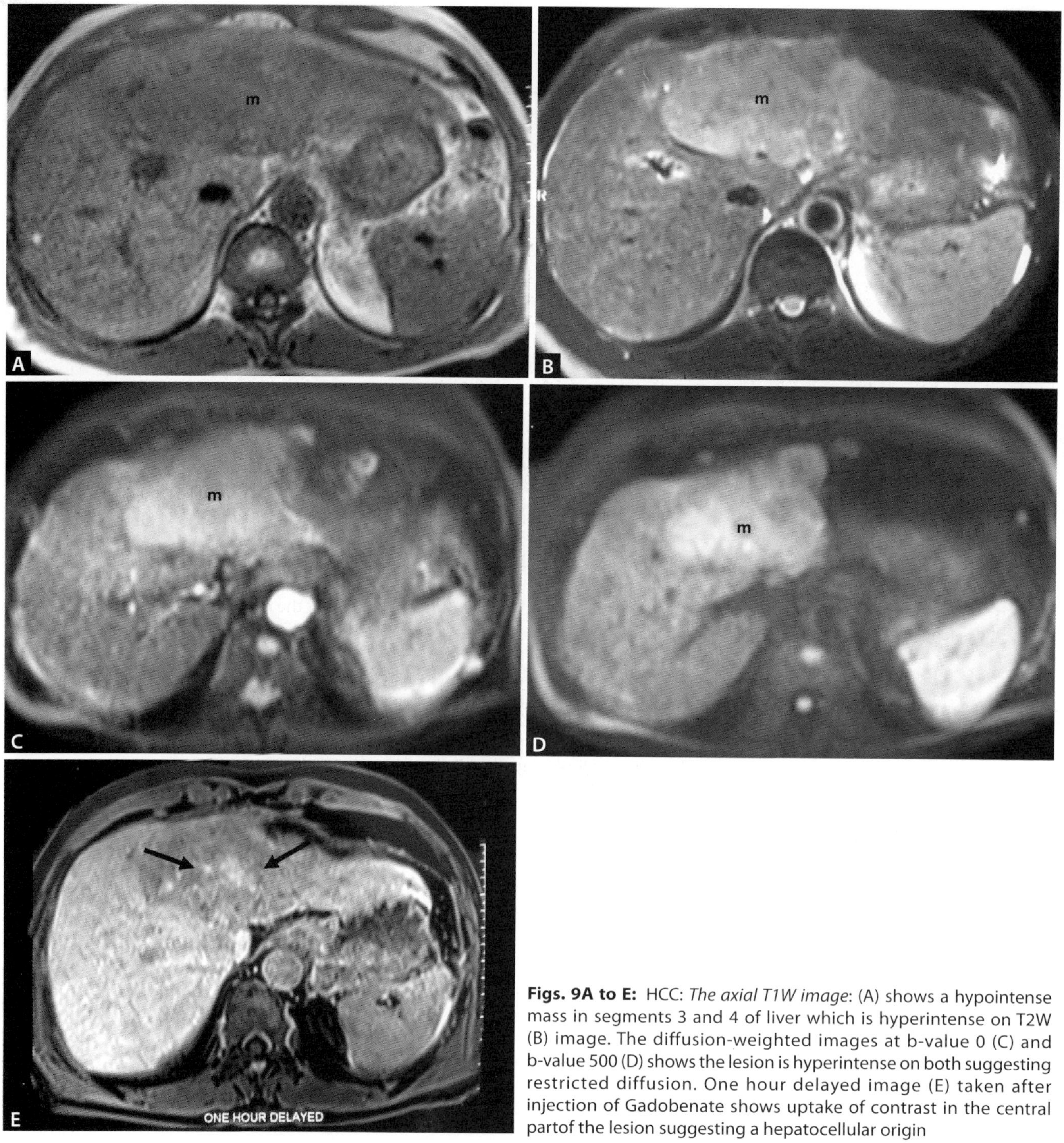

Figs. 9A to E: HCC: *The axial T1W image*: (A) shows a hypointense mass in segments 3 and 4 of liver which is hyperintense on T2W (B) image. The diffusion-weighted images at b-value 0 (C) and b-value 500 (D) shows the lesion is hyperintense on both suggesting restricted diffusion. One hour delayed image (E) taken after injection of Gadobenate shows uptake of contrast in the central partof the lesion suggesting a hepatocellular origin

Differential Diagnosis of HCC

In a cirrhotic liver, regenerative nodules and dysplastic nodules are also common and these must be differentiated from HCC.[20,30] Regenerative nodules are usually isointense on both T1W and T2W images as they contain normal liver cells. They may be hyperintense on T1W images, which is due to the presence of protein, fat and copper **(Figs. 11A and B)**. Siderotic nodulesare hypointense on both T1W and T2W images, due to the presence of iron and fibrous content. They predominantly have portal venous blood supply and thus are isointense to normal liver on

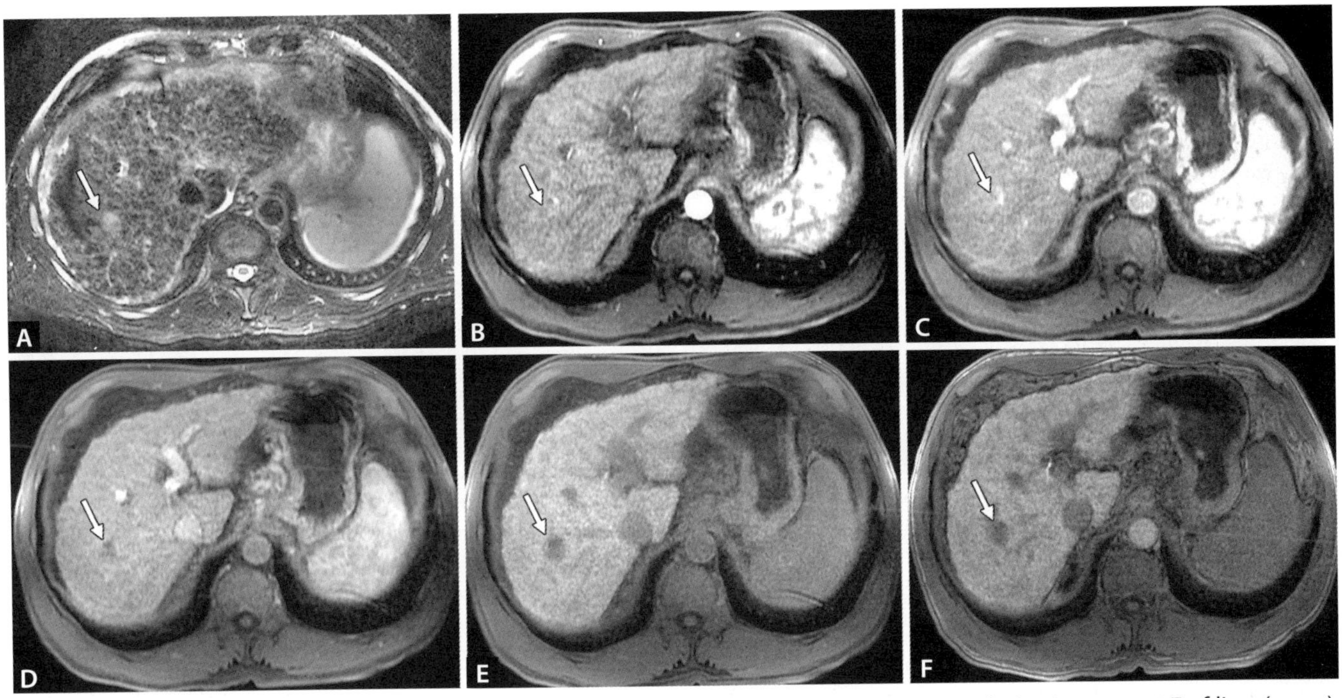

Figs. 10A to F: Gadoxetic acid-enhanced MRI. (A) T2W axial image showing a small hyperintense lesion in segment 7 of liver (arrow); (B) Arterial phase T1W image showing mild enhancement in the lesion (arrow); Venous (C) and Delayed (D) phase images showing contrast washout (arrow); Scans taken at 8 min (E) and 20 min (F) showing hypointense nature of the lesion (arrow) on hepatocyte phase suggesting no uptake of contrast by the lesion.
Courtesy: Dr Avinash Kambadakone, Dr Vinit Balyan, Massachusetts General Hospital, Boston.

Flowchart 2: Barcelona Clinic Liver Cancer (BCLC) staging system for hepatocellular carcinoma

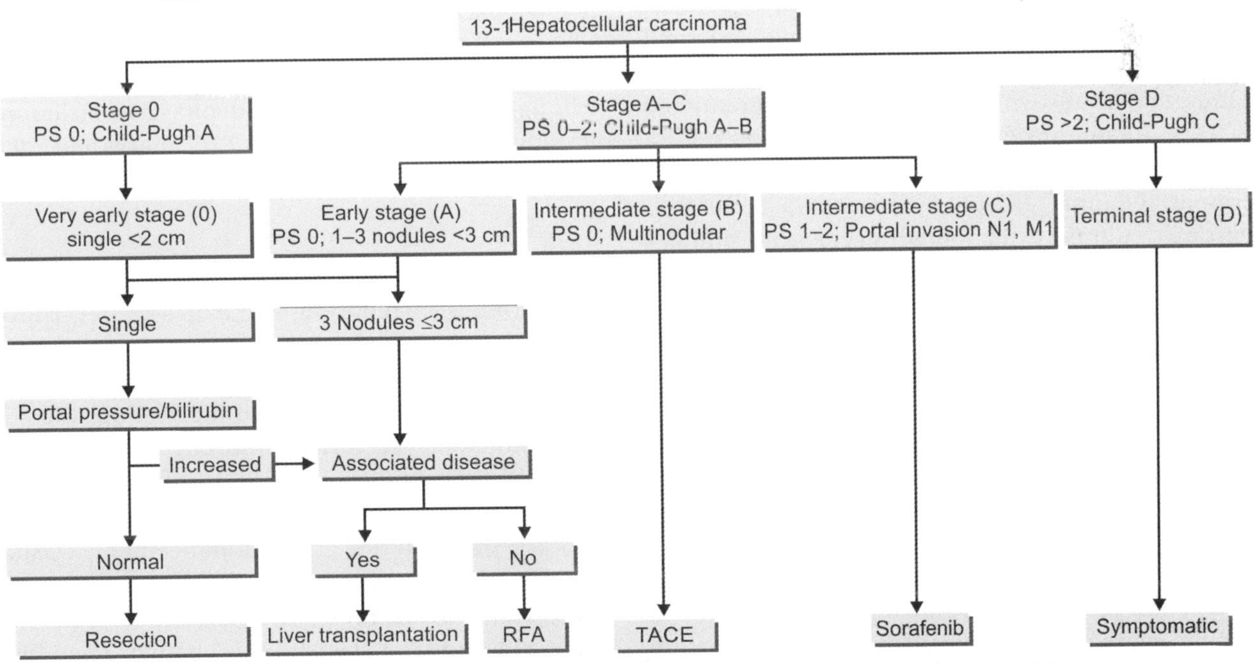

Abbreviations: M: Metastasis; N: Node stage; PS: Performance status; RFA: Radiofrequency ablation; TACE: Transarterial chemoembolization.

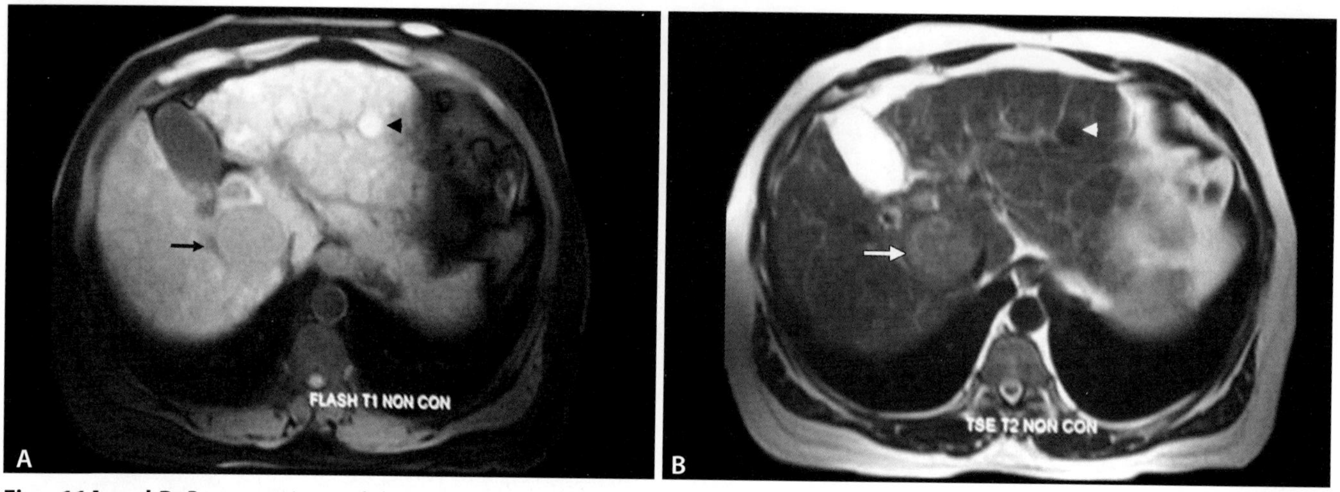

Figs. 11A and B: Regenerative nodule. Axial T1W image (A) shows a small hyperintense nodule (arrowhead) in left lobe which is hypointense on T2W image (B) suggestive of a regenerative nodule. In contrast to this, the segment 8 lesion (arrow) is hypointense on T1W image and mildly hyperintense on T2W image suggestive of HCC.

all three phases of CEMR. Dysplastic nodules, which are the precursors of HCC, are usually hyperintense on T1W and hypointense on T2W images. These too mostly (but not always) receive blood supply from portal veins and remain isointense on CEMR. A 'nodule within a nodule' appearance on T2W images (hyperintense focus in a hypointense nodule) is suggestive of HCC in a dysplastic nodule.[31] In doubtful cases, the features favoring HCC are size >2 cm, hyperintense T2W appearance, delayed washout, delayed enhancement of the capsule and rapid interval growth.

Other conditions which should to be differentiated from HCC include nodular regenerative hyperplasia (NRH), focal confluent fibrosis and nontumoros arterioportal shunt.[20] NRH is a non-neoplastic disease consisting of diffusely distributed regenerative nodules without associated fibrosis, occurring in noncirrhotic conditions like Budd-Chiari syndrome. These nodules are hyperintense on T1W images, hypo-to iso-intense on T2W images and often contain a central scar. They show arterial phase enhancement and differentiation from HCC is at times difficult. Focal confluent fibrosis may sometimes simulate tumors. It is often located in the anterior and medial segments of liver, and is wedge-shaped with base towards the liver capsule. It typically shows delayed enhancement, but occasionally arterial enhancement may be seen. The location of the lesion, shape and presence of atrophy with capsular retraction differentiate confluent fibrosis from HCC. Nontumoros arterioportal shunts are often seen in a cirrhotic liver. They are subcapsular, wedge shaped and do not produce mass effect. They are isointense on T1W and T2W scans, and show intense enhancement on arterial phase images, but become isointense on portal venous and delayed phase.

Other differentials include intrahepatic cholangiocarcinoma, hypervascular metastases, flash filling hemangiomas and angiomyolipoma (especially epithelioid variety).

Imaging features favoring HCC in a cirrhotic liver include lesions >2 cm, enhancement in arterial phase, washout of contrast in venous or equilibrium phase, peripheral capsule in delayed phase, restriction of diffusion, hyperintense signal on T2W images and interval growth.[20]

Liver Imaging Reporting and Data System

The liver imaging reporting and data system (LI-RADS) was developed to standardize the CT and MRI techniques, terminology, diagnosis and reporting of HCC and other liver lesions in patients with chronic liver disease.[32] The focal lesions are categorized into LR1 to LR5, with LR1 being definitely benign and LR5 being definitely HCC. Major findings included in this system for diagnosis of HCC are size, arterial phase enhancement, washout, capsule and threshold growth. There are many ancillary features and tie breaker rules, the detailed discussion of which is beyond the scope of this chapter. The LIRADS version 2014 is the latest and is shown in **Flowchart 3**. The accuracy is above 80%. Further modification and simplification of classification is underway.

Flowchart 3: Liver imaging reporting and data system (LI-RADS) classification of liver lesions in patients of chronic liver disease.

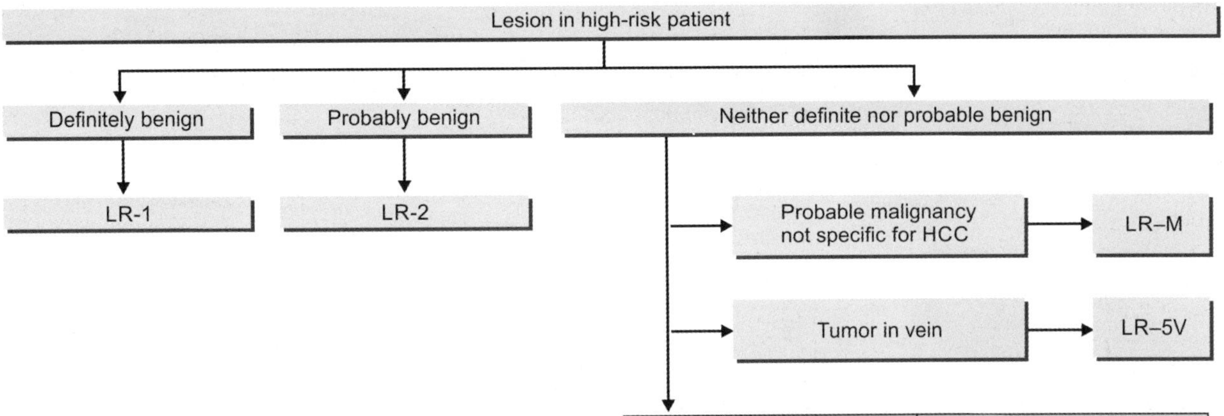

		Arterial phase hypo- or iso-enhancement		Arterial phase hyper-enhancement		
Diameter (mm)		<20	≥20	<10	10–19	≥20
Washout	None	LR–3	LR–3	LR–3	LR–3	LR–4
Capsule	One	LR–3	LR–4	LR–4	LR–4/5	LR–5
Threshold growth	≥ Two	LR–4	LR–4	LR–4	LR–5	LR–5

FIBROLAMELLAR HEPATOCELLULAR CARCINOMA

This is an unusual liver tumor found in young adults with a mean age of 25 years.[33,34] Patients do not have underlying cirrhosis nor are there any predisposing risk factors. It is frequently resectable and has a better prognosis than the usual HCC. The 5-year survival for fibrolamellar hepatocellular carcinoma (FLC) is 60% as compared to 30% for typical HCC. Serum AFP levels are typically normal. They usually present as a solitary large circumscribed mass that is partly or completely encapsulated. Satellite nodules are often seen. The major radiological clue to the diagnosis is the presence of central fibrous scar and central stellate calcification. Portal vein invasion, necrosis and hemorrhage are much less common than in typical HCC.[1,2]

On sonography, FLC is usually seen as a lobulated predominantly hyperechoic mass, although hypo and isoechoic forms have also been described **(Fig. 12A)**. Central hyperechoic nonshadowing areas with foci of shadowing correlate with the central scar and calcification within the scar. On unenhanced CT, FLC is a well-defined, lobulated and hypodense lesion. The central stellate calcification has been reported as a distinctive radiological feature and occurs in a high proportion (up to 68%) of these lesions **(Figs. 12A to D)**.[32] After intravenous contrast, FLC shows heterogeneous enhancement in the arterial and venous phases **(Figs. 12A to D)**. The scar does not show early enhancement but may enhance on delayed images.[2] On MRI, FLC is hypo- to isointense on T1W images and hyperintense on T2W images. The scar because of its fibrous nature, remains hypointense on T1- and T2-weighted images. The enhancement pattern on CEMR is similar to that seen on CT scans. On hepatobiliary phase, the lesion is hypointense to the surrounding liver parenchyma. The scar may be hyperintense. Although scar may be seen in other benign and malignant liver lesions, a large scar (>2 cm wide) along with fibrotic strands is more suggestive of FLC.[32]

The most important differential diagnosis of FLC is focal nodular hyperplasia (FNH). The central scar is hyperintense on T2W scans in FNH, but hypointense in FLC. Also, the scar of FLC shows calcification, but this is seen in <1.5% of cases of FNH. MRI with liver specific contrast agents is useful as FNH shows uptake of contrast in hepatobiliary phase unlike FLC.[1] The differentiation between the two is important as FNH is managed conservatively but FLC is treated surgically. Biopsy provides the diagnosis in difficult cases.[2] Other differentials include conventional HCC (differentiation is based on age, underlying liver disease, serum AFP levels) and intrahepatic cholangiocarcinoma (differentiation by enhancement characteristics, biliary dilatation).

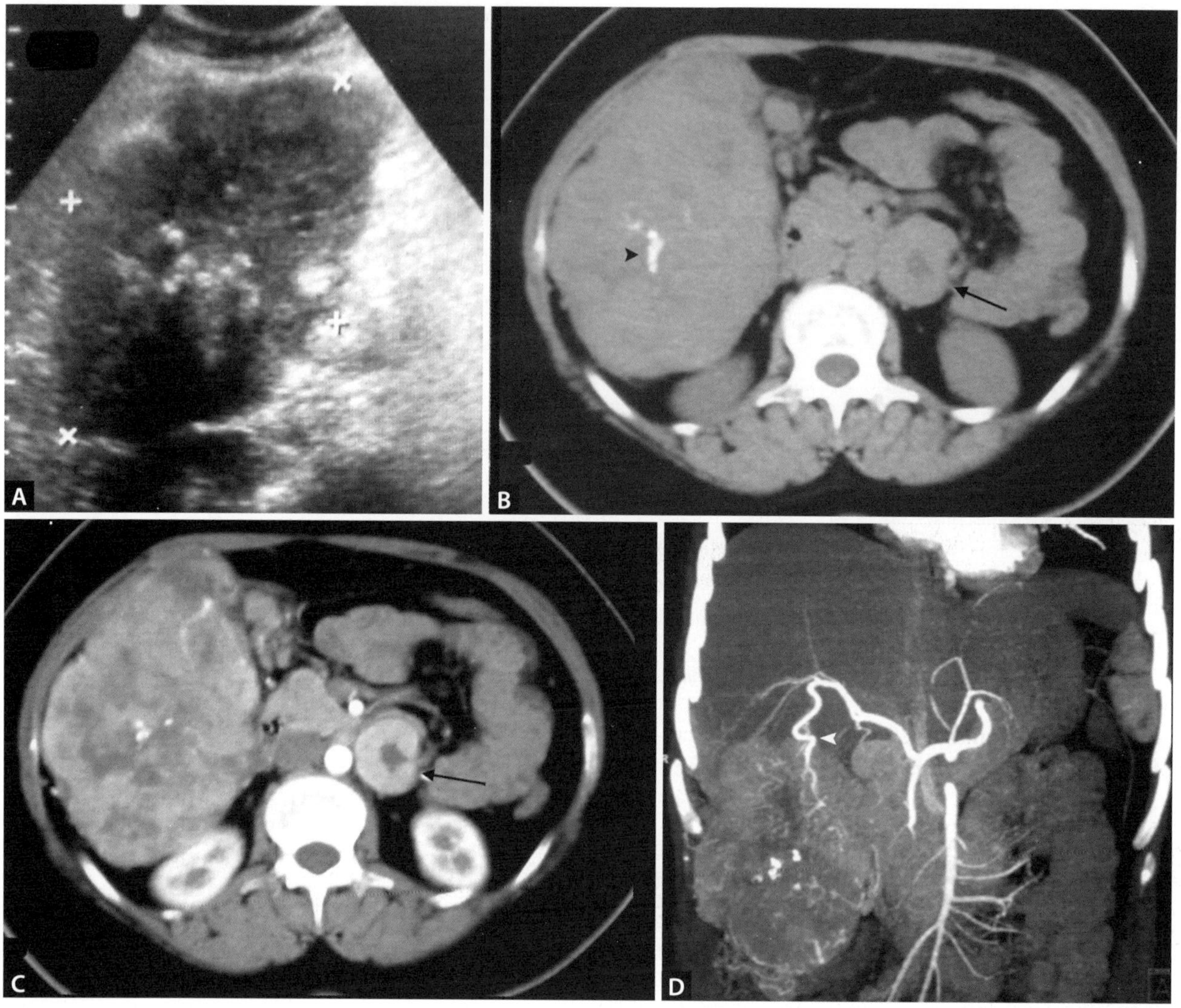

Figs. 12A to D: Fibrolamellar carcinoma: Ultrasonography (A) a hypoechoic mass in segment 6 of liver showing central calcification. Noncontrast CT scan; (B) hypodense mass in the liver with central calcification (arrowhead) and left para-aortic lymphadenopathy (arrow). Contrast-enhanced arterial phase CT image; (C) Heterogeneous enhancement with central scar showing calcification. The para-aortic node is showing intense enhancement (arrow). The CT maximum intensity projection image (D) shows a prominent feeder arising from the right hepatic artery (arrowhead).

Interventional Techniques

Many methods have been developed for the nonsurgical management of HCC employing angiographic and percutaneous techniques. These include hepatic arterial infusion chemotherapy and embolization and percutaneous techniques like ethanol ablation, and radiofrequency ablation. The details of these techniques are discussed in the chapter on Hepatic Intervention.

INTRAHEPATIC CHOLANGIOCARCINOMA

Intrahepatic cholangiocarcinoma is the second most common primary malignant hepatic tumor. It accounts for 10% of all cholangiocarcinomas and arises in small intrahepatic ducts. It has an increased incidence in patients with Caroli's disease, sclerosing cholangitis, intrahepatic calculi and inflammatory bowel disease. Cholangiocarcinoma typically produces extensive desmoplastic reaction.[2] Cirrhosis of liver may be a predisposing factor for intrahepatic cholangiocarcinoma (ICCA).

Patients present clinically with abdominal pain, anorexia and weight loss. Jaundice occurs only if major ducts are obstructed. A normal serum AFP may be helpful in suggesting ICCA rather than HCC.

Imaging

Sonographically, one or more hyperechoic, iso- or hypoechoic masses may be seen. Homogeneous hypoechoic pattern is the most common appearance **(Fig. 13)**. On Doppler USG the lesion is not very vascular. Dilated intrahepatic bile ducts distal to the mass are often seen.[1,2] On unenhanced CT, it is seen as a well-defined round to oval, hypodense mass. On multiphase contrast-enhanced CT, it typically shows thick irregular peripheral enhancement in the arterial or portal venous phase. A delayed central enhancement is often seen which may take 5–15 minutes and is thought to be due to the fibrous matrix of the tumor.[2] The mass may involve the portal vein branch with resultant atrophy of ipsilateral segment or lobe. The contralateral lobe may undergo hypertrophy. Hepatic capsular retraction, atrophy-hypertrophy complex and biliary dilatation adjacent to the mass are highly suggestive of ICCA (as these are rarely seen with HCC).[35] On MR imaging, the lesion appears hypointense on T1W and hyperintense on T2W images **(Figs. 14A to F)**. The central fibrous area may appear hypointense on T2W images. DWI shows restriction of diffusion. On CEMR, smaller lesions (2–4 cm) enhance homogeneously but those >4 cm show thick peripheral enhancement with centripetal progression **(Figs. 14A to F)**. On hepatobiliary phase (with gadoxetic acid or gadobenate dimeglumine) the lesion appears hypointense.[36] Occasionally, central fibrotic area may be hyperintense due to extracellular contrast retention. The primary angiographic finding in cholangiocarcinoma is serrated or serpiginous arterial infiltration. Large tumors

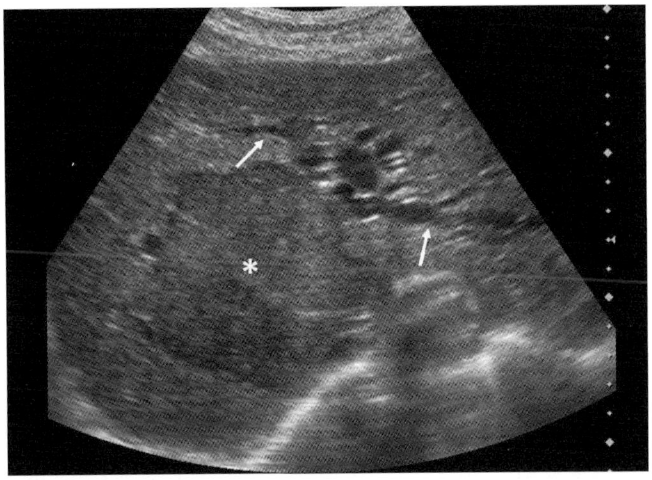

Fig. 13: USG of mass forming cholangiocarcinoma showing a large isohypoechoic mass in right lobe of liver (asterisk) with dilatation of biliary radicles (arrows).

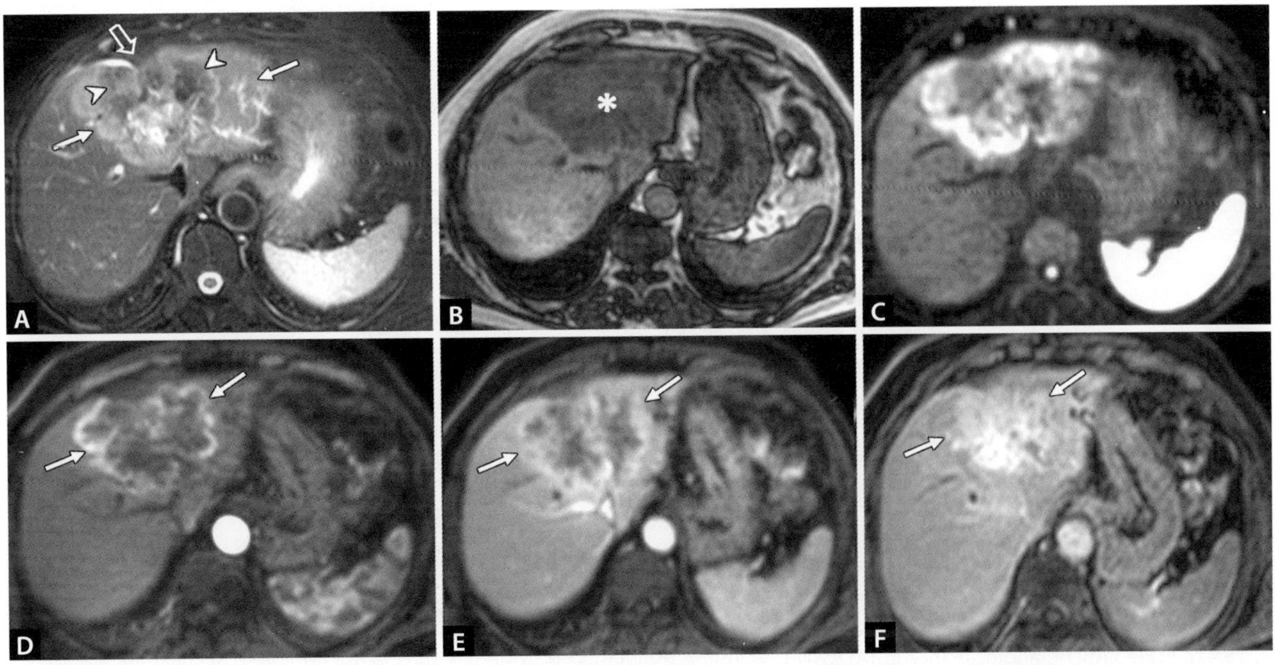

Figs. 14A to F: Mass forming cholangiocarcinoma. (A) Axial T2W fat-saturated image showing lobulated heterogeneous mass in left lobe of liver (arrows) with hypointense fibrotic areas (arrowheads) and retraction of capsule (block arrow); (B) Axial T1W image showing hypointense appearance of the lesion (asterisk); (C) Axial diffusion-weighted image (b-800) showing restriction of diffusion in the lesion; On contrast-enhanced images, the lesion shows thick smooth peripheral enhancement in arterial phase; (D) with gradual filling in of the lesion with contrast in venous; (E) Delayed; (F) Phases (arrows).

may be mildly vascular but in small tumors arterial encasement is the only abnormality.

The differential diagnosis include HCC, hemangioma and metastasis from gastrointestinal primary malignancy. The presence of capsular retraction, biliary dilatation, lobar or segmental atrophy, T2W hypointensity, peripheral thick band like enhancement in arterial phase and centripetal filling favour a diagnosis of ICCA. It is important to distinguish this tumor from HCC in a cirrhotic liver as patients with ICCA are taken off from the transplant list.

HEPATOCHOLANGIOCARCINOMA

Hepatocholangiocarcinoma (HCCA) is an uncommon biphenotypic malignancy.[33] It may be seen in patients of cirrhosis of liver and chronic viral hepatitis.[37] They have worse prognosis than HCC. The clinical presentation is nonspecific. Serum markers although not very helpful, diagnosis should be suspected if both AFP and CA19-9 are elevated. On imaging, morphological features of both HCC and ICCA are seen **(Figs. 15A to F)**.[38] The lesion may show peripheral enhancement in the arterial phase with retention of contrast in the venous and delayed phases. Washout of contrast and capsular retraction may also be seen. Thus, more often, the enhancement characteristics follow more of ICCA than HCC. Biliary dilatation is uncommon. The lesion may show restriction of diffusion on DWI. However, whenever there is overlap of imaging features of HCC and ICCA in a liver lesion, HCCA should be suspected. Biopsy is needed for confirmation. It is important to differentiate HCCA from HCC as liver transplantation should be avoided in HCCA due to high recurrence.

BILIARY CYSTADENOCARCINOMA

Biliary cystadenocarcinoma is a rare tumor of bile duct origin and often develops due to malignant transformation of biliary cystadenoma.[39] They are more commonly seen in females in the age of 40–60 years. The clinical presentation is nonspecific and patients may present with abdominal pain or bloating, lump, vomiting or jaundice.[33] Anorexia and loss of weight may be present. Tumor markers such as cancer antigen (CA) 19-9 and carcinoembryonic antigen (CEA), may be elevated in some cases, but are not helpful in making a diagnosis.

USG shows a variable-sized cystic lesion with multiple internal septations which appear thick and echogenic. Solid nodules may also be seen which may show internal vascularity. Contrast-enhanced CT or MRI shows the

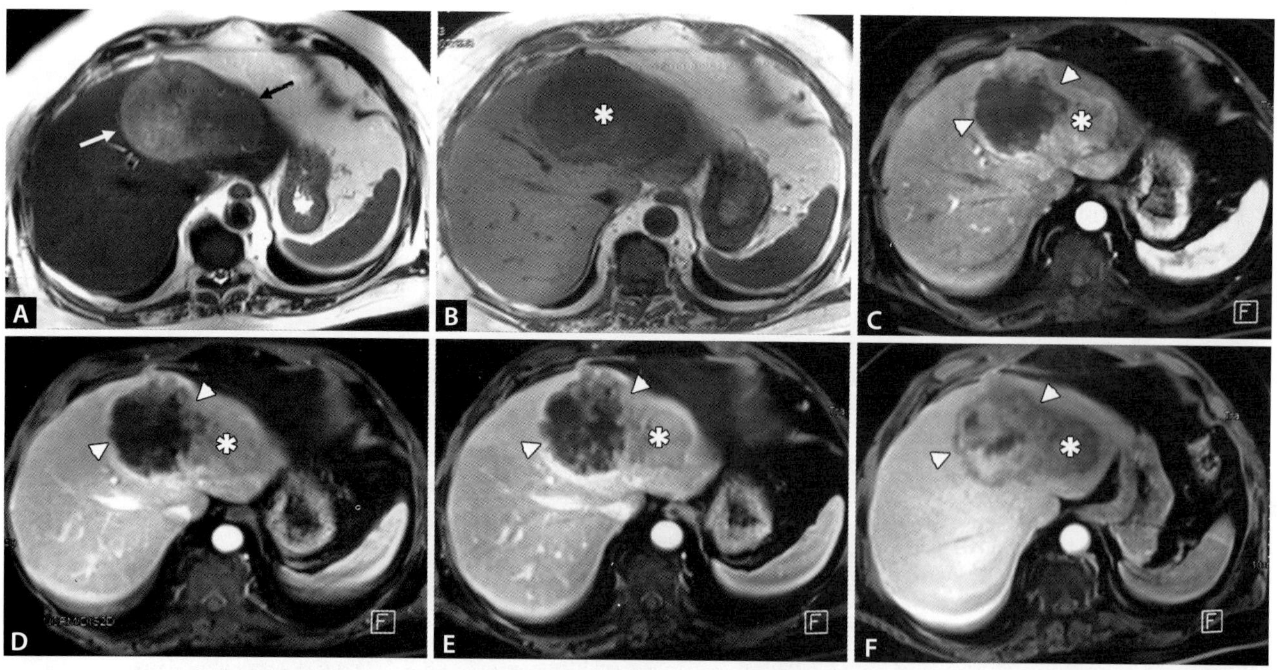

Figs. 15A to F: Hepatocholangiocarcinoma. (A) Axial T2W image showing a well-defined mass in the right lobe of liver with hyperintense (white arrow) and hypointense (black arrow) areas; (B) Axial T1W image showing homogeneous hypointense signal of the lesion; Dynamic contrast-enhanced T1W images showing the hepatocellular component (asterisk) with enhancement in arterial phase (C) and washout in venous (D) and delayed (E) phases with capsule formation (E). The cholangiocellular component (arrowheads) shows peripheral arterial enhancement (C) with gradual filling in of contrast in venous and delayed phases; (F) Axial T1W image in hepatobiliary phase shows hypointense hepatocellular component and retained contrast in cholangiocellular component due to fibrous matrix.

cystic lesion with enhancing thick septations **(Fig. 16)**. Enhancing solid nodules are seen which may show restriction of diffusion on DWI. Biliary communication or obstruction is usually not seen.

Differential diagnosis includes hydatid cyst and complicated liver cysts. Absence of enhancing septations and solid nodules may suggest that diagnosis but in most cases final diagnosis is possible only after surgical excision.

HEPATOBLASTOMA

Hepatoblastoma is the most common primary liver tumor of childhood.[34] It most commonly occurs in the first three years of life, whereas hepatocellular malignancies in children older than five years tend to be morphologically similar to those found in adults.

The most common presentation is a painless abdominal mass, however anorexia, weight loss, pain and jaundice can occur. Serum AFP levels are elevated in over 90% of patients.

Pathologically hepatoblastoma tends to be well defined, pseudoencapsulated, large, unifocal lesion. Less commonly multiple nodules or diffuse liver involvement may be seen. Calcification may be seen in up to one-third of patients.[2]

Imaging

The sonographic appearance of hepatoblastoma is of a large, inhomogeneous echogenic mass sometimes with calcification. Anechoic foci due to necrosis and a lobular pattern caused by septation may be seen.

CT most commonly demonstrates a well-defined hypodense mass with mild enhancement **(Figs. 17A and B)**.

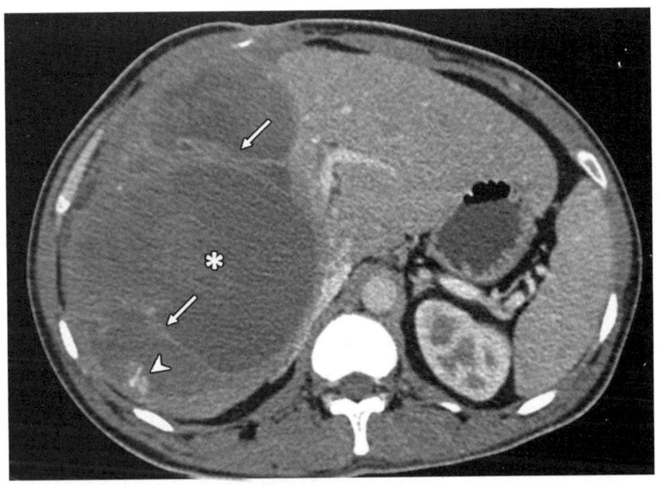

Fig. 16: Biliary cystadenocarcinoma. Contrast-enhanced CT scan showing a large cystic lesion in the right lobe of liver (asterisk) with thick enhancing septations (arrows) and enhancing mural nodule (arrow head).

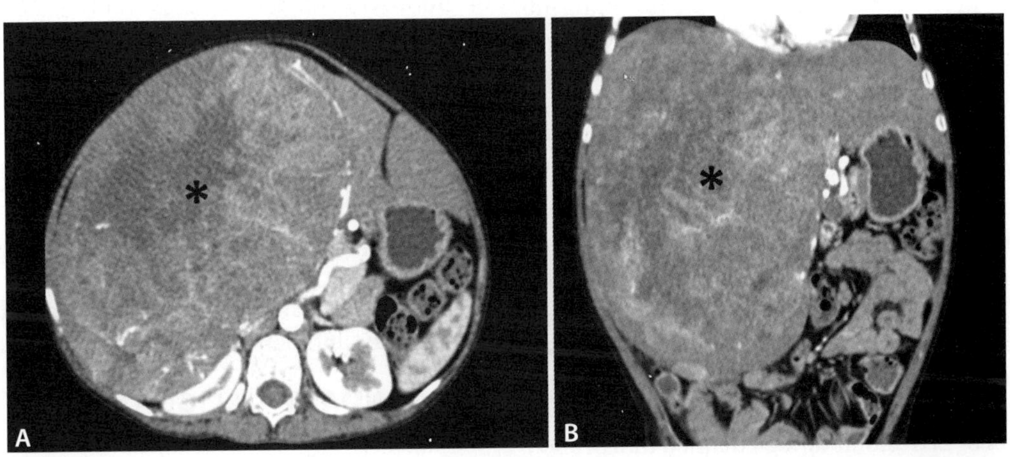

Figs. 17A and B: Hepatoblastoma. Axial (A) and Coronal (B) contrast-enhanced CT images showing a large mass replacing the right lobe of liver with central necrotic areas and peripheral enhancing areas in a 2-year-old child.

Involvement of portal vein and inferior vena cava (IVC) can be demonstrated. Three-dimensional reconstruction provides important information about vascular invasion. If this shows portal vein invasion and in very large lesions neoadjuvant chemotherapy is given to shrink the tumor away from portal vein and then surgical excision is done.[40] Lung metastasis is common at presentation and CT scan of the chest is routinely performed before treatment. On MRI hepatoblastoma is seen as a lobulated mass that is hypointense on T1W and hyperintense on T2W scans. Internal septa are seen as bands of low signal intensity. On CEMR, immediate diffuse enhancement followed by washout is noted. DWI sequence is useful to pick up additional lesions.

EPITHELIOID HEMANGIOENDOTHELIOMA

Epithelioid hemangioendothelioma is a rare tumor of vascular origin which develops almost exclusively in adults, with slight female predominance. Pathologically multiple tumors are usually present that tend to grow and coalesce to form confluent masses. They are typically distributed in the periphery of the liver. They have better prognosis than angiosarcoma. Metastasis is seen in about 30% cases. Adjacent capsular retraction and calcification are frequently seen.[41,42]

Imaging

Sonographically, epithelioid hemangioendothelioma (EHE) usually presents as multiple peripheral hypoechoic masses. Hyperechoic and heterogeneous appearance has also been described. On unenhanced CT scan, multiple peripheral low attenuation lesions are noted. Calcification is infrequently present **(Figs. 18A to D)**. After intravenous contrast it shows peripheral enhancement surrounding the low attenuation fibrous core. Retraction of the overlying capsule is a common, though nonspecific, finding and should raise the possibility of this diagnosis. Large tumors are often associated with compensatory hypertrophy of the uninvolved lobes due to slow growth of these masses.[2] On MRI the lesion is hypointense on T1W images with a thin peripheral dark rim. T2W images show heterogeneously hyperintense lesion with or without low signal intensity peripheral rim **(Figs. 18A to D)**. Target appearance may be seen (hyperintense center with hypointense rim). Moderate peripheral and delayed central enhancement may be seen on CEMR. MRI is better than CT scan in characterization of EHE. Lollipop sign defined by a branch of a portal vein or hepatic vein leading to the periphery of an enhancing mass has been described in EHE. Target sign is seen on T2W, contrast-enhanced T1W and on DWI (peripheral restriction and central free diffusion).

Differential diagnosis includes mass forming intrahepatic cholangiocarcinoma, atypical hemangioma, confluent hepatic fibrosis and metastasis. Presence of confluent masses, target appearance on T2W, early peripheral enhancement and late central enhancement, and capsular retraction help in making a diagnosis. Biopsy is however needed in difficult cases.

ANGIOSARCOMA

Angiosarcoma is a rare tumor usually seen in adults in the fifth to seventh decade and is more common in males.[34] The risk factors include exposure to thorotrast, vinyl chloride, arsenic and steroids. Most of the angiosarcomas are multiple. Solitary lesions are unencapsulated and may contain blood-filled cystic areas. Clinical presentation is with weakness, loss of weight and appetite and abdominal pain. Thrombocytopenia may develop due to sequestration of platelets in large tumors.[2] Spontaneous rupture may be seen in up to 25% cases.

Sonography shows multiple or single hyperechoic masses. Anechoic areas due to necrosis and hyperechoic areas due to fresh hemorrhage may be seen **(Figs. 19A to F)**. On unenhanced CT angiosarcoma has a nonspecific low attenuation appearance. When the etiology is thorotrast exposure, background of high density reticular thorotrast laden parenchyma is seen. Marked peripheral enhancement is noted after administration of contrast. The enhancement may show a peripheral spread, usually with inhomogeneity on delayed scans. Differentiation from hemangioma may be difficult.[1,2] Presence of focal enhancing areas with attenuation less than aorta and peripheral ring-like enhancement (instead of globular) suggests angiosarcoma. Angiosarcoma is hypointense on T1W and heterogeneously hyperintense on T2W MRI **(Figs. 19A to F)**.[43] Fluid levels may be present representing internal hemorrhage. Dynamic CEMR shows an enhancement pattern similar to that of hemangioma. However, heterogeneous appearance on T2W images is unusual for hemangiomas.

On angiography, hepatic arteries supplying an angiosarcoma are of normal size and may show displacement but not encasement. A tumor stain appears at the periphery of the tumor and persists for a prolonged period.

SECONDARY MALIGNANCIES METASTATIC DISEASE

The liver is second only to regional lymph nodes as a site for metastatic disease. It is far more common than

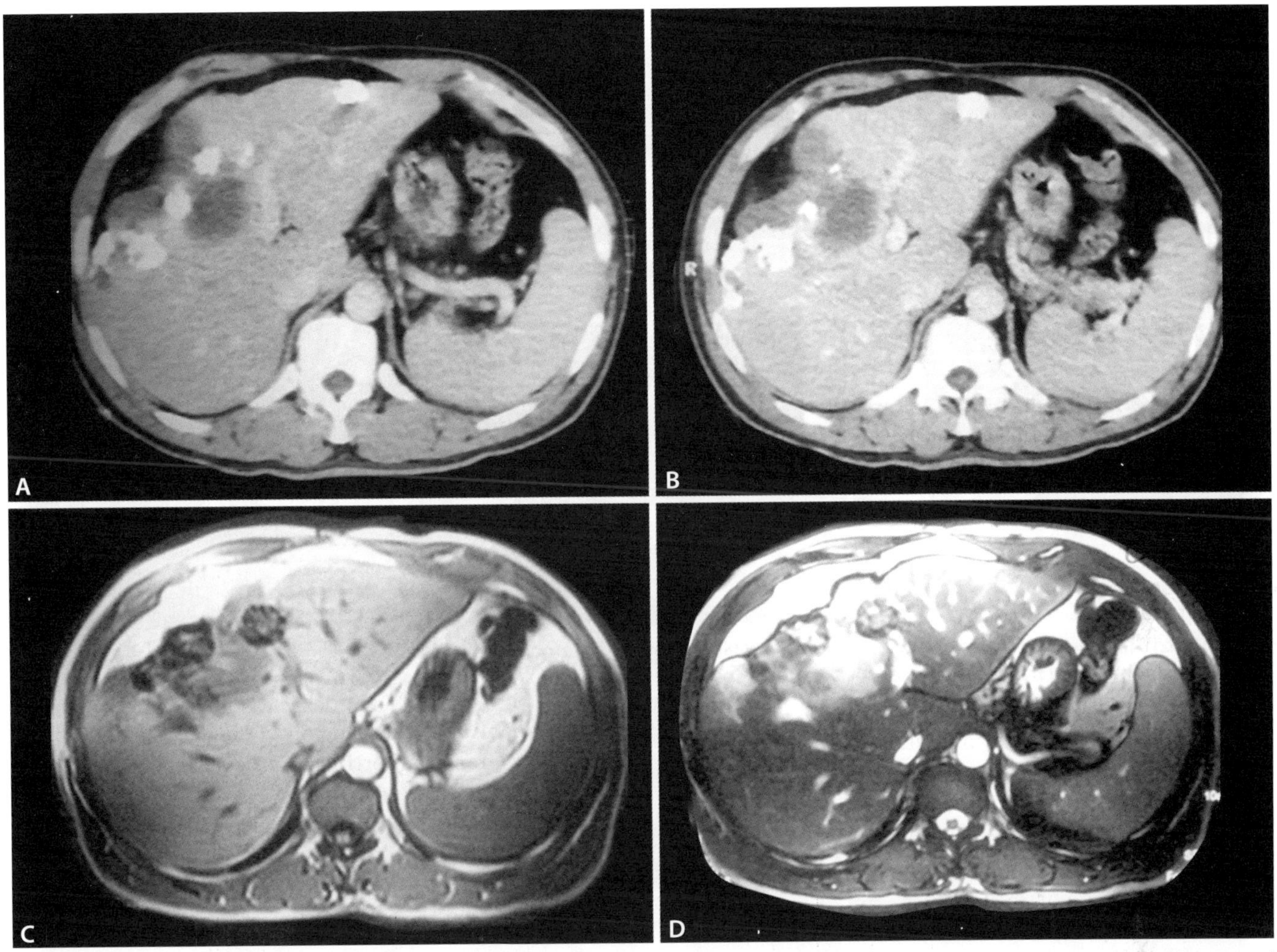

Figs. 18A to D: Epithelioid hemangioendothelioma: (A and B) CECT showing a hypodense mass in segments IVA and VIII with capsular retraction on the surface. Foci of calcification are seen in the lesion as well as another focus in the left lobe; (C) Axial gradient echo T1W scan shows that the mass is hypointense. The foci of calcification are markedly hypointense; (D) Axial T2W scan shows the mass is hyperintense with hypointense foci suggestive of calcification.

primary liver cancer. The colon, stomach, pancreas, and breast are the common primary sites. Metastases are more common in the right lobe of the liver. Although the presence of liver metastases is a poor prognostic factor, the use of aggressive regimes in some subgroups can result in a better outcome. Over the past decade there has been increasing acceptance of liver resection as the best treatment for colorectal metastases. Successful outcome depends on knowledge of the size, number and location of the tumor burden and accurate radiological assessment is essential to identify the subset of patients who would benefit from aggressive management.[1,2]

Many patients have hepatomegaly. Ascites, jaundice and varices may also be present. Liver function tests are normal in up to half of the patients and thus are unreliable for metastasis detection or follow-up. Thus, imaging is vital for diagnosis and follow-up of patients with liver secondaries.

Ultrasonography

This technique has variable sensitivity in detection of liver metastasis, ranging from 40–77%, and <20% for lesions under 1 cm.[44] Drawbacks include operator dependence, poor results in obese patients and in detecting small lesions near the dome and on the liver surface. Contrast-enhanced USG improves the accuracy of lesion detection.[1]

Hepatic metastases may be hypoechoic, hyperechoic, cystic or mixed echogenicity **(Figs. 20A to C)**. The most common pattern is hypoechoic with no distal shadowing or enhancement. This is produced by highly cellular and

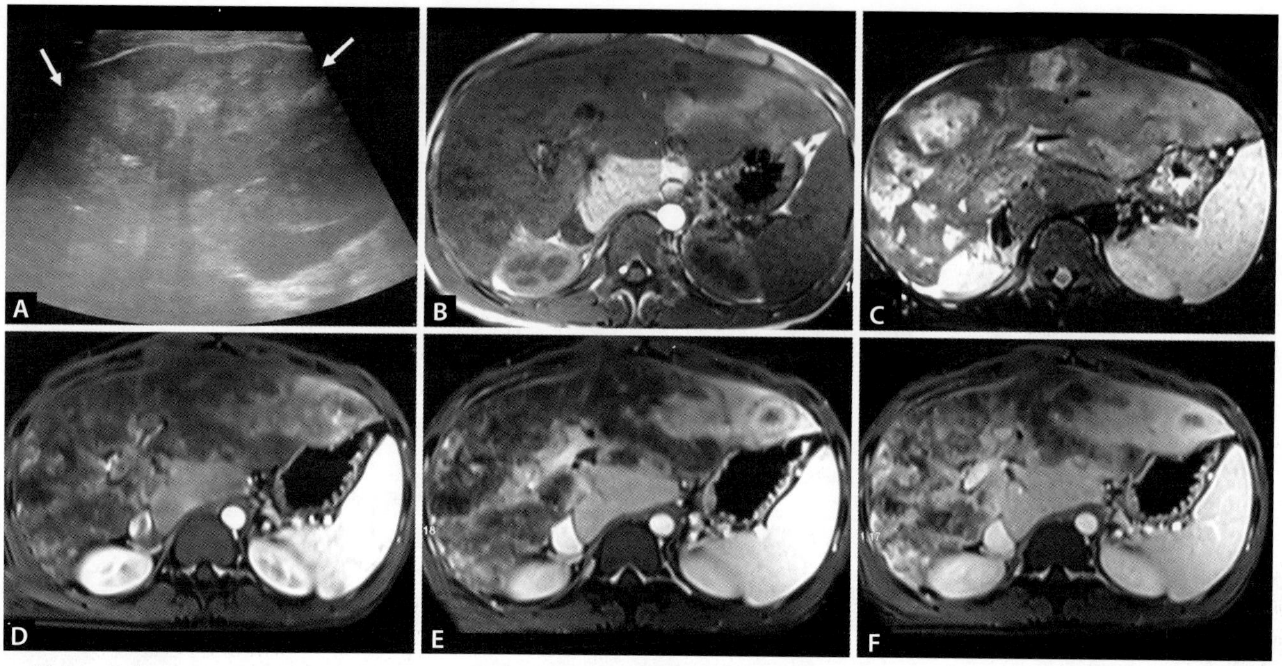

Figs. 19A to F: Angiosarcoma. (A) Ultrasonography showing multiple heteroechoic lesions in the liver (arrows); (B) Axial T1W image showing predominantly hypoechoic lesions replacing almost the entire liver; (C) Axial T2W fat-saturated image showing heterogeneous signal intensity of the lesions; Dynamic contrast-enhanced MRI in arterial (D), venous (E) and delayed (F) phases showing mild enhancement of the lesions in the arterial phase with gradual filling in of the lesions with contrast on venous and delayed phases.

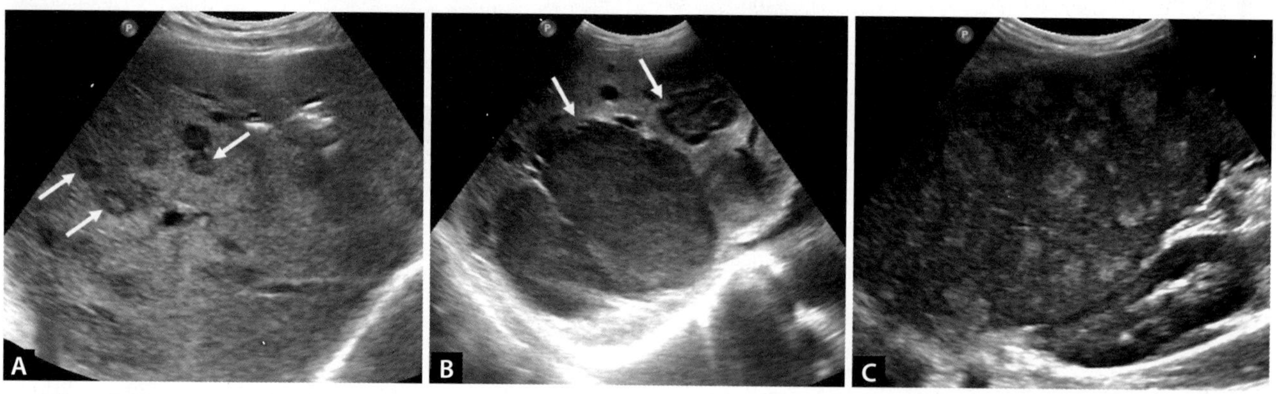

Figs. 20A to C: Metastases–Ultrasonography. (A) USG showing "target like" lesions (arrows) suggestive of metastases in a patient with lung carcinoma; (B) USG showing hypoechoic masses (arrows), which were metastases from carcinoma of colon; (C) USG of liver showing hyperechoic lesions suggestive of metastases in a patient with neuroendocrine tumor.

hypovascular lesions. Hyperechoic metastases are often seen with colonic and gastrointestinal malignancies and with vascular metastases from islet cell tumors, carcinoid, choriocarcinoma and renal cell carcinoma. They may be surrounded by a hypoechoic halo producing the bull's eye or target appearance **(Fig. 20)**. Presence of halo indicates an aggressive tumor and is commonly seen with bronchogenic carcinoma.[2] Calcification may be seen in mucinous metastases from colon and ovary. Cystic metastases are seen with adenocarcinoma of pancreas, ovary and colon.

On color Doppler imaging, metastases usually do not show intratumoral signal but a 'detour' pattern with a dilated portal vein meandering around the tumor nodules has been described. Intraoperative sonography is a very useful adjunct in patients who are candidates for surgical resection of metastases. It may show additional lesions in comparison with preoperative USG and CT scan.

Computed Tomography

The advent of multidetector CT has led to a lot of flexibility but has also added complexity to the imaging protocols for liver evaluation. Advantages include significant reduction in scan time, elimination of respiratory misregistration, improved Z axis resolution, better multiplanar and 3D reformats and it allows a more precise timing for evaluation of liver in different phases of contrast enhancement. It also helps in demonstration of a vein close to a lesion as this determines the response to radiofrequency ablation. Lesions in proximity to a vessel have higher chances of recurrence.

Since most metastases are hypovascular the usual protocol is to scan in the portal venous phase of enhancement **(Figs. 21A and B)**. Dual phase scanning may be useful for detection of metastases from hypervascular primaries such as renal cell carcinoma and islet cell tumors **(Figs. 22A and B)**. Although breast carcinoma metastases can be hypervascular, studies have not shown any added benefit of biphasic CT over portal phase CT for this indication.[2]

On unenhanced CT most metastases are hypodense to the liver parenchyma, whereas some are indistinguishable from normal liver. Small lesions are nodular and homogeneous, while larger lesions are more irregular, heterogeneous and with ill-defined margins. Calcification is common in mucinous GI tract carcinomas and in chemotherapeutically treated hypervascular lesions (e.g. carcinoid). After contrast administration, metastases from hypovascular tumors may have an enhancing rim that

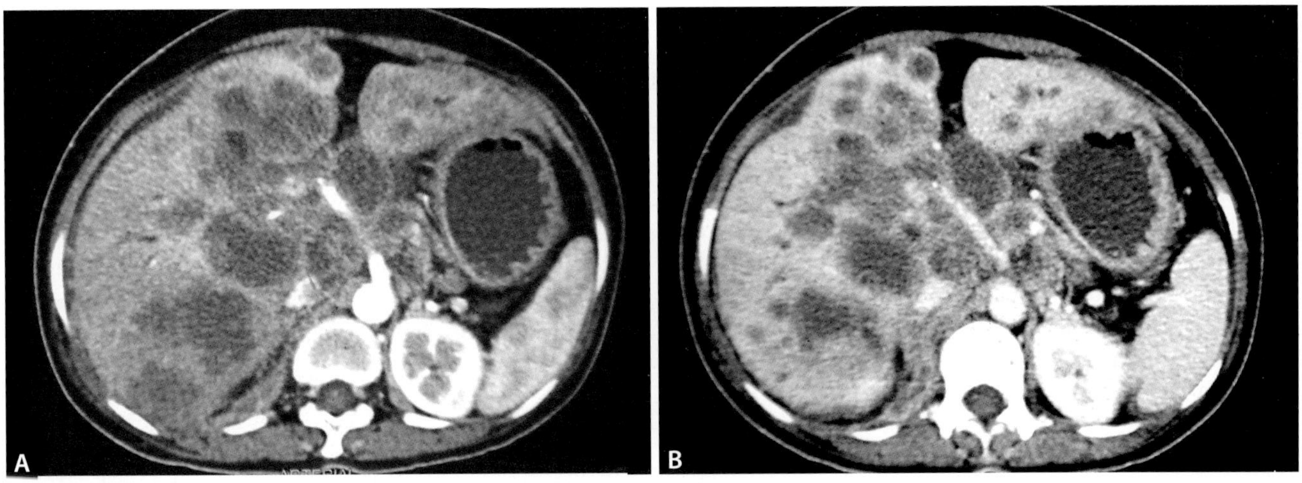

Figs. 21A and B: Hypovascular metastases: The contrast-enhanced arterial phase (A) and venous phase image (B) shows multiple hypodense lesions involving all segments of liver. The lesions do not show any enhancement in either of the phases.

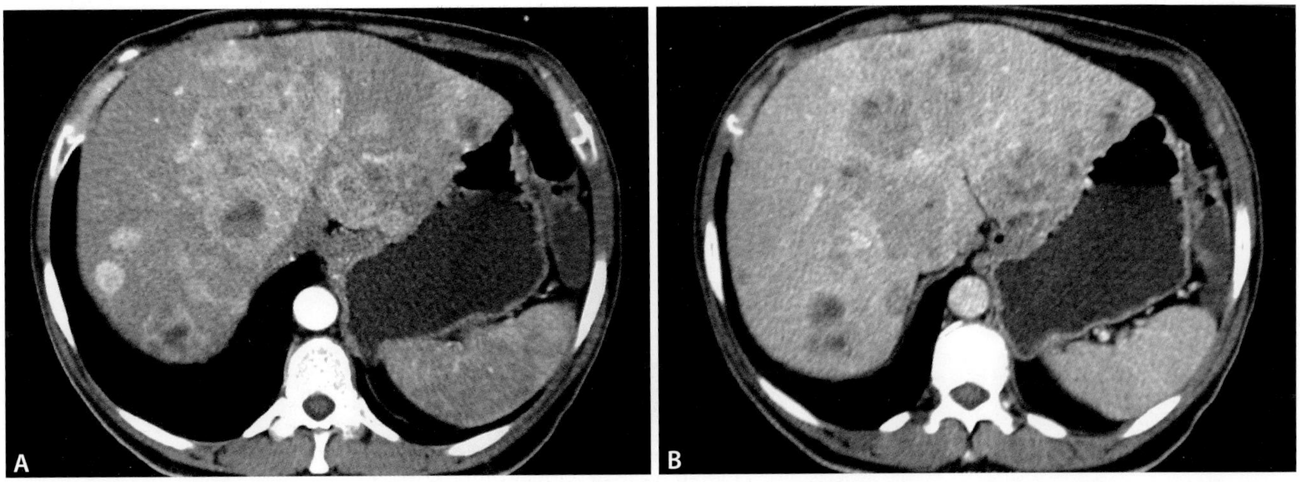

Figs. 22A and B: Hypervascular metastases: The contrast-enhanced arterial phase image (A) shows multiple intensely enhancing lesions in both lobes of a noncirrhotic liver with wash out seen in the venous phase (B).

can be seen during arterial phase and occasionally during portal phase **(Figs. 23A and B)**. Lesions that do not have an enhancing rim show little if any enhancement during the arterial phase and become hypoattenuating during the portal phase.

Hypervascular metastases show moderate-to-intense enhancement during the arterial phase that may persist during the portal phase. However, most show a rapid washout and become iso- or hypodense to surrounding liver.

Magnetic Resonance Imaging

Liver metastases like most other liver lesions are hypointense to normal liver on T1W images and hyperintense on T2W images **(Figs. 24A to C)**. The use of fat suppression on T2W sequences, particularly fast spin echo T2W scans, is important as it improves the detection of subcapsular lesions. Morphological features have been shown to be useful in differentiating metastatic lesions from common benign lesions such as hemangioma and cysts. Heterogeneous signal intensity and irregular or indistinct margins, smooth or irregular areas of high signal intensity surrounded by a ring of relatively lower signal intensity are said to be suggestive of metastatic disease. The acquisition of at least one sequence in the coronal plane is useful to evaluate the superior and inferior margins of the liver.

Six appearances of liver metastasis have been described on MRI.[2] Doughnut shape is usually seen with larger lesions, where the lesion is of low signal intensity on T1W images with central necrosis which has even lower signal. These lesions have target appearance on T2W image. Amorphous appearance is seen with heterogeneous masses with ill-defined margins. Peripheral halo is seen with some metastasis and represents either tumor infiltration or surrounding edema. Light bulb morphology, where the lesion is hyperintense on T2W images, is seen with cystic and hypervascular metastasis. Cauliflower appearance is typically seen with colorectal metastasis. Here the lesion has scalloped margins with enhancing periphery and internal septae.

Hypervascular metastases such as those from islet cell tumors, carcinoid and renal cell carcinoma are generally high in signal intensity on T2W images and show intense peripheral ring of enhancement immediately after gadolinium administration. This appearance may mimic hemangiomas. Dynamic serial gadolinium-enhanced MR is very helpful in differentiating these metastases from hemangiomas. Hemangiomas typically show early discrete nodular enhancement which shows a centripetal progression on delayed scans. Metastases often show a transient enhancement of the periphery with a peripheral washout on delayed scans. Enhancement of hypervascular metastases is better shown on MR than on CT images because of the higher sensitivity of MR to gadolinium chelates and the more compact bolus of contrast delivered to the hepatic parenchyma.[2] Hypovascular metastasis may show enhancing rim in arterial phase, with incomplete centripetal filling-in in delayed phase but remain hypointense in all the phases.

State-of-the-art MRI has a higher diagnostic accuracy and greater effect on patient management than CT scan. Diffusion weighted imaging is useful in detection of metastatic liver lesions.[27,45] Liver specific contrast agents such as gadobenate dimeglumine and gadoxetic

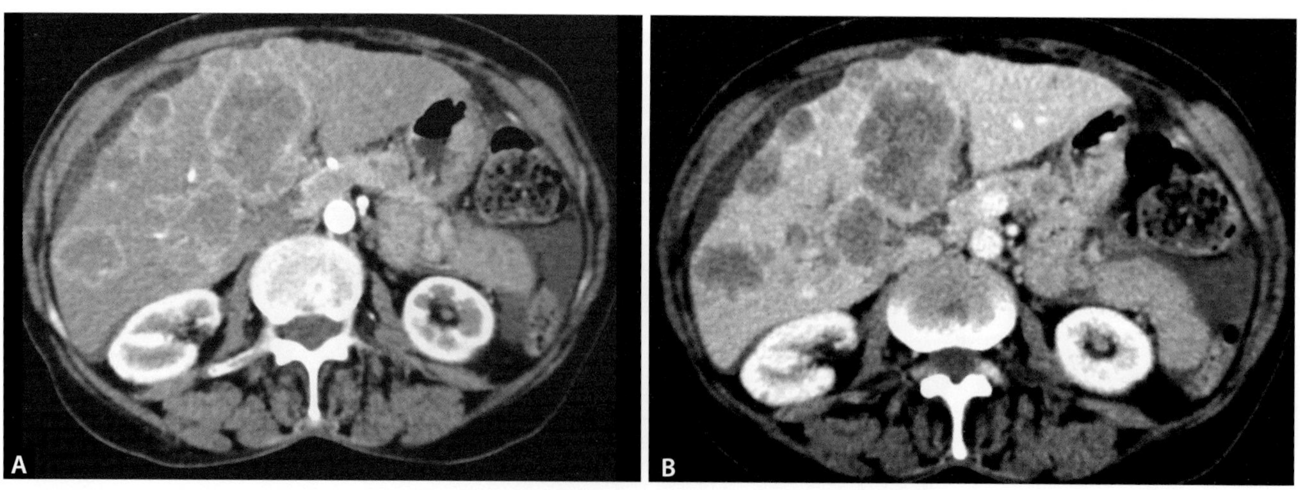

Figs. 23A and B: Rim-enhancing metastases. The contrast-enhanced arterial phase image (A) shows multiple rim-enhancing lesions with wash out seen in the venous phase image (B).

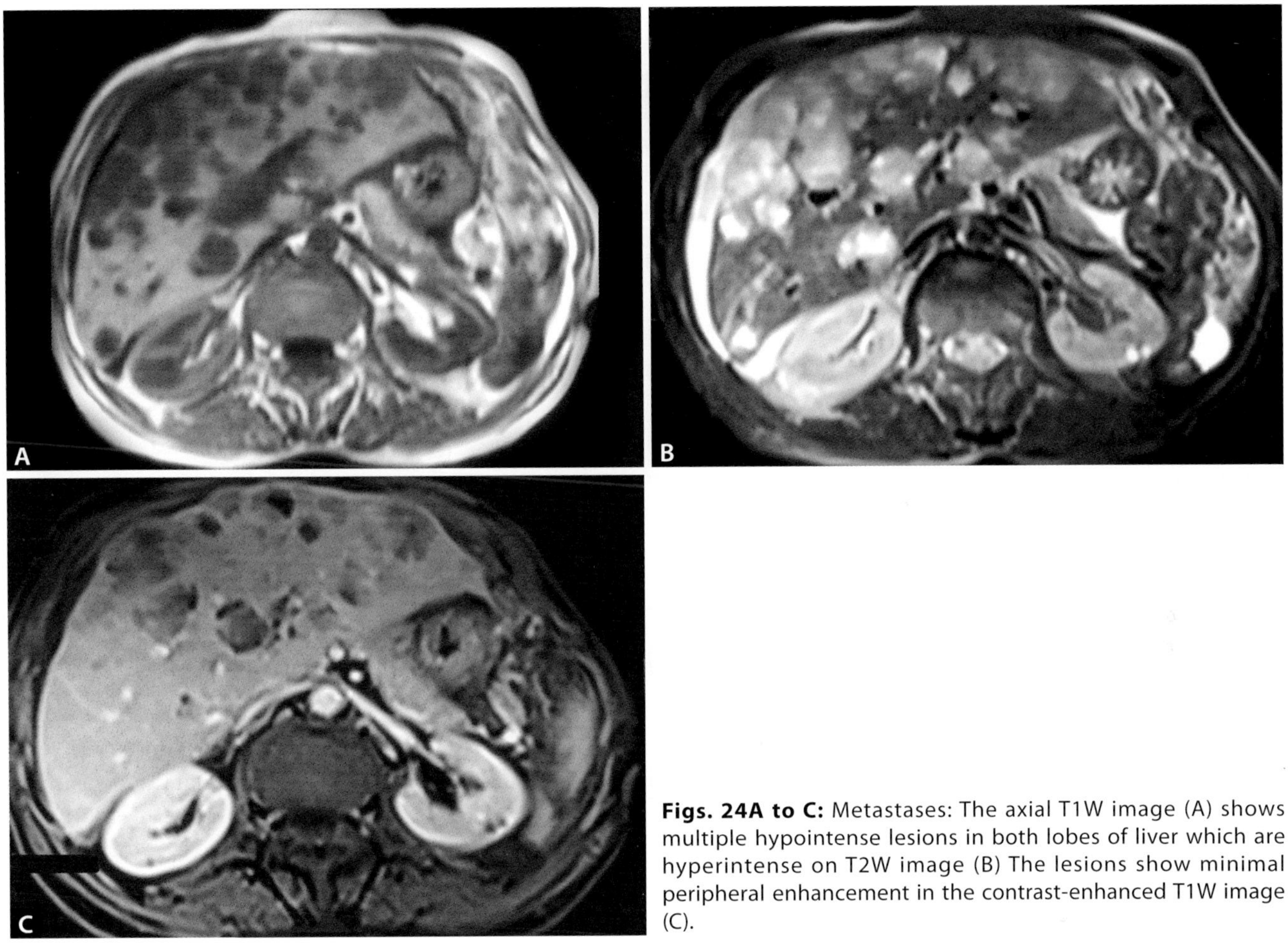

Figs. 24A to C: Metastases: The axial T1W image (A) shows multiple hypointense lesions in both lobes of liver which are hyperintense on T2W image (B) The lesions show minimal peripheral enhancement in the contrast-enhanced T1W image (C).

acid improve lesion detection in hepatobiliary phase.[46] Despite the marked improvement in the accuracy of detection and characterization of metastatic disease, a significant number of lesions are found at surgery that goes undetected on preoperative imaging. These include subcentimeter and subcapsular lesions.

Differential Diagnosis

Multifocal HCC is an important differential for hypervascular liver metastases. Presence of background chronic liver disease, a capsule on delayed images and absence of a primary malignancy may suggest a diagnosis. However, differentiation may sometimes be difficult and sampling may become necessary. Multiple inflammatory granulomas (like tuberculosis and sarcoidosis) appear hypodense or hypointense on contrast-enhanced imaging studies, similar to metastasis. They usually do not show peripheral rim enhancement in the arterial phase. Clinical and laboratory details, presence of enlarged nodes and splenic lesions may help in making a diagnosis. Pseudotumoral nodular steatosis may mimic metastases; however, MRI is useful in making the diagnosis. There is characteristic signal drop within or in the margin of the lesions on the opposed phase T1W images.[47]

LYMPHOMA

Primary hepatic lymphoma is rare and most often of non-Hodgkin's (diffuse large B-cell type) type.[48] Primary hepatic lymphoma is much more common in organ transplant recipients treated with cyclosporine and patients with AIDS. The most common appearance is that of a solitary large mass, which is hypodense on unenhanced CT and does not enhance significantly after intravenous contrast. Tumors are moderately low in signal intensity on T1W scans and mild-to-moderately hyperintense on T2W scans, with marked diffusion restriction and show mild heterogeneous enhancement on immediate contrast enhanced MR images **(Figs. 25A to D)**.[1,2]

Secondary liver involvement in lymphoma is more common than primary lymphoma and occurs both in

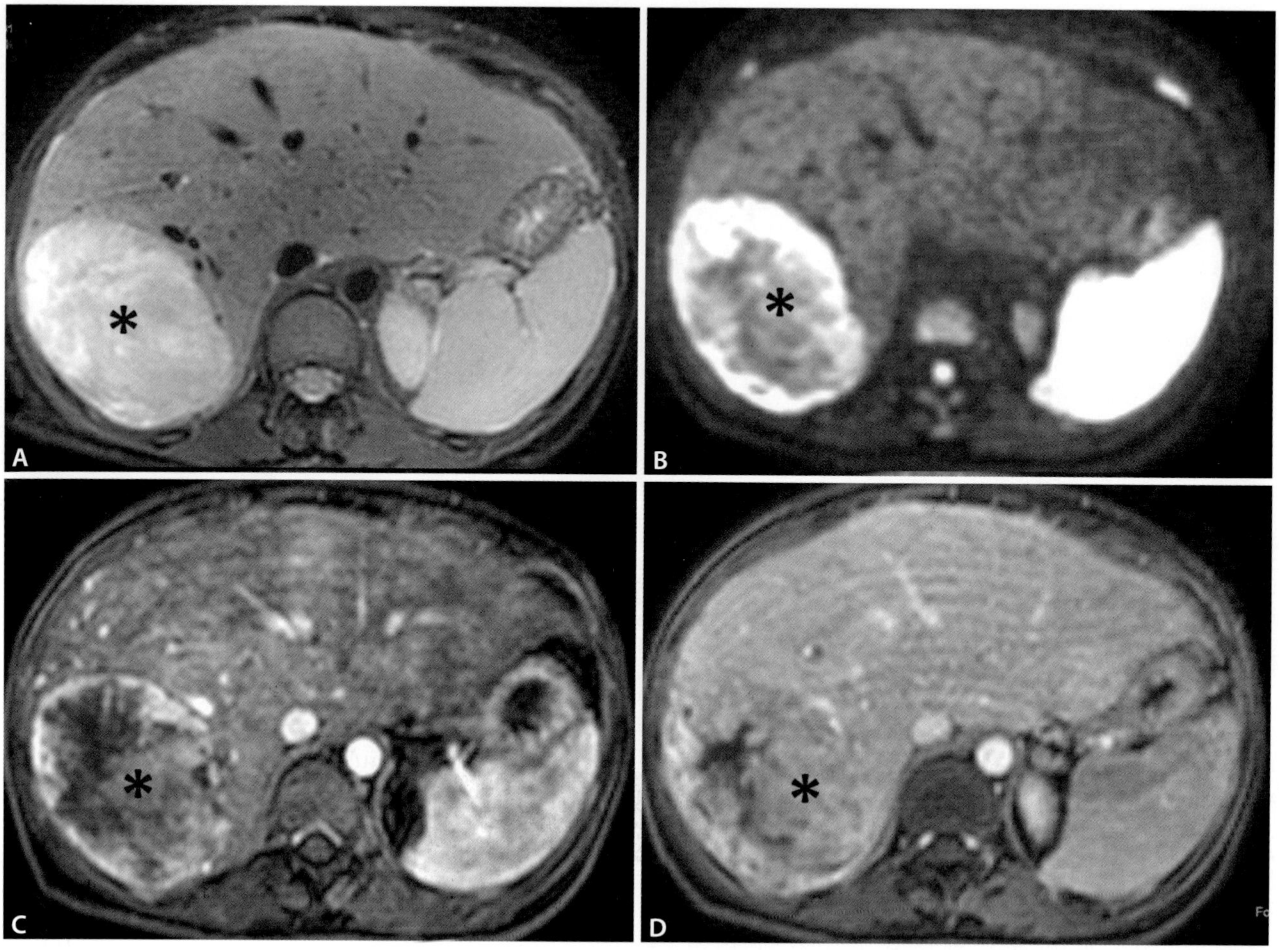

Figs. 25A to D: Primary hepatic lymphoma. (A) Axial T2W fat-saturated image showing well-defined hyperintense lesion in right lobe of liver (asterisk); (B) Diffusion-weighted image (b-800) showing restriction of diffusion within the lesion; Axial contrast-enhanced T1W image in arterial (C) and venous phases (D) showing heterogeneous contrast enhancement. Histopathology showed diffuse large B-cell lymphoma.

Hodgkin's disease and in non-Hodgkin's lymphoma. Diffuse infiltration is more common in Hodgkin's disease, whereas diffuse and nodular hepatic involvement is equally frequent in non-Hodgkin's lymphoma. Imaging findings are nonspecific and cannot be differentiated from other space occupying lesions.

PITFALLS IN THE DIAGNOSIS OF FOCAL LIVER LESIONS

Despite advances in imaging, there are several difficulties which can arise during the diagnosis of focal liver lesions.[46] Knowledge of these pitfalls is necessary for accurate diagnosis of liver lesions. Focal fatty infiltration or sparing may look like a focal lesion. But geographic nature of the lesion, presence of vessels within it and signal drop on opposed phase MRI assist in the diagnosis. Arterioportal shunts, which are sometimes seen in a cirrhotic liver, are seen as ill-defined areas of hyperenhancement in the arterial phase. There may be an adjacent enhancing small branch of portal vein. Isodense appearance on venous/delayed images, peripheral location and absence of discrete lesion on T2W images helps in its differentiation from HCC. Chronic superior vena caval obstruction results in opening up of collateral pathways and sometimes there are cavoportal collaterals which are seen as hyperenhancing area in the left lobe of liver in the arterial phase (hot spot sign). This may mimic hypervascular tumors of the liver. Focal confluent fibrosis is another entity which may mimic focal lesion in the liver. Presence of capsular retraction, location in segments 4, 7 or 8, wedge shape and enhancement in delayed phase suggest a diagnosis. Pseudotumor steatosis, as described above, is another entity which may cause difficulties in diagnosis.

30. Park YS, Lee CH, Kim JE, Shin S, Park CM. Differentiation of hepatocellular carcinoma from its various mimickers in liver magnetic resonance imaging: what are the tips when using hepatocyte-specific agents? World J Gastroenterol. 2016;22:284-99.
31. Roskams T, Kojiro M. Pathology of early hepatocellular carcinoma: conventional and molecular diagnosis. Semin Liver Dis. 2010;30(1):17-25.
32. Shah A, Tang A, Santillan C, Sirlin C. Cirrhotic liver: What's that nodule? The LI-RADS approach. J Magn Reson Imaging. 2016;43(2):281-94.
33. Ganeshan D, Szklaruk J, Kundra V, Kaseb A, Rashid A, Elsayes KM. Imaging features of fibrolamellar hepatocellular carcinoma. AJR. 2014;202:544-52.
34. Sunnapwar A, Katre R, Policarpio-Nicolas M, Katabathina V, Erian M. Imaging of rare primary malignant hepatic tumors in adults with histopathological correlation. J Comput Assist Tomogr. 2016;40:452-62.
35. Choi BI, Lee JM, Han JK. Imaging of intrahepatic and hilar cholangiocarcinoma. Abdom Imaging. 2004;29:548-57.
36. Kang Y, Lee JM, Kim SH, et al. Intrahepatic mass-forming cholangiocarcinoma: enhancement patterns on gadoxetic acid-enhanced MR images. Radiology. 2012;264(3):751-60.
37. Bhagat V, Javle M, Yu J, Agrawal A, Gibbs JF, Kuvshinoff B, Nava E, Iyer R. Combined hepatocholangiocarcinoma: case-series and review of literature. Int J Gastrointest Cancer. 2006;37(1):27-34.
38. Shetty AS, Fowler KJ, Brunt EM, et al. Combined hepatocellular-cholangiocarcinoma: what the radiologist needs to know about biphenotypic primary liver carcinoma. Abdom Imaging. 2014;39:310-22.
39. Lantinga MA, Gevers TJG, Drenth JPH. Evaluation of hepatic cystic lesions. World J Gastroenterol. 2013;19:3543-54.
40. Lu M, Greer ML. Hypervascular multifocal hepatoblastoma: dynamic gadolinium-enhanced MRI findings indistinguishable from infantile hemangioendothelioma. Pediatr Radiol. 2007;37:587-91.
41. Azzam RI, Alshak NS, Pham HP. AIRP best cases in radiologic-pathologic correlation: hepatic epithelioid hemangioendothelioma. Radiographics. 2012;32(3):789-94.
42. Lin J, Ji Y. CT and MRI diagnosis of hepatic epithelioid hemangioendothelioma. Hepatobiliary Pancreat Dis Int. 2010;9(2):154-8.
43. Bruegel M, Muenzel D, Waldt S, et al. Hepatic angiosarcoma: cross-sectional imaging findings in seven patients with emphasis on dynamic contrast-enhanced and diffusion-weighted MRI. Abdom Imaging. 2013;38(4):745-54.
44. Bartolotta TV, Taibbi A, Midiri M, et al. Focal liver lesions: contrast-enhanced ultrasound. Abdom Imaging. 2009;34(2):193-209.
45. Kandpal H, Sharma R, Madhusudhan KS, Kapoor KS. Respiratory-triggered versus breath-hold diffusion-weighted MRI of liver lesions: comparison of image quality and apparent diffusion coefficient values. AJR. 2009;192(4):915-22.
46. Chen L, Zhang J, Zhang L, et al. Meta-analysis of gadoxetic acid disodium (Gd-EOB-DTPA)-enhanced magnetic resonance imaging for the detection of liver metastases. PLoS One. 2012;7(11):e48681.
47. Vilgrain V, Lagadec M, Ronot M. Pitfalls in Liver Imaging. Radiology. 2016;278(1):34-51.
48. Dhamija E, Madhusudhan KS, Shalimar, Das P, Srivastava DN, Gupta AK. Primary hepatic diffuse large B-cell lymphoma: unusual presentation and imaging features. Curr Probl Diagn Radiol. 2015;44(3):290-3.

CONCLUSION

Malignant focal lesions of the liver are common and imaging plays a vital role in detection and characterization. MRI is superior to CT for characterizing liver lesions. Many lesions have classical imaging appearances and in combination with clinical features, help in making the correct diagnosis often obviating the need for tissue diagnosis. Liver-specific contrast agents are useful and have potential role in diagnosis. Knowledge of pitfalls in imaging helps to reduce the chances of misdiagnosis. Biopsy may be required in difficult cases after discussion in multidisciplinary group meeting.

REFERENCES

1. Lamba R, Faranazapir G, Corwin MT, Khatri VP. Diagnostic imaging of hepatic lesions in adults. Surg Oncol Clin N Am. 2014;23:789-820.
2. Ros PR, Erturk SM. Malignant tumors of the liver. In: Gore RM, Levine MS (Eds): Textbook of Gastrointestinal Radiology, 4th edition. Philadelphia: Saunders; 2015. pp.1561-607.
3. Bosman F, Carneiro F, Hruban R, Theise N (Eds). Tumors of the liver and intrahepatic bile ducts. In: WHO classification of tumors of the digestive system, IARC. Lyon; 2010.
4. Van Beers BE, Daire JL, Garteiser P. New imaging techniques for liver diseases. J Hepatol. 2015;62:690-700.
5. Dewall RJ. Ultrasound elastography: principles, techniques, and clinical applications. Crit Rev Biomed Eng. 2013;41: 1-19.
6. Kim SH, Kamaya A, Willmann JK. CT perfusion of the liver: principles and applications in oncology. Radiology. 2014; 272(2):322-44.
7. Agrawal MD, Pinho DF, Kulkarni NM, Hahn PF, Guimaraes AR, Sahani DV. Oncologic applications of dual-energy CT in the abdomen. Radiographics. 2014;34(3):589-612.
8. Gordic S, Puippe GD, Krauss B, Klotz E, Desbiolles L, Lesurtel M, Mullhaupt B, Pfammatter T, Alkadhi H. Correlation between dual-energy and perfusion CT in patients with hepatocellular carcinoma. Radiology. 2016;280:78-87.
9. GW ter Voert, L Heijmen, HWM van Laarhoven, A Heerschap. In vivo magnetic resonance spectroscopy of liver tumors and metastases. World J Gastroenterol. 2011;17(47):5133-49.
10. McGlynn KA, London WT. Epidemiology and natural history of hepatocellular carcinoma. Best Pract Res Clin Gastroenterol. 2005;19(1):3-23.
11. Fattovich G, Stroffolini T, Zagni I, Donato F. Hepatocellular carcinoma in cirrhosis: incidence and risk factors. Gastroenterology. 2004;127:S35-S50.
12. Llovet JM, Burroughs A, Bruix J. Hepatocellular carcinoma Lancet. 2003;362:1907-17.
13. Kudo M. Real practice of hepatocellular carcinoma in Japan: conclusions of the Japan Society of Hepatology 2009 Kobe Congress. Oncology. 2010;78(Suppl 1):180-8.
14. Tyson GL, El-Serag HB. Risk factors for cholangiocarcinoma. Hepatology. 2011;54(1):173-84.
15. Choi JY, Lee JM, Sirlin CB. CT and MR imaging diagnosis and staging of hepatocellular carcinoma: Part I. Development, growth and spread: key pathologic and imaging aspects. Radiology. 2014;272(3):635-54.
16. Taguchi K, Asayama Y, Aishima S, et al. Morphologic approach to hepatocellular carcinoma development in man: de novo or the so-called 'dysplastic nodule-carcinoma' sequence? Oncol Rep. 2002;9(4):737-43.
17. Hanna RF, Aguirre DA, Kased N, Emery SC, Peterson MR, Sirlin CB. Cirrhosis-associated hepatocellular nodules: Correlation of histopathologic and MR imaging features. Radiographics. 2008;28:747-69.
18. Bruix J, Sherman M, American Association for the Study of Liver Diseases. Managementof hepatocellular carcinoma: an update. Hepatology. 2011;53(3):1020-2.
19. NCCN guidelines Version 2.2016. Hepatocellular carcinoma. NCCN.org.
20. Willatt JM, Hussain HK, Adusumilli S, Marrero JA. MR imaging of hepatocellular carcinoma in the cirrhotic liver: challenges and controversies. Radiology. 2008;247:311-30.
21. Brannigan M, Burns PN, Wilson SR. Blood flow patterns in focal liver lesions at microbubble-enhanced US. Radiographics. 2004;24:921-35.
22. Salvatore V, Gianstefani A, Negrini G, Allegretti G, Galassi M, Piscaglia F. Imaging diagnosis of hepatocellular carcinoma: recent advances of contrast-enhanced ultrasonography with sonovue. Liver Cancer. 2016;5: 55-66.
23. Takahashi M, Maruyama H, Shimada T, Kamezaki H, Sekimoto T, Kanai F, Yokosuka O. Characterization of hepatic lesions (≤ 30 mm) with liver-specific contrast agents: a comparison between ultrasound and magnetic resonance imaging. Eur J Radiol. 2013;82(1):75-84.
24. Marrero JA, Hussain HK, Nghiem HV, et al. Improving the prediction of hepatocellular carcinoma in cirrhotic patients with an arterially-enhancing liver mass. Liver Transpl. 2005;11(3):281-9.
25. Filippone A, Blakeborough A, Breuer J, et al. Enhancement of liver parenchyma after injection of hepatocyte-specific MRI contrast media: a comparison of gadoxetic acid and gadobenate dimeglumine. J Magn Reson Imaging. 2010;31(2):356-64.
26. Xu PJ, Yan FH, Wang JH, Shan Y, Ji Y, Chen CZ. Contribution of diffusion-weighted magnetic resonance imaging in the characterization of hepatocellular carcinomas and dysplastic nodules in cirrhotic liver. J Comput Assist Tomogr. 2010;34(4):506-12.
27. Calistri L, Castellani A, Matteuzzi B, Mazzoni E, Pradella S, Colagrande S. Focal liver lesions classification and characterization: what value do DWI and ADC have? J Comput Assit Tomogr. 2016 [Epub ahead of print].
28. Glockner JF. Hepatobiliary MRI: current concepts and controversies. J Magn Reson Imaging. 2007;25:681-95.
29. Arslanoglu A, Seyal AR, Sodagari F, Sahin A, Miller FH, Salem R, Yaghmai V. Current guidelines for the diagnosis and management of hepatocellular carcinoma: a comparative review. Am J Roentgenol. 2016;207:W1-11.

CHAPTER **80**

Interventional Radiology in Treatment of Liver Tumors

Deep Narayan Srivastava, Shivanand Gamanagatti, Shashi Bala Paul

INTRODUCTION

Liver is among the most common sites for primary and secondary tumors. Hepatocellular carcinoma (HCC) represents more than 90% of the primary liver tumors and is the second important cause of cancer related death. Its incidence and mortality is on the rise world over.[1] Metastatic liver tumors are even more common particularly in cases of colorectal carcinoma where about 20% of the cases have metastases at the outset and about half of them are likely to develop during its course.[2] Surgery remains the first line of therapy for these patients and the options of resection or liver transplant provide best outcomes of 5-year survival ranging from 60% to 80%.[3] However, the vast majority of these patients are unsuitable for surgery due to the advanced disease at diagnosis, poor liver reserve and performance status. Furthermore, limited infrastructure, organ shortage and long waiting period denies timely liver transplantation in many.

Over the last two decades, a large number of radiological interventions consisting of either ablative techniques or angiographic procedures have evolved, which are effective in prolonging survival **(Tables 1 and 2)**. Being widely available, safe and efficacious, these minimally invasive

Table 1: Radiological interventions for liver tumors.

1. Percutaneous ablative techniques
Chemical ablation: • Ethanol • Acetic acid
Thermal ablation: • Radiofrequency ablation • Microwave ablation • Laser ablation • Cryoablation • High intensity focused ultrasound ablation
Nonthermal ablation: • Irreversible electroporation (IRE) or nano knife
2. Intra-arterial procedures
• Transarterial embolization • Transarterial chemoembolization (TACE) • Transarterial chemotherapy (TAC) • Transarterial rhenium/Yttrium therapy (TART)
3. Portal vein embolization

Table 2: Survival rate of various interventional techniques, surgical resection and liver transplantation for treatment of HCC.

			Survival (%)				
Procedure	***No. of patients***	***1st year***	***2nd year***	***3rd year***	***5th year***	***7th year***	***10th year***
Surgical resection	25066	88.2	78.4	69.5	54.2	42.0	29.0
Transplant	183	74.2	69.3	63.4	56.7	NA	NA
Ablation	27150	92.8	81.4	68.6	45.6	29.8	15.7
TACE	19569	77.8	59.0	44.2	24.2	14.0	6.5

techniques have become widely popular and have emerged as the alternative therapeutic options to surgery for both primary and secondary liver malignancies. This chapter focuses on the armamentarium of the currently available image-guided interventional treatments used in the management of liver tumors.

TREATMENT OF MALIGNANT TUMORS

Hepatocellular Carcinoma

The treatment of HCC depends on the stage of the disease, severity of liver function and the performance status of the individual. The Barcelona Clinic Liver Cancer (BCLC) staging **(Flowchart 1)** is the most validated and widely used staging for HCC. Besides staging the disease on the basis of these parameters, it also recommends the therapeutic options for all the different stages of HCC.[4] Amongst the interventional therapies, ablation and intra-arterial therapies are indicated for HCC of BCLC A and BCLC B/C stage respectively. Both these are termed locoregional therapies as they target exclusively the tumor tissue sparing the adjoining normal hepatic parenchyma.

Pretreatment Assessment for Locoregional Therapy

The evaluation includes laboratory studies, imaging and counseling of the patient. Laboratory studies include complete blood count, liver function tests, coagulation profile and AFP levels. Cross-sectional imaging by either multiphasic computed tomography (MPCT) or MRI is essential for staging of the disease. Treatment planning is done by careful appraisal of the imaging for the size, number and location of the tumors, presence of macrovascular (portal vein) invasion and extrahepatic disease. Holistic treatment needs to be done, which involves treating the tumor, the underlying tumor etiology (invariably is viral hepatitis) and the associated deranged liver function.

Percutaneous Ablative Therapy

Percutaneous ablation is the treatment recommended for unresectable early HCC. It aims at destroying the viable tumor tissue and creating a safety margin of 0.5–1 cm around. It is safe, easy to perform, well tolerated with very

Flowchart 1: The Barcelona Clinic Liver Cancer Staging System.

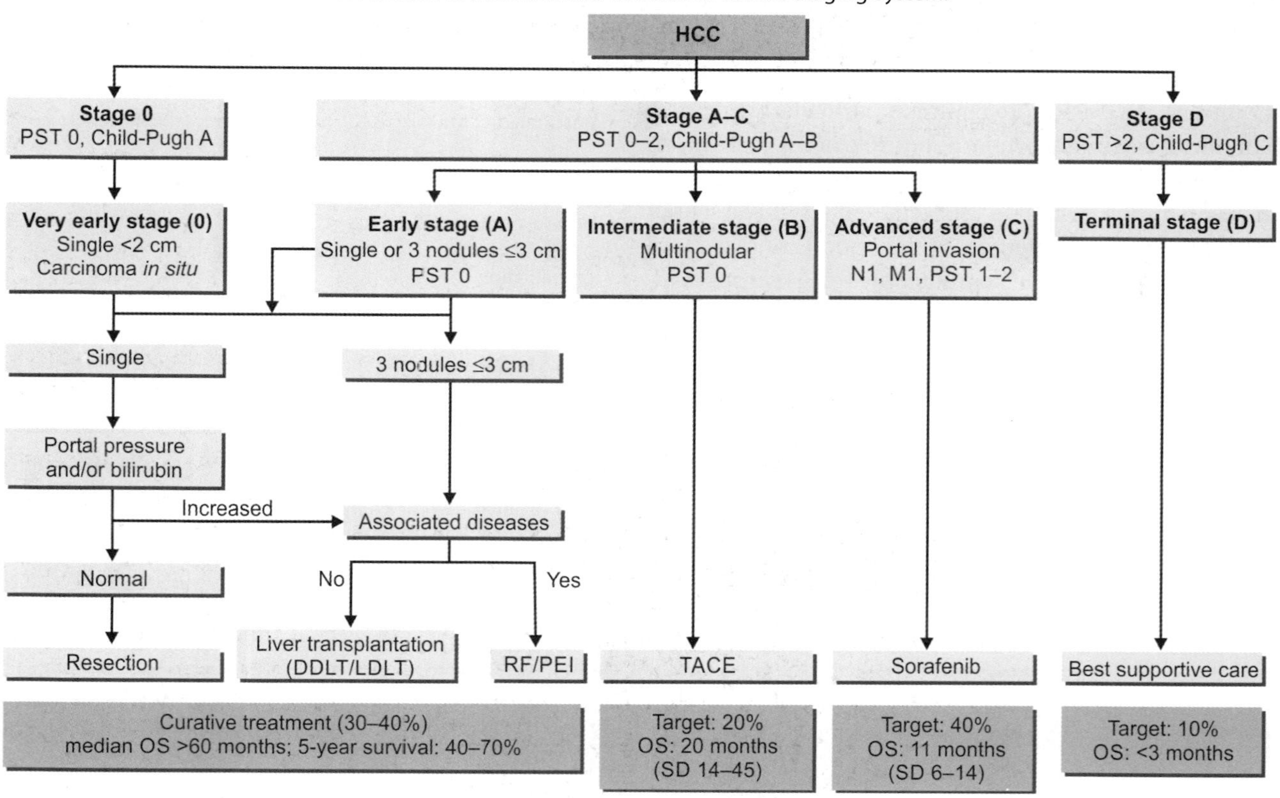

Abbreviations: HCC: Hepatocellular carcinoma; LDLT: Living donor liver transplantation; DDLT: Deceased donor liver transplantation; TACE: Transarterial chemoembolization; PEI: Percutaneous ethanal injection; RF: Radiofrequency; PST: Performance status; SD: Standard deviation.

low major and minor complication rate. The best outcome of complete response following ablation varies and is related to the size of the tumor (90–100% in tumors of 2 cm, 50% in the tumors of 5 cm).[5] Hence, the real benefit of therapy lies in treating early, small tumors.

Selection criteria for ablation: Ideal HCC patients for ablation are those who are Child-Pugh class A/B cirrhosis, have performance status of 0–1, tumor size smaller than 5 cm (ideal < 3 cm), well-defined intrahepatic with hepatic parenchyma all around, solitary or multiple (not more than 3 in number) with absence of vascular invasion and extrahepatic disease.

Absolute contraindications to ablation are, presence of intravascular invasion, tumor located less than 1 cm from the main biliary duct, intrahepatic biliary dilatation, exophytic tumor or uncorrectable coagulopathy. Relative contraindications are the presence of extrahepatic metastases, bilioenteric anastomosis, superficial lesions, lesions close to gallbladder or any part of gastrointestinal tract, ascites, low platelet count (<50,000/mm^3, pacemaker/defibrillator, hepatic failure.[6]

- *Chemical ablation:* Chemical ablation involves the use of percutaneous ethanal injection (PEI) of either ethanol or percutaneous acetic acid injection (PAI) into the tumor. PEI is the earliest technique which has been extensively studied and its role in treating small HCCs has been well-established.[7] It is inexpensive and can be readily performed with imaging guidance without the use of any special equipment.
  - *Mechanism of ethanol/acetic acid ablation:* Neoplastic and nonneoplastic tissue is made up of cellular, interstitial, and vascular compartments. Chemical agents with relatively low molecular weight, such as ethanol and acetic acid, when injected into the tumor, penetrates the cellular compartment remote from the point of injection, through the tumor interstitium. HCCs have extracellular volumes more than twice that of noncancerous liver. These factors result in a high interstitial fluid pressure and interstitial diffusion coefficient that favors easy diffusion of these low molecular weight agents.[8]

    As ethanol distributes through the tumor interstitium, its cytotoxic mechanisms are exerted through a combination of cytoplasmic dehydration, denaturation of cellular proteins, and small vessel thrombosis. These effects result in coagulative necrosis.

    The cytotoxic mechanisms of acetic acid are similar to those of ethanol, which include protein denaturation, dissolution of cellular basement membranes, and destruction of interstitial collagen.
  - *Technique of chemical ablation:* Percutaneous chemical ablation is usually performed with real-time ultrasound (US) guidance and local anesthesia. A 20–22 gauge end-hole or conical tip multi-side-hole needle is used. Infusion is performed slowly in 0.1– 0.2 mL aliquots with continuous US monitoring. When the tumor becomes echogenic, the needle is withdrawn while injecting local anesthetic agent for local pain relief **(Figs. 1A to D)**.
  - *Volume of alcohol and acetic acid injection:* Strength of the chemical agents used are 95% absolute alcohol (ethanol) or 50% acetic acid. The volume estimation is based on the volume of the tumor and a "surgical margin" of 1 cm beyond the periphery of the lesion. For PEI, the volume is calculated using formula: $V= 4/3\pi\ (r + 0.5)^3$, where V is the target volume of ethanol, r the radius of the lesion (in centimeters), and 0.5 for the correction for the additional "surgical margin". Multiple sessions are performed once or twice weekly and the number of treatment sessions varies according to the size of the lesion, the distribution of intralesional ethanol within the tumor and the condition of the patient.

    For PAI, the maximum total volume of acetic acid required to ablate the tumor is three times the maximum diameter of the tumor. This total dose is injected over multiple sessions (1–2 mL of acetic acid per tumor per session per week) under US guidance.
  - *Advantage of PAI over PEI:* Both PAI and PEI are effective in treating small HCC less than 3 cm. PAI has high diffusion capacity and because of this smaller volume of acetic acid and fewer treatment sessions are required to achieve the same degree of cell kill as that with ethanol.[9] PAI has an advantage of infiltrating the tumor septae and capsule of tumors, whereas ethanol is unable to do so. Due to this limitation, PEI is unable to ablate the small satellite nodules and create a safety margin. The local recurrence rate of the tumor is therefore higher in PEI than PAI [37% and 8%, respectively ($P < 0.001$)].[10]
  - *Complications:* PAI and PEI are safe procedures with low complication rate and no major complications. Minor complications in the form

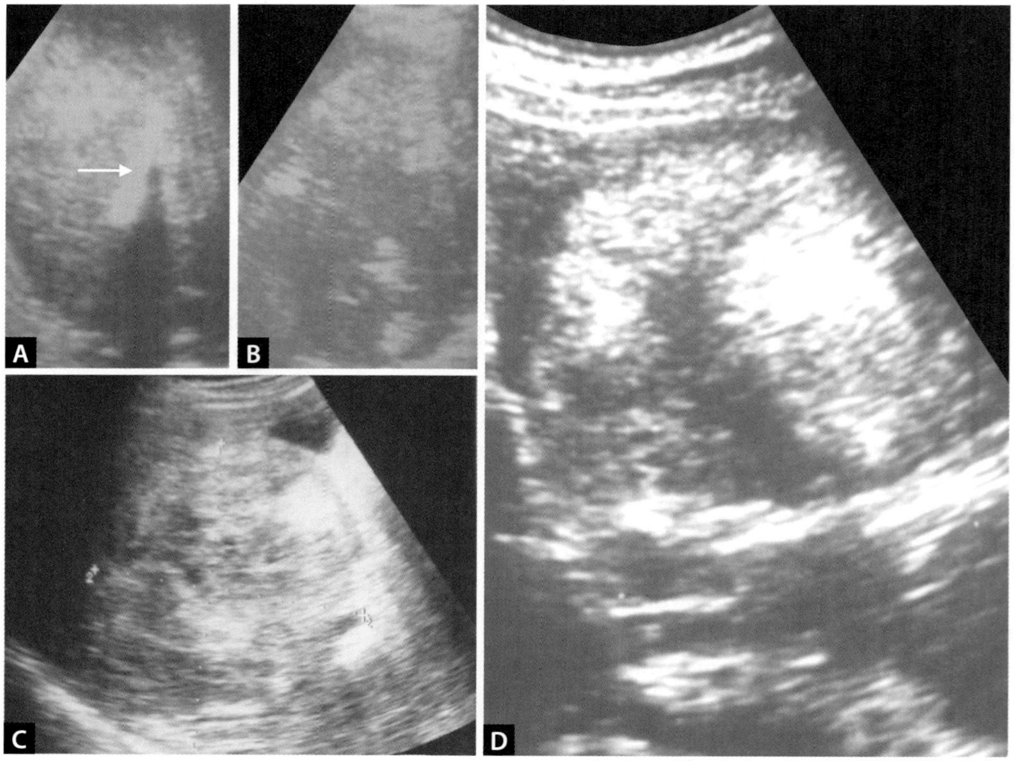

Figs. 1A to D: Percutaneous alcohol injection under ultrasound guidance in HCC: Alcohol is injected in the deepest portion (arrow) (A) followed by superficial portion (B) and (C) of the tumor with the help of a long needle (arrow). The perfused areas are seen as patches of hyperechogenicity (D).

of transient pain, fever, transient renal failure (with acetic acid) may be encountered. Rarely, transient hemoglobinuria may occur immediately following PAI and this clears on its own. Major complications are rare which include hemorrhage, liver necrosis and abscess formation. Although PEI is performed with a small-caliber needle, substantial hemorrhage has been reported. Therefore, correction of underlying coagulopathy should be performed to a target international normalized ratio of 1.4 or less and a platelet count of 50,000/mm.[1,2]

- *Thermal ablation:* There are four types of thermal ablative techniques namely: Radiofrequency ablation, microwave ablation, cryoablation and laser ablation (***see*** **Table 1**). Among these, radiofrequency ablation (RFA) is the most widely used. The first experiments with thermal ablation of living tissue were described by d´Arsonval as early as 1868, while the use of thermal ablation for treatment of malignant hepatic lesions was first shown by McGahan et al. and Rossi et al. in 1990.[11,12] Since then, the technique has evolved as the most popular ablative technique world over.
   - *Principle of RFA:* The goal of RFA is to induce thermal injury to the tumor tissue by electromagnetic energy deposition. The patient is a part of a closed-loop circuit which includes an RF generator, an electrode needle, and a large dispersive electrode (ground pads). Radiofrequency energy is delivered as an alternating current at a frequency of 375–500 kHz within the tumor producing ionic agitation around the needle tip because of the relatively high electrical resistance of the tissue in comparison to the metal electrodes. This ionic agitation produces frictional heat around the electrode with resultant coagulative necrosis. The thermal damage is dependent on the tissue temperature achieved and the duration of heating. A temperature of 50–55°C for 4–6 minutes produces irreversible cellular damage.
   - *Types of RFA electrodes:* There are various types of electrodes which have either monopolar or bipolar technology. The difference between the two technologies is elaborated in **Table 3**. Bipolar and multipolar technology is the latest advance in the technique of radiofrequency ablation. This has

Table 3: Monopolar versus bipolar RFA technology.

Monopolar system	*Bipolar system*
• Circuit is completed inside the patient (Patient is part of the complete circuit)	• Circuit is completed with the lesion
• Grounding pads are required	• No grounding pads
• Multiple lesions cannot be treated at same time	• Multiple lesions can be ablated at same time
• Arrhythmias may occur	

eliminated the need of a grounding pad and is also more effective in ablating large areas.[13,14]

The electrodes are broadly divided into the cooled tip or noncooled tip type depending upon the presence of the continuous cooling system. In the cooled tip type, there is continuous saline circulation through the electrode which produces cooling of the needle tip which prevents tissue charring. The heat is generated away from the electrode which results in coagulation necrosis of the tumor tissue.

Based upon the array configuration, the electrodes may be single, clustered, multitined or saline perfused **(Figs. 2A to F)**.

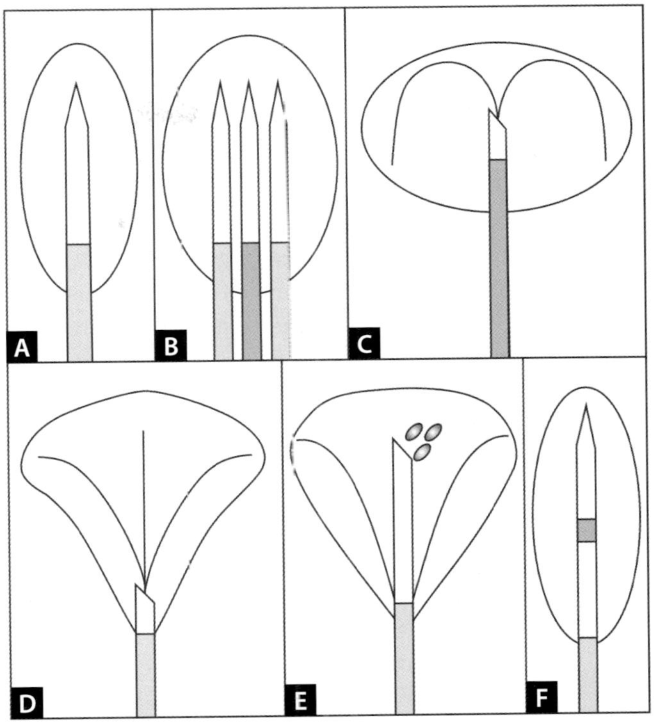

Figs. 2A to F: RFA electrode designs: (A) Monopolar single electrode; (B) Clustered electrode; (C) Tined electrode; (D) Multitined; (E) Saline perfused; (F) Bipolar single electrode.
Note: The area marked around each electrode represents the shape of ablating zone.

- *Patient selection:* RFA is ideally suited for smaller lesions less than 3 cm size. Although tumors up to 5 cm diameter can be ablated with RFA, but chances of complete ablation diminishes with increase in tumor diameter. The technique can also be used to treat multiple lesions and up to three lesions can be safely treated in single or multiple sittings. Lesions close to main branches of portal or hepatic veins are difficult to treat as continuous high blood flow in these vessels will have cooling effect because the thermal energy will be dissipated away, which is known as "heat sink effect". If the lesion is close to liver capsule or gallbladder, chances of peritonitis or cholecystitis respectively are high. For these reasons, lesions that do not have at least one centimeter of normal liver parenchyma separating it from the liver capsule, gallbladder, porta hepatis or major vessels are considered a relative contraindication for RFA. Such tumors close to critical structures require special procedures for ablation like saline instillation (5% dextrose water) or balloon occlusion of the larger vascular channel.[15]

  Contraindications are similar to the other ablative procedures, like—extrahepatic metastatic disease, tumor volume more than 30% of the total liver volume, sepsis, severe debilitation and uncorrectable coagulopathies.
- *Technique of RFA:* RFA is usually performed with real-time ultrasound (US) guidance or computed tomography guidance, under intravenous sedation and standard cardiac, pressure, and oxygen monitoring.[7] To perform a typical ablation with monopolar RFA system, two grounding pads are placed on the patient's thighs to begin with. The radiofrequency probe is electrically insulated in its proximal part while the short distal part near the tip is uninsulated from where the electric current is passed into the tumor. The electrode is inserted into the lesion under either US or CT guidance. The RF generator is set for the wattage, timer, and temperature as per the device instructions (vendor specific). A pulsed RF energy is applied for 15–30 minutes, which causes a rise of the temperature at the target site from 80°C to 110°C. Once there is ionic agitation within the tissue, the microbubbles are seen forming around the electrode which make the lesion echogenic

and obscures the tumor margins. After successful ablation, additional energy is applied during the withdrawal of the electrode under monitoring by real time ultrasound. This is done to prevent seeding of tumor cells in the probe track.

- *Post-RFA evaluation:* For immediate post RFA evaluation, contrast-enhanced sonography is useful for ascertaining the completeness of ablation. In situations of residual disease, reapplication of the radiofrequency electrode in the untreated area in the same sitting can be done to ensure complete response. Multiphasic CT of the liver within a few hours of the ablation is also helpful in gauging the completeness of ablation as well as evaluating any associated complications. However, the accuracy of immediate post RFA assessment scan is limited because of the presence of ablation-induced hyperemic rim around the ablated tumor tissue which mimics the appearance of residual viable tumor. The reactive hyperemia generally resolves in a months' time when more accurate assessment of tumor response can be made on imaging.
- *Complications:* RFA is a safe procedure with a mortality rate as low as 0.1–0.3% and the major complication rate of 2.2–3.1%. Minor complication rate ranges from 5% to 8.9%. Pain or fever is common and is usually self-limiting. Peritoneal hemorrhage, bile duct injury, hepatic abscess, intestinal perforation are some of the adverse outcomes rarely encountered.[16,17] Late complication of tumor seeding along the needle track is also known to occur but is highly uncommon (0.5–0.8%).
- *Limitations of RFA:* Complete tumor response is difficult to achieve in larger tumors more than 5 cm for which newer electrodes are coming into existence. Moreover combination of RFA with other available treatment modalities are being used for larger tumors with improved results.[18] Tumors adjacent to large blood vessels are difficult to treat due to the "heat-sink effect"—a perfusion-mediated tissue cooling reducing the extent of coagulation necrosis produced by thermal ablation.[19]

- *Microwave ablation:* Microwave ablation (MWA) uses electromagnetic waves generated from one or more thin microwave antennas that are applied directly to the tumor to create heat and friction that destroys the tumor.[20]

  The benefit of MWA over radiofrequency ablation (RFA) is the ability to do multiple ablations at the same time. MWA has the potential to destroy larger sized tumors faster and with less pain.
- *Cryoablation:* Cryoablation is another form of the ablative therapy in which the tumor is frozen and this results in cell death. The technique involves creation of an ice ball with subzero temperatures by circulating liquid nitrogen in a probe that is directly inserted into the tumor. As with other ablative therapies, CT, MR or ultrasound scanning provides precise guidance for the procedure. One of the major concerns of cryoablation is "Cryo shock", a fatal complication seen in large hepatic ablation occurring due to rapid release of cellular debris (inflammatory cytokine release) into the systemic circulation.[21] Cryoablation is more widely used in kidney, prostate, lung and bone than in liver tumors.
- *High-intensity focused ultrasound ablation:* High-intensity focused ultrasound (HIFU) is a noninvasive modality producing thermal ablation. The high frequency ultrasound beam is generated by ultrasound transducer which is arranged into a spherical form by an acoustic lens to create a focal point. The beam on reaching the focal point, delivers high temperature focused acoustic energy to the liver tumor producing tumor destruction at a temperature of 60°C.[22] General anesthesia is used and no needle placement within the tumor is required. HIFU is effective in tumors close to major vessels like inferior vena cava, portal or hepatic veins. Complete response can be achieved in 91% of tumors of <3 cm, and the 1 and 3 years survival rates are 87.7% and 62.4%, respectively.[22]
- *Laser ablation:* In this technique, the tumor is destroyed by the heat energy converted from light. Bare tip quartz fibers (300–600 μm) when inserted through multiple 21 gauge needles transmit laser light to the tumor. This light is absorbed and distributed within the tumor, converted to heat in the target tumor tissues and produce coagulation necrosis of the tumor. It is safe and highly effective in HCCs less than 4 cm and can also be used in patients with liver metastases.[23]
- *Nonthermal ablation—Irreversible electroporation:* Irreversible electroporation (IRE) is a new addition to the nonthermal ablative technique which is performed under CT guidance using short pulses of high voltage electrical energy through the electrodes for producing cellular damage in the tumor. Ninety pulses of 1000–3000 V/cm are delivered and a destabilizing electrical potential along the cell membrane is generated leading

to formation of permanent nanopores in the lipid bilayer. Cell death is incurred by irreversible disruption and increased cell permeability.[24] IRE is useful for treating hepatic tumors located close to the major vessels, bile ducts or hepatic veins.

Intra-arterial Procedures

Image-guided intra-arterial procedures are the most commonly used palliative treatment options for the patients of HCC as the vast majority have advanced disease at the outset which precludes the use of curative options. Being palliative in nature, the treatment invariably needs to be repeated in situations of disease progression or recurrences.

- *Transarterial chemoembolization (TACE):* TACE is used for treating patients of unresectable HCC of BCLC B stage,[4] unsuitable candidates for local ablative therapies of BCLC A stage and for downstaging the disease to make patients suitable for resection or transplant. Being palliative in nature, the primary goal of the therapy is to improve quality of life and prolong survival.

  The procedure of TACE is a combination of two steps—intra-artenal injection of chemotherapeutic drugs followed by embolization of the feeding supply to the tumor. In TACE, also called conventional TACE, the chemotherapeutic drug emulsion is prepared by mixing the chemotherapeutic drugs with lipiodol and the subsequent embolization is performed by either gelfoam pledgets or PVA particles **(Fig. 3)**.[25-27] This result in extensive necrosis of the hypervascular HCC as increased dose (up to hundred fold higher) of the chemotherapeutic agent is administered intra-arterially compared to systemic administration. The effect is further augmented by the additional embolization of the feeding arteries (branches from the hepatic arteries) causing ischemic necrosis of the tumor.

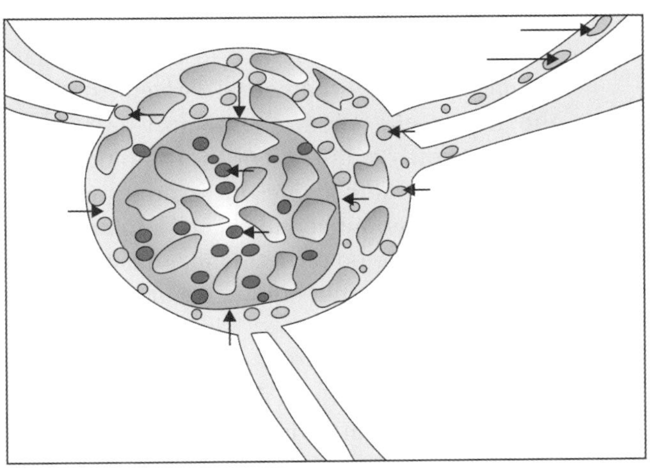

Fig. 3: Diagrammatic representation of transcatheter chemoembolization. Lipiodol is mixed with chemotherapeutic drug and is infused in hepatic artery followed by gelfoam embolization (long arrows) of the arterial branches. The dark area represents the tumor (small arrows).

  - *Agents used:* Doxorubicin, epirubicin alone or in combination with cisplatin are the commonly used chemotherapeutic agents. Lipiodol, mixed with chemotherapeutic drugs to prepare emulsion, is used as a drug carrier. This drug emulsion is selectively retained within the tumor cells resulting in increased exposure of the neoplastic cells to the chemotherapeutic agents and also enhances the visibility of the emulsion on fluoroscopy.
  - *Patient selection:* Ideal candidates are patients of BCLC B stage. These patients are those who have a preserved liver function (Child-Pugh class A, B), multinodular tumors without vascular invasion or extrahepatic spread. Patients who have reduced liver function or hepatic failure (Child-Pugh C), have to be excluded for this treatment since the liver function may further deteriorate due to ischemic damage of the unaffected liver tissue leading to acute liver failure.
  - *Benefit of arterial embolization:* Arterial embolization induces selective ischemia which results in tumor necrosis and enhances the cytotoxicity of the anti- chemotherapeutic agents. Gelfoam embolization creates hypoxic environment in the tumor bed and tissue hypoxia inhibits the active efflux of the chemotherapeutic drug by making transmembrane P-glycoprotein, an ATP-dependent pump ineffective.
  - *Technique* **(Figs. 4A to F)**: Chemoembolization is performed in the angiography suite, under aseptic precautions with the patient under conscious sedation and through the percutaneous route. To begin with, diagnostic mesenteric and celiac arteriograms are performed using various preshaped polyurethane catheter (4 or 5F) with the digital subtraction technique to determine the vascular anatomy, feeding tumor supply and the portal blood flow. The placement of the catheter tip in the feeding artery, as close to the tumor as possible, is the most important technical factor undertaken for maximizing the treatment effect on the tumor and minimizing damage to nontumor hepatic tissue. Superior mesenteric arteriogram

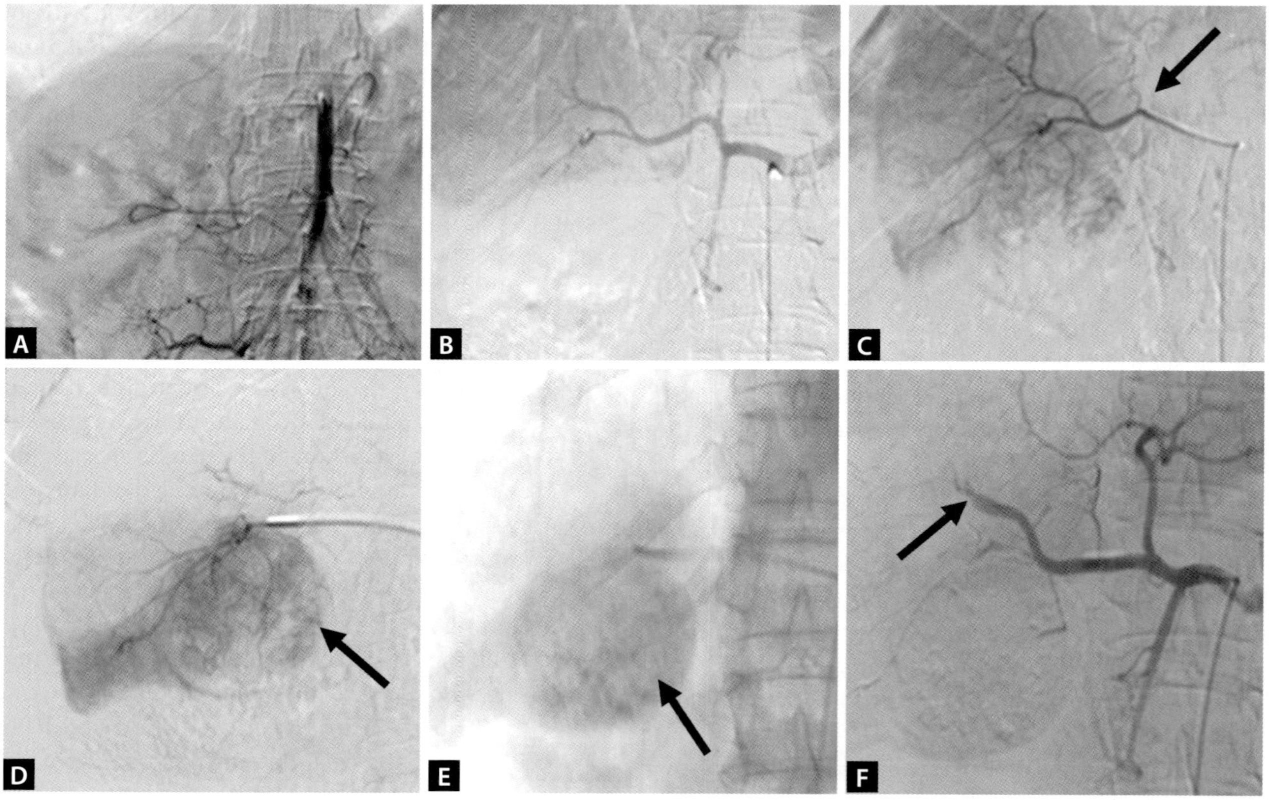

Figs. 4A to F: Various steps of angiographic technique of TACE: Initial SMA angiogram (A) performed to look for anomalous origin of hepatic artery, followed by celiac axis angiogram (B); Selective angiogram of the right hepatic artery (arrow) (C) showing abnormal tumor blush (arrow)(D), followed by injection chemotherapeutic emulsion into the tumor bed shows retention of lipiodol (arrow) (E) and stasis of blood flow (F) following gelfoam embolization (arrow).

is done for detecting the presence of any hepatic arterial supply (accessory and aberrant) arising from the vessel as well as foe evaluating the patency of the portal vein. Depending upon the hepatic arterial branches arising from celiac artery, selective arteriography of the common, left and right hepatic arteries as per the case is done. The peripheral part of the large tumor, surface tumors, stenosis or occlusion of the hepatic artery or previously treated tumors may develop supply from the extrahepatic sources like parietal arteries, phrenic, internal mammary or intercostal arteries. Unusual origins of the various arterial supply to the tumor may be encountered, like the gastroduodenal artery arising close to the origin of the middle or left hepatic artery, the right gastric artery arising from right or proper hepatic artery or the left hepatic artery arising from the left gastric artery. Use of microcatheter and sometimes coil embolization of these vessels is performed to protect the stomach and duodenum from potential reflux of the chemotherapeutic and embolic agents. Microcatheter, coaxial system helps to reach the tumor superselectively avoiding vessel spasm and dissection. After advancement of the microcatheter system to the appropriate segmental or subsegmental vessel supplying the tumor, the chemotherapeutic mixture is injected slowly at the rate of 1 mL/minute under continuous fluoroscopic observation avoiding reflux of chemotherapeutic agent into nontarget areas. There are no recommendations regarding the volume of emulsion to be injected with reference to the tumor size.

In case of multiple vascular feeders, the emulsion is injected into all the feeders superselectively in divided fractions. In case of significant arterioportal or arteriovenous shunting, a small amount of gelfoam is injected to block the shunt prior to the injection of chemotherapeutic emulsion. Subsequently, the feeding vessels are embolized by gelfoam pledgets to reduce the blood flow and also the wash out of chemotherapeutic agents into the systemic circulation.

If the tumor is very large in size, repeated sessions of TACE may be required to achieve complete response **(Figs. 5A and B)**. It is also important to search for any extrahepatic supply to the tumor in such cases.

- *Complications of TACE:* Postembolization syndrome is commonly encountered and is self-limiting. Major complications include hepatic insufficiency, liver abscess, ischemic complications (cholecystitis, bile duct necrosis, perforation of the alimentary tract), and renal dysfunction.

- *TACE using drug eluding beads (DEB-TACE):* The main target of TACE is to reduce systemic toxicity, increase the therapeutic efficacy and provide a sustained release of chemotherapy over time without damaging the healthy surrounding hepatic parenchyma. Recently, introduced novel technologies consisting of embolic microspheres have the ability to actively sequester doxorubicin hydrochloride from a solution and release it in a controlled and sustained fashion (DEB). They have been shown to substantially diminish the amount of chemotherapy that reaches the systemic circulation compared with lipiodol-based conventional TACE, thus significantly increasing the local concentration of the drug and achieving better tumor response rates.[28]
- *Transarterial radionuclide therapy (TART):* Hemodynamic principles and techniques of TART are similar to TACE. Internal radiotherapy by injection of isotopes like ^{131}Iodine+lipiodol, ^{188} Rhenium + lipiodol and ^{90} Yttrium (^{90}Y) into the hepatic artery has shown improvement in survival. ^{90}Y radioembolization can deliver extremely high levels of radiation (up to 150 Gy), with tolerable exposure to normal parenchyma. TART is a safe, effective and promising therapeutic option in patients with inoperable HCC **(Figs. 6A to E)**. The best candidate for TART is BCLC-Advanced stage C, i.e. HCC with portal vein tumor thrombosis (PVT).[29]

Combination Treatment

Currently, in cases with increased tumor burden or larger sized tumors, multimodality approach is being considered. The regional and local therapies are combined in the same patient to produce better results as compared to the use of single therapy.[30,31]

Ablative therapies of PEI or RFA are performed after the procedure of TACE in cases of small residual disease, TACE followed by oral chemotherapy is used for advanced HCC and in patients with postresection recurrence (s), RFA or TACE is undertaken frequently **(Figs. 7A to D)**.

Follow-up and response assessment after locoregional therapies for HCC

Clinical follow-up: Postprocedure, patients are followed up at 1–2 monthly intervals for the assessment of the liver function status and treatment side-effects if any. Liver and renal function tests, serum AFP (if elevated prior to treatment) and viral markers (depending upon the etiology of HCC) for monitoring of the hepatitis B or C activity status is undertaken. If a clinical suspicion of recurrence

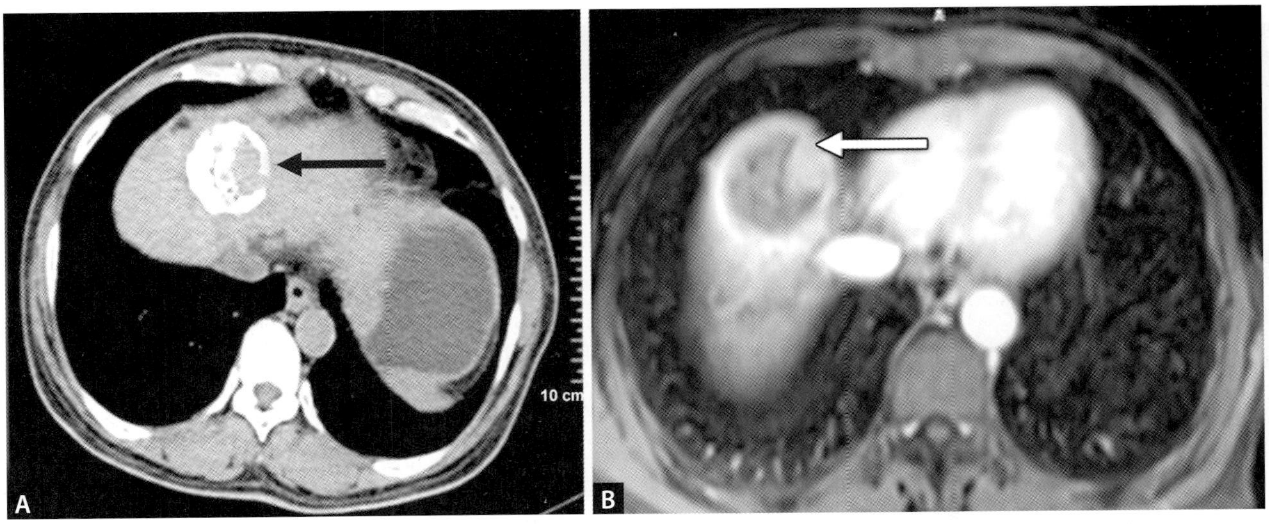

Figs. 5A and B: CT and MRI images of treated by TACE: Axial NCCT image (A) showing lipiodol defect on the medial aspect of the treated lesion (arrow). Postcontrast axial MR image (B) confirming the presence of enhancing component in the area of lipiodol defect (arrow) suggestive of partial response.

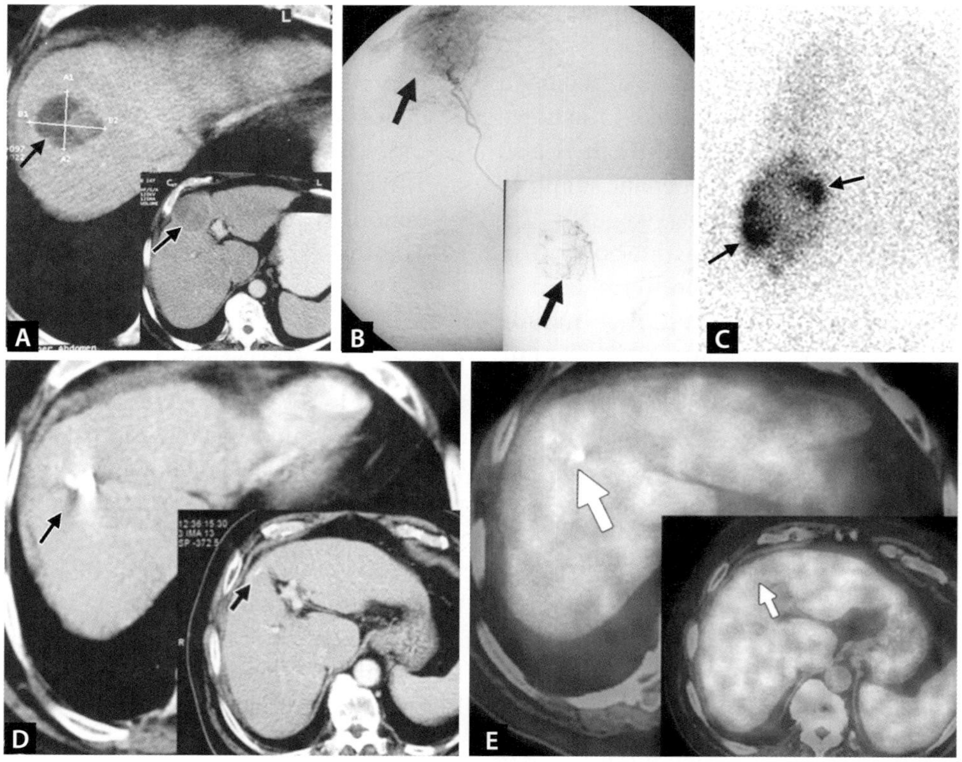

Figs. 6A to E: A 69-year-old man with two HCC lesions involving both lobes of the liver. Both lesions were completely ablated after two doses of ^{188}Re HDD iodized oil at three-monthly intervals. At the time of this writing, the patient was alive and ambulatory with normal serum AFP levels and no evidence of mass at 3-year follow-up CT: (A) Pretherapy axial contrast-enhanced CT shows two lesions (arrows): One each in segments IV and VIII; (B) Angiogram shows increased vascularity in both lesions (arrows); (C) Post-treatment ^{188}Re whole body scan shows radiotracer accumulation in the tumors (arrows), with faint visualization of lungs and no radiotracer uptake in the thyroid, gastrointestinal tract, or anywhere else; (D) Repeat CT obtained 3 months after the second dose shows complete disappearance of both lesions (arrows). Small radiopaque area in segment IV lesion (appearing to be enhancing HCC mass in larger arterial phase image) is actually a small amount of iodized oil, which was seen in all CT scanning phases (noncontrast, arterial, portal venous, and delayed); (E) Positron emission tomography/CT scan obtained 2 years after treatment also shows no evidence of residual or recurrent disease (arrows). Inset images show segment IV lesion.

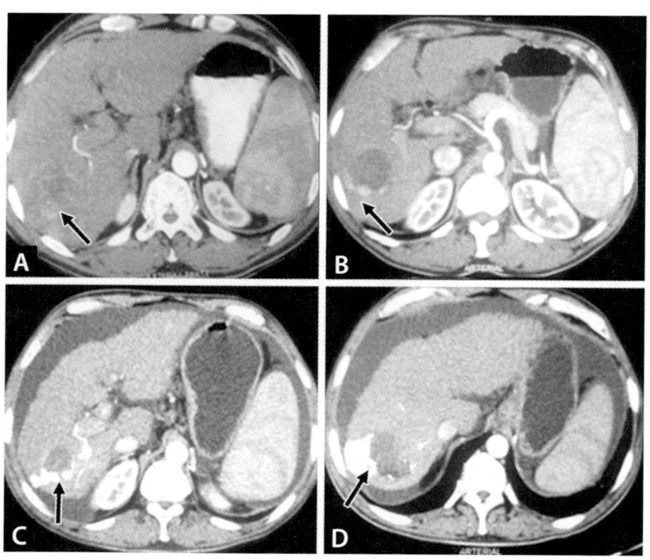

Figs. 7A to D: Combination treatment for HCC (RFA followed by TACE): Pre-RFA axial CT (arterial phase) image (A) showing arterial enhancing lesion (arrow) in segment VI treated by RFA. Post-RFA CT (arterial phase) image (B) showing peripheral nodular enhancing area (arrow) in segment VI lesion, which was subsequently treated by TACE. Post-TACE axial CT images (C and D) showing lipiodol deposition in the periphery of the lesion (arrows) corresponding to nodular enhancing area seen on image B. Findings are suggestive of complete response.

or disease progression arises on follow-up (features of decompensation or rise in AFP), imaging evaluation is asked for and the management done accordingly.

Imaging follow-up: Accurate assessment of tumor response is extremely important in oncology practice for prolonging survival. Imaging techniques of multiphasic CT and MR are generally recommended and lately, use of contrast-enhanced ultrasound (CEUS) has also been used with promising results.[32,33]

Due to the differences in the principles of imaging techniques, contrasts used, these modalities have some limitations, advantages and accuracies in the therapeutic assessment. Response evaluation entails detection of any viable tumor tissue which on contrast imaging techniques (CEUS, MPCT, MRI) is seen as an enhancing area at the tumor site, while the nonviable tissue lacks enhancement. One of the major limitations of MPCT is the difficulty in accurate assessment of the residual disease in post-lipiodol TACE patients. Lipiodol is radiodense and is seen as a hyperdensity in the tumor site on MPCT, the appearance that is similar to the hyperenhancing viable tumor tissue following contrast injection. This at times leads to masking of the small viable tissue on MPCT resulting in misinterpretation.

MRI has the highest accuracy in these patients as the assessment is not affected by the lipiodol presence.[34] Contrast sequences can be complimented with diffusion-weighted sequences (DWI) to improve the diagnostic accuracy. DWI helps to differentiate inflammatory enhancement (T2-shine through) from the viable tumor (diffusion restriction).[35] Evaluation by CEUS is also not hampered by the lipiodol presence and thus CEUS can diagnose even a small viable tissue with high accuracy.[36]

Multiphasic CT or MRI is done at 1, 3, 6 12 months post-procedure for detection of residual disease on the basis of mRECIST criteria.[37] Response assessment by this criterion is based on the percentage of necrosis, viable tumor tissue and not on the overall tumor size shrinkage. This is because the locoregional therapies produce tumor destruction and accurate interpretation of the viable and nonviable cells would give the true picture of efficacy of the therapy in the form of complete or partial response. According to the mRECIST criteria, tumor response is categorized as complete response (CR) is the disappearance of any intratumoral arterial enhancement in all target lesions, partial response (PR): >30% decrease in sum of diameters of all viable (enhancing) target lesions, progressive disease (PD) is >20% increase in the sum of diameters of all viable (enhancing) target lesions and any case that does not qualify for either PR or PD is stable disease (SD) **(Figs. 5 and 8)**.

If the imaging findings suggest PR or PD, then depending upon the disease stage at that point of time, the decision of further treatment is taken. When CR is achieved, the patient is kept under regular clinical and imaging follow-up. On MPCT/MRI, assessment of tumor morphology, resorption of ethiodized oil, overall liver size, development of new lesions or metastases is looked for.[38] Completely treated tumor invariably shrinks in size over period of time **(Figs. 9A to D)**.

Outcome of chemical ablation: PEI is highly effective in small HCCS of 3 cm size. Complete tumor response is encountered in about 80% of the cases and when the size increases to 5 cm, the complete response drops to 50%.[39] In Child's A with early HCC, a 5 years survival rate of 47–53% is seen following PEI.[40]

Limited studies on PAI are available. With PAI too, the response rates are better in small masses up to 3 cm. The local tumor recurrence rate is 51% at 1year and 74% at 3 years. The survival rate at 1 and 3 years is 84% and 51% respectively.[10] Combination of PEI or PAI with other treatments is being taken up for improving treatment outcomes of larger tumors.

Outcome of RFA: Like other techniques of ablation, the tumor response depends on the size, number and location of the tumor as well as the associated liver function. Several studies have reported the complete ablation rates of 80–90% in nodules <3 cm, 50–80% for 3–5 cm and as low as 25% in nodules >5 cm.[41] On comparing the outcome of RFA with surgical resection in multinodular HCC, a recent meta-analysis has shown a better survival benefit with resection than RFA, whereas in solitary small HCC of 2 cm, comparable results of RFA and resection have been observed.[42]

Outcome of transarterial chemoembolization: TACE is an effective procedure which produces significant tumor response and survival benefit despite tumor size in comparison to supportive care. A survival advantage of 82% and 63% for chemoembolization has been documented in comparison to 63% and 27% for supportive care at 1 and 2 years, respectively.[43,44] The largest Japanese cohort study has depicted a median survival of 34 months and a survival benefit at 1, 3, 5 and 7 years as 82%, 47%, 26% and 16%, respectively with negligible procedure-related mortality (0.5%).[45]

A study from India, TACE performed for relatively larger tumor size [up to16 cm (Mean size 6.6–3.92 cm], the cumulative survival rate at 1, 2 and 3 years was 66%, 47% and 36.4%, respectively.[46]

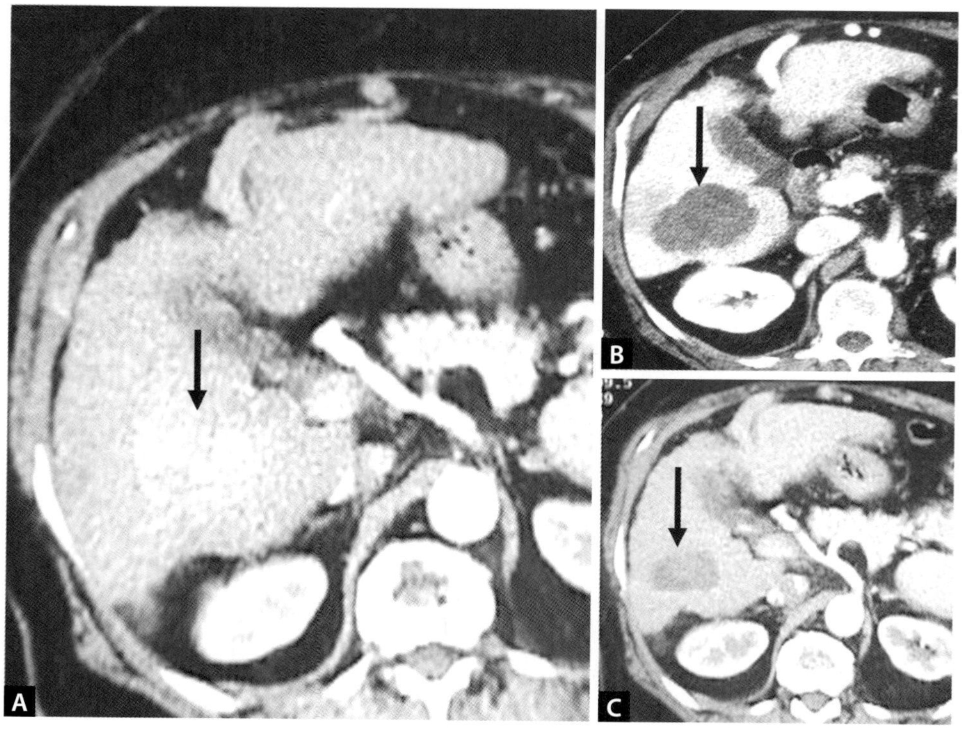

Figs. 8A to C: Preablation arterial phase CT liver showing vascular tumor (arrow, A) in segment VI, complete necrosis and reduction in size (arrow) at 1 year (B) and 2 years (C) after radiofrequency ablation. The patient died after two and half years due to hepatic failure secondary to advanced cirrhosis.

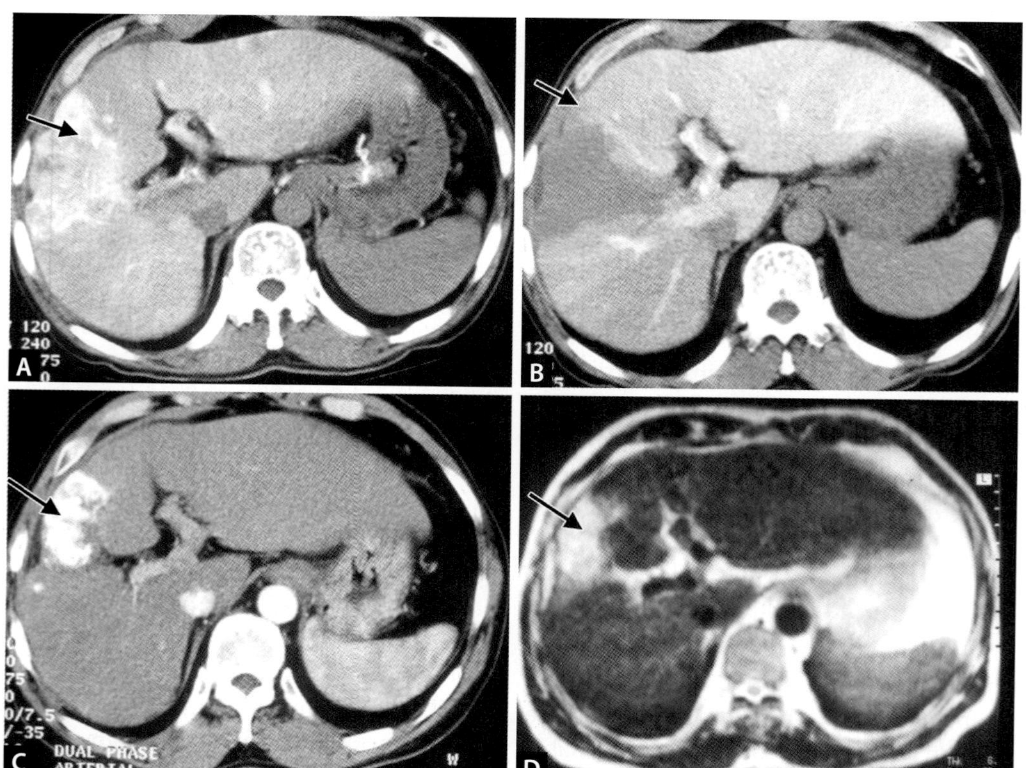

Figs. 9A to D: Pre- (A and B) and post-treatment CT (C) and MR (D) of liver showing vascular mass (arrows) in segments IV and V. The mass is reduced in size after TACE.

Outcome of DEB-TACE: As the DEB produce slow, sustained release of the chemotherapeutic drug, the liver toxicity as well as the systemic toxicity is less. Limited literature is available on long term follow-up. Improved local response and fewer treatment sessions are required with DEB-TACE in comparison to conventional TACE. Decreased frequency of postembolization syndrome with 100–300 mm versus 400–600 mm beads has also been documented. Less side effects leading to low hospitalization rates are seen.[47,48] In India, the biggest limitation of its use has been the high cost and limited availability.

Outcome of TART: As yet, there is limited evidence on the outcome of 90Y radioembolization in patients with unresectable hepatocellular carcinoma. The therapeutic efficacy essentially depends upon the radiation effects as opposed to the ischemia associated with chemoembolization or pure embolization. With 90Y, best outcomes occur in patients with preserved liver function (Child's A) regardless of PVT. Those with Child's B liver function and PVT, have poor outcomes.[29,49,50] The difference in survival between Child's A and B patients has been 17.2 months and 7.7 months; P= 0.002, respectively.[50] Rhenium used in one Indian multicentric trial depicted survival rates of 90.5% at 1 year and 30.5% at 3 years.[29]

Transcatheter arterial embolization (TAE): In this, tumor is embolized with intra-arterial temporary or permanent embolizing materials in single or multiple sessions. It has been proved to be a less effective palliative treatment especially for large and peripherally located HCC due to development of collateral circulation.

Transcatheter arterial embolization of the tumor may be done as an emergency procedure to reduce gastrointestinal hemorrhage in selected patients. Gastrointestinal hemorrhage from hepatocellular carcinoma (HCC) during the natural course of the tumor is unusual. The causes of massive intermittent gastrointestinal bleeding may be either due to varices or due to direct invasion of duodenum, transverse colon and stomach by the tumor. The variceal bleeding may be consequent to portal hypertension secondary to intra-tumoral arterioportal shunts **(Figs. 10A to D)**. These patients may respond well to TAE.[51] Some studies have shown that TAE is an effective method for palliative treatment in such patients.[51,52]

Portal Vein Embolization

Percutaneous portal vein embolization has become an important preoperative treatment in patients who undergo extensive liver resection due to hepatic malignancy. It is done when future liver remnant volume is less than 25% in case of normal back ground liver (less than 40% in case of cirrhotic patients). The aim is to occlude right portal vein either through ipsilateral or contralateral approach using various embolizing agents such as glue, PVA particles and coils. This results in compensatory hypertrophy of the future liver remnant and hence subsequent increase in the functional reserve of the liver and reduces postoperative hepatic failure. The procedure is done percutaneously using both ultrasound and angiography guidance. In normal livers, sufficient hypertrophy typically occurs within 2–4 weeks, whereas regeneration in patients with cirrhosis can take ≥4 weeks. This technique is mainly useful in noncirrhotic livers with malignant tumor confined to segments of one lobe **(Figs. 11A to D)**.[53]

Hepatic vein stenting: The association of Budd-Chiari syndrome and HCC is favored by two conditions. First, HCC can cause obstruction of the main hepatic veins or inferior vena cava due to endoluminal invasion by the tumor. This produces an acute or fulminant variant of Budd-Chiari syndrome, which has a poor prognosis. Second, HCC can develop in patients with chronic Budd-Chiari syndrome and accounts for 0.7% of all the cases of HCC. HCC is most common in patients with membranous obstruction of the vena cava. These patients can be managed effectively by combined interventional techniques; hepatic vein stenting or IVC dilatation to relieve the venous obstruction combined with transarterial chemoembolization for the hepatocellular carcinoma **(Figs. 12A to D)**.

TREATMENT OF METASTATIC DISEASES OF LIVER

Short of surgery, like HCC, interventional techniques of Ablation (commonly RFA) and intra-arterial chemotherapy is the standard treatment recommended for metastases to liver **(Figs. 13A to D)**.[54]

Transarterial administration of anticancer drugs (Doxorubicin, cisplatin, 5-FU, mitomycin C, irinotecan), either alone or as hepatic arterial infusion (HAI), or combined with embolization of feeding artery [transarterial chemoembolization (TACE)] or bland vascular embolization (TAE) is used **(Figs. 14A to D)**. TART with Rhenium-188-HDD-lipiodol has also been used in the management of multiple intrahepatic recurrences after radiofrequency ablation and surgery of hepatocellular carcinoma **(Figs. 15A to G)**.[55-57]

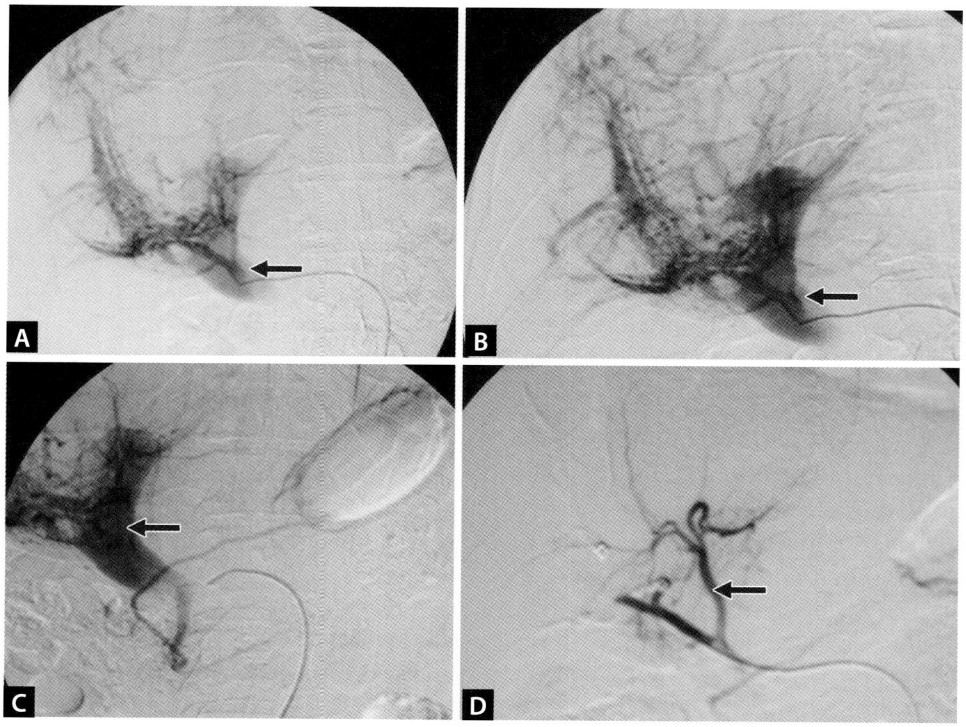

Figs. 10A to D: A 62-year-old male presented with massive upper gastrointestinal hemorrhage (GIH) due to variceal rupture secondary to intratumoral arterioportal shunts causing portal hypertension. The tumor (HCC) was embolized and GIH was stopped. Hepatic arteriograms (A to C) are showing tumor vascularity with simultaneous opacification of portal vein (arrows). The right hepatic artery branches were embolized with fiber steel coils. The postembolization angiogram is not showing opacification of portal vein; (D) The left hepatic artery was not embolized (arrow).

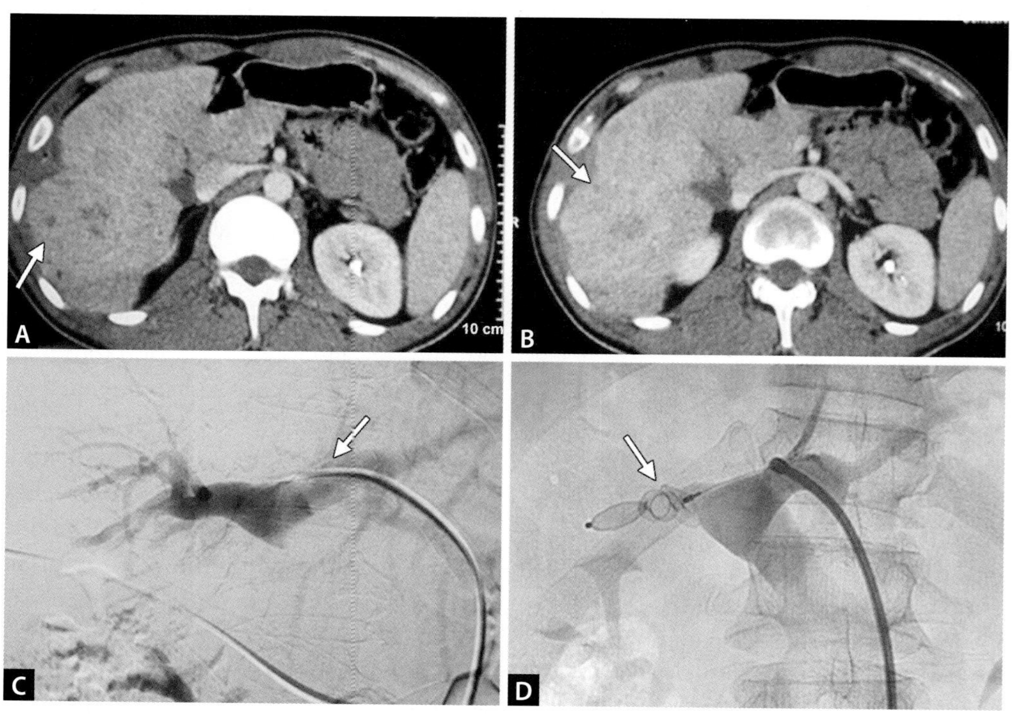

Figs. 11A to D: Right portal vein embolization for right lobe hepatocellular carcinoma planned for extended right hepatectomy: Axial CT images (A and B) showing large mass lesion in right lobe of liver (arrows), portal vein was accessed from left side (arrow) (C) and right portal vein was blocked using Amplatzer plug (arrow) (D).

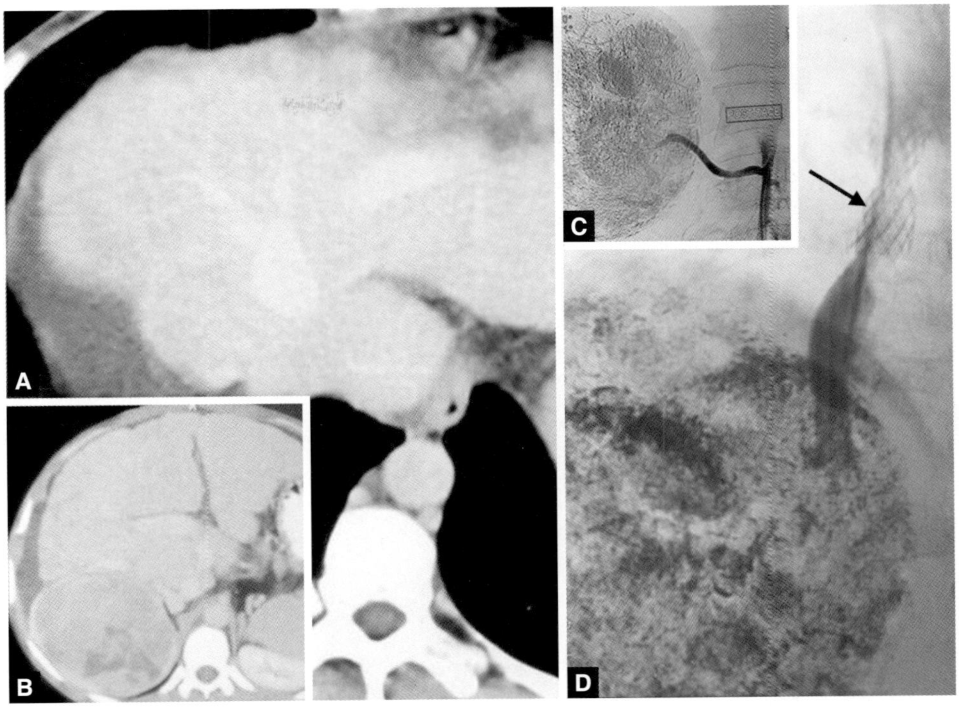

Figs. 12A to D: A 32-year-old male with HCC secondary to hepatic vein outflow tract obstruction (HVOTO) was treated with TACE and hepatic vein stenting. He developed lung metastases on one-year follow-up CT and is presently on systemic chemotherapy. Contrast-enhanced CT liver (A and B) showing right lobe HCC with HVOTO. The tumor was treated with chemoembolization (C) and HVOTO by right hepatic vein stenting (arrow) (D).

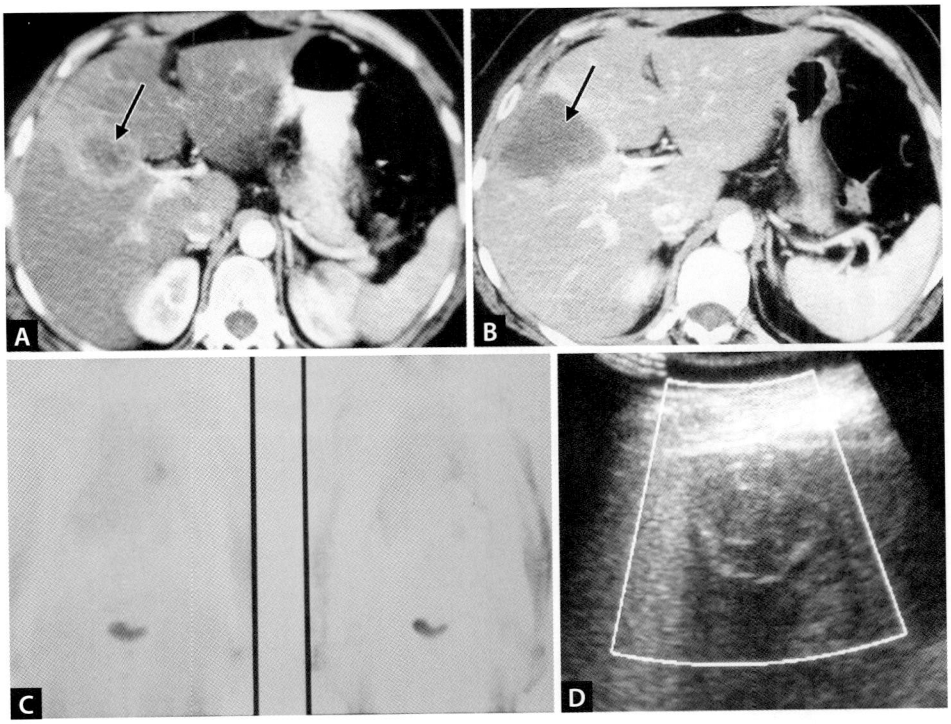

Figs. 13A to D: A 46-year-old female with single liver metastasis from carcinoma of breast (mastectomy done one year back) was treated with single session of RFA. Arterial phase CT (A) is showing single lesion (3.1 × 3 cm) in right lobe of liver (arrow). Post-PFA 3 months arterial phase CT (B) is showing complete ablation of tumor (arrow). Seven years follow-up PET (C) and color Doppler ultrasound (D) are normal.

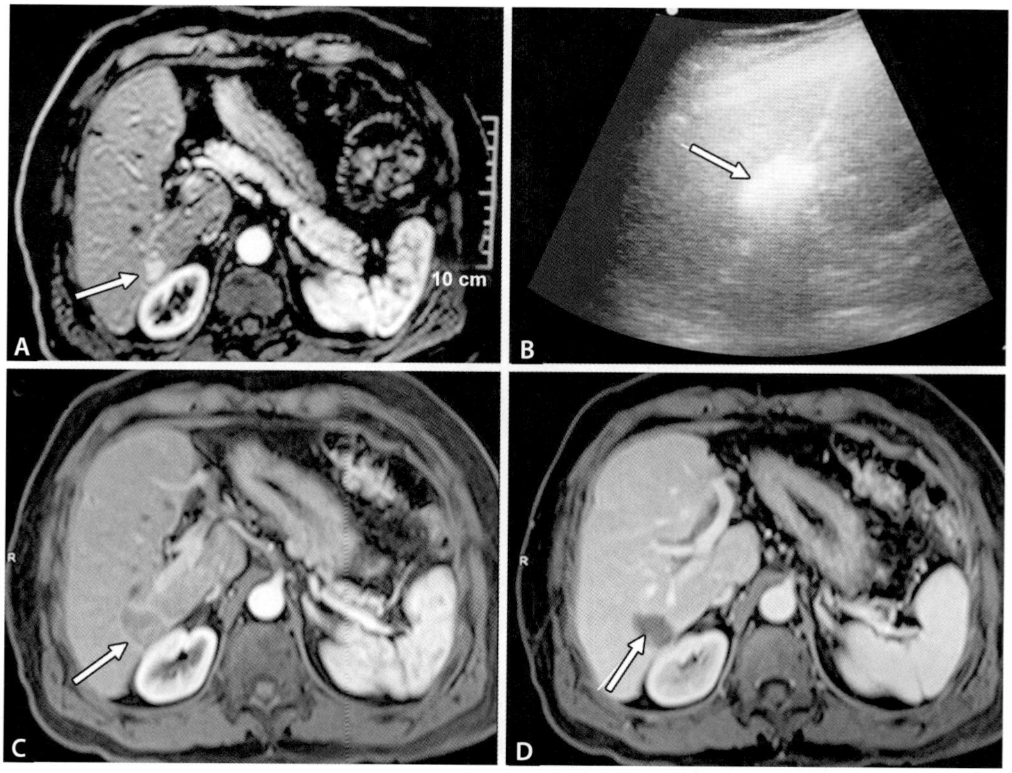

Figs. 14A to D: Radiofrequency ablation for hypervascular metastasis from neuroendocrine primary: Axial MR image (arterial phase) (A) showing small arterial enhancing lesion (arrow) in segment VI of liver which was ablated (arrow) under ultrasound guidance (B); Postablation axial MR images (C and D) showing complete necrosis of the lesion (arrows) suggesting complete response.

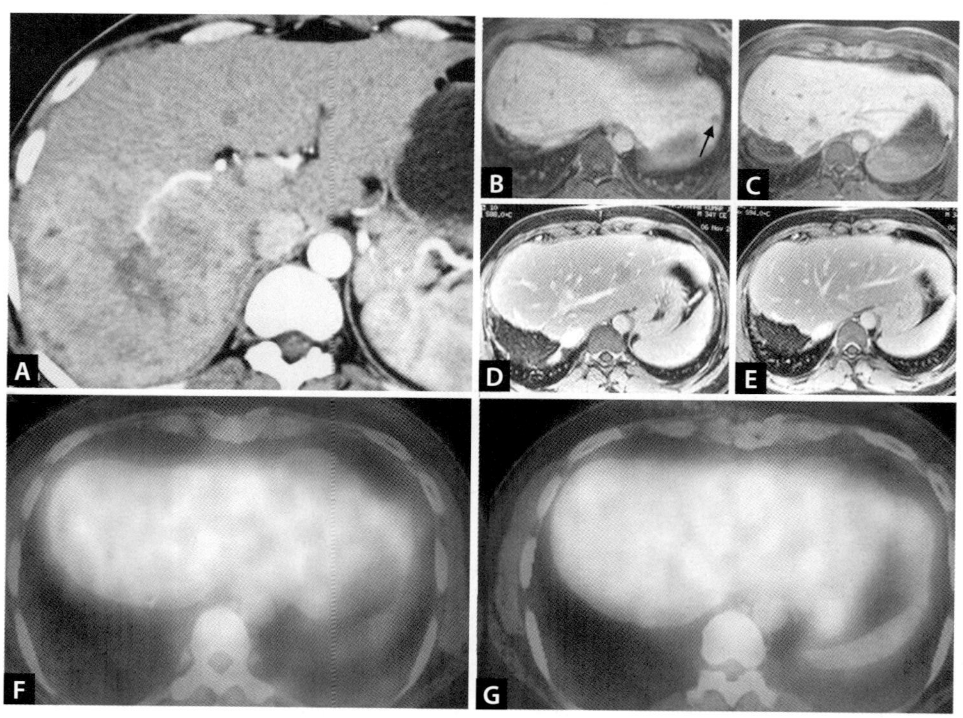

Figs. 15A to G: Arterial phase CT liver (A) is showing HCC in right lobe of liver. One year postright hepatectomy MR (B and C) is showing two metastatic deposits (arrow) in left lobe of liver. The lesions disappeared on follow-up MR (D and E) and PET/CT (F and G) after Re HDD[188] treatment.

TREATMENT OF BENIGN LIVER TUMORS

Hemangioma is the most common benign tumor of the liver. Cavernous hemangiomas are usually asymptomatic but may become symptomatic with rapid tumor enlargement. These patients may present with abdominal pain, fever, anemia, obstructive jaundice, hemobilia, spontaneous rupture with subsequent life-threatening hemorrhage, thrombocytopenia, hypofibrinogenemia and rarely portal hypertension either due to arterioportal fistula or pressure effect on portal vein.

Hepatic artery embolization using both temporary and permanent occluding material may be indicated in the management of symptomatic hemangiomas, causing pressure symptoms or at high risk of bleeding **(Figs. 16 and 17)**. Various studies have shown that TAE of hepatic

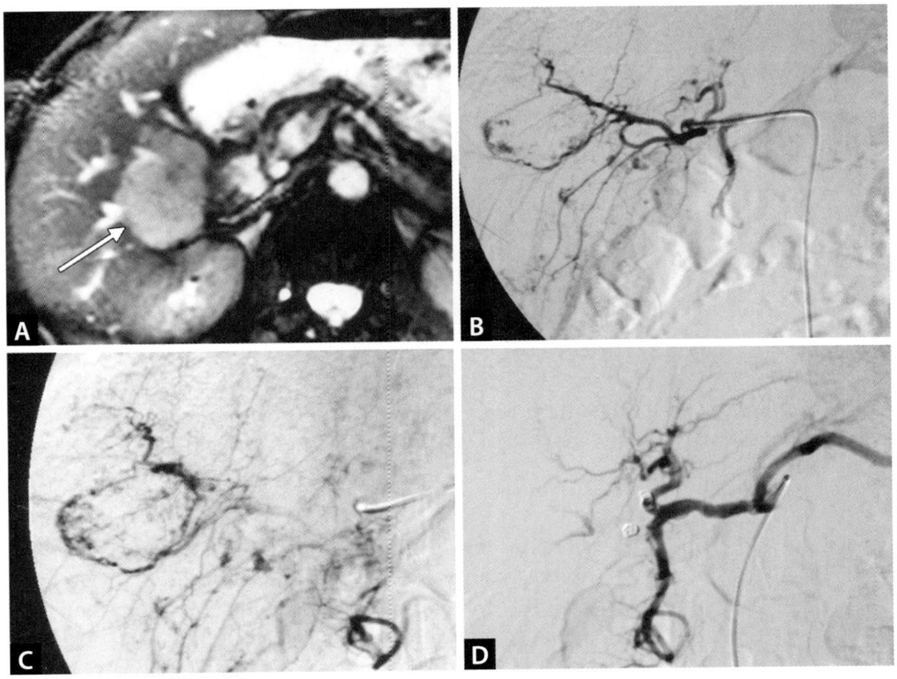

Figs. 16A to D: Large cavernous hemangioma of right lobe of liver extending up to porta hepatis causing recurrent pain and cholangitis was embolized: (A) MR image shows exophytic component of mass (arrow); (B and C) Hepatic artery angiograms show arterial supply from right hepatic artery; (D) Tumor was embolized with multiple steel coils and PVA particles. There was significant reduction in size of mass on follow-up imaging.

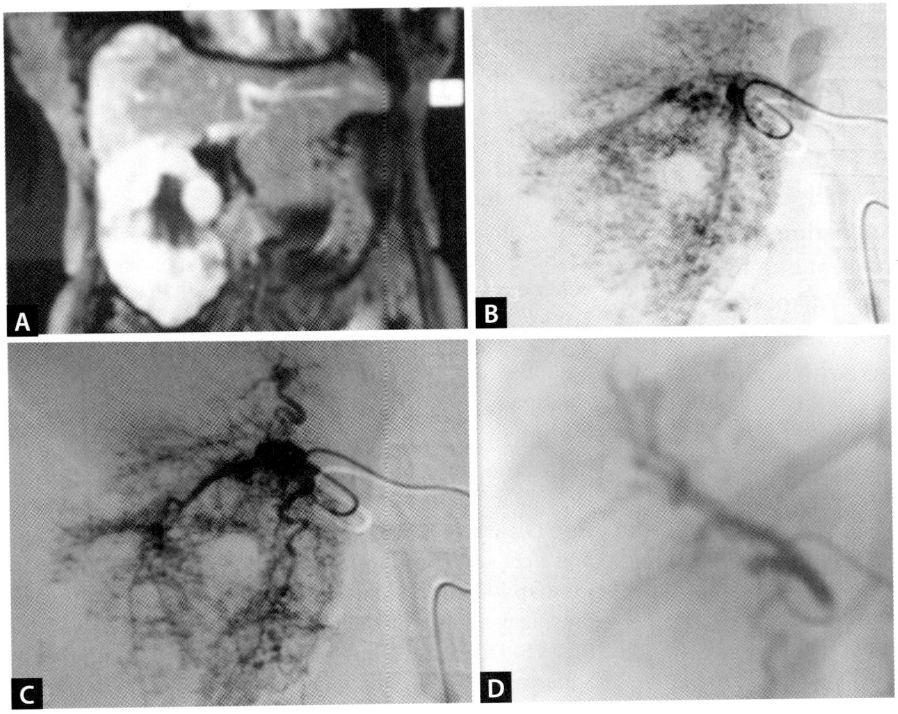

Figs. 17A to D: Large symptomatic pedunculated hepatic hemangioma was embolized preoperatively and surgically removed later: (A) Contrast MR image showing enhancing pedunculated mass in right lobe of liver with hypertrophied left lobe; (B and C) Right hepatic arteriogram showing large cavernous hemangioma with retrograde filling of portal vein; (D) Complete preoperative embolization of the tumor. The tumor was surgically removed with less blood loss.

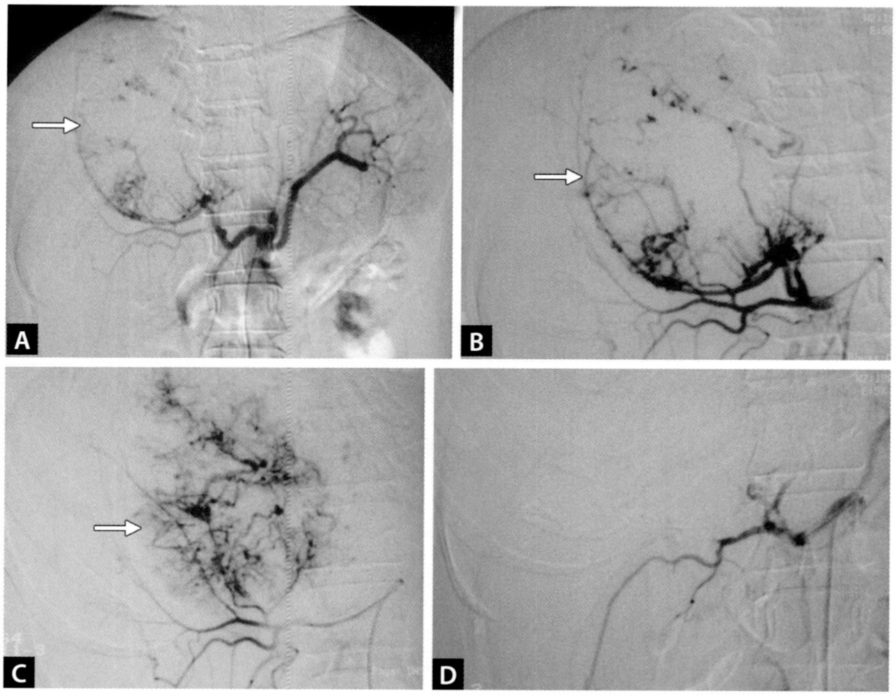

Figs. 18A to D: A 32-year-old female with hepatic adenoma left lobe of liver. Hepatic angiograms show (arrows) marked tumor vascularity (A to C). The tumor was embolized with gelfoam and the postembolization angiogram (D) is not showing tumor vascularity. Complete surgical removal of the tumor was done with less blood loss.

cavernous hemangioma is a useful procedure in the therapy of symptomatic hemangiomas.[58-60]

Preoperative embolization of focal nodular hyperplasia, hepatic adenoma or other vascular tumors may help in surgical removal of the tumor, by reducing intraoperative blood loss **(Figs. 18A to D)**.

CONCLUSION

Radiological interventions are established procedures and recommended therapeutic options for liver tumors. A variety of locoregional therapies are available which can be used in isolation or as a part of combination therapy. Treatment is based upon the clinical presentation, stage of the disease, liver function and the performance status of patient and varies from case-to-case. Decision and execution of treatment is a team work which aims at providing maximum patient benefit.

REFERENCES

1. International Agency for Research on Cancer: World Health Organization. GLOBOCAN 2012: Estimated cancer incidence, mortality, and prevalence worldwide in 2012. *http://globocan.iarc.fr* (Accessed January 20, 2015).
2. Lencioni R, Crocetti L, Cioni D, Della Pina C. Bartolozzi C. Percutaneous radiofrequency ablation of hepatic colorectal metastases: technique, indications, results, and new promises. Invest Radiol. 2004;39:689-97.
3. EASL-EORTC clinical practice guidelines: management of hepatocellular carcinoma. J Hepatol. 2012;56:908-43.
4. Llovet JM, Brú C, Bruix. Prognosis of hepatocellular carcinoma: the BCLC staging classification. Semin Liver Dis. 1999;19(3):329-38.
5. Livraghi T, Bolondi L, Buscarini L, et al. No treatment, resection and ethanol injection in hepatocellular carcinoma: a retrospective analysis of survival in 391 patients with cirrhosis. Italian Cooperative HCC Study Group. J Hepatol. 1995;22:522-6.
6. Foltz G. Image guided percutaneous ablation of hepatic malignancies. Semin Intervent Radiol. 2014;31:180-86.
7. Clark TW, Soulen MC. Chemical ablation of hepatocellular carcinoma. J Vasc Interv Radiol. 2002;13(9 Pt 2):S245-52.
8. Kapoor V, Thaete FL. Percutaneous ethanol and acetic acid ablation of hepatocellular carcinoma. Hepatocellular Cancer. Pages: 153-169. Publisher: Humana Press.
9. Ohnishi K, Nomura F, Ito S, Fujiwara K. Prognosis of small hepatocellular carcinoma (less than 3 cm) after percutaneous acetic acid injection: study of 91 cases. Hepatology. 1996;23: 994-1002.
10. Huo TI, Hiang YH, Wu JC, et al. Comparison of percutaneous and acid injection and percutaneous ethanol injection for hepatocellular carcinoma in cirrhotic patients. A prospective study. Scand J Gastroenterol. 2003;7:770-8.
11. Rossi S, Di Stasi M, Buscarini E, Cavanna L, Quaretti P, Squassante E, et al. Percutaneous radiofrequency interstitial

thermal ablation in the treatment of small hepatocellular carcinoma. Cancer J Sci Am. 1995;1(1):73-81.

12. McGahan JP, Gu WZ, Brock JM, Tesluk H, Jones CD. Hepatic ablation using bipolar radiofrequency electrocautery. Acad Radiol. 1996;3:418-22.
13. Goldberg SN, Grassi CJ, Cardella JF, Charboneau JW, Dodd GD 3rd, Dupuy DE, et al. Society of Interventional Radiology Technology Assessment Committee and the International Working Group on Image-guided Tumor Ablation. Image-guided tumor ablation: standardization of terminology and reporting criteria. J Vasc Interv Radiol. 2009;20 (Suppl 7):S377-90.
14. Seror O, N'kontchou G, Ibraheem M, Ajayon Y, et al. Large (> = 5.0—cm) HCCs: Multipolar RF ablation with three internally cooled bipolar electrodes initial experience in 26 patients. Radiology. 2008;248(1):288-96.
15. Yang W, Yan K, Wu GX, Wu W, Fu Y, Lee JC, et al. Radiofrequency ablation of hepatocellular carcinoma in difficult locations: Strategies and long-term outcomes. World J Gastroenterol. 2015;21(5):1554-66. doi: 10.3748/wjg.v21.i5.1554.
16. Livraghi T, Solbiati L, Meloni MF, et al. Treatment of focal liver tumors with percutaneous radiofrequency ablation: complications encountered in a multicenter study. Radiology. 2003;226:441-51.
17. Lahat E, Eshkenazy R, Zendel A, Zakai BB, Maor M, Dreznik Y, Ariche A. Complications after percutaneous ablation of liver tumors: a systematic review. Hepatobiliary Surg Nutr. 2014;3(5): 317-23.
18. Sheta E, El-Kalla F, El-Gharib M, Kobtan A, Elhendawy M, Abd-Elsalam S, Mansour L, Amer I. Comparison of single-session transarterial chemoembolization combined with microwave ablation or radiofrequency ablation in the treatment of hepatocellular carcinoma: a randomized-controlled study. Eur J Gastroenterol Hepatol; 2016.
19. Poch FG, Rieder C, Ballhausen H, Knappe V, Ritz JP, Gemeinhardt O, et al. The vascular cooling effect in hepatic multipolar radiofrequency ablation leads to incomplete ablation *ex vivo*. Int J Hyperthermia; 2016.pp.1-8.
20. Meloni MF, Chiang J, Laeseke PF, Dietrich CF, Sannino A, Solbiati M, et al. Microwave ablation in primary and secondary liver tumors: technical and clinical approaches. Int J Hyperthermia; 2016. pp. 1-10.
21. Kim GM, Won JY, Kim MD, Park SI, Lee DY, Shin W, et al. Cryoablation of hepatocellular carcinoma with high-risk for percutaneous ablation: safety and efficacy. Cardiovasc Intervent Radiol. 2016.
22. NG KK, Poon RT, Chang SC, et al. High-intensity focused ultrasound for hepatocellular carcinoma: a single center experience. Ann Surg. 2011;253:981-87.
23. Pacella CM, Bizzarri G, Francica G, Bianchini A, De Nuntis S, Pacella S, et al. Percutaneous laser ablation in the treatment of hepatocellular carcinoma with small tumors: analysis of factors affecting the achievement of tumor necrosis. J Vasc Interv Radiol. 2005;16(11):1447-57.
24. Davlos RV, Mir IL, Rubinsky B. Tissue ablation with irreversible electroporation. Annals Biomed Eng. 2005;33:223-31.
25. Tsochatzis EA, Germani G, Burroughs AK. Transarterial chemoembolization, transarterial chemotherapy, and intra-arterial chemotherapy for hepatocellular carcinoma treatment. Semin Oncol. 2010;37(2):89-93.
26. Davis CR. Interventional radiological treatment of hepatocellular carcinoma. Cancer Control. 2010;17(1):87-99.
27. Ramsey DE, Geschwind JH. New interventions for liver tumors. Semin Roentgenology. 2002;37:303-11.
28. Carter S, Martin Ii RC. Drug-eluting bead therapy in primary and metastatic disease of the liver. HPB (Oxford). 2009;11:541-50.
29. Kumar A, Srivastava DN, Chau TTM, et al. Inoperable hepatocellular carcinoma: transarterial 188Re HDD-Labeled iodized oil for treatment—prospective multicenter trial. Radiology. 2007;243:509-19.
30. Yamakado K, Nakatsuka A, Ohmori S, et al. Radiofrequency ablation combined with chemoembolization in hepatocellular carcinoma treatment response based on tumor size and morphology. J Vasc Interv Radiol. 2002;13:1225-32.
31. Yang M, Yuan JQ, Bai M, Han GH. Transarterial chemoembolization combined with sorafenib for unresectable hepatocellular carcinoma: a systematic review and meta-analysis. Mol Biol Rep. 2014;41:6575-82.
32. Lee JM, Yoon JH, Joo I, Woo HS. Recent advances in CT and MR imaging for evaluation of hepatocellular carcinoma. Liver Cancer. 2012;1:22-40.
33. Minami Y, Kudo M. Therapeutic response assessment of transcatheter arterial chemoembolization for hepatocellular carcinoma: ultrasonography, CT and MR imaging. Oncology. 2013;84(Suppl 1):58-63.
34. Guan Y-S, Sun L, Zhou X-P, Li X, Zheng XH. Hepatocellular carcinoma treated with interventional procedures: CT and MRI follow-up. World J Gastroenterol. 2004;10: 3543-8.
35. Yuan Z, Li WT, Ye XD, Peng WJ, Xiao XS. Utility of diffusion-weighted imaging to assess hepatocellular carcinoma viability following transarterial chemoembolization. Oncol Lett. 2014;8:831-6.
36. Liu M, Lin MX, Lu MD, Xu ZF, Zheng KG, Wang W, et al. Comparison of contrast-enhanced ultrasound and contrast-enhanced computed tomography in evaluating the treatment response to transcatheter arterial chemoembolization of hepatocellular carcinoma using modified RECIST. Eur Radiol. 2015;25:2502-11.
37. Riccardo Lencioni R, Llovet JM. Modified RECIST (mRECIST) assessment for hepatocellular carcinoma. Semin Liver Dis. 2010;30:52-60.
38. Chung JC, Naik NK, Lewandowski RJ, Deng J, Mulcahy MF, Kulik LM, et al. Diffusion-weighted magnetic resonance imaging to predict response of hepatocellular carcinoma to chemoembolization. World J Gastroenterol. 2010;16(25):3161-7.

39. Vilana R, Bruix J, Bru C, Ayuso C, Sole M, Rodes J. Tumor size determines the efficacy of percutaneous ethanol injection for the treatment of small hepatocellular carcinoma. Hepatology. 1992;16:353-7.
40. Lencioni R. Locoregional treatment of hepatocellular carcinoma. Hepatology. 2010;52:762-73.
41. Cucchetti A, Piscaglia F, Cescon M, Ercolani G, Pinna AD. Systematic review of surgical resection versus radiofrequency ablation for hepatocellular carcinoma. World J Gastroenterol. 2013;19:4106-18.
42. Duan C, Liu m, Zhang Z, Ma K, Bie P. Radiofrequency ablation versus hepatic resection for the treatment of early stage hepatocellular carcinoma meeting Milan criteria: a systematic review and meta-analysis. World J Surgl Oncol. 2013;11:190.
43. Llovet JM, Bruix J. Systematic review of randomized trials for unresectable hepatocellular carcinoma: chemoembolization improves survival. Hepatology. 2003;37:429-42.
44. Yamada R, Sato M, Kawabata M, Nakatsuka H, Nakamura K, Takashima S. Hepatic artery embolization in 120 patients with unresectable hepatoma. Radiology. 1983;148:397-401.
45. Takayasu K, Arii S, Ikai I, et al. Prospective cohort study of trans-arterial chemoembolization for unresectable hepatocellular carcinoma in 8510 patients. Gastroenterology. 2006;131:461-9.
46. Paul SB, Gamanagatti S, Sreenivas V, et al. Trans-arterial chemoembolization in patients with unresectable hepatocellular carcinoma: experience from a tertiary care centre in India. Indian J Radiol. Imaging. 2011;21:113-20.
47. Lammer J, Malagari K, Vogl T, et al. Prospective randomized study of doxorubicin-eluting-bead embolization in the treatment of hepatocellular carcinoma: results of the PRECISION V study. Cardiovasc Interv Radiol. 2010;33:41-52.
48. Prajapati HJ, Dhanasekaran R, El-Rayes BF, et al. Safety and efficacy of doxorubicin drug-eluting bead transarterial chemoembolization in patients with advanced hepatocellular carcinoma. J Vasc Interv Radiol. 2013;24:307-15.
49. Geschwind JF, Salem R, Carr BI, et al. Yttrium-90 microspheres for the treatment of hepatocellular carcinoma. Gastroenterology. 2004;127:S194-205.
50. Salem R, Lewandowski RJ, Mulcahy MF, et al. Radioembolization for hepatocellular carcinoma using Yttrium-90 microspheres: a comprehensive report of long-term outcomes. Gastroenterology. 2010;138:52-64.
51. Srivastava DN, Thulkar S, Sharma S, Pandey GK, Sahni P, Julka PK, Acharya SK. Therapeutic radiological interventional procedures in hepatocellular carcinoma. Indian J Gastroenterol. 2002;21:96-8.
52. Srivastava DN, Gandhi D, Julka PK, et al. Gastrointestinal hemorrhage in hepatocellular carcinoma management with transhepatic arterioembolization. Abdominal Imaging. 2000;25:1-6.
53. Madoff DC, Hicks ME, Vauthey JN, Charnsangavej C, Morello FA Jr, Ahrar K, et al. Transhepatic portal vein embolization: anatomy, indications, and technical considerations. Radiographics. 2002;22(5):1063-76.
54. Gunabushanam G, Sharma S, Thulkar S, Srivastava DN, et al. Radiofrequency ablation of liver metastases from breast cancer: results in 14 patients. J Vasc Interv Radiol. 2007;18(1):67-72.
55. Kumar A, Bal C, Srivastava DN, Thulkar SP, Sharma S, Acharya SK, et al. Management of multiple intrahepatic recurrences after radiofrequency ablation of hepatocellular carcinoma with rhenium-188-HDD lipiodol. Eur J Gastroenterol Hepatol. 2006;18(2):219-23.
56. Kumar A, Srivastava DN, Bal C. Management of postsurgical recurrence of hepatocellular carcinoma with Rhenium 188-HDD labeled iodized oil. J Vasc Interv Radiol. 2006;17(1):157-61.
57. Srivastava DN, Madhusudan KS. Oncologic Imaging. Ind J of Medical and Paediatric Oncology. 2008;29(1):65-6.
58. Srivastava DN, Sharma S, Yadav S, et al. Pedunculated hepatic haemangioma with arteriportal shunt - treated with angioembolization and surgery. Australasian Radiology. 1998;2:151-3.
59. Srivastava DN, Gandhi D, Seith A, Pande GK, Sahni P. Transcatheter arterial embolization in the treatment of symptomatic cavernous haemangioma of the liver: a prospective study. Abdominal Imaging. 2001;26:510-14.
60. Rammohan A, Sathyanesan J, Ramaswami S, Lakshmanan A, Senthil-Kumar P, Srinivasan UP, et al. Embolization of liver tumors: Past, present and future. World J Radiol. 2012;4(9):405-12.

CHAPTER 81

Imaging in Liver Transplant

Chandan Jyoti Das, Kumble S Madhusudhan, Deep Narayan Srivastava

INTRODUCTION

Liver transplantation is one of the boons in the history of medicine and has become the accepted treatment for patients with end stage liver disease with reported 1-year graft and patient survival rates of 80–95% and 5-year rates of 60–85%.[1] Unfortunately, there is inadequate availability of cadaveric liver grafts because of several limitations in organ donation, and hence transplantation of partial grafts from both living and deceased donors has become more popular in the last decade. There has been a paradigm shift in the various imaging techniques concomitant with the technical refinements in partial liver transplantation which allows precise as well as better understanding of donor and recipient anatomy prior to the transplantation.

Pretransplantation evaluation of the extent of liver disease, details of the vascular and biliary anatomy of potential recipients and donors are of paramount importance for successful liver transplantation. In this chapter, we will discuss the indications and contraindications of various types of liver transplantations, different surgical techniques and plethora of imaging modalities used for radiologic evaluation of donors as well as recipients. We also briefly discuss about imaging in various postoperative complications.

INDICATIONS AND CONTRAINDICATIONS FOR LIVER TRANSPLANTATION

The common indications for liver transplantation includes complications of cirrhosis, hepatocellular carcinoma, autoimmune hepatitis, chronic hepatitis B and C, cholestatic diseases like primary biliary cirrhosis and primary sclerosing cholangitis and metabolic diseases such as hemochromatosis and Wilson disease **(Table 1)**.[2]

Table 1: Common indications for liver transplantation.

• Cirrhosis with end stage liver disease and decompensation Hepatocellular carcinoma/hepatoblastoma
• Alchoholic liver disease
• *Hepatitis:* Autoimmune, chronic hepatitis B and C
• *Cholestatic diseases:* Primary biliary cirrhosis, primary sclerosing cholangitis
• *Metabolic diseases:* Hemochromatosis Wilson disease
• *Fulminant hepatic failure:* Viral/toxin/drug-induced

There are few absolute and relative contraindications for transplantation. The absolute contraindications include uncontrolled ongoing sepsis, active abuse of alcohol or other substance, extrahepatic malignancy, severe cardiopulmonary disease, hepatopulmonary syndrome with severe pulmonary hypertension, lack of a psychosocial support system and some variants of cholangiocarcinoma. The relative contraindications include age > 65 years, human immunodeficiency virus (HIV) infection, hepatocellular carcinoma (HCC) (not fitting in established criteria), morbid obesity and psychologic instability.

HOW TO SELECT PATIENTS?

Most of the patients have end-stage liver disease which is assessed by the model for end-stage liver disease (MELD) scoring system.[2,3] MELD is an objective way of assessing patients waiting for liver transplantation and is being used to prioritize the allocation of livers for transplantation. This scoring system, based on the patient's bilirubin, international normalized ratio (INR), and creatinine, was initially created to predict the 3-month mortality for patients with non HCC end-stage liver disease (ESLD) undergoing a Transjugular Intrahepatic Portosystemic Shunt (TIPS) procedure.[2,4] MELD scores range from 6 to 40, with 6 indicating the least sick patients and 40 indicating the sickest patients. It is generally thought that for liver transplantation wait-listing the patient should have at least 15 MELD points. Conversely it may be futile to contemplate transplantation for patients with MELD values closer to 40.

HEPATOCELLULAR CARCINOMA

Among patients with hepatocellular carcinoma (HCC), to be eligible for transplantation, the tumor must be grade 1 or grade 2, be solitary <5 cm, or may have up to 3 nodules with each < 3 cm, and there must be no extrahepatic metastases or evidence of macrovascular invasion. This is according to the Milan criteria which is accepted by most National deceased donor based transplant programs the world over.[5]

In the tumor, node, metastasis (TNM) staging system, T1 tumors may be any size as long as they do not extend into blood vessels. T2 tumors may be any size if they do extend into the blood vessels; they may also be classified as T2 if there are more than one and they are smaller than 5 cm. Tumors are characterized as T3 if larger than 5 cm. T4 tumors extend beyond the liver, except for the gallbladder. Transplant priority should be given to stage T2 disease because patients with T1 disease have high survival rates without transplantation, and those with T3 disease have a high rate of recurrence.[5]

Milan criteria is used for assessing transplant eligibility for small HCCs. According to Milan criteria, to be eligible for liver transplantation, patients with HCC should have a single tumor that is smaller than 5 cm or three or fewer tumors that are 3 cm or smaller. Similarly, the University of California San Francisco (UCSF) criteria is used for liver transplantation in patients with large tumors, i.e. they have a single tumor that is 6.5 cm or smaller or if three or fewer tumor nodules are present, with the largest being 4.5 cm or smaller. Recently, a cut off tumor volume of 115 cm^3 has been used for selecting candidates for transplantation showing enhanced accuracy of pretransplantation imaging.[6] Factors with high potential for recurrence after living donor liver transplantation (LDLT) include: a tumor larger than 6 cm, multiple nodules >3, disease that progresses after pretransplantation treatment, gross vascular invasion, and a tumor that is exposed to the liver surface.[7]

TYPES OF LIVER TRANSPLANTATION

Currently, there are 3 types of liver transplantation being performed: whole-liver cadaveric transplant, split-liver cadaveric transplant, and living donor liver transplant. Worldwide, the cadaveric or deceased donor liver transplantation (DDLT) is the most common type. It is also the most technically straightforward form of liver transplantation and has the advantages of full sized donor liver.

LIVING DONOR LIVER TRANSPLANTATION

Living donor liver transplant (LDLT) account for approximately 4.0% of the liver transplants performed in the last 10 years but accounts for more than 85% of the transplants being performed in our country. The advantages of LDLT include the elective nature of the procedure, good quality organ and lack of preservation injuries of the organ. The main disadvantage of this technique is the risk related to the healthy donor with a mortality risk of 0.15% to 0.20%, and postoperative complication rate of 20–40%. The residual donor liver must be more than 30% of the total donor hepatic volume to ensure adequate postoperative liver function, and the graft-to-recipient body weight ratio (GRWR) should be greater than 0.8 to minimize the risk of 'small-for-size' syndrome in the recipient.[8]

For an adult recipient, either a full-right or full-left hepatic graft (small adults < 50 kg) can be used. In the donor right hepatectomy, the liver is split on the right of the middle hepatic vein (MHV), close to Cantlie's line that connects the left border of the suprahepatic inferior vena cava (IVC) to the midpoint of the gallbladder fossa. Generally the MHV remains with the donor when the right side of the liver is harvested whereas it is harvested when left donor hepatectomy is performed.[9] Hence, variations in anatomy of the MHV are critical to the success of this operation and needs to be conveyed to the transplant surgeon beforehand. Left donor hepatectomy involves harvesting the MHV en-bloc to obtain an adequate sized-graft with good venous outflow as congestion of the paramedian segment (segment IV) in the recipient is avoided. As the right hepatic vein is dominant in most patients and caudate lobe usually remains in the donor, congestion of the remnant donor liver after removal of the MHV along with the left hemi liver usually is not clinically significant. The recipient left hepatic vein (LHV) and MHV can be enlarged and then anastomosed to the enlarged graft MHV-LHV confluence to provide unimpeded venous outflow to the graft after implantation. Left lateral segmentectomy (segments 2 and 3 with or without the caudate lobe) are suitable for children and smaller recipients (20–30 kg).[9,10]

Split-Liver Cadaveric Transplant is the least common type in which a single cadaveric liver is anatomically divided and transplanted into 2 recipients (usually one adult and 1 child).[10,11] The right lobe is given to an adult recipient whereas the left lateral segment is given to a child. Although this helps mitigate the shortage of deceased donor livers available, there are technical difficulties related to sharing of blood vessels/bile duct and a higher risk of complications in the adult recipient (bile leaks, cut surface bleeding, segment 4 necrosis). The most common cadaveric splitting technique involves a transection plane 1 cm to the right of the falciform ligament, resulting in a right extended graft (segments I and IV–VIII) used in adults, and a left lateral graft (segments II–III) for a pediatric recipient who are not larger than 30 kg. The common bile duct, main portal vein and inferior vena cava (IVC) are included in the right liver graft, and the main arterial trunk is part of the left liver graft. The biliary reconstruction of the left lateral graft usually entails a hepaticojejunostomy in the pediatric recipient.[10,11]

PREOPERATIVE IMAGING MODALITIES

Multidetector computed tomography (MDCT) and MRI are the workhorses of pretransplant imaging and has been used as complementary to each other in the evaluation of donor and recipient.

Multidetector Computed Tomography

Multidetector computed tomography (MDCT) is frequently used to evaluate the donor and recipient arterial as well as venous anatomy using intravenous contrast in the form of CT angiography (CTA). Donor liver fat content is also evaluated by unenhanced scan (by calculating the Hepatic attenuation index). Dual energy CT (DECT) scan has been increasingly used as virtual noncontrast image can be reconstructed from the set of enhanced images thus obviating the need of a true unenhanced scan reducing the dose of radiation. MDCT/CTA generates a huge amount of dataset which require dedicated postprocessing by vendor specific software for optimal evaluation of the anatomy—the hepatic arteries on three-dimensional or axial MIPs, the hepatic veins on axial MIPs, portal veins on coronal MIPs and volume renderings of the hepatic parenchyma. All these can be superimposed on one another for further delineation of the anatomy for the surgeons. MDCT should be judiciously used to reduce the radiation dose as donors are often young and healthy.

MR Imaging

MR imaging (MRI) coupled with magnetic resonance cholangiopancreatography (MRCP) is primarily performed to evaluate the biliary system. Hepatobiliary contrast agents such as Gd-BOPTA (Multihance, Bracco Diagnostics, NJ) can be used. The biliary tree is better seen on 3-dimensional heavily T2-weighted or 3-dimensional T1-weighted, postcontrast coronal oblique images. MRI can also be used to evaluate the hepatic parenchyma for characterizing incidental focal lesions and the degree of fatty infiltration.

Preoperative Imaging Evaluation

Recipient Evaluation

Imaging of the recipient liver should be performed as close to the time of transplantation as possible because tumors may grow rapidly, invade local structures, or metastasize, which may affect the stage of disease, management perspective, and surgical technique. Candidate eligibility is determined by the patient's MELD score to allow for candidate list prioritization based upon medical need. Imaging plays a pivotal role in the care of patients with HCC.[2] Imaging of the recipient consist of detailed evaluation and description of the arterial, portal venous and hepatic venous anatomy and the extent of tumor burden in HCC patients awaiting transplant.

For patients with liver lesions, the Organ Procurement and Transplantation Network (OPTN) or Liver Imaging Reporting and Data System (LI-RADS) criteria are used to characterize liver lesions as benign, suspicious for HCC, or definitely HCC.[12,13] The intrinsic signal intensity of the mass, enhancement and washout pattern, capsule appearance, and nodule architecture are frequently used to determine the likelihood that a nodule is HCC. Once the liver nodules are characterized, the Milan/UCSF criteria are used to determine transplant candidacy. Patients with HCC whose tumors are growing at a significant rate or who are expected to wait more than 6 months on the transplant list may be offered locoregional therapy, a practice known as "bridging to transplant". Occasionally. Some programs use down staging locoregional therapy for cases where the HCC lesions were beyond the standard listing criteria, provided there is no evidence of extrahepatic disease or macrovascular tumor invasion. In such patients there is a need for a 3-month waiting period post down-staging therapy (usually TACE/RFA) and re-imaging to see whether they fit the listing criteria before being considered for LT. This is accomplished by alcohol injection, thermal ablation (including radiofrequency and microwave ablation), transarterial radioembolization (TARE), and most commonly transarterial chemoembolization (TACE).[14] The choice of therapy is based on Barcelona Clinic Liver Cancer Staging (BCLC) Criteria, which take into account the number and size of HCC nodules, the patient's Child-Pugh score, and the patient's Eastern Cooperative Oncology Group (ECOG) performance status.[15] All the focal lesions should be described segment wise along with its relation with major vascular structures, the gallbladder, and central bile ducts because the outcome may be affected. If MDCT is indeterminate for a lesion characterization, contrast-enhanced MRI imaging should be performed to further characterize the lesion. It is also critical to perform CT chest and abdomen to exclude extrahepatic malignancy or spread.

Preoperative Imaging of the Living Donor Liver Transplantation Donor

Accurate preoperative depiction of donor anatomy is essential to determine the suitability of the donor so that hepatectomy may safely be performed without any risk to the donor and at the same time avoiding "small-for-size" syndrome in the recipient. This syndrome is characterised by poor bile production, delayed synthetic function, prolonged cholestasis, and intractable ascites and deranged coagulation which leads to septic complications and high mortality. To avoid small-for-size syndrome, the residual liver volume should exceed 30–35% of the total donor liver volume and the GRWR should be > 0.8 w.r.t the recipient.[16] Preoperative imaging of the living donor liver transplantation (LDLT) donor involves assessment of various features such as vascular and biliary anatomy for relevant variants, MHV anatomy, the hepatic parenchyma for degree of fatty infiltration, iron content, and focal hepatic lesions and last but not the least, calculation of liver volumes. Minor variations of anatomy can be tackled with advanced vascular surgical techniques.

In a study by Tsang et al. the various causes of donor unsuitability were recipient issues such as inadequate remnant volume (57.4%); steatosis (27.7%); a small-for-size graft (8.9%); and variations of biliary system (5%) hepatic artery (4%) and portal vein (1%) anatomy.[16]

Among the various imaging techniques, MDCT angiography is faster and more cost-effective than MR angiography and is used more often. Two-dimensional or three-dimensional reformations from MDCT in both arterial and portal venous phases provide the best methods of analysis. The MDCT protocol for liver donors vary with institutions. The protocol followed at our institution includes unenhanced CT followed by multiphase contrast-enhanced CT. In the unenhanced CT protocol, four 10 mm sections are obtained first followed by arterial and portal venous phase contrastenhanced CT. The details are given in **Table 2**.

Vascular Anatomy

Preoperative imaging of the hepatic artery, portal and hepatic veins involves identification of the vessels **(Figs. 1A to C)** and their variations and measuring the diameter at the site of the proposed anastomosis, since anastomosis of similar size decreases the risk of thrombosis or stenosis.

Hepatic Arteries

Normal hepatic arterial anatomy (Michel Type I) consisting of common hepatic artery arising from celiac axis and dividing into right and left hepatic artery is found in only 55% of the population.[17] Replaced right hepatic artery (RHA) from superior mesenteric artery (11%) and replaced left hepatic artery (LHA) from left gastric artery (10%) are other common variations.[17] The terms "aberrant" or "replaced" are used when the variant arteries substitute the normal artery whereas the variant artery that persists in addition to the normal one is termed "accessory." The most common arterial variant is an accessory right or left hepatic artery. As few of these variants are surgically relevant, hence variants should be mentioned in the report. A replaced or accessory RHA will affect right LDLT

Table 2: MDCT protocol for LDLT donor evaluation.

Phases	*Iodinated contrast material*	*Delay*	*kVp*
Unenhanced CT	—	—	120 kVp
Arterial phase	80–100 mL of with a concentration of 370 mg/mL @ 4–5 mL per second	30 Sec	100–120 kVp
Portal venous phase	80–100 mL of with a concentration of 370 mg/mL @ 4–5 mL per second	60–70 Sec	120 kVp

Abbreviations: MDCT: Multidetector computed tomography; LDLT: Living donor liver transplantation; CT: Computed tomography

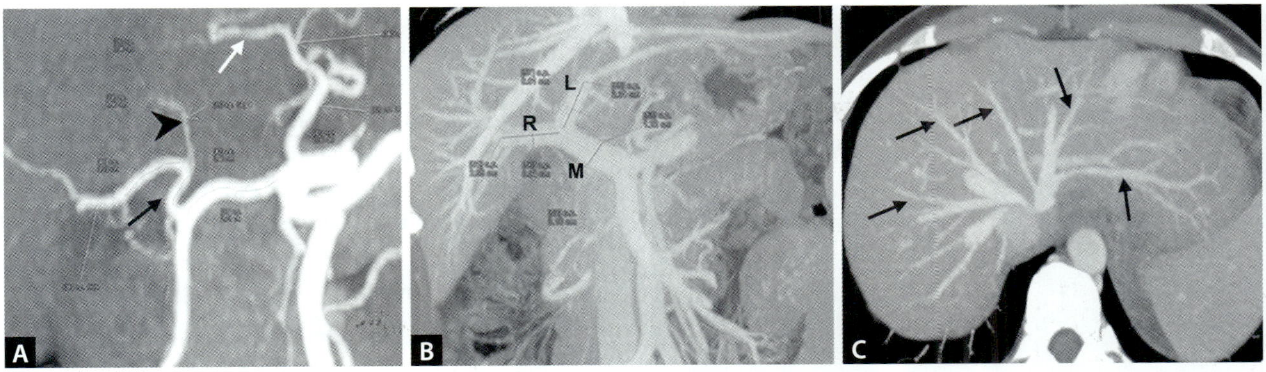

Figs. 1A to C: Preoperative work-up of liver donor: (A) CT scan in arterial phase showing right hepatic artery (black arrow) from celiac trunk and left hepatic artery (white arrow) from left gastric artery. Segment 4 branch (arrowhead) or middle hepatic artery is also seen. Caliber and length of the hepatic arteries should be measured. (B) Venous phase images showing densely opacified portal vein (M) with measurements of caliber and length of main as well as right (R) and left (L) branches. (C) Venous phase showing opacified hepatic veins and their tributaries (arrows) (segments 5 and 8 being important).

whereas a replaced or accessory LHA will affect full left or left lateral segment LDLT. Similarly, presence of middle hepatic artery (MHA) will affect both right as well as left LDLT. Diameter of RHA or LHA is also important as <2 mm diameter makes the future arterial anastomoses prone to thrombosis and microvascular techniques are often required.

Hepatic Veins

Hepatic venous variants are seen in 16–33% of the population and if not dealt with intraoperatively, these can lead to hepatic insufficiency in the donor or recipient if drainage to a liver segment is compromised.[18] Identification of the exact location and variation of the MHV is paramount for guiding surgical planning because the hepatectomy plane—which, in living donors, is to the right of the MHV along the gallbladder fossa—may be affected.[19] MDCT is frequently used to evaluate hepatic veins **(Fig. 2)**. The usual position of the MHV is between segments VIII and IV. The drainage of segment IVa and IVb should also be mentioned. It is important to determine if an accessory inferior right hepatic vein (RHV) as it is the most common venous variant. If there is accessory RHV(s) draining VI, VII and V, a separate anastomosis is needed to preserve drainage of these segments during a right LDLT. Similarly, the right lobe anterior sector segmental veins (V5 and V8) draining into MHV, need to be separately anastomosed to the recipient suprahepatic IVC to preserve drainage of these segments during right LDLT. This is especially needed when the right lobe graft is harvested without the MHV. When the right lobe graft is harvested with the MHV, in a MHV predominant system, care has to be taken to preserve the V4a tributary and terminal part of the MHV in the donor remnant liver.

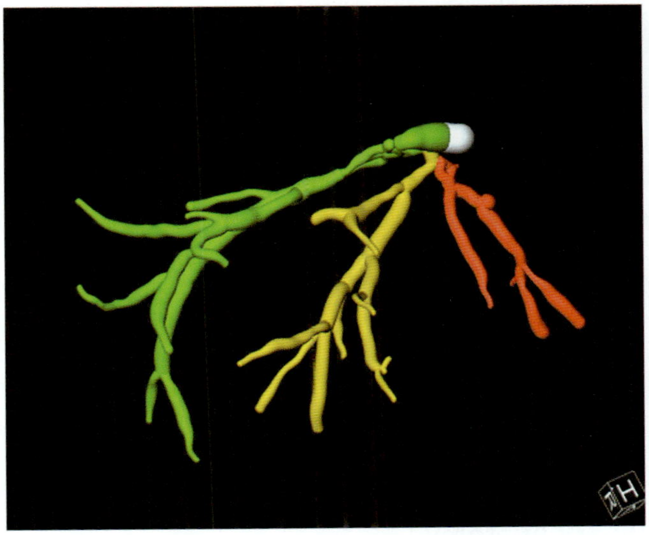

Fig. 2: Three-dimensional model of hepatic venous anatomy.

The most common venous variant is an accessory right inferior hepatic vein (RHV) and if its caliber is 5 mm or more, then a separate anastomosis to the IVC is performed to prevent hepatic congestion. The distance in the coronal plane between the accessory inferior RHV and the right hepatic vein is crucial for the surgeon while planning the graft implantation.[20]

Portal Veins

Portal venous anatomic variants are less common, although a few surgically relevant variations exist. 3D CT images can help to find out the variation easily **(Fig. 3)**.

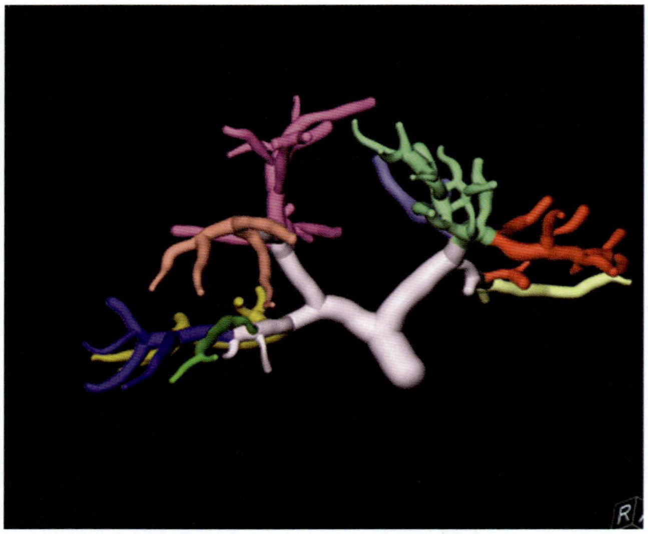

Fig. 3: Three-dimensional model of portal venous anatomy.

Few critical findings that can affect the transplant include left branch of portal vein (LPV) from right anterior branch of PV (RAPV) (affects Right LDLT, may be relative contraindication to donation) RAPV from LPV (affects left LDLT, may be relative contraindication to donation) and trifurcation into right posterior branch of PV (RPPV), RAPV, and LPV (affects both right and left LDLT; Right LDLT: must clamp and anastomose these separately; Left LDLT: RAPV from graft must be excluded).[21] There has been described association between portal venous and biliary system variants. Hence, if portal venous variants are identified, these should be examined closely to preclude associated biliary tree variations.[21]

Biliary Anatomy

A biliary anastomosis is usually between the donor common bile duct (CBD) and the recipient common hepatic duct (CHD) in a DDLT. Biliary variations are common seen in up to 33% of the population and if not identified preoperatively may result in biliary leaks and strictures leading to substantial morbidity or mortality in the donor and recipient in the postoperative period.[5] Biliary complications are the most common cause for morbidity after split and LDLT, occurring in up to 40% of patients.[21] Magnetic resonance cholangiopancreatography (MRCP) is useful for a detailed understanding of the biliary anatomy to prevent these types of complications.[22] Variations like right posterior hepatic duct (RPHD) or right anterior hepatic duct (RAHD) draining into left hepatic duct (LHD) are contraindication to left lobe donation whereas LHD draining into RAHD or RPHD are contraindication to right lobe donation. In order to prevent biliary complications and to be sure of the hilar ductal configuration during LDLT fluoroscopy-based intraoperative cholangiography (IOC) is essential before proceeding with the donor hepatectomy. IOC is repeated after graft removal to ensure there is no biliary leak and confirm that the calibre of the remnant ductal system is adequate.[22]

Liver Parenchyma

The final step of preoperative donor imaging is evaluation of the hepatic parenchyma to identify focal or diffuse liver disease (particularly steatosis), any incidental benign or malignant conditions that may preclude segmental donation and measurement of liver volumes **(Fig. 4)**.

Hepatic steatosis >30% precludes donation. NCCT findings consistent with this degree of steatosis include: hepatic density more than 10 HU lower than the spleen, hepatic density <40 HU and a hepatic-to-splenic density ratio of <0.8 **(Figs. 5A and B)**.[23] In MRI this degree of steatosis corresponds to 30% signal dropout on Dixon-type chemical shift imaging, with liver parenchymal signal drop-out normalized to the spleen. MR spectroscopy is considered to be better for estimating hepatic steatosis.

Finally, integrated software may be used to calculate the volume of the entire liver, the potential residual volume in the donor, and the potential volume in the recipient by performing virtual hepatectomy **(Figs. 6A to C)** from the MDCT data set. All the processed images of vascular tree, biliary system and liver parenchyma can be superimposed into a single presurgical liver model which can help as a guide map during surgery.

POSTOPERATIVE EVALUATION

Imaging of Post-transplant Complications

Multiple complications can be observed after liver transplantation. LDLT grafts recipient experience a higher rate of complications postoperatively as compared to recipients of whole-liver grafts. The role of imaging is to detect transplant related complication as well as to exclude other complications that can clinically mimic acute rejection. Postoperative evaluation starts USG plus Doppler daily for first week and twice weekly for next 2 weeks. Assessment of hepatic vein **(Figs. 7A to C)**, hepatic artery **(Figs. 8A and B)**, IVC and portal vein are performed along with their various flow parameters. Any abnormality in USG/Doppler—further evaluation with CT/MRCP which are complementary to US and is reserved as a problem solving modality. An understanding of the strengths and weaknesses of each

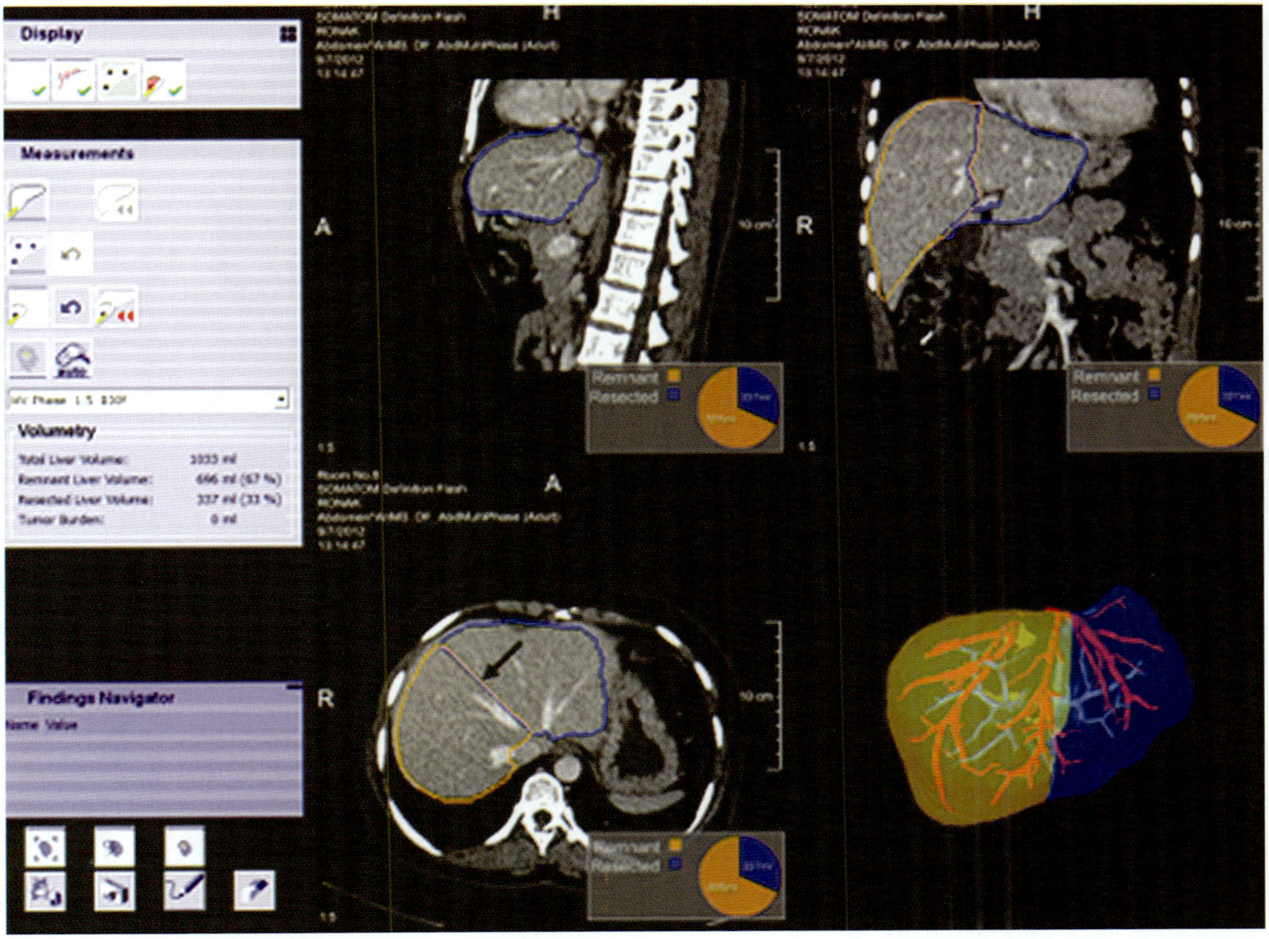

Fig. 4: Liver volumetry showing assessment of total liver volume using vendor specific software and generation of 3D model of liver. Note assessment of residual as well as donor liver volume separately by the software with line of division along the lateral margin of MHV (black arrow).

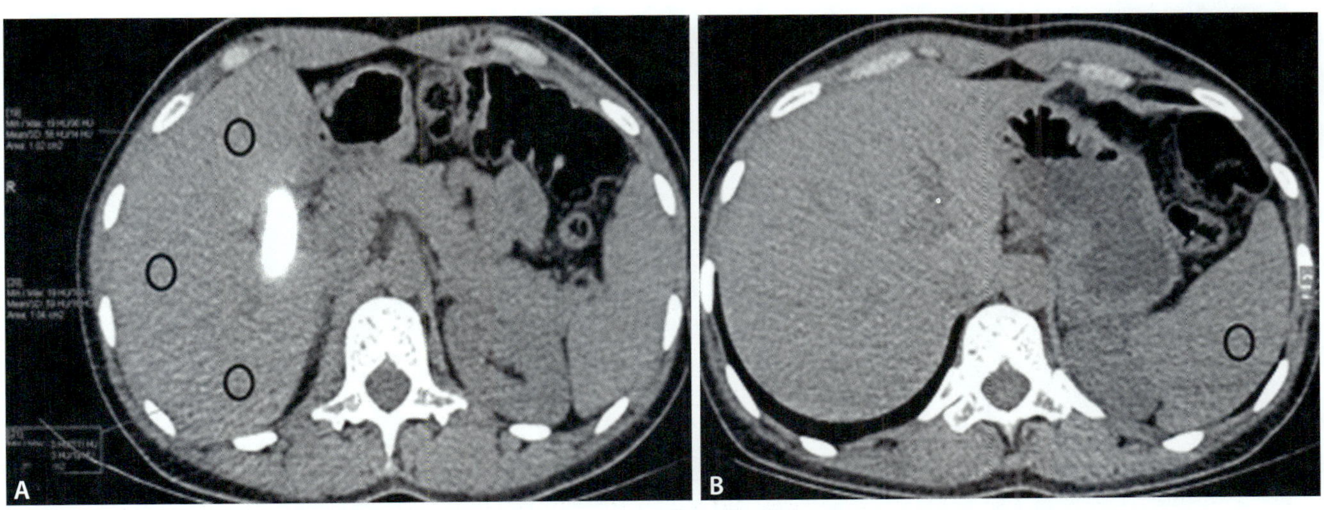

Figs. 5A and B: Liver attenuation index (LAI): Regions of interest (ROI) drawn on liver (25 ROI) and splenic (3 ROI) parenchyma avoiding vessels.

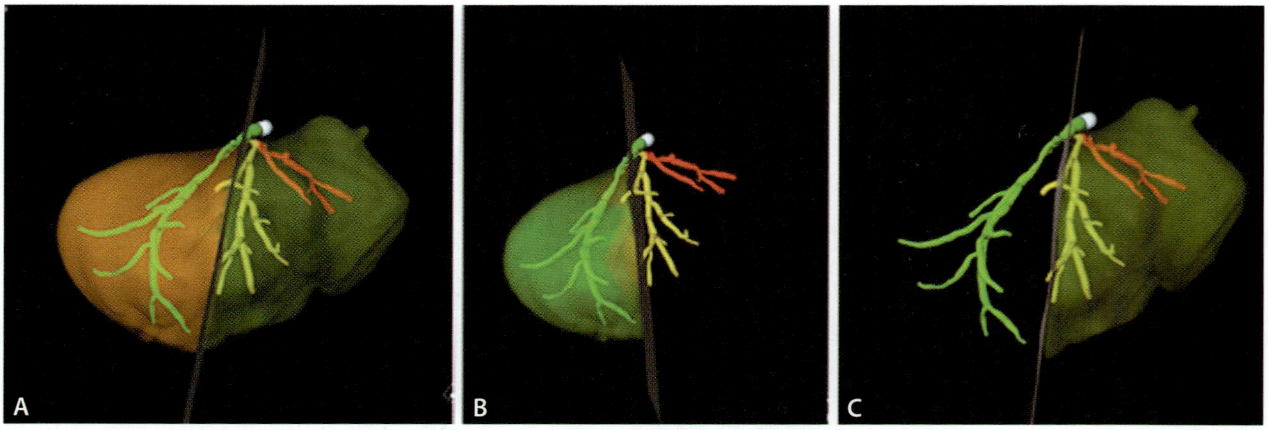

Figs. 6A to C: Virtual hepatectomy: Three-dimensional reconstructed CT images of the entire donor liver (A) showing the plane of hepatectomy which passes to the right of the middle hepatic vein, through segment VIII. The potential residual donor liver (B) and the donor segment (C) is also shown.

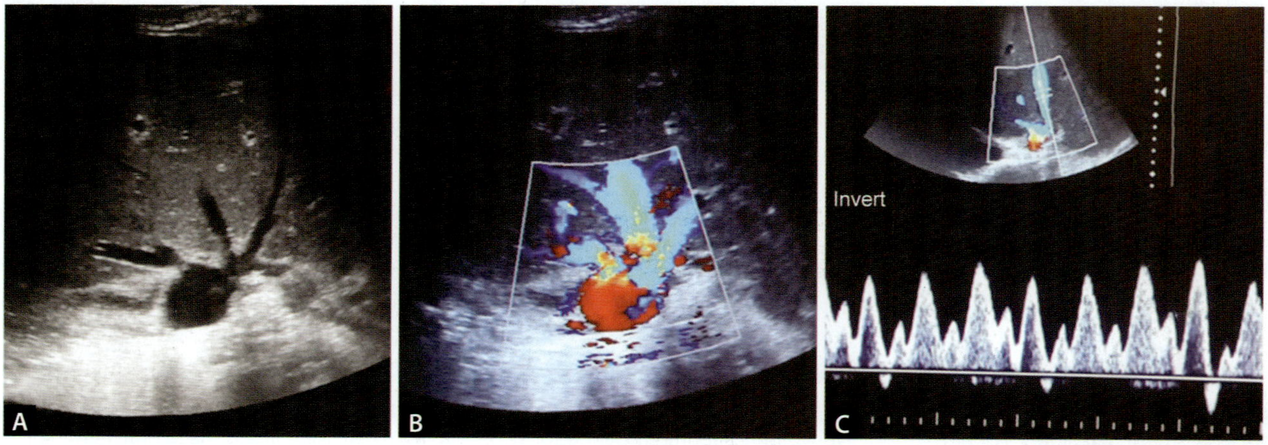

Figs. 7A to C: Postoperative ultrasonography: Hepatic veins. Grayscale (A), color flow (B) and Doppler trace (C) images show normal and patent hepatic veins and inferior vena cava.

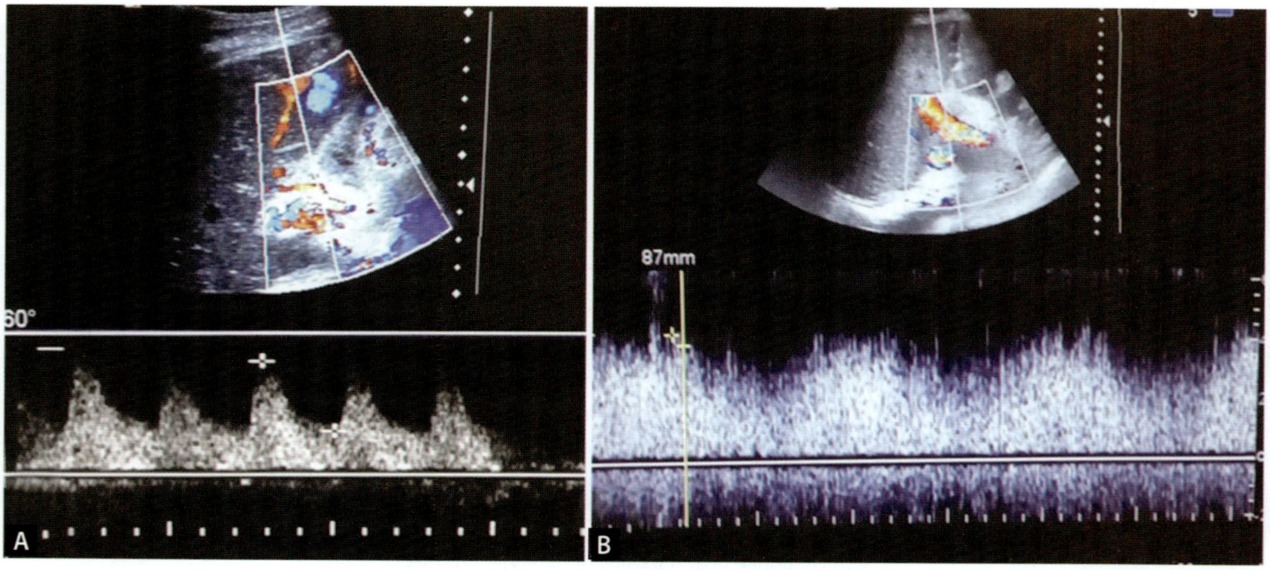

Figs. 8A and B: Postoperative ultrasonography: (A) Color Doppler image shows normal hepatic artery with low resistance flow. (B) Color Doppler image shows normal portal vein with undulating spectral waveform.

imaging modality will aid in early diagnosis and treatment. Knowledge of the location of various anastomosis is important because stenosis usually occurs in the anastomotic site.

Hepatic artery: Hepatic artery complications include thrombosis **(Figs. 9 and 10)**, stenosis, and pseudoaneurysm.[24] Hepatic artery thrombosis (HAT) and stenosis can lead to biliary ischemia leading to a nonanastomotic biliary stricture or a biloma. In orthotopic liver transplantation, the donor celiac axis is anastomosed to the recipient hepatic artery at either the bifurcation into left and right hepatic arteries or the origin of the gastroduodenal artery. In order to pre-empt and pick up HAT in the early post-transplant period (1st week post-transplant) serial Doppler sonographic evaluations are mandatory. In the event of any ambiguity, arterial patency has to be confirmed by CT angiography when required. The radiologist has a crucial role to play in the diagnosis as treatment usually consists of emergent thrombectomy or retransplantation.[25]

Portal venous: Portal vein complications include thrombosis and stricture **(Figs. 11A and B)** at anastomotic site.[26] In orthotopic liver transplantation, portal vein anastomosis is most often end to end between the donor and recipient portal veins. Complications may occur due to faulty surgical technique, discrepancy between

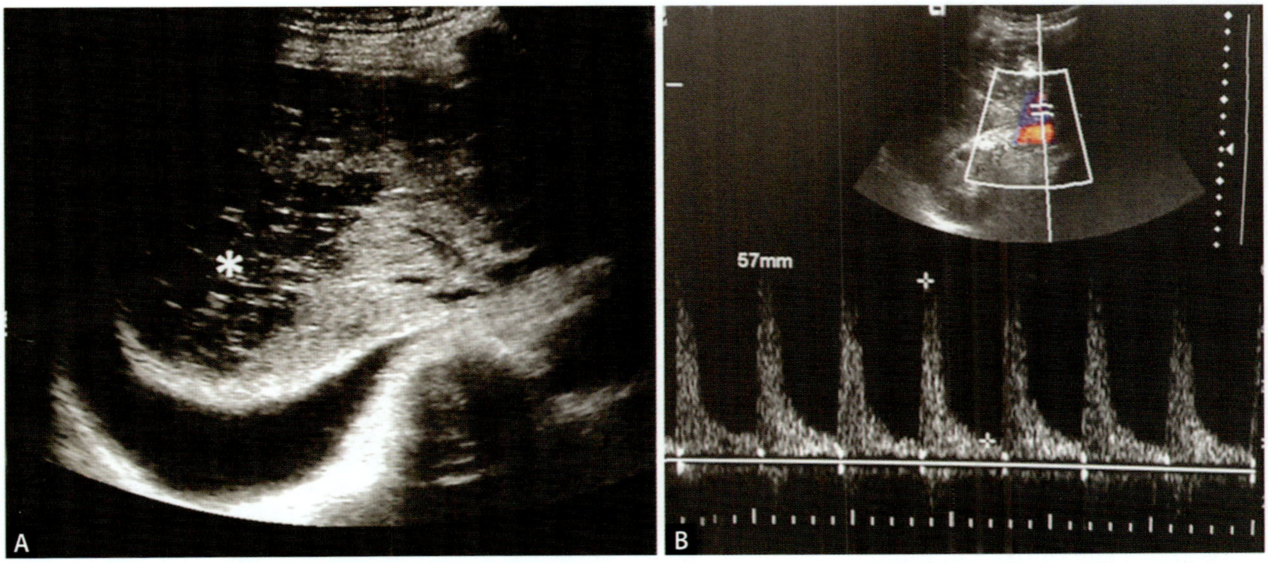

Figs. 9A and B: Hepatic artery thrombosis: Postoperative day 2 of a patient after cadaveric liver transplantation. (A) Grayscale ultrasonography shows a wedge-shaped hypoechoic area (asterisk) suggestive of infarct. (B) Color Doppler image at porta shows high resistance flow in hepatic artery proximal to the thrombosis.

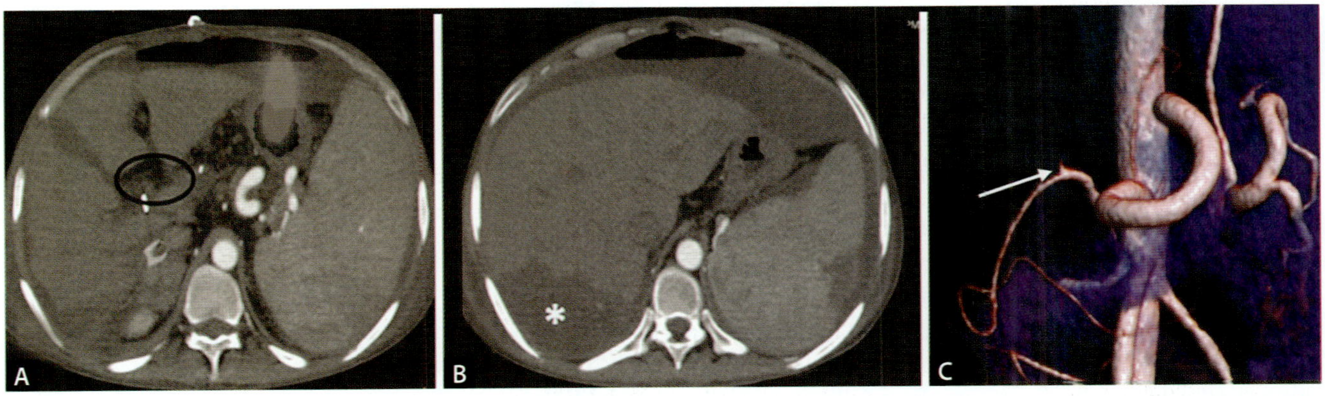

Figs. 10A to C: Hepatic artery thrombosis: CT angiography images show nonvisualization of hepatic artery at porta (ellipse in A) with hypodense area in right posterior segments suggesting infarct (asterisk in B). Volume-rendered image (C) shows abrupt cut-off of the hepatic artery with a small stump (arrow).

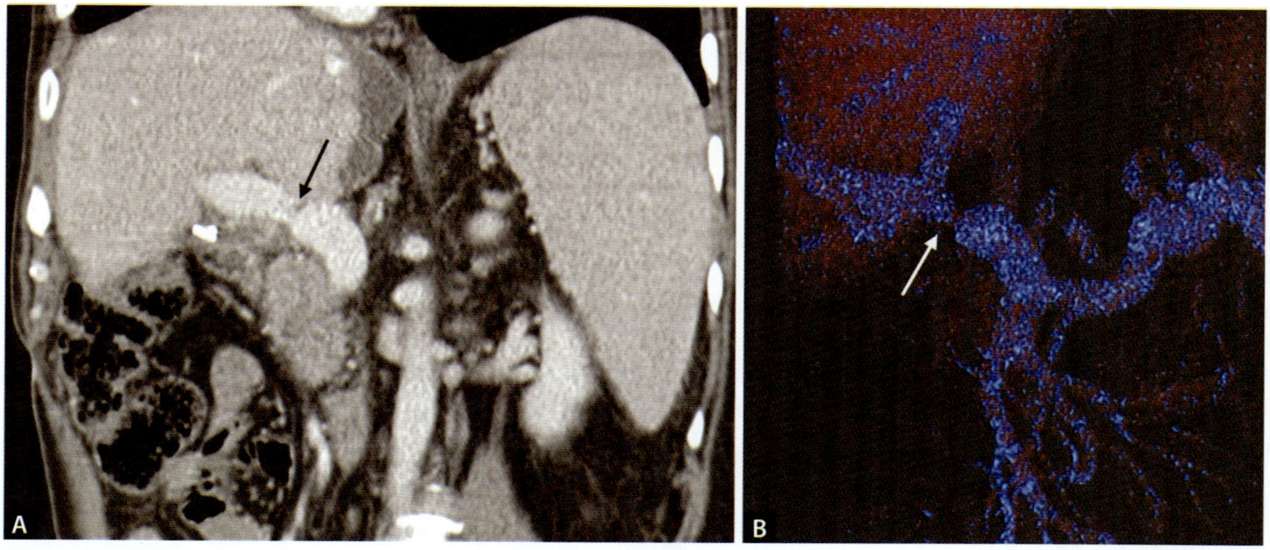

Figs. 11A and B: PV narrowing: Coronal (A) and volume rendered (B) contrast-enhanced CT images show short segment portal vein stenosis (arrow) with dilated splenic vein and splenomegaly, suggesting portal hypertension.

the calibres of the donor and recipient portal veins, hypercoagulable state, and history of previous thrombosis.

HV and IVC: Complications include IVC stenosis and thrombosis and hepatic vein stenosis.[27] Anastomosis of the donor and recipient IVCs can be end to end, with resection of the recipient retrohepatic IVC and anastomosis of the donor IVC superiorly and inferiorly to the recipient IVC. With living donor liver transplantation, the donor hepatic vein is anastomosed to the recipient IVC.[27] Strictures/kinking can occur in these levels of anastomosis and can affect the graft venous outflow.

Biliary tree: The most common types of biliary complications are bile duct stricture and bile leak causing biloma.[28] Other complications include bile duct obstruction, stone formation, biliary necrosis, and cholangitis. Biliary complications are more common with right-lobe liver donor transplantation. Scintigraphy is commonly used for the detection of bile leak whereas MRCP is very useful for bile duct obstruction. US has a lower sensitivity for detecting biliary complications.[29] Knowledge of the anastomotic site is important because stenosis may occur at this site **(Fig. 12)**. Non anastomotic strictures can occur in patients who have faced delayed graft hepatic artery stenosis or thrombosis and in whom immediate attempts at revascularization have failed. Biliary problems related to ischemic cholangiopathy are also more commonly observed in marginal deceased donor grafts especially from donations following cardiac death. The most common form of deceased donation in our country is donation after brain death (DBD).

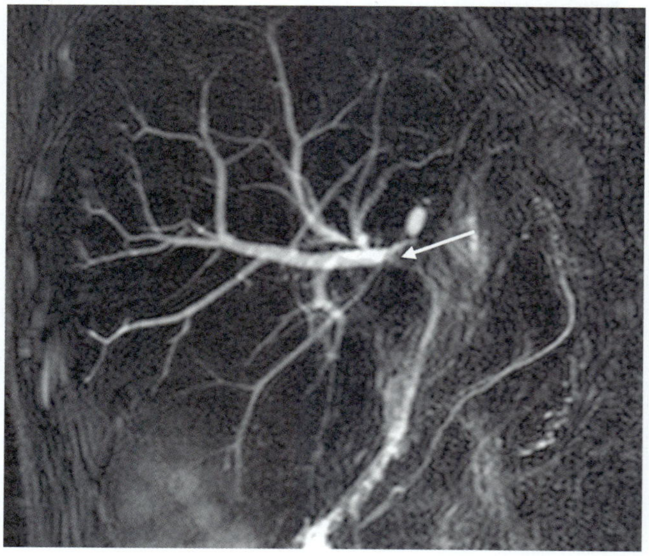

Fig. 12: Biliary stricture: MRCP in patient after right lobe liver donor liver transplantation showing short segment narrowing of bile duct (arrow) at the site of anastomosis with mild intrahepatic biliary radicle dilatation

Other complications include hematoma, abscess, infection, recurrent hepatitis, splenic infarct, recurrent malignancy, and post-transplantation lymphoproliferative disorder. Imaging also has an important role to play in their management.[30]

CONCLUSION

Preoperative imaging in potential liver transplant donor and recipient with CT and MRI is important for candidate selection and for preoperative evaluation of the liver parenchyma, vascular and biliary anatomy in the setting of LDLT. Multiphase liver CT is the modality of choice for pre-transplantation assessment of living donors and recipients whereas MRCP is commonly used for evaluation of biliary tree. Understanding the indications for transplantations and the common surgical techniques are important for a thorough assessment and can help the radiologist to craft a succinct and meaningful report **(Table 3)** which needs to be conveyed to the transplant surgeon. This report with the sets of reconstructed images and 3D model helps the surgeon perform liver transplant in a safe manner thus avoiding post-transplant complications. Imaging is also useful for the detection of various post-operative complications and long-term follow-up for transplant viability.[31]

Table 3: Checklist for living donor MDCT reporting.

Liver size (craniocaudal) • Any evidence of acute or chronic liver disease • Any focal lesions: Yes/No (If yes, describe the number, size, segment and nature of the lesions) • Any biliary obstruction or IHBD
Liver fat estimation (on unenhanced or VNC images): • Mean liver attenuation (in HU) • Mean splenic attenuation (in HU) • Liver attenuation Index (in HU) • Do the intrahepatic vessels appear hypoattenuated compared to the liver parenchyma: Yes/ No
Liver volume analysis: • Total liver volume (in cc) • Graft volume (in cc) • Donor remnant liver volume (in cc) • Donor remnant liver volume (in percentage of total liver volume)

Hepatic arterial anatomy:
• *Right hepatic artery (RHA)*:
  – Vessel of origin
  – Diameter at origin (in mm)
  – Length before first sectional division (in cm)
  – *Any vascular thrombus*: Yes/No (If yes, mention the degree of occlusion)
• *Left hepatic artery (LHA)*:
  – Vessel of origin
  – Diameter at origin (in mm)
  – Length before first sectional division (in cm)
  – *Any vascular thrombus*: Yes/No (If yes, mention the degree of occlusion)
• *Segment IV artery origin*: RHA/LHA/others (mention)
• *Any variant vascular anatomy*: Yes/No (If yes, specify according to Michael classification)
• *Accessory RHA/ LHA/ segmental artery (if any)*:
  – Vessel of origin
  – Diameter at origin (in mm)
  – Length before first division (in cm)

Portal venous anatomy:
• *Main portal vein (MPV)*:
  – Length before first division (in cm)
  – *Any evidence of portal hypertension*: Yes/ No
  – *Any thrombus*: Yes/No. If yes, mention the extent (length and degree of luminal compromise), duration (acute versus chronic), nature (bland vs. malignant) and presence of collaterals.
• *Right portal vein (RPV)*:
  – Length before first sectional division (in cm)
  – Diameter at origin (in mm)
  – *Any thrombus*: Yes/No
• *Left portal vein (LPV)*:
  – Length before first sectional division (in cm)
  – Diameter at origin (in mm)
  – *Any thrombus*: Yes/No
• *Any variant vascular anatomy*: Yes/No. If yes, specify according to Nakamura classification. If type C, mention the distance between the ostium of the right anterior and posterior sectional portal veins (in cm).
• Accessory RPV/LPV (if any)

Contd...

Contd...

Hepatic venous anatomy: • Diameters at IVC ostium in mm – Right hepatic vein (RHV) – Common middle hepatic vein (MHV) and left hepatic vein (LHV) stump (mention otherwise if separate) • *Any major (> 4 mm) segment V/ VIII tributaries into MHV*: Yes/ No. If yes, mention the number. • *Any major segment VI/VII drainage into segment V/VIII veins or MHV*: Yes/ No. If yes, describe. • *Any accessory inferior RHV*: Yes/ No. If yes, specify the number of veins and the vertical distance between these veins and the RHV in cm. • *Any thrombosis of IVC*: Yes/ No. If yes, mention the site, extent and nature.
Other abdominal organs: Normal/ abnormal. If abnormal, specify.
Ascites or lymphadenopathy: Yes/ No
Visualized lung bases and bone: Normal/abnormal. If abnormal, specify.

ACKNOWLEDGMENTS

Authors sincerely acknowledge Dr Peush Sahni, Dr Sujoy Pal and Dr Nihar Ranjan Dash from Department of Gastrointestinal Surgery, All India Institute of Medical Sciences (AIIMS), New Delhi, India.

REFERENCES

1. Ioannou GN. Development and validation of a model predicting graft survival after liver transplantation. Liver Transpl. 2006;12(11):1594-606.
2. United Network for Organ Sharing. National Data Report. *http://www.unos.org/*. Accessed September 23, 2016.
3. Koffron A, Stein JA. Liver transplantation: indications, pretransplant evaluation, surgery, and post-transplant complications. Med Clin North Am. 2008;92(4):861-88, ix.
4. Kamath PS, Wiesner RH, Malinchoc M, et al. A model to predict survival in patients with end-stage liver disease. Hepatology. 2001;33(2):464-70.
5. Singh AK, Cronin CG, Verma HA, Boland GW, Saini S, Mueller PR, Sahani DV. Imaging of preoperative liver transplantation in adults: what radiologists should know. Radiographics. 2011;31(4):1017-30.
6. Toso C, Trotter J, Wei A, et al. Total tumor volume predicts risk of recurrence following liver transplantation in patients with hepatocellular carcinoma. Liver Transpl. 2008;14(8):1107-15.
7. Woo HY, Jang JW, Choi JY, et al. Living donor liver transplantation in hepatocellular carcinoma beyond the Milan criteria. Liver Int. 2008;28(8):1120-8.
8. Marelli L, Grasso A, Pleguezuelo M, et al. Tumour size and differentiation in predicting recurrence of hepatocellular carcinoma after liver transplantation: external validation of a new prognostic score. Ann Surg Oncol. 2008;15(12):3503-11.
9. Woo HY, Jang JW, Choi JY, et al. Living donor liver transplantation in hepatocellular carcinoma beyond the Milan criteria. Liver Int. 2008;28(8):1120-8.
10. Tanaka K, Yamada T. Living donor liver transplantation in Japan and Kyoto University: what can we learn? J Hepatol. 2005;42(1):25-8.
11. Foster R, Zimmerman M, Trotter JF. Expanding donor options: marginal, living, and split donors. Clin Liver Dis. 2007;11(2):417-29.
12. Broering DC, Wilms C, Lenk C, et al. Technical refinements and results in full-right full-left splitting of the deceased donor liver. Ann Surg. 2005;242(6):802-12; discussion 812-3.
13. Rosenkrantz AB, Campbell N, Wehrli N, et al. New OPTN/UNOS classification system for nodules in cirrhotic livers detected with MR Imaging: Effect on hepatocellular carcinoma detection and transplant allocation. Radiology. 2015;274(2):426-33.
14. Liver imaging reporting and data system. Available at: *http://www.acr.org/quality-safety/resources/LIRADS*. Accessed May 24, 2016.
15. Prasad MA, Kulik LM. The role of bridge therapy prior to orthotopic liver transplantation. J Natl Compr Canc Netw. 2014;12:1183-91.
16. Forner A, Gilabert M, Gruix J, et al. Treatment of intermediate-stage hepatocellular carcinoma. Nat Rev Clin Oncol. 2014;11: 525-35.
17. Tsang LL, Chen CL, Huang TL, et al. Preoperative imaging evaluation of potential living liver donors: reasons for exclusion from donation in adult living donor liver transplantation. Transplant Proc. 2008;40(8):2460-2.
18. Michels NA. Blood supply and anatomy of upper abdominal organs. Philadelphia, PA: Lippincott, 1955.
19. Fan ST, Lo CM, Liu CL. Technical refinement in adultto-adult living donor liver transplantation using right lobe graft. Ann Surg. 2000;231:126-31.
20. Sahani D, Mehta A, Blake M, Prasad S, Harris G, Saini S. Preoperative hepatic vascular evaluation with CT and MR angiography: implications for surgery. RadioGraphics. 2004;24(5):1367-80.
21. Erbay N, Raptopoulos V, Pomfret EA, Kamel IR, Kruskal JB. Living donor liver transplantation in adults: vascular variants important in surgical planning for donors and recipients. AJR. 2003;181(1):109-14.
22. Sahani D, D'souza R, Kadavigere R, et al. Evaluation of living liver transplant donors: method for precise anatomic definition by using a dedicated contrast enhanced MR imaging protocol. Radiographics. 2004;24:957-67.

23. Itamoto T, Emoto K, Mitsuta H, et al. Safety of donor right hepatectomy for adult-to-adult living donor liver transplantation. Transpl Int. 2006;19(3):177-83.
24. Piekarski J, Goldberg HI, Royal SA, et al. Difference between liver and spleen CT numbers in the normal adult: its usefulness in predicting the presence of diffuse liver disease. Radiology. 1980;137:727-9.
25. Orons PD, Sheng R, Zajko AB. Hepatic artery stenosis in liver transplant recipients: prevalence and cholangiographic appearance of associated biliary complications. AJR. 1995; 165(5):1145-9.
26. Singh AK, Nachiappan AC, Verma HA, Uppot RN, Blake MA, Saini S, Boland GW. Postoperative imaging in liver transplantation: what radiologists should know. Radiographics. 2010;30(2):339-51.
27. Nghiem HV. Imaging of hepatic transplantation. Radiol Clin North Am. 1998;36(2):429-43.
28. Uzochukwu LN, Bluth EI, Smetherman DH, et al. Early postoperative hepatic sonography as a predictor of vascular and biliary complications in adult orthotopic liver transplant patients. AJR. 2005;185(6):1558-70.
29. Fulcher AS, Turner MA. Orthotopic liver transplantation: evaluation with MR cholangiography. Radiology. 1999;211(3): 715-22.
30. Zemel G, Zajko AB, Skolnick ML, Bron KM, Campbell WL. The role of sonography and transhepatic cholangiography in the diagnosis of biliary complications after liver transplantation. AJR. 1988;151(5):943-6.
31. Dupuy DE, Costello P. Cross-sectional imaging of liver transplantation. Semin Ultrasound CT MR. 1992;13(5):399-409.

CHAPTER 82

Imaging and Interventions in Hepatic Venous Outflow Tract Obstruction

Naveen Kalra, Ujjwal Gorsi, Niranjan Khandelwal

INTRODUCTION

Hepatic venous outflow tract obstruction, Budd-Chiari syndrome (BCS), is a rare disorder of hepatic venous outflow obstruction which may involve the hepatic veins, inferior vena cava (IVC) or both and is characterized by structural and functional abnormalities of the liver. It affects 1 in 100,000 population worldwide. The disease is more common in Northern India, South Africa and Japan as compared to the Western countries. The term 'Budd Chiari' was coined after George Budd, who reported three cases of hepatic vein thrombosis in 1845 and Hans Chiari, who described obliterating endophlebitis of the hepatic veins in 1899.[1]

BCS is classified into three types based on the level of venous occlusion.[2] In type I, involvement is at the level of IVC alone, in type II, it is at the level of hepatic veins and type III is the mixed type with involvement of both IVC and hepatic veins.

CLINICAL PRESENTATION

The clinical course of BCS is determined by the degree of hepatic venous outflow obstruction and the rapidity with which it develops. Usually the clinical presentation of the syndrome is nonspecific. Large and sudden blockage of veins results in acute BCS, which is characterized by severe abdominal pain, ascities, jaundice, tender hepatomegaly and rapidly developing hepatic failure over a period of few days to few weeks. Subacute BCS is the most common clinical type, has an insidious onset and may take as long as 3 months to become asymptomatic. The development is slow and during the period decompressive collaterals develop. Thus subacute BCS does not present with esophageal bleed. On the other hand, when there is still more insidious gradual venous outflow obstruction it leads to chronic BCS which is characterized by the development of postsinusoidal portal hypertension, prominent abdominal veins, upper GI bleed, pedal edema, ascities and large nodular liver developing over a period of several months. Acute BCS is mostly reported from western countries, whereas cases of chronic BCS are reported mainly from Japan, China, South Africa and India. Differentiation of acute and chronic forms of the disease is important for determining the prognosis and planning the treatment. In patients with acute form, the prognosis is poor with high mortality if not treated, whereas chronic form is less ominous and 50% patients are alive after five years.[3]

ETIOPATHOGENESIS

The BCS is classified as primary when the obstruction to hepatic venous outflow is due to a primary venous thrombosis, stenosis or web. It is classified as secondary when the obstruction is caused by extensive compression by tumor, cyst or abscess.[4] These lesions obstruct venous outflow by invasion of the lumen or by extrinsic compression. Most of the patients of BCS have an underlying inherited or acquired hypercoagulable state. Myeloproliferative disease is the most common thrombotic disorder detected. The other conditions associated with

BCS are JAK2 V617F mutation, Factor V Leiden mutation, oral contraceptive pills, pregnancy, antiphospholipid antibodies, paroxysmal nocturnal hemoglobinuria, protein C and S deficiency. JAK2 V617F mutation may be detected in 30–50% of patients with BCS.

The etiology of BCS also has geographical variation.[5] In Asian countries, the most common causes are web or membranous obstruction of the IVC (MOVC), pregnancy and infections, while in the West, primary myeloproliferative disorders, hypercoagulable states, steroidal contraceptives and tumors are responsible in majority of cases. While earlier studies from India found isolated IVC obstruction to be the most common disease type, recent studies found the combination of IVC and hepatic vein obstruction to be the most common type.[6] Rarely, BCS may occur due to malignant thrombosis of the IVC or main hepatic veins secondary to hepatic, renal and adrenal neoplasms.[7] Hepatocellular carcinoma can produce an acute fulminant variant of BCS by causing obstruction of the main hepatic veins or inferior vena cava due to endoluminal invasion by the tumor. However, in 30–50% of patients etiology remains unidentified.[5]

Initially when the hepatic veins occlude, the sinusoidal and portal pressures increase and there is hepatic congestion **(Fig. 1A)**. This increase in sinusoidal pressure leads to hypoxic injury to hepatocytes which results in noninflammatory centrilobular cell necrosis especially in perivenular zones. In case the hepatocyte damage is massive, the patient presents with fulminant BCS. In case the damage is insidious, the liver slowly develops fibrosis and later cirrhosis **(Fig. 1B)**. The patient will then present with portal hypertension and ascites.

Liver biopsy differentiates BCS from veno-occlusive disease (VOD) which is due to nonthrombotic obstruction of hepatic vessels by subendothelial swelling on account of injury of sinusoidal wall **(Fig. 1C)**. The cause of VOD is toxic agents and it is also associated with bone marrow transplantation. Cyclophosphamide is the most common causative agent. VOD is also known as sinusoidal obstruction syndrome.

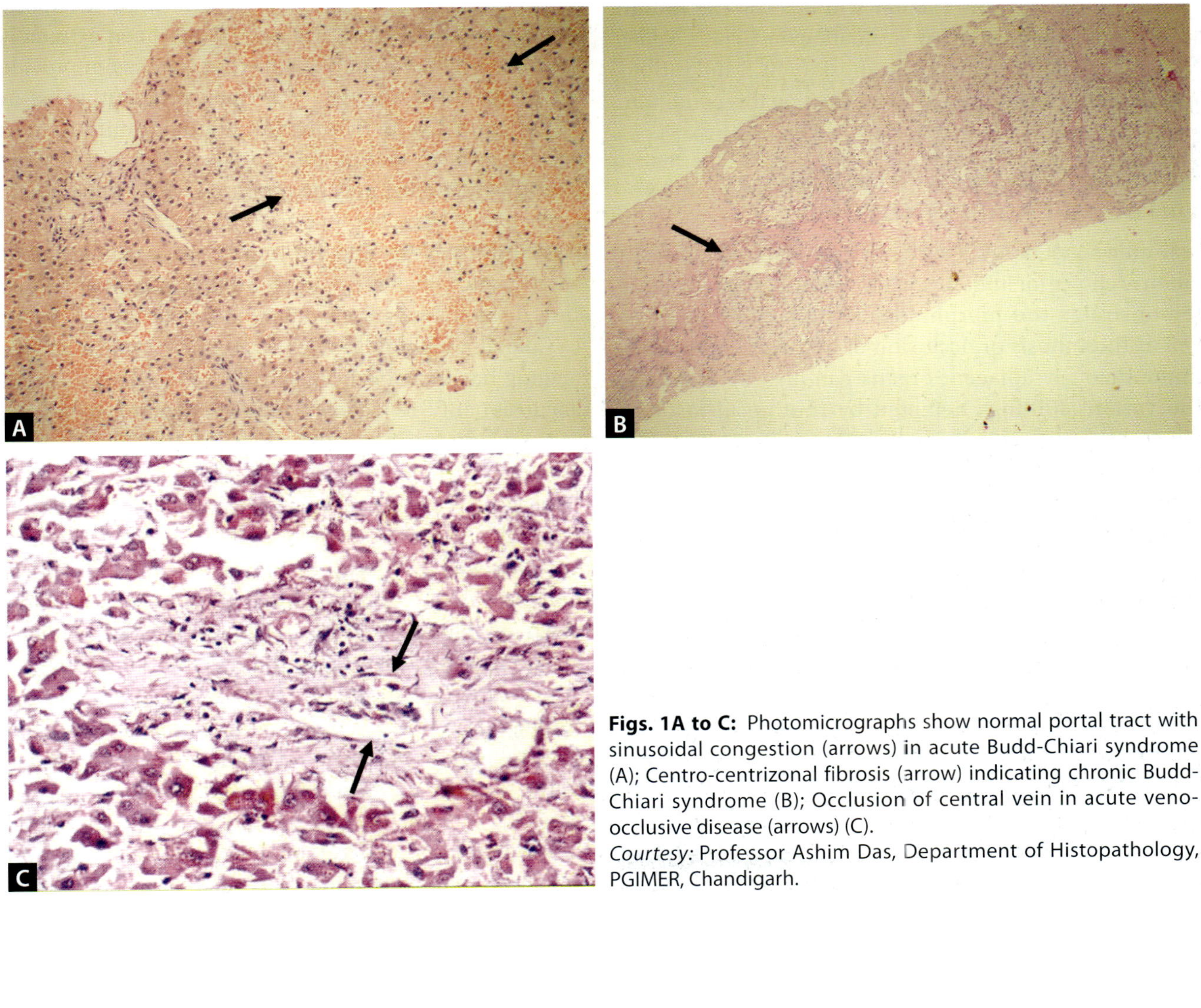

Figs. 1A to C: Photomicrographs show normal portal tract with sinusoidal congestion (arrows) in acute Budd-Chiari syndrome (A); Centro-centrizonal fibrosis (arrow) indicating chronic Budd-Chiari syndrome (B); Occlusion of central vein in acute veno-occlusive disease (arrows) (C).

Courtesy: Professor Ashim Das, Department of Histopathology, PGIMER, Chandigarh.

DIAGNOSTIC TECHNIQUES

The recent advances in imaging techniques have enabled delineation of the exact vascular abnormalities and their treatment resulting in better and improved survival rates in patients of BCS. The available therapeutic options include medical treatment; radiological interventional methods like balloon angioplasty, stent placement, transjugular intrahepatic portosystemic shunt (TIPS) and surgical treatment which includes portosystemic shunts and liver transplantation. Imaging thus plays a crucial role in diagnosis and management. Till recently, IVC venography, hepatic venography and liver biopsy alone or in combination were the definitive investigations available for anatomic and hemodynamic evaluation in patients of BCS, but these procedures are invasive and have risk of complications particularly in patients with coagulation abnormalities. Lately, several noninvasive imaging modalities like ultrasound, CT and MRI are being increasingly used in the diagnosis of BCS as they can depict the hepatic vascular anatomy accurately without catheterization and thereby guide management decisions. The current chapter will discuss the role of these newer investigations in evaluating the hepatic veins, IVC and liver parenchyma in diagnosis of BCS and various interventional techniques used for treating this condition.

EVALUATION OF HEPATIC VEINS IN BUDD-CHIARI SYNDROME

Real-time sonography is currently considered the investigation of choice for initial evaluation of BCS. The technique demonstrates the morphological hepatic changes as well as thrombosis or occlusion of hepatic veins or IVC. Simultaneously adjacent organs can also be assessed. The various findings depicted by routine ultrasound include hepatomegaly, heterogeneous liver and caudate lobe enlargement. In addition, findings that suggest hepatic vein thrombosis on ultrasound (US) include nonvisualization of confluence of hepatic veins with IVC, distorted or absent hepatic veins, stenosed hepatic veins with thick wall echoes **(Fig. 2A)**, hyperechoic hepatic veins **(Fig. 2B)**, portal vein thrombosis and ascities. Presence of comma shaped veno-venous intra-hepatic collaterals is considered a very reliable sign of BCS **(Fig. 2C)**.[8-13] Subcapsular venous collaterals may also be seen. In case only the hepatic vein occlusion is the cause of BCS, at least two of the hepatic veins must be blocked for clinically evident disease.[14]

Liver is generally enlarged but may be normal in size or shrunken in advanced cases of chronic BCS. Right lobe may show atrophy with hypertrophy of the left lobe. Echotexture of liver is homogenously hypoechoic in acute BCS and nonhomogeneous in chronic BCS. The surface of the liver may reveal fine nodularity due to cirrhotic changes. Caudate lobe enlargement is a common feature and a useful pointer towards the diagnosis, seen in 82–91% of the cases but is a nonspecific sign as it can be seen in cirrhosis due to other causes.[15]

Caudate lobe enlargement is explained by the fact that it has separate veins which are not affected by the thrombotic process and drain directly into the IVC just distal to the ostia of the main hepatic veins. This segment of the liver thus receives uninterrupted supply of hepatotropic agents like insulin. Caudate lobe drainage serves as an outflow for intrahepatic venous collaterals. It has been reported that visualization of a caudate vein >3 mm in diameter strongly suggests the diagnosis of BCS in an appropriate clinical setting.[16] The overall accuracy of ultrasound for detecting hepatic venous thrombosis has been found to be 70–87% in the literature.[11,17]

The normal diameter of the right and middle hepatic veins is less than 10 mm while that of the left hepatic vein is less than 9 mm.[18] Though US has been extremely useful for evaluation of hepatic veins, it does not provide any information about blood flow in hepatic veins or IVC or portal vein. The technique has limitations in cases of swollen and nodular, or shrunken and scarred liver in which veins may be obscured within the hepatic parenchyma. Detection of intraluminal webs, thrombosis or membranes is also limited. Poor delineation of extrahepatic collaterals and possibility of an inadequate study due to bowel gas are other limiting factors.

Color flow duplex Doppler US combined with real-time imaging has increased the sensitivity and specificity of diagnosis of BCS as it allows better visualization of hepatic veins by automatically adding flow information. Doppler waveform of hepatic veins in healthy individuals is a triphasic waveform (two negative waves and one positive) **(Fig. 3A)**.[19] Loss of the normal triphasic waveform is seen in BCS as well as in cirrhosis. Presence of flat waveform (uniphasic flow) without flutter or absent or reversed flow in hepatic veins are the most reliable signs of hepatic vein thrombosis **(Fig. 3B)**. Veins that may be nonvisualized on real-time ultrasound due to compression by hepatic nodules may reveal flow on color flow ultrasound and thus prove to be normal.[12] 3D ultrasound can also be used to show the entire morphology of the IVC and the hepatic veins.[18]

Magnetic resonance (MR) has also been used for evaluation of hepatic veins.[20] T2 weighted gradient echo

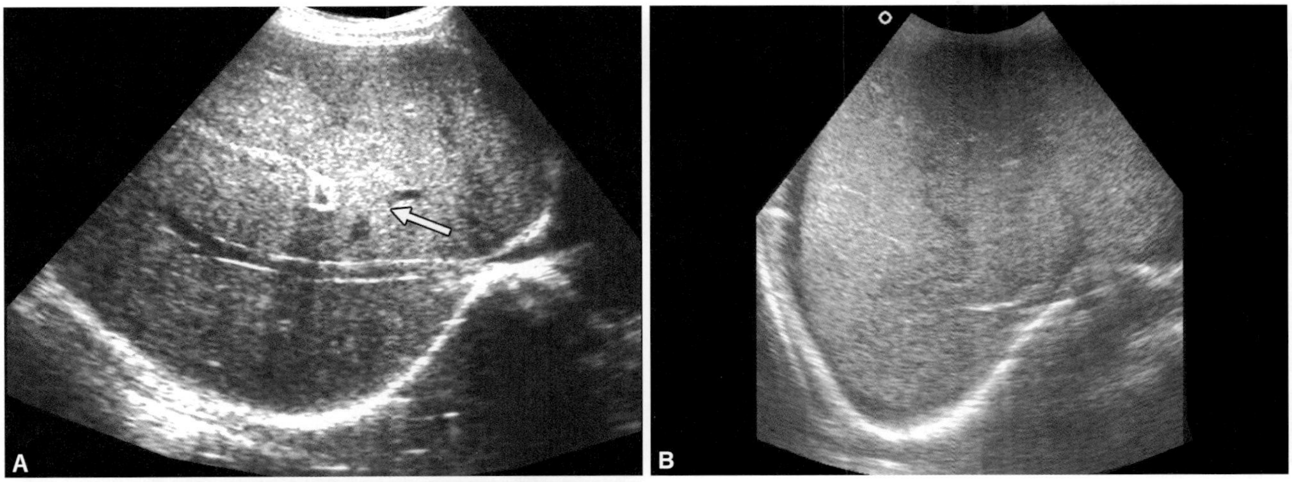

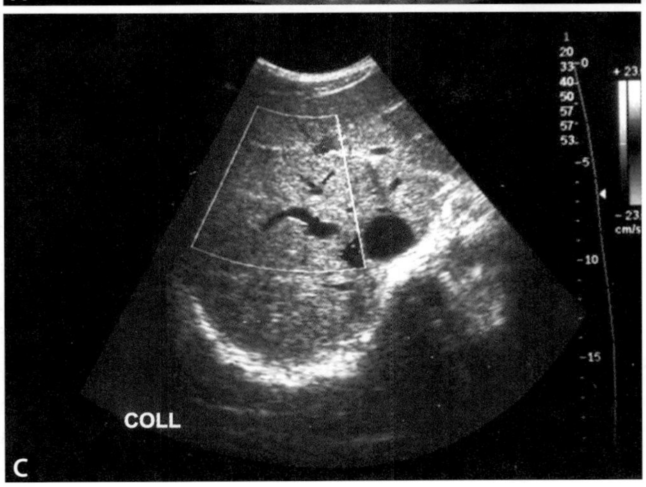

Figs. 2A to C: Transverse ultrasound section shows echogenic walls of the RHV suggestive of thrombosed RHV. MHV and LHV are not visualized. A comma-shaped intrahepatic collateral is seen (arrow) (A). Transverse ultrasound section shows echogenic cord-like RHV suggestive of thrombosed RHV. MHV and LHV are not visualized (B). Transverse ultrasound section in another patient of BCS shows multiple comma-shaped intrahepatic collaterals, nonvisualized hepatic veins and dilated IVC (C).

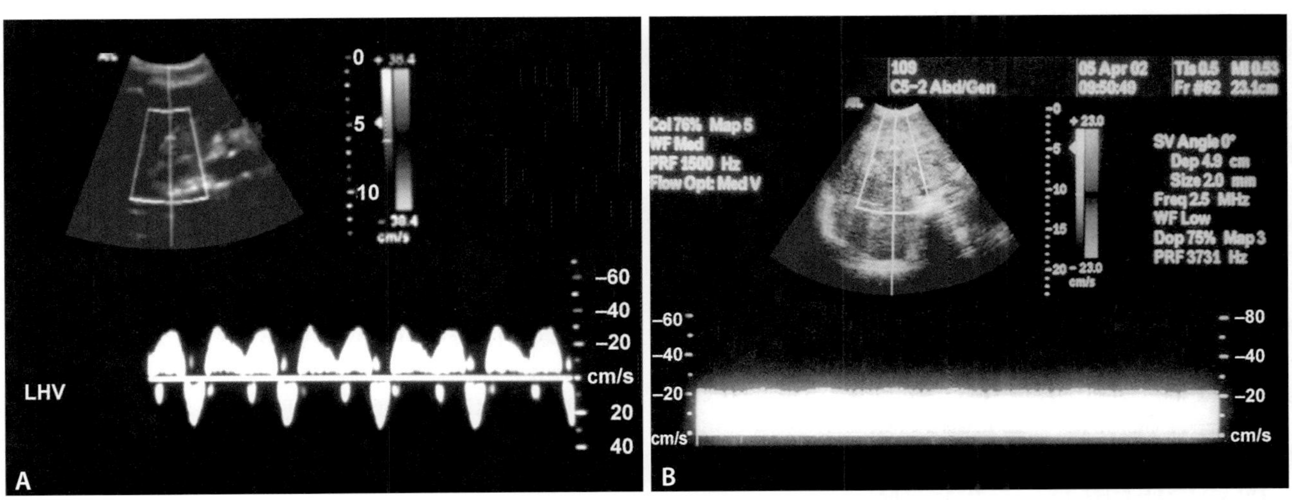

Figs. 3A and B: Normal pulsed Doppler tracing in the left hepatic vein (LHV) shows the triphasic waveform. The antegrade flow occurs during the ventricular systole and atrial diastole while retrograde flow occurs during the atrial systole (A); Doppler US with color box placed in the region of RHV and MHV in a patient of BCS shows no flow in RHV. MHV shows uniphasic flow (B).

sequence or multiphase contrast-enhanced images are needed for the evaluation of vessels and collaterals. MR has particular advantage of being able to show hepatic veins in three dimensions but its ability to determine the degree of flow is limited in the routine MR sequences. In our experience color flow Doppler US is superior to MR for evaluation of hepatic veins as the ostial narrowing can be better detected by US. The angiographic techniques used for delineation of the hepatic veins include IVC graphy with retrograde hepatic vein cannulation, percutaneous hepatography (injection of contrast in the hepatic parenchyma under fluoroscopy with serial filming to visualize the hepatic veins entering into IVC) **(Fig. 4)** and direct hepatic venography under US guidance. These techniques are the most definitive but are reserved for patients being considered for angioplasty or stent placement where exact delineation of the length of stenosed segment is mandatory for deciding the management. In BCS there is a collateral circulation between the tributaries of the hepatic veins which forms a 'spider web'. In the initial stage these collaterals are fine giving rise to a 'fine spider web'. With long standing BCS, these collaterals form a 'coarse spider web'.[21] Arteriography if performed in a patient with BCS would show larger diameter of the hepatic artery as compared to the splenic artery since the blood supply to the liver by the hepatic artery is increased.[22]

Scintigraphy and CT have also been used for the diagnosis of BCS. Scintigraphy may reveal increased uptake by caudate lobe and left lobe, patchy uptake of radionuclide in the rest of the liver giving the appearance of hot spots. On CT, presence of enlarged caudate lobe with low attenuation areas elsewhere in the liver, atrophy of right lobe, nonvisualization of hepatic veins and irregular surface of the liver may be seen. On CECT presence of patchy hepatogram, areas of linear, irregular or wedge-shaped hypoattenuation particularly in the peripheral portions of liver due to fibrosis and parenchymal destruction indicate hepatic venous thrombosis. Dynamic CT may demonstrate thrombus within the hepatic veins and comma shaped intrahepatic collaterals **(Fig. 5A)**. Presence of areas of hypoattenuation surrounded by areas of increased enhancement can simulate presence of intra-hepatic mass lesion. Although there is limited literature about the role of MDCT in BCS, the availability of volume imaging and 3D reconstructions **(Fig. 5B)** will provide a useful adjunct to axial images in the near future.[22]

EVALUATION OF INFERIOR VENA CAVA IN BUDD-CHIARI SYNDROME

Evaluation of IVC is an important and essential component of the imaging evaluation of a patient suspected to have BCS for two reasons. Firstly, IVC obstruction alone or in combination with hepatic vein obstruction may itself lead to BCS. Secondly, patency of IVC must be established before deciding upon the surgical procedure

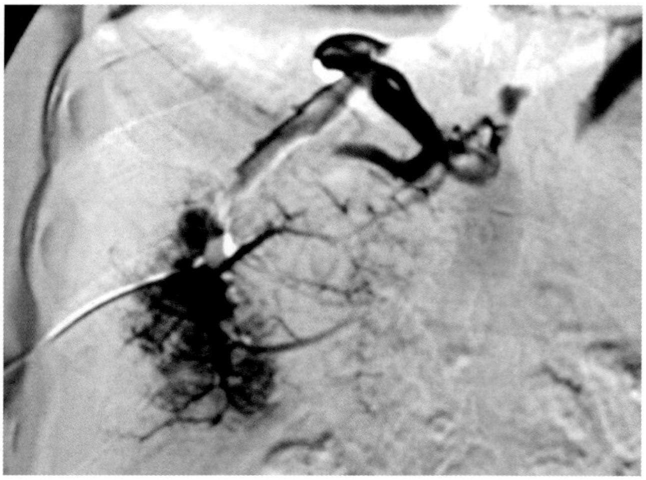

Fig. 4: Percutaneous hepatography shows nonopacification of the hepatic veins. There is filling up of multiple intrahepatic collaterals some of which have 'spider web' configuration.

to be undertaken such as portocaval/ mesocaval shunt when IVC is patent and mesoatrial shunt when IVC is obstructed.

Incidence of IVC obstruction in BCS varies from 33% to 56%.[23,24] IVC can be obstructed in its intrahepatic portion, suprahepatic portion or both. The causes of IVC obstruction are membranes, tumor thrombus and caudate lobe hypertrophy.[11,23,24] Suprahepatic obstruction is generally due to short segment stenosis or IVC webs. Intrahepatic IVC obstruction is most commonly due to compression from the enlarged caudate lobe. Chronic thrombosis of the IVC can evolve into calcification.[22]

Webs are visualized as dome shaped thin linear filling defects on contrast venography and MR angiography. On real-time imaging they appear as hyperreflective linear foci best seen in deep inspiration **(Figs. 6A to D)**. Whether these webs represent congenital lesions or they are the result of thrombotic process is an issue which remains disputed.[25] It seems quite plausible to assume that both IVC web and segmental stenosis actually represent the spectrum of same pathological process, i.e. thrombosis.

On real-time ultrasound, short segment stenosis is seen as an area of narrowing and the caliber of IVC is dilated proximal to the obstruction with loss of phasic variation with respiration **(Figs. 7A and B)**. Long segment narrowing of the IVC due to caudate lobe enlargement is well depicted. When the IVC obstruction is due to tumor thrombi, extension of the tumor into the IVC is well demonstrated. However, ultrasound is unable to determine the length of stenosis, webs can be missed and the hemodynamic significance of IVC narrowing cannot

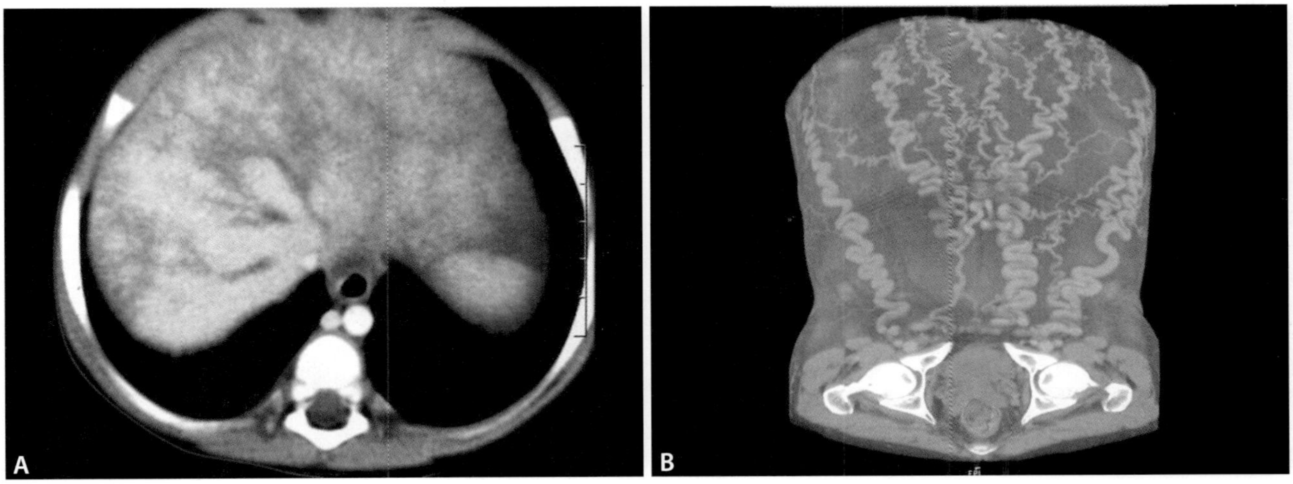

Figs. 5A and B: CECT in a patient of BCS shows patchy hepatogram: The right hepatic vein and middle hepatic vein are thrombosed while the left hepatic vein is not visualized (A); MDCT reconstructed image shows multiple parietal wall collaterals in a patient with type III BCS (B).

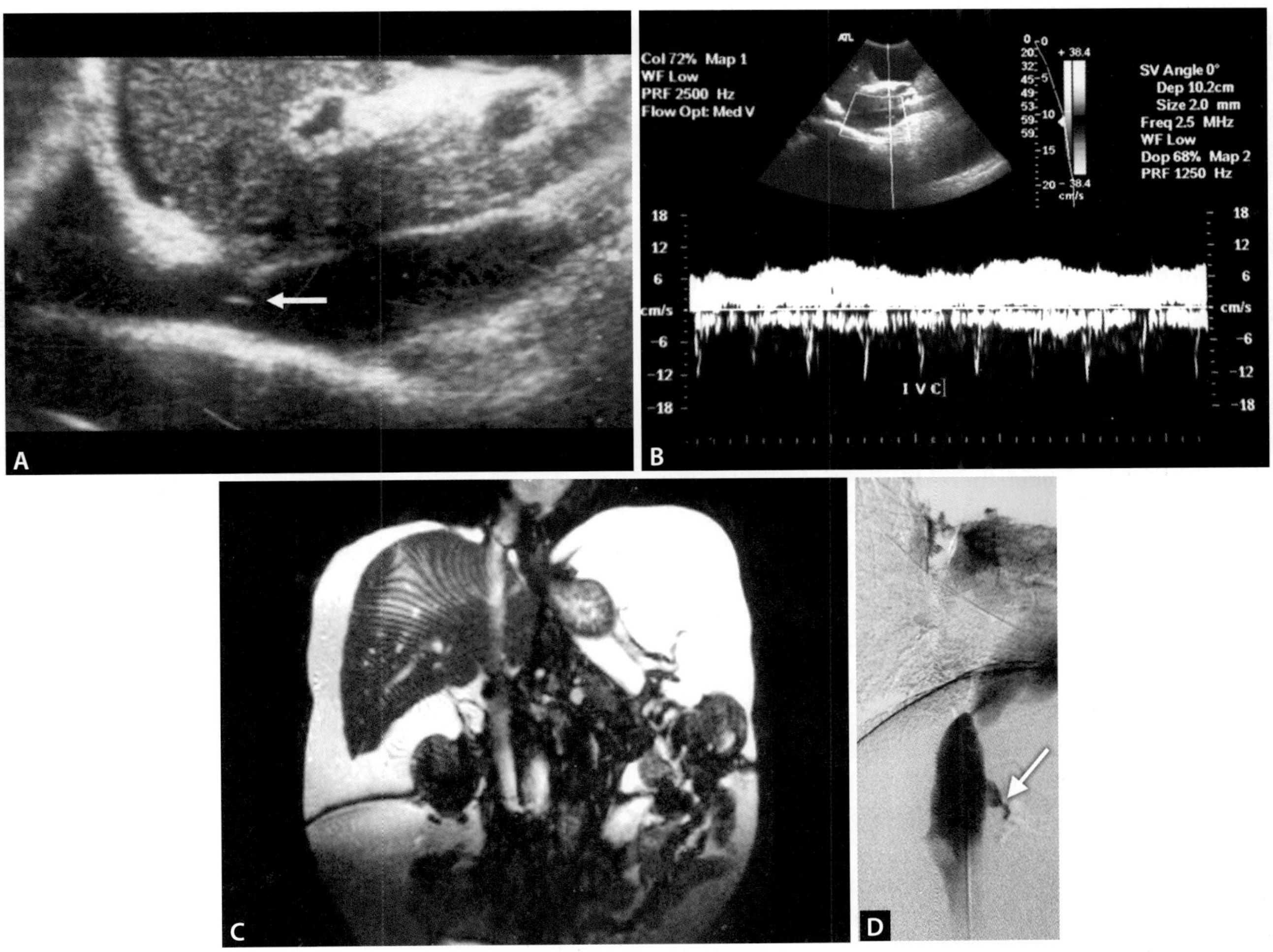

Figs. 6A to D: A 60-year-old male presenting with abdominal distention. Sagittal US showing echogenic linear area in IVC proximal to cavoatrial junction suggestive of a web in IVC (arrow) (A). There is uniphasic flow with fluttering seen in the IVC (B). Coronal FLASH flow sensitive MR image shows a hypointense linear signal in the IVC proximal to cavoatrial junction suggestive of a web in the suprahepatic portion (C). IVC graphy lateral view shows dome-shaped obstruction of suprahepatic IVC with a jet of blood flowing into right atrium confirming the presence of web. There is filling up of an intrahepatic collateral (arrow) (D).

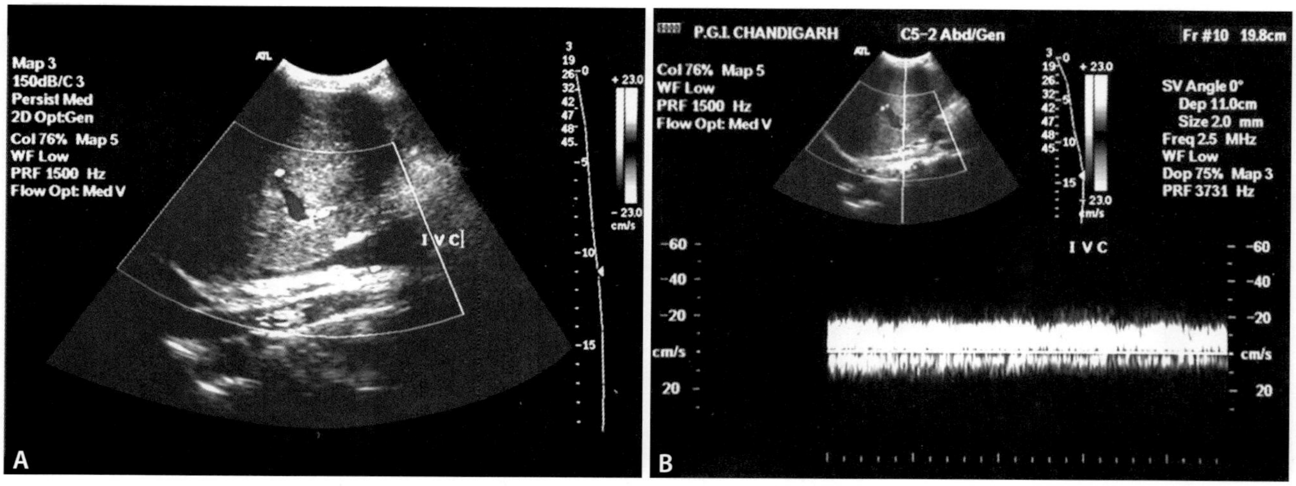

Figs. 7A and B: Dopplers show a smooth long segment narrowing in the intrahepatic portion of IVC with loss of the normal phasic variation and a uniphasic flow pattern.

be assessed. Possibility of poor study due to bowel gas is also a limiting factor.

Color Doppler US combined with real-time imaging is superior to grayscale imaging as it provides better assessment of IVC impairment by adding flow information. The normal flow pattern of IVC is a triphasic waveform. The flow abnormality can be seen in the form of either absent (IVC occlusion), reversed or uniphasic flow (stenosis).[12,26] Turbulent flow may be seen at the site of short segment stenosis.[26,27]

The IVC venography has been considered the gold standard for evaluation of inferior vena cava. However, in patients of BCS, it has certain limitations particularly for evaluation of hepatic veins. Diagnosis of hepatic vein occlusion is inferred when there is failure to cannulate the hepatic veins selectively at the time of catheterization. Thus, over diagnosis of hepatic vein thrombosis may result even when failure of cannulation is due to technical failure. The other limitations of IVC graphy include nonvisualization of IVC distal to obstruction due to diversion of contrast into the collaterals. Thus, in case of suprahepatic obstruction due to web/membrane visualization of IVC above and below the lesion may require double catheter study. Lastly the intrahepatic collaterals which form important parameters for diagnosis of chronic BCS are not detected with IVC graphy.

Recently MR venography has shown a great potential by overcoming many of the limitations of IVC venography. MR venography accurately depicts the site and cause of IVC obstruction with clear delineation of IVC both above and below the obstruction **(Fig. 8)**.[17,20] MR is excellent for detection of both intra- and extrahepatic collaterals, portal vein obstruction and detection of tumor thrombi within

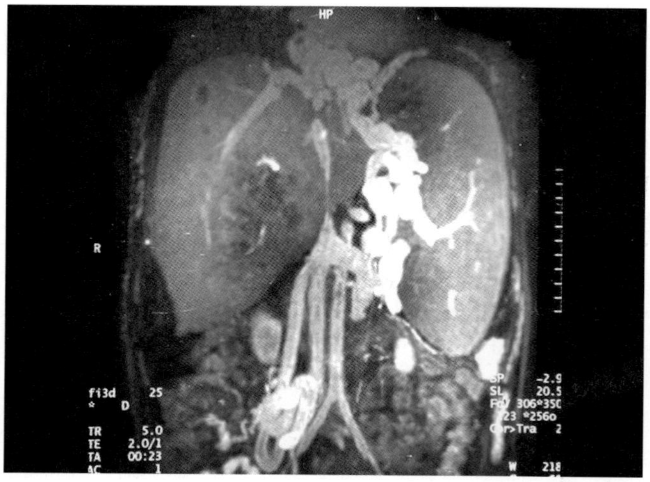

Fig. 8: Coronal contrast-enhanced MR venography shows long segment narrowing of IVC in intrahepatic portion with filling defect proximal to cavoatrial junction. There are multiple collaterals in the retroperitoneum and at the splenic hilum.

the IVC. Incidence of portal vein thrombosis in BCS is 5–20%.[26,27]

Five Types of Collateral Pathways Develop in Budd-Chiari Syndrome[28]

1. Left renal-hemiazygous pathways
2. Vertebrolumbar azygous pathways
3. Intrahepatic collaterals
4. Superficial abdominal wall collaterals
5. Inferior phrenic-pericardiophrenic collaterals.

Intrahepatic collaterals have been noted in 80–93% cases of BCS[12,27,29] and are seen as comma shaped bridging veno-venous collaterals which reveal flat waveform on color Doppler ultrasound.

ASSESSMENT OF LIVER PARENCHYMA IN BUDD-CHIARI SYNDROME

As a result of hepatic venous or IVC obstruction there is ischemic damage to the liver cells resulting in severe congestion, centrilobular necrosis followed by fibrosis and cirrhosis. In acute BCS, congestion predominates whereas patients of chronic BCS are more likely to develop cirrhosis and regenerative nodules.[24] Since the obstruction of the hepatic veins is usually asynchronous, liver biopsy may show areas of congestion and hyperplastic enlargement in the recently affected areas and fibrosis with atrophy in the older affected segments. As the distribution of the disease in the liver is inhomogeneous liver biopsy may even be normal.[30]

Development of regenerative nodules in BCS is known to occur in response to focal loss of portal perfusion and hyper arterialization in areas with preserved hepatic venous outflow.[22] Incidence of nodules greater than 5 mm have been seen on histology in 40–80% of patients.[27,31] Although the question of possible malignant transformation of the large regenerative nodule remains unsettled, it is generally believed that HCC is extremely rare in patients presenting with BCS due to hepatic venous obstruction alone. However, it may be co-existent in patients of BCS due to IVC obstruction particularly MOVC.[24] The obstruction may make the hepatocytes more susceptible to the action of environment carcinogens. HCC in BCS accounts for 0.7% of all cases of hepatocelluar carcinoma.[32] Differentiation of HCC from regenerative nodules is important. US and conventional CT are both poor modalities for detection of these nodules. On the other hand MRI and biphasic CT have been reported to be more reliable.[7,33,34]

Benign regenerative nodules which are hyperintense on T1WI and iso- to hypointense on T2WI are likely to be benign **(Figs. 9A and B)** compared to HCC nodules which are hypointense on T1WI and hyperintense on T2WI **(Figs. 10A and B)**. Multiple (>10) and small (<4 cm) lesions are suggestive of benignity.[7] On biphasic CT large regenerative nodules are markedly and homogeneously hyperattenuating on arterial phase images and remain slightly hyperattenuating on portal venous phase images.[22,34] On histopathology these nodules have normal or hyperplastic hepatocytes, arteries extending radially from the center of the nodule and a central scar in the larger nodules.[31,35] The imaging characteristics of this scar may be similar to those of the scar found in focal nodular hyperplasia on dynamic imaging.[31]

Liver biopsy has been used in the past to differentiate acute from subacute and chronic BCS. A liver biopsy is required only if radiological imaging is inconclusive.[36] Differentiation is important for deciding the plan of treatment. Acute BCS may be treated by infusion of thrombolytic substances at the site of block followed by stenting whereas, chronic BCS requires the creation of a shunt between the hepatic veins and portal vein by transjugular intrahepatic portosystemic shunt procedure. MRI and dynamic CT have shown potential to determine the chronicity of the hepatic changes.[17,37,38]

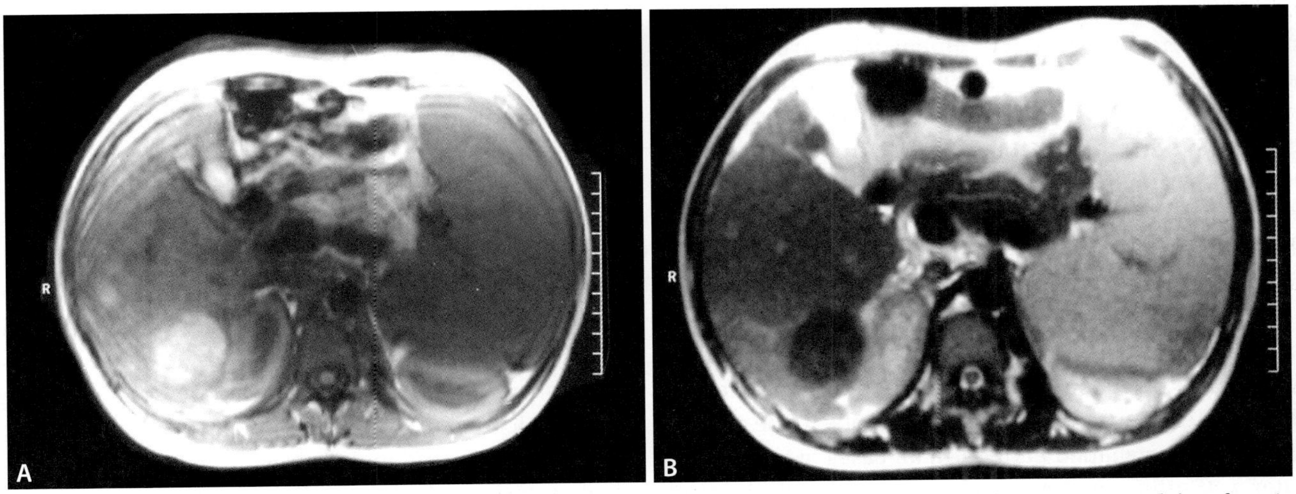

Figs. 9A and B: (A) Axial T1W FLASH image shows single large hyperintense nodule and multiple small hyperintense nodules of varying sizes in the liver. The hyperintensity of the nodules on T1WI is suggestive of their benign nature; (B) Axial T2W HASTE image at the same level depicts the hypointense signal of the large nodule. Smaller lesions are not seen, probably due to being isointense to the liver parenchyma.

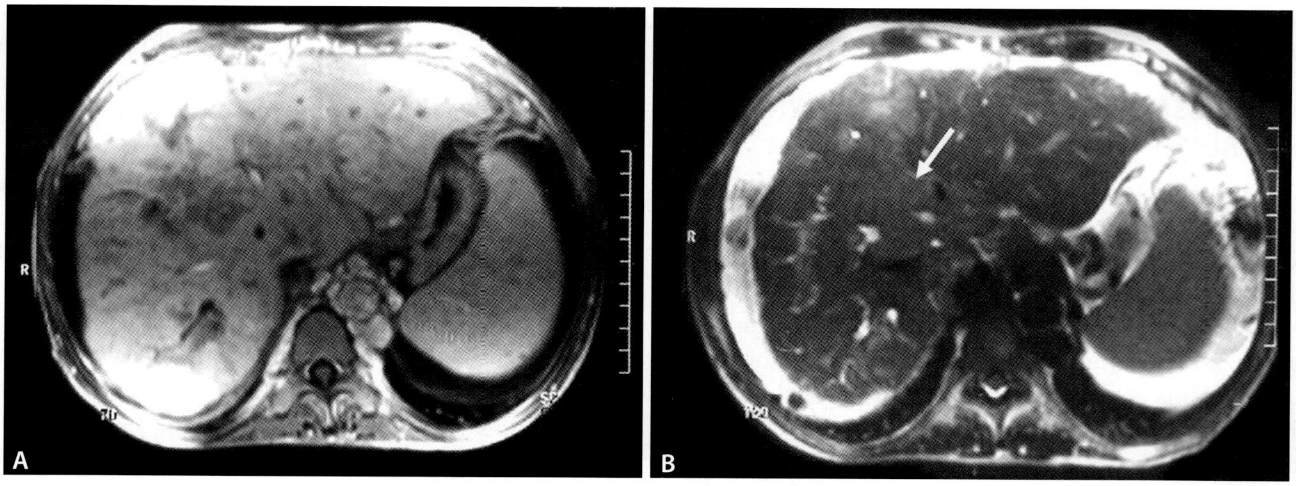

Figs. 10A and B: Axial T1W FLASH MR image at the level of hepatic veins shows irregular outline of liver with multiple ill-defined hypointense focal lesions in the liver. Ascites is seen (A); Axial T2W HASTE image at the same level shows that the lesions are isointense to hyperintense in signal (arrow). FNAC proved these lesions to be HCC (B).

A study by Noone et al.[17] has described the role of MRI in differentiation of acute, subacute and chronic BCS. In their experience in acute BCS there is decreased signal intensity on T1WI and heterogeneously increased signal intensity on T2WI peripherally with decreased enhancement of peripheral liver after gadolinium administration **(Figs. 11A to C)**. These changes were attributed to acutely increased tissue pressures and edema in the peripheral portions of the liver because of hepatic venous obstruction thus causing diminished inflow of blood. As the duration of disease increases there is reversal of flow in the portal vein and development of small collaterals permitting egress of blood. Thus in subacute BCS the signal characteristics on T1 and T2-weighted images are similar to those observed in patients with acute disease, however, periphery shows marked heterogeneous enhancement unlike to that seen in acute BCS. In chronic BCS there is no parenchymal edema and this stage is characterized by changes of fibrosis. Thus, there is no differential signal intensity and enhancement between peripheral and central liver. Using that criteria, in a study conducted at our institute 13 out of 20 cases of chronic BCS were correctly diagnosed with MRI **(Figs. 12A and B)**.[39]

Abnormal patterns of parenchymal enhancement have also been reported on triphasic helical CT in different stages of BCS in a study by Camera et al.[38] They found abnormal enhancement of the caudate lobe in the arterial phase, the 'fan shaped pattern', in all cases of acute BCS. Later a 'flip-flop' pattern develops in which the central liver becomes hypodense compared to the peripheral liver. On the other hand 'patchy pattern' of enhancement was seen in patients of subacute and chronic BCS.

In conclusion, ultrasound with color flow Doppler imaging is the modality of choice for initial diagnosis of BCS. When combined with MR and MRA, need for diagnostic IVC venography can be obviated which can be reserved for patients where surgical or radiological intervention is being contemplated. The role of dynamic helical CT in BCS also appears promising.

MANAGEMENT OF BUDD-CHIARI SYNDROME

The treatment modality for BCS is determined by the status of hepatocyte necrosis and the stage of the disease. Nonsurgical management of BCS such as radiological intervention alone or in combination with medical management is indicated in patients, where biopsy shows no evidence of hepatocyte necrosis.

The medical management includes treatment for ascites by diuretics or paracentesis and control of gastrointestinal bleeding with balloon tamponade or sclerotherapy. Systemic thrombolytic therapy has been shown to have varying outcome. Treatment with heparin alone has been followed by recanalization of thrombosed hepatic veins and of thrombosed portal vein when associated with thrombosed hepatic veins. Patients with fulminant disease who are not responding to systemic thrombolysis may benefit from local direct pharmacological and mechanical thrombolysis.[40]

Treatment of BCS by radiological intervention was first described in 1974 by Eguchi et al. who reported the successful balloon membranotomy for obstruction of the inferior vena cava.[41] The aim of the radiological

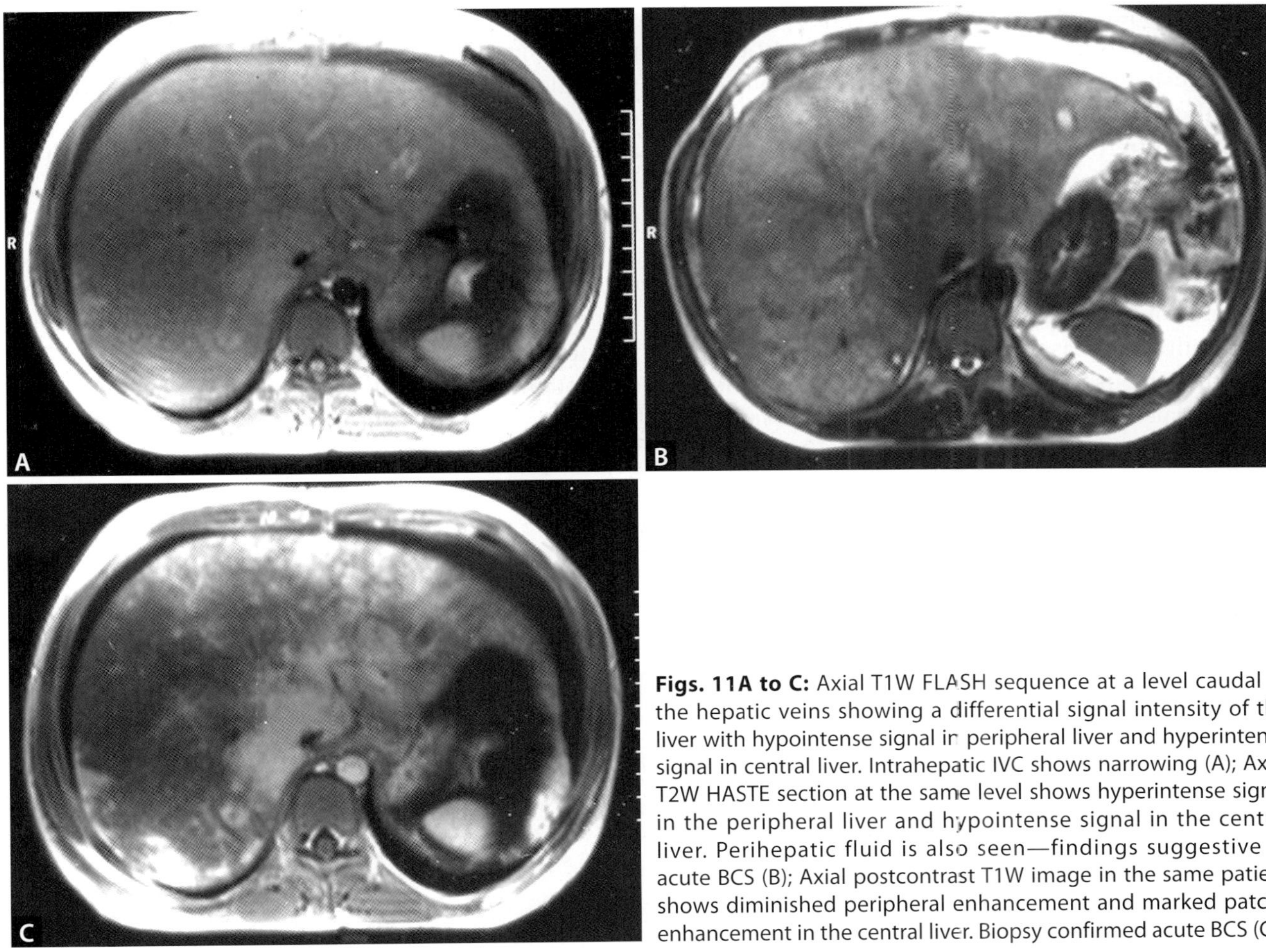

Figs. 11A to C: Axial T1W FLASH sequence at a level caudal to the hepatic veins showing a differential signal intensity of the liver with hypointense signal in peripheral liver and hyperintense signal in central liver. Intrahepatic IVC shows narrowing (A); Axial T2W HASTE section at the same level shows hyperintense signal in the peripheral liver and hypointense signal in the central liver. Perihepatic fluid is also seen—findings suggestive of acute BCS (B); Axial postcontrast T1W image in the same patient shows diminished peripheral enhancement and marked patchy enhancement in the central liver. Biopsy confirmed acute BCS (C).

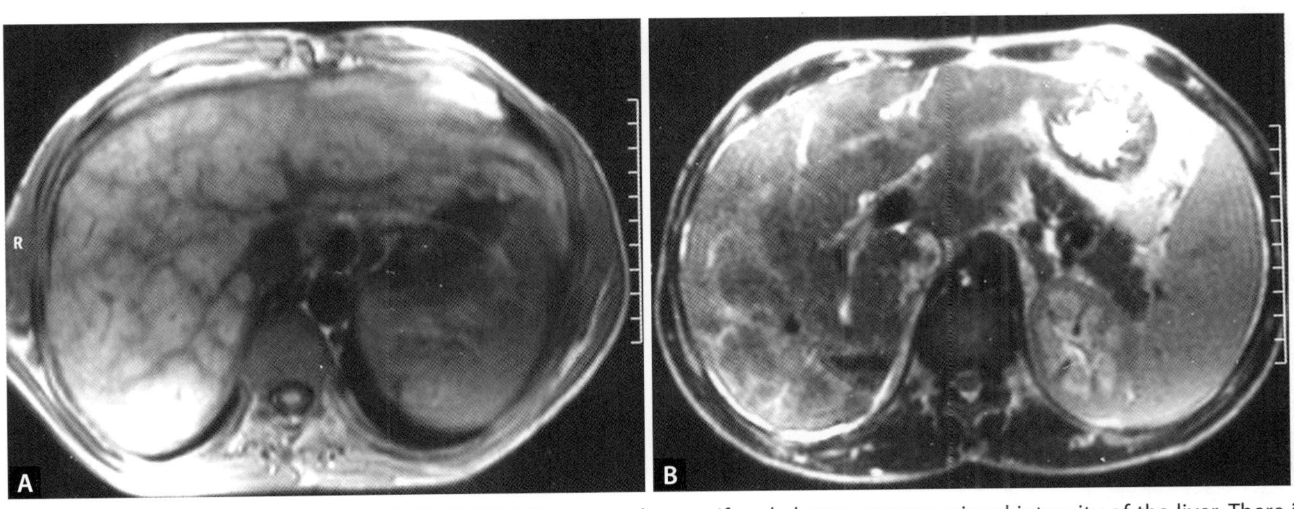

Figs. 12A and B: Axial T1W FLASH and T2W HASTE MR images show uniformly heterogeneous signal intensity of the liver. There is no differential SI of the peripheral or central liver seen. Hepatic veins are not visualized—a case of chronic BCS due to hepatic vein thrombosis and IVC stenosis.

interventions is the restoration of hepatic blood outflow by means of repermeation of the obstructed hepatic veins or IVC or by portosystemic shunting. The methods include balloon angioplasty, stent insertion and TIPS (transjugular intrahepatic portosystemic shunt). IVC interventions should preferably be done using the femoral route as negotiation across narrowed segments is easier when this route is used. The abnormal segment or web is crossed using a guide wire and then serial dilatation is done with a balloon catheter **(Figs. 13A to D)**. Stenting is rarely required due to the large lumen of the IVC. Balloon angioplasty is also used for short length stenosis of the hepatic veins. This results in immediate relief of the obstruction. However, the recurrence following this procedure is common. Griffith, et al.[42] in their study of 18 patients found that restenosis occurred in all patients treated with angioplasty when followed for longer than 10 months. The use of wall stents has resulted in better long-term patency rates of the order of 80–90% over a one year follow-up period **(Figs. 14A to F)**.[27,43,44] Baijjal, et al.[45] performed percutaneous angioplasty followed by primary stent placement in their study of 9 patients with IVC obstruction. There was residual stenosis of about 9–40% after the procedure. Revascularization was successful in all patients and the IVC remained patent during the follow-up period (3–31 months).

Surgical management of BCS is indicated in patients with features of congestion, hepatocyte necrosis and fibrosis on liver biopsy. Decompressive surgical shunts like portocaval and mesocaval shunts relieve the sinusoidal congestion and thus halt the ongoing hepatocyte necrosis. The rationale for the side to side portocaval shunts is to

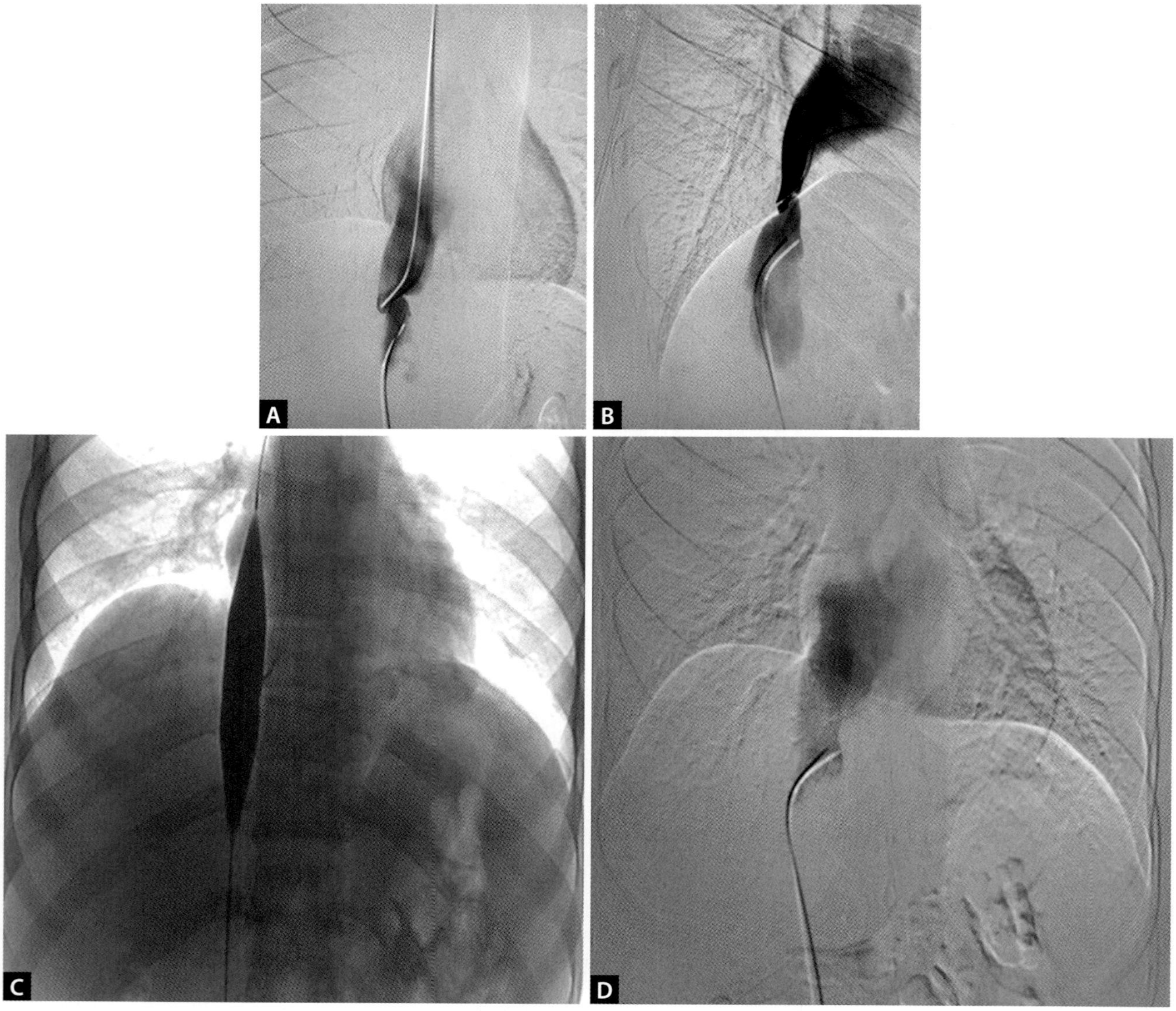

Figs. 13A to D: IVC venography in AP (A) and lateral (B) views with contrast injection from both the jugular and femoral access catheters showing a short segment stenosis of the IVC; The stenosis was crossed with a guidewire from the femoral access. Subsequently a balloon catheter was used for dilatation of the narrowing (C); Contrast injection through the femoral catheter shows no residual stenosis (D).

transform the portal vein into an outflow tract for the hepatic circulation. A portocaval or mesocaval shunt is successful if the portal vein minus infrahepatic IVC pressure is >10 mm Hg. If this pressure gradient is <10 mm Hg, these infrahepatic surgical shunts should not be done.[21] These shunts are associated with a 25% mortality

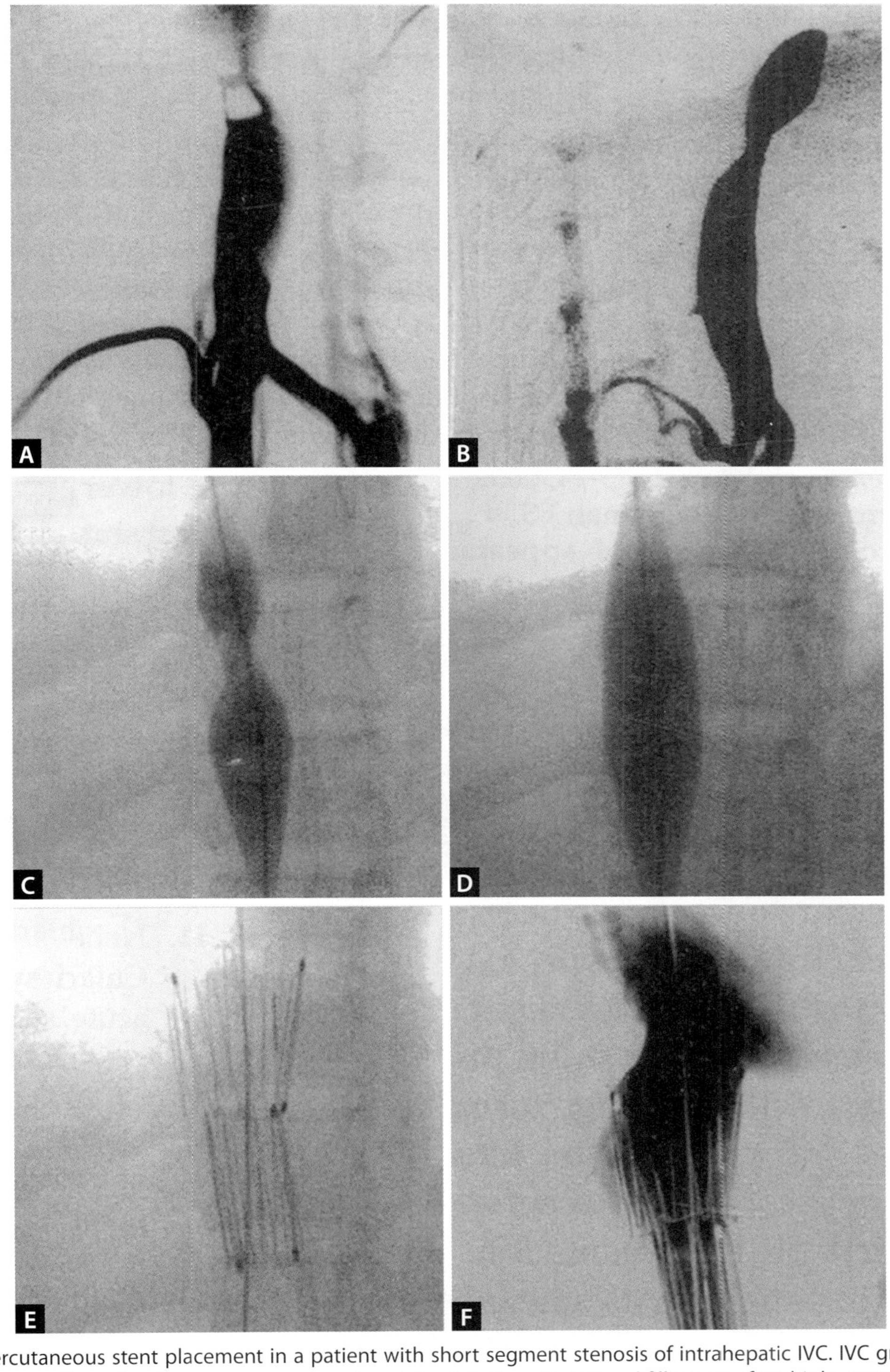

Figs. 14A to F: Percutaneous stent placement in a patient with short segment stenosis of intrahepatic IVC. IVC graphy images in AP (A) and lateral (B) views show the short segment narrowing of the intrahepatic IVC and filling up of multiple paravertebral collaterals. The stenosed segment was predilated with a balloon (C and D). This was followed by stent placement across the stenosis (E and F). Check angiogram shows free flow of contrast across the IVC into the right atrium.

rate and shunt thrombosis which may occur in 10–25% of patients. Stenosis of the shunt is a late complication and is amenable for percutaneous balloon dilatation with or without stenting **(Figs. 15A to C)**. In patients who have intrahepatic IVC abnormality these classical infrahepatic portocaval shunts do not work unless a stent is inserted in the IVC to correct the pressure gradient. Such patients require a suprahepatic shunt, i.e. mesoatrial shunt between the SMV and the right atrium. The criteria for the mesoatrial shunt are reduction of IVC diameter more than 75% or a caval atrial gradient exceeding 20 mm Hg.[46] These shunts are, however, associated with poorer results and a higher incidence of shunt thrombosis.

Successful treatment of BCS with TIPS was described in 1993 by Peltzer et al. and Ochs et al.[47,48] This involves the placement of an intrahepatic shunt connecting a hepatic vein stump through the liver to a branch of the portal vein **(Figs. 16A to D)**. The shunt can also be created between the suprahepatic IVC and the portal vein when no hepatic vein stump is available. The transcaval approach is also technically more feasible in BCS. This is because the liver is enlarged and the intrahepatic IVC is surrounded by liver

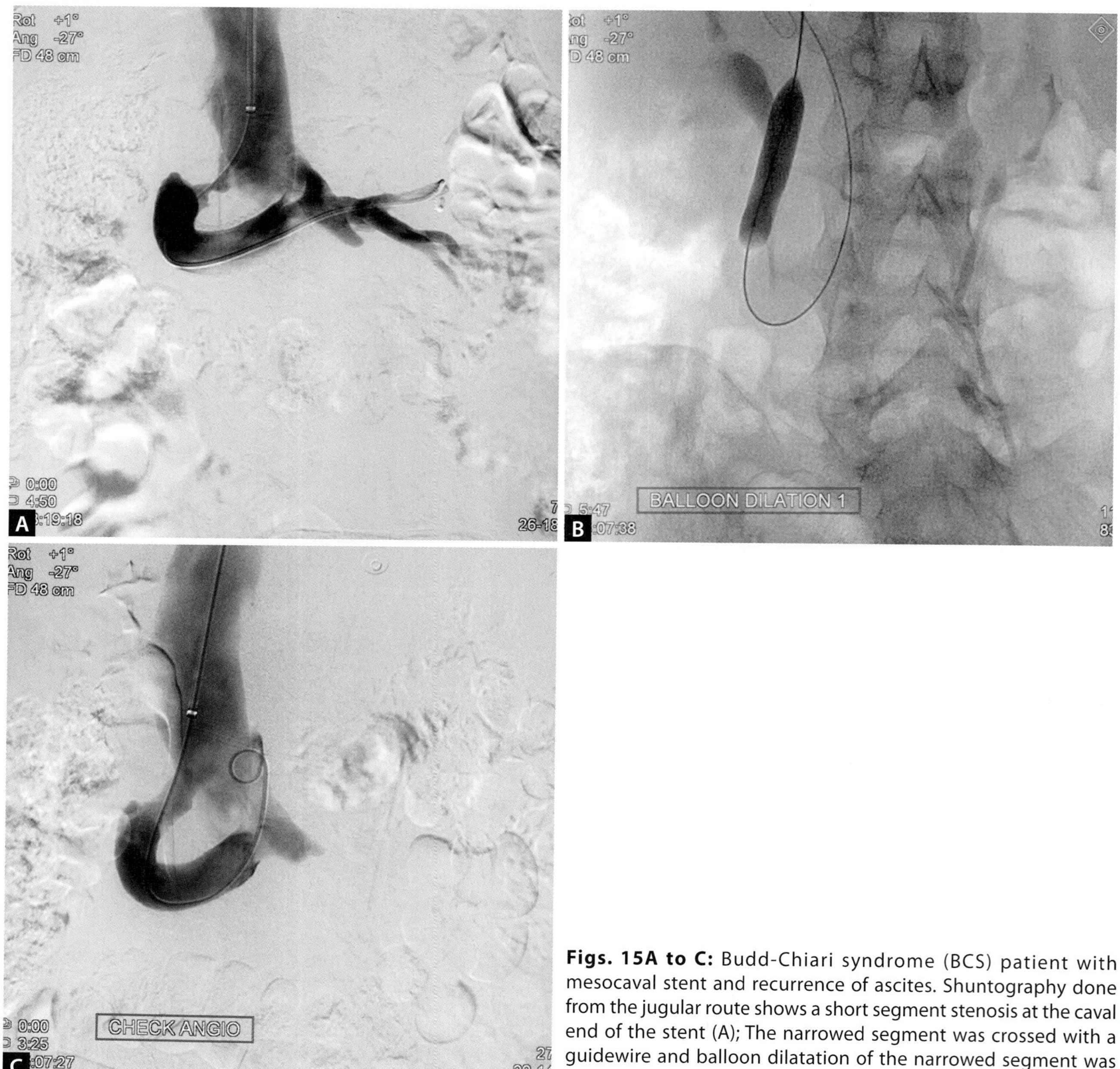

Figs. 15A to C: Budd-Chiari syndrome (BCS) patient with mesocaval stent and recurrence of ascites. Shuntography done from the jugular route shows a short segment stenosis at the caval end of the stent (A); The narrowed segment was crossed with a guidewire and balloon dilatation of the narrowed segment was done (B); Shuntography now shows no residual stenosis (C).

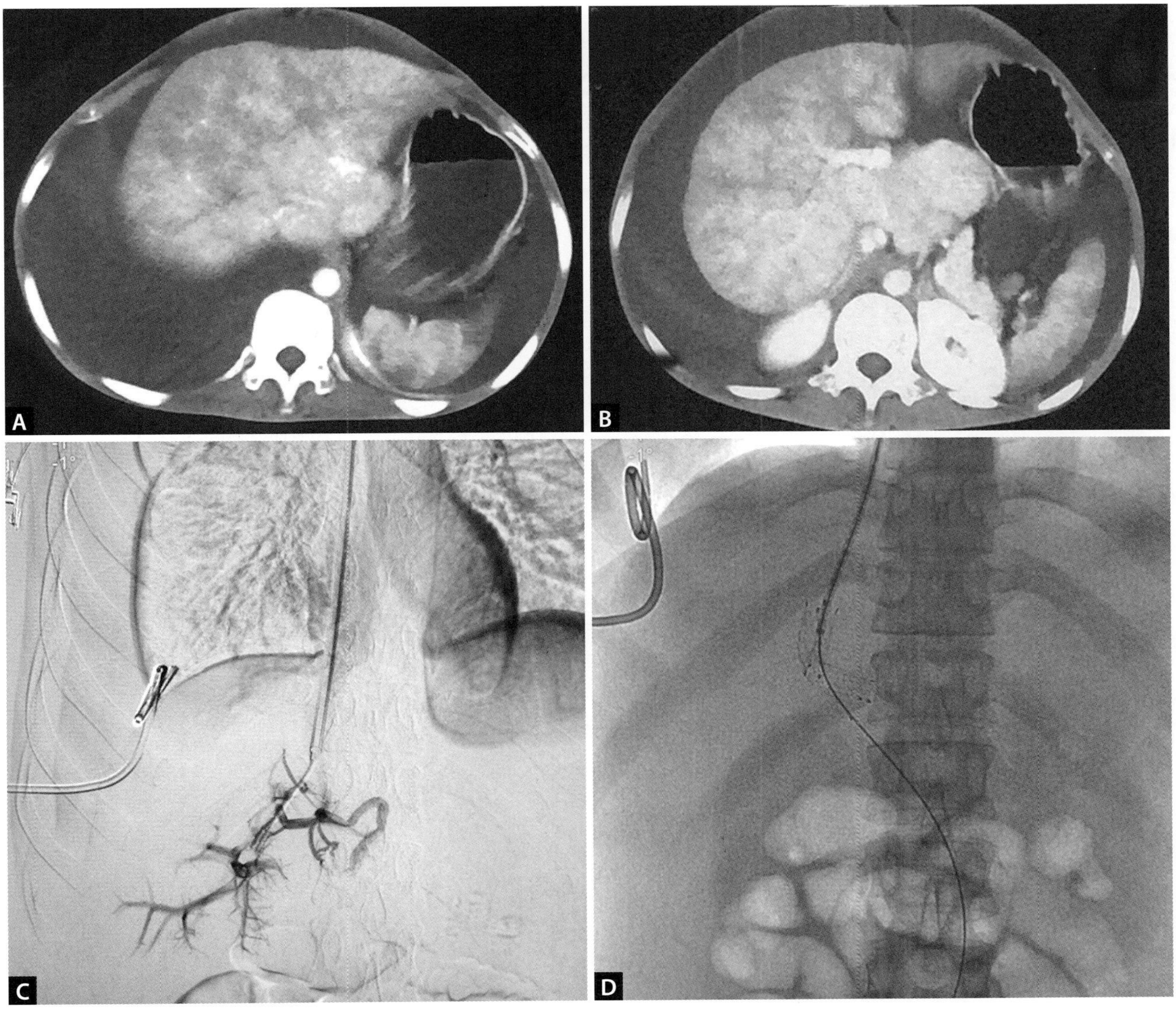

Figs. 16A to D: Contrast-enhanced CT scan showing mosaic attenuation of liver parenchyma with attenuated hepatic veins and normal caliber portal vein (A and B); there is gross ascites and right pleural effusion. Using the transjugular approach the hepatic vein stump was cannulated with a sheath. A puncture needle was advanced through the sheath and the liver parenchyma into the right branch of portal vein (C); Subsequently a calibrated pigtail catheter was advanced in the track. This was followed by balloon dilatation of the track. The stent was then placed in the track over an exchange guidewire (D).

parenchyma providing stability for the transcaval direct intrahepatic portosystemic shunt (DIPS). These shunts may be created using a transjugular approach but a combined percutaneous and transhepatic approach may also be required **(Figs. 17A to E)**. In BCS the liver parenchyma is also relatively soft unlike that in other causes of cirrhosis.[49] The primary patency rate of these shunts has also increased with the use of polytetrafluoroethylene (PTFE) covered stents. The advantages of TIPS are its minimal invasiveness and the lower mortality rate as compared with surgical shunting. In addition, intrahepatic caval stenosis can also be bypassed by using TIPS which is not possible with the surgical shunts. This essentially functions as a portoatrial shunt. The most frequent complication of TIPS is hepatic encephalopathy which can occur in up to 30% of patients but can be treated medically. Other complications include stenosis or occlusion requiring revision in about 70% of cases by 6 months, intraperitoneal bleed, liver failure and subcapsular hematomas. The 6- and 12-month patency rates were 100% and 85.7% respectively for stent graft compared with 16.7% and 0% for bare stents.[49] Surgical options are now usually reserved for patients with failed

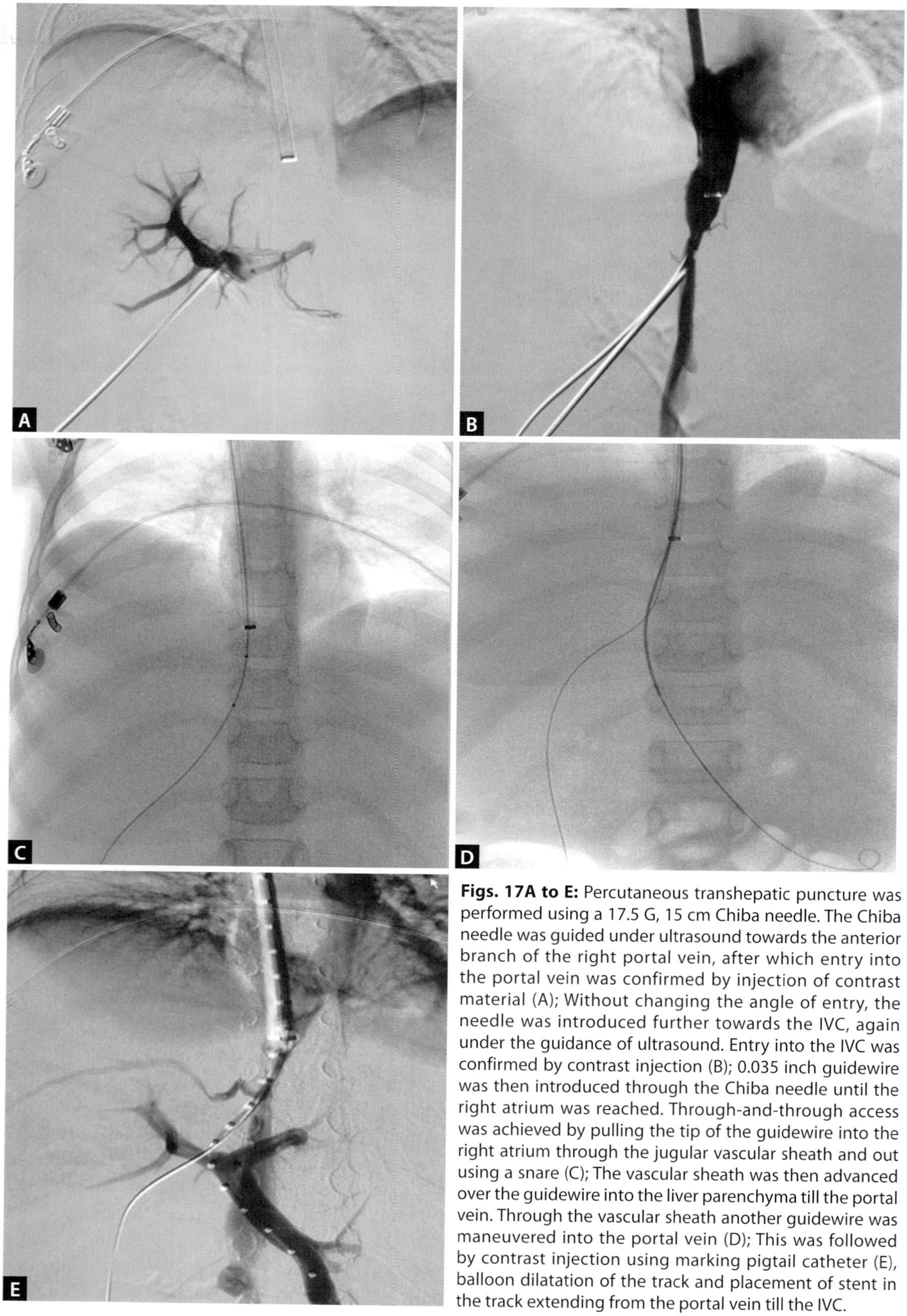

Figs. 17A to E: Percutaneous transhepatic puncture was performed using a 17.5 G, 15 cm Chiba needle. The Chiba needle was guided under ultrasound towards the anterior branch of the right portal vein, after which entry into the portal vein was confirmed by injection of contrast material (A); Without changing the angle of entry, the needle was introduced further towards the IVC, again under the guidance of ultrasound. Entry into the IVC was confirmed by contrast injection (B); 0.035 inch guidewire was then introduced through the Chiba needle until the right atrium was reached. Through-and-through access was achieved by pulling the tip of the guidewire into the right atrium through the jugular vascular sheath and out using a snare (C); The vascular sheath was then advanced over the guidewire into the liver parenchyma till the portal vein. Through the vascular sheath another guidewire was maneuvered into the portal vein (D); This was followed by contrast injection using marking pigtail catheter (E), balloon dilatation of the track and placement of stent in the track extending from the portal vein till the IVC.

radiological interventions. Some studies have suggested that an early use of TIPS in selected cases may have a survival advantage.[50,51] However, a study from India found that angioplasty and not TIPS, is of utility to the majority of BCS patients. The authors also reported that Child class and response to interventional treatment are important predictors of survival in BCS patients.[52]

It is imperative after any radiological intervention in BCS to continue long-term anticoagulant therapy in order to maintain the INR (international normalized ratio) around 2.5.[40,53] It is also important to have a regular three monthly follow-up in the first year using color Doppler. Subsequently the patients may be kept on a six monthly follow-up regimen.

The first liver transplant for BCS was performed in 1974. Liver transplantation is indicated for patients with fulminant hepatic failure, those who deteriorate after shunt procedure and in cirrhotics with end stage disease. In fact orthotopic liver transplantation is considered the only curative treatment for BCS.[43] Significant fibrosis and cirrhosis on liver biopsy with poor hepatocellular reserve can only be managed by transplantation. It is a useful option in patients with a hereditary thrombophilia state such as protein C, protein S, and antithrombin III deficiency which can be corrected with liver replacement. Ten-year survival rates up to 75% have been reported after liver transplantation.[27,54]

REFERENCES

1. Ferral H, Behrens G, Lopera J. Budd-Chiari syndrome. AJR. 2012;199;737-45.
2. Patil P, Deshmukh H, Popat B, et al. Spectrum of imaging in Budd-Chiari syndrome. J Med Imaging Radiat Oncol. 2012;56:75-83.
3. Mulholland JP, Fong SM, Kafaghi FA, et al. Budd-Chiari syndrome: Diagnosis with ultrasound and nuclear medicine calcium colloid liver scan following nondiagnostic contrast CT scan. Australas Radiol. 1997;41:53-6.
4. Sharma V, Aggarwal A, Singla R, et al. Giant Hemangioma causing Budd-Chiari syndrome. Journal of Clinical and Experimental Hepatology. 2014;4:380-1.
5. Mahmoud A, Elias E. Advances in hepatology—new approaches to the Budd-Chiari syndrome. J Gastroenterol Hepatol. 1996;11:1121-3.
6. Eapen CE, Mammen T, Moses V, et al. Changing profile of Budd-Chiari syndrome in India. Indian J Gastroenterol. 2007;26:77-81.
7. Vilgrain V, Lewin M, Vons C, et al. Hepatic nodules in Budd-Chiari syndrome: imaging features. Radiology. 1999;210:443-50.
8. Arora A, Sharma MP. Recent trends in the diagnosis and treatment of Budd-Chiari syndrome. J Assoc Physicians India. 1992;40:533-6.
9. Floyd JL. The radiographic gamut of Budd-Chiari syndrome. Am J Gastroenterol. 1981;76:381-7.
10. Menu Y, Alision D, Lorphelin JM, et al. Budd-Chiari syndrome: US evaluation. Radiology. 1985;157:761-4.
11. Powell-Jackson PR, Karani J, Ede RJ, et al. Ultrasound scanning and 99mTc sulphur colloid scintigraphy in diagnosis of Budd-Chiari syndrome. Gut. 1986;27:1502-6.
12. Chawla Y, Kumar S, Dhiman RK, et al. Various imaging diagnostics in Budd-Chiari syndrome, liver cirrhosis and carcinoma-Duplex Doppler sonography in patients with Budd-Chiari syndrome. J Gastroenterol Hepatol. 1999;14:904-7.
13. Makuuchi M, Hasegewa H, Yamazaki S, et al. Primary Budd-Chiari syndrome: ultrasonic demonstration. Radiology. 1984;152:775-9.
14. Musa Aydini, Yusuf Bayraktar. Budd-Chiari syndrome: etiology, pathogenesis and diagnosis. World J Gastroenterol. 2007;13(19):2693-6.
15. Lupescu IG, Dobromir C, Popa GA, et al. Spiral computed tomography and magnetic resonance angiography evaluation in Budd-Chiari syndrome. J Gastrointestin Liver Dis. 2008;17:223-6.
16. Bargallo X, Gilabert R, Nicolau C, et al. Sonography of the caudate vein: value in diagnosing Budd-Chiari syndrome. Am J Roentgenol. 2003;181:1641-5.
17. Noone TC, Semelka RC, Siegelman ES, et al. Budd-Chiari syndrome: spectrum of appearances of acute, subacute and chronic disease with magnetic resonance imaging. J Magn Reson Imaging. 2000;11:44-50.
18. XU K, Ren K, Chen Y, et al. Application and evaluation of non-invasive examination for Budd-Chiari syndrome. Chinese Medical Journal. 2007;120:91-4.
19. Ohta M, Hashizume M, Tomikawa M, et al. Analysis of hepatic vein waveform by Doppler ultrasonography in 100 patients with portal hypertension. Am J Gastroenterol. 1995;89:170-5.
20. Kane R, Eustace S. Diagnosis of Budd-Chiari syndrome: comparison between sonography and MR angiography. Radiology. 1995;195:117-21.
21. Kamath PS. Budd-Chiari syndrome: Radiologic findings. Liver Transplantation. 2006;12:S21-2.
22. Brancatelli G, Vilgrain V, Federle MP, et al. Budd-Chiari syndrome: spectrum of imaging findings. Am J Roentgenol. 2007;188:W168-76.
23. Datta DV, Saha S, Singh SA, et al. Chronic Budd-Chiari syndrome due to obstruction of the intrahepatic portion of the inferior vena cava. Gut. 1972;13:372-8.
24. Dilawari JB, Bambery P, Chawla Y, et al. Hepatic outflow obstruction (Budd-Chiari syndrome)—Experience with 177 patients and a review of the literature. Medicine (Baltimore). 1984;73:21-36.
25. Kage M, Arakawa M, Kojiro M, et al. Histopathology of membranous obstruction of the inferior vena cava in the Budd-Chiari syndrome. Gastroenterology. 1992;102:2081-90.
26. Bolondi L, Gaiani S, Li Bassi S, et al. Diagnosis of Budd-Chiari syndrome by pulsed Doppler ultrasound. Gastroenterology. 1991;100:1324-31.

27. Valla DC. Hepatic vein thrombosis (Budd-Chiari syndrome). Semin Liver Dis. 2002;22:5-14.
28. Cho OK, Koo JH, Kim YS, et al. Collateral pathways in Budd-Chiari syndrome. CT and venographic correlation. Am J Roentgenol. 1996;167:1163-7.
29. Clain D, Freston J, Kreel L, et al. Clinical diagnosis of Budd-Chiari syndrome. A report of six cases. Am J Med. 1967;43:544-54.
30. Janssen HL, Garcia-Pagan JC, Elias E, et al. Budd-Chiari syndrome: review by an expert panel. J Hepatol. 2003;38:364-71.
31. Maetani Y, Itoh K, Egawa H, et al. Benign hepatic nodules in Budd-Chiari syndrome. Radiologic-pathologic correlation with emphasis on the central scar. Am J Roentgenol. 2002;178:869-75.
32. Tanju S, Erden A, Ceyhan K, et al. Contrast-enhanced MR angiography of benign regenerative nodules following TIPS shunt procedure in Budd-Chiari syndrome. Turk J Gastroenterol. 2004;15:173-7.
33. Brancatelli G, Federle MP, Grazioli L, et al. Benign regenerative nodules in Budd-Chiari syndrome and other vascular disorders of the liver: radiologic-pathologic and clinical correlation. Radiographics. 2002;22:847-62.
34. Brancatelli G, Federle MP, Grazioli L, et al. Large regenerative nodules in Budd-Chiari syndrome and other vascular disorders of the liver: CT and MR imaging findings with clinicopatholgic correlation. Am J Roentgenol. 2002;178:77-883.
35. Cazals-Hatem D, Vilgrain V, Genin P, et al. Arterial and portal circulation and parenchymal changes in Budd-Chiari syndrome: a study in 17 explanted livers. Hepatology. 2003;37:510-9.
36. Valla DC. Prognosis in Budd-Chiari syndrome after reestablishing hepatic venous drainage. Gut. 2006;55:761-3.
37. Artia T, Matsunaga N, Kobayashi H. Budd-Chiari syndrome: Peripheral abnormal intensity of the liver on magnetic resonance imaging. Clin Radiol. 2000;55:640-2.
38. Camera L, Mainenti PP, Di Giacomo A, et al. Triphasic helical CT in Budd-Chiari syndrome: patterns of enhancement in acute, subacute and chronic disease. Clin Radiol. 2006;61:331-7.
39. Kalra N, Virmani V, Singh P, et al. Imaging of Budd-Chiari syndrome (electronic exhibit presented at the 109th Annual Meeting of the American Roentgen Ray Society, 2009 at Boston, USA).
40. Mukund A, Gamangatti S. Imaging and interventions in Budd-Chiari syndrome. World J Radiol. 2011;28:169-77.
41. Eguchi S, Takeuchi Y, Asano K. Successful balloon membranotomy for obstruction of the hepatic portion of the inferior vena cava. Surgery. 1974;76:837-40.
42. Griffith JF, Mahmoud AEA, Cooper S, et al. Radiological intervention in Budd-Chiari syndrome: techniques and outcome in 18 patients. Clin Radiol. 1996;51:775-84.
43. Lopez RR, Benner KG, Hall L, et al. Expandable venous stents for the treatment of the Budd-Chiari syndrome. Gastroenterology. 1991;100:1435-41.
44. Pisani-Ceretti A, Intra M, Prestipino F, et al. Surgical and radiologic treatment of primary Budd-Chiari syndrome. World J Surg. 1998;22:48-53.
45. Baijjal SS, Roy S, Phadke RV, et al. Management of idiopathic Budd-Chiari syndrome with primary stent placement: early results. J Vasc Interv Radiol. 1996;7:545-53.
46. Orloff MJ, Orloff MS, Daily PO. Long-term results of treatment of Budd-Chiari syndrome with portal decompression. Arch Surg. 1992;127:1182-7.
47. Peltzer MY, Ring EJ, LaBerge JM. Treatment of Budd-Chiari syndrome with a transjugular intrahepatic portosystemic shunt. J Vasc Interv Radiol. 1993;4:263-7.
48. Ochs A, Sellinger M, Haag K, et al. Transjugular intrahepatic portosystemic stent shunt (TIPS) in the treatment of Budd-Chiari syndrome. J Hepatol. 1993;18:217-25.
49. Gandini R, Konda D, Simonetti G. Transjugular intrahepatic portosystemic shunt patency and clinical outcome in patients with Budd-Chiari syndrome: covered versus uncovered stents. Radiology. 2006;241:298-305.
50. Liu L, Qi XS, Zhao Y, et al. Budd-chiari syndrome: current perspectives and controversies. Eur Rev Med Pharmacol Sci. 2016;20:3273-81.
51. Mancuso A. Budd-Chiari syndrome management: timing of treatment is an open issue. Hepatology. 2014;59:1213.
52. Shalimar, Kumar A, Kedia S, et al. Hepatic venous outflow tract obstruction: treatment outcomes and development of a new prognostic score. Aliment Pharmacol Ther. 2016;43:1154-67.
53. Faraoun SA, Boudjella Mel A, Debzi N. et al. Budd-Chiari syndrome: an update on imaging. Clin Imaging. 2016;40:637-46.
54. Mentha G, Giostra E, Majno PE, et al. Liver transplantation for Budd-Chiari syndrome: a European study on 248 patients from 51 centres. J Hepatol. 2006;44:520-28.

CHAPTER 83

Imaging Approach to Obstructive Biliopathy

Anjali Prakash, Rashmi Dixit

Imaging a patient with jaundice is done primarily to rule out obstruction of the bile ducts. This can be due to a block at any level, the hilar/perihilar level or at the low/mid duct level. The causes can be malignant, mainly due to pancreatic carcinoma, cholangiocarcinoma, metastasis, and gallbladder carcinoma. Among the benign cause of obstruction choledocolithiasis is the most common.

In a majority of patients, clinical findings such as age, pain, systemic symptoms such as itching, and biochemistry determines the type of jaundice. Breakdown of hemoglobin leads to formation of bilirubin which is conjugated in liver to form a water soluble compound, which is excreted in urine as urobilinogen. Presence of urobilinogen points to jaundice having a posthepatic cause or mechanical obstruction.

Imaging in a patient with obstructive biliopathy is required to answer the following questions, apart from documenting the presence of obstruction:

- Where is the obstruction? What is the anatomical level of obstruction?
- What is the cause of obstruction?
- If the cause is malignant, is it resectable? If unresectable, to decide the suitable route for palliative stenting.

IMAGING MODALITIES

Ultrasound

This is the initial modality to be used in a patient who presents with jaundice. It is cheap, noninvasive, easily available, does not use radiation, and dynamic evaluation is possible.

Dilated intrahepatic ducts are the imaging hallmark in a patient of obstructive jaundice. The bile ducts are seen as tubular structures adjacent to the portal vessels. The right and left ducts are routinely visualized at sonography **(Fig. 1)**. The intrahepatic ducts measure 2–3 mm centrally, the detection of the more peripheral intrahepatic ducts is seen with obstructive biliopathy **(Figs. 2A and B)**. The normal caliber of the common hepatic duct is considered up to 6 mm, in patients without history of biliary disease. There is an increase in diameter with increasing age and after cholecystectomy reaching up to 10 mm, however a ductal diameter of 7 mm or above is suspicious for

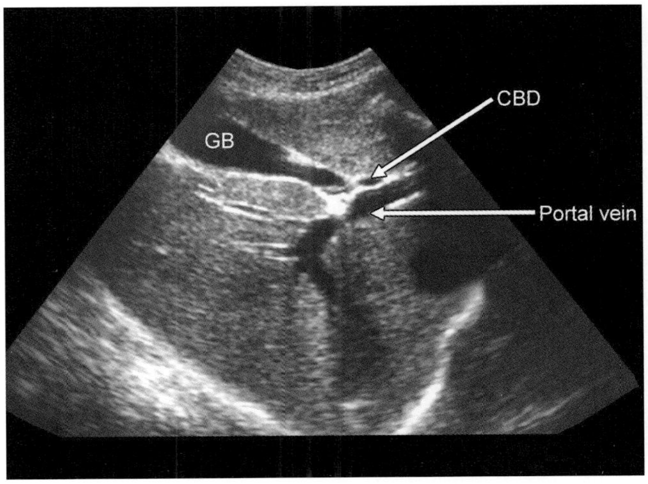

Fig. 1: Ultrasound of right hypochondrium-subcostal view-normal common bile duct (CBD) anterior to the portal vein.
Abbreviation: GB: Gallbladder

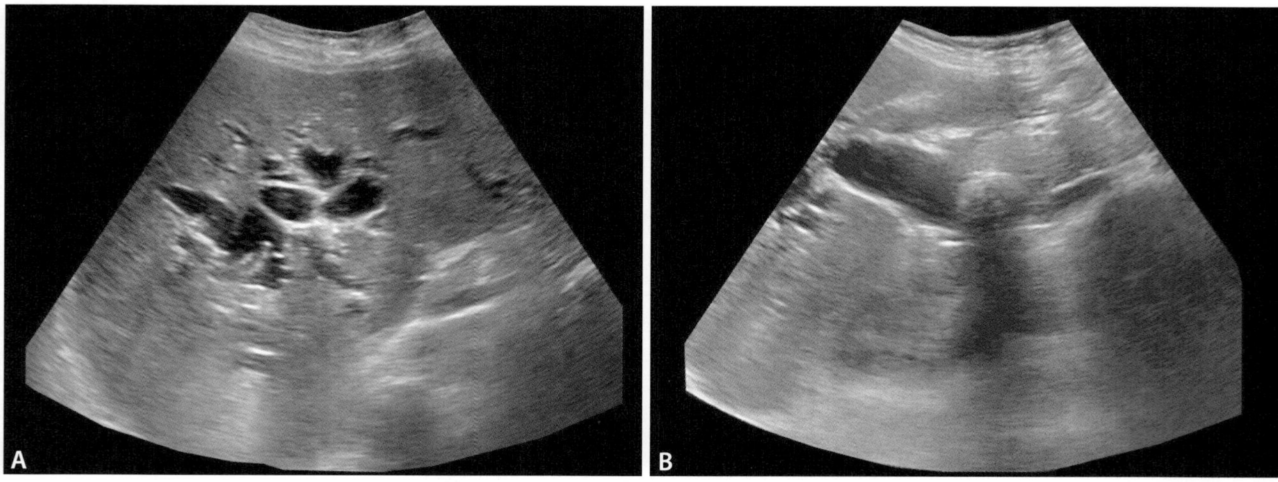

Figs. 2A and B: Ultrasound—dilated intrahepatic biliary radicals (A) in a case of choledocholithiasis (B), a large calculus is seen in common bile duct with distal shadowing.

obstruction and warrants a search for the cause.[1,2] In patients with history of cholecystectomy, a duct diameter of <4 mm has a high negative predictive value for choledocolithiasis.

In a majority of patients with obstructive biliopathy, bile duct dilatation will be seen on imaging. However, in a small percentage, there may be an obstruction without biliary duct dilatation. This may be seen in patients of choledocolithiasis, postoperative stricturing and sclerosing cholangitis. There is a time lag of 4–5 days after obstruction for the intrahepatic ducts to dilate after extrahepatic obstruction.[3] A dilated duct can be seen after passage of calculus. Not all dilated ducts imply obstruction, as in cases of choledochal cyst there is dilatation of duct but no obstruction.

The ultrasound technique should include (apart from a routine scan), a subcostal view in suspended inspiration; proximal common bile duct and porta hepatis are best seen on a subcostal view whereas distal common bile duct is best evaluated by using the epigastric window. An impacted calculus can be detected by slight rotation of the transducer. Ultrasound has certain limitations. Excessive bowel gas and body habitus may hamper visualization of the biliary system. The technique may be optimized[4] by:

- *Changing the patient position*: This will alter relative position of the bowel gas.
- *Compression of epigastrium*: This may displace bowel loops.
- Changing the sonographic window and the use of water in stomach and duodenum to provide an acoustic window may be used.
- Harmonic imaging increases the contrast between duct and the liver parenchyma with enhanced visualization of the lumen, wall and contents of the duct.

The reported sensitivity of ultrasound in defining the level of obstruction and cause ranges from 27% to 95% and from 23% to 88% respectively.[4,5] This wide variation underlines the fact that ultrasound is an operator-dependent modality.

Computed Tomography

Computed tomography (CT) is the imaging modality of choice in imaging a patient of obstructive jaundice, when a pancreaticobiliary malignancy is suspected.

The CT for a patient of obstructive jaundice should be a multiphasic study tailored to the clinical scenario and the ultrasound. It includes a late arterial phase, pancreatic phase at 45 seconds (whenever a pancreatic pathology is suspected), portal venous phase, and a delayed phase.

The CT helps to differentiate malignant from benign stricture. The zone of transition from a dilated to nondilated or non visualized duct provides the clue for the cause. Abrupt termination of the bile duct is a sign of malignancy whereas a gradually tapering duct indicates a benign process. Focal eccentric wall thickening of bile duct prior to obstruction is a sign of cholangiocarcinoma. There can be an associated mass lesion **(Figs. 3 to 6)**. Hyperenhancement of bile duct wall may be seen in both benign and malignant obstruction.[6]

In malignant obstruction, imaging has to determine resectability. In malignant hilar block, the proximal extent, i.e. extension into left/right hepatic ducts

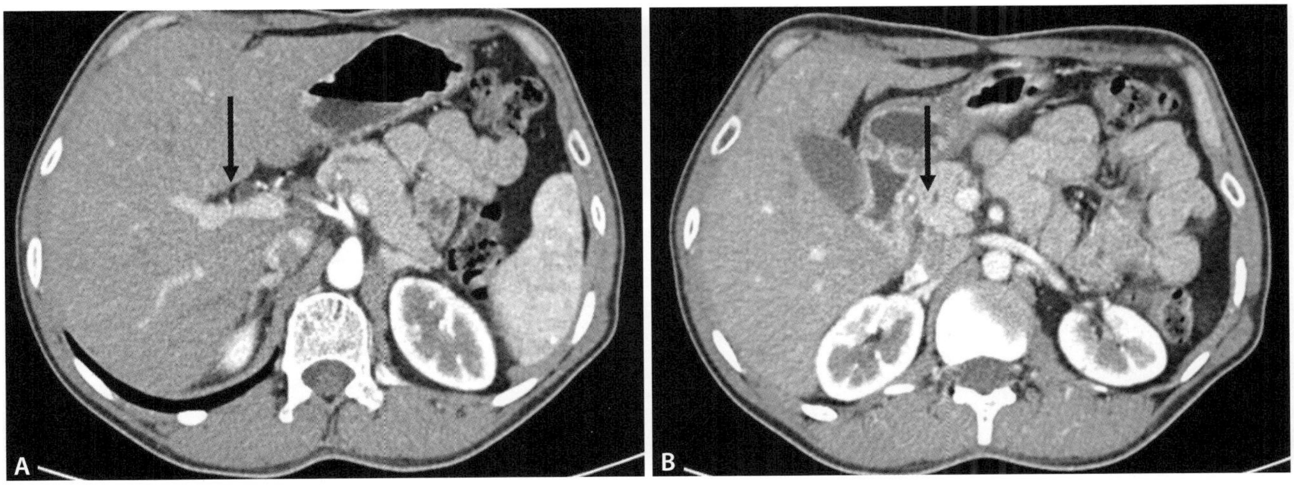

Figs. 3A and B: CT upper abdomen—normal caliber of CBD at porta hepatis (A), in the intrapancreatic part (B).

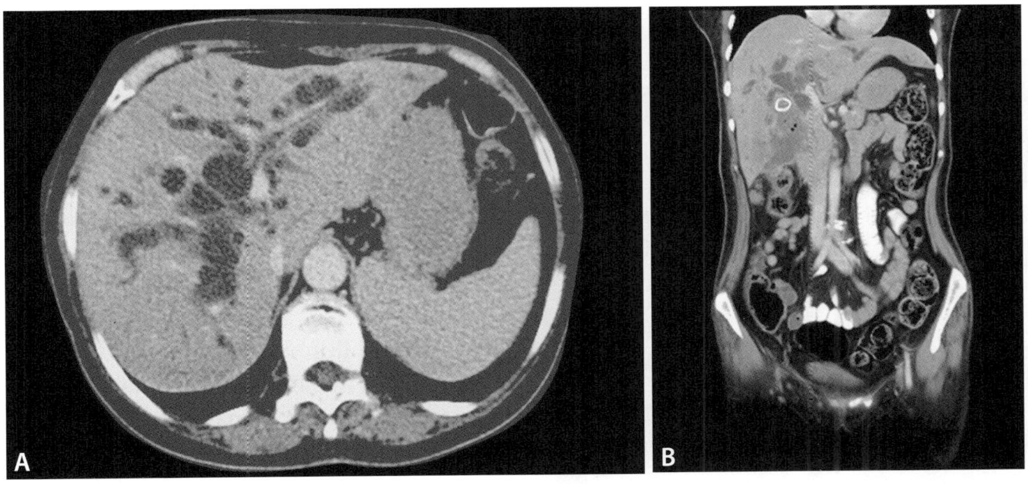

Figs. 4A and B: CT upper abdomen—axial (A) and coronal reformat (B). Intrahepatic biliary ductal dilation with a mass in the gallbladder fossa with cholelithiasis—a case of gallbladder malignancy.

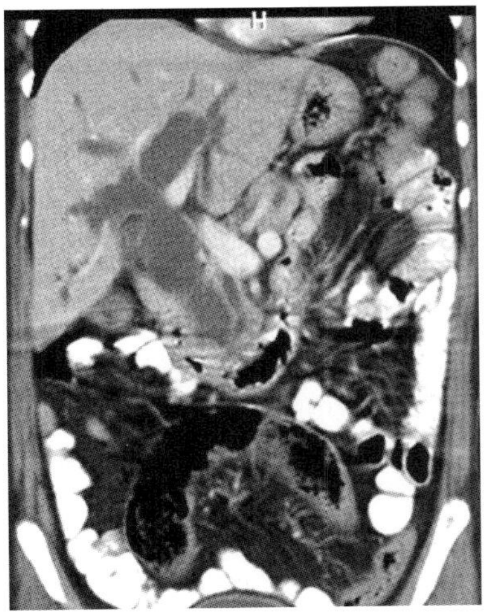

Fig. 5: CT coronal MPR—double duct sign—dilatation of both common bile duct and pancreatic duct in a case of carcinoma head of pancreas.

according to Bismuth classification, patency of portal veins, presence of secondaries needs to be evaluated. In malignant low obstruction due to periampullary or pancreatic carcinoma, the factors to be evaluated are the tumor size, vascular involvement, lymph node and hepatic metastasis. A meta-analysis has shown that CT has a higher accuracy than ultrasound and magnetic resonance imaging (MRI) in the diagnosis and in the determination of resectability of pancreatic cancer. CT does not have similar accuracy in assessing resectability of cholangiocarcinomas, it is limited in its ability in detecting small peritoneal deposits, secondaries in normal sized nodes and the intraductal extent of tumor.[7]

The CT may detect biliary calculi, if they are partially calcified or have bilirubinate in a sufficient quantity to

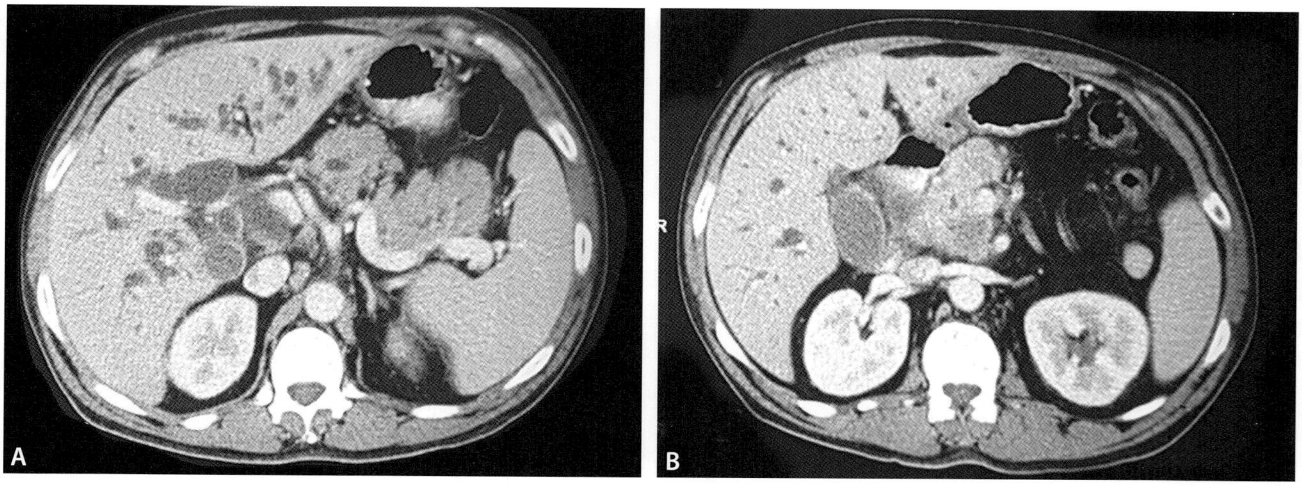

Figs. 6A and B: CECT abdomen-dilatation of intrahepatic duct (A), Common bite duct due to a hypoenhancing mass in head of pancreas (B).

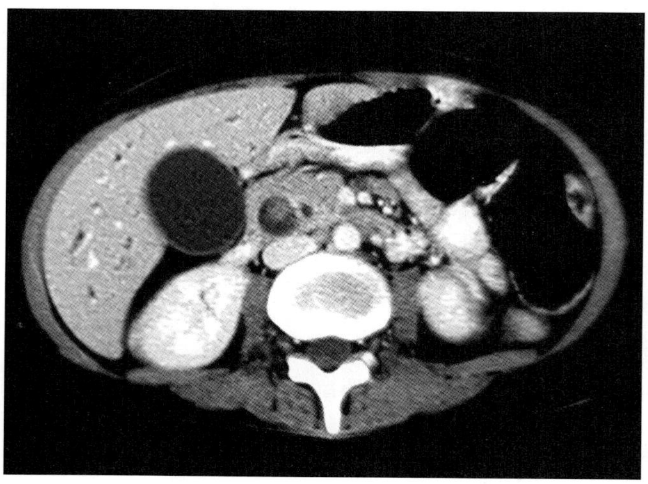

Fig. 7: CECT abdomen-calculus noted in common bile duct with upstream dilatation.

render them hyperattenuating **(Fig. 7)**. CT is insensitive to cholesterol calculi. Biliary stones are usually seen as soft tissue density or a ring like density surrounded by lower density bile. In cases of suspected biliary calculus, noncontrast CT is to be done as contrast may obscure the calculus. Thin sections with a collimation <2.5 mm and tube kvp at 140 kv may help in demonstrating biliary calculi. CT is not the preferred modality for detection of biliary calculi.

Computed tomography has a reported sensitivity of 96–100% in detection of obstruction and level of obstruction is identified in nearly all cases whereas cause is identified in 70%.[8] The drawback of CT is the use of radiation and the need for IV contrast.

COMPUTED TOMOGRAPHY INTRAVENOUS CHOLANGIOGRAPHY

This investigation was used to study the biliary ductal system. There is very limited availability of the contrast (available in a few countries only, not available in India) and as the contrast has certain amount of toxicity, the examination has limited indications, in some cases of live hepatic donation for transplantation, to evaluate biliary anatomy. Certain variants of biliary anatomy are contraindications in hepatic transplant.

Intravenous contrast that is preferentially excreted by liver is given by slow infusion followed by CT after 30 minutes. Opacification of bile ducts is noted. The contrast used is Meglumine iotroxate (Biliscopin™) which has a better safety profile, than other IV biliary agents. The technique requires normal liver function and fails in patients with elevated bilirubin levels. CT intravenous cholangiography (CT-IVC) is a functional study as there is excretion and passage of contrast into the bile ducts.[9,10]

Magnetic Resonance Cholangiopancreatography

Magnetic resonance imaging (MRI) and magnetic resonance cholangiopancreatography (MRCP) have emerged as a primary imaging modality for evaluating the biliary ducts and the pancreatic duct. The examination can be done in jaundiced patients unlike CT-IVC. Contrast material is not routinely required and there is no sedation required. It is the preferred modality in pregnant patients with suspected hepatobiliary disease as there is no radiation exposure.

The two most commonly used sequences are T2-weighted turbo spin echo sequence and 2D single shot fast spin echo (SSFSE). 3D respiratory triggered fast spin echo provides greater details with 3-4 minutes acquisition. Luminal abnormalities are better evaluated with thin slab images. Biliary calculi appear as signal void areas, irrespective of their chemical composition **(Figs. 8 and 9)**. The sensitivity of MRCP in detection of calculi is dependent on the size of the calculus. Sensitivity for small stones, i.e. <3 mm is less than 50%, this increases to 67–100% with calculi >10 mm in size.[11,12] A bile duct filled with calculi may also look like a stricture. Interpreting 3D maximum intensity projection (MIP) images alone without interpreting 2D acquisition may lead to overlooking of small calculi due to superimposition effects on MIP images.

Artefacts due to MR technique or in postprocessing may mimic pathology.Surgical clips or pneumobilia may look like a signal void. Indention by an adjacent artery; usually the right hepatic artery may mimic a stricture. All signal voids should be seen in at least two orthogonal planes for a confident diagnosis of calculus.

Sensitivity of MRI in differentiating benign and malignant stricture varies between studies (30–98%).[13,14] Malignant strictures are long due to infiltrative pattern of growth, irregular with asymmetric dilatation of the biliary radicals and there may be presence of a mass **(Fig. 10)**. Benign strictures are short in length, show gradual smooth tapering with a regular border.

The sensitivity decreases in patients with history of cholangitis or biliary intervention as inflammatory soft

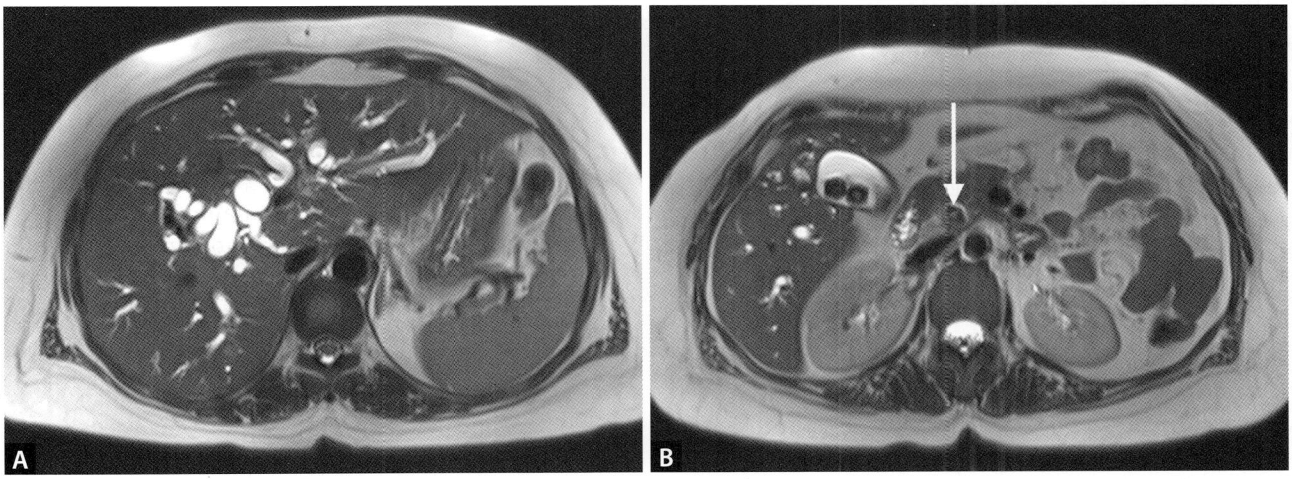

Figs. 8A and B: MRI-TRUE FISP sequence—dilated intrahepatic biliary radicals (A) in a case of cholelithiasis with choledocholithiasis. A large calculus is seen in common bile duct as a signal void (arrow marked in B).

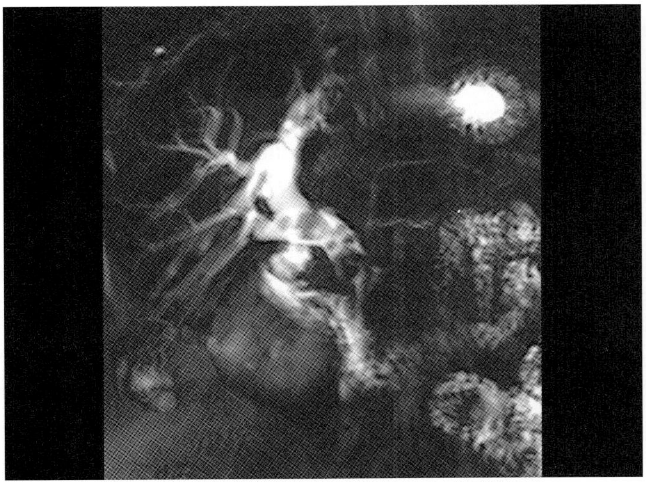

Fig. 9: MRCP-HASTE thick slab coronal—multiple calculi seen as signal voids in the common bile duct with dilatation of CBD and the intrahepatic bile ducts.

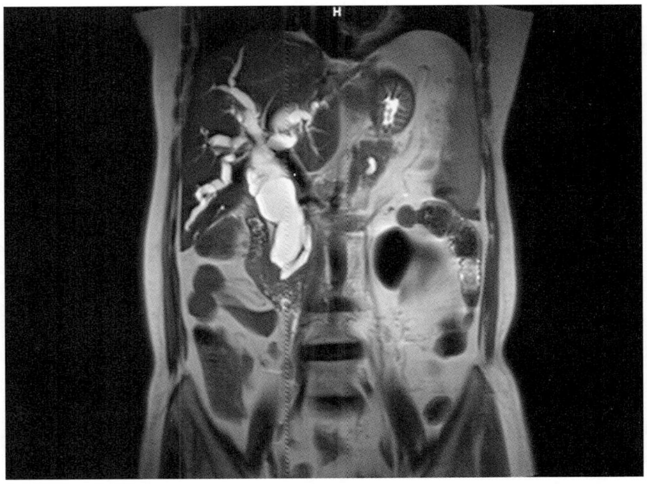

Fig. 10: MRI-T2W coronal image-dilatation of both common bile ducts, pancreatic duct in a case of pancreatic carcinoma.

tissue may mimic a mass. MRI and MRCP has a higher sensitivity than CT in determining nature of hilar stricture. Lesions at the ampulla may however, be missed.

The MRCP has an advantage over endoscopic retrograde cholangiopancreatography (ERCP) that it demonstrates biliary ducts above the level of stricture, which ERCP cannot. This can help guide a planned management with ERCP. MRCP is useful in patients with biliary enteric reconstructions. However, no functional information is provided and it has an inferior resolution to ERCP. The biggest drawback is that no therapeutic intervention is possible.

The MRCP has a reported accuracy of 96–100% for level and 90% for cause of obstruction.[13,14]

CONTRAST-ENHANCED MAGNETIC RESONANCE CHOLANGIOGRAPHY

T1W imaging is done after intravenous (IV) administration of contrast gadolinium ethoxybenzyl diethylenetriamine penta-acetic acid-Gd-EOB-DTPA/Gadobenate disodium. Imaging is done in the hepatobiliary phase. Thin sections are obtained to generate MIP images. The study fails in cases of raised serum bilirubin as there is poor excretion of contrast. This is used in cases of biliary leaks and choledochal cysts.

ENDOSCOPIC ULTRASOUND

This is performed by combined endoscopy and ultrasound. Endoscopes are introduced via transgastric or transduodenal route and using a water balloon system for acoustic coupling. The frequency range is between 7.5 MHz and 12 MHz, with a depth of penetration of 8–10 cm.

Endoscopic ultrasound (EUS) does not use radiation, unlike ERCP, is less invasive, can diagnose most causes of obstructive jaundice, and provide tissue sampling. However, EUS is not easily available, there is operator dependence. Presence of surgical clips, stents and aerobilia may hamper visualization. The most important drawback is that therapeutic option is not possible at the same time unlike in ERCP.

Endoscopic ultrasound is useful in detecting small biliary calculi, especially within non dilated ducts. It is equal to MRCP/ERCP in detection of calculi.

The EUS is used in the detection of pancreaticobiliary malignancies and in obtaining biopsy. It has a higher sensitivity than all other imaging modalities in the diagnosis of pancreatic tumors. This is especially useful in small (<3 cm) pancreatic tumors, those that will benefit from surgical resection. EUS has a reported sensitivity of 92% in T stage and 82% for N staging in pancreatic malignancy.[15] EUS is more accurate than CT and angiography in detecting invasion of portal vein, splenic vein and of the confluence. It has a similar sensitivity as dual phase CT in detection of pancreatic malignancy; however it is better in lesions less than 15 mm in size. These are the lesions most amenable to surgical resection.

The EUS has a sensitivity of 97% and a specificity of 88% in determining the cause of extrahepatic obstruction.[14,15]

FUNCTIONAL IMAGING

Scintigraphy-99mTc hydroxyiminodiacetic acid (HIDA) is the radiotracer used as it is excreted in bile. It is not a sensitive modality in assessing the level or cause of obstruction. The tracer may not be excreted in patients with high bilirubin level. This is not routinely used as MRCP/CT have higher resolution and provide comprehensive evaluation.

DIRECT CHOLANGIOGRAPHY

This includes endoscopic retrograde cholangiopancreatography and percutaneous transhepatic cholangiogram. Both investigations are invasive. There is a reported sensitivity of 100% in the detection of obstruction; these remain the gold standard for the evaluation and of biliary leaks and for subtle luminal changes. However, no extraluminal information can be obtained with either.

The ERCP is done after cannulation of the ampulla after a duodenoscope is introduced. Contrast is introduced in both biliary and pancreatic ducts. ERCP has a sensitivity of 90–96% and specificity of 98% in the detection of calculi.[14,16] There is reduced sensitivity in detection of small stones in a dilated bile duct. Air bubbles may be misinterpreted as calculi.Treatment in the form of sphincterotomy, balloon and basket removal of stones can be done via the same route.

The ERCP has a definite role in diagnosis and management of pancreaticobiliary tumors. Long strictures, with irregular margins, asymmetric dilatation and presence of mass point towards a malignant stricture.

Endoscopic tissue sampling like brush cytology, fine needle aspiration and forceps biopsy are available, with nearly 100% specificity though with moderate sensitivity (20–60%). Palliation of malignant obstruction can be done using a plastic or metal stent.

The ERCP carries significant morbidity (10%-pancreatitis) and a 0.4% mortality. The other drawbacks include cost of equipment, availability of trained personnel, need for conscious sedation. It is not possible to visualize ducts proximal to the obstruction. ERCP is now used for treatment and not for primary diagnosis.

Percutaneous Transhepatic Cholangiography

This has been almost completely replaced by MRCP/ERCP and is now used in transhepatic biliary intervention as a route for biliary decompression. The liver is punctured with a 22 gauge Chiba needle to enter an intrahepatic biliary duct after checking the coagulation profile. Contrast is then injected to opacify the biliary system and visualize the site of obstruction. The success of this procedure is dependent on the ducts being dilated, being almost 100% when the ducts are dilated and 75% in a nondilated system.[17,18]

The reported complication rate is <5%, and these are biliary leaks, bile peritonitis, hemobilia, sepsis, etc. PTC is reserved for patients with failed ERCP or to provide palliation in unresectable hilar tumors.

PET-CT

The index SUV (standardized uptake value) max, that measures glucose uptake shows a significant difference of value between benign and malignant causes of obstructive jaundice. Pancreatic cancer has a high uptake of the tracer, however tumors like infiltrating cholangiocarcinoma show low uptake. Combining PET with conventional imaging like CT, MRI increases the sensitivity and accuracy when compared with conventional imaging alone.[19]

INTRADUCTAL ULTRASOUND

This is done using a flexible, thin (2 mm) probe which is introduced via the endoscope into the pancreatic and biliary duct. The ducts are filled with fluid to provide acoustic coupling. The frequencies range from 12 MHz to 30 MHz providing high resolution but limited penetration. It is superior to EUS in evaluation of proximal biliary ducts. Intraductal ultrasound (IDUS) increases ability of ERCP in distinguishing benign from malignant cause of obstruction. A sessile tumor, size of tumor >10 mm and interrupted wall structure on IDUS favour malignancy. Heterogeneous and irregular bile duct thickening and invasion of vessels is seen in malignant obstruction. Lack of availability, operator expertise, low penetration remain a drawback.

IMAGING ALGORITHM IN OBSTRUCTIVE JAUNDICE

The American College of Radiology (ACR) has categorized patients with jaundice into three categories:[14]

1. High likelihood of mechanical obstruction. This has been further subdivided into benign and malignant obstruction
2. Low likelihood of obstruction
3. Intermediate likelihood.

The ACR has further suggested the most appropriate imaging modality in each scenario and ranked them on a scale of 0–10 with the most appropriate being.[10]

Imaging in a case of obstructive jaundice starts with transabdominal ultrasound. Once biliary dilatation is seen then the anatomical level of obstruction is to be determined. The differential diagnosis would be based on this and will guide further investigations **(Flowcharts 1 to 3)**.

In patients where choledocolithiasis is detected on ultrasound, ERCP is the next modality which is used for stone extraction. MRCP may be used to provide a roadmap to the endoscopist.If obstruction is found on ultrasound with history of biliary colic, and no cause is found, the second test should be MRI + MRCP.

Endoscopic ultrasound is to be done in patients in whom MRCP is normal, and especially in cases of nondilated ducts. If there is no clinical suspicion of

Flowchart 1: Imaging pathway in a case of jaundice with suspected biliary colic.

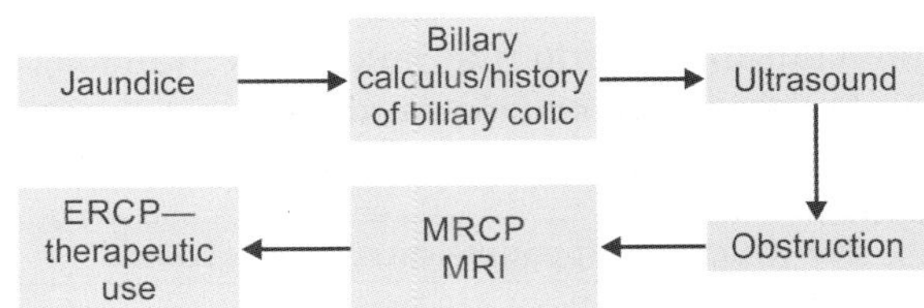

Abbreviations: MRCP: Magnetic resonance cholangiopancreatography; MRI: Magnetic resonance imaging.

Flowchart 2: Imaging pathway in a case of jaundice with suspected malignancy.

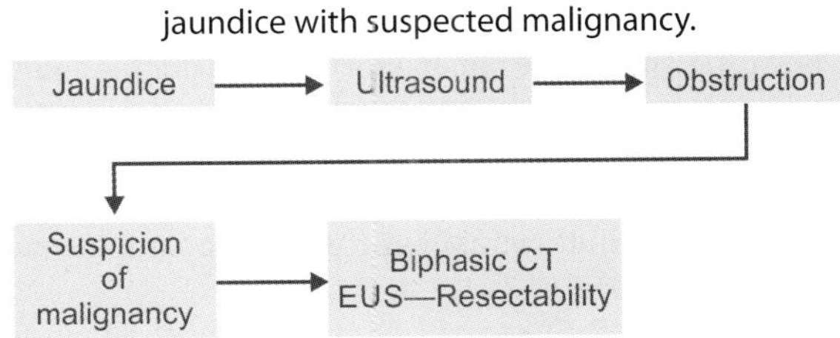

Abbreviations: CT: Computed tomography; EUS: Endoscopic ultrasound.

Flowchart 3: Imaging pathway in a case of jaundice with no features of obstruction on ultrasound.

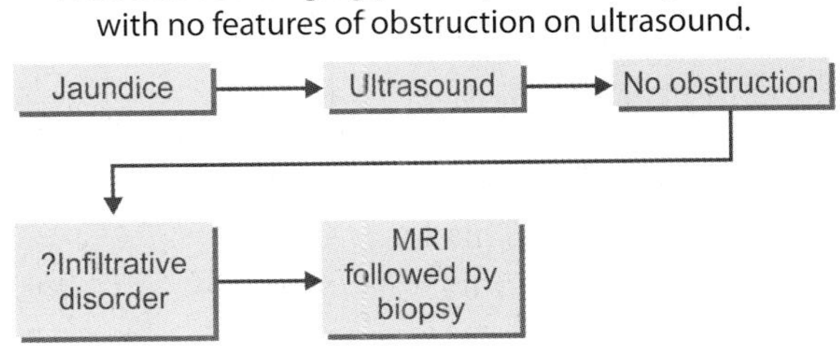

Abbreviation: MRI: Magnetic resonance imaging.

calculus or colic then ultrasound should be followed by a biphasic CT for assessing the point of obstruction, resectability and staging in cases of malignancy. EUS is also used to assess resectability by evaluating vascular involvement in cases of pancreatic head tumors and in periampullary malignancy. Image (by ultrasound and CT)-guided biopsy or fine needle aspiration can be done. In the cases where surgical resection is planned, a preoperative biopsy is not considered appropriate. In cases where palliation is being considered, biopsy is to be deferred till after decompression to prevent bile leaks. Direct cholangiography is reserved as a therapeutic option.

If no mechanical obstruction is found, an infiltrative disorder needs to be looked for on MRI, followed by biopsy.

CONCLUSION

Obstructive biliopathy is a common clinical problem. Four questions have to be addressed while imaging these patients (inset). The choice of the modality used depends on the clinical scenario, the modalities available, the local expertise, the institutional and referring physician's preference and patient criteria.

Obstructive biliopathy—imaging questions?
• Is there obstruction? • What is the level of the block? • What is the cause of obstruction? • If the cause is malignant, is it resectable?

REFERENCES

1. Bowie JD. What is the upper limit of normal for the common bile duct on ultrasound: how much do you want it to be? Am J Gastroenterol. 2000;95(4):897-900.
2. Horrow MM, Horrow JC, Niakosari A, et al. Is age associated with size of adult extrahepatic duct: Sonographic study. Radiology. 2001;221(2):411-4.
3. Rudralingam V, Sukumar SA. Imaging of the jaundiced adult. Imaging. 2013;22:51415473.
4. Turner MA, Fulcher AS. Gallbladder and biliary tract; normal anatomy and examination techniques. In: Gore RM, Levine MS (Eds). Textbook of gastrointestinal radiology, 2nd edition.Philadelpia. PA: WB Saunders; 2000.pp.1250-76.
5. Mittelstaedt CA. Ultrasound of the bile ducts. Semin Roentgenol. 1997;32:161-71.
6. Choi SH, Han JL, Lee JM, Lee KH, et al. Differentiating malignant from benign common bile duct stricture with multiphasic helical CT. Radiology. 2005;236:173-83.
7. Bipat S, Phoa SS, Van Delden OM, Bossuyat PM, et al. Ultrasonography, computed tomography and magnetic resonance imaging for diagnosis and determining resectability of pancreatic adenocarcinoma: a meta-analysis. J Comput Assist Tomogr. 2005;29:438-45.
8. Wyatt SH, Fishman EK. Biliary tract obstruction: the role of spiral CT in detection and definition of disease. Clin Imaging. 1997;21:27-34.
9. Ahmetoglu A, Kosucu P, Kul S, et al. MDCT cholangiography with volume rendering for the assessment of patients with biliary obstruction. AJR. 2004;183:1327-32.
10. Hyodo T, Kumano S, Kushihata F, Okada M, et al. CT and MR cholangiography: advantages and pitfalls in perioperative evaluation of biliary tree. Br J Radiol. 2012;85(1015):887-96.
11. Ishizaki Y, Wakayama T, Okada Y, Kobayashi T. Magnetic resonance cholangiography for evaluation of obstructive jaundice. Am J Gastroenterol. 1993;12:2072-7.
12. Kim JH, Kim MJ, Park SI, Chung JJ, Song SY, et al. Using kinematic MR cholangiopancreatography to evaluate biliary dilatation. AJR. 2008;190(2):396-405.
13. Romagnuolo J, Bardou M, Rahme, et al. Magnetic resonance cholangiopancreatography: a meta-analysis of test performance in suspected biliary disease. Ann Intern Med. 2003;139(7):547-57.
14. Lalani T, Couto CA, Rosen MP, Baker ME, Blake MA, et al. ACR Appropriateness Criteria® jaundice. [online publication]. Reston (VA), American College of Radiology (ACR); 2012.p.9.
15. Gress F, Hawes R, Savides T, et al. The role of EUS in the preoperative staging of pancreatic cancer: a large single center experience. Gastrointest Endosc. 1999;50:786-91.
16. Jailwala J, Fogel EL, Sherman S, Gottlieb K, et al. Triple tissue sampling at ERCP in malignant biliary obstruction. Gastrointest Endosc. 2000;51:383-90.
17. Ferrucci JT, Mueller PR, Harbin WP. Percutaneous transhepatic biliary drainage: technique, results and applications. Radiology. 1980;135:1-13.
18. Cotton PB, Speer AG. Risks and benefits of percutaneous transhepatic biliary drainage. Gastroenterology. 1987;93:667-8.
19. Wang S, Wu H, Wang Q, Zhou W, et al. 18F-FDG PET/CT in differentiating malignant from benign origins of obstructive jaundice. Hepatobiliary Pancreat Dis Int. 2015;14:516-22.

CHAPTER 84

Inflammatory Pathologies of the Biliary Tract

Anmol Bhatia, Ajay Gulati, Uma Debi

INFLAMMATORY CONDITIONS OF THE GALLBLADDER

Acute and chronic inflammatory conditions involving gallbladder are amongst the common causes of acute abdomen. Imaging helps in an early diagnosis and detection of complications in patients with gallbladder inflammatory disorders, thereby reducing morbidity and mortality. This part of the present chapter deals with chronic gallbladder inflammatory conditions. The acute inflammatory conditions have been covered in the chapter on nontraumatic acute abdomen.

Chronic Cholecystitis

Chronic cholecystitis is one of the most common inflammatory conditions of gallbladder and is seen to occur in the background of cholelithiasis in almost all of the patients. Patients usuall present with history suggesting recurring episodes of a ite cholecystitis and/or biliary colic, while few patie s may be totally asymptomatic previously.[1] There is associated gallbladder dysmotility as evidenced by poor gallbladder ejection fraction on ultrasound.

The most commonly seen findings on cross-sectional imaging include cholelithiasis and thickened gallbladder wall. The gallbladder is usually contracted, and pericholecystic inflammation is mostly absent **(Fig. 1)**.[2]

Complications related to chronic cholecystitis include:

- Acute cholecystitis **(Figs. 2A and B)**.
- Gallbladder malignancy.
- *Cholecystoenteric fistula:* This results in the passage of gallbladder calculi into the bowel loops resulting in bowel obstruction, which is termed as gallstone ileus. The passed out stones in the small bowel usually get stuck up in the terminal ileal loops near the ileocecal junction; they may however, be found in any location throughout the small bowel as well as in large bowel loops also.[3] Identification of Rigler's triad (which consists of gallstone in an abnormal/ectopic location, pneumobilia, and features of intestinal obstruction) on plain radiographs at times may be helpful in making the diagnosis. Rigler's triad, however, is seen in a small number of patients only.[3]

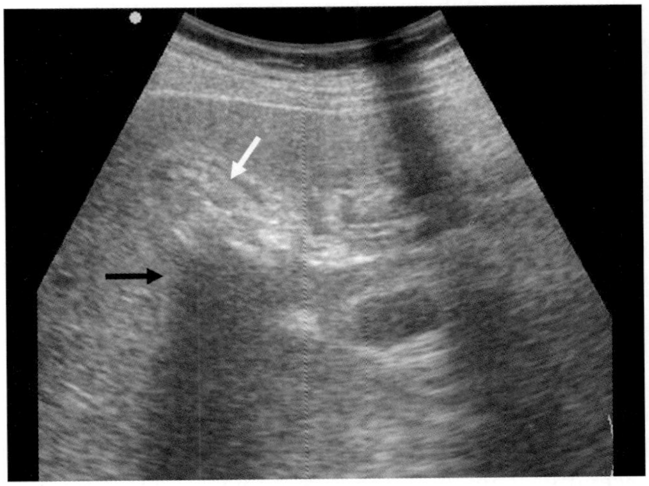

Fig. 1: *Chronic cholecystitis:* Ultrasound image showing contracted gallbladder with diffusely thickened wall (white arrow) and distal acoustic shadowing (black arrow) caused by multiple small calculi in its lumen.

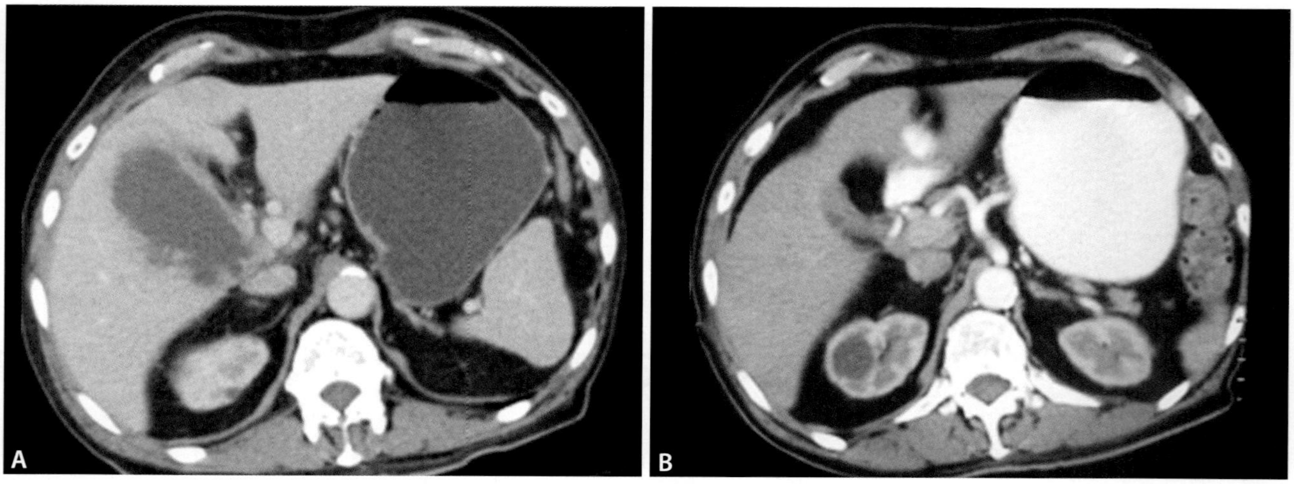

Figs. 2A and B: *Acute on chronic cholecystitis:* (A) Axial CECT image shows distended gallbladder with mural thickening and irregularity at places suggesting acute cholecystitis. Fat stranding is also seen in the adjacent fat; (B) Follow-up CT after 7 months shows shrunken gallbladder.

Xanthogranulomatous Cholecystitis

It is an inflammatory syndrome characterized by thickened gallbladder wall with intramural nodules,[4,5] which are formed by the occlusion and later on rupture of the Rokitansky–Aschoff sinuses. This leads to extravasation of bile into the wall inciting an inflammatory response, characterized histologically by the presence of fibroblasts, histiocytes, and multinucleated giant cells. Xanthogranulomatous cholecystitis is known to occur commonly in elderly population, but can occur across a wide range of age group.[6]

The most common findings on ultrasound (US) and computed tomography (CT) in xanthogranulomatous cholecystitis include gallbladder calculi and focal or diffuse gallbladder wall thickening. Inflammatory fat stranding may also be seen in pericholecystic region. Intramural hypoechoic areas on US and hypoattenuating nodules/bands on CT are highly specific for diagnosing xanthogranulomatous cholecystitis **(Figs. 3A to D)**.[5] Xanthogranulomatous cholecystitis many-a-times is a close mimicker of gallbladder carcinoma on US and CT,[4] while xanthogranulomatous cholecystitis is also associated with an increase in the risk of gallbladder malignancy.[4,6]

Complications encountered in xanthogranulomatous cholecystitis are gallbladder perforation, biliary fistula, liver abscess, stricture within the biliary ducts, and ascending cholangitis.[6] Open cholecystectomy is the preferred option in xanthogranulomatous cholecystitis due to adhesions and associated fibrosis, which make the laparoscopic surgery often unsuccessful.

INFLAMMATORY CONDITIONS OF THE BILIARY TREE

Imaging of biliary tract inflammation has undergone many changes in the last two decades. Due to availability of better diagnostic modalities and treatment options, some entities which were common before have become rare. Advances in cross-sectional imaging have led to an increase in the number of investigations for establishing the diagnosis. There has been evolution of new notions for the occurrence of the inflammatory pathologies affecting the biliary tree resulting in new entities that the radiologists need to know. This part of the present chapter aims to discuss these varying aspects of the biliary tract inflammation.

FIRST ASPECT: ENTITIES WHICH WERE COMMON IN THE PAST AND NOW RARELY SEEN

AIDS-related Cholangiopathy

The biliary tree is affected by human immunodeficiency virus (HIV) in patients having CD4 count of $<100/mm^3$, and the patients usually have pain in the right hypochondrium along with abnormal liver function tests, which are nonspecific. The alkaline phosphatase (ALP) level is elevated more than twenty times the normal value, while the bilirubin levels may be normal or show mild elevation. Abnormal liver function tests can occur due to a variety of causes which include drug-related reactions and hepatitis. Fever with chills may be indicative of systemic infection, whereas jaundice occurs only when there is severe hepatic

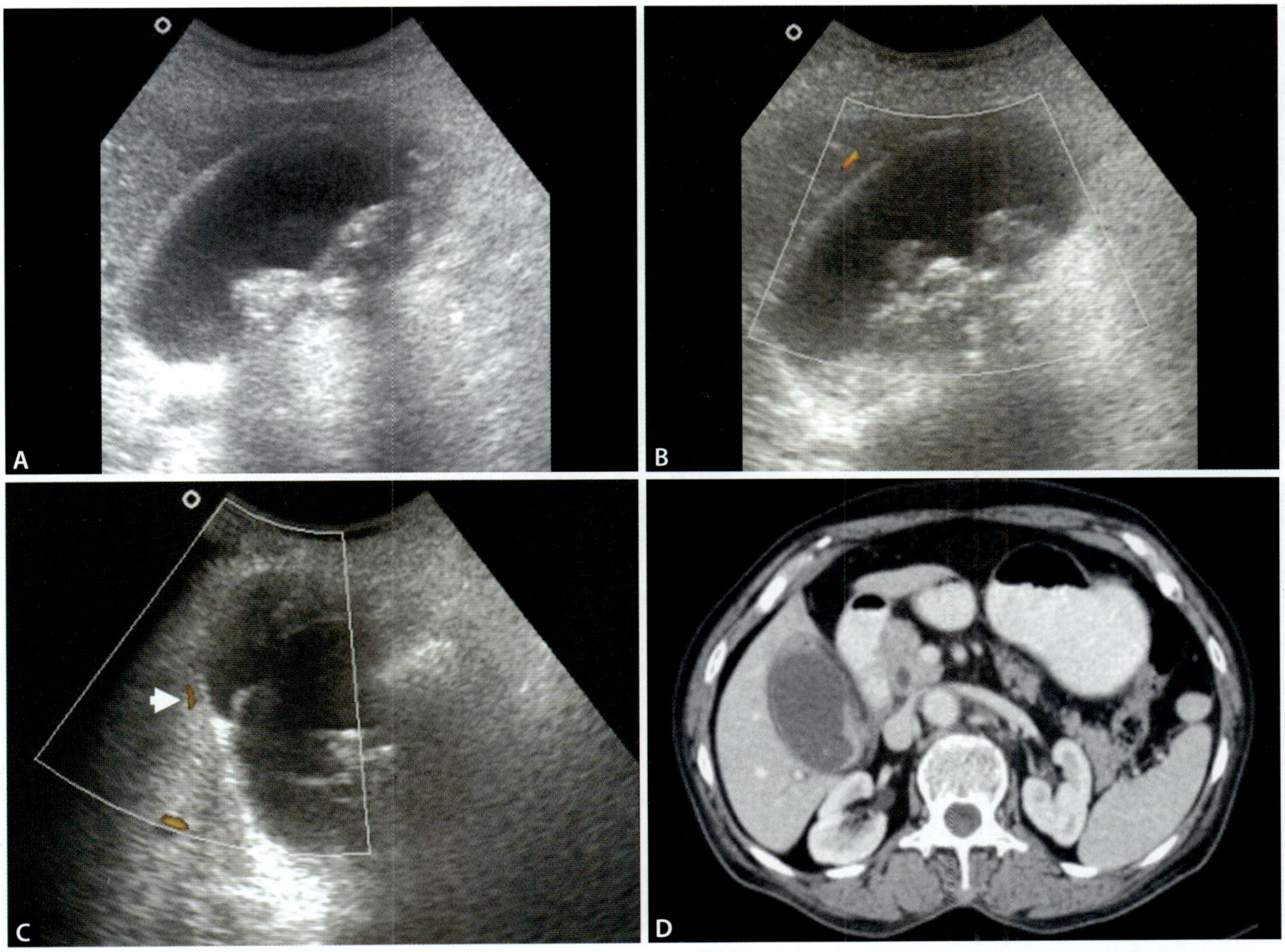

Figs. 3A to D: *Xanthogranulomatous cholecystitis:* (A) Grayscale ultrasound image showing cholelithiasis with thickened gallbladder wall. (B) Color Doppler (B) and power Doppler (C) images showing vascularity adjacent to the thickened wall (arrowhead in C). (D) Axial CECT image showing hyperattenuating inner wall and hypoattenuating outer wall. FNAC was suggestive of benign etiology with possible xanthogranulomatous foci.

dysfunction or significant common bile duct (CBD) obstruction. Imaging, therefore, has an important role to play to assess HIV patients suspected to have hepatobiliary involvement.[7,8]

Acquired immunodeficiency syndrome (AIDS) cholangiopathy is one of the causes of secondary sclerosing cholangitis due to opportunistic infections involving the biliary system, or damage to autonomic nerves or ischemia, but can also occur due to direct invasion of lining of the biliary tract by HIV.[7,8] In majority of the patients, no definite pathogen is isolated/identified; while a gamut of organisms have been implicated, which include *Mycobacterium avium* complex (MAC), herpes simplex virus, *Cryptosporidium parvum*, and cytomegalovirus. It needs to be differentiated from parenchymal liver processes such as MAC infection, for which imaging and biopsy need to be done to establish the diagnosis.[7-9]

Imaging features ***(Figs. 4A to E)*** *include*:

- Acalculous cholecystitis.
- Dilatation of intrahepatic and extrahepatic biliary ducts, predominantly involving left side ductal system.
- Irregular thickening and pruning of the CBD with areas of saccular dilatations.
- Papillary stenosis.

Diagnosis is confirmed by duodenal or ampulla biopsy, with the typical findings of biliary inflammation and the detection of involved organisms. The various treatment options available are sphincterotomy, stricture dilatation, and biliary stenting. Antimicrobial therapy is based on the specific pathogen involved.[7]

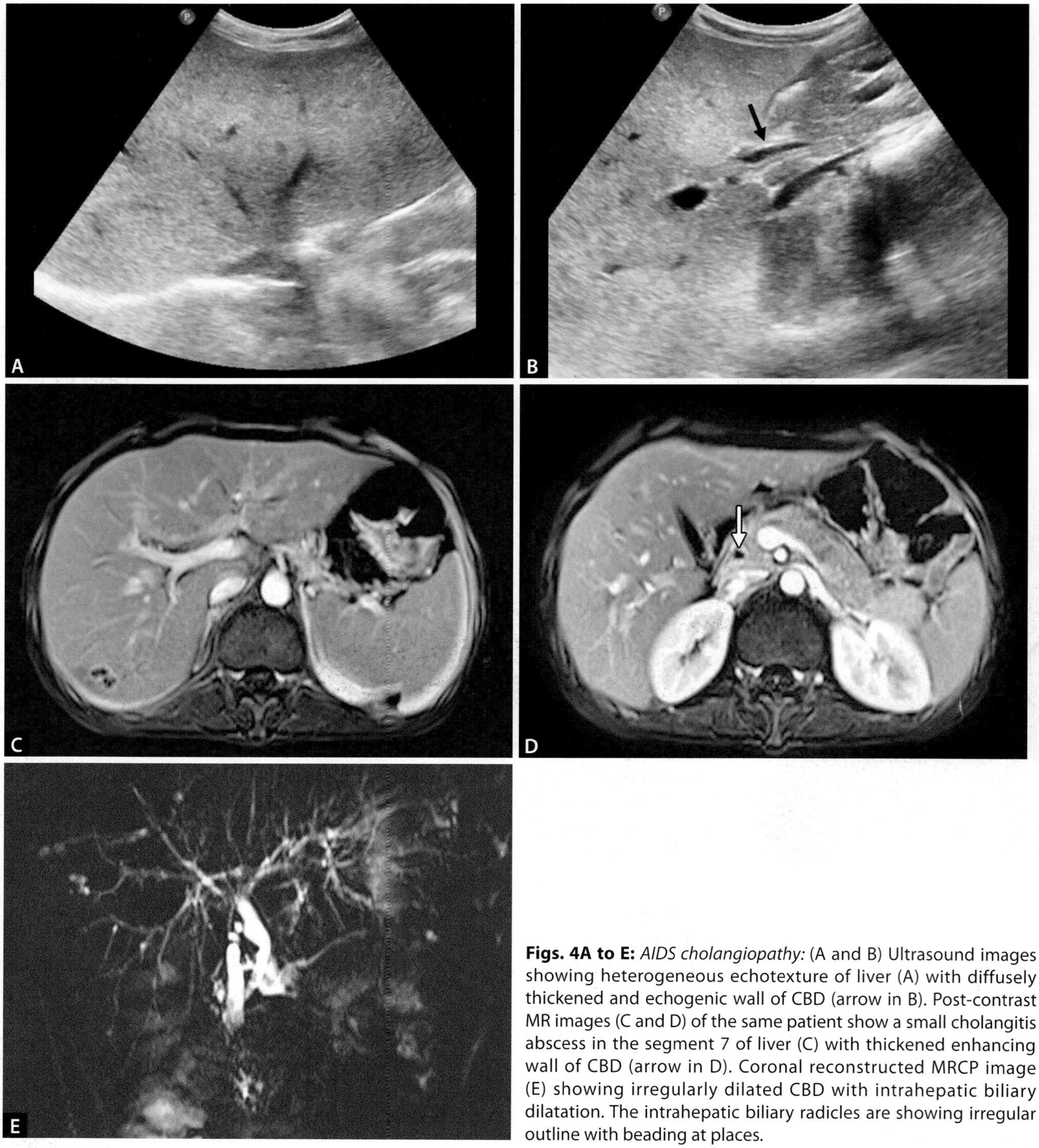

Figs. 4A to E: *AIDS cholangiopathy:* (A and B) Ultrasound images showing heterogeneous echotexture of liver (A) with diffusely thickened and echogenic wall of CBD (arrow in B). Post-contrast MR images (C and D) of the same patient show a small cholangitis abscess in the segment 7 of liver (C) with thickened enhancing wall of CBD (arrow in D). Coronal reconstructed MRCP image (E) showing irregularly dilated CBD with intrahepatic biliary dilatation. The intrahepatic biliary radicles are showing irregular outline with beading at places.

DISEASES KNOWN IN THE PAST WITH INCREASED DETECTABILITY IN THE PRESENT ERA

Primary Sclerosing Cholangitis

Primary sclerosing cholangitis (PSC) is an idiopathic, chronic, fibrosing inflammatory disorder affecting the biliary radicles leading to obstruction of bile ducts, cholestasis, progressing to biliary cirrhosis. It has a strong association with ulcerative colitis, which is seen in 70% of patients.[10] It is thought to be an autoimmune process due to its association with other autoimmune disorders including mediastinal fibrosis, Sjögren syndrome, and retroperitoneal fibrosis.[11,12]

Diagnostic criteria include:

- *Typical cholangiographic abnormalities:* Multifocal, intrahepatic strictures involving the biliary ducts alternating with normal-sized ducts producing a beaded appearance **(Figs. 5A and B)**.
- *Clinical, biochemical, and liver histology findings:* About 75% patients present with progressive fatigue, pruritus, or jaundice.[13] Elevated serum bilirubin and ALP is seen in most of the patients, with ALP rise at least three times the normal range.[13,14] Liver biopsy shows inflammatory fibrosis (nonspecific) involving the portal tracts with a scarcity of bile ducts. Therefore, the histology is considered for confirmation only in case there is a suspicion of PSC.
- *Excluding the secondary causes of sclerosing cholangitis:* This includes a gamut of disorders including chronic bacterial cholangitis following strictures or stones in the biliary system, parasitic infections, AIDS cholangiopathy, ischemia because of drugs like floxuridine or hepatic arterial thrombosis, intrahepatic cholangiocarcinoma, liver metastases, hepatobiliary surgery, as well as congenital disorders of the biliary system.

ERCP, which has been the gold standard for diagnosis of PSC, is associated with risk of cholangitis following bile stasis and biliary injury because of presence of sacculations with increased stiffness of the biliary system **(Figs. 6A and B)**. MRCP has been shown equivalent to ERCP for detecting and localizing the levels of obstruction in the biliary system, and can be helpful in establishing the diagnosis as well as help in planning for an intervention.[15]

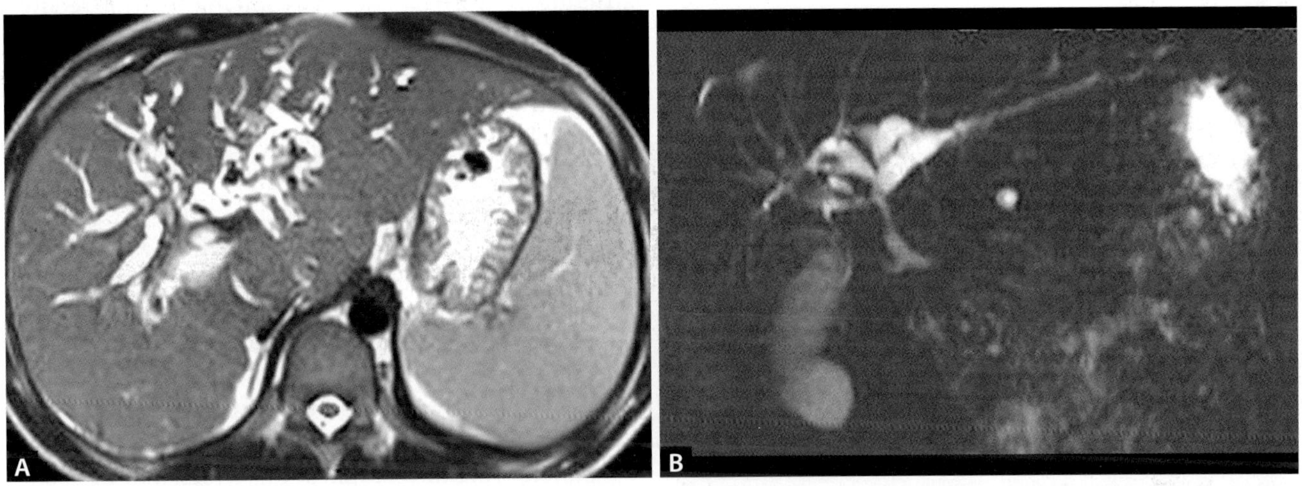

Figs. 5A and B: *Primary sclerosing cholangitis:* Axial T2-HASTE image (A) showing bilobar intrahepatic biliary dilatation. Coronal reconstructed MRCP image (B) showing multifocal strictures involving the biliary radicles with areas of dilatation.

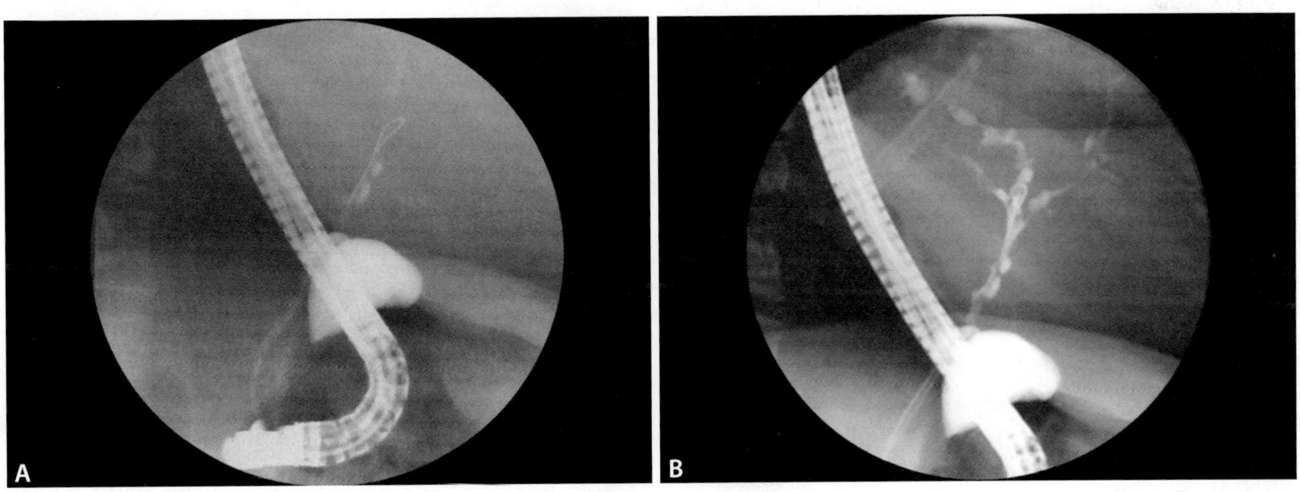

Figs. 6A and B: *Primary sclerosing cholangitis:* ERCP images (A and B) with guidewire showing multifocal segmental narrowing and dilated segments of the biliary ducts and CBD along with sacculations in CBD.

The role of MRI/MRCP in PSC imaging is to address the following three aspects:

1. *Evaluation of intrahepatic and extrahepatic components of biliary system:* The pressure created by the injected contrast during ERCP maximally distends the biliary ducts, thereby making minimal changes and narrowing due to strictures, particularly in the peripheral system to be evaluated, while for involvement of the ducts alone MRCP is likely to miss the minimal changes of PSC. But, if more central strictures are present which are obstructing the flow of contrast during ERCP, MRCP shows upstream ductal involvement.
2. *Morphologic findings in the liver parenchyma supporting PSC diagnosis:* Liver in later stages of PSC shows markedly prominent lobulations of caudate lobe, left lobe atrophy, regenerative nodules (predominantly central in location), and enlarged lymph nodes may be seen in perihepatic location.[12-14] Postcontrast late arterial phase imaging shows peripheral hyperenhancing areas which occur due to a transient hepatic attenuation difference. This indicates increase in the arterial flow compensating for the decreased flow from portal venous system in areas where there is obstruction of the biliary channels.[8,12,14] Hyperintensity can be seen on T2WI along the portal tracts, occurring due to combination of fibrosis, inflammatory infiltrate and lymphatics.[15] This may again show enhancement on postcontrast delayed phase scans.
3. *To diagnose cholangiocarcinoma:* MRI is also useful to detect cholangiocarcinoma, which is known to occur in 10-15% of PSC.[8] This tumor shows peripheral enhancement on arterial phase images with diffuse enhancement on delayed scans.

Secondary Processes Simulating PSC

These include ascending cholangitis occurring due to strictures, congenital anomalies of the bile duct, calculi, AIDS-related cholangiopathy, oriental cholangiohepatitis, and ischemia following iatrogenic insult or intra-arterial chemotherapy.

Nonsclerosing pathologies can also mimic PSC at ERCP, which include polycystic liver disease, metastases, cirrhosis, multifocal hepatocellular carcinoma (HCC) and cholangiocarcinoma. Cross-sectional imaging is therefore warranted to differentiate these nonsclerosing pathologies from PSC.

Ascending Cholangitis

It is caused by bacterial infection, usually by gram-negative enteric bacteria in an obstructed biliary system. The most common causes of obstruction include strictures, calculi, and papillary stenosis. Ascending cholangitis is a clinical diagnosis, and hence the role of imaging is find out the underlying cause of the obstruction. Also, findings of biliary enhancement on imaging help to corroborate with the clinical symptoms **(Fig. 7)**. Patients usually present with the Charcot triad of pain, fever and jaundice. Increased ductal pressure results in the injury of the walls of the ducts which leads to reflux infected bile into the portal triads, thereby forming liver abscess.[15]

Oriental Cholangiohepatitis

It is a parasitic infection of the biliary system in which the patients present with recurrent episodes of pain, fever, and jaundice. Endemic areas, like Southeast Asia, are most commonly affected where parasites like *Ascaris lumbricoides* and *Clonorchis sinensis* inhabit the biliary ducts and later on lead to ductal injury and formation of strictures.[15] It is considered synonymous with recurrent pyogenic cholangitis.

Imaging findings[15] include:

- Multifocal strictures with dilated intrahepatic bile radicles.
- Calculi within the intrahepatic biliary radicles **(Figs. 8A and B)**.
- Disproportionately dilated extrahepatic biliary system, which is not related to strictures or calculi.
- Branching pattern in a right-angled fashion, with reduced degree of arborization.
- Bile lakes or cholangiectasis.
- Primary pigmented stones (in 80% patients), liver abscess, and cholangiocarcinoma (in 2.5%–5.0% patients) are the complications which may be seen.

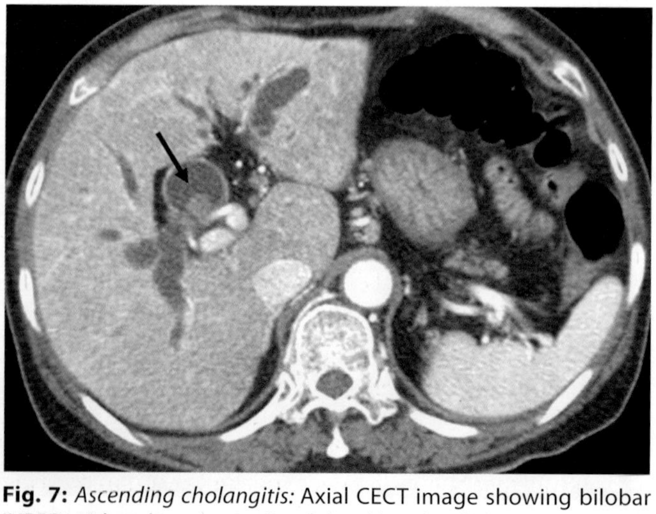

Fig. 7: *Ascending cholangitis:* Axial CECT image showing bilobar IHBRD with enhancing walls of the dilated radicles suggestive of cholangitis. In addition, there is presence of a calculus (arrow) in CHD.

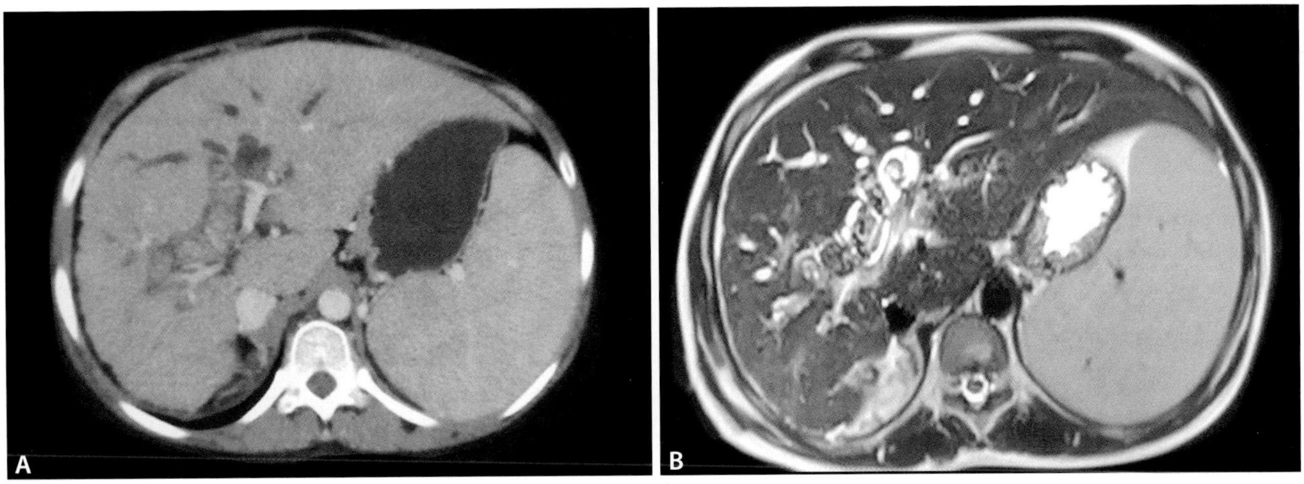

Figs. 8A and B: *Oriental cholangiohepatitis: An* 18-year-old female came with history of recurrent attack of abdominal pain, fever and jaundice. Axial CECT image (A) showing multiple large calculi within the dilated biliary ducts, which are seen signal voids within the ducts on axial T2WI (B).

Chemotherapy-induced Cholangitis

This usually is seen following intra-arterial infusion of chemotherapeutic drugs like floxuridine, in cases of liver metastases form colorectal cancer as a palliative treatment. This occurs due to a large amount of drug extraction during the first pass through the liver, leading to an inflammatory reaction as well as fibrosis around the portal triads mimicking PSC at imaging. Bile duct strictures are known to occur within 2 months of the initiation of the treatment and seen in up to 15% of patients. Strictures are seen at the division of the common hepatic duct (CHD), and distal common bile duct (CBD) is spared.[16]

NEW CONCEPTS

The era of autoimmune disease lead to evolution of the new insights in the inflammatory conditions of the biliary tract. Primary biliary cirrhosis (PBC) has been a well-known entity, but diseases which have been included in this list are autoimmune hepatitis, overlap syndromes, IgG4-related disease and eosinophilic cholangitis.

Primary Biliary Cirrhosis

Primary biliary cirrhosis (PBC) occurs due to inflammation of the medium and small sized biliary radicles/ducts, having components of acute as well chronic inflammation resulting in features of cholestasis clinically. It typically affects women (>90% of cases) between 30 and 65 years of age. Elevated antimitochondrial antibodies (more specific) and antinuclear antibodies (less specific) are characteristic findings in serology. It usually occurs in association with other autoimmune disorders, like inflammatory bowel disease, Sjögren's syndrome, calcinosis, raynaud phenomenon, esophageal dysmotility, sclerodactyly and telangiectasia (CREST) syndrome, etc.

Imaging is not needed in most of the cases of PBC. The biliary tract abnormalities are reflection of the secondary changes of developing cirrhosis. However, when there is a diagnostic dilemma, imaging may be helpful in providing valuable information. On MRI, a fairly specific periportal halo sign is best seen on postcontrast T1W-FS portal venous phase or delayed scans.[17] It is seen with less conspicuity on T2WI as a low signal halo surrounding a high-signal-intensity center.[17] Hepatocellular carcinoma may be seen as a complication in around 5% of patients.

Autoimmune Hepatitis and Overlap Syndromes

Overlap syndrome is defined as a combination of PBC and autoimmune hepatitis, or PSC and autoimmune hepatitis. Autoimmune hepatitis leads to a more inflammatory reaction than seen in cases of PBC or PSC, where there is more cholestasis. Chronic inflammation in cases of autoimmune hepatitis begins in the periportal region and breaches the periportal plate thereby extending into the adjacent parenchyma. Autoimmune hepatitis affects younger women (15–40 years old) population, 3–4 times than men.[18,19]

A diagnosis is established when the work-up for the different causes of hepatitis is negative and abnormal findings are seen on serology with raised ANA, anti-SMA, or antibody to LKM 1.[18] Liver biopsy is required as an adjunct to establish the diagnosis and assessing the degree of inflammation.

MRI shows areas showing increased enhancement in liver parenchyma in early stages of the disease; and later on the varying degrees of fibrosis, generalized volume loss, and locoregional lymphadenopathy.[19] Up to 18% of patients with autoimmune biliary disorder have two diseases simultaneously.[20] The greater degree of inflammation in cases of autoimmune hepatitis warrants the use of immunosuppressive treatment in the patients with overlap syndrome.[20]

IgG4-related Biliary Involvement

IgG4-related disorder includes cholangitis; inflammatory pseudotumor; and IgG4 hepatopathy, which includes portal inflammation and/or interface hepatitis, lobular hepatitis, obstruction of large bile ducts, portal sclerosis, and canalicular cholestasis.[21,22] It is seen in up to 88% of cases of autoimmune pancreatitis, and the bile ducts are seen to be commonly involved after the involvement of pancreas in IgG4-related disorder. Involvement of the biliary tree alone without the involvement of other organs is known to occur.

On cross-sectional imaging, the involved segments of the biliary tree show thickened walls with enhancement on contrast-enhanced scans, luminal narrowing, and stenosis. MRCP or ERCP shows the location and the degree of involvement and are useful in assessing the response to the treatment. Involvement of region of the porta with a soft tissue mass may simulate cholangiocarcinoma.[23]

Distinguishing between IgG4-related disease and overlap with primary sclerosing cholangitis may be challenging for the radiologist as the imaging findings in IgG4-related disease are not diagnostic. Clinically, primary sclerosing cholangitis occurs in the third to fourth decades and patients are typically less symptomatic than in IgG4-related sclerosing cholangitis, in which they have a more acute presentation of a smaller duration. Multifocal, short, band like strictures are seen in PSC, while the strictures of IgG4-related disease are typically long and show a continuity with segments of prestenotic dilatation. Isolated strictures involving the distal CBD only are also seen.[24] The soft tissue around the common bile duct is another important diagnostic finding **(Figs. 9A**

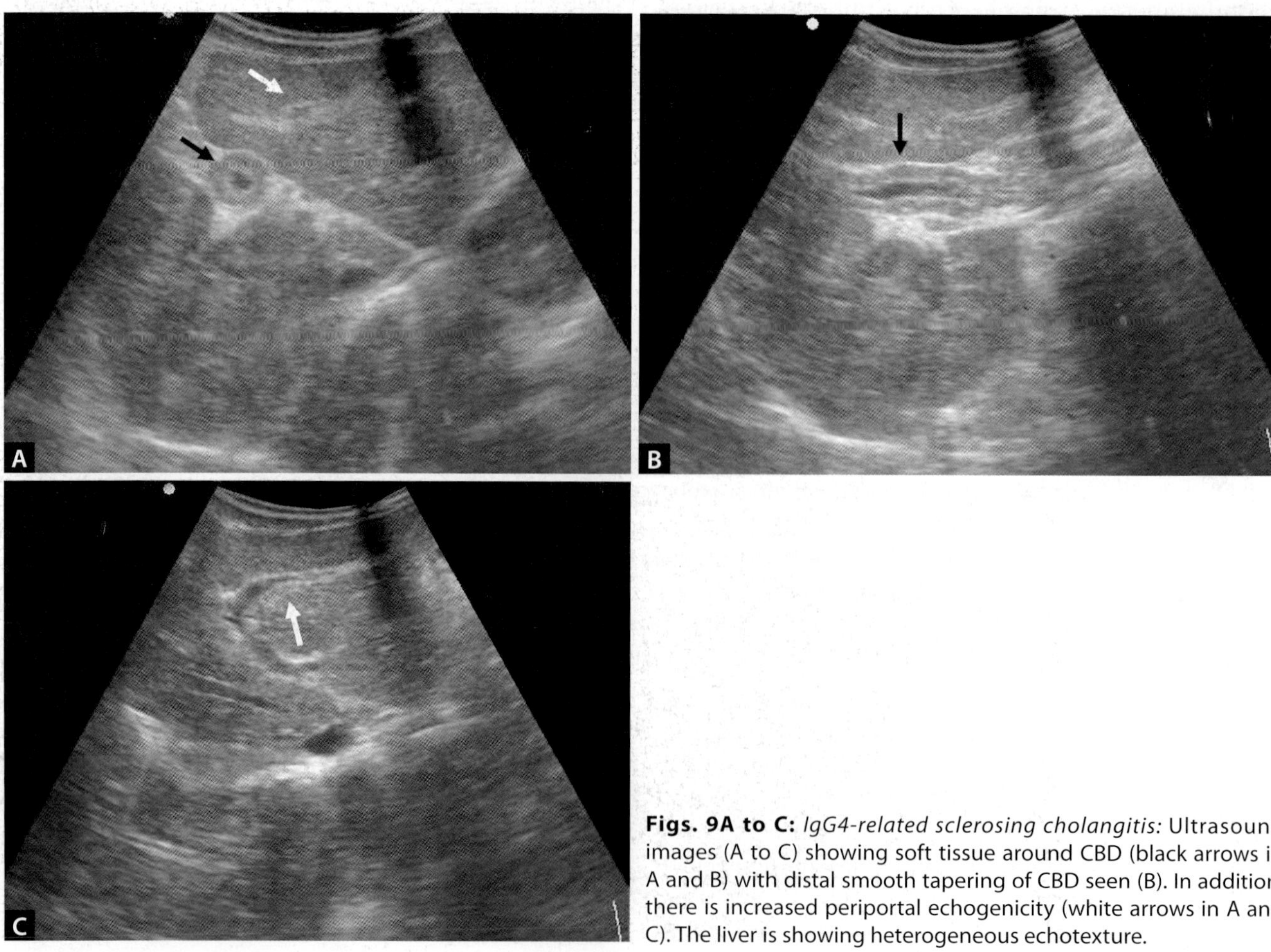

Figs. 9A to C: *IgG4-related sclerosing cholangitis:* Ultrasound images (A to C) showing soft tissue around CBD (black arrows in A and B) with distal smooth tapering of CBD seen (B). In addition, there is increased periportal echogenicity (white arrows in A and C). The liver is showing heterogeneous echotexture.

to C). The soft tissue in primary sclerosing cholangitis is present to a lesser extent than in IgG4-related cholangitis. The inflammatory reaction of IgG4-related disease is centrifugal with respect to the ductal lumen and is associated with tiny fibroinflammatory nodules, while that in PSC is centripetal and is associated with degeneration and destruction of lining of the biliary tree.[25]

IgG4-related inflammatory hepatic pseudotumors have been classified as either fibrohistiocytic or lymphoplasmacytic by Zen et al.[26] depending on the histopathology. Lymphoplasmacytic type is more strongly associated with IgG4-related disease.[26]

On CT, homogeneous delayed enhancement has been considered an important imaging finding of IgG4-related disease.[27] On MRI, the lesions are hyperintense on T2WI, and isointense to hypointense on T1WI with variable contrast enhancement patterns **(Figs. 10A to D)**.[28] The differential diagnosis on imaging can be hepatocellular carcinoma, lymphoma and cholangiocarcinoma.

Involvement of the gallbladder, manifests as diffuse acalculous cholecystitis **(Fig. 10B)**, which can be seen in up to 25% of patients with IgG4-related sclerosing pancreatitis having concurrent IgG4-related sclerosing cholangitis. Though the imaging appearance of acalculous cholecystitis is nonspecific, there is extramural involvement predominantly with associated subserosal inflammatory nodular changes in IgG4-related disease.

Eosinophilic Cholangitis

It is usually seen in cases of eosinophilic gastroenteritis with radiologic and histologic features suggesting cholecystitis, chronic hepatitis, or cholangitis **(Figs. 11A to C)**. The patients rapidly respond well with corticosteroids.[15]

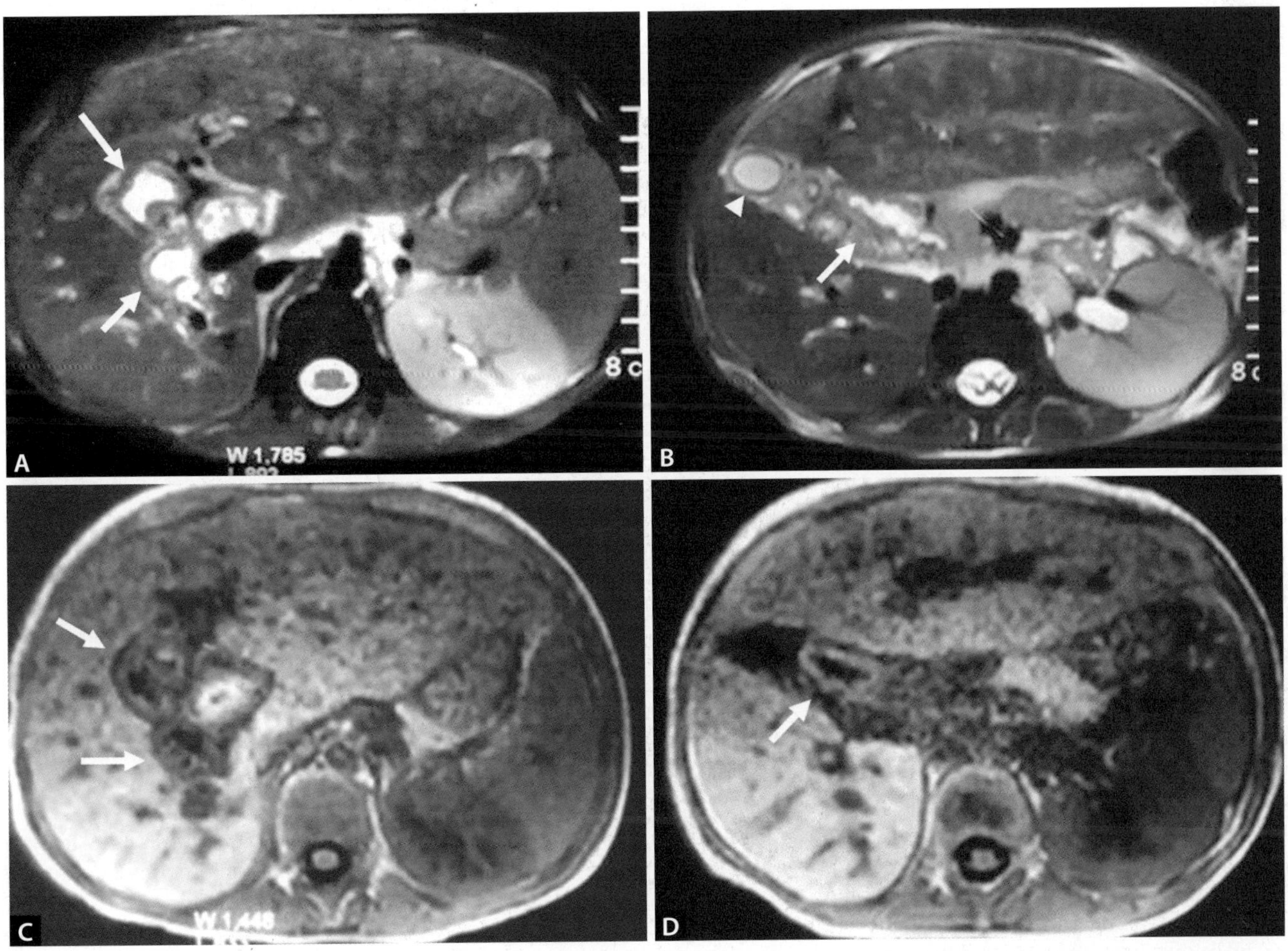

Figs. 10A to D: *IgG4-related sclerosing cholangitis:* MR images of the patient in Figure 9 showing diffusely heterogeneous signal intensity of the liver with increased periportal signal on T2WI (A and B). Soft tissue is seen around the biliary radicles (arrows in A and C) as well as around CBD (arrows in B and D) which is relatively hyperintense on T2WI (A and B) and isointense on T1WI (C and D). In addition, the wall of gallbladder is also thickened (arrowhead in B) suggesting acalculous cholecystitis.

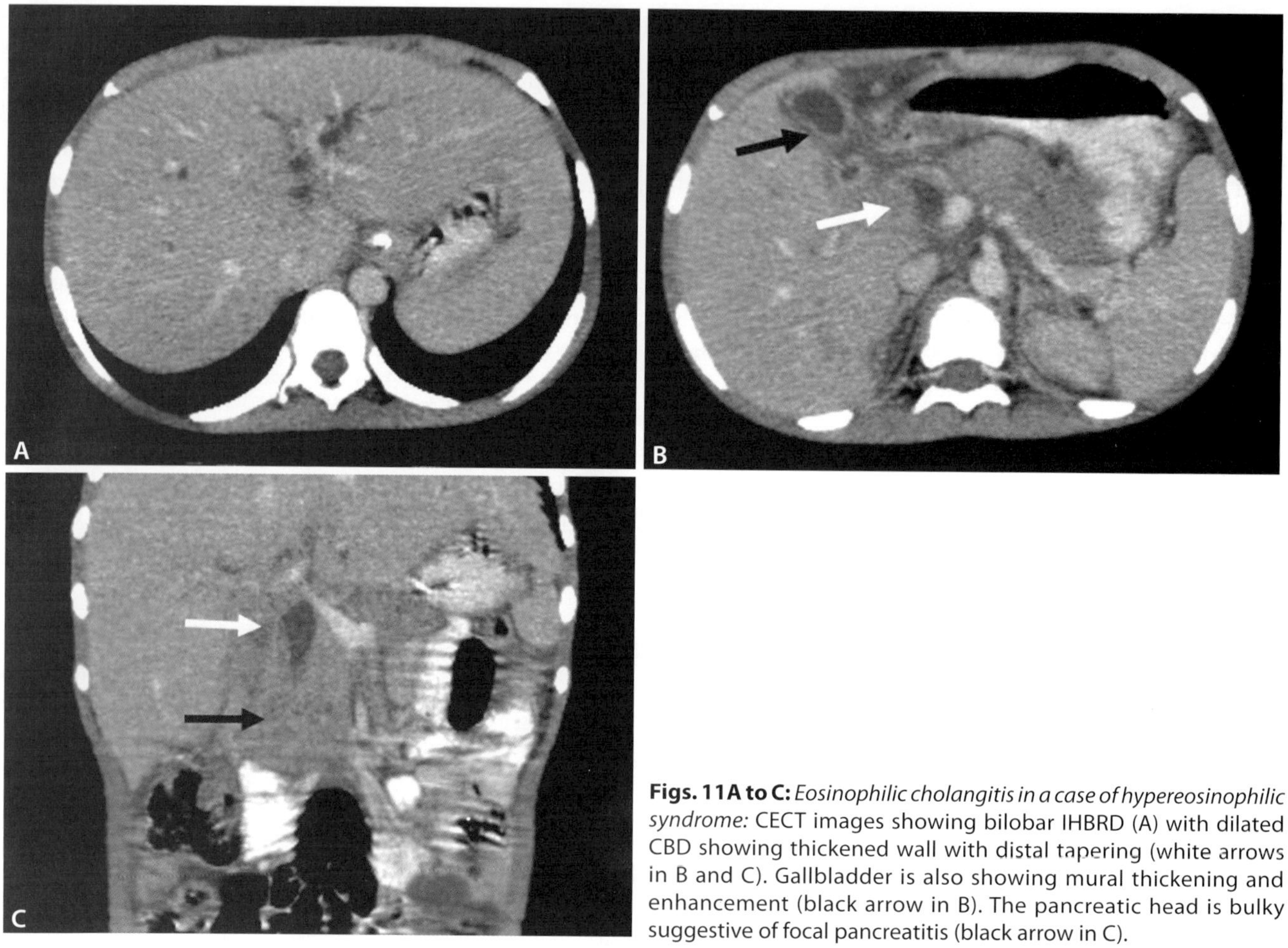

Figs. 11A to C: *Eosinophilic cholangitis in a case of hypereosinophilic syndrome:* CECT images showing bilobar IHBRD (A) with dilated CBD showing thickened wall with distal tapering (white arrows in B and C). Gallbladder is also showing mural thickening and enhancement (black arrow in B). The pancreatic head is bulky suggestive of focal pancreatitis (black arrow in C).

CONCLUSION

The gamut of biliary inflammatory disorders has changed and multiple etiologic factors for the inflammation of biliary tract have been proposed. Radiologists should be aware of these changing concepts regarding various pathophysiologic mechanisms and also understand the different approaches to imaging, as well as imaging findings of the various conditions involving the biliary tract.

REFERENCES

1. Raptopoulos V, Compton CC, Doherty P, et al. Chronic acalculous gallbladder disease: multi-imaging evaluation with clinical-pathologic correlation. AJR. 1986;147:721-4.
2. Yun EJ, Cho SG, Park S, et al. Chronic gallbladder carcinoma and chronic cholecystitis: differentiation with two-phase spiral CT. Abdom Imaging. 2004;29:102-8.
3. Bruljevac M, Busic Z, Cabrijan Z. Sonographic diagnosis of gallstone ileus. J Ultrasound Med. 2004;23:1395-8.
4. Chun KA, Ha HK, Yu ES, et al. Xanthogranulomatous cholecystitis: CT features with emphasis on differentiation from gallbladder carcinoma. Radiology. 1997;203:93-7.
5. Parra JA, Acinas O, Bueno J, Güezmes A, Fernández MA, Fariñas MC. Xanthogranulomatous cholecystitis: clinical, sonographic, and CT findings in 26 patients. AJR. 2000;174:979-83.
6. Roberts KM, Parsons MA. Xanthogranulomatous cholecystitis: clinicopathological study of 13 cases. J Clin Pathol. 1987;40:412-7.
7. Keaveny AP, Karasik MS. Hepatobiliary and pancreatic infections in AIDS: part II. AIDS Patient Care STDS. 1998;12:451-6.
8. Mahajani RV, Uzer MF. Cholangiopathy in HIV-infected patients. Clin Liver Dis. 1999;3:669-84.
9. Barthet M, Chauveau E, Bonnet E, et al. Pancreatic ductal changes in HIV-infected patients. Gastrointest Endosc. 1997;45:59-63.
10. Wiesner RH, LaRusso NF. Clinicopathologic features of the syndrome of primary sclerosing cholangitis. Gastroenterology. 1980;79:200-6.
11. Chapman RW, Jewell DP. Primary sclerosing cholangitis: an immunologically mediated disease? West J Med. 1985;143:193-5.
12. Crippin JS. Primary sclerosing cholangitis: etiology and immunology. Eur J Gastroenterol Hepatol. 1992;4:261-5.

13. Ueno Y, LaRusso NF. Primary sclerosing cholangitis. J Gastroenterol. 1994;29:531-43.
14. Lindor KD, Wiesner RH, MacCarty RL, Ludwig J, LaRusso NF. Advances in primary sclerosing cholangitis. Am J Med. 1990;89:73-80.
15. Vitellas KM, Keogan MT, Freed KS, et al. Radiologic manifestations of sclerosing cholangitis with emphasis on MR cholangiopancreatography. RadioGraphics. 2000;20:959-75.
16. Shea WJ Jr, Debas BE, Goldberg HI, Hohn DC, Ferrell LD, Kerlan RK. Sclerosing cholangitis associated with hepatic arterial FUDR chemotherapy: radiographic-histologic correlation. AJR. 1986;146:717-21.
17. Wenzel JS, Donohoe A, Ford KL III, et al. Primary biliary cirrhosis: MR imaging findings and description of MR imaging periportal halo sign. AJR. 2001;176:885-9.
18. Czaja AJ, Freese DK. Diagnosis and treatment of autoimmune hepatitis. Hepatology. 2002;36:479-96.
19. Bilaj F, Hyslop WB, Rivero H, et al. MR imaging findings in autoimmune hepatitis: correlation with clinical staging. Radiology. 2005;236:896-902.
20. Schramm C, Lohse AW. Overlap syndromes of cholestatic liver diseases and autoimmune hepatitis. Clin Rev Allergy Immunol. 2005;28:105-14.
21. Zen Y, Harada K, Sasaki M, et al. IgG4-related sclerosing cholangitis with and without hepatic inflammatory pseudotumor, and sclerosing pancreatitis-associated sclerosing cholangitis: do they belong to a spectrum of sclerosing pancreatitis? Am J Surg Pathol. 2004;28:1193-203.
22. Umemura T, Zen Y, Hamano H, et al. IgG4 associated autoimmune hepatitis: a differential diagnosis for classical autoimmune hepatitis. Gut. 2007;56:1471-2.
23. Vlachou PA, Khalili K, Jang HJ, Fischer S, Hirschfield GM, Kim TK. IgG4-related sclerosing disease: autoimmune pancreatitis and extrapancreatic manifestations. RadioGraphics. 2011;31:1379-402.
24. Nakazawa T, Ohara H, Sano H, et al. Cholangiography can discriminate sclerosing cholangitis with autoimmune pancreatitis from primary sclerosing cholangitis. Gastrointest Endosc. 2004;60:937-44.
25. Cheuk W, Chan JKC. IgG4-related sclerosing disease: a critical appraisal of an evolving clinicopathologic entity. Adv Anat Pathol. 2010;17:303-32.
26. Zen Y, Fujii T, Sato Y, Masuda S, Nakanuma Y. Pathological classification of hepatic inflammatory pseudotumor with respect to IgG4-related disease. Mod Pathol. 2007;20:884-94.
27. Naitoh I, Nakazawa T, Ohara H, et al. IgG4-related hepatic inflammatory pseudotumor with sclerosing cholangitis: a case report and review of the literature. Cases J. 2009;2:7029.
28. Anderson SW, Kruskal JB, Kane RA. Benign hepatic tumors and iatrogenic pseudotumors. RadioGraphics. 2009;29:211-29.

CHAPTER 85

Malignant Pathologies of Biliary Tree

Ujjwal Gorsi, Ajay Gulati, Mandeep Garg

INTRODUCTION

Biliary tract malignancies are the second most common hepatobiliary malignancy after hepatocellular carcinoma. These tumors can arise from any part of the biliary tract from smallest intra hepatic ductule to ampulla of Vater.[1] Most of the tumors that arise in biliary tree are adenocarcinomas as they occur as a consequence of malignant transformation of simple columnar epithelium which lines whole of the biliary tree and gallbladder.[2] Gallbladder cancer is the cancer arising from the gallbladder and the cystic duct. Cholangiocarcinoma can either be intrahepatic or extra hepatic. Cancer arising from the ampulla of Vater is included under the category of periampullary carcinomas which also include cancers arising from the terminal most common bile duct, head of pancreas and the duodenal bulb as they have similar clinical and radiological features and also the similar management.[3]

Patients with malignancies of biliary tree present clinically with symptoms of jaundice and right upper quadrant pain which are similar to many other benign conditions affecting the biliary tract. It is of paramount importance for the radiologist to be aware of imaging features of biliary tract malignancies so as to diagnose these tumors with certainty. In most of the instances, there is no single imaging test that will answer all clinical questions so multimodality imaging becomes necessary. The techniques routinely used to evaluate biliary tree pathologies include ultrasonography (USG), multidetector computed tomography (MDCT), magnetic resonance imaging (MRI) with magnetic resonance cholangiopancreatography (MRCP), endoscopic retrograde cholangiopancreatography (ERCP) and endoscopic ultrasound (EUS).

GALLBLADDER CARCINOMA

Gallbladder carcinoma is the cancer arising from gallbladder and cystic duct.[1] It is a notoriously lethal malignant tumor that is often discovered late.

Epidemiology

Gallbladder cancer is the seventh most common malignancy of the gastrointestinal tract and the most common malignant neoplasm of the biliary tree.[4] Some geographic areas have a high incidence of gallbladder cancer, including South America and India. The incidence of gallbladder cancer increases with age with more than 90% of patients being older than 50 years; the peak incidence is 70–75 years.[5]

In India, prevalence of gallbladder cancer is high in northern and northeastern states of Uttar Pradesh, Bihar, Orissa, West Bengal and Assam.[6] It is two times higher in women than men. In northern India cities, it is the most common digestive cancer in women.[7]

Risk Factors

Most common risk factor which is associated with gallbladder cancer is cholelithiasis with chronic inflammation and there are studies showing increase in risk of developing cancer as the size of stones increases.[8,9] Porcelain gallbladder is also a risk factor for developing gallbladder malignancy, however risk is not up to 22% which was reported in earlier studies[8] but between 7% and 15% as shown by newer studies.[10-12] Primary sclerosing cholangitis, congenital anomalous pancreaticobiliary duct junction and gallbladder polyps (solitary and symptomatic polyp >1 cm) are also associated with increased risk of developing gallbladder carcinoma. Other associations that are frequently implied include typhoid carrier state, chronic bacterial infections affecting gallbladder, and exposure to certain carcinogens.[8]

Pathological Features, Staging and Prognosis

Most carcinomas of the gallbladder are adenocarcinoma (85–90%) and can be papillary, tubular, mucinous, or signet cell type.[13] In gallbladder, most common location for the tumor to originate is fundus (60%) followed by body (30%) and neck (10%).[14] The gallbladder has unique anatomic features as its wall does not contain sub mucosa and at its hepatic attachment and along liver surface, there is no serosa. In addition, connective tissue of gallbladder is continuous with the interlobular connective tissue of the liver.[14] These anatomical features promote early local invasion into liver.

Gallbladder carcinoma is staged surgically by the depth of invasion, extension of disease into adjacent structures, involvement of lymph nodes, and presence of metastases by the American Joint Committee on Cancer TNM staging system **(Table 1)**.[15]

Strongest prognostic factor gallbladder cancer is tumor stage. In a study, about 2500 patients with gallbladder malignancy from hospital cancer registries were analyzed and survival was related to tumor stage. 5 year survival for Stage 0 patients was 60%, for Stage I patients 39%, 15% for Stage II patients, 5% for Stage III patients and only 1% for Stage IV patients.[16]

Table 1: TNM staging classification for gallbladder cancer (AJCC, 7th Edition).

TX	Primary tumor cannot be assessed
T0	No evidence of primary tumor
Tis	Carcinoma *in situ*
Tla	Tumor invades lamina propria
Tlb	Tumor invades muscular layer
T2	Tumor invades perimuscular connective tissue
T3	Tumor perforates serosa or directly invades the liver and/or one other adjacent organ
T4	Tumor invades main portal vein or hepatic artery or invades multiple extra hepatic organs
NX	Regional nodes cannot be assessed
N0	No regional nodal metastasis
N1	Metastasis to nodes along the cystic duct, common bile duct, hepatic artery and/or portal vein
N2	Metastasis to periaortic, pericaval, superior mesenteric artery, and/or celiac artery lymph nodes
M0	No distant metastasis
MI	Distant metastasis

Stage 0	Tis	N0	M0
Stage I	T1	N0	M0
Stage II	T2	N0	M0
Stage IIIA	T3	N0	M0
Stage IIIB	T1-3	N1	M0
Stage IVA	T4	N0-1	M0
Stage IVB	Any T	N2	M0
	Any T	Any N	M1

IMAGING MODALITIES

The USG is often the initial imaging modality for suspected gallbladder cancer and many times it is on USG that a diagnosis of clinically unsuspected gallbladder malignancy will be suggested. The diagnostic accuracy of USG in gallbladder cancer is more than 80%, but it main limitation is its inability to stage the tumor.[17] Endoscopic USG can illustrate the depth of tumor invasion better and thus can overcome this limitation. In addition it helps in characterizing polypoid lesions involving gallbladder.[18] Dynamic contrast enhanced MDCT or MRI with MRCP are most useful imaging modalities for better depiction of the tumor morphology as well as staging. MRI may differentiate adenomyomatosis or xanthogranulomatous cholecystitis from gallbladder cancer, which may not be possible with other modalities. MRCP provides more detailed information than ultrasound or CT about biliary involvement of the tumor. In addition, adding diffusion-weighted imaging to the standard MRI protocol may improve sensitivity for distinguishing gallbladder cancers from other benign gallbladder diseases, which present with wall thickening.[19]

Radiological Findings

Radiologic Evaluation of the Primary Tumor

On imaging, gallbladder carcinoma can present as three patterns echoing the similar histologic patterns: a mass replacing or obscuring the gallbladder (most common), Intra luminal polypoid mass and mural thickening or irregularity of the wall of the gallbladder.[20]

Carcinoma Manifesting as a Gallbladder Fossa Mass

Most common presentation of gallbladder carcinoma is a large mass obscuring or replacing the gallbladder. This pattern is seen in 40–65%.[20] A large mass in gallbladder fossa that fills the lumen of gallbladder or replaces it and is seen invading the adjacent liver parenchyma is likely to be a gallbladder carcinoma.[21]

On USG, heterogeneous hypoechoic mass is seen in gallbladder fossa. Hyper echoic foci may be seen with in this mass, which are commonly due to calculi but may also represent porcelain gallbladder or tumor calcifications.[22]

On noncontrast CT gallbladder carcinoma is hypodense.[23] On MRI, on T1-weighted sequences gallbladder carcinomas hypo- to isointense and hyperintense on T2-weighted sequences.[20] On CT or MRI, after contrast administration, in early arterial phase, periphery of the mass may show enhancement which can be intense and irregular. During portal venous and delayed phases, contrast enhancement may be retained in fibrous stromal components of gallbladder carcinoma **(Figs. 1A to C)**. This feature helps in differentiating this tumor from large hepatocellular carcinomas (HCC) which may occur near the gallbladder fossa as HCC shows contrast material washout.[24] Other differential diagnoses include intra hepatic cholangiocarcinoma and metastasis to gallbladder fossa.[25]

Carcinoma Manifesting as a Polypoid Mass

Gallbladder carcinoma can present as intra luminal polypoid mass in 25% of cases and is more likely to be confined to the gallbladder at the time of diagnosis. These lesions are usually homogeneous and can be hyperechoic, isoechoic or hypoechoic on sonography and do not cast an acoustic shadow aiding in differentiation from gallstones. Necrosis or calcification is uncommon and the tumor shows homogeneous enhancement **(Figs. 2A to D)**. Small polypoid malignancies can be indistinguishable from

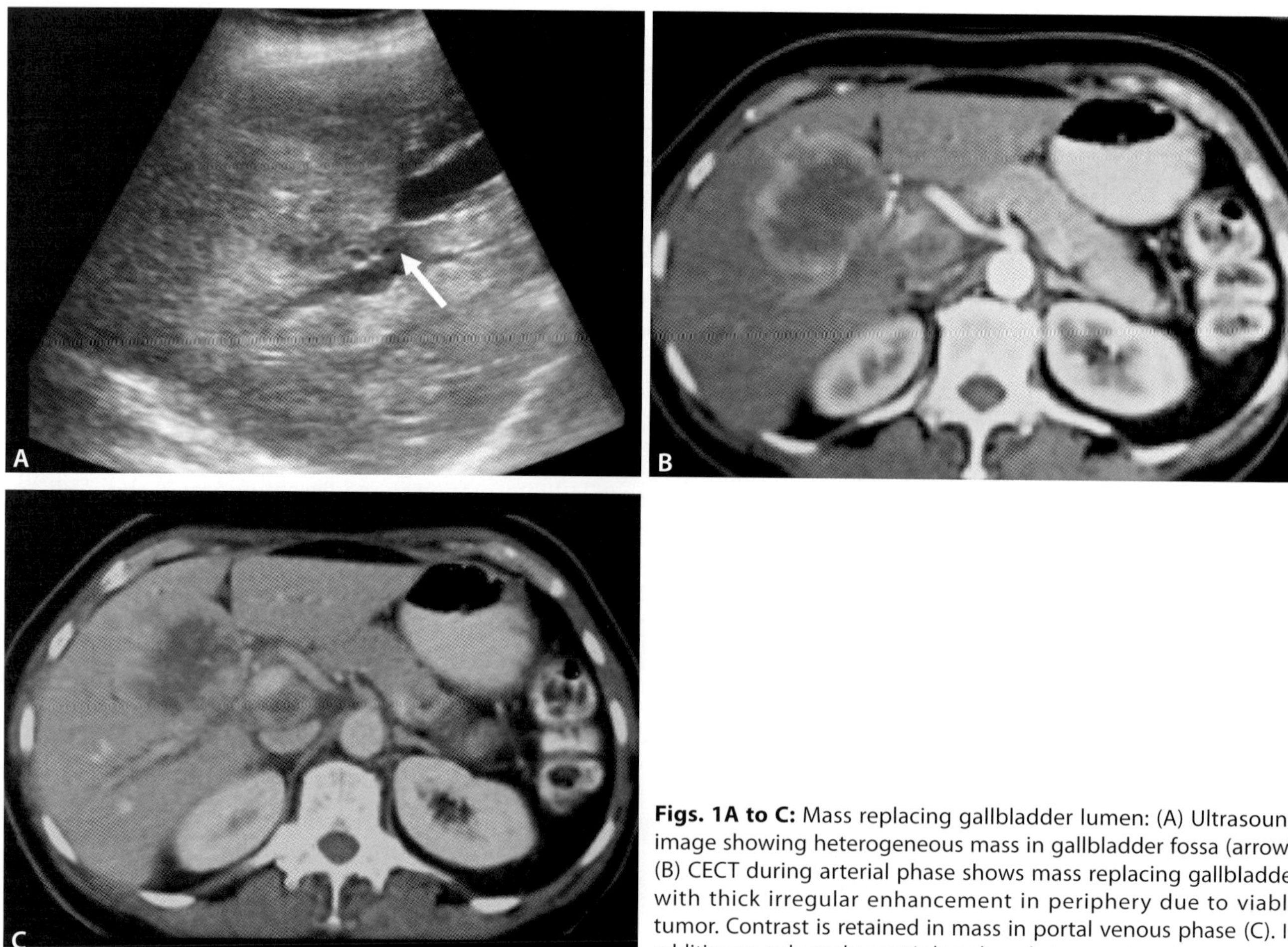

Figs. 1A to C: Mass replacing gallbladder lumen: (A) Ultrasound image showing heterogeneous mass in gallbladder fossa (arrow); (B) CECT during arterial phase shows mass replacing gallbladder with thick irregular enhancement in periphery due to viable tumor. Contrast is retained in mass in portal venous phase (C). In addition an enlarged necrotic lymph node is seen at porta.

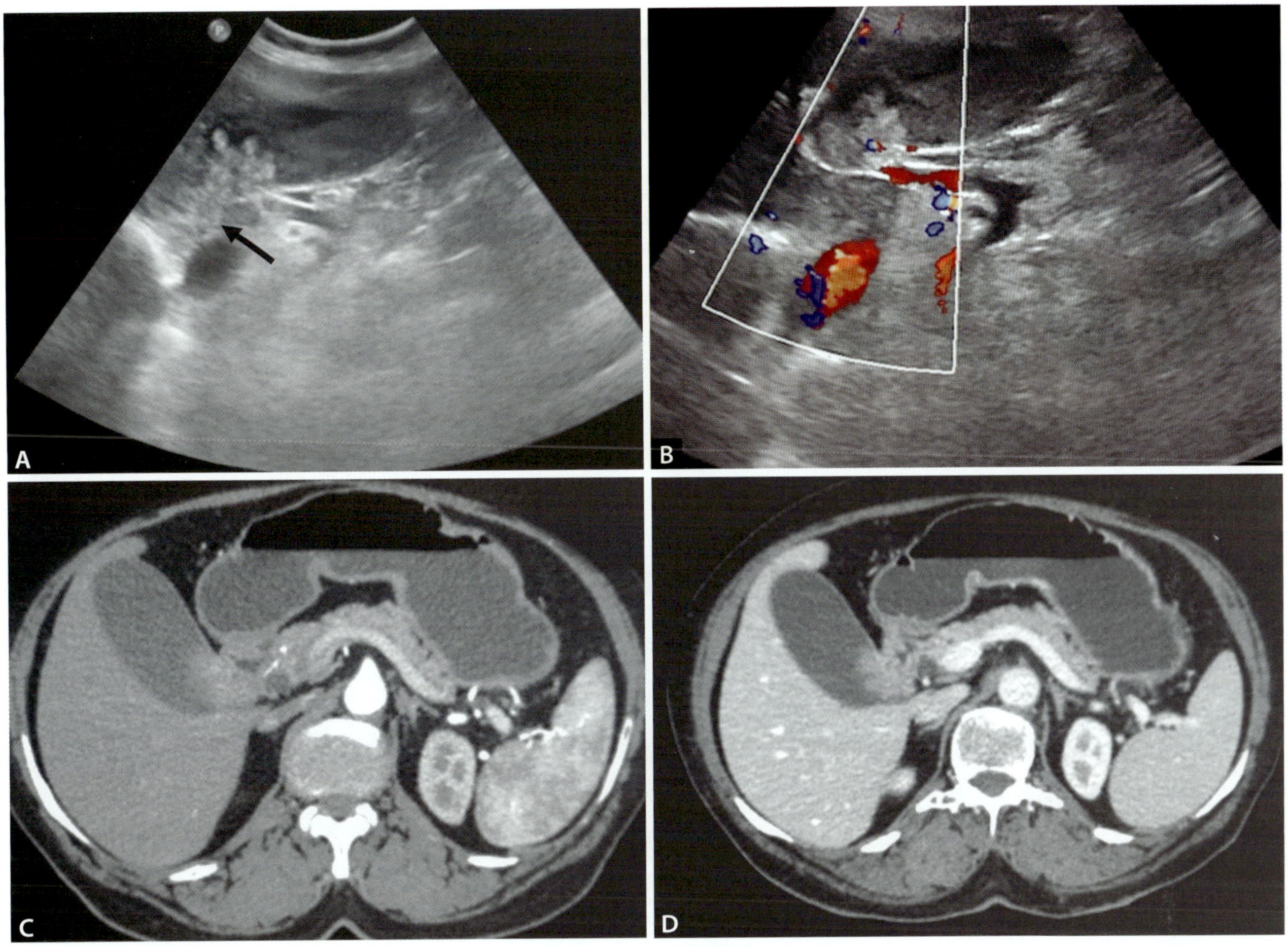

Figs. 2A to D: Intraluminal polyp: (A) Grayscale ultrasound image showing echogenic polypoid lesion in region of gallbladder neck (arrow) with no posterior acoustic shadow; (B) Color Doppler shows vascularity with in the lesion. CECT during arterial phase (C) and venous phase (D) shows homogeneously enhancing polypoid lesion with no arterial hypervasculairty and no extension outside the gallbladder.

cholesterol polyp, adherent noncalcified stone, adenoma, tumefactive sludge or blood clot. Polyps should be removed surgically if the size exceeds one cm, associated calculi are present, age of the patient is more than 50 years and the patient is symptomatic. Sludge is usually mobile when patient's position is changed, is more echogenic than tumor and does not show vascularity unlike tumor.[26]

Carcinoma Manifesting as Mural Thickening

The least common and most difficult to diagnose presentation of gallbladder malignancy is mural thickening which may be focal or diffuse.[27] The thickness of gallbladder wall up to 3 mm or less is considered normal and early lesions confined to the mucosa or slightly raised lesions are generally not picked up on ultrasound.[28] Gallstones can obscure subtle wall thickening associated with early malignancy. In general, benign entities, which include acute and chronic cholecystitis, adenomyomatosis, hepatitis, low protein states, inadequate distension and other causes, will cause diffuse mural thickening.[27] CT is inferior to ultrasound in depicting mucosal irregularity, mural thickening, and cholelithiasis however CT scores over ultrasound in evaluating the thickening of those portions of the gallbladder wall which are obscured by gallstones or mural calcification on USG.[28]

On contrast-enhanced MDCT, thick (>2.5 mm) and strong enhancement of the inner wall and irregular contour of the affected wall are considered significant predictors for malignancy while evaluating gallbladder wall thickening **(Figs. 3A to D)**.[29-31] When CT shows focal or irregular mural thickening of the gallbladder, careful inspection of the images should be done to look for bile duct dilation, local invasion,

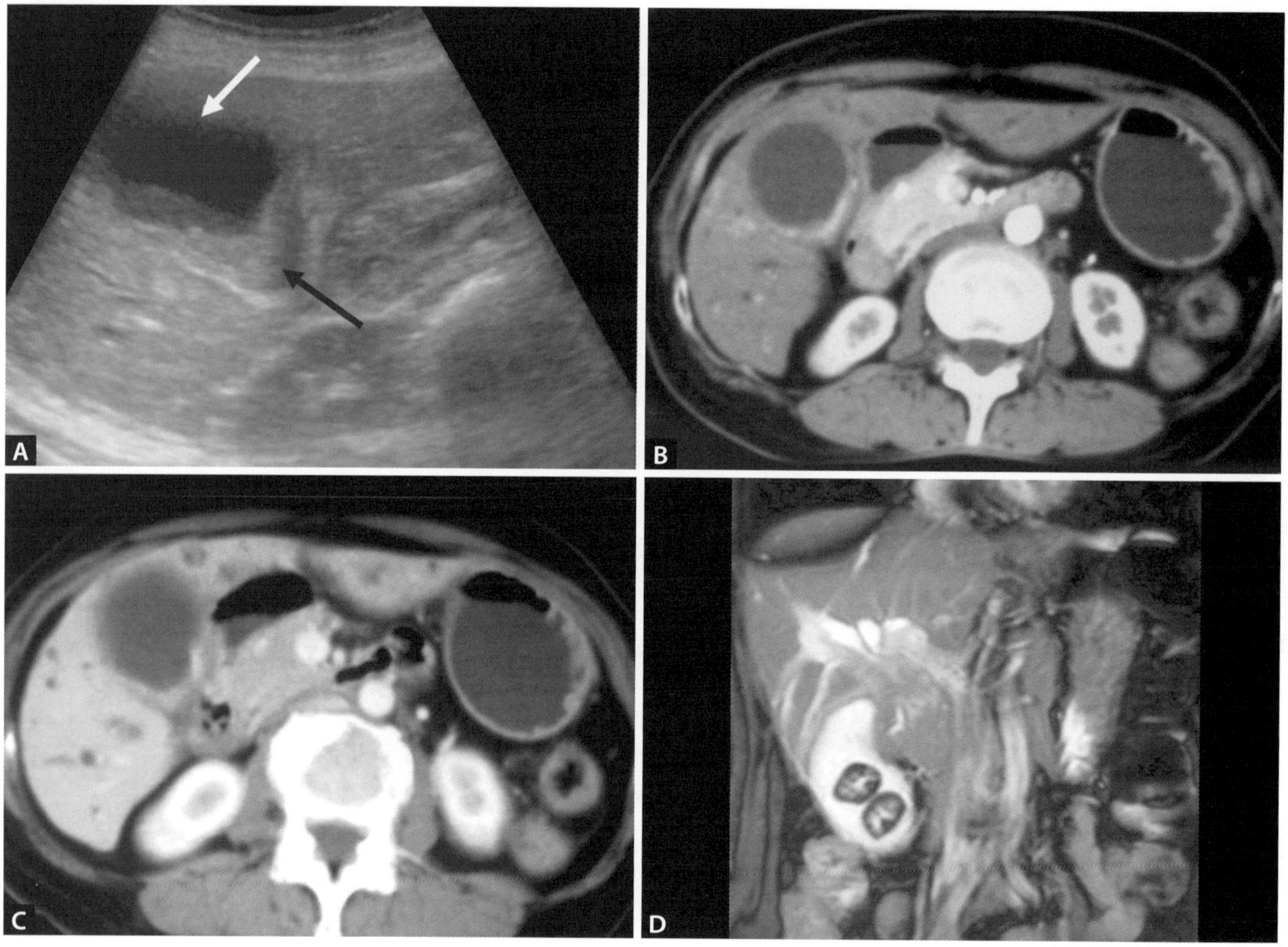

Figs. 3A to D: Asymmetric mural thickening: (A) Grayscale ultrasound image showing distended gallbladder (white arrow) and asymmetric irregular mural thickening involving gallbladder neck; CECT during arterial phase (B) and portal venous phase (C) shows layered pattern of enhancement of gallbladder wall thickening with hyperattenuating inner wall; (D) T2 axial TrueFisp coronal image depicting mural thickening in gallbladder neck and calculi in gallbladder.

lymphadenopathy or metastasis[30] as presence of these help in predicting malignancy. Multiplanar reformatted images of MDCT scans are valuable for demonstrating extent of gallbladder cancers as well as relationship with adjacent organs.[27]

On MRI mural thickening will be hyperintense on T2-weighted sequences. Studies have demonstrated that diffusion-weighted MRI can improve the diagnostic capability for gallbladder wall thickening or polypoid lesions by demonstrating high signal on high b value diffusion-weighted imaging and a lower apparent diffusion coefficient value of gallbladder cancers than that of benign gallbladder diseases.[19]

Pathways of Tumor Spread

Pathway of gallbladder cancer spread include: Direct invasion of the liver, hepatoduodenal ligament, duodenum, or colon; lymphatic spread to regional and retroperitoneal lymph nodes; intraductal tumor extension; hematogenous spread to the liver and peritoneal spread **(Fig. 4)**. Distant metastases are unusual.

Gallbladder carcinoma spreads most commonly by direct invasion of the liver.[32] Invasion of the gastro hepatic ligament may lead to biliary obstruction at the porta hepatis. Compression of common bile duct (CBD) by lymphadenopathy, intra ductal tumor growth and choledocholithiasis are other causes of biliary obstruction in a patient of gallbladder malignancy.

There is a rich lymphatic drainage of gallbladder which facilitates rapid spread to lymph nodes most commonly at the porta hepatis, peri pancreatic and para aortic region. In determining the T stage of gallbladder carcinoma, MDCT has a accuracy of up to 84%.[29] MDCT has accuracy of 85% in predicting respectability.[33] Sensitivity and specificity of

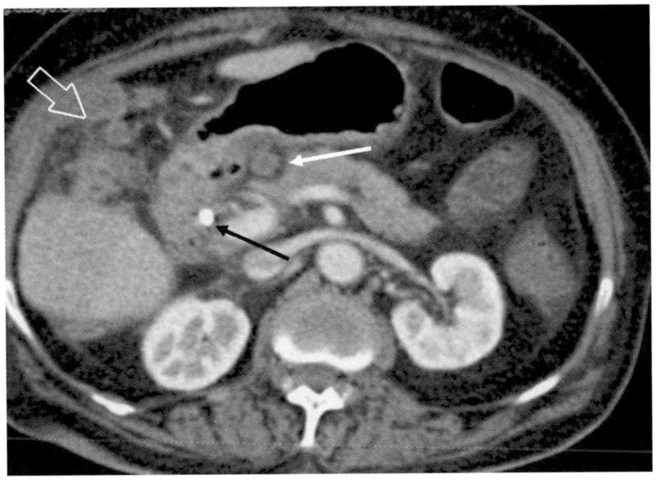

Fig. 4: CECT image showing multiple peritoneal deposits (block arrow) from a gallbladder carcinoma (not shown). Also seen is a metastatic necrotic peripancreatic lymph node (arrow). CBD stent is seen *in situ* (arrow).

multi phasic MRI with MRCP in detecting hepatic invasion, lymph node metastasis and bile duct invasion is 87.5% and 86%, 60% and 90%, and 80% and 100%, respectively.[34]

OTHER MALIGNANT GALLBLADDER NEOPLASMS

Metastasis to the gallbladder are rare but may occur. Among the most common primary malignant neoplasms which may present as gallbladder metastasis are melanoma, breast carcinoma, hepatocellular carcinoma, and lymphoma.[24] Most of the times it is not possible to differentiate between metastatic neoplasms and primary gallbladder carcinoma except that gallstones will be seen less frequently in patients with metastases.

Cholangiocarcinoma

Cholangiocarcinoma is a malignant tumor arising from the epithelium of bile duct which is usually diagnosed late and is associated with poor outcome.

Epidemiology

Cholangiocarcinoma is the second most common primary hepatobiliary malignancy after hepatocellular carcinoma. This malignancy has poor prognosis. 5-year survival rate is less than 5%.[35] Its incidence shows distinct geographic variation, with the highest prevalence in far east and Southeast Asia,[36] where liver fluke infection and choledocholithiasis are common. Men are affected more often then women with a male-to-female ratio of 1.3: 1. Most of the tumors are diagnosed between 50 and 70 years.[37]

Risk Factors

Risk factors for developing cholangiocarcinoma include primary sclerosing cholangitis (PSC), choledochal cyst, congenital hepatic fibrosis, hepatolithiasis, familial polyposis, liver flukes, chronic typhoid carriers and a history of exposure to thorotrast.[38] Patients who have cystic bile duct disorders (Caroli's disease and choledochal cyst) have a life time incidence of cholangiocarcinoma which may range from 6% to 30%.[39] A higher prevalence of positive anti-hepatitis C antibody is associated with this tumor. Cirrhotic patients have ten-fold higher risk of developing cholangiocarcinoma than the general population.[36,40]

Pathology and Classification

More than 95% of cholangiocarcinomas are adenocarcinoma originating from bile duct epithelium and are well or moderately differentiated adenocarcinomas. These tumors tend to have early perineural invasion and are often associated with desmoplastic reaction.[41]

Cholangiocarcinoma are classified based on their anatomical location as intrahepatic or extrahepatic cholangiocarcinoma with the later being more common. Intrahepatic cholangiocarcinoma is also called peripheral cholangiocarcinoma. A tumor that arises peripheral to the secondary bifurcation of the left or right hepatic duct is considered an intra hepatic cholangiocarcinoma. Extra hepatic cholangiocarcinomas are classified into hilar and distal tumors. Hilar cholangiocarcinomas occur at or near the primary biliary confluence where as distal cholangiocarinoma arise from extra hepatic bile duct above the ampulla of Vater.[27] Perihilar disease is most common and represents about 50%, of cholangiocarcinoma cases. Distal disease account for 40%, and intrahepatic disease less than 10% of cholangiocarcinoma cases.[42] From a treatment point of view, these types are considered as distinct entities. Intrahepatic tumors are treated with hepatectomy, hilar malignancies are managed with resection of the bile duct, preferably with hepatectomy where as extrahepatic tumors are treated similar to periampullary malignant neoplasms with pancreato duodenectomy.[27]

On the basis of morphology, cholangiocarcinoma are classified into three types:

1. Mass-forming type which often shows necrosis and fibrosis in the center and accompanying satellite nodules.
2. Periductal infiltrative type, which present as tumor growth along the bile duct longitudinally often resulting in concentric mural thickening and upstream

biliary tree dilatation and may be associated with dense fibroblastic reaction.

3. Intra ductal growing papillary cholangiocarcinoma which present as intra luminal papillary tumors which may involve intrahepatic or extrahepatic bile ducts. This tumor leads to obstruction and dilation of the bile ducts due to abundant much in production. The primary tumor is usually small but may result in multiple tumors involving adjacent segments of bile ducts as it can spread superficially along the mucosal surface.[43,44]

Radiological Findings

The imaging features of cholangiocarcinoma depend on tumor location and type.

Intrahepatic Cholangiocarcinoma

Mass-forming intrahepatic cholangiocarcinoma most commonly presnt on imaging as well-defined mass with irregular borders.[45,46] It lacks the fibrous capsule found in hepatocellular carcinoma (HCC). Peripheral intrahepatic cholangiocarcinoma are usually large at presentation because symptoms occur late. Ultrasonography reveals a hypoechoic, isoechoic or hyper echoic mass, which may be homogeneous or heterogeneous. Unenhanced CT reveals a hypodense solitary mass that may have satellite lesions. Focal intrahepatic biliary ductal dilatation, segmental atrophy and capsular retraction may be seen. On MRI, intrahepatic cholangiocarcinoma is hypointense on T1-weighted images and hyper intense on T2-weighted images.[47] On enhanced CT/MRI, the tumor may shows thin rim or thick band of peripheral and patchy enhancement in early phase corresponding to active tumor growth. The central area of the tumor, due to its fibrous composition, does not enhance during early phase but may show enhancement during the delayed phase, a feature which may help to differentiate it from HCC **(Figs. 5A to C)**.[48] The delayed enhancement may be bright enough to simulate hemangioma.

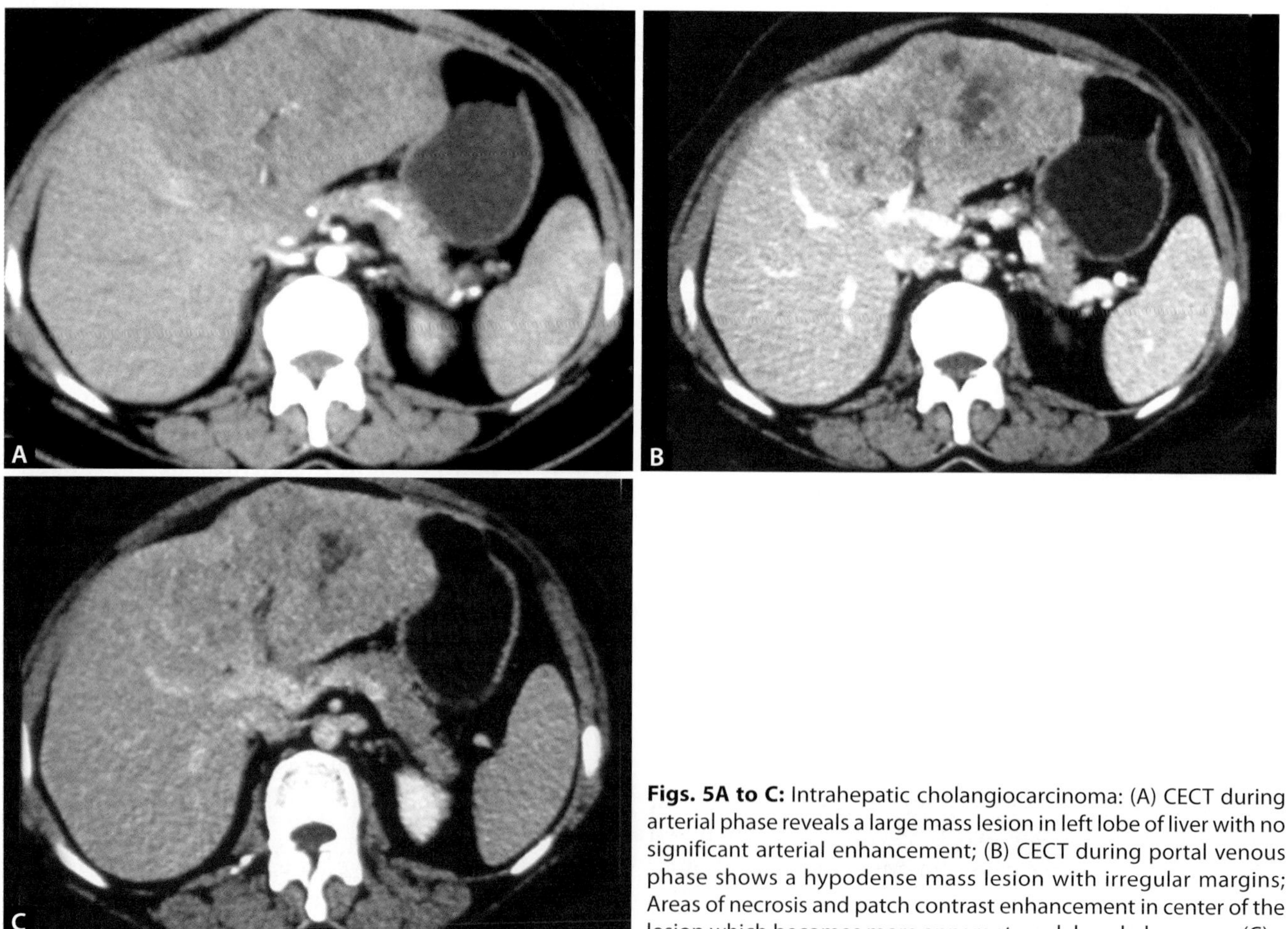

Figs. 5A to C: Intrahepatic cholangiocarcinoma: (A) CECT during arterial phase reveals a large mass lesion in left lobe of liver with no significant arterial enhancement; (B) CECT during portal venous phase shows a hypodense mass lesion with irregular margins; Areas of necrosis and patch contrast enhancement in center of the lesion which becomes more apparent on delayed phase scan (C).

Peripheral cholangiocarcinoma can also be of periductal infiltrating type or intra ductal polypoidal type and these may cause segmental bile duct dilatation and lobar atrophy **(Figs. 6A to C)**. Polypoidal (papillary) variant can occasionally produce abundant mucin similar to IPMT of the pancreas. This can result in gross dilatation of the bile duct. Demonstration of direct continuity of tumor with bile ducts helps differentiate this entity from biliary cystadenocarcinoma. Hypovascular metastases can have an enhancement pattern similar to that of peripheral cholangiocarcinomas. Absence of a known primary malignant neoplasm, relatively large tumor size, and bile duct dilation suggest a diagnosis of cholangiocarcinoma rather than metastases.[45]

Hilar Cholangiocarcinoma (Klatskin's tumor)

Hilar cholangiocarcinoma are usually periductal infiltrating type and most often arise at the primary confluence or in the proximal common hepatic duct. Sonographic findings include intrahepatic bile ductal dilatation with or without isolation of right and left sided ducts and lobar atrophy. Definite mass is rarely seen on US and demonstration of dilated intrahepatic ducts without any evidence of extrahepatic dilatation alone should raise the suspicion of hilar cholangiocarcinoma. Sometimes tumor may be seen on sonography as bile duct wall thickening and less commonly may be seen as a polypoidal lesion. The tumors are moderately echogenic, reflecting the fibrous nature of the tumor. MDCT with its multi planer abilities is superior to USG in identification of these small tumors.[49] Although the tumor appears hypodense to liver in both unenhanced and enhanced CT scans, the focally thickened bile duct wall due to infiltrating tumor may appear hyper dense to the liver in the arterial and portal venous phase. In keeping with their fibrous rich stroma, delayed enhancement can be seen 8–15 minutes after contrast injection.[50] Cholangiocarcinoma are isointense/hypointense on T1-weighted images while T2 signal varies from markedly hyperintense to only mildly increased signal in fibrous tumors. Lobar hepatic atrophy

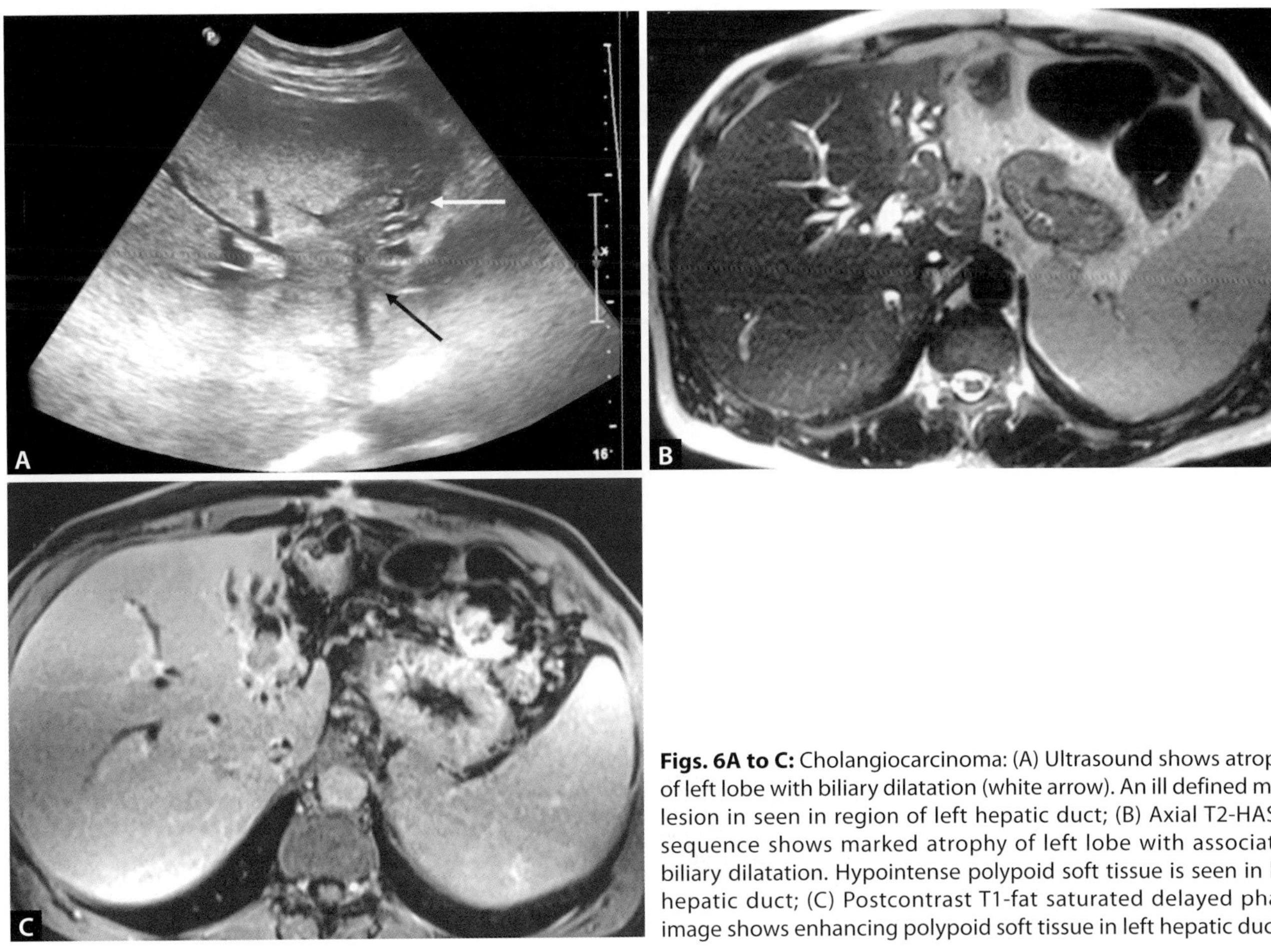

Figs. 6A to C: Cholangiocarcinoma: (A) Ultrasound shows atrophy of left lobe with biliary dilatation (white arrow). An ill defined mass lesion in seen in region of left hepatic duct; (B) Axial T2-HASTE sequence shows marked atrophy of left lobe with associated biliary dilatation. Hypointense polypoid soft tissue is seen in left hepatic duct; (C) Postcontrast T1-fat saturated delayed phase image shows enhancing polypoid soft tissue in left hepatic duct.

is seen in one fourth of patients with cholangiocarcinoma and this finding coupled with biliary dilatation is strongly suggestive of cholangiocarcinoma. Atrophy results from long standing biliary obstruction or portal venous involvement and results in crowding of dilated bile ducts and volume loss most often affecting the left lobe of liver.[48] Contiguous invasion of the liver parenchyma and hepatoduodenal ligament is frequent in Klatskin tumors. Lymph nodal metastases can be seen in peri portal and peri pancreatic regions. Retroperitoneal adenopathy, proximal intestinal obstruction and peritoneal dissemination occur in advanced stages. Diagnostic percutaneous transhepatic cholangiography (PTC) and ERCP are now less commonly employed for cholangiocarcinoma. The involved ducts appear stenosed with smooth shouldering or irregular tapering. MDCT and cholangiography provide complimentary information as superficial (mucosal) involvement is better assessed on direct cholangiography while submucosal/extra mucosal involvement and areas not opacified on cholangiography are better seen on CT. Contrast enhanced MRI with MRCP can provide most comprehensive tumor staging.[51] EUS with EUS-guided FNA is increasingly being used for characterizing biliary strictures and assessing extent of periductal involvement and lymph nodal metastasis.[52] Hilar cholangiocarcinomas are commonly periductal infiltrating type though intra ductal papillary tumor may also be seen. The intra ductal tumors are hyperdense on noncontrast CT (NCCT) images and are hypodense on postcontrast images as they lack fibrotic stroma. These tumors when multiple can be confused with calculi. Contrast enhancement in these tumors help in differentiating these tumors from stones.[53,54]

Nonresectability of hilar cholangiocarcinoma is suggested by:[55,56]

- Severe bilateral involvement of the secondary confluence
- Involvement of the main portal vein
- Involvement of both branches of the portal vein
- Bilateral involvement of the hepatic artery and portal vein
- Vascular involvement on one side of the liver and extensive bile duct involvement on the other side.

Perihilar cholangiocarcinoma are graded according to modified Bismuth-Corlette classification. The original Bismuth-Corlette system[57] classified perihilar cholangiocarcinoma into three types: type I, tumor distal to the confluence of the left and right hepatic ducts; **(Fig. 7)** type II, tumors involving the main biliary confluence and the main left or right ducts but not extending into the secondary level of ductal

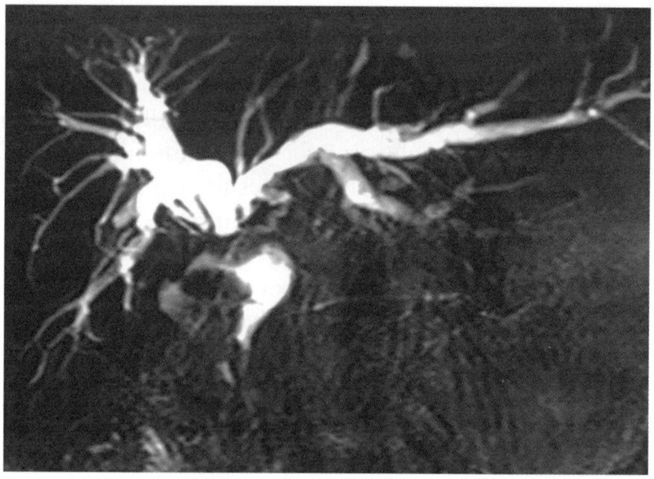

Fig. 7: Perihilar cholangiocarcinoma type 1: Coronal reconstructed MRCP image showing abrupt cut off of common hepatic duct with proximal biliary dilatation.

confluences; **(Figs. 8A and B)** type III, extension into the confluence of either the left or right hepatic ducts. The modified Bismuth-Corlette system[58] divided type III hilar cholangiocarcinoma into types IIIa and IIIb and added a type IV. Type IIIa is tumor extension beyond the confluence of the right hepatic duct into secondary biliary radicles, type IIIb involves similar extension into the left hepatic ductal system **(Fig. 9)**. Type IV signifies tumor extension to bilateral secondary biliary radicles **(Figs. 10A to C)**.

Distal Cholangiocarcinoma

Distal cholangiocarcinoma is the tumor arising from common bile duct between the origin of cystic duct and the ampulla of Vater. Tumors arising from ampulla are not included in distal cholangiocarcinomas.[44] These are usually small and have better prognosis than perihilar cholangiocarcinomas. Imaging features include biliary dilatation proximal to an abrupt obstruction. Mass itself is rarely demonstrated on imaging hence differentiation from benign strictures may not be possible. Cholangiocarcinoma should be suspected when abrupt obstruction of common bile duct is seen without visualization of a mass or calculus and the pancreas is normal in the absence of history of previous surgery. Carcinoma of the pancreas is more likely if the mass is seen near head of the pancreas.[59] Even with all imaging modalities, differentiating between benign and malignant biliary strictures is sometimes difficult. Longer and thicker involvement by the stricture, irregularity of lumen, asymmetric narrowing, hyper enhancement in portal venous phase, periductal soft tissue mass, and enlarged lymph node are associated with malignant

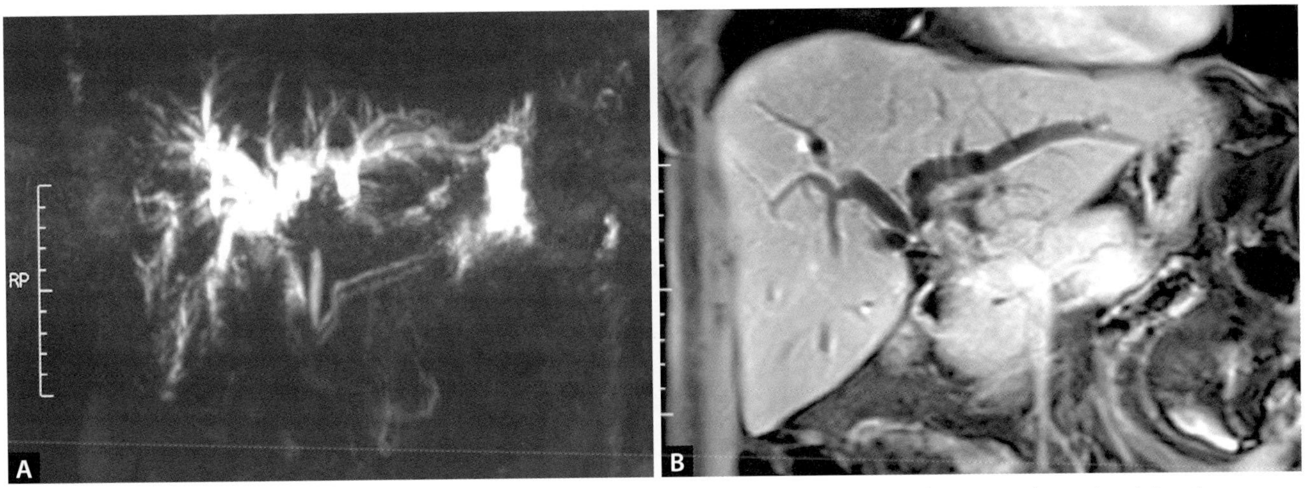

Figs. 8A and B: Perihilar cholangiocarcinoma type 2: (A) Coronal reconstructed MRCP image showing stricture involving the common hepatic duct and primary biliary confluence; (B) Postcontrast T1-fat saturated image showing ill defined poorly enhancing soft tissue at primary biliary confluence.

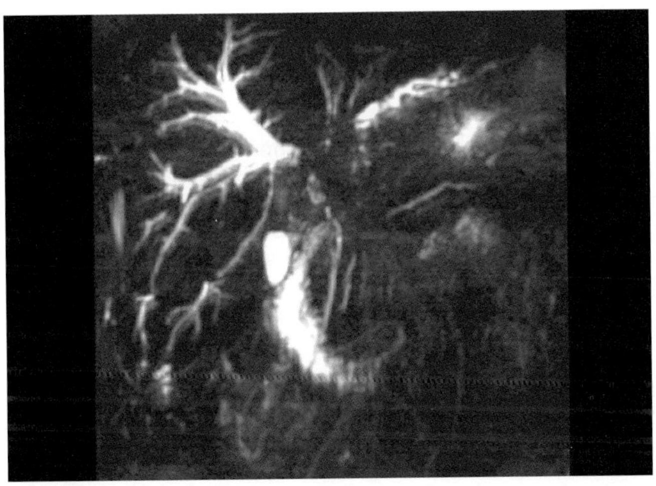

Fig. 9: Perihilar cholangiocarcinoma type 3b: Coronal reconstructed MRCP image showing stricture involving main biliary confluence and extending into left secondary confluence.

stricture.[60] ERCP and EUS are important for complete evaluation of these tumors. EUS-FNA is very useful to predict unresectability.[61]

Periampullary Carcinoma

Periampullary carcinomas are those tumors arising from or within 1 cm of the papilla of Vater and include ampullary, pancreatic, bile duct, and duodenal malignancies.[3] It is often impossible by imaging or even by histologic examination to know the origin of tumor with certainty. Patients with familial adenomatous polyposis have higher incidence of these tumors and are often preceded by duodenal or ampullary adenomas.[62] These tumors are usually of lower grade than proximal biliary malignancies. Periampullary tumors may not be seen on imaging, in which case a dilated common bile duct and dilated main pancreatic duct with abrupt termination in the head of pancreas is usually seen **(Fig. 11)**. Dilation of common bile duct is observed in 75% of cases, and pancreatic ductal dilation is seen in 67%.[62,63] On imaging if periampullary tumors are visualized they tend to be small and are likely to have a polypoidal growth pattern **(Fig. 12)**. Nodal and hepatic metastasis are rare at the time of diagnosis.

On T1-weighted images, periampullary tumors are usually hypo intense. On immediate postgadolinium T1-weighted images, these lesions will show low signal intensity due to their hypo vascular character compared with background pancreatic tissue.[63] On two minute delayed images, a thin rim of peripheral enhancement may be seen. ERCP though invasive will permit biopsy and stent placement. Sensitivity of EUS in detecting small periampullary tumor matches that of ERCP and is better than CT **(Fig. 13)**.[64] EUS shows the depth of invasion into the duodenum and local extension of the tumor. It may be the most accurate modality for assessing local staging of ampullary tumors.[65]

Malignant Cystic Bile Duct Neoplasms: Cystadenocarcinoma

Biliary cystadenoma and cyst adenocarcinoma are rare cystic neoplasms lined by mucin secreting columnar epithelium. They are usually seen in middle-aged women. Most cystadenomas and cyst adenocarcinomas are intrahepatic masses that are hypoechoic on ultrasound

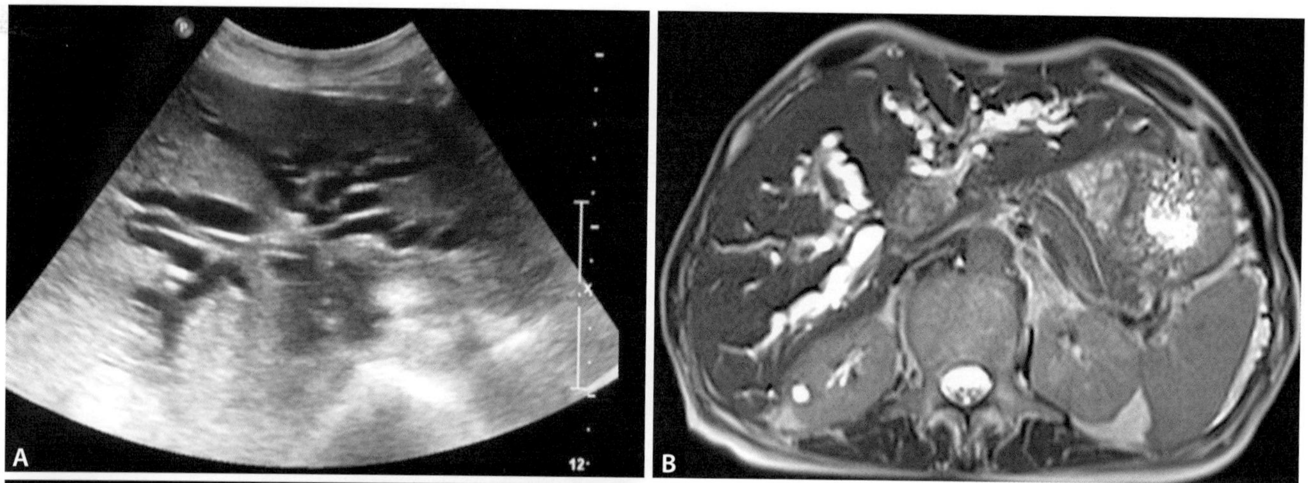

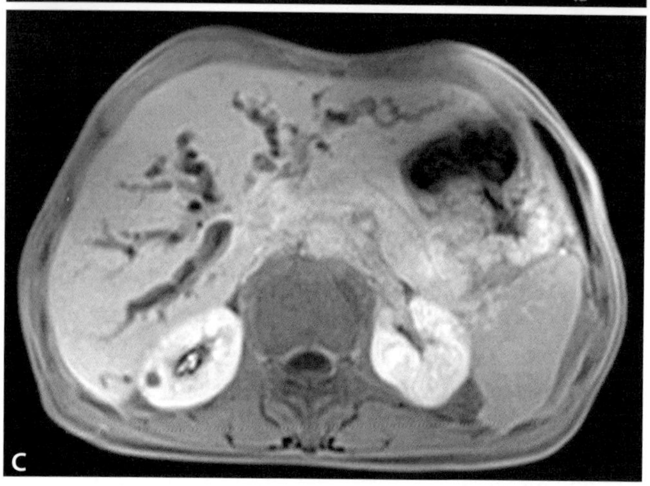

Figs. 10A to C: Perihilar cholangiocarcinoma type 4: (A) Ultrasound showing intrahepatic biliary dilatation in both lobes of liver with nonpatent primary and secondary confluence on both sides; (B) Axial T2-HASTE image showing heterogeneous hypointense mass lesion involving primary biliary confluence extending into right and left secondary confluence; (C) Postcontrast T1 delayed phase image showing enhancing infiltrating soft tissue.

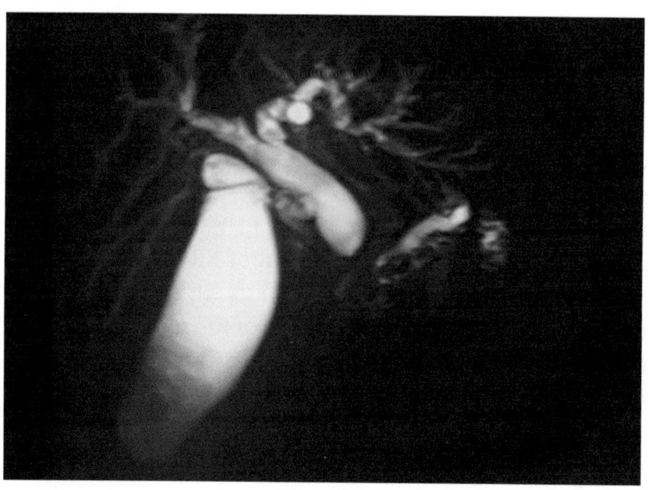

Fig. 11: Periampullary carcinoma: Coronal reconstructed MRCP image showing biliary dilatation with dilatation of both CBD and MPD (Double duct sign).

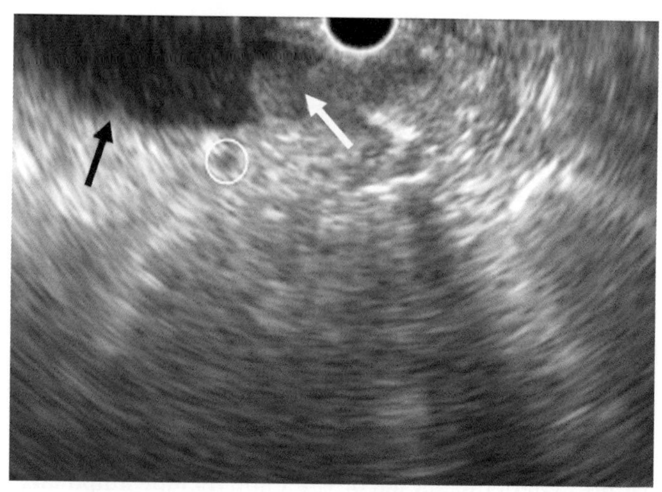

Fig. 12: Periampullary carcinoma: Endoscopic ultrasound image using linear EUS probe shows dilated CBD (black arrow) and polypoid hypoechoic mass in terminal CBD (white arrow). MPD (encircled) is not dilated. Findings are consistent with terminal bile duct cholangiocarcinoma.
Courtesy: Dr SS Rana, Department of Gastroenterology, PGIMER, Chandigarh, India.

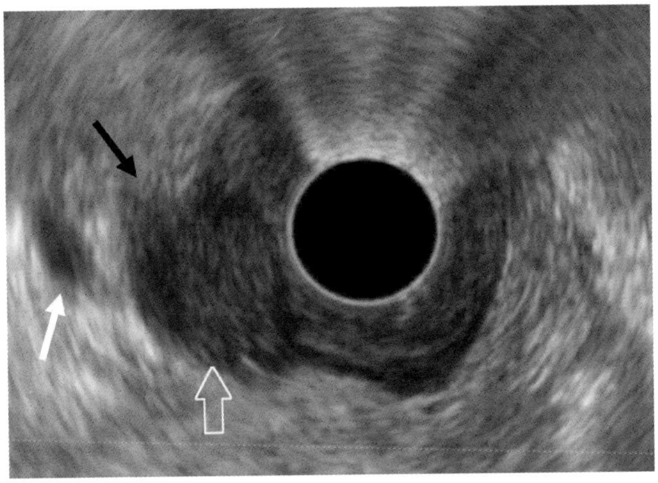

Fig. 13: Periampullary carcinoma: Endoscopic ultrasound (EUS) image using radial EUS probe shows dilated CBD (black arrow), dilated MPD (white arrow) and hypoechoic mass in ampulla (block arrow). Findings are consistent with ampullary carcinoma.
Courtesy: Dr SS Rana, Department of Gastroenterology, PGIMER, Chandigarh, India.

and are hypodense on CT. These cystic lesions can be unilocular or multilocular.[66] Mural nodules, papillary growths and septations are seen both in cystadenoma and cyst adenocarcinoma though cyst adenocarcinomas show papillary excrescences and solid portions more often.[66] The differential diagnosis of these tumors includes hepatic cysts, hydatid cysts, liver abscesses, cystic metastases, hematoma, cystic sarcomas, and choledochal cysts.[66]

OTHER MALIGNANT NEOPLASMS OF THE BILE DUCTS

In adults, metastasis, lymphomas, leiomyosarcomas, and carcinoid tumors can rarely occur in the bile ducts. Embryonal rhabdomyosarcoma is the second most common cause of jaundice in the pediatric population after choledochal cyst. Sonography and CT will show intra hepatic duct dilation and a soft tissue mass in the region of the common bile duct or porta hepatis. On MRCP, grape like filling defects are seen in dilated CBD which may show enhancement.[67]

CONCLUSION

Malignancies of the biliary tract are often discovered late. USG is the initial imaging modality whenever a biliary tree malignancy is suspected. MDCT with multi planer reformations, MRI with MRCP, ERCP and EUS all have a role to play in early detection, characterization, staging and preoperative planning of these highly lethal tumors. It is important for the radiologist to be aware of imaging features of malignant pathologies of biliary tree so as to play critical role in their management.

REFERENCES

1. Cleary SP, Dawson LA, Knox JJ, et al. Cancer of the gallbladder and extra-hepatic bile ducts. Curr Probl Surg. 2007;44:396-482.
2. Craig JR, Peters RL, Edmondson HA. Tumors of the liver and intra hepatic bile ducts. In: Atlas of Tumor Pathology. 2nd series. Fascicle 26. Washington, DC: Armed Forces Institute of Pathology; 1989.
3. Heinrich S, Clavien PA. Ampullary cancer. Curr Opin Gastroenterol. 2010;26(3):280-5.
4. Jemal A, Siegel R, Xu J, et al. Cancer statistics, 2010. CA Cancer J Clin. 2011;60:133-4.
5. Kiran RP, Pokala N, Dudrick SJ. Incidence pattern and survival for gallbladder cancer over three decades—an analysis of 10301 patients. Ann Surg Oncol. 2007;14:827-32.
6. Nanda Kumar A, Gupta PC, Gangadharn P, et al. Geographic pathology revisited: development of an atlas of cancer in India. Int J Cancer. 2005;116:740-54.
7. Dhir V, Mohandas KM. Epidemiology of digestive tract cancers in India IV. Gallbladder and pancreas. Indian J Gastroenterol. 1999;18:24-8.
8. Sheth S, Bedford A, Chopra S. Primary gallbladder cancer: recognition of risk factors and the role of prophylactic cholecystectomy. Am J Gastroenterol. 2000;95:1402-10.
9. Tazuma S, Kajiyama G. Carcinogenesis of malignant lesions of the gallbladder. The impact of chronic inflammation and gallstones. Langen becks Arch Surg. 2001;386:224-9.
10. Khan ZS, Livingston EH, Huerta S. Reassessing the need for prophylactic surgery in patients with porcelain gallbladder: case series and systematic review of the literature. Arch Surg. 2011;146(10):1143-7.
11. Schnelldorfer T. Porcelain gallbladder: a benign process or concern for malignancy? J Gastrointest Surg. 2013;17:1161-8.
12. Stephen AE, Berger DL. Carcinoma in the porcelain gallbladder: a relationship revisited. Surgery. 2001;129(6):699-703.
13. Henson DE, Albores Saavedra J, Corle D. Carcinoma of the gallbladder. Histologic types, stage of disease, grade and survival rates. Cancer. 1992;70:1493-7.
14. Albores Saavedra J, Henson DE. Tumors of the gallbladder and extra-hepatic bile ducts. Atlas of Tumor Pathology, Fascicle 22, 2nd Series. Washington, DC: Armed Forces Institute of Pathology, 1986.
15. Edge SB, Byrd DR, Compton CC, et al. AJCC Cancer Staging Manual, 7th ed. Chicago, Springer; 2010.pp.211-7.
16. Donohue JH, Stewart AK, Menck HR. The national cancer data base report on carcinoma of the gallbladder, 1989–1995. Cancer. 1998;83:2618-28.

17. Bach AM, Loring LA, Hann LE, et al. Gallbladder cancer: Can ultra sonography evaluate extent of disease? J Ultrasound Med. 1998;17:303-9.
18. Soyer P, Gouhiri M, Boudiaf M, et al. Carcinoma of the gallbladder: imaging features with surgical correlation. AJR. 1997;169:781-4.
19. Ogawa T, Horaguchi J, Fujita N, et al. High b-value diffusion-weighted magnetic resonance imaging for gallbladder lesions: Differentiation between benignity and malignancy. J Gastroenterol. 2012;47:1352-60.
20. Levy AD, Murakata LA, Rohrmann CA. Gallbladder carcinoma: radiologic-pathologic correlation. RadioGraphics. 2001;21:295-314.
21. Rodríguez-Fernádez A, Gómez-Río M, Medina-Benitez A, et al. Application of modern imaging methods in diagnosis of gallbladder cancer. J Surg Oncol. 2006;93:650-64.
22. Tsuchiya Y. Early carcinoma of the gallbladder: macroscopic features and sonography findings. Radiology. 1991;179:171-5.
23. Franquet T, Montes M, Ruiz de Azua Y, et al. Primary gallbladder carcinoma: imaging findings in 50 patients with pathologic correlation. Gastrointest Radiol. 1991;16: 143-8.
24. Yoshimitsu K, Honda H, Kaneko K, et al. Dynamic MRI of the gallbladder lesions: differentiation of benign from malignant. J Magn Reson Imaging. 1997;7:696-701.
25. Furlan A, Ferris JV, Hosseinzadeh K, et al. Gallbladder carcinoma update: multimodality imaging evaluation, staging, and treatment options. AJR. 2008;191:1440-7.
26. Wilbur AC, Sagireddy PB, Aizenstein RL. Carcinoma of the gallbladder: color Doppler ultrasound and CT findings. Abdom Imaging. 1997;22:187-9.
27. Choi BI, Lee JM. Neoplasms of the Gallbladder and Biliary Tract. In: Richard M Gore, Marc S Levine (Eds): Textbook of Gastrointestinal Radiology. 4th edn. Saunders Elsevier; 2015.pp.1402-26.
28. Onoyama H, Yamamoto M, Takada M, et al. Diagnostic imaging of early gallbladder cancers: retrospective study of 53 cases. World J Surg. 1999;23:708-12.
29. Kim SJ, Lee JM, Lee JY, et al. Accuracy of preoperative T-staging of gallbladder carcinoma using MDCT. AJR. 2008;190:74-8.
30. Kim SJ, Lee JM, Lee JY, et al. Analysis of enhancement pattern of flat from cholecystitis. AJR. 2008;191:765-71.
31. Sandhu MS, Yoganand K, Kalra N, et al. Radiological evaluation of the enhancement patterns of thickened gallbladder wall to differentiate benign from malignancy. PGIMER study.
32. Kondo S, Nimura Y, Kamiya J, et al. Mode of tumor spread and surgical strategy in gallbladder carcinoma. Langenbecks Arch Surg. 2002;387:222-8.
33. Kalra N, Suri S, Gupta R, et al. MDCT in the staging of gallbladder carcinoma. AJR. 2006;186:758-62.
34. Kaza RK, Gulati M, Wig JD, et al. Evaluation of gallbladder carcinoma with dynamic magnetic resonance imaging and magnetic resonance cholangiopancreatography. Australas Radiol. 2006;50:212-7.
35. Mosconi S, Beretta GD, Labianca R, et al. Cholangiocarcinoma. Crit Rev Oncol Hematol. 2009;69: 259-70.
36. Shaib Y, El-Serag HB. The epidemiology of cholangio-carcinoma. Semin Liver Dis. 2004;24(2):115-25.
37. Henson DE, Albores-Saavedra J, Corle D. Carcinoma of the extra hepatic bile ducts: histologic types, stage of disease, grade, and survival rates. Cancer. 1992;70:1498-501.
38. Sainani NI, Catalano OA, Holalkere NS, et al. Cholangio-carcinoma: current and novel imaging techniques. Radiographics. 2008;28:1263-87.
39. Tyson GL, El-Serag HB. Risk factors for cholangio-carcinoma. Hepatology. 2011;54:173-84.
40. Sorenson HT, Friis S, Olsen JH, et al. Risk of liver and other types of cancer in patients with cirrhosis: a nationwide cohort study in Denmark. Hepatology. 1998;28:921-5.
41. Khan ZR, Neugut AI, Ahsan H, et al. Risk factors for biliary tract cancers. Am J Gastroenterol. 1999;94:149-52.
42. DeOliveira ML, Cunningham SC, Cameron JL, et al. Cholangiocarcinoma: thirty-one-year experience with 564 patients at single institution. Ann Surg. 2007;245: 755-62.
43. Nakanuma Y, Sato Y, Harada K, et al. Pathological classification of intra hepatic cholangiocarcinoma based on a new concept. World J Hepatol. 2010;2:419-27.
44. Razumilava N, Gores GJ. Classification, diagnosis, and management of cholangiocarcinoma. Clin Gastroenterol Hepatol. 2013;11:13-21.
45. Heller SL, Lee VS. MR imaging of the gallbladder and biliary system. Magn Reson Imaging Clin N Am. 2005;13:295-311.
46. Choi BI, Lee JM, Han JK. Imaging of intra hepatic and hilar cholangiocarcinoma. Abdom Imaging. 2004;29:548-57.
47. Choi BI, Han KJ, Kim TK. Benign and malignant tumours of the biliary tract. In: Gazelle GC, Saini S, Meuller PR (Eds). Hepatobiliary and pancreatic radiology. New York, 1st edn, Thieme; 1998.pp.630-76.
48. Loyer FM, Chin H, DuBrow RA, et al. Hepato cellular carcinoma and intra hepatic peripheral cholangio carcinoma. Enhancement patterns with quadruple phasehelical CT. Radiology. 1999;212:866-71.
49. Choi BI, Lee JH, Han MC. Hilar cholangiocarcinoma. Comparative study with sonography and CT. Radiology. 1989;172:689-92.
50. Motohara T, Semelka RC, Bidar TR. MR cholangio pancreatography. RCNA. 2003;41:89-96.
51. Yeh TS, Jan YY, Tseng JH, et al. Malignant perihilar biliary obstruction: MRCP findings. Am J Gastroenterol. 2000;95:432-40.
52. Nguyen K, Sing JT Jr. Review of endoscopic techniques in the diagnosis and management of cholangiocarcinoma. World J Gastroenterol. 2008;14:2995-9.
53. Lee JW, Han JK, Kim TK, et al. CT features of intra ductal intra hepatic cholangiocarcinoma. AJR. 2000;175:721-5.
54. Kim JE, Lee JM, Kim SH, et al. Differentiation of intra ductal growing type cholangiocarcinomas at biliary MR imaging with MR cholangiography. Radiology. 2010;257:364-72.

55. Ahrendt SA, Pitt HA. Biliary tract. In: Townsend CM, Beauchamp RD, Evers BM, Mattox KL (Eds): SabistonTexbook of Surgery (17th edn) Philadelphia: Saunders Elsevier, 2004.pp.1112-43.
56. Manfredi R, Masselli G, Maresca G, et al. MR imaging and MRCP of hilar cholangiocarcinoma. Abdom Imaging. 2003;28:319-25.
57. Bismuth H, Corlette MB. Intra hepatic cholangioenteric anastomosis in carcinoma of the hilus of the liver. Surg Gynecol Obstet. 1975;140:170-8.
58. Bismuth H, Nakache R, Diamond T. Management strategies in resection for hilar cholangiocarcinoma. Ann Surg. 1992; 215:31-8.
59. Choi SH, Han JK, Lee JM, et al. Differentiating malignant from benign common bile duct stricture with multi phasic helical CT. Radiology. 2005;236:178-83.
60. Park MS, Kim TK, Kim KW, et al. Differentiation of extra hepatic bile duct cholangiocarcinoma from benign stricture: Findings at MRCP versus ERCP. Radiology. 2004;233:234-40.
61. Mohamadnejad M, DeWitt JM, Sherman S, et al. Role of EUS for preoperative evaluation of cholangiocarcinoma: a large single-center experience. Gastrointest Endosc. 2011;73:71-8.
62. Dittrick GW, Mallat DB, Lamont JP. Management of ampullary lesions. Curr Treat Options Gastroenterol. 2006;9:371-6.
63. Kim JH, Kim MJ, Chung JJ, et al. Differential diagnosis of peri ampullary carcinomas at MR imaging. Radiographics. 2002;22:1335-52.
64. Skordilis P, Mouzas IA, Dimoulios PD, Alexandrakis G, Moschandrea J, Kouroumalis E. Is endosonography an effective method for detection and local staging of the ampullary carcinoma? A prospective study. BMC Surg. 2002;2:1.
65. Kubo H, Chijiiwa Y, Akahoshi K, Hamada S, Matsui N, Nawata H. Pre-operative staging of ampullary tumours by endoscopic ultrasound. Br J Radiol. 1999;72:443-7.
66. Choi BI, Lim JH, Han MC, et al. Biliary cyst adenoma and cyst adenocarcinoma: CT and sonographic findings. Radiology. 1989;171:57-61.
67. Tireli GA, Sander S, Dervisoglu S, Demirali O, Unal M. Embryonal rhabdomyosarcoma of the common bile duct mimicking choledochal cyst. J Hepatobiliary Pancreat Surg. 2005;12:263-5.

CHAPTER 86

Biliary Interventions

Mandeep Kang, Naveen Kalra, Anupam Lal

INTRODUCTION

The past few decades have witnessed a revolution in minimally invasive surgeries and techniques with image guided interventions having emerged at the forefront of these developments. Percutaneous biliary interventions had their origin way back in 1921 when direct puncture of the gall- bladder was first performed to opacify the biliary tree. This was followed by reports describing percutaneous direct puncture of the biliary tree. The technique of percutaneous biliary drainage for the relief of obstructive jaundice was introduced in the 1970s[1-3] followed by percutaneous cholecystostomy in the 1980s.[4-6] The development of biliary stents has further enlarged the scope of percutaneous applications in the management of biliary diseases.[7-11]

In the present day, percutaneous biliary interventions include percutaneous transhepatic cholangiography (PTC) and biliary drainage (PTBD) for the diagnosis and management of biliary obstruction and percutaneous cholecystostomy. This route can also be used for percutaneous transhepatic cholangioscopy or biliary ultrasonography; biopsy of the biliary duct, cholangioplasty for benign biliary strictures and as an access for the removal of bile duct calculi, the application of intraluminal brachytherapy or radiofrequency ablation.

PERCUTANEOUS TRANSHEPATIC CHOLANGIOGRAPHY

Percutaneous transhepatic cholangiography (PTC) is a diagnostic procedure which involves placement of a fine needle into a peripheral biliary radicle under image guidance followed by contrast injection to opacify the biliary tree. The procedure is used for:[8,12]

- To define the level of obstruction in patients with obstructive biliopathy.
- To evaluate for presence of suspected choledocholithiasis.
- To determine the etiology of cholangitis.
- To evaluate suspected bile duct inflammatory disorders.
- To demonstrate the site of bile duct leak.
- As the preliminary step for draining the biliary tree (most common indication).

Although PTC has been shown to be an effective technique which reliably demonstrates the level of obstruction, it is more invasive and painful than endoscopic retrograde cholangiopancreatography (ERCP). It also involves the risk of significant complications such as hemoperitoneum and bile peritonitis. Hence, PTC is nowadays reserved for patients in whom an ECRP is not possible due to anatomy altering surgeries or following unsuccessful cannulation of the common bile duct.

Preprocedure Evaluation and Preparation

The initial workup of a patient with obstructive biliopathy includes a clinical evaluation with history taking, physical examination and pertinent laboratory tests. Cross sectional imaging such as ultrasonography, CT and MRI should be performed to provide information about the level of obstruction of the biliary tree and to determine the cause.

Coagulation parameters including prothrombin time, prothrombin time index (>75%) and the international normalized ratio (≤1.5) as well as platelet count (>50–75,000) should be checked prior to the procedure and corrected with fresh frozen plasma or platelets if deranged.

Antibiotics are routinely administered in all patients as bacteremia and sepsis can develop during the procedure. Broad spectrum antibiotics covering both gram-positive and gram-negative organisms should be started prior to the procedure. A venous access should be secured and an informed consent obtained after explaining the procedure completely to the patient and attendants.

Conscious sedation should be used for adequate pain control. Over dosage of the sedative should be avoided as the patient needs to follow the instructions of the operator such as breath holding. General anesthesia may however be required in selected cases.[12-14]

Technique

With the patient lying supine on the fluoroscopy table, the upper abdomen is cleaned and draped. The skin puncture site is anesthetized with a local anesthetic (2% lidocaine) up to the liver capsule. If the peripheral biliary radicles are dilated they can be punctured under ultrasonographic guidance. If not dilated, the procedure is performed under fluoroscopic guidance. Most PTCs are performed from the right mid-axillary approach through an intercostal space which is caudal to the costophrenic sulcus. This can be identified on fluoroscopy on deep inspiration. A 15 cm fine (22G) Chiba needle is advanced into the liver aiming for the right lateral aspect of the 12th thoracic vertebral body. After the stylet is removed, the needle is slowly withdrawn while injecting a small amount of contrast. When contrast is seen to opacify the biliary tree, needle withdrawal is stopped and cholangiography performed to delineate the biliary anatomy. If the first puncture is unsuccessful a second or third puncture can be made by changing the needle angulation once the needle tip is near the liver capsule.

The success rates for PTC are reported to be more than 90% in a dilated system and 67–80% in a nondilated system. Major complications are seen in 3.5–10% of procedures and include sepsis, cholangitis, bile leak, hemorrhage or pneumothorax.[12-15]

PERCUTANEOUS TRANSHEPATIC BILIARY DRAINAGE

Percutaneous transhepatic biliary drainage (PTBD) is a therapeutic procedure that consists of sterile puncture of a peripheral biliary radicle under image guidance followed by placement of a catheter or stent for internal or external drainage of bile. Percutaneous therapy of bile duct lesions is often a staged procedure, requiring multiple sessions to achieve the therapeutic goals.[8]

Indications for Biliary Drainage

The presence of cholestasis, whether due to benign or malignant etiology, predisposes to biliary infection. Secondly, protracted hyperbilirubinemia causes impairment of the renal function. The surgical morbidity and mortality rates are also high (40–60% and 15–25% respectively) in the setting of hyperbilirubinemia, therefore decompression should be done as early as possible in patients with obstructive biliopathy. Malignancy causing biliary obstruction is often unresectable at the time of diagnosis and palliative therapy is the only management option possible. A normalized liver function is also required for the administration of chemotherapy. Biliary drainage thus will not only normalize liver function, restore the physiological drainage of bile into the duodenum, prevent the development of cholangitis and sepsis but also improve the nutritional status and quality of life of the patient.[7,9,10]

Common causes of benign biliary obstruction include choledocholithiasis, sclerosing cholangitis, and inflammatory conditions such as pancreatitis, iatrogenic causes (post-laparoscopic cholecystectomy, liver transplantation or anastomotic strictures) and infections such as HIV infection, oriental and parasitic cholangitis.[15] The common causes of malignant biliary obstruction include gallbladder carcinoma, cholangiocarcinoma, carcinoma of the pancreas and metastatic disease.[10,16]

The indications include:

- To decompress the obstructed biliary tree
- To dilate benign biliary strictures
- To remove bile duct stones
- To divert bile from and stent bile duct defects
- To stent malignant strictures.

There are no absolute contraindications for the procedure. Deranged coagulation parameters are a relative contraindication and should be corrected prior to the procedure with platelets or fresh frozen plasma. The presence of gross ascites with presence of perihepatic fluid is also a relative contraindication which requires to be drained before performing a PTBD.[14,16]

PATIENT PREPARATION

The patient preparation and preprocedure work-up are as for PTC. The endoscopic route is preferred for drainage, particularly in lesions involving the mid or distal common bile duct (CBD) as it is associated with a decreased complication rate. However, with lesions involving the hilum, the percutaneous approach is associated with a higher success rate and is therefore preferred. In cases of failed ERCP or where ERCP is not possible due to anatomy altering surgeries, PTBD is the only approach available.[10,11,16,17]

Preprocedure Imaging

Cross-sectional imaging with contrast enhanced computed tomography (CECT) and magnetic resonance imaging (MRI) with magnetic resonance cholangiopancreatography (MRCP) should be performed prior to the procedure. These will help identify the level and cause of obstruction and aid in planning the approach to percutaneous management.[7,10] When there is obstruction beyond the hilum of the liver, only one access is required. The left system is accessed from an anterior, subxiphoid approach while the right is accessed from the midaxillary approach using as caudad an intercostal space as possible, well below the costophrenic sulcus. Whether to use a left or right approach is largely a matter of individual or institutional preference, when both sided biliary radicles are adequately dilated. When the drainage is required for a longer period of time, most patients are more comfortable with a subxiphoid catheter rather than a right intercostal catheter. Other advantages of a left approach include a less painful procedure which is technically easier to perform (limited respiratory excursion of the left lobe of liver in comparison to the right and a shorter route to be traversed through the hepatic parenchyma), decreased pleural complication rate and less likelihood of catheter dislodgement, again due to less respiratory excursion of the left lobe as well as the fact that the patient finds it easier to look after a percutaneous catheter which is in front of his/her eyes rather than on one side of the body. The disadvantage of the left approach is the increased radiation dose to the operator's hands.

In cases of hilar obstruction with isolation of the biliary radicles, careful assessment has to be done of the CECT/ MR as well as by preprocedure ultrasonography to assess the degree of biliary dilatation. One also has to look for obstruction of the secondary confluence, both right and the left as well as for multilevel isolation which may be present in the setting of metastatic disease. One also has to assess the approach to the segmental duct to be punctured for any mass or cyst in the path of the needle. At least 25–30% of the liver parenchyma should be drained with a single catheter as placement of multiple catheters increases the morbidity and mortality in a patient.[7,10]

If the procedure is done for palliative purposes for the relief of jaundice, drainage of one lobe is enough. However, in the presence of cholangitis, if drainage of one side does not relieve the symptoms, the other side will also need to be drained. In case of parenchymal atrophy of one lobe or segment, it is not useful to drain that lobe/segment as the procedure is unlikely to improve the hepatic function. In case of segmental isolated obstructions, if the patient is not in cholangitis, one should not drain that segment as once a drainage catheter is placed, it becomes virtually impossible to withdraw the access due to bacterial contamination and the patient will be left with an unneeded, potentially problematic catheter.[7,10,18]

Technique

The procedure is performed under conscious sedation with the patient placed supine on the fluoroscopy table. The first step of the procedure is performing a PTC. If the peripheral biliary radicles are sufficiently dilated, sonographic guidance may be used to puncture the selected segmental duct. After cleaning and draping the chosen puncture site, the skin is anesthetized by infiltrating with 2% lidocaine and a small skin incision given using a surgical blade. The underlying soft tissues should be dissected free as this will ease the subsequent drainage catheter insertion.[14] In a dilated system, a 18G puncture needle with a diamond tip is used to enter the selected biliary radicle as peripherally as possible.

Allowing a small amount of bile to drain after the puncture before injecting contrast is beneficial as it prevents over-distension of the biliary system which can result in bacteremia and sepsis. A little contrast is injected to opacify the biliary tree and to confirm that the needle tip is completely within the biliary system. If contrast is seen pooling at the puncture site, it signifies that the tip is within the parenchyma. If contrast is seen entering a tubular system with rapid dissipation, it denotes placement of the needle tip within a vascular structure. In both these situations, the needle has to be carefully repositioned. Once there is backflow of bile and contrast injection opacifies the biliary tree, a 0.032 or 0.035 inch hydrophilic guidewire is passed through the needle and manipulated into the biliary tree towards the liver hilum **(Figs. 1A to C)**.[10,14]

After safely anchoring the guidewire, the needle is withdrawn and a 4F or 5F sheath or cannula introduced. The slippy hydrophilic guidewire can then be exchanged for a stiffer (Teflon coated) guidewire over which a 7F or 8F drainage catheter can be placed after dilatation of the tract with fascial dilators **(Figs. 2A and B)**. If the tip of

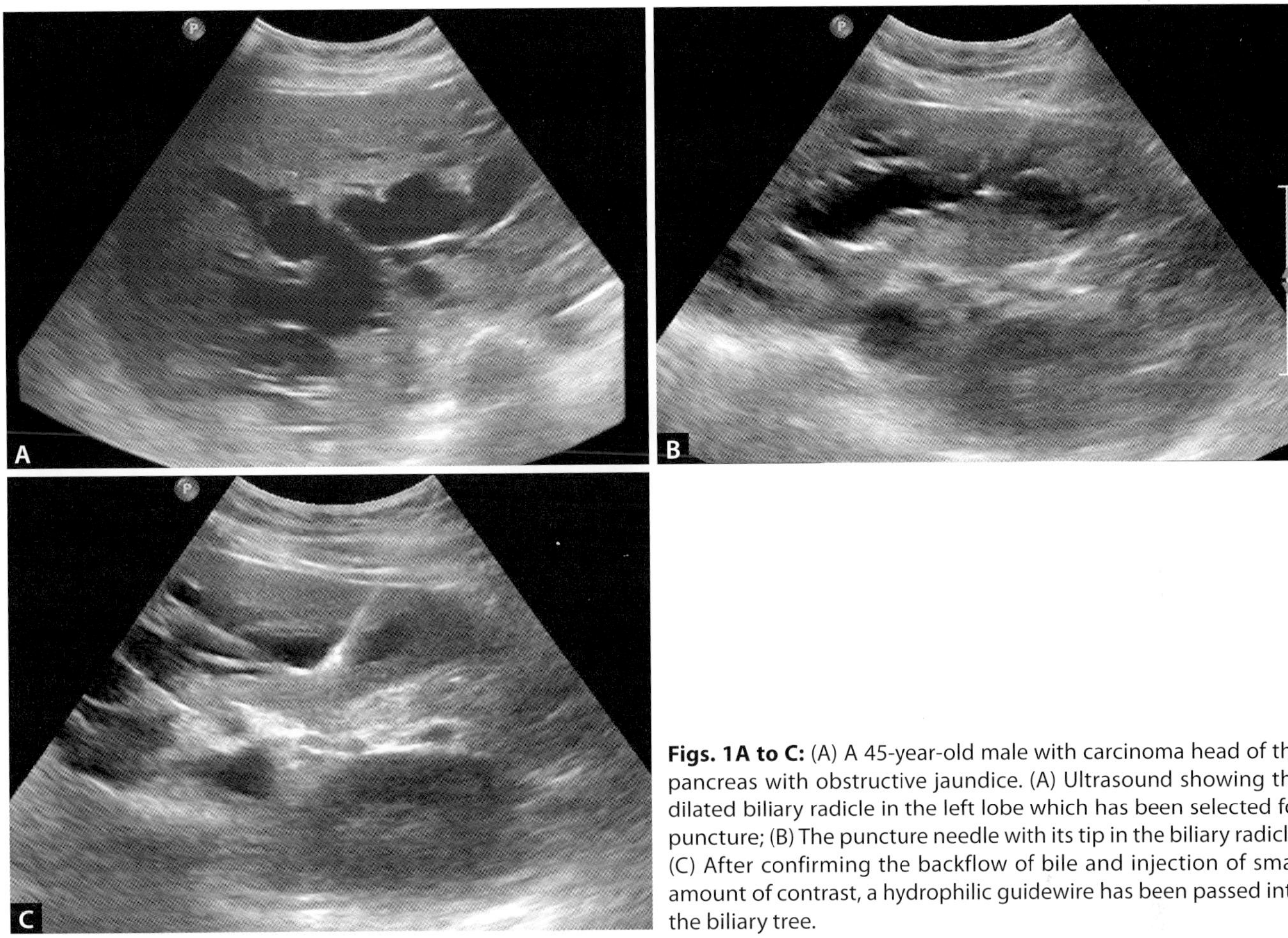

Figs. 1A to C: (A) A 45-year-old male with carcinoma head of the pancreas with obstructive jaundice. (A) Ultrasound showing the dilated biliary radicle in the left lobe which has been selected for puncture; (B) The puncture needle with its tip in the biliary radicle; (C) After confirming the backflow of bile and injection of small amount of contrast, a hydrophilic guidewire has been passed into the biliary tree.

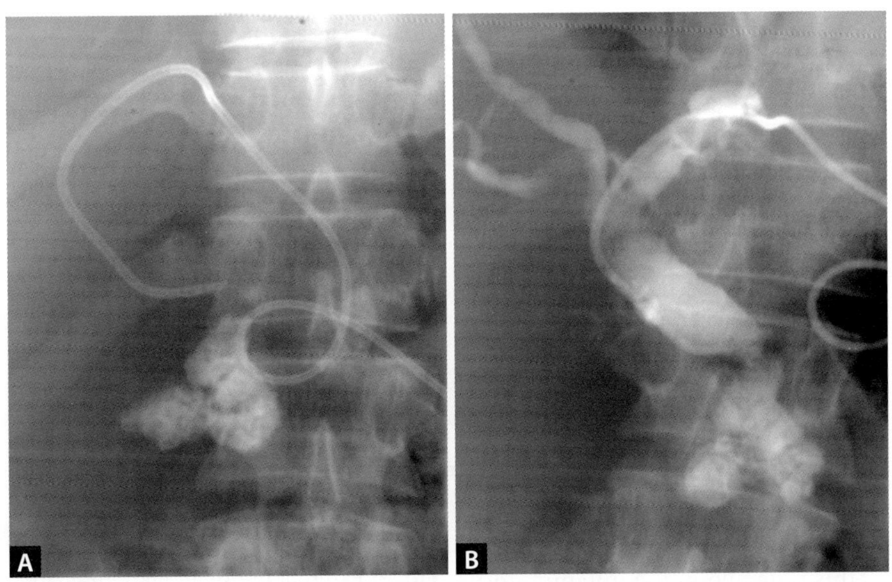

Figs. 2A and B: External biliary drainage: A 52-year-old male with chronic calcific pancreatitis with obstructive jaundice. (A) An 8F PTBD catheter has been placed via the left duct approach into the CBD for external drainage; (B) Cholangiogram shows a complete block of the distal CBD.

the catheter is in the CBD, a catheter of the pigtail type is placed. If the tip of the catheter is in an intrahepatic duct an angled catheter is selected. A self-locking catheter is usually used to prevent accidental slippage. The catheter should also be secured to the skin surface by using a suture or commercially available skin anchoring devices. The catheter is then attached to a drainage bag and left for gravity drainage.

Fluoroscopic Guidance

Fluoroscopic guidance can be used in patients with or without biliary dilatation for performing PTBD. There are two methods by which the procedure can be done. In the one step method, a 21G chiba needle is used for the puncture as for PTC. A 0.018" guidewire is then passed through the needle and manipulated into the biliary tree. The needle is then removed and a 4F percutaneous access set manipulated over the guidewire. The sheath of the access set allows passage of a 0.035" stiff guidewire and the rest of the procedure is as described under US guidance.[7]

In the two step method, a 22G chiba needle is used for puncture of the biliary radicle. After opacification of the biliary tree a second 18G puncture needle is used for re-puncture of a suitable biliary radicle.[14] This allows passage of a 0.035 guide-wire and the rest of the procedure is as described earlier.

Minimal contrast injection and minimal possible manipulation should be done on the initial day of procedure to place an indwelling catheter to avoid over distension of the biliary tree and cholangiovenous reflux.

Two points should be kept in mind while doing the procedure. The site of puncture of the biliary radicle should be as far as possible from the obstructing lesion so as to allow safe anchorage of the external drainage catheter. Also, a longer passage makes subsequent internal drainage easier to perform. Secondly, the puncture should not be done in deep inspiration as the liver will move caudad, thereby causing a difference in the level between the site of punctures of the skin surface and the liver. Therefore, the puncture should be performed in shallow inspiratory breath-hold.

Internal and External Drainage

Internal drainage should ideally be attempted 48–72 hours after the initial PTBD. This allows decompression of the biliary system and therefore, straightening of the course of the wire. Secondly, this time allows the inflammatory changes to subside, particularly the edema around the obstructing lesion.[3,10,19] Injection of contrast through the drainage catheter at this stage will demonstrate the true picture of the type of obstruction whether beak shaped, tapered or flat-shaped. The drainage catheter is replaced with a 4F or 5F angiographic or biliary manipulation catheter with a curved or angled tip over a stiff guidewire. The stiff guidewire is then changed for a soft, angled or J-tip hydrophilic guidewire. If the site of obstruction is beak shaped or tapered, the tip of the catheter is wedged into the beak and the soft hydrophilic guidewire is gently pushed through the obstruction. On the other hand, if the site of obstruction is flat or irregular it may be better to keep the catheter a little proximal to the obstruction and gently probe the area with the hydrophilic guidewire, while simultaneously rotating the tip of the angled catheter into different directions.[10,20]

Once the guidewire successfully crosses the stenosis, it is manipulated into the duodenum along with the catheter. The slippy guidewire is then exchanged for a stiff guidewire over which a 8.3F ring biliary catheter or 10F pigtail catheter is placed with the loop in the duodenum **(Fig. 3)**. Contrast injection to check that side holes are present both proximal and distal to the obstruction and no side-holes are within the hepatic parenchyma completes the procedure **(Figs. 4A and B)**. The catheter should initially be left to external biliary drainage while ensuring adequate hydration of the patient. It can be capped to allow internal drainage once the bile is clear from blood or debris and the patient is afebrile. Once the "capping test" is successful with no fever, pain or vomiting, the patient can be discharged to home with the instruction to open the cap and attach an external drainage bag in the event of any of the above complications, and to report back to the hospital as soon as possible.

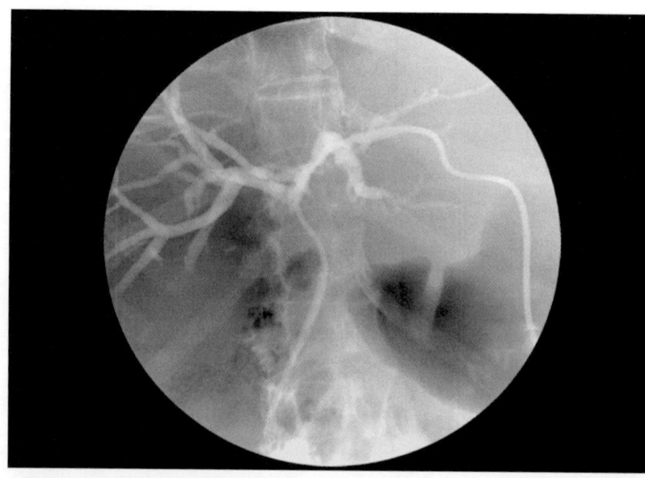

Fig. 3: External-internal biliary drainage: A 55-year-old female with carcinoma gallbladder with obstructive jaundice. Cholangiogram shows complete block of the common hepatic duct just distal to the confluence. An external-internal drainage has been instituted with the distal catheter tip placed in the second part of duodenum.

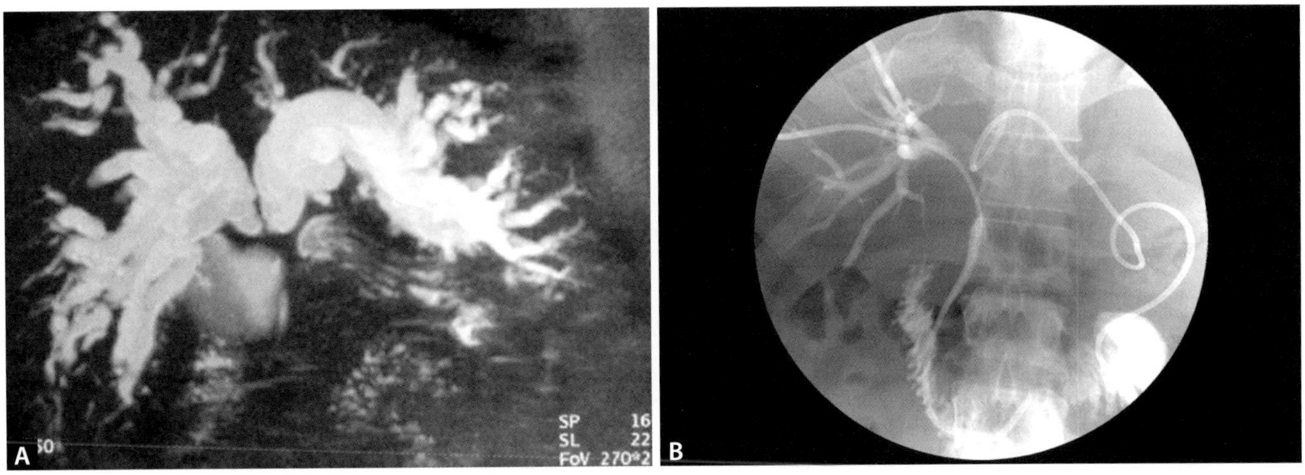

Figs. 4A and B: A 45-year-old male with carcinoma gallbladder with obstructive jaundice. (A) MRCP MIP image shows a hilar block with isolation of the biliary radicles; (B) An external-internal catheter has been placed in the right ductal system with its tip in the third part of duodenum. Check cholangiogram after the procedure confirms that side-holes are present both above and below the strictured segment. An external drainage catheter is seen in the left ductal system with its tip lying just proximal to the confluence.

Postprocedure Management

Patients who have undergone biliary drainage procedures require in-patient admission for at least 24 hours following the procedure. The patient needs to be closely monitored as the procedures can cause bacteremia and sepsis. Vital signs should be checked every 15 minutes for one hour, every 30 minutes for 2 hours, hourly thereafter for 4 hours, and then 6 hourly for 4 hours. Biliary output can range from 400 to 800 mL every 24 hours, so adequate hydration needs to be taken care of. Adequate analgesics need to be administered for controlling the post procedural pain. Appropriate antibiotics also need to be continued for at least 48 hours after the procedure.[14]

Follow-up of Biliary Catheters

Patients who have undergone percutaneous biliary drainage procedures require close monitoring and regular follow-up to be able to detect catheter migration or obstruction at an early stage. Bile output, color and body temperature should be recorded every day and a watch kept on the serum bilirubin and amylase levels. The normal daily output of bile is 400–800 mL and it is clear and yellow in color. Any decrease in the output, change in color or increased turbidity are signs of cholangitis. Regular sonographic examination to look for any dilated intra-hepatic radicles which denote undrained ducts or development of catheter obstruction should be performed. Some authors advocate daily, gentle, forward flushing of the catheter with 5–10 mL of normal saline or sterile water to prevent collection of debris which causes catheter blockage. Pericatheter leakage is usually due to occlusion of the catheter or dislodgement and requires flurosocopic evaluation and correction of the problem. Catheter blockage will also cause the serum bilirubin values to rise. Catheters should ideally be exchanged every 2–3 months to prevent blockage or breakage.[14]

Biliary Stenting

Biliary endoprostheses may be either plastic or metallic and various kinds of both types are available. An external drainage tube can be uncomfortable or of psychological disadvantage to the patient particularly in cases of malignant obstruction. An internal stent also prevents the complicationsofpericatheterbiliaryleakageorslippage.The disadvantage of stents is the need for performing a new procedure (PTBD or ERCP) in case of stent obstruction.

Metallic stents are used almost exclusively for the palliative management of unresectable biliary malignant obstruction. The major advantage of metallic stents is that they can be inserted in a contracted state through a small calibre tract and can achieve a large lumen (up to 10 mm) following expansion **(Fig. 5)**. They are available as self-expanding metallic stents (SEMS) or balloon-mounted stents. These stents are less prone to migration and show a better patency rate than plastic stents.[7,21,22] The disadvantages include the high cost and difficulty in removal. Plastic stents are cheap but have many disadvantages including early occlusion, frequent migration and a traumatic insertion procedure due to the large tract size required **(Fig. 6)**. Because of the large calibre, endoscopic insertion is done more frequently than the percutaneous route.[23,24]

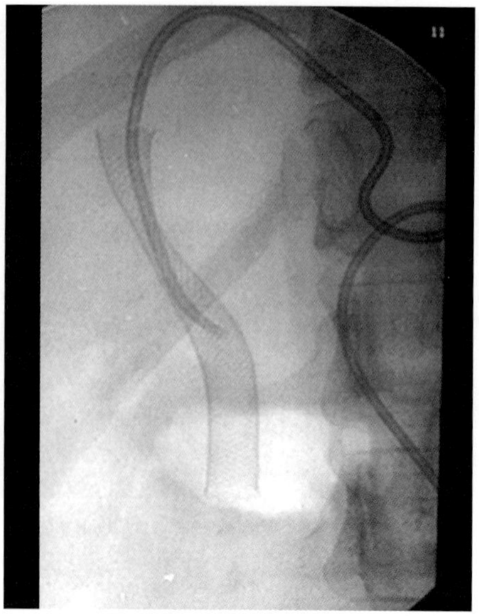

Fig. 5: (A) 63-year-old male with carcinoma head of the pancreas causing obstructive jaundice. A single, self-expanding metallic stent has been placed in the CBD.

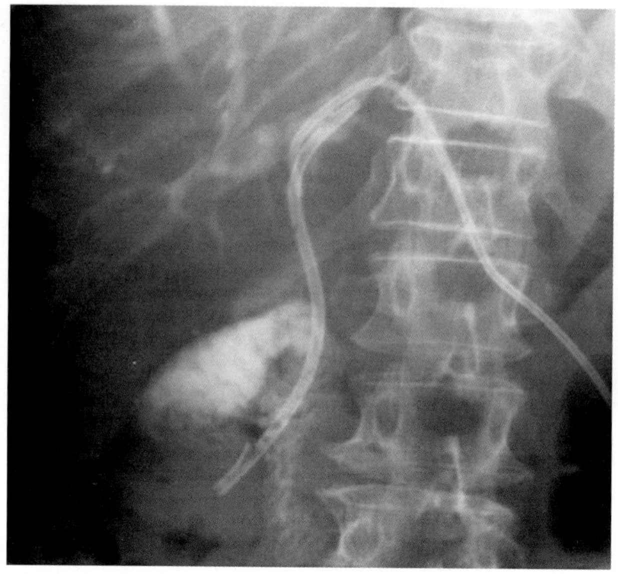

Fig. 6: A 58-year-old male with carcinoma head of the pancreas. A single plastic biliary stent has been placed across the stricture. An external drainage catheter has been left in place as a safety measure in the immediate postprocedure period.

Most physicians prefer to allow internal drainage for a few days prior to stent placement. However, if the passage through the stricture has been relatively atraumatic without significant hemorrhage or debris, stenting can be done in the same sitting as the internal external drainage.[25]

A super-stiff guidewire is passed through the internal-external drainage catheter and securely looped in the duodenum. The catheter is removed and an appropriate introducer sheath placed. If a self-expanding metallic stent is being used, some workers prefer to balloon dilate the stricture prior to stent deployment.[14] It is advisable to over-stent the stricture with the proximal and distal ends of the stent at least 1–1.5 cm beyond the strictures limits.[21] Once the stent is at the appropriate site, as evidenced by the position of the radio-opaque markers at the ends of the stent, it is deployed. Since SEMS have a thermal memory, they will gradually expand to their maximum width within 24 hours after deployment once they achieve body temperature. A safety 8F biliary drainage catheter is then placed with its tip within the stent and the guidewire removed **(Figs. 7A to E)**. The external drain is capped after 24 hours and if the patient tolerates the "capping", a check cholangiogram is performed to confirm adequate drainage through the stent, following which the external catheter is removed.[9,14]

A single stent normally suffices for short segment strictures in the CBD. For longer strictures, one may need to place two telescoped stents (one stent overlapping with the other). In cases of hilar obstruction, bilateral stents may be required which can be placed in either a 'T' or 'Y' configuration. When placing in a 'Y' configuration, it is advisable to place the lower ends of the stents at the same level in the common bile duct **(Figs. 8A and B)**.[7,26] This parallel arrangement may prevent complete expansion of the stents at the level of the liver hilum, so other workers advocate using a "stent within stent" deployment technique. In this technique, the second stent is placed through the mesh of the first stent.[27] This technique is also said to prevent displacement of the stents. The advantage of 'T' stenting is that only a single percutaneous access is required thereby decreasing the complication rate **(Figs. 9A and B)**. However, at times the stricture cannot be crossed to the contralateral side, thereby necessitating the second puncture.[28] No significant difference has been reported between using the 'T' or the 'Y' configurations in terms of rates of technical success, complications or stent patency.[28] Multiple stents may be required in cases of involvement of the secondary confluences (Bismuth type III or IV strictures).[7]

The reported patency rate for palliative metallic stents in malignant obstructions is about 50% at 6 months.[17] Stent blockage occurs because of tumor in growth through the mesh of the stent or tumor over growth at the ends of the stent, biliary sludge and debris.[10,17] In an effort to limit tumor ingrowth, covered stents coated with polyurethane,

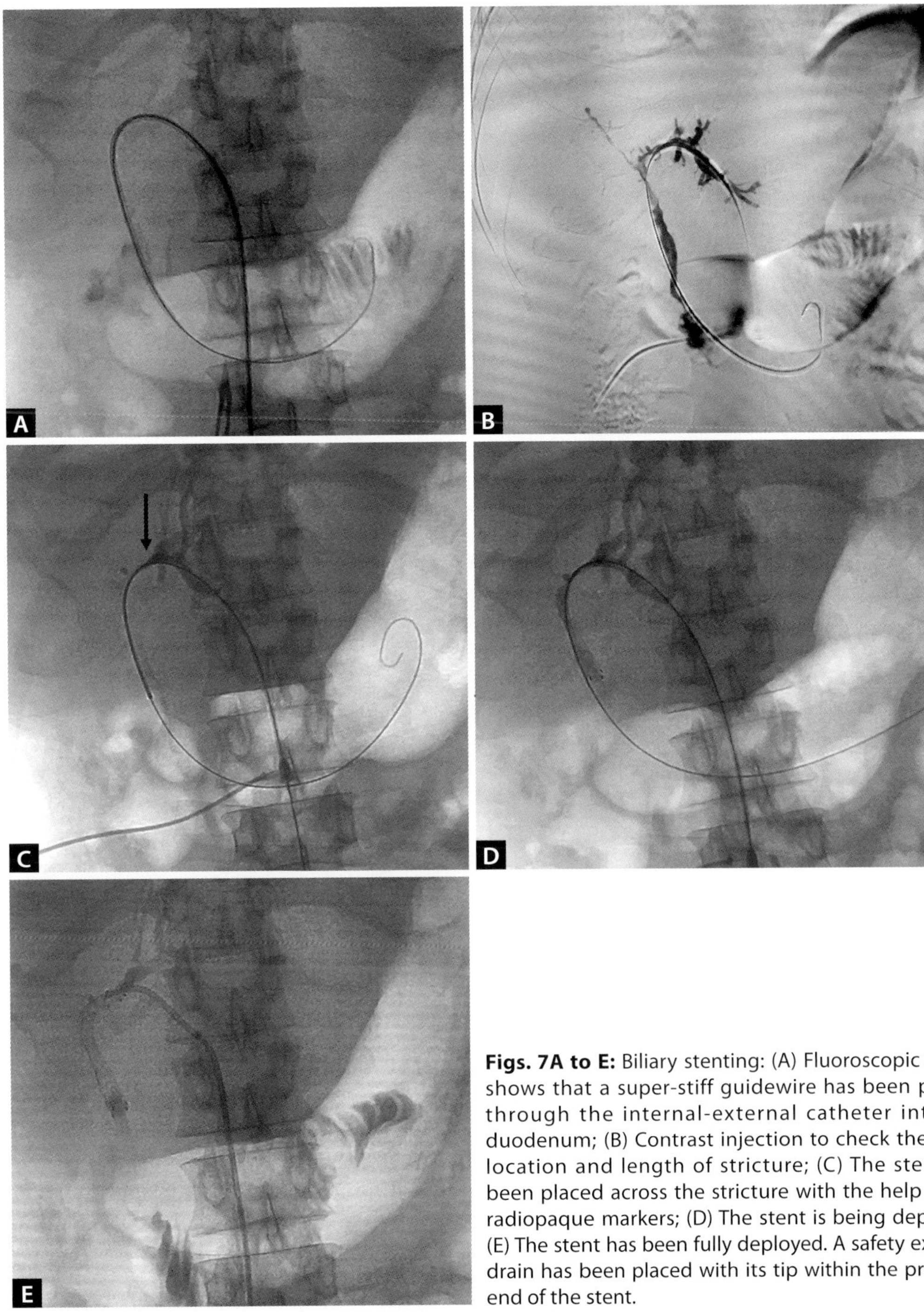

Figs. 7A to E: Biliary stenting: (A) Fluoroscopic image shows that a super-stiff guidewire has been passed through the internal-external catheter into the duodenum; (B) Contrast injection to check the exact location and length of stricture; (C) The stent has been placed across the stricture with the help of the radiopaque markers; (D) The stent is being deployed; (E) The stent has been fully deployed. A safety external drain has been placed with its tip within the proximal end of the stent.

silicone or expanded polytetrafluoroethylene (ePTFE) were developed. These stents are not integrated within the biliary wall and therefore, are prone for migration. Secondly, the openings of the side branches or cystic duct may be blocked by the stent, resulting in a higher complication rate of cholangitis, cholecystitis or pancreatitis.[29] Stent obstruction requires a repeat procedure with either placement of an internal—external drain or a fresh stent through the lumen of the obstructed stent.

Results and Complications of Biliary Drainage

Successful biliary drainage is defined as placement of a drainage tube or stent to provide continuous drainage of bile. The reported rates are 95% in dilated ducts and 70%

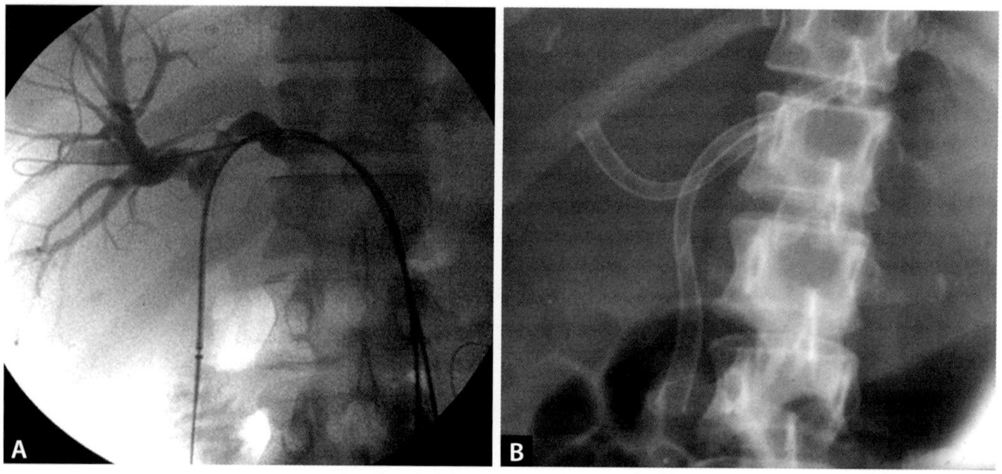

Figs. 8A and B: T-stenting in a 38-year-old female with hilar block due to carcinoma gallbladder. (A) An internal-external drain is present on the left side along with a left-to right drain. A stiff guidewire has been anchored in the right ductal system and a stent placed across the hilar stricture into the duodenum; (B) Two metallic stents have been placed across the hilar stricture in a "T" configuration.

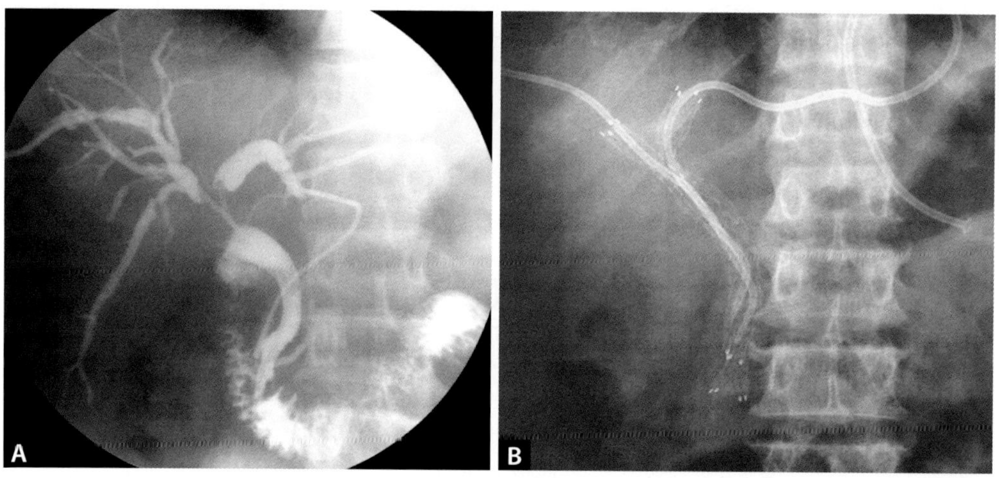

Figs. 9A and B: Y-stenting in a 58-year-old male with hilar obstruction due to cholangiocarcinoma. (A) Cholangiogram shows an internal-external drainage catheter placed via left and right ductal systems; (B) Two metallic stents have been placed parallel to each other in a "Y" configuration.

in non-dilated ducts for placement of external drainage catheters. Of these, about 90% of cases successfully undergo internal-external drain placement.[8]

The complication rate for PTBD can be substantial and depends upon the pre-procedure patient status and diagnosis. The rate is higher in cases with malignant obstruction, cholangitis or coagulopathy. Major complications include hemorrhage, shock due to injection of contrast medium or sudden biliary decompression, sepsis and bile peritonitis due to slippage of catheter. The hemorrhage may be due to venous or arterial injury. Hemobilia following the procedure is common and usually resolves within 48–72 hours but may require clamping of the catheter or change to a larger bore catheter.[25] If hemobilia persists, a CT angiogram should be done. If the scan shows a pseudoaneurysm or active extravasation of contrast, it can be managed with embolization. Pancreatitis can occur after internal-external drainage and may be due to edema of the common bile duct or obstruction of the main pancreatic duct by the catheter. Pneumothorax or pleural effusion can result from inadvertent transpleural puncture. Cholangitis can develop if there is blockage of the catheter or if some intrahepatic ducts remain undrained. The reported rate of major complications is 2.5–10% while the reported mortality is 0–3%.[7]

INTRALUMINAL PROCEDURES THROUGH PERCUTANEOUS TRANSHEPATIC BILIARY DRAINAGE

Various procedures can be performed using the access available through the percutaneous biliary drainage route. Diagnostic procedures include endobiliary tissue sampling for histopathological analysis. This can be done by using a cytological brush or endoluminal forceps through an 8F sheath after internal external drainage.[30]

Palliative therapies can be performed through the PTBD access route in an effort to improve the quality of life, life expectancy and stent patency. These include brachytherapy, radiofrequency ablation and photodynamic therapy. High dose rate intraluminal brachytherapy (ILBT) using Iridium-192 can be delivered selectively to the tumor whilst avoiding the side effect of external radiotherapy. This treatment can be offered in patients who have a single tumor with an overall stricture length of less than 6 cm and the absence of distant disease. The drainage catheter is replaced by the brachytherapy catheter over a stiff guidewire and positioned with its tip 1 cm beyond the distal end of the stricture. The unit is programmed to treat the stricture length and 1 cm beyond and proximal to the stricture **(Figs. 10A and B)**. Studies have shown a significant improvement in the quality of life when ILBT is combined with PTBD with improved stent patency.[31,32]

Similarly, a radiofrequency probe can be introduced through a sheath and the active part placed across the stricture **(Fig. 11)**. RF energy is applied in the range of 8–15 watts for 2 minutes at each level. The procedure has been shown to be safe, whether it results in improved stent patency requires further larger studies to be done.[33] Photodynamic therapy using laser has also been described.[34]

Percutaneous Transhepatic Cholangioplasty

Most benign biliary strictures are treated surgically with creation of biliary enteric anastomoses. A considerable number suffer recurrence of the stricture after surgical treatment and these are even more difficult to treat surgically. Balloon dilatation of these strictures is a therapeutic option. The technique consists of replacing the internal-external drainage catheter with a balloon catheter. The stricture is inflated with a 8–10 mm balloon for at least 10 minutes and a large diameter catheter is placed across the stricture to induce nonstenosed fibrosis **(Figs. 12A and B)**. It is recommended that three to six balloon inflations be performed at intervals of three weeks with upsizing of the drainage catheter at each sitting. Once cholangiograms show free flow of contrast across the stricture, the catheter is retracted proximal to the stricture and capped. The patient is monitored for a few days to ensure that the bile is flowing internally. The external catheter is removed if the patient remains asymptomatic. Success rates of 70–93% have been reported in literature.[35,36]

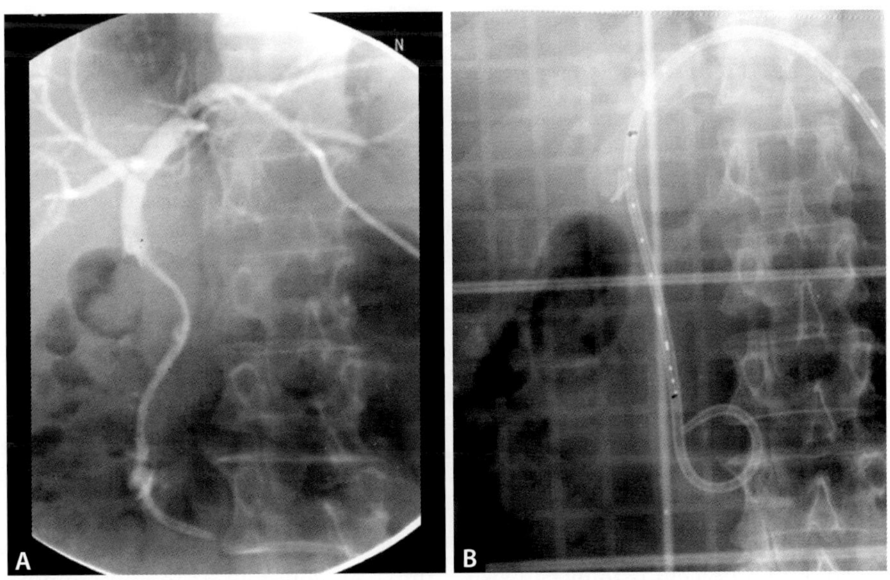

Figs. 10A and B: Intraluminal brachytherapy in a 41-year-old female with carcinoma gallbladder. (A) Cholangiogram after internal-external drainage demonstrates a 4 cm stricture in the mid CBD; (B) A 10 F pigtail catheter has been placed with its in the duodenum. Simulator film shows placement of the brachytherapy catheter within the pigtail catheter with its distal end 1 cm beyond the distal end of the stricture.

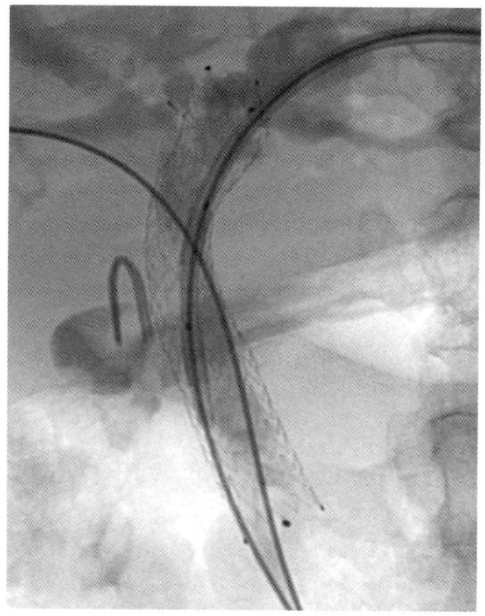

Fig. 11: Intraluminal radiofrequency ablation in a malignant hilar stricture. The radiofrequency probe has been placed through a sheath across the stricture.
Courtesy: Dr Shyamkumar N Keshava, Christian Medical College, Vellore, Tamil Nadu, India.

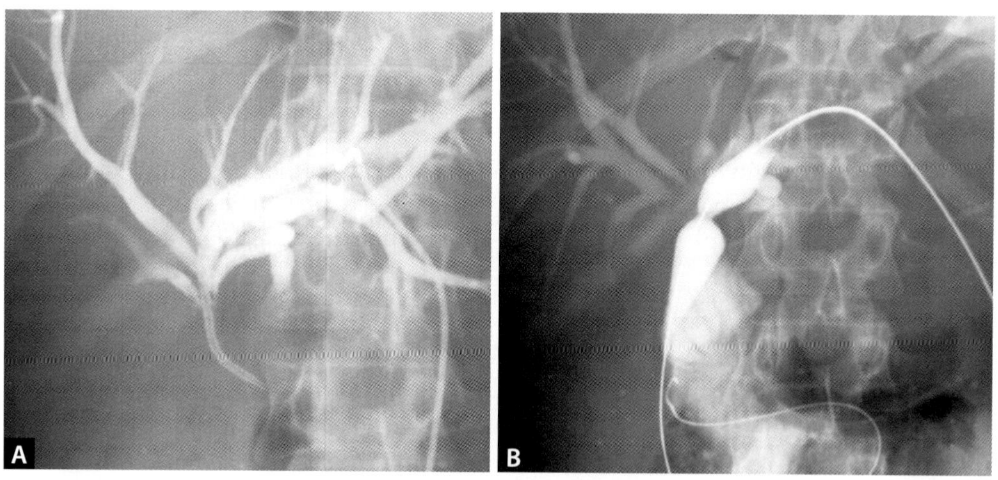

Figs. 12A and B: Balloon dilatation of a benign biliary stricture in a case of postoperative choledochojejunostomy stricture. (A) 8F drainage catheter has been placed across the stricture with its tip in the jejunal loop from the left duct approach; (B) Balloon catheter has been placed over the stricture and inflated. Note the "waist" formation in the balloon due to the tight stricture.

PERCUTANEOUS CHOLECYSTOSTOMY

Percutaneous cholecystostomy may be used as a temporizing measure in patients of acute cholecystitis who are critically ill and therefore cannot undergo surgery.[4-6,37] After the patient's condition is stabilized, cholecystectomy as the definitive treatment will still be required. However, in acalculous cholecystitis, percutaneous drainage may be the only treatment required. Cholecystostomy can also provide a means of accessing the biliary tree in patients with obstructive jaundice in whom the bile ducts are not dilated and the level of obstruction is distal to the insertion of the cystic duct.

Technique

The gallbladder is punctured under US guidance. There are two approach routes available for puncturing the gallbladder. The transhepatic route is usually preferred as the transperitoneal approach carried a greater risk of biliary leak with bile peritonitis. Using the transhepatic route, the gallbladder is punctured where it is fixed to the liver, generally at the junction between the cephalic and middle third of the body. In the transperitoneal approach, the gallbladder is punctured at the point where it lies closest to the anterior abdominal wall. The trocar technique is generally used for direct puncture while

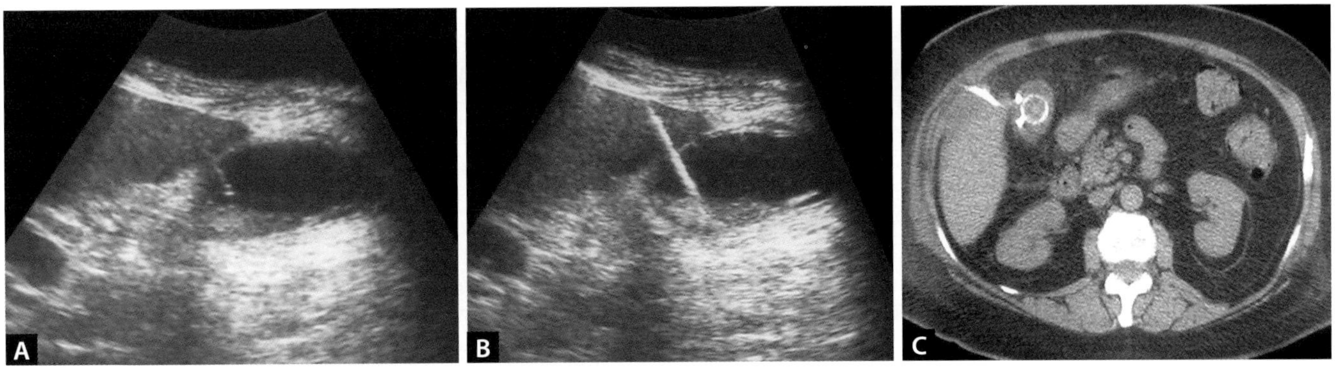

Figs. 13A to C: Percutaneous cholecystostomy in a case of empyema of the gallbladder. (A) Sonogram demonstrates the tip of the puncture needle in the lumen of the gallbladder placed via the transhepatic approach; (B) A stiff guidewire has placed and coiled in the lumen; (C) Follow-up CT axial image demonstrates the loop of the pigtail catheter in the lumen of the gallbladder.

the seldinger technique is preferred for the transhepatic route.

An 18G needle is used to puncture the gallbladder and sample collected for gram staining and culture. A small amount of contrast is then injected to opacify the gallbladder for the subsequent steps for which flurosocopic guidance is used. A J-shaped soft tip guidewire is then inserted through the needle and coiled within the lumen. After dilating the tract, a 7F or 8F catheter having an anchor mechanism or of the pigtail type is placed within the gallbladder lumen and sutured to the skin. The catheter is left to drain by gravity **(Figs. 13A to C)**.

If surgery is not considered as in acalculous cholecystitis, the catheter can be removed once the patient's signs and symptoms resolve and a sufficient time has elapsed for the tract to mature. This is said to be at least two weeks when the transhepatic route is used and three weeks when the transperitoneal approach is used. Removal of the catheter before tract maturation may result in leakage of bile and peritonitis.[38,39]

Complications

The complications which can occur following percutaneous cholecystostomy include bile peritonitis, hemobilia and gallbladder perforation. Vasovagal reaction due to tube placement can be managed with atropine. Hemorrhage can at times be fatal. Minimal manipulation should be done at the time of initial drainage to avoid complications.[40] Reported mortality rates range from 3% to 36% depending on the co-morbid conditions.[14]

CONCLUSION

In conclusion, percutaneous biliary procedures are a well-established method of management of patients with obstructive jaundice. PTBD and stenting offer a safe and effective method for the palliative treatment of malignant biliary obstruction. Newer intraluminal palliative techniques hold the promise of improvement in the patient's quality of life and improved stent patency rates. Percutaneous cholangioplasty is a safe and effective therapeutic procedure for benign biliary strictures. Percutaneous cholecystostomy is a life-saving management option in critically ill patients.

REFERENCES

1. Molnar W, Stockum AC. Relief of obstructive jaundice through percutaneous transhepatic catheter—a new therapeutic method. AJR. 1974;122:356-67.
2. Ferrucci JT Jr, Mueller PR, Harbin WP. Percutaneous transhepatic biliary drainage: technique, results and applications. Radiology. 1980;135:1-13.
3. Mueller PR, Van Sonnenberg E, Ferrucci JT Jr. Percutaneous biliary drainage: Technical and catheter related problems in 200 procedures. AJR. 1982;138:17-23.
4. Hamy A, Visset J, Likholatnikov D, et al. Percutaneous cholecystostomy for acute cholecystitis in critically ill patients. Surgery. 1997;121:398-404.
5. Lee KT, Wong SR, Cheng JS, et al. Ultrasound guided percutaneous cholecystostomy as an initial treatment for acute cholecystitis in elderly patients. Dig Surg. 1998;15:328-32.
6. Davis CA, Landercasper J, Gundrsen LH, et al. Effective use of percutaneous cholecystostomy in high risk surgical patients: techniques, tube management, and results. Arch Surg. 1999;134:727-31.
7. van Delden OM, Laméris JS. Percutaneous drainage and stenting for palliation of malignant bile duct obstruction. Eur Radiol. 2008;18:448-56.
8. Saad WEA, Wallace MJ, Wojak JC, Kundu S, Cardella JF. Quality improvement guidelines for percutaneous transhepatic cholangiography, biliary drainage, and percutaneous cholecystostomy. J Vasc Interv Radiol. 2010;21:789-95.
9. Tapping CR, Byass OR, Cast JEI. Percutaneous transhepatic biliary drainage (PTBD) with or without

stenting—complications, re-stent rate and a new risk stratification score. Eur Radiol. 2011;21:1948-55.
10. Madhusudan KS, Gamanagatti S, Srivastava DN, Gupta AK. Radiological interventions in malignant biliary obstruction. World J Radiol. 2016;8(5):518-29.
11. Pu LZCT, Singh R, Loong CK, de Moura EGH. Malignant biliary obstruction: Evidence for best practice. Gastroenterol Res Pract. 2016;Epub 2016 Feb11.
12. Harbin WP, Mueller PR, Ferrucci JT Jr. Transhepatic cholangiography: complications and use patterns of the fine-needle technique: a multi-institutional survey. Radiology. 1980;135(1):15-22.
13. Mueller PR, Harbin WP, Ferrucci JT Jr, et al. Fine-needle transhepatic cholangiography: reflections after 450 cases. AJR. 1981;136:85-90.
14. Rosenblatt M, Aruny JE, Kandarpa K. Transhepatic cholangiography, biliary decompression, endobiliary stenting and cholecystectomy. In: Handbook of Interventional Radiologic procedures, 3rd edn. Lippincott, Williams and Wilkins, Philadelphia, Kandarpa K, Aruny JE (Eds). PA. 2002;19106 USA.
15. Fidelman N. Benign biliary strictures: Diagnostic evaluation and approaches to percutaneous treatment. Tech Vasc Interv Radiol. 2015;18(4):210-7.
16. Baijal SS, Dhiman RK, Gupta S, et al. Percutaneous transhepatic biliary drainage in the management of obstructive jaundice. Trop Gastroenterol. 1997;18:167-71.
17. Tsetis D, Krokidis M, Negru D, Prassopoulos P. Malignant biliary obstruction: the current role of interventional radiology. Ann Gastroenterol. 2016;29:33-6.
18. Inal M, Akgül E, Aksungur E, Seydaoğlu G. Percutaneous placement of biliary metallic stents in patients with malignant hilar obstruction: unilobar versus bilobar drainage. J Vasc Interv Radiol. 2003;14(11):1409-16.
19. Madhusudan KS, Gamanagatti S, Gupta AK. Imaging and interventional in hilar cholangiocarcinoma: a review. World J Radiol. 2015;7:28-44.
20. Kücükay F, Okten RS, Yurdakal M, et al. Percutaneous management of malignant biliary disease: factors influencing the ability to overcome the stricture. Diagn Interv Radiol. 2011;17:169-73.
21. Lammer H, Hausegger KA, Fluckiger F, et al. Common bile duct obstruction due to malignancy: treatment with plastic versus metal stents. Radiology. 1996;201:167-72.
22. Moss AC, Morris E, MacMathuna P. Palliative biliary stents for obstructing pancreatic carcinoma. Cochrane Database Syst Rev. 2006;CD004200.
23. Moss AC, Morris E, Leyden J, MacMathuna P. Do the benefits of metal stents justify the costs? A systematic review and meta-analyses of trials comparing endoscopic stents for malignant biliary obstruction. Eur J Gastroenterol Heaptol. 2007;19:1119-24.
24. Mukai T, Yasuda I, Nakashima M, et al. Metallic stents are more efficacious than plastic stents in unresectable malignant hilar biliary strictures: a randomized controlled trial. J Hepatobiliary Pancreat Sci. 2013;20:204-22.
25. Inal M, Akgül E, Aksungur E, Demiryürek H, Yağmur O. Percutaneous self-expandable uncovered metallic stents in malignant biliary obstruction. Complications, follow-up and re-interventions in 154 patients. Acta Radiol. 2003;44:139-46.
26. Lee M, Dawson SC, Mueller PR, Saini S, Lu DS, Goldberg MA, Gazelle GS. Failed metallic biliary stents: causes and management of delayed complications. Clin Radiol. 1994;49:857-62.
27. Gwon D, Ko G, Kim JH, et al. Percutaneous bilateral metallic stent placement using a stent-in-stent deployment technique in patients with malignant hilar biliary obstruction. AJR. 2013;200:909-14.
28. Kim CW, Park AW, Won JW, Kim S, Lee JW, Lee SH. T-configured dual stent placement in malignant biliary hilar obstructions with a newly designed stent. J Vasc Interv Radiol. 2004;15:713-7.
29. Gwon D, Ko G, Yoon H, et al. Safety and efficacy of percutaneous Y-configured covered stent placement for malignant hilar biliary obstruction: a prospective pilot study. J Vasc Interv Radiol. 2012;23:528-34.
30. Xing GS, Geng JC, Han XW, Dai JH, Wu CY. Endobiliary brush cytology during percutaneous transhepatic cholangiodrainage in patients with obstructive jaundice. Hepatobiliary Pancreat Dis Int. 2005;4:98-103.
31. Aggarwal R, Patel FD, Kapoor R, Kang M, Kumar P, Sharma S. Evaluation of high-dose rate intraluminal brachytherapy by percutaneous transhepatic biliary drainage in the palliative management of malignant biliary obstruction—a pilot study. Brachytherapy. 2013;12: 162-70.
32. Chen Y, Wang XC, Yan ZP, et al. HDR-192 Ir intraluminal brachytherapy in treatment of malignant obstructive jaundice. World J Gastroenterol. 2004;10:3506-10.
33. Mizandari M, Pai M, Xi F, et al. Percutaneous intraductal radiofrequency ablation is a safe treatment for malignant biliary obstruction: feasibility and early results. Cardiovasc Interv Radiol. 2013;36:814-9.
34. Lee TY, Cheon YK, Shim CS. Current status of photodynamic therapy for bile duct cancer. Clin Endosc. 2013;46:38-44.
35. Fidelman N. Benign biliary strictures: Diagnostic evaluation and approaches to percutaneous treatment. Tech Vasc Interv Radiol. 2015;18(4):210-7.
36. Gwon Dl, Ko GY, Ko HK, Yoon HK, Sung KB. Percutaneous transhepatic treatment using retrievable covered stents in patients with benign biliary strictures: mid-term outcomes in 68 patients. Dig Dis Sci. 2013;58(11):3270-9.
37. Boggi U, DiCandio G, Campatelli A, et al. Percutaneous cholecystostomy for acute cholecystitis in critically ill patients. Hepatogastroenterology. 1999;46(25):121-5.
38. Kiviniemi H, Makela JT, Antio R, et al. Percutaneous cholecystostomy in acute cholecystitis in high risk patients: an analysis of 69 patients. Int Surg. 1998;83(4):299-302.
39. Hatjidakis AA, Karampekios S, Prassopoulos P, et al. Maturation of the tract after percutaneous cholecystostomy with regard to the access route. Cardiovasc Interv Radiol. 1998;21:36-40.
40. Pang KW, Tan Ch, Loh S, et al. Outcomes of percutaneous cholecystostomy for acute cholecystitis. World J Surg. 2016;02 (Epub ahead of print).

Acute Pancreatitis: Imaging and Interventions

Kumble S Madhusudhan, Raju Sharma

INTRODUCTION

Acute pancreatitis (AP) is defined as acute inflammation of pancreas. The inflammation may extend beyond the pancreas to the surrounding fat and other organs as well and infrequently results in a systemic inflammatory response syndrome and organ failure. Mild type of pancreatitis is seen in about 80% patients and the severe variety in 20%.[1] Severe acute pancreatitis has high mortality reaching up to 30%.[2] The incidence of acute pancreatitis is rising due to increase in the incidence of obesity, gallstone disease and alcoholism.[3] Hence, early recognition and diagnosis of this condition is critical for judicious management. Recently, there has been a change in the terminology related to this disease and awareness of the features of revised classification and the role of radiologist in diagnosis and management is important.

PATHOPHYSIOLOGY

Pancreas secretes many enzymes; autodigestion of pancreatic parenchyma by these enzymes results in acute pancreatitis.[4] In normal pancreas, this is prevented by various natural defence mechanisms in pancreas. Whenever, there is pancreatic injury (e.g. alcohol) or increase in ductal pressure (e.g. gallstone), there is increase in secretion of activated proteolytic enzymes (trypsin, amylase, lipase) and increased permeability which result in increased concentration of these enzymes within the parenchyma **(Fig. 1)**. This leads to autodigestion of the pancreatic parenchyma and peripancreatic regions. A vicious cycle is initiated with more destruction of pancreatic cells and more release of enzymes.[4] This incites inflammation and increases cytokine production which is responsible for systemic manifestations. Lipase results in fat necrosis and saponification of peripancreatic fat.

ETIOLOGY

The two common causes of acute pancreatitis are alcohol intake and gallstone disease. These two together constitute 70–80% of cases of acute pancreatitis.[5] Other uncommon causes include abdominal trauma, drugs (azathioprine, tetracycline, thiazides), iatrogenic (post-endoscopic interventions), hypercalcemia, hyperlipidemia, tumors (periampullary carcinoma) and infections (mumps, coxsackie B virus). No cause is identified in about 10–15% cases (idiopathic).[5]

REVISED ATLANTA CLASSIFICATION

The original Atlanta classification was presented in the year 1992 to classify the types of pancreatitis, its severity and complications and was mainly based on clinical criteria.[6] Since then, there has been improvement in understanding of the disease, imaging techniques and treatment options. Also, the classification was inadequate, ambiguous and did not include radiological criteria. Thus there was a need for revising the classification which was done in 2012 **(Flowchart 1)**.[7] For the radiologists, the important aspect is the different morphological types of pancreatitis and CT criteria for various named fluid collections.[8] This revised classification is specific for acute pancreatitis and does not apply to chronic pancreatitis, acute on chronic pancreatitis and groove pancreatitis, which have different pathophysiology and outcome.

The following are the salient features of the revised Atlanta classification **(Flowchart 1)**:

Diagnosis

The diagnosis of AP is made when any two of the following three features are fulfilled:

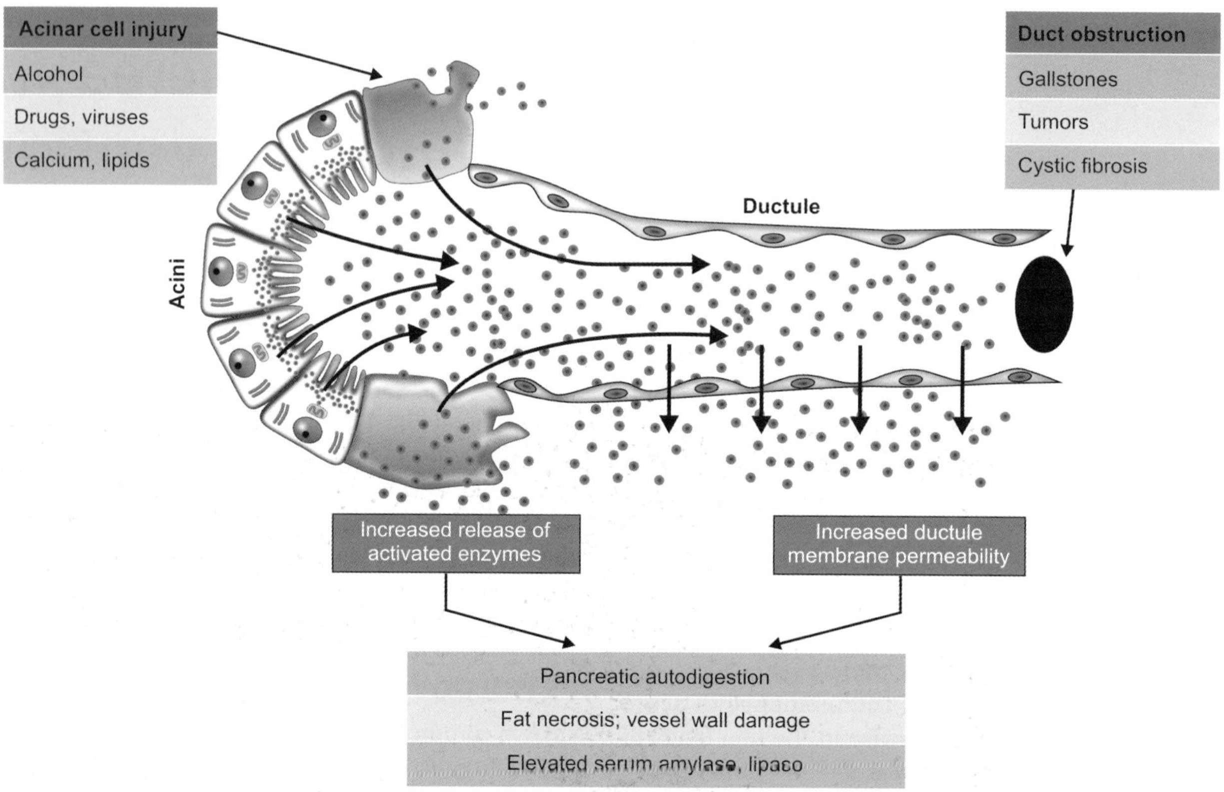

Fig. 1: Schematic diagram showing the pathophysiology of acute pancreatitis.

Flowchart 1: The nomenclature used in revised Atlanta classification.

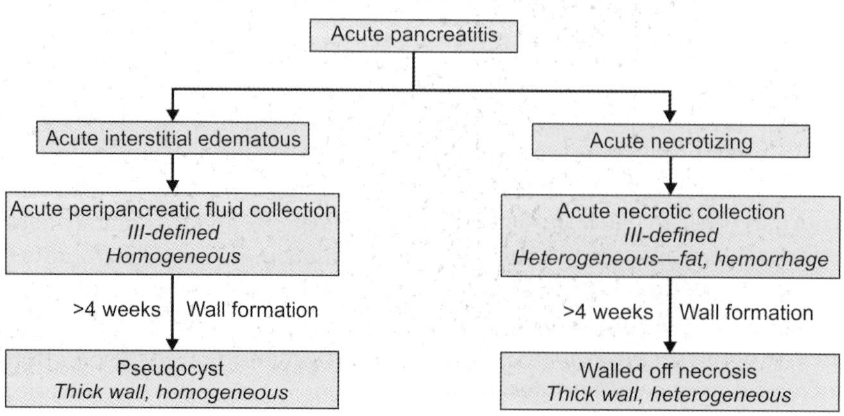

1. Characteristic pain of acute pancreatitis (epigastric pain, radiating to the back)
2. Elevated serum amylase or lipase levels more than at least three times the normal levels
3. Typical imaging features of acute pancreatitis.

Thus acute pancreatitis is often a clinical diagnosis (when first two features are fulfilled) and imaging is needed only when clinical features are atypical.

Types of Acute Pancreatitis

Acute interstitial edematous pancreatitis (AIEP): In this type, there is inflammation in and around the pancreas, with or without fluid collections. However, no pancreatic or peri-pancreatic necrosis is seen. This has good prognosis and has a mortality under 3%.[9]

Acute necrotizing pancreatitis (ANP): This, as the name suggests, is associated with pancreatic and/or peripancreatic necrosis. This has variable prognosis, ranging from complete recovery to mortality, which is seen in up to 30% cases.

Phases of Acute Pancreatitis

Acute pancreatitis is divided into two phases due to biphasic clinical course. *Early phase* occurs in first week and is associated with systemic inflammatory response syndrome (SIRS) or multiorgan failure which may cause mortality.[2] In *late phase* (after first week), there are other complications such as infection or sepsis which are common causes of mortality. Imaging plays an important role in the late phase of the disease.

Nomenclature

The terminology has now been defined to allow uniformity among the radiologists and referring clinicians **(Figs. 2A to D)**.[5]

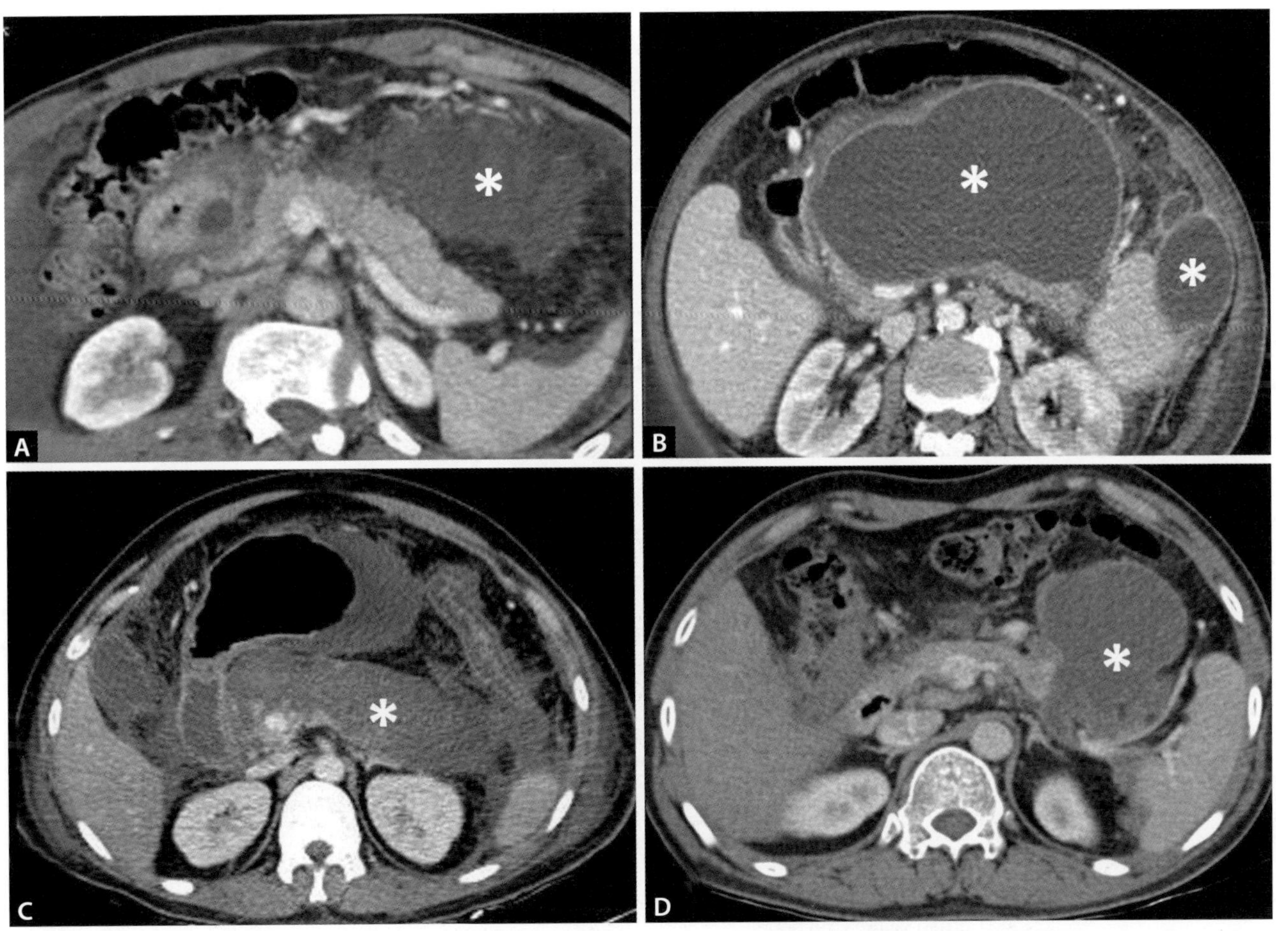

Figs. 2A to D: Nomenclature of collections (asterisks) according to revised Atlanta classification on contrast-enhanced CT scan: (A) Acute peripancreatic fluid collection; (B) Pseudocyst; (C) Acute necrotic collection; and (D) Walled-off necrosis.

Acute peripancreatic fluid collection (APFC): This is seen in AIEP and is defined as simple fluid collection in peripancreatic location with ill-defined walls and homogeneous low density appearance and limited by fascial planes or peritoneal reflections. This is seen less than 4 weeks from the onset of the disease.

Acute necrotic collection (ANC): This is seen in ANP and is a heterogeneous ill-defined collection of fluid within or around the pancreas. This is seen less than 4 weeks from the onset of the disease.

Pseudocyst: This is seen after 4 weeks of illness in the setting of acute edematous pancreatitis and is seen as a well-defined homogeneous low density fluid collection with well-defined wall.

Walled-off necrosis (WON): This is ANC after 4 weeks duration and is seen as a heterogeneous thick-walled collection.

It is important to understand that these terms have relevance in disease management. After 4 weeks, there is walling off of the collection with liquefaction in case of WON which determines successful intervention. Also, by convention, acute peripancreatic fluid collection (APFC) and pseudocyst are not seen in acute necrotizing pancreatitis (ANP) and acute necrotic collection (ANC) and WON are not seen in acute interstitial edematous pancreatitis (AIEP). The terms like pancreatic pseudocyst, phlegmon, pancreatic abscess and hemorrhagic pancreatitis are not used anymore.

Classification of Severity

Based on severity (clinical and on imaging), acute pancreatitis can be divided into mild, moderately severe and severe **(Table 1)**. *Mild pancreatitis* is not associated with organ failure or any local or systemic complications. *Moderately severe pancreatitis* is defined when there is transient organ failure (lasting < 48 hours) or local/systemic complications in the form of symptomatic collections or systemic inflammatory response syndrome (SIRS) requiring prolonged hospital stay or interventions. *Severe pancreatitis* is characterized by persistent organ failure (for > 48 hours) with or without local or systemic complications. This has prognostic importance as almost all patients of mild pancreatitis recover in a week whereas patients with severe pancreatitis have high morbidity and mortality.[10] However, the correlation is not absolute. About 5% of patients with mild pancreatitis may have significant complications with mortality of 1–2% and about 30% of severe pancreatitis may have a benign course.[9]

Table 1: Classification of severity of acute pancreatitis.

Severity of acute pancreatitis	
Mild	No organ failure/local complications
Moderately severe	Local complications and/or organ failure < 48 hours
Severe	Organ failure > 48 hours

IMAGING TECHNIQUES

Imaging plays an important role in the management of patients of acute pancreatitis. However, it is not done routinely in all patients of pancreatitis. Further, timing of imaging is also important.

Indications (Table 2)

As discussed above, the diagnosis of acute pancreatitis can often be made clinically. Imaging is needed when the abdominal pain is not typical or when serum amylase level elevation is borderline. Here, imaging will help in confirming or excluding a diagnosis of acute pancreatitis.[11]

In AIEP, imaging after diagnosis is not necessary as most patients have an unremarkable self-limiting course. Only when complications are clinically suspected, imaging is needed during the course of the disease. In ANP, imaging is often needed, usually in the first week, to define the extent of necrosis. Subsequently, imaging is done when complications are suspected, patient is not improving, there is organ failure, drop in hemoglobin, gastrointestinal bleed or features of sepsis. Imaging thus plays a role in severity assessment, evaluation of complications and guiding management.[8]

Plain Radiography

Plain radiography has a very limited role in the diagnosis of acute pancreatitis. It may show sentinel dilated jejunal/

Table 2: Indications for imaging.

Indications for imaging in acute pancreatitis
Doubtful/inconclusive clinical diagnosis *Interstitial edematous pancreatitis:* • Organ failure • Local complications *Necrotizing pancreatitis:* • Initial baseline scan (after 5–7 days) • Persistent organ failure or SIRS • Fever/elevated leukocyte count • Patient deterioration • Requirement of interventions • Gastrointestinal bleed/Hb drop

Abbreviation: SIRS: Systemic inflammatory response syndrome.

duodenal loop in the left hypochondrium due to ileus. Other signs include colon cut-off (dilated large bowel till splenic flexure), gasless abdomen, obliteration of left psoas shadow and elevated hemidiaphragm.[12] Calcifications may be seen in a patient with chronic calcific pancreatitis. More important role of abdominal radiograph is in excluding other causes of acute abdomen such as bowel perforation and acute small bowel obstruction.

Ultrasonography

Ultrasonography (USG) is often the initial investigation of choice in patients with acute abdomen. Normal pancreas shows intermediate echogenicity uniformly; it may appear hyperechoic due to fatty infiltration, which typically happens with age. The normal thickness of pancreatic parenchyma is about 20–25 mm in head and tail regions and 15–20 mm in the body region.[13] The normal pancreatic duct is less than 3 mm in size and shows smooth outline.

Frequently, due to extensive inflammation (especially in ANP) and ileus, pancreas is not visualized and diagnosing acute pancreatitis is difficult.[14] Although USG has lower sensitivity and specificity for diagnosis of acute pancreatitis, its major advantage is that it is radiation free and may be repeated whenever needed. It mainly helps in detection of gallstones, bile duct calculi, biliary obstruction and assessing the extent of liquefaction of collections which help in planning drainage procedures.[15] USG is also useful in guiding diagnostic and therapeutic interventions. Additional advantages include that it can be used in children and in bedside assessment of acute pancreatitis.[15]

Computed Tomography

Computed tomography (CT) scan occupies the centre stage of imaging in acute pancreatitis and has high accuracy (80-90%).[14] It is performed as a contrast-enhanced CT (CECT) scan after injecting intravenous-iodinated contrast agent and acquiring scans in the portal venous phase (60–70 seconds) after the beginning of contrast injection. An arterial phase (25–30 seconds) is acquired, whenever there is suspicion of gastrointestinal or extraluminal hemorrhage, pancreatic mass or mesenteric ischemia.[5] Pancreatic phase (40–50 seconds) has been suggested by some instead of portal venous phase as the pancreas enhances most during this phase.[16] In patients with renal failure or those with allergy to iodinated contrast agents, non-contrast CT or MRI may be done. Oral contrast is usually not necessary, when the patient presents with acute abdomen. However, during follow-up, positive oral contrast helps in evaluation of bowel loops and differentiate a distended fluid-filled bowel from fluid collection. Plain scans are usually not necessary, although it may help in detecting calcification and hemorrhage. The scan is done from the level of diaphragm to symphysis pubis initially. Subsequent follow-up scans may be limited to upper abdomen (diaphragm to iliac crest). Coronal and sagittal reformats are useful in defining the extent of inflammation and collections. Normal pancreas appears as homogeneously enhancing tissue with smooth outline. There may be lobulations uncommonly. As age progresses, fatty infiltration may be seen in the parenchyma.

The CT scan should be typically performed after atleast 72 hours of onset of pain as parenchymal necrosis is well-defined by this time. A CT scan done in very early stage of the disease may miss necrosis and will not accurately assess the severity.CECT is also the modality of choice when pancreatitis occurs in patients over 40 years of age to exclude a possible tumor causing secondary pancreatitis.

Magnetic Resonance Imaging

The role of MRI in acute pancreatitis is limited. The long scan times needed and difficulty in breath-holding in these sick patients often results in poor image quality. Faster sequences may still provide answers in select situations. Further, the high cost, need for MR compatible monitors in critically ill patients and limited availability has resulted in limited usage.[15] Specific indications include patients with renal failure or allergy to iodinated contrast agents, children and pregnant patients. It is also used in the evaluation of biliary tree for presence of any obstructing calculus, to assess for liquefaction of a necrotic collection prior to planning drainage and in evaluation of communication of pancreatic duct with collection. Diffusion weighed imaging (DWI) may help in differentiation of infected from sterile necrotic collection. Non-contrast MRI with DWI is better than non-contrast CT scan and should be preferred wherever possible.

The typical sequences include T1W gradient echo (in-phase and opposed phase), T2W spin echo-fat saturated, thick slab T2W rapid recovery and DWI sequences **(Table 3)**. Oral contrast is not necessary. Intravenous gadolinium is necessary when evaluating necrotizing pancreatitis, to assess the extent of necrosis.

IMAGING APPEARANCE

Acute Interstitial Edematous Pancreatitis

On USG, the pancreas appears hypoechoic and bulky **(Fig. 3)**. There may be a hypoechoic rim of inflammation

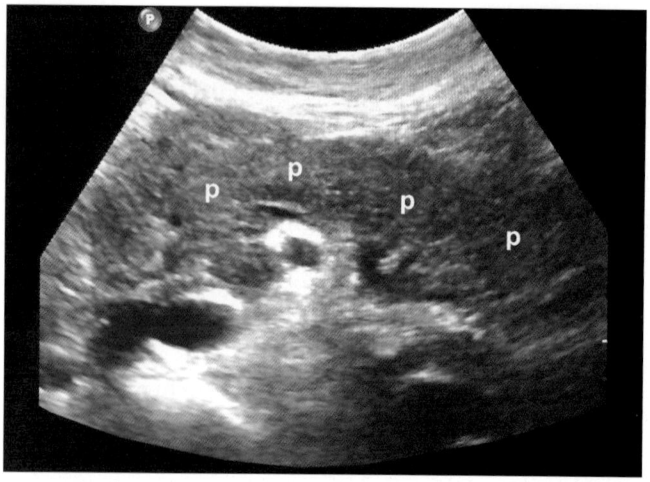

Fig. 3: Ultrasonography of a patient with acute interstitial edematous pancreatitis showing diffusely bulky and hypoechoic pancreas (p).

Table 3: MRI sequences used in the evaluation of acute pancreatitis.

MRI sequences	
Axial T1W	Anatomy; pancreatic edema
Axial T2W FSE–FS	Pancreatic/peripancreatic edema; liquefaction of collections
Coronal T2W–FS	Pancreatic/peripancreatic edema; liquefaction of collections CBD
Axial SSFP	Vascular assessment
DWI	Infected necrosis; debris in collection
MRCP	Biliary tree and pancreatic duct evaluation
Contrast enhanced T1W–FS	Evaluation of pancreatic necrosis

Abbreviations: FSE: Fast spin echo; FS: Fat-suppressed; CBD: Common bile duct; SSFP: Steady-state free precession; DWI: Diffusion-weighted imaging; MRCP: Magnetic resonance cholangiopancreatography.

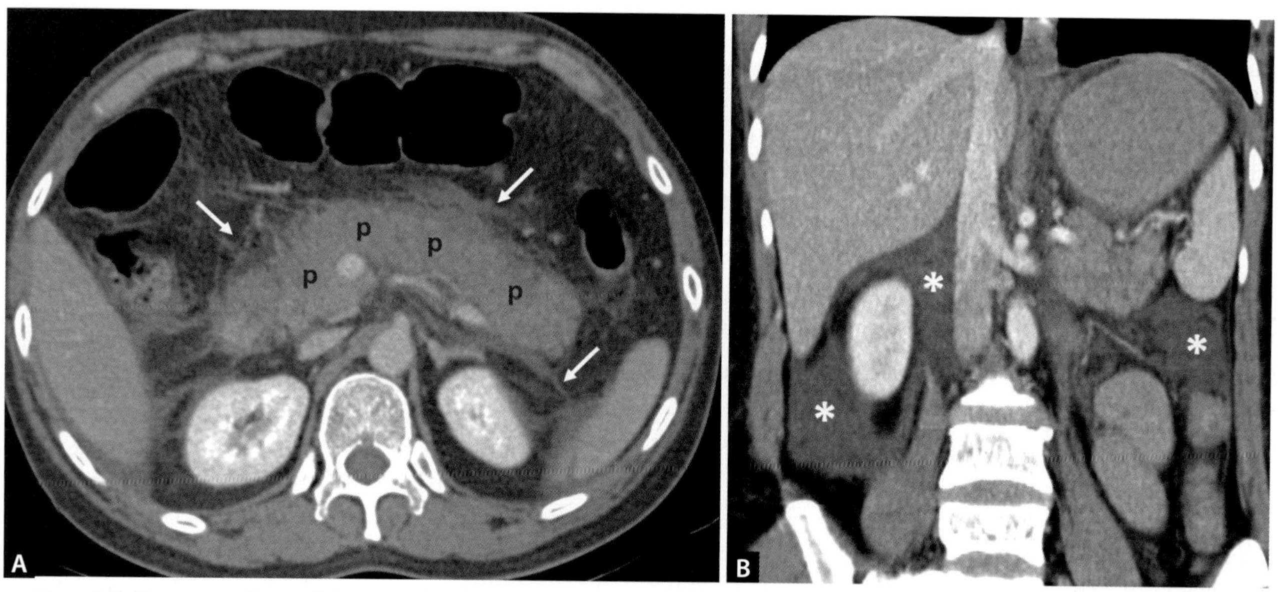

Figs. 4A and B: Contrast-enhanced CT scan of a patient with acute interstitial edematous pancreatitis: Axial (A) and coronal (B) images show diffusely bulky pancreas (p) with peripancreatic fat stranding (arrows). Acute peripancreatic fluid collections are seen in the coronal image (asterisks).

or fluid around the pancreas. Fluid collections may be seen in the peripancreatic regions. Abnormal pancreas is seen in 33–90% of patients of acute pancreatitis.[17]

Contrast-enhanced computed tomography shows diffuse or focal (20%—head or tail) enlargement of the pancreas with mild heterogeneous contrast enhancement **(Figs 4A and B)**.[5] Non-enhancing areas are not seen in the parenchyma. The lobulated outline of pancreatic parenchyma may be lost. There is soft tissue stranding and hypodensity in the peripancreatic fat with thickening of anterior pararenal and lateroconal fascia. There may be associated fluid collections (APFC), seen as ill-defined homogeneous low density areas, ascites and pleural effusion, often left sided. The pancreatic duct is usually normal, unless acute inflammation occurs in the background of chronic calcific pancreatitis. As the disease progresses, most of the patients (80%) improve without any complications. About 10-20% progress to form pseudocysts after about 4 weeks of illness, which also resolve in most patients.[18] In some patients, pseudocyst may result in symptoms when intervention becomes necessary. Secondary infection is very rare.

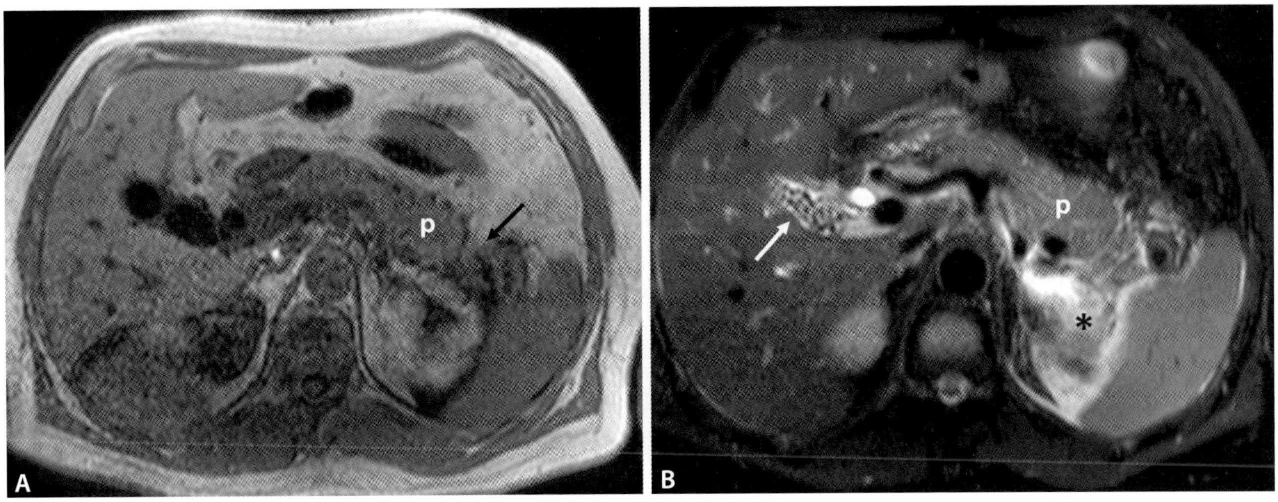

Figs. 5A and B: MRI in a patient with acute interstitial edematous pancreatitis: Axial T1-weighted (A) and T2-weighted fat saturated (B) images showing bulky body and tail of pancreas (p) with peripancreatic inflammation (hypointense on T1W—black arrow; hyperintense on T2W—asterisk). Note gallstones in B (white arrow).

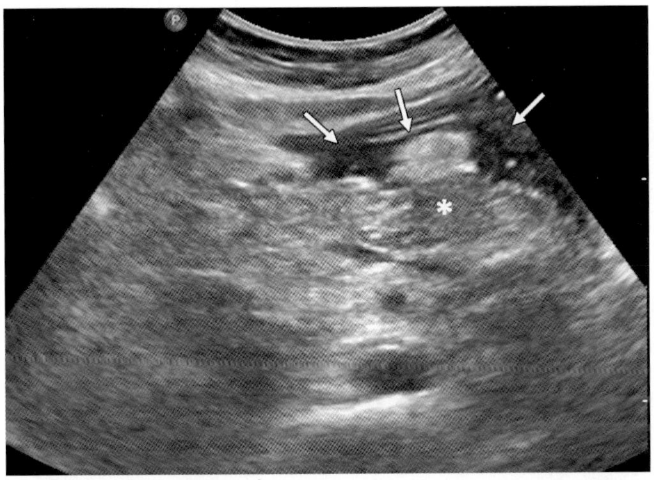

Fig. 6: Ultrasonography of a patient with acute necrotizing pancreatitis showing diffusely bulky and heteroechoic pancreas with hypoechoic area in the body (asterisk) and peripancreatic collection with debris (arrows).

MRI also shows diffusely bulky and edematous pancreas appearing hypointense on T1-weighted and hyperintense on T2-weighted images **(Figs. 5A and B)**.[19] Fluid collections may be seen in the peripancreatic region. Otherwise, inflammation is seen as ill-defined feathery hyperintense areas on T2-weighted images in peripancreatic regions. Thickening of anterior pararenal and lateroconal fascia is seen with hyperintense signal on T2W. Associated findings include gallstones, calculi in common bile duct with biliary dilatation and dilated pancreatic duct in cases of acute inflammation occurring in the background of chronic pancreatitis. DWI may show restriction of diffusion of the entire pancreas.

Acute Necrotizing Pancreatitis

Ultrasonography is less sensitive in the evaluation of ANP. Depending on the extent of necrosis, pancreas may be variably visualized. There may be fluid collections, appearing hyperechoic or isoechoic, in the lesser sac, perinephric and paracolic regions **(Fig. 6)**. In later stages, hypoechoic fluid collection may be seen in these areas.

In ANP, CECT is critical in defining the extent of parenchymal necrosis as it determines prognosis. The scans should ideally be done between 5 and 7 days after the onset of the disease.[19] In addition to the features of AIEP, non-enhancing areas suggesting necrosis are seen in the parenchyma **(Figs. 7A and B)**. On MRI, the necrotic tissue is frequently hypointense on both T1- and T2-weighted images prior to liquefaction **(Figs. 8A and B)**. Similar to CT, parenchymal necrosis shows no contrast enhancement. The collections seen in the peripancreatic regions are heterogeneous and often contain areas of fat. They are ill-defined initially (ANC) and gradually get walled-off and liquefy over 4 weeks (WON). Since it is a necrotic collection, it acts as a nidus for secondary infection to develop. Presence of infection is suggested when air-foci are seen in the collection on CECT scan.

The necrosis can be of three types according to the revised Atlanta classification. They include pancreatic necrosis only, peripancreatic necrosis only and combined pancreatic-peripancreatic necrosis.[5,19]

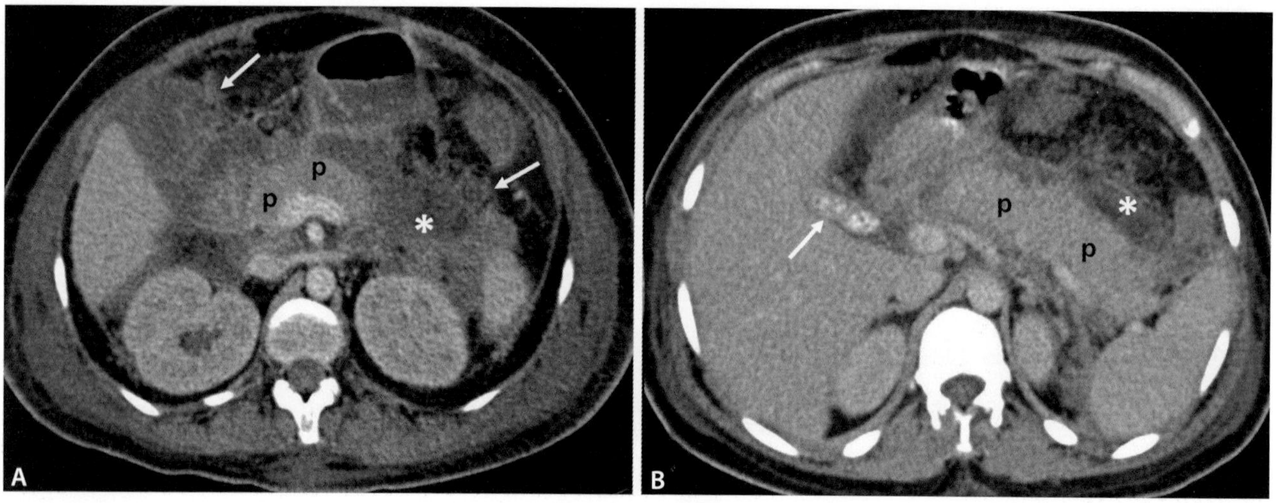

Figs. 7A and B: Contrast-enhanced CT scan of a patient with acute necrotizing pancreatitis: (A) Axial image showing pancreatic (asterisk) and peripancreatic (arrows) necrosis with areas of fat density. Normal enhancing pancreas (p) is seen; (B) Axial image showing normal enhancing pancreas (p) with isolated peripancreatic necrosis (asterisk). Note calcified calculi in the gallbladder (arrow in B).

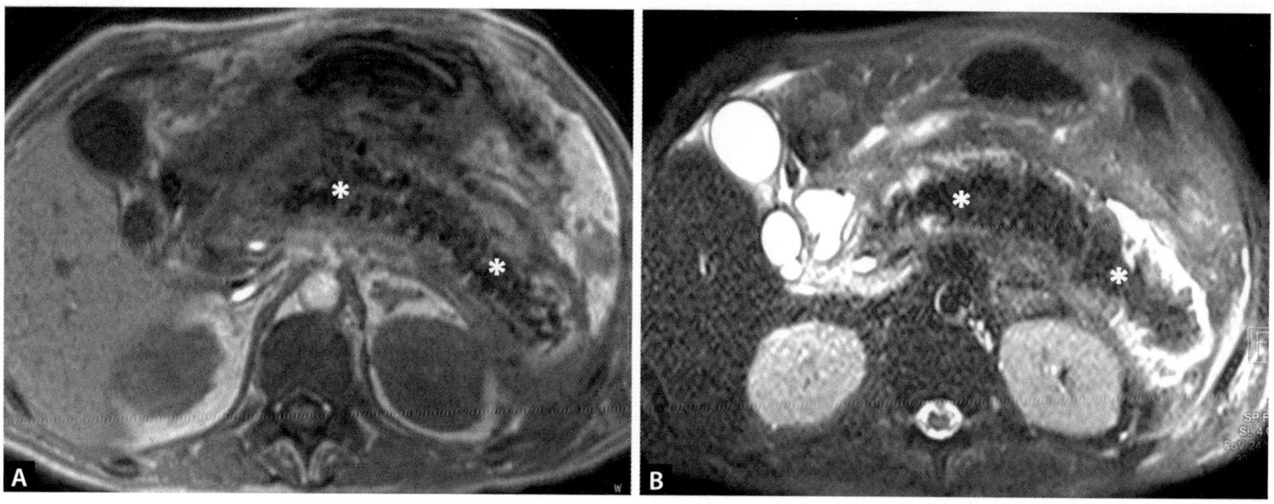

Figs. 8A and B: MRI in acute necrotizing pancreatitis: Axial T1-weighted (A) and T2-weighted fat saturated (B) images showing diffusely bulky pancreas with hypointense necrotic area (asterisks) and peripancreatic fat stranding.

Pancreatic necrosis alone is the least common type, seen in less than 5% of cases. Here, the necrosis is confined to the pancreatic parenchyma and appears as a hypoenhancing/non-enhancing area **(*see* Fig. 2C)**. The extent of necrosis has prognostic significance and is a part of CT severity index (vide infra). The necrosis usually liquefies as it evolves and may show a defined wall, when it is called walled of pancreatic necrosis. This, depending on the size may resolve spontaneously, may persist or may undergo complications (infection, hemorrhage, mass effect) at which point intervention becomes necessary.

Peripancreatic necrosis is the second most common type of finding, where necrosis is limited to peripancreatic regions. This is typically seen as heterogeneous areas of low density (usually 20–40 HU) on CECT, with areas of fat, hemorrhage or soft tissue density within **(Fig. 7B)**.[8] The usual locations include lesser sac, perinephric and paracolic regions. Initially they are called acute necrotic collection which gradually liquefies and in about four weeks becomes walled-off necrosis. However, liquefaction may be difficult to identify on CT and USG or MRI may be needed. A recent study suggested that volume of

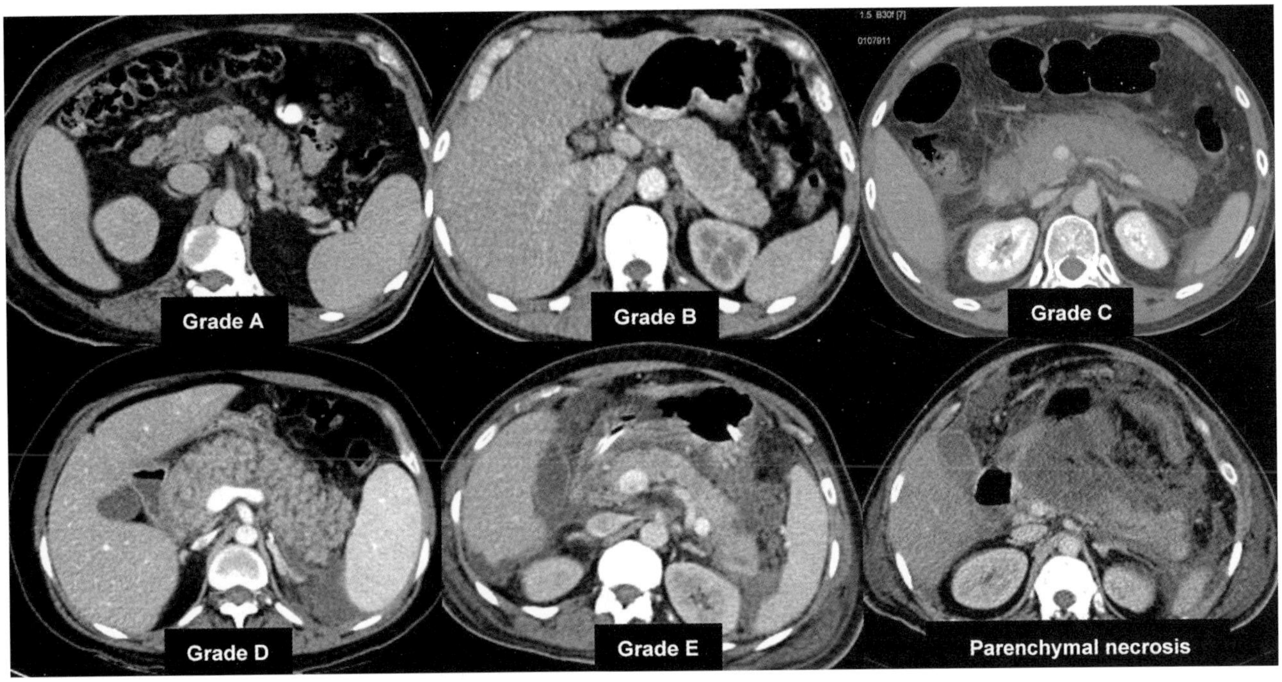

Fig. 9: Balthazar grade and CT severity index.

extrapancreatic necrosis has prognostic significance and a volume greater 100 mL is associated with higher incidence of organ failure and infection and poor prognosis.[20]

Combined pancreatic and peripancreatic necrosis is the most common type of necrosis seen in about 80% of patients. The imaging features are a combination of both the types described earlier **(Fig. 7A)**.

Table 4: CT severity index.

CT grade	*CT finding*	*Score*
A	Normal pancreas	0
B	Pancreatic enlargement	1
C	Pancreatic and peripancreatic inflammation	2
D	Single peripancreatic fluid collection	3
E	2 or more fluid collections ± gas	4
% Necrosis		*Score*
0		0
<30%		2
30–50%		4
>50%		6

SEVERITY ASSESSMENT SCORES

Various clinical scores are used in the assessment of severity of acute pancreatitis as they help in determining prognosis. The clinical scores have modest accuracy and include Marshall scoring, Ranson's scoring and bedside index for severity in acute pancreatitis (BISAP).

There are various radiological scoring systems available to predict the severity of acute pancreatitis.[21] The scores used by the radiologist are Balthazar grade and CT severity index (CTSI) **(Fig. 9)**.[22] Balthazar graded acute pancreatitis from A to E **(Table 4)**. CT severity index includes the extent of parenchymal necrosis, giving 2 points for <30% necrosis, 4 points for 30–50% necrosis and 6 points for >50% necrosis in addition to Balthazar grade. A CTSI score of 7–10 suggests poor prognosis, 4–6 intermediate and 1–3 indicates good prognosis. This scoring has high correlation with clinical outcome with a sensitivity of 71% and specificity of 93%.[23] A modified CTSI was suggested by Mortele et al,[24] which is defined in **Table 5**. Studies, however, have suggested no significant difference between CTSI and modified CTSI in terms of prognostication of the disease.[23] Another scoring system by de Waele et al,[25] which relies mainly on extrapancreatic findings such as ascites, pleural effusion, retroperitoneal inflammation and mesenteric inflammation [Extra Pancreatic Inflammation on CT (EPIC) score], has limited clinical utility. Recent comparative studies have shown that CT scoring systems are similar to clinical scoring systems in accurately predicting severity of acute pancreatitis.[10,26] However, a study quantifying the extrapancreatic necrosis in patients with ANP showed significant correlation of its volume with clinical outcome.[20]

COMPLICATIONS

Acute pancreatitis is associated with wide range of complications which can broadly be classified into vascular and non-vascular complications **(Table 6)**.[18]

Nonvascular Complications

Symptomatic collections are the most common complication of acute pancreatitis. These collections may be acute peripancreatic collections, pseudocysts or walled-off necrosis.[18] Symptoms develop when these collections get infected or when they compress adjacent structures **(Figs. 10A to C)**. Infection commonly occurs in necrotic collection, and is seen as a fluid density area with air foci within. However, air in infected necrosis is seen in about 20–40% cases.[27] Further, air foci may occur due to prior intervention or fistulous communication with the bowel. In the absence of air foci, diagnosis of secondary infection is done based on clinical suspicion or needle aspiration. Collections may be seen at variable locations with common locations being peripancreatic region, perisplenic, perigastric, perihepatic, paracolic and perinephric areas. Rarely, they may be seen in the mediastinum, within the spleen or liver and in the psoas muscle. Ascites is also commonly seen. The revised Atlanta classification defines five types of collections, acute peripancreatic fluid collection, acute necrotic collection, pseudocyst, walled-off necrosis and post-necrosectomy pseudocyst **(*see* Fig. 2A to D)**. Other terms such as pancreatic abscess, phlegmon and collection are not used. Pancreatic abscess is same as infected necrosis, but the latter terminology is better and has implications in drainage.

Table 5: Modified CT severity index.

Imaging feature	***Score***
Pancreatic inflammation	
Normal pancreas	0
Intrinsic pancreatic abnormalities with or without inflammatory changes in peripancreatic fat	2
Pancreatic or peripancreatic fluid collection or peripancreatic fat necrosis	4
Pancreatic necrosis	
None	0
≤ 30%	2
> 30%	4
Extrapancreatic complications	
One or more of pleural effusion, ascites, vascular complications, parenchymal complications, or gastrointestinal tract involvement	2

Table 6: Complications of acute pancreatitis.

Vascular	***Nonvascular***
Arterial: • Pseudoaneurysms • Rupture (Contrast extravasation) *Venous*: • Acute thrombosis (SV, SMV, PV) • Collateralization—varices	*Collections*: • Infected necrosis • Walled off necrosis/ pseudocyst Bowel necrosis/perforation Pancreatic ascites Pancreatic fistula

Abbreviations: PV: Portal vein; SMV: Superior mesenteric vein; SV: Splenic vein.

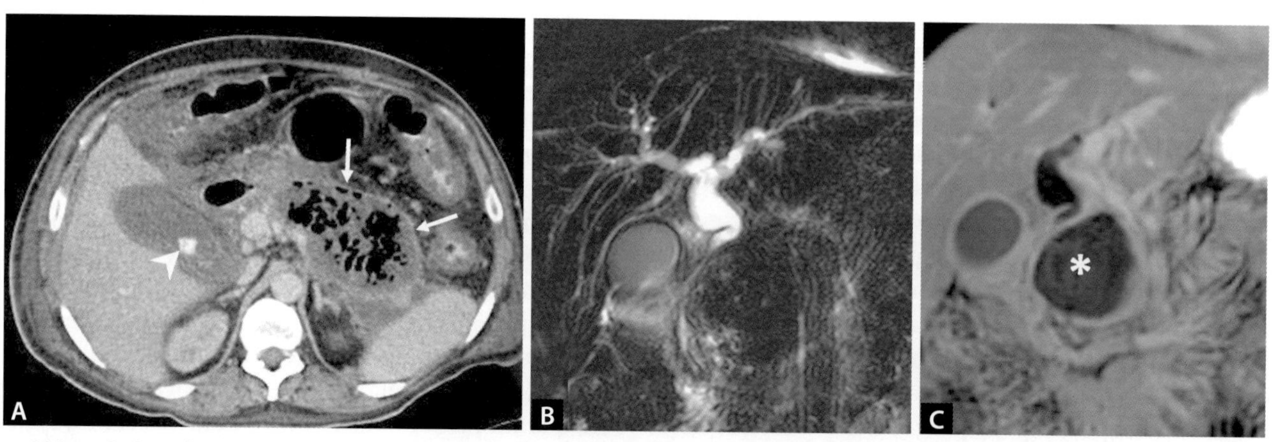

Figs. 10A to C: Complications—collections: (A) Axial contrast-enhanced CT image showing necrotic collection in the pancreatic bed—lesser sac region with multiple air foci suggesting secondary infection (arrows). Gallstone is also seen (arrowhead). (B and C) MRCP (B) and coronal contrast-enhanced T1W (C) images showing walled-off necrosis in the head of pancreas (asterisk) causing compression of distal common bile duct with proximal dilatation.

Acute peripancreatic fluid collection (APFC) is seen in AIEP, in the first 4 weeks of illness. It is seen on CECT as ill-defined homogeneous low density areas, often with feathery margins. On MRI, it is seen as an ill-defined homogeneous, non-encapsulated hyperintense area on T2-weighted images and hypointense area on T1-weighted images. This is an exudative fluid collection and contains only fluid and inflammatory cells without necrosis. It may or may not have communication with side branches of pancreatic duct. It resolves spontaneously in most patients and intervention is not necessary. It must be differentiated from ascites which is seen in perihepatic, perisplenic and pelvic regions.

Pseudocyst is the collection which is seen in AIEP, after four weeks. This develops from an APFC, when it forms a wall around it. Thus, no necrosis is seen within it. On CECT, it is seen as a well-defined homogeneous low density collection with relatively thick walls. On MRI, it is seen as homogeneously hyperintense on T2W images. No restriction of diffusion is seen. Imaging may or may not show communication of the pseudocyst with pancreatic duct. The collection contains pancreatic juice and high amylase, which helps in making a diagnosis in difficult situations. Most of the pseudocysts resolve and infection is rare. Intervention is needed only if they are symptomatic.

Acute necrotic collection (ANC) is seen in ANP, in the initial four weeks of the disease. This may be seen in the pancreas or peripancreatic region. This develops as a result of leak of pancreatic enzymes which results in fat necrosis and saponification. Unlike APFC, it is seen as an ill-defined heterogeneous density area, often with foci of fat and/or hemorrhage within on CECT. But, early in the stage of the disease, prior to fat necrosis, it may appear homogeneous, and is difficult to differentiate from APFC. MRI is useful as the collections are seen as variable signal intensity (hyperintense and hypointense areas) on T2W images. DWI often shows diffusion restriction. As time progresses, ANCs may resolve spontaneously (20%), get infected (20%) or develop into walled-off necrosis (60%). Resolution of ANC is size dependent, majority of those less than 2 cm resolve spontaneously and most of those larger than 5 cm persist.[28]

Walled-off necrosis (WON) develops from ANC in ANP after 4 weeks. As the name suggests, there is a thick non-epithelial wall formed around the necrotic collection. The collection, depending on the extent of liquefaction, may be homogeneous or heterogeneous. Although, on CECT, it appears as homogeneous or heterogeneous collection with thick walls, the extent of liquefaction is difficult to assess. MRI or USG is helpful for this. USG shows the liquefied portion as anechoic area with internal echoes **(Figs. 11A to D)**. On MRI, the liquefied component appears as hyperintense on T2W and the necrotic component as iso-hyperintense on T1W and hypointense on T2W images **(Figs. 12A and B)**. Intervention is frequently needed for this collection. When a WON is fully liquefied, it may mimic pseudocyst on imaging. This differentiation is important as it has management implications. Pseudocyst is seen only in extrapancreatic location, associated with AIEP, and may be associated with dilated pancreatic duct due to compression, unlike WON where duct is necrosed and is decompressed due to drainage into the collection. Sometimes the term *disconnected duct syndrome* is used where a collection is formed due to necrosis of the pancreatic duct in the neck or body region **(Fig. 13)**. This seen in up to 30% of patients of ANP and is usually treated by either drainage or pancreatic resection.

Post-necrosectomy pseudocyst develops as a long-term complication after surgical necrosectomy of the pancreatic/peripancreatic necrosis. This may be seen either in the pancreas or in extrapancreatic location. This occurs as a result of disconnected duct syndrome due to necrosis in the head and body of pancreas. After necrosectomy, there is oozing of pancreatic juice from tail to form a collection at the site of necrosectomy, resulting in pseudocyst. On imaging, it is similar to the pseudocyst described above. Intervention is needed if symptomatic.

Infected necrotic collection is diagnosed on CECT scan when there are air foci in the collection **(Fig. 10A)**. In the absence of air foci, DWI or aspiration may help in making a diagnosis.

Bowel ischemia and necrosis are a rare but serious complications of acute pancreatitis.[29] They are seen typically in patients of ANP due to extension of inflammation along the mesentery to involve the vessels in the mesentery and walls of the bowel. Transverse colon and splenic flexure are the most common sites.[30] The involved bowel segment shows circumferential wall thickening with maintained stratification on CECT scan **(Figs. 14A and B)**. As the inflammation progresses, bowel necrosis and perforation may occur which is seen as pneumoperitoneum and extraluminal leak of oral contrast on CECT scan. Other complications include bowel obstruction and ileus.

Pancreatic fistula is a complication which develops as a result of necrosis of pancreatic ductal walls. This results in leak of pancreatic secretions causing persistence of collections. Such collections have high amylase levels on sampling. Management involves endoscopic stenting or surgery.

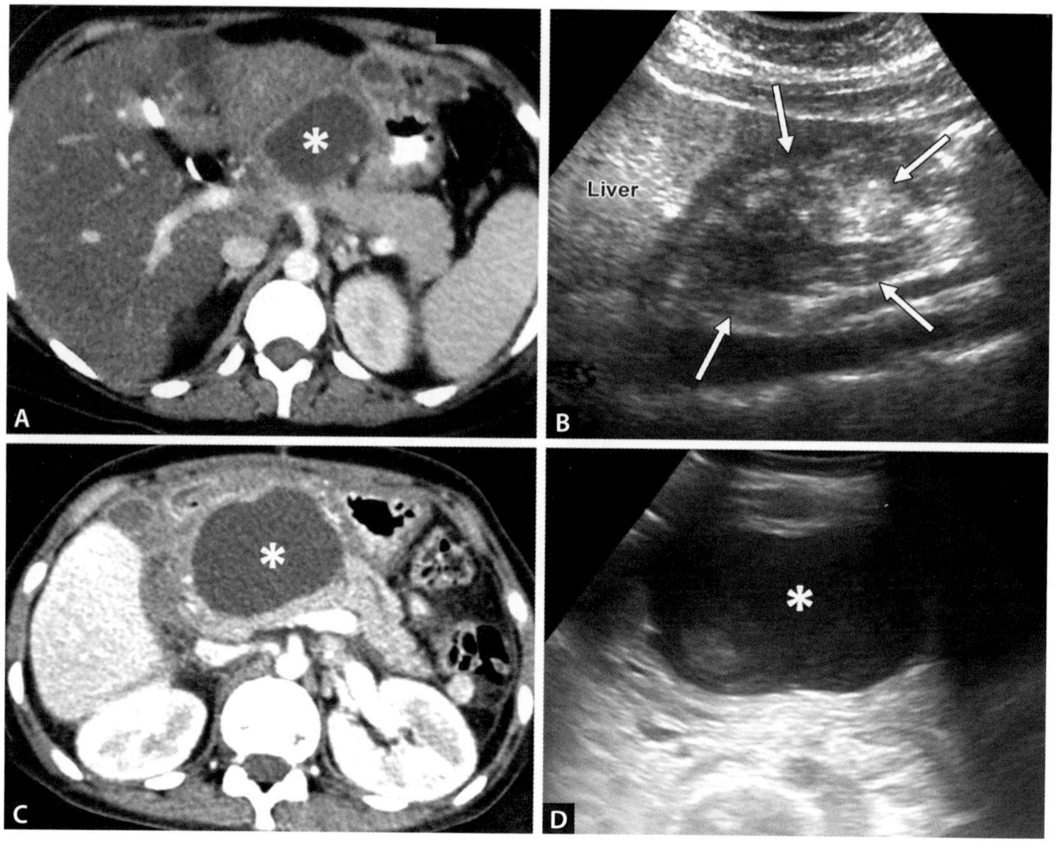

Figs. 11A to D: Assessment of liquefaction by ultrasonography: (A and C) Contrast-enhanced CT scans show similar looking walled of necrosis (asterisks). However, ultrasonography shows one is solid looking and not liquefied (arrows in B) and the other is fully liquefied (asterisk in D).

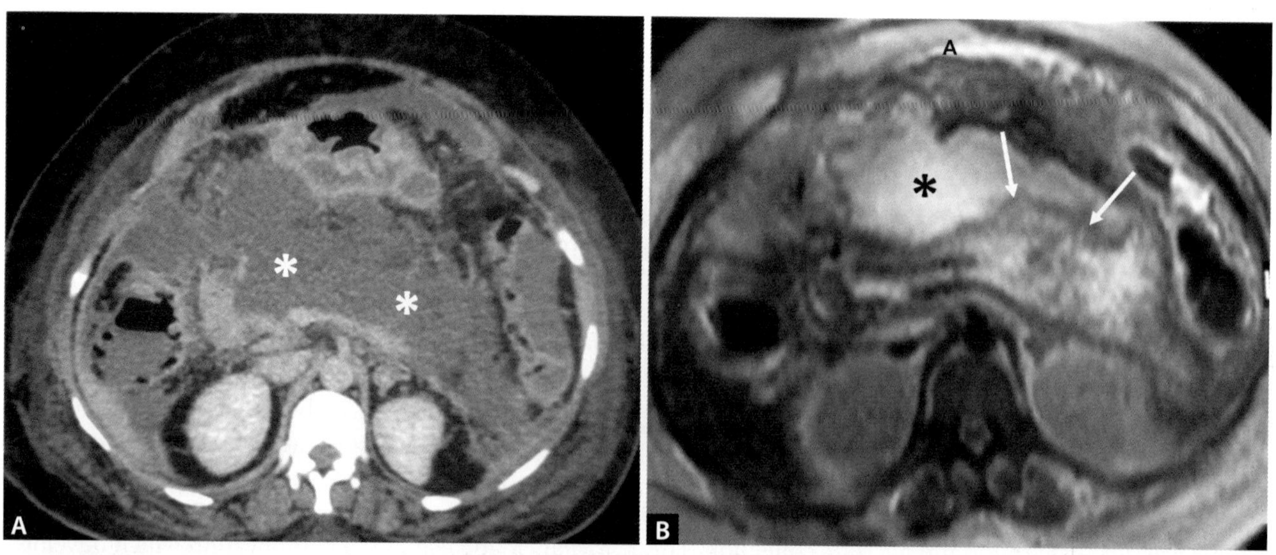

Figs. 12A and B: Assessment of liquefaction by MRI: (A) Contrast-enhanced CT scan shows large relatively homogeneous necrotic collection without definitive information on liquefaction (asterisks). (B) However, T2W-MR image shows both liquefied (asterisk) and non-liquefied (arrows) areas.

Other abdominal complications include cholecystitis, pancreatic duct strictures and splenic infarcts. Extra-abdominal complications are also seen, most common being pleural effusion. This is mostly reactive but may be gross causing respiratory symptoms. Lungs may show non-cardiogenic pulmonary edema in severe cases. Rarely, there may be fat embolism and patient may present with neurological symptoms.

Vascular Complications

Vascular complications may involve arterial or venous structures. Involvement of arteries may result in arteritis and erosion of the arterial wall by pancreatic enzymes which may lead to formation of pseudoaneurysms, rupture and thrombosis. Arterial hemorrhage and pseudoaneurysms are seen in up to 5% of patients with acute pancreatitis and are usually solitary.[31] It most commonly involves the splenic artery (60–65%; **Fig. 15A**), followed by the gastroduodenal artery (20–25%; **Figs. 15B and C**).[32] Other arteries involved include left gastric, hepatic, inferior pancreaticoduodenal and gastroepiploic arteries. Since these pseudoaneurysms are prone to rupture, which has very high mortality, immediate management is necessary. CT angiography (from dome of diaphragm to iliac crest) should be done in all cases where there is gastrointestinal bleed, hypotension or drop in hemoglobin. On imaging, plain CT scan may be done to show hemorrhage (high density area) in the collection **(Figs. 16A and B)** or in the adjoining bowel loops. The angiography images show a variable-sized smooth or irregular contrast filled out pouching from an artery or its branch. Sometimes the feeding artery may not be clearly seen due to spasm. Pseudoaneurysms with a very narrow neck may not opacify in the arterial phase, and may fill in the venous phase. Hence, both arterial and venous phases are needed in the evaluation of hemorrhage in patients of acute pancreatitis.[32]

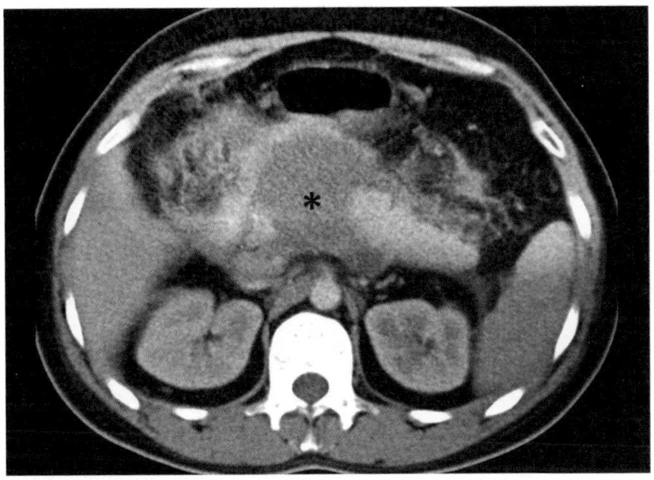

Fig. 13: Axial contrast-enhanced CT scan in a patient with ANP showing full thickness necrosis of pancreatic neck and body with walled-off collection (asterisk), suggesting disconnected duct syndrome.

Venous complications most commonly include thrombosis of splenic vein, portal vein and superior mesenteric vein which may result in formation of perigastric and splenic hilar collateral venous channels and portal hypertension. Splanchnic vein thrombosis is seen in about 2% patients of acute pancreatitis and about half of the patients with ANP.[33,34] Splenic vein thrombosis is the most common, accounting for over 80% of the cases. Diagnosis is mostly made on CECT. In the initial stage, thrombosis is seen as filling defect within the enhancing splenic vein **(Figs. 17A and B)**. Subsequently, as the thrombosis evolves, there is complete obstruction

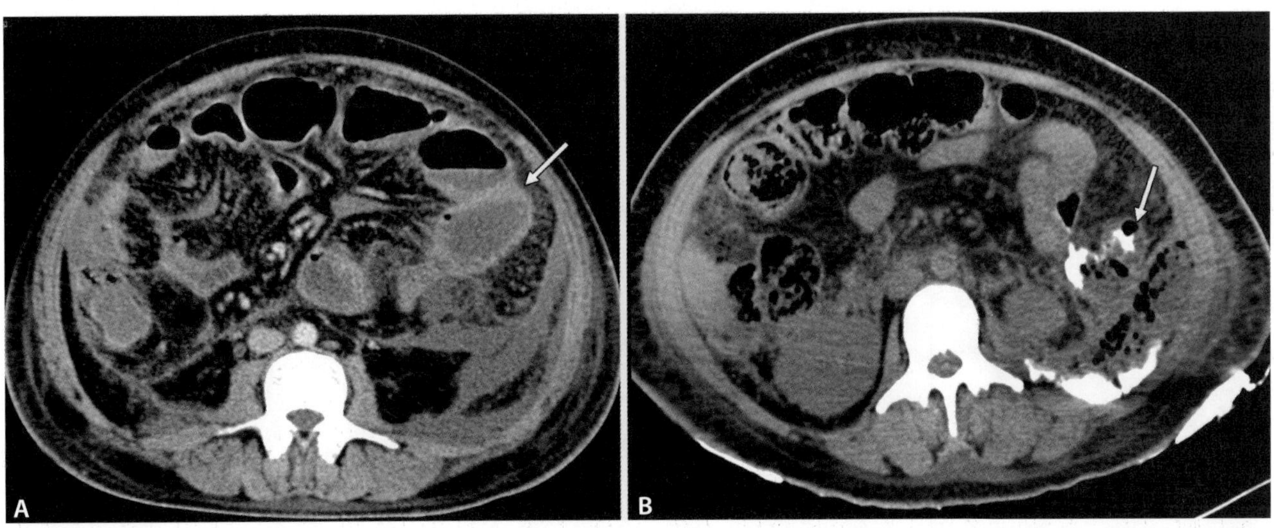

Figs. 14A and B: Bowel necrosis: (A) Axial contrast-enhanced CT scan shows circumferential thickening of descending colon (arrow). After drainage of paracolic collection percutaneously, there was feculent discharge in the drain; (B) Tubogram performed by injection of contrast into the drainage catheter shows contrast in the descending colon (arrow) suggesting perforation and fistula.

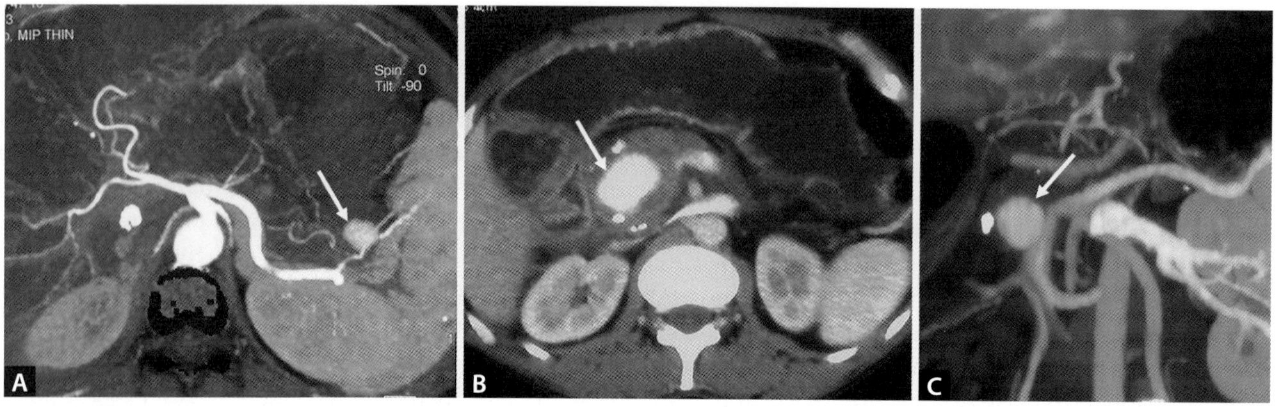

Figs. 15A to C: Pseudoaneurysm: (A) Maximum intensity projection (MIP) of CT scan in arterial phase shows a pseudoaneurysm arising from distal splenic artery (arrow); (B and C) Axial and coronal MIP contrast-enhanced CT images show a pseudoaneurysm in the region of head of pancreas, arising from gastroduodenal artery (arrow).

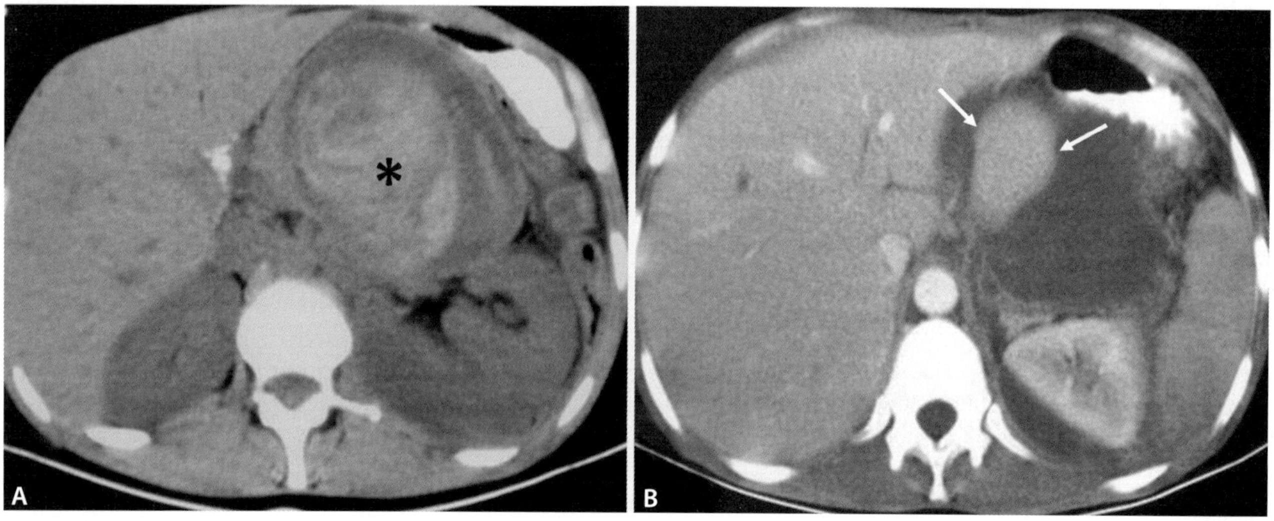

Figs. 16A and B: Pseudoaneurysm: (A) Noncontrast CT scan showing hyperdensity (asterisk) within a peripancreatic collection suggesting acute hemorrhage; (B) Late arterial phase CT scan showing an oval pseudoaneurysm (arrows) arising from splenic artery.

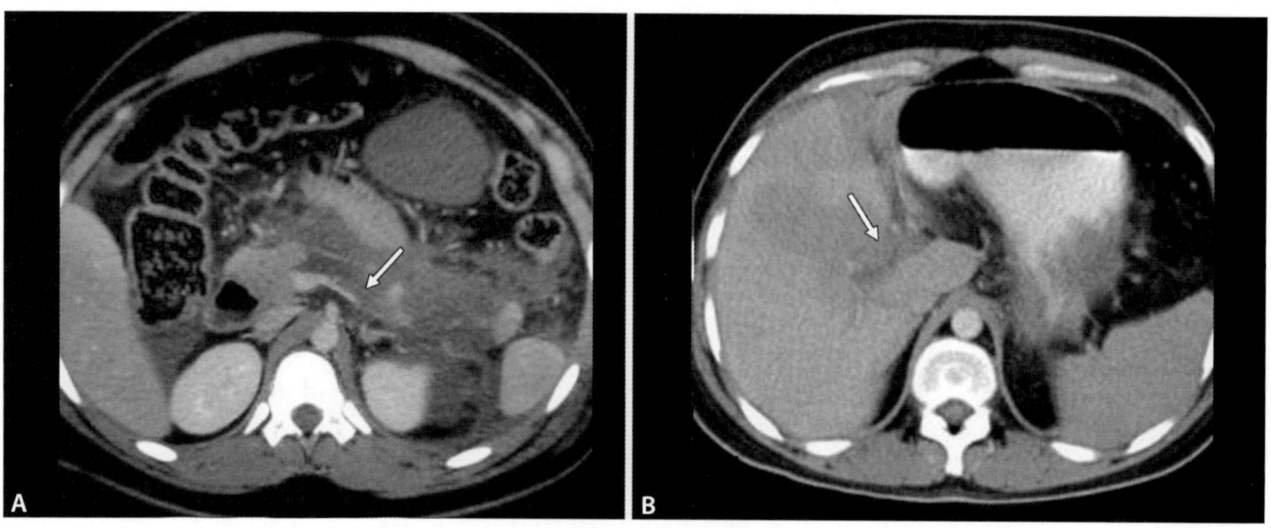

Figs. 17A and B: Venous thrombosis: (A) Contrast-enhanced CT scan showing a case of necrotizing pancreatitis with thrombosis of splenic vein seen as hypodense filling defect with in its lumen (arrow); (B) Contrast-enhanced CT scan in a case of acute pancreatitis showing non-enhancement of portal vein (arrow) suggesting thrombosis.

of the vein with opening up of short gastric and omental collaterals. Splenomegaly and splenic infarcts may also be seen. There may be thrombosis of the main portal vein and superior mesenteric vein which may be replaced by collaterals.

MANAGEMENT

Management of patients of acute pancreatitis involves multiple disciplines with a team approach. The gastroenterologists, gastrointestinal surgeons and radiologists all play an important role. In patients with AIEP and ANP, initial management is mostly conservative with the role of radiologist being in imaging, whenever necessary. The management involves nutritional support (oral for AIEP and enteral for ANP), fluid resuscitation, pain control and mobilization.[35] ERCP may be done when there is biliary obstruction, calculi or cholangitis. There is no role for prophylactic antibiotics. In resolving phase, if there is a persistent pseudocyst (in AIEP) causing symptoms, it is usually managed by endoscopic or surgical cystogastrostomy. Percutaneous drainage may be needed occasionally. Radiological interventions play an important role in managing patients of ANP presenting with complicated collections and hemorrhage.

Radiological Interventions

Radiological interventions are broadly classified into vascular and nonvascular procedures.

Non-vascular procedures form the major bulk of radiological interventions in patients with acute pancreatitis. This predominantly involves drainage of collections. It is important to understand that any collection seen in acute pancreatitis does not need drainage. Specific indications for drainage include infection, mass effect, symptoms, non-improvement or deterioration of symptoms and large collections (>5 cm) which are persistent (>6 weeks).[36] A sterile collection should not be drained unless it is causing symptoms like pain, abdominal distension, vomiting or jaundice **(Fig. 10B)**. Secondary infection is mostly seen with necrotic collection, in up to 33% cases and is typically seen between 2nd and 4th week of onset of illness.[37] This occurs mostly due to translocation of microbia from the bowel into the collection.[38] Diagnosis of infected collection is based on clinical (fever, persistent/new organ failure) and lab parameters (leukocytosis) and by imaging (air within the collection on CECT; **Fig. 10A**). Although diagnostic aspiration of fluid may help in detection of infection, it is not routinely practiced due to high false negative rate (20–25%).[39] Mass effect due to collections may result in gastric outlet obstruction (due to duodenal compression), biliary dilatation (due to compression of bile duct), hydronephrosis (compression of ureters) and portal hypertension with multiple venous collaterals (compression of splenoportal axis).[16] It is important that a retroperitoneal route is used for drainage of collections and traversing the bowel should be avoided as it is unsafe and may give false positive results due to contamination. DWI and FDG-PET (with labeled autologous leukocytes) may be useful in differentiation of sterile and infected necrosis. Infected necrosis is associated with high morbidity and mortality (25–70%).[40]

An infected necrotic collection should always be drained.[36] However, the timing of drainage is important for its success. Usually, collections begin to liquefy after 3–4 weeks of the onset of illness. Hence, drainage should be planned after this time. This may be confirmed by either USG or MRI whenever possible as CECT is a poor investigation for assessment of liquefaction. There are various approaches used for drainage of collections in acute pancreatitis **(Fig. 18)**. Most common and the preferred approach is through the retroperitoneum, typically through the anterior pararenal space. This approach is associated with less complications, allows better drainage by gravity and the same tract can be used when endoscopic or minimally invasive surgical necrosectomy is done. Other approaches used include transgastric, paraspinal, transperitoneal and transhepatic. Mediastinal collections should be drained through paraspinal extrapleural approach. Saline injection may be necessary for avoiding lung or pleural puncture. The technique of drainage used is either the Seldinger technique or trocar technique. The imaging guidance used is either USG or CT scan **(Figs. 19A to D)**. When the collection is deep seated, in the

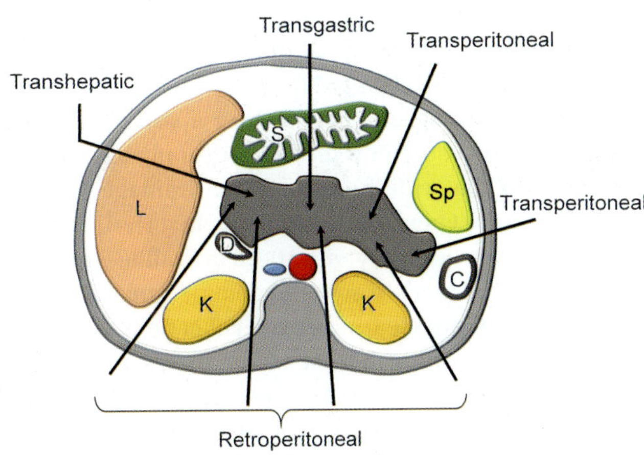

Fig. 18: Schematic diagram showing various approaches used to drain pancreatic collection.
Abbreviation: C: Colon; D: Duodenum; K: Kidneys; L: Liver; S: Stomach; Sp: Spleen.

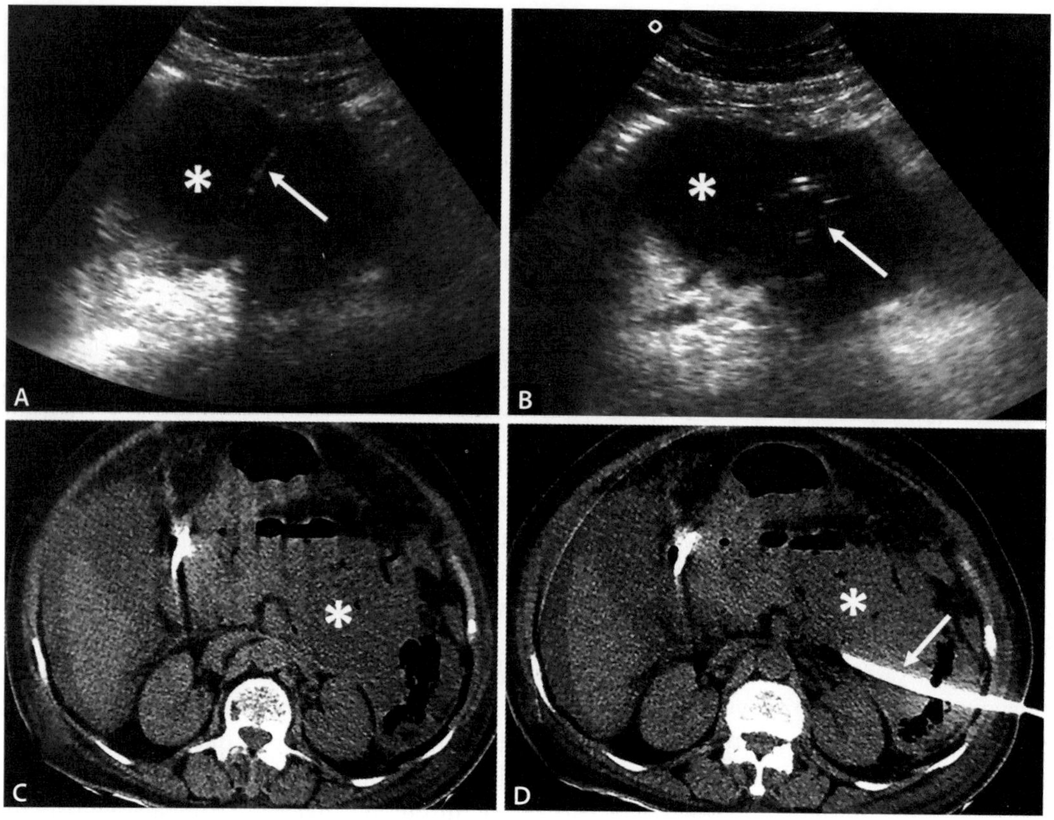

Figs. 19A to D: (A and B) Ultrasound-guided drainage of lesser sac collection (asterisk). Trocar with pigtail catheter is seen in A (arrow) with pigtail catheter in position in B (arrow); (C and D) CT-guided drainage of collection (asterisk). A lesser sac collection is seen with air pockets in C and catheter inserted in D (arrow).

lesser sac—anterior pararenal space and retroperitoneal approach is needed or when there is extensive air in the collection, CT guidance is preferred. In cases where the collection is visible on USG and liquefied, in sick patients when bedside procedure is needed and in superficial collections, USG guidance should be used.

The size of drainage catheter initially used is 10/12F. Subsequently, this needs serial upgradation through 16F, up to 20 or 24 F **(Figs. 20A to D)**. Once the initial catheter is inserted, exchanges are done over a stiff guidewire. Usually, Malecot catheter is preferred over pigtail catheter as the former has wide holes to allow drainage of thick necrotic debris. Once the catheter is inserted, regular flushing atleast twice a day with 10–20 mL saline is needed to allow free drainage. In some patients, simple drainage alone is sufficient in clearing all the collections. In rest of the patients, collections persist and further interventions in the form of percutaneous endoscopic necrosectomy, surgical necrosectomy or video-assisted retroperitoneal debridement are needed (*step-up approach*).

Other interventions performed in patients of acute pancreatitis include drainage of ascites, drainage of pleural effusion and percutaneous cholecystostomy (for biliary decompression).

Vascular interventions mostly involve embolization of pseudoaneurysms.[41] This can be done by three different approaches. Firstly, through the endovascular route, which is most commonly used. Second is the percutaneous approach, done for pseudoaneurysms within solid organs and superficial locations. Last is the endoscopic ultrasonography (EUS) guided route used when the previous two approaches fail or are not possible. Endovascular embolization has over 90% technical and clinical success rates in treatment of pseudoaneurysms of acute pancreatitis. But ongoing inflammation may be a problem and may result in recurrence. Coils are the most commonly used embolizing agents. Other agents used include glue n-butyl cyanoacrylate (nBCA) and thrombin. The latter is used often with percutaneous or EUS approaches.

The *endovascular* embolization is usually done through transfemoral route. It is important that a CT angiogram is done in all these cases as it will help to identify the source artery responsible for bleeding and

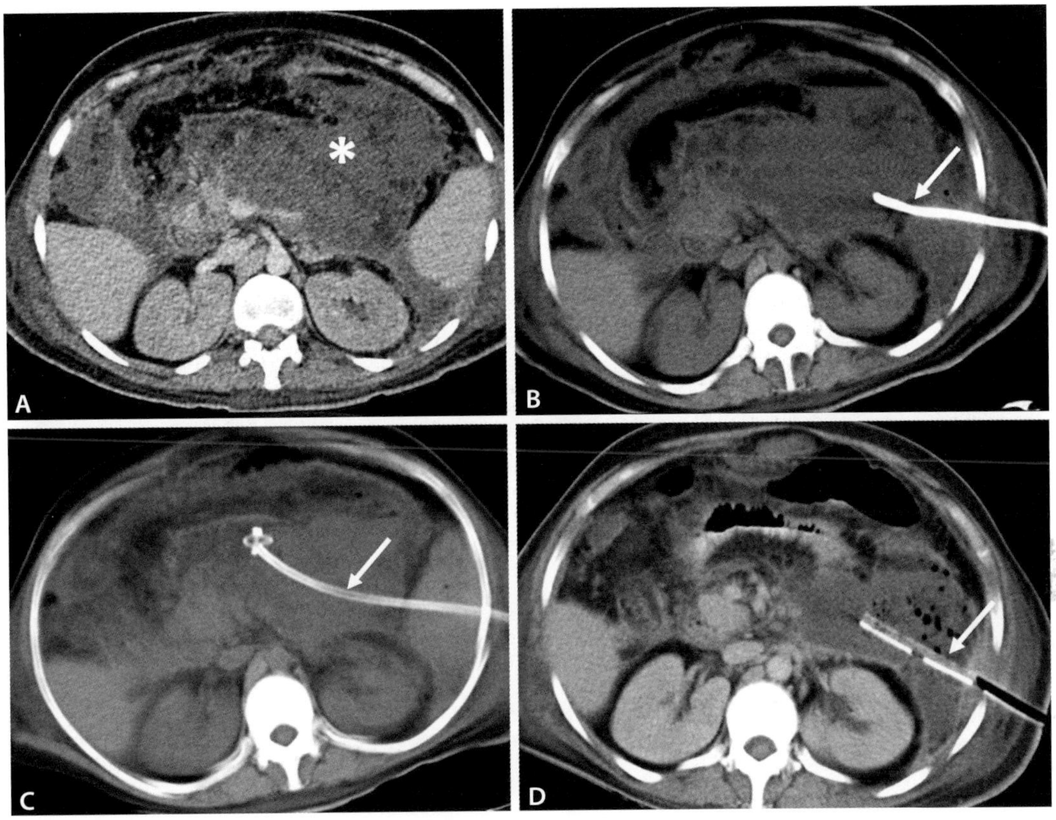

Figs. 20A to D: Serial upgradation of catheters under CT guidance: (A) Contrast-enhanced CT image showing necrotic collection in lesser sac (asterisk); (B) Collection with 12F pigtail catheter *in situ* (arrow); (C) Catheter upgraded to 16F Malecot catheter (arrow); (D) 20F drainage catheter within the collection (arrow).

also identify anatomical variations. This will reduce the time of the procedure and radiation exposure. When the source artery is known, the artery is catheterized using a 5F catheter (RC1; Cook). After initial angiogram acquired with catheter tip placed in proximal larger arteries (celiac, hepatic, splenic or superior mesenteric origin), distal catheterization of smaller arteries is done with microcatheter to avoid injury to the arteries. Once the neck is identified, embolization procedure should be done. It is important to note that gastroduodenal, splenic, left gastric and hepatic arteries have collateral circulation and hence 'sandwich' technique of embolization should be used **(Figs. 21 and 22)**. Here, embolization of segment of artery distal to the neck of pseudoaneurysm and proximal to it is done so that there is no refilling from collaterals. This will isolate the pseudoaneurysm from the systemic circulation and thrombosis ensues. Microcoils (platinum coils) with fibers are used for embolization through either 'anchor' technique (anchoring the tip of microcoil into a smaller branch) or 'scaffolding' technique (using a stiffer coil initially like steel coils). They cause thrombosis by causing mechanical obstruction and due to the presence of thrombogenic fibers. n-BCA may also be used in specific situations like when optimal catheterization of the artery is not possible, when there are multiple feeders to the pseudoaneurysm or when there is coagulation derangement.[42] In *percutaneous* approach, the pseudoaneurysm is directly punctured using a 21G/22G needle under USG guidance.[41] Once the backflow of blood is confirmed, the embolic agent (thrombin or n-BCA) is injected under USG guidance. Thrombosis of the pseudoaneurysm occurs immediately and can be confirmed with color Doppler.

RADIATION EXPOSURE

Patients of acute pancreatitis, especially ANP, undergo multiple CT scans during the course of their admission which significantly increases radiation exposure. In a study by Ball et al. it was shown that the median number of CT examinations in patients of ANP was five and mean effective dose was 63 mSv.[43] Patients who underwent DSA were further exposed to more radiation. They also suggested that management decisions infrequently followed the CT scan. Thus it is important to avoid unnecessary CT scans

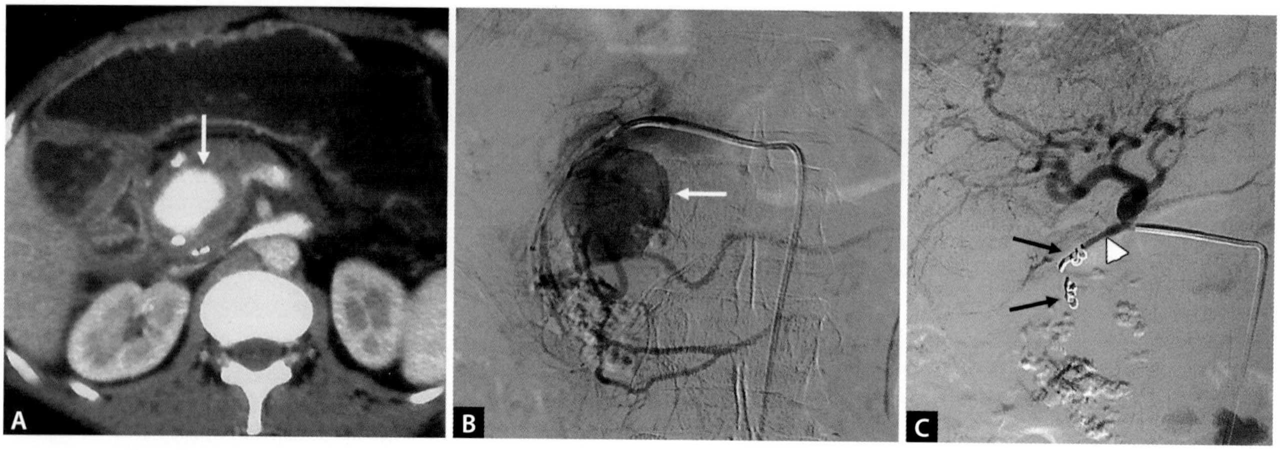

Figs. 21A to C: Embolization: (A) Contrast-enhanced CT scan shows a pseudoaneurysm arising from gastroduodenal artery (GDA, arrow); (B) Digital subtraction angiography (DSA) of gastroduodenal artery shows the pseudoaneurysm (arrow); (C) DSA after proximal and distal coiling (arrows) of GDA (arrowhead) shows complete embolization of the pseudoaneurysm.

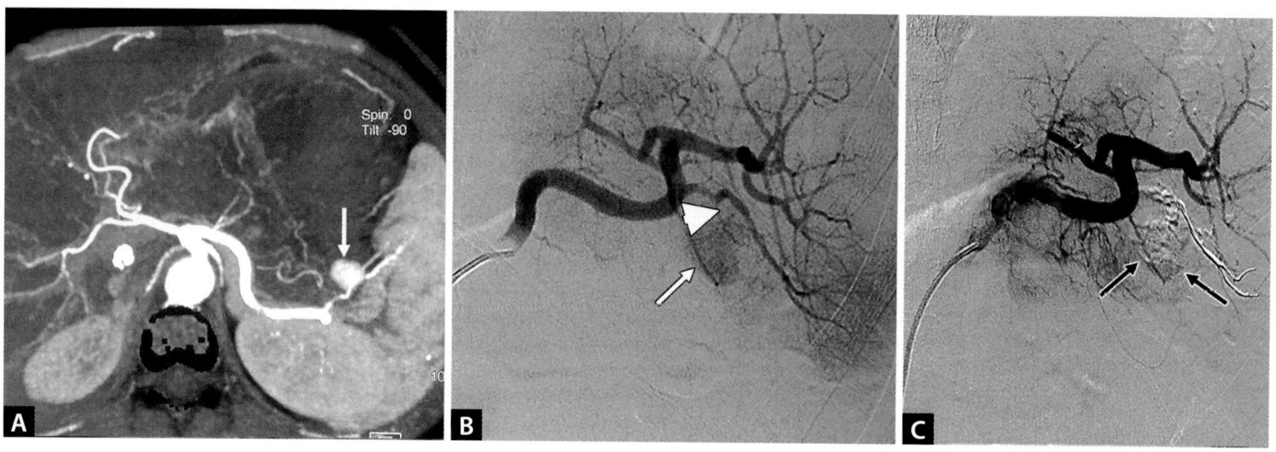

Figs. 22A to C: Splenic artery pseudoaneurysm: (A) MIP-CT image in arterial phase showing a contrast filled outpouching (arrow) in the distal splenic artery, (B) DSA of splenic artery shows the pseudoaneurysm (arrow) arising from distal branch of splenic artery (arrowhead). (C) DSA after embolization with combination of coils and glue shows complete obliteration of the pseudoaneurysm (arrows).

in patients of acute pancreatitis. Alternate modalities like USG or MRI which are free of radiation should be used, wherever possible. Even during follow-up CT scan, low kV (100 kV) helps in reducing radiation dose. CT-guided procedures may be performed under low kV with scan area limited to the region of interest. Awareness of this problem and methods to reduce it is critical to prevent significant radiation exposure.

ADVANCES IN IMAGING

Ultrasound elastography may be a simple radiation-free tool to diagnosis acute pancreatitis. In patients with acute pancreatitis, there is increase in pancreatic stiffness. Measurement of pancreatic stiffness on sonoelastography may be a helpful bedside technique to diagnose acute pancreatitis in difficult cases. A recent study has shown that acoustic radiation force impulse (ARFI) is an accurate non-invasive tool in diagnosing acute pancreatitis and is comparable to CECT scan.[44]

Contrast-enhanced USG (CEUS) is being used in assessment of areas of necrosis in patients with ANP with accuracies equal to contrast enhanced CT scan.[45] The sensitivity and specificity of CEUS for diagnosing acute pancreatitis are 90% and 99% respectively. Thus it is a cost-effective method and can be used in patients where iodinated contrast agents cannot be used. The limitations are same as those for B-mode USG.

CT perfusion is a new imaging technique which has application in evaluation of acute pancreatitis. Perfusion CT (PCT) involves continuous acquisition of sections through the pancreas over a period of 2–3 minutes after intravenous contrast injection. The acquired images are then processed to generate various perfusion parameters. In acute pancreatitis, the role of perfusion CT is in the predicted severe variety. PCT done early in the course of the disease (within 48 hours) shows areas of hypoperfusion which on follow-up show necrosis.[46] Thus, perfusion CT is helpful in predicting the areas of necrosis prior to their development and may open new therapeutic options to prevent this ominous development.

Dual energy CT scan (DECT) has been shown to be useful in evaluation of pancreatic diseases. In patients with acute necrotizing pancreatitis, DECT in portal venous phase may help in assessment of areas of hypoperfusion and necrosis in the pancreatic parenchyma with improved contrast to noise ratio.[47] DECT thus may have potential in better identifying and defining necrotic areas.

All these advanced techniques are in the early stages of research and more evidence is needed to use them in routine practice.

SUMMARY

Acute pancreatitis is a disease with high morbidity. Early detection is important for judicious management. Knowledge of the revised Atlanta classification helps understanding the disease and defining various stages and terms uniformly. Imaging should be done only when indicated and whenever possible, modalities without radiation should be used. Diagnosis of various complications often requires high index of suspicion. Radiologist plays a critical role in both diagnosing these complications and in managing them, wherever necessary.

REFERENCES

1. Wu BU, Banks PA. Clinical management of patients with acute pancreatitis. Gastroenterology. 2013;144(6):1272-81.
2. Banks PA, Bollen TL, Dervenis C, et al. Classification of acute pancreatitis-2012: revision of the Atlanta classification and definitions by international consensus. Gut. 2013;62:102-11.
3. Lankisch PG, Apte M, Banks PA. Acute pancreatitis. Lancet. 2015;386(9988):85-96.
4. Elfar M, Gaber LW, Sabek O, Fischer CP, Gaber O. The inflammatory cascade in acute pancreatitis: relevance to clinical disease. Surg Clin N Am. 2007;87:1325-40.
5. Bollen TL. Acute pancreatitis: international classification and nomenclature. Clin Radiol. 2016;71:121-33.
6. Bradley III EL. A clinically based classification system for acute pancreatitis. Summary of the International Symposium on Acute Pancreatitis, Atlanta, GA, September 11 through 13, 1992. Arch Surg. 1993;128:586-90.
7. Banks PA, Bollen TL, Dervenis C, et al. Classification of acute pancreatitis 2012: revision of the Atlanta classification and definitions by international consensus. Gut. 2013;62(1):102-11.
8. Thoeni RF. The revised Atlanta classification of acute pancreatitis: its importance for the radiologist and its effect on treatment. Radiology. 2012;262(3):751-64.
9. Singh VK, Bollen TL, Wu BU, et al. An assessment of the severity of interstitial pancreatitis. Clin Gastroenterol Hepatol. 2011;9(12):1098-103.
10. Bollen TL, Singh VK, Maurer R, et al. A comparative evaluation of radiologic and clinical scoring systems in the early prediction of severity in acute pancreatitis. Am J Gastroenterol. 2012;107:612-9.
11. Bharwani N, Patel S, Prabhudesai S, et al. Acute pancreatitis: the role of imaging in diagnosis and management. Clin Radiol. 2011;66(2):164-75.
12. Merkle EM, Gorich J. Imaging of acute pancreatitis. Eur Radiol. 2002;12(8):1979-92.
13. Sirli R, Sporea I. Ultrasound examination of the normal pancreas. Med Ultrasound. 2010;12(1):62-5.
14. Turkvatan A, Erden A, Turkoglu MA, Secil M, Yener O. Imaging of acute pancreatitis and its complications. Part 1: Acute pancreatitis. Diagn Interv Imaging. 2015;96(2):151-60.
15. Bollen TL, van Santvoort HC, Besselink MG, et al. Update on acute pancreatitis: ultrasound, computed tomography, and magnetic resonance imaging features. Semin Ultrasound CT MR. 2007;28(5):371-83.
16. O'Connor OJ, McWilliams S, Maher MM. Imaging of acute pancreatitis. AJR. 2011;197(2):W221-5.
17. Balthazar EJ. Acute pancreatitis: assessment of severity with clinical and CT evaluation. Radiology. 2002;223:603-13.
18. Turkvatan A, Erden A, Turkoglu MA, Secil M, Yuce G. Imaging of acute pancreatitis and its complications. Part 2: Complications of Acute Pancreatitis. Diagn Interv Imaging. 2015;96(2):161-9.
19. Theoni RF. Imaging of acute pancreatitis. Radiol Clin N Am. 2015;53:1189-208.
20. Meyrignac O, Lagarde S, Bournet B, et al. Acute pancreatitis: extrapancreatic necrosis volume as early predictor of severity. Radiology. 2015; 276:119-28.
21. Delrue LJ, De Waele JJ, Duyck PO. Acute pancreatitis: radiologic scores in predicting severity and outcome. Abdom Imaging. 2010;35:349-61.
22. Balthazar EJ, Robinson DL, Megibow AJ, et al. Acute pancreatitis: value of CT in establishing prognosis. Radiology. 1990;174:331-6.
23. Bollen TL, Singh VK, Maurer R, et al. Comparative evaluation of the modified CT severity index and CT severity index in assessing severity of acute pancreatitis. AJR. 2011;197:386-92.
24. Mortele KJ, Wiesner W, Intriere L, et al. A modified CT severity index for evaluating acute pancreatitis: improved correlation with patient outcome. AJR. 2004;183:1261-5.
25. De Waele JJ, Delrue L, Hoste EA, et al. Extrapancreatic inflammation on abdominal computed tomography as an early predictor of disease severity in acute

pancreatitis: evaluation of a new scoring system. Pancreas. 2007;34:185-90.

26. Sharma V, Rana SS, Ravi SK, et al. A study of radiological scoring system evaluating extrapancreatic inflammation with conventional radiological and clinical scores in predicting outcomes in acute pancreatitis. Ann Gastroenterol. 2015;28:397-402.
27. van Baal MC, Bollen TL, Bakker OJ, et al. The role of routine fine-needle aspiration in the diagnosis of infected necrotising pancreatitis. Surgery. 2014;155(3):442-8.
28. Kloppel G. Acute pancreatitis. Semin Diagn Pathol. 2004;21(4): 221-6.
29. Gardner A, Gardner G, Feller E. Severe colonic complications of pancreatic disease. J Clin Gastroenterol. 2003;37:258-62.
30. Van Minnen LP, Besselink MG, Bosscha K, et al. Colonic involvement in acute pancreatitis: a retrospective study of 16 patients. Dig Surg. 2004;21:33-8. discussion 39-40.
31. Mortele KJ, Mergo PJ, Taylor HM, Wiesner W, Cantisani V, Ernst MD, Kalantari BN, Ros PR. Peripancreatic vascular abnormalities complicating acute pancreatitis: contrast-enhanced helical CT findings. Eur J Radiol. 2004;52(1):67-72.
32. Kirby JM, Vora P, Midia M, Rawlinson J. Vascular complications of pancreatitis: imaging and intervention. Cardiovasc Intervent Radiol. 2008;31:957-70.
33. Easler J, Muddana V, Furlan A, et al. Portosplenomesenteric venous thrombosis in patients with acute pancreatitis is associated with pancreatic necrosis and usually has a benign course. Clin Gastroenterol Hepatol. 2014;12(5):854-62.
34. Harris S, Nadkarni NA, Naina HV, et al. Splanchnic vein thrombosis in acute pancreatitis: a single-center experience. Pancreas. 2013;42(8):1251-4.
35. Working Group IAP/APA Acute Pancreatitis Guidelines. IAP/APA evidence-based guidelines for the management of acute pancreatitis. Pancreatology. 2013;13.1-15.
36. Bharwani N, Patel S, Prabhudesai S, Fotheringham T, Power N. Acute pancreatitis: the role of imaging diagnosis and management. Clin Radiol. 2011;66:164-75.
37. van Santvoort HC, Bakker OJ, Bollen TL, et al. A conservative and minimally invasive approach to necrotising pancreatitis improves outcome. Gastroenterology. 2011;141(4):1254-63.
38. Fritz S, Hackert T, Hartwig W, et al. Bacterial translocation and infected pancreatic necrosis in acute necrotising pancreatitis derives from small bowel rather than from colon. Am J Surg. 2010;200(1):111-7.
39. Rodriguez JR, Razo AO, Targarona J, Thayer SP, Rattner DW, Warshaw AL, et al. Debridement and closed packing for sterile or infected necrotizing pancreatitis: insights into indications and outcomes in 167 patients. Ann Surg. 2008;247:294-9.
40. Shyu JY, Sainani NI, Sahni VA, et al. Necrotizing pancreatitis: diagnosis, imaging, and intervention. Radiographics. 2014;34:1218-39.
41. Madhusudhan KS, Venkatesh HA, Gamanagatti S, Garg P, Srivastava DN. Interventional Radiology in the Management of Visceral Artery Pseudoaneurysms: A Review of Techniques and Embolic Materials. Korean J Radiol. 2016;17(3):351-63.
42. Madhusudhan KS, Gamanagatti S, Garg P, Shalimar, Dash NR, Pal S, Peush S, Gupta AK. Endovascular Embolization of Visceral Artery Pseudoaneurysms Using Modified Injection Technique with N-Butyl Cyanoacrylate Glue. J Vasc Interv Radiol. 2015;26(11):1718-25.
43. Ball CG, Correa-Gallego C, Howard TJ, Zyromski NJ, House MG, Pitt HA, Nakeeb A, Schmidt CM, Akisik F, Lillemoe KD. Radiation dose from computed tomography in patients with necrotizing pancreatitis: how much is too much? J Gastrointest Surg. 2010;14(10):1529-35.
44. Göya C, Hamidi C, Hattapoğlu S, Çetinçakmak MG, Teke M, Degirmenci MS, Kaya M, Bilici A. Use of acoustic radiation force impulse elastography to diagnose acute pancreatitis at hospital admission: comparison with sonography and computed tomography. J Ultrasound Med. 2014;33(8):1453-60.
45. Ardelean M, Şirli R, Sporea I, Bota S, Martie A, Popescu A, Danila M, Timar B, Buzas R, Lighezan. Contrast-enhanced ultrasound in the pathology of the pancreas: a monocentric experience. Med Ultrason. 2014;16(4):325-31
46. Yadav AK, Sharma R, Kandasamy D, Bhalla AS, Gamanagatti S, Srivastava DN, Upadhyay AD, Garg PK. Perfusion CT: can it predict the development of pancreatic necrosis in early stage of severe acute pancreatitis? Abdom Imaging. 2015;40(3):488-99.
47. Yuan Y, Huang ZX, Li ZL, Song B, Deng LP. The value of dual-source dual-energy CT with iodine overlay in the diagnosis of acute necrotizing pancreatitis. Sichuan Da Xue Xue Bao Yi Xue Ban. 2012;43(4):597-600.

CHAPTER 88

Chronic Pancreatitis and its Variants

Anupam Lal, Manphool Singhal, Mandeep Kang

INTRODUCTION

Pancreatitis, the acute form is the most common benign condition affecting the pancreas, and in most cases, it resolves without significant structural or functional impairment. In contrast, chronic pancreatitis (CP) is a progressive fibro-inflammatory disease. This results in irreversible structural changes in the pancreas with progressive loss of the lobular morphology, deformation of the large ducts and changes in the arrangement and composition of the islets. These changes ultimately manifest as ductal obstruction, destruction of acini and the islets of Langerhans, causing loss of exocrine and endocrine functions. Patients may present with abdominal pain, nausea, vomiting, weight loss, diarrhea, and diabetes. The classic clinical triad of CP is exocrine and endocrine pancreatic dysfunction with recurrent episodes of abdominal pain.

ETIOPATHOGENESIS

The risk-factors associated with CP are multi-factorial, including environmental factors (alcohol, tobacco and nutrition), hereditary (mutations), ductal obstruction and autoimmune causes. In adults, the most common etiology attributed to CP is alcohol consumption (70–80% cases).[1] Development of CP is linked/associated with the dose and duration of alcohol consumption; however, recent epidemiological studies and animal experiments suggest that alcohol alone is not sufficient to induce CP and other environmental and genetic factors also play important role. Overall, less than 10% of heavy alcohol consumers develop alcohol-induced CP, nevertheless consumption of lesser quantities may also lead to pancreatic injury and may have an impact on the progression of the disease.[2,3]

Malnutrition remains the most common cause of CP in general population worldwide.[1] Among the hereditary causes, cystic fibrois and mutation of trypsinogen gene are well recognized. Pancreatic or periampullary neoplasms, sphincter of oddi dysfunction, ampullary stricture and congenital lesions like abnormal pancreaticobiliary junction and pancreatic divisum are also important causes of CP. Other causes of CP include hypercalcemia, hyperparathyroidism and hyperlipidemia. Whatever be the cause, the end result is pancreatic fibrosis, which usually takes several years to develop.

In children, the cause of CP is not ascertained in most cases hence labelled as idiopathic (up to 30% of cases). It is thought that hereditary and tropical pancreatitis is responsible for the majority of cases of chronic childhood pancreatitis.[4]

CLASSIFICATION OF CHRONIC PANCREATITIS

Large Duct Pancreatitis versus Small Duct Pancreatitis

There are two pathological subtypes of chronic pancreatitis: *Large duct* and *small duct pancreatitis*, which represent two ends of the same spectrum but have different pathological and radiological features and thus their management also varies.

Large duct pancreatitis is characterized by dilatation and dysfunction of the large ducts (MPD >7 mm) and diffuse pancreatic calcifications. These manifestations are easily recognizable on the imaging. Men are usually more commonly affected as compared to females. Clinical presentation is steatorrhea and abdominal pain. Treatment with replacement of pancreatic enzymes is not effective and the patients usually require surgical or endoscopic drainage to alleviate symptoms.

On the other hand, *small duct pancreatitis* (MPD <3 mm) occurs more in women and is usually not associated with pancreatic calcification. Imaging is essentially normal; therefore, a high index of suspicion is needed for diagnosis. Abdominal pain is the predominant symptom and steatorrhea is rare. Patients may respond to replacement of pancreatic enzymes. Traditionally, radical pancreatic resectional procedures have been carried out for small duct CP. The longitudinal V-shaped excision of the ventral pancreas has also shown promising results for diffuse small duct CP.[5]

CP may also be classified according to major predisposing risk factors as either (1) toxic-metabolic, (2) idiopathic, (3) genetic, (4) autoimmune, (5) recurrent and severe acute pancreatitis, or (6) obstructive (TIGAR-O system).[6]

Radiologically, three major forms of CP are recognized:

1. *Calcifying chronic pancreatitis:* It is characterized by acinar destruction and perilobular fibrosis with acute and chronic inflammatory cells, leading to pancreatic paronchymal calcification and intraductal calculi. Etiopathogenesis to begin with is precipitation of proteinaceous material in the pancreatic ducts, which form protein plugs that subsequently calcify. Subsequent to the site of obstruction (by protein plugs or fibrosis) the pancreatic duct and smaller pancreatic ductules dilate. The main pancreatic duct shows a chain-of-lakes appearance due to alternating stenoses and dilatation. In approximately half of patients with chronic calcific pancreatitis, the pancreatic parenchyma may contain cuboidal epithelium lined cysts containing pancreatic enzymes of varying sizes (several millimeters to 5 cm). Clinically, this form presents as recurrent episodes of abdominal pain. Alcohol and tobacco are implicated for this form of CP. Other forms of calcifying CP can be hereditary, tropical, idiopathic, and senile.
2. *Obstructive chronic pancreatitis:* This form of CP is due to persistent obstruction of the pancreatic duct (tumor or ductal stricture) leading to atrophy of the distal pancreas. The prominent histologic changes are periductal fibrosis and subsequent ductal dilatation. These changes can either be focal or diffuse depending upon the site of pancreatic ductal obstruction. Focal changes in this form are much more common than other forms of CP. Diffuse changes occur when pancreatic duct or ampulla is obstructed. Intraductal calculi are rare. The pancreatic duct is dilated, and the pancreas is normal in size, atrophic, or focally and/or globally enlarged. Abdominal pain is usually absent, though occasionally the patients present with acute pancreatitis.
3. Autoimmune pancreatitis (AIP) is part of a chronic systemic sclerosing disease characterized by lymphoplasmacytic inflammatory process involving the pancreas and other organs. AIP unlike other forms of CP shows focal, segmental or diffuse narrowing of MPD and non-visualization of side branches on ERCP. The narrowing can also be seen in the lower end of common bile duct (CBD) causing biliary dilatation. On imaging, it may appear as diffuse (duct destructive) or as pseudotumoral lesions.

DIAGNOSIS

Evaluation of CP usually needs a battery of tests. Biochemical investigations are used to assess the endocrine and exocrine function of the pancreas. Fecal elastase 1 (FE 1) is one of the commonly used indirect methods but has low sensitivity.[7] Tubed secretin test is a direct method which involves prolonged intubation and serial collection of pancreatic juice after hormonal stimulation. It is considered as a reference standard for the evaluation of exocrine function of pancreas.[8]

Radiological investigations are primarily used for evaluation of structural changes and complications of CP.

Imaging Modalities

Usually a combination of imaging is required with different imaging modalities having their own advantages and limitations and the role of imaging is to help confirm the diagnosis, assess disease severity, detect complications, and provide a "road map" for interventional procedures.

Abdominal Radiographs

Abdominal radiographs are not routinely done for the evaluation of CP. Often pancreatic calcifications are incidentally detected on radiographs done to rule out other causes for abdominal pain and thus the diagnosis

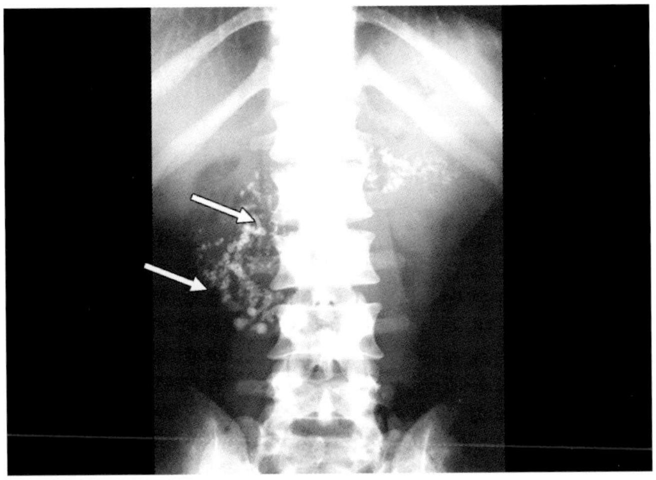

Fig. 1: Chronic calcifying pancreatitis: Plain radiograph abdomen showing calcifications along the course of pancreas. Note a pancreatic stent *in situ* (arrows).

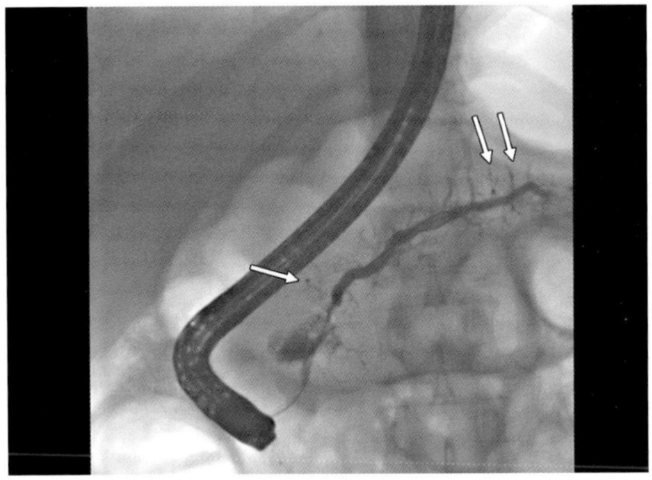

Fig. 2: Endoscopic retrograde cholangio-pancreatography (ERCP): Early changes of chronic pancreatitis showing mild irregularity of side branches (arrows). Main pancreatic duct (MPD) is not dilated.

suspected. CP is manifested on abdominal radiographs as multifocal calcifications typically seen across the spine along the course of pancreas **(Fig. 1)**. Since calcifications are usually seen in the advanced cases and only in certain types of CP, radiographs are not a sensitive investigation. Typical pancreatic calcifications, however if seen on radiographs are pathognomonic of CP.

Endoscopic Retrograde Cholangio-pancreatography

Endoscopic retrograde cholangio pancreatography (ERCP) is considered as the gold standard for the diagnosis of CP because of its superior spatial resolution and its ability to depict the ductal system in distended state. Side branch abnormalities in early CP may be detected. ERCP is an invasive procedure and has inherent procedure-related complications; hence this modality is mostly used with intent of therapeutic interventions. On ERCP, diameter of normal main pancreatic duct (MPD) varies with the region of pancreas—up to 4 mm in head, 3 mm in body and 2 mm in tail region. Side branches join the MPD at right angles in alternating fashion. Early CP is seen on ERCP in the form of irregularity and dilatation of side branches **(Fig. 2)**. These changes are more severe along with dilatation, loss of normal tapering and irregularity of MPD as the disease progresses **(Fig. 3)**. In advanced stages, alternate dilatation and stenosis of MPD can give the appearance of chain of lakes **(Figs 4 and 5)**.

The Cambridge classification of CP based on ERCP is used to group patients into equivocal, mild, moderate or marked type. The status of MPD, side branches, presence of calculi and ductal strictures are taken into account in Cambridge classification.[9]

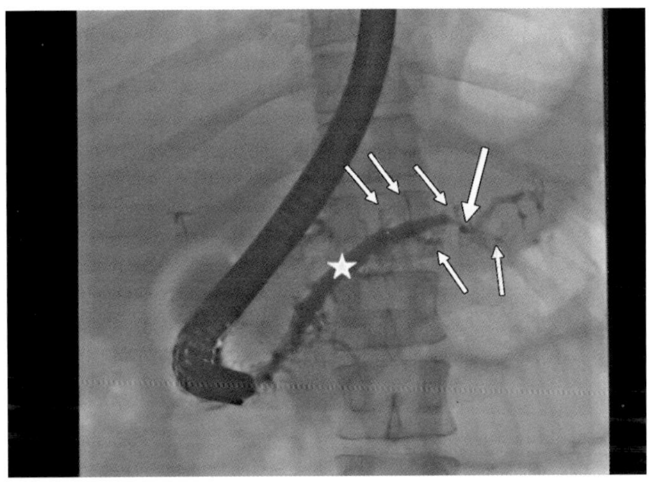

Fig. 3: ERCP: MPD is dilated (star). Note narrowing of MPD in tail region (long arrow) and multiple abnormal side branches (arrows).

Cambridge Classification

Score 1 (Cambridge Class 0)

- Severity: normal
- Good quality ERCP/US or CT visualizing whole gland without abnormal signs.

Score 2 (Cambridge Class 0)

- Severity: equivocal
- ERCP: <3 abnormal branches

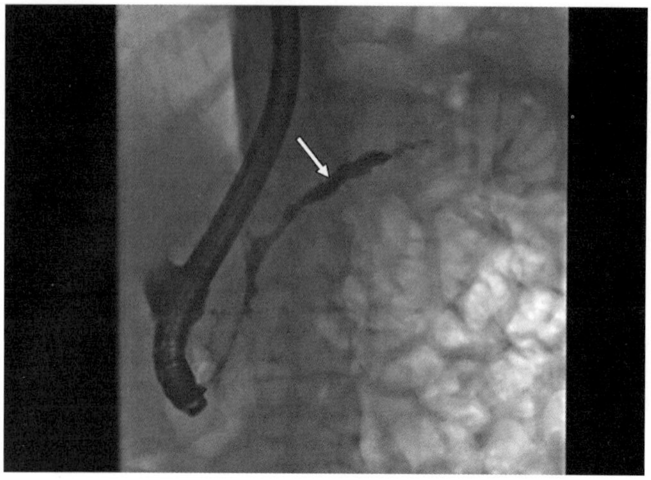

Fig. 4: ERCP: MPD (arrow) showing multiple strictures and irregular dilatation with truncated and abnormal side branches.

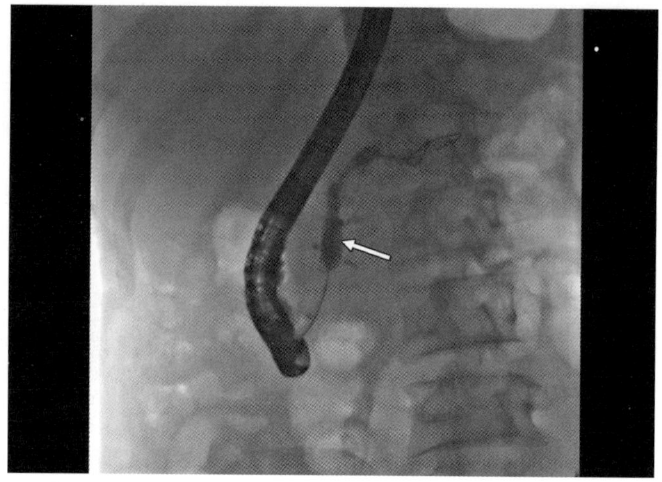

Fig. 5: ERCP: Multiple strictures of MPD (chain of lakes appearance). Note abnormally dilated side branches in head region and non-opacification of side branches in body and tail region.

- *US/CT*: abnormal sign—main pancreatic duct 2 to 4 mm diameter, gland 1 to 2 × normal.

Score 3 (Cambridge Class I)

- Severity: mild
- *ERCP*: 3 or more abnormal branches
- *US/CT*: 2+ abnormal signs: cavities <10 mm, duct irregularity, focal acute necrosis, parenchymal heterogeneity, increased echogenicity of duct wall, contour irregularity of head/body.

Score 4 (Cambridge Class II)

- Severity: moderate
- ERCP: >3 side branches plus abnormal main duct
- US/CT: as score 3.

Score 5 (Cambridge Class III)

- Severity: severe
- ERCP: all of above, plus 1 or more of: large cavity >10 mm, intraductal filling defects, duct obstruction (stricture), duct dilation or irregularity
- US/CT: all of above, plus 1 or more of: large cavity >10 mm, intraductal filling defects, duct obstruction (stricture), duct dilation or irregularity, calculi/pancreatic calcification, contiguous organ invasion.

ERCP is also helpful in diagnosing other obstructive causes of CP such as ampullary lesions, intraductal neoplasms and congenital anomalies such as pancreatic divisum **(Figs 6A and B)** or annular pancreas.

Ultrasonography

Trans-abdominal sonography: It is usually the first and initial imaging modality as most patients present with abdominal pain or discomfort. Sonographic evaluation is often challenging due to obscuration of pancreas by bowel gases. Maneuvers such as distending the stomach with water, changing position of patient and visualizing the tail of pancreas through splenic window are helpful. It is also important that the patient should be fasting adequately to reduce bowel gases.

USG appearance of pancreas varies with the stage of CP. In early stage, pancreas appears heterogeneous due to focal areas of intervening hypoechogenicity which are areas of focal inflammatory changes **(Fig. 7)**. At this stage only with a very high index of suspicion, the diagnosis can be suggested. In moderate-to-severe stages the changes become more marked and appreciable in most cases. In advanced disease, the changes of CP are easily appreciated in the form of irregular dilated main pancreatic duct (MPD) with pancreatic and intraductal calculi and associated atrophy of pancreas **(Fig. 8)**. USG is useful for detection of complications like pseudocysts, venous thrombosis or arterial pseudoaneurysms.

Endoscopic ultrasound (EUS): Pancreas by the virtue of its location proximal to lumens of stomach and duodenum allows EUS to obtain high-resolution imaging without interference by bowel gas, which usually is the limiting factor for comprehensive evaluation by trans-abdominal USG. EUS allows recognition of early changes and several other features of CP which cannot be appreciated with other imaging modalities **(Fig. 9)**. These include hyperechoic margins of the pancreatic duct, subtle lobularity of the parenchyma, small cystic changes in the parenchyma, and side branch duct ectasia.[10] Currently, EUS is considered

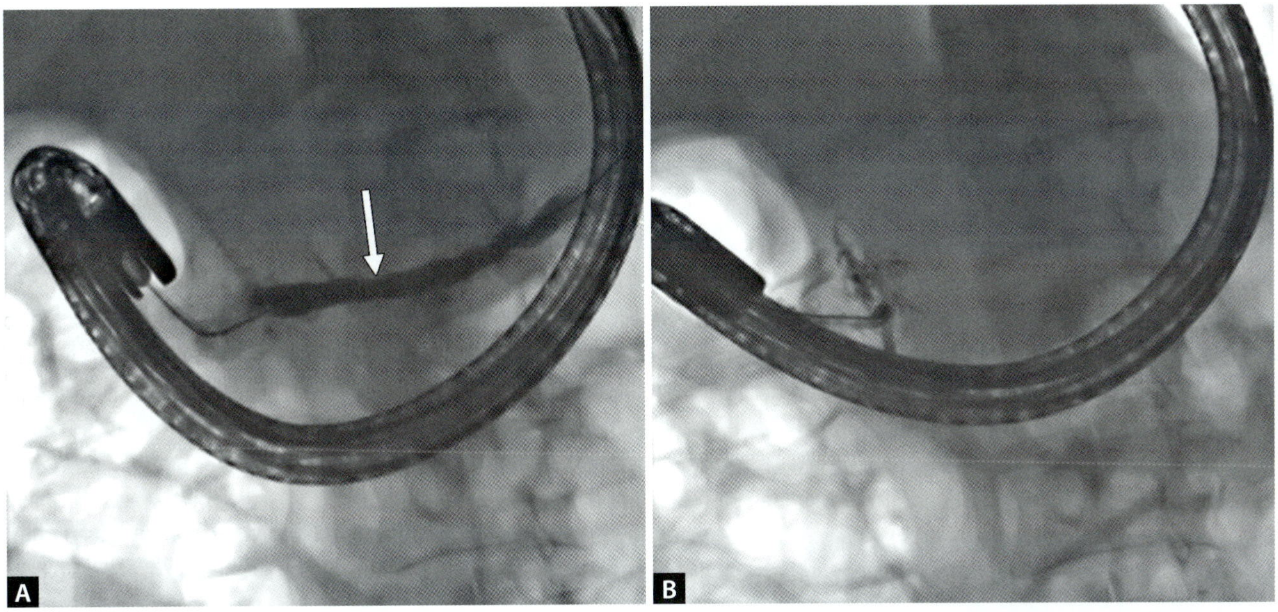

Figs 6A and B: Pancreatic divisum, ERCP Images (A and B). Cannulation of minor papilla (A) shows opacification of entire dorsal duct which is mildly dilated (arrow) with truncation of some side branches. Cannulation of major papilla shows only part of ventral duct draining part of head and uncinate process of pancreas. Also note the long route taken by the endoscope required for cannulation of minor papilla.

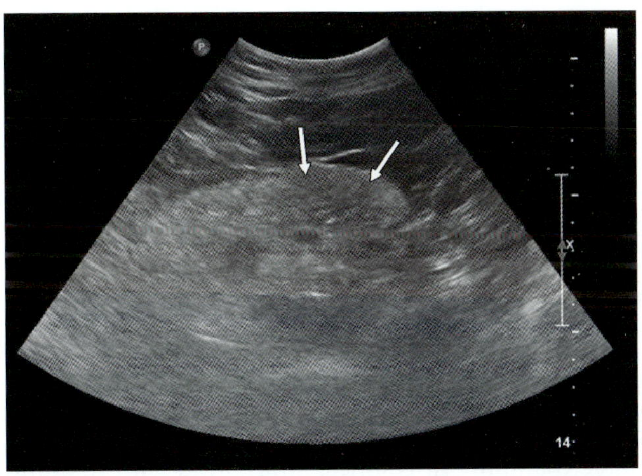

Fig. 7: Early chronic pancreatitis: Transabdominal USG image showing subtle ill-defined hypoechoic areas in pancreatic body (arrows).

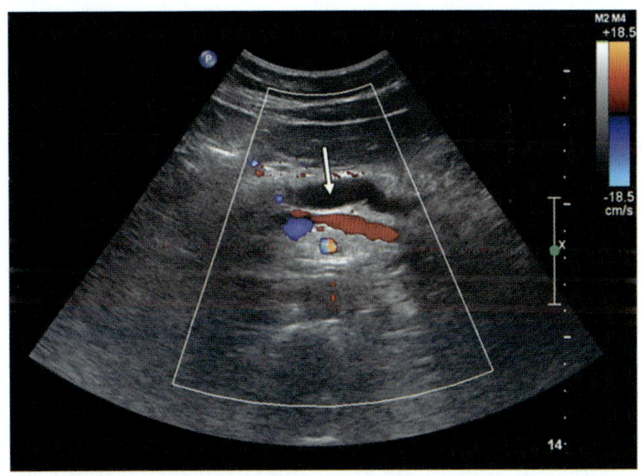

Fig. 8: Advanced changes of chronic pancreatitis: USG with color Doppler shows dilated MPD (arrow) with atrophy of pancreas.
Abbreviation: MPD: Main pancreatic duct.

to be the best imaging modality which can detect early chronic pancreatitis.[11]

Ultrasound elastography has also been used to evaluate the extent of fibrosis (stiffness) of pancreas and can be used along with trans-abdominal and endoscopic ultrasound. Retroperitoneal location of pancreas and close proximity to aorta (effect of aortic pulsations) are major hindrance for evaluation of pancreas with elastography. With advancing technology and improvement in equipment design, elastography may become a very useful imaging modality for early detection of chronic pancreatitis such as parenchymal edema recognized as change of tissue stiffness.[12] Also, elastography may contribute to early detection of pancreatic cancer in patients with CP.

Computed Tomography

Computed tomography (CT) is the imaging modality of choice for the evaluation of CP. The pancreatic calcifications

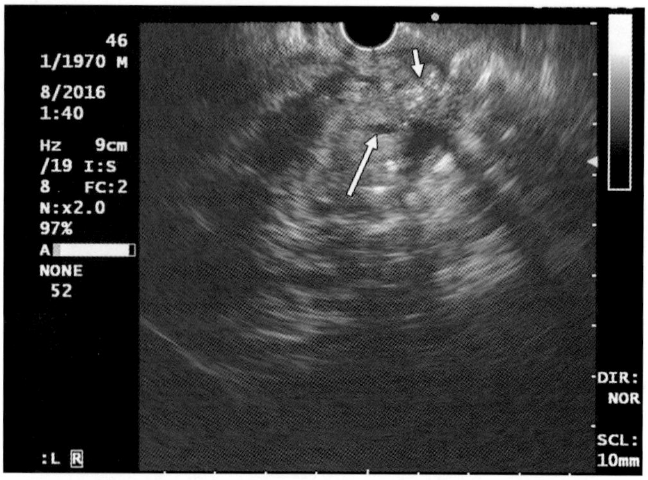

Fig. 9: Chronic pancreatitis: EUS image showing calcifications (arrow) in pancreatic head and mildly dilated MPD (long arrow).

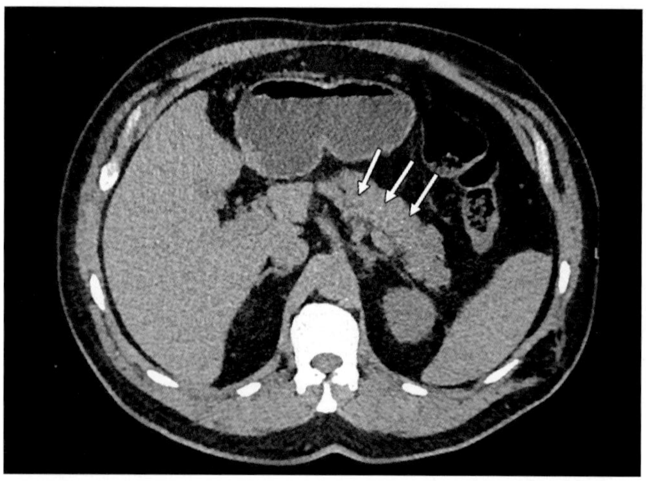

Fig. 10: Alcohol-induced chronic pancreatitis: CT axial image showing subtle pancreatic calcifications (arrows) in pancreatic body and tail region.

are best seen on CT **(Fig. 10)**. It also plays a pivotal role in follow-up after medical or/and surgical treatment. The complete evaluation of CP on CT is optimally done using a multiphase protocol which includes unenhanced scan, arterial phase and a parenchymal phase scan. Pancreatic calcifications/calculi are detected on unenhanced scan and detection of arterial complications and arterial mapping are done using the arterial phase. Pancreatic parenchymal and ductal evaluation, pseudocysts and focal lesions are best evaluated using the parenchymal phase scans.

Normal pancreas on CT appears as a homogeneous structure with smooth lobulated borders. Inflammation in pancreas leads to focal or diffuse hypodensity and surrounding fat stranding. The characteristic features of

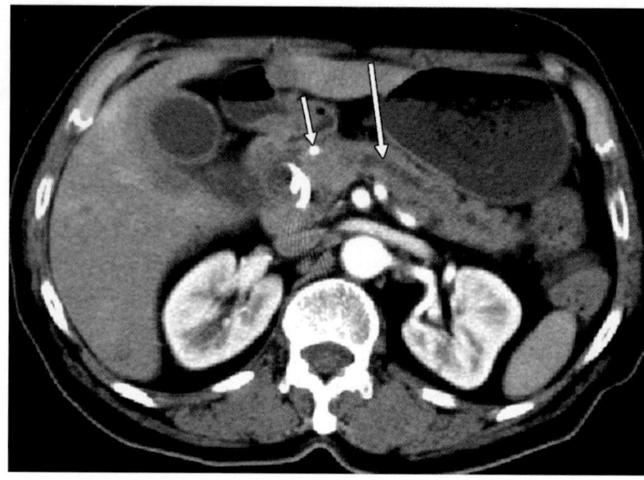

Fig. 11: Chronic pancreatits, CT axial image showing calcification (arrow) and dilated MPD (long arrow). An inflammatory mass is seen in head region obstructing the MPD. Note biliary stents *in situ*.

CP are atrophy of pancreas, ductal dilatation and multiple parenchymal and intraductal calcifications.[13] In the early stage of CP, the MPD and side branches changes are not noticeable on CT and the contrast enhancement is also relatively homogeneous. With disease progression multifocal fibrotic changes lead to heterogeneity of enhancement as the normal parenchyma enhances earlier in the venous phase, whereas the fibrotic areas show delayed enhancement.

The pancreatic head is the most common location of parenchymal calcifications. The calcification can vary in size and morphology and the degree of calcification is directly proportional to the duration of the disease. Calcifications are seen early in alcoholic CP and certain hereditary pancreatitis as compared to obstructive CP.[13] Alcohol-related CP shows calcification in 20–40% of patients and it is usually seen after 5–10 years.[3] The MPD shows segments of stenosis alternating with dilatation containing multiple calculi of varying sizes and irregular morphology **(Figs 11 and 12)**. In patients with cystic fibrosis having CFTR mutations, the calcifications appear late and they are smaller when compared to other genetic mutation. The stones in genetic mutation-related CP other than cystic fibrosis are usually round or oval in shape measuring more than 2–3 cm. On CT, they have a typical appearance with hypodense center and hyperdense periphery which is due to the lack of calcium in the center. It is often referred to as Bull's eye stone.[14] These stones are usually arranged linearly within the dilated MPD. The above features of multiple large round to oval bull's eye stones should point towards the diagnosis of

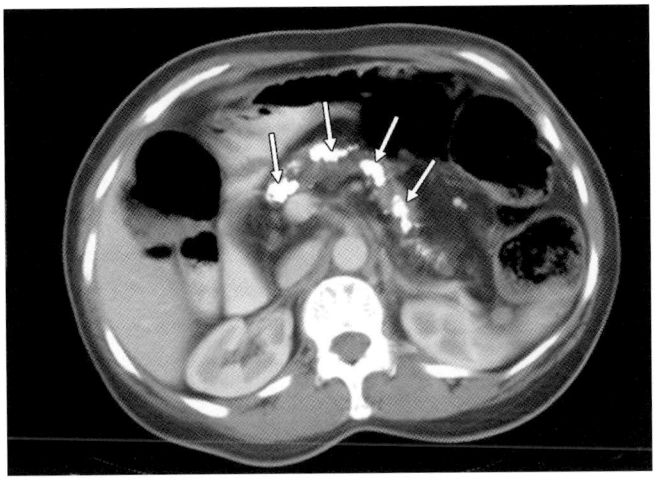

Fig. 12: Chronic pancreatitis—CT axial image: Large pancreatic ductal calculi (arrows) with atrophy and fatty replacement of pancreas.

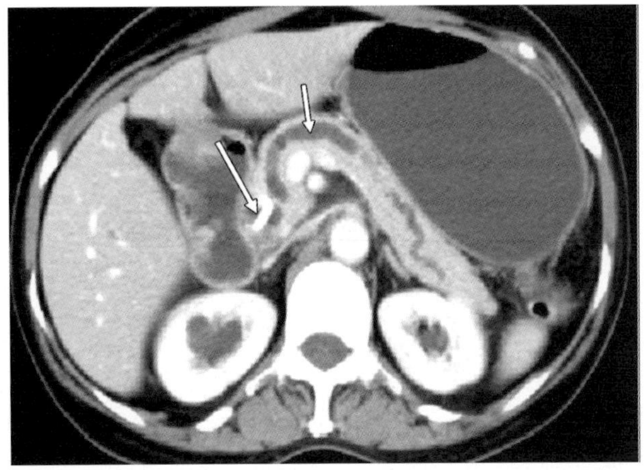

Fig. 13: CT image showing ill-defined hypoenhancing lesion at ampulla (periampullary CA) obstructing the MPD (arrow). Note biliary stents *in situ* (long arrow).

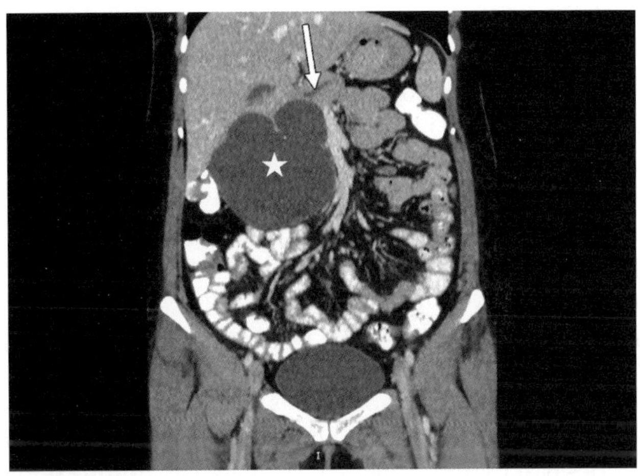

Fig. 14: CT coronal reformatted image: Large mucinous cystadenoma (star) causing pancreatic ductal obstruction (arrow).

CP secondary to genetic mutations. Tropical pancreatitis which is predominantly a disease of developing countries also presents with parenchymal atrophy, ductal dilatation and large calculi which can reach up to 5 cm in size and can extend into side branches.[15] This finding is in contrast to alcoholic CP in which calcifications are small and speckled. CT in this scenario has an edge over MRI in giving a specific diagnosis.

In patients with obstructive CP the MPD is dilated, however, parenchymal or intraductal calcifications are usually not seen. Another important role of CT is to evaluate the cause for obstructive CP. Focal lesions such as pancreatic adenocarcinoma, periampullary carcinoma, and rarely non-functioning neuroendocrine tumors can lead to MPD obstruction and cause repeated attacks of pancreatitis eventually presenting as CP **(Fig. 13)**. Cystic tumors of pancreas such as serous, mucinous and intraductal tumors can also cause obstructive form of CP **(Fig. 14)**. CT is very helpful in characterising these solid tumors and to some extent cystic tumors.

Pancreatic divisum is one of the common congenital causes for CP for which the modality of choice is MRI. However, in advanced stages CT can recognize the changes due to pancreatic divisum. The inflammatory, fibrotic changes and the ductal changes are limited to the dorsal part of pancreas whereas the ventral pancreas appears normal.

CT has the ability to evaluate the complications related to CP. The prevalence of pancreatic pseudocysts in chronic pancreatitis is 20% to 40%.[16] Pancreatic pseudocysts most commonly arise in patients with alcoholic chronic pancreatitis (70–78%).[17] Pseudocysts are cystic lesions with a wall and usually they are well defined. They can be seen in peripancreatic region, intraperitoneal, retroperitoneal or even in remote locations like chest. In CP, pseudocysts are generally formed during the evolution of peripancreatic fluid collections after an episode of pancreatitis **(Fig. 15)**. Pseudocysts are closely mimicked by retention cysts which occur in pancreas as a result of obstruction to MPD or side branch by calculi or as a result of fibrosis. The resulting cystic lesions are seen on CT as non-enhancing well-defined lesions and they are not necessarily associated with an acute episode of pancreatitis. Pseudocysts along with peripancreatic inflammation can involve the venous structures in the vicinity leading to phlebitis and thrombosis. These complications can be seen in splenic, superior mesenteric and portal vein

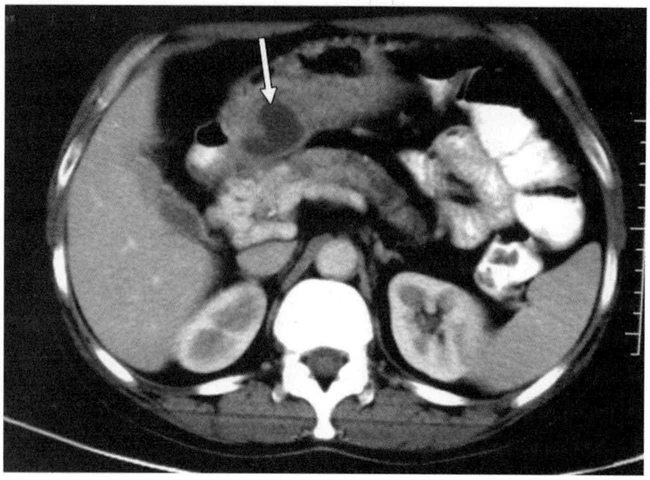

Fig. 15: CT image showing a duodenal intramural pseudocyst (arrow). Changes of chronic pancreatitis are evident.

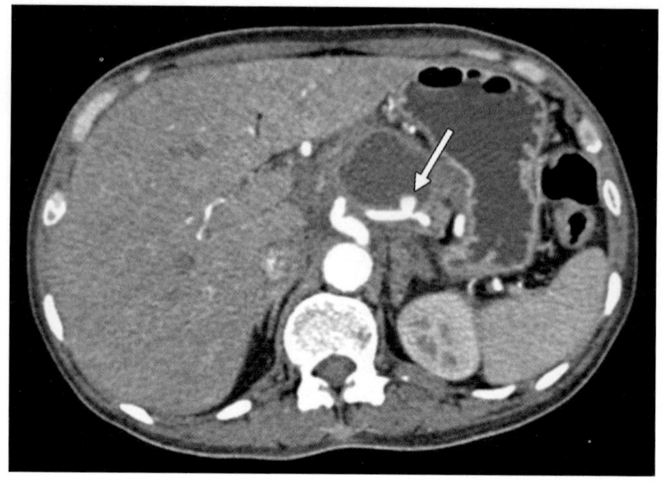

Fig. 16: Chronic pancreatitis: CT axial image showing splenic artery pseudoaneurysm (arrow) projecting into pseudocyst.

and are seen as filling defects or occlusion on contrast-enhanced CT. The resulting portal hypertension which is usually limited to left side (segmental portal hypertension) can lead to the development of multiple collaterals. When the inflammation involves the arteries in the vicinity, it can cause formation of pseudoaneurysms **(Fig. 16)**. In CP, gastroduodenal, pancreaticoduodenal and splenic arteries are the most common to be involved. They can rupture and bleed into peritoneal cavity, bowel or biliary system and present an acute emergency. Sometimes they are detected on routine imaging in which case they have to be treated at the earliest to prevent catastrophic complications. Pseudoaneurysms are best seen on arterial phase CT scan when the concentration of contrast in arteries is at its peak. They can be missed on routine portal venous scan which makes the arterial phase acquisition important in this scenario.

Sometimes in CP, pancreatic fistula can develop with the peritoneal cavity or even pleural cavity. It can occur secondary to rupture of pseudocyst. On CT, they are seen as ascites or pleural effusion, however, the actual fistula site may not be demonstrated on CT scans. Biliary complications due to CP can manifest as fistula or inflammatory strictures which are better evaluated with MRCP.

Evidence from several case-control, cohort, and record linkage studies confirms that patients with CP are at increased risk of pancreatic cancer, although only about 5% of patients with common forms of pancreatitis will develop pancreatic cancer. Patients with early onset of pancreatitis, as in HP, have a high risk of developing pancreatic cancer.[18] Pancreatic carcinoma in patients with CP can mimic inflammatory mass forming chronic pancreatitis, focal AIP and groove pancreatitis. Reliable distinction between these lesions on imaging is quite challenging and is not always possible. Advances in CT techniques in the form of perfusion CT have added another dimension to the diagnostic capability of CT scanners. Perfusion CT is novel technique in which scans of a particular area are acquired in quick succession. The data collected is postprocessed and the contrast dynamics of the given area is depicted as color coded maps. Perfusion parameters such as blood flow and blood volume can be quantified. There are promising reports in which researchers have used perfusion CT to differentiate pancreatic carcinoma from mass forming chronic pancreatitis.

Lack of information on the exocrine function of pancreas, limited contrast resolution and exposure to radiation are the most important limitations of CT. Also CT does not have specific imaging characteristics in most cases on the basis of which an etiologic factor can be identified.

Magnetic Resonance Imaging

MRCP has replaced ERCP for the diagnostic imaging of biliary and pancreatic ducts. In MRCP, heavily T2 weighted sequences are used to image fluid-filled structures. MR has the additional advantage of having excellent contrast resolution without using ionizing radiation.

Normal pancreas is the most T1 hyperintense structure in abdomen due to the presence of proteinaceous secretion within the gland **(Fig. 17)**. T1 fat saturated sequence is a very sensitive sequence for the identification of any focal lesion within the pancreas as many of the focal lesions

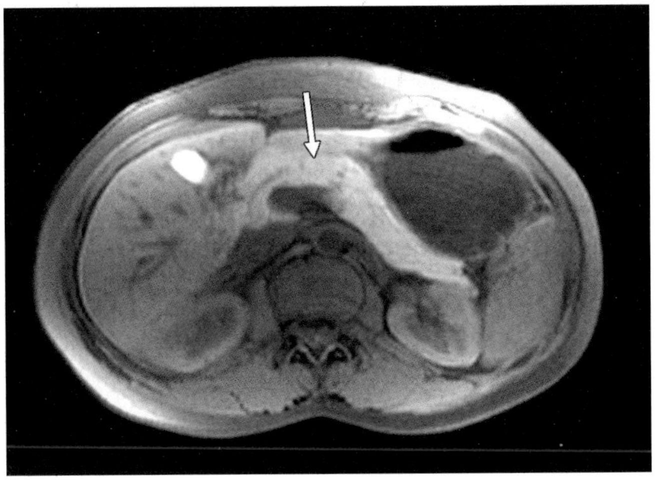

Fig. 17: T1 fat saturated MR image showing homogeneous hyper intense signals of pancreas (arrow).

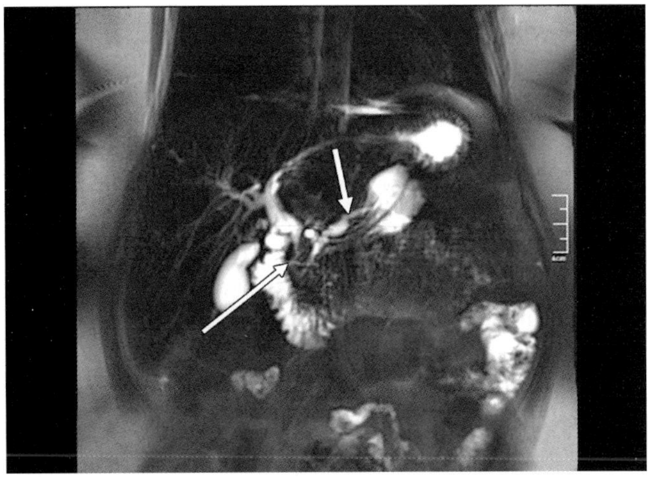

Fig. 18: Chronic pancreatitis: MRCP image showing multiple strictures (arrow) with irregular dilatation of MPD (arrow). Note stricture at lower end of CBD (long arrow).

appear hypointense and they are easily recognized. Similarly any inflammation in pancreas leads to drop in signal on T1 weighted sequences.

In early stages of CP, because of the inflammation and onset of fibrosis there is drop in T1 signal. The gland may be heterogeneous because of focal areas of inflammation and fibrosis. There is heterogeneous and delayed enhancement in the post-contrast images because of fibrosis and this delayed enhancement compared to the normal pancreas is considered as an early marker of CP.

The ductal changes are better visualized on MRCP as compared to CT scan; however, subtle side branch changes can be missed. The ductal findings of early disease can range from normal looking MPD to mild irregularity of MPD and side branches **(Fig. 18)**. With progression of disease, there is progressive glandular atrophy and poor enhancement in portal venous phase and increased enhancement in delayed phase. Severe ductal changes in the form of irregular dilatation of both MPD and side branches along with interposed strictures give the appearance of chain of lakes on MRCP. MR is also good in depicting the associated complications such as pseudocysts and fistula. Intraductal calcifications are seen as filling defects in the hyperintense background of fluid. The sensitivity of MR for small calcification is limited when compared to CT scan.

MR is excellent modality to detect ductal abnormalities such as pancreatic divisum **(Fig. 19)**, and any solid or cystic focal lesion causing obstructive type of CP. It can also differentiate CP from other mimics like intraductal papillary mucinous neoplasms (IPMN) and other variants such as groove pancreatitis and AIP.

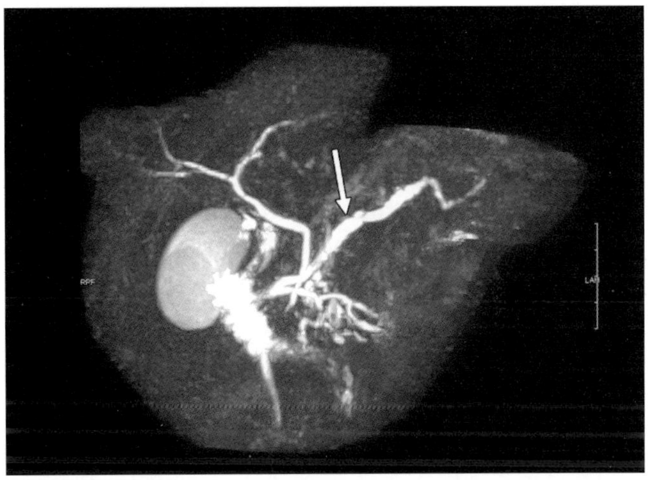

Fig. 19: Pancreatic divisum: MRCP image showing the main pancreatic duct (arrow) crossing horizontally the CBD and opening into minor papilla.

It is challenging to differentiate mass-forming chronic pancreatitis from pancreatic adenocarcinoma even on MRI. 'Duct penetrating sign' on MRCP, which means that a normal or smoothly stenotic MPD is seen to penetrate the mass, has been reported to be associated with inflammatory mass rather than carcinoma.[19] It has a reported sensitivity of 85% and specificity of 96%. Recently, diffusion weighted imaging (DWI) has been used to accurately differentiate mass-forming pancreatitis from carcinoma.[20] The role of 5-fluorodeoxyglucose-positron emission tomography (FDG-PET) in this scenario still remains controversial.

One of the major limitations of MRCP in the evaluation of CP is the lack of functional information and inability to image the ductal system in distended state. This drawback can be overcome by using secretin and acquiring serial MR images which is known as secretin enhanced MRCP or secretin stimulated MRCP (S-MRCP).[21] Secretin causes transient increase in the tone of sphincter of Oddi and increased secretion of bicarbonate-rich fluid. Patient should be fasting for 4–6 hours and a negative oral contrast is administered 30 minutes before the study to suppress the signals from pre-existing fluid in the duodenum. Baseline images are taken and secretin is injected as a slow intravenous injection to prevent the side effects. After injection, T2-weighted images are acquired every 30 seconds for a period of 15 minutes. This leads to the dilatation of MPD and the maximum dilatation occurs at 2–5 minutes after which the sphincteric tone decreases and MPD diameter comes to baseline after 10 minutes. The pancreatic secretions can be seen in the duodenum and can be graded in quantitative or semi-quantitative manner and reflect the exocrine function of the pancreas. The MPD should show an increase of at least 1 mm compared to baseline in patients with normal sphincter, absence of which would imply impaired ductal compliance. In normal pancreas the side branches are not visualized after secretin, whereas in patient with early CP because of subtle fibrosis, the side branches can show dilatation which are not otherwise seen on conventional MRCP. This is an important advantage of S-MRCP as it distends the MPD so that even the subtle abnormalities are better shown akin to ERCP. For the same reason, it is superior to conventional MRCP in delineating ductal anomalies such as pancreas divisum.

The exocrine function can be graded as follows: fluid confined to duodenal bulb is grade 1, confined to first and second part of duodenum is grade 2 and fluid reaching into the third part is grade 3. Grade 3 is considered normal and grades 1 and 2 are considered as impaired exocrine function. This quantification is found to consistently correlate with fecal elastase 1 values. Thus s-MRCP has the capability to provide both the structural and functional information which is crucial for the management of these patients.

Diffusion weighted imaging (DWI) is also used for the evaluation of CP using the apparent diffusion coefficient (ADC) values.[20] ADC of pancreas in patients with CP was found to be less than in normal patients. It is because of the decreased exocrine reserve of pancreas leading to decreased water diffusion and fibrosis which can by itself restrict diffusion. ADC values can potentially be used as an indicator of fibrosis and its extent in patients with CP which can be used to predict the outcome in patients who undergo surgery. Furthermore, DWI may be combined with S-MRCP to study the increase in ADC with the administration of secretin which increases secretion and hence promotes water diffusion.[21,22] In normal patients, the ADC is expected to increase in the early part of the s-MRCP study. This can be a potential method of quantification of exocrine function of pancreas in future.

MISCELLANEOUS TYPES OF CHRONIC PANCREATITIS

Autoimmune Pancreatitis

Autoimmune pancreatitis (AIP) is a pancreatic involvement in IgG4-related diseases which have been recently recognized as a distinct identity in the year 1995 by Yoshida et al.[23] It accounts for about 10% of all cases of chronic pancreatitis. On histology, lymphoplasmacytic infiltration is seen around the veins and ducts sparing the arterioles. Awareness of imaging features is of paramount significance for radiologists as correct diagnosis obviates unnecessary delay in treatment and surgeries. Accurate diagnosis is thus desirable as the disease responds dramatically to immune-suppressive therapy (mostly steroids). Diagnosis is usually established by typical imaging findings supplemented with raised serum immunoglobulin G4 (IgG4) levels and histopathology.

Men are affected twice as frequently as women with varying age of presentation (14 to 77 years), however, most patients at presentation are about 50 years of age.[24] AIP characteristically almost never presents with typical acute episodes of pancreatitis. Patients may present with jaundice, abdominal pain and weight loss, and diabetes mellitus.[24]

Various extra-pancreatic manifestations associated with AIP are biliary system (68–88%), where it presents with smooth strictures of biliary system (seen in up to 90% of patients), bowel (about 17%) (most commonly, ulcerative colitis), salivary glands (sialadenitis-12 to 16%), kidneys (4–35%) and retroperitoneal fibrosis (3–8%).[25] Strictures of more proximal bile ducts are also known and may resemble primary sclerosing cholangitis and therefore distinction of both is important as strictures due to AIP demonstrates dramatic response to steroid therapy while those of sclerosing cholangitis show a poor response to steroid treatment. Pulmonary involvement may be seen in the form of parenchymal nodules and infiltrates or mediastinal lymphadenopathy. Autoimmune prostatitis may be seen as an infrequent extra-pancreatic manifestation. Renal parenchymal involvement in the form of small peripheral cortical nodules, round lesions, well-defined wedge-shaped lesions, or diffuse patchy involvement may be seen and are important supporting clue for diagnosing autoimmune pancreatitis.[25]

Based on the current understanding, AIP has two distinct subtypes: *Type 1* is known as lymphoplasmacytic sclerosing pancreatitis (LPSP), which is characterized by elevated serum IgG4 levels, abundant infiltration with IgG4 positive cells and extrapancreatic involvement. *Type 2* is known as idiopathic duct centric pancreatitis (IDCP). LPSP is more common in Eastern countries whilst IDCP is more common in the Western world. Typical feature of IDCP is the presence of granulocyte epithelial lesions (GEL). Unlike type 1, IDCP usually does not have elevated serum levels of IgG4 and infiltration by IgG4-positive cells. In addition, extrapancreatic involvement is not seen in IDCP except that it can be associated with inflammatory bowel disease. Recurrence is common in AICP but rare in IDCP.

The Japan Pancreatic Society criteria based on imaging features: Serology or histopathology is one of the most commonly used criteria for the diagnosis of AIP. Various serological tests suggested are: serum gamma globulin, IgG4, antilactoferrin antibody (ALA), anti-carbonic anhydrase II antibody (ACA II), anti-smooth muscle antibody (ASMA), and antinuclear antibody (ANA).[26]

In 2011, an International Consensus Diagnostic Criteria (ICDC) was developed based on the various existing and commonly used criteria. ICDC is considered to be the most sensitive and specific criteria for diagnosing AIP. ICDC is based on the imaging features of pancreatic parenchyma, ducts, serology, involvement of other organs, histology and response to steroid therapy.

CT scan is the diagnostic modality of choice and on imaging three distinct patterns (diffuse, focal and multifocal) have been described.[27] *Diffuse pattern* which is the most common type is seen as featureless or sausage-like pancreas because of the loss of lobular architecture **(Figs 20 to 22)**. The involved pancreas is homogeneous and the MPD is either non-dilated or diffusely narrowed which is a characteristic finding in AIP. Calcification is rare unlike other types of chronic pancreatitis. There can be a hypoattenuating rim with associated fat stranding and foreshortening of pancreatic tail. The rim shows a characteristic delayed enhancement. On ERCP, characteristic finding is focal, segmental or diffuse narrowing and irregularity of MPD. MRI can show a mildly enlarged pancreas with loss of signal intensity on T1-weighted images and mild hyperintensity on T2-weighted images. After contrast administration the involved part of the pancreas shows delayed enhancement. The rim around the pancreas is hypointense on both T1- and T2-weighted images and shows delayed enhancement. MRCP can show features similar to ERCP and it can also show associated strictures in biliary tree.

The *focal* type of AIP can present as a focal mass lesion on all imaging modalities mimicking carcinoma pancreas. Even the clinical presentation may simulate and confuse with pancreatic cancer as some of these patients may have elevated carcinoembryonic antigen and cancer antigen 19-9 levels. Focal type can also present with upstream dilatation of MPD, however, the dilatation is less severe when compared to carcinoma pancreas. Delayed enhancement in AIP is another feature which differentiates it from carcinoma pancreas.

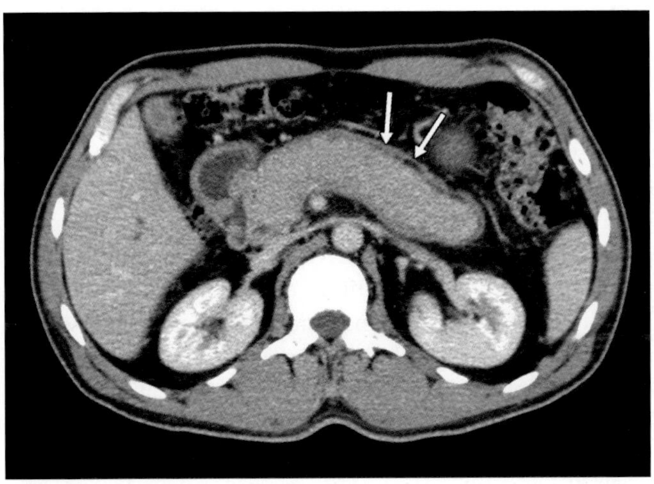

Fig. 20: Autoimmune pancreatitis: Axial CT image showing diffusely enlarged pancreas with loss of lobulations and peripheral hypoenhancing rim (arrows).

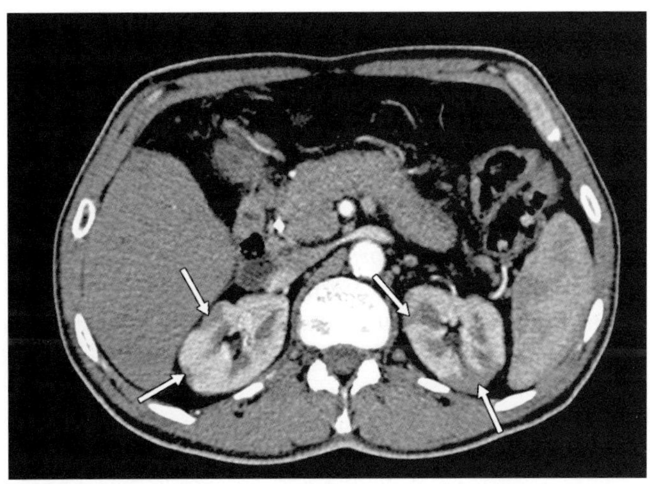

Fig. 21: Autoimmune pancreatitis: Axial CT image showing multple hypoenhancing wedge-shaped lesions in both kidneys (arrows).

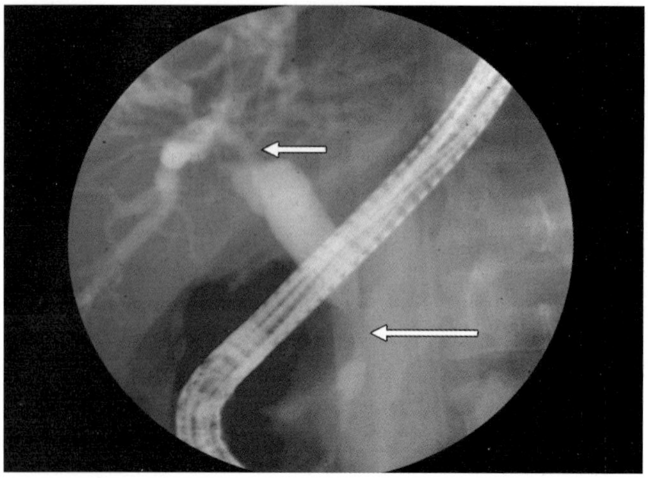

Fig. 22: Autoimmune pancreatitis: Endoscopic retrograde cholangiopancreatography (ERCP) image showing a hilar (arrow) and lower common bile duct (CBD) (long arrow) stricture.

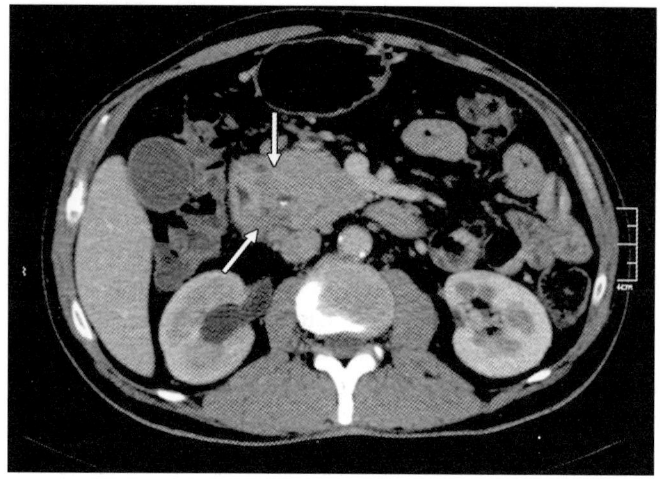

Fig. 23: Groove pancreatitis: CT axial image showing hypoenhancing sheet-like soft tissue in pancreaticoduodenal groove (arrows). Note presence of tiny cysts within this soft tissue and mildly bulky head of pancreas.

Positron emission tomography with 2-[fluorine 18] fluoro-2-deoxy-d-glucose can be useful, if imaging is equivocal and there is need to differentiate autoimmune pancreatitis from pancreatic cancer. On PET, AIP demonstrates heterogeneous pattern with multofocal areas of uptake in the pancreas. Extra-pancreatic uptake in lachrymal or salivary gland, biliary system, retroperitoneal space, or prostate gland provide important clue to diagnosis.[28]

Groove Pancreatitis

Groove pancreatitis is a rare type of CP which is localized to the pancreaticoduodenal groove. Exact etilogy is not known but factors such as duodenal ulcer, gastric resection, duodenal wall cysts, pancreatic heterotopia, pancreatic ductal obstructions have been implicated. Groove pancreatitis, cystic dystrophy of duodenum and paraduodenal wall cysts have many features in common and hence they are collectively categorized as paraduodenal pancreatitis.

Two forms of groove pancreatitis have been recognized: *"segmental"* and *"pure" form.* Typically the former involves the head of pancreas with formation of scar tissue within the groove, while in latter only groove is affected sparing the pancreatic head.[29] Patients usually present with duodenal and biliary obstruction. Biliary strictures are seen in majority (50% of cases).[29]

On imaging a soft tissue density is seen within the pancreaticoduodenal groove that usually shows delayed enhancement (fibrosis) and small cystic lesions along the medial wall of the duodenum **(Fig. 23)**. MR imaging is superior for characterization of these findings and post-gadolinium scans may show delayed enhancement of the mass.[30]

Groove pancreatitis may mimic pancreatic malignancy. Displacement of gastroduodenal artery towards pancreatic head, with associated cystic changes of duodenal wall which occurs in groove pancreatitis and abrupt cut-off of MPD which occurs in carcinoma pancreas can be helpful in differentiation.

Chronic Pancreatitis in Cystic Fibrosis

There is chloride channel CFTR gene mutation in cystic fibrosis (autosomal recessive inherited disease). This leads to dysfunction of chloride channels which fail to add enough fluid in pancreatic glandular secretions causing inspissations of secretions, obstruction to the flow within pancreatic ducts and triggers the disease process.

In pediatric population, cystic fibrosis is the most common cause of exocrine pancreatic insufficiency with occurrence of one in 2500 children.[31,32] Clinical presentation are failure to thrive, fat intolerance, abdominal pain, bloating, and flatulence.[32] Glucose intolerance is quite common (seen in up to 50% of cases); however, transformation to frank diabetes mellitus is noted in 13% only.[32] Presentation in form of acute pancreatitis is rare.[33] Histopathologic evaluation demonstrates inflammation in the pancreas with widespread loss of acinar cells, fatty replacement of the pancreatic parenchyma and interstitial fibrosis. The severity of exocrine dysfunction usually correlates with degree of pancreatic fatty infiltration.

Pancreatic calcifications indistinguishable from those in other forms of chronic pancreatitis may be seen. USG may show atrophic pancreas with increased echogenicity secondary to fatty replacement. On CT, fat replacement with or without pancreatic atrophy is the most common and a characteristic finding **(Figs 24 and 25)**.[34] Other findings include calcification, cysts and ductal strictures, beading, and dilatations. Acute pancreatitis are rarely seen. Pancreatic cystosis is a rare manifestation of cystic fibrosis, where the entire pancreas is replaced by multiple cysts of varying sizes. On MR imaging and MR cholangiopancreatography, findings are the same and thus preferred in children due to lack of radiation exposure.

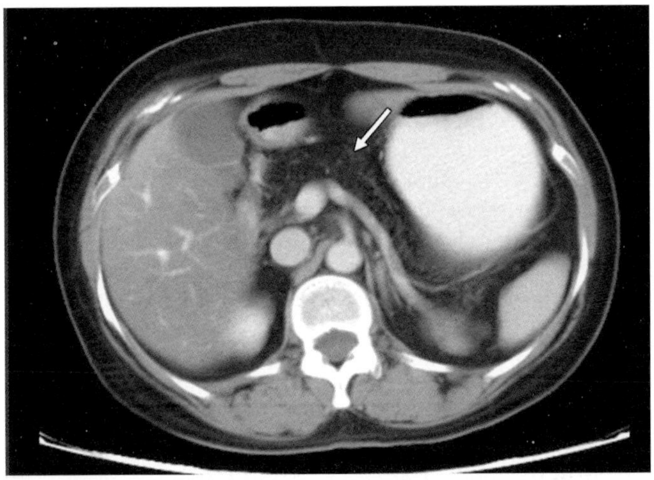

Fig. 24: Chronic pancreatitis in cystic fibrosis: CT image showing diffuse lipomatous transformation of pancreas (arrow).

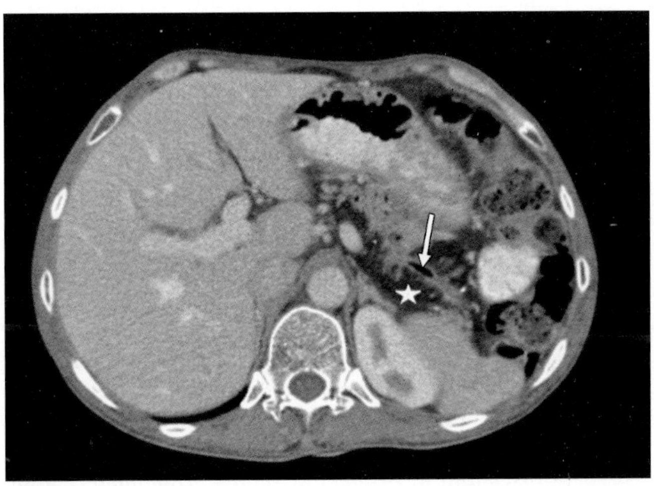

Fig. 25: Chronic pancreatitis in cystic fibrosis: CT image showing focal dilatations of MPD (arrow) and fatty transformation of pancreas (star). Note changes of CP in side branches.

Hereditary Pancreatitis

Hereditary pancreatitis is an autosomal dominant disease that occurs due to mutation of the cationic trypsinogen gene (PRSS1) that leads to increased auto-activation of trypsinogen.[35,36]

Children between the ages of 5–10 years are commonly affecte where it presents with epigastric pain.[37] Hereditary pancreatitis is an uncommon cause of recurrent and chronic pancreatitis (less than 1%) and should be suspected in any patient who has suffered at least two unexplained attacks of acute pancreatitis.[35,38]

In its chronic form are: significant pancreatic atrophy, pancreatic calcifications, and calculi are seen.

Hereditary pancreatitis is associated with more than 50 fold increased risk of development of pancreatic cancer which otherwise is low in other form of CP (15–25-fold increased risk).[39]

Tropical Chronic Pancreatitis

Tropical chronic pancreatitis (TCP) has a typical geographic distribution and usually restricted to countries having tropical climate. Protein energy malnutrition, pancreatic ductal anomalies, food toxicities (chronic cyanide toxicity from cassava), and genetic predisposition (SPINK 1 N34S mutation and CFTR mutation) are implicated in its etiology.[40] TCP affects young population (mean age–12.5 years) with a slightly male predilection (male-to-female ratio, 1.6–5:1).[41] It is characterized by large intraductal calculi and development of insulin-requiring diabetes mellitus within 10 years of onset in about two thirds of patients (fibrocalculous pancreatic diabetes).[42] Ketosis is rare in these individuals but there is higher incidence of pancreatic malignancy, which most frequently occurs in the pancreatic body and tail.[43] There is no association with alcohol consumption, biliary tract disease, and biochemical or structural predisposing factors for pancreatitis.

Chronic Pancreatitis and Pancreatic Adenocarcinoma

Association of pancreatic cancer and chronic pancreatitis is seen only in 1–2% of cases.[44] On imaging, it may be difficult to differentiate a focal mass of CP from pancreatic carcinoma **(Fig. 26)**. One should suspect pancreatic malignancy when an abnormal contour bulge or change in the morphology in the form of mass effect and alteration or disappearance of pre-existing calcification is detected in the setting of CP. Duct penetrating sign in this setting is useful in distinguishing an inflammatory mass from malignancy. Findings that favor diagnosis of carcinoma

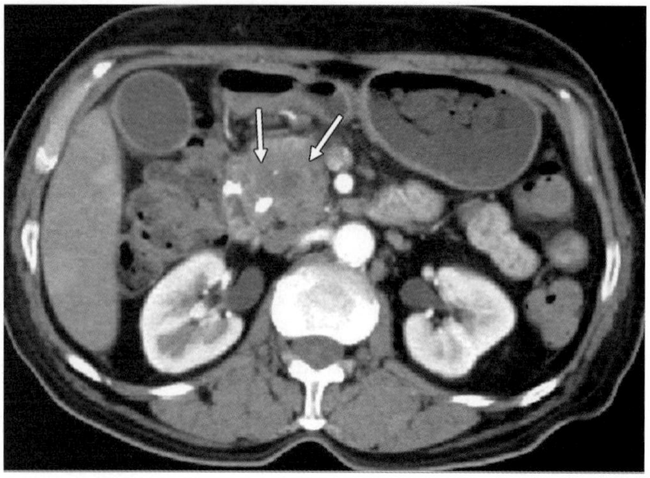

Fig. 26: Malignant change in CP: Pancreatic head show multifocal calcifications consistent with chronic pancreatitis. There is marked atrophy of pancreatic body and tail and contour deformity of head. An ill-defined hypodense lesion (arrows) is seen in pancreatic head which was confirmed to be adenocarcinoma on FNAC.

pancreas are: grossly dilated MPD, locoregional or distant lymphadenopathy, metastases, and vascular encasement or invasion.

Pancreatic perfusion CT can generate perfusion parameters which help in this distinction. The blood flow and blood volume are reduced in both inflammatory mass and carcinoma, the values usually are much lower in carcinoma than in inflammatory mass. Diffusion weighted imaging is also emerging as a helpful tool, in which carcinoma is shown to have a more marked diffusion restriction. FDG-PET CT has also been used for the same purpose with varying degree of success.

ACKNOWLEDGMENT

Professor SK Sinha, Department of Gastroenterology, Postgraduate Institute of Medical Education and Research (PGIMER), Chandigarh, India for ERCP images.

REFERENCES

1. Owyang C. Chronic pancreatitis. In: Yamada T (Ed). Textbook of Gastroenterology. Philadelphia, Pa: Lippincott Williams & Wilkins; 2003.p.2062.
2. Lankisch MR, Imoto M, Layer P, DiMagno EP. The effect of small amounts of alcohol on the clinical course of chronic pancreatitis. Mayo Clin Proc. 2001;76:242-51.
3. Dufour MC, Adamson MD. The epidemiology of alcohol-induced pancreatitis. Pancreas. 2003;27:286-90.
4. Vaughn DD, Jabra AA, Fishman EK. Pancreatic disease in children and young adults: evaluation with CT. RadioGraphics. 1998;18(5):1171-87.
5. Yekebas EF, Bogoevski D, Honarpisheh H, et al. Long-term Follow-up in Small Duct Chronic Pancreatitis: A Plea for Extended Drainage by "V-Shaped Excision" of the Anterior Aspect of the Pancreas. Annals of Surgery. 2006;244(6):940-8.
6. Etemad B, Whitcomb DC. Chronic pancreatitis: diagnosis, classification, and new genetic developments. Gastroenterology. 2001;120(3):682-707.
7. Brydon WG, Kingstone K, Ghosh S. Limitations of faecal elastase-1 and chymotrypsin as tests of exocrine pancreatic disease in adults. Ann Clin Biochem. 2004;41(1):78-81.
8. Bian Y, Wang L, Chen C, et al. Quantification of pancreatic exocrine function of chronic pancreatitis with secretin-enhanced MRCP. World Journal of Gastroenterology: WJG. 2013;19(41):7177-82.
9. Sarner M, Cotton PB. Classification of pancreatitis. Gut. 1984;25(7):756-9.
10. Seicean A. Endoscopic ultrasound in chronic pancreatitis: Where are we now? World Journal of Gastroenterology: WJG. 2010;16(34):4253-63. doi:10.3748/wjg.v16.i34.4253.
11. Ito T, Ishiguro H, Ohara H, et al. Evidence-based clinical practice guidelines for chronic pancreatitis 2015. J Gastroenterol. 2016; 51(2):85-92.
12. Kawada N, Tanaka S. Elastography for the pancreas: Current status and future perspective. World Journal of Gastroenterology. 2016;22(14):3712-24.
13. Luetmer PH, Stephens DH, Ward EM. Chronic pancreatitis: reassessment with current CT. Radiology. 1989;171(2): 353-7.
14. Graziani R, Frulloni L, Cicero C, Manfredi R, Ambrosetti MC, Mautone S, Pozzi Mucelli R. Bull's eye pattern of pancreatic-duct stones on multidetector computed tomography and gene-mutation-associated pancreatitis (GMAP). Radiol Med. 2012;117(8):1275-86.
15. Barman K, Premalatha G, Mohan V. Tropical chronic pancreatitis. Postgraduate Medical Journal. 2003;79(937):606-15.
16. Arthet M, Bugallo M, Moreira LS, Bastid C, Sastre B, Sahel J. Management of cysts and pseudocysts complicating chronic pancreatitis. A retrospective study of 143 patients. Gastroenterol Clin Biol. 1993;17:270-6.
17. Ammann RW, Akovbiantz A, Largiader F, Schueler G. Course and outcome of chronic pancreatitis. Longitudinal study of a mixed medical-surgical series of 245 patients. Gastroenterology. 1984;86:820-8.
18. Raimondi S, Lowenfels AB, Morselli-Labate AM, Maisonneuve P, Pezzilli R. Pancreatic cancer in chronic pancreatitis; aetiology, incidence, and early detection. Best Pract Res Clin Gastroenterol. 2010;24(3):349-58.
19. Ichikawa T, Sou H, Araki T, Arbab AS, Yoshikawa T, Ishigame K, Haradome H, Hachiya J. Duct-penetrating sign at MRCP: usefulness for differentiating inflammatory pancreatic mass from pancreatic carcinomas. Radiology. 2001;221(1):107-16.
20. Sandrasegaran K, Nutakki K, Tahir B, Dhanabal A, Tann M, Cote GA. Use of diffusion-weighted MRI to differentiate chronic pancreatitis from pancreatic cancer. AJR. 2013;201(5):1002-8.

21. Manfredi R, Pozzi Mucelli R. Secretin-enhanced MR Imaging of the Pancreas. Radiology. 2016;279(1):29-43.
22. Wathle GK, Tjora E, Ersland L, Dimcevski G, Salvesen ØO, Molven A, Njølstad PR, Haldorsen IS. Assessment of exocrine pancreatic function by secretin-stimulated magnetic resonance cholangiopancreaticography and diffusion-weighted imaging in healthy controls. J Magn Reson Imaging. 2014;39(2):448-54.
23. Yoshida K, Toki F, Takeuchi T, Watanabe S, Shiratori K, Hayashi N. Chronic pancreatitis caused by an autoimmune abnormality: proposal of the concept of autoimmune pancreatitis. Dig Dis Sci. 1995;40(7):1561-8.
24. Kim KP, Kim MH, Song MH, Lee SS, Seo DW, Lee SK. Autoimmune chronic pancreatitis. Am J Gastroenterol. 2004;99(8):1605-16.
25. Takahashi N, Kawashima A, Fletcher JG, Chari ST. Renal involvement in patients with autoimmune pancreatitis: CT and MR imaging findings. Radiology. 2007;242(3):791-801.
26. Khalili K, Doyle DJ, Chawla TP, Hanbidge AE. Renal cortical lesions in patients with autoimmune pancreatitis: a clue to differentiation from pancreatic malignancy. Eur J Radiol. 2008;67(2):329-35.
27. Kawamoto S, Siegelman SS, Hruban RH, Fishman EK. Lymphoplasmacytic sclerosing pancreatitis (autoimmune pancreatitis): evaluation with multidetector CT. RadioGraphics. 2008;28(1):157-70.
28. Ozaki Y, Oguchi K, Hamano H, et al. Differentiation of autoimmune pancreatitis from suspected pancreatic cancer by fluorine-18 fluorodeoxyglucose positron emission tomography. J Gastroenterol. 2008;43(2):144-51.
29. Stolte M, Weiss W, Volkholz H, Rösch W. A special form of segmental pancreatitis: "groove pancreatitis." Hepatogastroenterology. 1982;29(5):198-208.
30. Irie H, Honda H, Kuroiwa T, et al. MRI of groove pancreatitis. J Comput Assist Tomogr. 1998;22(4):651-5.
31. Witt H. Chronic pancreatitis and cystic fibrosis. Gut. 2003;52(suppl 2):ii31–ii41.
32. Gore MD, Fernbach SK. Pancreatic insufficiency and cystic fibrosis. In: Gore RM, Levine MS, Laufer I (Eds). Textbook of gastrointestinal radiology. Vol 2. Philadelphia, Pa: Saunders; 1994.pp.2187-92.
33. De Boeck K, Weren M, Proesmans M, Kerem E. Pancreatitis among patients with cystic fibrosis: correlation with pancreatic status and genotype. Pediatrics. 2005;115(4):e463–e469.
34. Soyer P, Spelle L, Pelage JP, et al. Cystic fibrosis in adolescents and adults: fatty replacement of the pancreas—CT evaluation and functional correlation. Radiology. 1999;210(3):611-5.
35. Efthimiou E, Crnogorac-Jurcevic T, Lemoine NR, Brentnall TA. Inherited predisposition to pancreatic cancer. Gut. 2001;48(2):143-7.
36. Steinberg WM, Barkin J, Bradley EL 3rd, DiMagno E, Layer P. Workup of a patient with familial pancreatic cancer. Pancreas. 1999;18(3):219-24.
37. Efthimiou E, Crnogorac-Jurcevic T, Lemoine NR Brentnall TA. Inherited predisposition to pancreatic cancer. Gut. 2001;48(2):143-7.
38. Ellis I, Lerch MM, Whitcomb DC. Consensus Committees of the European Registry of Hereditary Pancreatic Diseases, Midwest Multi-center Pancreatic Study Group, International Association of Pancreatology. Genetic testing for hereditary pancreatitis: guidelines for indications, counseling, consent and privacy issues. Pancreatology. 2001;1(5):405-15.
39. Ghaneh P, Costello E, Neoptolemos JP. Biology and management of pancreatic cancer. Gut. 2007;56(8):1134-52.
40. Bhatia E, Choudhuri G, Sikora SS, et al. Tropical calcific pancreatitis: strong association with SPINK 1 trypsin inhibitor mutations. Gastroenterology. 2002;123(4):1020-25.
41. Balakrishnan V, Sauniere JF, Hariharan M, Sarles H. Diet, pancreatic function, and chronic pancreatitis in south India and France. Pancreas. 1988;3(1):30-5.
42. Petersen JM. Tropical pancreatitis. J Clin Gastroenterol. 2002;35(1):61-6.
43. Chari ST, Mohan V, Pitchumoni CS, Viswanathan M, Madanagopalan N, Lowenfels AB. Risk of pancreatic cancer in tropical calcifying pancreatitis: an epidemiologic study. Pancreas. 1994;9(1):62-6.
44. Levine E. Carcinoma of the pancreas presenting as acute pancreatitis: CT diagnosis. Gastrointest Radiol. 1981;6(1):29-33.

CHAPTER 89

Pancreatic Cancer Imaging

Ankur Goyal, Raju Sharma

INTRODUCTION

Pancreatic cancer is an aggressive malignancy with dismal prognosis. Strategically located deep in the retroperitoneum, it can potentially involve many crucial arteries, veins and nerves catering to liver, spleen, stomach and bowel.[1] Ductal adenocarcinoma is the most common nonendocrine pancreatic malignancy. After colorectal malignancies, pancreatic carcinoma is the second most common malignancy of the gastrointestinal tract. Pancreatic adenocarcinoma is the fourth most common cause of cancer-related deaths in the US. There have been lot of advances in the imaging and surgical management of pancreatic malignancies. Nevertheless, patient survival is dismal owing to early lymphatic and perineural spread.[2] Pancreatic carcinoma has a propensity to spread via celiac and mesenteric neural plexus and this results in preclinical dissemination.

The clinical presentation is vague, thus contributing to delay in diagnosis. The patients usually present with abdominal pain, anorexia, weight loss, nausea and jaundice. Age of presentation is middle age or elderly. Jaundice is a common presenting symptom in tumors of pancreatic head region whereas lesions of the body and tail present with abdominal pain and weight loss. Pancreatic carcinoma should also be suspected in diabetic patients with unusual manifestations such as late age of onset, abdominal symptoms and continuing weight loss.[3] It is important to differentiate ampullary cancers from the ductal adenocarcinomas, since the former have a much better prognosis and longer survival.[4] The serum levels of CA 19-9 are often elevated. Activating mutations in k-ras oncogene are present in more than 90% cases.[5]

The risk factors for pancreatic cancer include cigarette smoking, alcohol, high body mass index, chronic pancreatitis and occupational exposure to chemicals. Recently, there has been substantial increment in knowledge of the molecular biology of the disease. R0 surgical resection (negative margins) is the only treatment modality which can prolong survival in these patients; though even with surgery, mean patient survival is 2 years and thus long-term survival is lacking. Whipple surgery is a major intervention and is associated with postoperative morbidity. Thus, imaging is very important to diagnose malignancy and also to assess resectability. Accurate preoperative staging is essential for optimal management.

IMAGING MODALITIES

Multidetector computed tomography (MDCT) is the investigation of choice for diagnosis and staging of pancreatic cancer.[6] Thin sections, multiplanar reformation and high spatial resolution enable accurate delineation of tumor extent on MDCT. Transabdominal sonography may also detect larger lesions and depict local invasion, however the accuracy is much less. Magnetic resonance imaging (MRI), endoscopic ultrasound (EUS) and positron emission tomography–CT (PET-CT) are also useful in the diagnostic assessment of pancreatic malignancy.

Sonography

Ultrasound (US) abdomen is the most commonly used initial imaging modality for evaluation of abdominal pain and jaundice. It not only diagnoses obstructive jaundice but also localizes the level of obstruction and helps in suggesting the cause. Common benign diseases such as cholelithiasis and choledocholithiasis may be easily diagnosed. Though small pancreatic lesions may be easily missed on US, larger lesions can usually be seen and secondary evidence such as pancreatic ductal dilatation may also be evident. US can also provide real-time guidance for percutaneous sampling; although endoscopic route is preferred. Disadvantages are operator dependence and proper evaluation of pancreas may not be feasible because of obesity or bowel gas.

Multidetector Computed Tomography

Helical CT on a scanner with multiple rows of detector (16 or more) is the workhorse for workup of patients with suspected pancreatic cancer. A dedicated protocol is essential to accurately detect and stage pancreatic cancers **(Flowchart 1)**. The examination starts with neutral oral contrast given over 15–30 minutes for gastroduodenal distension. This enables proper visualization of the pancreas and ampullary region. Intravenous nonionic iodinated contrast is injected via rapid bolus at 4 mL/s using a pressure injector and a biphasic breath-hold acquisition is done.

The first acquisition is done in the late arterial/pancreatic phase, usually 40–50 seconds from the start of contrast injection. If contrast triggering is used, then typically a delay of 20–25 secs is optimal, after the threshold attenuation is reached in the region of interest (ROI) (descending thoracic aorta in this case). The rapid contrast injection produces intense enhancement of the normal pancreas in this phase and thus the hypovascular ductal carcinomas are demonstrated well. The pancreatic phase scan should include the liver and pancreas (upper abdomen). Hypervascular lesions (like neuroendocrine tumors), hypervascular liver metastases, as well as flow-related phenomena (arterial hyperenhancement in case of pancreatic cancer liver metastases) are well seen in the late arterial phase. Subtle surrounding perivascular infiltration is also well seen.[7]

The second acquisition is portal venous phase at 60–70s from the start of contrast injection and covers the entire abdomen and pelvis. The portal venous system is well opacified and the splanchnic viscera show homogeneous parenchymal contrast enhancement (CE). Former enables assessment of vascular involvement while the latter enables detection of hypoenhancing liver metastases. The scan coverage in this phase may include chest as well for complete staging.

Careful analysis of thin sections and three dimensional (3D) reconstructions on a workstation is key to accurate imaging assessment. Coronal and curved multiplanar reformations help to evaluate the status of common bile duct and pancreatic duct in relation to the tumor **(Figs. 1A to D)**. Postprocessing of volumetric dataset serves to highlight local invasion along blood vessels.

Flowchart 1: MDCT protocol for pancreatic cancer imaging

500 mL neutral oral contrast (water)

↓

100 mL IV contrast (≥300 mg iodine/mL) at 4 mL/s

↓

Pancreatic phase acquisition of upper abdomen
(at 40–50 s from start of injection or 25 s delay after trigger)

↓

Portal venous phase (Abdomen and pelvis)
(60–70 s from start of injection or 15–20 s delay after first scan)

Magnetic Resonance Imaging

The MRI has similar accuracy to MDCT in staging of pancreatic cancers with the advantage of absence of radiation exposure.[8] The excellent contrast resolution more than makes up for the lower spatial resolution than MDCT. High resolution fast imaging of pancreas has become feasible owing to multichannel coils, parallel imaging, higher magnetic field strength (3T) and other advancements in MRI technology.

Fat-supressed (FS) T1-weighted (T1W) images demonstrate the normally hyperintense pancreatic parenchyma very well. Pancreatic cancers are hypointense on T1W, intermediate signal on T2W and show diffusion restriction on diffusion-weighted MR imaging (DW MRI). The latter manifests as retained high signal on the high b-value image and dark signal on the apparent diffusion coefficient (ADC) map. ADC map also enables quantification and pancreatic carcinoma is associated with lower ADC values compared with remaining parenchyma.[9] Heavily T2W sequences like HASTE employed in MR cholangiopancreatography (MRCP) enable exquisite demonstration of pancreatic and biliary ducts enabling detection of subtle areas of narrowing. Similar to CT, multiphasic scanning after contrast administration enables detection of pancreatic

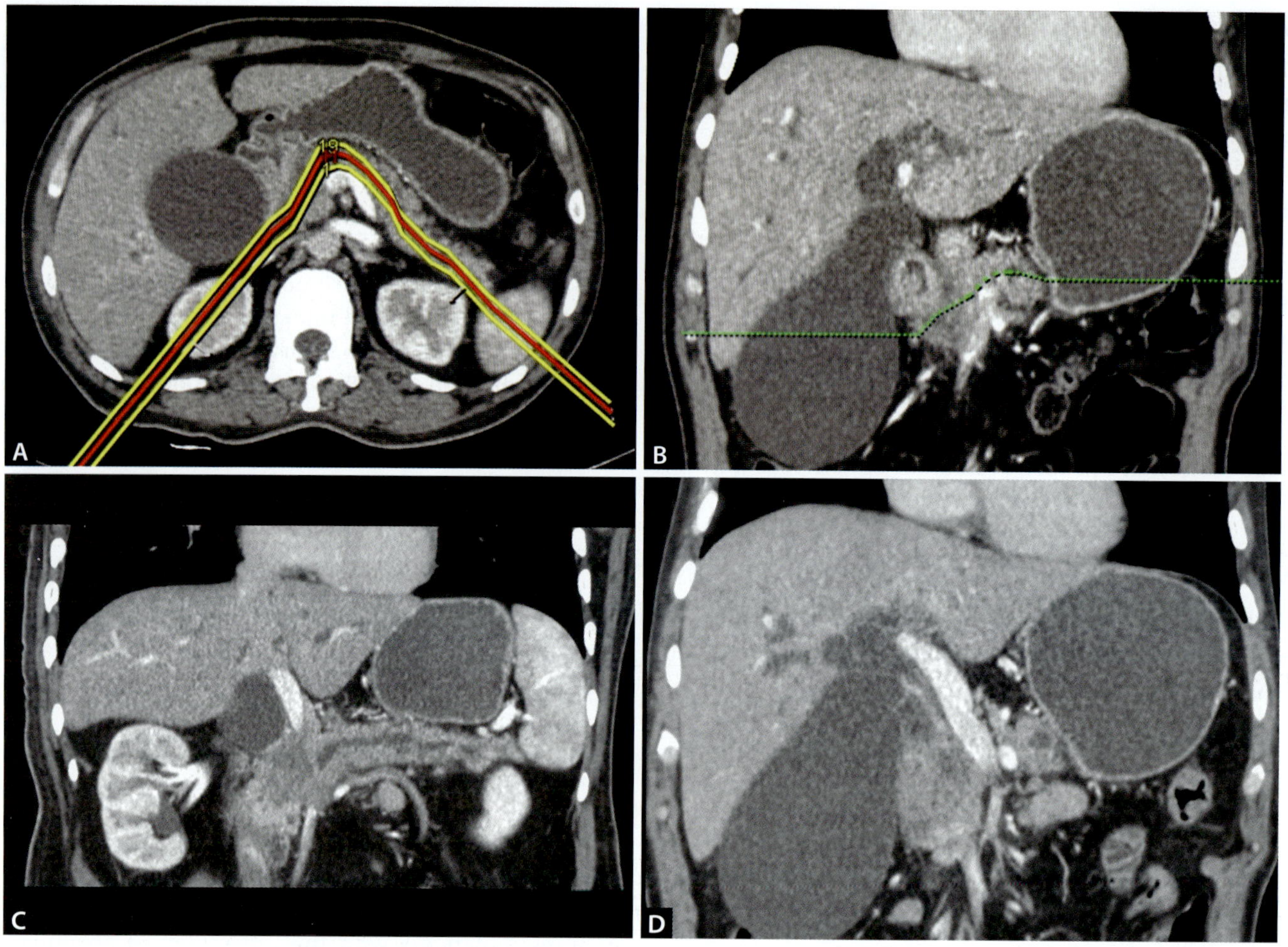

Figs. 1A to D: Utility of curved multiplanar reformations (MPR): Axial (A) and coronal (B) CT images demonstrate the planning of curved MPR along the pancreas. Resultant image (C) depicts the hypodense mass in the head with abrupt cut-off and upstream dilatation of pancreatic duct. Curved MPR better delineates the mass in relation to pancreatic duct in a single image compared to orthogonal coronal image (D).

cancer in the late arterial phase and accurate staging in the portal venous phase. Ideally, MRI for evaluation of pancreatic cancer should include post-contrast multiphasic acquisition. However, noncontrast MR sequences can provide sufficient information in majority of the cases; and thus MRI is the modality of choice in patients with renal insufficiency where contrast administration is undesirable.

Magnetic resonance imaging is also a problem solving modality in case of small lesions and subtle liver metastases. The latter are best detected on diffusion-weighted MRI (DWI) **(Figs. 2A and B)**. DW MRI is useful in detection of small lesions as well as post-therapy response assessment. Absence of exposure to ionizing radiation is another advantage of MRI. Disadvantages include high cost, limited availability and long examination time.

Endoscopic Techniques

Side-viewing endoscopy is often employed for evaluation of periampullary malignancies, especially when small mass is not visible on CT or MRI but there is ductal dilatation.

Endoscopic ultrasound (EUS) may aid in detection of small lesions, may depict subtle vascular involvement and nodal spread, as well as guide sampling **(Figs. 3A and B)**. The advantage of this route of sampling is that the needle track falls within the field of surgical resection. The role of EUS is complimentary to CT for staging.[3] However, it is invasive and not widely available.

Endoscopic retrograde cholangiopancreatography (ERCP) with brush cytology is indicated when no mass is seen on imaging and stenting is to be done for palliation. Nowadays, ERCP is done only with the purpose of biliary decompression.

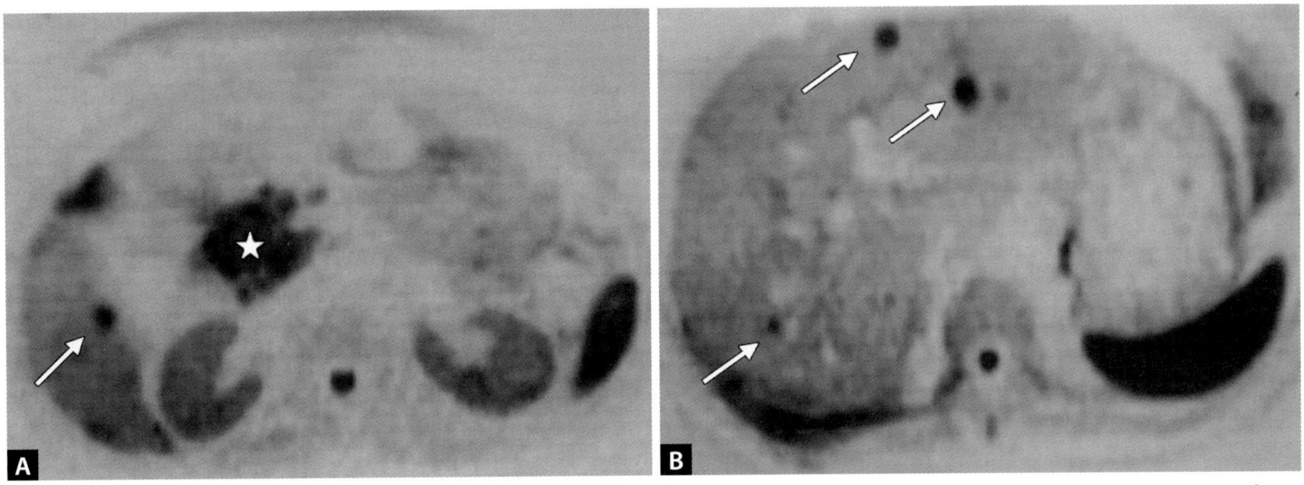

Figs. 2A and B: Utility of diffusion-weighted MRI in detecting small liver metastases. Contrast-inverted high b-value (1000 s/mm^2) axial DW images (A and B) depict marked restriction of diffusion in the pancreatic head mass (asterisk) and multiple small liver metastases (arrows).

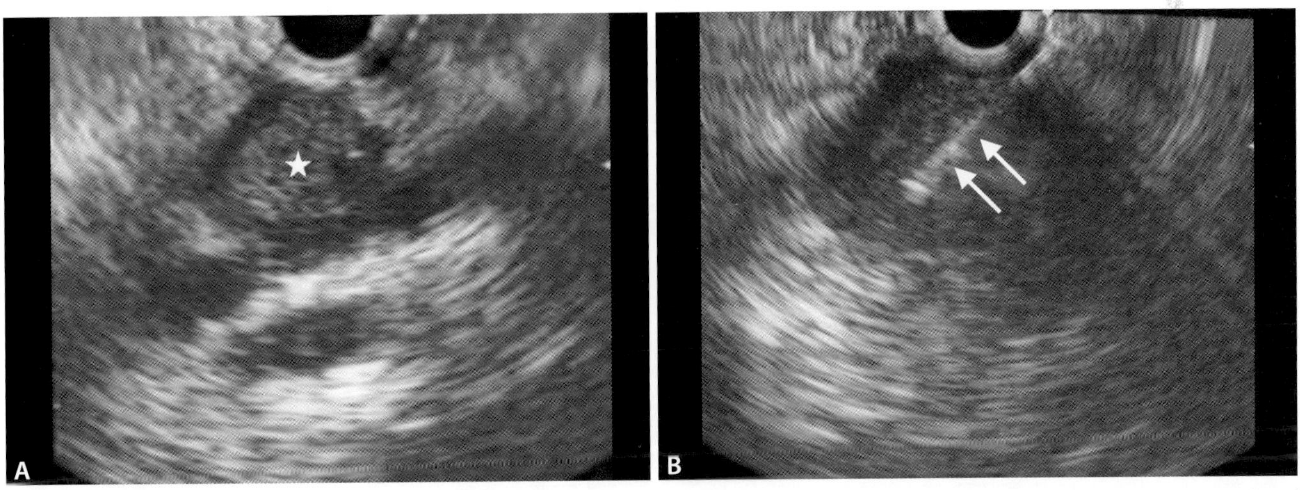

Figs. 3A and B: Endoscopic ultrasound (EUS) in evaluation of pancreatic carcinoma: EUS image (A) clearly shows the pancreatic head mass (asterisk) and (B) depicts sampling using EUS guidance (arrows denote the needle).

Positron Emission Tomography–Computed Tomography

Functional positron emission tomography (PET) imaging may be used as per institutional preference, in high-risk patients to detect metastases; but it is not a substitute for diagnostic CT/MRI.[3] It may be more helpful in follow-up assessment where post-therapy alterations may pose problems. It may prove useful in identifying unexpected sites of recurrence. However, the exact role of this modality in evaluation of pancreatic carcinoma is still evolving.

Recent Advances

Ultrasound elastography is a new technique which may be employed for detection of pancreatic cancers. Owing to deep location and small size of pancreas, elastography has been considered difficult and less reliable. However, it is a promising modality for distinction between benign and malignant lesions and for screening in high-risk patients.[10] It can be performed through transabdominal or endoscopic routes. Contrary to shear wave elastography (SWE), strain elastography requires application of external pressure. Manual compression is however not effective for pancreas and strain generated by aortic pulsations is used instead. Thus it requires the probe, pancreas and aorta to be in the same line.[10] Also, pancreatic body can be well evaluated but not head and tail regions. SWE can be performed for the entire pancreas but not currently available via endoscopic route.[10] Pancreatic adenocarcinoma appears as hard heterogeneous lesion while chronic pancreatitis is soft and heterogeneous.[10,11] Neuroendocrine tumors are seen as hard homogeneous lesions.

Contrast-enhanced USG (CEUSG) employs microbubble contrast media which are excreted via lungs and thus can be used in patients with renal dysfunction. This is especially useful along with EUS to confirm areas of abnormality. Ductal adenocarcinoma commonly appears as hypoenhancing lesion relative to the surrounding pancreas.[12] Mass-forming chronic pancreatitis is isoenhancing or hyperenhancing while neuroendocrine tumors are hyperenhancing.[12]

Perfusion CT involves scanning the region of interest (pancreas) multiple times over a short span after rapid bolus contrast injection. In addition to color coded maps, many quantitative parameters such as blood flow, blood volume, mean transit time, time to peak, etc. are generated which are more representative of the contrast kinetics and vascularity of the lesion. This technique has a potential role in detection of small isodense pancreatic lesions **(Figs. 4A to D)**[13] and in assessment of post-therapy response. The basis of the latter use is that chemotherapeutic agents target tumor neo-angiogenesis and thus reduction in vascularity indicates response to therapy. Perfusion CT parameters, (especially blood flow) may also help to differentiate adenocarcinoma from mass forming chronic pancreatitis (MFCP).[14] The main drawback is increased radiation exposure.

Dual-energy CT scanners enable generation of virtual noncontrast images from a single acquisition. Also, lower keV dataset can be generated which offers superior contrast resolution while higher keV images have better signal-to-noise ratio (SNR) **(Figs. 5A to D)**.[15]

The *DW MRI* is now part of routine abdominal MR protocols in most of the institutions worldwide. The

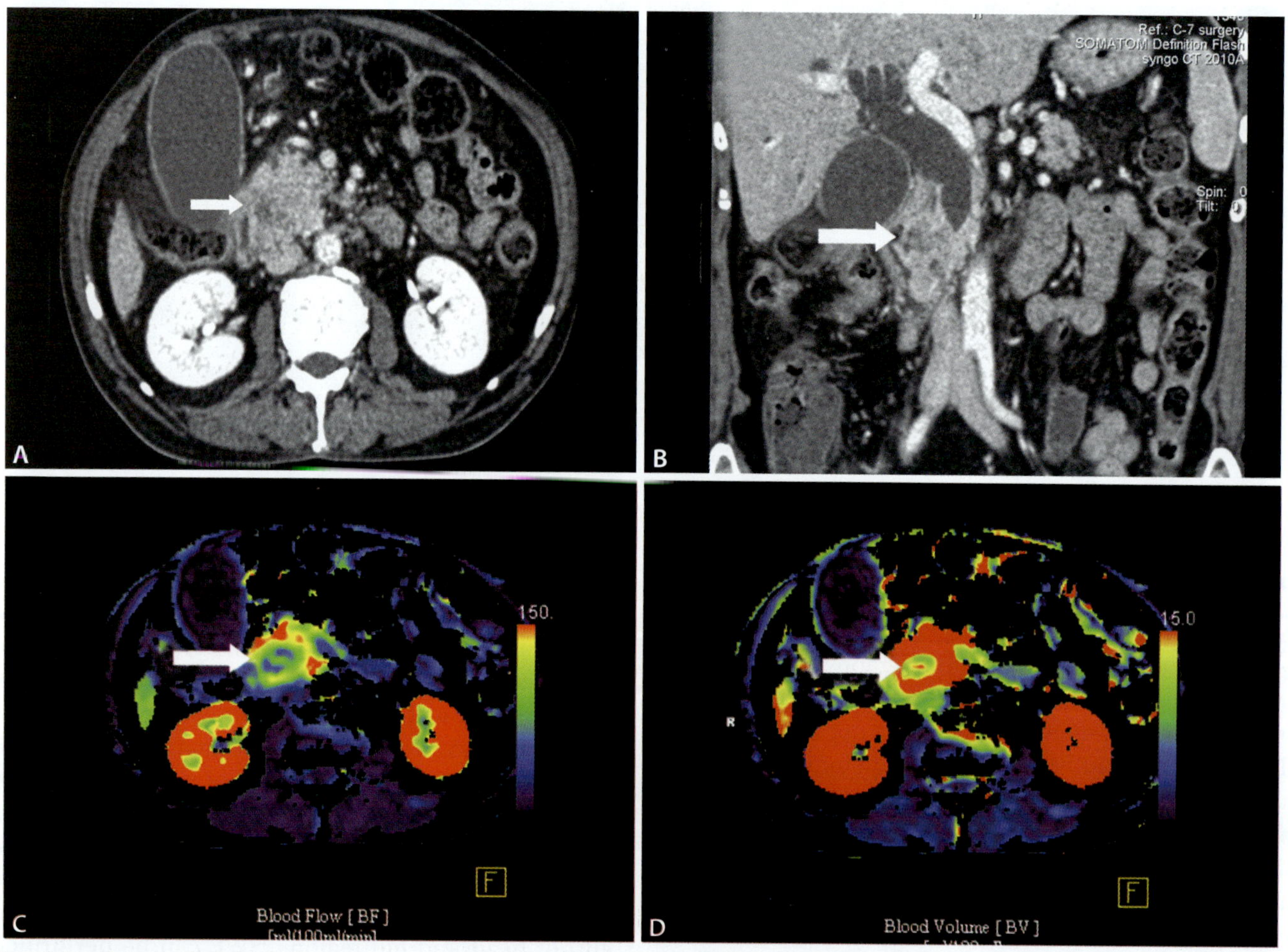

Figs. 4A to D: Role of perfusion CT in isodense masses: Axial (A) and coronal (B) contrast-enhanced CT images show an ill-defined mass in pancreatic head, which is mildly hypodense to the surrounding parenchyma (arrows) with dilated common bile duct. Axial blood flow (C) and blood volume (D) color maps (derived from perfusion CT) enable a much clearer depiction of hypovascular mass, distinct from adjacent parenchyma (arrows).

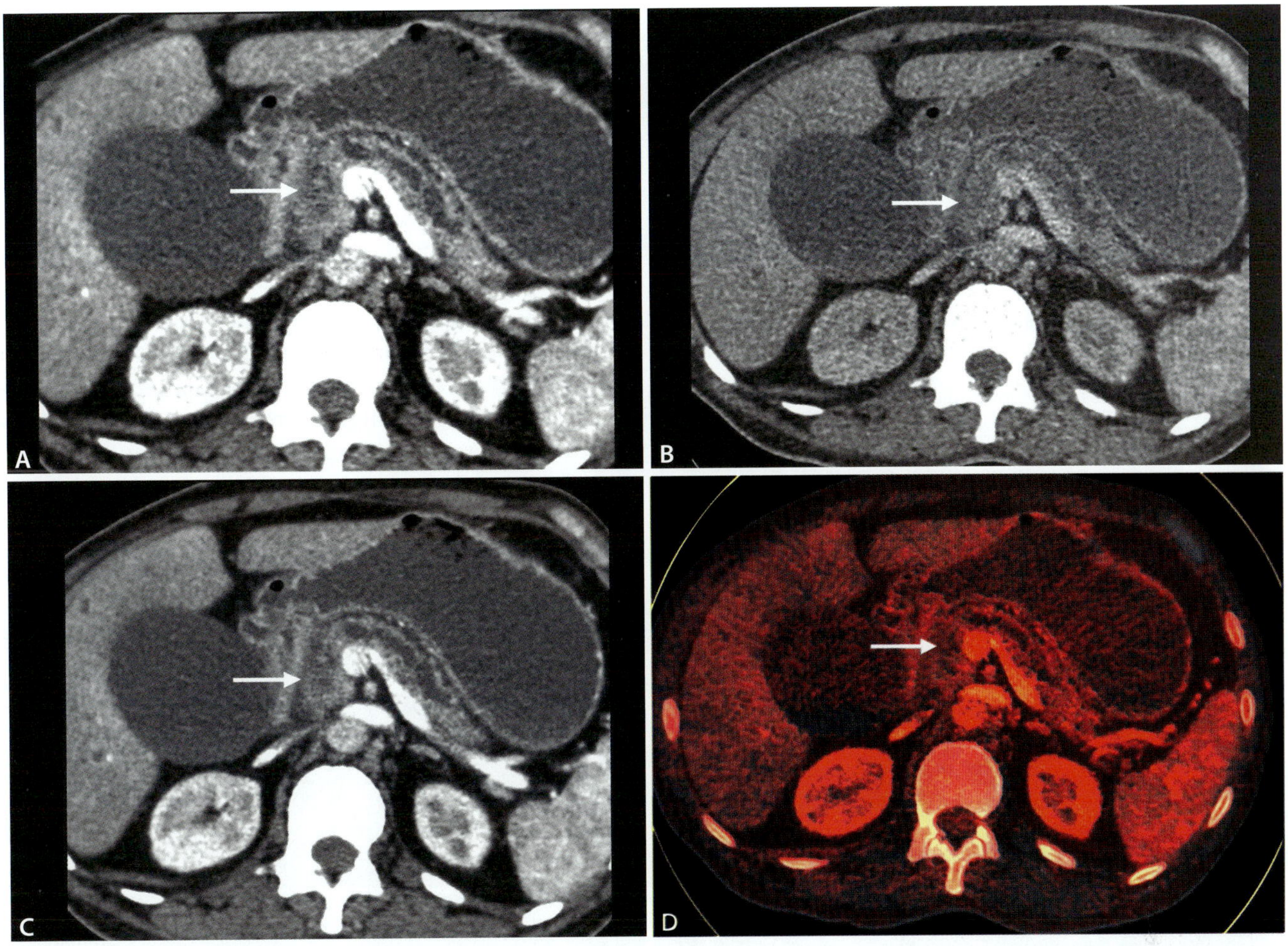

Figs. 5A to D: Dual-energy CT (DECT) in pancreatic mass evaluation: Axial monochromatic CECT images generated from dual-energy dataset: 70 keV image (A) gives better demonstration of mass (arrow) compared to 100 keV image (B), however is noisy. Optimal contrast image (C) derived by mixing of the datasets yields high contrast as well as low noise. Iodine map (D) depicts the hypodense mass distinct from the enhancing parenchyma as well as cut-off of pancreatic duct.

simple way of quantifying the diffusion restriction is based on the monoexponential model which generates a single ADC value based on combination of both diffusion and perfusion effects. Recently, biexponential-based estimation of the intravoxel incoherent motion (IVIM) parameters has been employed, with generation of separate diffusion and perfusion metrics. Perfusion fraction (f) has been shown to be markedly reduced in pancreatic ductal adenocarcinomas[16-18] and postulated to be superior than diffusion in differentiating from mass-forming chronic pancreatitis.[16,17] Another method which has been proposed is the non-Gaussian kurtosis model, which takes into account tissue heterogeneity (kurtosis effects).[9] Corrected diffusion coefficient (D_k) has been found to have highest accuracy for differentiation of adenocarcinoma and remaining pancreatic parenchyma.[9]

IMAGING FINDINGS (TABLE 1)

Pancreatic cancers are solid scirrhous tumor with reduced perfusion compared to normal parenchyma. They are infiltrative and incite surrounding inflammation and desmoplastic reaction. These lesions tend to obstruct and constrict the ductal structures, causing jaundice and pancreatitis. Pancreatic head is the most common location (60–70% cases) and thus biliary obstruction is frequent in pancreatic adenocarcinomas. Head is the part of pancreas to the right of SMV while body is to the left. Also, head lesions are detected at a relatively earlier stage because of biliary obstruction, whereas body and tail lesions may grow large before producing significant symptoms. Thus, lesions in the body and tail region are large at presentation and have areas of necrosis/hemorrhage within. Pancreatic carcinoma commonly metastasizes to the liver, peritoneum, lungs and bones.

Table 1: Imaging features of pancreatic carcinoma.

• *Sonography*: – Solid – Hypoechoic – Irregular ill-defined margins – Usually no demonstrable internal vascularity
• *CT*: – Mildly enhancing lesion which appears hypodense relative to brightly enhancing normal pancreatic parenchyma – Contour bulge
• *MRI*: – T1 hypointense mass against background hyperintense *pancreas*: – Diffusion restriction – Mass enhances less than surrounding parenchyma in pancreatic phase
• *Secondary signs*: – Upstream pancreatic ductal dilatation with/without atrophy – Contour bulge (in larger lesions) – Local infiltration – Biliary dilatation in head lesions

Pancreatic cancers are usually solid hypoechoic on ultrasound and upstream ductal dilatation (diameter of pancreatic duct >2 mm) may be seen **(Figs. 6A to D)**. Margins are ill-defined and irregular. On color Doppler examination, no significant internal vascularity is seen. Larger lesions may have necrosis within and show infiltration of surrounding structures. Lesions in the pancreatic head often result in biliary dilatation **(Figs. 6A to D)**.

On the late arterial phase CT or MRI, the masses are hypodense in more than 90% cases **(Figs. 7A to D)**.[19] In addition to the attenuation difference, larger masses also produce a contour bulge of the pancreas **(Figs. 7A to D)**, and the fat planes with adjacent structures may be lost. 5–10% of the pancreatic carcinomas are isodense to the surrounding parenchyma **(Figs. 7A to D)** and thus difficult to detect based on attenuation values.[20] The

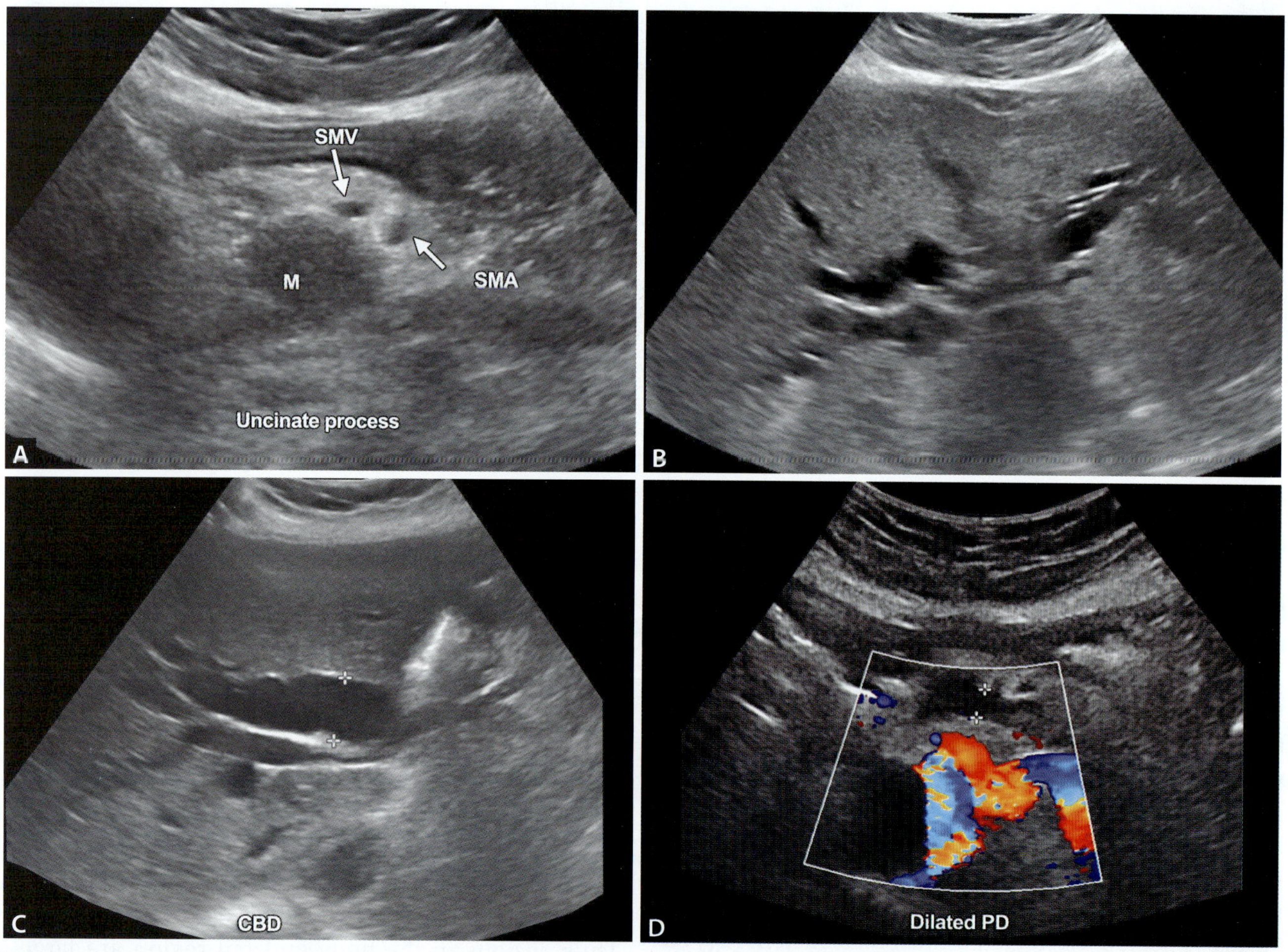

Figs. 6A to D: Sonography in pancreatic cancer: Gray-scale ultrasound image (A) shows solid hypoechoic mass lesion in the head and uncinate process of pancreas (M) with irregular margins. Superior mesenteric vessels (SMA and SMV) are seen separately; USG image (B) shows bilobar intrahepatic biliary radical dilatation and (C) depicts dilated common bile duct (cursors); Color Doppler image (D) shows dilated pancreatic duct (PD) (cursors).

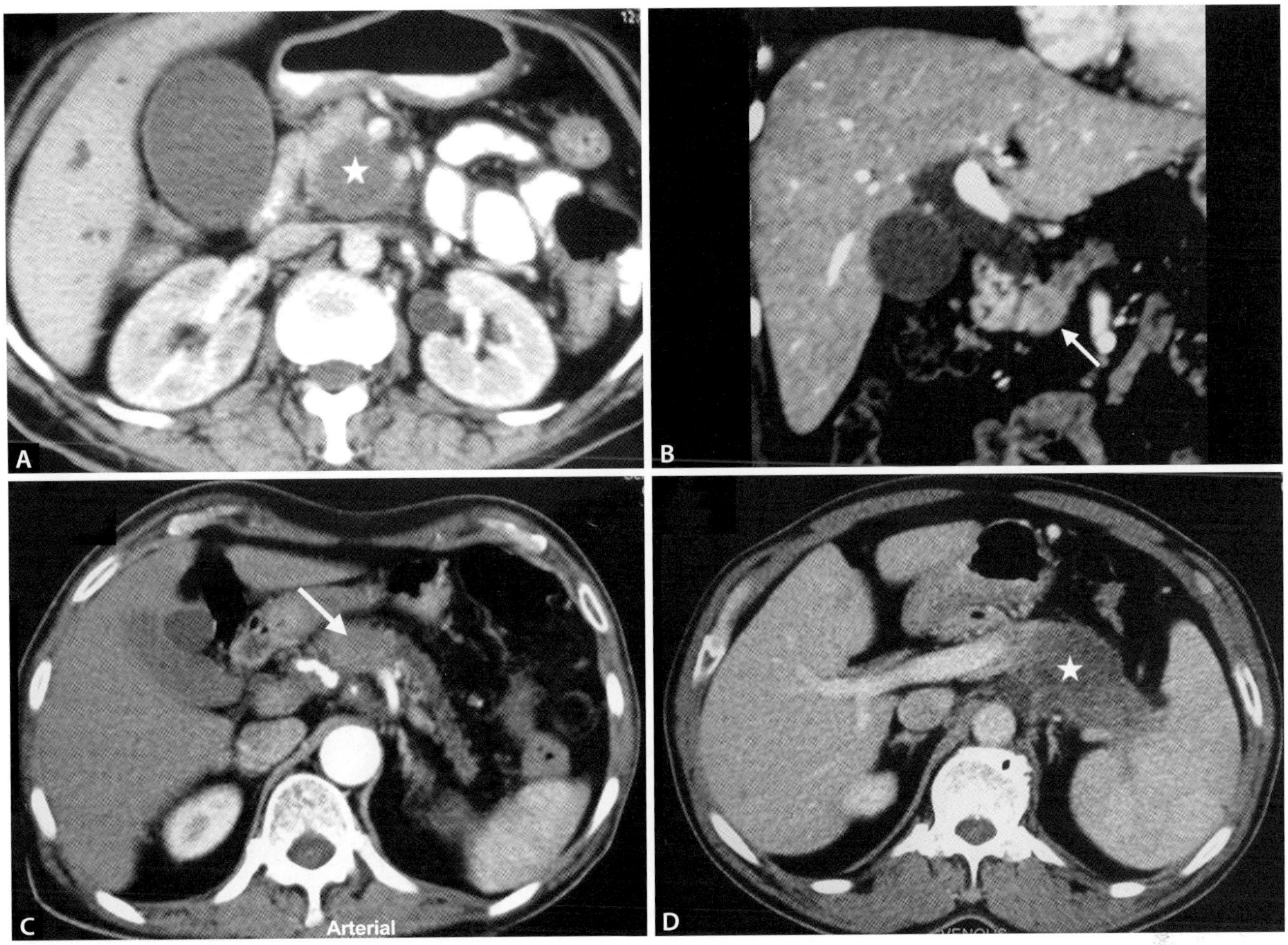

Figs. 7A to D: CT images of different patients showing pancreatic carcinoma with variable morphology in different locations. Axial CECT image (A) shows a hypodense mass lesion in the uncinate process of pancreas (star), abutting the superior mesenteric artery. Coronal CECT image (B) shows isodense mass lesion in the pancreatic head (arrow) with atrophy of distal pancreatic parenchyma and pancreatic ductal prominence. Axial CECT image (C) demonstrates isodense mass in the neck of pancreas (arrow) without contour bulge, but with pancreatic ductal dilatation. Axial CECT image (D) shows large hypodense mass lesion in the distal body and tail of pancreas with areas of necrosis within (star).

problem is further compounded because these isodense cancers are frequently small (<2 cm) and may not deform the pancreatic contour.

MRI is useful in such cases with lesion being hypointense on T1W FS images, against background hyperintense parenchyma. MRI may visualize up to 79% of isodense pancreatic lesions **(Figs. 8A to D)**.[19] T2W images depict the mass as having intermediate signal intensity and are not much helpful in demonstrating the mass; but heavily T2W images depict ductal dilatation and obstruction quite well. Calcification is unusual in pancreatic adenocarcinoma. Pancreatic adenocarcinomas show heterogeneous diffusion restriction on DW MRI and their ADC values are lower than surrounding parenchyma **(Figs. 9A to E)**. Addition of DWI to conventional sequences increases the sensitivity of detection of pancreatic cancer.[21]

The secondary findings include dilatation of the pancreatic duct with or without biliary dilatation **(Fig. 10)**. Biliary dilatation occurs in case of lesions located in the pancreatic head as well as may occur due to metastatic lymph node enlargement compressing the suprapancreatic portion of common bile duct. The pancreatic duct may be abruptly cut off with upstream dilatation and may be the only clue to diagnosing small isodense and non-contour deforming lesions **(Figs. 10A to D)**.[22] *Double duct sign* is seen in cancers located in the pancreatic head and represents dilatation of both pancreatic and biliary ducts due to obstruction of both PD and adjacent intrapancreatic part of common bile duct **(Fig. 11)**. Long standing lesions may cause distal parenchymal atrophy as well.

Rarely, pancreatic cancer may present as single or multiple episodes of acute pancreatitis, secondary to

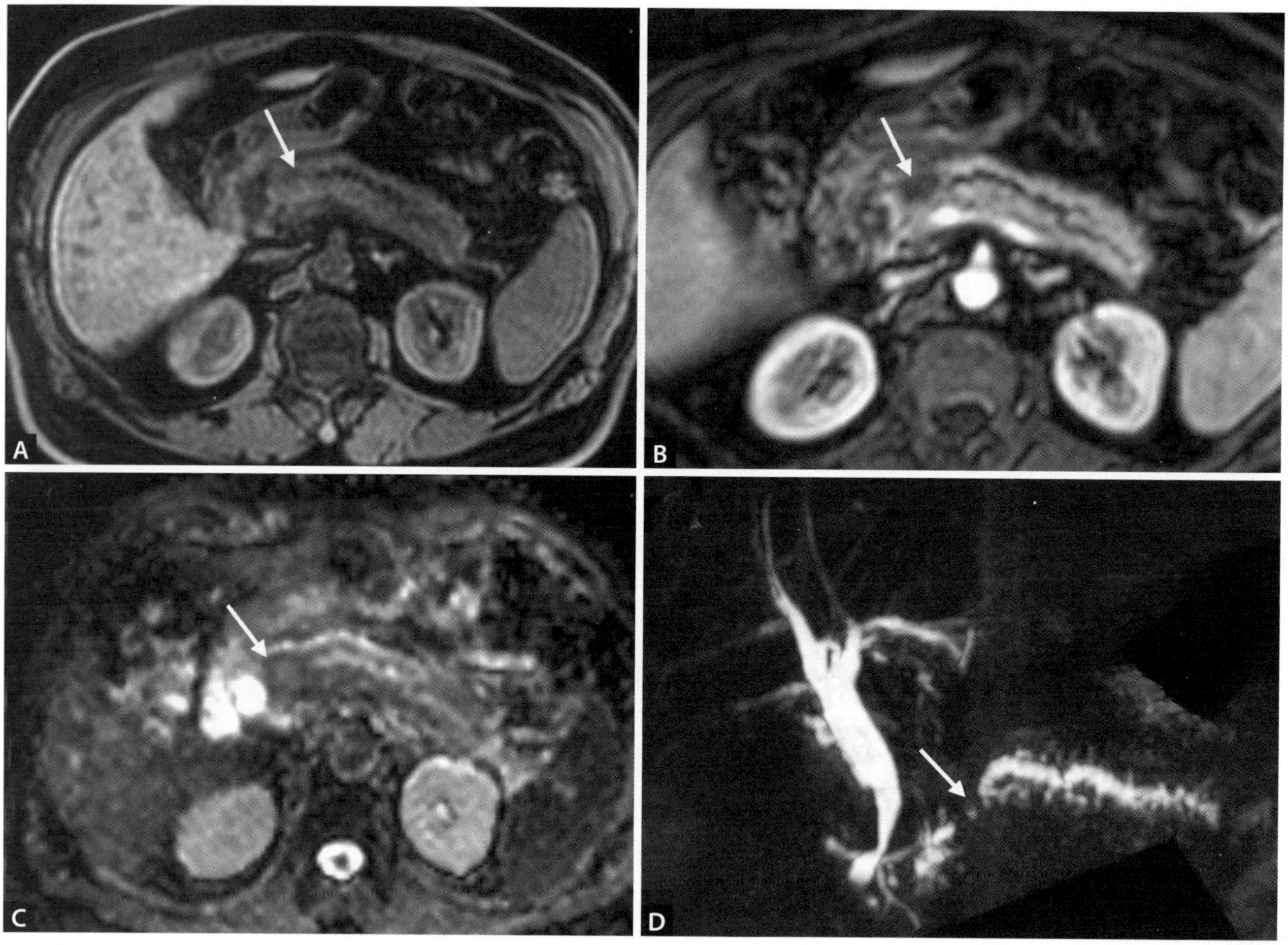

Figs. 8A to D: Utility of MRI in small lesions. Axial T1-weighted (T1W) fat-supressed (FS) image (A) shows an ill-defined small isointense mass in the pancreatic head-neck region (arrow) which is hypoenhancing compared to rest of parenchyma on postcontrast pancreatic phase imaging (B), with pancreatic ductal dilatation. Axial apparent diffusion coefficient (ADC) map (C) shows the lesion is dark (arrow), suggesting restricted diffusion. Projectional MRCP image (D) depicts abrupt cut-off of the main pancreatic duct (arrow). There is diffuse irregular dilatation of main pancreatic duct and side branches due to background chronic pancreatitis.

ductal obstruction.[23] In these cases, inflammatory changes predominate and may mask the underlying lesion. Disproportionate enlargement of the head, significant dilatation of the pancreatic duct with abrupt change in caliber, focal pancreatitis distal to obstruction and recurrent pancreatitis in the absence of risk factors may raise the suspicion of an underlying malignancy **(Figs. 12A and B)**. Many times, the lesion may be diagnosed only on follow-up scans when the inflammatory changes have subsided.[23]

Both pancreatic phase and venous phase images are important for accurate assessment of staging. A characteristic feature of liver metastases from pancreatic adenocarcinomas is flow-related phenomenon, seen on the late arterial phase images **(Figs. 13A to D)**. This can either be in the form of thin peripheral contrast enhancement around hypodense metastases or perfusion abnormalities like transient hepatic attenuation difference. Liver metastases are best detected on T2W and diffusion-weighted MR sequences. Peritoneal dissemination is suggested by the presence of ascites, omental thickening and peritoneal nodularity. Peritoneal nodules are better visualized on DW MRI and PET-CT **(Figs. 14A to C)**.

PANCREATIC CANCER VARIANTS

Other than ductal adenocarcinoma, there are few rare variants which constitute around 10% of the pancreatic tumors.[24]

Acinar cell carcinoma is also a malignant epithelial tumor with slightly better prognosis and has a propensity

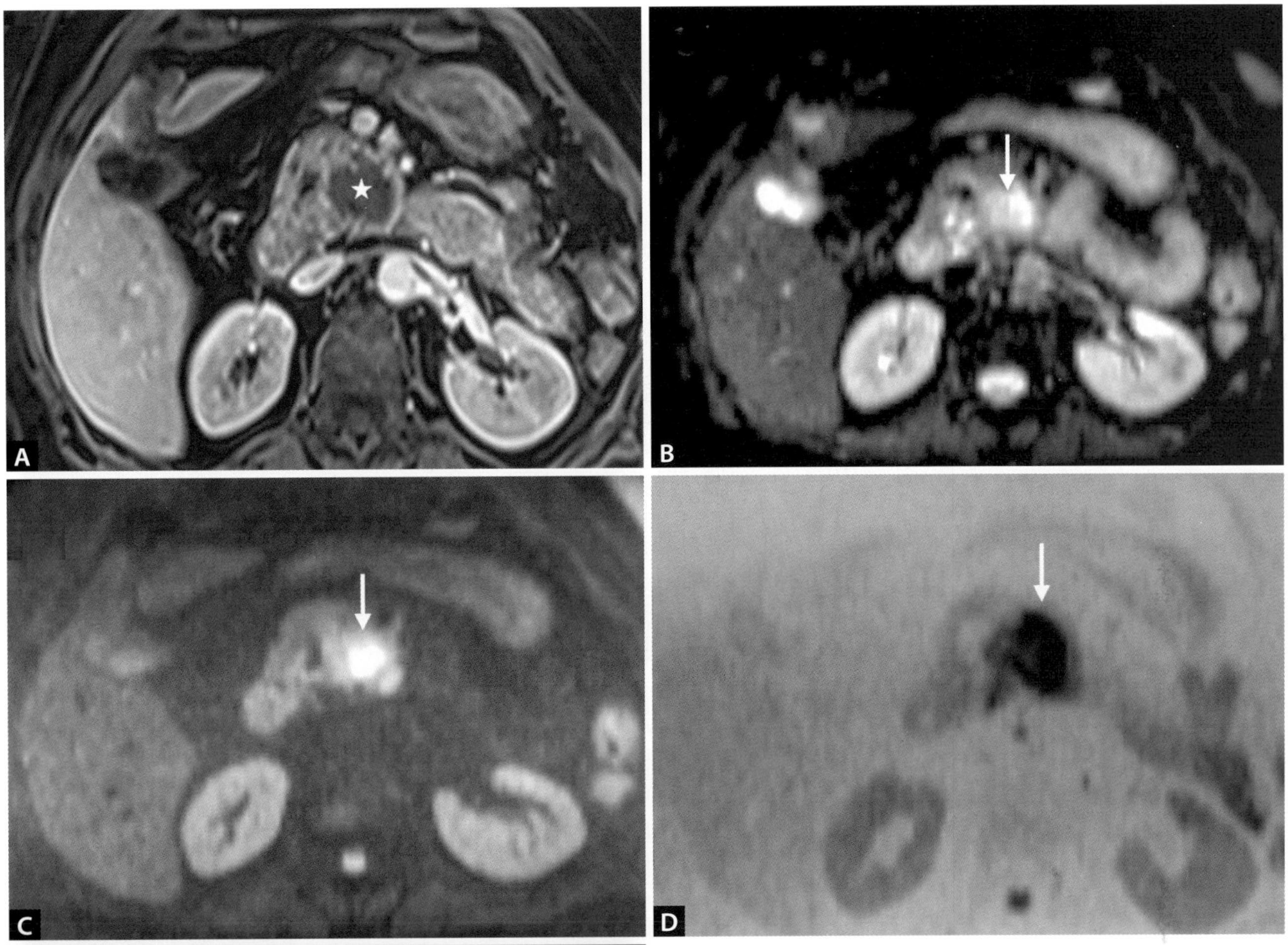

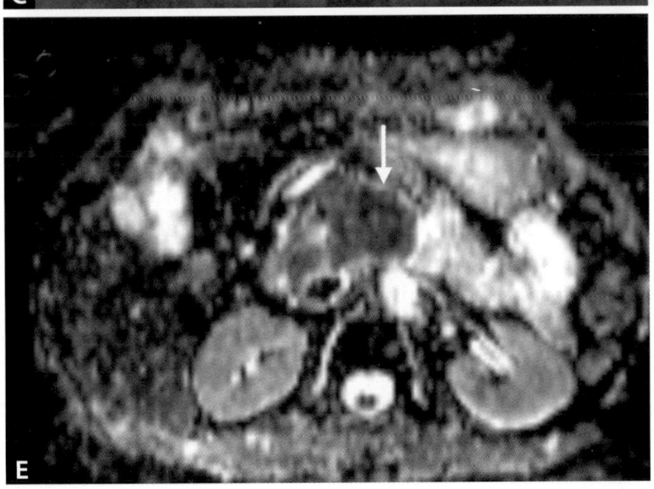

Figs. 9A to E: DW MRI in pancreatic cancer. Axial contrast-enhanced MR image (A) shows hypointense mass in the uncinate process of pancreas (star). Axial DW image at b0 (B), b500 (C), contrast-inverted image at b 1000 s/mm^2 (D) and ADC map (E) depict severe heterogeneous diffusion restriction in the mass (arrow). There is retention of signal on the high b-value image.

to metastasize to lymph nodes and liver. Jaundice is usually not seen. These tumors are solid, can reach large size, and do not cause ductal dilatation even in advanced stage. Similar to adenocarcinomas, these are hypoenhancing; but in contrast, they show well-defined margins.

Mucinous colloid carcinoma also has better prognosis than adenocarcinoma. It shows T2 hyperintensity owing to mucin within. Adenosquamous carcinoma has both glandular and squamous components and is a histological diagnosis with worse prognosis. Anaplastic carcinomas

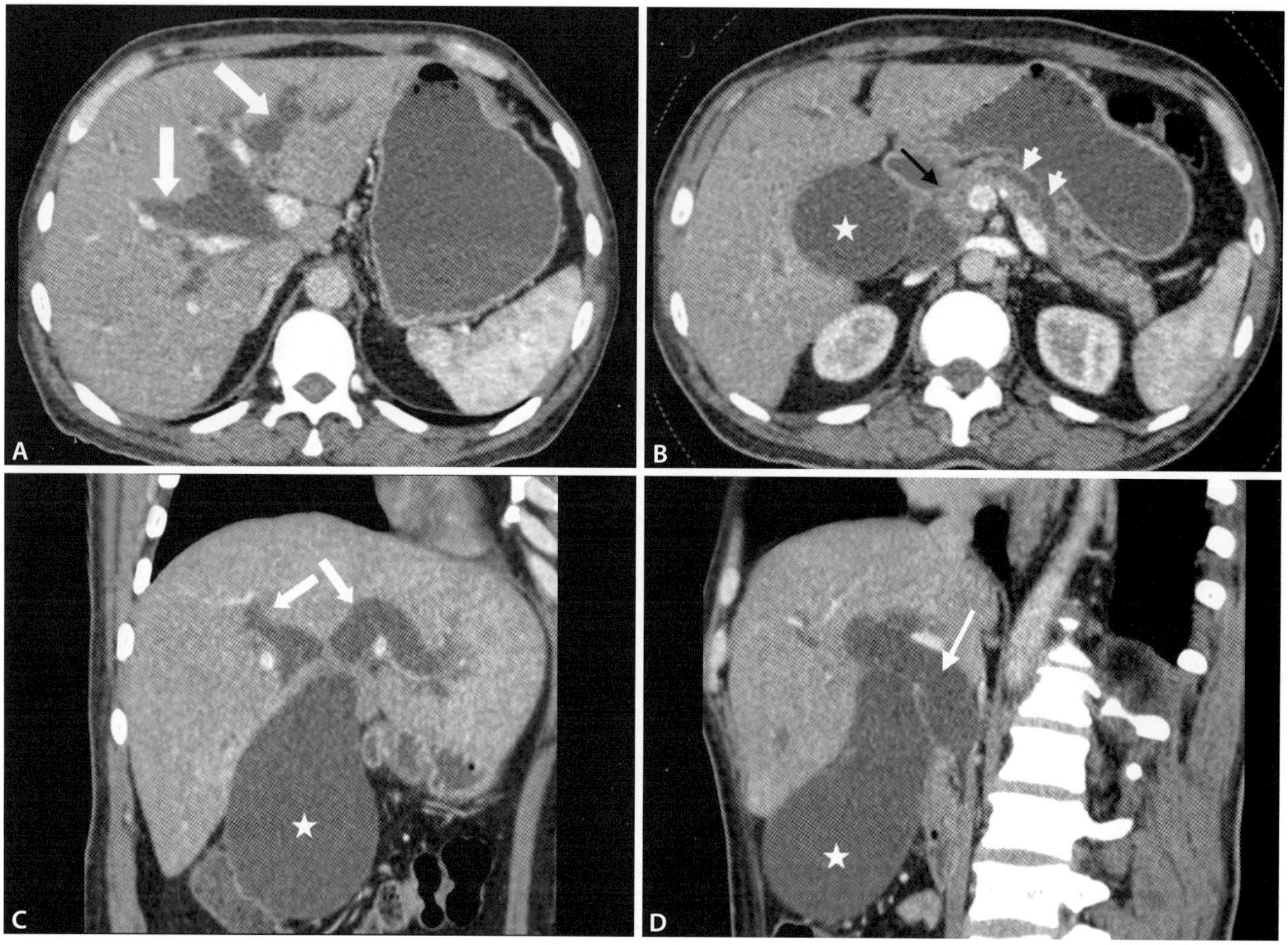

Figs. 10A to D: Secondary findings in pancreatic cancer: Axial (A and B), oblique coronal (C) and oblique sagittal (D) CT images in the pancreatic phase show dilatation of intrahepatic biliary radicals (solid arrows), common bile duct (white arrows), gallbladder (star) and pancreatic duct (arrowheads). These secondary signs help in the detection of small isodense mass in the pancreatic head (black arrow).

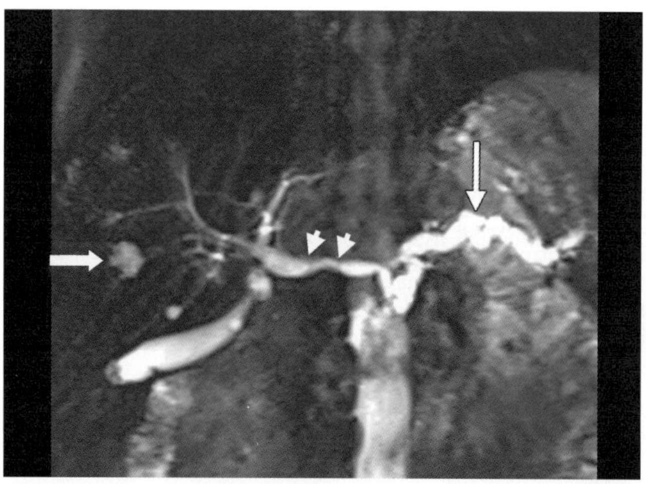

Fig. 11: Projectional MRCP image shows dilatation of both pancreatic (arrow) and biliary ducts (arrowheads) along with mild dilatation of intrahepatic biliary radicals. Few cholangiolar abscesses are also seen in the right lobe (solid arrow) due to obstructive cholangitis.

are large tumors, common in the tail of pancreas. They may show marked contrast enhancement and have central areas of necrosis, and thus may mimic neuroendocrine tumors. These are aggressive lesions which usually present with lymphadenopathy and metastases.

DIFFERENTIAL DIAGNOSES

Focal pancreatitis (including autoimmune type) is an important diagnostic consideration especially because secondary changes of upstream ductal dilatation or atrophy may be seen.[25] *Mass-forming chronic pancreatitis (MFCP)* is chronic inflammation usually involving the pancreatic head. History of repeated episodes of acute abdomen and presence of calcifications indicates underlying chronic calcific pancreatitis. Pancreatic duct in the latter shows long smooth narrowing or irregular beaded appearance. The "Duct penetrating sign" refers to nonobstructed attenuated duct, which traverses the mass

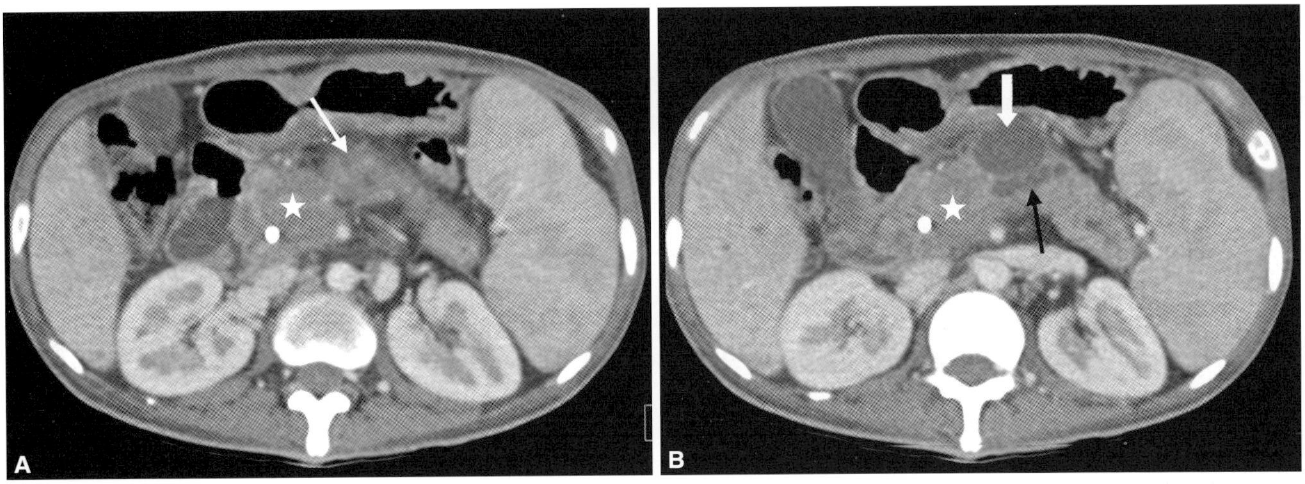

Figs. 12A and B: Pancreatic cancer causing acute pancreatitis with biliary stent in situ. Axial CECT images depict bulky heterogeneous mass in the pancreatic head region (star) with heterogeneity in the proximal body (white arrow). Former was ductal adenocarcinoma while latter was focal pancreatitis secondary to obstruction. Note is made of peripancreatic fat stranding in (A), peripancreatic fluid collection (solid arrow) and pancreatic ductal dilatation (black arrow) in (B).

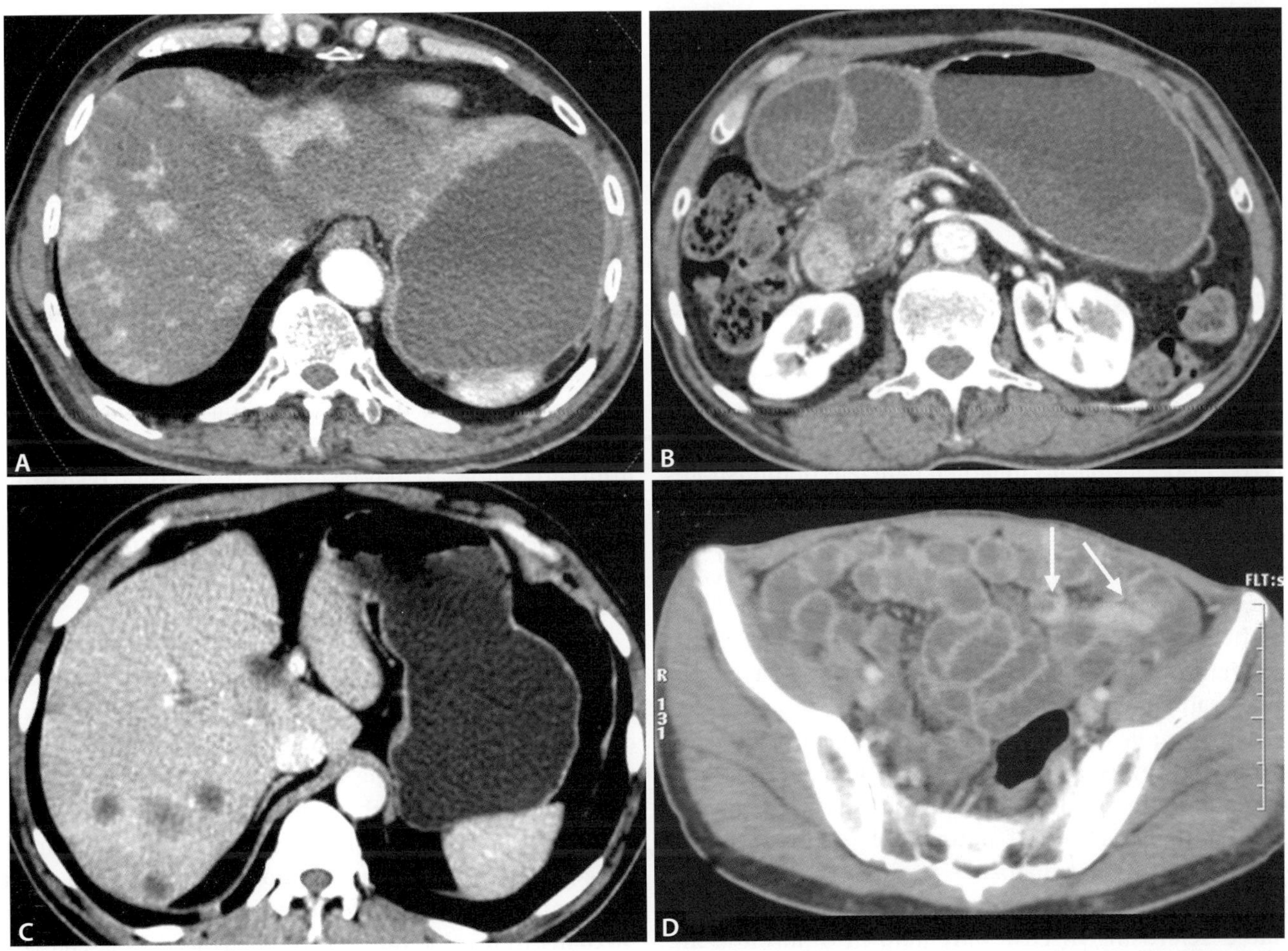

Figs. 13A to D: Liver and peritoneal metastases in pancreatic carcinoma. Late arterial phase axial CT image (A) shows multiple liver lesions with surrounding hyperenhancement and transient hepatic attenuation difference. Axial CT image at lower level (B) depicts a large heterogeneous pancreatic head mass. Axial CT image in a different patient (C) shows multiple hypodense liver metastases in the venous phase. Same patient as (C) also showed multiple areas of eccentric bowel wall thickening (arrows in D), suggesting serosal metastases.

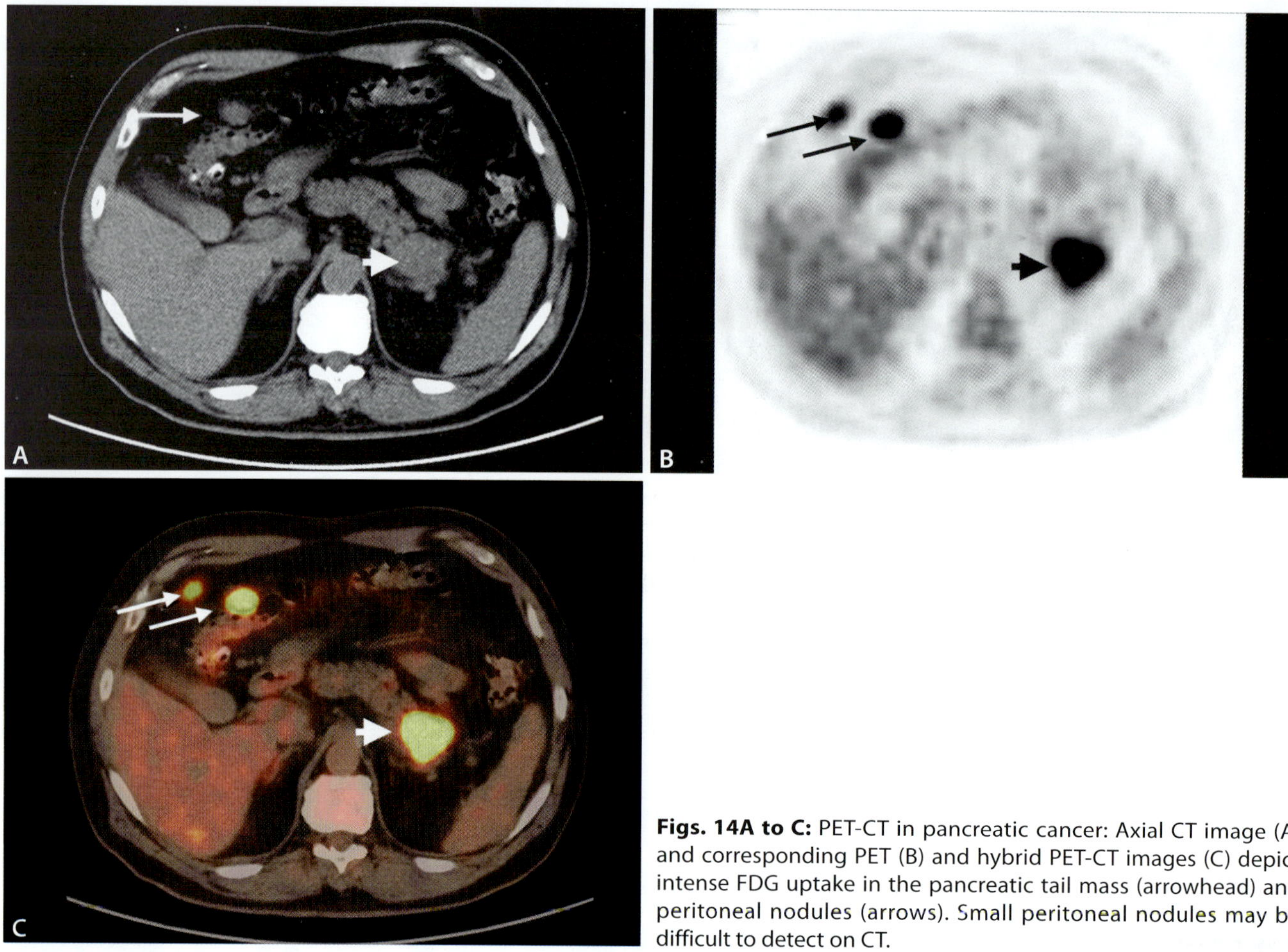

Figs. 14A to C: PET-CT in pancreatic cancer: Axial CT image (A) and corresponding PET (B) and hybrid PET-CT images (C) depict intense FDG uptake in the pancreatic tail mass (arrowhead) and peritoneal nodules (arrows). Small peritoneal nodules may be difficult to detect on CT.

instead of getting cut-off and is used to differentiate an inflammatory pancreatic mass from malignancy **(Figs. 15A to D)**.[26] Also, chronically inflamed pancreas demonstrates greater enhancement than tumor in the pancreatic phase imaging. Ratio of the diameter of dilated pancreatic duct to the maximum width of the abnormal part of gland greater than 0.5 favors carcinoma. DW MRI and perfusion CT can also help to differentiate focal chronic pancreatitis from malignancy.[14,27] EUS may be helpful in these cases and guided sampling may be done.

Autoimmune pancreatitis is characterized by elevated serum IgG4 levels and is treated with steroids and does not require surgery. The focal form can mimic malignancy on imaging. Absence of pancreatic duct dilatation, diffuse involvement, halo-like peripancreatic smooth hypodensity and extrapancreatic manifestations of IgG4-related sclerosing disease may help in differentiating from carcinoma.[27] The pancreatic and biliary ducts may show irregular wall thickening and enhancement.[28] Homogeneous enhancement (similar to surrounding parenchyma) and duct penetrating sign may help in differentiating mass-forming autoimmune pancreatitis from carcinoma.[29] It may be noted that diffusion restriction with low ADC values can be seen in autoimmune pancreatitis also due to dense lymphoplasmacytic infiltration and thus ADC values overlap with that of pancreatic malignancy.[29]

Paraduodenal/Groove pancreatitis is a type of chronic focal inflammation localized to the space between the pancreatic head and the second part of duodenum. It is seen more often in middle aged men with history of alcohol abuse. Imaging appearance is in the form of ill-defined sheet-like thickening and bulky pancreatic head with delayed enhancement. There is a pure form which affects only the pancreatoduodenal groove and a segmental form which affects the groove and may extend medially to involve the pancreatic head. Cystic changes may be seen especially in the medial duodenal wall along with duodenal wall thickening **(Figs. 16A to C)**.[30] Thus, it comes in the differential diagnosis of periampullary and

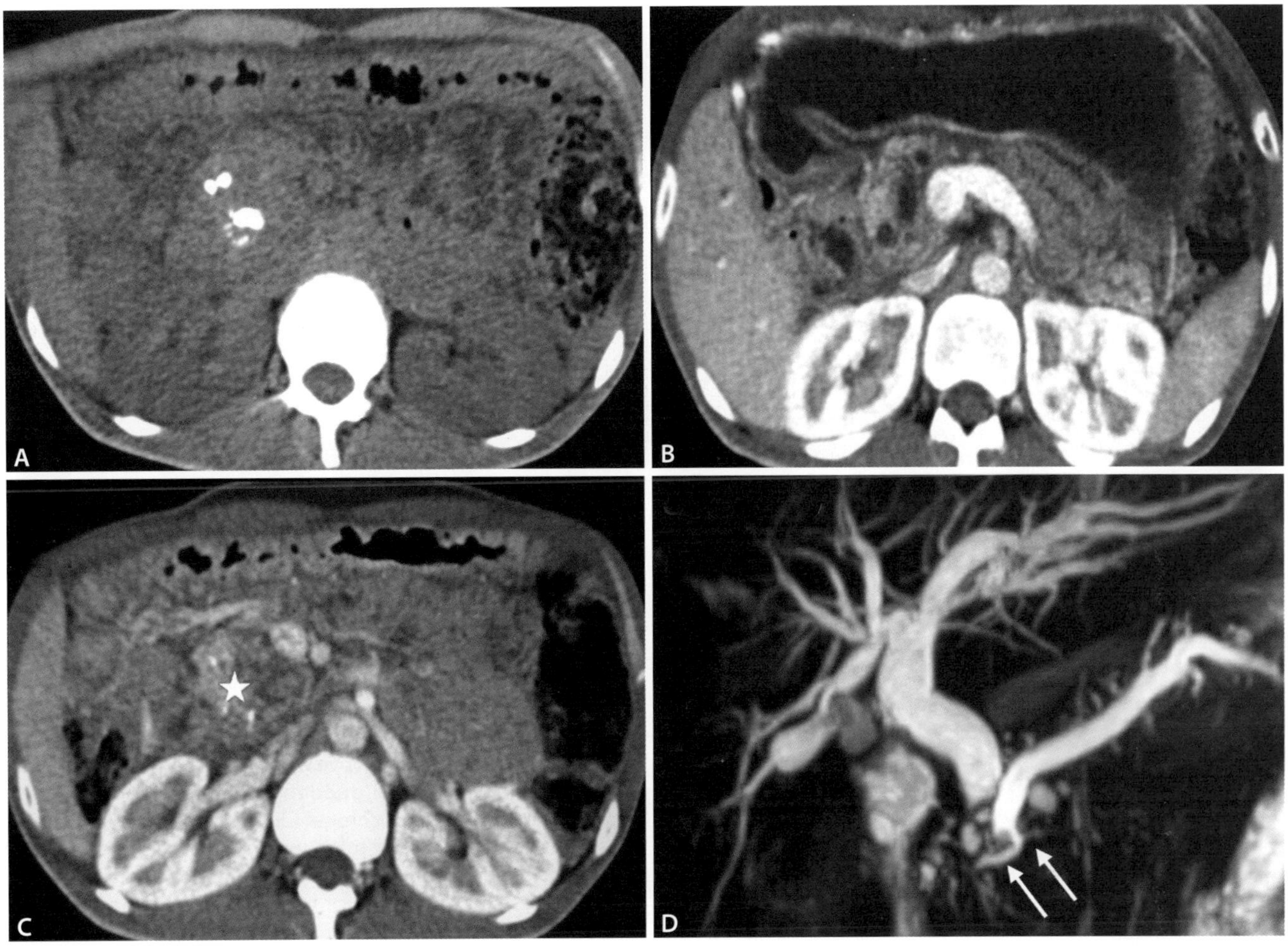

Figs. 15A to D: Mass-forming chronic pancreatitis: Axial noncontrast CT image (A) depicts multiple foci of calcification in the region of pancreatic head. Axial CECT images (B and C) show bulky heterogeneously enhancing head (star) with dilated pancreatic and common bile ducts. However, there is no abrupt cut-off of the ducts and the narrowed pancreatic duct can be seen to course through the head region (arrows in D), suggesting duct penetrating sign. EUS sampling confirmed focal chronic pancreatitis.

pancreatic head malignancies. Pancreatic ductal dilatation is usually not seen.

Despite all imaging advancements and even with sampling, focal pancreatitis may be difficult to differentiate from carcinoma and they may occasionally coexist. Relatively spared pancreatic parenchyma in the background of atrophic gland in chronic pancreatitis may also mimic pancreatic malignancy.

Neuroendocrine tumors are usually small in size and show hypervascularity on the pancreatic phase imaging. Ductal dilatation is uncommon, as opposed to pancreatic carcinomas. Nonfunctional neuroendocrine tumors are large and heterogeneous with areas of necrosis and calcification within **(Figs. 16A to C)**. They may appear similar to ductal adenocarcinomas in the body and tail region because the latter also have large heterogeneous appearance. *Cystic pancreatic tumors* also come in the list of differentials in this scenario.

Metastases to pancreas are not common and most of these patients have metastatic lesions elsewhere in the body also. Primary malignancies which can metastasize to the pancreas include lung, breast and renal carcinomas and melanomas. Metastases can be solitary, multiple or diffuse infiltrating. Usually, they are multiple and well-defined but may mimic pancreatic carcinoma when occur singly. Enhancement characteristics are similar to the primary lesion (hypervascular in renal carcinomas and melanomas).

Lymphomatous involvement of the pancreas occurs frequently by direct infiltration from adjacent enlarged lymph nodes and is more common in non-Hodgkin's lymphoma. Other manifestations include single/multiple

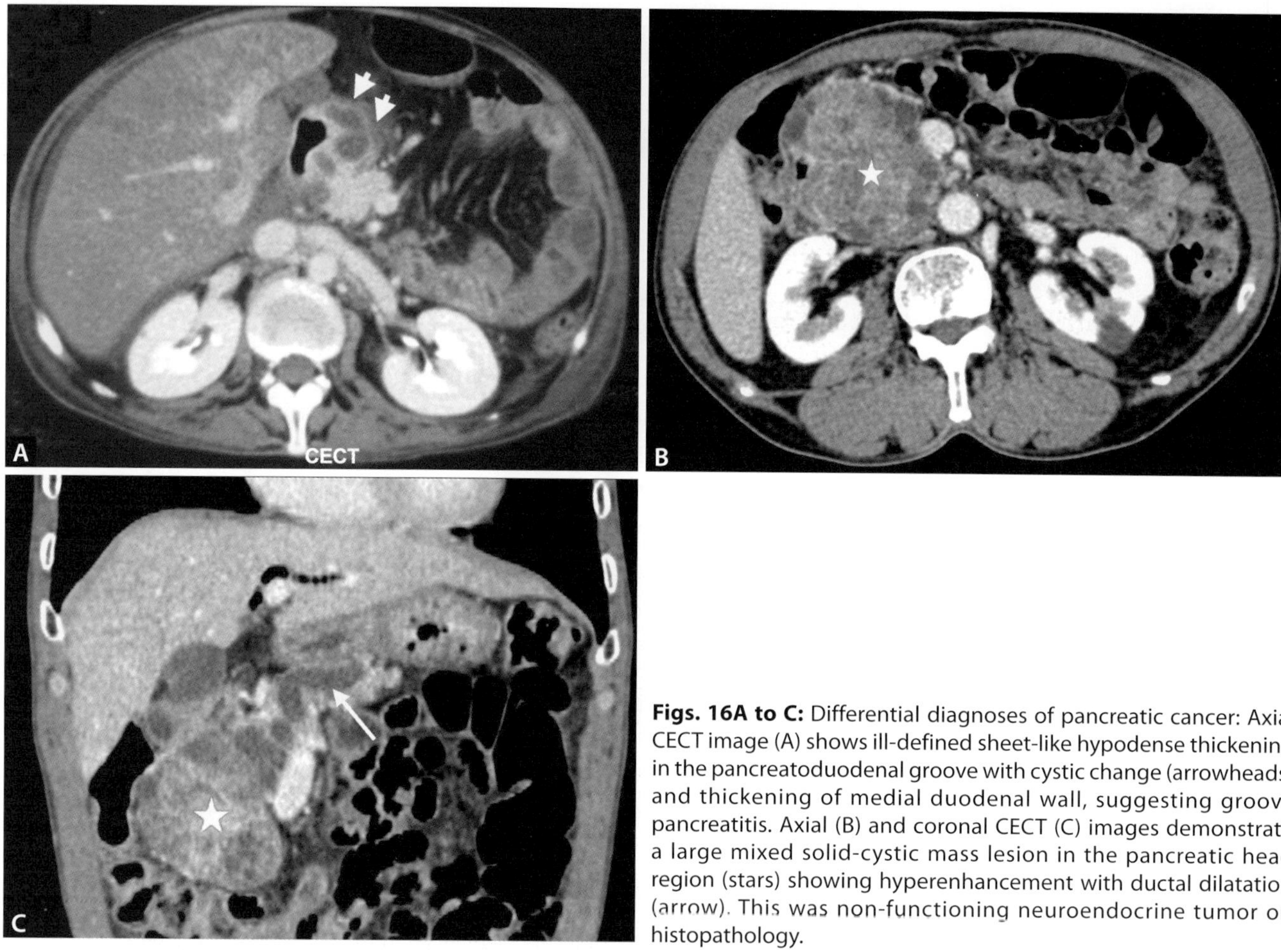

Figs. 16A to C: Differential diagnoses of pancreatic cancer: Axial CECT image (A) shows ill-defined sheet-like hypodense thickening in the pancreatoduodenal groove with cystic change (arrowheads) and thickening of medial duodenal wall, suggesting groove pancreatitis. Axial (B) and coronal CECT (C) images demonstrate a large mixed solid-cystic mass lesion in the pancreatic head region (stars) showing hyperenhancement with ductal dilatation (arrow). This was non-functioning neuroendocrine tumor on histopathology.

homogeneous focal masses showing little contrast enhancement. Ductal dilatation is infrequent, as is necrosis and calcification. Pancreatic head is commonly involved and diffuse involvement of the entire pancreas may also occur.

Occasionally *gastrointestinal tumors* from the stomach and duodenum may also mimic the imaging appearance of pancreatic cancer. *Tuberculosis* is another confounder, especially in developing countries.

STAGING OF PANCREATIC CANCER

After diagnosis, the next step is to assess the resectability of the lesion and also patient's suitability for pancreaticoduodenectomy. Surgery is beneficial only if R0 resection (negative margins on pathology) is possible. Thus, it is important to avoid unnecessary laparotomy in rest of the patients since there is little survival benefit. The criteria to determine resectability rely more on specificity than sensitivity to avoid denying the benefit of surgery to potentially resectable patients. CT and MRI are equally accurate in the staging of pancreatic cancers.

The spread of pancreatic cancer depends on its location. Anteriorly located head lesions spread towards gastroduodenal and common hepatic arteries while posterior lesions cause early involvement of SMV-PV and replaced/ accessory right hepatic arteries (arising from SMA). SMV is more commonly involved in head lesions, compared to SMA. This is because SMV is nearer to the head and also because arteries have thick muscular walls compared to thin walls of veins. Tumors located in the uncinate process have a propensity to grow along jejunal branches of SMA and SMV and thus perineural spread is common. Tumors located in the body and tail region have a tendency to infiltrate splenic vessels and hilum of the spleen. In advanced cases, stomach, gallbladder and duodenum may also get involved.

There are three categories as per National Comprehensive Cancer Network (NCCN) criteria: resectable, borderline resectable and unresectable **(Table 2)**.[3,31] Location of the tumor and vascular involvement are the important determining factors for categorization. It is important to note that arterial encasement (contact >180 degrees or half the arterial circumference in cross-section) is an important criterion of unresectability of the pancreatic mass.[32] Infiltration of the surrounding structures (stomach, transverse colon, spleen, etc.) does not make the tumor unresectable, though surgery becomes more extensive.[31]

The lesion is *resectable* **(Figs. 17A and B)** if there is neither extrapancreatic infiltration nor distant metastases. Thus there is a clear fat plane separating the tumor from main arteries (celiac axis, common hepatic artery CHA and superior mesenteric artery SMA). The contact with the surrounding veins (superior mesenteric vein SMV and portal vein PV) is also absent or there is just abutment (≤180 degrees contact without contour irregularity). No venous encasement or tumor thrombus is seen.

Unresectable tumors **(Figs. 18A to F)** either have distant metastases (including nonregional lymphadenopathy) or local invasion. Liver and peritoneal cavity are the common sites of metastases. Arterial invasion is in the form of encasement (contact >180 degrees circumference) of SMA, celiac axis or contact with first jejunal branch of SMA. Unresectable venous involvement includes unreconstructible SMV-PV due to infiltration/occlusion or contact with the most proximal draining jejunal branch into SMV.

Borderline resectability **(Figs. 19A to C)** in terms of venous involvement includes encasement or abutment of

Table 2: Imaging criteria of resectability of pancreatic carcinoma.

	Arterial	*Venous*
Resectable	No arterial contact with tumor	No contact or only abutment of SMV-PV without irregularity and distortion
Borderline resectability	• Tumor contact with CHA without extension to celiac axis proximally or hepatic artery bifurcation distally (so as to allow for surgical reconstruction) • SMA abutment • Variant arterial anatomy with tumor contact • Celiac axis abutment in pancreatic body/ tail lesions* • Celiac axis encasement without involvement of aorta and with intact uninvolved GDA*	• Encasement or abutment of SMV-PV with contour irregularity or venous thrombosis but suitable vessel available proximal and distal for surgical reconstruction • Tumor contact with IVC
Unresectable	• Encasement of SMA, celiac axis • Celiac axis abutment in pancreatic head lesions • Extensive encasement of CHA (surgical reconstruction not possible) • Contact with first jejunal branch of SMA • Any contact with aorta	• Unreconstructible SMV-PV due to infiltration/occlusion • Contact with the most proximal draining jejunal branch (into SMV)

* Some institutions may consider these criteria to indicate unresectable disease.
Distant metastases, including nonregional lymphadenopathy also make the disease unresectable.

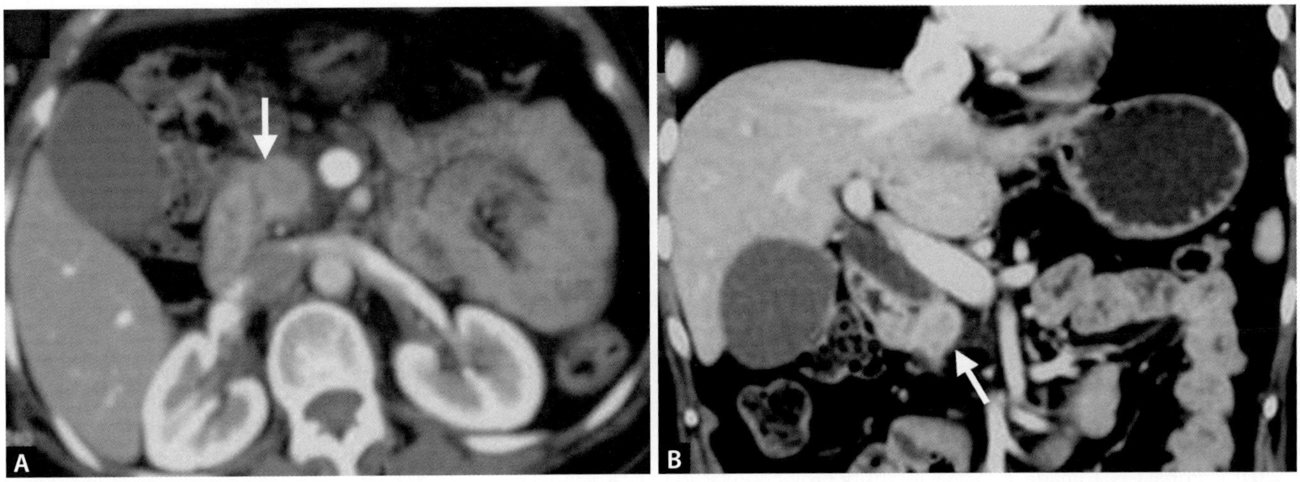

Figs. 17A and B: Resectable pancreatic cancer: Axial (A) and coronal (B) CECT images shows small pancreatic head mass (arrows) with clearly maintained fat planes with superior mesenteric vessels.

short-segment SMV-PV (usually up to 2 cm) with contour irregularity or venous thrombosis but amenable to surgical reconstruction. The prerequisite for reconstruction is that the two venous ends should have single lumen and thus branches cannot be attached to a single lumen.[1] Arterial involvement criteria are tabulated in **Table 2**.

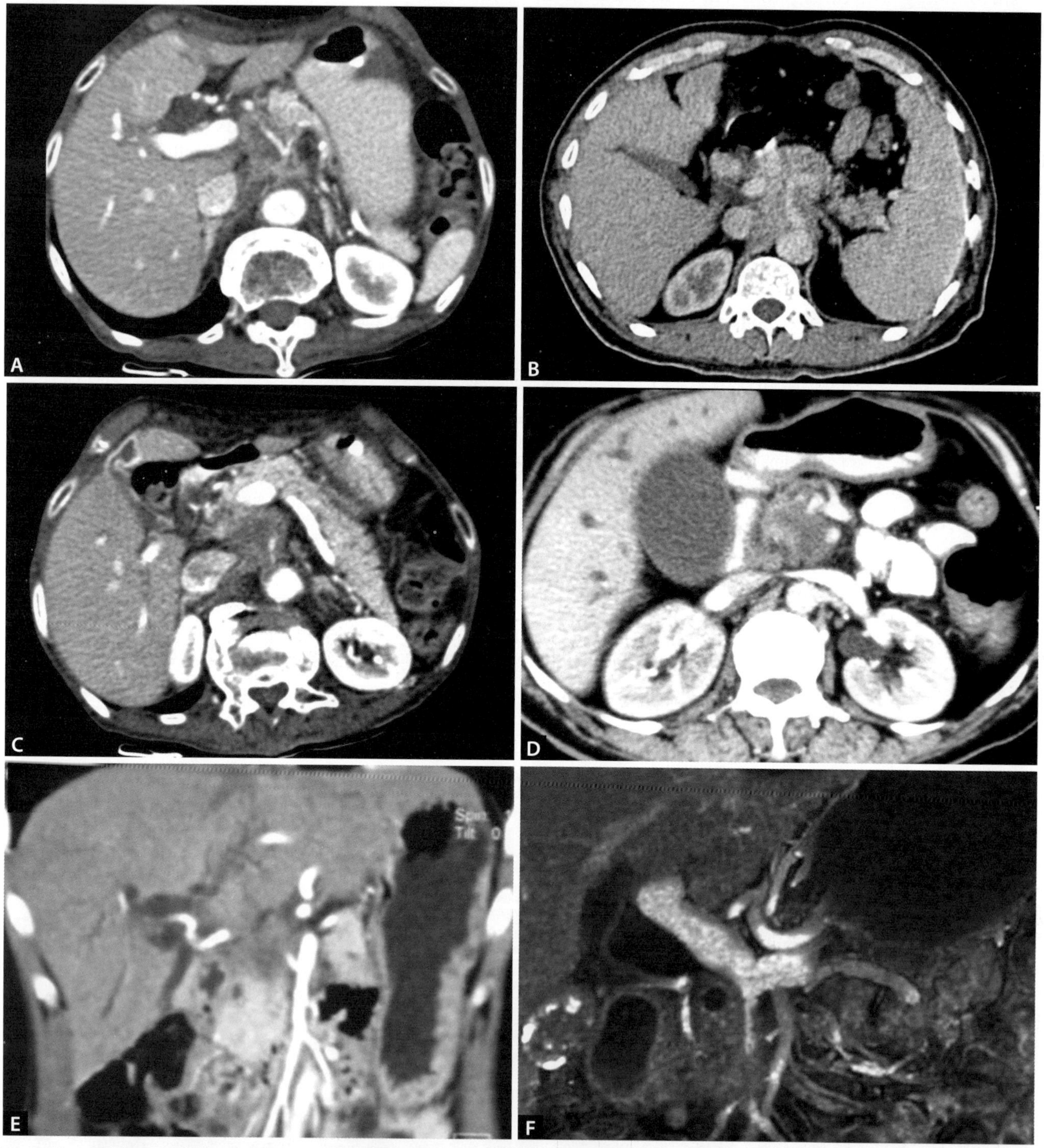

Figs. 18A to F: Unresectable pancreatic cancer: Axial CECT images depict encasement of celiac artery and common hepatic artery (A), encasement of celiac trunk and contact with aorta (B), encasement and irregular narrowing of SMA (C) and encasement of both SMA and SMV (D). Coronal CECT image, maximal intensity projection (MIP) in late arterial phase (E) depicts tumor encasement of replaced right hepatic artery (arising from SMA). Coronal MIP image generated from postcontrast MR images (F) shows encasement with irregularity of SMV with extension up to the jejunal branch, precluding surgical reconstruction.

Identifying variant vascular anatomy is also important and should be conveyed to the surgeon. Tumor contact with variant vessels (replaced right hepatic artery from SMA, low origin of CHA from celiac axis with abnormal course inferior to portal vein, high insertion of jejunal branches on SMV near PV confluence) can make resection/reconstruction difficult.[33]

Few authors have tried to correlate the appearance of venous contact of the tumor to the likelihood of successful R0 resection.[34-36] Latter is successful in those having smooth mass effect or unilateral focal mass effect with narrowing of SMV-PV. Patients with bilateral narrowing and circumferential encasement have high probability of positive surgical margins. Encasement of SMV leads to 'tear-drop' shape of the vein and suggests unresectability **(Figs. 20A to D)**.[37] Dilated peripancreatic vessels has been suggested to indicate surrounding local invasion.[38]

Metastatic lymph nodes can be identified by size criteria (>1 cm in short axis), morphology (round shape) and/or presence of central hypodensity (necrosis). Unequivocal lymph node enlargement beyond the extent of Whipple resection (i.e. except celiac axis) makes the mass unresectable. For lesions in the pancreatic head and neck, nodes along celiac axis, peripancreatic and periportal regions can be removed during surgery.[39] For body and tail cancers, nodes along CHA, celiac trunk, splenic vessels and splenic hilum come in the operative field. If nodal involvement is confirmed at surgery, then adjuvant chemotherapy is indicated.

The overall accuracy of MDCT in predicting resectability of pancreatic cancer is 88–93%.[40] The problem areas include microscopic peritoneal implants and metastases to normal-sized lymph nodes.[41] Former are even more difficult to detect in the absence of ascites. Some centers routinely perform laparoscopy just prior to surgery to detect these peritoneal metastases. In cases of mismatch between surgery and imaging, metastases were found to be the most common cause of unresectability, rather than local invasion.[1] CT is very accurate in diagnosing unresectable disease (89–100% positive predictive value);

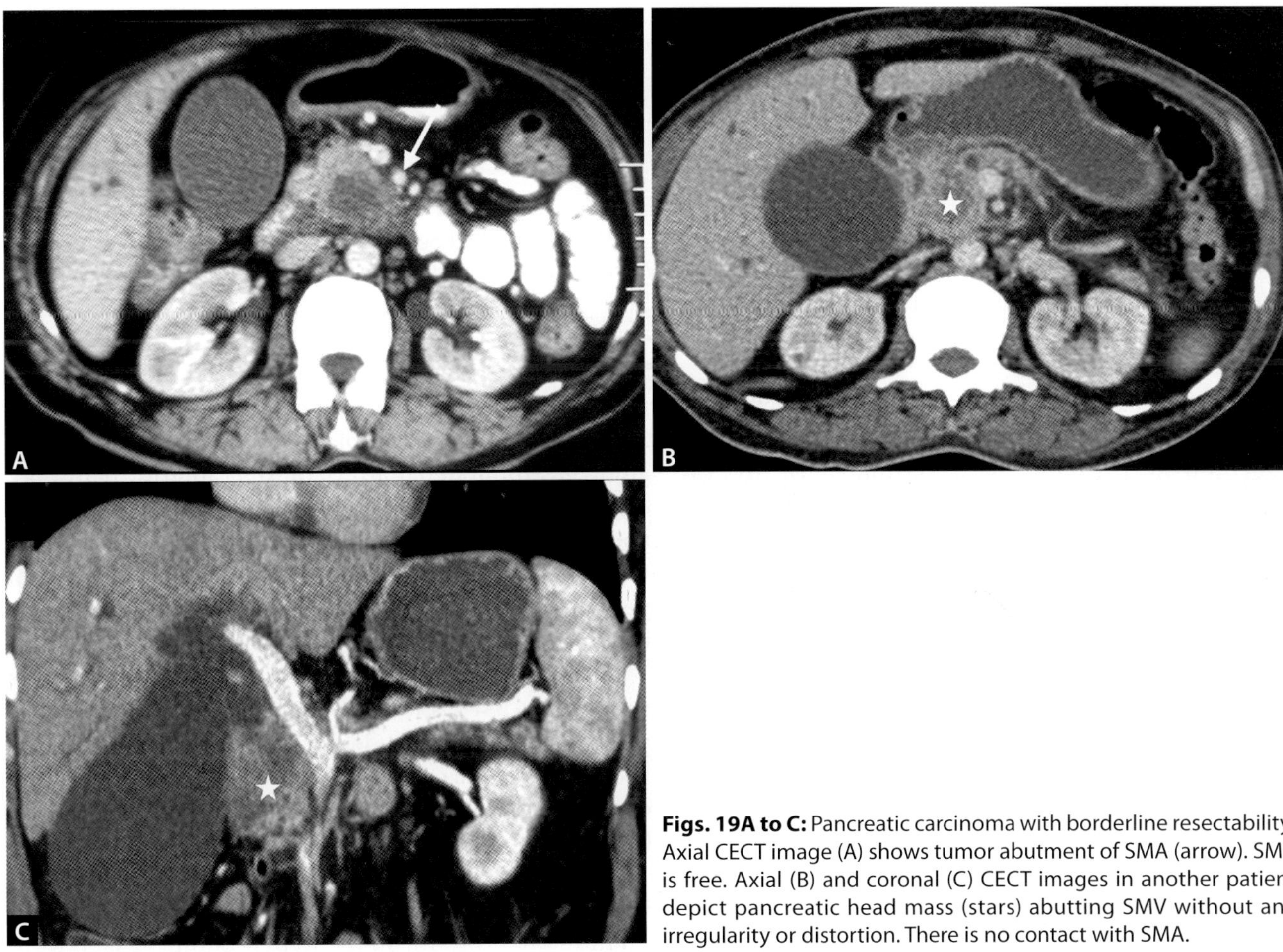

Figs. 19A to C: Pancreatic carcinoma with borderline resectability: Axial CECT image (A) shows tumor abutment of SMA (arrow). SMV is free. Axial (B) and coronal (C) CECT images in another patient depict pancreatic head mass (stars) abutting SMV without any irregularity or distortion. There is no contact with SMA.

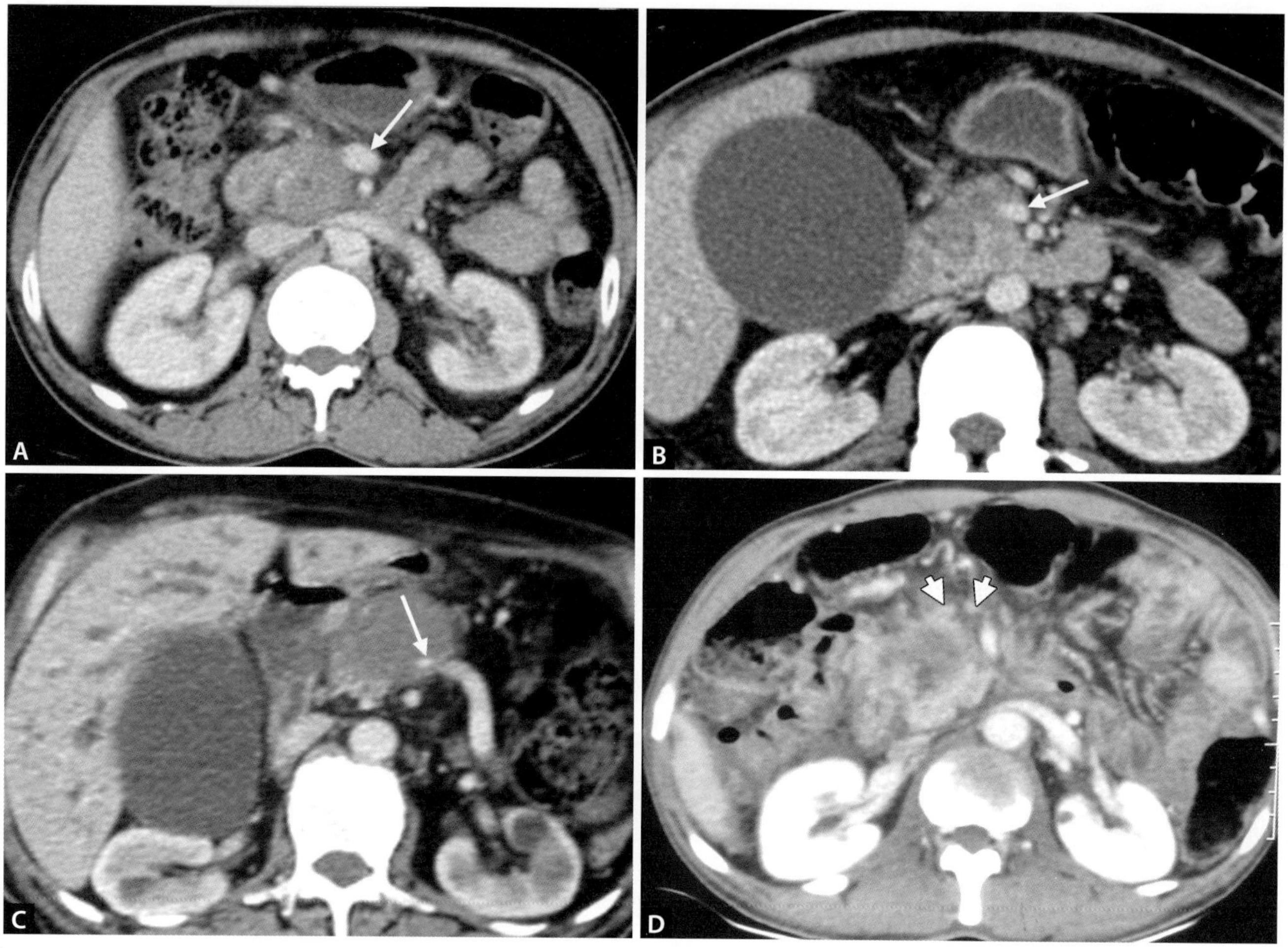

Figs. 20A to D: Spectrum of SMV involvement in pancreatic carcinoma: Axial CECT images show abutment of SMV (arrow) (A), encasement of SMV (arrow) with deformed contour (B), irregular narrowing of SMV (arrow) due to complete encasement (C) and nonvisualization of SMV (D) due to complete thrombosis and presence of collaterals (arrowheads).

however, accuracy is lower for predicting resectability (45–79%).[42]

Perineural invasion is a hallmark of ductal adenocarcinomas, although it may be seen in ampullary cancers and cholangiocarcinoma as well.[43] Perineural invasion may be suggested on CT when there is direct soft tissue infiltration along a known perineural pathway and has poor prognosis. The most common route of spread is along the plexus pancreaticus capitalis for cancers of the pancreatic head and uncinate process.[44] Plexus pancreaticus capitalis 1 (posterior hepatic plexus) extends from the right celiac ganglion, courses behind the portal vein up to upper medial border of uncinate process.[44] This is involved in pancreatic head lesions. Plexus pancreaticus capitalis 2 extends from SMA plexus, courses along posteroinferior pancreaticoduodenal artery and jejunal trunk of SMV, reaching up to the uncinate process. This plexus is usually involved in cancers of the uncinate process. Anteriorly located tumors of the head region may infiltrate along gastroduodenal artery plexus (anterior pathway), extend to plexus of CHA and hepatoduodenal ligament, and reach the right celiac ganglion and SMA plexus.[24] Literature regarding radiologic-pathologic correlates of perineural invasion is lacking but this has the potential to become an important criterion of unresectability.

Tumor node metastasis (TNM) staging system is not widely used since management depends on the resectability criteria as delineated above. However, it is used to assess the clinical prognosis and generate survival data.[31] The latest TNM staging system is shown in **Table 3** (American Joint Committee on Cancer AJCC, 7th edition).

The EUS may also be helpful in suggesting vascular invasion. The features suggesting vascular invasion include loss of normally hyperechoic vessel wall,

Table 3: TNM Staging (AJCC 4th edition) of pancreatic carcinoma.

T-stage	
TX:	Primary tumor cannot be assessed
T0:	No evidence of primary tumor
Tis:	Carcinoma *in situ*
T1:	Tumor limited to the pancreas, 2 cm or less in the greatest dimension
T2:	Tumor limited to the pancreas, >2 cm in the greatest dimension
T3:	Tumor extends beyond the pancreas but without involvement of celiac axis or SMA
T4:	Tumor involves the celiac axis or SMA
N-stage	
NX:	Regional lymph nodes cannot be assessed
N0:	No regional lymph node metastasis
N1:	Regional lymph node metastasis
M-stage	
MX:	Distant metastasis cannot be assessed
M0:	No distant metastasis
M1:	Distant metastasis
Stage 0:	Tis N0 M0
Stage IA:	T1 N0 M0
Stage IB:	T2 N0 M0
Stage IIA:	T3 N0 M0
Stage IIB:	T1-3 N1 M0
Stage III:	T4 Any N M0
Stage IV:	Any T Any N M1

vessel irregularity/occlusion and direct visualization of intravascular thrombus.[45]

SAMPLING

The EUS-guided FNA of biopsy is preferred over CT/USG-guided percutaneous sampling because of better yield, safety and lower risk of peritoneal seeding. When clinicoradiologic findings are typical, then biopsy proof is not mandatory and an equivocal biopsy should not delay surgery in patients suspected to have pancreatic cancer. Nevertheless, tissue diagnosis is necessary before neoadjuvant therapy and in patients with unresectable disease. Sampling of equivocal lymph nodes can also be done under EUS guidance.

Staging laparoscopy may be beneficial in patients deemed resectable by CT but otherwise at increased risk for dissemination. The additional lesions (usually peritoneal metastases) detected on preoperative laparoscopy may alter the management in 4–15% patients.[46]

BIOMARKERS

The most validated and studied biomarker is CA 19-9, but is nonspecific, being elevated in multiple hepatobiliary and pancreatic malignancies. It may also be elevated in any biliary obstruction and infections. It is a poor biomarker for screening but has value as prognostic marker and shows correlation with staging and survival.

k-ras gene mutations are common in patients with pancreatic carcinoma and are associated with poor prognosis.[47] Detection of k-ras mutations in the peripheral blood may indicate tumor burden and serve as prognostic biomarker.[47]

FOLLOW-UP IMAGING

Clinical follow-up is recommended every 3–6 months for the first 2 years after surgery and annually thereafter. CA 19-9 and CT can be done annually for detection of recurrence.

For locally advanced or metastatic disease on treatment (chemotherapy and/radiotherapy), serial CT follow-up is advised. Routine portal venous phase acquisition is sufficient, unless surgery is contemplated; for which dedicated pancreatic protocol is required.[3] Conventionally, size of the target lesions has been the main criterion of response evaluation.[24] Whether the lesion has become resectable comes next.

Early detection of nonresponders (to chemotherapy and/radiotherapy) is the key research area, considering the cost and toxicity associated with these therapies. This becomes even more relevant because change in size takes considerable time. Functional imaging modalities like PET-CT, perfusion CT/MRI and diffusion MRI may have a role in early response assessment. Treatment induces necrosis, and thus is expected to reduce the metabolic activity [indicated by standardized uptake values (SUV)] on PET scan, reduce the perfusion parameters and increase the apparent diffusion coefficient (ADC) values on DW MRI. However, differentiating post-treatment changes from viable tumor is difficult. This becomes even more challenging because treatment induces inflammatory changes which may mimic tumor infiltration on conventional imaging and also show increased metabolic uptake. DW MRI and perfusion imaging may have a role in this scenario. Comparison with previous imaging is also of paramount importance in these cases.

Assessment of resectability postneoadjuvant therapy is difficult because post treatment inflammation and fibrosis may mimic local vascular infiltration. Thus, the imaging accuracy decreases in detecting resectable disease.[39] This poses a practical problem in patients who receive neoadjuvant therapy after being diagnosed to have borderline resectable disease on initial CT. It has been found that radiological downstaging to resectable disease is rare (0.8%), though a significant proportion (66%) of such patients are actually found to have resectable disease at surgery.[48] Thus International Study Group of Pancreatic Surgery (ISGPS) recommends that in all patients with neoadjuvant therapy, exploratory laparotomy with attempted resection should be done, provided there is no progression on follow-up imaging.[49]

STRUCTURED REPORTING

Following a structured format for reporting pancreatic multiphasic CT examinations enables better evaluation of pancreatic cancer and optimal surgical planning.[50] Surgeons find it easier to understand the objective terms used in structured reporting format and are more likely to have all the information needed for surgical planning from these structured reports.[50] A sample structured reporting template for reporting suspected pancreatic malignancies is given in **Table 4**. The main problem with narrative reporting is that some of the key descriptors may be missing and the standardized lexicon may not be used, thus contributing to ambiguity in management.

CONCLUSION

Early detection, accurate characterization and staging is essential for optimal management of pancreatic cancer, and imaging plays a crucial role. Sonography is frequently performed as the first investigation for evaluation of these patients. Both MDCT and MRI perform equally well in the detection and staging of pancreatic malignancies with CT being the most validated modality owing to faster acquisition and high spatial resolution. MRI is equally accurate and may have an edge in case of smaller lesions, demonstrating relationship with ducts and in cases where intravenous contrast cannot be given. DW MRI is very sensitive in detection of liver metastases. EUS provides limited but detailed

Table 4: Structured reporting format for suspected pancreatic malignancy.

Pancreatic lesion present: Y/N	• Location—head/neck/body/tail • Size • Enhancement relative to pancreas (in pancreatic phase)—hypo/iso/hyper • Misc—necrosis/calcification/none • Contour bulge—yes/no • Confined to pancreas with clear fat planes—yes/no • PD dilatation—yes with atrophy/yes without atrophy/no • Biliary dilatation—yes/no • GB status • Diagnosis—adenocarcinoma/others (specify differentials)
Status of arteries	• Arterial contact—yes/no • Celiac axis—no contact/abutment/encasement • CHA—no contact/abutment/encasement Surgically reconstructible—yes/no • SMA—no contact/abutment/encasement Surgically reconstructible—yes/no • Contact with first jejunal branch of SMA—yes/no • GDA—involved/free • Aorta—involved/free • Variant arterial anatomy with tumor contact—yes/no • Significant atherosclerosis at origin of celiac axis/SMA—yes/no
Status of veins	• Venous contact—yes/no • Least distance to SMV • SMV—no contact/abutment/encasement Surgically reconstructible—yes/no • Contact with the most proximal draining jejunal branch (into SMV)—yes/no • PV—no contact/abutment/encasement Surgically reconstructible—yes/no • Length of venous involvement • Contact with IVC—yes/no
• Adjacent structure infiltration • Adenopathy—yes/no (site) • Metastases—yes/no (liver/peritoneal/others—specify) • Ascites—yes/no	
ADV- EUS +/– sampling/MRI	

Flowchart 2: Imaging and management protocol in a patient suspected to have pancreatic malignancy.

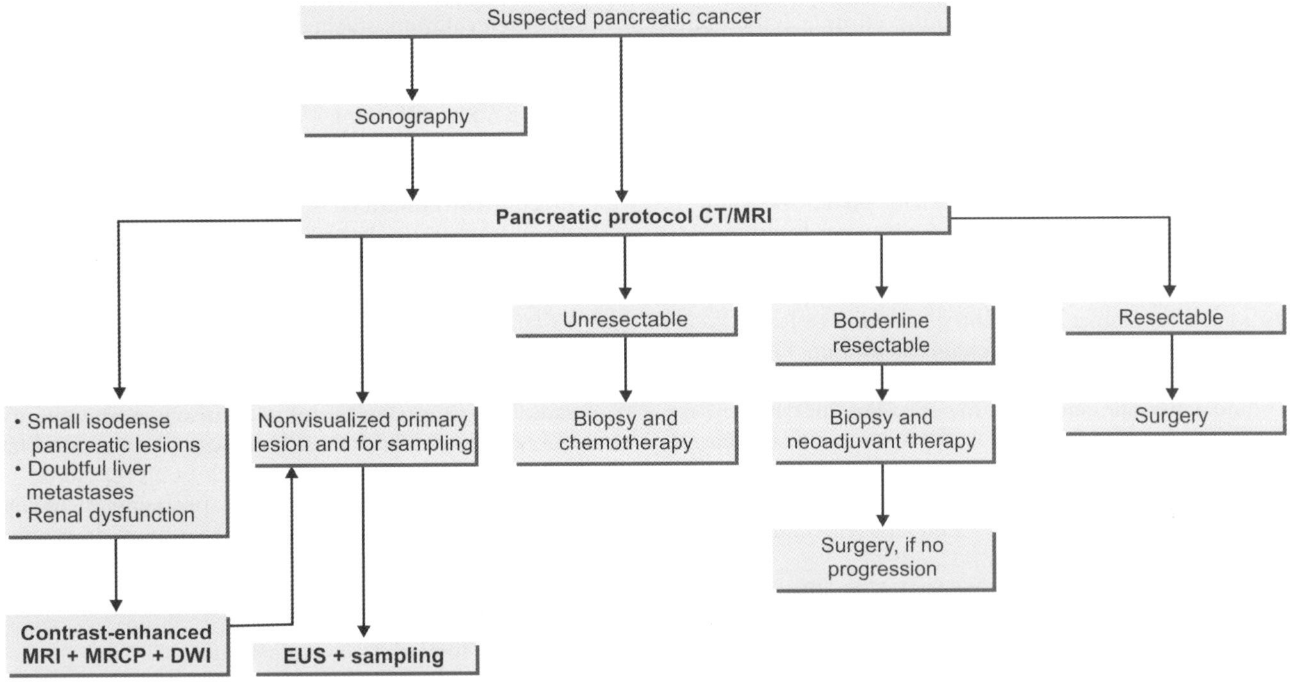

information and plays a role in image-guided sampling. **Flowchart 2** shows imaging and management algorithm in a patient suspected to have pancreatic malignancy. Structured reporting improves evaluation and provides accurate assessment of the status of vessels, and better communication with the surgeon.

NCCN panel recommends that all diagnostic and surgical management decisions must involve multidisciplinary consultations in high volume centers. Imaging also plays a role in post-therapy response assessment and this is the field of active research, especially on newer and functional imaging modalities.

REFERENCES

1. Tamm EP, Balachandran A, Bhosale PR, Katz MH, Fleming JB, Lee JH, et al. Imaging of pancreatic adenocarcinoma: update on staging/resectability. Radiol Clin North Am. 2012;50(3):407-28.
2. Jeffrey RB. Pancreatic cancer: radiologic imaging. Gastroenterol Clin North Am. 2012;41(1):159-77.
3. NCCN Clinical Practice Guidelines in Oncology. Pancreatic Adenocarcinoma. Version 1.2016. nccn.org.
4. Allema JH, Reinders ME, van Gulik TM, van Leeuwen DJ, Verbeek PC, de Wit LT, et al. Results of pancreaticoduodenectomy for ampullary carcinoma and analysis of prognostic factors for survival. Surgery. 1995;117(3):247-53.
5. Almoguera C, Shibata D, Forrester K, Martin J, Arnheim N, Perucho M. Most human carcinomas of the exocrine pancreas contain mutant c-K-ras genes. Cell. 1988;53(4):549-54.
6. Kinney T. Evidence-based imaging of pancreatic malignancies. Surg Clin North Am. 2010;90(2):235-49.
7. Kaneko OF, Lee DM, Wong J, Kadell BM, Reber HA, Lu DSK, et al. Performance of multidetector computed tomographic angiography in determining surgical resectability of pancreatic head adenocarcinoma. J Comput Assist Tomogr. 2010;34(5):732-8.
8. Schima W, Ba-Ssalamah A, Goetzinger P, Scharitzer M, Koelblinger C. State-of-the-art magnetic resonance imaging of pancreatic cancer. Top Magn Reson Imaging TMRI. 2007;18(6):421-9.
9. Kartalis N, Manikis GC, Loizou L, Albiin N, Zöllner FG, Del Chiaro M, et al. Diffusion-weighted MR imaging of pancreatic cancer: A comparison of mono-exponential, bi-exponential and non-Gaussian kurtosis models. Eur J Radiol Open. 2016;3:79-85.
10. Kawada N, Tanaka S. Elastography for the pancreas: Current status and future perspective. World J Gastroenterol. 2016;22(14):3712-24.
11. Iglesias-Garcia J, Larino-Noia J, Abdulkader I, Forteza J, Dominguez-Munoz JE. EUS elastography for the characterization of solid pancreatic masses. Gastrointest Endosc. 2009;70(6):1101-8.
12. Gonçalves B, Soares JB, Bastos P. Endoscopic Ultrasound in the diagnosis and staging of pancreatic cancer. GE Port J Gastroenterol. 2015;22(4):161-71.
13. Klauss M, Stiller W, Fritz F, Kieser M, Werner J, Kauczor HU, et al. Computed tomography perfusion analysis of pancreatic carcinoma. J Comput Assist Tomogr. 2012;36(2):237-42.

14. Yadav AK, Sharma R, Kandasamy D, Pradhan RK, Garg PK, Bhalla AS, et al. Perfusion CT—can it resolve the pancreatic carcinoma versus mass forming chronic pancreatitis conundrum? Pancreatol Off J Int Assoc Pancreatol IAP Al. 2016.
15. Klauss M, Stiller W, Pahn G, Fritz F, Kieser M, Werner J, et al. Dual-energy perfusion-CT of pancreatic adenocarcinoma. Eur J Radiol. 2013;82(2):208-14.
16. Kang KM, Lee JM, Yoon JH, Kiefer B, Han JK, Choi BI. Intravoxel incoherent motion diffusion-weighted MR Imaging for characterization of focal pancreatic lesions. Radiology. 2013;270(2):444-53.
17. Klauss M, Lemke A, Grünberg K, Simon D, Re TJ, Wente MN, et al. Intravoxel incoherent motion MRI for the differentiation between mass forming chronic pancreatitis and pancreatic carcinoma. Invest Radiol. 2011;46(1):57-63.
18. Re TJ, Lemke A, Klauss M, Laun FB, Simon D, Grünberg K, et al. Enhancing pancreatic adenocarcinoma delineation in diffusion derived intravoxel incoherent motion f-maps through automatic vessel and duct segmentation. Magn Reson Med. 2011;66(5):1327-32.
19. Kim JH, Park SH, Yu ES, Kim M-H, Kim J, Byun JH, et al. Visually isoattenuating pancreatic adenocarcinoma at dynamic-enhanced CT: frequency, clinical and pathologic characteristics, and diagnosis at imaging examinations. Radiology. 2010;257(1):87-96.
20. Prokesch RW, Chow LC, Beaulieu CF, Bammer R, Jeffrey RB. Isoattenuating pancreatic adenocarcinoma at multi-detector row CT: secondary signs. Radiology. 2002;224(3):764-8.
21. Park MJ, Kim YK, Choi S, Rhim H, Lee WJ, Choi D. Preoperative detection of small pancreatic carcinoma: value of adding diffusion-weighted imaging to conventional MR imaging for improving confidence level. Radiology. 2014;273(2):433-43.
22. Goodman M, Willmann JK, Jeffrey RB. Incidentally discovered solid pancreatic masses: imaging and clinical observations. Abdom Imaging. 2012;37(1):91-7.
23. Shanbhogue AKP, Fasih N, Surabhi VR, Doherty GP, Shanbhogue DKP, Sethi SK. A clinical and radiologic review of uncommon types and causes of pancreatitis. RadioGraphics. 2009;29(4):1003-26.
24. Sharma R, Kandasamy D. Imaging of pancreatic cancer. In: Garg PK (Eds). ECAB clinical update—pancreatic tumors. 2013th edn. Elsevier Health Sciences.
25. Lee H, Lee JK, Kang SS, Choi D, Jang KT, Kim JH, et al. Is there any clinical or radiologic feature as a preoperative marker for differentiating mass-forming pancreatitis from early-stage pancreatic adenocarcinoma? Hepatogastroenterology. 2007;54(79):2134-40.
26. Ichikawa T, Sou H, Araki T, Arbab AS, Yoshikawa T, Ishigame K, et al. Duct-penetrating sign at MRCP: usefulness for differentiating inflammatory pancreatic mass from pancreatic carcinomas. Radiology. 2001;221(1):107-16.
27. Coakley FV, Hanley-Knutson K, Mongan J, Barajas R, Bucknor M, Qayyum A. Pancreatic imaging mimics: Part 1, imaging mimics of pancreatic adenocarcinoma. AJR. 2012;199(2):301-8.
28. Sahani DV, Sainani NI, Deshpande V, Shaikh MS, Frinkelberg DL, Fernandez-del Castillo C. Autoimmune pancreatitis: disease evolution, staging, response assessment, and CT features that predict response to corticosteroid therapy. Radiology. 2009;250(1):118-29.
29. Choi SY, Kim SH, Kang TW, Song KD, Park HJ, Choi YH. Differentiating mass-forming autoimmune pancreatitis from pancreatic ductal adenocarcinoma on the basis of contrast-enhanced MRI and DWI findings. Am J Roentgenol. 2016;206(2):291-300.
30. Blasbalg R, Baroni RH, Costa DN, Machado MCC. MRI features of groove pancreatitis. AJR. 2007;189(1):73-80.
31. Al-Hawary MM, Francis IR, Chari ST, Fishman EK, Hough DM, Lu DS, et al. Pancreatic ductal adenocarcinoma radiology reporting template: consensus statement of the Society of Abdominal Radiology and the American Pancreatic Association. Radiology. 2014;270(1):248-60.
32. Callery MP, Chang KJ, Fishman EK, Talamonti MS, William Traverso L, Linehan DC. Pretreatment assessment of resectable and borderline resectable pancreatic cancer: expert consensus statement. Ann Surg Oncol. 2009;16(7):1727-33.
33. Lall CG, Howard TJ, Skandarajah A, DeWitt JM, Aisen AM, Sandrasegaran K. New concepts in staging and treatment of locally advanced pancreatic head cancer. AJR. 2007;189(5):1044-50.
34. Ishikawa O, Ohigashi H, Imaoka S, Furukawa H, Sasaki Y, Fujita M, et al. Preoperative indications for extended pancreatectomy for locally advanced pancreas cancer involving the portal vein. Ann Surg. 1992;215(3):231-6.
35. Raptopoulos V, Steer ML, Sheiman RG, Vrachliotis TG, Gougoutas CA, Movson JS. The use of helical CT and CT angiography to predict vascular involvement from pancreatic cancer: correlation with findings at surgery. AJR. 1997;168(4):971-7.
36. Chun YS, Milestone BN, Watson JC, Cohen SJ, Burtness B, Engstrom PF, et al. Defining venous involvement in borderline resectable pancreatic cancer. Ann Surg Oncol. 2010;17(11):2832-8.
37. Hough TJ, Raptopoulos V, Siewert B, Matthews JB. Teardrop superior mesenteric vein: CT sign for unresectable carcinoma of the pancreas. AJR. 1999;173(6):1509-12.
38. McNulty NJ, Francis IR, Platt JF, Cohan RH, Korobkin M, Gebremariam A. Multidetector row helical CT of the pancreas: effect of contrast-enhanced multiphasic imaging on enhancement of the pancreas, peripancreatic vasculature, and pancreatic adenocarcinoma. Radiology. 2001;220(1):97-102.
39. Pietryga JA, Morgan DE. Imaging preoperatively for pancreatic adenocarcinoma. J Gastrointest Oncol. 2015;6(4):343-57.
40. Li H, Zeng MS, Zhou KR, Jin DY, Lou WH. Pancreatic adenocarcinoma: the different CT criteria for peripancreatic major arterial and venous invasion. J Comput Assist Tomogr. 2005;29(2):170-5.
41. Sai M, Mori H, Kiyonaga M, Kosen K, Yamada Y, Matsumoto S. Peripancreatic lymphatic invasion by pancreatic

carcinoma: evaluation with multidetector row CT. Abdom Imaging. 2010;35(2):154-62.
42. Brennan DDD, Zamboni GA, Raptopoulos VD, Kruskal JB. Comprehensive preoperative assessment of pancreatic adenocarcinoma with 64-section volumetric CT. Radiogr Rev Publ Radiol Soc N Am Inc. 2007;27(6):1653-66.
43. Makino I, Kitagawa H, Ohta T, Nakagawara H, Tajima H, Ohnishi I, et al. Nerve plexus invasion in pancreatic cancer: spread patterns on histopathologic and embryological analyses. Pancreas. 2008;37(4):358-65.
44. Deshmukh SD, Willmann JK, Jeffrey RB. Pathways of extrapancreatic perineural invasion by pancreatic adenocarcinoma: evaluation with 3D volume-rendered MDCT imaging. Am J Roentgenol. 2010;194(3):668-74.
45. Yusoff IF, Mendelson RM, Edmunds SEJ, Ramsay D, Cullingford GL, Fletcher DR, et al. Preoperative assessment of pancreatic malignancy using endoscopic ultrasound. Abdom Imaging. 2003;28(4):556-62.
46. Pisters PW, Lee JE, Vauthey JN, Charnsangavej C, Evans DB. Laparoscopy in the staging of pancreatic cancer. Br J Surg. 2001;88(3):325-37.
47. Tao L, Zhang L, Xiu D, Yuan C, Ma Z, Jiang B. Prognostic significance of K-ras mutations in pancreatic cancer: a meta-analysis. World J Surg Oncol. 2016;14:146.
48. Katz MHG, Fleming JB, Bhosale P, Varadhachary G, Lee JE, Wolff R, et al. Response of borderline resectable pancreatic cancer to neoadjuvant therapy is not reflected by radiographic indicators. Cancer. 2012;118(23):5749-56.
49. Bockhorn M, Uzunoglu FG, Adham M, Imrie C, Milicevic M, Sandberg AA, et al. Borderline resectable pancreatic cancer: a consensus statement by the International Study Group of Pancreatic Surgery (ISGPS). Surgery. 2014;155(6):977-88.
50. Brook OR, Brook A, Vollmer CM, Kent TS, Sanchez N, Pedrosa I. Structured reporting of multiphasic CT for pancreatic cancer: potential effect on staging and surgical planning. Radiology. 2015;274(2):464-72.

CHAPTER 90

Cystic Pancreatic Tumors and Neuroendocrine Tumors of Pancreas

Jyoti Kumar, Alpana Manchanda, Sapna Singh

CYSTIC PANCREATIC TUMORS

Cystic pancreatic tumors are a diverse group of lesions with different clinical presentation, histology, biologic behavior and prognostic implications. Imaging plays a key role in stratifying the risk in these patients, and hence, deciding upon the treatment options and appropriate follow-up strategy. Most of these tumors are picked up incidentally and increasing use of cross-sectional imaging techniques and their improved resolution have led to a 20-fold increase in the incidental detection of these lesions.[1] This has led to an increase in surgery for these tumors. In many instances, these resected lesions turn out to be benign and the surgery is actually unjustified.[2] Few of these tumors, especially when large, have characteristic imaging features that can aid in differentiation of these cystic masses. However, smaller lesions can have indeterminate findings on imaging and management protocols may still be confusing.[3]

Imaging Modalities

Both multidetector computed tomography (MDCT) and magnetic resonance imaging (MRI) are widely used in characterizing the cystic lesions of pancreas. MDCT is usually the primary modality of investigation with high spatial and temporal resolution. Its wide availability and ease of interpretation are the other advantages. CT also shows calcification within lesions to a greater advantage than MRI. In various studies, the accuracy of MDCT (56–85%) has been found to be comparable to MRI in characterizing cystic pancreatic lesions.[4–6]

Magnetic resonance imaging (MRI), on the other hand, has superior soft tissue and contrast resolution. Hence, it is an excellent technique to assess internal morphological features of cystic tumors, especially small cystic tumors measuring <3 cm.[7] Three-dimensional magnetic resonance cholangiopancreaticography (MRCP) is an effective tool in detecting communication of the lesion with the pancreatic duct. Sainini et al. showed a higher accuracy of MR in revealing ductal communication as compared to CT (100% versus 75% sensitivity).[7] As MR does not involve radiation, it is the preferable modality for follow-up of young patients with cystic pancreatic tumors.[8]

Endoscopic ultrasound (EUS) is an excellent technique to depict internal morphology of cystic lesions, showing internal septations and nodularity to a greater advantage, and hence assessing the aggressiveness of the pathology. It also enables sampling of fluid and solid contents of the lesion.[9] However, this is an invasive technique and highly operator dependent. It allows limited evaluation of the pancreatic tail region. It is used predominantly when CT and MR findings are indeterminate and in asymptomatic cysts as symptomatic cysts would anyways warrant a resection.

Clinical Presentation

Most of these cystic tumors are picked up incidentally during work-up for other nonrelated conditions.[9] Symptomatic cystic tumors mostly present with abdominal lump and pain. Jaundice and pancreatitis may result from biliary/pancreatic ductal communication. If it is an advanced cystic malignancy, patients may present with symptoms of pain, weight loss or jaundice.[3,9]

Classification

Cystic tumors of pancreas may be classified into relatively common cystic tumors and rare cystic tumors **(Table 1)**. The common cystic tumors may be serous cystadenoma, mucinous neoplasms (mucinous cystic neoplasm and intraductal papillary mucinous neoplasm) or solid pseudopapillary neoplasm. The rare cystic tumors include lymphangioma, teratoma, paraganglioma or solid tumors which have undergone cystic degeneration such as adenocarcinoma, neuroendocrine tumors and metastases.[10]

Morphological Classification

On the basis of imaging appearances, pancreatic cystic lesions can be classified into four major categories—unilocular appearance, microcystic lesion, macrocystic lesion and cysts with solid component **(Figs. 1A to D) (Table 2)**.[10]

Unilocular cysts include cysts with no internal septation, calcification or nodularity. Although inflammatory pseudocysts are the prototype example, cystic tumors that may uncommonly have a unilocular appearance are intraductal papillary mucinous neoplasms (IPMNs) and serous cystadenoma. Since pseudocysts are the most common cystic lesions of pancreas, correlation with history of acute or chronic pancreatitis is of paramount importance. Microcystic lesions are cysts with internal septations resulting in formation of mutiple tiny cysts which are usually more than 6 in number and <2 cm in size. The main example of a microcystic lesion is serous cystadenoma. Macrocystic lesions are multilocular cysts with fewer loculi (<6 cm) which are larger in size (>2 cm). The characteristic example of a macrocystic lesion is mucinous cystic neoplasm (MCN) and side branch IPMN. Cystic lesions with a solid component may be unilocular or multilocular. Mucinous cystic neoplasms or intraductal papillary mucinous neoplasm may have this appearance.[10]

Serous Cystadenoma (Table 3)

Serous cystadenoma accounts for 1–2% of exocrine pancreatic tumors. About 80% of these lesions occur in older women, with an average age of 65 years.[11-13] There is a slight preponderance of these tumors in the head region but they can be seen to occur throughout the pancreas. These lesions are mostly asymptomatic, and hence can become large at presentation. The larger lesions may result in mass effect and nonspecific abdominal discomfort.

Table 1: Classification of cystic pancreatic tumors.

Common Cystic Tumors • Serous cystadenoma • *Mucinous neoplasms*: – Mucinous cystic neoplasm – Intraductal papillary mucinous neoplasm • Solid pseudopapillary neoplasm
Rare Cystic Tumors • Lymphangioma • Teratoma • Paraganglioma • Cystic degeneration of solid tumors such as adenocarcinoma, neuroendocrine tumors and metastases

Table 2: Morphological classification of cystic pancreatic tumors.

• Unilocular • Microcystic • Macrocystic • Cystic lesions with solid component

Table 3: Key points of serous cystadenoma.

• Mostly in older women; average age 65 years • Increased incidence in von Hippel-Lindau disease • Typically microcystic in appearance with lobulated outline • Central scar seen in 30% cases and when seen is pathognomonic • Only hypervascular cystic tumor of pancreas • Benign tumor with no malignant potential

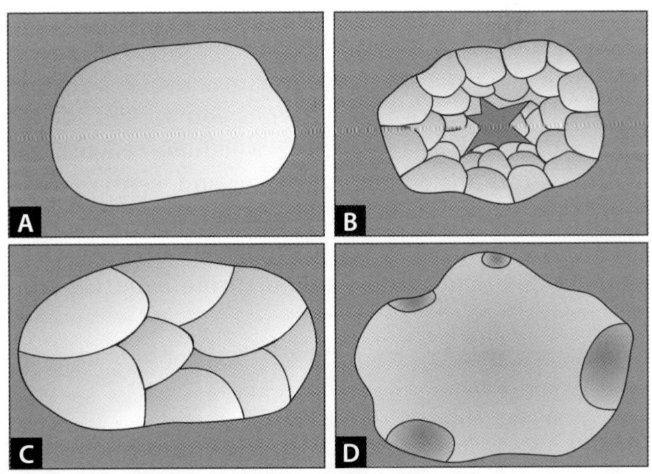

Figs. 1A to D: Morphological classification of cystic lesions: (A) Unilocular cyst with no internal septations; (B) Microcystic appearance with formation of multiple small cysts (>6 in number, <2 cm in size); (C) Macrocystic lesion with larger and fewer cysts; (D) Cyst with solid mural nodule.

Since these are benign lesions with no malignant potential, surgery is not indicated unless the large size (>4 cm) of the lesion mandates surgery because of its mass effect and resultant symptoms or rapid growth (approximately

2 cm/year).[14-16] In cases of von Hippel-Lindau disease, there may be an increased incidence of serous cystadenomas.[14]

These are typically microcystic lesions showing a honey-comb appearance on gross inspection. These are well-circumscribed lesions with lobulated outline and are not encapsulated. These fine external lobulations result from the larger cysts in the periphery of the lesion in this microcystic tumor. These lesions may have a central scar with or without stellate calcification. Although seen in only 30% of serous cystadenomas, it is considered pathognomonic when present.[9]

On ultrasound, these lesions are seen as lobulated lesions with hypoechoic cysts and hyperechoic fibrous component. Calcification may be seen within the fibrous scar when present. However, the lesion may appear solid due to multiple interfaces of the septations within the lesion.[3]

On CT, the lobulated microcystic appearance can be appreciated. Central stellate scar with calcification may be seen **(Fig. 2)**. The lesion may have a solid appearance because of the tiny size of these cyst separated by multiple septations. On contrast administration, the septae and scar enhance avidly with persistent enhancement on delayed images. Absence of ductal obstruction or invasion of surrounding structures confirms the benign nature of these lesions as these tumors displace surrounding structures rather than invade them.

MRI can aid in delineating the microcystic appearance of these tumors to a greater advantage when these are seen as high signal intensity structures on T2-weighted images **(Figs. 3A to C)**. The fibrous component is seen as hypointense on T1- and T2-weighted images. On contrast administration, the scar and septae show intense enhancement on the arterial phase with persistent enhancement on the delayed images, which helps to differentiate these tumors from hypervascular neuroendocrine tumors of pancreas which show washout on delayed images.[3]

Uncommonly, serous cystadenomas may have a macrocystic or oligocystic appearance (in less than 10% of cases) **(Fig. 4)**.[10] In these cases, mucinous cystic neoplasm is a close differential. In a study by Cohen-Scali et al. presence of a combination of any 3 of the following imaging features could help distinguish between the two entities with a specificity of 100%—location in head region, lobulated outline, wall thickness <2 mm and absence of wall enhancement. These findings favor the diagnosis of serous cystadenoma.[17]

Mucinous Cystic Neoplasm (Table 4)

Mucinous cystadenoma accounts for approximately 2.5% of exocrine pancreatic tumors.[18] Mucinous cystic neoplasms are most frequently encountered in middle-aged women

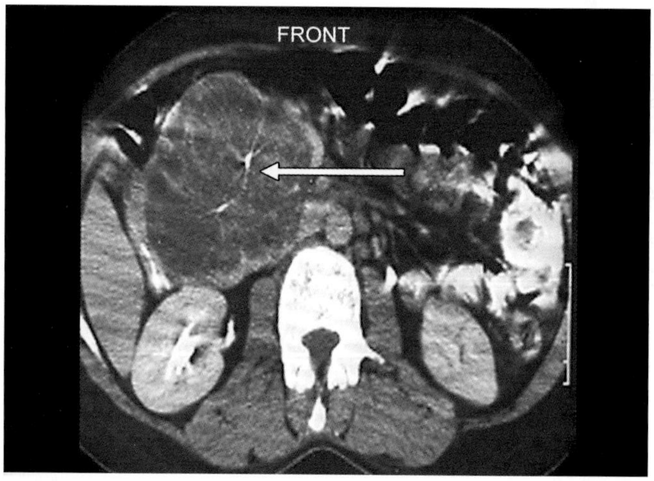

Fig. 2: Serous cystadenoma in a 62-year-old woman: Axial CECT image reveals a microcystic lesion with lobulated outline in the pancreatic head region. Central scar with stellate calcfication (arrow) is seen in this case which is pathognomonic for the lesion.

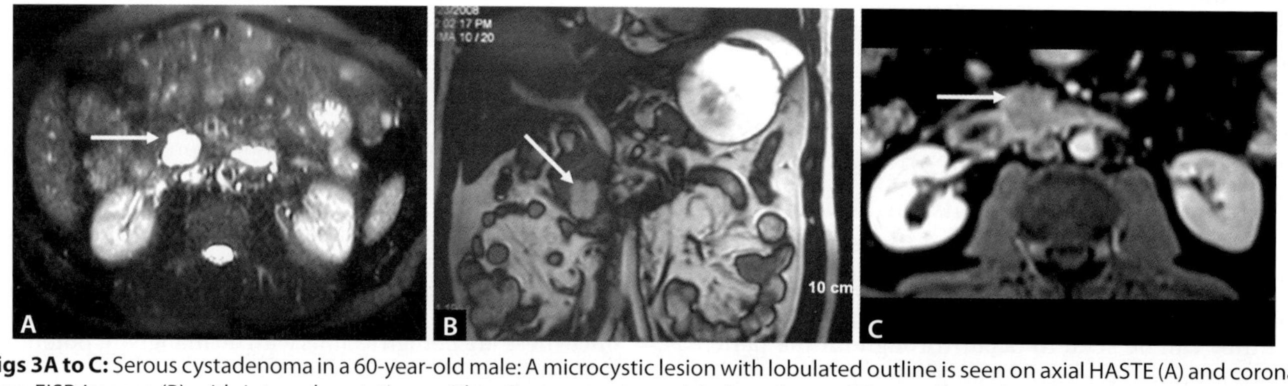

Figs 3A to C: Serous cystadenoma in a 60-year-old male: A microcystic lesion with lobulated outline is seen on axial HASTE (A) and coronal True FISP images (B) with internal septations within. Postcontrast arterial phase image (C) reveals subtle enhancement of the septae
Abbreviations: HASTE, Half-fourier acquisition single-shot turbo spin-echo; True FISP, True fast imaging with steady state precession.

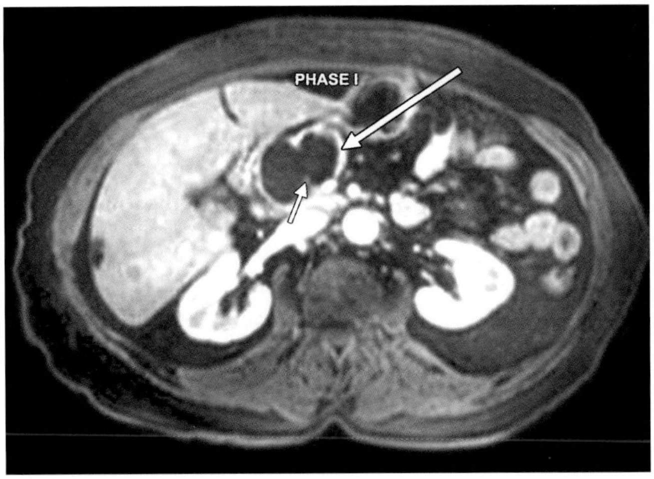

Fig. 4: Macrocystic serous cystadenoma in a 55-year-old man: A lobulated macrocystic lesion is seen in the head region of pancreas (long arrow) on this axial T1-weighted postgadolinium MR image. Thin septal enhancement (short thin arrow) is seen.

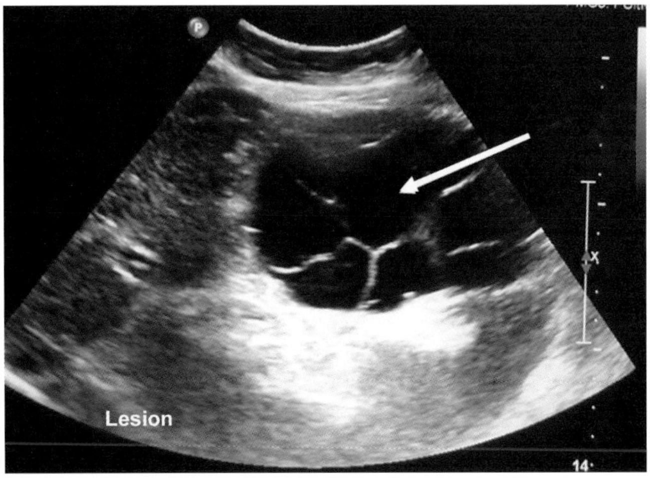

Fig. 5: Mucinous cystic neoplasm in a 52-year-old woman: US images shows a well-marginated macrocystic mass arising from the pancreatic tail.

Table 4: Key points of mucinous cystic neoplasm.

- Almost exclusively in women
- Average age 50 years, slightly lesser than serous cystadenoma
- Typically macrocystic in appearance with smooth outline
- Curvilinear calcification is considered specific for the diagnosis
- Thick wall, mural or septal calcification and internal enhancing soft tissue component are predictive of malignancy
- Unlike IPMNs which are also macrocystic, there is no ductal communication

with an average age of 50 years, slightly lesser than that of serous cystadenomas. These are known to occur almost exclusively in women with a frequency of approximately 99.7%.[3,19]

Patients may be symptomatic due to mass effect caused by the neoplasm although they are asymptomatic in 75% cases.[20] These neoplasms have a malignant potential and hence are considered surgical lesions. On histology, these could range from benign mucinous cystadenoma, borderline mucinous cystic tumor, mucinous neoplasm with carcinoma *in situ* to a frankly malignant mucinous cystadenocarcinoma. The stromal elements of these tumors are similar to ovarian stroma unlike IPMNs which have ductal origin stroma. Sampling of the lesion may not be an accurate method of differentiating between benign and malignant lesions as different parts of the lesion may have different configuration of epithelium.[21]

These neoplasms are most commonly macrocystic in appearance. On ultrasound, a well-circumscribed multicystic mass is often seen which may have septations, mural nodules or calcification **(Fig. 5)**. Rarely, debris or hemorrhage may be seen within these cysts.[3]

On CT, these are well-defined encapsulated lesions with smooth outline **(Fig. 6)**. Calcification may be seen along the septae or wall of the lesion **(Fig. 7)**. This may be seen in approximately 15% of cases. Curvilinear calcification along the wall of the lesion is considered specific for this diagnosis.[22] On contrast administration, the wall is seen to enhance along with septae and mural nodules. In a study by Procacci et al.[23] the following imaging features were predictive of malignancy—thick wall, mural or septal calcification and internal enhancing soft tissue component.

MR can better delineate the internal morphology of the lesion. On T2-weighted imaging, the lesion is usually seen as hyperintense fluid-filled multiloculated lesion with hypointense wall. The signal intensity of the cyst, however, may be variable due to proteinaceous contents of the cyst. The wall and septations enhance on contrast administration, more so on the delayed images due to fibrous nature of the wall **(Figs. 8A and B)**. If the lesion results in pancreatic ductal obstruction, concomitant pancreatitis may result which may be seen as glandular atrophy, ductal dilatation and decreased signal on T1-weighted images with delayed enhancement.[3,24]

Side branch IPMNs are a close-imaging differential diagnosis. Patient demographics and absence of ductal communication in MCNs can help in differentiating the two entities. Although they do not communicate with ductal system, they can result in ductal obstruction, especially when aggressive. MCNs are most commonly encountered in body and tail region of pancreas wheras the uncinate process is the typical location of side branch IPMN.[9,21]

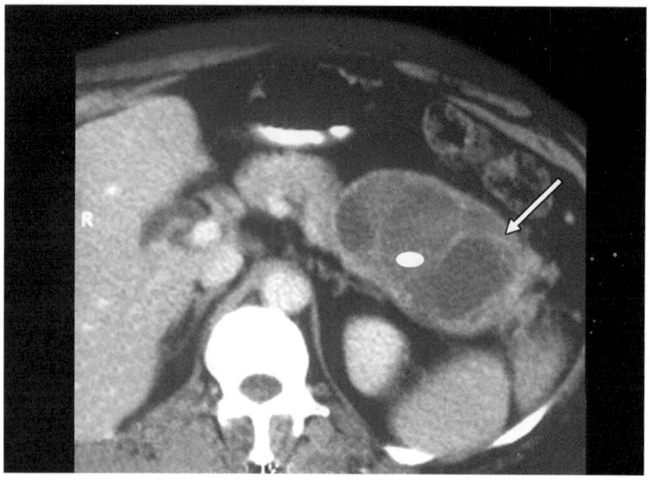

Fig. 6: Mucinous cystic neoplasm in a 51-year-old woman: Axial CECT image depicts a well-circumscribed macrocystic lesion in pancreatic tail (arrow) with variable attenuation of the internal contents of the cyst (dot) which could be due to proteinaceous contents.

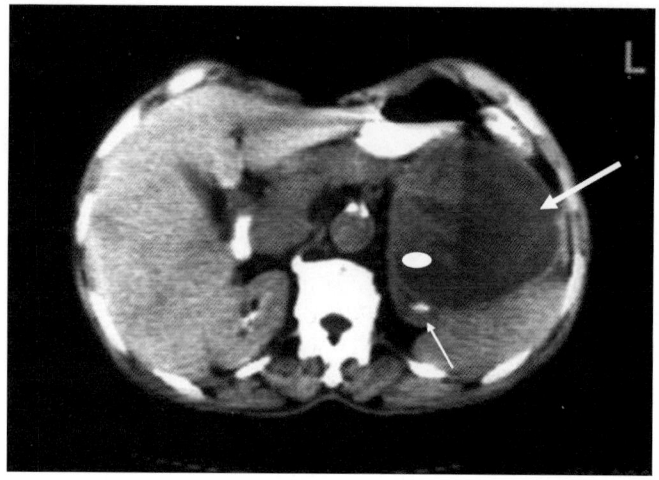

Fig. 7: Mucinous cystic neoplasm in a 48-year-old woman: CECT image showing a unilocular thin-walled cystic mass in the pancreatic tail (arrow) with small peripheral calcification in the inferior part of the cyst (short thin arrow).

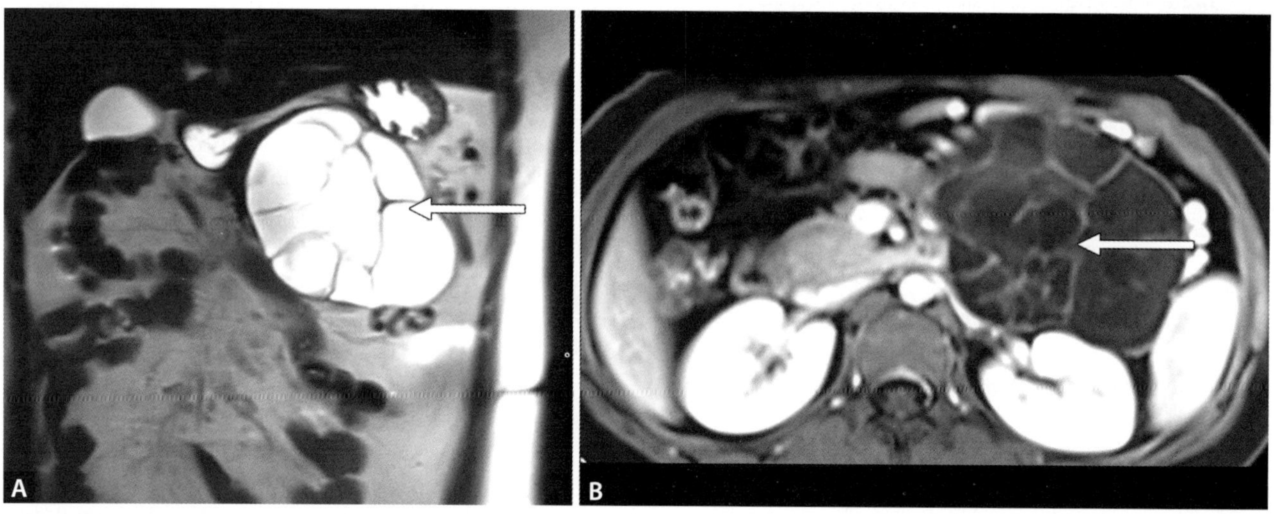

Figs. 8A and B: Macrocystic neoplasm in a 52-year-old woman: Coronal HASTE (A) and axial postgadolinium (B) images reveal a well-circumscribed macrocystic neoplasm in the tail region of pancreas with enhancing septae.

Intraductal Papillary Mucinous Neoplasm (Table 5)

Intraductal papillary mucinous neoplasms (IPMNs) are also mucinous tumors arising from ductal epithelium and may be main duct, side branch or mixed type. 70% of these lesions are encountered in men with a mean age of 65 years.[25,26]

These lesions have a variable degree of aggressiveness with risk of malignancy being higher in main duct and mixed type IPMNs than side branch IPMNs.[27,28] The pathological spectrum ranges from benign adenomas to invasive carcinomas.

Table 5: Key points of intraductal papillary mucinous neoplasm.

- 70% are seen in men with an average age of 65 years
- Can be main duct, side branch or combined type
- Side branch IPMNs present as cystic pancreatic lesions
- Uncinate process is the classical site of side branch IPMN
- Communication with pancreatic duct is pathognomonic of this cystic tumor
- Copious mucin extruding from bulging papilla on endoscopy is highly suggestive
- Side branch lesion of size >3 cm, main duct component, enhancing soft tissue, enhancing MPD wall and dilatation of CBD are pointers towards aggressive nature.

Abbreviations: MPD: Main pancreatic duct; CBD: Common bile duct.

Main duct IPMN does not fall into the category of a cystic pancreatic neoplasm and mainly presents as ductal dilatation. It is the side branch IPMN which generally presents as a pleomorphic cystic lesion communicating with the pancreatic duct. The cystic lesion is actually the mucin distended side branch which is affected by the pathology. Communication with pancreatic duct is the most important imaging feature which is in contrast to other cystic neoplasm of pancreas. Serous cystadenoma, mucinous cystic neoplasm or solid pseudopapillary neoplasm generally do not show any communication with the pancreatic duct.[21]

On ultrasound, main duct IPMN is seen as dilatation of pancreatic main duct **(Fig. 9)** whereas a well-defined cystic mass may be seen in the case of a side branch IPMN. Communication of the cystic lesion with pancreatic duct cannot be appreciated on ultrasound in most cases. Other ancillary features such as mural nodularity, mucin globules or septations may be seen on ultrasound depending on the aggressive nature of the lesion. As ultrasound features are most often nonspecific, further imaging is required to evaluate these lesions.[3,21]

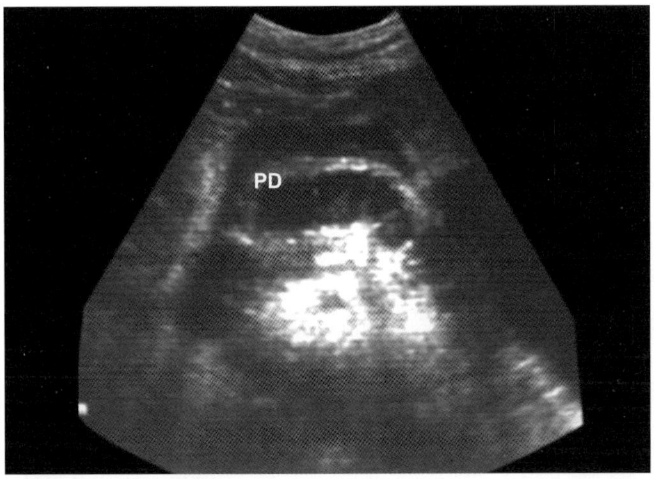

Fig. 9: Main duct IPMN in a 55-year-old male: US image depicts a markedly dilated main pancreatic duct with few-filling defects within.

On CT, a side branch IPMN appears as a pleomorphic cystic lesion most often in the uncinate process, which is the classical site **(Figs. 10A and B)**. Communication with pancreatic duct is best seen on curved multiplanar reformatted images. Main duct IPMN is seen as diffuse or segmental dilatation of the pancreatic duct **(Fig. 11)**. Septations, and filling defects may be seen within the dilated duct **(Figs. 12A to C)**. The filling defects may either be mucin globules or soft tissue component associated with a more aggressive lesion; these may be differentiated using contrast-enhanced imaging, where soft tissue enhances and mucin globules do not enhance.[3,21]

MRI with MRCP remains the modality of choice to depict communication of the lesion with the pancreatic duct. The side branch lesion is seen as hyperintense on T2-weighted images and hypointense on T1-weighted images. In main duct IPMN, the duct is dilated with no obvious obstructive lesion or narrowing. The duct may be dilated diffusely or only involving a segment. Papillary bulging may be evident due to copious mucin production by the tumor.[12] Copious mucin extruding from a bulging papilla seen on correlative endoscopic examination is

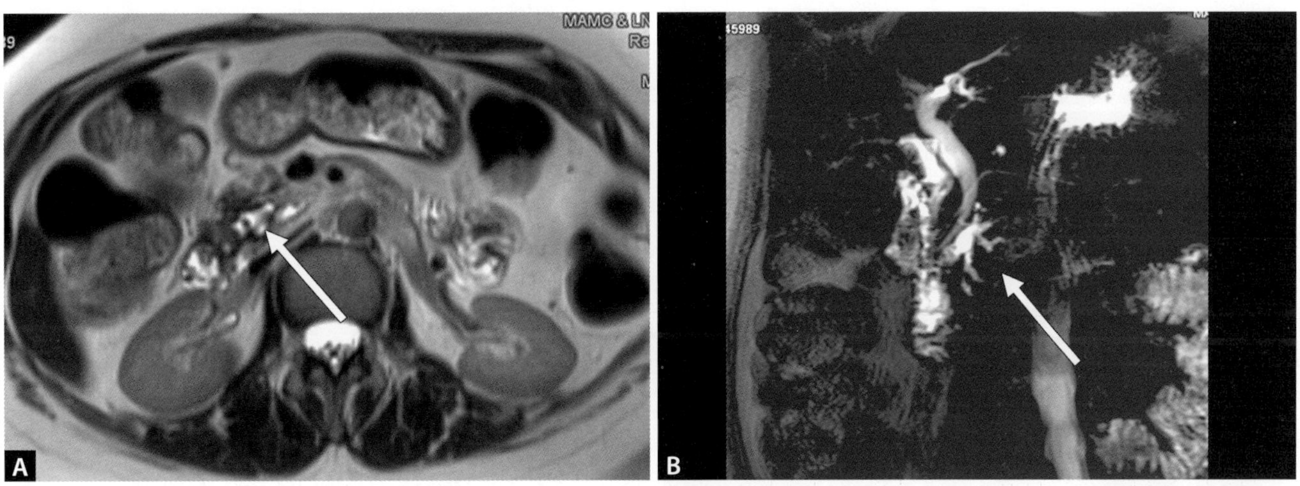

Figs. 10A and B: Side branch IPMN in 56-year-old woman: Axial HASTE image (A) reveals multiple cystic lesions in the region of head and uncinate process (arrow). On rare thick slab coronal image (B), multiple dilated side branches (arrow) are seen in pancreatic head region communicating with the pancreatic duct.

considered highly suggestive of the diagnosis.[29] Combined duct IPMNs are seen as dilatation of both main pancreatic duct and its side branches.

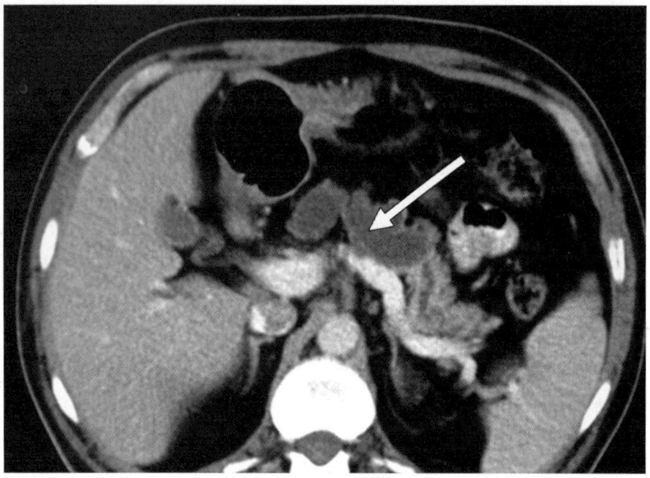

Fig. 11: Main duct IPMN in a 55-year-old male: There is segmental dilatation of the main pancreatic duct (arrow) in the pancreatic body region in this case of segmental main duct IPMN.

Various features on imaging can be the pointers towards the aggressive nature of the pathology. These include main duct dilatation >10 mm, diffuse or multifocal involvement of main pancreatic duct, cystic lesion of size more than 3 cm in case of a side branch lesion, increasing size of these cystic lesions, presence of enhancing soft tissue component or enhancing MPD wall, and dilatation of common bile duct.[3]

Main duct IPMN can be confused with chronic pancreatitis, which can also have duct dilatation and parenchymal atrophy. Presence of irregular beaded appearance of duct with stricture formation and presence of ductal calculi favor the diagnosis of chronic pancreatitis. Bulging papilla and enhancing nodules within the lesion are pointers to the diagnosis of IPMN.

Solid Pseudopapillary Neoplasm (SPN) (Table 6)

This is a rare pancreatic tumor with approximately 1000 cases reported in literature.[30] This is seen to occur mostly

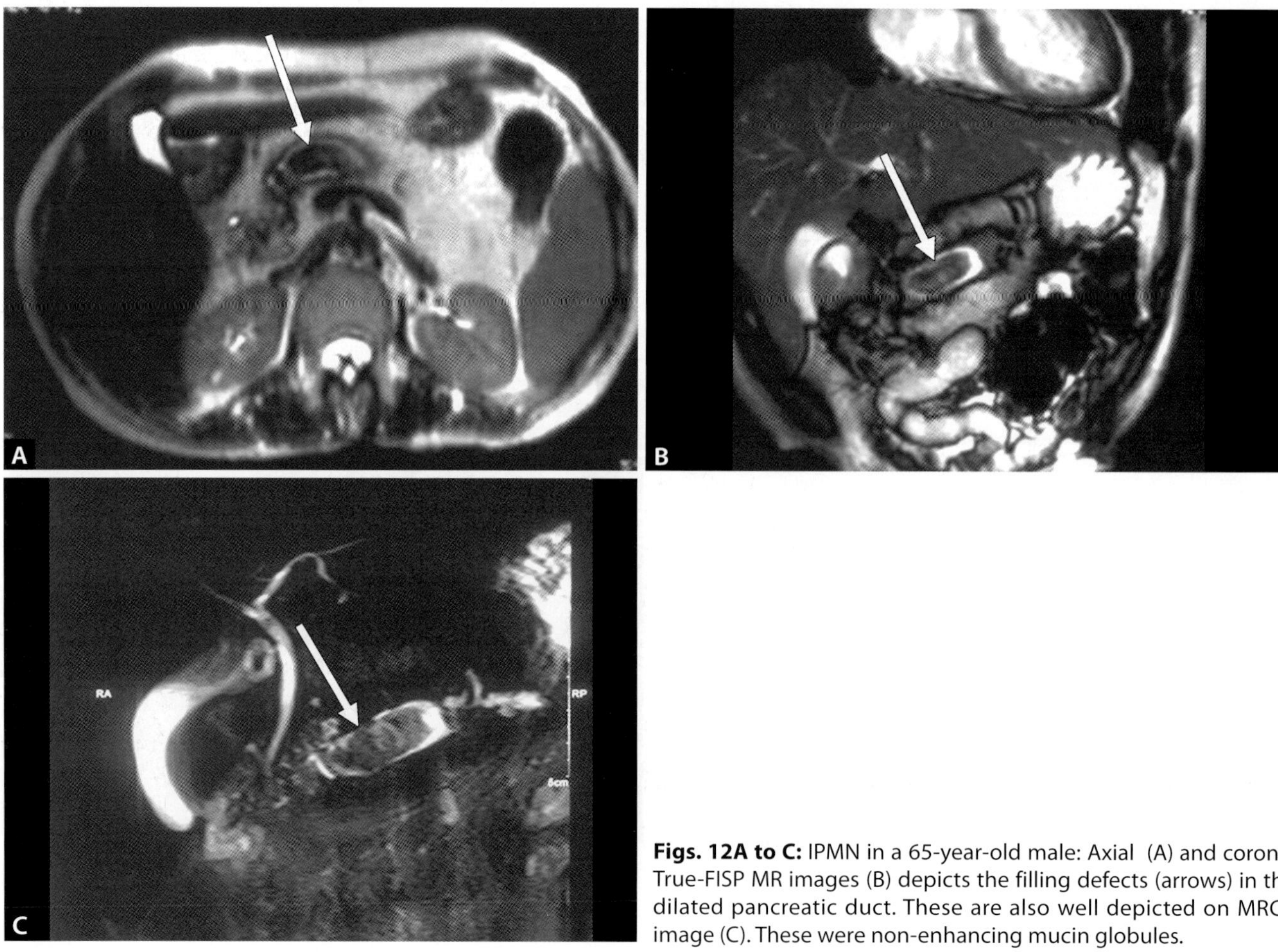

Figs. 12A to C: IPMN in a 65-year-old male: Axial (A) and coronal True-FISP MR images (B) depicts the filling defects (arrows) in the dilated pancreatic duct. These are also well depicted on MRCP image (C). These were non-enhancing mucin globules.

Table 6: Key points of solid pseudopapillary neoplasm.

• Mostly seen in young women with a mean age of 25 years • Encapsulated lesion • Combination of solid and cystic components • Areas of hemorrhage commonly seen • Tumors with low malignant potential and vascular invasion and metastastic disease can be seen in aggressive cases • Survival rates are as high as 96% even with solid pseudopapillary carcinoma after complete surgical resection

in young women with a mean age of 25 years.[31] It is seen most often in the tail region of pancreas.[32]

This tumor is mostly asymptomatic and usually detected when large in size. The average size at detection is 9.3 cm.[33] Larger masses may present with symptoms due to mass effect. These are tumors with low malignant potential and vascular invasion and metastastic disease can be seen in aggressive cases. Treatment is generally surgery and survival rates are as high as 96% even with solid pseudopapillary carcinoma.[3]

On imaging, SPN is a well-demarcated encapsulated lesion. Ultrasound features are nonspecific with a large complex attenuation mass with or without through transmission **(Fig. 13)**.

On CT, these are seen as well-defined encapsulated masses which have a combination of solid and cystic components **(Fig. 14)**. Areas of hemorrhage are commonly seen. The capsule and solid component enhance on contrast administration.[31]

Areas of hemorrhage can be better seen on MR imaging, appearing hypointense on T2-weighted images and hyperintense on T1-weighted images.[31] Hemorrhagic and cystic degeneration is mostly seen in the central part of the lesion while solid component is seen at the periphery. The capsule can be seen as hypointense on T1- and T2-weighted images, which is a key feature on imaging. On contrast administration, solid portions are seen to progressively enhance.[3] Cantisani et al. reviewed 19 cases of SPN and found early and intense enhancement of the capsule which blends with the rest of the solid component during later phases,[34] in most cases of SPN.

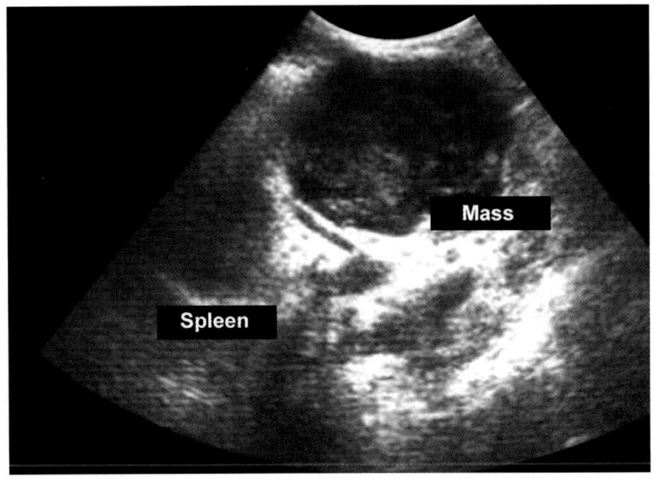

Fig. 13: Solid papillary epithelial neoplasm in a 32-year-old woman: Transverse sonogram image showing a mixed solid cystic mass in the pancreatic tail.

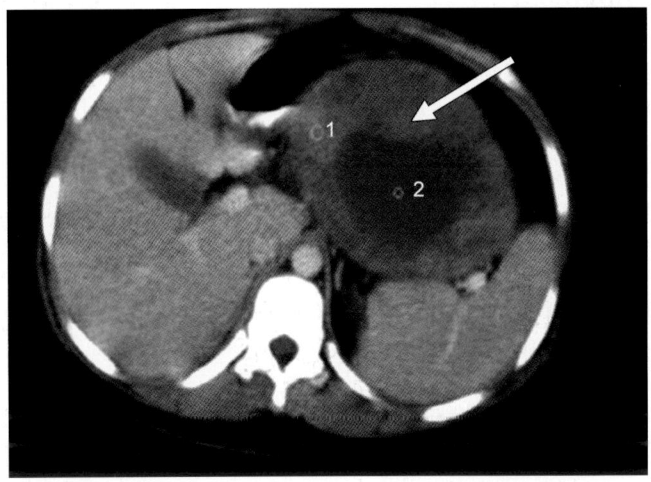

Fig. 14: Solid pseudopapillary neoplasm in a 32-year-old woman: Axial CECT image depicts a large well-circumscribed heterogeneous mass (arrow) with internal necrotic component in the region of pancreatic tail.

UNCOMMON CYSTIC PANCREATIC TUMORS

Cystic Endocrine Tumors

Endocrine tumors are discussed in detail in the latter half of the chapter.

These are usually solid tumors which may undergo cystic or necrotic degeneration. Most of these cystic lesions are the nonsyndromic variety and if syndromic, they are the noninsulin producing tumors. These are generally larger at presentation than the solid variants. One fourth of these cases may be associated with multiple endocrine neoplasia type 1 (MEN I) and the rest are usually sporadic.[35]

These are mostly seen in the body and tail region of pancreas. Solid component of these masses can show hypervascular enhancement on imaging in the arterial phase although this may not be seen in all cases.

Cystic Metastases

Cystic metastases to pancreas most often arise from renal cell carcinoma and lung carcinoma. These are usually seen in late stages of disease when hematogenous metastases are also found at multiple other sites. An exception here is metastases from renal carcinoma where isolated pancreatic metastases have been encountered.[36]

Cystic Teratoma

Cystic teratoma is a very rare tumor with only few cases reported in literature. They can have varied imaging appearances as they can be composed of up to 3 germinal layers. Teratomas are generally well-defined lesions with a variable internal appearance. These could range from predominantly cystic to mixed cystic solid to pure soft tissue masses. They may have fatty elements and areas of calcification. Various studies have shown that although these masses may abut vascular or biliary structures, they generally do not result in invasion or obstruction of these structures.[37,38]

Lymphangiomas

Although lymphangiomas are benign tumors, they may be locally invasive. Less than 1% of lymphangiomas may be seen in abdomen as most of them are encountered in neck and axilla.[39]

These are mostly seen in women with no age predilection. These are usually seen as multiloculated cystic lesions which may abut the pancreas or may be attached to pancreas by a pedicle **(Fig. 15)**. Hemorrhage or infection can occur within the cysts leading to complex attenuation or signal intensity.[3]

Endoscopic Ultrasound (EUS)/EUS-guided Fluid Characteristics of Cystic Lesions

In the evaluation of pancreatic cystic lesions, when the diagnosis is indeterminate on cross-sectional imaging, endoscopic ultrasound can be done to further characterize the internal morphology of these lesions. The diagnostic accuracy of endoscopic ultrasound has been found to be variable in various studies. The largest prospective study by by Brugge et al.[40] reported an accuracy of 50% in detecting septations and mural soft tissue on endoscopic ultrasound.

The additional benefit of EUS is guided fine needle aspiration of cyst fluid that may be done along with the diagnostic procedure. Although it increases the risk of certain complications such as pancreatitis and hemorrhage, it generally carries a favorable benefit to risk ratio.[41]

On fluid analysis, thick viscous fluid with high mucin content is seen in mucinous neoplasms (MCNs and IPMNs) while the fluid is thin and clear in serous cystadenoma.

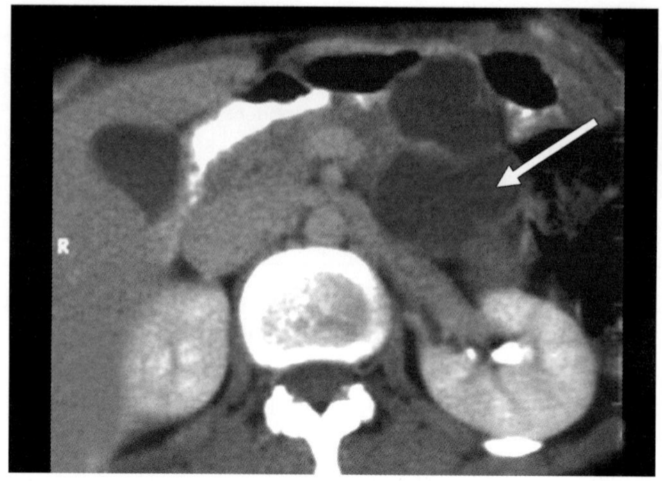

Fig. 15: Lymphangioma in a 30-year-old woman: CECT image shows a well-circumscribed multicystic mass (arrow) with thin septations within abutting the pancreatic tail.

The amylase levels may be raised in IPMNs (>2000 u/mL) as they involve the pancreatic ductal system and are typically low in serous cystadenomas (<250 U/L) and mucinous cystic neoplasms. Level of carcinoembryonic antigen (CEA) is raised in mucinous neoplasms (generally more than 192 mg/mL) and low in SCA (generally less than 5 ng/mL); hence CEA is used as tumor marker to differentiate between mucinous and non-mucinous cystic tumors. Other tumor markers such as CA 125 and CA 72-4 are raised in malignant transformation of mucinous neoplasms. Presence of glycogen is a specific marker for SCA.[3,8]

Management Guidelines

The treatment approach is usually selective, weighing the benefit-risk ratio in each patient. Various factors such as patient's age, tumor location and associated comorbidities need to be considered before a decision is made regarding patient management strategy. Surgery is generally indicated when there is a confident diagnosis of mucinous cystic neoplasm, IPMN with main duct component, side branch IPMN with features suspicious for malignancy, solid pseudopapillary neoplasm and serous cystadenoma when its size is larger than 4 cm or when it is symptomatic.[31] For asymptomatic SCA, annual imaging surveillance is generally considered optimal. Cystic lesions without septations/nodules can be followed up at 6 months and 1 year and then annually for 3 years. Cystic lesions with complex features can be followed up at more closer intervals.[3] On follow-up imaging, increasing cyst size, development of complex features within these cysts or new onset symptoms in this period are worrisome features that may point towards malignant transformation and resection may be considered in good surgical candidates.[31]

PANCREATIC NEUROENDOCRINE TUMORS (TABLE 7)

Pancreatic neuroendocrine tumors (pNETs) are rare tumors and account for only 1–2% of pancreatic neoplasms.[42] Since they are known not to arise from islet cells but from ductal cells that undergo endocrine differentiation, the term islet cell tumors is no longer preferred.[43] These are mostly seen between 40 and 60 years of age.[44]

These tumors may or may not be associated with symptoms due to hormone production, and hence, may be termed functioning and nonfunctioning respectively. The common functioning tumors may be insulinoma, gastrinoma, glucagonoma, VIPoma and somatastainoma.[44] While functioning tumors present with various hormonal symptoms, nonfunctioning tumors present with clinical features of mass effect or due to systemic metastases. Hence, functioning tumors are small at presentation, whereas non-functioning tumors are larger at presentation. It is these larger tumors that have a greater propensity to undergo necrotic/cystic change. Extensive cystic change with a thin peripheral rim can be encountered in 5-10% of cases.[44,45] They may be sporadic or associated with various syndromes such as multiple endocrine neoplasia I, von-Hippel Lindau syndrome, neurofibromatosis and tuberous sclerosis.[46]

As per the WHO 2010 classification system, these have been graded into well-differentiated grade 1 and grade 2 tumors and poorly differentiated grade 3 tumors. This grading has been done based on their mitotic count and cell proliferation (measured as Ki-67 labeling index).[47]

On US examination, these may be seen as well-defined hypoechoic masses. The larger tumors may be more heterogeneous with necrotic/cystic change. Presence of peripancreatic nodes and liver metastases are pointers towards malignancy. Hypervascular pattern may be noted on contrast-enhanced US.[44]

At CT, pNETs are well-circumscribed hypervascular tumors which enhance brightly on late arterial phase images **(Figs. 16A to C)**. However, they may not always be hypervascular, especially the nonfunctioning tumors.[45] Larger tumors can undergo necrotic/cystic degeneration. Cystic appearing neuroendocrine tumors can be differentiated from other cystic lesions of pancreas on the basis of the hypervascular nature of the peripheral rim. This hypervascular rim may be seen in 90% of cystic pNETs in a study by Ligneau et al.[48] In various studies, it has been shown that arterial phase images have a higher sensitivity for detecting pNETs (83–89%) than venous phase images (11–76%).[49,50] However, some tumors may only be seen on venous phase images.[44] Calcification may also be seen in pNETs and is more frequent in nonfunctioning tumors.[45] Lymph node and liver metastases may be seen in malignant pNETs and these are also hypervascular in nature, and hence, more appreciable on arterial phase images.[44]

On MRI, pNETs appear hypointense to the pancreatic parenchyma on T1-weighted images and hyperintense on T2 WI. Tumors with more fibrous content may have intermediate or hypointense signal on T2-WI. pNETs are generally seen as hypervascular masses with homogeneous, heterogeneous or rim enhancement. Heterogeneous/rim enhancement is seen in necrotic tumors. Liver metastases are hypointense on T1 and hyperintense on T2 WI. Liver and lymph node metastases may also show prominent enhancement. With liver specific contrast agents, these metastases are seen as hypointense lesions on hepatocyte phase imaging.[44,51]

If these cross-sectional modalities are unable to depict these tumors, then endoscopic US and nuclear imaging studies may be performed. Sensitivity with endoscopic US may be as high as 94% although, it has poorer performance in the tail region of pancreas.[52]

Nuclear medicine studies can depict the primary tumor, evaluate metastases and also receptor status for planning therapy. Nuclear imaging scans are based on the expression of somatostatin receptors in these tumors, and Octreotide is the most commonly used somatostatin analog. Scintigraphy techniques using octreotide include planar imaging as well as single photon emission computed tomography (SPECT). Octreotide scans have highest sensitivity for gastrinomas and lowest sensitivity for insulinomas depending upon the expression of somatostatin receptors.[45] PET scan has better spatial resolution than scintigraphy. Octreotide is conjugated

Table 7: Key points of pancreatic neuroendocrine tumors (pNETs).

- Rare tumors, mostly seen between 40–60 years of age
- May be functioning or non-functioning
- Hypervascular tumors which enhance brightly on arterial phase imaging
- Calcification may be seen and is more frequent in nonfunctioning tumors
- Peripancreatic nodes and liver metastases are pointers towards malignancy
- Metastases are also hypervascular in nature

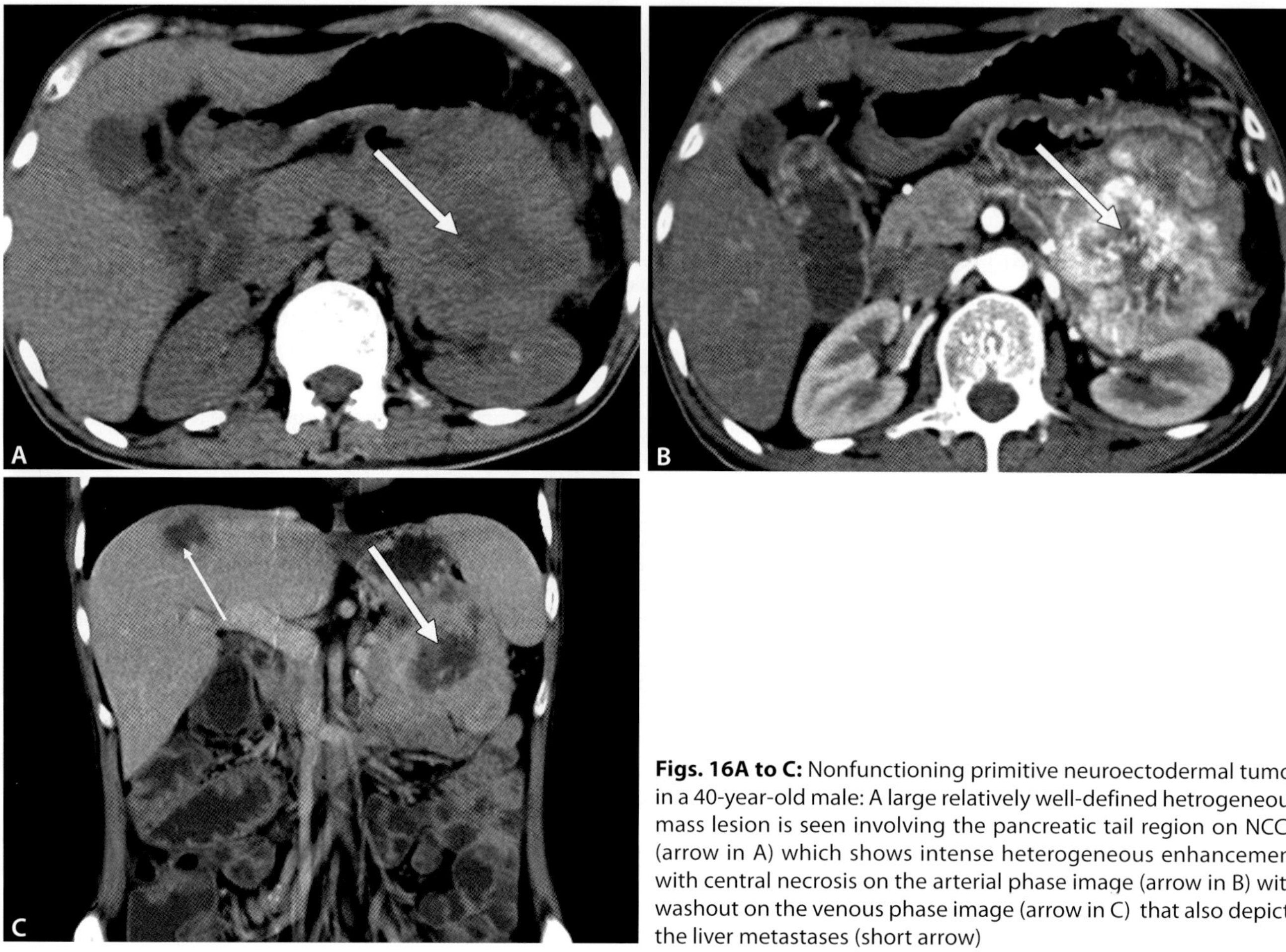

Figs. 16A to C: Nonfunctioning primitive neuroectodermal tumor in a 40-year-old male: A large relatively well-defined hetrogeneous mass lesion is seen involving the pancreatic tail region on NCCT (arrow in A) which shows intense heterogeneous enhancement with central necrosis on the arterial phase image (arrow in B) with washout on the venous phase image (arrow in C) that also depicts the liver metastases (short arrow)

with the chelator tetra-azacyclododecanetetra-acetic acid (DOTA) and is used for imaging as well as therapy of pNETs. Ga^{68} DOTA-TOC (DOTA-tyrosine-3-octreotide) and Ga^{68} DOTANOC (DOTA-1-NaI-octreotide) (DOTA-NOC) are the most frequently used analogs for depiction of the primary tumor as well as metastases.[44]

Specific Features of Various pNETs (Table 8)

Insulinomas are the most common functioning tumors and account for more than 40% of functioning endocrine tumors of pancreas. These are usually smaller than other functioning as well as nonfunctioning tumors of pancreas due to the dramatic clinical symptomatology associated with these tumors. Most of these tumors (90%) are less than 2 cm in size and 40% are even smaller than 1 cm.[53] Since they are discovered early, they also usually carry the best prognosis. The characteristic Whipple's triad of their presentation includes the following symptoms: low blood glucose level, symptoms of hypoglycemia and relief of symptoms on administering glucose.[54] These are evenly distributed through the head, body and tail region of pancreas. Multiple lesions may be seen with MEN1 syndrome.[44]

Gastrinomas are the second most common functioning pNETs after insulinomas. These are mostly encountered in pancreatic head region and have an average size of 3–4 cm. These are most often seen in the gastrinoma triangle region, which is bounded by the following three points—junction of cystic and common bile duct, junction of 2nd and 3rd parts of duodenum and junction of neck and body of pancreas **(Fig. 17)**. Their somatostatin receptor concentration is also high and hence these are more readily depicted on nuclear imaging techniques than insulinomas. Gastrin levels in these patients are usually markedly elevated to more than 1000 pg/mL resulting in increased gastric acid production and peptic ulcer disease. Zollinger-Ellison syndrome refers to a triad of a gastrinoma, increased secretion of gastric acid and peptic

Table 8: Classification of pNETs.

• *Non-functioning pNETs*: – Generally larger in size as they present late with features of mass effect or systemic metastases – Evenly distributed throughout pancreas • *Functioning pNETs*: – *Insulinomas*: • Most common functioning tumors • Characteristic Whipple's triad with low blood glucose, symptoms of hypoglycemia and relief of symptoms on administering glucose • Evenly distributed through head, body and tail region • Multiple lesions in MEN 1 syndrome – *Gastrinomas*: • Second most common • Most often seen in gastrinoma triangle • Zollinger Ellison syndrome constitutes a triad of gastrinoma, increased gastric acid production and peptic ulcers in unusual locations – *Glucagonomas*: • Third most common pNET • Mostly in pancreatic body and tail region • Present with 4D syndrome—dermatitis, deep vein thrombosis, diabetes and depression – *VIPomas*: • Rare tumors; pancreatic or extrapancreatic in origin • Mostly seen in tail region • WDHA syndrome—watery diarrhea, hypokalemia amd achlorhydria – *Somatostatinoma*: • Rare tumors • Can present with diabetes mellitus, diarrhea, steatorrhea, weight loss

ulcers in unusual locations (e.g. postbulbar duodenum, jejunum). Up to 60% of these tumors may be malignant.[44,55]

Glucagonomas are the third most common pNETs. These are usually large at presentation with an average size of 5–6 cm. These are most often seen in pancreatic body and tail region. Most of these tumors are malignant. Clinically, they present with 4D syndrome which includes dermatitis, diabetes, deep vein thrombosis, and depression.[44,53]

VIPomas are rare tumors that can be pancreatic or extrapancreatic in origin. Extrapancreatic tumors may arise from sympathetic ganglia of the retroperitoneum or mediastinum and even from stomach, small bowel, colon and liver. Symptoms result from excessive production of Vasoactive Intestinal peptide (VIP), a hormone that is not normally secreted by the pancreas. VIP prevents intestinal reabsorption and promotes intestinal secretion of water and electrolytes and these patients then present with watery diarrhea, hypokalemia and achlorhydria (WDHA syndrome). Most of these tumors are seen in tail region and are malignant tumors with an average size of approximately 5 cm.[44,56]

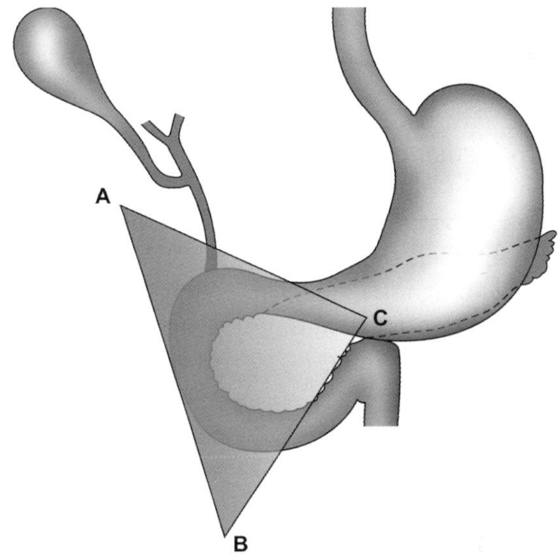

Fig. 17: Gastrinoma triangle region: This region is bounded by the following three points—junction of cystic and common bile duct (A); junction of 2nd and 3rd parts of duodenum (B); and junction of neck and body of pancreas (C).

Somatostatinomas are rare tumors which can present with diabetes mellitus, steatorrhea, diarrhea, weight loss. Other hormones that may very rarely be produced by these functioning pNETs are adrenocorticotropic hormone, serotonin, growth hormone, and calcitonin.[44]

Nonfunctioning tumors may secrete pancreatic polypeptide, and have no associated hormonal symptoms. These are more common than functioning endocrine tumors of pancreas. They are seen evenly distributed throughout the pancreas. These are generally larger than functioning tumors as they present late with features of mass effect. These have greater propensity for necrotic and cystic degeneration. Calcification may also be seen in these tumors.[44,57]

Poorly differentiated endocrine cancers are extremely rare tumors and carry a prognosis much worse than well-differentiated tumors. The tumors usually are fatal within 1 year of detection. They are mostly seen in elderly men. On imaging, they are ill-defined masses with local invasion and distant metastases at presentation. They are mostly seen in the pancreatic head region. On nuclear imaging, octreotide scan has lower sensitivity for these cancers as they have poor expression of somatostatin receptors whereas FDG-PET scan can yield better results.[44]

CONCLUSION

Cystic tumors of pancreas can have overlapping imaging features. Patient demographics and few salient morphological features can help to narrow differential diagnosis on imaging. Endoscopic US and cyst aspiration may prove useful in indeterminate lesions.

Pancreatic neuroendocrine tumors can have a varied presentation but similar imaging features. They are generally indolent in behavior except for poorly differentiated endocrine cancers. Somatostatin analog nuclear imaging techniques can help us narrow our differential diagnosis, and also enable receptor-guided therapy as these confirm the presence of soamtostatin receptors on these tumors.

REFERENCES

1. Khalid A, Brugge W. ACG Practice Guidelines for the Diagnosis and Management of Neoplastic Pancreatic Cyst. Am J Gastroenterol. 2007;102:2339-49.
2. Allen PJ, Jaques DP, D'Angelica M, et al. Cystic lesions of the pancreas: selection criteria for operative and nonoperative management in 209 patients. J Gastrointest Surg. 2003;7(8): 970-7.
3. Dewhurst CE, Mortele KJ. Cystic lesions of the pancreas: Imaging and Management. RCNA. 2012;50:467-86.
4. Laffan TA, Horton KM, Klein AP, et al. Prevalence of unsuspected pancreatic cysts on MDCT. American Journal of Roentgenology. 2008;191(3):802-7.
5. Procacci C, Biasiutti C, Carbognin G, et al. Characterization of cystic tumors of the pancreas: CT accuracy. Journal of Computer Assisted Tomography. 1999;23(6):906-12.
6. Martin RCG, Klimstra DS, Brennan MF, Conlon KC. Solid-pseudopapillary tumor of the pancreas: a surgical enigma. Annals of Surgical Oncology. 2002;9(1):35-40.
7. Chang MK, Kyung SK, Jin SC, Kim H, Woo JL, Byong RK. Solid pseudopapillary tumor of the pancreas suggesting malignant potential. Pancreas. 2006,32(3).276-80.
8. Jani N, Hani BM, Schulik RD, Hruban RH, Cunningham C. Diagnosis and management of cystic lesions of the pancreas. Diagnostic and therapeutic endoscopy. 2011; *doi: 10.1155/2011/478913.*
9. Sahani DV, Kambadakone A, Macari M, Takahashi N, Chari S, Fernandez-del Castillo C. Diagnosis and management of cystic pancreatic lesions. AJR. 2013;200:343-54.
10. Sahani DV, Kadavigere R, Saokar A, Fernandez-del Castillo C, Brugge WR, Hahn PF. Cystic pancreatic lesions: A simple imaging-based classification system for guiding management. Radiographics. 2005;25:1471-84.
11. Fernandez-del Castillo C, Warshaw AL. Cystic tumors of the pancreas. Surg Clin North Am. 1995;75:1001-16.
12. Kalb B, Sarmiento JM, Kooby DA, Adsay NV, Martin DR. MR imaging of cystic lesions of pancreas. Radiographics. 2009;29:1749-65.
13. Solicia E, Capella C, Kloppel G. Tumors of the exocrine pancreas. (3rd series, fasc. 20) In: Rosai J, Sorbin L (Eds). Atlas of tumor pathology. Armed Forces Institute of Pathology, Washington, DC; 1997.pp.31-144.
14. Kanno A, Satoh K, Hamada S, et al. Serous cystic neoplasms of the whole pancreas in a patient with von Hippel-Lindau disease. Intern Med. 2011;50:1293-8.
15. Buck JL, Hayes WS. From the Archives of the AFIP. Microcystic adenoma of the pancreas. Radiographics. 1990;10:313-22.
16. Colonna J, Plaza JA, Frankel WL, et al. Serous cystadenoma of the pancreas: clinical and pathological features in 33 patients. Pancreatology. 2008;8:135-41.
17. Cohen-Scali F, Vilgrain V, Brancatelli G, et al. Discrimination of unilocular macrocystic serous cystadenoma from pancreatic pseudocyst and mucinous cystadenoma with CT: initial observations. Radiology. 2003;228:727-33.
18. Scott J, Martin I, Redhead D, et al. Mucinous cystic neoplasms of the pancreas: imaging features and diagnostic difficulties. Clin Radiol. 2000;55:187-92.
19. Crippa S, Roberta S, Warshaw A, et al. Mucinous cystic neoplasms of the pancreas is not an aggressive entity: lessons from 163 resected patients. Ann Surg. 2008;247: 571-9.
20. Sarr MG, Murr M, Smyrk TC, et al. Primary cystic neoplasms of the pancreas: neoplastic disorders of emerging importance: current state-of-the-art and unanswered questions. J Gastrointest Surg. 2003;7(3):417-28.
21. Sidden CR, Mortele KJ. Cystic tumors of the pancreas: Ultrasound, computed tomography, and magnetic resonance imaging features. Semin US CT and MRI; 2007. pp.339-56.
22. Loftus EV, Olivares-Pakzad BA, Batts KP, et al. Intraductal papillary-mucinous tumors of the pancreas: clinicopathologic features, outcome and nomenclature. Gastroenterology. 1996; 110:1909-18.
23. Procacci C, Carbognin G, Accordini S, et al. CT features of malignant mucinous cystic tumors of the pancreas. Eur Radiol. 2001;11:1626-30.
24. Zhong N, Zhnag L, Takahashi N, et al. Histological and imaging features of mural nodules in mucinous pancreatic cysts. Clin Gastroenterol Hepatol. 2011;10:192-8.
25. Ohashi K, Murakami Y, Maruyama M. Four cases of mucin producing cancer of the pancreas on specific findings of the ampulla of Vater. Prog Dig Endosc. 1982;20:348.
26. Kawamoto S, Horton KM, Lawler LP, et al. Intraductal papillary mucinous neoplasm of the pancreas: can benign lesions be differentiated from malignant lesions with multidetector CT? Radiographics. 2005;25:1451-68.
27. Tanaka M. Intraductal papillary mucinous neoplasm of the pancreas: diagnosis and treatment. Pancreas. 2004;28(3): 282-8.
28. Taouli B, Vilgrain V, Vullierme M, et al. Intraductal papillary mucinous tumors of the pancreas: helical CT with histopathologic correlation. Radiology. 2000;217:757-64.
29. Barral M, Soyer P, Dohan A, Laurent V, Hoeffel C, Fishman EK, Boudiaf M. Magnetic resonance imaging of cystic pancreatic lesions in adults: an update in current diagnostic features and management. Abdominal imaging. 2014;39:48-65.

30. Casadei R, Santini D, Calculli L, et al. Pancreatic solid-cystic papillary tumor: clinical features, imaging findings and operative management. JOP. 2006;7:137-44.
31. Choi JY, Kim MJ, Kim JH, et al. Solid pseudopapillary tumor of the pancreas: typical and atypical manifestations. AJR. 2006;187:178-86.
32. Morgan DE. Cystic lesions of the pancreas. Semin Roentgenol. 2009;44(4):255-65.
33. Balthazar EJ, Subramanyam BR, Lefleur RS, et al. Solid and papillary epithelial neoplasm of the pancreas: Radiographic, CT, sonographic, and angiographic features. Radiology. 1984;150:39-40.
34. Cantisani V, Mortele KJ, Levy A, et al. MR imaging features of solid pseudopapillary tumor of the pancreas in adult and pediatric patients. AJR. 2003;181:395-401.
35. Horton KM, Hruban RH, Yeo C, et al. Multi-detector row CT of pancreatic islet cell tumors. Radiographics. 2006;26:453-64.
36. Eidt S, Jergas M, Schmidt R, et al. Metastasis to the pancreas: an indication for pancreatic resection. Langenbecks Arch Surg. 2007;392:539-42.
37. Koomalsingh KJ, Fazylov R, Chorost MI, et al. Cystic teratoma of the pancreas: presentation, evaluation and management. JOP. 2006;7:643-6.
38. Seki M, Ninomiya E, Aruga A, et al. Image-diagnostic features of mature cystic teratomas of the pancreas: report on two cases difficult to diagnose preoperatively. J Hepatobiliary Pancreat Surg. 2005;12:336-40.
39. Koenig TR, Loyer EM, Whitman GJ, et al. Cystic lymphangioma of the pancreas. AJR. 2001;177:1090.
40. Brugge WR, Lewandrowski K, Lee-Lewandrowski E, et al. Diagnosis of pancreatic cystic neoplasms: a report of the cooperative pancreatic cyst study. Gastroenterology. 2004; 126(5):1330-6.
41. Frossard JL, Amouyal P, Amouyal G, et al. Performance of endosonography-guided fine needle aspiration and biopsy in the diagnosis of pancreatic cystic lesions. American Journal of Gastroenterology. 2003;98(7):1516-24.
42. Eriksson B, Oberg K. Neuroendocrine tumours of the pancreas. Br J Surg. 2000;87:129-31.
43. Oberg K. Genetics and molecular pathology of neuroendocrine gastrointestinal and pancreatic tumors (gastroenteropancreatic neuroendocrine tumors). Curr Opin Endocrinol Diabetes Obes. 2009;16:72-8.
44. Lewis RB, Lattin GE, Paal E. Pancreatic endocrine tumors: radiologic-clinicopathologic correlation. Radiographics. 2010;30.
45. Kartalis N, Pozzi Mucelli RM, Sundin A. Recent developments in imaging of pancreatic neuroendocrine tumors. Ann Gastroenterol. 2015;28(2):193-202.
46. Metz DC, Jensen RT. Gastrointestinal neuroendocrine tumors: pancreatic endocrine tumors. Gastroenterology. 2008;135:1469-92.
47. Rindi G, Arnold R, Bosman FT, et al. Bosman FT, Carneiro F, Hruban RH, Theise ND. WHO classification of tumors of the digestive system, 4th edn. Lyon: IARC Press; Nomenclature and classification of neuroendocrine neoplasms of the digestive system; 2010.pp.13-4.
48. Ligneau B, Lombard-Bohas C, Partensky C, et al. Cystic endocrine tumors of the pancreas: clinical, radiologic, and histopathologic features in 13 cases. Am J Surg Pathol. 2001;25(6):752-60.
49. Fidler JL, Fletcher JG, Reading CC, et al. Preoperative detection of pancreatic insulinomas on multiphasic helical CT. AJR. 2003;181(3):775-80.
50. Gouya H, Vignaux O, Augui J, et al. CT, endoscopic sonography, and a combined protocol for preoperative evaluation of pancreatic insulinomas. AJR. 2003;181(4): 987-92.
51. Thoeni RF, Mueller-Lisse UG, Chan R, Do NK, Shyn PB. Detection of small, functional islet cell tumors in the pancreas: selection of MR imaging sequences for optimal sensitivity. Radiology. 2000;214(2):483-90.
52. Zimmer T, Scherübl H, Faiss S, Stölzel U, Riecken EO, Wiedenmann B. Endoscopic ultrasonography of neuroendocrine tumours. Digestion. 2000;62(suppl 1): 45-50.
53. Mansour JC, Chen H. Pancreatic endocrine tumors. J Surg Res. 2004;120(1):139-61.
54. Whipple AO, Frantz VK. Adenoma of islet cells with hyperinsulinism: a review. Ann Surg. 1935;101(6): 1299-1335.
55. Zollinger RM, Ellison EH. Primary peptic ulcerations of the jejunum associated with islet cell tumors of the pancreas. Ann Surg. 1955;142(4):709-23; discussion, 724-8.
56. Ghaferi AA, Chojnacki KA, Long WD, Cameron JL, Yeo CJ. Pancreatic VIPomas: subject review and one institutional experience. J Gastrointest Surg. 2008;12(2): 382-93.
57. Hruban RH, Pitman MB, Klimstra DS. Tumors of the pancreas. In: Silverberg SG, Sobin LH (Eds). AFIP atlas of tumor pathology, 4th edn. Washington, DC: American Registry of Pathology, 2007.

CHAPTER 91

Nontraumatic Acute Abdomen

Mandeep Kang, Anmol Bhatia, Anindita Sinha

INTRODUCTION

Acute abdomen is defined as a clinical syndrome characterized by acute abdominal pain of sudden onset.[1] Patients with an acute abdomen comprise the largest group presenting to the surgical emergency department.[2] Identification of patients who require surgery is crucial for timely management and reducing the associated morbidity and mortality. Acute abdomen may be due to variety of diseases which may involve the gastrointestinal system, biliary tree, solid viscera or genitourinary system. Acute appendicitis is the most common cause of an acute abdomen, particularly in young adults. In a review of 10,682 patients presenting with an acute abdomen, acute appendicitis accounted for 28% of cases, followed by acute cholecystitis (9.7%), small bowel obstruction (4.1%), gynecologic disorders (4%), acute pancreatitis (2.9%), renal colic (2.9%), peptic ulcer disease (2.5%), cancer (1.5%), diverticular disease (1.5%) and a variety of less common conditions (9%).[3] In about one-third of cases, the cause of the abdominal pain remains indeterminate or nonspecific. On account of the considerable overlap of symptoms and signs in an acute abdomen, the clinical accuracy for the specific diagnosis is low, ranging from 50% to 65%.[4] This limitation emphasizes the importance of imaging in the diagnostic work-up of the acute abdomen.

The various imaging modalities available for investigating the acute abdomen include plain films, contrast studies, ultrasound (US), computed tomography (CT), and magnetic resonance imaging (MRI). The choice of the initial modality to be used should be guided by the disease suspected on clinical grounds, for example, plain radiographs continue to be the initial imaging modality in cases of intestinal obstruction and perforation.[2] Contrast examinations have a limited role. An upper GI series with water soluble contrast may be performed in cases of suspected perforation or a contrast enema may be required to confirm a colonic obstruction.

Ultrasound is the ideal screening modality for suspected hepatobiliary disease or for suspected pelvic pathology such as ectopic gestation or acute pelvic inflammatory disease (PID). It is also indicated for the initial evaluation of a patient with right lower quadrant pain especially in young women.[5] In cases of suspected intestinal obstruction, it may at times be difficult to differentiate between mechanical obstruction and paralytic ileus on plain radiographs. US is of special value in such a situation as it demonstrates increased peristalsis in cases of mechanical obstruction, whereas presence of dilated, atonic loops suggest the diagnosis of paralytic ileus. US is also helpful in localizing intra-abdominal abscesses, particularly in the solid viscera.

The introduction of multidetector computed tomography (MDCT) has impacted imaging of all organs of the body, especially the abdomen.[6] Because of the greater speed of Zee-Axis coverage and thinner sections with 3D reconstruction now available, MDCT has become the imaging modality of choice for evaluation of the acute abdomen. It provides a comprehensive view of all the intra-abdominal solid and hollow viscera, as well as the peritoneum, mesentery, lymph nodes and retroperitoneum. Data can be acquired in different phases making MDCT an ideal modality for evaluation of suspected mesenteric ischemia or vascular disorders such as abdominal aortic aneurysms. Low dose unenhanced CT has replaced excretory urography as the screening method of choice for the evaluation of renal colic in most centers.[6] Recent improvements in resolution and development of faster breath-hold sequences have drastically increased the utility of MRI in evaluation of the gut.[7] However, MRI is still not routinely used for evaluation of an acute abdomen except in situations where iodinated contrast cannot be administered or in pregnant patients.

COMPUTED TOMOGRAPHY TECHNIQUE

The technique used for acquisition of the image data set is of paramount importance for accurate diagnosis and should be tailored according to the most likely clinical diagnosis. Oral contrast is routinely administered to all patients in the form of 800–1000 mL of 2% iodinated contrast or dilute barium solution over a period of 45 minutes prior to the study. Negative oral contrast (plain water) is preferred in suspected mesenteric ischemia to adequately distend the bowel lumen. Oral contrast is withheld in patients with renal, ureteric or biliary calculi or patients in whom CT angiography is contemplated such as aortic dissection, aneurysm rupture, etc. Per rectal contrast is given in patients with suspected pelvic or large bowel pathology. Intravenous contrast, preferably nonionic iodinated contrast, helps in better depiction of inflammatory as well as neoplastic pathology, enables differentiation of lymph nodes from vessels and detection of vascular complications. 100–120 mL of contrast is injected at a rate of 2.8–3.5 mL/second and images routinely obtained in the portal venous phase at a delay of 70 seconds. Arterial phase imaging or dual energy scanning can be added, depending on the most likely clinical diagnosis. Scanning should be performed from the domes of the diaphragm to the pubic symphysis using a slice thickness of 5–10 mm which can be retrospectively reconstructed to thinner sections for various 3D reconstructions.

Plain Radiographs in Evaluation of the Acute Abdomen

Plain radiographs still remain an important initial investigation in the evaluation of a patient with acute abdomen. Interpretation of these radiographs represents a formidable challenge to the radiologist, as the findings may be nonspecific, confusing or even misleading at times.[2] Abdominal plain films are of greatest value in cases of hollow viscus perforation and intestinal obstruction.

Perforation

In the past, a minimum three film radiographic series was recommended for evaluation of an acute abdomen. This included a supine film of the abdomen and erect radiographs of the abdomen and chest **(Figs. 1A to C)**. More recently, it has been demonstrated that the erect film of the abdomen can be eliminated from the initial series without significant loss of the diagnostic information.[8] The upright chest film is ideal for demonstrating free air as the X-ray beam strikes the hemidiaphragms tangentially at their highest point and at an optimal exposure. Classical studies have shown that as little as 1 mL of free air can

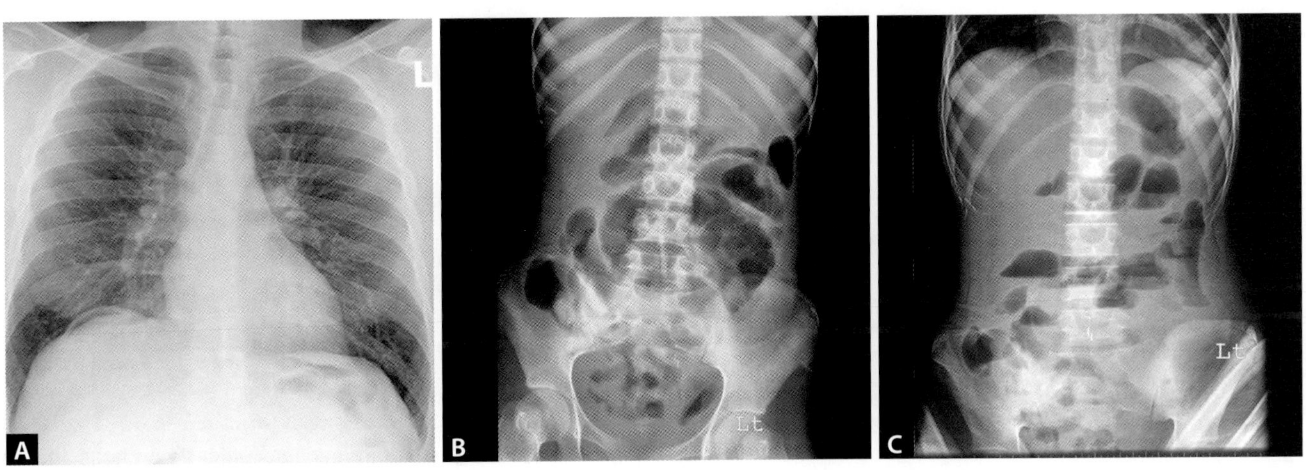

Figs. 1A to C: Abdominal series (Three views of the abdomen): (A) Chest X-ray reveals absence of free air under the domes of diaphragm; (B) Supine film shows dilated jejunal and ileal loops with no air in the large bowel; (C) Erect film demonstrates multiple air-fluid levels in a case of distal small bowel obstruction.

be detected below the right hemidiaphragm provided the patient has been in an erect position for at least 10–15 minutes prior to obtaining the radiograph.[9,10] The chest radiograph may also reveal chest diseases such as pneumonia, pulmonary or myocardial infarction which may mimic an acute abdomen. If the patient cannot sit or stand up a left lateral decubitus film will demonstrate air between the opacity of the liver and the abdominal wall. If the patient is too ill to roll over, a cross-table lateral view of the abdomen is obtained **(Fig. 2)**.

Various signs of pneumoperitoneum can be seen even on supine films if carefully searched for. The signs include "Rigler's or "double wall" sign describing visualization of both the mucosal and serosal aspect of the bowel wall due to presence of intra- and extraluminal air **(Fig. 3)**. The falciform ligament may be outlined by air in the epigastrium just to the right of the midline. The "football" sign is due to presence of large quantity of air which fills the peritoneal cavity. The lateral umbilical ligaments may be visualized in the lower abdomen known as the "inverted V" sign. Free air in morrison's pouch may be seen as an oval radiolucency in the subhepatic region. The right upper quadrant may appear radiolucent due to air collecting between the anterior surface of liver and the abdominal wall. The under surface of the central part of the diaphragm may be visualized—the "cupola" sign.[11] Retroperitoneal perforation of a duodenal ulcer results in air outlining the renal or psoas shadows **(Fig. 4)**. Large bowel may also perforate into the retroperitoneal space resulting in mottled extraluminal air lucencies. Plain films are inferior to CT for the detection of free intraperitoneal air. Supine abdominal films may detect free air in only about 60% of the cases, whereas CT can reliably detect even small amounts of free air which is usually seen just beneath the anterior abdominal wall or in the peritoneal recesses. Viewing the scan at wide window settings (lung window) increases the sensitivity of CT for the detection of free air.[9]

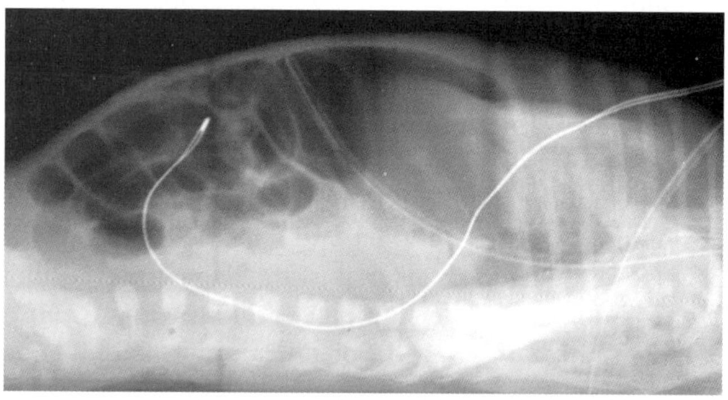

Fig. 2: Cross-table lateral view of a premature neonate reveals free intraperitoneal air in a case of necrotizing enterocolitis.

Intestinal Obstruction

The diagnosis of intestinal obstruction may be correctly suggested on the basis of plain films alone in nearly 80% of the cases. Additional imaging with US and CT is required in equivocal cases and also to determine the level and cause of obstruction.

In mechanical obstruction, plain films reveal dilated, gas-filled bowel loops with air-fluid levels proximal to the obstruction with collapsed loops with absence of air distal

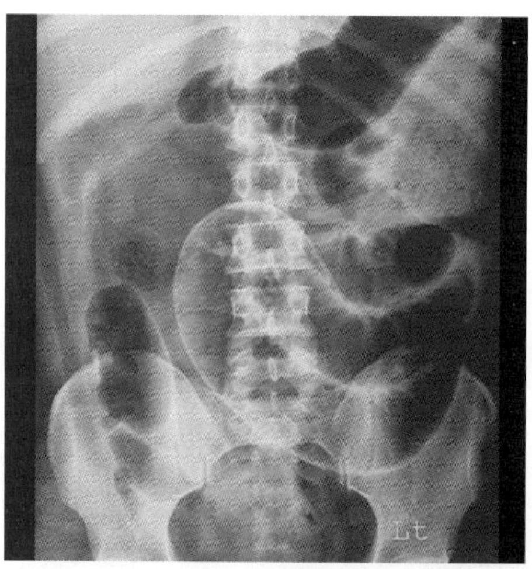

Fig. 3: X-ray abdomen, supine film. Both the inner and outer walls of the small bowel loop are visualized due to the presence of free intra-peritoneal air. Air is also seen in the subhepatic region (Morrison's pouch).

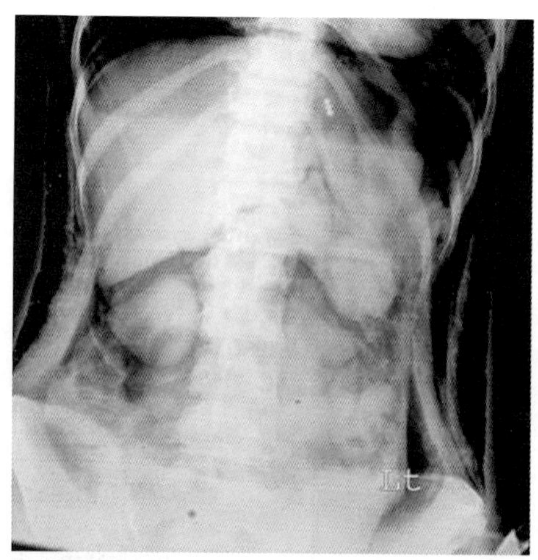

Fig. 4: Plain radiograph abdomen, erect film shows large amount of free air in the upper abdomen. In addition, air is also seen outlining the right kidney signifying retroperitoneal perforation of a duodenal ulcer.

to the obstruction **(Figs. 1A to C)**. Dilatation of both small and large bowel loops from stomach to rectum indicates a diagnosis of paralytic ileus. It may not always be possible to differentiate between mechanical obstruction and paralytic ileus. A lateral view to look for air in the rectum may aid in the differentiation, however CT or contrast studies may be required in equivocal cases.[2,9]

Distinction between small and large bowel loops on plain films is based on the central position of the small bowel, presence of valvulae conniventes in the jejunum and tubular featureless appearance of the ileum. The dilated loops measure between 3 cm and 5 cm. The valvulae conniventis form thin, 1–2 mm complete rings at intervals of 1 mm. In contrast, the large bowel loops are located peripherally, usually measure more than 5 cm in diameter and display haustral markings that are incomplete, 2–3 mm wide and occurring at intervals of 1 cm.[12] The erect film in a normal person usually displays 2–3 fluid levels in the small bowel which does not exceed 3 cm in caliber. Dilated fluid-filled loops of small bowel may be identified as oval or round soft tissue densities.[2] At times the bowel loops proximal to the site of obstruction may get completely filled with fluid resulting in a gasless abdomen. When a tiny amount of gas accompanies a large amount of intraluminal fluid, small gas bubbles get trapped between the valvulae conniventis resulting in the "string-of-beads" sign[2] **(Fig. 5)**. This appearance is virtually diagnostic of mechanical obstruction as it is never seen with paralytic ileus.

Strangulating obstruction is a mechanical obstruction caused when two limbs of a loop are incarcerated within a hernia so as to cause vascular compromise by compression of the mesenteric vessels. Presence of thumb-printing due to submucosal edema or hemorrhage should suggest ischemia in the loops. If left untreated, the ischemia may progress causing breach of the mucosa, intramural air, air in the mesenteric and portal veins and frank perforation which are all ominous signs.

Intramural air in the form of parallel streaks of gas along the bowel wall or as rings may also be seen in infants with necrotizing enterocolitis. This appearance should not be confused with the bubbly appearance of pneumatosis coli which is a benign condition affecting the colon in adults.

The causes of intestinal obstruction vary with the age of the patient. In neonates and infants, the usual causes of obstruction are congenital conditions such as hypertrophic pyloric stenosis, duodenal stenosis or atresia, ileal atresia, etc. Duodenal atresia shows the typical "double-bubble" sign. In young children, intussusception or Ladd's bands are common causes of obstruction. Intussusception may be seen as a mass-like soft tissue shadow with a crescent of gas surrounding the leading edge. A barium examination will reveal the coil-spring appearance of the intussuscipiens with the "claw" sign **(Fig. 6)**.

In adults, adhesions and hernias account for more than 80% of small bowel obstructions. Other causes include an intraluminal obturation by neoplasm, gallstone or bezoar or a volvulus due to twisting of the gut around its mesentery. Sigmoid volvulus is generally seen in the older age group. The distended ahaustral sigmoid loop assumes an inverted "U" shape with its apex under either dome. The opposed inner walls of the loops appear as a

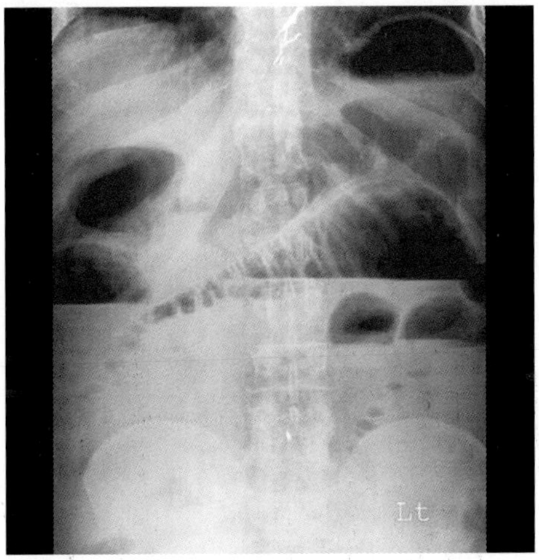

Fig. 5: X-ray abdomen, erect view shows multiple air-fluid levels in the proximal jejunal loops with "string of beads" sign.

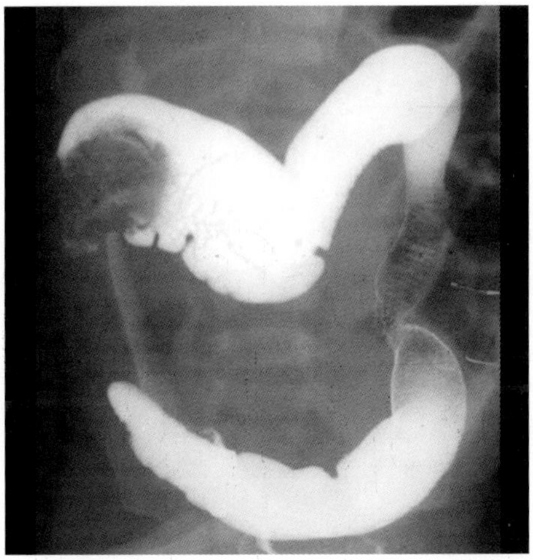

Fig. 6: Barium enema in a case of large bowel obstruction shows a crescentic intraluminal filling defect in the hepatic flexure with a soft tissue mass due to ileocolic intussusception.

single line giving the "coffee bean" appearance **(Fig. 7)**. Cecal volvulus generally occurs in younger individuals. The cecum twists and inverts so that its pole and appendix lie in the left upper quadrant.

In mechanical large bowel obstruction, the small bowel loops also dilate if the ileocecal valve is incompetent. However, if the ileocecal valve is competent, it can result in gross gaseous distension of the cecum with the attendant dangers of ischemia and perforation.

MISCELLANEOUS CONDITIONS

Apart from perforation and intestinal obstruction, plain films may sometimes reveal important findings which may clinch the diagnosis or indirectly suggest the possible diagnosis such as:

- Presence of intramural and intraluminal gas in patients of gangrenous cholecystitis.
- Presence of air in the biliary tree with small gut obstruction due to gallstone ileus caused by erosion of the gallstone into the duodenum.
- Presence of localized duodenal ileus (sentinel loop), dilated transverse colon with "colon cut-off" in case of acute pancreatitis.
- Presence of extraluminal mottled gas in patients with abdominal abscess.
- Presence of soft tissue mass with obliteration of properitoneal fat line in the right lower quadrant and scoliosis with convexity to the left in patients of acute appendicular abscess.
- Presence of gas in the perinephric region in cases of emphysematous pyelonephritis.
- Presence of intestinal pneumatosis or portomesenteric air in mesenteric ischemia.

ROLE OF CROSS-SECTIONAL IMAGING IN SPECIFIC DISEASE ENTITIES

Acute Appendicitis

In the majority of patients, the clinical picture is typical and patients undergo laparotomy without any imaging. Imaging is needed only in equivocal cases or when the clinical diagnosis is in doubt. In about one-third of patients, presentation of acute appendicitis is atypical. Conversely, other conditions may also mimic appendicitis resulting in a false negative laparotomy rate of 20% which rises to 35–45% in young women of reproductive age in whom distinction from acute PID and other gynecological conditions such as torsion of ovarian cyst is difficult on clinical grounds alone.[13] On plain radiography, although the presence of an appendicolith strongly suggests appendicitis, it is visualized on properly exposed radiographs in only 14% of all patients with appendicoliths **(Fig. 8)**.[8] At barium enema, lack of appendiceal visualization and presence of a cecal mass impression are nonspecific findings and not definitely diagnostic of appendicitis. Filling of the appendix up to its bulbous tip virtually excludes appendicitis, however, the appendix may not fill completely in up to one-third of normal individuals.[14] US is the screening modality of choice for initial evaluation in suspected appendicitis, followed by CT in selected cases. Graded compression sonography using high frequency linear transducers is a highly accurate technique with a sensitivity of 80–93%, specificity

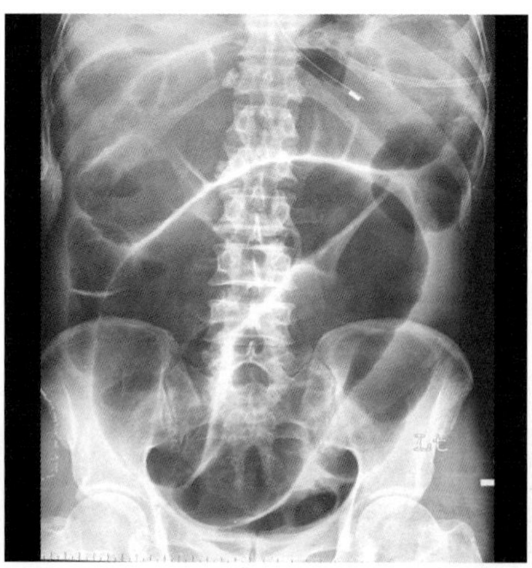

Fig. 7: X-ray abdomen, supine view shows a hugely dilated a haustral loop arising from the pelvis with the "coffee-bean" sign in a case of sigmoid volvulus.

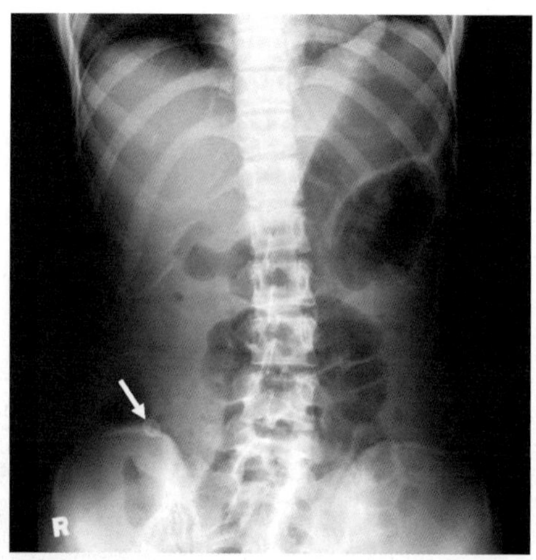

Fig. 8: X-ray abdomen showing a paucity of gas in the right side with an appendicolith (arrow).

of 94–100% and an accuracy of 95–97% for the diagnosis of acute appendicitis.[15] Another technique for improving visualization of retrocecal appendix in obese or muscular patients is posterior manual compression of right lower quadrant in anterior or anteromedial direction using the left hand with simultaneous anterior graded compression by transducer. Turning the patient from supine position to left oblique lateral decubitus position also displaces cecum, terminal ileum and appendix medially on to the psoas muscle and reduces the depth of the lateral portion of the retrocecal area, thereby improving visualization of retrocecal appendix.[16]

The US criteria for a normal appendix are presence of a compressible, tubular, blind-ending structure filled with fluid, gas or feces, originating from the base of the cecum having a wall thickness of 2 mm or less and diameter of 6 mm or less. The sonographic diagnosis of acute appendicitis is based on one or more of the following: direct visualization of a concentrically layered, aperistaltic, noncompressible appendix with an anteroposterior diameter >6 mm, or echogenic incompressible periappendicular inflamed fat with or without an appendicolith **(Fig. 9)**. On color Doppler, increased flow signals in the appendiceal wall or periappendicular space allow confirmation of the diagnosis. Perforation should be suspected if there is loss of symmetry of the concentric layers of the wall or a right lower quadrant fluid collection without visualization of inflamed appendix. However, inconclusive US studies may be seen in a right lower quadrant phlegmon or abscess without a visible appendix, retrocecal inflamed appendix, cecal edema or terminal ileum thickening, distal or tip appendicitis with a normal proximal appendix, obesity and if there is pain limiting compression. A false-positive sonogram may be seen in Crohn's disease, cecal diverticulitis and salpingitis.

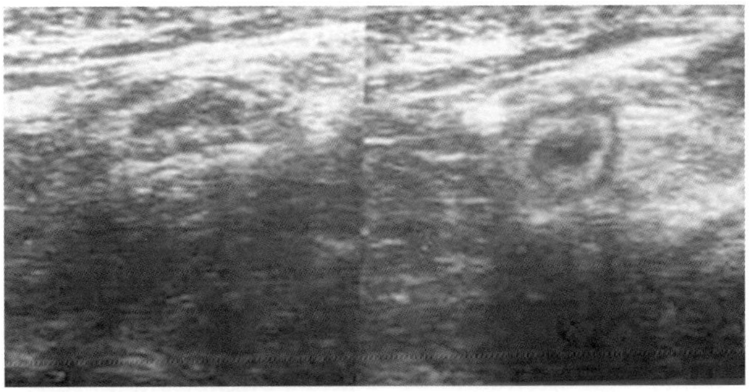

Fig. 9: Longitudinal and transverse sonograms showing the classical target lesion in the right iliac fossa due to inflamed, incompressible appendix with thickened walls.

Helical CT using thin sections (4–5 mm) has a higher reported sensitivity of 90–100%, specificity of 91–99% and accuracy of 94–98% compared to US.[17] CT signs of appendicitis include visualization of an abnormal appendix with a distended lumen, thickened and enhancing wall or an appendicolith, periappendicular inflammatory changes in the form of fat stranding, phlegmon, fluid, abscess or adenopathy, cecal changes like circumferential mural thickening of cecum and terminal ileum, cecal apical thickening or the "arrow head" sign which results due to funneling of contrast medium on both sides of the inflamed cecal apex coming to a point at the occluded orifice of the appendix **(Figs. 10 and 11)**. As the "arrowhead" sign highlights extension of inflammation to the upper portion of cecum, it may identify patients who require more than standard ligation appendectomy. CT is also of special value in suggesting an alternative diagnosis in patients who do not have appendicitis. MRI is a good

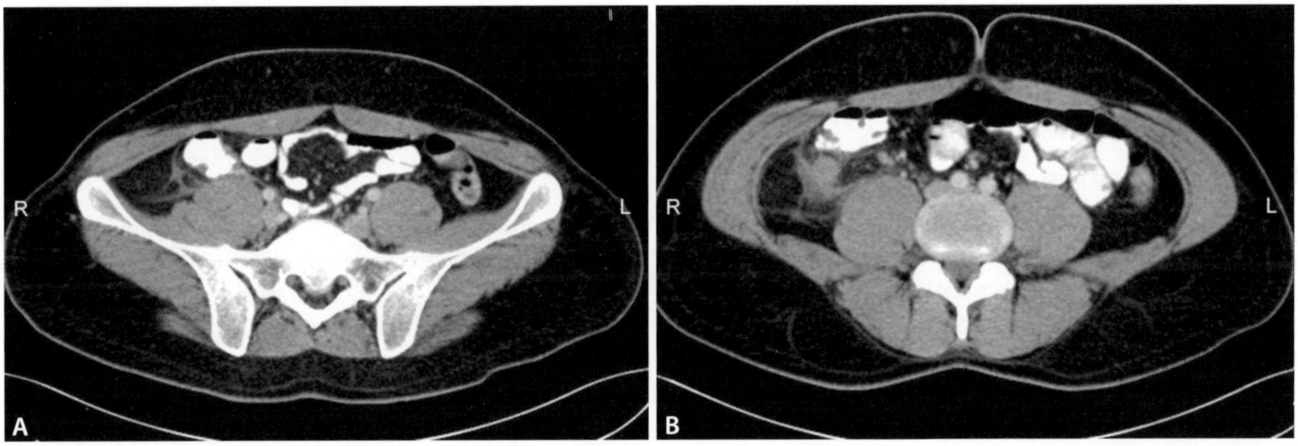

Figs. 10A and B: CECT abdomen, axial sections: (A) A thin streak of oral contrast is seen to enter the base of the appendix; (B) The appendix shows mural thickening with stranding in the surrounding fat in a case of acute appendicitis.

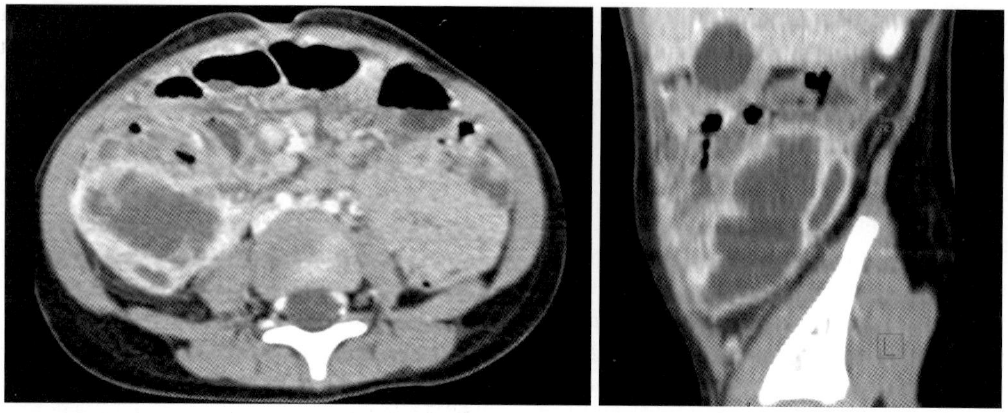

Fig. 11: Acute appendicitis: Axial and sagittal reconstructed CT images demonstrating a large, irregular collection with thick enhancing walls in the right iliac fossa posterior to the cecum which is displaced anteromedially. A tubular structure with enhancing walls is seen posterior to this collection representing the inflamed appendix.

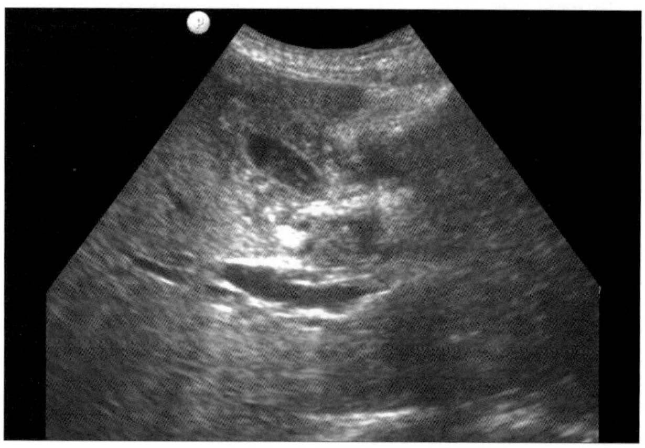

Fig. 12: Ultrasound image showing small calculi in the gallbladder with diffusely thickened walls in a case of acute cholecystitis. US Murphy's sign was positive.

imaging modality in pregnant patients and pediatric population, in whom ionizing radiation is of high concern. MRI has demonstrated high specificity and sensitivity for appendicitis in pediatric and pregnant patients, with nearly 100% sensitivities reported for both populations.[18]

Acute Cholecystitis

Sonography is the primary imaging modality of choice for evaluating acute inflammatory conditions of the gallbladder. Acute cholecystitis is associated with gallstones in 90–96% of patients with a calculus causing cystic duct obstruction being the most common cause. Sensitive sonographic features are positive Murphy's sign (in 96% of patients with acute cholecystitis), calculi (in 95%) and a thickened gallbladder (GB) wall (in 73%).[19] However, these signs are not specific and may occur in other conditions such as chronic cholecystitis, pancreatitis, cirrhosis or hepatitis. Other sonographic signs include distension of the gallbladder (GB), edematous wall, mucosal irregularity, intramural gas and/or pericholecystic collection **(Fig. 12)**. Doppler sonography improves diagnostic confidence in acute cholecystitis by revealing mural hypervascularity **(Fig. 13)**.

The CT may be used as an adjunct to US if sonography is inconclusive, especially in acalculous cholecystitis or when complications such as perforation or emphysematous cholecystitis are suspected.[20] CT findings of acute cholecystitis include wall thickening, pericholecystic stranding, GB distension, pericholecystic fluid, subserosal edema, high attenuation bile and sloughed membranes, gas or septations within the gallbladder **(Fig. 14)**.[21] As the inflammatory response in calculous and acalculous cholecystitis is similar, the CT appearance of inflammation is similar in both. MRI can be a valuable complement to US and CT in demonstrating impacted calculi in the gallbladder neck or cystic duct which are often difficult to detect on US. Also, conditions causing acalculous cholecystitis like adenomyomatosis, gallbladder polyp, malignant neoplasm or other cancers can be depicted on MR.[22]

Complications of acute cholecystitis include the following:

- *Empyema*: It occurs when pus fills the distended and inflamed GB, typically in diabetic patients. On US and CT, pus resembles sludge. Heavily T2WI are sensitive in demonstrating purulent bile as a dependent hypointense layer relative to normal bile.
- *Gangrenous cholecystitis*: Gangrenous cholecystitis is an advanced, severe form of acute cholecystitis, seen more commonly in elderly men. It results from marked

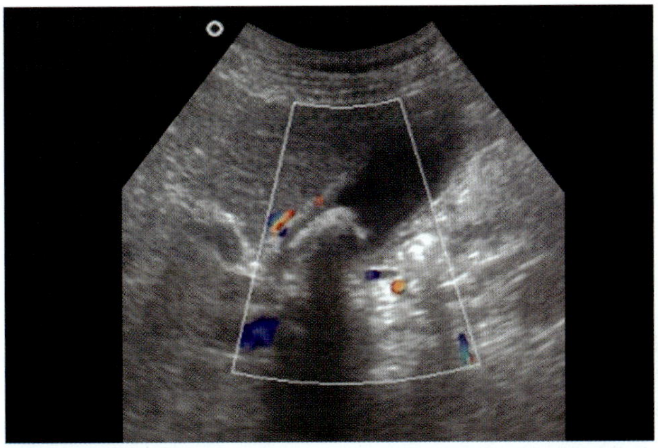

Fig. 13: Ultrasound (color Doppler) image showing cholelithiasis with increased vascularity in the gallbladder wall.

distension of the GB with resultant increase in tension in the wall. Associated inflammation leads to ischemic necrosis. US reveals heterogeneous or striated thickening of GB wall or intraluminal membranes representing desquamated mucosa. US findings typical of uncomplicated acute cholecystitis may be absent in this subset of patients. Gallbladder wall thickness may be <3 mm or Murphy's sign may be absent due to denervation of the GB wall.[23] CT features consist of intraluminal membranes, irregular wall, pericholecystic fluid/abscess and lack of mural enhancement.

- *Gallbladder perforation*: Gallbladder perforation is most often a complication of acute gangrenous cholecystitis. As blood supply is poor in the region of fundus, this is the most common site of perforation. Perforation can be classified into three types:
  a. Acute free perforation into peritoneal cavity,
  b. Subacute perforation with pericholecystic abscess, and
  c. Chronic perforation with a cholecystoenteric fistula.[24] Subacute perforations are the most common. Following perforation, US, CT and MR show complex pericholecystic fluid collections and the wall of GB can appear focally disrupted **(Fig. 15)**.[7]
- *Emphysematous cholecystitis*: Emphysematous cholecystitis is a rare form of acute cholecystitis seen in patients with diabetes and peripheral atherosclerotic disease. The majority of patients are between 50 and 70 years. US demonstrates intraluminal and intramural gas as highly echogenic foci. CT is the most sensitive and specific imaging modality to identify gas in the lumen or wall **(Fig. 16)**.[25]
- *Hemorrhagic cholecystitis*: It can complicate acute calculous or acalculous cholecystitis, and the patient presents with acute biliary colic, jaundice, melena, and hematemesis.[25] It needs to be differentiated from other causes of gallbladder hemorrhage, which include trauma, tumors, and coagulopathy states. Ultrasound shows echogenic or heterogeneous material within the gallbladder lumen or wall, which are seen as high-attenuation contents on CT. MRI can be quite helpful in the diagnosis. Subacute blood products are generally hyperintense on both T1WI and T2WI because of the presence of extracellular methemoglobin.[26] Complications of hemorrhagic cholecystitis include gallbladder wall perforation and associated potentially life threatening hemoperitoneum.[26]

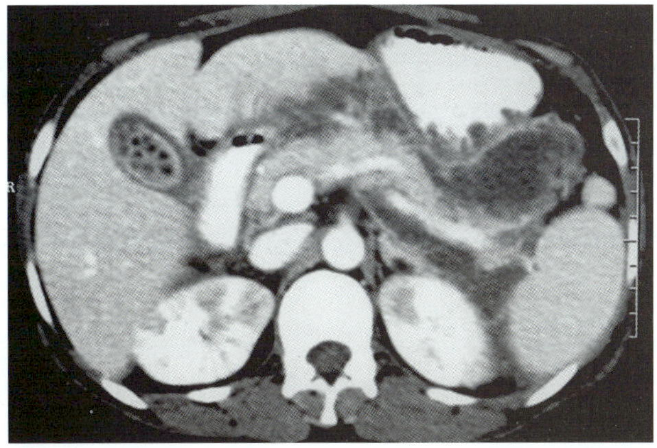

Fig. 14: Axial CECT abdomen. The gallbladder has thick, enhancing walls with a hypodense rim of pericholecystic fluid. The lumen is filled with high density bile resulting in the calculi appearing as filling defects. Note the loss of peripancreatic fat planes with a large collection in the lesser sac due to associated pancreatitis.

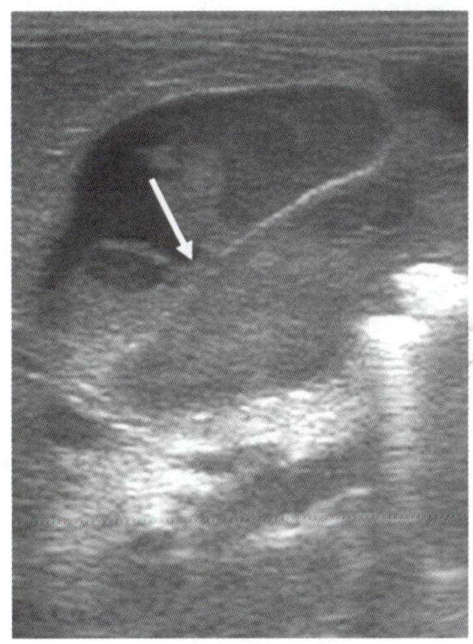

Fig. 15: Ultrasound image showing a rent in the gallbladder wall (arrow) with a large collection adjacent to the rent in a case of gallbladder perforation.

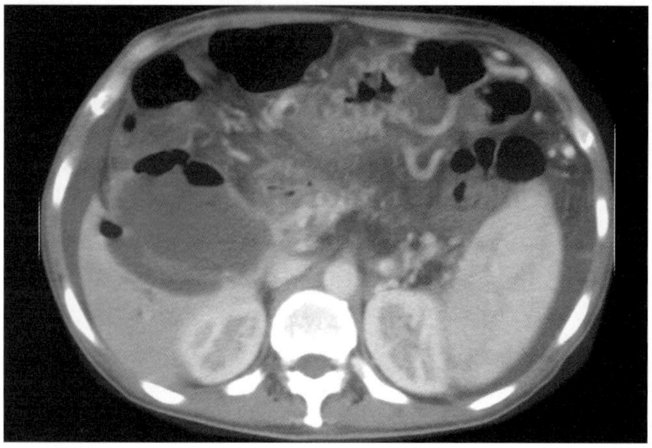

Fig. 16: Axial CECT image showing grossly distended gallbladder with intramural air foci suggestive of emphysematous cholecystitis.

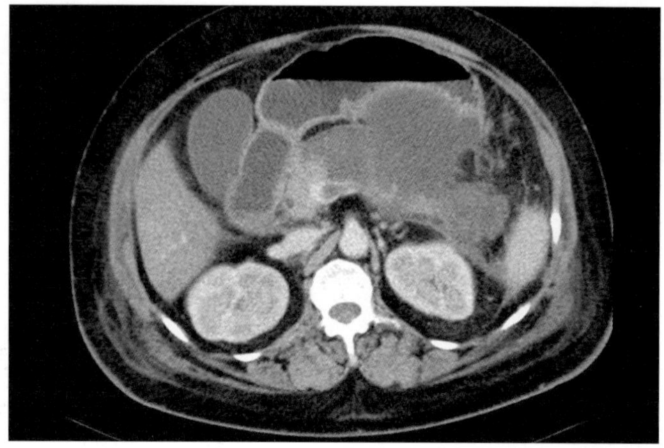

Fig. 17: Acute necrotizing pancreatitis grade E. The body and tail of the pancreas are hypodense with only a small amount of normally enhancing parenchyma seen in the head of pancreas. There are extra-pancreatic collections with a hypodense filling defect in the portal vein due to thrombosis (CTSI-10).

Acute Pancreatitis

Acute pancreatitis is an acute inflammatory process of the pancreas which may range in severity from a mild parenchymal edema to severe necrotizing pancreatitis with variable involvement of other regional tissues or remote organ systems. Most of the patients with the mild form of the disease have an uneventful recovery, however the cases with severe pancreatitis show significant mortality and morbidity with development of failure of various organ systems and require aggressive management.

The diagnosis of acute pancreatitis is usually made on clinical grounds supported by laboratory data. The role of imaging is to confirm the diagnosis, stage the severity of disease and detect complications such as infection, pseudocyst formation or vascular involvement. Ultrasound may reveal an enlarged, hypoechoic pancreas in the early stages with presence of peripancreatic fluid. It may also detect the presence of cholelithiasis or choledocholithiasis which is a major etiological factor for acute pancreatitis. It can also be used in the follow-up of acute fluid collections or pseudocysts particularly after percutaneous catheter drainage.

Contrast-enhanced CT is the modality of choice not only to confirm the diagnosis or detect extra-pancreatic intra-abdominal disease, but also to stage the severity of disease which is required for prognostication.[27] It is also highly accurate for the detection of necrosis and complications **(Fig. 17)**. The various grading systems, complications related to pancreatitis as well as pancreatic interventions will be dealt with in detail in a later chapter.

MR has also been reported to have similar accuracy to MDCT for the diagnosis of acute pancreatitis and assigning a severity index. The presence of hyperintensity in the pancreatic parenchyma on noncontrast T1 and T2 weighted images signifies the presence of hemorrhagic pancreatitis. Fat suppressed noncontrast sequences are used to detect hemorrhagic peripancreatic collections, both these situations signify a more severe form of pancreatitis.[28]

Intra-abdominal Abscess

A localized collection of pus can occur anywhere in the abdomen including the parenchyma of solid organs, in the peritoneal or extra-peritoneal spaces. Early detection, accurate localization and prompt drainage are the mainstay of successful management. US is an excellent modality for the detection of visceral abscesses and is also useful for screening for intraperitoneal abscesses, like in the post-operative patient.[29] Abscesses appear as a rounded, complex fluid collection with irregular walls, posterior acoustic enhancement, low level internal echoes, septations or debris **(Figs. 18A and B)**. A fluid-fluid level may be seen. At times, the abscess may have a solid appearance. Color Doppler demonstrates peripheral hypervascularity.

Computed tomography has a high sensitivity and specificity with an overall accuracy of 95% for the detection of intra-abdominal abscesses.[30] CT will show a low attenuation fluid collection with mass effect and peripheral rim enhancement with or without gas bubbles or an air-fluid level. MDCT allows accurate delineation of

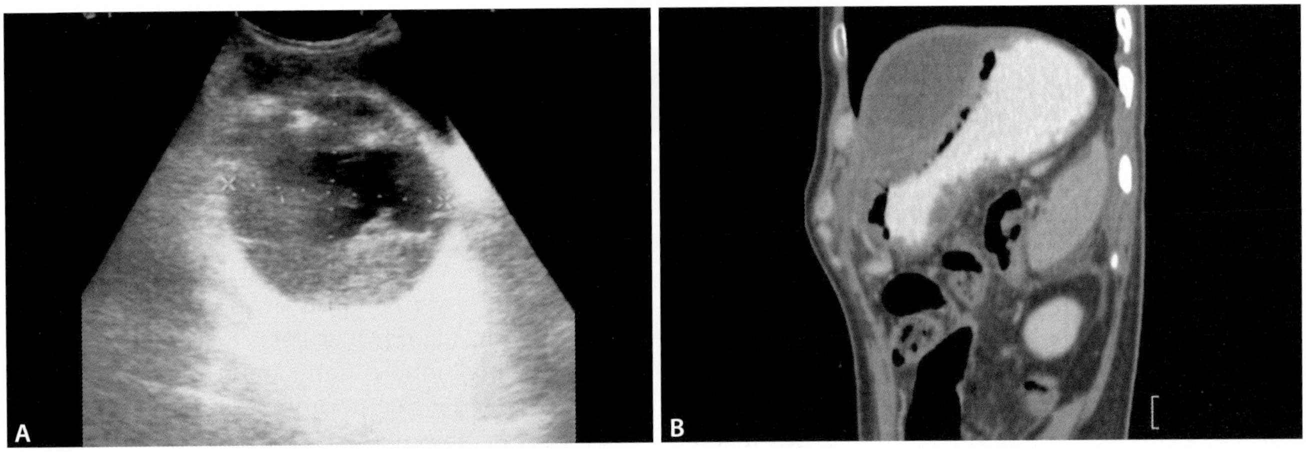

Figs. 18A and B: (A) The ultrasound of the pelvis shows a rounded fluid collection with internal echoes, debris and septations with posterior acoustic enhancement in a case of postoperative abdominal abscess; (B) Coronal MPVR image shows a large, left subphrenic, low-attenuation fluid collection elevating the left hemidiaphragm. The transpleural approach had to be employed for percutaneous drainage of this abscess.

the complex anatomy which may exist in intra-abdominal collections and thus enables proper planning of a safe approach route for percutaneous catheter drainage **(Figs. 18A and B)**.

Intestinal Obstruction

Imaging studies such as US and CT are required to confirm the clinical diagnosis of obstruction (made on the basis of clinical findings and plain X-ray appearance), differentiate between mechanical obstruction and paralytic ileus and for determining the level and cause of mechanical obstruction. CT is also useful for detecting an obstruction not visualized on plain films, e.g. closed loop obstruction. More importantly, CT can detect complications like strangulation which require emergent surgery.

The CT diagnosis of bowel obstruction is based on the presence of dilated loops (small bowel >2.5 cm, large bowel >5 cm) with air-fluid levels proximal to a transition zone with collapsed distal bowel. Minimal mural thickening with enhancement may at times be seen at the transition zone in cases of adhesions **(Fig. 19)**.[31] The "small bowel feces" sign refers to the presence of gas bubbles mixed with particulate matter in dilated loops proximal to the site of obstruction. This is a less common but reliable indicator of mechanical obstruction. Gas filled loops, mesenteric vessels and fat may be seen in the inguinal canal or other sites of external hernias. Circumferential mural thickening of the dilated bowel loops with increased attenuation in the mesentery or bowel wall denotes the presence of strangulation. An internal hernia can be diagnosed if a cluster of dilated small bowel loops which appears to be enclosed in a sac is seen in an ectopic location (e.g. lesser sac or anterior to transverse colon) with crowding and twisting of the mesenteric vessels. A markedly dilated, fluid filled bowel segment with abrupt tapering ends denotes a closed loop obstruction. These show relatively little dilatation of the proximal bowel and are at greater risk for strangulation. Fixed radial distribution of several dilated small bowel loops with stretched and prominent mesenteric vessels converging towards the point of torsion (whirl sign) with mesenteric edema indicates a small bowel volvulus **(Fig. 20)**. A target appearance on cross-section with a bowel-within-bowel appearance on longitudinal scans suggests a diagnosis of intussusception. Mesenteric fat and vessels can be identified within the mass and the lead point if present **(Fig. 21)**. Enteroenteric intussusceptions without proximal dilatation that are less than 3.5 cm in length

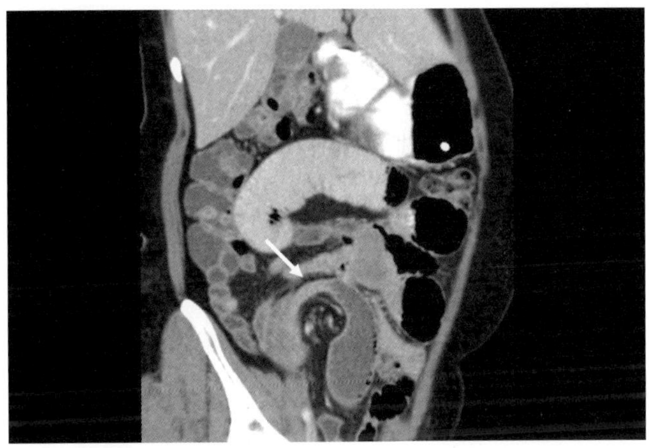

Fig. 19: Oblique MPR image showing abrupt angulation of an ileal loop with minimal mural thickening (arrow) at the site of postoperative adhesion in a case of small bowel obstruction.

are probably not significant in adults. Intussusceptions involving the colon that are 4 cm in length or longer, have proximal dilatation or mural thickening should be carefully evaluated for an underlying neoplasm. Foreign bodies, gallstones and bezoars can all cause obstruction and can be readily identified on CT. CT has a sensitivity of 90–96%, specificity of 91–96% and overall accuracy of 90–95% for the diagnosis of high grade obstruction.[1,32] CT enterography with neutral oral contrast is also helpful in cases of partial small bowel obstruction demonstrating the exact site and the cause of obstruction **(Figs. 22A and B)**. It helps in improved visualization of mucosal lesions as compared with conventional CT.[33] Fast MRI has also been shown to be sensitive (95%), specific (100%) and accurate (96%) in the setting of small bowel obstruction.[34]

Bowel Perforation

Gastrointestinal (GI) tract perforation can be caused by peptic ulcer disease, foreign body, appendicitis, bacterial enteritis, Crohn's disease, diverticulitis, bowel ischemia, obstruction or malignant neoplasms. Some studies have reported US to be a more sensitivity modality than plain radiography for the diagnosis of pneumoperitoneum.[35] Sonographic findings of perforated hollow viscus include demonstration of free air as echogenic spots or lines with posterior ring-down artifacts that shift with change in patient position, enhancement of the peritoneal stripe, echogenic free peritoneal fluid and decreased peristalsis.[36] When patient is in supine position, the reverberations are seen between anterior surface of

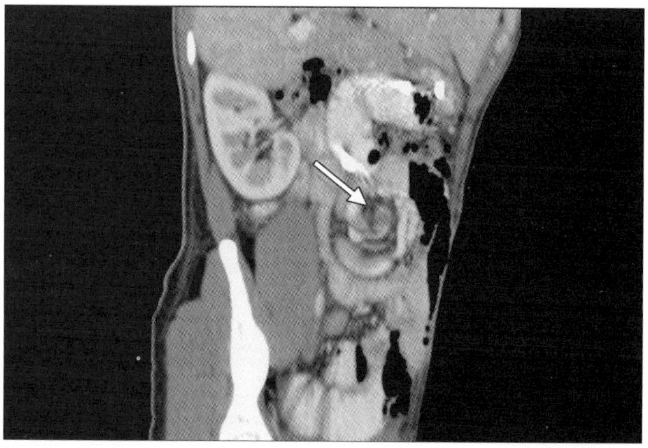

Fig. 20: Oblique MPR image showing midgut volvulus with presence of whirl sign (arrow).

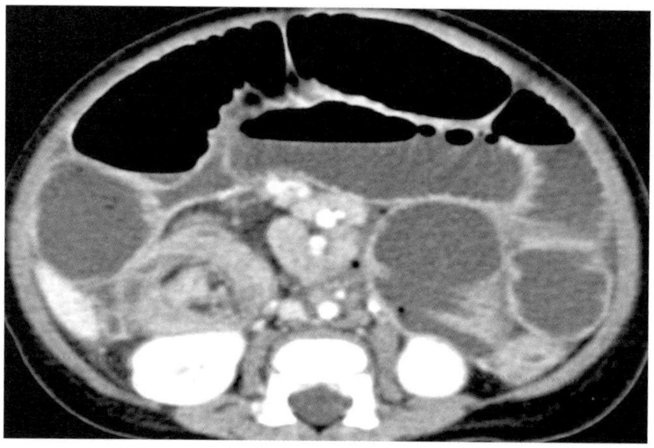

Fig. 21: Axial CECT section demonstrates a 4 × 5 cm, heterogeneous mass in the right lumbar region showing a target appearance with mesenteric fat and vessels within the lesion suggestive of intussusception. The proximal small bowel loops are dilated.

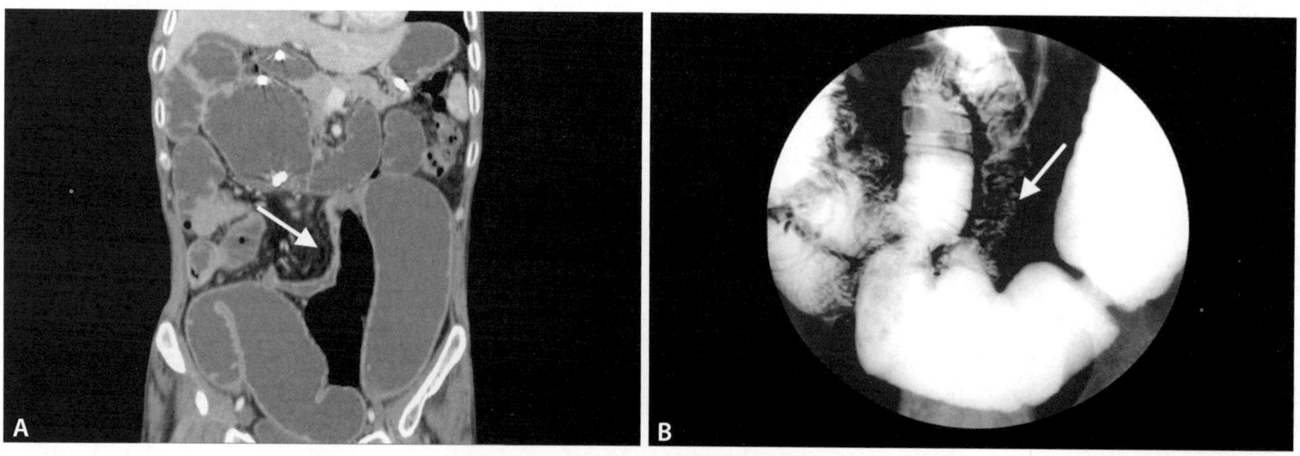

Figs. 22A and B: (A) CT enterography coronal MPR image showing a long segment distal ileal stricture (arrow) causing obstruction with dilatation of the proximal small bowel loops; (B) Barium enteroclysis done subsequently confirms the stricture (arrow) in a case of tuberculosis.

left lobe of liver and anterior abdominal wall. Shifting phenomenon is seen on rolling the patient to left lateral position as free air rises to the highest portion of the right hypochondrium. Enhancement of peritoneal stripe refers to increased echogenicity and thickening of the peritoneal stripe due to free intraperitoneal air with associated dirty shadowing.

The CT is superior to both plain films and US for the detection of presence, cause and site of perforation. Preoperative localization of the site of perforation is beneficial for the surgeon, with the laparoscopic approach currently being used for most surgical procedures instead of open surgery. Extraluminal contrast extravasation, when seen, is pathognomonic. Other direct signs are the presence of extraluminal air or discontinuity of the bowel wall. Inflammatory changes may also be seen at the site of perforation. CT images should be assessed in wide window settings to distinguish free air from fat density. Careful analysis of anterior peritoneal surfaces of liver and mid-abdomen as well as of peritoneal folds should be done, so as not to overlook a small amount of extraluminal air. The site of colonic perforation may be predicted by the site of extraluminal contrast leakage, concentrated bubbles of air in close proximity to the bowel wall, focal interruption of bowel wall, segmental bowel wall thickening, ill-defined mass, adjacent fat stranding and extraluminal fluid **(Figs. 23A and B)**. A large amount of intraperitoneal air usually indicates gastroduodenal perforation, except for bowel perforation caused by obstruction or an endoscopic procedure.[37] The location of air also helps in determining the site of perforation. Air in the lesser sac can be seen in posterior perforation of stomach or duodenum, or less commonly, from perforation of transverse colon. Free air confined to the intra-hepatic ligamentum teres is commonly due to gastroduodenal perforations. Air trapped in the mesenteric folds is found in colon and small bowel perforation, but seldom in gastric perforation. Retroperitoneal air is caused by perforation of extraperitoneal sites of gastrointestinal tract, viz. descending and horizontal parts of duodenum, ascending and descending colon, sigmoid colon and rectum.

Mesenteric Ischemia

Bowel ischemia or infarction is a common but complex disorder with a plethora of primary causes and a wide range of clinical and pathological manifestations. Acute mesenteric ischemia is therefore a diagnostic challenge particularly in view of its high mortality rate which ranges from 50% to 90% depending upon the cause and degree of bowel wall damage. Acute occlusion of the superior mesenteric artery (SMA) due to embolus is the most common cause of mesenteric ischemia accounting for nearly 50% of cases.[38] The manifestation may range from a self-limiting superficial ischemia involving the watershed zones to a diffuse ischemic injury to the entire bowel—"shock bowel" which requires immediate surgical intervention.[39] Plain films reveal the characteristic thick-walled dilated loops with thumb-printing in only 20–30% of cases.[40] Intramural air or portomesenteric air is also rarely visualized on the plain radiograph.

Multidector computed tomography (MDCT) angiography is the modality of choice for the evaluation of bowel ischemia with a sensitivity approaching that of angiography. The most common finding of mesenteric

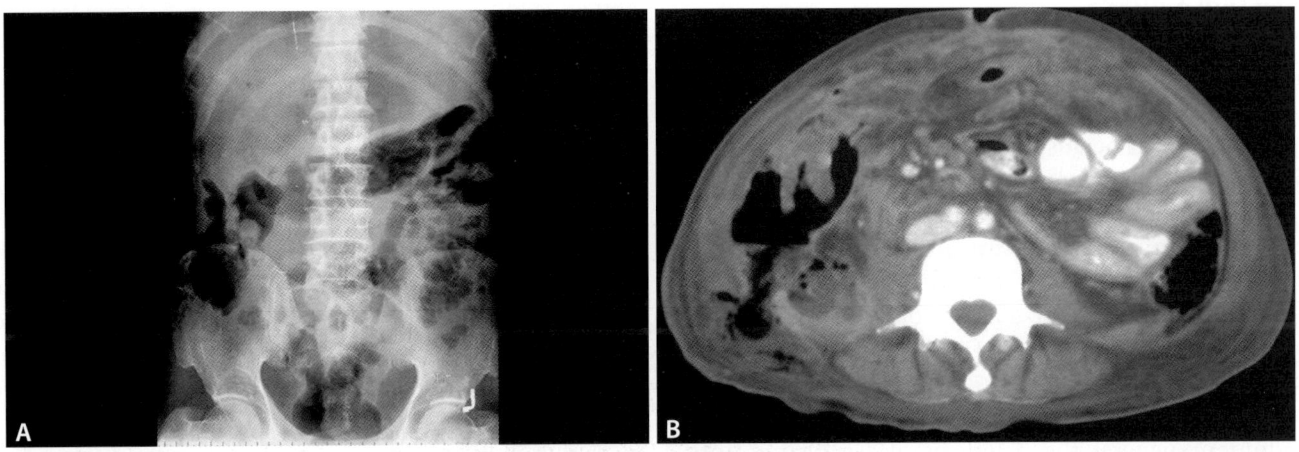

Figs. 23A and B: (A) Plain radiograph of the abdomen shows extraluminal, mottled air lucencies in the right iliac region denoting perforation of a hollow viscus; (B) Axial CECT section reveals an ill-defined mass involving the cecum with discontinuity of the lateral cecal wall. A large amount of extraluminal air is seen adjacent to the perforation with extension of inflammation into the right gluteal region and formation of an abscess. This was a case of carcinoma cecum with perforation.

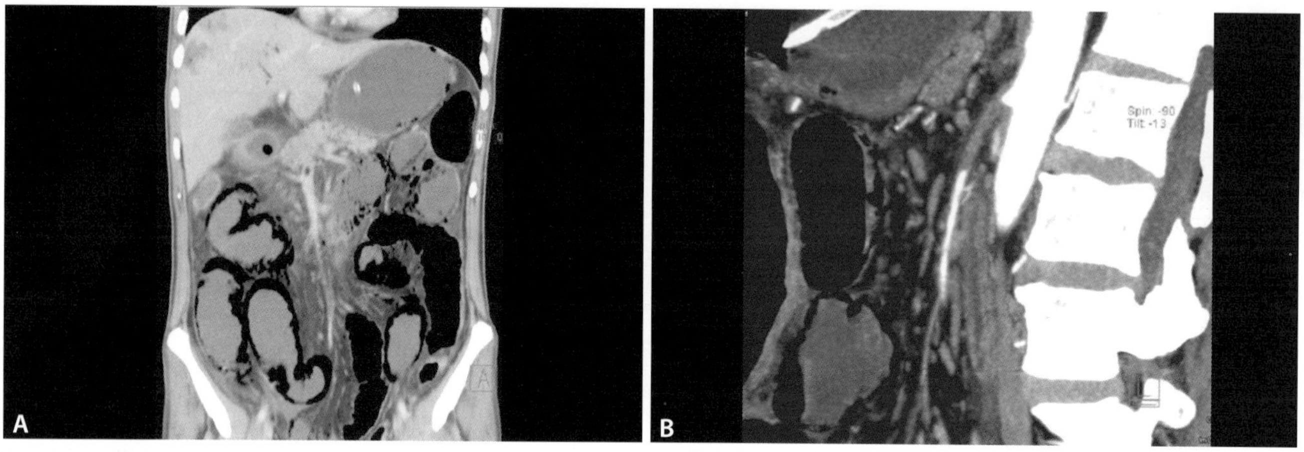

Figs. 24A and B: Mesenteric ischemia—CT angiography: (A) The small bowel loops are dilated with thinned-out walls and gross pneumatosis. Air is also seen in the mesenteric veins and the portal radicles in the liver. Note the irregular, nonenhancing hypodense areas in the periphery of the liver due to infarcts; (B) Sagittal MIP image demonstrates the occlusion of the proximal superior mesenteric artery.

ischemia is bowel wall thickening though this feature strongly depends on the degree of bowel distension. In complete arterial occlusion, there can be absence of the normal enhancement of the bowel wall. Conversely, in nonocclusive ischemia there can be abnormal persistent mural enhancement. The target sign is seen when there is hyperenhancement of the mucosa and submucosa due to hyperemia and hyperperfusion with mural edema.

Luminal dilatation with air-fluid levels can be seen in 56–91% of cases. Pneumatosis and portomesenteric gas are less common but more specific findings of ischemia being present in 6–28% and 3–14% of cases respectively **(Figs. 24A and B)**.[38,39] The presence of pneumoperitoneum or focal peritonitis signifies perforation.

Vascular Causes

Vascular conditions that may present as acute abdomen include rupture of an aortic aneurysm, spontaneous aortic occlusion, acute hemorrhage and hepatic or splenic vascular occlusion. Aneurysmal dilatation of the abdominal aorta is rare before the age of 50 with average age at the time of diagnosis being 65–70 years. Most abdominal aortic aneurysms are true aneurysms and occur below the level of renal arteries. An abdominal aortic aneurysm is defined as an aortic diameter of 3 cm or more while a diameter of 5.5 cm or more warrants urgent intervention.[41] Presence of a pulsatile mass and sudden hypotension in the clinical setting of acute pain abdomen suggests the diagnosis of a ruptured aortic aneurysm. Although US may detect the aneurysm as well as the associated thrombus and hematoma, frequently the entire aorta cannot be evaluated due to overlying bowel

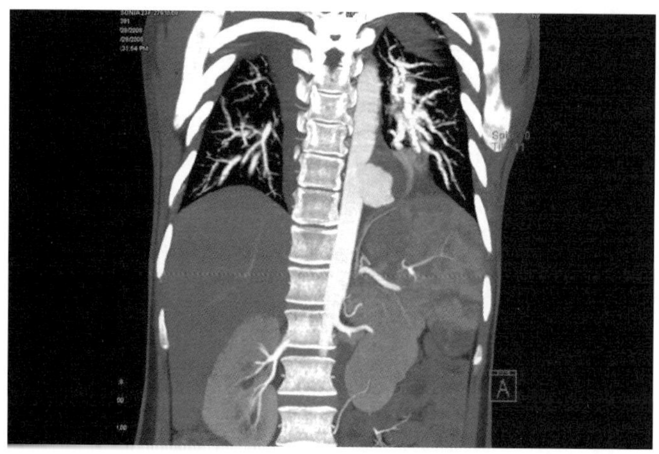

Fig. 25: CT angiography: MIP image shows an irregular, sac-like lobulated outpouching from the wall of the thoracoabdominal aorta due to a mycotic pseudoaneurysm in a case of infective endocarditis. There is associated thrombus as well as a peripheral rim of hyperdensity because of the surrounding hematoma.

gas or body habitus. Multidetector CT is the modality of choice for evaluation of acute aortic syndrome. The most common finding of rupture of aortic aneurysm is a retroperitoneal hematoma adjacent to the aneurysm **(Fig. 25)**. Other CT features may include active extravasation of contrast, extension of periaortic blood into perirenal or pararenal spaces or the psoas muscle or peritoneal cavity. Signs predictive of impending rupture are:

- Draped aorta sign—seen with contained leak. The posterior wall of aorta cannot be defined due to close application and lateral 'draping' of the aneurysm around the adjacent vertebral bodies.[42]

- Increase in aneurysm size—a patient with a very large aneurysm (>7 cm diameter) who presents with acute aortic syndrome has a high likelihood of aneurysmal rupture. Also, a rate of enlargement of >10 mm/year warrants surgical repair.
- Thrombus-to-lumen ratio—this ratio decreases with increasing aneurysm size. A thick circumferential thrombus is protective against rupture.
- Focal discontinuity in intimal calcification.
- Hyperattenuating crescent sign due to hemorrhage in either the peripheral thrombus or aneurysm wall.

Acute abdominal hemorrhage may result due to ruptured aneurysm in a case of polyarteritis nodosa, ruptured tumor (usually renal cell carcinoma) or in a patient on anticoagulant therapy. Noncontrast CT demonstrates a hyperdense collection at the site of hemorrhage. MDCT angiography can accurately delineate the site and cause of hemorrhage.

Rare causes of acute abdomen include hepatic vein thrombosis (acute Budd-Chiari syndrome) and portal vein thrombosis. US in the acute phase may show liver enlargement, partial or complete inability to visualize hepatic veins, intraluminal hepatic vein echogenicity or thrombosis, marked narrowing of intrahepatic IVC and ascites. Color Doppler is the technique of choice for initial evaluation. Absence of flow or flow in an abnormal direction in all or part of the hepatic veins may be seen. CT and MR are complimentary techniques for definitive diagnosis which provide a more complete evaluation of the hepatic parenchyma, hepatic veins and IVC.

Pelvic Disease

The various entities that have to be additionally thought of while evaluating a young female in the reproductive age group presenting with acute abdomen are ruptured ectopic pregnancy, PID, twisted ovarian cyst and complications of early pregnancy, etc.

- Signs of a ruptured ectopic pregnancy on ultrasound include an inhomogeneous adnexal mass, pelvic fluid or hematoma, decidual reaction without intrauterine gestation sac, in the presence of a positive pregnancy test. Visualization of an echogenic adnexal ring separate from the ovary that has prominent peripheral flow on color Doppler is highly suggestive of ectopic gestation. Corpus luteum is a useful guide while looking for an ectopic pregnancy and is usually seen in the ipsilateral ovary in 70–85% cases.[43] Using transvaginal ultrasound, the live embryo can be detected in up to 17% of all ectopic pregnancies.
- Fibroids may present with acute pain if there is torsion or degeneration of a submucosal or subserosal fibroid. On imaging, uterine enlargement with a focal mass or contour deformity are seen. Degenerated fibroids may have a cystic appearance.
- Ovarian torsion usually occurs in children and is attributed to excessive mobility of the ovary. In adults, a cyst or mass, frequently a cystic teratoma, is present in the ovary undergoing torsion. Sonographic findings include an enlarged ovary with peripherally distributed follicles, an associated cyst or mass, with diminished or absent central venous flow on Doppler. On CT or MR, deviation of the uterus to the twisted side, obliteration of fat planes and an enlarged ovary displaced from its adnexal location is seen **(Fig. 26)**. Contrast enhanced CT may show surrounding enhancing blood vessels due to congestion.
- Hemorrhage into a corpus luteal or follicular cyst may manifest with abrupt onset of pelvic pain. If the cyst ruptures, associated hemoperitoneum can be life threatening. On imaging, hemorrhagic ovarian cysts can mimic a variety of solid and mixed solid-cystic masses. A fluid-fluid level may be present. On CT, high attenuation components are usually seen due to hemorrhage.
- Pelvic inflammatory disease (PID) is among the common causes of acute pain in young women. In the early stage of PID, US may demonstrate a small amount of fluid in the cul-de-sac or endometrial canal. On CT, there may be stranding in the parapelvic fat, thickening of the uterosacral ligament and ovarian enlargement with oophoritis. In advanced stages,

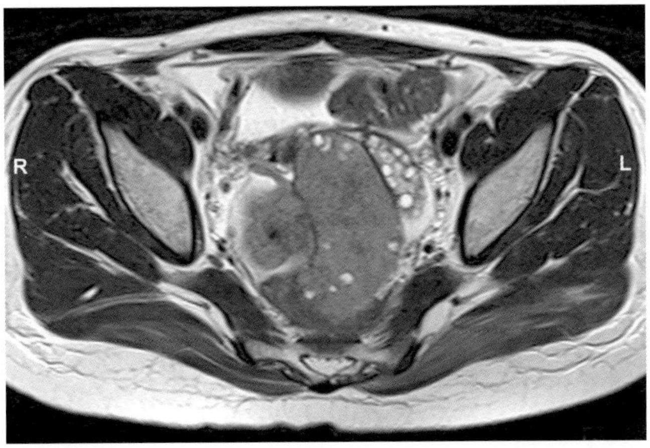

Fig. 26: Ovarian torsion: Axial MR T2WI shows an enlarged right ovary with peripheral follicles displaced into the midline. Note the adjacent normal left ovary.

there is development of pyosalpinx or tubo-ovarian abscess.

- Ovarian vein thrombosis (OVT) should be suspected as a cause of abdominal pain in the postpartum period, in women with PID, recent abdominal surgery, malignancy or known hypercoagulable state. Pregnancy increases the risk for venous thrombosis due to stasis, alteration in coagulation factors and by nearly tripling the diameter of the ovarian veins. In 90% of cases, the right ovarian vein is involved due to dextrotorsion of the uterus.[44] Ovarian vein thrombosis (OVT) may be diagnosed by US, CT or MRI, however CT is the modality of choice and demonstrates a low attenuation thrombus in lumen of ovarian vein.[44]

MISCELLANEOUS

Diverticulitis

The tetrad of left lower quadrant pain and tenderness, fever and leukocytosis is the classic presentation of diverticulitis. Diverticular disease of the colon affects 65% of the Western population by the age of 65 years, and diverticulitis eventually develops in up to 25% of individuals with diverticulosis.[45] Findings on barium enema include diverticulae, muscular wall hypertrophy, intramural or extramural mass effect on the barium column, colonic obstruction or peritoneal extravasation of contrast material, such as with fistula or sinus tract formation. The full extent of peritoneal involvement cannot be estimated on barium examination, hence it has largely been replaced by CT for imaging of suspected diverticulitis. Findings on CT include diverticulae, muscular wall hypertrophy, symmetrical mural thickening >4 mm, pericolonic fat stranding, phlegmon, extraluminal gas bubbles, extravasation of contrast in case of perforation and paracolic abscess formation. Adequate distension and opacification of the colon by contrast material administered per-rectally is the cornerstone of an optimal CT evaluation and helps to distinguish true inflammatory wall thickening from apparent wall thickening due to incomplete luminal distension. The differential diagnosis includes carcinoma: presence of enlarged lymph nodes, mural thickening >1.5 cm and an abrupt change from normal to abnormal colon favors carcinoma over diverticulitis.[46]

Toxic Megacolon

Toxic megacolon is an acute transmural fulminant colitis which can occur as a complication of any colitis but is most commonly seen with ulcerative colitis (1.6–13% of cases). Plain radiographs show marked colonic dilatation (>8 cm) particularly of the transverse colon as this is the least dependent part of the large bowel in the supine position. The wall has a shaggy appearance with mucosal islands or pseudopolyps with absence of haustra due to profound inflammation and ulceration. There may be air-fluid levels and small bowel dilatation. CT shows the distended colon filled with air, fluid and blood with a distorted or absent haustral pattern and irregular, nodular wall.[47] There may be presence of intramural air or blood. The prognosis is poor in the presence of perforation and complications.

Acute Pyelonephritis

Acute pyelonephritis is the bacterial or fungal infection of the renal parenchyma and collecting system. Presenting features include flank pain, dysuria and high grade fever with rigors. On US, renal enlargement, decreased visualization of sinus fat secondary to compression, loss of corticomedullary differentiation, focal poorly marginated hypoechoic areas representing interstitial edema or complications like abscesses may be seen. Harmonic imaging and contrast—enhanced ultrasound can increase the conspicuity of renal parenchymal abnormalities in acute pyelonephritis.[48]

The CT is the imaging modality of choice and can reveal calculi, obstruction, renal enlargement, striated nephrogram, ill-defined, wedge-shaped areas of decreased attenuation radiating from the papillae to the cortical surface, abscess, thickening of Gerotas' fascia and perinephric stranding **(Fig. 27)**. Emphysematous pyelonephritis usually occurs in patients with poorly controlled diabetes with the most common infecting organism being *Escherichia coli*. Presence of air in the renal parenchyma is pathognomonic of this condition.

Acute Urinary Colic

Impacted ureteric stone is the most common cause of acute post-renal obstruction. US is useful for the detection of small/radiolucent calculi missed on plain films. Secondly, direct visualization of the effects of these calculi on the urinary tract is also possible. However, because pelvicaliectasis may be mild to negligible in acute obstruction, US may miss up to one-third of acute obstructions. Color Doppler US helps demonstrate absence of the normal urinary jet on the obstructed side. Unenhanced helical CT has emerged as an attractive modality in the diagnostic workup of urinary tract disease. NCCT KUB is performed rapidly, without patient preparation and without risk of contrast reaction. It can provide information about size, localization and chemical composition of the stone. In addition to direct stone visualization, secondary CT signs of urinary obstruction, including ureteral dilatation, perinephric or periureteric fat stranding, blurring of renal sinus fat and ureteral wall edema, are usually present to confirm the diagnosis even after recent stone passage.[49]

Acute Epiploic Appendagitis, Omental Infarction

Epiploic appendages are fat-containing peritoneal out-pouchings that arise from cecum to rectosigmoid junction, along the serosal surface of the colon. These are 0.5–5.0 cm long and contain fat and small vessels. Epiploic appendagitis is due to torsion of an epiploic appendage leading to venous occlusion and ischemia. It is usually associated with obesity, hernia and unaccustomed exercise. The condition manifests as acute left lower quadrant pain, predominantly in males in the 4th-5th decades of life. On US, a hyperechoic, incompressible mass delineated by a hypoechoic ring is seen at the point of maximum tenderness. The lesions are hyperechoic due to their fat content or hemorrhagic necrosis. CT features include an oval, fat attenuation lesion less than 5 cm in diameter that abuts the anterior or anterolateral serosal aspect of the colonic wall, surrounded by inflammatory changes.[50] A hyperattenuating rim corresponding to the hypoechoic ring on US is seen on CT due to swollen serosa covered by fibrinoleukocyte exudate.

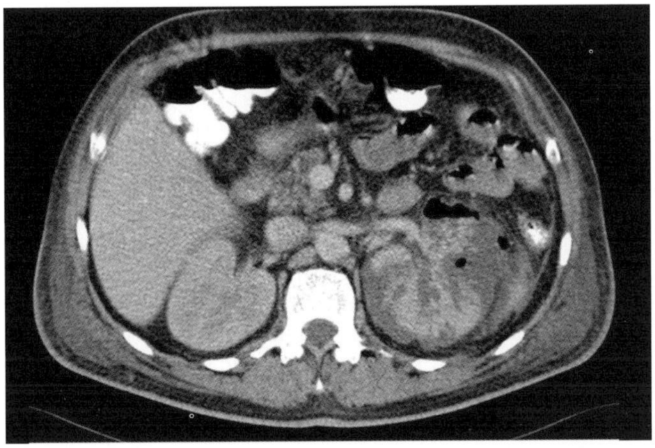

Fig. 27: Axial CT image shows multiple, irregular, linear, hypodense areas in the left kidney due to pyelonephritis. A hypodense area with an air-fluid level is seen in anterior cortex suggestive of renal abscess. In addition, perinephric collection with air is also visualized.

Omental infarction commonly involves the inferior aspect of right side of omentum. It is characteristically situated between the anterior abdominal wall and the transverse or ascending colon, corresponding in location to the greater omentum. Predisposing factors include obesity, strenuous activity, congestive heart failure, digitalis administration, recent abdominal surgery and abdominal trauma. Pain is localized to the right lower or upper quadrant and the presumptive diagnosis is usually appendicitis. Both US and CT show an ovoid, soft tissue mass just beneath the anterior abdominal wall. The infarcted omental fat is hyperechoic on ultrasound and appears heterogeneous with no enhancement on CT.

Although omental infarction may resemble acute epiploic appendagitis on CT, it lacks the hyperattenuating ring seen in the latter. Moreover, omental infarction is larger than epiploic appendagitis which is often less than 5 cm. Omental infarction is commonly located next to the cecum

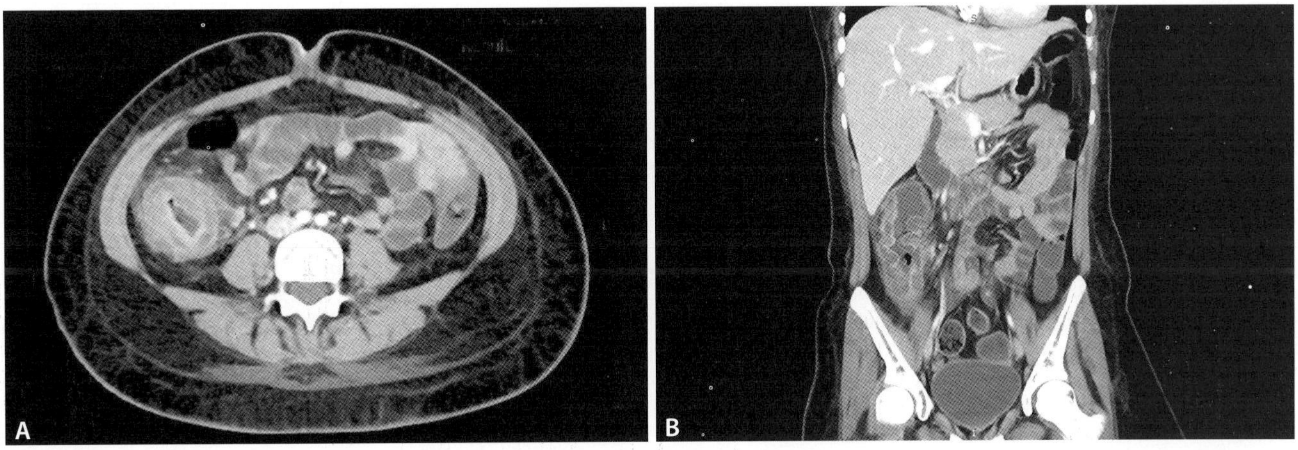

Figs. 28A and B: Neutropenic colitis: (A) Axial and (B) Coronal images demonstrate the gross mural thickening in the cecum and ascending colon.

and ascending colon whereas acute epiloic appendagitis is usually located adjacent to sigmoid colon.[50]

Acute Abdomen in Neutropenic Patients

Neutropenic enterocolitis and acute graft versus host disease are common causes of acute abdominal pain in immunocompromised patients and patients with allogenic bone marrow transplants. Cecal wall thickening and involvement of the right side of the colon is the most common finding in neutropenic colitis **(Figs. 28A and B)** with the greatest degree of thickening being found in *Clostridium difficile* colitis.[51] In acute graft versus host disease, bowel wall thickening and abnormal mucosal enhancement are common, with small bowel being most commonly affected.[52]

REFERENCES

1. Gore RM, Thakrar KH, Wenzke DR, et al. The acute abdomen. In: Gore RM, Levine MS (Eds). Textbook of Gastrointestinal Radiology, 4th edition. Philadelphia: Elsevier-Saunders; 2015.pp.2255-69.
2. Field S, Morrisom I. The acute abdomen. In: Sutton D (Ed). Textbook of Radiology and Imaging, 7th edition. Edinburgh: Churchill Livingstone; 2003.pp.663-90.
3. de Bombal FT. Introduction. In: de Bombal FT (Ed). Diagnosis of acute abdominal pain, 2nd edition. Churchill Livingstone: Edinburgh, 1991.
4. Balthazar EJ, Chako AC. Computerized tomography in acute gastrointestinal disorders. Am J Gastroenterol. 1990;85:1445-52.
5. Macari M, Balthazar EJ. The acute right lower quadrant: CT evaluation. Radiol Clin N Am. 2003;41:1117-36.
6. Kundra V, Silverman P. Impact of mutlislice CT on imaging of acute abdominal disease. Radiol Clin N Am. 2003;41:1083-93.
7. Lomas DJ. Technical developments in bowel MRI. Eur Radiol. 2003;13:1058-71.
8. Mirvis SE, Young JWR, Keramati B, et al. Plain film evaluation of patients with abdominal pain: Are three radiographs necessary? AJR. 1986;147:501-3.
9. Morrison ID, McLaughlin P, Maher MM. Current status of imaging of the gastrointestinal tract: Imaging techniques and radiation issues. In: Adam A, Dixon AK, Gillard JH, Schaefer CL, Prokop CM (Eds). Grainger and Allison's diagnostic Radiology Edinburgh: Churchill Livingstone; 2015.pp.593-609.
10. Miller RE, Nelson SW. The roentgenological demonstration of tiny amounts of free intra-peritoneal gas: experimental and clinical studies. AJR. 1971;112:574-85.
11. Rubesin SE, Levine MS. Radiologic diagnosis of gastrointestinal perforation. Radiol Clin N Am. 2003;41:1095-115.
12. Messmer JM, Levine MS. Gas and soft tissue abnormalities. In: Gore RM, Levine MS (Eds). Textbook of gastrointestinal radiology, 4th edition. WB Saunders Company; 2015. pp.178-96.
13. Bongard F, Landers DV, Lewis F. Differential diagnosis of appendicitis and pelvic inflammatory disease. Am J Surg. 1985;150:90-96.
14. Rao PM, Rhea JT, Novelline RA, et al. Helical CT technique for the diagnosis of appendicitis: Prospective evaluation of a focused appendix CT examination. Radiology. 1997;140:139-44.
15. Gaitini D, Beck-Razi N, Mor-Yosef D, et al. Diagnosing acute appendicitis in adults: accuracy of color Doppler sonography and MDCT compared with surgery and clinical follow-up. AJR. 2008;190:1300-6.
16. Lee JH, Jeong YK, Park KB, et al. Operator dependent techniques for graded compression sonography to detect the appendix and diagnose acute appendicitis. AJR. 2005;184:91-7.
17. Poortman P, Lahle PNM, Schoemaker CMC, et al. Comparison of CT and sonography in the diagnosis of acute appendicitis: A blinded prospective study. AJR. 2003;181:1355-9.
18. Romero M, Buxbaum JL, Palmer SL. Magnetic Resonance Imaging of the gut: A primer for the luminal gastroenterologist. Am J Gastroenterol. 2014;109: 497-509.
19. Uggowitzer M, Kugler C, Schramayer G, et al. Sonography of acute cholecystitis: comparison of color and power Doppler sonography in detecting a hypervascularized gallbladder wall. AJR. 1997;168:707-12.
20. Blankenberg F, Wirth R, Jeffry BR Jr, et al. Computed tomography as an adjunct to ultrasound in the diagnosis of acute a calculous cholecystitis. Gastrointestinal Radiol. 1991;16:149-53.
21. Fidler J, Paulson EK, Layfield L. CT evaluation of acute cholecystitis: Findings and usefulness in diagnosis. AJR. 1996;166:1085-8.
22. Watanabe Y, Nagayama M, Okumura A, et al. MR imaging of acute biliary disorders. Radiographics. 2007;27: 477-95.
23. Bennett GL, Rusinek H, Lisi V, et al. CT findings in acute gangrenous cholecystitis. AJR. 2002;178:275-81.
24. Morris BS, Balpande PR, Morani AC, et al. The CT appearances of gallbladder perforation. BJR. 2007;80:898-90.
25. Gore RM, Yaghmai V, Newmark GM, et al. Imaging benign and malignant disease of the gallbladder. Radiol Clin North Am. 2002;40:1307-23.
26. Smith EA, Dillman JR, Elsayes KM, Menias CO, Bude RO. Cross-sectional imaging of acute and chronic gallbladder inflammatory disease. AJR. 2009;192:188-96.
27. Balthazar EJ, Ranson JHC, Naidich DP, Megibow AJ, Caccavak R, Cooper MM. Acute pancreatitis: prognostic value of CT. Radiology. 1985;156:767-72.
28. Stimac D, Miletic D, Radic M. The role of NEMRI in early assessment of acute pancreatitis. Am J Gastroenterol. 2007; 102(5):997-1104.
29. Joseph AEA, MacVicar D. Ultrasound in the diagnosis of abdominal abscess. Clin Radiol 1990;42:154-6.

30. Go Hl, Baarslaq HJ, Vermeulen H, Laméris JS, Legemate DA. A comparative study to validate the use of ultrasonography and computed tomography in patients with post-operative intra-abdominal sepsis. Eur J Radiol. 2005;54(3):383-7.
31. Federle MP, Anne VS. Small bowel obstruction. In: Federle MP (Ed). Diagnostic Imaging—Abdomen, 1st edition Amirsys Inc, Utah, 2004.
32. Canon CL. Gastrointestinal Tract. In Lee JKT, Sagel SS, Stanley RJ, Heiken JP (Eds). Computed body tomography with MRI correlation, 4th edition Lippincott Williams and Wilkins, Philadelphia PA, 2006.
33. Ilangovan R, Burling D, George A, Gupta A, Marshall M, Taylor SA. CT enterography: review of technique and practical tips. BJR. 2012;85:876-86.
34. Beall DP, Fortman BJ, Lawler BC, et al. Imaging bowel obstruction: a comparison between fast magnetic resonance imaging and helical computed tomography. Clin Radiol. 2002;57(8):719-24.
35. Chen SC, Wang HP, Chen WJ, et al. Selective use of ultrasonography for the detection of pneumo-peritoneum. Acad Emerg Med. 2002;9:643-5.
36. Jones R. Recognition of pneumo-peritoneum using bedside ultrasound in critically ill patients presenting with acute abdominal pain. Am J Emerg Med. 2007;25:838-41.
37. Furukawa A, Sakoda M, Yamasaki M, et al. Gastrointestinal tract perforation: CT diagnosis of presence, site and cause. Abdom Imaging. 2005;30:524-34.
38. Rha SE, Ha HK, Lee S, et al. CT and MR imaging findings of bowel ischemia from various primary causes. Radiographics. 2000;20:29-42.
39. Wiesner W, Khurana B, Ji H, Ros PR. CT of acute bowel ischaemia. Radiology. 2003;226:635-50.
40. Ha HK, Rha SE, Kim AY, et al. CT and MR diagnosis of intestinal ischaemia. Seminars in US, CT and MRI. 2000;21(1):40-55.
41. Scott RA, Ashton HA, Kay DN. Abdominal aortic aneurysm in 4,237 screened patients: prevalence, development and management over 6 years. Br J Surg. 1991;78:1122-5.
42. Rakita D, Newatia A, Hines JJ, et al. Spectrum of CT findings in rupture and impending rupture of abdominal aortic aneurysms. Radiographics. 2007;27:497-507.
43. Condous G, Okaro E, Khalid A, et al. The accuracy of transvaginal ultrasonography for the diagnosis of ectopic pregnancy prior to surgery. Hum Reprod. 2005;20:1404-9.
44. Heavrin BS, Wrenn K. Ovarian vein thrombosis: A rare cause of abdominal pain outside the peripartum period. J Emerg Med. 2007;34:67-9.
45. Rao PM, Rhea JT, Novelline RA, et al. Helical CT with only colonic contrast material for diagnosing diverticulitis: Prospective evaluation of 150 patients. AJR. 1998;170: 1445-9.
46. Chintapalli KN, Esola CC, Chopra S, et al. Pericolic mesenteric lymph nodes: An aid in distinguishing diverticulitis from cancer of the colon. AJR. 169:1253-55,1997.
47. Imbriaco M, Balthazar EJ. Toxic megacolon: role of CT in evaluation and detection of complications. Clin Imaging. 2001;25:349-54.
48. Kim B, Lim HK, Choi MH, Woo JY, Ryu J, Kim S, et al. Detection of parenchymal abnormalities in acute pyelonephritis by pulse inversion harmonic imaging with or without microbubble ultrasonographic contrast agent: Correlation with computed tomography. J Ultrasound Med. 2001;20:5-14.
49. Sourtzis S, Thibeau JF, Damry N, et al. Radiologic investigation of renal colic: unenhanced helical CT compared with excretory urography. AJR. 1999;172:1491-4.
50. Singh AK, Gervais DA, Halin PF, et al. Acute epiploic appendagitis and its mimics. Radiographics. 2005;25:1521-34.
51. Iain D, Kirkpatrick C, Greenberg HM. Gastrointestinal complications in the neutropenic patient: Characterization and differentiation with abdominal CT. Radiology. 2003;226:668-74.
52. Kalantari BN, Mortelé KJ, Cantisani V, et al. CT features with pathologic correlation of acute gastrointestinal Graft-Versus-Host disease after bone marrow transplantation in adults. AJR. 2003;181:1621-5.

CHAPTER 92

Imaging in Abdominal Trauma

Atin Kumar, Shivanand Gamanagatti, Chandrashekhara SH

INTRODUCTION

Blunt abdominal trauma in isolation accounts for 5% of trauma mortality and further contributes 15% to mortality as part of polytrauma.[1] Excessive bleeding accounts for 80–90% of acute deaths from abdominal injury. In recent years, advances in cross-sectional imaging coupled with image-guided interventional therapy have made significant contributions in enabling nonsurgical management of blunt abdominal trauma in hemodynamically stable patients.

A radiologist must have a detailed understanding of the patterns of injury, imaging appearance of traumatic injuries, assessment of hemodynamic status, and common image artifacts. The imaging evaluation must take place within the context of systematic and orderly resuscitation of the patient.

Abdominal trauma can be blunt or penetrating. Blunt trauma accounts for approximately two-thirds of abdominal injury patients. Motor vehicle accidents account for up to 80% of blunt trauma with the remainder being caused by falls, assault and industrial accidents. Penetrating injuries commonly result due to gunshot injuries and stab wounds.

The spleen, liver and kidneys are the most frequently injured organs in order of frequency followed by small bowel/mesentry, bladder, colon, diaphragm, pancreas and major vessels. There are multiple organs involved simultaneously in many patients.[2]

Up to two-thirds of the abdominal trauma patients have a significant injury to other systems as well and these injuries may take precedence for both diagnosis and treatment.

Radiology plays an important role in the diagnosis and management of abdominal trauma patients. This has become even more relevant in the last two decades because there is an increasing trend towards conservative management of most solid abdominal organ trauma. The emergence of imaging as a strong marker for extent of injury has made the surgeons more comfortable with a trial of nonoperative management of these patients and has improved the outcome.

The various imaging modalities used and their current role is discussed below.

PLAIN RADIOGRAPHY

Plain radiography of abdomen is not routinely recommended in an abdominal trauma patient. It is insensitive for the detection of hemoperitoneum as intraperitoneal volume of greater than 800 cc is usually necessary for the demonstration of classic plain radiographic signs, e.g. "dog ear" or "bladder ear" sign when there is accumulation of intraperitoneal blood in the pouch of Douglas. According to Advanced Trauma Life Support (ATLS) guidelines, chest radiograph and pelvic radiographs are recommended as adjunct to primary survey and resuscitation of an abdominal trauma patient.

The chest radiograph, besides being required for detecting chest injuries, can also detect pneumoperitoneum. It is possible with optimal radiographic technique to demonstrate as little as 1 cc of free air on an upright chest radiograph. However in this setting it is often not possible to obtain the radiograph in upright position The supine chest radiograph which is usually done is not that sensitive for detecting pneumoperitoneum. The pelvic radiographs are done to detect pelvic fractures in suspected pelvic injuries.

ULTRASONOGRAPHY

Sonography is commonly used for the initial assessment of abdominal trauma. Abdominal ultrasound in cases of major trauma is usually performed with a FAST (Focussed Assessment with Sonography in Trauma) examination. It provides a fast overview of the abdomen to detect free fluid which indicates hemoperitoneum and visceral organ injury in this setting. The FAST scan should be completed within few minutes with an aim to primarily search for free intraperitoneal fluid and screen organs for injury. While parenchymal organ injuries may be detected, search for such injuries should not delay the examination specially in the setting of suspicion of hemorrhage. Following standard views are recommended:

- Transverse view of epigastrium to detect pericardial fluid and injury to left lobe of liver.
- Longitudinal view of right upper quadrant for right lobe of liver, right kidney and Morison's pouch and perihepatic free fluid.
- Longitudinal view of left upper quadrant for spleen, left kidney and perisplenic free fluid.
- Longitudinal views of bilateral flanks to look for free fluid in paracolic gutters.
- Transverse and longitudinal views of suprapubic region for urinary bladder and free fluid in pelvis and pouch of Douglas.
- Bilateral longitudinal thoracic views for pleural effusion.

The reported sensitivity of FAST for detection of free intraperitoneal fluid ranges from 64% to 98% and specificity from 86% to 100%.[3] The false negative rate of FAST is on an average 15% for free fluid detection. Negative FAST should be interpreted as indicative of the absence of hemoperitoneum, not the absence of intra-abdominal injury. However, it should be remembered that the sensitivity of FAST for free fluid is less than that of CT. A negative FAST should be viewed with suspicion if the finding is not commensurate with the patient's clinical presentation. On the other hand, a positive FAST does not necessarily mandate laparotomy. Hemodynamically stable patients with positive FAST should have their injuries staged with CT, giving them the benefit of nonoperative management whenever possible. FAST is not reliable for assessment of the retroperitoneum.

The sensitivity of ultrasound for detection of liver injury ranges from 0.15 to 0.883 and it misses an average of 15% injuries to liver. The sensitivity for splenic injuries is reported to be between 37% and 85% with an average false negative rate of more than 50%. Sensitivity for renal and pancreatic injuries is less than of liver and spleen and even lesser for bowel and mesenteric injuries. The sensitivity for pericardial effusion is high (97–100%).[3] Hence, ultrasound as a modality to detect abdominal injuries is not recommended.

In a technically successful examination, hemoperitoneum **(Fig. 1)** is visualized as a lenticular collection in the subphrenic space, triangular in Morison's pouch and ovoid in the pelvis.

Recently contrast enhanced ultrasound (CEUS) has been used for improving the detection of solid abdominal organ injuries. It has been shown to detect hepatic, splenic and renal injuries including vascular injuries **(Figs. 2A to C)**. However, the assessment of bowel, mesentery and retroperitoneum is not possible. Hence, it can be used as an alternative to contrast-enhanced computed tomography (CECT) for use in low energy localized trauma in patients with contraindication to CT contrast. It may also be useful in follow-up of patients to monitor the organ injury especially in pediatric patients where radiation dose is a concern.[4]

Ultrasound has certain limitations as the technique is operator dependent and may be limited by excessive bowel gas (especially in post-traumatic paralytic ileus).

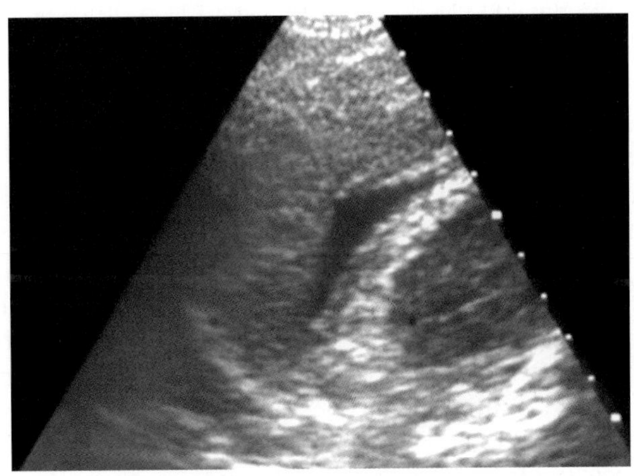

Fig. 1: Axial ultrasound image shows free fluid in hepatorenal pouch.

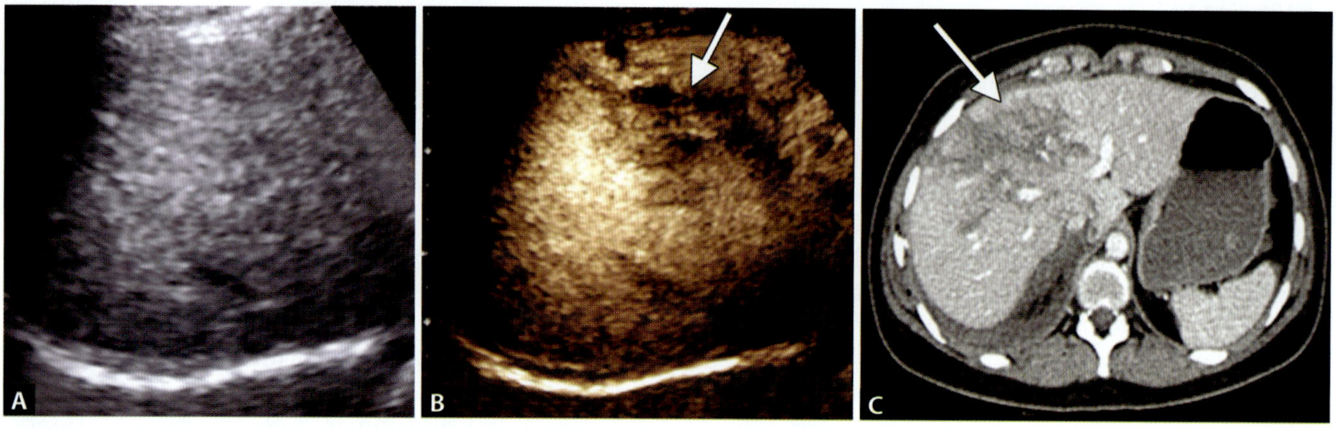

Figs. 2A to C: Contrast-enhanced ultrasound of right hypochondrium (B) shows the hypoechoic linear lacerations within the right lobe of the liver (arrow). These were not well appreciated on the grayscale ultrasound (A). CECT axial scan (C) also clearly shows multiple lacerations (arrow).

It may also be limited by open wounds and bandages and by subcutaneous emphysema.

COMPUTED TOMOGRAPHY

Computed tomography (CT) is now firmly established as the principal imaging modality for diagnostic evaluation of abdominal trauma. It is useful in detecting otherwise occult injuries to both intra-abdominal and retroperitoneal structures and grading the severity of specific parenchymal injury. Associated injuries of head and chest, etc. can also be evaluated. According to American College of Radiology (ACR) guidelines, if the initial CT abdomen of a stable patient is negative, then the patient can be safely discharged from the emergency department without a period of observation.[5]

Computed Tomography Technique

Meticulous attention to scanning technique is essential. Scans should be done expeditiously and care should be taken to avoid artifacts and repeat scanning. Current MDCT scanners have significantly reduced the scan time with less motion artifacts besides providing excellent quality reconstructions in coronal and sagittal planes. Administration of intravenous iodinated contrast material is mandatory as it makes detection and location of parenchymal contusions and hematoma more conspicuous, identifies great vessels and provides information regarding integrity of organs or extent of the injury. MDCT protocols vary from institution to institution but typically involve imaging at sub-mm slice thickness, 60–70 seconds after initiating an injection of 100–120 mL of 300 mg/dL low osmolar intravenous contrast medium at 2.5–3.0 mL per second. This phase is best for parenchymal injury detection and is often the only phase done. Careful evaluation of the images is done on the console immediately after acquisition of this phase. If, there is evidence of a contained vascular injury (pseudoaneurysm or fistula) or active contrast extravasation, a localized repeat phase is taken immediately to confirm the same. If the scan shows renal injury then a delayed scan after 5–10 minutes during urographic phase is essential to detect collecting system injuries.[6] Some centers include an arterial phase (25–30 sec after start of contrast injection) to better delineate vascular injuries. However routine use of dual phase (arterial and venous) is not advocated due to concern of radiation. Presently arterial phase is obtained mainly in selected indications—pelvis radiograph showing displaced fracture of the pelvic ring and in patients with severe mechanisms of injury.

Computed tomography (CT) cystography may be done in specific situations like hematuria with no renal injury seen on CT or hematuria along with pelvic fracture.[2] It is done by instillation of approximately 300–400 mL of diluted (1:10) iodinated contrast into bladder via Foley's catheter or suprapubic catheter. A delayed phase with passive filling of urinary bladder by renal contrast excretion is not a substitute for the same.

Oral contrast is not administered in the setting of acute trauma in most trauma centers across the world.[2,6] It has a potential use for detecting bowel injuries by showing extravasated oral contrast. But, presence of pneumoperitoneum or pneumoretroperitoneum is an indirect marker for the same. Also usually there is not enough time available at hand to administer oral contrast. Rectal contrast is used occasionally in specific situations to detect colorectal injuries in patients with perineal lacerations and penetrating flank or back wounds.[6]

Viewing on bone window for detecting subtle fractures and upper sections with lung windows for unsuspected pneumothorax, lung contusion or free peritoneal gas should be done.

MAGNETIC RESONANCE IMAGING

Currently, magnetic resonance imaging (MRI) does not play much role in the initial evaluation of the acutely injured patient. MRCP may be useful in detecting biliary transection. MR imaging is useful only for niche indications in hemodynamically stable patients. It has been shown to be useful in detection of pancreatic injuries. The pancreatic parenchymal lacerations and contusions are sometimes better demonstrated on MRI than CT in the acute setting. However, CT remains the first modality for evaluation. If, there are equivocal findings on CT pertaining to pancreatic parenchymal injury, then MRI can subsequently be done to aid in the diagnosis. Moreover involvement of main pancreatic duct is also better characterized on MRI (and MRCP) which is important for deciding management.[7]

DIGITAL SUBTRACTION ANGIOGRAPHY

With recent trend towards nonoperative management of abdominal trauma patients, digital subtraction angiography (DSA) with embolization has been increasingly used in the management of post-traumatic hemorrhage. Angiographic embolization is indicated when CT shows evidence of vascular injury (pseudoaneurysm, arteriovenous fistula) and in active contrast extravasation as an alternative to surgery. It has also been used in controlling bleeding in patients with high grade (IV and V) liver and spleen injuries especially in hemodynamically stable patients with falling hematocrit.

IMAGING AND MANAGEMENT PROTOCOLS

When a patient of suspected abdominal trauma presents to the emergency department, the initial evaluation and assessment is done as per the ATLS guidelines. Chest and pelvic radiograph along with FAST ultrasound are considered as an adjunct of this primary survey and resuscitation. The subsequent management and further role of imaging is dependent upon the hemodynamic stability of the patient. As per the ACR guidelines/ appropriateness criteria (first published in 1996 and subsequently updated in 2012)[6] the patients are divided into following categories:

Category A: Patients who remain hemodynamically unstable after initial evaluation and resuscitation. The further management and imaging protocol in this group is outlined in **Flowchart 1**.

Category B: Patients who are hemodynamically stable either at presentation or get stabilized after resuscitation. The imaging and management protocol in this group is outlined in **Flowchart 2**.

Category C: Patients of abdominal trauma who have hematuria. This group requires some modification of imaging workup which is outlined in **Flowchart 3**.

Flowchart 1: Hemodynamically unstable patient. Imaging and management protocol in Category A patients.

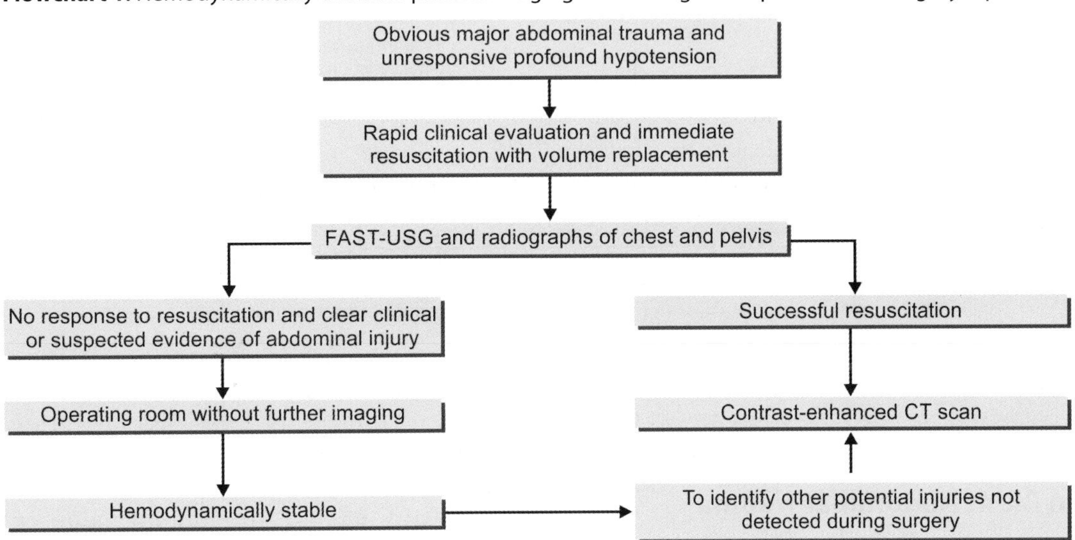

Abbreviation: FAST-USG: Focused assessment with sonography for trauma-ultrasound.

Flowchart 2: Hemodynamically stable patient. Imaging and management protocol in Category B patients.

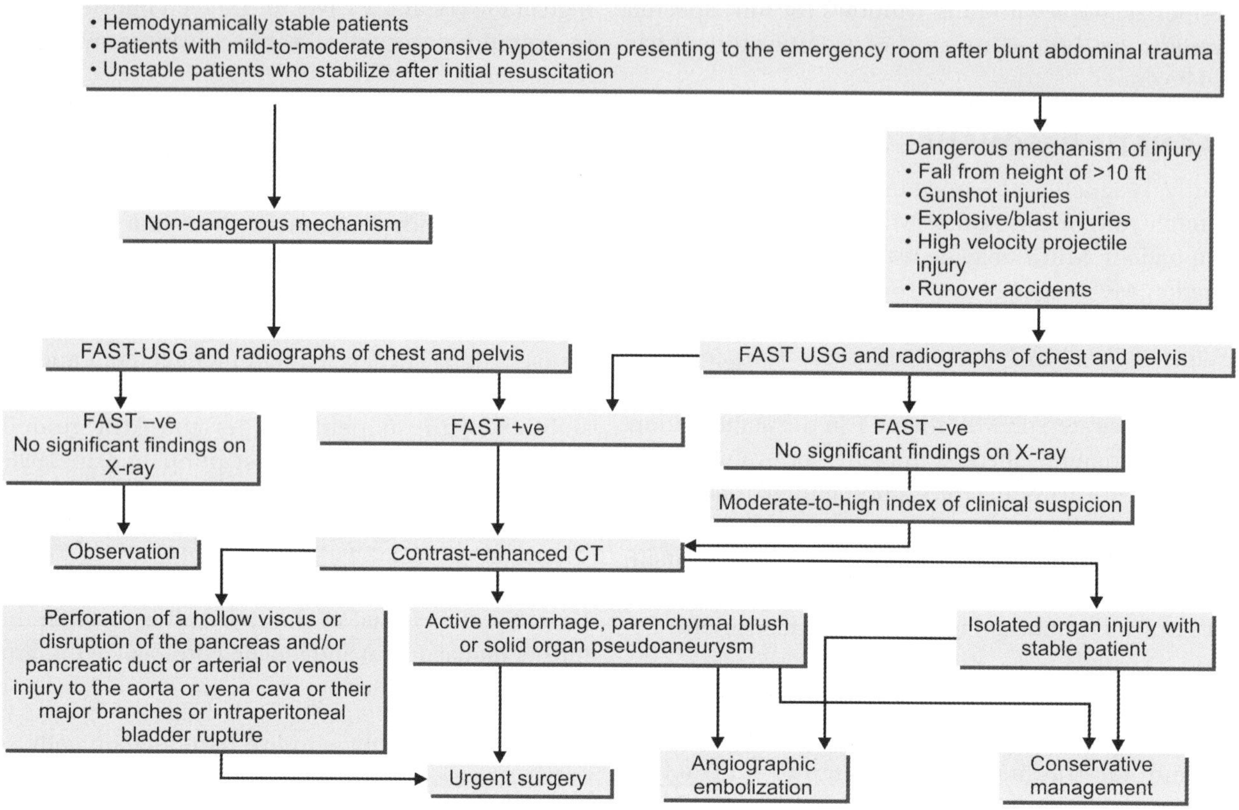

Flowchart 3: Suspected lower urinary tract injury. Imaging and management protocol in category C patients.

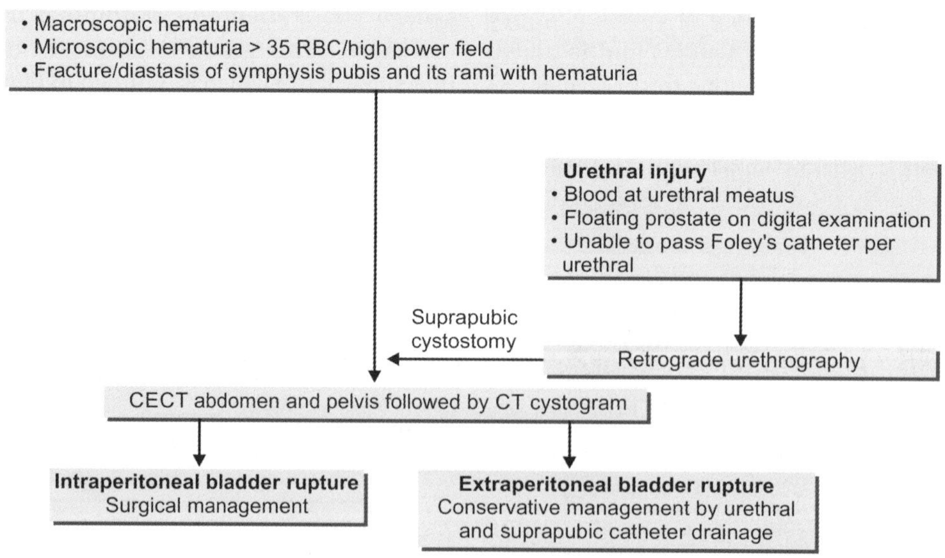

DIAGNOSTIC IMAGING

CT Signs in Blunt Abdominal Trauma

- *Hemoperitoneum:* Blood collects in the peritoneum following injury to the liver, spleen, bowel or mesentery. CT is sensitive in detecting intra-abdominal or pelvic hemorrhage. Non-clotted blood typically has an attenuation value of 30–45 HU whereas clotted blood has attenuation values between 45–70 HU. However a quarter of patients may have HU value less than 20 HU. Therefore hemoperitoneum may not be distinguishable from ascites, extravasated small intestinal fluid from bowel perforation or from intraperitoneal urine from ruptured urinary bladder. Detection of fluid within the abdomen in a suspected patient of abdominal trauma is considered as hemoperitoneum unless proven otherwise. It should however be remembered that in women of child bearing age small amounts of intraperitoneal fluid may be a normal finding. Detection of fluid in each paracolic gutter indicates that at least 200 mL of blood must be present in each gutter. CT visualization of blood in the abdomen and pelvis corresponds with amounts greater than 500 mL.

- *Sentinel clot sign:* Clotted blood adjacent to the site of injury is of higher attenuation (45–70 HU) than unclotted blood which flows away **(Figs. 3A and B)**. When source of intraperitoneal bleed is not evident or in the situation of multiple organ injuries, the location of highest attenuating blood clot is a clue to the most likely source.
- *Interloop fluid:* Triangular fluid collection(s) between the leaves of mesentery are important indicators of bowel or mesenteric injury. Hemoperitoneum from liver or spleen injury typically does not form such collections, but instead tracks from the upper abdomen along the paracolic gutters into the pelvis. When interloop fluid is of low attenuation (< 15 HU), bowel injury is suspected and when it is of high attenuation (> 30 HU), mesenteric hematoma is likely.
- *Hemodynamic status:* There are a combination of CT findings which give valuable morphological information that correlates with the intravascular volume and cardiac output. Hypoperfusion complex is a gamut of visceral and vascular manifestations which signify the presence of clinical shock in the patient **(Figs. 4A to C)**. They are outlined in **Table 1**.[8]

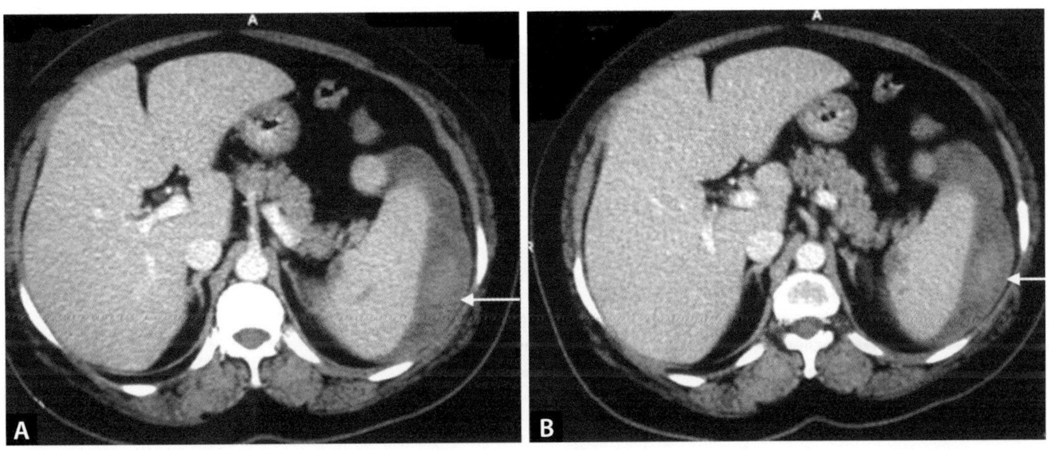

Figs. 3A and B: Axial CECT scans show hemoperitoneum in perisplenic region. Note the presence of higher density clotted blood adjacent to the spleen (arrows)—the 'sentinel clot sign'.

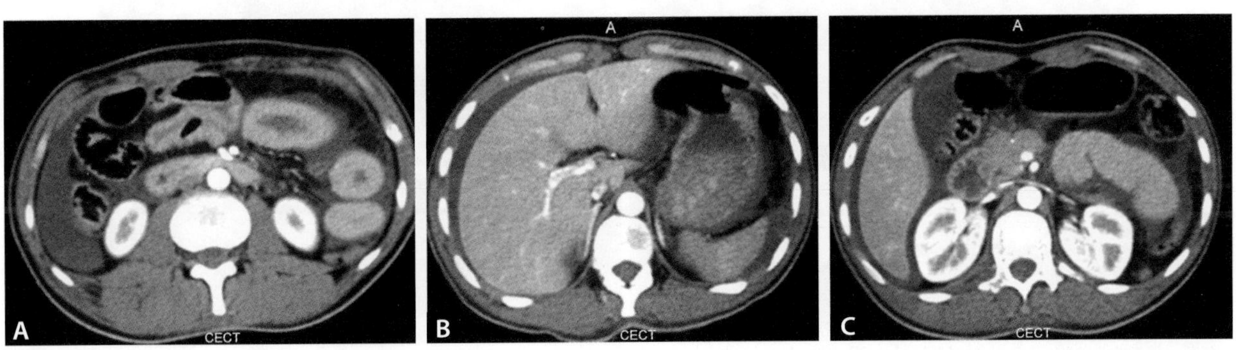

Figs. 4A to C: Hypoperfusion state (shock bowel). Axial CECT scan through midabdomen (A) shows diffuse thickening and hyperenhancement of jejunal loops. Note the presence of hemoperitoneum. Axial scan through adrenals (B) show hyperenhancing bilateral adrenal glands. Axial scan through kidneys (C) show flat IVC.

- *Vascular injuries:* Vascular injuries are classified as free/uncontained and contained vascular injuries. The uncontained vascular injury is seen as active arterial contrast extravasation which is defined as leakage of intravascular contrast from vessel into surrounding extravascular tissues. The active contrast leak appears as a poorly marginated high attenuation contrast density (85–350 HU) seen outside the confines of a vessel **(Figs. 5A and B)**. It may be lobulated or may be spreading. It is usually surrounded by a hematoma. The extravasation appears more hyperdense than clotted blood which has HU values in the range of 45–70. On a repeat delayed scan, the active contrast leak can show change in shape (spreading). The attenuation may either increase or decrease. The contained vascular injuries (pseudoaneurysm or arteriovenous fistula) are seen as contrast outpouching which is usually rounded and well marginated **(Figs. 6A and B)**. It is typically of same attenuation as the adjacent major artery or aorta. On the delayed phase it does not change in shape and the attenuation parallels the attenuation of the adjacent artery or aorta. The vascular injuries must be actively looked for as they (especially uncontained) signify active arterial bleeding in the patient at the time of CT scanning. Detection of these injuries is often an indicator for surgical/angiographic intervention.

Table 1: CT signs for hypoperfusion complex.

Vascular signs	***Visceral signs***
Diminished caliber of IVC: AP diameter less than 9 mm on 3 slices of intrahepatic IVC, at and 2 cm below renal veins	*Hollow visceral abnormalities*: • Increased bowel wall mucosal enhancement, gastric dilatation
Diminished caliber of aorta: AP diameter less than 1.3 cm, 2 cm above, at and below renal arteries	*Solid visceral abnormalities*: • Intense adrenal gland enhancement (greater than IVC) • Renal cortical enhancement (greater than that of aorta) • Dark spleen • Only pancreatic parenchymal enhancement

- *Pneumoperitoneum:* It is a sign of perforated hollow viscus, but may also occur following pneumothorax and mechanical ventilation. Small amount of air is easily detectable under the right hemidiaphragm on erect chest radiograph. CT is the most sensitive investigation for detection for free peritoneal air. In order not to miss small amounts of free air the images should be viewed on lung window settings. It may be detected on CT over the liver and anteriorly in the mid abdomen **(Fig. 7)**. Bubbles of free air may be trapped between the leaves of the mesentery or in the peritoneal recesses.
- *Contusion/hematoma:* The contusion/hematoma within the parenchyma of solid abdominal organs appears as focal, poorly marginated areas of low attenuation representing edema, hemorrhage and necrotic tissue **(Fig. 8)**. Subcapsular hematomas are characterized by their lenticular configuration and flattening of the adjacent parenchyma. The compression of underlying parenchyma helps to differentiate subcapsular location of hematoma from free intraperitoneal fluid or blood. Acute hematomas show increased density (40–60 HU) relative to the adjacent normal liver parenchyma at unenhanced CT.
- *Laceration:* Lacerations are seen as nonenhancing linear or branching areas usually at the periphery of

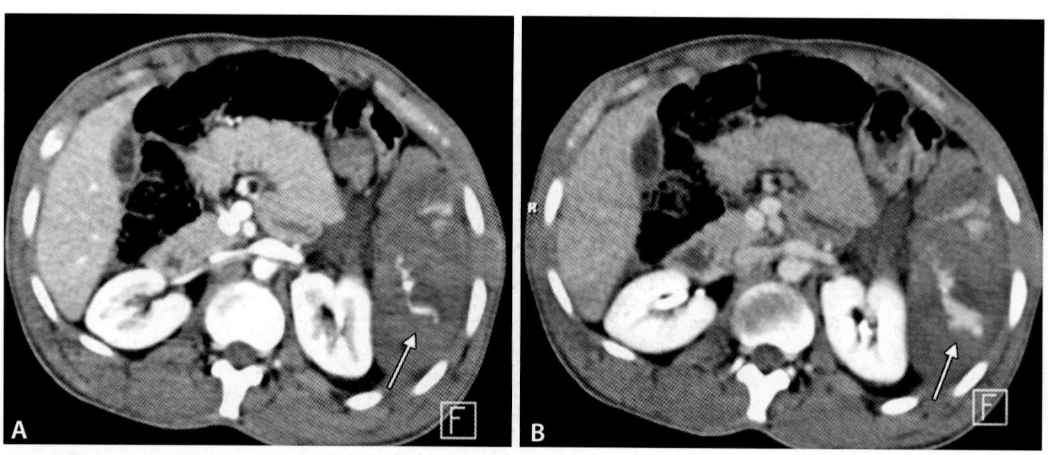

Figs. 5A and B: CECT abdomen axial image through the level of spleen (A) shows an irregular contrast density (arrow) in the region of splenic bed. The spleen is showing a large hematoma. The delayed image (B) acquired immediately after the first scan shows the contrast density to be spreading and changing in shape (arrow) confirming active contrast extravasation.

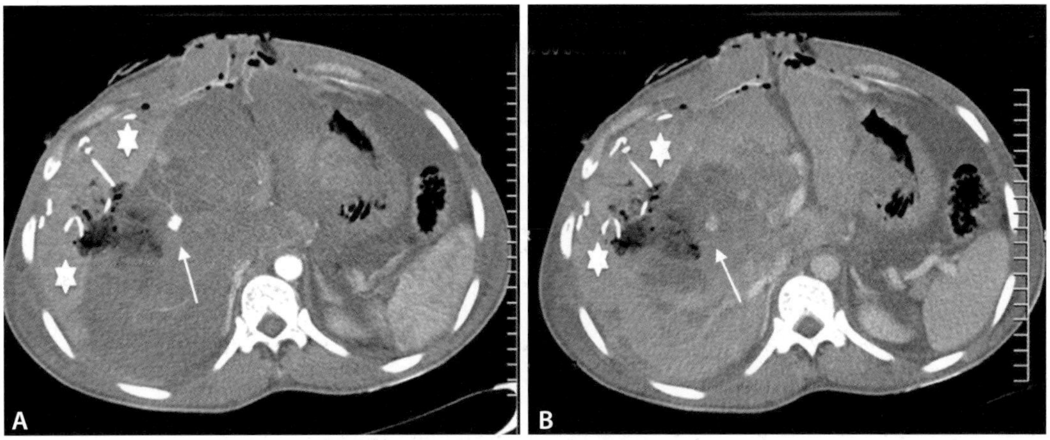

Figs. 6A and B: CECT abdomen axial image through the level of liver in a patient who underwent an urgent damage control surgery with perihepatic packing (A) shows a well-marginated, rounded-contrast density lesion (arrow) in the liver which is of same density as the aorta. On the delayed image (B) acquired immediately after the first scan, the lesion (arrow) maintains the same shape but shows decrease in attenuation paralleling the attenuation of the aorta. Note the presence of a large perihepatic hematoma (stars in A and B) with surgical packs.

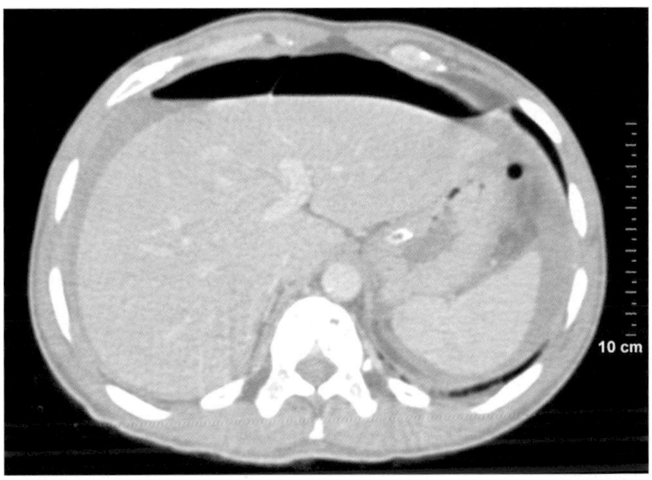

Fig. 7: Axial CECT scan through upper abdomen in lung window settings shows pneumoperitoneum anterior to liver.

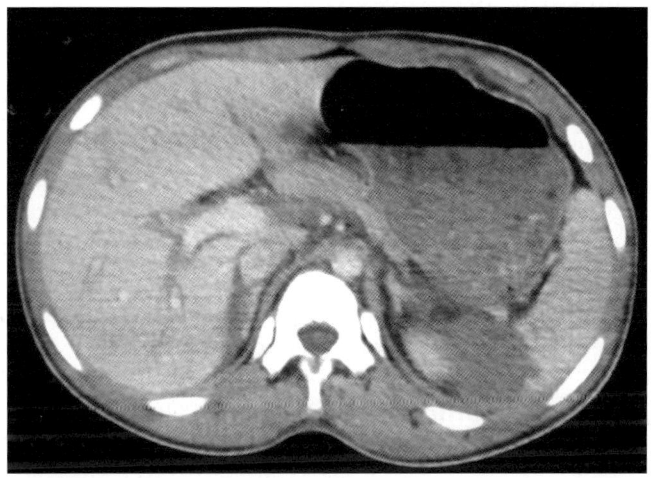

Fig. 8: Axial CECT scan through upper abdomen shows a splenic parenchymal hematoma.

the parenchyma **(Fig. 9)**. They are commonly multiple and may involve different areas including different segments. Lacerations decrease in size and number with time. When delayed phase images are taken, the lacerations appear to 'fill-in' from the periphery and become less visible.

- *Infarction/devascularization:* Infarct appears as a well-demarcated wedge-shaped area of low attenuation which remains unchanged on delayed images. It may decrease in size or remain unchanged on follow-up scans. Devascularization occurs secondary to vascular pedicle injury. The entire organ or a large segment does not show enhancement **(Fig. 10)**. Often the occluded major artery is also seen.

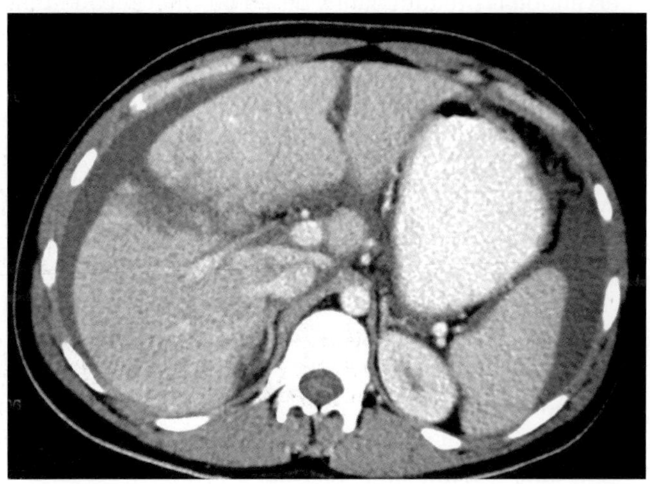

Fig. 9: Axial CECT scan shows a linear liver laceration

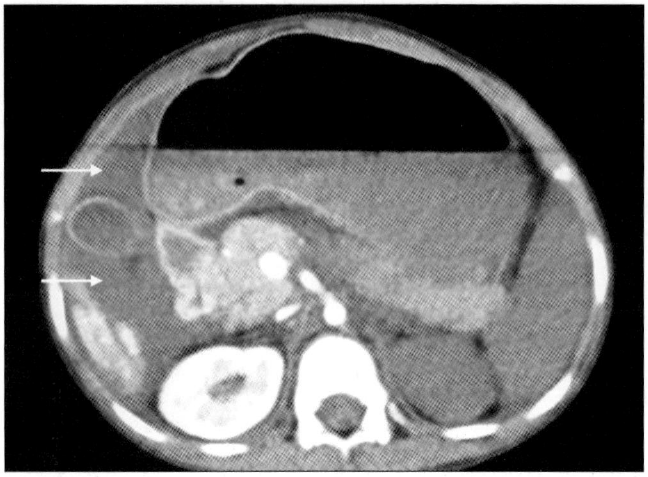

Fig. 10: Axial CECT scan shows nonenhancing and left kidney spleen (devascularized) (arrows).

Computed Tomography Staging of Abdominal Injuries

Most of the organs in the abdomen are staged according to the American Association for Staging in Trauma (AAST) grading system. It is a surgical grading but can be very well correlated with CT. All organ injuries should be staged accordingly as it is an important marker for extent of injury and deciding further course of management. Majority of the injuries to the liver, spleen and kidneys can be managed nonoperatively. However, the higher grade injuries require a close observation and often surgical intervention.

Computed Tomography Signs for Operative/ Angiographic Intervention

As already discussed, most abdominal injuries are currently treated by nonoperative management. The surgical intervention is predominantly based on clinical condition of the patient. The CT grading aids the trauma surgeon to monitor the patient. The higher grade injury *per se* is not an indication for surgical intervention but are more likely to be associated with an unstable hemodynamic condition of the patient which may require surgery or angiography. However, there are few CT findings which when seen may warrant a surgical repair. These are:

- Pneumoperitoneum—signifies full thickness bowel injury (exclude other causes as described later)
- Pancreatic transection—with involvement of pancreatic duct
- Diaphragmatic injury
- Intraperitoneal rupture of urinary bladder
- Mesenteric hematoma/vascular injury
- Renal pelvic injury.

Table 2: AAST organ injury scale for Spleen.

*Grade**	*Description*
Grade I	*Hematoma:* Subcapsular, <10% surface area *Laceration:* Capsular tear, <1 cm in parenchymal depth
Grade II	*Hematoma:* Subcapsular, 10–50% surface area; intraparenchymal, <5 cm in diameter *Laceration:* Capsular tear, 1–3 cm in parenchymal depth, not involving a trabecular vessel
Grade III	*Hematoma:* Subcapsular, >50% surface area or expanding; ruptured subcapsular or parenchymal hematoma; intraparenchymal hematoma >5 cm or expanding *Laceration:* >3 cm in parenchymal depth, involving trabecular vessels
Grade IV	*Laceration:* Involving segmental or hilar vessels producing major devascularization (>25% of spleen)
Grade V	*Hematoma:* Completely shattered spleen *Laceration:* Hilar vascular injury that devascularizes spleen

*Advance one grade for multiple injuries up to grade III

Abbreviation: AAST, American Association for the Surgery of Trauma.

The following CT features when seen are relative indications for either a surgical or angiographic intervention:

- Grade 4/5 liver injuries
- Grade 4/5 splenic injuries
- Vascular injuries—uncontained (active contrast extravasation) or contained (pseudoaneurysm or arteriovenous fistula).

SPLEEN

Spleen is the most commonly injured organ following blunt abdominal trauma. It is the most vascular organ of the body containing approximately 500–600 mL of blood. Although it may occur as an isolated injury, most patients with splenic trauma have associated intra-abdominal injuries.[9] The AAST splenic injury grading scale is depicted in **Table 2**.[10]

However, this AAST injury grading score is based on appearance of the spleen at surgery. CT may not be able to correctly show all the above features and hence there may be limitations in accurately grading the splenic injuries. Moreover the AAST grading does not take into account vascular injuries on CT. Marmery et al.[10] have proposed a modified splenic injury grading system taking into account the findings of active splenic hemorrhage and vascular injuries on CT. According to their modified grading system, active intraparenchymal and subcapsular splenic bleeding, splenic vascular injury (pseudoaneurysm or arteriovenous fistula) and shattered spleen should be classified as Grade IVa and active intraperitoneal bleeding as Grade IVb. There is no Grade V in their classification. It has now been well established that the presence of active hemorrhage and vascular injuries is predictive of the need for splenic artery transcatheter embolization or splenic surgery. The authors compared their modified grading with the AAST splenic injury grading scale and found it to be a better predictor for surgical or angiographic intervention in patients of splenic trauma (grade IV patients).

- Arterial phase, if obtained, shows vascular injuries better and they may sometimes be difficult to detect on venous phase alone.[9] However, it is important to evaluate spleen on portal venous phase of CT as heterogeneous enhancement in the arterial phase can simulate injury. If the arterial phase has not been obtained and the venous phase shows suspicion of a vascular injury then, as already stated above, another immediate delayed phase should be obtained. This will help to confirm vascular injury and also differentiate between contained and uncontained injury.
- Delayed phase may also be useful in differentiating a laceration from a splenic cleft.[9,11] When delayed phase images are taken, the lacerations appear to 'fill-in' from the periphery and become less visible. In contrast, splenic clefts remain unchanged in appearance on delayed phase images besides having smooth or rounded margins.

Splenic artery embolization (SAE) has now been established as an effective tool to aid in the nonsurgical management of splenic injuries. Currently grades 4 and 5 injuries **(Fig. 11)** and those showing vascular injuries (active leak or pseudoaneurysms) are indications for SAE **(Figs. 12A and B)**. Selected cases of grade 3 with large hemoperitoneum who may be transiently responding to resuscitative efforts can also benefit by SAE. The embolization aims to reduce the perfusion pressure to the spleen by blocking the arterial supply. However development of collaterals from pancreatic circulation prevents clinically significant infarction thereby preserving splenic function. SAE has been shown to have beneficial effect on hematocrit drop and fluid requirements of the patient besides decreasing the length of hospital stay.[12,13]

LIVER AND BILIARY TRACT

The liver is the second most frequently injured solid abdominal organ after spleen.[2] The right lobe is injured

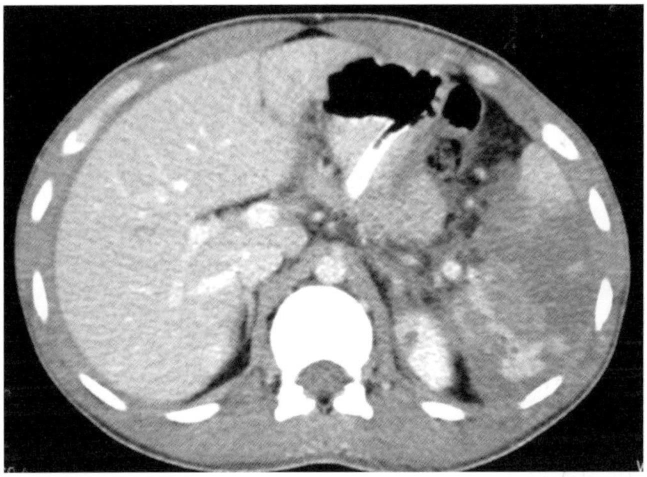

Fig. 11: Axial CECT scan through the spleen shows a shattered splenic parenchyma consistent with grade V injury.

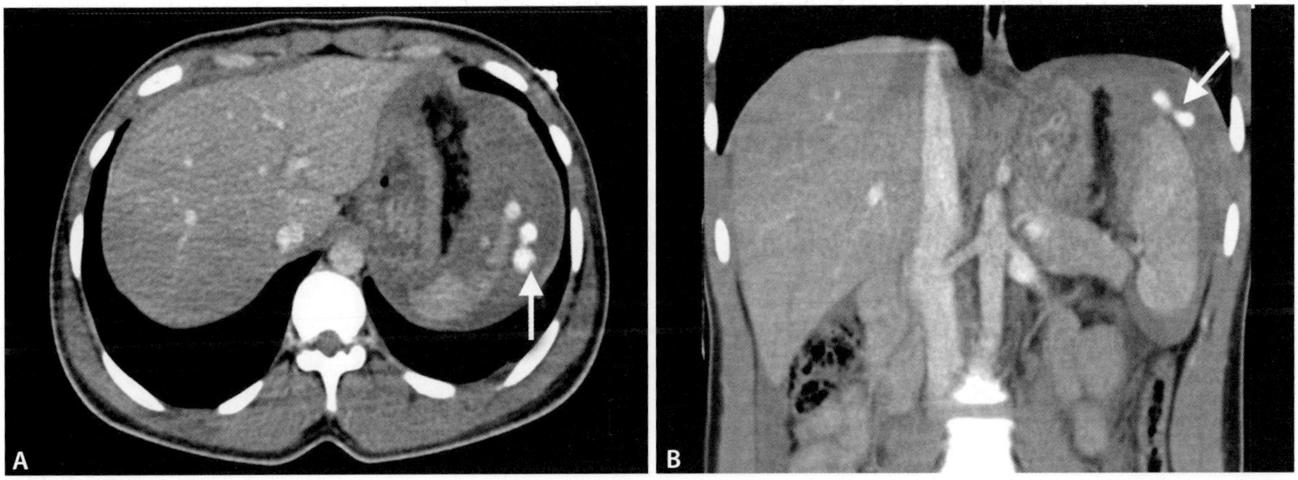

Figs. 12A and B: CECT axial (A) and coronal reformatted (B) images shows active contrast extravasation (arrows) from the spleen into peritoneum. The upper pole of the spleen shows a laceration. There is hemoperitoneum in perisplenic region.

more frequently and severely than the left and posterior segments are more frequently injured than anterior. As with spleen, CT is currently the diagnostic modality of choice for the evaluation of blunt liver trauma in hemodynamically stable patients. The AAST liver injury grading system is depicted in **Table 3.**[10]

- Majority (80%) of liver injuries cause hemoperitoneum. The finding of integrity of the liver capsule is important because it correlates with the amount of blood loss. Few specific features of liver injuries are discussed below. The subcapsular hematomas are located most commonly in the anterolateral aspect of right lobe of liver **(Figs. 13A and B)**.
- Laceration is the most common type of liver injury. They frequently course along the vascular planes (portal vein branches and hepatic veins) and fissures (ligamentum teres and venosum), which are anatomic weak zones. They can be classified as superficial (≤ 3 cm in depth) or deep (> 3 cm).
- Periportal tracking is seen as low density areas along the portal vein branches. When accompanied by an adjacent parenchymal laceration, it indicates blood tracking along the periportal connective tissue **(Fig. 14)**.[14] It may also be secondary to distension of periportal lymphatic vessels due to increased central venous pressure of any cause most commonly following vigorous intravenous fluid replacement.
- Major hepatic venous injury should be suspected if CT shows lacerations or hematomas extending into one or more major hepatic veins or IVC. If detected, it is an indicator for surgical treatment.
- Uncommonly intrahepatic or subcapsular air may be seen up to 2 days after the injury, and it is attributed to necrosis rather than infection.
- Hemobilia is seen as high attenuating material in the gallbladder or biliary channels **(Figs. 15A and B)**. It is caused when persistent arterial hemorrhage elevates intrahepatic pressure leading to parenchymal necrosis and blood spilling into the biliary tree and gut.
- Intraperitoneal bile leak and peritonitis can occur secondary to disruption of biliary system by trauma. Bile leaks are seen as relatively low attenuation fluid

Table 3: AAST organ injury scale for liver.

*Grade**	*Description*
Grade I	*Hematoma:* Subcapsular, <10% surface area *Laceration:* Capsular tear, <1 cm in parenchymal depth
Grade II	*Hematoma:* Subcapsular, 10–50 % surface area; intraparenchymal, < 10 cm in diameter *Laceration:* 1–3 cm in parenchymal depth, <10 cm in length
Grade III	*Hematoma:* Subcapsular, >50% surface area or expanding; ruptured subcapsular or parenchymal hematoma; intraparenchymal hematoma > 10 cm or expanding or ruptured *Laceration:* >3 cm in parenchymal depth
Grade IV	*Laceration:* Parenchymal disruption involving 25–75% hepatic lobe or 1–3 Couinaud segments
Grade V	*Laceration:* Parenchymal disruption involving >75% hepatic lobe or > 3 Couinaud segments *Vascular:* Juxtahepatic venous injuries (i.e. central major hepatic veins or retrohepatic vena cava)
Grade VI	*Vascular:* Hepatic avulsion

*Advance one grade for multiple injuries up to grade III

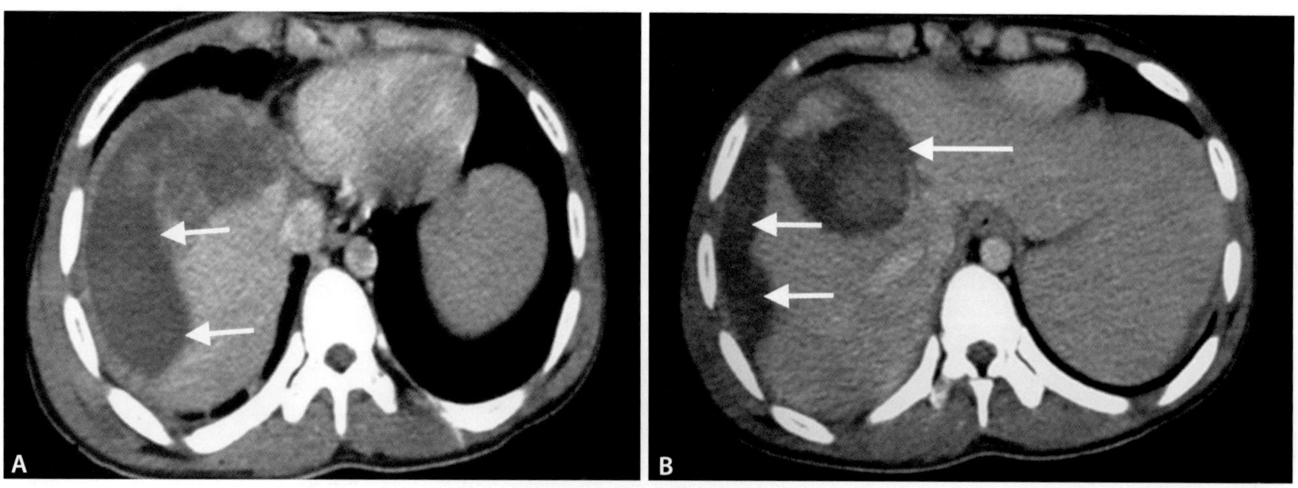

Figs. 13A and B: Axial CECT scans show a large subcapsular liver hematoma (small arrows in A and B) caused due to rupture of a parenchymal hematoma (long arrow in B).

collections as compared to hemoperitoneum. These may be intrahepatic or extrahepatic, diffuse, focal or encapsulated (biloma).[14]

With the current concept of nonsurgical conservative management being employed in majority of patients of liver injury including those with severe grades, there is increased frequency of delayed complications visualized on follow-up CT. These include:[14]

- *Delayed hemorrhage:* Secondary to rupture of pseudoaneurysm formed by a biloma or secondary to an initially minimal but expanding injury.
- *Hepatic artery pseudoaneurysm and hemobilia:* A pseudoaneurysm is formed when the arterial continuity is disrupted and blood extravasates into a parenchymal hematoma with formation of a fibrous tissue capsule. They appear as focal rounded enhancing lesions paralleling the attenuation of arterial blood in all phases. When the pseudoaneurysm ruptures into biliary system it leads to hemobilia and subsequent drainage into duodenum can lead to hematemesis or melena. These pseudoaneurysms should be treated early and angiographic embolization is the modality of choice.
- *Abscess:* Usually seen in follow-up of high grade liver injuries. It is visualized as fluid containing focal lesion with air bubbles or air-fluid levels. The treatment of choice is percutaneous catheter drainage.
- *Biliary complications:* Biliary leaks are usually self-limiting with no definitive treatment required. Hepatic scintigraphy and MRCP may be helpful in detecting bile leaks. Bile leak into a hematoma may cause necrosis of surrounding liver tissue leading to formation of biloma which on CT appears as low attenuating well circumscribed collection. Enlarging or symptomatic bilomas can be treated with percutaneous catheter drainage with or without ERCP guided endobiliary stent placement. Bile leak into peritoneal cavity leads to biliary peritonitis which may be suspected on CT if peritoneal thickening and enhancement is seen with increasing amount of low attenuation fluid.

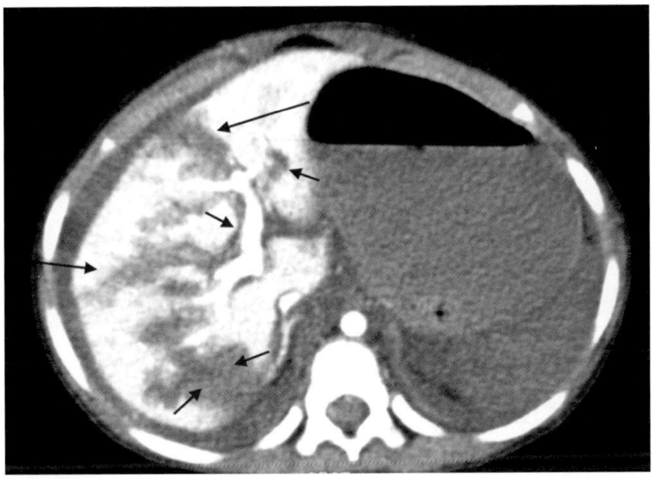

Fig. 14: Axial CECT scan though liver shows periportal fluid tracking (small arrows). The liver shows multiple lacerations (long arrows) and contusion.

Follow-up CT is usually not required in low grade injuries unless patient's clinical status demands so. However in high grade injuries (grades IV or V), due to increased incidence of delayed complications a follow-up ultrasound is usually required and should be done between 7 days to 10 days after injury.[15] Contrast-enhanced ultrasound, if available, can improve the

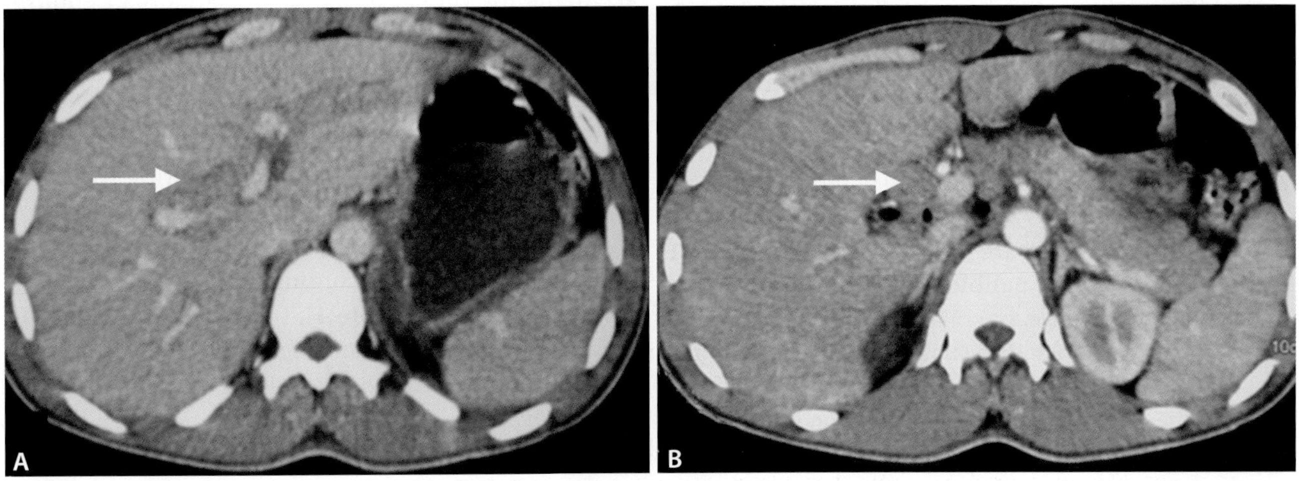

Figs. 15A and B: Axial CECT scans through upper abdomen show hyperdensity within intrahepatic bile ducts (arrow in A) and within the CBD (arrow in B) suggesting hemobilia.

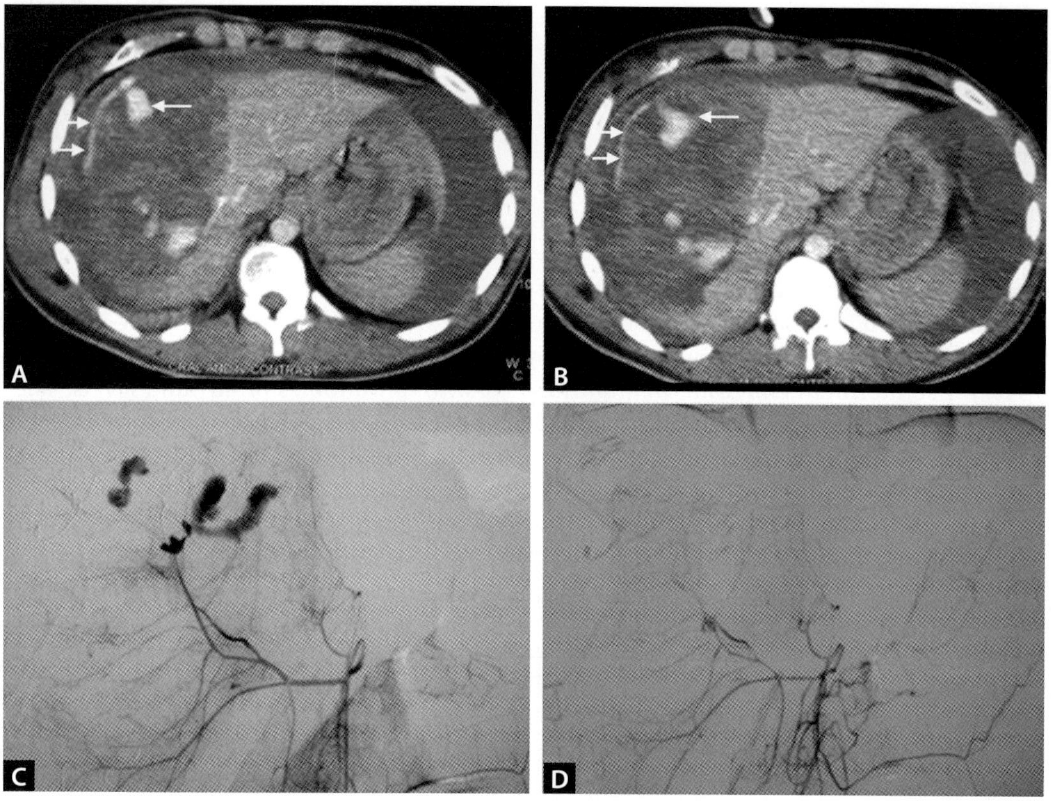

Figs. 16A to D: Axial CECT scans (A and B) show active contrast extravasation within liver parenchyma (arrows) extending into peritoneal space (small arrows). DSA image (C) of selective hepatic artery injection shows active contrast extravasation. Post coil embolization (D), the extravasation has stopped.

diagnostic accuracy. CT scan may be required in selected complicated cases.

Hepatic artery embolization (HAE) has also been increasingly used in the management of liver injuries.[15] It is indicated when CT shows presence of a vascular injury in the form of active contrast extravasation or pseudoaneurysm **(Figs. 16A to D)**. It can also be done prophylactically for grades 4 and 5 injuries and has been shown to decrease morbidity and mortality. The dual blood supply to the liver from hepatic artery and portal venous system helps in this regard wherein the hepatic artery or its branches can be sacrificed without much risk of infarction.

Gallbladder injuries are unusual. CT findings of ill-defined contour of gallbladder, wall thickening, intraluminal hemorrhage, or collapsed lumen, especially in the presence of pericholecystic fluid suggests primary gallbladder injury in patients with abdominal trauma. Injuries to the extrahepatic bile ducts are uncommon and occur at the points of fixations, i.e. where the hepatic ducts enter the liver and where common bile duct enters the pancreas. The diagnosis is most often made at surgery.

PANCREAS

The pancreas is the least commonly injured solid organ, accounting for 3–12% of all abdominal injuries.[16] This injury occurs after a sudden force that compresses the pancreatic neck against lumbar spine, e.g. in motor vehicle accidents in adults and bicycle accidents in children. Pancreatic injuries are difficult to diagnose. The presence of abdominal pain, leukocytosis and hyperamylasemia is nonspecific and frequently not present.

CT has been shown to have sensitivity and specificity of about 85% for detection of pancreatic injuries. The routine venous phase which is acquired for rest of the abdomen is often sufficient to diagnose pancreatic injuries. The injuries are classified according to the AAST grading for pancreatic injuries **(Table 4)**.[17] The following points are most relevant for clinical management:

- Presence of a laceration involving the pancreatic duct. However, the pancreatic duct may not often be seen. When a central laceration is seen extending for more than 50% of anteroposterior or craniocaudal width of the pancreatic parenchyma, then it is presumed to

Table 4: AAST organ injury scale for pancreas.

*Grade**	*Description of injury*
Grade I	Minor contusion without duct injury Superficial laceration without duct injury
Grade II	Major contusion without duct injury or tissue loss Major laceration without duct injury or tissue loss
Grade III	Distal transaction or parenchymal injury with duct injury
Grade IV	Proximal transaction or parenchymal injury involving ampulla
Grade V	Massive disruption of pancreatic head

*Advance one grade for multiple injuries up to grade III

involve the main pancreatic duct. Hence, it is required to quantitate the depth of laceration as a percentage of parenchymal width.[16,18]

- *Location of the laceration:* It most commonly involves the region of pancreatic neck **(Fig. 17)**. Within the neck region, it is important to describe whether it is to the right or left of superior mesenteric artery (SMA). If the laceration (greater than 50%) or transection is seen to the right of SMA then it is managed by a Whipple's surgery. If it lies to the left of SMA, then a distal pancreatectomy is done.[18]
- Large lacerations and hematomas in the head of pancreas are managed with Whipple's surgery **(Fig. 18)**.
- Often the direct evidence of injury to pancreas is not visualized on CT especially when done within 24–48 hours of injury. Indirect CT signs of pancreatic injury include focal or diffuse enlargement of the gland, fluid in the peripancreatic fat, around the SMA, in the transverse mesocolon and lesser peritoneal sac, fluid separating pancreas from the splenic vein, and thickening of left anterior renal fascia. In a patient with suspected pancreatic injury in whom the initial CT scan shows a normal pancreas, a follow-up thin section CT scan within 24–48 hours of injury may show an injury not evident initially.

Recent studies have shown increasing role of MRI with MRCP in the diagnosis of pancreatic injuries. MRI has been shown to increase the diagnostic confidence for detection of parenchymal contusions and lacerations especially the involvement of the main pancreatic duct which is essential for planning treatment **(Figs. 19A and B)**.[5] Endoscopic retrograde cholangiopancreatography (ERCP) may also be needed for confirmation but its role is mainly limited to pancreatic ductal stenting for treatment of ductal injury.

Major complications can result following pancreatic trauma, e.g. pancreatic fistula, intra-abdominal abscess, pseudocyst formation **(Fig. 20)**, hemorrhage, acute recurrent pancreatitis, etc.

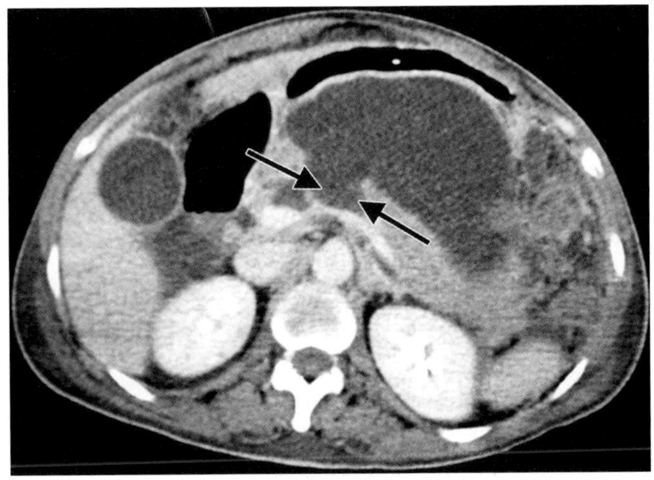

Fig. 17: Axial CECT scan through pancreas shows a laceration/transection involving neck/proximal body of pancreas (arrows) with a large collection seen anterior to pancreas.

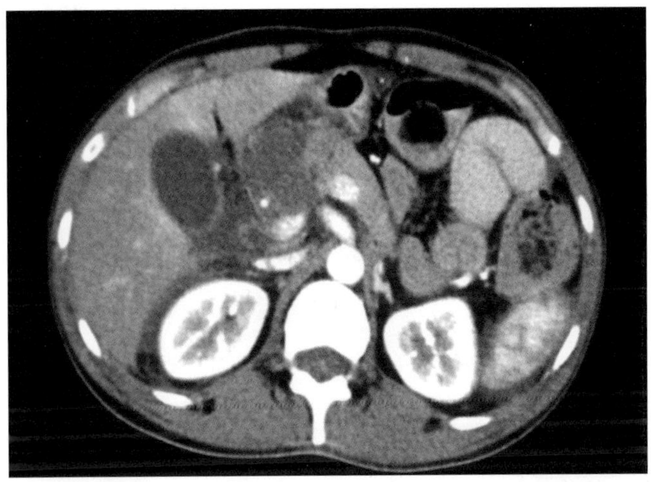

Fig. 18: Axial CECT scan shows a contusion involving the head of pancreas.

URINARY TRACT

Urinary tract injuries are outside the purview of this book and will be described in detail in a forthcoming book in this series on 'Urogenital Imaging'.

Adrenal

With the increasing use of CT, adrenal injuries are now recognized as the most common retroperitoneal injury.[19] It is usually associated with injury to other organs especially liver and kidneys. Adrenal hemorrhage due to

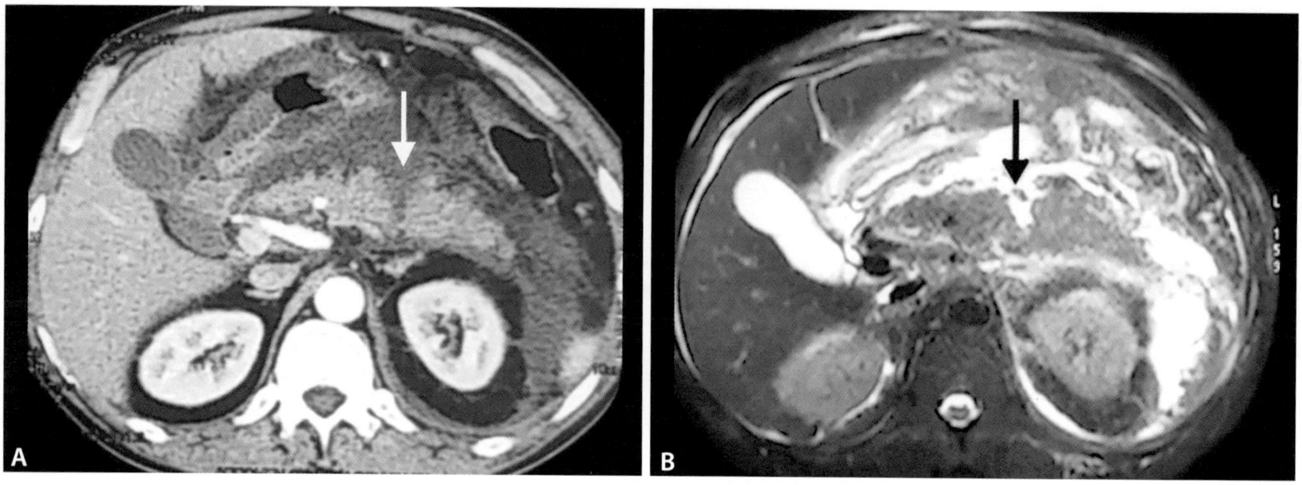

Figs. 19A and B: CECT axial scan (A) at level of pancreas shows a laceration (arrow) involving the distal body of the pancreas. The laceration extends to more than 50% of parenchymal depth, hence it is likely involving the main pancreatic duct. Note the surrounding inflammatory changes of pancreatitis. HASTE axial MRI image (B) at same level clearly shows the pancreatic laceration (arrow) with surrounding inflammatory changes.

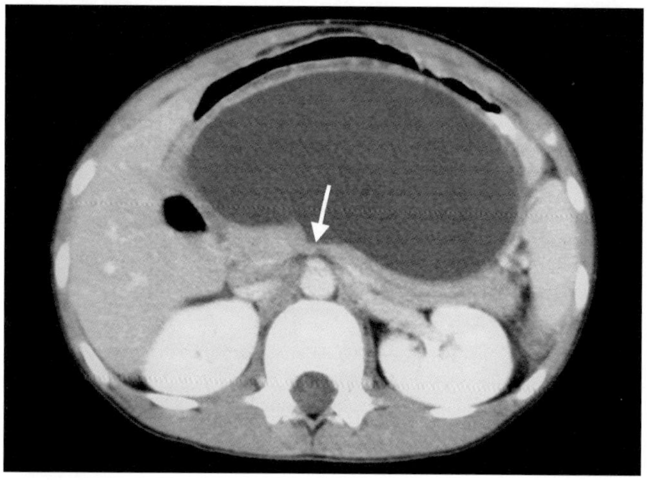

Fig. 20: Axial CECT scan at level of pancreas shows a large pseudocyst anterior to pancreas with a beak-shaped extension (arrow) in the neck of pancreas representing partial transection of pancreas.

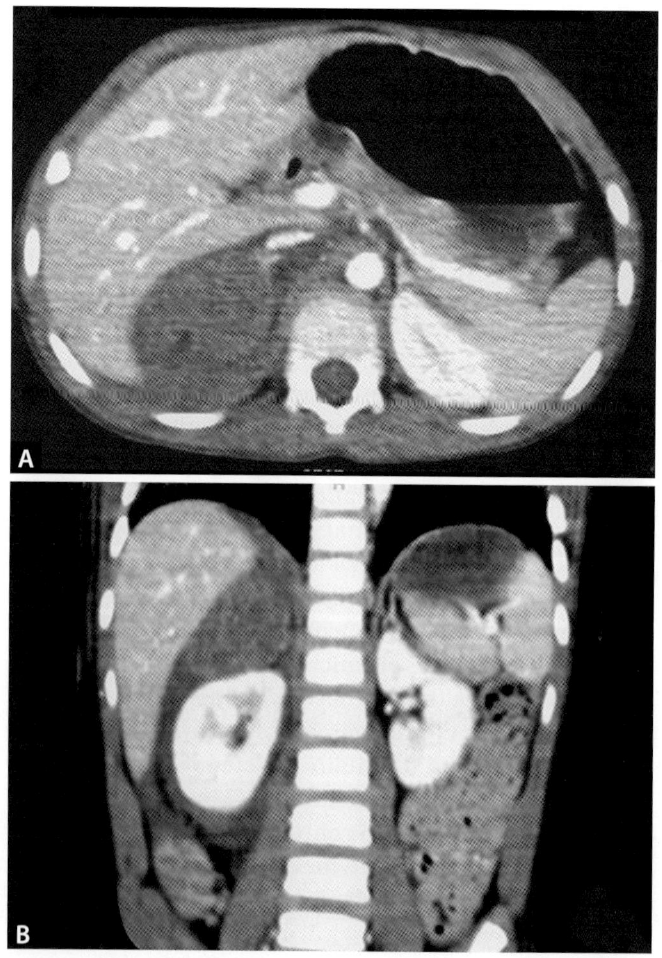

Figs. 21A and B: Axial (A) and coronal reformat (B) CECT scans show a right adrenal hematoma.

trauma is unilateral in more than 90% of cases and usually the right adrenal gland is involved. The mechanism of injury may be compression of the adrenal gland between the liver and spine. On CT, adrenal hematoma appears as round to oval homogeneous density mass (40–75 HU) that replaces all or a portion of the normal adrenal gland **(Figs. 21A and B)**. In addition there may be stranding of the periadrenal fat that extends to the upper pole of the kidney and apparent thickening of the ipsilateral diaphragmatic crus due to adjacent hemorrhage.[19] A post-traumatic cyst or calcification may be seen as a sequel on long-term follow-up. Adrenal hemorrhage is of little clinical significance, particularly when it is unilateral.[20] Rarely bilateral adrenal hemorrhage has been shown to precipitate adrenal insufficiency.[21]

HOLLOW VISCUS, OMENTAL AND MESENTERIC INJURY

The diagnosis of intestinal injury is one of the most difficult and controversial aspects of trauma care. The symptoms may be delayed for many hours. If not surgically repaired it may lead to bleeding and leakage of gastrointestinal contents into the peritoneal cavity or retroperitoneum, leading to peritonitis or sepsis. The plain radiographs of the abdomen are relatively insensitive in detecting bowel injury. Rupture of a hollow viscus may produce free air either in the peritoneal cavity or retroperitoneum. Additional findings of free intraperitoneal fluid may be seen. MDCT is the diagnostic modality of choice for detection of bowel and mesenteric injuries and has been shown to be more sensitive and specific than clinical examination, diagnostic peritoneal lavage and abdominal ultrasound.[22] The signs of bowel injury are frequently subtle. The most specific signs of bowel injury are:[22-24]

- Pneumoperitoneum or pneumoretroperitoneum,
- Extravasation of oral contrast material (if administered)
- Low attenuating fluid between loops
- Bowel wall discontinuity **(Figs. 22A to C)**.

Retroperitoneal air tends to localize near the site of injury, often accompanied by fluid, either blood or intestinal. The presence of these signs usually mandates urgent laparotomy. All the above signs, though highly specific, are not as sensitive.[24] Also care must be taken to exclude other causes of extraluminal contrast (bladder injury) and extraluminal air (mechanical ventilation, pneumothorax, chest injury, peritoneal lavage prior to CT, Foley's catheter in a intraperitoneal bladder rupture). Another important consideration is 'pseudopneumoperitoneum' which leads to false positive diagnosis. It refers to trapped air between the parietal peritoneum and the abdominal wall. So, it is actually extraperitoneal, but can be confused as intraperitoneal on images. It is seen in patients with pneumothorax and pneumomediastinum especially on positive pressure ventilation where the air dissects and extends caudally beneath the abdominal wall. Careful evaluation of the CT images especially with coronal and sagittal reconstructions often helps in localizing this air to be extraperitoneal.

It should also be remembered that absence of pneumoperitoneum does not rule out bowel perforation. This can occur due to multiple causes like very early imaging post-trauma, spontaneous healing of perforation, paralytic ileus causing failure of gas to escape from intestine, or reabsorption of small quantity of gas through the peritoneal lining. Hence, other suggestive signs should also be looked for. Often the clinical signs on abdominal examination alone can warrant exploratory laparotomy.

Less specific signs of bowel injury include:[22-24]

- Peritoneal fluid without a known cause,
- Focal bowel wall thickening greater than 3 mm
- Mesenteric infiltration, thickening or hematoma
- Abnormal bowel wall enhancement **(Figs. 23A and B)**.

Patients manifesting these signs may have bowel perforation requiring surgery, a less severe bowel contusion or hematoma that may be managed without surgery or no bowel injury at all. It must be remembered that diffuse bowel wall thickening may also be noted in fluid overload or in hypoperfusion state (shock bowel) wherein it would have other accompanying features of hypoperfusion complex as detailed earlier in this chapter 8. There can be various abnormal patterns of bowel wall enhancement secondary to trauma:

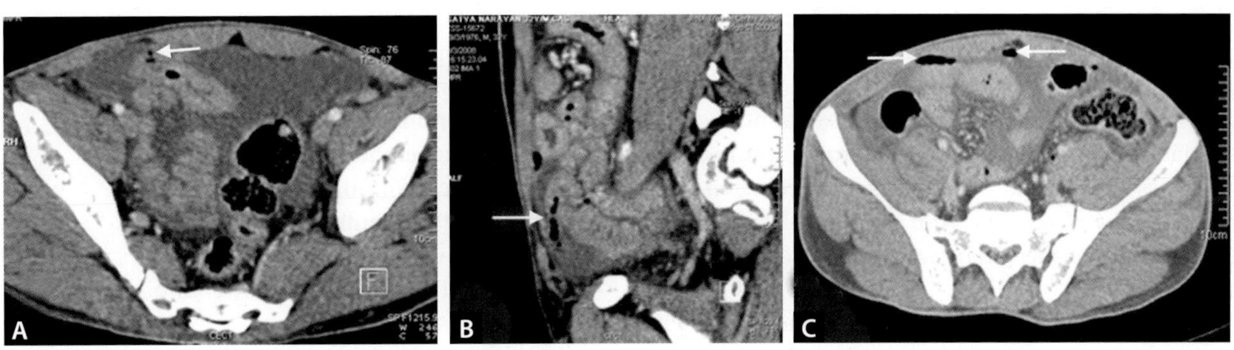

Figs. 22A to C: Axial (A) and sagittal reformat (B) images of CECT shows a focal defect in wall of ileum (arrows) with air extending outside bowel lumen. An axial section at a different level with changed window settings shows the presence of pneumoperitoneum (arrows).

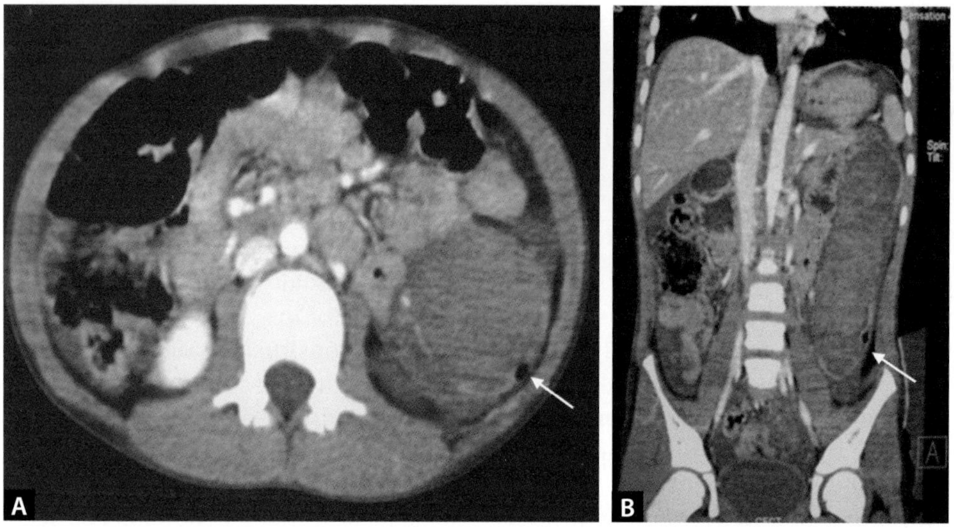

Figs. 23A and B: Axial (A) and coronal reformat (B) CECT scans of abdomen show entire descending colon distended with hyperdense contents representing hematoma with thinned out abnormally enhancing walls and air within the wall (arrow in A and B) suggesting colonic injury.

- Increased enhancement as in hypoperfusion state (due to increased vascular permeability with interstitial leakage of contrast)
- Patchy and irregular enhancement due to wall injury
- Decreased or absent enhancement due to ischemia.

Blunt injuries to the stomach are uncommon. The second and third parts of duodenum are the most frequently injured portion of small bowel as they are fixed.[22] Duodenal hematoma has a characteristic appearance on CT scan. In the absence of duodenal perforation, focal thickening or high attenuating mass in the duodenal wall, possibly associated with retroperitoneal fluid, is suggestive of intramural hematoma. Blunt injuries of the small intestine are most commonly seen at the points of fixation (ligament of Treitz and terminal ileum) but may occur anywhere along the length of the small intestine. Blunt colonic injuries are rare.

The mesentery and omentum are most often associated with injuries elsewhere in the abdomen and pelvis. Avulsion of the superior mesenteric artery and vein occurs most commonly near their origin, because of shearing effect. Massive hemorrhage can result from rupture or tear of these vessels. Vascular thrombosis and occlusion by an intimal flap may also result from trauma. CT scan can be used to determine the extent and location of mesenteric injury.

Mesenteric injury has certain specific and nonspecific features on MDCT.[22,23] The specific CT features of mesenteric vascular injury are:

- Active contrast extravasation within mesentery

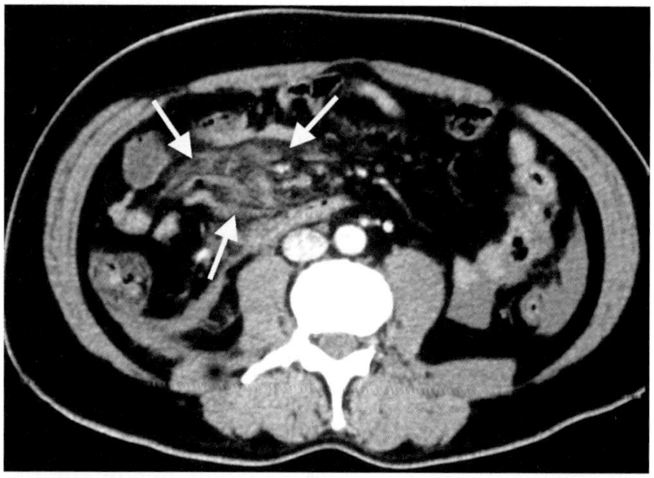

Fig. 24: Axial CECT scan through lower abdomen shows infiltration and hematoma (arrows) in mesenteric root representing mesenteric injury.

- Beaded appearance of mesenteric vessels
- Abrupt termination of mesenteric vessels.

The relatively nonspecific findings include:

- Mesenteric hematoma **(Fig. 24)**
- Mesenteric infiltration
- Bowel wall thickening
- Abnormal wall enhancement secondary to ischemia
- Increased fluid within the bowel lumen
- Pneumatosis intestinalis.

It must be remembered that some of these signs may also be seen in bowel injury alone without concomitant mesenteric injury.

DIAPHRAGM

Diaphragmatic rupture and subsequent herniation of abdominal contents into thorax is nine times more common on left side than right due to the protective effect of the liver.[1] On the right side most injuries to the diaphragm go unrecognized during the acute phase. In the interval phase, the abdominal viscus may not have herniated or the patient may have acclimatized to the presence of abdominal contents in the thorax. In the later phase, obstruction or strangulation presents with severe abdominal or chest pain. The injury may also be evident at a later stage in those patients who were earlier on positive pressure ventilation and extubated later.

Chest radiograph may diagnose diaphragmatic rupture if the following specific signs are visualized:

- Visualization of bowel loops or solid masses above the diaphragm
- Loss of the normal diaphragmatic contour
- Detection of a nasogastric tube above the left hemidiaphragm.

The diagnosis may also be suspected on chest radiograph if a combination of following nonspecific signs is visualized:

- Indistinct or elevated hemidiaphragm **(Fig. 25A)**
- Pleural effusion
- Atelectasis with shift of the mediastinum to the contralateral side
- Hemothorax
- Pneumothorax
- Lower rib fractures.

Contrast studies (barium meal or enema) can be used to clearly delineate the herniation.

The advent of MDCT with multiplanar reconstructions has significantly improved the sensitivity of CT in detecting diaphragmatic injuries.[25] The various CT signs which are seen in diaphragmatic rupture are:

- Focal diaphragmatic discontinuity or elevation
- Focal diaphragmatic thickening (retraction)
- Herniated abdominal contents into thorax
- 'Collar' sign—narrowed waist of a herniated intra-abdominal organ due to compression at the neck (diaphragm tear)
- 'Dependent viscera' sign—herniated intra-abdominal contents abutting the posterior thoracic wall without intervening diaphragmatic slip **(Figs. 25A and B)**.

Amongst the above features the 'dependent viscera' sign and the 'collar' signs are reported to be 100% specific.[1] CT is unreliable in diagnosing diaphragmatic tears before herniation. MRI also has been reported to be highly sensitive in detecting diaphragmatic rupture.

RETROPERITONEUM

The most frequently injured retroperitoneal structures include the adrenals, pancreas, great vessels, gastrointestinal tract, genitourinary tract and musculoskeletal system.[1,2] Inability to account for

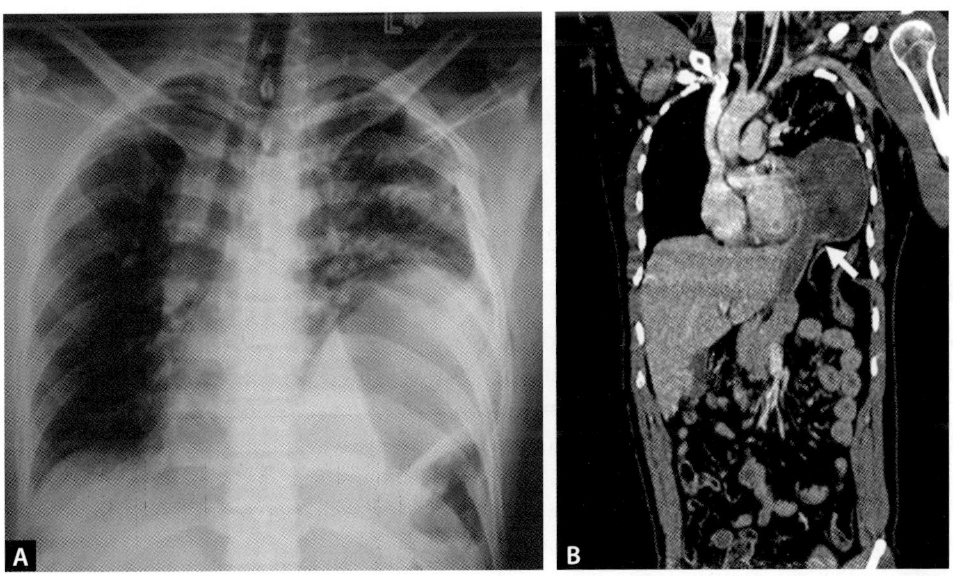

Figs. 25A and B: Chest radiograph PA view (A) shows opacity in left lower zone with smooth convex upper margin and air lucencies within. Coronal reformatted CECT image (B) shows clearly the diaphragmatic defect (arrow) with stomach herniating through it into the thorax.

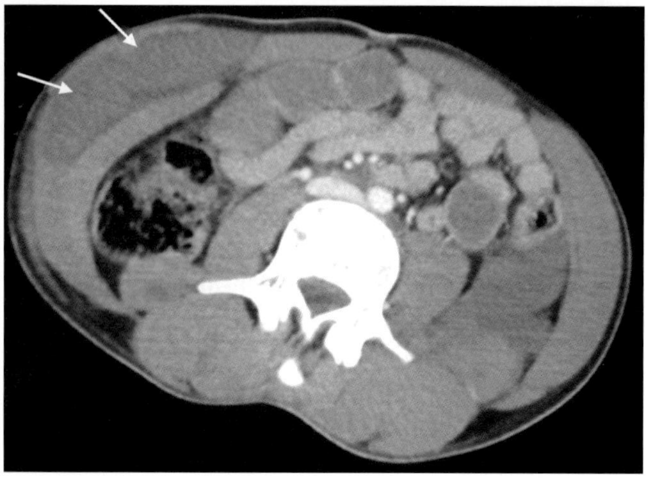

Fig. 26: Axial CECT scan through midabdomen shows a large abdominal wall hematoma (arrows).

blood loss either in the chest or abdomen in a patient with ongoing transfusion requirements should dictate angiographic investigation. The potential for simultaneous angiographic embolization of actively bleeding vessels is well documented and may be lifesaving since opening the retroperitoneum to control bleeding is associated with high mortality.

ABDOMINAL WALL INJURY

Abdominal wall injuries are easily overlooked if not specifically looked for. Most common are bruises, which appear on CT as skin thickening and soft tissue infiltration of subcutaneous fat. Intramuscular hematomas may be seen **(Fig. 26)**. Tearing of lateral abdominal wall or rectus abdominis is an unusual occurrence that results in subcutaneous hematoma and occasionally bowel herniation. Morel Lavallee lesion representing internal degloving injury is seen on CT as separation of skin from the subcutaneous with intervening fluid collection.

PENETRATING ABDOMINAL TRAUMA

Traditionally, almost all stab and gunshot wounds to the abdomen used to undergo surgical exploration. With increasing interest in nonoperative management of penetrating injuries, CT has become important in evaluating extent of injury in selected hemodynamically stable patients. The most important information required by the surgeon is whether or not there is a breach of the peritoneum by the penetrating wound. If the wound is deep then it is important to look for solid organ laceration, bowel perforation, retroperitoneal hematoma, and hemoperitoneum. It is often difficult to detect small perforations of the bowel that result in only small amounts of peritoneal fluid on CT. In contrast to stab wounds, gunshot wounds are potentially complex injuries and depend upon the type of weapon, distance between the weapon and victim amongst others. CT is directly able to demonstrate the path of the bullet.

CONCLUSION

Diagnostic imaging technology has evolved considerably during the past decade and CT in particular has increased the sensitivity and specificity of imaging in abdominal trauma. Currently, CT is universally accepted as a valuable tool for evaluating hemodynamically stable patients. The value of CT in diagnosis of abdominal injuries can be optimized by using state of art MDCT scanners, maintaining adequate patient physiologic support and monitoring devices within the CT suite, using appropriate intravenous contrast, paying careful attention to CT technique and timely interpretation of CT images. However, CT must be considered as an adjunct to the clinical evaluation of the patient, which remains the most important criteria for guiding management of the patient with abdominal trauma. Increasing role of angioembolization in management of hepatic, splenic and pelvic injuries has widened the role of radiologist in successful nonsurgical management of these patients.

TAKE HOME KEY POINTS

- Chest and pelvic radiographs along with FAST ultrasound are done as initial investigations in all patients of suspected abdominal trauma.
- MDCT is done in patients for further evaluation depending upon the hemodynamic stability, mechanism of injury and findings of the initial radiological investigations.
- Role of radiologist is to detect and characterize the solid and visceral organ injuries and to grade them as per American Association for the Surgery of Trauma (AAST) grades.
- Most of the abdominal injuries are managed conservatively if the patient's condition remains hemodynamically stable.
- The few surgical indications which can be detected on CT should be carefully looked for and communicated to the surgeon. These include full thickness bowel injury, pancreatic transaction, intraperitoneal rupture of urinary bladder, diaphragmatic tear, mesenteric hematoma/vascular injury and renal pelvic injury.

- Other CT findings which require close monitoring of patient and would often require a surgical or angiographic intervention also need to be specifically looked for. These include uncontained vascular injury (depicted by active arterial contrast extravasation), contained vascular injury (pseudoaneurysm or arteriovenous fistula) and high grade (4/5) liver and splenic injuries.
- Angiographic embolization procedures are frequently used to aid the nonoperative management of patients with vascular injuries and high grade liver and spleen injuries.

REFERENCES

1. Stanescu AL, Gross JA, Bittle M, Mann FA. Imaging of blunt abdominal trauma. Semin Roentgen. 2006;41(3):196-204.
2. Soto JA, Anderson SW. Multidetector CT of blunt abdominal trauma. Radiology. 2012;265(3):678-93.
3. Korner M, Krotz M, Degenhart C, Pfeifer KJ, Reiser MF, Linsenmaier U. Current role of emergency US in patients with major trauma. Radiographics. 2008;28:225-44.
4. Cokkinos D, Antypa E, Stefanidis K, et al. Contrast-enhanced ultrasound for imaging blunt abdominal trauma—indications, description of the technique and imaging review. Ultraschall in Med. 2012;33(1):60-67. *https://acsearch.acr.org/docs/69409/Narrative/*
5. Stuhlfaut JW, Lucey BC, Varghese JC, Soto JA. Blunt abdominal trauma: utility of 5-minute delayed CT with a reduced radiation dose. Radiology. 2006;238(2):473-9.
6. Panda A, Kumar A, Gamanagatti S, Bhalla AS, Sharma R, Kumar S, Mishra B. Evaluation of diagnostic utility of multidetector computed tomography and magnetic resonance imaging in blunt pancreatic trauma: a prospective study. Acta Radiol. 2015;56(4):387-96.
7. Prasad KR, Kumar A, Gamanagatti S, Chandrashekhara SH. CT in post-traumatic hypoperfusion complex: a pictorial review. Emerg Radiol. 2011;18(2):139-43.
8. Boscak A, Shanmuganathan K. Splenic Trauma: What is New? Radiologic Clinics of North America. 2012;50(1):105-22.
9. Moore EE, Cogbill TH, Jurkovich GJ, et al. Organ injury scaling: spleen and liver (1994 revision). J Trauma. 1995;38:323-4.
10. Marmery H, Shanmuganathan K, Alexander M, Mirvis S. Optimisation of selection for nonoperative management of blunt splenic injury: Comparison of MDCT grading systems. AJR. 2007;189:1421-7.
11. Gamanagatti S, Rangarajan K, Kumar A, Jineesh. Blunt abdominal trauma: imaging and intervention. Curr Probl Diagn Radiol. 2015;44(4):321-36.
12. Parihar ML, Kumar A, Gamanagatti S, Bhalla AS, Mishra B, Kumar S, et al. Role of splenic artery embolization in management of traumatic splenic injuries: a prospective study. Indian J Surg. 2013;75(5):361-7.
13. Yoon W, Jeong YY, Kim JK, Seo JJ, Lim HS, Shin SS, et al. CT in blunt liver trauma. Radiographics. 2005;25:87-104.
14. Kumar R, Kumar A, Baliyan V, Bhalla AS, Sharma R, Gupta A, Kumar S, Misra MC. Correlating MDCT liver injury grade and clinical outcome in patients without significant extrahepatic injury. Indian J Surg. 2016;78:275.
15. Melamud K, LeBedis CA, Soto JA. Imaging of pancreatic and duodenal trauma. Radiologic Clinics of North America. 2015;53(4)757-71.
16. Moore EE, Cogbill TH, Malangoni MA, et al. Organ injury scaling II: Pancreas, duodenum, small bowel, colon and rectum. J Trauma. 1990;30:1427.
17. Kumar A, Panda A, Gamanagatti S. Blunt pancreatic trauma: a persistent diagnostic conundrum? World J Radiol. 2016;8(2):159-73.
18. To'o KJ, Duddalwar VA. Imaging of traumatic adrenal injury. Emerg Radiol. 2012;19:499.
19. Panda A, Kumar A, Gamanagatti S, Bhalla AS, Sharma R, Kumar S, Mishra B. Are traumatic bilateral adrenal injuries associated with higher morbidity and mortality?: a prospective observational study. J Trauma Manag Outcomes. 2015;9:6.
20. Francque SM, Schwagten VM, Ysebaert DK, et al. Bilateral adrenal hemorrhage and acute adrenal insufficiency in a blunt abdominal trauma: a case-report and literature review. Eur J Emerg Med. 2004;11:164-7.
21. Brofman N, Atri M, Epid D, Hanson JM, Grinblat L, Chughtai T, et al. Evaluation of bowel and mesenteric blunt trauma with multidetector CT. Radiographics. 2006;26: 1119-26.
22. Iaselli F, Mazzei MA, Firetto C, et al. Bowel and mesenteric injuries from blunt abdominal trauma: a review. Radiol Med. 2015;120:21.
23. Panda A, Kumar A, Gamanagatti S, Das R, Paliwal S, Gupta A, Kumar S. Can multidetector computed tomography detect the site of gastrointestinal tract injury in trauma?: a retrospective study. Diag Interv Radiol. 2016; 22...(ahead of print).
24. Panda A, Kumar A, Gamanagatti S, Patil A, Kumar S, Gupta A. Traumatic diaphragmatic injury: a review of CT signs and the difference between blunt and penetrating injury. Diagn Interv Radiol. 2014;20(2):121-8.
25. Barbiera F, Nicastro N, Finazzo M, et al. The role of MRI in traumatic rupture of the diaphragm. Our experience in three cases and review of the literature. Radiol Med. 2003;105(3): 188-94.

CHAPTER 93

Imaging of Peritoneum and Mesentery

Anju Garg, Anjali Prakash, Alpana Manchanda

The peritoneum is a thin, translucent, serous membrane made up of a single layer of mesothelial cells. It is supported by submesothelial connective tissue containing lymphatics, blood vessels, inflammatory cells like lymphocytes and plasma cells and a variable amount of fat. Just like the pleura, the peritoneum also has 2 layers—the *parietal peritoneum* lines the anterior, lateral and posterior walls of the peritoneal cavity and the *visceral peritoneum* which envelops the hollow and solid abdominal organs. Between these two layers lies the *peritoneal cavity*—a potential space containing a small amount of fluid which acts as a lubricant.[1] The peritoneal cavity is a closed continuous space in males, but in females, it communicates with the extraperitoneal compartment of the pelvis through the ostia of the fallopian tubes.[2]

EMBRYOLOGY

Knowledge of the developmental anatomy of the peritoneum, helps to understand the peritoneal ligaments, spaces and their relationship with the abdominal organs. The majority of the ligaments in the abdomen are formed from remnants of the ventral and dorsal mesenteries which suspend the primitive gut. The liver and its ligaments arise in the *ventral mesentery*. The anterior part of the ventral mesentery becomes the falciform, coronary and triangular ligaments and the posterior part of the ventral mesentery becomes the lesser omentum. The stomach, spleen and pancreatic tail and their ligaments develop in the *dorsal mesentery* of the foregut. At the level of spleen, the anterior part of the dorsal mesentery becomes the gastrosplenic ligament, and the posterior part of the dorsal mesentery becomes the splenorenal ligament **(Figs. 1A to C)**. Above the level of spleen the dorsal mesentery gives rise to gastrophrenic ligament and below the level of spleen it gives rise to the greater omentum (gastrocolic ligament).[3]

Below the level of the transverse colon, the ventral mesentery regresses while the dorsal mesentery forms the transverse mesocolon, small bowel mesentery and sigmoid mesocolon. During development, the duodenum, ascending and descending colon lose their mesenteries and become retroperitoneal.

ANATOMY OF THE PERITONEUM[4-7]

The peritoneum forms double layered folds, or ligaments, that interconnect the organs and viscera within the peritoneal cavity. The *peritoneal ligaments* are named according to the two major structures connected by them, e.g. splenorenal ligament or gastrohepatic ligament, etc. *Omentum* is a specialized ligament that attaches the stomach to other structures whereas *mesentery* is the ligament attaching the bowel to the posterior abdominal wall. These ligaments divide the peritoneal cavity into a number of compartments and recesses **(Figs. 2A and B)**.

The peritoneal ligaments carry vessels, nerves and lymphatics from the extraperitoneal spaces to the intraperitoneal organs. They act as boundaries for spread of pathological processes within the abdomen, but may also become conduits for spread of disease. They

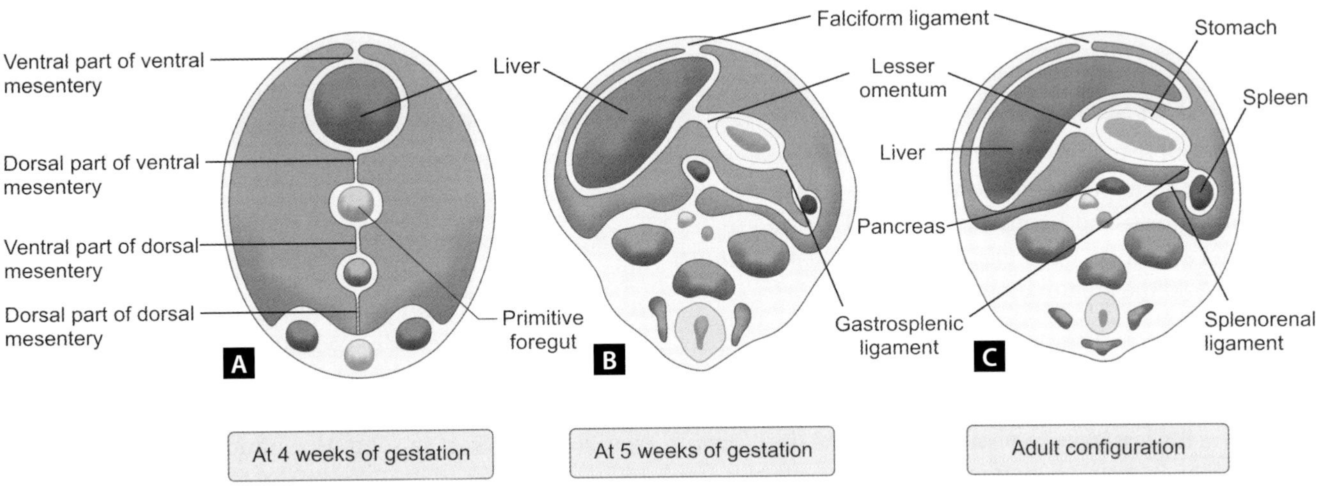

Figs. 1A to C: Embryologic development and rotation of the peritoneal structures to the eventual adult position. The ventral part of the ventral mesentery becomes the falciform ligament, the dorsal part of the ventral mesentery becomes the lesser omentum, the ventral part of the dorsal mesentery becomes the gastrosplenic ligament, and the dorsal part of the dorsal mesentery becomes the splenorenal ligament. The liver arises in the ventral mesentery, whereas the stomach, spleen and pancreatic tail develop in the dorsal mesentery. The liver fills and moves to the right side of the peritoneal cavity as it grows. The spleen moves to the left.

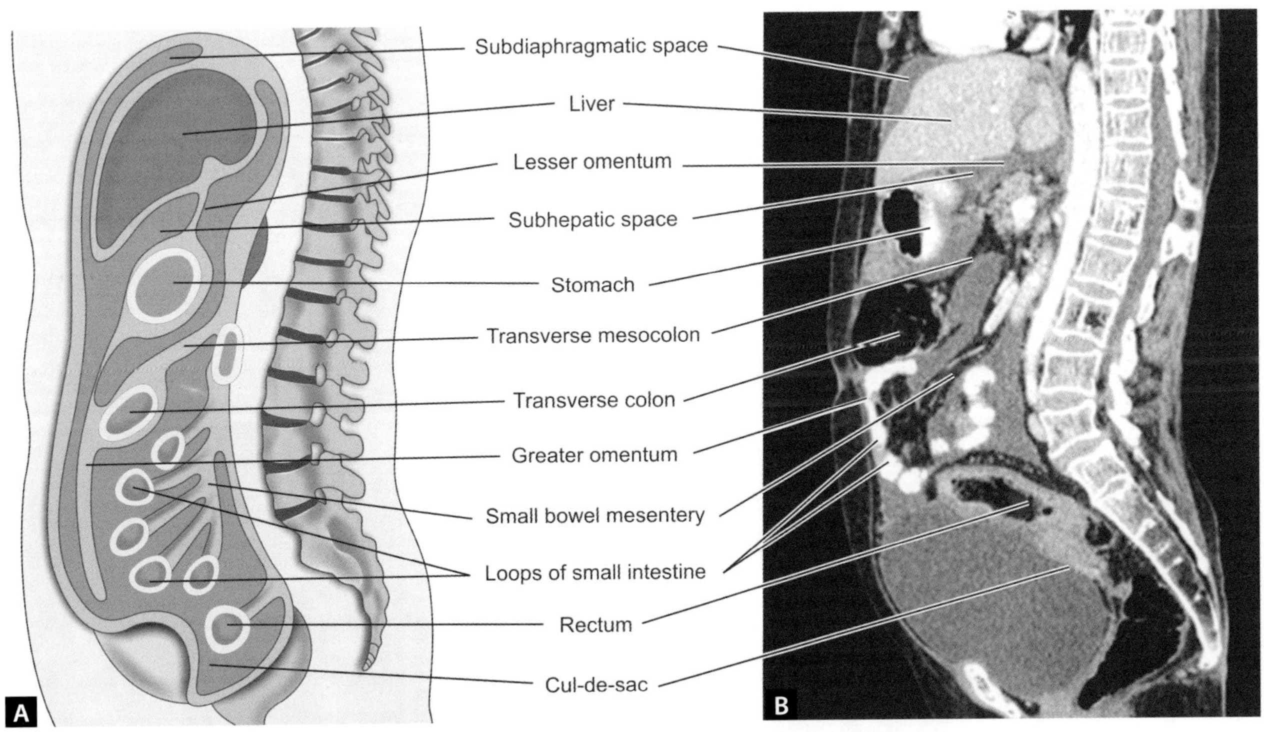

Figs. 2A and B: Sagittal illustration and corresponding sagittal CT scan in a patient with ascites, showing the peritoneal ligaments in the midline sagittal section.

are not directly visible on cross sectional imaging but can be identified by either their typical position, organ relationships, or by the anatomical landmarks provided by their constituent vessels. They may become directly visible when they get thickened by edema, inflammation or neoplastic infiltration or when they are outlined by air or fluid in the peritoneal cavity. They can be grouped into:

- Ligaments of the stomach
- Ligaments of the liver and spleen
- Ligaments attached to the small bowel

- Ligaments attached to the large bowel
- Ligaments of the pelvis.

Ligaments of Stomach

The peritoneal ligaments of the stomach include two main groups: Ligaments attached to the lesser curvature, the lesser omentum, and ligaments attached to the greater curvature which include gastrophrenic, gastrosplenic ligaments and the greater omentum.

Lesser omentum: The lesser omentum is formed by the gastrohepatic and hepatoduodenal ligaments **(Figs. 2A and B)**. *The gastrohepatic ligament (GHL)* is attached to the lesser curve of the stomach and the visceral surface of the liver and contains the coronary vein and left gastric artery **(Figs. 3A and D)**. The GHL can be involved by pancreatitis or metastatic disease from oesophageal, gastric, and biliary tumors. It is also the site for coronary varices. The *hepatoduodenal ligament (HDL)* attaches the first part of the duodenum to the liver and contains the portal vein, hepatic artery, common hepatic ducts, and part of the cystic duct **(Fig. 3D)**. It is a common site for spread of biliary and gall bladder neoplasms.

Greater omentum: It is also known as the *gastrocolic ligament* **(Figs. 2 and 3)**. It attaches to the greater curvature of the stomach and proximal part of duodenum. Its descending and ascending portion fuse to form a four layer vascular fatty apron which hangs down covering the small bowel. It has mostly fatty tissue with few gastroepiploic vessels. On CT, it is seen as a band of fatty tissue, just beneath the anterior abdominal wall and anterior to the stomach, transverse colon and small bowel. It is a mobile structure and has an important role in limiting spread of

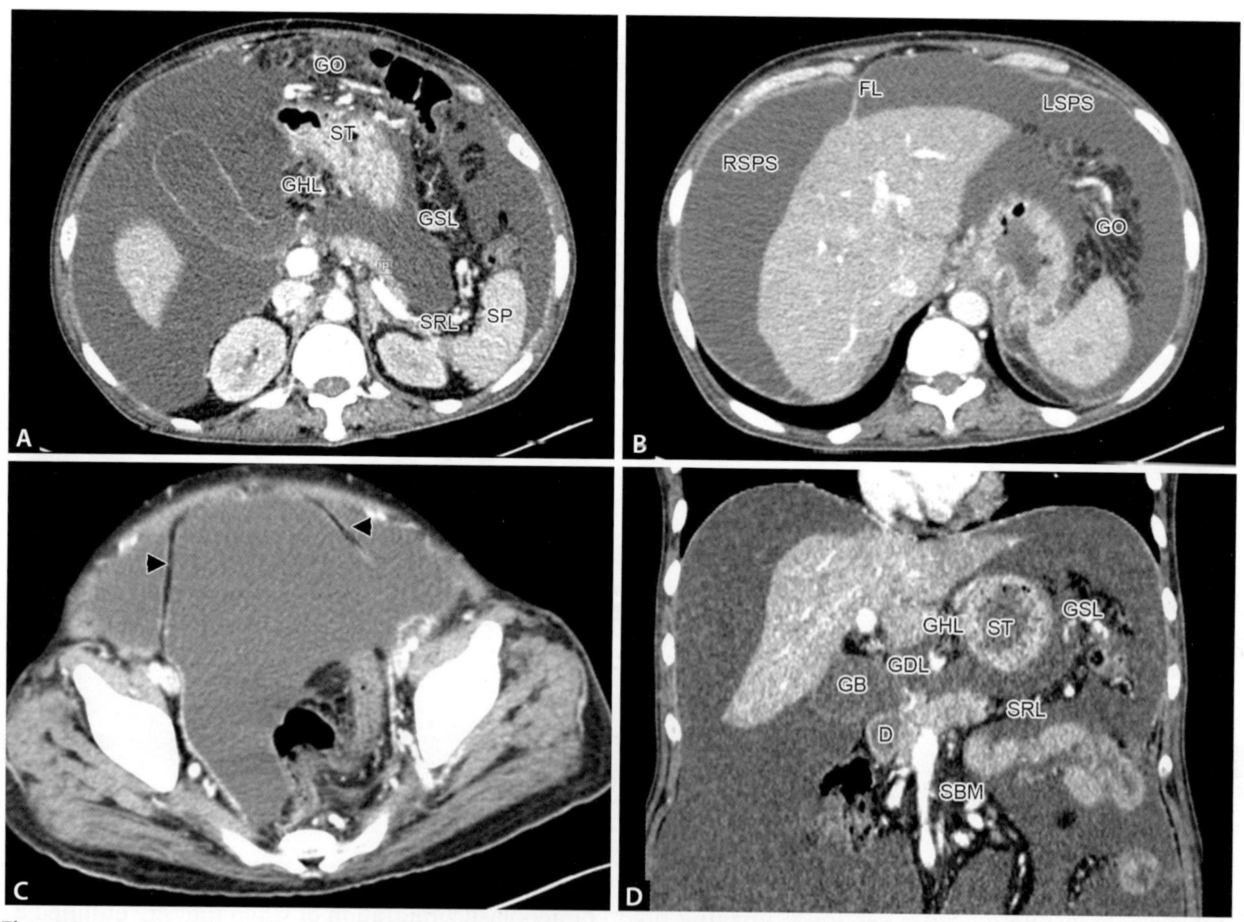

Figs. 3A to D: (A to C) Axial CECT and (D) Coronal scans showing the peritoneal ligaments in a 61-year-old man with peritoneal carcinomatosis with ascites, thickened enhancing peritoneum and omental nodularity.

Abbreviations: FL: Falciform ligament; GO: Greater omentum; GHL: Gastrohepatic ligament; GDL: Gastroduodenal ligament; GSL: Gastrospenic ligament; SRL: Splenorenal ligament; SBM: Small bowel mesentery; ST: Stomach; SP: Spleen; D: Duodenum; RSPS: Right subphrenic space; LSPS: Left subphrenic space; and Medial umbilical ligaments (arrowheads).

infections and confining injuries to the bowel. However, it is a common site of spread of metastatic peritoneal disease and is also commonly involved in tubercular peritonitis.

Gastrosplenic ligament: It attaches the greater curvature of the stomach to the spleen and contains the short gastric and left gastroepiploic vessels and lymphatics **(Figs. 3A and D)**. It is a leftward continuation of the greater omentum and is also in continuity with the splenorenal and phrenicocolic ligaments. The gastrosplenic ligament is a frequent route for spread of pancreatitis-related fluid and the vessels form a collateral route of venous flow in cases of splenic vein thrombosis.

Gastrophrenic ligament is attached to the posterior surface of the stomach. The attachment of the gastrophrenic ligament lies in apposition with the diaphragm, and frequently with the upper portion of the left suprarenal gland.

Ligaments of the Liver and Spleen

The peritoneal ligaments of the liver include the suspensory ligaments of the liver and lesser omentum. The suspensory ligaments of the liver include the falciform, coronary and triangular ligaments. The peritoneal ligaments of spleen include gastrosplenic and lienorenal ligaments.

Triangular and coronary ligaments: These are peritoneal attachments between the liver and the parietal peritoneum. The triangular ligaments are formed by fusion of the coronary ligaments and outline the bare area of the liver. The right triangular ligament is long and separates the right subphrenic space from the right subhepatic space while the left triangular ligament is short and does not compartmentalize the left subphrenic space.

Falciform ligament: It attaches the ventral surface of the liver to the anterior abdominal wall and contains the ligamentum teres, i.e. obliterated umbilical vein **(Fig. 3B)**. The recanalized paraumbilical vein is also found in the falciform ligament. It is an important site of peritoneal seeding of metastatic tumors which may be mistaken for hepatic metastases.

Splenorenal ligament: It is the connecting peritoneal reflection between the spleen and the left kidney. It contains the tail of the pancreas, splenic vessels, and small vessels to the retroperitomeum. Tumor spread and systemic portal collaterals can develop in this space.

Ligaments Attached to Small Bowel

Small bowel mesentery: It is a broad fan-shaped peritoneal fold that attaches the jejunum and ileum to the retroperitoneum and contains branches of the superior mesenteric vessels, lymph nodes, nerves and varying amounts of fat **(Figs. 2 and 4)**. The root of the mesentery extends from the ligament of Trietz to the ileocecal valve, a length of approximately 15 cm, whereas the intestinal border is 6–8 meters long, and so the mesentery is thrown into a number of folds **(Figs. 4A and B)**.

The small bowel mesentery is commonly involved by metastatic disease and infectious processes of the peritoneum. Inflammation and tumor from the pancreatic body or jejunum can involve the small bowel mesentery directly or by way of neurovascular plexus or lymphatics.

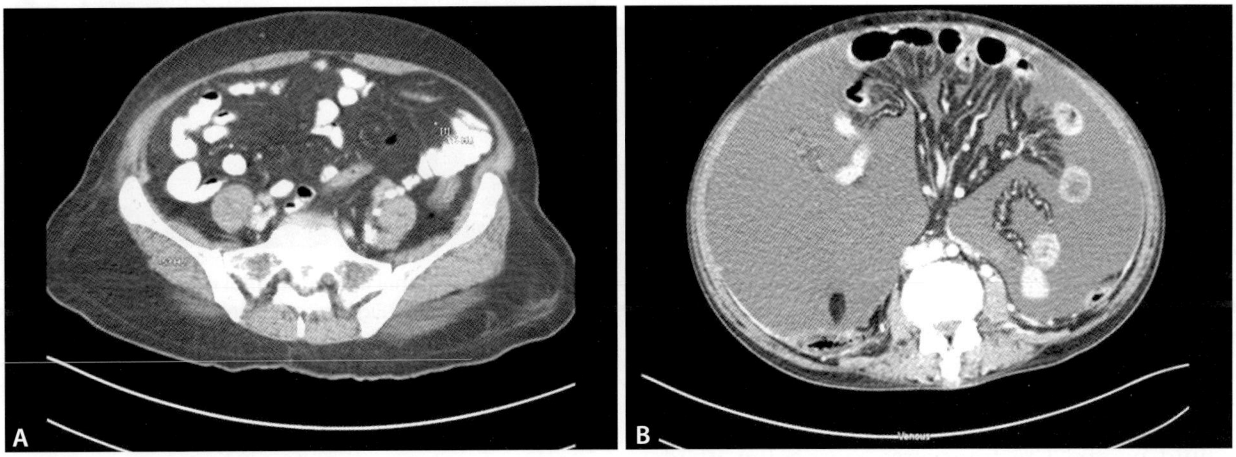

Figs. 4A and B: Axial CECT scans through abdomen in two different patients showing normal mesentery: (A) Mesentery is seen as diffuse fat density structure with mesenteric vessels within. The leaves of the mesentery cannot be made out separately; (B) In a patient with ascites, the leaves of the mesentery are separated by the ascitic fluid.

Rotational and fusion anomalies may lead to volvulus or internal hernias.

Ligaments Attached to Large Bowel

Transverse mesocolon: It is a peritoneal fold that attaches the transverse colon to the anterior surface of the pancreas **(Figs. 2 and 5)**. It contains the middle colic vessels and lymph nodes. Local extension of pancreatic head cancers occurs along the transverse mesocolon.

Sigmoid mesocolon: It is the peritoneal attachment of the sigmoid colon to the posterior pelvic wall **(Fig. 5C)**. It contains the hemorrhoidal and sigmoid vessels. It serves as a medial and caudal boundary for the spread of material from the left paracolic space. Acute diverticulitis, Crohn's disease and tumor of the sigmoid colon can involve the sigmoid mesocolon.

Phrenicocolic ligament: It attaches the proximal descending colon to the left hemidiaphragm. It separates the supramesocolic compartment from the left paracolic gutter. Pancreatic disease can spread via this ligament to involve the splenic flexure of the colon.

Table 1 lists the peritoneal ligaments, their attachments, contents and the major pathological processes involving these ligaments.

Ligaments of the Pelvis

The *broad ligaments* extend from the uterus to the pelvic sidewalls and envelop the parametria, fallopian tubes, ovaries, uterine vessels and ureters. These ligaments can be involved by inflammatory and neoplastic processes affecting the uterus, ovaries and fallopian tubes.

Round ligaments are the anterior suspensory ligaments of the uterus. They run lateral to the deep inferior epigastric vessels, enter the inguinal canal and insert on the labia majora. They contain lymphatic channels.

There are two paired *lateral and medial umbilical ligaments* and *one median umbilical ligament* in the midline. The lateral folds are formed by reflection of the peritoneum over the deep inferior epigastric vessels, the medial folds are peritoneal reflections over the obliterated umbilical arteries and the median fold lies over the obliterated urachus **(*see* Fig. 3C)**.

PERITONEAL SPACES[4,5,7]

The peritoneal ligaments divide the peritoneal space into multiple compartments and recesses. On imaging these spaces are visualized only when they are distended with fluid or air. The transverse mesocolon divides the peritoneal cavity into the supramesocolic and the inframesocolic compartments.

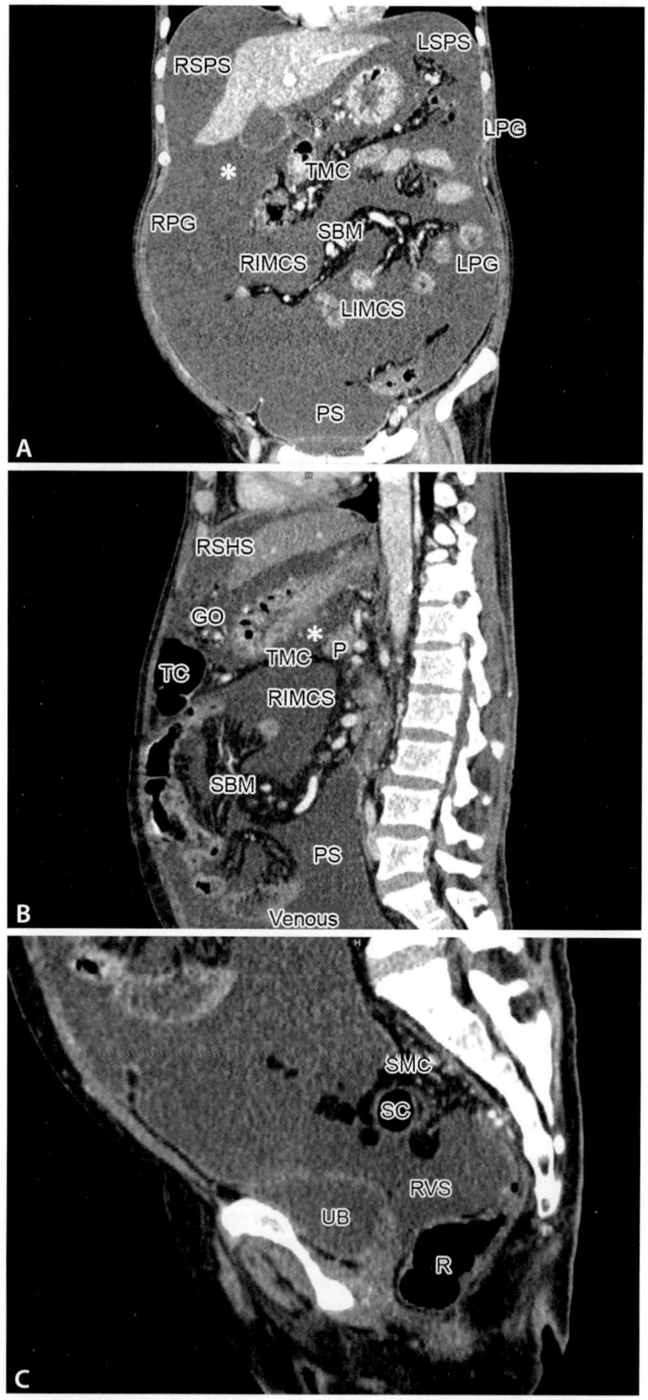

Figs. 5A to C: Coronal (A) and sagittal (B and C) reformats in the same patient as in Figure 2, showing the peritoneal spaces.
Abbreviations: RSPS: Right subphrenic space; LSPS: Left subphrenic space; RSHS: Right subhepatic space (* in A); Lesser sac (* in B); RPG: Right paracolic gutter; LPG: Left paracolic gutter; RIMCS: Right inframesocolic space; LIMCS: Left inframesocolic space; PS: Pelvic space; TMC: Transverse mesocolon; GO: Greater omentum; TC: Transverse colon; P: Pancreas; SC: Sigmoid colon; RVS: Rectovesical space; R: Rectum; SBM: Small bowel mesentery; SMC: Sigmoid mesocolon; UB: Urinary bladder.

Table 1: Peritoneal ligaments, attachments, contents and major pathological processes which involve these ligaments.

Peritoneal ligaments	***Attachments***	***Contents***	***Other relevant information***
• *Ligaments of stomach and duodenum*:			
– Attached to lesser curvature			
- Lesser omentum			
◆ Gastrohepatic ligament	Lesser curvature of the stomach and the visceral surface of liver	Coronary vein and left gastric artery	• Can be involved by pancreatitis or metastatic disease from esophageal, gastric, and biliary tumors • Can be a site for coronary varices
– Hepatoduodenal ligament	First part of duodenum and liver	Portal vein, hepatic artery, common hepatic ducts, and part of the cystic duct	• Common site for spread of biliary and gallbladder neoplasms
– Attached to greater curvature			
- Gastrosplenic ligament	Greater curvature of the stomach and spleen	Short gastric vessels	• Frequent route for subperitoneal spread of pancreatitis-related fluid
- Gastrophrenic ligament	Posterior surface of the stomach and diaphragm	Left inferior phrenic artery	
- Greater omentum	Greater curvature of the stomach and proximal part of duodenum	Fatty tissue with few gastro-epiploic vessels	• Common site of spread of metastatic peritoneal disease • Commonly involved in tubercular peritonitis • Important role in limiting spread of infections and confining injuries to bowel
• *Ligaments of liver and spleen*:			
– Triangular and coronary ligaments	Liver and the diaphragm	No vessels	• Right triangular ligament separates the right subphrenic space from the right subhepatic space • Left triangular ligament does not compartmentalize the left subphrenic space
– Falciform ligament	Ventral surface of the liver and the anterior abdominal wall	Ligamentum teres (obliterated umbilical vein) and recanalized paraumbilical vein	• Important site of peritoneal seeding of metastatic tumors
– Lesser omentum	As above		
– Ligaments of spleen			
- Splenorenal ligament	Spleen and left kidney	Tail of the pancreas, splenic vessels, and small vessels to the retroperitoneum	• Systemic portal collaterals can develop in this space • Renal and splenic neoplasm can spread
- Gastrosplenic ligament	As above		
• *Ligaments attached to small bowel*:			
– Small bowel mesentery	Jejunum and ileum and the retroperitoneum (root of mesentery extends from the ligament of Trietz to ileocecal valve)	Branches of superior mesenteric vessels, lymph nodes, nerves and varying amounts of fat	• Commonly involved by metastatic disease and infectious processes of peritoneum • Rotational and fusion anomalies may lead to volvulus or internal hernias
• *Ligaments attached to large bowel*:			
– Transverse mesocolon	Transverse colon and the anterior surface of the pancreas	Middle colic vessels and lymph nodes	Local extension of pancreatic head cancer
– Sigmoid mesocolon	Sigmoid colon and the posterior pelvic wall	Hemorrhoidal and sigmoid vessels	Serves as medial and caudal boundary for spread of material from left paracolic space. Can be involved by acute diverticulitis, Crohn's disease and tumor of the sigmoid colon
– Phrenicocolic ligament	Proximal descending colon and the left hemidiaphragm		Separates the supramesocolic compartment from left paracolic gutter

Supramesocolic space: It extends from the diaphragm to the transverse mesocolon. It includes the perihepatic spaces and the lesser sac. The perihepatic spaces consist of the subphrenic and subhepatic spaces which are right, left, anterior and posterior.

The *subphrenic space* lies adjacent to the lateral and superior portion of the liver, between the diaphragm and the abdominal wall. The right subphrenic space is limited medially by the falciform ligament, which separates it from the left subphrenic space **(Figs. 5A to C)**. Inferiorly it is continuous with the right subhepatic space and the right paracolic space. The left subphrenic space is located below and around the left lobe of liver and stomach. It is limited inferiorly by the phrenicocolic ligament.

The *right subhepatic space*, also known as the Morrison's pouch or hepatorenal space, lies adjacent to the gall bladder and duodenum, and extends posteriorly to the anterior surface of the right kidney **(Figs. 2 and 5)**. It is an important site of fluid collection as it is the most gravity dependant space. Medially it extends into the lesser sac through the foramen of Winslow. The *left subhepatic space* lies between the lateral segment of the left lobe of liver and the stomach.

The *lesser sac* also known as the *omental bursa*, lies behind the stomach, anterior to the pancreas **(Fig. 5)**. It is further subdivided by the reflection over the left gastric artery into 2 recesses—a smaller superior recess and a larger inferior recess. The *superior recess* surrounds the caudate lobe of the liver. It communicates with the subhepatic space through the foramen of Winslow that is located posterior to the free edge of the hepatoduodenal ligament. The larger *inferior recess* lies between the stomach and the anterior surface of the spleen and pancreas. Abnormalities of the pancreas, posterior wall of stomach, duodenum, caudate lobe and transverse colon may all extend into the lesser sac.

Inframesocolic space: The right and left inframesocolic spaces are separated by the root of the mesentery. The *left inframesocolic space* is larger and communicates freely with the pelvic spaces. The *right inframesocolic space* is limited inferiorly by the attachment of the small bowel mesentery to the cecum and does not communicate with the pelvis **(Figs. 5A and B)**.

Paracolic spaces: They lie lateral to the peritoneal reflections of the left and right side of the colon. The right space is larger and deeper than the left. It communicates freely with the right perihepatic space, whereas the left is partially limited by the phrenicocolic ligament. Both paracolic spaces communicate freely with the pelvic spaces **(Fig. 5A)**.

Pelvic Peritoneal Spaces

The pelvic cavity can be divided into the anterior and posterior paravesical spaces. The anterior paravesical space is divided by the medial umbilical folds, into lateral and medial compartments. On each side, the inferior epigastric artery divides the lateral pelvic compartments into lateral and medial inguinal fossae, the sites of direct and indirect inguinal hernias, respectively.

In males, the posterior paravesical space is subdivided into the *rectovesical* and *pararectal space* by the peritoneal coverings of the rectum and bladder. In females, peritoneal coverings of the uterus divide the rectovesical space into the *vesicouterine* and *rectouterine space* (cul-de-sac or pouch of Douglas). The rectouterine space is the most dependant portion of the pelvis in women while the rectovesical space is the most dependant portion of pelvis in men and these spaces are a common location for fluid, drop metastases and abscesses in women and men respectively **(Figs. 5A to C)**.[4]

PERITONEAL FLUID DYNAMICS

The peritoneal cavity contains a small amount of fluid—approximately 50–100 mL.[8] This fluid has a natural tendency to move inferiorly towards the pelvis due to gravity. However, due to the respiratory motion of the diaphragm, gravitational pull of the liver and peristalsis of bowel, there is an active flow of the peritoneal fluid laterally and upwards towards the diaphragm. It predominantly flows up the right paracolic gutter which is deeper and wider than the left to the subphrenic space where majority (about 90%) of the peritoneal fluid is cleared by the submesothelial lymphatics. These lymphatics are connected with lymphatics on the other side of the diaphragm. Thus, metabolic, infectious and neoplastic processes in the peritoneal cavity may pass through the diaphragm to the subdiaphragmatic lymph nodes.[9] Ascites and tumor cells may also pass through the lymphatics and produce an ipsilateral pleural effusion. As these lymphatics have unidirectional valves, pleural effusion cannot pass into the peritoneal cavity. There are some areas of fluid stasis in the peritoneal cavity namely ileocolic region, root of sigmoid mesentery and pouch of Douglas, which become important in harboring disease.

ASCITES

Ascites is the pathological accumulation of fluid in the peritoneal cavity. It can occur due to a large number of causes. Common causes are listed in **Table 2**. Ascitic fluid is traditionally characterized as either *transudate*—thin,

Table 2: Causes of ascites.

• *Hepatic*: – Cirrhosis, portal hypertension, Budd-Chiari syndrome, alcoholic hepatitis, fulminant hepatic failure
• *Cardiac*: – Congestive heart failure, constrictive pericarditis, cardiac tamponade
• *Renal*: – Nephrotic syndrome, renal failure
• Hypoalbuminemia
• *Infective peritonitis*: – Bacterial, tuberculosis, viral, fungal
• *Neoplasms*: – Primary neoplasms of abdominal organs—colon, pancreas, ovary, liver, etc. – Primary peritoneal malignancy – Metastatic peritoneal disease
• Trauma
• Blunt, penetrating or iatrogenic trauma to abdominal organs can lead to collection of blood, bile, chyle, urine, etc. depending on the organ involved

with a low protein count and low specific gravity and *exudate*—high protein count and specific gravity. It has been seen that the serum-ascites albumin gradient is more accurate in classification of the causes of ascites.[10]

The imaging appearance of ascites depends on the amount of fluid, its contents and whether it is free flowing or loculated. In uncomplicated *transudative* ascites which is usually free flowing, the fluid tends to collect in dependant areas like pelvic cul-de-sac, Morrison's pouch and paracolic gutters in early stages. Due to the suction effect of the diaphragm, fluid also accumulates in the subphrenic spaces. Larger amounts of fluid will fill the entire peritoneal cavity and displace the small bowel loops centrally. The fluid collection is shaped by the surrounding structures, forms acute angles where fluid borders organs and does not deform the normal shape of adjacent organs. Complicated ascites, i.e. exudative or loculated ascites is associated with adhesions, malignancy or infection. Loculated ascites is noncompressible and has rounded margins with mass effect and frequently displaces adjacent structures.

Ultrasound is a sensitive modality for detection, quantification, localization and characterization of ascitic fluid. As little as 0.8 mm of fluid has been detected in the pouch of Douglas by transvaginal scanning.[11] US can also be very helpful in differentiating transudative from exudative ascites. In patients with transudative ascites, the US appearances are predominantly those of anechoic, mobile fluid. Features associated with exudative ascites due to inflammatory or malignant causes include loculated fluid collections, particulate ascites, septa, and matted bowel loops with interposed fluid. US can also help determine whether identified fluid is free or loculated, as free ascites moves when the patient changes position.

CT is most sensitive to small amounts of fluid in the peritoneum which collects preferentially in the dependent regions. The CT density of intraperitoneal fluid can give a clue to the underlying etiology, transudative ascites density is approximately that of water (–10 to +10 HU), whereas exudative ascites density is greater than 15 HU and increases with increasing protein content, hemoperitoneum density is higher still (~45 HU) and chylous fluid density is <0 HU. Enhancement of the peritoneum may be seen on CECT in infective and neoplastic ascites. As CT provides a more complete evaluation of the abdomen and pelvis than sonography, other intra- or extra-abdominal CT features may give further evidence to the origin of the ascites (e.g. features of heart failure, features of cirrhosis, peritoneal catheter *in situ*, etc).

It is often difficult to characterize the nature and underlying cause of peritoneal fluid collections on basis of imaging alone and a diagnostic paracentesis may be required to sample the fluid. US can be used to guide aspiration for diagnostic or therapeutic purpose.

PNEUMOPERITONEUM

Normally there is no free air within the peritoneal cavity. The most common cause of a pneumoperitoneum is due to rupture of an abdominal viscus. Other causes are—postoperative status, patient on peritoneal dialysis, rupture of a cyst in pneumatosis intestinalis etc. It is important to be able to recognize the signs of a pneumoperitoneum on various imaging modalities and to be able to differentiate a true pneumoperitoneum from a pseudopneumoperitoneum. This has been discussed in detail elsewhere in the book.

INTERNAL HERNIAS

Internal hernia is the protrusion of a viscus through a normal or abnormal aperture in the peritoneum or mesentery, within the confines of the peritoneal cavity. This aperture can be congenital or acquired, such as postsurgical, post-traumatic or even postinflammatory. Congenital hernias may occur through a normal aperture, e.g. foramen of Winslow, or abnormal defects which arise from anomalies of internal rotation and peritoneal attachment.

Based on the location, Meyers traditionally classified these hernias as paraduodenal (53%), pericecal

(13%), foramen of Winslow (8%), transmesenteric and transmesocolic (8%), intersigmoid (6%), retroanastomotic (5%) and paravesical (7%—not a true internal hernia).[12] The most common internal hernias have been the paraduodenal hernias which are congenital hernias, however with the increasing surgical procedures being performed these days, the incidence of the acquired post-operative hernias is increasing.[13]

Clinically, internal hernias can have a variable presentation ranging from asymptomatic to mild colicky abdominal pain to acute intestinal obstruction. Imaging plays an important role in diagnosis as they are difficult to identify clinically. Imaging features on barium studies and CT include cluster of dilated/nondilated bowel loops in an abnormal location **(Figs. 6A and B)**, crowding of loops in a hernia sac and/or features of obstruction. CT may additionally show mesenteric vessel abnormalities as engorgement, twisting, or stretching of the vessels. **Table 3** lists the various hernias with their characteristic clinical and imaging findings.

PERITONEAL INFECTIONS AND INFLAMMATION

Peritonitis

Peritonitis is defined as a diffuse inflammation of the parietal and visceral peritoneum. It is most often caused by introduction of an infection into the otherwise sterile peritoneal environment through perforation of an abdominal viscus, but it may also result from other irritants, such as foreign bodies (such as talc or barium), bile from a perforated gallbladder or a lacerated liver, or gastric acid from a perforated ulcer. Gynecologic disease processes such as salpingitis may also cause peritonitis. Uncommonly, primary bacterial peritonitis may occur due to hematogenous spread of organisms in association with chronic liver or renal disease.

Clinically, patients may present with an acute or insidious onset of symptoms, limited and mild disease, or systemic and severe disease with septic shock. On imaging, there is presence of ascites which may be loculated or show presence of debris, septa or gas **(Fig. 7)**. US is superior to CT in demonstrating the nature of the ascitic fluid.[14] In association with ascites there is peritoneal and mesenteric thickening. The thickened peritoneum is seen to enhance on contrast administration, and is often smooth **(Fig. 8)**. In some cases evidence of the underlying primary pathology can be seen such as diverticulitis, appendiceal perforation, bowel ischemia, etc.

Peritoneal abscess is an infected fluid collection encapsulated by fibrinous exudate, omentum, and/or adjacent visceral organs. The majority of abscesses occur secondary to spread of infection from an adjacent infected organ or viscus, e.g. inflamed appendix, pancreatitis, diverticulitis, Crohn's disease, liver abscess, etc. Abscess formation may also occur as a complication of abdominal or pelvic surgery or penetrating trauma. The risk of abscess increases in cases of preoperative perforation of the hollow viscus, significant fecal contamination of the peritoneal cavity, bowel ischemia, as well as in the setting of immunosuppression.

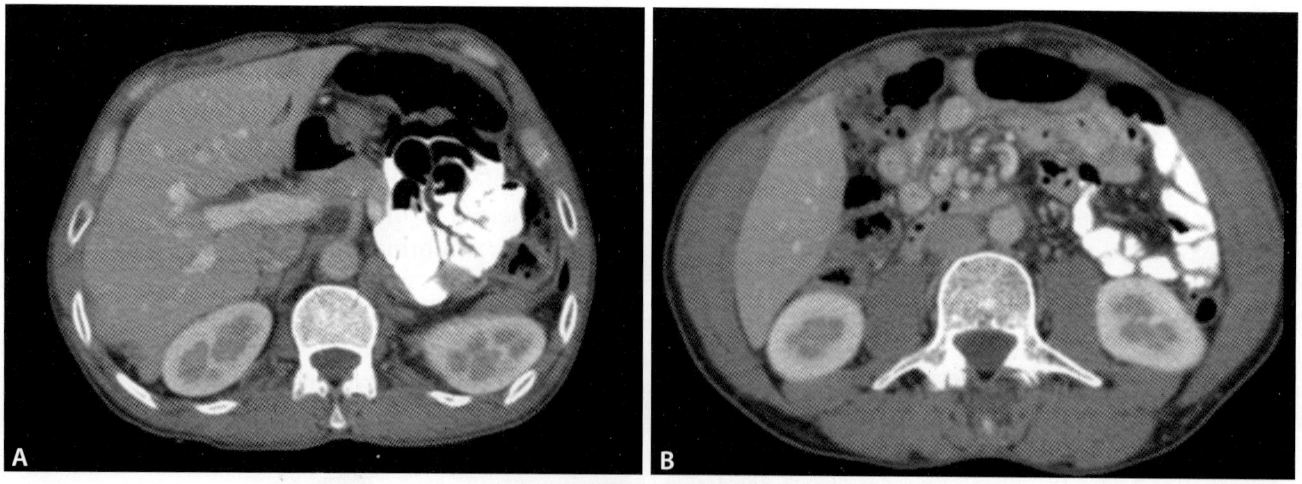

Figs. 6A and B: Left paraduodenal hernia in a 45-year-old man with chronic postprandial abdominal pain. Axial CECT image (A) shows a sac like mass of jejunal loops between stomach and pancreatic body. Section obtained at lower level (B) shows crowded and dilated mesenteric vessels.

Table 3: Internal hernias: Clinical and imaging features.

Type of hernia	*Congenital/Acquired site*	*Findings on plain radiographs and barium studies*	*CT findings*
Left paraduodenal	Congenital Through Landzert's fossa behind the fourth part of the duodenum	Cluster of jejunal loops in left hypochondrium, lateral to the 4th part of duodenum; may have mass effect indenting posterior wall of stomach or displacing transverse colon inferiorly	• Encapsulated cluster of dilated small-bowel loops between stomach and pancreas, behind pancreas itself, or between transverse colon and left adrenal gland • Inferior mesenteric vein displaced superoanteriorly in neck of hernia sac
Right paraduodenal	Congenital Through Waldeyer's fossa (representing a defect in the first part of the jejunal mesentery)	Clustered loops lateral and inferior to the 2nd part of duodenum; associated with nonrotation of small-bowel	• Encapsulated cluster of loops lateral and inferior to the 2nd part of duodenum; associated with small-bowel nonrotation • Superior mesenteric artery displaced anteriorly
Pericecal	Congenital/acquired Through a defect in the cecal mesentery and extending into the right paracolic gutter	Clustered small-bowel loops (usually distal ileal) posterior and lateral to the cecum in right paracolic gutter	Clustered small-bowel loops (usually distal ileum) posterior and lateral to the cecum in right paracolic gutter
Foramen of Winslow	Congenital Through Foramen of Winslow	Circumscribed loops medial and posterior to the stomach	Loops in the lesser sac between liver and inferior vena cava
Intersigmoid	Congenital/acquired Fossae/defects in and around sigmoid mesocolon	U- or C-shaped cluster of small bowel posterior and lateral to the sigmoid colon	U- or C-shaped cluster of small bowel posterior and lateral to the sigmoid colon
Transmesenteric	• Congenital in children through defect in small bowel mesentery • Acquired in adults associated with abdominal surgery	Variable, air within gastric remnant in postoperative cases; may simulate a left paraduodenal hernia	Small bowel lateral to colon; displaced omental fat with small bowel directly abutting abdominal wall
Retroanastomotic	Acquired Through a defect related to a surgical anastomosis	Variable	Variable

Source: Adapted from Martin LC, Markle EM, Thompson WM. Review of internal hernias: radiographic and clinical findings.[13]

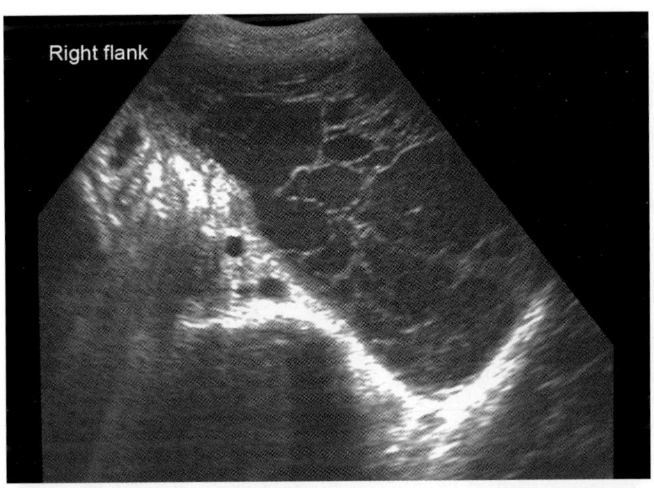

Fig. 7: Purulent peritonitis: Transverse US image through right flank shows ascites with peritoneal thickening and ascitic fluid. The fluid shows internal echoes characteristic of exudative nature and multiple septae within.

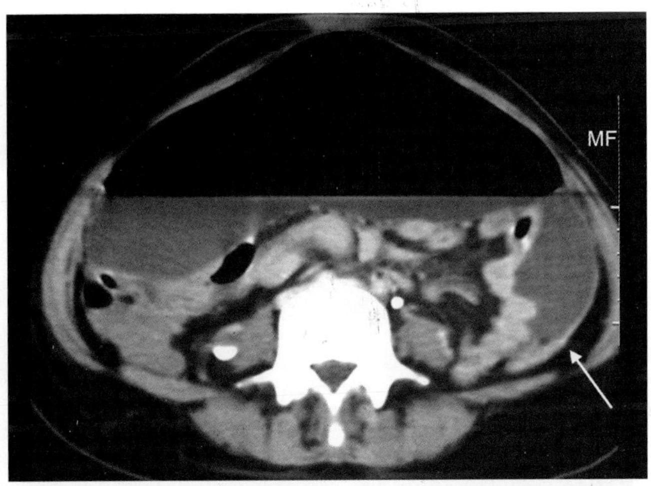

Fig. 8: Perforation peritonitis: CECT axial section through the abdomen, shows fluid in the peritoneal cavity with a large air fluid level. Smooth, enhancing, thickening of the peritoneal lining is seen (arrow).

Clinically patients present with fever, tachycardia, and symptoms localized to area of abscess, e.g. with a subphrenic collection, there may be shoulder tip pain, hiccups and unexplained pulmonary symptoms (pleural effusion, basal atelectasis). Sometimes clinical features may be minimal specially in immunocompromised patients.

The CT appearance of an abscess varies depending on its age. In early stages, it may appear as a mass with soft tissue attenuation values. As the liquefaction progresses, a central hypodense, nonenhancing area with a definable, enhancing wall is seen. Gas may be seen within the abscess cavity as multiple small bubbles or as an air fluid level **(Figs. 9 and 16B)**. Occasionally septations may be seen. There is thickening and obliteration of adjacent fat planes, mass effect on surrounding structures. Features of the predisposing cause of the abscess, e.g. acute appendicitis, Crohn's disease, or diverticulitis, etc. may be seen.

On US, an abscess is seen as a round or oval fluid collection with a well-defined irregular wall, with occasional internal septa or debris. Small pockets of air within the abscess cavity can be seen as echogenic foci with posterior reverberation artefact.[15] However, US detection of abscess is hampered by bowel gas, intra-abdominal fat, gas within the abscess cavity and in postoperative cases, there is limited availability of scanning surface. Thus, US has a low sensitivity in abscess detection. CT is the preferred modality and can confidently rule out intra-abdominal abscess if the CT examination is negative.

On MRI, abscesses are seen as well-defined fluid collection with low SI on T1W and high SI on T2W images. Adjacent inflammation can be seen as diffusely increased SI on T2W images.

Percutaneous aspiration is frequently required to confirm the presence of pus in a suspected abscess. Percutaneous drainage has become the widely accepted treatment for abdominal abscesses and can be done under US or CT guidance. US can be used for the follow-up evaluation of abscess under treatment.[7]

Tuberculous Peritonitis

The peritoneum and its reflections can also be commonly involved by tuberculosis. The mode of transmission may be hematogenous or lymphatic, reactivation of latent tuberculous foci in the peritoneum or peritoneal spill from tubercular salpingitis. Discharge of caseous material from diseased lymph nodes may also lead to tubercular peritonitis.

Classically, three forms of tuberculous peritonitis have been described.[16-18]

- *Wet ascitic type*: Seen in 90% cases characterized by large amount of free or loculated ascitic fluid. This may be accompanied by diffuse and smooth peritoneal thickening.
- *Fibrotic fixed type*: Characterized by mesenteric and omental thickening and matted bowel loops resembling masses, with formation of cocoon in some cases.
- *Dry or plastic type*: Predominant peritoneal and mesenteric thickening with caseous nodules, lymph node enlargement and dense adhesions.

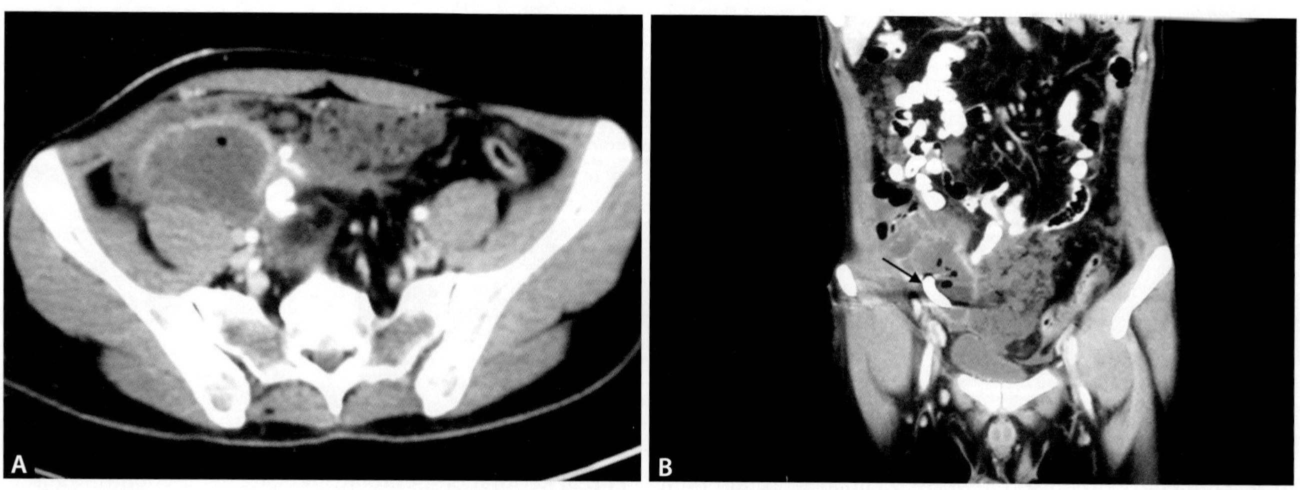

Figs. 9A and B: Appendicular abscess: CECT axial (A) and coronal scans (B) show a well defined hypodense collection with a thin peripheral enhancing rim in the right iliac fossa. Small gas bubbles are seen within the abscess. There is evidence of associated inflammatory changes in the adjacent fat. A drain can be seen in the abscess in (B) (arrow).

Imaging Features

Tubercular infection diffusely involves the peritoneum, mesentery and omentum. *Free or loculated ascites* is seen in 30–100% cases and is demonstrated by both ultrasound and CT.[19-21]

Ultrasound may show fine, multiple, complete or incomplete mobile strands of fibrin and debris in the ascites **(Fig. 10A)**. Peritoneal thickening and tiny nodules are better visualized in presence of ascites on US. On CT, usually high density (25–45 HU) ascitic fluid due to high fibrin content and cellular debris is characteristic of TB.[22] However ascites may be near water density, representing an earlier transudative stage of immune reaction. Fat fluid level, a feature of chylous ascites with supportive evidence of mesenteric adenopathy has been described in tuberculosis.[23] CT fails to show the multiple, thin interlacing septa in most patients **(Figs. 11A to C)**. Smooth, slight peritoneal thickening and/or pronounced enhancement are seen in presence of ascites on CT in almost all cases. Enhancement of peritoneal lining in patients with tubercular ascites has been described on delayed contrast-enhanced MRI.

Mesenteric involvement is seen as linear striations, vascular engorgement, nodular lesions, increased density at the root of mesentery, mesenteric thickening and loss of normal mesenteric configuration. On US the mesentery becomes echogenic as a result of increased fat deposition due to lymphatic obstruction. Presence of enlarged lymph nodes adds to the diagnosis of early tuberculosis **(Figs. 10A to C)**. Mesenteric nodular lesions may present as micro (<5 mm) or macro (>5 mm) nodules. Mesenteric abscess may form as result of extension of caseous material from diseased lymph nodes. Fixed loops of bowel and mesentery standing out as spokes radiating out from the mesenteric root are described as ultrasound 'stellate' sign. CT demonstrates the thickened mesentery by its increased vascularity and thickened strands and tethering of bowel loops forming an abdominal mass **(Figs. 11 to 12)**. 'Club sandwich sign' or the 'sliced bread' appearance is due to localized or focal ascitis between radially oriented bowel

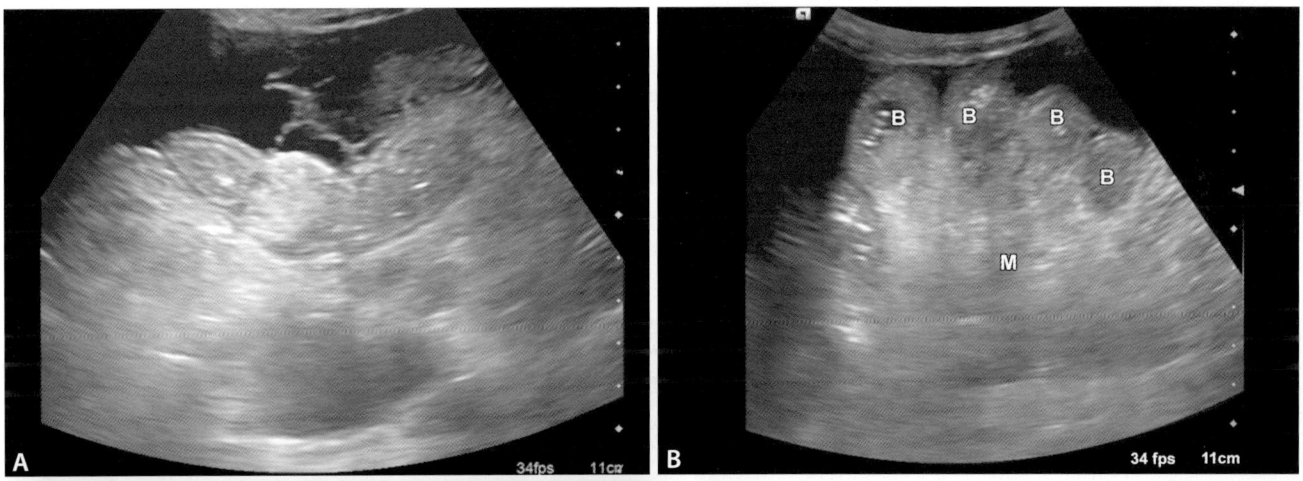

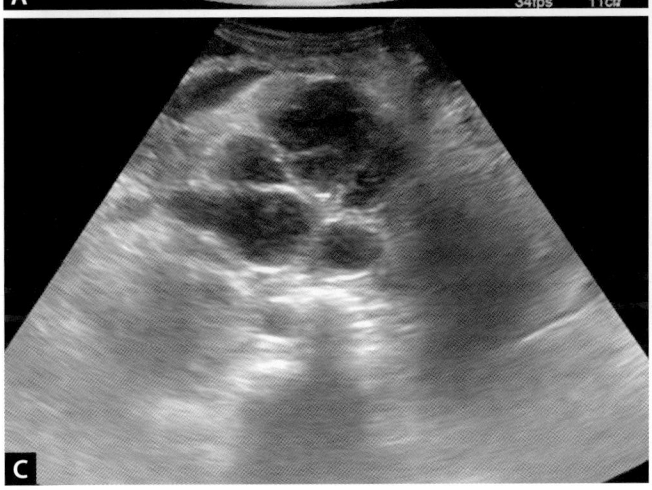

Figs. 10A to C: 40-year-old patient with peritoneal tuberculosis. Transverse transabdominal ultrasound shows (A) loculated ascites with thin fibrinous septae and posteriorly adherent bowel loops. (B) Thickened echogenic mesenteric leaves—"stellate" appearance (M) with bowel loops (B) suspended radially at the mesenteric edge and surrounding ascites. (C) Enlarged, variable sized, hypoechoic mesenteric nodes are also seen.

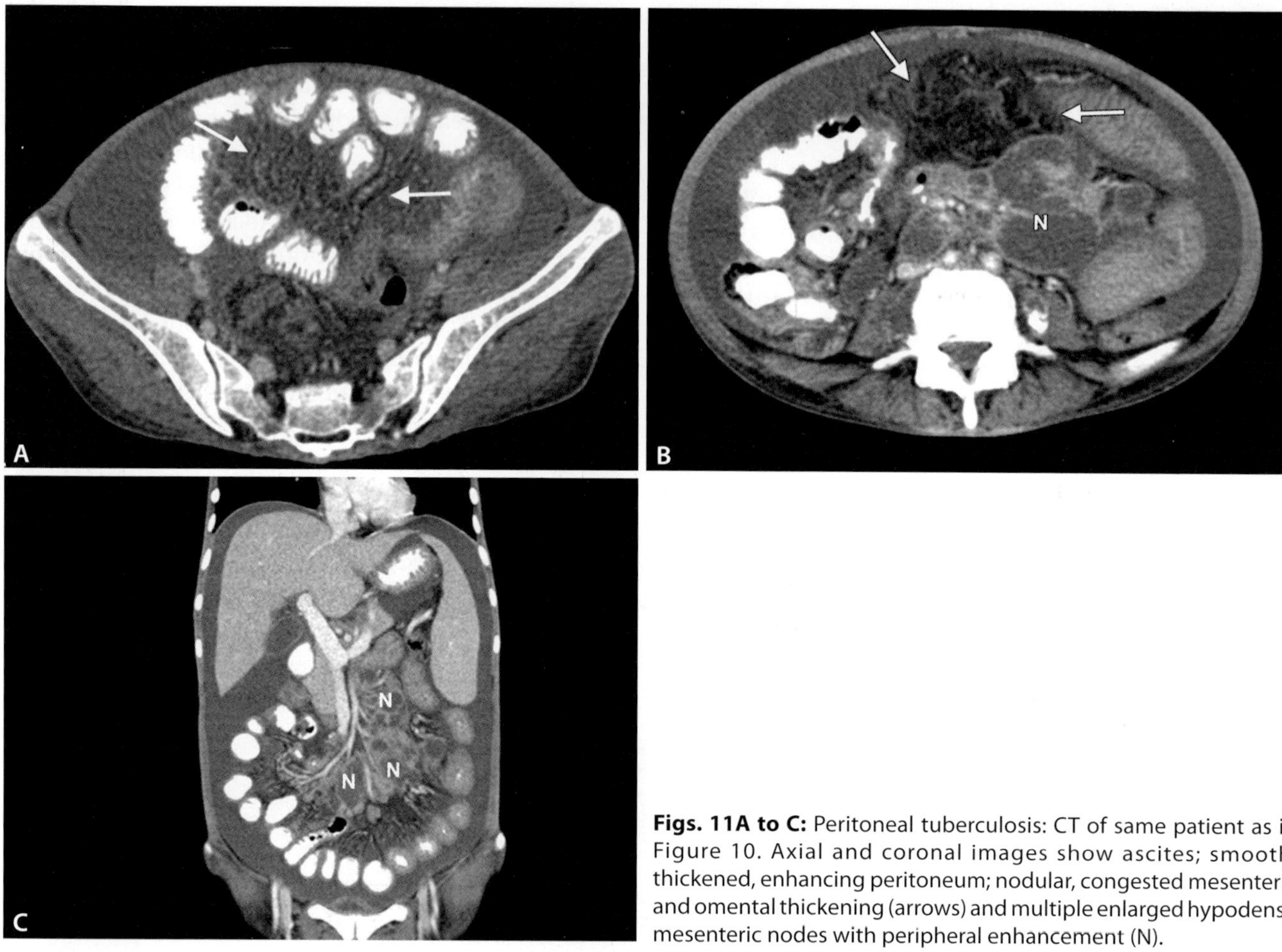

Figs. 11A to C: Peritoneal tuberculosis: CT of same patient as in Figure 10. Axial and coronal images show ascites; smooth, thickened, enhancing peritoneum; nodular, congested mesenteric and omental thickening (arrows) and multiple enlarged hypodense mesenteric nodes with peripheral enhancement (N).

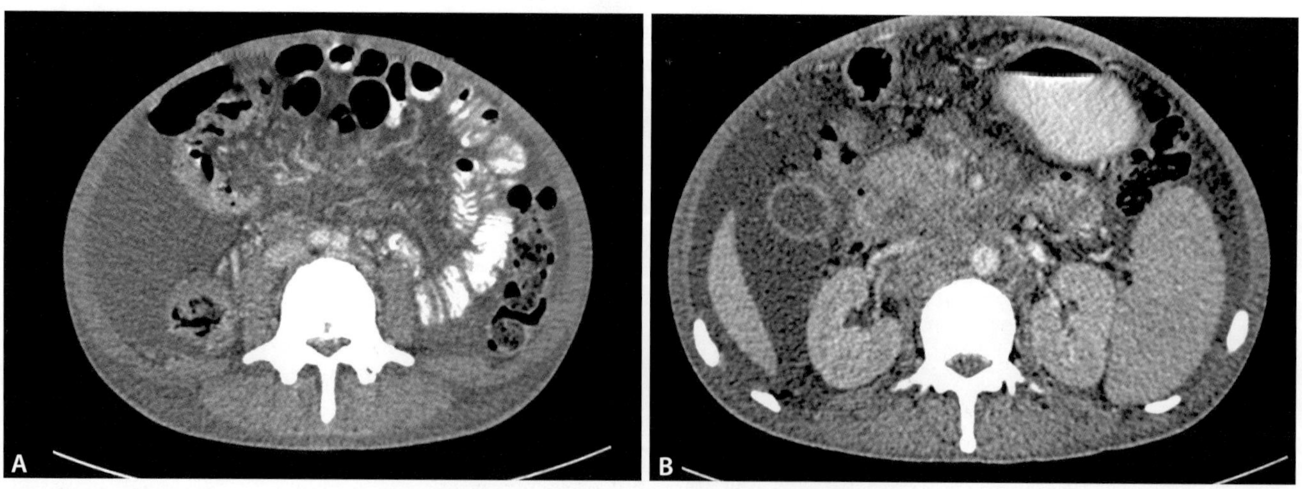

Figs. 12A and B: Tubercular peritonitis—wet ascitic type: CECT axial scans show the presence of ascites with small nodules and haziness in the mesentery and omentum (A); At a more cranial level (B), conglomerate caseous lymphadenopathy is seen in mesenteric and retroperitoneal regions.

due to local exudation from inflamed bowel or ruptured lymph nodes.

Omental thickening is a feature of both TB and peritoneal carcinomatosis and many different appearances 'nodular' 'smudged' or 'caked' have been described. The thickened omentum shows heterogeneous iso- to hyperintense signal on T2W sequences on MRI.[24] A marked degree of peritoneal enhancement is seen on enhanced CT and MRI **(Figs. 13 and 14)**. Sclerosing encapsulating peritonitis (abdominal cocoon) formation has also been described in tubercular involvement of peritoneum **(*see* Figs. 17A to D)**.

Associated features of intra-abdominal tuberculosis may also be present, such as thickening of the bowel wall, particularly the terminal ileum, focal abnormalities in the liver or spleen due to granulomas and occasionally adrenal pathology. Notably the chest radiograph is abnormal in only 50% of patients with tuberculous peritonitis.[25]

The *differential diagnosis* of tubercular peritonitis constitutes peritoneal carcinomatosis, mesothelioma, peritonitis and rarely lymphoma. A marked overlap exists between the imaging appearances of tubercular peritonitis and peritoneal carcinomatosis. Features favoring carcinomatosis are nodular implants with irregular thickening. Irregularly thickened outer contour of the infiltrated peritoneum favors malignancy, whereas a thin omental line, suggestive of a fibrous wall covering

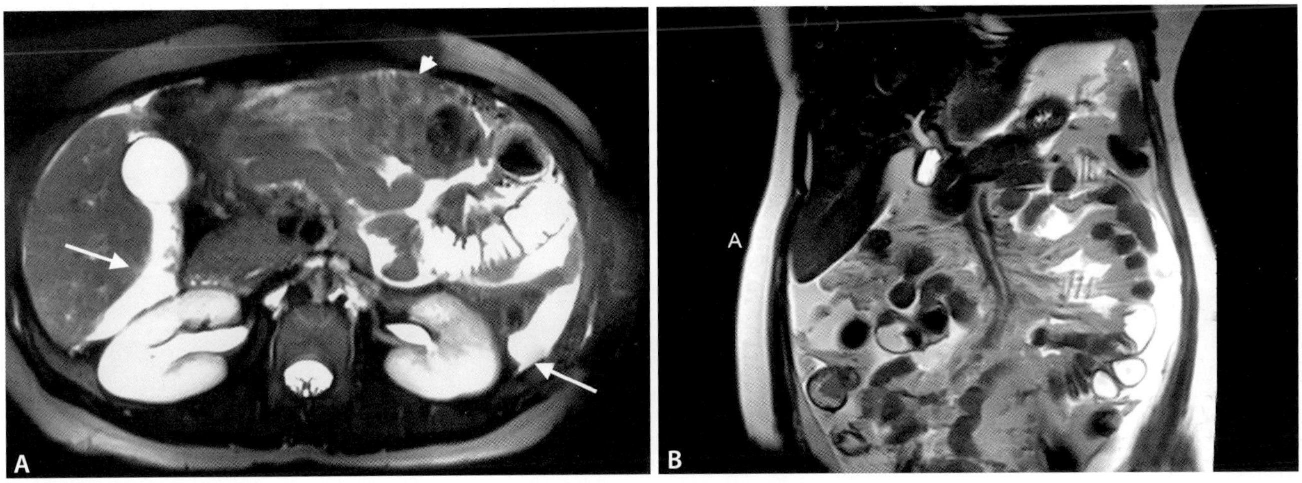

Figs. 13A and B: Peritoneal tuberculosis in 35-year-old woman with loss of weight and abdominal fullness for 1 month: (A) Axial T2W haste MR image shows presence of ascitic fluid in Morrison's pouch, left paracolic gutter (arrows) and in interloop regions. The omentum is thickened showing a heterogeneous soft tissue signal (arrowhead); (B) Coronal T2W haste MR image shows diffuse infiltration of the mesenteric fat by isointense soft tissue. Ascites is seen in the paracolic gutters and subhepatic space.

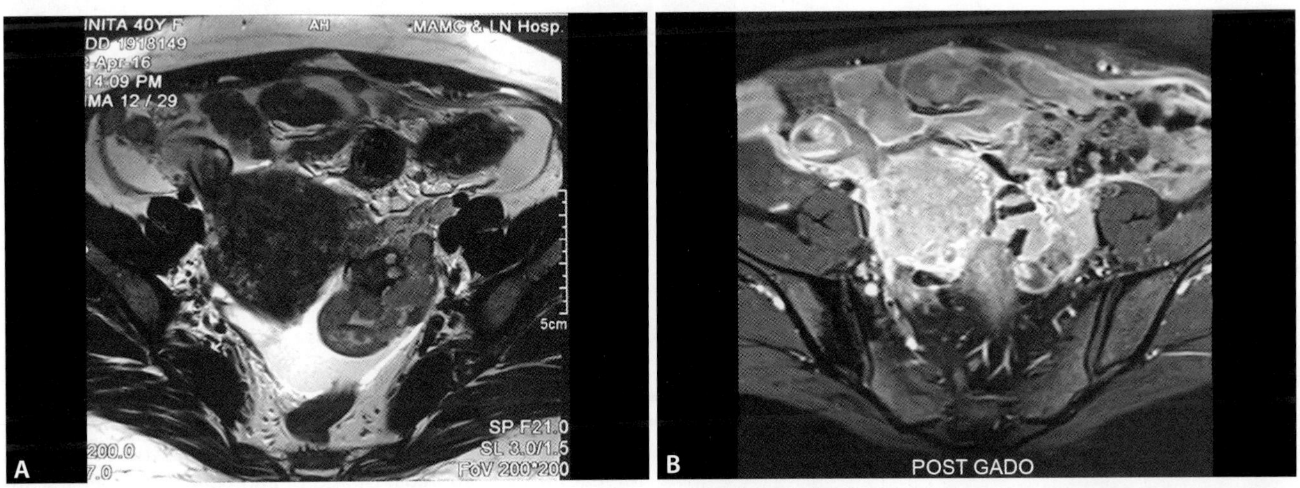

Figs. 14A and B: Peritoneal tuberculosis-same patient as in Figure 13: Axial T2W haste (A) and postcontrast (B) MR images show presence of ascites, clumped bowel loops, with thickened and enhancing serosa. Left tubo-ovarian was seen which also enhanced on the postcontrast scan. On laprotomy the bowel serosa and the adnexal mass were studded with multiple small granulomas, which were not identifiable individually on the MR images, but caused the intensely enhancing peritoneal lining.

the infiltrated omentum is more common in tubercular peritonitis.[26,27] However, a clinical background of malignancy along with laboratory investigations are often required to differentiate between them. Peritoneal mesothelioma shows multifocal peritoneal thickening of either sheet or nodular type which can be up to 3 cm in thickness, omental or mesenteric soft tissue masses, thick rigid septae between peritoneal leaves and fixed bowel loops with disproportionately small amount of ascites to the degree of tumor dissemination.

PERITONEAL HYDATIDOSIS

Peritoneal hydatidosis is an uncommon manifestation of hydatid disease and is almost always secondary to hepatic disease. It occurs as a result of traumatic or surgical rupture of a hepatic or splenic hydatid cyst. However, spontaneous, asymptomatic microruptures of hepatic cysts into the peritoneal cavity are not uncommon leading to peritoneal seeding. Primary hydatidosis is a rare entity accounting for just 2% of all intra-abdominal hydatid disease.[28]

Clinical picture: Most patients remain asymptomatic for years. Symptoms such as nonspecific pain, abdominal fullness, dyspepsia, anorexia, and vomiting arise due to enlarging abdominal cysts. Rupture of the cyst into the peritoneum may present as acute abdominal pain. Antigenic fluid released into the peritoneal cavity and absorbed into the circulation may present with acute allergic manifestations.[29]

Imaging features: Hydatid cysts can be well seen on US, CT and MRI. Cysts may be multiple and located anywhere in the peritoneal cavity **(Figs. 15A to C)**. The imaging appearances of hydatid cysts are similar to those in hepatic disease. Sometimes, peritoneal hydatid disease occupy the entire peritoneal cavity, simulating a multiloculated mass which is known as encysted peritoneal hydatidosis.[28]

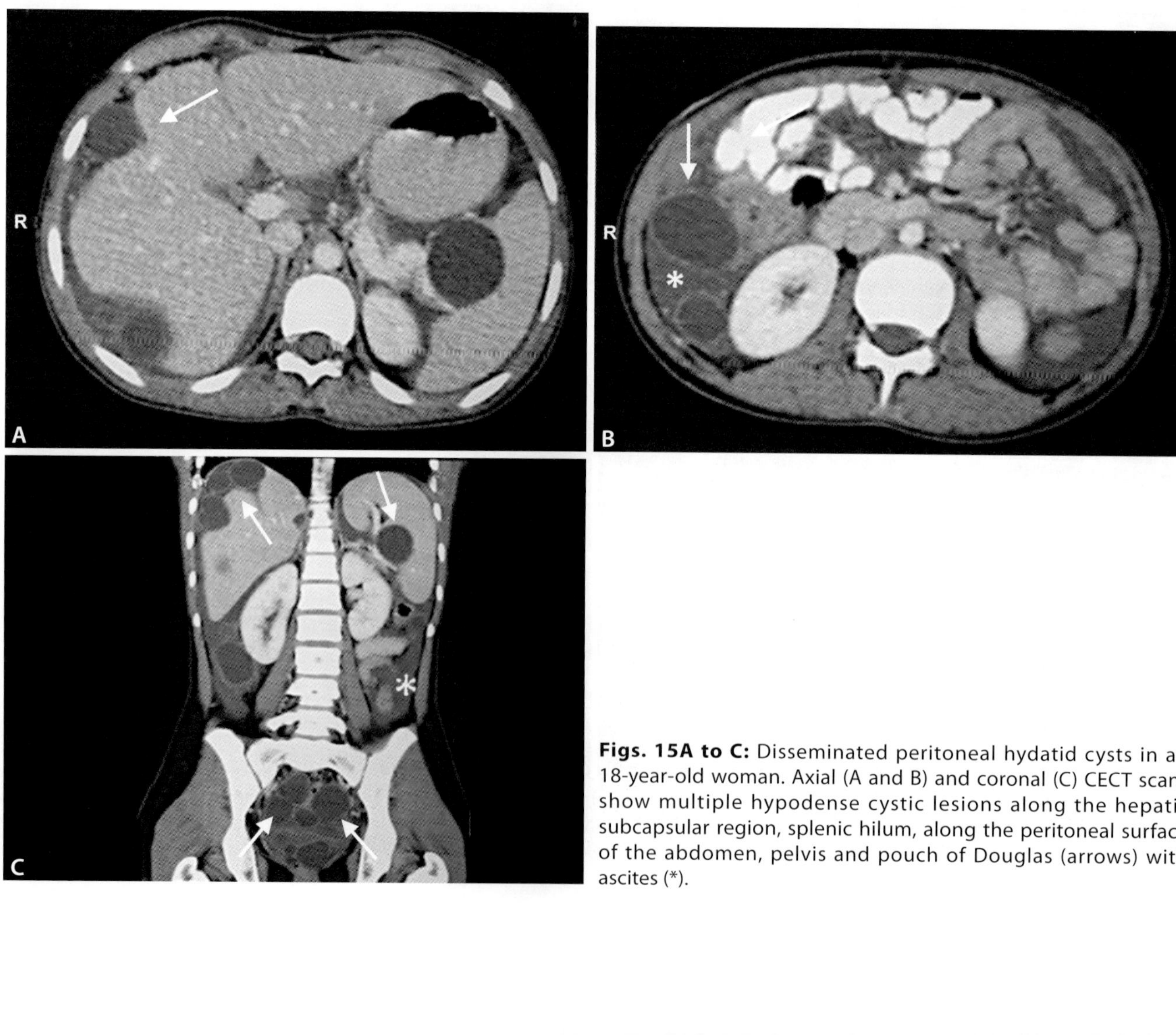

Figs. 15A to C: Disseminated peritoneal hydatid cysts in an 18-year-old woman. Axial (A and B) and coronal (C) CECT scans show multiple hypodense cystic lesions along the hepatic subcapsular region, splenic hilum, along the peritoneal surface of the abdomen, pelvis and pouch of Douglas (arrows) with ascites (*).

SECONDARY INFLAMMATORY PROCESSES

Inflammation of any part of the abdominal viscera may be accompanied by inflammatory change of the regional fatty tissue. This may progress to phlegmon formation, abscess or even generalized peritonitis. Appendicitis, diverticulitis, pancreatitis, inflammatory bowel disease, cholecystitis, etc. are conditions which commonly give rise to these localized inflammatory changes. They are best visualized on CT as soft tissue stranding of adjacent fat, fluid, phlegmon or abscess formation, sinus tracts and fistulas **(Figs. 16A and B)**.

Besides the above inflammatory changes, Crohn's disease may show other mesenteric abnormalities in the form of hypertrophied mesenteric fat (fibrofatty proliferation), engorged vasa recta (the comb's sign), and small mesenteric nodes. The presence of engorged vasa recta indicates active inflammation, whereas the fibrofatty proliferation can be seen even with quiescent disease.

Mesenteric edema is defined as diffuse increase in attenuation throughout the mesentery that obscures visualization of the blood vessels as they course through the mesentery, also termed as 'misty mesentery'. It may be secondary to various causes, including hypoalbuminemia, cirrhosis, nephrosis, heart failure, tricuspid disease, constrictive pericarditis, portal hypertension, portal vein thrombosis, mesenteric ischemia, vasculitis or trauma. On CT, mesenteric edema increases the density of the mesenteric fat from –100 to –160, which is similar to the density of subcutaneous fat, to values of –40 to –60.[30] On MRI, the mesentery shows abnormal signal. The mesenteric arteries and veins lose their sharp definition and are not clearly visualized as they course to the bowel. Associated ascites may be present and generalized subcutaneous and retroperitoneal fat haziness secondary to generalized edema can be seen. The extent and site of involvement gives a clue to the differential diagnosis.

SCLEROSING ENCAPSULATING PERITONITIS/ABDOMINAL COCOON

Sclerosing encapsulating peritonitis is a rare chronic inflammatory process of the peritoneum which is characterized by total or partial encasement of the small bowel within a thick fibrocollagenous membrane. Sclerosing encapsulating peritonitis (SEP) is most commonly associated with abdominal tuberculosis in our country. It can occur as a complication in patients who undergo continuous peritoneal dialysis. It has also been described in association with long-term β-blocker treatment, sarcoidosis, SLE, indwelling abdominal catheter, etc.[31] These conditions predispose patients to peritoneal irritation and inflammation which can lead to peritoneal fibroneogenesis. Sometimes no predisposing condition may be found for the SEP.

Clinically, patients may be asymptomatic or have abdominal distention, pain and vomiting that resolve spontaneously suggesting recurrent episodes of small bowel obstruction. A soft nontender mass may be felt at abdominal palpation. It is seen to be commoner in young adolescent girls.

Imaging features: A barium meal follow-through study may show a conglomeration of multiple bowel loops that appear

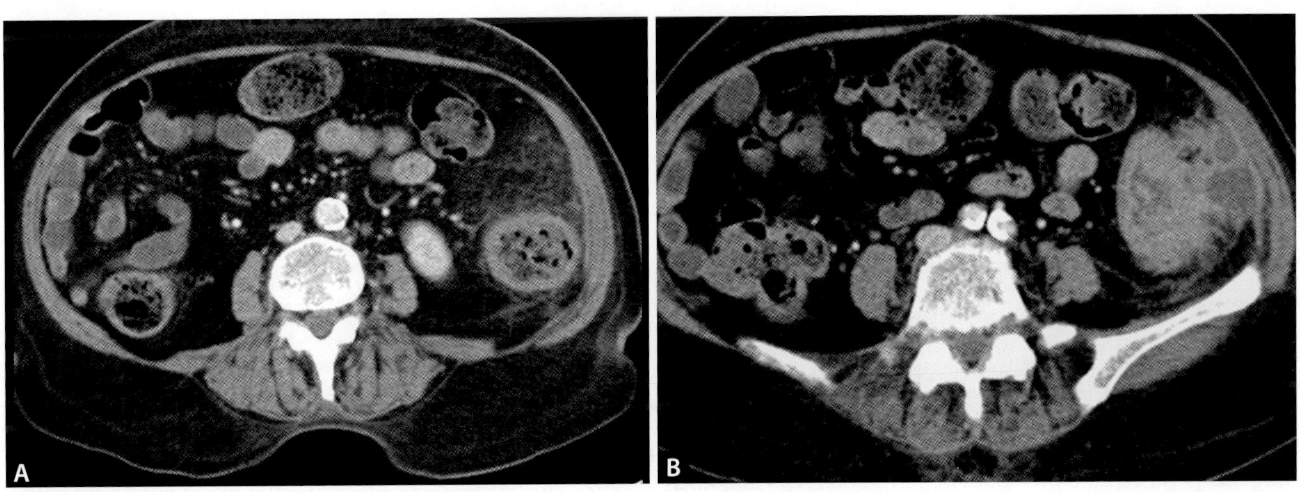

Figs. 16A and B: Acute diverticulitis showing local extension of inflammation: CECT axial scans (A) inflammatory fat stranding seen around the thickened segment of descending colon; (B) In another patient, there is formation of abscesses seen as rim enhancing hypodense masses in the left pericolonic region.

to adhere to each other with or without delayed passage of contrast material **(Fig. 17A)**. Characteristic sonographic findings include altered peristalsis, adherence of the bowel to the anterior abdominal wall and a membranous sac seen to encase the small bowel loops **(Fig. 17B)**. There is a concertina—like arrangement of small bowel loops with a narrow posterior base. The encapsulating membrane may be identified with high frequency linear probes.[32]

Contrast-enhanced computed tomography shows conglomeration of small-bowel loops in the central abdomen with a thick enhancing membrane surrounding the bowel, forming a saclike structure or a cocoon **(Figs. 17C and D)**. Small amount of fluid may be seen within the cocoon. Bowel loops may be of normal caliber or dilated. The fibrous membrane surrounding the bowel loops is best visualized on CT. CT also gives more accurate information on the degree of obstruction and the types of bowel loops involved. Multiple foci of linear calcification may develop or there can be diffuse peritoneal calcification.[33,34]

The most important differential diagnosis of SEP is from an internal hernia that also causes localized collection of small-bowel loops with symptoms of obstruction. However, there is no membrane like sac around the clustered small bowel loops in internal hernias. SEP may also be confused with congenital peritoneal encapsulation, which is characterized by a thin accessory peritoneal sac surrounding the small bowel.

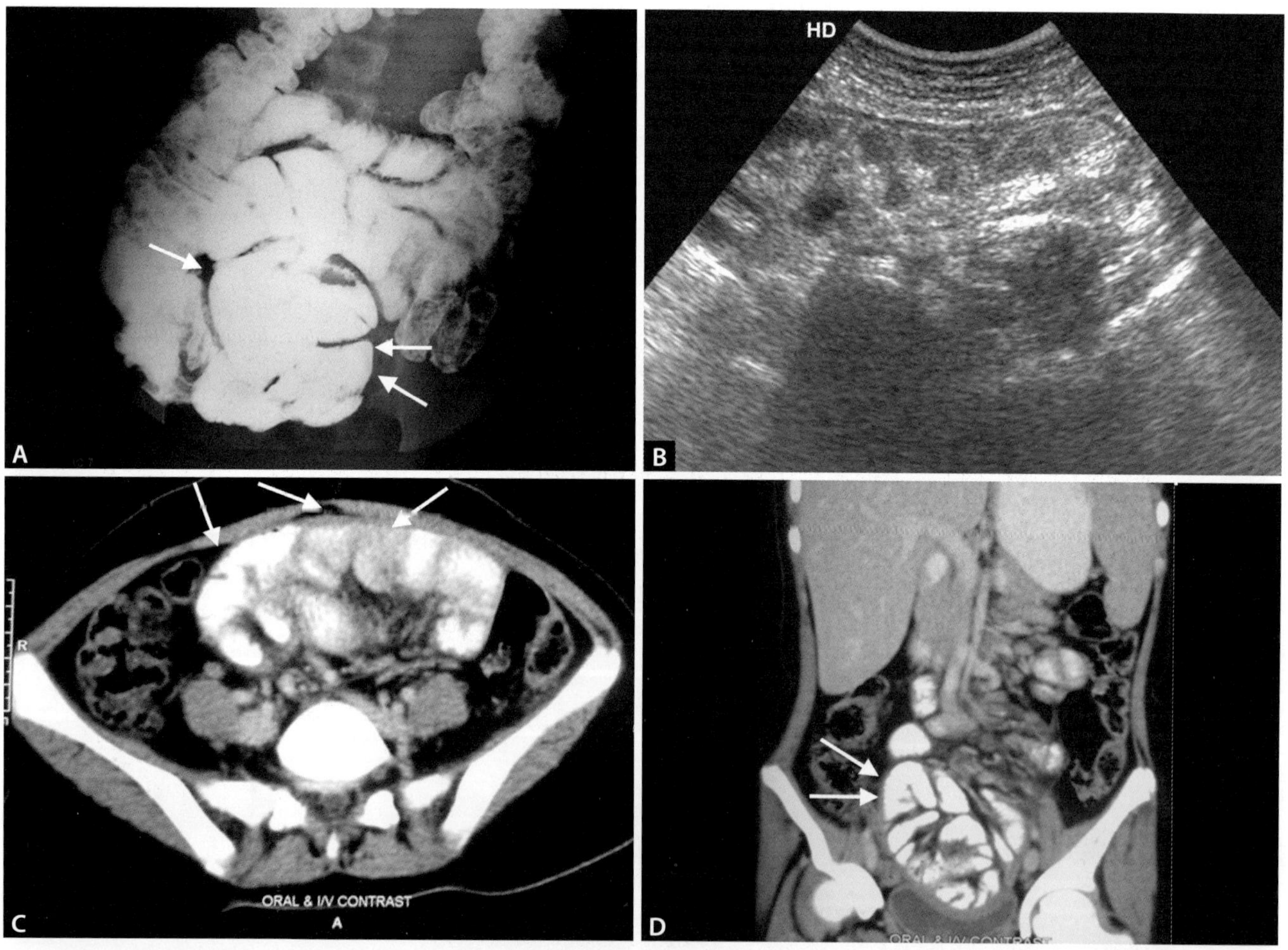

Figs. 17A to D: Sclerosing peritonitis: A 14-year-old girl with recurrent episodes of intestinal obstruction: (A) Barium meal follow through study shows clustered bowel loops in pelvis and lower abdomen (arrows); (B) Transverse US through lower abdomen show clumped bowel loops adherent to the anterior abdominal wall. An increased peristalsis was noted in the loops on real-time; Axial (C) and coronal (D) CECT scans show clumped small bowel loops in the lower abdomen with a thin surrounding membrane (arrows). Small mesenteric nodes are also seen.

SCLEROSING MESENTERITIS (MESENTERIC PANNICULITIS, MESENTERIC LIPODYSTROPHY, RETRACTILE MESENTERITIS)

Sclerosing mesenteritis is a rare, slowly progressive disorder characterized by nonspecific inflammation of the mesenteric fat. It usually involves the root of the small bowel mesentery, but may affect the transverse mesocolon, peripancreatic region, omentum, retroperitoneum or pelvis.[35]

Histologically, it has varying amounts of fibrosis, chronic inflammation, and fat necrosis. Depending on the predominant component it has been categorized into three subgroups:

1. Sclerosing/retractile mesenteritis when the fibrous component is dominant.
2. Mesenteric panniculitis when chronic inflammation predominates.
3. Mesenteric lipodystrophy, when fat necrosis is the predominant component.[36]

Although its exact cause remains unknown, various underlying possibilities have been suggested like prior surgery or trauma, ischemia, an autoimmune process or malignancy. An association with other idiopathic inflammatory disorders like retroperitoneal fibrosis, Reidel's thyroiditis, orbital pseudotumors and sclerosing cholangitis has been noted.

Clinical picture: It occurs more commonly in males and the average age of presentation is around 60 years. Patients present with abdominal pain, mass, obstructive symptoms or diarrhea or may even be completely asymptomatic.

Imaging Findings

The imaging findings reflect the underlying histology of the lesion. When the fibrous component is dominant, i.e. sclerosing type of mesenteritis, an infiltrative soft tissue mass with variable degree of enhancement is seen on CT. Central calcification or necrosis, radiating strands of soft tissue (desmoplastic reaction), small lymph nodes in the adjacent fat may all be seen **(Figs. 18A and B)**. There may be preservation of fat around the mesenteric vessels, a phenomenon that is referred to as the "fat ring sign".[37] On MRI, the signal intensity pattern is consistent with fibrosis, showing low signal intensity on both T1- and T2-weighted images. Sometimes a high signal on T2W image may be seen which correspons to myxomatous change or hypervascularity accompanying active proliferation of fibrosis. Secondary changes may be seen in the adjacent bowel as angulations by the fibrotic process in the mesentery, or edematous thickening due to obstruction of lymphatics and veins.[36]

In mesenteric panniculitis, CT may show subtle increase in attenuation with small nodes within it with no evidence of a mass. The term 'misty mesentery' may be used to describe this process as it is not specific for mesenteric panniculitis, but may also be seen in any infiltrating process in the mesentery like edema, hemorrhage, fibrosis or tumor. The 'fat-ring sign' can be seen in mesenteric panniculitis. A tumoral pseudocapsule, i.e. a peripheral band of soft

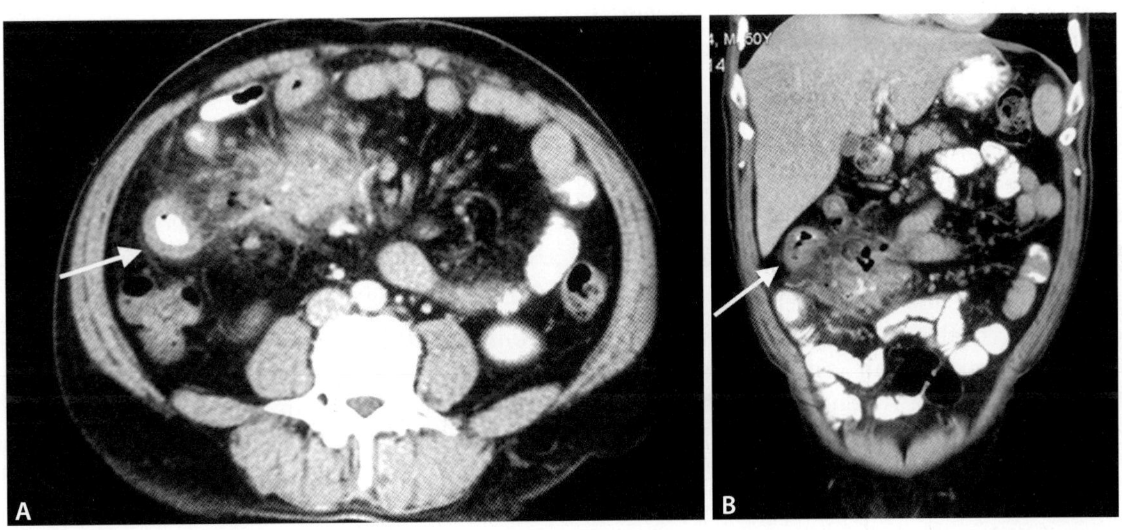

Figs. 18A and B: Sclerosing mesenteritis: Enhanced axial (A) and coronal (B) CT scans show an ill-defined soft tissue mesenteric mass with irregular, spiculated margins and thickening of adjacent jejunal loops (arrow). Small mesenteric lymph nodes are seen.

tissue attenuation, appearing hypointense on T2W MR images, may sometimes be seen separating the normal mesentery from the inflammatory process.

Differential diagnosis: Several conditions can mimic the CT appearance of sclerosing mesenteritis, including lymphoma, carcinoid tumor, carcinomatosis, primary mesenteric mesothelioma, and mesenteric edema.[38] Except for primary mesenteric mesothelioma, these conditions are considerably more common than sclerosing mesenteritis. Mesenteric panniculitis can be mimicked by mesenteric edema resulting from various conditions such as cirrhosis, hypoalbuminemia, heart failure, portal or mesenteric vein thrombosis, and vasculitis. Trauma can also result in edema and hemorrhage in the mesentery. Mesenteric edema secondary to systemic disease is often diffuse and coexists with generalized subcutaneous edema and ascites, which will not be present in patients with sclerosing mesenteritis. Also, the clinical history will often be the clue to the correct diagnosis. A biopsy is necessary for diagnosis and although results of the biopsy may suggest the diagnosis, surgical excisional biopsy is often required for complete histologic analysis.

ACUTE EPIPLOIC APPENDAGITIS

Epiploic appendages are visceral peritoneal outpouchings that arise from the serosal surface of the colon, containing fat and blood vessels. Acute epiploic appendagitis occurs due to torsion or venous thrombosis of the vein, leading to ischemic or hemorrhagic infarction of epiploic appendages. It is seen to be associated with obesity and unaccustomed exercise.

Clinical picture: Acute epiploic appendagitis occurs in the 4th to 5th decades of life, and is more common in males than females. Patients present with abdominal pain and rebound tenderness that correlates with the site of infarcted appendage. Clinical picture mimics that of acute appendicitis or diverticulitis. However, laboratory parameters are generally normal. Epiploic appendagitis is usually self limited and resolves spontaneously.

Imaging features: On CT, the infarcted epiploic appendage is seen as a pericolic, oval to round lesion of fat attenuation with a hyperdense rim, less than 5 cm in size, surrounded by inflammatory changes. A central hyperattenuating dot or line may be seen corresponding to a thrombosed vessel **(Fig. 19)**. Mild reactive thickening of the adjacent colonic wall may be seen.[39] On ultrasound, a small, noncompressible hyperechoic mass surrounded by a hypoechoic rim, representing the inflamed visceral

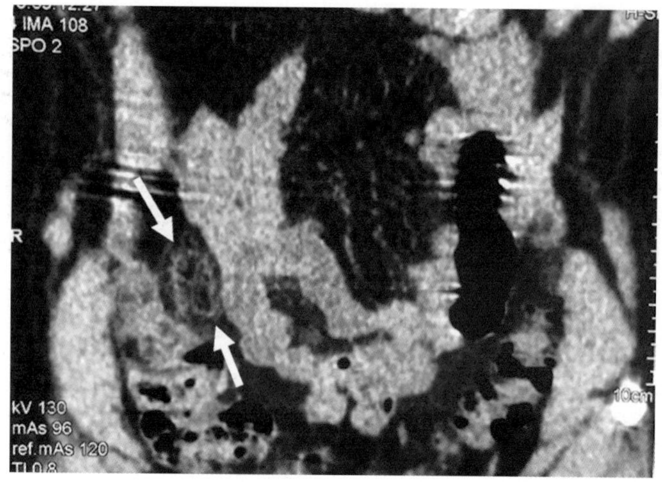

Fig. 19: Epiploic appendagitis: Coronal CECT shows a pericolic oval lesion of fat attenuation with a hyperdense rim (arrows). A central line seen within represents the thrombosed vein. There is associated inflammatory stranding seen in the adjacent fat.

peritoneum, may be seen at the site of maximum tenderness. T1- and T2-weighted MR images show a focal lesion with the signal intensity of fat. Contrast-enhanced T1-weighted MR images show an enhancing rim around the oval fatty lesion.

The differential diagnosis of acute epiploic appendagitis presenting as an inflammatory fatty lesion associated with an acute abdomen include acute omental infarct, acute diverticulitis, sclerosing mesenteritis and occasionally a primary tumor or metastases that involve the mesocolon.[40]

OMENTAL INFARCTION

Omental infarction (OI) occurs due to vascular compromise, torsion or venous thrombosis, of the greater omentum. It can be primary or secondary. Primary omental infarction is generally right-sided and is related to the tenuous blood supply to the right edge of the greater omentum. Secondary omental infarction occurs due to vascular insult after trauma, surgery or inflammation of the greater omentum and it is located near the site of the initial insult. Unaccustomed exercise, straining or coughing can precipitate this condition.[40]

Clinical findings: Primary OI is more common in children. Obesity is an important risk factor. Patients present with subacute onset of pain most often localized in the right upper or lower quadrant without any other gastrointestinal symptoms. There can be mild leucocytosis. Establishing a preoperative diagnosis of OI is difficult as it often mimics acute appendicitis or cholecystitis. The management is conservative.

Imaging features: On CT, it appears as a fatty, large (>5 cm) encapsulated mass, with soft-tissue stranding adjacent to the ascending colon. Early or mild infarction may manifest as ill-defined, mild haziness. It is classically located between the anterior abdominal wall and the ascending or transverse colon **(Fig. 20)**. Swirling of vessels may be seen in omental torsion. At US, omental infarction may appear as a focal area of echogenic, noncompressible fat that corresponds to the site of focal tenderness.[40]

MESENTERIC LYMPHADENOPATHY

The mesentery contains multiple small lymph nodes which may get enlarged in a number of disease processes notably infective, inflammatory and neoplastic **(Table 4)**. Normal mesenteric lymph nodes may now be routinely identified at the mesenteric root and throughout the mesentery on US, CT and MRI, and are generally <5 mm in short axis diameter. The size of the nodes alone does not always reflect disease, the number and distribution of lymph nodes is also important. Lymph nodes greater than 6 mm in short axis diameter or a group of 3 or more clustered together in one anatomic location are taken as abnormal.[41,42]

Tuberculous Lymphadenitis

Lymphadenopathy in abdominal tuberculosis usually occurs in mesenteric, peripancreatic, periportal, and para-aortic groups of lymph nodes. It can occur through lymphatic spread, hematogenous route or direct spread from adjacent infected organs. The nodes may vary from increased number of normal-sized nodes to massive conglomerates with matting, the latter resulting from adhesions due to periadenitis. Pathologically tuberculous infection of a lymph node follows a spectrum from early exudative to caseous to late fibro-calcification phases.

On sonography, the lymph nodes are seen either as discrete or conglomerate masses. Enlarged nodes show central hypoechoic areas with a mixed heterogeneous echotexture, in contrast to homogeneously hypoechoic nodes seen in lymphoma **(*see* Fig. 10C)**. Heterogeneity of echo pattern in nodes of a single anatomic subgroup, prior to treatment is strongly suggestive of tuberculosis, rather than lymphoma. Larger areas of caseation may coalesce with adjacent nodes, resulting in larger collections. Lymph nodes may be adherent to intra-abdominal vasculature and a fibrous reaction surrounding clusters of nodes maybe seen as increase in background echogenicity.[43,44]

On CT the multicompartmental localization of nodes with relative sparing of the retroperitoneal compartment is the most characteristic feature of tuberculosis. On unenhanced scans, the nodes may display low attenuation values < 30 HU or soft tissue attenuation values similar to muscle. Four different patterns of nodal enhancement have been described by Pombo et al.[45]

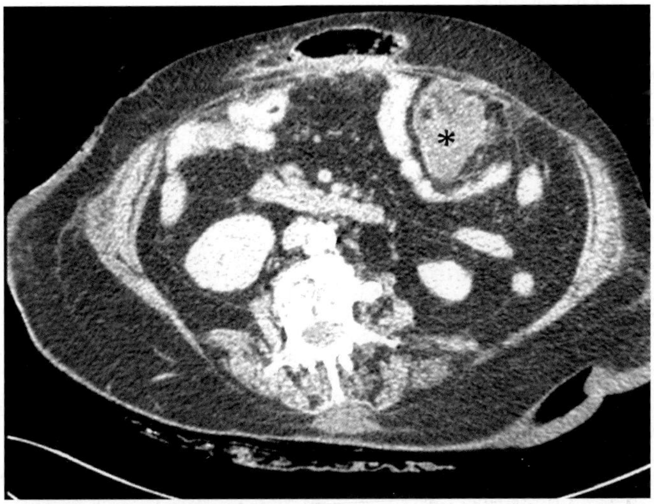

Fig. 20: Omental infarction: A 60-year-old patient with complaint of pain abdomen 6 days after undergoing abdominal surgery. CECT axial scan shows a hypodense, heterogeneous soft tissue mass with focal fatty areas within and adjacent fat stranding between the anterior abdominal wall and the transverse colon (*). A pocket of air is seen in the subcutaneous tissue due to dehiscence of the distal sutures.

Table 4: Causes of mesenteric lymphadenopathy.

Infective processes: • Tuberculosis • Mesenteric adenitis syndrome • Celiac disease • Intestinal infection—Yersinia • Mycobacterium avium-intracellulare (MAC) infection • HIV • Whipple's disease
Inflammatory lesions: • Local inflammatory processes such as acute appendicitis, diverticulitis, pancreatitis, etc. • Crohn's disease • Mesenteric panniculitis • Connective tissue disorders—rheumatoid arthritis, scleroderma, SLE, etc. • Others
Neoplastic processes: • Lymphoma • Metastatic disease • Kaposi's sarcoma
Miscellaneous: • Castleman's disease • Sarcoidosis • Amyloidosis, etc.

- Peripheral enhancement, the most frequent pattern, is characterized by peripheral rim enhancement, with or without low attenuation center. This pattern is seen in younger patients and reflects significant central liquefactive or caseous necrosis and a highly vascular perinodal inflammatory reaction which is relatively diagnostic for tuberculosis, although not pathognomic **(*see* Figs. 11A to C)**.
- Inhomogeneous enhancement is also a frequent manifestation of tubercular adenitis, due to intranodal granulomas and relatively less necrosis than in nodes that show peripheral enhancement **(*see* Figs. 12A and B)**.
- Homogeneous contrast enhancement represent a less frequent manifestation. These are indistinguishable from untreated lymphomatous nodes and are seen in patients with infection with mycobacterium avium intracellulare and AIDS.
- Nonenhancing nodes.

Magnetic resonance imaging shows majority of nodes to be hypointense on T1 and hyperintense on T2-weighted images when compared to abdominal muscle, with a few demonstrating a rim which is hypo- on T1W and hyperintense on T2W images. Minority of nodes are hypo- to isointense on both T1 and T2 weighted images. The varying signal intensity on T2W images is explained on the stage of evolution of the disease—the central T2 hyperintensity reflects caseous necrosis while central T2 hypointensity denotes presence of paramagnetic free radicles secreted from phagocytic cells. On contrast-enhanced images, different enhancement patterns, including peripheral, heterogeneous and less frequently homogeneous enhancement may be seen, similar to CT.[46,47]

With the institution of appropriate treatment, nodal masses tend to show a transient increase in size for 3–4 weeks followed by a gradual reduction in overall dimensions. Focal calcification may occur in nodal and omental masses and collections, which may be clustered along the periphery or may be central in location.

Tubercular adenitis may be confused with nodes of lymphoma and metastatic disease, and clinical and radiological differentiation may be difficult. Lymphoma nodes have a different anatomical distribution and near homogenous enhancement pattern prior to treatment. Caseation and calcification are highly suggestive of tubercular etiology.[48]

Lymph nodes with hypodense centers are also seen in metastatic malignancy, lymphoma after treatment, inflammatory conditions (such as Crohn's disease), pyogenic infection and Whipple's disease, however, other imaging findings and clinical features are helpful in diagnosis Lymphatic involvement is also a common feature in patients with AIDS. The nodes in these are usually located in mesenteric and retroperitoneal region. Nonenhanced low attenuation nodes may be seen in AIDS.

Primary Mesenteric Adenitis

Primary mesenteric adenitis consists of right-sided mesenteric adenopathy without any associated identifiable inflammatory process. Although it has been termed as primary, it is thought that the enlarged nodes arise from an infective process (e.g. *Yersinia sp*) causing a terminal ileitis that may or may not be seen on imaging.

Clinically patients present with nonspecific abdominal pain which maybe acute or chronic, often mimicking appendicitis. US and CT will show clustered, discrete, moderately enlarged nodes in the right lower quadrant with a short axis diameter of generally <10 mm. Occasionally, thickening of the terminal ileum may also be seen **(Figs. 21A and B)**.[49]

This is a self limiting condition, which resolves on conservative treatment. The most important differential diagnosis is acute appendicitis, as enlarged reactive nodes may often be seen in the right lower quadrant in appendicitis. The identification of a normal appendix on imaging favors primary mesenteric adenitis.[50]

Neoplastic Lymphadenopathy

Lymphoma is the most common cause of neoplastic mesenteric lymph node enlargement. Non-Hodgkin's lymphoma involves the mesenteric nodes along with the retroperitoneal para-aortic nodes. Approximately 30–50% cases of NHL spread to the mesenteric nodes, commonly from the retroperitoneal nodes.[51] The enlarged nodes can show three patterns of involvement—in the mesenteric root, scattered throughout the peripheral mesentery or a mixed root-peripheral pattern **(Figs. 22A and B)**. In early cases, the lymph nodes may be small and discrete, but they progressively increase in size to form coalescent conglomerate masses. As they are soft tumors, they tend to grow around the vessels and the bowel without causing pressure effect. On CT images, lymphomatous nodes are seen as multiple round, mildly enhancing, homogeneous masses that often surround mesenteric arteries and veins. Pretreatment calcification is rare. Associated peritoneal and mesenteric involvement can be seen.[35]

Metastatic involvement of mesenteric nodes can occur from GI malignancies, however is rare from tumors of genitourinary or extrabdominal malignancies.

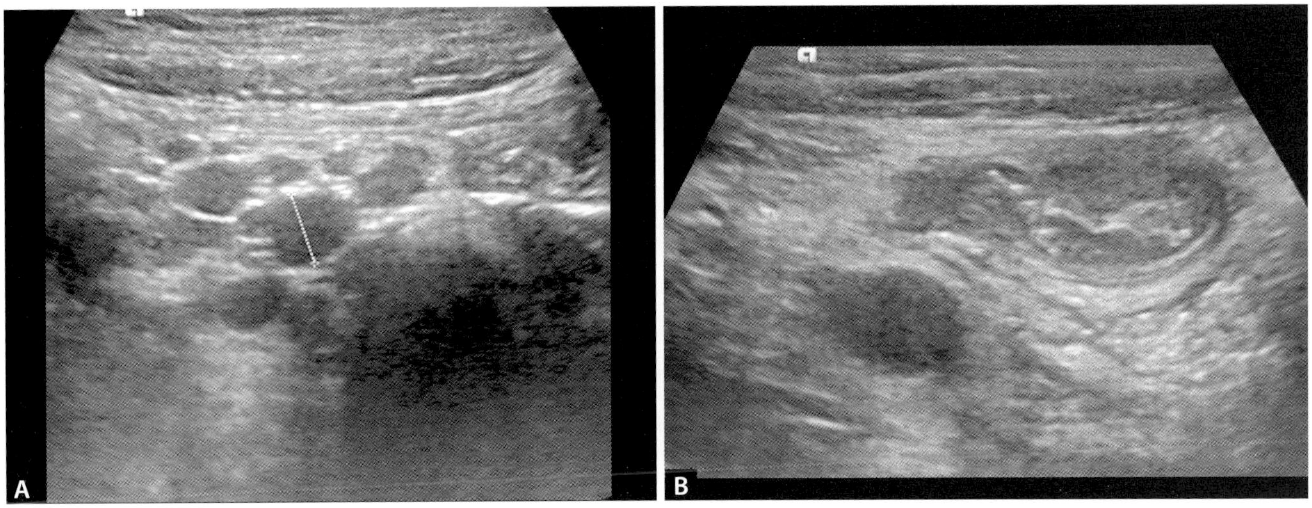

Figs. 21A and B: Mesenteric adenitis in a 10-year-old boy presenting with pain in right iliac fossa: (A) US shows multiple small nodes in the right iliac fossa; (B) A more caudal scan shows a thickened distal ileal loop.

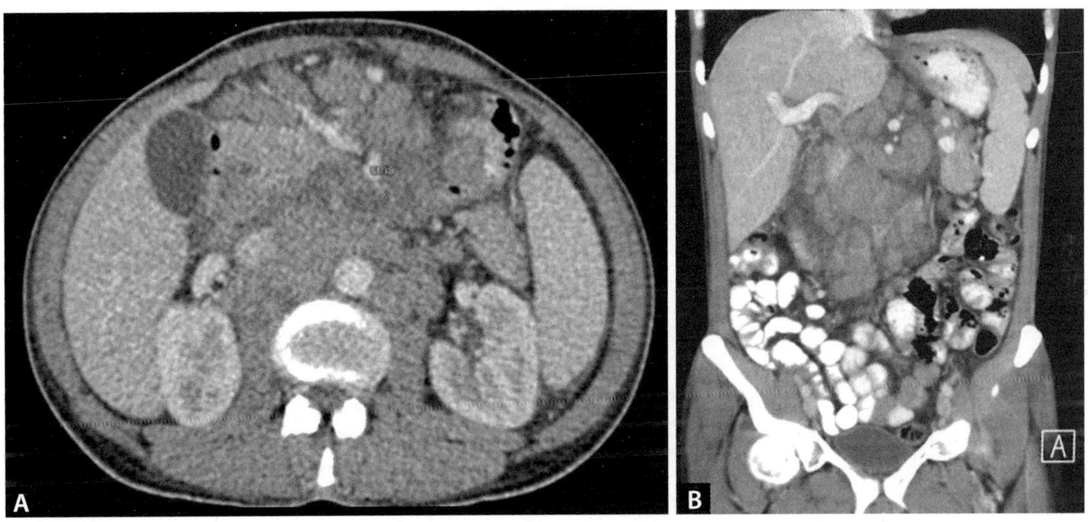

Figs. 22A and B: Lymphoma: CECT axial (A) and coronal (B) scans show multiple homogeneously enhancing mesenteric and retroperitoneal lymph nodes in a 45-year-old man with non-Hodgkin's lymphoma.

Kaposi's sarcoma is a low grade mesenchymal tumor seen in patients of AIDS involving the blood and lymphatic vessels. Mesenteric lymphadenopathy is seen as homogenously enhancing, large nodes, measuring 3–5 cm in short axis diameter. They may coalesce to form large masses. Associated lymphadenopathy may be seen in the porta hepatis, retroperitoneum and pelvis. Bowel, spleen and liver involvement may occur.[35]

PRIMARY PERITONEAL NEOPLASMS

The peritoneum can be involved by both, primary and secondary neoplastic disease, with metastatic involvement being much more common than primary tumors. Primary peritoneal tumors are defined as tumors with primary manifestation in the peritoneum in the absence of a visceral site of origin.[52]

They are uncommon lesions which arise from the mesothelial cells, submesothelial mesenchymal cells and uncommitted stem cells. As they share a common anatomic site of origin, they have similar clinical manifestations. Patients frequently present with abdominal discomfort and distention, gastrointestinal complaints, and, less commonly, pelvic pain or a palpable mass. **Table 5** lists the primary tumors that can involve the peritoneum.

Table 5: List of primary tumors of peritoneum.

• Primary malignant mesothelioma
• Cystic mesothelioma
• Primary peritoneal serous carcinoma
• Desmoplastic small round cell tumor
• Desmoid tumor/Mesenteric fibromatosis
• Inflammatory myofibroblastic pseudotumor
• Primary peritoneal lymphoma
• *Benign mesenchymal tumors*: – Hemangioma – Lymphangioma – Lipoma – Leiomyoma – Nerve sheath tumor – Gastrointestinal stromal tumors (GIST) – Leiomyomatous pertonealis disseminata
• *Malignant mesenchymal tumors*: – Liposarcoma – Leiomyosarcoma – Fibrosarcoma – Angiosarcoma – Malignant fibrous histiocytoma – Synovial sarcoma – GIST – Nerve sheath tumors
• Others

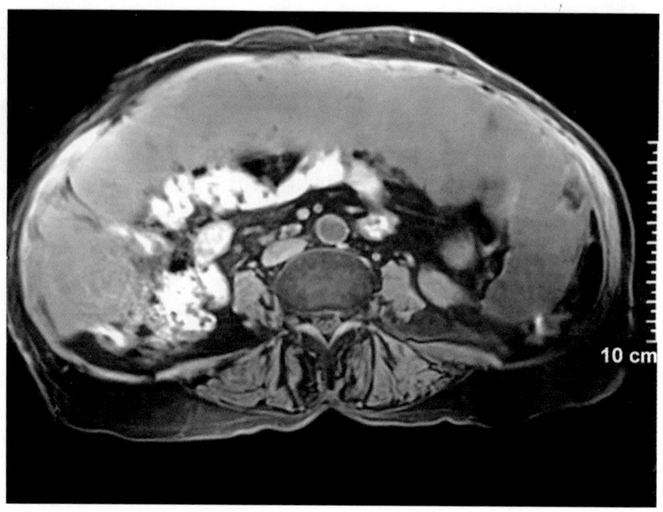

Fig. 23: Peritoneal mesothelioma: 57-year-old woman presenting with abdominal discomfort and distension. T2W MR image shows a thick characteristic 'omental cake' appearance.

PERITONEAL MALIGNANT MESOTHELIOMA

Malignant mesothelioma is an aggressive tumor arising from serous membranes of pleura, peritoneum, pericardium and tunica vaginalis. Peritoneal mesotheliomas account for 10–15% of all mesotheliomas.[53] They can be classified into two subtypes—the diffuse form which is highly aggressive and the localized or focal form which is amenable to surgery and has a good prognosis.

Clinical picture: Similar to pleural mesotheliomas, peritoneal malignant mesotheliomas are also associated with asbestos exposure, and usually develop in individuals exposed to higher levels of asbestos, as compared to pleural mesotheliomas. The majority of malignant mesotheliomas occur in men, with a median age at presentation of 60 years, whereas in women, the mean age is 50 years.[54] Patients present with abdominal pain, abdominal distention, nausea, anorexia, and weight loss. Intestinal obstruction may occur with advanced disease.

Imaging features: In the *diffuse* form of the disease, there is sheet-like thickening of the peritoneum, leading to an irregular and nodular thickening of the peritoneum. There is associated moderate amount of ascites and omental caking **(Fig. 23)**. In the *localized* form there are heterogeneous, solid intraperitoneal masses. The margins are often irregular. The ascites is small in amount and may be loculated. Local invasion can be seen into the abdominal wall, mesentery, liver, and other organs in both forms. Rarely calcification may occur. Mesenteric involvement can be seen as "pleated" or "stellate" appearance and sheet-like thickening can be seen to encase the small bowel loops in some cases. Generally, lymph node enlargement does not occur which is differentiating point from lymphomatosis and tubercular peritoneal involvement. Calcified pleural plaques and other asbestos-related changes such as pleural thickening and masses may be present within the chest.[55] CT radiographic findings of large tumor burden with significant bowel distortion or the presence of a small bowel obstruction is predictive of incomplete resectability. MRI imaging may quantify the extent of disease more accurately.

The role of positron emission tomography (PET) scan is not well-defined and may have some limited use in the detection of recurrent disease.[56] Biopsy is required to establish a diagnosis and can be performed under imaging guidance or surgically. Ascitic fluid cytology has a variable sensitivity of 32–76% with the major limitation being difficulty in distinguishing benign from malignant lesions.[57] Cytoreductive surgery (CRS) with hyperthermic intraperitoneal chemotherapy (HIPEC) have become the more widely adopted methods of treatment for peritoneal mesothelioma, however are associated with significant morbidity. Studies using novel molecular targets such as sphingosine kinase are under process to develop targeted therapies.[58]

Differential diagnosis: The presence of peritoneal masses with or without ascites in the abdominal cavity is most suggestive of peritoneal carcinomatosis in the majority of patients. However, when a sheet like thickening is seen, the diagnosis of a primary mesothelioma must be kept in mind. Other differentials to be considered are tuberculous peritonitis—shows a smooth peritoneum with mild thickening and marked enhancement; lymphomatous peritonitis—which shows marked mesenteric and retroperitoneal lymphadenopathy; and sarcomatous peritonitis—which is characterized by heterogeneous, bulky, hypervascular masses with a variable amount of ascites.[7]

MULTICYSTIC MESOTHELIOMA/ PERITONEAL INCLUSION CYST/ MULTILOCULAR INCLUSION CYST

Multicystic mesothelioma is a benign, multilocular cystic tumor that most commonly arises from the pelvic surface of the peritoneum. There is an ongoing debate regarding the origin of this entity. It is considered by some authors to be a mesothelial neoplasm as it can recur locally and may rarely show malignant transformation, while others consider it to be non-neoplastic, reactive mesothelial proliferation.[59]

Clinical features: It is most commonly seen in premenopausal women. It occurs much less commonly in men with an older age of presentation. Clinically, it can present with chronic or intermittent lower abdominal or pelvic pain, abdominal distension, tenderness, mass, and pressure symptoms like dyspareunia, urinary hesitancy, or constipation. It is very commonly associated with a history of prior abdominal surgery, endometriosis or PID which supports the reactive, non-neoplastic origin.

Imaging features: Ultrasound is often the first modality in detection of these lesions. They are seen as large, multi-septated, cystic structures which are in close contact with the ovaries and uterus. They are frequently anechoic, but sometimes may show internal echoes due to debris or hemorrhage. The ovary may sometimes be completely surrounded by the cystic mesothelioma. Septations may be complete, incomplete, of varying thickness, and maybe nodular or polypoid **(Figs. 24A to C)**. Unilocular and multifocal cysts may also be seen. In men, multicystic mesothelioma typically arises from the peritoneal surface along the superior margin of the bladder or in the retrovesical space.[55]

CT and MRI are useful in defining the exact extent of the lesion and for identifying presence of multiple cysts. Large mutiseptated cyst with fluid attenuation can be seen on CT, while MR shows homogeneous fluid signal intensity that is hypointense on T1 and hyperintense on T2W images. The septations enhance with contrast administration.

Differential diagnosis: Pseudomyxoma peritonei in the early stages, lymphangioma, complex loculated ascites, and cystic ovarian neoplasms can all be considered in the differential diagnosis of multicystic mesothelioma.

PRIMARY PERITONEAL SEROUS CARCINOMA

Primary peritoneal serous carcinoma is an epithelial tumor of the peritoneum, arising from the extraovarian mesothelium and is histologically similar to its ovarian counterpart. This tumor occurs in postmenopausal women and an association with BRCA1 gene has been demonstrated.[60]

Imaging features: Ascites, peritoneal nodules and thickening, and omental nodules and masses are the most common cross-sectional imaging features of primary peritoneal serous carcinoma. A minority of patients have either no ascites or only a small amount at initial presentation. Calcifications within peritoneal and omental nodules representing psammoma bodies maybe seen in 30% cases **(Fig. 25)**.[55] The criteria for diagnosing primary peritoneal serous carcinoma are that:

- Both ovaries should be normal
- Involvement of extraovarian sites should be greater than involvement of ovarian surface
- Ovarian involvement should only be limited to surface epithelium.

However, histological confirmation is required to differentiate from metastatic ovarian disease and make a correct diagnosis.

DESMOPLASTIC SMALL ROUND CELL TUMOR

Desmoplastic small round cell tumor (DSRCT) is a rare aggressive malignancy occurring in adolescents and young adults. Histologically it is composed of small, round, blue cells, a group that includes Wilms tumor, neuroblastoma, Ewing sarcoma, primitive neuroectodermal tumor, and rhabdomyosarcoma. DSRCT most often develops as a primary tumor of the peritoneal cavity but can also arise in other sites including pleura, bone, testes, or salivary glands.[61]

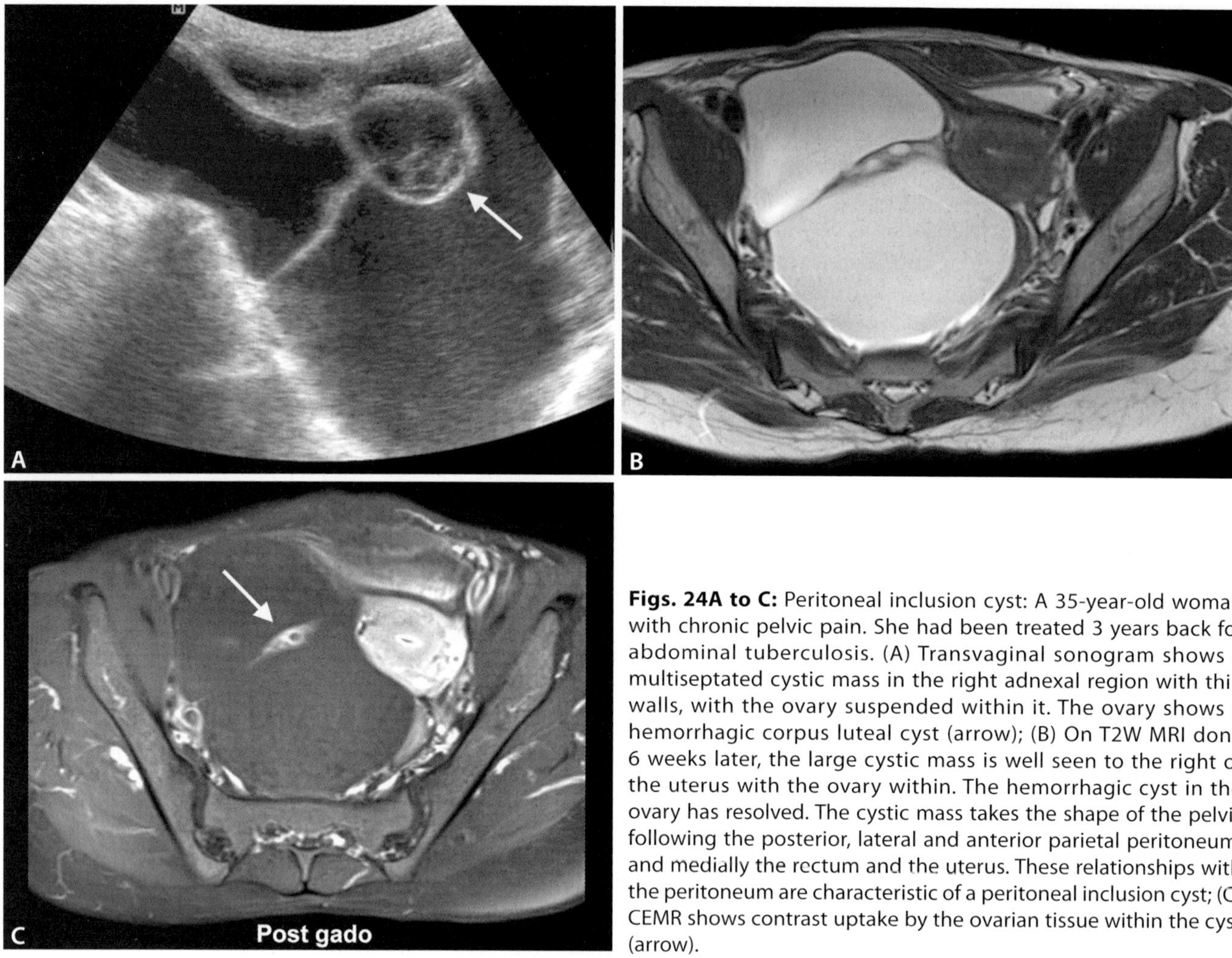

Figs. 24A to C: Peritoneal inclusion cyst: A 35-year-old woman with chronic pelvic pain. She had been treated 3 years back for abdominal tuberculosis. (A) Transvaginal sonogram shows a multiseptated cystic mass in the right adnexal region with thin walls, with the ovary suspended within it. The ovary shows a hemorrhagic corpus luteal cyst (arrow); (B) On T2W MRI done 6 weeks later, the large cystic mass is well seen to the right of the uterus with the ovary within. The hemorrhagic cyst in the ovary has resolved. The cystic mass takes the shape of the pelvis following the posterior, lateral and anterior parietal peritoneum, and medially the rectum and the uterus. These relationships with the peritoneum are characteristic of a peritoneal inclusion cyst; (C) CEMR shows contrast uptake by the ovarian tissue within the cyst (arrow).

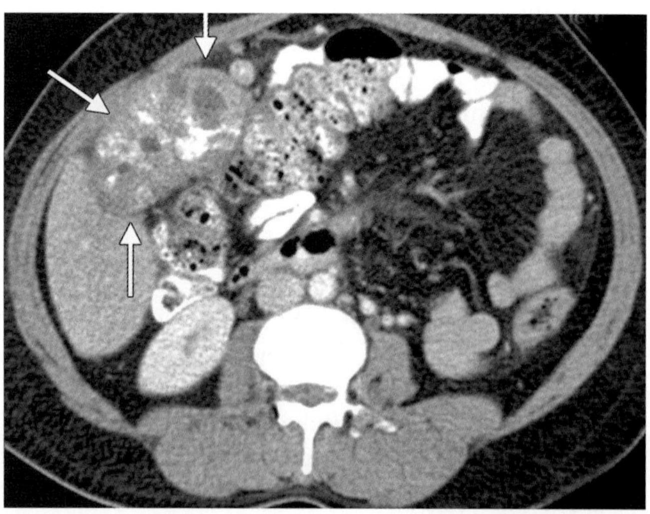

Fig. 25: Papillary serous carcinoma: A large well defined, enhancing, peritoneal mass is seen in the subhepatic region (arrows) with psammomatous calcification and few nonenhancing necrotic areas.

Clinical features: The mean age of presentation of DSRCT is of 22 years (range, 5–30 years) with a marked male preponderance. The most common signs at presentation are an intra-abdominal mass, abdominal pain and increased abdominal girth.[61]

Imaging features: It is characterized by bulky, peritoneal masses in the omentum or paravesical region, which are heterogeneous, or have central low-attenuation areas on CT, suggestive of intratumoral necrosis or hemorrhage. The masses vary in size from 3 cm to 22 cm **(Fig. 26)**. When multiple masses are present, nearly all patients have a single dominant mass (>10 cm), usually in the retrovesical or retrouterine space. They may also show small, punctate calcifications. Ascites is frequently present. At MR imaging, the tumors are typically heterogeneous in signal intensity but predominantly hypointense on T1-weighted sequences and hyperintense on T2-weighted sequences.

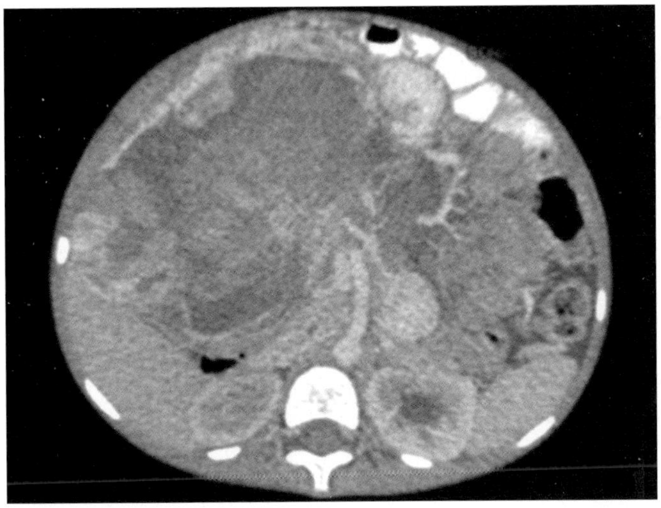

Fig. 26: Desmoplastic round cell tumor in a 15-year-old boy. CECT axial scan shows a large necrotic mass in the mesentery.

Imaging after intravenous administration of gadolinium shows heterogeneous enhancement. Lymph nodal metastases and hematogenous metastasis to the liver, lung, and bone may occur.[62]

DSRCT is FDG-avid with a mean standardized uptake value of 11.1 (range, 3.7–15.0) and FDG PET/CT has been shown to enable accurate detection of lesions with a sensitivity of 96.1% and specificity of 98.6%, but its role in assessment of treatment response and follow-up of DSRCT has not yet been defined.[63]

Well-differentiated papillary mesothelioma, adenomatoid tumor, primary peritoneal serous borderline tumor and solitary fibrous tumor are uncommon tumors of the peritoneum.

DESMOID TUMOR/MESENTERIC FIBROMATOSIS

Desmoids are locally aggressive fibrous tumors with a tendency to recur. Desmoids can be intra-abdominal, in the abdominal wall, or extra-abdominal. The mesentery is the most common site of involvement. Most cases are sporadic but approximately 10–15% occur in patients with familial adenomatous polyposis (FAP), particularly those with Gardener's syndrome. More than 80% of patients with FAP have a history of previous abdominal surgery, whereas only 10% of sporadic mesenteric fibromatosis have had abdominal surgery.[35]

Clinical features: Desmoids may occur at any age but have a peak incidence in the third decade with a predilection for the female sex. Clinically, they may be asymptomatic or may present with abdominal pain or intestinal obstruction due to mass effect on the small or large bowel.[64]

Imaging features: Focal masses with well-defined or infiltrative margins can be seen within the mesentery **(Figs. 27A to C)**. The internal features depend on the relative content of collagen and myxoid stroma within the tumor mass. On US, these tumors have variable echogenicity, appearing as masses of low, medium, or high echogenicity with smooth, defined margins. On CT, they can be seen as well-circumscribed homogeneous masses that may be isodense or hyperdense relative to muscle. Some cases show heterogeneous masses with infiltrative outer margins. Masses with high myxoid content may appear hypodense. On MRI, low to intermediate SI is seen on T1W images and intermediate SI on T2W images. Contrast enhancement is also variable as the myxoid component does not enhance. Some lesions that do not enhance on CT may show enhancement on MRI.[65]

Due to the close association with vital structures, resection of the tumor may not be possible, in which cases systemic therapy with or without surgical excision should be considered. FAP—associated mesenteric desmoids, are more likely to be unresectable or lead to significant morbidity, including perioperative hemorrhage, short-bowel syndrome, intestinal ischemia, obstruction, or fistula formation. Also, desmoid tumors have a tendency to recur, even after complete surgical resection. Therefore, conservative management has been recommended whenever possible, using analgesia and minimally invasive therapy as needed and recently, radiotherapy and chemotherapy have been used in the management of desmoid tumors.[66]

Differential diagnosis: On the basis of imaging findings, desmoid tumors are difficult to differentiate from gastrointestinal stromal tumor and other malignant neoplasms of the mesentery, such as lymphoma, metastatic disease, and soft-tissue sarcoma. They may closely resemble lymphoma whenever the lesions manifest with well-defined margins, homogeneous attenuation, and involvement of adjacent small bowel segments. GISTs more commonly have areas of hemorrhage and necrosis, which are seen as focal areas of hypoattenuation.

INFLAMMATORY MYOFIBROBLASTIC PSEUDOTUMOR

Inflammatory myofibroblastic pseudotumor (IMP) is a rare solid tumor of mesenchymal origin, which may originate

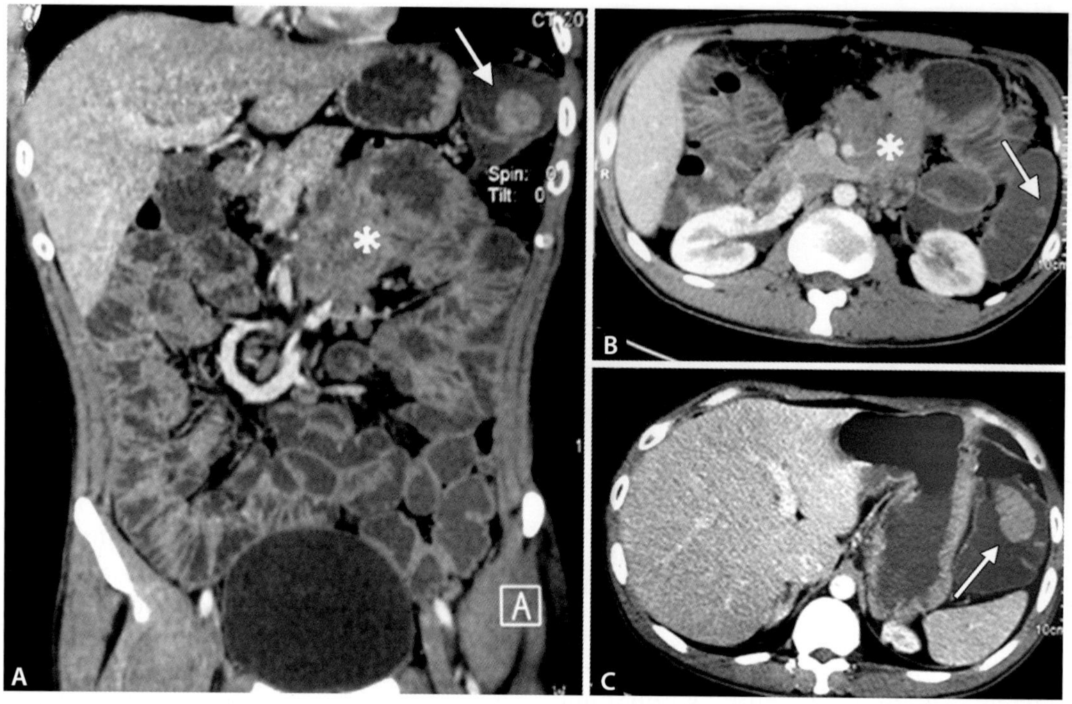

Figs. 27A to C: Desmoid tumor in a 31-year-old man with familial adenomatous polyposis: CECT coronal (A) and axial (B and C) scans show an irregular, heterogeneous mass with infiltrative margins in the mesentery (*). Multiple polypoid lesions can be seen in the large bowel (arrows).

in virtually any anatomic site but is most often found in the lung, mesentery, and omentum. It was originally thought to be inflammatory or reactive in origin, but on the basis of more recent cytogenetic studies, it is now considered a neoplasm of intermediate biologic behavior.[67]

Clinical features: This tumor is most commonly seen to affect children and young adults, with a slight tendency to occur more frequently in girls. The clinical symptoms are nonspecific and depend on the site of origin. The most common presenting symptom is abdominal pain due to mass effect. A minority of patients present with systemic signs and symptoms suggestive of infection.[68] Most inflammatory myofibroblastic tumors demonstrate benign behavior and are cured with resection. Yet, a propensity for local recurrence and even multifocal regional recurrence has also been shown, particularly in the omentum and mesentery.

Imaging features: At CT, inflammatory myofibroblastic pseudotumor typically manifests as a bulky, well-demarcated, homogeneous or heterogeneous, spherical or multilobulated mass **(Figs. 28A and B)**. A few cases may show central calcifications. Contrast enhancement is variable and includes early peripheral enhancement due to vascular tissue and delayed central enhancement of fibrotic components. Large tumors may demonstrate hypoattenuating, nonenhancing areas that represent central necrosis. These tumors rarely show aggressive growth patterns such as circumferential growth around vessels and extension into the bowel with mural infiltration and ulceration.[68,69]

At MR imaging, IMP is hypointense on T1-weighted images and hyperintense on T2-weighted images, although tumors with a great deal of fibrotic stroma may be dark on both T1- and T2-weighted images. On postcontrast scans, there is heterogeneous enhancement of the tumor mass. Delayed contrast enhancement of fibrotic components may be seen.[70] FDG-PET shows nonspecific increased uptake of radiotracer by inflammatory myofibroblastic tumor, similar to other malignancies.[71]

LEIOMYOMATOSIS PERTONEALIS DISSEMINATA/DIFFUSE PERITONEAL LEIOMYOMATOSIS

Leiomyomatosis peritonealis disseminata is a rare, benign disorder characterized by innumerable smooth muscle nodules throughout the peritoneal cavity. These nodules are derived from metaplasia of the submesothelial cells.

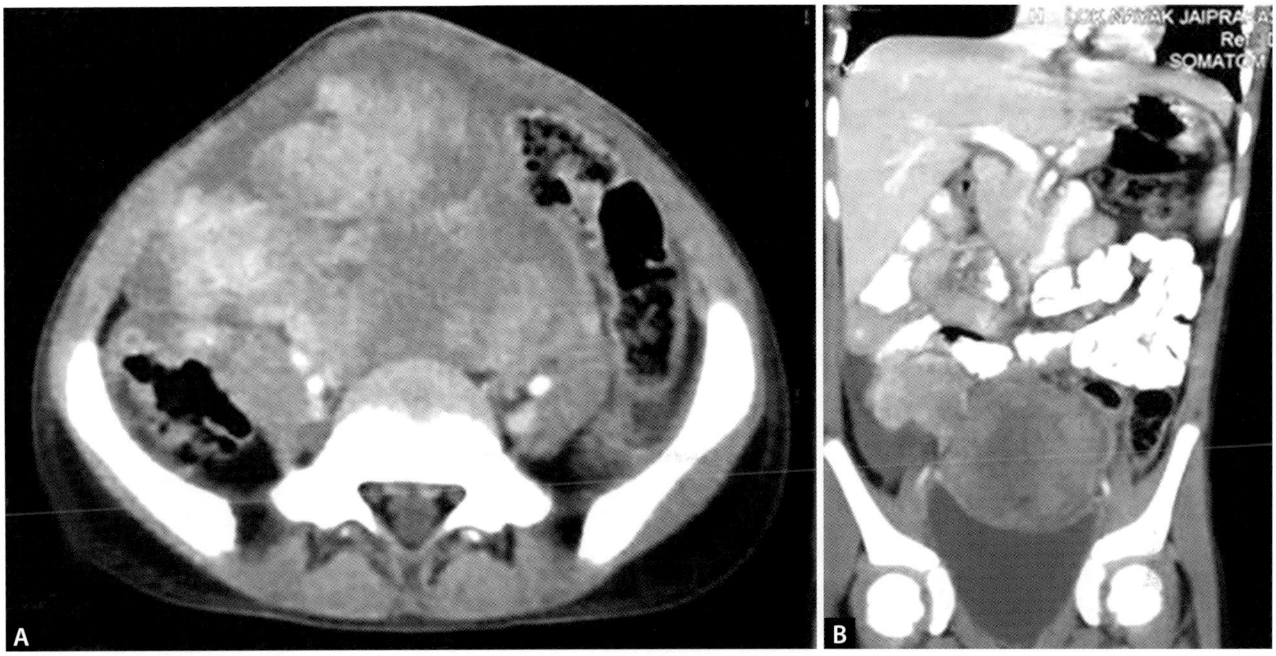

Figs. 28A and B: Inflammatory myofibroblastic tumor in a 7-year-old girl: CECT axial (A) and coronal (B) images show a large well circumscribed, multiloculated, heterogeneously enhancing mass in the lower abdomen displacing the bowel loops superiorly and laterally. Associated ascites is present.

Clinical features: Leiomyomatosis peritonealis disseminata is almost always seen in women. It may be associated with high estrogen states, caused by pregnancy and oral contraceptive use, but rarely may occur in postmenopausal women, and even in men.[72] It is often discovered incidentally during surgery or imaging examinations of women who have uterine leiomyomas. The clinical course is often benign, with spontaneous regression of the leiomyomas or regression can occur after withdrawal of hormonal stimulus. In rare cases, sarcomatous degeneration of the tumor nodules, may occur.[73]

Imaging features: CT and MRI show numerous well-circumscribed, variable-sized solid masses in the peritoneal cavity. Heterogeneous attenuation is seen on CT. The masses enhance similarly to uterine leiomyomas. On MR imaging, the masses are isointense relative to muscle on T1-weighted sequences and low signal intensity on T2-weighted sequences with heterogeneous enhancement, similar to uterine leiomyomas, as seen on CT.[55]

MISCELLANEOUS MESENCHYMAL TUMORS

Mesenchymal tumors include benign entities such as leiomyoma, lipoma, neurofibroma and malignant tumors such as leiomyosarcoma, liposarcoma, fibrosarcoma, mesothelioma, and hemangiopericytoma. Imaging findings are nonspecific. Benign tumors are usually well ciurcumscribed and localized whereas malignant tumors have indistinct or infiltrative margins with invasion into surrounding structures. Lipomas and liposarcomas are more distinctive due to their characteristic features of fat containing masses.

LYMPHATIC MALFORMATION/ LYMPHANGIOMA

Lymphatic malformations (LMs) are rare nonmalignant masses consisting of fluid-filled channels or spaces thought to be caused by the abnormal development of the lymphatic system. Abdominal LMs occur most commonly in the mesentery, followed by the omentum, mesocolon, retroperitoneum and abdominal viscera.[74,75]

Clinical features: Although LMs can occur at any age, they are seen more commonly in infants and young children.[75] Abdominal pain and distension are the common presenting features. Rarely, patients may present with acute abdominal pain due to complications like torsion, infarction or intestinal obstruction.

Imaging features: LMs are thin-walled unilocular or multilocular cystic masses containing serous or chylous fluid. On US, these lymphatic malformations are seen as cystic, unilocular or multilocular masses with echogenecity varying from anechoic to hypoechoic depending on the internal content **(Figs. 29 and 30)**. CT shows enhancing cyst wall and internal septae with homogenous, low attenuation fluid content. The attenuation of the fluid may have negative values in the presence of chyle. MRI also shows similar findings with low signal intensity on T1W and high on T2W images. The presence of hemorrhage or infection in the cysts may change the CT attenuation or MR signal pattern. Calcification is uncommon.[74]

Differential diagnosis: Large mesenteric lymphangiomas need to be differentiated from ascites. The presence of septa, compression of the adjacent intestinal loops and lack of fluid in the dependant peritoneal recesses helps to establish a diagnosis of lymphangioma. Other differentials to be considered are benign ovarian neoplasms and peritoneal inclusion cysts. Duplication cyst or mesothelial cyst are uncommon.

SECONDARY PERITONEAL NEOPLASMS

Secondary neoplasms are the most common malignancies involving the peritoneum. The dissemination of tumor

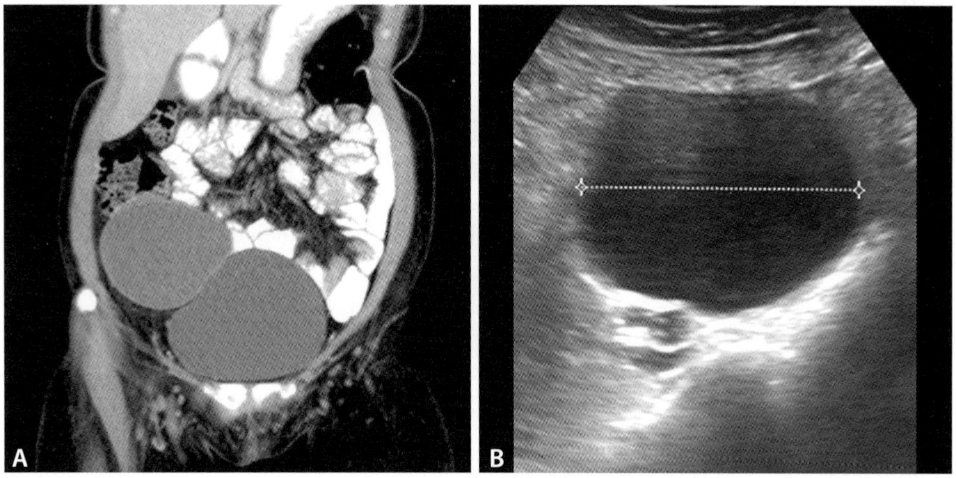

Figs. 29A and B: Mesenteric cyst in a 34-year-old woman with chronic pain in right iliac fossa. Coronal CT image (A) and US scan (B) show an anechoic, unilocular thin-walled cyst in the peritoneal fat.

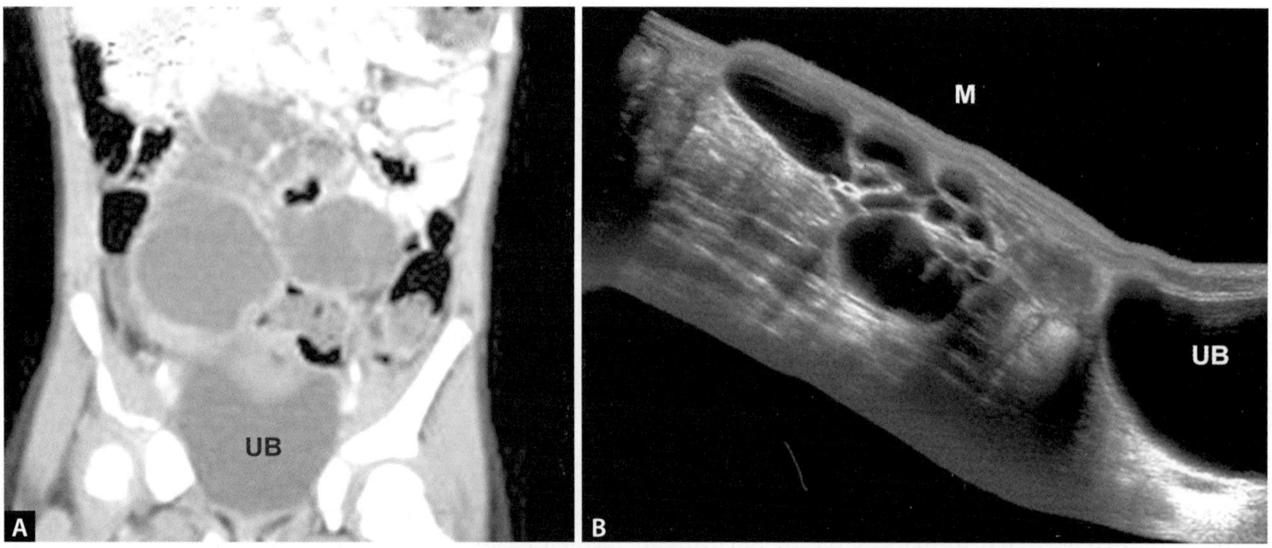

Figs. 30A and B: Mesenteric lymphangioma: (A) CECT coronal image shows a multiloculated cystic mass in the mesentery with enhancing septae; (B) Longitudinal section US, panoramic image, shows the whole extent of the mesenteric lymphangioma as a multiloculated cystic mass (M) with varying sized cysts.
Abbreviation: UB: Urinary bladder.

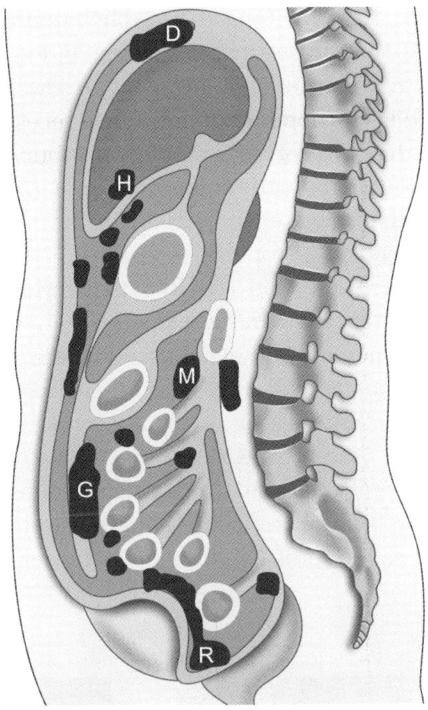

Fig. 31: Sagittal schematic illustration of the abdomen and pelvis showing common locations of peritoneal deposits. Commonly involved sites include greater omentum (G), rectouterine pouch (R), subdiaphragmatic region (D), subhepatic region (H) and small bowel mesentery (M).

cells within the peritoneal cavity can occur by several mechanisms: (a) intraperitoneal seeding, (b) direct invasion, (c) embolic hematogenous dissemination, and (d) lymphatic permeation.

Intraperitoneal seeding occurs most commonly from gastrointestinal and ovarian tumors due to intramural tumor growth and invasion through bowel wall or extension through the peritoneal lining of organs like ovary, pancreas or liver. Seeding can also occur due to iatrogenic spillage of tumor cells into the peritoneal cavity during biopsy or surgery. These tumor cells are carried by the peritoneal fluid and disseminated throughout the peritoneal cavity. They get preferentially deposited in the areas of fluid stasis, i.e. pouch of Douglas in women, rectovesical space in men, distal small bowel mesentery near the ileocecal junction, the sigmoid mesocolon, the right paracolic gutter, Morrison's pouch and the right subdiaphragmatic space **(Fig. 31)**[76] and these areas should be carefully examined in all cases when evaluating for metastic disease. Two unusual sites of peritoneal carcinomatosis are the umbilicus and the ovaries; such metastases are respectively called Sister Mary Joseph's nodule and Krukenberg tumors. Ovarian carcinoma is the most common tumor to spread by this mechanism. Gastric, pancreatic, colonic, biliary and endometrial tumors also spread through intraperitoneal seeding.

Direct invasion: Intra-abdominal primary malignancies can directly invade into the leaves of mesentery along the mesenteric vessels or through ligamentous attachments to involve adjacent organs. Pancreatic, gastric, biliary, colonic, hepatic, splenic and ovarian tumors may spread in this way. Small bowel carcinoid tumor commonly invades the mesentery. Lymphoma and tumors arising from retroperitoneal structures may spread directly to the root of the small bowel mesentery along its retroperitoneal attachment.

Hematogenous spread: Tumor emboli from malignant melanoma, lung or breast carcinoma and sarcomas may spread to the mesentery by hematogenous spread. These tumors usually involve the antimesenteric margins of the small bowel producing soft issue nodules that may cause bowel obstruction and/or intussusception.

Lymphatic extension: Lymphatic dissemination plays a minor role in spread of gastrointestinal malignancies to the peritoneum, but it is the main pathway for spread of lymphomas to mesenteric lymph nodes. Chronic lymphocytic leukemia may also spread through the lymphatics and produce large mesenteric nodal masses which encase the branches of abdominal aorta-celiac trunk, superior and inferior mesenteric arteries without causing vascular compression.

PERITONEAL CARCINOMATOSIS

Peritoneal carcinomatosis is the malignant tumor seeding of the peritoneum with the most common primaries being the ovarian, gastric and colorectal malignancies. Other less common primary sites include pancreas, uterus, kidney, bladder and melanoma.

Patients with peritoneal carcinomatosis may be asymptomatic at the onset, but may progress to abdominal distension from ascites, or nausea, vomiting and abdominal pain from bowel obstruction.

Imaging features: The classic feature of peritoneal carcinomatosis is *tumor nodules* studding the peritoneal surfaces. A fibrotic response can occur as the tumor grows along the peritoneal surface or invades into the subperitoneal tissues, replacing the omental fat with tumor and fibrosis which produces the gross appearance of *omental caking* **(Fig. 32)**. Peritoneal carcinomatosis can also exhibit a *sheet-like growth* pattern encircling and encasing intraperitoneal viscera producing an appearance similar

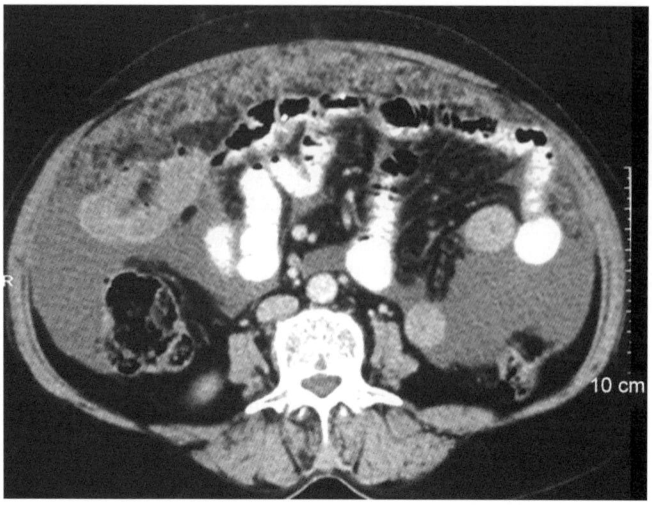

Fig. 32: Peritoneal carcinomatosis in a 65-year-old woman with ovarian malignancy. Enhanced axial CT scan shows thickening and nodular infiltration of the omentum with ascites.

to malignant mesothelioma. A variable amount of ascites may accompany the peritoneal seeding, but is not always present. Calcification can be seen in the peritoneal deposits from serous papillary ovarian carcinoma **(Figs. 33A to C)**, rarely gastric carcinomas, or in metastases after chemotherapy. Adenocarcinoma with abundant mucin and signet ring cell morphology is the most frequent tumor type seen on histopathology.

On US, the ascitic fluid seen in patients with peritoneal carcinomatosis may be anechoic or may contain echogenic particulate matter, which reflects proteinaceous exudate. Tumor nodules on peritoneal surfaces appear as hypoechoic nodules or sheet like masses **(Figs. 34A and B)**.[77] The omentum with tumor infiltration appears as an echogenic, plaque like structure either floating in the ascitic fluid or it may be adherent to the anterior abdominal wall or serosal surface of the bowel.

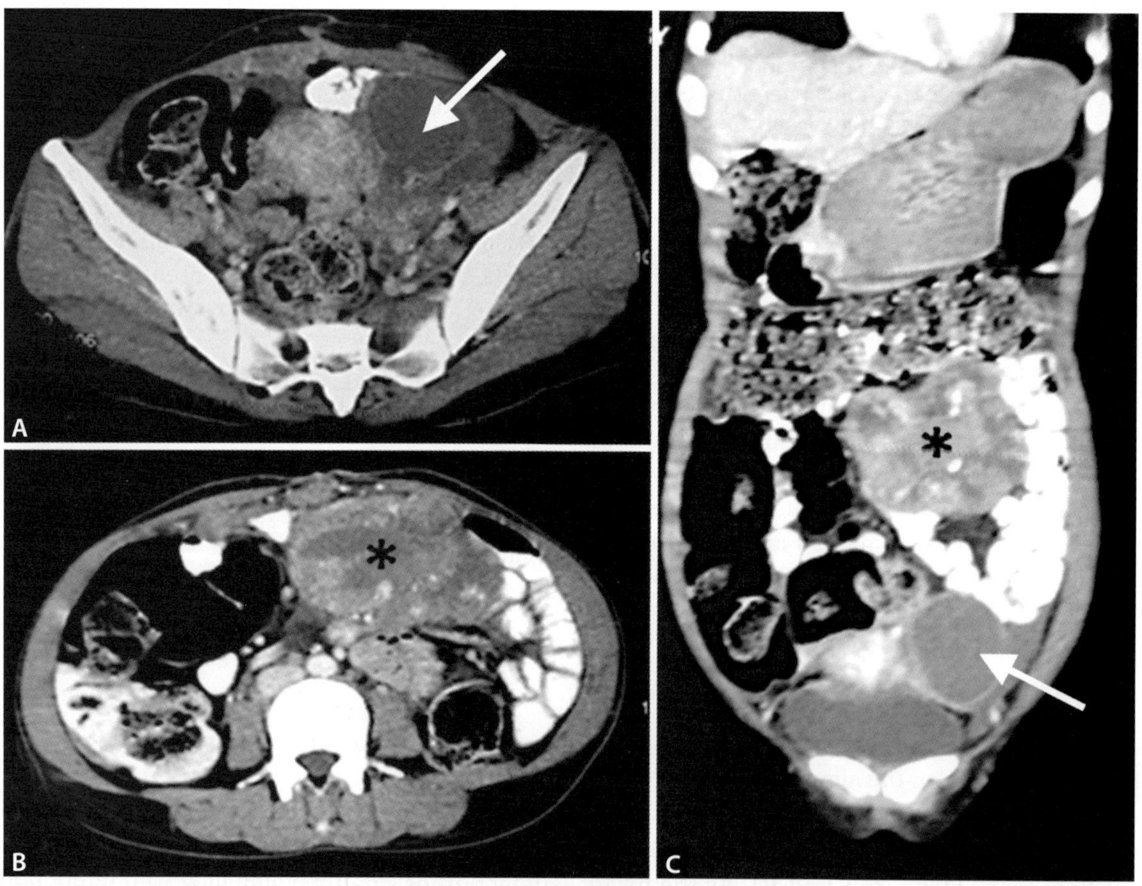

Figs. 33A to C: Peritoneal carcinomatosis from ovarian mucinous adenocarcinoma in a 45-year-old woman. Axial (A and B) coronal (C) CECT scans show a solid-cystic mass lesion in the left adnexa (arrow). There is an associated large heterogeneously enhancing solid mass lesion (*) in the mesentery with foci of calcification within.

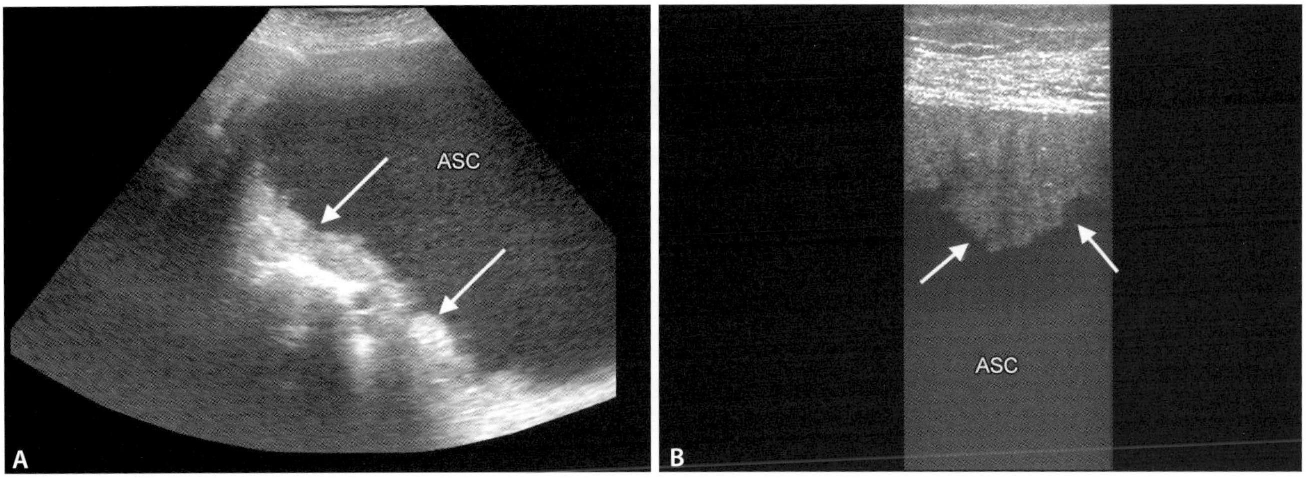

Figs. 34A and B: Peritoneal carcinomatosis with metastatic peritoneal deposits: (A) Transverse US image of right flank shows a large amount of ascites with fine internal echoes and multiple small peritoneal implants along the right paracolic gutter: (B) High frequency US image in a different patient shows an irregular solid hypoechoic mass projecting within the ascitic (ASC) fluid from the anterior peritoneal margin (arrows).

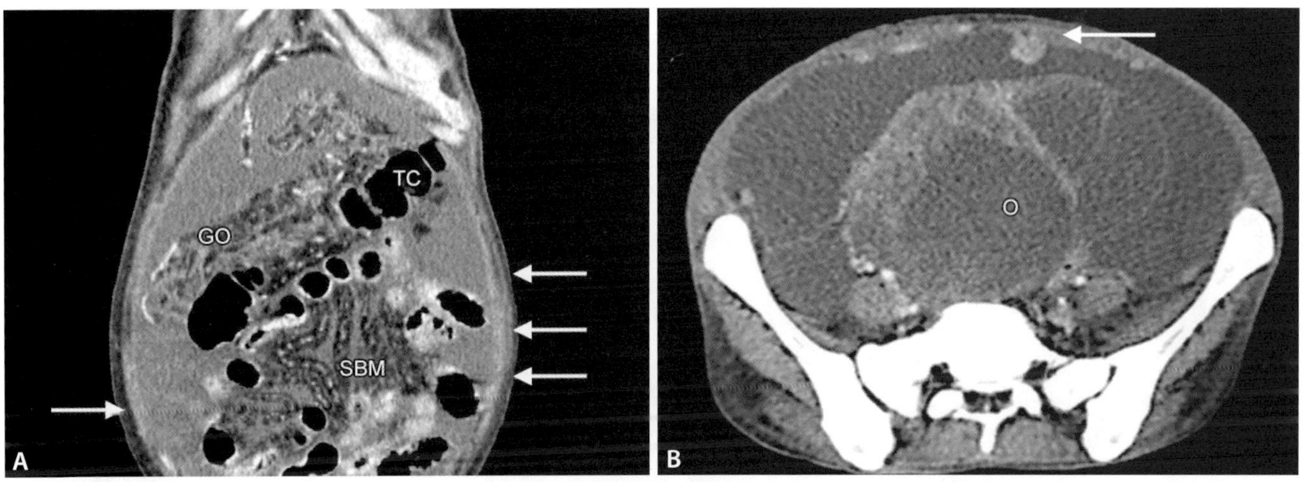

Figs. 35A and B: Peritoneal carcinomatosis in a 65-year-old woman with ovarian malignancy: Coronal (A) and axial (B) CECT scans show ascites with nodular enhancing peritoneum (arrows), thickened and nodular greater omentum (GO), and a stiffened small bowel mesentery (SBM); Ovarian mass (O).

Multidetector computed tomography (MDCT) is the optimal technique for detecting the presence, location and extent of peritoneal carcinomatosis with reported overall diagnostic accuracy of 94%, specificity of 92% and sensitivities between 75% and 81%. However, CT sensitivities for detection of smaller nodules, less than 1 cm, is much lower.[78] The parietal peritoneum shows smooth, nodular or plaque like thickening which enhances on postcontrast scans **(Figs. 35A and B)**. As the tumor infiltrates the small bowel mesentery, it becomes stiff and loses its normal undulations. There is a characteristic straightening of the mesenteric vasculature producing a 'pleated' appearance on CT images. A 'stellate' pattern of mesenteric involvement may occur when the tumor infiltrates the perivascular spaces, causing the vessels within the mesentery to appear denser than the surrounding fat and appears like stars in the sky on axial CT scans. Nodular or diffuse thickening can occur along the serosal surface of the bowel, leading to small bowel obstruction.[38]

Magnetic resonance imaging (MRI) can improve the detection of small peritoneal implants. These are best seen on contrast-enhanced T1-weighted images with fat suppression. Peritoneal carcinomatosis enhances slowly after intravenous administration of gadolinium and images should be obtained 5–10 minutes after injection. The normal peritoneum has an enhancement similar to that of liver. An abnormal enhancement should be suspected when peritoneum enhances more than liver or shows associated thickening, nodularity or mass. Typically, omental and mesenteric masses are of low T1-weighted and mixed T2-weighted signal intensity compared with surrounding soft tissues **(Figs. 36A and B)**. A combination of DWI and conventional sequences improves the accuracy for detection.[79]

Fluorodeoxyglucose (FDG) PET/CT is another promising modality for evaluation of peritoneal implants. Metastatic foci appear as round, oval, or globular areas of increased activity on FDG-PET.[80] One of the primary limitations of FDG PET/CT is that benign infectious or inflammatory peritoneal conditions may be FDG avid and therefore may mimic malignant peritoneal disease. Other sources of false-positive FDG PET/CT findings in the peritoneal cavity include physiologic bowel activity, motion artefact at the diaphragm, and urinary excretion of FDG.[81]

The evolution of cytoreductive surgery and hyperthermic intraperitoneal chemotherapy in the treatment of malignant peritoneal deposits has made it essential to have an extremely accurate preoperative assessment of the overall disease burden, and the exact sites of involvement in specific areas of the peritoneum. Analysis of imaging findings need to be done on a site to site basis, and presence, type and size of the deposits reported so as to be able decide on the feasibility and extent of surgery.[82]

Differential diagnosis: There are several non-neoplastic and neoplastic conditions that may mimic peritoneal carcinomatosis on imaging. The most important differential is the involvement of the peritoneum by tuberculosis, which is very common in our country. The differentiating points have been discussed above. Other differentials include lymphomas, sarcomatous involvement of the peritoneum **(Table 6)** and primary peritoneal malignancies such as mesothelioma. Primary peritoneal mesothelioma may be indistinguishable from carcinomatosis when the predominant imaging findings are multifocal peritoneal nodules and omental involvement ranging from finely infiltrated fat to

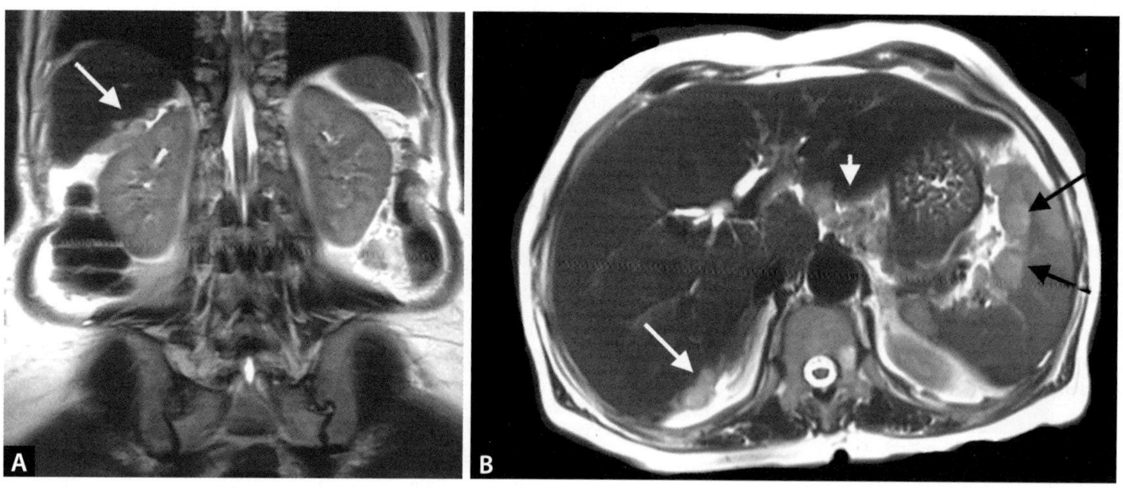

Figs. 36A and B: Peritoneal deposits: MR T2W images show multiple intermediate intensity nodular deposits in the Morrison's pouch (white arrows), gastrohepatic ligament (arrowhead) and perisplenic region (black arrows) in a case of colonic adenocarcinoma.

Table 6: Main differentiating features between peritoneal carcinomatosis, lymphomatosis and sarcomatosis.

	Peritoneal carcinomatosis	***Peritoneal lymphomatosis***	***Peritoneal sarcomatosis***
Peritoneal lesions	Multiple small nodules	Bulky homogeneous masses	Bulky heterogeneous masses
Lymphadenopathy	Lymph nodes around primary mass	Diffuse enlarged lymph nodes	None
Ascites	++	+	+/–

Source: Cabral FC, Krajewski KM, Kim KW, et al. Peritoneal lymphomatosis: CT and PET/CT findings and how to differentiate between carcinomatosis and sarcomatosis[92]

omental caking. A history of asbestos exposure favors mesothelioma.

PSEUDOMYXOMA PERITONEI

Pseudomyxoma peritonei (PMP) or 'jelly belly' is a specific type of peritoneal neoplasia resulting from peritoneal implants of columnar epithelium associated with progressive accumulation of mucinous ascites. It is most commonly seen with rupture of a benign or malignant mucin producing tumor of the appendix or ovary and occasionally pancreas, stomach, colon or urachus. The relationship between appendiceal and ovarian mucinous tumors has long been observed and a controversy exists as to whether in patients with pseudomyxoma peritonei and synchronous manifestation of ovarian and appendiceal tumors, the ovarian tumors are primary or secondary as the ovarian tumors are frequently seen to occur on the right side or are bilateral. Results of several clinical, histopathological and immunohistochemical studies strongly suggest that in these patients ovarian tumor deposits are almost always metastases of an appendiceal primary.[83,84]

Two types of pseudomyxoma have been described. *Disseminated peritoneal adenomucinosis* is a benign entity which spreads along the peritoneal surfaces, and does not invade the stroma. It is seen in association with low-grade mucinous carcinomas of appendix that penetrate or rupture into the peritoneal cavity. The second type is *peritoneal mucinous carcinomatosis*, which occurs from high grade mucinous carcinomas of the gastrointestinal tract, gallbladder, pancreas, or ovary, and its clinical course is often fatal.[85]

Clinical features: It occurs more commonly in women than men. Patients typically complain of progressive abdominal pain, increasing abdominal girth, and weight loss. Small bowel obstruction can occur in later stages.

Imaging features: On sonography, pseudomyxoma peritonei is seen as echogenic ascites, with nonmobile echoes in the ascitic fluid, in contrast to echoes seen with other exudative ascites. Echogenic septations within representing the margins of the mucinous nodules can be seen.[86,87]

Focal or sheet-like echogenic masses can occur due to involvement of omentum and parietal peritoneum. Scalloping of the visceral surfaces of the abdominal organs, specially liver and spleen, is an important hallmark of PMP. This scalloping represents indentations of the margins of organs due to extrinsic pressure of the intraperitoneal mucinous implants.[86]

On CT, the mucinous nodules are seen as hypodense areas filling the peritoneal cavity. Soft-tissue attenuation masses may be seen representing solid tumor elements, fibrosis, or compression of the mesentery and mucin. There may be curvilinear or amorphous calcifications. Scalloping of margins of liver and spleen is well visualized on CT **(Figs. 37A and B)**.

The regions of the appendix and ovaries should be closely evaluated in all newly diagnosed cases of PMP. However in many cases, it may be impossible to identify the originating appendiceal mucinous low-grade neoplasm or

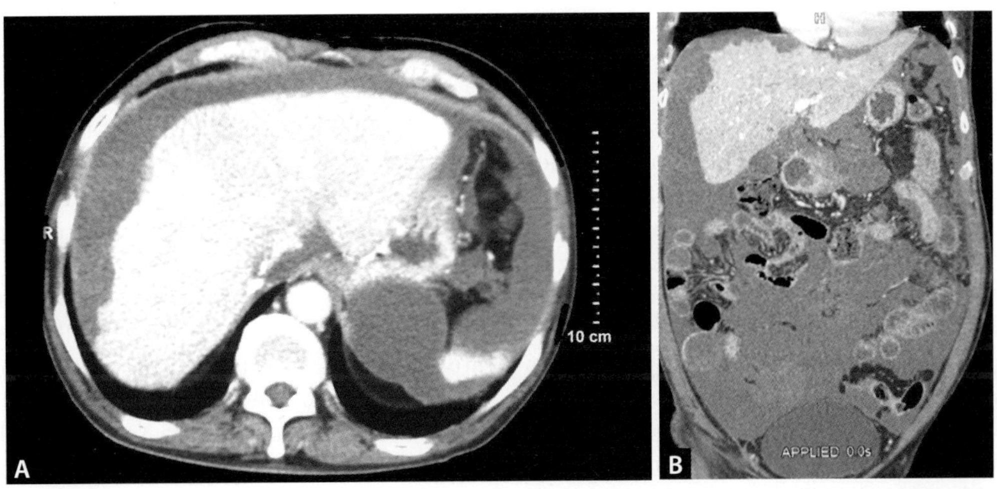

Figs. 37A and B: Pseudomyxoma peritonei from mucinous adenocarcinoma of appendix manifesting as increasing abdominal girth. Axial (A) and coronal (B) CECT scans show large locules of high density intraperitoneal fluid. Scalloping of the liver margins by the mucin locules can be very well seen.

cystadenocarcinoma. It may be difficult to differentiate adenomucinosis from mucinous carcinomatosis as they have overlapping findings. Carcinomatosis tends to involve thorax more commonly. Pleural effusions, pleural masses, enlarged mesenteric or retroperitoneal lymph nodes, omental caking and invasion into parenchymal organs are characteristically seen. In contrast, adenomucinosis does not invade visceral organs or spread by lymphatic or hematogenous routes.[88]

PERITONEAL LYMPHOMATOSIS

Peritoneal lymphomatosis is defined as the intraperitoneal spread of lymphoma. Lymphomatous involvement of the peritoneum maybe a primary or secondary process. *Secondary* involvement is more common, and can occur from nodal or extranodal non-Hodgkin lymphomas, such as small B-cell lymphoma, diffuse large B-cell lymphoma, or Burkitt lymphoma. *Primary* lymphomas of the peritoneum, also called body cavity-based lymphomas or primary effusion lymphomas, are uncommon and nearly exclusively found in immunocompromised patients, most of whom are infected with the human immunodeficiency virus.[89]

Imaging features: Diffuse thickening of peritoneal surfaces with multifocal nodules and masses that mimic peritoneal carcinomatosis can be seen. There can be associated ascites, peritoneal enhancement and thickening, omental caking, infiltration of the small bowel mesentery, and fine nodularity in the mesentery.[90] Enlarged lymph nodes, especially in the retrocrural region and in the small bowel mesentery are commonly seen in association with the mesenteric disease and should be a clue to the diagnosis. Associated GI involvement may also be seen in some cases.

In primary effusion lymphoma, the most common imaging manifestation is ascites without associated lymphadenopathy, organomegaly, or masses. In later stages, lymph node enlargement and nodular peritoneal thickening may occur, however, ascites remains the most predominant manifestation.[89,91]

The FDG-PET/CT has been shown to improve staging, evaluation of therapy response and earlier detection of recurrent disease in peritoneal lymphomatosis. FDG-PET/CT shows 2 patterns of glucose metabolism in peritoneal lymphomatosis—a nodular and a diffuse metabolic pattern. The FDG avidity in lymphoma is variable with aggressive and highly aggressive non-Hodgkin's lymphoma (NHL) and Hodgkin lymphomas showing high FDG avidity and indolent lymphomas showing an overall low-grade or no FDG uptake because of low metabolic activity. FDG-PET/CT not only has greater sensitivity than CT for depicting peritoneal involvement in subtle cases but it also has greater accuracy in identifying extranodal sites other than the peritoneum, even in the absence of CT findings. Due to its improved usefulness in distinguishing residual active lymphoma and benign fibrosis, FDG-PET/CT has been found valuable in assessment of treatment response.[92]

Sporadic Burkitt lymphoma is the most common form of NHL diagnosed in children younger than 15 years, accounting for 30–50% of cases.[93] It is a very aggressive B-cell lymphoma with a doubling time of only 24 hours, and thus needs to be diagnosed urgently. Burkitt lymphoma involving the peritoneum may appear as a large solitary mass or multiple abdominal masses **(Figs. 38A to C)**. Encasement of mesenteric vessels is a characteristic feature. Large tumors may show central necrosis. Associated peritoneal thickening or nodularity along the liver capsule and peritoneal reflections may be noted. Omental caking is not a feature of Burkitt lymphoma. Intrinsic involvement of the gastrointestinal tract is common, which is seen as bowel wall thickening or mural masses. Other solid organs like liver, spleen, kidneys and pancreas may be involved either intrinsically or by direct invasion by the peritoneal masses. Malignant ascites is found in 25% of cases of abdominal Burkitt lymphoma. Enlarged abdominal lymph nodes may be seen.[67]

Peritoneal lymphomatosis is treated nonsurgically, and often shows dramatic improvement with chemotherapy, and therefore its early and precise diagnosis is of utmost importance.

PERITONEAL SARCOMATOSIS

Peritoneal sarcomatosis or the disseminated intraperitoneal spread of sarcoma occurs most frequently from intra-abdominal sarcomas like malignant gastrointestinal stromal tumors (GIST), leiomyosarcomas or liposarcomas, by direct seeding of the peritoneal cavity. Metastases to peritoneum from extremity sarcomas are unusual and presumed to occur through the hematogenous route.

On imaging, peritoneal sarcomatosis may show focal, large soft-tissue masses, nodular infiltration, or confluent areas of increased attenuation within the mesentery and omentum **(Figs. 39A and B)**. Visceral deposits can occur and are seen as soft-tissue masses on serosal surfaces of the liver and spleen. Ascites is generally minimal and occurs late in the course of disease. GIST is the most common soft tissue sarcoma metastasizing to the peritoneum, seen in 21–45% cases of GISTs.[94,95]

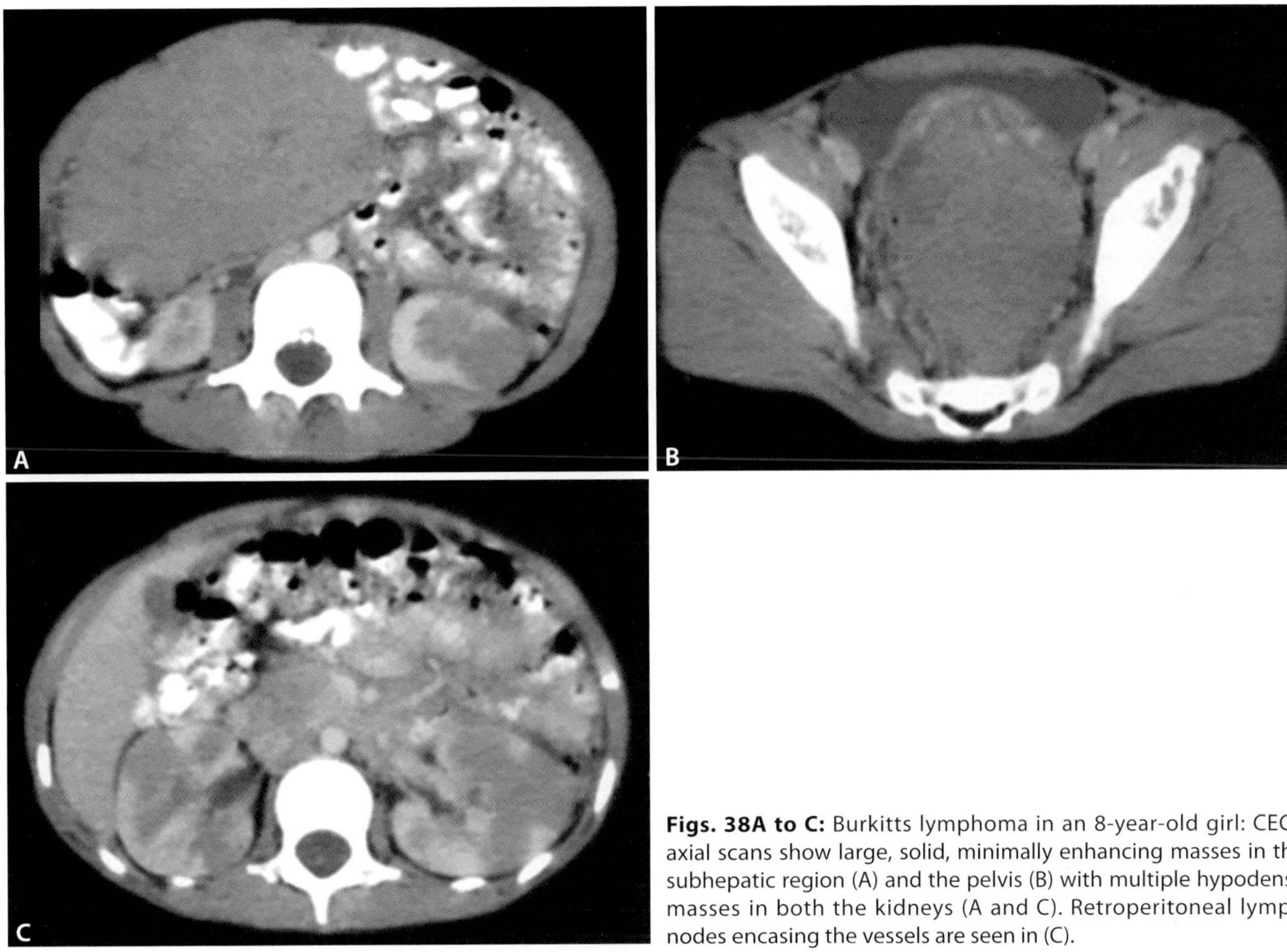

Figs. 38A to C: Burkitts lymphoma in an 8-year-old girl: CECT axial scans show large, solid, minimally enhancing masses in the subhepatic region (A) and the pelvis (B) with multiple hypodense masses in both the kidneys (A and C). Retroperitoneal lymph nodes encasing the vessels are seen in (C).

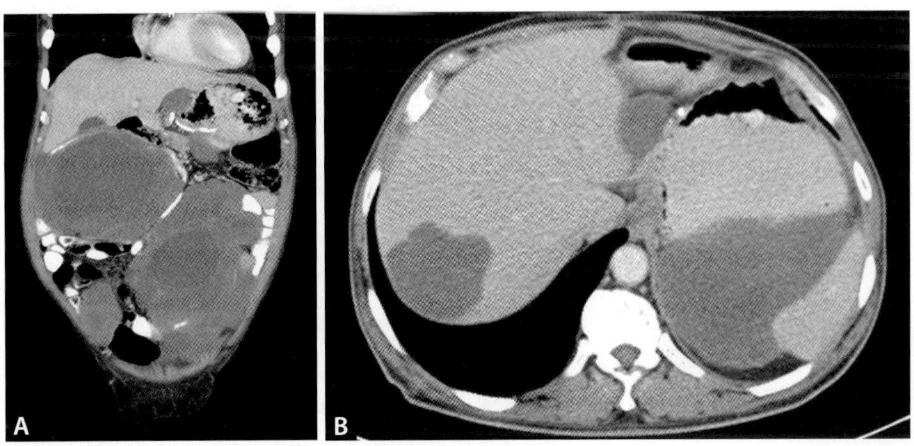

Figs. 39A and B: A 60-year-old man with gastrointestinal stromal tumor: Coronal (A) and axial (B) CECT images show bulky, heterogeneous peritoneal masses. Metastatic lesion seen in the liver on the axial scan (B). There is no evidence of ascites.

The peritoneal deposits in GIST are seen as large, discrete masses with necrosis with heterogeneous enhancement. Less commonly, diffuse hypervascular peritoneal involvement may occur with omental 'cake' formation. The hypervasculature nature of the metastases may lead to GI bleeding and hemoperitoneum.[93]

The appearance of peritoneal sarcomatosis may show overlap with carcinomatosis and lymphomatosis, although bulky heterogeneous masses, hypervascularity, minimal ascites, and hemoperitoneum are more characteristic of sarcomatosis. **Table 6** lists the main differentiating features between peritoneal carcinomatosis, lymphomatosis and sarcomatosis.

MESENTERIC CARCINOID (NEUROENDOCRINE TUMOR)

The small intestine is the most common location for gastrointestinal carcinoid tumors. Independent of site of origin, aggressive carcinoid tumors typically spread to the mesentery, mesenteric lymph nodes, liver, ovaries, and spleen.

Approximately 40–80% of gastrointestinal carcinoids spread to the mesentery, either by direct extension or through the local lymphatics.[96] The primary intestinal mass is often small and difficult to detect, the mesenteric tumor is usually discovered first. Secondary involvement of the mesentery leads to a desmoplastic reaction incited by local release of serotonin and other vasoactive substances.

Imaging features: CT/MR enterography is an appropriate imaging modality for evaluating patients suspected of having carcinoid tumors as it may show both the components of carcinoid tumor, the primary mural nodule and the secondary mesenteric mass.

Carcinoid tumor incites a strong desmoplastic reaction thought to be due to the effect of serotonin and other vasoactive peptides produced by the tumor. It is usually seen as a enhancing soft-tissue mass with linear bands radiating in the mesenteric fat **(Figs. 40A to C)**. Segmental thickening of adjacent bowel loops resulting from chronic ischemia or tumor infiltration as well as angulation can be

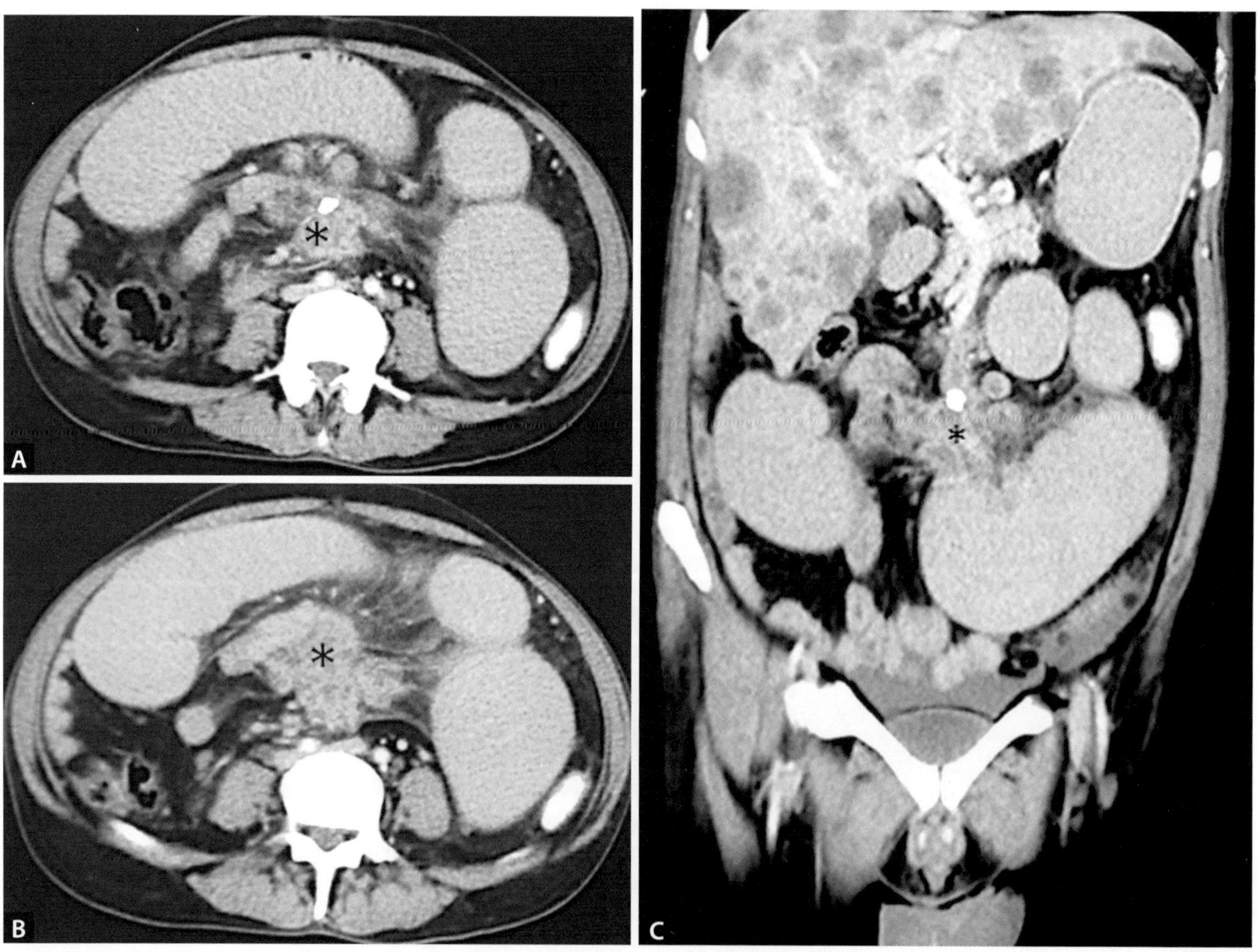

Figs. 40A to C: Metastatic carcinoid syndrome in a 42-year-old man: CECT axial (A and B) and coronal (C) scans show a heterogeneously enhancing mass in the mesentery (*) with a focus of calcification within and marked desmoplastic reaction in the adjacent mesentery, associated jejunal obstruction and dilated proximal jejunal loops. There are multiple hepatic metastases. Minimal ascites is seen.

seen. Dystrophic calcification may be seen in up to 40% of carcinoids on CT.[97] On MRI the lesions exhibit low T1 signal intensity, high T2 signal intensity and moderately intense gadolinium enhancement.[98] Functional imaging like octreotide scintigraphy and G-68 DOTANOC PET/CT play an important role in the diagnosis and management of these lesions.

CONCLUSION

Diseases of the peritoneum are common, but there is a considerable overlap in their imaging appearances. This often results in misinterpretation of the findings, and thus peritoneal diseases present a diagnostic challenge. With the appropriate clinical setting, CT and MRI substantially aid in the identification of peritoneal disease. Radiologists must be familiar with the anatomy of the peritoneal ligaments and spaces, and a knowledge of the various diseases that can involve the peritoneum, to provide an accurate interpretation of findings.

REFERENCES

1. Kim S, Kim TU, Lee JW, et al. The perihepatic space: comprehensive anatomy and CT features of pathologic conditions. Radio Graphics. 2007;27(1):129-43.
2. Standring S. Gray's anatomy: the anatomical basis of clinical practice, Peritoneum and peritoneal cavity, 39th edition. Churchill Livingstone; 2004.
3. Le O. Patterns of peritoneal spread of tumor in the abdomen and pelvis. World J Radiol. 2013;5:106-12.
4. DeMeo JH, Fulcher AS, Austin RF. Anatomic CT demonstration of the peritoneal spaces, ligaments, and mesenteries: normal and pathologic processes. Radiographics. 1995;15(4):755-70.
5. Tirkes T, Sandrasegaran K, Patel AA, et al. Peritoneal and retroperitoneal anatomy and its relevance for cross-sectional imaging. Radiographics. 2012;32:437-51.
6. Sharma M, Rai P, Rameshbabu CS, et al. Imaging of peritoneal ligaments by endoscopic ultrasound. Endosc Ultrasound. 2015;4(1):15-27.
7. Haaga JR, Pickhardt PJ. Peritoneum. In: Haaga JR, Dogra VS, Frosting M, et al. (Eds). CT and NRI of the whole body, 5th edition. Philadelphia, PA: Mosby. 2009:1675-1730.
8. Turnage RH, Li BD, McDonald JC. Abdominal wall, umbilicus, peritoneum, mesenteries, omentum and retroperitoneum. In: Townsend CM, Beauchamp RD, Evers BM, Mattox Kl (Eds). Sabiston Textbook of Surgery, 17th edition. Philadelphia, PA: Saunders; 2004.pp.1181-2.
9. Feldman GB, Knapp RC. Lymphatic drainage of the peritoneal cavity and its significance in ovarian cancer. Am J Obstet Gynecol. 1974;119:991-4.
10. Runyon BA, Montano AA, Akriviadis EA, et al. The serum-ascites albumin gradient is superior to the exudate-transudate concept in the differential diagnosis of ascites. Ann Intern Med. 1992;117(3):215-20.
11. Nicholas JE, Steinkampf MP. Detection of free peritoneal fluid by transvaginal sonography. J Clin Ultrasound. 1993;21:171-4.
12. Meyers MA. Dynamic radiology of the abdomen: normal and pathologic anatomy, 4th edition. New York, NY: Springer-Verlag; 1994.
13. Martin LC, Merkle EM, Thompson WM. Review of internal hernias: radiographic and Clinical findings AJR. 2006;186:703-17.
14. Edell SL, Gefter WB. Ultrasonic differentiation of types of ascitic fluid. Am J Roentgenol. 1979;133:111-4.
15. Gazelle GS, Mueller PR. Abdominal abscess: imaging and intervention. Radiol Clin North Am. 1994;32:913-32.
16. Batra A, Gulati MS, Sarma D, Paul SB. Sonographic appearances in abdominal tuberculosis. J Clin Ultrasound. 2000;28:233-45.
17. Leder RA, Low VHS. Tuberculosis of the abdomen. Radiol Clin North Am. 1995;33:691-705.
18. Burill J, Williams CJ, Bain G, et al. Tuberculosis: a radiological review. Radiographics. 2007;27:1255-73.
19. Hulnick DH, Megibow AJ, Nadiach DP, et al. Abdominal tuberculosis: CT evaluation. Radiology. 1985;157:199-204.
20. Lundstedt C, Nymon R, Brimsar J, et al. Imaging of abdominal tuberculosis. Abdominal manifestations in 112 patients. Acta Radiol. 1996;37:489-95.
21. Malik A, Saxena NC. Ultrasound in abdominal tuberculosis. Abdom Imaging. 2003;28(4):574-9.
22. Leder RA, Low VH. Tuberculosis of the abdomen. Radiol Clin North Am. 1995;33(4):691-705.
23. Anbarasu A, Upadhyaya A, Merchant SA, et al. Tuberculous chylous ascites: pathognomic CT findings. Abdom Imaging. 1997;22:50-1.
24. Joshi AR, Basantani AS, Patel TC. Role of CT and MRI in abdominal tuberculosis. Current Radiology Reports. 2014;2:66.
25. Healy JC, Reznek RH. The peritoneum, mesenteries and omenta: normal anatomy and pathological processes Eur Radiol. 1998;8:886-900.
26. Ha HK, Jung JM, Lee MS, et al. CT differentiation of tuberculous peritonitis and peritoneal carcinomatosis. Am J Roentgenol. 1996;167:743-8.
27. Rodriquez E, Pombo F. Peritoneal tuberculosis versus peritoneal carcinomatosis: distinction based on CT findings. J Comput Asst Tomogr. 1996;20(2):269-72.
28. Pedrosa I, Saíz A, Arrazola J, Ferreirós J Pedrosa CS. Hydatid disease: radiologic and pathologic features and complications. Radiographics. 2000;20(3):3795-817.
29. Acharya AN, Gupta S. Peritoneal hydatidosis: a review of seven cases. Tropical Gastroenterology. 2009;30(1):32-4.
30. Mindelzun RE, Brooke Jeffrey R, Lane MJ, Silverman PM. The misty mesentery on CT: differential diagnosis. AJR. 1996;167:61-5.
31. Demir MK, Akinci O, Onur E, et al. Case 108: sclerosing encapsulating peritonitis. Radiology. 2007;242(3):937-9.

32. Vijayaraghavan SB, Palanivelu C, Sendhilkumar K, Parthasarathi R. Abdominal cocoon: sonographic features. J Ultrasound Med. 2003;22:719-21.
33. Hur J, Kim KW, Park MS, Yu JS. Abdominal cocoon: preoperative diagnostic clues from radiologic imaging with pathologic correlation. Am J Roentgenol. 2004; 182:639-41.
34. Gupta S, Shirahatti RG, Anand J. CT findings of an abdominal cocoon. Am J Roentgenol. 2004;183(6):1658-60.
35. Auh YH, Kung S, Shih G. Mesentery. In: Haaga JR, Dogra VS, Frosting M, et al, (Eds). CT and MRI of the whole body, 5th edition. Philadelphia, PA: Mosby. 2009:1731-70.
36. Horton KM, Lawler LP, Fishman ER. CT Findings in Sclerosing Mesenteritis (Panniculitis): Spectrum of Disease. Radiographics. 2003;23:1561-7.
37. Valls C. Fat-ring sign in sclerosing mesenteritis. Am J Roentgenol. 2000;174:259-60.
38. Hamrick-Turner J, Chiechi M, Abbitt P, Ros P. Neoplastic and inflammatory processes of the peritoneum, omentum and mesentery: diagnosis with CT. Radiographics. 1992;12:1051-68.
39. Singh AK, Gervais DA, Hahn PF, Rhea J, Mueller PR. CT of acute appendagitis. Am J Roentgenol. 2004;183:1303-7.
40. Singh AK, Gervais DA, Hahn PF. Acute epiploic appendagitis and its mimics. Radiographics. 2005;25(6):1521-34.
41. Lucey BC, Stuhlfaut JW, Soto JA. Mesenteric lymph nodes: detection and significance on MDCT. Am J Roentgenol. 2005;184:41-4.
42. Lucey BC, Stuhlfaut JW, Soto JA. Mesenteric lymph nodes seen at imaging—causes and significance. Radiographics. 2005;25:351-65.
43. Jain R, Sawhney S, Bhargava DK, et al. Diagnosis of abdominal tuberculosis: sonographic findings in patients with early disease. AJR. 1995;165:1391-5.
44. Kedar RP, Shah PP, Shirde RS, et al. Sonographic findings in gastrointestinal and peritoneal tuberculosis. Clin Radiol. 1994;49:24-9.
45. Pombo F, Rodriquez E, Mato J, et al. Patterns of contrast enhancement of tuberculous lymph nodes demonstrated by CT. Clin Radiol. 1992;46:13-7.
46. De Backer AI, Mortele KJ, Deeren D, Vanschoubroeck IJ, De Keulenaer BL. Abdominal tuberculous lymphadenopathy: MRI features. Eur Radiol. 2005;15(10):2104-9.
47. Rocha ELD, Pedrassa BC, Bormann RL, et al. Abdominal tuberculosis: a radiological review with emphasis on CT and MRI findings. Radiol Bras. 2015;48(3):181-91.
48. Yang ZG, Min P, Sone S, et al. Tuberculosis versus lymphoma in the abdominal lymph nodes. Evaluation with contrast-enhanced CT. Am J Roentgenol. 1999;172:619-23.
49. Macari M, Hines J, Balthazar E, Megibow A. Mesenteric adenitis: CT diagnosis of primary versus secondary causes, incidence, and clinical significance in pediatric and adult patients. Am J Roentgenol. 2002;178:853-8.
50. Rao PM, Rhea JT, Novelline RA. CT diagnosis of mesenteric adenitis. Radiology. 1997;204:713-7.
51. Yenarkam P, Theni RF, Hanks D. Lymphoma of the mesentery. Radiology. 2007;242:628-31.
52. Mok SC, Schorge JO, Welch WR, Hendrickson MR, Kempson RL. Peritoneal tumors. In: Tavassoli FA, Devilee P (Eds). Pathology and genetics of tumours of the breast and female genital organs. Lyon, France: IARC. 2003;197-202.
53. Boffetta P. Epidemiology of peritoneal mesothelioma: a review. Ann Oncol. 2007;18:985-990.
54. Churg A, Cagle PT, Roggli VL. Tumors of the serosal membranes. Silver Spring, Md: ARP; 2006.
55. Levy AD, Arnáiz J, Shaw JC, Sobin LH. From the archives of the AFIP: primary peritoneal tumors—imaging features with pathologic correlation. Radiographics. 2008;28:583-607.
56. Cao Q, Lu M, Heath J, Hausner PF, Alexander HR, Dilsizian V, Chen W. 18F-FDG PET/CT in a recurrent diffuse malignant peritoneal mesothelioma. Clin Nucl Med. 2012;37:492-4.
57. Turner KM, Varghese S, Alexander HR. Surgery for peritoneal mesothelioma. Curr Treat Options Oncol. 2011;12:189-200.
58. Raza A, Huang WC, Takabe K. Advances in the management of peritoneal mesothelioma. World J Gastroenterol. 2014;7: 20(33):11700-12.
59. Ross MJ, Welch WR, Scully RE. Multilocular peritoneal inclusion cysts (so-called cystic mesotheliomas). Cancer. 1989;64:1336-46.
60. McLaughlin P, Flippone A, Maher MM. Neoplastic diseases of Peritoneum and Mesentery. AJR. 2013;200:W400-w420.
61. Zhang J, Xu H, Ren F, Yang Y, Chen B, Zhang F. Analysis of clinicopathological features and prognostic factors of desmoplastic small round cell tumor. Pathol Oncol Res. 2014;20(1):161-8.
62. Arora VC, Price AP, Fleming S, et al. Characteristic imaging features of desmoplastic small round cell tumor. Pediatr Radiol. 2013,43(1):93-102.
63. Magnan H, Abramson SJ, Price AP, et al. Positron emission tomography for response assessment in desmoplastic small round cell tumor. J Pediatr Hematol Oncol. 2013;35(5): e190-3.
64. Casillas J, Sais GJ, Greve JL, Iparraguirre MC, Morillo G. Imaging of intra- and extraabdominal desmoid tumors. Radiographics. 1991;11:959-68.
65. Azizi I, Bali M, Belkacem A, et al. MRI Features of mesenteric desmoids tumors in familial adenomatous polyposis. AJR. 2005;184:1128-35.
66. Shinagare AB, Ramaiya NH, Jagannathan JP, et al. A to Z of desmoids tumours. Am J Roentgenol. 201;197(6):W1008-14.
67. Chung EM, Biko DM, Arzamendi AM, et al. Solid tumours of the peritoneum, omentum, and mesentery in children: radiologic-pathologic correlation: from the radiologic pathology archives. Radiographics. 2015;35:521-46.
68. Aptel S, Gervaise A, Fairise A, et al. Abdominal inflammatory myofibroblastic tumour. Diagn Interv Imaging. 2012;93(5): 410-2.

69. Narla LD, Newman B, Spottswood SS, Narla S, Kolli R. Inflammatory pseudotumor. Radiographics. 2003;23(3): 719-29.
70. Sedlic T, Scali EP, Lee WK, Verma S, Chang SD. Inflammatory pseudotumors in the abdomen and pelvis: a pictorial essay. Can Assoc Radiol J. 2014;65(1):52-9.
71. Dong A, Wang Y, Dong H, et al. Inflammatory myofibroblastic tumor: FDG PET/CT findings with pathologic correlation. Clin Nucl Med. 2014;39(2):113-21.
72. Lausen I, Jensen OJ, Andersen E, Lindahl F. Disseminated peritoneal leiomyomatosis with malignant change in a male. Virchows Arch A Pathol Anat Histopathol. 1990;417:173-5.
73. Fulcher AS, Szucs RA. Leiomyomatosis peritonealis disseminata complicated by sarcomatous transformation and ovarian torsion: presentation of two cases and review of the literature. Abdom Imaging. 1998;23:640-4.
74. Levy AD, Cantisani V, Miettinen M. Abdominal lymphangiomas: imaging features with pathologic correlation. Am J Roentgenol. 2004;182:1485-91.
75. Merrot T, Chaumoitre K, Simeoni-Alias J, Alessandrini P, Guys JM, Panuel M. Abdominal cystic lymphangiomas in children. Clinical, diagnostic and therapeutic aspects: apropos of 21 cases. Ann Chir. 1999;53:494-9.
76. Meyers MA. Intraperitoneal spread of malignancies. In: Meyers MA (Ed). Dynamic Radiology of the Abdomen: Normal and Pathologic Anatomy, 5th edition. New York/ London: Springer. 2000.pp. 131-263.
77. Hanbridge AE, Lynch D, Wilson SR. US of the peritoneum. Radiographics. 2003;23/3:663-83.
78. Marin D, Catalano C, Baski M, et al. 64-section multi-detector row CT in the preoperative diagnosis of peritoneal carcinomatosis: Correlation with histopathological findings. Abdom Imaging. 2010;35:694-700.
79. Iafrate F, Ciolina M, Sammartino P, et al. Peritoneal carcinomatosis: imaging with 64-MDCT and 3T MRI with diffusion-weighted imaging. Abdom Imaging. 2012;37:616-27.
80. Soussan M, Des Guetz G, Barrau V, et al. Comparison of FDG-PET/CT and MR with diffusion-weighted imaging for assessing peritoneal carcinomatosis from gastrointestinal malignancy. Eur Radiol. 2012;22:1479-87.
81. Anthony MP, Khong PL, Zhang J. Spectrum of 18F-FDG PET/CT appearances in peritoneal disease. AJR. 2009;193:1646.
82. Tentes KA, Courcoutsakis N, Prasopoulos P. Combined cytoreductive surgery and perioperative intraperitoneal chemotherapy for the treatment of advanced ovarian cancer—clinical and therapeutic perspectives. In: Samir F (Ed). Ovarian Cancer—Clinical and Therapeutic Perspectives. New York: InTech; 2012.pp.143-67.
83. Seidman JD, Elsayed AM, Sobin LH, Tavassoli FA. Association of mucinous tumors of the ovary and appendix: a clinicopathologic study of 25 cases. Am J Surg Pathol. 1993;17:22-34.
84. Young RH, Gilks CB, Scully RE. Mucinous tumors of the appendix associated with mucinous tumors of the ovary and pseudomyxoma peritonei: a clinicopathological analysis of 22 cases supporting an origin in the appendix. Am J Surg Pathol. 1991;15:415-29.
85. Ronnett BM, Zahn CM, Kurman RJ, Kass ME, et al. Disseminated peritoneal adenomucinosis and peritoneal mucinouscarcinomatosis: a clinicopathologic analysis of 109 cases with emphasis on distinguishing pathologic features, site of origin, prognosis, and relationship to "pseudomyxoma peritonei." Am J Surg Pathol. 1995;19:1390-408.
86. Seshul MB, Coulam CM. Pseudomyxoma peritonei: Computed tomography and sonography. Am J Roentgenol. 1981;136:803-6.
87. Yeh HC, Shafir MK, Slater G, Meyer RJ, Cohen BA, Geller SA. Ultrasonography and computed tomography in pseudomyxoma peritonei. Radiology. 1984;153:507-10.
88. Bechtold RE, Chen MY, Loggie BW, Jackson SL, Geisinger K. CT appearance of disseminated peritoneal adenomucinosis. Abdom Imaging. 2001;26:406-10.
89. Levy AD, Shaw JC, Sobin LH. Secondary tumours and tumour-like lesions of the peritoneal cavity: imaging features with pathologic correlation. Radiographics. 2009;29:347-73.
90. Kim Y, Cho O, Song S, Lee H, Rhim H, Koh B. Peritoneal lymphomatosis: CT findings. Abdom Imaging. 1998;23:87-90.
91. Ferrozzi F, Tognini G, Mulonzia NW, Bova D, et al. Primary effusion lymphomas in AIDS: CT findings in two cases. Eur Radiol. 2001;11:623-5.
92. Cabral FC, Krajewski KM, Kim KW, et al. Peritoneal lymphomatosis: CT and PET/CT findings and how to differentiate between carcinomatosis and sarcomatosis. Cancer Imaging. 2013:13(2):162-70.
93. Swerdlow SH. International Agency for Research on Cancer, World Health Organization. WHO classification of tumours of haematopoietic and lymphoid tissues. Lyon, France: International Agency for Research on Cancer, 2008.
94. Katz SC, DeMatteo RP. Gastrointestinal stromal tumors and leiomyosarcoma. J Surg Oncol. 2008;97:350-9.
95. Burkill GJ, Badran M, Thomas JM. Malignant gastrointestinal stromal tumor: distribution, imaging features, and pattern of metastatic spread. Radiology. 2003;226:527-32.
96. Sheth S, Horton KM, Garland MR, Fishman EK. Mesenteric neoplasms: CT appearances of primary and secondary tumors and differential diagnosis. Radiographics. 2003;23:457-73.
97. Levy AD, Sobin LH. From the archives of the AFIP: Gastrointestinal carcinoids: Imaging features with clinicopathologic comparison. Radiographics. 2007;27:237-57.
98. Elsayes KM, Staveteig PT, Narra VR, et al. MRI of the peritoneum: spectrum of abnormalities. Am J Roentgenol. 2006;186:1368-79.

CHAPTER 94

Imaging of Spleen

Mukesh Kumar Yadav, Priyanka Naranje, Ekta Dhamija

INTRODUCTION AND ANATOMY

The spleen is an encapsulated organ located intraperitoneally in the left subdiaphragmatic region of the abdomen. Multiple ligaments support the spleen in its normal position. The important ones are gastrosplenic ligament and lienorenal ligament. Others are phrenicosplenic, splenocolic, pancreaticosplenic, phrenocolic, and pancreaticocolic ligaments. The capsule is penetrated at the hilus located anteromedially, by the splenic artery, splenic vein, lymphatics, and nerves. Within the spleen, the branches of arteries, veins, nerves, and lymphatics form a trabecular network.

The parenchyma of spleen has a unique arrangement of white pulp (25%) and red pulp (75%).[1] Splenic cords and vascular sinuses containing predominantly erythrocytes constitute the red pulp, whereas lymphatic tissue, macrophages and lymphocytes compose the white pulp area of spleen. Some of the normal variations in enhancement pattern of spleen seen on contrast-enhanced computed tomography (CT) as well as gadolinium enhanced magnetic resonance imaging (MRI) are attributed to this unique anatomy of the spleen.

The spleen arises from aggregations of mesenchymal tissue between the layers of the dorsal mesogastrium during the fifth gestational week giving a lobulated pattern of the fetal spleen. The principal function of the embryonic spleen is erythropoiesis, which increases from the first to mid-second trimester and subsequently reduces. In the later life, spleen filters the damaged or aged red blood cells, bacteria, antigen-coated cells and foreign particles. The spleen comprises the largest functional mass of lymphoid tissue in the body. It consumes the circulating platelets when there is splenomegaly and also functions as reservoir for platelets, releasing them in response to epinephrine.[1]

IMAGING MODALITIES

Plain Abdominal Radiographs

A plain radiograph of the abdomen normally shows the spleen below the left hemidiaphragm in upper quadrant, lateral to gastric bubble and superior to colon. Excessive gaseous distension of bowel loops may obscure the splenic density. Enlarged spleen will be seen as soft tissue opacity displacing the stomach medially and colonic gas inferiorly **(Fig. 1)**. Curvilinear or chunky calcifications may be identified on plain radiographs in the region of spleen in cases of calcified hydatid cyst, calcified wall of splenic artery aneurysms or calcified granulomas.

Ultrasonography (USG)

Sonography is a nonionizing, radiation free, noninvasive and inexpensive modality for evaluating the spleen. It is frequently the initial investigation tool used for suspected splenic pathology. Sonography is used for evaluating splenic size, shape, location, and multiplicity, especially in children. Characterization of focal splenic lesions, splenic size evaluation in portal hypertension and cases

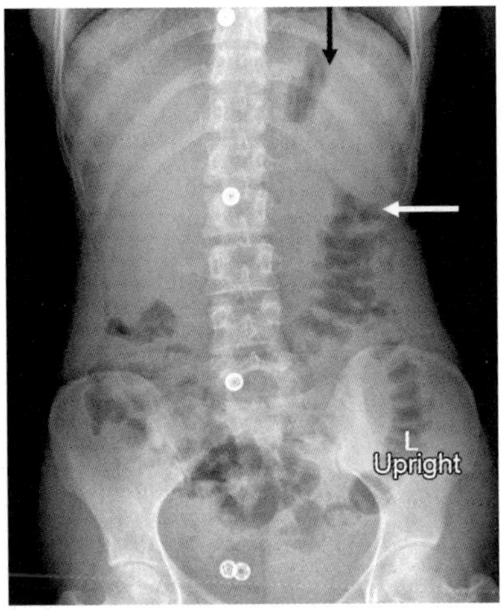

Fig. 1: Plain radiograph of abdomen shows indentation of splenic flexure (inferiorly) and greater curvature of stomach by soft tissue in left upper abdomen due to splenomegaly.

of extrahepatic portal venous obstruction (EHPVO) along with assessment of perisplenic collaterals, splenic vein assessment in cases of pancreatitis, identification of splenic arterial aneurysms, preoperative work-up and postoperative follow-up of cases requiring splenectomy and as a guidance tool for various interventions such as fine needle aspiration cytology (FNAC), biopsies or drainages, are other common indications for using ultrasound for spleen. Sonography is ideally suited to study the internal architecture of a focal mass within the spleen, and distinguish a solid from a cystic lesion. Diffuse splenic involvement in infections like tuberculosis, fungal infections or in sarcoidosis or in cases of lymphoma, ultrasound may reveal the abnormality better than computed tomography **(Figs. 2A and B)**. Some lesions are known to have characteristic sonographic morphology and this modality helps to narrow the differential diagnosis and triage patients for further imaging work-up. The major drawback of this technique is that it is highly operator dependent. The details of sonographic features of different pathologies will be discussed subsequently. Role of focused assessment of spleen in trauma (FAST) by USG cannot be over emphasized and is covered in the chapter on Abdominal Trauma.

Technique

The spleen is usually scanned in the supine or right decubitus position with a 3.5–5 MHz convex array transducer in the sagittal and oblique planes as well as transversely, mostly from an intercostal approach in suspended deep inspiration and end expiration. Sometimes due to deep inspiration, the lateral margin of the left lung obscures the visualization of spleen **(Fig. 2D)**. In such situation, either scanning in expiration **(Fig. 2E)** or scanning with a small foot print probe in intercostal space may be helpful. An attempt is made to localize the splenic hilum, which represents the mid portion of the spleen, and the scanning is done taking a swipe posterior and anterior to the visualized hilum. Color Doppler is useful to assess the splenic hilar vein and artery at the hilum.

On ultrasonography, normal spleen shows a homogeneous echotexture **(Fig. 2C)**. Its echogenicity is a little more than that of the kidneys **(Fig. 3)** and is isoechoic to slightly hyperechoic compared to the liver. Tubular anechoic tortuous structures on gray-scale at the hilum of spleen are the splenic vessels **(Fig. 2C)** and intrasplenic vessels are visualized on color Doppler imaging.

Elasticity of the spleen can be measured with the real-time elastography, which measures the stiffness of parenchyma and it can be utilized as a marker for portal hypertension in patients with chronic liver disease.[2]

Few studies on contrast-enhanced ultrasound (CEUS) have described its utility in spleen.[3-5] The European Federation of Societies for Ultrasound in Medicine and Biology (EFSUMB) Guidelines and Recommendations on the Clinical Practice of CEUS, updated in 2011, recommend several indications where CEUS may be utilized in the spleen.[6] These are:

1. To characterize inhomogeneity of splenic parenchyma or to characterize suspected lesions on conventional US
2. To characterize accessory spleens or splenosis
3. To confirm suspected splenic infarction
4. To detect malignant splenic lesions in oncologic patients when CT and/or MRI and PET are contraindicated or inconclusive
5. To evaluate the spleen in selected patients following trauma.

Computed Tomography

On a non-contrast CT (NCCT), a normal spleen reveals a homogeneous attenuation which is higher than the liver by 1–18 Hounsfield Unit (HU).[7] Normal HU of spleen is 40–60 HU. Splenic artery follows a tortuous course normally and splenic vein shows a straighter course and is usually located posterior to pancreatic body and tail.

For identification and characterization of focal lesion in the spleen or in trauma setting, contrast-enhanced computed tomography is frequently required.

Most often transient inhomogeneous splenic attenuation patterns are identified during the first

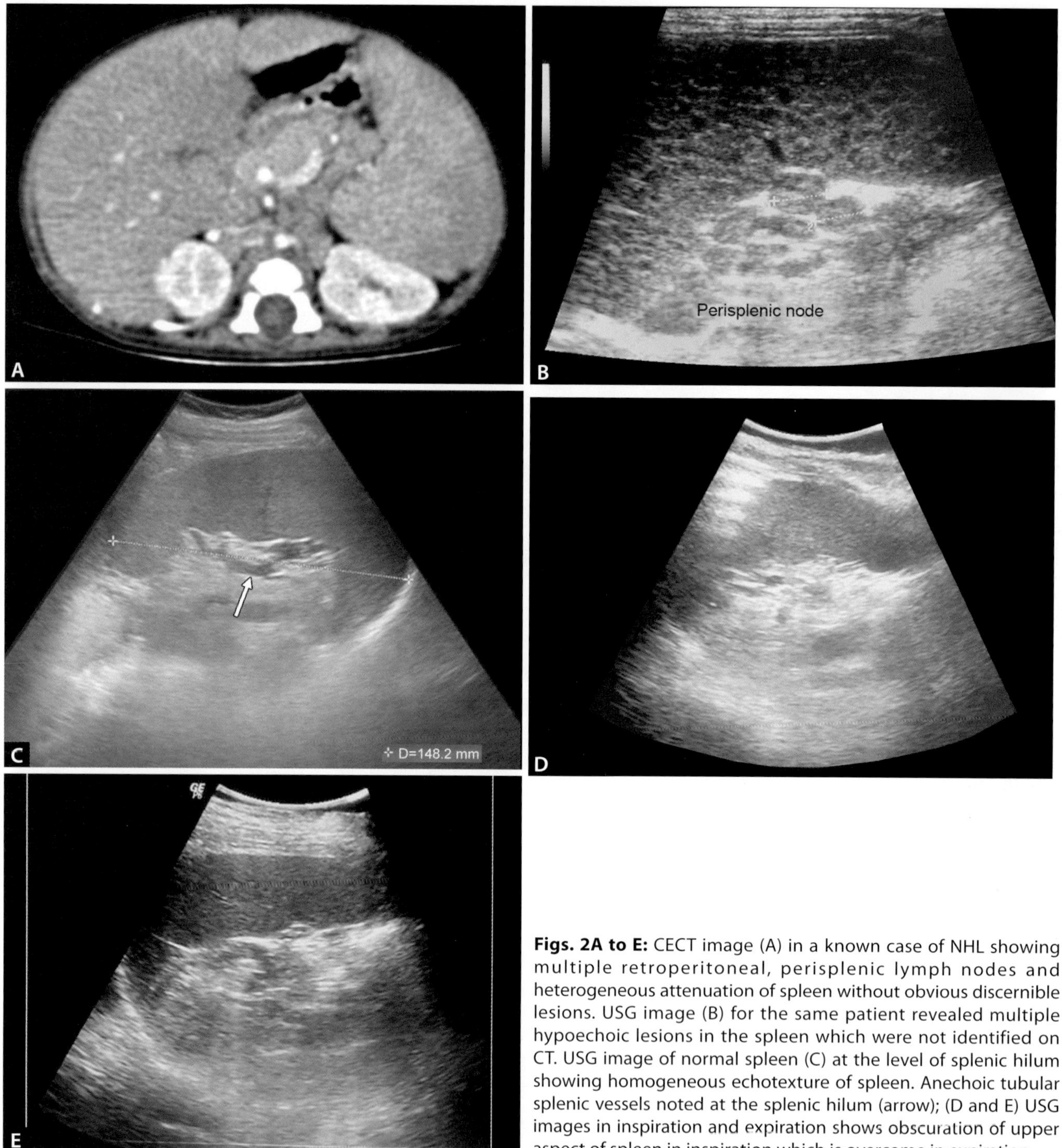

Figs. 2A to E: CECT image (A) in a known case of NHL showing multiple retroperitoneal, perisplenic lymph nodes and heterogeneous attenuation of spleen without obvious discernible lesions. USG image (B) for the same patient revealed multiple hypoechoic lesions in the spleen which were not identified on CT. USG image of normal spleen (C) at the level of splenic hilum showing homogeneous echotexture of spleen. Anechoic tubular splenic vessels noted at the splenic hilum (arrow); (D and E) USG images in inspiration and expiration shows obscuration of upper aspect of spleen in inspiration which is overcome in expiration

minute of contrast-enhanced CT, particularly with rapid intravenous injection of iodinated contrast media.[8] This is a normal flow phenomenon and must not be misinterpreted as an indication of focal abnormality. It is thought to be due to different blood flow rates through the cords of red pulp[9] and white pulp. As the internal architecture of the spleen develops, this phenomenon gets more evident in children older than 1 year. Frequently described heterogeneity patterns include: (1) archiform pattern, consisting of ring-like or zebra-stripe bands of alternating low and high attenuation (commonest pattern) **(Figs. 4A and B)**; (2) diffuse, mottled areas of heterogeneity; and

(3) focal areas of low density.[8] More homogeneous splenic enhancement is seen about approximately 70 seconds after commencement of the contrast injection. This heterogeneous splenic enhancement pattern can obscure pathologic lesions. With increasing age, the heterogeneous pattern is less often seen and in adults, several other factors may be responsible for the heterogeneous splenic enhancement, such as the liver disease, portal vein thrombosis, and congestive heart failure.[10]

CT angiography is performed for the detection of splenic artery aneurysms. Multiplanar reformation (MPR), maximum intensity projections (MIP) and volume rendered (VR) imaging help for complete morphological assessment of these aneurysms.

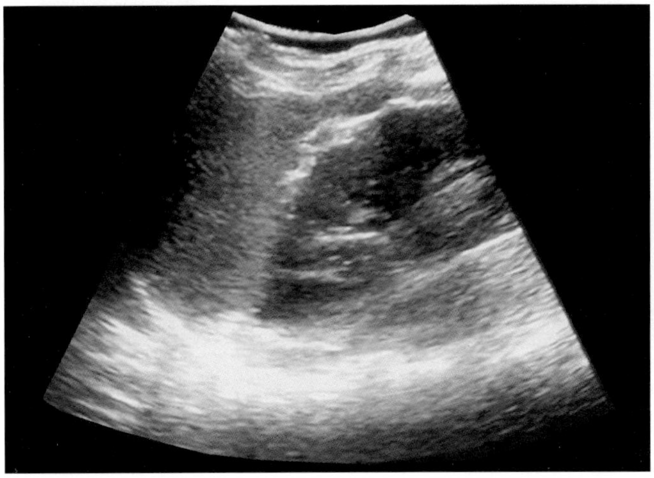

Fig. 3: USG images showing normal splenic echotexture as slightly more than the adjacent left kidney.

Magnetic Resonance Imaging

Magnetic resonance imaging (MRI) offers major advantages due to its high contrast resolution, lack of ionizing radiation and multiplanar capability. Technical advances in MR hardware and software have allowed the introduction of faster pulse sequences with significantly reduced motion artifacts that previously posed limitations to abdominal MR imaging. Indications for performing MRI for splenic pathology are mainly as a problem solving technique for focal splenic lesions or tumors, proliferative lymphatic diseases or in iron deposition conditions.

On MRI, normal adult spleen is T2 hyperintense relative to the liver **(Figs. 5A to D)**. On T1-weighted images (T1WI), the normal spleen shows lower signal intensity (SI) than that of liver and slightly greater SI than that of muscle. Such a signal intensity of spleen is attributed to large fractional heme content, which results in long T1 and T2 relaxation times.[11] However, in a neonate, due to the immaturity of the white pulp, the spleen is T1 as well as T2 hypo to isointense compared to the liver **(Figs. 6A and B)**. After 8 months of age as white pulp matures, the spleen becomes hyperintense on T2-weighted image (T2WI) relative to the liver and it maintains this appearance through adulthood.[12] On diffusion-weighted imaging, the spleen shows physiologically restricted diffusion **(Figs. 5A to D)**.[13]

Dynamic gadolinium-enhanced MR imaging has potential advantages over conventional MR imaging of the spleen because it can potentially provide differential contrast enhancement between splenic lesions and normal splenic tissue with greater contrast resolution compared with CT. Heterogeneous enhancement patterns of the normal spleen,

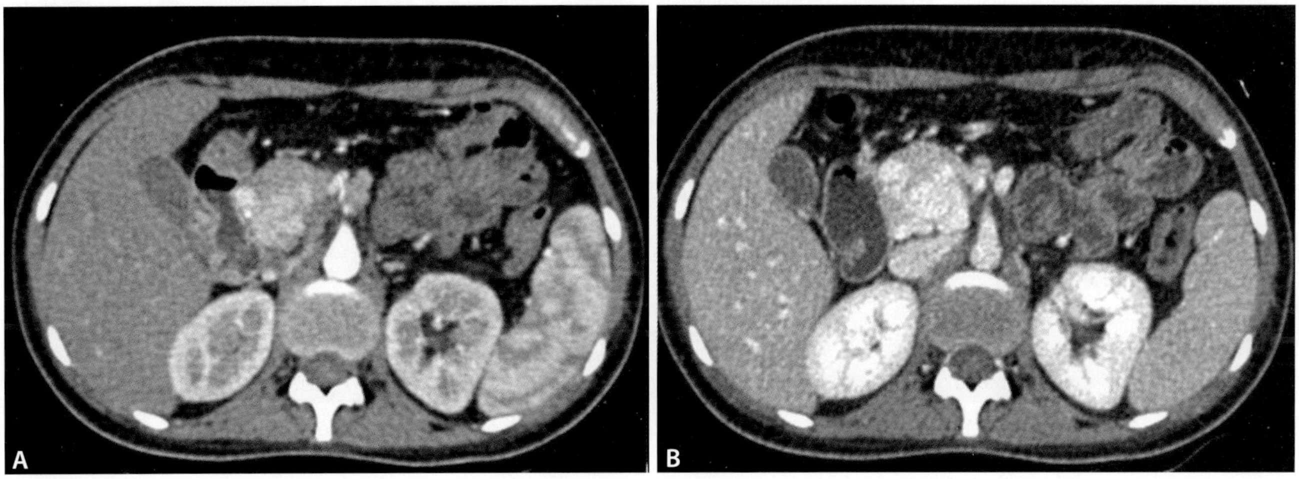

Figs. 4A and B: Contrast-enhanced CT images in arterial phase (A) showing normal Zebra-stripe/archiform enhancement pattern and venous phase (B) showing homogeneous enhancement.

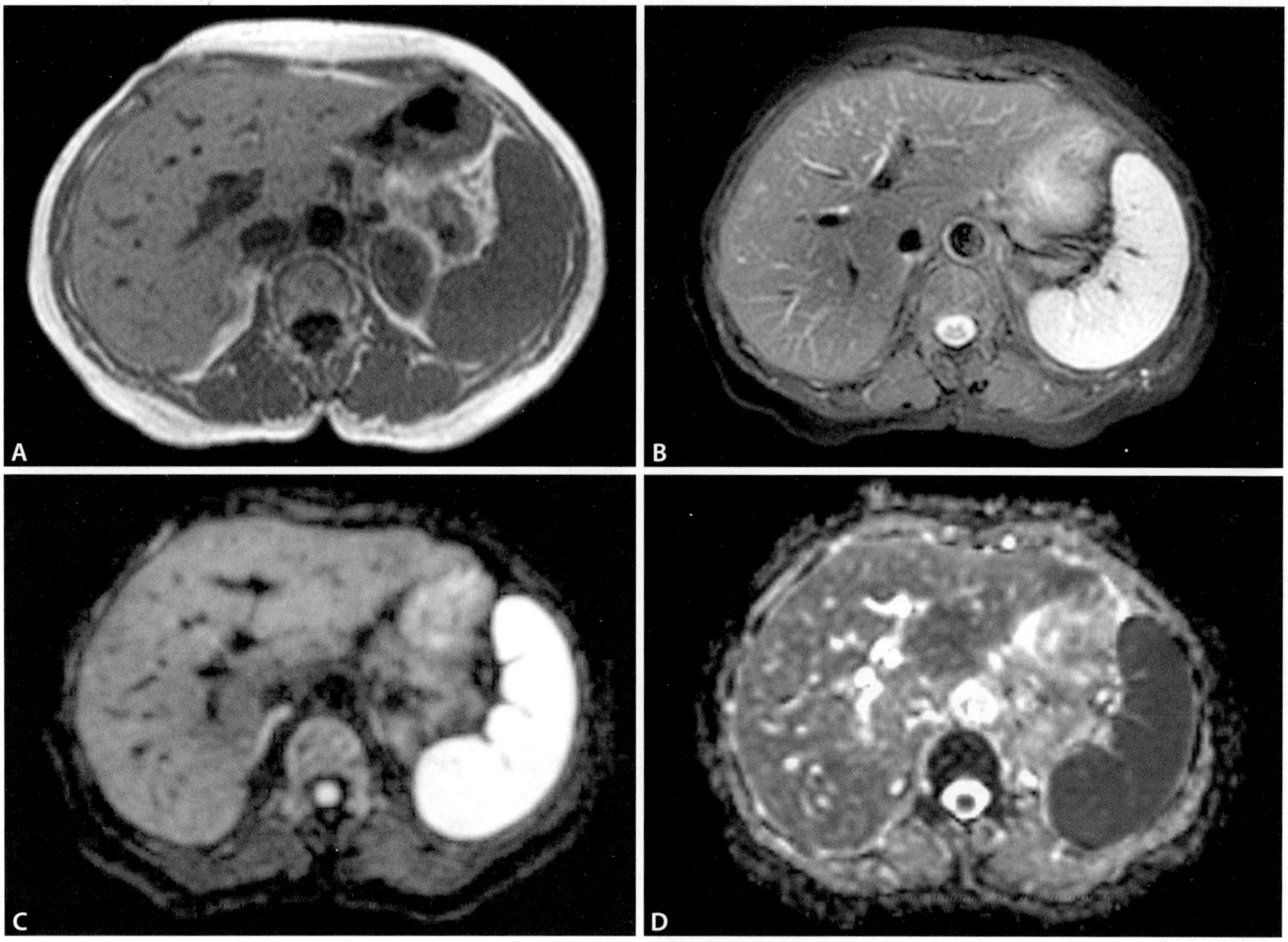

Figs. 5A to D: Axial T1WI (A), T2 WI (B), DWI- b 1000 (C), and ADC map (D) showing T1 hypointensity, T2 hyperintensity and restricted diffusion on DWI and ADC maps of normal spleen.

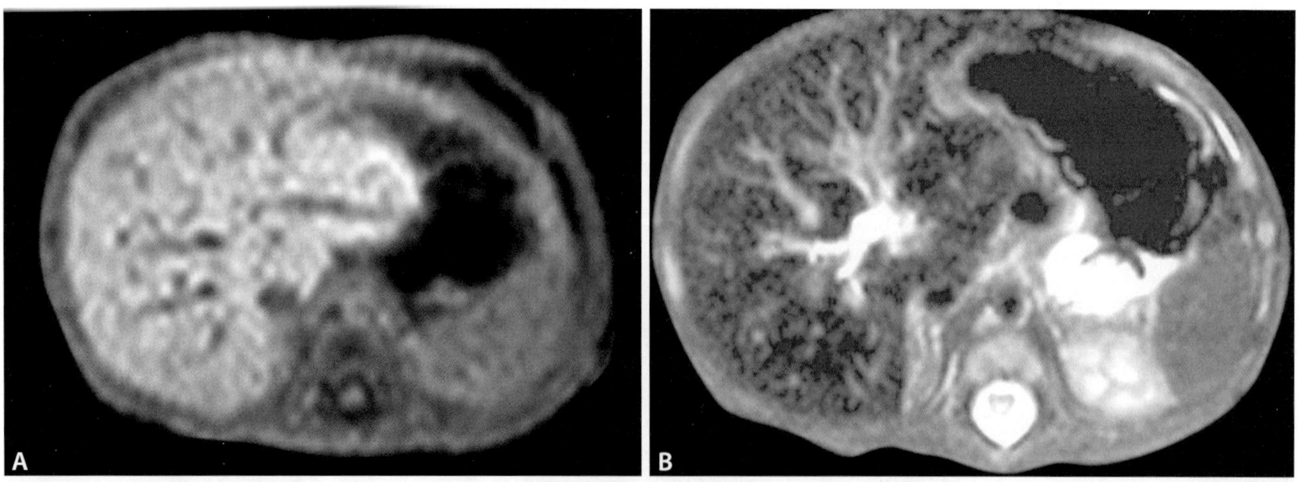

Figs. 6A and B: MRI T1WI (A) and T2WI (B) images showing normal hypointense spleen in a neonate.

seen commonly with early phase contrast-enhanced CT scans, are also seen with dynamic contrast-enhanced MRI **(Figs. 7A to C)**.

Scintigraphy

Scintigraphic splenic imaging involves the use of technetium-99m–labeled sulfur colloid. The tracer is taken up by the reticuloendothelial system and hence is helpful for the assessment of splenic congenital anomalies, e.g. splenic ectopia, accessory spleen, splenic hamartoma, etc.

Positron Emission Tomography/Computed Tomography (PET/CT)

It plays a role in evaluation of staging for lymphoma. Involvement of the spleen can be more accurately assessed using 18F- FDG PET or fused PET/CT.[14]

Angiography

The high quality of images provided by cross-sectional imaging techniques has led to a dramatic change in the indications for splenic artery angiography. This technique is now seldom used for diagnostic purpose; however, it is widely used for vascular interventions for the management of splenic artery aneurysms and traumatic splenic injuries. CT angiography and MR angiography offer excellent visualization of the spleen and its vessels for diagnostic purposes.

SPLENIC SIZE

On USG, the measurement of splenic length is done by measuring maximum distance on a longitudinal coronal view obtained at the level of splenic hilum, between the most inferolateral and the most superomedial points **(Fig. 2C)**. CT and MRI also readily allow for more standardized and reproducible measurement. Splenic volume can be readily measured with CT or MRI.

Normal splenic size in children and adolescents vary according to age and the upper limit of normal at various age range are given in **Table 1**. In normal adult, the spleen measures approximately 12 cm in length, 4 cm in thickness

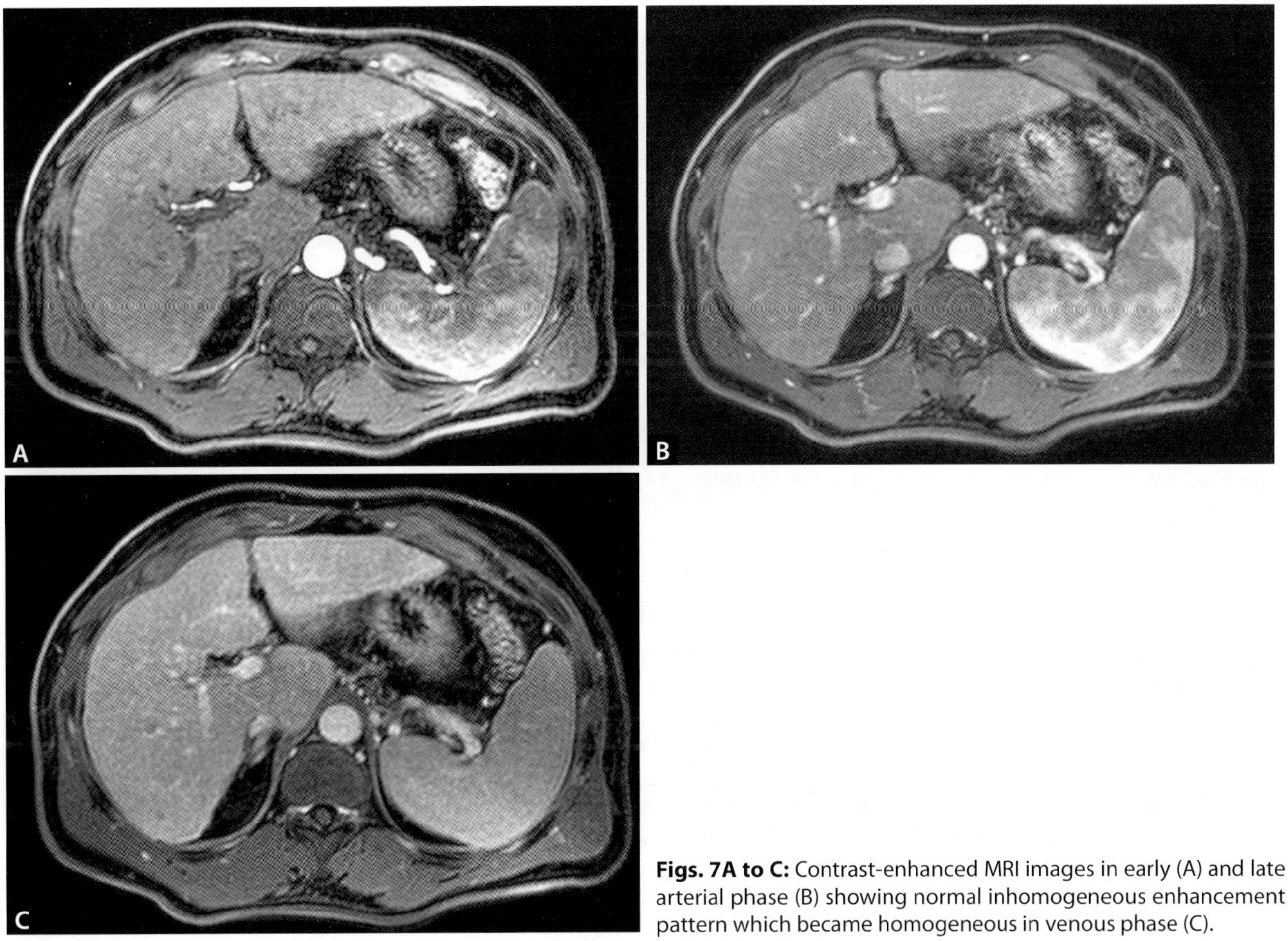

Figs. 7A to C: Contrast-enhanced MRI images in early (A) and late arterial phase (B) showing normal inhomogeneous enhancement pattern which became homogeneous in venous phase (C).

and 7 cm in anteroposterior (AP) diameter. However, due to high variability in the shape of the spleen, these measurements are not very useful in evaluating splenic size. A more precise approach for the estimation of splenic volume is the splenic index, a product of length, width and thickness of the spleen, expressed in centimeters **(Figs. 8A to C)**. Length is determined by summing the number of contiguous sections on which the spleen is visible or simpler is to measure the craniocaudal length in coronal reconstruction. Width is the longest AP splenic diameter in an axial image. Thickness is measured between the inner and outer borders of the spleen, at the level of the splenic hilum (normal splenic index is 120–480 cm^3).[15]

Table 1: Spleen Length in Children and Adolescents*.[16]

Group	No.	10th Percentile	Median	90th Percentile	Upper Limit
0–3 months	28	3.3	4.5	5.8	6.0
3–6 months	13	4.9	5.3	6.4	6.5
6–12 months	17	5.2	6.2	6.8	7.0
1–2 years	12	5.4	6.9	7.5	8.0
2–4 years	24	6.4	7.4	8.6	9.0
4–6 years	39	6.9	7.8	8.8	9.5
6–8 years	21	7.0	8.2	9.6	10.0
8–10 years	16	7.9	9.2	10.5	11.0
10–12 years	17	8.6	9.9	10.9	11.5
12–15 years	26	8.7	10.1	11.4	12.0
15–20 years (male)	5	9.0	10.0	11.7	12.0
15–20 years (female)	12	10.1	11.2	12.6	13.0

*All measurements are in centimeters.

NORMAL VARIANTS/DEVELOPMENTAL ANOMALIES

Various developmental anomalies are seen resulting from deficient fusion of separate splenic masses of the dorsal mesogastrium during embryogenesis. These include complete agenesis, persistent lobulations **(Fig. 9)**, clefts

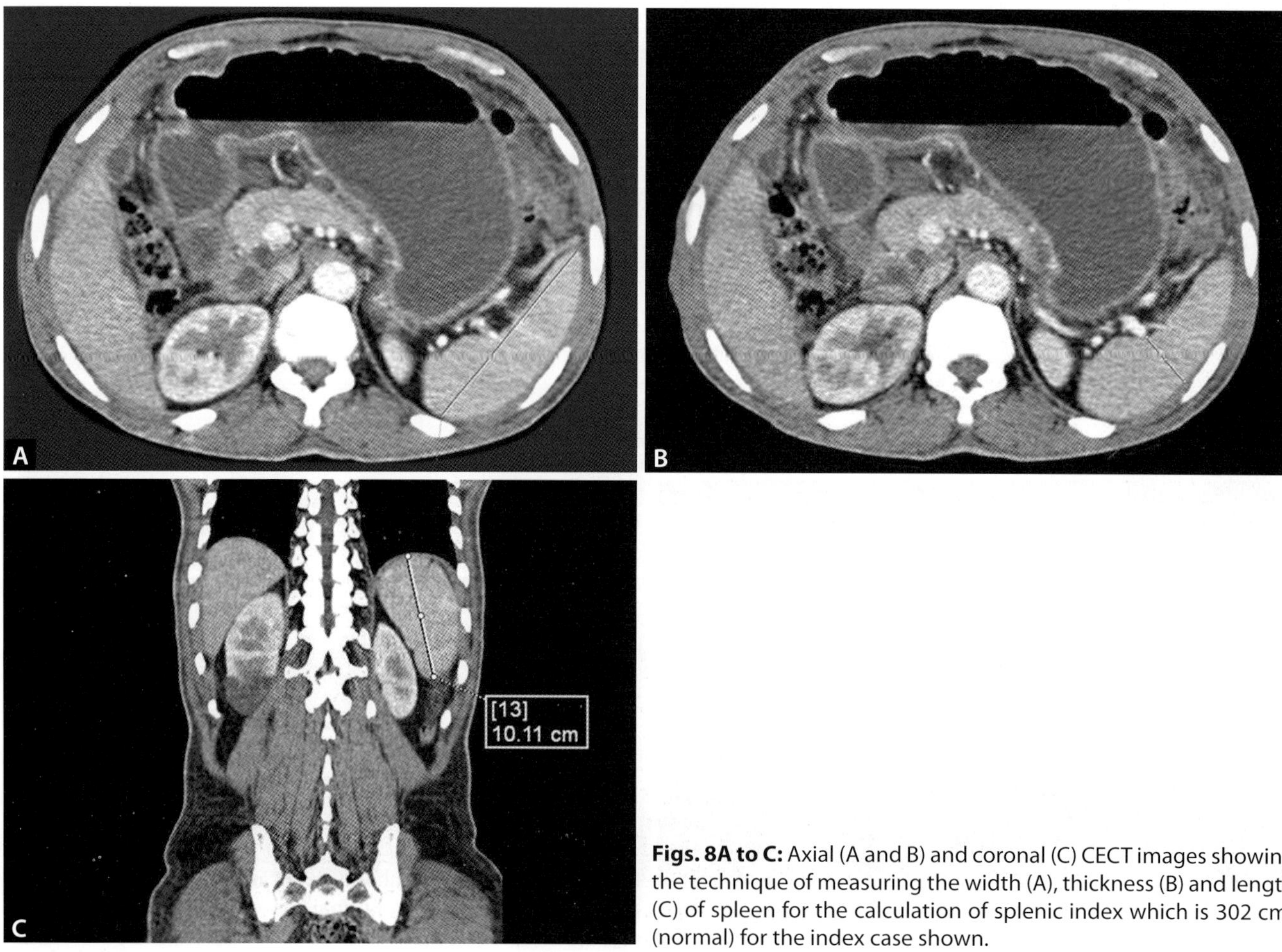

Figs. 8A to C: Axial (A and B) and coronal (C) CECT images showing the technique of measuring the width (A), thickness (B) and length (C) of spleen for the calculation of splenic index which is 302 cm^3 (normal) for the index case shown.

(Figs. 10A and B), notches, isolated small splenunculi and polysplenia.

Splenunculus/Accessory Spleen

Accessory spleen is the most frequent congenital abnormality of the spleen. They can be found virtually anywhere in the abdomen **(Figs. 11A and B)**, but the most common sites are hilus and vascular pedicle of the spleen, around tail of the pancreas, along the greater curvature of the stomach, greater omentum, mesentery, near left ovary or left testicle and in the pouch of Douglas.[17] Splenunculi are found in 10–44% of autopsies.[18] They are usually found incidentally on imaging done for unrelated reasons and generally require no treatment. The clinical significance of accessory spleen is that after splenectomy, the accessory spleen may dramatically enlarge and cause recurrence of symptoms if splenectomy was done for some hematologic or other disorders. Intrapancreatic location of accessory splenic tissue is also described, which may, if missed at surgery, be a cause of recurrence of the symptoms **(Figs. 11C and D)**. It enhances markedly in the arterial phase and is a rare differential diagnosis for neuroendocrine tumor of the pancreas. Splenunculi are usually six or fewer in number and they have histological features same as primary organ and has blood supply from a branch of the splenic artery.[17] They rarely exceed 2 cm in diameter and can be confused with splenic hilar or peripancreatic lymph nodes. Splenunculi can be identified on imaging modalities such as ultrasound, CT, or MRI, as of same attenuation or signal intensity as that of normal spleen **(Figs. 11E and F)** both before as well as after intravenous administration of contrast material but when there is doubt 99m Tc sulfur colloid liver-spleen scan is definitive.

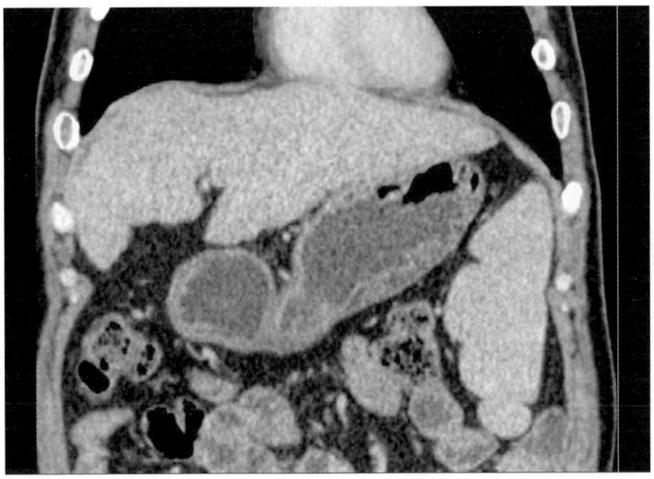

Fig. 9: Contrast-enhanced CT images (coronal reformat) showing prominent lobules of splenic tissue on medial and inferior aspect of spleen (suggesting persistence of fetal lobulations).

Ectopic splenic tissue can also be found due to acquired causes such as trauma (splenosis).

Wandering Spleen

Spleen changing its position within the abdomen due to ligamentous laxity, traumatic injury, maldevelopment of suspensory ligaments is referred to as wandering spleen. It may present as mobile unexplained mass in abdomen or may present with acute pain abdomen if torsion occurs.

It is thought to result from congenital abnormal fusion of the posterior mesogastrium.[19] Incidence of wandering

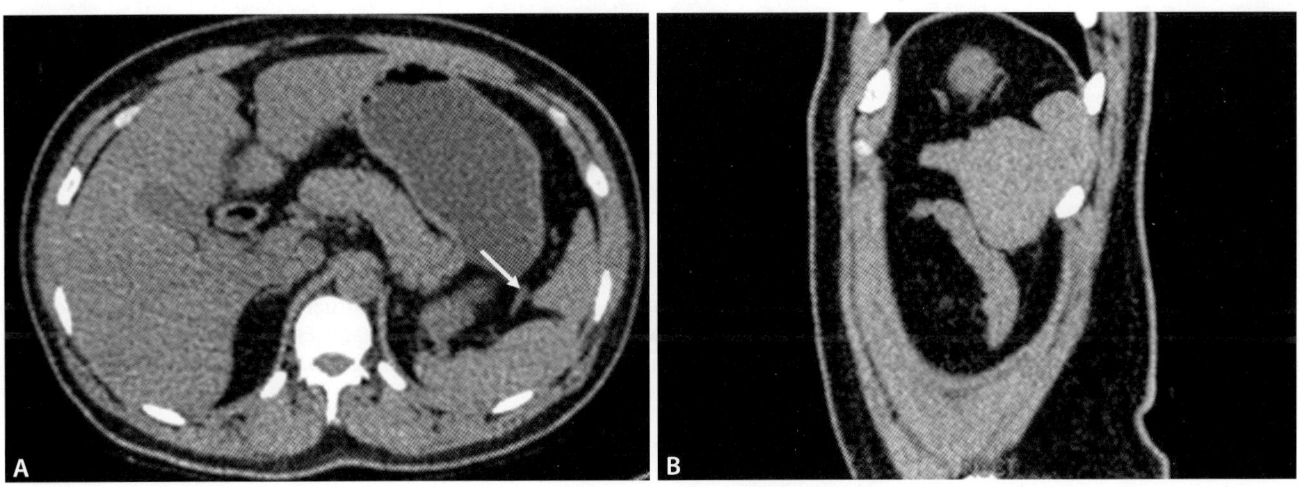

Figs. 10A and B: Non-contrast CT images [axial (A) and sagittal (B) reformat] showing splenic cleft (arrow). These may be confused with laceration in case of history of trauma.

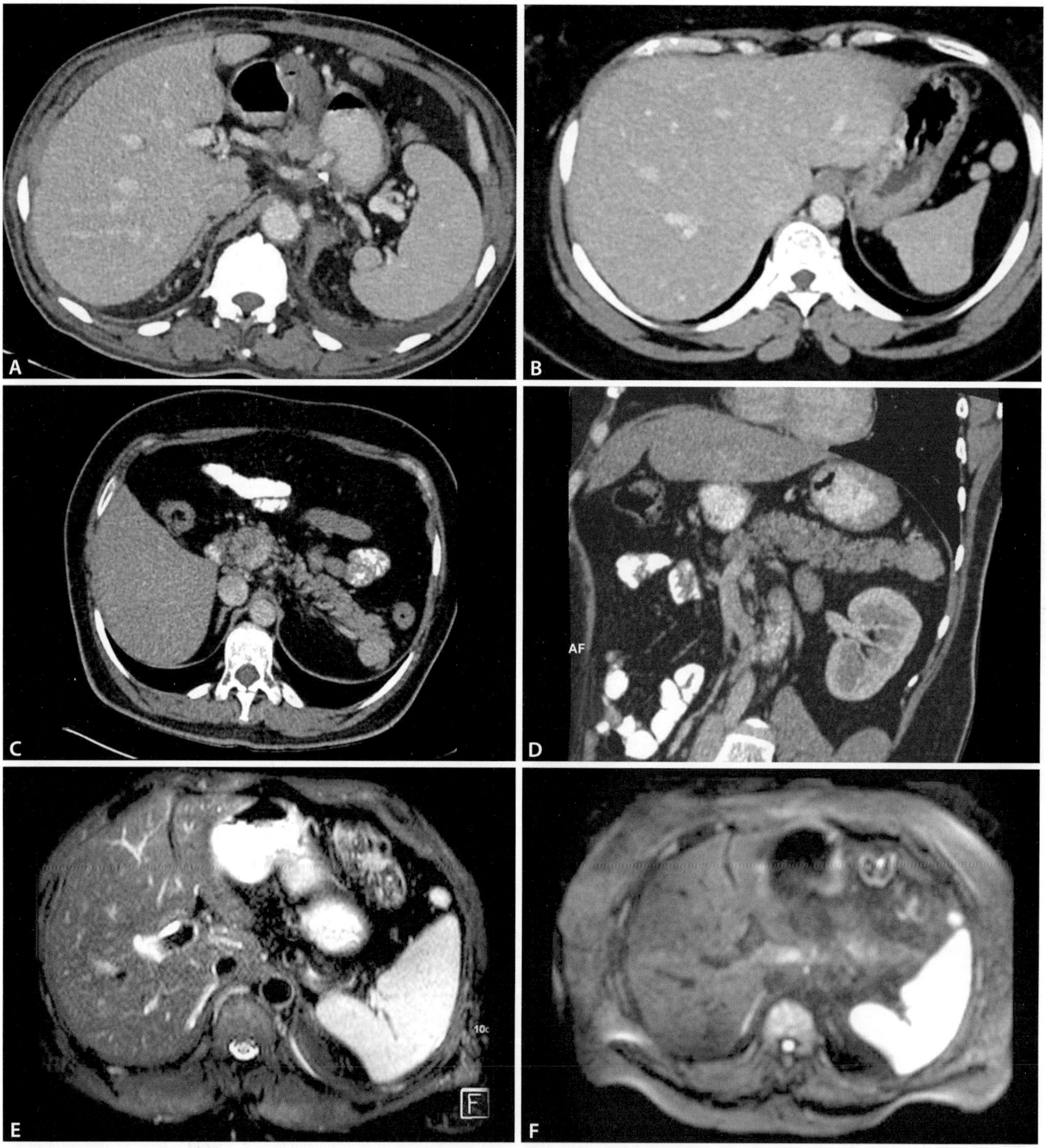

Figs. 11A to F: Axial contrast-enhanced CT images showing small rounded nodular well-defined structures having same enhancement as spleen at hilum (A), near pole (B) and within pancreatic parenchyma (C and D). Axial T2 WI MRI image (E) and b-1000 diffusion-weighted image (F) reveals splenunculus showing similar T2 hyperintensity and restricted diffusion respectively as adjacent normal spleen.

spleen is higher in multiparous women. On imaging, the changing position of the spleen can be determined on USG. CT **(Figs. 12A and B)** also can depict the same and in case of torsion may show a 'whorled appearance' of splenic pedicle. Splenic infarcts, ascites, pancreatic tail necrosis can also be identified.

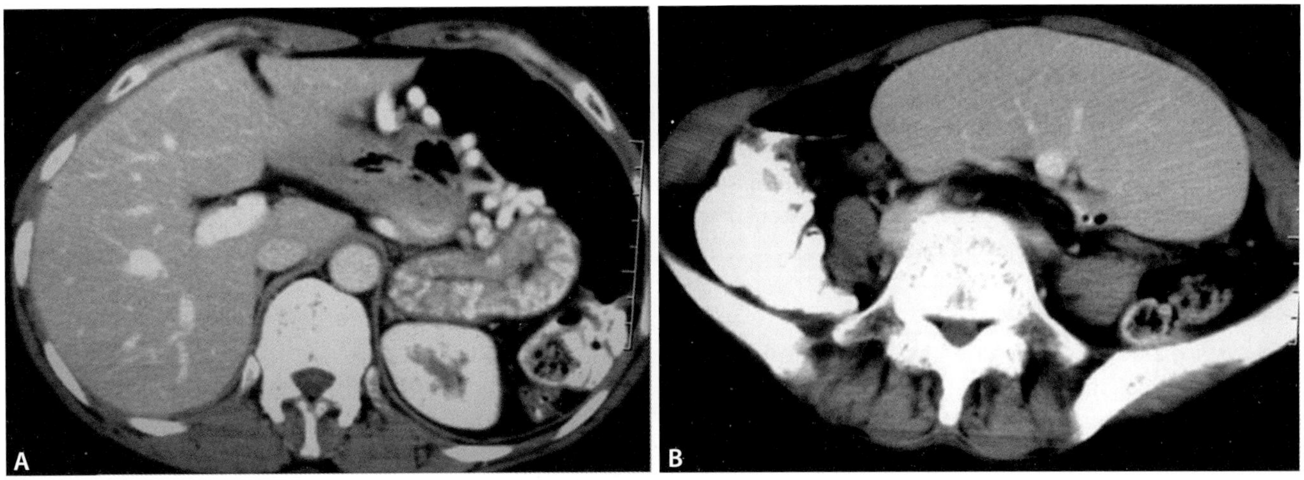

Figs. 12A and B: Axial contrast-enhanced CT showing absence of spleen in left upper abdomen (A) with centrally and inferiorly located spleen in lower abdomen (B). Follow-up USG revealed changing positions of spleen (not shown).

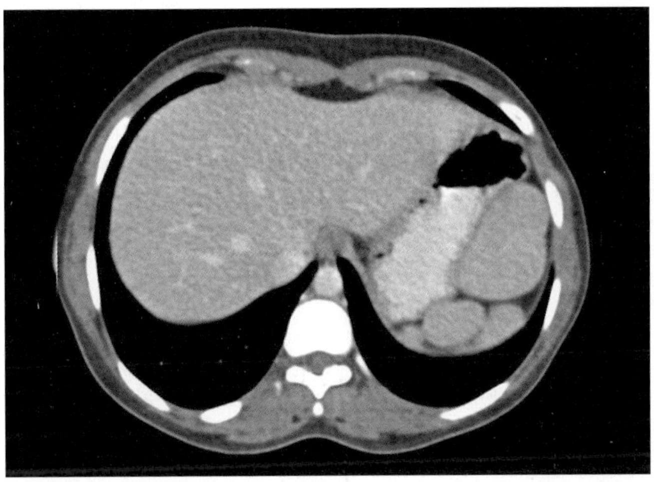

Fig. 13: Axial contrast-enhanced CT showing multiple small splenic masses in left subphrenic region suggestive of polysplenia.

Polysplenia

Presence of multiple splenules is known as polysplenia. It is seen in association with left-sided atrial isomerism syndrome and is more common in females than males. Patients with polysplenia may be asymptomatic or symptoms may occur due to congenital heart disease, biliary atresia or intestinal malrotation. On imaging, numerous small splenic masses are seen in the left **(Fig. 13)** or right hypochondrium.

Asplenia

Congenital absence of spleen is termed asplenia and it is seen in association with situs ambiguous. The condition is more common in males and association with congenital heart diseases is seen in 99–100% of the patients.[20]

CYSTIC LESIONS OF SPLEEN

The cystic lesions of the spleen can be primary (true) or secondary (pseudocyst) cysts, depending on the whether there is cellular or fibrous lining respectively.[21]

Primary cysts are divided into parasitic and non-parasitic. Primary non-parasitic cysts may be of epithelial origin (congenital cysts), such as epidermoid, dermoid, or transitional cell cysts, or of endothelial origin, such as lymphatic malformations and hemangiomas. Primary parasitic cysts include echinococcal cysts. Secondary/false or pseudocysts may form secondary to trauma, hematoma, infarction-degeneration or inflammation.

Congenital Cysts

Congenital or epithelial splenic cysts such as epidermoid, dermoid, or transitional cell cysts, account for about 25% of primary cysts of the spleen.[21] They are usually solitary, but can be multiple and are commonly seen in pediatric population and young adults. The exact etiopathogenesis of congenital splenic cysts is unknown. In general, these cysts are asymptomatic. Symptoms develop due to increase in size, trauma, hemorrhage, rupture or infection of the cyst.

When symptomatic, surgery in the form of partial or total splenectomy is the treatment of choice.

On USG, these cysts are generally anechoic, or may show fine internal echoes. CT shows splenic cysts as being characteristically spherical and well-defined lesions **(Figs. 14A to C)**. Attenuation value of near water and a thin or imperceptible nonenhancing wall are other features of a congenital cyst.[22] Internal debris, hemorrhage and peripheral calcifications of the cyst wall may give a more complex picture.

Epidermoid cyst **(Figs. 14D to G)** has a complex imaging appearance due to epithelial peripheral trabeculations causing thickening and irregularity of the posterior wall and due to presence of internal blood clots.

False Cyst (Pseudocyst)

False cysts/pseudocysts are lined by dense fibrous tissue which is often calcified and have no epithelial lining, and account for approximately 75% of the cysts of the spleen.[21] Trauma, infarction or infection are common causes. The most apparent etiologic factor is trauma. The majority of these cysts are solitary and asymptomatic. Cyst contains mostly blood and necrotic debris. It is often not possible to differentiate between primary and secondary cysts based on radiological appearance alone. Patient's history and clinical presentation may sometimes help to narrow the differential diagnosis.

Echinococcal Cyst

Splenic involvement by hydatid disease is uncommon. It can be seen in endemic areas. Clinical findings are nonspecific and patient may present with abdominal pain, fever and splenomegaly.

Ultrasonography demonstrates a cystic lesion which is either anechoic or with internal debris, membranes, daughter cysts or calcification depending upon the stage of cyst growth.

The three layers of hydatid cyst consist of the following:
1. The outer pericyst, composed of modified host cells that form a dense and fibrous protective zone.
2. Middle laminated layer, which is also referred to as ectocyst, allows passage of nutrients.
3. Inner germinal layer, where the scolices (the larval stage of the parasite) and the laminated membrane are produced. The true wall of the cyst is formed by this inner most germinal layer.

Daughter cysts are small spherical vesicles formed from rest of the germinal layer and contain the protoscolices. Cyst fluid secreted by the germinal layer is antigenic and may also contain scolices. When vesicles rupture within the cyst, scolices are mixed with cyst fluid and form white sediment known as hydatid sand.

Imaging features on USG, CT or MRI depend on stage of growth of the cyst, i.e. whether it is unilocular, have daughter vesicles, partially calcified or completely calcified signifying a dead parasite.

The ultrasonographic appearance of hydatid cysts are:
i. A well-defined anechoic cyst **(Fig. 15C)**.
ii. A well-defined anechoic cyst with hydatid sand.
iii. Detachment of the endocyst from pericyst resulting in "floating membranes" within the cavity.
iv. The honeycomb pattern due to presence of daughter cysts.
v. Calcification of either cyst wall or internal matrix. Partial calcification of the cyst does not always indicate the death of the parasite, nevertheless, densely calcified cysts may be assumed to be inactive.

Infected hydatid may give an appearance of abscess with thick irregular walls and internal debris and lose its characteristic sonographic appearance.

The CT scans show the cyst as a well-defined, round or oval cystic mass of near water density **(Figs. 15A to E)**. A multilocular appearance may be seen with the presence of multiple low attenuating daughter cysts. Detached membranes can be seen as curvilinear increased attenuation areas within the cyst. Homogeneous higher attenuation within the lesion is frequently encountered and may occur secondary to the formation of daughter cysts or as a result of the collection of dense debris (hydatid sand) within the cyst. Enhancement of internal septations may be seen with contrast administration. Calcification of cyst wall or internal septa is easily detected at CT.

Splenic hydatid cysts are T1-hypointense and T2-hyperintense on MRI. Collagen makes the pericyst appear T1 and T2 hypointense and this low signal intensity rim on T2WI has been proposed as a characteristic sign of hydatid cyst. MR also demonstrates daughter cysts as hypo to isointense on T1WI and isointense on T2WI relative to hyperintense hydatid fluid of the mother cyst. The floating membranes appear as low intensity structures within the degenerating cyst. Intraparenchymal rupture of the cyst appears as a defect in the low intensity rim. Thick calcifications may produce a signal void on MR imaging, however, are better demonstrated by CT.

INFECTIOUS DISEASES OF SPLEEN

Involvement of the spleen in systemic infectious processes is commonly seen in immunocompromised patients, and the prevalence has increased as a result of the increased use of steroids and chemotherapeutic agents and human immunodeficiency virus (HIV) infection.[11] Bacteria, fungi, and *Mycobacterium tuberculosis* are frequent agents. Splenic involvement can also occur in immune-competent hosts with cat scratch disease, granulomatous diseases

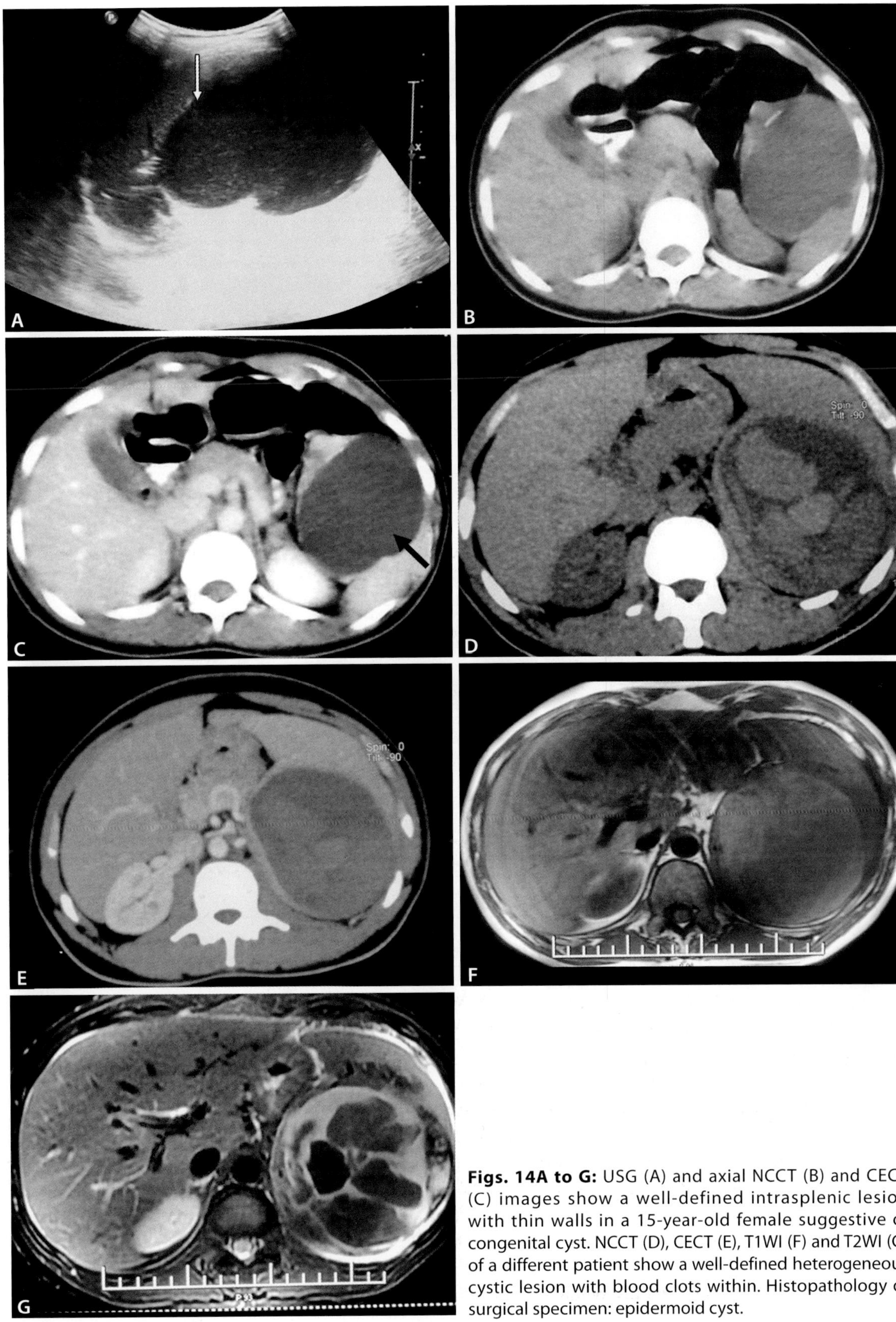

Figs. 14A to G: USG (A) and axial NCCT (B) and CECT (C) images show a well-defined intrasplenic lesion with thin walls in a 15-year-old female suggestive of congenital cyst. NCCT (D), CECT (E), T1WI (F) and T2WI (G) of a different patient show a well-defined heterogeneous cystic lesion with blood clots within. Histopathology of surgical specimen: epidermoid cyst.

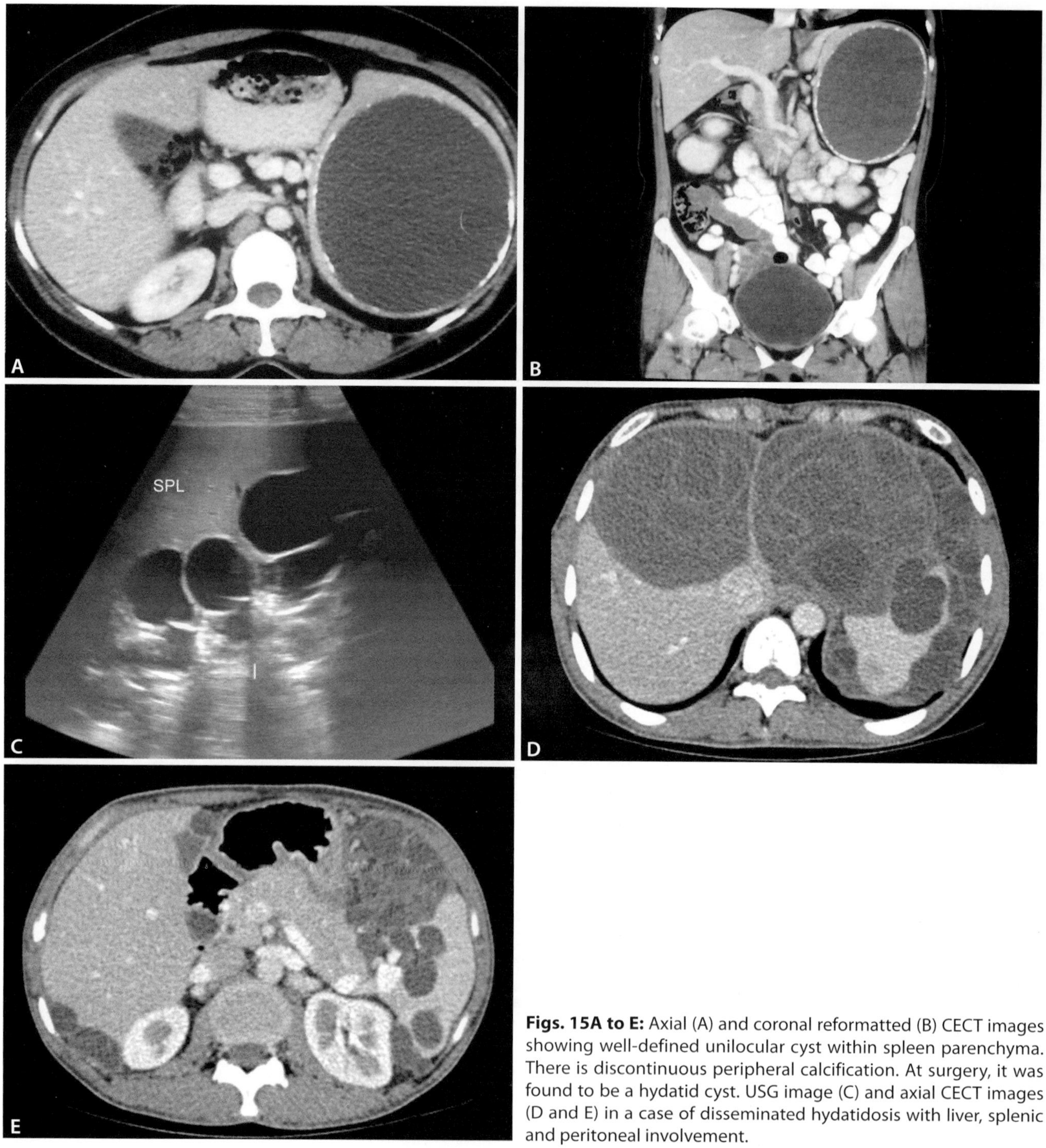

Figs. 15A to E: Axial (A) and coronal reformatted (B) CECT images showing well-defined unilocular cyst within spleen parenchyma. There is discontinuous peripheral calcification. At surgery, it was found to be a hydatid cyst. USG image (C) and axial CECT images (D and E) in a case of disseminated hydatidosis with liver, splenic and peritoneal involvement.

such as histoplasmosis, parasitic diseases such as hydatid cyst, and viral infections. Nonspecific splenomegaly can be seen in viral infections and enteric fever.

Splenic abscesses are localized collection of pus and they are found in 0.14–0.7% of autopsy cases.[23] It may be solitary, multiple, or multilocular. USG shows single or multiple hypoechoic to frankly anechoic lesions. Larger lesion may show internal echoes or septations. On CT and MR, the abscess appears as a lesion of fluid attenuation or signal intensity respectively and show peripheral enhancement on contrast administration when the capsule develops **(Figs. 16A and B)**.

Bacterial causes of splenic abscess include infection with aerobic organisms, commonly *Staphylococcus, Streptococcus, Escherichia coli* and *Salmonella*. The route of infection is mainly hematogenous (75%), penetrating trauma (15%) and prior splenic infarction (10%).[21] The factors leading to involvement of the spleen are metastatic infection (bacterial endocarditis, sepsis), contiguous infection (pancreatitis, periphrenic abscess), embolic noninfection events causing ischemia and superadded infection, trauma and immunodeficiency.[24]

On CT and MRI, the lesion shows thick, irregular, dense peripheral enhancing rim with internal nonenhancing area. Sometimes, air foci may also be seen within the bacterial abscesses. Peripheral enhancement of the wall of the abscess on a venous phase CT is less often seen than in liver abscesses. Post-gadolinium MRI is more sensitive to depict the rim enhancement.

Fungal abscesses are mainly seen in immunocompromised patients including post solid organ transplantation, patients on chemotherapy for malignancy or leukemia and children with immunodeficiency, such as chronic granulomatous disease. *Candida albicans, Aspergillus fumigatus,* and *Cryptococcus neoformans* are the commonly encountered fungi. Fungal infection of the spleen are mostly due to hematogenous spread and form microabscesses in the splenic parenchyma which may not be detectable on imaging at times even in the presence of disseminated infection and may only present with diffuse splenomegaly. When visible on CT, fungal abscesses are seen as multiple well-defined small hypoattenuating lesions and vary from few millimeters to 2 cm in size. Rim enhancement is usually not seen. Occasionally, CT may demonstrate a wheel within a wheel pattern/bulls-eye (e.g. Candidial infection) or a central focus of higher attenuation corresponding to ultrasound findings (echoic lesion with central hypoechoic nidus due to necrosis containing fungal elements). Histoplasmosis of the spleen demonstrates multiple scattered hypointense lesions on both T1 and T2WI on MRI **(Figs. 17A to D)**. Old granulomas can be calcified.

Splenic involvement is seen in 80–100% of autopsies of disseminated Tuberculosis since it has a rich network of reticuloendothelial cells.[25] Three forms of splenic involvement include splenomegaly, micronodular/miliary or macronodular form. USG may show normal spleen or mild heterogeneous echotexture whereas CT may demonstrate multiple low-density intrasplenic foci with nodules that range from 0.5 mm to 2.0 mm in diameter in the micronodular form of disease **(Figs. 18A to D)**. Macronodular form manifests as solitary or multifocal 1–3 cm sized lesions which are hypodense on CT **(Figs. 19A to F)**, and sometimes show peripheral rim of enhancement and may demonstrate calcification. MRI features vary depending on the stage of evolution of tuberculomas. A tuberculoma with central caseous necrosis appears as a centrally nonenhancing lesion with peripheral enhancement and this is one of their typical features. Such caseous necrosis might show hypointensity or hyperintensity on T2WI. The reason for the variable signal on T2WI is not clearly understood;

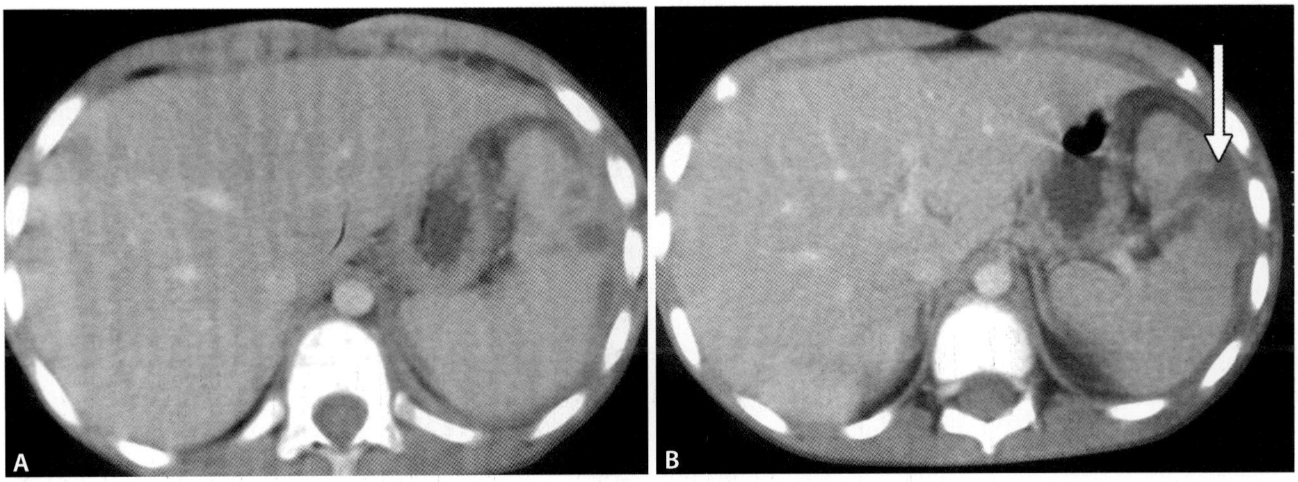

Figs. 16A and B: Axial CECT images (A and B) showing multiple small peripherally enhancing lesions in spleen suggestive of abscesses. Presence of perisplenic fluid (arrow) indicates rupture.

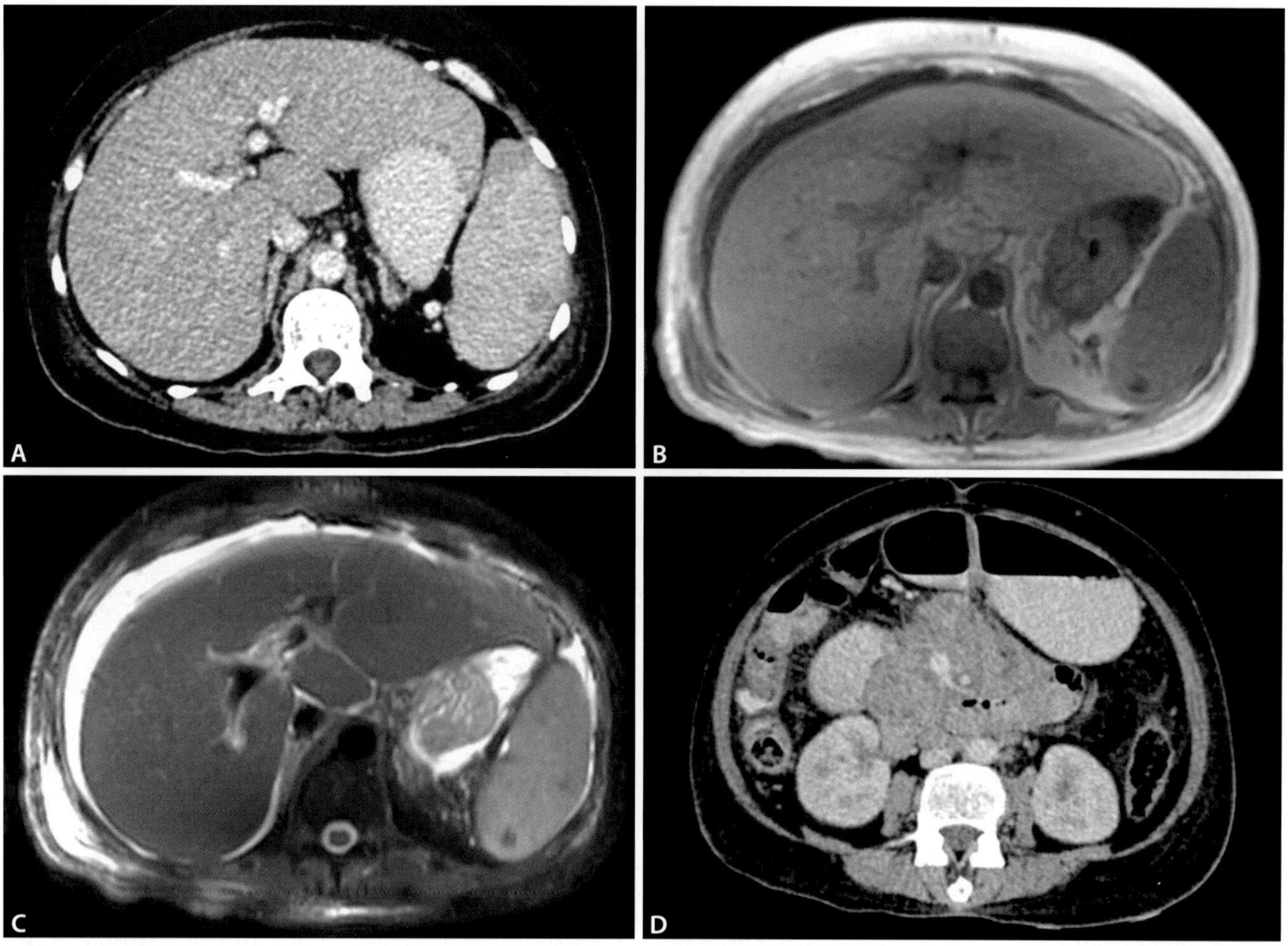

Figs. 17A to D: Axial CECT image (A) showing ill-defined focal lesions in spleen. Axial T1WI (B) and T2WI (C) shows hypointense lesions on both sequences. Axial CECT image (D) showing multiple lymph nodes with necrosis—Biopsy proven histoplasmosis.

however, internal hypointensity could suggest more solid caseation **(Fig. 19C)**.[26] Lesions with no central caseous necrosis may demonstrate gradual peripheral enhancement with complete fill-in of the lesions. Other imaging findings may be abdominal lymphadenopathy with low central attenuation, high-attenuation ascites with nodular peritoneal thickening, hepatomegaly, and pleural effusion. Other organ involvement or presence of necrotic lymph nodes makes a diagnosis of tuberculosis more certain.

It is difficult to distinguish between tubercular, pyogenic and disseminated fungal infections as well as leukemic and lymphomatous infiltration. Fine needle aspiration cytology (FNAC) from splenic focal lesions is required to reach a definitive diagnosis if there is no other focus of tuberculosis or in case of non-responders to treatment.

Splenic Infarcts

Splenic infarcts are a relatively common entity. It is usually secondary to arterial occlusion. The various recognized causes of spleen infarct are arterial embolism, massive splenomegaly secondary to myeloproliferative disorders or hematological malignancies, storage disorders, lymphoma, portal hypertension, torsion, infectious mononucleosis, etc. Imaging findings of splenic infarct depend upon the 'age of infarct'. On USG, it is seen as an ill-defined hypoechoic area in acute phase which progressively becomes more well defined. In later stage, secondary to fibrosis and calcification it may appear as hyperechoic area also. Splenic rupture and superimposed infection are complications seen in the areas of infarction.[9]

CT is the imaging investigation of choice for evaluation of splenic infarcts. Imaging should be performed in portal

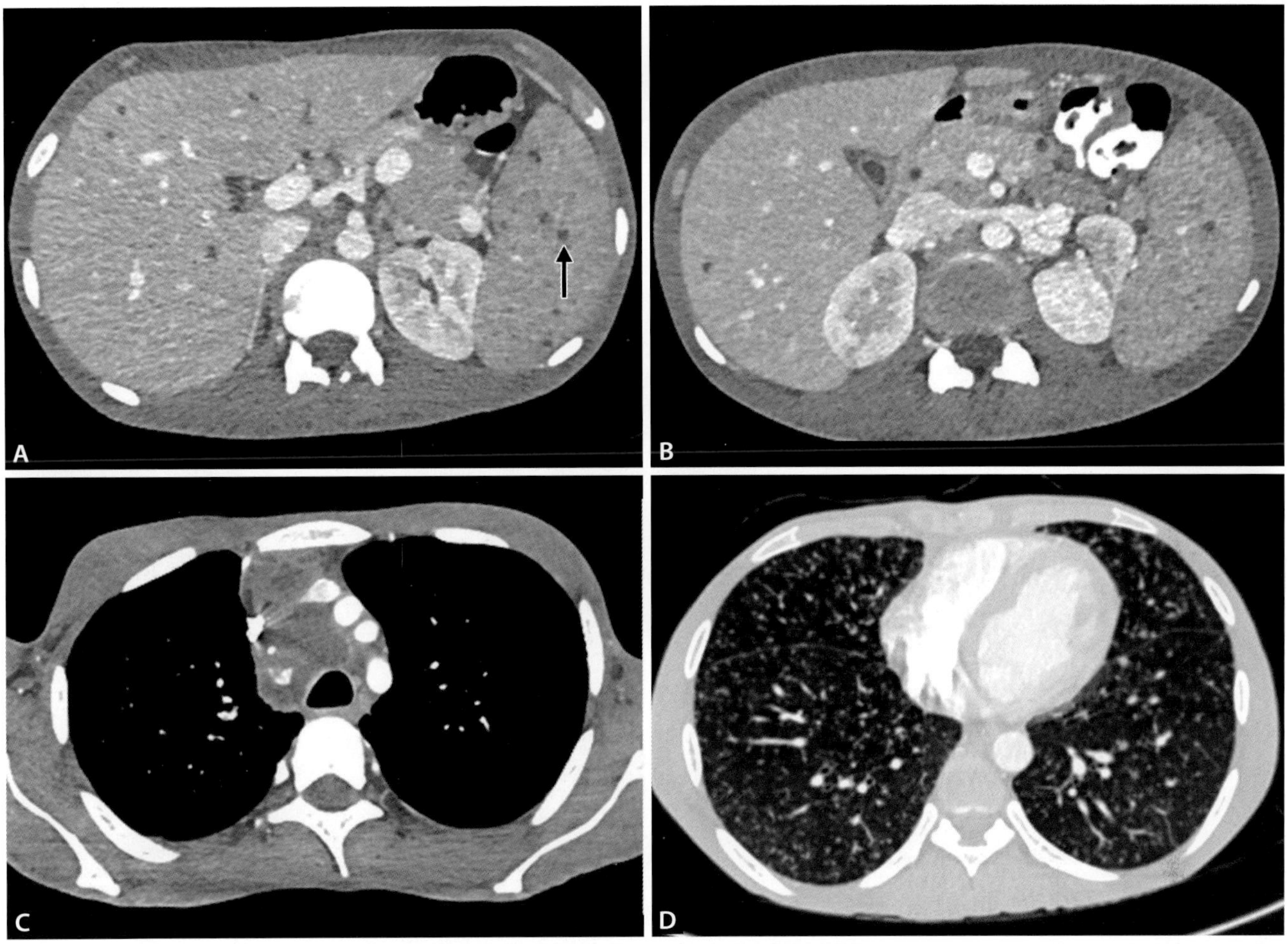

Figs. 18A to D: Axial CECT images (A and B) of 20-year-male patient with disseminated tuberculosis showing multiple diffusely scattered tiny hypodense lesions in spleen (arrow). Similar lesions also noted in liver and pancreas. Mediastinal (C) and lung window images (D) showing necrotic lymph nodes and miliary nodules respectively.

venous phase images, which reveal better depiction of the infarcted areas.

On CT, various imaging findings are described for infarcts. There are multiple, heterogeneous areas of patchy enhancement in acute phase. Typical peripheral, wedge-shaped nonenhancing or hypoenhancing area is seen with further progression with time **(Fig. 20A)**. Entire splenic parenchyma may not be enhancing, e.g. in splenic torsion. With time, the infarcted area may decrease and sometimes may vanish entirely or may remain as a cystic lesion (pseudocyst).

The MRI shows various signal intensity in splenic infarct based on its chronicity and composition. If infarct is hemorrhagic, it may appear as hyperintense on T1 as well as T2WI. Chronic infarcts will be relatively well defined; wedge shaped and usually have hypointense signal on T1WI and hyperintense signal on T2WI **(Figs. 20A to H)**.[27]

Trauma

Please refer to chapter on Abdominal Trauma for full discussion of splenic trauma.

Splenic Rupture

Splenic rupture most commonly occurs secondary to significant trauma. However, there are many uncommon cause of splenic rupture other than trauma.[28] This condition of atraumatic splenic rupture has been variously described as 'spontaneous', 'pathological' or 'occult' splenic rupture. Practically, it refers to rupture of spleen in the absence of any perceivable significant injury to

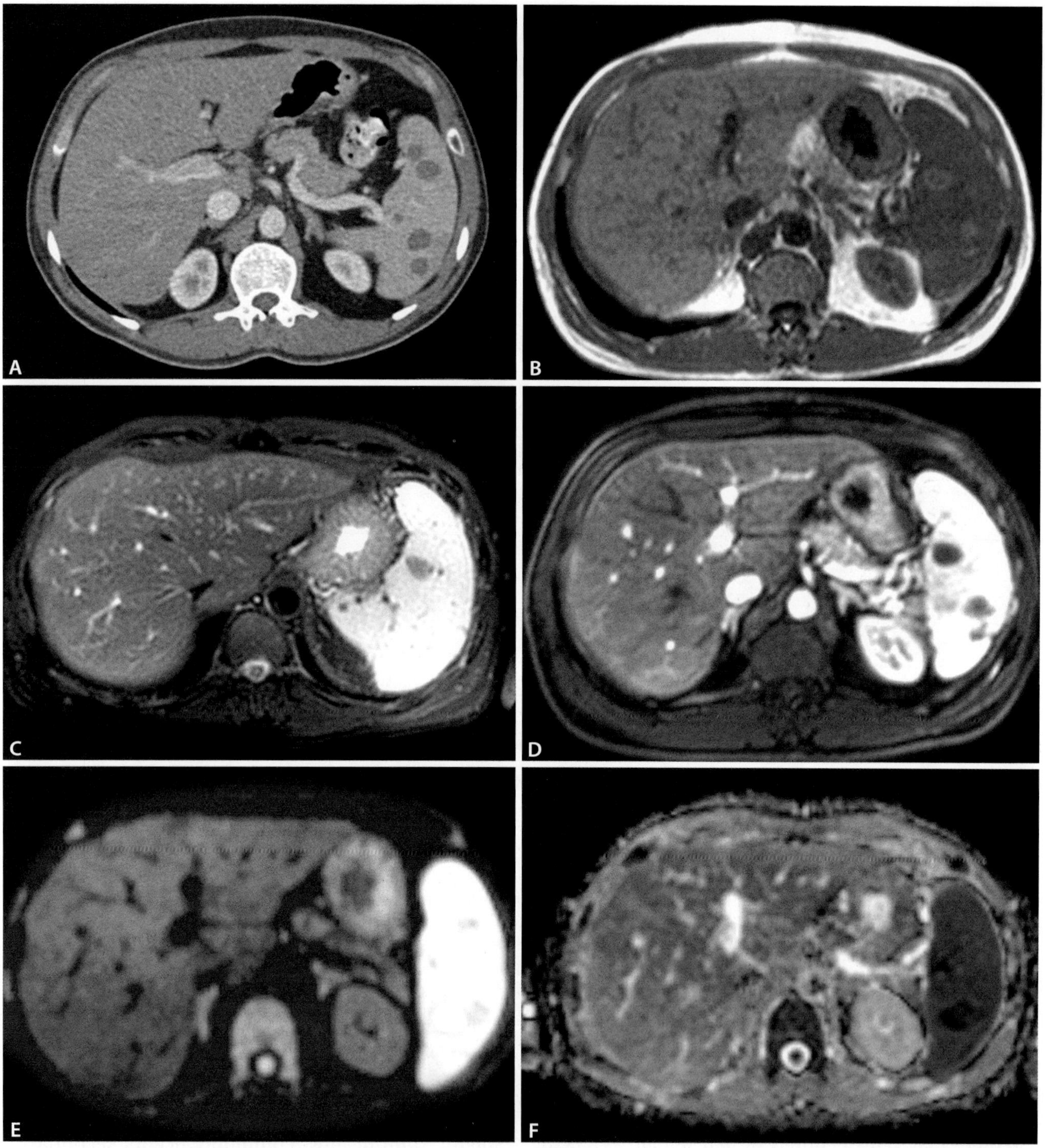

Figs. 19A to F: Axial CECT (A) image showing multiple large hypodense lesions in spleen. T1WI (B), T2WI (C), Postcontrast T1WI (D), DWI (E) ADC map (F) MRI images of patient with macronodular form of tuberculosis (FNAC proven).

spleen. Various causes of atraumatic splenic rupture are malaria, leukemia, lymphomas, secondary to pancreatitis, congestive splenomegaly, amyloidosis, infectious mononucleosis or splenic abscess, etc.

Exact pathogenesis of truly idiopathic splenic rupture (with causes unknown) is still not clear. Majority of these patients have associated splenomegaly. Imaging findings associated with splenic rupture are commonly similar

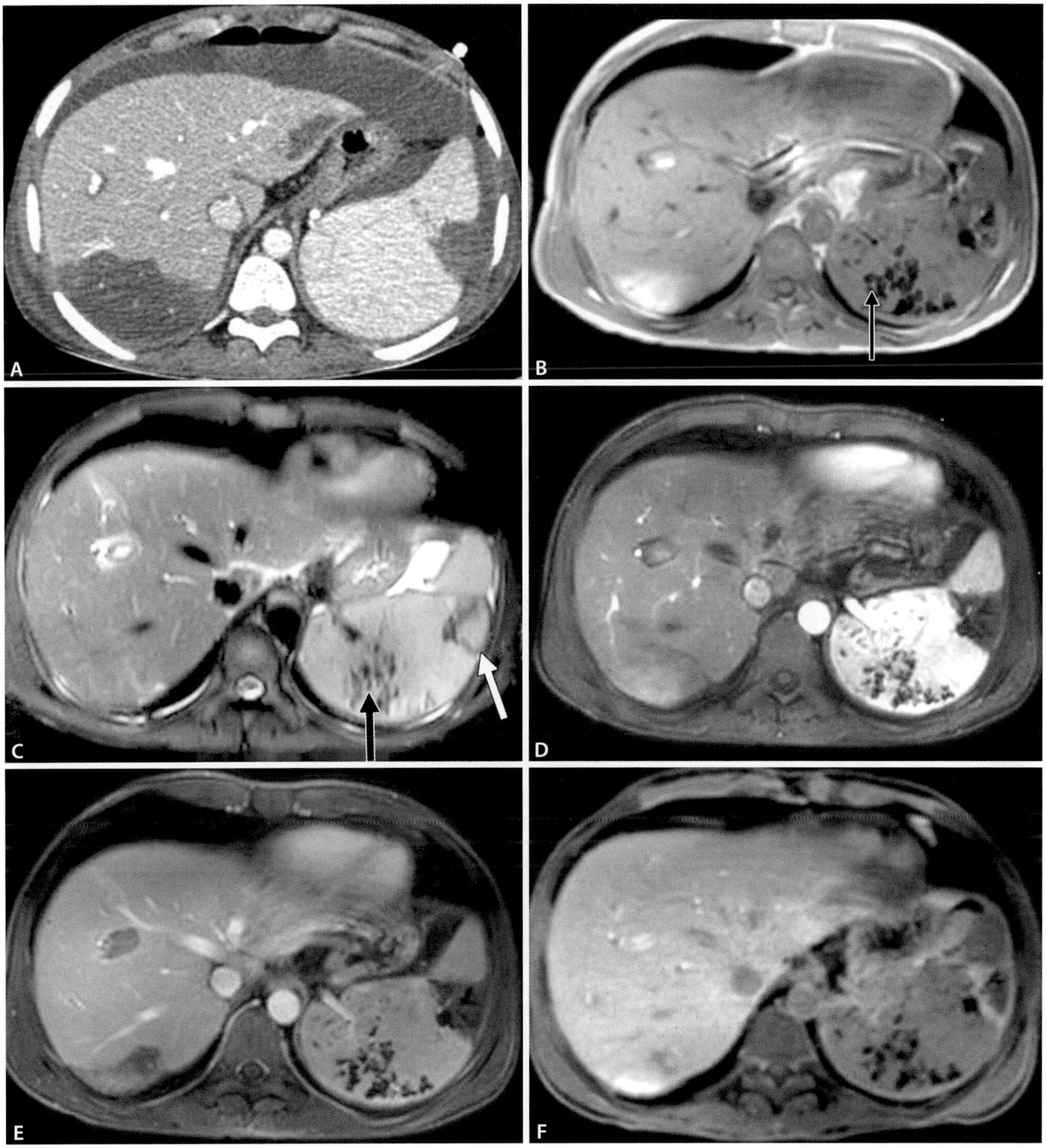

Figs. 20A to F

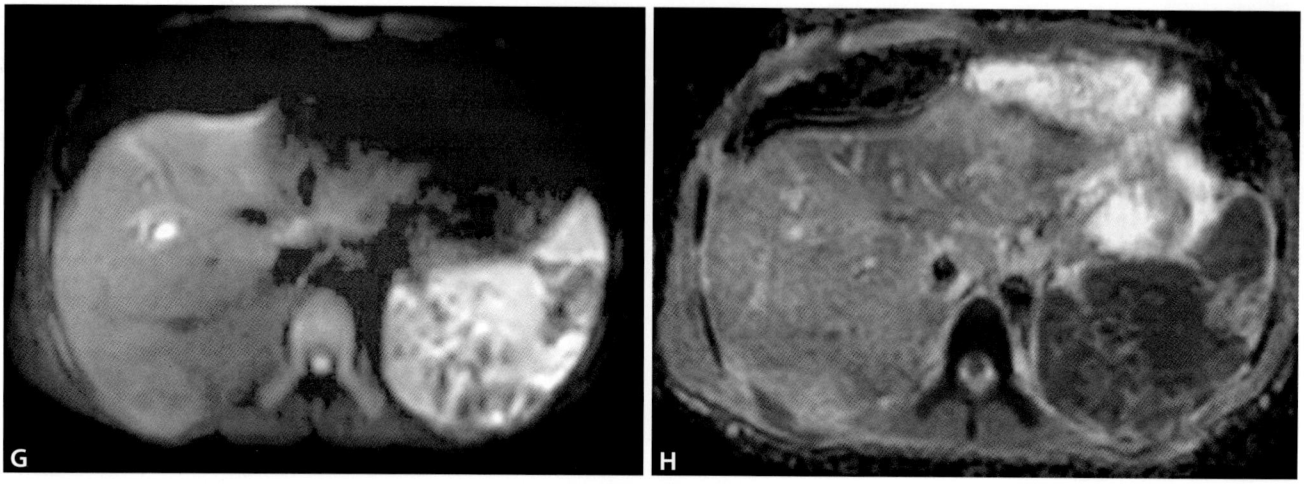

Figs. 20G and H

Figs. 20A to H: Contrast-enhanced CT scan (A) showing peripheral wedge-shaped hypodensity in spleen suggestive of infarct. Incidentally liver infarct is also seen. T1WI (hyperintense) (B) and T2WI (C) (hyperintense with hypointense rim) respectively showing peripheral wedge-shaped altered signal intensity (white arrow). Multiple T1 and T2 hypointense Gamna-Gandy bodies are also noted (black arrow). Arterial (D) venous (E) and delayed (F) MR images showing nonenhancing area with peripheral enhancement on delayed phase. DWI (G) and ADC map (H) showing no restriction (suggestive of chronic infarct—3 months).

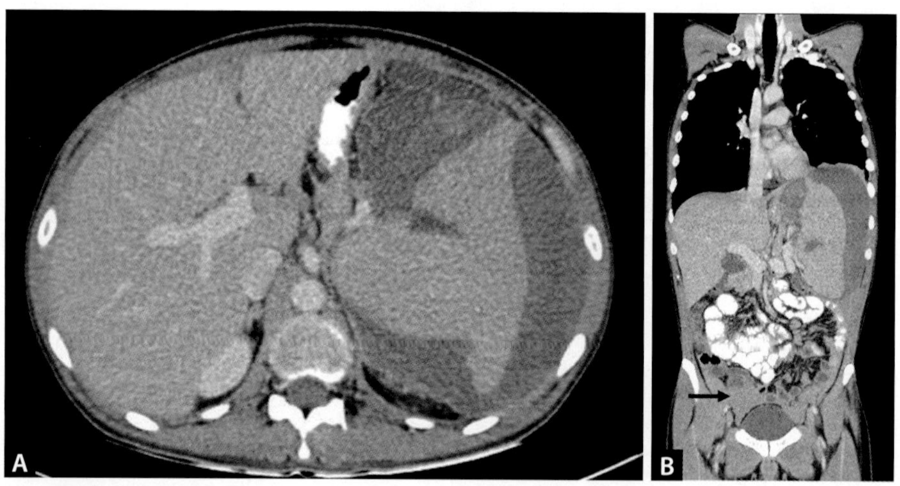

Figs. 21A and B: Axial (A) and coronal-reformatted (B) CECT images showing laceration in the medial margin of an enlarged spleen with perisplenic hematoma and hemoperitoneum (arrow) in a patient with high-grade fever and splenomegaly. No history of trauma was present suggestive of spontaneous splenic rupture.

to cases of post-traumatic splenic rupture, however, the incidence of splenomegaly is more common in these atraumatic patients. On USG, fluid with internal echoes is seen in perisplenic area and peritoneal cavity. Other findings may be subcapsular hematoma and hypoechoic splenic laceration. CECT will depict similar findings **(Figs. 21A and B)**. On arterial phase CT images, sometimes areas of active extravasation may be seen which signifies ongoing active bleed. MRI may be helpful in deciding the 'age' of hematoma. Majority of these patients are treated by surgery.

SPLENIC NEOPLASMS

Splenic neoplasms can be divided into benign and malignant neoplasms. Among the benign lesions, hemangioma, lymphangioma, hamartoma, littoral cell angioma, peliosis and inflammatory pseudotumors are common. Among the malignant lesions, metastasis, lymphoma and angiosarcoma are common entities.

Benign Neoplasms

Hemangioma

Hemangioma is the most common benign primary neoplasm of spleen with prevalence ranging from 0.3–14%.[29] Most hemangiomas are small in size and detected incidentally on imaging. When large, it may present with pain in left hypochondrium with presence of palpable non tender mass. Splenic hemangiomatosis may occur in cases with generalized angiomatosis, like Klippel-Trenaunay syndrome.[30] Spontaneous rupture may occur in 25% of the patients having large hemangiomas.[31]

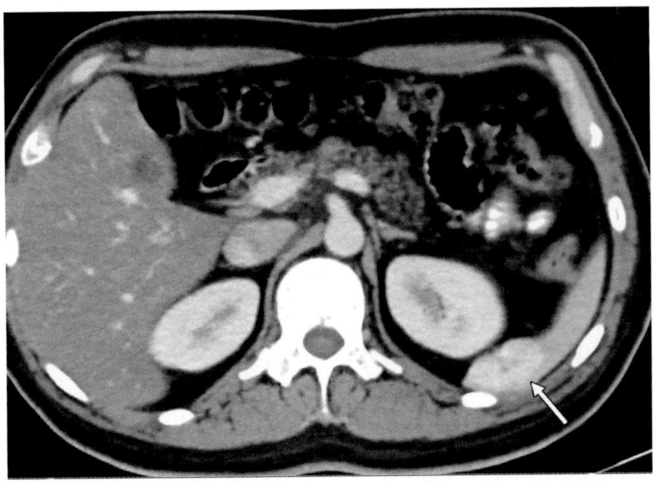

Fig. 22: Axial CECT showing an enhancing lesion in lower pole of spleen suggestive of hemangioma. Incidentally a metastatic lesion is seen in segment 5 of liver.

On USG, they are seen as echogenic solid or cystic lesions which are iso to hypodense on unenhanced CT. Hemangioma can be capillary and cavernous on histology. The cavernous hemangiomas have solid isodense component which show enhancement on contrast administration while cystic component remains hypodense **(Fig. 22)**. Peripheral punctuate calcification may be seen on CT. On MRI, the lesions are hyperintense relative to spleen on T2WI and hypo-to isointense on T1WI. After injection of gadolinium, three patterns of enhancement have been described: (a) immediate homogeneous enhancement which persists, (b) early peripheral enhancement with delayed uniform enhancement, and (c) peripheral enhancement which progresses centripetally with presence of enhancing central fibrous scar.[32]

Lymphangioma

Lymphangioma is a congenital malformation of lymphatic system that occurs most commonly in neck, mediastinum and retroperitoneum; rarely affecting the spleen.[33] Splenic lymphangiomas are asymptomatic in majority of patients and detected incidentally. Spleen may be normal in size or enlarged and shows presence of predominantly cystic masses. These lesions are seen as anechoic to hypoechoic well defined intrasplenic cysts on USG and hypodense lesions on CT; with few showing fine internal septations **(Figs. 23A and B)** or echogenic debris within. Thin calcification may be seen along the periphery.[34] The signal intensity on MRI corresponds to simple fluid; however, the

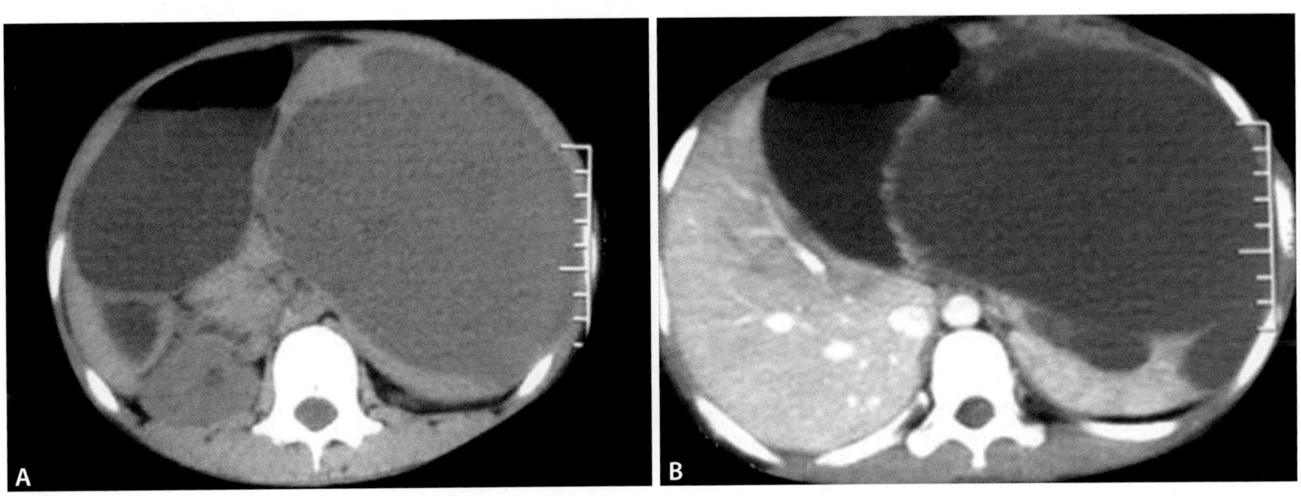

Figs. 23A and B: Axial NCCT (A) and CECT (B) images showing intrasplenic hypodense lesion with septations in a case of lymphangioma.

cysts containing hemorrhage and proteinaceous material demonstrate high signal intensity on T1WI.[35]

Hamartoma

Splenic hamartoma is rare benign neoplasm, which is composed of malformed red pulp elements without organized lymphoid follicles. Incidence in autopsy series is estimated to be 0.024–0.13%.[36] Most patients have no symptoms and the lesion is detected incidentally.

On USG, it is depicted as solid mass with homogeneous or heterogeneous echopattern showing intense vascularity on color Doppler owing to presence of red pulp within it. CT scan reveals homogeneous or heterogeneous low density or isodense masses causing contour deformity with or without presence of calcification and fatty component within. Persistent enhancement in delayed images has also been documented due to stagnation of contrast within the sinusoids of red pulp.[37] The lesion shows variable signal intensity on MRI depending upon the amount of fibrous content within it. The non-fibrous hamartoma is isointense on T1WI and hyperintense on T2WI and fibrous hamartoma shows iso to hyperintense signal on T1 and hypointense signal on T2WI. However, both variants show mild early enhancement after IV contrast and uniform enhancement on delayed phase.[38]

Littoral Cell Angioma

Littoral cell angioma (LCA) is a very rare neoplasm arising from cells lining the sinuses of splenic red pulp, the Littoral cells. It may be asymptomatic or may present with anemia or splenomegaly. Sonography reveals splenomegaly with heterogeneous echotexture and presence of multiple nodules which are of low or iso attenuation on non-contrast CT and demonstrate minimal delayed enhancement on post-contrast CT.[39] MRI depicts markedly hypointense signal on T1WI and T2WI due to presence of hemosiderin within the lesions.[32]

Peliosis

Peliosis is an uncommon condition, which is characterized by presence of blood filled spaces within the splenic parenchyma. It may occur in isolation or along with peliosis hepatis. Usually asymptomatic; rupture of the hemorrhagic cyst leading to intraperitoneal hemorrhage has been described. It may appear as echogenic or heteroechoic mass lesion in the left upper quadrant on USG which shows rapid enhancement on contrast-enhanced USG without any centripetal enhancement.[40] Non-contrast CT demonstrates hypodense lesions with fine internal septations which enhance significantly on contrast administration. Variable signal intensity is seen on MRI owing to blood products at different stages. Fluid-fluid level may be visualized within these cysts due to hematocrit effect.[41] Based on these imaging features, the differential diagnosis would include hemangiomatosis, angiosarcoma and lymphangioma.

Inflammatory Pseudotumor

Inflammatory pseudotumors, also known as inflammatory myofibroblastic tumor, are basically myofibroblastic neoplasms which result from unusual inflammatory response to any injury or infection. They may present with features of mass effect on surrounding structures or may remain asymptomatic. Imaging features include well circumscribed mass on USG with hetero or homogeneous enhancement on CT and there may be calcification within or a central scar which does not show enhancement. Diagnosis solely based on imaging is difficult and is mostly established after surgery.[35,39]

The other tumors like hemangioendothelioma, hemangiopericytoma, fibroma, lipoma, angiofibromas are extremely rare.

Malignant Neoplasms

Lymphoma

Spleen is affected in many hematological malignancies like lymphoma, leukemia, plasma cell malignancies; most common being Diffuse large B-cell lymphoma type of non-Hodgkin's lymphoma (NHL).[42] Hodgkin's lymphoma (HD) also involves the spleen in one third of patients when it is considered as nodal disease in contrast to NHL in which its infiltration is considered to be extranodal.[43] The lymphomatous involvement of spleen may be primary or secondary. Primary splenic lymphoma is rare, constituting approximately 1–2% of all lymphomas. DLBCL is the most common type in such patients[44] and magnetic resonance imaging (MRI).

On imaging, four patterns have been described: (a) homogeneous splenomegaly without any focal lesion; (b) diffuse infiltration with miliary lesions (less than 5 mm); (c) multiple focal nodular lesions (1-10 cm); and (d) large solitary mass. Li, et al. documented single large mass as the most common pattern.[44] Diffuse involvement may occur in normal sized spleen **(Fig. 25A)** and mild to moderate enlargement may represent reactive splenomegaly in 30% of cases.[45] However, marked splenomegaly almost always suggests infiltration.[46] Diffuse involvement of spleen is commonly seen in Hodgkin's disease due to predominant involvement of periarteriolar lymphoid sheath.[42,47] The nodules appear hypoechoic on ultrasound and hypoenhancing on contrast-enhanced CT **(Figs. 24A and B)**.[48] On MRI, the lesions are hyperintense on T2WI, iso to hypointense on T1WI and show reduced enhancement on contrast administration.[11]

18-FDG PET/CT is considered superior to CT in staging and restaging of lymphoma by virtue of detecting FDG avid normal sized nodes and detection of extranodal sites like liver, spleen **(Figs. 25A and B)** and bone marrow.[43] Sensitivity and specificity of CT, PET and PET/CT have been reported to be 91% and 96%, 75% and 99%, and 100% and 95%, respectively in a series of 111 patients.[49] Hence, for the staging of patients with FDG-avid, potentially curable lymphomas (e.g. diffuse large B-cell lymphoma and Hodgkin disease), PET is recommended routinely to delineate the disease extent more accurately and monitor response to therapy.[43] In lymphoma patients, the post-therapy inflammatory changes may persist for up to 2 weeks after chemotherapy alone and for up to 2–3 months or longer after radiation therapy or chemoradiotherapy. Thus to avoid false positive results, PET scans should not be performed for at least 3 weeks, and preferably 6–8 weeks, after completion of therapy.[50,51]

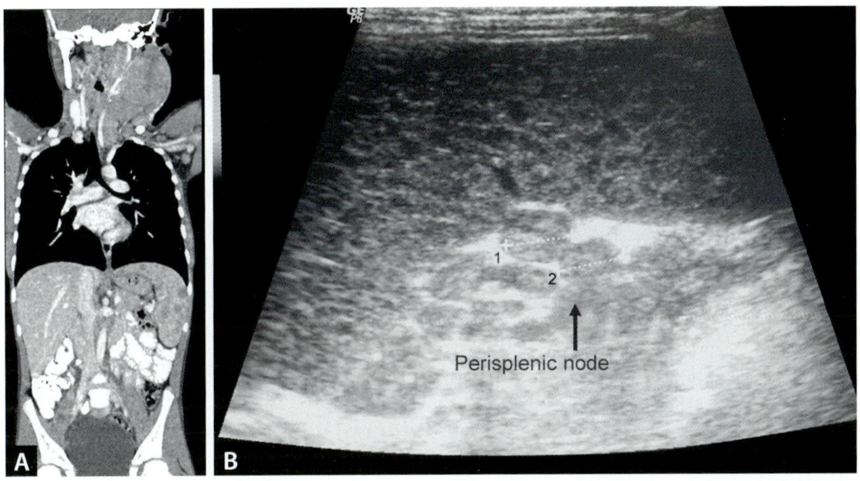

Figs. 24A and B: Coronal reformatted CECT image (A) showing bulky cervical lymphadenopathy and multiple lesions seen in the spleen in a case of Hodgkin's lymphoma. USG image (B) in a different patient of NHL showing multiple small hypoechoic nodular lesions diffusely distributed in the splenic parenchyma. Note is made of multiple homogeneous, non-necrotic perisplenic lymph nodes (arrow).

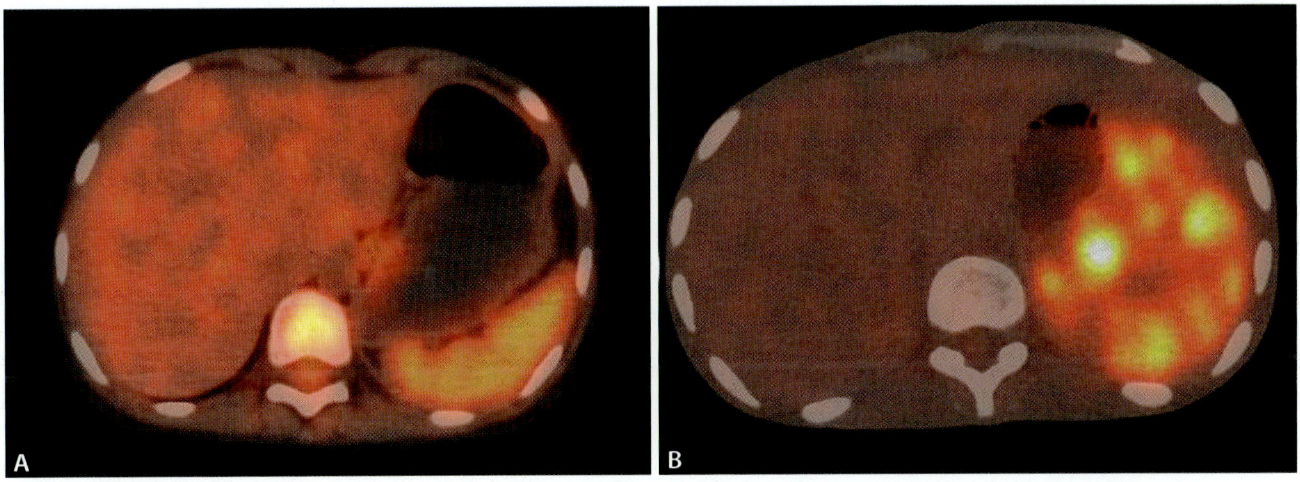

Figs. 25A and B: 18-F FDG PET-CT image showing diffuse involvement (A) and focal nodules (B) in patient of NHL as areas of avid uptake of FDG.

Angiosarcoma

Splenic angiosarcoma is a rare and aggressive neoplasm, which arises from the splenic vascular endothelium and the mesothelial cells of the sinusoids.[52] It is considered to be the most common primary non-lymphoid neoplasm of spleen with an estimated annual incidence of 0.14–0.25 cases per million persons.[53] The exact etiopathogenesis is unknown; although, it has been postulated that the benign splenic tumors such as hemangioma and lymphangioma may act as precursors. It presents with upper abdominal pain in 80% of patients and anemia in 75–81%.[52] Angiosarcoma of spleen is a fatal neoplasm and may present as splenic rupture in 13–32% of cases.[53] It is associated with high rate of metastases at the time of presentation (69–100%); liver being the most common site followed by lungs, lymph nodes and bone.[54] Early diagnosis and splenectomy is the treatment of choice with less defined role of chemoradiotherapy. Despite prompt measures, it has a dismal prognosis.

There is limited literature available on the imaging features of angiosarcoma in the form of anecdotal case reports and few case series. Splenomegaly with heterogeneous mass is seen in 60% cases on all imaging modalities.[55] On ultrasound, it appears as solid-cystic mass in an enlarged spleen with mixed echogenicity. CT demonstrates single or multiple masses, which show mixed attenuation and ill-defined margins. Nonenhancing areas represent necrosis and active contrast blush is seen in the areas of active bleeding. Areas of active hemorrhage appear hyperdense on non-contrast CT and the lesions may show peripheral enhancement after contrast administration.[55] On MRI, the nodules are hypointense on T1 and T2WI relative to splenic parenchyma; however, hyperintense signal may be seen due to presence of hemorrhage or necrosis within. Chronic hemorrhage leading to hemosiderin deposition causes reduction in signal intensity. The pattern of contrast enhancement includes peripheral nodular enhancement with nonenhancing areas due to necrosis or hemorrhage.[55]

Metastases

Splenic metastases occur mostly in the setting of multisystem metastatic disease. The prevalence ranges from 1.3% to 7.1%, reported in autopsy series.[56] It has been postulated that the relative lower incidence of splenic metastases is due to innate hostile environment for malignant invasion, the reticuloendothelial system inhibiting tumor cell seeding and lack of afferent lymphatics.[57] Agha Mohammadi, et al. reported gynecological malignancy to be the most common primary neoplasm followed by colorectal, lung and gastric cancer associated with splenic metastases.[58] The lesions are hypodense on imaging with majority being lobulated, well-defined, nonenhancing nodules on CT **(Figs. 26A to C)**.[59] On MRI, the lesions typically appear as hyperintense on T2WI and hypo- to isointense on T1WI.[11]

SPLENIC INTERVENTIONS FNAC AND BIOPSY OF SPLEEN

Fine needle aspiration cytology (FNAC) of spleen is a relatively safe procedure. Common indications of performing FNAC in spleen are infectious diseases, sarcoidosis and neoplastic conditions like metastases. Uncommonly, FNAC is also performed to rule out storage disorders, amyloidosis, hemophagocytic syndrome and primary splenic benign and malignant diseases. In India because of very high prevalence of tuberculosis, focal splenic lesions even in patients of a known malignancy may be infective in nature. This is a relatively common clinical scenario for performing FNAC to differentiate these two possibilities.

There is a reluctance to do guided interventions in spleen because of potential risk of hemorrhage that may necessitate urgent splenectomy. However, with the use of thinner gauge biopsy needles for splenic biopsy, the risk of complication is similar to risk associated with other large organ biopsies.[60]

Major indications of performing FNAC or biopsy in spleen are to evaluate a solid or cystic lesion or to evaluate splenomegaly of uncertain etiology. Most common indication for splenic biopsy is suspicion of lymphoma or presence of splenic lesion in a patient who is already known to have some primary malignancy apart from spleen.[61,62]

A significant percentage of patients of lymphomas (HD as well as NHL) have involvement of the spleen.[61] Another important consideration is that splenic involvement in lymphoma has got prognostic importance and overall treatment of the patient changes according to whether spleen is involved or not.

It is important to consider the fact that if metastasis is also present at some other site in addition to spleen, then it is advisable to obtain biopsy from these accessible sites.[63]

Whenever chances of bleeding are high, e.g. in presence of coagulopathy, it is advisable to obtain FNAC rather than core biopsy. FNAC is normally performed with 20–23 G Chiba needle **(Figs. 27A and B)**, which

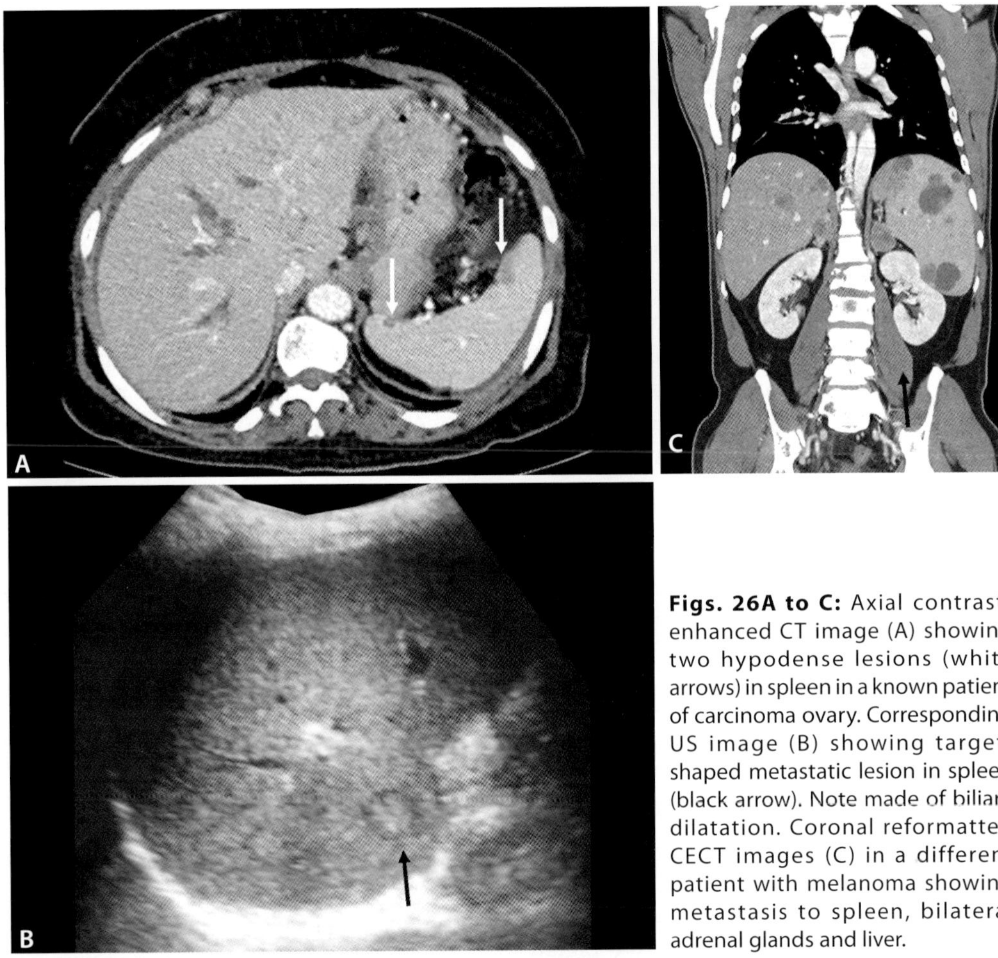

Figs. 26A to C: Axial contrast-enhanced CT image (A) showing two hypodense lesions (white arrows) in spleen in a known patient of carcinoma ovary. Corresponding US image (B) showing target-shaped metastatic lesion in spleen (black arrow). Note made of biliary dilatation. Coronal reformatted CECT images (C) in a different patient with melanoma showing metastasis to spleen, bilateral adrenal glands and liver.

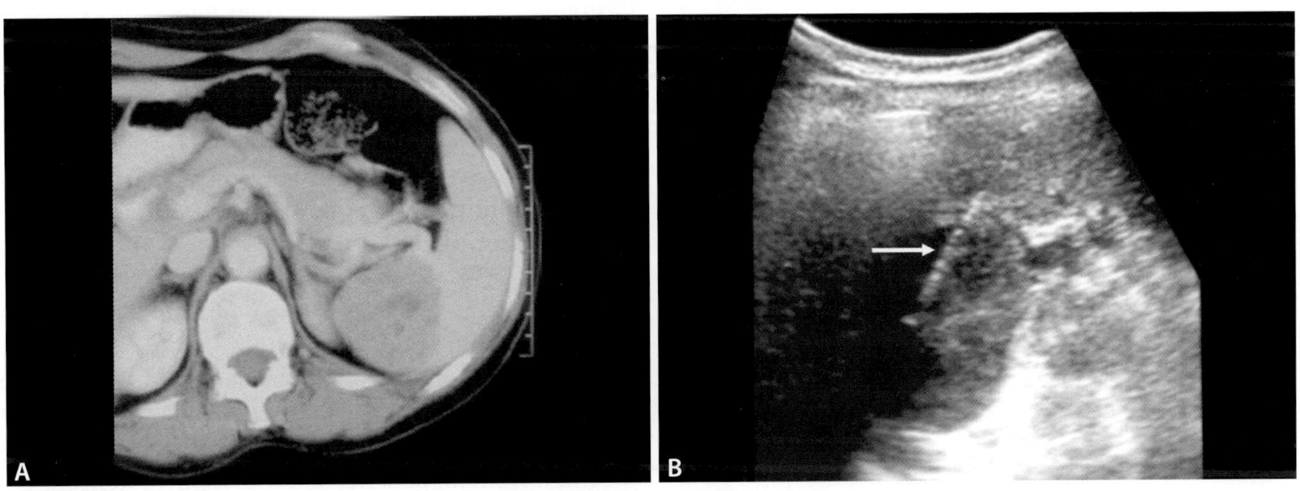

Figs. 27A and B: Axial CECT image (A) showing focal hypodense mass lesion in spleen. USG-guided FNAC procedure (B) showing echogenic needle *in situ* (arrow). FNAC was reported as NHL.

has safer profile compared to core biopsy which is done with 14–18 G needles. However, it is important to note that FNAC is not useful in evaluation of lymphoma because the obtained sample is usually insufficient to further subtype lymphomas. With the advent of specific targeted chemotherapeutic agents of different subtypes of lymphoma, it is essential to provide larger tissues to pathologist for subtyping, which directly results in better selection of chemotherapeutic regimen. Additional samples are taken for flow cytometry if lymphoma is one of the clinical possibilities.

Contraindications for splenic biopsy or drainage are uncorrectable coagulopathy, lack of safe access route and uncooperative patient. For biopsy, minimal caliber needle should be chosen which can give sufficient diagnostic yield so as to decrease chances of post-procedural bleed. It is advisable to traverse some normal splenic tissue before obtaining access to the target lesion in spleen to help decrease bleeding by way of tamponade effect. Frequent hemodynamic monitoring and placing the patient in left lateral decubitus is advisable.

Drainage

Drainage of splenic abscess is done uncommonly for tubercular, fungal or bacterial abscesses which are more common in patient with altered immunity status.[64]

The success rate of percutaneous drainage for splenic abscess is more than 80%[63,65,66] with reduced success in presence of loculations and multiple internal septations. Usually collections less than 3 cm^3 can be managed by single time needle aspiration only.[67] If lesion is bigger than 3 cm^3 then drainage is usually considered. Seldinger techniques as well as tandem trocar techniques, both are feasible for splenic drainage. Normally, 8–10 F pigtail catheters are selected, however, if on initial aspiration thick pus is aspirated it should be drained with bigger pigtail catheter (e.g. 12–14 F). Intermittent (every 8 hour) flushing of the catheter with 10 mL of saline helps in improving the patency of catheters. If the drainage from catheter drops to less than 10 mL/24 hr, white blood cell (WBC) counts return to normal and fever subsides, then catheter removal should be planned. Repeat USG screening is useful before removing catheter to rule put significant residual collection.

Ultrasonography guidance is better than CT for evaluating internal architecture of fluid collection/abscess in spleen as the thin internal septations are better seen on USG.

Splenic Artery Aneurysm and Intervention

In abdomen, only aorta and iliac artery aneurysms are more common sites of aneurysm than splenic artery.[68] With more frequent use of USG and CT, incidental splenic artery aneurysms are also seen more commonly.[69] The difference between true aneurysm and pseudoaneurysm is with respect to the adventitial layer of the wall; which is present in true aneurysm but absent in pseudoaneurysm. The exact etiopathogenesis of true aneurysm are not yet completely elucidated. The clinical settings in which it is seen include atherosclerosis, pregnancy, portal hypertension, cirrhosis and post liver transplant.[70-72] Inflammatory and infectious conditions, collagen vascular diseases, arterial fibrodysplasia are other conditions, which are associated with it. In pancreatitits, release of proteolytic enzymes may cause weakening of the wall of splenic artery with consequent pseudoaneurysm formation. Other causes of pseudoaneurysms are iatrogenic or accidental trauma and postoperative causes.[73]

A large majority of unruptured splenic artery aneurysms are clinically silent.[70] In contrast, ruptured splenic artery aneurysms are almost always symptomatic with pain abdomen, intestinal hemorrhage and hemodynamic instability as presenting features. Rupture rate has been described as approximately 2–3%.[74,75] Liver transplantation, pregnancy and portal hypertension are associated with increased frequency of rupture.[76] CECT scan is the most commonly used modality for diagnosing splenic artery aneurysms and pseudoaneurysms however, the gold standard for diagnosing these conditions still remains direct catheter angiography. If CECT is utilized, a meticulous evaluation of arterial phase images is vital which reveals a well-defined rounded intensely enhancing outpouching from the splenic artery **(Figs. 28A and B)** or its branch. Other findings which may be seen are presence of calcification in its wall, mural thrombosis in peripheral part of the aneurysm or extravasation of contrast in its vicinity or within the lumen of adjacent bowel loops. If aneurysm is large, it may be seen on USG or color Doppler **(Fig. 28C)**, however small aneurysms may be missed on USG/Doppler as frequently there is poor sonographic window in presence of pancreatitis and postoperative changes.

The treatment strategies for splenic artery aneurysm and pseudoaneurysms are quite different. If patient is symptomatic then treatment of splenic artery aneurysm should be done.[70] For asymptomatic patients, treatment should be contemplated for certain high risk factors like pregnant women, patients of cirrhosis, hypertension and liver transplantation.[77] Treatment is also recommended for asymptomatic aneurysms larger than 2 cm in those patients with life expectancy more than 2 years and having reasonable operative risk.[68,70]

The modality of treatment depends on many factors like clinical condition of the patient, location of aneurysm

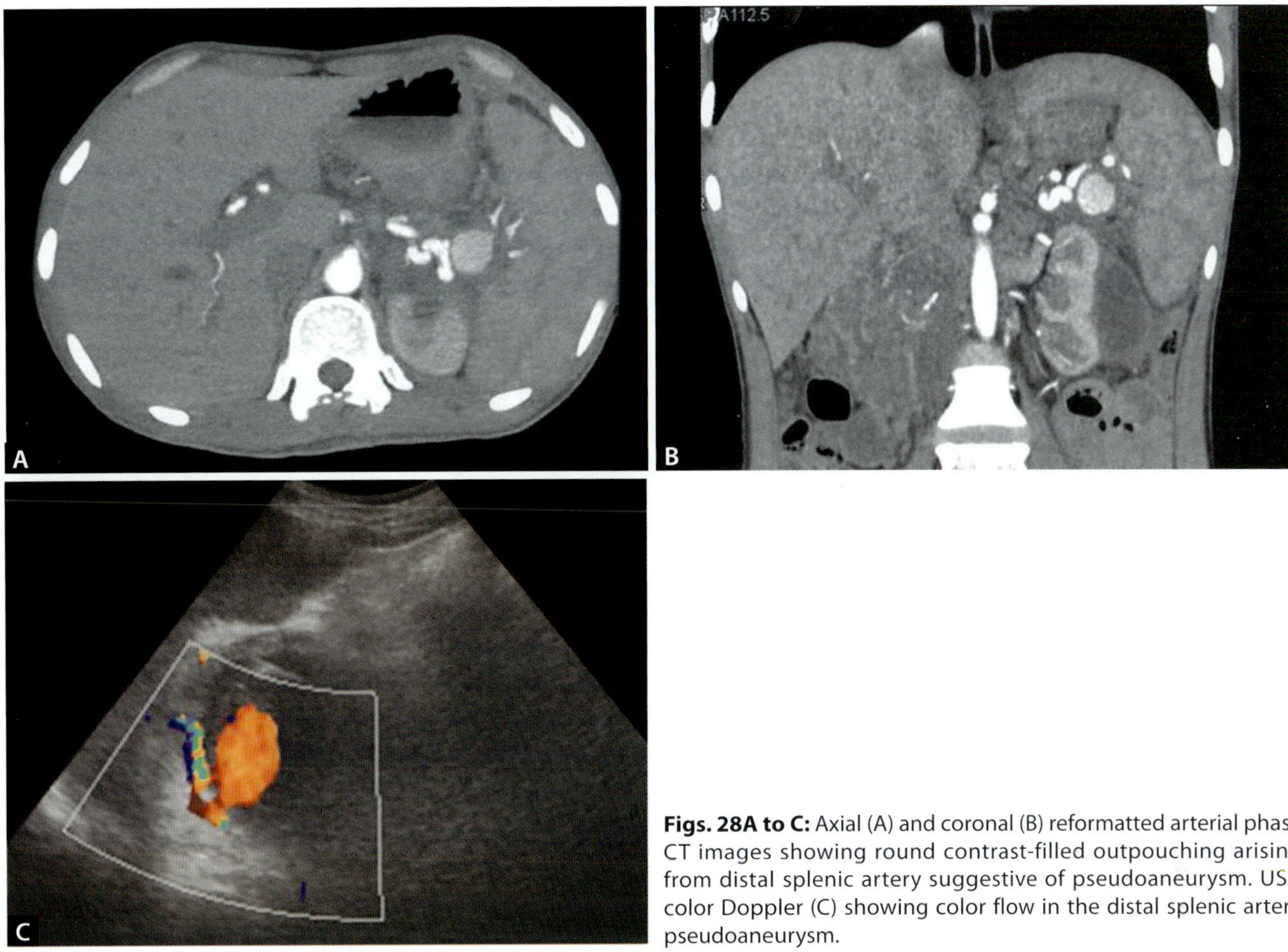

Figs. 28A to C: Axial (A) and coronal (B) reformatted arterial phase CT images showing round contrast-filled outpouching arising from distal splenic artery suggestive of pseudoaneurysm. USG color Doppler (C) showing color flow in the distal splenic artery pseudoaneurysm.

and operative risks associated in given scenario. Elective surgery is associated with more than 0.5% mortality rate; hence, patient selection and treatment modality selection are of paramount importance.[76] Previously, surgical treatment for proximal and middle splenic artery used to be simple excision with ligation of proximal and distal stumps; in which case short gastric arteries may help to preserve splenic supply through collaterization. Surgical treatment for distally located aneurysms is splenectomy.[77]

Endovascular repair of splenic artery aneurysm is more efficacious than open surgical treatment in short-term follow-up with lesser perioperative mortality. However, late complications and reintervention rate is more with endovascular repair as compared to open surgical repair.[78] Endovascular repair has also been found to be more cost effective for treatment of splenic artery aneurysms.[79] Acceptable success rates have been achieved with endovascular techniques using embolization with coils **(Figs. 29A and B)** and gel foam.[80]

Splenic artery embolization has also been used successfully for treatment of hypersplenism.[81]

Occasionally use of percutaneous thrombin has been shown to be successful if the patients are not good candidates for endovascular treatment.[82,83]

Miscellaneous Conditions

Sarcoidosis

Splenic involvement in sarcoidosis is much less common than lungs, mediastinum and eyes. However, when involved it may be seen on CT as multiple hypodense nodules in spleen, which may vary in shape and size. If the nodules increase with time these may also look like confluent masses. These nodules and masses are hypodense and show less enhancement as compared to splenic parenchyma.[84] On MRI, these show hypointense signal on T1 and T2WI as compared to background parenchyma with hypoenhancement on early arterial phase.[85] These nodules may show enhancement on

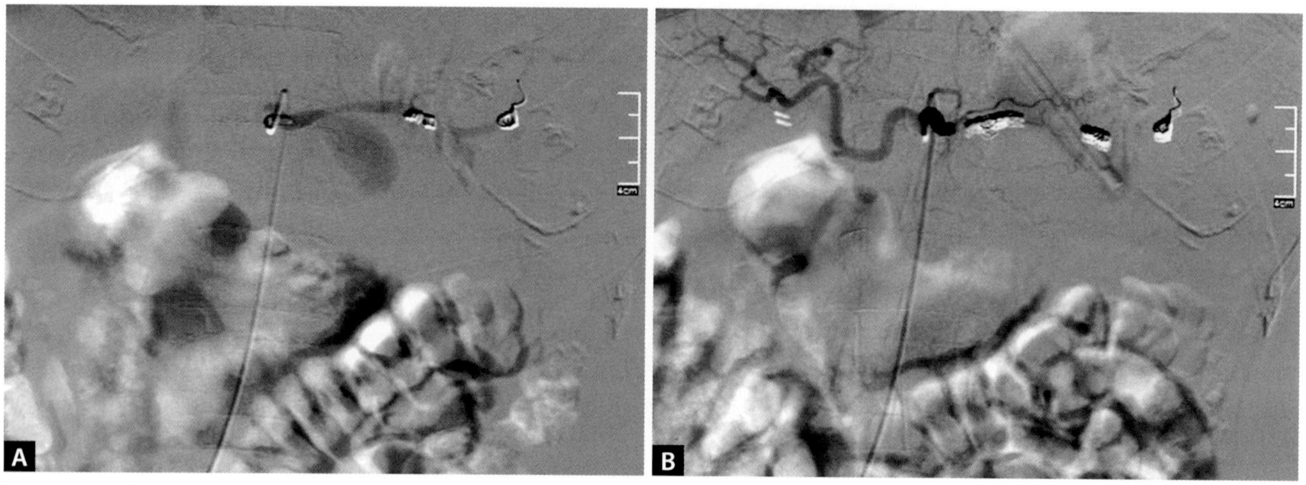

Figs. 29A and B: Angiogram (A) showing aneurysm in proximal part of splenic artery. Coils have been placed distal to splenic artery aneurysm. Incidentally, a coil is seen migrated in the distal most part of splenic artery. Coils have been placed proximal to aneurysm also to 'trap' the aneurysm (B).

delayed phase images **(Figs. 30A to E)**. Other common finding is hepatosplenomegaly.

Gamna Gandy Bodies

Histologically, these are small siderotic nodules which contain hemosiderin, calcium and fibrosis. These are commonly seen in clinical setting of portal hypertension.[86] Other conditions in which these are seen include portal vein or splenic vein thrombosis and hemolytic anemias. They are best seen on MRI as hypointense foci in all sequences **(Figs. 31A to D)**.[87] Their usual size is from few millimeters to up to one centimeter.

Gaucher's Disease

Gaucher's disease occurs due to deficiency of lysosomal enzyme glucocerebrosidase. This disease affects the skeleton, spleen and liver most dominantly. Majority of times the patient is already diagnosed before they reach the radiology department. Skeletal involvement is in form of osteopenia, osteoporosis and fractures. Spleen may be massively enlarged with frequent findings of focal lesions and infarcts. On CT, these focal lesions are hypodense and enhance less as compared to splenic parenchyma. On MRI, most of these lesions are hyperintense on T2WI although occasionally they may be hypointense on T2WI also. These are hypointense on T1WI with hypoenhancement as compared to splenic parenchyma.[88] Liver enlargement is less striking as compared to splenic enlargement.

Hemochromatosis

Hemochromatosis may be primary (due to increased absorption from GIT) or secondary (due to increased extravscular hemolysis). In primary form, liver involvement is much more as compared to spleen and in secondary form, the spleen is predominantly involved. The usual imaging feature on CT, is presence of increased attenuation involving these organs. On MRI these involved organs show decreased signal on T2WI due to susceptibility artifacts because of presence of iron in visceral organs.[89,90] Spleen is also hypointense on T2WI however the involvement of liver is much more in primary forms **(Fig. 32)**. Conversely spleen is more profoundly hypointense than liver if the etiology is secondary hemochromatosis. MR using gradient echo sequences is also used to quantify liver iron load in an attempt to avoid the need of repeated biopsies.

Amyloidosis

Pathologically in amyloidosis, there is abnormal accumulation of some fibrillar material in extracellular matrix in a wide variety of tissues in body. Based on the biochemical property of this fibrillar material, it can be divided into primary type (type AL, monoclonal proliferation) and secondary type (AA type, secondary to chronic inflammatory diseases). Both of these types can involve the spleen which may be diffuse (more commonly) or focal. Splenomegaly is quite uncommon.[91] Various imaging features are focal tumor like lesions,[92] diffuse low attenuation[91] and decreased enhancement. Occasionally, extensive focal splenic calcification has also been described in splenic involvement of amyloidosis.[93] On MRI, decreased signal on T2WI has been described.[94]

In conclusion, spleen is affected by a wide variety of disorders ranging from developmental abnormalities

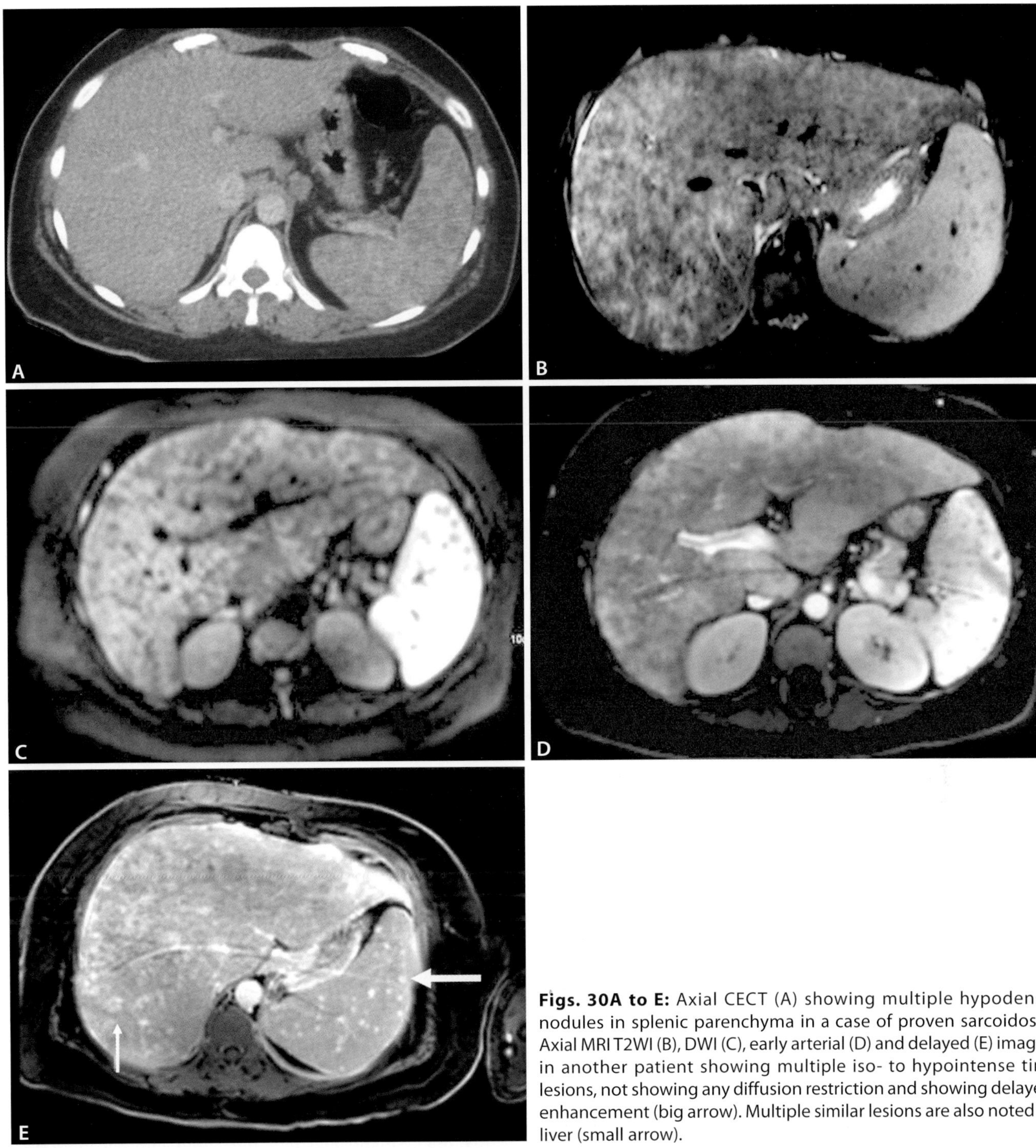

Figs. 30A to E: Axial CECT (A) showing multiple hypodense nodules in splenic parenchyma in a case of proven sarcoidosis. Axial MRI T2WI (B), DWI (C), early arterial (D) and delayed (E) images in another patient showing multiple iso- to hypointense tiny lesions, not showing any diffusion restriction and showing delayed enhancement (big arrow). Multiple similar lesions are also noted in liver (small arrow).

to storage disorders, infective, vascular and neoplastic pathologies. A thorough knowledge of available imaging modalities and judicious utilization of these is necessary for optimal patient care. USG and CT are the most commonly used imaging modalities for evaluation of splenic disorders. MRI can be used as a problem solving tool. FNAC, biopsy and splenic artery embolization are major interventions performed, which need meticulous planning using these imaging modalities. FNAC with or without cell block is a safe and useful procedure for diagnosis of focal splenic lesions, especially granulomatous diseases such as tuberculosis.

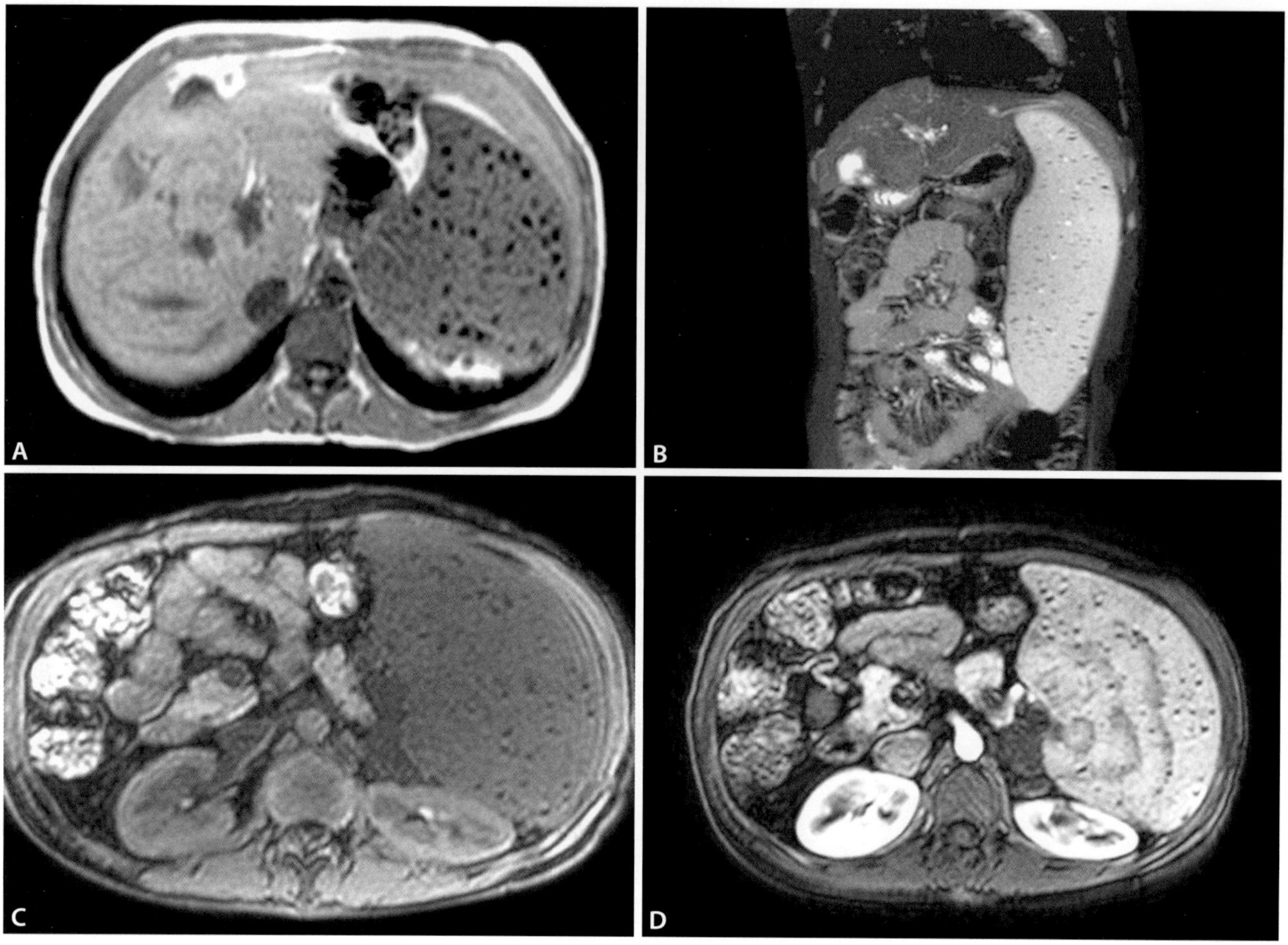

Figs. 31A to D: Axial T1WI (A), coronal T2WI (B), T1FS non-contrast (C) and post-contrast (D) MR images showing numerous hypointense tiny focal lesions in enlarged spleen on all sequences with no enhancement on postcontrast images suggestive of Gamna-Gandy bodies in a patient with portal hypertension.

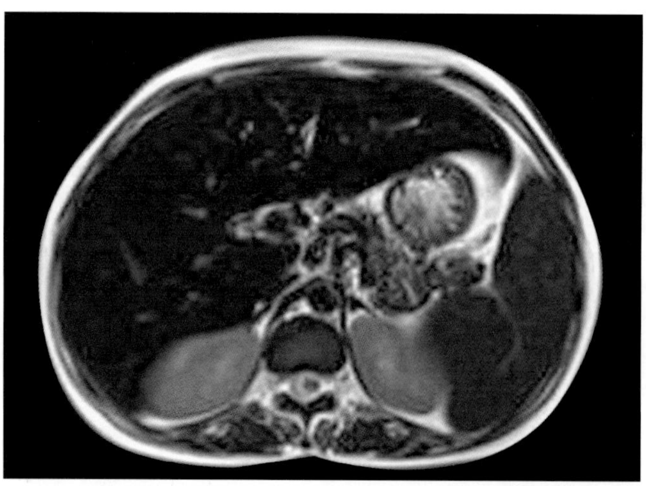

Fig. 32: Axial T2WI showing diffuse hypointense signal in spleen in a case of hemolytic anemia.

ACKNOWLEDGMENTS

Dr Raju Sharma, Dr Shivanand Gamanagatti and Dr Manisha Jana.

REFERENCES

1. Chadburn A. The spleen: anatomy and anatomical function. Semin Hematol. 2000;37(1 Suppl 1):13-21.
2. Hirooka M, Ochi H, Koizumi Y, Kisaka Y, Abe M, Ikeda Y, et al. Splenic elasticity measured with real-time tissue elastography is a marker of portal hypertension. Radiology. 2011;261(3):960-8.
3. Grzelak P, Augsburg L, Majos A, Stefanczyk L, Gorski P, Piotrowski W, et al. Diagnostic potential of contrast-enhanced ultrasound (CEUS) in the assessment of spleen and liver granulomas in the course of sarcoidosis. Pneumonol Alergol Pol. 2013;81(5):424-8.

4. Omar A, Freeman S. Contrast-enhanced ultrasound of the spleen. Ultrasound. 2016;24(1):41-9.
5. Miele V, Piccolo CL, Galluzzo M, Ianniello S, Sessa B, Trinci M. Contrast-enhanced ultrasound (CEUS) in blunt abdominal trauma. Br J Radiol. 2016;89(1061):20150823.
6. Piscaglia F, Nolsoe C, Dietrich CF, Cosgrove DO, Gilja OH, Bachmann Nielsen M, et al. The EFSUMB Guidelines and Recommendations on the Clinical Practice of Contrast Enhanced Ultrasound (CEUS): update 2011 on non-hepatic applications. Ultraschall Med. 2012;33(1):33-59.
7. Park YS, Park SH, Lee SS, Kim DY, Shin YM, Lee W, et al. Biopsy-proven nonsteatotic liver in adults: estimation of reference range for difference in attenuation between the liver and the spleen at nonenhanced CT. Radiology. 2011;258(3):760-6.
8. Donnelly LF, Foss JN, Frush DP, Bisset GS 3rd. Heterogeneous splenic enhancement patterns on spiral CT images in children: minimizing misinterpretation. Radiology. 1999;210(2):493-7.
9. Rabushka LS, Kawashima A, Fishman EK. Imaging of the spleen: CT with supplemental MR examination. Radiographics. 1994;14(2):307-32.
10. Urban BA, Fishman EK. Helical CT of the spleen. AJR. 1998;170(4):997-1003.
11. Elsayes KM, Narra VR, Mukundan G, Lewis JS Jr, Menias CO, Heiken JP. MR imaging of the spleen: spectrum of abnormalities. Radiographics. 2005;25(4):967-82.
12. Donnelly LF, Emery KH, Bove KE, Bissett GS 3rd. Normal changes in the MR appearance of the spleen during early childhood. AJR. 1996;166(3):635-9.
13. Yoshikawa T, Kawamitsu H, Mitchell DG, Ohno Y, Ku Y, Seo Y, et al. ADC measurement of abdominal organs and lesions using parallel imaging technique. AJR. 2006;187(6):1521-30.
14. Rini JN, Leonidas JC, Tomas MB, Palestro CJ. 18F-FDG PET versus CT for evaluating the spleen during initial staging of lymphoma. J Nucl Med. 2003;44(7):1072-4.
15. Spleen. In: Lee JKT, Sagel SS, Stanley RJ, Heiken JP (eds). Computed Body Tomography with MRI Correlation, 4th edn. Philadelphia: Lippincott Williams and Wilkins; 2006.
16. Rosenberg HK, Markowitz RI, Kolberg H, Park C, Hubbard A, Bellah RD. Normal splenic size in infants and children: sonographic measurements. AJR. 1991;157(1):119-21.
17. Radu CC, Mutiu G, Pop O. Accessory spleen. Rom J Morphol Embryol. 2014;55(3 Suppl):1243-6.
18. al-Ahmadi M, Brundage S, Brody F, Jacobs L, Sackier JM. Splenosis of the mesoappendix: case report and review of the literature. J R Coll Surg Edinb. 1998;43(3):200-2.
19. Costello P, Kane RA, Oster J, Clouse ME. Focal splenic disease demonstrated by ultrasound and computed tomography. J Can Assoc Radiol. 1985;36(1):22-8.
20. Fulcher AS, Turner MA. Abdominal manifestations of situs anomalies in adults. Radiographics. 2002;22(6):1439-56.
21. Zech CJ, Bartolozzi C, Baron R, Reiser MF (eds). Multislice-CT of the Abdomen. Springer. Verlag Berlin Heidelberg, 2012.
22. Dachman AH, Ros PR, Murari PJ, Olmsted WW, Lichtenstein JE. Nonparasitic splenic cysts: a report of 52 cases with radiologic-pathologic correlation. AJR. 1986;147(3):537-42.
23. Al-Hajjar N, Graur F, Hassan AB, Molnar G. Splenic abscesses. Rom J Gastroenterol. 2002;11(1):57-9.
24. Ooi LL, Leong SS. Splenic abscesses from 1987 to 1995. Am J Surg. 1997;174(1):87-93.
25. Tirumani SH, Ojili V, Gunabushanam G, Shanbhogue AK, Nagar A, Fasih N, et al. Imaging of tuberculosis of the abdominal viscera: beyond the intestines. J Clin Imaging Sci. 2013;3:17.
26. Murata Y, Yamada I, Sumiya Y, Shichijo Y, Suzuki Y. Abdominal macronodular tuberculomas: MR findings. J Comput Assist Tomogr. 1996;20(4):643-6.
27. Ito K, Mitchell DG, Honjo K, Fujita T, Uchisako H, Matsumoto T, et al. MR imaging of acquired abnormalities of the spleen. AJR. 1997;168(3):697-702.
28. Renzulli P, Hostettler A, Schoepfer AM, Gloor B, Candinas D. Systematic review of atraumatic splenic rupture. Br J Surg. 2009;96(10):1114-21.
29. Husni EA. The clinical course of splenic hemangioma with emphasis on spontaneous rupture. Arch Surg. 1961;83:681-8.
30. Louis TH, Sanders JM, Stephenson JS, Harbour LN, Ford KL 3rd. Splenic hemangiomatosis. Proc (Bayl Univ Med Cent). 2011;24(4):356-8.
31. Shinde J, Pandit S, Kolte S, Singh SP. Laparoscopic splenectomy for haemangioma of the spleen. J Minim Access Surg. 2014; 10(1):42-4.
32. Abbott RM, Levy AD, Aguilera NS, Gorospe L, Thompson WM. From the archives of the AFIP: primary vascular neoplasms of the spleen: radiologic-pathologic correlation. Radiographics. 2004;24(4):1137-63.
33. Yang F, Chen WX. Splenic lymphangioma that manifested as a solid-cystic mass: a case report. World J Gastroenterol. 2013;19(5):781-3.
34. Ioannidis I, Kahn AG. Splenic lymphangioma. Arch Pathol Lab Med. 2015;139(2):278-82.
35. Kaza RK, Azar S, Al-Hawary MM, Francis IR. Primary and secondary neoplasms of the spleen. Cancer Imaging. 2010;10: 173-82.
36. Lam KY, Yip KH, Peh WC. Splenic vascular lesions: unusual features and a review of the literature. Aust NZJ Surg. 1999; 69(6):422-5.
37. Ohtomo K, Fukuda H, Mori K, Minami M, Itai Y, Inoue Y. CT and MR appearances of splenic hamartoma. J Comput Assist Tomogr. 1992;16(3):425-8.
38. Yu RS, Zhang SZ, Hua JM. Imaging findings of splenic hamartoma. World J Gastroenterol. 2004;10(17):2613-5.
39. Giovagnoni A, Giorgi C, Goteri G. Tumours of the spleen. Cancer Imaging. 2005;5:73-7.
40. Davidson J, Tung K. Splenic peliosis: an unusual entity. Br J Radiol. 2010;83(990):e126-8.
41. Maves CK, Caron KH, Bisset GS 3rd, Agarwal R. Splenic and hepatic peliosis: MR findings. AJR. 1992;158(1):75-6.

42. Saboo SS, Krajewski KM, O'Regan KN, Giardino A, Brown JR, Ramaiya N, et al. Spleen in haematological malignancies: spectrum of imaging findings. Br J Radiol. 2012;85(1009):81-92.
43. Paes FM, Kalkanis DG, Sideras PA, Serafini AN. FDG PET/CT of extranodal involvement in non-Hodgkin lymphoma and Hodgkin disease. Radiographics. 2010;30(1):269-91.
44. Li M, Zhang L, Wu N, Huang W, Lv N. Imaging findings of primary splenic lymphoma: a review of 17 cases in which diagnosis was made at splenectomy. PLoS One. 2013;8(11):e80264.
45. Fishman EK, Kuhlman JE, Jones RJ. CT of lymphoma: spectrum of disease. Radiographics. 1991;11(4):647-69.
46. Guermazi A, Brice P, de Kerviler EE, Ferme C, Hennequin C, Meignin V, et al. Extranodal Hodgkin disease: spectrum of disease. Radiographics. 2001;21(1):161-79.
47. Bhatia K, Sahdev A, Reznek RH. Lymphoma of the spleen. Semin Ultrasound CT MR. 2007;28(1):12-20.
48. Manzella A, Borba-Filho P, D'Ippolito G, Farias M. Abdominal manifestations of lymphoma: spectrum of imaging features. ISRN Radiol. 2013;2013:483069.
49. de Jong PA, van Ufford HM, Baarslag HJ, de Haas MJ, Wittebol SH, Quekel LG, et al. CT and 18F-FDG PET for noninvasive detection of splenic involvement in patients with malignant lymphoma. AJR. 2009;192(3): 745-53.
50. Cheson BD, Pfistner B, Juweid ME, Gascoyne RD, Specht L, Horning SJ, et al. Revised response criteria for malignant lymphoma. J Clin Oncol. 2007;25(5):579-86.
51. Juweid ME, Stroobants S, Hoekstra OS, Mottaghy FM, Dietlein M, Guermazi A, et al. Use of positron emission tomography for response assessment of lymphoma: consensus of the Imaging Subcommittee of International Harmonization Project in Lymphoma. J Clin Oncol. 2007;25(5):571-8.
52. Hamid KS, Rodriguez JA, Lairmore TC. Primary splenic angiosarcoma. JSLS. 2010;14(3):431-5.
53. Badiani R, Schaller G, Jain K, Swamy R, Gupta S. Angiosarcoma of the spleen presenting as spontaneous splenic rupture: A rare case report and review of the literature. Int J Surg Case Rep. 2013;4(9):765-7.
54. Manouras A, Giannopoulos P, Toufektzian L, Markogiannakis H, Lagoudianakis EE, Papadima A, et al. Splenic rupture as the presenting manifestation of primary splenic angiosarcoma in a teenage woman: a case report. J Med Case Rep. 2008;2:133.
55. Thompson WM, Levy AD, Aguilera NS, Gorospe L, Abbott RM. Angiosarcoma of the spleen: imaging characteristics in 12 patients. Radiology. 2005;235(1):106-15.
56. Comperat E, Bardier-Dupas A, Camparo P, Capron F, Charlotte F. Splenic metastases: clinicopathologic presentation, differential diagnosis, and pathogenesis. Arch Pathol Lab Med. 2007;131(6):965-9.
57. Showalter SL, Hager E, Yeo CJ. Metastatic disease to the pancreas and spleen. Semin Oncol. 2008;35(2):160-71.
58. Agha-Mohammadi S, Calne RY. Solitary splenic metastasis: case report and review of the literature. Am J Clin Oncol. 2001; 24(3):306-10.
59. Senturk S, Karcaaltincaba M, Akata D. CT diagnosis of intrasplenic metastasis from ovarian carcinoma. Eur J Radiol. 2012;81(6):1094-9.
60. McInnes MD, Kielar AZ, Macdonald DB. Percutaneous image-guided biopsy of the spleen: systematic review and meta-analysis of the complication rate and diagnostic accuracy. Radiology. 2011;260(3):699-708.
61. Tam A, Krishnamurthy S, Pillsbury EP, Ensor JE, Gupta S, Murthy R, et al. Percutaneous image-guided splenic biopsy in the oncology patient: an audit of 156 consecutive cases. J Vasc Interv Radiol. 2008;19(1):80-7.
62. Lucey BC, Boland GW, Maher MM, Hahn PF, Gervais DA, Mueller PR. Percutaneous nonvascular splenic intervention: a 10-year review. AJR. 2002;179(6):1591-6.
63. Kang M, Kalra N, Gulati M, Lal A, Kochhar R, Rajwanshi A. Image guided percutaneous splenic interventions. Eur J Radiol. 2007;64(1):140-6.
64. Kamaya A, Weinstein S, Desser TS. Multiple lesions of the spleen: differential diagnosis of cystic and solid lesions. Semin Ultrasound CT MR. 2006;27(5):389-403.
65. Thanos L, Dailiana T, Papaioannou G, Nikita A, Koutrouvelis H, Kelekis DA. Percutaneous CT-guided drainage of splenic abscess. AJR. 2002;179(3):629-32.
66. Singh AK, Shankar S, Gervais DA, Hahn PF, Mueller PR. Image-guided percutaneous splenic interventions. Radiographics. 2012;32(2):523-34.
67. Sammon J, Twomey M, Crush L, Maher MM, O'Connor OJ. Image-guided percutaneous splenic biopsy and drainage. Semin Intervent Radiol. 2012;29(4):301-10.
68. Trastek VF, Pairolero PC, Joyce JW, Hollier LH, Bernatz PE. Splenic artery aneurysms. Surgery. 1982;91(6):694-9.
69. Rokke O, Sondenaa K, Amundsen S, Bjerke-Larssen T, Jensen D. The diagnosis and management of splanchnic artery aneurysms. Scand J Gastroenterol. 1996;31(8):737-43.
70. Abbas MA, Stone WM, Fowl RJ, Gloviczki P, Oldenburg WA, Pairolero PC, et al. Splenic artery aneurysms: two decades experience at Mayo clinic. Ann Vasc Surg. 2002;16(4):442-9.
71. Lee PC, Rhee RY, Gordon RY, Fung JJ, Webster MW. Management of splenic artery aneurysms: the significance of portal and essential hypertension. J Am Coll Surg. 1999;189(5):483-90.
72. Selo-Ojeme DO, Welch CC. Review: spontaneous rupture of splenic artery aneurysm in pregnancy. Eur J Obstet Gynecol Reprod Biol. 2003;109(2):124-7.
73. Tessier DJ, Stone WM, Fowl RJ, Abbas MA, Andrews JC, Bower TC, et al. Clinical features and management of splenic artery pseudoaneurysm: case series and cumulative review of literature. J Vasc Surg. 2003;38(5):969-74.
74. Stanley JC, Wakefield TW, Graham LM, Whitehouse WM Jr, Zelenock GB, Lindenauer SM. Clinical importance and management of splanchnic artery aneurysms. J Vasc Surg. 1986;3(5):836-40.

75. Trastek VF, Pairolero PC, Bernatz PE. Splenic artery aneurysms. World J Surg. 1985;9(3):378-83.
76. Mattar SG, Lumsden AB. The management of splenic artery aneurysms: experience with 23 cases. Am J Surg. 1995;169(6): 580-4.
77. de Perrot M, Buhler L, Schneider PA, Mentha G, Morel P. Do aneurysms and pseudoaneurysms of the splenic artery require different surgical strategy? Hepatogastroenterology. 1999;46(27):2028-32.
78. Hogendoorn W, Lavida A, Hunink MG, Moll FL, Geroulakos G, Muhs BE, et al. Open repair, endovascular repair, and conservative management of true splenic artery aneurysms. J Vasc Surg. 2014;60(6):1667-76 e1.
79. Hogendoorn W, Lavida A, Hunink MG, Moll FL, Geroulakos G, Muhs BE, et al. Cost-effectiveness of endovascular repair, open repair, and conservative management of splenic artery aneurysms. J Vasc Surg. 2015;61(6):1432-40.
80. Guillon R, Garcier JM, Abergel A, Mofid R, Garcia V, Chahid T, et al. Management of splenic artery aneurysms and false aneurysms with endovascular treatment in 12 patients. Cardiovasc Intervent Radiol. 2003;26(3):256-60.
81. Gu JJ, He XH, Li WT, Ji J, Peng WJ, Li GD, et al. Safety and efficacy of splenic artery coil embolization for hypersplenism in liver cirrhosis. Acta Radiol. 2012;53(8):862-7.
82. Puri S, Nicholson AA, Breen DJ. Percutaneous thrombin injection for the treatment of a post-pancreatitis pseudoaneurysm. Eur Radiol. 2003;13(Suppl 4):L79-82.
83. Krueger K, Zaehringer M, Lackner K. Percutaneous treatment of a splenic artery pseudoaneurysm by thrombin injection. J Vasc Interv Radiol. 2005;16(7):1023-5.
84. Hoeffel C, Bokemeyer C, Hoeffel JC, Gaucher H, Galanski M, Fornes P. CT hepatic and splenic appearances with sarcoidosis. Eur J Radiol. 1996;23(2):94-6.
85. Torres GM, Terry NL, Mergo PJ, Ros PR. MR imaging of the spleen. Magn Reson Imaging Clin N Am. 1995;3(1): 39-50.
86. Minami M, Itai Y, Ohtomo K, Ohnishi S, Niki T, Kokubo T, et al. Siderotic nodules in the spleen: MR imaging of portal hypertension. Radiology. 1989;172(3):681-4.
87. Sagoh T, Itoh K, Togashi K, Shibata T, Nishimura K, Minami S, et al. Gamna-Gandy bodies of the spleen: evaluation with MR imaging. Radiology. 1989;172(3):685-7.
88. Hill SC, Damaska BM, Ling A, Patterson K, Di Bisceglie AM, Brady RO, et al. Gaucher disease: abdominal MR imaging findings in 46 patients. Radiology. 1992;184(2): 561-6.
89. Housman JF, Chezmar JL, Nelson RC. Magnetic resonance imaging in hemochromatosis: extrahepatic iron deposition. Gastrointest Radiol. 1989;14(1):59-60.
90. Long JA Jr, Doppman JL, Nienhus AW, Mills SR. Computed tomographic analysis of beta-thalassemic syndromes with hemochromatosis: pathologic findings with clinical and laboratory correlations. J Comput Assist Tomogr. 1980;4(2): 159-65.
91. Kim SH, Han JK, Lee KH, Won HJ, Kim KW, Kim JS, et al. Abdominal amyloidosis: spectrum of radiological findings. Clin Radiol. 2003;58(8):610-20.
92. Liu TY, Chen SC, Wang LY, Chuang WL, Chang WY, Liu CS. Systemic amyloidosis presenting as splenic tumor. Gastrointest Radiol. 1991;16(2):137-8.
93. Kennan NM, Evans C. Case report: hepatic and splenic calcification due to amyloid. Clin Radiol. 1991;44(1):60-1.
94. Monzawa S, Tsukamoto T, Omata K, Hosoda K, Araki T, Sugimura K. A case with primary amyloidosis of the liver and spleen: radiologic findings. Eur J Radiol. 2002;41(3):237-41.

CHAPTER 95

Imaging of the Postoperative Abdomen

Mandeep Kang, Ujjwal Gorsi, Anmol Bhatia

INTRODUCTION

Recent advances in the understanding of the pathophysiology of disease processes has led to improved medical as well as surgical management. There have been substantial advances in the technique and type of surgical procedures being performed with an increasing trend towards minimally invasive techniques. This in turn has led to an increasing number of requests for radiological investigations for the evaluation of postoperative patients. These include the detection of complications both in the early (less than 4 weeks) and late phases (more than 4 weeks) as well as disease recurrence. To be able to recognize these complications, the radiologist needs to be familiar with the normal postoperative appearances of the surgery that has been performed as well as the complications that can occur after the procedure. It becomes critical here to be able to differentiate between what are the expected postoperative changes (relative to the temporal profile) and what findings constitute pathology, which in-turn can alter patient management.

In this chapter, we will address the basics of imaging of the postoperative abdomen, the general complications which may occur, the normal postoperative anatomy as well as specific complications which are peculiar to certain commonly performed surgical procedures.

IMAGING MODALITIES

Plain X-rays of the abdomen are commonly asked for in the immediate postoperative period and are useful for the detection of pneumoperitoneum, ileus or intestinal obstruction. Ultrasonography is often asked for to detect fluid collections or abscess or to look for biliary radicle dilatation after biliary procedures. The presence of surgical dressings on the abdominal wall and pneumoperitoneum or ileus in the immediate postoperative period limit its usefulness.[1] However, its portability as well as the use of non-ionizing radiation is of advantage particularly when children or young women have to undergo repeated imaging.

Helical CT is now the modality of choice for the radiological evaluation of the postoperative patient. Rapid acquisition is of advantage when critically sick patients need to be imaged. The ability to reconstruct multiplanar images is useful when complex postoperative anatomy has to be evaluated.

CT PROTOCOL

Positive water-soluble iodinated oral contrast should be used in most postoperative examinations, particularly when anastomotic leakage has to be ruled out. Any leakage of the water-soluble contrast into the peritoneal cavity will not have any deleterious effect on the patient. Oral contrast is also most useful for differentiating distended bowel loops from extraluminal fluid collections. Sick patients may not be able to tolerate larger volumes, administering between 500 to 1000 mL of oral contrast should be enough to achieve an optimal diagnostic study. If plain radiographs of the abdomen reveal evidence of bowel obstruction, oral contrast can be avoided as the fluid in the dilated bowel loops provides a natural contrast.

If suspected bowel ischemia or acute gastrointestinal bleeding is the clinical indication for the CT scan, one should perform a biphasic CECT with negative oral contrast. In both these clinical scenarios, performing dual energy CT is of benefit, both from the point of view of reducing the patient's radiation dose as well as improving the diagnostic accuracy. By using dual energy CT and generating virtual non-enhanced images, one can omit the pre-contrast acquisition which is generally performed to detect presence of hyperattenuation signifying bleed in the bowel lumen.[2] Subtle differences in the enhancement of ischemic bowel loops become more conspicuous with the use of iodine maps or quantitative measurements of the iodine content in the wall of the bowel.[3] Rectal contrast should be used particularly following colorectal surgery.

Intravenous iodinated contrast should be used in all patients, unless there is a specific contraindication such as deranged renal parameters or history of allergy to contrast. Besides the clinical scenarios mentioned previously where one should acquire a biphasic CECT, a single portal venous phase acquisition is adequate. The anatomical coverage should be from the domes of the diaphragm to the public symphysis, even if the surgery has been performed in the upper abdomen or pelvis. This is because both the compartments are interconnected and fluid may track along anatomical pathways from one to the other.[4] Secondly many new pathways come into existence because of defects in the mesentery created due to the surgical procedure and so fluid may track to a location remote from the surgical bed.

NORMAL RADIOLOGICAL FINDINGS IN THE POSTOPERATIVE ABDOMEN

Some amount of changes will occur following surgery which do not represent complications but are due to the procedure itself. Soft tissue stranding or patchy increased density will be seen in the subcutaneous fat around the incision site and in the intra-abdominal fat around the operative site. When the surgical procedure has involved significant handling of the bowel loops, these can show mural thickening or ileus **(Fig. 1)**. Subcutaneous emphysema may be seen in the anterior abdominal wall which may be extensive following laparoscopic procedures.[5]

Presence of free intraperitoneal air can pose a diagnostic dilemma to the radiologist as it can be due to the procedure itself or represent a complication such as an anastomotic leak or development of infection. Detection of pneumoperitoneum on plain radiographs formed the basis of initial literature. CT shows a much higher

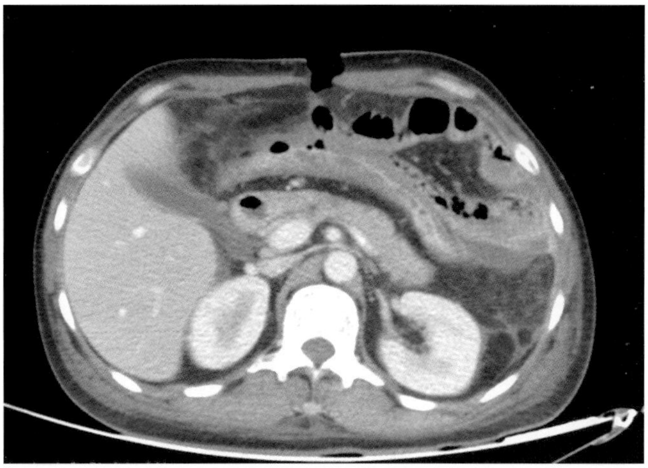

Fig. 1: A 42-year-old male underwent right hemicolectomy for carcinoma ascending colon. CECT axial image on postoperative day 4 shows diffuse mural thickening of the small bowel loops due to edema.

sensitivity for the detection of free intraperitoneal air in comparison to plain radiographs (87% on day 3 on CT versus 53% on X-ray).[6] Pneumoperitoneum is reported to be present in up to 44% of CT scans performed on the third postoperative day, decreasing with time to 30% of cases between days 14 and 18 following surgery. The volume does not usually exceed 10 mL but larger volumes up to 40 mL may be seen in some patients.[7]

Laparoscopic surgery involves insufflation of carbon dioxide to create an artificial pneumoperitoneum. Carbon dioxide is more rapidly absorbed than nitrogen which is the main component of room air. Therefore, the amount of postoperative free intraperitoneal air is less with laparoscopic surgeries in comparison to open surgeries and is expected to be completely resorbed by 48 hours. It may however be seen up to the 9th postoperative day on plain X-rays[8] and up to 2 weeks on CT.[5] Presence of pneumoperitoneum more than 7–10 days following open surgery and more than two days after laparoscopic surgery is a cause for concern. Individual cases normally require clinicoradiological correlation. If there is still a doubt, one can consider follow-up radiological evaluation as any increase in the volume of pneumoperitoneum over time is definitely due to a complication.[9] One must also remember that surgical drains or percutaneous catheter *in situ* also lead to free intraperitoneal air and their presence must be kept in mind while interpreting the significance of the pneumoperitoneum.

A picture of generalized fluid retention may be seen in the postoperative period as a result of hypoproteinemia,

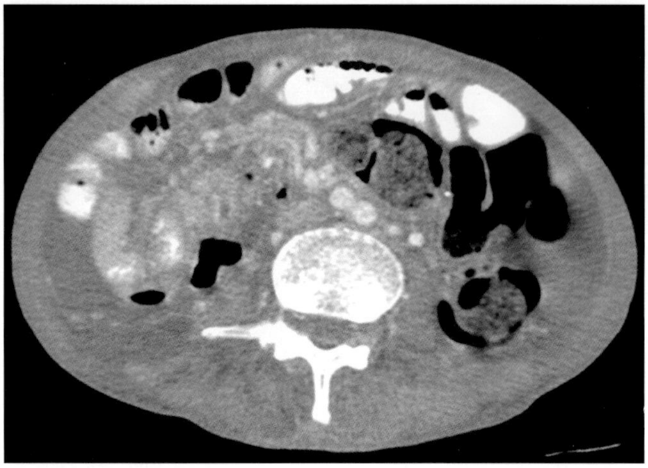

Fig. 2: A 53-year-old male underwent palliative distal gastrectomy with feeding jejunostomy for carcinoma distal stomach. CECT axial image on day 8 shows ascites with diffuse increased density of the mesentery with generalized edema of the subcutaneous fat.

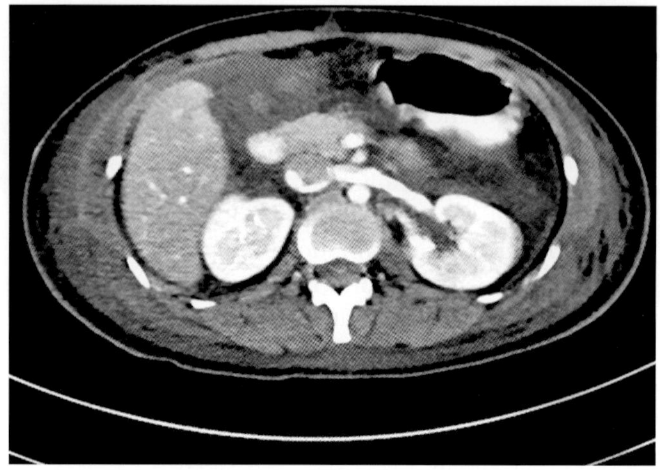

Fig. 3: A 28-year-old female postlaparoscopic cholecystectomy. CECT on day 4 following surgery shows mild peritoneal enhancement with fluid in the gallbladder fossa.

fluid retention and fluid overload. This is more commonly seen in patients with comorbidities, particularly, renal or cardiac problems. This may result in a "Wet" patient with combinations of pleural effusion, mild ascities and edema of the mesenteric or subcutaneous fat **(Fig. 2)**.[9] Due to the surgical procedure, there is some accumulation of blood, lymph and intraperitoneal fluid in the operative bed. These appear radiologically as unencapsulated, crescentric collections which do not anatomically displace any surrounding structures. These are generally absorbed spontaneously.[10] There may be mild peritoneal enhancement **(Fig. 3)**. Due to the decreased diaphragmatic excursion secondary to the pain associated with movement of the abdominal wall, some degree of bilateral basal passive atelectasis of the lungs is also expected in the immediate postoperative period.

Hemostatic compounds may be used by the surgeons to control intraoperative bleeding. The most commonly used is Surgicel, made of oxidized regenerated cellulose which may be left behind in the abdomen as it is bioabsorbable. On CT, it appears hypodense with a bubbly appearance, containing multiple gas foci which may be peripheral, located in the operative bed **(Fig. 4)**. This may be mistaken for an abscess, however Surgicel will not show any enhancement following contrast.[11]

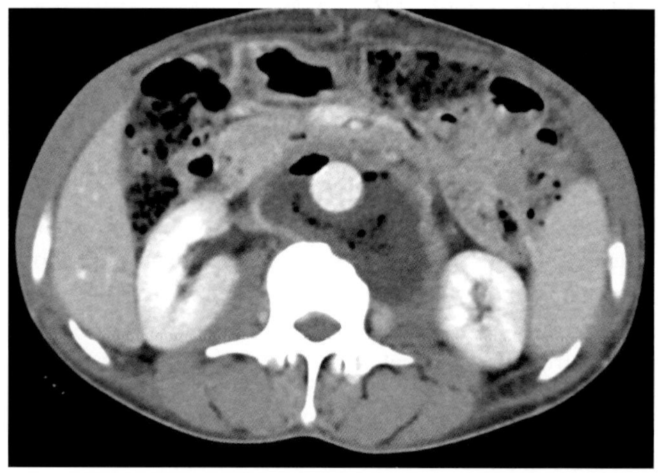

Fig. 4: A 70-year-old male underwent aortic aneurysm repair with graft placement. CECT axial image on postoperative day 3 shows Surgicel as a hypodense area with a bubbly appearance surrounding the graft with air foci.

POSTOPERATIVE COMPLICATIONS

Postsurgical complications are common as they are part of the inherent risk of the procedure. In the immediate post-operative period, they are commonly related to infections or the surgical technique. Later complications may occur due to the altered anatomy, or recurrence of the primary disease process.

Anastomotic Leak

Anastomotic leaks are common to all reconstructive gastrointestinal surgeries and have an incidence of 1–5% after upper gastrointestinal surgeries and of 5–10% following colon resections.[12] They are associated with a high mortality (up to 50%) and morbidity and therefore require prompt recognition and early treatment.[10] Leaks occur at the anastomotic margins due to devascularization leading to necrosis, and therefore usually manifest clinically within the first fortnight following the surgery. Clinical symptoms are usually of sudden onset and consist of fever, which may show spikes, intense abdominal pain with guarding and rebound tenderness, tachycardia and rising leukocyte counts. Fluoroscopic gastrointestinal studies using water soluble iodinated contrast have been shown to be useful for the detection and localization of leaks,[4,10] however helical CT with its multiplanar reformation capability is a better modality. It has been reported to confirm clinically suspected leaks in 48–100% of cases.[13] The hallmark of an anastomotic leak is extraluminal extravasation of oral or rectal contrast with air in the operative bed **(Fig. 5)**. At times oral contrast may not have had time to reach the anastomotic site due to the associated ileus. In this case, presence of loculated fluid with excess of extraluminal air in the surgical bed should raise the possibility of leak **(Figs. 6A and B)**.[14] At times, one can also seen disruption of the staple line at the anastomotic site.

Postoperative Abscess

Postoperative intra-abdominal abscesses are a serious complication associated with high morbidity and mortality rates of 10–40%.[10] They usually occur due to anastomotic leaks, in association with wound infections or operative contamination. Enteric pathogens such as *Klebsiella*, *E. Coli*, and *Proteus* are the usual causative organisms. Helical CT is reported to have a high accuracy of more than 90% for the detection of intra-abdominal abscesses.[10,15,16] On CT, these appear as a low attenuation fluid collection, spherical or ovoid in shape, which is usually well defined. They usually show a peripheral enhancing rim. Air foci, air-fluid levels or septations may be seen at times. There may be mass effect with distortion or displacement of adjacent structures. The abscess may be located in the surgical bed or at a remote location due to spread of inflammation along anatomical pathways in the peritoneal cavity or

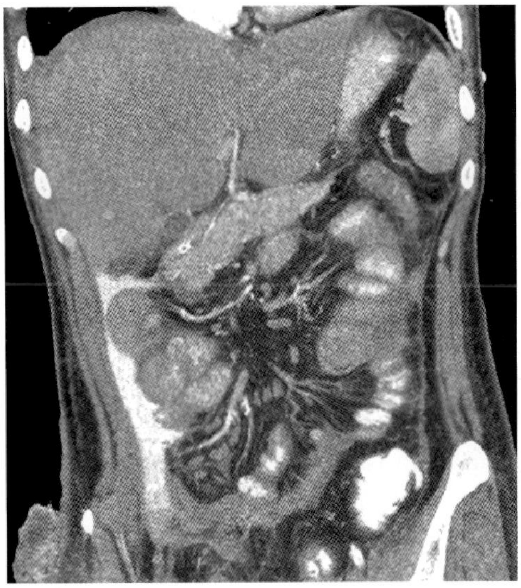

Fig. 5: A 27-year-old female underwent subtotal colectomy with endileostomy for a perforation at the hepatic flexure. Presented on day 3 following surgery with fever and pain abdomen. Coronal MPR demonstrates extraluminal oral contrast due to anastomotic leak.

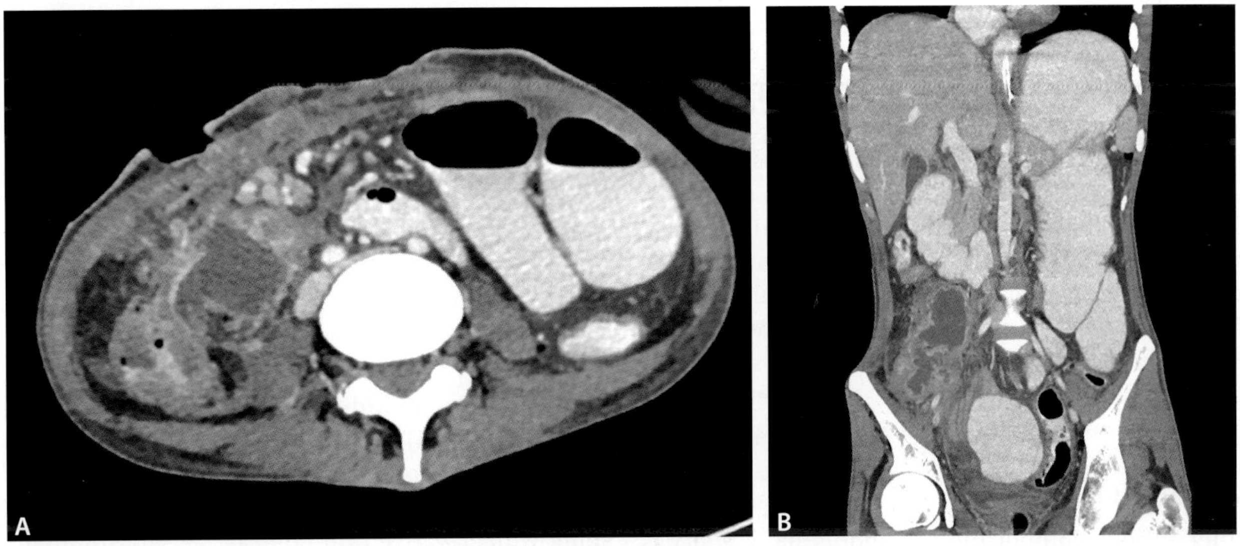

Figs. 6A and B: A 26-year-old female underwent ileal resection for bowel gangrene with end jejunostomy. Postrestoration of bowel continuity with jejunocolic anastomosis, presented on day 4 with high-grade fever and abdominal distension. (A) Axial CECT image shows a multiloculated collection with surrounding stranding adjacent to the anastomotic site. The ascending colon shows diffuse mural thickening. Note the thickening of the anterior abdominal wall with separation of the layers and few specks of air. (B) Coronal reconstructed image shows grossly dilated proximal jejunal loops.

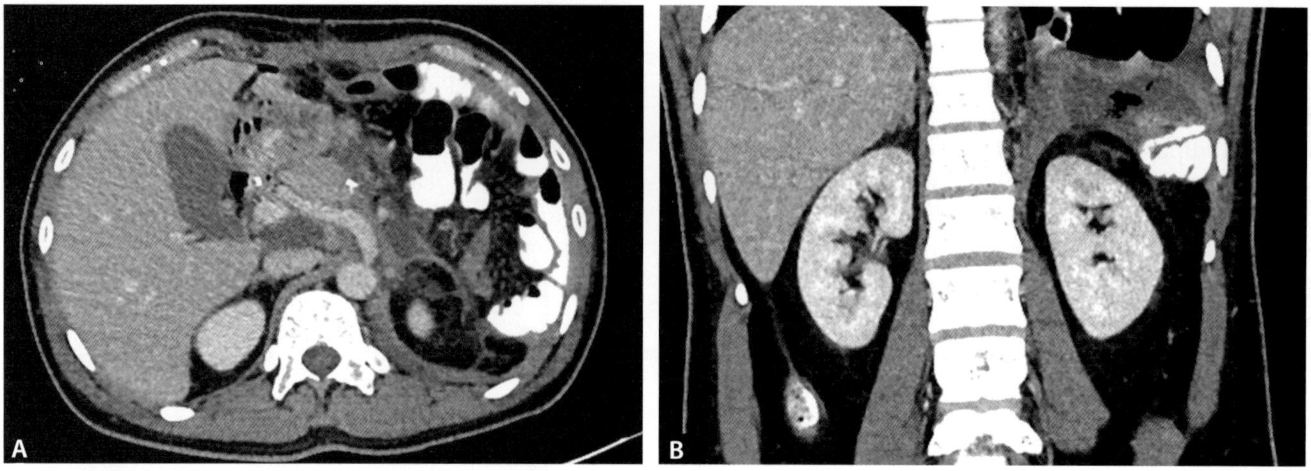

Figs. 7A and B: A 47-year-old male with gastric GIST underwent a total gastrectomy, distal pancreatectomy and splenectomy. Patient developed spiking fever on 7th postoperative day. (A) Axial CECT image shows small amount of fluid and fat stranding in the operative bed; (B) Coronal MPR demonstrates a fluid collection with specks of air and thick-enhancing rim in the left subphrenic space.

along the surgically created non-anatomic pathways and spaces.[4,10] As an example, the gastrosplenic and gastrocolic ligaments are transected during gastrectomy while the gastrohepatic ligament is partially transected. This creates a communication between the lesser sac, left sub-phrenic, gastrosplenic and gastrohepatic spaces. Hence, an anastomotic leak may cause a fluid collection or abscess in this newly created compartment with spread to the left sub-phrenic space **(Figs. 7A and B)**. Abscesses in the left subphrenic space usually have associated left pleural effusion and basal consolidation.[17] Inter-loop abscesses may be accompanied by paralytic ileus.[10]

Image-guided percutaneous catheter drainage is the preferred management option, and therefore, the initial CT report should mention the suitability for safe drainage of the abscess, especially regarding the location and access route. The true internal character of the abscess may not be evident on CT. Ultrasonography and MR are better at determining the degree of liquefaction and presence of septations which in-turn help predict whether this particular abscess will respond to percutaneous catheter drainage alone or will surgical intervention be required.[9,18] Percutaneous catheter drainage is also less likely to succeed, if the abscess is due to an anastomic leak, or if there is a fistulous communication with the bowel.[9,10]

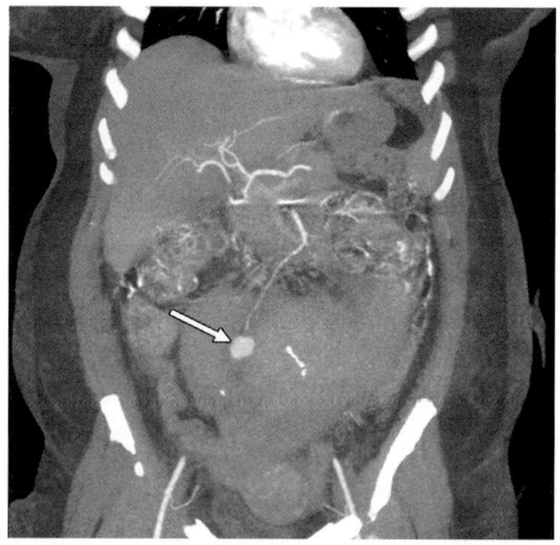

Fig. 8: A 56-year-old female underwent resection with end-to-end anastomosis for bowel gangrene. Presented with bleeding from main wound on fourth postoperative day. CT angiography coronal MIP image shows a 23 × 20 mm pseudoaneurysm arising from a branch of the superior mesenteric artery with surrounding hematoma.

Postoperative Bleeding

Another serious complication of abdominal surgery is hemorrhage which may be due to inadvertent vessel or organ injury, inadequate hemostasis or vascular ligation. In addition, in patients with obstructive jaundice or hepatic dysfunction, deficiency of vitamin K or coagulation factor may cause a hemorrhagic diathesis leading to this postoperative complication. Clinically, the patients present with signs of blood loss with falling hematocrit, tachycardia and hypotension. The surgical drains (if placed) may reveal bloody fluid or there may be oozing of blood through the incision site.[4,10,17] As mentioned previously, a biphasic CT scan should be done with negative oral contrast as intraluminal high attenuation can be masked by the positive oral contrast. A bleeding vessel may at times be seen on the CT showing active extravasation of the intravenous contrast **(Figs. 8 and 9)**. These patients may be managed by

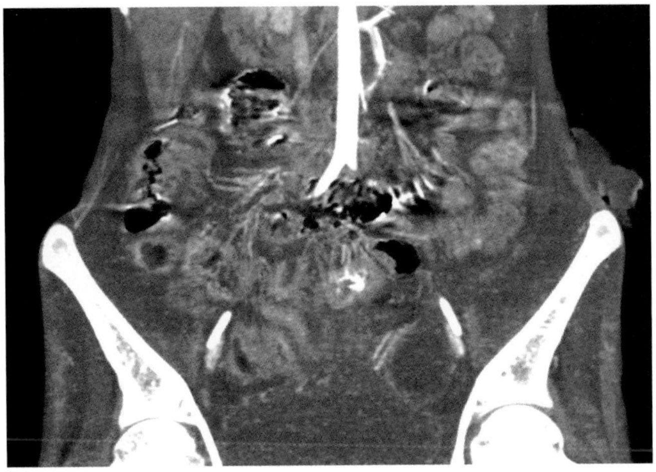

Fig. 9: A 32-year-old female who had undergone a right hemicolectomy for abdominal tuberculosis developed an enterocutaneous fistula. Presented with history of bleeding from site of fistula. CT angiography MIP image demonstrates high attenuation in the bowel lumen due to active extravasation of contrast from a branch of the superior mesenteric artery.

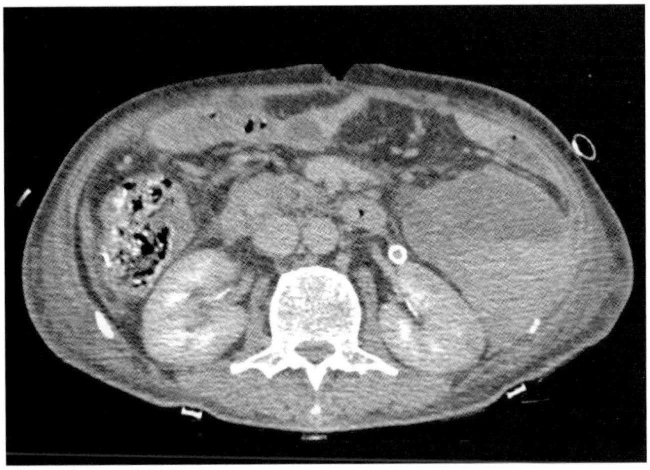

Fig. 10: A 42-year-old male underwent distal pancreatectomy with splenectomy. CECT axial image on postoperative day 4 shows a large hyperdense collection in the right lumbar region with a layered appearance consistent with acute hematoma.

endovascular embolization. Acute hematomas are hyperdense on CT with attenuation values between 20–60 HU with a layered appearance, with gradual decrease in density over time as hemoglobin is removed from the clot **(Fig. 10)**. Chronic hematomas have fluid attenuation and may be indistinguishable from other fluid collections. There can be mass effect on the adjacent structures depending upon their location and size. Postoperative hematomas involving the solid organs (spleen, liver or kidneys) are usually confined by the organ capsule. Therefore, they appear as crescentric collections in the subcapsular space with variable compression of the underlying parenchyma.

Anterior abdominal wall hematomas can occur due to injury to perforators in the subcutaneous fat during the placement of trocars in laparoscopic surgery. High attenuation collections in the subcutaneous fat with thickening of the abdominal wall muscles which appear hyperdense will be visualized on CT **(Fig. 11)**.[5]

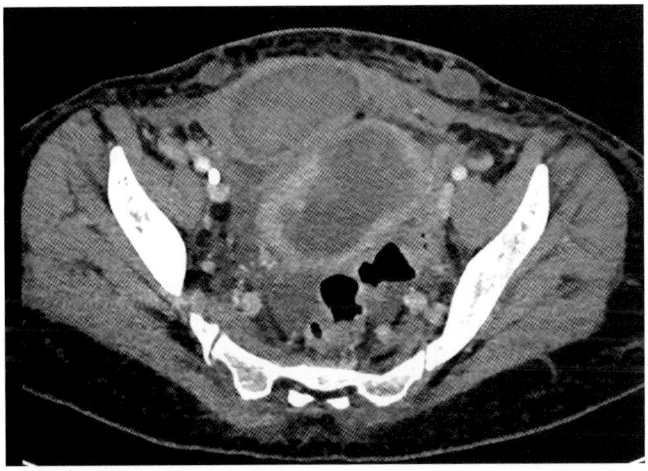

Fig. 11: A 22-year-old female underwent a cesarean section with development of postoperative sepsis. CECT on day 14 demonstrates a large hypodense collection in the right rectus sheath with few internal hyperdensities consistent with hematoma.

Anastomotic Strictures

Hold-up in the passage of contrast across the anastomotic sites on fluoroscopic examinations done in the immediate postoperative period is generally due to edema and resolves spontaneously over time. Nevertheless, anastomotic strictures may develop following surgical procedures due to ischemia and are more common when there has been an anastomotic leak. These can usually be managed with balloon dilatation, if an endoscopic approach is available.[19]

Postoperative Bowel Obstruction

Postoperative ileus is commonly seen in the early phase following abdominal surgery and may be due to excessive handling of the bowel loops during the procedure. It may later be a manifestation of inter-loop abscesses. Plain radiographs show mild dilatation of the small bowel loops. On CT, the small bowel is distended with fluid and air with no obvious transition point.[10] At times, there may be accompanying dilatation of the ascending and transverse

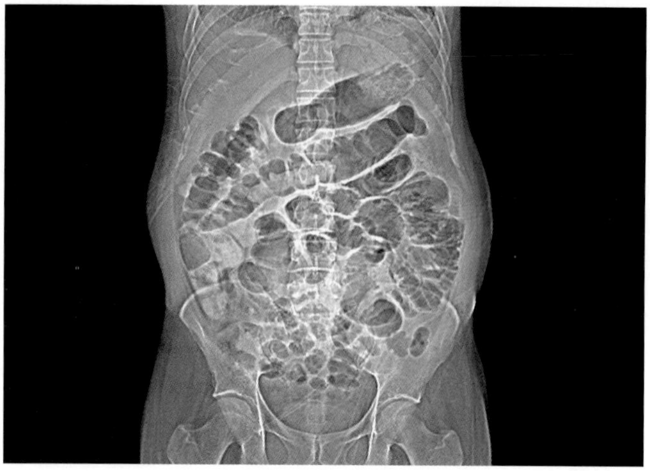

Fig. 12: A 38-year-old female developed abdominal distension on the second postoperative day following open cholecystectomy. Scout film prior to CT shows moderately dilated small bowel loops with dilatation of the ascending and descending colon and collapsed distal colon due to ileus.

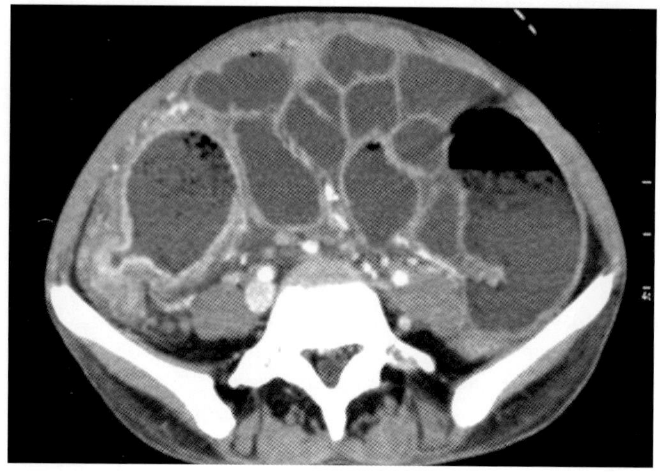

Fig. 13: A 38-year-male underwent a total colectomy with end ileostomy for ulcerative colitis. Presented with mechanical bowel obstruction two months after the surgery. CECT axial image shows gross dilatation of a small bowel loop with mottled air lucencies—the "small bowel feces" sign.

colon extending till the splenic flexure with collapse of the distal colon. This is said to be due to the increase in the intra-abdominal pressure resulting in collapse of the left colon which lies in a dependent position posteriorly **(Fig. 12)**.[20] Small bowel mechanical obstruction can occur in the postoperative period due to the formation of adhesions, internal hernias or incisional or port site hernias, volvulus, strictures or tumor recurrence. Adhesions can occur in more than 90% of patients who have undergone major abdominal surgery.[21] Internal hernias can occur when the surgical procedure has involved creating defects in the mesentery or mesocolon, for example following Roux-en-Y gastrojejunostomy.[19] Typical radiological features include dilated proximal small loops with collapsed loops distal to the transition zone. There may be particulate feculent matter seen in the small bowel loop just proximal to the point of obstruction known as the "small bowel feces" sign **(Fig. 13)**.[22] An abrupt transition with no identifiable cause is likely due to adhesions **(Fig. 14)**. A cluster of dilated loops may be seen in cases of internal hernias or volvulus. The mesenteric vessels may be engorged and demonstrate the "swirl" sign as the mesentery is pulled into an abnormal location.

One must carefully look for signs of ischemia in the obstructed loop as the management of the patient may be radically altered, if present. In brief, these include mural thickening which can give a stratified appearance, abnormal enhancement of the involved segment of bowel and soft tissue stranding or fluid in the subtending mesentery. The presence of pneumatosis in the involved segment of bowel or gas in the portal venous radicles are signs of irreversible ischemia.[23]

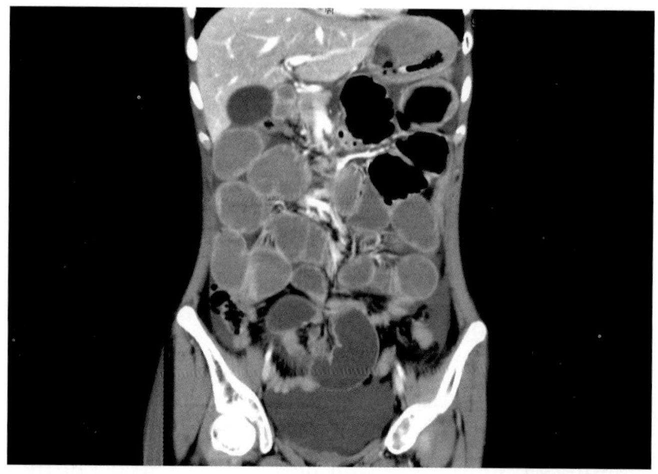

Fig. 14: A 35-year-old female postdistal pancreatectomy with splenectomy with abdominal distension and no passage of flatus. CECT reconstructed coronal image shows the dilated fluid-filled jejunal loops with an abrupt transition point beyond which the loops are collapsed. No obvious mass or stricture is seen at the transition zone, the cause of obstruction is most likely due to adhesions.

Large bowel obstruction is less common in the postoperative period but can lead to marked dilatation of the colon. As the cecum is the most distensible segment of the colon, it bears the brunt of the dilatation. In the presence of a competent ileocecal valve, thereby preventing decompression into the small bowel, there is a grave risk of cecal ischemia as well as perforation.[9]

Wound Complications

On CT, the surgical incision site can be easily recognized as an area of increased attenuation in the subcutaneous fat and muscles of the abdominal wall. Wound infection develops in about 5–10% of patients who undergo abdominal surgery generally due to contamination by anaerobic organisms.[10] The resultant inflammation can lead to necrosis and pus accumulation at the incision site, with the potential adverse sequelae of wound dehiscence, necrotizing fasciitis, incisional hernia formation, peritonitis and systemic sepsis. Various risk factors associated with increased incidence of wound infections include elderly patients, obesity, tobacco, drugs or alcohol abuse, and presence of comorbidities. The risk also depends upon the kind of surgery performed with abdominoperineal resections having a higher incidence.[26]

CT scan can detect the presence of wound infection even before it becomes clinically apparent as small collections of fluid and air in the subcutaneous fat and muscles of the abdominal wall at and around the incision site **(Fig. 15)**.[4,10] Unless this condition is recognized early and treated promptly, it can lead on to frank abscess formation and ultimately separation of the fascia at the incision and wound dehiscence. On CT, one needs to meticulously evaluate all the layers of the abdominal wall around the incision site, including the anterior and posterior fascial sheaths for evidence of any separation which portends dehiscence.[27]

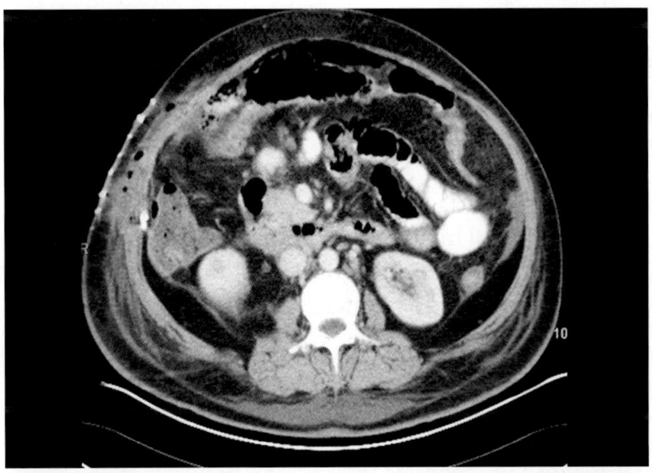

Fig. 15: A 41-year-old female underwent extended cholecystectomy for carcinoma gallbladder. Postoperative day 14 CECT shows thickening of the layers of the anterior abdominal wall at the incision site with multiple foci of air suggestive of wound infection.

Incisional Hernia

Despite improvements in surgical techniques, incisional hernias develop in about 3–30% of cases[24,28] with the incidence rising in the presence of wound infection.[29] It is also more common when median or paramedian vertical incisions are used in comparison to horizontal incisions as vertical incisions transect the muscular fibers rather than dissect along them. These transected muscles are rendered more prone to disruption in the presence of increased abdominal pressure.[10,30] Most incisional hernias develop within the first year following surgery but may manifest clinically much later. Clinical examination usually suffices to reach the diagnosis, however in the presence of obesity or a thick keloid, the abdominal wall defect may not be palpable. Secondly, the omentum is usually the initial content of the hernia and may not be palpable, if the sac has dissected between the layers of the abdominal wall. In this clinical setting, a CT may be asked for in order to find a cause for the patients symptoms and will establish the correct diagnosis.[24-26] Once bowel loops also herniate into the sac, they can get incarcerated and obstructed.

CT scans will show a defect in the layers of the abdominal wall with protrusion of omentum, a loop of small bowel or mesentery through it into the subcutaneous fat. Presence of stranding in the fat, small fluid collections or mural thickening of the herniated bowel loop are early changes that suggest strangulation.[25] Herniation may also occur at port sites following laparoscopy with a reported incidence of 0.5% with a higher risk associated with the use of trocars over 12 mm and large diameter ports.[5] Parastomal herniation may also occur along ileostomy or colostomy sites **(Figs. 16A and B)**.[10]

Retained Surgical Foreign Material

Unintended retention of a surgical material in a patient poses a serious risk of complications for the patient and lays the surgical team open for a malpractice suit. Usual operating theater procedures include repeated counts of all surgical material being used to prevent this complication, but it still occurs though the exact incidence is not known. Reports reveal that surgical sponges are the most often retained foreign object followed by instruments.[31] Septic or aseptic complications result due to the retained foreign object (RFO). If the RFO remains sterile, fibrosis occurs due to a foreign body response leading to adhesions or fistula formation. Retained surgical swabs are referred

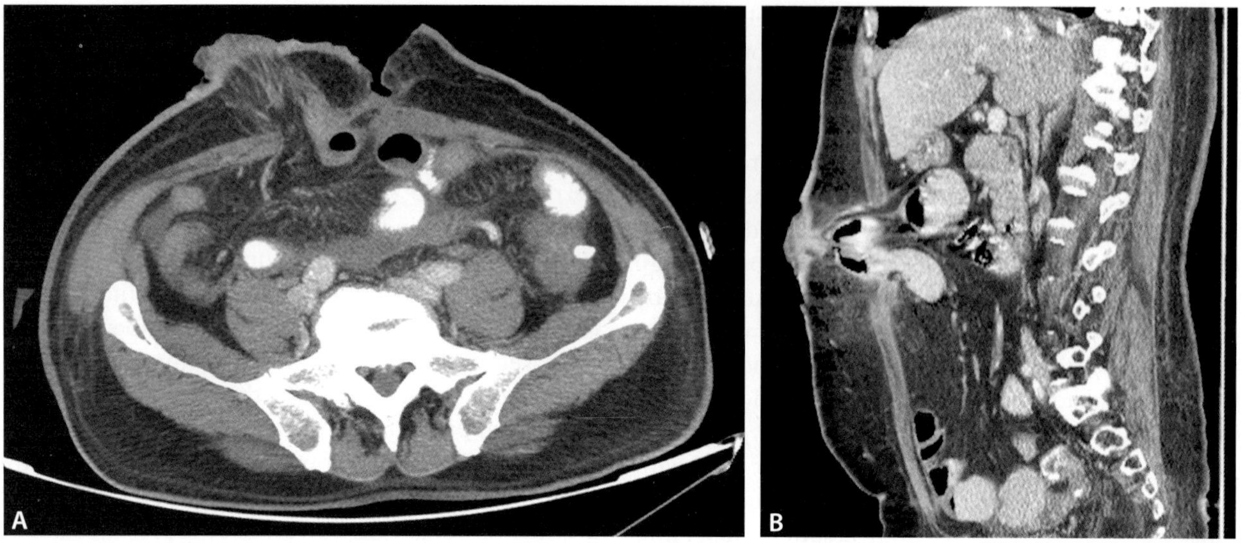

Figs. 16A and B: (A) Axial CECT image of a 78-year-old male showing a small parastomal hernia containing mainly omental fat and vessels; (B) Coronal MPR image of a 43-year-old female with a transverse colostomy with a large parastomal hernial sac containing small bowel loops.

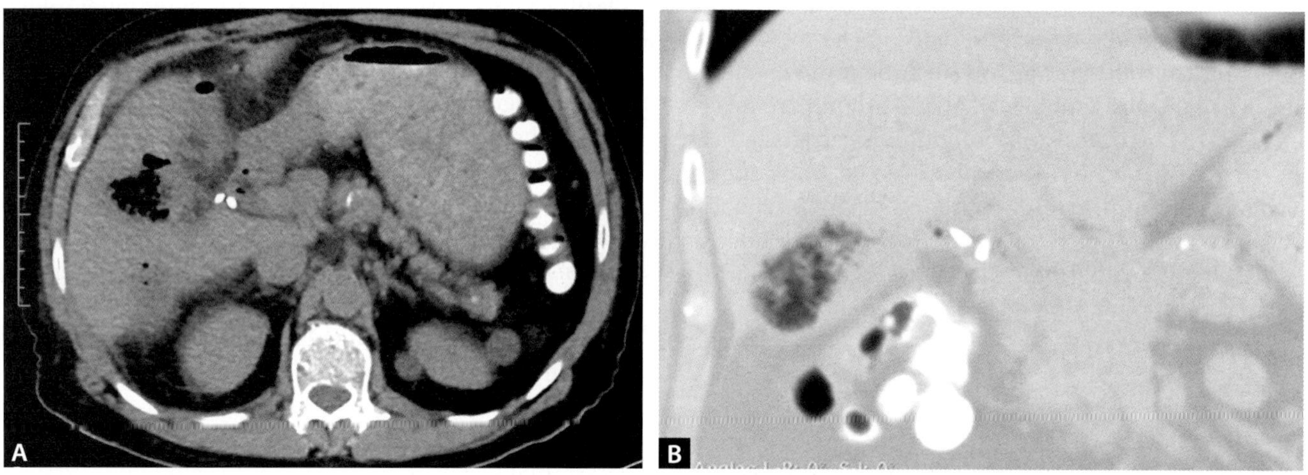

Figs. 17A and B: A 28-year-old female complained of intermittent right hypochondrial pain following a laparoscopic cholecystectomy. (A) CECT axial image shows an ill-defined hypodense area with multiple air foci adjacent to the surgical clips consistent with gossypiboma; (B) The internal whorled appearance is better appreciated on viewing at lung window settings.

to as gossypibomas or textilomas and appear on CT as well-defined soft tissue masses with a whorled texture and multiple internal foci of air **(Figs. 17A and B)**. Enhancement of the rim is seen following intravenous contrast. It is helpful to identify the wavy radiopaque markers which are now incorporated into most surgical sponges[9,32] which may be better appreciated on the scout image rather than the axial images. In the setting of infection, there is abscess formation with a loculated fluid collection often showing a thick enhancing rim. On MR imaging, retained sponges show an intermediate signal intensity on T1-weighted images similar to skeletal muscle. Internal high signal intensity fluid may be seen on T2-weighted images with low signal intensity structures having a whorled appearance.[31]

NORMAL POSTOPERATIVE ANATOMY AND COMPLICATIONS SPECIFIC TO PROCEDURE

It is beyond the scope of this chapter to discuss the normal postoperative anatomy of the myriad surgical procedures performed in the abdomen. This chapter will limit itself to discussing some of the most commonly performed surgical procedures.

Esophageal Surgeries

Esophageal resections are commonly performed for malignancy but may also be performed for benign strictures refractory to balloon dilatation. The Ivor Lewis esophagectomy involves resection of the diseased part of the mid and distal esophagus, and mobilization of the stomach which is then placed vertically inside the mediastinum after fashioning it into a tubular structure by resection of the greater curvature. This is then anastomosed with the esophagus in an end-to end or end-to-side manner. In case of disease involving the upper esophagus a neck dissection is also done and the esophagogastric anastomotic is created in the neck. These are usually accompanied with a pyloroplasty to drain the stomach as the vagus nerve is sacrificed during the procedure.[33]

Upper gastrointestinal contrast studies are routinely performed between 5–10 days postoperatively to look for any anastomotic leak before the patient is allowed oral intake. Water-soluble non-ionic contrast is preferred as it does not carry the risk of chemical pneumonia in case of aspiration.[34] Many authors advocate the use of repeating the study with dilute barium in case the first study is negative in order to increase the sensitivity.[35,36] A plain radiograph should be obtained prior to administering contrast so that any subtle difference in density in pleural effusions can be detected which denote leak. It also aids in differentiating between a small leak and a surgical clip. CT may be done, if the contrast study is negative but the patient is unwell and improves the sensitivity for the detection of anastomotic leaks.[36]

Major complications occur in about 20% of patients which can be grouped into general complications of a thoracotomy such as pneumonia, atelectasis and respiratory failure or specific to the esophageal surgery. There can be vascular injury leading to a hemothorax or injury to the thoracic duct leading to a chylothorax but the most common complication is an anastomotic leak which carries significant morbidity and mortality. The leak usually occurs early in the postoperative period (2–3 days) due to technical failure of the anastomoses. Leaks occurring later at around 3–7 days are usually due to ischemia of the anastomotic margins. The leak may occur from the esophagogastrectomy, from the margins of the stomach where the greater curvature has been resected or from the pyloroplasty, hence all these sites need to be carefully examined. A leak can lead to formation of an esophago-bronchial or esophagopleural fistula, mediastinitis and sepsis **(Fig. 18)**. These patients are also at increased risk for the subsequent development of strictures.[37]

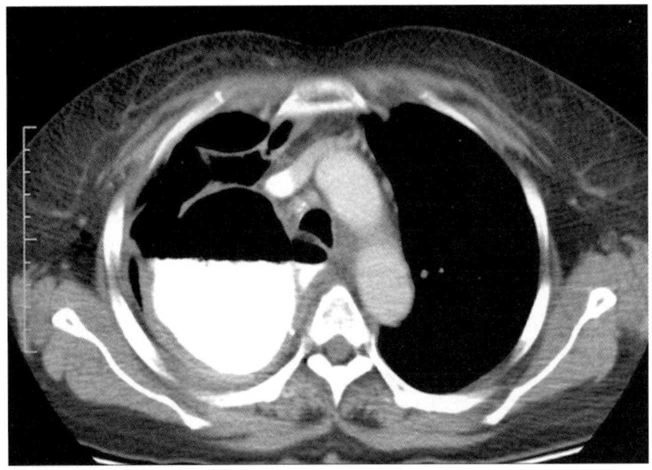

Fig. 18: A 42-year-old male underwent thoracoscopic assisted esophagectomy for carcinoma. Presented with complaints of chest pain, dyspnea and had tachycardia. CECT axial image demonstrates a leak from the esophagogastric anastomotic site with formation of a esophagopleural fistula.

Imaging has a similar role to look for anastomotic leaks following bypass procedures where colonic, jejunal or myocutaneous flaps are used. A more dreaded complication is ischemia of the conduit which is diagnosed endoscopically.

Surgeries of the Stomach and Duodenum

Gastric resections are commonly performed surgical procedures for malignancies involving the stomach or complicated peptic ulcer disease. In the Billroth I partial gastrectomy, the distal stomach is resected and an anastomosis created between the duodenum and proximal stomach. The Billroth II/Polya partial gastrectomy involves resection of the distal stomach, closure of the duodenal stump and creation of a gastrojejunostomy in an antecolic or retrocolic position. In a Roux-en-Y procedure, the bowel continuity after distal gastrectomy is restored through construction of a Roux loop. Direct anastomoses of the distal esophagus with a jejunal Roux loop is performed following total gastrectomy. A contrast fluoroscopic study is usually performed using water soluble contrast in the immediate postoperative period to rule out leakage. However, the study can detect subclinical leaks in 7% of cases which do not require any further surgical intervention. The study may also return false negative results with leaks identified on subsequent endoscopy.[38] Hence, some surgeons reserve the contrast study to cases where there is a clinical suspicion of leak. The afferent limb may not opacify with oral contrast, hence a CT examination should be done in case of clinical suspicion of duodenal stump blow-out.

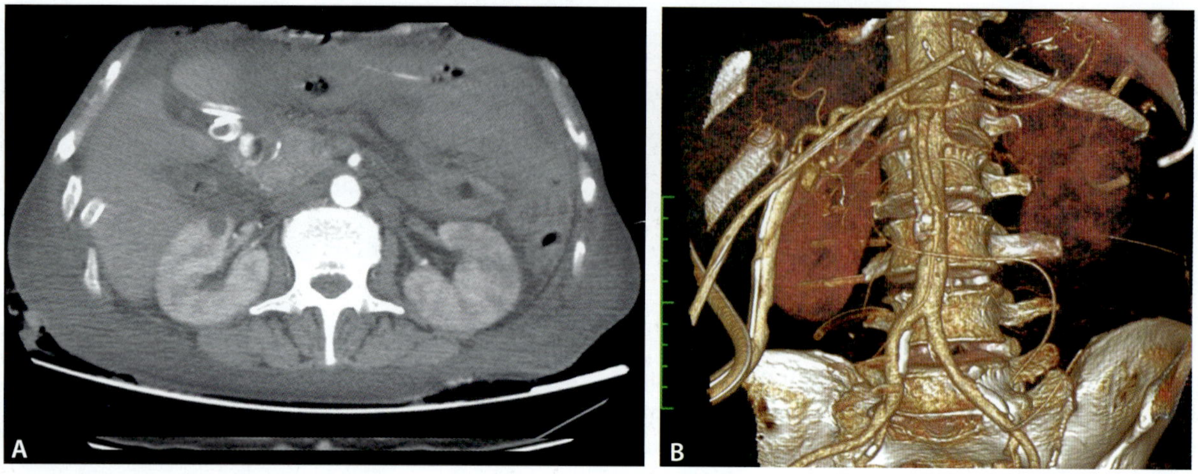

Figs. 19A and B: A 57-year-old male with gastric carcinoma, status postgastrectomy and Billroth II gastrojejunostomy. Had duodenal stump blow-out which was being managed conservatively with placement of a subhepatic drain. Now presented with bloody discharge from the drain. CT angiography (A) axial image shows active extravasation of intravenous contrast with pooling in the duodenum adjacent to the surgical drain; (B) Coronal volume-rendered image shows pseudoaneurysms arising from the gastroduodenal artery, probably due to leak of the pancreatic enzymes from the duodenal stump.

It may show complex, air/fluid collections in the region of the duodenal stump which can be identified by the surgical staples line **(Figs. 19A and B)**. Collections may also be seen in the subhepatic or peripancreatic spaces.[17]

The afferent loop may get obstructed due to adhesion or twisting of the bowel at the gastroenterostomy site. Acute obstruction can cause duodenal stump blow-out and is an emergent situation. CT can demonstrate the dilated, fluid-filled loop passing posterior to the superior mesenteric vessels to the left side. Obstruction to the outflow of bile usually results in associated dilatation of the biliary tree.[39]

Tumor recurrence becomes a more common cause for obstructive symptoms developing later in the time course after the surgery. CT is the imaging modality of choice in this situation and should be carefully evaluated for recurrence in the surgical bed or anastomotic site and any evidence of spread of disease to the lymph nodes, liver or peritoneum.[40] If the initial malignancy was a gastrointestinal stromal tumor, addition of an arterial phase to the imaging protocol is of benefit as these tumours are typically hypervascular.

Bariatric Surgery

Morbid obesity has shown an alarming increasing trend in its prevalence even in India over the last few years and has now reached epidemic proportions. A BMI over 25 kg/m^2 is considered overweight internationally. However, updated guidelines released by the Indian Council of Medical Research and the Ministry of Health and Family Welfare in 2012 considers a BMI over 23 kg/m^2 as overweight. This is due to a genetic tendency of Indians towards abdominal obesity with its attendant risk of life style diseases. Despite the morbidly obese forming a high-risk group, surgery for weight loss is offered to these patients as it reduces the long-term associated morbidity and improves life expectancy.[41]

Two kinds of procedures are used: malabsorptive procedures wherein the length of the absorptive surface is reduced by bypassing a segment of the small bowel. These are seldom used in isolation these days due to significant associated complications. Restrictive procedures aim to reduce the capacity of the stomach in order to induce early satiety. These include sleeve gastrectomy, vertical gastroplasty and laparoscopic adjustable gastric banding (LAGB). The Roux en Y gastric bypass (RYGB) and biliopancreatic diversion are combination procedures with both restrictive and malabsorptive components. Sleeve gastrectomy involves creating a narrow gastric tube along the lesser curvature by resecting 70–85% of the stomach along the greater curvature. In LAGB, an inflatable band is placed just below the gastroesophageal junction, thereby creating a small gastric pouch. The band is connected to a port in the anterior abdominal wall through which the volume of the band can be adjusted and therefore the degree of restriction. In the RYGB, a small gastric pouch is created in its proximal part and anastomosed to a Roux loop. The rest of the stomach and duodenum forms the biliopancreatic limb which is also anastomosed to the Roux loop. The length of the Roux loop determines the degree of malabsorption with more distal loops having more malabsorptive effect.[42]

Early in the postoperative period, a contrast fluoroscopic examination is usually performed to rule out anastomotic leaks. Following sleeve gastrectomy, most of the leaks occur from the proximal end, close to the gastroesophageal junction. CT is required for evaluation of the biliopancreatic limb in RYGB procedures. It is also the best modality for investigating a patient with suspected efferent loop obstruction, which may be due to adhesions, strictures, internal hernias or incisional hernias. Three types of internal hernias can occur following RYGB procedures:

a. Through the defect created in the transverse mesocolon when a retrocolic anastomosis has been created. Multiple, dilated small bowel loops will be seen superior to the transverse mesocolon, rather than the single anastomotic Roux loop on CT.
b. Through the defect created in the small bowel mesentery due to the jejunojejunostomy. In this case, a cluster of loops will be seen located beneath the anterior abdominal wall with absence of any intervening omental fat. The colon may be centrally displaced.
c. Through the defect in the mesentery posterior to the Roux loop (Peterson type).[43] Characteristically, there will be a cluster of small bowel loops in the left upper abdomen with shift of the superior mesenteric vessels to the left.

The gastric band placed in LAGB may migrate away from the gastroesophageal junction. The usual orientation of the balloon is at 45°, with migration it takes up a more vertical or horizontal position ("O" sign), which will be evident on plain radiographs.[44] A contrast swallow will confirm dilated stomach above the band. If the migration remains unrecognized or untreated, it may lead to gastric necrosis.

Small Bowel

Surgeries on the small bowel are commonly performed for resection of diseased segments or resections of segments which are required to be used as a conduit elsewhere. As mentioned earlier, the most common immediate postoperative complication is an anastomotic leak which is best evaluated by a CT after oral intravenous contrast. Delayed complications such as intestinal obstruction or recurrence of disease are usually evaluated with a combination of fluoroscopic contrast studies and cross-sectional imaging such as CT or MR enteroclysis or enterography.

Blind Pouch Syndrome

Side-to-side small bowel anastomoses or incorrectly performed end-to-side anastomoses can result in the formation of a blind pouch which is an enlarged, blind-ended, aperistaltic small bowel loop. These usually manifest late after surgery with features of malabsorption or due to complications such as perforation or bleeding. A dynamic investigation such as fluoroscopic enteroclysis will demonstrate the preferential filling of the blind pouch with dilatation of the loop. CT will demonstrate a saccular structure filled with oral contrast in close relation to surgical clips/staples.

Ileal Pouch-Anal Anastomoses (IPAA)

A total proctocolectomy is the definitive treatment for patients with ulcerative colitis or familiar adenomatous polyposis (FAP). This is followed by creation of an ileal pouch which is anastomosed to the anal canal, thus maintaining continence by preserving the anal sphincter. The ileal reservoir is created from the terminal ileum in a J, S or W manner of which the J-shape is the most commonly performed.[45] The pouch is usually allowed to heal by performing a proximal temporary ileostomy with restoration of the bowel continuity after 8-12 weeks. Routine fluoroscopic contrast studies are performed before closure of the ileostomy to rule out any leaks. CT may be done, if there is clinical suspicion of an abscess or obstruction.

Pouchitis is a non-specific inflammation of the pouch with uncertain etiology which can affect upto half the patients. The usual clinical presentation is with diarrhea, bleeding and tenesmus. The radiologic features are non-specific with dilatation of the pouch, mural thickening, mucosal enhancement and stranding in the surrounding fat.[46]

Large Bowel

Various kinds of resections of the large bowel are performed for both benign and malignant diseases. The right hemicolectomy involves resection of the right colon and terminal ileum with an ileotransverse colon anastomosis. In the extended right hemicolectomy, the transverse colon is also resected to varying extents. In a left hemicolectomy, the left colon including the splenic flexure and proximal sigmoid colon are resected. A Hartmann's procedure involves closing off of the rectum and sigmoid colon after a diverting colostomy after distal colectomy when a primary anastomosis is not considered safe. This rectal stump can later be reattached to the distal colon. At times, instead of closing off the stump, a distal mucous fistula is created by bringing the stump upto the anterior abdominal wall. Anterior resection consists of resecting the sigmoid colon and varying part of the rectum with a colorectal anastomosis. When the upper rectum is resected above the peritoneal reflection, it is termed a high anterior resection while in the low or extended

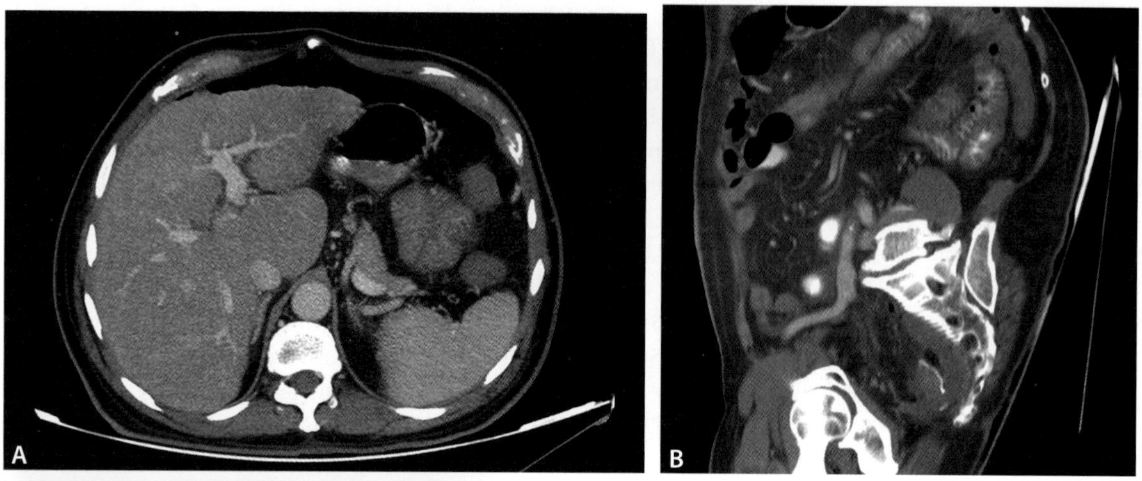

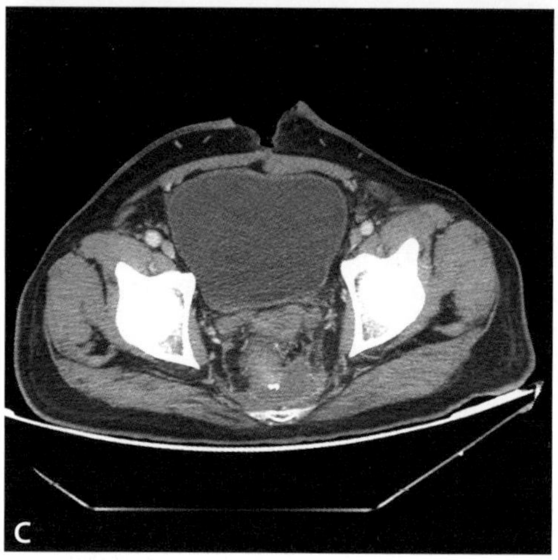

Figs. 20A to C: A 68-year-old male postextended low anterior resection for carcinoma rectum had fever with abdominal distension. CECT (A) axial image shows a large pneumoperitoneum beneath the anterior abdominal wall; (B) Oblique MPR and (C) Axial images reveal a displaced staple with a collection showing specks of air posterior to the rectum due to an anastomotic leak—the double-barrel sign.

low anterior resection, the middle or distal rectum are also resected. Abdominoperineal excision of the rectum involves resection of the anal canal as well. Restorative proctocolectomy involves resection of the entire colon and rectum with formation of an ileal pouch.

Some surgeons routinely ask for fluoroscopic contrast studies to rule out anastomotic leaks. These are most often posterior in location after procedures involving the rectum and may cause anterior displacement of the rectum (3–5 cm from the anterior sacral margin). The patient must be fluoroscoped again after being asked to void as some leaks may become evident only after emptying the rectum.[25]

CT may be asked for in the early postoperative period, if there is clinical suspicion of an anastomotic leak, abscess, fistula or bowel obstruction. Rectal contrast should always be administered prior to the scan. The "double rectum" sign has been described in rectal anastomotic leaks. This is due to the anteriorly displaced rectum with a fluid collection in the presacral space due to the leak **(Figs. 20A to C)**.[25,47] Other signs of leaks are frank extravasation of the rectal contrast, air within or outside the bowel wall, fluid collections, disruption of the staple line and pneumoperitoneum.

Diversion Colitis

Once the temporary colostomy has to be taken down with restoration of bowel continuity, a fluoroscopic contrast study is normally asked for by the surgeon prior to closure. The unused segment often appears nondistensible with diffuse mucosal nodularity or even punctuate ulcerations. The exact etiology is unclear, however, the colon returns to normal once the bowel continuity is restored with resumption of the fecal stream through it.[25]

HEPATOBILIARY SURGERIES

Curative liver surgeries are performed for many benign and malignant liver diseases. The type of surgery depends on the nature and location of the disease and expertise of the surgeon.[48] Most common indications for liver resections are malignancies such as colorectal metastasis, hepatocellular carcinoma (without underlying cirrhosis), neuroendocrine metastasis, cholangiocarcinoma, benign diseases such as hepatic adenomas, symptomatic cysts, intrahepatic biliary calculi and traumatic hepatic lacerations.[49]

Surgical Procedures

Hepatectomies are divided into anatomical and non-anatomical resections. Anatomical resections involve removing contiguous hepatic segments whereas non-anatomical resections are wedge resections which are usually small and peripheral. A standardized nomenclature for anatomical resections has been proposed by the Brisbane 2000 Terminology of Hepatic Anatomy and Resection.[50] Right hepatectomy involves resection of segments 5, 6, 7, and 8, that is, removing the entire liver parenchyma to the right of the middle hepatic vein. Extended right hepatectomy involves additional resection of segment 4 in addition to right lobe. Left hepatectomy involves resection of segments 2, 3, and 4, that is, resection of liver parenchyma to the left of the middle hepatic vein. Extended left hepatectomy involves additional resection of segments 5 and 8. Monosegmentectomy is resection of a single segment, whereas bisegmentectomy involves resection of two contiguous segments. Nonanatomical resections are suitable for small peripheral lesions.[48]

Normal Postoperative Imaging Features

Small fluid collections, hematomas or bilomas can be routinely observed in the early postoperative period and generally regress over a period of few weeks. In addition metallic surgical clips, extra-luminal gas accumulation, and pleural effusions are also routine findings on imaging. Thrombosis of the portal branch stump can also be seen in the early postoperative period. In addition, a linear band of low attenuation may be observed adjacent to the resection margins. This finding is transient and is possibly due to accumulation of bile or blood, or devascularized parenchyma.[48]

Late Postoperative Period

The volume of the remaining liver rapidly increases up to 100% during 6 months to 1 year; with up to 60% in the first 7 days following the surgery.[51,52] After right hepatectomy, the left and caudate lobes hypertrophy and shift to the right. There is upward displacement of the right kidney, hepatic flexure, and small bowel loops with posterior displacement of the IVC. After left hepatectomy, there is hypertrophy of right and caudate lobes, right kidney is usually displaced caudally and stomach or colon occupy the left hepatic fossa. Transient splenic enlargement during initial 6 months after liver resection may be observed.[53]

EARLY POSTOPERATIVE COMPLICATIONS

The most frequent early postoperative complications are fluid collections, vascular thrombosis and biliary injuries. Fluid collections are usually adjacent to resection margins, and correspond to seromas, hematomas (50%), bilomas (25%), or infected collections (25%).[48]

Vascular Thrombosis

Thrombosis of a single hepatic vein is frequently seen after liver resections and is usually partial and seen close to the resection margins. Portal vein and hepatic artery thrombosis are rare, with segmental portal thrombosis more frequently observed than thrombosis of the main portal vein **(Fig. 21)**.[48]

Biliary Injuries

Biliary injuries can be bile leaks and biliary obstruction. Bile leak after hepatic surgery may originate from the site of a biliary-enteric anastomosis, or may be related to the removal of an external drainage tube, or to intraoperative bile duct injury.[54] Ultrasonography and MDCT may show fluid collections at the resection margin. MRCP may be used to identify the location and the nature of the leak.[54]

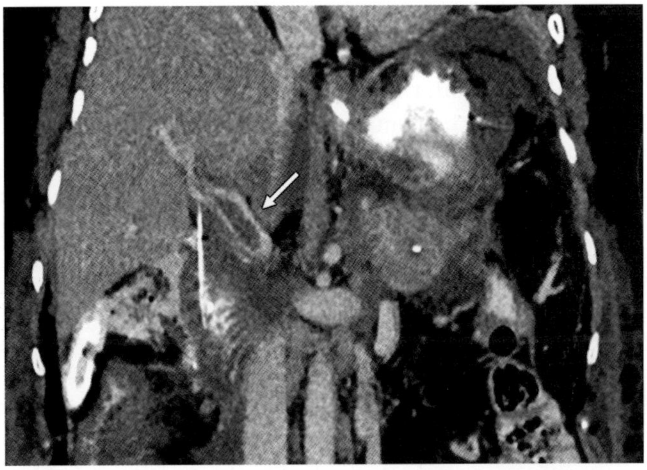

Fig. 21: A 61-year-old male underwent a left hepatectomy. CECT coronal MPR reveals a thrombus as a hypodense filling defect in the main portal vein (arrow).

Biliary obstruction results from postoperative fibrosis at the bile duct stump or inadvertent bile duct ligation. It is most frequently seen after biliary-enteric anastomosis, with obstruction of the Roux-en-Y loop.[55] Multidetector computed tomography (MDCT) will show dilated biliary tree with dilated fluid-filled Roux-en-Y loop.[48]

Intraoperative Diaphragmatic Injury

Diaphragmatic injuries are very rare and mostly seen after right hepatectomy. Right pleural effusion with increased pleural enhancement may be seen on MDCT. They may present with early small bowel obstruction, if the bowel herniates through the diaphragmatic defect.[48]

LATE POSTOPERATIVE COMPLICATIONS

Late complications after hepatic resection are disease recurrence and ischemic cholangitis. Follow-up MDCT or MR are performed depending on the nature of the resected hepatic tumor for the detection of tumor recurrence. Presence of segmental or subsegmental bile duct dilatation although nonspecific, may be suggestive of disease recurrence, even in the absence of a visible focal lesion.[48]

Ischemic cholangitis may occur after liver resection within several months to several years in cases of intraoperative arterial injury. The clinical presentation is nonspecific with jaundice and fever. Magnetic resonance cholangiopancreatography (MRCP) is the modality of choice and may show irregular and multiple bile duct stenoses with intra-hepatic bile duct dilatations.[48]

Laparoscopic Cholecystectomy

Laparoscopic cholecystectomy is the preferred procedure for patients with symptomatic gallstones. However, complications after laparoscopic cholecystectomy especially bile duct injuries, have been reported to be more common in comparison to open surgery.[56] USG, CT, ERCP, MRCP and radionuclide imaging have a role to play in evaluating the postoperative patient.[57–59] These investigations are complementary and the primary imaging technique to be used will depend on the clinical problem faced and availability.

Normal Appearances after Laparoscopic Cholecystectomy

- A small amount of fluid in the surgical bed is a common finding postoperatively during the first week. These fluid collections have no distinct or well-demarcated borders on CT.[60]
- Increased density in the abdominal wall fat at the site of the laparoscopic ports and small amounts of free pelvic fluid may also be seen.[61]
- The diameter of the CBD may increase post-cholecystectomy, with a maximal diameter of 13 mm identified.[62] When biliary dilatation is identified on postoperative imaging, correlation with preoperative imaging and current clinical features and biochemistry is required.

Complications

Major complications after cholecystectomy can be divided into biliary, vascular, and laparoscopic complications. Biliary complications include bile duct injury, biliary obstruction, and dropped stones.

Biliary Injury

Bile leakage secondary to bile duct injury is the most common complication of laparoscopic cholecystectomy.[63] Most leaks occur from the cystic duct stump. Some common mechanisms for the leak include dislodgement of clips from the cystic duct stump, laceration, transection or thermal injuries of the duct.[64] The initial assessment in these patients is usually with sonography or MDCT which may show peri-hepatic fluid. Hepatobiliary scintigraphy is a less commonly used method of evaluating patients with suspected bile duct injury, however, it has been claimed to be more sensitive and specific than sonography or CT in detecting bile leaks.[65] Although it is an invasive procedure, ERCP is useful as it can show the exact site of leak and successfully treat the leak using internal stents. Endoscopic retrograde cholangiopancreatogram (ERCP) is more likely to be successful, if the injury to the duct is < 5 mm, the injury is extra-hepatic, and there is no associated abscess or biloma.[66] Open surgery may be required, if the leak persists. MRCP is a non-invasive way of assessing the anatomy of bile ducts. The use of mangafodipir trisodium, a contrast agent that is primarily excreted via bile helps to both diagnose a bile leak and identify the source of the leak.[67]

Biliary Obstruction

Retained gallstones, misplaced surgical clips, fibrosis due to inflammation from adjacent clips, and thermal injury from cautery devices are causes of biliary obstruction **(Fig. 22)**.[66] Patients present with progressive postoperative obstructive jaundice. Ultrasound and MRCP detect duct dilatation and exclude CBD stones. ERCP is useful in confirming the diagnosis and may be therapeutic.

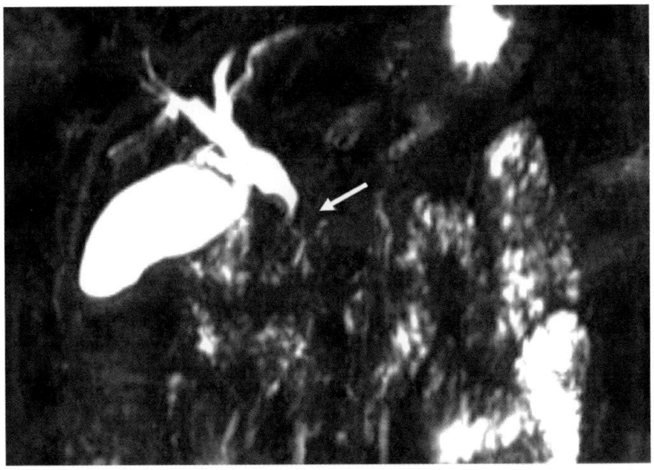

Fig. 22: A 25-year-old female underwent a laparoscopic cholecystectomy for gallstone disease. She presented with obstructive jaundice 6 months later. MRCP-MIP image shows a stricture (arrow) in the lower end of the CBD.

Stone Retention

Stone retention is an important complication of laparoscopic cholecystectomy, with an incidence between 1.1% and 7%.[68] Factors which predispose to retained stones are a long cystic duct pedicle and incomplete excision of gallbladder due to adhesions. Similarly, since the CBD is not explored during laparoscopic cholecystectomy, a gallbladder stone can migrate into the CBD in patients with patulous cystic duct when the gallbladder is pulled in a cephalad direction during cholecystectomy, causing biliary obstruction. In patients with suspected stone retention, MRCP is helpful in depicting these stones, while ERCP is both diagnostic and therapeutic.[64]

Dropped Gallstones

Spillage of gallstones occurs due to inadvertent entry into the gallbladder during dissection or at the time of gallbladder extraction through the port site. The majority of "dropped" gallstones are found in the right upper quadrant, but they may migrate to dependent areas (right paracolic gutter or pelvis).[69] Most remain asymptomatic, however, significant complications can occur since they cause a local foreign body reaction.[70] Abscess formation is the most common complication resulting from "dropped" stones and may develop months later following cholecystectomy.[69]

Vascular Injury

Injury to blood vessels during trocar insertion is responsible for peri or postoperative hemorrhage.[71] During dissection of Calot's triangle, the right hepatic artery is the most common vessel to be injured followed by the portal vein **(Figs. 23A to C)**.[70] Hepatic artery ligation may lead to the development of a delayed ischemic cholangiopathy. MRCP may show irregular ductal dilatation and stenosis.

Pancreatic Surgeries

Pancreatic resection surgeries for the tumors and chronic pancreatitis include Whipple and Beger's procedures as well as central and distal pancreatectomy, while drainage procedures include Puestow and Frey's operations.[72] Information regarding the type of surgery the patient has undergone as well as the interval between surgery and imaging is important for interpretation of postoperative scans.

Whipples procedure: This procedure involves resection of pancreatic head, jejunum, gastric antrum, and duodenum, followed by hepaticojejunostomy (HJ), pancreaticojejunostomy (PJ), and duodenojejunostomy (DJ) or gastrojejunostomy (GJ). The normal postoperative findings include the presence of these different anastomoses.[72] Following pancreatic head resection, the splenomesenteric venous junction and superior mesenteric vein will be seen to the right of the residual pancreatic parenchyma and in close proximity to the inferior vena cava posteriorly.

Beger's procedure: It involves resection of the pancreatic head with preservation of duodenum. PJ is done at two locations of the Roux-en-Y limb following pancreatic head removal. A sleeve of the pancreatic parenchyma is left behind along with duodenum ensuring the preservation of blood supply of the duodenum.[72]

Puestow procedure: It consists of side-to-side longitudinal PJ with MPD draining directly into a loop of jejunum. The Roux-en-Y loop following this surgery lies immediately anterior to pancreatic body or tail.[72]

Frey's procedure: It includes partial resection of pancreatic head and a longitudinal PJ, with an intact biliary duct.[72]

Central pancreatectomy: Part of the pancreatic body or neck is resected, followed by a Roux-en-Y PJ to the remaining pancreatic tissue in the distal part. The distal end of the pancreas, may, however be anastomosed to the stomach. The proximal cut end is sutured, and the Roux-en-Y bowel is seen at the level of the splenoportal confluence, separating apart the pancreatic head from its body and tail.

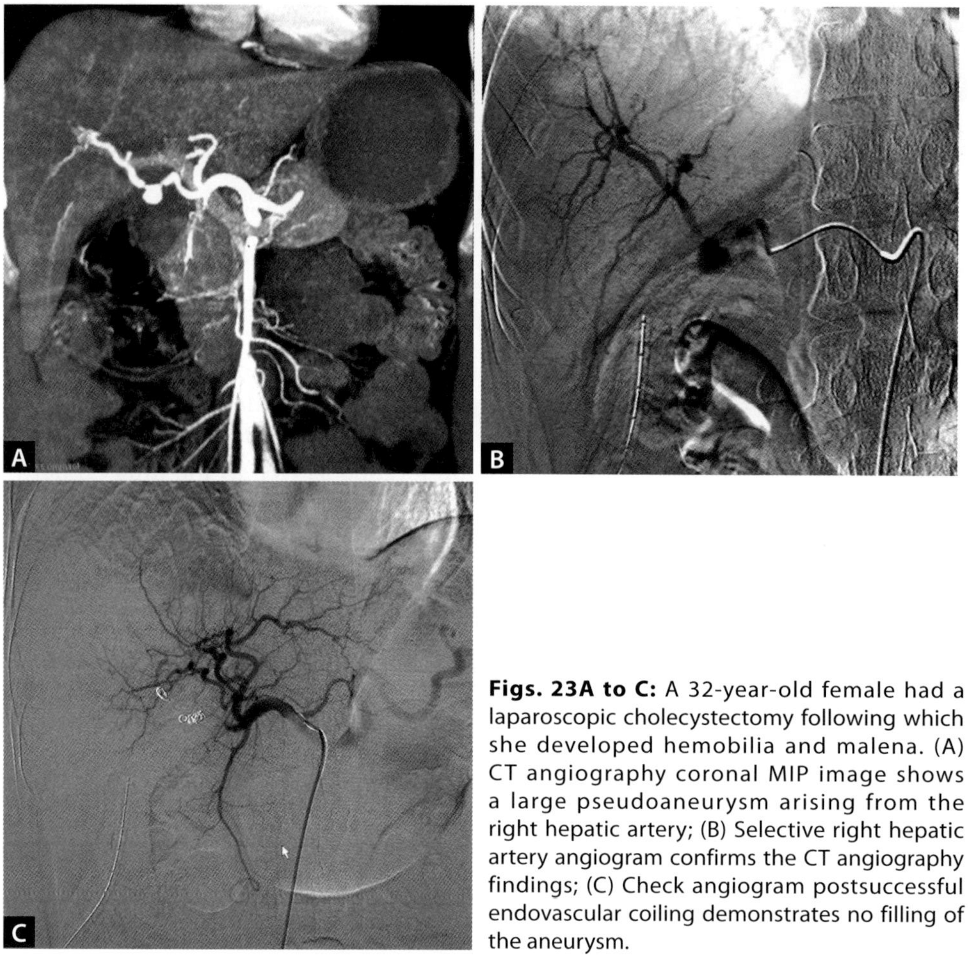

Figs. 23A to C: A 32-year-old female had a laparoscopic cholecystectomy following which she developed hemobilia and malena. (A) CT angiography coronal MIP image shows a large pseudoaneurysm arising from the right hepatic artery; (B) Selective right hepatic artery angiogram confirms the CT angiography findings; (C) Check angiogram postsuccessful endovascular coiling demonstrates no filling of the aneurysm.

Distal pancreatectomy: The pancreatic parenchyma lying to the left of SMV is resected, and the cut end is sutured to prevent pancreatic juice leakage. The pancreas thereby ends abruptly, and the surgical bed will not have any bowel related to the pancreas, stomach or duodenum, as against in the above described surgeries. As the blood supply to the tail of pancreas comes mostly from splenic artery branches, splenectomy becomes necessary at times along with distal pancreatectomy.

NORMAL POSTOPERATIVE FINDINGS

Several normal postoperative CT and MRI findings may be misdiagnosed as the disease process, hence, knowledge of normal postoperative appearances is highly essential.

- Pneumobilia (tends to persist) and periportal hepatic edema (usually resolves within a month) are universally seen. Air may be seen in the MPD also as a normal finding. However, pneumobilia should not be seen following surgeries in which there are no biliary anastomoses.[72]
- The afferent loop of bowel following Frey procedure which drains the biliary ducts and pancreas may be thick and edematous for the first three weeks following surgery, and should not be misdiagnosed as hemorrhage or ischemia.[72]
- Roux loop following the Puestow procedure lies between the body of the pancreas and stomach in the lesser sac, and may be falsely diagnosed to be a pancreatic mass or internal hernia.[72] The use of positive oral contrast for distending the bowel and changing the patient from a supine to a lateral decubitus position during CT, characteristic location as well as course of the Roux loop, and the presence of valvulae conniventes help in preventing a misdiagnosis.[73]
- Transient fluid collections in the surgical bed are common in the first month following surgery. The presence of air foci within these collections does not necessarily indicate infection but should raise the suspicion of a pancreatic fistula.[74–76]

- Reactive lymphadenopathy (nodes up to 1.5 cm in the short axis diameter) is seen up to two months after the surgery and regresses on follow-up imaging.[77]
- Perivascular cuffing around the celiac artery and its branches, and superior mesenteric artery is seen for up to 6 weeks following Whipple and Beger's procedures. This cuffing is inflammatory in nature in patients having negative surgical margins and should not be wrongly diagnosed as tumor recurrence. Follow-up imaging becomes necessary to distinguish between the perivascular cuffing and disease recurrence.
- Mild pancreatic duct dilation (1–2 mm in comparison to preoperative imaging) is an expected postoperative appearance, and does not correlate with subsequent pancreatitis.[72]
- There may be a cavity detected in the head of the pancreas after Frey's procedure, which may be falsely diagnosed as a pancreatic pseudocyst or cystic neoplasm.[72] This cavity usually decreases with time.

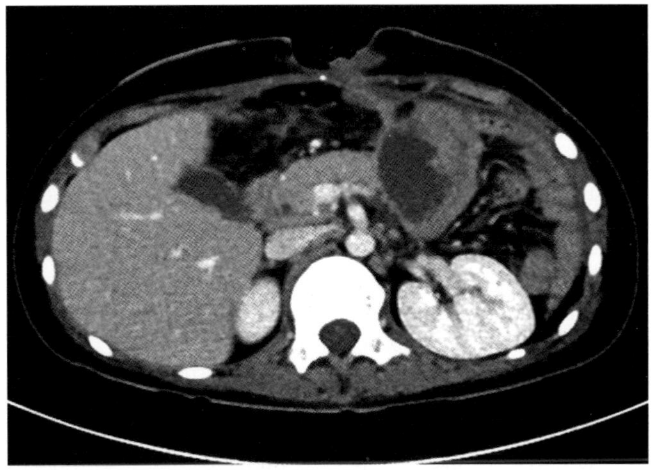

Fig. 24: A 38-year-old male underwent a distal pancreatectomy, gastrectomy and splenectomy for a desmoid tumor of the tail of pancreas. Presented with history of watery discharge from incision site. CECT axial image shows an irregular collection with thick enhancing wall in the region of the tail of pancreas with a fistulous track seen extending anteriorly to the anterior abdominal wall.

COMPLICATIONS

Minor complications are relatively more frequent (seen in 28–29% patients), as against major complications that may require surgical intervention or vascular embolization (seen in 11% patients).[72]

- *Delayed gastric emptying:* Seen in upto 50% of patients during the early postoperative course following pylorus preserving pancreatoduodenectomy.[78,79] Gastric outlet obstruction may also be seen due to narrowing of the gastric outlet.
- *Arterial complications:* Splenic artery and common hepatic artery pseudoaneurysms are known to occur after pancreatic surgery. Stenosis in the celiac artery can also be seen following pancreatic surgery, but is treated only when there are symptoms attributable to it, as isolated vessel stenosis is usually asymptomatic due to presence of rich collaterals between the celiac and SMA.
- *Thrombosis of portal vein and splenic infarction:* Due to postoperative pancreatitis or as a result of iatrogenic injury.
- *Pancreatic fistula and postoperative pancreatitis:* Detection of amylase-rich fluid after the 10th postoperative day in the drainage tube kept in the surgical bed raises the suspicion of a PJ fistula **(Fig. 24)**.[72]
- Extrahepatic CBD dilatation of >10 mm is abnormal and is likely due to ischemia of the distal CBD.[72]

CONCLUSION

A knowledge of the normal postoperative appearance following abdominal surgery is essential for the accurate interpretation of postoperative imaging. A two-way communication between the radiologist and his clinical colleagues is required so that the radiologist is aware of the exact nature of the procedure the patient has undergone. Helical CT with its multiplanar capability is the modality of choice for the detection and characterization of postoperative complications.

REFERENCES

1. Bader FG, Schröder M, Kujath P, Muhl E, Bruch HP, Eckmann C. Diffuse post-operative peritonitis: value of diagnostic parameters and impact of early indication for relaparotomy. Eur J Med Res. 2009;14(11):491-6.
2. Sun H, Xue HD, Wang YN, et al. Dual-source dual-energy computed tomography angiography for active gastrointestinal bleeding: a preliminary study. Clin Radiol. 2013;68(2):139-47.
3. Fulwadhva UP, Wortman JR, Sodickson AD. Use of dual-energy CT and iodine maps in the evaluation of bowel disease. Radiographics. 2016;36:393-406.
4. Ghahremani GG, Gore RM. CT diagnosis of post-operative abdominal complications. Radiol Clin North Am. 1989;27: 787-803.
5. Hindman NM, Kang S, Parikh MS. Common post-operative findings unique to laparoscopic surgery. Radiographics 2014;34:119-38.

6. Earls JP, Dachman AH, Colon E, Garrett MG, Molloy M. Prevalence and duration of postoperative pneumoperitoneum: sensitivity of CT vs left lateral decubitus radiography. AJR. 1993;161(4):781-5.
7. Gayer G, Jonas T, Apter S, et al. Postoperative pneumoperitoneum as detected by CT: prevalence, duration, and relevant factors affecting its possible significance. Abdom Imaging. 2000;25(3):301-5.
8. Hope WW, Herriford BT, Norton HJ, et al. Duration and clinical significance of radiographically detected "free air" after laparoscopic nephrectomy. Surg Laparosc Endosc Percut Tech. 2009;19(5):415-8.
9. Chalmers AG, Macafee D, Tolan DJM, Brittenden J. Introduction to the postsurgical abdomen. In: Brittenden J, Tolan DJM (Eds). Radiology of the post surgical abdomen. London: Springer-Verlag. 2012.pp.1-40.
10. Gore RM, Berlin JW, Yaghmai V, et al. CT diagnosis of post-operative complications. Semin Ultrasound CT MR. 2004;25(3):207-21.
11. Young ST, Paulson EK, McCam RC, Baker ME. Appearance of oxidised cellulose (Surgicel) on postoperative CT scans: similarity to postoperative abscess. AJR. 1993;160(2):275-7.
12. Bertelsen CA, Andreasen AH, Jørgensen T, Harling H. Danish Colorectal Cancer Group. Anastomotic leakage after anterior resection for rectal cancer: risk factors. Colorectal Dis. 2010; 12(1):37-43.
13. Nicksa GA, Dring RV, Johnson KH, Sardella WV, Vignati PV, Cohen JL. Anastomotic leaks: what is the best diagnostic imaging study? Dis Colon Rectum. 2007;50(2):197-203.
14. Power N, Atri M, Ryan S, Haddad R, Smith A. CT assessment of anastomotic bowel leak. Clin Radiol. 2007;62(1):37-42.
15. Burke C, Maura M, Molina PL. Interventional computed tomography. In: Lee J, Sagel SS, Stanley RJ (Eds). Computed Body Tomography. Philadelphia: Lippincott Williams & Wilkins; 2006.pp.95-144.
16. Kambadakone A, Mueller PR. Abdominal abscesses. In: Gore RM, Levine MS (Eds). Textbook of Gastrointestinal Radiology, 4th edn. Philadelphia: Elsevier-Saunders; 2015. pp.1254-78.
17. Kim KW, Choi BI, Han JK, et al. Postoperative anatomic and pathologic findings at CT following gastrectomy. Radiographics. 2002;22:323-36.
18. Kumar RR, Kim JT, Haukoos JS, et al. Factors affecting the successful management of intra-abdominal abscesses with antibiotics and the need for percutaneous drainage. Dis Colon Rectum. 2006;49:183-9.
19. Tolan DJM, Harris KM, Prasad D, Mehta SP. The stomach and duodenum. In: Brittenden J, Tolan DJM (Eds). Radiology of the post surgical abdomen. London: Springer-Verlag; 2012.pp.72-124.
20. Frager D, Rovno HD, Baer JW, Bashist B, Friedman M. Prospective evaluation of colonic obstruction with computed tomography. Abdom Imaging. 1998;23(2):141-6.
21. Dükstra FR, Niewenhuizen M, Reijinen MMPT, et al. Recent clinical developments in pathophysiology, epidemiology, diagnosis and treatment of intra-abdominal adhesions. Scand J Gastroenterol. 2000;232:52-9.
22. Berl S, Dawkins A, DiSantis D. The small bowel feces sign. Abdom Radiol. 2016;41(4):794-5.
23. Elsayes KM, Menias CO, Smullen TL, Platt JF. Closed-loop small bowel obstruction: diagnostic patterns by multidetector computed tomography. J Comput Assist Tomogr. 2007;31:697-701.
24. Ghahremani GG, Jimenez MA, Rosenfeld M, Rochester D. CT diagnosis of occult incisional hernias. AJR. 1987;148(1):139-42.
25. Weinstein S, Osei-Bonsu S, Aslam R, Yee J. Multidetector CT of the postoperative colon: Review of normal appearances and common complications. Radiographics. 2013;33:515-32.
26. Ogilvie JW, Ricciardi R. Complications of perineal surgery. Clin Colon Rectal Surg. 2009;22(1):51-9.
27. Smith-Behn J, Arnold M, Might J. Use of computerized tomography of the abdominal wall in the diagnosis of partial post-operative wound dehiscence. Postgrad Med J. 1986;62(732):947-8.
28. Zhang L. Incidence of abdominal incisional hernia in developing country: a retrospective cohort study. Int J Clin Exp Med. 2015;8(8):13649-52.
29. Itatsu K, Yokoyama Y, Sugawara G, et al. Incidence and risk factors for incisional hernia after abdominal surgery. Br J Surg. 2014;101(11):1439-47.
30. Brown SR, Goodfellow PB. Transverse versus midline incisions for abdominal surgery. Cochrane Database Syst Rev. 2005:CD005199.
31. Gayer G, Lubner MG, Bhalla S, Pickhardt PJ. Imaging of abdominal and pelvic surgical and postprocedural foreign bodies. Radiol Clin North Am. 2014;52:991-1027.
32. Manzella A, Filho PB, Albuquerque E, Farias F, Kaercher J. Imaging of gossypibomas: pictorial review. AJR. 2009;193: S94-101.
33. Orringer MB. Tumors, injuries and miscellaneous conditions of the esophagus. In: Greenfield LJ, Mulholland MW, Oldham KT, et al (Eds). Surgery: Scientific Principles and Practice. Philadelphia: Lippincott Williams & Wilkins; 2001.pp.692-735.
34. Tolan DJM, Harris KM, Prasad D, Mehta SP. The esophagus. In: Brittenden J, Tolan DJM (Eds). Radiology of the post surgical abdomen. London: Springer-Verlag; 2012. pp.41-71.
35. Swanson JO, Levine MS, Redfern RO, Rubesin SE. Usefulness of high density barium for detection of leaks after esophagogastrectomy, total gastrectomy and total laryngectomy. AJR. 2003;181:415-20.
36. Upponi S, Ganeshan A, D'Costa H, et al. Radiological detection of post-oesophagectomy anastomotic leak: a comparison between multidetector CT and fluoroscopy. Br J Radiol. 2008;81:545-8.
37. Rubesin SE. Postoperative esophagus. In: Gore RM, Levine MS (Eds). Textbook of Gastrointestinal Radiology, 4th edn. Philadelphia: Elsevier-Saunders; 2015.pp.449-61.
38. Lamb PJ, Griffin SM, Chandrashekar MV, Richardson DL, Karat D, Hayes N. Prospective study of routine contrast radiology after total gastrectomy. Br J Surg. 2004;91:1015-9.

39. Gayer G, Barsuk D, Hertz M, Apter S, Zissin R. CT diagnosis of afferent loop syndrome. Clin Radiol. 2002;57:835-9.
40. Tolan DJM, Harris KM, Prasad D, Mehta SP. The stomach and duodenum. In: Brittenden J, Tolan DJM (Eds). Radiology of the post surgical abdomen. London: Springer-Verlag; 2012.pp.72-126.
41. Carucci LR. Postoperative stomach and duodenum. In: Gore RM, Levine MS (Eds). Textbook of Gastrointestinal Radiology, 4th edn. Philadelphia: Elsevier-Saunders; 2015. pp.630-56.
42. Quigley S, Colledge J, Mukherjee S, Patel K. Bariatric surgery: a review of normal post-operative anatomy and complications. Clin Radiol. 2011;66(10):903-14.
43. Blachar A, Federle MP. Gastrointestinal complications of laparoscopic Roun-en-Y gastric bypass surgery in patients who are morbidly obese: Findings on radiography and CT. AJR. 2002;179:1437-42.
44. Pieroni S, Sommer EA, Hito R, et al. The "O" sign: a simple and helpful tool in the diagnosis of laparoscopic adjustable gastric band slippage. AJR. 2010;195:137-41.
45. Sandrasegaran K, Maglinte DD, Rajesh A, et al. CT findings for postsurgical blind pouch of small bowel. AJR. 2006;186:110-3.
46. Broder JC, Tkacz JN, Anderson SW, Soto JA, Gupta A. Ileal pouch-anal anastomosis surgery: imaging and intervention for post-operative complications. Radiographics. 2010;30(1):221-33.
47. Macklin CS, Brittenden J, Jayne D, Tolan DJM. The colon. In: Brittenden J, Tolan DJM (Eds). Radiology of the post surgical abdomen. London: Springer-Verlag; 2012. pp.255-93.
48. Mulé S, Colosio A, Cazejust J, Kianmanesh R, Soyer P, Hoeffel C. Imaging of the postoperative liver: review of normal appearances and common complications. Abdom Imaging. 2015;40(7):2761-76.
49. Guthrie JA, Salahudeen HM, Lodge JPA. The liver. In: Brittenden J, Tolan DJM (Eds). Radiology of the post surgical abdomen. London: Springer-Verlag; 2012. pp.187-226.
50. Terminology Committee of the International Hepato-Pancreato-Biliary Association. Terminology of liver anatomy and resections. HPB (Oxford). 2000;2:333-9.
51. Kele PG, de Boer M, van der Jagt EJ, Lisman T, Porte RJ. Early hepatic regeneration index and completeness of regeneration at 6 months after partial hepatectomy. Br J Surg. 2012;99(8):1113-9.
52. Zappa M, Dondero F, Sibert A, et al. Liver regeneration at day 7 after right hepatectomy: global and segmental volume trianalysis by using CT. Radiology. 2009;252(2):426-32.
53. Petrovai G, Truant S, Langlois C, et al. Mechanisms of splenic hypertrophy following hepatic resection. HPB (Oxford). 2013;15(12):919-27.
54. Hoeffel C, Azizi L, Lewin M, et al. Normal and pathologic features of the postoperative biliary tract at 3D MR cholangiopancreatography and MR imaging. Radiographics. 2006;26(6):1603-20.
55. Boraschi P, Donati F. Biliary-enteric anastomoses: spectrum of findings on Gd-EOB-DTPA-enhanced MR cholangiography. Abdom Imaging. 2013;38(6):1351-9.
56. Kaman L, Sanyal S, Behera A, Singh R, Katariya RN. Comparison of major bile duct injuries following laparoscopic cholecystectomy and open cholecystectomy. ANZ J Surg. 2006; 76(9):788-91.
57. Z'graggen K, Wehrli H, Metzger A, Buehler M, Frei E, Klaiber C. Complications of laparoscopic cholecystectomy in Switzerland: a prospective 3-year study of 10,174 patients. Swiss Association of Laparoscopic and Thoracoscopic Surgery. Surg Endosc. 1998;12:1303-10.
58. Hjelmqvist B. Complications of laparoscopic cholecystectomy as recorded in the Swedish laparoscopy registry. Eur J Surg Suppl. 2000;585:18-21.
59. Gorsi U, Gupta P, Kalra N, Kang M, Singh R, Gupta R, et al. Multidetector computed tomography evaluation of post cholecystectomy complications: A tertiary care centre experience. Trop Gastroenterol. 2015;36(4):236-43.
60. Quinn SF, Sangster W, Standage B, Schuman E, Gross G. Biliary complications related to laparoscopic cholecystectomies: Radiologic diagnosis and management. Surg Laparosc Endosc Percutan Tech. 1992;2(4):279-86.
61. Moran J, Del Grosso E, Wills JS, Hagy JA, Baker R. Laparoscopic cholecystectomy: imaging of complications and normal postoperative CT appearance. Abdom Imaging. 1994;19:143-6.
62. Feng B, Song Q. Does the common bile duct dilate after cholecystectomy? Sonographic evaluation in 234 patients. AJR. 1995;183:1559-66.
63. Lohan D, Walsh S, McLoughlin R, Murphy J. Imaging of the complications of laparoscopic cholecystectomy. Eur Radiol. 2005;15(5):904-12.
64. Desai NS, Khandelwal A, Virmani V, Kwatra NS, Ricci JA, Saboo SS. Imaging in laparoscopic cholecystectomy: what a radiologist needs to know. Eur J Radiol. 2014;83(6): 867-79.
65. Tripathi M, Chandrashekar N, Kumar R, et al. Hepatobiliary scintigraphy: an effective tool in the management of bile leak following laparoscopic cholecystectomy. Clin Imaging. 2004;28:40-43.
66. McGahan JP, Stein M. Complications of laparoscopic cholecystectomy: imaging and intervention. AJR. 1995;165: 1089-97.
67. Park M, Kim KW, Yu JS, et al. Early biliary complications of laparoscopic cholecystectomy: evaluation on T2-weighted MR cholangiography in conjunction with mangafodipir trisodium–enhanced 3D T1-weighted MR cholangiography. AJR. 2004;183:1559-66.
68. Glenn F. Retained calculi within the biliary ductal system. Ann Surg. 1974;179(5):528-39.
69. Jagadesham VP, Sheridan M, Lodge JPA, Brittenden J. The biliary tree. In: Brittenden J, Tolan DJM (Eds). Radiology of the post surgical abdomen. London: Springer-Verlag; 2012. pp.153-85.
70. Thurley PD, Dhingsa R. Laparoscopic cholecystectomy: postoperative imaging. AJR. 2008;191:794–801.

71. Shamiyeh A, Wayand W. Laparoscopic cholecystectomy: early and late complications and their treatment. Langenbecks Arch Surg. 2004;389:164-71.
72. Sandrasegaran K, Maglinte DD, Howard TJ, Lappas JC. Surgery for Chronic Pancreatitis: cross-sectional imaging of postoperative anatomy and complications. AJR. 2005;184:1118-27.
73. Yamauchi FI, Ortega CD, Blasbalg R, Rocha MS, Jukemura J, Cerri GG. Multidetector CT evaluation of the postoperative pancreas. Radiographics. 2012;32:743-64.
74. Coombs RJ, Zeiss J, Howard JM, Thomford NR, Merrick HW. CT of the abdomen after the Whipple procedure: value in depicting postoperative anatomy, surgical complications, and tumor recurrence. AJR. 1990;154:1011-4.
75. Hashimoto M, Koga M, Ishiyama K, et al. CT features of pancreatic fistula after pancreaticoduodenectomy. AJR. 2007;188:W323-7.
76. Hashimoto N, Yasuda C, Ohyanagi H. Pancreatic fistula after pancreatic head resection: incidence, significance and management. Hepatogastroenterology. 2003;50:1658-60.
77. Cullen JJ, Sarr MG, Ilstrup DM. Pancreatic anastomotic leak after pancreaticoduodenectomy: incidence, significance, and management. Am J Surg. 1994;168:295-8.
78. Mortelé KJ, Lemmerling M, de Hemptinne B, de Vos M, de Bock G, Kunnen M. Postoperative findings following the Whipple procedure: determination of prevalence and morphologic abdominal CT features. Eur Radiol. 2000;10:123-8.
79. Riediger H, Makowiec F, Schareck WD, Hopt UT, Adam U. Delayed gastric emptying after pylorus preserving pancreatoduodenectomy is strongly related to other postoperative complications. J Gastrointest Surg. 2003;7:758-65.

CHAPTER 96

Portal Hypertension: Imaging and Intervention

Shivanand Gamanagatti, Kumble S Madhusudhan

IMAGING OF PORTAL HYPERTENSION

INTRODUCTION

It is defined as increase in portal pressure above the normal range of 6–10 mm Hg or pressure gradient >5 mm Hg between portal and hepatic veins, as evaluated by hepatic vein cannulation. Portal hypertension is considered clinically significant, when the pressure gradient is more than 10–12 mm Hg.[1]

Portal hypertension is of hemodynamic importance, since it leads to range of complications such as gastrointestinal hemorrhage, ascites, portal-systemic encephalopathy, hepatorenal syndrome, hepatopulmonary syndrome, and spontaneous bacterial peritonitis.[2,3]

CAUSES OF PORTAL HYPERTENSION[4]

Causes of portal hypertension are divided into prehepatic, intrahepatic, and posthepatic causes **(Table 1)**.

ANATOMY OF PORTAL SYSTEM[5]

The liver has two sources of blood supply, 70% of blood flow is via the portal vein and remaining 30% is via hepatic artery. Portal blood is poorly oxygenated and has high content of chemicals absorbed from the gut, whereas hepatic arterial blood is rich in oxygen. Portal and hepatic blood merge within the portal sinusoids, which drain into hepatic veins and then to the systemic venous system, i.e. inferior vena cava (IVC).

The portal vein is formed by the confluence of the superior mesenteric vein (SMV) and splenic vein (SV) posterior to the neck of pancreas. It courses superiorly and laterally to enter the liver at the porta. Other tributaries include inferior mesenteric vein (IMV) and right and left gastric veins, which drain into portal circulation **(Fig. 1)**.

Work-up[6,7]

Laboratory Studies

Aimed at identifying the causes of cirrhosis (the most common cause of portal hypertension), Studies include **(Table 2)**.

Imaging Studies

- Duplex-Doppler ultrasonography[8-11]
- Ultrasound (US) is used as screening modality for evaluating portal hypertension, since it is a safe and cost-effective method. It helps in identifying the patency of portal vein, direction of portal flow (hepatopetal or hepatofugal), also helps in diagnosing cavernoma formation of main portal vein, splanchnic vein thrombosis.
  - *Limitations of US include*:
    - Reproducibility of findings is challenging.
    - Portal hemodynamics affected by several variables such as circadian rhythm, meals and medications.
    - Substantial inter-observer and intra-observer discrepancy.

Table 1: Causes of portal hypertension.

Prehepatic causes	*Intrahepatic causes*	*Posthepatic causes*
Caused by obstruction of the portal, splenic, or superior mesenteric veins. • Portal vein thrombosis/extrahepatic portal vein obstruction • Congenital origin, such as aplasia or hypoplasia • Infection, such as pylephlebitis • Splanchnic arteriovenous fistula	Caused by intrinsic diseases of the parenchyma • Cirrhosis due to various causes • Congenital hepatic fibrosis • Noncirrhotic portal fibrosis/Idiopathic portal hypertension	Caused by diseases obstructing the blood outflow from the liver • Budd-Chiari syndrome • Veno-occlusive disorder

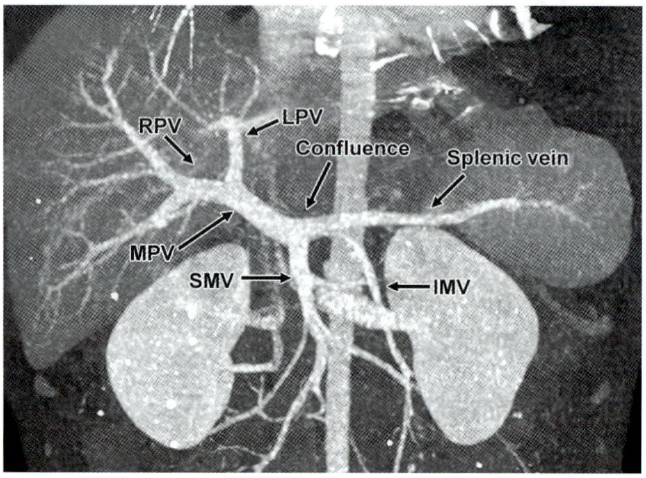

Fig. 1: Coronal 3D MIP image of CT portography showing anatomy of splenoportal axis.
Abbreviations: SMV, superior mesenteric vein; IMV, inferior mesenteric vein; MPV, main portal vein; RPV, right branch of portal vein; LPV, left branch of portal vein

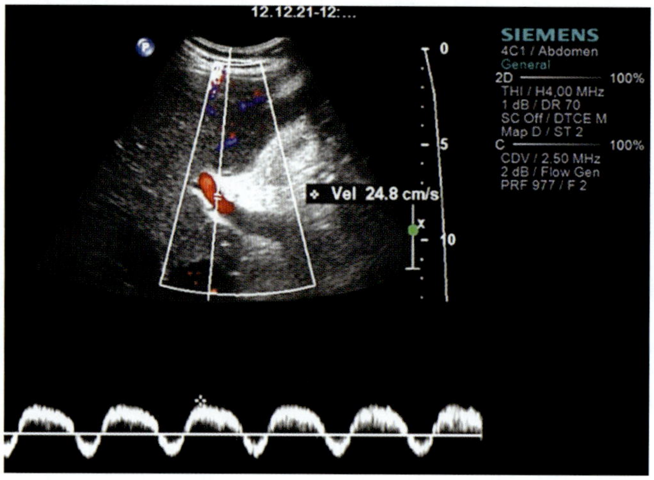

Fig. 2: Ultrasound Doppler image showing typical waveform of main portal vein exhibiting continuous hepatopedal (antegrade) flow with undulation due to respiratory and cardiac variation.

Table 2: Laboratory studies for the work-up of cirrhosis.

• Liver function tests • Prothrombin time • Albumin • Viral hepatitis serologies • Platelet count • Antinuclear antibody, antimitochondrial antibody, anti-smooth muscle antibody • Iron indices • Alpha-1 antitrypsin deficiency • Ceruloplasmin alone or along with 24-hour urinary copper in selective cases

Normal Doppler Findings of Portal Vein

The portal vein has a typical Doppler waveform and exhibits continuous hepatopetal (antegrade) flow. The normal flow velocity range is 15–18 cm/sec. Mild undulation due to respiratory and cardiac variation in the waveform is a common finding **(Fig. 2)**.

Technique of Doppler of Portal System

Doppler evaluation of splenoportal axis can be extremely challenging, due to the altered anatomy, blood flow conditions, bowel gas and the type of the changes that happen in a diseased liver. Doppler examination should be performed following overnight fasting, because bowel gas may interfere with evaluation of superior mesenteric vein and retroperitoneal collaterals.

Checklist of typical Doppler evaluation of splenoportal axis **(Figs. 3A to F)** consists of looking at the:

- Patency of hepatic veins
- Patency of IVC
- Liver size and echo-texture, any space occupying lesion
- Patency of splenoportal axis (MPV/splenic vein/SMV)
- Diameter of SPA (dilated/normal)
- Direction of flow (hepatopetal/hepatofugal)
- Respiratory variation of portal blood flow (present or absent)
- Collaterals (intrahepatic/extrahepatic)

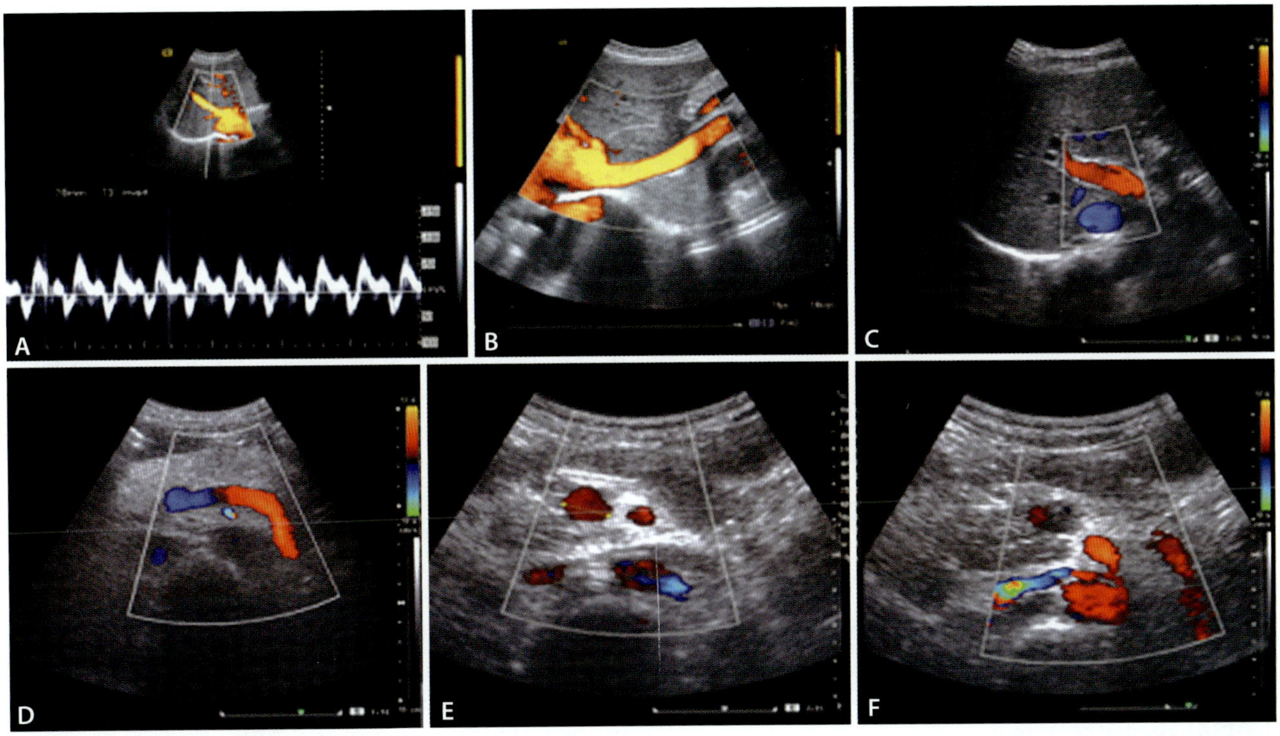

Figs. 3A to F: Power Doppler images showing normal Doppler findings to look at during scanning in setting of portal hypertension: (A) Patency of hepatic vein; (B) Patency of IVC; (C) Patency of MPV; (D) Patency of splenic vein; (E) Patency of SMV; (F) Patency of left renal vein (LRV).

- Splenic size (normal/enlarged)
- Ascites (present or absent)
- Patency of left renal vein.

Challenges of Doppler evaluation include:

- Acquiring a suitable angle of insonation
- Altered depth of the vessels
- Slow flow velocities due to disease process
- Amount of tissue movement due to respiration

In portal hypertension, a Doppler signal demonstrates a low frequency shift and low amplitude, and also, there is an increase in noise from tissue movement. Hence, it is very important to optimize the imaging parameters and sonographic technique to increase the frequency shift and to increase the signal amplitude.

Optimization of Sonographic Technique

Angle of Insonation

Single most useful adjustment that improves the Doppler signal quality is to decrease the angle of insonation. Ideally, the angle of insonation should be less than 60°. In routine clinical practice, it is difficult to achieve this angle due to restrictions related to vessel position, body habitus, ribs and gas.

Useful modifications for improving the angle include:

- Roll the patient into left lateral decubitus position to move the liver away from the ribs and move bowel gas
- Use a small footprint phased array transducer to visualize vessels through intercostal space.

Color Frequency

Current ultrasound machines come with transducers having multiple Doppler frequencies. This offers, the sonographer a chance to increase the frequency shift or increase the amplitude of the returning echoes depending on conditions within the body.

A higher incident frequency will produce a greater frequency shift but subject to higher rates of attenuation thereby decreasing penetration and reducing signal amplitude. Hence, when scanning deep abdominal vessels a lower frequency shift should be used to overcome problems of poor penetration.

Optimization of the Received Signal

The scale or pulse repetition frequency (PRF) needs to be set appropriately in order to optimize the display of Doppler signal received. In cirrhosis, blood flow states are very low, hence the scale (PRF) should be set low enough to display these small frequency shifts.

One can use the zoom facility that significantly improve resolution and frame rate by reconfiguring the beam forming for a smaller field of view.

Respiration

Smart use of respiration can be very helpful. Performing Doppler in arrested inspiration may hamper the detection of flow as the increase in intra-abdominal pressure can halt or even reverse the flow in diseased portal venous system. Hence, scanning should be done with arrested expiration or gentle respiration even if flow is not seen.

Presets

It is recommended to use vendor presets as a starting point and also it is advocated that each department generate a dedicated presets for abdominal vascular studies.

Pathophysiology of Doppler Findings in Portal Hypertension

Cirrhosis is a mixture of fibrosis and regeneration that alters the normal liver architecture. Cirrhosis leads to obstruction to blood flow in distal sinusoids due to perisinusoidal collagen deposition and fibrosis. This obstruction reduces flow from the portal veins and hepatic artery into the hepatic veins. This increases arterial resistance and leads to an increase in arterial flow into the portal vein via existing and new anastomoses that result from the fibrotic scarring. The net result of this obstruction to venous outflow and increase in arterial to portal vein flow manifests as increase in portal vein pressure, drainage of blood away from the liver (hepatofugal flow) via collateral pathways.

Ultrasound Criteria for Detecting Portal Hypertension

Portal Vein Diameter

Portal vein diameter is a luminal measurement made at the level where the portal vein enters porta. A portal vein diameter of 13 mm or more is abnormal and an indicator of portal hypertension. While it has good specificity, it has a sensitivity of only about 40% **(Fig. 4)**.

This lack of sensitivity is due to collateral pathways, which partially decompress the system. Portal vein size normally varies with respiration and loss of this variation can also be used to identify portal hypertension. Less than 20% variation in diameter with respiration is reported as having 80% sensitivity and 100% specificity.

Although this is a sensitive test for portal hypertension, in practice obtaining reliable and reproducible measurements can be difficult as many of these patients have poor ultrasound access and limited ability to comply with directions.

Flow Reversal or Hepatofugal Flow

This is relatively uncommon in the portal vein and is a poor marker for portal hypertension being seen in only 1–8% of cases of portal hypertension **(Fig. 5)**. When present, it is usually associated with a reduction in vein diameter. It is

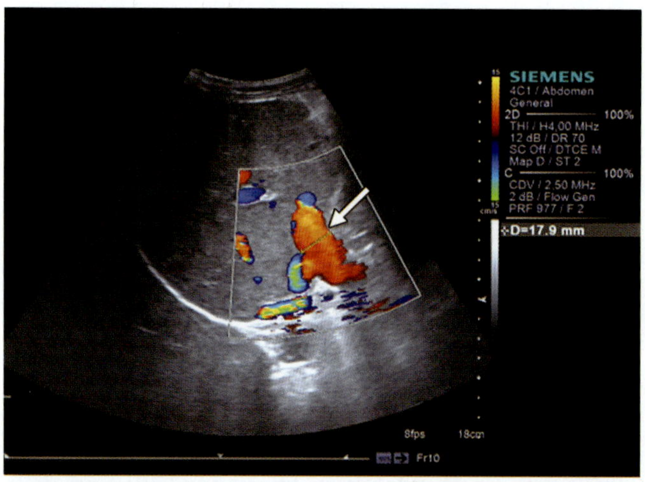

Fig. 4: Doppler ultrasound image showing dilated main portal vein (arrow) in a cirrhotic patient, which measures 17.9 mm at porta.

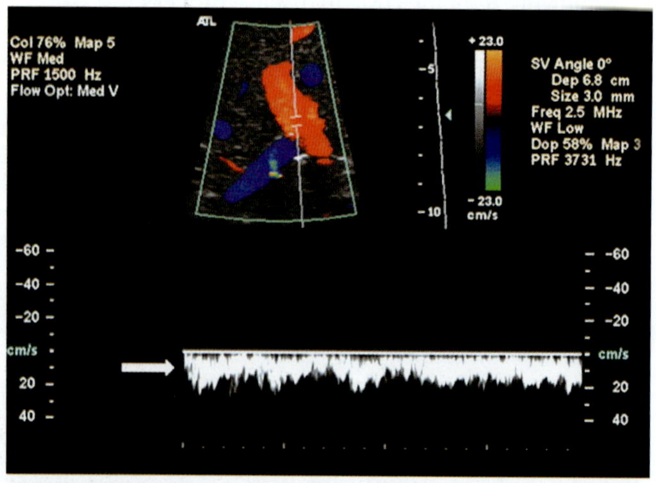

Fig. 5: Doppler ultrasound image showing dilated main portal vein with reversal of flow (arrow) on spectral waveform suggestive of hepatofugal flow.

highly dependent on the severity of the disease and the location of collaterals (if a paraumbilical collateral exists forward flow is usually maintained because the shunt is beyond the level of the portal vein).

Splenomegaly and Ascites

Splenomegaly develops in most, but not all cases, of portal hypertension however is of little use due to the large number of alternative causes **(Figs. 6A and B)**.

Ascites is not usually caused by uncomplicated portal hypertension. It is often secondary to underlying liver diseases with liver cell failure and is insensitive, as it tends to be a late complication.

Portosystemic Venous Collaterals

Collaterals have up to 90% sensitivity and excellent specificity for portal hypertension. Paraumbilical collaterals have a specificity of 100% for portal hypertension. Collaterals have predictable locations making them a very practical sign for the diagnosis of portal hypertension. Clues to their presence and location can also be found from changes in the flow patterns in the portal venous system.

The collaterals most frequently detected with ultrasound are the **(Figs. 7A to F)**:

- Paraumbilical
- Splenorenal
- Gastroesophageal.

Other, less common collaterals, such as mesenteric and pericholecystic **(Figs. 7A to F)**, may also be found.

Computed Tomography[12,13]

Computed tomography (CT) is not the prime diagnostic tool in patients with portal hypertension, usually done as second line technique to ultrasound with color Doppler imaging. Main limitation of CT scan include, unable to provide information about flow direction, portal flow rates or pressure gradients and radiation issue. CT findings practically depend upon morphologic changes rather than flow dynamic changes.

Indications for CT, in patients with known portal hypertension:

- To demonstrate the main collateral pathways
- To identify possible causes for portal hypertension
- To identify and characterize focal lesions like hepatocellular carcinoma (HCC).

Examination Technique

Multidetector computed tomography (MDCT) permits improved timing of contrast injection, excellent outlining of collateral pathways and better detection of accompanying liver lesions in patients with portal hypertension.

Scan parameters and protocols with respect to different MDCT scanners are mentioned in **Table 3**.

The amount of contrast to be used differs depending upon the iodine strength in contrast medium. If the iodine strength is 300 mg/mL, recommended amount is the range of 120–150 cc, whereas if iodine strength is 370 mg/mL, then amount only 80–100 cc. Also as a standard for liver imaging using MDCT, nonionic contrast medium is used with injection rate of 4–5 cc/sec, using pressure injector.

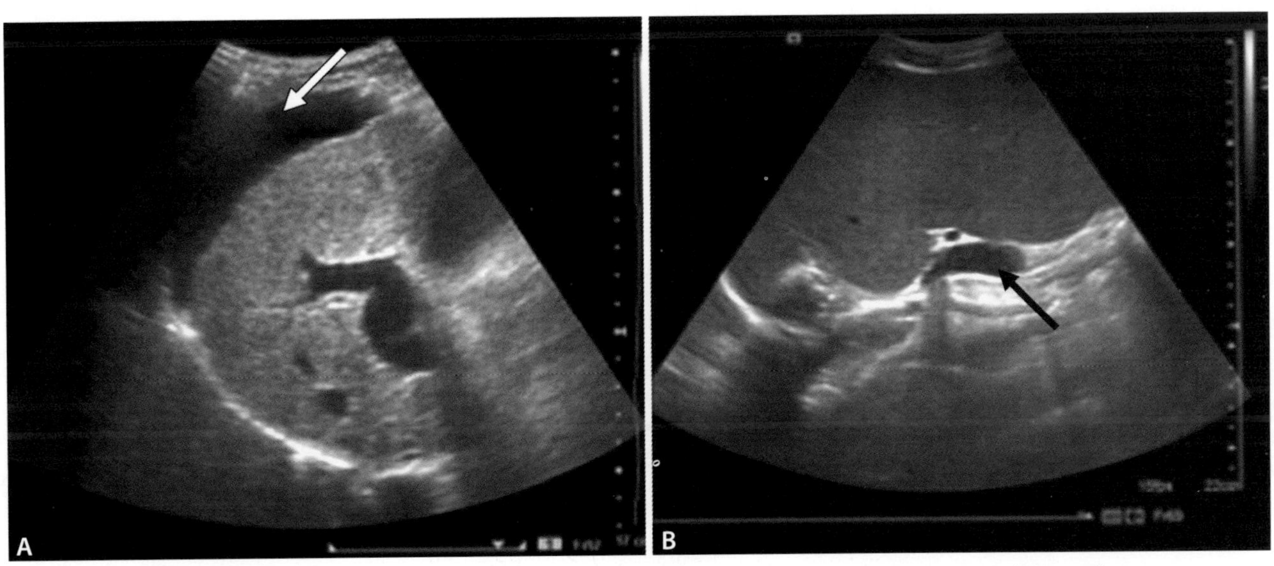

Figs. 6A and B: Ultrasound images of a cirrhotic patient showing shrunken liver with nodular surface, dilated splenoportal axis, splenomegaly (black arrow) and ascites (white arrow).

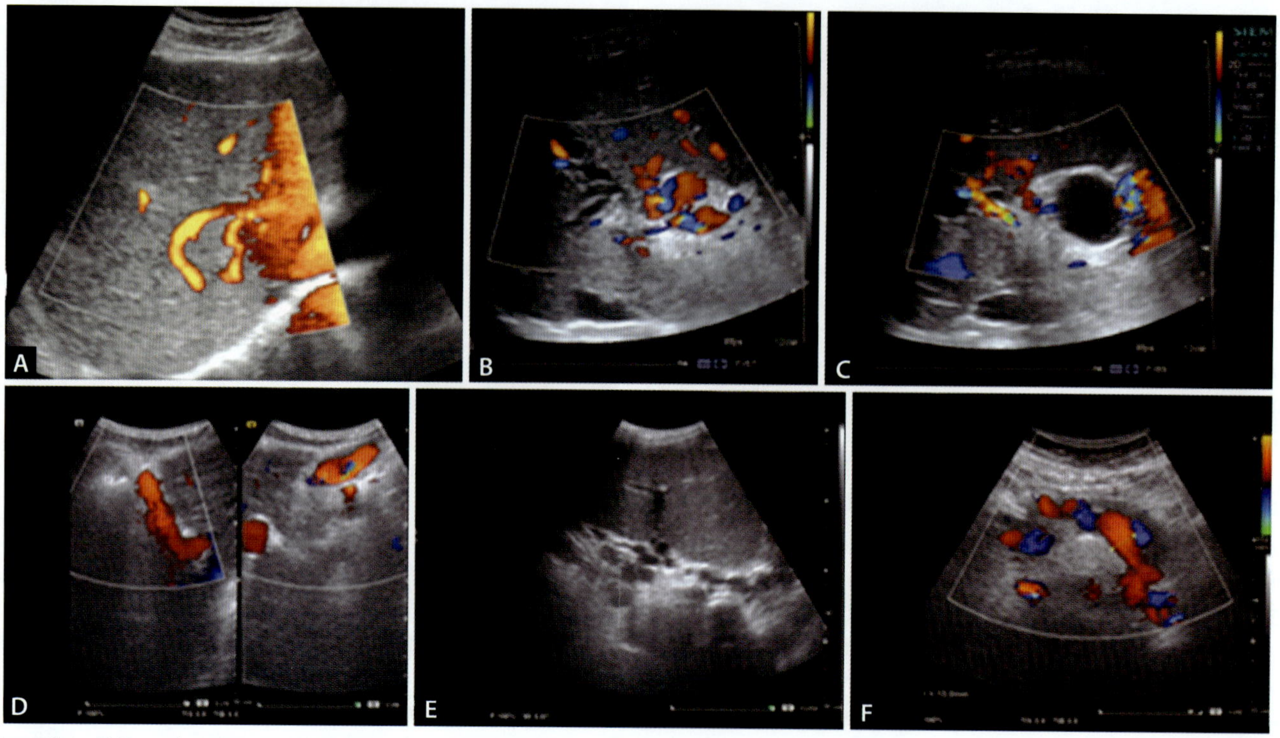

Figs. 7A to F: Doppler ultrasound images showing collaterals in various location; intrahepatic veno-venous collaterals (A), at porta (B), pericholecystic (C), paraumbilical (D), lienorenal location (E) and mesenteric location (F).

Table 3: Scan parameters and protocols with respect to different MDCT scanners.

Parameter	*4 channel*	*16 channel*	*64 channel*
Detector collimation (mm)	4 × 1.25	16 × 0.625	64 × 0.6
Slice thickness (mm) Arterial phase Venous phase	 1.25 1.25	 1 1	 1 1
Arterial delay	Bolus tracking/automated trigger Empircal delay: 25–30 sec		
Venous delay	65–70 sec	60 sec	50–60 sec

Therefore, it is important to customize the injection rate protocols and amount of contrast used depending upon the higher or lower iodine concentration contrast media.

Oral Contrast

The positive oral contrast interferes with evaluation of varices. Hence, it is suggested to use water as a negative contrast agent that helps in better depiction of varices. Patients are advised to take about 1–1.5 L water, 30 minutes before the start of CT examination; to distend the stomach and the proximal bowel loops.

Precontrast scans are generally not required; however, in patients with suspected HCC or hypervascularized liver lesions, may be useful if hemorrhage or calcifications are suspected. In case of dual energy scanner, virtual non-contrast images can be obtained from the arterial phase data without subjecting the patient to additional radiation for obtaining the unenhanced scan.

For optimal visualization of splenoportal axis, scanning should start 45–50 sec following contrast injection. In patients with portal hypertension, this time delay has to be increased up to 65–70 sec, because of slower opacification of the portal branches.

For suspected HCC, a multiphasic technique should be used with injection of 100 mL of contrast at a flow rate of 4–5 mL/s using a power injector.

Display Technique[13]

CT images are usually assessed based upon axial sections. In patients with portal hypertension because of development of complex collateral pathways further assessment using interactive cine display is very helpful and will resolve most of the fundamental diagnostic information.

In certain cases, multiplanar reformats (MPRs)/ volume-rendering techniques (VRTs) and in particular, thin slab maximum intensity projection (MIP) are valuable in better understanding of the collateral pathways **(Figs. 8A and B)**.

Magnetic Resonance Imaging[14-16]

- Provides morphologic information comparable to CT scan when ultrasound findings are inadequate.
- MRI angiography also helps in localizing and defining the extent of the presence of portosystemic collaterals **(Figs. 9A to D)**.

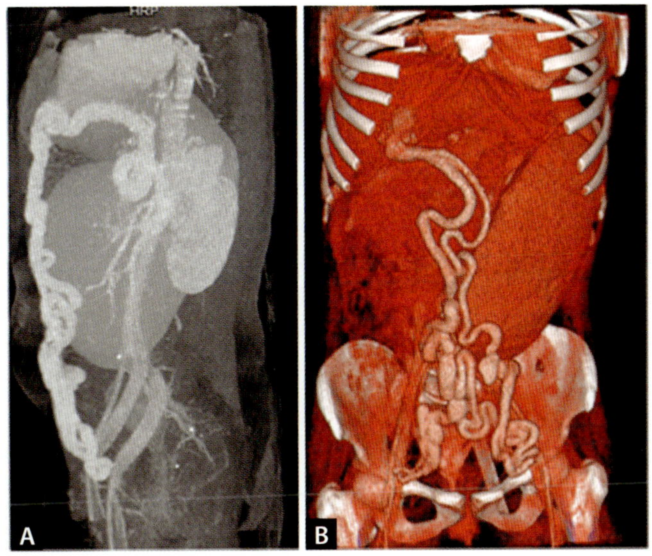

Figs. 8A and B: Thin slab MIP (Maximum Intensity Projection) (A) and VRT (Volume Rendered Technique) (B) images showing dilated tortuous paraumbilical vein, showing advantages of these techniques in understanding of the collateral pathways.

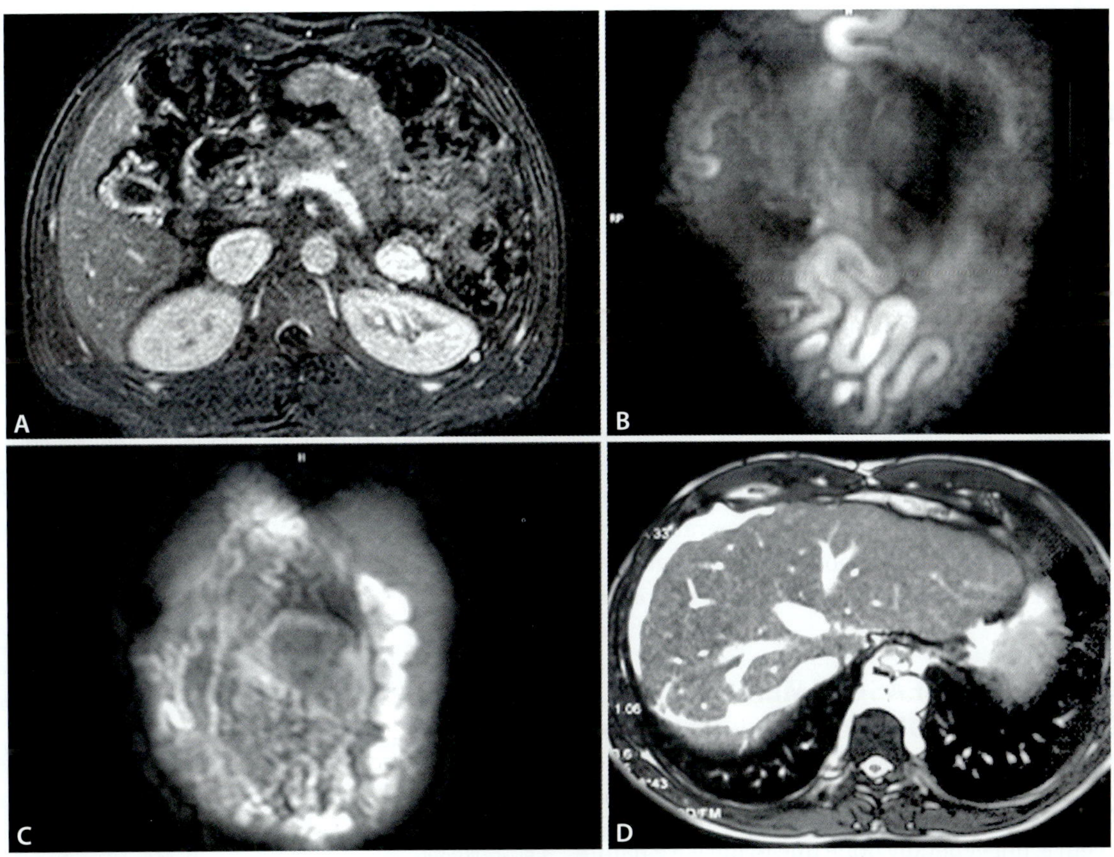

Figs. 9A to D: MR Images showing various collateral pathways; pericholecystic (A), paraumbilical (B), abdominal wall (C) and intrahepatic venovenous collaterals (D).

- Special MR techniques (like Phase contrast) also offer quantitative information about portal venous flow.

Magnetic resonance portography has few benefits over other imaging techniques used for evaluation of portal hypertension. Doppler ultrasonography is an inexpensive and noninvasive, provides quantitative information on portal blood flow, but it is operator dependent and may be unproductive when a proper acoustic window is not available. CT portography can demonstrate the portal venous system in a short time, but this technique is associated with ionizing radiation and requires administration of large amount of contrast material.

MR Technique

Nonenhanced MR angiography using time-of-flight (TOF) and phase-contrast (PC) techniques can demonstrate portal venous system, but is limited by its long data acquisition time, motion and flow artifact, and in-plane saturation.

However, contrast enhanced MR portography overcomes flow artifacts and saturation effects. MR portograms reconstructed by maximum-intensity projection postprocessing technique and source images, provide detailed information about the portal venous system **(Figs. 9A to D)**.

MR Protocol

MR imaging is performed with a 1.5-T superconducting magnetic unit using a torso-phased array coil. A 3D fast spoiled gradient recalled pulse sequence with minimum repetition time and echo time should be used. An optimized slab volume is placed in axial plane on coronal localizer extending from dome of diaphragm to inferior part of kidneys and the acquisition is performed during a single breath-hold period of 13–15 sec. An intravenous bolus of 0.2 mmol/kg of gadolinium is injected either using pressure injector or manually. Gadolinium injection was immediately followed by a 15-mL saline flush. Three repetitive acquisitions (performed within separate breath-hold of 13–15 sec) for portal venous phase imaging are obtained after a delay of 45–50 sec after start of contrast injection.

HEMODYNAMIC MEASUREMENT OF PORTAL PRESSURE[17]

Procedures (Figs. 10A and B)

- Portal pressure measurement by direct puncture of portal vein is not generally done due to invasive nature and also there is high risk of associated anesthetic and bleeding complications.
- However, most commonly indirect pressure measurement that closely matches the direct portal pressure is used, which is popularly known as hepatic venous pressure gradient (HVPG) measurement.
- In this procedure, through transfemoral route or more commonly through transjugular route, a Swan Ganz balloon catheter is placed into the right hepatic vein and free hepatic venous pressure (FHVP) is measured without inflating the balloon.
- In next step, the balloon is inflated using either diluted contrast or room air, occluding the hepatic vein outflow completely and occluded hepatic venous pressure or wedged hepatic venous pressure (WHVP) is measured **(Figs. 10A and B)**.
- The wedged pressure value minus free venous pressure value gives hepatic venous pressure measurement (HVPG).

Interpretation (Table 4)

- Normal hepatic vein pressure gradient (HVPG) is <5 mm Hg.
- Complications of portal hypertension such as variceal bleeding, ascites, or hepatorenal syndrome are seen when HVPG exceeds 10 mm Hg.

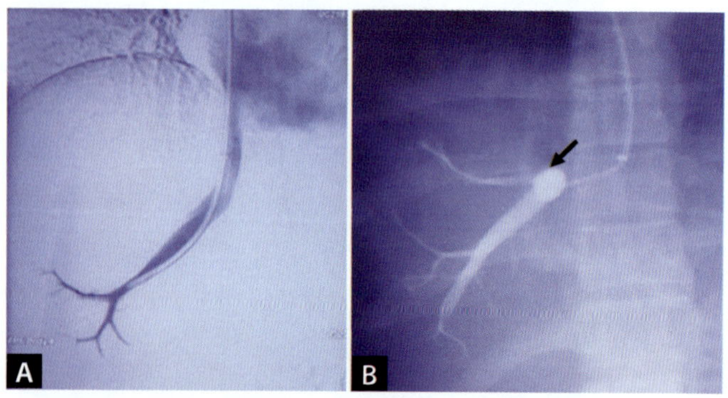

Figs. 10A and B: DSA spot images showing steps of HVPG measurement; Cannulation of the right hepatic vein (A) for measuring the free hepatic venous pressure (FHVP) followed by inflation of balloon catheter (B) (arrow) and measuring the wedged hepatic venous pressure (WHVP).

Table 4: Interpretation of HVPG findings.

Cause	*FHVP*	*WHVP*	*HVPG*
Prehepatic	Normal	Normal	Normal
Hepatic pre-sinusoidal	Normal	Normal to ↑	Normal to ↑
Sinusoidal	Normal	↑↑	↑↑
Post-sinusoidal	Normal	↑↑	↑↑
Post-hepatic	↑↑	↑↑	Normal to ↑

Abbreviations: FHVP, free hepatic vein pressure; HVPG, hepatic vein pressure gradient; WHVP, wedged hepatic vein pressure

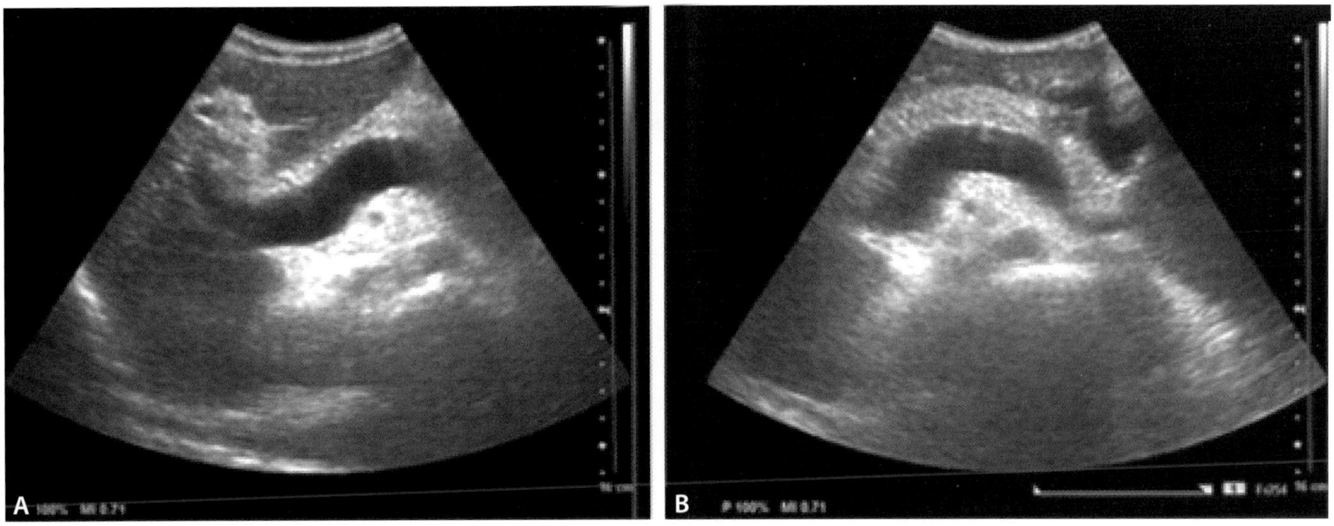

Figs. 11A and B: Ultrasound images showing dilated entire splenoportal axis: (A) Dilated MPV; and (B) Dilated splenic vein.

Table 5: Normal portosystemic communications **(Figs. 12A to D)**.

Lower esophagus	*Left gastric vein*	*Esophageal veins*
Rectum and anal canal	Superior rectal vein	Middle and inferior rectal vein
Umbilicus	Paraumbilical veins	Superior and inferior epigastric veins
Bare area of liver	Portal vein branches	Inferior phrenic vein
Retroperitoneum	Tributaries of splenic, pancreatic and colic veins	Renal, suprarenal, gonadal and paravertebral veins

Table 6: Gastroesophageal and ectopic varices **(Figs. 13 and 14)**.

Gastroesophageal varices	*Ectopic varices*
Esophageal	Duodenal
Paraesophageal	Jejunoileal
Gastric and perigastric	Colonic Pancreatic Mesenteric Vesical Pericholecystic Retroperitoneal Rectal/perirectal

- If there is HVPG <10 mm Hg and complications of portal hypertension are present, then one should suspect non-cirrhotic portal hypertension.

MORPHOLOGIC SIGNS OF PORTAL HYPERTENSION

Divided into Direct and Associated Signs

Direct Signs include, dilatation of splenoportal axis, i.e. main portal vein diameter >13 mm, splenic vein diameter >10 mm **(Figs. 11A and B)**. If there are adequate venous collaterals, SPA may not show significant dilatation.

Collateral Pathways[18,19]

In healthy human, congenitally originated connections exists between portal and systemic circulation **(Table 5)**. In the setting of portal hypertension, these connections get dilated leading to formation of varices at various sites within the body.

Table 7: Spontaneous shunts **(Figs. 15A to C)**.

Intrahepatic	*Transhepatic*	*Extrahepatic*
Rare	Recanalized paraumbilical vein	Gastrorenal Splenorenal Gastrocaval

These varices are divided into two groups **(Table 6)**:

1. Gastroesophageal varices
2. Ectopic varices

In long-term, these varices develop large spontaneous shunts **(Table 7)**, which are categorized into intrahepatic, transhepatic and extrahepatic shunts.

VARICES

Esophageal and Paraesophageal Varices

The most common varices encountered in portal hypertension are esophageal varices (50%). Esophageal

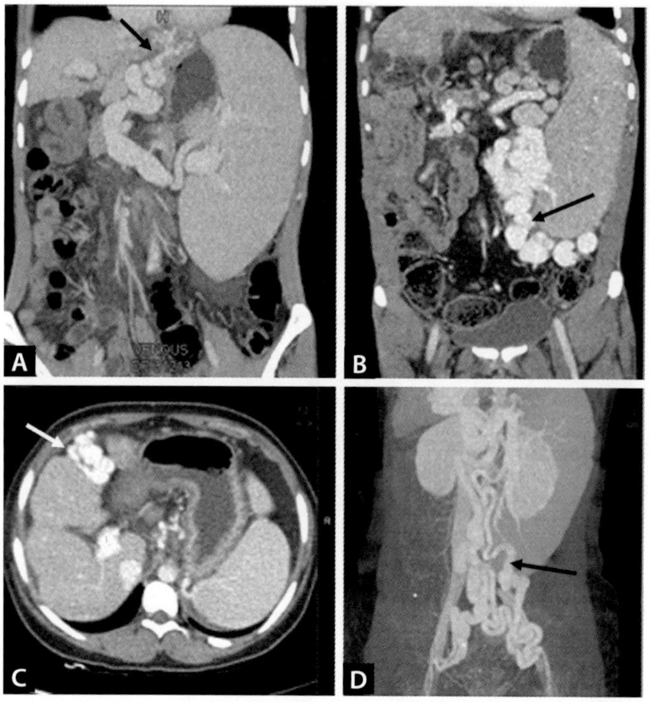

Figs. 12A to D: CT images showing various normal portosystemic communications; at lower end of esophagus (A), in retroperitoneum (B) and at umbilicus (paraumbilical veins) (C and D).

varices are located within the wall of the lower esophagus, whereas paraesophageal varices are located outside the esophageal wall. These are the most common varices to bleed in portal hypertension due to high pressure and high volume of blood that they carry and account for high mortality due to spontaneous hemorrhage.

Gastric and Perigastric Varices

Gastric varices are less common than esophageal varices (5–33%), drain either into the left renal vein through spontaneous gastrorenal shunt or directly into the IVC through a spontaneous gastrocaval shunt. Risk of bleeding is low as compared to esophageal varices but the severity of bleeding is much higher due to their large size.

Ectopic Varices

They account for 2–5% of variceal bleeding, have a 4-fold increased risk of bleeding as compared to esophageal varices and associated with high mortality rate. These varices are difficult to treat and there is no established standard treatment. When hemorrhage arises from these ectopic varices, it is challenging to control by any method, and the bleeding may be potentially lethal.

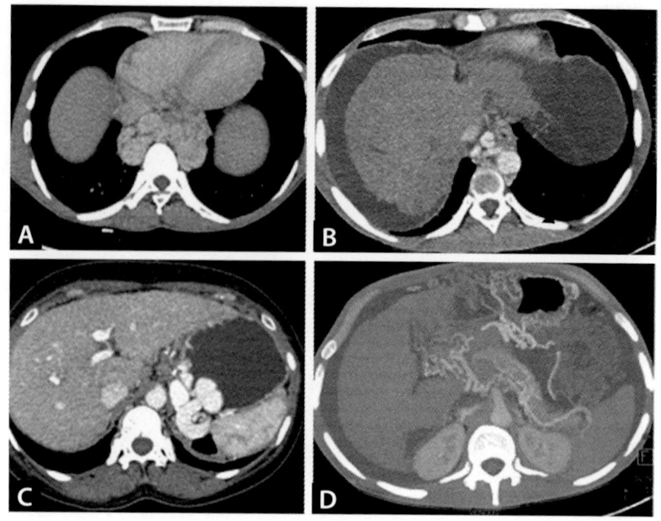

Figs. 13A to D: Axial CT images showing various gastroesophageal varices: Paraesophageal (A), Esophageal (B), Fundal (C) and Perigastric (D) locations.

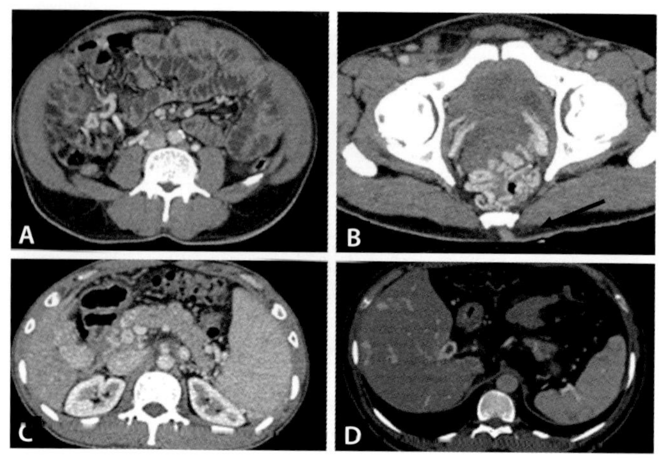

Figs. 14A to D: Axial CT images showing ectopic varices; colonic (A), rectal (B), pericholecystic (C) and pericholedochal locations (D).

Associated Findings

The most important associated findings in portal hypertension are splenomegaly and ascites. Other associated findings are small bowel edema, thickening of the gallbladder wall, increased density within mesenteric fat (misty mesentery) and omentum. In addition, patients with PHT especially those with hypersplenism have an increased incidence of splenic artery true aneurysms due to hyperkinetic circulation, which may be seen as incidental finding on imaging.

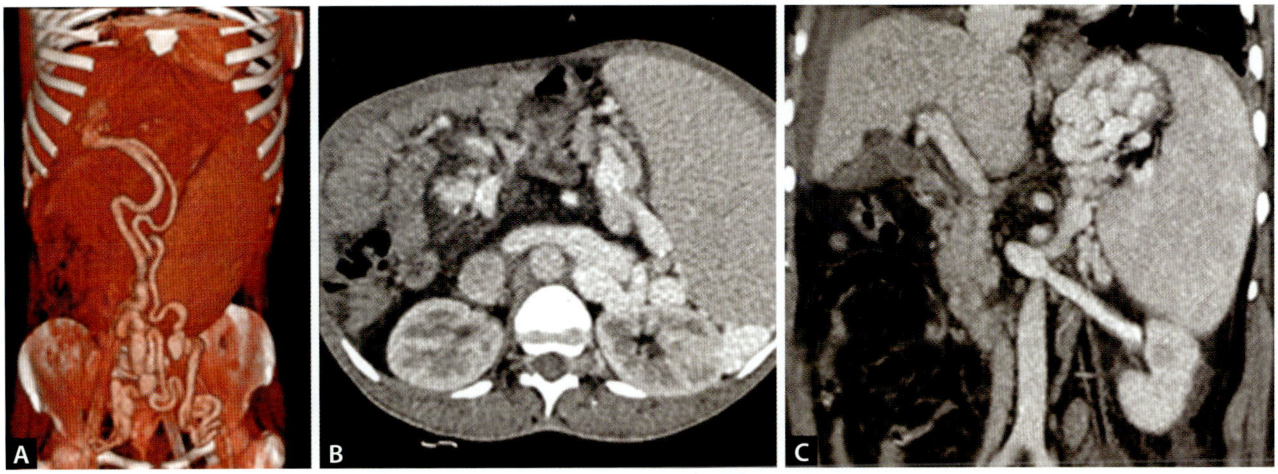

Figs. 15A to C: CT images showing spontaneous shunts; recanalized paraumbilical (Transhepatic shunt) (A), splenorenal (B), and gastrorenal (C) shunts.

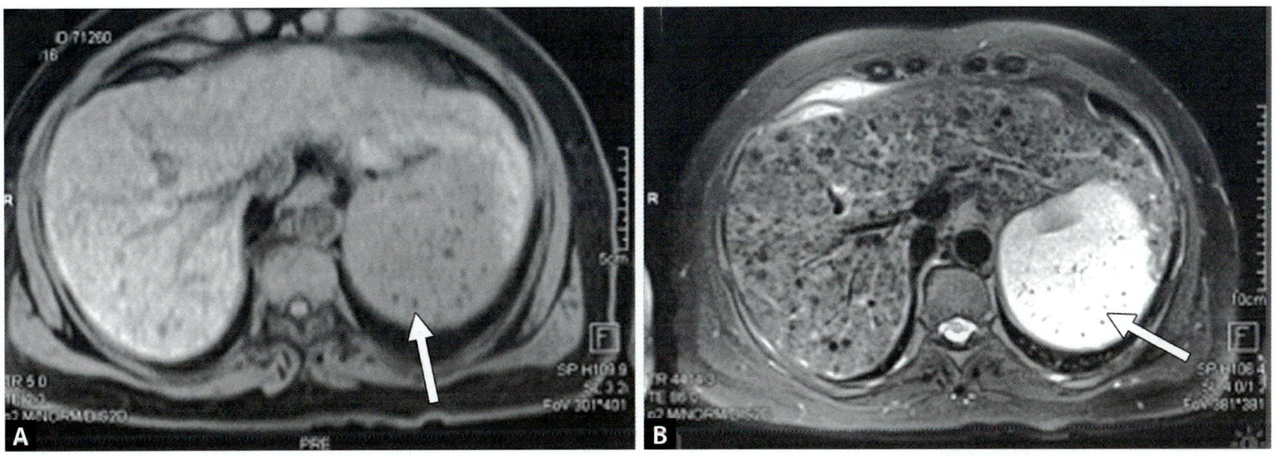

Figs. 16A and B: Axial T1W and T2W MR images (A and B) showing multiple low signal intensity foci (arrow) scattered in enlarged spleen in a cirrhotic patient.

Splenomegaly

Splenomegaly develops in most, but not all cases, of portal hypertension however is of little use due to the large number of alternative causes. The size of the spleen does not correlate with degree of portal hypertension. Also, if splenomegaly is absent, portal hypertension cannot be ruled out. Siderotic Gamna-Gandy nodules that represent small foci of perifollicular and trabecular hemorrhage may be seen as multiple faint hyperechoic foci on ultrasound or multiple faint calcifications on CT. They are seen as multiple low signal foci 3–8 mm in size on gradient echo sequences of MR images **(Figs. 16A and B)**.

Ascites is not usually caused by uncomplicated portal hypertension. It is often secondary to underlying liver diseases with liver cell failure and increase in sinusoidal pressure leading to an increase in fluid in the space of Disse with resultant ascites. In prehepatic PHT, liver function remains normal and ascites is minimal.

SPECIFIC SITUATIONS

Intrahepatic Portal Hypertension

Cirrhosis of Liver: Imaging features are described under diffuse liver diseases chapter.

Sonography can differentiate intrahepatic from extrahepatic portal hypertension in majority of cases and can also detect the presence of splenomegaly and ascites. Evaluation of the liver by ultrasound may reveal changes of cirrhosis such as coarsened echo texture with or without altered echogenicity, nodularity of liver surface, presence

Table 8: Causes of noncirrhotic portal hypertension.

- Extrahepatic portal venous obstruction (EHPVO)
- Noncirrhotic portal fibrosis (NCPF) or idiopathic portal hypertension (IPH)
- Nodular regenerative hyperplasia
- Partial nodular transformation
- Congenital hepatic fibrosis
- Schistosomiasis
- Peliosis hepatitis

Flowchart 1: Etiopathogenesis of extrahepatic portal venous obstruction and noncirrhotic portal fibrosis.

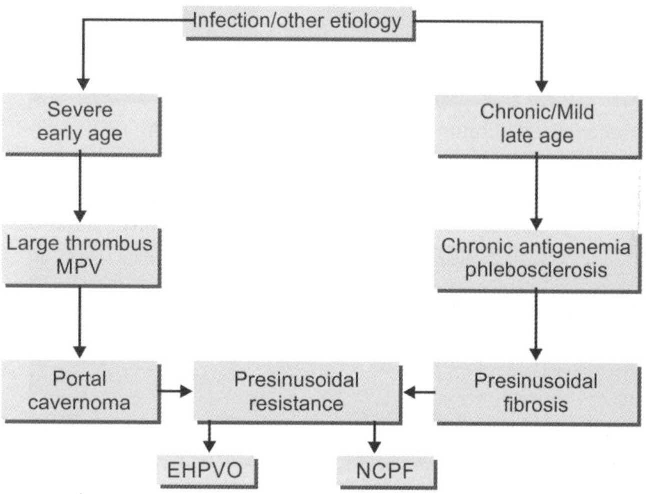

Abbreviations: EHPVO: Extrahepatic portal venous obstruction; MPV: Main portal vein; NCPF: Noncirrhotic portal fibrosis.

of regenerating nodules and reduction in the number of visible portal or hepatic veins. Reduction of liver size with a combination of segmental hypertrophy and atrophy in the form of caudate to right lobe ratio >0.65 and reduction of the transverse diameter of segment IV.

Noncirrhotic portal hypertension (NCPH): Includes a spectrum of diseases of diverse causes **(Table 8)**.

The most common causes of NCPH are non-cirrhotic portal fibrosis (NCPF) and extrahepatic portal vein obstruction (EHPVO). These constitute 1/3rd of all cases of portal hypertension (PHT) in India.[20,21]

The fundamental cause in both NCPF and EHPVO is thought to be vascular origin. However, the exact etiopathogenesis of the two conditions is not known, but a common pathway with different outcomes has been advocated and is depicted in **Flowchart 1**.

Basically, in a genetically susceptible patient, a trigger point such as infection or prothrombotic episode can incite thrombosis in portal system.

In EHPVO, a major thrombotic event in early life leads to occlusion of main portal vein with resultant cavernoma formation.

Table 9: Guidelines for the diagnosis of NCPF.

- Presence of splenomegaly
- Normal liver function tests
- Varices on upper GI endoscopy
- Patent portal and hepatic veins on Doppler
- Normal or mildly elevated wedged hepatic venous pressure (WHVP); and markedly elevated intrasplenic and portal vein pressure
- No evidence of cirrhosis on liver biopsy

Where as in NCPF, repeated events of microthrombi in later life leads to occlusion of small and medium sized venous cannels with resultant presinusoidal fibrosis.

Noncirrhotic portal fibrosis (NCPF): This condition was first described by Banti in late 19th century and was originally identified in India as an etiological factor of portal hypertension in mid-20th century.

NCPF is a seen in patients during their 3rd–4th decade of life and especially more common in individuals of low socioeconomic background.[20,21]

There are well-established guidelines for making diagnosis of NCPF **(Table 9)**.

Imaging findings include normal size liver with normal echogenicity, splenomegaly, patent hepatic veins, dilated splenoportal axis and presence of varices **(Figs. 17A to D)**. Few specific ultrasound findings are also described (which are difficult to document), such as echogenic thick-walled portal branches, narrowing or cuff of peripheral portal vein branches classically described as "withered tree" appearance.[21,22]

Management: Prognosis is generally excellent in NCPF, since, liver functions are well preserved. Main concern is usually prevention/control of variceal bleeding which is the major cause of death in these patients.

PREHEPATIC CAUSES

Extrahepatic Portal Vein Obstruction[23,24]

Definition

Extrahepatic portal vein obstruction (EHPVO), an important cause of upper GI bleeding in pediatric age group, caused by thrombotic event in early life resulting in cavernoma formation.

The disease process may involve only the main portal vein and its branches at porta, or may extend to involve the splenic vein and upper portion of the superior mesenteric vein. Splenoportal confluence is the most common site to get involved in this disease process; whereas entire SPA is involved in only 10% of cases.

The etiopathogenesis of EHPVO is not known in nearly 50% of patients. Possible causes include, neonatal sepsis,

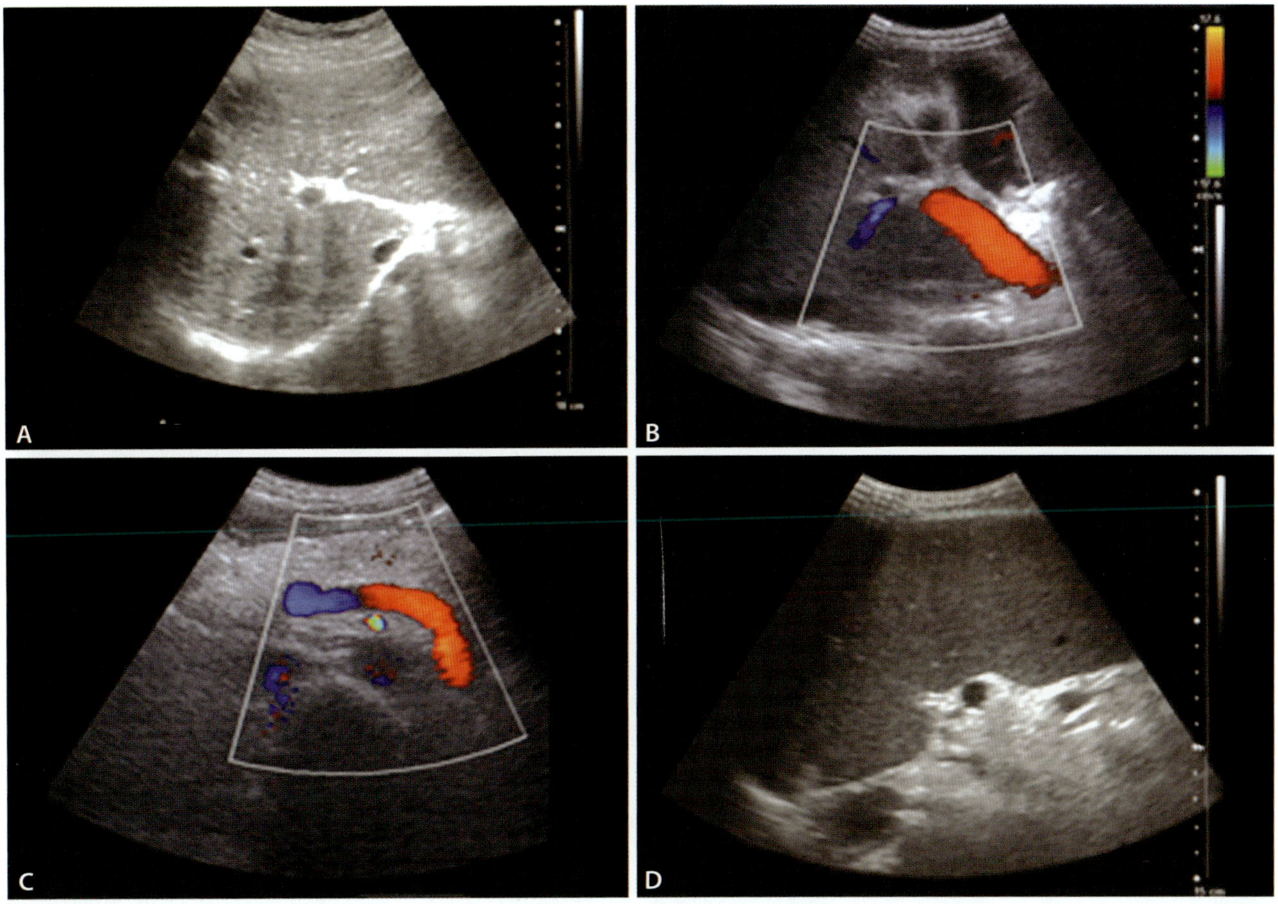

Figs. 17A to D: Ultrasound and Doppler images of noncirrhotic portal fibrosis (NCPF) patient showing normal size liver with normal echotexture (A), dilated MPV (B), splenic vein (C) and splenomegaly (D).

omphalitis, umbilical vein catheterization, dehydration, multiple exchange transfusions, and hypercoagulable states.

These patients may present anywhere between 6 weeks to adulthood with well-controlled variceal bleeding and massive splenomegaly. Generally, LFTs are normal in young patients with EHPVO. Infrequently, these patients may present with jaundice due to portal biliopathy. Hemodynamically, wedged HVPG is normal since the block is (presinusoidal hepatic), however direct intrasplenic pressure is significantly increased in these patients.

Portal biliopathy refers biliary abnormalities (Intrahepatic/extrahepatic) either due to compression of bile ducts by prominent paracholedochal and epicholedochal varices or due to ischemic injury (stricture formation) **(Fig. 18)**. Although imaging biliary abnormalities have been described in 80–100% of cases, but only a few patients present with jaundice or pain.[25]

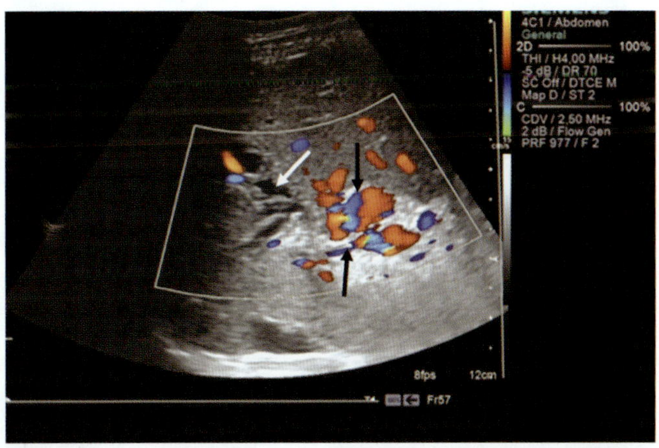

Fig. 18: Doppler ultrasound image showing multiple collaterals at porta (black arrow) replacing the main portal vein (MPV) with dilatation of intrahepatic biliary radicles suggestive of portal biliopathy (white arrow).

Imaging modalities: Currently the ultrasonography with Doppler is best imaging modality to evaluate EHPVO patients **(Fig. 18)**. Invasive, direct splenoportography provides information about the portal venous system to identify the site of obstruction, extent of disease and extent of collateral circulation, however this procedure is obsolete

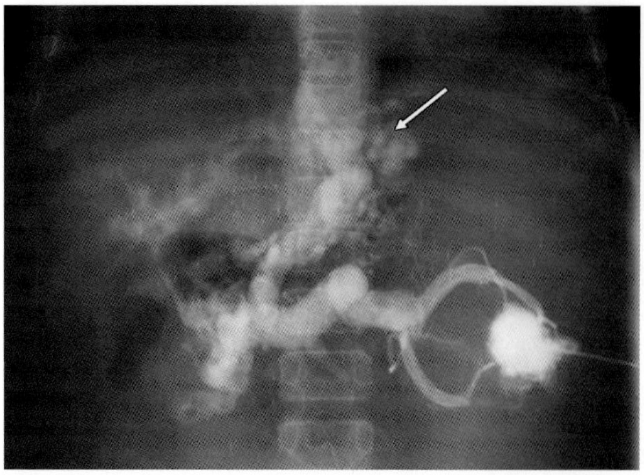

Fig. 19: Spot image of direct splenoportography showing patent and dilated splenoportal axis with varices supplied by the left gastric vein (arrow).

these days **(Fig. 19)**. The more advanced techniques like computed tomographic portography and MR portography of the upper abdomen, are performed only if Doppler is of suboptimal quality **(Figs. 20A to D)**.

Imaging findings: Main portal vein is replaced by echogenic fibrosis and multiple collaterals around the porta classically described as cavernoma formation **(Figs. 21A and B)**. Sometime, one may see recanalized portal vein or dominant collateral at porta. CT/MR portography are used as problem solving modalities when Doppler findings are inconclusive.

Treatment and Prognosis

Prognosis is generally good in EHPVO, since, liver functions are well-preserved. Main concern is usually prevention/

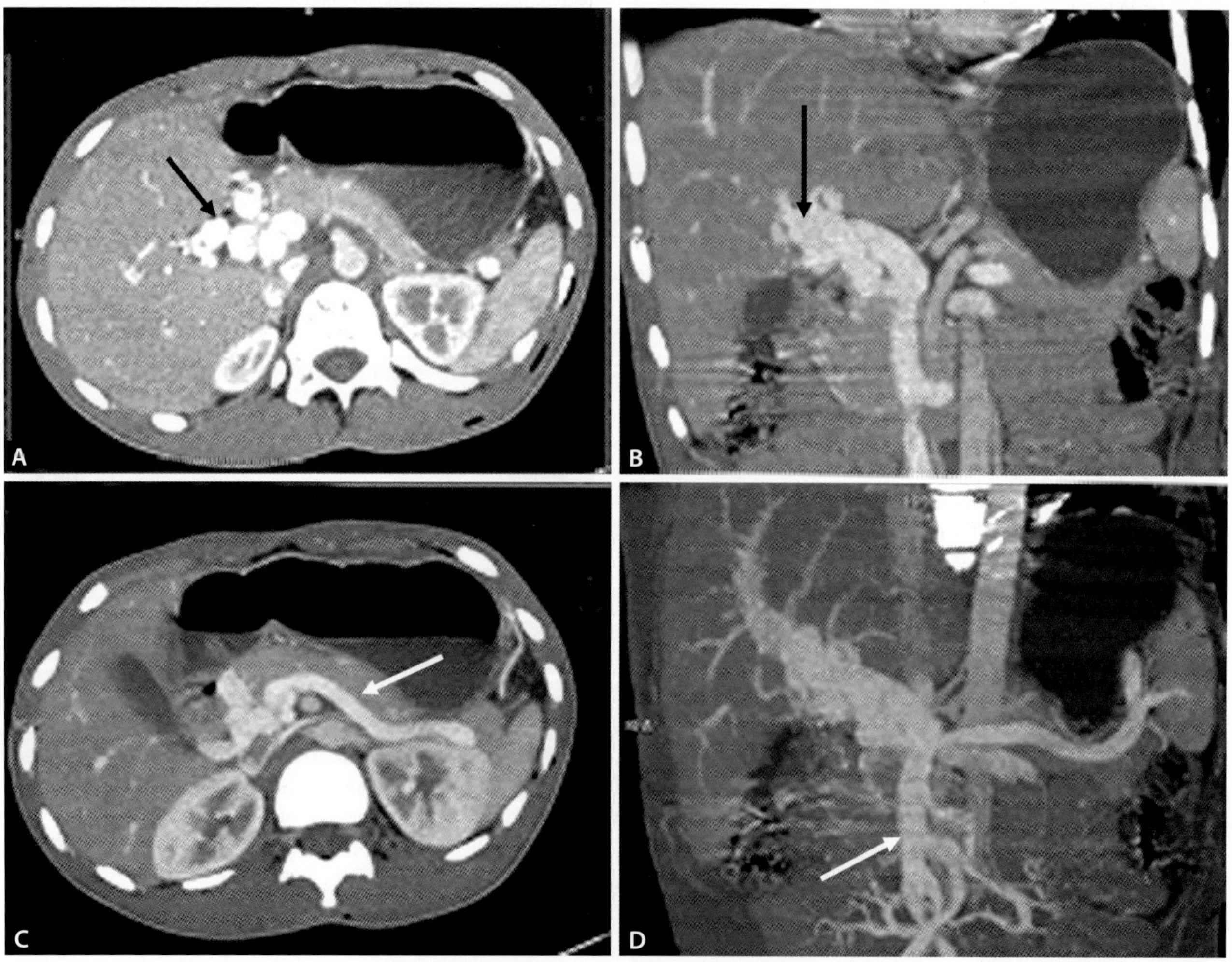

Figs. 20A to D: CT portography images showing multiple collaterals at porta (arrow) (A and B) replacing the main portal vein (MPV) with patent splenic (C) (arrow) and superior mesenteric vein (D) (arrow).

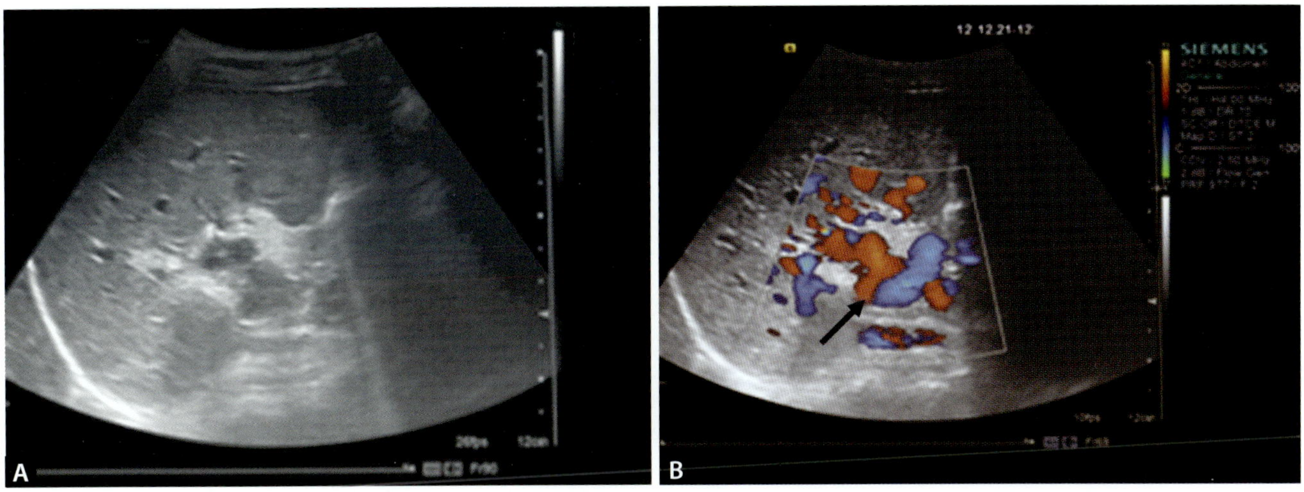

Figs. 21A and B: Doppler ultrasound images showing multiple collaterals at porta replacing the main portal vein (B) (arrow) with small size liver having normal echotexture (A).

control of variceal bleeding which is the major cause of death in these patients. Endoscopic therapy is the first line of treatment for variceal bleeding. However, surgery is reserved for patients with variceal bleeding who fail to respond to endoscopic management. Other indications for surgery include, patients with ectopic variceal bleeding, portal biliopathy and growth retardation.

Portal Vein Thrombosis[24,26,27]

Cirrhosis is an important risk for development of splanchnic vein thrombosis in cirrhotic patients, either due to development of portal venous hypertension or stasis of blood flow in portal circulation.

Other risk factors for development of acute portal vein include, infectious disease (e.g. sepsis, cholangitis, and pancreatitis), neoplasms, hypercoagulable states and surgery.

Contrast-enhanced CT/CT portal venography can exhibit a filling defect occludes the portal vein lumen either partially or completely **(Figs. 22A and B)**. Indirect signs include presence of cavernous transformation of the portal vein and the presence of portosystemic collateral vessels.

It is important to differentiate bland thrombus from malignant thrombus in cirrhotic patients. Bland thrombus will not enhance on post-contrast studies and will not distend the lumen **(Figs. 22A and B)**. Whereas malignant thrombus, distends the lumen and shows enhancement similar to primary lesion, classically described as "Threads-streaks" **(Figs. 23A and B)**. Malignant lesion

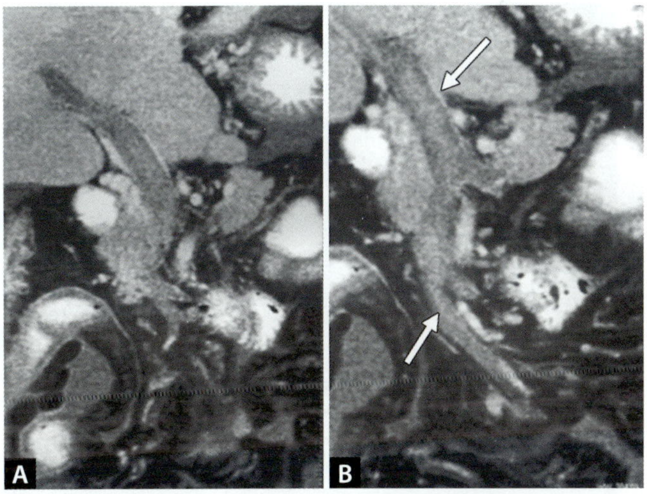

Figs. 22A and B: Coronal thin slab MIP image showing long segment non-enhancing filling defect (A) within the main portal vein extending into superior mesenteric vein (B) (arrows).

shows diffusion restriction on diffusion-weighted MR imaging.

Left-sided Portal Hypertension

Left sided portal hypertension (LSPH) is a special form of portal hypertension that occurs due to obstruction of the splenic vein in isolation and presents with bleeding from isolated gastric varices. The main cause of LSPH is splenic vein thrombosis and pancreatic disease is the most common etiology. This entity is usually thought in situation of gastrointestinal bleeding with normal liver function and unexplained splenomegaly. At times, LSPH

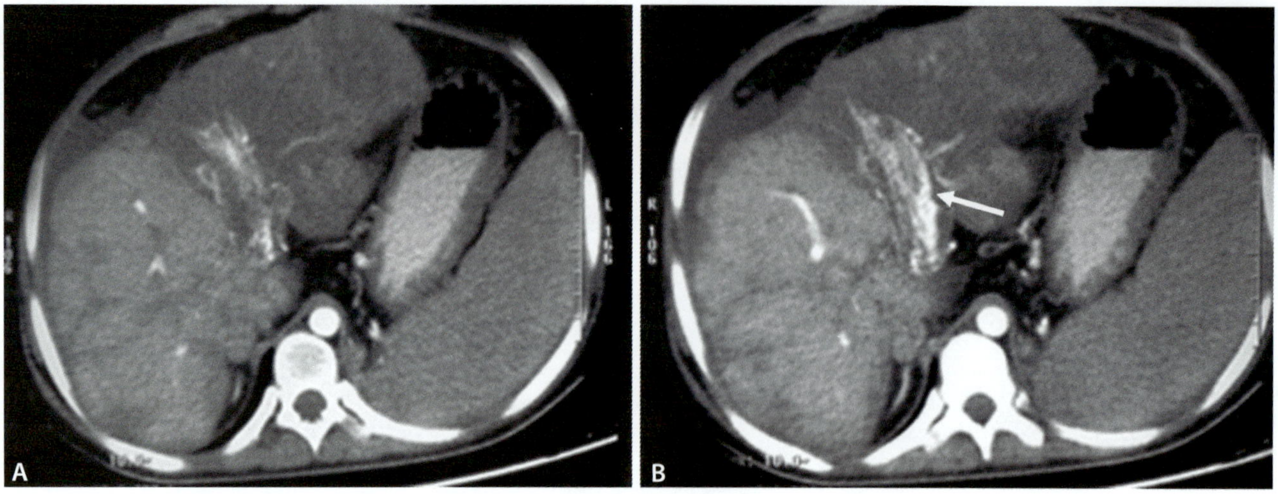

Figs. 23A and B: Axial CT images in arterial phase showing large infiltrative mass in left lobe of liver (A) with enhancing tumor thrombus in left portal vein (B) giving streaks and thread appearance (arrow).

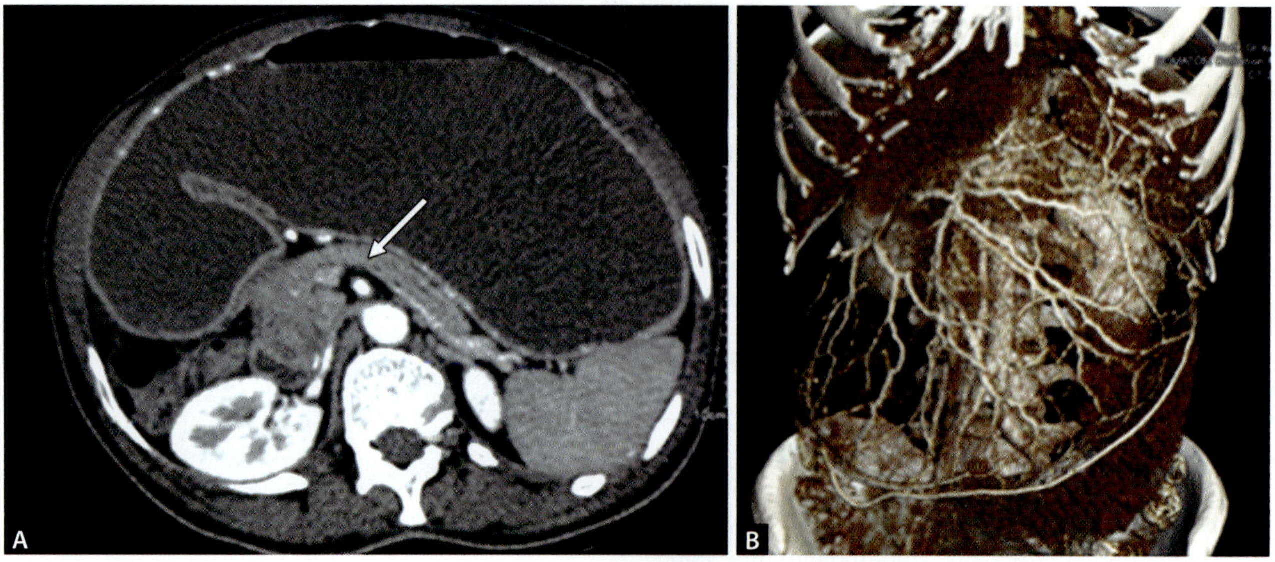

Figs. 24A and B: Axial CT (A) and coronal VRT (B) images showing severely attenuated and splenic vein (arrow) and is replaced by extensive collaterals around the stomach (B).

may be difficult to diagnose on both endoscopically and radiologically. On imaging, there is thrombosis or severe attenuation of splenic vein with extensive collaterals all around the stomach **(Figs. 24A and B)**. If repeated gastric variceal bleeding complicates this condition, splenectomy is considered.[28]

Splanchnic Arterioportal Fistula

Arterioportal fistula (APF) is rare, occurring mainly from a ruptured pseudoaneurysm communicating with portal system either due to iatrogenic cause or due to penetrating trauma. This entity is encountered increasingly, due to rising numbers of percutaneous transhepatic procedures. The predominant symptoms are due to complications of portal hypertension, most commonly variceal bleeding. Angiography remains the gold standard **(Figs. 25A to C)**. However, duplex ultrasonography is a useful screening tool. CT angiography helps in pretreatment planning such as artery involved, level of communication, diameter of communication and to see the extent of varices.

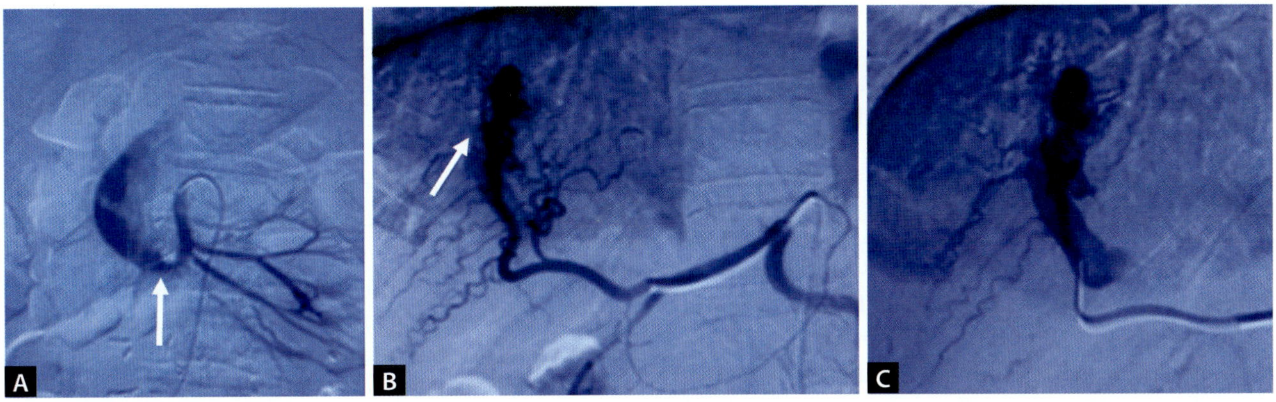

Figs. 25A to C: DSA spot images (A to C) showing fistulous communication between superior mesenteric artery and superior mesenteric vein (A) (arrow). Fistulous communication between right hepatic artery and right portal vein suggestive of arterioportal fistula (B and C) (arrow) as a prehepatic causes of portal hypertension.

In broad, surgery is the treatment of choice for large extrahepatic fistula, whereas embolization is ideal for intrahepatic fistulas and small extrahepatic fistula. Embolization is also beneficial for patients with comorbidities who carry high risk of surgical mortality. Main goal of treatment is to occlude the fistula and maintain the arterial flow.[29]

Posthepatic Causes

Budd-Chiari Syndrome: Imaging findings and interventions are described in detail in separate chapter.

RADIOLOGICAL INTERVENTIONS IN PORTAL HYPERTENSION

INTRODUCTION

The role of radiologists in the management of portal hypertension (PHT) had been confined to its diagnosis and treatment planning. However, with the advancements in the field of interventional radiology various minimally invasive techniques have evolved in the management of portal hypertension and its complications such as recanalization techniques, shunt creation and variceal bleeding control. Thus, with these technical advances, there is a shift in role of radiologist from diagnosis to the management of portal hypertension.

The management of portal hypertension and its complications requires multi-modality approach including medical and endoscopic management and surgical and nonsurgical (minimally invasive radiological techniques) methods to reduce portal pressure. Surgical methods carry significant morbidity and mortality in these groups of patients.

Table 10: Radiologic interventions in portal hypertension.

Interventions in portal hypertension
Interventions that reduce portal blood pressure: • Transjugular intrahepatic portosystemic shunts (TIPS) • Recanalization of hepatic venous outflow • Partial splenic embolization • Recanalization of occluded/thrombosed portal veins or tributaries • Occlusion of arterioportal shunts (congenital/acquired) • Revision of occluded surgical or radiological shunts
Interventions to control the symptoms of PHT: • Percutaneous transhepatic variceal embolization • Balloon-occluded retrograded transvenous obliteration of gastric varices (BRTO)
Occlusion of surgical or radiologic shunts in refractory encephalopathy

Interventions in Portal Hypertension

Primary aim is to reduce the portal pressure and thereby reduce the complications related to PHT such as variceal bleed, ascites, hydrothorax, and hepatorenal syndrome.

Secondary aim (In cases where it is difficult to bring down the portal pressure) is to deal with the complications of PHT such as esophageal and gastric varices, refractory ascites and encephalopathy.

The radiologic interventions in PHT are broadly categorized in **Table 10**.

Transjugular Intrahepatic Portosystemic Shunts

Transjugular intrahepatic portosystemic shunts (TIPS) involve the creation of a low resistance conduit between the portal vein and hepatic vein by deploying an intra-hepatic stent. The procedure is done under fluoroscopic and ultrasound guidance, under conscious sedation or general anesthesia depending upon patients' condition. Prophylactic antibiotics may be given and coagulation defects have to be corrected prior to the procedure.

Technique: The procedure starts with puncture of right internal jugular vein for venous access under sonographic guidance. A 10F long vascular sheath is placed across the right heart into the inferior vena cava. Initial cavogram is obtained to look for the status of inferior vena cava and the ostium of hepatic vein. Diagnostic angiographic catheter is then introduced into one of the hepatic veins (preferably right hepatic vein). At this stage, baseline hepatic vein wedge pressure is obtained using balloon catheter occluding the hepatic vein outflow. After getting access into right hepatic vein, this catheter is exchanged with a long metallic cannula with 7F vascular sheath over the metallic guidewire. This metallic cannula is then wedged against the hepatic vein wall close to the ostium and gentle contrast study is done to look for retrograde visualization of intrahepatic portal vein branches. USG or direct transhepatic portography may also be used to visualize the portal vein and branches in difficult cases with distorted anatomy. Then using a combination of coaxial system of 16G metallic cannula with 7F sheath and 21G Chiba needle with 4F catheter, hepatic parenchyma is entered through hepatic vein wall. Using either fluoroscopic landmark of portal vein or USG guidance, access into the portal vein is done using 21G Chiba needle with 4F catheter loaded over it. This is the most critical step of TIPS that, utmost care should be taken not to breach the liver capsule to prevent life-threatening intraperitoneal bleed. The preferable site of portal vein puncture is at the portal vein bifurcation or within 2 cm of portal vein bifurcation. Once portal vein access is obtained, portogram is obtained to look for splenoportal axis anatomy and variceal status. The parenchymal tract is dilated using angiographic balloon catheters (diameter 8–10 mm) and specially designed TIPS stent (uncovered segment in portal vein and covered segment in hepatic parenchyma and hepatic vein) is deployed to maintain the patency of the tract. PTFE (polytetrafluoroethylene)-covered stents are preferred over bare stents as they showed improved long-term patency of the shunt and prevent porto-biliary fistula.[30-32] Customized TIPS stent graft has a small uncovered part (2 cm), which is to be kept in the portal vein to promote good inflow and avoid portal vein thrombosis **(Figs. 26A to E)**.

The established indication for TIPS is in the management of patients with cirrhosis and portal hypertension complicated by recurrent/refractory variceal bleeding and refractory ascites. Refractory acutely bleeding varices and complicated chronic/acute Budd-Chiari syndrome are among the optional indications **(Table 11)**.[33]

Absolute contraindications for TIPS placement include congestive cardiac failure, severe pulmonary hypertension, unrelieved biliary obstruction, pre-existing hepatic encephalopathy, etc. **(Table 12)**.[34]

Variceal bleeding is a major cause of death in cirrhotic patients and correlates with portal hypertension. Many studies have demonstrated the efficacy of TIPS in controlling and preventing massive life-threatening variceal hemorrhage. It is recommended to reduce the HVPG below 12 mm Hg in controlling variceal bleeding. TIPS is also beneficial in preventing bleeding from hypertensive gastropathy.[34]

Refractory ascites reflects severe portal hypertension and advanced liver dysfunction and is associated with very poor outcome and survival. TIPS will decrease the need for repeated large volume paracentesis in patients with refractory ascites. However, in view of poor functional status of such patients and the higher risk of hepatic encephalopathy, TIPS is recommended for those who are intolerant to repeated paracentesis. Similarly in cases of refractory hepatic hydrothorax, TIPS is only recommended to those whose effusion is not controlled by diuretics and sodium restriction. In cases of Budd-Chiari syndrome TIPS or direct intrahepatic portosystemic shunt (DIPS) is recommended in cases with moderate severity and those who failed to respond to anticoagulation.[33]

Complications of TIPS

Immediate complications are procedure related; such as hematoma, arrhythmia, stent displacement, bilhemia and shunt thrombosis. Uncommon life-threatening complications include hemoperitoneum, cardiac failure, liver ischemia and sepsis. Chronic complications include congestive cardiac failure, portal vein thrombosis, chronic recurrent encephalopathy, TIPSitis and TIPS dysfunction. TIPS dysfunction is defined as loss of decompression of portal system due to occlusion or stenosis of the shunt. The best indicator of it is reappearance of symptoms such as variceal bleeding and ascites and can be demonstrated by imaging.

Recanalization of Hepatic Venous Outflow (Budd-Chiari Syndrome)

Budd-Chiari syndrome is a heterogeneous group of disorders characterized by hepatic venous obstruction

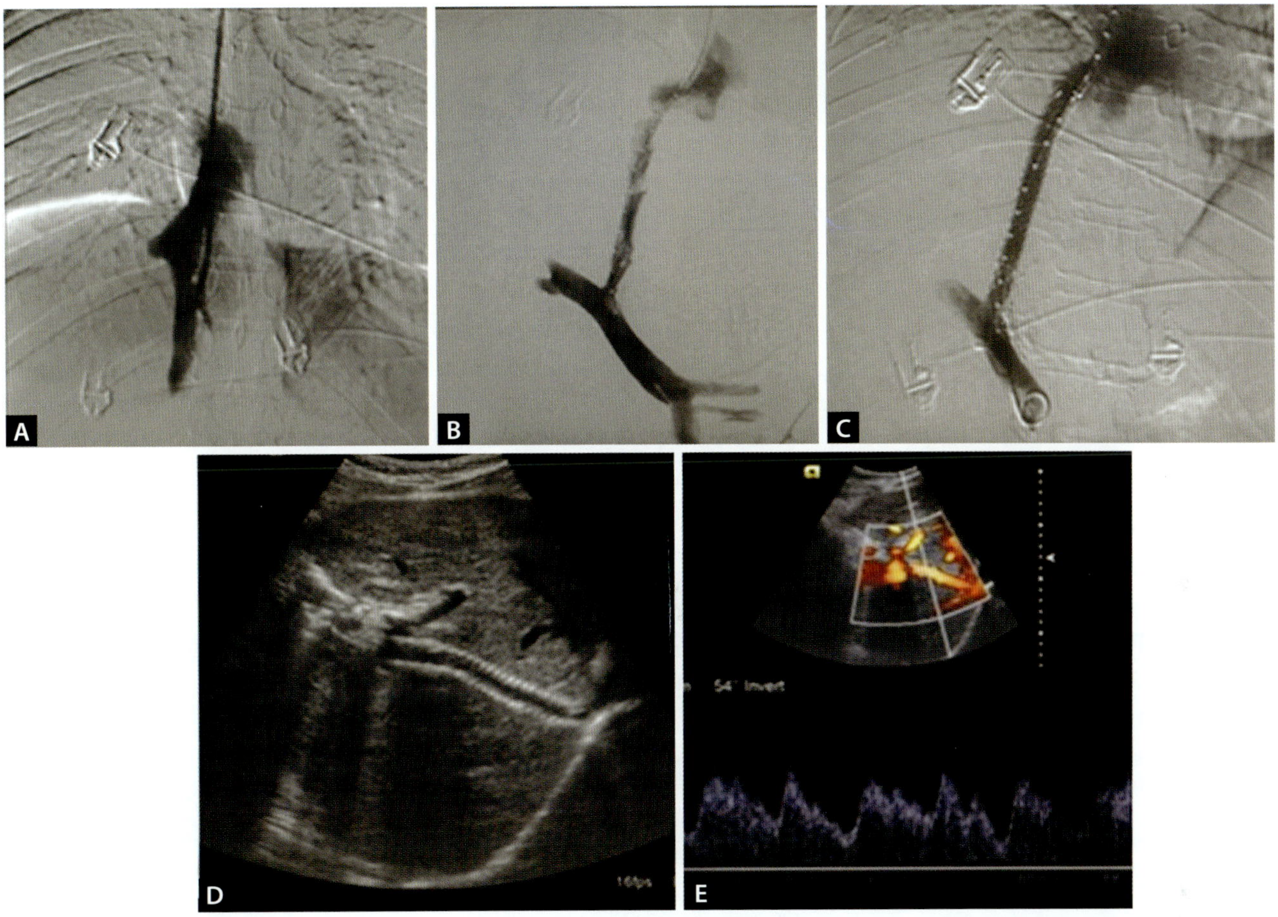

Figs. 26A to E: TIPS performed in a cirrhotic patient with uncontrollable variceal bleeding: (A) Initial cavogram showing normal caliber IVC and hepatic vein; (B) A parenchymal tract is made from the hepatic vein to the portal vein; (C) Post-TIPS venogram showing freeflow of contrast through the stent graft; (D and E) USG and color Doppler showing TIPS stent with optimal flow.

Table 11: Indications for TIPS.

• Refractory cirrhotic ascites
• Refractory acutely bleeding varices
• Portal hypertensive gastropathy
• Bleeding gastric varices
• Refractory hepatic hydrothorax
• Hepatorenal syndrome
• Budd-Chiari syndrome
• Veno-occlusive disease
• Hepatopulmonary syndrome

Table 12: Contraindications of TIPS.

Absolute
• Right-sided heart failure
• Biliary tract obstruction
• Uncontrolled infection
• Pulmonary hypertension
• Chronic recurrent disabling hepatic encephalopathy
• Hepatocellular carcinoma involving hepatic veins
Relative
• Severe liver failure (Pugh score >12)
• Portal vein thrombosis
• Multiple hepatic cysts

at the level of hepatic veins, inferior vena cava (IVC) or right atrium. Hepatic venous outflow increases sinusoidal pressure, portal hypertension and decreased liver perfusion which in turn leads to progressive liver failure. The manifestations can range from fulminant acute liver failure to chronic liver disease depends on factors such as extent and acuteness of obstruction and adequacy of remaining collateral circulation. The etiology of obstruction in western population is primarily thrombosis (bland or tumor). Membranous web like obstruction of hepatic veins and IVC is seen commonly in Asian population.

Medical therapy including anticoagulation for preventing recurrence and extension of thrombosis and measures to control ascites and gastrointestinal bleeding has poor long term outcomes. Surgical options in BCS include creation of a portosystemic shunt and

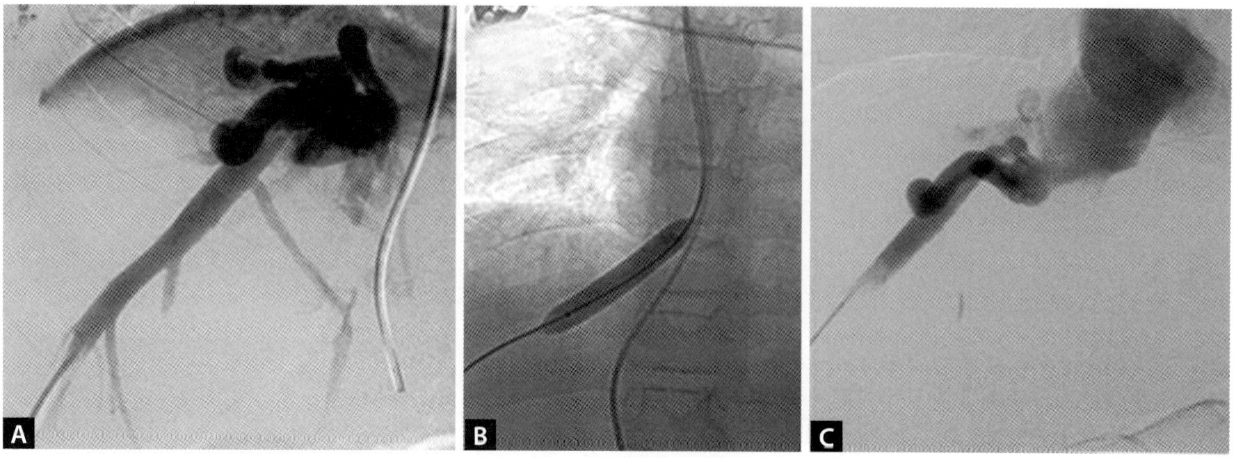

Figs. 27A to C: Hepatic vein angioplasty in a patient with Budd-Chiarri syndrome: (A) Hepatic venogram (percutaneous approach) shows complete occlusion at the ostium with multiple venous collaterals; (B) Balloon angioplasty of the stenosed ostium; (C) Postangioplasty hepatic venogram showing freeflow of contrast into IVC.

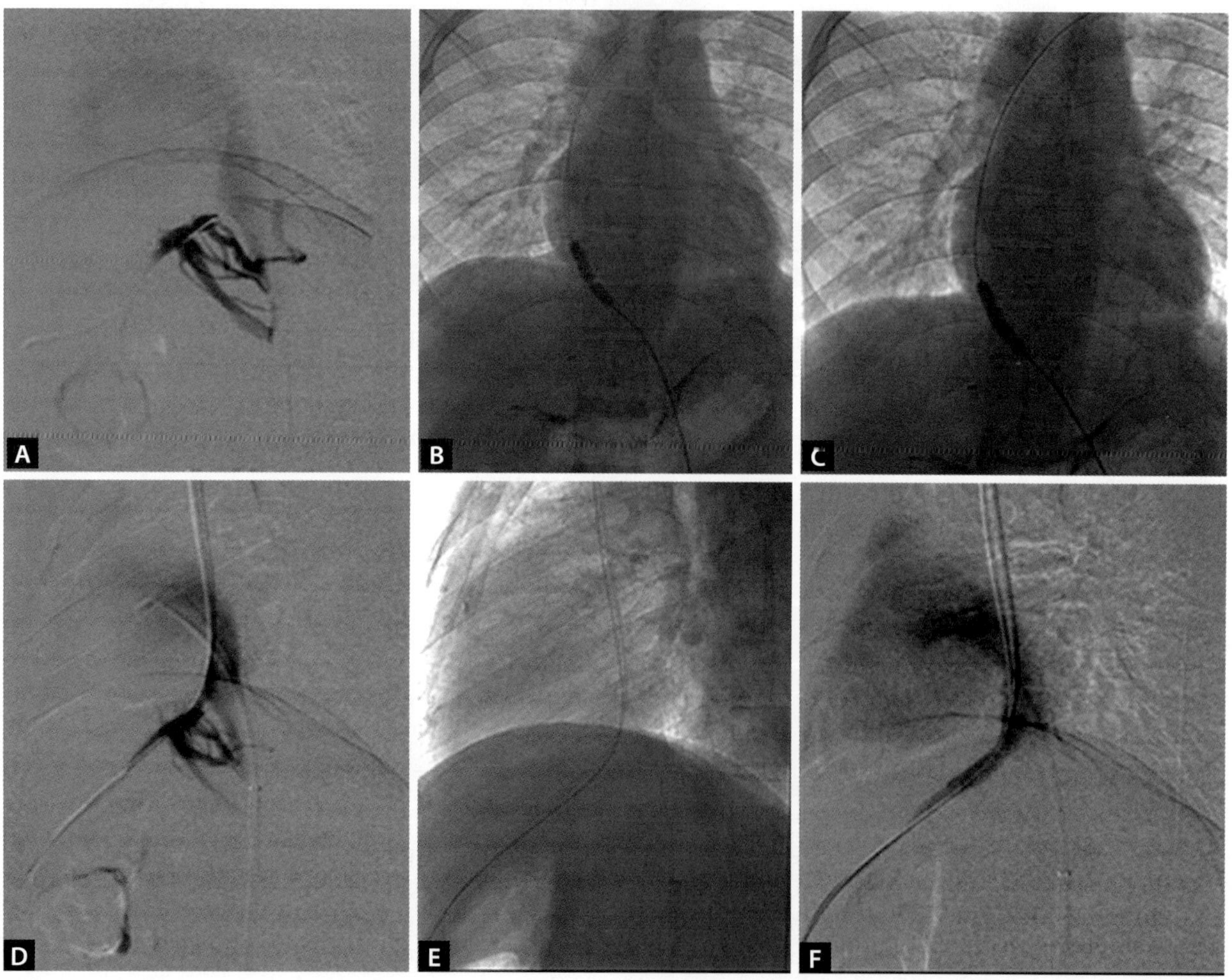

Figs. 28A to F: Hepatic vein stenting: (A) Hepatic venogram showing stenosis at ostium with multiple collaterals; (B and C) Balloon angioplasty; (D) Postangioplasty showing residual stenosis with persistent collaterals; (E and F) Stent deployment and subsequent study showing freeflow of contrast with disappearance of collaterals.

liver transplant. Portosystemic surgical shunts can only partially decompress the portal system and feasibility liver transplant depends largely on availability of donor.

Percutaneous techniques in BCS include transluminal balloon angioplasty of hepatic veins and or IVC and stent placement. Percutaneous interventions can restore physiologic hepatic venous outflow and help in resolution of venous congestion, improvement in hepatic function and arresting hepatic destruction. Hepatic venous recanalization techniques are feasible if the occlusion is short segment with large patent segment.

Transjugular approach is preferred for approaching the hepatic veins. Once the hepatic venous ostium is accessed, attempt is made to negotiate a guidewire across the stenosis followed by balloon angioplasty of the narrowed segment. Transjugular approach may fail in cases with tight stenosis at the ostium. Percutaneous transhepatic approach is preferred is such cases which involves USG-guided puncture of patent segment of hepatic veins and negotiating the guidewire across stenosis into the IVC. The guidewire is then snared through the transjugular route and procedure is completed by transjugular route to avoid making larger tracts in the liver. Successful angioplasty is seen as freeflow of contrast across the stenosis, reduction in pressure gradients and collapse of intrahepatic venovenous collaterals **(Figs. 27A to C)**. Metallic stents are deployed in cases of insufficient response and rapid re-stenosis following balloon angioplasty **(Figs. 28A to F)**. Good medium-term outcome is noted following angioplasty provided adequate anticoagulation is maintained.[35,36]

Inferior vena cava stenosis secondary to liver congestion in BCS get resolved after successful venous decompression procedures. However, primary caval stenosis that occludes hepatic venous outflow has to be addressed by IVC angioplasty. IVC angioplasty is performed by femoral or jugular approach **(Figs. 29A to D)**. Caval stenting is needed if angioplasty fails.

Long segment occlusion of hepatic veins is difficult to reopen and have higher chances of re-occlusion and this subgroup of patients require creation of a portosystemic shunt. TIPS and DIPS are being increasingly performed in such scenario with gratifying results.[37,38]

Partial Splenic Embolization

Partial splenic embolization (PSE) is performed to decrease portal venous inflow, thereby decreasing the portal pressure. It is performed by super-selective catheterization of splenic arterial branches and embolization using polyvinyl alcohol particles **(Figs. 30A to D)**. PSE is efficacious in reducing the episodes

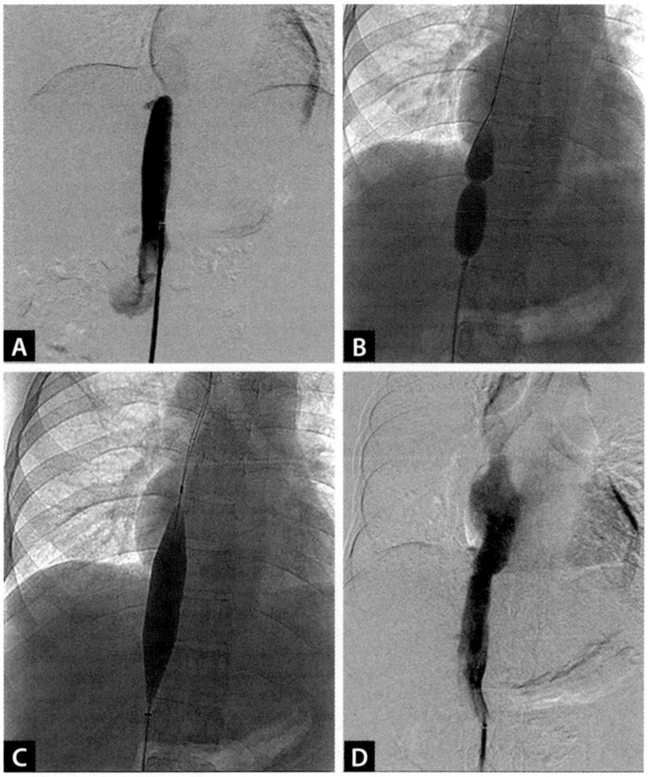

Figs. 29A to D: IVC angioplasty: (A) Cavogram showing total occlusion below cavo-atrial junction; (B and C) Angioplasty using balloon catheter; (D) Postangioplasty cavogram showing freeflow of contrast into right atrium.

of variceal bleeding. It also helps in decreasing splenic size and in improving hematologic parameters and hepatic protein synthesis.[39] PSE is an safe, simple and effective alternative for splenectomy in hypersplenism.[40] It causes partial necrosis of splenic parenchyma with minimal risk of complications such as liver abscess and sepsis. Splenic artery embolization can also be used in management of bleeding gastric varices secondary to splenic vein thrombosis.[41]

Recanalization of Occluded/thrombosed Portal Veins or Tributaries

Portal hypertension can be caused by obstruction of portal vein or its tributaries. It can be due to inflammatory stenosis, bland thrombus or due to tumor infiltration. In both benign and malignant conditions, patients present with variceal bleeding, ascites or abdominal pain. These symptoms can be relieved by recanalization occluded vessels, which can be achieved by angioplasty and stenting through transjugular, transhepatic or transsplenic route.[42,43] Anastomotic strictures of portal vein can also be treated by angioplasty **(Figs. 31A to D)**.

Occlusion of Arterioportal Shunts (Congenital/Acquired)

Arterioportal shunts can cause portal hypertension by increased portal flow. Etiology of arterioportal shunts may be congenital malformation, trauma, tumors, aneurysms and surgery or hepatic interventions. Such patients may rarely present with gastrointestinal bleeding, ascites, heart failure and splenomegaly. Transarterial embolization of feeding arteries by coils, glue or other closure devises depending on the size of the fistula is the preferred treatment in such cases **(Figs. 32A to D)**.[44]

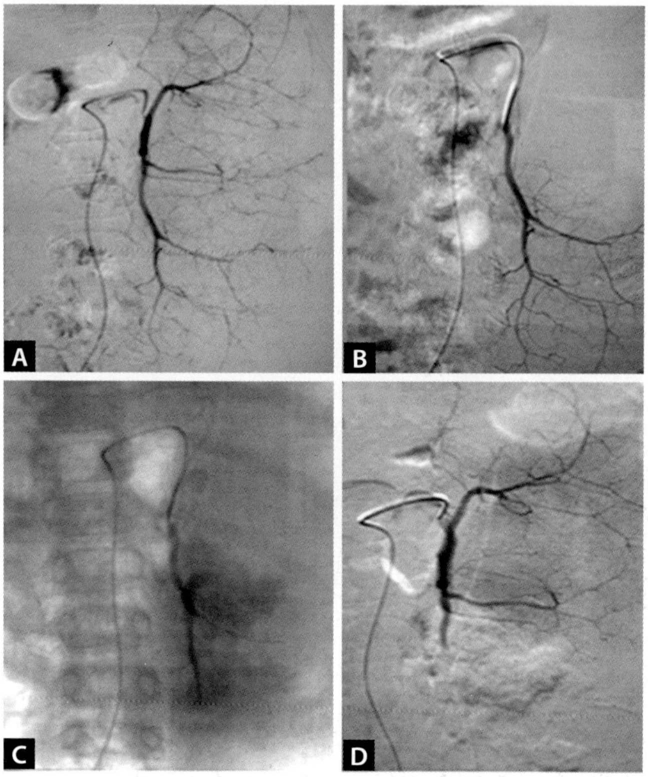

Figs. 30A to D: Partial splenic embolization in a patient with hypersplenism: (A) Splenic arteriogram showing parenchymal branches; (B) Selective run of lower branch of splenic artery; (C) Embolization of lower part of spleen using PVA particles; (D) Post-embolization study showing decreased perfusion in lower part.

Revision of Occluded Surgical or Radiological Shunts

Surgically created portosystemic shunts for portal hypertension may be complicated by thrombosis and occlusion. Surgical treatment of such cases is difficult and carries a high morbidity. Occluded leno-renal shunts and mesocaval shunts can be successfully recanalized by endovascular route **(Figs. 33A to E)**.[45,46]

Percutaneous Transhepatic (or Trans-splenic) Variceal Embolization

Percutaneous transhepatic variceal embolization was introduced as technique to manage bleeding esophago-gastric varices by Lunderquist and Vang in 1974.[47] Subsequent studies had shown excellent immediate success rate of 70–90%. Recurrent bleeding rate of 30–65% was noted in those studies since the procedure alone do not address the basic issues of portal hypertension and hepatic insufficiency.[48-52] Subsequently the procedure was recommended in acute settings when the variceal bleeding was not controlled by endoscopic sclerotherapy, vasopressin infusion and balloon tamponade.[53] It can also be used in the management of bleeding gastric varices, which are difficult to localize by endoscopy.[54,55]

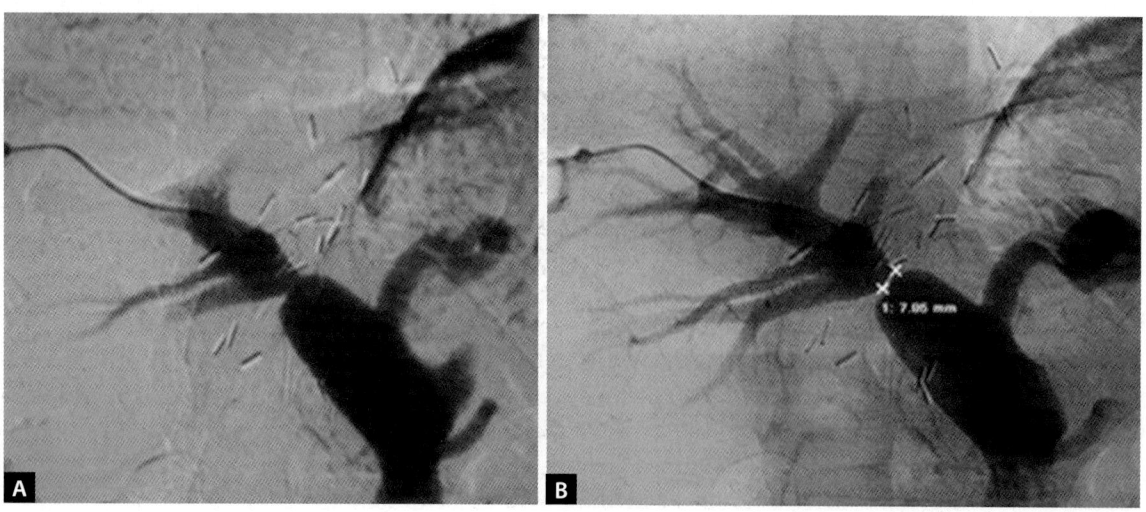

Figs. 31A and B

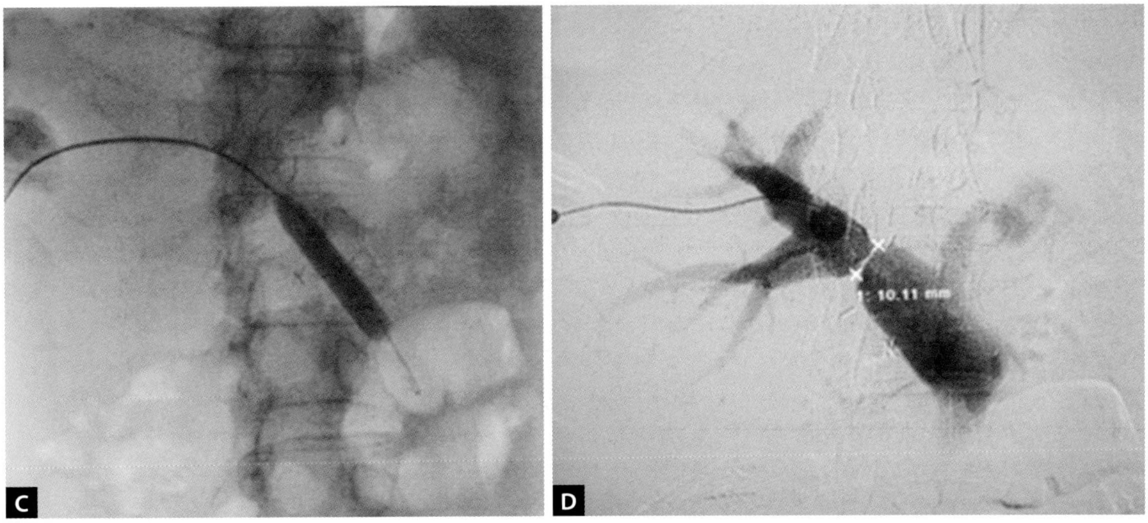

Figs. 31C and D

Figs. 31A to D: Recanalization of anastomotic stricture of portal vein: (A and B) Portogram showing stricture at anastomotic site; (C) Balloon dilatation of the stricture; (D) Postangioplasty run showing improvement in stricture.

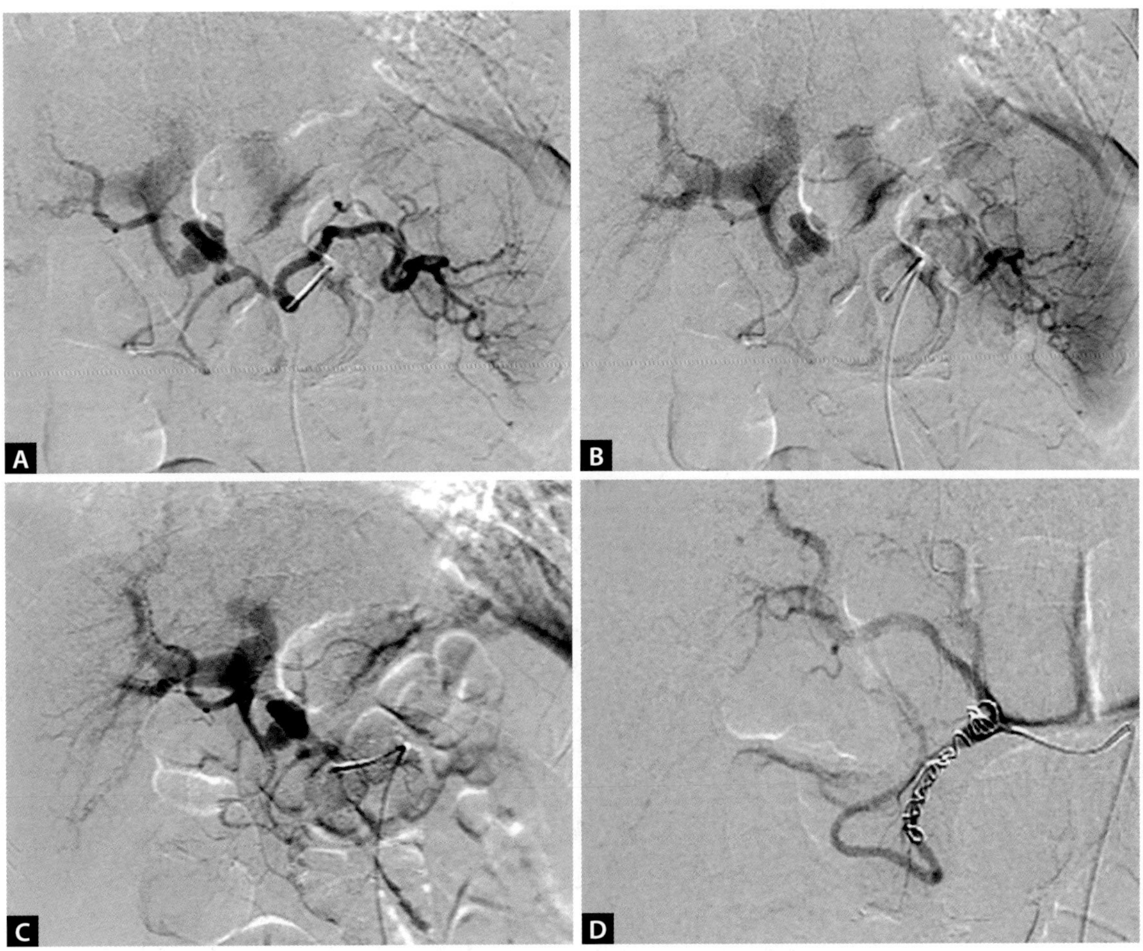

Figs. 32A to D: Occlusion of arterioportal shunts: (A and B) Celiac angiogram showing pseudoaneurysm of gastroduodenal artery communicating with portal vein; (C) Selective hepatic angiogram prior to embolization showing pseudoaneurym; (D) Postembolization study showing complete isolation of pseudoaneurysm and disappearance of abnormal shunt.

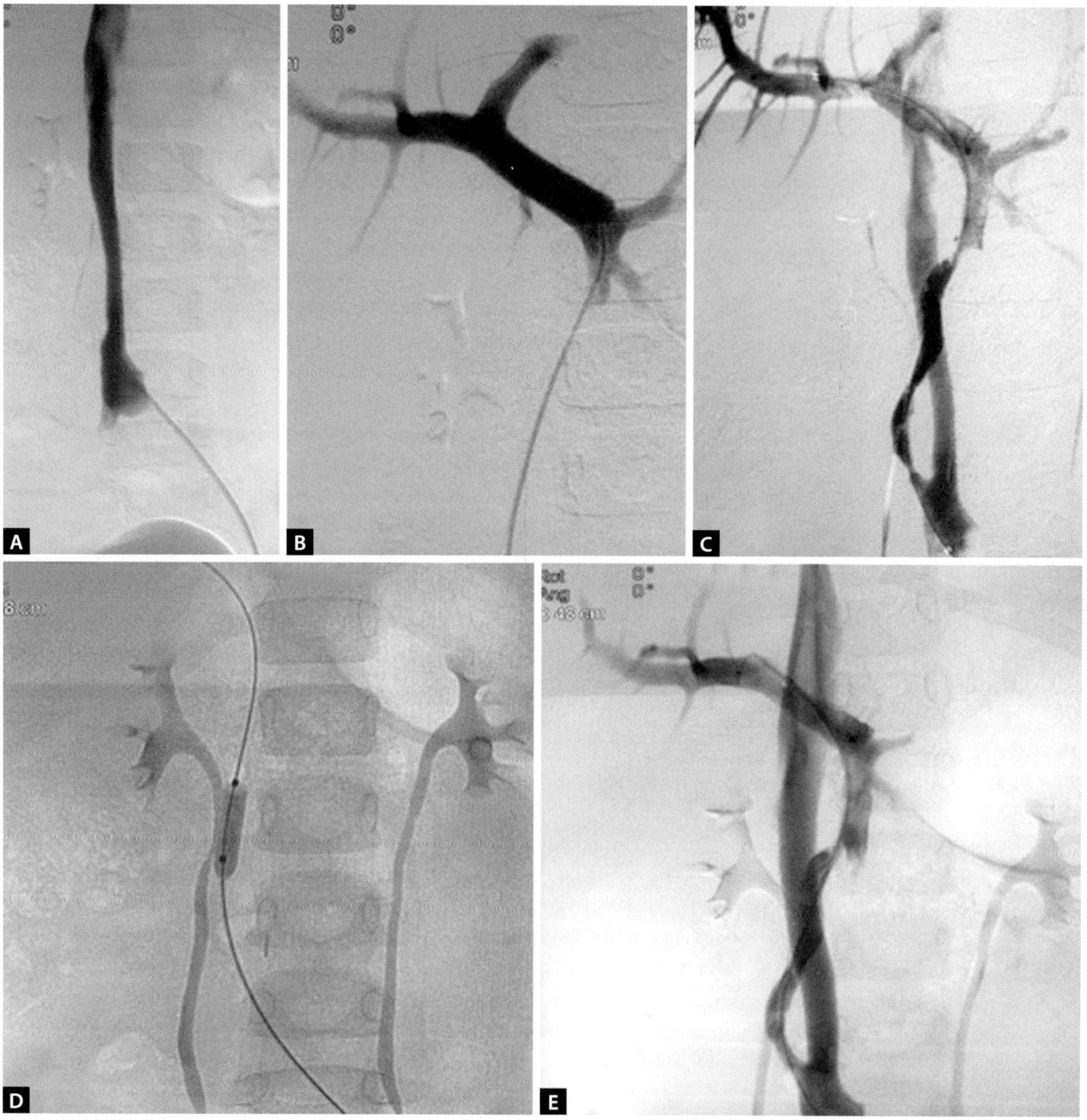

Figs. 33A to E: Mesocaval shunt revision: (A) Cavogram showing normal IVC; (B and C) Portogram done after advancing the catheter into portal vein through mesocaval shunt showing stenosis in the shunt; (D) Balloon dilatation of stenosis; (E) Subsequent portogram showing improved flow of contrast through the shunt.

The technique starts with percutaneous transhepatic puncture of the intrahepatic branch of portal vein with ultrasound or fluoroguidance and advancement of catheter into the splenic vein. Diagnostic splenoportography is then performed to delineate the feeding veins, varices and draining veins. The common veins feeding the gastric varices are the left gastric, short gastric and posterior gastric veins. Subsequently, the feeding vein is selectively catheterized and venography is performed to assess the size of the varices, velocity of flow and the size of gastrorenal shunt. On the basis of these data variceal sclerotherapy is performed with cyanoacrylate mixed with lipiodol. In cases with large gastrorenal shunts with rapid venous drainage, the gastrorenal shunts has to be occluded with angiographic balloon catheter prior to sclerotherapy. The track in the hepatic parenchyma is embolized using gelfoam and steel coils at the end of the procedure **(Figs. 34A to D)**.

Variceal embolization can also be done with transsplenic route in which the access into portal system is through splenic vein and rest of the procedure being same. The transsplenic route is especially helpful in cases with pre-existing portal vein thrombosis.[56]

Balloon-occluded Retrograded Transvenous Obliteration of Gastric Varices (BRTO)

Patients of portal hypertension are often complicated by bleeding from esophagogastric varices. Although less

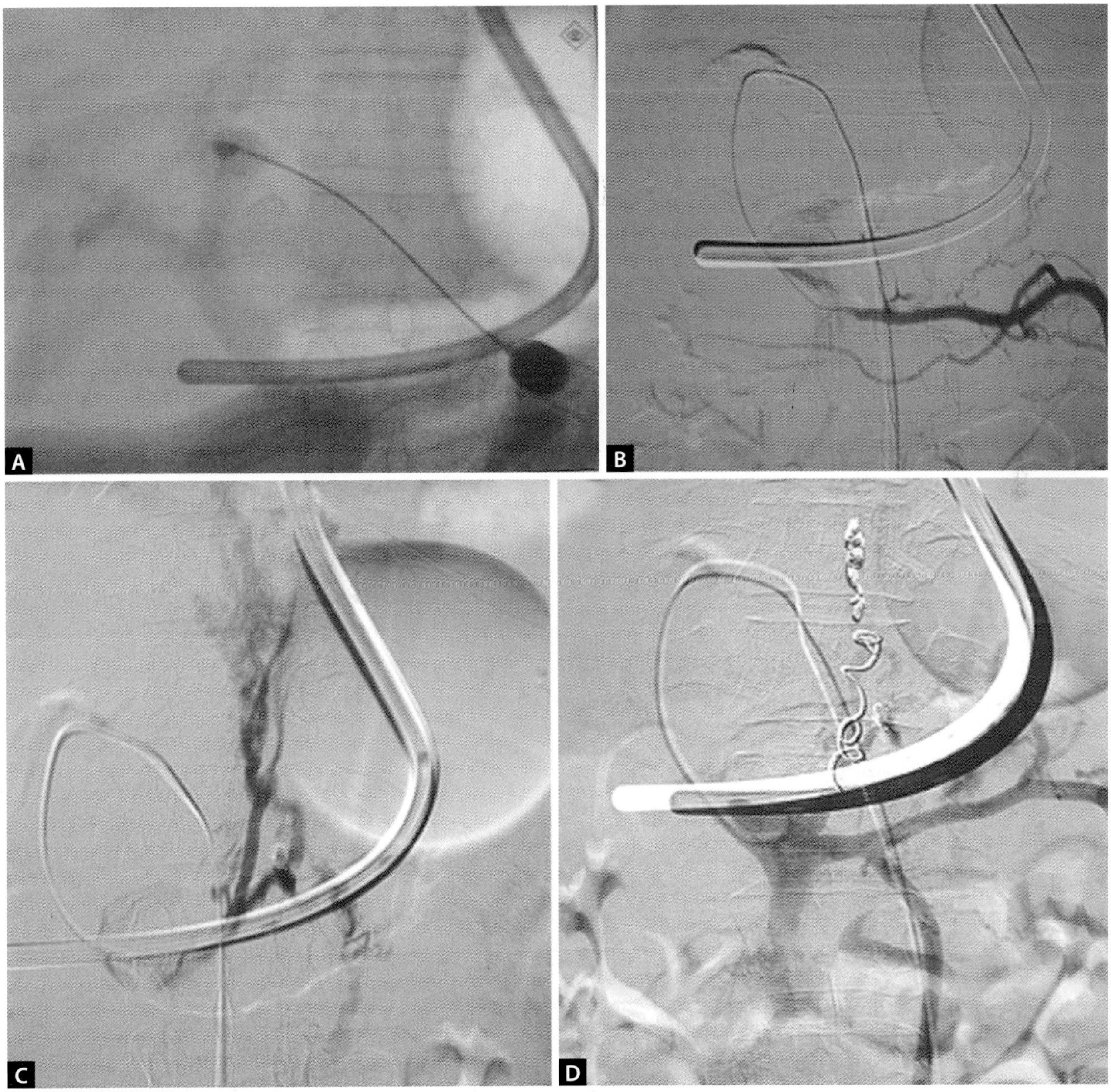

Figs. 34A to D: Percutaneous transhepatic variceal embolization: (A and B) Percutaneous transhepatic portogram showing portal vein and branches; (C) Selective angiogram of coronary vein is showing gastric varices; (D) Feeding vein is occluded by deploying stainless steel coils.

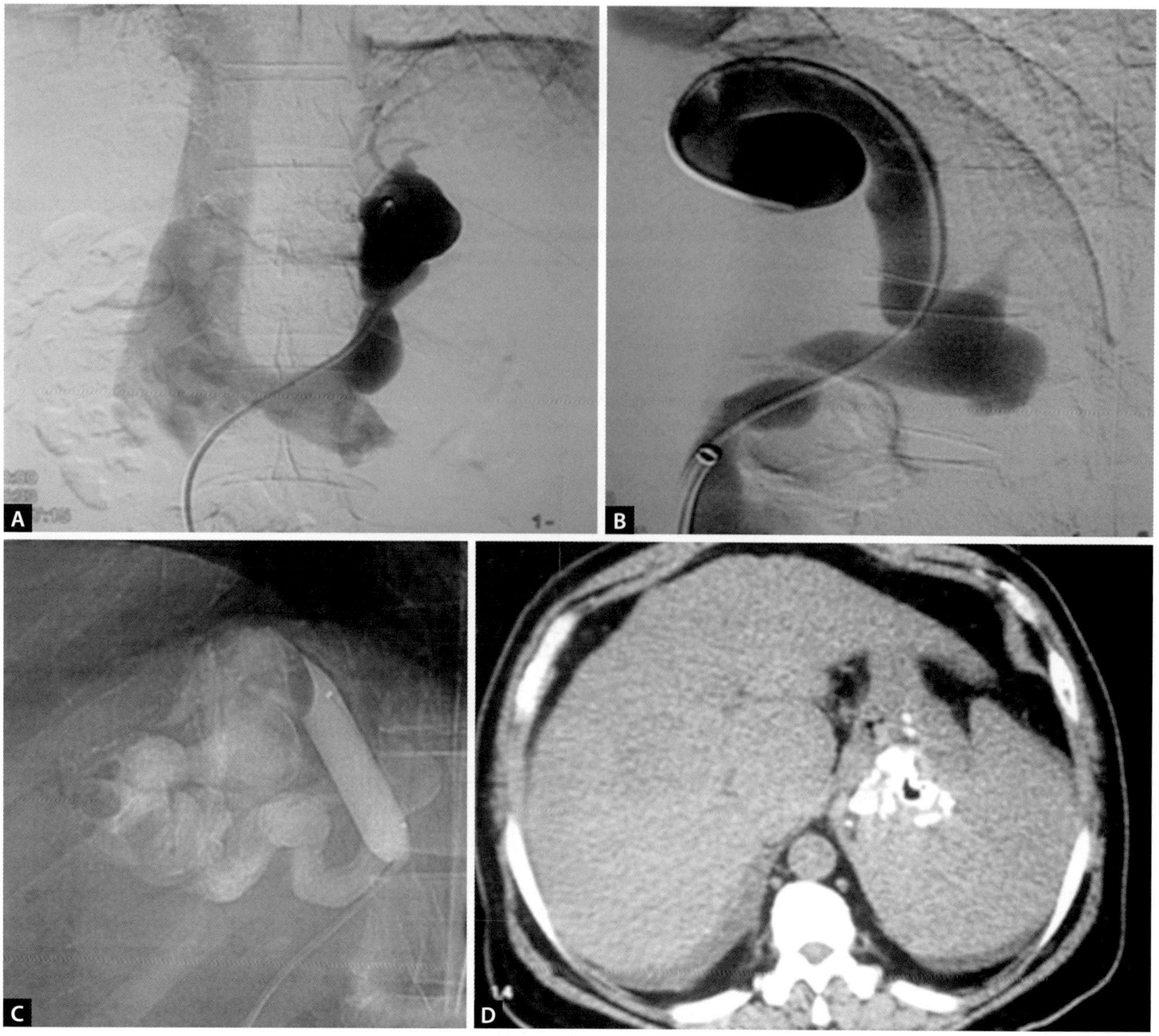

Figs. 35A to D: Balloon-occluded retrograded transvenous obliteration of gastric varices (BRTO): (A and B) Fundic gastric varices are approached through large gastrorenal collaterals of left renal vein; (C) Sclerosing agent (STS) mixed with lipiodol is injected into the varices with the balloon inflated and kept for about 3 hours; (D) Follow-up NCCT scan is showing lipiodol cast formation within the varices in fundal region of stomach.

common, gastric variceal rupture often leads to profuse bleeding and are difficult to manage with endoscopic and surgical technique.[57] BRTO is a novel technique in the management of gastric varices with major gastrosystemic shunts. It involves obliteration of gastric varices using sclerosants after occluding the communicating shunts with angiographic balloon catheter.

Contrast-enhanced computed tomography (CECT) of the abdomen is commonly performed for planning the procedure. The diameter of major shunts is assessed using CECT to calculate the size of balloon catheter which can occlude it. Gastrorenal shunt is commonly encountered. Other shunts such as gastrocaval and gastro-pericardiophrenic are also rarely seen.

The procedure is commonly performed with an access through right femoral vein. After cannulating the left renal vein, guidewire is advanced into left adrenal vein which is a common channel to gastrorenal shunt. Along the guidewire the balloon catheter is advanced into the shunt and inflated so as to block the shunt. Contrast study through the catheter is done to see the opacification of gastric varices. Some of the varices may show leaking

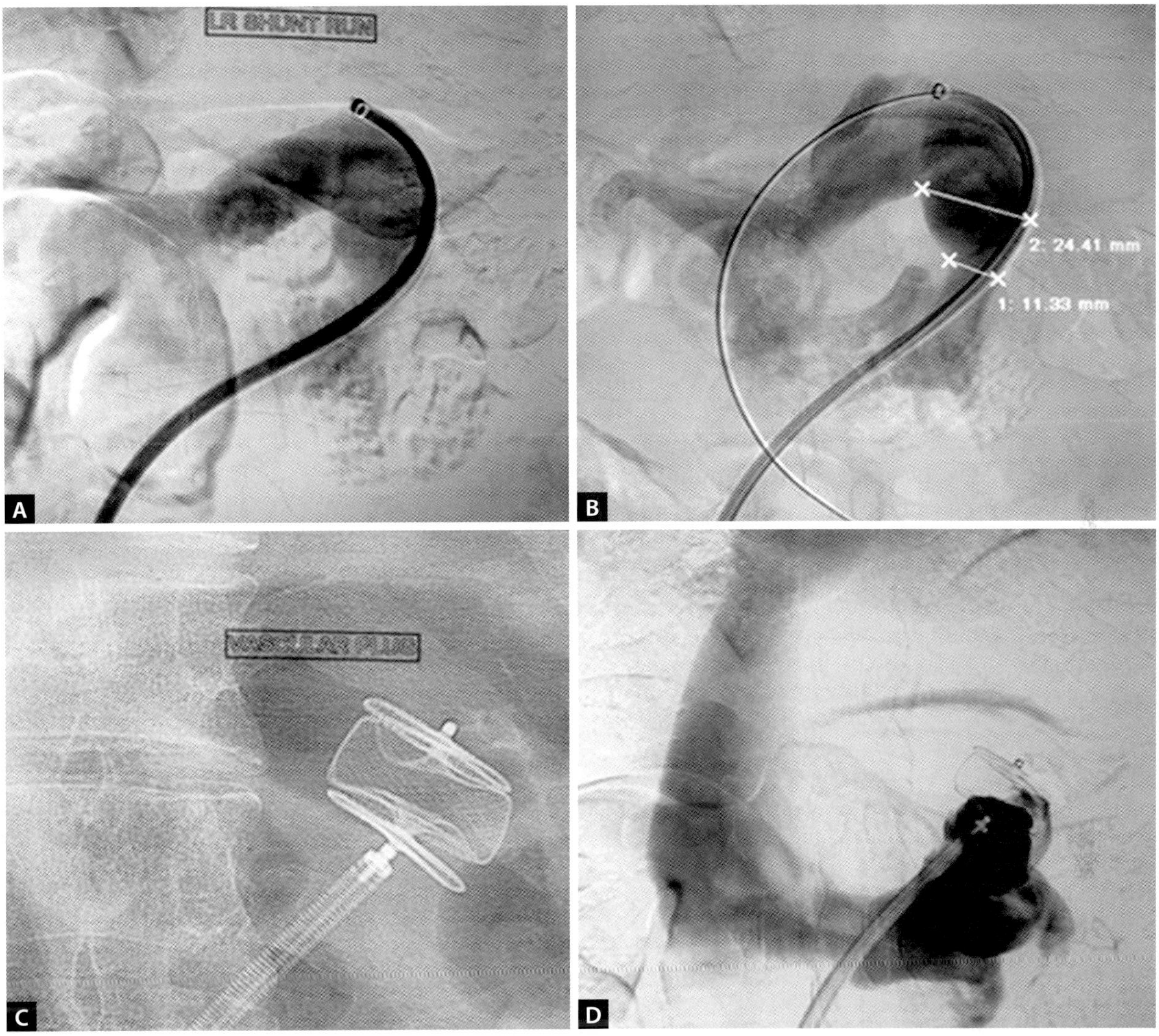

Figs. 36A to D: Occlusion of surgical shunts in refractory encephalopathy: (A and B) The surgically created lienorenal shunt for the extrahepatic portal vein obstruction (EHPVO) was accessed through left renal vein. Contrast study showing the large patent shunt, diameter is approximately 11 mm; (C) Deployed vascular plug (16 mm diameter) at the level of shunt close to the renal vein; (D) Post-shunt closure contrast showing complete closure of the shunt and patent left renal vein.

collaterals which can be dealt by deploying microcoils or gelfoam pledgets after selective catheterization. Subsequently, the sclerosant mixed with contrast (e.g. 5% ethanolamine oleate with lipiodol or sodium tetradecyl sulfate with contrast medium like iomeron) is injected into the varices through the balloon catheter. The angiographic balloon is kept inflated for a variable time ranging from 1 hours to 24 hours for adequate thrombosis to occur in the varices. After a period of time to allow thrombi formation, the hemolyzed blood with the remaining sclerosant is aspirated and balloon is deflated and catheter removed. If freeflow of blood is seen in aspirate, supplemental dose of sclerosant can be injected. Amount of sclerosant and duration of application is up to the discretion of the radiologist and it varies with the size and extent of varices. Rarely varices may show multiple shunts and balloon occlusion of all the shunts would be required in such cases. CT scan is performed after 2–4 days for immediate response. Follow-up with CT or endoscopy every 3–6 months is done depending on different patient factors **(Figs. 35A to D)**.

Since the introduction of the technique by Kanagawa et al, BRTO has been widely performed as a minimally invasive technique to manage gastric fundal varices.[58] The technique has an excellent efficacy of 81–100% and relapse rate of 0–10% reported in literature.[59-64] Complications reported include technique related errors like coil migration, balloon malposition and extension of thrombus outside the varices. Renal failure secondary to hemolysis is a known complication with the use of ethanolamine oleate and can be prevented by administration of haptoglobin. Development of ascites, pleural effusion, hepatic encephalopathy and worsening of esophageal varices are also observed in occasional patients depending on their preprocedure functional status.[64]

Occlusion of Surgical or Radiologic Shunts in Refractory Encephalopathy

In occasional patients of advanced cirrhosis the surgical porto-systemic shunts (or TIPS) can cause or aggravate hepatic encephalopathy. In such scenarios, therapeutic occlusion of the shunts can be achieved by surgical or endovascular route. Endovascular route is preferred because of its minimally invasive nature favored in a sick patient. Using endovascular approach different occlusion devices are used depending on the size of shunt vessels. Large lumen shunts are closed with larger devices such as Amplatzer vascular plugs **(Figs. 36A to D)**.

REFERENCES

1. Kumar A, Sharma P, Sarin SK. Hepatic venous pressure gradient measurement: time to learn! Indian J Gastroenterol. 2008;27(2):74-80.
2. Peck-Radosavljevic M, Trauner M, Schreiber F. Austrian Society of Gastroenterology and Hepatology. Austrian consensus on the definition and treatment of portal hypertension and its complications. Endoscopy. 2005;37(7):667-73. Review
3. Sanyal AJ, Bosch J, Blei A, Arroyo V. Portal hypertension and its complications. Gastroenterology. 2008;134(6):1715-28.
4. DeLeve LD, Valla DC, Garcia-Tsao G. American Association for the Study Liver Diseases. Vascular disorders of the liver. Hepatology. 2009;49(5):1729-64.
5. Schmidt S, Demartines N, Soler L, Schnyder P, Denys A. Portal vein normal anatomy and variants: implication for liver surgery and portal vein embolization. Semin Intervent Radiol. 2008;25(2):86-91. doi: 10.1055/s-2008-1076688.
6. Brůha R, Petrtýl J. Evaluation and treatment of portal hypertension. Cas Lek Cesk. 2016;155(2):22-6.
7. Procopet B, Cristea VM, Robic MA, Grigorescu M, Agachi PS, Metivier S, et al. Serum tests, liver stiffness and artificial neural networks for diagnosing cirrhosis and portal hypertension. Dig Liver Dis. 2015;47(5):411-6.
8. Zwiebel WJ. Sonographic diagnosis of hepatic vascular disorders. Semin Ultrasound CT MR. 1995;16(1):34-47.
9. Görg C, Riera-Knorrenschild J, Dietrich J. Colour Doppler ultrasound flow patterns in the portal venous system. Br J Radiol. 2002;75;919-29.
10. Kruskal JB, Newman PA, Sammons LG, Kane RA. Optimizing Doppler and colour flow US: application to hepatic sonography. Radiographics. 2004;24:657-75.
11. Wachsberg RH, Bahramipour P, Sofocleus CT, Barone A. Hepatofugal flow in the portal system: pathophysiology, imaging findings and diagnostic pitfalls. Radiographics. 2002;22:123-40.
12. Kang HK, Jeong YY, Choi JH, Choi S, Chung TW, Seo JJ, et al. Three-dimensional multi-detector row CT portal venography in the evaluation of portosystemic collateral vessels in liver cirrhosis. Radiographics. 2002;22(5):1053-61. Review.
13. Calhoun PS, Kuszyk BS, Heath DG, Carley JC, Fishman EK. Three-dimensional volume rendering of spiral CT data: theory and method. Radiographics. 1999;19:745-64.
14. Prince MR, Grist TM, Debatin JF (Eds). Portal Venous System. 3D Contrast MR Angiography, 3rd edn. New York: Springer-Verlag; 2003.pp.171-84.
15. Leyendecker JR, Rivera E, Washburn WK, Johnson SP, Diffin DC, Eason JD. MR angiography of the portal venous system: techniques, interpretation, and clinical applications. Radiographics. 1997;17:1425-43.
16. Kim HC, Bae SH, Choi CS, Kim EA, Kim IJ, Cho SY, Yun KS. MR portography. J Korean Radiol Soc. 1994;31(6): 1121-5.
17. Bosch J, Abraldes JG, Berzigotti A, García-Pagan JC. The clinical use of HVPG measurements in chronic liver disease. Nat Rev Gastroenterol Hepatol. 2009;6(10):573-82.
18. Sharma M, Rameshbabu CS. Collateral pathways in portal hypertension. J Clin Experimen Hepatol. 2012;2(4):338-52.
19. Arora A, Rajesh S, Meenakshi YS, Sureka B, Bansal K, Sarin SK. Spectrum of hepatofugal collateral pathways in portal hypertension: an illustrated radiological review. Insights into Imaging. 2015;6(5):559-72. doi.10.1007/s13244-015-0419-8.
20. Bissonnette J, Rautou PE, Valla DC. Idiopathic non-cirrhotic portal hypertension: An update. Presse Med. 2015;44(10):1009-15.
21. Arora A, Sarin SK. Multimodality imaging of obliterative portal venopathy: what every radiologist should know. Br J Radiol. 2015;88(1046):20140653.
22. Sarin SK, Kumar A, Chawla YK, Baijal SS, Dhiman RK, et al. Members of the APASL Working Party on Portal Hypertension. Noncirrhotic portal fibrosis/idiopathic portal hypertension: APASL recommendations for diagnosis and treatment. Hepatol Int. 2007;1(3):398-413.
23. Arora A, Sarin SK. Multimodality imaging of primary extrahepatic portal vein obstruction (EHPVO): what every radiologist should know. Br J Radiol. 2015;88:1052.
24. Rajesh S, Mukund A, Arora A. Imaging diagnosis of splanchnic venous thrombosis. Gastroenterol Res Pract. 2015;2015:101029.
25. Baskan O, Erol C, Sahingoz Y. Portal biliopathy, magnetic resonance imaging and magnetic resonance cholangiopancreatography findings: a case series. Gastroenterol Rep (Oxf). 2016;4(1):68-72.

26. Chawla YK, Bodh V. Portal vein thrombosis. J Clin Exp Hepatol. 2015;5(1):22-40.
27. Yerdel MA, Gunson B, Mirza D, et al. Portal vein thrombosis in adults undergoing liver transplantation: risk factors, screening, management, and outcome. Transplantation. 2000;69(9):1873-81.
28. Köklü S, Coban S, Yüksel O, Arhan M. Left-sided portal hypertension. Dig Dis Sci. 2007;52(5):1141-9. Epub 2007 Mar 24. Review.
29. Lumsden AB1, Allen RC, Sreeram S, Atta H, Salam A. Hepatic arterioportal fistula. Am Surg. 1993;59(11):722-6.
30. Angermayr B, Cejna M, Koenig F, Karnel F, Hackl F, Gangl A, et al. Survival in patients undergoing transjugular intrahepatic portosystemic shunt: ePTFE-covered stentgrafts versus bare stents. Hepatol Baltim Md. 2003;38(4):1043-50.
31. Bureau C, Pagan JCG, Layrargues GP, Metivier S, Bellot P, Perreault P, et al. Patency of stents covered with polytetrafluoroethylene in patients treated by transjugular intrahepatic portosystemic shunts: long-term results of a randomized multicentre study. Liver Int Off J Int Assoc Study Liver. 2007;27(6):742-7.
32. Cejna M, Peck-Radosavljevic M, Thurnher SA, Hittmair K, Schoder M, Lammer J. Creation of transjugular intrahepatic portosystemic shunts with stent-grafts: initial experiences with a polytetrafluoroethylene-covered nitinol endoprosthesis. Radiology. 2001;221(2):437-46.
33. Boyer TD, Haskal ZJ, American Association for the Study of Liver Diseases. The role of transjugular intrahepatic portosystemic shunt in the management of portal hypertension. Hepatol Baltim Md. 2005;41(2):386-400.
34. Boyer TD. Transjugular intrahepatic portosystemic shunt: current status. Gastroenterology. 2003;124(6):1700-10.
35. Fisher N, McCafferty I, Dolapci M, Wali M, Buckels J, Olliff S, et al. Managing Budd-Chiari syndrome: a retrospective review of percutaneous hepatic vein angioplasty and surgical shunting. Gut. 1999;44(4):568-74.
36. Cura M, Haskal Z, Lopera J. Diagnostic and interventional radiology for Budd-Chiari syndrome. Radiogr Rev Publ Radiol Soc North Am Inc. 2009;29(3):669-81.
37. Michl P, Bilzer M, Waggershauser T, Gülberg V, Rau HG, Reiser M, et al. Successful treatment of chronic Budd-Chiari syndrome with a transjugular intrahepatic portosystemic shunt. J Hepatol. 2000;32(3):516-20.
38. Ochs A, Sellinger M, Haag K, Nöldge G, Herbst EW, Walter E, et al. Transjugular intrahepatic portosystemic stent-shunt (TIPS) in the treatment of Budd-Chiari syndrome. J Hepatol. 1993;18(2):217-25.
39. Koconis KG, Singh H, Soares G. Partial splenic embolization in the treatment of patients with portal hypertension: a review of the english language literature. J Vasc Interv Radiol. 2007;18(4):463-81.
40. Alwmark A, Bengmark S, Gullstrand P, Joelsson B, Lunderquist A, Owman T. Evaluation of splenic embolization in patients with portal hypertension and hypersplenism. Ann Surg. 1982;196(5):518-24.
41. Saugel B, Gaa J, Phillip V, Schmid RM, Huber W. Splenic artery embolization in a woman with bleeding gastric varices and splenic vein thrombosis: a case report. J Med Case Reports. 2010;4(1):247.
42. Yamakado K, Nakatsuka A, Tanaka N, Fujii A, Isaji S, Kawarada Y, et al. Portal venous stent placement in patients with pancreatic and biliary neoplasms invading portal veins and causing portal hypertension: initial experience. Radiology. 2001;220(1):150-6.
43. Shan H, Xiao X-S, Huang M-S, Ouyang Q, Jiang Z-B. Portal venous stent placement for treatment of portal hypertension caused by benign main portal vein stenosis. World J Gastroenterol. 2005;11(21):3315-8.
44. Vauthey JN, Tomczak RJ, Helmberger T, Gertsch P, Forsmark C, Caridi J, et al. The arterioportal fistula syndrome: clinicopathologic features, diagnosis, and therapy. Gastroenterology. 1997;113(4):1390-401.
45. López-Medina A, Peiró J, Gonzalez de Garay M, Antoñana MA, Sustacha J, Grande D. Treatment of occluded distal splenorenal shunts with endovascular stents: a report of two cases. Cardiovasc Intervent Radiol. 2001;24(3):194-7.
46. Lorenz JM, Funaki B, Denison G. Balloon dilatation of a distal splenorenal shunt in a child. AJR. 2005;184(6):1915-6.
47. Lunderquist A, Vang J. Transhepatic catheterization and obliteration of the coronary vein in patients with portal hypertension and esophageal varices. N Engl J Med. 1974; 291(13):646–9.
48. Bengmark S, Börjesson B, Hoevels J, Joelsson B, Lunderquist A, Owman T. Obliteration of esophageal varices by PTP: a follow-up of 43 patients. Ann Surg. 1979;190(4):549-54.
49. Benner KG, Keeffe EB, Keller FS, Rösch J. Clinical outcome after percutaneous transhepatic obliteration of esophageal varices. Gastroenterology. 1983;85(1):146-53.
50. Lunderquist A, Börjesson B, Owman T, Bengmark S. Isobutyl 2-cyanoacrylate (bucrylate) in obliteration of gastric coronary vein and esophageal varices. AJR. 1978;130(1):1-6.
51. Smith-Laing G, Scott J, Long RG, Dick R, Sherlock S. Role of percutaneous transhepatic obliteration of varices in the management of hemorrhage from gastroesophageal varices. Gastroenterology. 1981;80(5 pt 1):1031-6.
52. L'Herminé C, Chastanet P, Delemazure O, Bonnière PL, Durieu JP, Paris JC. Percutaneous transhepatic embolization of gastroesophageal varices: results in 400 patients. AJR. 1989;152(4):755-60.
53. Sos TA. Transhepatic portal venous embolization of varices: pros and cons. Radiology. 1983;148(2):569-70.
54. Kwak HS, Han YM. Percutaneous transportal sclerotherapy with N-butyl-2-cyanoacrylate for gastric varices: technique and clinical efficacy. Korean J Radiol Off J Korean Radiol Soc. 2008;9(6):526-33.
55. Tian X, Wang Q, Zhang C, Liu F, Cui Y, Liu F, et al. Modified percutaneous transhepatic variceal embolization with 2-octylcyanoacrylate for bleeding gastric varices: long-term follow-up outcomes. AJR. 2011;197(2):502-9.

56. Gong GQ, Wang XL, Wang JH, Yan ZP, Cheng JM, Qian S, et al. Percutaneous transsplenic embolization of esophageal and gastro-fundal varices in 18 patients. World J Gastroenterol. 2001;7(6):880-3.
57. Sarin SK, Lahoti D, Saxena SP, Murthy NS, Makwana UK. Prevalence, classification and natural history of gastric varices: a long-term follow-up study in 568 portal hypertension patients. Hepatol Baltim Md. 1992;16(6):1343-9.
58. Kanagawa H, Mima S, Kouyama H, Gotoh K, Uchida T, Okuda K. Treatment of gastric fundal varices by balloon-occluded retrograde transvenous obliteration. J Gastroenterol Hepatol. 1996;11(1):51-8.
59. Hirota S, Matsumoto S, Tomita M, Sako M, Kono M. Retrograde transvenous obliteration of gastric varices. Radiology. 1999;211(2):349-56.
60. Matsumoto A, Hamamoto N, Nomura T, Hongou Y, Arisaka Y, Morikawa H, et al. Balloon-occluded retrograde transvenous obliteration of high risk gastric fundal varices. Am J Gastroenterol. 1999;94(3):643-9.
61. Koito K, Namieno T, Nagakawa T, Morita K. Balloon-occluded retrograde transvenous obliteration for gastric varices with gastrorenal or gastrocaval collaterals. AJR. 1996;167(5):1317-20.
62. Kiyosue H, Mori H, Matsumoto S, Yamada Y, Hori Y, Okino Y. Transcatheter obliteration of gastric varices: Part 2. Strategy and techniques based on hemodynamic features. Radiogr Rev Publ Radiol Soc North Am Inc. 2003;23(4):921-37; discussion 937.
63. Ninoi T, Nishida N, Kaminou T, Sakai Y, Kitayama T, Hamuro M, et al. Balloon-occluded retrograde transvenous obliteration of gastric varices with gastrorenal shunt: long-term follow-up in 78 patients. AJR. 2005;184(4):1340-6.
64. Arai H, Abe T, Takagi H, Mori M. Efficacy of balloon-occluded retrograde transvenous obliteration, percutaneous transhepatic obliteration and combined techniques for the management of gastric fundal varices. World J Gastroenterol. 2006;12(24):3866-73.

CHAPTER 97

Percutaneous Nonvascular Gastrointestinal Tract Interventions

Shivanand Gamanagatti, Deep Narayan Srivastava, Chandrashekhara SH

In the treatment of patients suffering from gastrointestinal tract diseases various therapeutic interventional techniques have been developed using percutaneous routes. These are:

- Percutaneous gastrostomy
- Percutaneous jejunostomy
- Esophageal stenting
- Gastroduodenal stenting
- Colorectal stenting
- Percutaneous enterocutaneous fistula closure.

PERCUTANEOUS GASTROSTOMY

Its procedure is used to provide nutritional support for patients with swallowing disorders. Enteral feeding is preferred in those with adequate small-bowel function to absorb sufficient water, electrolytes, and nutrients from a normal or elemental diet.[1-3]

Enteral feeding may be can be provided through various tubes placed either through nose or percutaneously. Nasogastric tube placement either blind approach or fluoroscopic approach is naive technique; also patients poorly tolerate this intubation when considered for long duration.[4] Nasogastric or nasojejunal tubes are usually used for short term duration.

For long-term feeding, tubes are placed directly into the stomach or jejunum percutaneously by fluoroscopic/endoscopic/surgical gastrostomy or jejunostomy technique.

Surgical gastrostomy involves an abdominal incision usually performed under general anesthesia and is associated with significant morbidity; Majority of patients undergoing some form of enteral feeding are poorly nourished, hence surgical wound may not heal properly leading to seepage and morbidity.[5,6]

Gauderer et al. described the percutaneous endoscopic gastrostomy (PEG) technique in 1980.[7] In PEG, the stomach is punctured percutaneously and, with the aid of a gastroscope, a string is brought up out of the patient through the mouth. The feeding tube is attached to the string and is pulled downward into the stomach and out through the anterior gastric and abdominal wall. PEG has fewer complications than surgery as it is performed under IV sedation instead of general anesthesia.

Percutaneous transgastric jejunostomy, another alternative to surgery, is a method that uses the Seldinger technique. In this technique, under image guidance a feeding tube is placed in the stomach and sometime up to the jejunum.[8-10]

Indications

Nutritional support: For patients with swallowing disorders, like abnormal peristalsis associated with cerebrovascular accidents, anoxic brain damage, degenerative central nervous system disease, trauma, and neurosurgery. It can be used to provide enteral nutritional support for patients with anorexia nervosa, severe depression, and advanced malignancy.

Decompression of the stomach or small intestine patients with chronic small-bowel obstruction may benefit from drainage with large-bore (24- to 28-French) gastrostomy tubes, which obviates long-term nasogastric suction. This indication is more common in patients with chronic intestinal obstruction secondary to carcinomatosis.

Other Indications

Innovative use of percutaneous gastrostomy has been reported in few unusual clinical settings, like retrograde dilatation of a gastroplasty stoma constructed for weight reduction in morbidly obese patients, to divert bile into the duodenum in patients with an external biliary drainage catheter where attempts to internalize the catheter are unsuccessful and in prolonged ileus after major surgery.

Contraindications

In cases of massive ascites, gastric varices, total gastrectomy and abnormal coagulation parameters.

Hardwares

The procedure requires following hardwares:

- 18G needle
- Suture anchoring set
- J guidewire 0.038 inch
- Superstiff guidewire
- Gastrostomy tube (18-24F).

Technique (Figs. 1A to E)

Preprocedure preparation includes overnight fasting. Procedure is performed under local anesthesia. If the nasogastric tube is already in place or else under fluoroscopic guidance a 5F angiographic catheter is passed into the stomach, after administration of 40 mg butylscopolamine (Buscopan), the stomach is totally distended with 750–1200 mL atmospheric air so that anterior wall of the stomach abuts the abdominal wall.

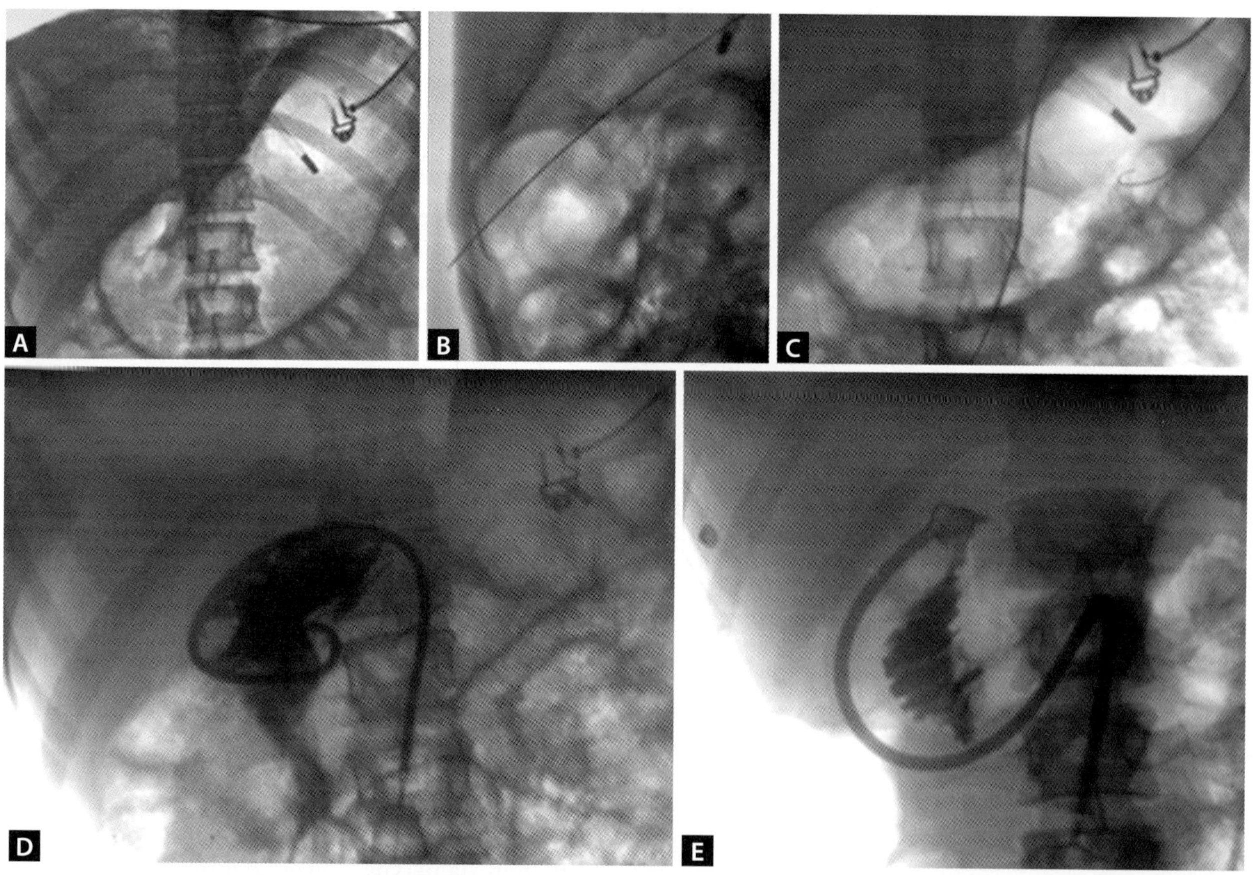

Figs. 1A to E: Fluoroscopic spot images showing technique of gastrostomy; initially stomach was distended (A and B) after injecting room air through nasogastric tube, followed by puncturing of the distended stomach using the 18G needle preloaded with T-fastener followed by passage of the guidewire (C) and retraction of T-fastener so as to retract the stomach wall against the abdominal wall and serial dilatation of the tract, finally placement of the either pigtail or malecot large bore catheter as gastrostomy tube (D and E).

Then, puncture is made halfway between the greater and lesser curvatures of the stomach at the junction of the upper 2/3rd and lower 1/3rd (to avoid the arterial injury) with an 18 G needle, preferably in lateral projection. Following gastric puncture, iodinated contrast medium is injected to see the precise needle location. Once satisfied with needle position, T-fastener present (preloaded) inside the needle is subsequently pushed into the gastric lumen (Cope gastrointestinal suture anchor set; Cook, Bloomington, MA) by using the stiff guidewire that comes with suture anchor set. The needle is then withdrawn out of the stomach leaving the T-faster in place. Now, T-fastener is retracted tightly so that the anterior wall of stomach closely approximates the abdominal wall and T-faster is then sutured to the abdominal wall. The stiff guidewire is still inside the stomach and the stomach wall is retracted to the anterior abdominal wall with suture anchor, the tract is dilated over the guidewire serially using Seldinger technique. Preferably larger bore catheter like 18F–20F Malecot catheter or loop forming pigtail catheter is inserted as gastrostomy tube. Next day, iodinated contrast study is done, prior to start of feeding.

Sutured T-fasteners are mostly removed after 10–15 days, to fall inside the stomach lumen.[11,12]

Technical Difficulty

- Different angiographic catheters can be used to negotiate through the stomach and duodenum.
- In difficult situations, gastric puncturing can be done under CT guidance.
- If access is lost after tract dilatation, patient may complain of gastric leak. It is advisable to give antibiotic and supportive care.[13]

Complications

- *Minor complications:*
  - Pain, fever
  - Wound contamination
  - Pericatheter seepage
  - Tube dislodgement
- *Major complications:*
  - Hemorrhage requiring blood transfusion or other intervention
  - Peritonitis
  - Aspiration pneumonitis

Feeding through percutaneous gastrostomy is associated with gastroesophageal reflux and aspiration in some patients. It is better to advance the tube beyond duodenal cap into jejunum.

Tips to Avoid Complications[14]

- Puncturing site should be proper to avoid arterial injury.
- Prior oral barium would help to opacify colon; help to deliniate colon and stomuch.
- Keeping the stomach fully distended during procedure
- Ascites if present need to be drained prior to the procedure.

PERCUTANEOUS JEJUNOSTOMY

Gray, described the fluoroscopic percutaneous jejunostomy in 1987 and was later revised by Coleman in 1990.[15,16]

Main concern of this procedure is technical difficulties like:

- Puncture of the mobile and collapsed jejunum
- Difficulty in supporting the location of the jejunum during the catheter placement.

Ultrasound or CT guidance can be used to puncture the jejunum, thus avoiding the colon. Care has to be taken not to transverse more than one jejuna loop.

Indications

In cases, where percutaneous gastrostomy is not be possible due to unfavorable position of the stomach or because of previous partial or total gastrectomy.

Other indications included diversion of success from a leaking anastomosis after esophagectomy and access to a limb of a Roux-en-Y anastomosis to facilitate biliary interventions.

Technique (Figs. 2A to D)

General preparation should include overnight fasting and, whenever possible, insertion of a nasogastric tube. Interposition of colon or liver between the stomach and the anterior abdominal wall should routinely be excluded by both sonographic and fluoroscopic assessment of the upper abdomen. Procedure is performed under local anesthesia.

A 120 cm long, jejunal tube is used to catheterize the duodenum or proximal jejunum through the nose. After administration of 40 mg butylscopolamine (Buscopan), the proximal jejunum was opacified with dilute, iodinated, aqueous contrast material and distended. Using the 18G needle preloaded with suture anchor set (Cope gastrointestinal suture anchor set; Cook, Bloomington, MA), one of the jejunal loop which is close to anterior abdominal wall is punctured under fluoroscopy and ultrasound. Following bowel puncture, iodinated contrast

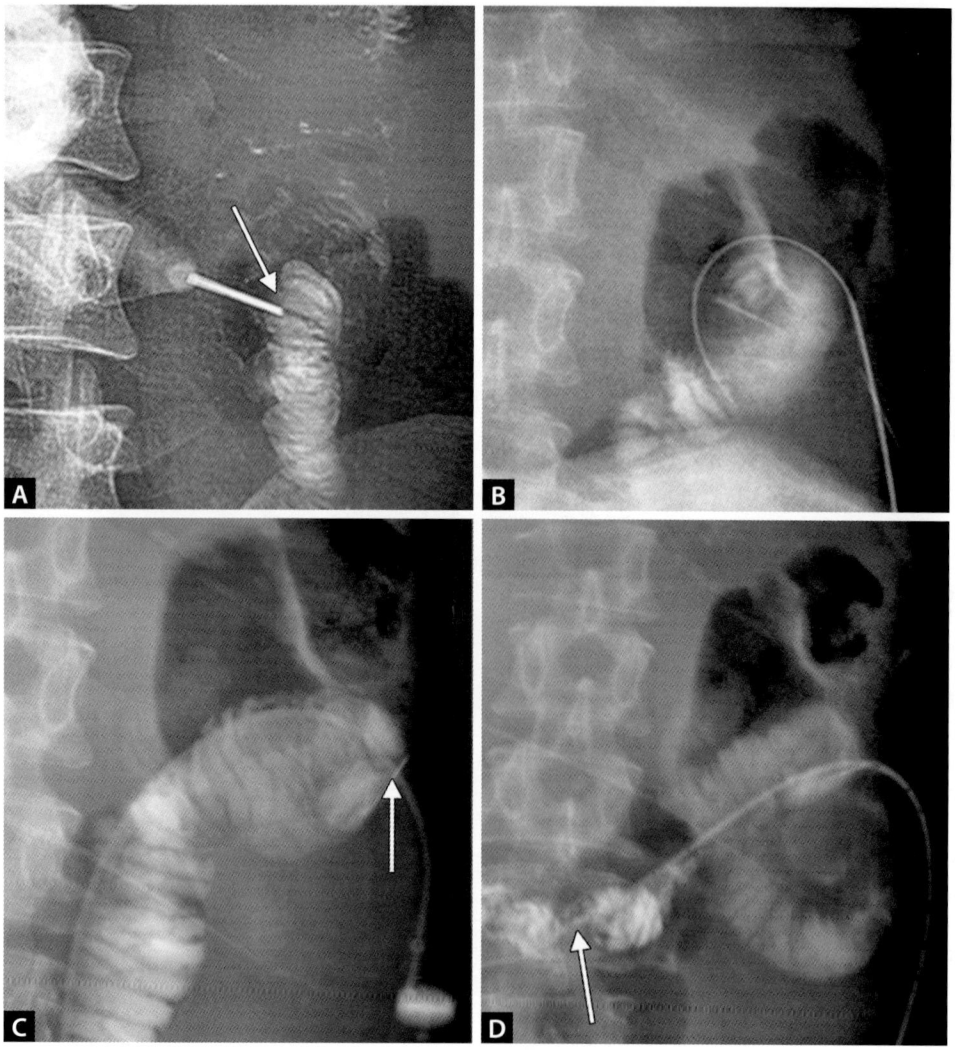

Figs. 2A to D: Technique of percutaneous jejunostomy. Jejunal loop is punctured and the correct needle position is checked by contrast injection (A) (arrow). The T-fastener mounted in the needle is then pushed into the jejunum using the stiff guidewire that comes with suture anchor set (B). The needle is withdrawn and the T-fastener retracted and sutured to the abdominal wall (C) (arrow). The tract is dilated over the guidewire serially using Seldinger technique till the desired size of catheter to be inserted (D) (arrow).

medium is injected to see the precise needle location (***see* Figs. 1A to E**). Once needle position is confirmed inside the bowel lumen, rest of the steps is similar to gastrostomy technique as described above (vide supra). Next day, iodinated contrast study is done, prior to start of feeding. Sutured T-fasteners are mostly removed after 10–15 days, to fall inside the jejunal lumen.[1-3]

Complications

Are same as in case of percutaneous gastrostomy.

ESOPHAGEAL STENTING

The palliation of esophageal cancer was first described by Celestin in 1959, through a plastic stent inserted at laparotomy.[17] Whereas endoscopic esophageal plastic stent insertion was described by Atkinson in 1970.[18] Endoscopic placement of esophageal metallic stent was first introduced in 1983 by Frimberger.[19]

Indications

The main purpose of esophageal stenting is restoring oral feeding and improve quality of life. Stents are used primarily in patients with advanced or inoperable malignant esophageal obstruction and in those patients in whom surgery is contraindicated.

Other indications are:

- Anastomotic tumor recurrence following surgery
- Malignant esophageal fistula

- Primary or secondary tumors within the mediastinum causing extrinsic esophageal compression
- Esophageal perforation (iatrogenic/traumatic)
- *Benign esophageal strictures:* As a last option, if the patient condition is high risk for surgery. Benign esophageal strictures are caustic ingestion, esophageal surgery, radiotherapy, etc. Esophageal stenting is indicated in refractory benign stenosis after 5 repeated endoscopic dilations and for long stenosis (>2 cm).[20] Uncovered metallic stents should be avoided in benign strictures due to risk of incarceration.

Types of Stents

- Metallic—Nitinol stents
- Partially covered stents—better embedding and achoring
- Fully covered stents—chances of migration are high; used for benign conditions
- Uncovered self-expandable metallic stent (SEMS)—tumor ingrowth is major problem.

Stent Designs

Esophageal stents are available in covered and uncovered forms. The covered stents are coated with plastic lining either from inside or outside.

The main benefit of uncovered stent is less chances of migration, particularly through the gastroesophageal (GE) junction. But they have high chances of blockage due to tumor in-growth. Current practice of esophageal stenting is to use covered stent in setting of esophageal cancer. Majority of esophageal stents are placed under endoscopic guidance. However, esophageal stenting is also performed under fluoroscopic guidance, which allows accurate positioning. In market, various types of esophageal stents are available **(Fig. 3)**.[21]

Stent Selection

Across the GE junction, it is desirable to use an uncovered stent (Flamingo/Gianturco stent), to reduce the chances of stent migration. When stent is placed across GE junction, majority of patients will develop reflux and may lead to aspiration. Hence, it is recommended to use medicines prophylactically to reduce reflux symptoms.

Currently, anti-reflux stents (Gianturco, FerX-Ella and Choo stents) are also available to place stents across the GE junction, which prevent GE reflux.

For treating stricture located high, close to cricopharynx, more flexible stent (Ultraflex) should be used. However, it is important to remember that, patient will complain of foreign body sensation, if the stent is placed across the cricopharynx.

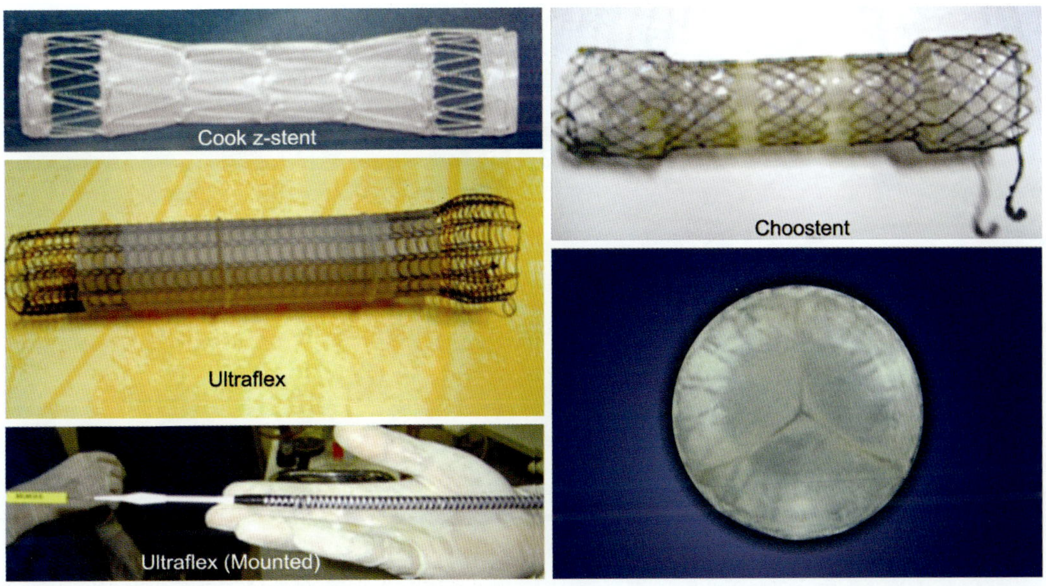

Fig. 3: Various designs of stents: Gianturco-Z stent (Cook). This is made from stainless steel and a polyethylene covering with barbs on the outside or uncoated flared ends to prevent migration. Ultraflex (Boston Scientific Ltd). This stent is made from a knitted Nitinol mesh and is available in both uncovered and covered. It has the weakest radial force but greater flexibility. These stents may be best for tortuous and upper third strictures. *Choostent (Diagmed)*: This is a polyurethane-covered stent made from Nitinol and has a retrievable attached thread. These stents also come with an internal distal anti-reflux valve.

They also have increased risks of perforation, proximal migration, and poor tolerance.[20] For the management of refractory benign stricture, retrievable stents are recommended.

Technique (Figs. 4 and 5)

Before the start of the procedure, patient is given thin barium suspension for fluoroscopic study to localize the abnormal segment and length of stricture. Once abnormal segment is localized, it is important to desensitize the pharyngeal mucosa prior to the procedure by local anesthesia using lidocaine aerosol spray. Under fluoroscopy, combination of a diagnostic angiographic catheter and a hydrophilic guidewire is introduced, attempt is made to cross the strictured segment. Once the strictured segment is crossed, the hydrophilic guidewire is exchanged with stiff metallic guidewire. Then strictured segment is dilated using either balloon catheter or surgical bougie over the metallic guide wire. Based the length of abnormal segment on preliminary barium study, a covered stent usually 4–5 cm longer than strictured segment is selected to cover the entire abnormal segment and to keep the proximal and distal ends of the stents in normal segments of the esophagus **(Fig. 3B)**. Prior to insertion of stent, delivery system is lubricated with lidocaine jelly. Then delivery system is negotiated over the metallic guidewire and appropriately placed across the abnormal segment under fluoroscopy. Stent is deployed by uncovering the outer sheath of delivery system, while holding the pusher handle in place. Once the stent is positioned, the delivery system and metallic guidewire are withdrawn. Patient is given thin barium suspension again to confirm the stent location and patency.[22]

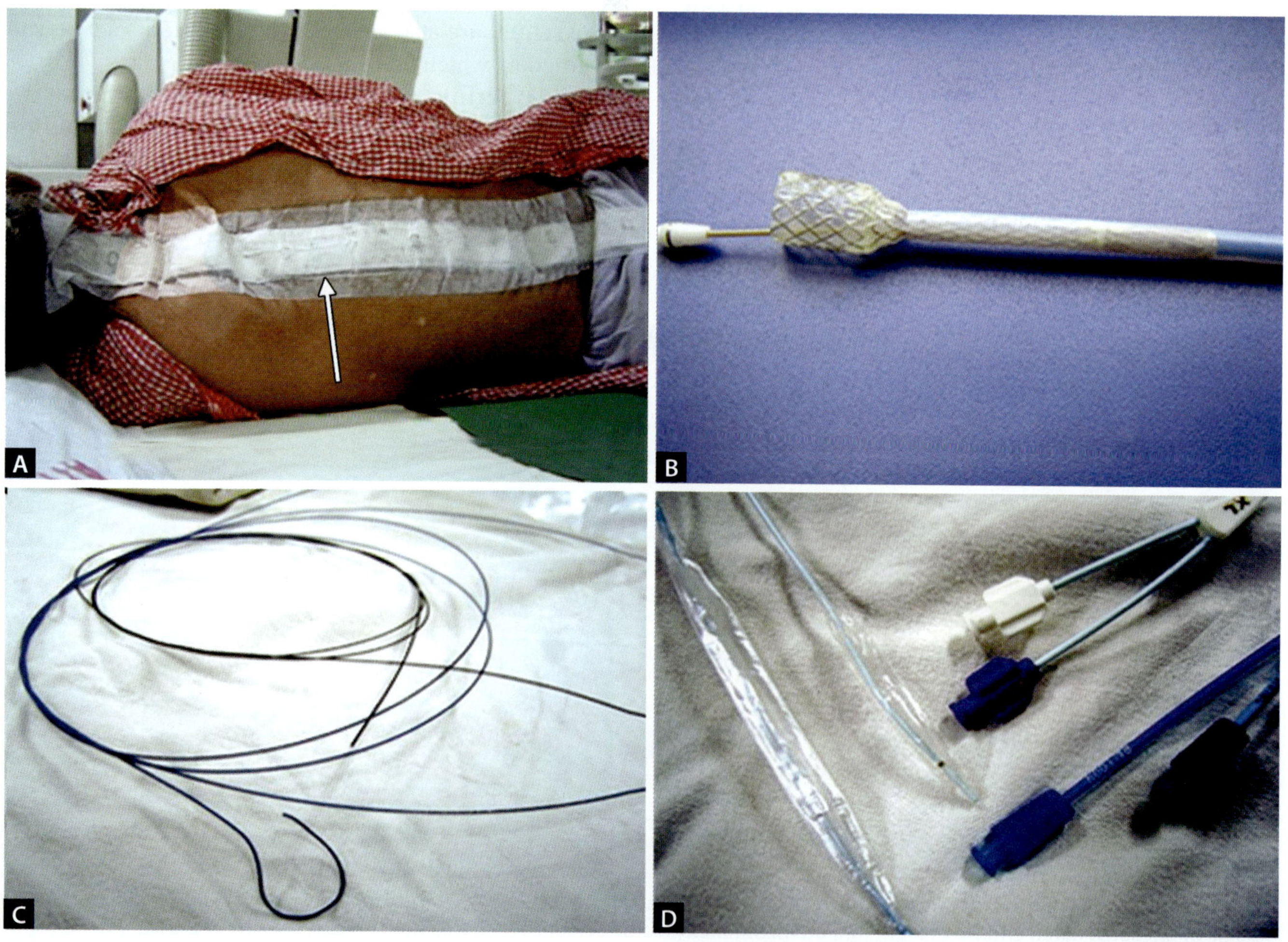

Figs. 4A to D: The preparation of esophageal stenting. Metallic marker pasted over the back of the patient (A) (arrow). Delivery system loaded with self-expandable fully covered metallic stent (partially released). (B) Metallic and terumo guidewire; (C) and Balloon catheter (D).

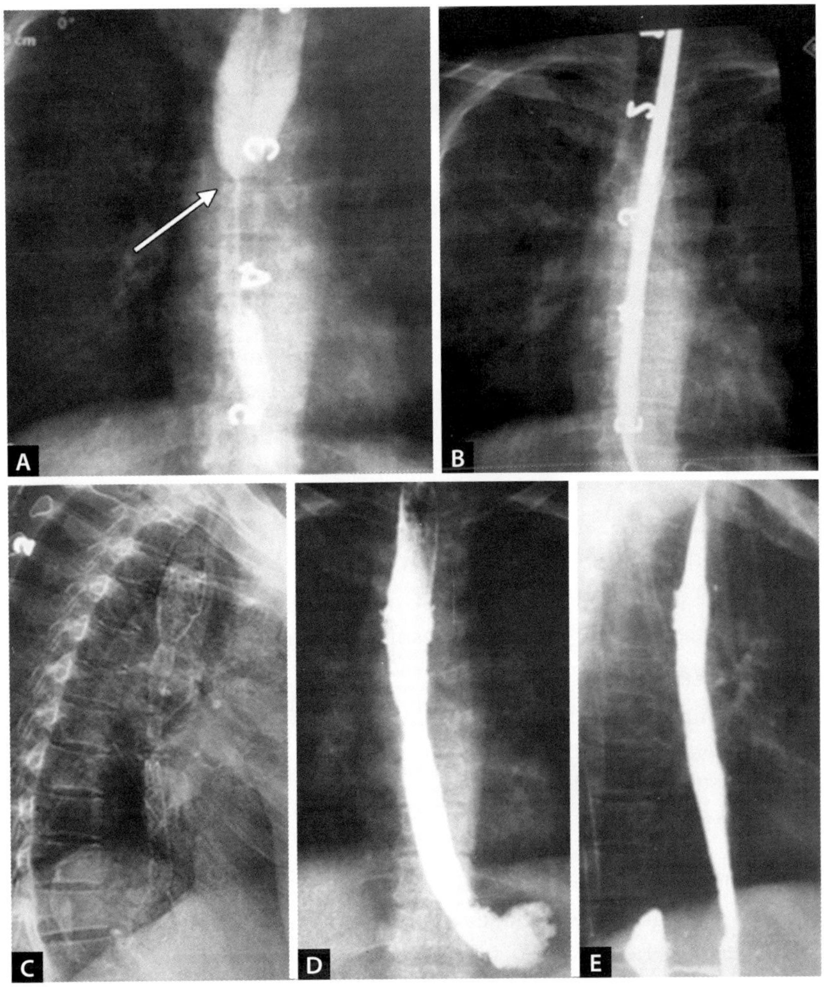

Figs. 5A to E: Technique of esophageal stenting. Barium swallow shows irregular narrowing in mid third of thoracic esophagus with proximal hold up of barium column (A) (Arrow). Dilatation of the stricture with bougie (B). Completely deployed Choostent seen *in situ* (*Note:* Lead markers placed on the patient's back for exact localization of stricture) (C). Esophagogram showing freeflow of contrast across the stent (D and E).

Postprocedure Care

After the procedure, patients are allowed to take clear fluids and kept on a soft diet for few days, then shifted to a semi-solid diet. Progressive change in diet is recommended after stent placement. It is imperative to tell the patients not to take grassy, unprepared vegetables and meat.

Patients are evaluated immediately after stent placement and every month thereafter. Patient's symptomatic improvement is assessed based on dysphagia score.

Complications

Early Complications

Early chest pain is the major-minor complication, that settles with analgesics. Major complications such as hemorrhage and perforation are uncommon. Bleeding occur more in stents extending above the level of the aortic arch because left subclavian artery and aortic arch are close to esophagus.[20]

Late Complications

Re-intervention following stent placement is due to tumor in-growth with uncovered stents and tumor over growth with covered stents. Other late complications include hemorrhage, stent migration and stent fracture.

Guidelines for Esophageal Stenting

- Uncovered stents are selected for gastroesophageal junction strictures and covered stents for non-gastroesophageal junction strictures.

- Covered stents should be used for esophageal fistulas.[14]
- SEMS are used commonly for palliation of dysphagia in advanced esophageal carcinoma.
- Partially covered stents are used for malignant esophageal fistula and strictures caused by villous tumors.
- Plastic stents can be used for benign strictures and removed after 4–16 weeks to prevent epithelial hypertrophy and stent incarceration.
- Plastic stent delivery system is wider and stiffer than SEMS. Hence, dilatation before stent insertion may increase the complication rates.
- Antireflux stents have similar efficacy of SEMS with benefit in gastroesophageal reflux.
- Combined stent and brachytherapy is a safe palliative option in patients with inoperable advanced esophageal carcinoma.[20]

MDCT in Esophageal Stent Evaluation

- Stent evaluation using CT is usually performed using water as oral contrast. Positive contrast material is used to evaluate perforation, fistula and collections
- Noncontrast CT scan evaluates stent position, location and stent fractures.
- MDCT can identify the complications such as:
  - Esophageal perforation, seen as periesophageal air pockets, adjacent collection and leakage of oral contrast.
  - Stent leakage, stent fracture, tracheal compression by the stent and stent migration.[20]
- MDCT also helps in identifying tumor overgrowth (tumor growth at either ends of the stent) and tumor ingrowth (through the struts of uncovered stent) as a long-term complications or as progression of disease process.

GASTRODUODENAL STENTING

Patients with cancers of stomach/duodenum usually present with symptoms of gastric outlet obstruction such as nausea, vomiting, electrolyte discrepancy, under nutrition, and signs of dehydration.[23]

Patients with unresectable tumors/poor surgical candidates are offered palliative treatment to relieve symptoms of gastric outlet obstruction by placement of stenting across the gastroduodenal area. The ideal gastroduodenal stent should possess enough radial and axial force with good flexibility to overcome tortuosity.[24]

Indications

- Gastric, duodenal malignant obstructions caused by unresectable tumors either by primary tumors or by secondary involvement by the cancers of adjacent organs such as gallbladder and pancreas.
- Patients with tumor recurrence who had surgical anastomosis and present with symptoms of gastric outlet obstruction.[25]
- *Benign gastroduodenal strictures:* As a last option, if the patient condition is high risk for surgery.

Contraindications

- Presence of perforation
- Additional distal or multisegment intestinal obstruction due to extensive peritoneal carcinomatosis.

Available Devices

Unlike esophageal stenting, uncovered stents are more suitable for malignant gastroduodenal strictures compared to covered stents due to less chances of migration and longer patency.[26,27]

Various stent designs available in the market, however, more commonly used stents is Wall stent **(Fig. 2)**, because of its flexibility to overcome the tortuosity and good radial force. One of the main concern of this stent is foreshortening after deployment to the extent of 40–50%.

Endoscopic versus Fluoroscopic Placement

Routinely, endoscopic approach is used for placing the gastroduodenal stents. However, fluoroscopic approach can also be used with nearly similar technical success rate.[28] Technical failure rates is low (<5%), usually due to unable to cross the stricture.

Precise stent positioning is better done under fluoroscopy rather than endoscope alone. There are reports in literature who reported higher technical rate with fluoroscopic guidance than with endoscopic approach.[29,30]

Technique (Figs. 6A to D)

Oral contrast study, using either iodinated or thin barium suspension), is performed prior to the stenting to look for location and length of abnormal segment. Because of long-standing obstruction the stomach hugely distended and stretched out, that makes procedure difficult due to buckling of the catheter system inside the stomach.

Hence, nasogastric suction is recommended prior to stent placement that not only assist manipulation of deliver system and also helps in preventing aspiration during the procedure.

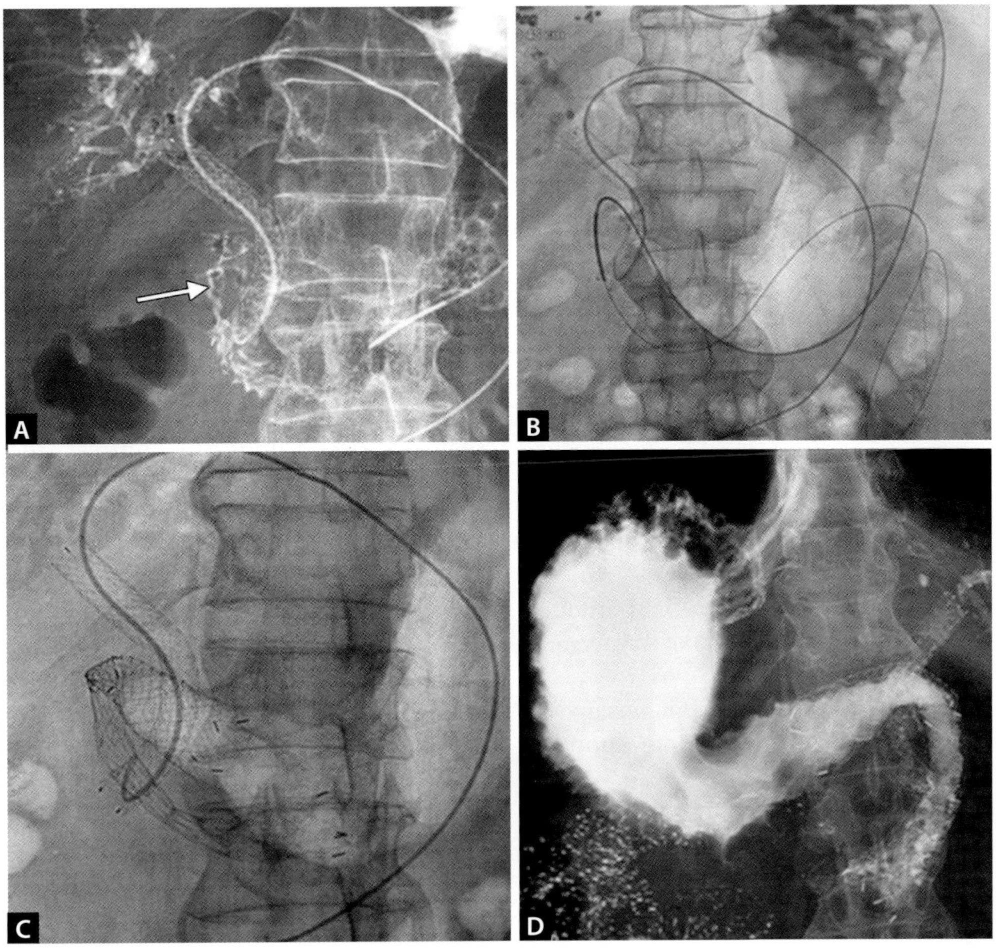

Figs. 6A to D: Technique of duodenal stenting. Contrast study showing narrowing of D2 segment, proximal to ampulla (A) (arrow), Guidewire negotiated across the stricture (B), Completely deployed Wall stent seen *in situ* (C) and barium study showing freeflow of contrast across the stent (D).

Technique of gastroduodenal stenting is similar to esophageal stenting as described above. Initial pharyngeal anesthesia is done using lidocaine spray, followed by negotiating the stricture using catheter and hydrophilic guidewire combination. Once the stricture is crossed, hydrophilic guidewire is exchanged with superstiff metallic guidewire usually of 260-300 cm. Then stent of appropriate size based on preliminary contrast study is advanced over the metallic guidewire. Technique of stent deployment is similar to esophageal stenting. In case of difficulty in negotiating delivery system across the stomach, right lateral decubitus positioning helps by unfolding the tortuous anatomy. It is recommended to "overstent" the stricture segment to include at least 2 cm distal and 2 cm proximal normal segments to prevent recurrence of obstruction by tumor ingrowth. Usually, stents are not dilated using balloon after stent placement, since these stents mostly expand over next few days.[31]

In difficult situations like simultaneous biliary and duodenal stenting, it is better to do prior biliary decompression through percutaneous transhepatic approach.[26] Newly designed duodenal metal stent, which has central unfixed structure helps in tackling the problems of biliary and duodenal stenting. [32]

Postprocedure Care

A follow-up upper gastrointestinal study is usually performed the next day to look for patency and location. Postprocedure instructions to the patient are similar to esophageal stenting.

Clinical success of the procedure is usually assessed by relief of symptoms of gastrointestinal obstruction. Clinical failure rate is nearly 10% inspite of technical success is usually due to distal obstruction.[33,34]

Guidelines for Duodenal Stents[20]

- Self-expandable metallic stent (SEMS) are standard of care for malignant duodenal stenosis, when surgery is not possible.
- No clear guidelines for the duodenal stenting in benign strictures.
- Biliary decompression is done prior to duodenal stenting in case of biliary dilatation.[26]

MDCT in Duodenal Stent Evaluation[20]

- Stent evaluation using CT is usually performed using water as oral contrast.
- Oral positive contrast material is used in suspected cases of perforation, fistula and collection.
- Perforation is seen as retroperitoneal or intraperitoneal free air on CT. The free gas at distal tip of stent should raise the suspicion of perforation.
- Stent fracture is seen as buckling of stent and may be associated with incomplete or complete duodenal obstruction.
- Multidetector computed tomography (MDCT) also helps in finding out the cause for post-stent duodenal bleed.

Complications

Complications are infrequent and potential complications include pain, perforation, migration, hemorrhage and food impaction. Post stent chemotherapy reduce the chances of tumor in growth and prolong the patency, but increase the rate of stent migration.[26,35] Migration is rare with uncovered stents.

COLORECTAL STENTING

Indications

The primary indications for colorectal stenting include:[33]

- Colorectal stenting is done as temporary procedure to decompress the colon in patients with an acute obstruction who have potentially resectable malignancy to allow bowel preparation followed by surgical resection.
- More commonly, long-term stenting is done as palliative procedure to relieve symptoms of colonic obstruction in patients with unresectable malignancy.

Contraindications

- Clinical or radiologic evidence of perforation
- More proximal lesions within the colon.

Technical Considerations

Various stent designs available in the market, however, more commonly used colonic stents are Wall stent, Ultraflex stent, and Memotherm stent.[36-39]

Stenting can be performed either endoscopic route or fluoroscopic route or combined.

Prior to the procedure, water-soluble contrast enema is performed to look for location and length of abnormal segment. Based upon the contrast study findings the suitable device can be selected.

Technique of stent placement is similar to esophageal or gastroduodenal stenting, first step is to cross the strictured segment using catheter-guidewire combination. Once the stricture is crossed, hydrophilic guidewire is exchanged with superstiff metallic guidewire usually of 260–300 cm. Then stent of appropriate size based on preliminary contrast study is advanced over the metallic guidewire. Technique of stent deployment is similar to esophageal/gastroduodenal stenting.

It is recommended to "overstent" the stricture segment to include at least 2 cm distal and 2 cm proximal normal segments to prevent recurrence of obstruction by tumor ingrowth. Long lesions may require two stents.[33]

Postprocedure Follow-up

A water-soluble contrast enema study is done following the procedure look for patency and leakage.

Patients with unresectable malignancy are kept on placed on a low-residue diet and advised to take lubricant laxative to prevent probability of stent obstruction.

Complications

Complications are rare and are usually minor such as pain and temporary bleeding, which do not require any treatment. Major complications include perforation, persistent hemorrhage, stent migration, and restenosis.[26]

Guidelines for Colonic Stents

- Uncovered self-expanding metallic stents are used in colonic stenting
- Colonic stenting is used as palliative procedure for malignant colonic stenosis

- Colonic stenting can also be used as bridge to surgery to relieve obstruction.
- It is associated with less stoma rate, lesser complications, shorter hospital stay and less morbidity.
- The role of SEMS in benign colonic stenosis is controversial. They have limited role in diverticular disease and radiation-induced stenosis.[20]

MDCT in Colonic Stent Evaluation[20]

- Stent evaluation using CT is usually performed using water as oral contrast.
- It helps in evaluating site of obstruction and number of sites of colonic obstruction. Colonic stenting is not preferred in multiple sites of obstruction.
- CT helps to rule out perforation both before and after colonic stenting. Colonic perforation may be seen as pneumoperitoneum and adjacent fluid collection.
- CT may show marked colonic edema suggesting colonic ischemia in patients with post stent colonic dilatation.
- During follow-up scans, tumor ingrowth within stenting can be demonstrated on CT.

PERCUTANEOUS ENTEROCUTANEOUS FISTULA CLOSURE WITH N-BUTYL-2-CYANOACRYLATE

Enterocutaneous fistulae usually occur as complications of complex alimentary tract surgery but may also arise spontaneously in patients with inflammatory bowel disease or after trauma or radiation therapy.[40,41] Gastrointestinal fistula are classified into high output and low output fistulas, based on amount of output from fistula per day. Most fistulae that originate in the duodenum, jejunum, and ileum are classed as high-output and

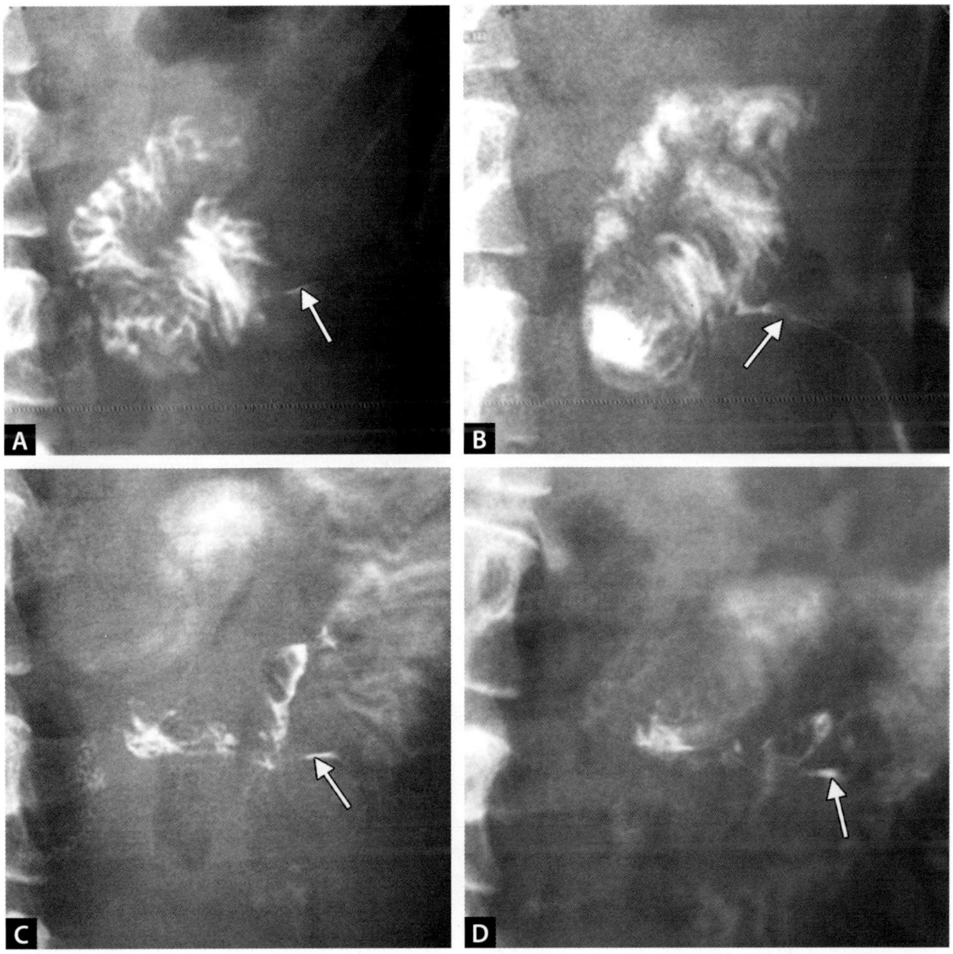

Figs. 7A to D: Technique of enterocutaneous fistula closure with glue. Contrast study to show outline and length of the fistulous tract (arrow) (A and B). Following glue injection, the cast of glue outlining the fistulous tract is seen (arrow) (C and D). The tract was completely obliterated on follow-up.

may drain as much as 4,000 mL of intestinal contents per day.

The problems posed by such fistula include massive lossesoffluid, electrolytes, and nutrients are formidable and, frequently, management is complicated by the presence of one or more intra-abdominal abscesses. Currently, most authors recommend a trial of conservative management before surgical therapy is attempted; accurate fluid and electrolyte replacement and prevention of malnutrition are combined with attempts to reduce the drainage of intestinal contents by nasogastric intestinal intubation.[41-44] Although this approach is occasionally successful, both the quantity and quality of bowel effluent and the presence of ongoing infection usually prevent the development of a mature, fibrous, external tract and spontaneous closure.

Radiologic involvement in the care of patients with enterocutaneous fistulae has largely been limited to opacification of the fistulous tract and identification of the morbid anatomy.[45] However, recent technical advances in interventional radiology techniques have made the treatment of low output fistula closure more practically feasible. The glues have been used successfully in the closure of fistulas in various locations such as pancreas, biliary and gastrointestinal.[46,47]

Mechanism of Action of the Glue (N-butyl-2-cyanoacrylate)

Glue polymerizes and produces a cast immediately, when it comes in contact with body fluids. Usually it is used in endovascular or surgical procedures. Mild inflammatory reaction is seen within 24 hours. By end of one week, inflammatory reaction is minimal.[48]

Prerequisites

- Fistula should be low output
- The fistulous tract should be short in length (longer the tract lesser the chances of success)
- Tract should be linear, nonbranching
- No associated abscess cavity
- Nonepithelialized tract (if the tract is epithelialized, it is traumatized the tract to make the surface raw).

Technical Consideration

Percutaneous closure of fistulous tract is performed as an outpatient procedure and no anesthesia is required.

Preparation

Before the procedure, it is advisable to administer intravenous antibiotics covering gram-negative gastrointestinal flora. The potency (i.e. "stickiness") of glue requires dilution prior to its use. Dilution of glue is usually done by mixing with lipiodol that delays polymerization and improves visibility during injection under fluoroscopy.

Various combination of dilution (range: 1:1 to 1:3) has been suggested. If the mixture is too strong that causes premature polymerization and catheter occlusion whereas very dilute mixture increases the risk of distal embolization. 5% dextrose solution is used to flush the catheter and to prevent the risk of polymerization inside the catheter.

Technique (Figs. 7A to D)

After obtaining the contrast fistulogram study, the fistulous tract is catheterized either with angiographic catheter (4F) or using venflon (18–20G). The catheter should be advanced close the inner opening of fistula. After flushing the catheter with 50% dextrose solution, the diluted glue preparation (1:1 or 1:2) is injected, starting from inside and gradually withdrawing the catheter outside, while continuously injecting the glue.

After the procedure, recatheterization of the tract is not done; otherwise the glue may get dislodged. If the fistula has not closed, another session of glue injection is tried. Sometime we may need 3–4 session to close the tract depending upon the length, diameter and degree of epithelialization of the tract.

REFERENCES

1. Yang ZQ, Shin JH, Song HY, Kwon JH, Kim JW, Kim KR, Kim JH. Fluoroscopically guided percutaneous jejunostomy: outcomes in 25 consecutive patients. Clin Radiol. 2007;62(11):1061-5; discussion 1066-8. Epub 2007 Sep 4.
2. van Overhagen H, Ludviksson MA, Laméris JS, Zwamborn AW, Tilanus HW, Dees J, Hansen BE. US and fluoroscopic-guided percutaneous jejunostomy: experience in 49 patients. J Vasc Interv Radiol. 2000;11(1):101-6.
3. Cope C, Davis AG, Baum RA, Haskal ZJ, Soulen MC, Shlansky-Goldberg RD. Direct percutaneous jejunostomy: techniques and applications—ten years experience. Radiology. 1998;209(3):747-54.
4. Miller KS, Tomlinson JR, Sahn SA. Pleuropulmonary complications of enteral tube feedings, two case reports: review of the literature and recommendations. Chest. 1985;88:230-3.
5. Wasiljew BK, Ujiki GT, Beal JM. Feeding gastrostomy: complications and mortality. Am J Surg. 1982;143:194-5.
6. Shellito PC, Malt RA. Tube gastrostomy: technique and complications. Ann Surg. 1985;201:180-95.
7. Gauderer WL, Ponsky JL, Izant AJ. Gastrostomy without laparotomy: percutaneous endoscopic technique. J Pediatr Surg. 1980;15:872-5.
8. Ho CS. Percutaneous gastrostomy for jejunal feeding. Radiology. 1983;149:595-6.

9. Tao HH, Gillies AR. Percutaneous feeding gastrostomy. AJR. 1983;141:793-4.
10. Wills JS, Oglesby JT. Percutaneous gastrostomy. Radiology. 1983;149:449-53.
11. Brown AS, Mueller PA, Ferrucci JT. Controlled percutaneous gastrostomy: nylon T-fastener for fixation of the anterior gastric wall. Radiology. 1986;158:543-5.
12. Cope C. Suture anchor for visceral drainage. AJR. 1980;135: 402-3.
13. Kessel D, Robertson I. Interventional Radiology: A survival guide, 3rd edn. Churchil Livingstone Elsevier; 2011. pp.325-30.
14. Kaufman JA, Michael JL (Eds.). The requisites: Vascular and interventional radiology, 2nd edn. Elsevier Saunders, Philadelphia, PA; 2014.pp.425-50.
15. Celestin LR. Permanent intubation in inoperative cancer of the esophagus and cardia. Ann R Coll Surg Eng. 1959;25:165-70.
16. Atkinson M, Ferguson R. Fibre-optic endoscopic palliative intubation of inoperable oesophogastric neoplasms. BMJ. 1997;1:266-7.
17. Gray RR, Ho CS, Yee A, et al. Direct percutaneous jejunostomy. AJR. 1987;149:931-2.
18. Coleman CC, Coons HG, Cope C, et al. Percutaneous enterostomy with the Cope suture anchor. Radiology. 1990;174: 889-91.
19. Frimberger E. Expanding spiral: a new type of prosthesis for the palliative treatment of malignant oesophageal stenosis. Endoscopy. 1983;15:213-4.
20. Malgras B, Lo Dico R, Pautrat K, et al. Gastrointestinal stenting: Current status and imaging features. Diagn Interv Imaging. 2015;96(6):593-606.
21. Lee SH. The role of oesophageal stenting in the non-surgical management of oesophageal strictures. Br J Radiol. 2001;74(886):891-900. Review.
22. Neyaz Z, Srivastava DN, Thulkar S, Bandhu S, Gamanagatti S, Julka PK, Chattopadhyaya TK. Radiological evaluation of covered self-expandable metallic stents used for palliation in patients with malignant esophageal strictures. Acta Radiol. 2007;48(2):156-64.
23. Patton JT, Carter R. Endoscopic stenting for recurrent malignant gastric outlet obstruction. Br J Surg. 1997;84:865-6.
24. Wei Zhong Zhou, Zheng Qiang Yan. Stenting for malignant gastric outlet obstruction: Current status. Gastrointest Interv. 2014;3:65-8.
25. Klose KJ. Nitinol prostheses for the treatment of inoperable malignant esophageal obstruction. J Vasc Intervent Radiol. 1994;5:899-904.
26. Shi D, Qiu Xm, Feng Ty. Current status of metal stents for malignant gastro-Duodenal obstruction. J Gastroint Dig Syst. 2013;3:140. doi: 10.4172/2161-069X.1000140.
27. Woo SM, Kim DH, Lee WJ, Park KW, Park SJ, et al. Comparison of uncovered and covered stents for the treatment of malignant duodenal obstruction caused by pancreaticobiliary cancer. Surg Endosc. 2013;27: 2031-9.
28. Spinelli P, Cerrai FG, Dal Fante M. Endoscopic treatment of upper gastrointestinal tract malignancies. Endoscopy. 1993; 25:675-8.
29. de Baere T, Harry G, Ducreaux M, et al. Self-expanding metallic stents as palliative treatment of malignant gastroduodenal stenosis. AJR. 1997;169:1079-83.
30. Pinto IT. Malignant gastric and duodenal stenosis: palliation by peroral implantation of a self-expanding metallic stent. Cardiovasc Intervent Radiol. 1997;20:431-4.
31. Lopera JE, Brazzini A, Gonzales A, Castaneda-Zuniga WR. Gastroduodenal stent placement: current status. Radiographics. 2004;24(6):1561-73. Review.
32. Moon JH, Choi HJ, Ko BM, Koo HC, Hong SJ, et al. Combined endoscopic stent-in-stent placement for malignant biliary and duodenal obstruction by using a new duodenal metal stent (with videos). Gastrointest Endosc. 2009;70: 772-7.
33. Mauro MA, Koehler RE, Baron TH. Advances in gastrointestinal interventions: the treatment of gastroduodenal and colorectal obstructions with metallic stent. Radiology. 2000;215:659-69.
34. Kaw M, Singh S, Gagneja H, Azad P. Role of self-expandable metal stents in the palliation of malignant duodenal obstruction. Surg Endosc. 2003;17:646-50.
35. Park CI, Kim JH, Lee YC, Jahng J, Youn YH, et al. What is the ideal stent as initial intervention for malignant gastric outlet obstruction? Dig Liver Dis. 2013;45:33-7.
36. Rey JF, Romanczyk T, Greff M. Metal stents for palliation of rectal carcinoma: a preliminary report of 12 patients. Endoscopy. 1995;27:501-4.
37. Spinelli P, Dal Fante M, Mancini A. Rectal metal stents for palliation of colorectal malignant stenosis. Bildgebung. 1993; 60(Suppl 1):48-50.
38. Mainar A, Tejero E, Maynar M, et al. Colorectal obstruction: treatment with metallic stents. Radiology. 1996;198:761-4.
39. Saida Y, Sumiyama Y, Nagao J, et al. Stent endoprosthesis for obstructing colorectal cancers. Dis Colon Rectum. 1996;39:552-5.
40. Edmunds LH Jr. Williams GM, Welch CE. External fistulas arising from the gastrointestinal tract. Ann Surg. 1960; 152:445-71.
41. Fischer JE. The management of high out-put intestinal fistulas. Adv Surg. 1975;9:139-76.
42. Reber HA, Roberts C, Way LW, Dunphy JE. Management of external gastrointestinal fistulas. Ann Surg. 1978;188:460-7.
43. Blackett RL, Hill GL. Postoperative external small bowel fistulas: a study of a consecutive series of patients treated with intravenous hyperalimentation. Br J Surg. 1978;65:775-8.
44. Soeter PB, Ebeid AM, Fischer JE. Review of 404 patients with gastrointestinal fistulas. Ann Surg. 1979;190:189-202.
45. Miller WT, Sullivan MA. Roentgenologic demonstration of sinus tracts and fistulae. AJR. 1969;107:812-7.
46. Lee YC, Na HG, Suh JH, et al. Three cases of fistulae arising from gastrointestinal tract treated with endoscopic injection of histoacryl. Endoscopy. 2001;33:184-6.
47. Seewald S, Brand B, Omar S, et al. Endoscopic sealing of pancreatic fistula by using N-butyl-2-cyanoacrylate. Gastrointest Endosc. 2004;59:463-70.
48. Suga T, Akamatsu T, Kawamura Y, et al. Actual behaviour of N-butyl- 2-cyanoacrylate (histoacryl) in a blood vessel: a model of the varix. Endoscopy. 2002;34:73-7.

Section 4

Genitourinary Imaging

CHAPTER 98

Current Status of Conventional Techniques in Urogenital Imaging

Naveen Kalra, Manavjit Singh Sandhu

BACKGROUND

The history of uroradiology dates back to July 11, 1896 when MacIntyre, Glasgow first reported the X-ray demonstration of a renal calculus in a patient.[1] Subsequently, urologists developed cystography, retrograde pyelography and retrograde urethrography within a span of next 15 years. In 1929, Moses Swick[2] introduced a successful intravenous urographic contrast agent called uroselectan (5-iodo-2-pyridone N acetic acid) which ushered in intravenous urography (IVU) that became an integral part of the urological work-up of patients. Plain X-ray of kidney, ureter and bladder (KUB) and intravenous urography (IVU) continued to be used as the primary imaging techniques for the diagnostic evaluation of urinary tract for several years **(Figs. 1A to C)**. However, recently with the development of ultrasound (US), computed tomography (CT) and magnetic resonance imaging (MRI), there are now several techniques in the diagnostic armamentarium of the uroradiologist. While a multimodality approach is often required to come to a final conclusion, the strengths and weaknesses of each technique must be known so that both conventional and newer techniques can be used to the maximum benefit of

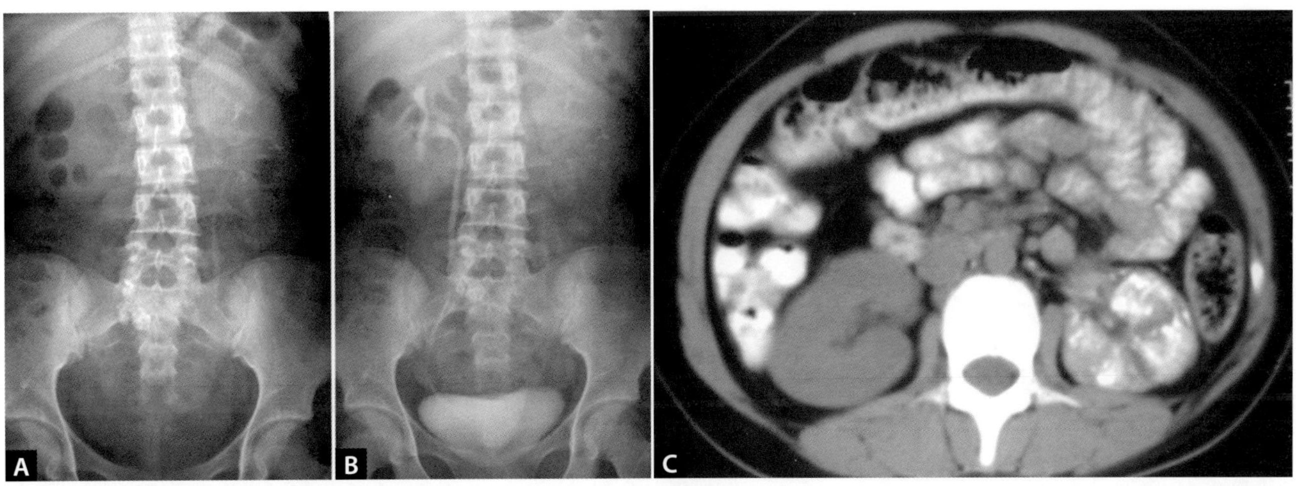

Figs. 1A to C: (A) Plain radiograph of the abdomen shows extensive calcification in the left kidney and along the course of left ureter as a result of tuberculosis infection; (B) IVU shows no contrast excretion into the calyceal system on the left side. The right kidney and ureter are normal; (C) Nonenhanced axial CT section shows extensive parenchymal calcification in the left kidney.

patients. Availability, cost effectiveness and radiation dose are some of the other important factors determining the choice of the imaging modality while investigating various clinical problems. This chapter will discuss the current status of conventional radiological procedures vis-à-vis the newer techniques in common clinical situations.

Patients suspected to have urolithiasis may present with acute flank pain, hematuria or recurrent urinary tract infections. A plain film of the abdomen (X-ray KUB) is usually the first radiological investigation performed in these patients. However, the diagnostic accuracy of plain film for the detection of urinary tract calculus depends on the chemical composition of the stone, its size, location, overlying bowel gas shadows and technical quality of the film. Levine et al.[3] in their study of 178 patients found that plain radiographs had a sensitivity of only 45% for detecting ureteral calculi which marginally increased to 59% when the plain films were retrospectively reviewed with CT as the standard of reference. However, plain films are still good as baseline study and for follow-up of stone disease post-treatment.

Recently, ultrasound on account of its simplicity, freedom from radiation and ready availability has been proposed as an alternative technique when used in combination with KUB for diagnostic evaluation of patients presenting with acute flank pain. In a prospective study conducted by Lewis-Jones et al., X-ray KUB and ultrasound provided similar information as that obtained by IVU in 81.4% of patients. Considering the cost effectiveness, the authors concluded that KUB and US could replace IVU in patients of renal colic. In a series of 180 patients, Dalla Palma et al. showed a 95% negative predictive value of the KUB/US combination indicating that IVU was unlikely to be helpful, if the KUB/US tests were negative.[5] While US is highly sensitive for detection of dilated collecting system, it has several limitations. Calculi smaller than 5 mm can be easily missed and ureteral stones that are seen in association with undilated collecting system cannot be detected.

In the last decade, unenhanced. CT has rapidly gained popularity for investigating a patient of renal colic, and there are several studies which have reported high sensitivity and specificity (95–97%) for detection of renal and ureteral calculi.[6,7] CT detects virtually all stones regardless of their composition. In a study of 20 patients by Smith et al.,[8] 5 patients had shown calculi on both IVU and CT, 6 had a stone that was detected only on CT and one patient had a stone that was not detected either on CT or IVU. With the availability of fast spiral CT scanner, the technique is specially useful in the emergency setting. There are many centers where plain films and IVU have been replaced by helical CT in patients presenting with flank pain and hematuria. In addition the extent of perine-phric edema seen on CT has been used to predict the degree of ureteral obstruction and chances of spontaneous passage of ureteral stone with an accuracy of 94%.[9] Thus, in centers where there is free access to spiral CT, unenhanced CT has actually replaced plain films and IVU for diagnosis of stones in the urinary tract. KUB and ultrasound may be used as the initial screening modality which is followed by spiral CT if the KUB and US are negative **(Figs. 2A and B)**. However, IVU is still the best investigation if CT is not available. The KUB/US combination has also been compared to spiral CT. In a prospective study of 66 patients, the KUB/US combination had a sensitivity of 79% for detecting ureteric stones.

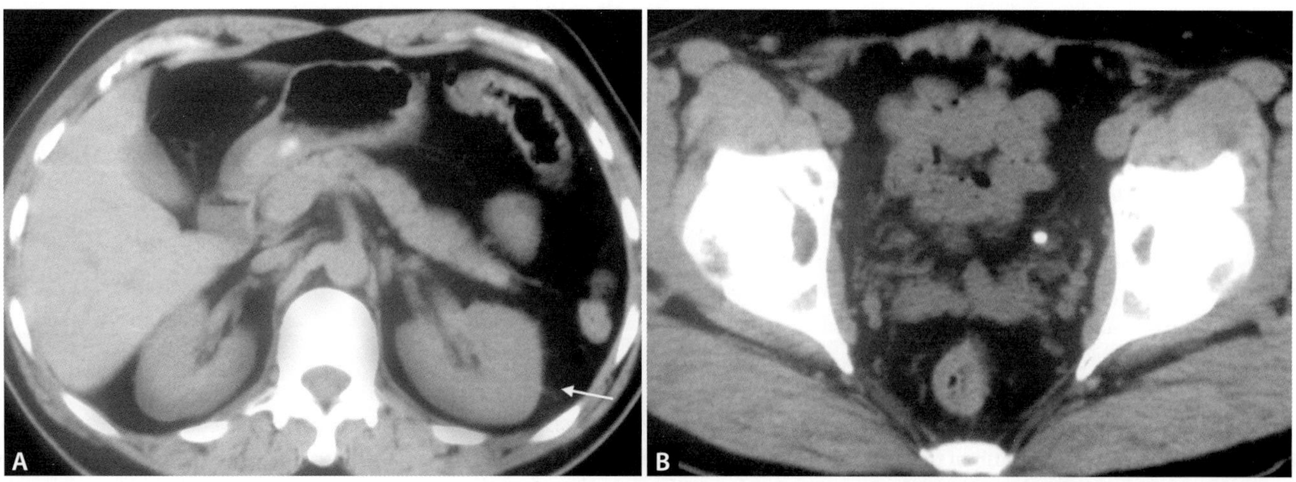

Figs. 2A and B: Nonenhanced axial helical CT sections of a patient with renal colic and normal X-ray KUB and US. (A) The left kidney is enlarged with mild perinephric stranding (arrow); (B) A small calculus is seen in the left lower ureter.

However, all the missed cases had spontaneous passage of stone, and it was concluded that CT would not add useful information after a negative KUB/US study.[10]

Radiation dose is one of the major factors which influences the choice of appropriate imaging modality. The radiation dose of unenhaced CT is greater than that of IVU even though patients with obstruction may require more number of radiographs than those without obstruction. The low dose CT protocol for stone detection proposed by Liu et al.[7] still results in approximately double the effective dose equivalent in comparison with IVU (2.8 mSv for CT, 1.33 mSv for conventional IVU).

Painless hematuria is another major urological problem which needs evaluation of both renal parenchyma and urothelium to rule out urinary tract malignancy. Traditionally IVU has been used as the baseline investigation in these patients. IVU is a time tested technique which is most acceptable to the urologist as it gives a global view of the renal parenchyma and the collecting system. However, with advent of helical CT and CT/MR urography the exact place of IVU in this clinical setting is again under question and there is no universal agreement about the first imaging modality to be used in patients with hematuria. The American Urological Association Best Practice Policy Guidelines include either IVU or CT urography as the initial imaging test for asymptomatic microscopic hematuria.[11] In addition, the American College of Radiology has rated IVU and CT urography equal as to their appropriateness for evaluation of patients with hematuria.[12] In patients with hematuria due to renal parenchymal disease, US is the best imaging modality for evaluating renal volume and morphology.

It is generally agreed that imaging with US/CT/MRI is superior to IVU for detection and characterization of renal masses. In addition a urogram or retrograde pyelogram may be required to visualize the urothelium of the renal collecting system and the ureters in patients when there is suspicion of urothelial neoplasm. CT urography is an evolving technique wherein three-dimensional (3D) coronal reconstruction of contrast enhanced CT images is achieved using the maximum intensity projections **(Fig. 3)**. McNicholas et al.[13] found no significant differences in the ability of CT urography and IV urography in opacifying the calcyces, pelvis and ureter and opined that CT urography has the potential for evaluating the urothelium. Chow et al.[14] concluded that CT urography in conjunction with the axial images is a single examination which alone may be required for the work-up of patients with hematuria as it is capable of imaging both the parenchyma and the collecting system. On the other hand, Hattery and King[15] have reported their experience of CT urography and found 10% of urinary tract abnormality were either better or only detected by IVU compared to 5 mm axial sections and CT urography. The authors listed several examples, such as pyeloureteritis cystica, papillary necrosis and transitional cell carcinoma where CT urography may not provide the high quality images needed for diagnosis. The authors supported the notion that CT with digital reformatted images does not provide sufficient detail for evaluation of subtle urothelial neoplasms. Cowan et al.[16] compared CT urography with retrograde pyelography for the detection of urothelial carcinoma in 106 patients. The only false-negative CT urogram was a small urothelial tumor that was not detected in an unopacified segment. From the aforesaid, it is clear that as refinement of CT urography continues, IVU will be replaced by CT urography subject to availability and affordability.

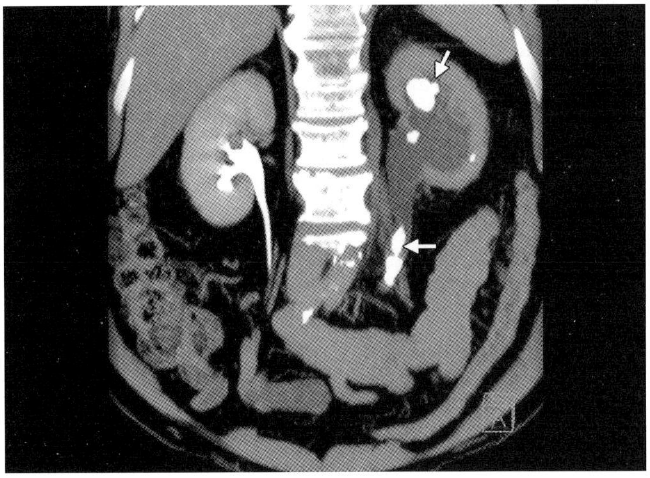

Fig. 3: CT urography in the pyelogram phase showing good opacification of the calyceal system and ureter on the right side. There is presence of left hydroureteronephrosis with renal and ureteric calculi (arrows).

IVU is the only modality to detect early changes in renal calyces in tuberculosis, papillary necrosis, etc. US, CT and MRI may be totally normal in these early cases. Hence, in a suspected case of urinary tract TB, IVU is the first imaging modality for diagnosis and subsequent follow-up.[17] However, it is always advisable to intergrate IVU with cross-sectional imaging in patients with suspected tuberculosis.

Children presenting with repeated attacks of UTI have been traditionally investigated with IVU and cystourethrography. The aim of imaging is to diagnose any underlying congenital renal anomaly that may predispose to recurrent urinary tract infections and detect the presence of renal scarring and vesicoureteric reflux. Recent studies have shown that diagnostic yield of IVU in this clinical setting is unacceptably low (8.3%)[18] and the abnormalities detected rarely change the management. Risks of IVU in terms of radiation and possibility of adverse reaction to contrast media outweigh its benefits and there is thus a strong case for withdrawal of routine IVU as a screening test in patients with recurrent UTI. Renal scintigraphy using ^{99m}TcDMSA is superior to IVU for detection of renal scarring. Despite many proponents of radionuclide cystography (RNC), conventional contrast voiding cystourethrography (VCUG) continues to be the gold standard for detecting and grading of the vesicoureteric reflux (VUR) on account of false-negative studies and poor grading accuracy of radionuclide cystography.[19] RNC has a much lower radiation dose than VCUG, but the low spatial resolution cannot identify the anatomic abnormalities of the urethra, bladder and ureters. RNC is recommended for follow-up of VUR and for screening the asymptomatic siblings of patients with VUR. Initial evaluation of VUR in girls may be done with RNC but in boys RNC is inadequate as anatomic imaging of urethra and bladder can only be done with VCUG.

In children and pregnant patients being investigated for obstructive uropathy, MR urography also has the potential to replace IVU due to the absence of radiation exposure **(Figs. 4A and B)**. Using T2-weighted (static-fluid urography) and contrast enhanced dynamic T1-weighted sequences (excretory urography), images of sufficient diagnostic quality can be obtained in infants with oral sedation.[20] Blandino et al. in 2001[21] in their study of 115 patients found that the speci-ficity of MR urography in detecting hydronephrosis was 98% and the accuracy in revealing the level of obstruction was 100%. The sensitivity of detecting stones, strictures and congenital ureteropelvic junction obstructions was 68.9%, 98.5% and 100%, respectively. The sensitivity of detecting ureteral calculi is technique dependent, with higher sensiti-vity being reported for excretory urography than for static-fluid urography.[22]

In patients of renal trauma, IVU and renal arteriography were the main diagnostic tools in the past. With introduction of US and CT, IVU is no longer used in these patients and CT is considered the technique of choice for detection and characterization of renal injuries and for assessment of vascular status.

Angiography is reserved for patients who require interventional treatment, such as embolisation of traumatic pseudoaneurysm or AV fistula. Contrast cystography, micturating cystourethrography and retrograde urethrography continue to be the techniques of choice for diagnosing bladder and urethral injuries and urethral strictures **(Figs. 5A and B)**.

Pretransplant work-up of renal donor used to include IVU and conventional angiography. Precise information of number of ureters, site of joining in case of duplication of ureter and vascular anatomy is mandatory before donor selection. The reported sensitivity and specificity of MDCT angiography for the detection of accessory renal arteries, prehilar branching and venous anomalies are 88% and 98%, 100% and 97% and 100% and 97%, respectively. In one of the studies, CT findings agreed with surgical findings for accessory renal arteries, prehilar branching and venous anomalies in 94%, 93% and 98% of patients respectively.[23]

At times before pelvic surgery for bladder, uterus, ovaries, etc. the surgeon needs exact relationships of the lower ureters in the surgical field or involvement of ureters by the pelvic pathology to reduce the chances of ureteral

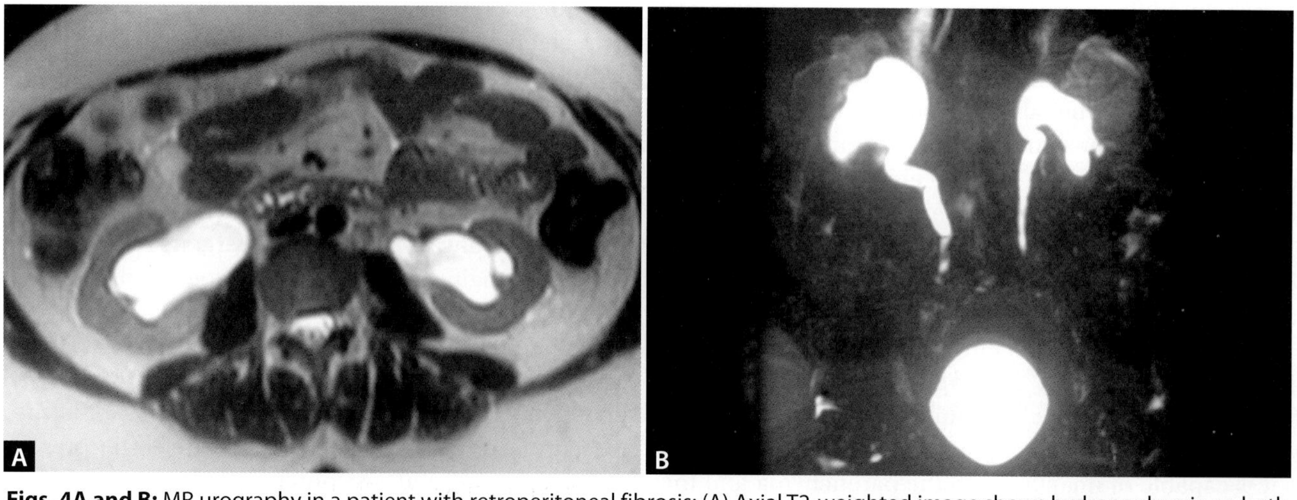

Figs. 4A and B: MR urography in a patient with retroperitoneal fibrosis: (A) Axial T2-weighted image shows hydronephrosis on both sides; (B) Static-fluid MRU image shows hydroureteronephrosis on both sides with medially deviated ureters.

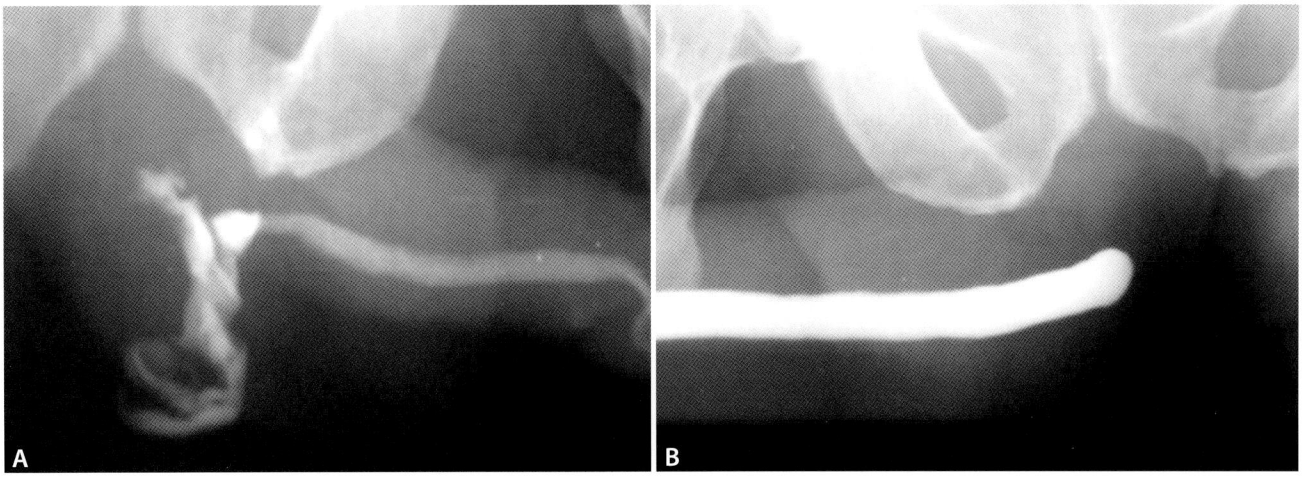

Figs. 5A and B: (A) Retrograde urethrography (RGU) in a patient following pelvic trauma shows contrast extravasation from the bulbar urethra; (B) Follow-up RGU in the same patient shows stricture at the level of bulbar urethra.

injury. However, IVU should not be used routinely before hysterectomy but should be performed in patients with large pelvic masses or known pelvic cancer.[24]

CONCLUSION

To conclude it appears that conventional uroradiology continues to play an important but limited role in urogenital imaging. Nonenhanced helical CT has nearly replaced conventional uroradiology for evaluation of urinary tract calculi. However, in countries such as ours, a blanket substitution may not be feasible due to cost factor and availability. CT and MR urography at present cannot fully substitute contrast urography although CT urography is the current heir apparent to IVU. Technical improvements in CT urography like reduction in radiation exposure and MR urography like faster imaging time and consistent image quality are required to further enhance the utility of CT and MR urography in the future.

REFERENCES

1. Maclntyre J. Photograpy of renal calculus: Description an adjustable modification in the focus tube. Lancet. 1896;2:118.
2. Swick M. Visualization of the kidney and urinary tract on roentgenograms by means of intravenous administration of a new contrast: Uroselectan. Klin Wochenschr. 1929;8:2087.
3. Levine JA, Neitlich J, Verga M, et al. Ureteral calculi in patients with flank pain: correlation of plain radiography with unenhanced helical CT. Radiology. 1997;204:27-31.
4. Lewis-Jones HG, Lamb GH, Hughes PL. Can ultrasound replace the intravenous urogram in preliminary investigation of renal tract disease? A prospective study. Br J Radiol. 1989;62:977-80.
5. Palma DL, Stacul F, Bazzocchi M, et al. Ultrasound and plain film versus intravenous urography in ureteric colic. Clin Radiol. 1993; 47:333-6.
6. Boulay I, Holtz P, Foley WD, et al. Ureteral calculi: Diagnostic efficacy of helical CT and implications for treatment of patients. AJR. 1999;172:1485-90.
7. Liu W, Esler SJ, Kenny BJ, et al. Low dose non-enhanced helical CT of renal colic: Assessment of ureteric stone detection and measurement of effective dose equivalent. Radiology. 2000; 215:51-4.
8. Smith RC, Rosenfield AT, Choe KA, et al. Acute flank pain: Comparison of non-contrast enhanced CT and intravenous urography. Radiology. 1995;194:789-94.
9. Boridy IC, Kawashima A, Goldman SM, et al. Acute ureterolithiasis: Nonenhanced helical CT findings of perinephric edema for prediction of degree of ureteral obstruction. Radiology. 1999;213:663-7.
10. Ripolles T, Agramunt M, Errando J, et al. Suspected ureteric colic: Plain film and sono-graphy vs unenhanced helical CT. A prospective study in 66 patients. Eur Radiol. 2004;14:129-36.
11. Grossfeld GD, Litwin MS, Wolf JS Jr, et al. Evaluation of asymptomatic microscopic hematuria in adults: The American Urological Association best practice policy. II. Patient evaluation, cytology, voided markers, imaging, cystoscopy, nephrology evaluation, and follow-up. Urology. 2001;57: 604-10.
12. Choyke PL, Bluth EI, Bush WH Jr, et al. Radiological investigation of patients with hematuria. American College of Radiology, ACR Appropriateness Criteria, 2005.
13. McNicholas MMJ, Raptopoulos VD, Schwartz RK, et al. Excretory phase CT urography for opacification of the urinary collecting system. AJR. 1998;170:1261-7.
14. Chow LC, Sommer FG. Multidetector CT urography with abdominal compression and three dimensional reconstruction. AJR. 2001;177: 849-55.

15. Hattery RR, King BF. Invited Commentary. Radiographics. 2001;21:822-3.
16. Cowan NC, Turney BW, Taylor NJ, et al. Multidetector computed tomography urography for diagnosing upper urinary tract urothelial tumor. BJU Int. 2007;99;1363-70.
17. Palma DL. What is left of IV urography? Eur Radiol. 2001;11: 931-9.
18. Little MA, Johnson DBS, O'Callaghan JP, et al. The diagnostic yield of intravenous urography. Nephrol Dial Transplant. 2000;15:200-4.
19. Kass EJ, Kernen KM, Carey JM. Paediatric urinary tract infection and the necessity of complete urological imaging. BJU Int. 2000;86:94-6.
20. Riccabona M, Simbrunner J, Ring E, et al. Feasibility of MR urography in neonates and infants with anomalies of the upper urinary tract. Eur Radiol. 2002;12:1442-50.
21. Blandino A, Gaeta M, Minutoli F, et al. MR pyelography in 115 patients with a dilated renal collecting system. Acta Radiol. 2001;42:532-6.
22. Silverman SG, Leyendecker JR, Amis SE Jr. What is the current role of CT urography and MR urography in the evaluation of the urinary tract? Radiology. 2009;250: 309-23.
23. Namasivayam S, Small WC, Kalra MK, et al. Multidetector-row CT angiography for preoperative evaluation of potential laparoscopic renal donors: How accurate are we? Clin Imag. 2006;30:120-6.
24. Mushlin AI, Thornbury JR. Intravenous pyelography: The case against its routine use. Annals of Int Med. 1989;111:58-70.

CHAPTER 99

Ultrasound of Urogenital Tract: Techniques and Normal Appearances

Anju Garg

Ultrasonography is an indispensable modality for morphological evaluation of the urogenital tract. It is accurate, safe, does not require exposure to ionizing radiation or normal renal function for image production. With modern instrumentation, bedside sonography and guided procedures can be performed on even the most seriously ill patients.

KIDNEYS AND URETERS

Technique

A 3–5 MHz sector/linear transducer is used to scan the urinary tract. Although no specific preparation is required for scanning the kidneys, fasting optimises the visualization. Evaluation of the renal vessels is augmented by adequate patient hydration and a full bladder is essential for visualising the lower ureters, vesicoureteric junction and the bladder. The kidneys are scanned in the supine or lateral decubitus position. Varying the degree of respiration can help in complete evaluation of the kidneys. The left kidney is more difficult to visualize because gas in small bowel and splenic flexure interfere with the anterior or anterolateral approach. A posterolateral approach often gives a good visualization of left kidney. Scanning in prone position is rarely required in adults, except for renal guidance procedures, but in young children it remains a useful approach.

Some of the common indications for evaluating the upper urinary tract are:

- Evaluation of collecting system obstruction
- Evaluation of suspected or known nephrolithiasis
- Evaluation of cystic renal disease
- Detection of a renal or perirenal mass lesion
- Characterization of a renal mass lesion
- Guidance for diagnostic or therapeutic interventional procedures.

Normal Sonographic Appearance

The kidneys lie retroperitoneally on either side of the spine enclosed in fascial layers. The adult kidney is reniform in shape with a smooth outline. It is surrounded by a fibrous capsule which demarcates it from the surrounding perirenal fat. The cortex forms the outer part of renal parenchyma surrounding the medulla which is made up of renal pyramids arranged around the renal sinus **(Fig. 1)**.

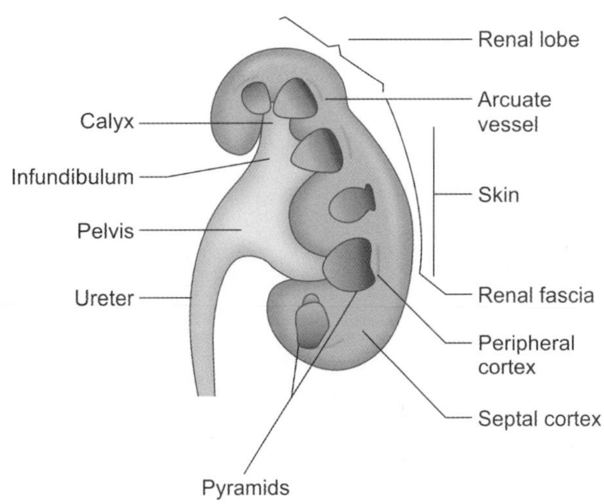

Fig. 1: Diagram depicting the normal sectional anatomy of kidney.

On sonography, the cortex has a fine homogeneous texture with a reflectivity less than that of the adjacent liver and spleen **(Figs. 2A and B)**, but the degree of differentiation is to some extent dependent on the equipment. However, if the renal cortex is brighter than the liver, it strongly suggests the presence of disease. Medullary pyramids are seen as echopoor oval areas evenly distributed around the inner margin of the cortex. Arcuate vessels mark the true corticomedullary junction and can be seen as punctuate echogenic foci **(Fig. 3A)** in approximately 25% of patients.[1] The **cortical thickness** is the distance between the capsule and the outer margin of the medullary pyramid while **parenchymal thickness** is the distance between the capsule and the margin of the sinus **(Fig. 3B)**. It is often easier and more consistent to measure the parenchymal thickness.

The renal sinus contains the calyces, infundibulum, a portion of the renal pelvis, fibrous tissue, fat, vessels and lymphatics. On US, the renal sinus appears as a central hyperechoic area, largely because of its fat content. When collapsed, the collecting system merges with the echoes of the renal sinus. However, in well-hydrated patients it may be slightly distended with echo free urine.

The **neonatal kidney** is sonographically more echogenic than that of the older infant and adults **(Fig. 4)**. Echogenicity is equal to or greater than the adjacent liver. It assumes the adult appearance by 2–3 months of age.[2] Other differences are tabulated in **Table 1**.

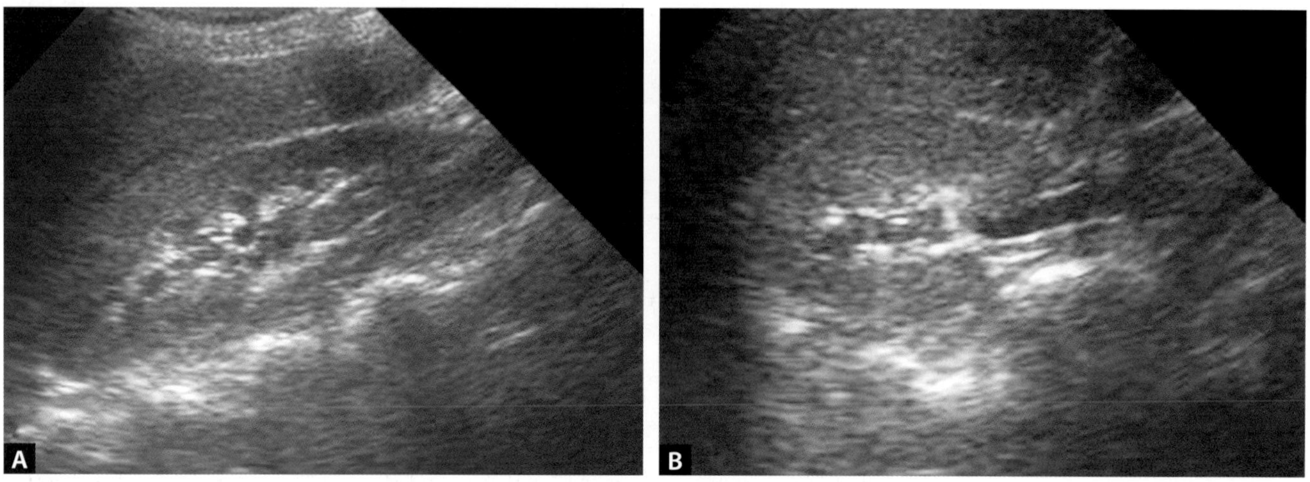

Figs. 2A and B: Normal kidney: (A) Sagittal view showing cortex and hypoechoic pyramids with bright central sinus echoes; (B) Transverse view at level of renal hilum.

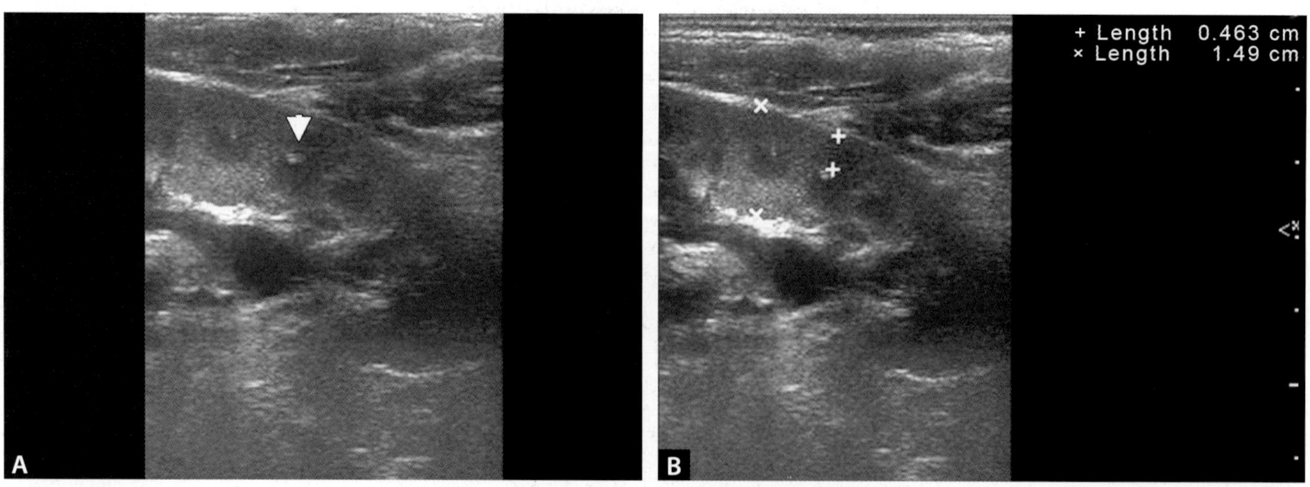

Figs. 3A and B: Corticomedullary differentiation. (A) Echogenic arcuate vessel (arrowhead) seen at corticomedullary junction; (B) Cortical thickness (++) and parenchymal thickness (××).

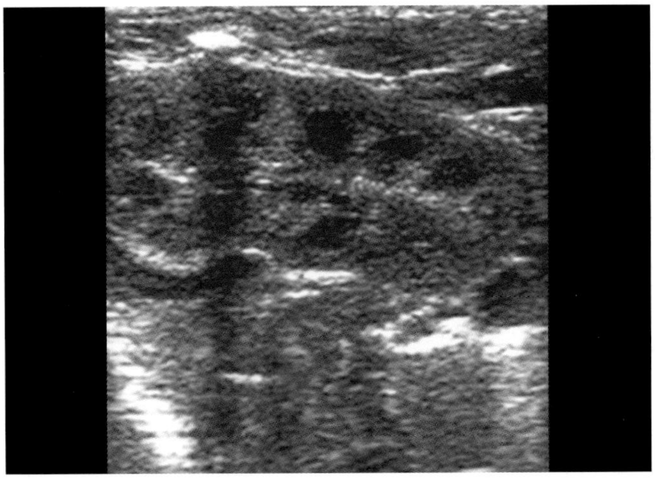

Fig. 4: Normal neonatal kidney. The cortex of the kidney is relatively thin and moderately reflective. The medullary pyramids appear disproportionately large and are very poorly reflective. Only minimal renal sinus structures are seen.

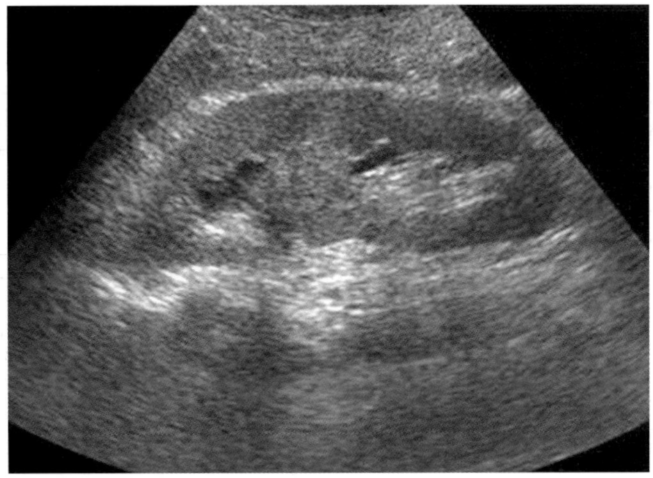

Fig. 5: Duplex collecting system. Sagittal sonogram shows central parenchyma separating the upper and lower moieties. There is mild dilatation of upper moiety.

Table 1: Differences between neonatal and adult kidney.

	Neonatal	*Adult*
Contour	Lobed	Smooth
Cortex reflectivity	++	+
Medullary reflectivity	–	–
Sinus	Echo poor	Echogenic
Collecting system	Apparent	Inapparent

Table 2: Normal kidney length in adults (cm).

	Adult female	*Adult male*
Left kidney	11 (9.9–12.1)	11.5 (10.4–12.6)
Right kidney	10.7 (9.5–12)	11.2 (10.1–12.4)

The determination of renal size with US is more accurate than with intravenous urography because the kidney is imaged without magnification and contrast induced osmotic diuresis. As a result renal size is approximately 15% smaller**.** Renal size is related to sex, age and built of the patient. The length of the normal adult kidney is usually 10–12 cm but can range from 7 to 14 cm in patients with normal renal function **(Table 2)**. Length can also vary in the same individual depending on the state of hydration.

On sonography the longest cranio-caudal length is imaged by rotating the probe around its vertical axis.[3] Care must be taken to measure the longest length as it is easy to get a false low measurement due to the ellipsoid shape of the kidney. For more accurate measurement of renal size, a renal volume assessment can be made, either by measuring the area of kidney in serial slices and subsequently calculating the volume or by using the modified 3D ellipsoid formula. The precise value is probably not as important as consistency so that changes in volume over a period of time can be measured. Emamian et al.[4] measured the renal size in 665 healthy adult volunteers and showed that the parenchymal volume of the right kidney is smaller than the left. Possible explanation for this could be as follows: (1) The spleen is smaller than the liver and so there is more space for left kidney growth and (2) The left renal artery is shorter than the right and therefore, increased blood flow on the left results in an increase in renal volume.

Normal Variations

The kidneys may vary in **position** due to ptosis or an ectopic location. The most common site for the ectopic kidney is the pelvis, where it may be difficult to detect, as it can be obscured by bowel gas. **Renal duplication** is common and spans a range from complete to minimal. However, sonography may only show an elongated kidney perhaps with separation of the renal sinus into two parts **(Fig. 5)**. A double pelvis may be visualised when the collecting system is distended. Residual **fetal lobulations** may be seen. A **dromedary hump** can be seen sometimes which is a bulge along the lateral border of the left kidney due to moulding by the adjacent spleen **(Fig. 6)**.

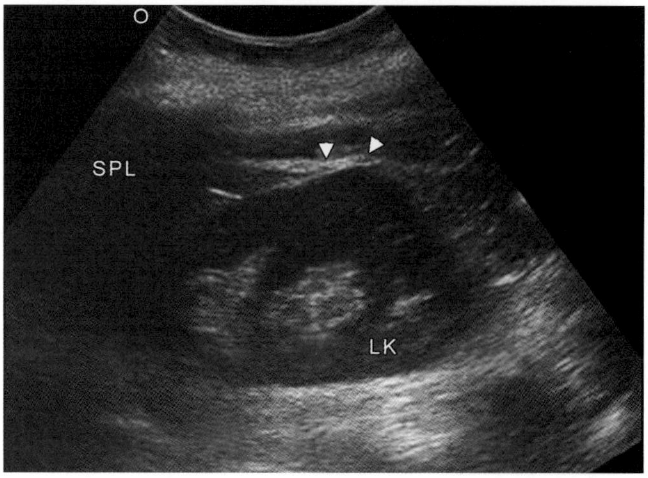

Fig. 6: Dromedary hump seen as a focal bulge along the lateral aspect of the left kidney (arrowheads).

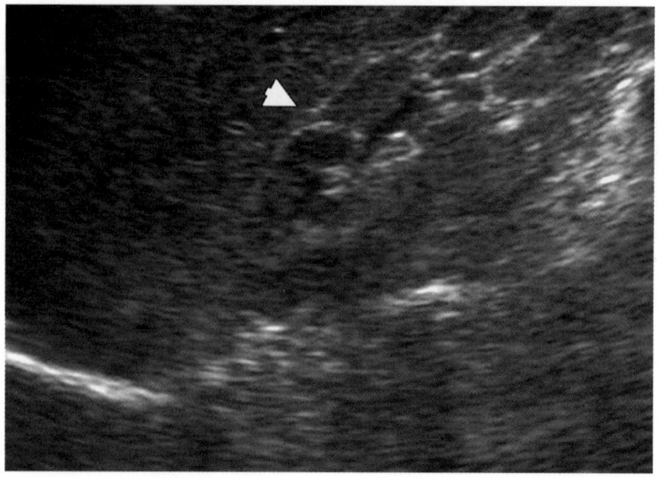

Fig. 7: Anterior junction line. Sagittal sonogram demonstrating the echogenic line (arrowhead) that extends from the renal sinus to the perinephric fat.

A **hypertrophied column of Bertin** is a normal variant and represents unresorbed polar parenchyma from one or both of the 2 subkidneys that fuse to form the normal kidney.[5] Sonographic criteria to diagnose a hypertrophied column of Bertini include isoechogenicity and continuity with rest of the renal cortex, lack of mass effect, indentation of renal sinus laterally, generally less than 3 cm in size with a normal vascular pattern on Doppler. Occasionally it may be difficult to differentiate a small avascular tumour from a hypertrophied column of Bertini when further investigations maybe required.

A wedge-shaped echogenic defect or an echogenic line, the **intervesicular fissure or parenchymal junctional defect**, may sometimes be seen running obliquely from the sinus to the capsule in upper anterior or lower posterior part of the kidney **(Fig. 7)**. It was thought to represent connective tissue at the junction of the development of anterior and posterior components of the kidney. However, subsequent reassessment suggests that this line represents an extension into the parenchyma of hilar/sinus fat in patients with a deep renal sinus, rather than a true plane of fusion between embryological components.[6] It may mimic a scar or rarely a small echogenic tumor.

The **renal sinus thickness** is normally equal to the parenchymal thickness. However, it may vary depending on the fat content of the sinus. An increase in fat content of the renal sinus can occur in obese individuals, in renal sinus lipomatosis, and in cases of parenchymal atrophy. It is decreased in neonates and in cachectic patients.

A mild distension of the collecting system can occur due to physiological filling. This can be seen in a fluid loaded subject,a patient on diuretics, diabetics, recovery phase of acute tubular necrosis, single kidney, neonatal kidney and patients with an overdistended bladder.

Doppler Evaluation

The renal arteries arise from the aorta, slightly below the origin of the superior mesenteric artery. The right renal artery (RRA) arises from the anterolateral aspect of the aorta and then passes posterior to the IVC as it courses towards the right renal hilum. The left renal artery (LRA) arises from the lateral or posterolateral aspect of the aorta and follows a posterolateral course to the left renal hilum. Accessory renal arteries may arise from the aorta in as many as 20% individuals, either superior or inferior to the main renal artery. The renal arteries typically divide into anterior and posterior divisions that lie anterior and posterior to the renal pelvis, respectively. These divisions give rise to the segmental arteries which branch further within the renal sinus, forming interlobar arteries that penetrate the renal parenchyma. These terminate in arcuate arteries that curve around the corticomedullary junction giving rise to cortical branches.

Each renal vein is formed from tributaries that coalesce in the renal hilum. The left renal vein passes anterior to the aorta and posterior to SMA, to enter the left side of IVC. The right renal vein, which is shorter, extends directly to the IVC from the right renal hilum.

Technique

With the patient supine, the RRA can be identified arising approximately 1 cm below the origin of the SMA. Occasionally, LRA can be identified at its origin from the posterolateral or lateral surface of aorta. Both renal veins and their junction with the IVC can usually be demonstrated in this plane. In slim patients it is occasionally possible to follow the renal artery and vein into the hilum of the kidney. The right and left posterior oblique positions can also be used to identify the vessels in the midline. Throughout the course of examination of renal vessels, colour Doppler is frequently switched on to confirm the nature and direction of flow. The optimum pulse repetition frequency is selected to detect moderate flow velocities, although it may need to be modified to detect high velocities if a stenosis with aliasing of colour signals is present. With the system set to detect low or moderate flow velocities, flow can be identified in almost all patients in the vessels at the renal hilum. Angling of the probe medially from the right or left flank will allow assessment of the intrarenal vessels. Though the hilar and interlobar vessels are demonstrated in all patients, the arcuate and striate arteries may be seen only in slimmer patients. Power doppler can show smaller vessels with slow flow, though with loss of directional information **(Fig. 8)**. The use of ultrasound contrast material can further enhance visualization of parenchymal vessels.

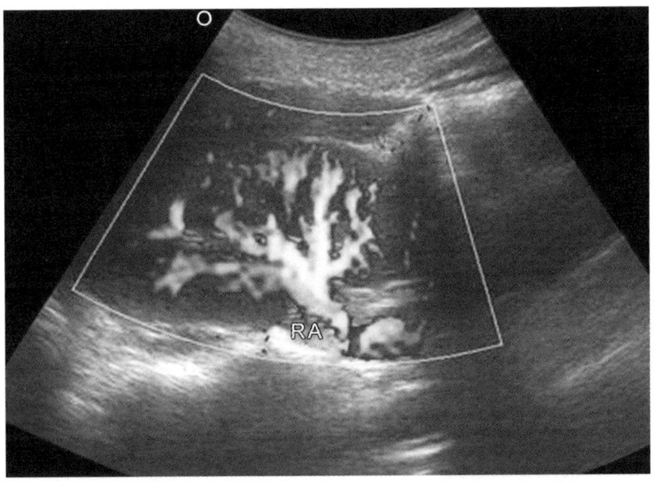

Fig. 8: Power Doppler image of the renal vasculature.
Abbreviations: RA: Renal artery.

Normal Doppler Pattern

The typical spectral pattern of the renal artery is shown in **Figure 9A**. There is a rapid systolic upstroke, which is occasionally followed by a secondary slower rise to peak systole. Subsequently there is a gradual diastolic decay but with persistent forward flow in diastole.[7] Spectral indices are measured in the renal artery at proximal, middle and at the hilum. Normal range of values is shown in **Table 3**. Further, indices should also be measured in the intrarenal vessels at the superior, middle and inferior pole of the kidney. The RI and PI values measured in healthy subjects show a significant dependence on age and the area sampled. The values in the main artery are higher than in the more distal smaller arteries and they are lowest in the interlobular arteries **(Fig. 9B)**.

Table 3: Normal renal indices[7].

Index	*Range*
Pulsatility index (PI)	0.7–1.4
Resistance index (RI)	0.56–0.7
Peak systolic velocity (PSV)	60–140 cm/sec (<180)
Renal artery/aorta ratio (RAR)	<3.5
Acceleration time	0.04–0.05 sec
Acceleration index	2.5–3.8 m/sec^2

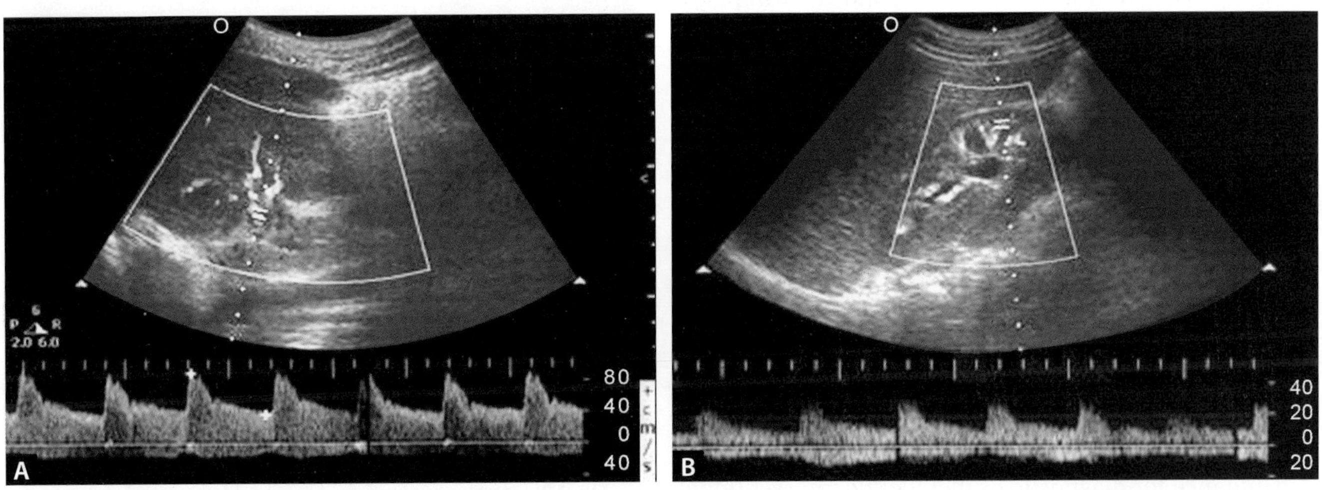

Figs. 9A and B: (A) Normal renal spectral pattern. The normal renal artery spectral waveform shows a steep systolic peak and a smooth downslope to diastole; (B) Spectral waveform in an intrarenal vessel showing lower velocities.

The renal vein spectra are often different for right and left veins. The RRV is short and often mirrors the pulsatility of the IVC, while the left, particularly if it is sampled to the left of the SMA, may show only slight variability of flow velocities.

Indications

- Renovascular hypertension
- Characterisation of mass lesions.
- Differentiation between obstructive and nonobstructive hydronephrosis
- Evaluation of transplant kidney
- Renal vein thrombosis
- Miscellaneous, e.g. trauma, AVM, etc.

Ureters

The ureter is a long (30–34 cm) mucosal lined tube varying in diameter from 2–8 mm.[8] The normal ureters are usually difficult to visualise as they are thin, collapsed structures. However, dilated ureters can be imaged in their proximal and distal parts. The proximal ureters are best visualised in a coronal oblique view, using the kidney as a window. An attempt can be made to follow the ureter upto the bladder using the same approach. The distal ureters can be seen suprapubically through the full bladder.

URINARY BLADDER AND URETHRA

Technique

Examination of the bladder necessitates a well filled bladder for its detailed evaluation and for the study of entire pelvic cavity. The urinary bladder is scanned transabdominally using 3–5 MHz transducers or transperineally using 7–10 MHz transducers. Endocavitary high frequency probes (transrectal/transurethral) can give excellent detail of the bladder wall. The full bladder and postmicturition residual volume can be calculated using the formula for a prolate ellipsoid (0.523 × length × width × height).

Common **indications** for sonography of the lower urinary tract are as follows:

- Determination of the existence and rate of urine flow through the vesicoureteric junction in patients with dilated ureters
- Determination of pre- and post-void bladder volume
- Detection of bladder calculi or mass
- Detection and quantification of bladder wall thickening
- Guidance for diagnostic or therapeutic interventional procedures

Normal Sonographic Appearance

The normal distended bladder is an anechoic structure occupying the midline of the true pelvis. It is triangular in the sagittal plane and oval in the transaxial plane. It has thin walls (less than 3 mm in the distended state and 5–6 mm when nondistended), which are regular and smooth. The ureteric orifices appear as small focal thickenings of the bladder base. Transabdominal evaluation of the ureteral jets is helpful to assess for any proximal obstruction. On grayscale, a stream of low level echoes can be seen entering the bladder from the ureteric orifice. Density differences between the jet and bladder urine allow its sonographic visualization.[9] Doppler evaluation improves the detection of ureteric jets **(Fig. 10)**. Depending on the state of hydration, the jet frequency may vary from less than 1 per minute to continuous flow; however, both sides should be symmetrical in a healthy individual. Detection of these jets excludes complete ureteric obstruction and establishes renal function.

Transrectal and transurethral scanning can evaluate the layers of the bladder wall and evaluate the extent of a mass lesion through tissue planes in and around the urinary bladder. Guidance for biopsy can also be better provided with endocavitary probes.

Urethra

The posterior male urethra can be best evaluated by the endorectal route. Penile urethra can be visualised through the penile shaft using a 7–10 MHz linear probe after filling the penile urethra with gel or fluid. The normal penile urethra is seen as an anechoic tubular structure when distended.

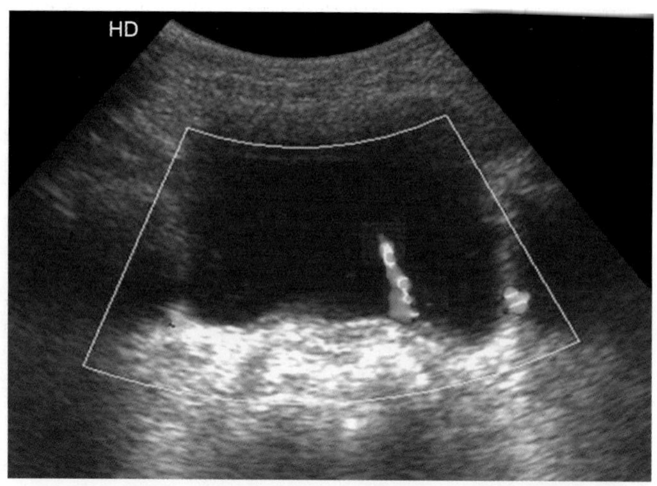

Fig. 10: Doppler evaluation showing a left ureteric jet on a transverse sonogram of the urinary bladder.

The female urethra can be visualized on transabdominal scanning in 35% of the patients and in 100% of the patients with a catheter in place. It can also be well identified in all patients by translabial or endovaginal scanning with the probe placed at the introitus or just partially inserted into the vagina. It is seen throughout its length as a short anechoic channel **(Fig. 11)**.

PROSTATE AND SEMINAL VESICLES

Technique

The prostate and seminal vesicles can be examined sonographically via the transabdominal (TAS) and the transurethral (TRUS) routes. Transabdominally, a 3–5 MHz sector probe is used with the full bladder acting as an acoustic window. The prostate is visualized posterior to the bladder in both axial and sagittal planes. A 5–7.5 MHz specially designed probe with a multiplanar facility is used for TRUS. The most commonly used commercially available probes fire from the end and can be used for both transrectal and transvaginal imaging. The bladder should be empty and a cleansing enema may be given. The patient is examined in the left lateral decubitus position with the knees flexed. The probe is lubricated and covered by a rubber balloon or condom. It is then inserted gently into the rectum. Sagittal and axial scans are obtained by rotating the probe through 90°.

In the sagittal plane, the gland is systematically surveyed from right to midline to left; while in the axial plane, cranial to caudal viewing is done from a plane just superior to the prostate (showing the seminal vesicles) to the apex of the prostate caudally.

Prostatic volume can be calculated on TAS and TRUS by using the prolate ellipsoid formula (0.523 × length × width × height). The volume measured can be converted to weight because the specific gravity of prostatic tissue is 1, thus 1 mL of prostate tissue is equal to 1 gram.

The presence of anal or rectal strictures or advanced rectal carcinoma may disallow the transrectal method. In these cases transperineal evaluation approach can be used. However, it is compromised by beam scattering artifacts. A transurethral route has also been used to visualize the prostate. It needs specially designed probes and is an invasive technique.

Common **Indications** for sonograhic evaluation of the prostate are:

- To quantify prostate volume
- Assessment of a palpable nodule
- Evaluation of infertile patients
- Guided prostatic biopsy.

Normal Sonographic Appearance

The normal prostate gland is shaped like a pyramid and lies posteroinferior to the bladder **(Fig. 12)**. The base of the prostate lies adjacent to the bladder and apex adjacent to the membranous urethra. It measures approximately 4 cm in length (cephalocaudal), 4 cm in transverse diameter and 3 cm in height (anteroposterior); the normal volume (weight) ranges from 20–25 mL (g). The border of the prostate appears sharply defined, except at the posterolateral margins where the neurovascular structure enters the prostate gland.

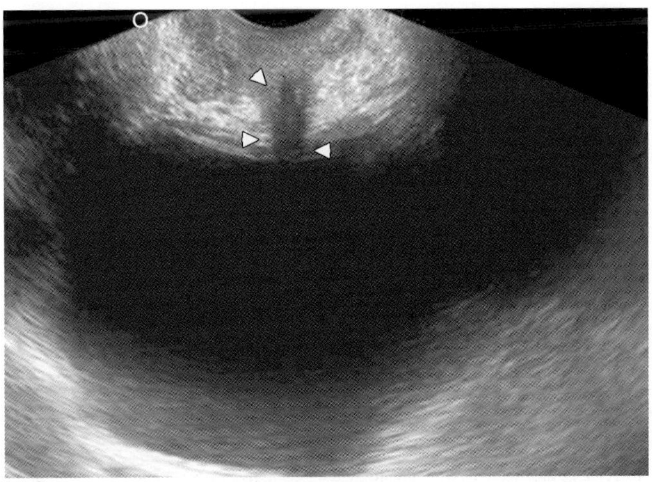

Fig. 11: Translabial ultrasound of the female urethra showing the hypoechoic tubular urethra (arrowheads) extending from the bladder.

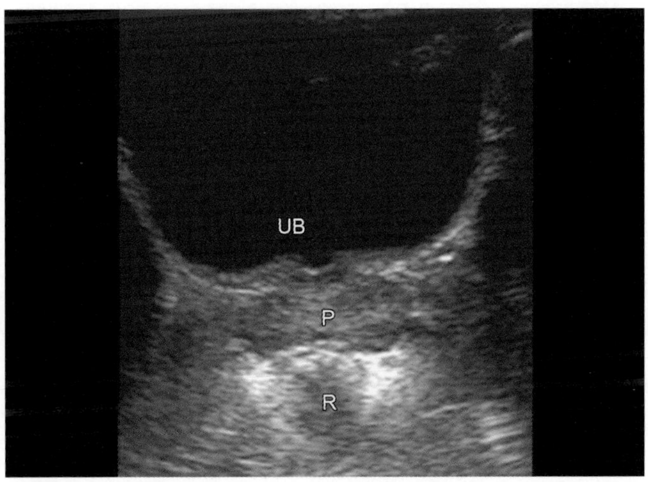

Fig. 12: Normal prostate. Transabdominal axial scan shows the prostate (P) between the urinary bladder (UB) and the rectum (R).

The prostate glandular structure can be divided into three zones, peripheral, transition and central **(Fig. 13)**. More than 80% of prostate cancers arise in the peripheral zone (PZ), which contain 70% of the prostate glandular elements. The central zone surrounds the ejaculatory ducts and is the site of the primary lesion in less than 10% of cases. The transition zone (TZ), the site of development of benign prostatic hyperplasia (BPH), contains 10% of the glandular elements (although up to 80% in cases of BPH) and is the site of origin for less than 20% of prostate cancers.

On TRUS, axial scans show the gland as a homogeneous bean shaped structure with well defined margins. It is often difficult to distinguish the PZ from the inner gland in a young male. In older men, with benign prostatic hyperplasia (BPH), the surgical capsule becomes more evident as a thin hypoechoic line between the PZ and inner gland **(Figs. 14A and B)**. The PZ is more uniform

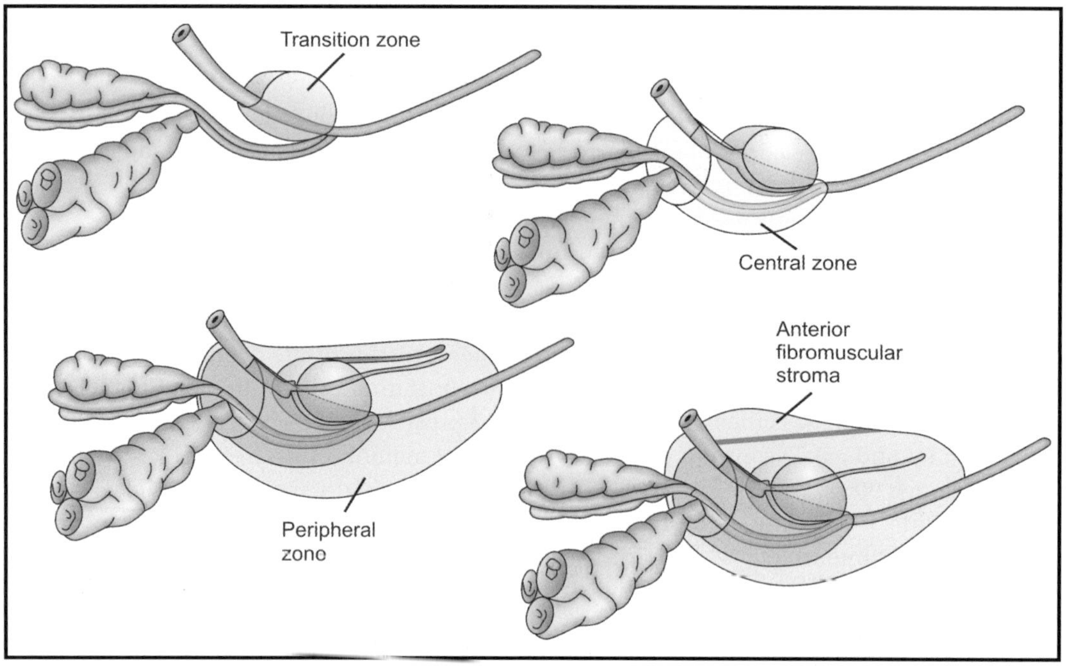

Fig. 13: Zonal anatomy of prostate.

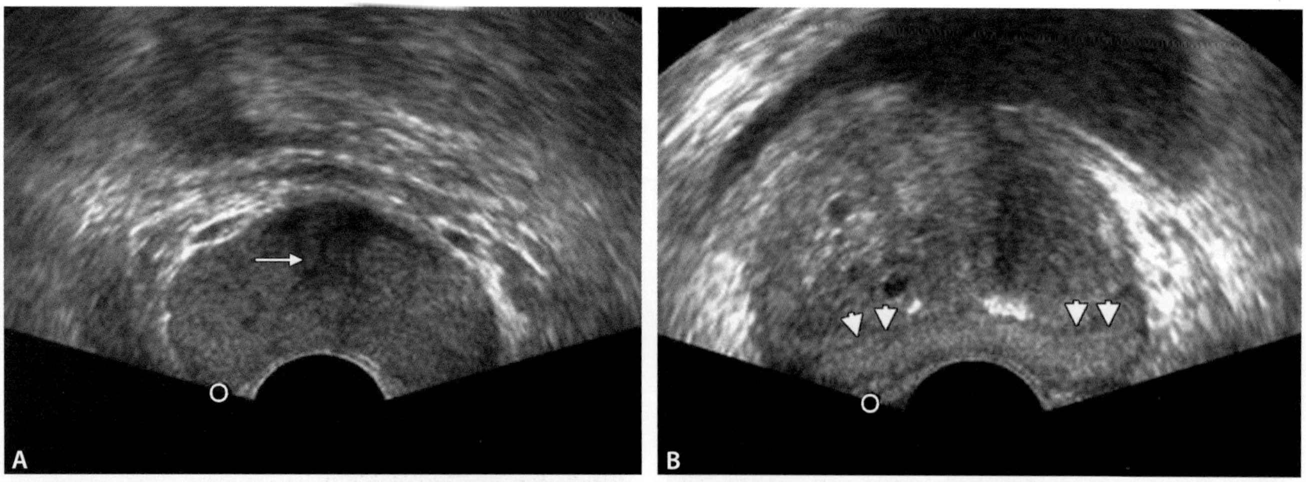

Figs. 14A and B: Transrectal axial sonograms of prostate at midgland level. (A) In a young male note the normal hypoechoic muscular internal sphincter (arrow); (B) In an older male with BPH. The more echogenic PZ is seen posteriorly compressed by the anterior enlarged TZ. The surgical capsule (arrowheads) is well seen as a thin hypoechoic line between PZ and TZ.

in texture and slightly more echogenic. This echogenicity is taken as the standard and echogenicity in other areas of the gland is compared to that of the PZ.[10] The posterior urethra and its surrounding smooth muscle and glandular area appear relatively hypoechoic and can be quite prominent measuring upto 2 cm in diameter. The urethra and ejaculatory ducts may be identified. At the level of verumontanum, the ejaculatory ducts and urethra merge. Near the apex of the gland most of the tissue is the peripheral zone.

In the sagittal plane, the most parasagittal images of the gland show only PZ tissue with uniform echotexture in young men. With BPH, the transition zone may extend laterally, compressing the PZ posteriorly. At the base of the gland, the seminal vesicles immediately adjoin the central and peripheral zones. In the midsagittal section the collapsed urethra is seen as an echogenic line surrounded by the hypoechoic smooth muscle forming the internal urethral sphincter. The ejaculatory ducts can be seen coursing through the CZ from the seminal vesicles and joining the urethra at the verumontanum.

With color **Doppler**, particularly using the power mode, the prostate is seen as a very vascular structure. The capsular and urethral arteries are easily seen, and branches to the inner gland and peripheral zone are usually very prominent.

The **seminal vesicles** are seen as paired, relatively hypoechoic, symmetric structures cephalad to the base of the prostate **(Fig. 15)**. They are imaged in the long axis on the axial images and in cross-section on sagittal images. They are up to 1 cm in width, but occasionally they may be very large in normal men.[11] Cysts representing the remnants of the Wolffian and Müllerian ducts are not uncommon in this region.

Normal Variants

Benign ductal ectasia is seen in older men due to atrophy and dilatation of peripheral prostatic ducts. They are seen either singly or grouped, radially oriented, 1–2 mm in diameter, tubular structures in the peripheral zone, starting at the capsule and radiating towards the urethra.[10] Their significance lies in that they can be mistaken for a cancerous lesion.

Prostatic calcification and corpora amylacea are frequently seen in the older age group of patients as bright echogenic foci or areas in the prostate. Corpora amylacea are proteinaceous debris in dilated prostatic ducts and are most commonly seen in the periurethral glands along the surgical capsule **(Fig. 16)**, but can occur anywhere in the prostatic gland. They can be very dense, thus causing marked attenuation of the sound beam. However, they are usually not palpable.

SCROTUM

Technique

A high frequency (7.5–15 MHz) linear array transducer is used to scan the scrotum. The examination is done with the patient in supine position, thighs are adducted and a towel or sheet is placed underneath the scrotum and held taut. This supports the scrotum and eases the examination. Alternatively, the scrotal sac maybe supported by the examiner's hand. Palpation prior to and during scanning is useful specially if a small mass is suspected. The scrotum

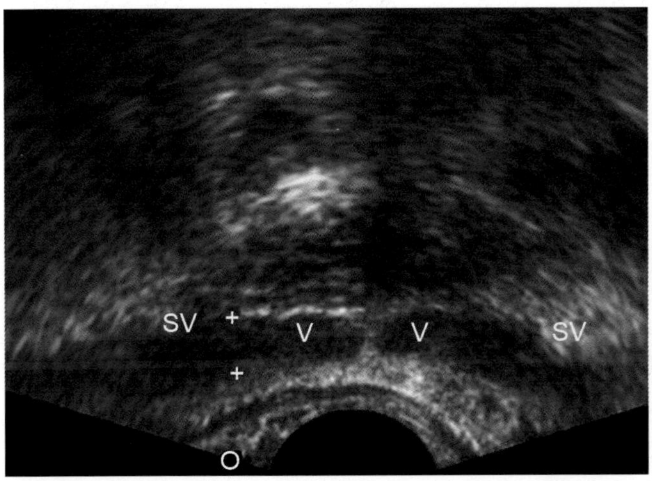

Fig. 15: Transrectal ultrasound (TRUS): Axial image above base of prostate showing the seminal vesicles (SV) and vas (V).

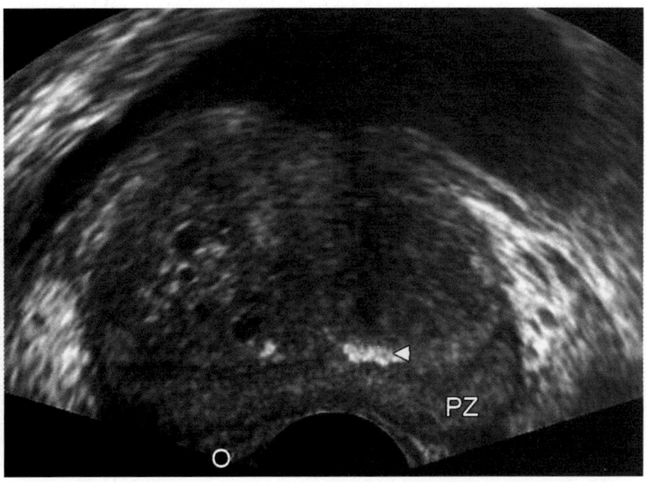

Fig. 16: Corpora amylacea seen as echogenic foci (arrowhead) just anterior to the surgical capsule.

is scanned by direct contact after application of a suitable gel. Both testes are visualized in the transverse and sagittal planes. If possible, a transverse scan showing both testes for comparison should be obtained using a dual image or extended field of view technique. Scanning from the opposite side helps in identification of small lesions.

Normal Appearances

The testis is an ovoid organ measuring 3–5 cm in length, 2–4 cm in width and 3 cm in anteroposterior diameter. Each testis weighs 12.5–19 g. Testicular size and weight decrease with age.[12,13] It is surrounded by a dense fibrous capsule, the tunica albuginea. It comprises of 200–300 lobules separated by thin septae **(Fig. 17)**. Seminiferous tubules from each lobule converge into large collecting tubules and form the rete testis adjacent to the mediastinum (which is a longitudinal condensation of fibrous tissue on one side of the testis). Efferent ductules from the rete testis exit the testis over its upper half to form the epididymis. The epididymis lies closely applied to the testis in the long axis with two expansions–the head at the upper pole and the tail at the lower pole. The vas, a tubular structure, is a continuation of the epididymal tail and runs upwards from the lower pole parallel to the epididymis to form the spermatic cord. The cord, testis and epididymis are enveloped by a thin membrane, the tunica vaginalis, which is reflected back onto the scrotal wall posteriorly.

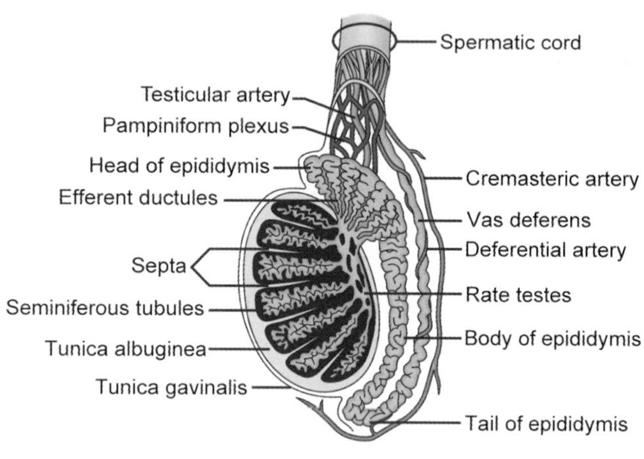

Fig. 17: Normal intrascrotal anatomy.
Source: Sudakoff GS, Quiroz F, Kaarcaaltincaba M, Foley WD. Scrotal ultrsonography with emphasis on the extratesticular space: Anatomy, embryology and pathology. Ultrasound Quarterly 2002;18:255-73.

Sonographically, the **testis** is seen as an organ of homogeneous granular echotexture with medium level echoes surrounded by an echogenic capsule **(Fig. 18A)**. The mediastinum is seen as a thin echogenic band on the same side as the epididymis with fine hypoechoic strands of septa radiating from it into the testicular parenchyma. The appearance of the medistinum testis varies according to the amount of fibrous and fatty tissue present. It is best visualsed between the ages of 15-60 years.[13] The **epididymis** is of varying reflectivity with the head being isoechoic or slightly hyperechoic to the adjacent testis, measuring approximately 10–12 mm in diameter and lying lateral to the superior pole of the testis, while the main body is hypoechoic measuring less than 4 mm in diameter and lies along the posterolateral aspect of testis.[14] The tail, appendix epididymis and appendix testis are most often identified sonographically as separate structures when a hydrocele is present. The **appendix testis**, a remnant

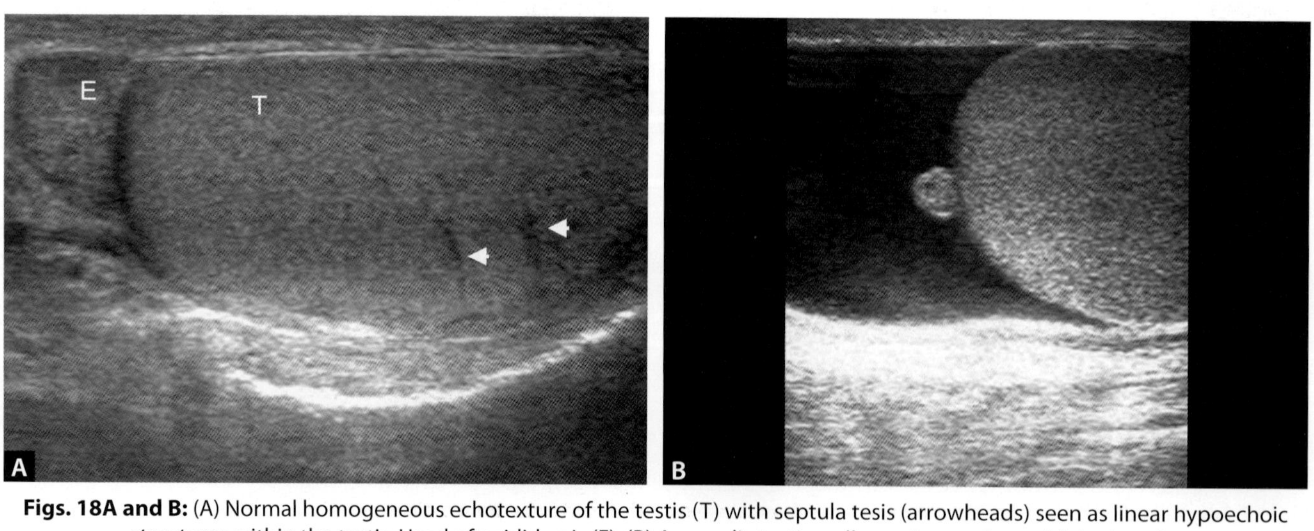

Figs. 18A and B: (A) Normal homogeneous echotexture of the testis (T) with septula tesis (arrowheads) seen as linear hypoechoic structures within the testis. Head of epididymis (E); (B) Appendix testis well seen in a patient with hydrocele.

of the paramesonephric duct is a small ovoid structure located most commonly on the superior pole of the testis **(Fig. 18B)** or in the groove between the testis and the head of the epididymis and is seen in almost 80% of testes.[15]

The **vas** is more difficult to identify, but may be seen as a fine hypoechoic tubular structure with a hyperechoic lumen running along the epididymis. The **spermatic cord** consists of the vas deferens; the cremasteric, deferential and testicular arteries; a pampiniform plexus of veins; the lymphatics and the nerves of the testis. Sonographically, the normal spermatic cord is difficult to distinguish from the adjacent soft tissues of the inguinal canal, but its position can be identified by the pulsations of the testicular artery within it.

The **scrotal sac** is composed of several layers that are derived from the skin, abdominal wall muscles and the peritoneum (tunica vaginalis). The **tunica vaginalis** is derived from the peritoneum and is a closed pouch folded around the testis. The inner or visceral layer of the tunica vaginalis covers the testis, epididymis and the lower portion of the spermatic cord, while the outer or parietal layer lines the walls of the scrotal pouch and is attached to fascial coverings of the testis. A small amount of fluid is normally present between these two layers, specially in the polar regions and between the epididymis and testis. Sonographically, the layers of the normal scrotal wall cannot be identified separately and are seen as a 5–7 mm thick hyperechoic stripe.

Indications

- Evaluation of acute scrotal pain
- Evaluation of scrotal enlargement
- Evaluation of infertility
- Localization of undescended testis
- Evaluation of scrotal trauma
- Detection of occult tumor in patients with known metastases.

Doppler Evaluation

The main arterial supply to the testis is from the testicular artery which arises from the mid abdominal aorta and passes into the scrotum via the inguinal canal along with cremasteric artery and deferential artery. The testicular artery forms a network of capsular branches over the testis which pass through the tunica albuginea and form another network in the testicular substance. The pampiniform plexus of draining veins is formed around the upper half of the testis. This drains into the testicular vein. The right testicular vein drains into the IVC, while the left drains into the left renal vein.

On color Doppler, the normal testis shows little flow in the testicular tissue, but larger centripetal and centrifugal vessels are seen in the lobular septa and around the capsule. A prominent transmediastinal artery may sometimes be seen traversing the testis. The velocity waveforms of the normal capsular and intratesticular arteries show high levels of antegrade diastolic flow throughout the cardiac cycle, reflecting the low vascular resistance of the testis **(Fig. 19)**. In a study of normal subjects, peak systolic flow velocities in intratesticular arteries, including capsular arteries, ranged from 4 to 23.4 cm/sec (mean 10.8), end-diastolic velocities ranged from 1.6 to 9.2 cm/sec (mean 3.8) and RI from 0.46 to 0.78 (mean 0.64).[16] Supratesticular arterial waveforms vary in appearance. Two main types of waveform exist: A low resistance waveform (testicular artery and its branches) and a high resistance waveform with a sharp, narrow systolic peak and little or no diastolic flow which is believed to reflect the high vascular resistance of the extratesticular tissues (branches of cremasteric and deferential arteries). The pampiniform venous plexus is seen as a network of venous channels (less than 2 mm in width) around the upper half of the testis, generally on the same side as the epididymis and vas.

Indications

- Testicular inflammation—acute and chronic
- Testicular torsion
- Varicocele
- Testicular tumors.

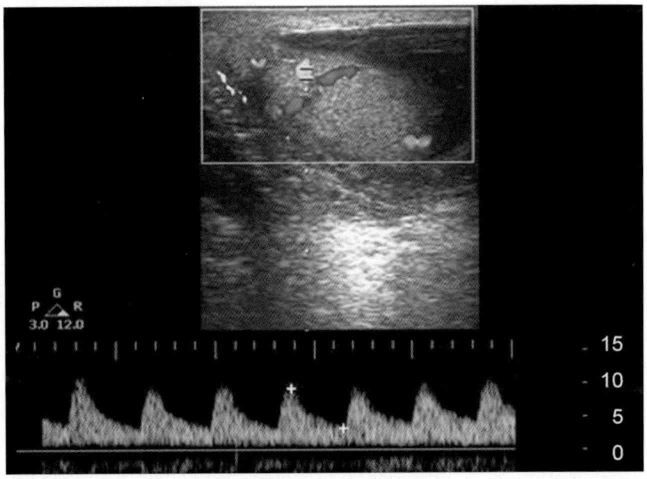

Fig. 19: Spectral waveform of the testicular artery showing typical low impedance flow.

PENIS

Technique and Normal Appearance

Sonographic examination of the penis is performed with the patient in the supine position, with the penis lying on the anterior abdominal or supported with towels between the thighs, using a high frequency (7.5–15 MHz) linear array transducer. Examination is performed in transverse and longitudinal planes, starting at the level of the glans and moving towards the base of the penis. A transperineal approach maybe used to assess the base of the penis.

The penis contains three longitudinal columns of erectile tissue: the paired dorsal corpora cavernosa and the ventral corpus spongiosum. The urethra passes through the corpus spongiosum. The deep cavernosal arteries run centrally through the length of each corpus cavernosum with dorsal arteries lying superficially. The dorsal vein of the penis lies between the two dorsal arteries.

The corpora cavernosa are seen as two circular structures adjacent to each other, of medium echogenicity with the deep arteries lying medially within them on the transverse section **(Fig. 20)**. The normal cavernosal artery diameter ranges from 0.3–1 mm (mean 0.3–0.5 mm),[17] with a peak systolic velocity of 10–15 cm/sec in the flaccid state.[18] The corpus spongiosum is often compressed and is difficult to visualize optimally from the ventral aspect. It is more hypoechoic with the urethra seen as an anechoic central area within it. The tunica albuginea is seen as a hyperechoic capsule surrounding the periphery of the corporal structures.

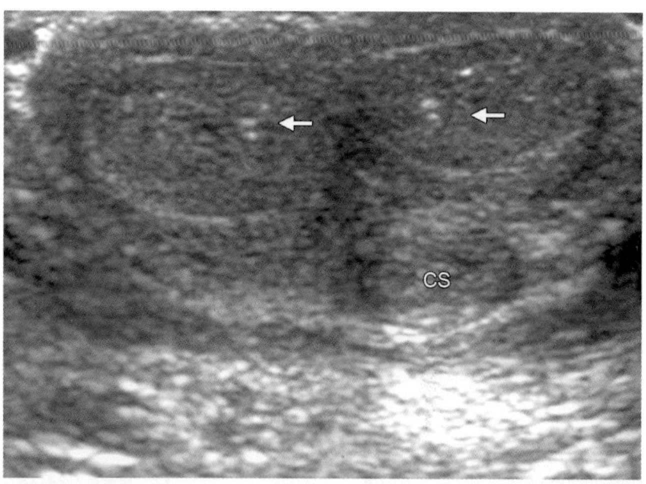

Fig. 20: Normal penile sonogram. Transverse section through the mid shaft shows the paired dorsal corpora cavernosa and the ventral corpus spongiosum (CS). The deep arteries are seen as echogenic foci in the corpora cavernosa (arrows).

Indications

- Penile masses
- Trauma
- Urethral strictures
- Peyronie's disease
- Impotence.

UTERUS AND ADNEXA

Technique

Sonographic evaluation of the uterus and the adnexa can be done by the transbdominal (TAS) and transvaginal (TVS) routes. They are complementary techniques and both are used extensively in evaluation of the female pelvis. The **transabdominal** scan is performed with 3.5–5 MHz sector transducer, with a full bladder as an essential prerequisite. The urinary bladder is considered adequately full when it covers the entire fundus of the uterus. Overdistension is to be avoided as it may distort the anatomy and may push the pelvic organs beyond the focal zone of the transducer.

Imaging of the uterus is performed in both sagittal and axial planes. The adnexa are imaged by scanning obliquely from the contralateral side, although in many cases good visualization may be achieved by scanning directly over the adnexa.

The limitations of this technique are as follows:
- Patients unable to fill the bladder
- Patients with retroverted uterus in whom fundus may be beyond the focal zone of the transducer
- Limited resolution.

Transvaginal scanning affords improved resolution of the pelvic organs. Specially designed probes of 5–8 MHz frequency are used for this procedure. The bladder should be empty. However, a minimal distension may be required if the uterus is severely anteflexed.

The patient is positioned supine with the knees flexed and hips slightly elevated. The probe is prepared as for TRUS and inserted gently into the vagina till the uterus is identified. The uterus is imaged in its longitudinal axis, first sweeping from left to right. Short axis images are then obtained. The relative position of the uterus can be inferred by the orientation of the probe that best images the uterus, e.g. if the uterus is best imaged with a posterior inclination, the uterus is retroflexed and vice versa. For imaging the cervix, the transducer should be withdrawn to the mid vaginal level.

The ovaries are imaged by tilting the transducer to either side of the midline in the transverse section. The internal iliac vessels can be identified as anechoic tubular structures along the pelvic side walls. The ovaries usually lie anterior and medial to these vessels.

Limitations of this technique are as follows:
- Limited field of view
- Vaginal atrophy may disallow examination.

Normal Appearances

The uterus lies between the bladder anteriorly and rectosigmoid posteriorly **(Fig. 21)**. Its size and shape vary throughout life related to age, hormonal status and parity. The infantile or prepubertal uterus has an inverse pear-shaped appearance with a disproportionately larger cervix occupying up-to one-half to two-thirds the size of the uterus **(Fig. 22)**. In the immediate neonatal period the uterus is slightly larger and shows an echogenic endometrium, because of residual maternal hormonal stimulation. A small amount of endometrial fluid may also be seen in 25% of neonatal uteri.[19] There is little growth of the prepubertal uterus from infancy till about 8 years of age when the uterus gradually increases in size till puberty when it attains a pear-shaped appearance with the body of the uterus becoming approximately double the cervix. The normal postpubertal or adult uterus varies considerably in size. The maximal dimensions of the nulliparous uterus are approximately 8 cm in length by 5 cm in width and 4 cm in AP diameter. Parity increases the normal dimensions by more than 1 cm in each dimension[20] **(Table 4)**. After menopause the uterus atrophies with the most rapid decrease in size occurring in the first ten years following the cessation of menstruation.

The uterus usually assumes a position that is both anteverted and anteflexed **(Fig. 23)**. The degree of bladder filling alters the lie of the uterus; on transvaginal scanning with an empty bladder the uterus is angled forwards from the lie of the vagina, whereas a full bladder straightens the uterus. In case of retroverted or retroflexed uterus, the fundus lies posteriorly. It is often not possible to distinguish between retroversion and retroflexion on sonography so the general term retroposition is used. On transabdominal scanning the deeper portions of the fundus may be difficult to delineate and may even appear abnormal because of shadowing from the intervening body and cervix. Transvaginal scanning gives an excellent visualization of the retropositioned uterus as the probe can be directed posteriorly.[21]

The uterus consists of an external serosa (perimetrium), a middle muscle layer (myometrium) and the internal mucosa (endometrium). The perimetrium is not visible on ultrasound examination, although subserosal veins may be seen as a normal variant. On sonography the myometrium has three layers. The inner myometrium (or the subendometrial halo) appears as a thin hypoechoic area surrounding the echogenic

Table 4: Uterine size.

	Length (cm)	*Width (cm)*	*AP diameter (cm)*
Neonates	2.3–4.6		0.8–2.1
2–11 years	2–4	–	0.5–1
Adult	8–9	5–6	4–5
Postmenopausal	3.5–6.5		1.2–1.8

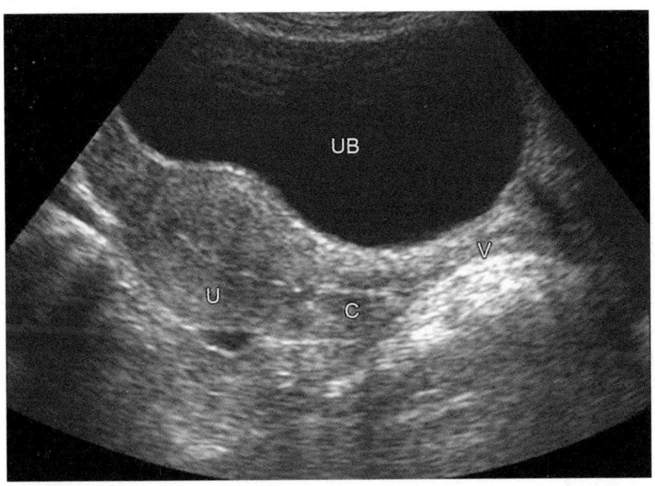

Fig. 21: Normal uterus (U), cervix (C) and vagina (V) on a transabdominal sagittal scan. Central linear echo representing apposed surfaces of vaginal mucosa (V).

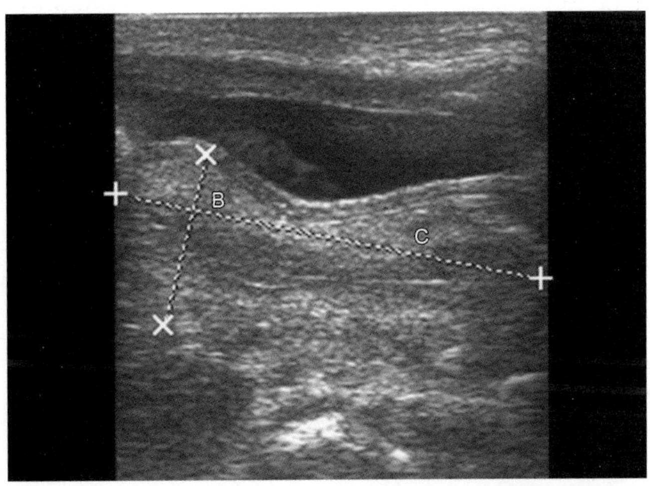

Fig. 22: Normal neonatal uterus—sagittal scan. Inverse pear-shaped with cervix (C) having greater width than body (B) of uterus.

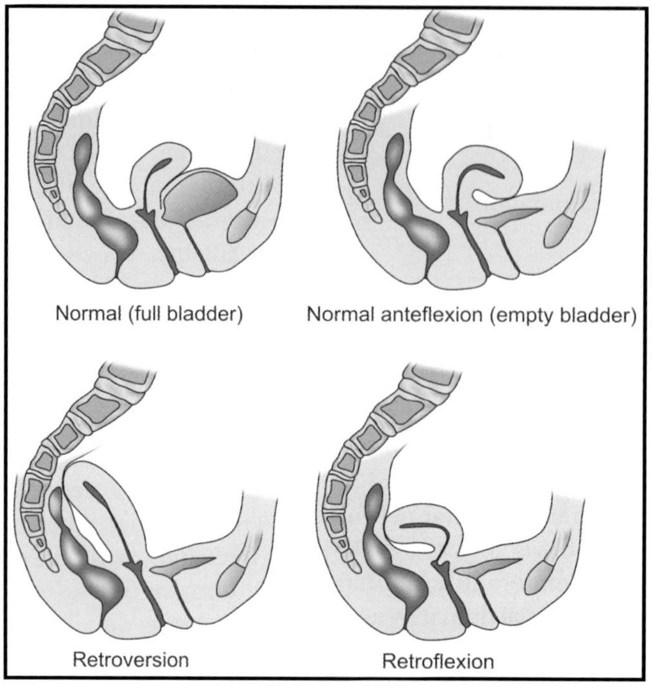

Fig. 23: Alterations in uterine position. The normal position of uterus in most women is anteverted with a mild degree of anteflextion. In retroversion, the long axis of the uterus and cervix points more posteriorly than the long axis of the vagina. In retrofexion, the body of the uterus is angled posteriorly relative to the cervix.

endometrium. The intermediate layer is the thickest and has a uniformly homogeneous low to moderate echogenicity. The thin outer layer is less echogenic and separated from the intermediate layer by the arcuate vessels, which can be visualized on ultrasound as small anechoic foci in the periphery of the uterus. Calification may be seen in the arteries in postmenopausal women. Sometimes small highly echogenic foci may be seen in the inner layer of myometrium. These small, single or multiple, nonshadowing foci are thought to represent dystrophic calcification related to previous instrumentation like dilatation and curettage or endocervical biopsy.[22]

The normal endometrial cavity is seen as a central echogenic line as a result of specular reflection from the interface between apposing surfaces of the endometrium. It should be straight or smoothly curved. The sonographic appearance of the endometrium varies during the menstrual cycle and has been correlated with histology.[23] The appearance during the various phases of the menstrual cycle has been given in **Table 5 and Figures 24A to C**. The endometrium is best measured on the midline sagittal scan of the uterus. The measurement is taken from the proximal to the distal interfaces between the subendometrial halo that surrounds the endometrium and the more echogenic endometrium. This is the double layer thickness.

In postmenopausal women, the normal sonographic endometrial appearance varies according to presence or absence of hormonal replacement therapy (HRT). Additionally, the type of HRT (i.e. continuous, combined or sequential) is important.[24] In asymptomatic postmenopausal women not receiving HRT, several reports suggest endometrial thickness should not exceed 4 mm, whereas others use 8 mm as the upper normal value. For women receiving HRT, the sonographic appearance of the endometrium depends on whether the patient takes continuous estrogen or a combination of estrogen and progesterone (either continuously or sequentially). Sequential HRT results in monthly withdrawal bleeding and cyclic endometrial thickening. At mid cycle, maximal endometrial thickness frequently exceeds 8 mm and in

Table 5: Appearance of endometrium in a normal menstrual cycle.

Date of cycle	*Phase*	*Thickness (mm)*	*Appearance*
1–4	Menstrual phase	1–4	Small amounts of fluid may be seen endovaginally Thin interrupted central echo.
5–14	Proliferative phase	4–8	Central hyperechoic line with surrounding thin hypoechoic band
	Periovulatory	6–10	Trilayered appearance; the hypoechoic band becomes more prominent with thin echogenic lines on either side
15–28	Secretory phase	8–16	Thick Echogenic with through transmission.

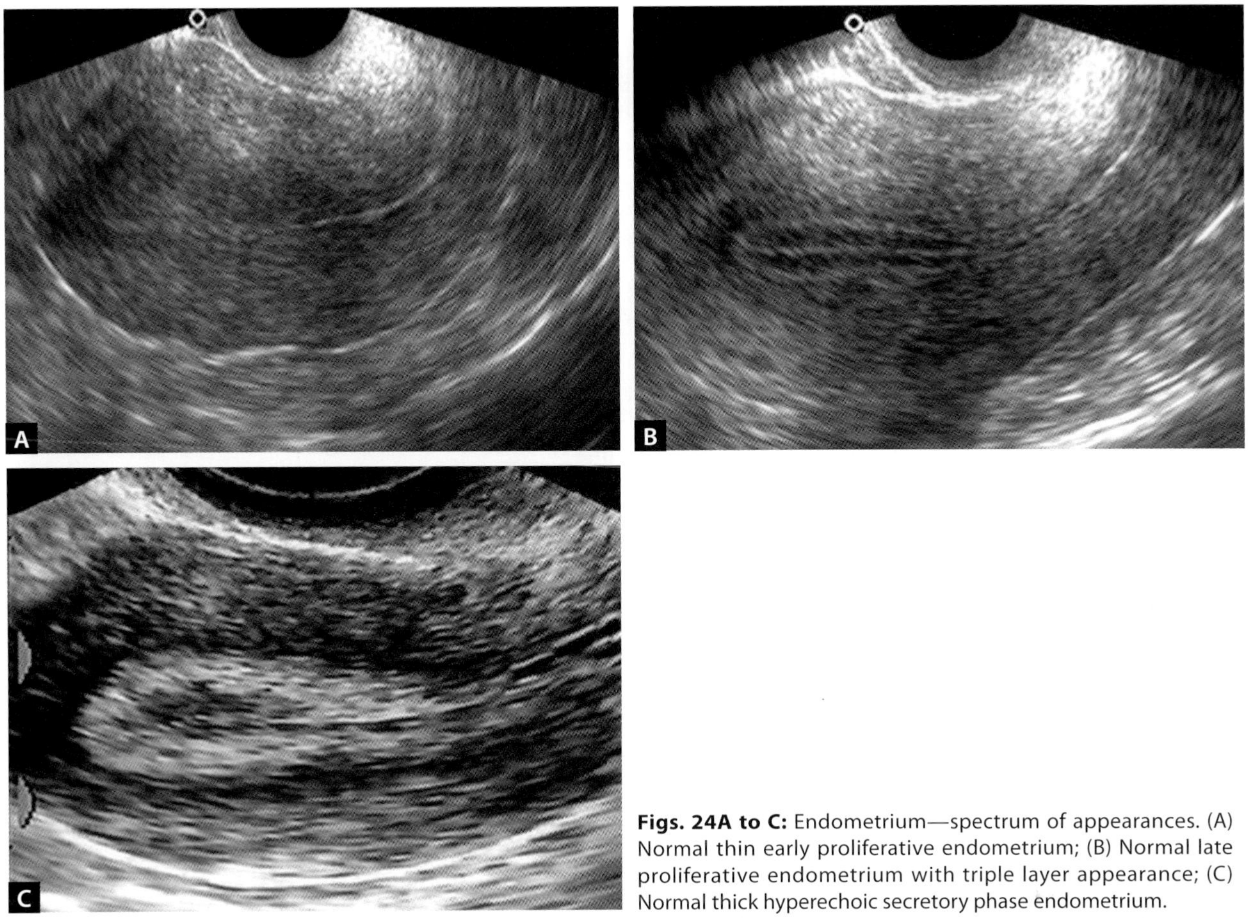

Figs. 24A to C: Endometrium—spectrum of appearances. (A) Normal thin early proliferative endometrium; (B) Normal late proliferative endometrium with triple layer appearance; (C) Normal thick hyperechoic secretory phase endometrium.

some cases may approach 15 mm. In these women, it is important to do a follow-up scan. In women taking either continuous estrogen or continuous estrogen and progesterone the maximal endometrial thickness is 8 mm and cyclic endometrial changes should not occur. Postmenopausal women may often have a trace of fluid (approximately 1 mm in thickness) in the endometrial cavity due to cervical stenosis.[24]

Sonohysterography can be done to visualize the intracavitary anatomy and any pathology within the cavity. The endometrial cavity is distended with fluid introduced via a self-retaining catheter, prior to transvaginal sonography. The fluid within the cavity gives an excellent visualization of any pathology within the cavity and also differentiates between intracavitary versus extracavitary pathology **(Figs. 25A and B)**.

CERVIX AND VAGINA

The **cervix** is better visualized by transvaginal sonography as a tubular structure of homogeneous echogenicity **(Fig. 26)**. The mucus within the endocervical canal usually appears as an echogenic interface which may become hypoechoic during the periovulatory period as the fluid content increases. Retention (nabothian) cysts of the cervix are commonly seen during routine sonography. They may vary in size from a few mm to four cm. They may be single or multiple and usually diagnosed incidentally, although they may be associated with chronic cervicitis.

The **vagina** runs anteriorly and caudally from the cervix between the bladder and rectum. It is best seen on the mid sagittal transabdominal scans as a collapsed hypoechoic tubular structure with a central hyperechoic line representing the apposed surfaces of the vaginal mucosa **(Fig. 21)**. In patients who have had a hysterectomy, the vaginal cuff should not be mistaken for a mass. The normal upper limit of the AP diameter of the vaginal cuff is 2.1 cm.[25]

ADNEXA

The adnexae consist of the ovaries, the fallopian tubes, ligaments and vessels. The **ovaries** most commonly lie lateral to the uterus (usually within a few centimeters)

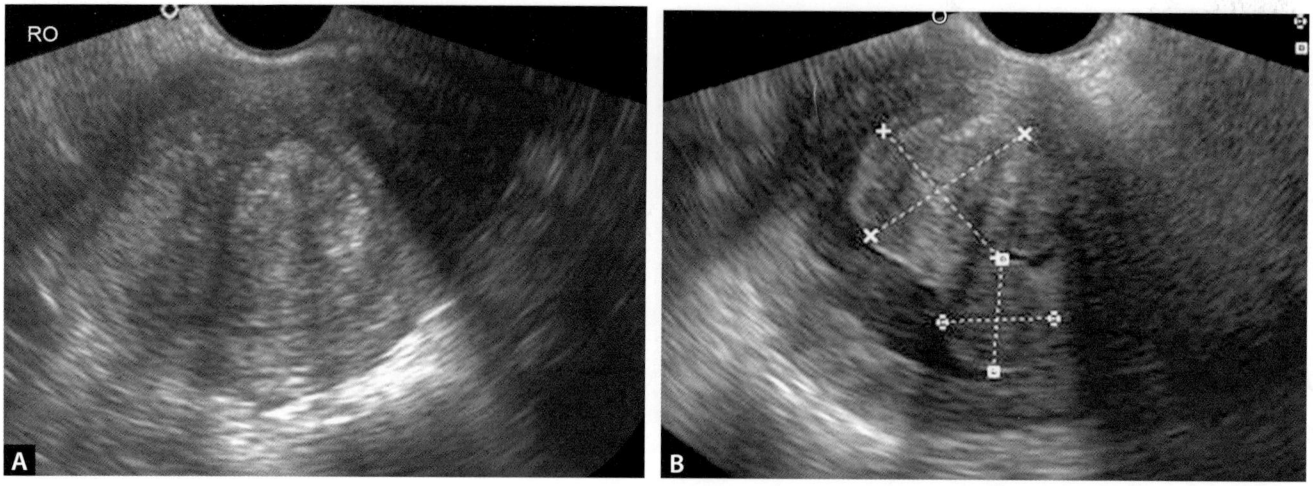

Figs. 25A and B: Sonohysterography. (A) Transvaginal scan shows hyperechoic masses within the uterus; it is not possible to determine their relation with the endometrium; (B) On instillation of intracavitary saline, 2 well-defined masses (within calipers) are seen projecting into the endometrial cavity—Submucous fibroids.

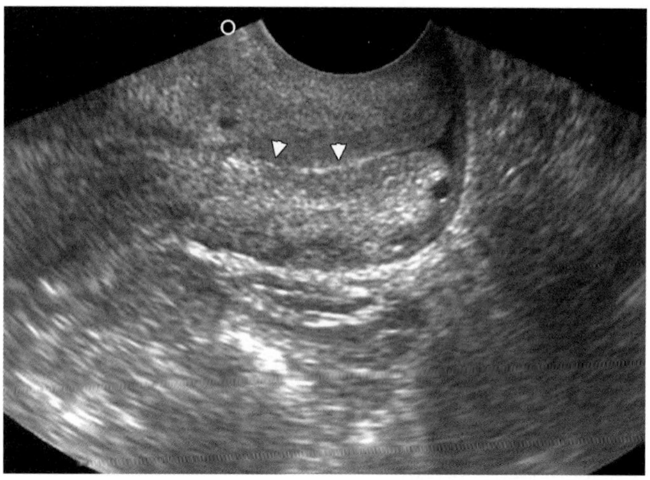

Fig. 26: The normal cervix as seen on sagittal transvaginal scan, with a central echogenic line (arrowheads) representing the cervical canal. Two small Nabothian cysts are seen.

at about the level of the cornua. Variations are common and insignificant. A relatively constant relationship of the ovaries is their location anterior to internal iliac vessels, which serves as a useful landmark for the ovaries particularly during TVS.

The ovaries are typically seen as oblong structures with a relatively homogeneous echotexture. Well-defined small anechoic follicles may be seen peripherally in the cortex. By day 8 or 9 of the menstrual cycle, one follicle becomes dominant and reaches upto 2–2.5 cm in size and the others become atretic **(Figs. 27A and B)**. Nondominant follicles are usually less than 14 mm in diameter. Following ovulation, a corpus luteum develops which can commonly be seen as a hypoechoic or isoechoic structure preipherally within the ovary **(Fig. 27C)**, but may show a very varied sonographic appearance. Sometimes, it may form a cyst and become very large **(Fig. 28)**. Its irregular walls and low level internal echoes with low impedance Doppler signals may be a cause for concern. However, unless a pregnancy occurs, the corpus luteum involutes towards the end of the cycle, so that a repeat scan 2–6 weeks later will usually resolve the dilemma.

Because of the variability in shape, **ovarian volume** is considered the best method for evaluating the ovarian size ($0.523 \times \text{length} \times \text{width} \times \text{AP diameter}$). For this measurement any cyst larger than 1 cm in diameter is excluded. In the first 2 years of life the ovarian volume ranges between 1–3 cc (largest in the first 3 months). It remains relatively stable upto 5 years of age and then gradually increases upto menarche when the mean volume is 4.2 ± 2.3 cc with an upper limit of 8 cc.[26] The normal ovarian volume ranges from 6 to 15 cc in an average adult female.[27] The two ovaries should be approximately equal in volume, neither should be more than twice the volume of the other.

Small echogenic, nonshadowing foci may sometimes be seen in a normal ovary, which are thought to be due to specular reflection from tiny unresolved cysts below the spatial resolution of the ultrasound machine.[28]

The **postmenopausal ovaries** may be difficult to recognise sonographically as they are relatively small and do not contain follicles **(Fig. 29)**. Wolf et al.[29] in a study of 290 postmenopausal ovaries known to be present, using both transabdominal and transvaginal sonography,

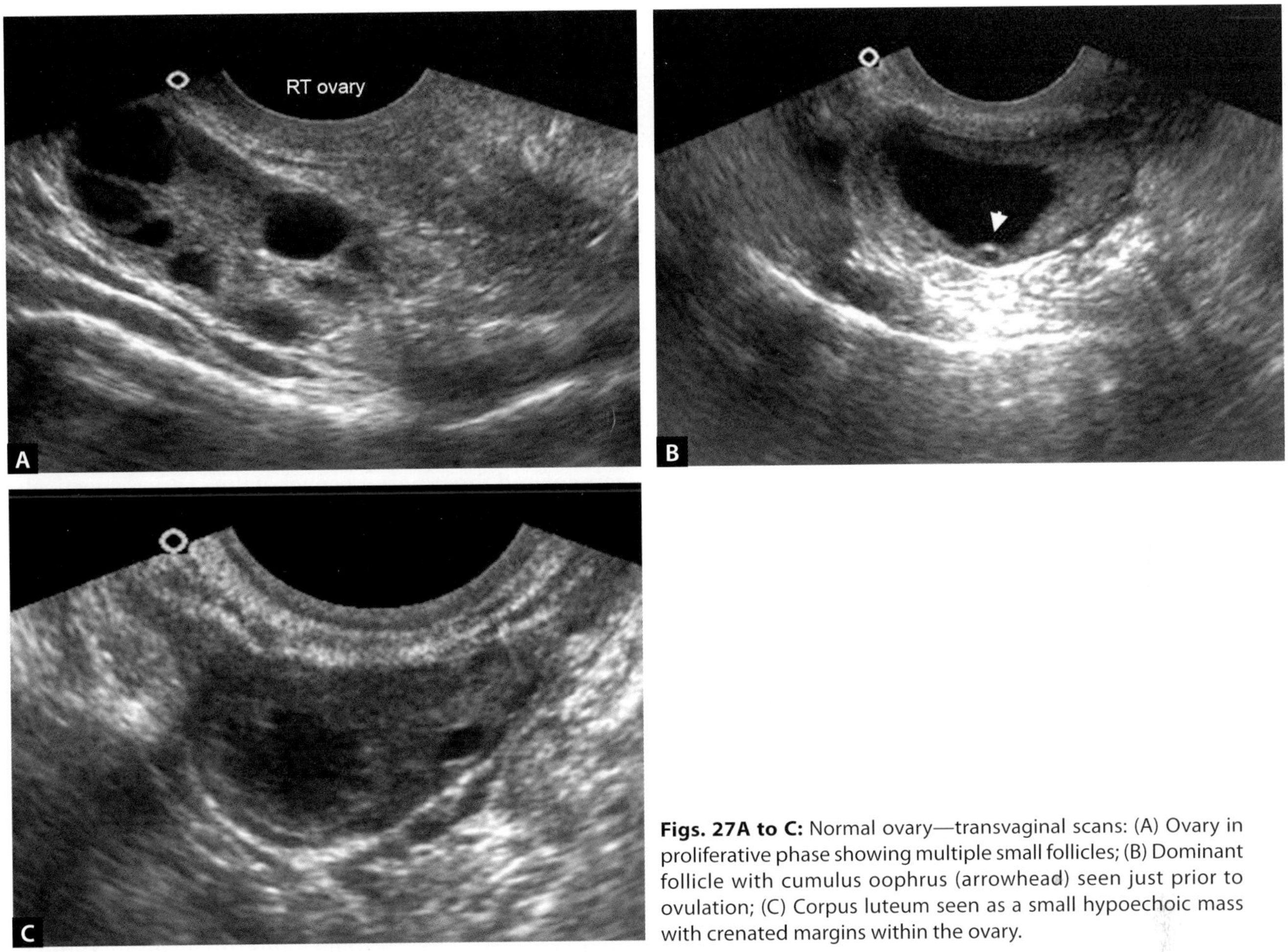

Figs. 27A to C: Normal ovary—transvaginal scans: (A) Ovary in proliferative phase showing multiple small follicles; (B) Dominant follicle with cumulus oophrus (arrowhead) seen just prior to ovulation; (C) Corpus luteum seen as a small hypoechoic mass with crenated margins within the ovary.

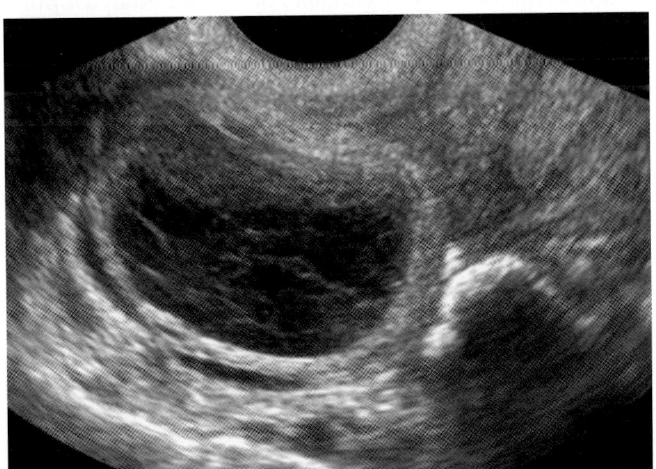

Fig. 28: Hemorrhagic corpus luteum cyst: Characteristic reticular pattern of internal echoes seen within the cyst.

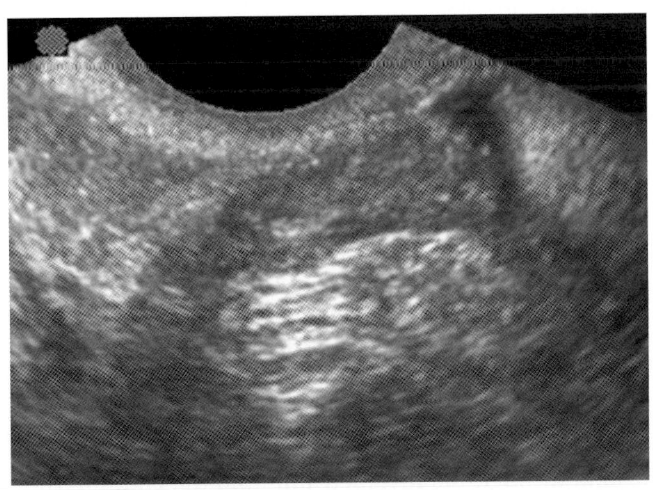

Fig. 29: Postmenopausal ovary: Small in size with no follicles, often difficult to identify.

visualized only 40% of ovaries transvaginally and 58% transabdominally. Using both techniques resulted in 68% visualization. Mean postmenopausal ovarian volume ranges from 1.2 to 5.8 cc, with the volume decreasing in size with increasing age. An ovarian volume of more than 8 cc is definitely abnormal. Small anechoic cysts (less than

3 cm) may be seen in upto 15% of post menopausal ovaries and are not related to age, length of time since menopause or hormone use. These cysts can disappear or change in size overtime.[29]

The non-distended fallopian tubes are difficult to see on ultrasound. Delineation of the tubes is possible if intraperitoneal fluid is present in the cul-de-sac or if they are distended by saline/contrast agent. Sonosalpingography can be done to establish the patency of the fallopian tubes by instilling fluid or contrast agent into the uterus and then visualizing sonographically its passage through the tubes, or presence of fluid in the pouch of Douglas. The use of color Doppler in conjunction with ultrasound contrast improves the sensitivity of the technique in the detection of tubal spill.

The posterior cul-de-sac (pouch of Douglas) is the most posterior and inferior reflection of the peritoneal cavity located between the rectum and vagina. Small quantities of fluid in the cul-de-sac is a normal finding in asymptomatic women and can be seen in all phases of the menstrual cycle.

Indications for Evaluation of Uterus and Adnexa

- Menstrual disorders
- Post-menopausal bleeding
- Pelvic inflammatory disease
- Pelvic mass
- Infertility
- Guided procedures.

Doppler Evaluation

The blood supply to the uterus is via the uterine artery, a branch of the internal iliac artery. The uterine artery enters the uterus at the cervicocorporal junction and ascends along the lateral aspect of the uterine body to the cornua. At the cornua an adnexal branch originates that supplies the ipsilateral ovary and anastomoses with the ipsilateral ovarian artery. The uterine arteries anastomose through the anterior and posterior arcuate arteries which are located in the outer one-third of the myometrium. The endometrium is supplied by branches of the uterine arteries. Radial arteries arise from the arcuate vessels and extend through the myometrium upto the endometrium where they form (i) the basal arteries which supply the basalis layer of endometrium and (ii) the spiral arteries which supply the functional layer of endometrium. The spiral arteries are responsive to hormonal changes similar to the endometrium.

The ovarian arteries arise from the abdominal aorta and enter the pelvis through the infundibulopelvic ligament. They reach the ovaries through the hilus via the mesovarium. After supplying the ovary, terminal branches anastomose with branches of the uterine artery.

The uterine and ovarian vessels can be identified on color Doppler. The course of the uterine artery is ideally suited for transvaginal assessment with ideal geometry for Doppler signal recording. It is also possible to record Doppler signals transabdominally with an empty bladder when the uterus is anteverted. The ovarian arteries are more difficult to assess as they run a transverse course through the pelvis. The branches of the uterine artery extending towards the ovary can be identified in the broad ligament and the superior aspect of the ovary respectively. Because of their tortuosity, only short segments of the arteries are usually identified in any scan plane. The lowest possible filter, with a high color gain should be used to detect slow flow.

During the reproductive years of a normal female both color and duplex Doppler patterns change concomitant with grey scale changes.[30]

The general pattern of uterine blood flow throughout the menstrual cycle is that perfusion increases in response to rising plasma oestrogen and progesterone and decreases with periovulatory fall in estrogen. The typical spectral waveform shows a high resistance pattern characterized by high flow velocity with an early diastolic notch **(Fig. 30)**. The normal values are given in **Table 6**. Endometrial vascularity can also be evaluated by Doppler sonography. The extent of vascular penetration into the

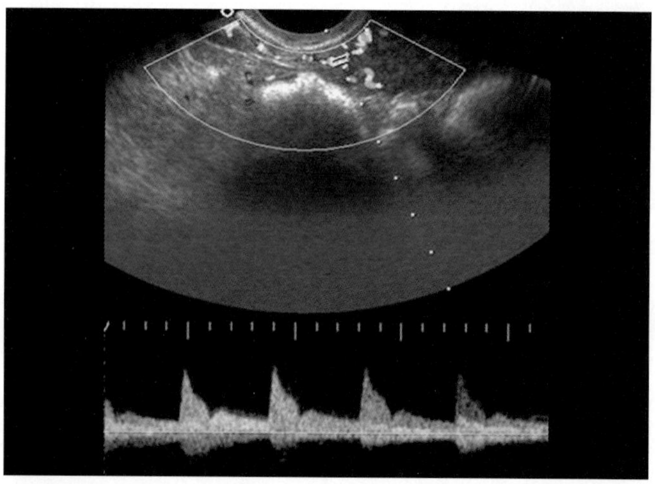

Fig. 30: Normal spectral waveform of the uterine artery characterized by a high flow velocity, a post-systolic notch and low diastolic flow.

endometrium correlates well with successful conception and it is possible to see variations in the depth of vascular penetration before, during and after the mid-cycle.

The ovarian arterial supply also exhibits different flow characteristics during different phases of a normal menstrual cycle. In general, the index value is high during the early follicular phase, progressively decreases till the early luteal phase and then rises again in the late luteal phase[31] **(Table 6)**. Differences in flow characteristics may also be seen between the dominant and non-dominant ovaries. In the ovary containing the dominant follicle, continuous diastolic flow may be seen by the early luteal phase. In contrast, both diastolic flow and cyclical changes may be absent in the non dominant ovary.

Doppler ultrasound can demonstrate the neovascularity within the wall of the corpus luteum. Demonstrable color flow surrounding the developing dominant follicle becomes more apparent as the midcycle approaches and continues around the corpus luteum until the late luteal phase. In the event of pregnancy both the low resistance flow and the color flow to the corpus luteum may remain until the eleventh week of amenorrhea.[30]

Indications

- Characterization of uterine/ovarian masses.
- Infertility and assisted reproduction.

Three-dimensional Sonography

Three-dimensional imaging has several obvious benefits that relate to an improved spatial orientation and the demonstration of multiplanar views, of which the coronal plane is particularly useful[32] **(Fig. 31)**. It offers a more objective and reproducible measurement of volume and vascularity of the region of interest and an improved assessment of normal and pathological pelvic organs through further post-processing modalities, including tomographic ultrasound imaging and various rendering modalities. It also has the benefit of offering reduced scanning time, the option of teleconsultation and storage of images for re-evaluation.

There are different types of 3D acquisition, manual, sensor-based and automatic. For manual acquisitions the user moves the probe during the data acquisition. The smoothness and speed at which the probe is moved should be constant. Since the time for post-processing depends on the acquired number of frames, it is recommended to start with a high frame rate. Low frame rates result in fewer acquired frames for the 3D dataset, which results in more intensive post-processing (interpolation). Manual acquisitions are much more user dependant and are unable to be used for measurement. When performing sensor-based acquisitions a transmitter is used to generate a pulsed electromagnetic field, which is detected by a sensor attached to the transducer. As the sweep is done the position information is detected and used to calculate a 3D data set. Automatic acquisitions are more uniform and consistent due to the ultrasound system driving the movement of the acoustic array. The anatomy is acquired as a dataset and each anatomical scan plane can be rotated on the X, Y or Z axis to obtain the optimal image, allowing for more accurate 2D and volume measurements.

Indications

- Diagnosing congenital uterine malformations **(Fig. 32)**.
- Accurate volume measurement, e.g. endometrial, ovarian cysts and follicles, tumour masses, prostate.
- Exact localization of pathology—intrauterine fibroid, IUCD, etc.

Table 6: Variation in Doppler indices in the uterine and ovarian arteries.

	*RI OVA**	*PI OVA**	*PI UTA*
Early proliferative	0.65–0.7	1.8–2.2	1.67± 0.22
Late proliferative/ Ovulation	0.55–0.6	1.0–1.3	1.89 ± 0.4
Luteal	0.6–0.65	1.3–1.8	1.23 ± 0.67
Postmenopausal	0.6–1.0	1.3–4.0	1.8–3.8

Abbreviations: RI: Resistance index; PI: Pulsatility index; OVA: Ovarian artery; UTA: Uterine artery.

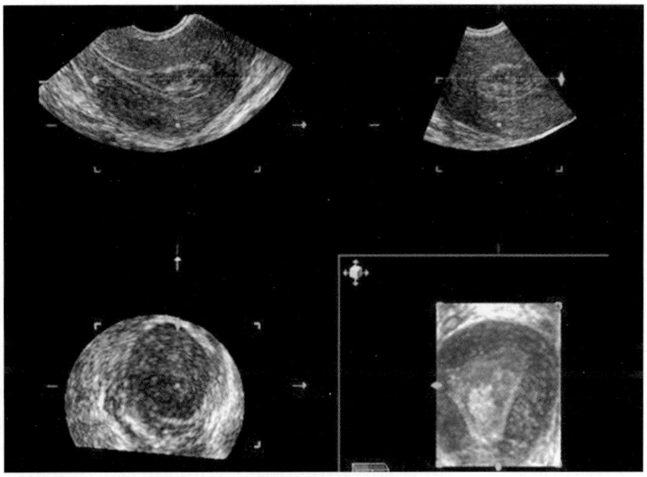

Fig. 31: 3D ultrasound permits collection and review of data obtained from a volume of tissue in multiple imaging planes and allows visualization of the third or coronal plane of the uterus.

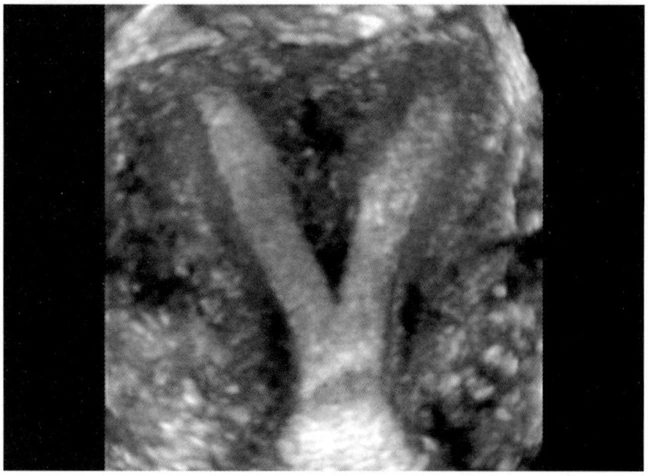

Fig. 32: 3D reconstructed coronal view showing a subseptate uterus.

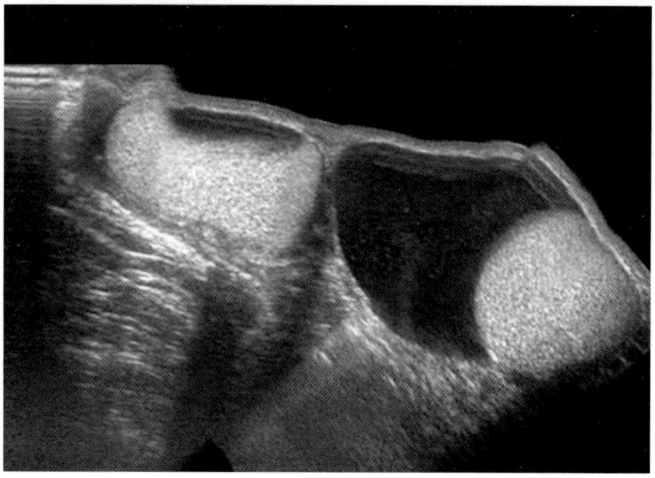

Fig. 33: EFOV image of the scrotum showing left hydrocele with normal left testis, along with the normal right testis.

- Characterisation of adnexal masses.
- Extent of tumor infiltration into adjacent tissues/organs.
- 3D power Doppler can aid in characterization of vessel morphology.

Extended Field of View Imaging[33]

Overcomes the drawback of limited field of view of sonography, enabling the visualization of large fields of view in a single image. This technology is now available in most of the modern equipments. The technique is relatively simple and requires only a steady sweep of the transducer over the concerned area to acquire the data. The extended field of view (EFOV) image is then reconstructed automatically by the computer. Although EFOV plays its most important role in the evaluation of relatively superficial structures, e.g. in evaluation of scrotal masses and establishing their relation with the testes **(Fig. 33)**, it can also help in localization and orientation of lesions in the abdomen and pelvis. Doppler EFOV allows a panoramic visualization of vascularity in mass lesions, helping in their characterization. Transvaginal EFOV is also possible to illustrate the relation of smaller pelvic masses with the uterus and ovaries in a single image. EFOV images are comparable to CT/MRI images as it provides a panoramic view.

Image enhancement tools like **spatial compound imaging** and **tissue harmonic imaging** can add to the diagnostic confidence. Spatial compound imaging is a technology by which the unwanted speckle and clutter or "noise" can be reduced, thus giving better contrast resolution and clearer borders. Tissue harmonic imaging takes advantage of nonlinear propagation of ultrasound in tissue. It diminishes low frequency , high amplitude noise and improves imaging of technically difficult patients.

Elastography[34]

Elastography is a recently introduced ultrasound imaging technique that evaluates the elasticity of tissue. Neoplastic tissue has a greater cell density leading to increase in hardness. Elastography shows promising results in the evaluation of prostate cancer.[35]

Contrast-enhanced Ultrasonography (CEUS)

Contrast agents can help delineate vascular structures and enhance Doppler signals from small volumes of blood making it possible to image organ and lesion perfusion in real time.[36] Gas-filled microbubbles are used as ultrasound contrast agents. They are in the size range of 1–4 microns in diameter and can be administered intravenously. There are two forms of CEUS, untargeted CEUS, which is used in echocardiography and targeted CEUS, which is a disease/organ specific technique and can be used in cases of inflammatory or malignant lesions of the liver, prostate, kidney, uterus, ovaries and other organs. However, targeted CEUS has not yet been approved for clinical use. If these microbubble-based techniques are successful, future application will likely expand to include detection and staging of malignancies, as well as monitoring response to therapy.[37]

CONCLUSION

Ultrasound remains the first line investigation when evaluating the urogenital tract. Other than its inherent advantages of lack of ionizing radiation and low cost, it gives an excellent visualization of the organs of the urogenital tract. With the addition of Doppler, the vascular pattern and morphology can also be very well evaluated. The introduction of contrast agents has made it possible to interrogate even the slow flow areas. Multiplanar and surface rendered images are possible with 3D technology. However, it is essential to recognize that operator skill, regardless of the equipment used, ultimately determines the final benefit of ultrasound in patient care.

REFERENCES

1. Zagoria RJ. An Introduction to Radiologic methods. In Genitourinary Radiology. The Requisites; (2nd Edn). Mosby; 2004.pp.1-50.
2. Swischuk LE. Genitourinary Tract and Adrenal Glands. In Imaging of the Newborn, Infant & Young Child. (5th Edn) Lippincott Williams & Wilkins; 2004.pp.590-724.
3. Allan Paul. The normal kidney. In Meire HB, Cosgrove D, Dewbury KC, Tarrant P (Eds). Abdominal and General Ultrasound Edinburgh. Churchill Livingstone; 2001. pp.515-27.
4. Emamian SA, Nielsen MB, Pedersen JF, et al. Kidney dimensions at sonography: Correlation with age, sex and habitus in 665 adult volunteers. AJR. 1993;160:83-6.
5. Yeh HC, Halton KP, Shapiro RS, et al. Junctional parenchyma. Revised definition of Hypertrophied Column of Bertin, Radiology. 1992;185:725-32.
6. Dalla Palma L, Bazzichi M, Cressa C, et al. Radiological anatomy of the kidney revisited. Br J Radiol. 1990;63:680-90.
7. Dubbins PA. The kidney. In: Allan PL, Dubbins PA, Pozniak M, Mc Dicken WN (Eds). Clinical Doppler Ultrasound. Churchill Livingstone; 2000.pp.169-90.
8. Thurston W, Wilson SR. The Urinary Tract. In: Rumack CM, Wilson SR, Charboneau JW (Eds): Diagnostic ultrasound, 3rd edition. Elseiver Mosby; 2005.pp.321-93.
9. Price CI, Adler RS, Rubin JM. Ultrasound depiction of differences in density: Explanation of ureteric jet phenomenon and implications for new ultrasound applications. Invest Radiol. 1989;24:876-83.
10. Bree RL, Toi A. The Prostate. In: Rumack CM, Wilson SR, Charboneau JW (Eds). Diagnostic ultrasound, 3rd edn. Elseiver Mosby; 2001.pp.395-424.
11. Rickards D, Hare C. The lower urinary tract. In: Meire HB, Cosgrove D, Dewbury KC, Farrant P (Eds). Abdominal and General Ultrasound. Edinburgh: Churchill Livingstone; 2001.pp.585-611.
12. Krone KD, Caroll BA. Scrotal Ulatrasound. RCNA. 1985;23: 121-39.
13. Rifkin MD, Foy PM, Goldberg BS. Scrotal Ultrasound: Acoustic characteristics of the normal testis and epididymis defined with higher resolution superficial scanners. Med Ultrasound. 1984;8:91-7.
14. Gorman B, Caroll BA. The Scrotum. In: Rumack CM, Wilson SR, Charboneau JW (Eds): Diagnostic ultrasound, 3rd edn. Elseiver Mosby; 2001.pp.849-88.
15. Johnson KA, Dewbury KC. Ultrasound imaging of the appendix testes and appendix epididymis. Clinical Radiology. 1996;51:335-7.
16. Middleton WD, Thorne DA, Melson GL. Colour Doppler ultrasound of the normal testis. AJR. 1989;152:293-7.
17. Benson CB, Doubilet PM, Vickers MA. onography of the male genital tract. AJR. 1989;153:705-13.
18. Schwartz AN, Wang KY, Mark LA, et al. Evaluation of normal erectile function with color flow Doppler sonography. AJR. 1989;153:1155-60.
19. Siegel MJ. Pediatric gynaecologic sonography. Radiology. 1991;170:593-600.
20. Salem S, Wilson SR. Gynaecologic Ultrasound. In: Rumack CM, Wilson SR, Charboneau JW (Eds). Diagnostic ultrasound, 3rd Edn. Elseiver Mosby; 2001.pp.527-87.
21. Coleman BG, Arger PH, Grumbach K, et al. Transvaginal and transabdominal sonography: Prospective comparison. Radiology. 1988;168:639-43.
22. Burks DD, Stainken BF, Burkhard TK, et al. Uterine inner myometrial echogenic foci: Relationship to prior dilatation and curettage and endocervical biopsy. J Ultrasound Med. 1991;10:487-92.
23. Forrest TS, Elyaderani MK, Muilenburg MI. Cyclic endometrial changes: US assessment with histologic correlation. Radiology. 1988;167:233.
24. Laing FC, Douglas MD, et al. Gynecologic ultrasound. RCNA. 2001;39(3):523-40.
25. Schoenfield A, Levavi H, Hirsch M, et al. Transvaginal sonography in postmenopausal women. J Clin Ultrasound. 1990;18:350-8.
26. Orsini LF, Salardi S, Pilu G, et al. Pelvic organs in premenarchal girls: Real-time ultrasonography. Radiology. 1984;153:113-6.
27. Van Nagell JR Jr. Higgins RV, Donaldson ES, et al. Transvaginal sonography as a screening method for ovarian cancer. Cancer. 1990;65:573-7.
28. Muradali D. Colgin T, Hayeems E, et al. Echogenic ovarian foci without shadowing: Are they caused by psammomatous calcifications? Radiology. 2002;224:429-35.
29. Wolf SI, Gosink BB, Feldesman MR, et al. Prevalence of simple adnexal cysts in postmenopausal women. Radiology. 1991;180:65-71.
30. Applebaum M in The menstrual cycle, menopause, ovulation induction and *in vitro* fertilization. Copel JA, Reed KL (Eds). Doppler ultrasound in Obstetrics and Gynaecology. 1994;71-86.

31. Dubbins PA. The female pelvis. In: Allan PL, Dubbins PA, Pozniak MA, et al (Eds). Clinical Doppler Ultrasound. Churchill Livingstone; 2000. pp. 237-58.
32. Pretorirus DH, Borok NN, Coffler MS, et al. Three Dimensional Sonography in Obstetrics and Gynaecology. RCNA. 2001;39(3): 499-521.
33. Henrich W, Fuchs I, Schmider A. Transvaginal and Transabdominal Extended Field of View (EFOV) and Power Doppler EFOV Sonography in Gynecology: Advantages and Applications. Journal of Ultrasound in Medicine. 2002;21: 1137-44.
34. Ophir J, et al. Elastography: A quantitative method for imaging the elasticity of biological tissues. Ultrason Imaging. 1991;13(2):111-34.
35. Pallwein L, Fauscher F, Mitterberger M. Value of contrast enhanced ultrasound & elastography in imaging of prostate cancer. Curr Opin Urol. 2007;17(1):39-47.
36. Burns PN. Microbubble Contrast for Ultrasound Imaging: Where, How and Why. In: Rumack CM, Wilson SR, Charboneau JW (Eds). Diagnostic ultrasound, 3rd Edn. Elseiver Mosby; 2001. pp. 55-76.
37. Halpern EJ. Contrast-Enhanced Ultrasound Imaging for Prostate Cancer. Rev Urol. 2006;8(Suppl):S29-S37.

CHAPTER 100

Computed Tomography of Urogenital Tract: Techniques and Normal Appearances

Sapna Singh, Veena Chowdhury

INTRODUCTION

With the advent of the modern, cross-sectional imaging modalities of computed tomography (CT) and magnetic resonance imaging (MRI) and refinement in their techniques, the kidney is a much better understood organ as CT has enlarged the capacity to visualize the genitourinary tract noninvasively. The anatomical characteristics of the kidney and perirenal region can be accurately and consistently visualized. Further perfusion of the kidney can also be studied. Therefore, CT is a vital component of a uroradiologic diagnosis and plays a valuable role in evaluating patients with renal masses, renal cystic disease, renal infections, renal trauma and flank pain of unknown etiology. It is unsurpassed in evaluating lesions containing fat or calcium.

Helical CT has overcome the limitations of conventional CT (CCT) and is now the standard CT technology. It allows rapid volumetric assessment of the kidneys and is highly accurate in the evaluation of renal masses and blood vessels. 3D postprocessing capabilities allow the assessment of the renal vascular pedicle noninvasively by CT angiography. Gapless volume scanning and improved resolution in the Z-axis during the excretory phase enables improved visualization of the renal collecting system and ureters, resulting in a better demonstration of intraluminal and extraluminal pathology.[1] Thus, helical CT enables an improved characterization of renal lesions, reducing the diagnosis of indeterminate masses and thus, facilitating a better theraupetic management.

NORMAL RENAL STRUCTURE AND CT ANATOMY OF KIDNEYS

The retroperitoneum is divided into three compartments namely the anterior pararenal, posterior pararenal and the perinephric spaces. The perinephric space contains the kidneys, renal vessels, the adrenals, the IVC and lower aorta, perinephric fat and the renal collecting system. Each kidney is about 11 cm in length, 6 cm in breadth and 3 cm in anteroposterior dimension. The left kidney is little longer, narrower and is higher in position.The kidney itself, has an internal medulla, external cortex and an outer capsule. The capsule is surrounded by perinephric fat, which is enveloped by the renal fascia. The renal fascia is in two layers, the anterior and posterior, which are named Gerota's fascia and the fascia of Zuckerkandl, respectively.

The renal fascia fuses superiorly with the diaphragmatic fascia and laterally with the lateroconal fascia, inferiorly the layers of renal fascia fuse weakly with the iliac fascia and blend loosely with the periureteric connective tissue. The inferior apex of the compartment remains open towards the iliac fossa. The weakest point of the perinephric compartment through which urine or perinephric effusions escape most easily is at the inferomedial angle adjacent to the ureter. The posterior renal fascia fuses medially with the psoas and the quadratus lumborum fascia.[2,3]

On axial scanning, the kidney appears smooth and oval with an anteromedial break in the region of hilum where the vascular pedicle enters. The renal hilum is at the level

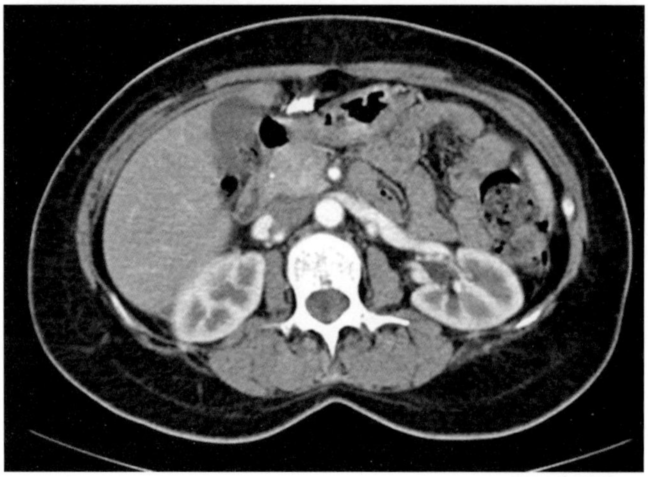

Fig. 1: Contrast-enhanced axial scan CT showing the longer left renal vein crossing anterior to the aorta and entering the inferior vena cava at the level of the uncinate process of the pancreas.

of L1-2 vertebra on the right side and is 1–2 cm higher on the left side. The renal vascular pedicle lies anterior to the pelvis and it may not be always possible to differentiate renal artery and vein on conventional scannings. The renal veins are usually larger than the renal artery and the longer left renal vein crosses anterior to the aorta and enters the inferior vena cava at the uncinate process of the pancreas **(Fig. 1)**. The aorta and superior mesenteric artery may pinch the left renal vein which causes the left renal vein to appear larger than the right.

NORMAL CT ANATOMY OF THE PELVIS

The pelvis contains the bony structures and within it the soft tissue structures including the ureters, urinary bladder, vascular structures, male and female genital organs. The ureters are best seen after intravenous administration of iodinated contrast material. At the level of the sacral promontory, the ureters are located anteromedial to the psoas major and anterior to the common iliac artery or lateral to the external iliac artery. The ureters then course medially and posteriorly to the external iliac arteries until they reach the midportion of the internal obturator muscle. At this level they course anteromedially to reach the trigone of the urinary bladder **(Figs. 2A to D)**. The configuration of the urinary bladder depends on the degree of filling and imaging is greatly improved when the bladder is fully distended. In the distended state, bladder wall is 1–3 mm thick. Partial volume artifacts may obscure a small area of the fundus and base of the bladder. Peritoneal reflections extend from the fundus of the bladder to the rectum in males, while in females; the peritoneum is first reflected onto the uterus and then to the rectum. These peritoneal reflections form small cul-de-sacs, which are the earliest site of small collections in pelvic inflammatory disease.

The prostate appears on CT scans as a homogeneous well-marginated soft tissue structure, 2–4 cm in length located just beneath the symphysis pubis immediately anterior to the rectum **(Fig. 3)**. Anteriorly prostate is anchored to the pubis with ligaments and posteriorly Denonvilliers fascia separates it from the rectum.The size of the gland increases with advancing age. The seminal vesicles lie posterior to the urinary bladder and superior to the prostate. They are separated by a wedge shaped layer of fat from the posterior wall of the bladder forming the seminovesical angle **(Fig. 4)**.

Female pelvic viscera is constituted by the uterus, fallopian tubes, ovaries, cervix and vagina. The vagina, urethra and rectum are bounded laterally by ligaments of the levator ani muscle. Prior to scanning, the lumen of vagina should be demarcated by inserting a tampon.[2] The uterine cervix appears as a transverse oval soft tissue structure with a diameter not exceeding 3 cm and is sharply demarcated from surrounding fat. The cross sectional diameter of a normal uterus in a reproductive age group female should be <5 cm **(Fig. 5)**. The uterine cavity is visible as a T-shaped structure after administration of IV contrast media. The broad ligaments are two fibrous sheets extending laterally from the uterus to the pelvic side wall and covered on their anterior and posterior surfaces by peritoneum.[3] They are not routinely seen on CT unless outlined by ascites. Between the leaves of the broad ligaments, are the parametrium, uterine artery, fallopian tube and round ligament. The round ligaments demarcate the superolateral border of the uterus and ascend anterolaterally over the external iliac vessels, pass through the inguinal canal and insert in the labia major. The triangular cardinal ligaments are located at the base of the broad ligament and fan out from their attachments at the cervix to insert on fascia covering the pelvic diaphragm. The uterosacral ligaments arise in continuity with the cardinal ligaments and pass posterolaterally around the rectum to insert on the sacrum.[3] The ovarian fossa is located between the external iliac vessels laterally and the pelvic ureter posteriorly. The ovaries, which are normally 3 × 1.5 cm in size are variable in position **(Fig. 6)**.

MULTIDETECTOR CT

Multidetector CT (MDCT) is the most recent advance in CT technology. Also known as multislice, multichannel or multisection CT, it uses a multiple row detector array instead

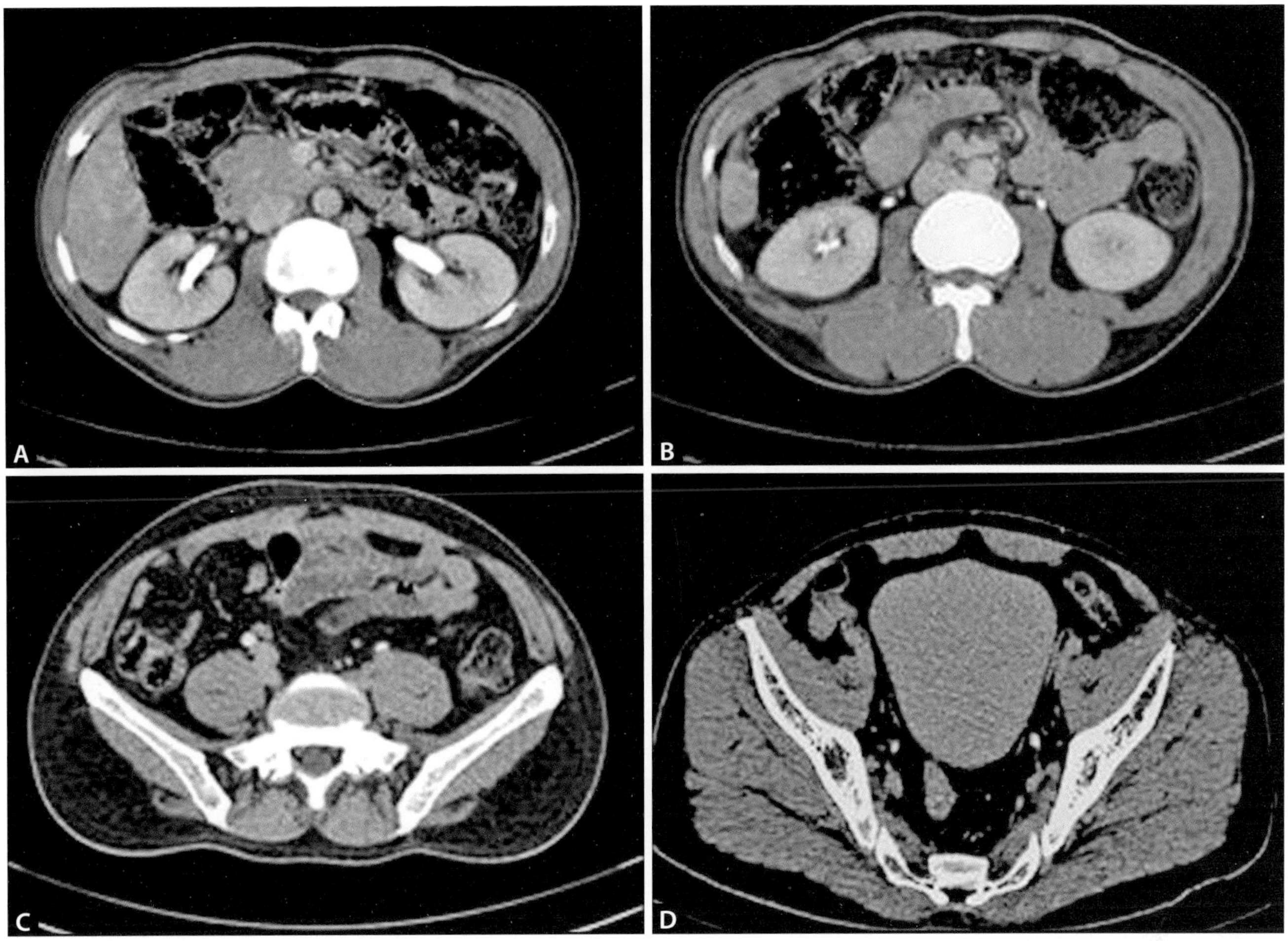

Figs. 2A to D: Transverse CT images obtained with a multidetector row CT scanner showing the normal anatomy progressing from superior to inferior (A) The renal pelvis; (B) Upper ureters; (C) Mid ureters and (D) Distal ureters.

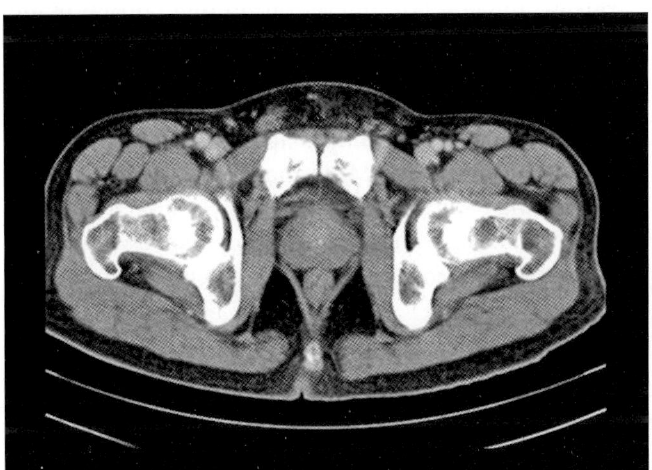

Fig. 3: Axial CT scan showing the normal prostate as a homogeneous well-marginated soft tissue 2–4 cm in length located beneath the symphysis pubis anterior to the rectum.

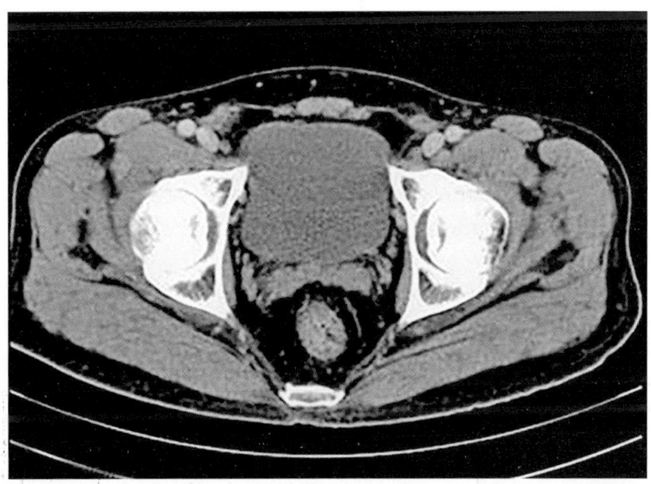

Fig. 4: Axial CT scan showing the seminal vesicles which lie posterior to the urinary bladder and separated by wedge-shaped layer of fat from the posterior wall of the bladder forming the seminovesical angle.

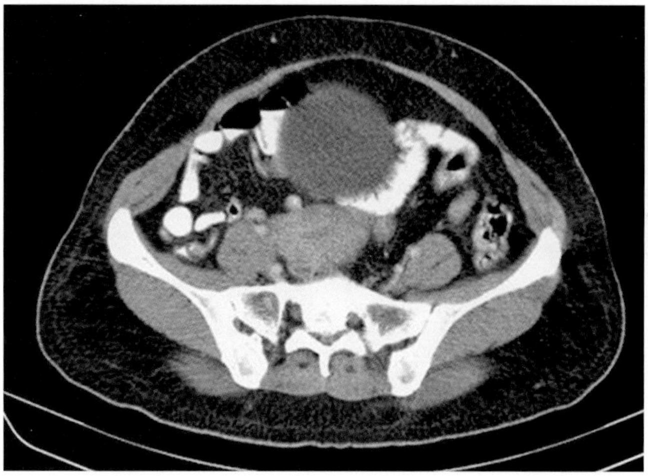

Fig. 5: Axial CT scan showing the normal uterus posterior to the bladder.

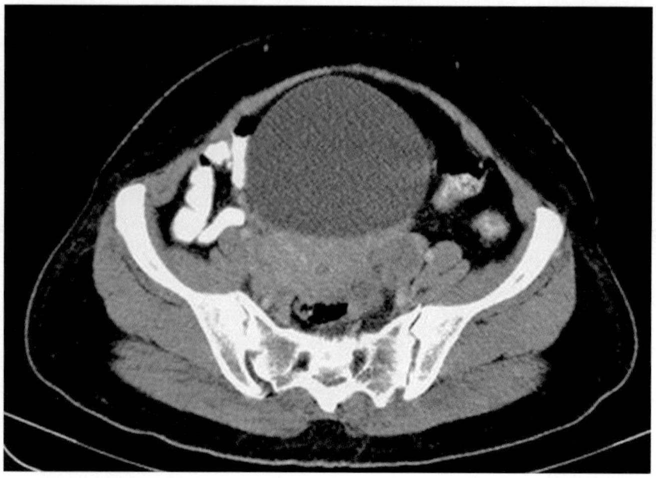

Fig. 6: CT scan showing the normal uterus and a cyst in the left ovary.

of the single row detector array used in single slice helical CT.[4] These new CT scanners with reduced gantry rotation times (0.5 sec or less for one 360° rotation) allow 2–25 times faster scan times than helical CT with the same or better image quality.[5] The faster scan times result in decreased breath hold times with reduced motion artifact and more diagnostic images. Increased volume coverage is combined with thinner slice thickness to obtain better quality volume data sets for three dimensional (3D) images. MDCT allows images to be obtained in multiple phases of renal parenchymal enhancement and excretion in the collecting system after administration of a single bolus of intravenous (IV) contrast material. Detection and characterization of small renal masses, display of the arterial and venous supply similar to conventional angiography and demonstration of the collecting system using different 3D display technique are possible with MDCT.[6]

Advantages of Renal Multidetector Row CT

The main advantages of MDCT are faster scanning time, increased volume coverage and improved spatial and temporal resolution.[7]

Increased Diagnostic Images

As MDCT uses multiple rows of detector, it allows for registration of more than one channel per gantry rotation whereas single detector helical CT allows registration of only one channel of image information of the scanned body part per gantry rotation.[8]

Increased Temporal Resolution

Current MDCT scanners have very fast gantry rotation time that is equal to or less than 0.4 seconds. Decreased gantry rotation time provides reduced scanning times and increased coverage along the Z-axis. Therefore, image acquisitions in multiple phases of renal parenchymal enhancement and contrast excretion in the collecting system after administration of a single bolus of IV contrast media are possible.[9]

Isotropic Data Acquisition and Increased Spatial Resolution

Isotropic data acquisition is defined as obtaining images with equal voxel size in three axes. MDCT scanners permit acquisition of thin sections with isotropic voxel size. Their effective section thickness is between 0.75 and 1.6 mm. MDCT scanners permit reconstruction of images at various thicknesses different from that chosen before the scan.[9] Isotropic imaging minimizes the importance of patient positioning and obviates obtaining axial, coronal and sagittal planes directly. Increased temporal resolution and acquisition of thin slices with isotropic voxel allows excellent quality MPR images to be obtained and 3D rendering of virtually any plane.[10] Optimal imaging of the renal hilar anatomy requires small slice widths and isotropic or near-isotropic data sets which can be achieved on MDCT scanners.[11]

EXAMINATION TECHNIQUE AND IMAGING PROTOCOLS OF MULTIDETECTOR ROW CT OF THE KIDNEY

Imaging protocols and parameters vary depending on the type of MDCT scanner (number of detectors and name of manufacturer). Every imaging department should optimize its imaging protocols and parameters.

The CT examination phases of the kidney are precontrast (noncontrast), corticomedullary, nephrographic and excretory (delayed or urographic) phases.

Noncontrast CT

Noncontrast scans are obtained to locate the kidneys, evaluate urolithiasis, detect acute hematoma and obtain baseline density measurements of renal masses.[12] Noncontrast CT is accepted as primary imaging to detect urinary calculi.

Contrast-enhanced CT Oral Contrast Medium

In the evaluation of urolithiasis, dense oral contrast medium in the bowel can make detection of ureteral stones more difficult. In addition, for 3D CT angiography, positive oral contrast medium should not be given in order to improve postprocessing image quality and to avoid major overlay in postprocessed images.[13] Some investigators suggest drinking 500–750 mL of water over a 15-20 minutes period before the start of a renal CT examination and do not advocate the use of oral contrast medium for renal MDCT.[14]

Administration of Intravenous Contrast Medium

For the contrast-enhanced phases, the optimal timing depends on the volume of the contrast medium, the rate of its administration and patient's cardiac output. The difference between the start of contrast medium injection and the start of scanning is referred to as delay time. 100–120 mL of nonionic contrast medium is sufficient at an infusion rate of 2–3 mL per second for routine renal imaging. Contrast is injected through an 18-gauge catheter placed in the antecubital vein.

PHASES OF RENAL ENHANCEMENT/ MULTIPHASIC HELICAL CT

Normal CT Nephrogram

The first perfusion phase, the cortical nephrogram or the **corticomedullary phase (CMP)** becomes visible 25–80 seconds after contrast administration. When contrast material enters the cortical capillaries and peritubular capillary spaces and filling of the lumina of the proximal cortical tubules starts, the renal cortex is distinctly differentiated from the unenhanced medulla **(Fig. 7)**.[15,16]

The second phase, the tubular nephrogram or **nephrographic phase** begins **90–120** seconds after contrast injection and includes the passage of contrast material through the renal tubule system.[15,16] During this phase the corticomedullary differentiation disappears and the renal parenchyma enhances homogeneously **(Fig. 8)**.

The third phase, the **excretory phase** (EP) begins 3–5 minutes after contrast administration and begins when contrast material is excreted into the collecting system **(Fig. 9)**.

Corticomedullary Phase

The advantages of corticomedullary phase (CMP) include differentiation of normal variants of renal

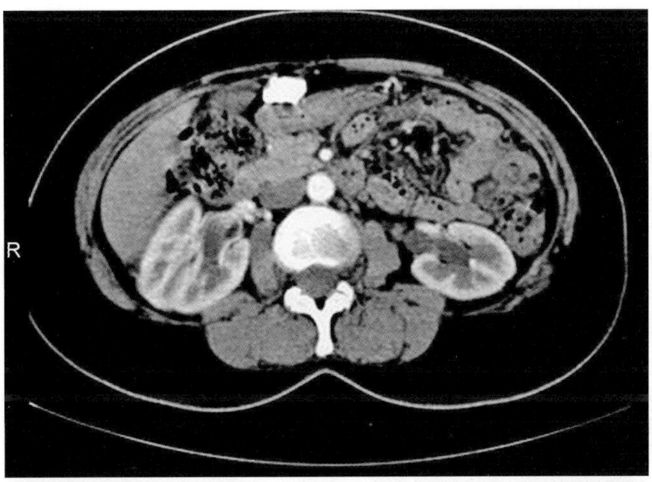

Fig. 7: Contrast-enhanced scan of the kidney in the corticomedullary (CM) phase showing dense cortical enhancement, the renal cortex is distinctly differentiated from the unenhanced medulla.

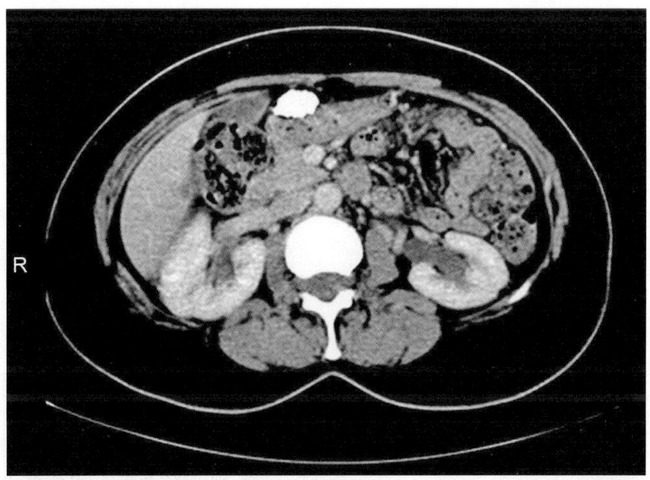

Fig. 8: CECT of the kidney in the nephrogram phase showing dense homogeneous parenchymal enhancement and disappearance of the corticomedullary differentiation during this phase.

parenchyma from renal masses and better depiction of tumor hypervascularity improving the characterization of solid renal mass lesions **(Figs. 10A to C)**. However, assessing the CMP alone may result in clinically significant errors[17] as small hypovascular tumors of the renal medulla may be missed since they are not sufficiently enhanced and hypervascular cortical renal cell carcinomas may enhance to the same degree as the normal cortex and may be missed. Thus imaging of the kidney during CMP should be completed by scanning the kidney during nephrographic phase (NP).

Nephrographic Phase

This is considered the optimal phase for the detection and characterization of renal masses, in particular of small renal masses <3 cm providing both homogeneous enhancement of cortex and medulla and lesion enhancement.[18] Lesion enhancement >20 HU which is considered sufficient proof for a malignant mass may be delayed and not visualized until the nephrographic phase (NP) **(Figs. 11A and B)**. Homogeneous enhancement of NP also provides the visualization of renal infarction, traumatic parenchymal lesions and acute pyelonephritis.

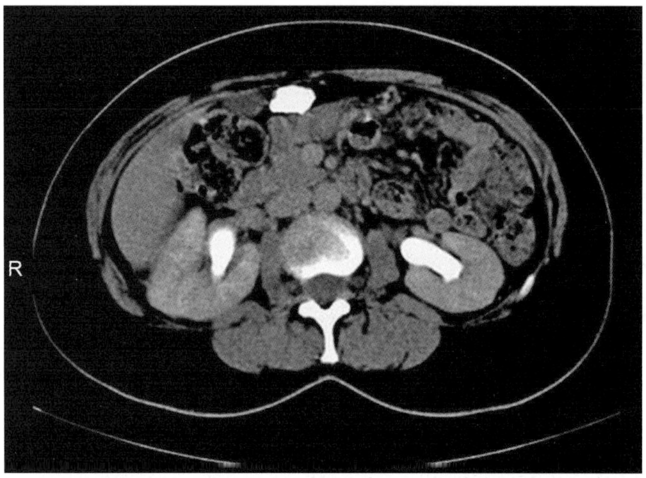

Fig. 9: Excretory phase or the delayed phase (5 minutes) axial CT image demonstrating calyceal opacification.

Pathological CT Nephrogram

Helical CT enables an improved depiction of renal pathology caused by abnormal vascular perfusion and/or reduced tubule transit rates.

Impaired renal perfusions with focal reduction of the nephrogram include renal infarction, blunt renal trauma and acute pyelonephritis. In blunt renal trauma, lack of the nephrogram is a feature of devascularization of renal parenchyma which may be segmental/total depending on the localization of the vessel injury **(Fig. 12)**. In acute pyelonephritis, hypoperfusion is combined with reduced tubule transit rates due to inflammatory obstruction. Delayed perfusion of the renal tubule system is visualized as a striated nephrogram of the infiltrated parenchyma. An initially reduced density and slowed temporal progression of the three phases of the nephrogram is caused by significant stenoses of the main renal artery, acute obstruction of the renal vein and acute ureteral obstruction. A bilaterally reduced density and persistence of the nephrogram is observed in shock due to diminished glomerular filtration rate and tubular stasis caused by severe systemic hypotension.

Excretory Phase

The excretory phase (EP) (the delayed or urographic phase), used to evaluate renal collecting system and ureters, begins 3 minutes after the start of contrast

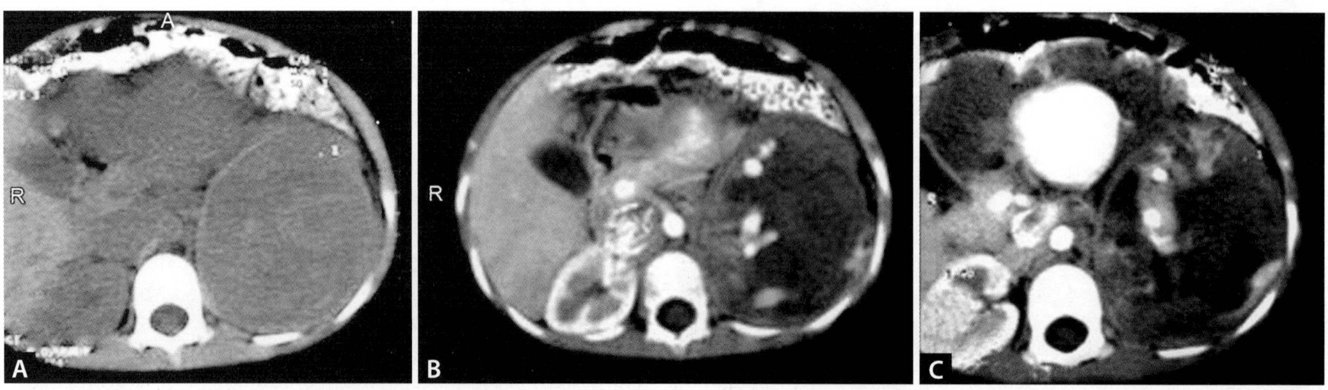

Figs. 10A to C: (A) Noncontrast axial CT showing a large hypodense mass with no differential density replacing the left kidney; (B and C) The corticomedullary phase shows multiple tortuous feeder vessels depicting tumor hypervascularity. Thrombus is also seen in IVC—Wilm's tumor.

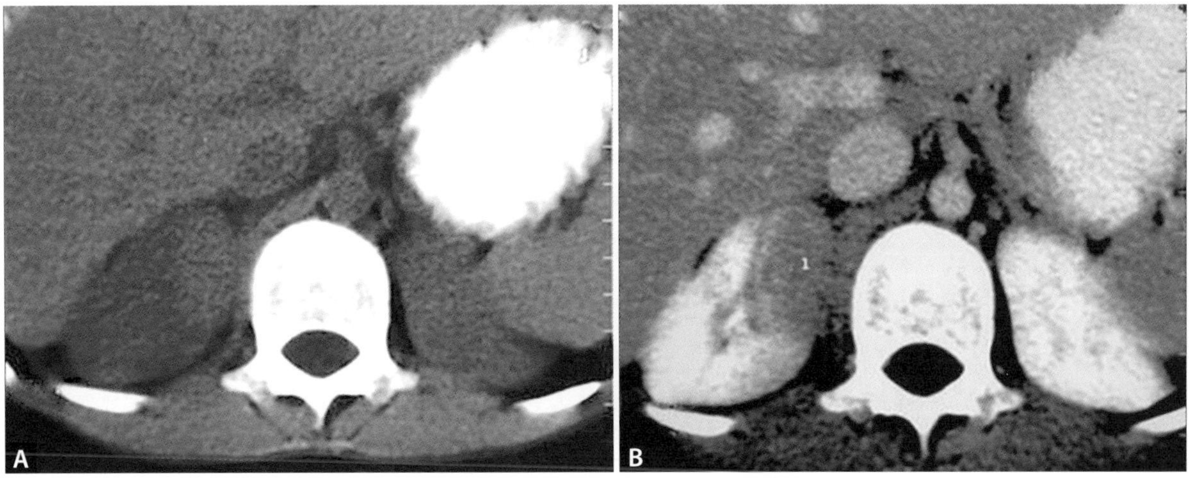

Figs. 11A and B: Noncontrast CT scan: (A) Showing an indeterminate mass in the right kidney. Nephrogram phase of renal enhancement; (B) Demonstrating significant enhancement > 20 HU suggestive of malignant mass.

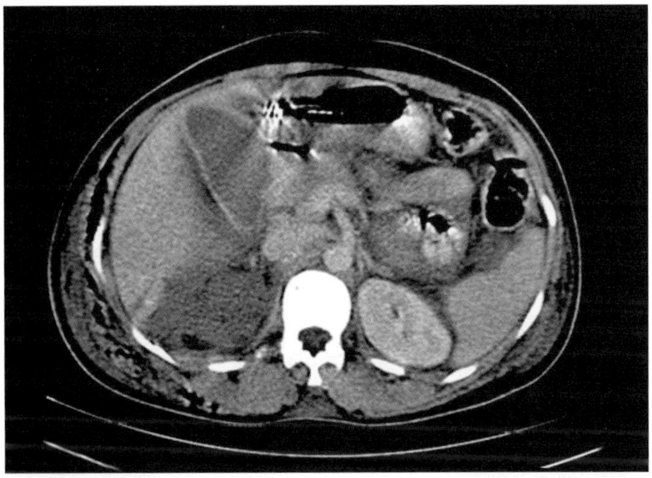

Fig. 12: Contrast-enhanced axial scan of the kidney showing lack of nephrogram on the right side suggesting devascularization of the renal parenchyma in a case of trauma. The normal nephrogram with homogeneous enhancement of the renal parenchyma is seen on the left side.

medium injection. In this phase, while the intensity of the nephrogram declines, excretion of the contrast medium permits opacification of the calyces, renal pelvis, and ureters. The opacification of the renal collecting system allows the depiction of intraluminal pathology.

Thus, Multiphasic HCT is the preferred technique in the evaluation of the kidney in clinically suspected/known renal disease.[19] It includes an unenhanced scan as well as scanning after rapid bolus injection (3-4 mL/sec) of contrast (100-120 mL/300 mg/mL) during both CMP and NP and/or EP respectively. Scan parameters include 120 kV, 220-280 mA, a collimation of 3-5 mm, a reconstruction interval of 2-4 mm and a pitch of 1.5 during a scan acquisition time of one breath-hold.

IMAGE PROCESSING AND POSTPROCESSING TECHNIQUES

Four main 3D visualization techniques currently are used on clinical 3D workstations: MPR, maximum intensity projections (MIP), shaded surface displays (SSD) and a volume-rendering technique (VRT).

Multiplanar Reformation

Multiplanar reformation (MPR) is the postprocessing technique used most commonly and represents simple reordering of the image voxel. A known limitation of MPR is the visualized structures must be in the same plane. Because most structures of interest are not within a single plane, a MRP cannot be created that demonstrates an entire structure **(Figs. 13A and B)**. As structures course in and out of the MPR, pseudostenoses are created. To solve this problem, curved planar reformation (CPR) are used. CPR have a single voxel thick tomogram, but it is capable of demonstrating an uninterrupted longitudinal cross-section as the display plane curves along the structure of interest.[20] CPR images can be obtained manually by drawing a line over a structure of interest or it can be produced automatically or semiautomatically by dedicated software. CPR provide the most useful luminal assessment (such as of blood vessels, airways, bowel and ureters) and are useful in improving the visualization of vessels of small diameter or tortuous anatomy such as the ureters **(Fig. 14)**.[21] CPR have an important limitation in that they are highly dependent on the accuracy of the curve.

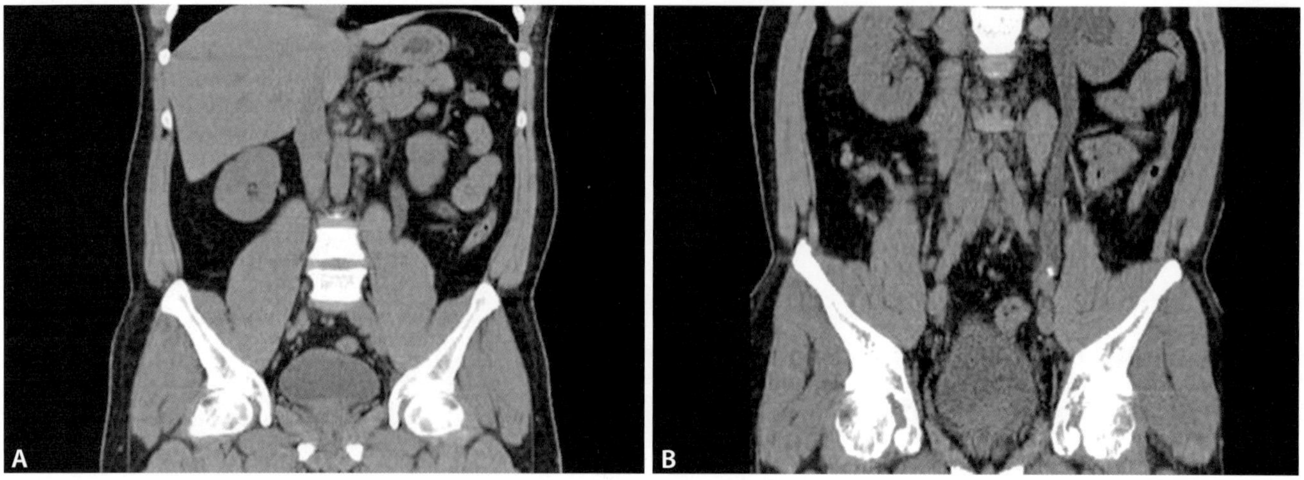

Figs. 13A and B: (A) Coronal MPR image demonstrating only a small segment of the left ureter in its mid portion; (B) Curved multiplanar reformation displaying a left ureteric calculus, the consequent hydronephrosis and the entire dilated ureter proximal to it in a single image regardless of opacificaion.

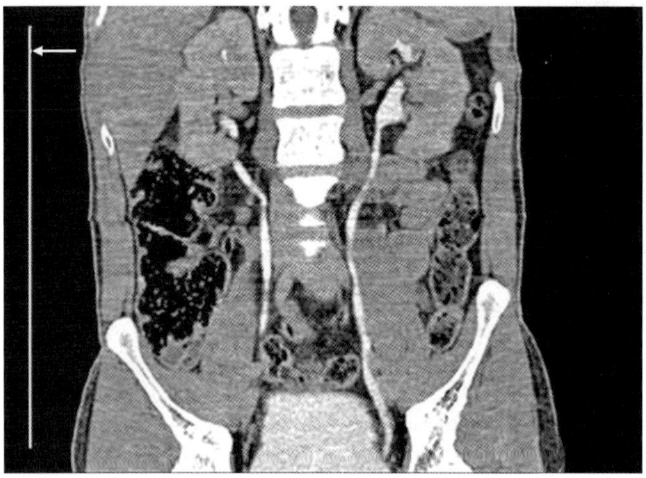

Fig. 14: Curved multiplanar reformation (CPR) image after contrast opacification of the pelvicalyceal system showing an uninterrupted course of the left ureter in its entirety as this technique displays all voxel values on the curve randomly drawn by the operator.

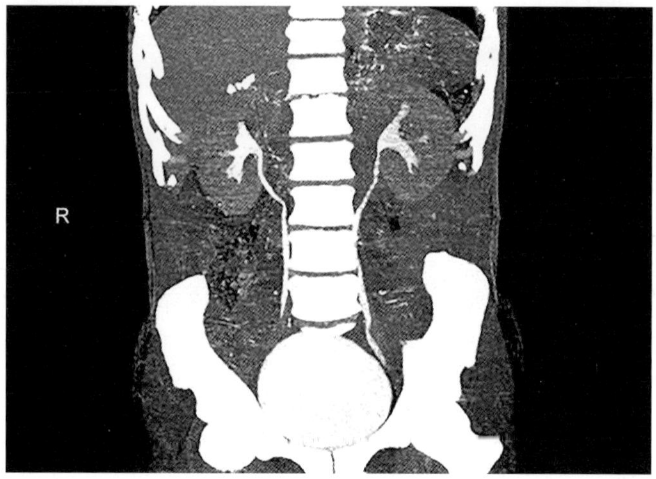

Fig. 15: Maximum intensity projection (MIP) in the exceretory phase demonstrating the normally opacified calyces, the ureters and the bladder. This technique displays the maximum voxel value along a line of viewer's projection through a given volume.

Maximum Intensity Projection

Maximum intensity projection (MIP) displays the maximum voxel intensity along a line of viewer projection in a given volume. High density structures, such as contrast filled vessels and the collecting system, are demonstrated nicely in images, such as angiograms or urograms **(Fig. 15)**. The main disadvantage of MIP is that it obscures the area of interest by high density material, such as bone, calcium and oral contrast medium. With the MIP technique, a 3D effect can be obtained with rotational viewing of multiple projections, but it lacks depth orientation.[14]

Shaded Surface Displays

Shaded surface displays (SSD) enables accurate 3D representations of anatomy, relying on the grayscale to encode surface reflections from an imaginary source of illumination. SSD images are limited by their dependence on user-selected threshold setting.

Volume-rendered Technique

With this technique, all attenuation values within a voxel are used to obtain the final image (each voxel contributes brightness, color and opacity to the final image). Anatomic structures with different levels of opacity (e.g. renal parenchyma, renal veins and arteries and the collecting system) can be demonstrated simultaneously **(Fig. 16)**. Volume-rendered technique (VRT) is an excellent 3D technique for presentation that provides a roadmap for surgery and summary picture for the referring physician.[22] The most important limitation of VRT is its need for more powerful computers and costly workstation. Using editing techniques, structures overlaying the area of interest can be removed for better visualization and desired orientation **(Figs. 17 and 18)**.

MULTIDETECTOR CT UROGRAPHY

Multidetector CT urography (MDCTU) may be defined as the examination of the urinary tract by MDCT in the excretory phase following intravenous administration.

Indications of CT Urography

- Calculi
- Renal tumors
- Urothelial tumors
- PUJ obstruction
- Congenital anomalies.

Calculi

It has been established unequivocally that currently MDCT is the most sensitive and specific test for the diagnosis of urinary tract calculi.[23] MDCTU can not only detect calculi but also accurately determine the level of obstruction **(Figs. 19A and B)**. MDCTU has an advantage over IVU that is, the ability to exclude extraurinary pathologies that may mimic calculi.[24] MDCT can also detect calculi in unusual positions such as in calyceal divertculae and is more accurate than IVU for detecting presence, size and location of urinary tract calculi. MDCTU also has the IVU advantage of demonstrating physiologic information, gained from the degree of delayed excretion, which was considered an index of severity of obstruction. Hydronephrosis, hydroureter, ipsilateral renal enlargement, perinephric and periureteral fat stranding, perinephric fluid, ureter rim sign and ureterovesical edema are secondary signs of obstructing calculi **(Figs. 20A to C)**. The presence of "soft time rim sign", namely, a circumferental rim of soft tissue attenuation surrounding a calcification is a reliable indicator that the calcification in question represents a calculus within the ureter. Calculi associated with a "soft tissue rim sign" have a mean size of 4 mm.[25,26] Conversely, a "comet tail sign" namely a linear or curvilinear soft tissue structure extending from an abdominal/pelvic calcification, has been stated to represent a phlebolith.

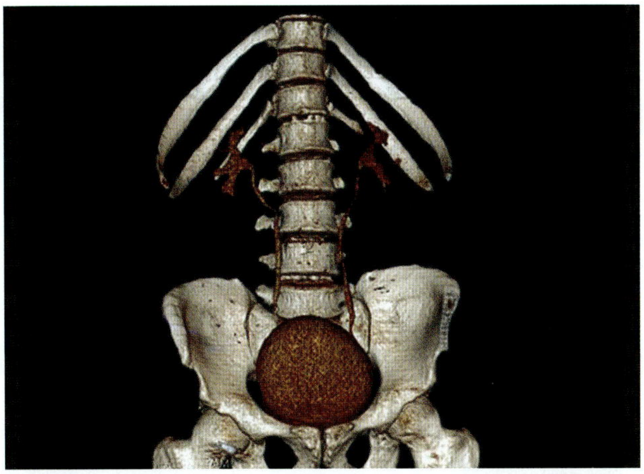

Fig. 16: Volume rendering technique (VRT) displaying the entire urinary tract. This technique takes the entire volume of data and displays anatomic structures with different levels of opacity/attenuation.

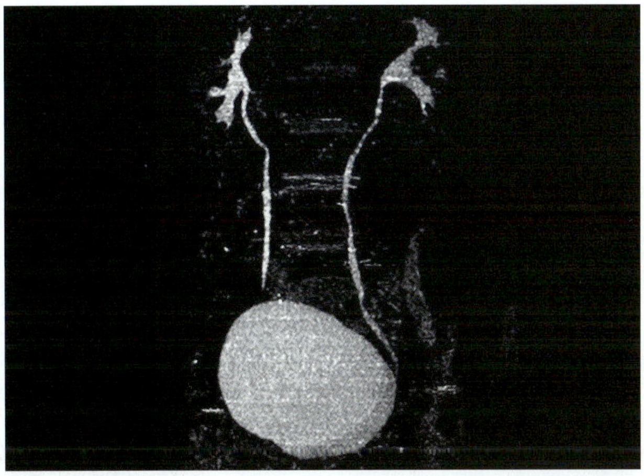

Fig. 17: Normal CT urogram image using maximum intensity projection (MIP) with bone editing displaying the entire urinary tract.

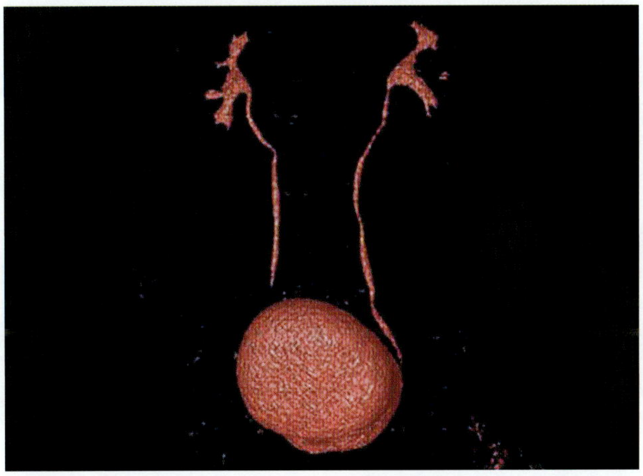

Fig. 18: Normal CT urogram image using volume rendering with bone editing displaying the entire urinary tract.

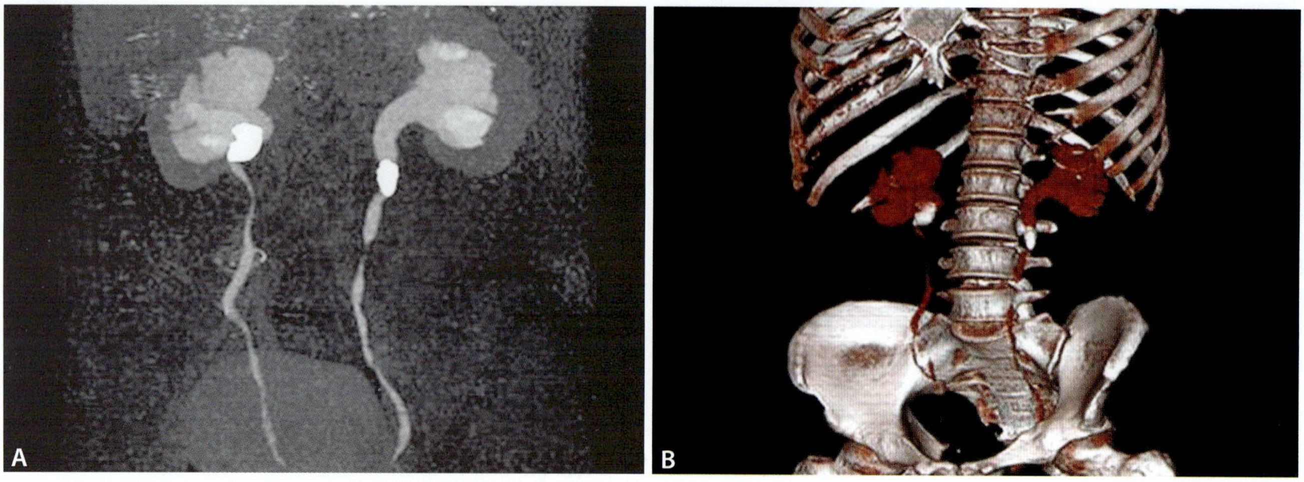

Figs. 19A and B: CT urogram using MIP technique (A) depicting a calculus at the pelviureteric junction on the right side and a calculus in the proximal left ureter. There are backpressure changes on both sides. VRT image (B) displaying the same.

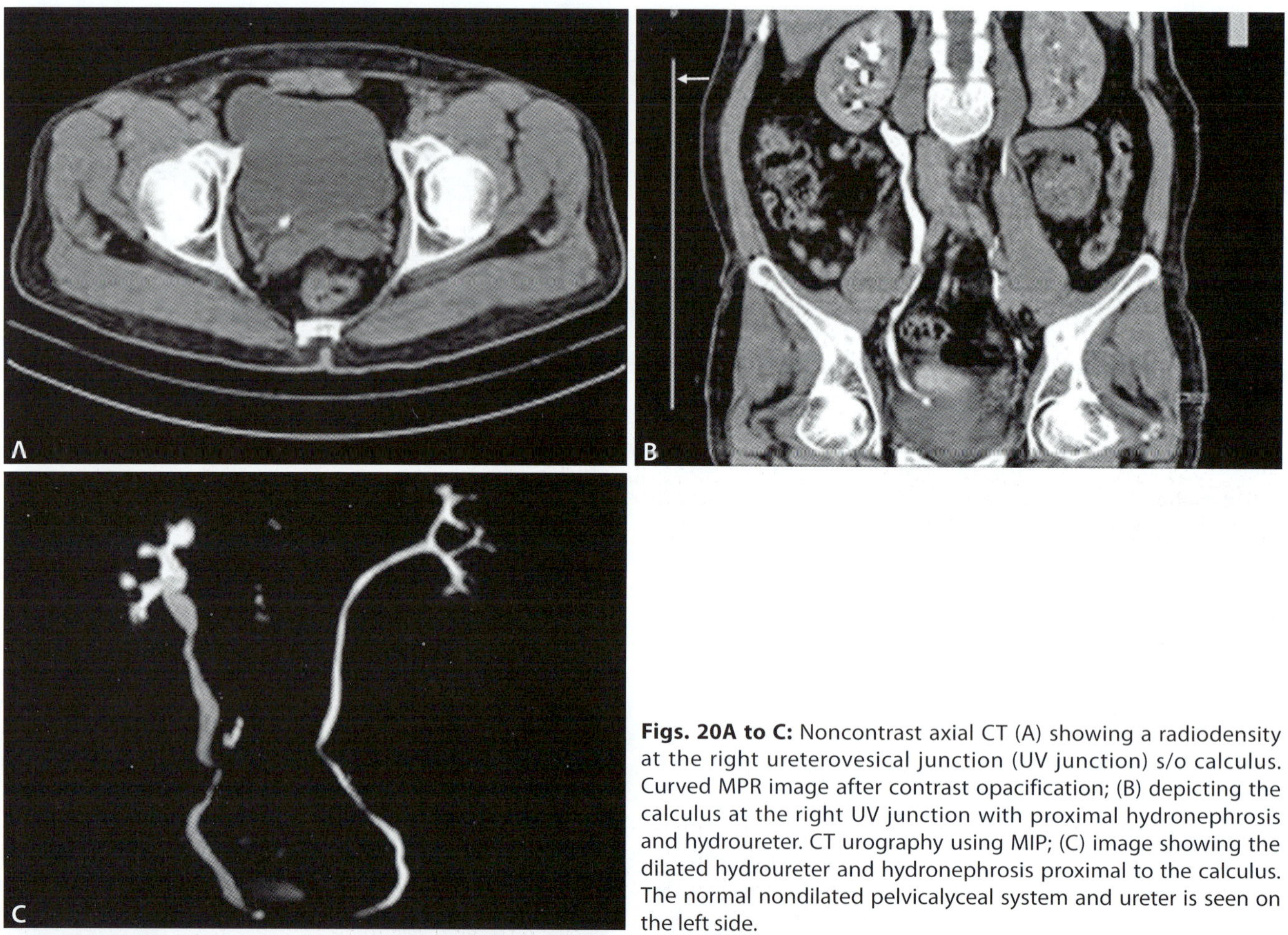

Figs. 20A to C: Noncontrast axial CT (A) showing a radiodensity at the right ureterovesical junction (UV junction) s/o calculus. Curved MPR image after contrast opacification; (B) depicting the calculus at the right UV junction with proximal hydronephrosis and hydroureter. CT urography using MIP; (C) image showing the dilated hydroureter and hydronephrosis proximal to the calculus. The normal nondilated pelvicalyceal system and ureter is seen on the left side.

Renal Tumors

MDCTU is an appropriate imaging test for the detection and characterization of renal masses. The initial unenhanced CT is obtained to serve as the baseline for measurements of enhancements on the nephrographic phase images.[27] Most renal cell cancers are solid, with attenuation greater than 20 HU on unenhanced CT.[28] Lesion enhancement greater than 20 HU is considered highly suspicious of a malignant lesion. The location of the tumor may also be helpful in the diagnosis and characterization of solid renal masses. Renal cell carcinoma is frequently located at the periphery or near the corticomedullary junction of the kidney as it originates in the renal cortex, while transitional cell carcinoma extends into the kidney from the renal pelvicalyceal system and occurs more centrally in the kidney.[29] These features are well-demonstrated by MDCT. Renal tumors with nephron sparing surgery require a precise depiction of the tumor and its relation to the collecting system **(Figs. 21A to C)**. MDCT urogram demonstrates not only the pelvicalyceal system as in conventional urography but also renal, perirenal and vascular tissues.

Urothelial Tumors

Transitional cell carcinoma is the most common malignant neoplasm of the urotheluim. Many urologists believe that intravenous urography is still the gold standard for evaluating the urothelium, however, it has been reported in the literature to have detection rates for urothelial neoplasms of only 43–64%.[30] In the early stages, these neoplasms are seen as subtle filling defects or mural thickening. A filling defect in the renal pelvis or ureter can be caused by a neoplasm, calculus, clot, mycetoma or vascular impression. MDCTU has shown increased sensitivity and specificity for detecting urothetial tumor compared with retrograde ureterography, an imaging test

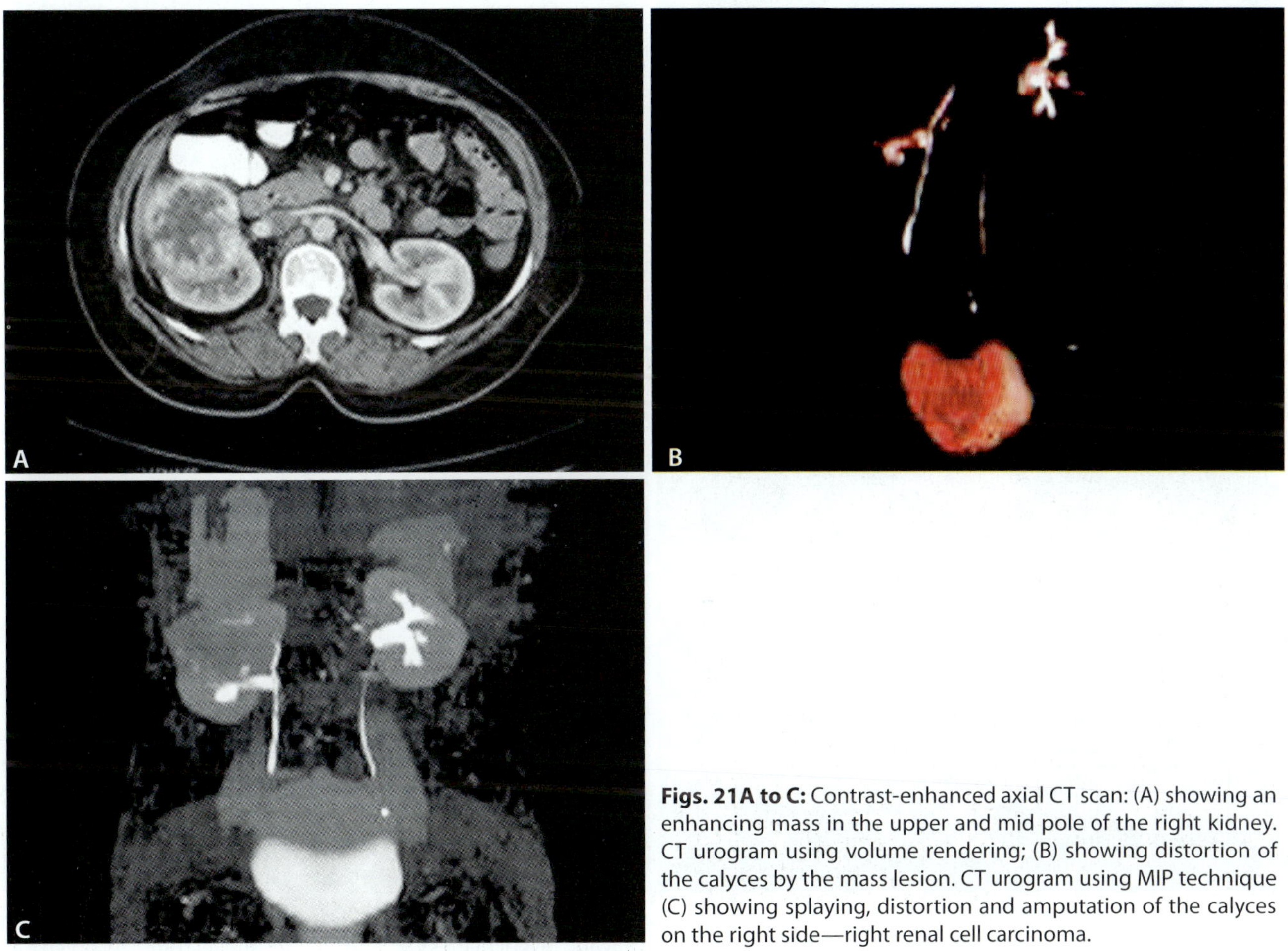

Figs. 21A to C: Contrast-enhanced axial CT scan: (A) showing an enhancing mass in the upper and mid pole of the right kidney. CT urogram using volume rendering; (B) showing distortion of the calyces by the mass lesion. CT urogram using MIP technique (C) showing splaying, distortion and amputation of the calyces on the right side—right renal cell carcinoma.

assumed to be superior to IVU in evaluating the collecting system and ureters.[31] A recent study suggests that MDCTU is an accurate means for detection and staging of upper urinary tract TCC with accuracy for peritumoral invasion with positive and negative predictive values of 88.8 and 87.5% respectively.[32] One of the main advantages of MDCTU over IVU includes identification of intrinisic and extrinsic causes of ureteric obstruction including mural thickening with short segment malignant strictures retroperitoneal masses or lymphadenopathy retroperitoneal fibrosis, benign ureteric strictures and iatrogenic causes.[33] It can also show ureteic infiltration in malignant pelvic masses (**Figs. 22A to D**).

Cystoscopy remains the "gold standard" for evaluating the urinary bladder but MDCT urogram is playing an important role in the detection of bladder urothelial neoplasms (**Figs. 23A and B**). As with urothelial tumors of the upper urinary tract, bladder neoplasms present as a filling defect, a focal mass or an area of focal bladder wall thickening (**Fig. 24**).[34] In a study a sensitivity of 93% and specificity of 99% has been quoted for MDCTU in detecting bladder neoplasms, when compared with cystoscopy.[35]

Pelviureteric Junction Obstruction

In patients with pelviureteric junction (PUJ) obstruction the success rate of endopyelotomy depends on whether there are crossing vessels at the UPJ. The sucesss rate is only 42% in patients with a crossing vessel and 80% if no crossing vessel is present. A combination of CT angiography with CT urography demonstrates the crossing vessel in relation to the renal pelvis very well.[36]

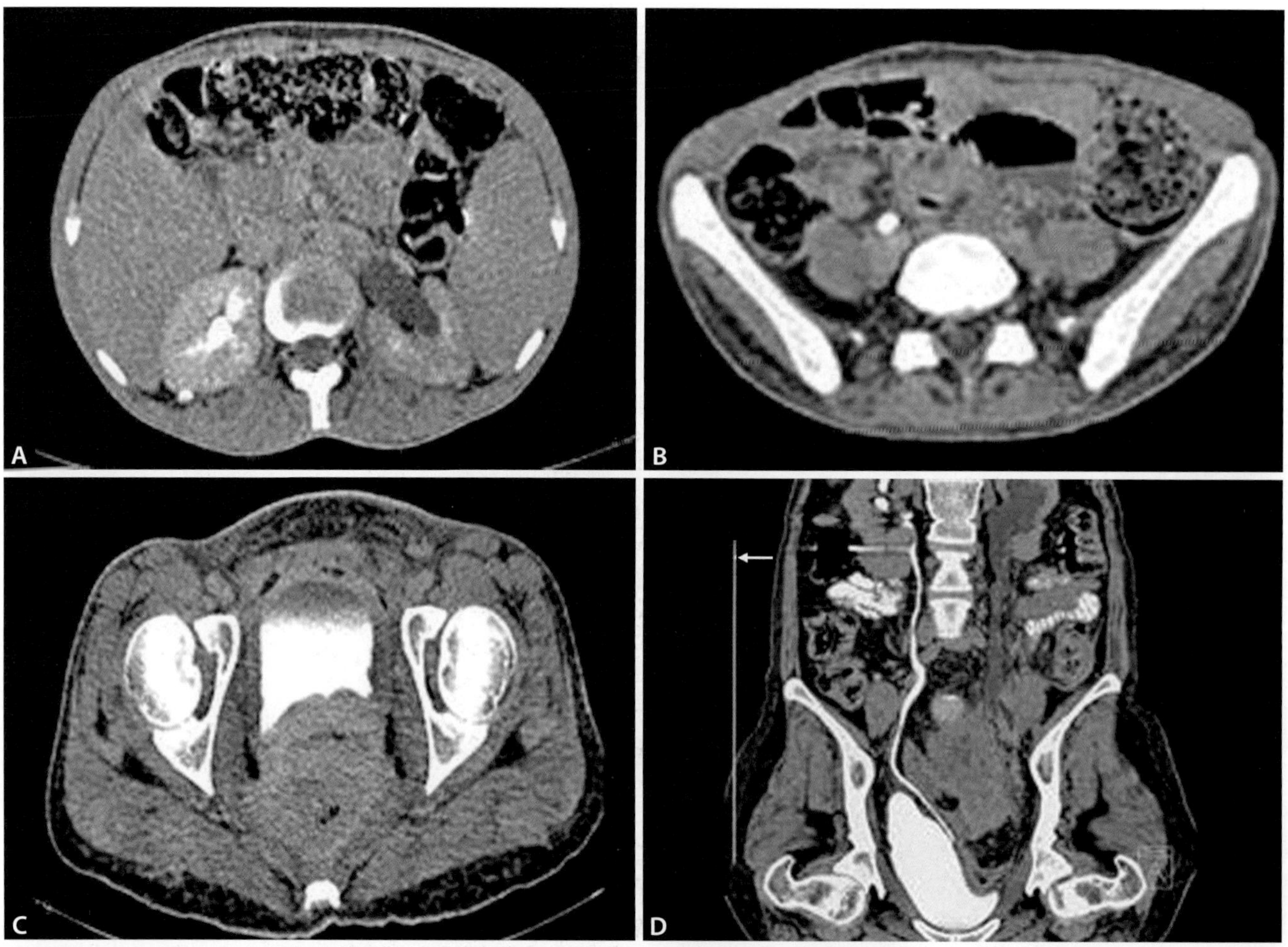

Figs. 22A to D: Contrast-enhanced axial scans of the abdomen showing left hydronephrosis (A) dilated left ureter; (B) Consequent to carcinoma cervix which has infiltrated the left ureter. The mass is also showing loss of planes with the bladder and rectum; (C) Curved MPR image; (D) Depicting the infiltration of the left ureter by cervical mass and proximal hydroureteronephrosis with delayed opacification of the pelvicalyceal system on the left side. The normal well-opacified pelvicalyceal system and ureter is seen on the right side.

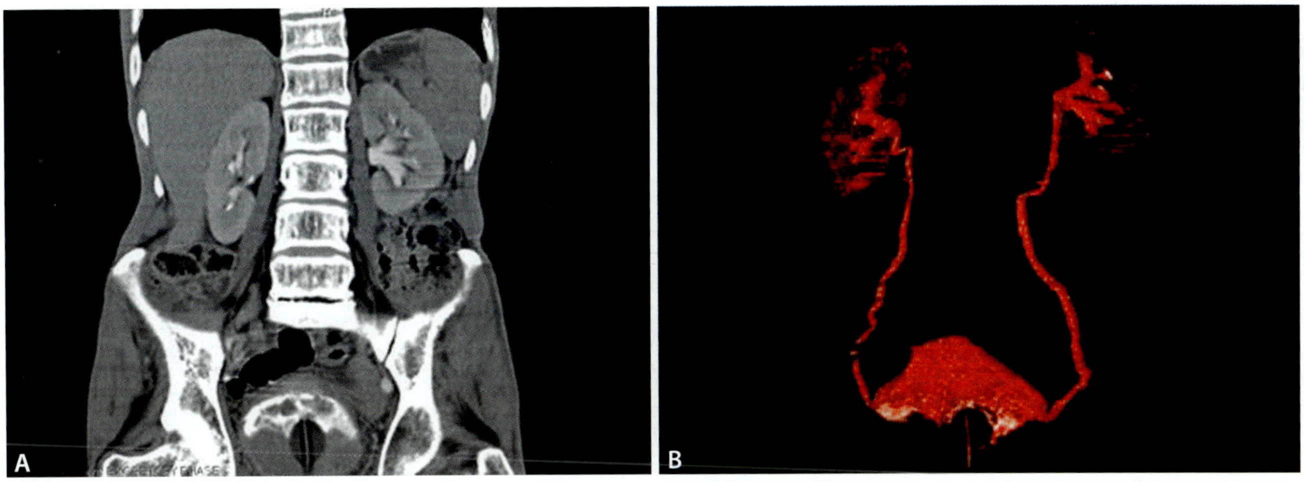

Figs. 23A and B: Coronal MPR image: (A) Revealing diffuse circumferential thickening of the bladder base with hydronephrosis seen in both kidneys (left > right). Foley's bulb is seen *in situ*. VRT image (B) showing the mass at the bladder base with backpressure changes on both sides, more marked on the left side—Carcinoma bladder.

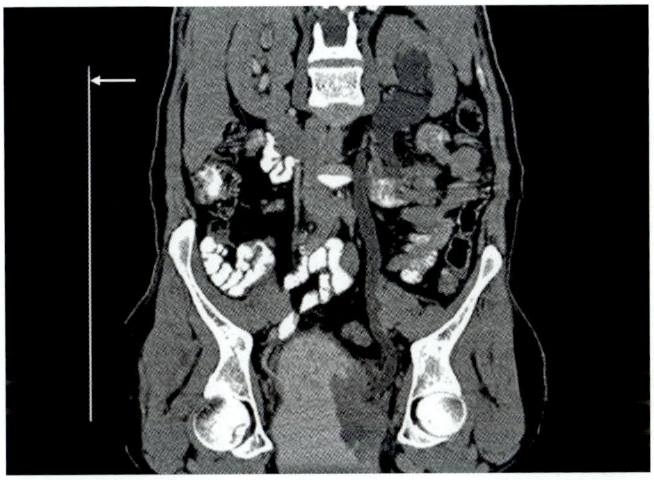

Fig. 24: Curved MPR image depicting a mass involving the left lateral wall of the urinary bladder with involvement of the left ureterovesical junction and consequent left hydroureteronephrosis and delayed opacification of the left side as compared to the normal contralateral right side—Carcinoma bladder.

Congenital Anomalies

In congenital lesion such as retrocaval ureter, not only does CT urography demonstrate the ureteric compression but also the IVC which is the cause for the retrocaval ureter. Ureteral duplication is another congenital anomaly **(Figs. 25A to C)**. The entire course of both upper and lower moiety must be demonstrated as well as the ectopic opening. Often the upper moiety with lower ectopic opening is hydronephrotic with a hydroureter. MCDTU has ability to demonstrate both functioning and nonfunctioning components.[37] MDCT can also display anomalies, such as crossed fused ectopia, horseshoe kidney and renal ectopia **(Figs. 26A to C)**.

MDCTU Protocol

The most commonly used MDCTU protocol comprises a three-phase protocol, which consists of an initial unenhanced phase, a second phase following the administration of nonionic contrast material (100–150 mL of 300 mg/mL iodine concentration at a rate of 2–4 mL/second) acquired following 90–100 sec delay, also known as the nephrographic phase. This phase is followed by pyelographic phase contrast that is taken 12–15 minutes following contrast to evaluate the urothelium from the pelvicalyceal system to the bladder.[23] A fourth phase protocol consists of two excretory phases (5 mintues and 7.5 minutes) to optimize ureteric distension and opacification. However, because of radiation dose a three-phase protocol is considered sufficient.

Split Bolus MDCT Urography with Synchronus Nephrographic and Exceretory Phase Enhancement

Chai and colleagues have proposed the use of a split bolus technique in place of a single intravenous injection to facilitate a two phase protocol, namely an unenhanced series of images and a second phase in which nephrographic and pyelographic phases are

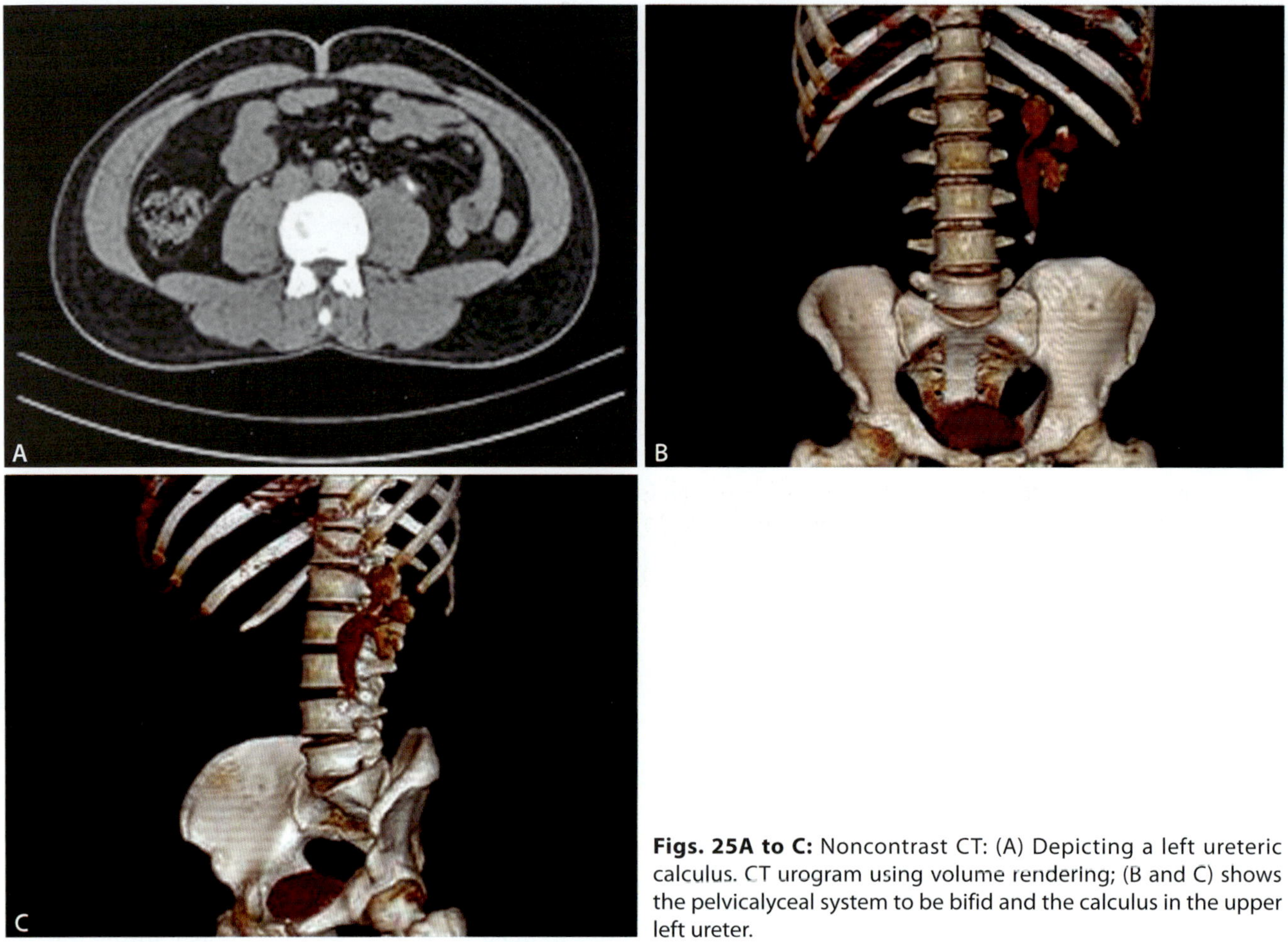

Figs. 25A to C: Noncontrast CT: (A) Depicting a left ureteric calculus. CT urogram using volume rendering; (B and C) shows the pelvicalyceal system to be bifid and the calculus in the upper left ureter.

simultaneously acquired called the "nephropyelographic" phase.[38] With this protocol, after the initial noncontrast administration, 30 CC of nonionic contrast material is infused intravenously and the patient is removed from the CT table. The patient is encouraged to walk for 10 minutes. 10–15 minutes later, the patient is placed in the CT table in the prone-position. A dynamic contrast-enhanced CT is then performed following the administration of an additional 100 cc of nonionic contrast material (300 mg/mL injected at 2 cc/second) following a delay of 100 seconds. Thus in a single "nephropyelographic phase" acquisition, the renal paremchyma (nephrographic phase) and the collecting system, ureters and bladder (pyelographic phase) are assessed. The main objective with MDCT urography is to detect all possible causes of hematuria while using the lowest possible radiation dose to the patient. The split bolus technique has the potential to reduce both radiation dose and the number of images generated by MDCT urography.[39]

Techniques to improve urinary tract distension and opacification have been done to achieve adequate opacification and distension of the pelvicalyceal system and ureters.

Compression

Analysis of various data have suggested that the percentage of nonvisualized segments reached upto 25% which is not significantly different from CT urography without compression. External compression is not recommended in patients with abdominal pain or in patients with history of urinary tract obstruction, radical cystectomy, recent surgery and aortic aneurysm. The benefits are outweighed by the added inconvenience and discomfort to the patient. Thus compression is not advocated in most of the centers.

Saline Infusion

It has been seen that saline infusion did not significantly improve ureteric distension or opacification and may

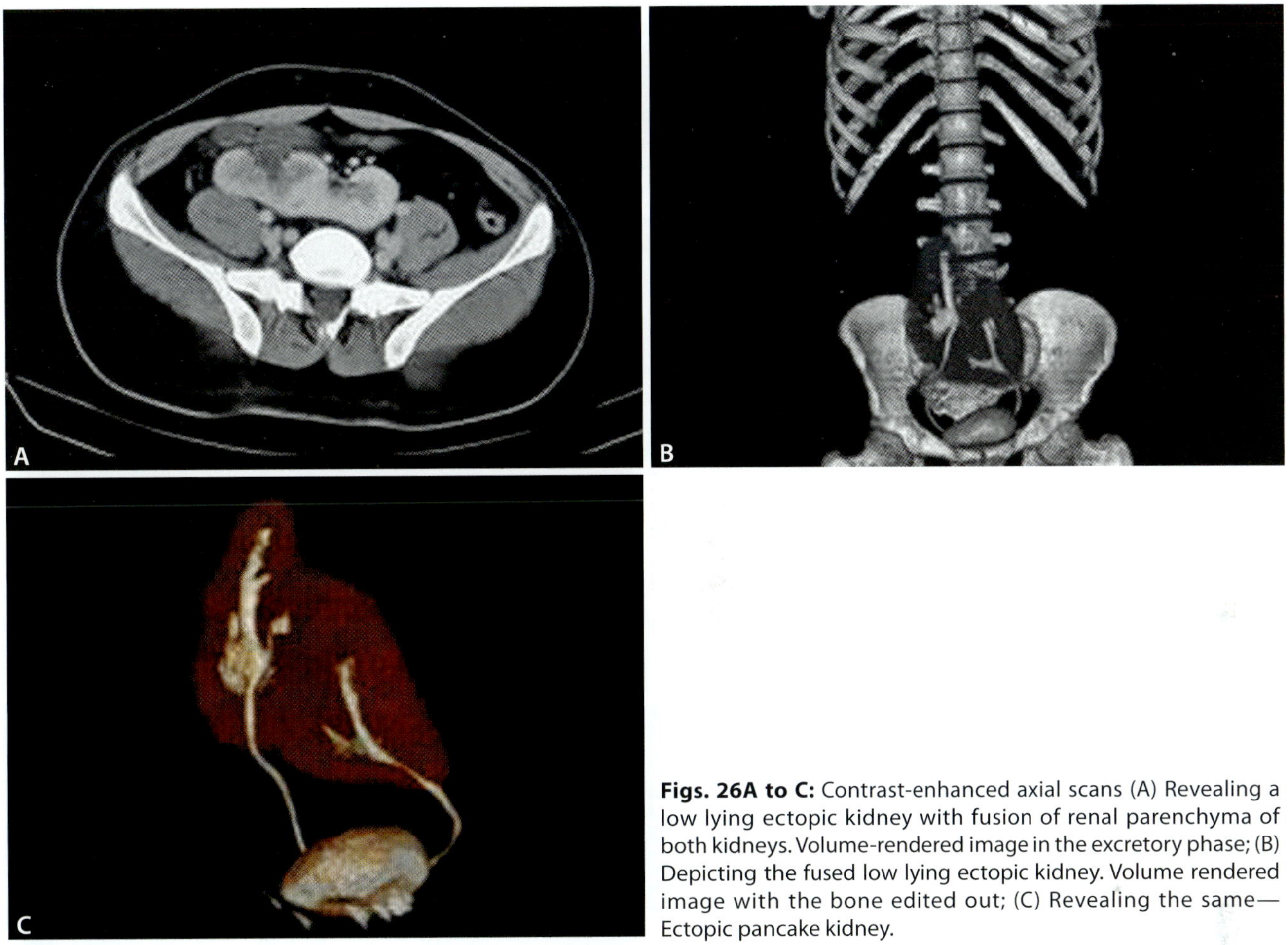

Figs. 26A to C: Contrast-enhanced axial scans (A) Revealing a low lying ectopic kidney with fusion of renal parenchyma of both kidneys. Volume-rendered image in the excretory phase; (B) Depicting the fused low lying ectopic kidney. Volume rendered image with the bone edited out; (C) Revealing the same—Ectopic pancake kidney.

simulate ureteric peristalsis in certain cases.[40] Thus saline infusion is usually not included in the MDCTU protocol.

Diuretic Administration

Proponents of low dose diuretic administration have recommended that the diuretic be administered 1 minute before contrast administration. The administration of intravenous diuretic has been reported to increase ureteric distension.

Patient Positioning

It has been reported that MDCTU performed with the patient in the prone position achieved higher opacification of the mid and distal ureters than supine scanning.[41]

Image Interpretation

Interpretation of MDCTU involves review of a large number of images, which includes comparison of unenhanced and enhanced images for presence of calculi and for degree of contrast enhancement which is particularly important for characterization of renal masses. The importance of the state of the art user friendly workstations cannot be overemphasized. MPR and MIP images are most commonly used and are very useful in the evaluation of the ureter and in localizing the exact level of the abnormality. These reformats are also useful in the characterization of urinary tract anomalies.

Thus MDCTU can be used as a "one stop imaging test" for the entire urinary tract.

MULTIDETECTOR CT IN RENAL MASSES

MDCT is accepted as the state of art technology in staging renal cell carcinomas (RCCs) due to its ability to obtain multiple scans through the area of interest. The multiphasic HCT with small and overlapping sections provides increased sensitivity in detection and better characterization of small RCCs and accurate staging of RCCs due to diagnosis of venous tumor extension. For optimal evaluation of a renal mass with MDCT, multiphase imaging is necessary.[28] For all renal imaging, the use of thin (5 mm or less) collimation is essential.[42] Preliminary non-contrast scans are used to detect calcifications and allow quantification of enhancement on the postcontrast scans.

The first phase of contrast enhancement is the **cortico-medullary phase** that is essential for accurate staging of RCC. Maximal opacification of the renal arteries and veins allows confident diagnosis of venous extension of tumoral tissue. In evaluation of renal mass special attention is given to visualization of renal vein and IVC junction. Venous extension is shown best during the corticomedullary phase **(Figs. 27A to C)**. The most specific sign of venous extension is the presence of a hypodense, filling defect within the vein **(Figs. 28A to C)**. A sudden change in caliber of the renal vein and the presence of a clot within collateral veins are useful ancillary signs. Direct continuity of the thrombus with the primary tumor and heterogeneous enhancement of the thrombus with contrast indicate tumoral thrombus. Accurate demonstration of the arterial anatomy is useful in selected cases to plan nephron sparing surgery.

The **nephrographic phase** is the most useful for detecting renal masses and for characterizing indeterminate lesions. A small lesion can be detected that may blend with the cortex on corticomedullary images. As most RCCS have a rich vascular supply they enhance significantly after contrast administration on the nephrographic phase. Enhancement value of more than 20 HU is considered suspicious for malignancy **(Figs. 29A and B)**.[43] Some less vascular RCC masses enhance 10–20 HU and this level of enhancement is seen more frequently with cystic RCC. Sometimes this level of enhancement can be seen in some benign lesions such as complicated cysts.[43]

The excretory phase is useful to delineate the relationship of a centrally located mass with the collecting system better and to define potential involvement of the calyces and the renal pelvis.[28] This phase is useful for detecting transitional cell carcinoma. Measurement of

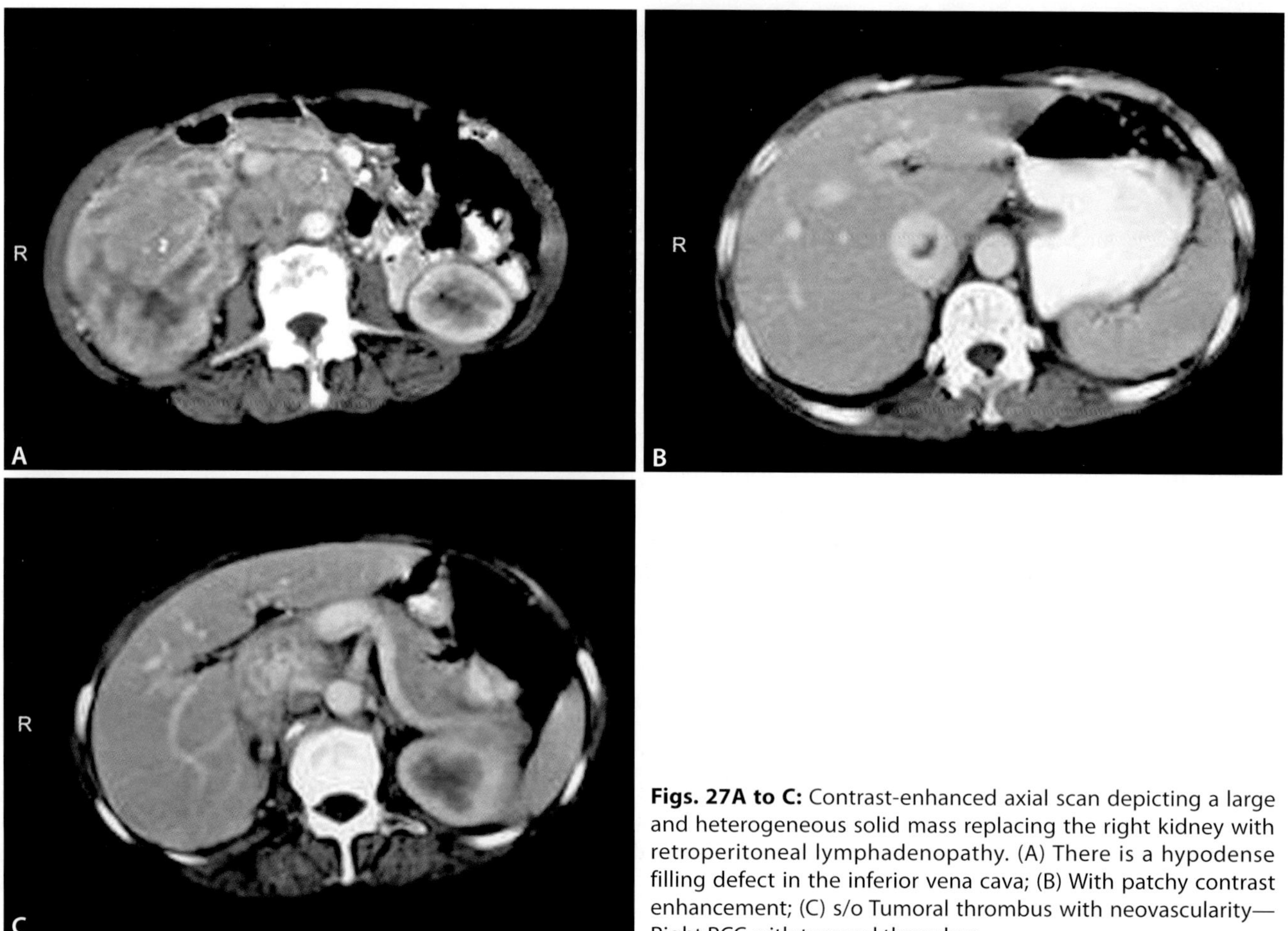

Figs. 27A to C: Contrast-enhanced axial scan depicting a large and heterogeneous solid mass replacing the right kidney with retroperitoneal lymphadenopathy. (A) There is a hypodense filling defect in the inferior vena cava; (B) With patchy contrast enhancement; (C) s/o Tumoral thrombus with neovascularity—Right RCC with tumoral thrombus.

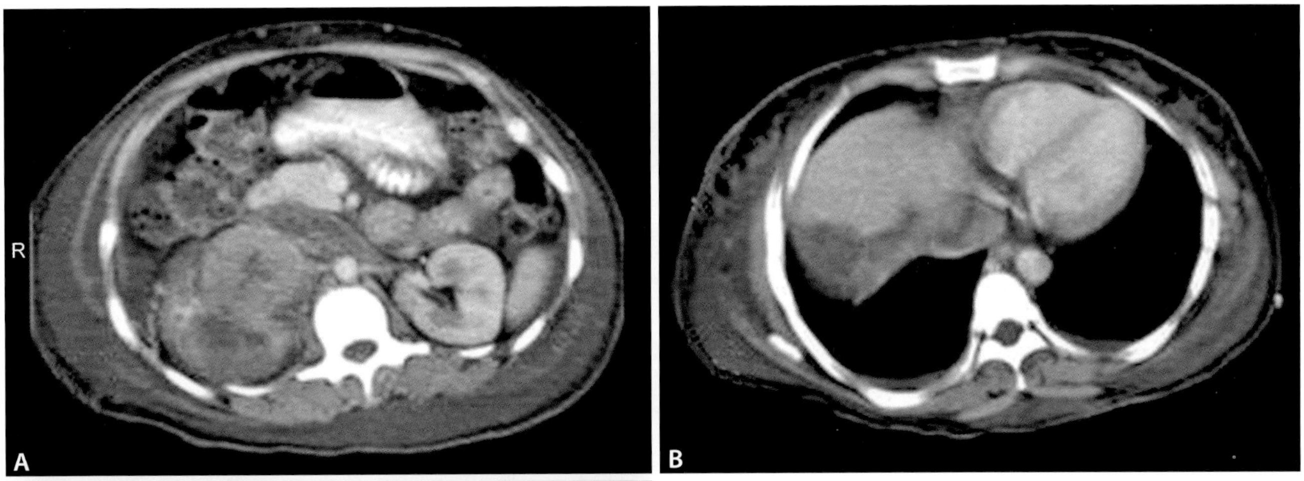

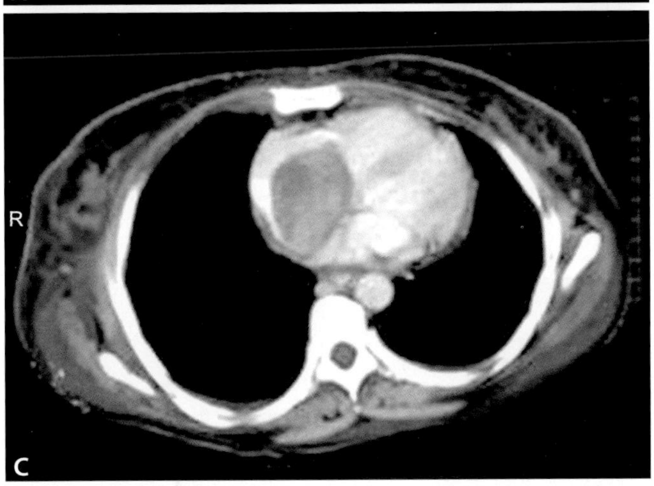

Figs. 28A to C: Corticomedullary phase of contrast enhancement phase showing a large heterogeneous mass in the right kidney with thrombus in the right renal vein (A). Extension of the thrombus into the IVC (B). The right atrium is seen (C).

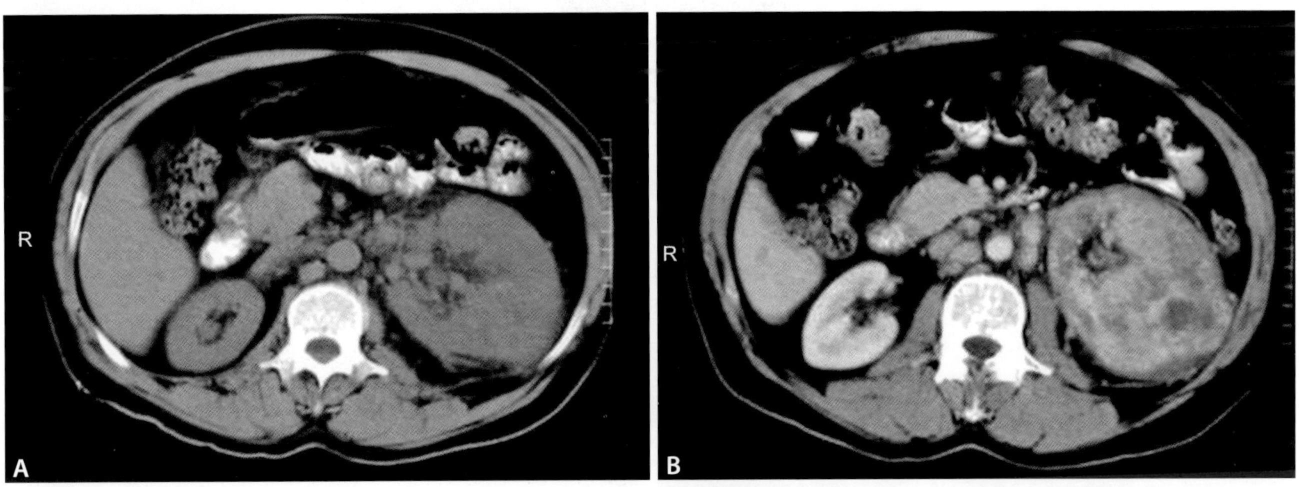

Figs. 29A and B: Noncontrast axial scan (A) showing an indeterminate ill-defined mass in the left kidney. Contrast-enhanced scan in the nephrogram phase (B) shows enhancement of the lesion > 20 HU consistent with a malignant mass.

wash out of contrast material from a lesion at 15 minutes may allow differentiation between hyperdense cysts and renal neoplasm.[44] A decrease of 15 HU or more is consistent with a tumor. Alternately, a hyperdense renal cyst shows no change in density between corticomedullary and delayed phase images.[44]

There dimensional CT combined with CT angiography has the potential to provide all the critical information needed to plan the required surgical procedure. The images can be viewed in multiple planes and orientations to define the tumour and its relationship to the renal surface, the collecting system and adjacent organs.[28] A 3D CT angiogram can display the renal arterial and venous anatomy.

MDCT IN BLUNT RENAL TRAUMA

When examining trauma patients MDCT involving fast volume scanning requires less patient cooperation and creates fewer arti-facts. A nonenhanced scan is essential followed by enhanced multiphasic HCT data acquisition. The CMP (Corticomedullary phase) images are best suited to visualize injury of the renal arteries including non-occlusive intimal injury of the main renal artery and renal vein thrombosis. Rapid image acquisition also allows distinguishing extravasations of contrast material due to active hemorrhage visualized during the CMP, from urine extravasations due to rupture of the renal collecting system. Bright enhancement close to the density of nearby arteries within a laceration or around an injured kidney during the CMP phase of CT scanning indicates either contained or active hemorrhage. A contained hemorrhage or pseudoaneurysm is well-circumscribed and contained within the renal parenchyma or laceration **(Figs. 30A to C)**. Active hemorrhage is ill-defined or flame or waterfall shaped with an associated fresh hematoma which often shows dependent or circumferential layering of older and fresh hemorrhage.[45]

During the nephrographic phase, renal parenchymal injuries and nonperfused parenchymal injuries are best assessed **(Figs. 31A and B)**. The EP images enable to detect

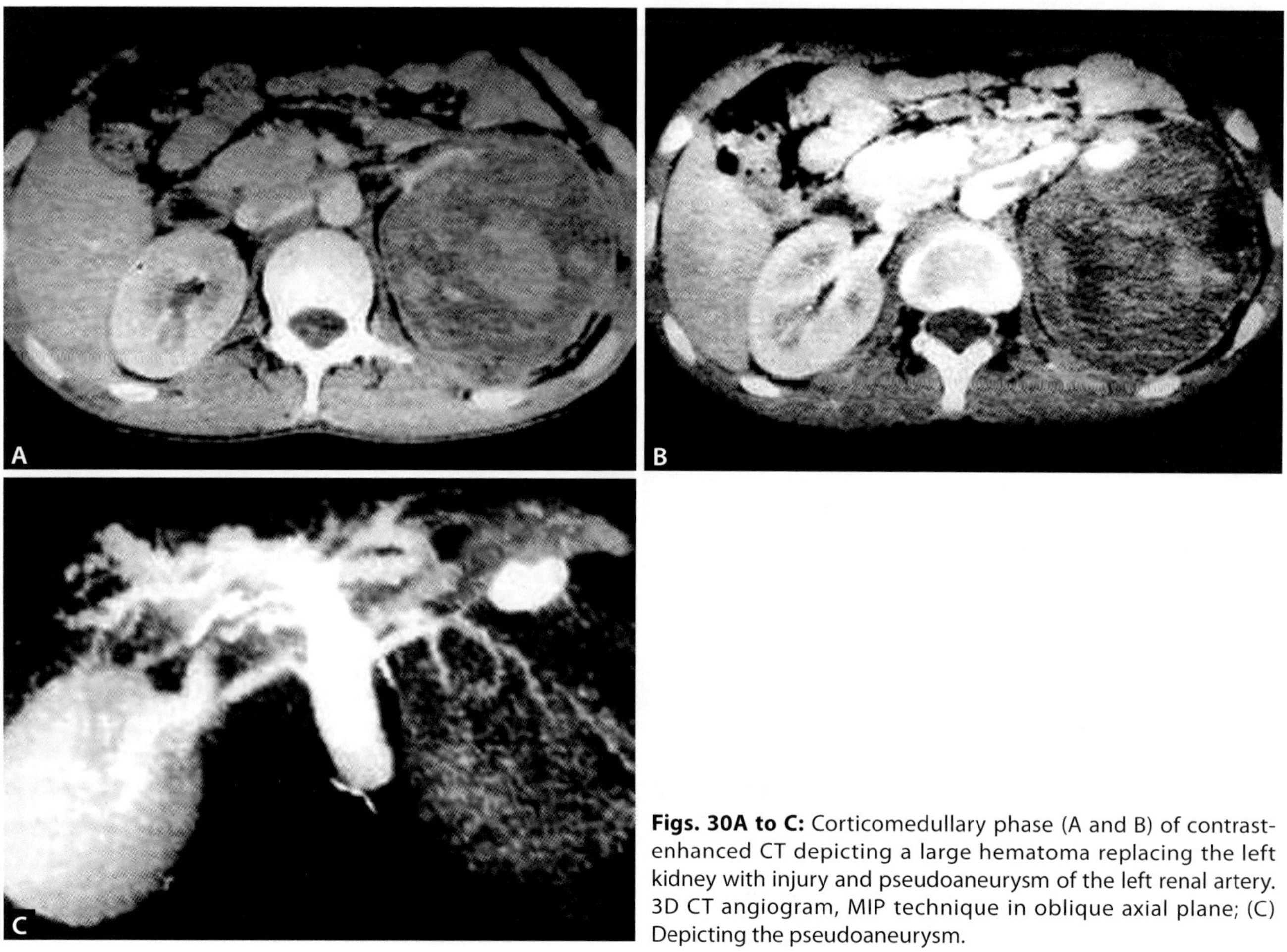

Figs. 30A to C: Corticomedullary phase (A and B) of contrast-enhanced CT depicting a large hematoma replacing the left kidney with injury and pseudoaneurysm of the left renal artery. 3D CT angiogram, MIP technique in oblique axial plane; (C) Depicting the pseudoaneurysm.

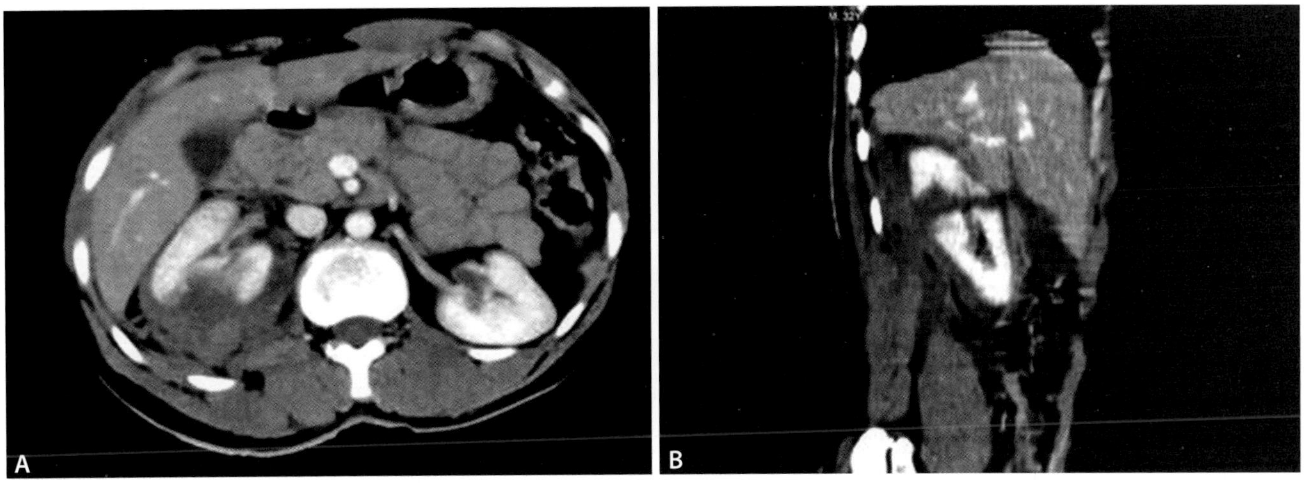

Figs. 31A to B: Nephrogram phase image (A) showing laceration of the right renal parenchyma with perinephric hematoma. Sagittal MPR image (B) depicting the fracture of the right kidney.

contrast extravasation caused by rupture of the renal collecting system. Delayed images (10–15 minutes) are obtained to evaluate for urinary contrast extravasations **(Figs. 32A and B)**. Multiplanar reconstructions [MPR] provide better demonstration of complex injuries of the renal parenchyma and improves the demonstration of the size of the hematomas and urinomas.

If bladder injury is a clinical concern (gross hematuria or pelvic ring fracture) a cystogram or CT cystogram should be performed. CT cystography is capable of distinguishing intraperitoneal, extraperitoneal or combined bladder rupture.[46] For CT cystography once the abdominal CT is complete a retrograde instillation of dilute iodine based contrast (10–12 mL of 300 strength contrast in 500 mL normal saline) is done and the pelvis is scanned again when the bladder is fully distended taking care to include the entire urinary bladder.

MDCT IN EVALUATION OF FLANK PAIN AND URINARY CALCULI

Unenhanced CT has been demonstrated to be the most accurate and efficient diagnostic imaging means to evaluate urinary lithiasis. Fielding et al. have reported a 98% sensitivity and 100% specificity.[47] Niall et al. have reported a sensitivity of 100% and specificity of 92% in detection of urolithiasis.[48] Using MDCT, thin collimation (3–5 mm) noncontrast scans are obtained through the abdomen from the superior aspect of the kidneys (or from the dome of the liver) through the inferior aspect of bladder base or pubic symphysis within seconds. Regardless of their calcium content, almost all urinary tract calculi are radiopaque on noncontrast scans. Reconstructed images such as MPR and CPR are useful in demonstrating the exact location of stones and their relationship to the ureter. Noncontrast CT is also helpful in detecting nonobstructing calculi in patients who have hematuria. Stone size is the single most reliable indicator of stone passage and can be measured accurately on CT **(Fig. 33)**.[49]

The most specific diagnostic finding of urolithiasis is the identification of a stone within the ureter. The second important finding is the "rim sign," seen as 1–2 mm of soft tissue thickening around the stone secondary to ureteral wall edema at the site of stone impaction. **(Fig. 34)**.[50] Other secondary CT findings of urolithiasis are dilatation of the ureter or collecting system, asymmetric enlargement or decreased density of the kidney, and perinephric stranding. Renal edema from obstruction results in loss of the hyperdense pyramid (white pyramid sign) and the attenuation of the parenchyma on the obstructed side is 5–14 HU less than on the normal side, an objective finding of obstruction **(Fig. 35)**.[51]

Some degree of uretral edema and thickening can be seen if a stone already has passed into the bladder. To decide whether or not a distal ureteral stone is in the ureterovesical junction or in the bladder, prone position imaging can be useful.

Pelvic phleboliths, arterial vascular calcification, calcified vas deferens and a calcified appendicolith can be considered a differential diagnosis of ureteric calculi. Phleboliths often show a central lucency, whereas true calculi are as dense or more dense at the center than at the periphery. Another useful sign for diagnosing phlebolith is the comet-tail sign, which is a linear or curvilinear soft

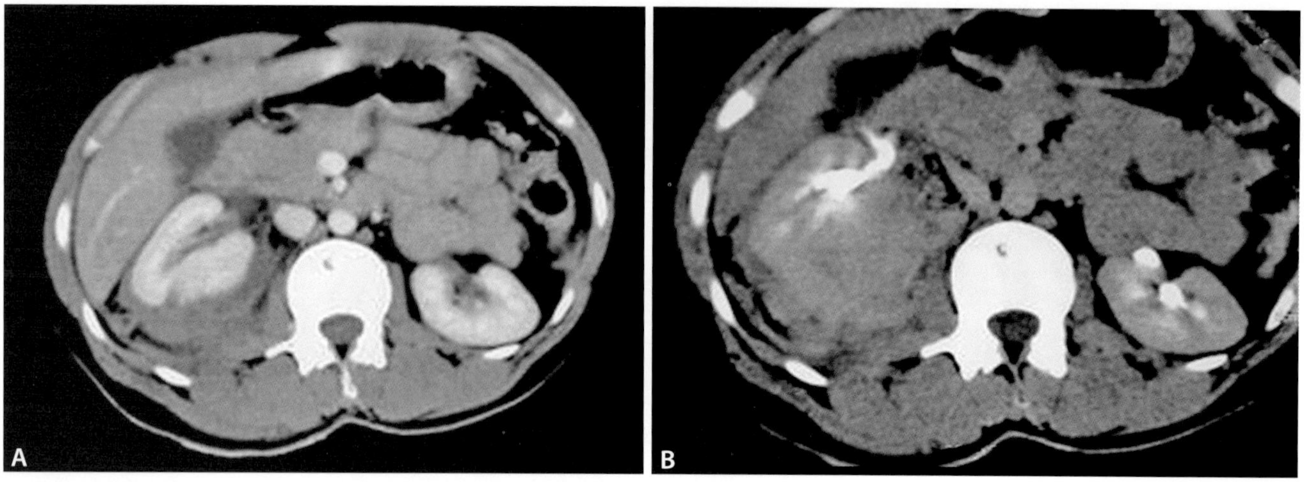

Figs. 32A and B: CT in the nephrogram phase (A) depicting a perinephric hematoma on the right side. Excretory phase image; (B) depicting the opacified pelvicalyceal system and extravasation of contrast in the perinephric hematoma suggesting rupture of the pelvicalyceal system.

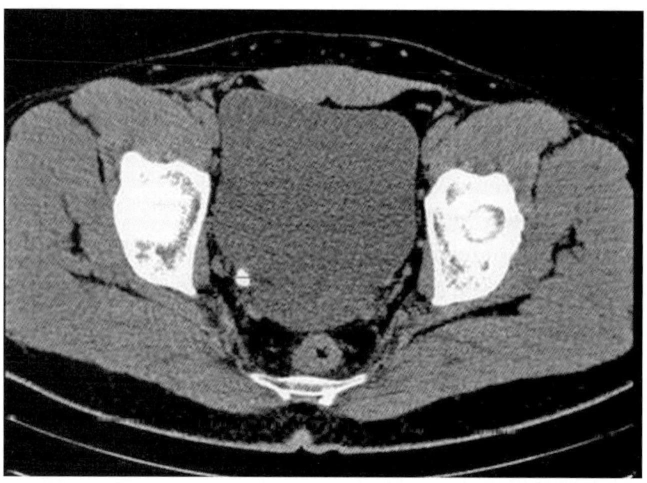

Fig. 33: Noncontrast CT shows a radiodense focus at the right uretero vesical junction suggestive of a calculus. The calculus is measuring 6 mm in size.

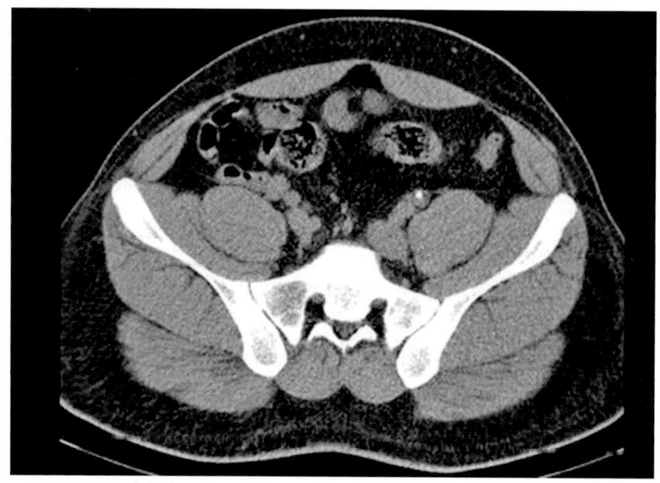

Fig. 34: Noncontrast CT scan showing a calculus in the midureter with a soft tissue rim around it consistent with the "rim sign" seen in a calculus.

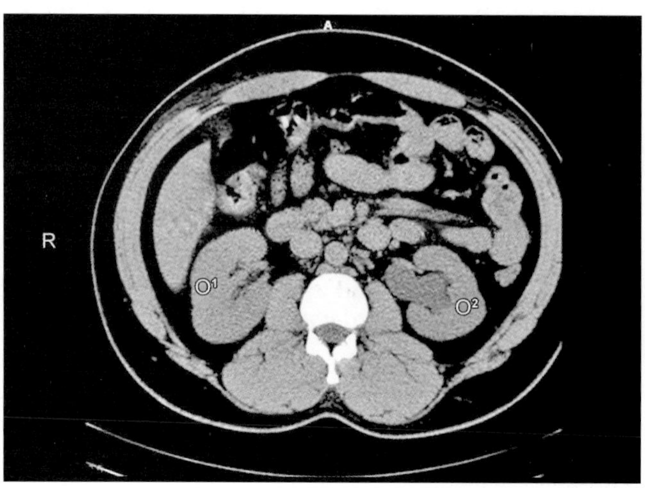

Fig. 35: Noncontrast CT showing a hydronephrotic left kidney with attenuation of the renal parenchyma on the left side 10 HU less than that of the contralateral right side, an objective finding of obstruction on the left side.

tissue structure represented by the noncalcified vessel, extending from an abdominal or pelvic calcification; its positive predictive value for phlebolith is 100%.

Another advantage of CT is its ability to detect nongenitourinary and nonstone disease which may be the cause of pain such as appendicitis, diverticulitis biliary colic, etc.[52]

MDCT IN RENAL INFECTIONS

MDCT is more useful than IVU or ultrasonography for the assessment of renal infection.[53] The main purpose of renal imaging is to obtain information regarding the nature and extent of the disease process and to identify any significant complications such as gas forming infection, abscess and urinary obstruction.[54]

The diagnosis of acute pyelonephritis is based on clinical and laboratory finding in most cases and routine imaging, therefore, is unnecessary. When a definite diagnosis of acute renal infection is not established or patients present with recurrent episodes of infection, renal imaging is indicated because of an increased possibility of stones, obstruction, abscess, or a congenital anomaly. After noncontrast CT, a contrast-enhanced study is essential, including angionephrographic or corticomedullary and nephrographic phases, for a complete evaluation of patients who have renal inflammatory disease to demonstrate alterations in the renal parenchymal perfusion and excretion of contrast material that may occur as a result of the inflammatory process.[54] The most common CT finding of acute pyelonephritis is ill-defined, wedge-shaped lesions of decreased attenuation radiating from the papilla to the cortical surface, with or without swelling. This finding may be subtle in the corticomedullary phase. This perfusion abnormality is detected best in the nephrographic phase. Another characteristic finding of acute pyelonephritis is a striated nephrogram on contrast-enhanced CT, consisting of linear bands of alternating hypoattenuation and hyperattenuation oriented parallel to the axes of the tubules and collecting ducts. **(Figs. 36A to C)**.[55]

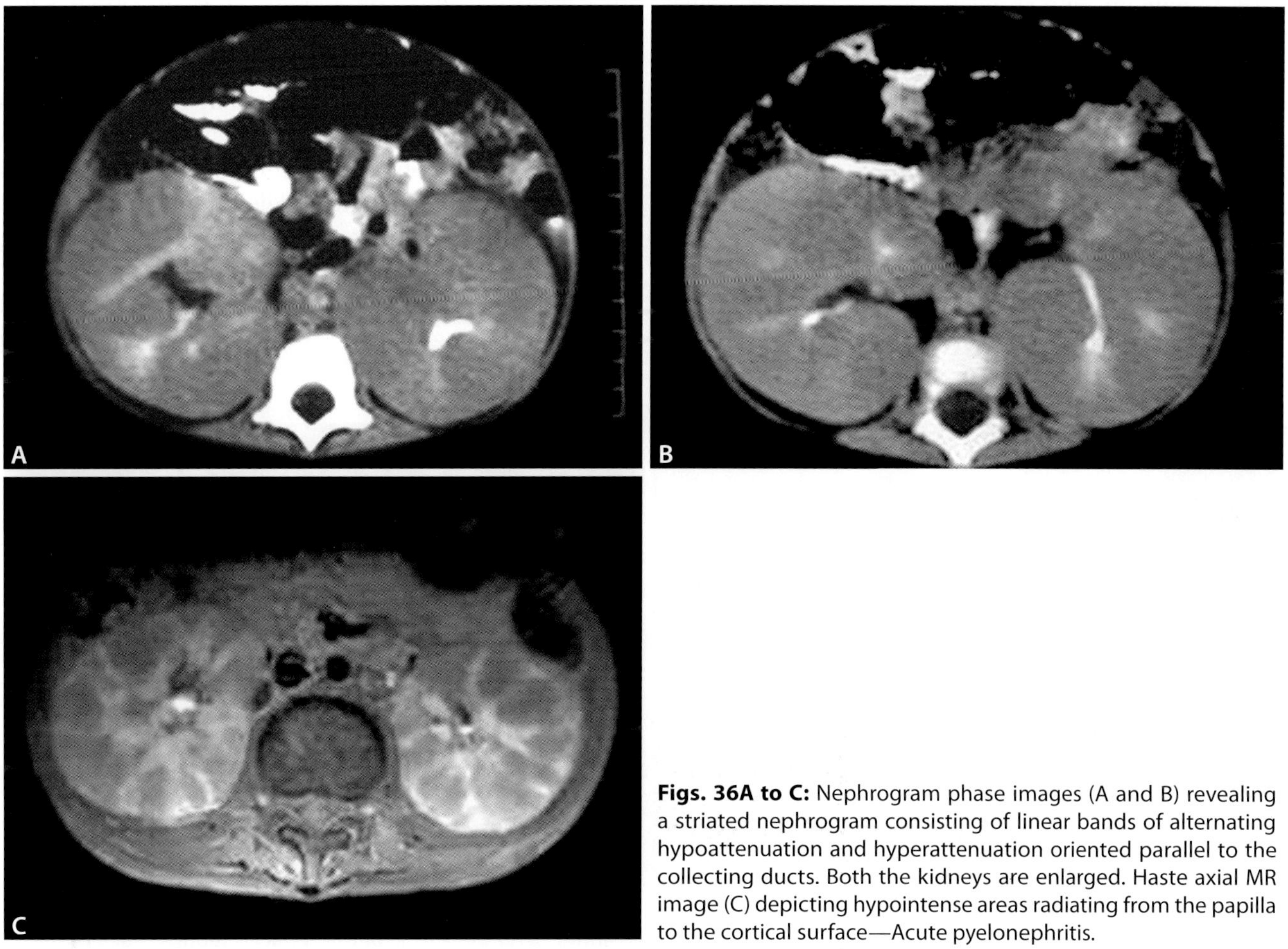

Figs. 36A to C: Nephrogram phase images (A and B) revealing a striated nephrogram consisting of linear bands of alternating hypoattenuation and hyperattenuation oriented parallel to the collecting ducts. Both the kidneys are enlarged. Haste axial MR image (C) depicting hypointense areas radiating from the papilla to the cortical surface—Acute pyelonephritis.

Diminished concentration of contrast material in the tubules, caused by tubular obstruction by inflammatory cells and debris, ischemia and interstitial edema, results in this characteristic CT finding. Other useful secondary CT findings of acute pyelonephritis are global or focal enlargement of the kidney, thickening of the pelvicalyceal wall, obliteration of the renal sinus and perinephric fat planes, focal calyceal obliteration, and thickening of the fascia of Gerota.[56] Scarring resulting from pyelonephritis may be demonstrated by MDCT as focal thining of the cortex or extensive contour abnormalities. VRT images may be useful for demonstrating focal defects resulting from abscess foci related to pyelonephritis.

HELICAL CT FOR LOWER URINARY TRACT AND PELVIS

Oral contrast opacification of small and large bowel is essential to perform a diagnostic pelvic CT. Patients drink 450mLofwatersolublecontrastmedium10–12hoursbefore the examination to opacify the large bowel and 450 mL, 45 minutes preceding the study to opacify pelvic small bowel. In patients with suspected ovarian cancer, pelvic inflammatory disease, endometriosis, diverticulitis or rectal cancer 200 mL water soluble contrast enema may be ideal to delineate disease extent. Intravenous contrast medium is used to opacify the bladder and ureter, enhance solid tumor components of bladder and ovarian cancer, endometrial sarcoma and gestational trophoblastic disease, differentiate iliac vessels from lymph nodes, enhance myometrium and visualize the endometrial cavity. With current high resolution fast CT scanners an optimum contrast enhancement technique uses mechanical injector to give 150 mL of 60% contrast at the rate of 2 mL/second.

A standard pelvic CT scan consists of contiguous 8–10 mm sections from the level of the symphysis pubis cephalad to the iliac crest. This protocol optimizes parenchymal enhancement as well as vascular opacification for lymph nodes metastasis detection. In cancer staging or abdominopelvic mass evaluation, sections are then taken at 1–1.5 cm intervals from the iliac crest to the diaphragm to screen for hydronephrosis and metastatic disease. At the end of the abdominal study additional 2–5 mm sections may be taken through pelvic tumor or small masses to define local extension better and eliminate the problem of volume averaging of mass and normal adjacent structures. Delayed thin sections through the pelvis delineate the interface between a mass and the contrast filled bladder and pelvic ureters **(Figs. 37A and B)**.

Measurement of the volume of an organ can be readily calculated by tracing the organ of interest with an electronic computer cursor and summating the surface area measure-ments obtained on the individual scans. This area is then multiplied by the slice thickness to determine the segmental volume. The total volume of the organ to be measured is com-puted by the addition of all segmental volumes. CT of the pelvis, in either males or females, usually is obtained in conjunction with CT, of the abdomen. Incidental gynecologic finding are visualized more frequently now, because the adnexa, for example, are better seen with MDCT than on single-slice CT. This improvement results largely from the decrease in partial-volume averaging. Suspected local or systemic disease in

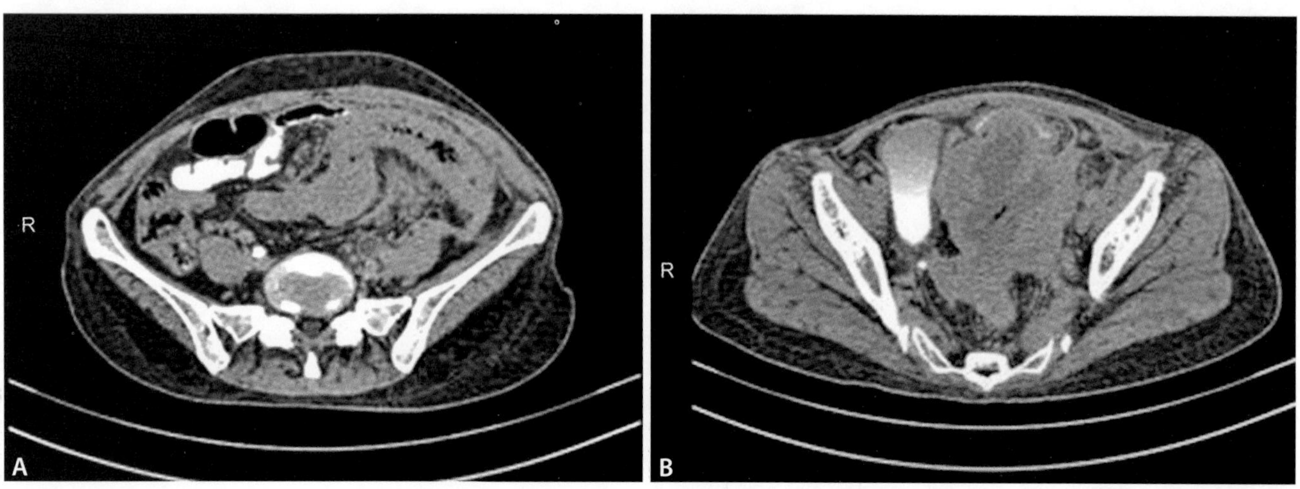

Figs. 37A and B: Contrast-enhanced axial scans in a case of carcinoma cervix showing the mass in the cervix with normal opacified right ureter. The left ureter is infiltrated by the mass and shows absence of contrast opacification.

the pelvis that prompts CT evaluation can affect the adnexa or uterus, and these abnormalities now can be seen better with MDCT. CT also plays a leading role in the aspiration or drainage of fluid collections such as pus or blood.

MDCT has been used successfully for staging and treatment planning of cervical and ovarian malignancy. CT has an advantage over clinical examination for staging, particularly for detecting ascites, metastases to the liver and pelvic and para-aortic lymph node involvement.[57] In the past, inability to resolve abnormalities smaller than 1 cm has been cited as a disadvantage of CT, but resolution is much improved with new MDCT technology and partial-volume averaging is significantly decreased. Ultrasound had been claimed to be superior to CT for staging ovarian cancer, because scanning occurs in both transverse and longitudinal planes; however, two-dimensional and three-dimensional reconstructions are now available with new MDCT technology. Coronal, sagittal and obliqaue multiplanar reconstruction (MPRs) are performed using the source data obtained in the axial plane and can be used to evaluate the complex female pelvic anatomy. In addition to its capability of multiplanar imaging, CT is superior to ultrasound in detecting tumor adherence to bowel, retroperitoneal lymphadenopathy and peritoneal implants. Further more, oncologists may be more familiar with cross-sectional anatomy as seen with CT as opposed to ultrasound.

Evaluation of female pelvic vasculature has included MDCT of fibroids after uterine artery embolization and of pelvic arteriovenous malformations after embolization.

CT ANGIOGRAPHY (CTA) OF RENAL ARTERIES

ThediagnosticaccuracyachievedbyCTAoftherenalarteries is highly dependent on the selection and acquisition of imaging parameters and optimization of contrast injection. The quality of CTA of renal arteries is maximized by minimizing collimation, reconstruction interval and table feed. Because of the small diameter of the vessels of interest and their parallel or near parallel course to the imaging plane thin nominal section thickness of 1.25 mm and overlapping reconstruction are necessary. An individually timed bolus injection of 150 mL of contrast material (300 mg/mL) with flow rate of 4 mL/sec provides scanning during the plateau phase of contrast enhancement and improves the quality of CTA. Indications for CTA of renal arteries include the preoperative assessment of number and course of renal arteries in renal donors, assessment of renal vessels crossing the ureteropelvic junction prior to repair of obstruction, the evaluation of renal artery involvement in abdominal aortic aneurysms, the detection of renal artery aneurysms and the evaluation of occlusive renal artery disease. MDCT of the kidney allows delineation of size, number and course of the renal arteries and vein, evaluation of the renal parenchyma and collecting system and diagnosis of unsuspected conditions that precuide organ donation. CT angiography can depict 100% of the main renal arteries and veins.[58]

The region of interest for scan volume is determined by the initial topogram/axial scans. Conventionally, the region between the superior mesenteric artery and lower border of L3 is chosen so as to include sites of origin of accessory renal arteries. Delay time is determined through prior time density curves of dynamic scanning and patient is instructed for breath holding. Maximum intensity projection (MIP)/shaded surface display (SSD) modes are used. SSD clearly depicts the complex vascular anatomy since it is the best technique for assessing regions of overlapping vessels and vessel origins in relationship to aneurysms of the abdominal aorta. However, SSD cannot display attenuation values of structures which are not within the threshold range and is therefore unable to show intravascular contrast and pathologies such as thrombus and calcification. Further, SSD over or underestimates stenosis depending on the defined threshold. In contrast to SSD, MIP images are not threshold dependent, preserve attenuation information and make structures that do not lie in a single plane visible in their entirety very similar to conventional angiograms **(Fig. 38)**. MIP is currently the technique of choice for CTA and is a reliable method for displaying accessory renal arteries. Superimposition of vessels may interfere but this may be overcome by

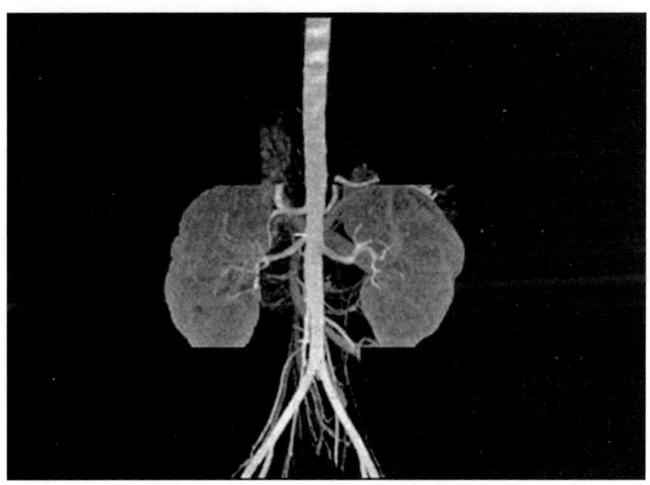

Fig. 38: CT angiography using MIP technique depicting the normal renal arteries on both sides.

generating multiple images in different projections which can be rotated about an axis to visualize three dimensional vascular relationships.[59]

Volumerenderingtechnique(VRT)avoidsextensiveloss of information that is inherent in SSD and MIP by retaining all CT data and summing the contributions from all voxels along a line from any viewing angle along the data set. Depth, surface and relative X-ray attenuation are all conveyed with VRT **(Fig. 39)**. Adjacent structures to vessels can be displayed and the 3D data set can be interactively modified in any orientation to optimize depiction of the renal vascular anatomy **(Fig. 40)**.[60]

VIRTUAL CYSTOSCOPY/ENDOSCOPY

Over the last few years the technique of virtual cytoscopy/endoscopy has been significantly refined and clinically tested. A volumetric dataset is acquired, the images are computer rendered to generate 3D images. Special software then allows navigation through the bladder. Virtual cystoscopy may prove to be useful for detecting bladder lesions greater than 5 mm. Virtual endoscopic techniques may provide ureteral "flythroughs" allowing the observer to have a ureteroscopic view point of the urinary tract.[60]

CT examination includes unenhanced scanning covering the entire urinary tract, contrast-enhanced scanning covering the abdomen and pelvis at a scan delay of 100–120 seconds and dedicated scanning for bladder evaluation. IV contrast material is administered in a power injector at a dose of 2 mL/kg of body weight at a rate of 3 mL/sec to a maximum of 150 mL. After the first two scans are obtained the patient gets down from the CT machine and is asked to report to the CT room when he or she feels a desire to void (90–140 minutes after IV injection of contrast material) and delayed CT is performed for bladder evaluation. Immediately, before the CT examination, all patients are asked to take supine and prone positions four times to obtain adequate mixing of the contrast material and urine in the bladder. Adequate mixing is obtained when high attenuation fills the entire bladder lumen homogeneously and there is no fluid- fluid level caused by unopacified urine. The CT data is then transferred to a workstation for reconstructing virtual cystoscopy and multiplanar reconstruction images. The interactive navigation and interpretation of 3D virtual reality imaging is performed.

Virtual cystoscopy has advantages over multiplanar reconstruction and source CT images.[61] First, virtual cystoscopy is dedicated for evaluating the mucosal surface of the bladder and therefore, can detect superficial lesions missed by multiplanar reconstruction or source CT images. Second, virtual cystoscopy can allow the operator to navigate the muscosal surface of the bladder in various projections.[62] A major advantage of virtual cystoscopy is its noninvasive nature. It is not associated with the risk of local infection, bladder perforation stricture or scarring.[63,64] It can be taken as a tool for initial screening of patients with hematuria and more accurate patient selection for invasive cystoscopy.

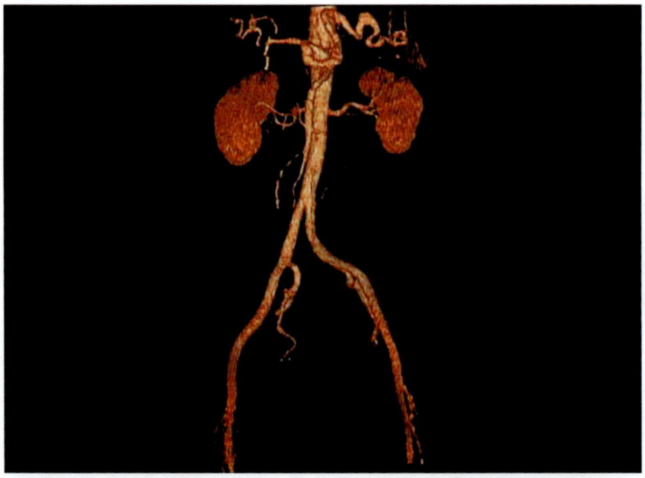

Fig. 39: CT angiography using VRT technique depicting the normal renal arteries on both sides.

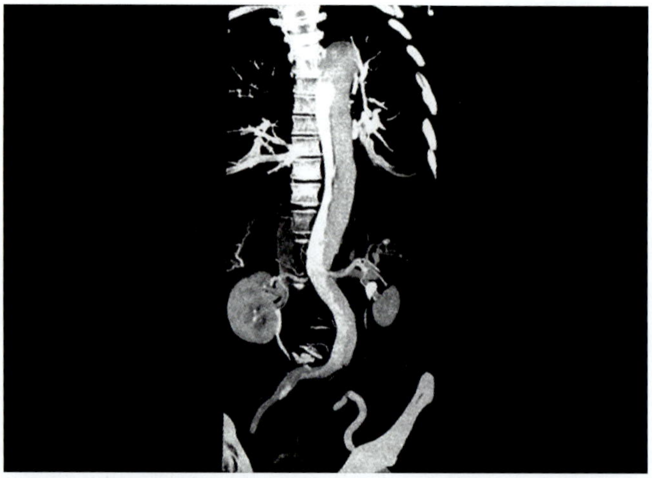

Fig. 40: CT angiography using volume-rendering technique depicting fusiform aneurysm of the aorta with dissection. The true lumen opacified with contrast and the non-opacified false lumen are clearly seen. The renal arteries are however normal.

In conclusion for every practicing radiologist an adequate knowledge of 3D anatomy of the urogenital system, a clear understanding of its physiology and that of contrast media is required. Improvements in scanner technology, coupled with affordable and powerful computer graphic systems have resulted in superb image generation and visualization tools for the radiologist and the clinician. Although the advanced visualization techniques do not actually create new anatomic data above and beyond the source cross-sections, using these tools to display the data in new ways that more closely simulate natural 3D scenes may create additional new visual information about the patient. The current challenge is to prove that the additional effort and expense are justified by improving patient care through more accurate diagnosis, improved patient outcome and improved communication with the referring physician.

REFERENCES

1. Schreyer HH, Uggowitzer MM, Ruppert-Kohlmayr A. Helical CT of the urinary organs. Eur Radiol. 2002;12:575-91.
2. Moss AA, Gamsu G, Genant HK. Computed Tomography of the Body with Magnetic Resonance Imaging. Philadelphia: WB Saunder Co. 1992;2(3):20.
3. Haaga JR, Lanzieri CF, Sartoris D, et al. Computed Tomography and Magnetic Resonance Imaging of the Whole Body. St Louis: CV Mosby Co., 1994;3(2):35-8.
4. Mc Collough CH, Zink FE. Performance evaluation of a multislice CT system. Med Phy. 1999;26:2223-30.
5. Rydberg J, Buck Walter KA, Caldemeyer KS, et al. Multisection CT: Scanning techniques and clinical applications. Radiographics. 2000;20:1787-806.
6. Kocakoc E, Bhatt S, Dogra VS. Renal Multidetector Row CT. Radiol Clin N Am. 2005;43:1021-47.
7. Napoli A, Fleischmann D, Chan FP, et al. Computed tomography angiography: State of the art imaging using multidetector row technology. J Comput Assist Tomography. 2004;28:S32-45.
8. Rydberg J, Liang Y, Teague SD. Fundamentals of multichannel CT. Radiol Clin North Am. 2003;41:465-74.
9. Foley WD. Special focus session. Multidetector CT: Abdominal visceral imaging. Radiographics. 2002;22:701-19.
10. Kalra MK, Maher MM, D'souza R, et al. Multidetector computed tomography technology: Current status and emerging developments. J Comput Assist Tomogr. 2004;28 (suppl 1):S2-6.
11. Lawler LP, Jarret TW, Corl FM, et al. Adult ureteropelvic junction obstruction: Insights with three dimensional multidetector row CT. Radiographics. 2005;25:121-34.
12. Tunaci A, Yekeler E. Multidetector row CT of the kidneys. Eur J Radiol. 2004;52:56-66.
13. Wintersperger BJ, Nikolaou K, Becker CR. Multidetector row CT angiography of the aorta and visceral arteries. Semin Ultrasound CT MR. 2004;25:25-40.
14. Sheth S, Fishman EK. Multidetector row CT of the kidneys and urinary tract: Techniques and applications in the diagnosis of benign diseases. Radiographics. 2004;24(2):20.
15. Yuh BI, Cohan RH. Helical CT for detection and characterization of renal masses. Semin Ultrasound CT MRI. 1997;18:82-90.
16. Saunders HS, Dyer RB, Shifrin RJ. The CT nephrogram: Implications for evaluation of urinary tract disease. Radiographics. 1995;15:1069-85.
17. Szolar DH, Kammerhuber F, Altziebler S, et al. Multiphasic helical CT of the kidney: increased conspicuity for detection and characterization of small (<3 cm) renal masses. Radiology. 1997;202:211-7.
18. Urban BA. The small renal mass: What is the role of multiphasic helical scanning. Radiology. 1997;202:22-3.
19. Garant M, Bonaldi UM, Taourel P, et al. Enhancement patterns of renal masses during multiphasic helical CT acquisitions. Abdom Imaging. 1998;23:431-6.
20. Rubin GD. 3-D imaging with MDCT. Eur J Radiol. 2003;45 (Suppl 1):S37-41.
21. Cademartiri F, Luccichenti G, Van Der Lugt A, et al. Sixteen row multislice computed tomography: Basic concepts, protocols and enhanced clinical applications. Semin Ultrasound CT MR. 2004;25:2-16.
22. Lockhart ME, Smith JK. Technical considerations in renal CT. Radiol Clin N Am. 2003;41:863-75.
23. Nolte Ernsting C, Cowan N. Understanding multislice CT urography techniques: many roads lead to Rome. Eur Radiol. 2006;16:2670-86.
24. Sourtzis S, Thibeau JF, Damry N, et al. Radiologic investigation of renal colic: Unenhanced helical CT compared with excretory urography. AJR. 1999;172:1491-4.
25. Bell TV, Fenlon HM, Davison BD, et al. Unenhanced helical CT criteria to differentiate distal ureteric calculi from pelvic phleboliths. Radiology. 1998;207:363-7.
26. Guest AR, Cohan RH, Korobkin M, et al. Assessment of the clinical utility of rim and comet tail signs in differentiating ureteral stones from phleboliths. AJR. 2001;177:1285-91.
27. Maher MM, Kalra MK, Rizzo S, et al. Multidetector CT urography in imaging of the urinary tract in patients with hematuria. Korean J Radiol. 2004;5:1-10.
28. S heth S, Scatarige JC, Horton KM, et al. Current concepts in the diagnosis and management of renal cell carcinoma: Role of multidetector CT and three dimensional CT. Radiographics. 2001;21:S237-54.
29. Browne RF, Meehan CP, Colville J, et al. Transitional cell carcinoma of the urinary tract: Spectrum of imaging findings. Radiographics. 2005;25(6):1609-27.
30. Caoili EM, Cohan RH, Korobkin M, et al. Urinary tract abnormalities: Initial experience with multidetector row CT urography. Radiology. 2002;222:353-60.
31. Cowan NC, Turney BW, Taylor NJ, et al. Multidetector computed tomography for diagnosing upper urinary tract urothelial tumour. BJU Int. 2007;99:1363-70.

32. Fritz GA, Schoellnast H, Deutschmann HA, et al. Multiphasic multidetector row CT (MDCT) in detection and staging of transitional cell carcinomas of upper urinary tract. Eur Radiol. 2006;16:1244-52.
33. Kalra MK, Maher MM, Sahani DV, et al. Current status of multidetector computed tomography urography in imaging of the urinary tract. Curr Probl Diagn Radiol. 2002;31:210-21.
34. Dillman JR, Caoili EM, Cohan RH. Multidetector CT urography: A one stop renal and urinary tract imaging modality. Abdom imaging. 2007;32:519-29.
35. Turney BW, Willatt JM, Nixon D, et al. Computed tomography urography for diagnosing bladder cancer. BJU Int. 2006; 98(2):345-8.
36. Kim JK, Cho KS. CT urography and virtual endoscopy: Promising modalitiies for urinary tract evaluation. BJR. 2003;76:199-209.
37. Kohli A. Has the time come to write the EPITAPH for the intravenous urogram? Ind J Radiol Imaging. 2005;15:161-4.
38. Chai RY, Jhaveri K, Saini S, et al. Comprehensive evaluation of patients with hematuria on multislice computed tomography scanner, protocol design and preliminary observations. Australas Radiol. 2001;45:536-8.
39. Chow LC, Kwan SW, Olcott EW, et al. Split bolus MDCT urography with synchronous nephrographic and excretory phase enhancement. AJR. 2007;189:314-22.
40. Sudakoff GS, Runn PP, Hellman RS, et al. Opacification of the genitourinary collecting system during MDCT urography with enhanced CT digital radiography: Nonsaline versus saline bolus. AJR. 2006;186:122-29.
41. McNicholas MMJ, Raptopoulos VD, Schwartz RK, et al. Excretory phase CT urography for opacification of the urinary collecting system AJR. 1998;170:1261-7.
42. Zagoria RJ. Imaging of small renal masses: A medical success story. AJR. 2000;175:945-55.
43. Sliverman SG, Lee BY, Seltzer SE, et al. Small (< or = 3 cm) renal masses: Correlation of spiral CT features and pathologic findings. AJR. 1994;163:597-605.
44. Macari M, Bosniak MA. Delayed CT to evaluate renal masses incidentally discovered at contrast-enhanced CT: Demonstration of vascularity with deenhancement. Radiology. 1999;213:674-80.
45. Willkmann JK, Roos JE, Platz A, et al. Multidetector CT: Detection of active hemorrhage in patients with blunt abdominal trauma. AJR. 2002;179:437-44.
46. Morgan DE, Nallamala LK, Kenney PJ, et al. CT cystography: Radiographic and clinical predictors of bladder rupture. AJR. 2000;174:89-5.
47. Fielding JR, Steele G, Fox LS, et al. Spiral computerized tomography in the evaluation of acute flank pain: A replacement for excretory urography. J Urol. 1997;157: 2071-3.
48. Niall O, Russell J, Mac Gregor R, et al. A comparison of noncontrast computerized tomography with excretory urography in the assessment of acute flank pain. J Urol. 1999; 161:534-7.
49. Olcott EW, Sommer FG, Napel S. Accuracy of detection and measurement of renal calculi: In vitro comparison of three dimensional spiral CT, radiography and nephrotomography. Radiology. 1997;204:19-25.
50. Heneghan JP, Dalrymple NC, Verga M, et al. Soft tissue "rim" sign in the diagnosis of ureteral calculi with use of unenhanced helical CT. Radiology. 1997;202:709-11.
51. Georgiades CS, Moore CJ, Smith DF. Differences of renal parenchymal attenuation for acutely obstructed and unobstructed kidneys on unenhanced helical CT: A useful secondary sign? AJR. 2001;176:965-8.
52. Smith RC, Verga M, Mc Carthy S, et al. Diagnosis of acute flank pain: Value of unenhanced helical CT. AJR. 1996;166: 97-101.
53. Akbar SA, Mortele KJ, Baeyens K, et al. Multidetector CT urography: Techniques clinical applications and pitfalls. Semin ultrasound CT MR. 2004;25:41-54.
54. Kawashima A, Le Roy AJ. Radiologic evaluation of patients with renal infections. Inf Dis Clin North Am. 2003;17:433-56.
55. Kundra V, Silverman PM. Impact of multislice CT on imaging of acute abdominal disease. Radiol Clin North Am. 2003;41:1083-93.
56. Kawashima A, Sandler CM, Goldman SM, et al. CT of renal inflammatory disease. Radiographics. 1997;17:851-66.
57. Pannu HK, Bristow RE, Montz FJ, et al. Multidetector CT of peritoneal carcinomatosis from ovarian cancer. Radiographics. 2003;23(3):687-701.
58. Rankin SC, Jan W, Koffman CG. Noninvasive imaging of living related kidney donors: Evaluation with CT angiography and gadolinuim-enhanced MR angiography. AJR. 2001;177: 349-55.
59. Chow LC, Rubin GD. CT angiography of the arterial system. Radiol Clin North Am. 2002;40:729-49.
60. Kim TS Chung JW, Park JH, et al. Renal artery evaluation: Comparison of spiral CT angiography to intra-arterial DSA. J Vasc Inter Radiol. 1998;9:553-9.
61. Kim JK, Park SY, Kim HS, et al. Comparison of virtual cystoscopy, multiplanar reformation and source CT images with contrast material filled bladder for detecting lesions. AJR. 2005;185:689-96.
62. Bernhardt TM, Schmidl H, Philipp C, et al. Diagnostic potential of virtual cystoscopy of the bladder. MRI vs CT preliminary report. Eur Radiol. 2003;13:305-12.
63. Merkle EM, Wunderlich A, Aschoff AJ, et al. Virtual cystoscopy based on helical CT scan datasets: Perspectives and limitations. BJR. 1998;71:262-7.
64. Bernhardt TM, Rapp Bernhardt U. Virtual cystoscopy of the bladder based on CT and MRI data. Addom Imaging. 2001;26:325-32.

CHAPTER 101

MRI of Urogenital Tract: Techniques and Normal Appearances

Paramjeet Singh, Sameer Vyas

INTRODUCTION

With recent advances in technology, MR imaging has emerged as single most important modality for evaluation of urogenital tract. The high spatial resolution, intrinsic tissue contrast, short scan time, elimination of motion artifacts and more extensive coverage of abdomen and pelvis provide better detection and characterization of anatomy and pathology of the urogenital tract.[1-5] It has become as an alternative technique to CT scan in view of its multiplanar capability, lack of ionizing radiation and angiographic capabilities.[6,7] In addition MR contrast agents (gadolinium-based) are considered relatively safer as compared to iodinated contrast agents. However, they are also associated with few risk factors which include nephrotoxicity, anaphylactic reaction, reaction at the injection site and nephrogenic systemic sclerosis (NSF).[8] NSF is most important delayed reaction seen as scleroderma-like fibrosing condition, especially in patients who have deranged renal functions. Spectroscopic studies especially in prostate are useful for detection and differentiation of malignant from benign pathologies by noninvasively providing the chemical assay of the assessed tissue. Diffusion weighted imaging (DWI) and dynamic contrast enhancement MR imaging holds good promise in the evaluation of cancers of kidneys, urinary bladder, prostate and female genital tract. High field strength imaging (i.e. 3T) is still in infancy in abdominal applications but is likely to play a greater role in future. Malignant lymph node detection also has improved significantly with new contrast agents, such as iron-based particles.

KIDNEY

Renal MRI has evolved as an alternative or complementary imaging modality to intravenous urography, ultrasonography and computed tomography. It is primarily used as an additional tool of renal imaging in a number of situations. It can be used for evaluation and characterization of renal masses and fluid collections. Internal tissue characters of masses, i.e. presence of fat, necrotic areas or hemorrhage in a cyst or mass can often be better assessed on MRI.[1] Small renal masses can be also diagnosed due to signal alteration produced by them. Because of multiplanar imaging capability, MRI has a definite role for staging of masses. This allows better definition of lesions at the renal poles, i.e. differentiating a renal mass from a supra-renal mass as well as demonstrating the tumor extension in a better way and allowing better surgical planning. Small tumor detection may be aided by fat suppression combined with gadolinium administration. Evaluation of renal vessels by MR angiography is useful in assessing cephalad extension of renal tumors into renal veins and inferior vena cava and evaluation of renal artery pathology. MRI is an alternative modality in patients with equivocal findings on CT or in whom the use of iodinated contrast material is contraindicated because of an increased risk of adverse reactions or nephrotoxicity, MR contrast media like gadolinium DTPA are dialyzable and are relatively safe in patients with compromised renal function or even overt renal failure. However, NSF is a concern in patients with low glomerular filtration rate (GFR <30 mL/min/1.73 m^2)

particularly nonionic linear chelates. MR contrast agents are freely excreted by kidneys and reflect GFR and tubular absorption and thus MR pyelography can be used as an alternative technique to intravenous pyelography for demonstrating pelvicalyceal system.

Techniques and Recommended Imaging Sequences

The MR pulse sequences and the precise imaging parameters depend upon the available equipment and the clinical problem in question. Usually both T1 and T2-weighted sequences are performed in the axial plane in combination with sections in coronal and sagittal planes.[3] The spin echo technique usually incorporates flow compensation and respiratory gating to reduce artifacts but gradient echo images (GRE) are preferred due to short examination time allowing breath hold images, thus providing better quality images. T2 fast spin echo (FSE) imaging has more or less replaced the conventional spin echo T2 imaging. Good quality T2-weighted images of high resolution can be obtained in a short-time using these techniques. In addition, in- and opposed-phase breath hold T1-weighted gradient echo sequences provide an excellent anatomic detail of the retroperitoneum and detection of intracellular lipid.[1] Gradient echo fast low-angle shot (FLASH) sequences are used for obtaining sections of the kidneys after contrast administration in corticomedullary, nephrographic and excretory phase, and provide information equivalent to the CT scan. Dynamic MR imaging following administration of a contrast agent also referred as MR renography has emerged as imaging modality of choice in suspected renal diseases as it provide comprehensive evaluation of renal anatomy and physiology.[1,3] It allows the visualization of contrast material within distinct time phase in different intrarenal regions and the signal intensity changes of cortex and medulla can be plotted in a time density curve. Cortical enhancement which primarily reflects renal perfusion is seen earliest, followed by medullary enhancement which reflects mainly glomerular filtration rate, and lastly the enhancement of the collecting system that represents the functional status of the renal tubules.

Normal Appearances

Renal MRI provides separate visualization of the renal cortex and medulla on both T1 and T2-weighted images **(Figs. 1A and B)**. T1-weighted images show good corticomedullary differentiation with cortex being usually higher in signal intensity compared to the medulla. On T2-weighted images, the renal cortex appears slightly hypointense to medulla.[3] This is due to the fact that cortex contains less water than the medulla thus has a longer T1 time. The sinus fat at the renal hilum appears bright on both T1- and T2-weighted images. The calyces are generally not well-visualized on MRI but if distended with urine appear dark on T1 and bright on T2 WI. The renal arteries, renal veins, aorta and inferior vena cava are seen as tubular structures that are free from intraluminal signal, although flow related artifacts may cause high signal in these vessels. The renal capsule can be seen as a hypointense line and the pararenal and perirenal fat appears bright. The arterial phase images (20 seconds) provide good corticomedullary differentiation, followed by the venous phase (nephrographic phase; 70 seconds) which are best for detection and characterization of renal masses, and lastly the delayed phase (excretory phase; 180 seconds) delineating the collecting system **(Figs. 2A to D)**.

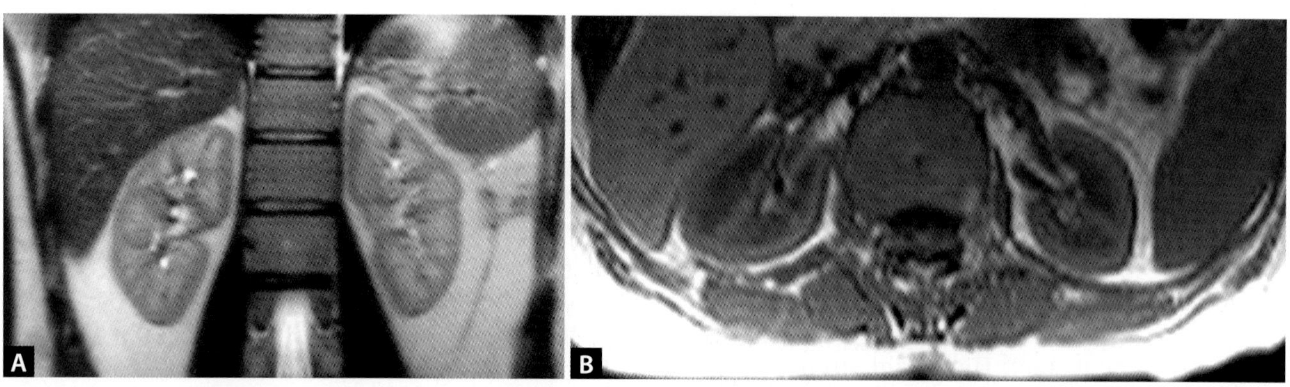

Figs. 1A and B: Coronal T2 HASTE (A) and axial T1 gradient echo FLASH (B) images showing good corticomedullary differentiation. The medulla is bright on T2WI compared to cortex. The renal sinus is also bright due to fat and urine. The T1WI show lower signal of the medulla and sinus shows bright fat. The pararenal fat is bright on T1 and intermediate in signal on T2 images.

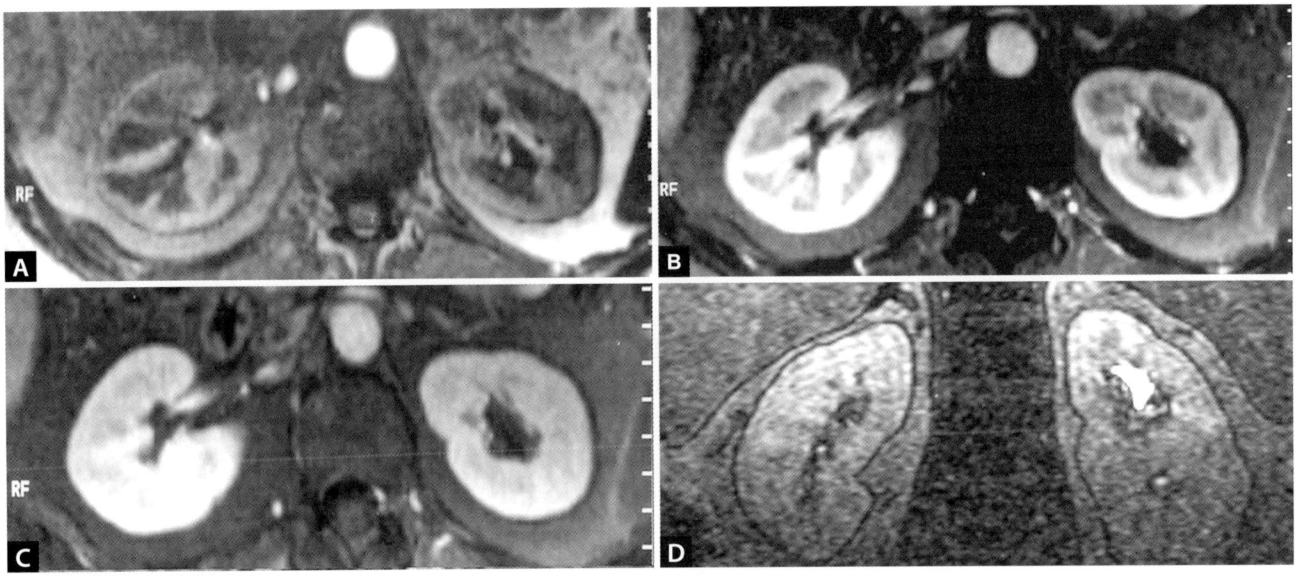

Figs. 2A to D: Postcontrast dynamic axial (A to C) and coronal (D) T1 FLASH images. The kidneys show maximal cortical enhancement in arterial phase with good corticomedullary differentiation (A). There is progressive opacification of medulla (B and C) with blurred corticomedullary differentiation in venous phase and subsequent appearance of contrast into the pelvicalyceal system (D).

MR Urography

MR urography constitutes the evaluation of the collecting system and urinary tract. It is based on the principle that simple fluids, such as urine have very long T2-relaxation time and heavily T2-weighted pulse sequence generate images with high signal intensity from static fluid in the collecting whereas lower signal intensity from parenchymal tissue is suppressed.[4] It is performed using heavily T2-weighted images, such as rapid acquisition with relaxation enhancement (RARE) and half fourier acquisition single-shot turbo spin-echo (HASTE) sequences.[5] These sequences are extremely fast and are performed in one breathhold. The fat in the background is suppressed. This is useful in patients where use of ionizing radiation or iodinated contrast material is to be avoided. However, this technique does not provide information about the renal function and may not visualize a non-dilated system. A T1-weighted gadolinium enhanced 3D FLASH sequence is used after a contrast injection of 0.1 mmol/kg and multiple thin sections are obtained. These are processed with maximum-intensity-projection to produce images similar to conventional contrast urography and provide quantitative functional as well as high resolution anatomical information **(Figs. 3 and 4)**. Low doses of a diuretic agent can be administered before the examination for better filling of the pelvicalyceal system.

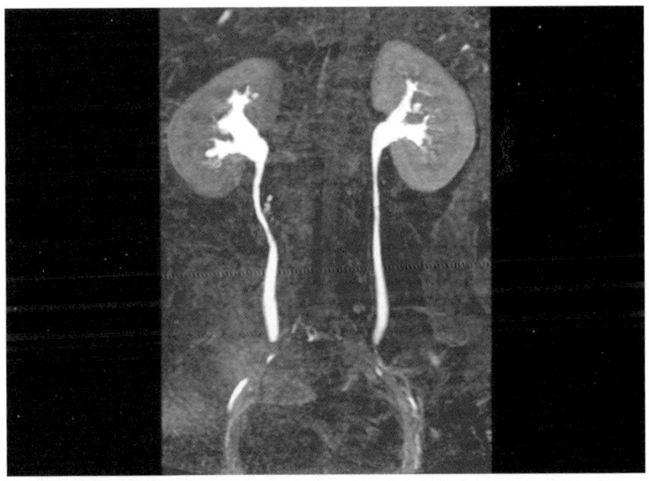

Fig. 3: MR urography, T1 FLASH coronal image showing excellent outlining of the pelvicalyceal system and the ureters by excretion of injected gadolinium contrast.

Renal Angiography and Venography

Contrast-enhanced MR angiography (CEMRA) is accurate and safe technique for evaluation of renal vessels **(Figs. 5A to C)**. This technique is independent of flow related phenomenon, assesses the true lumen of vessels and has high spatial resolution.[6] Noncontrast MRA techniques, such as gradient time of flight (TOF), TRUE FISP or phase contrast (PC) techniques render the flowing

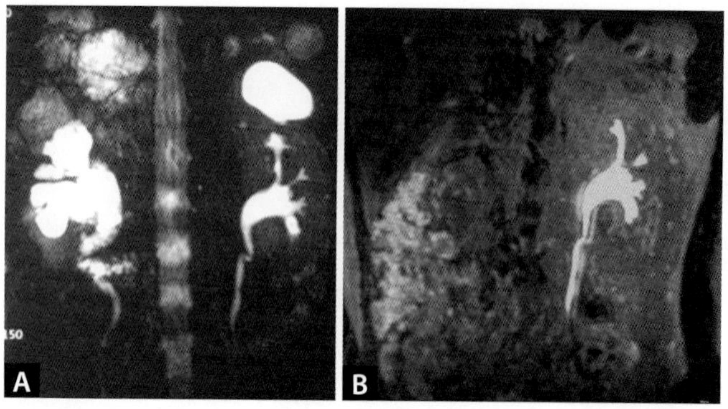

Figs. 4A and B: Bright fluid (RARE) urogram (A) and gradient contrast excretory urogram (B). Left kidney shows normal appearance of pelvicalyceal system on fluid sensitive sequence (A) and shows normal function with actively excreted contrast opacifying pelvicalyceal system on gradient contrast MR urography (B). The right kidney is not functioning due to long-standing malignant proximal ureteric obstruction (B) while accumulated urine in left PCS Is outlined in A.

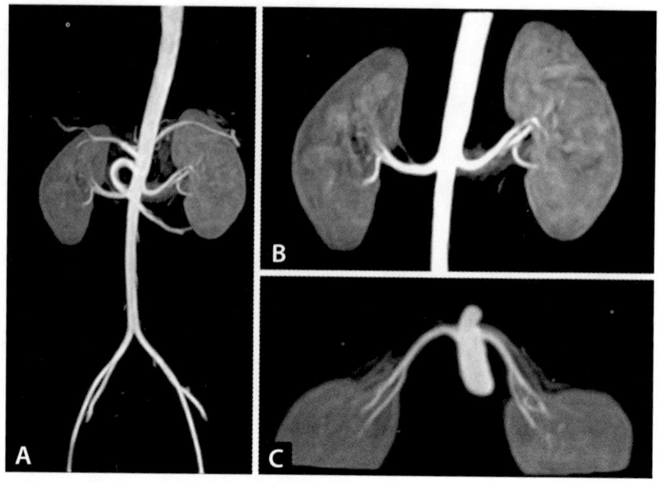

Figs. 5A to C: 3D contrast-enhanced angiogram coronal (A and B) and axial (C) maximum intensity projections showing normal appearance of abdominal aorta and renal arteries. Both the main arterial trunks and segmental branches are outlined.

blood bright **(Figs. 6A to C)**. However, these techniques have multiple limitations, such as signal loss due to turbulence at the stenosis, over estimation of stenosis due to turbulent jets leading to signal loss, bright signal of fresh thrombus, motion artifacts, non-visualization of small vessels and poor quality due to slow flow.[7] CEMRA is performed during the first pass of contrast, yields arterial detail and later images help in visualization of venous anatomy. An ultra-fast 3D T1 gradient echo sequence-like FLASH is used to obtain rapid thin slices (1–2 mm) which are reconstructed as maximum intensity projection to yield angiographic images **(Figs. 5 and 6)**.

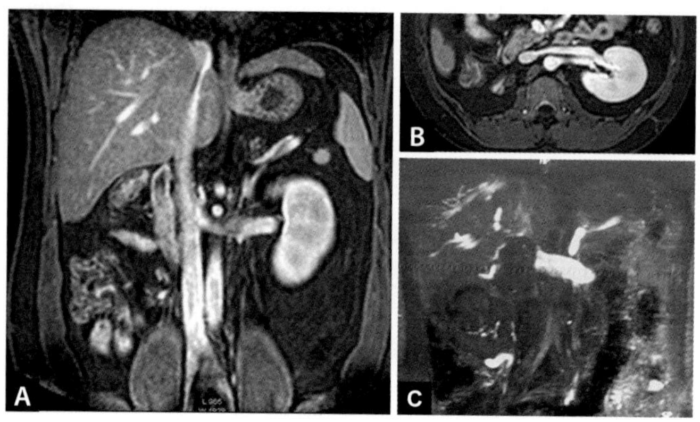

Figs. 6A to C: TRUE FISP coronal (A) and axial (B) images showing normal left renal vein lying anterior to the left renal artery (B). The vena cava in its entire extent is also shown. (C) Left renal vein is obstructed and expanded due to tumor thrombus on a contrast-enhanced venographic image.

URINARY BLADDER

Ultrasonography and CT are the primary imaging modalities for evaluation of the urinary bladder. MR plays a limited role in bladder imaging, mostly as a modality for staging of bladder tumors. Its multiplanar capability allows better visualization of tumors located at the bladder base and dome. The exquisite contrast resolution of MRI coupled with multiplanar imaging permits accurate staging of bladder malignancy.[9] MR has also been used for diagnosing fistulas involving the bladder and assessment of the underlying associated abnormalities.

Technique and Recommended Sequences

Phased array coils produce better resolution than the torso coils and have improved the tumour staging capability of MR imaging. They can also show invasion of the bladder wall while body coil can only show gross extravesical extension of tumours. Both T1- and T2W imaging are essential. The T1 SE and T2 FSE are normally used to image bladder in axial, coronal and sagittal planes.[10] It is important to orient the plane perpendi-cular to the tumor for accurate staging. Lateral walls are best evaluated on axial sections. Sagittal images are essential in evaluating the dome, the base and the anterior and posterior walls of the bladder. Coronal images are complementary in the evaluation of the dome and base of the bladder and also show the lateral walls in good details. T1WI best demonstrate extension of the tumor into perivesical fat which normally appears bright. T2WI are most useful for showing invasion of muscular wall and disruption of serosa as these structures show intermediate to low-signal intensity on T2-weighted images and invasion by intermediate intensity tumor can be better appreciated. Pelvic lymph node metastasis is best assessed on T1WI. An endoluminal coil can be used to assess small tumors at the posterior wall, bladder base or bladder neck. These allow better resolution, signal-to-noise ratio and field of view.

Normal Appearance

The urinary bladder is clearly demonstrated on MRI regardless of the degree of bladder distension. Since both urine and the muscles have a relatively long T1-relaxation time, both show low signal intensity on T1WI. In contrast to this, the T2-relaxation time of urine and smooth muscles are markedly different, enhancing differentiation between the two on T2WI in which urine appears extremely bright, while bladder wall is hypointense **(Figs. 7A and B)**. It is important to differentiate the normal low intensity of the bladder wall from the chemical shift artifact caused by different resonant frequency of the hydrogen nuclei of the urine and fat. The chemical shift artifact depends on the direction of the frequency encoding. On axial images, it is seen as a dark band along the lateral wall of one side of the bladder, and a bright stripe along the opposite wall. On sagittal or coronal images the artifact is seen along the base and dome of the bladder. This artifact should not be misinterpreted as bladder pathology. Dynamic contrast enhanced imaging using a fast gradient sequence allows differentiation of tumors from uninvolved bladder wall in most cases if the imaging is completed within 90 seconds as the normal bladder wall enhances later.[9]

PROSTATE GLAND

Prostate gland is a pyramidal fibromuscular gland which surrounds the urethra from the bladder base to the urogenital diaphragm. It has a thin true capsule, surrounded by fibrous sheath of pelvic fascia. Between these two layers lies the periprostatic venous plexus. Posterior to the prostate, lie the paired seminal vesicles. The ejaculatory ducts pierce the upper part of the posterior surface of the prostate gland and open into the prostatic urethra at the lateral margin of the prostatic utricle. The prostate gland can be subdivided into two major divisions—the peripheral gland and the central gland. The central gland in turn consists of periurethral glandular tissue, transitional and central zones. MRI has a unique ability to delineate the zonal anatomy of the prostate gland.[11] The zonal anatomy is of clinical importance, as most carcinoma arises in the peripheral zone, whereas benign prostatic hypertrophy affects the transition zone.[12] The relationship of the zones of the gland normally changes with age. In young men the central gland predominantly consists of central zone, whereas in older men with benign prostatic hyperplasia, most of the central gland is transitional zone. The prostate is described conventionally in terms of sextants, based on division of the gland into thirds in the craniocaudal direction (base, midgland and apex), and then into left and right side. Since surgery is potentially curable in a tumor confined to the gland, it is important to diagnose the extracapsular tumor spread, seminal vesicle and other adjacent visceral involvement and pelvic lymphadenopathy. The primary role of MRI is not for tumor detection, but for staging diagnosed cancer.

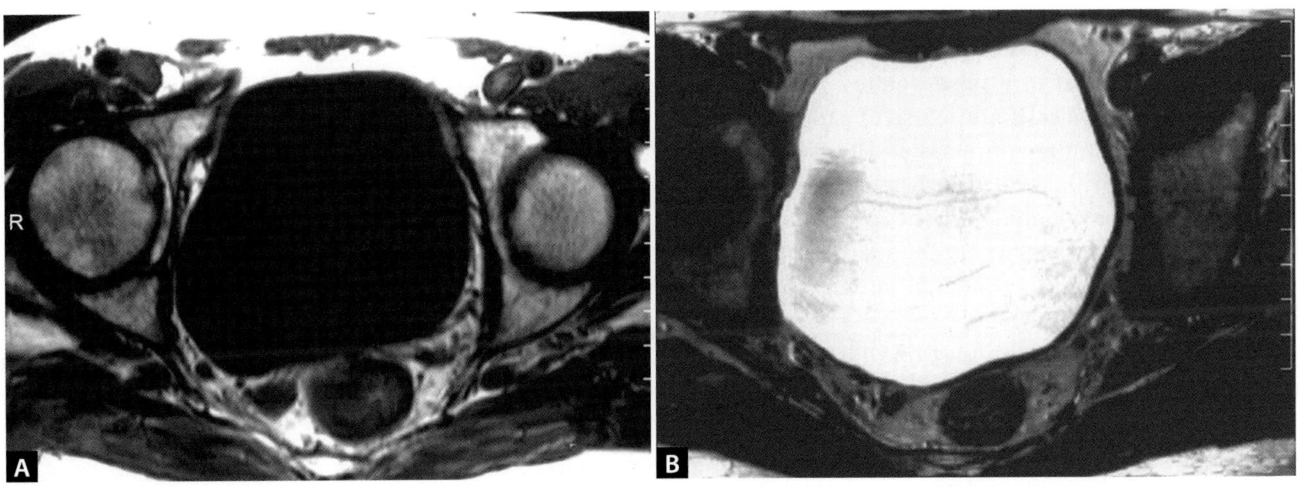

Figs. 7A and B: T1- and T2-weighted fast spin-echo axial sections (A and B) with phased array coil showing normal distended urinary bladder. The urine appears hypointense on T1 with intermediate signal bladder wall (A). The urine appears bright on T2 with low-signal wall (B). The paravesicle fat appears bright on T1 and intermediate signal on T2. The pelvic side walls, rectum and fat planes are well seen.

In addition, it helps in cancer localization, in treatment planning and post-treatment follow-up.[13] MR spectroscopic examination is helpful for showing normal and altered tissue metabolism. Functional MR techniques on 3T MRI, such as diffusion-weighted images (DWI) and dynamic contrast-enhanced MR imaging (DCEMRI) have evolved as promising new technique in evaluation of prostate cancer. Multimodality MR imaging which includes T2-weighted images, functional imaging and spectroscopic imaging may be able to accurately characterize and stage the carcinoma.

Technique and Recommended Sequences

MRI provides one-stop examination for detailed evaluation of prostate gland, periprostatic and pelvic anatomy. The results of prostate imaging using body coil are not very satisfactory. The combined use of an endorectal coil with a pelvic phased-array coil markedly improves image quality. A balloon mounted endorectal coil placed in the rectum provides the best contrast and spatial resolution for prostate imaging and the pelvic phased array coil provide good pelvic coverage and simultaneously assess pelvic side walls and lymphadenopathy. Axial spin-echo T1-weighted images are obtained of the entire pelvis, i.e. from aortic bifurcation to the symphysis pubis for detection of the nodal disease.[13] High spatial resolution (thin sections with a small field of view) T2-weighted fast spin echo sections in the axial, coronal and sagittal planes of the prostate and seminal vesicles are useful for tumor detection, localization and staging. Axial T2WI is important in differentiating peripheral and central zones whereas coronal and sagittal images are useful to assess the base and apex of the gland, pelvic muscles, rectum and seminal vesicles. Prostate imaging should not be performed for atleast 4–8 weeks (preferably 6 weeks) of a biopsy, as hemorrhage can lead to a false-positive and negative interpretation of cancer. Routine use of gadolinium and fat suppression is not recommended. However, contrast may be used in evaluation of prostatic infections and abscesses. However, enhancement of prostate cancer during the first pass of contrast with fast dynamic imaging has indicated its potential in detecting cancer, especially more aggressive cancers. MR spectroscopy is performed by chemical shift imaging with point resolved spectroscopy (PRESS) voxel excitation and band selective inversion with gradient rephrasing for water and lipid suppression.[13] Diffusion imaging with value from 0 to 800 have been applied to obtain data and create ADC maps which show restriction in high cellularity of tumors. For dynamic contrast-enhanced MR imaging, the data can be evaluated in a semiquantitative (contrast arrival, time to peak, peak enhancement and wash-in-washout gradient) or quantitative approach using pharmacokinetic modeling method.

Normal Appearance of Prostate on MRI

The appearance of prostate on MRI varies depending on the type of coil and technique used. On T1WI the zonal anatomy cannot be appreciated well and the gland is of uniform low signal intensity but post biopsy hemorrhage is better seen in these images. T1WI also show cysts and abscesses well. The zonal anatomy is well-demonstrated on T2WI, where the peripheral zone is seen as a relatively bright area compared to the central gland **(Figs. 8A and B)**.[12] It is surrounded by a thin uninterrupted hypointense line comprising true prostatic capsule. The anterior fibromuscular stroma is dark on all pulse sequences **(Fig. 9)**. The central and transitional zones are of intermediate signal intensity due to sparse glandular elements. These cannot be differentiated from each other but in older men the transitional zone stands out due to hypertrophy. The verumontanum may be seen on T2WI, where it has high signal intensity. The periprostatic fat is hyperintense on both T1 and T2WI and allows easy assessment of periprostatic spread of growth. The pelvic bone marrow shows high signal. The

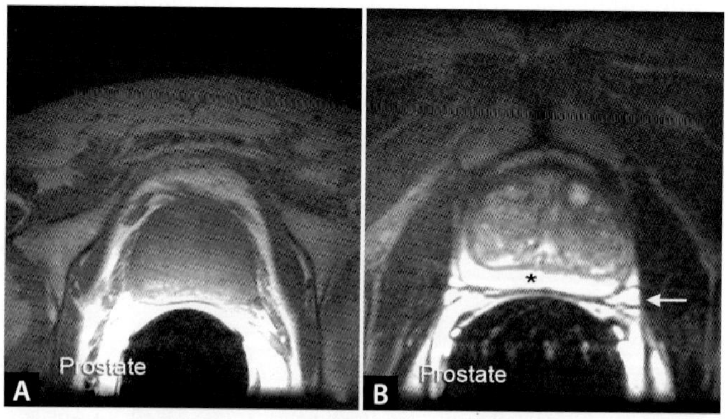

Figs. 8A and B: T1- (A) and T2- (B) weighted axial sections of prostate using endorectal coil. The zonal anatomy of prostate is not made out on T1 but the gland contour is well-outlined against bright periprostatic fat. The neurovascular bundle (arrow) is seen at 5 and 7 o'clock positions. T2-weighted image (B) shows zonal anatomy, i.e. hyperintense peripheral gland (*) and heterogeneous central zone due to hyperplastic changes. The bright nodule represents glandular hyperplasia and dark areas being stromal hyperplasia. The surgical and anatomical capsules are seen as hypointense structures. The near-field signal amplification is seen in proximity of the coil.

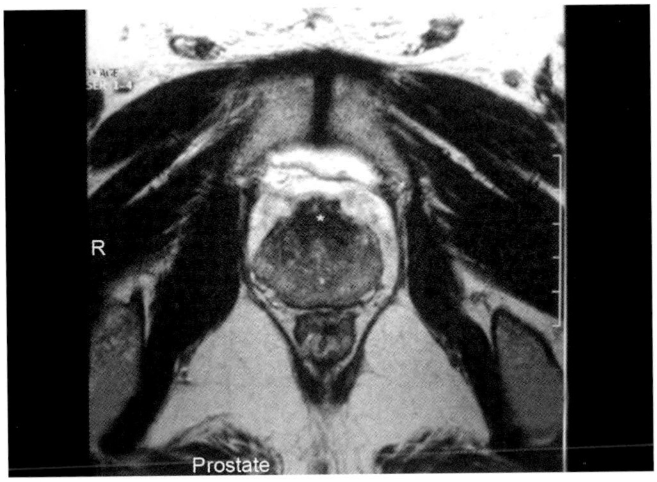

Fig. 9: T2-weighted axial section in a young adult. The gland does not show central and peripheral zone distinction or any hyperplastic central gland changes. The fibromuscular stroma anteriorly appears hypointense.

neurovascular bundles are seen at 5 and 7 o'clock position on axial images and are outlined by periprostatic fat, pelvic fascia and muscles. [12] The seminal vesicles are well seen on axial and coronal images **(Figs. 10A and B)** and appear bright on T2WI due to the water content. Loss of signal in these structures indicate invasion by malignancy. The prostate volume can be assessed on MR images by using the ellipsoid formula (half the product of maximum crani-ocaudal, anteroposterior and transverse dimensions). The vas deferens and seminal vesicles are seen well on axial and coronal images. Prostate spectroscopic examination shows relative concentrations of citrate, creatinine, choline and polyamines within contiguous voxels. Normal prostate tissue contains high levels of citrate **(Fig. 11)**.[13] High-field strength imaging may improve the quality of the spectra.

UTERUS AND OVARIES

MRI is now recognized as an important modality in evaluation of the female pelvis. Multiplanar capability, higher contrast resolution and lack of significant motion degradation of image in pelvis make MRI an imaging modality of choice for imaging female pelvis. In benign pelvic diseases, ultrasonography remains the most appropriate initial investigation because of its universal availability, lower cost and ease of operation. MRI is reserved as a problem solving technique for the patients in whom ultrasound is suboptimal or equivocal. MRI has become the imaging modality of choice for the diagnosis of congenital uterine anomalies (complex mullerian duct anomalies and ambiguous genitalia) and evaluation of the uterine and cervical malignancy. [14] It is useful in selected cases of leiomyoma prior to the myomectomy, assess response to medical therapy, and in search for submucosal lesions in infertile patients. It is the modality of choice for diagnosis of adenomyosis, and for staging endometrial and cervical malignancy.[15] Leiomyomas are most accurately detected as well as localized (subserosal, submucosal, intramural or cervical) by MRI.

It is the most sensitive imaging technique for the diagnosis of endometriosis and can replace laparoscopy for monitoring response after therapy and when laparoscopy is contraindicated. It is recommended as a problem solving modality in the evaluation of cystic ovarian lesions, especially dermoids. However, its role in staging ovarian cancer is controversial and needs further evaluation.

Technique and Recommended Sequences

Imaging is performed in supine position with an empty bladder after fasting for atleast 4 hours to limit bowel motion. A variety of receiver coils (body coil allowing better coverage and endoluminal coil for better anatomical depiction) have been used for pelvic imaging but the phased array coils provide the best results. Both T1- and T2-weighted sequences are necessary to evaluate the uterus and vagina. T1-weighted images using spin echo sequence provide excellent organ outline and help in tissue characterization and in evaluation of the nature of fluid collections. Alternatively gradient echo imaging can be done for dynamic studies, useful for staging pelvic malignancies. T2-weighted images are necessary to identify the uterine and vaginal zonal anatomy, and to depict intrauterine pathology.[15] FSE is the recommended T2 sequence. The appearance of uterus on gadolinium enhanced T1-weighted images depends on the phase in which images are acquired. Axial and sagittal planes are both useful for evaluation of the uterus.

It is necessary to use both T1- and T2-weighted spin-echo sequences to identify and evaluate the ovaries. Both transverse and coronal planes are optimal for identification of the ovaries and for confirming that a mass originates in the adnexa rather than the uterus. Chemical shift imaging with fat and water suppression is useful for differentiating lipid and blood products and fat suppressed sequences are useful for the diagnosis of dermoids. A fat suppressed T1WI is helpful in suspected cases of endometriosis.

Normal MR Appearance

On T2-weighted images, three distinct uterine zones can be differentiated in women of reproductive age[14] **(Fig. 12)**.

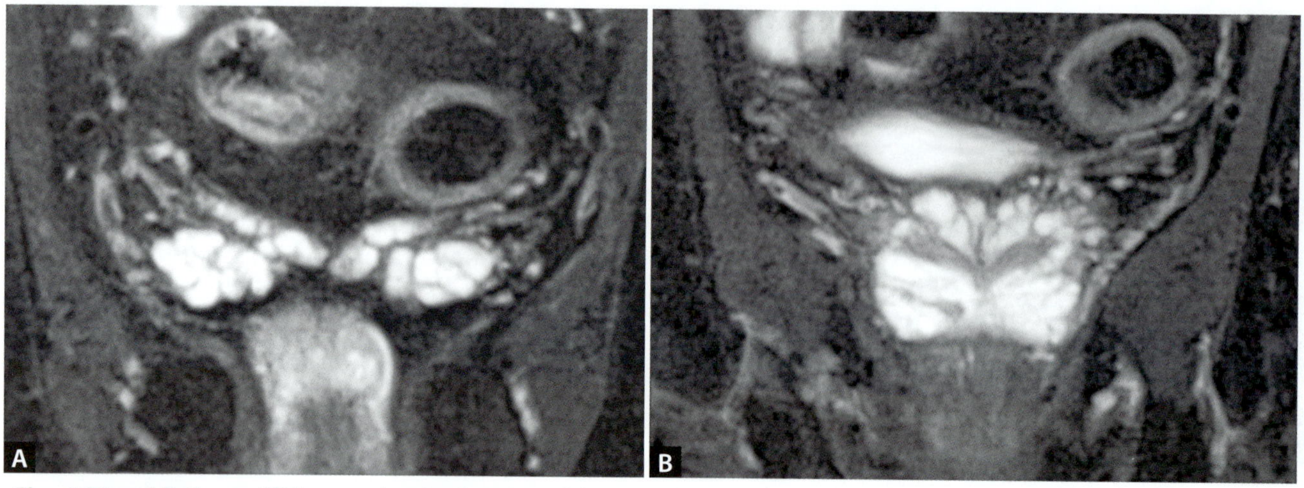

Figs. 10A and B: Coronal T2 images showing junction of the vas deferens and the seminal vesicle (A) both appearing normally bright due to fluid. More anteriorly the ejaculatory ducts are seen approaching the verumontanum, where they open into the urethra.

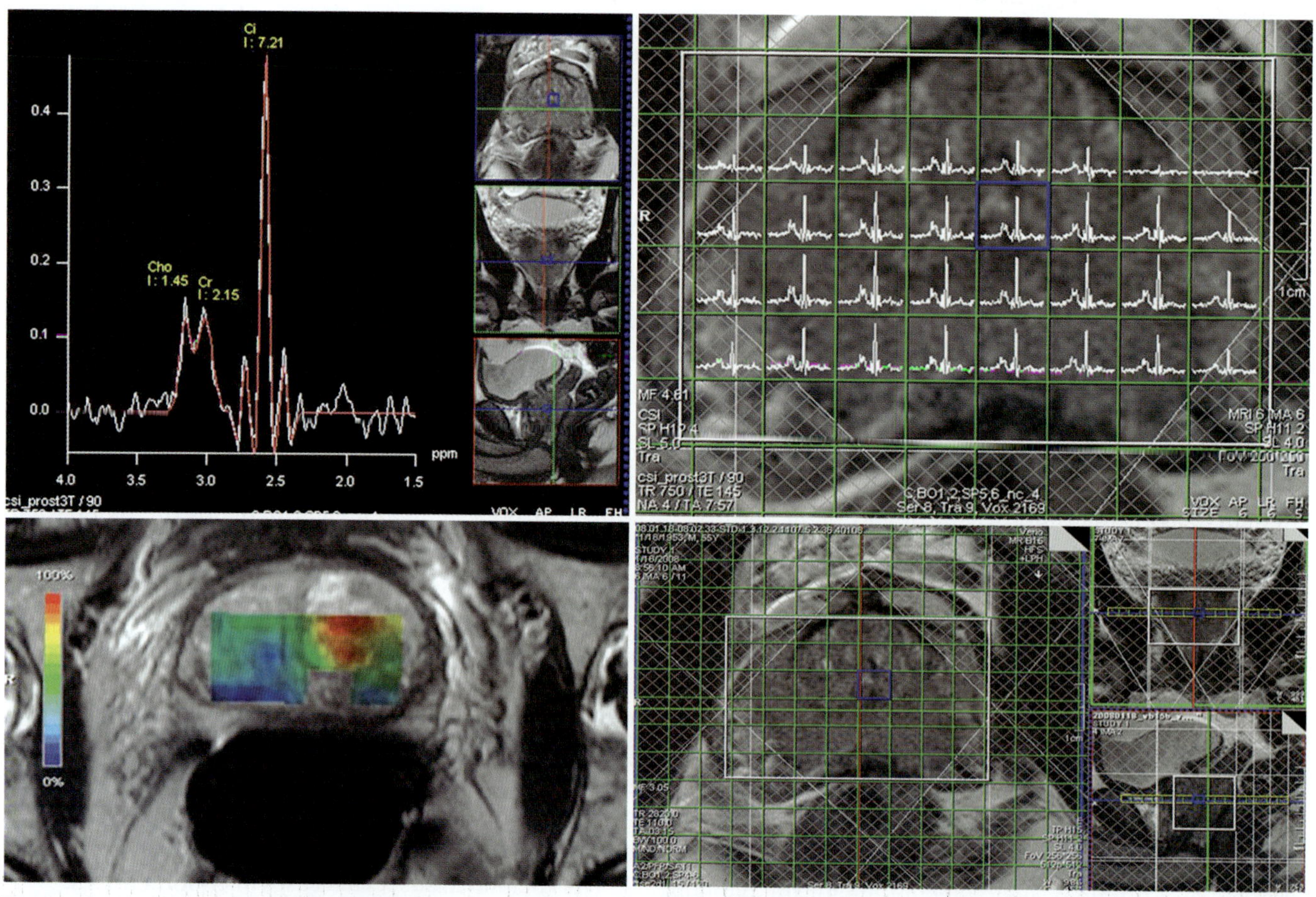

Fig. 11: Proton MR spectroscopic imaging (3D CSI- voxel size 8 x 8 x 8, spin echo TE 145, TR 750, total acquisition time 7.57 min). Spectra from normal prostate tissue shows dominant citrate peak at 2.6 ppm and choline/creatinine complex at 3–3.2 ppm. Metabolite map (lower left) and spectral map (upper right) seen overlaid on the T2 axial image. Volume selection (lower right) with presaturation slabs is to suppress periprostatic fat.

The endometrium represents central high signal intensity portion of the uterus. The endometrial thickness depends on phase of menstruation. It is thinnest immediately after menstruation and thickest during the midsecretory phase (3–7 mm). The low signal intensity middle layer is the junctional zone and represents the inner myometrium. The thickness of junctional zone is less than 8 mm. The outer medium signal intensity represents the outer myometrium. The zonal anatomy is important to assess the depth of the myometrial invasion of the endometrial carcinoma. On T1-weighted images, uterus is seen as an organ with medium to low signal intensity. Uterus is small with indistinct zonal anatomy in postmenopausal women.

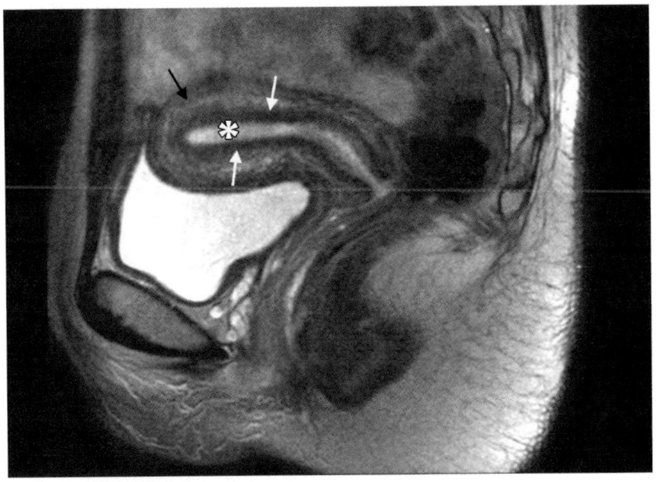

Fig. 12: T2-weighted sagittal image of pelvis showing normal anatomy of anteverted and anteflexed uterus. Endometrium (*) appears as a bright signal stripe. Junctional zone (white arrow) appears hypointense compared to outer myometrium (black arrow). The uterine isthmus and internal os are seen. The external os of cervix is seen projecting into vaginal fornices.

The cervix shows four layers on T2-weighted images.[14] The central high signal intensity represents mucus, which is surrounded by high-signal intensity endocervix. The hypointense fibrous stroma surrounds the endocervix and is continuous with the junctional zone **(Figs. 13A and B)**. The outer intermediate signal intensity corresponds to smooth muscles and is continuous with the outer myometrium. The vagina has three layers on T2-weighted images. The central high-signal intensity represents mucus-fluid complex, middle low signal intensity represents submucosa and muscularis and outer high signal intensity representing vaginal venous plexus.

On MRI, normal ovaries can be identified in 85% of the women of reproductive age. They are identified by following the course of the gonadal vessels or round ligament.[15] On T1-weighted images, the ovaries are seen as low or medium signal intensity structures, and on T2WI, they show low-signal intensity central stroma and high-signal intensity follicles and functional cyst of varied sizes **(Figs. 14A and B)**. A low intensity rim around ovaries represents fibrous capsule.

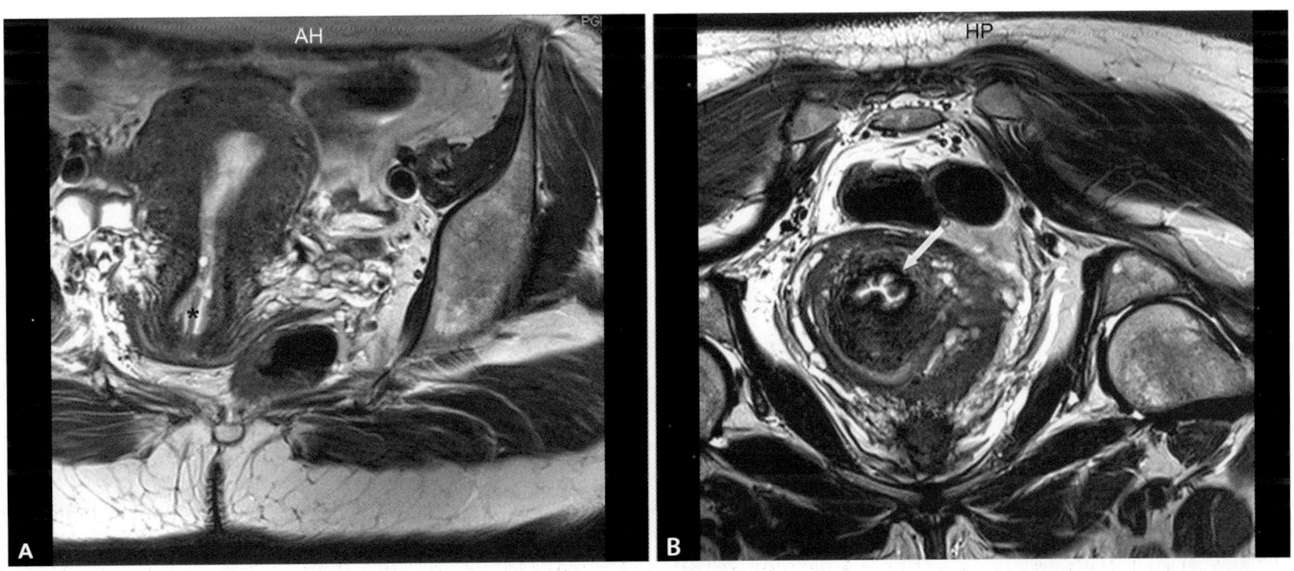

Figs. 13A and B: Coronal (A) and axial views (B) showing high signal endocervix and mucosal folds (*), and lower signal fibrous stroma (white arrow) which continues with the junctional zone. The outer layer is intermediate in signal and continues with outer myometrium.

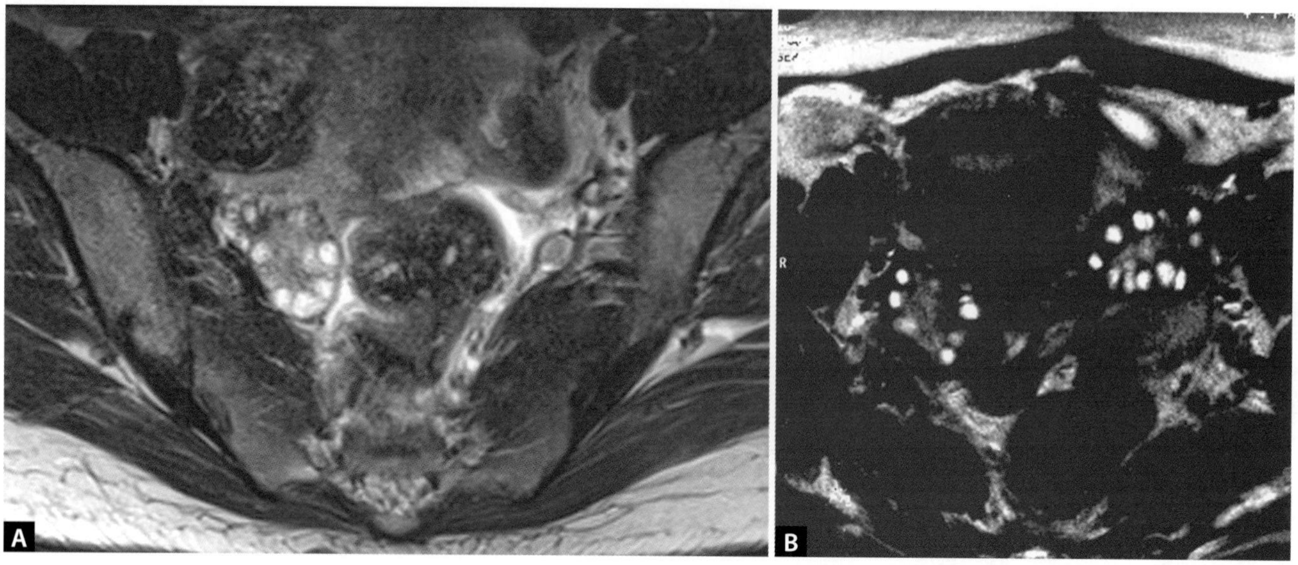

Figs. 14A and B: T2-axial fast spin echo section with a phased array coil shows excellent details of ovarian anatomy. Note the peripherally distributed hyperintense cysts and relatively low signal ovarian stroma.

PELVIC LYMPH NODES

MR imaging plays an important role in staging, accurate treatment and assessing prognosis of genitourinary cancers within the pelvis by allowing detailed evaluation of primary tumor along with pelvic lymph node.[16] The pelvic nodes are seen in relation to major pelvic vessels and are anatomically divided into the common iliac, external iliac, internal iliac and inguinal chains. MRI is useful for detection, localization and characterization of pelvic lymph nodes. The nodes are hypointense on T1WI and hyperintense on T2WI. Currently, MR imaging uses size criteria, presence of central necrosis and enhancement pattern in differentiating benign from malignant lymph nodes. MR lyphangiography using ultrasmall supraparamagnetic iron oxide (USPIO) is an evolving technique for characterization of nodal function independent of size.[16]

REFERENCES

1. Zhang J, Pedrosa I, Rofsky NM. MR technique for renal Imaging. Radiol Clin North Am. 2003;41:877-907.
2. Huang AJ, Lee VS, Rusinek H. MR Imaging of renal function. Radiol Clin North Am. 2003; 41:1001-17.
3. Pedrosa I, Rofsky NM: Kidneys. Edelman RR, Hessslink JR, Zlatkin MB, Crues III JV: In Clinical Magnetic Resonance Imaging. Saunders; 2006.pp.2792-862.
4. Kawashima A, Glockener JF, King BF. CT urography and MR urography. Radiol Clin North Am. 2003;41:945-61.
5. Grattan-Smith JD, Jones RA. MR Urography: Technique and results for the evaluation of urinary obstruction in the pediatric population. Magn Reson Imaging Clin of North Am. 2008; 16:643-60.
6. Michaely HJ, Schoenberg SO, Rieger JR, Reiser MF. MR angiography in patients with Renal Disease. Magn Reson Imaging Clin of North Am. 2005;13:131-51.
7. Leiner T, Michaely H. Advances in contrast-enhanced MR angiography of the renal arteries. Magn Reson Imaging Clin of North Am. 2008;16:685-96.
8. Thomsen HS, Marckmann P, Logager VB. Update on Nephrogenic Systemic Fibrosis. Magn Reson Imaging Clin of North Am. 2008;16:551-60.
9. Taveras N, Demas BE, Hricak H. MR imaging of bladder neoplasms. Urol Radiol. 1990;12:27-33.
10. Mallampati GK and Siegelman ES. MR imaging of the bladder. Magn Reson Imaging Clin of North Am. 2004;12:545-56.
11. Somford DM, Futterer JJ, Hambrock T, and Barentsz JO. Diffusion and perfusion MR imaging of the prostate. Magn Reson Imaging Clin of North Am. 2008;16:685-96.
12. Akin O, Hricak H. Imaging of Prostate Cancer. Radiol Clin North Am. 2007;45:207-22.
13. Rajesh A, Coakley FV. MR imaging and MR Spectroscopic imaging of prostate cancer. Magn Reson Imaging Clin of North Am. 2004;12: 557-80.
14. Brown MA, Sirlin CB. Female pelvis. Magn Reson Imaging Clin of North Am. 2005;13:381-96.
15. Aubel S, Wozney P, Edwards RP. MRI of female uterine and juxtauterine masses: Clinical application in 25 patients. Magn Reson Imaging. 1991;9:485-91.
16. Kim JY, Harisinghani MG. MR imaging staging of pelvic lymph nodes. Magn Reson Imaging Clin of North Am. 2004;12:581-6.

CHAPTER 102

Current Status of Nuclear Medicine in Urinary Tract Imaging

Rakesh Kumar, Shamim Ahmed Shamim, Rama Mohan Reddy

INTRODUCTION

Renal structure can be investigated in great detail with X-ray method, ultrasound and even with MRI, but functional evaluation of renal and urinary tract need complementary nuclear medicine technique. With the advent of gamma-camera imaging and high-quality radiopharmaceuticals has greatly facilitated the advances in radionuclide studies of the urinary tract. The techniques of renography, renal scanning, clearance studies, and voiding cystography have reached a point where a wealth of information is available to the nephrologist and urologist conversant with their capabilities and limitations. Besides being highly sensitive, these procedures are noninvasive, simple, rapid, nontoxic and allow acquisition of information often unavailable from other sources. Using these techniques, it has now become possible to assess split renal function in various renal and urinary tract disorders, evaluate kidney size in advanced azotemia, detect the presence of kidneys which are poorly functioning, evaluate renal perfusion, obtain a differential diagnosis of the upper urinary tract dilatation, diagnose urinary tract obstruction, detect intrarenal space-occupying lesions and monitor the renal function in renal failure.

A spectrum of nuclear medicine techniques are now available for the investigation of patients with nephro-urological disorders. These can be broadly classified into four categories: (i) dynamic renography, (ii) renal cortical scintigraphy, (iii) radionuclide cystography and voiding cystography and (iv) clearance studies, i.e. GFR estimation, ERPF estimation, etc. Various interventional techniques like diuresis and captopril/losartan have further improved the diagnostic capability of obstruction and renovascular hypertension simultaneously using radionuclide studies.

RADIOPHARMACEUTICALS

The various radiopharmaceuticals used in the evaluation of kidneys are classified into 2 groups. The first group consists of those which are rapidly eliminated by the kidneys and thus enabling the evaluation of renal function and urine drainage. ^{99m}Tc-LLEC, ^{99m}Tc-MAG-3, ^{99m}Tc-DTPA, ^{99m}Tc-GHA and ^{123}I-OIH are included in this group and with the exception of GHA, these agents are not used for static imaging because a few minutes after intravenous injection, they appear very briefly in the renal parenchyma before they are excreted. The second group includes radiopharmaceuticals, which are concen-trated in the renal parenchyma for a sufficiently long time, thus enabling detailed mapping of the renal parenchyma. Included in this group are ^{99m}Tc-DMSA, and ^{99m}Tc-GHA. Note that ^{99m}Tc-GHA is included in both the groups because approximately 10–15% of the injected dose is retained in the renal parenchyma while 65% of the injected dose is eliminated in the urine within 6 hours of being injected.

^{99m}Tc-MAG-3

Currently, ^{99m}Tc-MAG-3 (mercapto-acetyl-triglycine) is most commonly used renal radiopharmaceutical. It is cleared principally through active tubular transport.[1] Plasma clearance is in the order of 300 mL/min, approximately 60% that of ^{123}I-OIH,[2,3] and after 3 hours, approximately 90% of the injected dose can be recovered in the urine. It is more extensively protein bound than ^{123}I-OIH (88% versus 65%) and therefore its volume of distribution is lower than that of ^{123}I-OIH. Since the tubular secretion eliminates it and has a high initial renal uptake, the kidney to background ratio provided by this tracer is high. Moreover, the speedy excretion facilitates good temporal resolution. ^{99m}Tc-MAG-3 is a superior agent for renal dynamic scintigraphy but a practical limitation to its extensive use is the relatively high cost.

^{99m}Tc-LLEC

Metabolite of the brain perfusion tracer ECD (ethyl cystine dimer). LLEC has similar good imaging properties and higher renal clearance than MAG-3. Ethylene cystine can exit as four different stereoisomers D, D-EC, L, L-EC, syn D, L-EC, and anti D, L-EC. Labeling EC with ^{99m}Tc does not required boiling. Highest labeling yield is obtained at pH of 10–12 (97%). Like OIH and MAG-3 the secretion of ^{99m}Tc-LLEC occurs in proximal tubule.[4] D, D-EC has highest and faster renal clearance while L, L-EC has lower renal excretion and higher tissue retention.[4,5] Protien binding of D, D-EC is 28% and L,L-EC has 50%. Production of D, D-EC form, however, demands HPLC purification, a drawback for clinical use. The clearance of LLEC is about 75%. The disadvantage of EC is unknown amounts of different stereoisomers and forms produced by the different labeling kit, which have different excretion.

^{99m}Tc-DTPA

^{99m}Tc-DTPA (di-ethylene-triamine-penta-acetic acid) has been the tracer of choice for dynamic renal scintigraphy for almost three decades. However, it is now being replaced by ^{99m}Tc-MAG-3 and ^{99m}Tc-LLEC in many centers for the reasons stated above. It is excreted primarily by glomerular filtration, at a rate which is slightly lower than inulin, approximately 90 mL/min.[6,7] This lower rate of filtration is probably because of protein binding, the amount of which differs according to the formulation. A maximum concentration in kidneys is achieved usually by three minutes after intravenous injection. This is the best agent for renal dynamic study and estimation of GFR in same sitting.

^{123}I-OIH

^{123}I-OIH (orthoiodohippurate) is of use for dynamic renal scintigraphy because of its high uptake by renal tubules followed by the rapid excretion in the urine.[8] The excretion pattern is similar to para-aminohippuric acid (PAH), which is the standard for the measurement of effective renal plasma flow (ERPF). Approximately 20% of PAH is eliminated by glomerular filtration and 80% by tubular secretion, with an extraction ratio of approximately 0.9:1.0.[5] The extraction ratio of ^{123}I-OIH is approximately 85% that of PAH.

^{99m}Tc-GHA

^{99m}Tc-GHA (glucoheptonate) is rapidly taken up by the kidneys and by one hour, 8–10% of the initial tracer activity starts showing in the kidneys and almost 40% of the administered dose is eliminated by the urine.[9] Static renal scintigraphy is possible at approximately 2 hours or more after injection. Uptake of GHA occurs principally by active renal tubular transport and to a lesser extent by glomerular filtration and the tracer retained within the kidney is associated with cells of the proximal convoluted tubules.[10] Thus, it is possible to perform adequate dynamic renal imaging with rapid visualization of renal parenchyma, collecting system, pelvis, ureter and bladder. However, in children with obstructive diseases, some tracer may be retained within the pelvicalyceal system causing interference in the imaging of functional renal parenchyma leading to false interpretation of the study; therefore, late imaging should be used in such cases. Hepatobiliary system is an alternate route of excretion of GHA, and in patients with severe renal failure, late images at 4–6 hours may demonstrate tracer activity in the bowels.

^{99m}Tc-DMSA

^{99m}Tc-DMSA (dimercapto-succinic acid) is currently the agent of choice for cortical static renal scintigraphy both in planar and SPECT studies. The renal uptake of this agent is about 50% of the injected dose at 1 hour and about 70% at 24 hours after injection.[11] One hour or more postinjection, the tracer is found principally in the proximal convoluted tubules with very minimal activity elsewhere in the kidney. In most patients, therefore, excellent images of renal cortex can be obtained approximately 4 hours after injection of ^{99m}Tc-DMSA. Here again, patients with obstructive pathology may have tracer retention within the pelvicalyceal system leading to false interpretation. In such a case, delayed imaging upto 24 hours postinjection is recommended so that the tracer in the urine is allowed for elimination.

IMAGING TECHNIQUES

Renal Dynamic Scintigraphy

This refers to serial continuous imaging following intravenous injection of radio-tracer. It encompasses three principal techniques: (a) dynamic renography, (b) diuretic renography and (c) captopril renography.

Dynamic Renography

Patient preparation: Patient should be well-hydrated before study. Patients should be encouraged to drink fluids prior to the study. Before the examination begins, the patients are asked to empty their bladder. In suspected cases of obstruction, when patients cannot void or in children with VUR, a bladder catheter (Foley's type) should be inserted. The bladder should be allowed to drain through the catheter throughout the entire duration of the study. Intravenous line is established to avoid extravasations of the tracer, which may yield erroneous interpretation.

Radiopharmaceuticals ^{99m}Tc-MAG-3, ^{99m}Tc-DTPA, ^{99m}Tc-LLEC, ^{99m}Tc-GHA or ^{123}I-OIH can all be used in performing dynamic renal scintigraphy. The dose administered is given in **Table 1**.

Imaging: Patients are examined in the supine position with the gamma-camera placed underneath the examination table viewing the kidney and bladder area. In this position, the distance from the skin to each of the kidneys is approximately the same and for calculation of the left/right renal uptake ratio, depth correction is not critical. In renal transplants, however, the camera is placed anteriorly over the patient in supine position, viewing the allograft and bladder. In children, appropriate immobilization should be attained during acquisition. Once the patient is appropriately positioned, a rapid intravenous bolus of the tracer is injected and simultaneously the acquisition is started. One frame per two seconds is recorded for one minute, followed by one frame per 15 seconds for duration of 20–30 minutes.

Interpretation: A dynamic renal study is evaluated for the parenchymal phase, the cortical transit time, and the urine drainage phase.

- *Parenchymal phase:* Evaluating this phase is very critical. During the first few minutes of the dynamic study, after the initial vascular distribution of the tracer and before its appearance in the renal collecting system, the tracer is concentrated in the renal parenchyma. At this point there is progressive decrease in the blood level of the tracer with increasing concentration in the parenchyma till a peak is reached where maximum concentration has been attained. After this, the tracer appears outside the renal parenchyma with progressive decrease in levels within the parenchyma, marking the beginning of the drainage phase. The parenchymal phase is usually visualized 60–120 seconds after the IV injection and provides the following information:
  - Relative and absolute size of the functional renal parenchymal units
  - Total renal function (kidney/background ratio)
  - Relative or split renal function (right versus left)
  - Overall renal morphology and redistribution of functioning parenchyma
  - Position of the renal units.

  The relative renal size can easily be estimated through simple visual observation. Renal dimensions in longitudinal and transverse planes can be measured with a calibrated system or by imaging a radioactive ruler placed beside the patient. Parenchymal phase shows the position of the renal units. A qualitative estimate of the renal function can be obtained by visually evaluating the ratio of the renal and background activity. Normally, very little tracer activity should be present in the background, the blood pool and the liver during the parenchymal phase. If a high level of tracer activity is noted within these regions, then the renal uptake shall be low indicating a poor renal function. Split renal function can be assessed visually and also by calculating the individual renal uptake as a fraction of the total renal uptake from renal regions of interests (ROIs). Placement of ROIs should be strictly over the parenchymal region but under certain special circumstances, such as hydronephrosis, this may be difficult. Background ROIs should be placed with caution since this step is usually performed manually and different sizes and positions produce different results. This is a particular problem when

Table 1: Different radiopharmaceutical and their doses.

Radiopharmaceutical	*Dose (mCi/kg)*	*Minimum dose (mCi)*	*Maximum dose (mCi)*
^{99m}Tc-MAG-3	0.100	0.5	10.0
^{99m}Tc-DTPA	0.100	0.5	8.0
^{99m}Tc-GHA	0.100	0.5	8.0
^{123}I-OIH	0.010	0.1	0.5
^{99m}Tc-LLEC	0.100	0.5	10.0

renal function is low and/or there is presence of severe hydronephrosis.

Information about intrarenal distribution of radiotracer can be obtained during the parenchymal phase. Hydronephrosis is usually seen as a "photon deficient" area within the renal pelvis. Depending on the severity of hydronephrosis, the cortical uptake appears as a rim of varying size. It is important to note that absence of a photon deficient area within the renal outline does not rule out hydronephrosis. Reduction or absence tracer activity in a relatively large portion of the kidney, such as a malfunctioning upper pole in a duplex kidney, trauma, tumor, or cyst can be traced.

- *Cortical transit time:* Cortical transit time refers to the time interval between the intravenous injection of the radiotracer and its first appearance within the renal collecting system. Normally, this is about 3–6 minutes. A normal cortical transit time indicates that renal parenchymal function is not compromised, even in the presence of dilatation of the pelvicalyceal system. Conversely, therefore, the poorer the renal function, the longer is the cortical transit time. As the tracer is eliminated into the renal pelvis, there is gradual decline in the parenchymal activity. Even if the cortical transit time appears to be within the normal range, it is important to determine if it is associated with a decrease of tracer activity from the renal cortex. Cortical retention of tracer activity indicates renal dysfunction. A number of conditions may prolong the cortical time. These include ureteral obstruction, acute and chronic pyelonephritis, nephrotoxicity, trauma, renal artery stenosis, renal vein thrombosis, acute tubular necrosis and allograft rejection.
- *Drainage phase:* Drainage phase comprises of the passage of the radiotracer from the pelvicalyceal system through the ureter into the bladder. Usually, after 20 minutes of the study, much of the tracer would leave the renal parenchyma. At this time, minimal or no tracer should be visible in the renal collecting system. Time activity curves are generated from ROI over an entire kidney and reveal a peak time at 4–7 minutes with subsequent decrease to 30–50% of the peak activity at 15 minutes. Time activity curves should always be interpreted along with careful evaluation of images in the parenchymal phase and drainage phase, keeping in mind the cortical transit time. Normal cortical transit time can be seen with complete cortical clearance of tracer at 20 minutes along with a time activity curve that shows a delayed peak and a high-residual value. Such a pattern indicates delayed drainage without parenchymal dysfunction and is almost always without any clinical significance. The possibility of a vesicoureteric reflux of tracer during the drainage phase should also be kept in mind in order to be able to differentiate it from outflow tract obstruction.

Normal Dynamic Renal Study

There is an intense and rapid concentration of tracer in the renal parenchyma at 1–3 minutes postinjection. Subsequently, the tracer passes into the renal calyces and pelvis by 3–6 minutes. Ureters may be visualized in normal patients and in those with slow ureteral transit time. However, a dilated ureter with or without obstruction is always visible. The renal parenchyma is usually completely cleared of radiotracer by 20 minutes but a small residual amount may sometimes be present and is usually of no clinical significance. This residual tracer usually clears spontaneously with change in the patient's position or after the patient voids. The bladder is seen 3–6 minutes after injection and there is a progressive increase in tracer concentration with time. The background activity is usually a reflection of blood clearance of tracer or rather the renal extraction of tracer from the blood pool, which rapidly decreases with time in a patient with normal renal function. The dynamic acquisition can be terminated at 15–20 minutes, when there is no retention of tracer within the pelvicalyceal system or ureters **(Figs. 1A to C)**. If at the end of the initial 20 minutes, there is evidence of tracer retention, then the patient should be asked to get up and move for a few minutes (a small child should be picked up for a few minutes) to encourage postural drainage. An additional image is recommended to determine the tracer clearance, which, if adequate, should be considered normal, and the outflow tract not obstructed. A diuretic renogram is indicated if an obstruction is present or suspected.

Diuretic Renography

Furosemide causes a rapid diuretic response that drains out tracer from dilated nonobstructed system. In significant outflow tract obstruction, tracer in the renal area may decrease slowly or fail to decrease or even increase in response to a diuretic challenge. The urine flow is dependent not only on the function and amount of renal parenchyma, but also on the ability of the parenchyma to respond to a diuretic. Drainage is directly proportional to urine flow and inversely proportional to the volume of the renal pelvis and ureters. The poorer the function, the longer is the time of drainage. Compliance and volume of the pelvicalyceal system are also important

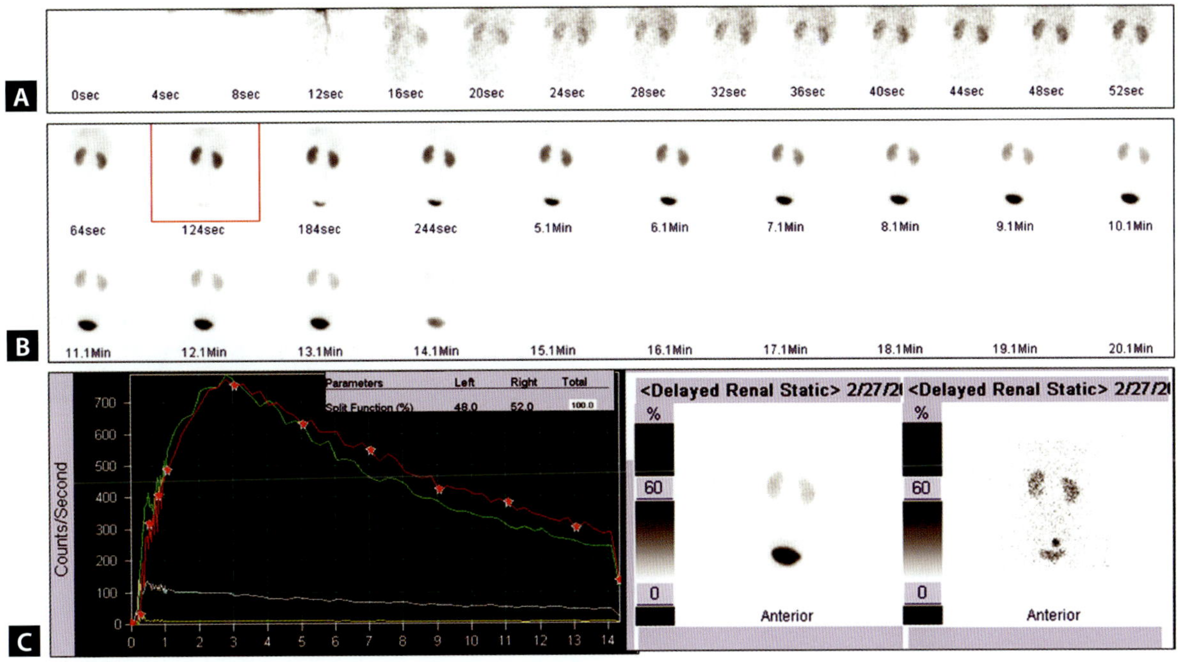

Figs. 1A to C: Normal ^{99m}Tc-LLEC scan: Normal dynamic function images with prompt symmetric radiotracer perfusion (A), uptake and rapid clearance (B). Normal time activity curves with steep uptake slope, distinct peak, and rapid clearance with normal early and delayed static images (C).

in that a large flaccid renal pelvis usually causes slow drainage of radiotracer. There are several factors that can limit the usefulness of diuretic renography. Severe hydroureteronephrosis may partly or wholly mask the effect of a diuretic on the emptying of the renal pelvis. Other factors include poor response of the renal parenchyma to the diuretic, poor delivery of the diuretic to the kidneys, bladder over distension, complex pelvic surgeries, prune-belly syndrome and ectopic kidney.

Imaging: Diuretic renography can be performed using the same radiopharmaceuticals mentioned earlier. It is crucial to ensure that tracer has filled the renal pelvis and postural drainage has not occurred before the diuretic is administered. The diuretic can be administered 15 minutes postinjection or simultaneously with the radiotracer. Forced hydration is recommended as a method to differentiate obstruction from nonobstruction in diuretic renography. The diuretic effect is usually seen within 1-2 minutes after administration of furosemide. Patients with intermittent hydronephrosis who complain of intermittent flank pain may have reproduction of pain on administration of diuretic. In some cases with otherwise balanced drainage and urinary flow, a diuretic may cause rapid over distension of the renal pelvis resulting in the disruption of the status of the system. It is important to note that in patients with urinary diversions, even in the absence of obstruction, flow dynamics may be slow, making the diagnosis of obstruction difficult. Overlap of kidney and an ileal or colonic diversion may give rise to confusing images. Imaging in various projections, removal or replacement of external urine collecting devices and attempts at postural drainage may sometimes be helpful.

Interpretation: Careful evaluation of the dynamic renal study preceding a diuretic administration is important during interpretation. In the absence of obstruction, rapid and complete washout of radiotracer occurs from the pelvicalyceal system **(Fig. 2)**. On the other side of the spectrum is an obstructed system with slow or no drainage of radiotracer following a diuretic challenge **(Figs. 3 and 4)**. Interpretation of intermediate diuretic renographic patterns is difficult. Usually, the images obtained prior to and after a diuretic injection are compared. A cinematic display verifies whether the patient moved during acquisition or not.

The diuretic washout $T_{1/2}$ is estimated by using an exponential interpolation between the point on the initial descent of the time activity curve and another point on the down slope while the curve is decaying monotonically. The diuretic $T_{1/2}$ should be only one of the several factors, which are considered while assessing urinary obstruction. Although there may be many variations in the time of diuretic injection and subsequent time of acquisition

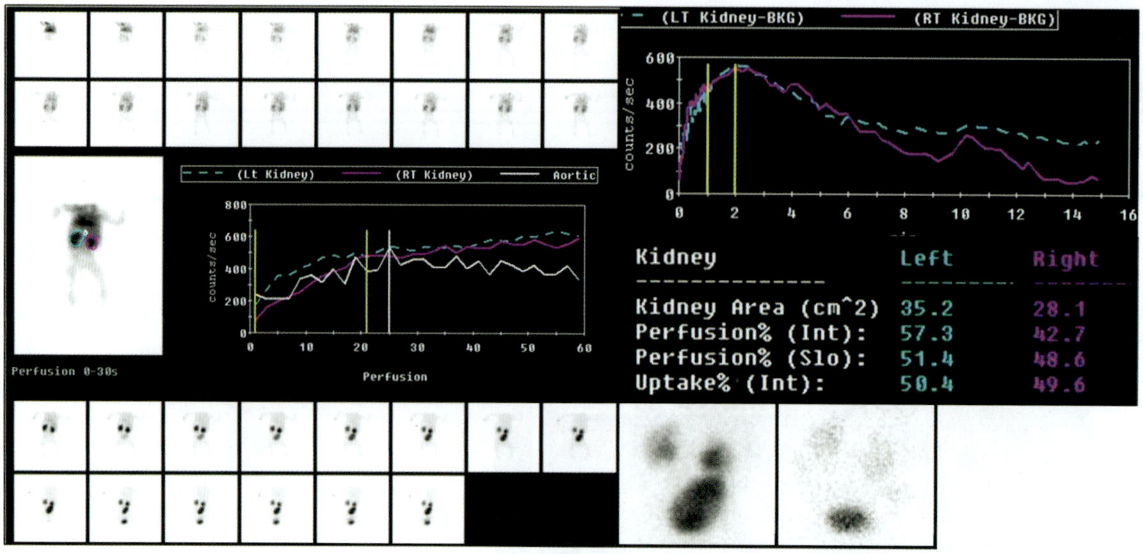

Fig. 2: ^{99m}Tc-LLEC scan in nonobstructive hydronephrosis: Dynamic and static renal images showing initial photopenia which is filling-up and nonobstructed clearance, findings are consistent with nonobstructed hydronephrosis.

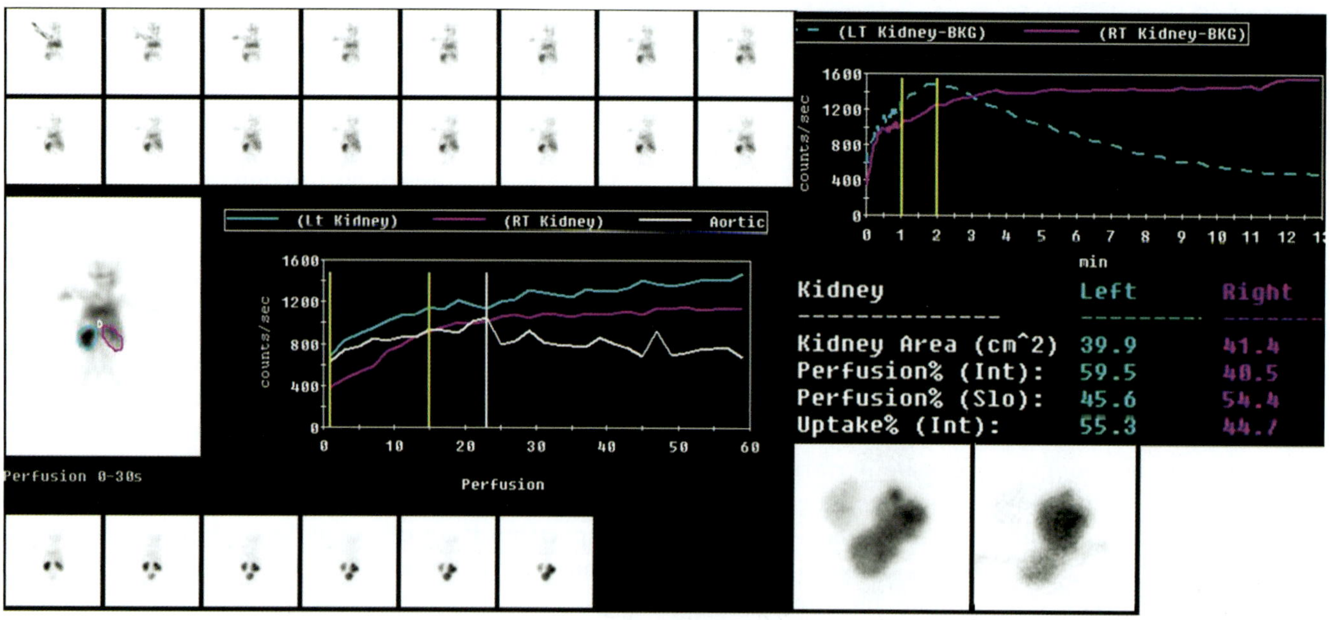

Fig. 3: ^{99m}Tc-LLEC scan in obstructed hydronephrosis: Progressive filling of enlarged dilated collecting system is seen on right side, whereas the left kidney clears normally. Time activity curves shows washout on the left side and obstructed pattern on right side. Early and delayed static images showing persistent activity in dilated PCS without clearance on right side.

following a diuretic response, the overall sensitivity of a diuretic renography for the detection of obstruction in children has been estimated at 93%.[12]

Drainage pattern of renogram: O' Reilly et al. (1978) classified patients on the basis of the renogram curve of ^{99m}Tc-DTPA with diuretic.[13]

- *Response I:* Normal initial renography and remained so after diuretics
- *Response II:* Obstructive initial renography and remained so after diuretics
- *Response IIIa:* Obstructive initial renography and showed rapid clearance after diuretics.

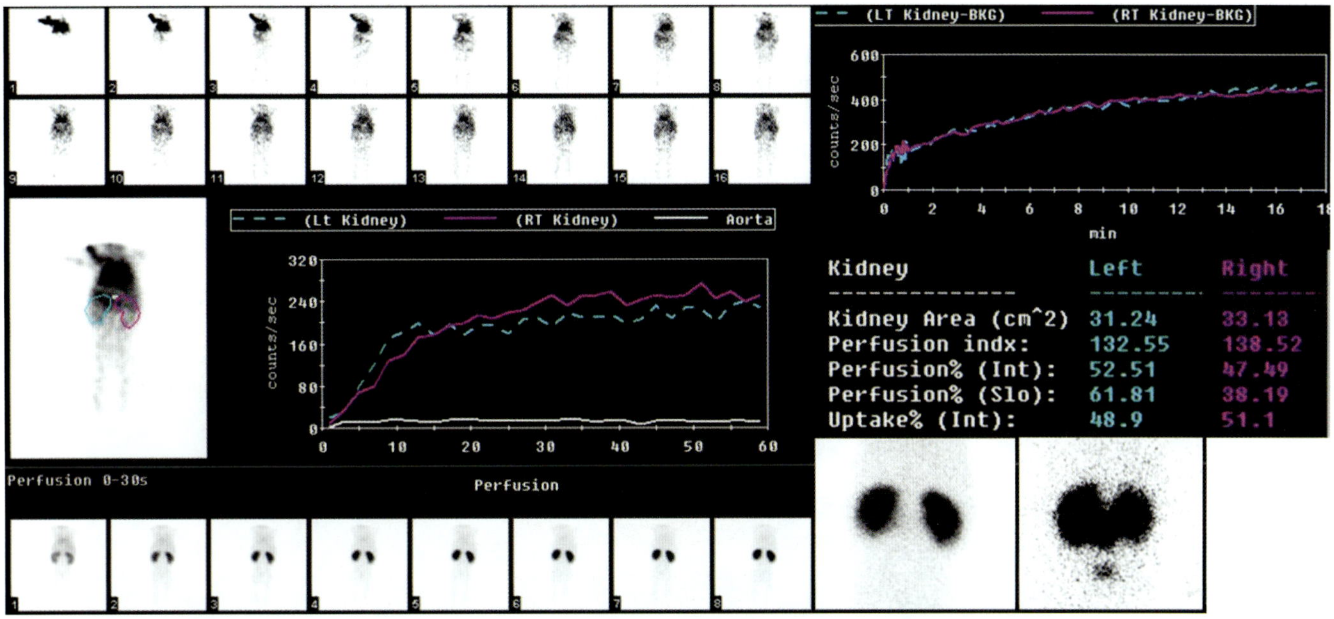

Fig. 4: ^{99m}Tc-LLEC scan in bilateral pelvic–uretric junction obstruction: Dynamic images showing progressive filling of enlarged dilated collecting system is seen on both side. Time activity curves shows obstructed pattern on both side. Early and delayed static images showing persistent activity in dilated PCS.

- *Response IIIb:* Obstructive initial renography and showed mild/partial clearance after diuretics
- *Combined:* Many centres go for combined approach.

Captopril Renography

Secondary hypertension is more common in children and renal disease is perhaps the most common cause in this group. In a study conducted by Londe S et al. in 1978,[14] 563 pediatric patients with secondary hypertension were evaluated. 78% had renal abnormalities and 12% had renal artery disease. Secondary hypertension may be caused less frequently by endocrinal, cardiovascular or nervous system disorders. The renal causes of hypertension are infarction, postpyelonephritic scarring and post-traumatic lesions, which are easily diagnosed by conventional renal scintigraphy. A dynamic study usually shows the affected kidney to be smaller with lesser uptake than the contralateral normal kidney. The more severe the affliction, the lower is the renal uptake of tracer. ^{99m}Tc-DMSA scintigraphy in patients with renovascular hypertension typically reveals renal asymmetry. The affected kidney is smaller and shows lesser tracer uptake than the normal one. In the presence of unilateral renal artery stenosis, there may be reduced renal perfusion and function on the affected side. However, sometimes the same kidney may remain adequately perfused and owing to the auto regulation mechanism the radionuclide study may remain normal in a significant number of cases. Thus conventional radio-nuclide studies are not reliable screening tests for the diagnosis of renovascular hypertension and that angiotensin converting enzyme (ACE) inhibitor renal scintigraphy is a markedly improved technique.

ACE inhibitors, such as captopril block the formation of angiotensin II, producing dilatation of efferent arterioles and a fall in transcapillary pressure gradient. This causes a significant decrease in GFR of the kidney with renal artery stenosis that can be easily diagnosed by renography.[15-19] Initially ^{99m}Tc-DTPA was used, but subsequent experience has shown that both glomerular and tubular agents can be used.[16] For ensuring that captopril absorbs well, the patients should not take solid food atleast four hours before the study. Enalapril another agent has a distinct advantage over captopril as this can be administered intravenously and therefore does not depend on the variations of absorption in the gastrointestinal tract. Caution should be taken about the potentially serious hypotensive episodes following intravenous enalapril. Significant hypotension is also seen after a single dose of captopril, and therefore, the patient should be well-hydrated and an intravenous access maintained throughout the study. Blood pressure should be monitored every 5–15 minutes. Diuretics may exaggerate the hypotensive effect and therefore its use should be avoided in conjunction with captopril renography.

A baseline study is obtained followed by a repeat examination either one-hour after oral captopril (1 mg/kg, up to 50 mg), or 15 minutes after intravenous enalapril (0.03 mg/kg). Some authors obtain the initial study with an ACE inhibitor and repeat later without the ACE inhibitor only if the first study is abnormal. Since the primary effect of ACE inhibitor is decreased GFR, studies using glomerular agents show decreased extraction of tracer and delayed visualization of the collecting system whereas with tubular agents prolonged retention of the tracer is seen. Moreover, detection of cortical retention of tracer is easier to appreciate than focal decreased extraction, tubular agents are probably more effective than glomerular agents in the detection of segmental renal artery stenosis. The typical findings of a positive captopril study are an increase in differential renal uptake, increase in cortical transit time, prolongation of time to peak and retention of tracer in the renal parenchyma **(Figs. 5A and B)**. The most

A

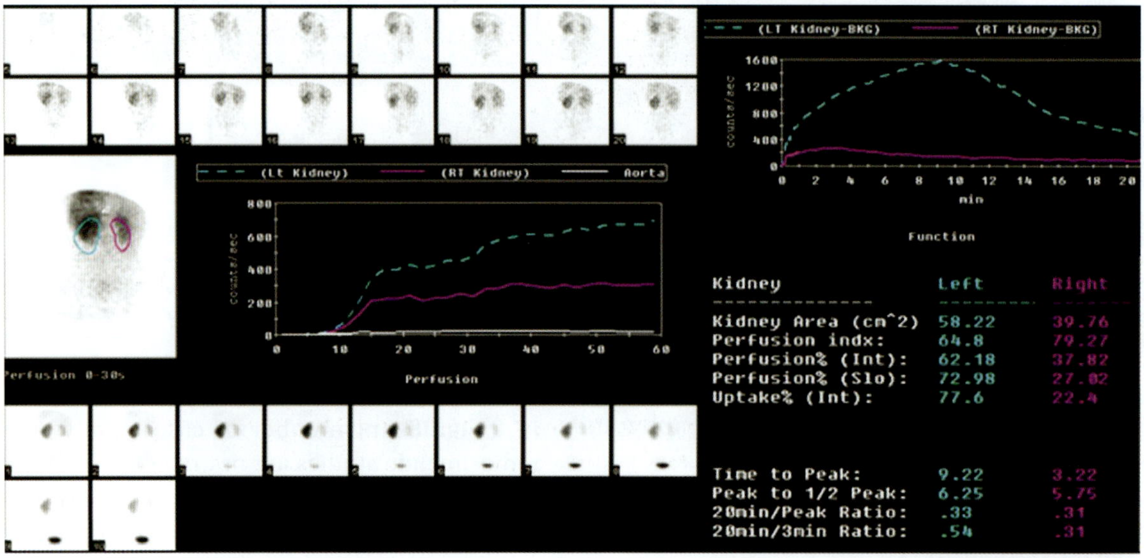

B

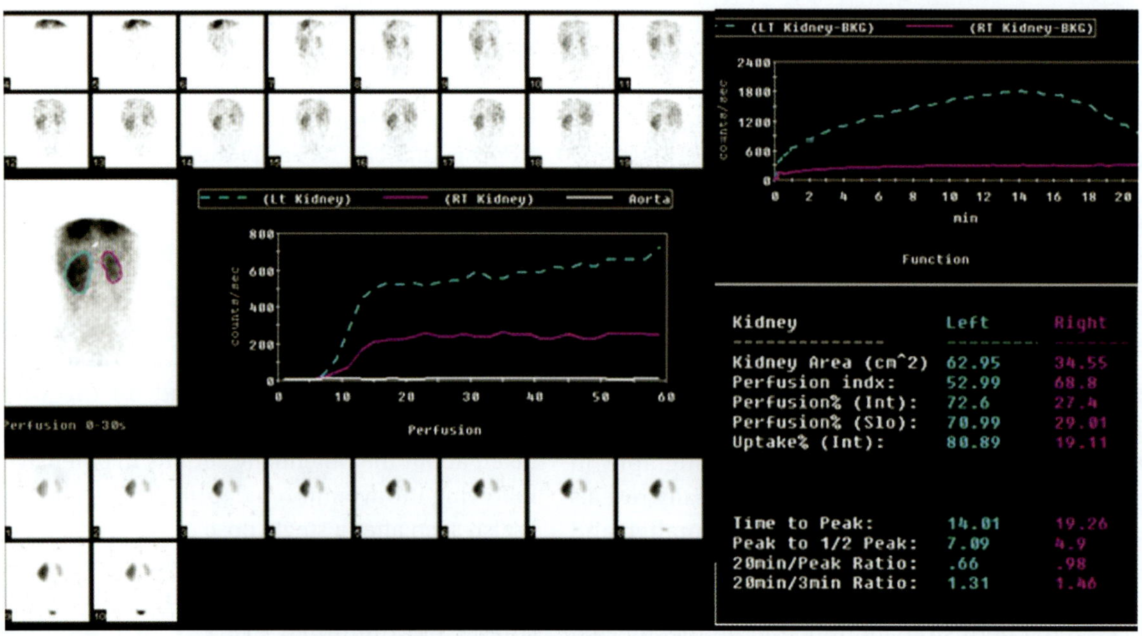

Figs. 5A and B: Positive captopril study with ^{99m}Tc-LLEC: Baseline study (A) showing normal functioning left kidney and impaired functioning right kidney. Captopril study (B) showing retention of radiotracer on left side and further impairment of function on right side with retention as well.

important parameter however is the split renal uptake. In patients with bilateral renal artery stenosis, the narrowing is usually asymmetrical and so is the effect of ACE inhibitor on each kidney. Cases in which captopril does not induce scintigraphic changes are usually indicate the failure of revascularisation or nephrectomy.[20-23]

Cortical Scintigraphy/Static Renal Scintigraphy

^{99m}Tc-DMSA is administered intravenous by a dose of 0.04–0.05 mCi/kg (1.5–1.9 MBq/kg) with a minimum of 0.3 mCi (11.1 MBq) and a maximum of 3 mCi (111 MBq). Imaging is started about 3–4 hours after injection. Planar magnified and SPECT images can be acquired.

Imaging Techniques

Planar renal scintigraphy: Patient is examined supine with the gamma-camera placed posterior recording 300,000–500,000 counts using a high resolution or preferably a ultrahigh-resolution collimator on a 256 × 256 matrix. Left and right posterior oblique projections are acquired which sometimes prove useful in the identification of cortical defects. Split renal uptake can be calculated by placing ROIs over posterior images. In cases of renal duplication, the upper and lower moieties can be outlined and differential renal function ascertained.

Magnified renal scintigraphy: Pinhole magnification or zoomed acquisition is mandatory in neonates and infants and may be useful in identification of cortical defects in older children and adults. Cortical defects following pyelonephritis, infarction, duplication and fetal lobulation can be distinguished more frequently with pinhole magnification as compared to parallel hole high-resolution collimators since the former with an internal diameter of 2 mm provide images which have higher spatial resolution than the latter. Posterior and posterior oblique projections are usually acquired.

SPECT: Mapping of regional functional parenchyma is best done with ^{99m}Tc-DMSA SPECT. The surface and volume rendered SPECT images permit a superior overall view of the functional anatomy of the kidneys. Using the modern multi-headed SPECT cameras, acquiring 120 images over 360° on a 128 × 128 matrix usually requires 15–20 minutes. Proper sedation is mandatory in acquiring SPECT images.

Radionuclide Cystography

This has been accepted as the technique of choice for evaluation and follow-up of children with urinary tract infection and reflux. The estimated gonadal radiation dose is one-hundredth of the voiding cystouretherography. Radionuclide cystography is more sensitive than voiding cystography in detecting vesicoureteric reflux. Other parameters like residual urine volume, bladder volume at the time of reflux and the rate of clearance of refluxed urine can also be calculated. The only disadvantage of radionuclide cystography is poor anatomical resolution of the bladder and urethra.

Clinical Applications

In urology practice, the most important clinical areas, where radionuclide studies may be of particular importance in patient management, can be considered under the following headings:

- Urinary tract obstruction
- Urinary tract infection
- Renovascular hypertension
- Congenital anomalies
- Renal failure
- Renal transplant evaluation.

Urinary tract obstruction: Radionuclide studies may be necessary to establish or confirm the diagnosis of obstruction, to ascertain its site or level, to determine its extent or severity or to measure how well the obstructed kidney is functioning.[24] In addition, radionuclide studies may be needed in other situation when any change in the function or condition of the kidney, or of the site and severity of obstruction, is to be determined if desirable clinically to assess patients prognosis and in differential diagnosis of urinary obstruction. In the differential diagnosis of urinary obstruction, diuretic renography is of immense value especially in those patients with a nonobstructed dilated collecting system associated with indeterminate flow curve **(Fig. 2)**. Injection of diuretic is essential, if obstruction at the pelviureteric junction is suspected, as this diagnosis can only be confirmed at high urine flow rate. However, one of the major drawbacks of diuretic renography is a large number of indeterminate results in poorly functioning kidneys. Some progress has been made in this regard by correcting furosemide response for level of renal function. Estimation of renal output efficacy (ROE), which is calculated by a technique independent of variations in uptake rate by the kidneys, provides an accurate diagnosis of renal outflow obstruction in patients with significantly impaired renal function.[25]

Urinary tract infection: Renal infection may be clinically obvious, but can be easily overlooked. Clinically, it is frequently difficult or impossible to differentiate infection of the bladder and ureters from the acute renal parenchymal infection. The lack of sensitivity of intravenous urography (IVU) and ultrasonography in the demonstration of early renal infection is wellknown. ^{99m}Tc-DMSA is valuable in the identification of renal damage due to early pyelonephritis. Even in the absence of urographic or ultrasonographic abnormalities, regional parenchymal uptake of DMSA may be altered in acute pyelonephritis. ^{99m}Tc-DMSA is also useful to quantify the degree of renal damage to follow the progress of antibiotic therapy, and to assess recovery and/or residual renal damage.

Imaging with ^{99m}Tc-DMSA facilitates detection of cortical scarring of pyelonephritis **(Figs. 6A to C)**. Unlike urography, cortical scarring can detect cortical defects that do not deform the renal outline or the collecting system. In the detection of renal scars ^{99m}Tc-DMSA scan is more sensitive (96%) and specific (98%) as compared with IVU.[26] Besides, in patients with chronic pyelonephritis with uncontrolled hypertension, demonstration of a severe segmental scar on a DMSA scan may guide the surgeon in undertaking partial nephrectomy **(Figs. 7 and 8)**.

One of the most common and routinely employed procedures in children with urinary tract infection is the direct radionuclide cystogram (DRCG) and urine flowmetry (UFMT) in conjunction with cortical scanning **(Figs. 9 to 11)**. In the diagnosis of vesicouretic reflux this procedure is much superior and the radiation exposure to the patient is much less as compared to micturating cystourethrogram (MCU).[27]

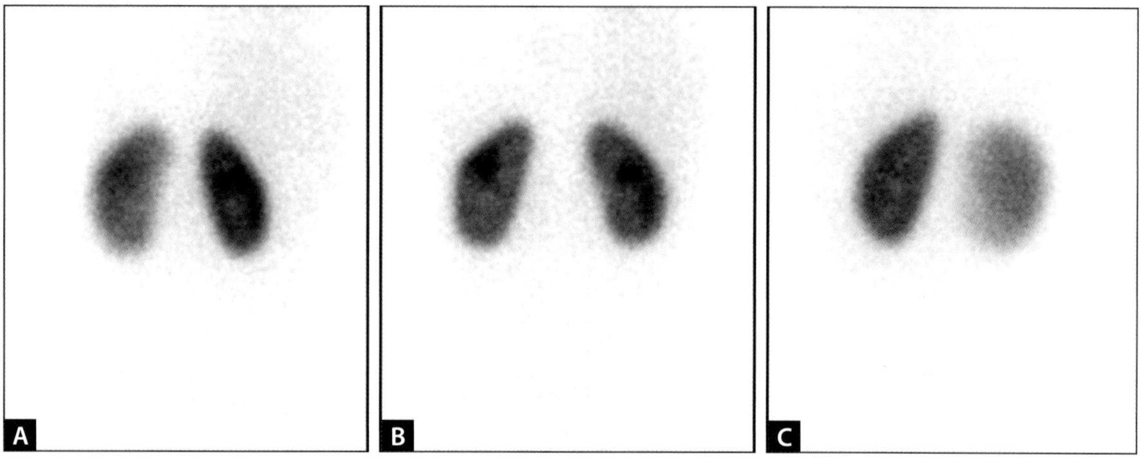

Figs. 6A to C: Normal ^{99m}Tc-DMSA scan: Bilateral kidneys are normal in size with smooth cortical outline and normal function. (A) Right posterior oblique; (B) Posterior; (C) Left posterior oblique.

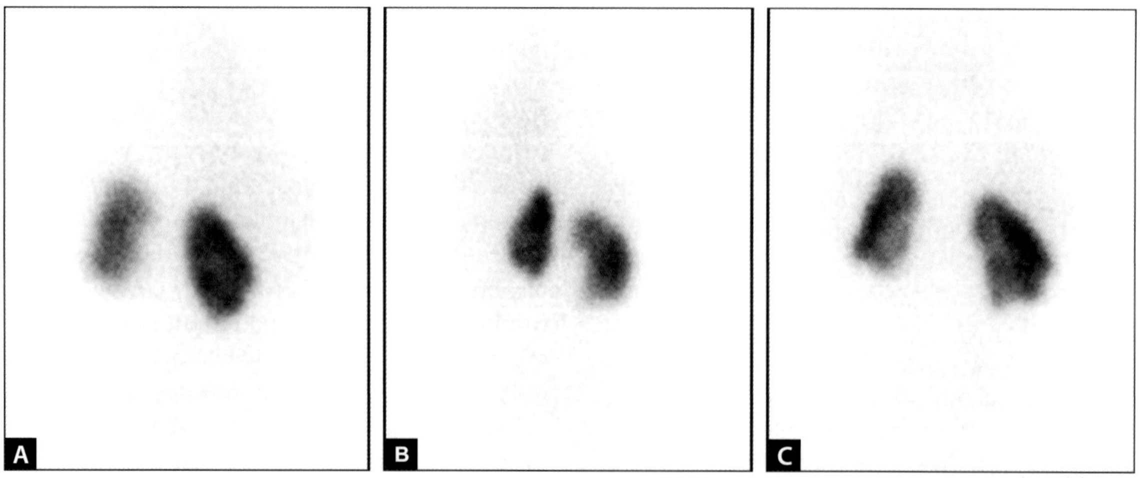

Figs. 7A to C: ^{99m}Tc-DMSA study in patient with bilateral vesicouretic reflux. All three views of ^{99m}Tc-DMSA scan show cortical break suggestive of renal scarring (multiple on left side and lower polar on right side). (A) Right posterior oblique; (B) Posterior; (C) Left posterior oblique.

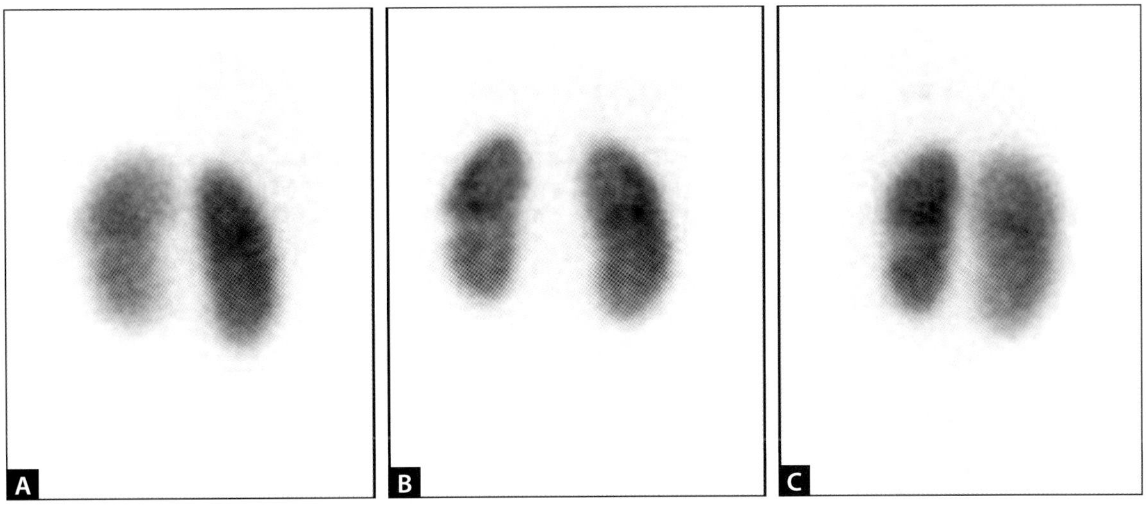

Figs. 8A to C: ^{99m}Tc-DMSA study in patient with left vesicouretic reflux. All three views of ^{99m}Tc-DMSA scan show cortical break in left kidney suggestive of left renal scarring. (A) Right posterior oblique; (B) Posterior; (C) Left posterior oblique.

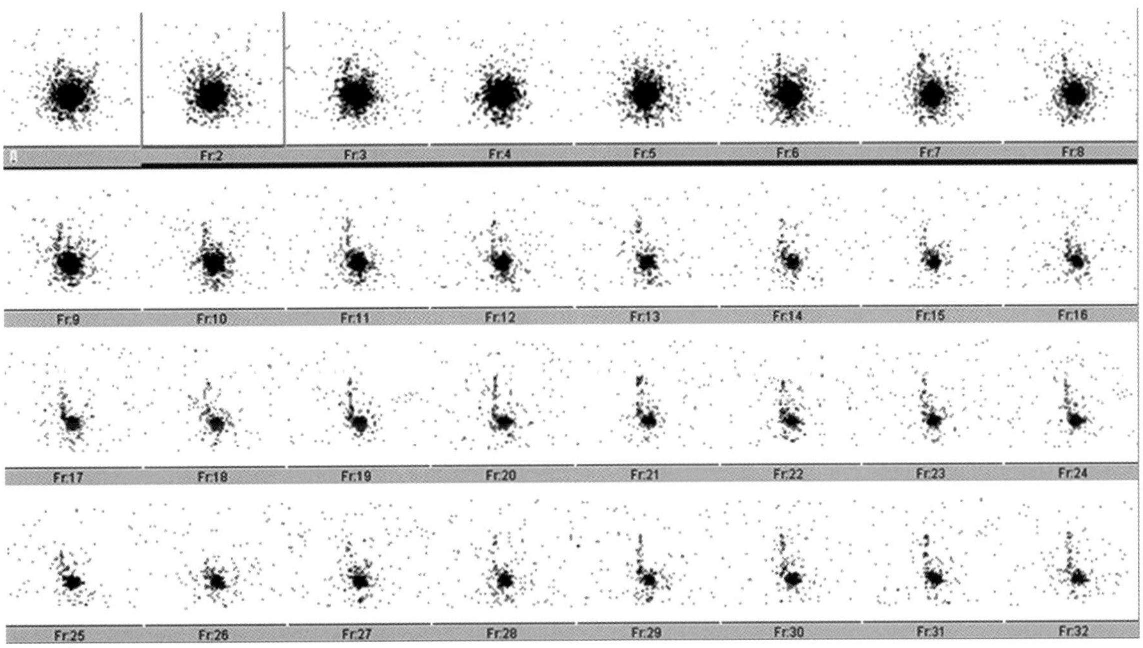

Fig. 9: DRCG study: Dynamic images showing vesicoureteral reflux of radiotracer from bladder into left ureter (grade II).

Renovascular hypertension: Renovascular hypertension is the most common cause of secondary and potentially curable hyper-tension. In spite of the problems associated with the routine renogram, availability of gamma-camera computer system has made meaningful preintervention renal assessment possible in such patients. This test as a follow-up procedure for evaluating the result of percutaneous angioplasty or surgery on the function in the affected kidney of the patients with renovascular disease is an extremely significant but often neglected application.

A major approach to the nuclear medicine diagnosis of the renovascular hypertension has been the introduction of captopril, an angiotensin converting enzyme (ACE)-inhibitor. The concept for the use of ACE-inhibitors in the differential diagnosis of the renovascular hypertension arose from the observation that patients with bilateral renal artery stenosis (RAS), or patient with solitary kidney having RAS had a tendency of developing acute renal failure when treated with these drugs. The theoretical basis for complication of ACE-inhibitor therapy and the

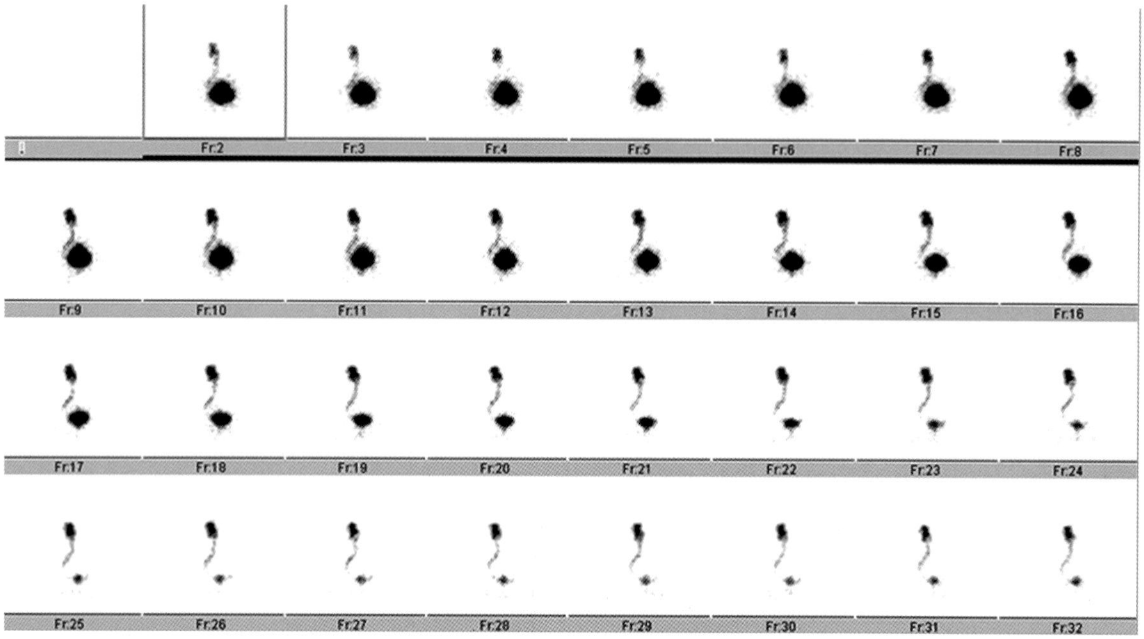

Fig. 10: DRCG study in unilateral reflux: Dynamic images showing vesicoureteral reflux of radiotracer from bladder into left ureter (grade III).

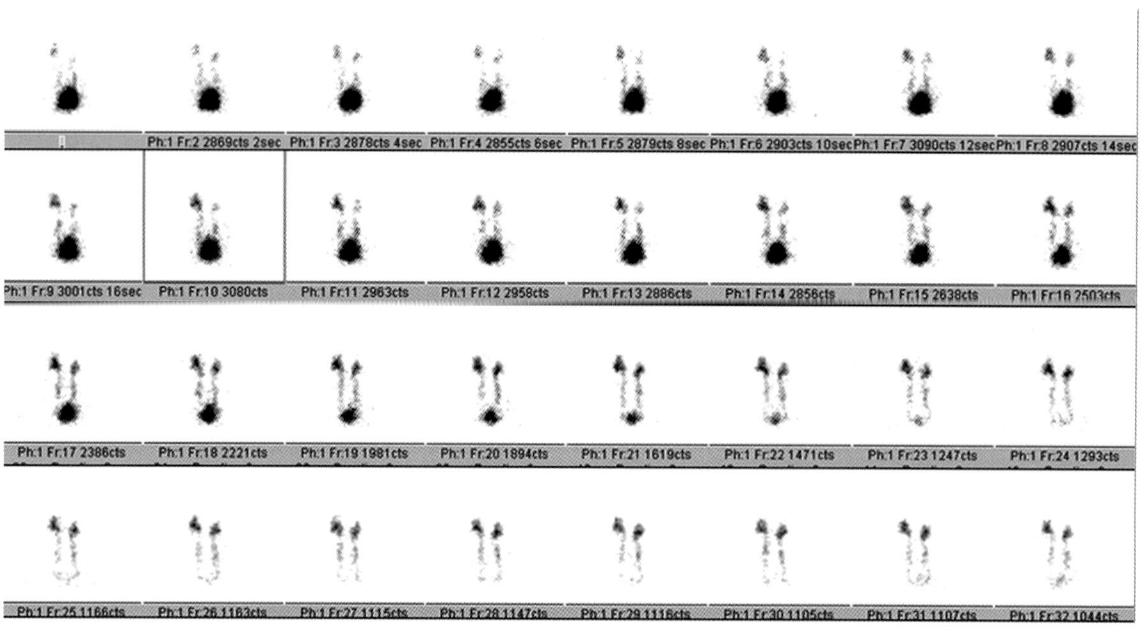

Fig. 11: DRCG study in bilateral vesicoureteral reflux: Dynamic images showing vesicoureteral reflux of radiotracer from bladder into both ureters (grade III).

rationale for the captopril renography test are essentially the same. The renin–angiotension system is thought to be a compensatory mechanism by which the kidney maintains perfusion, when it is subjected to low perfusion pressure, as may result distal to a renal artery stenosis. ACE-inhibitors act to block the step where angiotensin I is converted to angiotensin II, and as a result prevent the subsequent increase in the efferent arteriolar tone. In the absence of this compensatory mechanism, the glomerular filtration rate (GFR) drops significantly in the affected kidney.[16-19] A normal base line study followed by unilateral decreased in split renal function are the hallmark of unilateral renovascular hypertension **(Fig. 5)**. Wide-spread application of the captopril renography and improved surgical techniques as well as perfection of the catheter techniques for percutaneous transluminal angioplasty, has caused tremendous excitement in the field of renovascular disease, and resulted in sudden repopularization of radioisotope renography.

Congenital anomalies: Renal radionuclide studies are helpful in the diagnosis and functional evaluation of a spectrum of congenital disorders. Serial evaluation of the parenchymal and drainage function may be essential in patients with polycystic kidneys, and in medullary sponge kidneys. Radionuclide investigations have a definite "functional" edge over the urography in the management of ectopic kidneys, horseshoe-shaped kidney, cross ectopias, or malrotated kidneys.[28,29] Radionuclide studies are useful in the evaluation of regional cortical renal function in patients with duplications of the ureters and renal pelvis. Preoperative and serial postoperative functional as well as morphologic evaluation of the kidney, upper urinary tracts, and the urinary bladder can be effectively done in patients with posterior urethral valves by the renal dynamic, DMSA cortical imaging and DRCG-IFMT studies. Functional evaluation of the kidney and the urinary bladder by radionuclide studies in patients with neurogenic bladder has also been very well established.

Renal failure: The radionuclide studies in renal failure provide information about renal perfusion, the handling of the renal agent by the kidneys and if urine flow through the collecting system. Significant renal function has been reported on radionuclide studies in a large percentage of the patients with nonfunctioning kidneys seen on intravenous urography. The result is still better when ^{99m}Tc-DMSA is used for renal imaging.

Radionuclide clearance studies provide valuable information and help in monitoring glomerular or tubular function in nephropathies of various origins, the most important being the diabetic nephropathy. Kidney disease in diabetic patients has a devastating effect on survival, most evident in those with juvenile onset disease. It has been advocated that in such patients, the prospective monitoring of diminishing renal function should include precise measurement of GFR by radionuclide techniques combined with determination of fractional clearance of high molecular weight proteins. This is particularly significant when the effects of treatment on the early proteinuric phase of the diabetic nephropathy are being estimated.[30,31] The considerable loss of glomerular filtration capacity at this stage is undetected by inverse creatinine measurement, which remains an important tool for monitoring the late stage of nephropathy, when metabolic correction is likely to be ineffective.

Renal transplant evaluation: Radionuclide techniques offer rapid, effective and noninvasive means for the correct diagnosis of many of the ischemic, immunological and mechanical complications of the renal transplantation. Renal perfusion and function studies using ^{99m}Tc-DTPA or ^{99m}Tc-MAG-3 offer comprehensive evaluation of the renal blood flow, function and drainage **(Figs. 12A and B)**. Many techniques have been described for establishing the cause of acute renal failure in the transplant patients, especially for the diagnosis of acute rejection and acute tubular necrosis (ATN) **(Fig. 13)**. Some of the surgical complications like urinary obstruction, urinary extravasations, urinoma, nonurinary pelvic collections, e.g. hematoma or lymphocele and vesicoureteric reflux (VUR) can be diagnosed on radionuclide studies. Despite the relative merits and demerits of the radionuclide studies vis-a-vis other noninvasive diagnostic modalities, nuclear medicine has made an impact in clinical practice in at least three ways:

1. By reducing the number of invasive biopsies in transplant patients.
2. Diagnosing or confirming acute rejection very early for prompt treatment.
3. By being able to reassure the transplant surgeon regarding the viability of the allograft in uncomplicated ATN with prolonged period of oliguria or anuria. With improved techniques and increasing availability of the renal transplantation procedures at many more centers around the country, nuclear medicine is bound to have a crucial role in evaluation and management of renal transplant.[32,33]

Management of a clinical nephrourological problem can be best done by a multi-disciplinary approach. The various diagnostic modalities like X-ray, CT, US, magnetic resonance spectroscopy and nuclear medicine often support and complement each other.[34] However, radionuclide techniques have the most important "functional edge" over many other diagnostic methods. With further refinements in technology, instrumentation and radiopharmaceuticals, nuclear medicine destined to improve more in future.

Measurement of Renal Function

Glomerular filtration rates Renal function can be assess by clinical methods using blood-urea nitrogen (BUN) and serum creatinine level but these are relatively crude process, as significant decreased in function must occur before changes in BUN and creatinine are seen. Other factors which affect creatinine level are diet, difference in muscle mass and certain medication.

A
B
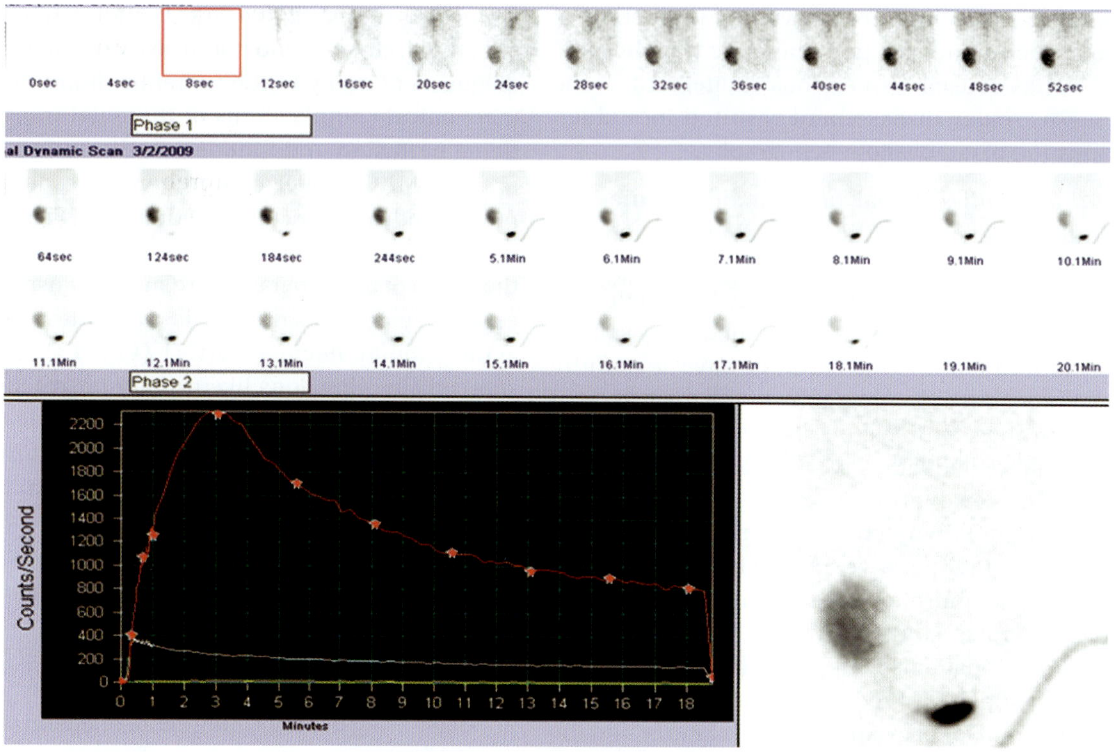

Figs. 12A and B: ^{99m}Tc-LLEC scan in normal functioning transplanted kidney. (A) Dynamic images show normal perfusion and uptake with prompt clearance; (B) Time activity curve shows steep uptake slope, distinct peak and rapid clearance.

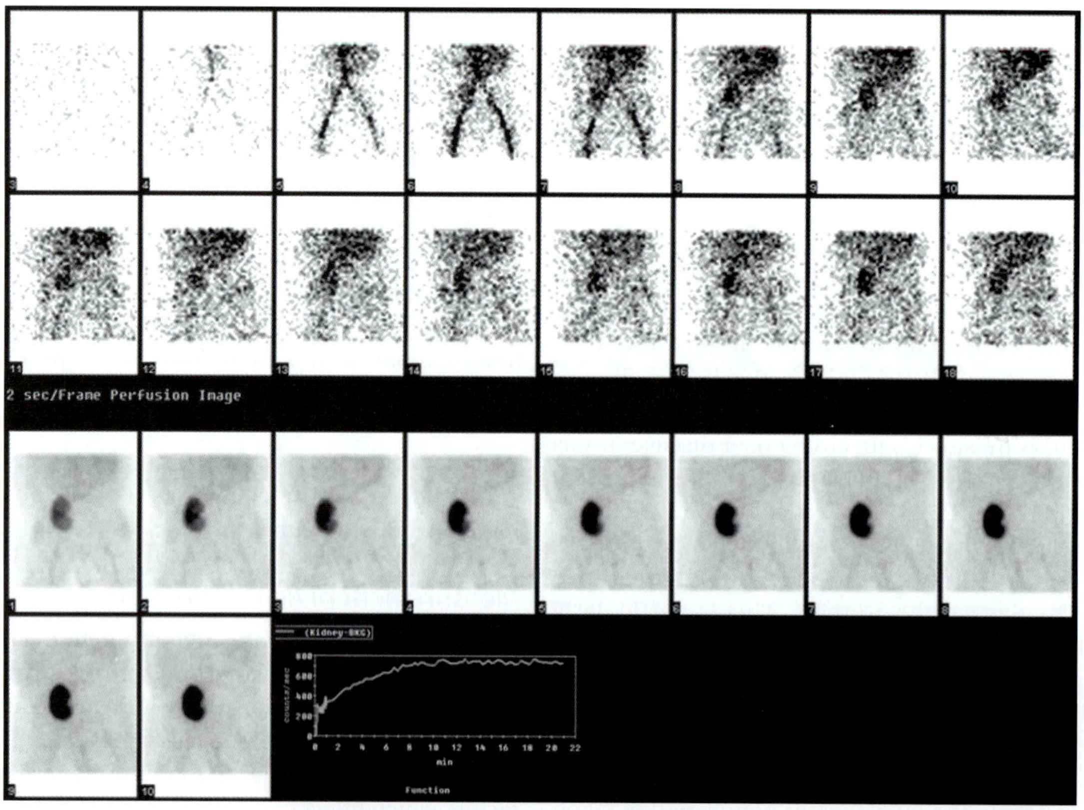

Fig. 13: ^{99m}Tc-LLEC scan in vasomotor nephropathy (ATN). Baseline images show normal perfusion and uptake but significant retention. Time activity curve not going down consistent with ATN.

GFR is the clearance rate of substance that is excreated from the body by glomerular filtration and not secreted or reabsorbed by tubules, the model molecule for this is inulin. Those substance has complete first pass extraction through kidney are used to calculate renal plasma flow (RPF). Para-amino hippurate is about 90% extracted and can be used for calculation of RPF. As it is not completely excreated the term effective renal plasma flow (ERPF) is used.

Many radiopharmaceuticals are used to calculate GFR; these include ^{99m}Tc-DTPA and ^{131}I-iothalamate. In India, ^{99m}Tc-DTPA is manly used for GFR calculation. Initially, multiple blood sample techniques were used, but now two blood sample technique most commonly used. Blood samples are taken at 1 hr and 3 hr after injection. Normal GFR value is approximately 106 ± 27 for adult. In small children adult level GFR reach at about 2-year of age.

Effective renal plasma flow (ERPF) ERPF is another parameter of renal of renal function. As inulin clearance is gold standard for GFR calculation, PAH is used for the calculation of ERPF. Measurement with PAH is accurate, but this method needs continuous infusion which is inconvenient and lack of precision. The radiolabeled form of hippuric acid, ^{131}I OIH and I-123 OIH, has been used to quantify ERPF. The urinary clearance of ^{131}I OIH is about 85% of the PAH. Currently, ^{99m}Tc-MAG-3 is commonly used for ERPF calculation. Plasma clearance of ^{99m}Tc-MAG-3 is 30–40% lower than that of OIH, but the ratio between their plasma clearance is identical at normal and reduced renal function.[35,36] For accurate calculation of ERPF need multiple blood samples but in clinical practice it is difficult to take multiple blood samples. Several methods have been published to assess the plasma clearance of ^{99m}Tc-MAG-3 using single blood sample.[36,37] Blood sample at 44 minutes has shown to reproducible within 19 mL/min.

Positron Emission Tomography: Computed Tomography (PET-CT)

A PET-CT is a relatively new nonimaging modality which provides functional/metabolic and structural details in the same setting. At present, 2-deoxy-2-[18F]-fluorodeoxyglucose ([18F]-FDG) is most commonly used for PET/ PET-CT imaging throughout the world. ([18F]-FDG is a radiolabeled analogue of glucose and as such it is able to detect altered glucose metabolism in various disease conditions. Frequently, there is a significant increase in glucose metabolism in cancer cells compared with that in the surrounding tissues. The role of FDG-PET in the initial staging, monitoring response to the therapy, and management of many types of cancer has been well documented.[38] There are relatively few FDG-PET reports describing its role in assessing primary urologic tumors at their sites of origin due to the potential problem of tracer excretion through the kidneys. The usefulness of FDG-PET-CT has been documented in the detection of distant metastasis from these malignancies.[39,40] In recent years, however, special PET-CT techniques have been evolved over the time to make PET-CT imaging possible in patients with primary kidneys and urinary bladder cancers. Moreover, the introduction of other PET radiotracers, such as C11-choline and C11-acetate, the role of this technique in patients with urologic cancer and especially in those with prostate cancer has been enhanced.[41] The main role of PET-CT in urologic malignancies is initial diagnosis and staging, evaluation of treatment response and detection of recurrent/metastatic disease.

Renal Cancer

Despite significant uptake and excretion through the kidneys, FDG has been used in the diagnosis and management of renal cell carcinoma (RCC). Bachor et al.[42] studied 29 patients with solid renal masses and found that PET was positive in 20 (77%) of 26 patients of RCC. PET was false-positive in an angiomyolipoma, a pericytoma, and a pheochromocytoma. Ramdave et al.[43] evaluated the accuracy of FDG-PET for staging and management of 17 patients with known or suspected RCC. PET and CT had an accuracy of 94%. In addition, PET detected pulmonary metastases in two patients. Miyakita et al.[44] compared biologic characteristics of RCC with FDG and concluded that PET-positive tumors had higher tumor grade and increased GLUT-1. Kumar et al.[45] showed good results in 28 solid renal masses of which 10 were primary (nine malignant, one benign) and 18 were metastatic renal tumors. FDG-PET accurately depicted 23 of 27 (85%) malignant renal 27 masses. Of the 10 primary renal tumors **(Fig. 14)**, FDG-PET was true positive in eight of nine (89%), true 28 negative in one and false-negative in one. In addition to the characterization of primary tumors, FDG-PET was valuable in 31 primary staging and altered treatment in 30% of patients (3 of 10). Of the 18 metastatic renal 32 masses, FDG-PET was positive in 15 (83%) masses. For detection of recurrent and distant disease, PET was found to have an accuracy of 100% in detecting local recurrence and metastases as compared CT which had accuracy of 88% **(Fig. 15)**. Majhail et al.[46] evaluated FDG-PET in the detection of distant metastases in 24 patients with RCC. FDG-PET results were compared with those abstracted with biopsy in 33 lesions. Overall sensitivity, specificity, and PPV of FDG-PET were 64%, 100% and 100%, respectively.

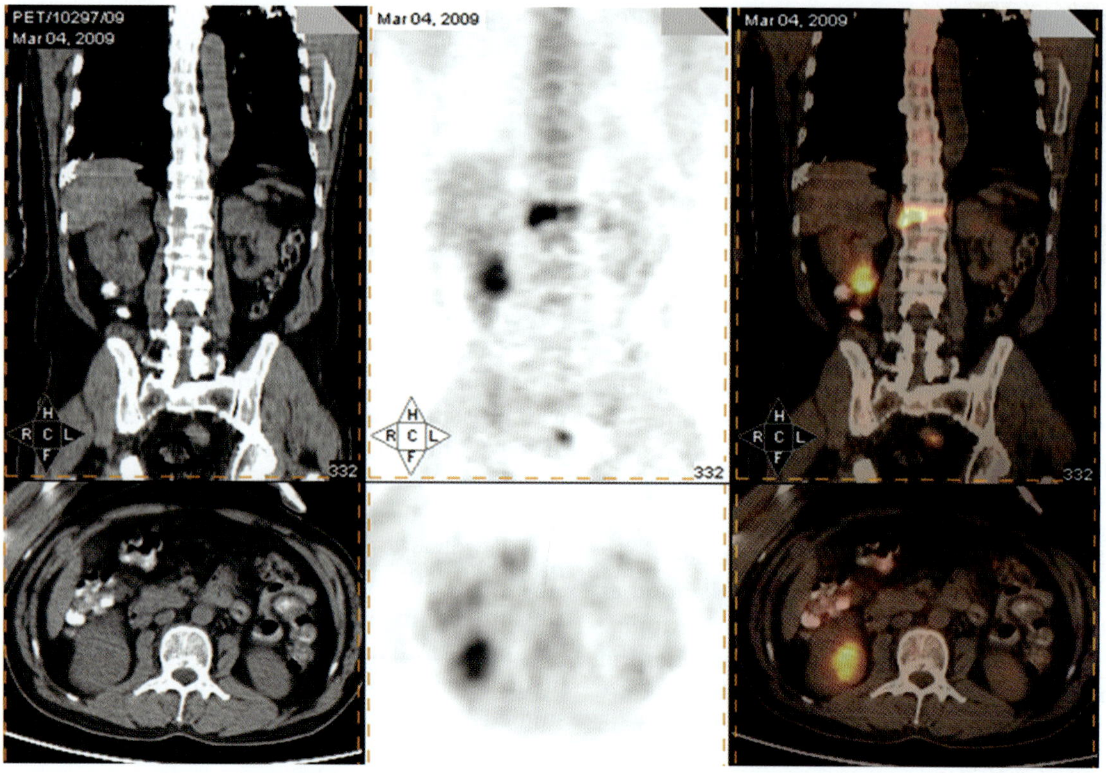

Fig. 14: ^{18}F-FDG PET-CT study: Coronal and axial sections of CT, PET and PET-CT showing soft tissue mass at lower pole of right kidney. Note FDG uptake in T12.

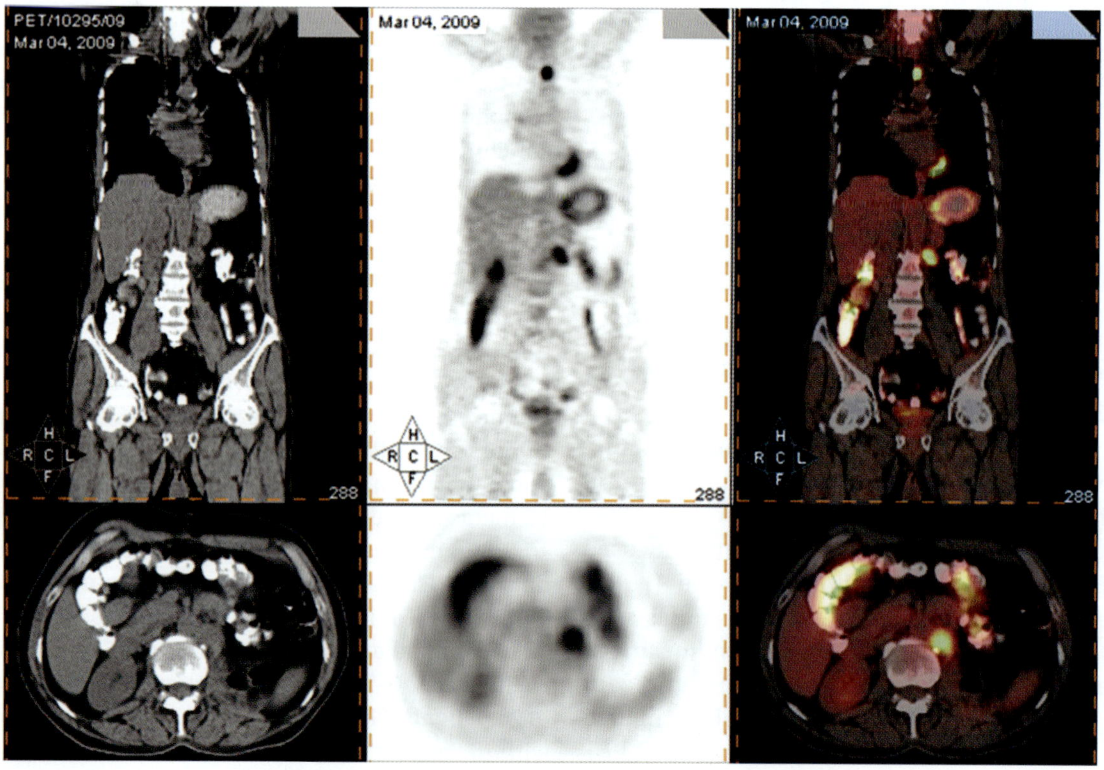

Fig. 15: ^{18}F-FDG PET-CT study: Coronal and axial sections of CT, PET and PET-CT showing soft tissue mass in left renal bed suggestive local recurrence.

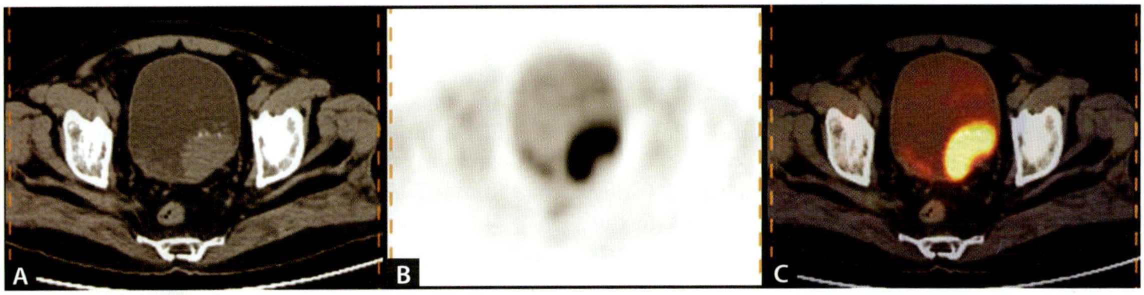

Figs. 16A to C: ^{18}F-FDG PET-CT study: Axial sections of CT, PET and PET-CT showing soft tissue mass in urinary bladder suggestive primary bladder cancer.

Urinary Bladder Cancer

Previously, FDG-PET was thought to have limited use in diagnosis and management of bladder cancer. However, with modified techniques (after injection of diuretic and delayed imaging) it is possible to image primary as well as recurrent urinary bladder cancer **(Figs. 16A to C)**. Kosuda et al.[47] studied 12 patients with FDG-PET for the evaluation of recurrent or residual disease. PET identified 100% (17 of 17) of distant metastases (lung, bones, and remote lymph nodes) and 67% (2 of 3) of local lymph nodes. Heicappell et al.[48] also had similar detection rate of 67% for local lymph node involvements. Ahlstrom et al.[49] attempted to improve the accuracy of PET by using C11-methionine, which has no urinary excretion. The authors reported a sensitivity of 78% (18 of 23) and there was good correlation of tracer uptake and tumor stage.

In conclusion, PET-CT has shown very encouraging results in a limited number of studies, and has also demonstrated a good sensitivity for initial staging in patients with renal and bladder cancer. FDG-PET seems to be superior to conventional imaging modalities for detecting local disease and recurrence, and distant metastases.

REFERENCES

1. Berkhin EF, Humphreys MH. Regulation of tubular secretion of organic compounds. Kindney Int. 2001;59:17-30.
2. Bubek B, Brandau W, Steinbacher M. Tc-99m labeled renal function and imaging agent. II. Clinical evaluation of Tc-99m MAG-3. Nucl Med Biol. 1988;15:109-18.
3. Jafri RA, Britton KE, Nimmon CC. Tc-99m MAG-3: A comparison with I-125 and I-131 OIH, inpatients with renal disorders. J Nucl Med. 1988;29:147-58.
4. Gutsche HU, Scheffler M, Muller-Surr R, et al. Micropuncture study on filtration and reabsorp-tion of technium-99m L, L-Ethylenedicysteine in rats, In: Taylor A, Nally JV, Thomsen H (Eds). Radionuclides in nephrourology. Society of Nuclear Medicine, Reston, Virbinia. 1997.pp.160-4.
5. Taylor A, Hansen L, Eshima D, et al. Comparison of ^{99m}Tc-LL-EC in rats and humans. J Nucl Med. 1997;38:821-6.
6. Atkins HL, Cardinale KG, Eckelman WC, et al. Evaluation of Tc 99m DTPA prepared by three different methods. Radiology. 1971;98:674-77.
7. Cohen ML, Smith FGJ, Mindell RS, Vernier RL. A simple reliable method of measuring glomerular filtration rate using single low dose iothalamate I-131. Pediatrics. 1969;43:407-15.
8. Chervu LR, Freeman LM, Blaufox MD. Radiopharmaceuticals for renal studies. Semin Nucl Med. 1974;4:3-22.
9. Arnold RW, Subramanian G, McAfee JG Blair BJ, Thomas FD. Comparison of Tc-99m com-plexes for renal imaging. J Nucl Med. 1975;16:357-67.
10. Lee HB, Blaufox MD. Mechanism of renal concentration of Tc99m-glucoheptonate. J Nucl Med. 1985;26:1308-13.
11. Enlander D, Weber PM, dosRemedios LV. Renal cortical imaging in 35 patients: Superior quality with Tc 99m-DMSA. J Nucl Med. 1974;15:743-9.
12. Meller St, Eckstein HB. Renal scintigraphy: Quantitative assessment of upper urinary tract dilatation in children. J Paeditr Surg. 1981;16:123-6.
13. O'Reilly PH, Testa HJ, Lawson RS, Farrar DJ, Charlton EG. Diuresis renography in equivocal urinary tract obstruction. Br J Urol. 1978;50:76-80.
14. Londe S. Causes of hypertension in the young. Pediatr Clin North Am. 1978;25:55-66.
15. Blaufox MD, Fine EJ, Heller S, Hurley J, Jagust M, Li Y, Mann SJ, Pickering TG, Zanzonico P, Zhang CG. Prospective study of simultaneous orthoiodohippurate and diet hylenetriamine-penta-acetic acid Captopril renography. The Einstein/Cornell Collaborative Hypertension Group. J Nucl Med. 1998;39(3):522-8.
16. Majd M, Potter BN, Guzzeta PC, Ruley EJ. Effect of captopril on efficacy of renal scintigraphy in detection fo renal artery stenosis. J Nucl Med. 1983;24:23-7.
17. Sfakianakis GN, Sfakiankis E. Lasix captopril renography in the diagnosis of renovascular hypertension. Contrib Nephrol. 1990;79:219-27.
18. Consensus Report on Captopril Renogram in Renovascular Hypertension. JNM. 1996.pp.1876–82.
19. Wenting GJ, Tan-Tjiong HI, Derkx FH. Split renal function after captopril in unilateral renal artery stenosis. BMJ. 1984;288:886-90.

20. Dondi M. Captopril renal scintigraphy with Tc99m-MAG-3 for detection renal artery stenosis. Am J Hypertens. 1991;4:737S-40S.
21. Arendshorst WJ, Brannstrom K, Ruan X. Actions of angiotensin II on the renal microvasculature. J Am Soc Nephrol. 1999;Suppl 11:S149-61.
22. Kumar R, Padhy Ajit Kumar, Machineni, Sriram Padey Anil Kumar, Malhotra A. Individual kidney GFR in the interpretation of non-diagnostic curves on captopril renography. Nucl Med Comm. 2000;21:637-43.
23. Setaro JF, Chenn CC, Hoffer PB, Black HR. Captopril renography in the diagnosis of renal artery stenosis and the prediction of improvement with revascularisation: The Yale vascular center experience. Am J Hypertens. 1991;4:698S-705S.
24. Padhy AK, Gopinath PG, Basu AK: Role of ^{99m}Tc-DTPA renal study in children with upper urinary tract dilation. Indian J Med Res. 1985;82:238-47.
25. Chaiwatanrat T, Padhy AK, Bomanji J, Nimmon CC, Sonmezoglu K, Britton KE. Validation of renal output efficiency as an objective quanti-tative parameter in the evaluation of upper urinary tract obstruction. J Nucl Med. 1993;34:845-8.
26. Sfakianakis GN, Damoulaki-Sfakianaki E. Nuclear medicine in pediatric urology and nephrology. J Nucl Med. 1988;29: 1287-300.
27. Padhy AK, Gopinath PG, Mitra DK, et al. Direct radionuclide cystogram (DRCG) and urine flowmetry in the evaluation of patients with VUR and/or associated obstructive/ neurogenic pathology of lower urinary tract in children. Indian J Paeditr. 1989;56:423.
28. Sfakianakis GN. Nuclear medicine in congenital urinary tract anomalies. In: LM Freeman (Ed). Nuclear Medicine Annual1991: New York: Raven Press, 1991.pp.129-92.
29. Kumar R, Ritesh Gupta, Malhotra A. Nephroptosis: GHA scan as a diagnostic modality. Clin Nucl Med. 2000;25:473-4.
30. Bell EG, Blaufox MD. Clinical application of renal Imaging. In EJ (Eds): Diagnostic Nuclear Medicine. Gottschalk A, Potchen Baltimore: Williams and Wilkins Co. 1976. pp.476-91.
31. Viberti GC, Bilous RW, Mackintosh D, Keen H. Monitoring Glomerular function in diabetic nephropathy: A prospective study. Am J Med. 1983;74:256-64.
32. Padhy AK, Gopinath PG, Mehta SN, et al. Significance of transplant perfusion index in the diagnosis of acute rejection—experience in live-related renal transplant recipients. Indian J Med Res. 1989;90:113-23.
33. Hilson AJW, Maisey MN, Brown CE, et al. Dynamic renal transplant imaging with ^{99m}Tc-DTPA (Sn) supplemented by a transplant perfusion index in the management of renal transplants. J Nucl Med. 1978;19:994-1000.
34. Padhy AK, Gopinath PG, Mehta SN, et al. Tc-99m renal transplant scintigraphy in the diagnosis of urinoma. Clin Nucl Med. 1989;14:769-71.
35. Bubeck B, Brandau W, et al. Pharmacokinetics of technetium-99m-MAG-3 in humans. J Nucl Med. 1990;3:1285-93.
36. Russell CD, Thorstad BL, et al. Quantation of renal function with technetium-99m MAG3. J Nucl Med. 1988;29:1931-3.
37. Relling M, Nielsen BV, et al. Renal and extrarenal clearance of ^{99m}Tc-MAG-3: A comparison with I-125 OIH and Cr-51-EDTA inpatients repre-senting all levels of glomerular filtration rate. Eur J Nucl Med. 1995;22:1379-84.
38. Kumar R, Zhuang H, Alavi A. PET in the management of urologic malignancies. Radiol Clin North Am. 2004;42(6):1141-53.
39. Seltzer MA, Barbaric Z, Belldegrun A, Naitoh J, Dorey F, Phelps ME, et al. Comparison of helical computerized tomography, positron emission tomography and monoclonal antibody scans for evaluation of lymph node metastases in patients with prostate specific antigen relapse after treatment for localized prostate cancer. J Urol. 1999;162:1322-8.
40. Hofer C, Laubenbacher C, Block T, Breul J, Hartung R, Schwaiger M. Fluorine-18-fluoro-deoxyglucose positron emission tomography is useless for the detection of local recurrence after radical prostatectomy. Eur Urol. 1999;36:31-5.
41. Oyama N, Miller TR, Dehdashti F, Siegel BA, Fischer KC, Michalski JM, et al. 11C-acetate PET imaging of prostate cancer: Detection of recurrent disease at PSA relapse. J Nucl Med. 2003;44:549–55.
42. Bachor R, Kotzerke J, Gottfried HW, Brandle E, Reske SN, Hautmann R. Positron emission tomography in diagnosis of renal cell carcinoma. Urologe A. 1996;35:146-50.
43. Ramdave S, Thomas GW, Berlangieri SU, Bolton DM, Davis I, et al. Clinical role of F-18 fluoro-deoxyglucose positron emission tomography for detection and management of renal cell carcinoma. J Urol. 2001;166: 825-30.
44. Miyakita H, Tokunaga M, Onda H, Usui Y, Kinoshita H, et al. Significance of 18F-fluoro-deoxyglucose positron emission tomography (FDG-PET) for detection of renal cell carcinoma and immunohistochemical glucose transporter 1 (GLUT-1) expression in the cancer. Int J Urol. 2002,9.15-8.
45. Kumar R, Chauhan A, Lakhani P, Xiu Y, Zhuang H, Alavi A. F18-FDG-PET in characterization of solid renal masses. Mol Imaging Biol. 2005;7(6):431-9.
46. Majhail NS, Urbain JL, Albani JM, Kanvinde MH, Rice TW, Novick AC, et al. F-18 fluoro-deoxyglucose positron emission tomography in the evaluation of distant metastases from renal cell carcinoma. J Clin Oncol. 2003;21:3995-4000.
47. Kosuda S, Kison PV, Greenough R, Grossman HB, Wahl RL. Preliminary assessment of fluorine-18 fluorodeoxyglucose positron emission tomography in patients with bladder cancer. Eur J Nucl Med. 1997;24:615-20.
48. Heicappell R, Muller-Mattheis V, Reinhardt M, Vosberg H, Gerharz CD, Muller-Gartner H, et al. Staging of pelvic lymph nodes in neoplasms of the bladder and prostate by positron emission tomography with 2- [(18)F]-2-deoxy-D-glucose. Eur Urol. 1999;36:582-7.
49. Ahlstrom H, Malmstrom PU, Letocha H, Andersson J, Langstrom B, Nilsson S. Positron emission tomography in the diagnosis and staging of urinary bladder cancer. Acta Radiol. 1996;37:180-5.

CHAPTER 103

Current Status of Urographic Contrast Media

Sumedha Pawa, Gaurav S Pradhan

INTRODUCTION

Iodinated radiographic contrast media are used widely for imaging of the genitourinary system. These are required for urography and for direct intraluminal studies of the genitourinary tract, such as urethrography, cystography, retrograde pyelography and loopograms. Their use is essential when CT scan examinations are performed to detect or to characterize renal masses and for CT staging of renal adenocarcinoma.[1] Contrast media are also required for diagnostic and therapeutic angiography.

The compounds used as contrast media in radiological practice should have the basic requirement of effective contrast-enhancement properties and complete inertia towards biological substrates which exert no impact on the physiology of the organs and tissues with which they come into contact. Since contrast media are used for diagnostic purposes, they are expected to have better safety profiles and higher risk margins as compared to regular therapeutic agents. In addition, the elimination needs to be quick and complete.[2-4]

DEVELOPMENT OF CONTRAST MEDIA

The long search for a contrast medium featuring the ideal qualities, began in the 1920s, following the advent of the first iodinated compound, sodium iodide. Since then, research has developed along two parallel and complementary lines which characterise all pharmaceutical research: increased efficacy and reduced toxicity.

Binding iodine to organic molecules marked the first breakthrough in the development of safer contrast media, making it possible to obtain a threefold reduction of iodine toxicity compared with sodium iodide, an inorganic salt. However, the development of the first organic agent-uroselecton, did not mark increased efficacy in terms of contrast enhancement, as each molecule bound to only one iodine atom. An initial increase in efficacy and reduced toxicity was achieved with uroselecton B, a bisodium salt with two iodine atoms. A further step forward in terms of efficacy was attained with the development of diodone, with 2 iodine atoms and 2 particles in solution.

Acetrizoic acid, a tri-iodinated compound was introduced in the early 1950s.[5] Strategies to improve efficacy and safety are demonstrated by modifications of the first tri-iodinated contrast medium, acetrizoate. It was suggested that the presence of a hydrogen atom on the tri-iodinated benzene ring provides better ability to bind protein than substitution of the hydrogen atom. An increase in protein binding ability is hypothesized to incite anaphylactoid reactions. In diatrizoate, exchange of accetamido unit for the unsubstituted hydrogen of acetrizoate leads to higher biologic tolerance.[6]

In the seventh decade of last century, all water soluble contrast media were salts of iodinated fully substituted benzoic acid derivatives. These organic acids have three hydrogen atoms replaced by iodine atoms and three hydrogen atoms replaced by simple side chains. For every three iodine atoms in solutions, two particles exist one anion and one cation in the ratio of 3:2.

Further strategies to decrease general toxicity have been to decrease both iconicity and osmotoxicity by replacing the ionizing carboxyl group (i.e. $COO^- Na^+$ and $COO^- Mg^+$) with hydrophilic structures that could be covalently bound to the benzene ring to get a nondissociating (nonionic) water soluble contrast medium molecule. In 1969, Almen suggested that nonionic molecules could reduce osmolality.[7] The first major breakthrough along these lines was the historic introduction, by Almen of the ratio 3 nonionic monomer, metrizimide released in 1977.[8] This generation of low osmolar contrast media (LOCM) now in widespread clinical use includes iopamidol, iobitridol, iohexol and ioversol.[9] In the 1980s and 1990s, there has been an ongoing development of nonionic isotonic dimers. These agents are consequence of further applications of principles to increase iodine atoms per molecule, increase hydrophilicity, lower osmotoxicity and eliminate ionicity.[9]

TYPES OF RADIOGRAPHIC CONTRAST MEDIA

Contrast media are characterized as ionic or nonionic and as monomers or dimers. Ionic media break down into charged particles when entering a solution such as blood.[10] The iodinated benzene ring contains the ionizing carboxyl group with a cation, usually sodium or meglumine. The carboxyl groups ionize in solution, making the agents water soluble. Because these compounds dissociate into ions in water and contain only one iodinated benzene ring, they are referred to as ionic monomeric agents. Commonly used contrast material anions are diatrizoate and iothalamate. In solution, the negatively charged contrast anions are conjugated with one of two positively charged cations: sodium or methylglucamine (also called meglumine). In some contrast agents only one of these two cations is used, whereas in others both are used in combination.[1]

Ionic monomers have a relatively high osmolality (>1400 mosmol/kg at 50–76% by weight concentrations) because each molecule which contains three iodine atoms dissociate into two particles in solution (ratio 3:2).

Amongst ionic monomers, meglumine iothalamate, sodium iothalamate and meglumine and sodium diatrizoate preparations are available in India.

Of the many lower-osmolality contrast agents introduced, nonionic monomers are the most popular. In nonionic monomers the tri-iodinated benzene ring is made water soluble by the addition of five or six hydrophilic hydroxyl groups to organic side chains placed at 1,3, and 5 positions. Because there is no carboxyl group, nonionic monomers do not ionize in solution. Nonionic contrast agents have the desirable property of being soluble in water (hydrophilic) and yet do not dissociate in solution. They have relatively low osmolality (500–700 mosmol/kg) at comparable iodine concentrations. Each nonionic monomer molecule contains three iodine atoms per one particle in solution (ratio = 3:1). The nonionic monomers currently in use in India include Iohexol, Iopromide, Ioversol and Iopamidol.

Ionic dimers are formed by joining two ionic monomers together and eliminating one of the carboxyl groups. These agents therefore, contain six iodine atoms for every two particles in solution (ratio of 6:2). The only commercially available ionic dimer is ioxaglate. It has concentration of 59% (320 mg iodine/mL) and a relatively low osmolality of 600 mosmol/kg at comparable iodine concentrations. Due to its viscosity, it is not manufactured at higher concentrations. Ionic oxaglate has been used more widely for peripheral arteriography than for intravenous studies. Nonionic dimers such as iotrol and iodixanol consist of two joined nonionic monomers. These substances contain six iodine atoms for every one particle in solution (ratio of 6:1) and therefore for a given iodine concentration they have the lowest osmolality of all the contrast agents (approximately 300 mosmol/kg). At approximating 60% by weight concentration they are iso-osmolar with plasma.[1] However, it results in higher viscosity and greater resistance to cathetar injection.[9]

Therefore, there are four types of contrast media used clinically—high osmolar ionic monomers, low osmolar ionic dimers, low osmolar non-ionic monomers and iso-osmolar non-ionic dimers. They are available at various iodine concentrations and have different physicochemical properties (osmolality, ions content, hydrophilicity, pH and viscosity). All contrast media are distributed in the extracellular space, they do not cross an intact blood-brain barrier and all are excreted through kidney.[4]

Ionic dimer is not available in India, while the nonionic dimer iodixanol was introduced in India in 2002.

The ratio of iodine atoms to dissolved particles is significant property of contrast media. It describes the association between imaging effect (attenuation of X-rays) and the osmotoxic effect of the media. The ratio represents number of iodine atoms divided by number of particles of the contrast medium in solution. Since more iodine means better X-ray attenuation and fewer particles of contrast medium mean a lower osmotoxic effect, a higher ratio is desirable.[11] Agents with a ratio of 1.5 (3:2) have been termed high-osmolar contrast media (HOCM). This group consists of ionic monomers, e.g. sodium iothalamate, meglumine iothalamate, sodium diatrizoate and meglumine diatrizoate. Agents with a ratio of 3 (3:1) have been termed low osmolar contrast media (LOCM) which include nonionic monomers like iohexol, iopamidol, ioversol etc. and ionic dimer called ioxaglate. Agents with a ratio of 6 (6:1) are termed isotonic contrast media (IOCM) which are nonionic dimers, e.g. iodixanol, iotrolan.[9]

PHARMACOKINETICS OF EXTRACELLULAR IODINATED CONTRAST AGENTS

X-ray contrast media molecules have very low lipid solubility and extremely low chemical reactivity with body fluids and they range in molecular weight from 600 to 1650. Molecules of this type distribute throughout the extracellular spaces of the body. There is no evidence of any substantial penetration of these contrast media molecules through the cell membrane or into the interior of viable cells, with the single exception of the proximal tubular cells of the kidney. Theoretically, the differences in the molecular weight and size between the monomeric and the dimeric contrast agents could lead to slightly slower distribution rates into the extracellular space for the larger dimers. This effect, however, appear to be quite small and is probably not clinically important, though the increased renal intratubular viscosity effects of the isotonic dimers are yet to be fully assessed.[12,13]

When the contrast media molecules reach the systemic circulation, the molecules rapidly distribute across capillary membranes to reach an equilibrium (except an intact blood-brain barrier).[14] The surge in intravascular osmolality for the hypertonic agents, including the LOCM, during the first phase of distribution, causes sudden shift of fluid across capillary membranes towards the intravascular hypertonic compartment. As the contrast medium molecules pass through the capillary bed, there is rapid movement through capillary pores into the interstitial, extracellular space, as well as glomerular filtration into the renal tubules.

The clearance of X-ray contrast media is primarily by means of glomerular filtration and renal clearance. Although older media such as iodopyracet (Diodrast) were excreted by means of both glomerular filtration and tubular secretion, none of the currently employed molecules are reabsorbed or secreted by the renal tubules. Under normal physiologic conditions, nearly 100% of the contrast medium is eliminated through the kidney and the instantaneous rate of removal is equal to the plasma iodine concentration times the glomerular filtration rate.

Less than one percent is excreted through other routes including bile, liver, small and large intestines, tears, saliva and sweat. Vicarious excretion through extrarenal routes occurs most commonly in association with a renal insult or renal failure.

The clearance of contrast media molecules is usually described by the half-time for the renal clearance portion of plasma decay curves. The half-time (the time required for elimination of 50% of the agent from the body) in patients with normal renal function is 1–2 hours for each of the four groups of contrast media.[9] In the total absence of renal function, the extracellular concentration of iodine will approach a value given by the total iodine injected divided by the extracellular volume, which is approximately 200 mL/kg of body weight.

In patients with renal failure, the issue has been debated, whether patients with renal failure must undergo emergent dialysis after examination in which contrast medium is used. No definitive studies have addressed this issue. Since contrast agents are not protein bound and possess relatively low molecular weights, they are readily dialyzable. Approximately one-third of either HOCM or LOCM will have already been naturally eliminated through extrarenal routes before dialysis can be set up and begun.[9]

PHYSICOCHEMICAL PROPERTIES OF CONTRAST MEDIA

The biocompatibility of iodine and its physical properties (k edge at photon energy of 33 kEq) allow the safe intravascular injection of large volumes at high concentration. All the other chemical elements in the molecules serve only to carry, or protect the iodine on the benzene ring. It is the iodine in the radiographic beam and the volume distribution of the contrast material that provide optimal contrast enhancement for imaging.[15]

The ideal contrast medium must exhibit low molecular toxicity. The contrast medium solution should have physicochemical properties (osmolality, viscosity) as close as possible to those of blood and its formulation should be free of substances interfering with physiological homeostasis.

Water Solubility, Hydrophilicity and Osmolality

Solubility of ionic compounds depends on their formation of salts in solution. The presence of charged groups while increasing the water solubility also increase the intrinsic molecular toxicity. The presence of ions (charged groups) in solution increases the conductivity of body fluids and changes the overall electrolyte balance.

Hydrophilicity: Nonionic compounds are made water soluble by their high hydrophilicity attributable to the presence of numerous hydroxyl groups on the molecule. This further decreases their protein-binding and tissue-binding propensities and makes them more biologically inert.

Osmolality: The osmolality of any solution is a measure of the number (not size) of dissolved particles, whether ions, molecules, or aggregates, in a liter.

Except for the newest iso-osmotic agents, many of the LOCM used for urography have osmolalities that range between 483–844 mosmol/kg H_2O, whereas those of commonly used HOCM range approximately between 1400 and 1515 mosmol/kg H_2O.[16] Greater osmolality increases the potential for tissue damage by contrast agents. The hyperosmolality of solutions is responsible for the sudden and drastic drawing of water from the cellular and interstitial spaces towards plasma, thereby producing local effects; such as heat and pain. The high osmolality of the contrast medium solution can induce systemic effects, such as vasodilation, alteration to the permeability of vessel endothelia, hyper-volemia and osmotic diuresis.[5] For urography and to some extent for CT scanning some degree of osmotic diuresis is necessary to distend the urinary tract optimally. With HOCM the osmotic diuretic effect is strong. The lower osmotic effect of LOCM, however is not a significant disadvantage because of a higher iodine concentration achieved in the urine.

Viscosity

When the contrast-medium is injected into a vessel at a high rate, a substantial slowing in the blood flow in the vessel is observed during administration, which is commensurate with the viscosity of the solution.[17] A lower viscosity is required for agents that have to be rapidly injected intravascularly. With increasing concentrations of any contrast agent, the viscosity increases. The viscosity is largely controlled by the composition of the side chains on the molecules. With conventional ionic compounds, the meglumine side chain helps to achieve water solubility and biologic tolerance but also increases the viscosity.

Contrast medium solutions today feature either reduced viscosity and high hyperosmolality at medium-high concentrations (300 mg/mL) (ionics); or reduced viscosity and limited hyperosmolality (nonionics); or high viscosity and iso-osmolality (nonionic dimers).

Viscosity also plays a role at the level of the nervous system, as a direct correlation has been observed between viscosity of solution and magnitude of damage to the blood-brain barrier.[18] If associated with high viscosity, isotonicity of radiopaque solutions also produces unwanted effects at renal level.

Pharmaceutical Characteristics: The Role of Formulation

Elements in the formulation (e.g. chelating agents, buffering agents, counter-ions) have a role in inducing adverse effects.

Diatrizoate compounds cause significant reduction in ionic calcium because of chelating agents (e.g. sodium citrate) which are mixed with the contrast material for the purpose of stabilization of the solution. Calcium supplemented solutions have been developed. Sodium EDTA was replaced with calcium-sodium EDTA.

Nonionic compounds produce little or no decrease in ionic-serum calcium because of absence of chelating additives. Potential undesirable cardiovascular side effects can be avoided by use of nonionic contrast media. These also may be preferred in patients with hypertensive cardiovascular disease who are taking calcium channel blockers.

ADVERSE REACTIONS TO CONTRAST MEDIA

Adverse effects of contrast media are believed to be primarily related to their (i) osmotoxicity, (ii) chemotoxicity, (iii) ion toxicity, and (iv) dose. Other factors, such as viscosity and lipophilicity may also play a role. Osmotoxic effects include pain and discomfort, vasodilatation with hypotension and rigidification of red blood cells. Chemotoxicity may be directly responsible for the release of vasoactive substances that cause allergy-like symptoms. High dosages that disturb the ionic and osmotic balance in the body will elicit adverse reactions without exhibiting a direct interaction with other molecules.[19]

Chemotoxicity of contrast media is believed to increase as the number of carboxyl groups increase and the number of hydroxyl groups decrease. Ion toxicity occurs when ionic sustances (either the ionic contrast medium anion itself, the cation it is conjugated with, or ionic components in additives) interfere with cellular functions.[20]

Intravascular contrast media have rare adverse events and generally classified as either chemotoxic or idiosyncratic. Idiosyncratic (i.e. anaphylactoid) reactions are unpredictable and are not dependent on the dose of the contrast agent. Most anaphylactic reactions are related to discharge of active mediators. On the other hand, chemotoxic effects are related to dose of contrast agents, their physiological characteristics (i.e. sodium content, calcium-binding properties, viscosity and osmolality) and molecular toxicity. Chemotoxic effects are more common in medically unstable or debilitated patients.[4]

Guidelines on Prevention and Management of Acute Reactions

Acute reactions to contrast agents are divided into minor, intermediate and severe life threatening reactions. The minor events include mild urticarial, pruritis, flushing headache, arm pain, nausea and vomiting. These events are usually mild, self-limiting, of short interval and does not generally require any specific treatment. Intermediate reactions include more severe above events, moderate degrees of bronchospasm and hypotension. Such events very often respond to appropriate symptomatic therapy. Severe life threatening reactions include severe presentation of minor and intermediate reaction symptoms, unconsciousness, convulsions, severe bronchospasm, edema of larynx, severe cardiac dysrhythmias and arrest, pulmonary edema, cardiovascular and pulmonary collapse. Low osmolar contrast media has at least five to six times less prevalence of adverse events as compared to high osmolar contrast media. There are very rare fatal reactions.[4]

While ionic contrast agent was the only available option, prophylactic corticosteroid was indicated to patients who suffered systemic moderate or severe contrast agent reaction, allergy or asthma requiring medical attention. Use of such routine prophylaxis is now debated following the exclusive use of nonionic contrast agents in most radiodiagnosis departments in the developed world.[4] A study conducted by the European Society of Urogenital Radiology[21] revealed that even though asthma was considered a significant risk factor only 48% of the survey respondents gave corticosteroid prophylaxis in such patients. It is relatively safe and inexpensive to administer a very short course of steroids but it needs to be used prudently in patients with systemic infection, active tuberculosis, peptic ulcer and diabetes mellitus.[22,23] However, severe adverse events may occur even in patients who receive both low osmolar contrast media and prophylactic corticosteroid.[21,24]

The safety committee for contrast agents has recommended that nonionic media should be administered in patients with higher risk (earlier systemic contrast medium reaction, either severe or moderate, allergy or asthma necessitating medical treatment).[24] After injection of contrast medium, patient should be continuously observed for 20–30 minutes and emergency resuscitation drugs should be available. If there is a risk of leakage or absorption of contrast agent into the circulation during extravascular applications, precautions similar to intravascular injection should be implemented.[4] Guidelines on prevention of generalized contrast medium reactions in adults are shown in **Table 1**.[21]

Acute serious reactions need to be immediately treated by the radiologist. If feasible, intravascular contrast agents are avoided among patients who are at high risk of these reactions.[21] Nonionic agents should be preferred in the presence of a resuscitation event, if the examination is absolutely essential. Patient should be explained about the potential adverse reactions.[21] A quick and appropriate treatment helps recovery in majority of patients who suffer from severe anaphylaxis **(Table 2)**.[4]

Every radiologist should be able to effectively assess and treat adverse reactions to contrast media. The first line resuscitation equipment and drugs such as sphygmomanometer, oxygen, one-way mouth "breather" apparatus, β_2-agonist metered dose inhaler, atropine, antihistaminic, adrenaline 1:1000, IV fluids—Ringer's solution or normal saline and anticonvulsant drugs (like diazepam) should be freely accessible wherever contrast agents are injected.[25]

Table 1: European Society of Urogenital Radiology (ESUR) guidelines on prevention of generalized contrast medium reactions in adults.[21]

A.	*Risk factors for reactions:* Previous generalized contrast medium reaction, either moderate (e.g. urticaria, bronchospasm, moderate hypotension) or severe (e.g. convulsions, severe bronchospasm, pulmonary edema, cardiovascular collapse) Asthma Allergy requiring medical treatment
B.	*To reduce the risk of generalized contrast medium reactions:* Use non-ionic agents
C.	*Premedication is recommended in high risk patients (defined in A):* When ionic agents are used When non-ionic agents are used, opinion is divided about the value of premedication *Recommended premedication:* Corticosteroids *Prednisolone 30 mg orally or methylprednisolone 32 mg orally 12 hours and 2 hours before contrast medium.* Corticosteroids are not effective if given less than 6 h before contrast medium *Antihistamines H_1 and H_2 may be used in addition to corticosteroids, but opinion is divided.* Remember for all patients: *Have a trolley with resuscitation drugs in the examination room* Observe patients for 20–30 min after contrast medium injection *Extravascular administration:* When absorption or leakage into the circulation is possible, take the same precautions as for intravascular administration

Table 2: Simple guidelines for first line treatment of acute reactions to contrast media.[4]

• *Nausea/vomiting:* – *Transient*: Supportive treatment – *Severe, protracted*: Appropriate antiemetic drugs should be considered
• *Urticaria:* – *Scattered, transient*: Supportive treatment including observation – *Scattered, protracted*: Appropriate H_1–antihistamine intramuscularly or intravenously should be considered. Drowsiness and/or hypotension may occur – *Profound*: Consider adrenaline 1:1000, 0.1–0.3 mL (0.1–0.3 mg) intramuscularly in adults, 0.01 mg/kg intramuscularly up to 0.3 max. in children. Repeat as needed
• *Bronchospasm:* 1. Oxygen by mask (6–10 L/min) 2. β_2- Agonist metered dose inhaler (2–3 deep inhalations) 3. Adrenaline **Normal blood pressure** *Intramuscular*: 1–1000, 0.1–0.3 mL (0.1–0.3 mg) (use smaller dose in a patient with coronary artery disease or elderly patient) *In pediatric patients: 0.01 mg/kg up to 0.3 mg max.* Decreased blood pressure *Intramuscular*: 1:1000, 0.5 mL (0.5 mg), (In pediatric patients, 0.01 mg/kg intramuscularly)
• *Laryngeal edema:* 1. Oxygen by mask (6–10 L/min) 2. Intramuscular adrenaline (1:1000), 0.5 mL (0.5 mg) for adults, repeat as needed
• *Hypotension:* – *Isolated hypotension*: 1. Elevate patient's legs 2. Oxygen by mask (6–10 L/min) 3. Intravenous fluid: rapidly, normal saline or lactated Ringer's solution 4. If unresponsive: adrenaline: 1:1000, 0.5 mL(0.5 mg) intramuscularly, repeat as needed – *Vagal reaction (hypotension and bradycardia)*: 1. Elevate patient's legs 2. Oxygen by mask (6–10 L/min) 3. Atropine 0.6–1.0 mg intravenously, repeat if necessary after 3–5 min, to 3 mg total (0.04 mg/kg) in adults. In pediatric patients give 0.02 mg/kg intravenously (max. 0.6 mg per dose) repeat if necessary to 2 mg total. 4. Intravenous fluids: rapidly, normal saline or lactated Ringer's solution
• *Generalized anaphylactoid reaction:* 1. Call for resuscitation team 2. Suction airway as needed 3. Elevate patient's legs, if hypotensive 4. Oxygen by mask (6–10 L/min) 5. Intramuscular adrenaline (1:1000), 0.5 mL (0.5 mg) in adults. Repeat as needed. In pediatric patients 0.01 mg/kg to 0.3 mg (max. dose) 6. Intravenous fluids (e.g. normal saline, lactated Ringer's) 7. H_1-blocker, e.g. diphenhydramine 25–50 mg intravenously

Guidelines on Late Adverse Reactions

Late adverse reactions to intravascular iodinated contrast media are defined as reactions occurring 1 hour to 1 week after contrast medium injection. The reactions include symptoms such as nausea, vomiting, headache, itching, skin rash, musculoskeletal pain and fever. Their prevalence remains uncertain and their pathophysiology is not fully understood.[26] Major proportion of such reactions is not related to the contrast agent. At the same time, an incidence of allergy-like dermal reaction is well known in ~2% of those injected with contrast agents. Delayed reactions are likely to be more common after nonionic dimers. Those patients that have a previous history of reaction and are on interleukin-2 treatment are predisposed to late skin reactions. Most such late skin reactions resolve within a week and are therefore self-limiting. Similar to other drug induced dermal reactions, management is largely symptomatic.[24]

Guidelines on Renal Adverse Reactions

The term contrast medium induced nephropathy refers to the reduction in renal function induced by contrast media. It implies impairment in renal function (an increase in serum creatinine by more than 25% or 44 µmol/ L) occurred within 3 days following the intravascular administration of contrast media in the absence of alternative etiology.[27]

The patients at highest risk for developing contrast induced acute renal failure are those with pre-existing renal impairment (>132 μmol/L) particularly when the reduction in renal function is secondary to diabetic nephropathy.[27,28] Diabetes mellitus per se without renal impairment is not a risk factor.[28] Risk of contrast medium induced nephropathy increases with multiple injections within consecutive three days or with significantly large doses of contrast media. Nephrotoxicty increases if contrast media is administered intra-arterially in aorta proximal to origin of renal arteries or directly in renal blood vessels.[27]

Occurrence of contrast medium induced nephropathy can be reduced through various recommended measures.[29,30] They include dilution of bolus of contrast through volume expansion including infusion of normal or half strength saline solution intravenously, administration of sodium bicarbonate, mannitol, pharmacological management, replacement of high osmolar ionic contrast agent with low osmolar or iso osmolar nonionic contrast media, gadolinium based contrast agents in place of iodine based contrast media for CT and radiography, performing hemodialysis quickly after administration of contrast and prolonging intervals (more than 48 hours) between intravascular administration of contrast media.

At present it is unclear whether there is a difference in nephrotoxic potential between low osmolar nonionic monomeric and iso-osmolar nonionic dimeric contrast media. At the same time, it is strongly evidenced that patients having risk factors can suffer nephropathy from any contrast media.[4]

Even though hemodialysis is able to remove iodinated contrast agents, it is not efficacious in averting contrast nephrotoxicity.[31] The contrast media safety committee concluded that hemodialysis is not protective against contrast medium induced nephropathy for kidneys that are functioning poorly.

While hemodialysis is ineffective, hemofiltration has been shown to be efficacious in decreasing the incidence of this adverse reaction in patients with advanced renal dysfunction undergoing intravascular contrast procedures.[30]

Among patients with high predisposition for contrast medium induced nephrotoxicity, gadolinium-based contrast media has been recommended for radiology procedures instead of iodinated contrast media. But, this endorsement is unsafe since gadolinium based contrast media are harmful to kidneys particularly at dosages more than that applied for MRI procedures (≥0.3 mmol/kg). Additionally, in most cases, gadolinium based contrast medium will not provide diagnostic radiologic information if approved intravenous doses up to 0.3 mmol/kg are injected. These agents are not primarily approved for radiographic examinations. Due to higher nephrotoxicity of gadolinium based contrast agent as compared to iodinated contrast media in equivalent attenuating dose, the contrast media safety committee does not endorse use of gadolinium based contrast media for radiographic examinations. However, if there is no impairment of renal function, gadolinium based contrast agents can be used in patients with a previous history of severe generalized adverse event to iodinated contrast media and in case of scheduled thyroid treatment with radioactive iodine.[32]

Contrast media may reduce renal function and therefore should be used carefully in diabetic patients being treated with metformin to avoid development of lactic acidosis.[33] At the same time, there is no conclusive evidence of contrast media developing metformin induced lactic acidosis in patients with normal serum creatinine (<132 mmol/L). Therefore, serum creatinine should be checked before infusion of contrast agents in diabetics receiving metformin. If the serum creatinine level is within normal range, the examination can be performed after stopping metformin. The regular prescribed dosage of metformin can be restarted after two day if the serum creatinine continues to remain within normal limits. Injection of contrast agent needs to be deferred for 2 days after stopping metformin if there is an elevated serum creatinine after the administration.[33]

Guidelines on Prevention and Management of Extravasation of Contrast Media

Usage of fast flow intravenous contrast injection in CT examinations has raised incidence of extravasation of contrast media and may result in accumulation of large volume within a short period of time leading to significant damage of tissue. In cases, where automated power jnjector is used, careful choice of appropriate sized cannula that is placed in a suitable vein (except on the dorsum of the hand) helps avoid extravasation. Luckily there are no long term effects of most extravasations. But extravasations may cause ulceration and severe skin necrosis. Extravasation of large volumes may give rise to compartment sydrome.[24]

EVALUATING THE PATIENT BEFORE CONTRAST MEDIA INJECTION AND IDENTIFYING GROUPS AT INCREASED RISK FOR ADVERSE CONTRAST REACTIONS

The patient should be questioned about any previous administration of contrast medium. If there is a history of adverse reaction, the nature of the event must be investigated. If the reaction was idiosyncratic and mild, premedication should be instituted and low-osmolality contrast material subsequently should be used. If the reaction was idiosyncratic and moderate or severe (significant respiratory reaction) an alternate study, such as sonography or MR imaging, should be considered. For example, contrast-enhanced MR imaging can be performed to evaluate the kidneys for renal masses, because MR imaging contrast agents are entirely different from iodinated radiographic contrast agents and there is no known cross-reactivity. Non-idiosyncratic adverse events of nausea or vomiting are not considered regular indications for corticosteroid premedication or even use of nonionic contrast media.[1]

It is important to know whether the patient has cardiac disease, renal insufficiency, diabetes mellitus, or asthma. Currently or recently taken medications should be known, because contrast material injection may have to be delayed in patients receiving metformin and may have to be monitored closely in patients who have had interleukin-2. Also, adverse reaction may be more difficult to recognize appropriately or treat in patients who are taking beta adrenergic blockers.[1]

Patients who previously have had adverse contrast media events have been found to be at highest risk. Adverse reactions to ionic contrast media were approximately four times as common in patients who had previous adverse reactions.[34] Katayama et al.[35] found that total adverse reactions and severe adverse reactions to any type of contrast agent occurred five to six times as frequently in patients with prior adverse reactions to contrast media in comparison with patients who had been exposed previously to contrast material and who had no adverse reaction. Conversely, the total and severe adverse reaction rate in patients receiving contrast media for the first time was 1.2–1.4 times that of patients who previously had received contrast material without difficulty.

Many other groups have been identified as being at increased risk of having a contrast reaction. As compared to general population, asthmatics have increased risk of 1.2–2.2. Patients with allergies to substances other than contrast material are 1.5–3 times more likely to have an adverse event.[34,35]

In a postmarketing suveillance study of Iopromide's prevalence of acute reactions[2], it was observed that intravenous administration was associated with a higher adverse drug reaction (ADR) as compared with intra-arterial use. Dose or concentration of contrast media IV or IA was apparently not correlated with the incidence of ADRs. Severe ADRs were reported among 0.02% of patients. Higher rate of ADRs was reported among patients of 18–50 years of age as compared to patients of greater than 50 years of age group; with the highest rate reported among patients of 18-30 years of age group.[2] Higher immune-competence among younger population was thought to be responsible for higher rate of ADRs among the younger age group, suggesting that such ADRs may involve an immune-mediated process. Lack of definite association of ADRs with dose or concentration of contrast medium or with total dose of iodine supports such an immune mediate theory. Females suffered significantly higher rate of ADRs than males. Even though, this observation peaked up in the 18–50 years of age group, it was true up to 70 years of age.[2] Rising prevalence of allergic diseases including asthma in recent times may be correlated with the existence of environmental estrogens, which would support the postulation that contrast media reactions are increased in the presence of high estrogen levels.[36]

Race may be an associated risk factor: in the UK, people of Mediterranean origin and Indian subcontinent have a significantly higher risk as compared to the native population.[10]

AGGRAVATION OF DISEASES BY CONTRAST MEDIA

Many disease processes can be aggravated by contrast media. These include cardiac disease (aggravation of arrhythmias, precipitation of angina or congestive heart failure), pheochromocytomas (hypertensive crisis), myasthenia gravis (acute worsening of respiratory symptoms of myasthenia), uncontrolled hyperthyroidism (thyroid storm), sickle cell anemia (sickle cell crisis), and paroxysmal nocturnal hemoglobinuria.

Guidelines on the Use of Iodinated Contrast Media in Patients with Thyroid Disease

Small amounts of free iodine present in radiographic water soluble contrast media may cause thyrotoxic crisis in patients with multinodular goiter and thyroid autonomy or with Graves' disease, especially if they live in iodine deficient areas or if they are elderly. The free iodide in contrast media may saturate iodine uptake and interfere with nuclear medicine diagnostic procedures and treatment for up to 2 months. Prophylaxis is not mandatory but prophylactic treatment may be prescribed by an endocrinologist in high risk patients particularly those from areas with deficiency of dietary iodine.[37]

Guidelines on the Use of Contrast Media in Patients with Catecholamine-producing Tumors (Pheochromocytomas and Paragangliomas)

Secretion of catecholamines by pheochromocytomas and paragangliomas may be continuous or intermittent.

Typical clinical presentations include hypertension resistant to regular antihypertensive treatment and intermittent precipitation of crisis including flushing or pallor, sweating, headace and attacks of hypertension. Crisis occurs when tumors release catecholamines. It may be spontaneous or may be precipitated by drugs, such as contrast media. The contrast media safety committee recommended that under referring physician's supervision, α and β-adrenergic blockade should be given to these patients with orally administered drugs before intravenous contrast administration. A nonionic agent should always be used in these patients.[24]

Guidelines on Interaction between Contrast Media with Other Drugs and Clinical Tests

The contrast media safety committee recommended that radiologists should be aware of patient's drug history and proper record should be kept for the contrast medium injection (time, dose and name). Patients taking drugs like hydralazine, interleukin-2, metformin, β-blocker, non-steroid anti-inflammatory drugs, cisplatin, cyclosporine, and aminoglycosides should get special attention before contrast media administration. Additionally, contrast media should not be mixed in syringes or tubes with other drugs. Biochemical analysis should be avoided for blood or urine, collected within 24 hours of injection of contrast medium. Administration of contrast media may interfere with some isotope studies and such an administration should be avoided for minimum 24 hours before labeling red blood cells for isotope studies and before isotope bone scanning.[38]

Guidelines on the Use of Iodinated Contrast Media during Pregnancy or Lactation

In general, intravenous contrast material should be avoided, when possible, in pregnant women so as to eliminate any theoretic adverse effects on the fetus. Since nonionic agents are, in general, better tolerated, their use is preferred over conventional ionic agents in pregnant women.

The radiation dose associated with examinations that require intravascular contrast material may be a more significant risk to the fetus than the contrast medium itself. Other tests not requiring the use of ionizing radiation should be considered unless there is no satisfactory alternative.

Teratogenic or mutagenic effects have not been reported after use of iodinated contrast media. Thyroid function of fetus/neonate may be suppressed by administration of free iodine in radiographic contrast medium. If iodinated contrast agent has been administered during pregnancy, neonatal should be checked for thyroid function during the first week. The contrast media safety committee recommended this check as mandatory; however, thyroid check is done routinely in many countries as part of neonatal screening. Discontinuing breastfeeding after contrast administration is unnecessary since only small amount of iodinated contrast agent given to lactating mother reaches the milk and a significantly smaller proportion is aborbed from baby's intestines.[39]

SELECTIVE VERSUS UNIVERSAL USE OF NONIONIC CONTRAST MATERIAL

Various organizations, including the American College of Radiology (ACR), the American College of Cardiology (ACC), and the Society of Cardiovascular and Interventional Radiology (SCVIR), have formulated guidelines to assist institutions in establishing a policy of limited use of low osmolality contrast media. In general, the guidelines recommend that low osmolality agents be administered to patients with previous contrast reactions, asthma and allergies and patients with those underlying diseases that may be aggravated by contrast media administration. The ACR also suggests that low osmolality contrast media be administrated to patients who are at increased risk for aspiration, severely debilitated, very anxious about the contrast procedure; noncommunicative (so that the existence of any pertinent history cannot be ascertained), or who specifically request low osmolality agents.[40] Many institutions also selectively administer these agents to patients with elevated serum creatinine levels.[41]

It can be difficult consistently to limit use of low osmolality agents to a selected group of patients. This is because some of the recommended guidelines can be interpreted differently by different individuals. Also, there is tendency for physicians directly involved in injecting the contrast media and monitoring patients after injection to use the better tolerated nonionic agents increasingly to reduce patient discomfort or the likelihood of a reaction. There is also a tendency for low-risk patients to choose nonionic agents when they are allowed specifically to select the type of contrast material that they are to receive.

STRATEGIES FOR CLINICAL USE: COST CONTAINMENT

It is universally acknowledged that if the LOCM was not so expensive, a complete switch to ionic or nonionic LOCM would have occurred years ago. Significant concerns persist regarding not only cost but liability. Professional liability is related to the somewhat hostile medicolegal problems today and often stands in opposition to the physician's obligation to follow the prudent course of choosing the best drug or therapy for the patient. A 'universal switch' strategy has extremely burdensome financial implications; therefore, any strategy for use must be rational yet dynamic. The most challenging task is to develop tactics for identification of patients considered to be at risk for the administration of any contrast media. Estimations of patient risk are derived from a variety of sources. Most physicians can recognize seriously ill and unstable patients. However, not all at-risk patients are always readily identified. In emergency situations or when adequate assessment or pretreatment with steroids is not possible, all patients are best served by LOCM. At the same time, concerted efforts should be made to decrease the waste of contrast material and to make every attempt to limit the dose and volume of contrast for any given study.

The ultimate decision on choice of contrast rests with organized medicine, public policy makers, the individual patient and treating physician. A basic understanding of contrast media, choice of agents, risks of administration and premedication regimens for high-risk patients, is beneficial in helping patients prepare for their examinations.

Physicians will need to continue being informed advocates, familiar with the science, yet sensitive to the economic implications of the decisions they make for choice of contrast media based on cost to best serve the interests of their patients.[15]

Finally, inspite of all considerations about the selection of contrast media and care taken about various risk factors outlined above, before an intravascular contrast study, it is not possible to opine confidentally how the patient will ultimately react to contrast media. Therefore, considering the medi-colegal aspects, it is advisable that a performa outlining the availability of various contrast media, their possible reactions, and the cost should be made available to the patient, also one must discuss directly with the patient/his relatives on these issues before planning a study, and an informed consent signed by the patient his relatives is mandatory.

REFERENCES

1. Cohan RH, Ellis JH. Iodinated Contrast Material in Uroradiology—Choice of Agent and Management of Complications. Rad Clin North Am. 1997;24(3):471-91.
2. Kopp AF, Mortele KJ, Cho YD, et al. Prevalence of acute reactions to Iopromide: Postmarketing surveillance study of 74,717 patients. Acta Radiol. 2008;8:902-11.
3. Katzberg RW. "Acute reactions to urographic contrast medium: Incidence, Clinical Characteristics, and relationship to history of hypersensitivity": A commentary. Am J Roentgenol. 2008;190:1431-2.
4. Thomsen HS. European Society of Urogenital Radiology (ESUR) guidelines on the safe use of iodinated contrast media. Eur J Radiol. 2006;60:307-13.
5. Del Favero C (Ed). Contrast Media: A multifactorial Approach. Intramed Communications; 1997.
6. Lasser E, Farr RS, Fujimagari T, et al. The significance of protein binding of contrast media in roentgen diagnosis. Am J Roentgenol. 1962;87:338-60.
7. Almen T. Contrast agent design: Some aspects of synthesis of water-soluble contrast agents of low osmolality. J Theo Biol. 1969;24:216-26.
8. Almen T, Boijsen E, Lindell SE. Metrizamide in angiography. I. Femoral angiography. Acta Radiol Diagn. 1977;18:33-8.
9. Katzberg RW. Urography into the 21st Century: New Contrast Media, Renal Handling, Imaging Characteristics, and Nephrotoxicity. Radiology. 1997;204:297-312.
10. Peter Dawson. Adverse reactions to intravascular contrast agents: Routine prophylaxis is not supported by evidence. BMJ. 2006;333:663-4.
11. Almen T. Visipaque: A step forward—A historical review. Acta Radiol. 1995;36(Suppl 399):2-18.
12. Dobroto M, Powell CJ, Holtz E. Biochemical and morphological effects of contrast media on the kidney. Acta Radiol. 1995;36:196-203.
13. Jakobsen JA. Renal effects of iodixanol in healthy volunteers and patients with severe renal failure. Acta Radiol. 1995;36(suppl 399):191-5.
14. Rapport SI, Levitan H. Neurotoxicity of X-ray contrast media: Relation to lipid solubility and blood brain barrier permeability. Am J Roentgenol. 1974;122:186-94.
15. McClennan BL, Stolbery HO. Intravascular contrast media: Ionic versus nonionic: Current status. Rad Clin North Am. 1991;29(3):437-54.
16. Segal AJ. Optimizing urography. World J Urol. 1998;16(1):3-8.
17. Morris TW, Kern MA, Katzberg RW. The effects of media viscosity on haemodynamics in selective arteriography. Invest Radiol. 1982;7:70-6.
18. Wycherley AG, Sage MR, Evill CA. Contrast media viscosity: a contributing factor in blood-brain barrier damage following intracarotid contrast injection? Australas Radiol. 1986;30:96-8.
19. Weinmann HJ, Platzek J, Schirmer H, et al. Contrast media: future aspects. Eur Radiol. 2005;15(Suppl 4):70-3.
20. Almen T. The etiology of contrast medium reactions. Invest Radiol. 1994;29(Suppl 1):S37-45.
21. Morcos SK, Thomsen HS, Webb JAW. Contrast Media Safety Committee of the European Society of Urogenital Radiology. Prevention of generalized reactions to contrast media: a consensus report and guidelines. Eur Radiol. 2001;11:1720-8.
22. Thomsen HS, Bush WH. Treatment of the adverse effects of contrast media. Acta Radiol. 1998;39:212-8.
23. Dunnick NR, Cohan RH. Cost, corticosteroids, and contrast media. AJR. 1994;162:527-9.

24. Thomsen HS (Ed). Contrast media: Safety issues and ESUR guidelines. Heidelberg: Springer Verlag; 2006.
25. Thomsen HS, Morcos SK. Members of Contrast Media Safety Committee of European Society of Urogenital Radiology (ESUR). Management of acute adverse reactions to contrast media. Eur Radiol. 2006;14:476-81.
26. Webb JAW, Stacul F, Thomsen HS, Morcos SK. Members of the Contrast Media Safety Committee of the European Society of Urogenital Radiology (ESUR). Late adverse reactions to intravascular iodinated contrast media. Eur Radiol. 2003;13:181-4.
27. Morcos SK, Thomsen HS, Webb JAW. Members of contrast media safety committee of the European Society of Urogenital Radiology (ESUR). Contrast media induced nephrotoxicity: a consensus report. Eur Radiol. 1999;9:1602-13.
28. Rudnik MR, Goldfarb S, Wexler L, et al. Nephrotoxicity of ionic and nonionic contrast media in 1196 patients: a randomized trial. Kidney Int. 1995;47:254-61.
29. Thomsen HS, Morcos SK. Members of Contrast Media safety committee of European Society of Urogenital Radiology (ESUR). In which patients should serum-creatinine be measured before contrast medium administration? Eur Radiol. 2005;15:749-54.
30. Morcos SK. Prevention of contrast media nephrotoxicity—The story so far. Clin Radiol. 2004;59:381-9.
31. Morcos SK, Thomsen HS, Webb JAW. Members of the Contrast Media Safety Committee of European Society of Urogenital Radiology (ESUR). Dialysis and contrast media. Eur Radiol. 2002;12:3026-30.
32. Thomsen HS, Almen T, Morcos SK. Members of Contrast Media Safety Committee of European Society of Urogenital Radiology (ESUR). Gadolinium-containing contrast media for radiographic examinations: a position paper. Eur Radiol. 2002;12:2600-5.
33. Thomsen HS, Morcos SK. Members of Contrast Media Safety Committee of European Society of Urogenital Radiology (ESUR). Contrast media and metformin. Guidelines to diminish the risk of lactic acidosis in non-insulin dependent diabetics after administration of contrast media. Eur Radiol. 1999;9:738-40.
34. Shehadi WH. Adverse reactions to intravascularly administered contrast media: A comprehensive study based on a prospective survey. Am J Roentgenol. 1975;124:145-52.
35. Katayama H, Yamaguchi K, Kozuka T, et al. Adverse reactions to ionic and nonionic contrast media. A report from the Japanese Committee on the safety of contrast media. Radiology. 1990;175:621-8.
36. Narita S, Goldblum RM, Watson CS, et al. Environmental estrogens induce mast cell degranulation and enhance Ig E-mediated release of allergic mediators. Environ Health Perspect. 2007;115:48-52.
37. Molen AJvd, Thomsen HS, Morcos SK. Members of Contrast Media Safety Committee of European Society of Urogenital Radiology (ESUR). Effect of iodinated contrast media on thyroid function in adults. Radiol. 2004;14:902-6.
38. Morcos SK, Thomsen HS, Exley CM. Members of Contrast Media Safety Committee of European Society of Urogenital Radiology (ESUR). Contrast Media: Interaction with other drugs and clinical tests. Eur Radiol. 2005;15:1463-8.
39. Webb JAW, Thomsen HS, Morcos SK. Members of Contrast Media Safety Committee of European Society of Urogenital Radiology (ESUR). The use of iodinated and gadolinium contrast media during pregnancy and lactaion. Eur Radiol. 2005;15:1234-40.
40. Manual on Iodinated Contrast Material. Reston, VA, American College of Radiology; 1991.
41. Cohan RH, Ellis JH, Dunnick NR. Use of low-osmolar agents and premedication to reduce the frequency of adverse reactions to radiographic contrast media: A survey of the society of Uroradiology. Radiology. 1995;194:357-64.

CHAPTER 104

Tubercular Infection of the Urinary Tract

Ashu Seith Bhalla, Arun Kumar Gupta, Raju Sharma

INTRODUCTION

Tuberculosis (TB) of the urinary tract is not uncommon in India. A multicentric study carried out in 1973 under Indian Council of Medical Research showed an incidence of 10–34%, of all patients presenting with various urological diseases.[1] The **genitourinary** system is one of the most common sites of involvement by extrapulmonary **tuberculosis**, accounting for 15–20% of infections outside the lungs.[2] Approximately 4–8% of patients with pulmonary **tuberculosis** will develop clinically significant **genitourinary** infection.[3] There is an increasing concern world over with the onset of HIV epidemic and the emergence of multidrug resistant strains in the last two decades. TB occurs in approximately 10% of patients with AIDS and involves at least one extrapulmonary site in nearly 50% of the patients, with kidneys being the most commonly involved genitourinary site.[4]

Urinary tract TB is an important clinical problem because of its nonspecific clinical presentation and progression to renal failure if undiagnosed and untreated. It is also a diagnostic problem because of variable imaging features which often resemble many other lesions. The disease is predominant between second and fourth decades of life being distinctly low in children, and less prevalent in fifth and sixth decades. The disease shows a male predominance.

PATHOGENESIS

Renal tuberculosis results from hematogeneous dissemination of the tubercle bacilli from a primary infection elsewhere. Past or concurrent pulmonary lesion is the most common primary lesion, followed by bone and joint tuberculosis. There is a latent period of 5–20 years between the original pulmonary infection and the appearance of clinical renal disease. This explains the low incidence of disease in children. The organisms may involve both kidneys in the initial phase, and are lodged in the glomerular and peritubular capillary bed. The subsequent course of the infection is determined by virulence of the organisms and host-resistance factors. Most of the initial lesions heal without sequelae, and only one or a few progress to clinically or radiologically apparent abnormalities. This happens when the bacilli erode out of their initial vascular location and spill into the tubules. This results in granuloma formation along the nephron. Granuloma, caseous necrosis, and cavitation represent stages of progression of the infection. This may communicate with the pelvicalyceal system, and the infection further spreads to the ureter and urinary bladder. The pelvicalyceal and ureteral involvement appears as mucosal ulcerations, focal or generalised dilatation or cicatrisation. Fibrosis and calcium depositions represent healing. The pattern of progression and healing is variable and produces asymmetric histologic, microscopic and radiological findings unique to each patient. If the hydronephrotic kidney becomes nonfunctioning, extensive dystrophic (putty like) calcification may form a cast of the kidney, referred to as autonephrectomy. Nonfunctioning kidneys in TB may be due to autonephrectomy or as a sequelae of obstruction **(Fig. 1)**. Important complications of renal TB

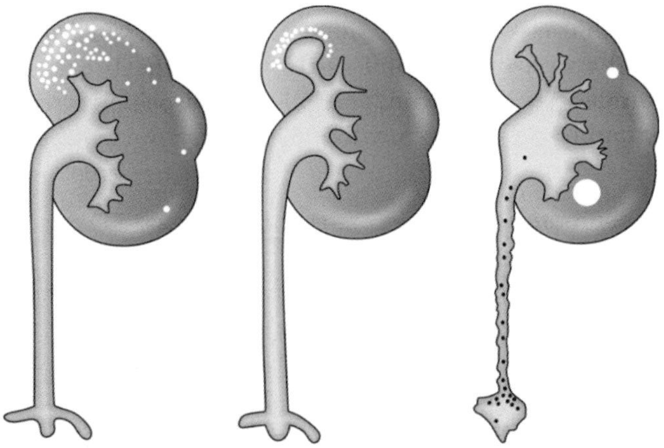

Fig. 1: Schematic diagram showing stages of progression of the disease.

include perinephritis, perinephric abscess, fistulae and psoas abscesses.

CLINICAL PICTURE

Frequency of urination, burning, dysuria or urgency are the most common presenting symptoms. Nearly 50% of the patients at sometime during the course of the disease have hematuria. Dull or chronic renal pain, even acute colic is not uncommon. Constitutional symptoms like fever, weight loss, fatigue are present in about 50% of the patients. Obstructive uropathy, and chronic cystitis are not uncommon with TB.[5,6] Patients may develop fistulae particularly in lower urinary tract involvement. The physical examination is often insignificant. Diagnosis of TB should be considered in patients with recurrent urinary tract infection that is not responding to appropriate therapy for typical pathogens.

LABORATORY INVESTIGATIONS

Pyuria which is sterile when cultured on standard media is characteristic. Presence of red blood cells in urine is frequent. The diagnosis is established by demonstration of acid-fast bacilli (AFB) on microscopic examination of urine, urine culture or growth of tubercle bacilli in inoculated guinea-pigs. However, urine culture for acid-fast bacilli is positive in nearly 33%, while soluble antigen fluorescent antibody (SAFA) test is strongly positive in only 13%, and weak or nonreactive in 87% of the patients. Also, routine AFB culture is cumbersome involving a delay of 6–8 weeks with a false-negative rate of 10-20%, using LJ media. Newer techniques for recovery of mycobacteria from urine specimens include BACTEC 460 and using the automated Mycobacteria Growth Indicator Tube system (MGIT 960), with mean time of positivity of 20 days.[7] As an alternative, polymerase chain reaction (PCR) technique or US-guided fine needle aspiration cytology (FNAC) can be used. PCR is highly sensitive (up to 94%), provides a quicker diagnosis but has a relatively poor specificity.[8] FNAC is useful in those with a negative culture to define granulomatous nature of the visible lesions.

CYSTOSCOPY

Visualization of tubercle, ulcer or retracted ureteric orifice strongly suggest the diagnosis. Generalized cystitis with reduced capacity is almost diagnostic. Biopsy from ulcer, tubercle or inflammatory lesion, particularly in absence of positive urine culture may provide the only diagnostic evidence of the disease.

RADIOLOGICAL EXAMINATION

A key role is often played by the radiologist in the diagnosis of the disease. The balance between local progress and healing of the disease process manifests many abnormal imaging features. Since demonstration of the typical calyceal, ureteral and vesical abnormalities is critical to establish the diagnosis of tuberculosis, conventional radiological studies remain the procedures of choice, while ultrasonography (US) and computerized tomography (CT) have a limited role. Essentially, early findings are best detected on intravenous urogaphy (IVU) while ultrasonography and CT are useful for late or chronic changes. US and CT are especially valuable in the evaluation of areas of mass effect and of the nonvisualized kidney at IVU.[9] MRI had not found a place in the diagnostic protocol for evaluation till recently. However, MRI can be useful too in evaluation of the nonfunctioning kidney and focal lesions. A study by Navarro et al. found that Intravenous urography provided the diagnosis in 85% of cases. The average interval between onset of symptoms and diagnosis was 15 months. They in fact state that the current use of imaging studies other than urography and the finding of other microorganisms in urine culture can delay the diagnosis.[10] The most valuable radiologic feature of genitourinary tuberculosis is the multiplicity of abnormal findings. Whenever a imaging pattern of chronic renal inflammatory disease is recognized, particularly in the setting of periureteric or peripelvic fibrosis, tuberculosis must be considered.[11]

Plain Films

Plain radiograph of abdomen is an important initial examination before IVU and may provide valuable information such as calcification or evidence of skeletal involvement. Small, enlarged or normal renal size; presence of scarring or focal bulge are all nonspecific findings. Deposition of calcium in an attempt to heal and limit the pathological process often provides a diagnostic clue. Calcification is of two types: (i) amorphous granular associated with granulomatous masses, and (ii) dense punctate calcification representing healed tuberculoma. It varies from a few minute areas to a cast of entire kidney **(Figs. 2 and 3)**. The lobar distribution of calcification is quite specific for renal TB. Tubercular calcification of ureter is not as common as renal calcification, and calcification of bladder is relatively rare.[12] Plain films may also reveal an evidence of skeletal tuberculosis in hip, sacroiliac joint or spine with or without a paraspinal abscess and calcification of abdominal lymph nodes. A coexisting focus of extrarenal TB elsewhere ranges from 23% to 53% in various series. Chest X-ray is abnormal in about 50% of the patients. However, active pul-monary tuberculosis is seen in only 5–10% with most patients showing sequelae of past infection.

Intravenous Urography

Even though miliary tubercles involve both kidneys, disease progression and hence radiological abnormalities are confined to a single kidney in over 70% of the patients. Intravenous urography (IVU) is a very useful modality to detect early features of urinary tract tuberculosis.[13,14] However, the diagnosis can be made with certainity on urography only if the lesion has ulcerated into the calyx. Hence, IVU may be normal in symptomatic renal tuberculosis in the initial stages when the bacilli are lodged in glomerulus and peritubular capillary bed. IVU is essential to assess the extent and severity of involvement, to monitor the response to treatment and to look for complications.

Kidney

The earliest urographic abnormality is the loss of definition of a minor calyx producing an indistinct feathery outline, irregularity of the surface of one or more papillae or calyces with normal renal size and contour **(Fig. 4)**. Progressive involvement of renal parenchyma occurs in three forms, which occur singly or in combination. First is coalescence of granulomas leading to unifocal or multifocal mass lesions. These may enlarge overall renal length or increase thickness of renal substance and cause displacement of adjacent collecting system. Caliectasis occurs with irregularity in contour indicating erosion of the pyramids and cortical necrosis. Depending on the necrosis, a cavity with irregular walls communicates with a deformed calyx **(Figs. 5 and 6)**. Radiographic appearance of this form simulates papillary necrosis of other origins. The second form seen in advanced renal tuberculosis is parenchymal surface scarring over retracted papillae and dilated calyces. This may be focal or diffuse involving the entire kidney and occurs due to tissue loss leading to fibrosis. Associated calcification or calculi maybe seen. Radiographic identification of calcification associated with renal TB is becoming less common. Calculus disease is rapidly becoming the most frequent form of calcification associated with renal TB.[15] Due to pelvic scarring the calculi formed also tend to take on this deformed shape. Upward pointing renal pelvic calculi may be seen due to 'hiked up' pelvis **(Figs. 7A to C)**.[15]

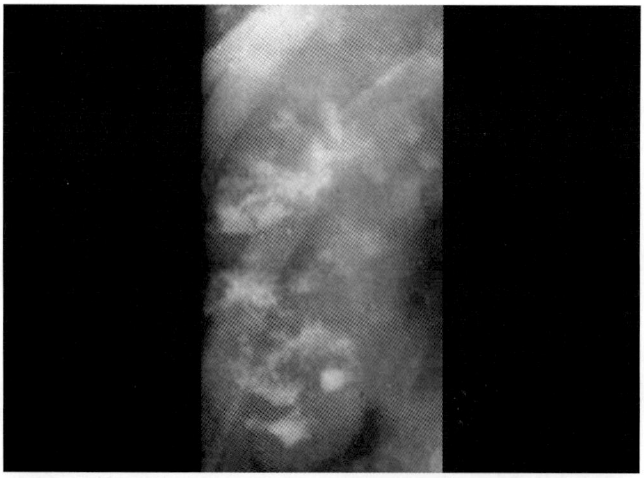

Fig. 2: Plain radiograph abdomen showing amorphous granular calcification involving the right kidney.

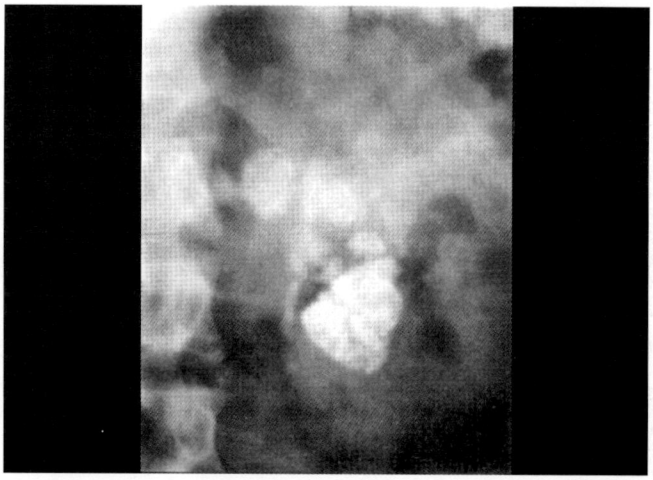

Fig. 3: Extensive calcification involving the entire left kidney with no function on intravenous urography—autonephrectomy.

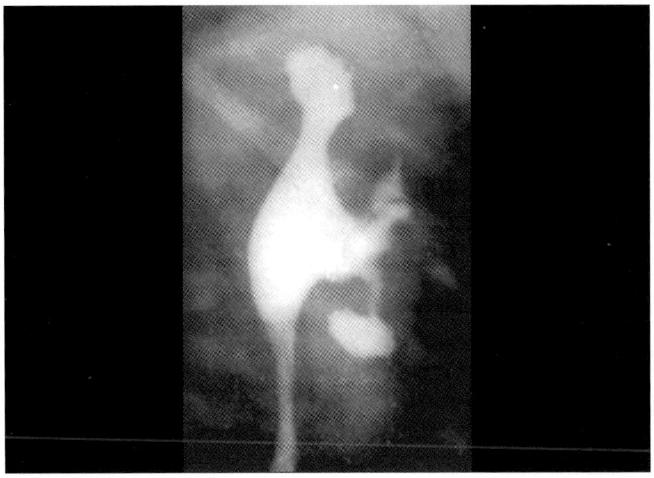

Fig. 4: IVU reveals marked dilatation of the inferior calyx with loss of sharpness and fuzziness of its outline. Rest of the calyces are also dilated.

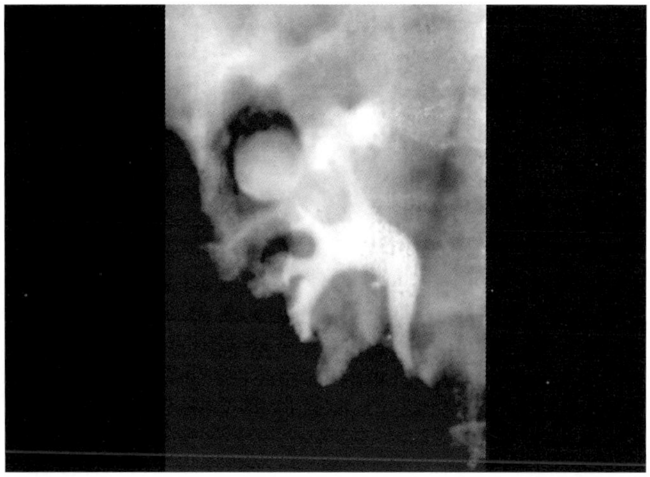

Fig. 5: IVU shows a large cavity communicating with a dilated, irregular superior calyx.

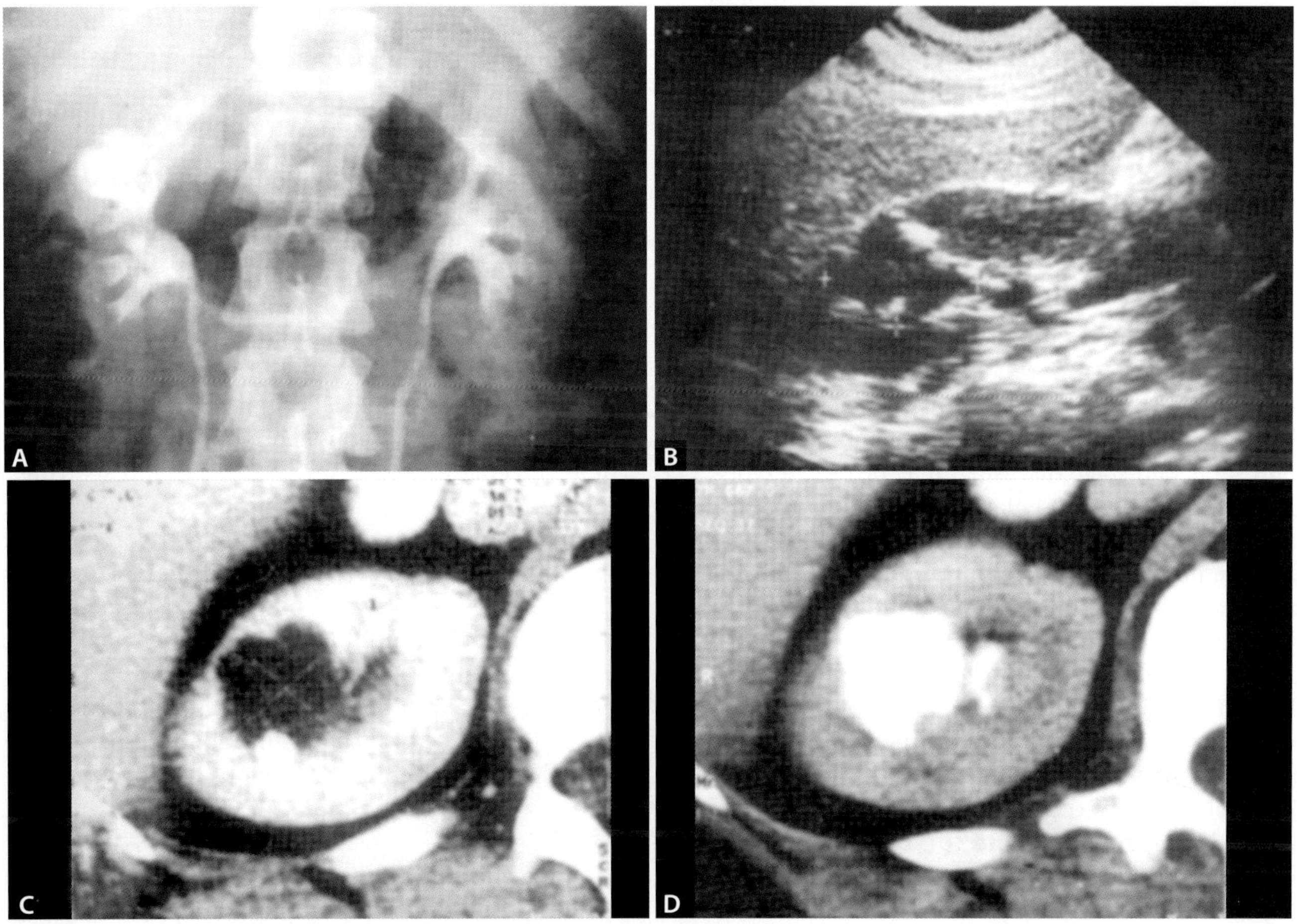

Figs. 6A to D: (A) IVU reveals a large cavity communicating with the superior calyx of right kidney; (B) US shows a hypoechoic focal lesion in the upper polar cortex with an echogenic rim; (C) CT confirms the presence of the cavity seen on IVU and US, with pooling of contrast on delayed images; (D) due to communication with the pelvicalyceal system.

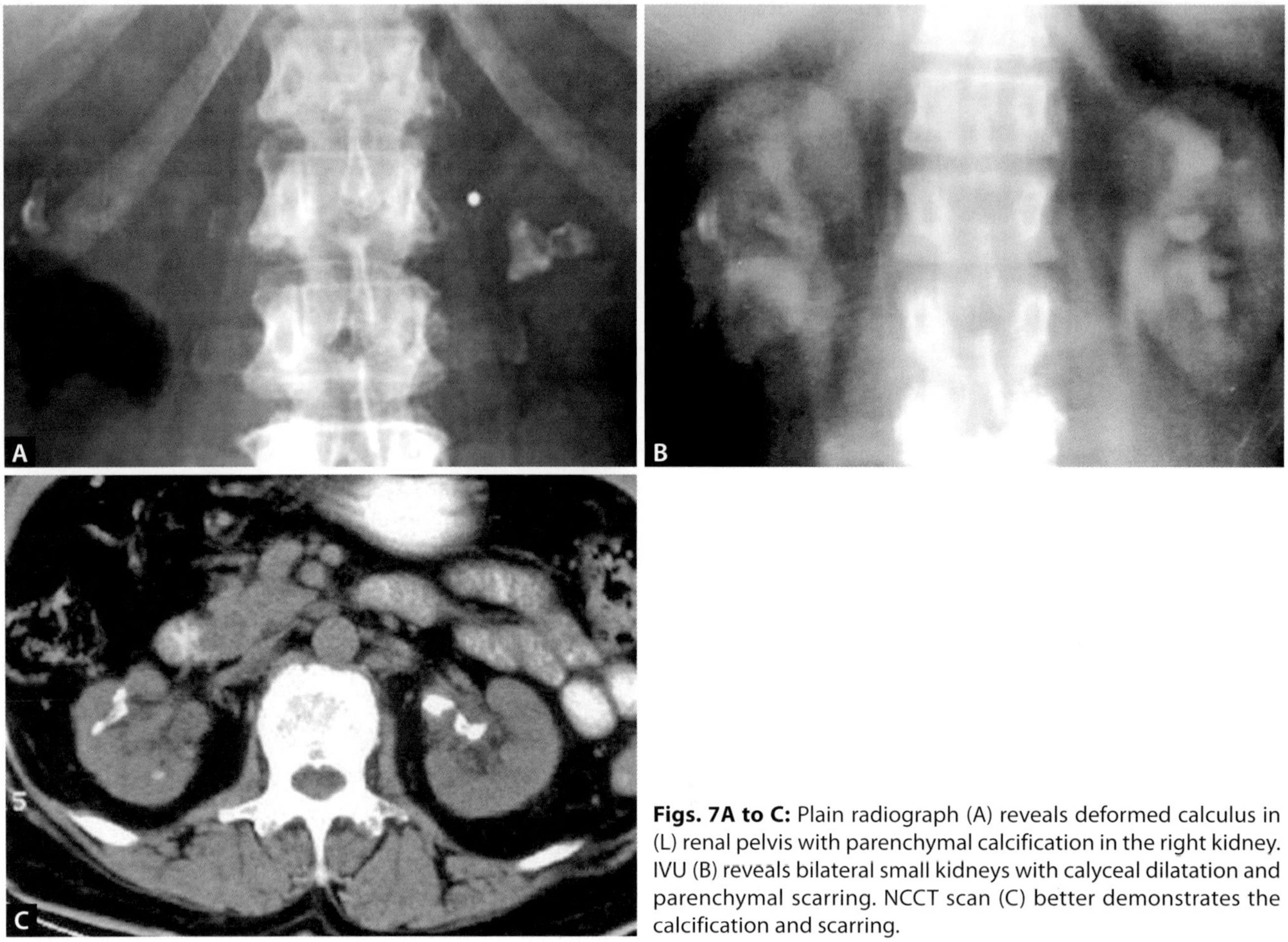

Figs. 7A to C: Plain radiograph (A) reveals deformed calculus in (L) renal pelvis with parenchymal calcification in the right kidney. IVU (B) reveals bilateral small kidneys with calyceal dilatation and parenchymal scarring. NCCT scan (C) better demonstrates the calcification and scarring.

Impaired excretion of contrast is seen in either of these two forms. A third form is autonephrectomy, which represents end stage disease. It may be of two types: (1) caseo-cavernous type-enlarged sac filled with caseous material, with or without calcification **(Fig. 8)**.[15] This can simulate xanthogranulomatous pyelonephritis; (2) calcified shrunken nonfunctioning kidney.

Following the drainage of a cavity into the collecting system, there is spread of infection to other parts of the urinary tract. Subsequent stimulation of scirrhous reaction causes stenosis and obstruction of parts of the collecting system. The common sites of strictures being the neck of a calyx, pelvi-ureteric junction and lower end of the ureter **(Figs. 9 and 10)**. Depending on the site of narrowing there is dilatation of a single calyx (hydrocalyx) or regional hydrocalycosis or generalized dilatation of the pelvicalyceal system. A completely stenosed infundibulum or calyx may lead to failure of contrast excretion by the involved parenchyma (phantom calyx). A tiny infundibular stump (amputated calyx) may be seen in such cases. The renal pelvis may be dilated or may show filling defects due to caseous debris and granulation tissue. The involvement progresses to fibrosis with scarring. If the inferior margin of the renal pelvis is involved with resultant cephalic retraction, a characteristic deformity called the "hiked up pelvis" results. In addition, deformity of the pelvicalyceal system may be caused by traction from a strictured infundibulum or parenchymal fibrosis kinking the pelvis (Kerr's kink) and involving areas not directly affected by tuberculous ulcerations. Occasionally, obstruction can be of such a high grade and so prolonged that marked hydronephrosis develops **(Fig. 11)**.[16]

Ureter

Ureteral involvement is almost always secondary to renal TB with spread of infection by bacilluria. In the early stages there is dilatation resulting from atony and prolonged bacilluria. With progression of the disease, irregular segments of ureter are seen due to mucosal ulcerations. Further necrosis of ureteral musculature is accompanied

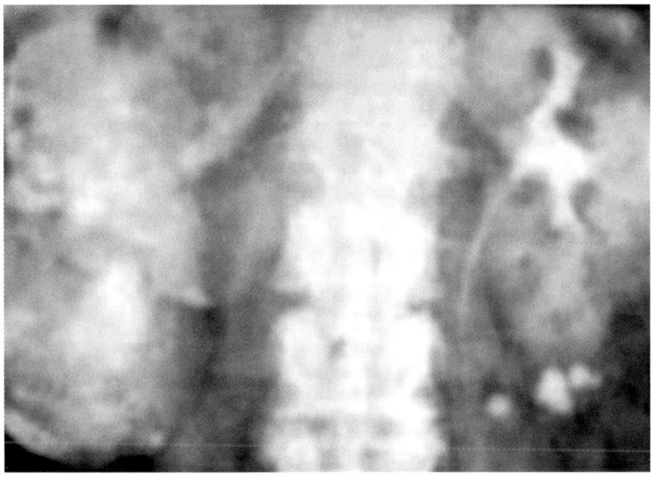

Fig. 8: IVU slowing an enlarged, sac-like poorly functioning right kidney—Advanced disease of caseocavernous type.

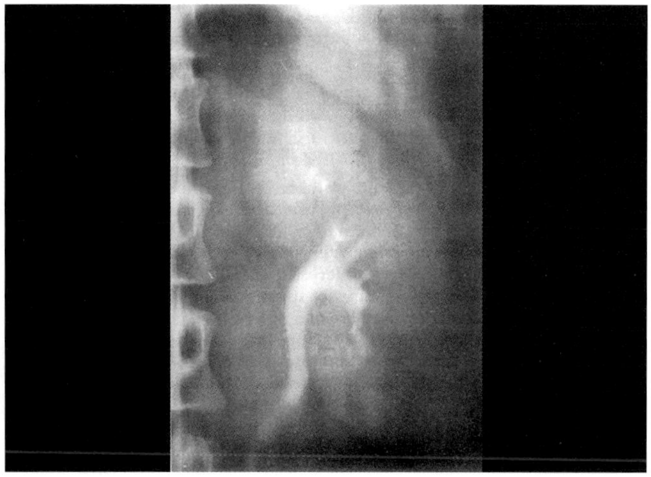

Fig. 9: IVU shows irregularity of the superior calyx with intrarenal reflux and infundibular narrowing.

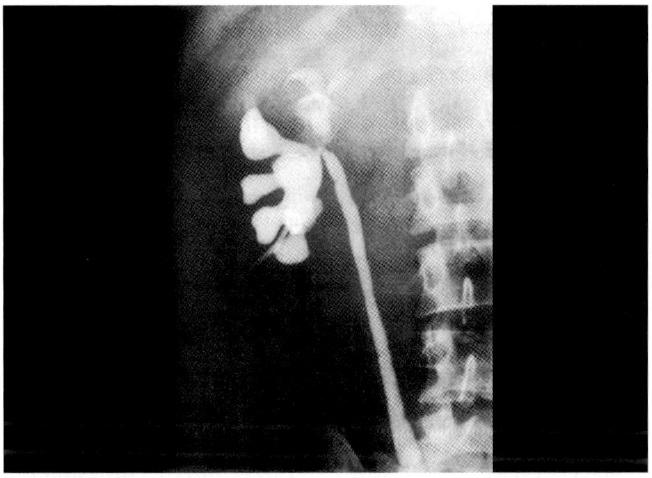

Fig. 10: Nephrostogram showing deformed and contracted renal pelvis with proximal dilatation of the pelvicalyceal system. Superior calyx is communicating with an irregular cavity and there is infundibular stenosis. Ureter is also dilated due to lower end stricture.

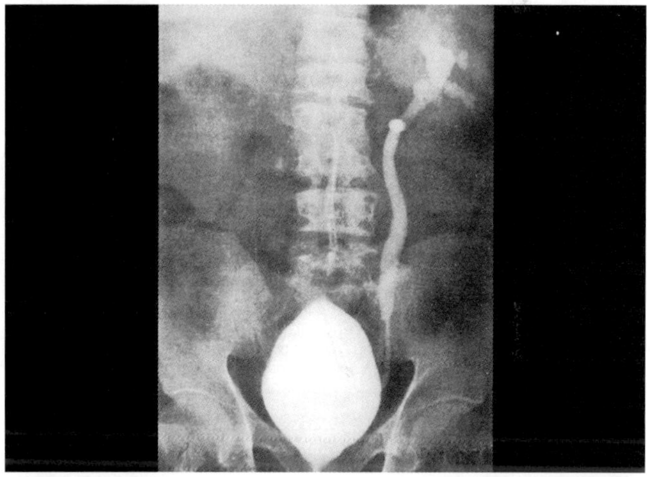

Fig. 11: IVU showing long irregular stricture involving lower end of left ureter with hydroureter, hydronephrosis and infundibular stenosis of inferior calyx of left kidney. Also note changes of tuberculosis involving L2–L3 vertebrae.

by fibrosis resulting in stricutre formation. The ureteric segments which are more superficially involved may heal without stricture formation. This produces a beaded or corkscrew appearance of the ureter.[17] Ureteral strictures have been reported in 10–56% of patients with urinary tract TB. The terminal segment of the ureter is most commonly involved **(Fig. 11)**. However, any part may be involved with multiple strictures seen in 19% cases. In later stages, severe thickening of the wall produces a rigid shortened ureter with narrow lumen termed as "pipe stem ureter." Renal damage secondary to ureteral strictures may be more severe than the effect of the original parenchymal involvement. Dilatation and stenting of the ureter may restore ureteral patency and salvage a kidney.

Urinary Bladder

Urinary bladder is involved later in the course of the disease in upto one-third of patients of urinary tract TB. Use of bacillus Calmette-Guérin therapy for bladder cancer can cause symptomatic tubercular infections of the lower genitourinary tract.[5] Tubercular cystitis leads to edema of the bladder mucosa. Large tuberculomas in vesical wall can manifest radiologically as filling defects simulating carcinoma.[18] Advanced disease leads to irregular contracture with thick walls and reduction of bladder capacity - the "thimble bladder" **(Figs. 12 and 13)**. Fibrosis in the region of the trigone produces gaping of the ureterovesical junction resulting in free vesicoureteric reflux.

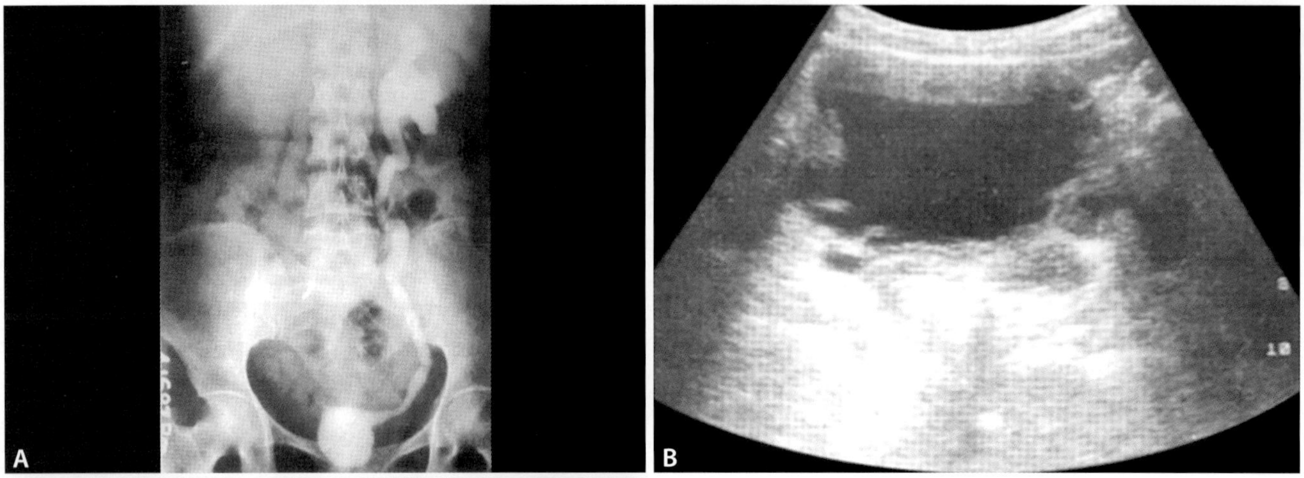

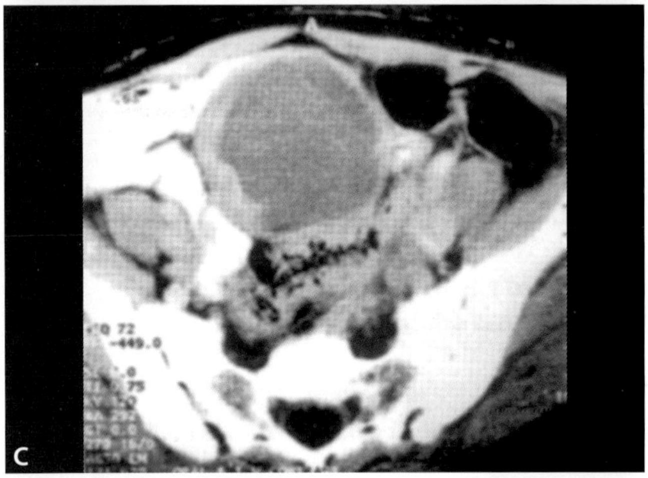

Figs. 12A to C: Urinary bladder TB: (A) IVU reveals a small capacity (thimble) urinary bladder, ureteral stricture with proximal hydroureter and hydronephrosis on left side. Right kidney is nonfunctioning; (B) US shows irregular, asymmetric wall thickening of the urinary bladder with trabeculations. A left adnexal mass is also seen posterior to the bladder; (C) CT shows a similar appearance of the urinary bladder.

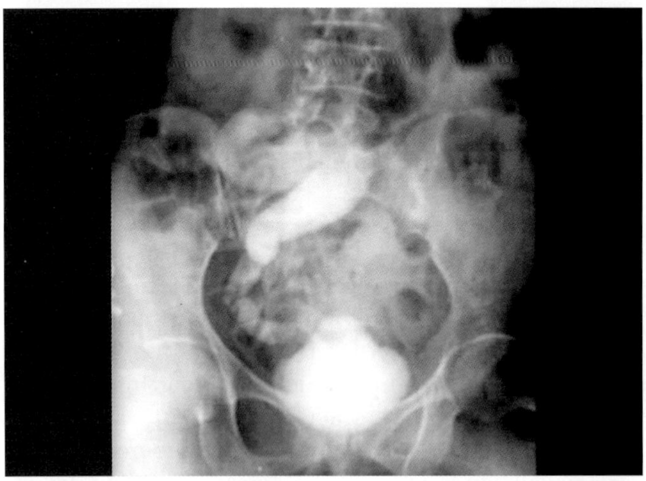

Fig. 13: MCU study reveals a small capacity bladder with reflux into a dilated, tortuous right ureter.

Urethral TB

Tuberculosis of the male urethra is uncommon and usually occurs secondary to renal infection. It may also be associated with prostatic abscess, periurethral abscess or fistula formation. It may result in a nonspecific stricture almost always in the bulbomembranous urethra that is indistinguishable on imaging from strictures due to other causes.

Retrograde Pyelography

Retrograde pyelography is particularly indicated in a patient with nonfunctioning kidney to demonstrate ureteric obstruction and cavitation in the kidney.

Ultrasonography

Ultrasound is not used as the primary imaging modality for diagnosis of urinary tract TB, as it is unable to show early calyceal changes and does not provide information about renal functional status. However, carefully performed sonogram can show a spectrum of morphological abnormalities.[19,20] The role of sonography is also to provide guidance for the interventional procedures of percutaneous nephrostomy (PCN), antegrade dilatation of ureteral stricture and drainage of the perinephric abscess.

Kidney

A focal renal lesion of varying echogenicity is a frequently encountered sonographic abnormality. In the early stages US demonstrates papillary lesions as areas of hypoechogenicity or hypoechoic foci with echogenic walls or echogenic nonshadowing lesions **(*see* Fig. 6B)**.[21] A sloughed calyx is seen as an echogenic flap separated from the normal calyceal wall **(Fig. 14A)**. Large liquefying conglomerate cavities or dilated calyces formed as a result of infundibular stricture appear as hypoechoic nodules or masses. The communicating tract from a cavity appears as a sonolucent track entering the dilated calyx **(Fig. 14B)**. Heterogeneous echotexture of the parenchyma or normal appearing parenchyma may be seen in diffuse involvement **(Figs. 15A and B)**. Such patients show poor excretory function on IVU and CT. Following pelvicalyceal system involvement, US may characteristically show uneven caliectasis without renal pelvis dilatation. It may also demonstrate hydronephrosis, parenchymal calcification, and perinephric abscess **(Figs. 16A and B)**.

Xuefang Rui et al.[22] reviewed sonographic features of 258 cases of renal tuberculosis. In this series of 258 cases, 152 cases were correctly diagnosed as renal tuberculosis by B-mode ultrasonography, and these were classified under six types: type I: nephrectasia type (23 cases); type II: hydrops type, (21 cases); type III: empyema type (13 cases); type IV: inflammatory and atrophy type (15 cases); type V: calcification type (34 cases); type VI: mixed type (46 cases).

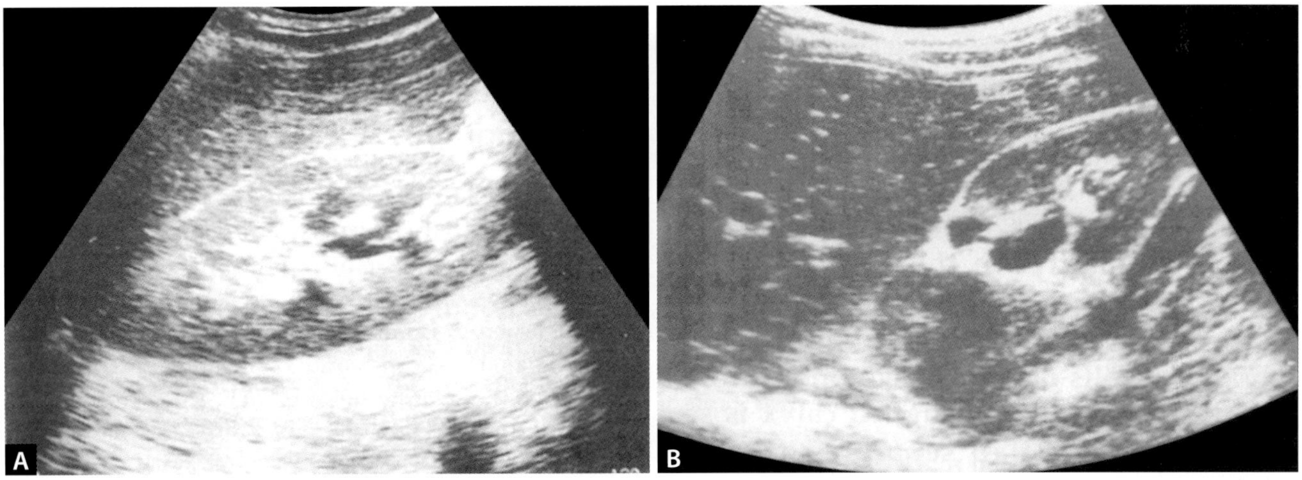

Figs. 14A and B: (A) US showing echogenic papillary sloughing in the middle calyx of the right kidney; (B) US of another patient reveals an anechoic cavity in the renal cortex with a sonolucent track connecting the cavity and the pelvicalyceal system.

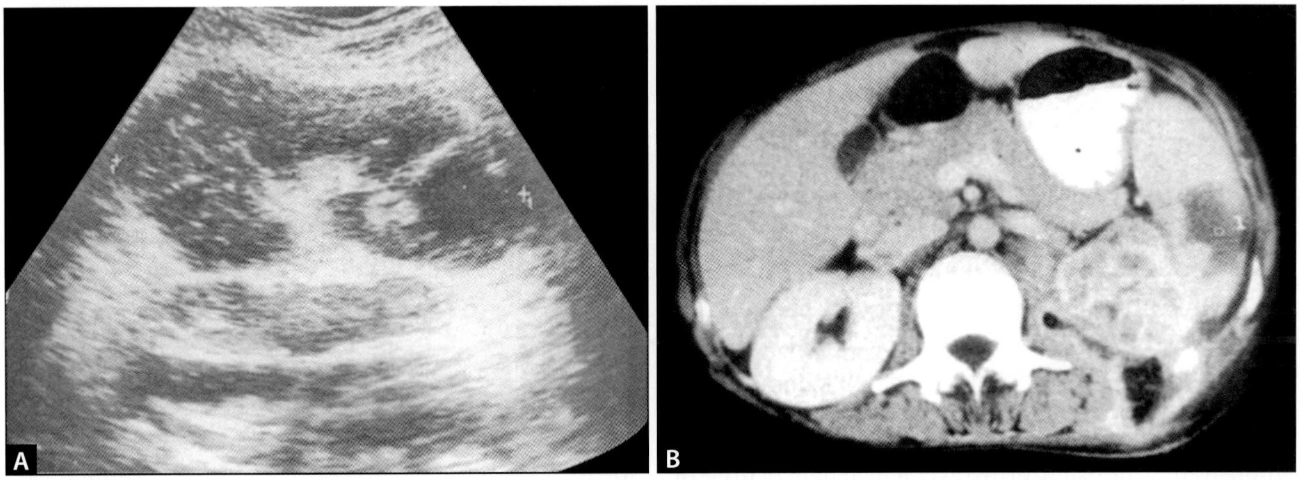

Figs. 15A and B: (A) US shows an enlarged heterogeneous left kidney with an anechoic cavity in the lower pole; (B) Contrast-enhanced CT of the same patient reveals poorly functioning heterogeneous left kidney with hypodense areas within. An irregular hypoattenuating splenic abscess and inflammatory changes in the left posterior renal space, left psoas and posterior parietes are also seen.

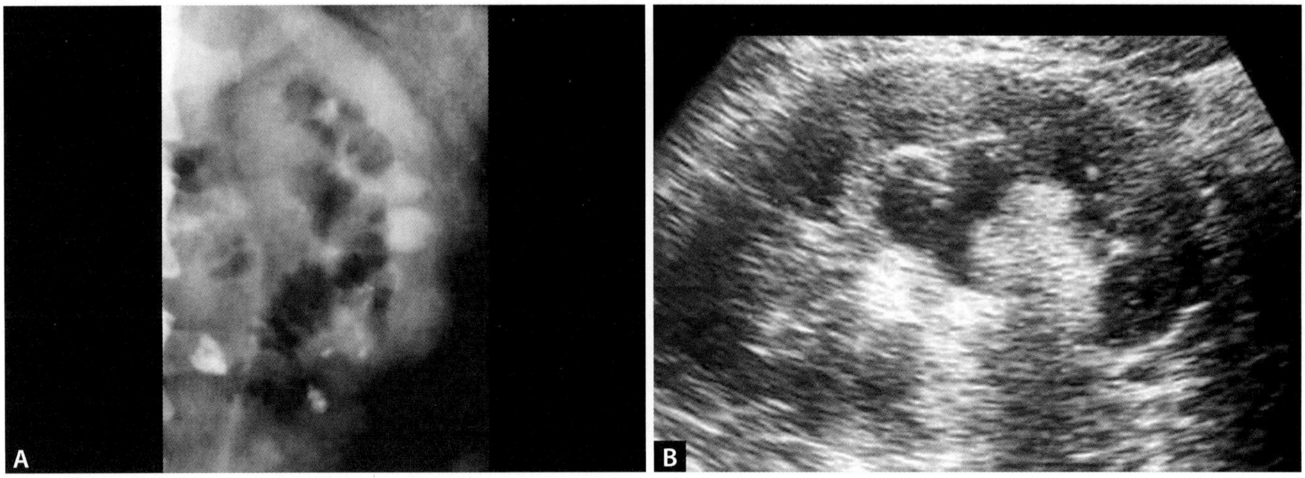

Figs. 16A and B: IVU (A) and US (B) of left kidney of a 28-year-old male reveals uneven caliectasis with calcification within.

In type I (nephrectasia), the renal capsule was very irregular. In the renal parenchyma and renal sinus, there were one or several anechoic zones, of different sizes with irregular margins and some nebulous light spot echoes within. The type II (hydrops type) also showed an irregular renal capsule. The renal pelvis and calyces were distended, within which there was an anechoic zone, similar to hydronephrosis. However, the inner wall was rough and uneven. In most cases, the ureter was involved and appeared thickened.

Ureter

US does not play a significant role in the acute phase. It is useful in assessment and follow up of back pressure changes and adjoining retroperitoneal disease.

Urinary Bladder

US may detect focal irregularity or thickening of the bladder wall with reduced capacity. Distension of the bladder may be necessary to gauge the bladder capacity accurately. The deformed bladder shape and focal abnormalities are also better appreciated following distension **(Fig. 12B)**.

Computed Tomography

Computed tomography is indicated only in patients with strong clinical suspicion but normal or equivocal findings on urography and ultrasonography. Multidetector CT (MDCT) with its multiple reconstructions is useful in demonstrating the extent of involvement, length of ureteric stricture, adjoining retroperitoneal disease and associated spinal or solid organ involvement.

Kidney

CT may show a spectrum of findings including multiple small poorly enhancing nodules, uneven caliectasis and calcification **(Figs. 17A to C)**. Similar to US the pelvis is typically not distended **(Figs. 18A to D)**. Isolated cortical involvement by focal lesions is well-demonstrated on CT. A cavity is well delineated with pooling of contrast in the delayed images **(Fig. 6C)**. Compared to US, CT is also able to provide better visualization of retroperitoneal structures, more detailed information on presence and pattern of calcification and functional status of the kidney **(Figs. 18 to 20)**. In poorly functioning kidneys the nephrogram effect is much better seen on CT than on IVU.

Ureter

Thickening of the renal pelvis or ureter is highly suggestive of tuberculosis and can be readily identified on CT **(Fig. 19D)**.

Urinary Bladder

CT offers no significant advantage in the evaluation of bladder involvement except for detection of faint calcification and demonstration of adjacent genital tract disease **(Figs. 12C and 20D)**.

MRI

MRI description of urinary tract TB is limited to sporadic reports. MRI with MR urography can be used to evaluate poorly or nonfunctioning kidney, especially the obstructive form for demonstration of ureteric involvement. MRI also demonstrates the renal parenchymal changes well, while MR urogram details the pelvicalyceal involvement

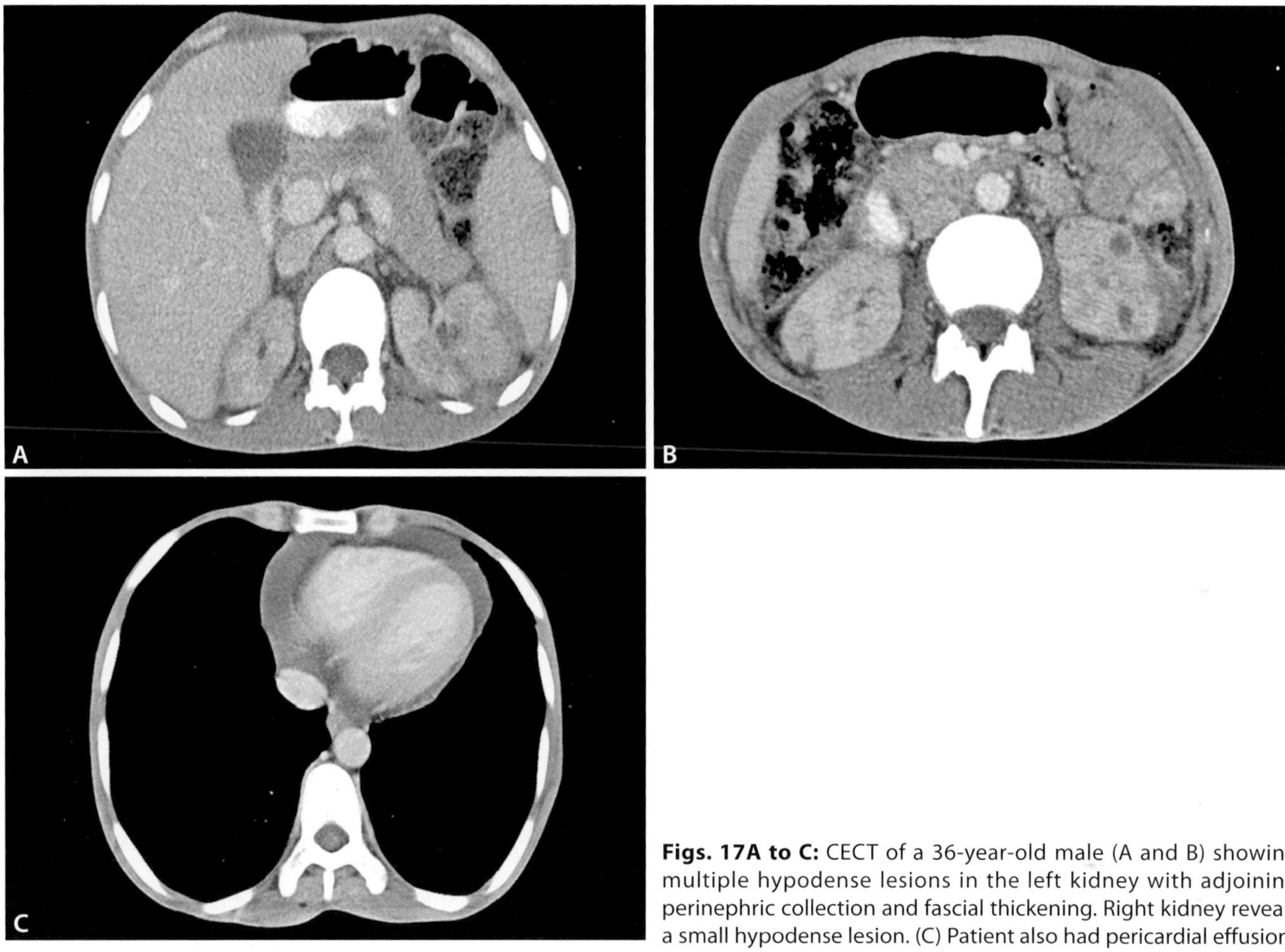

Figs. 17A to C: CECT of a 36-year-old male (A and B) showing multiple hypodense lesions in the left kidney with adjoining perinephric collection and fascial thickening. Right kidney reveals a small hypodense lesion. (C) Patient also had pericardial effusion.

(Figs. 21 and 22). Time-resolved dynamic contrast-enhanced MR urography can be used for the evaluation of ureteral peristalsis.[23]

COMPLICATIONS

The prominent complications include perinephric inflammation/abscess formation including psoas abscesses **(Figs. 22A to E)**. Fistulae or sinus tracts may develop into adjacent tissues or viscera **(Figs. 23 and 24)**.

Differential Diagnosis

The differential diagnosis of urinary TB can be varied depending upon the form of involvement. Early renal TB can simulate papillary necrosis. Focal lesions resemble other infections or even neoplasms. Calcification and extensive inflammation can mimic xanthogranulomatous pyelonephritis. Similarly urinary bladder involvement may be confused with neoplastic involvement.

In conclusion, diagnosis of urinary tract tuberculosis is based on a high index of clinical suspicion supported by a collective evaluation of microbiological, radiological and endoscopic features. While individual radiological features of urinary tract TB can be seen in other diseases such as papillary necrosis due to other causes, infections and neoplasms; the key to diagnosis is pattern recognition. Also, follow-up excretory urography at regular intervals is useful both for assessment of therapeutic response, and for an early detection of the complications.

Genitourinary Tuberculosis in HIV

The impact of HIV epidemic on the incidence and clinical presentation of genitourinary TB is largely unknown. Navarro et al.[10] evaluated clinical and epidemiological characteristics of patients diagnosed with genitourinary TB at their center over the last 10 years, found that of the 45 patients analyzed, 33% had a coexisting disease (14 were infected by human immunodeficiency virus). In

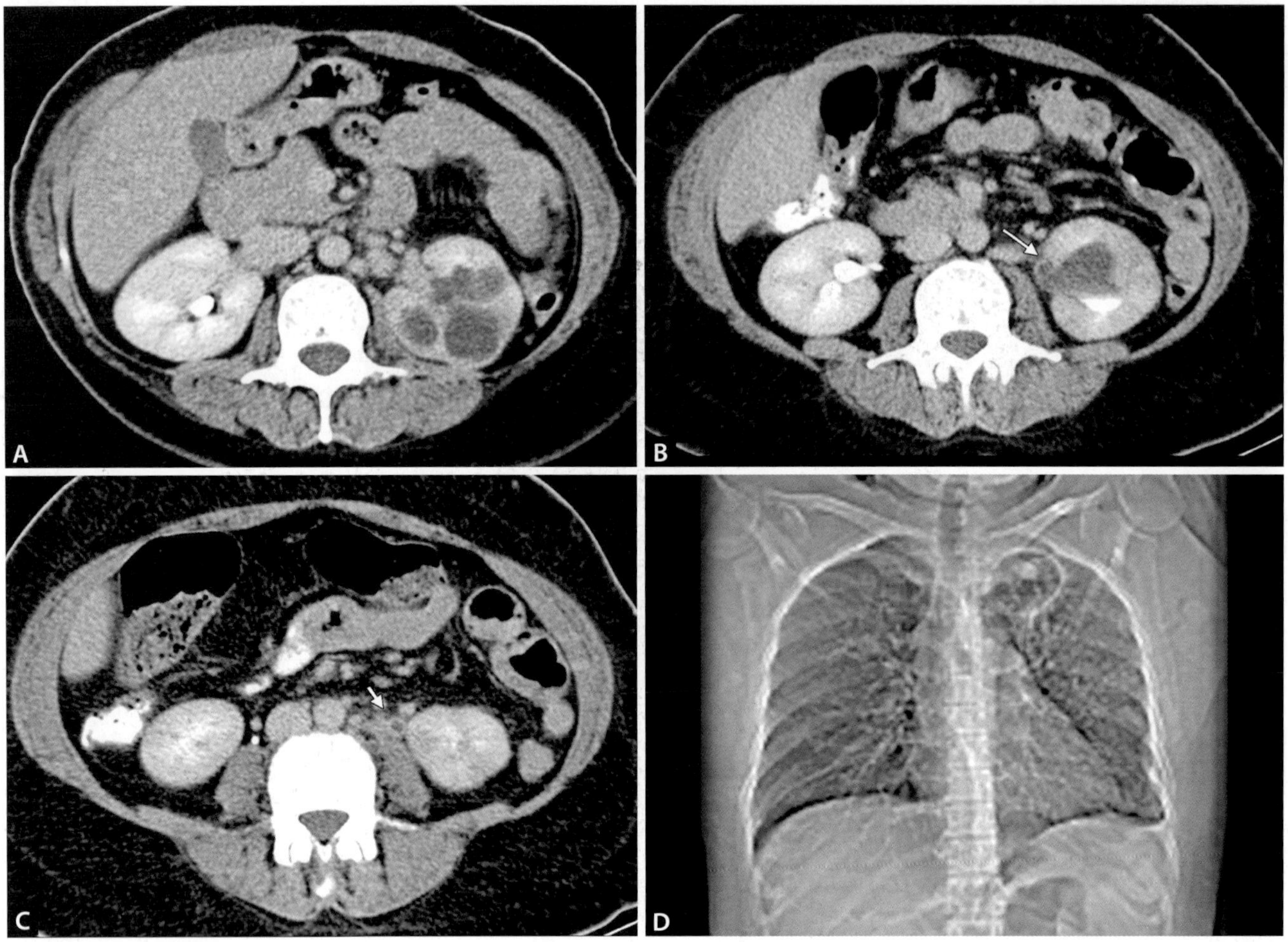

Figs. 18A to D: CECT of a young girl reveals a poorly functioning (L) kidney with hydronephrosis. Small retroperitoneal nodes are present (A), Renal pelvis is contracted with a thickened wall (arrow) (B); The ureteric wall is also thickened (small arrow) (C); Topogram (D) reveals a cavity in the left upper lobe of lung.

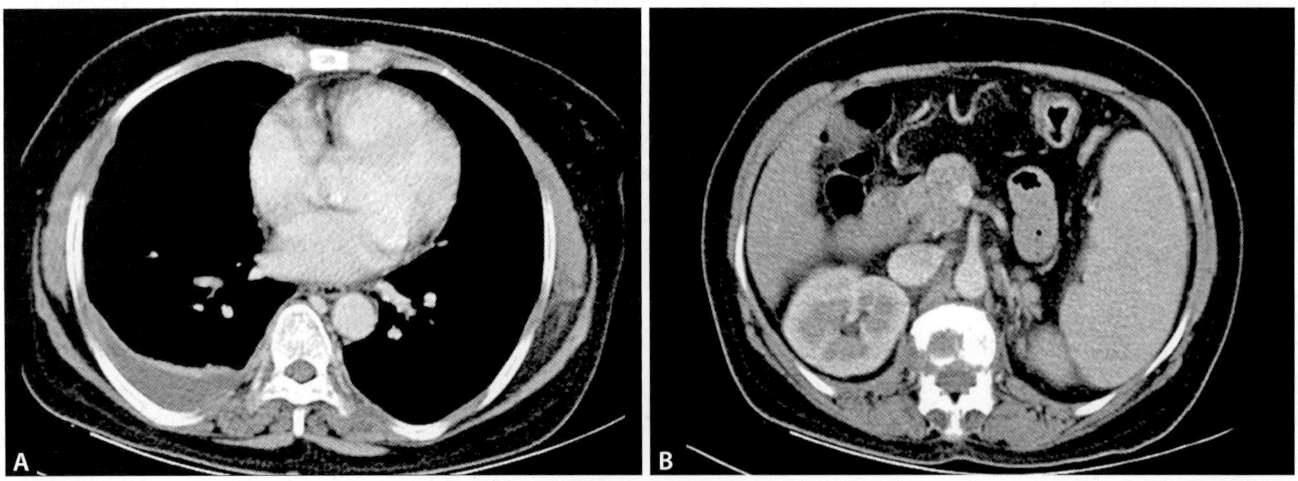

Figs. 19A and B

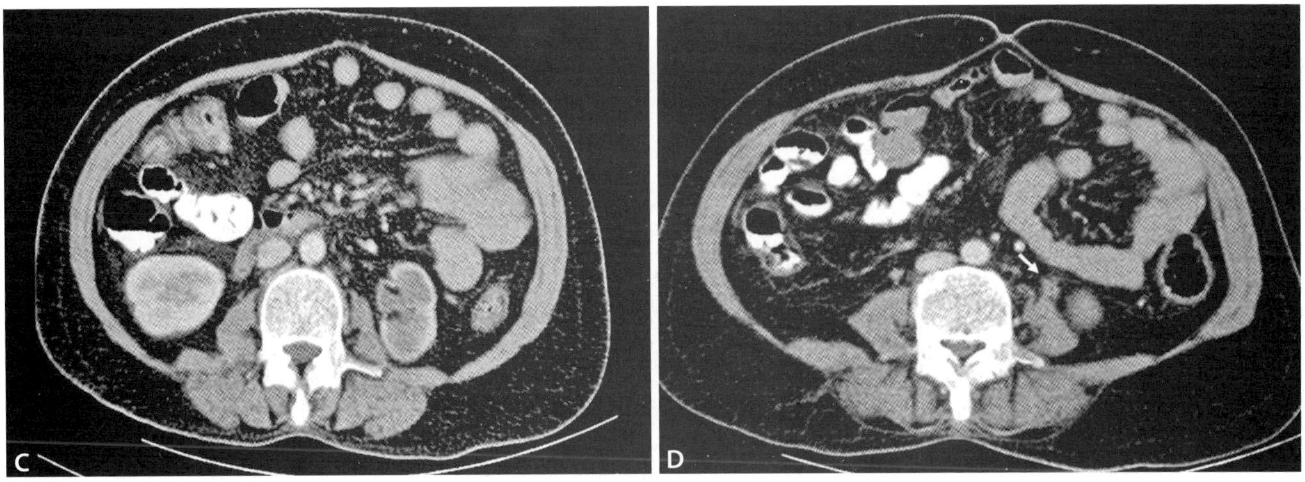

Figs. 19C and D

Figs. 19A to D: CECT of a 43-year-old female reveals right pleural effusion (A); destruction of L2 vertebra (B); left kidney is shrunken with hydronephrosis, scarred pelvis and parenchymal thinning (C); wall thickening of ureter (arrow) is present (D).

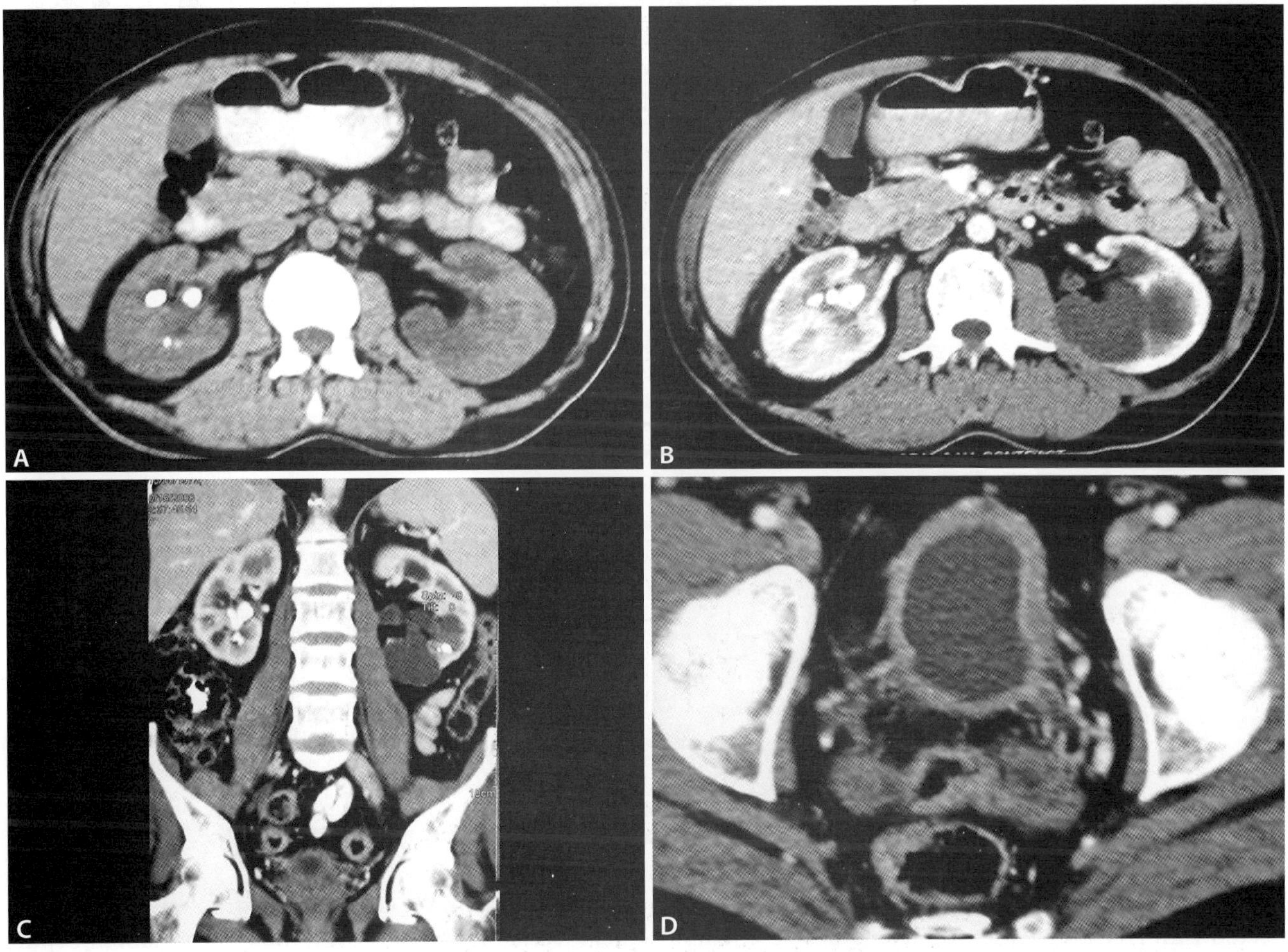

Figs. 20A to D: MDCT axial (A and B) and coronal (C) show a large cavity with irregular caliectasis and calcification involving the lower pole of left kidney. Right kidney has calculi. Scan through pelvis (D) reveals urinary bladder thickening with enlarged heterogeneous seminal vesicles.

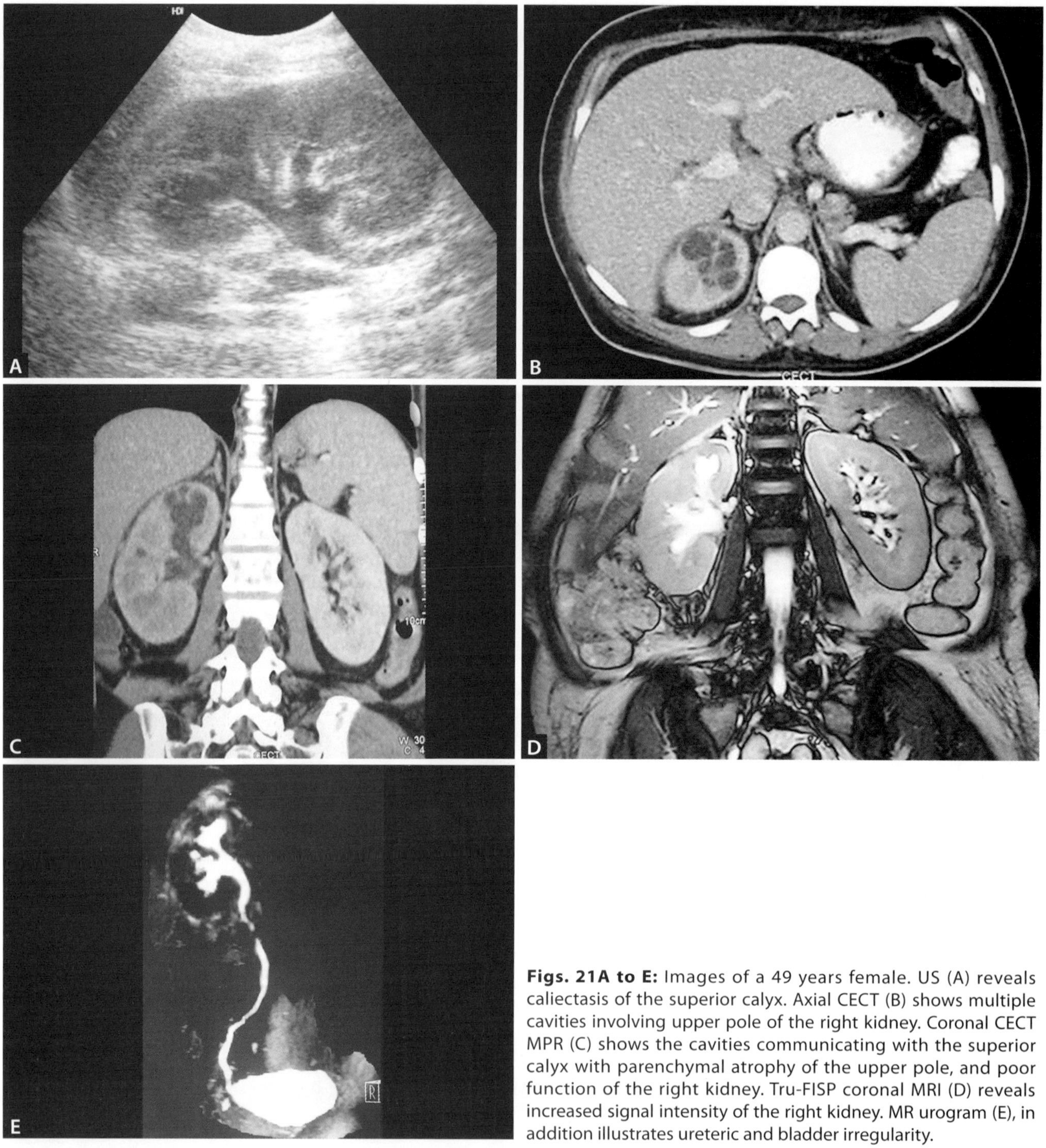

Figs. 21A to E: Images of a 49 years female. US (A) reveals caliectasis of the superior calyx. Axial CECT (B) shows multiple cavities involving upper pole of the right kidney. Coronal CECT MPR (C) shows the cavities communicating with the superior calyx with parenchymal atrophy of the upper pole, and poor function of the right kidney. Tru-FISP coronal MRI (D) reveals increased signal intensity of the right kidney. MR urogram (E), in addition illustrates ureteric and bladder irregularity.

a retrospective study from USA, case records of 16 patients infected with HIV and genitourinary TB were compared with those of 8 patients without HIV infection diagnosed with genitourinary TB. Data abstracted from records included demographics, symptoms, signs, laboratory and radiologic findings, and in-hospital mortality. Of 1,282

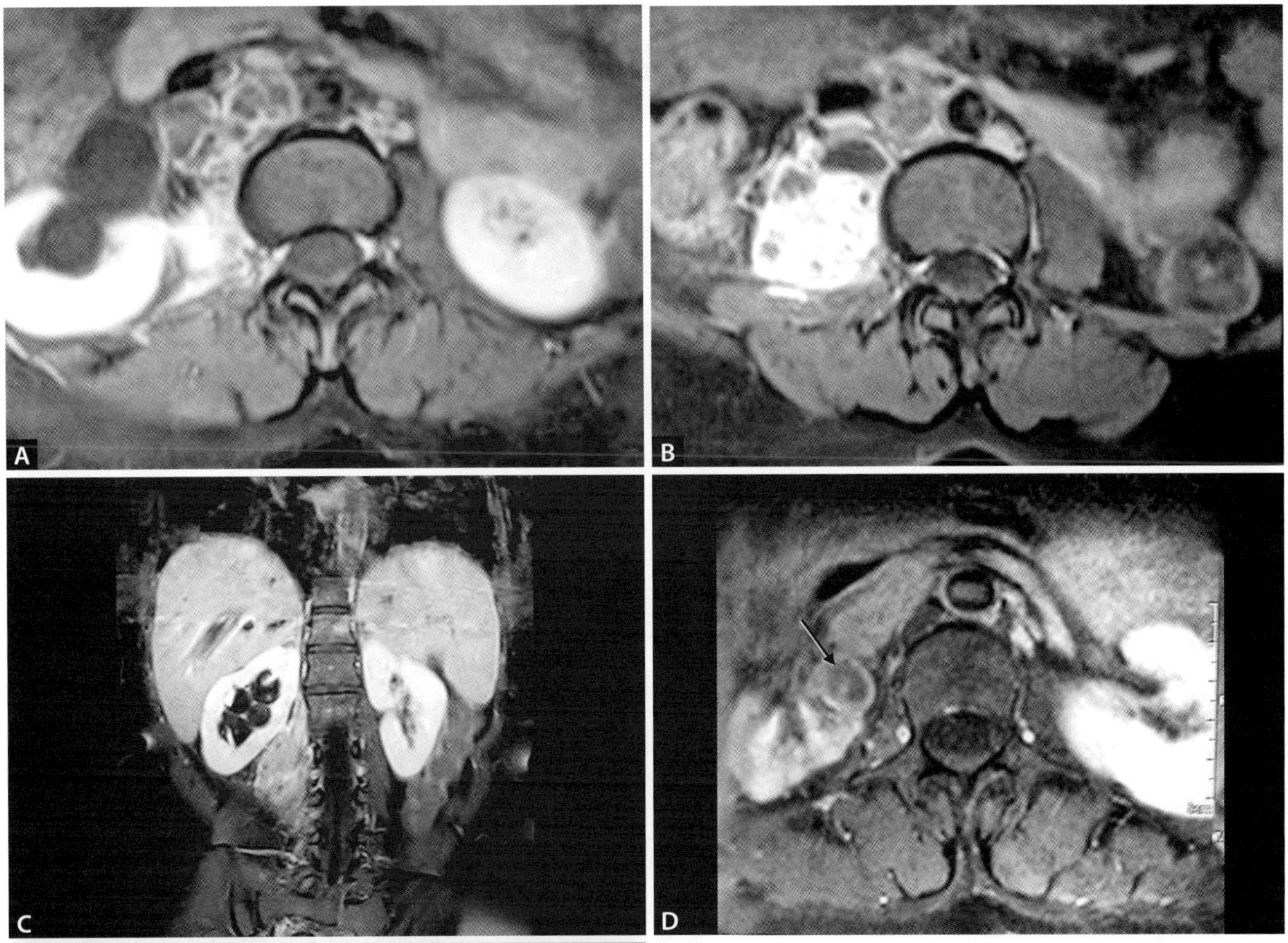

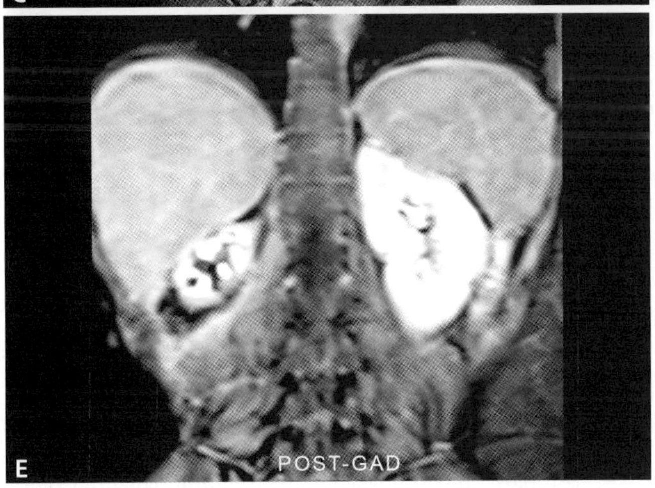

Figs. 22A to E: Serial gadolinium-enhanced MR images of a 28-year-old woman of multidrug-resistant tuberculosis. Axial (A and B) and coronal (C) postgadolinium images reveal necrotic retroperitoneal nodes with right psoas abscess encasing the ureter and causing hydronephrosis. MR scan obtained 8 months after second line ATT (D and E) shows reduction of the lymphadenopathy and psoas abscess. The right kidney is however shrunken and has a rim-enhancing lesion in the renal cortex suggesting an abscess (arrow).

patients with tuberculosis, 24 patients had positive urine cultures for *Mycobacterium tuberculosis.* HIV infection was present in 16 patients (75%). Patients infected with HIV were younger (mean age, 39.1 +/- 6.2 versus 53.9 +/- 17.2, P = 0.047) but did not differ significantly in clinical presentation from patients who did not have HIV infection.[24,25]

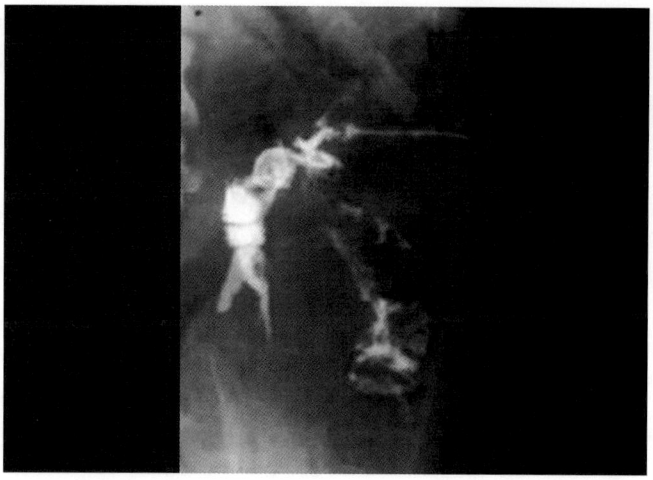

Fig. 23: Sinogram performed in a 28 years man with a chronic discharging (L) lumbar sinus reveals opacification of the pelvicalyceal system.

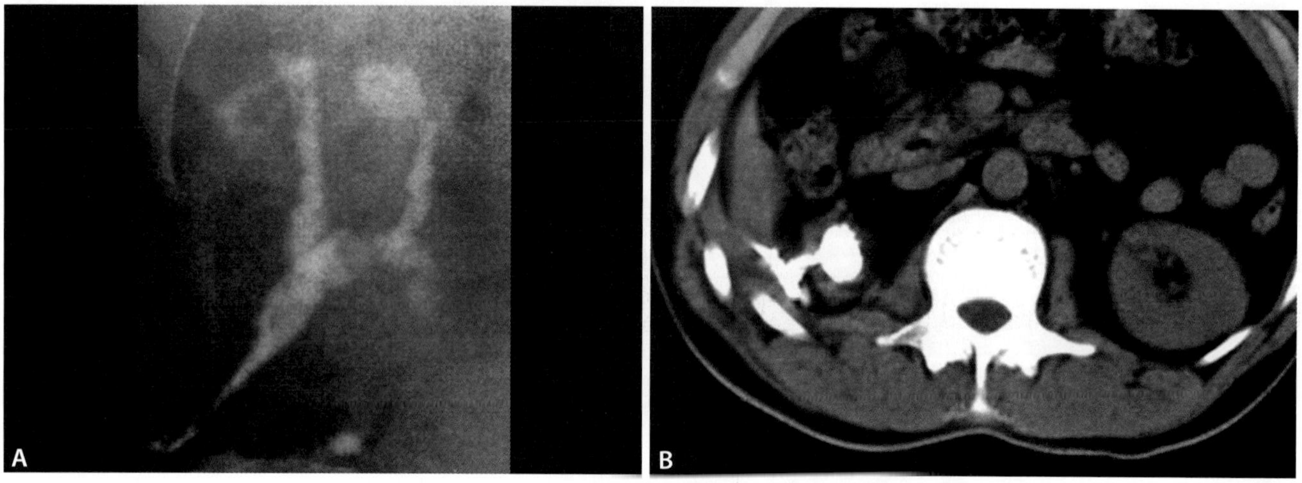

Figs. 24A and B: Sinogram (A) and CT sinogram (B) of a different patient show a shrunken right kidney, with sinus tract extending from the calyces to the skin.

REFERENCES

1. Colabawalla BN. Diagnostic evaluation in renal tuberculosis. Indian J Surg. 1978;40:109-12.
2. World Health Organization. Stop TB annual report 2001 Geneva, Switzerland: World Health Organization; 2002.
3. Leder RA, Low VH. Tuberculosis of the abdomen. Radiol Clin North Am. 1995;33:691-705.
4. Naidich DP, Garay SH, Leitman BS, Mc Gauley DI. Radiographic manifestations of pulmonary disease in the acquired immunodeficiency syndrome. Semin Roentgen. 1987;12:14-30.
5. Wise GJ, Shteynshlyuger A. An update on lower urinary tract tuberculosis. Curr Urol Rep. 2008;9(4):305-13.
6. Wise GJ, Marella VK. Genitourinary manifestations of tuberculosis. Urol Clin North Am. 2003;30(1):111-21.
7. Chan DS, Choy MY, Wang S, Sng LH An evaluation of the recovery of mycobacteria from urine specimens using the automated Mycobacteria Growth Indicator Tube system (BACTEC MGIT 960). J Med Microbiol 2008;57(Pt 10):1220-2.
8. Hemal AK, Gupta NP, Rajeev TP, et al. Poly-merase chain reaction in clinically suspected genitourinary tuberculosis: Comparison with intravenous urography, bladder biopsy and urine acid fast bacilli culture. Urology. 2000;56(4): 570-4.
9. Premkumar A, Lattimer J, Newhouse JH. CT and sonography of advanced urinary tract tuberculosis. AJR. 1987;148:65-9.
10. Navarro-Vilasaró M, Font B, Sala M, Prera A, Malet A, Mariscal D, Segura F. Genitourinary mycobacteriosis: Retrospective study of 45 cases in a general hospital. Enferm

Infecc Microbiol Clin. 2008;26(9):540-45. Article in Spanish, abstract in PubMed.
11. Goldman SM, Fishman EK, Hartman DS, Kim YC, Siegelman SS. Computed tomography of renal tuberculosis and its pathological correlates. J Comput Assist Tomogr. 1985;9:771-6.
12. Hyup S. Urogenital tuberculosis. In Pollack HM, McClennan BL (Eds): Clinical Urography Textbook (2nd Edn) Philadelphia: WB Saunders Co. 2000;2:1193-228.
13. Dalla Palma L. What is left of IV urography? Eur Radiol. 2001;11(6):931-9.
14. Kollins SA, Hartman GW, Carr DT, et al. Roentgenogrpahic findings in urinary tract tuberculosis: a 10-year review. Am J Roentgenol. 1974;121:487-96.
15. Merchant SM. Tuberculosis of the genitourinary system. In: Diagnostic Radiology and Imaging, 2nd edition. New Delhi: Jaypee Brothers Medical Publishers (P) Ltd; 2003,1997. pp.627-56.
16. Narayan AS. Overview of renal tuberculosis. Urology 1982;19:231-7.
17. Wasserman NF. Inflammatory disease of the ureter. Radiol Clin North Am 1996;34(6):1131-56.
18. Camilien LD, Boyce JG. Diagnostic imaging of gynecological disease—the clinicians view. Urol Radiol 1991;13:3-8.
19. Das KM, Indudhara R, Vaidyanathan S. Sonographic features of genitourinary tuberculosis. AJR. 1992;158:327-9.
20. Schaffer R, Becker JA, Goodman J. Sonography of tubercular kidney. Urology. 1983;22:209-11.
21. Fan ZM, Zeng QY, Huo JW, et al. Macronodular multi-organs tuberculoma: CT and MR appearances. J Gastroenterol. 1998;33(2):285-8.
22. Xuefang Rui, Xin-De Li, SongLiang Cai, Geming Chen and Baisen Cai Ultrasonographic diagnosis and typing of renal tuberculosis. International Journal of Urology. 2008;15:135-9.
23. Kim S, Jacob JS, Kim DC, Rivera R, Lee VS. Time-resolved dynamic contrast-enhanced MR urography for the evaluation of ureteral peristalsis: initial experience. J Magn Reson Imaging. 2008;28(5):1293-8.
24. Nzerue C, Drayton J, Oster R, Hewam-Lowe K. Genitourinary tuberculosis in patients with HIV infection: Clinical features in an inner-city hospital population. Am J Med Sci. 2000;320(5):299-303
25. Becker JA. Renal tuberculosis. Urol Radiol. 1988;10:25-30.

CHAPTER **105**

Nontubercular Infections of the Urinary Tract

Naveen Kalra, Ajay Kumar

INTRODUCTION

With the availability of US, CT, MRI, nuclear medicine and advances in interventional radiology, diagnosis and management of the renal and perirenal infections have undergone dramatic changes. Plain X-ray and intravenous urography (IVU) have a declining role whereas ultrasonography (US), computed tomography (CT) and magnetic resonance imaging (MRI) play a vital role in detection and delineation of the extent of renal infectious diseases.

The diagnosis of pyelonephritis is based on typical clinical features and laboratory findings.[1,2] Radiological imaging is generally not performed in uncomplicated cases. However, indication of early imaging in suspected cases of urinary tract infection (UTI) includes unusual severe symptoms, high-risk patients (elderly, diabetics or immunocompromised and patient not responding to intravenous antibiotics within 72 hours).[3] The main objectives of imaging in UTI are (i) to detect the conditions that must be cured immediately, i.e. pyonephrosis, abscesses to preserve renal function and to avoid septic condition, (ii) to search for primary etiological cause of UTI, i.e. obstruction, vesicoureteral reflux (VUR), diabetes, cyst infection.[1,2]

Plain X-ray may provide diagnostic information, such as presence of abnormal gas collection in the renal or perirenal area **(Fig. 1)** in patients with emphysematous pyelonephritis and renal abscess or stag-horn calculus in a patient suspected to have pyonephrosis. IVU has a limited role and can exclude congenital anomalies which are important risk factors in patients of recurrent urinary tract infections. Certain conditions like papillary necrosis and early tuberculosis may be diagnosed only on IVU.[4]

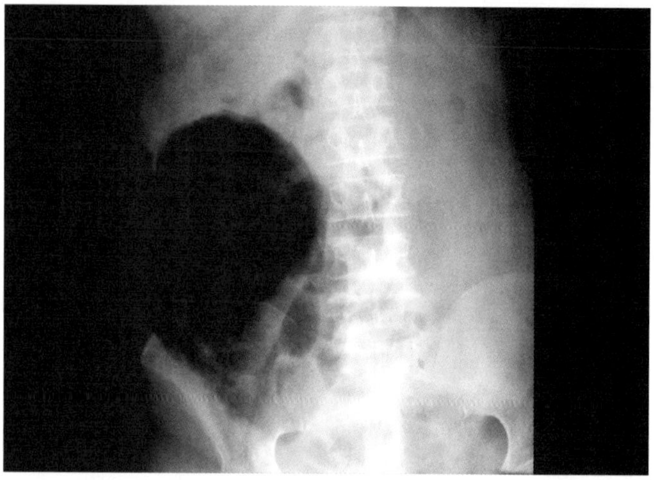

Fig. 1: Plain X-ray abdomen showing a large loculus of air overlying the right renal area in a diabetic patient with extensive emphysematous pyelonephritis.

Ultrasonography has 98% sensitivity in detection of hydronephrosis[5] and is of particular value in patients of renal failure in whom use of contrast media may be hazardous. Extrarenal fluid collections are easily detected, and it is the ideal guiding modality for various interventional procedures such as nephrostomy or cyst aspiration. Limitations of the ultrasound include its inability to detect the subtle changes of microabscesses,[6] small calculi,[7] and papillary necrosis.

CT is the gold standard for diagnosis as well as for delineating the extent of renal infective diseases.

MRI is being increasingly used as an effective modality for both medical and surgical diseases of kidney especially in pregnant women, in patients with renal failure where iodinated contrast cannot be used and in diabetics.[3] The cost and limited availability precludes its routine use, although it provides information similar to CT.

Radionuclide studies with cortical scintigraphy agents, such as ^{99m}Tc DMSA and glucoheptonate have been shown to be the most sensitive techniques for the diagnosis of acute pyelonephritis and detection of the renal scars in reflux nephropathy.[8]

Renal infections can be divided into acute and chronic infections. Acute infections include acute pyelonephritis and its various complications, such as focal bacterial nephritis (FBN), renal abscess, emphysematous pyelonephritis, papillary necrosis and pyonephrosis. Chronic renal infections include chronic pyelonephritis, reflux nephropathy, xanthogranulomatous pyelonephritis, malacoplakia, squamous metaplasia, cholesteatoma.

ACUTE PYELONEPHRITIS

Acute pyelonephritis refers to an inflammatory process affecting the collecting system and the renal interstitium. Inflammation is usually bacterial but may be fungal or viral. *Escherichia coli*, *Proteus* and *Klebsiella* are the common offenders when transmission of infection occurs by the ascending route. Hematogenous infections occur especially in drug addicts and patients with endocarditis. They are usually staphylococcal in origin. Predisposing factors include prolonged catheter drainage, reflux, obstruction, congenital anomalies, diabetes and pregnancy. Ninety percent of urinary tract infections occur as a single attack with 10% being recurrent.[3] Pyelonephritis is more common in sexually active women and there is also a peak increase in men over 60 years due to urinary stasis secondary to prostatic hyperplasia.[3]

Pathology

The affected kidney is enlarged due to edema, and there are multiple foci of inflammation which are characteristically patchy and may lead to microabscesses. With treatment, focal areas of inflammation usually resolve completely, but in the presence of diabetes or other risk factors and inadequate treatment, the infection progresses to result in bacterial nephritis which may be focal or diffuse and may further progress to renal and perirenal abscess.

Radiology

Imaging is usually not required for uncomplicated cases of acute pyelonephritis. The role of IVU in acute pyelonephritis has rapidly diminished. It is used when CT is not readily available. About 75% of all affected uncomplicated patients have normal urograms. Only 25% of cases of acute pyelonephritis will have positive IVU findings.[1,3] IVU may show global or focal renal enlargement with decreased, delayed, and persistent nephrogram. Pelvicalyceal system may show minimal dilatation or attenuation of the calyces. In severe cases, the picture may resemble renal vein thrombosis or replacement of the renal tissue with tumor. Ultrasound reveals focal or diffuse enlargement of the kidney with low level echoes and loss of corticomedullary (CM) differentiation. The advent of newer and more user friendly US contrast agents has helped better demonstrate areas of poor perfusion related to nephritis. Power Doppler is superior to color Doppler in defining extent of hypoperfusion. USG is considered the modality of choice for pregnant patients.[3] Biphasic/triphasic CECT is superior to both USG and IVU in detecting perinephric fluid collection, obstruction, renal enlargement and inflammatory masses. The CT nephrogram (at 20–45 sec) is felt to be superior in depicting the full extent of the disease and in general defines the abnormalities of acute pyelonephritis the best. Secretory phase (after 2 min) is useful to detect any sloughed papilla or fungus balls. The sensitivity and specificity of CT is about 86.8% and 87.5%, and of USG is 74.3% and 6.7%, respectively.[3] CECT may reveal wedge-shaped areas of decreased attenuation radiating from papilla due to hypoperfusion in an enlarged kidney **(Fig. 2)**. The transverse areas of alternate bands with

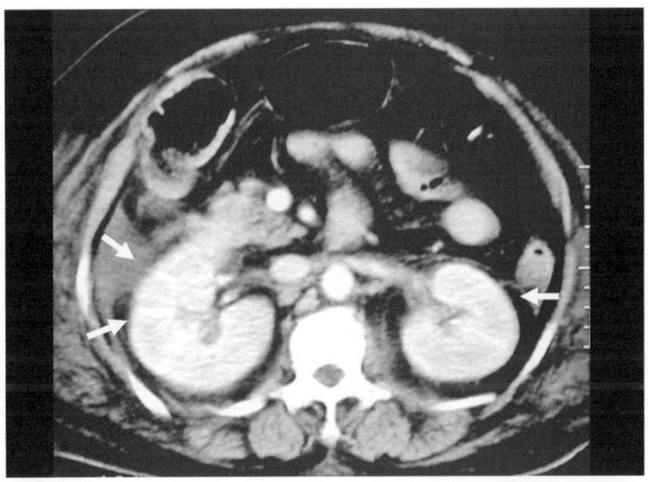

Fig. 2: Contrast-enhanced CT scan shows bilateral enlarged kidneys with striated nephrogram (arrows) suggestive of acute pyelonephritis. There is presence of perinephric stranding and thickening of Gerota's fascia and lateral conal fascia.

increased and decreased density represent microstriations due to vasoconstriction and renal edema. Dalla-Palma et al.[9] have described the role of delayed CT in outlining the true extent of renal infection. Three types of changes were seen on delayed scans: (a) a delayed nephrogram with streaky, wedge-shaped or round high density areas seen at the same site as the reduced density on early scans, (b) focal staining or a hyperdense rim surrounding abscesses and (c) focal areas of increased density distant from the low density areas seen on early scans. These features made it possible to better define the actual extent of infection. Scintigraphic techniques are considered superior to US and IVU for the diagnosis of acute pyelonephritis.[10] Renal cortical scintigraphy with ^{99m}Tc DMSA reveals wedge-shaped cortical defects. On MR imaging the affected area has low-signal on T1WI and increased signal on T2WI with loss of CMD. MRI features of pyelonephritis mimic those of CT. MRI may also help in differentiating acute infection from chronic scar. The potential pitfalls of MR imaging are in patients with gas forming infections and calculi with the inability of MR to distinguish between the two.[3]

ACUTE FOCAL BACTERIAL NEPHRITIS

An IVU reveals presence of a focal renal mass which on follow-up IVU may reveal an area of focal scarring due to healing opposite a normal or clubbed calyx. US reveals hypoechoic poorly defined mass with internal echoes **(Fig. 3A)**. The mass will be echogenic if there is hemorrhage.

CT shows focal low density area with patchy enhancement **(Fig. 3B)**. Lack of well-defined wall and central low density differentiates it from the renal abscess. Changes of acute pyelonephritis may be seen in the rest of the kidney, which may not have been detected on IVU or ultrasound.

RENAL AND PERIRENAL ABSCESS

Renal and perirenal abscess usually develops as a complication of focal bacterial pyelonephritis but may result from haematogenous infection or superadded infection in a renal cyst or direct involvement of the perinephric space from pancreas, colon, and retroperitoneum. Plain X-ray abdomen in a case of renal abscess shows renal enlargement, rotation, displacement, presence of mottled gas in the renal areas, and loss of psoas outline. IVU generally shows poorly or nonfunctioning kidney with calyceal attenuation and compression due to mass affect **(Figs. 4A and B)**. US may reveal a well-defined complex mass with good sound transmission **(Figs. 5A and B)**. Bright echoes with dirty distal shadowing are seen in the presence of air. However, these findings are nonspecific and may be seen in infected, hemorrhagic cysts or necrotic neoplasms.

CT is the gold standard to assess the renal as well as extrarenal extent of the renal abscess. Changes in the renal contour, parenchymal density, enhancement pattern and perinephric abnormalities such as thickening of the Gerota's fascia, psoas muscle involvement are best seen on CT **(Fig. 6)**. Presence of nonenhancing poorly marginated area of decreased attenuation may be seen during the earlier course of renal abscess **(Fig. 5B)**. This may be surrounded by an area of decreased enhancement

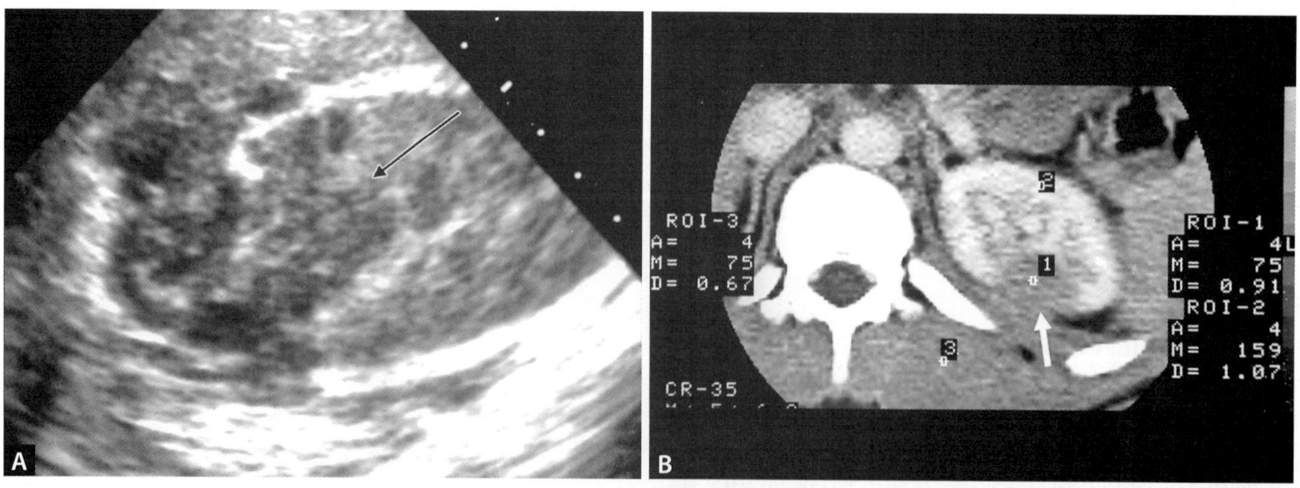

Figs. 3A and B: (A) Longitudinal ultrasound scan of the kidney showing poorly defined hypoechoic lesion with low level internal echoes in the upper polar region (arrow) which was due to focal bacterial nephritis; (B) Contrast-enhanced CT scan of another patient showing a focal low density area with patchy enhancement in the posterior aspect of upper pole of left kidney (arrow).

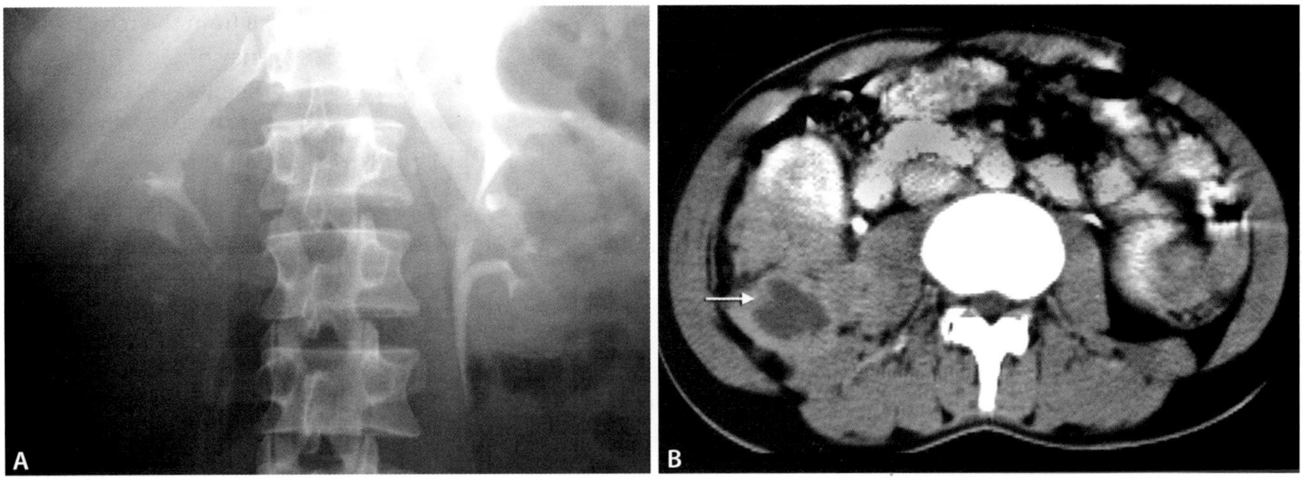

Figs. 4A and B: (A) IVU showing a mass impression on the collecting system of the upper pole and pelvis due to a right renal abscess. The lower group of calyces are not visualized. The psoas shadow on the ipsilateral side is also obliterated; (B) Contrast-enhanced CT scan of the same patient showing an absent nephrogram in the lower pole with a liquefied collection in the perinephric space (arrow) extending medially into the right psoas muscle.

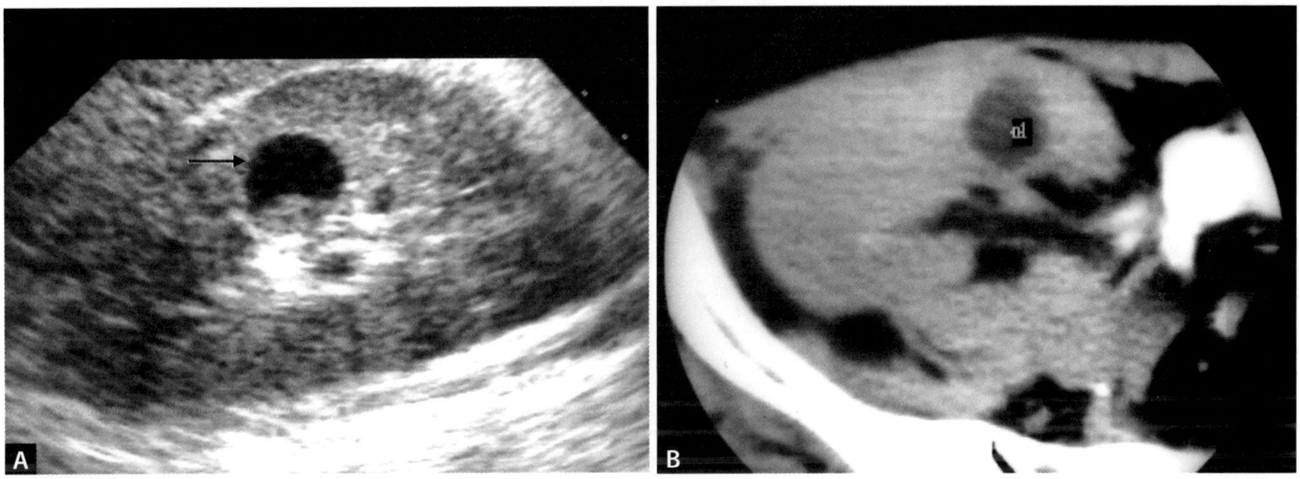

Figs. 5A and B: (A) Longitudinal ultrasound scan of the transplant kidney shows an anechoic lesion with internal debris in the interpolar region (arrow) suggestive of abscess; (B) Contrast-enhanced CT scan of the same patient shows a well-defined hypodense lesion in the anterior parenchyma with minimal peripheral contrast enhancement.

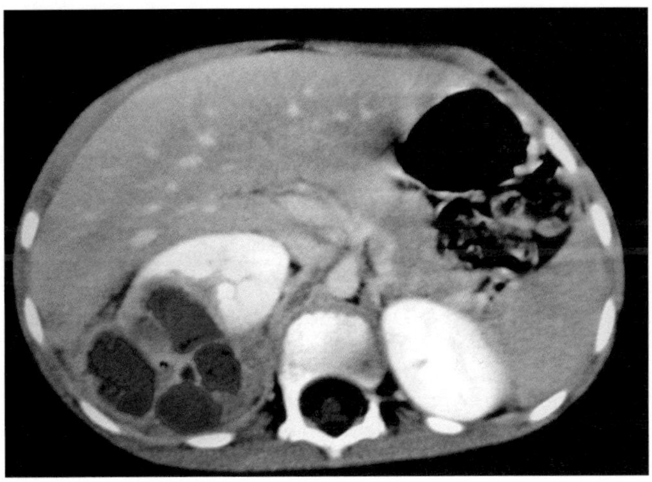

Fig. 6: Contrast-enhanced CT scan showing multiple low density lesions with rim enhancement in the right kidney suggestive of renal abscess with extension into the perinephric space.

due to presence of infected renal parenchyma. Later in the course of the disease, renal abscess appears as a sharply marginated area of low attenuation due to necrosis surrounded by a peripheral enhancing rim indicating a mature abscess **(Fig. 6)**. On MRI, a renal abscess is seen as a hypointense lesion on T1WI and a hyperintense lesion on T2WI. On gadolinium administration the lesion shows peripheral enhancement **(Figs. 7A to C)**. Differential diagnosis includes segmental renal infarct, metastasis, lymphoma, trauma, and renal vein thrombosis. Percutaneous drainage has decreased the mortality with a success rate of 85–95%.[11]

EMPHYSEMATOUS PYELONEPHRITIS

Emphysematous pyelonephritis (EPN) indicates severe renal infection with gasforming organisms characterized by presence of gas in the collecting system or renal parenchyma. It is commonly seen in diabetics and patients with ureteral obstruction. Radiologically emphysematous pyelonephritis can be divided into two types: Type I which is less common (33%), has parenchymal destruction and shows streaky/mottled gas in interstitium of renal parenchyma radiating from medulla to cortex, crescent of subcapsular/perinephric gas with no fluid collection. Type II is more common (66%) and shows bubbly/loculated intrarenal gas, renal/perirenal fluid collections and gas within the pelvicalyceal system. Prognosis wise former has worse prognosis having 69% mortality with the latter having mortality of only 18%.

Plain X-ray can demonstrate air specks in renal area in over 85% of cases. However this is frequently misinterpreted as bowel gas. There can be diffuse mottled appearance over the renal shadow with radially oriented air within, corresponding to renal pyramids. The crescent shaped air indicates the extension into perinephric space suggesting the advanced stage. IVU is rarely performed these days, but when performed, reveals a poorly functioning or nonfunctioning kidney. US examination reveals dense echoes with dirty shadowing in intrarenal infection. If the gas enters the perinephric space, there will

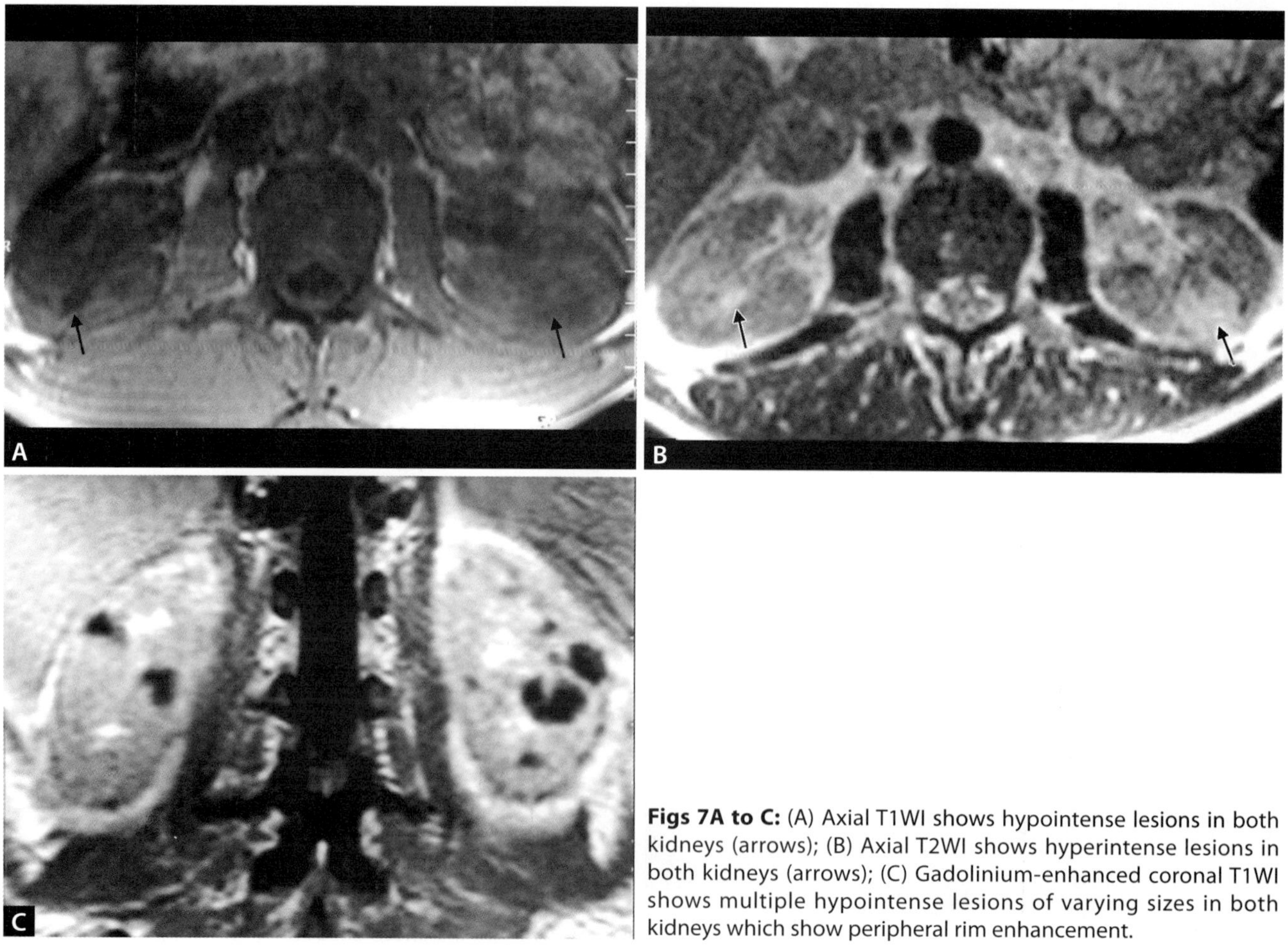

Figs 7A to C: (A) Axial T1WI shows hypointense lesions in both kidneys (arrows); (B) Axial T2WI shows hyperintense lesions in both kidneys (arrows); (C) Gadolinium-enhanced coronal T1WI shows multiple hypointense lesions of varying sizes in both kidneys which show peripheral rim enhancement.

be nonvisualization of kidney (gassed out kidney). CT is ideal to assess the renal as well as perirenal extent **(Fig. 8)**. It detects the presence of air, its precise location within the kidney as well as its extension into the perirenal or pararenal compartments of the retroperitoneal space. The role of MRI is limited as gas appears as an area of signal loss which cannot be differentiated from calculi, renal calcification and flowing blood on T1- and T2WI.

PYONEPHROSIS

Pyonephrosis is the term used to describe infection in an obstructed collecting system with suppurative destruction of the renal parenchyma. Obstruction may be due to renal calculi, stricture or tumor. US is the modality of choice to detect dilated collecting system which contains dependent echoes and shifting debris **(Fig. 9A)**. Plain X-ray of the abdomen may show enlarged kidney with or without stones. IVU shows a nonfunctioning kidney. CT is ideal to show intrarenal changes and the perirenal extension. High density of urine in the dilated system should suggest infection **(Figs. 9B and C)**. Thickening of the renal pelvic wall may be detected both on US or CT. Ultrasound guided aspiration may be performed to confirm the diagnosis as well as obtain specimen for culture and sensitivity. Percutaneous nephrostomy may also be performed under US guidance to provide immediate decompression of the collecting system as an adjunct prior to definitive surgery. In case of fungal pyonephrosis, direct infusion of amphotericin B may be accomplished through the PCN catheter. This may be preferable to systemic amphotericin which is more toxic.

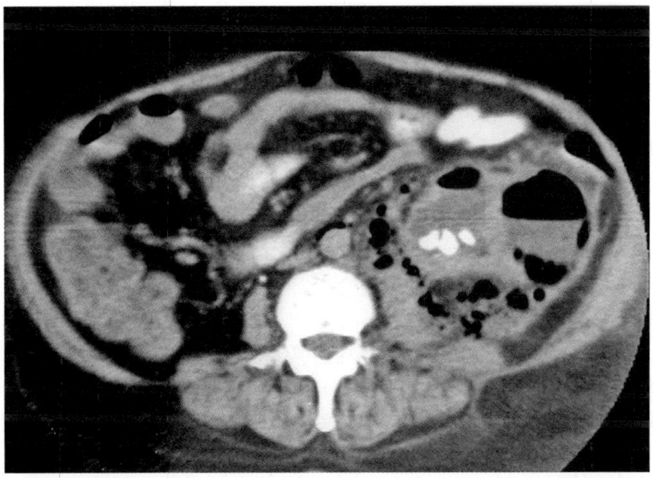

Fig. 8: Contrast-enhanced CT scan showing left renal calculi and dilated collecting system with dense urine suggestive of pyonephrosis. In addition extensive collection of air is seen in the renal parenchyma and perinephric space with extension around the aorta due to emphysematous pyelonephritis.

CHRONIC PYELONEPHRITIS

Chronic pyelonephritis refers to the chronic inflammation of the kidney characterized by cortical scarring overlying the involved calyx (usually polar). Entire collecting system may be involved resulting in small kidney with clubbed calyces **(Fig. 10)**. The opposite kidney may enlarge due to compensatory hypertrophy. Inflammation is generally patchy and the uninvolved areas of parenchyma may hypertrophy to cause mass effect (pseudotumor) which may require scintigraphy for confirmation. Differential diagnosis includes fetal lobulation, ischemia and hypoplastic kidney. In ischemia the adjacent calyx is normal. In fetal lobulation, the scars are in between the calyces. In congenital hypoplastic kidney the number of calyces are less than five.

REFLUX NEPHROPATHY

Reflux nephropathy results from combined effects of the vesicoureteric reflux and bacterial infection. The disease process begins in infancy and childhood, and is more common in females. Due to incompetent papillary duct orifices, there is intrarenal reflux of infected urine which leads to destruction of the tubules and subsequent scarring. Despite the low radiation dose to the patient during radionuclide cystogram, studies have suggested that fluoroscopic voiding cystourethrogram is a better technique to detect and grade the degree of reflux which is an important factor to determine the future treatment planning in these children.[12] In a child with repeated attacks of urinary tract infection, US is still considered the best screening tool to detect obstructive uropathy—an important factor placing the child at risk for recurrent infections and subsequent postinfectious nephropathy. Renal cortical scintigraphy is the best technique to detect renal scarring. Doppler US and power Doppler may be as useful as DMSA scanning for the detection of scarring. Dacher et al.[13] showed that power Doppler US could be used to detect acute pyelonephritis in children. They demonstrated peripheral triangular areas of decreased renal perfusion in these patients. Presence of vesicoureteric reflux needs to be excluded in all these children.

FAT PROLIFERATION IN THE KIDNEY

Sinus fat may increase as a normal phenomenon in an aging kidney, renal sinus lipomatosis (RSL) or it may completely replace the renal parenchyma which is

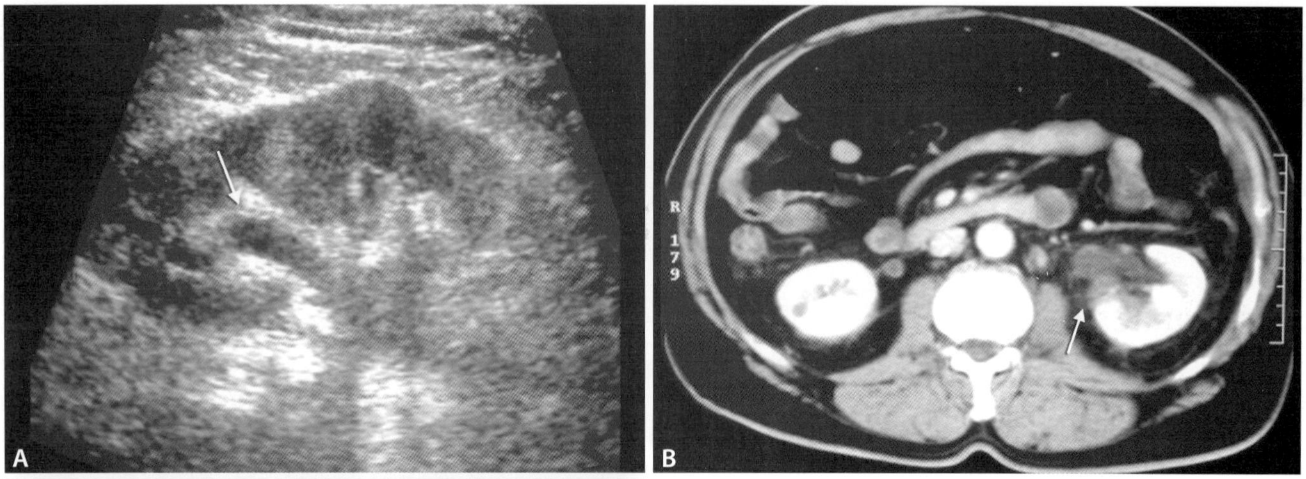

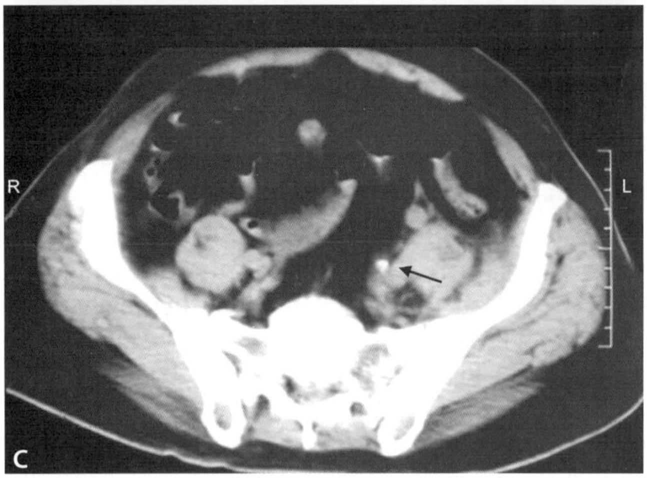

Figs. 9A to C: (A) Longitudinal ultrasound scan of right kidney showing dilated collecting system filled with echogenic material and thickened echogenic uroepithelium (arrow) suggestive of pyonephrosis; (B) Contrast-enhanced CT scan shows hydronephrosis of left kidney with presence of high density urine and perinephric and periureteric stranding (arrow); (C) Caudal axial section in the same patient shows a left lower ureteric calculus (arrow).

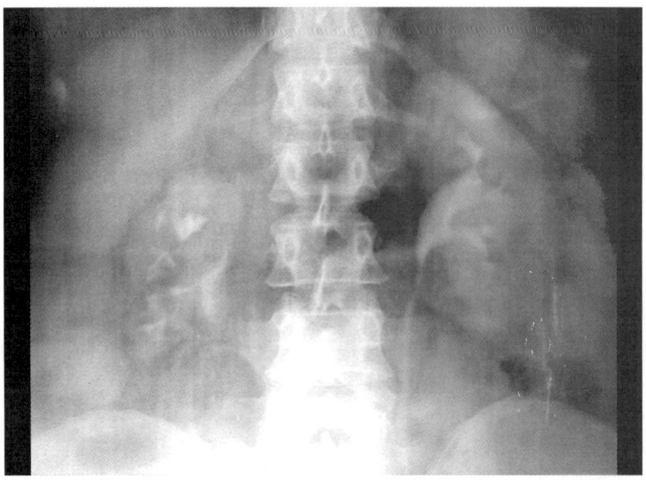

Fig. 10: Excretory urogram showing small irregular right kidney with dilated and distorted calyces and thinned out parenchyma, especially opposite the polar calyces.

destroyed by chronic inflammation (renal replacement lipomatosis).

RSL is usually seen in patients with extrarenal pelvis. The calyces are stretched and elongated, but there is no hydronephrosis and kidneys are otherwise normal. Differentiation from a parapelvic cyst may require ultrasonography which shows extensive echogenicity in case of RSL whereas parapelvic cyst is sonolucent. On CT, RSL may mimic parapelvic cyst and hydronephrosis **(Fig. 11)**.

In renal replacement lipomatosis, plain film frequently reveals calculi. IVU may show absent or poor excretion of contrast with stretched calyces. CT confirms the presence of fat in an atrophic kidney containing calculi. US also shows increased echogenicity indicating fat. Differential diagnosis includes fatcontaining tumors, such as angiomyolipoma.

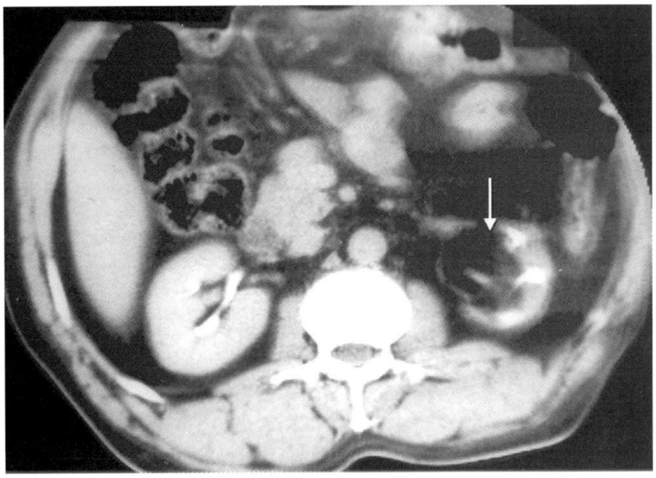

Fig. 11: Contrast-enhanced CT scan shows an enlarged renal sinus (arrow) with fat attenuation on the left side suggestive of renal sinus lipomatosis. The fat attenuation differentiates renal sinus lipomatosis from parapelvic cyst.

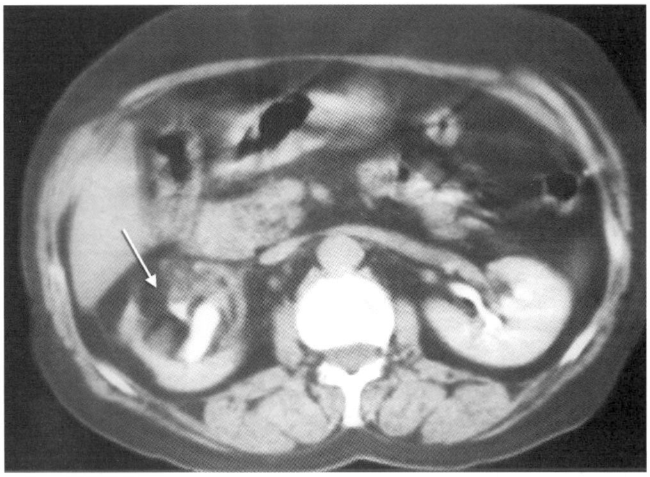

Fig. 12: Contrast-enhanced CT scan shows right renal calculi with a well-defined mass lesion with multiple fat attenuation areas (arrow) characteristic of xanthoma cell collection in a case of xanthogranulomatous pyelonephritis.

XANTHOGRANULOMATOUS PYELONEPHRITIS

Xanthogranulomatous pyelonephritis (XGPN) is a rare chronic granulomatous inflammation of the kidney usually seen in patients who have stones and obstruction. The disease is characterized by destruction and replacement of the renal parenchyma with lipidladen macrophages which are para-aminosalicylic acid (PAS)-positive (xanthoma cells). The condition is more common in women frequently presenting with mass in the renal area. Two types of the disease, i.e. focal and diffuse have been described. Pathologically depending on the extent, three stages have been described: in stage I, kidney alone is involved; in stage II, there is extension into Gerota's fascia; and in stage III, perinephric spaces are also involved.

Imaging features include presence of staghorn calculus and/or also small calcifications scattered throughout the kidney which may be detected on plain X-ray or CT. IVU reveals evidence of a focal mass (tumefactive type), or diffusely enlarged nonfunctioning kidney. Presence of lucent areas on X-ray and nonenhancing cystic areas on CT corresponding to the xanthoma cell collection is characteristic **(Fig. 12)**. Renal vein may be thrombosed. Perinephric extent is best seen on CT. US findings include multiple anechoic or hypoechoic areas with central echogenic foci corresponding to the fine calcification. Small cystic collection due to cortical abscesses may be seen. Differential diagnosis from pyonephrosis, tuberculosis, cystic carcinoma, and lymphoma may at times be difficult.

HIV-ASSOCIATED NEPHROPATHY

HIV can affect any organ of the body and the kidneys have been increasingly shown to be involved by a variety of disease processes in HIV infection. Kidneys may be involved as a collapsing glomerulopathy (HIVAN) or due to secondary infections by bacteria or opportunistic organisms, such as *Pneumocystis carinii* and cytomegalovirus. HIV-associated nephropathy (HIVAN) is a serious disorder which results in rapidly progressive renal failure. It manifests histologically as focal glomerulosclerosis and as membranous, membranoproliferative, and mesangial proliferative glomerulonephritis.[14] Imaging reveals renal enlargement (>13 cm) with increased echogenicity on US. However, Atta et al.[15] found that only renal echogencity and not kidney size has diagnostic utility for HIVAN. On CECT enlarged kidneys with striated nephrogram are seen.[16,17] On unenhanced CT scans, hyperattenuating medulla may be seen as a result of dilated protein filled tubules. Imaging findings may suggest the diagnosis of HIVAN, but it should be confirmed on histology. *Pneumocystis carinii* infection results in punctate areas of calcification within the renal parenchyma similar to those seen with cytomegalovirus or *Mycobacterium avium intracellulare* (MAI).[18]

RENAL PAPILLARY NECROSIS

Most common cause of renal papillary necrosis is analgesic abuse and diabetes. The other causes include urinary tract infection (UTI), renal vein thrombosis, obstruction, dehydration, and sickle cell disease. IVU remains the best technique for demonstrating the changes of papillary necrosis. Presence of extracalyceal contrast, ill-defined calyx, contrast outlining sloughed papillae (ring sign), and filling defect in the calyx or calcification of the papilla may be seen. The sloughed papillae may pass down the collecting system and ureter, and present radiological picture of obstruction.

MALACOPLAKIA

Malacoplakia is a rare granulomatous inflammatory disease seen almost exclusively in women who present with repeated attacks of UTI. Bladder and ureter are most frequently affected. Radiological features include enlarged poorly functioning kidney with presence of filling defect in the bladder and the ureter, similar to the changes seen in pyeloureteritis cystica, or transitional cell carcinoma. Strictures may also form, thus tuberculosis is an important differential diagnosis. Renal involvement results in focal or multiple masses indistinguishable from renal cell carcinoma or XGPN on US, CT or IVU. Diagnosis is usually based on pathology which reveals van Hanseman cells and Michaelis Gutman bodies in the nodular deposits.

SQUAMOUS METAPLASIA

Squamous metaplasia is the replacement of normal transitional cell epithelium by squamous epithelium as a result of infection. The condition is characterized by the presence of multiple linear radiolucencies in the ureter due to mucosal thickening resulting in so called "tree barking" or "Corduroy appearance" in IVU or RGU.

The term, cholesteatoma is used when there is a filling defect in the collecting system due to sloughed keratinized material. The filling defect on CT has a high attenuation value due to small punctate calcification which differentiates the condition from carcinoma and other causes of filling defects such as sloughed papillae, radiolucent stones, and fungus ball.

Fungal and *parasitic infections* of the kidney are rare, occurring generally in patients with impaired immune status such as diabetics, renal transplants and other chronic infections and on prolonged steroid therapy. Infection by *Candida, Aspergillus, Cryptococcus,* and *Mucor* has been described. Presence of bilateral poorly functioning/non-functioning enlarged kidneys with multiple low density areas located both in the cortex and medulla on CT should raise the possibility of the diagnosis of mucormycosis.[19] Both *Aspergillus* and *Mucor* are angioinvasive fungi and cause thrombosis of the large as well as small arteries which results in infarction and necrosis of the affected organs. The infection usually occurs by hematogenous route resulting in multiple abscesses which appear as low density areas in the renal parenchyma, and there may be perinephric spread **(Fig. 13)**.

PARASITIC INFECTION

Schistosoma usually affects the bladder causing calcification. Renal pelvic striations may be seen. Intrarenal hydatids are rare and appear as focal cystic masses which are usually thick walled and irregular, and may show calcification of crushed eggshell pattern **(Figs. 14A to C)**.

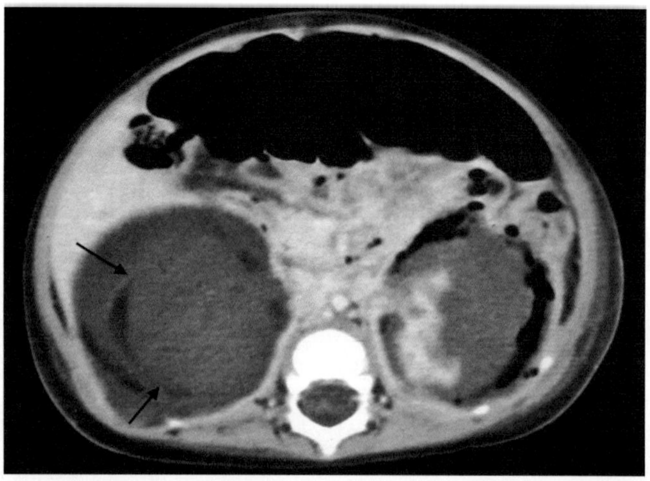

Fig. 13: Contrast-enhanced CT scan of a 2-year-old child with proven mucormycosis who presented with renal failure. The right kidney is enlarged and nonfunctioning (arrows) with evidence of perinephric collection. The left kidney shows functioning renal parenchyma on the medial aspect with presence of air in the perinephric space.

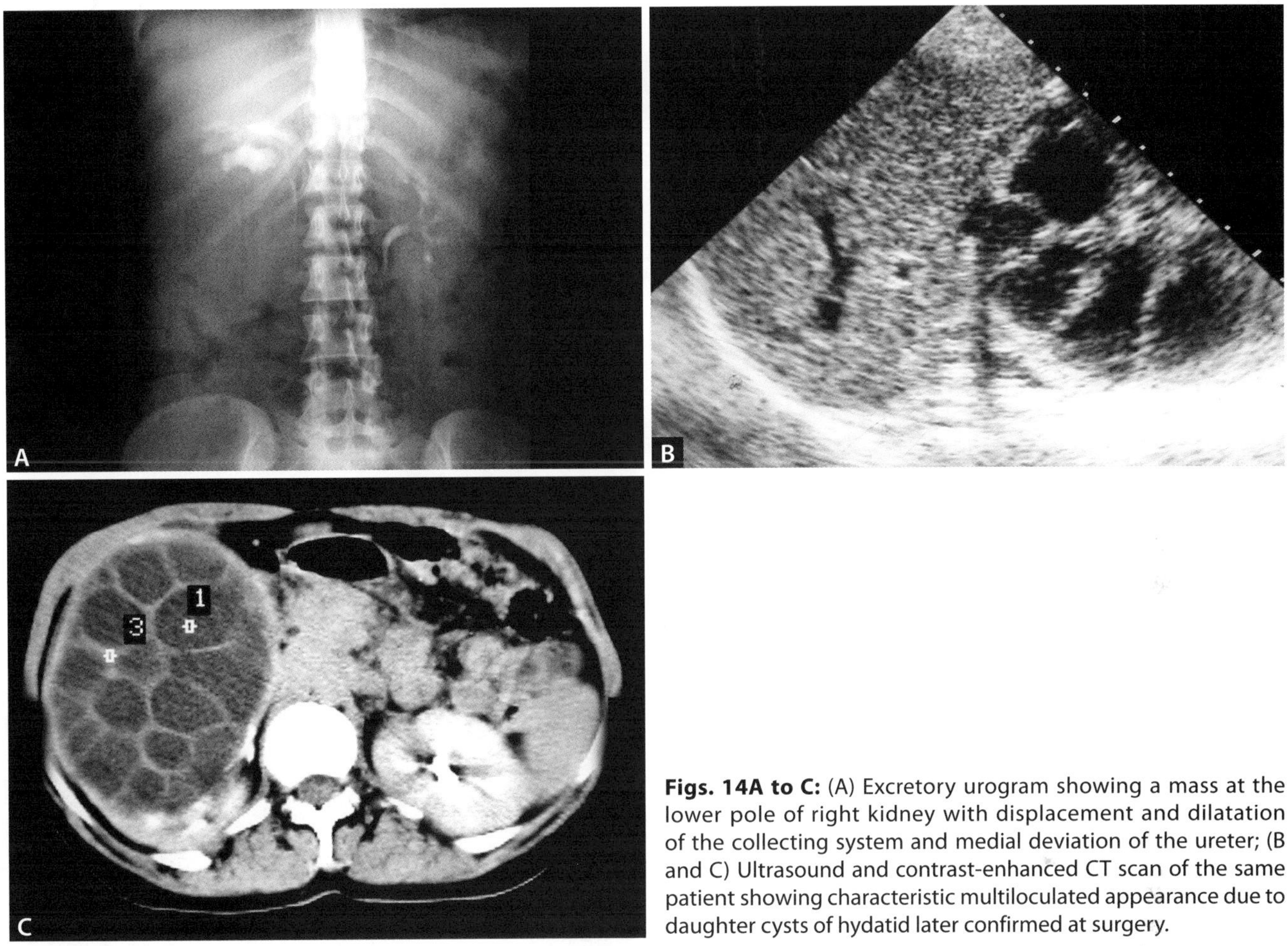

Figs. 14A to C: (A) Excretory urogram showing a mass at the lower pole of right kidney with displacement and dilatation of the collecting system and medial deviation of the ureter; (B and C) Ultrasound and contrast-enhanced CT scan of the same patient showing characteristic multiloculated appearance due to daughter cysts of hydatid later confirmed at surgery.

REFERENCES

1. Kawashima A, Sandler CM, Goldman SM. Imaging in acute renal infection. BJU International. 2000;86(Suppl 1):70-9.
2. Bjerklund Johansen TE. The role of Imaging in urinary tract infections. World J Urol. 2004;22:392-8.
3. Stunell H, Buckley O, Feeney J, et al. Imaging of acute pyelonephritis in the adult. Eur Radiol. 2007;17:1820-8.
4. Merenich WM, Popky GL. Radiology of renal infection. Med Clin N Am. 1991;75:425-69.
5. Ellenbogen PH, Schieble FW, Talner LB, et al. Sensitivity of gray scale ultrasound in detecting urinary tract obstruction. AJR. 1978;130:731-3.
6. Wicks JD, Thornbury JR. Acute renal infections in adults. Radiol Clin N Am. 1979;12:245-60.
7. Laing FC, Jeffrey RB (Jr), Wing VW. Ultrasound versus excretory urography in evaluating acute flank pain. Radiol. 1985;154:613-6.
8. Conway JJ. The role of scintigraphy in urinary tract infection. Semin Nucl Med. 1998;18:308-19.
9. Dalla-Palma L, Pozzi-Mucelli R, Pozzi-Mucelli F. Delayed CT in acute renal infection. Semin Ultrasound CT MR. 1997;18:122-8.
10. Talner LB, Davidson AJ, Lebowitz RL, et al. Acute pyelonephritis—can we agree on terminology? Radiol. 1994;192:297-305.
11. Van Sonnenberg E, D'Agostino HB, Sanchez RB, et al. Percutaneous abscess drainage. Radiol. 1992;184:27-9.
12. Kass EJ,Kernen KM, Carey JM. Paediatric urinary tract infection and the necessity of complete urological imaging. BJU Int. 2000;86:94-6.
13. Dacher JN, Pfister C, Monroc M, et al. Power Doppler sonographic pattern of acute pyelonephritis in children: comparison with CT. AJR. 1996;166:1451-5.
14. Symeonidou C, Standish R, Sahdev A, et al. Imaging and histopathologic features of HIV-related renal disease. Radiographics. 2008;28:1329-54.
15. Atta MG, Longenecker JC, Fine DM, et al. Sonography as a predictor of human immunodeficiency virus-associated nephropathy. J Ultrasound Med. 2004;23:603-10.
16. Kuhlman JE, Browne D, Shermak M, et al. Retro-peritoneal and pelvic CT of patients with AIDS: Primary and secondary involvement of the genitourinary tract. Radiographics. 1991;11:473-83.
17. Miller FH, Parikh S, Gore RM, et al. Renal manifestations of AIDS. Radiographics. 1993;13:587-96.
18. Bray HJ, Lail VJ, Cooperberg PL. Tiny echogenic foci in the liver and kidney in patients with AIDS: Not always due to disseminated *Pneumocystis carinii*. AJR. 1992;158:81-2.
19. Chugh KS, Sakhuja V, Gupta KL, et al. Renal mucormycosis: computerized tomographic findings and their diagnostic significance. Am J Kidney Dis. 1993;22(3):393-7.

CHAPTER 106

Pathology of Renal Tumors

Kusum Joshi

INTRODUCTION

Cancer of the kidney amounts to 2% of the total human cancers and occur in both adults and children, although the frequency of the cancer types is quite different in the two populations. Although renal tumors can be completely removed surgically, hematgenous spread may occur at an early stage of the disease. The pattern of somatic mutations in kidney tumors has been investigated extensively and has been incorporated, along with histopathology, in the classification of kidney tumors.

Currently, the recent WHO classification (2004) is most acceptable for use and incorporates the cytogenetic features where required.

Since the prevalence of renal tumors is distinctly different in adults and children, the following discussion will be under the subheadings of adult renal tumors and pediatric renal tumors. The following discussion is not a complete review of all types of adult and pediatric renal tumors, but rather a discussion on the common and important ones and those peculiar to the kidney.

ADULT RENAL TUMORS

Renal Cell Tumors

Renal cell carcinoma (RCC) is the most common malignant tumor to arise in the kidney and is responsible for 2% of all new cancers diagnosed, representing 85% of all primary renal neoplasms in adults **(Fig. 1)**. Renal cell carcinoma is a group of malignancies arising from the epithelium of the renal tubules. A male predominance exists with a male to female ratio of 1.6:1.0 and the peak incidence occurs in the sixth and seventh decades of life. In rare cases, RCC can also occur in children and adolescents. A study from India quotes that renal tumors constitutes 10.64% of all the malignant tumors of male urogenital tract or 1.51% of all the male cancers. The mean age of the cases for renal cell carcinoma was 50.3 years in this Indian study. An increased incidence of RCC is associated with end-stage renal disease and with acquired cystic kidney disease. The classic triad of presenting symptoms include hematuria, pain, and flank mass, but nearly 40% of patients

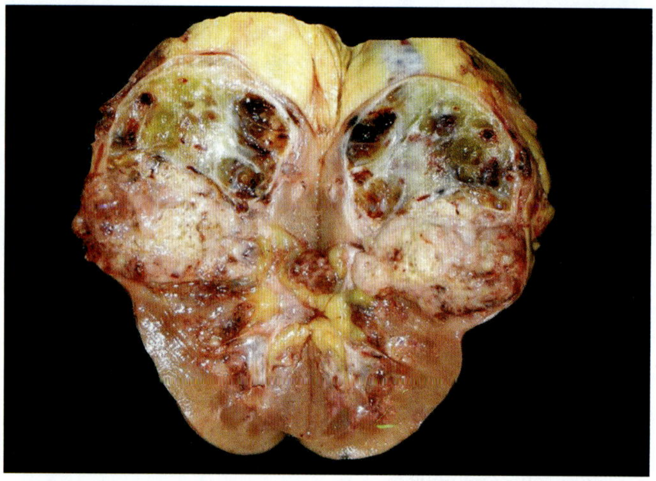

Fig. 1: Variegated gross appearance of renal cell carcinoma.

lack all of these and present with systemic symptoms, including weight loss, abdominal pain, anorexia, and fever. Normocytic anemia unrelated to hematuria occurs in about 33% of cases. Hepatosplenomegaly, coagulopathy, eleva-tion of serum alkaline phosphatase, trans-aminase, and α2-globulin concentrations may occur in the absence of liver metastases and may resolve when the renal tumor is resected. Systemic amyloidosis of the AA type occurs in about 3% of patients. Renal cell carcinoma may induce para-neoplastic endocrine syndromes, including hypercalcemia of malignancy (pseudohyperparathyroidism), erythrocytosis, hypertension, and gynecomastia. Hypercalcemia without bone metastases occurs in approximately 10% of patients and in nearly 20% of patients with disseminated carcinoma. RCCs have been regarded as a single entity in the past; however, cytogenetic and molecular studies have proven conclusively that these are group of distinguishable entities, as seen from **Table 1**.

Clear Cell (or Nonpapillary or Conventional) Renal Cell Carcinoma

This is the most common form of RCC, comprising 60% of cases. Male preponderance of 2:1 is seen and mean age at presentation is 61 years. Clear cell RCCs are solitary and randomly distributed cortical tumors which arise at equal frequency in either of the kidney. Multicentricity and/or bilaterality occur in less than 5% of cases. Clear cell RCCs are typically globular tumors which commonly protrude from the renal cortex as a rounded, bosselated mass. The interface of the tumor and the adjacent kidney is usually well demarcated, with a "pushing margin" and pseudocapsule. Diffuse infiltration of the kidney is uncommon. The average size is 7 cm in diameter. Clear cell RCC appears golden yellow because of the rich lipid content of its cells; cholesterol, neutral lipids, and phospholipids are abundant. Cysts, necrosis, hemorrhage, and calcification are

Table 1: WHO histological classification of renal tumors.

Renal Cell Tumors • Clear cell renal cell carcinoma • Multilocular clear cell renal cell carcinoma • Papillary renal cell carcinoma • Chromophobe renal cell carcinoma • Carcinoma of the collecting ducts of Bellini • Renal medullary carcinoma • Xp11 translocation carcinomas • Carcinoma associated with neuroblastoma • Mucinous tubular and spindle cell carcinoma • Renal cell carcinoma, unclassified • Papillary adenoma • Oncocytoma **Metanephric Tumors** • Metanephric adenoma • Metanephric adenofibroma • Metanephric stromal tumor **Nephroblastic Tumors** • Nephrogenic rests • Nephroblastoma • Cystic partially differentiated nephroblastoma **Mesenchymal Tumors** **Occurring Mainly in Children** • Clear cell sarcoma • Rhabdoid tumor • Congenital mesoblastic nephroma • Ossifying renal tumor of infants **Occurring Mainly in Adults** • Leiomyosarcoma (including renal vein) • Angiosarcoma • Rhabdomyosarcoma	• Malignant fibrous histiocytoma • Hemangiopericytoma • Osteosarcoma • Angiomyolipoma • Epithelioid angiomyolipoma • Leiomyoma • Hemangioma • Lymphangioma • Juxtaglomerular cell tumor • Renomedullary interstitial cell tumor • Schwannoma • Solitary fibrous tumor **Mixed Mesenchymal and Epithelial Tumors** • Cystic nephroma • Mixed epithelial and stromal tumor • Synovial sarcoma **Neuroendocrine Tumors** • Carcinoid • Neuroendocrine carcinoma • Primitive neuroectodermal tumor • Neuroblastoma • Pheochromocytoma **Hematopoietic and Lymphoid Tumors** • Lymphoma • Leukemia • Plasmacytoma **Germ Cell Tumors** • Teratoma • Choriocarcinoma **Metastatic Tumors**

commonly present. About 50% of clear cell RCCs are stage 1 and 2 and less than 5% are stage 4. Invasion of perirenal and sinus fat and/or extension into the renal vein occurs in about 45% of cases. Clear cell RCC mostly metastasize hematogenously through the vena cava primarily to the lungs.

Clear cell RCC is architecturally diverse, with solid, alveolar and acinar patterns, being the most common. If the alveolar and acinar structures dilate, they produce microcystic and macrocystic patterns. The carcinomas typically contain a regular network of small thin-walled blood vessels. The cytoplasm is commonly filled with lipids and glycogen, giving the appearance of a clear cytoplasm surrounded by a distinct cell membrane. Usually, the nuclei are condensed and hyperchromatic. Sarcomatoid change occurs in 5% of tumors and is associated with worse prognosis. Clear cell RCCs frequently react with antibodies to brush border antigens, low molecular weight cytokeratins, CK8, CK18, CK19, AE1, Cam 5.2 and vimentin. The majority of clear cell RCCs react positively for RCC marker, CD10 and epithelial membrane antigen. MUC1 and MUC3 are consistently expressed. Electron microscopic features resembling the proximal tubule can be found, i.e. brush border formation and basal infoldings **(Fig. 2)**.

Multilocular Cystic Renal Cell Carcinoma

This tumor is composed entirely of numerous cysts, the septa of which contain small groups of clear cells indistinguishable from grade 1 clear cell carcinoma. There is male predominance with male: female ratio of 3:1 and age range of 20-76 years with a mean of 51 years. These tumors have excellent prognosis. Multilocular cystic RCC consists of a well-circumscribed mass ranging in size from 25 to 130 mm and is composed of small and large cysts filled with serous or hemorrhagic fluid separated from the kidney by a fibrous capsule **(Fig. 3)**. The cysts are usually lined by a single layer of epithelial cells or occasionally by several layers of cells and even form papillae or may altogether lack an epithelial lining. The lining cells may be flat or plump and their cytoplasm ranges from, clear to pale. The nuclei almost always are small, spherical, and have dense chromatin (Fuhrman grade 1 or 2).

Papillary (or Chromophilic) Renal Cell Carcinoma

These tumors usually arise from the proximal tubule and comprise 7–14% of RCC cases. Papillary renal cell tumors can be divided into adenomas and carcinomas. Papillary adenomas are tumors with papillary or tubular architecture of low nuclear grade and 5 mm in diameter or smaller. Papillary adenomas are the most common neoplasms of the epithelium of the renal tubules. Autopsy studies have found that papillary adenomas increase in frequency in adulthood from 10% in patients younger than 40 years to 40% in patients older than 70 years. Papillary adenomas are well circumscribed, yellow to grayish white nodules as small as less than 1 mm in diameter in the renal cortex occurring just below the renal capsule. Usually, papillary adenomas are solitary, but occasionally they are multiple and bilateral. When they are numerous, this has been termed as "renal adenomatosis". Papillary adenomas have tubular, papillary, or tubulopapillary architecture. They are considered as a putative precursor of papillary renal cell

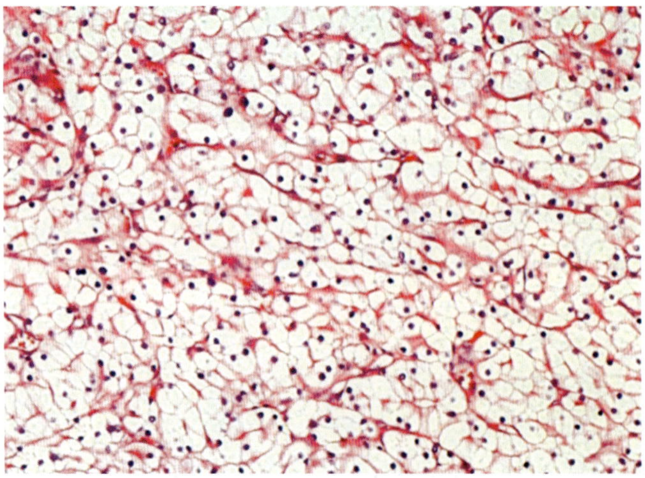

Fig. 2: Photomicrograph showing clear cell with grade 1 nuclei in a classical case of renal cell carcinoma.

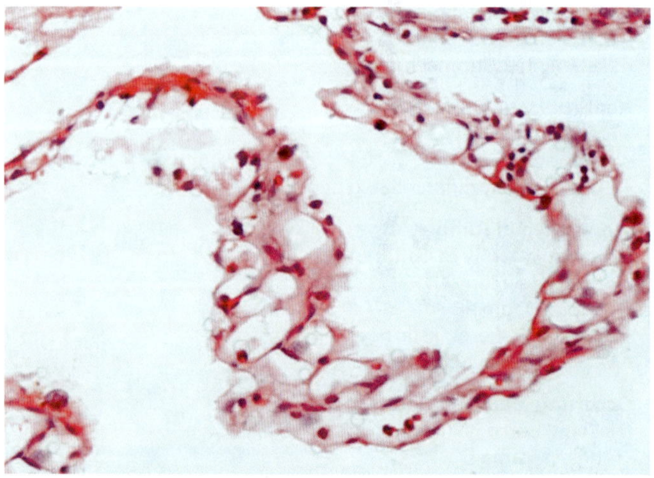

Fig. 3: Multilocular cystic renal cell carcinoma showing clear tumor cells in the septum.

carcinoma (PRCC). Bilateral and multifocal tumors are more common in PRCC than in other renal parenchymal malignancies. The tumor papillae contain a delicate fibro-vascular core and aggregates of foamy macrophages and cholesterol crystals may also be present. Occasionally, the papillary cores are expanded by edema or hyalinized connec-tive tissue. Solid variants of PRCC consist of tubules or short papillae resembling glomeruli. Hemosiderin granules may be present in macrophages, stroma and tumor cell cytoplasm. Two morphological types of PRCC have been described:

Type 1 tumors: They have papillae covered by small cells with scanty cytoplasm, arranged in a single layer on the papillary basement membrane **(Fig. 4)**.

Type 2 tumor cells: They are often of higher nuclear grade with eosinophilic cytoplasm and pseudostratified nuclei on papillary.

Type 1 tumors are more frequently multifocal. Sarcomatoid dedifferentiation is seen in approximately 5% of PRCC and has been associated with both type 1 and type 2 tumors. Cytokeratin 7 (CK 7) expression has been reported for PRCC however, this is more frequently observed in type 1 (87%) than type 2 (20%) tumors. For both conventional and papillary RCC, there has been discovery of both hereditary and sporadic cases. The common characteristics of hereditary RCC are the appearance of multiple and bilateral tumors and an early age of onset. There is no specific grading system for PRCC and the Fuhrman system is accepted as applicable to both clear cell renal cell carcinoma and PRCC.

Chromophobe Renal Cell Carcinoma

The tumor cells resemble and exhibit antigen profile of the intercalated cells type B from the cortical collecting duct. It comprise 6–11% of renal epithelial tumors. The mean age of presentation is in the sixth decade, with age range of 27–86 years, and the incidence in men and women is roughly equal. Mortality is less than 10%. Chromophobe RCC (CRCC) consists of solid tumor nodules with a slightly lobulated surface. In unfixed specimens the cut surface is homogeneously light brown or tan turning light grey after formalin fixation. The majority of CRCCs are stage T1 and T2 (86%) whereas only 10% show extension through the renal capsule into surrounding adipose tissue, and only 4% show involvement of the renal vein. In general, the growth pattern is solid, sometimes glandular, with focal calcifications and broad fibrotic septa. In contrast to clear cell renal cell carcinoma, many of the blood vessels are thick-walled and eccentrically hyalinized. The perivascular cells are often enlarged. Chromophobe renal cell carcinoma is characterized by large polygonal cells with transparent slightly reticulated cytoplasm with prominent cell membranes **(Fig. 5)**. These cells are commonly mixed with smaller cells with granular eosinophilic cytoplasm. The eosinophilic variant of chromophobe carcinoma is purely composed of intensively eosinophillic cells with prominent cell membranes. The cells have irregular, often wrinkled, nuclei and some are binucleated. Nucleoli are usually small and perinuclear halos are common.

Another diagnostic hallmark is a diffuse cytoplasmic staining reaction with Hale's colloidal iron stain. Ultrastructurally, the cytoplasm is surrounded by glycogen

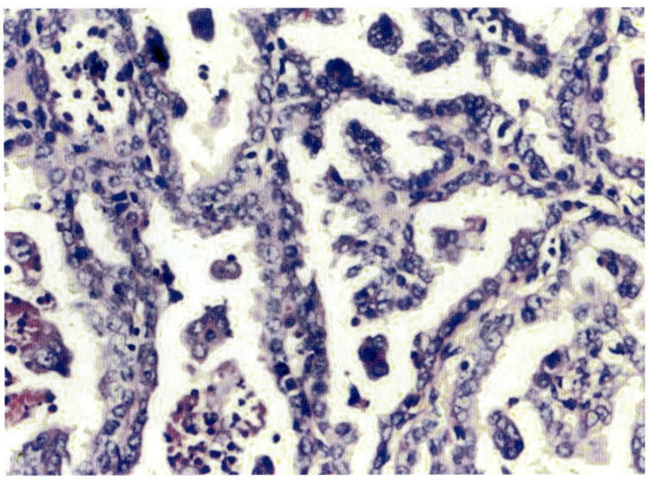

Fig. 4: Photomicrograph of papillary (type 1) renal cell carcinoma.

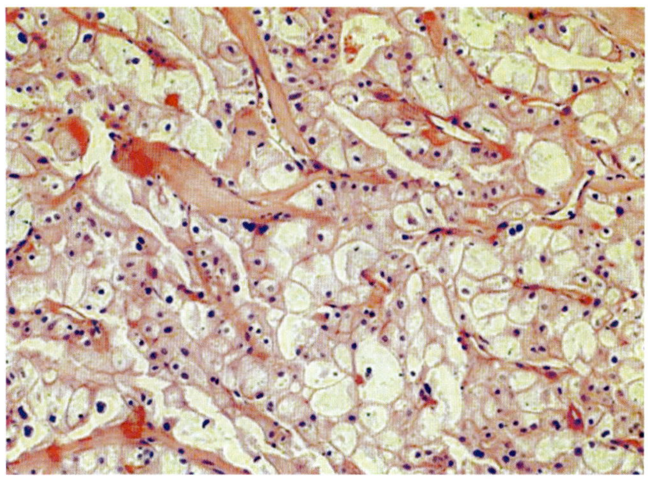

Fig. 5: Microscopic appearance of chromophobe carcinoma showing plant like cells with perinuclear clearing of cytoplasm .

deposits and numerous, sometimes invaginated, vesicles. Chromophobe RCC is positive for carbonic anhydrase C, but does not express band-3 protein.

Collecting Duct (Duct Bellini) RCC (CDC)

This subtype comprises 1% of all RCCs. It is a malignant epithelial tumor thought to be derived from the principal cells of the collecting duct of Bellini. Over 100 cases have been described and there is a wide age range from 13–83 years (mean, about 55) with a male to female ratio of 2:1. Upper tract imaging often suggests urothelial carcinoma and patients may occasionally present with positive urine cytology. Collecting duct carcinomas are usually located in the central region of the kidney. When small, origin within a medullary pyramid may be seen. These tumors typically have a firm gray-white appearance with irregular borders and their size varies from 2.5 to 12 cm. Some tumors grow as masses within the renal pelvis and areas of necrosis, satellite nodules and gross renal vein invasion may be present. Collecting duct carcinomas often display infiltration of perirenal and renal sinus fat. About one third of patients have metastases at presentation to the regional lymph nodes, lung, liver, bone and adrenal gland. The prototypic collecting duct carcinoma has a tubular or tubulopapillary growth pattern in which irregular angulated glands infiltrate renal parenchyma and are associated with a desmoplastic stroma. Criteria for diagnosing collecting duct carcinoma have been proposed. Major criteria include location in a medullary pyramid (small tumors), typical histology with irregular tubular architecture and high nuclear grade, inflammatory desmoplastic stroma with numerous granulocytes, reactive with antibodies to high molecular weight cytokeratin, reactive with ulex europaeus agglutinin 1 lectin and absence of urothelial carcinoma. Minor criteria include central location (large tumors), papillary architecture with wide, fibrous stalks and desmoplastic stroma, extensive renal, extrarenal, and lymphatic and venous infiltration, intratubular epithelial atypia adjacent to the tumor.

Solid, cord-like patterns and sarcomatoid features may be encountered. The sarcomatoid change is a pattern of dedifferentiation similar to that seen in other types of renal carcinoma. The cells of collecting duct carcinoma usually display high grade (Fuhrman 3 and 4) nuclear features. The cells may have a hobnail pattern of growth and the cytoplasm is generally eosinophilic; however, glycogen is usually inconspicuous in collecting duct carcinoma. Both intraluminal and intracytoplasmic mucin may be seen. High molecular weight keratins (34βE12, CK19) are commonly present and coexpression of vimentin may be seen. There is variable immunostaining for CD15 and epithelial membrane antigen. The CD10 and vinculin stains are negative. Lectin histochemistry, usual ulex europaeus agglutinin-1 and peanut lectin are commonly positive.

Renal Medullary Carcinoma

This is a rapidly growing tumor of the renal medulla associated almost exclusively with sickle cell trait. With few exceptions these are seen in young people with sickle cell trait between ages 10 and 40 years (mean 22 years) and chiefly in males by 2:1. These are poorly circumscribed tumors ranging in size from 4–12 cm and arising centrally in the kidney. Most of them show extensive hemorrhage and necrosis. A reticular growth pattern and a more compact adenoid cystic morphology are the common features. The cells are eosinophilic with clear nuclei and usually with prominent nucleoli. The sheets of cells can have squamoid or rhabdoid quality. Neutrophils are often admixed with the tumor and the advancing margins are often bounded by lymphocytes. Keratin AE1/AE3 is nearly always positive as is EMA but typically less strongly so. The prognosis is poor and the mean duration of life after surgery has been 15 weeks.

Renal Carcinomas Associated with XP11.2 Translocations/TFE3 Gene Fusions

These carcinomas are defined by several different translocations involving chromo-some Xp11.2, all resulting in gene fusions involving the TFE3 gene. These carcinomas predominantly affect children and young adults, though a few older patients have been reported. The ASPL-TFE3 carcinomas characteristically present at advanced stage. Renal carcinomas associated with Xp11.2 translocations are mostly tan-yellow, and often necrotic and hemorrhagic. The most distinctive histopathologic appearance is that of a carcinoma with papillary architecture comprised of clear cells; however, these tumors frequently have a more nested architecture, and often feature cells with granular eosinophilic cytoplasm. The ASPL-TFE3 renal carcinomas are characterized by cells with voluminous clear to eosinophilic cytoplasm, discrete cell borders, vesicular chromatin and prominent nucleoli. Psammoma bodies are constant and sometimes extensive, often arising within characteristic hyaline nodules. The PRCC-TFE3 renal carcinomas generally feature less abundant cytoplasm, fewer psammoma bodies, fewer hyaline nodules, and a more nested, compact architecture. The most distinctive immunohistochemical feature of these tumors is nuclear immunoreactivity for TFE3 protein. Only about 50% express epithelial markers such as cytokeratin and EMA by immunohistochemistry, and the labeling is often focal. The tumors consistently label for the RCC marker antigen and CD10. Ultrastructurally, Xp11.2-associated carcinomas most closely resemble clear cell renal carcinomas. Very little is known about the clinical behavior of these carcinomas. While the ASPL-TFE3 renal carcinomas usually present at advanced stage, their clinical course thus far appears to be indolent. However, a recent study by Argani et al. of 28 Xp11 translocation RCC in patients over the age of 20 years gives a somewhat different picture. Patients ranged from ages 22 to 78 years, with a strong female predominance (F : M = 22 : 6). Five of six patients with 1 or more years of follow-up developed hematogenous metastases, with 2 dying within the first year of diagnosis.

Mucinous Tubular and Spindle Cell Carcinoma

This is a recently described rare entity of low aggressive biological behavior, mostly reported in females of any age. It is a well circumscribed tumor, usually located in the medulla and is composed of elongated interconnected tubules, with cords of epithelial cells and interspersed with low grade spindle cell areas. The cells have a bland, monomorphic appearance and stroma can be focally myxoid. It has an ultra-structural resemblance to the Loop of Henle and is nick-named as a "Loopoma".

Renal Cell Carcinoma—Unclassified

Renal cell carcinoma, unclassified is a diagnostic category to which renal carcinomas are assigned when they do not fit readily into any of the other categories. Sarcomatoid change has been found to arise in all types of carcinoma in the classification, as well as in urothelial carcinoma of the renal pelvic mucosa. Since there is no evidence that renal tumors arise *de novo* as sarcomatoid carcinomas, it is not viewed as a type of its own, but rather as a manifestation of high grade carcinoma of the type from which it arose. Occasionally, the sarcomatoid elements overgrow the antecedent carcinoma to the extent that it cannot be recognized; it is appropriate to assign such tumors to renal cell carcinoma, unclassified.

Papillary Adenoma

These tumors are 5 mm or smaller in diameter, of lobular or papillary architecture and of low nuclear grade. These are the most common renal neoplasms, often found incidentally in autopsy studies, particularly in older individuals and in patients on hemodialysis or patients of acquired renal cystic disease. They may be multiple. Microscopically, most tumors are type I, although rare type II tumors are also seen. Karyotypic aberrations of loss of Y chromosome or trisomy of chromosome 7 and 17 have been identified.

Renal Oncocytoma

This subtype is thought to arise from the distal nephron and comprises 5% of RCC and shows a male-to-female ratio of 2.5:1. Oncocytoma is a benign renal epithelial neoplasm composed of large cells with mitochondria-rich eosinophilic cytoplasm, thought to arise from intercalated cells **(Fig. 6)**. Oncocytomas are well-circumscribed, nonencapsulated neoplasms that are classically mahogany-brown and less often tan to pale yellow. A central, stellate scar may be seen in up to 33% of cases but is more commonly seen in larger tumors. Hemo-rrhage is present in up to 20% of cases but grossly visible necrosis is extremely rare. Characteristically, these tumors have solid compact nests, acini, tubules, or microcysts. Often there is a hypocellular hyalinized stroma. The predominant cell type is round to polygonal with densely granular eosino-phillic cytoplasm, round and regular nuclei with evenly dispersed chromatin, and a centrally placed nucleolus. A smaller population of cells with scanty granular cytoplasm, a high nuclear: cytoplasmic ratio, and dark hyperchromatic nuclei may also be observed. Several cases of oncocytosis (Oncocytomatosis) have been reported in which the kidneys have contained a large number of oncocytic lesions with a spectrum of morphologic features, including oncocytic tumors, oncocytic change in benign tubules, microcysts lined by oncocytic cells and clusters of

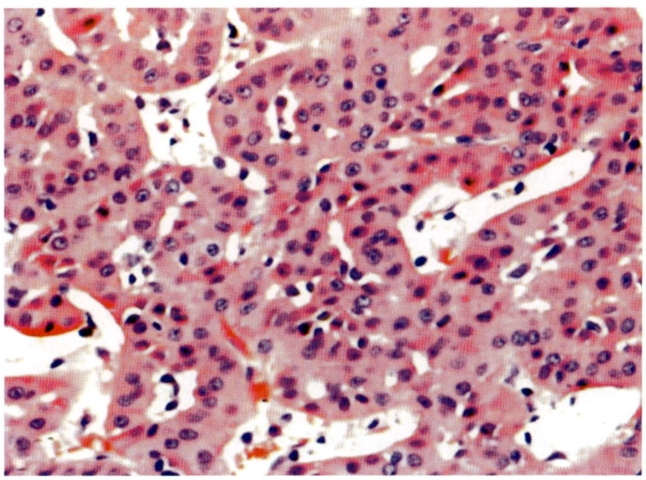

Fig. 6: Microscopic appearance of oncocytoma; cells have abundant granular eosinophilic cytoplasm and monomorphic nuclei.

oncocytes within the renal interstitium. Ultrastructurally, the cytoplasm is packed with numerous mitochondria. Renal oncocytomas originate in the intercalated cells type A of the cortical collecting tubule, which is substantiated by the shared expression of carbonic anhydrase C and band-3 protein.

MOLECULAR/GENETIC FEATURES OF RENAL CELL CARCINOMA

Although the primary classification of renal cell carcinoma is based on histomorphologic criteria, there is molecular genetic evidence that each is an oncogenetically distinct entity. For example, more than 90% of clear cell renal carcinomas harbor mutations and/ or deletions of the von Hippel-Lindau tumor suppressor gene located on the short arm of chromosome 3. In contrast, the majority of papillary carcinomas have trisomies of chromosomes 7, 16 and 17, and subsets of these tumors have been identified with mutations in the c-met gene. Chromophobe cell carcinomas consistently show abnormalities of chromosomes 1, 2, 6, 10, 13, 17, and 21, whereas some oncocytomas demonstrate a -Y, -1 karyotype and others have translocations involving 11q13.

Clear Cell Renal Cell Carcinoma

The most frequently encountered RCC subtype is characterized by loss of (part of) the short arm of chromosome 3 due to (a) deletion(s) or unbalanced translocation(s). Regions frequently lost are 3p12–14, 3p21- 22, and 3p25–26. Loss of at least two of these regions is necessary for kidney cells to develop into common type renal cell carcinoma, and loss of 3p21 is obligatory. Additionally, it was found that allelic losses in adenomas occurred in either 3p25 or 3p12–14, whereas those in carcinomas occurred in 3p21 together with losses in 3p25 or 3p12–14, or both. The most relevant RCC-related gene within 3p25–26 is the von Hippel-Lindau (VHL) gene. The von Hippel-Lindau tumor-suppressor gene was identified in 1993. In von Hippel-Lindau disease, one VHL allele is inherited with a mutation. Associated focal lesions, such as renal-cell carcinoma, arise from the inactivation or silencing of the remaining normal (wild-type) VHL allele. Defects in the VHL gene also appear to be responsible for about 60% of the cases of sporadic clear cell RCC, which represents a major portion of all cases of RCC.

Papillary Renal Adenomas and Carcinomas

Trisomy or tetrasomy 7, trisomy 17 and loss of chromosome Y are the commonest karyotypic changes in PRCC. Most of them are characterized by a unique combination of autosomal trisomies with trisomy 17. Papillary adenomas specifically show a -Y, +7, +17 chromosomal pattern as well as trisomy 3 or gain of the long-arm of chromosome 3, probably reflecting malignant transformation. Trisomy of chromosomes 12, 16, 20 as well as loss of the extracopy of chromosome 17 or loss of 17p are associated with progression from the adenoma into the carcinoma stage, i.e. papillary RCC. The high incidence of loss of the Y chromosome in combination with the strong male preponderance is suggestive of the loss of specific sequences harboured on the Y chromosome which probably is crucial for developing this subtype.

A small subset of papillary RCC is characterized by X;1 autosome translocations. The t(X;1)(p11.2;q21), resulting in a fusion of the transcription factor TFE3 on the X chromosome, with a novel gene, designated PRCC, on chromosome 1, appears to be a specific primary anomaly characterizing a distinct subgroup of papillary RCC with common RCC like features as clear cytoplasm. These tumors mostly occur in children and young (male) adults.

Renal Oncocytoma

One group is defined by (variant) translocations involving 11q13, and one with specifically defined numerical anomalies, in particular loss of chromosomes 1, and Y/X. The finding of mitochondrial DNA changes and the loss of Y/X in both renal oncocytoma and chromophobe carcinoma might indicate progression from renal oncocytoma to chromophobe renal cell carcinomas through additional chromosome losses, and explaining the occasional malignant behavior of renal oncocytomas.

Chromophobe Renal Carcinomas

They show multiple losses of entire chromosomes, i.e. loss of chromosomes 1, 2, 6, 10, 13, 17, 21, and the Y or X chromosome, leading to a low chromosome number.

Collecting Duct Carcinomas

These tumors do not show consistent chromosomal abnormalities as yet. Probably involvement of the short arm of chromosome 8, loss of the long arm of chromosome 13 as well as loss of part of the long arm of chromosome1q32 are related to poor prognosis. Loss of chromosomal material seems to be a defining characteristic for all distal nephron tumors.

Sarcomatoid Transformation in RCC

This variant represents the highest form of dedifferentiation and can in principle be derived from all the basic cell types.

Cytogenetic data on sarcomatoid RCC is scarce, some tumors show structural abnormalities of chromosomes 1, 5, 16, and 19 and losses of 3p, 4(q), 6q, 8p, 9, 13, 14, 17p, and gain of 5, 12, and 20 as well as TP53 mutations.

NUCLEAR GRADING

Several systems have been proposed over the years for the grading of renal tumors. Of these, one proposed by Fuhrman et al. is the most widely used **(Table 2)**.

Pathological Staging

This can be done either by AJCC (2002) method detailed below or by the WHO TNM staging system (2004) **(Table 3)**. The stage designation can be preceded by "pT" to highlight that it is a pathological stage rather than clinical stage.

Table 2: Fuhrman nuclear grading system in renal cell carcinoma.

Grade	Nucleus	Nuclear size (μ)	Nucleoli
1	Round, uniform	10	Absent/ inconspicuous
2	Slightly irregular	15	Evident
3	Very irregular	20	Large and prominent
4	Bizarre and multilobated	>20	Prominent, chromatin clumped

AJCC Staging

Stage Ia : 4 cm or less, organ confined
Stage Ib : > 4–7 cm, organ confined
Stage II : >7 cm, organ confined
Stage IIIa : Spread to perinephric tissue, including renal sinus, but confined within Gerota's fascia
Stage IIIb : Gross tumor in renal vein or its main branches or IVC below diaphragm
Stage IIIc : Gross tumor in IVC above diaphragm
Stage IV : Tumor beyond Gerota's fascia

METANEPHRIC TUMORS

Metanephric adenoma is a highly cellular epithelial tumor composed of small, uniform, embryonic-appearing cells **(Fig. 7)**. It occurs in children as well as adults, mostly in the fifth and sixth decades of their life. There is a 2:1 female preponderance. Almost 50% of metanephric adenoma are incidental findings with others presenting with polycythemia, abdominal or flank pain, mass, or

Table 3: TNM classification of renal cell carcinoma (WHO).

TNM classification					
T – Primary tumor		N – Regional lymph nodes			
TX	Primary tumor cannot be assessed	NX	Regional lymph nodes cannot be assessed		
T0	No evidence of primary tumor	N0	No regional lymph node metastasis		
T1	Tumor 7 cm or less in greatest dimension, limited to the kidney	N1	Metastasis in a single regional lymph node		
T1a	Tumor 4 cm or less	N2	Metastasis in more than one regional lymph node		
T1b	Tumor more than 4 cm but not more than 7 cm	M – Distant metastasis			
T2	Tumor more than 7 cm in greatest dimension, limited to the kidney	MX	Distant metastasis cannot be assessed		
T3	Tumor extends into major veins or directly invades adrenal gland or perinephric tissues but not beyond Gerota fascia	M0	No distant metastasis		
T3a	Tumor directly invades adrenal gland or perinephric tissues but not beyond Gerota fascia	M1	Distant metastasis		
T3b	Tumor grossly extends into renal vein(s) or vena cava or its wall below diaphragm	**Stage grouping**			
T3c	Tumor grossly extends into vena cava or its wall above diaphragm	Stage I	T1	N0	M0
T4	Tumor directly invades beyond Gerota fascia	Stage II	T2	N0	M0
		Stage III	T3 T1, T2, T3	N0 N1	M0 M0
		Stage IV	T4 Any T Any T	N0, N1 N2 Any N	M0 M0 M1

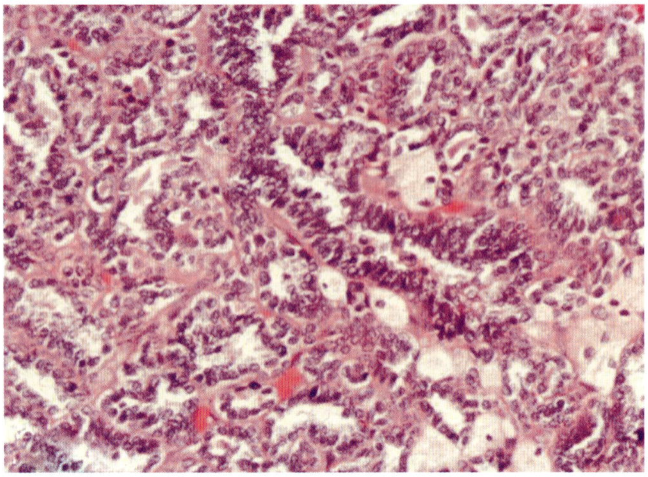

Fig. 7: Microscopic appearance of metanephric adenoma showing small embryonic acini.

hematuria. Grossly, size ranges from 30 to 60 mm in diameter. The tumors are typically well-circumscribed but not encapsulated. The cut surfaces vary from gray to tan to yellow and may be soft or firm. Foci of hemorrhage and necrosis are common; calcification is present in approximately 20%, and small cysts in 10%. Metanephric adenofibromas are typically solitary tan partially cystic masses with indistinct borders. Histology shows that metanephric adenoma is a highly cellular tumor composed of tightly packed small, uniform, round acini with an embryonal appearance. Long branching and angulated tubular structures also are common. The stroma ranges from inconspicuous to a loose edematous stroma. Hyalinized scar and focal osseous metaplasia of the stroma are present in 10–20% of tumors. Approximately 50% of tumors contain papillary structures, usually consisting of tiny cysts into which protrude blunt papillae reminiscent of immature glomeruli. Psammoma bodies are common and sometimes numerous. Metanephric adenofibroma is a composite tumor in which nodules of epithelium identical to metanephric adenoma are embedded in sheets of moderately cellular fibroblast like spindle cells. Variable amounts of hyalinization and myxoid change are present. Angiodysplasia and glial, cartilaginous, and adipose differentiation occur occasionally. The epithelial component consists of small acini, tubules and papillary structures, as described above in metanephric adenoma. Psammoma bodies are common and may be numerous. Immunohistochemical studies of metanephric adenoma have given variable results. Positive reactions with a variety of antibodies to cytokeratins have been reported, as have positive reactions with antibody to vimentin. Positive intranuclear reactions with antibody to WT-1 are common in metanephric adenoma.

MESENCHYMAL RENAL TUMORS OCCURRING IN ADULTS

Although a large number have been described (see classification above), the ones included in the description below are specific for the kidney.

Angiomyolipoma

These are distinctive tumors composed of variable combinations of abnormal vasculature, smooth muscle and adipose tissue, as the name suggests. Angiomyolipoma (AML) forms 1% of all resected specimens. Most are found within the kidney, but extrarenal sites include liver, lungs, lymph node and retroperitoneal tissue. About 80% of patients with tuberous sclerosis develop AML, whereas about one fourth of all AMLs occur in patients of tuberous sclerosis. In nontuberous sclerosis patients, it has a female preponderance (4:1). An AML belongs to a family of lesions characterized by proliferation of perivascular epithelioid cells (PEC). The etiology and pathogenesis of the neoplasm are unknown. The different frequency of AML in females and males in the surgical series, the onset of AML after puberty and the frequent progesterone receptor immunoreactivity in AML suggest a hormonal influence. Grossly, AMLs are well demarcated but not encapsulated **(Fig. 8)**. They vary in color from yellow to pinktan, depending on the relative proportions of the various tissue components and may mimic a clear cell RCC or a leiomyoma. Although AMLs may be large, they bulge into rather than infiltrate the perirenal fat. Most AMLs are solitary, but multiple tumors may be present, particularly in association with tuberous sclerosis. Microscopically, most tumors contain at least focal areas of adipose tissue,either mature or resembling lipoblasts. The smooth muscle cells appear to emerge from blood vessel walls in a radial fashion. The smooth muscle cells are most frequently spindle cells but may appear as rounded epithelioid cells. Rarely, striking degrees of nuclear atypia (occasionally with mitotic activity and multinucleation) may be observed in these cells, raising the possibility of malignancy. Some AMLs that are often located subcapsularly and composed almost entirely of smooth muscle cells (capsulomas) resemble leiomyomas. Cells associated with thin-walled, branching vessels may show a pattern similar to lymphangioleiomyoma. The blood vessels are thick-walled and lack the normal elastic content of arteries, and may mimic a vascular malformation. Prominent cystic change

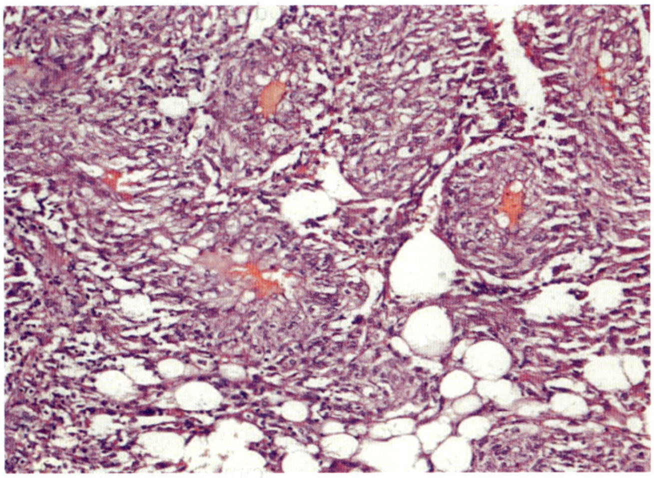

Fig. 8: Photomicrograph of angiomyolipoma of kidney reveals perivascular epithelioid smooth muscle cells along with mature adipocytes.

may very rarely be present in AML. Immunoprofile reveals a coexpression of melanocytic markers (HMB45, HMB50, CD63, tyrosinase, Mart1/Melan A and microophthalmia transcription factor) and smooth muscle markers (smooth muscle actin, muscle-specific actin and calponin); CD68, neuron-specific enolase, S-100 protein, estrogen and progesterone receptors, and desmin may also be positive, whereas epithelial markers are always negative. Coexpression of melanocytic and smooth muscle markers in myoid-appearing and lipid-distended cells supports the unitary nature of AML being a neoplasm with ability for phenotypic and immunotypic modulation. Ultrastructural evidence of melanogenesis is reported, and rarely melanin pigment can be abundant.

Epithelioid Angiomyolipoma

This variant of AML is potentially malignant. Tumors are usually large, with infiltrative growth pattern and are composed either exclusively or dominantly of polygonal cells with densely eosinophilic cytoplasm. Variable degrees of nuclear atypia and multinucleated cells are seen. Cells may have a clear cytoplasm. Population of short spindle cells are often present. Hemorrhage and necrosis is more common than in the classic variant. IHC reveals expression of HMB 45, HMB 50, Melan A and variable SMA or muscle specific actin. Allelic loss of chromosomal arm of 16p occurs similar to AML.

Juxtaglomerular Cell Tumor

These are rare tumors, first described by Robertson et al. in 1967. The tumor is generally small (2-3 cm), arising in the cortex, solitary and well encapsulated. The histological picture is variable. There are sheets of round to polygonal cells with slightly eosinophilic cytoplasm and distinct cell borders. Glomus like appearance, hemangiopericytomatous areas, ductal and papillary patterns, and areas of spindle cells are seen. PAS stain reveals granular cytoplasm. An IHC with anti-rennin antibodies is confirmatory, and electron microscopy shows distinctive membrane bound rhomboid to polygonal granules.

Renomedullary Interstitial Cell Tumor

Renomedullary interstitial cell tumors are incidental autopsy findings in adult, and are reported to be present in nearly 50% of men and women. About half the patients who have one renomedullary interstitial cell tumor have more than one. They are asymptomatic and while renomedullary interstitial cells play a role in regulation of blood pressure, renomedullary interstitial cell tumors have no clear influence on blood pressure. Almost all renomedullary interstitial cell tumors are 1–5 mm in diameter and appear as white or pale gray nodules within a renal medullary pyramid. Microscopically, the renomedullary interstitial cells are small stellate or polygonal cells in a background of loose faintly basophilic stroma reminiscent of renal medullary stroma. At the periphery, renal medullary tubules often are entrapped in the matrix. Interlacing bundles of delicate fibers usually are present. Some renomedullary interstitial cell tumors contain deposits of amyloid.

Nephroblastoma [Wilms' Tumor (WT)]

The tumor has a peak incidence between 2 years and 5 years and is the most important consideration except during the first 3 months of life.

The WT1 gene, located on chromosome 11p13 is consistently involved in genesis of WAGR (WT associated with aniridia, genital abnormalities and mental retardation) and Denys–Drash syndrome (WT with pseudohermaphroditism and glomerulopathy). However, WT1 gene is probably normal in 50% of sporadic cases of WT. WT2 gene locus maps on chromosome 11p15.

Abnormal substances in the blood or urine of patients of WT include von Willebrand factor, erythropoietin, rennin and neuron specific enolase, which may contribute to coagulopathy, polycythemia and hypertension in these patients. Rarely, they occurs in extrarenal sites. Metastasis is generally restricted to regional lymph nodes, lungs, and liver. Metastatic sites other than these (i.e. bone or brain) are unusual and should suggest alternative diagnoses.

PEDIATRIC RENAL TUMORS

The major pediatric renal neoplasms with their relative prevalence are as follows:

Nephroblastoma (Wilms' tumor)	85%
Mesoblastic nephroma	3%
Clear cell sarcoma of kidney	3%
Rhabdoid tumor	2%
Miscellaneous	7%
Xp11.2 renal carcinoma	
Papillary renal carcinoma	
Metanephric stromal tumor	
Metanephric adenofibroma	
Renal medullary carcinoma	
PNET	
Renal neuroblastoma	
Angiomyolipoma	
Lymphoma	

Gross Features

Most tumors are unicentric. However, multicentric masses in a single kidney and bilateral primary lesions can be seen rarely. Wilms' tumors are usually solitary rounded masses sharply demarcated from the adjacent renal parenchyma by a peritumoural fibrous pseudocapsule. They are mostly pale grey or tan appearance and of a soft consistency, although they may appear firm and whorled if a large fraction of the lesion is composed of mature stromal elements. Polypoid protrusions of tumor into the pelvicaliceal system may occur resulting in a "botryoid" appearance. Cysts may be prominent. The pathological staging relies on the identi-fication of penetration of the renal capsule, involvement of renal sinus vessels, positive surgical margins, and positive regional lymph nodes. Bilateral WTs are designated as stage V and their prognosis is determined by the stage of the most advanced tumor and by the presence or absence of anaplasia.

Microscopic Features

Most tumors have a triphasic appearance with variable components of blastemal, stromal and epithelial lineage **(Fig. 9)**. Biphasic and monophasic lesions are also often observed. While most of these components represent stages in normal or abnormal nephrogenesis, non renal elements, such as skeletal muscle and cartilage occur **(Fig. 10)**. The blastemal cells are small, round or oval with scanty cytoplasm, closely packed, and mitotically active. They have overlapping nuclei containing evenly distributed, slightly coarse chromatin, and small nucleoli. They occur in several distinctive patterns, such as diffuse, nodular, organized, serpentine and basaloid patterns. The diffuse blastemal pattern is characterized by a lack of cellular cohesiveness and an aggressive pattern of invasion into adjacent connective tissues and vessels. An epithelial component of differentiation is present in most nephroblastomas. This pattern may be manifested by primitive rosette-like structures, tubules and papillae. Heterologous epithelial differentiation may occur, the most common elements being mucinous and squamous epithelium. A variety of stromal patterns may occur and may cause diagnostic difficulty when blastemal and epithelial differentiation, are absent. Smooth muscle, skeletal muscle and fibroblastic

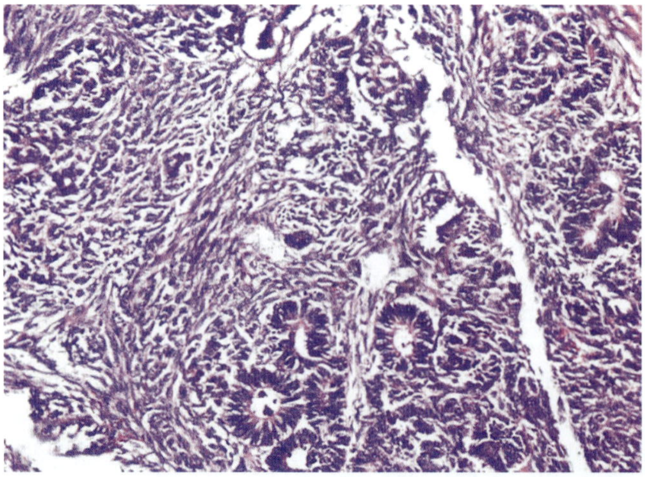

Fig. 9: Photomicrograph of nephroblastoma (Wilms' tumor), showing a triphasic pattern with blastemal, epithelial and stromal areas.

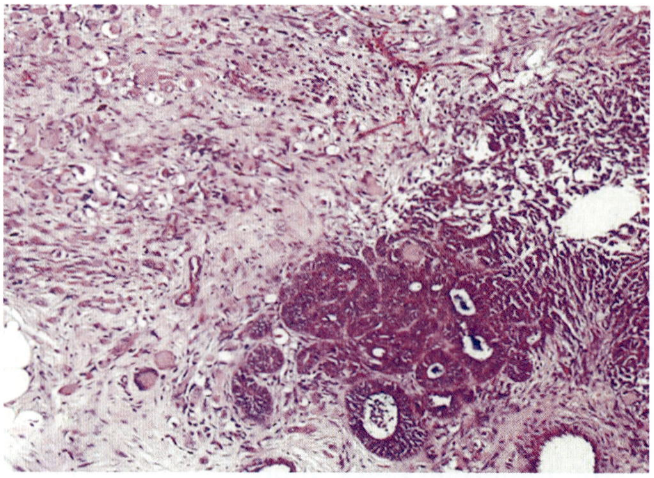

Fig. 10: Heterologous skeletal muscle differentiation in Wilms' tumor, along with epithelial and blastemal areas.

differentiation may be present. Skeletal muscle is the most common heterologous stromal cell type and large fields of the tumor often contain this pattern. Other types of heterologous stromal differentiation include adipose tissue, cartilage, bone, ganglion cells, and neuroglial tissue. Postchemotherapy changes include necrosis, xanthomatous histiocytic foci, hemosiderin deposits and fibrosis. There is often maturation of blastoma, epithelial, and stromal components, with striated muscle being the most frequent. Some tumors may show complete necrosis and are considered to be low risk.

Anaplasia

Approximately 5% of nephroblastomas are associated with an adverse outcome and are recognized pathologically because of their "unfavorable" histology due to the presence of nuclear anaplasia. Histologic diagnosis of anaplasia requires pesence of multipolar polyploid mitotic figures, marked nuclear enlargement and hyperchromasia. Anaplasia is most consistently associated with poor prognosis when it is diffusely distributed and when at advanced stages. For these reasons, pathologic distinction have been made between focal anaplasia and diffuse anaplasia. IHC reveals that blastemal cells regularly express vimentin, and may also show focal expression of neuron specific enolase, desmin, and cytokeratin Expression of WT-1 is not present in all nephroblastomas, and may be present in various other tumors. In nephroblastomas, it is confined to the nucleus and correlates with tumor histology: Areas of stromal differentiation and terminal epithelial differentiation show very low levels or no expression of WT-1, whereas areas of blastemal and early epithelial differentiation show high levels of WT-1.

Nephrogenic Rests

Nephrogenic rests are abnormally persistent foci of embryonal cells that are capable of developing into nephroblastomas. Nephrogenic rests are encountered in 25–40% of patients with nephroblastoma, and in 1% of infant autopsies. Nephrogenic rests are classified into perilobar (PLNR) and intralobar (ILNR) types. Nephroblastomatosis is defined as the presence of diffuse or multifocal nephrogenic rests. PLNRs are sharply circumscribed and located at the periphery. They may be dormant or mayregress. They may also undergo active proliferative overgrowth, resulting in hyperplastic nephrogenic rests, which can be almost impossible to distinguish from nephroblastoma. Rarely, PLNRs may trans-form into diffuse hyperplastic perilobar nephroblastomatosis. ILNRs are typically located in the central areas of the lobe, are poorly circumscribed and composed of stromal elements as well as epithelial tubules. ILNRs may be dormant, regress, or undergo hyperplasia. Nephroblastmatosis increases the chance of developing into a nephroblastoma.

Cystic Partially Differentiated Nephroblastoma (CPDN)

Rarely, Wilms' tumor may be composed entirely of cysts with delicate septa. Within the septa are small foci of blastoma, immature-appearing stromal cells, and primitive or immature epithelium. Such tumors are called "cystic partially differen-tiated nephroblastoma" (CPDN). This tumor is a multilocular cystic neoplasm of very young children, composed of epithelial and stromal elements, along with nephroblastomatous tissue. When no nephroblastomatous elements are found, the term "cystic nephroma" has been applied. CPDN is more common in males, and occurs below 2 years of age. Grossly, the tumor is large and multicystic, separated from the remaining kidney by a fibrous pseudocapsule. Microscopically, the cysts are lined with flattened, cuboidal, or hobnail epithelium **(Fig. 11)**. The septa contain undifferentiated and differentiated mesenchyme, blastema, and nephroblasto-matous epithelial elements. Skeletal muscle, cartilage, fat and myxoid mesenchyme may be present. In the papillonodular variant of CPDN papillae/nodules protrude into the cysts. The epithelial components consist mainly of mature and immature

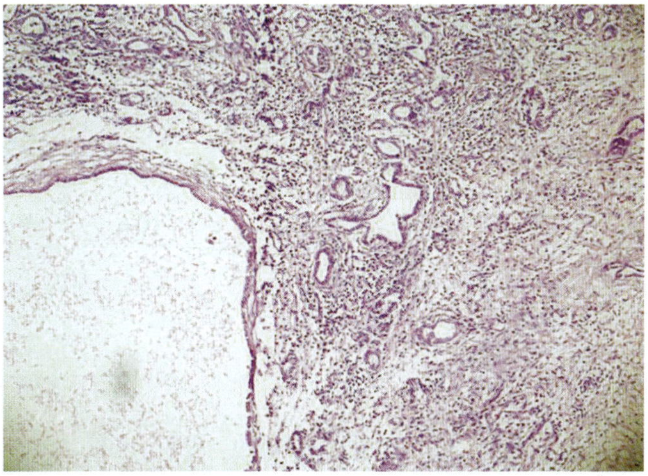

Fig. 11: Photomicrograph of cystic partially differentiated nephroblastoma, showing epithelial and blastemal elements within the wall of a cyst.

microscopic cysts resembling cross sections of tubules and stubby papillae resembling immature glomeruli. The importance of recognizing CPDN is to know that it is a low grade, potentially malignant tumor when diagnosed and not to miss the diagnosis by inadequate sampling.

Congenital Mesoblastic Nephroma (CMN)

This is the most common congenital renal tumor and occurs in infancy, presenting with an abdominal mass. Congenital mesoblastic nephroma (CMN) is a low-grade fibroblastic sarcoma. Gross appearance varies from firm and whorled to soft and cystic. Classic CMN (24% of cases) is morphologically identical to infantile fibromatosis of the renal sinus, composed of interlacing fascicles of fibroblastic cells with collagen deposition, and infiltration into the renal parenchyma **(Fig. 12)**. Cellular CMN (66% of cases) has microscopic features akin to infantile fibrosarcoma, These tumors show sheets and poorly formed fascicles with high mitotc activity. Mixed CMN (10% of cases) has features of both classic and cellular CMN within the same tumor. These tumors are immunoreactive for vimentin and actin, and negative for CD34. Cellular CMN but not classic CMN demonstrates a specific chromosome translocation, t(12;15)(p13;q25), which results in a fusion of the ETV6 and NTRK3 genes. Interestingly, the same chromosome translocation and gene fusion present in cellular CMN was first identified in infantile fibrosarcoma, and is not present in infantile fibromatosis. Hence, the analogy between cellular CMN and infantile fibrosarcoma and between classic CMN and infantile fibromatosis appears appropriate.

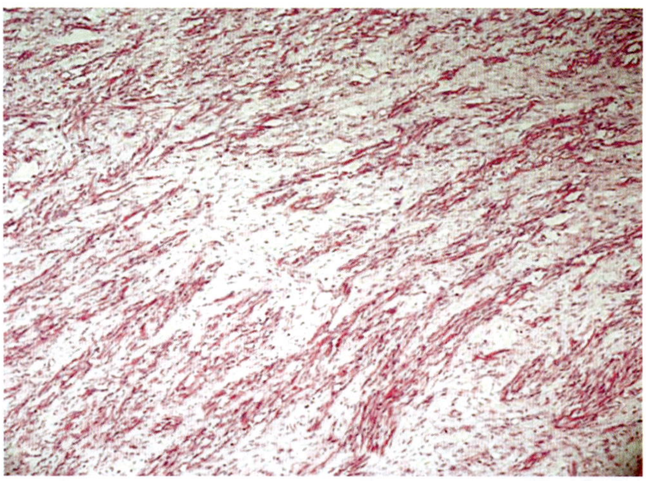

Fig. 12: Microscopic appearance of congenital mesoblastic nephroma shows fibroblastic cells with intervening collagen.

Clear Cell Sarcoma of Kidney

Clear cell sarcoma of the kidney (CCSK) is a rare pediatric renal sarcoma with a propensity to metastasize to bone and hence the proposed name "bone metastasizing renal tumor of childhood". It comprises approximately 3% of malignant pediatric renal tumors. The mean age at diagnosis is 36 months, with a male to female ratio of 2:1. On gross examination, it is a large tumor, present in the renal medulla, unencapsulated but circumscribed, soft, mucoid, and focally cystic. Microscopically, classic pattern of CCSK consists of nests or cords of cells separated by fibrovascular septa. The cord cells may be epithelioid or spindled, and are loosely separated by extracellular myxoid material that mimics clear cytoplasm. Nuclei are round to oval-shaped, have fine chro-matin, and lack prominent nucleoli. The septa may be thin, regularly branching "chicken-wire" capillaries, or thickened sheaths of fibroblastic cells surrounding a central capillary. CCSK can be myxoid or sclerosing. Rarely, the tumor can be anaplastic. Immunoprofile reveals vimentin and BCL2 to be reactive, no reaction with CD34, S100 protein, desmin, MIC2 (CD99), cytokeratin, and epithelial membrane antigen.

Rhabdoid Tumor

Rhabdoid tumor comprises approximately 2% of all pediatric renal tumors. It is a highly invasive and malignant neoplasm of young children. The mean age at diagnosis is approximately 1 year, and approximately 80% of patients are diagnosed in the first 2 years of life. Grossly, the tumors are typically large, hemorrhagic, necrotic and invasive. Microscopically, it is composed of sheets of cells with vesicular chromatin, prominent red nucleoli, and hyaline intracytoplasmic inclusions. Vascular invasion is usually extensive. A subset of tumors may be composed predominantly of primitive undifferentiated small round cells, but on closer inspection small foci of cells with diagnostic cytologic features can be identified. IHC shows strong vimentin labeling and focal but intense labeling for EMA. Ultrastructurally, the cytoplasmic inclusions reveal whorls of intermediate filaments having a diameter of 8–10 nm.

SUGGESTED READING

1. Argani P, Olgac S, Tickoo SK, Goldfischer M, Moch H, Chan DY, et al. Xp11 Translocation Renal Cell Carcinoma in Adults: Expanded Clinical, Pathologic, and Genetic Spectrum. Am J Surg Pathol. 2007;31:1149-60.

2. Argani P, Beckwith JB. Renal Neoplasms of Childhood. In Sternberg's Diagnostic Surgical Pathology. Carter D, Greenson JK, Oberman HA, Reuter V, Stoler MH, (Eds). Philadelphia. Lippincott Williams and Wilkins; 2004. pp.2001-33.
3. Cohen HT, McGovern FJ. Renal Cell Carcinoma. N Engl J Med. 2005;353:2477-90.
4. Eble JN, Sauter G, Epstein JI, Sesterhenn IA (Eds). World Health Organization Classification of Tumors. Pathology and Genetics of Tumors of the Urinary System and Male Genital Organs. Lyon: IARC Press; 2004.
5. Iliopoulos O, Eng C. Genetic and clinical aspects of familial renal neoplasms. Semin Oncol. 2000; 27:138-49.
6. Kim WY, Kaelin WG. Role of VHL gene mutation in human cancer. J Clin Oncol. 2004; 22:4991-5004.
7. Murphy WM, Beckwith JB, Farrow GM. Tumors of the kidney bladder, and related urinary structures. Atlas of tumor pathology, AFIP 1994; 3rd series, fascicle 11.
8. Reuter VE, Tickoo SK. Adult renal tumors. In: In Sternberg's Diagnostic Surgical Pathology 4th edition. Carter D, Greenson JK, Oberman HA, Reuter V, Stoler MH, editors. Philadelphia: Lippincott Williams and Wilkins; 2004. pp.1955-99.
9. Suzigan S, Lopez-Beltran A, Montironi R, Drut R, Romero A, Hayashi T, et al. Multilocular cystic renal cell carcinoma: A report of 45 cases of a kidney tumor of low malignant potential. Am J Clin Pathol. 2006;125:1-6.
10. Wang KL, Weinrach DM, Luan C, Han M, Lin F, Teh BT, et al. Renal papillary adenoma: A putative precursor of papillary renal cell carcinoma. Hum Pathol. 2007;38:239-46.

CHAPTER 107

Pathology of Gynecological Malignancies

Radhika Srinivasan

INTRODUCTION

The female genital tract consists of the uterus and cervix, vagina, vulva, bilateral fallopian tubes and ovaries. Among the malignancies affecting the female genital tract, cancer of the uterine cervix is the most frequent malignancy in our country with an age-adjusted incidence of 20–25 per 100,000 women. This is followed by a nearly equal incidence of cancer of the ovary and of the uterus (endometrium). Cancer of the vulva is less common and cancers of the fallopian tube and of the vagina *per se* are rare.

In general, carcinoma is the most common type of cancer to affect all these organs. Sarcomas are less frequent but do occur in the uterus, cervix, vagina and vulva. Rarely other malignancies such as primary lymphoma and melanomas also are known to involve the genital tract. Germ cell neoplasms and sex cord stromal tumors uniquely affect the ovary and are second to carcinomas in their frequency of occurrence.

Below is an overview of the major neoplasms of the ovary, fallopian tube, uterus, cervix and vulva.

NEOPLASMS OF THE OVARY

General comments: Ovarian carcinoma accounts for the greatest number of deaths from malignancies of the female genital tract. In the West, it is the 5th leading cause of cancer associated mortality. Generally, it occurs in older women (5th/6th decade). In India, the peak is seen almost a decade earlier. Familial ovarian cancer is due to mutations in *BRCA1* or *BRCA2* gene. Other syndromes such as Lynch type II syndrome are also associated with familial ovarian cancer. Ovarian cancer spreads commonly to the contralateral ovary, peritoneal cavity and the para-aortic and pelvic lymph nodes and the liver. With intra-abdominal spread, ascites develops commonly. Omental and peritoneal deposits also occur. An umbilical metastasis may be the first manifestation of the disease. Lung, pleura and distant metastases also occur. The spread of borderline tumors is mainly in the form of peritoneal implants, which may be invasive or non-invasive; spread to lymph nodes and other organs are also known.

Tumors of the ovary are classified based primarily on the tissue/cell of origin. Thus, we have tumors derived from the:

i. Ovarian surface epithelium, further divided into benign, borderline and malignant.
   a. Serous
   b. Mucinous
   c. Endometrioid
   d. Mixed
   e. Malignant mixed Müllerian tumor (MMMT)
ii. *Germ cells*:
   a. Dysgerminoma
   b. Teratoma
   c. Endodermal sinus tumor
   d. Mixed germ cell tumors
iii. *Sex cord*:
   a. Granulosa cell tumor
   b. Fibroma-thecoma

c. Sertoli-Leydig cell tumor
d. Others
iv. Germ cell-sex cord-stromal tumors
v. Metastatic tumors

Ovarian Surface Epithelial Tumors

These neoplasms constitute the most common ovarian tumors and may be further classified based on the specific cell types as serous, mucinous, endometrioid, mixed and unclassified **(Table 1)**.

Table 1: Immunohistochemical phenotype of ovarian neoplasms.

Tumor type	*Immunophenotype*
Surface epithelial tumors	
• Serous tumors	CA125, CK7+/CK20-
• Mucinous tumors	CK7+, CK20+ in 50%
• Endometrioid tumors	CK7+, CK20-
Germ cell tumors	
• Dysgerminoma	PLAP, CD117, OCT4
• Carcinoid tumor	NSE, Chromogranin and other secretory products
Sex cord stromal tumors	Inhibin alpha, Calretinin, Melan-A, CD99
Endometrial stromal sarcoma	CD10+, Caldesmon –ve

Serous Tumors

Serous tumors make up about 1/4th of all ovarian tumors and mostly occur in adults. Approximately 30–50% are bilateral **(Figs. 1A and B)**.

Gross appearance: Grossly, these tumors have a solid as well as cystic component. The cystic areas are filled with serous fluid and usually have papillary excrescences. Careful inspection of the outer surface is required as sometimes there may be papillary excrescences on outer surface. Benign serous tumors may be uniloculated or multiloculated with thin septae and smooth inner and outer surface. Papillary excrescences may be seen, but usually are focal and small in size. Borderline tumors usually are also cystic but tend to have larger areas (>10%) covered by papillary excrescences. Malignant tumors are characterized by solid tumors with variable cystic component. The solid areas are usually friable with papillations and show variable degrees of necrosis and hemorrhage.

Microscopic appearance: The cell type of serous tumors resemble the normal tubal epithelium and is cuboidal to low columnar epithelium lining the cysts and papillae. In about 1/3rd cases, psammoma bodies (calcific concretions with concentric lamination) are seen. A morphological spectrum of proliferation exists in these tumors. At one

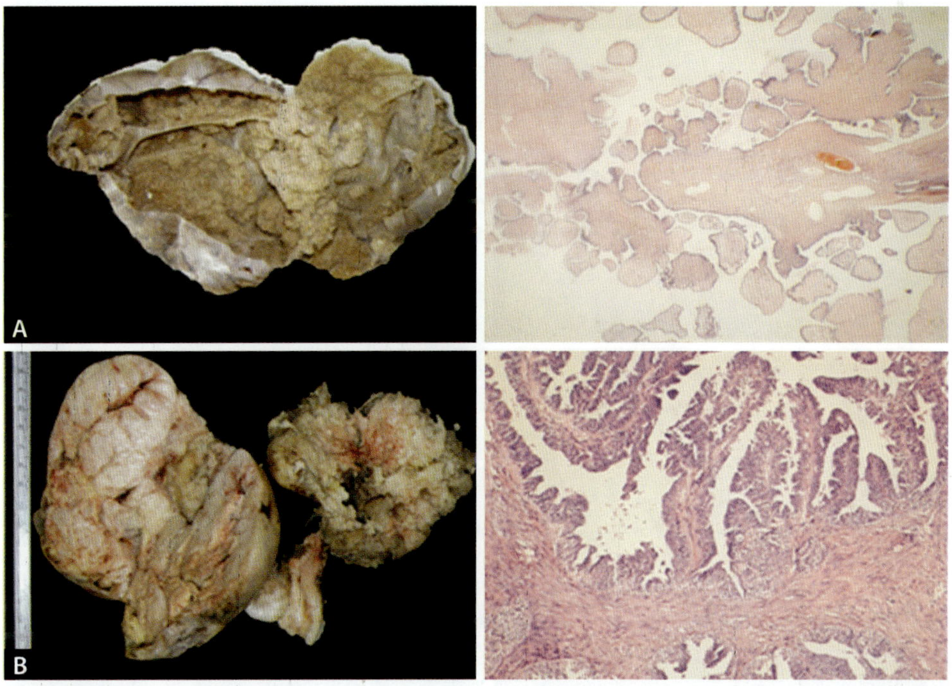

Figs. 1A and B: (A) Borderline serous tumor: Gross and microscopy. Grossly, a large cystic tumor, uniloculated with multiple papillary excrescences are seen. Microscopically, the hierchical papillae are lined by serous epithelial cells showing mild atypia. There is no stromal invasion; (B) Papillary serous carcinoma of the ovary: Gross and microscopy. Grossly, a predominantly solid tumor with friable areas and areas of necrosis and hemorrhage.

end of the spectrum is the benign serous cystadenoma, in which the cyst and papillae are lined by a single layer of cells without any complexity in the architecture or invasion. At the other end is the papillary serous cystadenocarcinoma characterized by nuclear atypia, invasion and architectural complexity. In between are the tumors designated borderline tumors which show proliferation and nuclear atypia but lack the stromal invasion. Tumors which show minimal areas of invasion are placed in the 'microinvasive carcinoma' category. Serous tumors with a significantly fibrous stroma are referred to as cystadenofibroma. These tumors also have benign, borderline and malignant categories as described above.

Mucinous Tumors

Mucinous neoplasms are less common than serous neoplasms and are bilateral in only 10–12% cases. As in serous tumors, mucinous cystadenoma, borderline mucinous tumors and mucinous cystadenocarcinomas are recognized **(Figs. 2A and B)**.

Gross appearance: Mucinous neoplasms usually present as multiloculated cystic tumors. The cysts contain thick viscous mucin. Malignant tumors have larger solid areas and typically areas consisting of smaller cystic spaces filled with mucinous material.

Microscopic appearance: The lining epithelium is tall, columnar and resembles the mucinous lining of the endocervix or the intestine. Benign tumors are lined by a single layer of cells. Papillae and villiform projections into the cystic spaces are also present. The cystic spaces show mucinous material. Foci of inflammatory reaction to the mucin may also be seen. Borderline tumors show greater degree of cellular proliferation and complexity of architecture. Stromal invasion should however be absent for a diagnosis of this type of neoplasms. Tumors with intraepithelial carcinoma and with stromal microinvasion are also recognized. In mucinous cystadenocarcinomas, frank stromal invasion, architectural complexity and nuclear atypia are evident. Mucin may leak into the adjacent ovarian stroma giving rise to an inflammatory reaction comprising of neutrophils, lymphocytes and even giant cells. Mucinous tumors may be associated with a condition called '*pseudomyxoma peritoneii*', wherein the peritoneal cavity is filled with thick, gelatinous mucoid material resulting in adhesions between the organs. Careful microscopic evaluation of this material is required to distinguish the relatively benign *peritoneal adenomucinosis* (lacking or with a few strips of benign appearing mucinous epithelium) from the frankly malignant mucinous carcinomatosis.

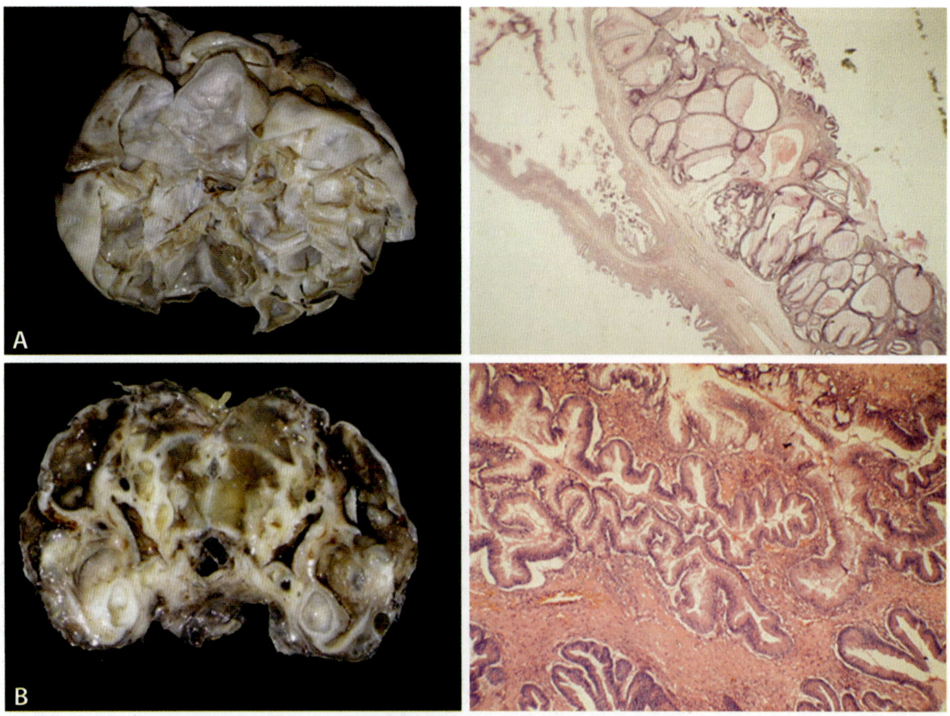

Figs. 2A and B: (A) *Borderline mucinous tumor*: Gross and microscopy. Grossly, a multicystic tumor, the cysts filled with gelatinous mucoid material and microscopically complexity of architecture and mild cytological atypia are seen; (B) *Mucinous carcinoma*: Gross and microscopy. Grossly, multicystic tumor with thick septae, the cystic spaces filled with mucoid material along with areas of hemorrhage and necrosis. Microscopically, frank stromal invasion is present.

The subgroup of mucinous tumors with a prominent stromal component is designated as mucinous adenofibroma/mucinous cystadenofibroma and mucinous adenocarcinofibroma, if malignant.

Exceptionally, mucinous adenocarcinomas may contain mural nodules with sarcoma-like nodules comprising of numerous giant cells, true sarcoma or anaplastic carcinoma.

Borderline mucinous tumors are known to have an association with long standing endometriosis.

Endometrioid Tumors

Endometrioid carcinoma comprises 10–25% of all primary ovarian carcinomas. Coexistent endometriosis may be demonstrated in 10–20% cases.

Gross appearance: These neoplasms may be solid or cystic. The contents tend to be hemorrhagic. Visible papillae are absent.

Microscopic appearance: These tumors resemble the usual endometrial adenocarcinoma with glandular spaces lined by tall columnar epithelium with eccentric nuclei. Squamous metaplasia is usually present.

Benign and borderline endometrioid tumors are recognized. These tumors generally have a prominent stromal component **(Figs. 3A to C)**.

Synchronous endometrioid tumors of the uterus may be present and their frequency varies from 15 to 30%.

Clear Cell Adenocarcinoma of the Ovary

Clear cell adenocarcinoma of the ovary shows a spongy, cystic tumor with variable hemorrhage and necrosis.

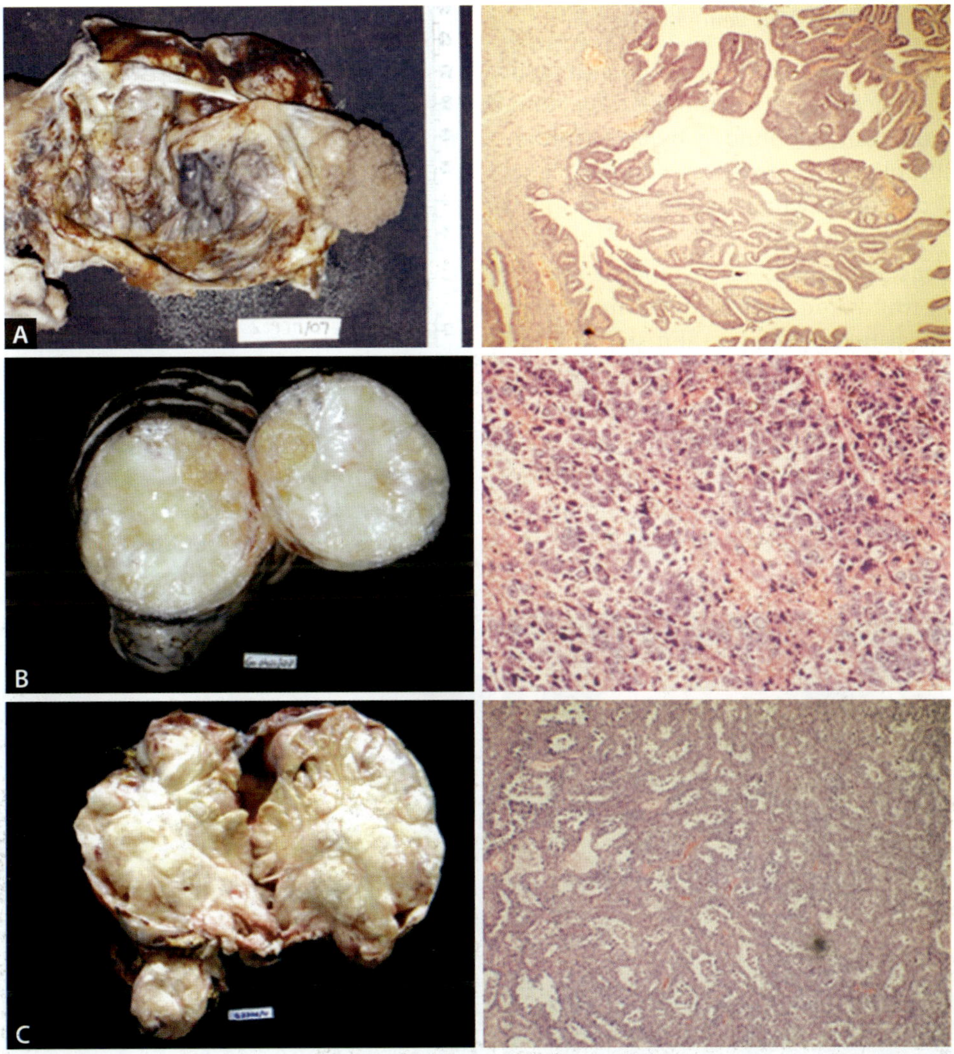

Figs. 3A to C: (A) Endometrioid carcinoma of the ovary arising in an endometriotic cyst. Note the thick-walled cyst with a solid area showing papillary excrescences. Microscopy shows papillae and glands lined by tall columnar endometrioid type of epithelium; (B) Endometrioid carcinoma of ovary showing a solid tumor with areas of necrosis. Microscopically, a moderately differentiated tumor is noted; (C) Clear cell carcinoma of ovary, gross and microscopy. Glands lined by cells with a clear cytoplasm and pleomorphic nuclei are seen.

Microscopically, tubular-cystic, papillary and solid patterns of growth may be seen. The cores of the papillae often exhibit prominent hyalinization. The tumor cells are large, pleomorphic and have prominent nucleoli. Some of the nuclei protrude into the lumina resulting in a 'hobnail' configuration. The cytoplasm is clear and may exhibit PAS positive diastase-resistant hyaline globules.

A high association of clear cell carcinomas with pelvic endometriosis is seen and sometimes these tumors are seen to arise directly from endometriotic cysts. These patients are in their 5-6th decades and have a poor prognosis.

Brenner's Tumor

Brenner's tumor constitutes between 1 and 2% of all ovarian neoplasms. These tumors are usually unilateral, solid tumors and appear whitish or yellow white.

Microscopic appearance: They consist of solid and cystic epithelial nests of epithelial cells resembling transitional epithelium or urothelium surrounded by an abundant stroma which is fibroblastic. There is a great resemblance to the 'Walthard' cell nests which are common in the mesosalpinx. The cytoplasm is clear and nuclei may show grooves. Cystic areas and mucinous metaplasia may be present. If papillary fronds and nuclear atypia are present, in addition to typical benign areas, then such tumors are referred to as *Proliferating Brenner's tumor*. Marked nuclear atypia signals malignancy. When both benign and malignant areas are recognized in a Brenner's tumor, it is designated as *malignant Brenner's tumor*. Tumors without a recognizable benign morphological component are designated as *transitional cell carcinomas*.

Malignant Mixed Müllerian Tumor (MMMT)

This tumor resembles its uterine counterpart. *MMMT homologous variety* is also called carcinosarcoma. The carcinomatous component may appear serous, endometrioid, squamous or clear cell type. The heterologous variety shows diverse sarcomas, such as chondrosarcoma, osteosarcoma, rhabdomyosarcoma or angiosarcoma. The prognosis of this tumor is extremely poor.

Germ Cell Tumors

Germ cell tumors constitute approximately 20% of all ovarian neoplasms and occur predominantly in children and young adults. Approximately 95% of these are mature cystic teratomas, whereas the rest are malignant.

Dysgerminoma

Dysgerminoma constitutes approximately 5% of all malignant ovarian tumors and 5-6% of all malignant tumors in children; approximately 5% occur in dysgenetic gonads. It is bilateral in 15% cases. Dysgerminomas are also the most common component of mixed germ cell neoplasms. Metastasis occurs to the contralateral ovary, lymph nodes and to the peritoneal cavity **(Figs. 4A and B)**.

Gross appearance: Dysgerminoma is usually a large tumor, encapsulated with a smooth outer surface. The cut surface is solid, gray white with foci of hemorrhage and necrosis.

Microscopic appearance: The tumor cells are arranged in well defined nests separated by thin fibrous septae infiltrated with lymphocytes. A granulomatous reaction is not uncommon. The tumor cells are uniform with large

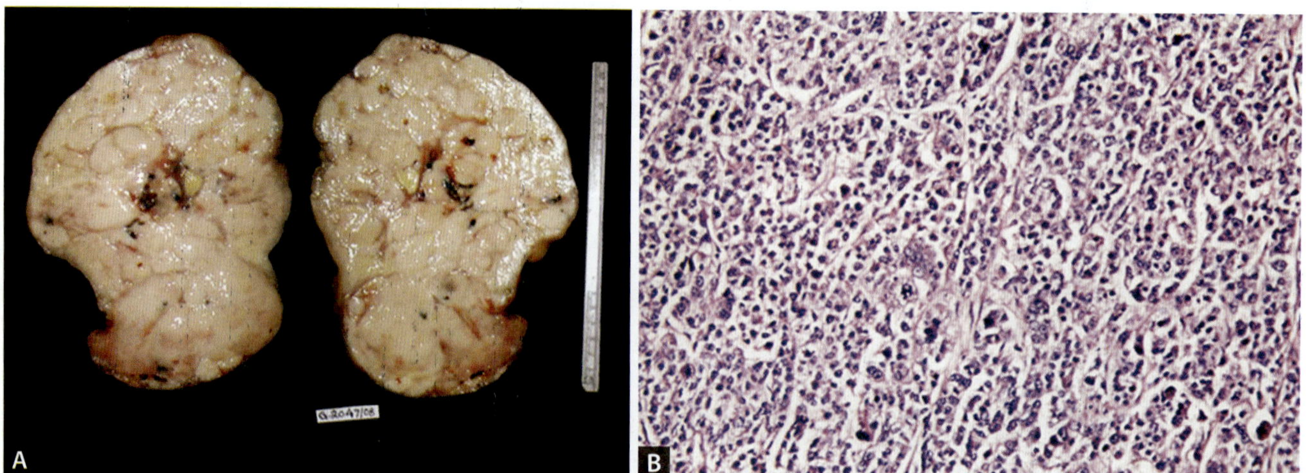

Figs. 4A and B: *Dysgerminoma*: Grossly, a solid, fleshy tumor is seen. Microscopically, nodules of tumor cells separated by fibrous septae showing lymphocytic infiltration.

nuclei and characteristically have one or more prominent nucleoli and abundant clear to finely granular cytoplasm containing glycogen. Dysgerminoma (in about 3% cases) may show scattered hCG positive syncytiotrophoblastic cells, which may be accompanied by elevated serum hCG levels. Sometimes, there is marked anaplasia when they are designated *anaplastic dysgerminomas.*

Yolk Sac Tumor (Endodermal Sinus Tumor)

Yolk sac tumor (endodermal sinus tumor) is a neoplasm of children and young adults.

Gross appearance: The tumors are large and on cut surface, have a variegated appearance with areas of necrosis, hemorrhage and cystic change.

Microscopic appearance: The appearance is variable. A variety of patterns are recognized such as microcystic pattern, polyvesicular vitelline pattern and hepatoid pattern. Schiller-Duval bodies are a characteristic feature of this tumor. Intracytoplasmic hyaline globules, which are PAS positive and diastase resistant and are immune-reactive for alphafetoprotein are also noted. The serum AFP is a good tumor marker for this entity.

Embryonal carcinoma is less common in the ovary as compared to the testis. It is usually a component of mixed germ cell neoplasms.

Primary ovarian choriocarcinoma is an exceedingly rare tumor and is morphologically similar to their uterine counterpart.

Immature Teratoma

This is a malignant tumor composed of a mixture of adult and embryonal tissues derived from all the three germ cell layers.

Gross appearance: Immature teratoma is composed of solid and cystic areas.

Microscopic appearance: The main component is primitive neuroepithelium. Primitive mesodermal element is also common. Endodermal derivatives resembling the intestine, liver, etc may be seen in variable amounts. Immature teratomas are graded (described by Norris, et al.) as:

Grade I: Abundance of mature tissues intermixed with loose mesenchymal tissue with occasional immature focus.

Grade II: Fewer mature tissue; rare foci of neuroepithelium with mitoses but not exceeding three low magnification fields.

Grade III: Few or no mature tissue; numerous neuroepithelial elements occupying four or more low magnification fields.

Thorough microscopic examination is required for proper grading. Further, immature teratomas may also be part of mixed germ cell neoplasms.

Mature Cystic Teratoma

These tumors are the most common ovarian benign neoplasm. Typically, they are cystic containing cheesy sebaceous and keratinous material and grossly evident hair. There is a solid nipple like area referred to as the 'Rokitansky's protuberance, where teeth may be seen. It is important to take sections from this area as a variety of tissues are represented in this area. Variable amounts of fat, cartilage and bone may be identified grossly.

Microscopic appearance: These tumors are characterized by tissues from all the three germ cell layers, which are mature. Thus, skin with pilosebaceous units, adnexae, neuroglial tissue derived from the ectoderm are very common followed by the respiratory epithelium with adjoining cartilage and intestinal tissue representing the endoderm derived tissues. Bone, fat, cartilage representing mesoderm derived tissue may all be present in variable amounts.

Rarely, malignancy can arise in a pre-existing mature cystic teratoma in about 2% cases. The most common malignancy is squamous cell carcinoma followed by carcinoid tumor and adenocarcinoma.

Carcinoid Tumor and Strumal Carcinoid

Carcinoid tumors of the ovary are uncommon and may represent metastases from elsewhere, part of a teratoma or as a primary neoplasm. Approximately one-third are associated with the carcinoid syndrome. Primary carcinoid carry a good prognosis.

Gross appearance: They have a smooth outer surface and their cut surface is solid, tan to yellow and homogeneous.

Microscopic appearance: The morphology is similar to carcinoids elsewhere with an insular, trabecular or solid growth patterns. The tumor cells are uniform with fine chromatin. Strumal carcinoid is a tumor that combines features of a carcinoid tumor with struma ovarii.

Sex Cord Stromal Tumors

These constitute approximately 5% of all ovarian neoplasms. The major tumors in this category are shown in **Figures 5A to C**.

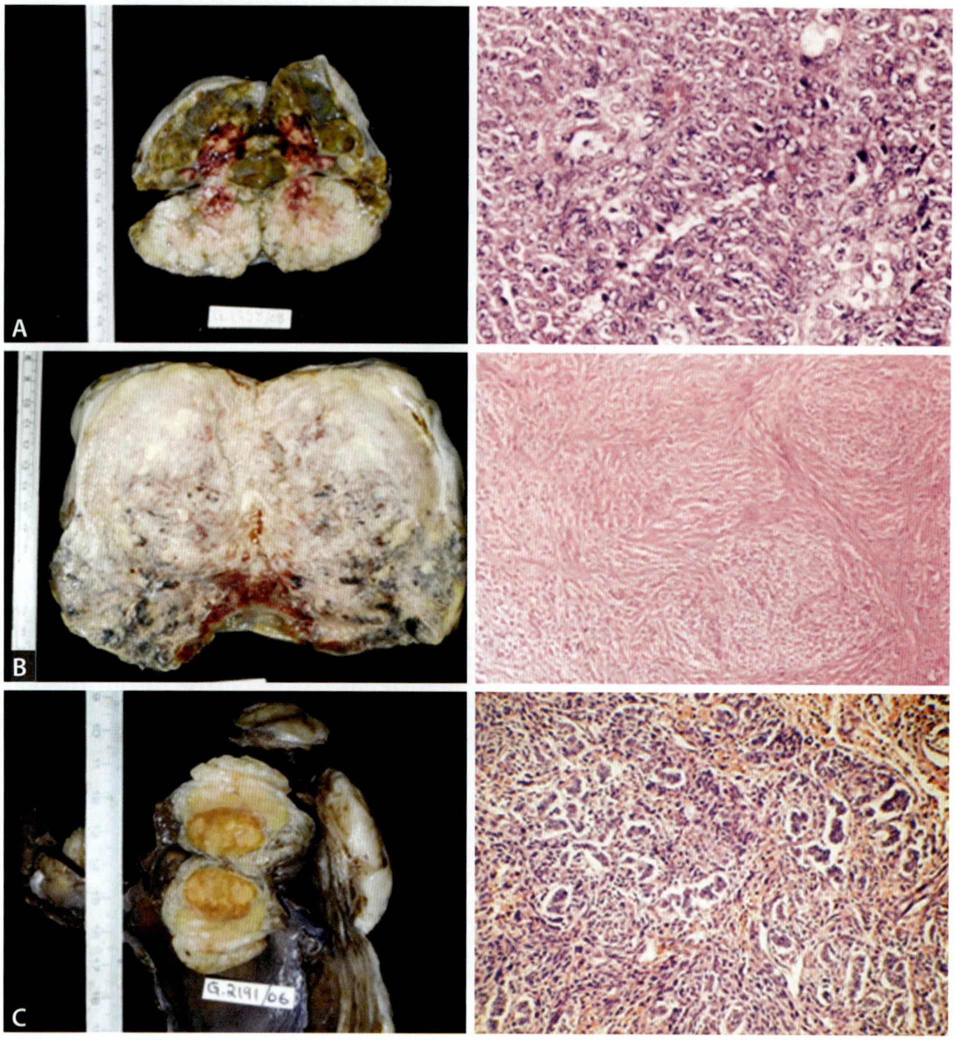

Figs. 5A to C: *Sex cord stromal tumors of the ovary*: (A) Granulosa cell tumor. Grossly, a solid tumor with areas of hemorrhage and necrosis. Microscopically, diffuse sheets of cell with oval, elongated nuclei which show grooving; (B) *Fibroma*: Grossly, a solid firm tumor and microscopically, spindle cell tumor with collagenization; (C) Sertoli-Leydig cell tumor with a characteristic yellow appearance grossly. Microscopically, Sertoli cells forming abortive tubules and Leydig cells with abundant eosinophilic cytoplasm is seen.

Granulosa Cell Tumor

Adult granulosa cell tumor is usually detected in the child bearing age and 3/4th of them are associated with hyperestrinism. The excessive estrogens may lead to a clinical presentation of precocious puberty in children, metrorrhagia in adults and in postmenopausal women. Some tumors are hormonally inactive, whereas the others may be androgenic.

Gross appearance: These tumors are encapsulated with a smooth-lobulated outline and a predominantly solid cut surface. The color may be gray or yellow, if leutinized. Cystic change may be present.

Microscopic appearance: There is a variety of growth patterns such as microfollicular, macrofollicular, trabecular, insular, watered-silk, solid and diffuse (sarcomatoid). Numerous typical 'Call-Exner' bodies may be seen. The nuclei typically show grooves resulting in a 'coffee bean' appearance. Serum inhibin is a useful tumor marker.

Juvenile Granulosa Cell Tumor (JGCT)

Juvenile granulosa cell tumor (JGCT) is tumor that presents in 80% of cases in the first two decades of life. Most patients present with isosexual precocity. There is a diffuse or macrofollicular growth pattern with pools of intrafollicular secretion, large tumor cells showing nuclear atypia and a variable but often high mitotic activity. The tumor cells are luteinized.

Thecoma, Fibroma and Other Tumors

These tumors often have an overlapping morphology and are sometimes referred to as fibrothecomas.

Thecomas present after menopause, are usually unilateral and varies in size. It has a well-defined capsule and is a solid tumor. The cut surface is solid with a few cysts and is yellow in color. Microscopically, it is composed of fascicles of spindle cells with moderate amount of cytoplasm. The intervening tissue shows collagen and hyaline plaque formation. Thecoma cells contain abundant intracytoplasmic fat.

Fibromas are common ovarian tumors, usually unilateral and occur after puberty. Grossly, fibromas are solid white tumors. Microscopically, they are composed of closely packed spindle cells with intervening hyalinization and collagenization. Cellularity is variable.

Sertoli-Leydig Cell Tumor

As the name suggests, these tumors are composed of a mixture of cells resembling the male Sertoli-Leydig cells. They are uncommon tumors constituting <0.1% of ovarian neoplasms. They are seen in young patients and rare after menopause. Nearly 50% show signs of androgen excess. This is manifested as defeminization with amenorrhea and breast atrophy and later by masculinization (voice deepening, clitoral hypertrophy). Some tumors may not have demonstrable endocrine effect, whereas others may secrete estrogen and progesterone.

Gross appearance: They are solid tumors with a variable cystic component.

Microscopic appearance: They may be well differentiated, intermediate or poorly differentiated (sarcomatoid) or pure Sertoli cell tumors. Heterologous elements such as liver, skeletal muscle, cartilage, etc. may be identified. A retiform variant is also identified.

The prognosis of this tumor is usually good and correlates with the stage and the degree of differentiation.

Metastatic Tumors

The ovary is a common site for metastatic tumors. Over half of metastases are bilateral. The most common primary sites are the breast, uterus, stomach, colon and gallbladder (in India). The eponym Krukenberg tumor is used to designate an ovarian neoplasm, usually bilateral, characterized by multinodular enlargement of the ovaries and microscopically by a diffuse infiltration by signet ring cells containing abundant neutral and acidic mucins in a cellular fibroblastic stroma. Lymphatic tumor emboli are often seen.

CARCINOMA OF THE FALLOPIAN TUBE

Primary fallopian tube carcinoma is rare accounting for 1% of primary genital tract malignancies. Most patients are postmenopausal. Nulliparity is common. Recent studies have shown a strong association of this cancer with carriers of *BRCA1* and *BRCA2* mutation. In developed countries, prophylactic salpingo-oophorectomy is carried out in such women **(Fig. 6)**.

Gross appearance: The tube is enlarged and has fibrous adhesions. The fimbriated end of the tube may be open or closed; a fact of prognostic significance. The cut surface shows a solid or papillary tumor filling and expanding the tubal lumen.

Microscopic appearance: All major types of carcinomas known to occur in the ovary are seen in the tube as well. The most common type is the papillary serous type. Other types include endometrioid, clear cell, sero-mucinous and transitional carcinomas.

The prognosis depends on the stage of the tumor (77% for stage I tumors vs 20% for stage III).

MALIGNANT TUMORS OF THE UTERUS

These include tumors of the endometrium and of the myometrium. Endometrial cancers include endometrial carcinoma, endometrial stromal sarcoma and malignant mixed Müllerian tumors (MMMT). Leiomyosarcoma arises from the smooth muscle of the myometrium.

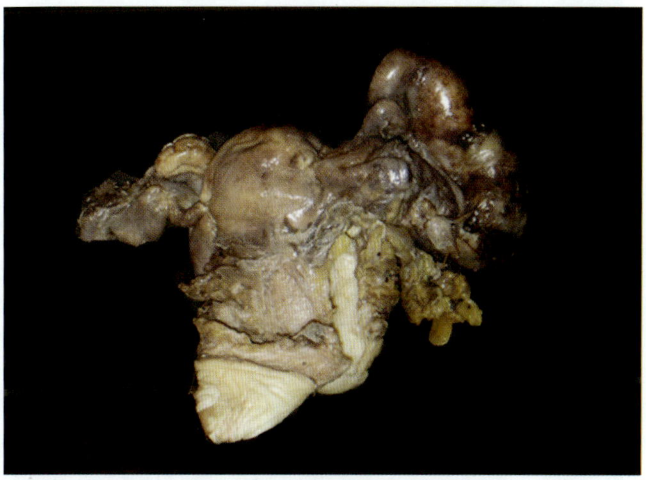

Fig. 6: Fallopian tubal carcinoma showing nodular expansion of the left tube by the tumor.

Endometrial carcinoma is the most common gynecological malignancy in developed countries. It typically occurs in elderly postmenopausal women. Based on the pathogenesis, two distinct types are noted: *Type I*, which occurs in a background of excess estrogenic stimulation and develops against a background of endometrial hyperplasia; and *Type II*, which occurs *de novo*. Obesity, hypertension, diabetes and nulliparity are risk factors for type I carcinomas. Other predisposing conditions include polycystic ovarian disease (PCOD), dysfunctional uterine bleeding (DUB), long-standing estrogen users, tamoxifen usage and those with functioning granulosa cell tumors.

Type I: Endometrioid Adenocarcinoma

Gross appearance: These tumors may be seen as a polypoidal, predominantly exophytic growth arising from the uterine cavity or as diffusely infiltrating tumors.

Microscopic appearance: They are like the usual adenocarcinomas and are divided into grade I–III tumors based on their degree of differentiation. The most important aspect in the evaluation of a uterine neoplasm especially endometrial adenocarcinoma is the depth of myoinvasion. The second aspect is to evaluate the vertical extent of involvement and to evaluate the involvement of the cervix. These pathological features are important in FIGO staging, which is a surgicopathological staging. Squamous metaplasia is often noted. Other types of metaplasias are also associated with endometrial adenocarcinoma.

Type II: Carcinoma

This category includes *serous carcinoma* and *clear cell carcinoma*. In contrast to type I carcinoma, these tumors are highly aggressive and occur in older women. Serous carcinoma represents a highly aggressive tumor characterized by a complex papillary growth pattern. The lining cells show moderate to severe pleomorphism and atypia with mitotic figures and sometimes psammoma bodies. Usually deep myoinvasion is present. However, it may remain confined to a polyp or remains intramucosal.

Clear cell carcinoma is composed of large clear cells with distinct cellular margins and abundant cytoplasm containing abundant glycogen. Papillary and glandular differentiation is present. Hobnailing of tumor cells may be seen. Hyaline bodies are also seen.

Endometrial Stromal Tumors

These tumors occur in the 5th decade of life and present clinically with vaginal bleeding **(Figs. 7A and B)**.

Gross appearance: They may present as sharply circumscribed nodule with no permeation of the surrounding tissue, when they are designated *endometrial stromal nodule. Low grade endometrial stromal sarcomas* (ESS) show diffuse permeation of the myometrium and

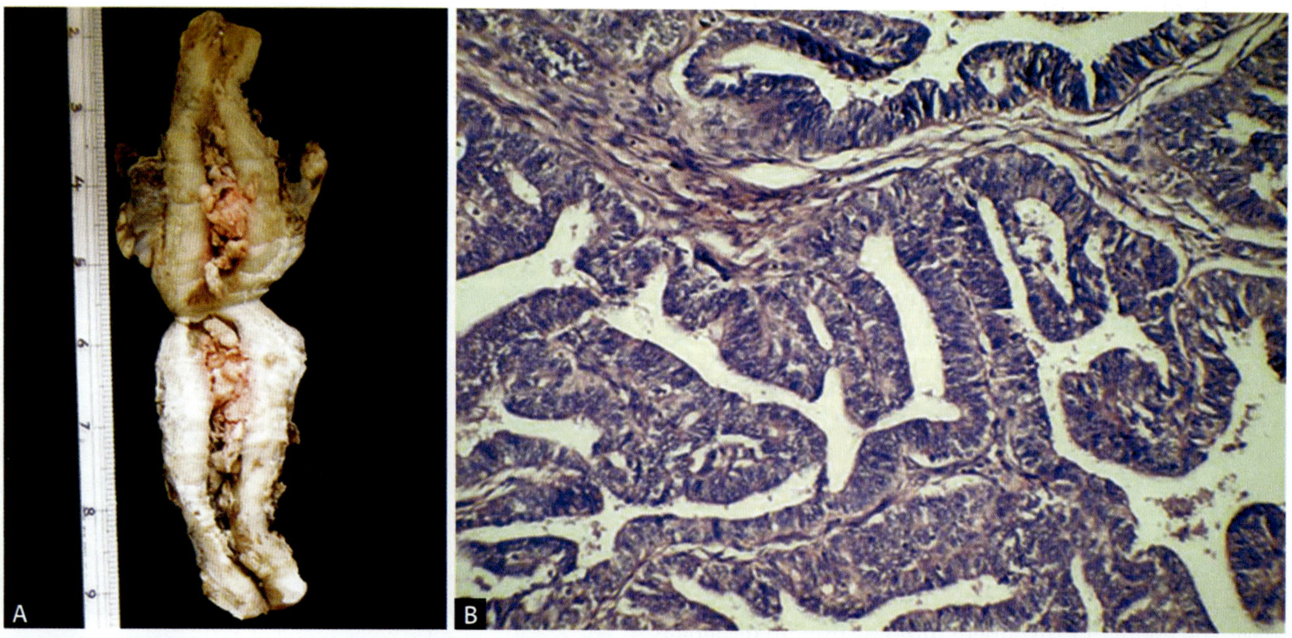

Figs. 7: *Carcinoma endometrium*: Grosssly, there is a friable tumor seen filling the uterine cavity with superficial myoinvasion (A). Microscopy shows a typical endometrioid carcinoma (B).

show small nodules on the cut surface. Permeation into the veins and lymphatics may be identified grossly as yellowish, ropy ball-like masses filling dilated channels. ESS can also present as solitary polypoid masses.

Microscopic appearance: These tumors are composed of small ovoid cells resembling the endometrial stromal cells. They are individually enveloped by reticulin fibers. The tumors show numerous finely dispersed small vessels resembling the endometrial spiral arterioles; the tumor cells typically encircle these blood vessels. Low-grade ESS usually has a low mitotic activity. Some tumors may show differentiation towards both smooth muscle and endometrial stromal cells. If each component is around 30%, then the tumor is designated *a combined smooth muscle-stromal tumor* **(Figs. 8A and B)**.

In contrast to low grade ESS, *high grade ESS* show necrosis, high mitotic activity and obvious nuclear atypia and are aggressive neoplasms.

MMMT Carcinosarcoma

MMMT are always seen in postmenopausal women. They present with uterine bleeding and enlargement.

Gross appearance: They present as soft, polypoidal masses filling the cavity with areas of hemorrhage and necrosis.

Microscopic appearance: The characteristic feature of an MMMT is an admixture of carcinoma and sarcoma-like elements. The carcinoma resembles endometrioid, clear cell or papillary serous types. The sarcomatous component may be homologous or heterologous in nature. Homologous refers to a sarcoma resembling endometrial stromal sarcoma or a spindle cell sarcoma resembling leiomyosarcoma or fibrosarcoma. Heterologous elements may be chondrosarcoma, osteosarcoma or rhabdomyosarcoma in nature. These tumors must be regarded primarily as carcinomas rather than sarcomas based on immunohistochemical and ultrastructural studies.

MMMTs are highly aggressive neoplasms. Extension into the pelvis, lymphatic and vascular permeation and blood-borne metastases are common. Extension of the tumor to the serosa and beyond is a sign of even worse prognosis.

Müllerian Adenosarcoma

This is a distinctive type of tumor and usually presents in the elderly as a bulky polypoidal growth filling the endometrial cavity. Microscopically, it shows a combination of epithelial and stromal elements. The epithelial component has a benign appearance whereas the stromal component is malignant and resembles a sarcoma. *Müllerian adenosarcoma with a sarcomatous overgrowth (MASO)* is an aggressive variant of this neoplasm with a poor prognosis **(Figs. 9A and B)**.

Leiomyosarcoma

Leiomyosarcoma occurs in older women and grossly is seen as a large fleshy intramural mass with submucous and subserosal extension. Areas of hemorrhage and necrosis are always present.

Microscopic appearance: These tumors are highly cellular with large areas of coagulative tumor necrosis. Cellular

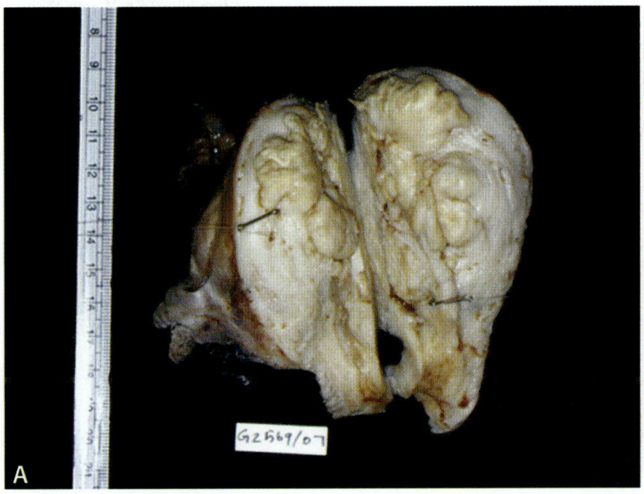

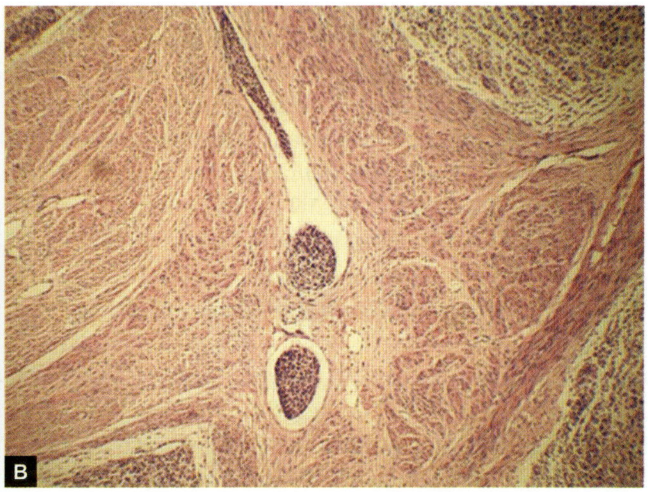

Figs. 8A and B: *Endometrial stromal sarcoma, low grade*: Grossly, there is an infiltrative tumor in the endomyometrium (A). Microscopically, infiltrating nests of tumor cells are seen in the lymphatics of the myometrium, a characteristic feature of this tumor (B)

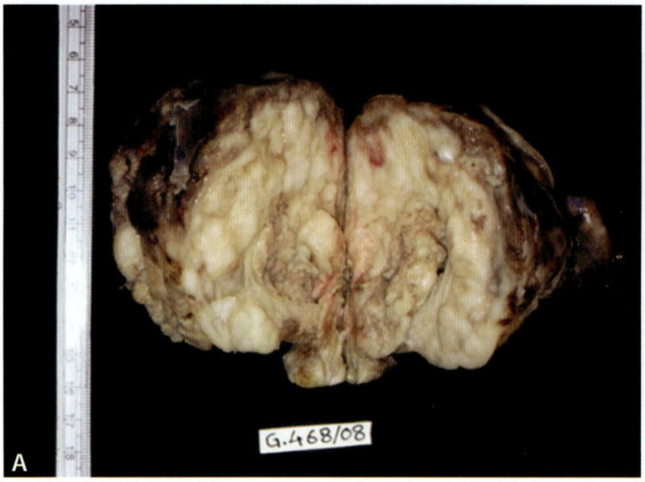

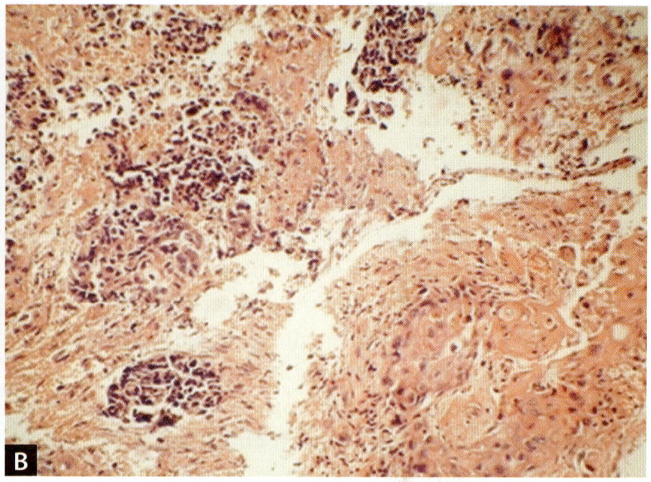

Figs. 9A and B: *Malignant mixed Müllerian tumor of the uterus*: Grossly, a large polypoidal, infiltrative tumor distorting the uterine cavity is seen (A). Microscopically, there is an admixture of epithelial and mesenchymal elements (B).

atypia is obvious and mitoses are numerous (>10/10 high power field). They must be distinguished from cellular and atypical leiomyomas by using histopathological criteria. *Epithelioid and myxoid variants* of leiomyosarcoma are known **(Figs. 10A to C)**.

CARCINOMA OF THE UTERINE CERVIX

The cervix is the lower part of the uterus and consists of the endocervix and the ectocervix. The former contains the endocervical canal and the ectocervix continues with the vagina. The ectocervix is covered with stratified squamous epithelium whereas the endocervix is covered by columnar mucin secreting endocervical epithelium. The junction of these two epithelia is called the *squamocolumnar junction (SCJ)*. During puberty and reproductive years of a woman, the squamo-columnar junction moves up and the epithelium between the old and the new SCJ is referred to as the '*transitional zone*' (TZ). It is important to remember that most cervical carcinomas originate in the transitional zone. Cervical cancer also has a well defined pre-cancerous state referred to *cervical intraepithelial neoplasia or CIN* which is graded from CIN I to CIN III. These lesions can be detected in a Papanicolaou smear and forms the basis for screening for cervical cancer **(Figs. 11A to D)**.

The association of *human papilloma virus* infection with cervical cancer and precancer is now well established. Out of the several oncogenic HPV types that are associated with cervical cancer, the most important genotypes are HPV 16 and 18 which together account for nearly 75% of the cancers. These are also referred to as high-risk HPV types. Screening programs for cervical cancer now also include testing for these high-risk HPV genotypes.

Invasive Cervical Carcinoma

Gross appearance: These tumors may be polypoid, predominantly exophytic tumors with a cauliflower-like appearance or may be endophytic, deeply infiltrative resulting in a hard cervix, which is only slightly enlarged. In the evaluation of a surgical specimen, it is important to note the extent of circumferential involvement as well as the upper and lower limits of the tumor. The depth of stromal involvement is also an important aspect. As cervical cancer spreads locally into the parametrium, this also needs careful evaluation.

Microscopic appearance: Squamous cell carcinoma is most common followed by adenocarcinoma. Other uncommon types include adenosquamous, verrucous, warty, glassy cell, adenoid-cystic, neuroendocrine and small cell carcinoma. The squamous cell carcinomas may be keratinizing or nonkeratinizing and may be well, moderately or poorly differentiated.

Adenocarcinoma also shows a varied morphology. Endocervical, endometrioid and other subtypes are recognized.

Carcinomas constitute nearly 99% of all malignancies of the cervix. The remaining 1% is made up of a large variety of neoplasms.

Botryoid rhabdomyosarcoma of the cervix is a variant of embryonal rhabdomyosarcoma and presents in children and adolescents as a myxoid polypoid mass covered by attenuated epithelium. This tumor arises in the vagina and less often in the cervix.

Microscopic appearance: The tumor cells are small, ovoid to spindle-shaped and form a dense layer beneath the

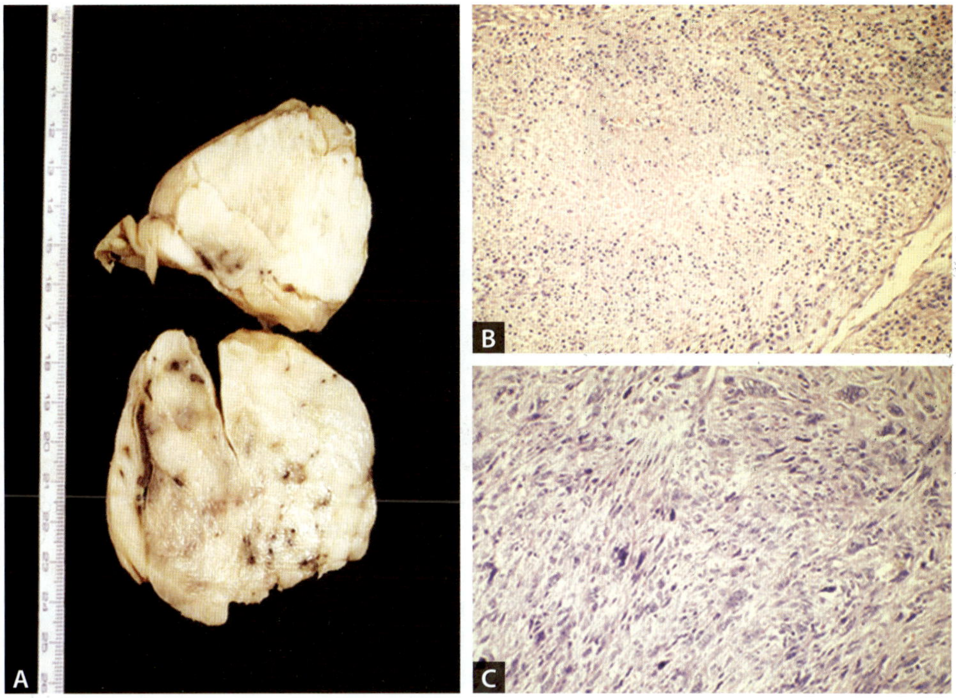

Figs. 10A to C: *Leiomyosarcoma uterus*: Grossly, a fleshy tumor is seen replacing the normal myometrium (A). Microscopically, coagulative necrosis and diffuse cytological atypia is noted (B and C).

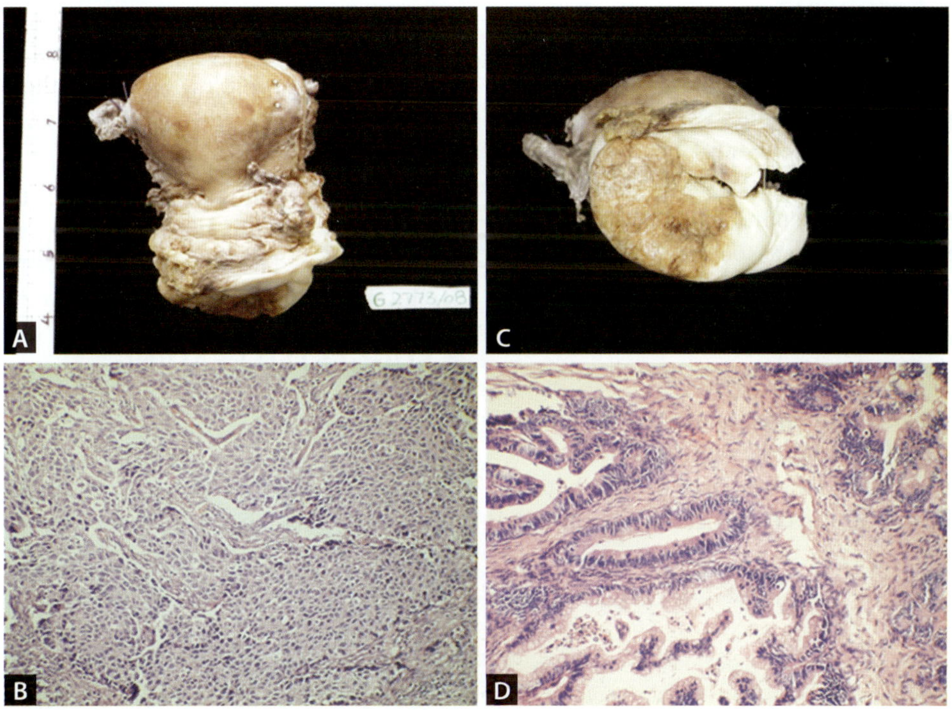

Figs. 11A to D: *Carcinoma cervix*: Gross picture of a resected specimen of carcinoma cervix showing an infiltrative growth involving the cervical lips circumferentially. (A and B) The bottom panel shows a squamous cell carcinoma on the left (C) and an adenocarcinoma on the right, the two principal histological types of invasive carcinoma (D).

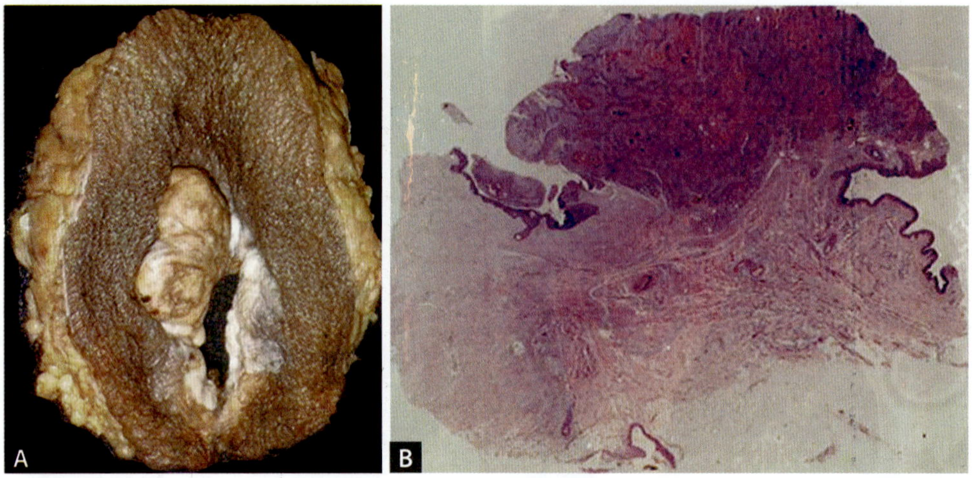

Figs. 12A and B: *Vulval carcinoma*: Grossly, the tumor is seen involving the right labia and extends to the clitoris (A). Microscopically, it shows a typical squamous cell carcinoma (B).

surface lining epithelium called *the 'cambium' layer.* The stroma is loose and myxoid with hypercellular and hypocellular areas. The nuclei are hyperchromatic and mitoses is variable. The tumor cells are positive for myogenic markers such as desmin and myogenin.

MALIGNANT TUMORS OF THE VULVA

Squamous Cell Carcinoma

Squamous cell carcinoma accounts for nearly 95% of all malignancies. On the basis of epidemiologic and virologic studies, it is proposed that there are two types of vulval carcinoma; one is HPV negative and occurs in older women and shows a typical keratinizing squamous cell carcinoma microscopically; second is HPV positive and occurs in younger women with associated VIN and has a basaloid or warty histology **(Figs. 12A and B)**.

Gross appearance: The tumor frequently arises in the labia majora but may involve the labia minora and clitoris.

Microscopic appearance: Squamous cell carcinomas are typically keratinizing. Other subtypes are also known.

Vulvar cancer spreads to the regional inguinal lymph nodes. Tumors located in the clitoris can show bilateral node involvement and also involve the deep nodes. Lately, the technique of sentinel lymph node biopsy (similar to breast cancer) has been introduced and practiced as a staging criterion and guide to management for vulvar carcinoma.

Vulvar Paget's Disease

Paget's disease is a malignant tumor of the vulva that clinically presents as a crusting, erythematous, scaling rash on the vulva. A biopsy shows large pale tumor cells forming solid nests or a continuous layer along the basement membrane. These cells are positive for mucin and immunohistochemically for MUC1 and MUC5AC, the latter in striking contrast to the breast. The cells are positive for EMA, CEA keratins and GCDFP-15, a marker of apocrine differentiation. The incidence of an underlying invasive carcinoma varies from 0–30% in vulvar Paget's disease.

SUGGESTED READING

1. Female Reproductive System in Rosai and Ackerman's Surgical Pathology, 9th edition. Mosby, Elsevier (Elsevier India); 2004; Vol. 2:1483-737.
2. Kurman RJ (Ed). Blaustein's Pathology of the Female Genital tract, 5th edition. New Delhi: Springer-Verlag; 2004.

CHAPTER 108

Imaging in Renal Tumors

Anjali Prakash

INTRODUCTION

Renal neoplasms that occur in adults constitute a heterogeneous group of tumors with characteristic histology and variable clinicobiological profile. The 2004 WHO classification[1] categorises neoplasms on basis of cell of origin and histopathology. Most renal tumors arise from the parenchyma, refered to as renal cell tumors, with a much smaller number arising from the collecting system and the mesenchyme.

A new classification system proposed in 2006 at Heidelberg subdivides renal cell tumor into benign and malignant parenchymal neoplasm and limits subcategory to the most commonly documented abnormalities **(Table 1)**.

BALLS VERSUS BEANS

A useful strategy for the evaluation of renal masses is to divide them on the basis of their growth pattern into ball type or bean type masses. This concept was developed by Hartman and Ros (Oral Communication, October 2006) **(Figs. 1A and B)**. Most renal masses like cysts, renal cell carcinomas, angiomyolipoma, metastasis, oncocytoma grow by expansion. These masses are shaped similarly to spheres or balls and they displace and compress, rather than invade normal structure. As these masses enlarge, they expand from normal parenchymal margins, either peripherally to the kidney or into renal sinus. Other renal lesions like transitional cell carcinoma, squamous cell, infiltrating carcinoma, lymphoma, renal medullary carcinoma grow along the latticework of normal renal parenchyma. Infiltrating lesions swell the area of involved parenchyma, but do not deform the shape. The kidney retains the 'bean' shape. These are difficult to detect radiologically since little mass effect is associated.

Imaging Modalities

Plain Films

Renal mass may be visible as a soft tissue shadow with displacement of retroperitoneal fat. Calcification can also be detected on plain film. Pattern of calcification may help in differentiating benign from malignant masses. Eighty percent of peripheral calcifications are seen in renal cysts, in 20% they are noted in malignant lesions. Renal masses that contain central, irregular calcifications are usually malignant **(Fig. 2)**.

Skeletal metastasis may also be detected. They appear as lytic expansile foci. Multiple osteomas or bone islands are another abnormality associated with renal mass, particularly in patients with tuberous sclerosis.

Intravenous Urograms

Excretory urography lacks specificity for accurately characterizing a lesion. Expansile masses cause contour abnormalities, calcyeal splaying, stretching and draping. Infiltrating renal mass produce little parenchymal mass effect and maybe seen as a filling defect in the collecting system.

Table 1: WHO classification of kidney tumors,

Familial Renal Cancer
Renal Cell Tumors *Malignant*: • Clear cell renal cell carcinoma • Multilocular clear cell renal cell carcinoma • Papillary renal cell carcinoma • Chromophobe renal cell carcinoma • Carcinoma of the collecting ducts of Bellini • Renal medullary carcinoma • Xp11 translocation carcinomas • Carcinoma associated with neuroblastoma • Mucinous tubular and spindle cell carcinoma • Renal cell carcinoma unclassified *Benign*: • Papillary adenoma • Oncocytoma
Metanephric Tumors • Metanephric adenoma • Metanephric adenofibroma • Metanephric stromal tumors
Mixed Mesenchymal and Epithelial Tumors • Cystic nephroma • Mixed epithelial and stromal tumor • Synovial sarcoma
Nephroblastic Tumors • Nephrogenic rests • Nephroblastoma • Cystic partially differentiated nephroblastoma
Neuroendocrine Tumors • Carcinoid • Neuroendocrine carcinoma • Primitive neuroectodermal tumor • Neuroblastoma • Pheochromocytoma
Other Tumors • Mesenchymal tumors • Hematopoietic and lymphoid tumors • Germ cell tumors • Metastatic tumors

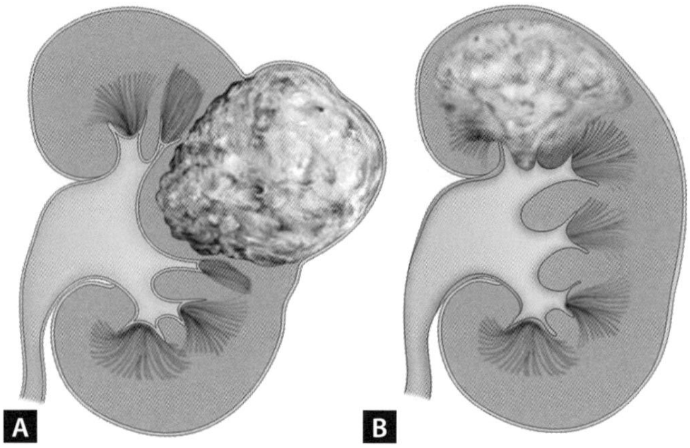

Figs. 1A and B: Ball versus Bean concept: (A) Ball type mass grows exophytically, with a contour deformity. (B) Bean type mass uses renal parenchyma as framework for growth with maintained reniform shape. Sinus fat and collecting system elements may be destroyed.

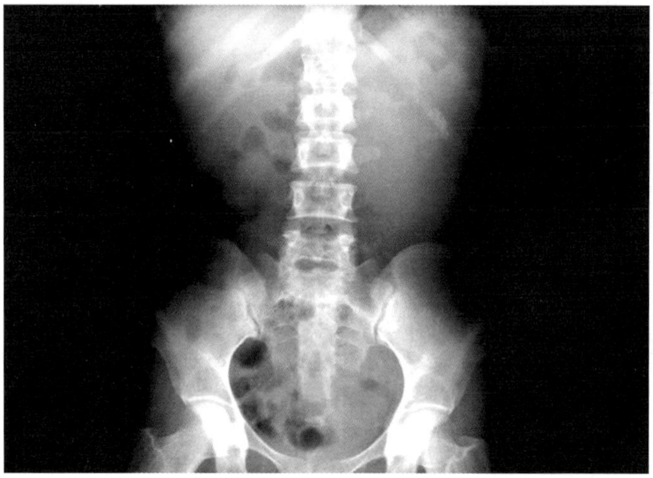

Fig. 2: Plain film showing soft tissue mass with amorphous calcification in left renal fossa.

Ultrasound

Ultrasound is very useful for detection of renal masses and characterizing them as solid or cystic. Ultrasound may also be useful when computed tomography (CT) pseudoenhancement is noted, leading to a simple renal cyst being mischaracterized as solid mass. Color Doppler sonography can evaluate renal vein and intravenous contrast (IVC) for presence of thrombus. The vascular flow within a renal mass, identified by color and power Doppler is strongly associated with clear cell carcinoma. The vascular distribution at power Doppler potentially could add information in differentiation of small solid renal masses. Peripheral or mixed peripheral and penetrating patterns are seen in all renal cell carcinomas (RCCs) and some benign angiomyolipomas (AMLs) and oncocytomas, whereas intratumoral focal and penetrating pattern is characteristic of angiomyolipomas.

Computed Tomography

Computed tomography (CT) is accurate in detection, characterization and staging of renal masses. Multidetector computed tomography (MDCT) allows fast, multiphase and high resolution imaging. Comprehensive evaluation of renal masses requires a dedicated CT protocol. For characterization of a renal mass, CT is done before and after administration of IVC. The different phases of renal enhancement [arterial (15–20 sec delay), corticomedullary (35–80 sec), nephrographic (85–180 sec) and excretory (3 min or more)], need to be evaluated.

The nephrographic phase is ideal for detection of masses as there is maximal and homogeneous parenchymal enhancement. This allows better delineation of renal masses which do not enhance to the same level as the renal parenchyma. During imaging in corticomedullary phase, small renal masses may be indistinguishable from renal medulla. During excretory phase, masses may be same attenuation as the parenchyma which has de-enhanced.

Imaging in corticomedullary phase may help in characterizing pseudotumors, such as hypertrophy of column of Bertin. Careful attention is to be given to enhancement that is identified as unequivocal and not due to pseudoenhancement which is elevated Hounsfield unit (HU) measurement of cyst due to image reconstruction algorithm. It may be useful to adopt gallbladder or a simple cyst (when present) as internal reference standard for HU measurement. An increase in attenuation of 10 HU or more in a lesion measuring at least 2 cm in diameter indicates enhancement. As enhancement is transient, washout of contrast is also useful. If an area of enhancement decreases subjectively or quantitatively (at least 10 HU), neoplasm is suspected. This is called "de enhancement".

CT urography is beginning to replace intravenous urogram (IVU) as the imaging examination of choice to detect upper urinary tract tumors.

Magnetic Resonance Imaging

MRI is useful for characterization of renal masses. This is especially useful in patients in whom iodinated contrast is contraindicated.

The protocol to be used includes a coronal HASTE, axial T2-weighted gradient and spin echo with fat suppression, axial dual echo in phase and opposed phase gradient echo T1 images and 3D fat-suppressed GRE T1 images before and after IVC followed by a coronal 3D fast gradient echo sequence with fat suppression after the dynamic series to display renal venous anatomy and IVC, MR imaging is valuable for distinct renal lesions. On magnetic resonance imaging, hemorrhagic cysts have high signal on T1WI. The combination of high signal on T1 and lack of enhancement are diagnostic for hemorrhagic cyst. T2-weighted images are useful in distinguishing a simple renal cyst from other lesions. A homogeneous hyperintense lesion on T2 with a thin wall and no enhancement is a renal simple cyst. All 3 phases of renal excretion are obtained after contrast and subtraction images may be obtained to determine, percentage of enhancement. In and opposed phase images help in detecting intratumoral fat.

MR urogram is indicated in patients with suspected collecting system disease.

Angiography

Renal angiography, once a basic element in the diagnosis of renal masses, is of little value now. CT and MR angiography give excellent vascular mapping of the kidney and have replaced catheter angiography for this diagnosis. Angiography may be an alternative to open biopsy in diagnosis of infiltrating renal neoplasm. Hypo and avascular lesion are usually urothelial malignancies.

Retrograde and Antegrade Pyelography

Retrograde and antegrade pyelography may be used for small urothelial tumors, for better mucosal detail.

RENAL CELL CARCINOMA[23]

Renal cell carcinoma, also called hypernephroma, pathologically adenocarcinoma is the most common primary renal malignancy in adults. It accounts for 85% of all malignant renal tumors and about 3% of all diagnosed neoplasms.

Renal carcinoma occurs more commonly in males, in the 5th to 7th decades. Most are sporadic; some may be associated with syndromes, such as von Hippel–Lindau (VHL). Risk factors include smoking, exposure to petroleum and asbestos. Usually RCC is unilateral, two percent are bilateral and nine percent are multicenteric in the same kidney. Bilateral and multicenteric tumors arise in patients of VHL syndrome, familial RCC and in patients on long term hemodialysis.

RCC is nowadays most commonly incidentally discovered (30%). These are often smaller and of lower grade and staging. RCC may however present with symptoms like flank pain (37%), hematuria and palpable mass; weight loss, anorexia, fever, GI or neurological symptoms or paraneoplastic syndromes. Superficial tumors can invade and breach the renal capsule and directly involve perirenal fat, adrenal gland and adjacent organs. Metastasis often occurs in regional nodes, invasion of cisterna chylii can lead to hilar and supraclavicular nodes. RCC has a propensity for venous thrombi. Systemic dissemination can take place into liver, bone, adrenal, opposite kidney or brain in decreasing order of frequency.

RCC is composed of different histological subtypes with different disease progression and metastatic potential.

Clear cell RCC is the most common type accounting for 75% of RCCs. They typically appear as variegated, expansile, cortical masses with areas of necrosis, hemorrhage, cystic change and calcification (15%). These show hypervascularity. Clear cell RCC, have the greatest metastatic potential and show hematogenous metastasis to lung, liver and bones. There is also a propensity of clear cell RCC for lymphatic and late and unusual sites of metastasis.

Papillary RCC, characterized by papillary or tubopapillary histologic architecture accounts for 10–15% of RCC. It presents at 40–50 years of age and is a slow growing tumor. They appear as homogeneous, hypovascular, soft tissue cortical masses with foci of calcification. A low tumor to aorta enhancement ratio or tumor to normal renal parenchyma enhancement ratio is highly indicative of papillary RCC. Papillary RCCs frequently show necrosis and hemorrhage.

Chromophobe RCC, a recently classified subtype of RCC, represents 5% of renal cell cancers and is characterized by large, pale cells with prominent cell membranes. They occur as solitary cortical masses. Bilateral and multicentric chromophobe RCCs are found in association with oncocytomas and Birt–Hogg–Dube syndrome. The tumor is typically large at presentation, homogeneous without necrosis or hemorrhage. The mass is relatively hypovascular. The chromophobe type is associated with the least malignant potential and best prognosis.

Multicystic renal cell carcinoma (MCRCC) is a recently described, rare subtype of RCC. The term is used to describe a cystic RCC with a small volume (25% or less) of neoplastic clear cells in the cyst. MCRCC typically manifests as multiseptated cystic masses with thin septations on imaging. Distinction from other cystic masses is difficult.

IVU

An RCC, on IVU appears as an expansile contour bulge. Since the tumor grows by expansion, the tumor usually displaces and distorts the calyces **(Fig. 3)**. Increased distance between calyx and cortex is a sensitive sign. Occasionally an RCC grows predominantly outward and no detectable mass effect is exerted on the calyceal system. RCC's that extend either exclusively anteriorly or posteriorly may be difficult to be detected on IVU as the mass contour is superimposed by normal kidney. Other signs on IVU of RCC are secondary to mass effect and the need for increased vascular perfusion. This is in the form of notching of renal pelvis and ureter as a result of enlarged ureteric and renal pelvic vessels which are enlarged to feed a hypervascular RCC. Focal or diffuse hydronephrosis may result due to a large RCC which leads to compression of major calyces, the renal pelvis and upper ureter. Decreased or absent function may be noted. The finding of globally decreased function with a renal mass is suggestive of RCC.

Less commonly, an RCC grows by infiltration rather than expansion and in these cases; malignant stricturing of the collecting system occurs, secondary to encasement and invasion of the urothelium.

Small RCCs are undetectable by IVU. One-third of mass lesions less than 3 cm in diameter, cannot be detected with IVU. A normal IVU in patients with clinical evidence of RCC should be supplemented with CT, ultrasound (US) or MRI. The detection of mass on IVU is nonspecific and needs further imaging for characterization.

Ultrasound

Renal adenocarcinoma is detected as a well encapsulated solid mass. It may have poorly defined margins. The reflectivity of the mass is similar to that of adjacent parenchyma, although texture is heterogeneous or is of reduced reflectivity. Tumors that are hyperechoic with echogenicity similar to renal sinus fat occur and account for one third of tumors under 3 cm in diameter, these mimic angiomyolipoma. Features that suggest a malignancy is an echopoor rim and small cysts within the tumor. The echopoor rim is due to a peudocapsule of compressed renal tissue and this is not seen in AML. As tumor grows, inhomogeneity of its appearance increases due to hemorrhage and necrosis **(Fig. 4)**. The echopattern of the tumor does not reflect the histological type of tumor. Papillary tumors, which are usually low grade, are of increased reflectivity.

If the tumor is cystic, it presents as a unilocular cystic mass in about 50% of such cases. Features, such as irregular thickened walls, echoes and calcification favor

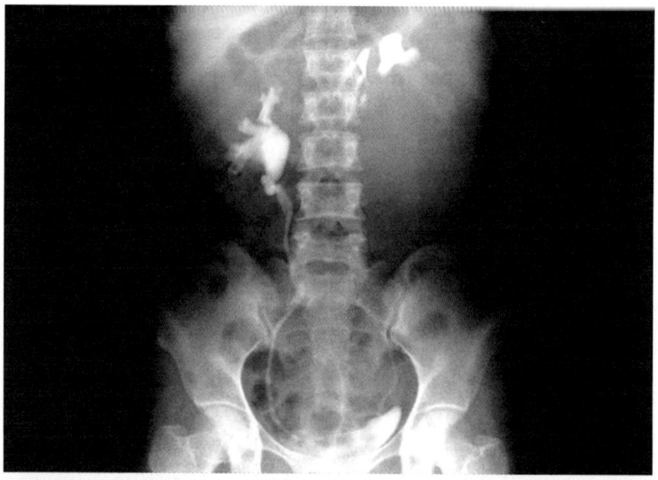

Fig. 3: IVU showing compression and displacement of calyces on the left. There is focal hydrocalyx of the upper pole—Renal cell carcinoma.

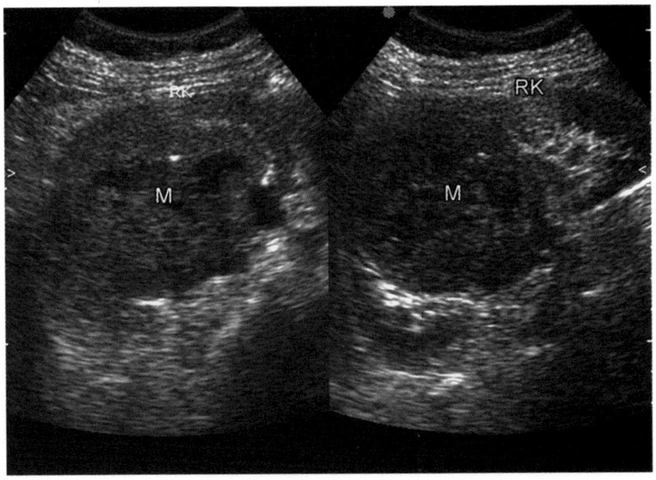

Fig. 4: Ultrasound: Transverse and longitudinal sonogram of the right kidney shows a large well-defined heterogeneous mass arising from the upper pole right kidney—Renal cell carcinoma.

malignancy. In 30%, the appearance is of a multilocular cystic mass with intervening solid areas, which may calcify. In remaining 20% there is a solid mass within the wall of cyst.

Doppler

An abnormal Doppler signal can be seen in the ipsilateral renal artery as an increase in velocity, spectral broadening and turbulence. These findings may also be seen in some inflammatory lesions making it nonspecific **(Figs. 5A and B)**.

Intraoperative ultrasound is being used in nephron sparing surgery to delineate exact extent of the mass and venous thrombi.

Computed Tomography

On unenhanced CT, renal cell carcinomas may be hypodense, isodense or hyperdense to the unenhanced renal parenchyma. They are often heterogeneous, with one or more low density central areas, the mass distorts the margin of the kidney in a majority (94%) of cases, irrespective of tumor size. The presence of calcification is also noted in approximately 25% and CT is the most sensitive modality for the depiction of parenchymal calcification. The calcification of RCC may be punctate, amorphous, linear or peripheral **(Figs. 6A and B)**. A zone of relative radiolucency surrounding the tumor or 'halo sign' may be noted. This represents the compressed ischemic renal parenchyma around the tumor—'Pseudocapsule'.

Following contrast administration, renal cell carcinomas reveal inhomogeneous enhancement to a lesser degree than normal parenchyma with an indistinct parenchymal interface **(Figs. 7A to D)**. Clear cell carcinomas enhance to a greater degree than other subtypes of malignant lesions, especially papillary carcinoma.

Most renal carcinomas are solid with an attenuation of atleast 20 HU on precontrast scans. An increase in attenuation of more than 10 HU after contrast suggests a solid mass and enhancement of more than 20 HU indicates malignancy **(Figs. 8A to D)**. Heterogeneous enhancement correlates with the presence of acellular regions within the tumor, but does not correlate with grade. Cystic and necrotic change is seen in clear cell type, whereas papillary and chromophobe are more homogeneous **(Fig. 9)**.

There, often is renal vein invasion and the thrombus may extend into the IVC (30%). CT is specific for renal vein invasion by tumor thrombus with specificity of 98%.[2] A hypodense filling defect outlined by contrast in the renal vein on CT using corticomedullary or nephrographic phase is diagnostic for thrombus **(Fig. 10)**. CT for detection of thrombus requires thin (<5 mm) slices at level of renal vein after pressure injection of contrast. Renal vein enlargement and displacement are not accurate signs for venous invasion, as it may be enlarged due to high flow and displaced due to bulk of tumor.

Heterogeneous enhancement of thrombus on nephrographic phase is further diagnostic for tumor thrombus. The flow of unenhanced blood from pelvis may be mistaken for IVC thrombus. In these cases delayed images may be needed for further characterization. Tumor thrombus may extend into IVC, often enlarging the caliber of the IVC. There may be bland thrombus inferior to the tumor thrombus in the IVC, as a result of occlusion of the lumen.

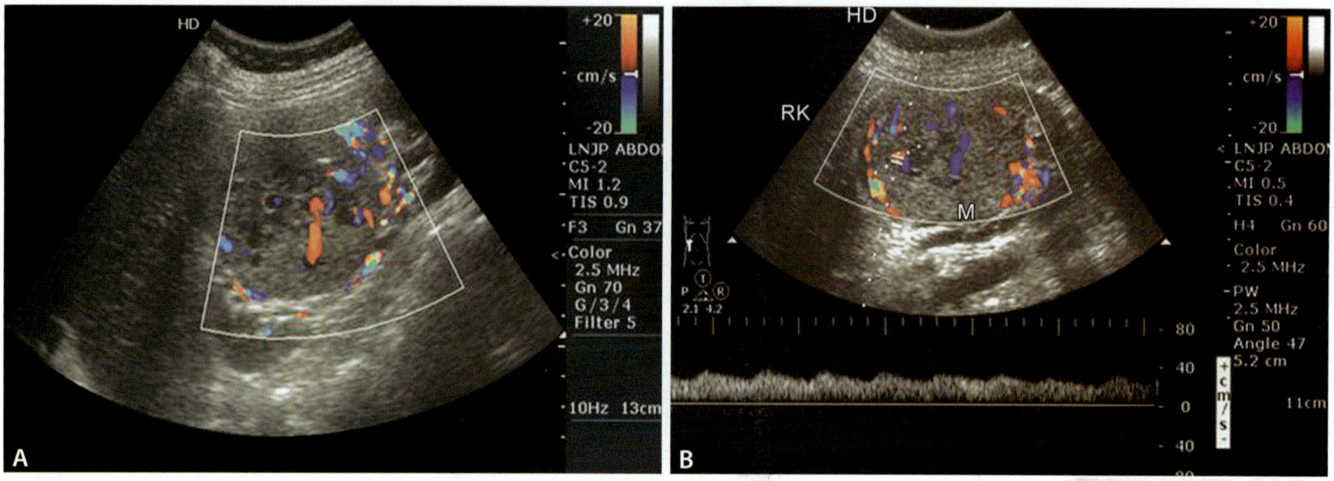

Figs. 5A and B: Color Doppler (A) and spectral trace (B) show vascularity within and surrounding the mass.

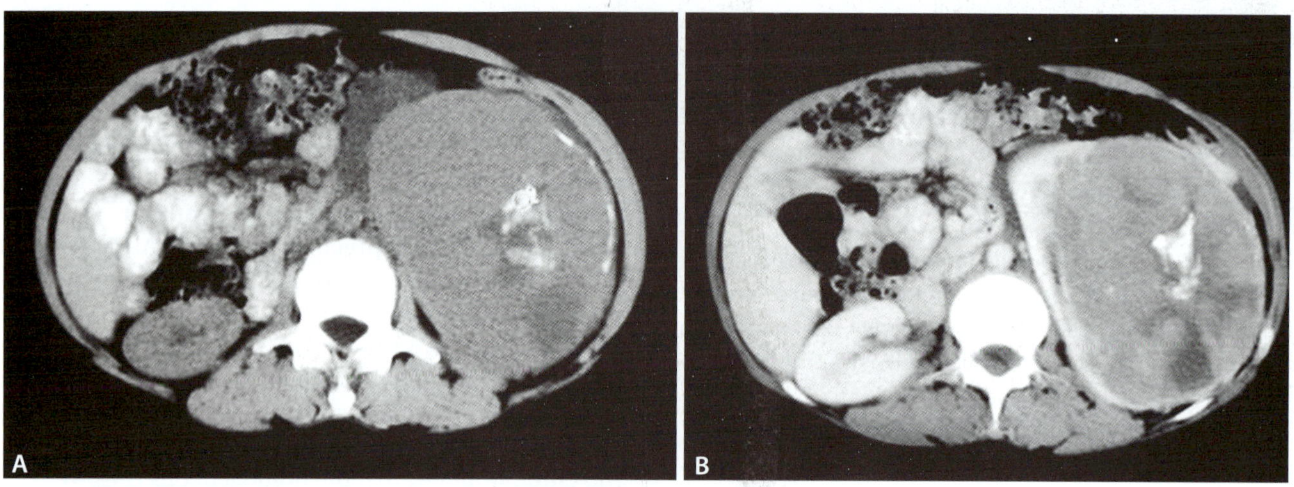

Figs. 6A and B: NCCT and contrast-enhanced computed tomography (CECT) showing a large enhancing left renal mass with peripheral and central coarse calcification in the left kidney.

Metastatic adenopathy in the retroperitoneum, associated with RCC has poor prognostic significance. The criterion of 1 cm as a threshold has proved to be unsuccessful in differentiating reactive nodes from metastatic adenopathy. Lymph nodes greater than 2 cm are always malignant. Nodes, less than 1 cm may contain metastasis.

Magnetic Resonance Imaging

Diagnosis is made on visualization of a contour disrupting mass, small RCCs are undetectable on MRI. RCC is typically mildly hypointense to the renal cortex on T1-weighted images and mildly high signal on T2-weighted images. Most RCCs have a hypointense 'pseudocapsule' on TIW (25%) and T2W (60%) at the periphery of tumor on SE images **(Figs. 11A and B)**. Interruption of this pseudocapsule correlates with advanced stage. Fat saturated images are also recommended as there is a signal drop in AMLs and rare for RCC to contain fat.

Based on T1-weighted images, a 15–20% enhancement on scans 3–5 minutes after gadolinium is considered diagnostic. When a diagnostic dilemma of enhancement is seen on CT scan, MR imaging is helpful. Subtraction (gadolinium-enhanced fat-suppressed T1-weighted images-unenhanced fat-suppressed T1-weighted image) is an easy, reliable method. However, it is necessary for subtraction, to have accurate corregisteration of enhanced and unenhanced MR images. It is recommended that all MR sequences be obtained during an end expiratory breath-hold which is more reproducible. It may also be

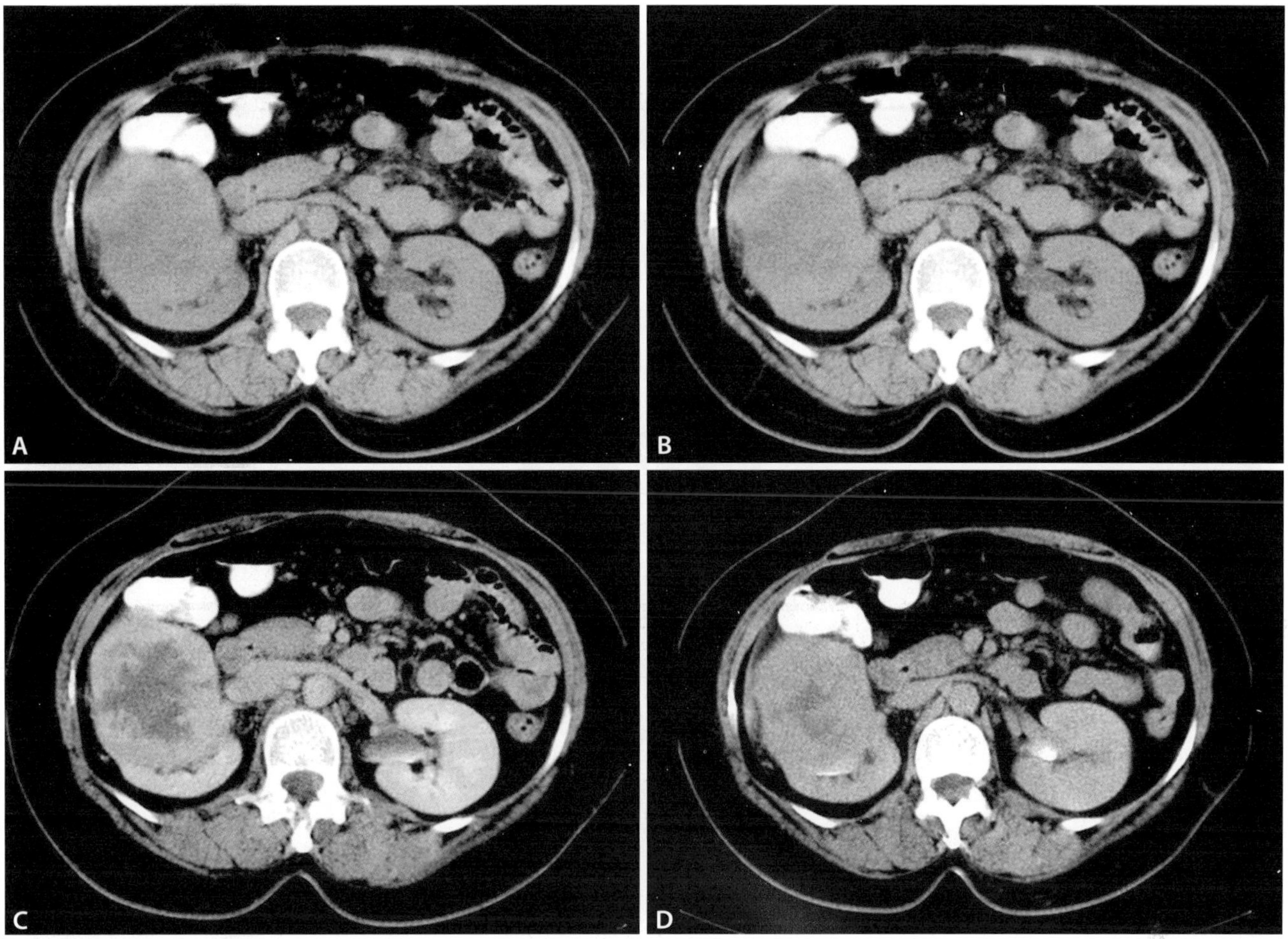

Figs. 7A to D: CT features of renal cell carcinomas in 4 phases: (A) Noncontrast, (B) Corticomedullary, (C) Nephrographic, (D) Excretory phases. Figures show a right renal mass with mixed enhancement pattern containing enhancing soft tissue and low attenuation areas representing necrosis or cystic change arising from the anterior renal cortex. The mass is best demarcated on nephrographic phase and shows "de enhancement" in the later phase.

difficult to detect enhancement on CT in a heavily calcified mass. MR imaging is helpful as calcification not being seen and any enhancement will be detected. MRI is useful in patients for whom iodinated intravascular contrast is contraindicated **(Figs. 12A to D)**. Multiplanar capability of MRI is helpful in evaluation of vascular thrombosis. GE sequences are used to assess thrombus by depicting flowing blood via a bright signal as opposed to a thrombus which is low signal intensity. GE images maybe helpful in cases with marked caval compression by tumor masses.

Various studies have correlated MRI appearance of renal masses with pathology. An MRI classification system has been proposed to predict the histological subtype and nuclear grade. This is based on certain characteristics like lesion size, peripheral vs central location, T2 signal intensity and degree of enhancement of the lesion, the presence of subvoxel fat on CSI, intratumoral necrosis, retroperitoneal vascular collaterals, vascular thrombosis. Clear cell RCC frequently demonstrates signal intensity similar to renal parenchyma on T1-weighted images and increased signal on T2-weighted images. Loss of signal intensity within the solid portions of clear cell RCCs on opposed phase images as compared to in phase images is due to cytoplasmic fat and is seen in upto 60% of these tumors **(Figs. 13A to H)**. Central necrosis is common and is typically seen as homogeneous hypointense on T1WI and moderately high signal on T2WI.Clear cell RCCs tend to be hypervascular with heterogeneous enhancement during arterial phase. Retroperitoneal collaterals and renal vein thrombosis are predictive of high grade clear cell RCC. Papillary RCC demonstrate low signal intensity on T2-weighted images due to presence of hemosiderin,

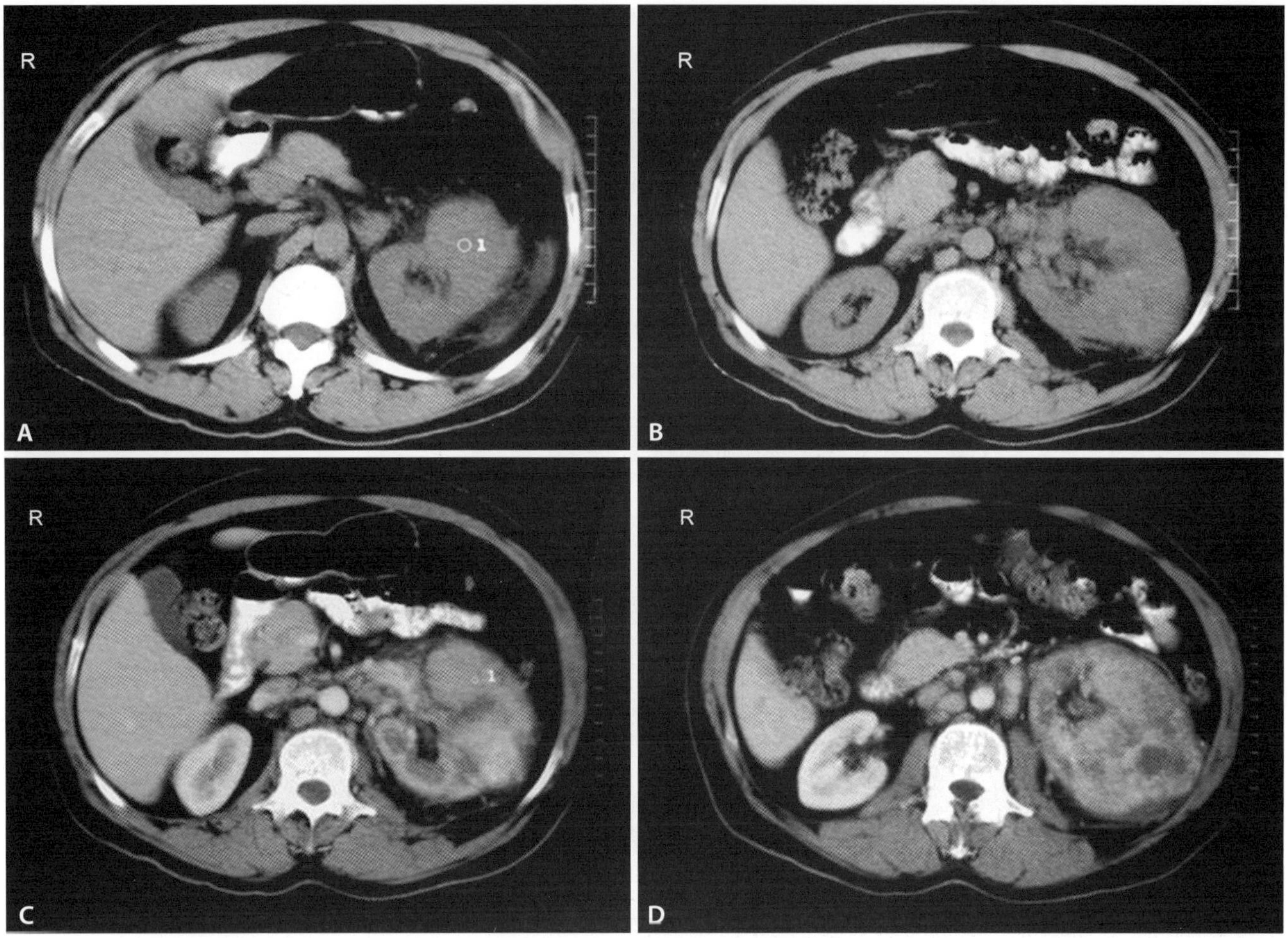

Figs. 8A to D: CT Pre- (A and B) and postcontrast (C and D) shows solid left renal mass with increase in attenuation of 20 HU—Malignant etiology (RCC).

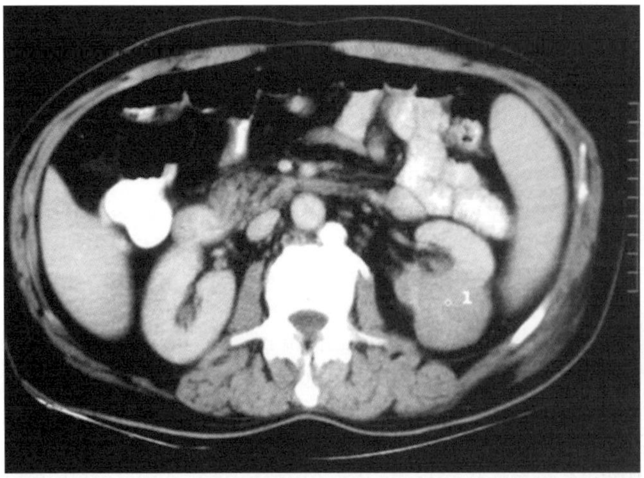

Fig. 9: CT abdomen shows a small hypodense well-defined cortical mass with no fat density. Possibility of small neoplasm (?papillary RCC) is to be considered.

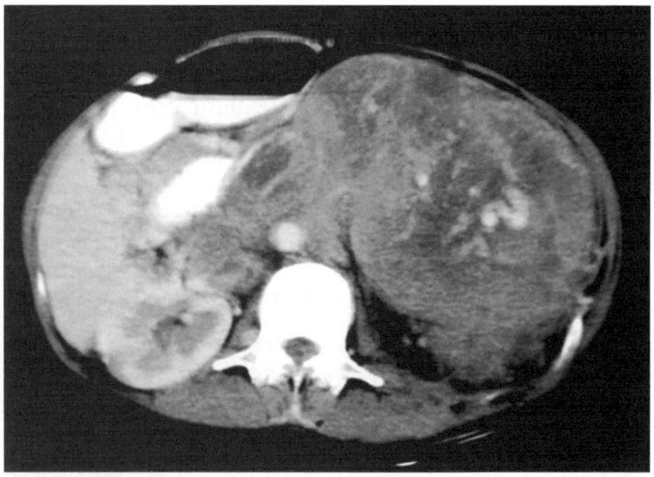

Fig. 10: CECT abdomen shows a large mass in the left kidney with neovascularity, definite extension into perinephric space, left renal vein and IVC—RCC.

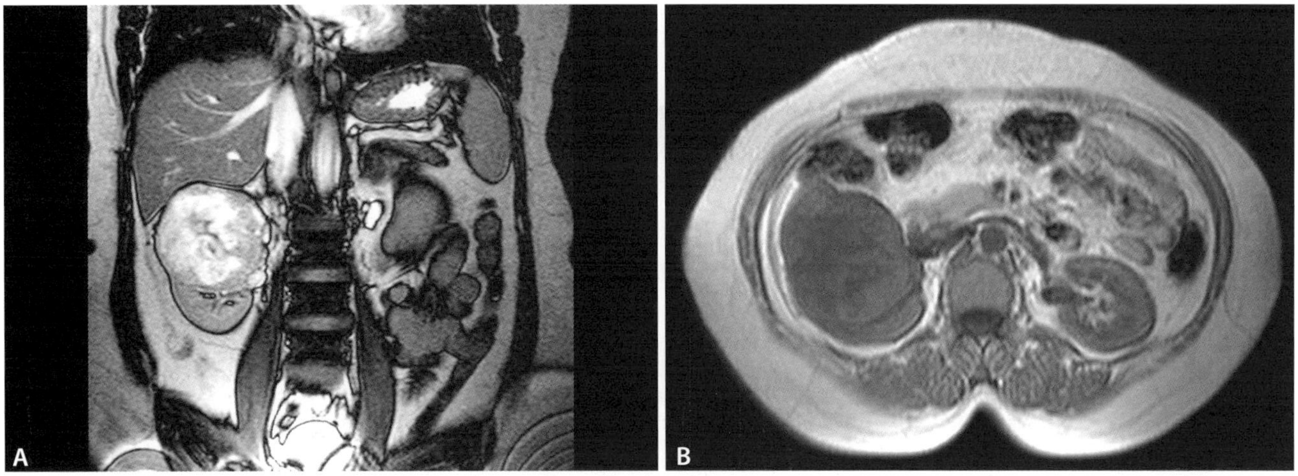

Figs. 11A and B: Renal cell carcinoma—MRI: (A) TRUE FISP coronal and (B) T1WI axial showing a well-circumscribed mass hypointense on T1 and hyperintense on T2 arising from upper pole of right kidney. IVC appears normal. Necrotic change is noted appearing hyperintense on T2W images.

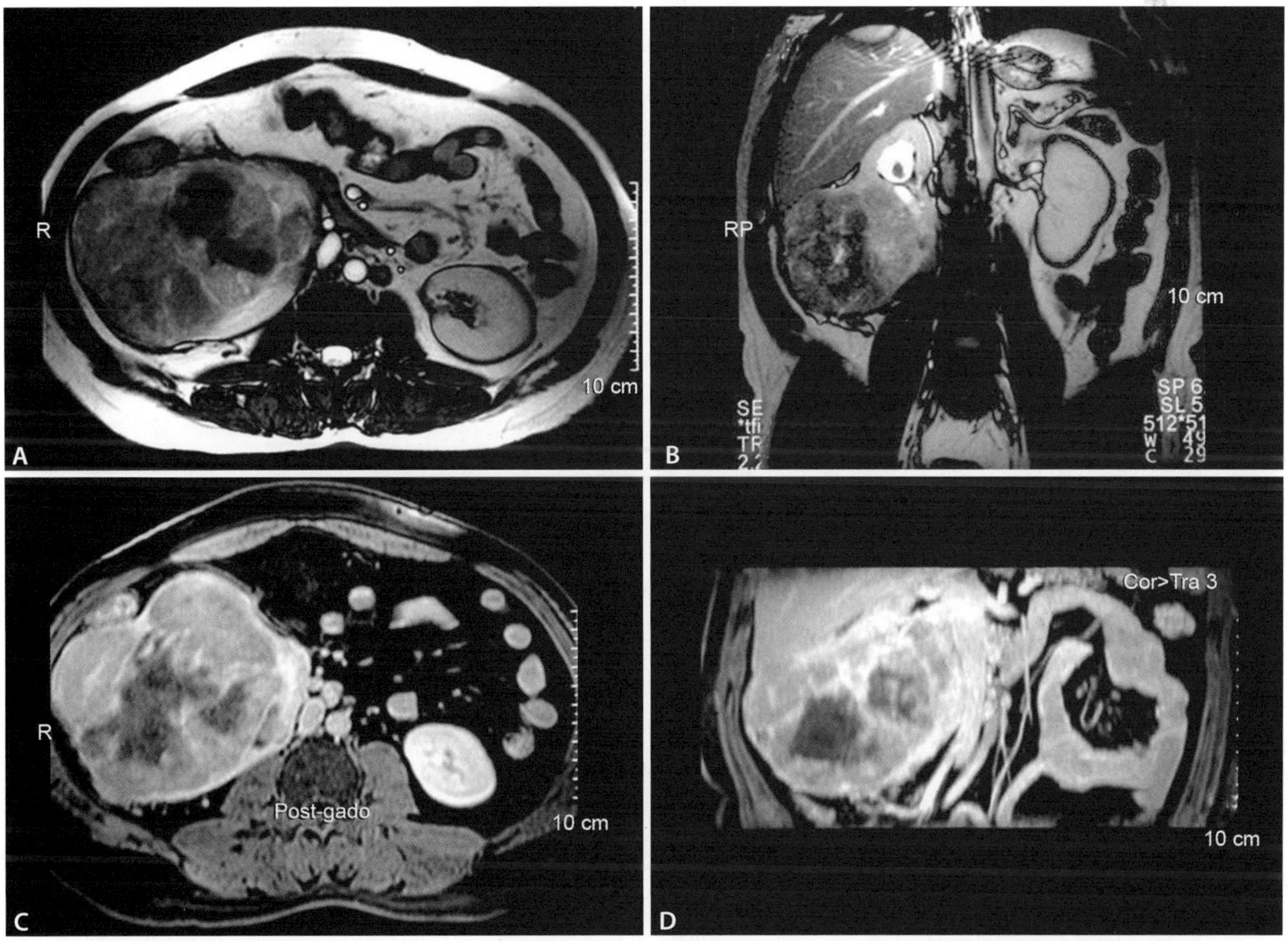

Figs. 12A to D: Magnetic resonance imaging: TRUE FISP axial (A) and coronal (B) showing mixed intensity right lower renal polar mass with areas of hemorrhage and well-defined "peudocapsule" TI postgadolinium axial (C) and MPR (D) shows enhancing soft tissue component of the mass.

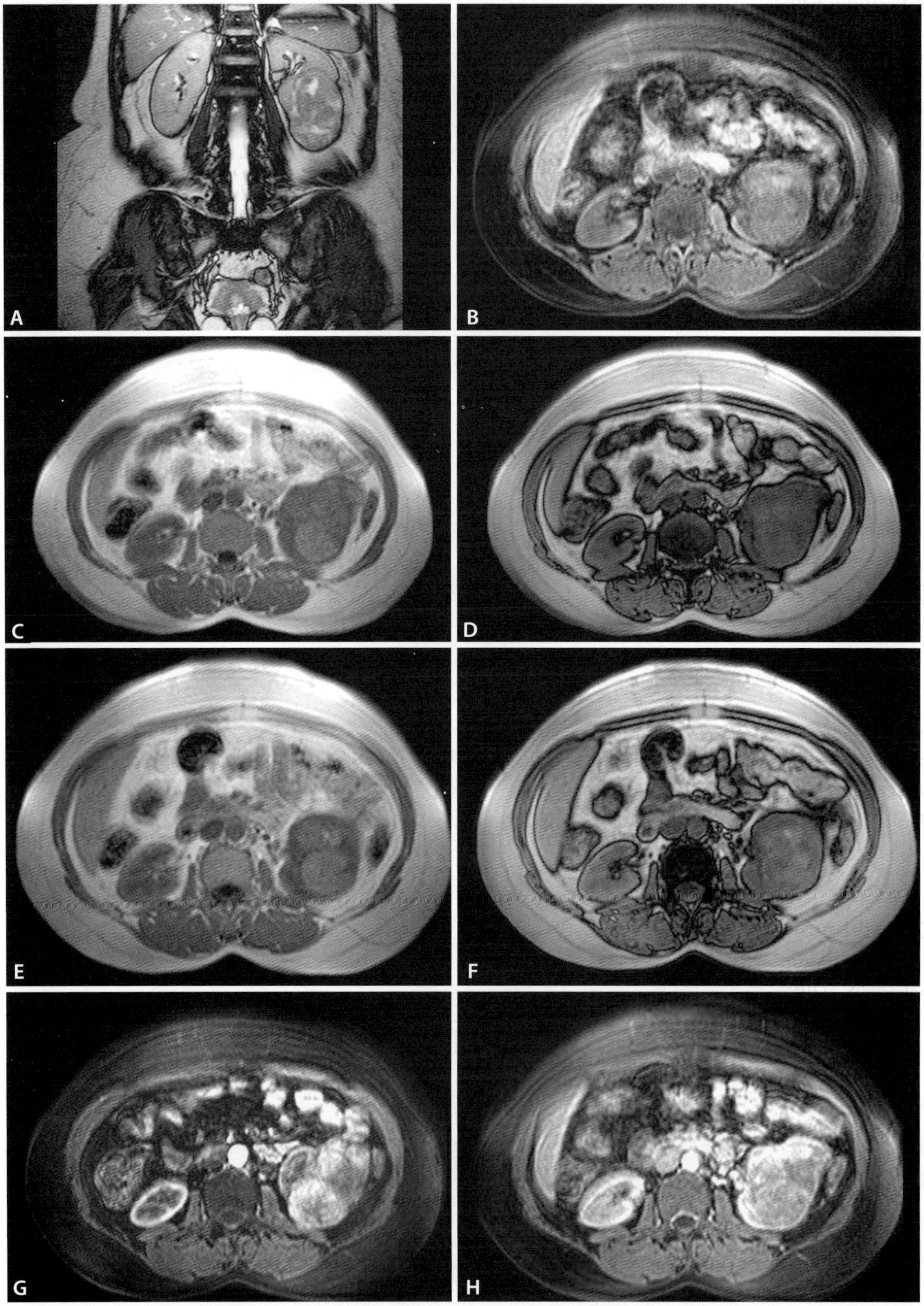

Figs. 13A to H: MRI T2 TRUE FISP coronal (A), TI VIBE axial (B), T1 in phase (C and E), opposed phase (D and F) TI axial post-gado (G and H): A solid-enhancing mass is seen in left kidney, hypointense on T1, hyperintense on T2, with a drop in signal intensity on opposed phase images compared to in phase images. Note lack of "India Ink" effect on opposed phase—clear cell RCC.

small size, peripheral location and low level enhancement. High-grade papillary RCC have a more complex appearance with hemorrhage and necrosis. Enhancing papillary projections at periphery of a cystic hemorrhagic mass are seen.[3,4]

Recent studies have shown a promising role of diffusion imaging in evaluation of renal masses. A decrease in ADC values is suggestive of malignant etiology.[5]

Angiography

Angiography, is only very occasionally indicated preoperatively for vascular mapping, especially if nephron sparing surgery is being contemplated for small neoplasm, multiple and bilateral neoplasm or tumors in horseshoe kidney. Most RCCs are hypervascular with presence of tumor vessels which are irregular, tortuous and distributed randomly.

Angioinfarction has a limited role, in large tumors and as palliative procedure to control pain, hematuria in inoperable/unfit for surgery patients.

Nuclear Scintigraphy

Flurodeoxyglucose-positron emission tomography (FDG-PET) has a reported sensitivity for detection of renal malignancy in the range of 40–94%.[6] Normal renal excretion of FDG may decrease contrast between tumor and normal renal parenchyma. False-positive results have also been seen in patients with benign inflammatory process of the kidney or benign tumors. Flurodeoxyglucose-positron emission tomography may have a role in evaluating distant metastasis and in the differentiation between recurrence and post-treatment changes.

Staging of Renal Cell Carcinoma[7-11]

Staging is a critical component of evaluation of a patient with renal mass. The staging and histological grading affects the survival and the therapeutic approach. Five-year survival rates vary from 95% for T1 to 20% for T4. Currently the most commonly used staging system is the TNM system of the American Joint Committee on Cancer **(Table 2)**. The patient's overall stage is determined by the American Joint Committee on Cancer stage groupings **(Table 3)**.

It is impossible to differentiate between stage I and stage II RCC with CT and MRI. Some signs like stranding of perinephric fat fascial thickening, obliteration/blurring of fat, adrenal involvement, visible collaterals are considered suggestive for extracapsular spread. Perinephric stranding may result from edema, congestion and obliteration of fat may be due to mass effect. The most reliable imaging sign of RCC spread is the presence of discrete perinephric mass >1 cm in diameter **(Fig. 14)**. This is usually of not much significance other than prognostication, since radical nephrectomy is the treatment for both, except when there is a solitary kidney or bilateral tumors. The presence of an intact pseudocapsule, composed of compressed normal renal parenchyma and fibrous tissue seen best on T2WI, suggests lack of perinephric invasion.

Table 2: TNM staging for renal cancer.

T	***Primary tumor***
TX	Primary tumor cannot be assessed
T0	No evidence of primary tumor
T1	Tumor ≤7 cm in greatest dimension, limited to the kidney
T1a	Tumor ≤4 cm in greatest dimension, limited to the kidney
T1b	Tumor >4 cm but ≤7 cm in greatest dimension, limited to the kidney
T2	Tumor >7 cm in greatest dimension, limited to the kidney
T3	Tumor extends into major veins or invades adrenal gland or perinephric tissues, but not beyond Gerota's fascia
T3a	Tumor directly invades adrenal gland or perirenal and or renal sinus fat, but not beyond Gerota's fascia
T3b	Tumor grossly extends into the renal vein or its segmental (i.e. muscle-containing) branches or the vena cava below the diaphragm
T3c	Tumor grossly extends into the vena cava above the diaphragm or invades the wall of the vena cava
T4	Tumor invades beyond Gerota's fascia
N	***Regional lymph nodes***
NX	Regional lymph nodes cannot be assessed
N0	No regional lymph node metastasis
N1	Metastasis in a single regional lymph node
N2	Metastasis in >1 regional lymph node
M	***Distant metastasis***
MX	Distant metastasis cannot be assessed
M0	No distant metastasis
M1	Distant metastasis

Table 3: Stage grouping for renal cancer.

Stage I	T1, N0, M0
Stage II	T2, N0, M0
Stage III	T1, N1, M0 T2, N1, M0 T3, N0, M0 T3, N1, M0
Stage IV	T4, N0, M0 T4, N1, M0 Any T, N2, M0 Any T, any N, M1

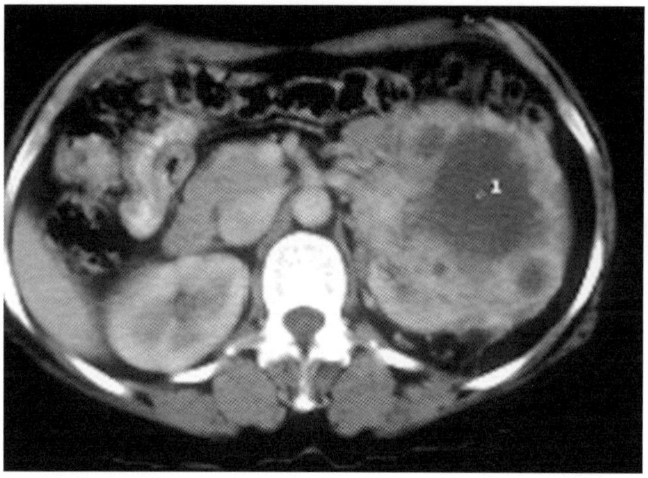

Fig. 14: Computed tomography: A large left renal mass with definite extension into the perinephric space—stage II.

Stage III includes invasion of renal vein, IVC, adrenal or regional adenopathy. Surgical planning for these patients depends on accurate preoperative staging. If tumor extends only into subdiaphragmatic cava, then a flank approach is sufficient. If it extends beyond this, then thoracoabdominal approach has to be followed. MRI is more sensitive for vascular invasion than CT and the diagnosis is aided by multiplanar ability of MRI. It is more sensitive, for IVC wall invasion and to confirm tumor thrombus **(Figs. 15A to C)**. On the right side it may be difficult to distinguish between intraluminal tumor thrombus and extrinsic caval compression caused by a large primary tumor or enlarged lymph nodes. Gradient echo images may detect a low-signal defect within the high signal lumen of IVC.

Based on nodal size criteria alone, MRI and CT are similar in sensitivity and specificity for metastatic adenopathy. False- positive rates of 58% have been reported, however, when a size criterion of 1 cm is used, owing to reactive or other benign nodal disease. These false-positives are more frequent in patients with tumor involvement of the renal vein and tumor necrosis. Ultrasmall supramagnetic iron oxide particles have shown promise in differentiating metastatic nodes from normal nodes. A normal node will take up this particle and create a drop in T2 signal, whereas no drop in signal is seen in metastatic nodes.

CT has a high negative predictive value for adrenal involvement from RCC. It has been suggested that only when the adrenal gland is not identified, not displaced or enlarged on CT, adrenal is said to be involved.

Stage IV cancer involves distant metastasis or spread to other organs;8 except the adrenal. Metastatic disease involves lung, liver, bone or brain. RCC <3 cm rarely metastasize. A renal mass may appear to invade the liver or spleen, when it is actually distorting the margin without direct invasion **(Figs. 16A to C)**. A chest radiograph is essential for the work-up. A chest CT to be done if the radiograph is abnormal or the local disease is advanced. RCC is associated with hypervascular liver metastasis, particularly from clear cell RCC. Portal venous phase imaging detects 90% of metastasis. Bone metastases are usually lytic. Bone scan is performed only in patients with bone pain or raised alkaline phosphatase. Bone scan may be negative as the lytic metastasis produce little osteoblastic reaction. MRI may be more sensitive to CT in detection of unsuspected bony metastasis, because of bone marrow imaging capability.

The overall accuracy of MR staging is comparable or superior to CT. It has advantages over CT in the evaluation of tumor vascular extension, differentiation of perihilar vessels from nodes and the assessment of direct tumor extension into other organs **(Figs. 17A and B)**. MRI is an excellent staging modality when the CT findings are equivocal.

Follow-up

Most recurrences occur within 3 years with a median relapse time of 1–2 years. Tumor diameter, T stage, nuclear grade are important determinants for recurrence. For imaging surveillance,CT is the modality of choice for local recurrence as well as distant metastasis. Baseline CT and follow-up CT at 6 months interval is recommended. Normal structures may migrate into the renal fossa after nephrectomy and may simulate recurrent tumor. The liver, ascending colon, 2nd part of duodenum, pancreatic head and small bowel may migrate into the right side. The most likely site of recurrence of tumors is in the nephrectomy site or adjacent structures **(Fig. 18)**. Solid organ recurrence also occurs in liver, contralateral kidney or adrenal. Flurodeoxyglucose-positron emission tomography may also play a role in follow up with a high positive predictive value.

Stages I and II are treated surgically with a partial or radical nephrectomy. Stage III lesions are usually treated with radical nephrectomy with extirpation of tumor filled veins, tumor thrombectomy and local lymph node excision. Patients with stage IV are treated palliatively. Renal sparing surgery is now becoming a widely accepted method for removing small cancers. Although partial nephrectomy is offered to patients of bilateral tumors or solitary kidney, it is now being offered to all patients with renal lesions less than 4 cm even in the setting of a normal

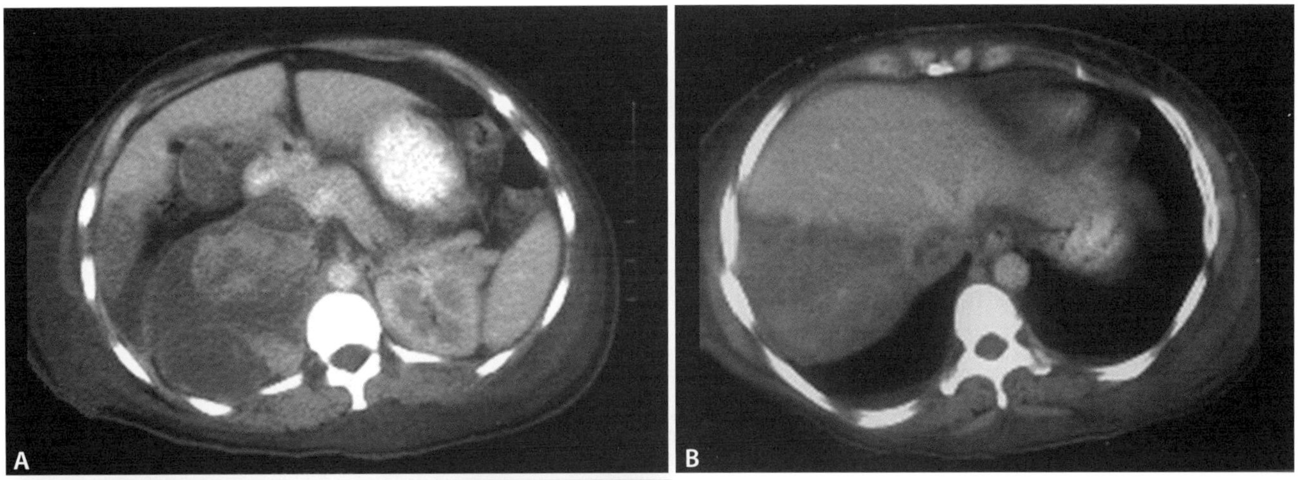

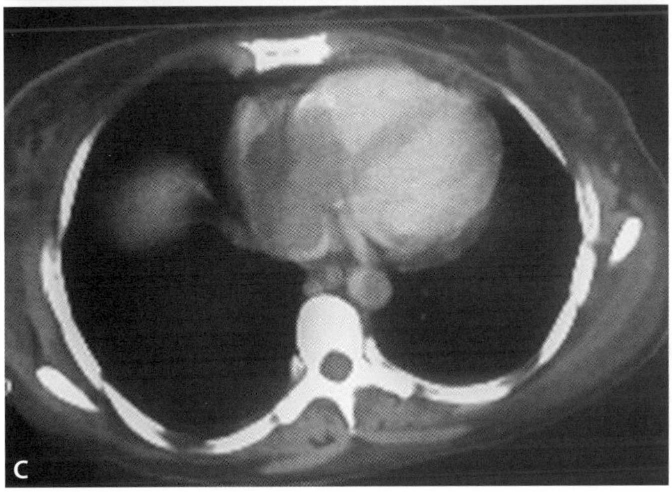

Figs. 15A to C: *Renal cell carcinoma*: CT shows a complex solid cystic mass with an intraluminal filling defect seen in the renal vein which is enlarged (A); A more cephlad section shows the enhancing thrombus within the IVC and a consequent to this, a perfusion deficit in liver (B); The thrombus is seen to extend into the right atrium (C).

contralateral kidney. These patients have a decreased risk of chronic renal insufficiency and proteinuria. Image-guided percutaneous radiofrequency ablative therapies are also being used. This is to treat patients who are high-risk for surgery and to preserve renal function in multifocal disease. The central tumors are more difficult to ablate than the peripheral exophytic ones.[12]

UROTHELIAL TUMOR

Transitional Cell Carcinoma

Urothelial tumors are less common in the upper urinary tract than renal cell carcinoma. However, transitional cell carcinoma (TCC) is the second most common renal neoplasm in adults. It is most common in urinary bladder, followed in frequency by ureter and pelvis. They may be bilateral in 10% and multicentric in 20–44%. This known multifocality warrants that the entire collecting system must be evaluated in patients with upper tract TCC because of high prevalence of tumor in the lower tract.

The risk factors for TCC include NSAID abuse, tobacco use or some occupational exposure. The incidence of TCC is more common in males, in the seventh decade. They commonly present with hematuria and flank pain. Hematogenous spread is less common than RCC, but lymphatic spread occurs earlier. High grade tumors are more common in upper tract than the urinary bladder. It has been suggested that stage rather than tumor grade is the main prognostic factor for urothelial tumor of the upper tract.

Intravenous Urogram

This is the primary investigative modality. The findings include a filling defect outlined by excreted contrast. The filling defect may be in pelvis (35%) or calyces (26%). 'Stipple sign' may be seen due to trapping of contrast in the interstices of a papillary growth. There may be obstruction of kidney with non opacification of the collecting system (phantom calyx) due to extensive areas of parenchymal

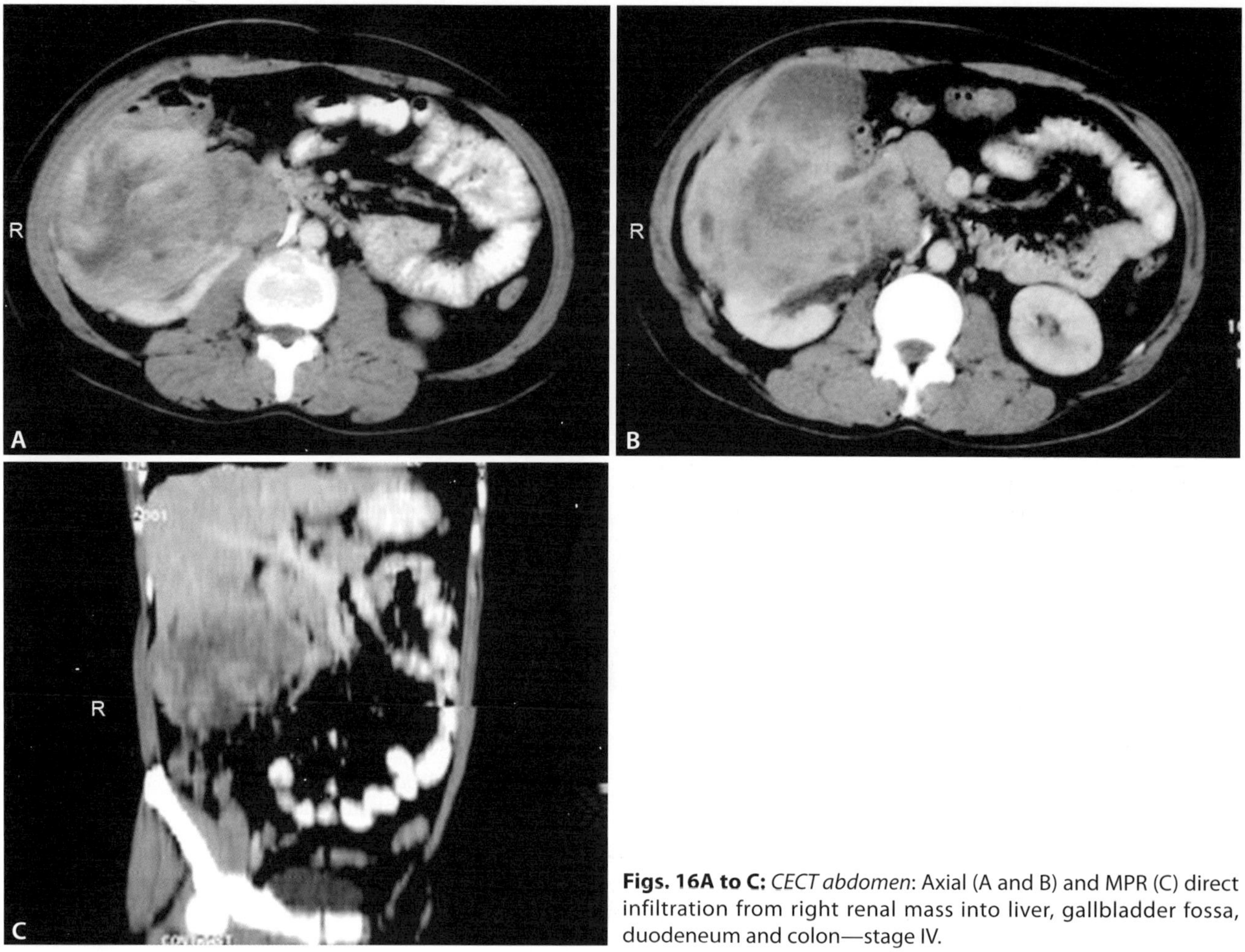

Figs. 16A to C: *CECT abdomen*: Axial (A and B) and MPR (C) direct infiltration from right renal mass into liver, gallbladder fossa, duodeneum and colon—stage IV.

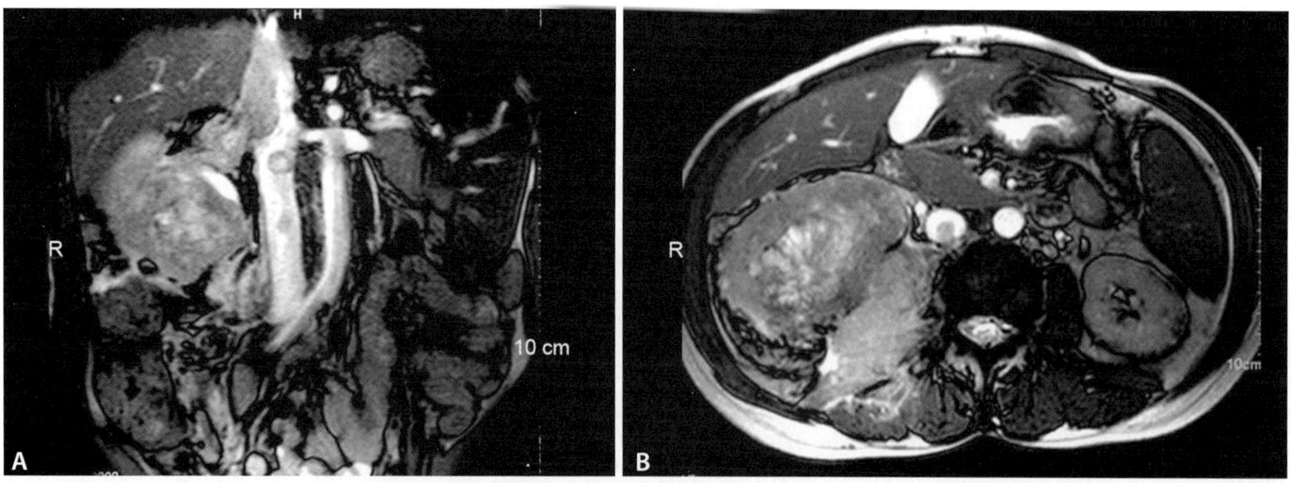

Figs. 17A and B: T2 TRUE FISP coronal (A) axial (B) extension of the renal mass into right renal vein which is enlarged and into the IVC. Direct infiltration into the psoas is also noted.

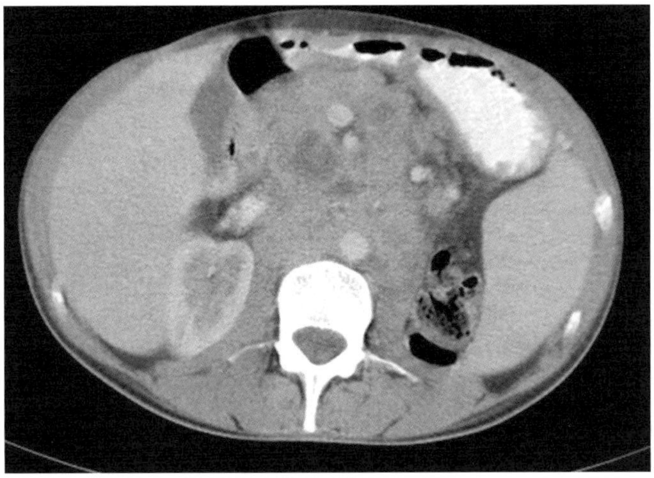

Fig. 18: CT abdomen in a postoperative case of RCC, presenting 1 year later with metastatic retroperitoneal lymphadenopathy.

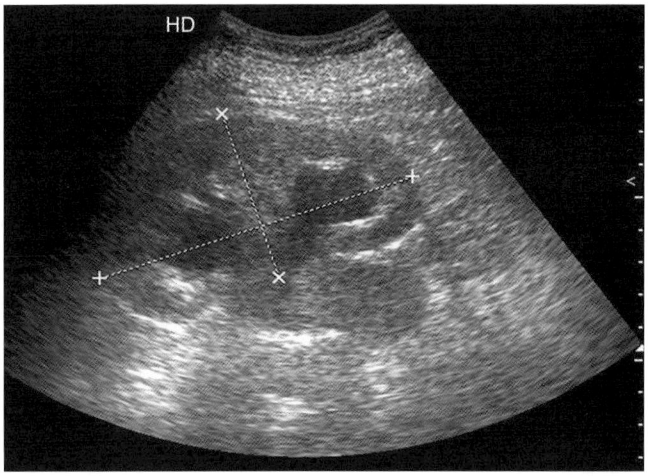

Fig. 19: Longitudinal sonogram of the left kidney shows a solid lesion in the renal pelvis and upper ureter with consequent hydronephrosis—Transitional cell carcinoma.

infiltration. Calices may be amputated or obliterated due to malignant infundibular structuring. Calices may be distended with tumor—"Oncocalices".

None of the signs on IVU are pathgnomic and can be simulated by a blood clot, radiolucent stone and granuloma.

Retrograde or percutaneous antegrade pyelography may be useful in such situations to delineate the site of obstruction and to obtain brush biopsy.

Ultrasonography

A large TCC is seen as an iso- to hypoechoic solid mass separating the central sinus echoes. A small TCC may not be detected on USG. Focal enlargement of renal cortex suggests infiltration of renal parenchyma. Other non specific findings include hydronephrosis, pyelocalyceal wall thickening. USG can help differentiate a radiolucent calculus from a tumor. It cannot differentiate from a blood clot unless followed up to show change **(Fig. 19)**.

Computed Tomography and Magnetic Resonance Imaging[13-15]

Computed tomography and MRI urography have increased the diagnostic confidence; however mucosal detail is still best seen on IVP and RGP. For CT or MRI evaluation, images should be obtained to include images in excretory phase (3–5 minutes after injection) to show a low attenuation mass involving the collecting system or ureter, as outlined by concentrated dense contrast.

There are three appearances on CT of a small TCC, the most common is of a small hypodense lesion in the renal collecting system, the lesion has a soft tissue attenuation (<40 HU), less than most renal calculi, the attenuation of TCC is slightly lower than a blood clot, but higher than urine. TCC will enhance approx 10–50 HU, with the enhancement being less than renal parenchyma. This mild enhancement helps differentiate it from blood clot and calculi **(Figs. 20A to C)**. In the kidney, TCC is usually more central than RCC, owing to the origin in the urothelium. TCC does not commonly involve the renal vein, though rare cases of IVC involvement have been reported. The central mass expands the kidney symmetrically and with centrifugal extension preserves the shape. The soft tissue component in the renal sinus obliterates and displaces intervening fat to merge with the renal parenchyma, an appearance described as 'faceless' kidney.[16] This is similar to the appearance on CT of a duplicated system.

TCC may present as a locally aggressive infiltrative renal mass, margins being ill defined. Involvement of renal parenchyma may be seen as a hypoenhancing mass involving parenchyma or heterogeneous abnormal hypoenhancement disrupting the normal parenchyma. A different appearance is thickening of collecting system, urothelium or ureteral wall. The thickening may be asymmetric or eccentric which may cause focal obstruction.

MR appearance of TCC is of a small focal lesion involving renal pelvis or calyceal system. TCCs are typically isointense relative to renal medulla on T1WI, making the detection of small tumors virtually impossible. Larger infiltrative tumors may obliterate the fat in the renal sinus. This may be appreciated on T1WI. Bright signal intensity due to urine in the collecting system on T2-weighted images provide

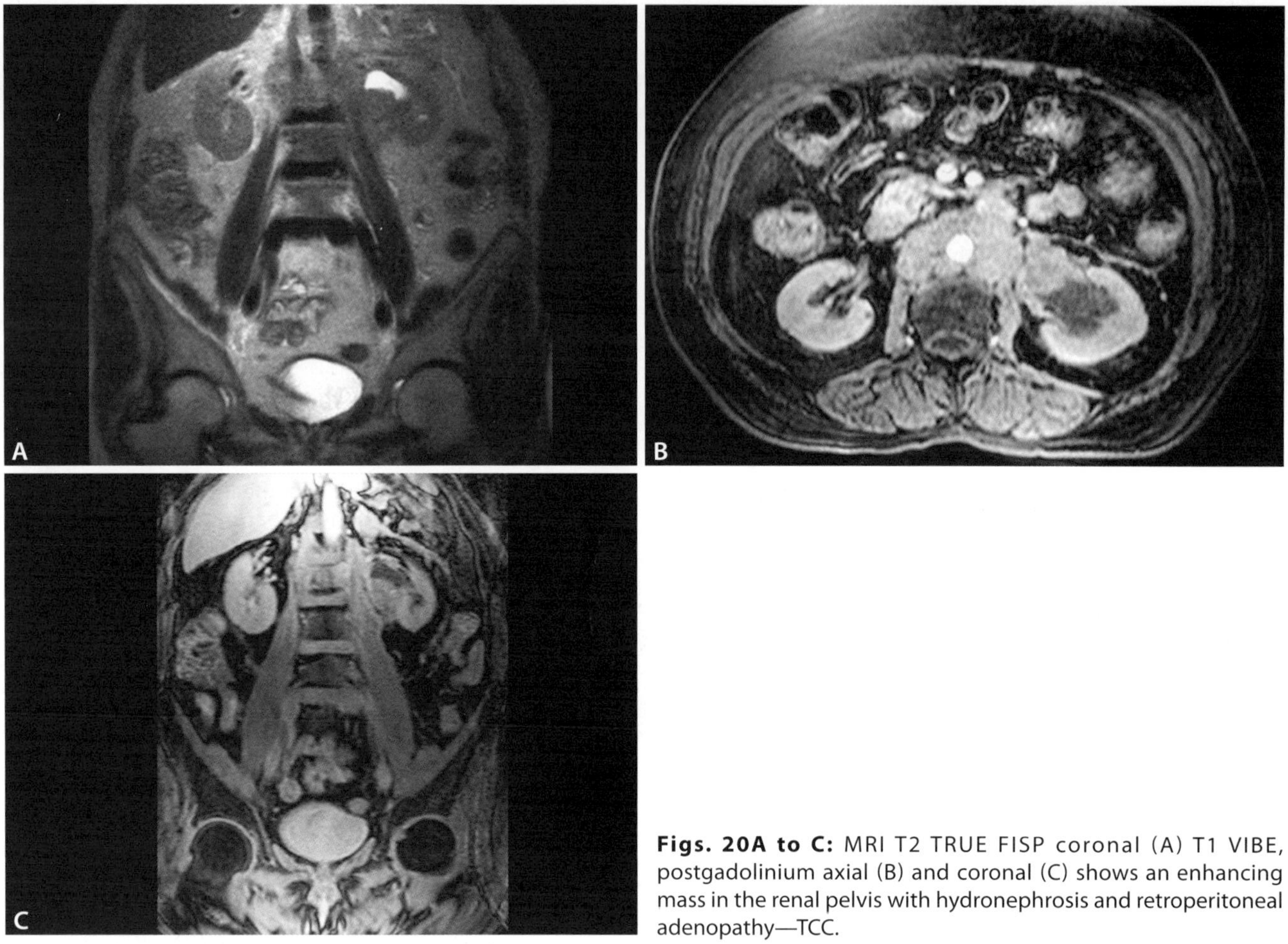

Figs. 20A to C: MRI T2 TRUE FISP coronal (A) T1 VIBE, postgadolinium axial (B) and coronal (C) shows an enhancing mass in the renal pelvis with hydronephrosis and retroperitoneal adenopathy—TCC.

excellent soft tissue contrast for detection of TCCs which are seen as hypointense filling defects. Infitrative TCCs may be seen on single shot T2WI as intermediate signal intensity mass infiltrating the renal parenchyma. Enhancement of a focal filling defect in the collecting system is strongly suggestive of TCC.[6] A cup-shaped dilatation of the ureter just distal to a focus of TCC in the ureter may be seen which is called as "chalice/goblet" sign.[17]

Staging

Staging of TCC in upper urinary tract has different prognostic indications **(Table 4)**. Carcinoma in situ and tumors limited to submucosa have best prognosis. Tumors beyond subepithelial tissue (stage II) and muscularis (stage III) have worse prognosis. CT cannot accurately distinguish T1 (limited to oroepithelium and lamina propria) from T2 (extending into musularis propria). Indications of stage III disease are parenchymal involvement or peripelvic and periureteral fat involvement.

Focal infiltrative renal lesion may mimic RCC or tuberculosis. TCC tends to be more centrally located and is more likely to expand the kidney centrifugally, while preserving the shape, the coexistence of a stone is a pointer towards SCC. A small area of parenchymal infiltration with papillary necrosis, is a major clue suggesting TB.

Squamous Cell Carcinoma

Squamous cell carcinoma of the renal pelvis is relatively rare tumor. It is highly aggressive, with a poor clinical prognosis. Chronic infection and calculi are implicated in its etiology. It often involves the renal parenchyma and perinephric tissue and may present with metastasis. Intravenous urography may reveal nonvisualization, hydronephrosis, a central mass or a pelvicalyceal filling defect seen in 83% of patients. In cross sectional imaging, this cannot be differentiated from transitional cell carcinomas. Pointers towards the diagnosis of SCC include the fact that SCC grow fast and rapid progression on sequential studies favor SCC. As SCC

Table 4: Staging of transitional cell carcinoma.

AJCC	*Disease extent*	*TNM*
0	Noninvasive papillary carcinoma	Ta
I/A	Carcinoma invading the subepithelial tissues	T1
II/B	Invasion of the muscularis	T2
III/C	Extension beyond the muscularis into peripelvic or periureteric fat or extension into the renal parenchyma	T3
IV	Invasion of adjacent organs or extension into perinephric fat (or any nodal or distant metastasis)	T4

develops following metaplasia due to chronic inflammation, in up to 50% cases renal calculus is noted.

Collecting Duct Carcinoma (Bellini Duct Carcinoma/Renal Medullary Carcinoma)[18,19]

This is a rare tumor arising from the cells lining the epithelium of the distal collecting tubule. The mean age of presentation is mid-fifties with complaints of hematuria. It is an aggressive tumor with poor prognosis. On CT, it is solid or complex-solid and cystic mass in the central portion of the kidney. Slightly hyperdense on CECT, it enhances less than renal parenchyma. On MRI, it is isointense on T1WI and appears hypointense on T2, which suggests the diagnosis. It has a right kidney predilection (82%). Renal medullary carcinoma is similar and arises from calyceal epithelium, in or near the renal papilla, from which it grows in an infiltrative pattern. It is seen in young African-American children and adults, seen exclusively with patients of sickle cell trait and commonly has metastasis at time of presentation.

Renal Sarcoma[3]

Renal sarcomas arise from the renal parenchyma or the capsule. They are most common in patients more than 40 years of age and they present with hematuria, abdominal distention, weight loss or pain. Leiomyosarcoma is the most common type of renal sarcoma, comprising half of all renal sarcoma. It is commonly located in the retroperitoneum or the perinehric space. On CT these tumors are heterogeneous with variable enhancement pattern. Liposarcoma of the kidney arises from the renal capsule and appears as a large retroperitoneal mass with macroscopic fat.

Lymphoma

Renal lymphoma is usually a part of systemic disease and associated with adenopathy or involvement with other organs, such as liver and GIT. Extranodal spread of lymphoma often affects the genitourinary system with the kidneys, being most commonly involved organ. Non-Hodgkin's lymphoma is more common than Hodgkin's lymphoma in renal involvement.

Renal involvement is often asymptomatic, detection usually occurs at imaging studies. The incidence at autopsy being as high as 41.6%. Despite the high prevalence, imaging studies demonstrate involvement in only 3–8% of patients.

Renal lymphoma has a variety of imaging appearances depending on the pattern of tumor proliferation. Malignant lymphocytes reach the renal parenchyma by means of hematogenous spread and proliferate within the interstitium, using nephrons, tubules and blood vessels as scaffolding for further growth. If it follows this infiltrative pattern, kidneys enlarge, maintaining the reniform shape. In many cases there is focal proliferation giving rise to single or more commonly bilateral renal expansile masses. Some tumors spread by means of contiguous extension from the retroperitoneal disease, penetrating the renal capsule. Renal involvement is usually bilateral, in form of nodules or diffuse infiltration, bulky single tumor, invasion from perirenal disease or microscopic invasion.

IVU is insensitive and findings when present occur late in the disease. On IVU, renal lymphoma may present as diffuse enlargement or multiple masses. Hydronephrosis or hydroureter may be seen due to displacement or obstruction to renal pelvis or ureter by lymph nodes. Poor function occurs due to diffuse and extensive involvement.

Ultrasonography[20] reveals hypoechoic solid lesions. Lymphoma masses tend to form by large number of uniform cells. This results in a homogeneous, nearly anechoic appearance on US. This may mimic renal cysts, but there is no through transmission and subtle low level echoes may be seen. This sonographic pattern is unique to renal lymphoma **(Figs. 21A and B)**. It may also detect hydroureteronephrosis, adenopathy and other foci in liver and spleen. The sinus fat surrounding the central pelvicalyceal echoes may completely disappear. Large retroperitoneal nodes may be seen encasing the vessels.

CT is more sensitive than ultrasound in detection of renal lymphoma. There are few common presentations.[21-23] The most common (50–60%) being of multiple focal masses which have attenuation similar or only slightly less

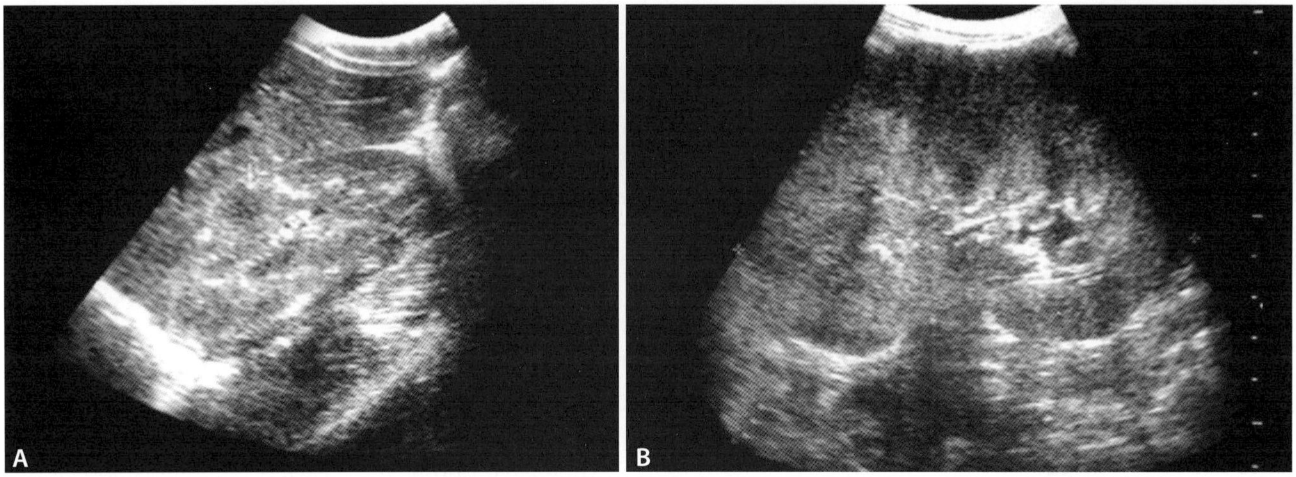

Figs. 21A and B: USG bilateral renal enlargement with poorly defined hypo/anechoic nodules giving a homogeneous appearance—Lymphoma.

than renal parenchyma on unenhanced images **(Figs. 22A and B)**. Nephrographic phase contrast CT is essential as many lesions are small and affect the medullary part of the kidney and may be missed on CM phase. After IVC, it enhances less than normal parenchyma. Heterogeneity and necrosis may be seen with larger lesions. Calcification is usually not seen, unless there has been therapy. Invasion into renal vein and IVC is rare.

Renal lymphoma manifests as solitary mass in 10–25% of patients. They characteristically demonstrate less enhancement following IVC differentiating them from RCC.

Contiguous involvement to kidneys or perinephric space from large retroperitoneal masses is the second most common pattern (25–30%). Perinephric involvement is noted in approximately one-third of patients, most of whom also have parenchymal involvement **(Fig. 23)**.

Another appearance of renal lymphoma in a perinephric ring of soft tissue is noted around the kidney without a focal parenchymal lesion; the soft tissue is of low attenuation, compresses the renal parenchyma without significant impairment of renal function.

Diffuse renal enlargement may be seen in the infiltrative form **(Fig. 24)**. There is a low attenuation mass expanding the kidney with predominent involvement of the renal medulla, with relative sparing of cortical margins. This is more common in Burkitt's lymphoma, either disseminated or limited to the kidneys. Heterogeneous enhancement of the kidneys, with loss of normal differential enhancement is seen.

Lymphoma can affect the renal sinus preferentially. CT shows, the normal sinus fat is replaced by homogeneous soft tissue mass. The mass usually causes encasement of the renal vessels leading to poor enhancement.

Massive retroperitoneal adenopathy is often coexistent with renal lymphoma.

The morphological appearance of lymphoma on MRI is similar to that on CT. Renal lymphoma is slightly hypointense to renal parenchyma on unenhanced T1-weighted images and mildly hyperintense on T2-images. There is mild heterogeneous enhancement on post-gadolinium images, the enhancement being less than that of the normal parenchyma.

Primary renal lymphoma is extremely rare, due to lack of lymphatic tissue within the kidney. The tumor is aggressive and shows bilateral renal involvement in majority of cases. The tumor is usually a B-cell non-Hodgkin's lymphoma and affect patients who are middle aged or older. Rapid improvement and decrease in renal size is noted following the initiation of chemotherapy. In chronic lymphatic leukemia, kidney may be involved in 90% of cases and is associated with membranous glomerulonephritis.

In suspected cases of lymphoma fine needle aspiration cytology (FNAC) or biopsy may be indicated for differentiating from other tumors. The distinction is important as lymphoma is usually treated medically.

Renal Metastasis[23]

Renal metastasis is present in approximately 10–20% of patients, in setting of other metastatic disease. Most renal metastasis are hematogenous, although a few may be due to direct invasion (adrenal, colonic and pancreas). The most common site of primary, being lung, colon,

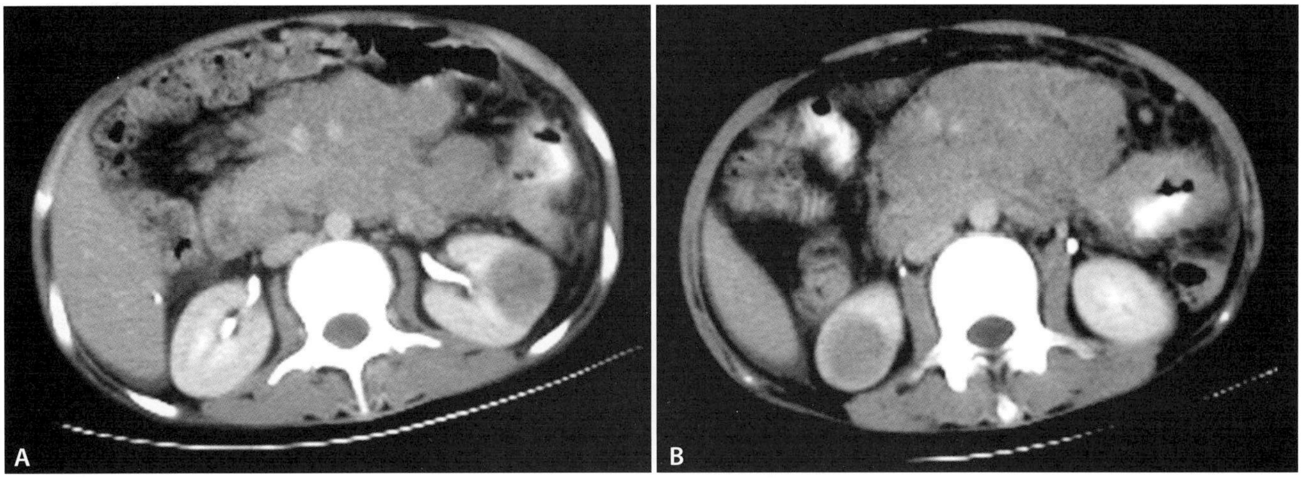

Figs. 22A and B: Contrast-enhanced CT showing well-defined focal hypodense masses in both kidneys with significant retroperitoneal adenopathy and bowel thickening—A case of lymphoma.

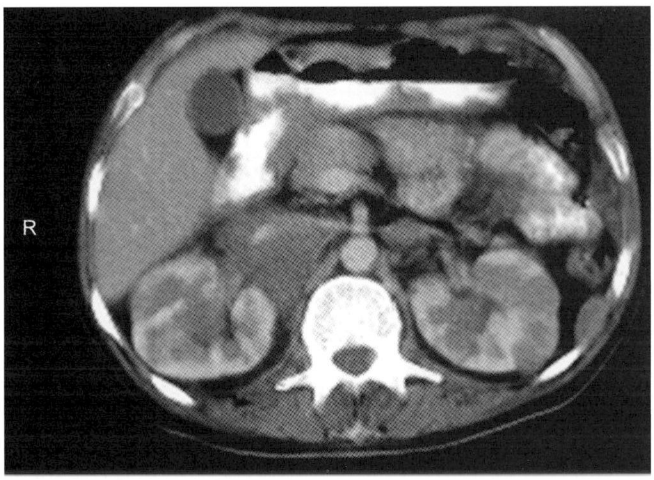

Fig. 23: *Renal lymphoma*: CECT shows multiple nodules in both kidneys with perirenal disease on the right side.

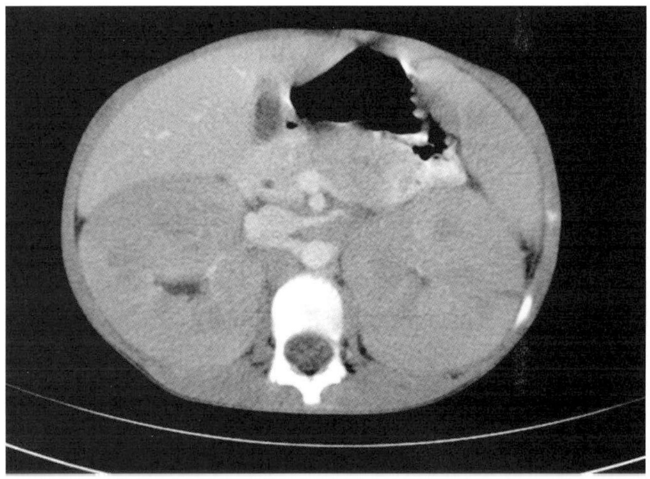

Fig. 24: *CT abdomen*: Bilateral kidneys are enlarged with loss of corticomedullary differentiation—A case of Burkitt's lymphoma.

breast, melanoma and reproductive organ malignancies. Melanoma, when present frequently metastasizes to kidney.

Metastasis are usually asymptomatic, may rarely present as hematuria.

On ultrasonography, they may be seen as hypoechoic lesions. On CT, the common appearance is of bilateral renal masses, though solitary renal metastasis are not uncommon. The lesions measure 20–44 HU on enhanced CT and have minimal enhancement after IVC of 5–15 HU. Large solitary renal metastasis disrupt renal cortical margins, may be associated with breast, lung or colon carcinomas. Direct involvement of perinephric space by metastasis, representing usually lymphatic spread is noted in metastasis from melanoma and lung carcinoma. Hemorrhagic renal metastasis is seen in melanoma and pheochromocytomas.

There may be a diagnostic dilemma between RCC versus metastasis **(Figs. 25A and B)**. Renal metastasis are usually bilateral (50%), solitary metastasis may resemble RCC, which however has no necrosis. Hyperenhancement and renal vein involvement favors RCC. The margination of metastasis is often less well defined than in RCC.

Oncocytoma

Renal oncocytoma is a benign solid non-fat containing renal mass, accounting for about 5% of renal cortical neoplasm. It is a benign renal epithelial tumor, arising from proximal tubule with many characteristics of RCCs. Oncocytomas are histologically composed of large cells

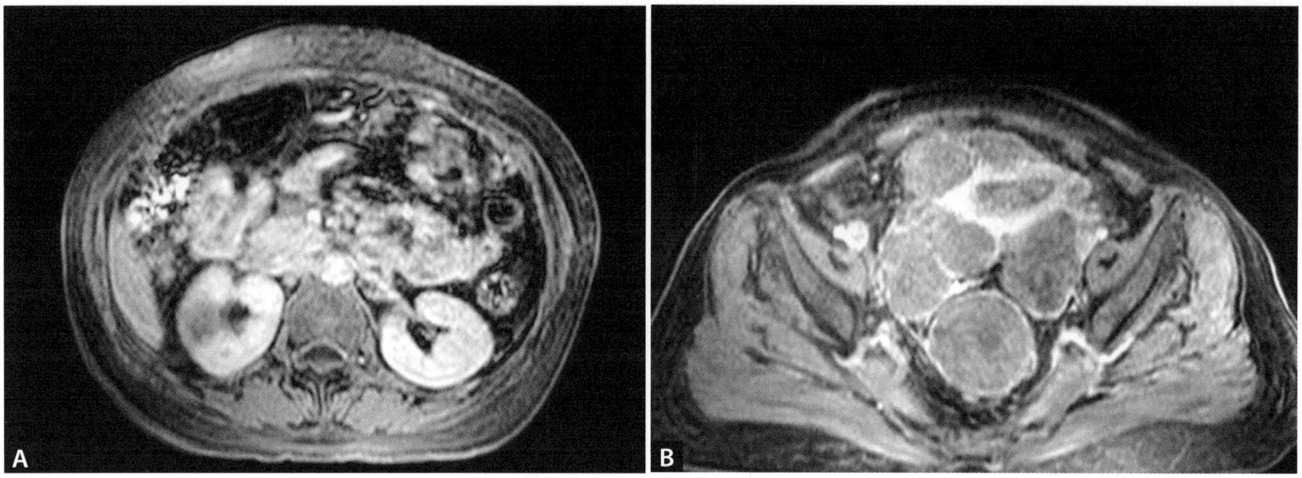

Figs. 25A and B: MRI T1 vibe postcontrast a focal poorly enhancing mass in the right kidney (A), renal metastasis from disseminated ovarian malignancy (B).

(oncocytes) with mitochondria rich cytoplasm. The appearance of a typical oncocytoma cannot be reliably differentiated from RCC.[3,24,25]

Most oncocytomas are asymptomatic (80%), but few may present with hematuria pain or mass. The peak age of incidence is in the seventh decade with a male preponderance. The incidence of oncocytomas is higher in incidentally discovered renal masses, as compared with patients who have urinary symptoms. They may be quite large at time of presentation. Oncocytoma appear as well demarcated, unencapsulated, fairly homogeneous renal cortical tumors. Bilateral multiple oncocytomas are seen in hereditary syndromes of renal oncocytosis.

Ultrasonography may show a central stellate scar within a solid hematogenous mass. On CT, they are solid, well-marginated tumors, slightly hypodense to renal parenchyma on unenhanced images. Some may exhibit a central low attenuation scar seen with branched appearance. However, central necrosis with RCC may mimic this. Renal capsular pathological invasion into perinephric fat occurs in 11%. There should be no adenopathy or vascular invasion. The presence of a central scar, absence of calcification or necrosis and hemorrhage suggests the diagnosis, though there is no specific CT finding to differentiate oncocytoma from RCC and surgery is usually performed for these **(Fig. 26)**.

The MRI appearance is of a hypo- to isointense (22%) mass on T1W images with high signal on T2WI, enhancing homogeneously after IV gadolinium and may exhibit spokewheel pattern of enhancement. The central scar, if present is hypointense on T2 vis-a-vis hyperintensity of necrotic RCCs on T2W images. A spokewheel pattern of feeding arteries associated with a homogeneous

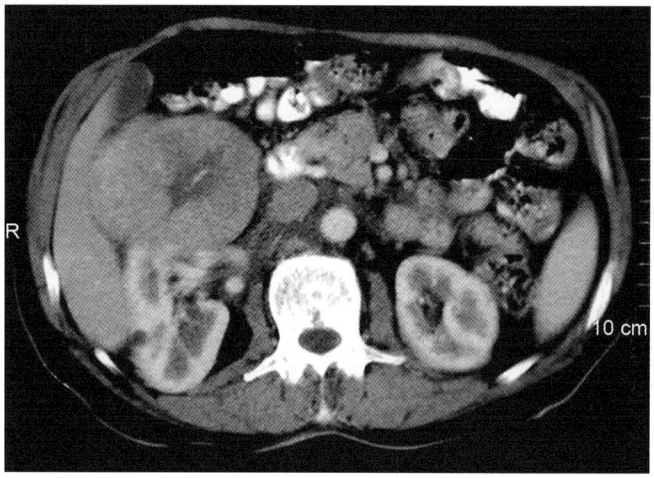

Fig. 26: *Computed tomography*: Well-defined, homogeneously enhancing mass right renal with a central scar—Oncocytoma.

nephrogram is a characteristic finding on catheter angiography.

In absence of previously and documented oncocytoma or stability of lesion, nephron sparing surgery is done.

Renal Adenomas

Papillary adenomas are the most common renal epithelial neoplasm. According to autopsy series, approximately 40% of patients above the age of 70 harbor renal adenoma. Papillary adenoma are also found in patients with acquired renal cystic disease and in those undergoing long-term hemodialysis. They are seen in about 15% of kidneys at autopsy and usually occur as cortical sub-capsular tumors less than 1 cm. They are indistinguishable from RCCs. According to some authors, renal adenoma is an earlier stage of evolution of renal cell carcinoma. By definition, papillary adenomas measure 5 mm or less.[26,27]

Metanephric adenoma is a benign neoplasm with a peak age in 5th-6th decades. Polycythemia, a characteristic finding seen in 10% disappears after surgery. Metanephric adenoma typically occurs as a well-defined, unencapsulated, solitary solid mass. Metanephric adenomas display hypovascularity and delayed, minimal enhancement.

MIXED EPITHELIAL AND STROMAL TUMORS[3,26]

This comprises of tumors previously referred to as hamartoma, adult mesoblastic nephroma. They are seen almost exclusively in perimenopausal women, most patients receiving estrogen therapy. Most present incidentally and are believed to be a hormonally dependent tumor. Mixed epithelial and stromal tumors (MESTs) are characterized by variegated imaging patterns including complex cysts, mixed solid cystic masses that show delayed and heterogeneous enhancement. On MR imaging, the degree of delayed enhancement and T2 hypointense signal is dependent on the stromal component.

CYSTIC NEPHROMA

These are rare benign neoplasms that also show a female preponderance. Most patients are asymptomatic. Cystic nephromas are predominantly unilateral, well circumscribed cystic lesions with thin septations. Hemorrhage or urinary obstruction may be caused by the prolapse of the cystic mass into the renal pelvis.

ANGIOMYOLIPOMA

These benign lesions are mesenchymal neoplasms (hamartomas), representing excess growth of mature fat, smooth muscle and thick walled blood vessels, the amount of each component being variable. AMLs are now grouped under a family of tumors characterized by the proliferation of perivascular epitheloid cells (PEComas).[28]

Tuberous sclerosis is the most commonly associated syndrome. Multiple and bilateral angiomyolipomas should suggest the diagnosis of TS. Approximately 80% of patients with TS have angiomyolipoma, only 20% of cases of angiomyolipomas, subsequently are diagnosed TS. Angiomyolipomas may rarely be associated with NF-I, von Hippel–Lindau or ADPKD. TS associated AML are asymptomatic, young patients without sex predilection. AML associated with TS are often multiple, bilateral and larger at the time of presentation. These are also likely to grow and be symptomatic. They may be sporadic tumors, commonly detected in females in 5–7th decades.

AML may originate from the cortex or the medulla. The tumor is usually well defined and calcification and necrosis. They appear as large, heterogeneous masses with varying amount of macroscopic fat, intralesional aneurysms and hypervascular soft tissue. Angiomyolipomas are composed of thick walled inelastic blood vessels, risk of intratumoral and perinephric hemorrhage is higher in lesion >4 cm diameter.

Plain abdominal radiography may show distinctive radiolucency, within a large soft tissue mass with lot of fat, in 10% of patients. Ultrasonography reveals highly, echogenic circumscribed mass (more echogenic than central fat). It may appear as echogenic fat within a tumor or isolated foci of echogenicity **(Figs. 27 and 28)**. If fat content is less or admixed with hemorrhage, the echogenicity of tumor is diminished and may appear as any other renal mass. Recent work has suggested that 32% of renal carcinomas are also highly reflective, although there are other pointers towards RCC, such as hyporeflective rim or focal small spotty areas of reduced central reflectivity. Another feature that helps in distinguishing an angiomyolipoma from a small RCC is posterior shadowing, seen in approximately 30% of AML, but is not seen in small hyper-reflective renal carcinomas.

CT is the most accurate imaging technique for detection and characterization of angiomyolipomas.[29,30] The lesions show low attenuation with fat measurements and presence of gross fat being typical for these. The ROIs are typically less than -10 HU. Thin slices are necessary to demonstrate fat in small AMLs because of volume averaging. Higher specificity may be obtained with threshold measurements of –15 to –30 HU. The fat may be interposed with solid components. A subset of lesions will not meet fat attenuation criteria due to volume averaging or hemorrhage, others are fat poor and rarely a well-differentiated RCC can mimic this appearance. CT pixel mapping,[31] over a region of interest within the tumor may be useful to detect small quantities of fat. With pixel mapping, three to six contiguous pixels with negative HU averaging below –20 HU indicates intratumoral fat **(Figs. 29 to 31)**.

The presence of typical AML in the contralateral kidney helps in the diagnosis. AMLs are usually well-marginated, but do not have a true capsule, the lesion is usually at the margin of the kidney and may expand beyond as a small hypodense wedge-shaped defect in the renal parenchyma. This wedge-shaped defect is diagnostic

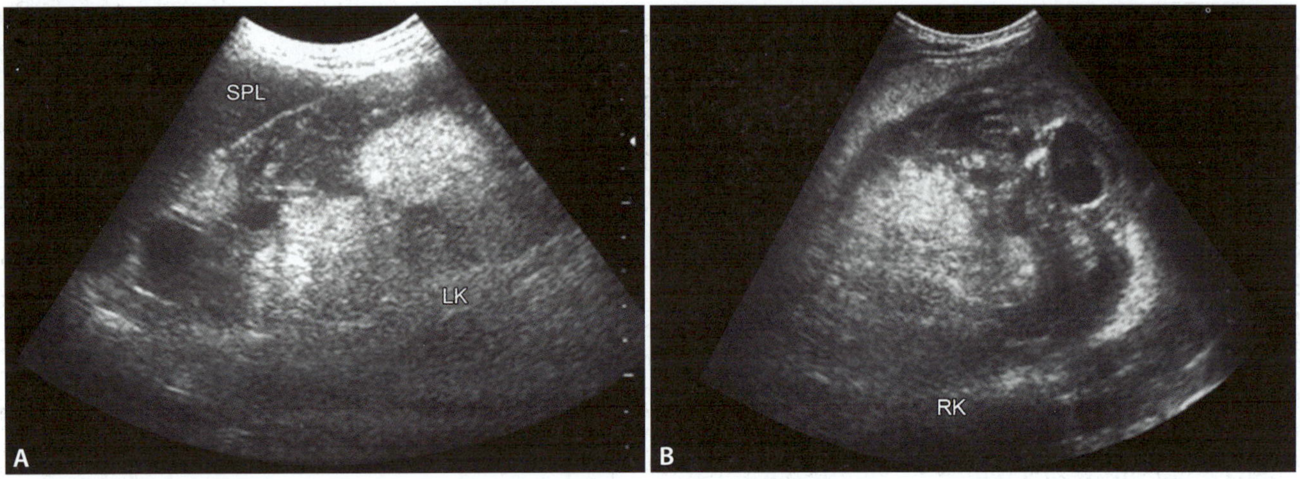

Figs. 27A and B: Multiple well-defined homogeneously hyperechoic lesions with no perilesional halo in both left and right kidneys—Angiomyolipomas.

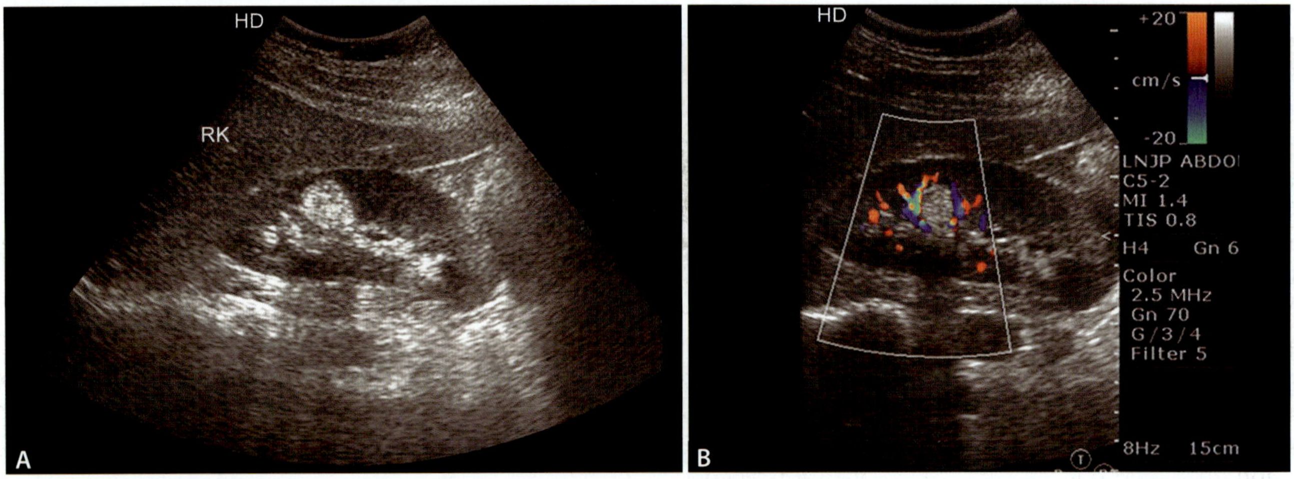

Figs. 28A and B: USG (A) and color Doppler (B) show a small well-defined hyperechoic lesion in the right kidney with peripheral vascularity—Angiomyolipoma.

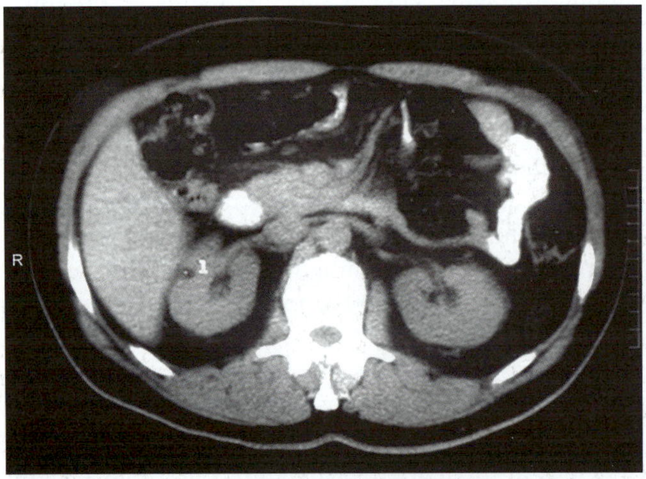

Fig. 29: CT shows a small pinhead lesion in right kidney with fat attenuation S/o AML.

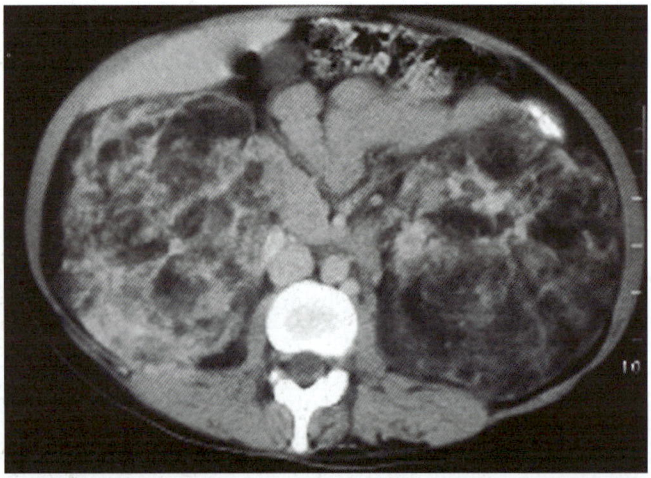

Fig. 30: CECT showing large heterogeneous soft tissue masses in both kidneys with fat density scattered throughout and enlarged vessels—A case of tuberous sclerosis.

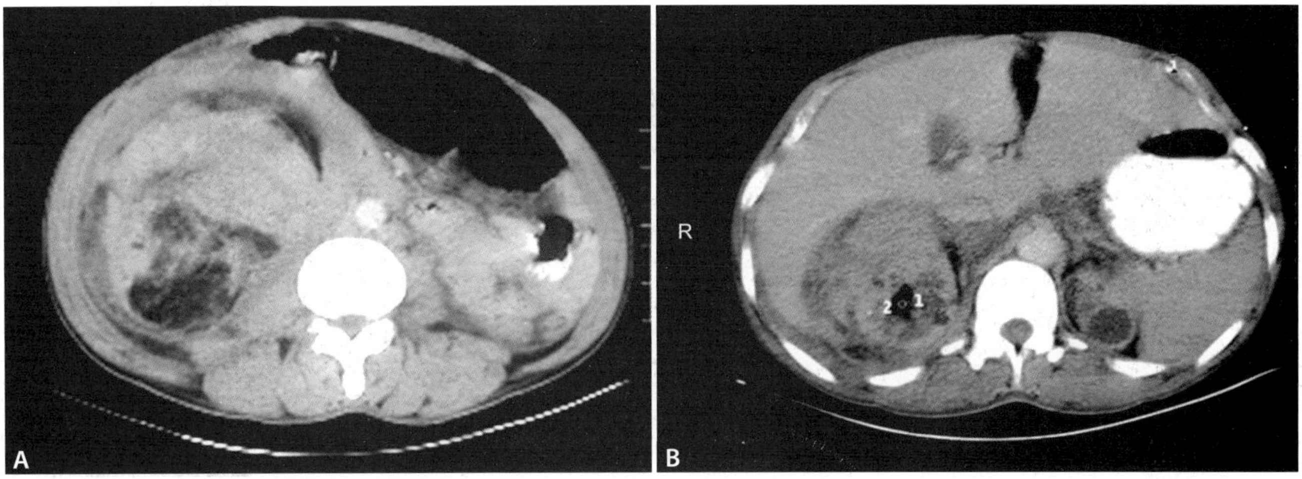

Figs. 31A and B: CT showing bilateral large fat attenuation lesions with enhancing soft tissues and perilesional hemorrhage—AML

of angiomyolipoma. These lesions are vascular, large vessels may be identified. Intratumoral aneurysms may be present and AML's exhibit moderate enhancement after IVC. Homogeneous and prolonged enhancement is a valuable predictor for differentiating AML with minimal fat from RCC.

MRI will also demonstrate fat component of an angiomyolipoma. On MRI, AMLs have a characteristic high T1-signal and on fat saturated images exhibit a drop in signal. The use of in-phase and opposed phase imaging is also helpful in the diagnosis of angiomyolipoma. In AML, a characteristic India ink artifact is seen at the interface between the mass and the normal renal parenchyma on opposed phase T1 images, whereas the central part of the lesion does not demonstrate changes in signal intensity compared with in phase images. This is useful in very small lesions in which direct comparison with T1 images with and without fat suppression may be difficult **(Figs. 32A to F)**. The appearance of AML on T2-weighted images is variable and depends on bulk fat present in the lesion. An AML composed of predominantly fat would demonstrate homogeneous high-signal at T2 single shot images. Lipid poor angiomyolipomas are frequently hypointense on T2-weighted images. This may help to differentiate from RCC which will be T2 hyperintense.[32]

Angiography may demonstrate multiple aneurysms and onion layer appearances. Approximately 58–75% of these lesions grow with time. Growth of an isolated AML without TS is less than those with TS and multiple lesions. Annual follow-up is recommended for asymptomatic lesions <4 cm. For larger lesions, due to risk of hemorrhage, semiannual evaluation is suggested. Even small AMLs may rarely bleed. For large symptomatic lesions embolization may decrease risk of hemorrhage.

Pathological differentiation between a well-differentiated liposarcoma from a angiomyolipoma may be difficult, unless radiological appearance is considered.[33] Liposarcomas, are rare, seen in older patients, are larger at time of diagnosis and are centered at perinephric space or capsule rather than intraparenchymal like AML. They are hypovascular, without enlarged vessels and aneurysms. The renal parenchymal defect in AML as stated earlier is not seen in well-differentiated liposarcomas, which will displace, compress and distort the kidney, but will not invade renal parenchyma. It is important to assess the relationship of fat to remainder of tumor, such that fat is intratumoral and not perirenal fat engulfed by a growing RCC.

PNET OF THE KIDNEY

This is a highly aggressive renal neoplasm, belonging to the Ewing's family of tumors. Patient is usually a young adult. Although radiological features, such as presence of tumor thrombus, proximity to neural foramina have been described,[34] diagnosis is based on histology and immunocytohistochemistry.

Biopsy[2,3,35]

Traditionally, percutaneous biopsy has played a limited role in evaluation of all solid renal tumors. This procedure is usually reserved for patients with known extra-renal malignancy and a solitary renal mass. This will enable differentiation from RCC, which is to be treated surgically, from a solitary metastasis which can be treated non-surgically. Percutaneous biopsy is to be avoided in renal infiltrating neoplasms, as there is a risk of needle track seeding, especially in transitional cell carcinomas.

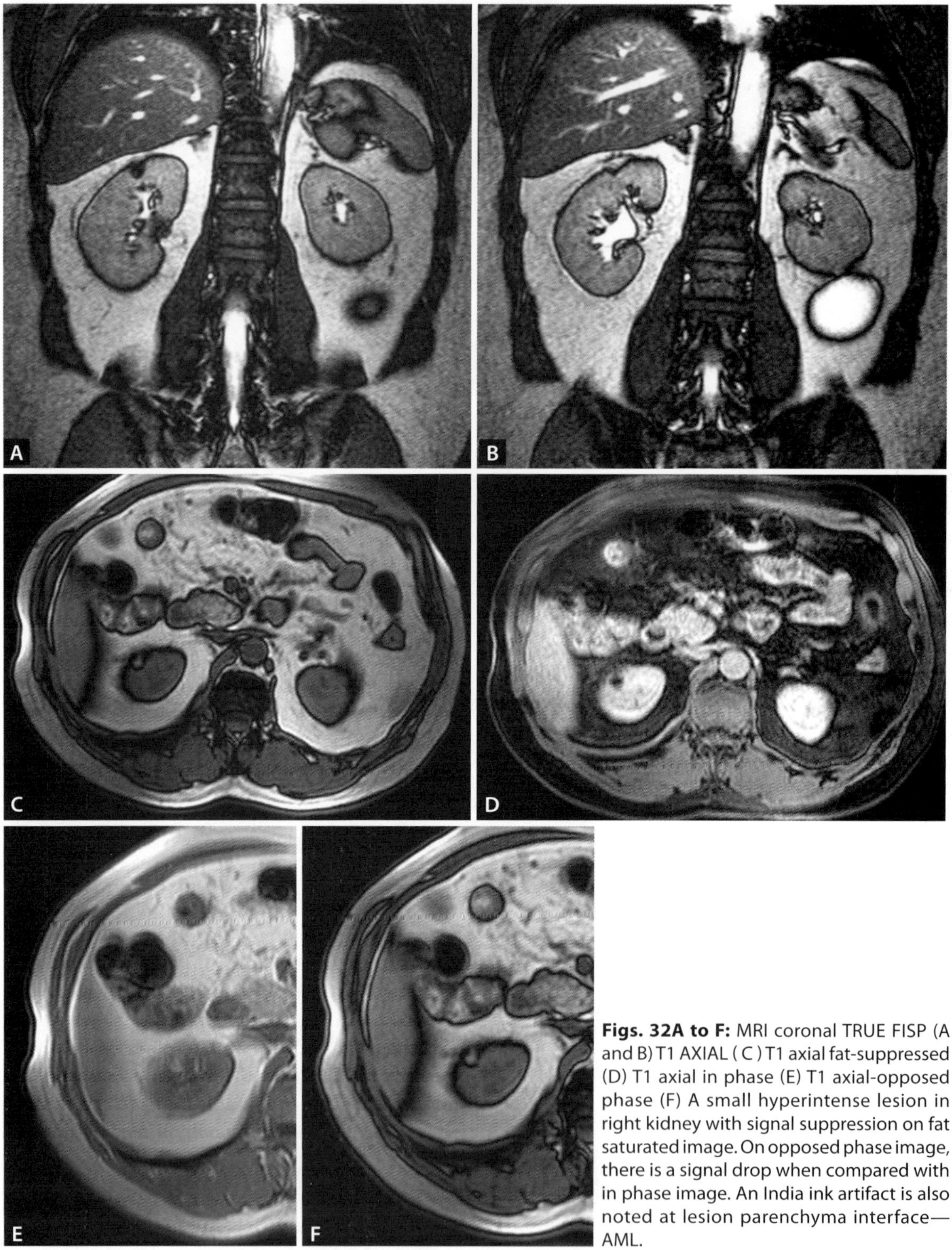

Figs. 32A to F: MRI coronal TRUE FISP (A and B) T1 AXIAL (C) T1 axial fat-suppressed (D) T1 axial in phase (E) T1 axial-opposed phase (F) A small hyperintense lesion in right kidney with signal suppression on fat saturated image. On opposed phase image, there is a signal drop when compared with in phase image. An India ink artifact is also noted at lesion parenchyma interface—AML.

Percutaneous biopsy should not be relied upon completely to differentiate between benign and malignant tumors. This is especially so for differentiation of oncocytoma and RCCs, for some RCCs contain oncocytic components that are indistinguishable from those in benign oncocytoma. The results may be inconclusive in excluding RCC. Recent studies have, however shown that image guided biopsy of a solid enhancing renal mass is a highly diagnostic procedure. When percutaneous renal mass biopsy is indicated, it has been shown that core needle biopsy is more accurate than FNACs.

Incidental Solid Renal Mass

The increased incidence of incidental renal masses with cross sectional imaging poses problems to the radiologist and the physician. When encountering a renal mass, a benign lesion like angiomyolipoma needs to be excluded. Differentiation from a RCC is necessary. CT, thin section CT, for small lesions and MRI including chemical shift imaging may be required. Hyperattenuating enhancing lesions may represent other benign tumors like, oncocytoma, metnephric adenoma.

If a large >3 cm solid mass is discovered, renal cell carcinoma (provided there is no fat on CT/MR protocols) is the most probable diagnosis and surgery is recommended. If the tumor is 1–3 cm in size, RCC is most likely though percutaneous biopsy may be required. Very small lesions <1 cm are more likely to be benign; thin sections (<3 mm) may help. Obsevation and follow up CT/MR at 3–6 months, then at 12 months and then yearly may be done.[36]

CT is the imaging modality of choice for evaluating renal tumor. When a proper technique is used CT provides a high degree of accuracy in detecting renal mass. Certain imaging features and enhancement pattern may help distinguish various subtypes of renal tumors. It also provides diagnostic information for treatment planning and follow up. MR imaging is a rapidly evolving tool, currently valuable as a problem-solving tool.

REFERENCES

1. Eble JN, Sauter G, Epstein JI, Sesterhenn IA (Eds). World Health Organisation Classification of Tumors: Pathology and Genetics of Tumors of the Urinary System and Male Genital Organs. Lyon, France: IARC Press; 2004.
2. Welch TJ, LeRoy AJ. Helical and electron beam CT scanning in the evaluation of renal vein. Involvement in patients with renal cell carcinoma. J Comput Assist Tomogr. 1997;21(3):467-71.
3. Pedrosa I, Sun MR, Spencer M, et al. MR imaging of renal masses: correlation with findings at surgery and pathologic analysis. Radiographics. 2008;28:985-1003.
4. Pedrosa I, Chou MT, Ngo L, et al. MR classification of renal masses with pathological correlation. Eur Radiol. 2008;18:365-75.
5. Zang J, Tehrani YM, Wang C, et al. Renal masses: characterisation with diffusion weighted MR imaging—a preliminary experience. Radiology. 2008;247(2):458-64.
6. Ramdave S,Thomas GW, Berlangieri SU, et al. Clinical role of F18 flurodeoxyglucose positron emission tomography for the detection and management of renal cell carcinoma. Urol. 2001; 166(3):825-30.
7. Zhang J, Lefkowitz RA, Bach A. Imaging of kidney career. Radiol Clin North Am. 2007;45:119-47.
8. Maki DD, Birhbaum BA, Chakraborty DP, et al. Renal cyst pseudo enhancement: Beam hardening effects on CT numbers. Radiology. 1999;213(2):468-72.
9. Johnson CD, Dunnick NR, Lohan RH, et al. Renal adenocarcinoma: CT staging of 100 tumors. Am J Roentgenol. 1987;148: 59-63.
10. Levine E. Renal cell carcinoma: Radiological diagnosis and staging. Semin Roentgenol. 1987;22:248.
11. Hallscheidt PJ, Bock M, Riedasch G, et al. Diagnostic accuracy of staging renal cell carcinomas using multidetector row computed tomography and magnetic resonance imaging: a prospective study with histopathological correlation. J Comput Assist Tomogr. 2004;2833-39.
12. Boss A, Clasen S, Kuczyk M, et al. Image guided radiofrequency ablation of renal cell carcinoma. Eur Radiol. 2007;17:725-33.
13. Gatewood OM, Goldman SM, Marshall FF, et al. Computerised tomography in the diagnosis of transitional cell carcinoma of the kidney. J Urol. 1982;127(5):876-87.
14. Parienty RA, Ducellier R, Pradel J, et al. Diagnostic valve of CT number in pelvicaliceal filling defects. Radiology. 1982;145(3): 743-47.
15. Leo ME, Petrou SP, Barrett DM. Transitional cell carcinoma of the kidney with vena caval involvement: Report of 3 cases and a review of the literature. J Urol. 1992;148(2 Pt 1):398-400.
16. Hulnick DH, Bosniak MA. 'Faceless kidney' CT sign of renal duplicity. J Comput Assit Tomogr. 1986;10:771-72.
17. Daniels RE. The Goblet Sign (3rd). Radiology. 1999;210:737-38.
18. Peyromaure M, Thiounn N, Scotte F, et al. Collecting duet carcinoma of the kidney: A clinicopathological study of 9 cases. J Urol. 2003;170:1138-40.
19. Swartz MA, Karth J, Schneider DT, et al. Renal medullary carcinoma: Clinical pathological immunohistochemical and genetic analysis with pathogenetic implications. Urology. 2002; (6016):1083-89.
20. Ruchman RB, Yeh HC, Mitty HA, et al. Ultrasonographic and computer tomographic features of renal sinus lymphoma. J Clin Ultrasond. 1988;16:35-40.
21. Reznek RH, Mootoosamy I, Webb JA, et al. CT in renal and perirenal lymphoma: A further look. Clin Radiol. 1990;42(4): 233-38.
22. Urban BA, Fishman EK. Renal Lymphoma: CT patterns with emphasis on helical CT. Radiographics. 2000;20:197-212.
23. Choyke PL, White EM, Zemen RK, et al. Renal metastasis: Clinicopathological and radiological correlation. Radiology. 1992;159(6):1229-34.
24. Quinn MJ, Harlman DS, Friedman AC, et al. Renal oncocytoma: New observations. Radiology. 1984;153:49-53.
25. Dyer R, Disantis MD, Mc clennan BL. Simplified approach for evaluation of the solid renal mass in adults. Radiology. 2008; 247(2):331-43.

26. Prasad SR, Surabhi VR, Menias CO, et al. Benign renal neoplasms in adults: Cross-sectional imaging findings. AJR. 2008;190:158-64.
27. Kiyoshima K, Oda Y, Nakamura T, et al. Multicenteric papillary renal cell carcinoma associated with renal adenomatosis. Pathol int. 2004;54:266-72.
28. Prasad SR, Mino Kneudson M, Narra VR, et al. Neoplasms of the perivascular epitheloid cell including the abdomen and pelvis: Cross sectional imaging findings. J Comput Assist Tomogr. 2007;31(5):688-96.
29. Bosniak MA, Meigbow AJ, Hulnick DH, et al. CT diagnosis of renal angiomyolipomas: The importance of detecting small amounts of fat. Am J Roentgenol. 1988;151(3):497-501.
30. Silverman SG, Mortele KJ, Tuncali MD, et al. Hyperattenuating renal masses: Etiologies, pathogenesis and imaging evaluation. Radiographics. 2007;27:1131-43.
31. Takahashi K, Honda M, Okubo RS, et al. CT pixel mapping in the diagnosis of small angiomyolipomas of the kidneys. J Comput Assist Tomogr. 1993;17:98-101.
32. Isreal GM, Bosniak MA. Pitfalls in renal mass evaluation and how to avoid them. Radiographics. 2008;28:1325-38.
33. Israel GM, Bosniak MA, Slywotzky CM, et al. CT differentiation of large exophytic renal angiomyolipomas and perirenal liposarcoma. Am J Roentgenol. 2002;179(3):769-73.
34. Chu WC, Reznikov B, Lee YN, et al. PNET of the kidney—a rare renal tumor in adolescents with seemingly characteristic radiological features. Paediatr Radiol. 2008;38(10):1089-94.
35. Maturen KE, Ngheim HV, Caoili EM, et al. Renal mass core biopsy: Accuracy and impact in clinical management. Am J Reontgenol. 2007;188:563-70.
36. Silverman SG, Israel GM, Herts BR, Richie JP. Management of the incidental renal mass. Radiology. 2008;249(1):16-31.

CHAPTER 109

Imaging of Urinary Bladder and Urethra

Anupam Lal, Paramjeet Singh

ANATOMY

Urinary Bladder

The urinary bladder is a musculomembranous sac which acts as a reservoir for the urine; and its size, position and relations vary according to the amount of fluid it contains. The empty bladder assumes the form of a flattened tetrahedron and when distended with fluid it becomes round or oval in shape. In adults, the normal bladder capacity is highly variable but is usually between 500 and 600 mL. The normal wall of the bladder is smooth and should be regular and uniform in thickness (typically 2–3 mm in fully distended bladder) not exceeding 6 mm in adults.

The bladder lies in the anterosuperior portion of the pelvic cavity which is separated anteriorly from the pubic rami by the fatty Retzius' space. Superiorly, the bladder is enveloped by peritoneum, which continues posteriorly and is then reflected onto the anterior surface of the rectum (anterior surface of uterus in females). The bladder is surrounded by perivesical fat; laterally, it is bordered by the obturator internus muscles and inferiorly by the prostate gland. The superoanterior portion of the bladder, the apex, is attached to the anterior abdominal wall by the median umbilical ligament, a remnant of the urachus. The posteroinferior wall, referred to as the base, is continuous with the bladder neck. The urinary bladder wall consists of smooth muscle, lamina propria, submucosa and mucosa. The muscular component of the bladder wall is composed of longitudinal and circular smooth muscle bundles that form distinct layers near the bladder neck.

The mucous membrane is loosely attached to the muscular coat. It is made of multilayered transitional epithelium. Contracted bladder gives it a wrinkled or folded appearance. The 'trigone' is a small triangular area, immediately above and behind the internal orifice of the urethra, the mucous membrane is adherent to the muscular coat and is always smooth. The anterior angle of the trigone is formed by the internal orifice of the urethra and posterolateral angles by the orifices of the ureters. A ridge of muscle, the interureteric ridge, extends between the ureteral orifices and forms the posterior aspect of the trigone. In the contracted bladder the ureteric orifices are about 2.5 cm apart and about the same distance from the internal urethral orifice; however, in distended bladder these increase in measurement to about 5 cm.

The bladder is attached to the pelvic wall by the endopelvic fascia which is strengthened by the pubovesical and rectovesical ligaments.

The bladder is supplied by superior, middle and inferior vesical arteries from the anterior trunk of the internal iliac artery. Small visceral branches to the bladder also arise from the obturator and inferior gluteal arteries with additional supply from the vaginal and uterine arteries in the female. The venous drainage is through a venous plexus on fundus near the prostate and the inferior surface draining into hypogastric veins. Lymphatic drainage is primarily to the external iliac lymph nodes.

Urethra

The urethra is composed of mucous mem-brane, supported by a submucous tissue which connects it with the various structures through which it passes.

Male Urethra

The length of male urethra varies from 17.5 to 20 cm. In relaxed state, it has a double curve, and consists of anterior and posterior portions, each of which is subdivided into two parts. The extention of anterior urethra is from the external meatus to the inferior edge of the urogenital diaphragm and it passes through the corpus spongiosum. On the basis of clinical and imaging findings, the anterior urethra is divided into the penile (or pendulous) and bulbous parts at the peno-scrotal junction. The fossa navicularis (1–1.5 cm long) is formed by the termination of pendulous portion in the glans penis. The "sump" of the bulbous urethra is the dilated proximal portion of the bulbous urethra and portion of the bulb just proximal to the sump assuming a conical shape at the bulbomembranous junction is known as the "cone." Periurethral Littré glands of anterior urethra are more numerous at the dorsal aspect of the penile urethra and in the bulbous urethral sump. Within the urogenital diaphragm on each side of the membranous portion of the posterior urethra are two pea-sized Cowper glands. The ducts (2 cm long) empty on either side of midline into the bulbous urethral sump.

The posterior urethra is divided into two parts as prostatic and membranous urethras. The most dilatable and widest part of the canal is the prostatic urethra, which is about 3–3.5 cm long and it runs through the prostate from its base to its apex almost vertically, lying nearer its anterior than its posterior surface; the canal is wider in the middle than its extremity and narrowest below where it joins the membranous portion and assumes spindle-shape. Urethral crest is a longitudinal ridge of smooth muscle on the posterior wall of the posterior urethra extending from the bladder neck to the membranous urethra. It continues into the verumontanum, an ovoid mound lying in the posterior wall of the prostatic urethra measuring 15–17 mm in length and about 3 mm in height.

Prostatic utricle is in the center of the verumontanum, which is a small saccular depression that is a vestigial remnant of the müllerian duct. The orifices of the paired ejaculatory ducts are seen just distal and lateral to the utricle. The prostatic glands empty directly into the prostatic urethra via multiple small openings that surround the veru-montanum. The prostatic urethra then tapers distally into the membranous urethra, which is approximately 1–1.5 cm long and ends at the inferior aspect of the urogenital diaphragm.

The membranous urethra is the shortest, least dilatable and, with the exception of the external orifice, the narrowest part of the canal. It extends downward and forward, with a slight anterior concavity, between the apex of the prostate and the bulb of the urethra, perforating the urogenital dia-phragm about 2.5 cm below and behind the pubic symphysis.

The proximal (internal) urethral sphincter extends from the bladder neck through the prostatic urethra above the verumontanum. Although it is similar to the detrusor muscle, it has different neurogenic innervation. The distal (external) sphincter has both intrinsic and extrinsic components. The "intrinsic" urethral sphincter is a concentric muscular structure and lies in the distal third of the prostatic urethra below the mound of the verumontanum and surrounds the membranous urethra. Both the internal and intrinsic sphincters are composed of smooth muscle and function as muscles that maintain passive continence. The internal sphincter functions as the primary continence sphincter and the intrinsic sphincter as the secondary continence sphincter. The extrinsic sphincter is a paraurethral, striated, voluntary muscle with contributions from the levator ani complex. The sphincter surrounds the membranous urethra and is involved in active continence.

Female Urethra

The female urethra is 4 cm long and extends from the bladder neck at the urethrovesical junction to the vestibule, where it forms the external meatus between the labia minora. It is placed behind the symphysis pubis, imbedded in the anterior wall of the vagina and its direction is obliquely downward and forward; it is slightly curved with the concavity directed forward. Its diameter when undilated is about 6 mm. It perforates the fascia of the urogenital diaphragm and its external orifice is situated directly in front of the vaginal opening and about 2.5 cm behind the clitoris. Many small periurethral glands open into the urethra. Distally, these glands group together on either side of the urethra (Skene glands) and empty through two small ducts to either side of the external meatus. The proximal part of the urethral wall is made up of two layers of smooth muscle (inner longitudinal and outer circular) that are contiguous with the smooth muscle of the bladder neck. The outer portion of the urethra is composed of striated muscle, which, in the upper two-thirds of the urethra, is primarily circular and extends proximally to blend with the bladder base. The lower portion of the urethra is situated very next to the anterior vaginal wall and surrounded by the urethrovaginal sphincter extending above the urogenital diaphragm to the inferior pubic ramus.

IMAGING MODALITIES

Various imaging modalities available for imaging of the urinary bladder and urethra include the following:

- Plain films
- Retrograde urethrography (RGU)
- Voiding cystourethrography (VCUG)
- Cystography
- Urodynamic studies
- Ultrasonography (US)
- Computed tomography (CT)
- Magnetic resonance imaging (MRI)
- Radionuclide imaging.

Plain Films

The role of plain films is in the detection of radiopaque calculi or foreign bodies, calcification, abnormal gas pattern and in identification of soft tissue and the bony abnormalities. A plain radiograph or fluoroscopic examination is mandatory before starting the contrast studies to identify any radiopacity (calculi, calcification or foreign body) that may be obscured with contrast subsequently. Radiolucent foreign bodies can be seen if these get encrusted with calcium. Causes of bladder wall calcification include tuberculosis, tumors, radiation cystitis, cyclophosphamide induced cystitis, alkaline incrustation cystitis, amyloidosis and schistosomiasis.[1] Bladder neoplasms may be suggested on detection of stippled calcification.

In emphysematous cystitis, the plain film typically shows gas within the bladder lumen and irregular streaky radiolucencies within the bladder wall. The presence of gas within the ureter may be seen in the setting of emphysematous pyeloureteritis or emphy-sematous pyelonephritis. Plain films may occasionally be helpful for the detection of metastases, spinal abnormalities in cases of neurogenic bladder and diastasis of the pubic symphysis in patients with exstrophy/ epispadias anomaly.

Retrograde Urethrography

Retrograde urethrography is indicated in the evaluation of urethral injuries, strictures and fistulas and is considered to be the best initial modality for urethral and periurethral imaging in men. The procedure starts with placing patient in a supine 45° oblique position. The penis should be kept over the proximal thigh and directed laterally with moderate traction. Discomfort experienced during balloon inflation should be explained to the patient and reassured. Then, 20–30 mL of 60% iodinated contrast material is injected under fluoroscopic guidance through the 16- or 18-F Foley catheter (having the bulb gently inflated in fossa navicularis) so that the anterior urethra is filled. Spasm of the external urethral sphincter may prevent filling of the deep bulbar, membranous and prostatic urethras. So, slow and gentle pressure is usually needed to overcome this resistance. Spot radiographs are obtained when there is visual confirmation of contrast material flowing into the bladder. During RGU opacification of the prostatic ducts, Cowper ducts and periurethral Littré glands is often, but not necessarily, associated with urethral inflammatory and stricture disease.[2] If the integrity of the urethral mucosal lining is disrupted by increased pressure during contrast material injection, intravasation of contrast material with opacification of the corpora and draining veins may occur **(Fig. 1)**.

Voiding Cystourethrography

Voiding cystourethrography (VCUG) is the most commonly used method in the evaluation of the posterior male urethra and female urethra. Voiding urethrography is done after filling bladder with contrast material using transurethral or suprapubic catheter. Spot radiographs of the bladder and urethra are taken when patient voids under fluoroscopic observation after the removal of transurethral catheter. The bladder neck opens widely

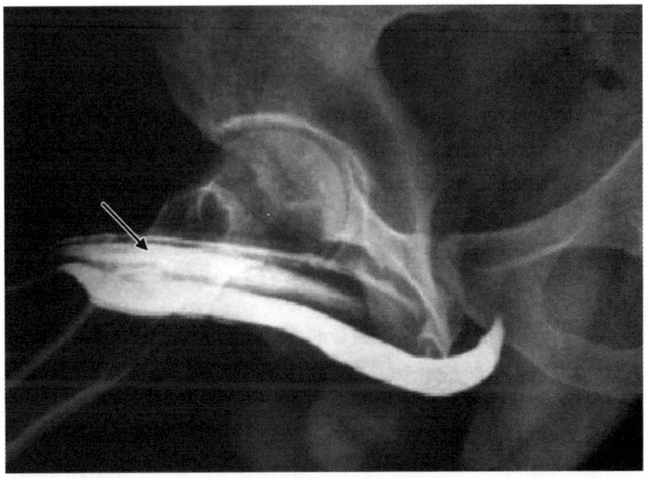

Fig. 1: Retrograde urethrography image showing opacification of the corpora (arrow) and draining veins due to increased pressure of injection.

during active voiding and assumes funnel shaped in both male and female patients by means of the internal sphincter mechanism. In male patients, the proximal bulbar urethra has a less conical appearance and verumontanum appears elongated. The membranous urethra is the narrowest segment between these parts of the urethra, however, it can dilate up to 6 or 7 mm in diameter during voiding.[2] Voiding cystourethrography fails to demonstrate certain abnormalities of the male anterior urethra as the normal anterior urethra is not fully distended to the degree seen at RGU. The anterior part of the urethra is best studied with a retrograde study and the posterior part with a voiding study.

Cystography

Cystography (excretory, retrograde and suprapubic) is a well-established modality for urinary bladder evaluation. The best cystogram is obtained by the retrograde method. Meglumine salts of diatrizoate and iothalmate are now universally used for cystography. Solution of 15% is generally adequate for cystography. In the excretory cystogram, bladder can be evaluated simultaneously along with upper urinary tracts, but it is not possible to recognize the presence of reflux.

In patients with renal failure having lesions in the bladder, retrograde cystography has a role. Cystography and micturating cystography is indicated for demonstration of the ability of the bladder to contract and control of the micturation, with assessment of vesical diverticulae and anatomic abnormalities of the bladder neck and urethra. However, the examination is contraindicated in presence of acute infections of the bladder and urethra.

Contrast cystogram can distinctly demonstrate intraluminal calculi, hematomas, tumors **(Fig. 2)** and wall irregularities. In traumatic injury of the bladder, cystogram depicts the type of bladder rupture (extraperitoneal or intraperitoneal), in addition to detection of pelvic fractures.

Extrinsic compression of the bladder can be produced by pelvic hematoma or lipomatosis resulting in appearance of bladder that has been referred to as "teardrop bladder". In such pathologies, ultrasound and CT play an important role in evaluating the cause of extrinsic compression.

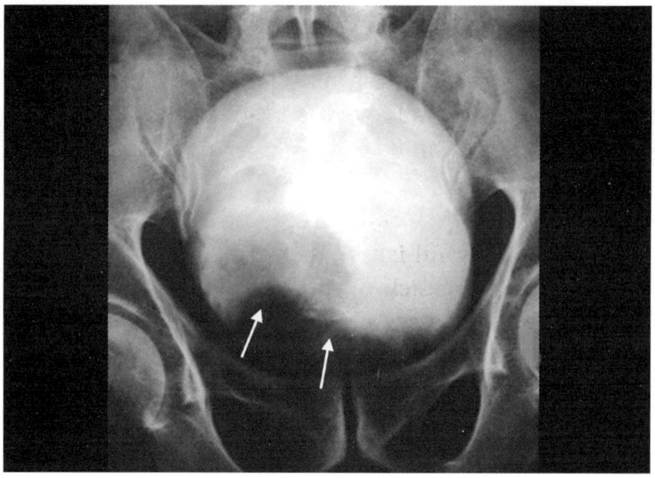

Fig. 2: Excretory cystogram showing irregular lobulated filling defect (arrows) at bladder base due to malignant growth.

Urodynamic Studies of the Lower Urinary Tract

The most definitive way of finding the source of symptoms involving the lower urinary tract, including the bladder and the urethra is urodynamic studies. These tests evaluate the function of storing and releasing urine and help to localize the anatomic or neurologic source of symptoms, such as leakage, frequent urination, problems starting a stream, dribbling, painful urination, problems completely emptying the bladder and recurrent urinary tract infections. The types of tests that are administered depend on the patient's symptoms and may include one or more of the tests like uroflowmetry, cystometry, electromyelogram, pressure studies for stress incontinence, VCUG, video urodynamics and assessment of postvoid residual urine, etc.

Ultrasonography

Real time US is a versatile modality in the detection of bladder lesions, and is frequently employed as the primary imaging modality for its evaluation. US of the urinary bladder can be carried out by transabdominal, endorectal or endovaginal approach. However, transabdominal approach is the simplest and the easiest. Bladder must be examined when it is comfortably distended. In the majority of patients this means a volume of about 350 mL. The bladder appears as a thin-walled smooth anechoic structure almost rectangular in configuration on transverse scanning with no intravesical filling defects.

Bladder US is used to assess the following:

- *Bladder wall anatomy*:
  - Thickening of the wall and focal abnormalities
  - Presence of trabeculation
  - Diverticulae
- Capacity of the bladder and postmicturation residual volume
- Anatomy of bladder base and urethral opening
- Distal ureteric anatomy
- Intravesical filling defects and extraluminal masses causing bladder compression.

Radiolucent calculi, which may be missed on plain radiographs, are easily picked up on US. Blood clots and sediments are usually freely mobile within the lumen. In obese patients and those with peritonitis in whom palpation of the bladder is difficult, ultrasound is very useful in determining whether the bladder is full enough to allow safe suprapubic catheterization. Transrectal US (TRUS) is useful in defining the plane between the prostate, seminal vesicles and the bladder, in posterior wall masses. Ultrasound cystodynamogram can be performed in patients with symptoms of voiding disorders.

Sonography of the urethra has mostly been used for diagnosis of urethral diverticula and strictures and is usually performed by using a broadband 5–10 MHz linear array for transpenile or transperineal scanning and a broadband curved array (5–9 MHz) for transvaginal or transrectal scanning. A 12.5 MHz, 6.2-F, catheter-based transducer on an intravascular US machine is used for endourethral sonography. Disadvantages of this technique include a single use urethral catheter, the need for a dedicated expensive intravascular US machine and limited field of view.

Sonourethrography has been shown to be accurate, sensitive and specific for the diagnosis and assessment of penile and bulbar urethral strictures. Retrograde urethrography and sonourethrography are equally efficacious in detection of anterior urethral strictures **(Fig. 3)**. Further characterization of strictures in terms of length, diameter and periurethral pathologies, like spongiofibrosis and false tracts, is done with greater sensitivity using sonourethrography as compared with RGU, with the added benefit of lower incidence of complications.[3]

Computed Tomography

The role of CT is in identification of size and number of distal ureteric, vesical or urethral calculi, pelvic trauma and in staging of vesicle or urethral malignancy.

On CT scan, the urinary bladder is seen as a homogeneous midline structure of water density. The size and configuration varies greatly depending on the amount of urine present. The outer margin of the bladder wall is smooth and usually well-delineated by the perivesical fat. Although urine is of near water density, the bladder wall has soft tissue attenuation. In contrast-enhanced CT (CECT) scan, opacified urine usually occupies the dependent portion of the bladder and unopacified urine layers above it. However, this relationship may be reversed in patients with glycosuria or infectious debris in the bladder, where the unopacified urine may have higher specific gravity than the excreted opacified urine.[4] Scans obtained before and

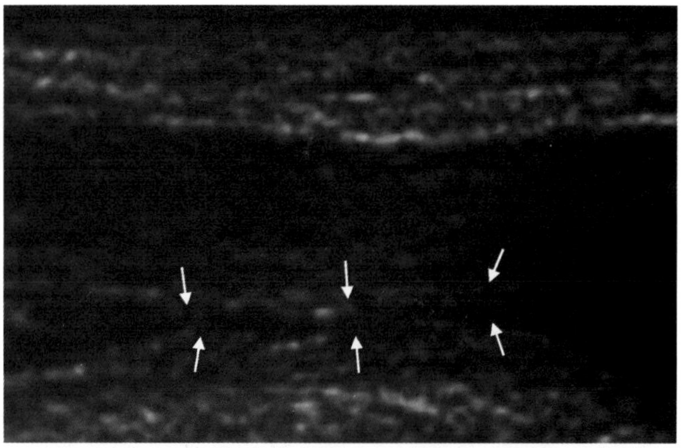

Fig. 3: Sonourethrogram showing a stricture (arrows) of penile urethra.

after administration of contrast medium can detect subtle vesical and perivesical abnormalities. Dense opacification of the lumen may obscure small tumors or calculi and can produce scan artifacts which degrade the image **(Figs. 4A and B)**. In the male pelvis, the seminal vesicles are seen posterior to the urinary bladder, cephalad to the rectum. They are oval to tear shaped structures. A small amount of fat is usually present between posterior wall of the urinary bladder and the seminal vesicle. This relationship may be distorted by a distended rectum or when the patient is prone. The prostate gland is located just posterior to the symphysis pubis and anterior to the rectum. Masses seen on intravenous urography compressing or displacing the bladder are readily evaluated by CT. True masses are easily distinguished from bladder impression produced by the bowel loops present in the pelvis, if the loops are adequately filled with contrast material. Alteration in the shape of the bladder can be produced by retroperitoneal fibrosis, pelvic lipomatosis, hematoma and lymphoceles, etc. In these benign conditions, CT reveals elevation and narrowing of the bladder (pear-shaped bladder).

Contrast-enhanced CT with delayed imaging or retrograde bladder filling (CT cystography) has been shown to be highly accurate and equivalent to conventional cystography in the detection of bladder rupture.[5]

Magnetic Resonance Imaging

Magnetic resonance imaging is reserved in congenital anomalies for cases of intersex anomalies or complex genitourinary anomalies, in cases where internal organs evaluation is essential. Magnetic resonance imaging is superior to contrast studies as it may demonstrate diverticula that are not seen on radiographic contrast-enhanced studies or inflammatory infiltration around the

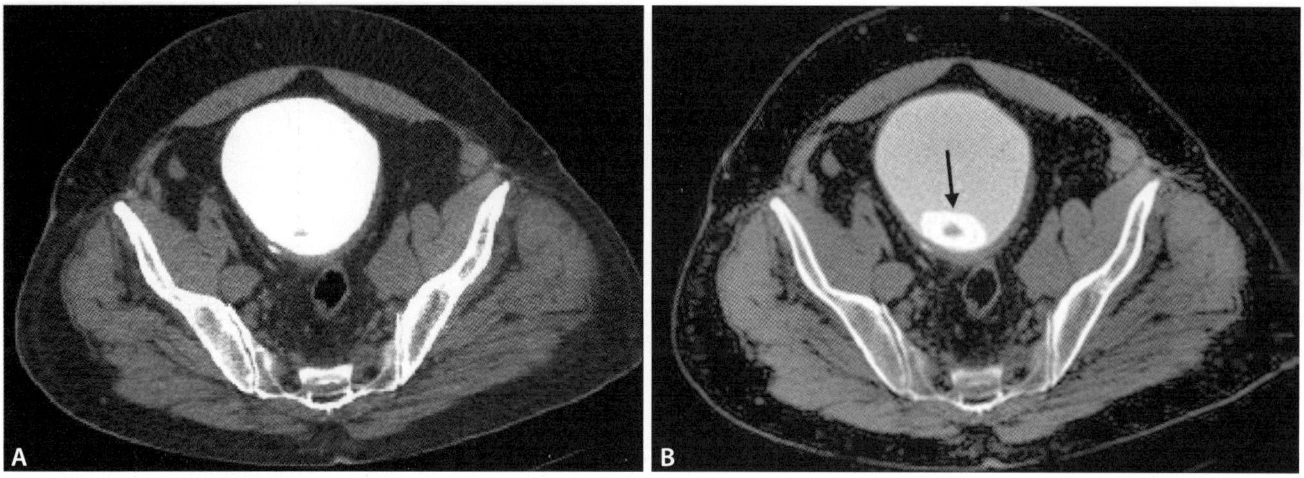

Figs. 4A and B: Bladder calculus: Dense opacification of bladder in CT axial image completely obscuring the calculus (A), which is visualized (arrow) in wide window setting (B).

urethra and presence of a periurethral abscess or sinus tract. It is very helpful in assessing the cases of trauma for presence and extent of anterior or posterior urethral injury and predicting the occurrence of complications. On MRI, fistula is seen as a direct communicating channel with an adjacent organ. MRI imaging is used for local staging in urethral tumors.[6]

Magnetic resonance images provide an excellent information about the anatomy and pathology of the urinary bladder. Both T1- and T2-weighted spin echo (SE) sequences are useful in bladder imaging. On T1-weighted images, muscle layer has an intermediate signal intensity equal to that of skeletal muscle and on T2-weighted images it shows low signal intensity **(Fig. 5)**. Proton density weighted images can sometimes be used to distinguish the mucosa and lamina propria from the muscle layer, because of higher signal intensity showed by the mucosa and lamina propria.

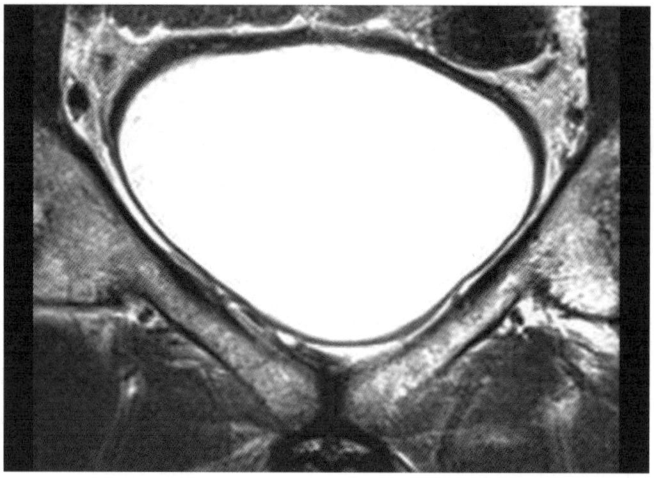

Fig. 5: Magnetic resonance: Coronal T2 image of urinary bladder. Note low signal intensity of detrusor muscle.

Fast SE sequences provide superior quality in T2-weighted MR images with a threefold to fivefold reduction of examination time compared with conventional SE sequences. At the moment, fast SE is the state of art for obtaining T2-weighted images of the pelvis. Three-dimensional (3D) techniques with offline reconstruction of high resolution images in any arbitrary plane are also very useful. The introduction of short TR (<10 msec) gradient echo sequences that use a preparation pulse, such as turbo fast low angle shot (FLASH), snapshot FLASH and magnetization prepared rapid gradient echo (MP-RAGE) and fast spin echo (FSE) sequences significantly reduce imaging time without compromising signal to noise ratio. For T1-weighted 3D imaging, the use of an MP-RAGE sequence has been described. Also, use of phased array multicoils and endorectal coils improves resolution. Dynamic contrast-enhanced MR provides the best information to help differentiate malignant from benign lesions.

Development of oral intestinal MR contrast agents, such as ferrite particles has improved the delineation of small bowel loops and para-aortic region.

The urethra can be evaluated obliquely along its course or in orthogonal planes (axial, sagittal and coronal). Both T1- and T2-weighted imaging are often needed to evaluate the male and female urethra. In male patients, axial plane is used for the best evaluation of the membranous urethra and coronal or sagittal plane is used assessing the relation between the membranous and bulbous urethra (particularly in cases of trauma). For imaging of the anterior urethra, the patient is placed in the supine position and the penis should be positioned anteriorly and taped to the abdominal wall beneath the surface coil **(Fig. 6)**. In female patients, axial images are essential.[7]

A combination of axial and sagittal or coronal imaging may be helpful for evaluation of a urethral diverticulum or spread of urethral cancer.

A desirable thin section for imaging the urethra is 3–5 mm thickness and a small intersection gap (1–2 mm). Surface coils or endovaginal or endorectal coils are used to improve the signal-to-noise ratio. Although endocavitary coils may improve the spatial resolution, the small field of view may limit the area of imaging and degradation of image quality due to high signal intensity in the near field. Use of intravenous contrast media is beneficial in selected cases, particularly in patients with extensive tumors or inflammation.

Radionuclide Imaging

Radionuclide cystography has been accepted as the technique of choice for evaluation and follow-up of children with urinary tract infection and reflux. The advantages being simplicity, lower radiation dose and no catheterization needed. Radionuclide cystography is more sensitive than voiding cystography in detecting vesicoureteric reflux; however, this has poor anatomical resolution than the conventional VCUG. Direct and indirect radionuclide cystography are interesting alternatives to the radiograph technique and are integrated into the process of diagnosis and follow-up of vesicoureteral reflux.[8]

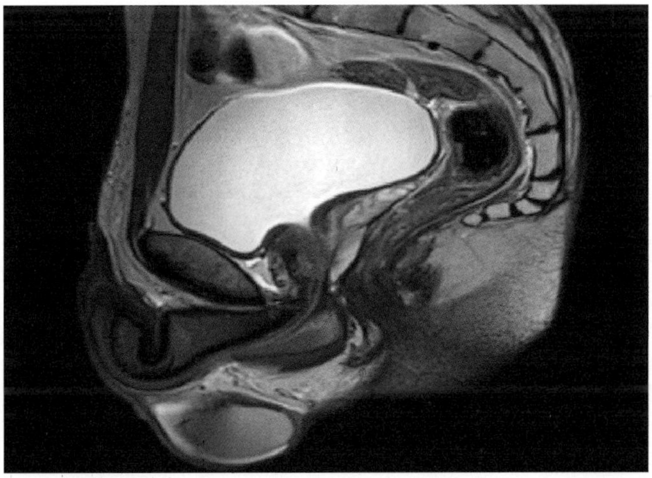

Fig. 6: Magnetic resonance: Sagittal T2 image showing the entire extent of urethra.

SPECIFIC DISEASES OF THE URINARY BLADDER

Bladder Diverticulae

Bladder diverticulae refer to pouch like eversion or evagination of the bladder wall. These may be congenital, but are more commonly acquired as a result of bladder outlet obstruction. Congenital bladder diverticulae develop as a result of herniation of bladder mucosa through the detrusor muscle, usually at a location slightly above and lateral to the ureteric orifice (Hutch diverticuli). These may vary from small to quite large and may cause either obstruction of, or reflux into the ipsilateral ureter. Diverticulae are sites of urinary stasis and thus lead to infection.

On cystogram, bladder diverticulae are seen as outpouchings from the bladder which may show persistence of contrast in the postmicturition phase. On US these appear as well-defined, thin-walled fluid containing structures communicating with the bladder lumen. The most important use of US is to detect the complications, i.e. stone or tumor in the diverticulum, which is not always possible to assess on cystography or endoscopy.

Urachal Anomalies

In fetal life, the urachus connects the dome of the bladder to the allantoic duct and develops from the superior portion of the urogenital sinus. It lies in space of Retzius behind the abdominal wall and anterior to the peritoneum. Normally, it obliterates before birth forming the fibrous median umbilical ligament. Incomplete obliteration leads to persistent urachus in one of the following four types:

	Urachal anomalies	*Entity*
1.	Completely patent urachus	Vesicocutaneous fistula between bladder and umbilicus
2.	Patent caudal portion opening into the bladder	Vesicourachal diverticulum
3.	Patent cephalic portion opening into the umbilicus	Urachal sinus
4.	Midportion is patent, both cephalic and caudal ends closed	Urachal cyst

In the newborn, patent urachus is diagnosed when there is leakage of urine from the umbilicus. Retrograde injection of contrast into umbilical orifice can directly demonstrate patent urachus. It may also fill up during voiding cystourethrogram, best demonstrated in the lateral projection. Urachal cyst is not delineated on conventional urography studies. An urachal diverticulum is identified as urine filled anterosuperior protrusion of the bladder dome on cystography.

In adults the urachal diverticulum may be complicated with infection or malignancy **(Figs. 7 and 8)**. Urachal anomalies can be delineated on US, CT and MRI. Ultrasonography reveals a tubular, anechoic structure in the lower, mid anterior abdominal wall. Magnetic resonance imaging is very helpful as it permits multiplanar imaging especially in the sagittal plane.

Exstrophy

Exstrophy of the bladder is a spectrum of defects in the formation of the anterior abdominal wall caused by varying degrees of failure of midline fusion of mesodermal tissue below the umbilicus. Classical exstrophy includes epispadias, separation of pubic bones (more than 10 mm) and communication of bladder with the anterior skin surface **(Fig. 9)**. On excretory urography, there is a wide lateral curve of the pelvic portion of the distal ureters, which then turn upwards and medially, passing through the bladder wall in a perpendicular direction. Cystogram is performed in postoperative follow-up of these patients.

Other Anomalies

Other major anomalies include, bladder agenesis and hypoplasia which are associated with urethral and other congenital anomalies, which when severe may even be incompatible with life. Duplication of the bladder may be partial or complete with two separate bladders, lying side by side separated by a peritoneal fold. Each bladder receives the ipsilateral ureter and empties into a separate urethra. This can be associated with anomalies of the gastrointestinal tract, genital system and lower spine. Anatomy of duplication can be well-demonstrated on US and MRI.

Neurogenic Bladder

Neurogenic bladder dysfunction may be caused by spinal dysraphism, cord compression or cord injury. Cystography is very helpful in diagnosis of neurogenic bladder. Ultrasonography is also useful to assess bladder size, shape, volume, post void residue, renal parenchymal changes and secondary calculi.

In the condition called as detrusor-external sphincter dyssynergia (DSED), contraction of the external sphincter occurs involuntarily at the same time as detrusor contraction thus impeding urinary flow and resulting in bladder outlet obstruction. In this condition bladder is often vertically oriented, with an irregular contour with trabeculation; frequently with multiple diverticulae and is referred to as "Christmas tree" or "pine tree" bladder. On VCUG, there may or may not be vesicoureteral reflux. In detrusor areflexia VCUG often reveals a smooth, thin-walled bladder with increased capacity, occasionally up to several liters and extending high into the abdomen. Significant postvoid residue is seen in both these conditions.

Infections

Acute Cystitis

Acute cystitis due to bacterial infection is most commonly the result of transurethral infection and is common in females. *Escherichia coli* is the most common pathogen.

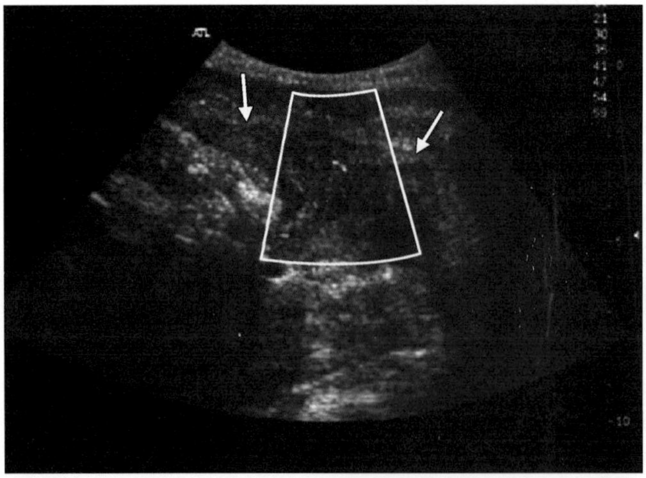

Fig. 7: Urachal diverticulum (arrow) complicated with infection: Ultrasonography image showing thickening of diverticular wall with increased vascularity.

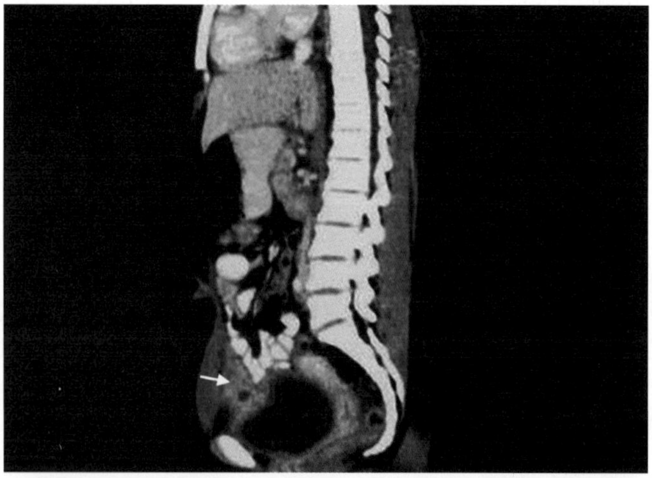

Fig. 8: Sagittal 3D reformatted CT image of the same patient as in Figure 7 showing thickening and enhancement of urachus.

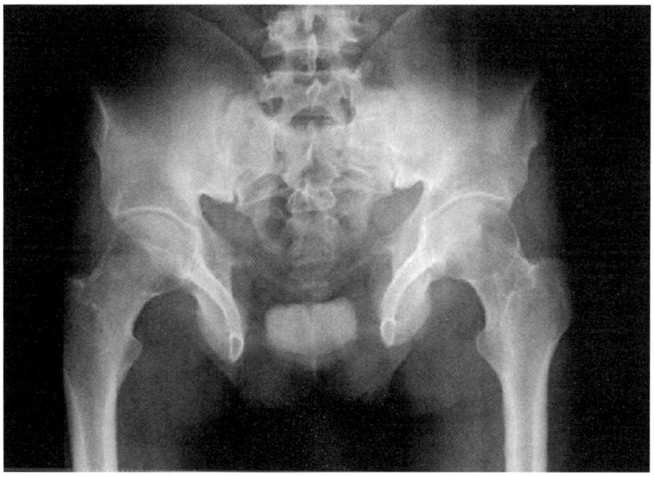

Fig. 9: Exstrophy of bladder: Radiograph showing diastasis of pubic symphysis.

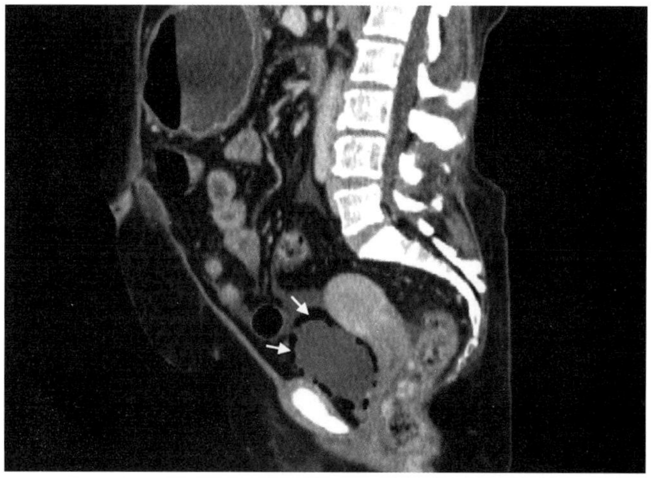

Fig. 10: Emphysematous cystitis: Sagittal reformatted CT image showing air pockets (arrows) within the bladder wall.

Cystography is contraindicated in acute infection. Ultrasonography is the most useful modality allowing evaluation of the upper tracts as well as the bladder. On US, cystitis show thickened and less distinct bladder wall with internal echoes or debris. Cobblestone appearance of bladder wall can be seen in severe bladder edema due to acute cystitis. Contour irregularity due to bladder mucosal edema can also be seen in radiation cystitis, cyclophosphamide cystitis and eosinophilic cystitis, and these can be associated with hemorrhage.

Emphysematous cystitis is almost always seen in diabetic or immunocompromised patients and *E. coli* is the most common pathogen **(Fig. 10)**.

Chronic Cystitis

The hallmark of chronic cystitis is thickening, calcification and irregularity of the bladder wall associated with trabeculation and often diminished bladder capacity. Tubercular infection of the bladder has been discussed in detail in the chapter on Tubercular Infection of the Urinary Tract.

Cystitis Cystica

Cystitis cystica is a benign condition commonly seen in women with recurrent or chronic cystitis, or in chronically irritated bladders, such as those catheterized for long periods or with calculus disease of the bladder. Multiple round contour defects at the bladder base can be seen in cystitis cystica and malakoplakia, on cystogram and US.

Malakoplakia

Malakoplakia is an uncommon granulomatous response to an infection of the urinary tract, predominantly with *E. coli*. Submucosal granulomas containing macrophages with inclusion bodies known as 'Michaelis-Gutmann bodies' are characteristic. It may affect any part of the urinary tract. Radiographically, these are seen as single or multiple mural filling defects especially in the trigone and bladder base. Accompanying bladder wall thickening may also be seen, simulating carcinoma.

Schistosomiasis

Schistosomiasis or bilharziasis is a parasitic infection caused by *Schistosoma hematobium*, producing polypoidal bladder wall thickening, which is nonspecific in appearance. In late stages fibrosis leads to a small capacity bladder with focal or curvilinear dense wall calcification.

Extravesical Processes

Appendicitis, diverticulitis and pelvic abscesses may produce reactive thickening of the bladder wall and mucosal irregularities.

Bladder Tumors

Primary bladder tumors are mostly epithelial in origin, less than 10% arising from a nonepithelial source. All epithelial tumors are malignant, majority being transitional cell type with SCC and adenocarcinoma being relatively uncommon. Nonepithelial tumors may be benign (e.g. leiomyoma, fibroma) or malignant (e.g. leiomyosarcoma and rhabdomyosarcoma). Various other primary tumors or masses may occur, including pheochromocytoma, hemangioma, leukoplakia, lymphoma and endometriosis. The bladder can also rarely be the site of metastases. The staging system most often used for bladder cancer is the TNM system (Adapted from: International Union Against Cancer (UICC). tumor nodes metastasis (TNM) classification of malignant tumors. 5th ed. Geneva (CH):UICC; 1997).

Ta	Noninvasive papillary carcinoma
Tis	Carcinoma *in situ*
T1	Invades subepithelial connective tissue
T2	Muscular invasion
T2a	Inner half
T2b	Outer half
T3	Invades perivesical tissues
T3a	Microscopic disease
T3b	Macroscopic disease
T4	Invades adjacent organs, pelvic-abdominal wall
T4a	Prostate, uterus or vagina
T4b	Pelvic or abdominal wall
N1	Single lymph node <2 cm
N2	Single lymph node >2–5 cm, multiple <5 cm
M0	No distant metastasis
M1	Distant metastasis.

The clinical staging (with deep fractioned transurethral resection) is much less accurate in staging invasive (Stages T2-T4) tumors. Cystogram cannot detect an early growth, extent of extravesical spread or status of the adjacent organs **(Fig. 11)**.

Although the intravesical position of many tumors can be visualized on US, an accurate assessment of the depth of penetration of the bladder wall cannot be done with US **(Fig. 12)**. The diagnostic accuracy of the transabdominal US for depth of infiltration ranges from 55 to 95%. Perivesical invasion cannot be frequently determined, however, extravesical spread may be recognized by the asymmetry due to infiltration.

Tumors involving the posterior bladder wall and neck; prostate and seminal vesicles may be visualized better with transrectal approach. Finally, none of the ultrasound methods optimally assesses the regional nodal status.

Computed tomography plays a major role in staging of carcinoma of the bladder rather than detection of the primary neoplasm. However, CT is not accurate for the early stages and its reliability increases with more advanced disease **(Fig. 13)**. Computed tomography has limited value in early disease as it cannot differentiate between the various layers of the bladder wall and cannot therefore distinguish lesions limited to the lamina propria (T1) from those invading the superficial (T2) and deep (T3a) muscles. So, CT is useful for detecting extravesical extension characterized by poor definition of the outer aspect of the bladder wall with an increase in density of the perivesical fat. Tumor involvement of the pelvic side wall is characterized by a soft tissue mass extending into the obturator internus muscle or by strands of soft tissue extending from the main tumor mass to the pelvic wall.

Tumor invasion of the seminal vesicles need to be considered if the seminal vesicle angle is obliterated by soft tissue mass. Caution should be exercised in interpretation of this finding as the normal seminal vesicle angle may be lost in over distended rectum or if the patient is scanned in prone position. Computed tomography is useful in detecting lymph node metastases, involvement being judged by the size of the node. Nodes greater than 10 mm in short axis are considered malignant. The obturator and external iliac lymph nodes are involved first. Computed tomography has limited accuracy in detecting perivesical infiltration and lymph node metastasis in invasive bladder

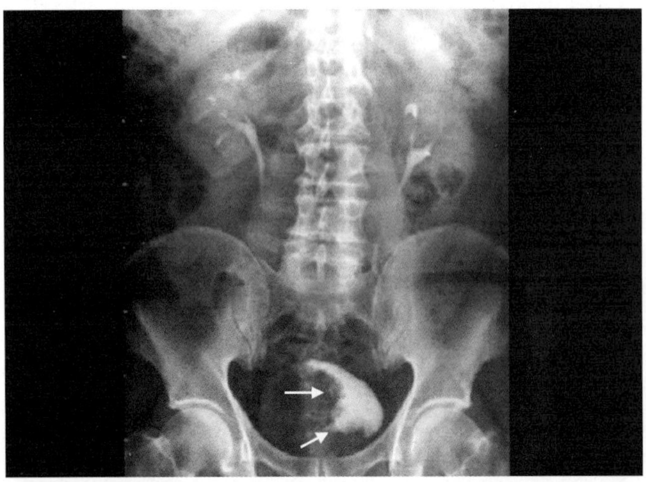

Fig. 11: Transitional cell carcinoma (TCC) of bladder: Intravenous urograms image showing large polypoidal filling defects (arrows) within the bladder.

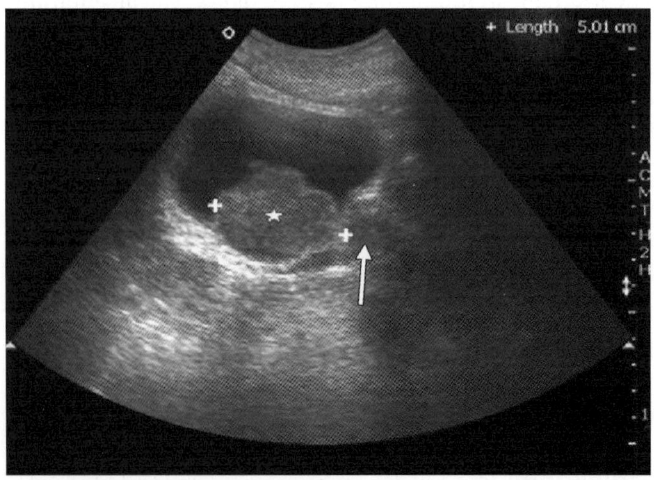

Fig. 12: Transitional cell carcinoma of bladder: Ultrasonography image showing intraluminal polypoidal mass within the bladder with invasion of left ureter (arrow).

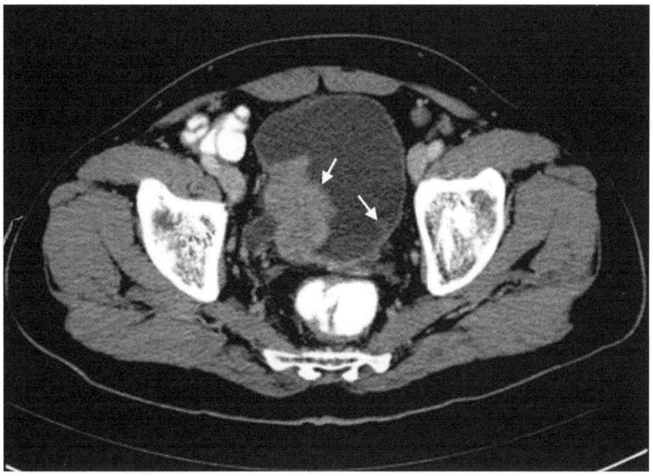

Fig. 13: Transitional cell carcinoma of bladder: Computed tomography axial image showing a large polypoidal growth (arrow) along right lateral wall and base of bladder causing ureteric obstruction. A small tumor is also seen along left lateral wall (arrow).

carcinoma[9,10] (accuracy of CT varies from 40 to 90% for staging, 65–85% for detection of perivesical extension and 65–97% for lymph node detection).

On MR, T1-weighted images are the best sequences for evaluating tumor extension into the adjacent bright fat, lymphadenopathy detection and bone marrow involvement.[11] There is better delineation of bladder cancer from urine with T2-weighted images. When compared with two-dimensional T1-weighted SE imaging, three-dimensional MP-RAGE imaging improved bladder carcinoma staging by 15%.[12] When compared with SE, fast SE sequences significantly reduced acquisition time by 3- to 5-fold without compromising T2-weighted image quality.[13] Presently, fast SE is state of the art for obtaining T2-weighted images of the pelvis. Contrast administration and fast dynamic imaging improves the ability of MRI to detect and stage bladder cancers. Most carcinomas enhance intensely following intravenous contrast material administration. Tumor tissue generally enhances earlier (average 6.5 s) than postbiopsy granulation tissue (13.5 s).[14]

Magnetic resonance imaging is the most accurate staging technique in invasive tumors. T2-weighted or contrast enhanced T1-weighted sequences are needed to evaluate the infiltrating component of the tumor. Visualization of the low signal intensity line on T2-weighted images representing the uninvolved bladder wall between the tumor and perivesical fat is an important feature in MRI staging, differentiating stage T3a from stage T3b. Stage T3b disease is indicated by disruption of the low signal intensity muscle layer of the bladder, irregularity of the outer bladder wall and perivesical stranding **(Figs. 14 to 17)**.

Multiplanar imaging helps in demonstration of direct tumor invasion into adjacent organs. Uterine or vaginal invasion is assessed using sagittal image. Assessment of invasion of the seminal vesicles is also facilitated by use of the sagittal image, invasion being demonstrated by an increase in size, decrease in signal intensity on T2-weighted images and obliteration of the angle between seminal vesicle and the posterior bladder wall.

Rectal and prostate infiltration is seen as direct tumor extension with a high signal intensity on T2-weighted images. Because of multiplanar imaging capability, MR is especially useful for evaluation of tumors at the bladder dome or base.

Lymph nodes are imaged with T1 weighted images as these have lower signal intensity than the surrounding fatty tissue. Magnetic resonance imaging with ultrasmall superparamagnetic iron oxide agents have shown potential for detecting metastases in normal size nodes and in differentiating reactive enlarged nodes from those with metastases.[15]

All modalities have limitation in determining extent of tumor growth in the muscle layer of the bladder wall, i.e. differentiation between stages T2 and T3a. This problem can be overcome by the use of endorectal surface coils or phased-array multicoils in combination with IV contrast agents or T2-weighted fast SE sequences which could differentiate stage T2 from stage T3 tumors.

Other newer imaging modalities like fluorescence cystoscopy, optical coherence tomography and narrow-band imaging are under evaluation and may prove useful in staging of early bladder cancer.[16] Virtual cystoscopy may allow noninvasive tumor diagnosis, treatment planning and surveillance.

Because of urinary stasis and chronic inflammation, there is a 2–10% increased incidence of carcinoma that develops within bladder diverticula.[17] Most neoplasms of bladder diverticulum are of urothelial origin. By definition the detrusor muscle is absent in diverticula; therefore, tumors often have invaded the perivesical fat at the time of diagnosis **(Fig. 18)**. A narrow diverticular neck or unusual location can preclude adequate visualization at cystoscopy; therefore, imaging has an important role in identifying such occult neoplasm.

Most urachal carcinoma are mucin-producing adenocarcinomas of the juxtavesical segment of the urachus.[18] Diagnosis is often facilitated by the characteristic midline location of the mass anterosuperior to the bladder,

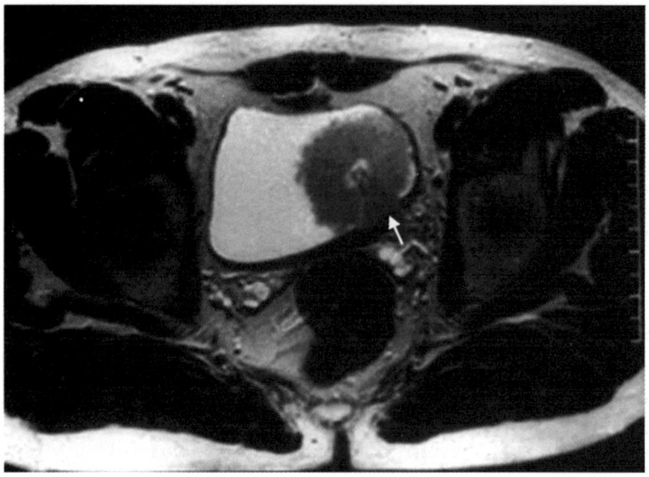

Fig. 14: Transitional cell carcinoma of bladder: Axial T2-weighted image of a papillary transitional cell carcinoma shows a intraluminal mass which is intermediate in signal intensity. The pedicle is clearly seen (arrow). The muscle wall is not infiltrated. Perivesical enlarged vessels are noted adjacent to the tumor on left side.

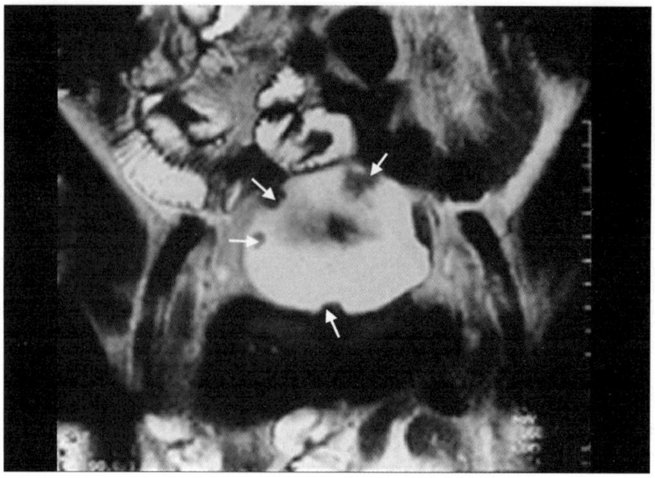

Fig. 15: Transitional cell carcinoma of bladder: Coronal T2-weighted image showing superficial masses in diffuse multifocal cancer (arrows) which appear relatively hypointense compared to bright urine. There is no perivesical extension.

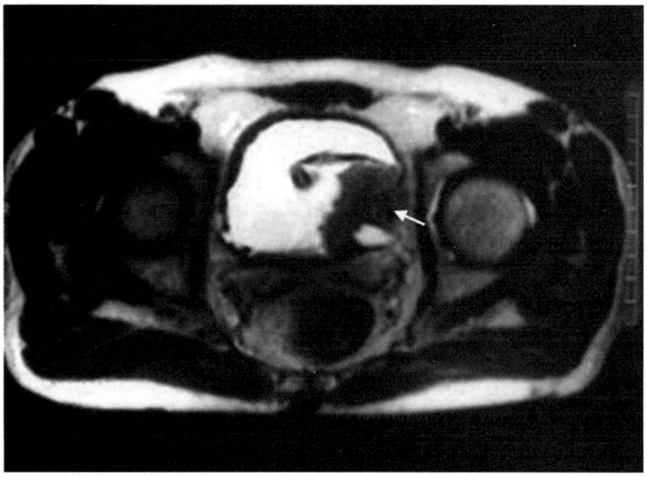

Fig. 16: Transitional cell carcinoma of bladder: T2 axial section shows left posterolateral wall tumor (TCC) with deep muscle infiltration leading to ureteric obstruction. Early perivesical spread is seen as stranding of fat along left posterolateral aspect (arrow).

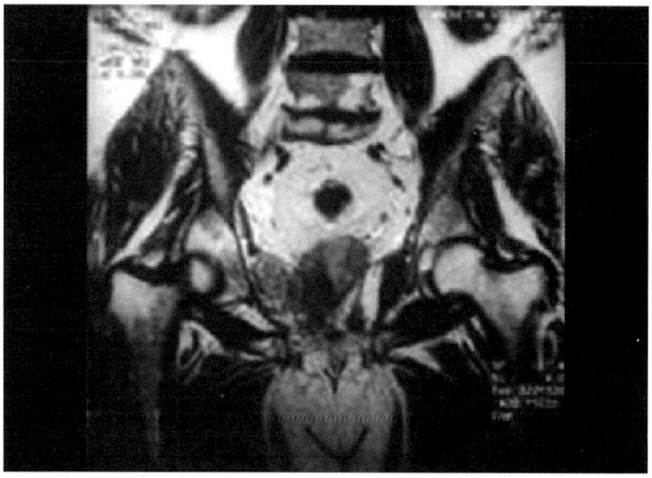

Fig. 17: Transitional cell carcinoma of bladder: Stage T4 disease with infiltration of the right pelvic side wall muscles by bladder cancer. Note normal marrow signal of the pelvic bones on this T1 image.

which is optimally delineated in the sagittal and coronal planes **(Fig. 19)**.

Chronic stasis and inflammation predispose to SCC. Schistosomiasis (bilharziasis) is associated with a higher incidence of vesical SCC.

SPECIFIC DISEASES OF URETHRA

Gonococcal and Nongonococcal Urethritis

Gram-negative diplococcus, *Neisseria gonorrhea* is associated with the gonococcal urethritis. Common organism of nongonococcal urethritis is *Chlamydia trachomatis*, accounting for 30–50% of cases. Purulent urethral discharge is the most common presentation of patients with gonococcal urethritis. Nongonococcal urethritis is usually associated with scanty urethral discharge. The acute gonococcal or non gonococcal urethritis is diagnosed by means of clinical and laboratory findings. Imaging studies are not necessary in non-complicated urethritis. Complications are more common and ominous with gonococcal urethritis than with nongonococcal with urethral stricture, periurethral abscess and fistula.

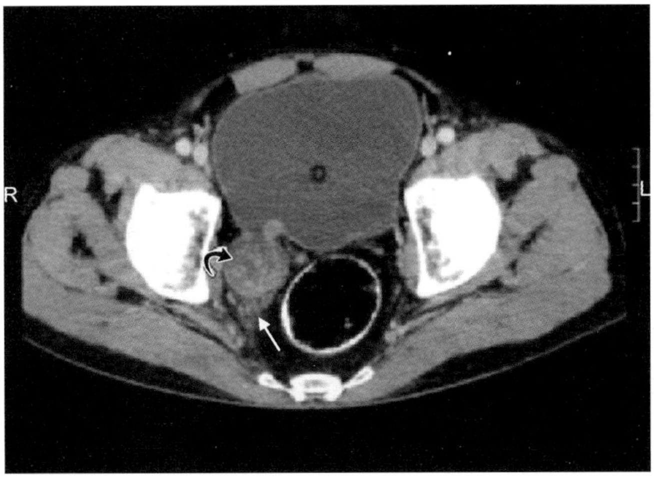

Fig. 18: Transitional cell carcinoma of bladder diverticulum: Axial CT image shows an enhancing mass almost completely filling the bladder diverticulum (curved arrow) along right posterolateral wall. Note extravesical extension of the tumor (arrow).

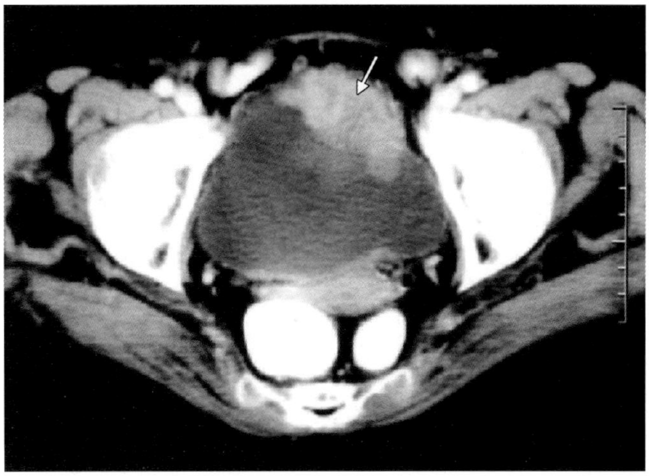

Fig. 19: Urachal carcinoma: Axial CT image showing a polypoid tumor mass (arrow) along the anterosuperior aspect of bladder.

The urethral stricture in typical gonococcal urethritis is seen as an irregular several centimeters long narrowing of urethra in urethrography **(Fig. 20)**. An estimated 15% of men with gonococcal urethritis develop stricture, in a span of 20–30 years between infection and the onset of obstructive symptoms.[19] Hard fibrous scars are present at the distal part of the bulbous urethra in 70% of patients. The causative factors of scar formation in this region are poor flushing by urination and the predominance of Littré glands in this area. Urethrography may show associated Littré glands dilatation. Narrow, elongated, asymmetric, irregular, or absent opacification of normal cone shaped proximal membranous urethra means involvement of the membranous urethra by stricture (seen in more than 90% of cases).[20] This information is of paramount importance to the urologist because iatrogenic incontinence of distal sphincter may develop if surgical treatment involves cutting of the scar tissue.

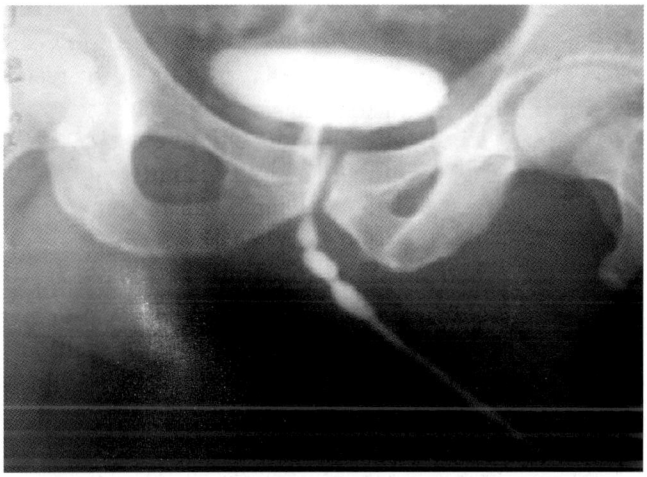

Fig. 20: Gonococcal urethral stricture: Retrograde urethrography image showing a panurethral stricture.

Periurethral abscess arises initially when a Littré gland becomes obstructed by inspissated pus or fibrosis **(Fig. 21)**. Gram-negative rods, enterococci and anaerobes are the most common infecting organisms. Periurethral abscess is a life-threatening infection of the male urethra and periurethral tissue and frequently a sequelae of gonococcal infection, urethral stricture disease, or urethral catheterization. Communication between urethra and periurethral abscess results in pseudodiverticulum formation. Because the tunica albuginea of the penis prevents the dorsal spread of infection, the abscess tracks ventrally along the corpus spongiosum, where it is confined by the Buck fascia. However, extensive necrosis of the subcutaneous tissue and fascia may occur once Buck fascia perforates. Rapid diagnosis and treatment are essential. Imaging studies may be indicated if the diagnosis is not established clinically. An abscess draining into the urethra may be demonstrated at urethrography. Ultrasonography can demonstrate the presence of periurethral abscess. Computed tomography and MR imaging can be used to assess the extent of the periurethral abscess and complications, such as fasciitis and Fournier gangrene.

Urethroperineal fistulas most often occur as a sequel of periurethral abscess. Generally there is contraction of the initial abscess cavity from healing fibrosis resulting in only a narrow fistulous tract from the urethra to the

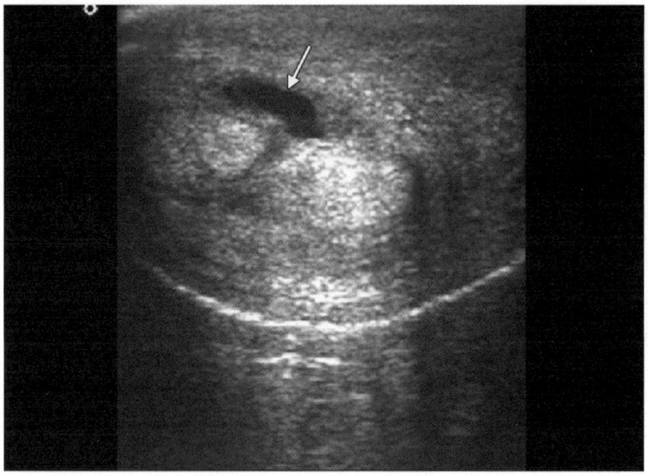

Fig. 21: Periurethral abscess: Ultrasonography image shows an abscess cavity (arrow) in relation to the penile urethra.

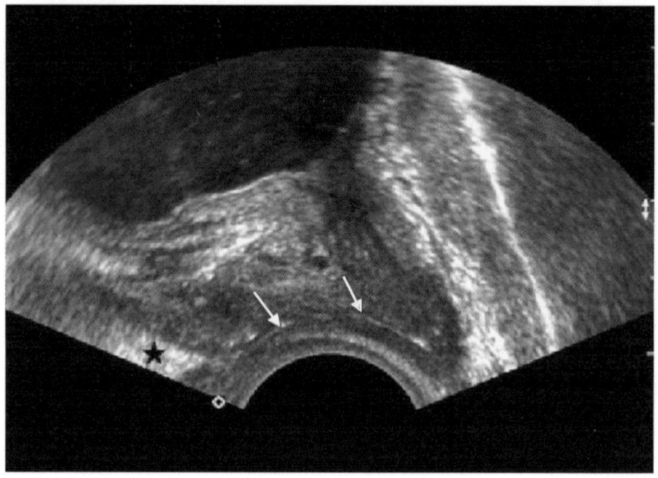

Fig. 22: Rectourethral fistula in a young male who had tuberculous prostatic abscesses and presented with pneumaturia: Transrectal US image shows the echogenic fistulous tract (arrows) between the rectum (star) and the prostatic urethra.

perineum and subsequently urination occurs through the perineal fistulas, resulting in the so-called "watering can perineum".[21] Urethroperineal fistulas are usually the result of tuberculosis and schistosomiasis infections.

Condyloma Acuminata (Venereal Warts)

Condyloma acuminata are caused by viral infection resulting in soft, sessile, squamous papillomas on the penile glans and shaft and the prepuce. Involvement of urethra occurs in 0.5–5% of male patients. Occasionally, warts may extend to the prostatic urethra and bladder. The diagnostic procedure of choice is VCUG. However, the diagnosis is often not suspected until RGU has been performed. Typically multiple papillary filling defects are seen in the anterior urethra.

Tuberculosis

Genital tuberculosis is usually a descending infection from upper urinary tract. Up to 70% of patients show associated prostatic involvement. Prostatorectal and prostatoperineal urethral fistulas may result in rupture of prostatic abscess into periprostatic structure **(Fig. 22)**. Urethral discharge and associated involvement of the epididymis, prostate and other parts of the urinary system is seen in acute phase. However, diagnosis becomes difficult in chronic phase as obstructive symptoms develop secondary to urethral strictures. Numerous fistulas develop in perineal and scrotal region in tuberculous urethral strictures which result in watering-can perineum. Retrograde urethrography typically demonstrates an anterior urethral stricture and associated multiple prostatocutaneous and urethrocutaneous fistulas. Similantaneous fistulography may be useful for assessing the entire urethra.

Urethral Strictures

Most urethral strictures are the result of infection, instrumentation, or other iatrogenic causes. Strictures in the anterior urethra may be due to trauma (external injury, instrumentation) ,inflammation (e.g., infection, balanitis xerotica obliterans), or congenital. The most common external cause of traumatic stricture is straddle injury. Iatrogenic trauma to the urethra may result in pressure necrosis at fixed points in the urethra from indwelling catheters **(Fig. 23)**. Instrumentation-related strictures usually occur in two common places which are: bulbomembranous and penoscrotal junctions.

Alternatively, posterior urethral stricture is often an obliterative process that occurs as a result of urethral distraction or disruption caused by either trauma or surgery **(Fig. 24)**. Posttraumatic posterior urethral stricture is often associated with resultant displacement of the urethral axis, which results in obliteration from intervening fibrosis. Iatrogenic stricture of the prostatic posterior urethra ("bladder neck contracture") usually occurs after transurethral resection of the prostate or open radical prostatectomy.[22]

Urethral Diverticulum

Acquired diverticulae more commonly occur in the females. It occurs most commonly in the midurethra and on the posterolateral wall rather than on the anterior

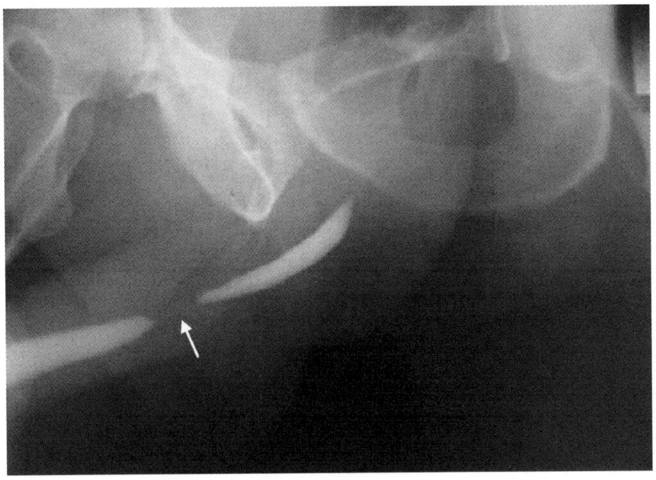

Fig. 23: Post-traumatic anterior urethral stricture: Retrograde urethrography image showing a penile urethral stricture due to instrumentation for transurethral resection of prostate.

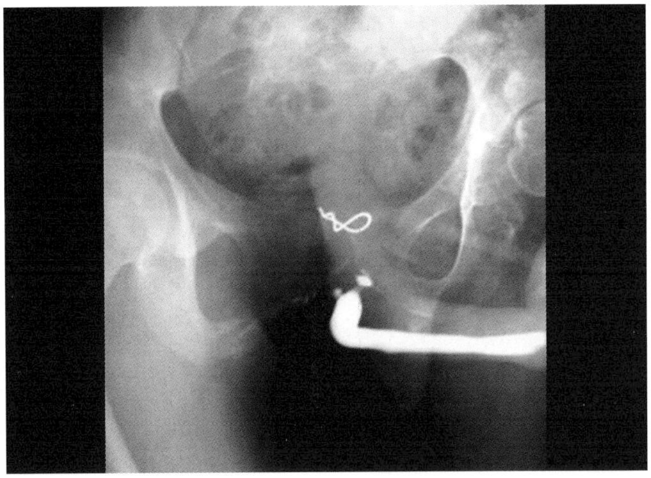

Fig. 24: Post-traumatic posterior urethral stricture: Retrograde urothrography image showing a tight posterior urethral stricture at membranous urethra due to pelvic trauma.

wall. Inflammation or repeated minor trauma to skene (periurethral) glands can result in dilation followed by rupture and diverticulae formation. Associations include—ductal remnant (Wolffian/Mullerian);cloacal epithelium. 1.4% of women with stress incontinence have been reported to have diverticulae.[23] Surgery for incontinence is another common cause due to periurethral fascial disruption during bladder neck suspension surgery resulting in focal posterior urethral prolapse.The diagnosis is usually made with VCUG (accuracy of 65%[24]) or cross-sectional imaging **(Fig. 25)**.

Ultrasonography can demonstrate a relatively anechoic paraurethral structure with internal debris or surrounding inflammatory changes. Magnetic resonance imaging is more sensitive than VCUG and double balloon urethrography in the detection of urethral diverticula, particularly in the detection of narrow-neck noncommunicating urethral diverticula.[25] The differential diagnosis includes vaginal cyst (Gartner duct, paramesonephric or müllerian duct cyst, epithelial inclusion cyst), ectopic ureterocele, endometrioma and urethral tumors.[26]

Urethral diverticula may be complicated by infection, stone formation and malignant degeneration. The most common malignancy arising from diverticulae being adenocarcinoma.

Urethral Calculi

Most urethral calculi are secondary due to expulsion from the bladder during voiding (migrant calculi). Rarely when there is stasis like within a diverticulum or proximal to a stricture, primary stone formation occurs. These are identified in the baseline preprocedural plain radiograph as radioopacities and as filling defects in RGU **(Figs. 26A and B)**.

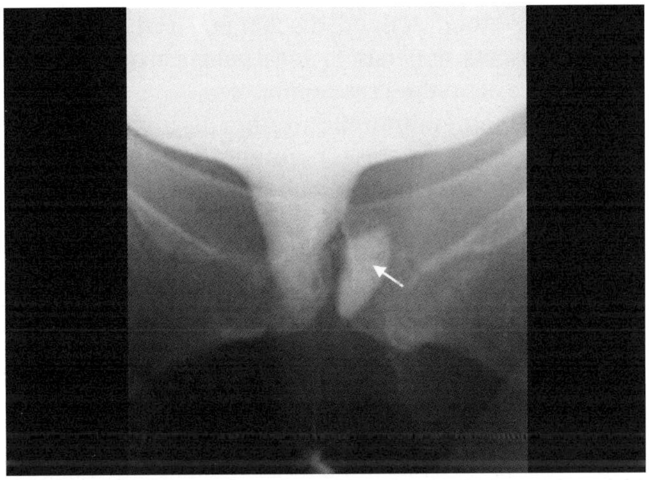

Fig. 25: Urethral diverticulum in an elderly female: Voiding cystourethrography image showing the urethral diverticulum (arrow).

Tumors of the Male Urethra

Benign urethral malignancies are quite rare originating from epithelial or mesenchymal cells and presenting as filling defects, with tissue diagnosis often being necessary to establish the correct diagnosis. Malignant tumor incidence is <1% of all urologic malignancies, usually occuring above 50 years of age. The most common presenting symptom is a mass in the perineum or along the urethral shaft with or without obstructive voiding

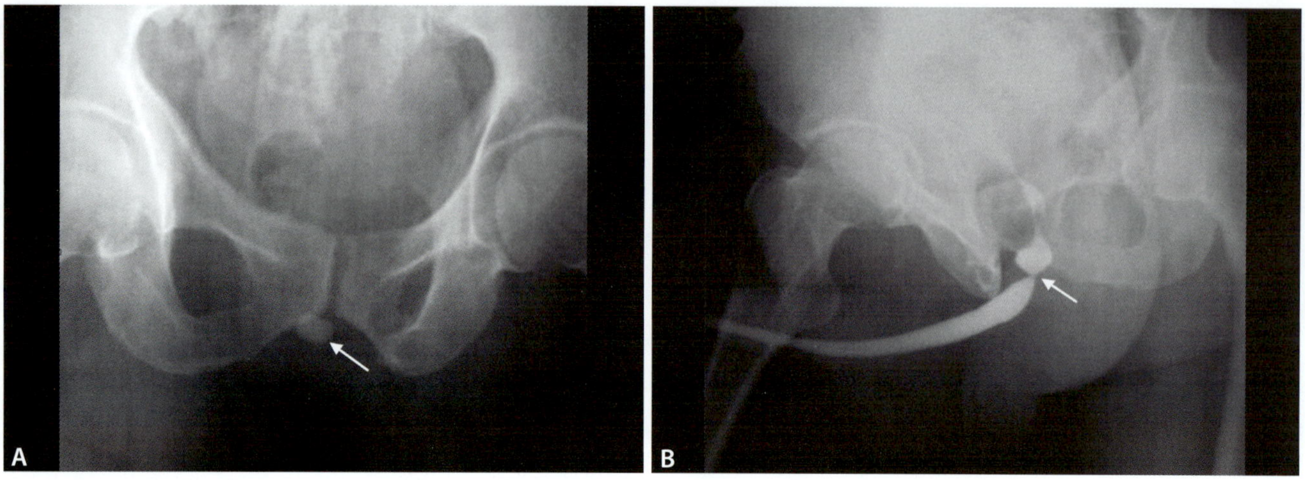

Figs. 26A and B: Urethral calculus: (A) Radiograph showing a calculus (arrow) in expected location of prostatic urethra; (B) RGU image showing the stricture (arrow) at bulbar urethra distal to the impacted calculus. Note the calculus is obscured by injected contrast.

symptoms. Urethral stricture or bleeding, obstructive symptoms, blood stained discharge, urethral fistula, perineal abscess, or persistent local pain in an elderly man is suggestive of urethral carcinoma.

The bulbomembranous urethra is involved most frequently (60% of cases), followed by the penile (30%) and the prostatic segment (10%).[27] 80% of male urethral carcinomas are SCC, 15% are TCC and 5% are adenocarcinoma or undifferentiated carcinoma. The histologic subtype of urethral cancers also varies according to anatomic location. Squamous cell carcinoma constitutes 90% of penile, 80% of bulbomembranous and 10% of prostatic malignancies. In contrast, transitional cell subtype predominates in the prostatic segment (90%); with only 10% occurence in each of the other segments **(Figs. 27 and 28)**. Adenocarcinoma (10% cases in the bulbomembranous segment) arises from the Littré or Cowper glands. 25% of urethral malignancy patients give a positive history for STDs, while half the patients have urethral strictures.

Male urethral carcinoma can spread by direct extension to adjacent structures or metastasize to regional lymph nodes. Stage I urethral tumor is confined to the subepithelial connective tissue. Stage II tumor invades the corpus spongiosum, prostate, or periurethral muscle. Stage III tumor invades the corpus cavernosum and bladder neck or beyond the prostatic capsule. Stage IV tumor invades other adjacent organs. Lymph node drainage is into the inguinal group (superficial and deep) and occasionally, into the external iliac lymph nodes. Tumors of the posterior urethra most commonly spread to the pelvic lymph nodes. Bulbomembranous segment cancers can invade the urogenital diaphragm, prostate as also the perineal and scrotal skin. Hematogenous dissemination is uncommon until advanced local disease is present or in primary TCC of the prostatic urethra. Anterior subtype has a better outlook due to its operability which posterior malignancies lack on account of local spread and distant metastasis.

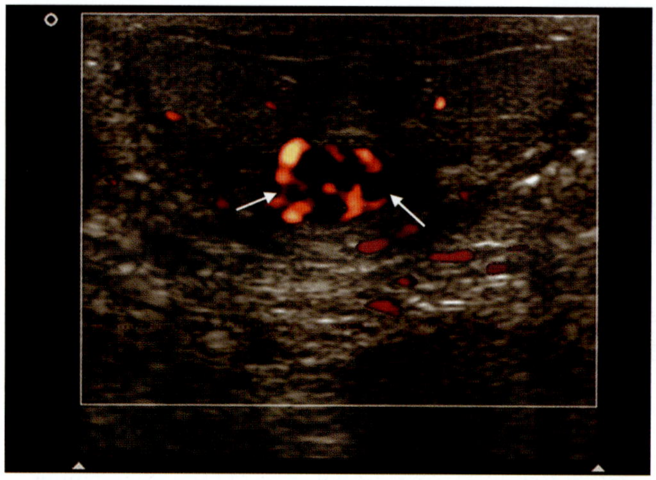

Fig. 27: Urethral TCC in an elderly male: US power Doppler image shows a hypoechoic hypervascular mass (arrows) at penile urethra.

The diagnosis of urethral tumors is usually suggested clinically at physical examination. Urethrography can be a useful adjunct, usually finding being focal irregular urethral narrowing. The common MR finding is a mass with relatively decreased signal compared to the normal corporal tissue in both T1- and T2-weighted sequences. Magnetic resonance imaging can depict invasion of the corpora cavernosa and is used for determining exact tumor site, size and local invasion.[28]

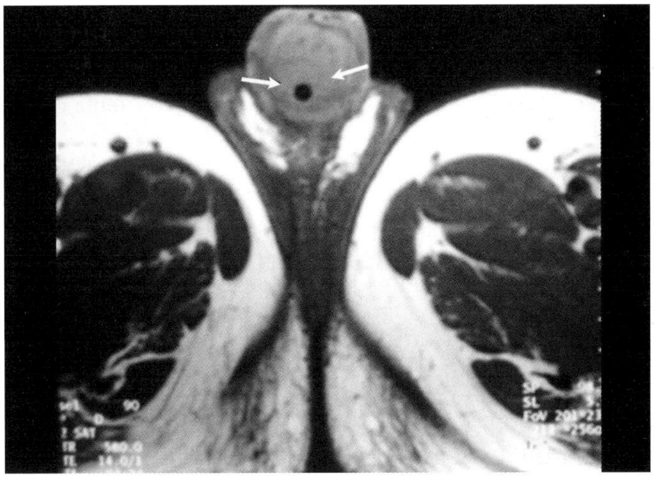

Fig. 28: Urethral SCC: Contranst-enhanced magnetic resonance axial image showing a hypoenhancing periurethral mass (arrow) of penile urethra. Note, the urethral outline can be clearly made due to presence of urinary catheter.

Tumors of the Female Urethra

Although carcinoma of the female urethra is more common than that of the male urethra, with a female-to-male ratio of 4:1, it accounts for less than 0.01% of all malignancies occurring in women. Most patients are over 50 years old. Causes associated with the development of urethral cancers in women include chronic irritation, urinary tract infection and proliferative lesions, such as caruncles, papillomas, adenomas, polyps and leukoplakia of the urethra. Most common symptoms include bleeding, frequent micturition, obstruction and a palpable mass or induration. Female urethral cancer is categorised as "anterior" or "entire" urethral cancer.[27] Anterior subtype involves exclusively the distal third of the urethra and account for 46% of urethral tumors. Entire urethral carcinomas tend to be high grade and locally advanced, most commonly being of the squamous cell subtype (60% of patients), followed by transitional cell (20%),adenocarcinoma (10%), undifferentiated type and sarcoma (8%), lastly melanoma (2%). Local extension of the primary lesions into the bladder neck, vagina, or vulva is not uncommon and therefore, differentiation of the primary urethral lesions from those of the vulva or vagina may be difficult.

The primary diagnosis is clinical. Contrast study demonstrates irregular decrease in the urethral calibre. Magnetic resonance imaging is quite accurate in evaluating local spread in 90% of cases. These tumors appear hypointense on T1-weighted images and relatively hyperintense on T2-weighted images. Tumor extent is best evaluated on sagittal T2-weighted images.

Metastatic Tumors of Urethra

Secondary urethral tumours are rare. Urethral instrumentation or cystectomy can cause local seeding; these lesions are appearing as multifocal small mucosal nodules during urethrography. Local spread of prostatic, rectal, testicular or spermatic cord malignancy may involve the corpus spongiosum, causing marked urethral narrowing and irregularity. Blood borne metastases to the corpora are occasionally seen with melanoma, prostatic, bladder, colonic, testicular and renal malignancies.

REFERENCES

1. Pollack HM, Banner MP, Martinez LO, Hodson CJ. Diagnostic considerations in urinary bladder wall calcification. AJR. 1981;136:791-7.
2. McCallum RW. The adult male urethra: normal anatomy, pathology, and method of urethrography. Radiol Clin North Am. 1979;17:227-44.
3. Choudhary S, Singh P, Sundar E, Kumar S, Sahai A. A comparison of sonourethrography and retrograde urethrography in evaluation of anterior urethral strictures. Clin Radiol. 2004; 59:736-42.
4. Kim SH, Han MC. Reversed contrast-urine levels in urinary bladder: CT findings. Urol Radiol. 1992;13:249-52.
5. Chan DP, Abujudeh HH, Cushing GL Jr, Novelline RA. CT cystography with multiplanar reformation for suspected bladder rupture: experience in 234 cases. AJR. 2006;187:1296-302.
6. Ryu J, Kim B. MR imaging of male and female urethra. Radiographics. 2001;21:1169-85.
7. Tan IL, Stoker J, Zwamborn AW, Entius KA, Calame JJ, Laméris JS. Female pelvic floor: endovaginal MR imaging of normal anatomy. Radiology. 1998;206:777-83.
8. Piepsz A, Ham HR. Pediatric applications of renal nuclear medicine. Semin Nucl Med. 2006;36:16-35.
9. Jinzaki M, Tanimoto A, Shinmoto H, Horiguchi Y, Sato K, Kuribayashi S, Silverman SG. Detection of bladder tumors with dynamic contrast-enhanced MDCT. AJR. 2007;188:913-8.
10. Baltaci S, Resorlu B, Yagci C, Turkolmez K, Gogus C, Beduk Y. Computerized tomography for detecting perivesical infiltration and lymph node metastasis in invasive bladder carcinoma. Urol Int. 2008;81:399-402.
11. Lee JK, Rholl KS. MRI of the bladder and prostate. AJR. 1986;147:732-6.
12. Barentsz JO, Jager G, Mugler JP 3rd. Staging urinary bladder cancer: value of T1-weighted three dimensional magnetization prepared-rapid gradient echo and two dimensional spin-echo sequences. AJR. 1995;164:109-15.
13. Barentsz JO, Ruijs SH, Strijk SP. The role of MR imaging in carcinoma of the urinary bladder. AJR. 1993;160:937-74.
14. Barentsz JO, Jager GJ, van Vierzen PB. Staging urinary bladder cancer after transurethral biopsy: value of fast

dynamic contrast-enhanced MR imaging. Radiology. 1996;201:185-93.
15. Deserno WM, Harisinghani MG, Taupitz M, et al. Urinary bladder cancer: preoperative nodal staging with ferumoxtran-10-enhanced MR imaging. Radiology. 2004;233:449-56.
16. Goh AC, Lerner SP. Application of new technology in bladder cancer diagnosis and treatment. World J Urol. 2009. [Epub ahead of print]
17. Dondalski M, White EM, Ghahremani GG, et al. Carcinoma arising in urinary bladder diverti-cula: imaging findings in six patients. AJR. 1993;161:817-20.
18. Sheldon CA, Clayman RV, Gonzalez R, et al. Malignant urachal lesions. J Urol. 1984;131:1-8.
19. DiSantis DJ. Inflammatory conditions of the urethra. In: Pollack AH, McClennon BL (Eds). Clinical Urography, 2nd edn. Philadelphia, Pa: Saunders; 2000.pp.1041-57.
20. Gallentine ML, Morey AF. Imaging of the male urethra for stricture disease. Urol Clin North Am. 2002;29:361-72.
21. Sharfi AR, Elarabi YE. The 'watering-can' perineum: presentation and management. Br J Urol. 1997;80:933-6.
22. Pansadoro V, Emiliozzi P. Iatrogenic prostatic urethral strictures: classification and endoscopic treatment. Urology. 1999;53:784-9.
23. Fortunato P, Schettini M, Gallucci M. Diverticula of the female urethra. Br J Urol. 1997;80:628-32.
24. Keefe B, Warshauer DM, Tucker MS, Mittel-staedt CA. Diverticula of the female urethra: diagnosis by endovaginal and transperineal sonography. Am J Roentgenol. 1991; 156:1195-7.
25. Daneshgari F, Zimmern PE, Jacomides L. Magnetic resonance imaging detection of symptomatic non-communicating intraurethral wall diverticula in women. J Urol. 1999;161:1259-61.
26. Hahn WY, Israel GM, Lee VS. MRI of female urethral and periurethral disorders. Am J Roentgenol. 2004;182:677-82.
27. Donat SM, Cozzi PJ, Herr HW. Surgery of penile and urethral carcinoma. In: Walsh PC, Reitik AB, Vaughan ED, Jr, Wein AJ (Eds). Campbell's urology, 8th edn. Philadelphia, Pa: Saunders; 2002.pp.2983-99.
28. Vapnek JM, Hricak H, Carroll PR. Recent advances in imaging studies for staging of penile and urethral carcinoma. Urol Clin North Am. 1992;19:257-66.

CHAPTER 110

Imaging of the Prostate Gland

Paramjeet Singh, Anupam Lal

INTRODUCTION

Any abnormality in the prostate gland is a common cause of urinary symptoms in elderly men. Two such important diseases of aging men are carcinoma and hyperplasia of the gland. In addition, a number of congenital and inflammatory pathologies also affect the gland. The advent of modern cross-sectional imaging techniques such as ultrasonography (US) and magnetic resonance imaging (MRI) has made it possible to directly visualize the prostate, assess its size accurately and also evaluate any suspicious lesion that may warrant a biopsy.

ANATOMY

The prostate is a chestnut-shaped gland surrounded by a fibrous capsule. Proximally its base is adjacent to the bladder neck, and distally its apex lies on the urogenital diaphragm. The seminal vesicles are paired saccular structures lying posterosuperiorly and in continuity with ampullae of the vasa efferentia as they taper medially towards the prostate. The urethra traverses the gland in an angular manner. Detailed anatomic dissection of the prostate reveals zonal anatomy, whereby the prostate is divided into four glandular zones surrounding the prostatic urethra: The peripheral zone, transition zone, central zone, and the periurethral glandular area.[1] In the normal gland, sonography can rarely identify these zones unless a pathologic condition is present. On sonography, it is useful to separate the prostate into a peripheral zone and the inner gland which encompasses the transition and central zones and the periurethral glandular area. A nonglandular region on the anterior surface of the prostate is termed the anterior fibromuscular stroma.[2] The peripheral zone, the largest of the glandular zones occupies the posterior, lateral and apical regions of the gland and contains approximately 70% of the prostatic glandular tissue and is the site of most prostate cancers. It surrounds the distal segment of prostatic urethra and is separated from the transition zone and central zone by the surgical capsule, which is often hyperechoic as a result of corpora amylacea or calcification. The transition zone, in the normal patient contains approximately 5% of the prostatic glandular tissue and is the exclusive site of origin of benign prostatic hyperplasia. It is seen as two small glandular areas located adjacent to the proximal prostatic urethra and continues with periurethral glandular tissue encircling the proximal urethra. The periurethral glands form about 1% of the glandular volume and are embedded in the longitudinal smooth muscle of the proximal urethra, also known as the internal prostatic sphincter. The central zone constitutes approximately 25% of the glandular tissue and is located at the prostatic base. The ducts of the vas deferens and seminal vesicles enter the central zone, and the ejaculatory ducts pass through it. The central zone is relatively resistant to disease processes and is the site of origin of only 5% of prostate cancers.

Prostate is supplied by the prostatic arteries which are branches of prostaticovesical arteries arising from the internal iliac arteries on each side. The prostatic artery gives rise to urethral and capsular arteries. The urethral artery supplies about one-third of the prostate while the capsular branches supply the remainder of the gland. Neurovascular bundle containing cavernous nerve from pelvic plexus passes posterolateral to the gland.

Most often the prostate is elliptical in shape, and using the formula for a prolate ellipse (0.523 × transverse × anteroposterior × cephalocaudal diameter), prostatic volume can be calculated. The normal prostate gland volume in the adult is approximately 20 cm^3.

IMAGING MODALITIES[3]

Ultrasonography

The prostate can be imaged sonographically by transabdominal, transperineal, transurethral and transrectal approaches. Correlative studies have shown that volumetric evaluation of the prostate with suprapubic ultrasound is accurate and that a gram of prostate tissue is equivalent to 1 cm^3. The suprapubic approach allows for gross evaluation of the prostate size but does not offer images of sufficient quality to visualize the zonal anatomy. Transperineal method is compromised by beam scattering but may be useful in patients following abdominoperineal resection. Transurethral approach using 7.5–10 MHz transducer affords enhanced visualization of the transitional zone but has poor resolution of the peripheral zone and is an invasive technique. Transrectal ultrasonography (TRUS) is currently the preferred method because of its ability to demonstrate the zonal anatomy, the ejaculatory ducts and seminal vesicles. The most commonly used commercially available probes (with a transducer frequency ranging from 5 to 8 MHz) fire from the end and the longitudinal and axial scans are obtained by rotating the transducer through a 180° axis. Other probe designs include 360° radial scanners paired with end viewing probes for a sagittal image and paired side viewing axial and sagittal probes. The advantages of end-viewing probe designs include patient convenience, ease of use, and biopsy capability at the time of the diagnostic examination. The central and peripheral zones form the bulk of prostate gland and appear uniformly hyperechoic with only subtle differentiation in their echogenicity. The hypoechoic peri-urethral area corresponds to the transitional zone. Seminal vesicles appear slightly less echogenic than prostate. Grayscale ultrasound relies on morphology and echogenicity for detection of pathology. To improve ultrasound as an imaging modality of the prostate, many new technologies, such as color and power Doppler, three-dimensional ultrasound of the prostate and contrast-enhanced ultrasound has been developed. In addition, treatment modalities using high intensity focused ultrasound (HIFU) for the treatment of BPH and localized prostatic cancer have been developed.[4]

Computed Tomography

The prostate appears as homogeneous dense structure on computed tomography. Though computed tomography (CT) provides a rough assessment of prostatic size and contour, it is not possible to differentiate normal from hyperplastic gland or detect the cancer when it is confined within the prostate gland.

Magnetic Resonance Imaging

Magnetic resonance imaging (MRI) allows detailed visualization of normal zonal anatomy of the prostate, the prostatic capsule, periprostatic structures and also pelvic lymph nodes.

On T1W images, the zonal anatomy is not very clear and the gland is of uniform low-signal intensity. T1W images are useful for detection of hemorrhage (post-biopsy) and to differentiate cyst from an abscess. Internal architecture of the prostate is best appreciated on T2W image. The peripheral zone has high-signal intensity while the central and transitional zones have relatively low-signal intensity. However, central and transitional zones cannot be differentiated from each other, and both together are termed as central gland **(Fig. 1)**. In young men, the central gland predominantly consists of central zone. In older men, with prostatic hyperplasia most of the central gland consists of transitional zone. The anterior fibromuscular

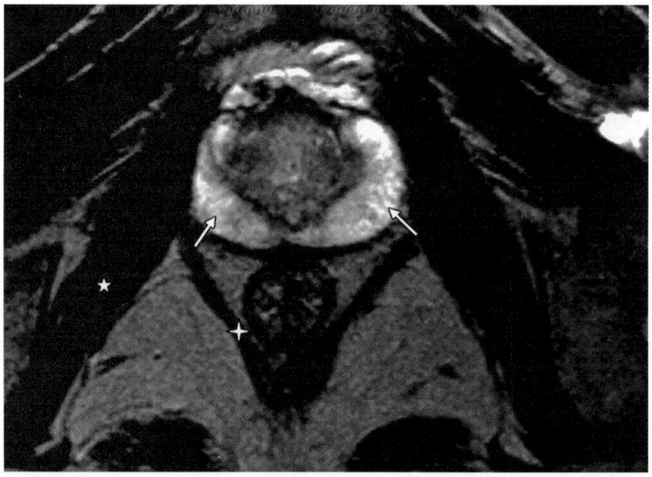

Fig. 1: Transverse T2-weighted image of prostate showing hyperintense peripheral zone (arrows) and relatively hypointense central gland. The obturator internus (star) and levator ani (cross) muscles are seen as hypointense structures.

stroma is dark on all pulse sequences. Seminal vesicle fluid appears bright on T2W image while the walls are hypointense. The periprostatic fat is hyperintense on both T1WI and T2WI and allows easy assessment of periprostatic spread of growth.

BENIGN PROSTATIC HYPERPLASIA

Enlargement of the prostate gland is common in older men; however, the gland size does not always correlate with symptoms of prostatism. Benign prostatic hyperplasia (BPH) starts in the form of nodules in the transition zone which enlarge in size and number, eventually impinging on the adjacent central and peripheral zones.

Ultrasonography

The sonographic appearance of benign prostatic hyperplasia is varied and depends on the histopathologic changes. Distinct nodules or diffuse enlargement can be present in the transition zone, the periurethral glandular tissue, or both. The typical sonographic feature of BPH is enlargement of the inner gland, which appears relatively hypoechoic to the peripheral zone. The border between central and peripheral gland which is indistinct in young men, becomes more distinct due to presence of BPH **(Fig. 2)**. The echo pattern of central gland depends on the admixture of glandular and stromal elements. Nodules may be fibroblastic, fibromuscular, muscular, hyperadenomatous, and fibroadenomatous.[4] Depending on the combination; the nodules may appear either isoechoic, hyperechoic or hypoechoic. Calcifications may also be seen in the central zone.

Because the growth of the gland is primarily anterior, the volume or weight cannot be estimated well by digital palpation. Prostatic ultrasound provides an accurate and reproducible method to determine the prostatic volume and the effect of the hyperplasia on the anterior urethra that correlates with the symptoms of prostatism.

Magnetic Resonance Imaging

T2W endorectal coil imaging of the prostate allows differentiation of glandular (high signal intensity) from the stromal component (low to intermediate signal intensity) in BPH. Surrounding central and peripheral zones are compressed forming a pseudocapsule around the hyperplastic gland (corresponding to the surgical capsule) **(Figs. 3A and B)**. On T1WI, nodules of BPH are isointense

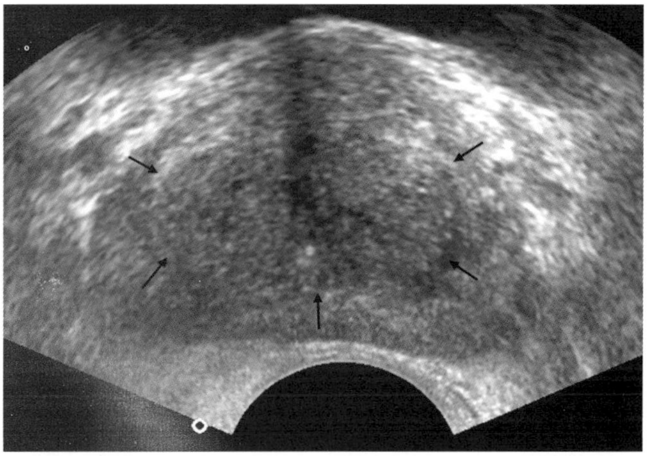

Fig. 2: Benign prostatic hyperplasia (BPH): Transrectal US shows enlarged heterogeneous central gland (between arrows).

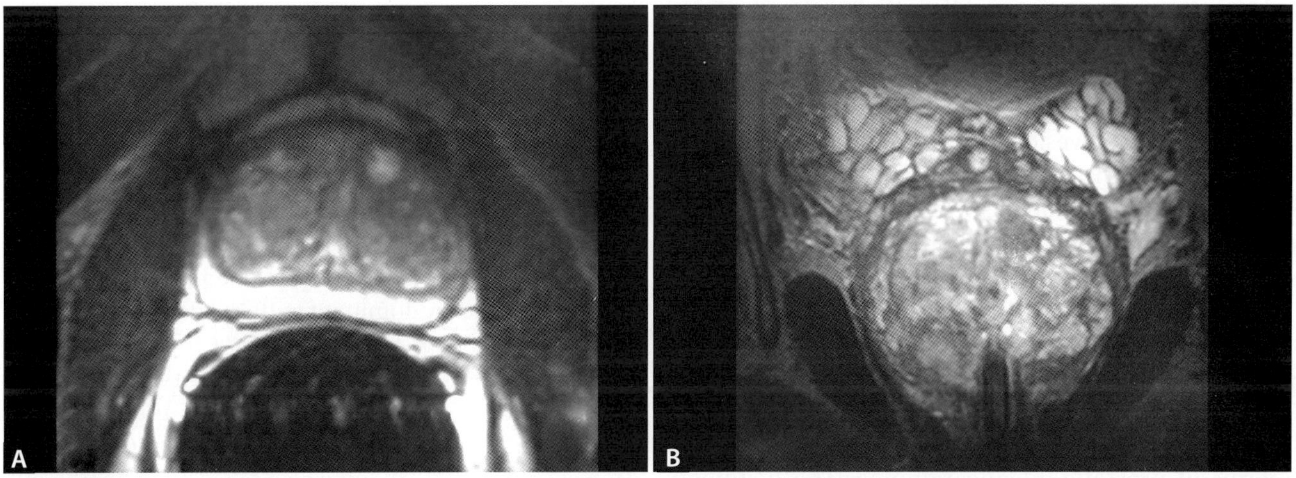

Figs. 3A and B: T2-weighted axial image (A) shows zonal anatomy, i.e. hyperintense peripheral gland and heterogeneous central zone due to hyperplastic changes. The bright nodule represents glandular hyperplasia and dark areas being stromal hyperplasia. The surgical and anatomical capsules are seen as hypointense structures; (B) Coronal T2 section shows changes of BHP with enlarged TZ nearly totally effacing the central zone.

with the remainder of prostate. MR imaging provides excellent resolution of internal prostatic anatomy, the information with respect to the ratio of glandular to stromal tissue in the prostate and an accurate estimate of prostate volume; however, is not routi-nely used in patients with BPH because of high cost and limited availability.

Other Imaging Modalities

Intravenous urography (IVU) is no longer routinely performed and is generally performed to evaluate other associated symptoms like hematuria, pyuria, and urinary calculi. Retrograde and voiding cystourethrography can provide anatomic information regarding bladder neck contracture, residual tissue, and urethral stricture disease in postprostatectomy patients. CT is hardly ever indicated for uncomplicated BPH as it provides little relevant information, other than prostatic volume determination.

PROSTATE CANCER

Cancer of the prostate is the most common cancer and ranks as the second most common cause of cancer death in men.[5] Adenocarcinoma is the most common histologic type, encountered in approximately 95% of patients. Around 70% of the prostatic cancer originates in the peripheral zone, 10–20% in the transitional zone, and 5–10% in the central zone. Multicentricity of the tumor is quite common. Approximately 30–46% men above 50 years of age may harbor a cancer focus but less than 20% of those develop clinical disease which is largely related to variability in aggressiveness. Imaging has little role in early detection of cancer but has a vital part in local and distant staging of the disease **(Table 1)**. Diagnostic tests for local staging must aim to differentiate organ confined disease from locally invasive disease extending beyond capsule (ECS) into periprostatic fat, lymphatics and vessels (stage 3) or adjacent organs (stage 4). Due to proximity, invasion of seminal vesicles and bladder base superiorly, membranous urethra distally and rarely rectum posteriorly should be looked for. Patients with metastatic disease fare worst and a lymph nodal and distant metastasis work-up is part of routine evaluation.

Confined disease (T2) is treated with surgery or radiotherapy while extracapsular spread or SV invasion (T3) is treated with radiation and/or hormonal therapy **(Table 2)**. The Gleason scoring system, which was first described in 1966, is based on the architectural growth patterns of prostatic adenocarcinoma. The histologic patterns are grouped into five grades, which are viewed as a continuum. It was found that tumors behaved more like the "average" grade rather than the highest grade present; therefore, Gleason developed a "score" based on the grade of the predominant pattern added to the grade of the second most prevalent pattern.[6] Clinical staging with digital rectal examination (DRE), serum PSA and biopsy tumor grade (Gleason score) remains the standard of practice though it under stages ECS in up to 30–60% cases.[7] However, definitive therapy also takes into consideration patient's life expectancy, his general health, tumor prognostic factors and presence of metastasis. Particularly, patients at increased risk for metastatic disease (Gleason

Table 1: Prostate adenocarcinoma—TNM staging classification.

Stage	***Extent of cancer***
T1	Clinical localized: Tumor not palpable on digital rectal examination
T1a	Focal tumor (≤5% of resected tissue on TURP) and low grade
T1b	Diffuse tumor (>5% of resected tissue on TURP) and high grade
T2	Clinically localized: Tumor palpable
T2a	Tumor involves ≤0.5 lobe
T2b	Tumor involves >0.5 lobe
T2c	Tumor involves both lobes
T3	Locally invasive beyond prostatic capsule: Tumor palpable
T3a	Unilateral extracapsular extension
T3b	Bilateral extracapsular extension
T3c	Seminal vesicle invasion
T4	Invades adjacent tissue (e.g. bladder, rectum, levator ani muscles)
N/M	Metastatic disease
N 1–4	Metastases to lymph nodes
M 1	Distant metastases

Table 2: Treatment decisions by prostate cancer stage.

Stage	***Possible treatment options***
T1 Gleason score 2–4	Consider watchful waiting
T1 Gleason score 5–10	Radical prostatectomy, XRT
T2b Gleason score <8 and PSA <20 ng/mL	Radical prostatectomy, XRT
T2b, Gleason score 8–10 or PSA >20 ng/mL	Radical prostatectomy or XRT
T2c	Radical prostatectomy or XRT
T3–4	XRT or hormonal therapy, if patient not candidate for radiation
N 1–4	XRT and hormonal therapy
Local recurrence	Consider XRT, if surgical failure, hormonal therapy
Metastatic disease	Palliative XRT, hormonal therapy

score 8–10, serum PSA >20 ng/mL or clinical stage T3–4) must undergo imaging work-up before definitive therapy.[7] On the other hand, patients with intermediate risk (Gleason score 5–7 and PSA 10–20) need further elucidation of prognostic factors by newer techniques estimating metabolic information, i.e. spectroscopy, angiogenesis by color Doppler and perfusion imaging and cellularity, i.e. diffusion imaging.

Transrectal Ultrasonography

Initially considered as a primary screening test for prostatic cancer, the role of transrectal ultrasonography (TRUS) has now been replaced by prostate specific antigen (PSA) and digital rectal examination (DRE). TRUS alone has limited potential to identify prostatic cancer because of frequent multifocality of cancer within the prostate, the variable sonographic appearance of prostatic tumors, the poor specificity of focal ultrasonic abnormalities, and the substantial percentage of isoechoic prostate cancers which cannot be differentiated from adjacent benign tissues with imaging.[8] Color Doppler and power Doppler have been added to TRUS in an attempt to increase the sensitivity and specificity of prostate ultrasound and ultrasound-guided biopsy. Preliminary reports suggest that increased vascularity in a prostatic lesion correlates with high-grade cancer and can suggest the lesion to be biopsied **(Fig. 4)**.[9] The indications for TRUS in patients with known or suspected prostate cancer are as follows:

- Evaluation of the patient with an abnormal digital rectal examination
- Evaluation of the patient with abnormal laboratory test results indicative of prostate cancer, including PSA, acid phosphatase, or other evidence of metastatic disease
- Guidance for biopsy
- Monitoring response to treatment for prostate cancer.

Against the background of normal peripheral zone glandular tissue, small prostatic cancer usually appears hypoechoic because of closely packed cells in the tumor nodule. Larger tumors may appear isoechoic or hyperechoic. This appearance may be caused by a desmoplastic response of surrounding normal tissue or due to infiltration of the neoplasm into a background of benign prostatic hyperplasia.[7] When an isoechoic tumor is present, it can be detected by presence of secondary signs including glandular asymmetry and capsular bulging. When the cancer totally replaces an entire zone or the entire gland, its identification becomes difficult. Such diffuse lesions must be identified based on the expected echogenicity of the area examined rather than its relation to surrounding structures. Periprostatic extension may be suspected when there is disruption of capsule echogenicity, and irregularity or bulging of the capsular margin **(Fig. 5)**. Seminal vesicle extension can be defined sonographically by enlargement, cystic dilatation, asymmetry, anterior displacement, hyperechogenicity, and loss of the seminal vesicle beak. A comparison from the other normal side can be helpful. Because of the high frequency transducers and thus limited depth of penetration, TRUS does not permit pelvic lymph node assessment. Sensitivity of TRUS for local extension into the capsule or seminal vesicles in different studies range from as high as 90% and as low as 40–60% and specificities for invasion range from 46–90%, depending on the size of primary tumor.[10,11]

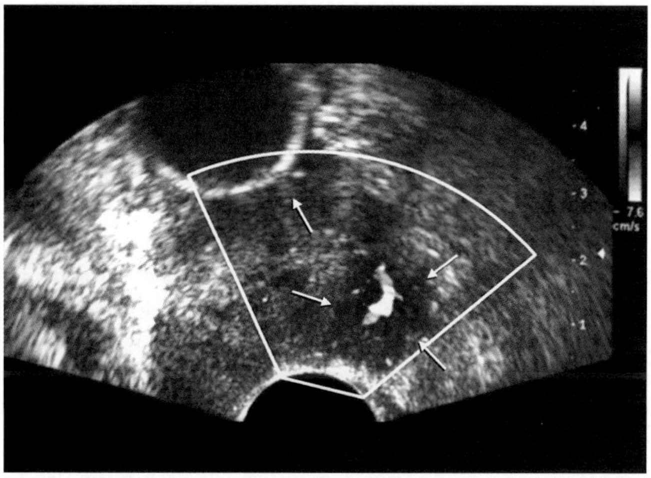

Fig. 4: Carcinoma prostate: Transrectal US with color Doppler shows increased vascularity within the tumor mass (arrows) in left PZ.

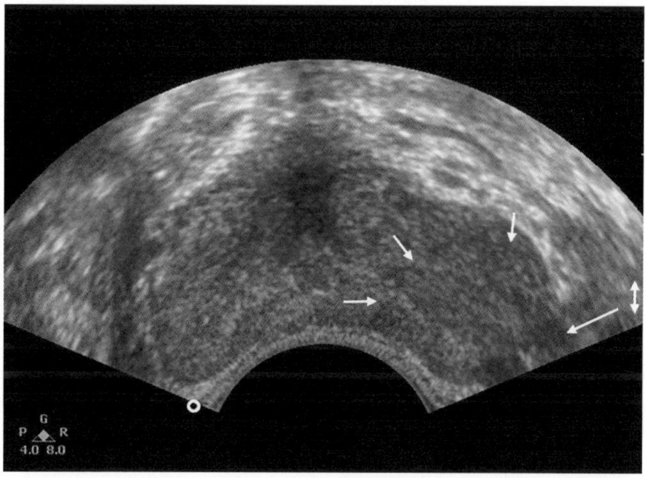

Fig. 5: Carcinoma prostate: Transrectal US image shows large hypoechoic mass in left PZ (arrows) with extracapsular extension (long arrow).

Newer developments in TRUS equipment over the past decade include the use of power Doppler, higher frequencies, broad band-width technologies, harmonic, contrast harmonic, and pulse inversion imaging. All these improvements may enhance detection of subtle focal sonographic abnormalities within the prostate. Ultrasonic contrast agents can aid visualizations of subtle alterations in prostatic echotexture by high-lighting changes in microvasculature. It is possible that Doppler's techniques and contrast agents have the potential to reveal prognostic information about cancer in individual patients by differentiating high-grade from low-grade tumors.[9]

Computed Tomography

Computed tomography (CT) has a limited role in the evaluation of patients with prostatic cancer. Although it can accurately evaluate lymph node and distant metastases and is inaccurate in local staging of the tumor nor helps in biopsy.[10]

Magnetic Resonance Imaging

Most prostatic cancers show low signal intensity relative to normal peripheral zone on T2WI **(Fig. 6)**. Central zone cancer detection is problematic due to fibrous stroma having low signal. Tumors with large mucin content, however, may be hyperintense. Low-signal intensities are also seen in bacterial or granulomatous prostatitis, postbiopsy hemorrhages and prostatic hyperplasia. The proposed sensitivity, specificity, positive- and negative-predictive values, and overall accuracy of MR imaging in the detection of cancer of prostate and of local extracapsular disease in different studies have a wide range of estimates (e.g. 64–98% accuracy has been reported).[11-16] A very high accuracy is precluded by (*a*) the frequency of microscopic regions of capsular invasion that are below even the best spatial resolution of MR imaging, (*b*) the wide differential diagnosis for the findings that frequently connote tumor, and (*c*) the inescapable technical difficulties relating to patient motion, postbiopsy changes, and other factors. As a very general rule, local staging of prostate tumor on the basis of transrectal MR imaging findings will be correct in approximately three-quarters of cases. Currently MRI is the imaging modality of choice for preoperative staging of the prostate cancer. It is more advantageous than ultrasound in detecting local invasion in form of capsular disruption or irregular bulging. Infiltration of low-signal intensity prostatic carcinoma into high-signal intensity seminal vesicles on T2WI can be detected prior to alteration in their size and contour. MRI can also evaluate involvement of the periprostatic neurovascular bundle in form of asymmetry **(Figs. 7A and B)**. The NVB if uninvolved can be spared during surgery. Faster sequences with high resolution like turbo spin echo, use of endorectal coil and multiplaner imaging improve staging.

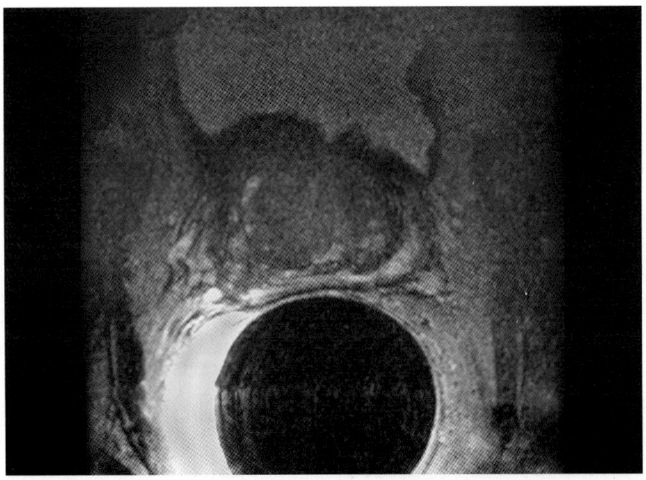

Fig. 6: Low-signal infiltrating cancer of the right posterolateral peripheral zone is seen on this endorectal coil axial T2 section of prostate gland.

Newer advances in MR imaging of the prostate include diffusion/perfusion imaging and MR spectroscopy. Normal spectra on Proton MR spectroscopic imaging (MRSI) show choline/creatinine, polyamines and citrate. Peripheral zone shows highest citrate concentration due to glandular elements. A reduction in citrate/polyamines and increase in choline resulting in high Ch–Cr/cit ratio is seen in cancers due to high phospholipids cell membrane turn over in proliferating malignant tissue **(Figs. 8 and 9)**. Sensitivity and specificity in cancer detection goes up to 91 and 95% respectively when MRSI is combined with routine MR imaging. Assessment of tumor volume, ECE, correlation with Gleason score, cancer detection in patients with prior negative biopsies and risk prediction are all improved with MRSI.[17] However, postbiopsy areas, fibrous stroma of hyperplastic nodules and prostatitis may yield false positive results.

Diffusion imaging may reveal restriction of diffusion in cancers ($1.30–1.35 \times 10^{-3}$) due to high cellularity vs benign tissue ($1.60–1.96 \times 10^{-3}$) particularly in peripheral zone which normally shows higher ADC. Central zone may show variable diffusion. DWI currently suffers from low SNR and needs to be compared with other techniques.[18] Dynamic contrast-enhanced MR imaging, assesses neoangiogenesis a hallmark of higher grade tumors. The data can be evaluated in a semiquantitative (contrast arrival, time-to-peak, peak enhancement and

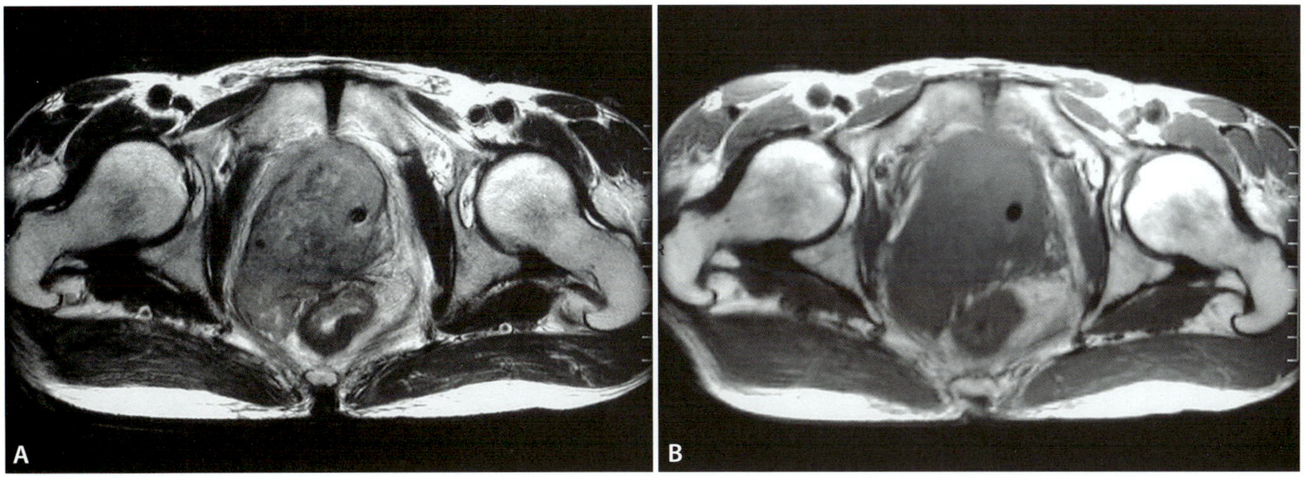

Figs. 7A and B: Axial T2 (A) and T1 (B) sections of prostate in a case of cancer. Extracapsular extension of cancer through the right neurovascular bundle is seen replacing the normal periprostatic fat.

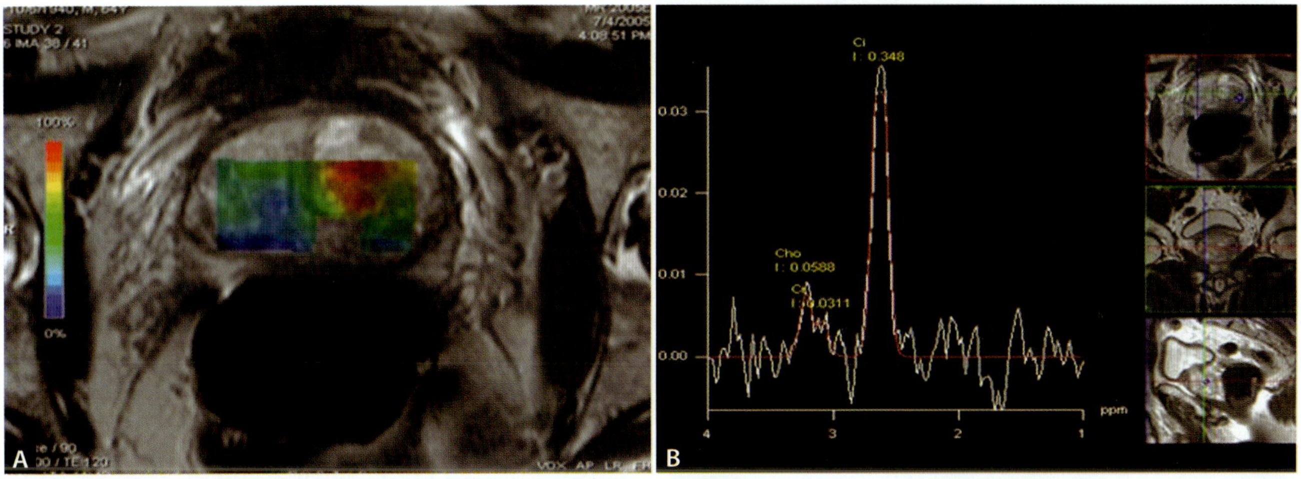

Figs. 8A and B: Proton MR spectroscopic imaging. Normal spectrum of prostate tissue shows dominant citrate peak at 2.6 ppm and choline/creatinine complex at 3–3.2 ppm.

wash-in-washout gradient) or quantitative approach using pharmacokinetic modeling method. It has been shown to detect 93% clinically important cancers.[18] It has lower sensitivity for central gland cancers and should be read along with T2WI. It is particularly important in assessing tumor recurrence.

A combination of these newer techniques (multiparametric imaging with image overlay) has potential to improve the yield of prostate cancer detection and staging, but require further validation. High field 3T imaging offers greater SNR and dynamic range facilitating these newer applications.

Positron Emission Tomography

The positron emission tomography (PET) scanning using various pharmaceuticals such as [18F] deoxyglucose, carbon-11 labeled choline and [11C] acetate has been used for both primary and metastatic prostatic cancers but the experience is largely experimental. FDG has limitations for evaluation of prostate cancer patients and therefore alternative tracers are being investigated. To date, the best results have been obtained with 11C-choline and 11C-acetate PET, which seem to demonstrate similar values in this field. At present, the only clinical indication for imaging prostate cancer with 11C-choline-PET is evaluation of suspected recurrence after treatment.[19]

EVALUATION OF THE METASTASES

Bone scintigraphy is a sensitive method for detecting bone metastases and should be a routine part of the staging process **(Fig. 10)**. However, the bone scan has little specificity, and abnormal (hot) areas must be further

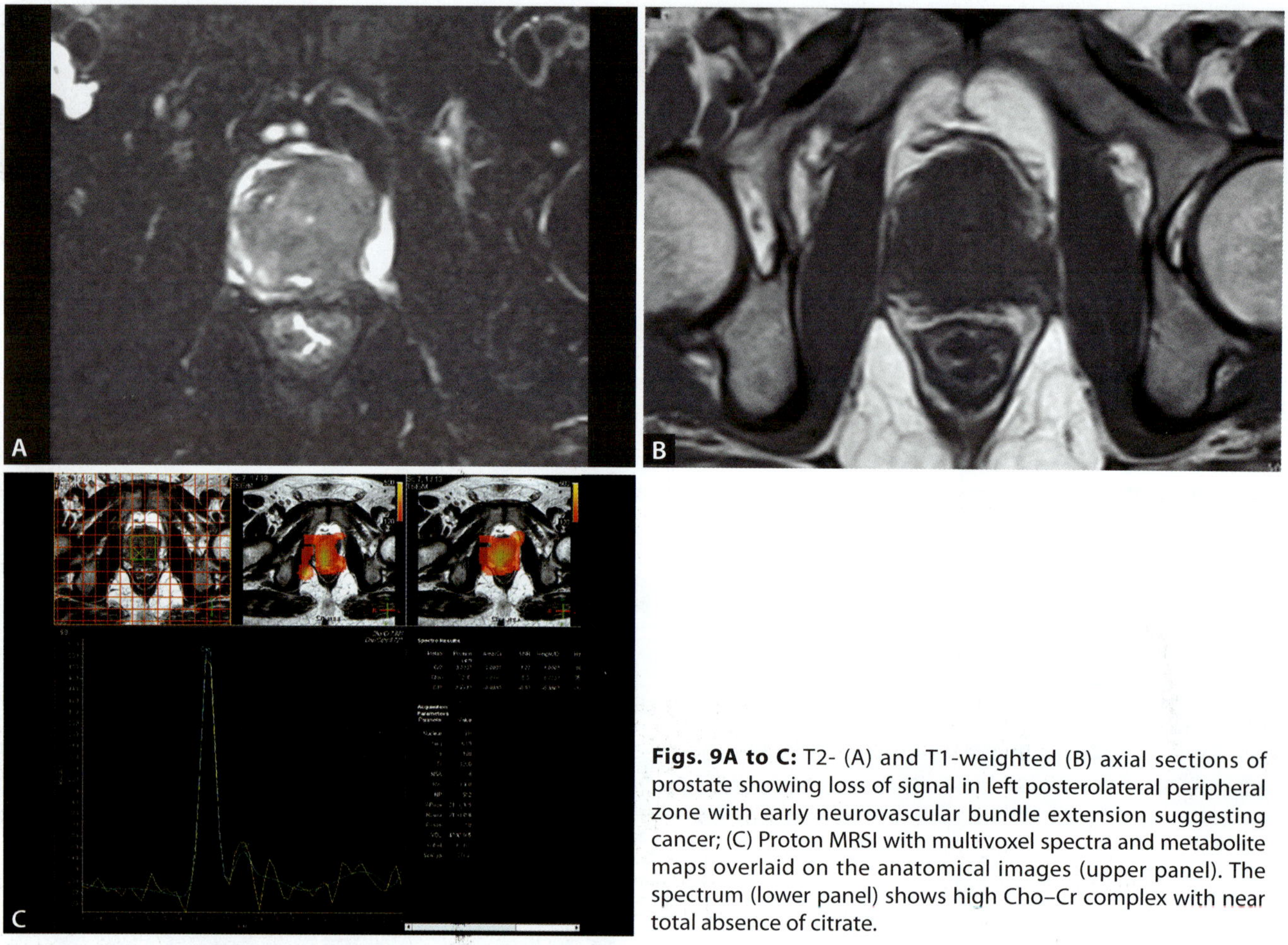

Figs. 9A to C: T2- (A) and T1-weighted (B) axial sections of prostate showing loss of signal in left posterolateral peripheral zone with early neurovascular bundle extension suggesting cancer; (C) Proton MRSI with multivoxel spectra and metabolite maps overlaid on the anatomical images (upper panel). The spectrum (lower panel) shows high Cho–Cr complex with near total absence of citrate.

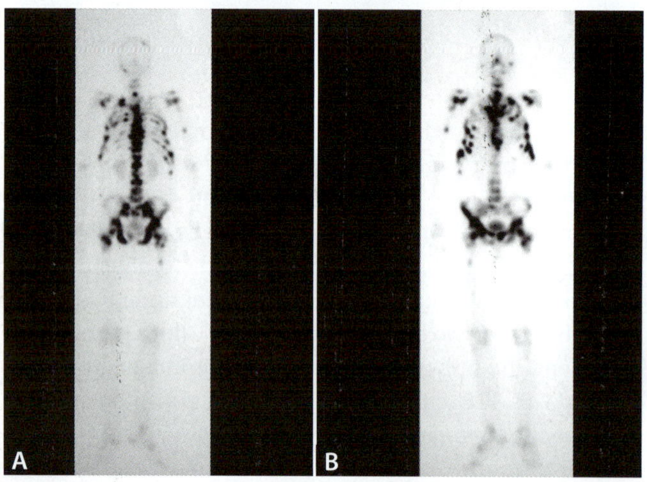

Figs 10A and B: Nuclear scan anterior and posterior views showing multiple osteoblastic metastatic deposits involving axial skeleton from cancer prostate (A) Posterior views; (B) Anterior view.

studied radiographically to allow differentiation between metastases and benign disorders such as fractures, degenerative arthritis and Paget's disease. MRI has shown to be more sensitive than radionuclide scan in detection of skeletal metastases **(Figs. 11A and B)**. A chest radiograph remains essential for evaluation of the intrathoracic metastases.

PROSTATITIS AND PROSTATIC ABSCESS

Acute focal or diffuse suppurative inflammation of the prostate (acute prostatitis) occurs most commonly due to ascent of bacteria from the urethra, less often by descent from the upper urinary tract or bladder, and occasionally by lymphogenous or hematogenous spread from a distant focus of infection. The common pathogens are those which cause urinary tract infection such as *E. coli, Klebsiella, Proteus, Pseudomonas,* etc. Chronic prostatitis

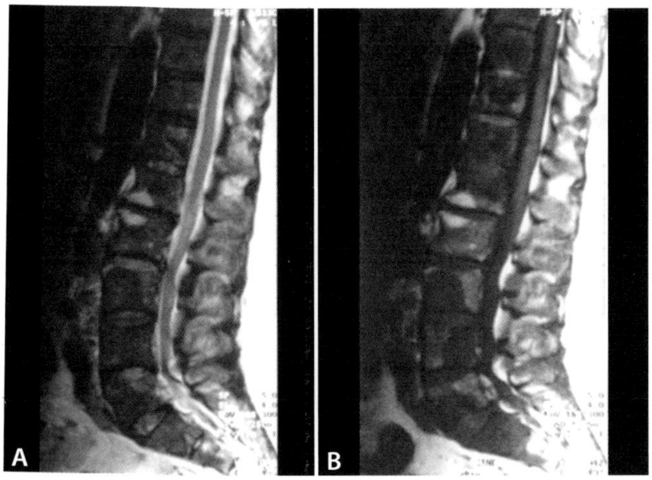

Figs. 11A and B: T1SE and T2TSE sagittal scans showing blastic marrow deposits appearing hypointense on T1 and T2 images involving dorsolumbar spine.

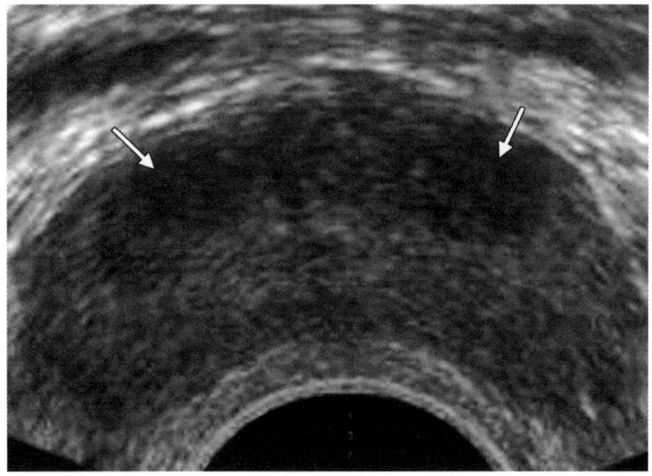

Fig. 12: Acute prostatitis with developing abscesses: Transrectal US show hypoechoic areas within the central gland (arrows).

is caused in much the same way and by the same bacterial pathogens as the acute prostatitis, however, it may be associated with certain abacterial pathogens such as *Chlamydia* or *Mycoplasma* organisms. In acute prostatitis, generally the glands are hypoechoic. Color Doppler shows a very vascular focus in areas of prostatitis, mimicking carcinoma. The development of an anechoic mass with or without internal echoes suggests the development of an abscess **(Fig. 12)**, which on color Doppler shows a highly vascular wall. The abscess cavity may also contain air due to gas producing organisms **(Fig. 13)**. In doubtful cases contrast-enhanced MRI can show the abscess cavity with enhancement of its wall **(Figs. 14A to C)**. Sonographic findings of chronic prostatitis include focal masses of different degrees of echogenicity, ejaculatory duct calcifications, capsular thickening or irregularity, and periurethral glandular irregularity. In addition, dilatation of periprostatic veins and distended seminal vesicles may be seen. Chronic granulomatous prostatitis can mimic sonographic features of prostatic carcinoma. Solitary or multiple diffuse large or small hypoechoic zones may be seen.

MRI appearance of chronic or granulomatous prostatitis can mimic prostatic carcinoma; however, low-signal intensity areas that do not deform the contour favor the diagnosis of chronic prostatitis.[20] Granulomatous prostatitis does not show contrast enhancement whereas prostatic carcinoma does. MRI is very helpful in suspected prostatic abscess since abscess has very high-signal intensity on T2WI and shows intense enhancement of its walls on contrast studies.

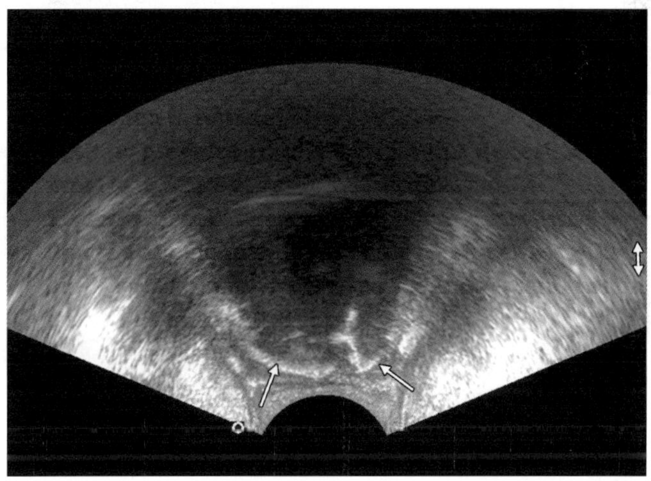

Fig. 13: Prostatic abscesses: Transrectal US shows large prostatic abscesses containing air (arrows).

PROSTATIC CYSTS

Midline prostatic cysts can be Müllerian duct cysts or utricle cysts. Müllerian duct cysts do not contain sperms and can cause infertility due to compression of the ejaculatory ducts. Utricle cysts contain sperms but unlike former do not extend beyond prostate **(Figs. 15 and 16)**. The paramidline cysts are Wolffian cysts, seminal vesicle cysts or ejaculatory duct cysts which contain sperms. Associated Wolffian duct anomalies, i.e. renal anomalies may be seen in these patients. Peripheral cysts are acquired retention cysts and may be associated with BPH. Cowper's gland cysts are also acquired cysts associated with urogenital diaphragm. Cystic

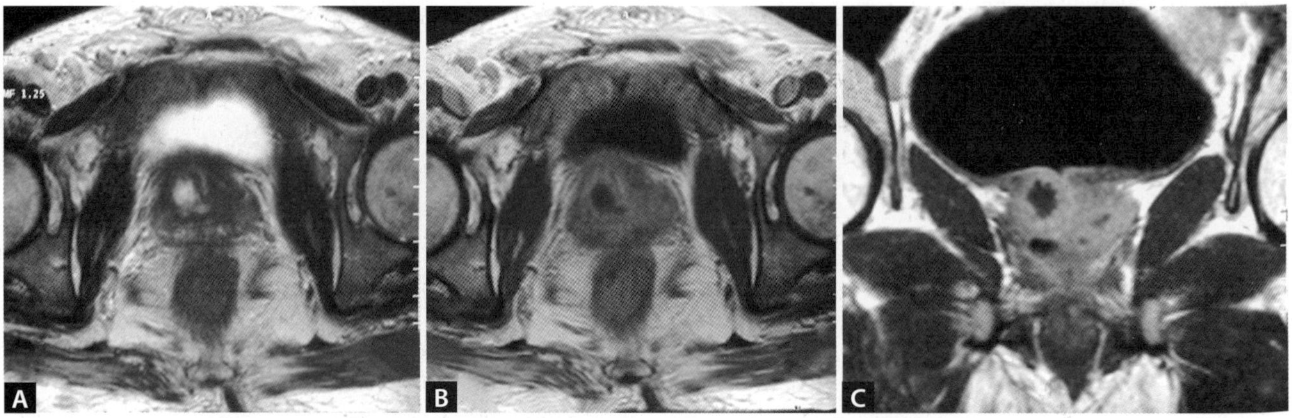

Figs. 14A to C: T2 axial (A), T1 postcontrast axial (B) and coronal (C) sections show a bacterial intraprostatic abscess appearing hyperintense on T2 and showing enhancing peripheral margins in the right half of the gland.

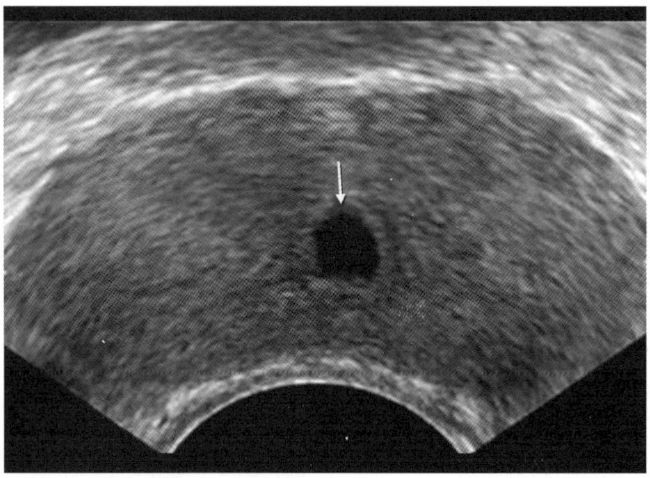

Fig. 15: Prostatic utricle cyst: Transrectal US shows the utricular cyst (arrow) in midline.

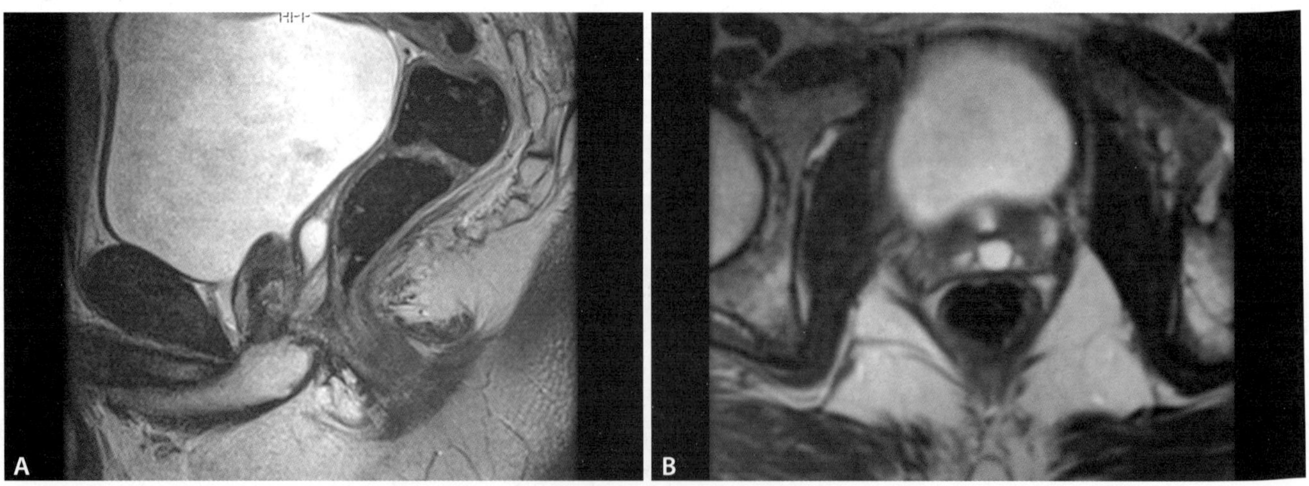

Figs. 16A and B: T2 sagittal and axial images (A and B) show a Müllerian duct cyst on posterior aspect of the prostate appearing hyperintense. Note the extension beyond the capsular margin.

lesions appear smooth walled, hypoechoic on USG and hyperintense on T2WI unless complicated by infection or hemorrhage.[21]

REFERENCES

1. McNeal JE. The zonal anatomy of the prostate. Prostate. 1981; 2:35-49.
2. Kaye KW, Richter L. Ultrasonographic anatomy of normal prostate gland: Reconstruction by computer graphics. Urology. 1990;35:12-7.
3. Amiel GE, Slawin KM. Newer modalities of ultrasound imaging and treatment of the prostate. Urol Clin North Am. 2006;33: 329-37.
4. Shinohara K, Scardino PT, Carter SS, Wheeler TM. Pathologic basis of the sonographic appearance of the normal and malignant prostate. Urol Clin North Am. 1989;16:675-91.
5. Jemal A, Siegel R, Ward E, Murray T, Xu J, Thun MJ. Cancer statistics 2007. CA Cancer J Clin. 2007;57:43-66.
6. Gleason DF. Histologic grading of prostate cancer: A perspective. Hum Pathol. 1992;23:237-79.
7. Yu KK, Hricak H. Imaging prostate cancer. Radiol Clin North Am. 2003;38:59-85.
8. Clements R. The role of transrectal ultrasound in diagnosing prostate cancer. Curr Urol Rep. 2002;3:194-200.
9. Inahara M, Suzuki H, Nakamachi H, Kamiya N, Shimbo M, Komiya A, et al. Clinical evaluation of trans-rectal power doppler imaging in the detection of prostate cancer. Int Urol Nephrol. 2004;36:175-80.
10. Rifkin MD, Dähnert W, Kurtz AB. State of the art: Endorectal sonography of the prostate gland. Am J Roentgenol (AJR). 1990; 154:691-700.
11. Hamper UM, Sheth S, Walsh PC, Holtz PM, Epstein JI. Carcinoma of the prostate; value of transrectal sonography in detecting extension into the neurovascular bundle. Am J Roentgenol. 1990;155:1015-9.
12. Chelsky MJ, Schnall MD, Seidmon EJ, Pollack HM. Use of endorectal surface coil magnetic resonance imaging for local staging of prostate cancer. J Urol. 1993;150:391-5.
13. Jager GJ, Barentsz JO, de la Rosette JJ, Rosenbusch G. Preliminary results of endorectal surface coil magnetic resonance imaging for local staging of prostate cancer. Radiologe. 1994;34: 129-33.
14. Bartolozzi C, Menchi I, Lencioni R, et al. Local staging of prostate carcinoma with endorectal coil MRI: Correlation with whole-mount radical prostatectomy specimens. Eur Radiol. 1996;6:339-45.
15. Fütterer JJ, Engelbrecht MR, Jager GJ, Hartman RP, King BF, Hulsbergen-Van de Kaa CA, et al. Prostate cancer: Comparison of local staging accuracy of pelvic phased-array coil alone versus integrated endorectal-pelvic phased-array coils. Local staging accuracy of prostate cancer using endorectal coil MR imaging. Eur Radiol. 2007;17:1055-65.
16. Beyersdorff D, Taymoorian K, Knösel T, Schnorr D, Felix R, Hamm B, Bruhn H. MRI of prostate cancer at 1.5 and 3.0 T: Comparison of image quality in tumor detection and staging. Am J Roentgenol. 2005;185:1214-20.
17. Kurhanewicz J, Vigneron D. Advances in mR spectroscopy of the prostate Mag Reson Imaging Clin N Am. 2008;16:697-710.
18. Somford DM, Futterer JJ, Hambrock T, Barentsz JO. Diffusion and perfusion MR Imaging of the prostate. Mag Reson Imaging Clin N Am. 2008;16:685-95.
19. Farsad M, Schiavina R, Franceschelli A, Sanguedolce F, Castellucci P, Bertaccini A, et al. Positron-emission tomography in imaging and staging prostate cancer. Cancer Biomark. 2008;4:277-84.
20. Shukla-Dave A, Hricak H, Eberhardt SC, Olgac S, Muruganandham M, Scardino PT, et al. Chronic prostatitis: MR imaging and 1H MR spectroscopic imaging findings: initial observations. Radiology. 2004;231:717-24.
21. Parsons RB, Fisher AM, Bar-Chama N, Mitty HA. MR imaging in male infertility. Radiographics. 1997;17:627-37.

CHAPTER 111

Renal Cystic Diseases

Veena Chowdhury

INTRODUCTION

Renal cystic diseases have continued to remain a diagnostic challenge for the radiologists despite the recent advances in imaging technology. Cystic disease of the kidney can be divided into two broad categories: congenital and developmental or acquired disorders. The congenital disorders include autosomal dominant and autosomal recessive polycystic disease, tuberous sclerosis, von Hippel–Lindau disease and medullary sponge kidney.[1] Statistically, most cystic lesions of the kidney are simple benign cortical cysts with classic imaging characteristics. Sometimes, these masses cannot be diagnosed because of overlap in appearance between benign and malignant lesions. Masses with calcification, high attenuation or high signal intensity or thin septations are probably benign and need a follow-up, while a multiloculated lesion with enhancing walls or nodularity suggests an aggressive nature and requires surgery. Therefore, it becomes a very important for the radiologist to make the critical differentiation between atypical benign cysts and cystic tumors.[2]

EMBRYOLOGY

The kidneys and ureters develop from the intermediate mesoderm. The permanent kidney or metanephros develops following the contact of the metanephric diverticulum or ureteric bud with the metanephric mesoderm. During the fourth week of gestation, a dorsal bud of the metanephric diverticulum grows out of the mesonephric duct into the mass of metanephric mesoderm; thus, during the fifth week of gestation, the metanephros is induced to develop meta-nephric tubules in its caudal portion. The tip of the ureteric bud becomes the renal pelvis and calyces. The metanephric collecting tubules then develop from the renal calyces. The blind end of the collecting tubules then induce clusters of mesenchymal cells to develop into metanephric tubules of the nephron. Further development of the permanent kidney occurs through both, the growth in the absolute number of nephrons and via the gradual ascent and rotation of the kidney.

The developmental process initially begins as a solid mass of cells which later cannulates to form the lumen. Most congenital cystic disorders are the result of an arrest in cannu-lation and communication at various stages of development.[3]

CLASSIFICATION

Renal cystic diseases comprise of a diverse set of developmental, heritable and acquired disorders. An awareness about the pathology of each cystic disease is of immense help in the understanding of the corresponding radiological images. Because of the diversity of etiology, histology and clinical presentation, no single universally accepted classification exists, but a practical working classification composed of major categories and most clinically significant renal cystic diseases is given in **Table 1**:[4-6]

Table 1: Classification of renal cystic diseases.

Nongenetic	*Genetic*
1. *Acquired disorders*:	1. *Autosomal dominant*:
a. Simple renal cysts; typical, atypical, complicated.	a. Autosomal dominant polycystic kidney disease
b. Acquired cystic disease in renal failure and hypokalemia	b. Tuberous sclerosis complex
c. Multilocular cystic nephroma	c. Von Hippel–Lindau disease
d. Hydronephrotic multicystic kidney	d. Medullary cystic disease
2. *Developmental disorders*:	e. Glomerulocystic disease
a. Multicystic dysplastic kidney	2. *Autosomal recessive*:
b. Pyelocalyceal cysts	a. Autosomal-recessive polycystic kidney disease
3. *Miscellaneous cystic disease*:	b. Nephrophthisis
a. Cystic renal carcinoma	
b. Inflammatory cysts	

Bosniak Classification System

To characterize cystic lesions of the kidney in 1986 Bosniak developed a classification system based on CT features, recognizing four basic types:

1. Category I lesions are simple cysts of water density (0–20 HU), sharply defined from the adjacent renal parenchyma with no perceptible wall thickness. They are homogeneous and do not show calcification or contrast enhancement **(Fig. 1)**.
2. Category II lesions are minimally complicated benign cysts and are of three types:
   a. Cysts with thin delicate calcification in the wall or septum.
   b. Cysts containing one or two nonenhancing thin internal septae (<1 mm wall thickness) with no thickened elements. Presence of delicate calcification can be seen in septated cysts **(Fig. 2)**.
   c. Hyperdense cysts showing uniform, nonenhancing high attenuation on a noncontrast CT examination. If a lesion with attenuation value of 50–90 Houns-field units is large (>3 cm), irregular, inhomogeneous or has any other noncystic characteristics, it cannot be considered as a category II lesion and should be evaluated surgically to exclude renal carcinoma or should be followed up at three monthly intervals to ensure that the lesion is not growing or changing.

   Lesions falling into category I and IIa and b are considered benign and do not require follow-up.
3. Category III lesions are masses with more numerous or thickened septae (>1 mm), thick wall, thick and irregular calcification or multiloculated lesions. Surgical management is indicated in these cases. Approximately half of these lesions may prove to be benign, e.g. aggregates of simple cysts, multilocular cystic nephroma, lymphangioma or hydatid disease.
4. Category IV lesions have more obviously malignant characteristics, such as inhomogeneity, solid elements, wall thickening, or enhancing components and are regarded as unequivocally malignant, requiring standard surgical management **(Fig. 3)**.

   Diagnosis and management is clear in category I and IV lesions but difficult in category II and III lesions. Computed tomography helps differentiate these two.[6]

In 1993, Bosniak revised the classification system to include a subset of minimally complicated lesion with dense calcifications under category 2 which could be managed with follow-up. The risk of malignancy in these lesions is approximately 5%. All imaging strategies are based on the principles of Bosniak classification.[7]

IMAGING MODALITIES

Conventional Radiography

Plain radiography and excretory urography (EU) are indirect imaging modalities. EU has the additional advantage of assessing the gross functional status of the kidney. Cystic masses of the kidney often reveal:

a. Abnormality of the renal contour or adjacent fascial planes, displacement of bowel loops or splaying of ribs.
b. Curvilinear or rim calcification in cyst wall.
c. Filling defects in the opacified cortex during the nephrographic phase of urography.
d. Splaying and distortion of opacified collecting system **(Fig. 4)**.

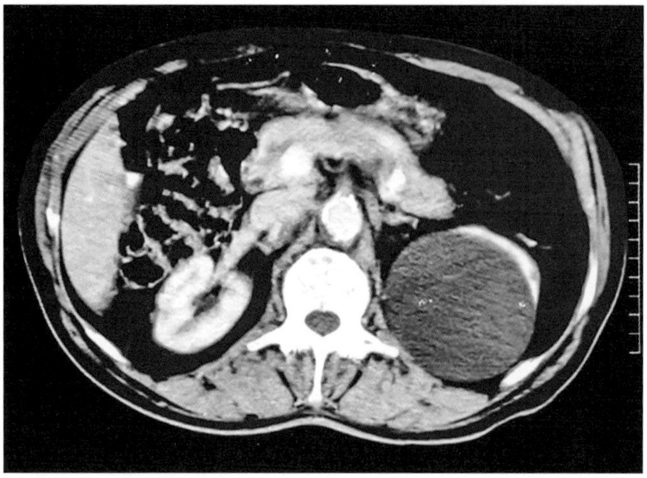

Fig. 1: Contrast-enhanced CT showing multiple simple cysts and a large smoothly marginated lesion of homogeneous fluid density in left kidney with cortical "beak" sign typical of simple cyst.

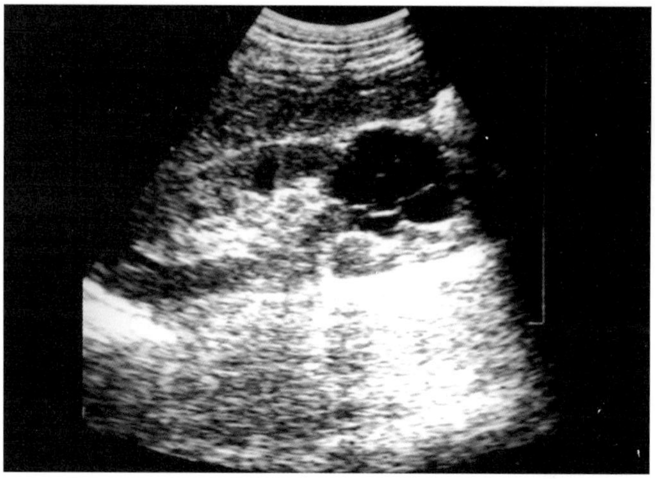

Fig. 2: Grayscale sonogram of right kidney showing a complicated cyst with few thin internal septations (Bosniak's category II lesion).

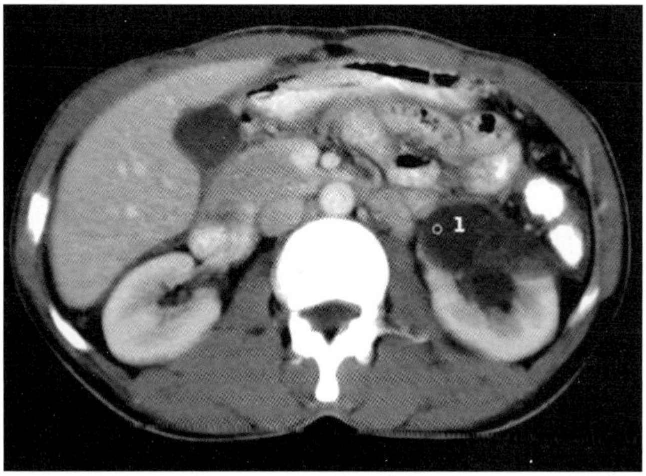

Fig. 3: CECT showing a multiloculated cystic mass arising from left kidney with nodular mural thickening and irregularity causing splaying and attenuation of pelvicalyceal system (1)—Cystic RCC (Bosniak's category IV lesion).

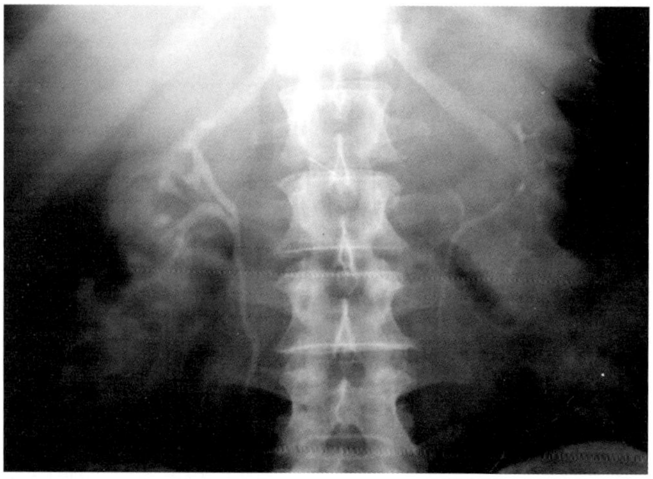

Fig. 4: Excretory urogram showing enlarged kidneys with splaying and stretching of pelvicalyceal system (spidery calyces) in a patient with polycystic kidney disease.

Ultrasonography

Grayscale, real-time sonography is the primary imaging modality for evaluation of renal cystic disorders. It is a noninvasive, multiplanar direct imaging modality, which requires no patient preparation, and unlike excretory urography it shows the mass lesion itself, along with changes in the renal parenchyma and tubular anatomy. It can almost always differentiate a cystic from a solid mass and simple cyst from cystic dysplasias associated with complications. However, obesity and excessive bowel gas can obscure the kidneys.

Tissue harmonic imaging is useful for identifying isoechoic lesions and small renal cysts which may be indistinguishable from normal renal parenchyma on the fundamental mode. Color Doppler flow imaging and Duplex Doppler sonography can aid in determining the presence or absence of vascularity and flow patterns which provide a clue regarding the benign versus malignant nature of renal cystic masses.

Computed Tomography

Computed tomography (CT) is the main modality for imaging and characterizing cystic renal lesions.

A lesion that contains fluid and has no blood supply remains water dense after contrast administration but solid tumors appear relatively dense in contrast to enhancing parenchyma. Enhancement depends upon the dose and rate of administration of iodinated contrast and the timing of imaging. The unenhanced CT, corticomedullary phase, nephrographic phase and excretory phase are obtained. The nephrographic phase is the most valuable for detecting mass lesions less than 3 cm which include clinically insignificant renal cysts and renal cell carcinomas.

A change of less than 10 HU from pre- to postcontrast images is considered typical of a benign cyst. Very rarely, cystic tumors may enhance less than 10 HU. Majority of pathologic lesions are more than 15 HU. An enhancement between 10 and 15 HU is considered suspicious but not diagnostic of a tumor. However, morphological features, such as wall thickening or nodule make the lesion suspicious even without enhancement especially in the case of papillary cancers.

Spiral CT and multislice helical CT have improved the detection and characterization of renal masses smaller than 10 mm. This is of great significance in patients with very small cysts which may contain foci of malignancy as in von Hippel–Lindau disease. Differentiation of angiomyolipomas (AML) from RCC in small lesions with minimal fat is best possible with helical CT. Excellent 3D reconstructions using maximum intensity projection (MIP), surface shaded display (SSD) or volume rendering techniques depict the cysts precisely.[5-7]

Magnetic Resonance Imaging

Multiplanar imaging capability and angiographic capabilities with excellent soft tissue contrast resolution have made magnetic resonance imaging (MRI) a useful method for evaluating the kidneys. The high field strengths, breathhold imaging, fat suppression techniques and use of MR contrast agents help in differentiating tumor from cysts. The multiplanar imaging capability of MRI makes it easier to assess polar lesions and coronal images make it simple for the urologist to visualize the relative position of a small lesion if a wedge resection or partial nephrectomy is to be planned. MR contrast agents do not have significant nephrotoxicity, hence can be used in patients with renal failure or iodinated contast sensitivity. MRI has a limitation in evaluating cystic lesions with calcification.

Conventional spin–echo sequences may be used for evaluating the kidneys. T1- and T2-weighted images are acquired in the axial planes and often in the coronal and sagittal planes as well. The newer fast imaging sequences reduce motion artifacts. Gradient-echo fast low angle shot (FLASH) sequences acquired during a single breath-hold are very useful for evaluating renal lesions.[2,8]

Angiography

Prior to the advent of newer imaging modalities like US, CT and MRI, angiography was commonly used for evaluation of renal mass lesions. However, in the present era, it is mainly indicated for interventional procedures of vascular and mass lesions of the kidney. It also serves as a "road map" before renal sparing surgery. Treatment of actively bleeding tumors, such as angiomyolipomas can be done through selective angiography by embolization of the intrarenal supply of the tumor.[9]

Cyst Puncture/Cystography

The radiologist plays a key role in the conclusive diagnosis of cystic renal lesions since percutaneous cyst aspiration under US or CT guidance is therapeutic in simple cystic lesions and the biochemical and cytological examination of cyst fluid aids in the differentiation of complex cysts.

SIMPLE RENAL CYST

A renal cyst is a dilated fluid-filled segment of a nephron or collecting tubule, which represents the most common renal mass in an adult, occurring in 50% of the population over the age of 50 years. A cystic kidney contains three or more cysts.[4]

Pathology

The pathologic characteristics of a simple nephrogenic cyst include one or more chambers lined by low cuboidal or flattened epithelium; a 1–2 mm thick fibrous wall; and a serous fluid content that is clear, slightly yellow, and may contain a small amount of protein. Uncommonly, thin septa divide the cyst into multiple chambers that may or may not communicate with each other. Calcium may deposit in the wall or septa of a simple nephrogenic cyst in the absence of any complication such as hemorrhage or infection.[10]

Although it is believed that simple cysts are acquired due to either tubular obstruction or medullary interstitial fibrosis, their exact pathogenesis is unknown. Occasionally, solid renal tumors may obstruct the tubules of adjacent normal parenchyma resulting in tubular dilatation and secondary cyst formation. Such cysts have been referred to as sentinel cysts. Therefore whenever a simple cyst is detected, the adjacent parenchyma should be carefully evaluated for the presence of an adjacent solid mass.

Clinical Features

Most cysts are asymptomatic especially when small. Large cysts may present as palpable mass, flank discomfort/pain, occasionally with hematuria or hypertension, proteinuria or polycythemia. Renal function is generally preserved in the host kidney regardless of size or position of the cyst.

Imaging Features

Excretory urography with tomography can detect renal cysts with a diameter of 2 cm or greater. Simple uncomplicated cysts present as round, smooth, radiolucent filling defect in the nephrogram and frequently show a beak at the interface of the cyst with the rest of the parenchyma, and there is absence of any definable wall. Large or centrally located cysts distort and splay the collecting structures. Sometimes, even abscesses and hypovascular renal cell carcinomas resemble simple cysts on urography; therefore, further investigation of the cystic mass by ultrasound becomes necessary.[10]

Sonographic studies show simple cysts to be round and uniformly echo-free internally, with a well-defined posterior wall and strong acoustic shadowing. One or more thin, delicate septations may be present **(Figs. 5 and 6)**. If these features are present, a simple cyst can be diagnosed and no further follow-up or intervention is required, provided there are no complicating clinical features to suggest the possibility of other significant lesion. On Doppler examination simple cysts show lack of color flow.

Computed tomographic scans shows cysts to be masses of water density (0–20 HU) sharply defined from the adjacent renal parenchyma with no perceptible wall thickness. They are homogeneous and do not show calcification or enhancement after intravenous contrast is administered.

Lesions that fulfill these criteria are simple cysts which do not require further intervention. When a renal lesion is not entirely cystic by strict US or CT criteria, a dedicated thin-section CT examination of the kidneys before and after IV contrast administration should be undertaken. For minimizing the errors in measurement created by partial volume averaging, the slice thickness should be less than half the diameter of the lesion. Enhancement is identified as an increase of at least 10 HU over baseline. Helical CT scanning, which allows for rapid continuous scanning of the kidneys during a single breath-hold, also helps in reducing the potential for errors of interpretation due to breathing misregistration.[10,11]

Sampling of fluid from a cystic renal lesion is easily accomplished percutaneously with ultrasound or CT guidance.

On MR imaging, simple cysts contain fluid that appears as uniformly low signal intensity on T1- and high-signal intensity on T2-weighted sequences **(Figs. 7A and B)**. MR diagnosis is based on the same morphologic criteria used to assess lesions by CT. As calcification is not detected on an MR scan, the modality is less effective in evaluating one of the key features distinguishing atypical lesions.[7,8]

Complicated Simple Renal Cyst

A simple cyst may be complicated by:

- Hemorrhage
- Infection
- Rupture
- Neoplasia.

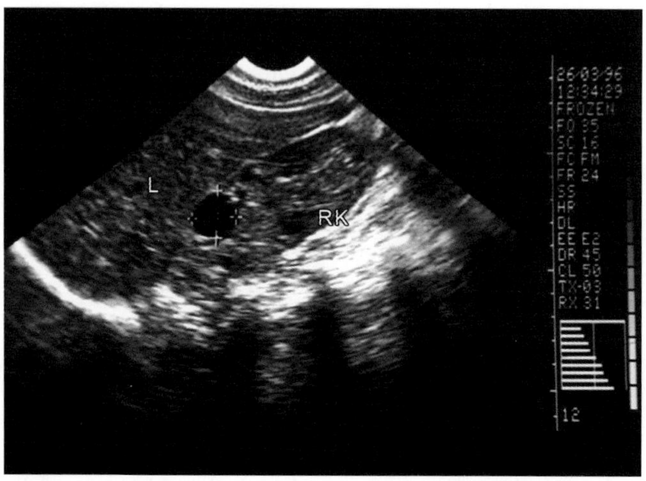

Fig. 5: US of kidney showing a well-marginated anechoic lesion with distal enhancement—Simple cortical cyst.

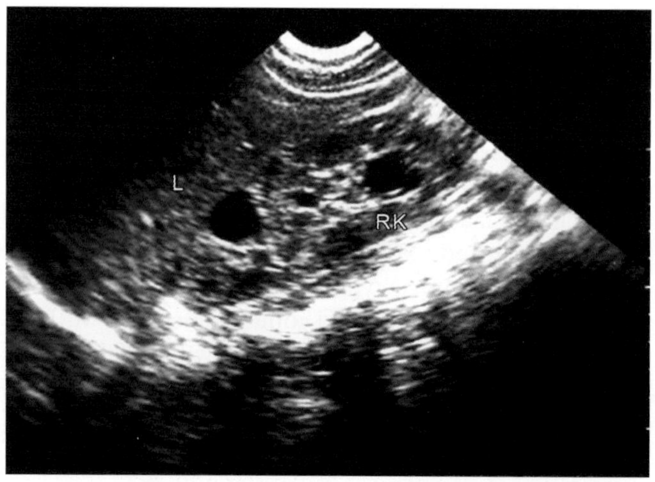

Fig. 6: Sonogram showing multiple simple cysts in the right kidney.

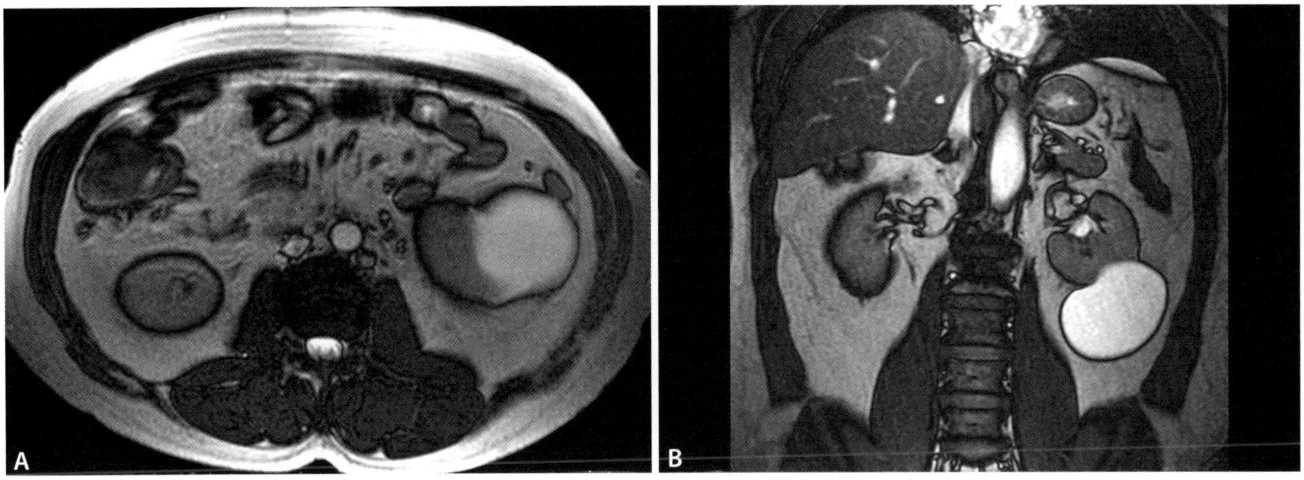

Figs. 7A and B: TRUE FISP axial (A) and coronal (B) MR images reveal a homogeneous sharply marginated lesion with imperceptible wall thickness and high signal arising exophytically from the left kidney—An exophytic simple cortical cyst.

Hemorrhagic Cyst

It refers to any cystic renal mass filled primarily with blood. It may result from hemorrhage into a simple cyst or organization of a liquefied hematoma. Approximately 6% of simple cysts are complicated by hemorrhage, which is usually the result of trauma, varicosities in the cyst wall or a bleeding diathesis.

Imaging features: On excretory urography, a hemorrhagic cyst presents as a lucent mass. In cases of trauma, the mass may communicate with the collecting system. In chronic cases, thick calcified walls may be present. An acute hemorrhagic cyst may be impossible to differentiate from an uncomplicated simple cyst on US. With chronicity, internal echoes are seen which represent debris and clot. Later, a thick calcified wall may be seen and the cyst may become multiloculated.

When acute hemorrhage into a cyst has occurred, CT reveals a homogeneous hyperdense mass measuring 70–90 HU, which appears relatively hypodense on postcontrast scans (flip-flop phenomenon) **(Fig. 8)**. As the blood liquefies and organizes, there may be a decrease in attenuation and increase in wall thickness with heterogeneous internal contents due to clot and debris.

On MRI variable signal intensity patterns may be seen in hemorrhagic cysts depending on the hemoglobin degradation products present. The methemoglobin in a hemorrhagic cyst alters its appearance, so that the lesion has an intermediate to high signal intensity on T1-weighted images. Signal intensity on T2-weighted images varies depending on whether or not the red cell lysis has occurred. The overlapping, variable signal intensities of

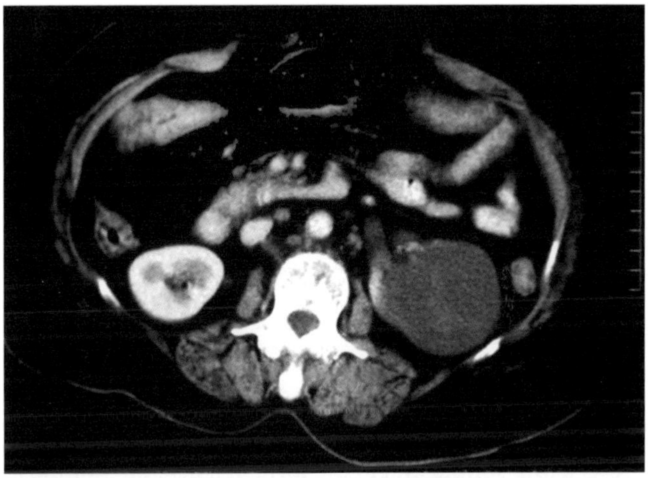

Fig. 8: Contrast-enhanced CT showing thin-walled septated hyperdense cystic lesion with an exophytic component arising from left kidney—Complicated hemorrhagic cyst.

hemorrhagic cysts and tumors with hemorrhage blur the distinction between benign and malignant cystic masses. MR diagnosis is based on the same morphologic criteria used to assess lesions by CT.[4,7]

Infected Cyst

A cyst may become infected by the following routes:

- Hematogenous dissemination
- Vesicoureteric reflux
- Surgical manipulation
- Cyst puncture.

Flank pain and fever may occur but symptoms may not be present.

Pathology: Infected cysts often have markedly thickened walls that are occasionally calcified. Their contents consist of varying amounts of inspissated pus and fluid as well as calcified and noncalcified debris.

Imaging features: EU demonstrates a mass with thick walls. Rarely, an air-fluid level may be seen when the cyst is infected by a gas-forming organism. Sonography reveals a cystic mass with thick walls along with internal echoes. Gas transmits the sonographic beam poorly and is suspected when intense specular echoes and ill-defined shadowing are recognized.

CT reveals cyst with thick walls, internal septations, debris fluid level, airfluid level and an inhomogeneous appearance of the cyst fluid **(Figs. 9A and B)**. On MRI, an infected cyst is more intense than a simple uncomplicated cyst but will usually appear less intense than a subacute hemorrhagic cyst, although it may be indistinguishable from a chronic hemorrhagic cyst.

Cyst Rupture

It is an uncommon complication of a simple renal cyst. Cyst rupture may be clinically silent or may be accompanied by severe pain and abdominal tenderness. Hematuria is common and the condition is usually diagnosed on the basis of EU, which often demonstrates the collecting system com-municating with the cyst.

US and CT can demonstrate fluid or blood in the perinephric and retroperitoneal spaces. Management in such cases is conservative.

Carcinoma in Wall of a Pre-existing Cyst

Rarely, a carcinoma arises from the epithelial lining of a pre-existing simple cyst in the form of a discrete nodule at the base of the cyst.

Imaging features: The cyst fluid provides an excellent acoustic window for visualizing the tumor nodule on sonography. CECT demonstrates focal wall thickening or a discrete tumor nodule that often enhances. MRI may reveal a focal mass or wall thickening. On angiography, it may be recognized as a focal blush in a larger hypovascular mass.

ATYPICAL SIMPLE CYSTS

Occasionally, simple cysts are atypical in their radiographic or clinical presentation. In these differentiation from cystic neoplasms, infectious diseases and other renal cystic disorders may be difficult.

Calcified Cyst

About 1–3% of cysts are calcified and the calcification is usually peripheral and curvilinear. US is unreliable owing to shadowing and reverberation artifacts due to calcification **(Fig. 10)**. CT is the most sensitive method of detecting calcification within a cyst however, a confident radiological diagnosis of a calcified simple cyst from a cystic RCC is often extremely difficult and may be achieved only after careful histological examination.

Hyperdense Cyst

Hyperdense cyst is a homogeneous, cystic appearing mass measuring 50–100 HU on unenhanced scans and demonstrating no significant contrast enhancement. It is thought to represent hemorrhage into a cyst while other explanations for a hyperdense cyst include high protein content, high viscosity and solidified colloid. Careful examination is required because some hyperdense masses may be secondary to either a primary or a secondary

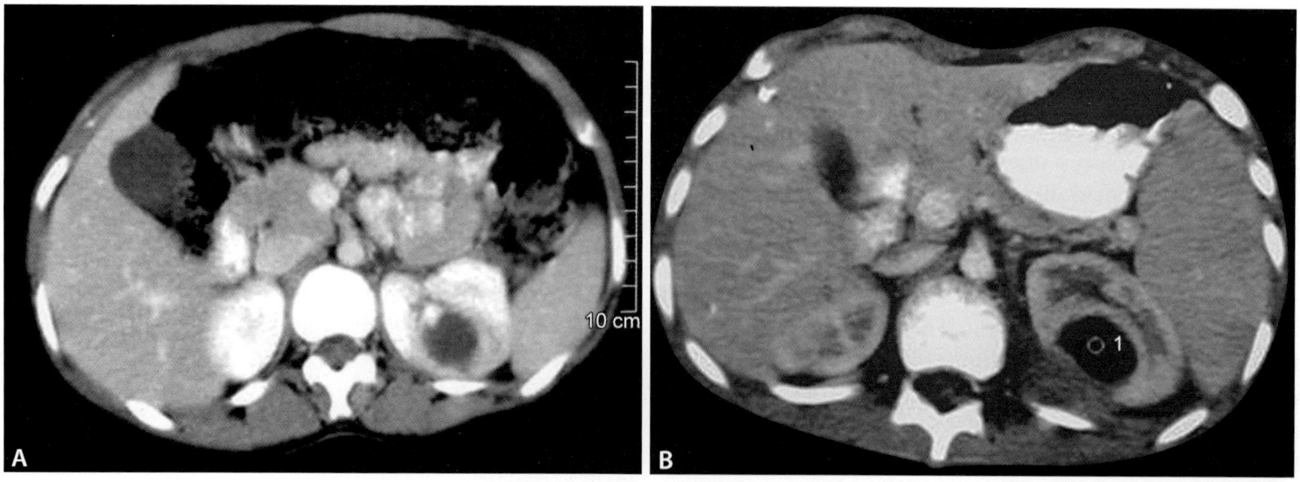

Figs. 9A and B: Contrast-enhanced CT scans: (A) Hypodense cystic lesion in the left kidney with inhomogeneous appearance of the cyst fluid; (B) Another case showing a hypodense cystic lesion in the left kidney with involvement of the ipsilateral psoas muscle (1)—Infected renal cysts.

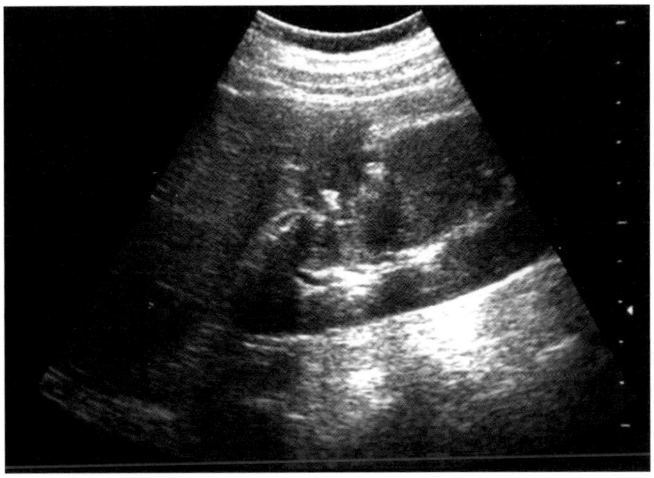

Fig. 10: Grayscale sonogram shows peripheral curvilinear calcification causing distal shadowing in a complicated cyst.

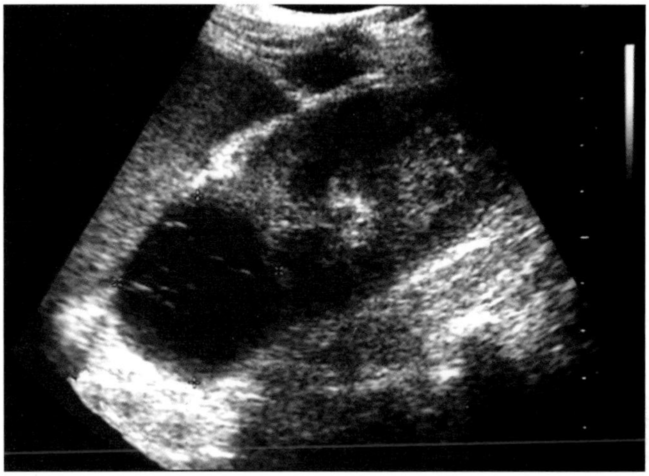

Fig. 11: US image showing multiseptated complex cystic mass within upper pole of left kidney distorting the renal contour and central sinus echoes—Atypical septated cystic metastases from carcinoma lung.

neoplasm. A measurement or washout of contrast material from a lesion at 15 minutes allows differentiation between hyperdense cysts and renal tumor. There is no change in hyperdense cysts while tumors show a decrease in attenuation or "de-enhancement".

Septated Cysts

Occasionally one or more septa are identified within a renal cyst, which may be a manifestation of two adjacent cysts sharing a common wall or a cyst, complicated by hemorrhage or infection. A septated cyst can be considered nonsurgical if the septae are 1 mm or less without any associated nodu-larity. The presence of multiple, thick septae should mandate further evaluation to rule out a cystic neoplasm **(Fig. 11)**.

Multiple Simple Cysts

They may occur in one or both kidneys and are often misdiagnosed as bilateral polycystic kidney disease. Features favoring the diagnosis of multiple simple cysts against PCKD are normal renal function, absence of family history and absence of cysts in other organs.

Localized Cystic Disease

These represent dilated ducts and tubules which vary in size from a few millimeters to several centimetres. Between the cysts, normal renal parenchyma without neoplastic or dysgenetic stroma is seen. On sonography, multiple small cysts often present as one large multiloculated mass. Individual smaller cysts are often recognized in the parenchyma adjacent to the main multiloculated mass **(Figs. 12A to C)**. The most important differential diagnosis is a multiloculated neoplasm which can be differentiated by the absence of capsule between the cluster of cysts and normal parenchyma and the presence of several small parenchymal cysts not contained within the main cluster of cysts. These findings are best appreciated on CT.[12]

POLYCYSTIC KIDNEY DISEASE

Autosomal Dominant Polycystic Kidney Disease (ADPKD) (Potter Type III)

An ADPKD is the most common of the hereditary diseases (1:1000). It is a systemic hereditary disorder with characteristics like cyst formation in ductal organs, particularly the kidney and liver, and gastrointestinal, cardiovascular and musculoskeletal abnormalities.

About 85% of cases are due to a dominant gene located on the short arm of chromosome 16 (the ADPKD-1 gene) whereas 5–10% of cases are due to an abnormal gene located on the long arm of chromosome 4 (the ADPKD-2 gene), which causes a milder form of the disorder.[4,5]

Patients with a positive family history of ADPKD and no imaging evidence of renal cysts can be further evaluated using gene-linkage analysis. It is proposed that the disorder results from failure of union of the branches of ureteral bud with metanephros, which deprived of the organizing influence from cysts.

Pathology

There is cystic dilatation of nephrons involving all segments from proximal convoluted tubule to collecting

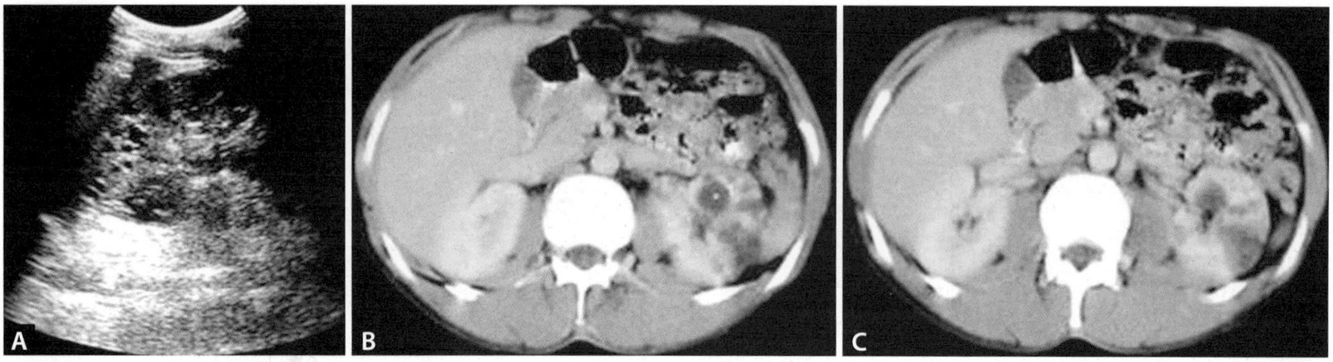

Figs. 12A to C: Sonogram showing (A) multiple small cysts in the upper pole of the left kidney seen as a multiloculated mass. Contrast enhanced CT scans (B and C) revealing multiple cysts in the upper pole of the left kidney separated by enhancing bands of renal parenchyma—Unilateral localized cystic disease.

duct due to epithelial hyperplasia leading to redundancy and predisposing to cyst formation.

With minimal disease, the kidneys are normal in size with smooth surface but with increase in the size and number of cysts, the kidneys are asymmetrically enlarged with bosselated surface contour; however, the reniform shape is maintained.

Although multiple bilateral renal cysts are the most important manifestation, ADPKD is really a systemic disease and is associated with many other organ abnormalities, including intracranial aneurysms, cardiac valvular abnormalities, liver and pancreatic cysts and colonic diverticulae.[4]

Clinical Features

Most affected individuals present in the fourth or fifth decade with flank pain, palpable masses, hypertension, hematuria, urinary tract infection, proteinuria or polycythemia. Progressive azotemia ensues as renal parenchyma is destroyed and renal failure occurs in most patients by the age of 60 years. Complications include superimposed infection, cyst hemorrhage, uric acid stones and hypertension.

Imaging Features

In a patient with a family history of ADPKD, screening for the disease with sonography, CT or MR imaging often helps to establish the diagnosis. Ultrasound is the modality of choice for primary evaluation of most patients with suspected ADPKD.

Plain films reveal bilateral enlarged kidneys with lobulated margins causing displacement of surrounding structures like colonic flexures. Calcification may be curvilinear or amorphous and presence of renal calculi often signifies superimposed infection. The "nephrogram" phase of the EU is characterized by numerous, smoothly marginated radiolucencies throughout the cortex and medulla, which have been likened to the appearance of "Swiss cheese". An appearance of spidery collecting system with stretched and crescentric calyces may be noted.

On US, cysts of varying sizes are noted in enlarged kidneys with a lobulated outline **(Figs. 13A and B)**. Similar cysts may be seen in liver, pancreas and the spleen. Antenatal diagnosis is possible on demonstration of enlarged cystic kidneys, ascites and hepatomegaly. The presence of atleast two renal cysts (unilateral or bilateral) in individuals, at risk and younger than 30 years, may be considered sufficient to establish a diagnosis. Among the patients aged 30–59 years, the presence of at least two cysts in each kidney may be required and among those aged 60 years and above, at least four cysts in each kidney should be present.[4]

The sensitivity of CT scan is greater than that of ultrasound in detecting renal cysts and thus, may establish the diagnosis at an earlier age and more definitively **(Figs. 14 and 15)**. On MRI, the renal cysts are hypointense on T1 weighted and hyperintense on T2 weighted images, with infected and proteinaceous cysts showing inter-mediate signal intensities **(Figs. 16 and 17)**.

Autosomal Recessive Polycystic Kidney Disease (ARPKD) (Potter Type I)

Of all the renal cystic diseases, ARPKD is the most common heritable disease manifesting in infancy and childhood. The two constant features of ARPKD are involvement of the liver and kidney. Its frequency has been reported as between 1 in 6000 and 1 in 55000 births, and the responsible gene has been mapped to chromosome 6.[13]

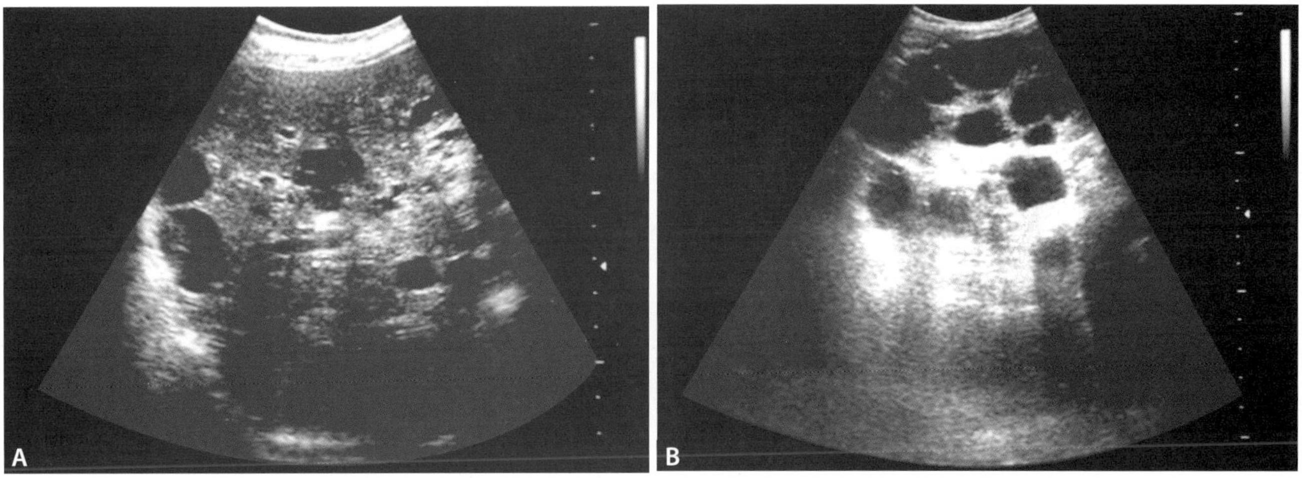

Figs. 13A and B: Sonography showing multiple noncommunicating cysts of varying sizes replacing the renal parenchyma and distorting the central sinus echoes—ADPKD. Cysts are also seen in the liver.

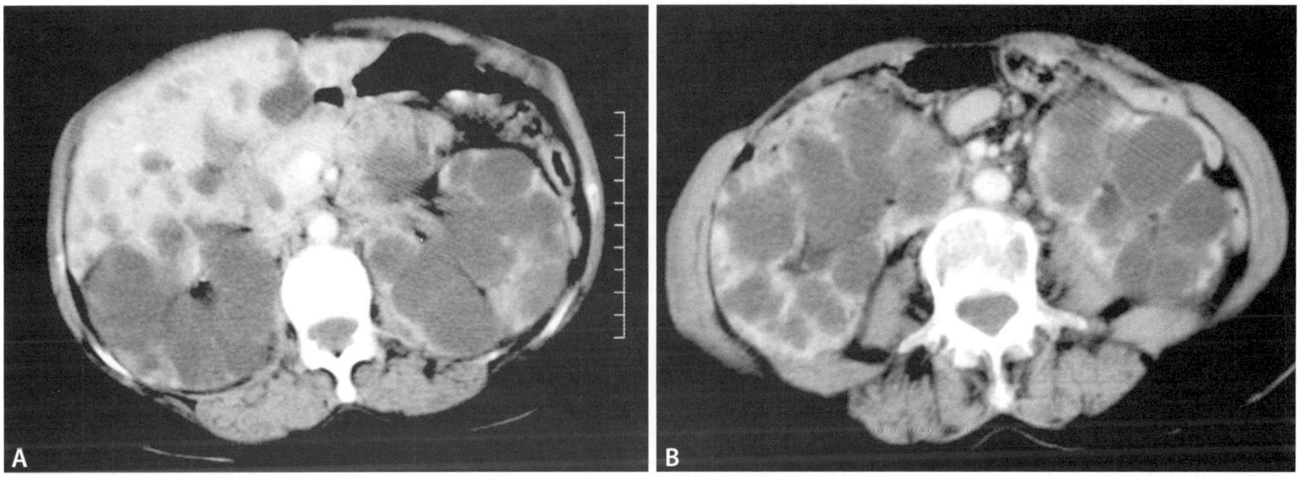

Figs. 14A and B: Contrast-enhanced CT scans revealing multiple noncommunicating cysts in both kidneys. Cysts are also seen in the liver—ADPKD.

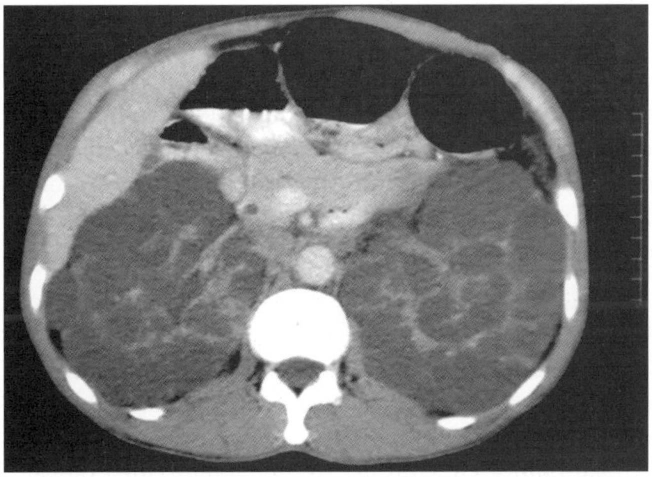

Fig. 15: CECT scan in another case showing multiple non-communicating cysts in both kidneys—ADPKD.

Clinicopathologic Features

An ARPKD is a disease of tubular malformation and ectasia. In the kidney, the disorder manifests as nonobstructive collecting duct ectasia, usually in a bilaterally symmetric fashion with enlargement of the kidneys. Fibrosis develops in the renal interstitium resulting in impairment of renal function and consequent hypertension, dilute urine and renal failure. The liver shows hepatic fibrosis and biliary ectasia.

The perinatal form of ARPKD is the most common, and it usually presents with severe renal failure and bilateral renal enlargement. In infancy or childhood the hepatic abnor-malities secondary to congenital hepatic fibrosis predominate with milder renal disease. Portal hypertension can result due to severe periportal fibrosis. Marked cystic dilatation of the intrahepatic biliary

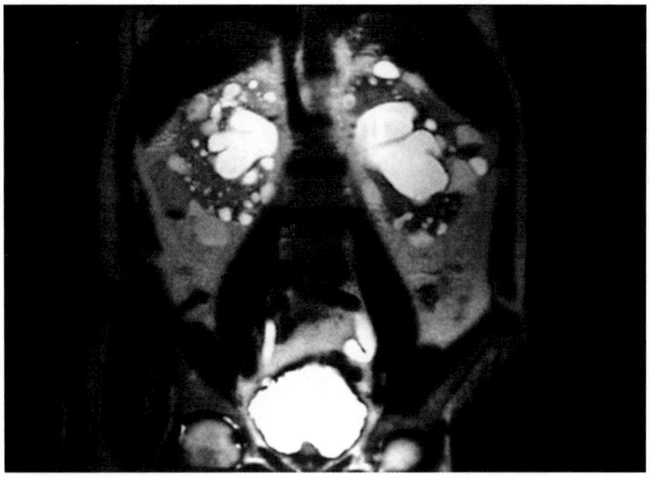

Fig. 16: T2W coronal MR image showing both kidneys to be enlarged with multiple cysts of varying sizes having fluid signal intensity studding the renal parenchyma of both kidneys consistent with polycystic kidney disease. Note is also made of bilateral hydronephrosis and back pressure changes in the bladder due to bladder outflow obstruction.

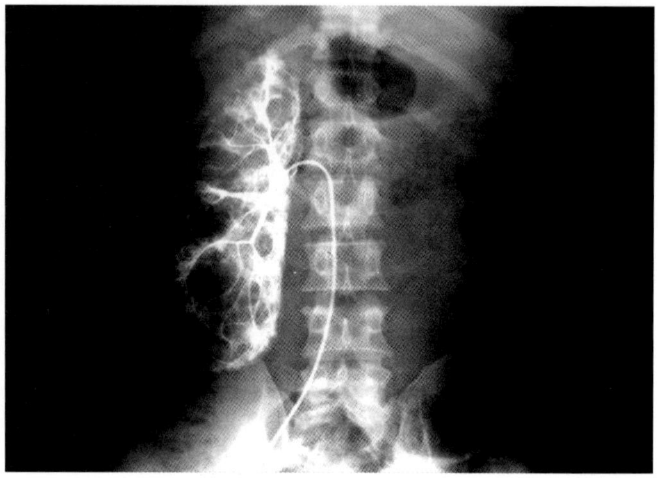

Fig. 17: Selective renal angiogram in a case of polycystic kidney disease showing avascular areas with splaying of the normal renal vessels around consistent with cysts.

ducts "Caroli's disease" is also associated with ARPKD. Generally, the hepatic and renal involvements are inversely proportional to each other in individual patients.[13]

Imaging Features

Antenatal diagnosis of ARPKD can be made. Bilateral symmetrically enlarged kidneys with severe oligohydramnios and a nondistended fetal bladder with thoracic cage compression are typical features seen in the third trimester.[5]

In neonates and infants with moderate to severe renal disease, the kidneys are smoothly enlarged. Plain films reveal abdominal distension with centrally placed gas filled bowel loops. With severe kidney disease, the baby may be born with pulmonary hypoplasia and a small thorax with evidence of pneumothorax.

On US, the kidneys are smoothly enlarged and diffusely echogenic with loss of corticomedullary differentiation. The bladder is usually small.

On unenhanced CT, the kidneys are smooth, enlarged and low in attenuation. Focal liver cysts and features of portal hypertension may be present. Recently bilateral renal calcifications have been reported on CT and the degree of calcification is related to the severity of renal disease.[14] After IV contrast administration, the kidneys show a "striated nephrogram", which represents accumulation of contrast material in the dilated tubules. On MR imaging, there is increased signal intensity of the renal parenchyma on T2-weighted images.

MEDULLARY SPONGE KIDNEY

Medullary sponge kidney (MSK) is an uncommon, benign cystic disorder of the renal medulla characterized by dilatation of the terminal portion of the collecting ducts (ducts of Bellini). The disorder is typically bilateral, although it may be unilateral or rarely involves only one pyramid. Its true prevalence in the general population is unknown but is estimated to be 1 in 5000 persons.[4]

Clinicopathologic Features

Renal size is normal to slightly enlarged with a smooth renal contour. It is characterized by dilatation of the papillary portions of the ducts with presence of small intraluminal calcification. Calcification is either due to distal renal tubular acidification defect or due to urinary stasis in the dilated collecting ducts.

Patients usually present in the third or fourth decade with renal colic, hematuria, dysuria and fever. Male/female ratio is 2:1. The association of MSK with other rare diseases suggests a hereditary pattern. It is associated with congenital hemihypertrophy, Ehlers-Danlos syndrome, parathyroid adenoma, Caroli's disease, Marfan's syndrome and ADPKD.[4]

Imaging Features

The diagnosis of MSK is made with EU, which shows a characteristic pattern of medullary nephrocalcinosis with multiple discrete calculi clustered in the renal pyramid on plain films. On contrast administration, the cystically dilated collecting ducts appear as clusters of small rounded opacities in the papillae, which may become distorted with splaying of the calyceal cups **(Fig. 18)**.

Ureteral obstruction may result when calculi are extruded into the collecting system. A brush or fan appearance of discrete linear densities may be seen. On sonography, the medulla may be hyperechoic from calcific deposits. Occasionally, cystic cavities and hydronephrosis may be detected.

CT scan is sensitive in the detection of medullary nephrocalcinosis, but insensitive in diagnosing MSK because there are many causes of medullary nephrocalcinosis.

MEDULLARY CYSTIC DISEASE

It is a rare disease process which is characterized by progressive renal failure, renal tubular atrophy, secondary glomerular sclerosis and cysts of the renal medulla and corticomedullary junction.[15]

Clinical Features

This disease complex can be divided into two distinct groups according to the age of onset and mode of inheritance. In the juvenile form inherited as an autosomal recessive disorder, the children present with hyposthenia, anemia and growth retardation and it is associated with ophthalmologic and neurologic abnormalities, congenital hepatic fibrosis and related dysplasia. The adult form presents in the 2nd–4th decades, typically with no extrarenal manifestations and is inherited as an autosomal dominant mode. Both of these forms progress to renal failure; hematuria typically is not present.

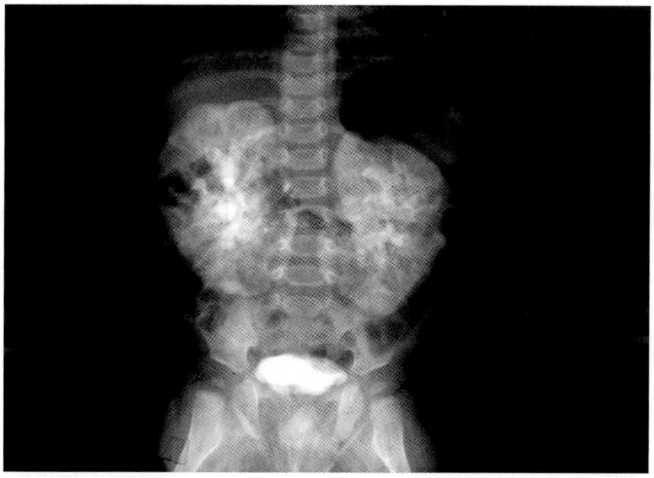

Fig. 18: Excretory urogram in a child with medullary sponge kidneys showing enlarged kidneys with medullary nephrocalcinosis and characteristic "Swiss cheese" nephrogram.

Imaging Features

Plain film shows normal to small kidneys with no calcifications. EU shows poor visualisation of normal to small kidneys with a smooth contour.

On USG, small fluid filled medullary cavities and smooth kidneys of increased echogenicity are noted.[15] CT demonstrates kidneys that are bilaterally small and smooth with presence of cysts in the medulla and corticomedullary junction.

MULTICYSTIC DYSPLASTIC KIDNEY (POTTER TYPE II)

Multicystic dysplastic kidney (MCDK) is a developmental and nonhereditary anomaly with multiple, smooth nonfunctioning and non-communicating cysts. It is one of the most common abdominal masses found in the newborn and is typically unilateral, other-wise asymptomatic. The bilateral form of MCDK is usually associated with congenital gastrointestinal and cardiac abnormalities. This form has a poor outcome due to accompanying oligohydramnios and pulmo-nary hypoplasia.[16]

Pathology

The kidney consists of multiple cysts which are held together by connective tissue with little or no normal renal parenchyma. Most often, there is atresia of the ureter and renal pelvis (pyeloinfundibular atresia). The hydronephrotic form is seen if incomplete but severe obstruction occurs early in nephrogenesis resulting in a dilated renal pelvis.

Potter described two subtypes of renal dysplasia depending on the size of renal cysts. In Potter type II a the kidney is enlarged due to polymorphic and multilocular cysts while in Potter type II b the kidney is smaller. These two types can be differentiated on sonography.[3]

Imaging Features

The diagnosis is made most often with antenatal or neonatal sonography. MCDK can be diagnosed *in utero* from as early as 15 weeks. A paraspinal mass with internal cysts of varying shapes and sizes without identifiable communication is seen and the renal pelvis and ureter are usually not visible. Oligohydramnios with bilateral MCDK is a poor prognostic sign **(Figs. 19A and B)**.

A hydronephrotic MCDK tends to have a more reniform shape and a dilated renal pelvis should be seen. Doppler waveforms have been reported to be markedly abnormal in MCDK with a reduced peak systolic frequency shift or no diastolic flow present. In the older child or

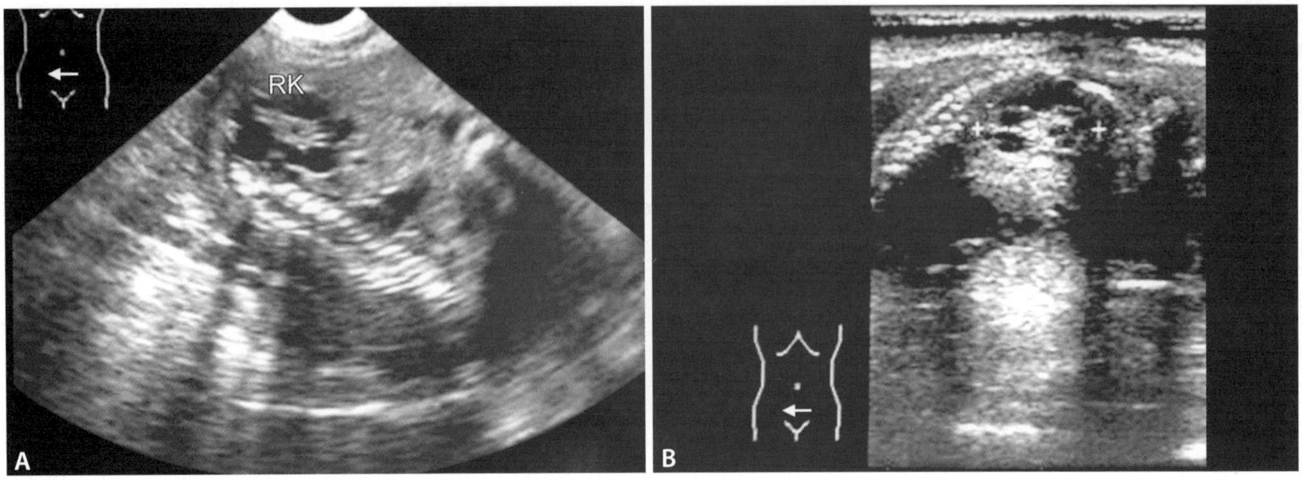

Figs. 19A and B: Antenatal sonogram showing multiple noncommunicating cysts in an enlarged fetal kidney—Multicystic dysplasia.

adult, radiographic studies show nonfunctioning kidney with evidence of ring calcification(s) in the renal region **(Figs. 20 and 21)**. Radio-nuclide scan is used to assess the functional activity when the diagnosis is in question. ^{99m}Tc mercaptoacetyltriglycine uptake is seen in an obstructed kidney but not in MCDK.[4]

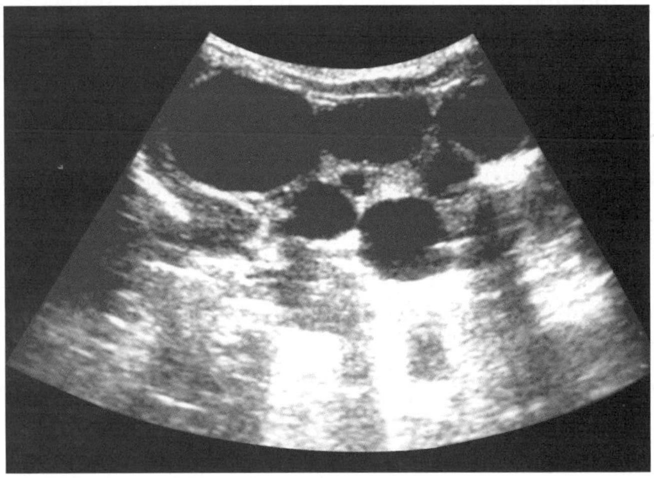

Fig. 20: US of right kidney in a 4 year old child shows multiple cysts of varying sizes distorting the reniform contour—MCDK.

CYSTIC DISEASE ASSOCIATED WITH RENAL NEOPLASM

Acquired Cystic Kidney Disease (ACKD)

An ACKD is characterized by the formation of multiple renal cysts in patients with endstage renal disease, who have no history of hereditary cystic disease. It is seen in 40–50% of patients on long term hemodialysis. After 3–5 years of dialysis, the prevalence of ACKD is 40–60%, rising thereafter to reach 90% between 5 and 10 years on dialysis.[4]

Multiple, bilateral small cysts that involve both the renal cortex and medulla are seen. ACKD is also associated with an increased incidence of renal neoplasms. Factors causing renal cyst and tumor formation in end-stage renal disease are unknown but the two are interrelated. It is postulated that with progressive destruction of functioning renal tissue cystogenic substances accumulate and cause hypertrophy and hyperplasia of epithelial cells. The tubular epithelium proliferates and cystic dilatation of tubules occurs. Subsequently there is a continuum from single layered epithelial cysts to multilayered cysts to renal cell carcinomas. Tumors can be both multiple and bilateral.[8,17,18]

Clinical Features

Most patients with ACKD are asymptomatic; however, increase in hemoglobin due to raised erythropoetin levels, hematuria and renal neoplasia, may be seen.

Imaging Features

On US, bilateral small kidneys with increased echogenicity and multiple cysts are seen **(Fig. 22)**. Solid or complex renal tumors may also be diagnosed **(Figs. 23A and B)**. CT reveals small kidneys with multiple cysts; cyst wall calcification is common. High density cysts and renal tumors are easily diagnosed and CT is the most useful study for ACKD.[19]

On MRI, simple cysts can be distinguished from hemorrhagic cysts (high SI on both T1 and T2WI). Furthermore, solid tumors showing inhomogeneous signal intensity more than that of renal parenchyma on T2WI can be well delineated.

von Hippel–Lindau Disease (VHL)

This is a relatively rare autosomal dominant disorder caused by an abnormal gene on short arm of chromosome 3.

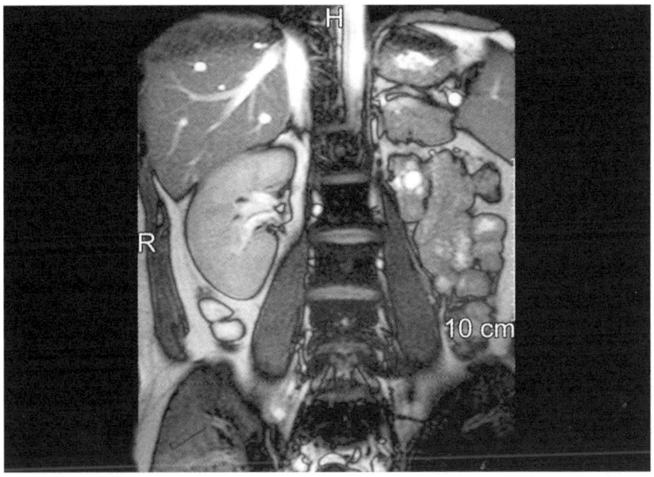

Fig. 21: Coronal TRUE FISP MR images reveal a small dysplastic left kidney replaced by multiple noncommunicating cysts showing hyperintensity on T2W image with compensatory hypertrophy of right kidney—Adult MCDK.

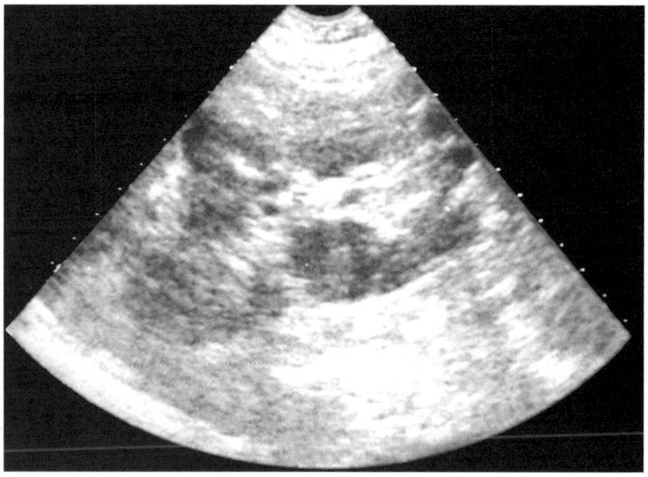

Fig. 22: US in a patient with chronic renal failure on long-term hemodialysis showing shrunken echogenic kidney with loss of corticomedullary differentiation and multiple small cortical cysts—ACKD.

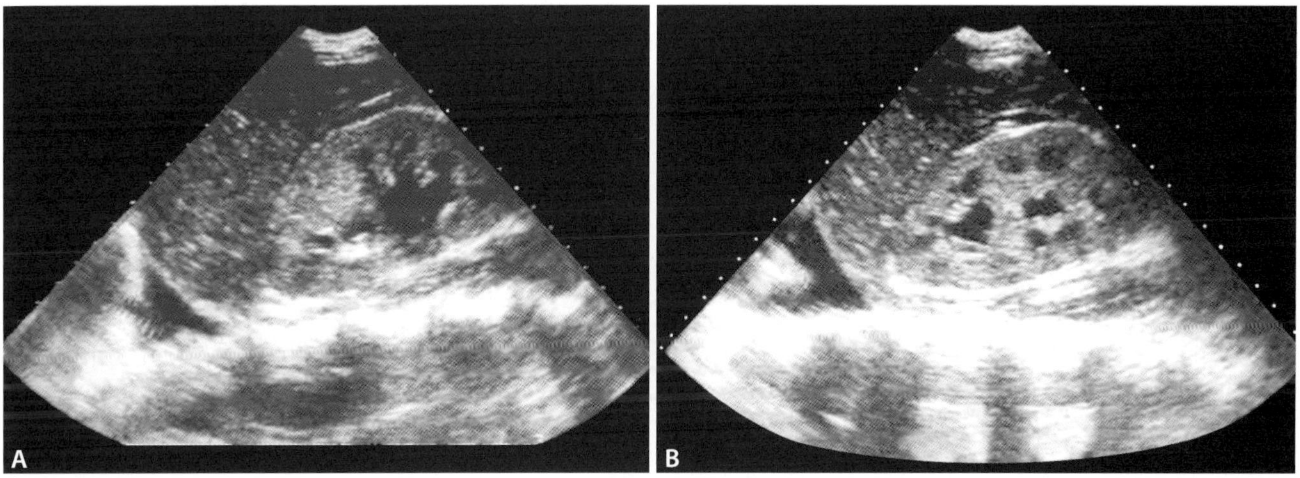

Figs. 23A and B: USG of a patient with renal failure showing shrunken echogenic kidneys with multiple small cortical cysts. Hydronephrosis is seen in the right kidney.

This disorder is associated with hemangioblastomas of the CNS, retinal angiomatosis, pheochromocytomas and cysts and tumors of the kidney and pancreas and papillary cystadenomas of the epididymis. Clinically, the patient presents with abdominal mass, flank pain and haematuria.[20]

Pathology

Bilateral, multiple small cortical cysts are seen without causing renal enlargement. Extensive disease can mimic ADPKD. Bilateral and multifocal renal cell carcinomas are also noted.

Imaging Features

On EU, renal cortical cysts are seen bilaterally, causing distortion of the renal architecture. USG is highly sensitive for detection of renal cysts; however, small renal tumors may not be seen. CT is more sensitive than USG for the detection and characterization of renal masses and small, solid renal masses can be precisely defined **(Fig. 24)**.

MR imaging is indispensable for the diagnosis of neurological neoplasms seen in patients with VHL. Furthermore, small RCCs can be detected on CEMR. Large tumors can be evaluated and characterized on nonenhanced scans and tend to be more heterogeneous.[21]

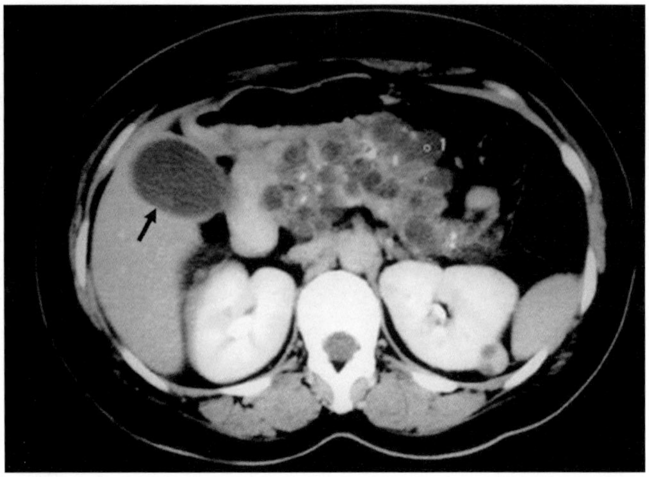

Fig. 24: CECT sections showing a solid enhancing mass and cyst in the left kidney with multiple cysts and calcifications in the pancreas—von Hippel-Lindau disease.

TUBEROUS SCLEROSIS (TSC)

It is a genetically transmitted neurocutaneous syndrome with sporadic occurrence. Genetic markers have been identified at *9q34*(TSCI) and *16p13*(TSCZ) although they account for only 50% of TSC families. The true incidence of TSC is difficult to measure though its birth incidence ranges from 1 per 5800 to 1 per 10,000. It has an autosomal dominant mode of inheritance and is characterized by mental retardation, seizures and cutaneous lesions. This disorder is associated with multiple hamartomas in the brain (cortical tubers), retina, skin, heart (rhabdomyomas), kidney (angiomyolipomas) and other organs.[22]

Renal cystic disease also occurs in TSC and the occurrence of both angiomyolipomas and renal cysts is virtually diagnostic of TSC. Angiomyolipomas are benign masses consisting of varying amounts of abnormal blood vessels, smooth muscle and fat.

Imaging Features

On abdominal radiographs, lucency suggesting fat within an AML can occasionally be detected. On EU, the findings vary with the size and number of renal cysts and the presence of AMLs. Multiple nonopacifying renal masses causing distortion of the collecting system are seen. On sonographic examination, multiple renal cysts and AMLs, showing hyperechoic reflections may be seen.[23]

On CT, fat containing AMLs with low attenuation values and intralesional hemorrhage may be noted along with renal cysts **(Figs. 25A and B)**. MR imaging aids in diagnosing AML's by showing high signal intensity on both T1- and T2-images.[8]

CYSTS OF RENAL SINUS

Peripelvic cysts, parapelvic cysts, parapelvic lymphatic cysts and parapelvic lymphangiectasia have been used variably to describe cysts of the renal sinus **(Fig. 26)**. The term renal sinus cyst is preferred for fluid filled masses in the renal sinus, either solitary or multiple, that are usually detected as an incidental finding in the older patients. Diagnosis may be incidental or during investigation of hematuria/hypertension.

Features are nonspecific and the treatment is cyst puncture.[6]

MISCELLANEOUS CYSTIC DISEASE

Inflammatory

Hydatid Cysts

The kidney can also be involved by hydatid disease; the patient is usually asymptomatic until the cyst has grown large enough to cause pressure symptoms or rupture.

Imaging Features

Plain radiography may reveal a localized bulge on the renal contour or evidence of calcification in a degenerated cyst; which may be eggshell or sunburst in appearance. On EU, an intact cyst with a complete pericyst is seen as filling defect in the kidney. When there is reposition of the pericyst, there is interposition of contrast medium between the ectocyst and pericyst. There is interposition of contrast medium between the ectocyst and pericyst producing the "goblet or wine glass or Surraco's sign". In the open type, when there is a communication between the hydatid cyst and collecting system, the contrast medium gives a mottled appearance and may also produce the "crescent sign".[6]

On US, calcific cysts or hydatid sand may be seen. Parallel echogenic stripes formed when membranes of dead daughter cysts become adherent, are very suggestive of hydatid cyst. CT shows unilocular, low attenuation cyst or daughter cysts arranged within the mother cyst, giving a rosette appearance **(Figs. 27A to C)**.

Pyogenic Cyst

These are usually secondary to acute pyelonephritis. Excretory urography reveals filling defects or irregular cavities communicating with the pelvicalyceal system. On sonography, thick walled cystic lesions with low level internal echoes are seen. CECT shows low attenuation masses with rim enhancement and thickening of perirenal fascia.

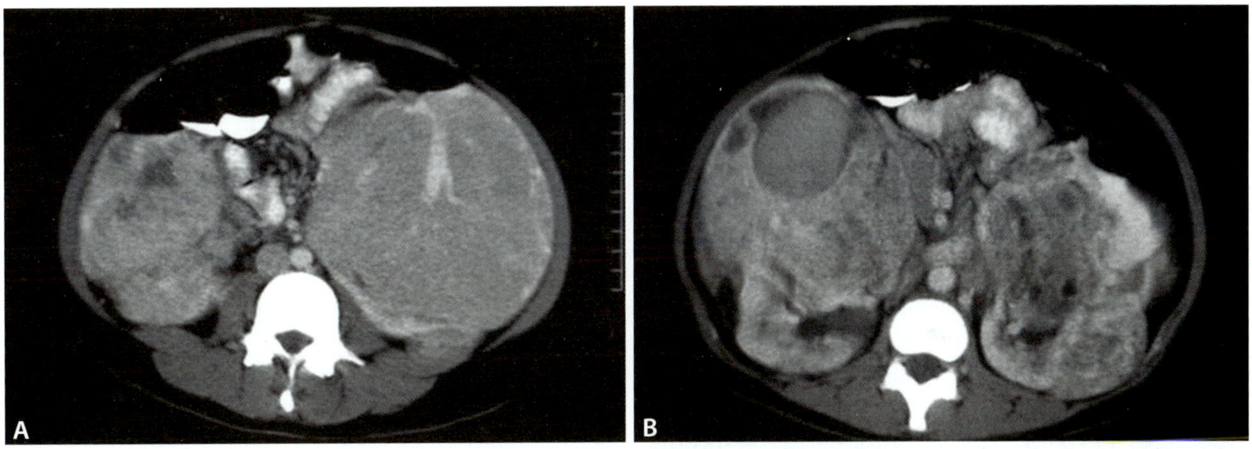

Figs. 25A and B: Contrast-enhanced CT scan showing heterogeneous masses involving both the kidneys. The masses show fat attenuation values and cystic areas within. The lesions show intralesional vacularity—Bilateral angiomyolipomas.

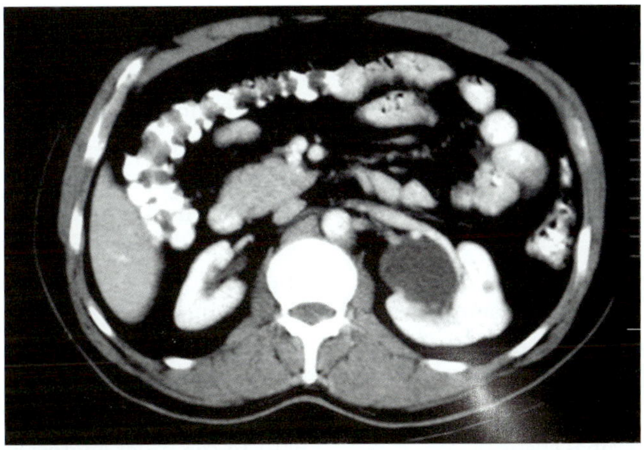

Fig. 26: Contrast-enhanced CT scan showing a solitary fluid-filled lesion in the renal sinus detected as an incidental finding in this patient—Parapelvic cyst.

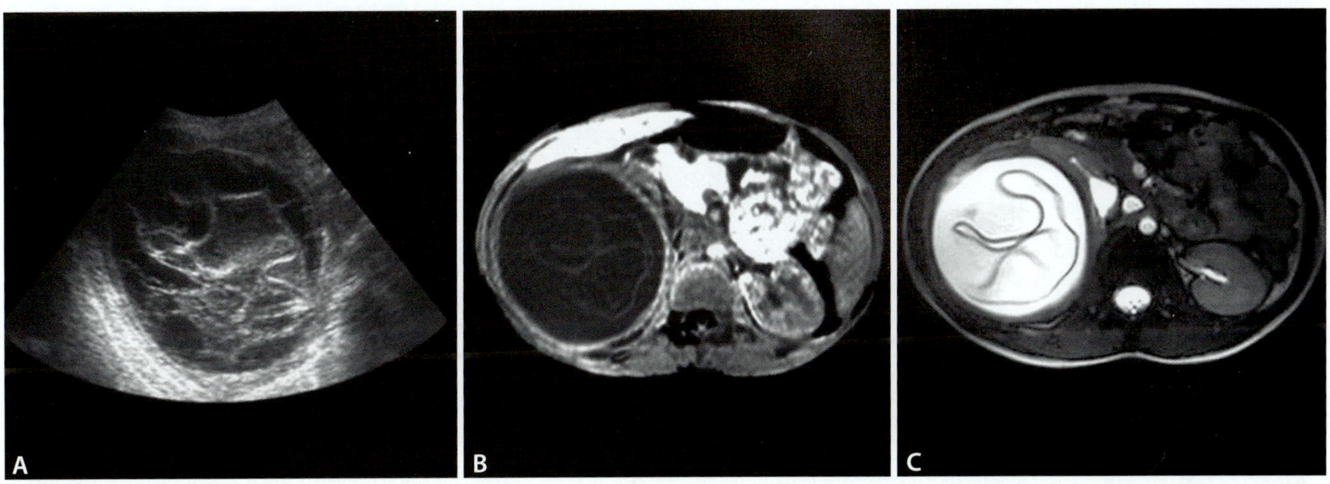

Figs. 27A to C: Sonogram (A) showing a cyst replacing the right kidney with multiple serpentine linear structures/membranes within s/o ruptured hydatid cyst. T1W MR axial image (B) showing the cyst replacing the right kidney. The cyst is hypointense on T1. T2W MR image (C) shows the cyst to have high signal. The membranes are seen as linear areas of low signal within—Ruptured hydatid cyst of the right kidney.

Tuberculous Cysts

The most common route of spread of Mycobacterium TB to the kidney is hematogenous seeding from the lungs. A tuber-culous focus is usually located in the renal cortex and may develop a communication with the tubular system and the pyramids, which can rupture into the calyces.

EU reveals extensive calcification and papillary necrosis with multiple irregular cavities. End-stage tubercular kidneys usually do not excrete contrast medium at urography. On US, multiple renal cavities can be seen.

Focal calyceal changes are seen on CT as calyceal enlargement, pericalyceal areas of early cavitation, infundibular strictures and loss of perirenal fat planes. Late features of calcification or hydronephrosis secondary to strictures may be seen.

Pleuricystic Kidney Disease

It applies to entities when one or more renal cysts are present in syndromes of multiple malformations. The degree of renal cyst formation in each syndrome is variable and reflects different responses to the underlying abnormality.

Glomerulocystic Disease

This is a rare congenital disease with characteristics like dilatation of Bowman's space and adjacent tubules. The kidneys are enlarged with multiple small cortical cysts leading to progressive renal failure.[6] This is not a familial entity and is not related to other renal cystic diseases.

Microcystic Disease

Infants with congenital nephrotic syndrome can have cystic dilatation of proximal convoluted tubules. However, no discernible radiological changes are noted.

CYSTIC RENAL CELL CARCINOMAS

They are seen in 5–10% cases of RCC. Four patterns are commonly seen and these are intrinsic multilocular growth, cystic necrotic tumor, unilocular cystadenocarcinoma and tumor found within a cyst wall. The most common appearance is that of a macrocystic multilocular cyst with large or small cystic components. This appearance is indistinguishable from a complicated cyst or benign multilocular cystic nephroma on sonography and CT **(Figs. 28A to C)**. However, the microcystic multilocular RCC appears solid on sonography and CT because of the small size of the cystic spaces which is less than 5 mm in diameter **(Figs. 29A to C)**. Rarely, unilocular renal cell carcinoma may occur **(Figs. 30A and B)**. Papillary renal cell carcinoma a subtype of renal malignancy can appear as a homogeneous hyperattenuating mass.

Another cystic type of RCC occurs when a solid lesion outgrows its blood supply and becomes necrotic. This is seen as a hemorrhagic complex cystic mass. The imaging appearances depend on the degree of necrosis present.[24]

In conclusion, any fluid-filled renal mass not fulfilling the imaging criteria of an uncomplicated cyst should be considered a cystic lesion. When multiple features are present the mass should be managed in accordance with to the most aggressive finding. Most multiloculated

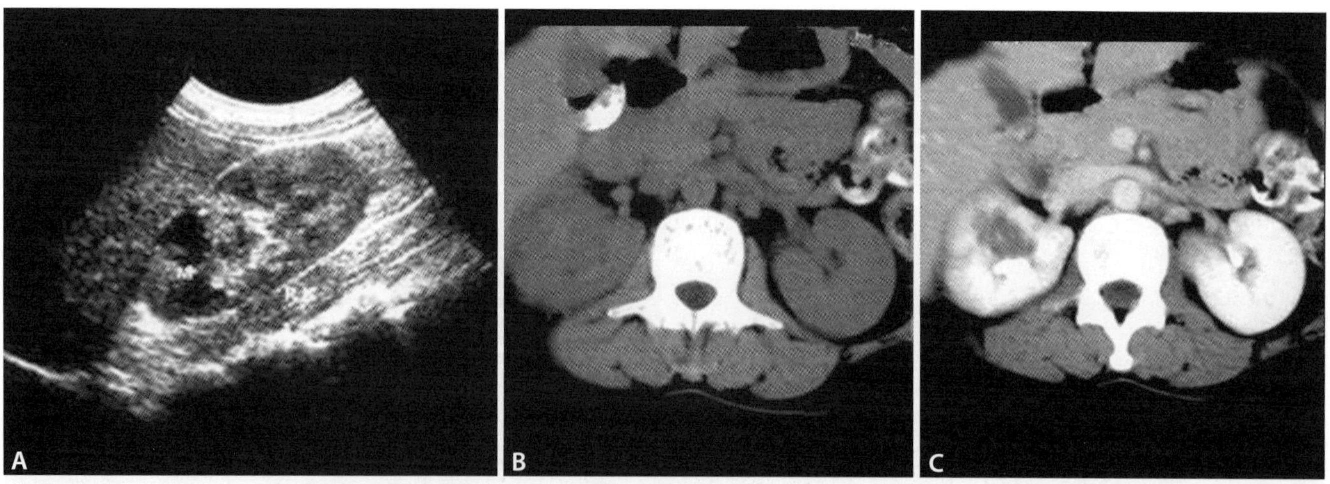

Figs. 28A to C: Sonogram (A) showing a complex cystic mass in the upper pole of the right kidney with thick septations. Noncontrast CT (B) showing an ill-defined hypodense mass in the right kidney. Contrast enhanced CT scan in the nephrogram phase (C) showing significant enhancement of the cystic lesion (enhancement >20 HU) consistent with a malignant cystic neoplasm.

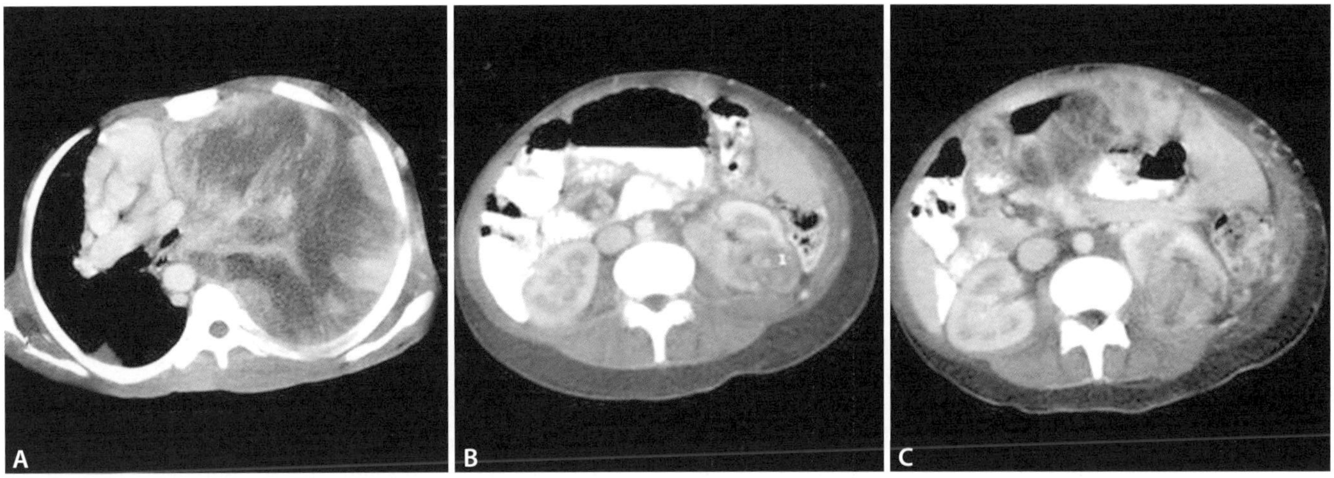

Figs. 29A to C: Contrast-enhanced CT scan of the chest revealing pulmonary sarcoma (A) with collapse of the left lung. (B and C) showing a solid appearing hypodense lesion in the left kidney—Renal metastasis.

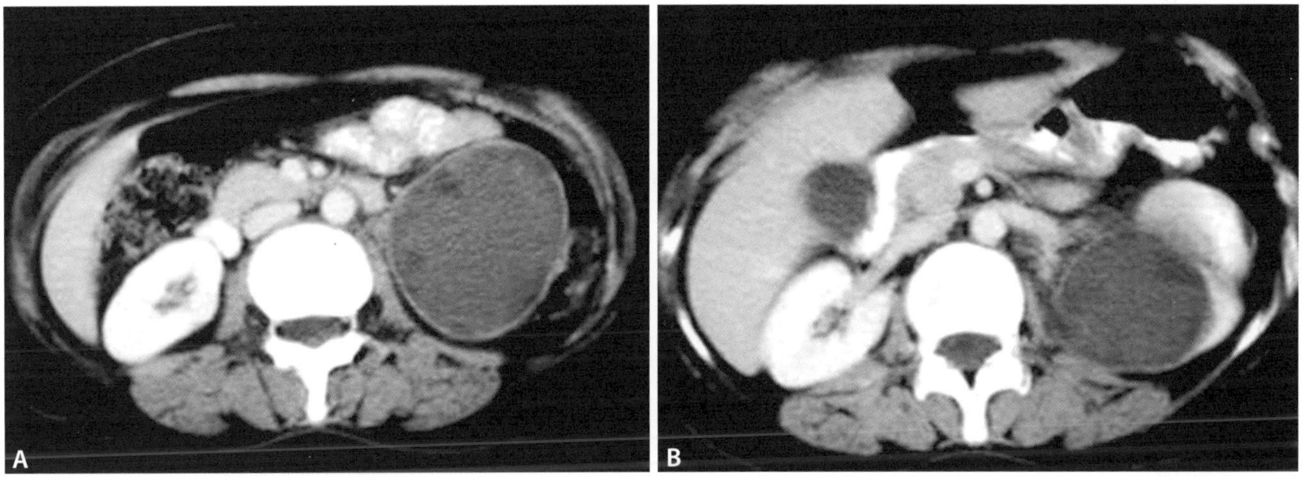

Figs. 30A and B: Contrast-enhanced CT scan showing a unilocular cyst in the left kidney. The cyst has inhomogeneous fluid content and shows solid elements within—Cystic RCC (L) kidney.

cystic masses with wall thickening, nodularity or enhancement would require surgery to establish a final diagnosis.

REFERENCES

1. Tantravahi JR, Steinman TI: Acquired cystic kidney disease. Seminars in Dialysis. 2000;13(5):330-4.
2. J Stuart Wolf: Evaluation and management of solid and cystic renal masses. Journal of Urology. 1998;159:1120-33.
3. Friedmann W, Vogel M, Dimer JS, et al. Prenatal differential diagnosis of cystic kidney disease and urinary tract obstruction: anatomic, pathologic, ultrasonographic and genetic findings. Eur J Obs and Gyn and Rep Biol. 2000;89:127-33.
4. Levine E, Hartman DS, Meilstrup JW, et al. Current concepts and controversies in imaging of renal cystic diseases. UCNA. 1997;24(3):523-43.
5. Thomsen HS, Levine E, Meilstrup JW, et al. Renal cystic diseases. Eur Radiol .1997;7:1267-75.
6. Hartman DS: Cystic disease. In: Pollack HM (Ed), Clinical urography. Philadelphia: WB Saunders; 1990.pp.1059-185.
7. Bosniak MA. Problems in radiological diagnosis of renal parenchymal tumors. Urol Clin North Am. 1993;20:217-30.
8. Gladys M, Torres, Pablo R Ros. Kidney. In: Stark DD, Bradley WG (Eds), Magnetic Resonance Imaging, 2nd edition. Mosby Year-Book, Inc; 1999.
9. Reichard EAP, Roubidoux MA, Dunnick NR. Renal neoplasms in patients with renal cystic diseases. Abdom Imaging. 1998;23:237-48.
10. Davidson AJ, Hartman DS, Choyke PL. Radiologic assessment of renal masses: Implications for patient care. Radiology. 1997;202:297-305.
11. Levine E. The Kidney. In: Haaga JR (Ed), Computed Tomography and Magnetic Resonance Imaging of the Whole Body, 3rd edition. Mosby-Year Book, Inc; 1994.

12. Hwang DY, Lee JG, Kim SH, et al. Unilateral renal cystic disease in adults. Nephrol Dial Transplant. 1999;14:1999-2003.
13. Lonergan GJ, Rice RR, Suarez ES. Autosomal recessive polycystic kidney disease: Radiologic-pathologic correlation. AFIP Archives Radiographics. 2000;20:837-55.
14. Lucaya J, Enriquez G, Nieto J. Renal calcifications in patients with autosomal recessive polycystic kidney disease. Prevalence and cause. AJR Am J Roentgenol. 1993;160:359-62.
15. Rego JD Jr, Laing FG, Jeffrey RB. Ultrasonic diagnosis of medullary cystic disease. J Ultrasound Med. 1983;2:43.
16. Mentser, Mahan J, Koff S. Multicystic dysplastic kidney. Pediatr Nephrol. 1994;8:113.
17. Henson JHL, Al-Hilli A, Penry JB. The development of acquired renal cystic diseases and neoplasia in a chronic haemodialysis patient. Br J Radiol. 1985;58:1215-7.
18. Diana L. Farmer. Urinary tract masses. Seminars in Pediatric Surgery. 2000;9(3):109-14.
19. Levine E, Grantham J, Slusher S. CT of acquired cystic kidney disease and renal tumors in long-term dialysis patients. AJR. 1984;142:125-31.
20. Choyke PL, Glenn GM, Walther MM. von Hippel-Lindau disease: Genetic, clinical and imaging features. Radiology. 1995;194:629.
21. Rominger M, Kenney P, Morgan D. Gadolinium-enhanced MR imaging of renal masses. Radiographics. 1992;12:1097-16.
22. Povey S, Burley M, Attwood J. Two loci for tuberous sclerosis: one on 9q34 and one on 16p13. Ann Hum Genet. 1994;58:107.
23. Durham DS. Tuberous sclerosis mimicking ADPKD. Aust NZJ Med. 1987;17:71.
24. Ooi GC, Sagar G, Lynch D. Cystic renal cell carcinoma: radiological features and clinico-pathological correlation. Clin Rad. 1996;51:791.

CHAPTER 112

Renovascular Hypertension

Niranjan Khandelwal, Anupam Lal, Manphool Singhal

INTRODUCTION

Hypertension, defined as blood pressure of 140/90 mm Hg or more, is a common medical problem affecting as much as one-third of the population. It is a leading cause of mortality and morbidity. In most cases (93–94%) hypertension is idiopathic and is labeled as essential hypertension. In a minority of patients, a specific etiology can be identified and such patients are said to have secondary hypertension. The major etiologies implicated in this category include renovascular, renal parenchymal, endocrine and neurologic with renovascular hypertension being the most common. Its prevalence is estimated at 1–5% of the general hypertensive population.[1,2]

Renovascular hypertension (RVH) denotes the casual relationship between a renal artery stenosis (RAS) and its clinical consequences, namely hypertension or renal failure.[3] It is also defined as hypertension that improves or resolves after correction of renal artery stenosis.[4]

Diagnosing renovascular hypertension is important because treatment of renal artery stenosis may cure patient's hypertension. Renal artery stenosis is also an important cause of ischemic nephropathy and end stage renal disease (ESRD) which can be prevented by early and appropriate intervention.[5-7] Also in view of the widespread use of angiotensin-converting enzyme (ACE) inhibitors, it is important to exclude the presence of RAS, as these agents may precipitate renal failure in the presence of bilateral renal artery stenosis or stenosis of renal artery in a solitary functioning kidney.

PATHOPHYSIOLOGY

Renal artery stenosis causes a decrease in perfusion pressure and glomerular filtration rate (GFR) by decreasing the hydrostatic pressure in the afferent arterioles. Regardless of the cause of stenosis, the accompanying reduction in intrarenal arterial pressure is sensed by the juxtaglomerular apparatus of the afferent arterioles. The renin angiotensin aldosterone system is triggered in an attempt to maintain glomerular filtration pressure. Renin secreted by juxtaglomerular apparatus of the kidney, converts plasma angiotensinogen to angiotensin I. This is converted by angiotensin-converting enzyme in the lungs to angiotensin II. Angiotensin II is a potent vasoconstrictor and increases blood pressure by direct effect on arterioles and by stimulating aldosterone secretion leading to salt and water retention. Angiotensin II also causes vasoconstriction of the efferent arterioles in an attempt to restore glomerular filtration to normal.

In patients with unilateral renal artery stenosis increased levels of angiotensin II causes not only vasoconstriction of afferent arterioles of the affected kidney but also a decrease in GFR and sodium excretion by the contralateral kidney. The nonaffected kidney also demonstrates marked decrease in renin secretion. Increased blood pressure ultimately results in pressure natriuresis from the contralateral kidney resulting in the classic 'high renin–normal volume' pattern of unilateral RAS.[8,9]

In patients with bilateral stenosis or a solitary kidney with renal artery stenosis the entire mass of nephrons is ischemic, resulting in increased renin, excess angiotensin II and aldosterone, which by counterregulatory mechanisms, decrease renin production. Since pressure natriuresis cannot occur from either kidney, there is volume retention. The overall picture in bilateral renal artery stenosis is a mixed one with both renin and volume factors typically being involved. Because of volume overload, these patients are prone to recurrent sudden 'flash' pulmonary edema.[8,9]

If RAS is untreated, prolonged exposure of renal vasculature to vasopressor agents may alter renal hemodynamics and result in nephrosclerosis, and subsequent removal of offending RAS does not relieve hypertension. This is called 'renoprival effect' and is indicated clinically by inability of the kidney to excrete sodium and water. Recently 'azotemic renovascular disease' is the preferred term for these changes as changes in the effected are not necessarily due to ischemic changes.[10] In animal models it has shown that due to critical renal artery stenosis oxidative stress pathways develops with stimulation of tissue fibrogenic pathways leading to acute tubular injury and subsequent irreversible interstitial fibrosis-fibrogenic cascade.[11-14] It is imperative therefore that renovascular hypertension is diagnosed and treated prior to these irreversible changes.[8]

ETIOLOGY OF RENAL ARTERY STENOSIS

Renal artery stenosis may be broadly categorized as atheromatous or nonatheromatous. The various causes are listed in **Table 1**.

Table 1: Causes of renovascular hypertension.

I. Renal Artery Stenosis
• Atherosclerosis
• Fibromuscular dysplasia
• Nonspecific aortoarteritis/Takayasu's arteritis
• Vasculitis
• Dissection
• Vasospasm
• Coarctation syndrome
• Neurofibromatosis
• Congenital rubella
• Syphilitic arteritis
• Tuberous sclerosis
• Extrinsic compression
• Middle aortic syndrome
• William's syndrome
II. Other Causes of Renovascular Hypertension
• Aneurysm of renal artery
• Renal artery embolus
• AVF—renal artery
• Irradiation
• Renal transplant
• Trauma

Atherosclerosis, fibromuscular dysplasias and in our subcontinent, nonspecific aortoarteritis (Takayasu's disease) account for most of the cases. Chugh et al[15] found that nonspecific aortoarteritis was responsible for 61% of patients, fibromuscular dysplasia for 28% and atherosclerosis for 8% patients with RVH in India. The incidence of atherosclerosis is rising in the urban population.[16]

Atherosclerosis

Atherosclerosis accounts for approximately two-thirds of patients of renal artery stenosis in the western world. It occurs more commonly in men over the age of 50 years. Obstruction usually results from aortic plaque engulfing the renal ostium (i.e. within 4 mm of aortic lumen). Less frequently plaque develops independently in the proximal third of the renal artery. The stenosis is often circumferential but may be eccentric and is commonly associated with calcification. Differentiation between proximal and ostial lesions is important because of their different response to angioplasty. Because atherosclerosis is a generalized process both renal arteries are frequently affected. If atheromatous lesions are left untreated there is a high probability of progression to complete occlusion.[17-19]

Fibromuscular Dysplasia

Fibromuscular dysplasia (FMD) has only been recognized for the past 30 years or so but accounts for almost a third of the patients with of renovascular hypertension according to western literature. It typically occurs in young women. It may involve any layer of the artery and is classified as intimal, medial or adventitial.[20,21]

- *Intimal fibroplasia*: There is concentric accumulation of collagen beneath the internal elastic membrane which causes focal smooth stenosis usually in the mid-portion of renal artery. It is more common in children and is progressive.
- *Medial dysplasia*: This is the most common type of dysplasia and accounts for approximately 95% cases.
  - *Medial fibroplasia*: This is the most common type of medial dysplasia in which there is replacement of smooth muscle by collagen. These alternate with small areas of dilatation due to aneurysm formation and result in the classic 'string of beads'

appearance. It is more common in women of 20–50 years of age and is progressive. It usually responds to angioplasty **(Figs. 1A and B)**.

- *Perimedial fibroplasia*: Collagen infiltrates outer layer of media. A beaded appearance similar to medial fibroplasia is seen but the 'beads' are smaller as aneurysms do not develop.
- *True medial hyperplasia*: Uncommon media is replaced by hyperplastic smooth muscle and fibrous tissue. A tubular smooth narrowing of the vessels is seen on angiography.
- *Medial dissection*: Also uncommon. A new channel is formed in the outer one- third of the media with visualisation of a false channel in media on angiography.

- *Adventitial dysplasia*: Collagenous infiltrate surrounds the adventitia, producing a tubular smooth narrowing on the angiogram.

FMD is not confined to renal arteries but is also seen in visceral and peripheral arteries. It also involves the carotid and vertebral arteries, but tends to spare the intracranial vessels.

Nonspecific Aortoarteritis/Takayasu's Arteritis[22-24]

Nonspecific aortoarteritis also known as Takayasu's disease is a granulomatous arteritis that commonly involves the aorta and its major branches. In the acute phase the media and adventitia are filled with giant cells and granulomata. Destruction of the entire vascular wall and progressive adventitial fibrosis lead to luminal narrowing, occlusion, dilatation or formation of aneurysms. The disease tends to affect young females (mostly less than 35 years of age) particularly from south-east Asia and India. In the active stage the disease is associated with clinical features like fever and increased sedimentation rate. Hypertension in Takayasu's disease may be caused by coarctation of aorta or main renal artery stenosis **(Fig. 2)**.

It may be classified into four types:

Type I : Narrowing of aortic arch or great vessels arising from arch.

Type 2 : Descending thoracic and upper abdominal aorta involvement.

Type 3 : Involvement of aortic arch vessels, abdominal aorta and major branches.

Type 4 : Pulmonary artery involvement.

Middle Aortic Syndrome[25-27]

A rare syndrome of diffuse narrowing of abdominal aorta often affects visceral and renal arteries. It typically occurs in young patients, most often in the second decade. Various etiologies, including chronic inflammatory aortitis, atherosclerosis, neurofibromatosis and cystic medial necrosis are implicated. According to some authors, there is no clear distinction between this condition and nonactive Takayasu's disease. The renal arteries are commonly affected by long stenosis.

SCREENING FOR RENOVASCULAR HYPERTENSION

Hypertension is common but RVH is not, therefore screening should be reserved for patients at moderate to high-risk for RVH. The following criteria have been proposed, in the presence of which prevalence of RVH is 20–30%:[8,9]

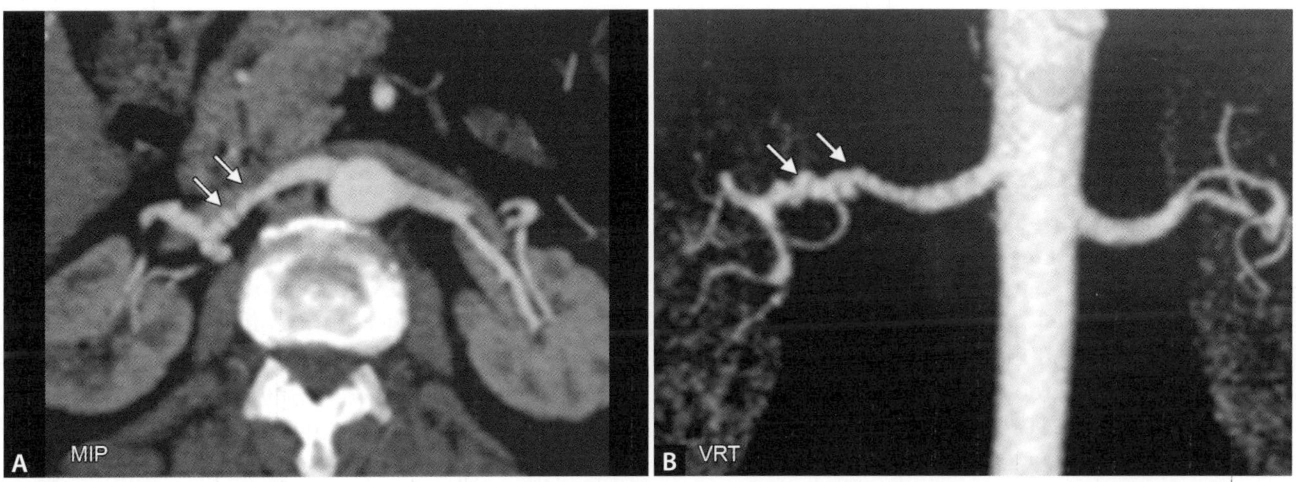

Figs. 1A and B: CT angiography images (MIP and VRT) showing classical 'string of beads' appearance (arrows) involving right renal artery and its divisions in a case of fibromuscular dysplasia (medial fibroplasia).

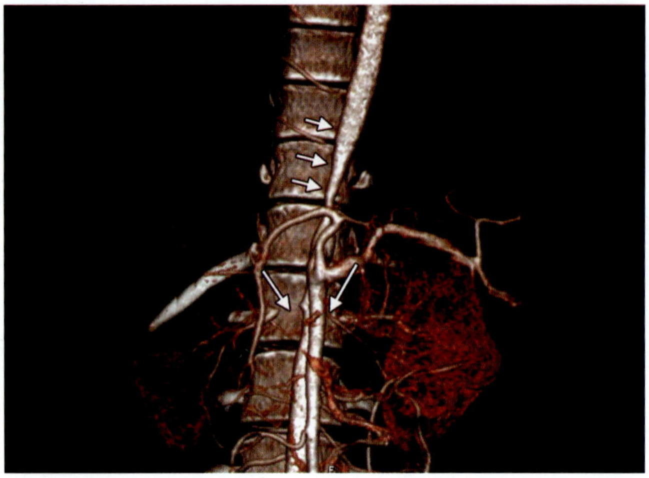

Fig. 2: CTA (VRT) image showing narrowing of abdominal aorta (arrows) and near total occlusion of bilateral renal artery (long arrows) in a case of Takayasu's aortoarteritis.

Clinical

- Patients presenting with accelerated/malignant hypertension
- Hypertension uncontrolled by triple drug therapy
- Onset of hypertension less than 20 years or more than 50 years of age, or a sudden worsening of their condition
- Unilateral small kidney discovered with any clinical study
- Impairment of renal function after treatment with an Angiotensin converting enzyme (ACE) inhibitor
- Patients with long history of smoking
- Patients with symptoms of peripheral vascular disease.

Physical signs that suggest RVH include the following:

- Abdominal or flank bruit (systolic or diastolic)
- Grade 3 or 4 fundoscopic changes of hypertension.

Laboratory tests that may indicate renovascular disease include as follows:

- Blood urea nitrogen >20 mg/dL
- Serum potassium <3.4 mEq/L
- Proteinuria

There is no perfect screening test for the detection of renovascular hypertension. The situation is further complicated by the fact that the presence of renal artery stenosis (RAS) may not always indicate a causal relationship. Not every RAS leads to renovascular hypertension and patients with essential hypertension may also develop RAS. The degree of stenosis that causes renovascular hypertension has not been established although most investigators treat stenosis measuring 50% or greater.[28,29] Physiologically, RAS is defined as inadequate renal blood flow leading to reduction in GFR and loss of renal parenchyma, hence it becomes prudent to establish the functional significance of RAS before proceeding to revascularization.[30]

Clinical and Biochemical Tests

Clinical/nonradiological tests that have been used for the diagnosis of RVH include plasma renin activity, ACE inhibitor challenge test, aspirin challenge test, and 24 hours ambulatory blood pressure monitoring.

IMAGING MODALITIES FOR ASSESSMENT OF RAS

In the clinically suspected patients having RAS as a cause of RVH, it becomes necessary to identify those patients, preferably through noninvasive methods, who have truly hemodynamically significant RAS and can benefit from interventional or surgical revascularization.[31-33]

Radionuclide renal scintigraphy, especially with ACE inhibitors is highly sensitive and accurate in detection of unilateral RAS but its accuracy decreases in patients suffering from bilateral RAS or azotemia and in patients with single functioning kidney.[34]

Doppler ultrasound is widely available and performed imaging modality for determination of renal size, morphology and allows direct evaluation of the renal arteries as well as transrenal Doppler waveform analysis, but it remains operator dependent.

Intravascular ultrasound (IVUS) is the best modality for the correct evaluation of stenosis and plaque morphology, but it being invasive and expensive it is unlikely to become a screening modality.[35]

Computed tomography angiography (CTA) with the advent of multidetector CT (MDCT) and contrast-enhanced magnetic resonance angiography (CE-MRA) are widely used for the initial evaluation of RAS with sensitivity and specificity equivalent to digital subtraction angiography (DSA).[36] However after published reports of nephrogenic systemic fibrosis (NSF) following gadolinium-based contrast agent in patients with deranged renal functions, CE-MRI as a screening test is being avoided.[37,38] It is of great importance that radiologists be aware of this serious disease and exercise caution when considering the use of Gd-based contrast media in patients with moderate (glomerular filtration rate <60 mL/min/1.73 m^2) to severe (glomerular filtration rate <15 mL/min/1.73 m^2) renal disease. In this situation various other MR techniques which can assess renal arterial morphology, perform functional measurements of arterial flow and parenchyma perfusion without the administration of gadolinium are being investigated and found useful in patients with deranged renal functions. These techniques are non-contrast studies, such as time-of-flight (TOF), phase contrast (PC), steadystate free precession (SSFP), and arterial spin labeling (ASL).[38] These advancements explains why renal MRI is evolving as the first-line imaging modality for the evaluation of renovascular disease.

An ideal renal artery imaging study should answer the following questions:[39]

- Localization and number of arteries
- Characterization of renal stenosis, including etiology of stenosis, localization, and poststenotic dilatation
- Hemodynamic and functional significance of the stenosis
- Further pathologies or variants that might have an influence on treatment planning.

Radionuclide Renal Scintigraphy

Radionuclide imaging of the kidney is the most widely performed screening test for the diagnosis of renovascular hypertension I^{131} orthoiodohippurate (OIH) was used in the past. Currently technetium 99m (^{99m}Tc) diethylenetriamine pentaacetic acid (DTPA) and mercaptoacetic triglyceride (MAG 3) are commonly used for isotope renography.[8]

The standard renogram reflects the salt and water retention on the ischemic side by demonstrating slow transit and excretion of radiotracer. The classic appearance is that of a small kidney with decreased uptake and delayed tracer transit and excretion. In its original form the test had an unacceptably high rate of both false-positives and false-negatives and was not significantly better than hypertensive urography hence was not used.[40] An incidental observation by Majd et al. in 1983[41] led to the emergence of captopril renography which has since become the standard screening test in the diagnosis of this condition. Captopril renal scintigraphy can be used as a screening test, to establish the hemodynamic significance of RAS, to predict the outcome of revascularization and in the follow-up after successful revascularization.

Principles of Angiotensin-converting Enzyme Inhibitor (Captopril) Scintigraphy

In a patient with a significant RAS the efferent arterioles of the glomeruli are constricted by angiotensin II to maintain glomerular filtration pressure in the face of diminished afferent arteriolar pressure. Administration of ACE inhibitor decreases this angiotensin related constriction of efferent arterioles which reduces glomerular filtration and hence urine flow. ACE inhibitor does not affect GFR in patients with normal renal arteries or those with essential hypertension.[8]

Protocol

ACE inhibitor scintigraphy is performed 1 hour after the oral dose of 25 mg of captopril or 15 minutes after an intravenous dose of 0.04 mg/kg of enalpril maleate. Patients are well-hydrated, are taken off antihypertensive medication 2–5 days prior to the study according to the half life. Resting blood pressure is monitored. After a baseline study, the scan is repeated 30 minutes after administration of ACE inhibitor. Time–activity curves are generated from renal cortex and pelvis.

Results

A positive result is said to be present if there is a decrease in uptake and delayed clearance by the affected kidney on the post-captopril study compared to the baseline study or if there is exaggeration of the baseline asymmetry between the normal and abnormal kidney in patients with unilateral RAS **(Fig. 3)**.

The exact findings depend on the radioisotope used. 99mTc DTPA is mainly excreted by glomerular filtration and captopril causes a decrease in renal uptake and excretion. On the other hand OIH I^{131} and MAG 3 are excreted predominantly by tubular secretion so that captopril administration predominantly acts by prolonging transit

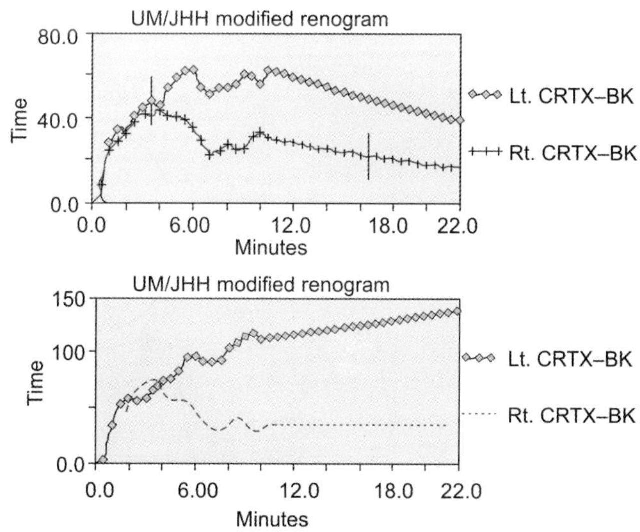

Fig. 3: Pre- (above) and postcaptopril (below) radionuclide renograms generated from cortical activity demonstrate asymmetric peak activity and cortical retension on the left side with exaggeration of abnormality on the postcaptopril scan.

time through the kidney. There is little difference reported in literature in the ability of various radiotracers to detect RVH. However, MAG 3 produces good images even in patients with impaired renal function.[42]

The overall sensitivity and specificity of the test exceeds 90% in most series with a few exceptions.[43] Advantages include low cost, relative reliability, and noninvasive nature. A positive captopril renography may suggest a cure or improvement in blood pressure after intervention. It may also be used in the follow up of patients after intervention.[44] Disadvantages and pitfalls include low sensitivity in patients with azotemia or underlying renal dysfunction and, in patients with bilateral RAS. Branch artery stenosis cannot be diagnosed. It has a low spatial resolution and provides functional not anatomic data. In patients who develop severe hypotension in response to captopril, bilateral symmetric parenchymal retention may be seen (false-positive). Symmetrical retention even in the absence of hypotension is usually a false-positive finding.[8,42] Presence of pelvic retention may complicate interpretation of cortical retention and scintigraphy must be interpreted with caution in the presence of pelvic retention.[45]

Ultrasound

A normal appearance of the kidneys on ultrasound does not exclude a significant unilateral or bilateral renal artery stenosis. Renal size and shape may be normal unless the stenosis is greater than 60% when a small decrease in size may be found.[46]

Color Doppler Flow Imaging (CDFI)

The advent of Doppler and more recently contrast-enhanced Doppler have provided important diagnostic tools in the evaluation of renal artery stenosis.[8]

Two approaches are used with Doppler ultrasound. The first is the direct visualization and interrogation of the stenotic segment of the renal artery. The second is an assessment of the arterial waveform distal to the stenosis within segmental renal vessels **(Fig. 4)**.

Direct Approach

This requires evaluation of the entire main renal artery, spectral traces are then obtained from areas of stenosis identified on color Doppler. The aorta is also interrogated and peak systolic velocity (PSV) obtained at the level of renal origins. An anterior or anterolateral approach usually allows insonation of both the arteries. A coronal approach can be used when bowel gas is present **(Fig. 5)**. The criteria used to diagnose significant stenosis or occlusion of a renal artery is as follows:[3,8,47]

- An increase in peak systolic velocity (Thresholds commonly applied in current literature to diagnose RAS include PSV (max) in the renal artery >150–180 cm/sec. **Fig. 6**).
- Renal artery/aortic ratio (RAR ratio) >3.5 calculated as:

$$\frac{\text{PSV max renal arteries}}{\text{PSV aorta at the origin of renal arteries}}$$

- Turbulent flow in the poststenotic area
- Visualization of the renal artery without detectable Doppler signal, a finding that indicates occlusion.

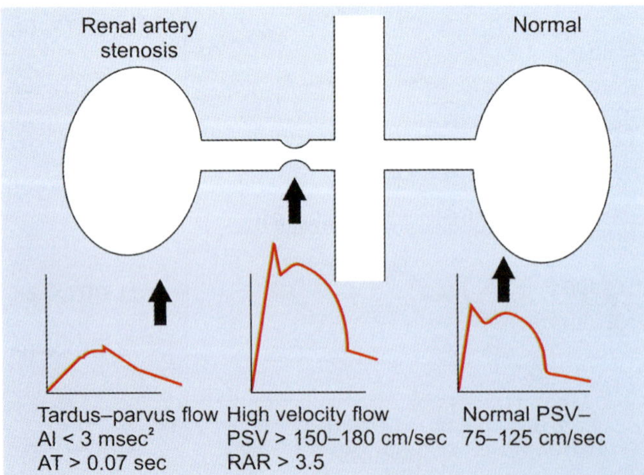

Fig. 4: Renal artery Doppler tracings showing the normal renal artery trace on the left side. On the right side high velocity at the site of stenosis and 'tardus–parvus' waveform is seen distal to the stenosis.

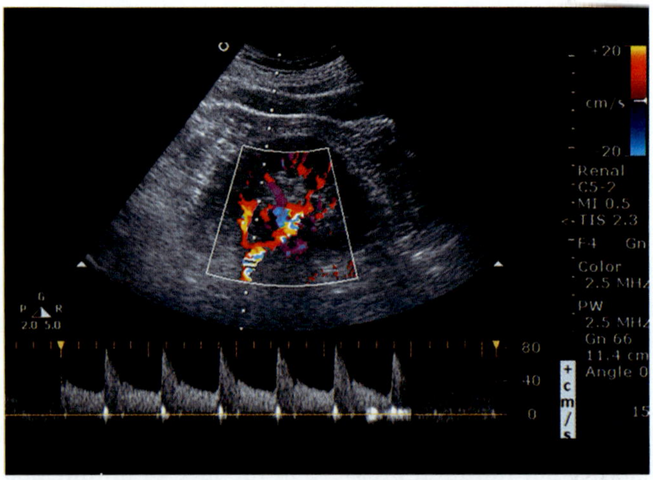

Fig. 5: Color Doppler image through coronal approach show normal spectral trace of main renal artey.

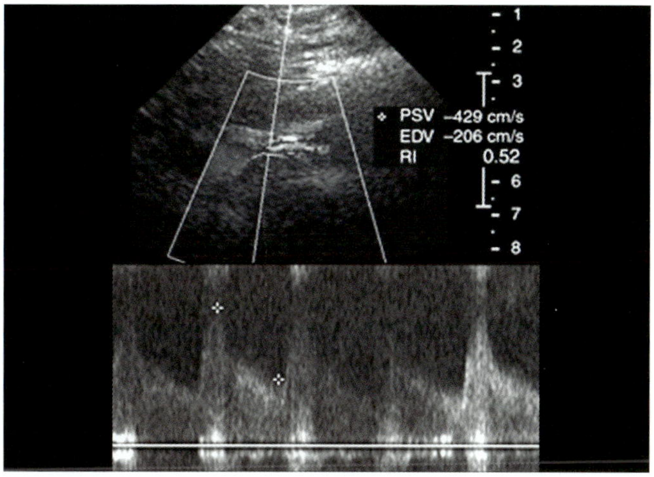

Fig. 6: Spectral trace at the site of stenosis of renal artery shows increased peak systolic velocities.

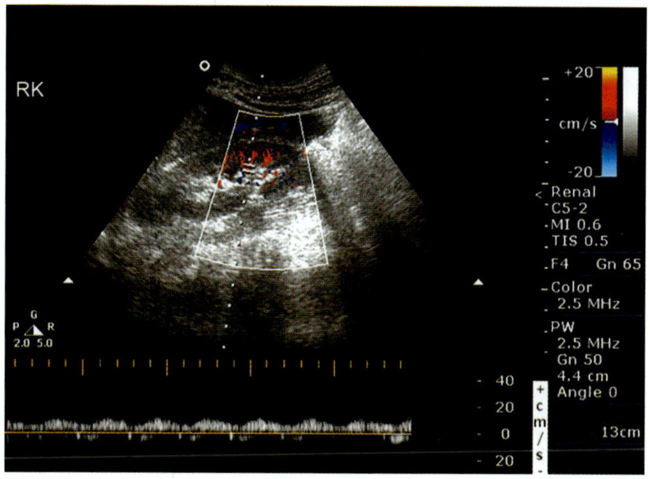

Fig. 7: Color Dopper image showing 'parvus–tardus' waveform in interlobar artery due to main renal artery stenosis.

Although theoretically simple in practice these measurements often cannot be obtained, as main renal arteries may not be visualized in up to 42% cases. The procedure is time consuming and operator dependent. Accessory renal arteries (present in upto 40% cases) may not be visualized. Branch artery stenosis cannot be diagnosed. In cases of renal artery occlusion collaterals may be sampled. The use of sonographic contrast media like Levovist has been found to enhance the visualization of main renal vessels resulting in higher technical success rates.

Indirect Approach

Arterial waveforms from the segmental renal arteries from the upper, mid and lower poles are evaluated. The normal waveform from these vessels shows a steep systolic upstroke with a peak in early systole referred to as early systolic peak (ESP). The early systolic acceleration seems to be the best predictor of RAS and should be measures along the initial portion of the systolic rise and should not include the late compliance peak.[48,49] In contrast the waveform in patients with RAS lacks both these features and is known as 'tardus-parvus' waveform. Tardus refers to the slowed systolic acceleration and parvus refers to the low amplitude of the systolic peak **(Fig. 7)**.

There are two quantitative measurements that are used (i) the acceleration time (AT) (ii) the acceleration index (AI). Acceleration time is the time from start of systole to peak systole and a value greater than 0.07 sec is significant. 'AI' is the slope of the systolic upstroke which is reduced to less than 3 m/sec^2 in significant RAS. Some authors have shown that simple pattern recognition of 'tardus-parvus' waveform is more accurate than calculation of 'AT' and 'AI'.[50] The waveform may also demonstrate a decrease in resistive index (RI) and pulsatility index.[51] Administration of captopril in individuals with significant RAS produces measurable changes in Doppler waveform which increases the degree of pulsus tardus and decreases the RI.[52]

These criteria only detect stenosis of greater than 70–80% reliably. The shape of the waveform is not simply related to the pressure drop across the stenosis but also compliance of renal arteries.[37] Coexisting parenchymal disease may also affect the waveform due to changes in peripheral resistance. The technique also cannot distinguish between high grade stenosis and complete occlusion with collateral flow. Tardus parvus waveform may also be produced by abdominal coarctation.[53]

Doppler sonography may also be used to predict the outcome of therapy for RAS.[54] A 'RI' of more than 80 probably identifies patient with RAS in whom angioplasty or surgery will not improve renal function or blood pressure.

The sensitivity of Doppler US when compared with DSA has varied significantly ranging from as high as 92% to as low as 50%. Recent studies indicate a specificity of 91–95%.[8]

CT Angiography

Computed tomography angiography (CTA) offers a noninvasive technique for obtaining angiographic images. The advent of spiral CT and more recently multidetector CT (MDCT) has revolutionized computed tomography and CTA. MDCT has made possible the acquisition of isotropic data with high spatial and temporal resolution;

this coupled with new softwares is providing angiograms comparable to catheter angiography. Data acquisition with MDCT is acquired craniocaudally with section thickness of 1mm with a pitch of 1.5 after an intravenous injection of 90–150 mL of contrast medium (300 mg I/mL) at the rate of 3–6 mL/sec using bolus tracking techniques.[36]

The axial images are reconstructed in multiple planes using multiplanar reconstruction (MPR), maximum intensity projection (MIP) or real time volume rendering techniques (VRT) for morphological evaluation of kidneys and main renal arteries **(Fig. 8)**.

The sensitivity of CTA in identifying main renal arteries has been 100%; accessory arteries are also almost always detected with any area of narrowing. The sensitivity and specificity for diagnosis of RAS has ranged between 90–95%[36, 55-57] CTA is more sensitive than Doppler ultrasound for detection of stenosis of main renal arteries (96 versus 63%) but specificity of the two techniques is similar (88 versus 89%).[44]

CTA can demonstrate the wall of the aorta unlike angiography which only visualizes the lumen of the vessel, important in cases of atherosclerosis **(Fig. 9)** and also aortoarteritis **(Fig. 10)** where the lumen may appear angiographically normal in places but may show vessel wall involvement in cross-sectional studies. It easily demonstrates the extent of plaque projecting into the vessel lumen, aiding in determining the form of intervention planned, such as angioplasty versus primary stent placement.[58] CTA has high efficacy for diagnosis of ostial stenosis—the most difficult place to evaluate during arteriography and improves the differentiation between ostial and truncal stenosis. MDCT CTA can also detect collaterals in the presence of renal artery occlusion **(Fig. 11)**. Unlike MR angiography, CTA can also be used to examine the patency of vessels that have been dilated by intravascular stents.[59] In a recent study MDCT produced interpretable multiplanar images of the renal artery even with a metallic stent in place and was adequate for determining stent patency; however, intrastent diameter was underestimated in most patients as compared to catheter angiography.[60]

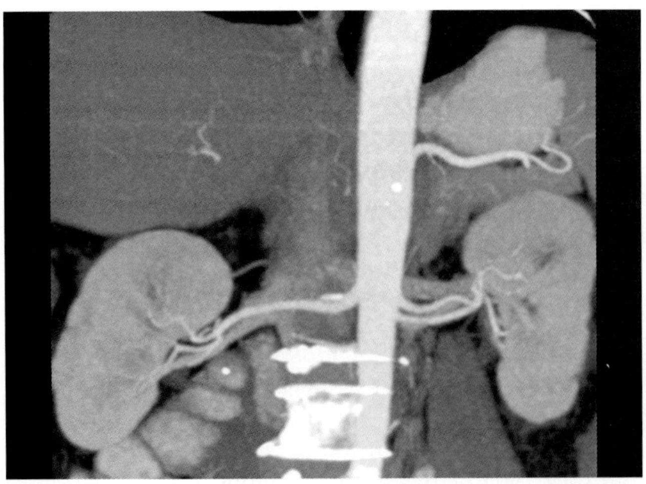

Fig. 8: MDCT angiographic image (MIP) showing normal caliber single renal artery on right side and two on left side.

Disadvantages with CTA include relatively high cost and use of large amount of iodinated contrast medium precluding its use in renal insufficiency. Mural calcification in the aorta or renal artery may result in overestimation of stenosis. In various series the overestimation of the renal artery stenosis varied from 3–7%.[57]

Magnetic Resonance Angiography

Magnetic resonance angiography (MRA) has the ability to visualize renal arteries non-invasively with or without the use of contrast medium. The CE-MRA is the preferred technique for the detection of RAS.[61] However, with the reports of nephrogenic systemic fibrosis the use of gadolinium is restricted for the patients having deranged renal functions.[37] In such cases noncontrast enhanced MR imaging of renal arteries should be done.[38]

It is essential to mention here that before analysis of renal arteries morphological assessment of kidneys in respect of their size, corticomedullary differentiation, and presence of any mass lesion or abnormalities of collecting system should be done.

Contrast-enhanced MRA (CE-MRA)

Recent advances in the magnetic resonance gradient hardware with availability of 3.0 T, acquisition of isotropic data with submillimeter resolution is allowing the detection of renal artery narrowing with high accuracy.[62,63] Moreover, it is now possible to demonstrate the functional consequences of RAS, such as a decline in renal perfusion and glomerular filtration.[64]

Intravenous gadolinium is used in a dose of 0.1–0.3 mmoles/kg with bolus tracking. With the advent of 3.0T the amount of contrast can be reduced because of increase in T1 of tissue. Entire acquisition is performed during a single breath hold. In patients unable to withhold breath for long time parallel imaging technology provides high resolution images with shorter acquisition times. Three-dimensional contrast MRA overcomes the limitations of noncontrast MRA. As a result renal arteries are assessed in their entirety, including the major segmental branch vessels, as well as small accessory renal arteries. In addition, speed, operator

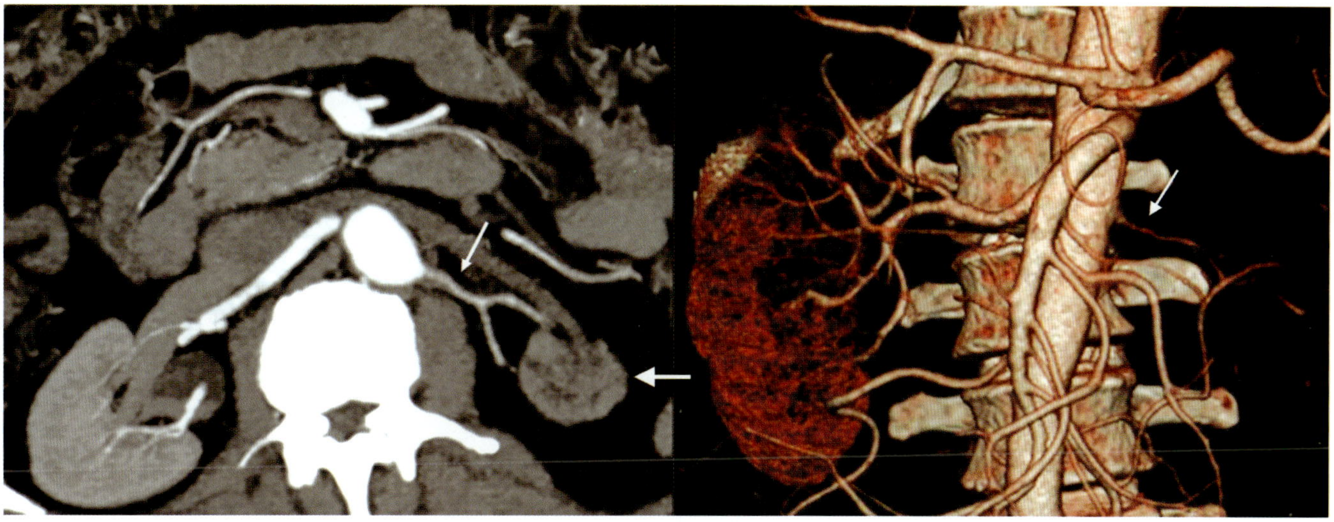

Fig. 9: CTA (MIP and VRT) images showing atherosclerotic narrowing of left renal artery (arrows) with asymmetric mural thickening renal artery near the ostium. Note atrophy of left kidney (thick arrow).

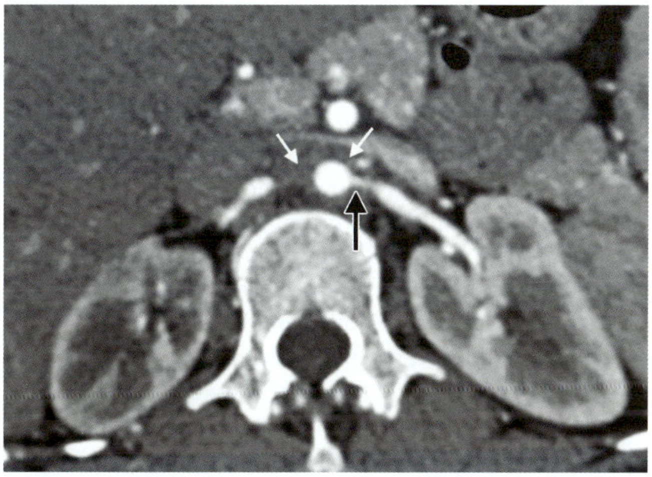

Fig. 10: Takayasu's aortoarteritis: CTA (MIP image) showing symmetric circumferential mural thickening of aorta at the origin of renal arteries (white arrows) with stenosis of renal arteries (black arrow).

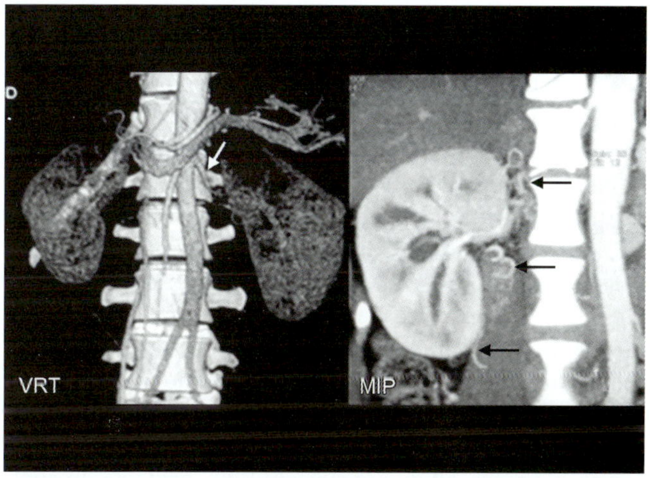

Fig. 11: CTA (VRT and MIP) images showing complete occlusion of right renal artery. The left renal artery in normal (white arrow). MIP image shows normal size of the right kidney and multiple arterial collaterals (black arrows) perfusing the kidney.

independence, high spatial and contrast resolution and lack of side effects have contributed to making 3D contrast MRA a well-suited screening alterative for detection of renovascular disease. The technique has sensitivities of 93–100% and a specificity of 90–100% **(Figs. 12A and B)**.

In several centers contrast enhanced MRA is complemented by 3D-PC acquisition. Areas of hemodynamically significant stenosis are detected by their associated turbulence seen as a signal void on 3D-PC images. The presence of a signal void at or immediately downstream from a stenosis suggests pressure drop across the stenosis. For 3D-PC MRA to be optimally sensitive to turbulent flow echo time should be approximately 8 ms and velocity encoded value (VENC) should be kept at 25–50 cm/sec.

The major advantages of MRA are absence of ionizing radiation, production of arteriographic images that unlike CTA are not affected by calcified plaques. Images can be viewed in multiple planes with facilities for temporal processing as well. Phase contrast studies can provide information about blood flow velocity also (as phase is related to time).

The drawbacks of MRA include its high cost and limited availability. Artifacts caused by motion and bowel peristalsis also tend to reduce usefulness of the study.

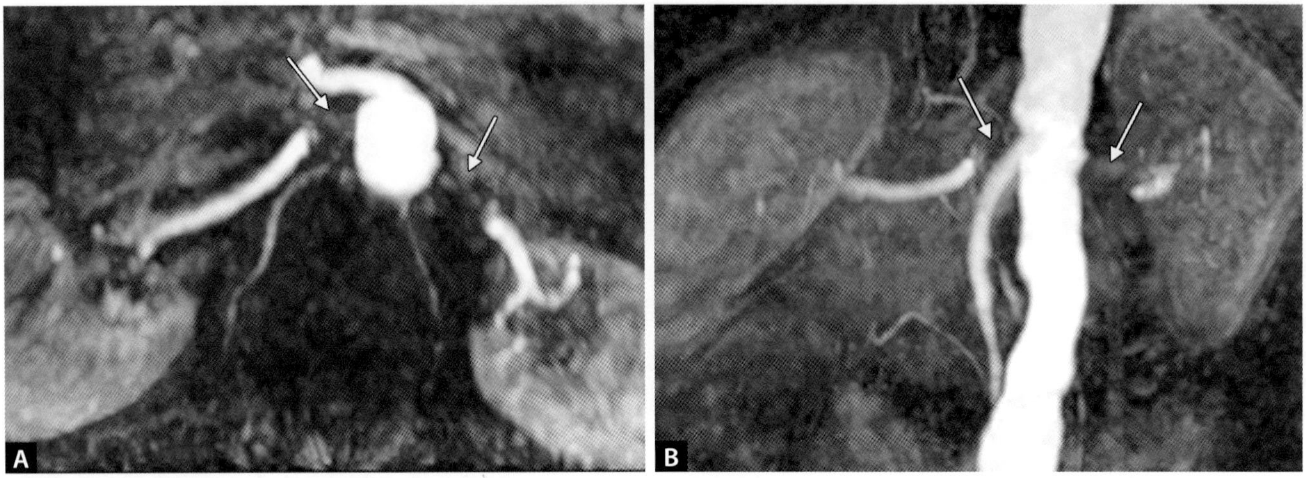

Figs. 12A and B: CE-MRA (MIP axial and coronal images) showing severe stenosis of bilateral renal arteries near origin (arrows)

The MRI is also being evaluated in acquiring the functional data that can provide comprehensive assessment of renal morphology and renal function prior to any intervention.[64] Dynamic contrast-enhanced (DCE)-MRI is fastly emerging technique in which fast repetitious imaging of the kidney is performed using first pass of the contrast agent. In the recently published series from different centers significant correlations between raising serum creatinine levels and decreasing renal perfusion parameters are found indicating that renal first pass perfusion may reflect, atleast to a certain degree, renal function.[63,65] In an another study significant reduction of the cortical perfusion and medullary perfusion and of the accumulation of contrast media in the medulla were found in patients with renal failure.[66] The DCE-MRI can evaluate the kidneys after the placement of stents which otherwise cannot be assessed due to susceptibility artifacts. In such situations demonstration of normal perfusion parameters proves the patency of stent.[63]

Noncontrast-enhanced MR Imaging of the Renal Arteries

Since the established link between gadolinium-based contrast agents and nephrogenic systemic fibrosis in patients suffering from severe renal insufficiency CE-MRA is not considered safe in such patients. Various noncontrast MRA techniques have evaluated, such as time of flight (TOF), phase contrast (PC), steady-state free-procession (SSFP), and arterial spin labeling (ASL).

Time of Flight-Magnetic Resonance Angiography (TOF MRA)

Signal in TOF MRA is produced by unsaturated blood flowing into the plane of imaging (flow related enhancement). TOF MRA is not an useful technique for the evaluation of renal arteries because of the following reasons:

- It tends to overestimate the degree of stenosis, in particular 2D techniques do not compensate for vessel tortuosity and therefore tend to overestimate vessels stenosis,
- Loss of signal in slow flow when vessel in oriented in axial plane (in-plane saturation),
- Inherently a slow technique requiring several minutes, causing breathing related degradation or extremely long scan times for signal averaging, and
- Poor visualization of the distal arterial segment where flow is slow.

Phase-contrast (PC) MRA

Phase-contrast (PC) MRA depicts not only the morphologic nature of a stenosis, but also provides quantitative analysis of flow dynamics in RAS.[67] Combining phase contrast with cardic gating, a 2D velocity map can be obtained, which is termed as "quantitative" or "q" flow.[68] With this flow maps similar to Doppler ultrasound can be generated and analyzed.

Steady-state Free Precession Magnetic Resonance Angiography

Three-dimensional steady-state precession (SSFP) is the most promising noncontrast bright blood technique for evaluation of renal arteries as it is intrinsically fast, high in signal-to-noise ratio (SNR), and flow compensated in all the three axis.[38] In the recent reported studies this sequence has 100% sensitivity and 100% negative predictive value.[69-71] Based on these studies SSFP either breath hold or navigator-gated can be performed as a first line MRA technique to rule out RAS especially in patients in risk of NSF. If SSFP is negative for high grade RAS (>50%), RAS can be excluded without using any gadolinium based contrast agents, vie-a-versa if SSFP is positive, then further studies (CE-MRI, DSA, CTA) can be done for better delineation of stenosis.[38]

Arterial Spin Labeling

Arterial spin labeling (ASL) uses blood as an endogenous contrast agent to obtain angiograms with an advantage to obtain tissue perfusion as well. The perfusion parameters are being investigated and initial reports suggest a good correlation with scintigraphy.[72]

Renal Angiography

Conventional angiography (or digital subtraction angiography) is the gold standard against which all other modalities for diagnosing renal artery stenosis are compared. Intraarterial DSA results in reliable depiction of main renal arteries and branch vessels, with less contrast material and with use of smaller lumen catheters than conventional angiography. Angiography plays a limited role as the preliminary screening test for RAS; however, all patients proceeding to percutaneous treatment of RAS initially undergo diagnostic angiography as part of the procedure.[8]

Angiographic evaluation should include aortography and bilateral selective renal arteriography. The initial aortogram is necessary to evaluate the renal artery ostia, identifying accessory renal arteries and avoid mistaking guide wire induced arterial spasm for fixed disease.

Flush aortography is usually adequate to demonstrate main renal arteries and any proximal renal stenosis. When intrarenal or branch artery stenosis are suspected selective injections are necessary. Because the origin of right renal artery is anterolateral and left renal artery is posterolateral an ostial lesion may be missed on an AP aortogram due to overlap by the opacified aorta, superimposition of intrarenal vessels may also mask stenosis. Depending on the site of stenosis oblique/lateral view, cranial/caudal angulation or magnification views may be required to optimally delineate stenosis.[73-75]

Features of RAS on Arteriography

Atherosclerosis produces irregular circumferential or eccentric narrowing of the ostium or proximal third of the renal arteries. Bilateral disease is common and infrarenal aortic involvement usually exists **(Fig. 13)**.

FMD typically involves middle to distal renal arteries and less commonly intrarenal branches. Bilateral disease may be seen in about two-third of cases. The right kidney is affected more commonly than the left. The classic appearance of the common medial fibroplasia type of FMD is a string of beads. Other forms may show different morphologies as already discussed. With FMD aorta is usually disease free.

The morphological pattern of involvement in aortoarteritis shows racial and geographical differences.[76] In Japan thoracic aortic involvement is more common and neck vessels are most often involved.[77] In most other Asian countries abdominal aorta is most often affected particularly renal and subclavian arteries.[76] Pulmonary artery involvement is less frequently seen in Indian patients. Steno-occlusive lesions are the most common type of lesions found in the north Indian population, dilating lesions are less common.[76]

After a stenosis has been identified, its hemodynamic significance must be proved by one of the following criteria.[78]

- Reduction in luminal diameter ≥75%
- Systolic pressure gradient across the stenosis >15–25 mm Hg or >20% of aortic systolic pressure
- Evidence of collateral circulation into distal vessel
- Pharmacologic manipulation of collateral vessel flow (epinephrine restricts flow to the kidney and makes collaterals more apparent).

A stenosis with 50–75% reduction in luminal diameter may be hemodynamically significant but in such cases other signs must be sought. Pressure gradients are the most accurate indicator of hemodynamic significance.

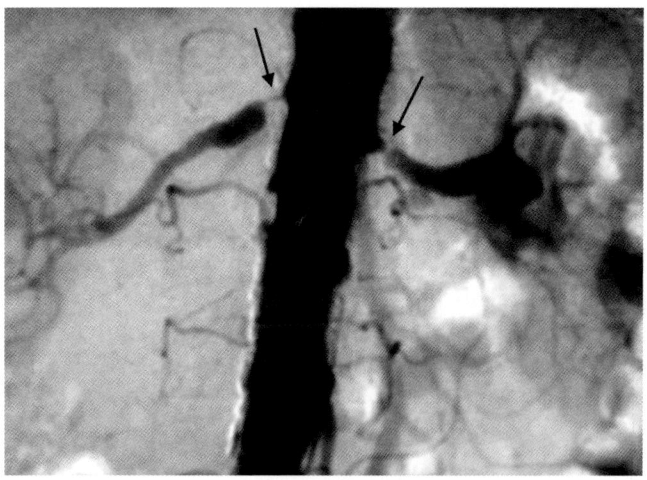

Fig. 13: DSA aortogram showing atherosclerotic stenosis (arrows) of bilateral renal arteries.

Advantages of conventional angiography/DSA include the high resolution of the technique making it the only modality capable of adequately visualizing branch renal artery stenosis. Pressure gradients can be measured to assess hemodynamic significance and selective renal catheterization may be followed by appropriate intervention in the same sitting.

Angiography is, however, not without limitations. It is expensive and invasive and carries the added risks that come with the use of iodinated contrast. Angiography only provides intraluminal information; no intramural information is gained about the vessel wall or plaques. There is a low but definite risk of complications which may be at the puncture site such as hematoma, pseudoaneurysm or at the level of renal arteries because of selective catheterization. The most serious of these are vessel dissection, arterial puncture and cholesterol embolization leading to renal failure. Transient decrease in renal function may occur in upto 5% patients.

In the future intravascular ultrasound or angioscopy may be useful in high-risk patients.[35,79]

TREATMENT

Atherosclerotic Disease

There are in principle three modes of treatment for renovascular hypertension—medical therapy, surgery and angioplasty. An antihypertensive drug by lowering the arterial pressure may further reduce renal perfusion pressure causing renal damage hence some type of revascularization is preferred.

Percutaneous Transluminal Renal Angioplasty (PTRA) and Stenting

Since PTRA was first reported by Gruntzig[80] in 1978 there has been a continuous refinement in technique and it has generally been accepted as a valuable first line therapy for RVH. Renal artery stenting has further extended the role of PTRA and both techniques can be considered complementary. Percutaneous techniques offer a minimally invasive alternative to surgery and properly performed are not preclusive of future surgical treatment.[81]

PTRA is best suited to discrete tight concentric, short segment stenosis located away from ostium and branches of renal arteries. Eccentric, long segment and calcified lesions, occlusion in tortuous vessels, stenosis adjacent to an aneurysm and occlusion or stenosis with a thrombus increase the risk of complications and reduce the likelihood of success.

Indications: Percutaneous revascularisation of renal arteries is indicated for (i) refractory hypertension, (ii) preservation of renal function, (iii) prevention of 'flash' pulmonary edema especially in patients on calcium channel blockers, and (iv) preservation of renal artery patency.

PTRA and stenting are justified in selected patients who have both normal renal function and normal blood pressure because of the natural history of renal artery stenosis to progress and ultimately result in impaired renal function.[82]

Before PTRA is performed the salvage ability of the procedure must be established. The commonly used criteria are (i) residual function-single kidney GFR by radionuclide studies, (ii) kidney size of 8–9 cm, (iii) renal biopsy showing preservation of glomeruli and tubule, and (iv) presence of collateral circulation to intrarenal vessels confirmed by arteriography. Revascularization is usually not beneficial in patients with severe renal failure (S creatinine >4.0 mg/dL).[78]

Renal Artery Stenting

Angioplasty failure is an absolute indication for stenting. The criteria for angioplasty failure include residual stenosis of more than 30%, residual aortorenal pressure gradient of >20 mm Hg, acute occlusive, flow limiting dissection flap and late restenosis (recurrent stenosis >50%).[82]

In selected patients in whom the risk of intervention or anatomic considerations make a repeat procedure in the future unlikely primary stenting is justifiable. It should be the technique of choice for ostial atherosclerotic RAS[83] **(Figs. 14A to C)**.

Complications: Complication rate in PTRA varies from 3 to 6%. Complications include those related to the arteriographic procedure and those due to angioplasty and stenting.[81,82] These include renal artery injury, guidewire perforation of kidney, flow limiting renal artery dissection, renal artery thrombosis, renal artery rupture.

Stent-related complications include stent malposition, misdeployment of stent, endovascular infection, and cholesterol embolization.

Outcome: Success in renal revascularisation can be judged by the technical success of angioplasty and by the clinical response.[84,85]

Angiography is considered to be technically successful if the residual stenosis is <30%, at least 50% enlargement in arterial diameter as compared to preangioplasty diameter and pressure gradient of less than 20 mm Hg or reduction in pressure gradient by at least 15 mm Hg from the pretreatment gradient.

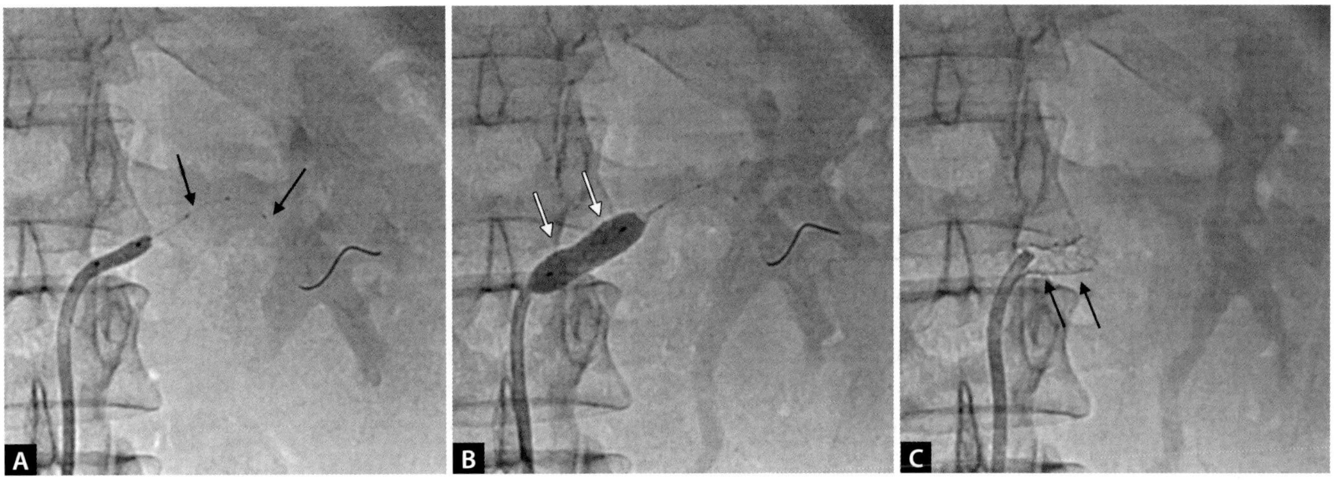

Figs. 14A to C: Stenting of left renal artery stenosis: The guidewire (arrows) is negotiated across the stenotic segment (A). The balloon expandable stent is deployed across the stenosis and inflated (arrows) (B), final position of the stent across the stenosis (arrows) (C). *Courtesy:* Department of Cardiology, PGIMER, Chandigarh, India.

Clinical results are judged as cured: diastolic blood pressure <90 mm Hg without medication, improvement: equal or reduced medication required to maintain the diastolic blood pressure below 90 mm Hg or a 15 mm Hg reduction in blood pressure with the same or reduced number of medicines, and failed: no change in blood pressure after the procedure.

In patients treated for renal salvage a reduction in serum creatinine levels of ≥20% may be considered successful treatment.

The results of PTRA depend on the type of lesion, indication for treatment, and factors such as age, coexistent essential hypertension and nephrosclerosis.

The results in FMD are uniformly good. Technical success is achieved in 90–100% patients. Hypertension is cured or improved in 98% patients.[82] Intimal FMD may require much greater pressures than medial fibroplasia type of FMD. Restenosis is uncommon in these patients and primary patency at 15 months is 92%.

For atherosclerotic lesions both angiographic and clinical results for nonostial stenosis are superior to those for ostial stenosis (within 2–10 mm of aortic lumen). Technical success occurs in 75–95% cases, although some authors have reported lower rates of 43% for nonostial lesions and 29% for ostial lesions. Long-term clinical benefit is seen in 76% patients with ostial lesions and 83% patients with nonostial lesions.[86] Van der Van et al. showed that PTA with stenting improved the outcome for ostial lesions.[83]

Lesser success can be expected in patients with bilateral RAS, generalized atherosclerosis, with heavily calcified or segmental artery lesion.

For renal salvage, the results are less favorable and improvement is seen in 40–60% cases.

Future Management of RAS

A paradigm shift in thinking in the treatment of RAS is being undertaken worldwide as conventional wisdom to dilate or stent the renal arteries having stenosis more than 50% was challenged in 2000, where no significant change was found in patients who had RAS and were treated either by medical antihypertensive therapy and angioplasty.[33] Based on this observation large trials such as STAR (The Dutch benefit of stent placement and blood pressure and lipid lowering for the prevention of progression of renal dysfunction caused by atherosclerotic ostial stenosis of renal artery) with 2 years follow-up, ASTRAL study (The large-scale angioplasty and stent for renal artery stenosis), CORAL study (Cardiovascular outcomes with renal atherosclerotic lesions) were undertaken and their final outcomes are expected soon.[87-89]

Takayasu's Arteritis/Nonspecific Aortoarteritis

The widespread nature of the disease and complexity of pathological changes in the vessel wall make surgical revascularization difficult. Graft occlusion is also common. These problems make percutaneous revascularization techniques extremely attractive.

Specific technical difficulties may be encountered during PTRA for aortoarteritis because of the tough noncompliant nature of the stenosis which is difficult to cross and resists repeated prolonged balloon dilatation. Patients may also develop hypotension and backache during the procedure.[85]

However, reports have shown high rate of technical success and frequently good clinical response.

Following angioplasty for any cause at least 3–6 months of follow up is required to assess durability of clinical response.

Surgical Therapy

Surgical revascularization is now indicated only in situations where PTRA fails or is contraindicated. Techniques include aortorenal, lienorenal, ileorenal arterial bypass, nephrectomy and autorenal transplantation.

Renal Artery Stenosis in Children[27,90]

Although RAS is uncommon in children the incidence is much higher in children with hypertension than in adults. About 4–20% of children with hypertension have RAS.

Causes

Fibromuscular dysplasia: The classical string of beads appearance is rarely seen with intimal fibroplasia being the most common type of lesion. The lesions are more often found in boys unlike adults. Branch artery stenosis is also more common.

Neurofibromatosis stenosis of proximal renal artery: These may be associated with hypoplasia of abdominal aorta.

Nonspecific aortoarteritis and middle aortic syndrome: They are other important causes.

Because of the higher incidence of RAS in children with hypertension patients with a strong clinical suspicion often undergo DSA.

PTRA is being used with increasing frequency in children; however, the success rate is lower than adults for two reasons— smaller size of vessels and more frequent vasospasm make children more difficult to angiogram and dilate. Adult FMD and atherosclerosis respond well to PTRA while children have a more fibrotic process that cannot be adequately dilated.

CONCLUSION

Diagnosis of renovascular hypertension is complex, because of the low prevalence and lack of strong causal relationship between renal artery stenosis and renovascular hypertension. Hence main aim should not to detect RAS of 50% or more in diameter but to identify stenosis which likely to get benefit from revascularization. Another concern is avoidance of unnecessary diagnostic angiography, especially in patients with renal failure.

Patients with a strong clinical suspicion are most often investigated by captopril renal scintigraphy or Doppler ultrasound. In good hands Doppler ultrasound proves to be cost effective with results near equal to scintigraphy. Patients with positive results may proceed directly to noninvasive angiography. However, patients with bilateral RAS or patient with significant renal impairment in addition to RVH may be missed if renal scintigraphy is the only screening test used.

The choice of the second screening test depends on local availability, expertise and patient's renal functional status. CTA/CE-MRA may be used, but after the insurgence of nephrogenic systemic fibrosis (NSF) in patients with deranged renal functions gadolinium based contrast agents should be avoided and so are the iodinated contrast agents for CTA. In such situations new MRI techniques, such as SSFP, ASL is being investigated with satisfactory results.

Angiography remains the gold standard for diagnosis. However, with advances in noninvasive imaging particularly MRA and CTA, angiography may only be necessary as a prerequisite for percutaneous intervention.

REFERENCES

1. Dunnick NR, Sfakianakis GN. Screening for renovascular hypertension. Radiol Clin North Am. 1991;29:497-50.
2. Silverman J, Friedman M, Van Allan R. Detection of main renal artery stenosis using phase contrast Cine MR angiography. AJR. 1996;166:1131-7.
3. Soulez G, Oliva VL, Turpin S, et al. Imaging of Renovascular Hypertension: Respective Values of Renal Scintigraphy, Renal Doppler US, and MR Angiography. Radiographics. 2000;20:1355-68.
4. Heaton CM, Farber JM. Magnetic resonance imaging of the renal arteries. Seminars in Interventional Radiology 2001;18:3-10.
5. National High Blood Pressure Education Program Working Group 1995 update on chronic renal failure and renovascular hypertension. Arch Intern Med. 1996;156:1938-43.
6. Rimmer JM, Gennai FJ. Atherosclerotic renovascular disease and progressive renal failure. Ann Intern Med. 1993;118: 712-9.
7. Jacobson HR. Ischemic renal disease: An overlooked clinical entity? Kidney Int. 1988;34:729-43.
8. Ahmad I, Ray CE. Diagnosing renovascular hypertension. Seminars in Interventional Radiology. 2001;18:11-21.
9. Pickering TG, Blumenfeld JD, Laragh JH. Renovascular hypertension and ischemic nephropathy. In: Brenner BM, ed. The Kidney. Philadelphia: WB Saunders, 1996. pp.2106-25.
10. Textor SC, Wilcox CS. Renal artery stenosis: A common, treatable cause of renal failure? Annu Rev Med. 2001;52:421-42.
11. Chade AR, Rodriguez-Porcel M Grande JP, et al. Distinct renal injury in early atherosclerosis and renovascular disease. Circulation. 2002;106:1165-71.

12. Chade AR, Rodriguez-Porcel M, Grande JP,et al. Mechanisms of renal structural alterations in combined hypercholesterolemia and renal artery stenosis. Arterioscler Thromb Vasc Biol. 2003;23:1295-01.
13. Nath KA, Croatt AJ, Haggard JJ, et al. Renal response to repetitive exposure to heme proteins: Chronic injury induced by an acute insult. Kidney Int. 2000;57:2423-33.
14. Vesna D. Garovic, MD, Stephen C, et al. Renovascular Hypertension and Ischemic Nephropathy Circulation 2005;112:1362-74.
15. Chugh KS, Jain S, Sakhuja V. Renovascular hypertension due to Takayasu's arteritis among Indian patients. Quarterly J Med. 1992;85:833-43.
16. Sharma S, Khosla A, Rajani M, et al. Coronary arteriographic profile in young north Indian patients with coronary heart disease. Asian Medical Journal.1989;32: 531-37.
17. Ram CV, Clagett GP, Radford LR. Renovascular hypertension, Semin Nephrol. 1995;15:152-74.
18. Schreiber MJ, Pohl MA, Navick MC. The natural history of atherosclerotic and fibrous renal disease. Urol Clin North Am. 1984;11:383-92.
19. Jaff MR, Olin JW. Atherosclerotic stenosis of the renal arteries. Tex Heart Inst J. 1998;25:34-9.
20. Harrison EG Jr, Mc Cormack LJ. Pathologic classification of renal arterial disease in renovascular hypertension. Mayo Clin Proc. 1971; 46:161-7.
21. Luescher TF, Lic JT, Stanson AW: Arterial fibromuscular dysplasia. Mayo Clin Proc. 1987;62:931.
22. Matsunaga N, Hayashi K, Sakamoto L, et al. Takayasu arteritis: Protean radiologic manifestations and diagnosis. Radiographics. 1997;17:579-94.
23. Keer GS. Takayasu's arteritis rheum. Dis Clin North Am. 1995;21:1041-58.
24. Lagneau P, Michel JB. Renovascular hypertension and Takayasu's disease. J Urol. 1985;134:876-9.
25. Conolly JE, Wilson SE. Middle aortic syndrome: Distal thoracic and abdominal coarctation, a disorder with multiple etiologies. J Am Coll Surg. 2002;194:774-81.
26. Sumboonnanonda A. Middle aortic syndrome clinical radiological findings. Arch Dis Child. 1992;64:501-5.
27. Greene JF, Fitzwater J, Burgers J. Arterial lesions associated with neurofibromatosis. Am J Clin Pathol. 1974;62:481-7.
28. Harden PN. Effect of renal artery stenting on progression of renovascular renal failure. Lancet. 1997;349:1133-6.
29. Van Jaarsveld BC. The Dutch renal artery stenosis intervention cooperative (DRASTIC) study. Abstract presented at the Interventional Society of Hypertension meeting, Amsterdam, The Netherlands, August 1998.
30. Preston RA, Epstein M. Ischemic renal disease: An emerging cause of chronic renal failure and end stage disease. J Hypertens. 1997;15:1365-77.
31. Dorros G, Jaff M, Muthiak L, et al. Four year-year follow-up of Palmaz-Schatz stent revascularization as treatment for atherosclerotic renal artery stenois. Circulation. 1998;98:642-7.
32. Watson PS, Hadjipetrou P, Cox SV, et al. Effect of renal artery stenting on renal function and size in patients with atherosclerotic renovascular disease. Circulation. 2000;102:1671-7.
33. van Jaarsveld BC, Krijen P, Pieterman H, et al. The effect of balloon angioplasty on hypertension in atherosclerotic renal-artery stenosis. Dutch Renal Artery Stenosis Intervention Cooperative Study Group. N Engl J Med. 2000;342:1007-14.
34. Huot SJ, Hansson JH, Dey H, et al. Utility of captopril renal scans for detecting renal artery stenosis. Arch Intern Med. 2002;162:1981-4.
35. De Scheerder I, De Man F, Herregods MC, et al. Intra-vascular ultrasound versus angiography for measurement of luminal diameters in normal and diseased coronary arteries. AM Heart J. 1994;127:243-51.
36. Willmann JK, Wildermuth S, Roos JE, et al. Aortoiliac and renal arteries: Prospective intraindividual comparison of contrast-enhanced three-dimensional MR angiography and multi-detector row CT angiography. Radiology. 2003;226:798-811.
37. Grobner T. Gadolinium. A specific trigger for the development of nephrogenic fibrosing dermopathy and nephrogenic systemic fibrosis? Nephrol Dial Transplant. 2006;21:1104-8.
38. Potthast S, Maki JH. Non-contrast-enhanced MR angiography of the renal arteries. Magn Reson Imaging N Am. 2008; 16:573-84.
39. Dellegrottaglie S, Sanz J, Rajajagopalan S. Technology insight: Clinical role of magnetic resonance angiography in the diagnosis and management of renal artery stenosis. Nat Clin Pract Cardiovasc Med. 2006;3:329-38.
40. Mitty HA, Shapiro RS, Parsons RB, et al. Renovascular Hypertension. Radiol Clin North Am. 1994;21:227-34.
41. Majd M, Potter BM, Guzzetta PC. Effect of captopril on efficacy of renal scintigraphy in detection of renal artery stenosis (abstract). J Nucl Med. 1983;24:23.
42. Fine EJ. Diuretic Renography and Angiotensin Converting Enzyme inhibitor renography. Radiol Clin North Am. 2001;39:979-95.
43. Van Jaarsrel B, Krijnen P, Derks F. The place of renal scintigraphy in diagnosis and treatment of renal artery stenosis, fifteen years clinical experience. Arch Intern Med. 1997;157:226-34.
44. Nally JV, Barton DP. Contemporary approach to diagnosis and evaluation of renovascular hypertension. Urol Clin North Am. 2001;28:781-91.
45. Krijnen P, Dei MY, Claessens RA. Interobserver agreement on captopril renography for assessing renal vascular disease. J Nucl Med. 2002;43:380-7.
46. Gutzman RP, Zierler RE, Issacson JA. Renal atrophy and arterial stenosis: A prospective study with duplex ultrasound. Hypertension. 1994;23:346-50.
47. Haan DC, Kroon AA, Flobbe K. Renovascular disease in patients with hypertension: Detection with duplex ultrasound. J Hum Hypertens. 2002;16:501-7.

48. Kliewer MA, Tupler RH, Carroll BA, et al. Renal artery stenosis: Analysis of Doppler waveform parameters and tardus-parvus pattern. Radiology. 1993;189:779-87.
49. Oliva VL, Soulez G, Lesage D, et al. Detection of renal artery stenosis with Doppler sonography before and after administration of captopril: Value of early systolic rise. AJR Am J Roentgenol. 1998;170:169-75.
50. Stavros AT, Packer SH, Yakes WF. Segmental stenosis of the renal artery Pattern recognition of the tardus and parvus abnormalities with duplex sonography. Radiology. 1992;184:487-92.
51. Schwerk B, Restrepo K, Stellwaag W. Renal artery stenosis grading with image directed Doppler US evaluation of renal resistive index. Radiology. 1996;190:785-90.
52. Rene PC, Oliva VI, Rao TB. Renal artery stenosis evaluation of Doppler US after inhibition of angiotensin converting enzyme with captopril. Radiology. 1995;196:675-9.
53. Bude O, Rubin M. Detection of renal artery stenosis with Doppler sonography: It is more complicated than originally though? Radiology. 1995;196:612-3.
54. Radermacher J, Charan A, Bleck J. Use of Doppler ultrasonography to predict the outcome of therapy for renal artery stenosis. N Engl J Med. 2001;344:410-6.
55. Olbricht CT, Paul K, Prokop M. Minimally invasive diagnosis of renal artery stenosis by spiral computed tomography angiography. Kidney Int. 1995;48:1332-7.
56. Galanski M, Prokop M, Charan A. Renal artery stenosis: Spiral CT angiography. Radiology. 1993;189:185-92.
57. Kaatce R, Beek F, Lange E. Renal artery stenosis detection and quantification with spiral CT angiography versus optimised digital substraction angiography. Radiology. 1997;205:121-7.
58. Halpern EJ, Rutter CM, Gardiner GA Jr. Comparison of Doppler US and CT angiography for evaluation of renal artery stenosis. Acta Radiol. 1998;5:524-32.
59. Harish A, Khatri P, Priyadarshini H, et al. Accuracy of 64-slice coronary CT angiography in predicting%age diameter stenosis. Indian Heart J. 2008;60:296-301.
60. Behar JV, Nelson RC, Zidar JP, et al. Thin-section multi detector CT angiography of renal artery stents. AJR. 2002;178:1155-9.
61. Schoenberg SO, Prince MR, Knopp MV, et al. Renal MR angiography. Magn Reson Imaging N Am. 1998;6:351-70.
62. Leiner T. Magnetic resonance angiography of abdominal and lower extremity vascukature. Top Magn Reson Imaging. 2005;16:21-66.
63. Michaely HJ, Sourbron S, Dietrich O et al. Functional renal imaging: An overview. Abdom Imaging. 2006. [epub ahead of print]
64. Leiner T, Michaely H. Advances in contrast-enhanced MR angiography of the renal arteries. Magn Reson Imaging N Am. 2008;16:561-72.
65. Michoux N, Montet X, Pechere A, et al. Parametric and quantitative analysis of MR renographic curves for assessing the functional behavior of the kidney. Eur J Radiol. 2005;54:124-35.
66. Michaely HJ, Herrmann KA, Nael K, et al. Functional renal imaging: Nonvascular renal disease. Abdom Imaging. 2007;32:1-16.
67. Debatin JF, Ting RH, Wegmuller H, et al. Renal artery blood flow: Quantitation with phase contrast MR imaging with and without breath holding. Radiology. 1994;190:371-8.
68. Schoenberg SO, Knopp MV, Londy F, et al. Morphologic and functional magnetic resonance imaging of renal artery stenosis: a multireader tricenter study. J Am Soc Nephrol. 2002;12:158-69.
69. Herborn CU, Watkins DM, Runge VM, et al. Renal arteries: comparison of steady-state free procession MR angiography and contrast-enhanced MR angiography. Radiology. 2006; 239:263-8.
70. Spuentrup E, Manning WJ, Bornert P, et al. Renal arteries: Navigator-gated balanced fast field-echo projection MR angiography with aortic spin labeling: Initial experience. Radiology. 2002; 225:589-96.
71. Katoh M, Buecker A, Stuber M, et al. Free-breathing renal MR angiography with steady-state free-precession (SSFP) and slab-selective spin inversion: Initial results. Kidney Int. 2004;66:1272-8.
72. Michaely HJ, Schoenberg SO, Ittrich C, et al. Renal disease: Value of functional magnetic resonance imaging with flow and perfusion measurements. Invest Radiol. 2004;39:698-705.
73. Verschuyl EJ, Kaalec R, Beek FJA. Renal artery origins best angiographic projection angles. Cardio Vasc Radiol. 1997;205:115-20.
74. Gerlock AJ, Goncharenki V, Oplis M, et al. Right posterior oblique: The projection of choice in aortography of hypertensive patients. Radiology. 1978;127:45-8.
75. Harrington DP, Levin DC, Garnic JC, et al. Compound angulation for the angiographic evaluation of renal artery stenosis. Radiology. 1083;146:829-31.
76. Sharma S, Rajani M, Talwar KK. Angiographic morphology in non specific aortoarteritis (Takayasu's arteritis) a study of 126 patients from north India. Cardiovasc Intervent Radiol. 1992;15:160-5.
77. Yamato M, Ceeky JW, Hiramatsu K, et al. Takayasu's arteritis; radiographic and angiographic findings in 59 patients. Radiology. 1986;161:329-34.
78. Valji K. Vascular and interventional radiology. Renal Arteries and Veins. WB Saunders. 1999;154-81.
79. Caramella N, Bisogni C, Laiolo E. Detection of accessory renal arteries with virtual vascular endoscopy of the aorta. Cardiovasc Intervent Radiol. 1999;22:1-6.
80. Gruntzig A, Khulmann K, Vetterr W. Treatment of renovascular hypertension with percutaneous transluminal dilatation of renal artery stenosis. Lancet. 1978;1:801-2.
81. Miller G, Ford K, Braun S. Percutaneous transluminal angioplasty versus surgery for renovascular hypertension. AJR. 1985;144:447-50.
82. Sanctis JTD. Renal artery Angioplasty and stenting. Seminars in Interventional Radiology. 2001;18: 23-35.

83. Van de Ver P, Kaatie R. Geutler Arterial stenting and balloon angioplasty in ostial atherosclerotic renovascular disease: A randomised trial. Lancet. 1999;353:282-6.
84. Sharma S, Saxena A, Talwar KK. Renal artery stenosis caused by nonspecific aortoarteritis (Takayasu's disease): Results of treatment with percutaneous transluminal angioplasty. AJR. 1992;158:417-22.
85. Martin LG, Cork RD, Kaufman SL. Long-term results of angioplasty in 110 patients with renal artery stenosis. J Vasc Interv Radiol. 1992;3:619.
86. Eldrup-Horgensen J, Harvey R, Sampson L. Should percutaneous transluminal renal artery angioplasty be applied to ostial renal artery atherosclerosis? J Vasc Surg. 1995;21:909-15.
87. Bax L, Mali WP, Buskens E, et al. The benefit of stent placement and blood pressure and lipid lowering for the prevention of progression of renal dysfunction caused by Atherosclerotic ostial stenosis of the renal artery. The STAR-study: rationale and study design. J Nephrol. 2003;16:807-12.
88. Mistry S, Ives N, Harding J, et al. Angioplasty and stent for renal artery lesions (ASTRAL trial): Rationale, methods and results so far. J Hum Hyperten. 2007;21:511-5.
89. Murphy TP, Cooper CJ, Dworkin LD, et al. The cardiovascular outcomes with renal atherosclerotic lesions (COREL) study: Rationale and methods. J Vasc Inter Radiol. 2005;16:1295-300.
90. Robinson L, Yedroye W, Reidy J. Saxton II Renal artery stenosis in children. Clin Radiol. 1991;44:376-82.

CHAPTER 113

Renal Parenchymal Disease and Renal Failure

Anupam Lal, Hina Arif Mumtaz

INTRODUCTION

Disorders of renal function are ubiquitous in contemporary practice of medicine. Kidney disease manifestations may vary from complete asymptomatic cases to life threatening emergencies. Insight into the causes and consequences of medical renal disease has progressively increased over the last decade, and radiological imaging has played a pivotal role in this improved understanding.

DEFINITION AND CLASSIFICATION OF RENAL FAILURE

The term renal failure encompasses the spectrum of diseases from acute and reversible to chronic and irreversible. It is broadly divided into two categories:

Acute Renal Failure

This is defined as a rapid deterioration in renal function characterized by progressive azotemia (best measured by serum creatinine) which may or may not be accompanied by oliguria (urine output <400 mL/d). The cardinal feature of acute renal failure (ARF) is a decline in glomerular filtration rate (GFR). There is sudden and often temporary loss of renal function, which is frequently reversible, with less than 20% cases ultimately requiring renal replacement therapy.[1] Imaging is, therefore, directed at identifying correctable causes of acute renal insult. Most common causes include acute tubular necrosis, severe dehydration, tubular blockade, infection and obstruction.

Chronic Renal Failure (CRF)

The diagnosis of chronic renal failure (CRF) implies a persistent abnormality in GFR with a wide range of causes. Slow progressive loss of kidney function over a span of years occurs, resulting in permanent kidney damage. Chronic kidney disease is defined as sustained kidney damage greater than 3 months duration resulting in a GFR of less than 60 mL/min/1.73 m^2.[2]

For purposes of diagnosis and management, renal failure can be divided into three categories:

1. *Prerenal*: Diseases caused by any process that decreases perfusion to kidneys in which the integrity of renal parenchymal tissue is preserved.
2. *Intrarenal*: Diseases affecting renal parenchymal tissue (which can be further divided into vascular, glomerular and tubular diseases).
3. *Postrenal*: Diseases associated with obstruction of the urinary tract or venous blood flow. It is also known as "surgical renal failure" as it is often amenable to correction.

This chapter is designed to give a contemporary insight of the intrarenal causes of acute and chronic renal failure—'Medical Renal Diseases'.

Various causes of acute and chronic renal failure are enumerated in **Flowcharts 1 and 2**.[1]

ROLE OF IMAGING IN RENAL FAILURE

Overlapping imaging findings are seen in renal failure. Comprehensive evaluation should be done in a particular

Flowchart 1: Causes of acute renal failure.

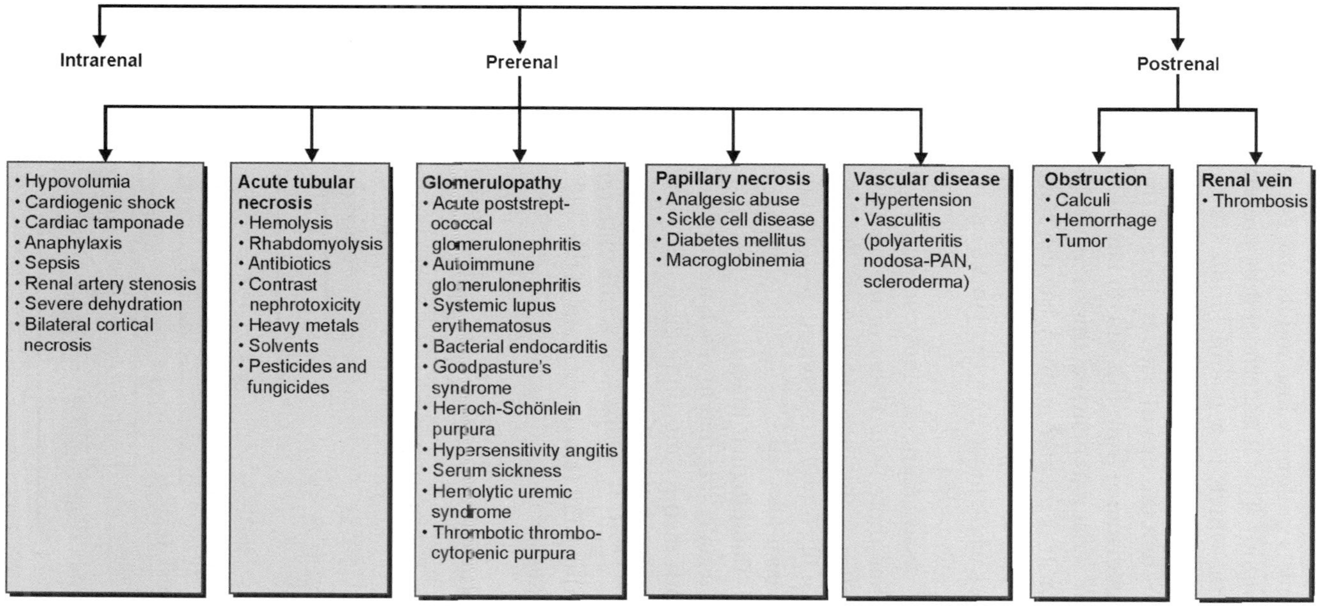

Flowchart 2: Causes of chronic renal failure.

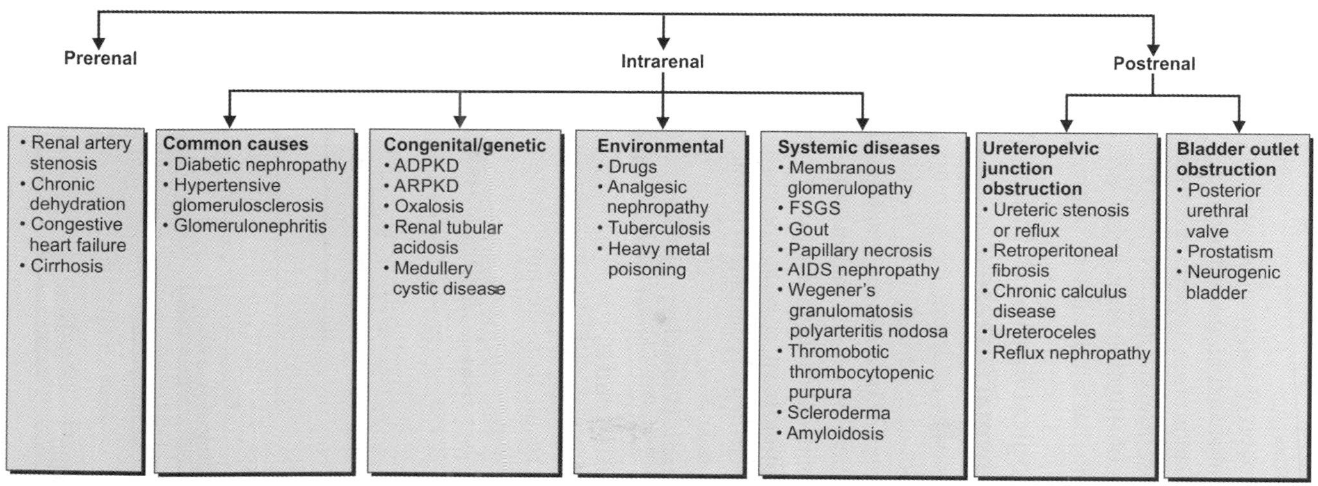

case which includes clinical profile, laboratory findings and histopathology along with imaging to arrive at a conclusive diagnosis.

The role of imaging in renal failure is to segregate the surgical and medical conditions resulting in renal insufficiency.[1] Goal for radiological studies in renal failure is as follows:

- Exclusion of correctable causes of acute renal failure (e.g. obstruction, thrombosis)
- Estimation of renal size to differentiate acute parenchymal disease from chronic parenchymal disease.

Once obstruction is excluded, prerenal, and postrenal causes of renal failures can be managed medically.

Radiological Approach to Renal Parenchymal Disease

Most diseases affecting the parenchyma of the kidney may produce lesions detectable only by electron or light microscopy, or by deranged renal function. However, some pathological processes manifest as renal morphological abnormalities and may be diagnosed by radiological imaging.

Morphological criteria are useful to categorize the wide spectrum of renal parenchymal diseases. Evaluation is done based on renal size, contour and laterality of involvement **(Flowchart 3)**. List of differential diagnosis of these morphological sets are given in **Table 1** and **Flowcharts 4 and 5**.

Renal size is an important diagnostic criterion. Large kidneys result from accumulation of fluid, deposition of protein, inflammatory or neoplastic infiltrates, glomerular or microvascular proliferation and cellular hypertrophy. Small kidneys result from loss of renal substance due to hypoplasia, necrosis, atrophy or fibrosis. Renal contour is another useful indicator. If a disease causes global reduction in renal mass, parenchymal bulk is uniformly lost and its size decreases with smooth contour. This is ascertained by preserved interpapillary line, which is a useful landmark for evaluating loss of renal parenchyma. Interpapillary line is drawn through the tips of papilla (base of the calyces) **(Fig. 1)**, the distance from this line to lateral surface of kidney is the renal parenchymal thickness which averages to 2.5–3 cm. It is greater at polar calyces ranging up to 3.5 cm. Distances less than 2 cm are suggestive of parenchymal loss while those greater than 3.5 cm indicate mass lesion or infiltration.[3]

Assessment of renal contour may show a deviation when there is focal loss or regional expansion. Laterality indicates nature of the disease. Bilateral renal lesions are usually found in systemic disorders in which total renal mass is affected.[4,5]

Radiological imaging in renal parenchymal disease is usually targeted to reach a set of differential diagnosis, with distinct morphological description. Bilateral large smooth kidney' constitutes to the group of acute renal parenchymal disease, while 'bilateral small smooth kidney' fall into description of chronic renal parenchymal disease.

Flowchart 3: Morphological criteria to categorize renal parenchymal disease (size, contour, laterality).

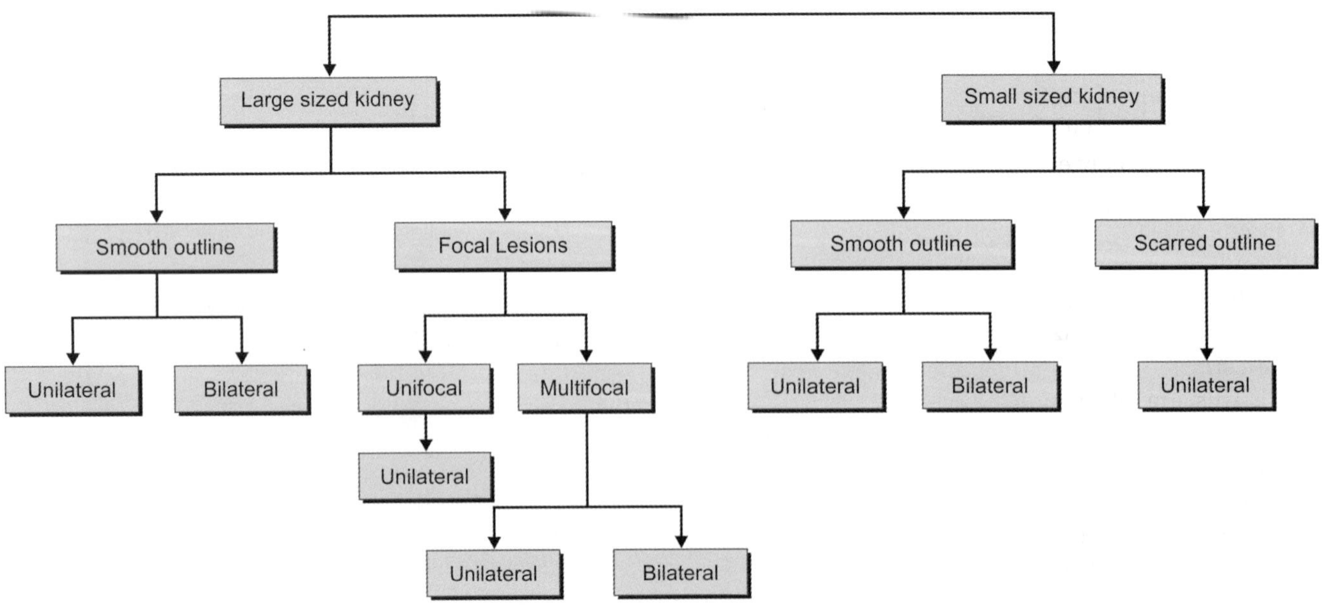

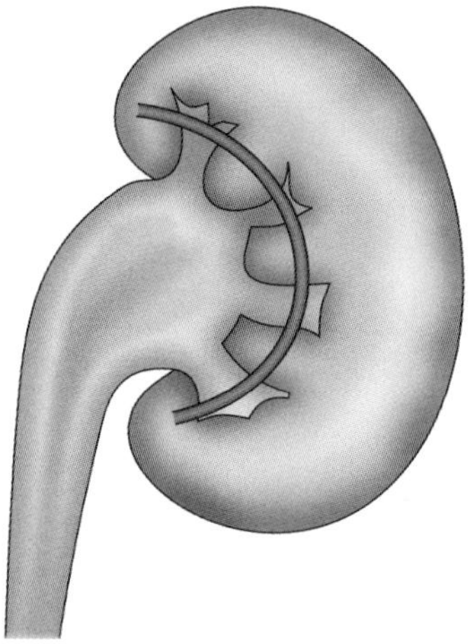

Fig. 1: Schematic diagram of normal interpapillary line: This line is drawn by joining the tips of renal papillae; smooth uninterrupted interpapillary line is seen in normal kidney.

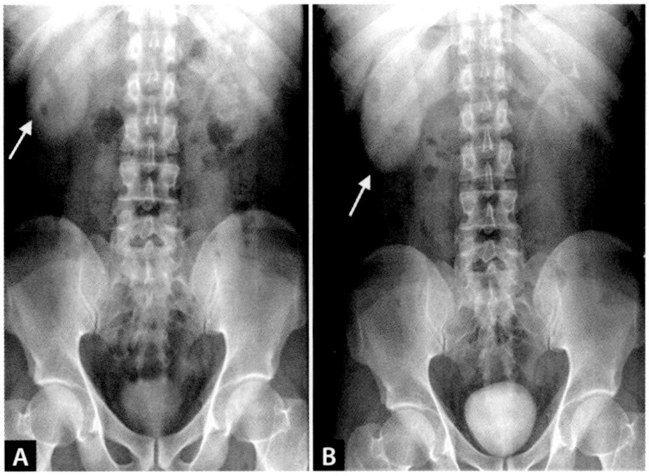

Figs. 2A and B: Increasing dense nephrogram: IVU shows increased nephrographic density (arrows) on 2-hour film as compared to 5-minute nephrographic phase. Patient had right-sided urinary obstruction, because of a small tumor near the right vesicoureteric junction.

Imaging Techniques

Recent advancements in all the fields of imaging have led to better evaluation of renal cases and their improved management. Imaging studies performed for evaluating the kidneys provide not only anatomic but also functional and metabolic information. To reach a diagnosis for a particular case, it is important to know the benefits and the limitations along with the diagnostic yield of each modality.

Plain Radiography and Urography

The plain film also known as KUB, has been used for years as the first step in the evaluation of the kidneys; however, it gives little significant information on its own. Role of plain radiography is to detect renal parenchymal calcification and calculi. Renal size and contour may be estimated if the renal outlines can be visualized. Renal size is approximately equal to 3–4 lumbar vertebral body height. Normal kidney measures 10–14 cm in men and 9–13 cm in women on conventional radiography and 1–2 cm less on ultrasonography. Generally, right kidney is smaller than the left by about 0.5 cm. In clinical setting, discrepancy in renal size of more than 2 cm is considered significant.[3]

In this era of cross-sectional imaging, urography is more of historic importance; however, interesting abnormal nephrographic patterns present in certain sets of diseases, were described by Fry and Cattell, which are:[6]

1. Immediate faint persistent nephrogram—chronic glomerular disease.
2. Increasingly dense nephrogram—acute renal obstruction, hypotension, renal ischemia, acute glomerular disease, intratubular obstruction and acute renal vein thrombosis **(Figs. 2A and B)**.
3. Immediate dense persistent nephrogram—acute tubular necrosis and severe inflammatory renal disease.

Striated nephrogram is a variant of obstructive nephrogram which may also be encountered in other conditions like pyelonephritis, polyarteritis nodosa (PAN), trauma and medullary cystic kidney disease. Prominent cortical nephrons are seen extending into the medulla as 'medullary rays'.

Ultrasonography

Ultrasonography is initial imaging modality for azotemia as it is noninvasive and readily differentiates between obstructive (surgical) and non-obstructive (medical) causes of renal failure **(Fig. 3A)**.[5] Renal sizes, cortical thickness, echogenicity of the kidneys and the presence or absence of hydronephrosis are easily assessed on ultrasonography. Renal size and parenchymal thickness are useful parameters to assess chronicity of renal disease **(Fig. 3B)**. Enlarged kidneys indicate an acute parenchymal lesion while contracted small kidneys suggest a chronic disease. Renal cortical echogenicity is an important indicator for the diagnosis of renal parenchymal disease. Normally the echogenicity of renal cortex is less than liver

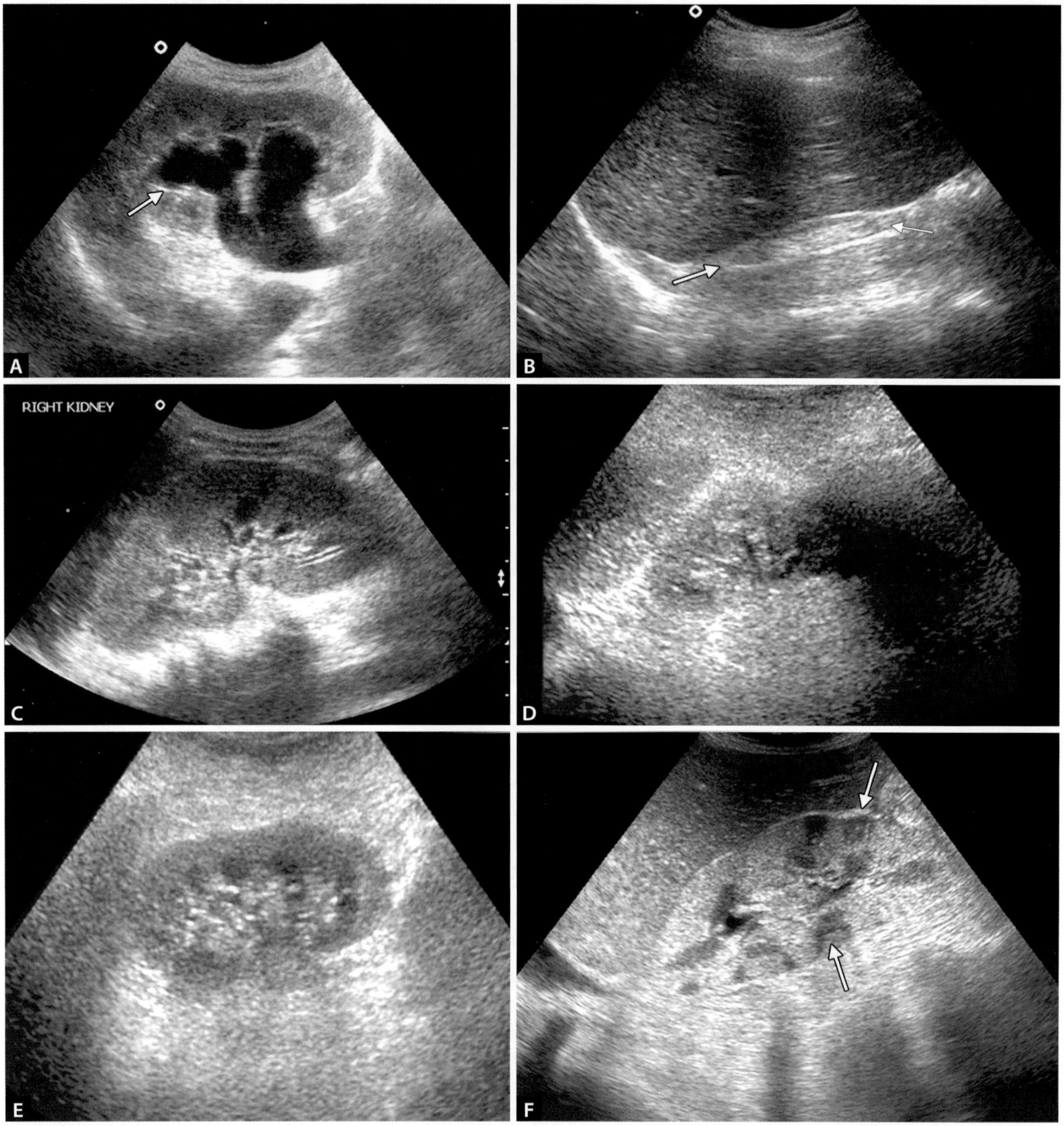

Figs. 3A to F: Obstructive renal failure in a man with distal ureteric calculus: (A) Longitudinal ultrasound image depicts marked dilatation of the pelvicalyceal system (arrow). Note the upper ureter is also dilated; (B) Chronic renal failure: Ultrasound image shows small smooth kidney with markedly decreased renal parenchymal thickness; (C to F) Acute renal parenchymal disease US images: (C) Slightly raised cortical echogenicity and lack of renal corticomedullary differentiation; (D) Markedly increased parenchymal echoes nearing to that of renal sinus resulting in loss of corticomedullary differentiation; (E) Hyperechoic renal cortex, relatively prominent renal medulla with accentuated corticomedullary differentiation; (F) Complicated pyelonephritis with multiple renal abscesses: Severely raised cortical echoes and few hypoechoic well-defined parenchymal lesions (abscesses)(arrows) with right pleural effusion.

or spleen; the demonstration of increased echogenicity of the renal cortex under standard scanning techniques may be useful in suggesting the presence of renal parenchymal (medical renal) disease. Renal corticomedullary differentiation may be preserved, obliterated or accentuated depending on the severity of renal cortical echoes[7,8] **(Figs. 3C to F)**.

Increased cortical echogenicity with preserved corticomedullary differentiation may be seen in glomerulonephritis, nephrosclerosis, amyloidosis, acute leukemia, ATN and Alport's syndrome while cortical echogenicity is decreased in lymphoma, acute pyelonephritis and renal vein thrombosis. Increased medullary echotexture is found in gouty nephropathy, medullary nephrocalcinosis and medullary sponge kidney. Interestingly, some authors recognize the altered state of hydration at the time of scanning as one of determining factors influencing the renal cortical echotexture of the patient.[8,9] An extracapsular hypoechoic rim of edema may surround the kidneys in renal failure. This finding when present is usually bilateral and is called as 'kidney sweat sign.'[10]

Ultrasound examination is also valuable for assessing the kidneys for follow-up of renal parenchymal disease. Changes in renal size, progression as well as resolution of the disease can easily be monitored on ultrasonography.

Color Doppler

Color Doppler is a handy, easily available and noninvasive tool for evaluation of renal blood vessels. Normal renal arterial branching pattern is well-appreciated on color flow imaging. Assessment of spectral wave pattern and flow indices of renal arteries can be done. Vascular resistance (Resistive index: RI) and pulsatility (Pulsatility index) along with absolute flow velocities of the main, intralobar and arcuate arteries may be calculated. Out of these indices, resistive index is most commonly used. It is calculated as:

$$\text{Resistive Index (RI)} = \frac{\text{Peak systolic velocity} - \text{Lowest diastolic velocity}}{\text{Peak systolic velocity}}$$

Normal resistive index is less than 0.7. Parenchymal diseases with tubulointerstitial or vascular involvement cause increased resistive index (>0.7), while glomerular diseases do not cause any significant increase in this parameter.[11] Elevated RI correlates with the severity of disease in SLE, HUS, diabetes and hepatorenal syndrome[5] **(Fig. 4)**.

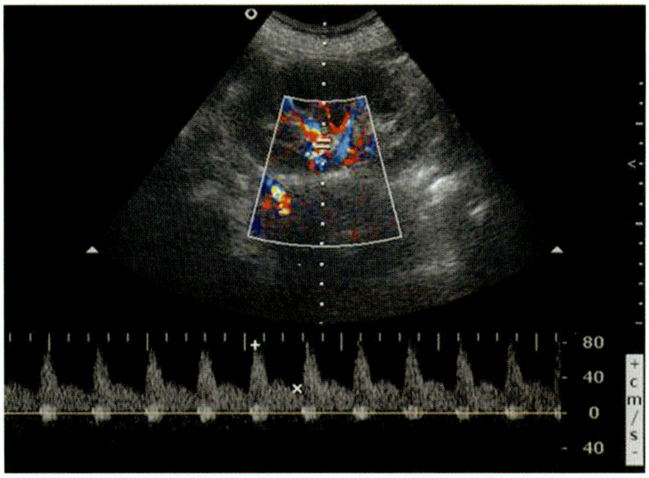

Fig. 4: Normal Doppler ultrasound: Doppler spectra obtained in the area of interlobar arteries show a sharp systolic peak and prominent antegrade flow during diastolic phase. Resistive index in this patient is 0.64, which is normal.

Computed Tomography

Computed tomography has a specific role in evaluation of renal failure. In acute renal failure noncontrast CT scan of kidneys may show parenchymal calcification. Renal parenchyma, however, appears homogenous in attenuation on NCCT. Various nephrographic patterns are demonstrated after the administration of contrast. Differential diagnosis of the nephrographic patterns used on urography is similarly applied to CT nephrogram. Excretory function can further be assessed on sequential dynamic imaging.[12]

Magnetic Resonance Imaging

Routine MRI evaluation of the kidney includes axial and coronal T1 weighted and T2 weighted spin echo sequences, with or without fat suppression. Corticomedullary differentiation (CMD) is distinctly seen on T1W and T2W images. In normal kidney, the cortex is slightly higher in signal intensity than the medulla on T1W images while renal medulla is hyperintense to cortex on T2W images **(Figs. 5A to D)**. In a normal well-hydrated kidney, sharp corticomedullary differentiation is seen on T1W sequence due to high signal of cortex as compared to medulla. Wide variety of renal medical diseases cause decrease in cortical signal and subsequent loss of CMD. Loss of corticomedullary differentiation on T1W spin echo sequences is a sensitive indicator of parenchymal diseases and correlates with elevated serum creatinine levels >3.0 mg/dL. Dynamic contrast enhanced T1 weighted sequences can also be done. CMD is lost on post-gadolinium dynamic MR

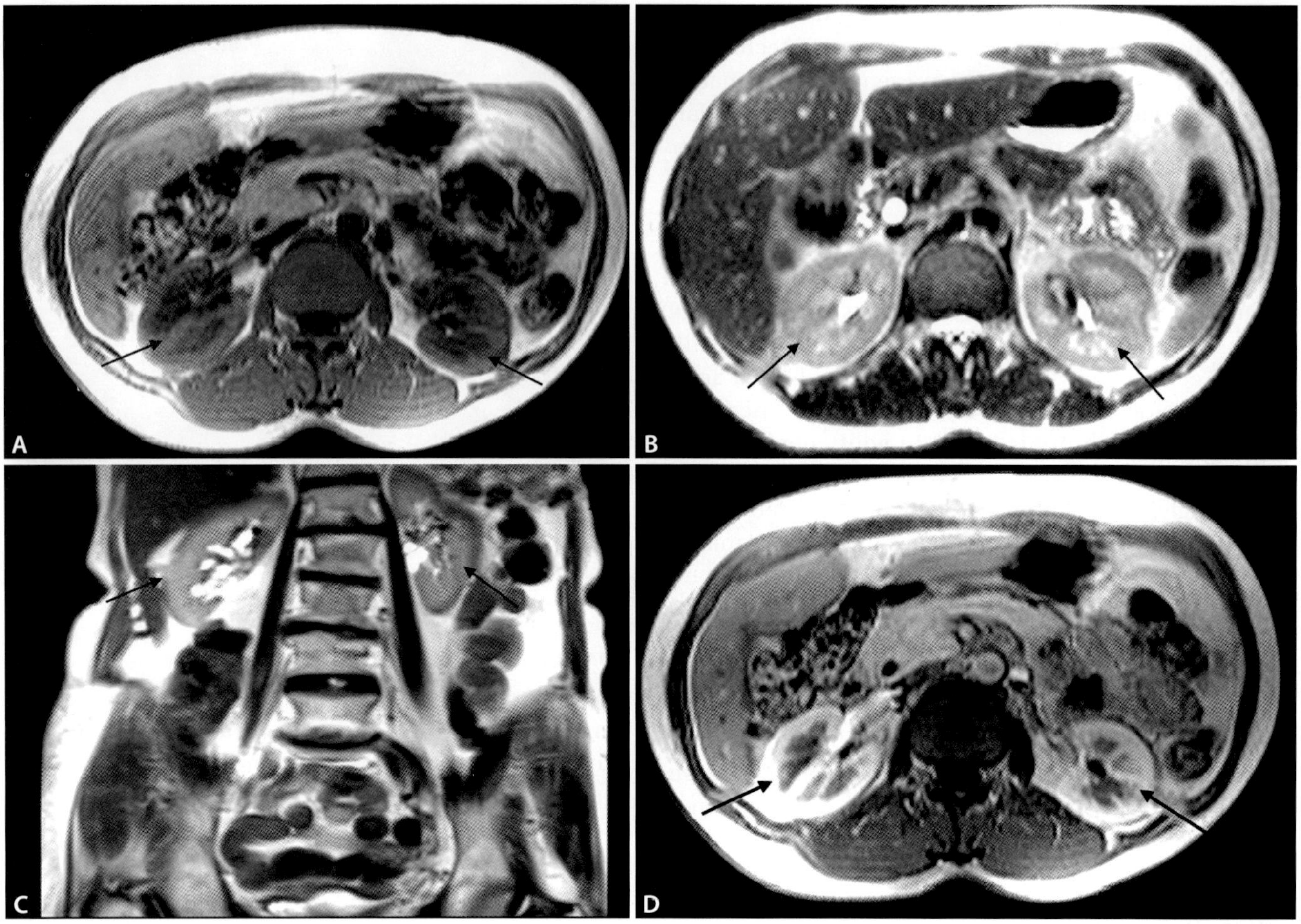

Figs. 5A to D: Normal spin echo magnetic resonance imaging findings: (A) T1W axial image shows corticomedullary differentiation resulting from high signal intensity of normal renal cortex and lower signal intensity of renal medulla (arrows); (B and C) T2W axial and coronal MR images depict the hyperintensity of normal renal medulla as compared to renal cortex (arrows); (D) Postgadolinium dynamic MR in cortical phase reveals the striking distinction between renal cortex and medulla (arrows).

imaging when serum creatinine is >8.5 mg/dL.[13] Some pilot studies are exploring the use of diffusion weighted MR imaging to demonstrate low values of ADC in renal cortex and medulla in patients of renal failure as compared to healthy volunteers.[14] When gadolinium was introduced as intravenous contrast agent for magnetic resonance imaging, it was initially regarded as nonnephrotoxic and was possibly recommended to replace iodinated contrast agents in patients at risk for acute renal failure. However, contrast induced nephropathy has been associated with gadolinium, especially in patients with advanced renal disease. Further research can clarify the renal effects of gadolinium in patients with renal insufficiency.[15]

Renal Angiography

Renal angiography has limited role in renal parenchymal disease as it is an invasive procedure and usually requires large amount of iodinated contrast medium. Characteristic appearances like aneurysmal dilatation of medium and small sized vessels on arteriography are seen in conditions like PAN, Wegener's granulomatosis and SLE. Pruned, tortuous vessels with slow flow with thinned renal cortex are demonstrated. Lucent or mottled nephrogram may be seen.

Renal artery stenosis is most accurately diagnosed on angiography and can be treated by angioplasty.[16]

Radionulceotide Imaging

Scintigraphy provides imaging based diagnostic information on renal structure and function. Radionucleotide agents are excreted by kidneys; hence, they should be judiciously employed in patients with renal failure. ^{99m}Tc-DTPA is excreted solely by the glomerular filtration, therefore it should not be used frequently. Tubular secretion of ^{99m}Tc-MAG3 and Hippuran I-131 occurs, hence these may be utilized in severe renal insufficiency.[17]

Contrast Medium-associated Nephropathy

The presence of renal failure may pose some limitations on the choice of an individual imaging modality. Iodinated contrast media may cause exacerbation of renal insufficiency.

Contrast medium-associated nephropathy (CAN) is one of the common causes of hospital acquired ARF. The exact mechanism of CAN is still unknown, but it is thought to be multifactorial.[18] CAN is defined as a rise of ≥0.5 mg/dL of serum creatinine (above a baseline value) within 48 hours of the administration of intravascular contrast material when no other cause of renal injury is readily apparent.[19] The rise in serum creatinine usually peaks at 3–5 days and return to baseline within 10–14 days. The most important risk factor is pre-existing renal insufficiency (serum creatinine >1.5–2.0 mg/dL), followed by diabetes mellitus, advancing age, congestive heart failure, dehydration, high dose of contrast media and furosemide. Adequate hydration, dose reduction and use of non-ionic contrast media are recommended as preventive measures.[5]

IMAGING IN RENAL PARENCHYMAL DISEASE

Acute Renal Parenchymal Disease

Radiographic appearance of 'Bilateral, large, smooth' kidneys is usually seen in the setting of renal failure of recent onset. When obstruction is ruled out a similar picture of enlarged smooth kidneys with normal or effaced collecting system is seen that indicates parenchymal disease of recent origin, which is possibly reversible. **Table 1** and **Flowchart 4** enumerate the causes of renomegaly based on morphological criteria.[4]

However, in some conditions certain characteristic appearances are seen imaging which shall be discussed in the next section of this chapter. Infections, cystic renal diseases, obstructions, renal vascular diseases and tumors are not included here, as they are covered in other chapters in this book.

Table 1: Causes of bilateral large smooth kidneys.[4]

Proliferative/necrotizing disorders:
• Acute glomerulonephritis
• Polyarteritis nodosa (microscopic form)
• Systemic lupus erythematosus
• Wegener's granulomatosis
• Allergic angitis
• Diabetic glomerulosclerosis
• Lung hemorrhage and glomerulonephritis (Goodpasture's syndrome)
• Anaphylactoid purpura (Henoch–Schonlein syndrome)
• Thrombotic thrombocytopenic purpura
• Focal glomerulonephritis associated with subacute bacterial endocarditis
Plasma cell dyscrasias:
• Multiple myeloma
• Waldenstrom's macroglobulinemia
• Amyloidosis
• Abnormal glycogen deposition
von Gierke's disease (Glycogen storage disease type I)
Abnormal lipid deposition:
• Fabry's disease
Abnormal fluid accumulation:
• Acute tubular necrosis
• Acute cortical necrosis
Leukemia
Acute interstitial nephritis
Acute blockage of tubules:
• Acute urate nephropathy
• Tamm–Horsfall protein
• Acute myeloma nephropathy
Acromegaly
Nephromegaly associated with cirrhosis, hyperalimentation and diabetes mellitus
Hemophilia
Homozygous-S disease:
• Tyrosinosis type I
• Infectious mononucleosis
• Autosomal recessive polycystic kidney disease
• Physiological response to contrast material and diuretics

Acute Tubular Necrosis

Acute tubular necrosis (ATN) is the most common reversible cause of renal failure. Renal hypoperfusion and ischemic injury (due to shock, severe dehydration, burns and crush injury) are the leading causes of ATN. The incidence of ATN related to nephrotoxic drugs (contrast media, aminoglycosides and other antibiotics) and agents (heavy metals, solvents and pesticides) is also rising. ATN is also commonly seen in the transplanted kidney.[20]

The pathogenesis of ATN is still debatable, but some authors have proposed that direct tubular damage is the primary event leading to necrosis of the epithelium and obstruction of the tubular lumen with cellular debris.[20]

Flowchart 4: Large kidney with focal lesion.[4]

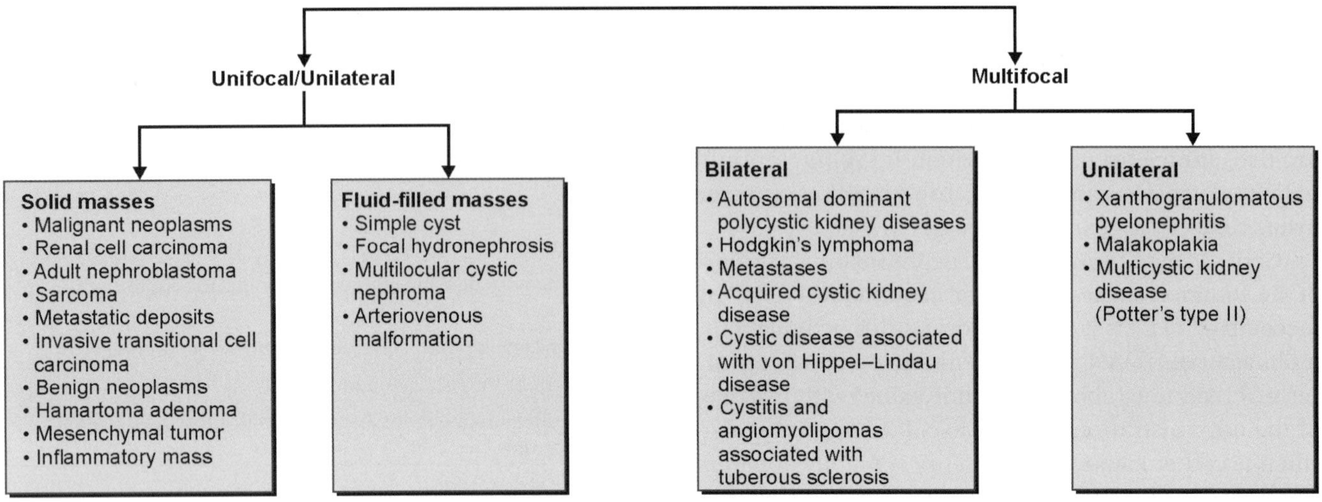

The oliguric (urine output <500 mL/day) or anuric phase usually begins less than 24 hours after the inciting incident and may last for 1–3 weeks. Dark urine and proteinuria may be present during this duration. It is followed by diuretic phase, a harbinger of renal recovery.[21]

Imaging Features

In ATN, both kidneys are enlarged and smooth in outline. Contrast enhanced studies are not recommended in ATN. If IV contrast is inadvertently given, persistent dense nephrogram is seen on urography which may persist for more than 24 hours. As tubules are filled with cellular infiltrates, contrast leaks into the interstitium through the damaged basement membrane; hence, faint or nonopacification of pelvicalyceal system occurs. Variable appearances of ATN on ultrasonography have been proposed by different authors, which are as follows:[22]

- Normal cortical and medullary echogenicity—ischemic ATN,
- Increase in cortical echogenicity with maintained corticomedullary differentiation—drug-related ATN,
- Normal cortical echogenicity with echogenic pyramids—associated with precipitation of Tamm-Horsfall protein .

Increased resistive index (>0.7) on Doppler imaging is present in majority of patients with ATN.[23]

Bilateral renomegaly with patchy nephrogram is seen on CT scan. Gadolinium enhanced MRI demonstrates compartmental renal involvement of cortex, inner and outer medulla and give complementary information about the pathological condition of the kidney. Perfusion abnormalities were also shown in experimentally induced ATN. Blood oxygen level dependent MRI (BOLD MRI) assesses intrarenal oxygen bioavailability which reflects tissue deoxyhemoglobin levels. Ischemia and hypoperfusion in ATN results[24] in reduced tissue oxygen bioavailability which is utilized to discriminate between acute rejection and acute tubular necrosis that may follow renal transplantation.[25]

Acute Cortical Necrosis

Acute cortical necrosis (ACN) is a rare form of acute renal failure which is characterized by ischemic necrosis of renal cortex, including renal column of Bertini with sparing of renal medulla, and thin rim of subcapsular cortex. Both kidneys are involved either diffusely or in patchy distribution; in both instances peripheral renal cortex is spared as it is supplied by the preserved capsular vessels.[5]

More than two-thirds of cases are associated with pregnancy and its complications—abruptio placenta, septic abortion and placenta previa. Other causes include severe trauma with shock, sepsis, transfusion reaction, severe dehydration, burns, peritonitis and toxins (e.g. snake venom). Although large numbers of conditions are associated with acute cortical necrosis, the pathophysiology unfortunately remains unclear. Ischemia following vasospasm is probably the initiating event which results due to constriction of small intracortical blood vessels. This may follow exposure to toxins, circulating hormones, or neural stimuli.[25]

Diffuse involvement of both the kidneys may result in complete renal failure requiring either dialysis or transplantation for survival, whereas patchy involvement leads to renal insufficiency.

Imaging Features

Imaging findings depend on the stage of illness. In the acute stage, urographic findings are nonspecific. Kidneys are diffusely enlarged with faint opacification of collecting system. For those surviving the early phase, smooth renal shrinkage occurs over several months. Radiographically, distinctive tram like or egg shell calcification of cortex may be seen which start appearing as early as 24 days after the onset of disease.[20]

On ultrasonography, enlargement of both kidneys and loss of the normal corticomedullary differentiation with a circumferential hypoechoic zone corresponding to the necrotic cortex is seen. Ultrasound is useful for follow up. Calcification of cortex causes dense cortical echoes with distal acoustic shadowing.

Specific appearance of acute cortical necrosis is described on contrast enhanced CT scan. The three diagnostic features are (a) enhancement of the medulla, (b) nonenhancement of the renal cortex, and (c) lack of excretion of contrast medium into the collecting system. Enhanced subcapsular cortex, the distinctive 'cortical rim sign' on contrast-enhanced CT scan suggests the sparing of the most peripheral region of renal cortex **(Figs 6A and B)**. 'cortical rim sign' is also seen in other conditions which result in hemodynamic derangement like renal infarction, renal vein thrombosis and ATN.[26-28]

MRI also shows these representative findings. Kidneys are enlarged in the early phase. Low signal intensity of the inner renal cortex and the columns of Bertin on every MR imaging sequence is the major characteristic finding of renal cortical necrosis. Swelling of both kidneys with increased signal intensity of the cortex on T2-weighted images instead of T1-weighted images is another feature of renal cortical necrosis at MR imaging. Later a thin rim of low signal intensity (T1WI and T2WI) may be seen along the border of kidneys due to calcification.[29]

Leukemia

Leukemia (predominantly lymphocytic leukemia) is the most common malignant cause of bilateral renal enlargement in children. Renal enlargement occurs due to infiltration of kidneys by leukemic cells. Usually, markedly large kidneys are seen; however, sometimes asymmetrical renal involvement or focal renal mass may be seen **(Figs. 7A and B)**.

Imaging Features

In leukemic infiltration of kidney, the nephrogram is faint and the collecting system is attenuated. Pelvicalyceal system is often filled with blood clots or uric acid stones which appear as filling defects.[20]

Acute Interstitial Nephritis

Acute interstitial nephritis (AIN) is an acute hypersensitivity reaction, mediated through immunologic mechanisms. It may result following an exposure to drugs or nonrenal infection (e.g. infectious mononucleosis). However, an idiopathic variety is also described. The most common cause of AIN are drugs, particularly methicillin, penicillin, amphotericin, NSAID, sulfonamides, phenytoin, and thiazide.[30]

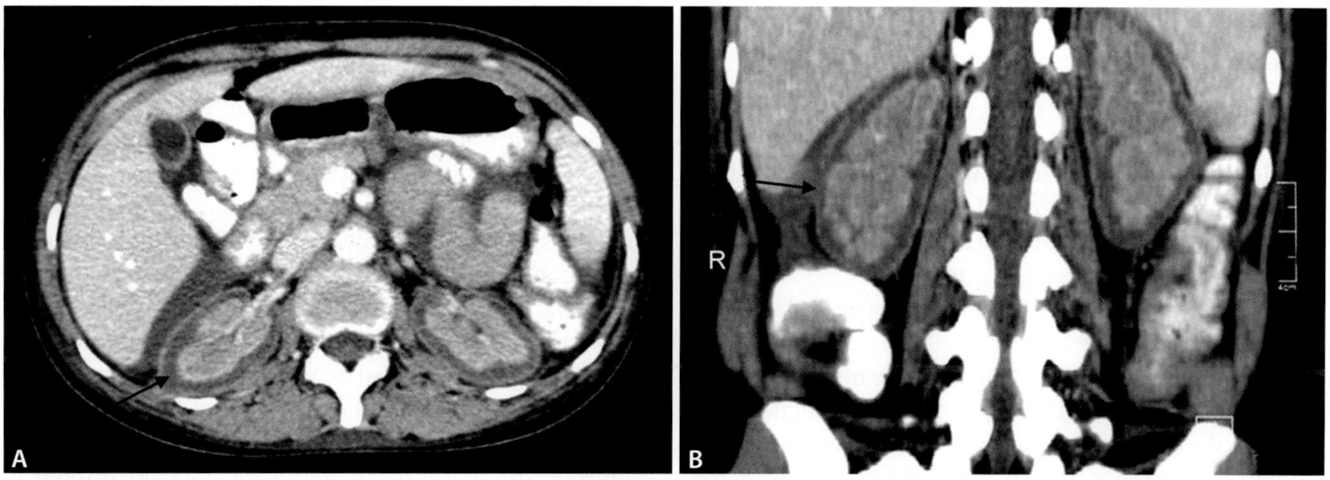

Figs. 6A and B: Acute cortical necrosis in a female patient with septic abortion: Axial and coronal postcontrast CT scans (corticomedullary phase) demonstrate absence of contrast enhancement in the cortex and relatively hyperdense medulla and subcapsular cortex, the characteristic 'cortical rim sign.'

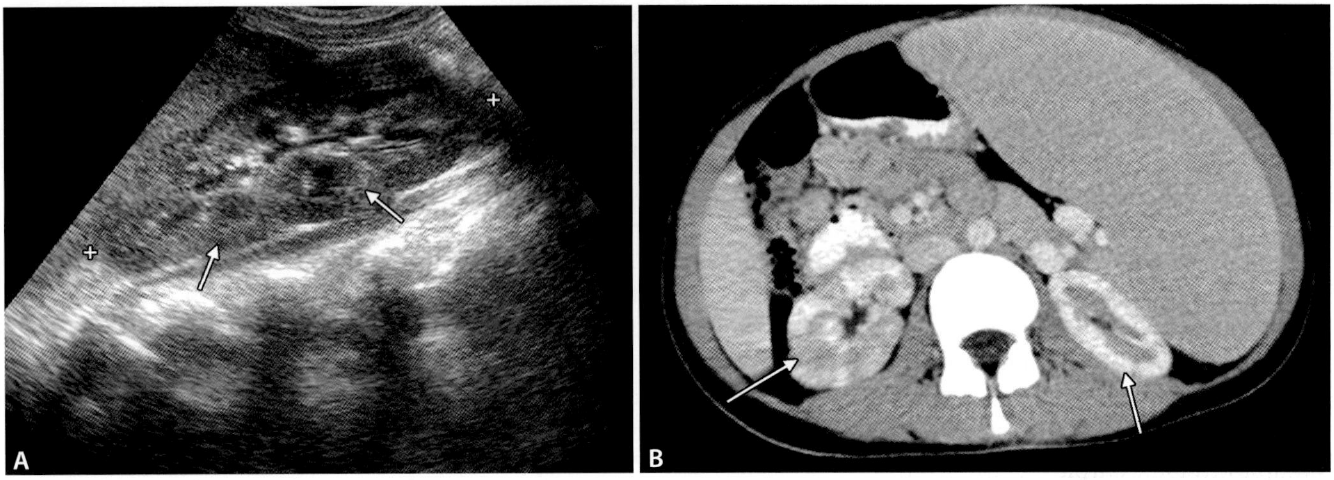

Figs. 7A and B: Renal manifestation of leukemia: (A) Ultrasonography of kidney shows focal, well-defined, hypoechoic masses; (B) CECT axial image in another patient also shows bilateral, multiple, focal hypodensities suggestive of leukemic deposits. Massive splenomegaly is also seen.

Fever, skin rashes, eosinophilia, oliguria and protienuria are the common clinical signs and symptoms of drug induced AIN which appear between 5 days and 5 weeks of exposure. Patient recovers with the withdrawal of the causative agent.[31]

Imaging Features

Bilateral renomegaly with diminished to normal opacification of collecting system is seen on urography. Ultrasound shows increased cortical echogenicity with renal enlargement. Enhanced uptake of Gallium citrate in the kidneys on renal scintigraphy is also reported.[30] Kidneys may become shrunken and irregular as the disease progresses to a chronic course. Calcification of renal papillae may occur in analgesic induced nephritis. Interstitial fibrosis leads to low signal intensity of renal cortex on T1W MRI.

Amyloidosis

Amyloidosis is a diverse group of diseases that have extracellular deposition of an insoluble fibrillar proteinaceous substance with a beta sheath configuration. Amyloidosis can be classified as follows:[32]

- *Primary Amyloidosis*: Without pre-existing or coexisting disease.
- Amyloidosis associated with multiple myeloma.
- Secondary or reactive amyloidosis associated with chronic infections (like tuberculosis, osteomyelitis, leprosy) chronic inflammatory disease (rheumatoid arthritis, ankylosing spondylitis) and malignancies (Hodgkin's lymphoma, renal cell carcinoma).
- Heredofamilial amyloidosis associated with familial mediterranean fever. Neurological, renal and cardiovascular involvement is seen.
- Localized amyloidosis without systemic involvement.
- Dialysis-related amyloidosis.
- Amyloidosis associated with aging.

Older men are more affected than women,[33] usually presenting with nonspecific symptoms like weight loss, fatigue and weakness.

Multiorgan involvement is present in more than 85% of cases. Kidney is affected in 80% patients with secondary amyloidosis and 35–40% patients with primary disease. Isolated involvement of the renal pelvis, ureter bladder, urethra, prostate seminal vesicle, and retroperitoneum can occur.[34]

Imaging Features

In acute phase bilateral renal enlargement is seen. Decrease in size occurs with progression of disease process, smooth outline is, however, maintained. Nephrogram is diminished with variable excretion into normal pelvicalyceal system. Cortical echogenicity is raised as seen in other parenchymal diseases. Rapid deterioration in renal function or sudden onset nephrotic syndrome indicates renal vein thrombosis, a complication of amyloidosis. Thrombosed renal vein is demonstrated on color Doppler, CT scan or MRI.

MRI shows reduced cortical signal intensity on T1 weighted images with subsequent loss of corticomedullary differentiation. Bilateral increased delayed uptake of Gallium 67 when other causes of abnormal gallium activity are excluded.[34]

Amyloidosis of Renal Pelvis

Isolated involvement of renal pelvis can occur in amyloidosis. Interesting radiological appearance of calcification or ossification in the amyloid deposits may be seen. These deposits are usually located in the submucosa of the pelvicalyceal system. A lucent band of mucosa separates the IV contrast density from calcification in the pelvis on IVU. Other causes for calcification of pelvicalyceal system are tuberculosis, leukoplakia primary carcinoma of renal pelvis and renal calculus.[34] Submucosal amyloid deposits appear hypo-intense on T1- and T2-weighted MR images.

Multiple Myeloma

Multiple myeloma is a plasma cell disorder which originates in the bone marrow and is characterized by involvement of the skeleton at multiple sites. The neoplastic plasma cells produce excess immunoglobulins and Bence-Jones proteins are characteristically present in the urine. Abnormal proteins precipitate in the renal tubules resulting in renal insufficiency in 30–50% of such patients.

Nausea, vomiting, anorexia, weight loss and progressive weakness are the presenting features. Nephrocalcinosis resulting from hypercalcemia, uric acid calculi, renal infections and amyloidosis may further complicate the illness.

Imaging Features

Urography shows enlarged smooth kidneys with faint opacification indicating impaired renal function. Collection system is attenuated. Injection of iodinated contrast media is hazardous in patients of multiple myeloma as it precipitates myeloma proteins in the renal tubules. Dehydration has to be avoided to reduce the risk of complications. Ultrasonography shows nephromegaly with reduced cortical echotexture. CT scan and radionucleotide study demonstrates impaired renal function.[21]

Paroxysmal Nocturnal Hemoglobinuria (PNH)

In PNH complement mediated erythrocyte damage results in hemolysis with release of hemoglobin in plasma. Hemolysis is precipitated by infections, drugs immunization and exercise. Patient presents with hemoglobinuria, iron deficiency anemia and venous thrombosis.

Imaging Features

Noncontrast CT may show high density of renal cortex due to hemosiderin pigments. Paramagnetic effects of hemosiderin results in markedly reduced signal in the cortex in both T1W and T2W images but it is more pronounced on T2W sequences. Similar imaging features are seen in intravascular hemolysis like in malfunctioning prosthetic valves, sickle cell anemia, hereditary spherocytosis and thalassemia.[35]

Chronic Renal Parenchymal Disease

In contrast to the capacity of kidney to regain back its function following acute renal insult, renal injury of more prolonged nature often leads to progressive and irreversible loss of nephrons. Such reduction in renal mass subsequently results in bilaterally small smooth kidneys. The uremic kidney shrinks globally reflecting the inherent tissue loss. Renal contour may be smooth or irregular. The echogenicity can be normal or increased. Radiological features, like those in acute renal parenchymal disease are overlapping in most of the causes of chronic renal parenchymal disease. However, some conditions show interesting radiological appearances and are discussed here. The various causes of bilateral small smooth kidneys are listed in **Flowchart 5**, the conditions leading to morphologically small, unilateral kidneys are also cited.[4] **Figures 8 to 11** show imaging in cases of chronic renal failure.

Renal Papillary Necrosis

Necroses of the renal papillae not only have many causes but also many radiological forms. Parenchymal diseases affecting the papillae and calyces are diagnosed on urography. In mild cases the kidney size and function are normal, and the abnormality is limited to the papillae only. In advanced disease, there is global shrinkage of kidney with impaired renal function. Most common cause of renal papillary necrosis is analgesic abuse nephropathy. Other causes are diabetes, sickle cell nephropathy, obstruction with infection, renal vein thrombosis, dehydration and prolonged hypotension.[5] (Pneumonic to remember causes of renal papillary necrosis—ADIPOSE: Analgesic nephropathy, diabetes, Infant in shock, Pyelonephritis, obstruction, sickle cell disease and ethanol).

In early papillary necrosis ischemia occurs in the renal papillae due to compression of the medullary vessels by inflammatory changes in the interstitium. If the phase of temporary spasm passes, normal circulation is restored and the involved tissues may recover. However, if ischemia continues and perfusion is not restored, irreversible coagulation necrosis, tubular fibrosis and lobar infarcts result.

Urographic findings during this period of early ischemic change are usually normal. On MDCT, the

Flowchart 5: Causes of small kidney.

Smooth

Unilateral
- Ischemia due to focal arterial disease
- Chronic infarction
- Renal vein thrombosis (late)
- Radiation nephritis
- Congenital hypoplasia
- Post-obstructive atrophy
- Post-inflammatory atrophy
- Reflux atrophy
- Partial nephrectomy

Bilateral
- Generalized arteriosclerosis
- Benign and malignant nephrosclerosis
- Atheroembolic renal disease
- Chronic glomerulonephritis
- Papillary necrosis
- Hereditary nephropathies
- Hereditary chronic nephritis (Alport's syndrome)
- Medullary cystic disease
- Amyloidosis (late)
- Arterial hypotension
- Cortical necrosis (late)

Scarred U/L
- Reflux nephropathy
- Lobar infarction

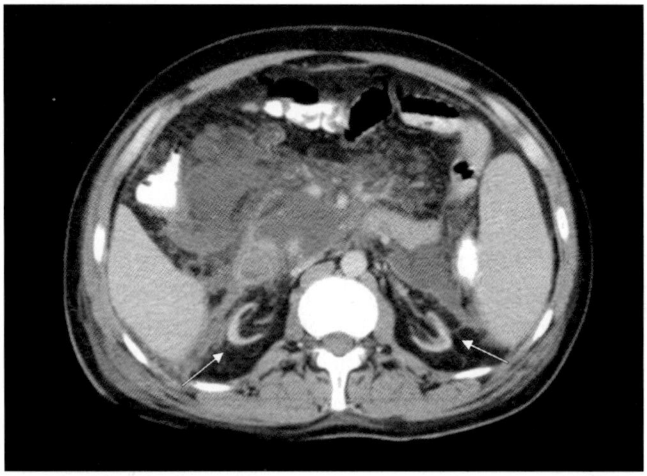

Fig. 8: End-stage renal disease: CECT axial image shows bilateral smooth shrunken kidneys in a patient of CRF with pancreatitis. Peripancreatic inflammatory fluid collections are also present.

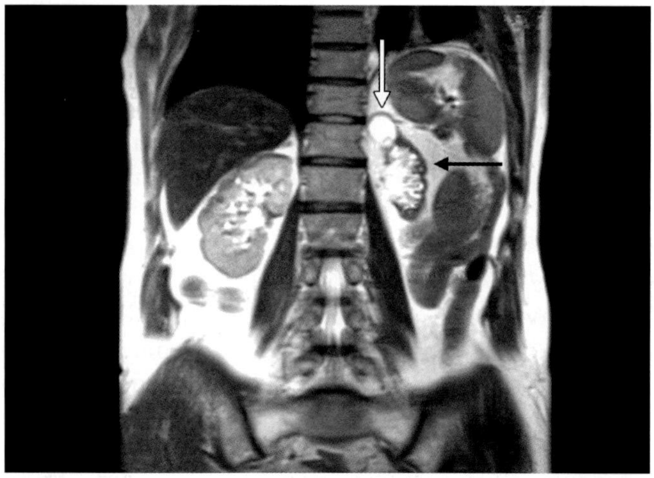

Fig. 9: Unilateral small smooth kidney: T2W coronal MR image reveals small, contracted left kidney with thinned renal parenchyma and indistinct CMD, subsequent to left renal artery stenosis (black arrow). Note made of simple cortical renal cyst in left upper pole (white arrow).

ischemic changes that lead to renal papillary necrosis can be demonstrated best on nephrographic phase as small, poorly marginated areas of diminished enhancement at the tip of the medullary pyramid.

In advanced stage of necrosis, clefts originate from the fornices and extend to the medullary pyramids and papillae, ultimately causing the papillae to slough **(Fig. 12)**. Caliceal deformities in renal papillary necrosis occur in three forms:

1. *Medullary*: Central necrosis takes place at the tip of the pyramid. Detachment of necrotic papillae starts in the central part of the calix, opening into a round or oval cavity.
2. *Papillary*: Detachment of necrotic papillae usually begins in the region of the caliceal fornices, and the resulting defect is triangular in shape also termed as lobster claw appearance.
3. *In situ*: When papillae fail to separate (necrosis in situ) calyces appear normal, they later calcify to give appearance of nephrocalcinosis.

In the healing phase, the papilla may epithelialize, and its tip takes a blunted appearance. In addition, shrinkage

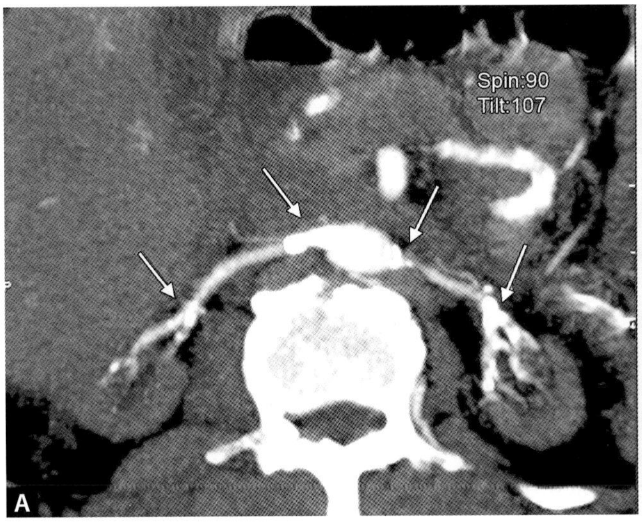

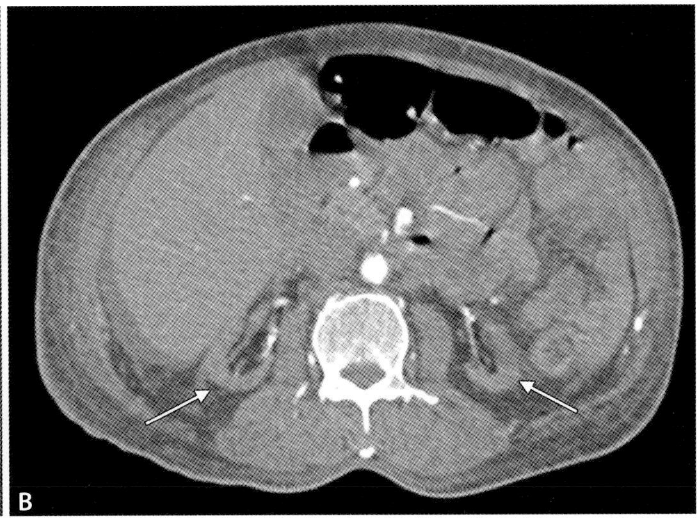

Figs. 10A and B: Bilateral small smooth kidneys: CT angiography (A) shows calcified artherothrombotic plaques involving both main renal arteries and their ostia (B) smooth globally shrunken kidneys, in a patient of severe bilateral renal artery stenosis. Mild perihepatic fluid is seen.

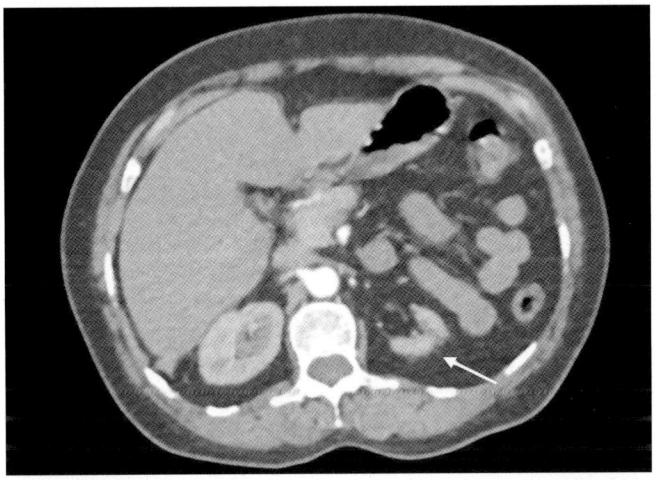

Fig. 11: Unilateral small scarred kidney: CECT axial image in cortical phase of enhancement shows small left kidney with irregular outline with parenchymal defect at interpolar region.

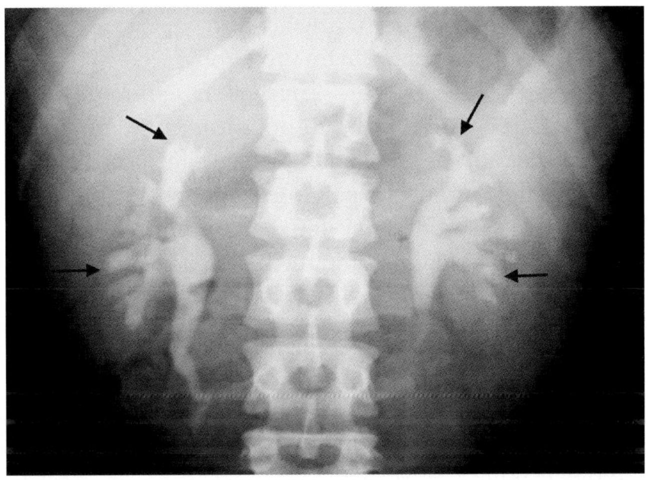

Fig. 12: Renal papillary necrosis: IVU film showing irregular and distorted calyces of both kidneys, with contrast excavation and formation of multiple cavities. Few amputated calyces are also seen.

of the kidney may occur with reduction of parenchymal thickness. This is the common sequel of renal papillary necrosis. Moreover, the loss of renal cortex is associated hypertrophy of the renal columns resulting in a typical irregular wavy renal outline.[36]

In advanced disease, after the sloughing of necrotic papillae, cavities are seen that are continuous with calices in renal medullary areas. Their differentiation with other cystic lesions in the renal medullae should be done (like hydronephrosis, congenital megacalices, parapelvic cysts, and caliceal diverticula).[37]

Alport's Syndrome

Alport's syndrome is progressive hereditary nephritis that manifests as hematuria and proteinuria, and is frequently associated with nerve deafness and variety of ocular abnormalities. It is often preceded by upper respiratory tract infections. Syndrome affects males more frequently than females. Progressive renal insufficiency occurs.

Imaging Features

Kidneys are severely shrunken in advanced stage, but maintain their smooth outline. Poor excretion of nephrographic contrast is noted. Renal echogenicity is increased on USG with loss of CMD. Hyperechogenicity due to nephrocalcinosis is present which is due to chronic glomerulonephritis. Non-specific pruning and tortuosity of interlobar arteries is seen on angiography.[37,38]

Benign and Malignant Nephrosclerosis

Nephrosclerosis affects the renal arterioles. The disease courses over many years but it rarely leads to kidney failure on its own. Malignant nephrosclerosis, however, progresses very rapidly and damages the arteries. These damaged arteries are unable to provide enough oxygen to the kidney tissues, resulting in kidney failure. The incidence of hypertensive nephrosclerosis increases with advancing age.[39]

Imaging Features

Kidneys are small and smooth in benign nephrosclerosis; occasionally shallow infarcts can be seen. Normal nephrographic opacification, and excretion into pelvicalyceal system is seen on urography.

On ultrasonography, increased central sinus echogenicity due to fat deposition may be seen. Subcapsular and perirenal hemorrhages may be detected as hypoechoic or anechoic fluid collections. High density fluid (blood) can be better detected on non-contrast CT scan. Blood degradation product may also be identified on MR imaging.[40]

Renal Osteodystrophy

A number of skeletal abnormalities may coexist in the metabolic bone disease due to renal failure. The primary radiologic bone changes reflect:

- *Deficiency in active form of vitamin D due to impaired renal function*: Rickets.
- *Impaired clearance of calcium leading to increased parathormone secretion*: Secondary hyperparathyroidism.

The spectrum consists of secondary hyperparathyroidism along with rickets, osteomalacia, osteosclerosis, and osteoporosis.

Inability of the kidney to adequately excrete phosphate, leads to hyperphosphatemia and increased osteoclastic activity. It can be categorized by resorption of bone at subperiosteal, cortical, subchondral, trabecular, endosteal, and subligamentous locations. Radiographic appearance of subperiosteal resorption has been described as a lacelike irregularity of the normal cortical margin, which may progress to areas of scalloping and spiculation. The earliest involvement is often seen along the radial aspects of the middle phalanges of the index and middle fingers, beginning in the proximal metaphyseal region. The terminal tufts may also demonstrate subperiosteal resorption. Additional sites of subperiosteal bone resorption include the upper medial tibia, humerus, and femur; superior and inferior ribs; and lamina dura **(Fig. 13)**.

Loss of trabecular sharpness occurs with trabecular resorption. This is well seen in the skull, described as a granular salt-and-pepper appearance, with loss of distinction between the inner and outer tables. Common sites of subchondral resorption are the distal clavicle and acromioclavicular joint, sacroiliac joint, sternoclavicular joint, symphysis pubis, and posterior patella **(Figs. 14A and B)**.[14] Osseous resorption may also occur at sites of ligamentous and tendinous attachments. Brown tumors are rare.

Osteosclerosis has a strong predilection for the axial skeleton, where cancellous bone predominates over cortical bone. In the vertebral bodies, bandlike areas of sclerosis involving the superior and inferior end plates with intervening normal osseous density are classically seen, which resemble the stripes on rugby jerseys called as rugger jersey spine.

Changes of rickets can be seen in children with a general delay in bone age, bowing of long bones, scoliosis, diffuse concave impressions at multiple vertebral end plates, basilar invagination of the skull, "triradiate pelvis" deformity and rachitic rosary. In children, epiphyseal displacement (slipped epiphysis) in children is also seen.

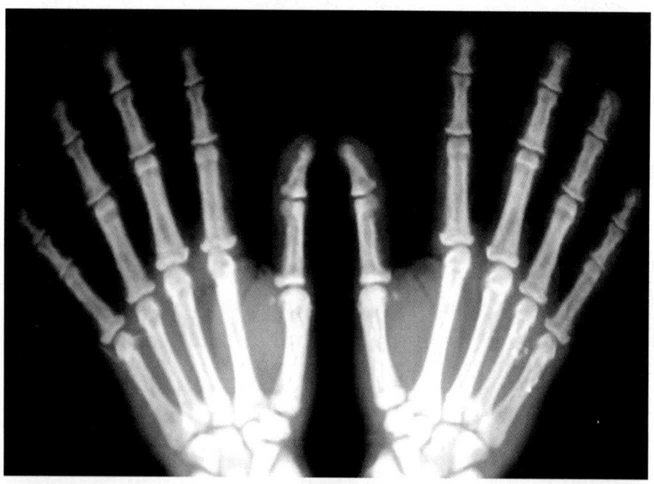

Fig. 13: Radiographs of hands in a patient of hyperparathyroidism in renal osteotrophy: Characteristic subperiosteal resorption phalanges including terminal tufts is seen. Subchondral and intracortical resorption is also seen.

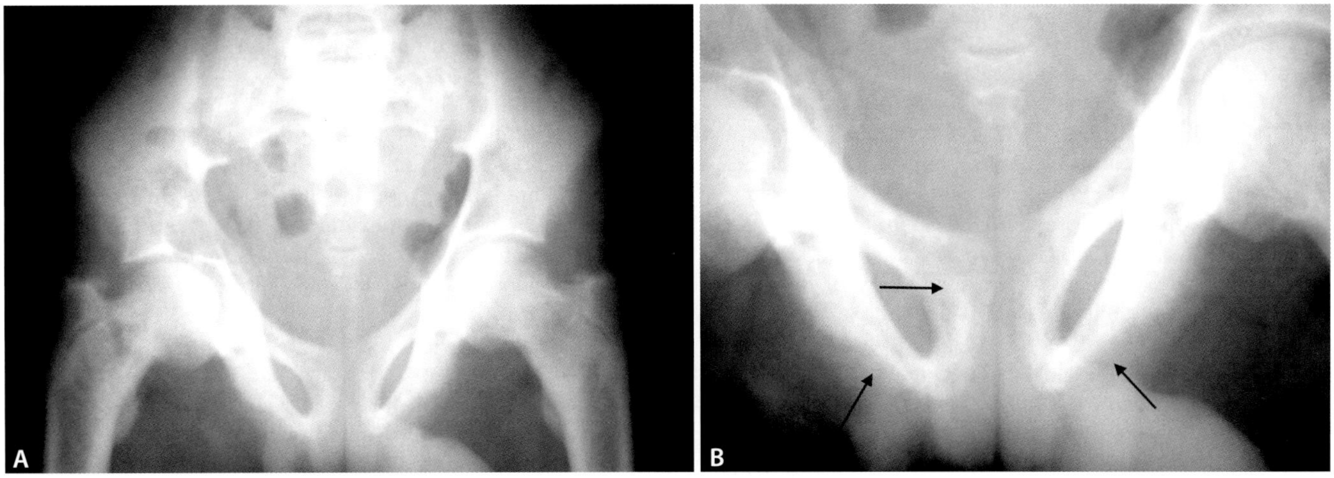

Figs. 14A and B: Renal osteodystrophy in a patient of tuberculosis: Anteroposterior view of pelvis shows osteopenic triradiate pelvis. Subchondral resorption of bone is seen at the pubis symphysis, ischial tuberosities, and sacroiliac joint (arrows).

Osteomalacia in adults may manifest as looser zones. Metastatic soft tissue and vascular calcification can be seen in ocular tissues, arteries, subcutaneous and periarticular soft tissues, and viscera.[41]

CONCLUSION

Imaging and management of renal failure continues to evolve with the development of newer imaging modalities and attainment of better cost effectiveness. Despite these achievements radiological imaging still has limitations in evaluation of renal parenchymal disease and renal failure. Radiological imaging techniques are rapidly expanding and are expected to grow even further. The future possibly holds improved methods to readily identify the causes of reversible acute renal failure and plan treatment strategies to combat chronic renal failure. The combination of better diagnostic methods and management strategies will lead to improved quality of life in patients with renal failure.

REFERENCES

1. PL Choyke, Zeiessman HA. Imaging of renal failure. In: Pollack HM, McClennan BL (Eds). Clinical Urography, 2nd edition. Philadelphia, PA: WB Saunders; 2000;3:3029-31.
2. National Kidney Foundation: K/DOQ1. Clinical practice guidelines for chronic kidney diseases: Evaluation, classification, stratification. Am J Kidney Disease 2002;1:39.
3. Friedenberg RM, Dunbar JS. Excretory urography. In: Pollack HM, McClennan BL (Eds). Clinical Urography, 1st edition. Philadelphia, PA: WB Saunders; 1990.2264-76,100-245.
4. Davidson AJ, Hartman DS. A systemic approach to Radiological Diagnosis of Renal Parenchymal Disease. In: Davidson AJ, Hartman DS (Eds). Radiology of Kidney and Urinary Tract, 2nd edition. Philadelphia, PA: WB Saunders; 1990.vol.1.pp.101-243.
5. Kim SH, Kim B. Renal Parenchymal Disease. In: Pollack HM, McClennan BL (Eds). Clinical Urography, 2nd edition. Philadelphia, PA: WB Saunders; 2000. vol.3.pp.2654-84.
6. Fry IK, Cattell WR. The nephrographic pattern during excretion urography. Br Med Bull. 1972;28:227-32.
7. Ritche WW, Vick CW, Glocheski SK, Cook DE. Evaluation of azotemic patients: Diagnostic yield of initial US examination. Radiology. 1998;167:245-7.
8. Hungtington DK, Hill SC, Hill MC. Sonographic manifestations of medical renal disease. Semin Ultrasound CT MR. 1991; 12:290-307.
9. Manley JA, O'Neill C. How echogenic is echogenic? Quantitative acoustics of the renal cortex. Am J Kidney Dis. 2001; 37:706-11.
10. Yasa NA, Peng M, Ralls PW. Perirenal lucency ('Kidney sweat'): A new sign of renal failure. AJR. 1999;173:1075-9.
11. Platt JF, Ellis JH, Rubin JM, et al. Intrarenal arterial Doppler sonography in patients with non-obstructive renal disease: Correlation of resistive index with biopsy findings. AJR. 1990;157:1223-7.
12. Saunder HS, Dyer BB, Shifrin RY, et al. The CT nephrogram: Implications of evaluation of urinary tract disease. Radiographics. 1995;15:1069-95.
13. Chung JJ, Semelka RC, Martin DR. Acute renal failure: Common occurrences of preservation of corticomedullary differentiation on MR images. Magn Reson Imaging. 2001;19:789-93.
14. Thoeny HC, Keyzer FD, Oyen RH, Peeters RR. Diffusion-weighted MR Imaging of Kidneys in Healthy Volunteers and Patients with Parenchymal Diseases: Initial Experience. Radiology. 2005;235:911-17.
15. Ledneva E, Karie S, Launay - Vacher V, Janus N, Deray G. Renal Safety of Gadolinium Based Contrast Media in Patients with Chronic Renal Insufficiency. 2009;250:618-28.
16. Abrams HA, Grassi CJ. Renal angiography in hypertension. In: Baums (Ed). Abrams Angiography: Vascular and Interventional Radiology, 4th edition. Boston, Little Brown; 1997.pp.1244-89.

17. Maisey M, Briton KE. Nuclear Imaging in Nephrology. In: Davidson AM, Cameron JS, Grunfeld JP, et al. In: Oxford textbook of clinical nephrology. 2nd edition. Oxford: Oxford University Press; 1998.pp.137-50.
18. Tublin ME, Murphy ME, Tessler FN. Current concepts in contrast media induced nephropathy, AJR. 1998;171:933-9.
19. Barrett BJ, Cariske EJ. Metanalysis of relative nephrotoxicity of high and low osmolality Iodinated Contrast Media Radiology. 1993;188:171-8.
20. Dunnick RN, Sandler CM, Newhouse JH, et al. Renal failure and medical renal disease, In: Textbook of Uroradiology. Lippincott Williams and Wilkins; 2001.pp.230-41.
21. Davidson A. Acute Renal Parenchymal Disease. In: Pollack HM, McClennan BL (Eds). Clinical Urography, 1st edition. Philadelphia, PA: WB Saunders; 1990.pp.2264-76.
22. Rosenfeld AT, Zeman RK, Cicchetti DV, et al. Experimental acute tubular necrosis: US Appearance Radiology. 1985;157:771.
23. Platt JH, Rubin JH, Ellis JH. Acute renal failure: Possible Role of Duplex Doppler US in Distinction between Acute Pre-renal Failure and acute tubular necrosis. Radiology. 1991;179:419.
24. Han F, Xiao W, Xu Y, et al. The significance of BOLD MRI in differentiation between renal transplant rejection and acute tubular necrosis. Nephrology Dialysis Transplantation. 2008;23:2666-72.
25. Gormsen H, Iverson P, Raaschou I. Kidney biopsy in acute anuria: with case of acute, bilateral cortical necrosis. Am J Med. 1955;19:209-11.
26. Jordan J, Low R, Jeffrey RB Jr. CT findings in acute renal cortical necrosis. J Comput Assist Tomogr. 1990;14:155-6.
27. Wang MT, Wu RH, Chen JC. CT Findings of Acute Renal Cortical Necrosis. Chin J Radiol. 2007;32:103-6.
28. Hnn L, Pfister RC. Renal subcapsular rim sign: New etiologies and pathologenesis. AJR. 1982;138:51-4.
29. Jeong JY, Kim SH, Lee HJ, Sim JS. Atypical Low - Signal - Intensity Renal Parenchyma: Causes and Patterns. Radiographics. 2002; 22:833-46.
30. Ten RM, Torres VE, Milliner DS, et al. Acute interstitial nephritis: immunologic and clinical aspects. Mayo Clin Proc. 1988;63:921.
31. Davidson AJ, Hartman DS. Diagnostic set: Large smooth, bilateral. In: Davidson AJ, Hartman DS (Eds). Radiology of Kidney and Urinary Tract, 2nd edition. Philadelphia, PA: WB Saunders; 1990.pp.157-86.
32. Sipe JD, Cohen AS. Amyloidosis. In: Fauci AS, Braunwald E, Isselbacher KJ, et al. (Eds). Harrison's principle of internal medicine. New York, McGraw-Hill; 1998.pp.1856-60.
33. Cohen AS: Amyloidosis. In: Pertersdrof RG, Adams RD, Braunwald E, et al. (Eds). Harrison's principle of internal medicine. NewYork, McGraw-Hill; 1983.pp.368-71.
34. Amendola RA. Amyloidosis of the urinary tract. In: Pollack HM (Ed). Clinical urography: An atlas and textbook of urologic imaging, Philadelphia, PA: WB Saunders; 1990. pp.2493-2500.
35. Kim SH, Han MC, Lee JS, Kim SP. Paroxysmal nocturnal hemoglobinuria: Case report of MRI and CT findings. Acta Radiol. 1991;32:315-6.
36. Jung DC, Kim SH, Jung S, Hwang S, Kim SH. Renal Papillary Necrosis: Review and Comparison of Findings at Multi-Detector Row CT and Intravenous Urography. Radiographics. 2006;26:1827-36.
37. Davidson A. Chronic renal failure. In: Pollack HM, McClennan BL (Ed). Clinical Urography, 1st edition. Philadelphia, PA: WB Saunders; 1990.pp.2279-90.
38. Chuang VP, Reuters SR. Angiographic features of Alport's syndrome: Hereditary nephritis. AJR. 1974;121:539-43.
39. Davidson AJ, Hartman DS. Diagnostic set: Small, Smooth, bilateral. In: Davidson AJ, Hartman DS (Eds). Radiology of Kidney and Urinary Tract, 2nd edition. Philadelphia, PA: WB. Saunders; 1990.pp.135-86.
40. Ono H, Ono Y. Nephrosclerosis and hypertension. Medical Clinics of North America. 1997;6:81.
41. Murphey MD, Sartoris D, Quale JL, Minim N, et al. Musculo-skeletal manifestations of chronic renal insufficiency. Radiographics. 1993;13:357-79.

CHAPTER 114

Renal Transplant

Ajay Gulati, Manavjit Singh Sandhu

INTRODUCTION

Renal transplantation as a treatment of choice is well established for patients with end-stage renal disease (ESRD) and leads to recovery of the normal renal function, cure of the uremic syndrome, and full rehabilitation from the renal disease. This has been made possible by improved surgical techniques, development of effective immunosuppressive medications, and better donor-recipient matching.

Renal function impairment of the transplant kidney can be secondary to parenchymal abnormality or due to surgical complications. Depending upon the clinical findings, appropriate diagnostic studies are carried out. Renal biopsy remains the definitive way to diagnose the parenchymal abnormalities.

TECHNIQUE

The transplanted kidney is usually placed extraperitoneally in patient's right iliac fossa with the pelvis lying anteriorly. In cadaveric renal transplants, an aortic patch (Carrel patch) is commonly removed with main renal artery. With live donors, only the main renal artery is harvested and anastomosed commonly in end-to-side manner with recipient's external iliac artery. The donor renal vein is always anastomosed end-to-side with external iliac vein. The current preferred method of re-establishing continuity of urinary tract is by creation of ureteroneocystostomy (commonly by using a submucosal tunnel to decrease the incidence of vesicoureteric reflux).[1,2]

Post-transplantation complications are characterized as either early or late. Early complications appear in the first few weeks and are generally due to surgical difficulties. Late complications appear some weeks later and are normally due to medical problems (usually due to immunosuppression or due to drug toxicity).

Early complications include acute rejection, acute tubular necrosis, hematoma, pyelonephritis, abscess, urinoma, acute ureteral obstruction and vascular complications. Late complications include chronic rejection, lymphocele, cyst formation, malignancies and opportunistic infections of transplant kidney.[3]

The greatest risk in the early post-transplant period is of early graft failure which presents with oliguria. To diagnose this early, there is a routine policy of clinical surveillance complemented with laboratory tests and imaging.[4]

COMPLICATIONS

Various complications of the renal transplant are as follows:

Acute Tubular Necrosis

Acute tubular necrosis (ATN) is caused by renal ischemia and presents with anuria immediately or within first few days after an initial diuresis. The patients remain constitutionally well and urine Na^+ is high. It is usually self-limiting with renal function returning to normal within few days to weeks. It is almost exclusively seen in cadaveric transplants.[4]

Rejection

Acute rejection remains one of the most serious and common complications. Virtually every patient experiences some degree of rejection, and differentiating rejection from other causes of graft dysfunction remains a challenging clinical problem.

Clinically, there are three distinct types of rejection: (i) hyperacute, (ii) acute, and (iii) chronic. Hyperacute rejection (due to circulating antibodies) usually occurs within hours to one or two days after the transplantation. It is characterized by the presence of fibrin thrombi in small arteries with cortical necrosis. The treatment is only the graft removal.

Acute rejection (mediated through CMI) is seen most frequently in first one-to-three weeks. It is characterized clinically by oliguria with systemic symptoms like pyrexia, hypertension, graft tenderness and swelling. The urine Na^+ is usually low (cf, ATN in which urine Na^+ is high). If diagnosed early, it may be reversed by steroids or by antibody therapy.[4]

Chronic rejection manifests as slow deterioration in renal function over a period of weeks or months. It does not respond to increased immunosuppressive therapy. Removal of the graft is required in majority of the patients.

Renal Artery Thrombosis

Renal artery thrombosis is a rare complication and results in loss of the graft. It is due to hyperacute or acute rejection and improper vascular anastomosis.

Renal Artery Stenosis

Renal artery stenosis is a well-recognized complication occurring in 3–12% of the transplants. It presents clinically as hypertension with or without deterioration of the renal function. Percutaneous transluminal angioplasty is the preferred mode of therapy with surgical correction reserved for the patients with unsuccessful angioplasty.

Pseudoaneurysm

Pseudoaneurysm is an uncommon complication which may present as hypertension because of the compression of the renal artery by the aneurysm.

Renal Vein Thrombosis

Renal vein thrombosis is rare but may by due to twisting or kinking at the time of surgery or secondary to thrombosis of the iliac veins.

Arteriovenous Fistula

Arteriovenous fistula (AVF) occurs most commonly after percutaneous needle biopsy. Most small fistulae close spontaneously, while large fistulae may require embolization or nephrectomy.

Peritransplant Fluid Collections

In the early postoperative period, the fluid collections around transplant kidney are hematoma, abscess or urinoma. Lymphocele generally occurs later (4–8 weeks after surgery).[5] Ultrasound-guided percutaneous aspiration can provide the definitive diagnosis.

Urinary Complications

These include urinary leak, obstruction, vesicoureteral reflux and nephrolithiasis. Urinary leak is the most frequent urinary complication in early postoperative period. This commonly occurs at the level of ureterovesical anastomosis secondary to ischemia of the distal ureter.

Urinary obstruction is commonly due to ureteric stricture in the distal one-third. It can also occur due to blood clot within the ureter or extrinsic compression by lymphoceles. The hydronephrosis can be due to obstruction or VUR. If RI >0.5, then hydronephrosis is generally due to obstructive causes.

Reflux is an important cause of recurrent urinary tract infections and makes the transplant at increased risk of pyelonephritis.

Calculi formation is a late complication of renal transplantation. It may occur *de novo* or as a result of hypercalcemia, hyperparathyroidism, steroid therapy, chronic infection, etc.[6-8]

Malignancy

Immunosuppressive therapy places the transplant recipient at 100 times the normal risk for developing cancers particularly of the skin, cervix, rectum, Kaposi's sarcoma and lymphoma.[6,7]

Post-transplantation lymphoproliferative disorder (PTLD), a potentially malignant process, is a complication that is associated with Epstein–Barr virus and occurs in approximately 1% of allograft recipients. The most common radiological feature is diffuse lymphadenopathy. In addition single or multiple extranodal masses can involve the liver, spleen, lung, CNS and GIT. It can even affect the graft itself with predilection for the renal hilum.[3,8,9]

Renal cell carcinoma also shows increased prevalence in transplant recipients with 90% occurring in the native kidneys and 10% in the transplant kidney.[8]

IMAGING TECHNIQUES

Impaired renal allograft function during the post-transplant period warrants an immediate and thorough evaluation to distinguish between the parenchymal and surgical complications.

The various imaging techniques and their indications are as follows:

Radiography

Plain Radiography

Plain radiographs are useful in demonstrating radiopaque calculi and gas in the renal parenchyma and collecting system in rare cases of emphysematous pyelonephritis.

Intravenous Urography

Intravenous urography was a useful study when ureteral obstruction or extravasation was suspected in a transplant recipient with adequate renal function. Presently it is not indicated because of the availability of ultrasonography and radionuclide imaging.

Cystography

Cystography is indicated to rule out vesicoureteral reflux in patients with persistent or recurrent urinary tract infection.

Radionuclide Imaging

Radio immunoassay (RIA) is the most useful modality for assessing the renal function both qualitatively and quantitatively while screening for common complications. Obtaining a baseline scan in the immediate postoperative period is extremely important.[5] Serial radionuclide scans allow early detection of rejection and can be used to monitor the recovery from ATN. The most common technique used is dynamic renal imaging using ^{99}Tc DTPA.[1]

Ultrasonography (US)

Sonography is a simple, inexpensive and readily available imaging modality that has become an essential component of the management of renal transplantation. High frequency transducers (5 MHz or higher) provide excellent details of the transplant kidney because of the superficial location. Several sonographic findings are seen in patients with graft dysfunction including enlargement of kidney, poor corticomedullary differentiation, reduced amplitude of sinus echoes and enlarged pyramids. Real-time ultrasonography combined with duplex Doppler or color and power flow imaging techniques is the most frequently used examination to evaluate worsening renal function in the post-transplantation period. Color Doppler is used to assess patency of vessels and detect any focal area of color aliasing which would indicate focal stenosis. Studies have shown that power Doppler sonography is superior to duplex Doppler sonography in screening patients with acute rejection. On spectral analysis, peak systolic velocity (PSV), acceleration time (AT), pulsatility index (PI) and resistive index (RI) are assessed. The upper limit of normal PSV in renal artery is 200–250 cm/s. The RI is considered to be normal if it is less than 0.7, indeterminate between 0.7 and 0.8 and elevated, if greater than 0.8 **(Figs. 1 and 2)**.

US also easily detects hydronephrosis and perinephric fluid collections **(Figs. 3 and 4)**. Minimal dilatation of the collecting system in the immediate postoperative period is acceptable and is usually due to edema at the ureteroneocystostomy site. Hydronephrosis may be secondary to the ureteral stricture or peritransplant fluid collections. Ultrasonography is sensitive for detection of the peritransplant fluid collections but it is not specific for fluid type, and aspiration of the fluid collection with ultrasound guidance is helpful in the management. US guidance minimizes the risk and discomfort of the percutaneous renal transplant biopsy. Vascular complications of transplantation, i.e. infarction, arteriovenous fistulae, pseudoaneurysms, arterial or venous thrombosis, and stenosis are readily identified by color and Duplex Doppler sonography **(Figs. 5A and B)**.[8,10-12]

A new technique for the quantification of vascularity based on the analysis of color Doppler images is described.[13] In this technique the velocity information obtained directly from cineloops is transferred to a computer for off-line analysis. This methodology is used in transplanted kidneys to assess parenchymal vascularity on the basis of percentage color pixel density and mean flow velocity in midkidney cross-sectional regions of interest and the distance from the most peripheral color pixels to the capsule of the kidney. In normally functioning transplants, the mean maximum color pixel density was 34.7+/– 13.4%, the mean flow velocity was 5.2 +/– 0.9 cm/second, and the mean distance to the capsule was 3.3 +/-1.1 mm. This technique can reliably detect allograft nephropathies.[13]

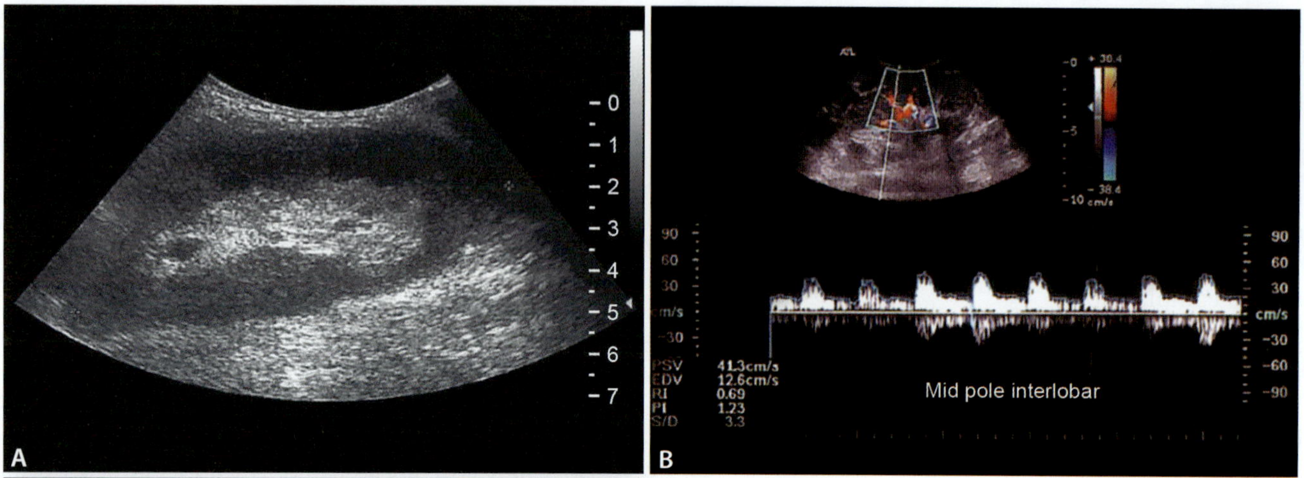

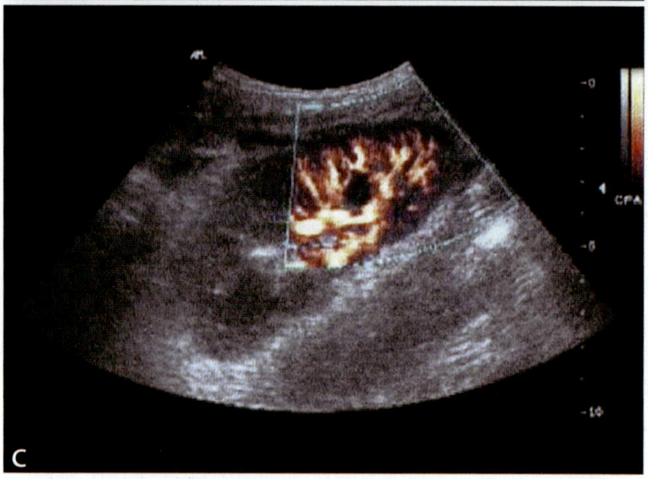

Figs. 1A to C: USG and Doppler images of the normal transplant kidney: (A) Grayscale sonogram showing normal size, outline, echogenicity, corticomedullary differentiation and pelvicalyceal system; (B) Duplex Doppler from interlobar artery shows normal low resistance flow with RI of 0.69 (<0.8) and PI of 1.23 (<1.5); (C) Power Doppler image shows normal cortical perfusion showing reaching up to the periphery of the renal cortex.

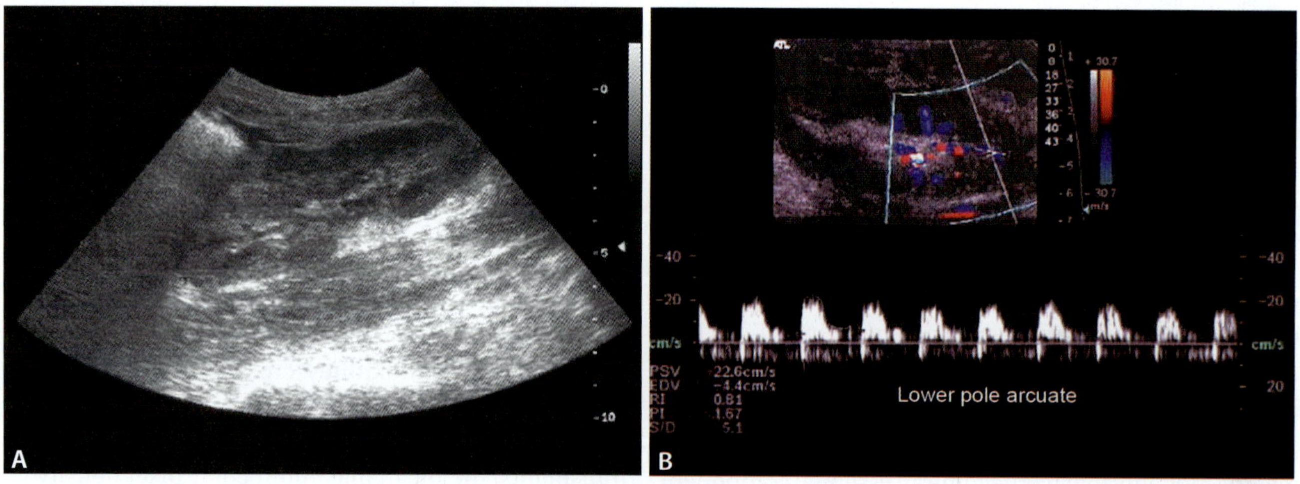

Figs. 2A and B

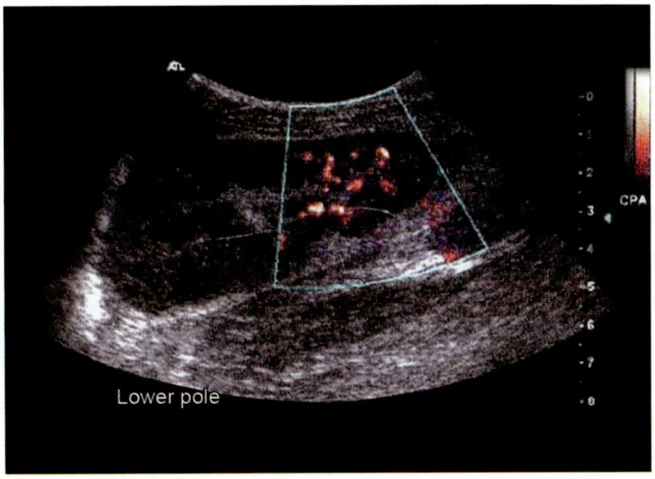

Fig. 2C

Figs. 2A to C: USG and Doppler images of the transplant kidney with acute rejection (confirmed on renal biopsy): (A) Gray-scale sonogram shows normal renal length and echogenicity with indistinct CMD and reduced renal sinus echoes; (B) Duplex Doppler from interlobar artery shows raised RI of 0.81and PI of 1.67; (C) Power Doppler image shows reduced cortical perfusion.

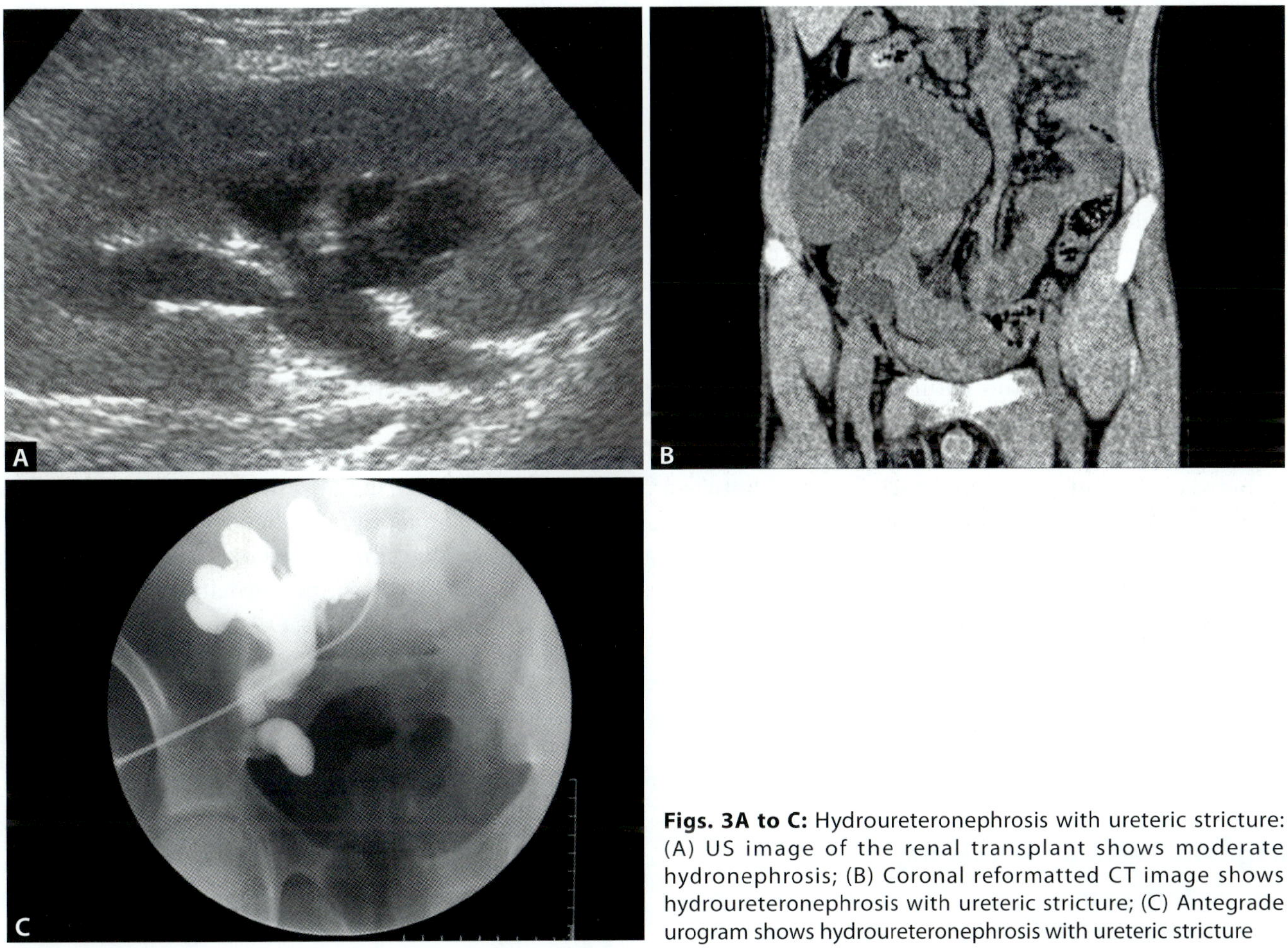

Figs. 3A to C: Hydroureteronephrosis with ureteric stricture: (A) US image of the renal transplant shows moderate hydronephrosis; (B) Coronal reformatted CT image shows hydroureteronephrosis with ureteric stricture; (C) Antegrade urogram shows hydroureteronephrosis with ureteric stricture

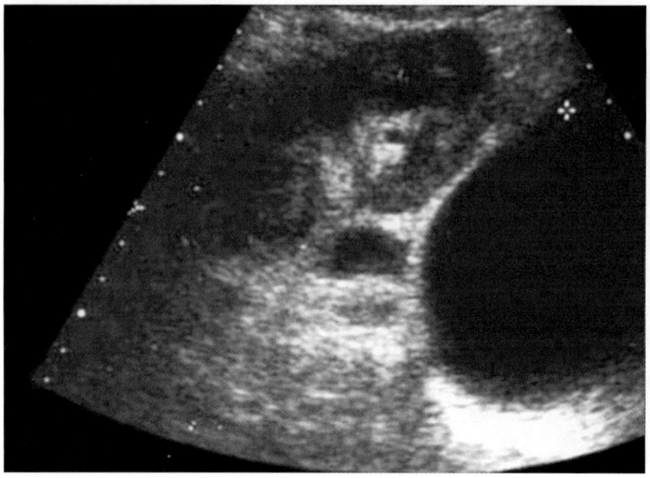

Fig. 4: Urinoma: Sagittal US image shows a large anechoic fluid collection seen posterior to the kidney. Note the dilatation of the ureter is attributable to the compression by the urinoma.

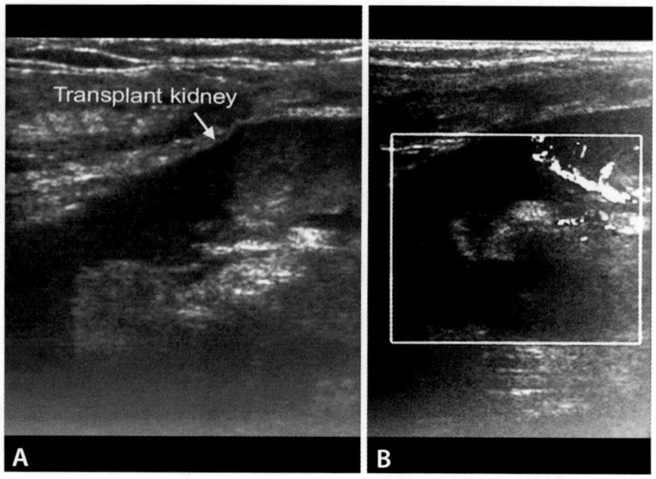

Figs. 5A and B: Renal Infarction: (A) US images shows well-demarcated hypodensity involving the renal parenchyma; (B) Power Doppler shows absence of flow in the involved renal parenchyma.

Computed Tomography

Helical computed tomography (CT) is an accurate, noninvasive technique which can depict parenchymal, perirenal, renal sinus, pyeloureteral and vascular diseases in renal transplant in great detail **(Figs. 6A to F)**. It helps differentiate acute rejection from obstructive uropathy, urinary fistula, perinephric fluid collections, mass lesions, etc. Dynamic CT has been used in the evaluation of physiological status of the renal transplants. It often delineates fluid collections and their anatomic relationship to adjacent structures better than USG. It can also distinguish the nature of fluid collections **(Fig. 7)**. Fresh blood in the form of hematoma has the highest attenuation value (55–66 HU), lymphoceles are between 10 and 20 HU, and the abscesses between 20 and 30 HU. In addition, drainage can be performed with CT guidance when USG cannot clearly define the relationship to the bowel **(Figs. 8 to 11)**. In assessing the complex problems such as detection of malignancy or sites of infection or sepsis, CT is the most useful modality. CT angiography with 3D reformatted images allows accurate imaging of the vascular diseases, such as stenosis, thrombosis, pseudoaneurysms and arteriovenous fistulae when US studies are inconclusive.

Magnetic Resonance Imaging

A magnetic resonance imaging (MRI) allows rapid global assessment of the renal transplant arterial system, renal parenchyma and peritransplant region. It can also detect or exclude various of the causes of renal transplant failure (e.g. stenosis or occlusion of transplant vessels, peritransplant fluid collections and ureteral obstruction).[14]

From the renal safety perspective, the lack of nephrotoxicity seen with the currently available gadolinium contrast media makes MRI a very useful and attractive alterative for evaluating renal transplant patients.[15]

A dynamic MRI performed with 3D fat saturated gradient echo T1-weighted sequence provides adequate information regarding the vessels and functional status of the transplant. HASTE T2-weighted acquisition also provides rapid assessment of the anatomy along with the detection of hydronephrosis, perirenal collections and malignancy, if present **(Figs. 12A and B)**.

The role of MRI in renal transplant dysfunction is rapidly evolving. Decreased or absent CMD on T1-weighted images is seen in majority of patients with acute rejection. However, this finding is not specific and can also be seen in allograft infection, cyclosporine toxicity and infiltrative or diffuse parenchymal diseases. On dynamic Gd-enhanced imaging, there is a blunted uprise and delayed peak in the cortical signal intensity curves. The medulla also show decreased enhancement in acute rejection.[15]

Preliminary reports indicate that phosphorus 31 MR spectroscopy may be useful in differentiating the rejection from other causes of the renal transplant failure. The use of MR spectroscopy for evaluating the phosphorus metabolism of allografts is still under development and has been reported to be useful. The long-term assessment of post-transplant renal prognosis with ^{31}P magnetic resonance spectroscopy has been recently evaluated and

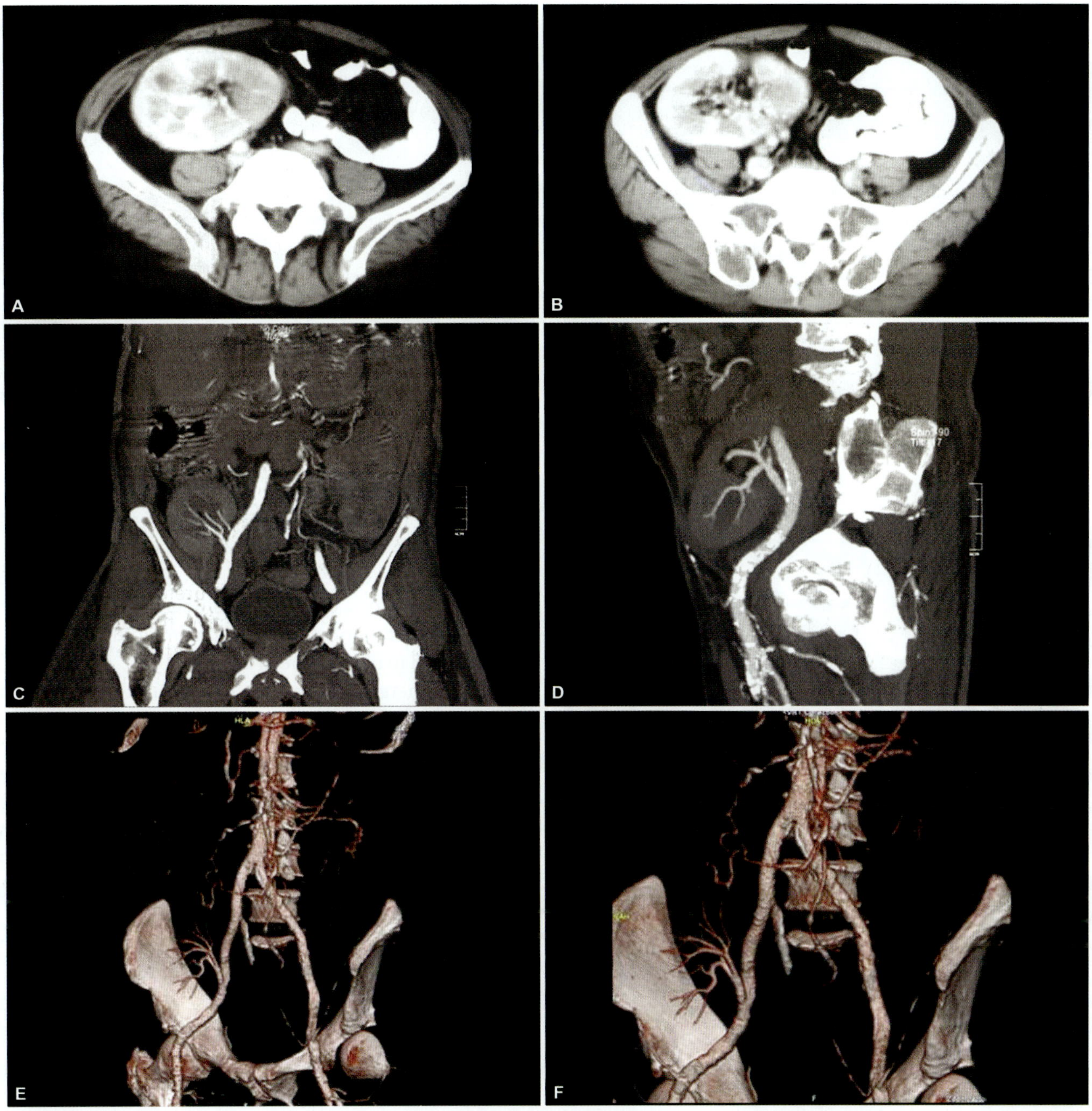

Figs. 6A to F: Normal transplant kidney: (A and B) Contrast-enhanced venous phase show uniformly enhanced parenchyma of the transplant kidney. Note made of a simple cyst; (C and D) Vascular MIP reformatted images depict the transplant renal artery anastomosed to the external iliac artery; (E and F) Volume-rendered images show the end-to-side anastomoses of the graft artery and the external iliac artery.

a beta-adenosine triphosphate/inorganic phosphate (beta-ATP/Pi) ratio above 1.2 suggests a high probability of 3-year renal survival, whereas a value over 2.5 indicates that the transplanted kidney could survive over 5 years.[16]

MRI is an excellent modality for screening of renal artery stenosis and other vascular complications **(Fig. 13)**. MRangiographicexaminationcanhelpinavoidingunnecessary catheter angiographies in majority of cases.

Angiography

Some important indications of renal transplant angiography are acute anuria, hypertension not responding to

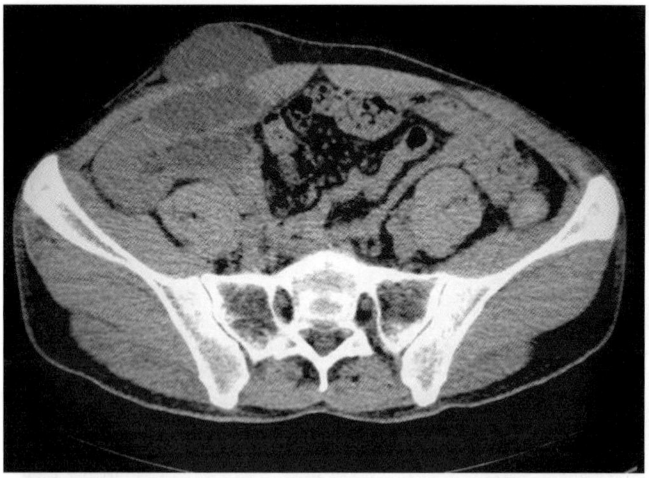

Fig. 7: Urinoma: NCCT KUB shows hydronephrosis with perinephric urinoma extending into the anterior abdominal wall.

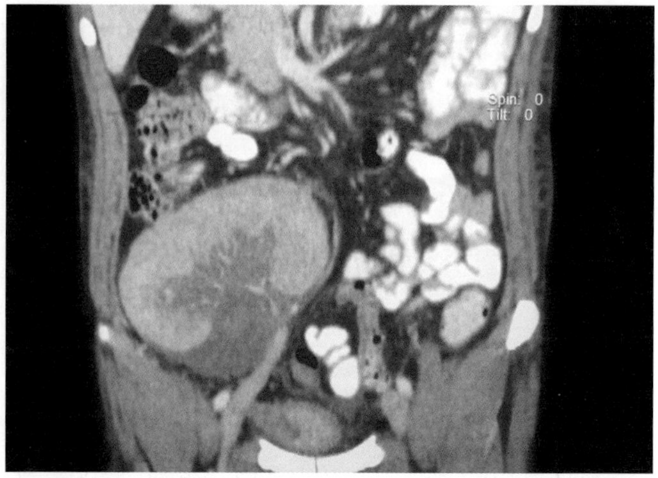

Fig. 8: PTLD involving renal transplant: Coronal reformatted CT image shows infiltrating mass in the renal hilum surrounding the graft pedicle.

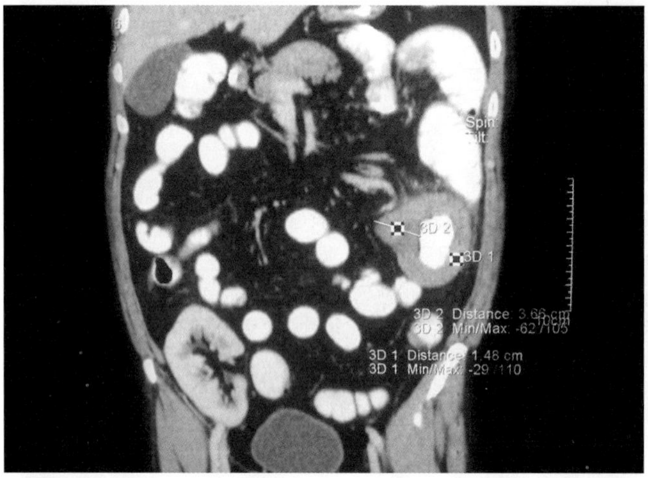

Fig. 9: Post-transplantation lymphoma: Coronal reformatted CT image shows homogeneous circumferential mural thickening involving the jejunum.

medication and functional deterioration of the allograft, in which confirmatory evidence of rejection or renal artery stenosis is necessary in order to proceed with the definitive surgery.[17,18] In acute rejection, there is a pruned-tree appearance secondary to the loss of second and third order branches. The arteriogram is essentially normal in acute tubular necrosis. In chronic rejection, arteriography demonstrates small graft size with irregularity, attenuation and occlusion of interlobar arteries and a patchy nephrogram secondary to the areas of cortical infarction.

Angiography is indicated in patients with hypertension not responding to the medical therapy. Angiography in such situation may demonstrate degree of renal artery stenosis. Percutaneous transluminal angioplasty can also be attempted to correct the arterial stenosis.

Transcatheter embolization is the treatment of choice for both symptomatic AVFs and enlarging pseudoaneurysms. Super-selective embolization performed with metallic coils minimizes the loss of functioning allograft tissue **(Figs. 14A to C)**. It allows the occlusion of targeted vessels in a precise and definitive manner, unlike embolization with particles that may reflux into nontargeted branches. Surgery is the treatment of last resort, with partial or total nephrectomy being the two options.

Percutaneous Interventional Techniques

Percutaneous interventional radiological techniques play an important role in management of the renal transplant patient and the timely use of these techniques may obviate surgery in some cases.

Antegrade pyelography is the most accurate and informative examination for the demonstration of ureteral stricture as well as the site of ureteral leak **(*see* Fig. 3C)**. Nephrostomy drainage catheter is placed in patients with urine leak and ureteral obstruction. Ureteral strictures can be dilated percutaneously by using angioplasty catheter, and indwelling ureteral stents left in place. Renal stone extraction through a percutaneous nephrostomy in a renal transplant patient can also be successfully accomplished.

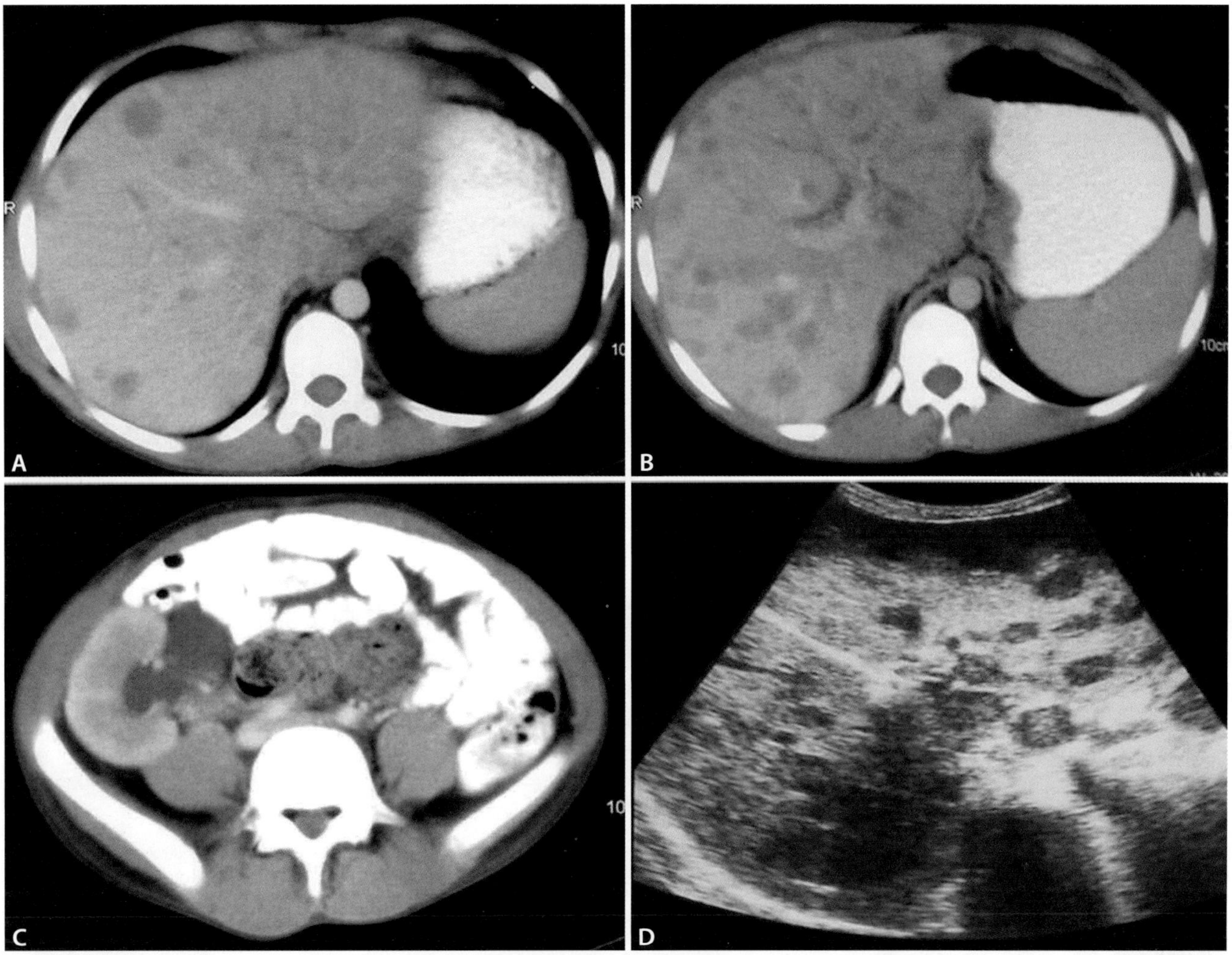

Figs. 10A to D: Hepatic PTLD: (A and B) Contrast-enhanced CT scan shows multiple hypodense lesions involving both the lobes; (C) CT scan at lower level shows hydronephrosis in renal transplant secondary to narrowing at ureterovesical anastomoses; (D) US image shows multiple well-defined hypoechoic lesions in the liver parenchyma.

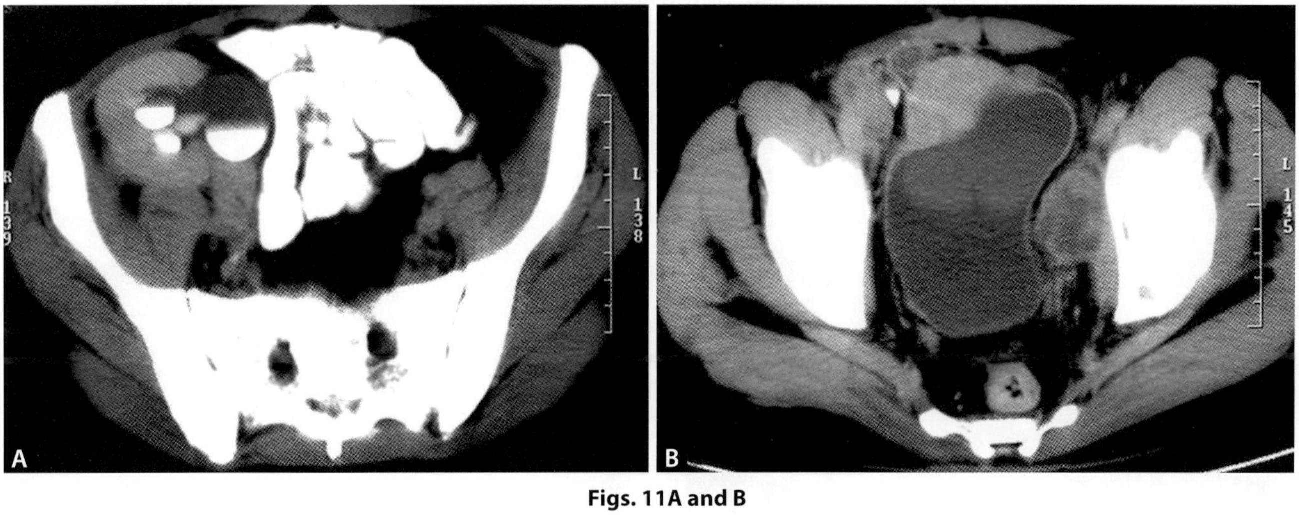

Figs. 11A and B

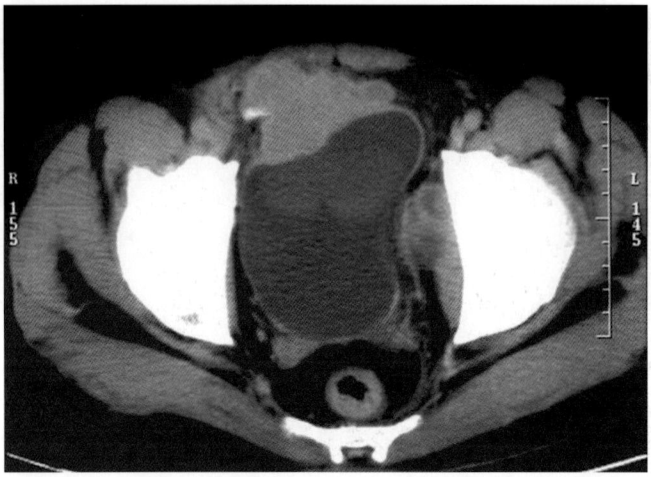

Fig. 11C

Figs 11A to C: Lymphoma in renal allograft recipient involving ureterovesical anastomoses: (A) Contrast-enhanced CT scan demonstrates hydroureteronephrosis; (B and C) Contrast-enhanced scans obtained at lower levels shows homogeneous soft tissue mass lesion at the ureterovesical anastomoses

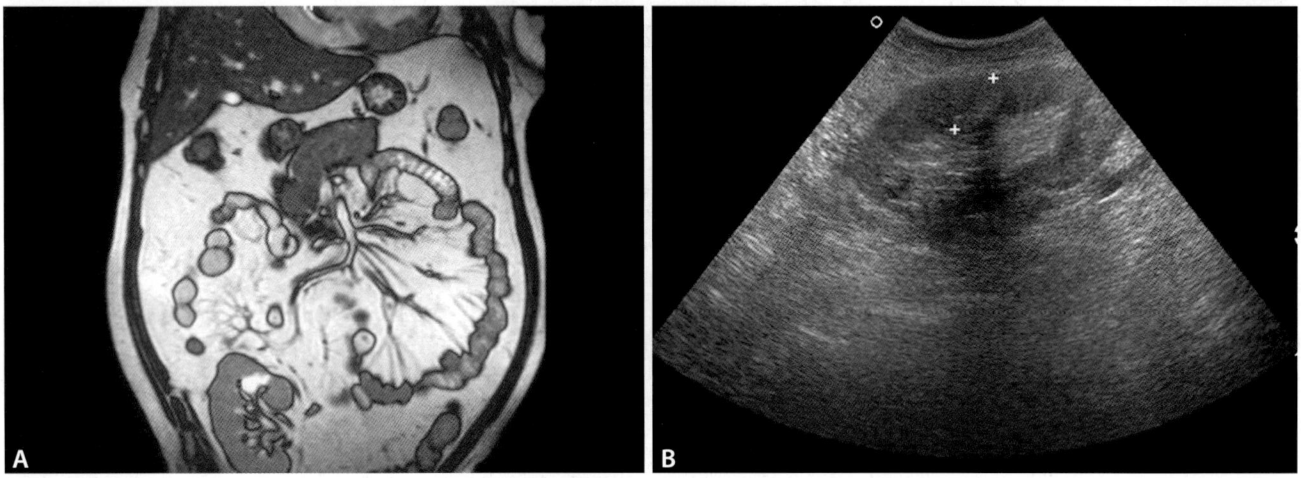

Figs. 12A and B: Renal cell carcinoma in a renal graft: (A) Coronal MR T2WI shows focal hyperintense lesion in the transplant kidney; (B) US image shows the lesion is iso- to hypoechoic to the renal parenchyma

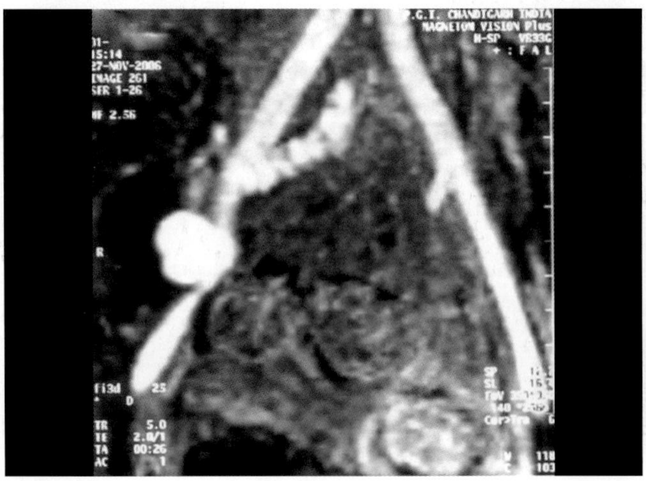

Fig. 13: Pseudoaneurysm: MIP reformatted MR angiogram depicts stenosis involving the external iliac artery with a pseudoaneurysm at the anastomotic site.

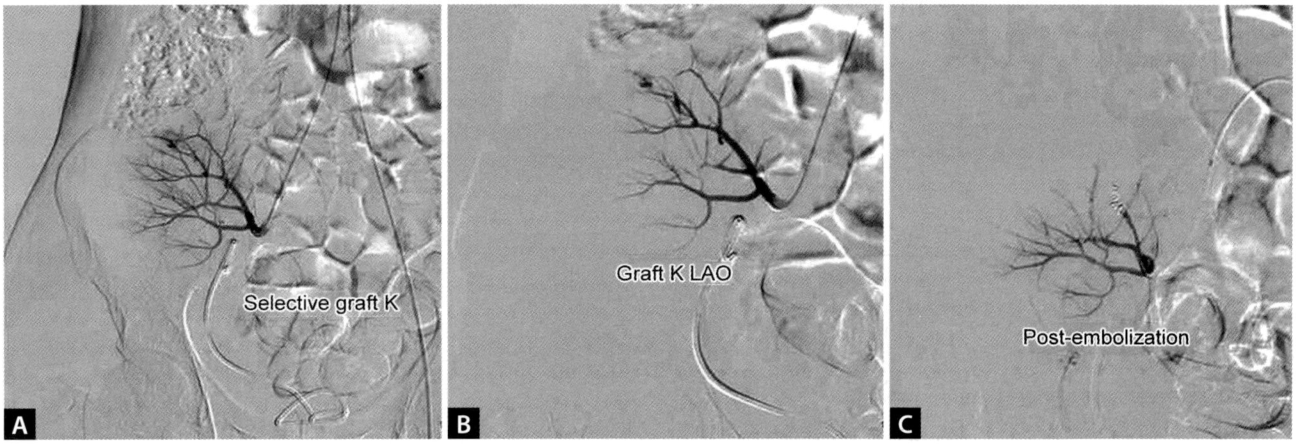

Figs. 14A to C: Transcatheter embolization of pseudoaneurysm: (A and B) Angiogram of transplant renal artery (AP and LAO projection) show a pseudoaneurysm in upper segmental artery; (C) Angiogram obtained after coil embolization shows successful obliteration of the aneurysm with preservation of the flow in the rest of the renal parenchyma.

ACKNOWLEDGMENTS

Sincere thanks to Dr Anupam Lal and Dr Manphool Singhal for contributing the images of the chapter.

REFERENCES

1. Rankin S. Renal parenchymal disease, including renal failure, renovascular disease (Ed) and transplantation. In: Grainger RG. Allison DJ (Eds). Diagnostic Radiology (5th edn): Churchill Livingstone (I): 851-5.
2. Oliver JH. Clinical indications, recipient evaluation, surgical considerations, and the role of CT and MR in renal transplantation. Radiol Clin N Am. 1995;33:435-44.
3. Sebastria C, Quiroga S, Boye R, Cantarell C, et al. Helical CT in renal transplantation: Normal findings and early and late complications. Radiographics. 2001;21:1103-17.
4. Sutton D. The kidneys and ureters. In: Kabala JE, Roobottom C (Eds). Textbook of Radiology and Imaging, 7th edn. Churchill Living Stone. 2014;2:982-6.
5. Brown ED, Chen YM, Wolfman NT, Ott DJ, et al. Complication of renal transplantation: Evaluation with US and Radionuclide Imaging. Radiographics. 2000;20:607-22.
6. Akbar SA, Jafri ZH, Amendola MA, Madrazp BL, et al. Complications of renal transplantation. Radiographics. 2005; 25:1335-56.
7. Kumar R, Wilson DD, Santa Cruz FR. Postoperative urological complications of renal transplantation. Radiographics. 1984;(4)3:531-47.
8. Langer JE, Jones LP, et al. Sonographic Evaluation of the renal transplant. Ultrasound Clin. 2007;2:73-88.
9. Sandhu MS, Kalra N, Sidhu R. Post-transplant lymphoproliferative disorder (PTLD) localised near the allograft mimicking a collection. Indian J of Radiol and Imaging. 2002;12:132-3.
10. O'neill WC, Baumgarten DA. Ultrasonography in renal transplantation. Am J Kidney Diseases. 2002;39:663-78.
11. Tublin ME, Dodd GD. Sonography of renal transplantation. Radiol Clin N Am. 1995;33:447-59.
12. Datta R, Sandhu M, Saxena AK, Sud K, et al. Role of duplex Doppler and power Doppler sonography with acute renal parenchymal dysfunction. Australasian Radiology. 2005;49: 15-20.
13. Gruenewald S, Skerrett D, Dolimier D, et al. Technique of colour Doppler quantification of vascularity in transplanted kidneys. J Clin Ultrasound. 2002;30:151-7.
14. Hohenwalter MD, Skowlund CJ, Erickson SJ, Hariharan S, et al. Renal transplant evaluation with MR angiography and MR Imaging. Radiographics. 2001;21:1505-17.
15. Pedrosa I, Rofsky NM. Kidneys. In: Edelman RR, Hesselink JR, Zlatkin MB, Crues JV (Eds): Clinical Magnetic Resonance Imaging, 3rd edition. Saunders (3 volume). 2006. pp. 2851-2.
16. Seto K, Ikechira H, Obata T, et al. Long-term assessment of post transplant renal prognosis with 31P magnetic resonance spectroscopy. Transplantation. 2001;72:627-30.
17. Orons PD, Zajko AB. Angiography and interventional aspects of renal transplantation. Radiol Clin N Am. 1995;33:461-71.
18. Kobayashi K, Censullo ML, Rossman LL, Kyriakides PN, et al. Interventional radiologic management of renal transplant dysfunction: Indications, limitations, and technical considerations. Radiographics. 2007;27:1109-30.

CHAPTER 115

Imaging of Obstructive Uropathy and Diseases of Ureter

Mahesh Prakash, Mandeep Kang

INTRODUCTION

Obstructive uropathy is a general term that describes obstructive changes in any part of the urinary tract. The renal structural and functional alterations caused by obstruction are termed as obstructive nephropathy.[1] Despite remarkable advances in diagnosis and treatment, obstruction remains a leading cause of damage to the urinary tract. Urinary obstruction affects patients of all ages and is responsible for thousands of hospital admissions and surgical procedures. Obstruction predisposes to urinary tract infection and renal failure. Early diagnosis and treatment of urinary obstruction can reverse the renal damage.

PATHOPHYSIOLOGY

When the ureter is acutely obstructed, the pressure of the collecting system proximal to the obstruction rises. Initially the renal blood flow (RBF) rises transiently, but over the next 6–12 hours, the RBF drops up to 30% due to increase of renal vascular resistance.[1] There are two mechanisms that come into play to temporarily decompress the nephron. First is pyelosinus and pyelovenous backflow and second is enhanced absorption of fluid from the tubules. Both mechanisms are responsible for continuing but reduced glomerular filtration. There is sufficient evidence to show that preglomerular arteriolar resistance develops in acute obstruction. This resistive index measure by Doppler has been used with variable success to confirm intrarenal vascular resistance in acute obstruction.[2,3] The elevated intrarenal resistance produces diminished diastolic flow eventually causing ischemia. The elevated intrarenal pressure also causes mechanical atrophy of tubules. After several days of total ureteric obstruction, less glomerular filtrate is produced so the intrapelvic pressure begins to fall. In 6–8 weeks time, the intrapelvic pressure returns to normal or subnormal levels however the glomerular filtration rate (GFR) is severely compromised.[4]

Relief of total but short lived obstruction leads to full restoration of the GFR. Longer period of total obstruction causes progressive nephron loss called obstructive atrophy.[1] Relief of obstruction that has already caused renal atrophy is followed by improvement in renal function but not to normal levels. The kidney often shrinks in size with blunting of the calyces and impaired ability of urinary concentration and acidification.[1] These semirecovered kidneys showing the anatomical and functional sequelae are said to exhibit postobstructive atrophy.

If the obstruction is partial and chronic, its effect to renal function is less predictable. Structural changes can occur in the medulla with impairment of the ability to concentrate urine. Sometimes, partial obstruction can exist for years without causing any functional impairment.

IMAGING OF ACUTE OBSTRUCTION

Intravenous urography (IVU), ultrasound (US), nuclear studies and computed tomography (CT) are the various modalities used for the assessment of urinary obstruction. The use of MR has been limited. IVU has conventionally been the initial imaging technique to evaluate possible renal obstruction. More recent studies however have shown the usefulness of ultrasound and noncontrast CT scan.

Plain X-ray

A single supine radiograph of the KUB region may reveal a radiopaque calculus as the cause of obstruction; however, nonradiopaque calculi cannot be detected.

Intravenous Urography

IVU historically has been the initial technique in evaluation of possible urinary obstruction with assessment of both the anatomical and physiological components of the kidney. The signs indicative of acute obstructive process are (i) prolonged dense nephrogram, (ii) renal enlargement, (iii) dilatation of the collecting system, (iv) delayed pyelogram, (v) ureteric dilatation, and (vi) pyelosinus extravasation.

If the obstruction is mild, then the nephrogram and calyceal opacification may be normal with minimal dilatation of the ureter. With more severe obstruction, the nephrogram is delayed in onset and becomes more dense and persistent **(Figs. 1A to D)**. The nephrogram may demonstrate faint radial striations due to contrast in the collecting ducts and tubules.[5] The kidney is often larger than normal. The opacification of calyces and ureter is delayed and depends upon the degree of obstruction. A completely obstructed kidney that has become anuric may not show any opacification of the collecting system; however once the opacification of the collecting system begins, additional radiographs are required to demonstrate the site of obstruction. For taking additional radiographs, the rule of eight can be helpful to prevent multiple exposures. If no contrast appears in the collecting system by 15 minutes after injection, there is little reason to obtain next film until two hours later.[6]

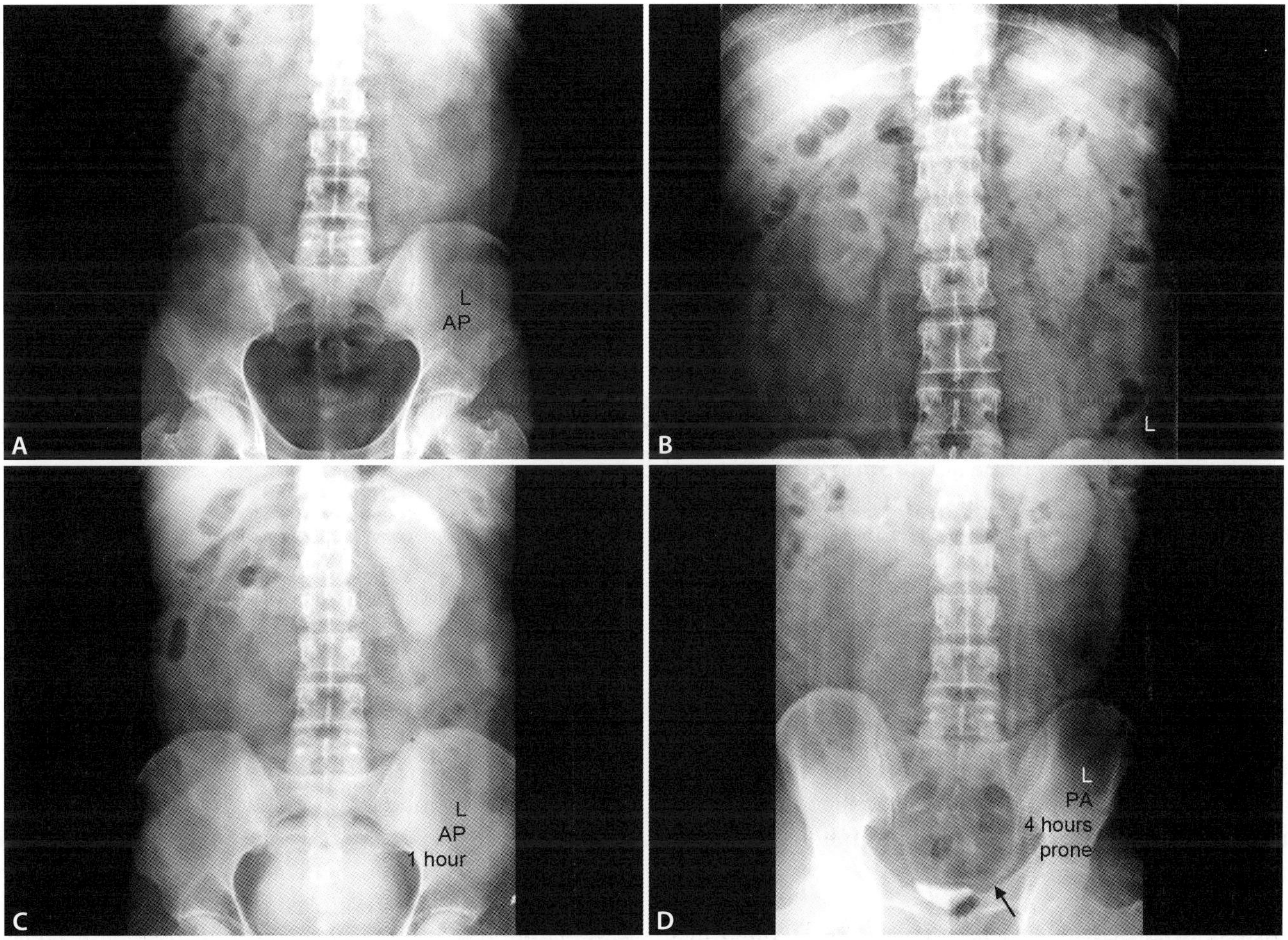

Figs. 1A to D: Serial IVU images of acute obstruction showing obstructing nephrogram. Plain film (A); five minute film (B); and 1 hour film (C) shows increasingly dense left nephrogram. Delayed (D) film well depicted the left lower ureter calculus as the cause of obstruction (arrow).

The collecting system and ureter are mildly dilated in acute obstruction. High obstructions cause more pelvicalyectasis then low ones. Extravasation of contrast medium from the kidney is demonstrated by IVU in up to 24% of obstructed patients.[7] Forniceal rupture occurs and opacified urine dissects through the tissues of the renal sinus. Minimal extravasation of contrast causes a smudged appearance of the calyces; however, when there is extensive leakage, contrast medium tracks around the renal pelvis and along the psoas muscles causing outlining of the ureter. Rarely, pyelolymphatic and pyelosubcapsular extravasation can occur. Unrelieved obstruction with continued extravasation of urine may result to a retroperitoneal collection called urinoma.[7] These collections are best visualized on USG, CT or MRI.

There has been a significant decline in the use of IVU as the dominant imaging technique in acute obstruction. This change has been driven by fear of contrast induced nephrotoxicity and by growth of renal sonography and particularly low-dose CT. The main drawback of IVU is that it can be time consuming because of the serial delayed films which may be required to be obtained until the level of obstruction is delineated. This may require many hours and repeated films. Acute side effects of iodinated contrast and contrast induced nephrotoxicity are also partly responsible for the decline in the use of IVU.[8]

Sonography

Conventional grayscale sonography is a good screening method for detecting subacute and chronic obstruction as demonstrated by pyelocaliectasis however in acute obstruction, pyelocaliectasis is minimal or absent. Another drawback is its inability to reliably distinguish mild hydronephrosis from normal or prominent extrarenal pelvis.[9] The routine gray-scale US misses approximately 30% of acute obstruction as pelvicaliectasis is usually mild to nonexistent. Grading of hydronephrosis as mild, moderate or severe is useful for descriptive purposes but it cannot be equated with either the presence or degree of obstruction. Urine debris levels or dependent echogenic material within the dilated collecting system have been reported in kidneys with pyonephrosis; however, a dilated pyelocalyceal system free of internal echoes does not rule out pyonephrosis.[6] If hydronephrosis is seen with dilated ureter, an attempt should be made to follow the ureter caudally to the point of obstruction.

Duplex and Color Doppler Sonography

Investigations with duplex and color Doppler ultrasound have yielded advances in three areas:

1. Distinguishing mild pyelectasis from prominent central renal blood vessels.
2. Detecting high grade acute ureteric obstruction through analysis of ureteral jets.
3. Establishing renal resistive index as an independent hemodynamic measure of urinary obstruction.

In certain cases normal renal vessels produce separation of the renal sinus echopattern which can mimic mild pelvicaliectasis. In this situation, color Doppler offers a quick and effective distinction between these two conditions. Normal ureteral jets are bilaterally symmetrical. The demonstration of ejection of the urine from ureter into urinary bladder excludes total obstruction.[10] The ureters with low-grade obstruction or nonobstructive ureterolithiasis may show normal or near normal ureteral jet pattern. Because of technical limitations and inconsistent findings in partial obstruction, evaluation of ureteral jets has limited clinical usefulness.

Resistive index (RI) is a measure of resistance to blood flow through the kidney and is defined as peak systolic velocity minus end diastolic velocity divided by peak systolic velocity. Normal intrarenal resistance in adults is less than 0.7. The RI may increase in acute obstruction **(Figs. 2A and B)**. The criteria suggested to diagnose obstruction include:[2,3]

1. Elevation above a threshold value.
2. Intrarenal RI difference of more than 0.06–0.10 with unilateral obstruction.
3. Abnormal RI response to diuretic challenge: there is increase of intrarenal RI with diuretic challenge in case of significant obstruction while normal kidneys with nonobstructive dilatation or partial obstruction show no change.

Computed Tomography

CT scan has emerged as an effective initial imaging tool in the evaluation of acute renal obstruction. CT scan adds value in the following conditions in the context of urinary obstruction:

1. Screening patients with acute flank pain.
2. Screening patients with azotemia who are strongly suspected as having obstruction.
3. Establishing the etiology of ureteral obstruction when other investigations have failed.

Previously, CT was not routinely used in the evaluation of ureteric obstruction because of ionizing radiation, need for intravenous contrast, increased expense and nonavailability in many institutions. Today, CT scan is widely available, very quick and can be done without contrast. Noncontract CT (NCCT) scan is useful in

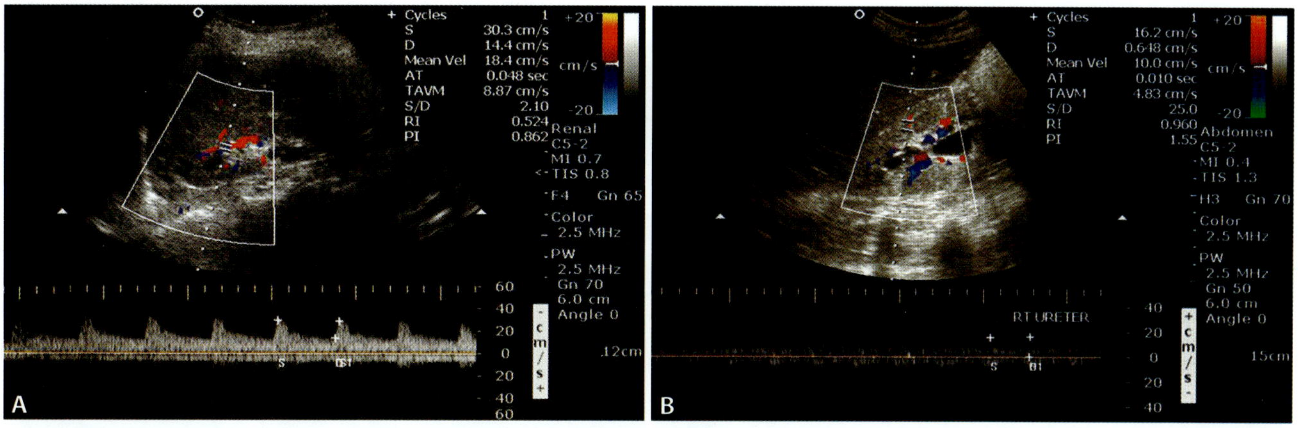

Figs. 2A and B: Doppler tracing of normal kidney (A) and in acute obstruction (B). The resistive index is increased in acute obstruction.

determining the presence or absence of obstruction and have higher sensitivity for detection of ureteric stones as compared with IVU.[11] The disadvantage of NCCT is higher radiation dose to patient however Tack et al. reported that low dose (30 mAs) NCCT gives a diagnostic quality image for detection of urinary stones and hence significantly reduces the radiation dose to patient[12] **(Figs. 3A and B)**. The secondary CT signs of obstruction that may be present in patients with ureteric stones are ureteral dilatation, pyelocaliectasis, perinephric stranding and renal enlargement.

The early corticomedullary differentiation is prolonged when contrast-enhanced CT is performed in acute obstruction. Gradual opacification of the medulla follows over minutes to hours, resulting in persistent homogenously dense or diffusely mottled nephrogram. If obstruction is unrelieved, the medullary pyramids may actually become more densely opacified then the cortex, creating the reverse corticomedullary nephrogram.

CT is extremely useful for diagnosing the cause of obstruction. Nonopaque filling defects in the renal pelvis or ureter seen on IVU deserve noncontrast CT to distinguish urate calculi from other lesions. Urate and xanthine stones always have high attenuation value.[13] CT is particularly useful in determining the etiology when IVU shows extrinsic ureteric obstruction. Lymphadenopathy, primary and secondary retroperitoneal malignancy, retroperitoneal fibrosis and perianeurysmal fibrosis are some of the common examples which can be easily visualized on CT. In a minority of patients, the cause of obstruction may not be seen as there may not be an intraluminal or periureteral mass. Secondary signs of obstruction include stranding of perinephric fat, dilatation of intrarenal collecting system, and unilateral increase in cortical thickness.[8]

Radionuclide Renography

The role of nuclear medicine in the evaluation of acute obstruction is limited. Use of technetium DTPA or MAG-3 permits evaluation of arrival, uptake, transit and elimination of radiopharmaceutical from the kidney. DTPA is a glomerular agent whereas MAG-3 operates by tubular secretion. MAG-3 is being increasingly used because of its better renal uptake even in the presence of in renal insufficiency. In obstruction, activity in the parenchyma may rise at a slower rate and persist for a longer time than the nonobstructed kidney. Activity in the collecting system also proceeds down the ureter at a slower rate.

Radionuclide renography however lacks precise anatomical delineation of obstruction as well as ability to define the cause of obstruction. Its major use is in the differentiation of a dilated nonobstructed system from a partially obstructed system. The diuretic renogram, using frusemide after DTPA or MAG-3 study can separate these two entities.[14] If the system is dilated but not obstructed, the collecting system activity washes out within 10 minutes after frusemide administration. If obstructed, no or partial response to the diuretic challenge is seen depending on the severity of obstruction.

Magnetic Resonance Imaging

At present, magnetic resonance imaging (MRI) has limited role to in the evaluation of urinary obstruction. Magnetic resonance urography (MRU) is an ideal technique in pregnancy, where there is contrast allergy, renal failure patients and if radiation dose is an issue. The level of obstruction is always identified.[15] Ureteric abnormalities are poorly defined especially if they are less than 4 mm in size and that includes stones. MR imaging remains more expensive and not readily available.

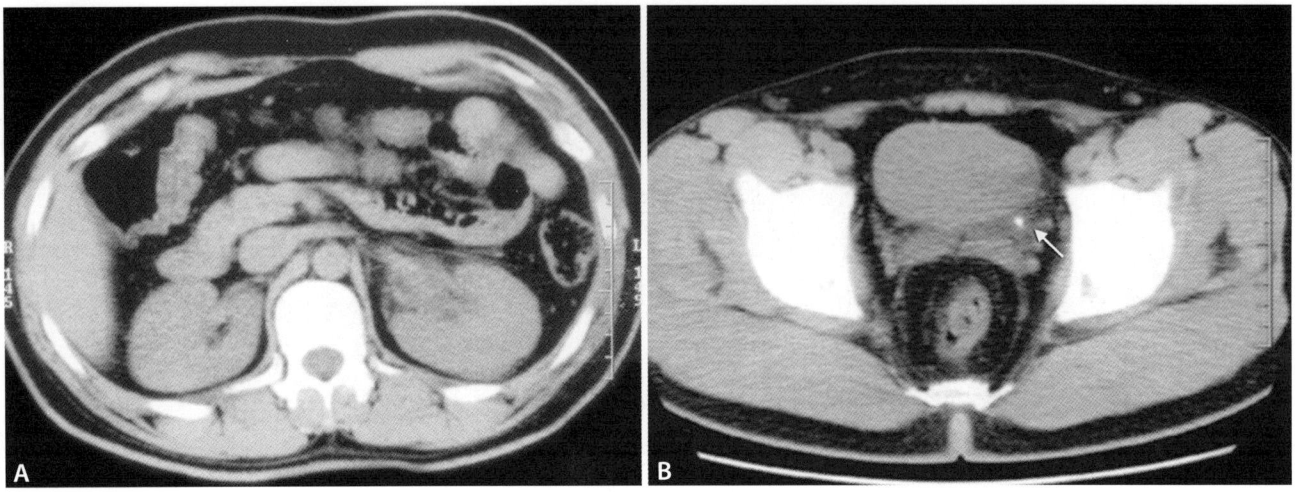

Figs. 3A and B: Low dose noncontrast CT scan (NCCT) of young male presented with acute loin pain. Axial section at the level of kidneys (A) shows minimal calyceal separation and perinephric stranding on left side and lower section at the level of bladder (B) shows obstructed calculus in lower ureter (arrow).

IMAGING OF CHRONIC OBSTRUCTION

The plain radiograph may reveal radiopaque stones that could be responsible for obstruction. A grossly hydronephrotic kidney may be visible as a soft tissue mass in the renal fossa.

Intravenous Urography

The urographic pattern varies in chronic obstruction.[16] The kidney size is small in untreated complete obstruction however long standing partial obstruction can result in enlargement of the collecting system and kidney. The obstructive nephrogram is usually not seen in cases of chronic obstruction as tubular concentrating ability and GFR are reduced. The nephrographic density may be normal, faint or none depending upon the residual functioning parenchyma. The renal parenchyma is usually atrophied. When parenchymal thickness is reduced to 1–2 cm, but the renal function is relatively preserved then calyceal crescents are sometimes seen during nephrogram **(Fig. 4A)**. The crescents are thin, curved collections of contrast denser than the nephrogram, located in the medulla. They represent realigned collecting tubules running perpendicular to their usual orientation.[17] They parallel the cortical margin of the ballooned calyces, located just 1–2 mm peripheral to the calyces. These crescents remain fixed regardless of patient position. The opacification of extremely thin parenchyma over the dilated calyceal sac produces a "rim" or shell nephrogram.

Chronic obstruction produces varying degree of pyelocalyceal dilatation. As contrast medium enters the dilated system, it glides to the dependent portion of calyces. With the patient supine, rounded puddles of contrast appear separated from the surrounding nephrogram by a boundary of nonradiopaque urine, this picture has been called the **ball pyelogram (Fig. 4B)**.

Chronic obstruction may lead to nonvisualized kidney on urogram. The ureter becomes dilated proximal to the obstructing lesion, elongated and tortuous, and in extreme cases it may resemble a segment of small intestine. This is called giant hydroureter or giant megaureter.

Sonography

Ultrasound is highly reliable in the detection of chronic ureteral obstruction by demonstrating pyelocaliectasis with reported sensitivities ranging from 93 to 100%.[18] The ureter is dilated proximal to the obstruction in most of the cases. Resistive index (RI) may be abnormal but it is less reliable in chronic obstruction then acute obstruction. Ultrasound may show false-positives as the collecting system may appear dilated in patients with extrarenal pelvis, vesicoureteric reflux, and persistent change due to obstruction that has been relieved.

Computed Tomography

CT shows the same findings as visualized on urography. Abnormal renal dimensions, varying degree of parenchymal thinning and pyelocaliectasis are seen. With moderate or severe hydronephrosis, urine-contrast layers in the dependent portion of the collecting system which are only occasionally demonstrated at IVU are commonly seen on CT. When the hydronephrosis is accompanied by parenchymal thinning, obstructive atrophy is diagnosed **(Figs. 5A and B)**. The CT version of

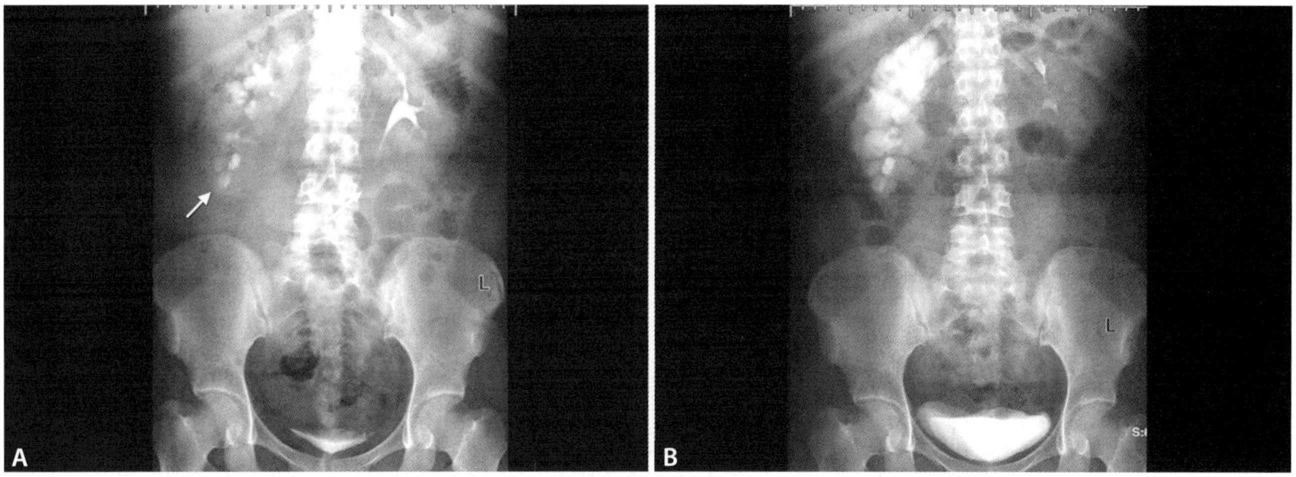

Figs. 4A and B: IVU study of chronic hydronephrosis due to ureteric stricture. An 11-minute film (A) shows crescents (arrow) and a 1 hour film (B) shows ball pyelogram.

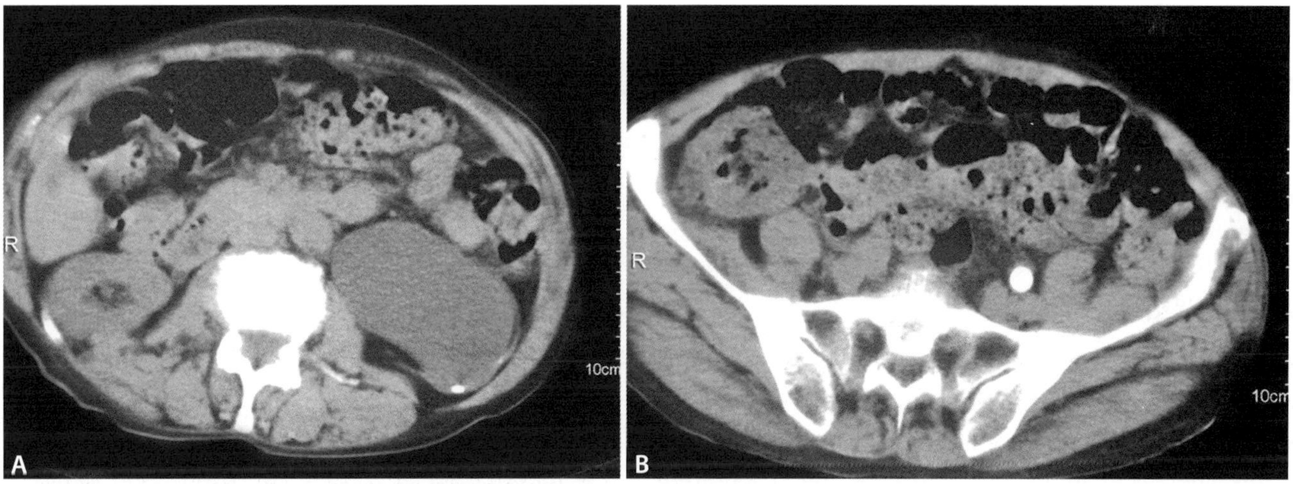

Figs. 5A and B: NCCT axial images shows gross hydronephrosis with obstructive atrophy and left renal calculus (A), lower sections shows obstructing calculus in lower ureter (B).

the shell or rim nephrogram is a thin band of opacified parenchyma surrounding the dilated pelvicalyceal system. Following relief of obstruction, the kidney may shrink remarkably as a manifestation of post-obstructive atrophy. Hydronephrosis with parenchymal signs of pyelonephritis, perinephric abscess or thickened renal pelvis can suggest pyonephrosis. CT is a modality of choice for demonstration, if the obstruction is caused by extrinsic process.[18] The concept of CT urography is attractive because both the renal parenchyma and urothelium can be evaluated at single comprehensive examination. CT urography is very useful in urinary obstruction as it simultaneously evaluates the functional status of the kidney, detects dilatation of the pelvicalyceal system as well as the level and cause of obstruction. The limitations of CT urography are the higher radiation dose and longer scan time.

Magnetic Resonance Imaging

The morphological characteristics of a chronically obstructed kidney may be demonstrated by MRI. The corticomedullary distinction usually seen on T1-weighted images may disappear because of atrophy or destruction of medulla. The dilated pelvicalyceal system is seen as hypointense region on T1- and hyperintense on T2-weighted images.

INVASIVE TECHNIQUES IN URINARY OBSTRUCTION

Antegrade Pyelography

This study is done by puncturing the collecting system percutaneously under fluoroscopy. Sonographic guidance facilitates placement of a small caliber needle into the intrarenal collecting system. Once correct placement is ensured by urine aspiration, contrast is injected under fluoroscopic control for opacification of the PCS and ureter. The usual indications are discussed further.[6]

1. To localize the collecting system before percutaneous nephrostomy or Whitaker test.
2. To pinpoint the level of obstruction in a dilated urinary system not adequately opacified by an IVU.
3. To opacify the urinary system after failed retrograde ureteropyelogram.
4. To obtain renal urine for bacteriological or cytological examination.

Retrograde Pyelography

This test is particularly valuable when IVU is suboptimal owing to poor renal function and in cases where IV contrast administration is contraindicated. Imaging with retrograde pyelography defines the level and degree of obstruction. It also clarifies whether the obstruction is intraluminal or not.

CAUSES OF OBSTRUCTION AND DISEASES OF URETER

In children, obstruction is commonly due to congenital causes whereas in adults most cases are due to acquired causes. Obstruction may also be classified by location as intrarenal, postrenal, supravesical or infravesical.

Congenital Ureteric Obstruction

Primary megaureter and obstruction associated with duplication are common causes of congenital ureteric obstruction. The major causes are given in **Table 1**.

Table 1: Congenital causes of ureteric obstruction.[6]

• UPJ obstruction
• Primary megaureter
• Ureterocele
• Ureteric valve
• Distal ureteric stenosis
• Ureteric atresia
• Circumcaval ureter

Ureteropelvic Junction Obstruction

Congenital obstruction of the ureteropelvic junction (UPJ) is a common anomaly of the urinary tract. It results due to deficiency and derangement of the ureteric smooth muscle fibers resulting in failure of normal peristalsis in the affected segment and subsequent functional obstruction. Males and the left side are commonly affected. Dilated renal pelvis and calyces are demonstrated on urography. Delayed radiographs are usually necessary for demonstrating the point of obstruction at UPJ. With long standing or high-grade obstruction the kidney may become nonfunctional. When there is insufficient contrast excretion or the ureter is not visualized, the diagnosis can be established by antegrade pyelography. Ultrasound usually shows hydronephrosis and dilated renal pelvis with a nondilated ureter. In patients with equivocal UPJ obstruction, diuresis renography and Whitaker procedure may be employed to assess functional obstruction.

Primary Megaureter

Primary megaureter or congenital megaureter is an uncommon entity probably caused by functional abnormality of the juxtavesical ureter, which is less distensible and fails to transmit normal peristalsis. Primary megaureter may be seen in both children and adults and typically remains asymptomatic in many cases.[19] Males are affected more than females. A characteristic beak-like configuration of the distal ureteral segment is seen on urography with proximal dilatation of ureter **(Fig. 6)**. The dilatation may extend proximally to calyces.

Primary megaureter may be associated with UPJ obstruction, contralateral renal agenesis and vesicoureteric reflux. Ultrasound readily detects PCS and ureteral dilatation. An MCU is required to determine whether vesicoureteric reflux is present or not. In the absence of reflux, the obstructive nature of the megaureter should be evaluated by diuretic urogram.

Ureterocele

The term ureterocele means saccular dilatation of the intramural portion of ureter as it passes through the bladder wall **(Fig. 7)**. It may be of two types—simple (orthotopic) and ectopic. The ureters of a simple ureterocele drain a nonduplex kidney and insert into the bladder at their normal position at the trigone. An ectopic ureterocele frequently occurs in a duplex kidney. Ureterocele typically appear on urography and cystography as smooth, rounded or ovoid filling defect in the bladder.

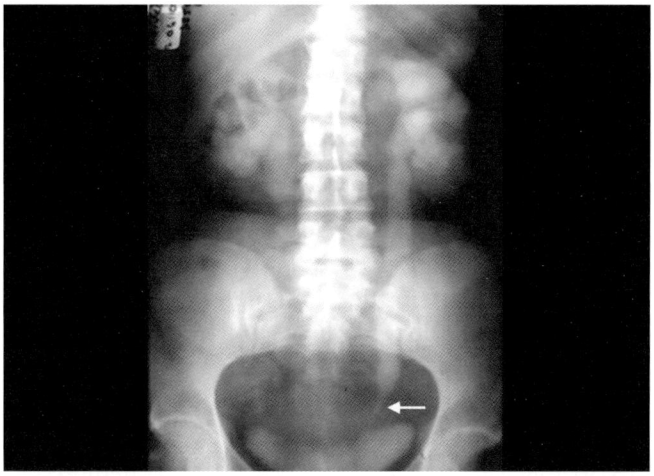

Fig. 6: Delayed IVU image (1 hour) shows bilateral hydroureteronephrosis with smooth tapering of lower ureter suggestive primary megaureter (arrow).

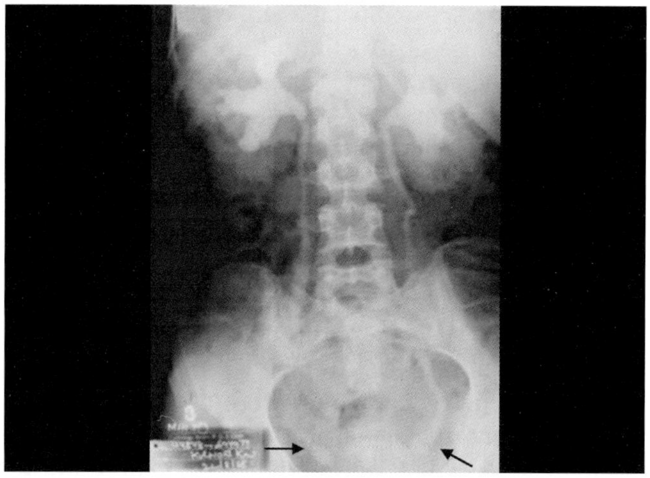

Fig. 7: IVU (30 min film) shows bilateral hydronephrosis with fusiform dilatation (arrows) of lower most portion of ureters suggestive of ureterocele.

Circumcaval Ureter

Circumcaval ureter results when the supracardinal vein persists and forms the major portion of the inferior vena cava. Embryonically, the subcardinal vein lies ventral to the ureter. The right ureter is carried medially by the migration of the subcardinal vein towards the developing IVC. The typical pattern on urography is a tortuous, dilated proximal right ureter and associated hydronephrosis. The proximal ureter has a characteristic reverse-J course before it crosses behind and around the IVC and then descends medial to the ipsilateral lumbar pedicle. The confirmation of the diagnosis can be made with CT, which shows the ureter passing posterior and medial to the IVC.

Acquired Ureteric Obstruction

The causes of acquired ureteric obstruction can be intraluminal or extraluminal.

Intraluminal Causes

Abnormalities may develop within the ureteral lumen without any attachment to the uroepithelial lining. The common causes are calculi, blood clots, tissue slough, fungus ball and foreign material.

Ureteric Calculus

Approximately 90% of urinary stones contain calcium (calcium oxalate, magnesium ammonium phosphate) and 10% are calcium free (uric acid, cystine and xanthine). Oxalate and cystine calculi are radiopaque; however, pure uric acid calculi are radiolucent on plain radiography. Calculi in the ureters can be difficult to visualize on plain X-rays in view of the fact that a third of the ureter may overlie bone. IVU is performed to establish whether or not a concretion seen on plain films lies in the urinary tract, if so, whether it is the cause of ureteric obstruction.

Stones, except for those composed of matrix are well seen on sonography. Strong echoes with a sharply marginated acoustic shadow are the distinguishing features that distinguish stones from other filling defects in the ureter.

Computed tomography plays a major role in the differential diagnosis of nonopaque filling defects in the ureter. Stones that are nonopaque (uric acid) or faintly opaque (cystine) are visualized as dense as calcium containing stones; however, their actual attenuation values are lower than calcium stones. Helical CT is of particular value in detecting acute obstruction caused by ureteric calculus. Noncontrast contiguous sections from kidney to bladder permit identification of the ureter as well as obstructing calculus.[20]

Blood clots: Blood clots in ureter are secondary to trauma, tumors, nephritis, vasculitis and bleeding disorders. Blood clots exhibit radiographic features that are common to other nonradiopaque lesions. The location of clot varies with time or with change in position of patient. When clot persists as a mass of fibrin, calcification may develop that resembles stones or uroepithelial tumors.[21] Sonography shows a mass-like filing defect with low level echoes. The CT attenuation value of clot varies with time. When the clot is fresh, its attenuation value exceeds that of soft tissue. Within a week its attenuation decreases. Blood clot does not enhance after intravenous contrast administration.

Tissue slough: Necrosed papilla and cholesteaotoma can slough and cause obstruction of ureter with proximal dilatation. Urography shows features of nonopaque filling defect. Calcium is sometime deposited along the periphery of a sloughed papilla. Sonography and CT demonstrate hypoechoic and hyperdense mass lesion, respectively.

Fungus ball: Most fungus balls or mycetomas are caused by *Candida albicans* and *Aspergillus*. Fungal infection of the urinary tract occurs in the setting of altered host resistance like HIV, steroid intake, severe debilitating disease and antineoplastic drug intake. The fungus balls fill the renal pelvis or ureter with a nonopaque mass. Sometime contrast material insinuates into the interstices of the mass causing lacelike radiodense pattern during IVU.[22] The fungus ball appears as an echogenic mass on sonography while CT shows soft tissue attenuation filling defects. Neither sonography nor CT can differentiate fungus ball from other intraluminal soft tissue.

Intramural Causes

Ureteral Tumors

Primary ureteral tumors are relatively rare, accounting for approximately 1% of all urinary tract tumors. Tumors arising from epithelium are commonest however they can arise from mesoderm. Males are affected more than females with the usual age of presentation being in the 5th–8th decades. The most common tumor of ureter is transitional cell carcinoma. Rare tumors include squamous carcinoma, adenocarcinoma, sarcoma and metastasis.

Transitional Cell Carcinoma

Transitional cell carcinoma (TCC) occurs more frequently in males and has a peak incidence in the seventh decade. Certain epidemiological factors have been associated with increased risk for development of transitional cell carcinoma. These include exposure to chemicals, dye, petroleum, rubber and cable industries. Tobacco, coffee, artificial sweetener, chronic inflammation and infection are additional risk factors. There is increased prevalence of TCC in analgesic and Balkan nephropathy. Squamous cell carcinoma occurs in older age and is generally associated with chronic infection and leukoplakia of urinary tract. Adenocarcinoma occurs in patients with severe infection and stone disease.

Radiological findings

IVU: The lesion appears as a smooth or lobulated, polypoidal filling defect in the ureter which maintains a constant relationship with the ureteric wall **(Figs. 8A and B)**. There is usually proximal obstruction dilatation of the ureter. The ureter just distal to the tumor is also often slightly dilated. The combination of distal margin of soft tissue mass invaginating into the distended segment of opacified ureter constitutes the Chalice or Bregman's sign.[23] This

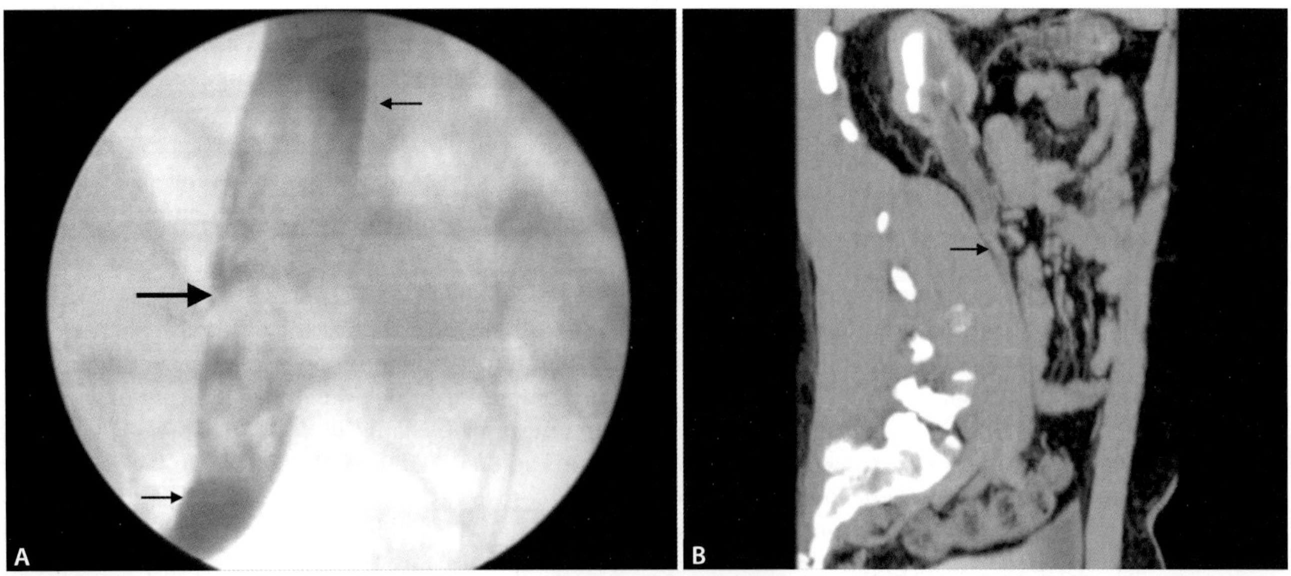

Figs. 8A and B: Transitional cell carcinoma (TCC) of ureter. Fluoroscopic spot of nephrostogram (A) shows irregular filling defect (thick arrow) in mid-ureter with dilatation of ureter (thin arrows) proximal as well as distal to the lesion (Bregman's sign). Another patient with TCC: Contrast-enhanced CT with sagittal reconstruction (B) showing circumferential mural thickening (arrow) of ureter with proximal hydroureteronephrosis. These findings may mimic inflammatory lesion of ureter.

sign is useful in distinguishing tumor from nonopaque stone as the ureter is not dilated distal to a stone.

Sonography: Tumors of the ureter may be seen as a soft tissue mass situated at the distal end of a slightly dilated ureter. USG examination does not reliably distinguish between ureteric tumor and blood clot.

CT: Computed tomography defines the contour and mural attachment of tumor following ureteral opacification. The tumor may enhance after intravenous contrast administration. The tumor may project into the ureteric lumen with circumferential or eccentric mural thickening. The lesion may infiltrate into the periureteric fat. CT is important in the staging of a documented ureteric tumor as it detects periureteral extension as well as lymph node enlargement.[24] MR may be used in patients in whom CT cannot be done.

Benign Tumors

Benign tumors of urothelium constitute approximately 20% of ureteral neoplasms. The most commonest is a papilloma which presents as a solitary filling defect attached to the ureter by a stalk.

Nonepithelial Tumors

Fibroepithelial polyp is the most common nonepithelial tumor. These typically occur in patients in the 20–40 years age group. The usual location is the proximal one-third of the ureter. The lesion is usually solitary but multiple lesions can rarely be seen. The lesion can present as a mobile, smooth, cylindrical, slightly mobile, filling defect. Sometimes the lesion can be frond like.

Secondary Tumors and Contiguous Infiltration

These are more common than primary ureteric tumors. Direct extension of tumor from primary sites such as cervix, prostate and bladder can cause ureteric obstruction. Malignant retroperitoneal lymphadenopathy also causes obstruction to the ureter. Some tumors invoke an intense periureteric desmoplastic reaction causing ureteric obstruction. In such cases, imaging may demonstrate a soft tissue mass like retroperitoneal fibrosis. Rarely, hematogenous malignant deposit can occur to the ureters. The common primaries responsible are melanoma, renal cell carcinoma, breast, lung and prostate.[25]

Inflammatory Lesions of Ureter

Inflammatory conditions of the ureter include a wide variety of disorders. Primary inflammation of the ureter is rare in the absence of systemic or regional disease in urinary tract, retroperitoneum, pelvis or peritoneum. Inflammation of ureteral wall may originate from inflammatory elements excreted in the urine, hematogenous embolism or contiguous spread from adjacent areas within the urinary tract and abdomen. The general responses of the ureter to inflammation are loss of ureteric peristalsis, dilatation, ulceration, irregularity, pseudopolyposis, edema and desmo-plasia leading to stricture and calcification.[26]

Radiological imaging radiology plays an important role in diagnosing and characterizing inflammatory conditions of the ureter. This information supplements that from other clinical diagnostic tools including urinalysis, urine culture, urine cytology and cystoureteroscopy.

Malakoplakia: It is a benign chronic granulomatous disorder more commonly seen in women than men. It can be seen at any level of the urinary tract but has a predilection for the bladder and lower ureter. It is seen in association with chronic *Escherichia coli* or *Proteus mirabilis* infection and is found more frequently in diabetics and immunosuppresed patients. On urography, the lesions are rounded to flat, coalescent filling defects lending an irregular contour to the ureteral margin.[27] Ureteric obstruction may be present. The imaging features overlap with ureteritis cystica but the lesions are usually rounder and the ureter is not dilated in the latter condition.

Ureteritis cystica: This disease entity is usually asymptomatic but may present with hematuria or symptoms of urinary tract infection. Histologically, this condition consists of multiple, small, subepithelial, fluid-filled cysts in the ureteric wall. Ureteritis cystica does not cause ureteric obstruction. The disease has a slight predilection for the upper ureter. The typical radiographic appearance is that of multiple, small, filling defects with scalloping of the ureteral margin. The differential diagnosis includes air bubbles, hemorrhage into ureteric wall, and papillary neoplasm.[28] The condition may or may not regress with treatment of the underlying inflammatory condition.

Leukoplakia: Leukoplakia is a rare inflammatory condition which more commonly involves the urinary bladder than the ureter. It results from squamous metaplasia of the urothelium and is frequently associated with chronic urinary tract infection or long standing stone disease. The imaging features include diffuse, irregular; filling defects. There may be ridging of the mucosa with ureteric dilatation. Differentiation from malakoplakia or ureteral malignancy is difficult on imaging.

Schistosomiasis: Schistosomiasis is a chronic indolent infestation caused by the trematode *Schistosoma hematobium*. The parasite lays its eggs in the veins of the bladder and lower ureter stimulating chronic inflammatory reaction resulting in cystitis and ureteritis and eventually scarring and calcification. Schistosomiasis commonly affects the bladder and ureteric involvement is seen in one-third of patients. The ureters are bilaterally asymmetrically involved with predominant involvement of the lower ureter. The disease usually affects a younger age group. Imaging findings are characteristic. Calcification of the ureter is seen in 75% of cases which is usually linear or tram-track in appearance. There is a characteristic deformity of the distal ureters consisting of medial and cephalic displacement which may resemble cow's horns.[29] There is varying degree of stenosis and dilatation and the ureter may show a beaded appearance which can resemble tubercular ureteritis.

Tubercular ureteritis: Tuberculosis of the urinary tract is usually due to hematogenous dissemination of Mycobacterium tuberculosis. Ureteral involvement is usually due to descending renal infection. The symptoms are nonspecific and include constitutional symptoms and lower urinary tract symptoms like frequency, dysuria, and suprapubic pain. The patients may present with hematuria and sterile pyuria. When the infection affects the ureteral wall, the first changes are those of ulceration and wall edema with thickening which progress to strictures and calcification. These changes may lead to proximal dilatation of the ureter and PCS. Plain films of abdomen may show evidence of ureteric calcification with or without calcification of the kidney. Characteristic urographic findings include alternating areas of dilatation and short strictures of the ureter (beaded appearance), long straight stricture (pipe-stem ureter) or isolated stricture **(Fig. 9)**. The ureter is shortened and straightened due to periureteral fibrosis.[30] The CT scan is useful in demonstrating ureteric wall thickening and presence of lymph nodes if any. The bladder may show poor distensibility owing to irritative spasm or fibrosis within the wall **(Figs. 10A and B)**.

Radiation ureteritis: Radiation can lead to early and late changes in the ureteric wall, ultimately leading to fibrosis and stricture. Fibrosis continues to develop long after radiotherapy has been completed. IVU may demonstrate mucosal irregularity and a short or long distal ureteric stricture. CT may demonstrate these findings as well as thickening and stranding of the wall of the ureter.

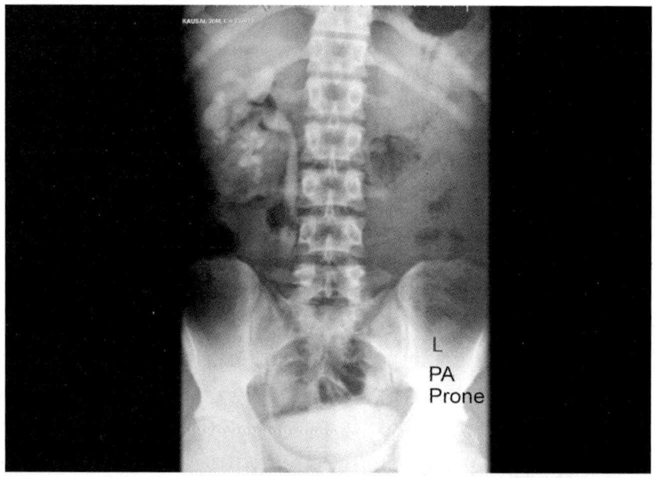

Fig. 9: IVU film (15 min) shows hydronephrosis, forniceal stenosis, cavitary changes in right kidney with ureteric narrowing. All these features suggest tubercular involvement of urinary tract.

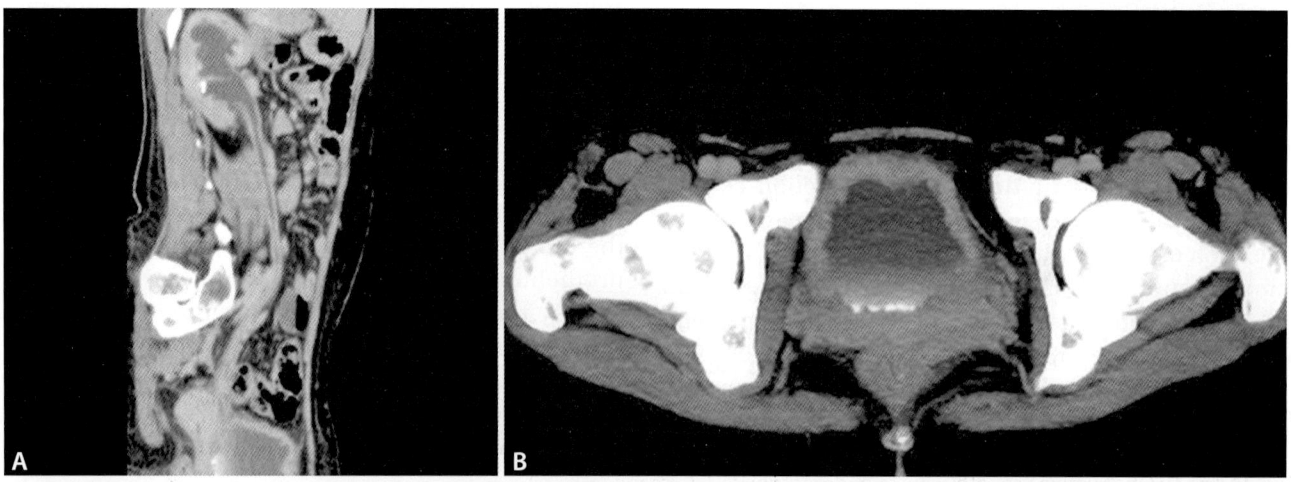

Figs. 10A and B: CT scan of urinary tract tuberculosis. Multiplanar reconstruction (MPR) (A) shows hydronephrosis of kidney with thickened ureteric wall (B) and irregular thickening of urinary bladder with reduced capacity.

Inflammatory Bowel Disease

Genitoureteric complications may occur in up to one-fourth of patients with inflammatory bowel disease. Obstruction due to direct ureteral involvement is the second most common complication, the first being nephrolithiasis. Ureteric involvement by Crohn's disease is usually at the level of the pelvic brim and the right ureter is more commonly involved.[31] On urography, the ureter shows a smooth area of narrowing with varying degree of obstruction. CT scan shows an inflammatory soft tissue mass with narrowing and mural thickening of the ureter.

Endometriosis: Ureteral involvement generally occurs in cases with widespread pelvic disease; however, cases of isolated ureteral involvement have been reported. Two forms of ureteral endometriosis have been described. Extrinsic involvement is four times more common than the intrinsic variety. The distal ureter is commonly involved. Ureteral involvement may result in narrowing of ureter, hydronephrosis and occasionally an intraluminal mass.[32] The stricture is usually smooth but abruptly tapered and may show medial sharp angulation. CT may demonstrate a soft tissue mass or endometrioma causing encasement of the ureter **(Figs. 11A to D)**.

Extrinsic Causes of Ureteral Obstruction

The extrinsic causes of ureteral obstruction are given in **Table 2**.

Retroperitoneal Fibrosis

Retroperitoneal fibrosis (RPF) is an important cause of obstructive uropathy leading to renal failure. It encompasses a range of diseases characterised by the presence of fibro-inflammatory tissue, which usually surrounds the abdominal aorta and iliac arteries and extends into the retroperitoneum to envelop neighbouring structures including the ureters. RPF may be idiopathic (Ormond's disease) or secondary to a wide variety of stimuli which includes both benign and neoplastic causes.

The classic triad of delayed renal contrast excretion with unilateral or bilateral (60% of cases) hydronephrosis and proximal hydroureter secondary to ureteral involvement, medial deviation of the middle-third of both ureters and tapering of the ureteral lumen at the L4–L5 vertebral level, though less frequently seen than previously thought is still useful in the identification of RPF. When there is insufficient contrast excretion on urography, retrograde or antegrade pyelography is required to demonstrate the

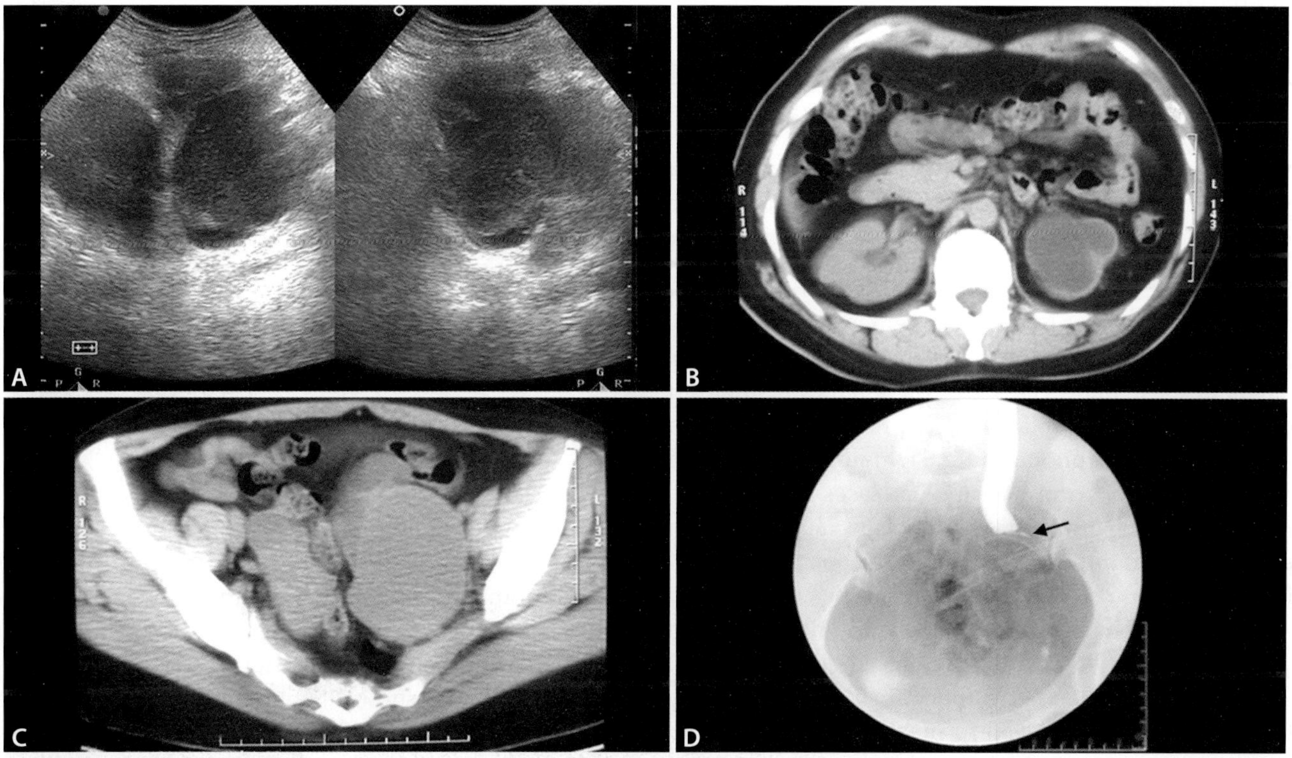

Figs. 11A to D: Obstructive uropathy due to endometriosis. USG image (A) shows complicated cyst with in left adnexa. CT scan axial scan at the level of pelvis (C) shows adnexal mass encasing lower ureter resulting obstructive atrophy of kidney (B). The nephrostogram (D) of the same patients shows displacement and stricture of lower ureter (arrow).

Table 2: Extrinsic causes of ureteral obstruction.[6]

Retroperitoneal tumors	Lymphoma, sarcoma, metastases, cysts
Pelvic tumors	Uterine leiomyomas, malignancies of cervix; ovary, bladder, prostate, colorectum
Retroperitoneal fibrosis	Idiopathic, secondary
Pelvic lipomatosis	
Pregnancy related	Hydronephrosis of pregnancy, ovarian vein thrombophlebitis, ovarian vein syndrome
Gynecologic conditions	Pelvic inflammatory disease, endometriosis, uterine prolapse, hydrocolpometra
Gastrointestinal diseases	Crohn's disease, diverticulitis, appendicitis, pancreatic and gastric malignancies
Miscellaneous	Amyloidosis, Reaction to foreign material (barium, surgical suture, etc.)

characteristic ureteral changes.[33] CT scan demonstrates sheet like soft tissue mass in retroperitoneum with encasement of ureters **(Figs. 12A to C)** CT may help in the identification of disease activity with the degree of soft-tissue enhancement correlating with the activity of the fibrotic process. Retroperitoneal fibrosis has signal characteristics similar to those of other fibrotic processes, with a tendency toward diffusely low signal intensity on T1-weighted MR imaging. T2 signal is a reflection of the degree of associated active inflammation (and thus edema) with high signal indicating early inflammatory phase of benign RPF or malignancy while low signal signifies chronic phase of benign RPF. Chronic, inactive fibrosis will have little edema and thus be visualized as having low signal on both T1- and T2-weighted imaging. This feature may also prove valuable in assessing a patient's response to treatment; decreasing T2-signal indicating a favorable therapeutic response.[33,34]

Retroperitoneal Neoplasms

Extraureteral malignancies causing obstructive uropathy are much more common than primary ureteral neoplasms. The ureter is very prone to involvement as it is near many structures in the retroperitoneum that frequently harbor malignancies. In many cases, obstruction may result from direct extension of neoplasms from primary sites like the bladder, prostate, endometrium, sigmoid colon, rectum and cervix **(Figs. 13 and 14)**. In other cases there may be metastasis to the periureteral tissues especially the lymph nodes by distant tumors which causes uropathy by direct infiltration of one or both the ureters or by compression and mechanical obstruction. Bulky lymph nodes seen in lymphomas may cause similar manifestations.

Primary retroperitoneal tumors arising in the vicinity of the ureters may also lead to mechanical obstruction. CT scores over sonography in the detection and possible classification of these tumors. Malignancies may incite an intense periureteral desmoplastic reaction resembling retroperitoneal fibrosis leading to ureteral obstruction. This is especially seen in metastases from carcinomas of lung, breast, pancreas, colon, stomach and sometimes lymphoma.[35] Patients who have received radiation therapy in the vicinity may also experience obstructive symptoms. This was initially thought to be due to radiation induced ureteric stricture but lately it has been realized that the ureter is relatively resistant to radiation. An obstruction in this case usually means that the tumor had involved the ureteral wall before radiation or there has been a recent relapse.

Pelvic Lipomatosis

It is an unusual disease resulting from proliferation of mature fibroadipose tissue in the pelvis. Usually seen in males, it may require surgery if it is causing obstructive uropathy by ureteral compression. Radiographic findings include relative hyperlucency of the pelvic cavity on plain radiographs. Contrast studies may show displacement and compression of rectosigmoid and urinary bladder leading to 'tear drop' or 'pear'-shaped bladder.[36] The distal ends of the ureters are displaced medially in the majority of cases with presence of hydroureter or hydroureteronephrosis. Identical appearance of the bladder can also be seen with pelvic lymphadenopathy, diffuse pelvic carcinomatosis, pelvic/perivesical liposarcoma and pelvic fibrosis (resembling retroperitoneal fibrosis).

Pregnancy-related Dilatation of Ureter

Variable degree of ureteral dilatation is often seen during pregnancy which is most marked in the third trimester with predominant involvement of the right side. In most of the cases the dilatation progressively disappears in the postpartum period. The ureteral segments below the pelvic brim do not show dilatation indicating that partial mechanical obstruction by the gravid uterus accounts for the major changes of hydroureter seen during pregnancy.

Sonography forms the initial and mainstay imaging modality in these conditions. If the sonographic findings

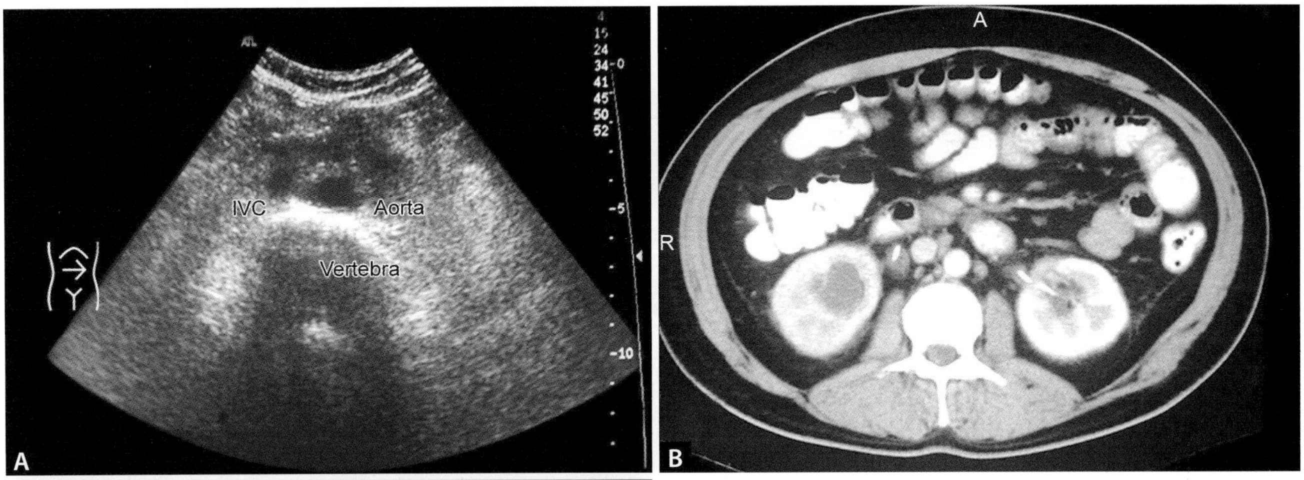

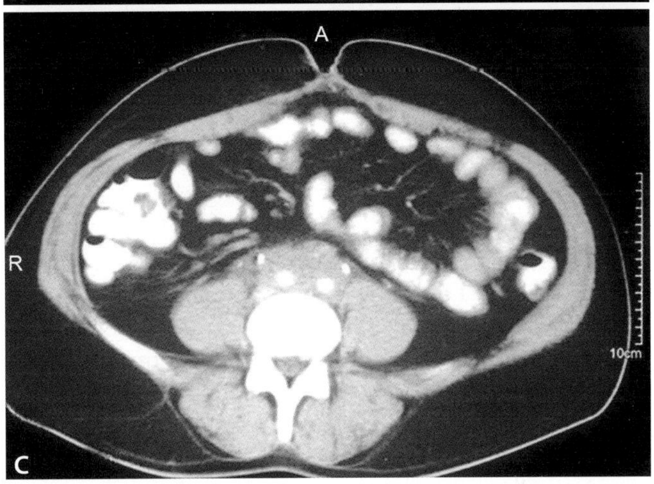

Figs. 12A to C: A young patient of idiopathic retroperitoneal fibrosis presented with obstructive uropathy. Ultrasound image (A) and contrast enhanced CT scan (B and C) show retroperitoneal mass encasing major vessels and bilateral ureter. Note made of bilateral DJ stents.

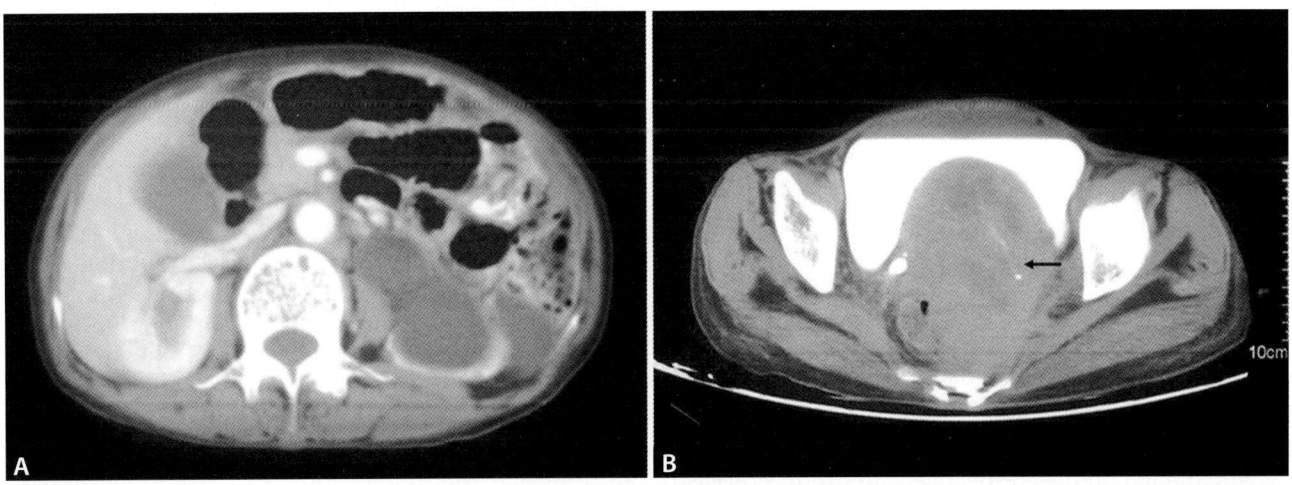

Figs. 13A and B: Carcinoma of cervix causing obstructive uropathy. Contrast-enhanced CT (CECT) axial section (A) shows obstructive atrophy of left kidney. Delayed section at the level of pelvis (B) shows large heterogeneous cervical mass causing encasement of lower ureter (arrow).

are equivocal, MR urography should be performed which can show tapered narrowing of the lumbar portion of the ureter which is being compressed by the gravid uterus against the iliac artery at the sacral promontory.[37] An obstructing calculus is usually above or below this level.

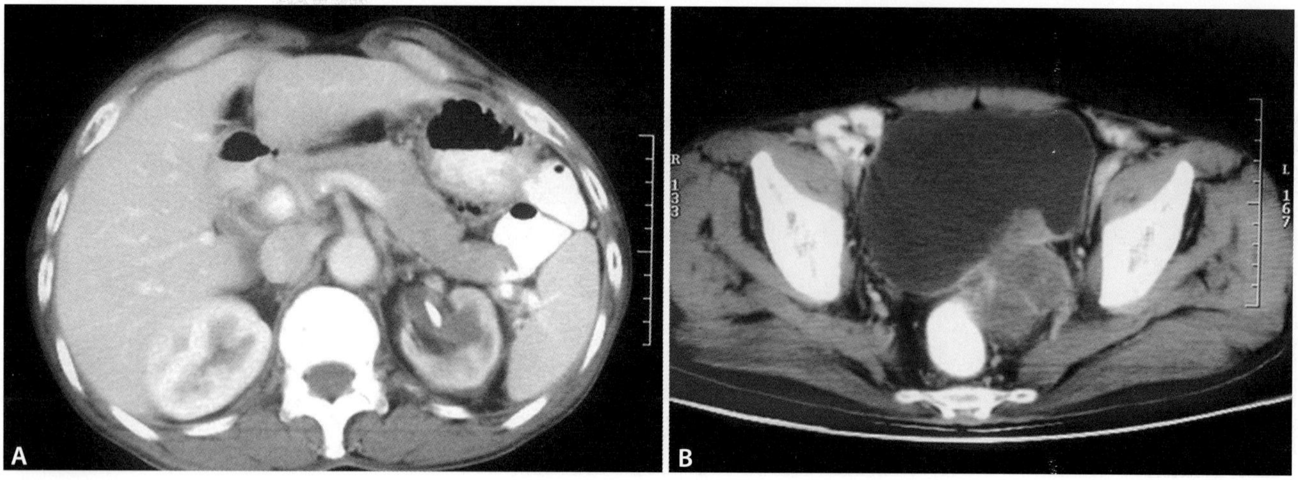

Figs. 14A and B: Ureteric obstruction caused by urinary bladder malignancy. Contrast CT axial section (A) shows left hydroureteronephrosis with large calculus in renal pelvis. Inferior section (B) shows large lobulated mass arising from urinary bladder with exophytic component causing left ureteric involvement.

Gynecological Causes

Various gynecologic causes disorders may cause extrinsic compression on the ureter leading to proximal dilatation of the urinary system. Tubo-ovarian abscesses in pelvic inflammatory disease (PID) may cause extrinsic ureteric compression or surround the ureter with inflammation leading to partial obstruction with lateral displacement of the ureter below the pelvic brim. Pneumohydronephrosis may rarely develop due to fistula formation between the abscess and the ureter. Uterine and bladder prolapse are important causes of reversible and preventable renal failure. Obstruction is usually bilateral and is often associated with UTI. Sonography along with IVU studies helps in the easy identification of the disease. Other gynecologic causes disorders like hydrometrocolpos and hydrocolpometra may also cause ureteral compression.

Gastrointestinal Diseases

Various diseases related to the GIT may lead to indirect involvement of the urinary tract by contiguous involvement of the ureters. Retroperitoneal extension of inflammation and fibrosis may occur in inflammatory bowel disease especially Crohn's disease as well as in complicated colonic diverticulitis with predominant involvement of the right and left ureters, respectively. In Crohn's disease, the ureter usually displays a sharply tapered, smooth area of narrowing over several centimeters leading to varying degree of obstruction. Pancreatic and appendiceal inflammation similarly may directly spread to the ureter, commonly on the right side leading to obstructive symptoms.

Miscellaneous Diseases of Ureter

Ureteral Injury

The causes of ureteric injury can be iatrogenic and external trauma. Radical hysterectomy, gynecological surgery and obstetric trauma are common causes of iatrogenic injury. Penetrating injury and fall from height are common causes for external trauma. Most surgically induced ureteric injuries go unsuspected at the time of injury, because they are often not a direct injury but the result of ischemia. Excretion intravenous urography may demonstrate extravasation of urine and hydronephrosis **(Figs. 15A and B)**. The complications of ureteric injury include hydronephrosis/pyonephrosis secondary to stricture, calculus formation, ureteric fistula, urinomas and renal failure.

Ureteral Herniation

Herniation of ureter is rare. Inguinal, femoral and sciatic hernias may include the ureter. Herniation of ureter can be recognized on urography, e.g. in sciatic herniation, the pelvic ureter extends laterally through the sacrosciatic notch, producing a hairpin shaped redundancy.[38]

Ureteral Fistula

The common causes of ureteral fistulae are penetrating trauma, complicated ureteral surgery and inflammatory or malignant disease.[39] Ureteral fistula usually presents with urinary tract infection and clinical evidence of flow through the fistula. The diagnosis of fistula is usually made by ureterography. Rarely, an ureteroenteric fistula may be demonstrated during contrast study of the gastrointestinal tract. CT may demonstrate the primary lesion and the fistulous tract.

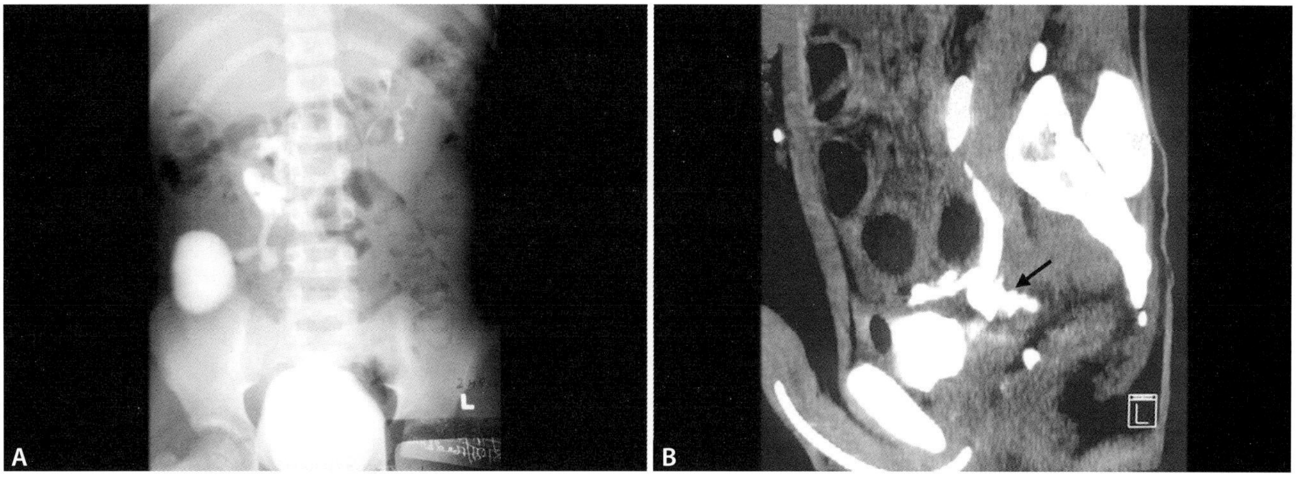

Figs. 15A and B: Ureteric trauma. Delayed IVU film (2 hours) (A) shows extravasation of contrast from right upper ureter; (B) CT reformation in another patient shows contrast leak from lower ureter suggestive of ureteric trauma (arrow).

REFERENCES

1. Hodson CJ. Experimental obstructive nephropathy in the pig.Br J Urol. 1969;41:5-20.
2. Tublin ME, Dodd GD III, Verdile VP. Acute renal colic; diagnosis with duplex Doppler US. Radiology. 1994;193:697-701.
3. Cronan JJ, Tublin ME. Role of resistive index in the evaluation of acute renal obstruction. AJR. 1995;164:377-8.
4. Wilson DR. Pathophysiology of obstructive nephropathy. Kidney Int. 1980;18:281-92.
5. Bigongiari LR, Davis RM, Nowak WG, et al. Visualization of medullary rays on excretory urography in experimental ureteric obstruction. AJR. 1977;129:89-93.
6. Talner LB. Urinary obstruction. In Grainger and Allison's Diagnostic Radiology, 3rd edition. Churchil Livingstone; 1997.
7. Bernardino ME, McClennan BL. High dose urography: incidence and relationship to spontaneous peripelvic extravasation. AJR. 1976;127:373-6.
8. Koelliker SL, Cronan JJ. Acute urinary tract obstruction: imaging update. Urologic Clinics of North America. 1997;24:571-81.
9. Kamholtz RG, Cronan JJ, Dorfman GS. Obstruction and the minimally dilated renal collecting system: US evaluation. Radiology. 1989;170:51-3.
10. Burge HJ, Middleton, WD, McClennan B, et al. Ureteral jets in healthy subjects and in patients with unilateral ureteric calculi: comparison with color doppler US. Radiology. 1975;180:437-42.
11. Smith RC, Rosenfield AT, Choe KA, et al. Acute flank pain: comparison of noncontrast enhanced CT and intravenous urography. Radiology. 1995;194:789-94.
12. Tack D, Sourtzis S, Delpierre I, et al. Low dose unenhanced mutidetector CT of patients with suspected renal colic. Am J Roentgenol. 2003;180:305-11.
13. Pollack HM, Arger PH, Banner MP. Computed tomography of renal pelvic filling defects. Radiology. 1981;138:645-51.
14. O'Reilly PH. Diuresis renography eight years later: an update. J Urol. 1986;136:993-9.
15. Hussain S,O'Mally M, Jara H. MR urography. Magn Reson Imaging North Am. 1997;5:95-106.
16. Elkin M. Obstruction and dilatation of urinary tract. In: Elkin M (Ed). Radiology of Urinary System. Little Brown: Boston; 1980.
17. Dunbar JS, Nogrady MB. The calyceal crescent: a roentgenographic sign of obstructive hydronephrosis. AJR. 1970;110:520-8.
18. Dunnick NR, Sandler CM. Textbook of Uroradiology, 3rd edition. Lippincot. press.
19. Pfister RC, Hendren WH. Primary megaureter in children and adults. Urology. 1978;12:160-6.
20. Dalrymple NC, Verga M, Anderson KR. The value of unenhanced helical computerized tomography in the management of acute flank pain. J Urol. 1998;159:735-40
21. Thomas J, Stey A, Abouker P. Calculi on blood clots. J Uro (Paris). 1976;82:496.
22. Margolin HN. Fungus infection of urinary tract. Semin Roentgenol. 1971;6:323-8.
23. Bergman H, Friedenberg RM, Sayegh V. New roentgenologic sign of carcinoma of ureter. AJR. 1961;86:707-10.
24. Kenney PJ, Stanley RJ. Coputed tomography of ureteral tumor. J Comput Assit Tomogr. 1987;11:102.
25. Winalski CS, Lipman JC, Tumeh SS. Ureteral neoplasms. Radigraphics. 1990;10:271.
26. Wasserman NF. Inflammatory disease of the ureter. Radiol Clin North Am. 1996;34:1131-56.
27. Elliot GB, Moloney PJ, Clement JG. Malacoplakia of urinary tract. AJR. 1972;116:830.
28. Menedez B, Sala X. Cystic pyeloureteritis: Review of 34 cases. Radiology aspects and differential diagnosis. Urology. 1997;50:31-7.

29. Young SW, Khalid KH, Farid Z et al. Urinary tract lesions of schistosoma hematobium. Radiology. 1974;111:81.
30. Royalance N, Penry JB, Davies ER et al. The radiology of tuberculosis of urinary tract. Clin Radiol. 1970;21:163.
31. Banner MP. Genitourinary complications of inflammatory bowel disease. Radiol Clin North Am. 1987;25:199.
32. Kane C, Dronin P. Obstructive uropathy associated with endometriosis. Amer J Obst Gynecol. 1985;151:207.
33. Cronin CG, Lohan DG, Blake MA et al. Retroperitoneal fibrosis: a review of clinical features and imaging findings. Am J Roentgenol. 2008;191:423-31.
34. Vaglio A, Salvarani C, Buzio C. Retroperitoneal fibrosis. Lancet. 2006;367:241-51.
35. Winalski CS, Lipman JC, Tumeb SS. Ureteral neoplasms. Radiographics. 1990;10:271.
36. Heyns CF. Pelvic lipomatosis: A review of its diagnosis and management. J Urol. 1991;146:267.
37. Grenier N, Pariente JL, Trillaud H et al. Dilatation of collecting system during pregnancy: physiologic vs obstructive dilatation. Eur Radiol. 2000;10:271-9.
38. Tsai PJ, Lin JT, Wu TT et al. Ureterosciatic hernia causes obstructive uropathy. Chin Med Assoc. 2008;71:491-3.
39. Moon SG, Kim SH, Lee HJ, et al. Pelvic fistulas complicating pelvic surgery or diseases: spectrum of imaging findings. Korean J Radiol. 2001;2:97-104.

CHAPTER 116

Urinary Tract Trauma

Atin Kumar, Shivanand Gamanagatti

INTRODUCTION

Approximately 10% of all traumatic injuries involve the urinary tract, most often the kidney.[1] Although trauma to the urinary tract is seldom the cause of death but serious morbidity can result if such injuries are missed. An accurate radiographic and imaging evaluation is important to determine the presence and extent of injury for the proper management of the patients. Evaluation of the urinary tract trauma should be integrated into the overall management of the trauma patient.

Blunt trauma accounts for 80–90% of all renal injuries.[1] These are primarily due to deceleration injuries in motor vehicleaccidents, falls or assault. In approximately 10–20% of the patients, penetrating injuries result due to gunshot or knife wounds. Pre-existing kidney lesions, e.g. renal tumors, hydronephrosis, polycystic kidney disease and horseshoe kidneys make the kidney more susceptible to the injury. In 80% of the patients with penetrating trauma and 75% of blunt trauma patients, associated injuries, e.g. splenic rupture, liver laceration and injuries to the small and large bowel are seen.[2] In about 50% of these patients, bone fractures are present. Iatrogenic causes, such as surgery, interventional procedures and biopsies are also associated with trauma to the urinary tract.

RENAL TRAUMA

Since the late 1980s, the prevailing techniques of imaging and clinical management of renal trauma have changed dramatically. Consensus has been building towards a conservative approach and successful clinical management must be based on an accurate assessment of the extent of injury.

Imaging Work-up in a Patient with Suspected Renal Trauma

Trauma to the kidney may be suspected to be minor or significant on the basis of clinical picture, nature and site of injury. An unstable patient may undergo no imaging work up if an immediate surgery is indicated on clinical grounds. In a clinically stable patient with abdominal trauma and with suspected abdominal organ injury and/or hypotension, kidneys are imaged as part of a standard abdomen and pelvic CT. The current globally accepted indications specifically for radiological evaluation of urinary tract in trauma patients are as follows:[2-5]

- Gross hematuria
- Microscopic hematuria with hypotension (BP <100 mm Hg at any time during evaluation)
- Injuries associated with renal injury, such as direct contusion or hematoma of flank soft tissues, fractures of lumbar spine, lower rib and transverse process
- Penetrating trauma with any degree of hematuria.

Earlier children with any degree of hematuria were also an indication for radiological evaluation, but recently there has been a trend to have an approach similar to adult patient. Renal imaging is not required in a patient with minor trauma having microhematuria without shock.

An approach to a patient having significant trauma can be outlined as shown in the algorithm **(Flowchart 1)**.

Role of Radiography (Plain Radiographs)

Widespread availability and use of CT and ultrasound has replaced abdominal radiography for evaluation of renal trauma. However radiographs have a role in the setting of penetrating abdominal trauma.

Role of Ultrasound

Specific visceral injuries are poorly assessed on ultrasonography. The value of sonography is primarily in rapid establishment of presence of hemoperitoneum in an unstable patient. In the setting of abdominal trauma it is usually done with focussed assessment with sonography in trauma (FAST) protocol. It is insensitive to detect retroperitoneal blood and renal parenchymal injuries.

Role of Intravenous Urography

The role of intravenous urogram (IVU) in suspected renal trauma is limited. It has been replaced by CT which is now easily available and is more sensitive than IVU for paren-chymal injuries, urinary contrast extravasation as well as for other abdominal injuries. However, IVU still has a role, depending on the preference of the surgeon, to establish gross function and evaluation of the uninjured contralateral kidney in hemodynamically unstable patients going for surgery and for urological evaluation of patients who are already in the operating room.[2,3] The technique followed is usually a tailored "single shot" study with a radiograph obtained 10 minutes after adminis-tration of intravenous contrast. However, if time and condition of patient permits, a precontrast plain radiograph and delayed radiographs may be taken for assessment of urinary contrast extravasation and for delayed function.

Role of CT

Contrast-enhanced CT scan is currently the investigation of choice for radiological evaluation of patients with blunt abdominal trauma.[4,5] It has replaced IVU for evaluation of renal trauma. The current trend of conser-vative management of blunt renal trauma has further enhanced the role of CT because 80% of renal injuries seen on CT are self-limiting. Helical CT avoids misregistration artifacts and allows a dual phase acquisition in two phases of renal enhancement. This technique distinguishes contrast

Flowchart 1: Imaging work-up in suspected renal trauma.

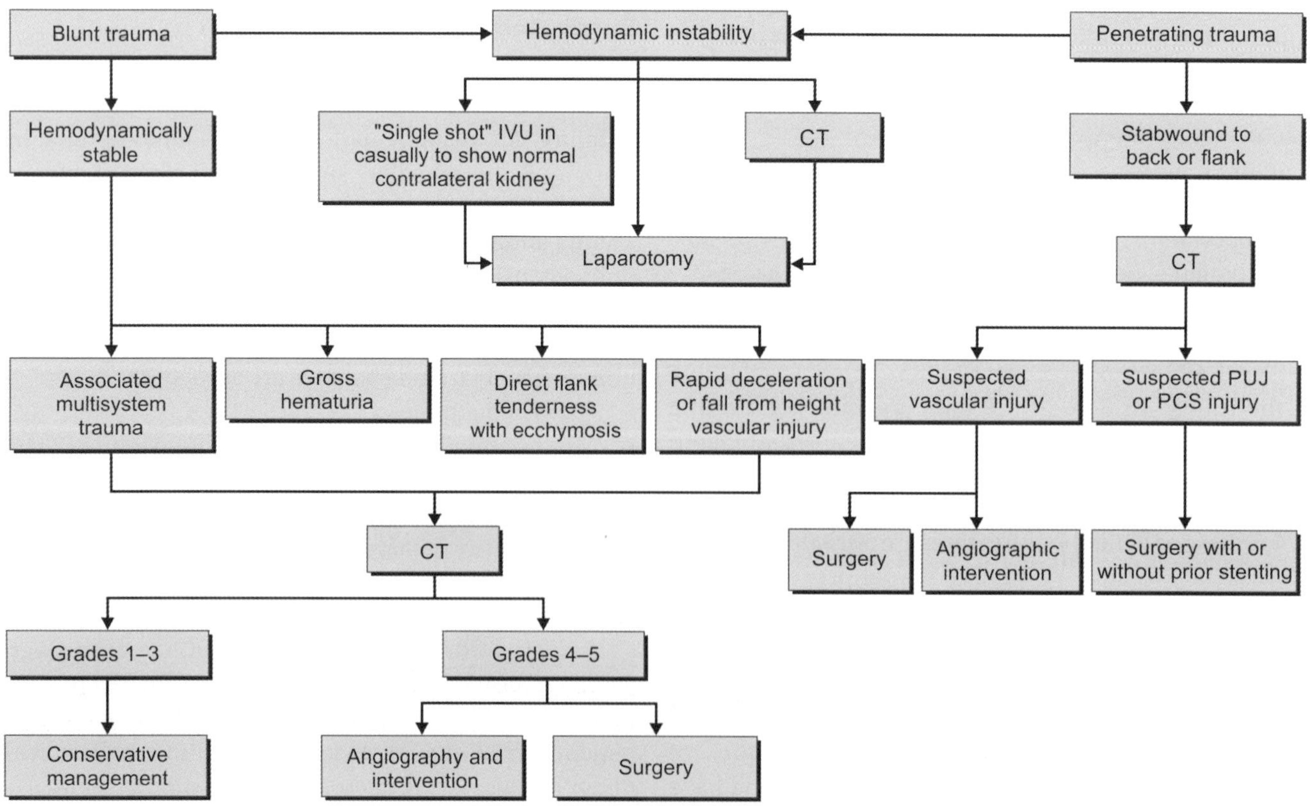

extravasation due to vascular injury (seen in the early images), from that due to pelvicalyceal injury (seen in the delayed images). Multislice CT has reduced the time required for CT evaluation still further and this is valuable in patients who are in need of immediate surgery.

CT accurately assesses all the criteria essential for management of renal trauma *viz.* extent of damaged nonviable tissue, amount of perirenal hemorrhage, extravasation of urine and evidence of renal pedicle or vascular injury.

CT technique: The technique needs to be tailored to the patient's specific condition.

- Noncontrast images of the kidney are optional.
- 100–150 mL of intravenous contrast is injected, ideally at a rate of 2–4 mL, using a pressure injector.
- The scanning parameters are variable depending upon the multislice capability of the scanner.
- The first set of images is obtained after 70–90 seconds delay.
- A second set of images is obtained after 3–5 min delay for detection of pelvicalyceal contrast extravasation.
- A further delayed set of images may be obtained after 10–15 min to delineate urinary contrast extravasation if there is significant perinephric or periureteric fluid.

Multiplanar reformatted images and three-dimensional images including CT urographic images can significantly aid in the evaluation.

Role of Angiography

CT can have characteristic findings in main renal artery occlusion or avulsion. Surgery can thus be undertaken solely on the basis of CT findings after blunt trauma.

The role of angiography is primarily in penetrating trauma with vascular injury suspected clinically or on CT. Also, late development of gross hematuria following blunt injury may signify an overlooked vascular injury or formation of a pseudoaneurysm. Catheter angiography accurately delineates the vessel changes which may occur due to injury, i.e. occlusion, laceration, pseudoaneurysm and AV fistula.

In this setting, there is an increasing role of therapeutic angiographic interventions as a nonsurgical therapy for transcatheter embolization of ongoing hemorrhage in renal trauma in hemodynamically stable patients and also for vascular complications of injury including post-traumatic pseudoaneurysms, arteriovenous fistulas, vascular stent placement for renal artery intimal injury and even thrombolysis of renal artery thrombosis.

Role of Retrograde Pyelography

Retrograde pyelography has a role in the specific setting of suspected renal pelvic, ureteropelvic junction or ureteral injury which has not been adequately excluded on CT. However, it is often not practically possible in emergent situation and also does not characterize renal injuries.

Role of Radionuclide Renal Scintigraphy

With widespread availability of CT, radionuclide scintigraphy is rarely used in acute trauma setting. It may have a role in demonstrating function of an injured kidney in patients allergic to iodinated contrast and in follow-up of repair of renovascular trauma.

Role of MRI

MRI may have a role in patients where CT is contra-indicated or not available. However, it is usually not practical in acute trauma setting. It can demonstrate renal parenchymal injuries as well as renal function after contrast administration.

Radiological Findings

The most commonly accepted classification of renal injuries is given by the American Association for the Surgery of Trauma based on the depth of injury and involvement of vessels or the collecting system.[6] It classifies the renal trauma into 5 grades as follows:

Grade 1

Grade 1 renal injuries account for approximately 75–80% of all renal injuries. They include:

- *Contusion*: Focal illdefined area of hypodensity which shows decreased enhancement as compared to adjacent normal renal parenchyma **(Figs. 1A and B)**. They are differentiated from infarct by the presence of some contrast enhancement as contrast from latter which has absent contrast enhancement. A global contusion may show a striated nephrogram, or spidery collecting system (due to parenchymal edema).
- *Subcapsular hematoma*: A non-expanding, hyper-attenuating (40–60 HU) fluid collection indenting the adjacent renal parenchyma **(Figs. 2A and B)**. It does not enhance on contrast administration.

Grade 2

Grade 2 renal injuries include:

- *Perinephric hematoma*: A nonexpanding ill-defined hyperattenuating fluid collection in perinephric space between the renal parenchyma and Gerota's fascia

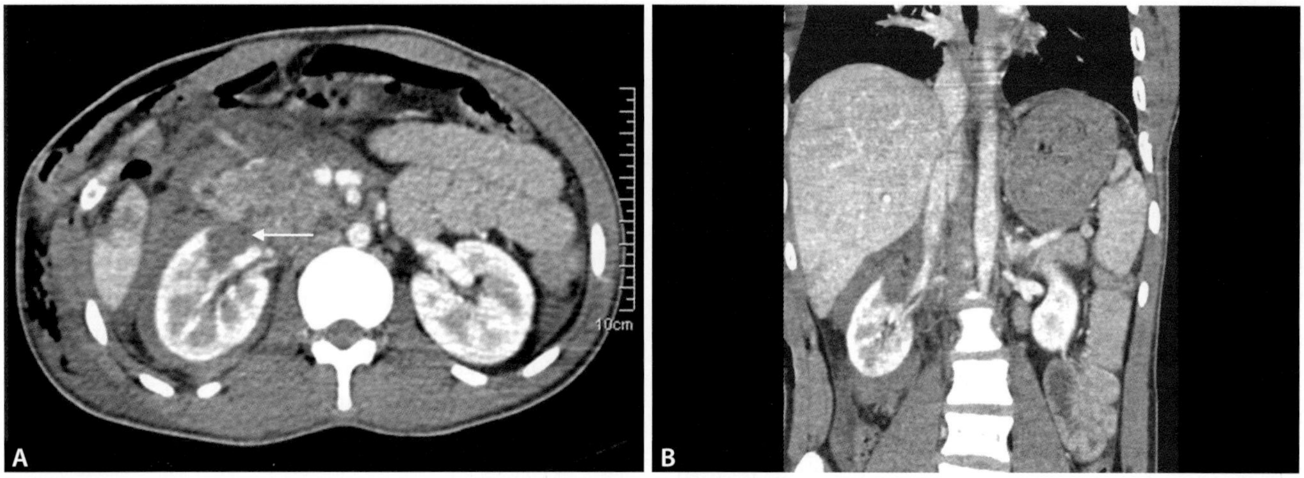

Figs. 1A and B: Axial (A) and multiformatted coronal (B) CECT shows a focal hypodense area (arrow) in anterior part of right kidney suggestive of contusion

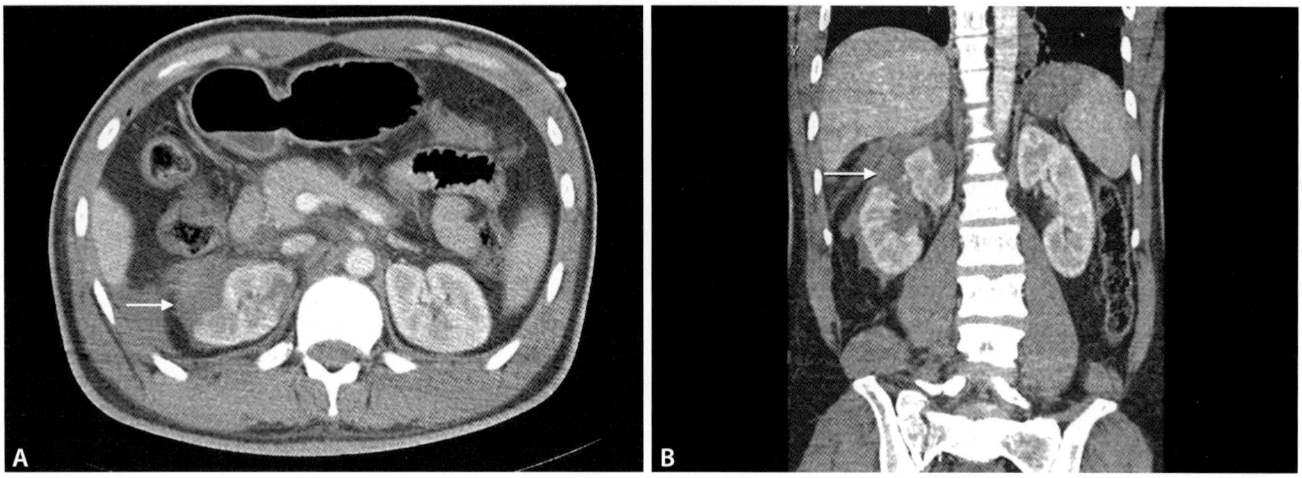

Figs. 2A and B: Axial (A) and multiformatted coronal (B) CECT shows a hyperdense nonenhancing subcapsular hematoma (arrows)

(Figs. 3A and B). It occurs after laceration of renal capsule.
- *Laceration*: A superficial (<1 cm deep), irregular or linear, low attenuation area within the renal parenchyma which may contain blood or clot. It does not enhance after contrast administration.

Grade 3

Grade 3 renal injuries include:
- *Lacerations*: >1 cm in depth but do not involve the collecting system **(Fig. 4)**.

Grade 4

Grade 4 renal injuries include:
- *Lacerations*: Deep lacerations extending through the kidney into the collecting system. It commonly leads to extravasation of urine and urinary contrast. Delayed phase CT in excretory phase is important to demonstrate urinary contrast extravasation **(Figs. 5A to D)**.
- *Vessel injury*: Injury to main renal artery or vein with contained hemorrhage.
- *Segmental infarction without associated laceration*: It occurs due to dissection, thrombosis or laceration of segmental arteries. Usually associated with other renal injuries. On CT it is seen as peripherally based, well circumscribed, wedge-shaped focal nonenhancing area through the renal parenchyma in a radial or segmental orientation **(Figs. 6A and B)**.

Grade 5

Grade 5 renal injuries include as follows:
- *Shattered kidney*: It refers to gross renal parenchymal disruption secondary to multiple renal lacerations

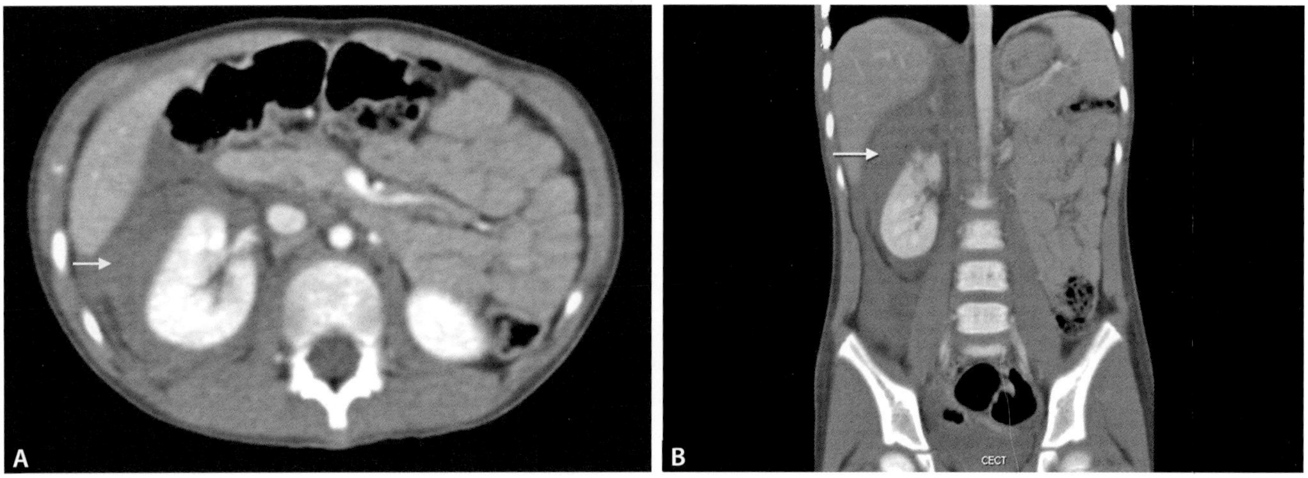

Figs. 3A and B: Axial (A) and multiformatted coronal (B) CECT shows perinephric hematoma (arrows) around right kidney.

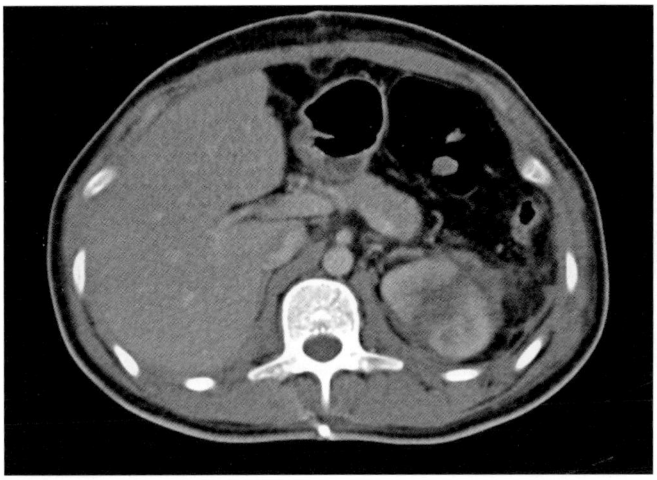

Fig. 4: Axial CECT abdomen shows a linear hypodense nonenhancing laceration involving upper pole of left kidney

associated with devitalized areas due to renal infarction **(Figs. 7A and B)**.

- *Devascularized kidney:*
  - Main renal artery may get thrombosed secondary to intimal tear following blunt renal trauma. It occurs due to stretching of the renal artery between the artery origin anchored to aorta and mobile kidney. It leads to global renal infarction **(Figs. 8A and B)**. CT reveals abrupt termination of renal artery after its origin with nonenhancing renal parenchyma except for a cortical rim sign which usually appears few days later and retrograde opacification of renal vein from IVC. Perinephric hematoma is characteristically absent in such cases. Renal angiography with thrombolysis may be done in selected cases, ideally within 12 hours after trauma or in a patient with only one kidney or bilateral renal artery thrombosis.
  - Renal artery may also get avulsed after blunt trauma. CT reveals global renal infarction with extensive medial perinephric hematoma with or without active arterial contrast extravasation.
  - Renal vein may get lacerated or thrombosed. CT reveals intraluminal thrombus with features of renal vein occlusion including increased size of kidney, diminished or delayed enhancement and delayed excretion **(Figs. 9A and B)**.
- *Ureteropelvic junction injuries*: Complete avulsion or partial tear. The injury occurs primarily in children who lack retroperitoneal fat to cushion the kidney during rapid deceleration. Usually the patient presents late with fever, flank pain and anuria. CT shows medial or circumferential urinoma with extravasation of urinary contrast into the urinoma on delayed phase images **(Figs. 10A and B)**. Partial tear can be differentiated from complete avulsion by presence of contrast within the distal ureter. Retrograde pyelography may be required for definitive diagnosis to demonstrate the distal ureter if CT or IVU fail to demonstrate distal ureteric filling.

Vascular Contrast Extravasation

It is seen as focal or diffuse areas of enhancement paralleling the attenuation of vessel seen within the parenchyma or in the perinephric hematoma **(Figs. 11A to C)**. It may be contained hemorrhage or pseudo-aneurysm which is well circumscribed and seen usually within a laceration. Active hemorrhage is illdefined, within an associated acute

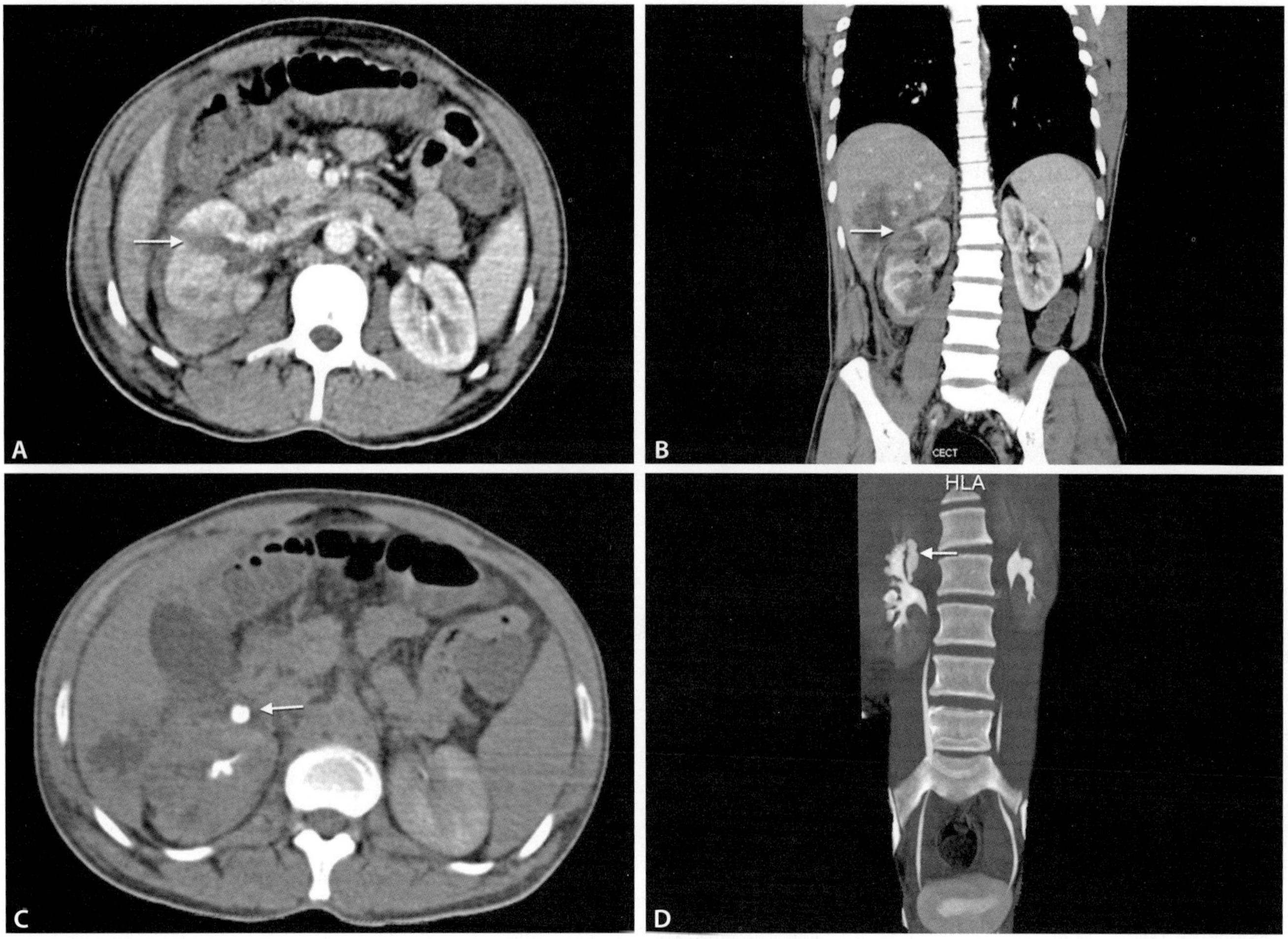

Figs. 5A to D: Axial (A) and multiformatted coronal (B) CECT shows a deep laceration (arrows) in upper pole of right kidney extending into pelvicalyceal system with perinephric hematoma. Delayed phase axial CT (C) shows contrast lying outside the kidney on its anterior aspect signifying urinary contrast extravasation. Reformatted coronal MIP image (D) clearly shows the extravasated contrast from upper calyceal injury.

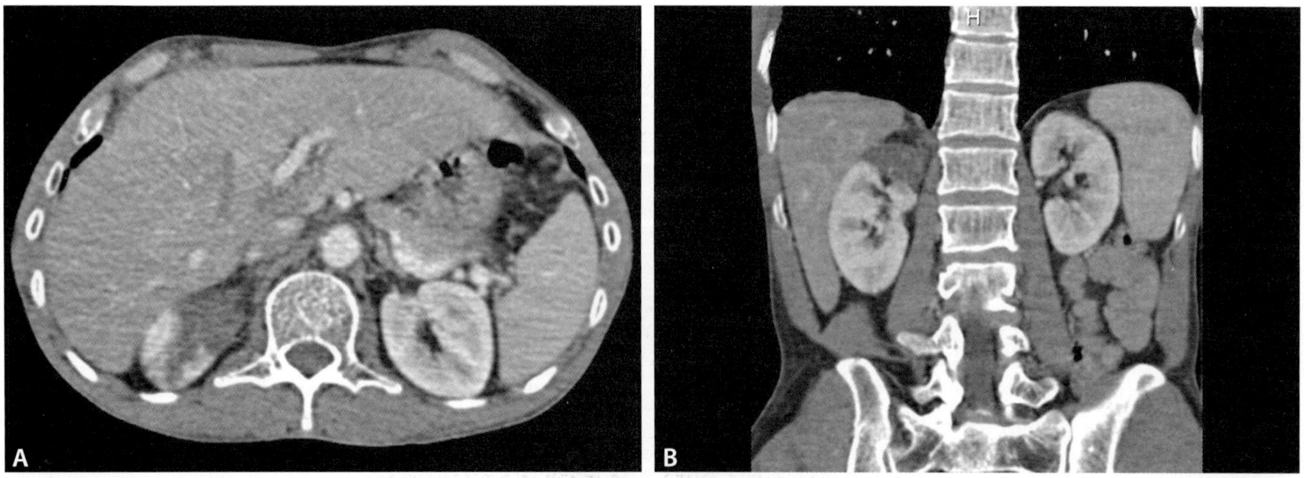

Figs. 6A and B: Axial (A) and multiformatted coronal (B) CECT shows a well-defined peripheral-based wedge-shaped nonenhancing area in upper pole of right kidney suggestive of a segmental infarct.

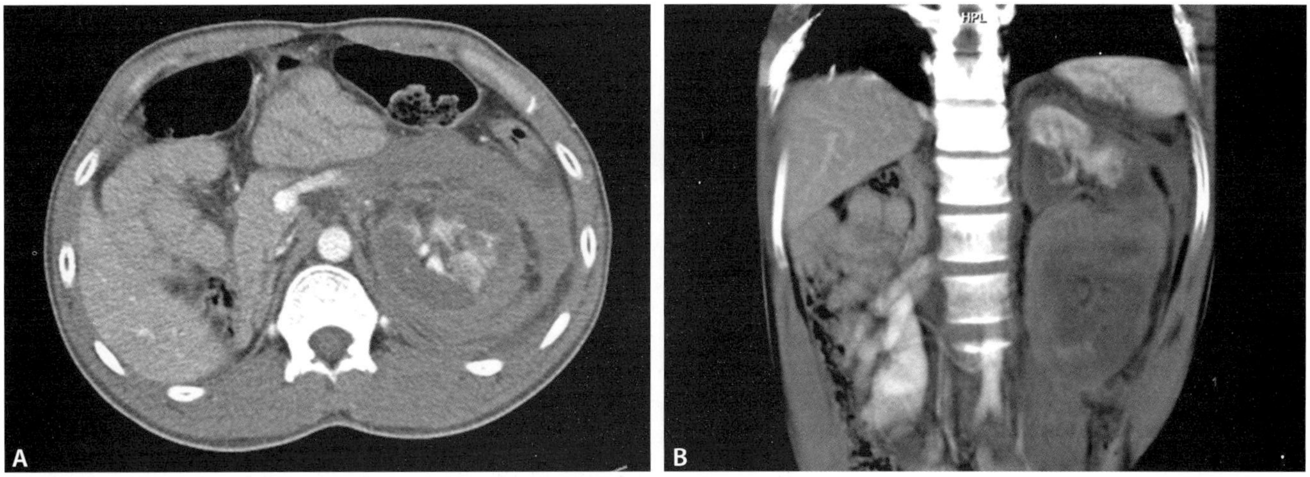

Figs. 7A and B: Axial (A) and multiformatted coronal (B) CECT shows completely shattered left kidney with large devitalized (nonenhancing) areas.

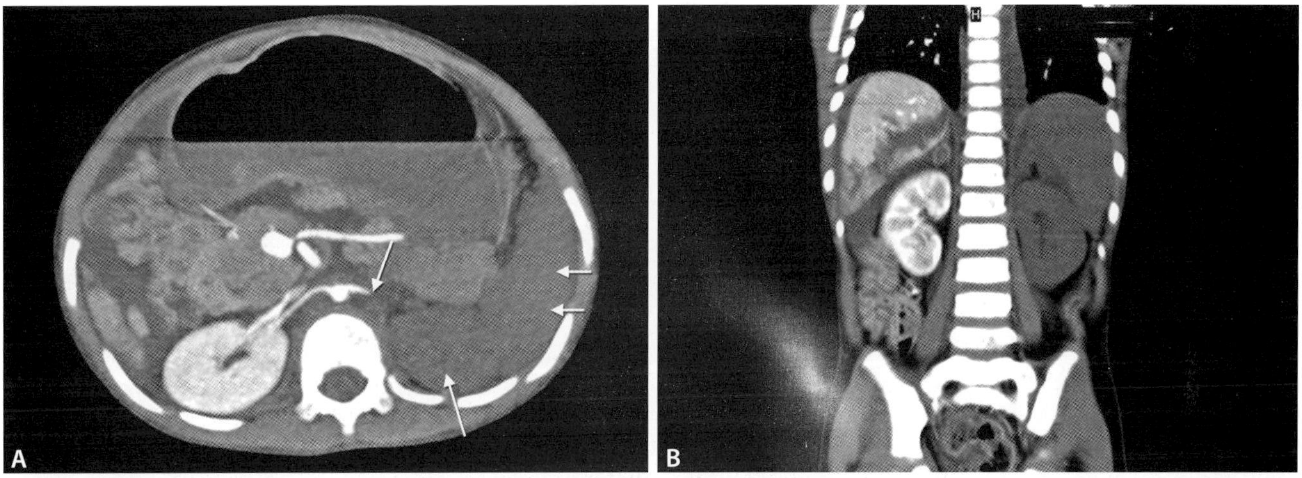

Figs. 8A and B: Axial MIP (A) and multiformatted coronal (B) CECT shows nonenhancing left kidney (long arrow) with abrupt termination of left renal artery (short arrow). Also note devascularized spleen (medium arrows) in (A) and large liver laceration (B).

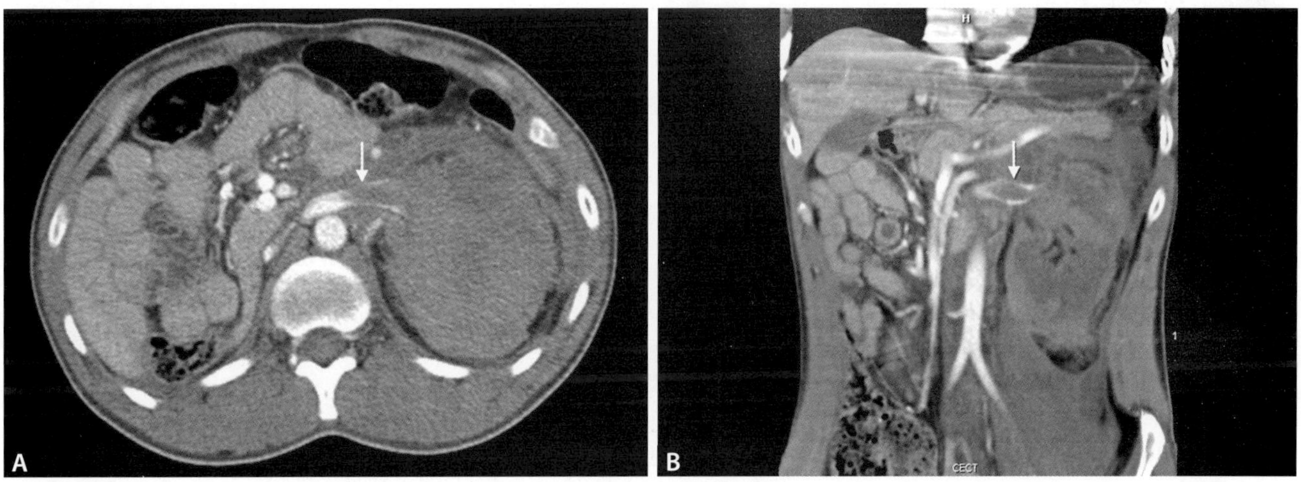

Figs. 9A and B: Axial (A) and multiformatted coronal (B) CECT shows an enlarged nonenhancing left kidney with large perinephric hematoma with a hypodense thrombus in the left main renal vein (arrows).

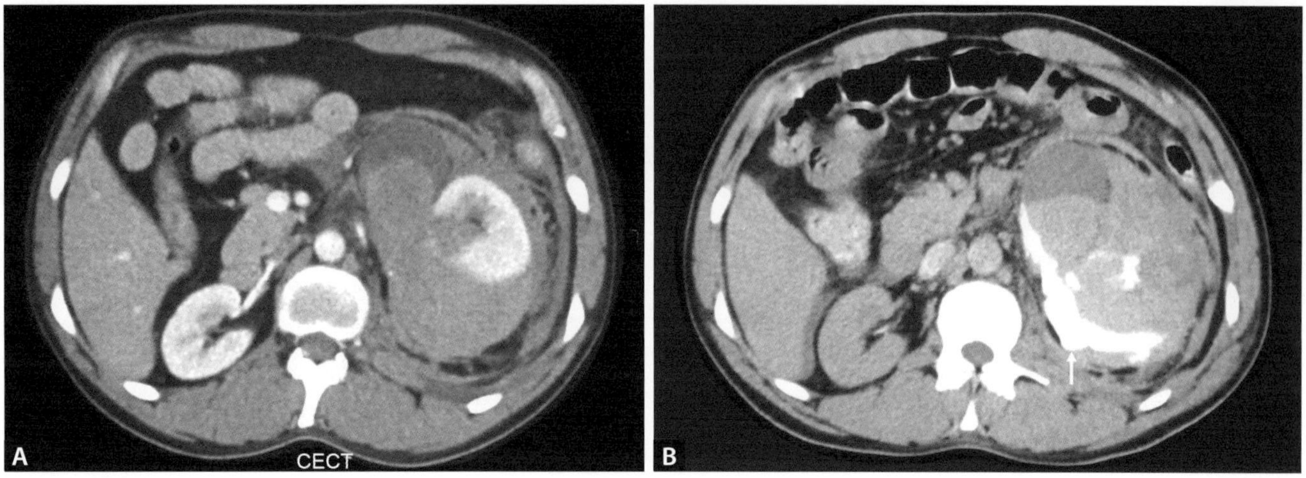

Figs. 10A and B: Axial CECT abdomen (A) shows extensive left perirenal hematoma/fluid collection. Delayed phase axial image (B) shows urinary contrast extravasation in medial perinephric space (arrow) signifying renal pelvic avulsion.

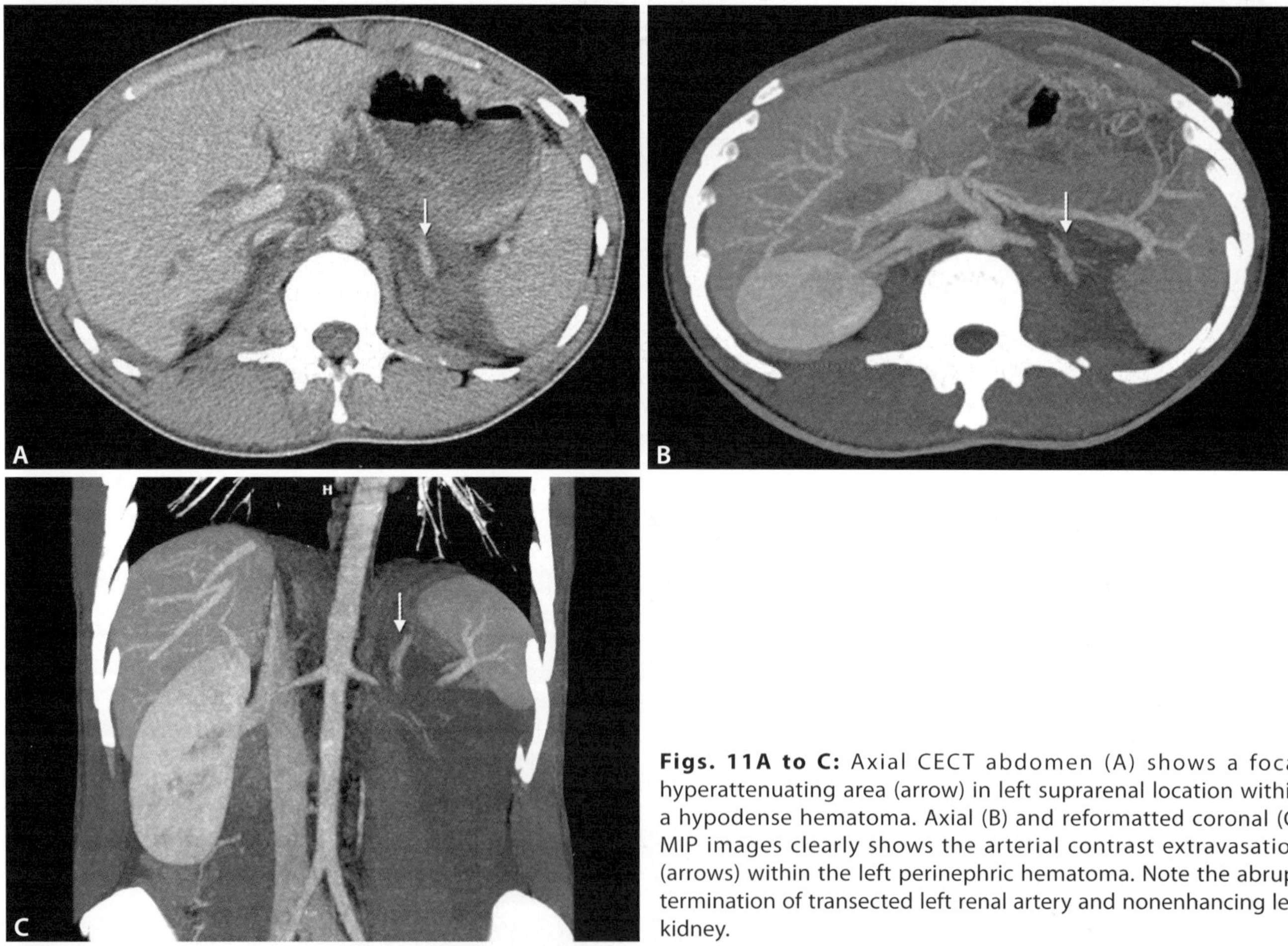

Figs. 11A to C: Axial CECT abdomen (A) shows a focal hyperattenuating area (arrow) in left suprarenal location within a hypodense hematoma. Axial (B) and reformatted coronal (C) MIP images clearly shows the arterial contrast extravasation (arrows) within the left perinephric hematoma. Note the abrupt termination of transected left renal artery and nonenhancing left kidney.

hematoma which tends to track into surrounding tissues on delayed phase images. When seen, it indicates the need for urgent surgical or angiographic intervention.

Renal Trauma with Pre-existing Abnormality

Kidney harboring a pre-existing abnormality is at more risk for injury in blunt abdominal trauma especially in children.[7] Hydronephrosis or extrarenal pelvis is at more risk of rupture. Cysts and tumors can also frequently hemorrhage after trauma. An ectopic or horseshoe kidney is also more prone to trauma, because it is less protected **(Figs. 12A and B)**.

Management of Renal Trauma

The classification of renal trauma into grades correlates with the need for surgery. In general the trend is towards nonoperative management for all but most severe injuries.[8] Grade 1–3 injuries, which constitute >90% of all renal injuries, are almost always managed conservatively. The only absolute indication for active intervention in these grade patients is presence of life-threatening active hemorrhage which may be dealt with angiographic embolization **(Figs. 13A and B)** or surgical exploration.[4] Most of grade 4 injuries can also be managed conservatively. Even large urinary extravasations resolve spontaneously on conservative management sometimes helped by percutaneous drainage of these collections with or without percutaneous nephrostomy and/or ureteric stent placement.[3,9] If they fail to resolve, surgical repair may be warranted. Grade 4 injuries with significant devitalized tissue (>50%) especially with concomitant injuries or urine leak usually require surgical debridement or repair to prevent later development of urinoma, abscess

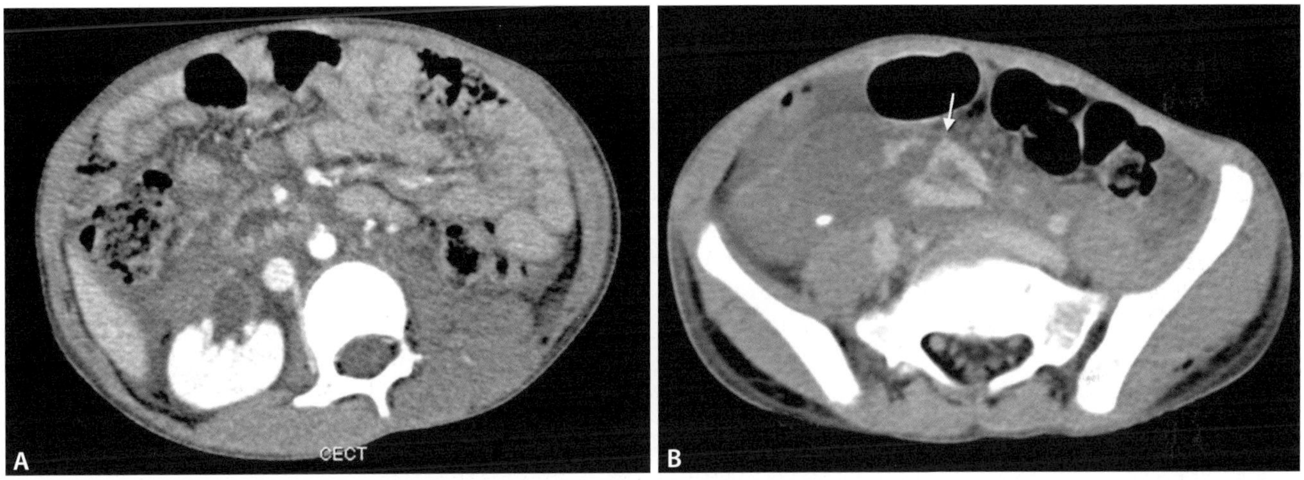

Figs. 12A and B: Axial CECT (A) at the level of kidneys shows left kidney is not present in left renal fossa. Axial image through the pelvis (B) shows extensive lacerations of ectopic left kidney (arrow).

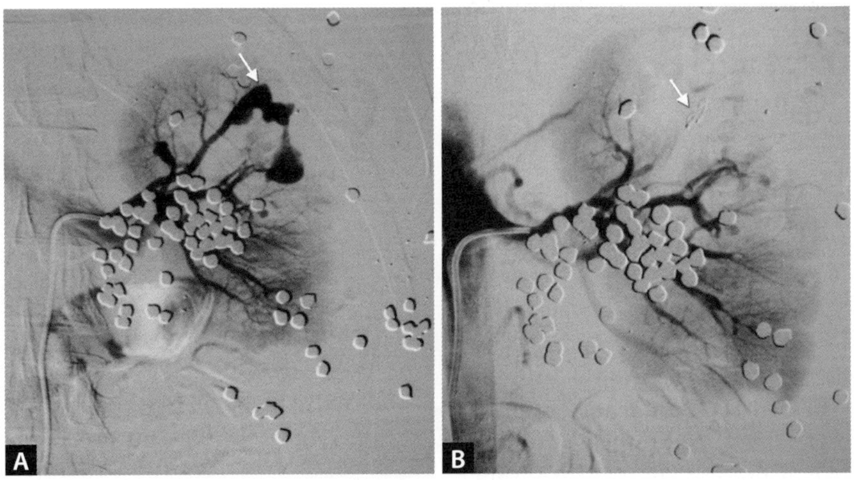

Figs. 13A and B: DSA image (A) of selective left renal artery injection in a patient injured with multiple pellets shows pseudoaneurysm formation with active bleed (arrow) in upper pole of left kidney; (B) The involved upper polar segmental branch was selectively embolized with coil (arrow) resulting in thrombosis of pseudoaneurysm.

or infection which may warrant nephrectomy. With aggressive monitoring and increasing use of angiographic embolisation and percutaneous drainage, overall <10% of grade 3–4 injuries require surgical intervention.[9] Grade 5 injuries with complete avulsion of ureteropelvic junction require surgical repair whereas partial tears may resolve on conservative management or stenting and proximal drainage.[2,3] Devascularization of kidney may be managed conservatively in a stable patient but requires nephrectomy in case of active bleed or major parenchymal disruption. Surgical repair or angiographic thrombolysis of acute renal artery thrombosis can be done to try to preserve the renal function but is shown to have best results usually within few hours of injury.[10] Renal hypertension developing weeks to months after renal trauma is a frequent finding which usually can be managed medically but may occasionally require nephrectomy.

To summarize, the only absolute indication for surgical exploration (or angiographic embolization) is life-threatening active hemorrhage.[4] Relative indications for operative management include the presence of (a) >50% of renal parenchyma devitalization, (b) arterial thrombosis, and (c) urinary extravasation which is not controlled by conservative management including proximal drainage and stenting.

URETERAL TRAUMA

Iatrogenic surgical trauma accounts for 95% of all ureteral injuries and usually occurs in association with gynecological procedures.[11] In gynecological surgery, majority of ureteral injuries are discovered postoperatively (84%) with an average delay of 65 days after the procedure. The patients present with flank pain, fever, hematuria and occasionally anuria. The emergence of endoscopic and laparoscopic surgery and endourological diagnostic and therapeutic interventions in the last two decades have further contributed to the increased incidence of iatrogenic ureteral trauma.[12] In urologic surgery, iatrogenic ureteral injuries occur in open surgery in 21% and 79% in endoscopic procedures. Recognition of the injury during surgery or the endoscopic procedure leads to immediate repair or placement of double J-stent for conservative management.

Gunshot wound, stabbing, and blunt trauma account for rest 5% of the ureteral injuries. Penetrating trauma to ureter is frequently associated with injuries to other organs.[13] Hematuria is usually present but may be absent. Blunt trauma in children with deceleration injury may occasionally lead to ureteral avulsion.

Imaging Work-up

Role of IVU

Traditionally IVU has been used as a follow up study to identify ureteric injury following trauma. However, with widespread avai-lability of CT, its role has become limited. IVU still has a role in the form of one-shot study in unstable patients who require emergency surgery.[14] IVU demonstrates extravasation at the site of injury or obstruction proximal to the site of injury **(Fig. 14)**. Patients in whom ureteral injury is missed, urinary extravasation, hydronephrosis and abscess formation can result. Demonstration of a mature fistulous tract or a large urinoma at a later stage is much more likely (90–100%). Hydronephrosis is seen at a later stage in 90% patients after ureteral injury. Ureteral avulsion may be diagnosed by contrast extravasation medial to the kidney.

Role of CT

Delayed phase CT has an important role in detection of ureter avulsion at UPJ in acute blunt trauma.[15] The diagnosis depends on demonstration of contrast extravasation medial to the kidney and lack of distal ureter opacification. CT is also useful in accurate assessment of the size of the associated peri-renal hematoma which helps the surgeon in deciding on the need for surgery.

Role of Antegrade and Retrograde Ureterograms

Ureterograms obtained *via* the antegrade or retrograde route are considered the gold standard for confirming the presence of ureteral injury. The ureterogram clearly defines the type and location of the injury as also its

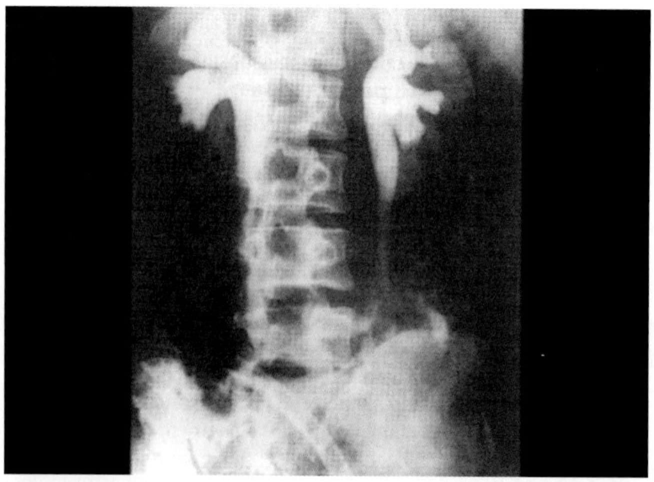

Fig. 14: IVU showing left ureteral injury with extravasation of contrast opposite L5 vertebra.

magnitude. Any associated fistulae and communicating urinomas are also delineated.

Classification

Ureteral injuries have been classified into following grades:[16]

Grade 1: Hematoma only
Grade 2: Laceration <50% of circumference
Grade 3: Laceration >50% of circumference
Grade 4: Complete tear <2 cm of devascularization
Grade 5: Complete tear >2 cm of devascularization

Management

Injuries detected during surgery are treated immediately by either surgical repair or endourologic interventions.[16,17] Injuries recognized later are treated by percutaneous nephrostomy for urinary diversion and antegrade or retrograde stent placement. Stenting may be preceded by balloon dilata-tion or endoureterectomy for strictures. In ureteral avulsion, stenting is coupled with drainage of urinoma which prevents fibrosis and facilitates passage of guide wire antegradely across the dehiscence. Fistulae are also managed with nephrostomy and stenting. Disruption of pelvic ureter can be managed by antegrade ureteroneocystostomy and stenting for 1–3 months for which a curved transjugular intrahepatic portosystemic shunt (TIPS) needle sheath can be used.

BLADDER TRAUMA

Bladder injury is relatively rare and constitutes only 2% of all abdominal injuries that require surgical repair. It may be due to blunt, penetrating or iatrogenic trauma. Majority of the patients of bladder trauma have associated fracture of pelvis most commonly of the anterior pubic arch.[18] A distended bladder is more prone to injury. The patient presents with suprapubic pain or tenderness and/or hematuria. In such cases the recommendation is to first exclude urethral injury by a retrograde urethrography (RGU) followed by insertion of a Foley's catheter. If a urethral injury is found, a suprapubic cystostomy is usually done. This is followed by cystography which may be conventional technique or CT cystography. However, with increasing use of CT scan, CT cystography has become the investigation of choice which can be done at the same sitting if the patient is undergoing CT scan for abdominal injuries.[19] Delayed scanning of the bladder after intravenous contrast administration so as to allow the contrast excreted by kidneys to opacify the bladder is no substitute for CT cystography as it has been shown to miss a significant number of bladder ruptures.[19,20] Conventional cystography may be done if CT is not available.

Cystography

Conventional Cystography

Technique

- 300–400 mL of dilute contrast is instilled into the bladder *via* the urethral (if urethral injury excluded) or the suprapubic route.
- The initial film is taken after 100 mL contrast is instilled to check gross extravasation.
- Films are then taken after the entire contrast is instilled.
- A postdrainage film excludes extravasation hidden by a distended bladder.

CT Cystography

The technique recommended is retrograde filling of the bladder with contrast (same as with conventional cystography) followed by a computed tomogram of the pelvis. With this technique, the diagnostic accuracy is comparable to that of conventional cystography. The CT cystography may be done at the time of initial examination simultaneously with acquisition of abdomen and pelvis after intravenous contrast administration. Postdrainage scans are not required. According to current recommendations, CT cystography should be done in all patients with known pelvic fractures or in patients with gross hematuria or severe pelvic trauma with no known pelvic fractures.

Classification

Blunt Trauma

A classification of bladder injury after blunt pelvic trauma has been described by Sandler et al.[18]

Type 1 : Bladder contusion
Type 2 : Intraperitoneal injury
Type 3 : Interstitial bladder injury
Type 4 : Extraperitoneal injury
A Simple
B Complex
Type 5 : Combined bladder injury.

Bladder contusion (type 1): This consists of a self-limiting, incomplete mural tear with localized echymosis. CT cystography is normal, showing a well-distended uniformly hyperattenuating thin-walled bladder with no contrast leakage. No specific therapy is required. A perivesical hematoma may be associated with major pelvic fractures even when no evidence of actual bladder tear is seen on cystography. Accumulated blood compresses upon the extraperitoneal part of the bladder narrowing it at the base. An "inverted tear drop" or "inverted pear sign" may be seen on cystogram.

Intraperitoneal injury (type 2): Intraperitoneal rupture usually occurs after a blow to the lower abdomen in the presence of distended bladder. Rupture occurs at the dome due to increased intravesical pressure. This is the weakest point of the bladder and also the peritonealized portion of the bladder wall. Urine will thus enter the peritoneal cavity. On cystography, contrast material may be seen outlining the abdominal viscera, loops of bowel, mesenteric folds, paracolic gutters or pouch of Douglas **(Figs. 15A and B)**. The contrast material may track to upper abdomen also. The locations of free intraperitoneal contrast are predictable with well-defined boundaries as compared to extra-peritoneal rupture.

Interstitial injury (type 3): This represents a dissecting rupture of the bladder wall without frank perforation. On CT cystography a mural hematoma/defect may be seen. Occasionally intramural contrast may be seen. But there is no contrast extravasation outside the bladder. Such defects may involve both extra- peritoneal and intraperitoneal portions of the bladder wall. Hence interstitial rupture was designated as a separate category in this classification.

Extraperitoneal injury (type 4): This is the most common injury to the bladder (80–90% of cases) and usually occurs in association with a fractured pelvis or in penetrating trauma. Earlier it was thought that the tear was caused by direct penetration of the bladder by bone fragments. However, now it is postulated that this type of injury may be either a type of bursting or shearing injury resulting from the force of pelvic ring disruption.

In **simple** (type 4A) extraperitoneal rupture, extravasation is confined to the perivesical space. On CT cystography, flame-shaped areas of extravasation are noted in the perivesical spaces and in the prevesical space (space of retzius) where it can track cranially upto umbilicus. The ill-defined contrast in the prevesical space is said to have a 'molar tooth' appearance.

A **complex** (type 4B) extraperitoneal rupture is diagnosed when contrast extravasation extends beyond the perivesical space into the scrotum, thigh, perineum, hip joint and anterior abdominal wall **(Fig. 16)**. It occurs secondary to rupture of urogenital diaphragm. Contrast may also track upwards into the paranephric spaces.

It is important to differentiate intraperitoneal rupture from extraperitoneal rupture of bladder because the former requires surgical repair where the latter is usually managed conservatively with foley's catheter placement.

Combined extra- and intraperitoneal bladder injury (type 5): An injury may result in rupture of both intraperitoneal and extraperitoneal portions of the bladder wall. On CT cysto-graphy, both patterns of contrast extra-vasation may be seen.

Penetrating Bladder Trauma

Injury may result from gunshot or knife wounds and may result in extraperitoneal, intraperitoneal or combined bladder injury. There is a high incidence of associated bowel or other visceral injury and exploratory surgery is required in virtually every patient.

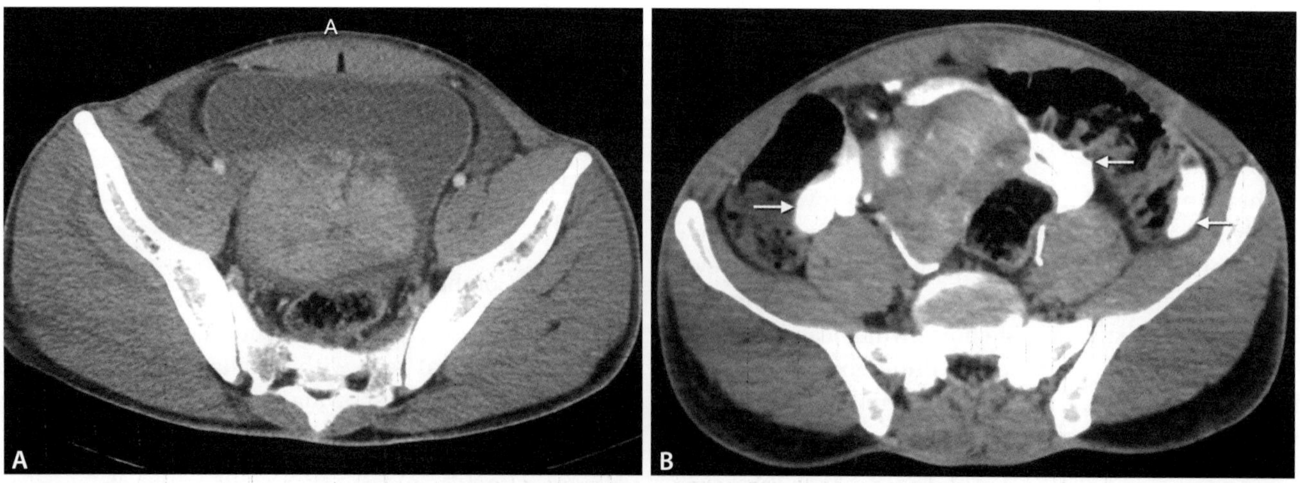

Figs. 15A and B: Axial CECT image (A) through urinary bladder shows a hyperdense clot within the bladder. Axial CT cystography image (B) shows extravasation of contrast outside the bladder in the peritoneal cavity outlining the bowel loops (arrows).

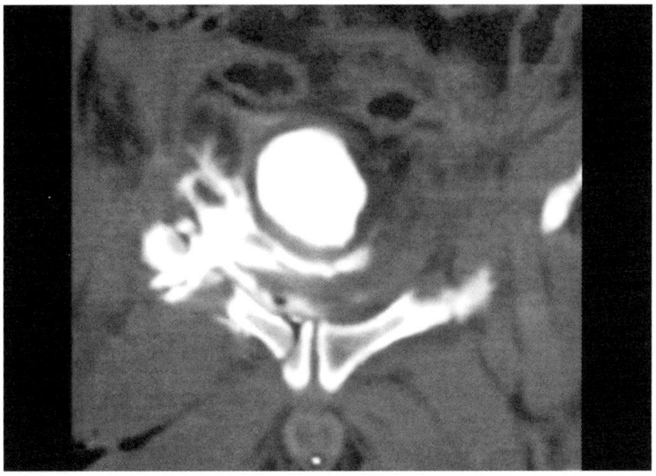

Fig. 16: Reformatted coronal MIP CT cystography image shows complex extraperitoneal rupture of urinary bladder with contrast lying in extraperitoneal spaces in perineum extending into right hip joint.

Iatrogenic Bladder Trauma

Bladder injuries may be due to urologic, gynecologic or obstetric procedures. Bladder perforations or vesicovaginal and vesicouterine fistulae may form. Cystography and hysterosalpingography help in the diagnosis. Migration of surgical devices like drains, catheters, contraceptives or orthopedic prostheses can sometimes perforate the bladder.

Management of Bladder Trauma

Type 1, 3 and 4 injuries are managed conservatively with placement of a Foleys catheter. However intraperitoneal rupture of bladder requires surgical repair. Hence, type 2 and 5 injuries are managed surgically.

URETHRAL TRAUMA

Posterior urethral injuries result from pelvic fractures and gunshot wounds. Injury associated with pelvic fracture mostly involves the urethra near the urogenital diaphragm. Anterior urethral injuries are much less common and are more commonly due to iatrogenic cause, straddle injury or gunshot wound. The lifelong consequences in males include incontinence, strictures and impotence. Female urethra injury is rare.

The clinical signs suggestive of urethral injury in a male patient with pelvic trauma include gross hematuria, blood at urethral meatus, inability to void, swelling or hematoma of the perineum or penis and a high riding prostate on per rectal examination associated with pelvic fracture.[21] The clinical signs in a female patient include difficulty in micturition, blood at meatus, hematuria, labial edema, vaginal bleeding or urine leak per rectum. If the above signs are present in a patient with pelvic trauma, urethrography should be done for evaluation of urethra before insertion of a Foley's catheter.

Radiology

The urethra is best evaluated with retrograde urethrography or voiding cystourethrography.

Technique of Urethrography

- Dynamic retrograde urethrography, ideally under fluoroscopy, is used for the evaluation of urethral injury
- Steep oblique films are obtained, at the end of injection of 25–30 mL of 50% contrast
- If the urethra appears intact, a catheter is passed into the bladder for cystography and a voiding urethrogram is obtained.

Blunt Urethral Trauma

Urethral injuries are classified anatomically as anterior or posterior urethral injuries. Posterior urethral injury occurs in 4–14% of patients with pelvic fracture and up to 20% of these have associated bladder laceration.[22] Anterior urethral injury commonly results from straddle pelvic injury secondary to the patient falling astride a blunt object or direct blow to the perineum. However, more commonly, anterior urethral injuries may be iatrogenic due to instrumentation.

Posterior Urethral Injuries Associated with Pelvic Fracture

- Commonly, prostatomembranous urethral injury above the urogenital diaphragm results.
- A high riding urinary bladder is seen on excretory urography. This is due to disruption of puboprostatic ligaments and hematoma in retropubic and perivesical spaces.
- Contrast extravasation will be seen adjacent to the posterior urethra and sometimes into the pelvic extraperitoneal space.

Anterior Urethral Injury

Straddle injuries resulting from the patient falling astride a blunt object or direct blow to the perineum may lead to anterior, mostly bulbous, urethral injuries. More commonly, anterior urethral injuries may be iatrogenic due to instrumentation. In partial rupture, extravasation of contrast occurs on urethrogram but continuity of the urethra is preserved. In complete rupture, no contrast is seen in the proximal urethra. Venous intravasation is seen commonly. Treatment is by suprapubic urinary diversion and delayed surgery.

Classification

Based on findings of urethrography, the following types of urethral injuries have been described by Goldman et al.[23] who have modified the initial classification given by Colapinto and McCallum.[24]

Type I
- Stretched, but intact posterior urethra is seen **(Fig. 17)**
- In this type of injury the prostate is detached from the urogenital diaphragm with an elevated bladder seen on cystography due to retropubic hematoma and rupture of puboprostatic ligaments
- No extravasation is seen on the urethrogram

Type II
- Seen in around 15% of cases
- Urethra is ruptured at the membrano-prostatic junction above the urogenital diaphragm which is intact **(Fig. 18)**
- Contrast extravasation is seen into the pelvic extraperitoneal space above the urogenital dia-phragm but not in the perineum

Type III
- Most common type
- Membranobulbous urethral rupture is seen with disruption of urogenital diaphragm
- Contrast extravasation both above and below urogenital diaphragm, i.e. into pelvis and the perineum **(Fig. 19)**

Type IV
- There is bladder neck injury with extension into the posterior urethra
- Contrast extravasation is seen in the pelvic extraperitoneal space with disruption of bladder neck **(Fig. 20)**

Type IVa
- Extraperitoneal bladder base injury simulating a bladder neck injury
- Radiologically indistinguishable from type IV injury

Type V
- Caused by straddle injury
- Anterior urethra, most commonly bulbous urethra, injury is seen which may be partial or complete
- Contrast extravasation is seen into the penile soft tissues **(Fig. 21)**.

Management of Urethral Trauma

Type 1 injuries are managed conservatively with placement of a urethral or suprapubic catheter. In general partial disruptions are also managed conservatively with supra-pubic or urethral catheterization whereas complete disruptions of the urethra are managed either by endoscopic realignment or delayed urethroplasty. Bladder neck injuries involve internal sphincter and hence are treated surgically to prevent development of incontinence. However, type IVa injury may be treated conservatively since it does not involve the bladder neck.

Evaluation before Delayed Urethroplasty

- A combined voiding cystourethrogram and a retrograde urethrogram is obtained.
- The bladder is filled with 30% dilute contrast through the suprapubic cystostomy.

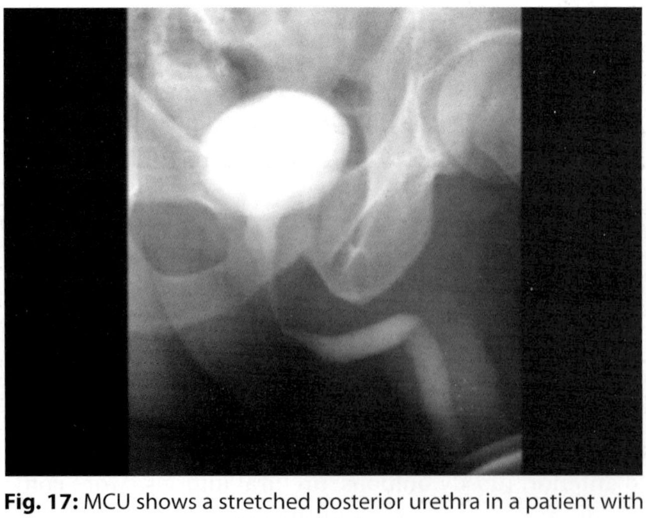

Fig. 17: MCU shows a stretched posterior urethra in a patient with multiple pelvic fractures.

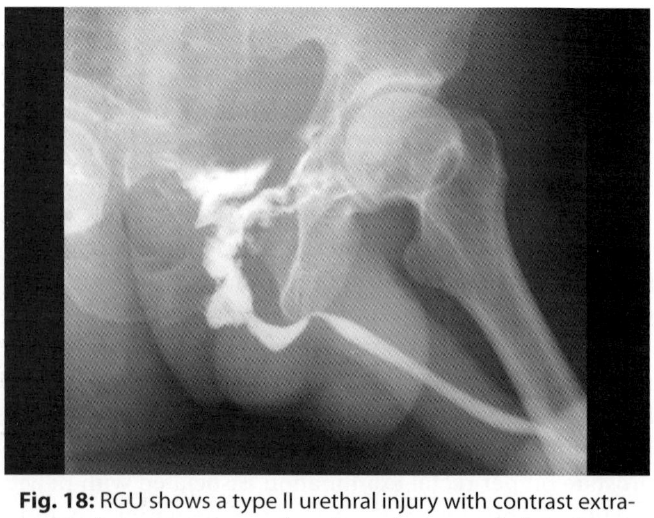

Fig. 18: RGU shows a type II urethral injury with contrast extravasation from posterior urethra above the urogenital diaphragm.

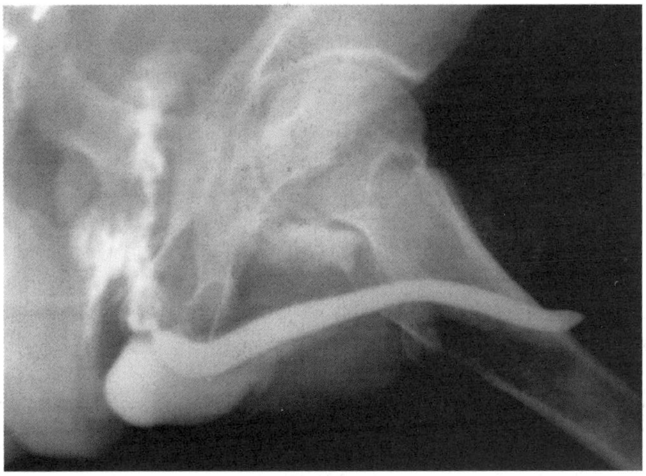

Fig. 19: RGU shows a type III urethral injury with contrast extravasation from posterior urethra both above and below the urogenital diaphragm.

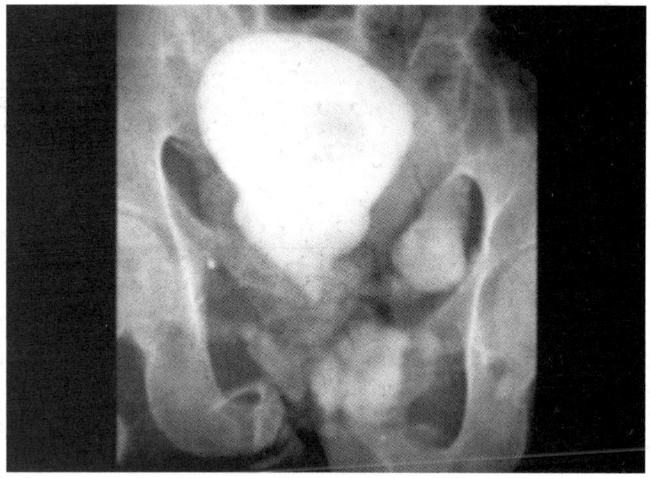

Fig. 20: MCU showing elongated injured bladder neck with contrast extravasation around the prostatic urethra.

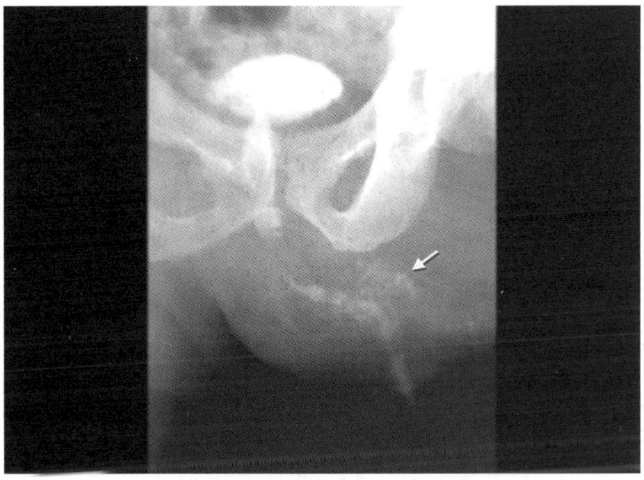

Fig. 21: RGU showing contrast extravasation in penile tissues from anterior urethral injury (arrow).

- The patient is then asked to void.
- A simultaneous retrograde urethrogram is performed.
- This technique demonstrates proximal and distal extent of the stricture. This enables the surgeon to decide between a transperineal and transpubic approach for urethroplasty.
- Recently reports have shown the potential of MRI to demonstrate length of the urethral injury along with amount of displacement of the prostatic apex. This information is helpful in preoperative planning of the surgical approach.

Penetrating Injury

Penetrating trauma to the urethra may be secondary to knife or gunshot wounds. The diagnosis is established by retrograde urethrography. Early surgery is the treatment of choice.

Iatrogenic Injury

Iatrogenic urethral injury may result from pelvic surgery, urethral instrumentation or indwelling catheters.

Female Urethra

Injury to the female urethra is rare because of its mobility. Excretory urography or cystourethrography may show extravasation of contrast at the site of rupture.

REFERENCES

1. McAninch JW. Renal injuries. In: Gillenwater JY, Grayhack JT, Howards SS, Duckett JW (Eds). Adult and Pediatric Urology, 3rd edn. St. Louis, Mo: Mosby; 1996.pp.539-53.
2. Kawashima A, Sandler CM, Corl FM, et al. Imaging of renal trauma: A comprehensive review. Radiographics. 2001;21:557-74.
3. Smith JK, Kenny PJ. Imaging of renal trauma. Radiol Clin N Am. 2003;41:1019-35.
4. Harris AC, Zwirewich CV, Lyburn ID, Torreggiani WC, Marchinkow LO. CT findings in blunt renal trauma. Radiographics. 2001;21:S201-S14.
5. Park SJ, Kim JK, Kim KW, Cho KS. MDCT findings of renal trauma. AJR. 2006;187:541-7.
6. Moore EE, Shackford SR, Patcher HL, et al. Organ injury scaling: Spleen, liver and kidney. J Trauma. 2001;50:195-200.
7. Pollack HM, Wein AJ. Imaging of renal trauma. Radiology. 1989;172:297-308.
8. Knudson MM, Maull KI. Nonoperative manage-ment of solid organ injuries:past, present and future. Surg Clin of N Am. 1999;79:1357-71.

9. Brandes SB, McAninch JW. Reconstructive surgery for trauma of the upper urinary tract. Urol Clin of N Am. 1999;26:183-99.
10. Peterson NJ. Genitourinary trauma. In: Feliciano DV, Moore EE, Mattox KL (Eds). Trauma (3rd ed). Stamford, Conn: Appleton and Lange; 1996.pp.661-94.
11. Assimos DG, Patterson LC, Taylor CL. Changing incidence and etiology of iatrogenic ureteral injuries. J Urol. 1994;152:2240-6.
12. Campbell EW Jr, Filderman S, Jacobs SC. Ureteral injury due to blunt and penetrating trauma. Urology. 1992;40:216-20.
13. Pitts JC, Peterson NE. Penetrating injuries of the ureter. J Trauma. 1981;21:978-82.
14. Lynch TH, Matnz-NL, Las, et al. European Association of urology: Guidelines on urological trauma. Eur Urol. 2005;47:1-15.
15. Kenney PJ, Panicek DM, Witanowski LS. Computed tomography of ureteral disruption. J Comput Assit Tomogr. 1987;11:480-4.
16. Bent C, Iyngkaran T, Power N, et al. Urological injuries following trauma. Clin Radiol. 2008;63:1361-71.
17. Lask D, Abarbanel J, Luttwak Z, et al. Changing trends in the management of iatrogenic ureteral injuries. J Urol. 1995;154:1693-5.
18. Sandler CM, Hall JT, Rodriguez MB, et al. Bladder injury in blunt pelvic trauma. Radiology. 1986;158:633-8.
19. Vaccaro JP, Brody JM. CT cystography in the evaluation of major bladder trauma. Radiographics. 2000;20:1373-81.
20. Power N, Ryan S, Hamilton P. Computed tomographic cystography in bladder trauma: pictorial essay. Can Assoc Radiol J. 2004;55(5):304-8.
21. Patel U. Lower urinary tract trauma. In: Patel U, Rickards D (Eds). Imaging and urodynamics of the lower urinary tract. London, England: Taylor and Francis; 2005.pp.115-21.
22. Kawashima A, Sandler CM, Wasserman NF, LeRoy AJ, King BF, Goldman SM. Imaging of urethral disease: A pictorial review. Radiographics. 2004;24:S195-S216.
23. Goldman SM, Sandler CM, Corriere JN Jr, et al. Blunt urethral trauma: A unified anatomical mechanical classification. J Urol. 1997;157:85-9.
24. Colapinto V, McCallum RW. Injury to the male posterior urethra in fractured pelvis: a new classification. J Urol. 1977; 118:575-80.

CHAPTER 117

Imaging the Adrenal Gland

Raju Sharma, Ashu Seith Bhalla, Arun Kumar Gupta

INTRODUCTION

Thomas Addison first described a clinical entity resulting from adrenal dysfunction in 1855, but it took nearly half a century for the scientific community to accept that adrenals are essential to life. Remarkable progress has since been made in defining the structure and function of the adrenal gland. Adrenal glands are small but their common involvement in many disease processes has made cross-sectional imaging modalities essential to detect abnormal morphological and functional alterations. Radiology also plays a critical role in the characterization of adrenal mass lesions. Therefore, it is important to first understand the normal anatomy and functional characteristics of the adrenal gland.

ANATOMY AND PHYSIOLOGY

The adrenal gland is named for its location adjacent to the kidney. It lies within perirenal fascia, embedded in perirenal fat. Each gland measures 3–5 cm in length, 2–3 cm in width, 5.0 mm in thickness and weighs around 3.5–5.0 g. Both glands differ in shape. The right adrenal is pyramidal in shape and its relations are liver laterally, upper pole of right kidney inferiorly, right crus of diaphragm posteromedially and inferior vena cava anteromedially. The left adrenal gland is crescent-shaped and its relations are upper pole of left kidney posterolaterally, left crus of diaphragm posteromedially, anteriorly stomach in upper two-third and pancreatic body with splenic vessels in lower one-third. Each adrenal gland receives its blood supply from three arteries, namely superior adrenal artery a branch of inferior phrenic, middle adrenal artery arising from descending aorta and inferior adrenal artery, a branch of renal artery. There is a single adrenal vein on either side, the right adrenal vein drains into inferior vena cava and left one into left renal vein.

The adrenal gland is made of an outer cortex that is derived from mesoderm and an inner medulla, derived from neural crest. The cortex forms almost 90% of total adrenal mass; the medulla contributes only 10%. The adrenal cortex is histologically comprised of three distinct zones—zona glomerulosa, zona fasciculata and zona reticularis from outside to inside. The adrenal cortex secretes three groups of steroid hormones. Zona glomerulosa constitutes 10–15% of the cortex and secretes mineralcorticoids, aldosterone being the most important. Zona fasciculata constitutes 80% of the cortex and secretes glucocorticoids, while zona reticularis contributing only 5–10% of cortex, secretes androgens. Zona glomerulosa is mainly involved in aldosterone biosynthesis whereas fasciculata-reticularis zone is the site for cortisol and androgen biosynthesis.

The adrenal medulla secretes epinephrine and norepinephrine, which form an integral part of sympathetic autonomic nervous system and play an important role in the regulation of vital functions and many metabolic processes.

IMAGING MODALITIES

A number of imaging modalities are available for evaluation of the adrenals. Before the advent of imaging modalities of US, CT and MRI, the radiological techniques available for evaluation of adrenals were plain X-ray abdomen, excretory urography, invasive techniques of perirenal air insufflation, adrenal venography and angiography. Most of these techniques have become obsolete. Angiography may be sometimes indicated to look for extra-adrenal pheochromocytoma in situations when metaiodobenzylguanidine (MIBG) scintigraphy is not available. Adrenal venous sampling may be recommended in patients with aldosteronism, both for distinguishing unilateral from bilateral disease and for localizing unilateral tumor. However, this technique is invasive, technically difficult to perform and requires long fluoroscopy time with resultant high radiation dose and needs hospitalization. Procedural complications include adrenal infarction, adrenal vein thrombosis, adrenal hemorrhage, hypotensive crises and adrenal insufficiency. Therefore, adrenal venous sampling is best reserved for patients with equivocal findings on cross-sectional imaging modalities.

Ultrasound is seldom used in imaging suspected adrenal pathology. CT and MRI remain the imaging modalities for evaluation of structural changes in the diseased adrenal whereas scintigraphy provides functional assessment of the gland. F-18 fluorodeoxyglucose positron emission tomography (F-18 FDG PET) has played an important role in defining physiological and pathological conditions of the adrenal glands. Integrated information obtained from anatomic and functional imaging is essential for characterization of adrenal disease.

Percutaneous biopsy of the adrenal lesion under USCT guidance has an accuracy of 80–90%. Minor complications include abdominal pain, hematuria or small pneumothorax. Major ones requiring treatment occur in 3–5% of the patients and include hemorrhage and pneumothorax.

Ultrasound

Despite availability of high-resolution real-time ultrasound (US) scanners, normal adrenal gland or small adrenal lesions remain difficult to be visualized on sonography, especially in obese patients. Therefore, ultrasonography is seldom indicated for adrenal lesion, although large adrenal mass may be detected incidentally during abdominal ultrasound examination. Ultrasound is, however, useful in evaluation of suspected adrenal hemorrhage in neonates. It may also be used as a screening modality in suspected pheochromocytoma, due to the easy availability of the examination. US guidance suffices for sampling of large adrenal lesions.

Computed Tomography

Computed tomography (CT) remains the first choice of imaging modality for evaluation of most of the adrenal diseases. The widespread availability of CT in clinical practice makes it an ideal noninvasive technique for evaluating adrenal gland morphology owing to the speed with which examination can be performed, its superior spatial resolution and quantification of contrast washout patterns.[1-3] The introduction of spiral CT and more recently multidetector-row helical CT (MDCT), has allowed rapid thin slice imaging of the adrenal glands during various phases of contrast enhancement. Small adrenal lesions can be detected and accurate density measurements of lesions can be done.

CT technique should be tailored according to the clinical indication. In general, when CT is used to study the adrenal glands the entire abdomen through the aortic bifurcation is scanned. This is helpful for staging or for evaluating possible ectopic adrenal lesions.[4] Five hundred milliliters of 2% of oral contrast is given 15 minutes prior to scanning to opacify the bowel loops. Oral contrast material is helpful so that unopacified loops of bowel are not confused as adrenal lesions. A nonenhanced CT examination should be done first. This may be followed by enhanced and delayed enhanced CT examination when required in a situation, where adenoma needs to be differentiated from metastasis.

While evaluating adrenal glands for suspected hyperplasia or adenoma, in a clinical setting of functioning tumors (e.g. Cushing's disease, Conn's syndrome, congenital adrenal hyperplasia), then thin sections are obtained through the adrenals. For these scans, intravenous contrast material is not required.[4]

In the search for pheochromocytoma, CT should be done from lower thorax to symphysis pubis. Pericardium is a rare site but can be easily included on CT. Large sporadic pheochromocytomas are easily detected on CT and contrast administration is usually unnecessary. However, syndromic pheochromocytoma may be small, multiple and extra-adrenal. In order to optimize visualization of tumors, contrast injection maybe necessary. It is debatable if IV contrast is safe in this setting. It is extremely rare for IV contrast to precipitate hypertensive crisis in patients of pheochromocytomas. Most authorities consider it unnecessary to give prophylactic alpha and beta adrenergic blockade prior to IV contrast.[5]

The adrenal gland has a characteristic inverted Y or V shape on CT and is seen as an anteromedial ridge with two posterior limbs, medial limb being shorter than the lateral limb and limbs have normally straight or concave outline **(Figs. 1A and B)**. The adrenal measurements on CT are taken as anteroposterior diameter from the tip of the anteromedial ridge to the posterior tip of the longest

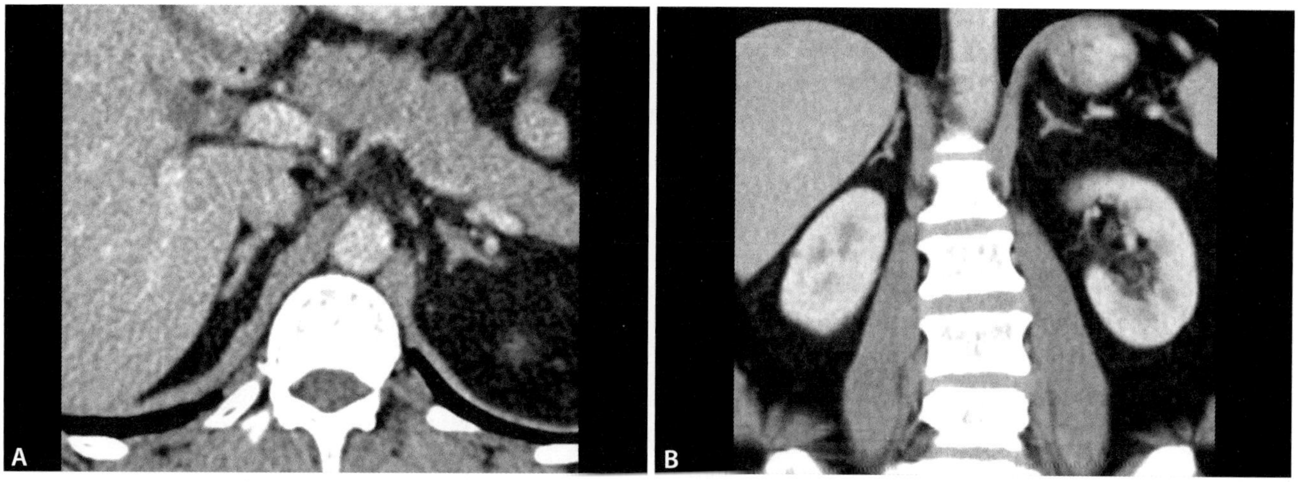

Figs. 1A and B: Axial (A) and coronal (B) CT images showing the normal adrenal glands.

limb, length by calculating the number of sequential scans in which the gland is visualized **(Fig. 2)**. The criteria for enlargement of adrenal are taken as length more than 4.0 cm, anteroposterior diameter of more than 3.0 cm and limb thickness of more than 6.0 mm or more than adjacent diaphragmatic crus. Besides these absolute measurements, any alteration in the contour, focal bulge, calcification, pattern of enhancement, CT attenuation values on nonenhanced, enhanced and delayed enhanced techniques, and displacement of surrounding structures should be evaluated.

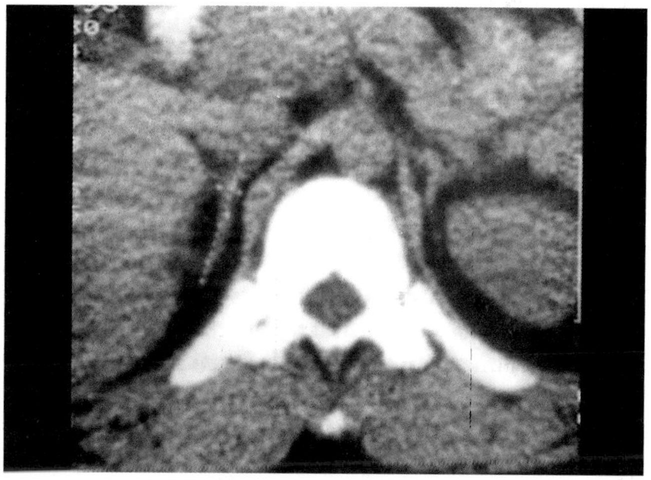

Fig. 2: Normal adrenal measurements: (1) Anteroposterior diameter and (2) Limb thickness.

Magnetic Resonance Imaging

The intention of most magnetic resonance imaging (MRI) techniques used so far has primarily been distinction of benign from malignant disease. The most reliable in this context is the combined use of in-phase and out-of-phase gradient-echo (GRE) techniques for adenoma vs metastasis distinction. The best approach is to use 2D or 3D gradient-echo sequences, without fat suppression. The only variation between sequences should be the echo-time (TE), with TE of 4.2–4.5 ms for in-phase imaging and TE of 2.2–2.7 ms for out-of-phase imaging at 1.5 T. On the newer MR systems, double echo (in phase and out of phase) sequences are available that allow more accurate comparison.[6] The normal adrenal cortex contains abundant lipid, which however, is not enough to be demonstrated on in-phase and out-of-phase imaging.

Serial postgadolinium gradient echo may also be used for benign vs malignant differentiation. The capillary-phase postgadolinium images are most useful.[7] As in the case of CT, the incidence of hypertensive crisis following gadolinium in suspected pheochromocytomas is extremely rare.[5]

T2-weighted images provide information on fluid-content of lesions. T2-weighted imaging hence is most useful in the search for pheochromocytomas which have a high fluid content. T2-weighted sequences also supplement benign vs malignant differentiation, although substantial overlap exists.[8] Normal adrenal gland may demonstrate cortico-medullary differentiation on T2WI.

As no single technique is more than 90% accurate, it is useful to combine in-phase and out-of-phase images with other techniques to increase confidence of lesion characterization, especially capillary-phase gadolinium enhanced imaging.[6,8]

Normal adrenal glands and small adrenal masses are well demonstrated on T1 weighted fat suppressed images **(Figs. 3A and B)**.[9] The demonstration of corticomedullary differentiation on either noncontrast T1W fat-suppressed

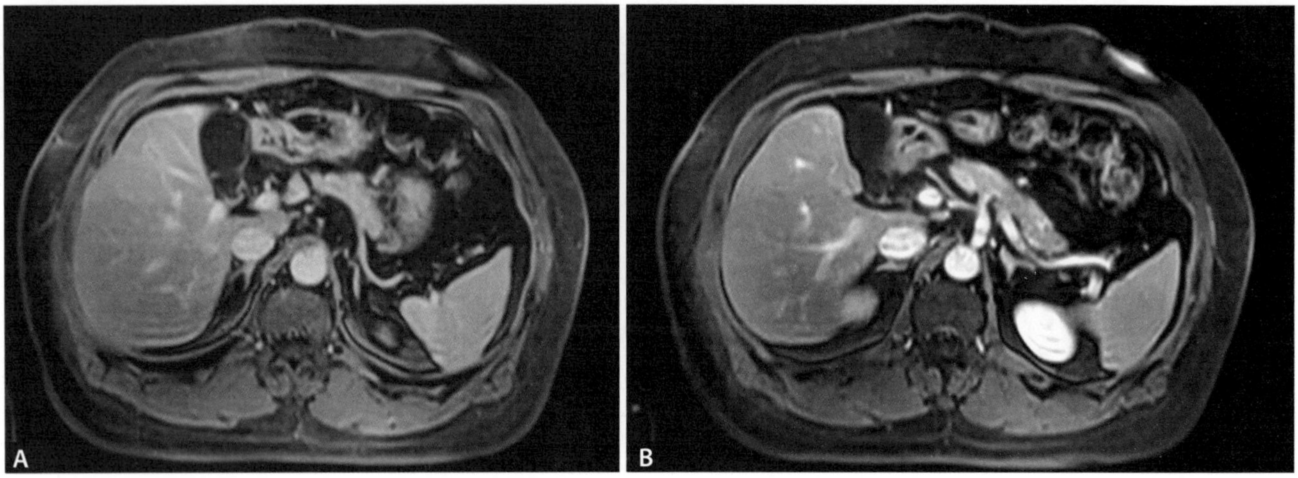

Figs. 3A and B: Gradient echo T1W axial images showing the normal inverted 'V' configuration of the adrenal gland.

images or immediate postgadolinium GE images is helpful in distinguishing adrenal from renal tumors.[10] Sagittal plane is more useful than coronal plane in this regard. The use of thin section 3D-GRE sequences in one plane of acquisition, allows reconstructions in other planes for defining tumor location.

Radionuclide Imaging

This technique is primarily used as a problem solving modality for lesions not adequately characterized on CT and MR imaging. It provides functional imaging of the adrenal cortex and medulla. Radiolabeled analogs of cholesterol, e.g. 75 Se selenomethyl norcholesterol, 59 NP beta-iodomethyl-19-norcholesterol can localize mass causing adrenal cortical dysfunction, the latter one is particularly useful in the work up for suspected aldosteronism. The advances made with CT and MRI have largely eliminated the use of 59 NP imaging for adrenal. Iodine-131 metaiodobenzylguanidine (MIBG) is concentrated in sympathoadrenal tissue and is used for imaging adrenal medullary lesion, especially to evaluate for pheochromocytoma and to screen the whole body for extra-adrenal pheochromocytoma.

Positron Emission Tomography

Recently positron emission tomography (PET) has become available as a possible tool for evaluating the adrenal. FDG-PET has shown promise in differentiating benign from malignant mass. However, in literature only limited data on the role of 18-FDG PET/PET-CT in characterization of adrenal lesions in oncology population is available, that too involving a relatively small sample size.[11] F18-FDG PET imaging has been found to be a reliable noninvasive imaging technique to differentiate benign from malignant adrenal masses. It has demonstrated a high-sensitivity, specificity and overall accuracy for detecting adrenal metastases in patients with malignancy.

The common causes of false positive adrenal lesions on F18-FDG PET imaging are benign adenomas and pheochromocytoma.[12,13] All the benign and malignant pheochromocytomas have been shown to accumulate F18-FDG, although uptake is found in a greater concentration in malignant as compared to benign pheochromocytoma.[12] The common causes of false negative F18-FDG PET results, are small size lesions, necrotic metastasis, and metastases from neuroendocrine tumors.[13] Small metastatic lesions can be missed because of the limited resolution of F18-FDG PET/PET-CT or the absence of sufficient tumor cells with increased glycolysis.

ADRENAL DISEASES

Diseases of the adrenal may become manifest as a result of hormone excess or deficiency. The adrenal diseases may be considered under the following three groups:

Group I : Adrenal hyperfunctional diseases.
Group II : Adrenal insufficiency.
Group III : Adrenal diseases with normal function.

Group I: Adrenal Hyperfunctional Diseases

Hyperfunctioning adrenal diseases occur either from the adrenal cortex (Cushing's syndrome, Conn syndrome, hyperandrogenism) or the adrenal medulla (pheochromocytoma). The clinical features depend on the type of hormone produced and its target organs.

Cushing's Syndrome

Cushing's syndrome is caused by adrenocorticotropic hormone (ACTH) overproduction in 75% of patients and by excess of cortisol production from adrenal neoplasms in 25%. ACTH overproduction results from either pituitary adenoma or from ectopic ACTH producing nonendocrine tumors. Ectopic ACTH producing nonendocrine tumors include bronchial carcinoid tumor, islet cell tumor of the pancreas, medullary carcinoma of thyroid, thymic carcinoid tumor and pheochromocytoma **(*see* Figs. 3A and B)**.

The diagnosis of Cushing's syndrome depends predominantly on the clinical features and biochemical findings. It presents an easily recognizable clinical picture of truncal obesity, moon facies, cutaneous striae, buffalo hump, hypertension, muscles weakness, fatigability, osteoporosis, profound emotional changes and amenorrhea in women.

Appropriate work-up of patients with Cushing's syndrome includes plasma cortisol and 24 hours urine for cortisol estimation followed by dexamethazone suppression test. The abnormal test establishes the diagnosis of Cushing's syndrome. The purpose of imaging is to identify the source of excess ACTH either from a pituitary tumor or an ectopic source and to detect or exclude adrenal mass. The adrenal appearances in Cushing's syndrome depend on the etiology of the syndrome. CT is the primary modality used in this setting. Visualization of adrenal pathology on CT is aided by the large amount of retroperitoneal fat that is usually present in these patients. MRI plays a secondary role.[14]

ACTH-dependent Cushing's Syndrome

This results from pituitary cause in 85% of patients and rest from ectopic ACTH secretion. The adrenals show changes of hyperplasia in the form of smooth thickened limbs or multiple small nodules of varying size involving one or both limbs. These changes may be seen in one or both adrenals **(Figs. 4 and 5)**. MRI signal intensity in adrenal hyperplasia closely follows that of the normal adrenal gland.

ACTH-independent Cushing's Syndrome

Adrenocortical adenoma: It accounts for 10–20% of patients with Cushing's syndrome. It is seen as a solitary, well-defined homogeneous mass, usually around 2-3 cm in diameter **(Figs. 6A to C)**. However, when large, it shows focal areas of necrosis and hemorrhage. These adenomas are larger than those seen in Conn's syndrome, and are usually lipid rich.[4] The contralateral gland is normal but occasionally atrophic. *Adrenal carcinoma* accounts for 10–15% of patients with Cushing's syndrome. Also, only 10% of adrenal carcinomas function to a level that results in *Cushing's* syndrome.[4] It is generally seen as a large mass often more than 6.0 cm, heterogeneous with areas of necrosis and calcification, with features of local invasion, regional lymphadenopathy and distant spread **(Figs. 7 and 8)**.

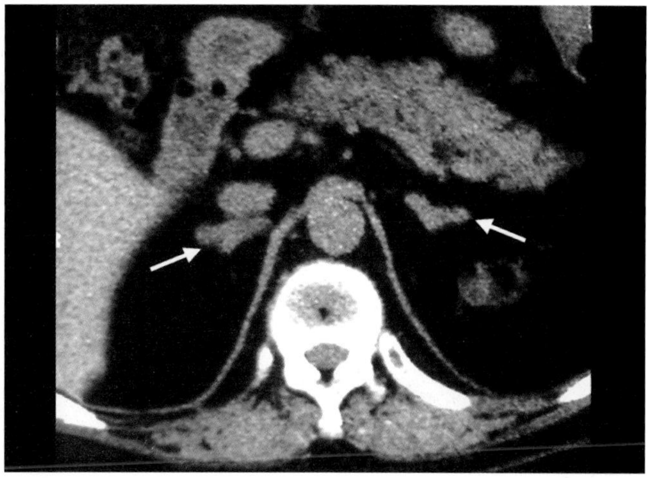

Fig. 4: NCCT of adrenal glands of a 20-year-old male patient presenting with Cushing's syndrome showing bilateral adrenal hyperplasia (arrows) with proliferation of perirenal and mesenteric fat.

Rockall et al.[15] while reporting findings in 37 patients with primary adrenal Cushing's syndrome found hyperfunctioning adenomas (n = 24) and functioning carcinomas (n = 10), accounted for 92% of cases. Adenomas had a significantly smaller mean size (3.5 vs 14.5 cm) and lower mean unenhanced CT attenuation value (11 vs 28 HU) than did carcinomas. The presence of necrosis, hemorrhage, and calcification favored a diagnosis of carcinoma. Six of ten carcinoma patients had metastases at presentation. Two adenomas were seen within a myelolipoma. Two adenomas were of uncertain malignant potential. Bilateral disease—primary pigmented nodular adrenal dysplasia (PPNAD) (n = 2) and ACTH-independent macronodular adrenal hyperplasia (AIMAH) (n = 1), had characteristic imaging features. In PPNAD, multiple tiny (2–5 mm) nodules were visible bilaterally, with no overall glandular enlargement and normal intervening adrenal tissue. In AIMAH, both glands were grossly enlarged and contained nodules up to 3 cm in diameter.

Aldosteronism

Aldosteronism (Conn's syndrome) is associated with excess of mineralocorticoids and characterized clinically

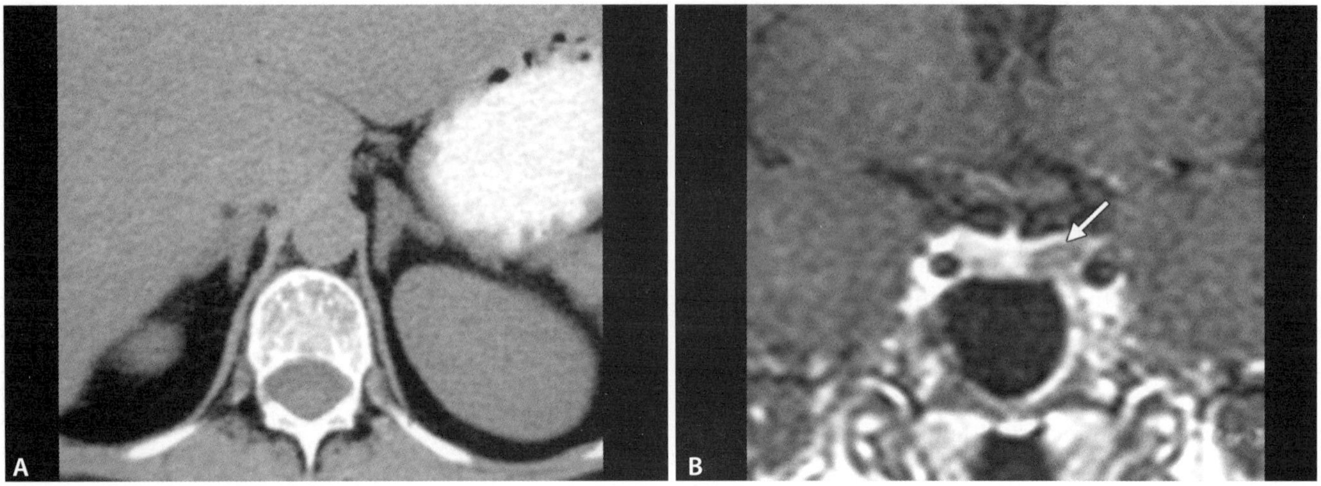

Figs. 5A and B: NCCT of adrenal glands (A) of a 32-year-old female patient presenting with Cushing's syndrome showing nodular, bilateral adrenal hyperplasia. Postcontrast T1W coronal image of MRI sella of the same patient (B) reveals a microadenoma on left side of anterior pituitary (arrow).

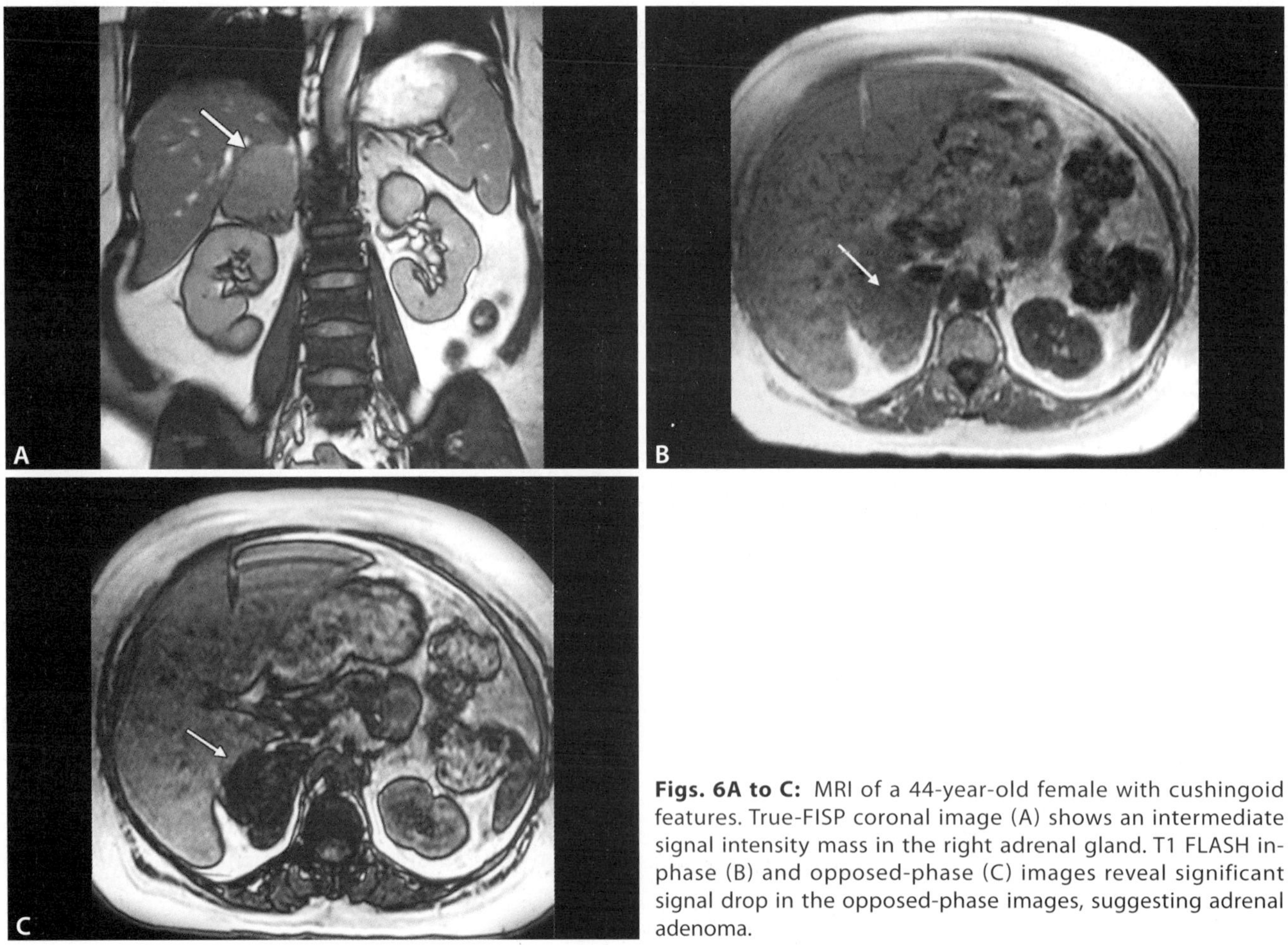

Figs. 6A to C: MRI of a 44-year-old female with cushingoid features. True-FISP coronal image (A) shows an intermediate signal intensity mass in the right adrenal gland. T1 FLASH in-phase (B) and opposed-phase (C) images reveal significant signal drop in the opposed-phase images, suggesting adrenal adenoma.

by hypertension, muscle weakness, polyuria, polydipsia and persistent hypokalemia. It is caused by adrenal adenoma in about 80% of patients while adrenal gland hyperplasia in the rest. Adrenal carcinoma is extremely rare, accounts for less than 1% of patients, as a cause of aldosteronism. In patients with unilateral adenoma, unilateral adrenalectomy is the treatment of choice. On the other hand, cases of bilateral adrenal gland hyperplasia are treated medically with pharmacological agents.[16] The imaging approach hence is to distinguish between these two entities.

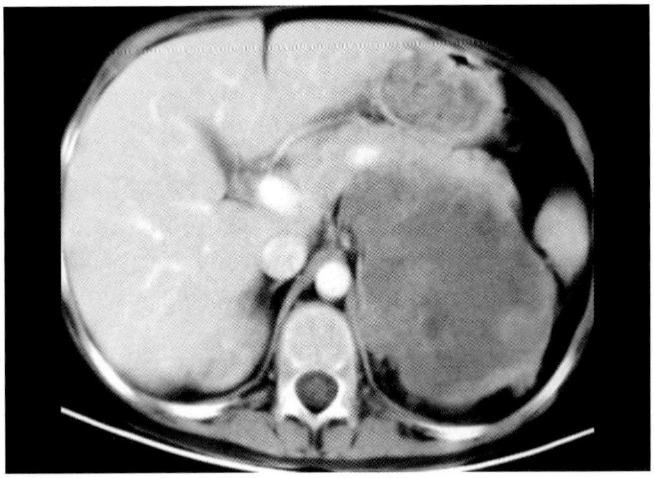

Fig. 7: Axial CECT of a 12-year-old boy with cushingoid features showing a heterogeneously enhancing mass arising from the left adrenal, suggesting adrenal carcinoma.

Aldosterone producing adenoma is small with a mean size of 1.6–1.8 cm and may have central low attenuation due to high lipid content **(Fig. 9)**. A dedicated CT examination with thin sections is required for localizing the adenoma.

If CT examination is inconclusive, adrenal cortical scintigraphy with NP-59 may be done. On NP-59 scintigraphy, both adrenals are normally visualized on 5th day or later, following injection of radiopharmaceuticals. Bilateral adrenal visualization before 5th day suggests adrenal gland hyperplasia while unilateral adrenal visualization before 5th day indicates an adenoma. If clinically strongly suspected and negative CT examination the other alternative study is adrenal venous sampling to determine lateralization of aldosterone secretion to one side suggesting adenoma or both sides suggesting bilateral hyperplasia. NP 59 scintigraphy has long procedural time of nearly two weeks with an accuracy of 71% in contrast to adrenal venous sampling with an accuracy of 95–100%.

Androgenital Syndrome

Androgenital syndrome is a consequence of excessive secretion of sex hormones. It causes virilization, feminization or precocious puberty depending upon the age and sex of the patient. The most common form is virilization, occurring in females.[4] The characteristic clinical features are amenorrhea, hirsuitism, clitoromegaly, deepening of voice.

The adrenal causes of androgen excess include congenital adrenal hyperplasia in children and virilizing

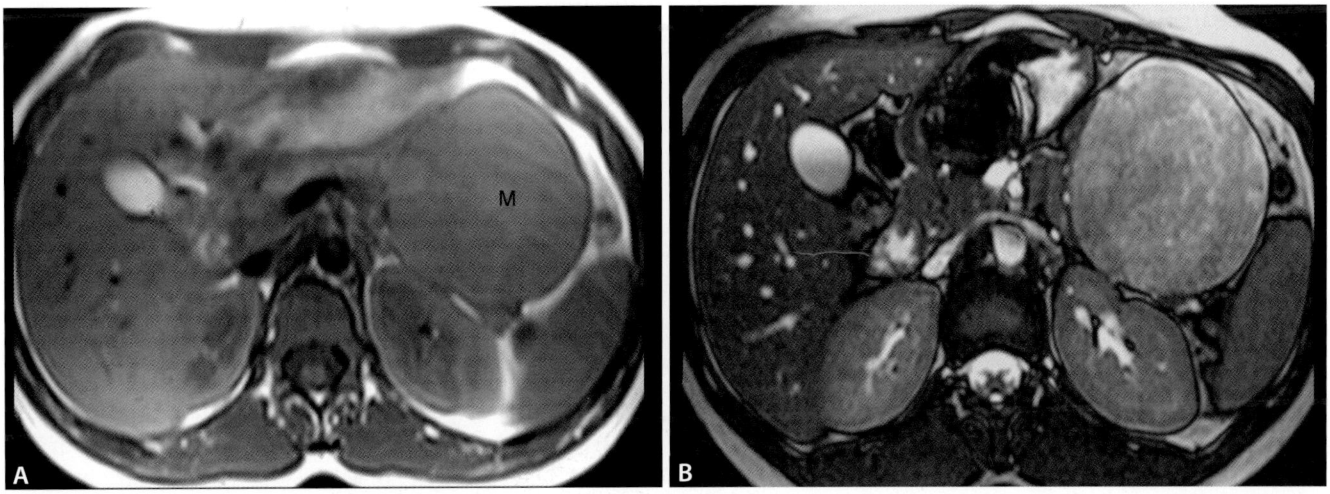

Figs. 8A and B: Axial T1W (A) and T2W (B) MR images of a 28-year-old female with clinical and biochemical features of Cushing's syndrome, reveal a well encapsulated mass (M), hypointense on T1W and heterogeneously hyperintense on T2W, arising from left adrenal gland. On biopsy, it was a carcinoma.

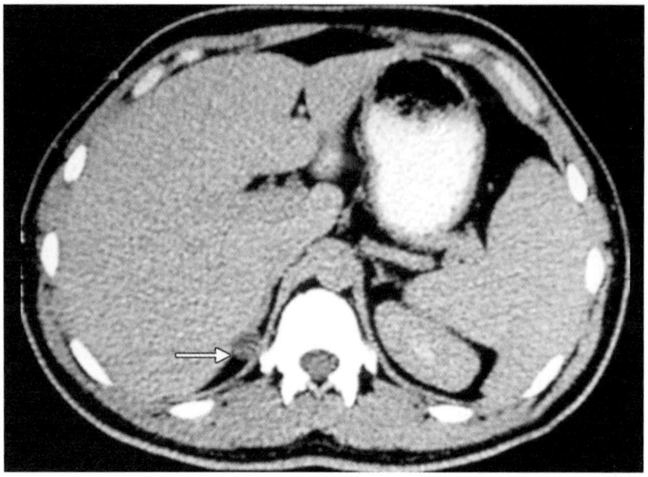

Fig. 9: NCCT of a 28-year-old male with hypertension shows a low attenuating nodule in the right adrenal (arrow) with attenuation value of 4HU. Conn's syndrome due to adrenal adenoma.

tumors (adenoma or carcinoma) in adults. Congenital adrenal hyperplasia (CAH) occurs due to deficiency of enzymes involved in the synthesis of steroid hormones. Each different enzyme deficiency results in a different form of congenital adrenal hyperplasia. The clinical manifestations are determined by the degree of deficiency of cortisol or aldosterone and by the biological properties of the biochemical intermediates that are formed and secreted in excess.

Androgen producing tumors are rare and include adenoma or carcinoma, and occur in both males and females at a later age. In general, in adults a higher proportion of malignant tumors result in adrenogenital syndrome than benign lesions.[4]

MRI is preferred to CT to image adrenals as well as ovaries particularly in children to detect tumors because of MRI being non-ionizing. CT is however often the initial and only modality performed in evaluation of suspected CAH, due to easy availability and short examination times **(Figs. 10 and 11)**.[17]

The tumors are usually more than 2.0 cm in size and show imaging characteristics described above **(Figs. 12A and B)**. Occasionally adrenal and gonadal venous sampling may be necessary to locate the source of excessive androgens.

Pheochromocytoma

Pheochromocytomas are catecholamine producing tumors which arise from ganglion cells anywhere in the autonomic nervous system. About 90% of pheochromocytomas originate in the adrenal medulla, while 10% are extra-adrenal, the common sites being paravertebral sympathetic ganglia, organ of Zuckerkandl, urinary bladder, neck or mediastinum. Ten percent of pheochromocytomas are bilateral and 10% are malignant. About 5–10% are inherited as autosomal dominant either alone or in combination with other abnormalities, such as multiple endocrine neoplasia, (MEN Type II or III), neurofibromatosis, von Hippel-Lindau's retinal and cerebellar hemangioblastomas.

Clinical features of hypertension, paroxysmal attacks of palpitation, headache, sweating and biochemical tests of plasma catecholamine levels and 24 hours urine vanillyl-mandelic acid level can provide the diagnosis. Imaging is required to locate the tumor. CT is the technique of choice to confirm adrenal mass. It is seen as soft tissue density mass with contrast enhancement on CECT **(Figs. 13A to C)**. On MRI, it is isointense or hypointense on T1 weighted image and extremely hyperintense on T2-weighted image. Although this finding is almost universally seen with pheochromocytomas, a percentage of adrenal metastases have overlapping findings.[4,6,18] Gadolinium-DTPA (diethylenetriamine penta-acetic acid) produces marked enhancement with slower wash out of contrast as compared to adenoma **(Figs. 14A to D)**. Pheochromocytomas show insignificant signal drop on out of phase GRE images. It may show variable necrosis but calcification in pheochromocytoma is rare **(Figs. 15A and B)**. The initial imaging findings in benign and malignant pheochromocytomas are nearly identical. Only the presence of metastases can clearly define a pheochromocytoma as malignant.[4]

CT and MRI can detect adrenal pheochromocytoma equally well. However, MRI is better for detecting extra-adrenal pheochromocytoma and recurrence after surgery. On sonography, pheochromocytoma is seen as well-defined hypoechoic mass which may show areas of necrosis or hemorrhage. The accuracy of ultrasonography in detecting pheochromocytoma is less than CT and MRI, particularly if the tumor is small and extra-adrenal.

In patients with strongly suspected pheochromocytoma, but no adrenal mass identified on CT or MRI, MIBG scintigraphy is the technique of choice to detect ectopic location and is also indicated for metastatic or locally recurrent disease. It is seen as focal areas of abnormal activity. The sensitivity of MIBG scintigraphy for detecting pheochromocytoma is 80–90% with a specificity of 90–100% but a positive MIBG scintigraphy should always be correlated with CT or MRI.

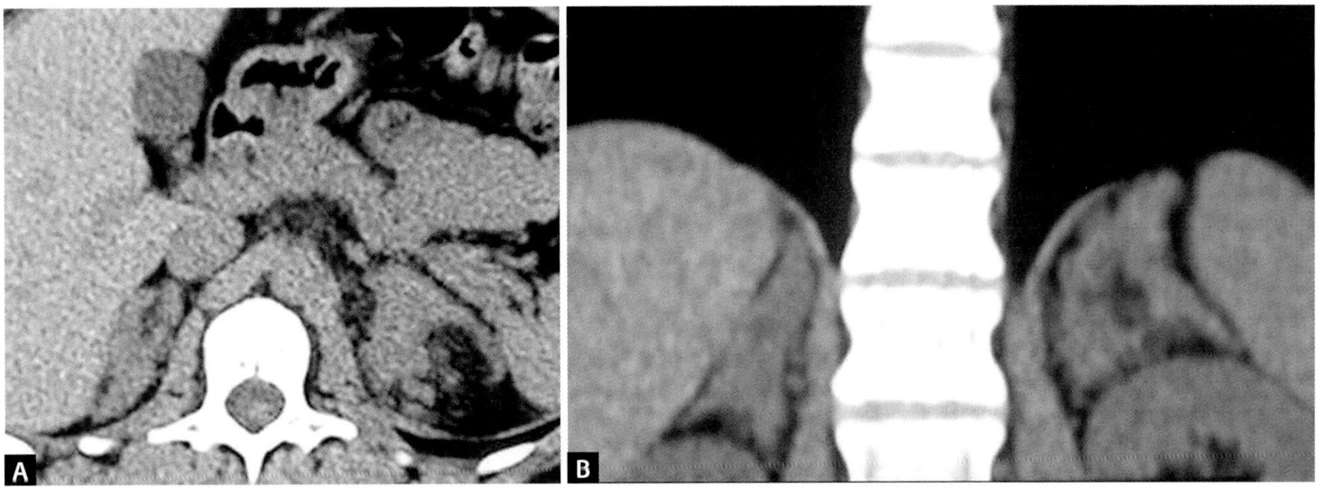

Figs. 10A and B: Axial (A) and coronal (B) NCCT scans of a 13-year-old girl with features of virilization show bilateral nodular adrenal hyperplasia.

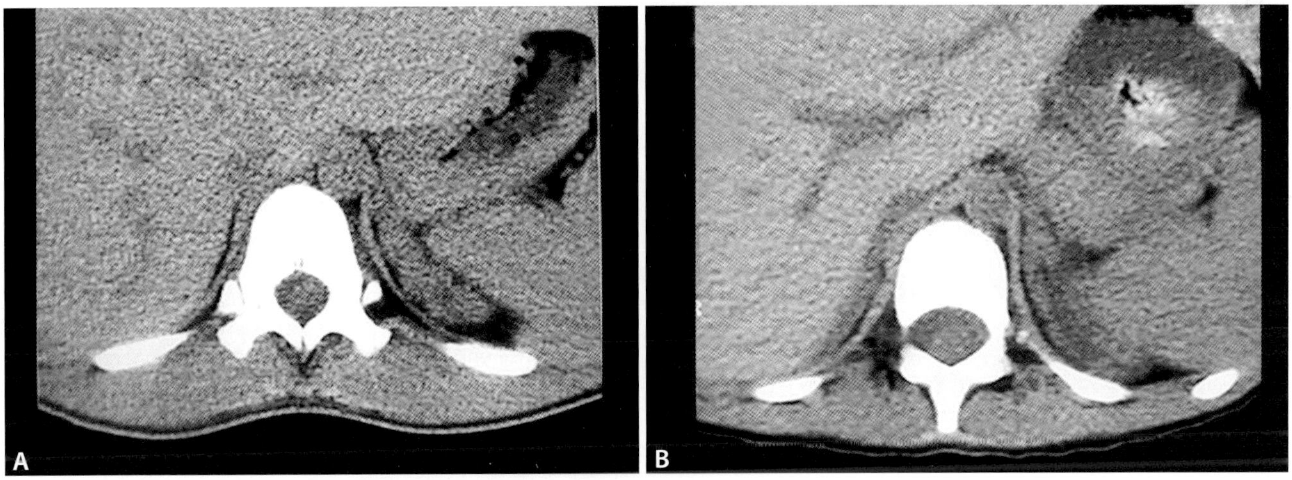

Figs. 11A and B: Axial NCCT of 11-year-old brother of the patient (A), presenting with precocious puberty and 5-year-old sister with virilization (B) also show features of congenital adrenal hyperplasia.

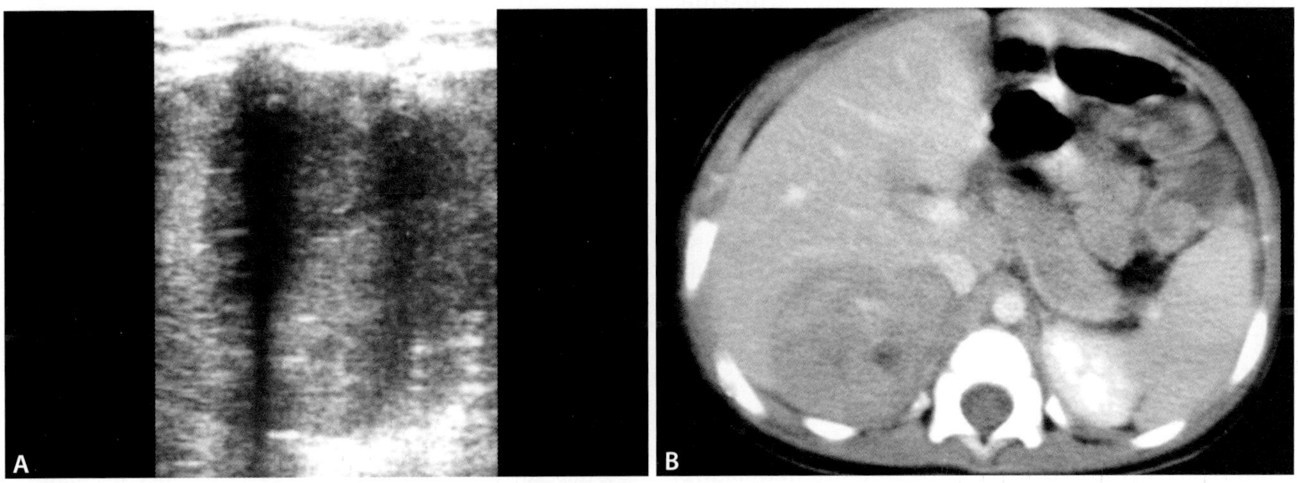

Figs. 12A and B: Ultrasound (A) and axial CECT (B) of a 1.5-year-girl child with feature of virilization show a large heterogeneous mass arising from the right adrenal, suggesting a carcinoma.

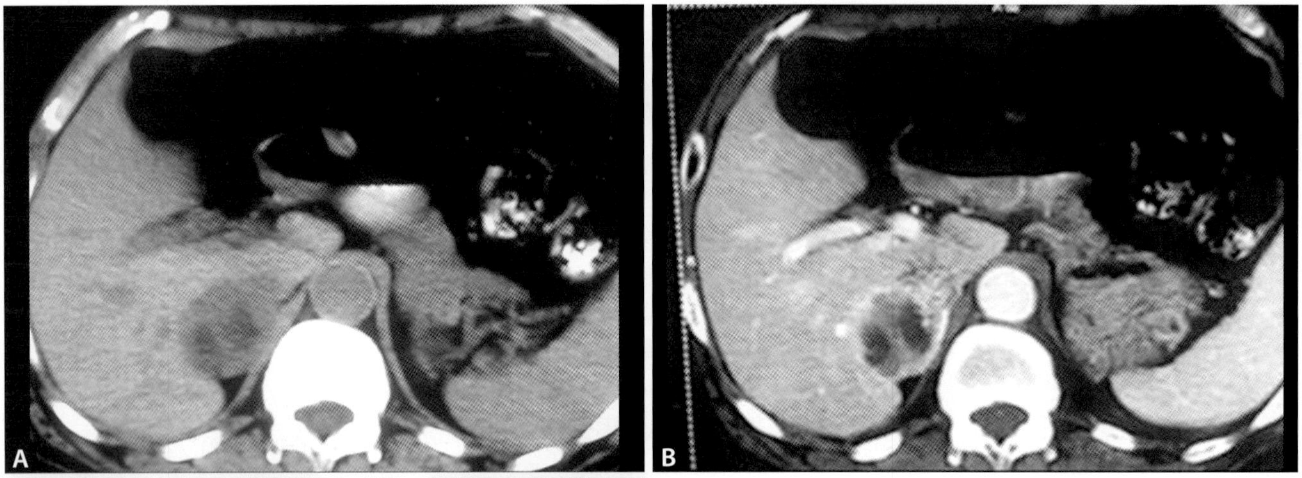

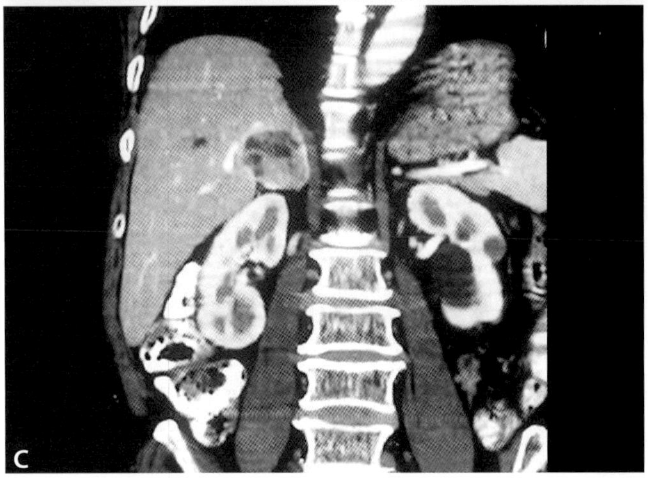

Figs. 13A to C: (A) NCCT scan of a young hypertensive male showing a mass in the right adrenal. Axial (B) and coronal (C) CECT reveal intense enhancement with central areas of necrosis.

Group II: Adrenal Insufficiency

Adrenal hypofunction refers to disorders of the adrenal cortex. It is classified as primary or secondary. Primary form is due to destruction of the adrenal cortex, while the secondary form results from pituitary causes. Usually, 85–90% of the adrenal cortex must be destroyed before the clinical syndrome manifests.[4] Primary adrenal insufficiency or Addison's disease presents with weakness, hypotension, weight loss with or without pigmentation.

The causes of Addison's disease include idiopathic atrophy, chronic granulomatous infections, e.g. tuberculosis, histoplasmosis, blastomycosis and adrenal hemorrhage. Other causes include autoimmune diseases and drugs.

Of the chronic infections, tuberculosis accounts for more than 60% of patients in India. This is in contrast to the west where idiopathic adrenal insufficiency accounts for almost 90% of the patients. CT is an important imaging modality to define size and morphology.[19] In patients with idiopathic atrophy, the glands are often too small to be identified **(Fig. 16)**. The CT morphology in tuberculosis includes bilateral asymmetrical adrenal enlargement with or without calcification or necrosis, small gland with calcification involving one or both adrenals, or small gland with no calcification **(Figs. 17 to 19)**. There may be evidence of associated pulmonary tuberculosis. Follow up studies in these patients on treatment, have shown reduction in size of the adrenals and presence of calcification **(Figs. 17A and B)**.

In histoplasmosis, adrenals may show bilateral asymmetrical enlargement but often normal configuration and usually no calcification **(*see* Figs. 14A to D)**. Histoplasmosis in India is not as rare as reported in the Indian literature. Because of lack of awareness and investigative facilities, many of these patients are probably treated for tuberculosis.

Bilateral adrenal hemorrhage is usually associated with anticoagulant therapy or with stress caused by

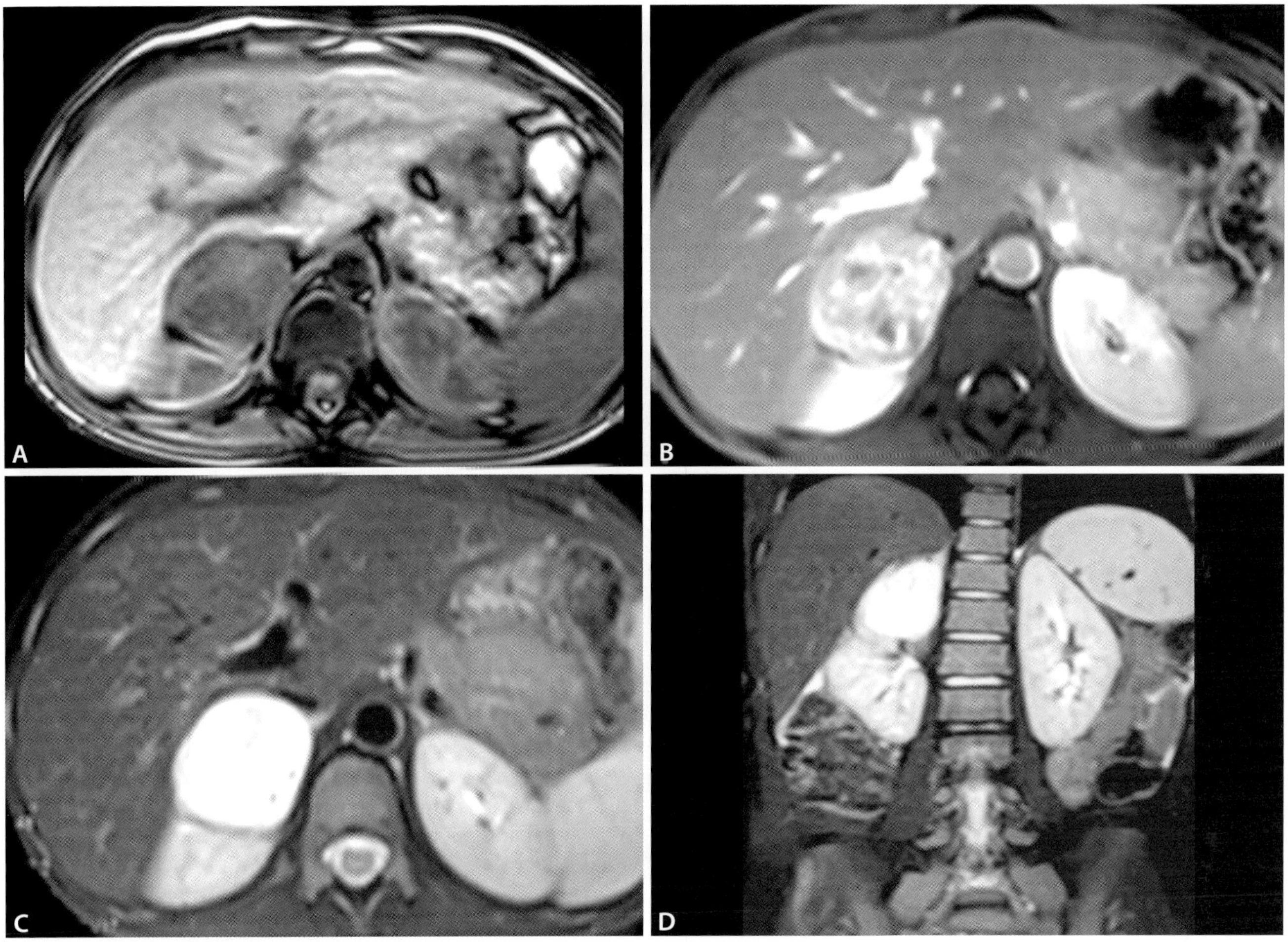

Figs. 14A to D: T1W pre- (A) and postgadolinium (B) axial images of 15-year-old male with hypertension reveal an intensely enhancing right adrenal mass. T2W axial (C) and coronal (D) images reveal the typical hyperintensity of a pheochromocytoma.

surgery, sepsis or hypotension. Less commonly, it is caused by trauma or hypoxia during delivery. CT may show asymmetrical adrenal enlargement with areas of high attenuation or blood-fluid level **(Fig. 20)**. Neonates, especially preterm infants may also show bilateral adrenal hemorrhage **(Fig. 21)**. Follow-up studies after appropriate treatment show diminution in size and decrease in attenuation thereby suggesting resorption **(Figs. 22A and B)**.

In the older child and adult, unilateral adrenal hemorrhage is usually caused by blunt abdominal trauma, and often involves the right adrenal. Unilateral adrenal hemorrhage has also been recently reported in patients undergoing liver transplantation. The excision of a segment of recipient's inferior vena cava necessitates ligation and division of right adrenal vein, this may result in venous infarction and hemorrhage in right adrenal. CT features are similar to those seen in bilateral hemorrhage.

Group III: Adrenal Diseases with Normal Function

A number of diseases may involve the adrenals which do not alter the adrenal function. Most of these disease entities are detected incidentally as adrenal mass or patients may present with vague abdominal pain or discomfort. These include nonfunctional adenoma or carcinoma, metastasis, lymphoma, neuroblastoma, adrenal cyst and myelolipoma. In some of these entities a specific diagnosis can be made from characteristic features on CT, e.g. adrenal cyst, myelolipoma. In some, CT may show nonspecific features but correlation with clinical features may suggest the possible etiology, e.g. neuroblastoma, metastasis.

Incidentaloma

These are adrenal nodules or masses discovered during imaging done for indications other than adrenal

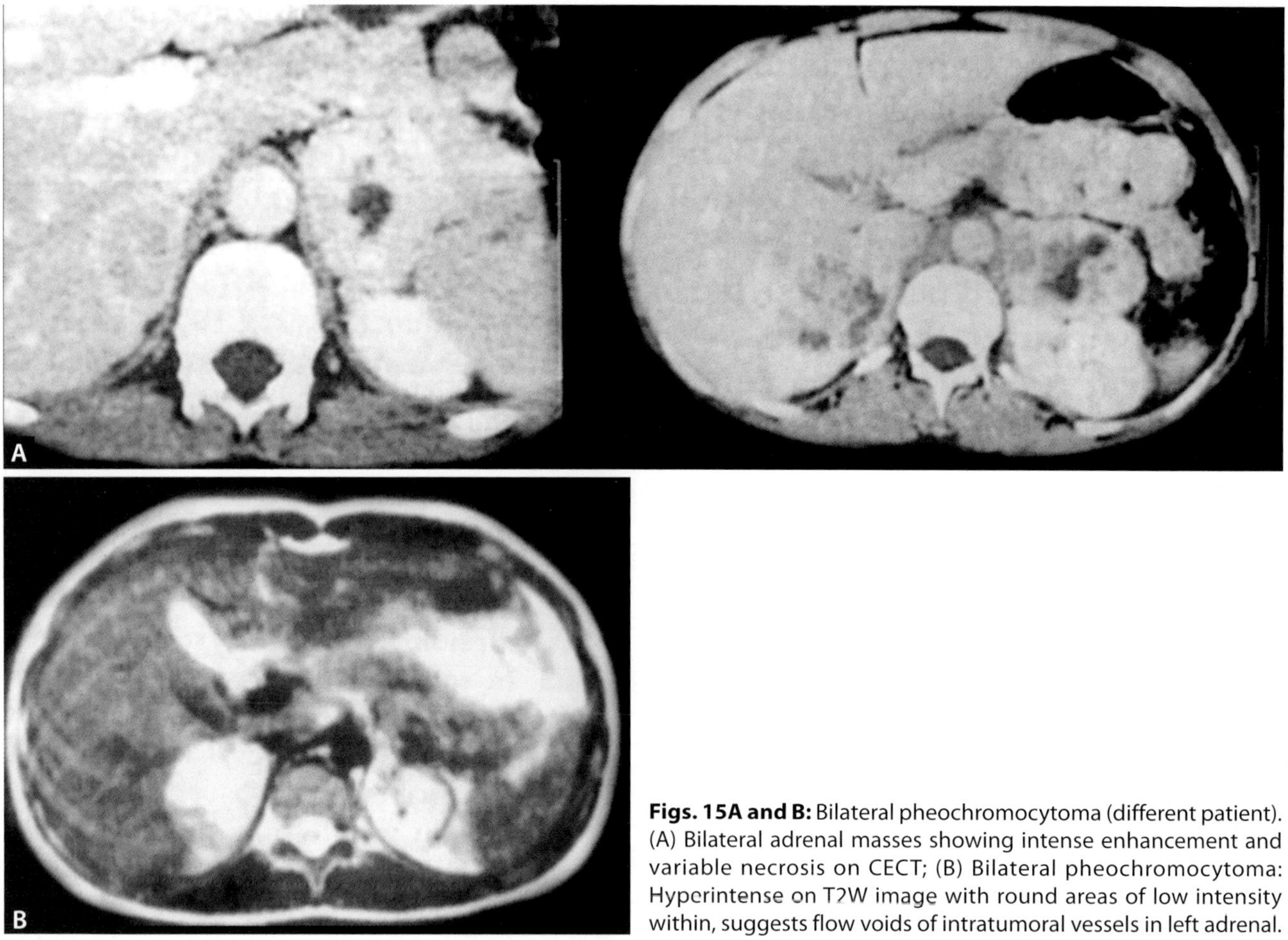

Figs. 15A and B: Bilateral pheochromocytoma (different patient). (A) Bilateral adrenal masses showing intense enhancement and variable necrosis on CECT; (B) Bilateral pheochromocytoma: Hyperintense on T2W image with round areas of low intensity within, suggests flow voids of intratumoral vessels in left adrenal.

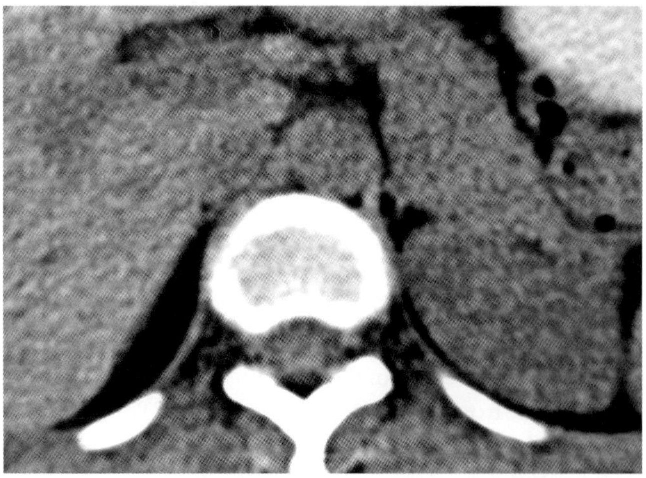

Fig. 16: NCCT scan of patient with Addison's disease showing bilateral atrophic adrenal glands.

disease **(Figs. 23 to 26)**. They are seen in 4-7% of the imaged population and majority of them are benign in the non-oncology population.[20,21] On the other hand, almost 50% of incidentally detected adrenal lesions in patients with known malignancy represent metastatic disease.[2,4] Characterization of such incidental masses remains an important clinical problem when a unilateral nonfunctional adrenal mass is present; the differential diagnosis rests between adenoma and carcinoma or metastasis. In a patient with known malignancy, it is very essential to differentiate such incidental adrenal mass as adenoma or metastasis because this will greatly affect patient's management and prognosis.

Adenoma versus Metastasis

- Adenomas are thought to represent non-neoplastic overgrowth of adrenocortical cells of zona fasciculata. They consist of cholesterol laden clear cells and contribute little to steroid production. The imaging features of functional and nonfunctional adenomas on CT or MRI are similar **(Figs. 23 to 26)** except the functional ones are usually smaller at the time of presentation than nonfunctional tumors. They account for almost 90% of all incidentalomas.[5]

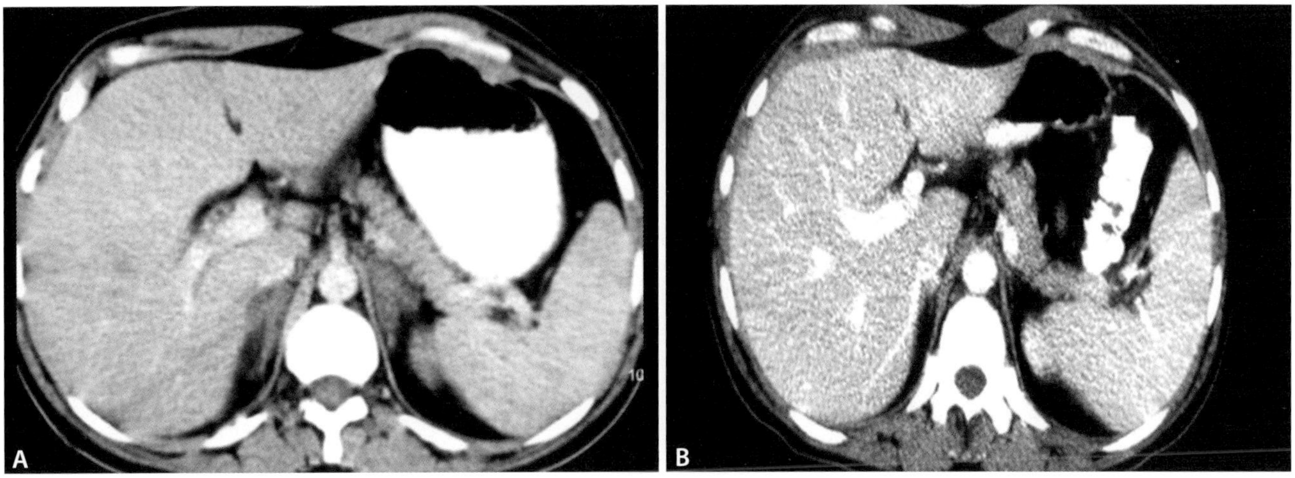

Figs. 17A and B: CECT scan (A) of a patient with fever and biochemical evidence of adrenal insufficiency shows bilateral asymmetric (left > right) enlargement of the adrenal glands. Few ill-defined focal are seen in the liver and spleen also suggesting disseminated tuberculosis. Patient was put on ATT. CECT obtained 1 year later (B) reveals small, atrophic adrenal glands.

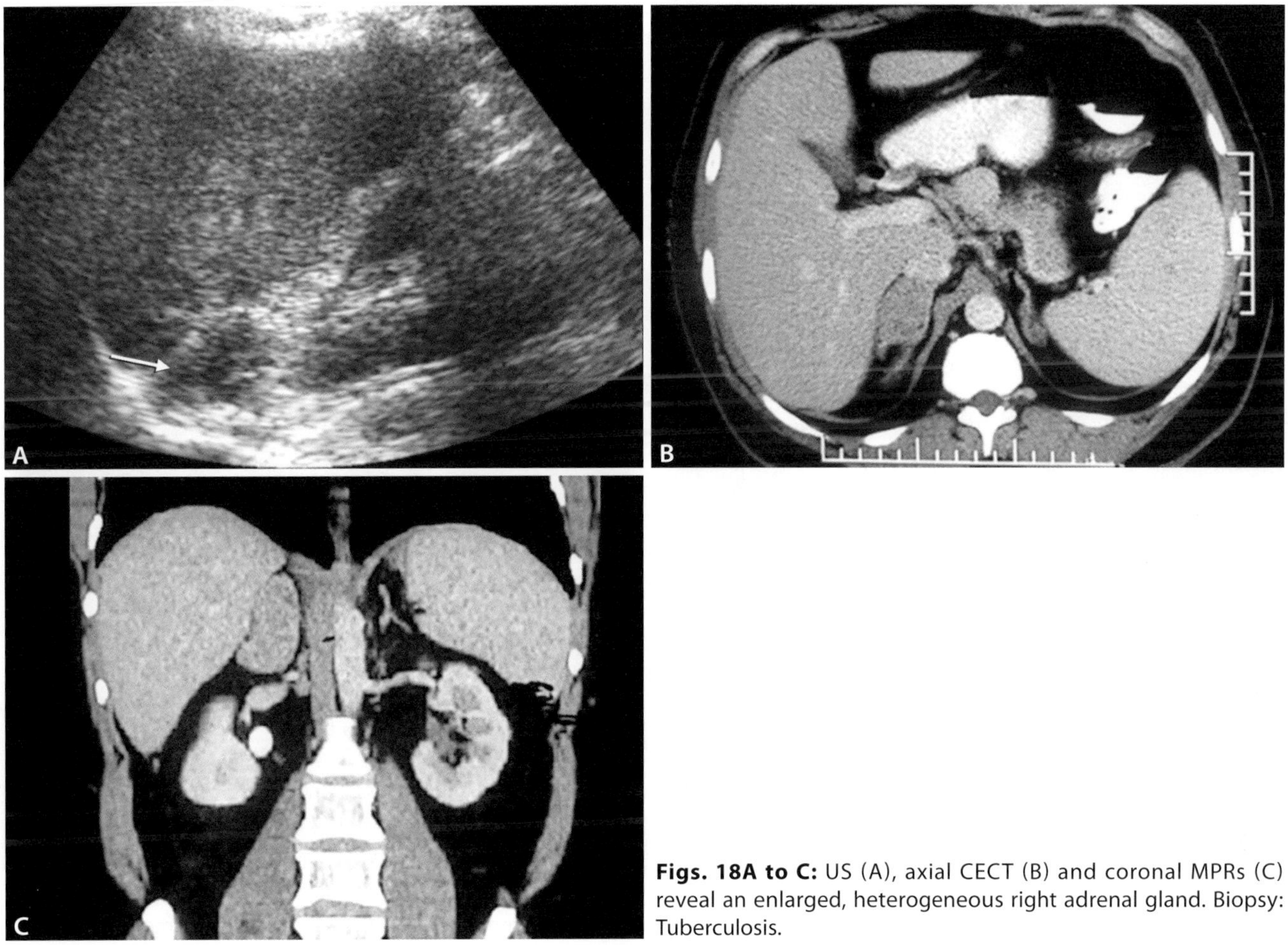

Figs. 18A to C: US (A), axial CECT (B) and coronal MPRs (C) reveal an enlarged, heterogeneous right adrenal gland. Biopsy: Tuberculosis.

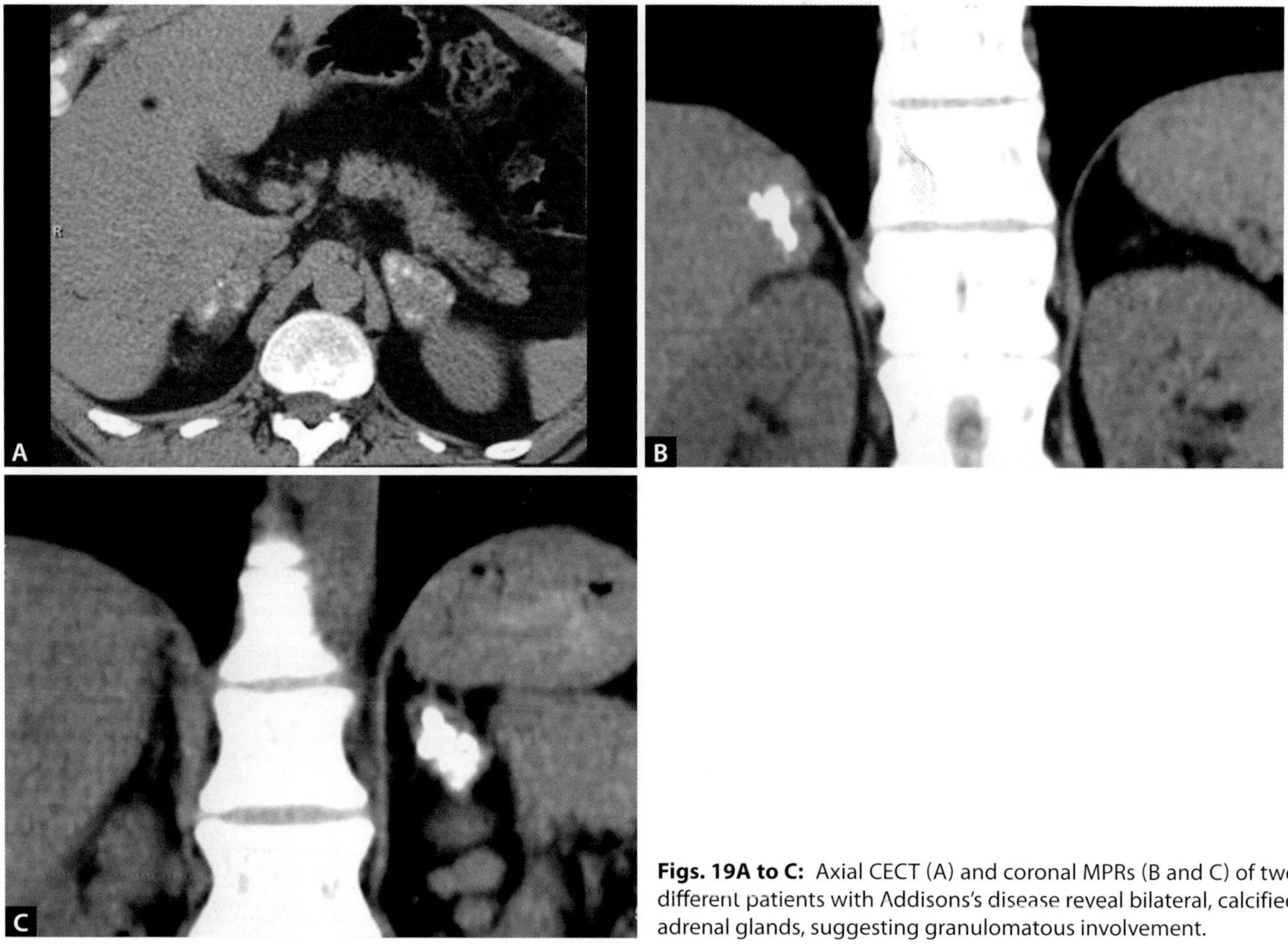

Figs. 19A to C: Axial CECT (A) and coronal MPRs (B and C) of two different patients with Addisons's disease reveal bilateral, calcified adrenal glands, suggesting granulomatous involvement.

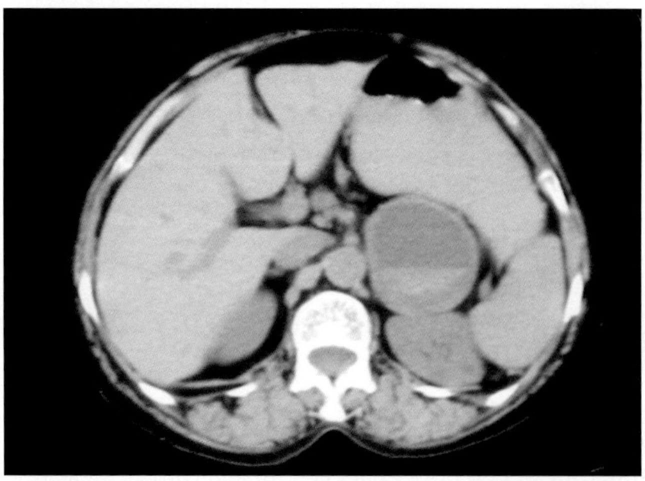

Fig. 20: Axial CT showing a low attenuating left adrenal mass with blood-fluid level suggestive of adrenal hemorrhage.

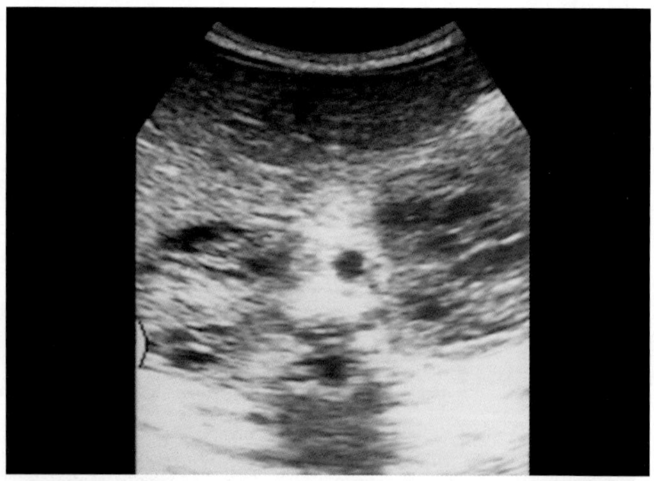

Fig. 21: US of a preterm neonate showing bilateral enlarged adrenal glands, suggesting adrenal hemorrhage.

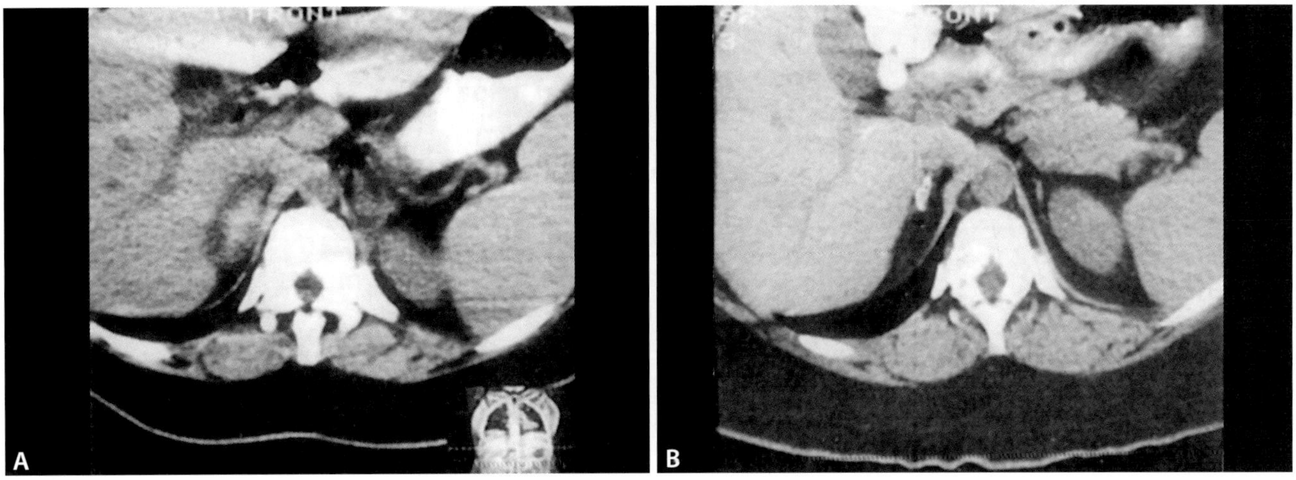

Figs. 22A and B: Adrenal hemorrhage: CT shows asymmetrically enlarged adrenals with heterogeneous attenuation but no calcification. Follow-up CT after 5 years shows small right adrenal with dense calcification and atropic left adrenal.

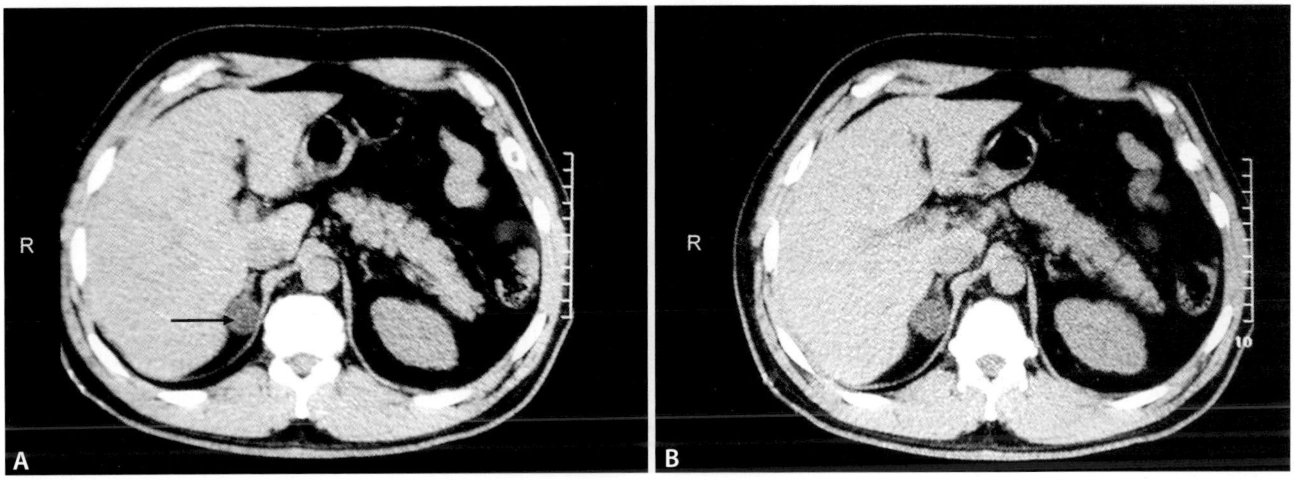

Figs. 23A and B: Adrenal adenoma: (A) NCCT shows a low attenuating well-defined mass in the right adrenal (arrow); The attenuation value was 6 HU (B).

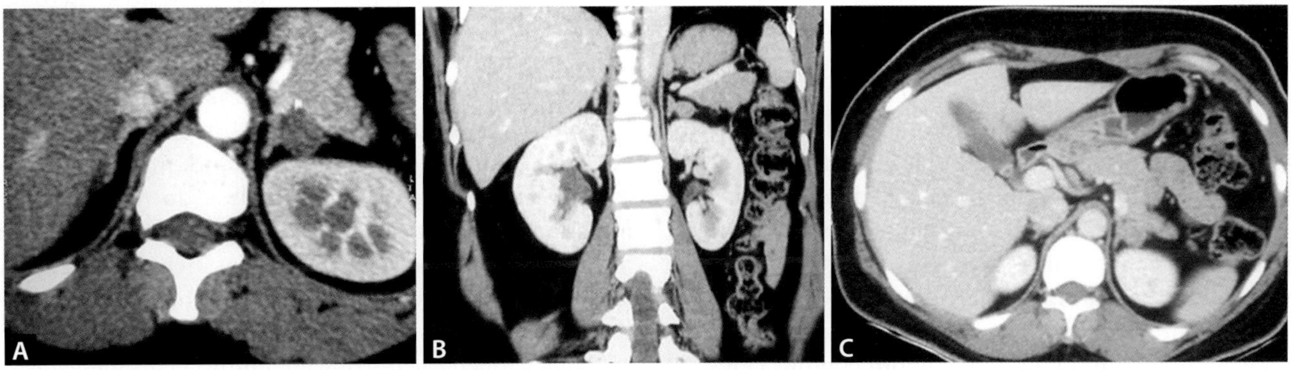

Figs. 24A to C: Adrenal adenoma: CECT (A) coronal MPR (B) and 15-minute delayed CT scan (C) show a mass in left adrenal gland which showed 65% washout on the delayed scan.

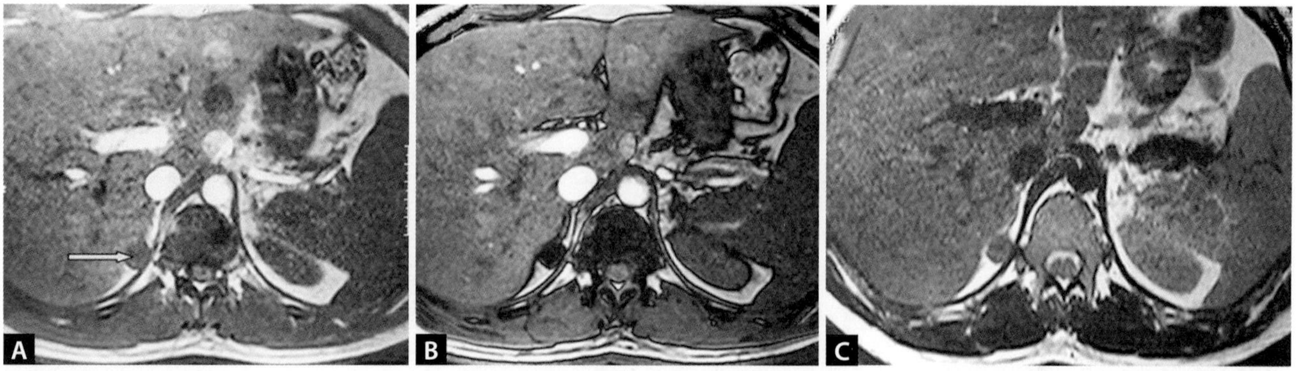

Figs. 25A to C: Incidentally detected adrenal adenoma: Gradient echo T1W in-phase image (A) shows a hypointense nodule in right adrenal (arrow) which shows marked signal loss on the opposed phase image (B). The lesion is hypointense on T2W scan (C) also.

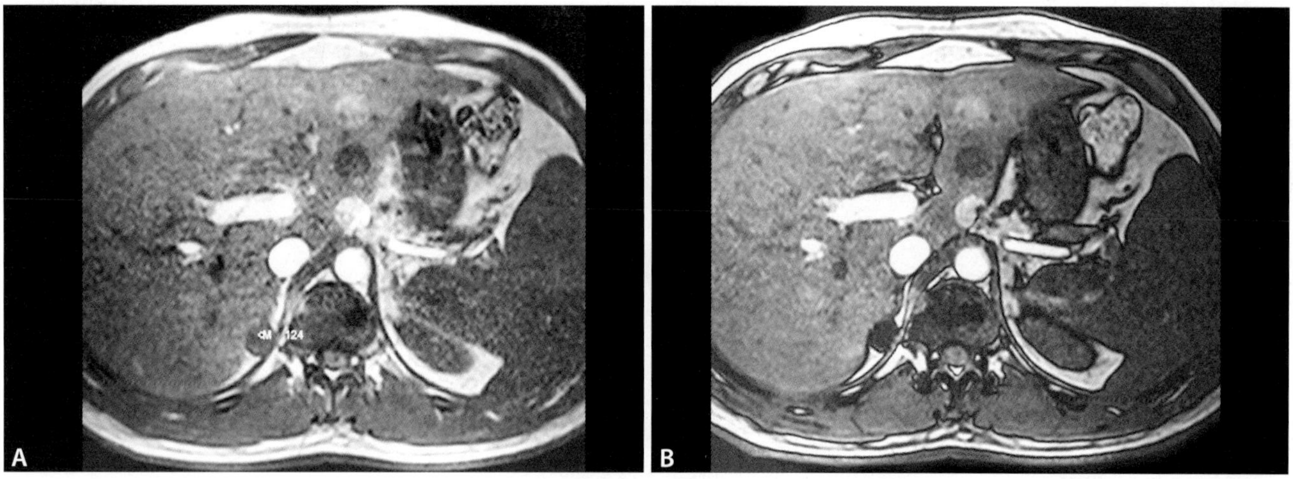

Figs. 26A and B: Adrenal adenoma: GRE T1W in-phase (A) and opposed phase image (B) showing drop in signal intensity of right adrenal lesion from 124 to 45 whereas spleen signal intensity changes from 83 to 80 only.

Tumors of the lung, kidney, breast, digestive tract, ovary and melanoma are the most common primary sites to metastasize to adrenals.[4,5] Metastases are well-defined with heterogeneous density and a thin irregular enhancing rim following intravenous contrast injection, commonly unilateral and usually larger than adenoma **(Figs. 27A to D)**. On MRI, they are hypointense on T1 weighted image and hyperintense on T2 weighted image, relative to liver intensity. It has been reported that 27% of patients with known malignancy have microscopic adrenal metastasis. However, the detection of an adrenal mass in a patient with known malignancy does not necessarily indicate metastatic disease and it may be a nonfunctional adenoma.

CT features of adenoma include size less than 5.0 cm and well-defined margins with smooth contour **(Figs. 23 and 24)**. Adrenal metastasis may show large mass with heterogeneous density and irregular shape **(Figs. 27A to D)**. However, these features are not specific. It has been also reported that size alone is a poor discriminator between benign adenoma and malignant mass.[5,6]

In recent years, several studies have reported two imaging criteria based on attenuation value and differences in vascular enhancement pattern to differentiate benign adenoma from adrenal metastasis.[2,20]

Adenomas have abundant intracytoplasmic fat and therefore show low attenuation on non-contrast CT **(Figs. 23A and B)**. On the other hand, metastases have little intracytoplasmic fat and thus do not show low attenuation. A large region of interest covering the adrenal mass should be used but should not include periadrenal fat for measuring attenuation value. It has been reported that a threshold of 10 HU has 71% sensitivity and 98% specificity for characterizing adenoma versus metastasis.[22] This specificity may be increased further if other features of size, shape and morphology are considered. Although 70% of adenomas have abundant lipid, the remaining are

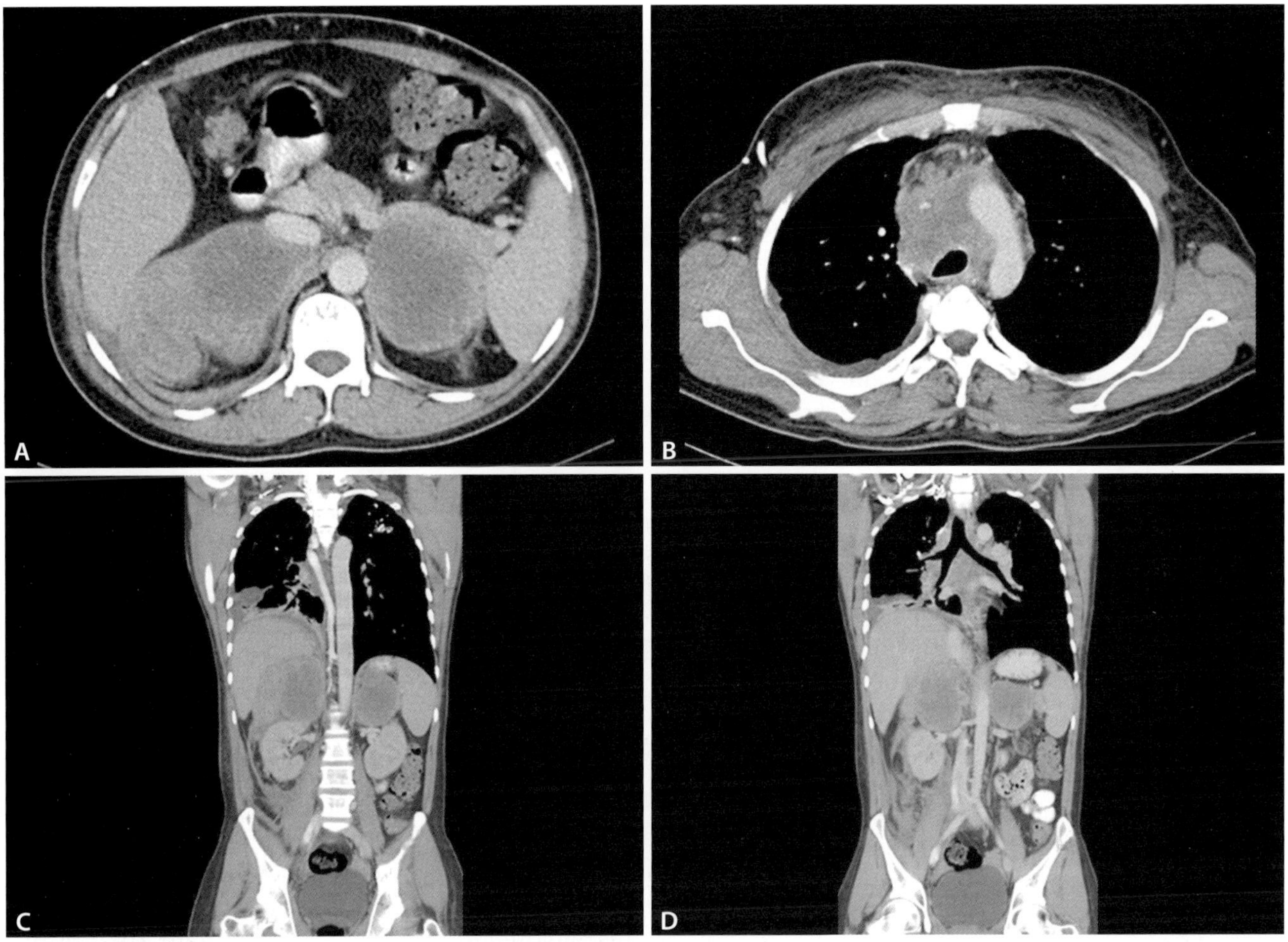

Figs. 27A to D: Adrenal metastases: CECT abdomen (A) shows bilateral solid adrenal masses. CECT chest (B) and coronal MPRs (C and D) show mediastinal adenopathy in a patient of bronchogenic carcinoma.

lipid poor and are difficult to characterize on a noncontrast scan.

If attenuation of the adrenal mass on noncontrast CT is 10 HU or less **(Figs. 9 to 23)**, the diagnosis is lipid rich adenoma and no further evaluation is required. If attenuation is more than 10 HU, the mass is indeterminate and requires further evaluation by contrast enhanced CT and 15 minutes delayed enhanced CT scan **(Figs. 24A to C)**.[23]

Adenomas enhance rapidly with intravenous contrast media and show rapid washout. Metastasis also enhance rapidly but the washout is delayed when compared to adenoma.[18,20] It has been speculated that this difference in enhancement wash out in nonadenoma is possibly due to disturbed capillary permeability, with prolonged retention of contrast in the effective extracellular space.

Adrenal masses with an attenuation value less than 30–40 HU on 15 minute delayed contrast enhanced CT are almost always adrenal adenomas.[1,24] In addition to the delayed CT attenuation itself, it is also possible to calculate the percentage wash-out of initial enhancement. The patient is first scanned without contrast, then again at 70 seconds, and then 15 minutes after contrast administration. Contrast wash-out can be quantified using Relative percentage wash out (RPW) and Absolute percentage wash out (APW) as follows:

$$RPW = 100 \times (\text{Enhanced HU} - \text{Delayed HU}) / \text{Enhanced HU}$$

$$APW = 100 \times (\text{Enhanced HU} - \text{Delayed HU}) / (\text{Enhanced HU} - \text{Non-enhanced HU})$$

If the APW is greater than 60% and the RPW is greater than 40%[20,23,24] lesion is labeled benign. This technique has a sensitivity of 88% and a specificity of 96% for the diagnosis of adenoma.[1,20] On the other hand, metastases and adrenocortical carcinoma have relative contrast retention on delayed contrast-enhanced CT.

It has been said that the relative washout percentage is more accurate for the differentiation of lipid poor adenomas from metastases than are the absolute attenuation values on delayed contrast enhanced scans.[25]

Dual energy CT: This is an emerging technique which has been used for determining bone mineral density and for evaluation of fatty liver. The difference in CT attenuation images acquired at 140 and 80 kVp is measured, and if the difference between the two kVp is more than 6 HU, it is suggestive of fat containing lesion.[2]

Magnetic resonance imaging: In recent years, MRI has become a problem solving modality for the characterization of indeterminate adrenal masses. When results on CT examination are equivocal, MRI is the next imaging modality for characterizing the lesion. Due to increased fluid content in adrenal cancer and metastases, these appear bright on T2 weighted MRI images. However, there is significant overlap between T1- and T2-weighted MRI images of adenoma and metastases. With the introduction of higher field strength magnets (1.5 T), chemical shift imaging and dynamic gadolinium enhanced MR imaging has shown promising results with adrenal gland lesions characterization. Confident diagnosis of adenomas on MRI requires the addition of chemical shift imaging to the protocol.

Chemical shift MR imaging has been used to differentiate adenoma from metastasis. This technique is based on the different resonance frequency rates of protons in fat and water molecules in a magnetic field. Two breath hold T1-weighted acquisitions are taken, first using a short echo time (TE 2.1 ms at 1.5 tesla) when the fat and water protons are out of phase and second in-phase acquisition using long echo time (TE 4.2 ms at 1.5 tesla). On most current MR scanners the in and opposed phase images can be obtained by one dual echo breath hold gradient echo sequence. The signal intensity on the in-phase image is derived from the signal of water plus fat protons while in the out of phase image, MR signal of water and lipid protons cancel each other out within a voxel. Therefore a mass containing intracellular lipid and water will show loss of signal in the out of phase images when compared with in-phase image **(Figs. 25A to C)**. Thus, adenoma appears darker on out of phase image than on in-phase image, while metastasis will show no significant signal loss on out of phase image and the signal intensity remains unchanged.[2,8,9]

The sensitivity and specificity ranging from 81% to 100% and 94% to 100% respectively on chemical shift MR imaging for differentiating adenoma from metastasis have been reported.[6,9,20] The loss of signal can be assessed visually using spleen as the internal control **(Fig. 26)**. The liver should not be used as the internal reference as it may also show signal loss on opposed phase image when there is steatosis.

The chemical shift change can also be detected by quantitative methods. Two ratios have been defined in CSI.

$$\text{SI Index} = \frac{(\text{Lesion IP}) - (\text{Lesion OP})}{(\text{Lesion IP})} \times 100$$

and

Adrenal to spleen ratio

$$\left[\frac{(\text{Lesion OP})/(\text{Spleen OP})}{(\text{Lesion IP})/(\text{Spleen IP})} - 1\right] \times 100$$

SI index of >16.5% and adrenal to spleen ratio of <0.71 is suggestive of adenoma/benign adrenal lesions. For a benign adrenal lesion characterization, the reported sensitivity and specificity using these two ratios were 87–100% and 92–100% respectively, whereas failure rate for diagnosis of lipid poor adenomas has been 13–17%.[20]

On dynamic MRI, contrast enhancement characteristics of adrenal masses is similar to that on CT with adenomas showing rapid contrast washout and metastases and carcinoma showing retention of contrast.

Diffusion-weighted MRI (DWI): It provides insight into water composition and cellularity in a tumor and may provide an additional tool to distinguish benign from malignant adrenal masses. Malignant tumors have an increased cellularity which manifests as restricted diffusion, and a decrease in the apparent diffusion coefficient. There are no major published studies specifically on the adrenal, but extrapolating from data on liver, kidney, etc., this may be a promising technique in the future to distinguish between benign and malignant masses.[2]

Positron emission tomography (PET): Due to the limitations of CT and MR imaging, functional imaging modalities like F-18 FDG PET are now increasingly used for further characterization of an adrenal lesion.

F-18-fluorodeoxyglucose positron emission tomography (F-18-FDG PET) is an imaging modality that permits acquisition of functional information and when fused with CT imaging, results in accurate localization and metabolic characterization of adrenal lesions. In PET-CT, 18-fluorodeoxyglucose is used as a glucose analog which is taken up preferentially by malignant cells because of their increased glucose metabolism. Due to relative lack of glucose-6-phosphatase in the cancer cells as compared to cells of normal tissues, there is a focal intracellular accumulation of FDG, resulting in high tumor uptake values as compared to the background uptake values. However, in literature only limited data on the role of 18-FDG PET/PET-CT in characterization of adrenal lesions in oncology population is available, that too involving a relatively small sample size.[11] The results of all these studies are encouraging and justify the use of PET for metastatic disease evaluation in cancer patients. Although, PET results are encouraging, several inherent problems are associated with FDG-PET imaging viz. small adrenal lesions are difficult to image owing to poor resolution, and uptake in other abdominal structures, such as renal pelvis, can obscure the adrenal gland.

18F-FDG uptake is taken as abnormal when it is higher than background liver uptake.[11,13] T. If a lesion shows F18-FDG uptake less than that of the liver, or shows uptake that is significantly higher than the liver, the study can be interpreted with high confidence unless the patient has pheochromocytoma, which can be excluded by biochemical markers.[13]

In evaluation of adrenal masses with F18-FDG PET/CT, combined information from the F18-FDG PET and unenhanced CT portions of a PET/CT study is more specific than F18-FDG PET information alone.[26] An SUV cut-off value of 3.1 has been used to differentiate malignant lesions and adenomas. PET data using a SUV cutoff of 3.1 to differentiate malignant adrenal masses from adenomas, yielded a sensitivity, specificity, positive predictive value and negative predictive value of 98.5%, 92%, 89.3%, and 98.9% respectively.[26]

Adrenal Carcinoma

Adrenal carcinomas are rare neoplasms, and are more common in women. They are usually larger than 10 cm at the time of presentation and are invasive. Only 10% are clinically functional which usually manifests as Cushing's syndrome, or virilization in females. CT or MRI show large solid masses with areas of degeneration and cystic changes, and 33% contain calcification **(Figs. 28 and 29)**.[2,5,20] They tend to be locally invasive, especially into adrenal or renal veins and inferior venacava. They are hypointense on T1- and hyperintense on T2-weighted scans **(Figs. 28D to F)** and show variable enhancement. Differential diagnosis includes adenoma, metastases, lymphoma, exophytic liver tumors, or upper polar renal masses.

Adrenal Lymphoma

Primary lymphoma of the adrenal gland is unusual, but its involvement in disseminated lymphoma is common. The latter is more often seen in non-Hodgkin lymphoma.[27] The most common presentation is diffuse bilateral enlargement of the gland, and the shape is usually maintained **(Figs. 30A to D)**. The tumor is hypovascular and shows only mild enhancement after contrast.

Adrenal Collision Tumor

This is a very rare entity characterized by coexistence of two contiguous but histologically different tumors. Both tumors may be malignant or one may be benign, other malignant or both may be benign. Imaging may show two distinct morphological features within the same mass. This entity should be suspected when only focal decrease in signal intensity of a mass is seen on opposed phase images or a focus of bright enhancement is seen within a mass which otherwise looks like an adenoma. Such an appearance may suggest a metastatic deposit within an adrenal adenoma.[5,28]

Adrenal Cyst

Adrenal cysts are rare and usually seen in females. They are derived from endothelium in 45% of patients and the rest are epithelial, parasitic or pseudocysts from prior hemorrhage. CT shows characteristically well-defined round low attenuating lesion suggesting fluid with rim enhancement **(Fig. 31A)**. Rim calcification may be noted **(Fig. 31B)**. The attenuation values may be mixed in the presence of debris or hemorrhage. On MR, adrenal cysts are hypointense on T1-weighted image and hyperintense on T2-weighted image. The complications of adrenal cysts include hemorrhage, infection and rupture.[20,29]

Myelolipoma

Myelolipoma is a benign tumor of the cortex, comprised of mature fat and hematopoietic elements. Patients are usually asymptomatic and the lesion detected incidentally. It accounts for about 7–15% of all incidentalomas. Imaging appearance may vary depending on which histological component is dominant. Ultrasonography and CT features are quite characteristic and diagnostic. Ultrasonography shows well-defined echogenic or heterogeneous adrenal mass, which may be associated with apparent posterior displacement of the diaphragm due to propagation speed artifact resulting from slow speed of sound through the fat. CT confirms presence of intratumoral fat **(Figs. 32A and B)**. Punctate calcification may be seen in 20% of cases.[4,5] MRI can also characterize the lesion by identification of presence of fat which appears hyperintense on both T1- and T2-weighted images, and shows loss of signal on fat suppression techniques **(Figs. 33A to D)**.[6] Marrow

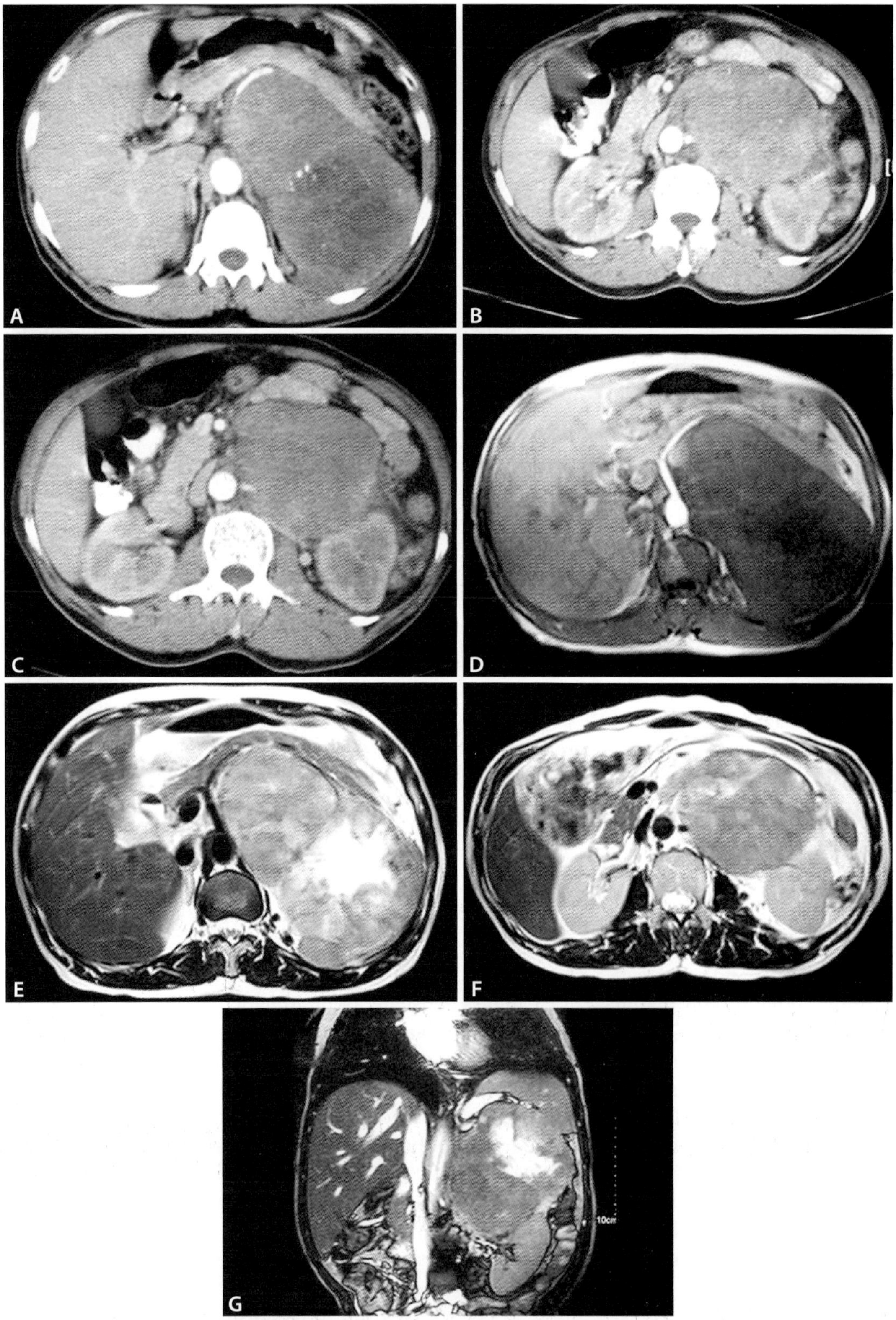

Figs. 28A to G: Adrenal carcinoma: Axial CECT (A to C) show a large left adrenal mass with foci of calcification and areas of necrosis, encasing the left renal artery and displacing the left kidney laterally. Axial T1W GRE image (D) shows a hypointense left-sided mass which is displacing the splenic artery anteriorly. The lesion is heterogeneously hyperintense on T2W scans (E and F). True FISP coronal image (G) shows the left suprarenal mass displacing the left kidney inferolaterally.

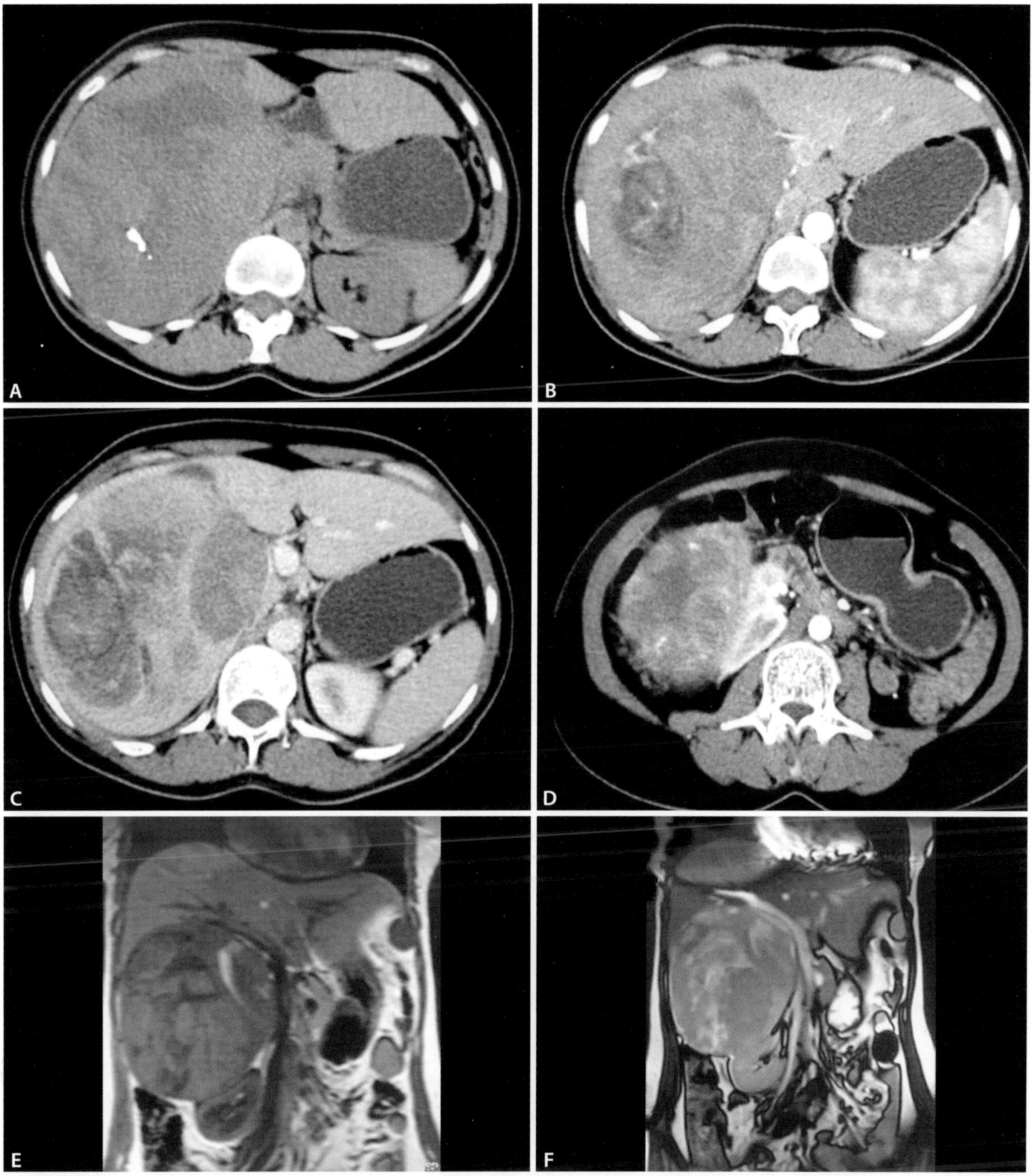

Figs. 29A to F: Adrenal carcinoma: Axial NCCT (A) and CECT (B to D) show a large right adrenal mass with foci of calcification. It mimics an exophytic liver mass. GRE T1W (E) and true-FISP coronal (F) MR images of same patient show the right adrenal mass displacing the kidney inferomedially.

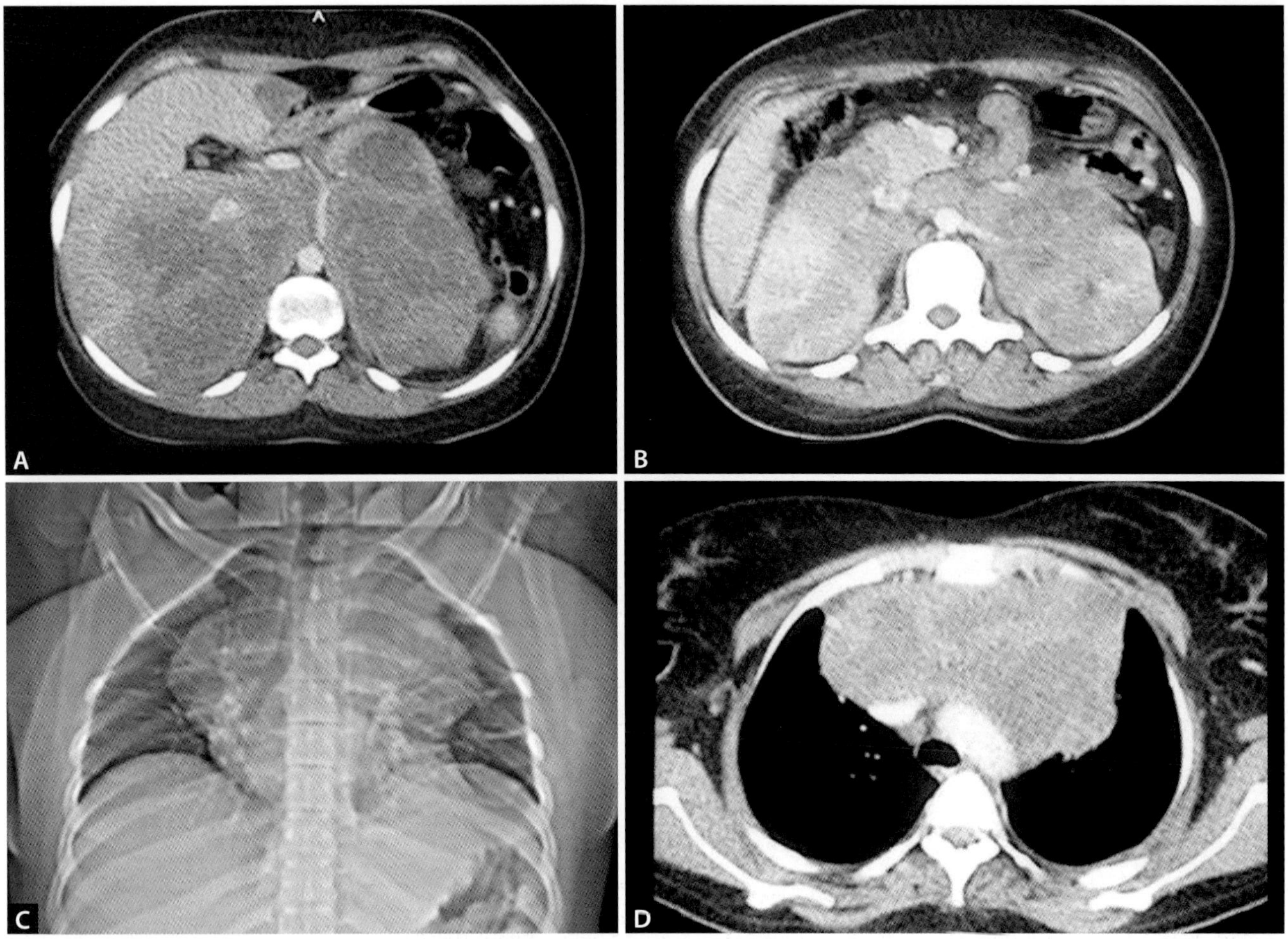

Figs. 30A to D: Adrenal involvement in non-Hodgkin's lymphoma: Axial abdomen CECT (A and B) show bilateral adrenal masses, retroperitoneal adenopathy and focal renal lesions. Chest radiograph (C) and CECT chest (D) show bulky mediastinal adenopathy.

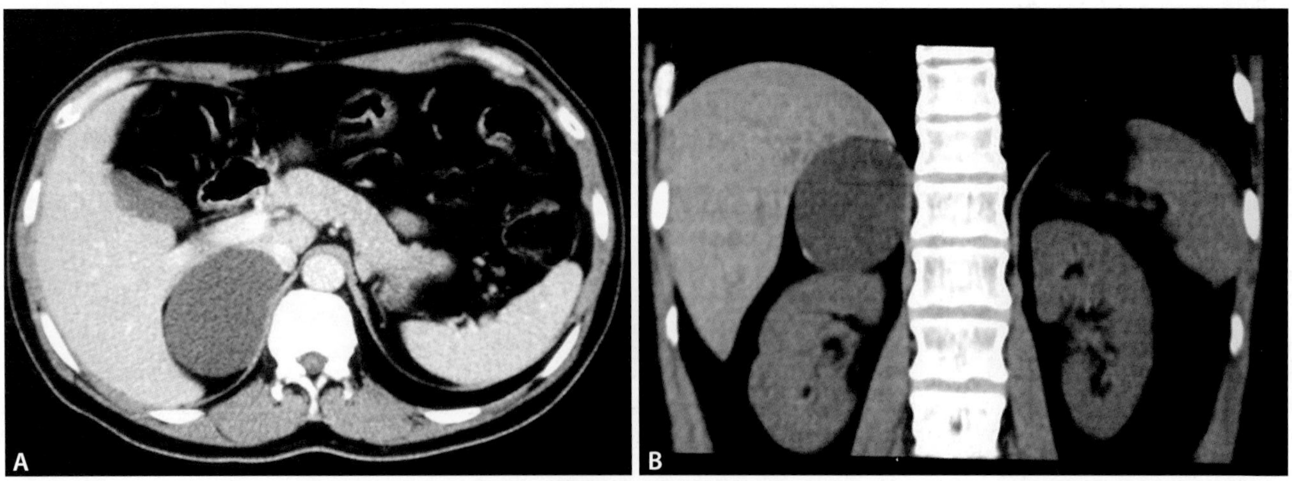

Figs. 31A and B: Adrenal cyst: Axial CT (A) and coronal MPR (B) show a fluid attenuating right adrenal mass with rim calcification.

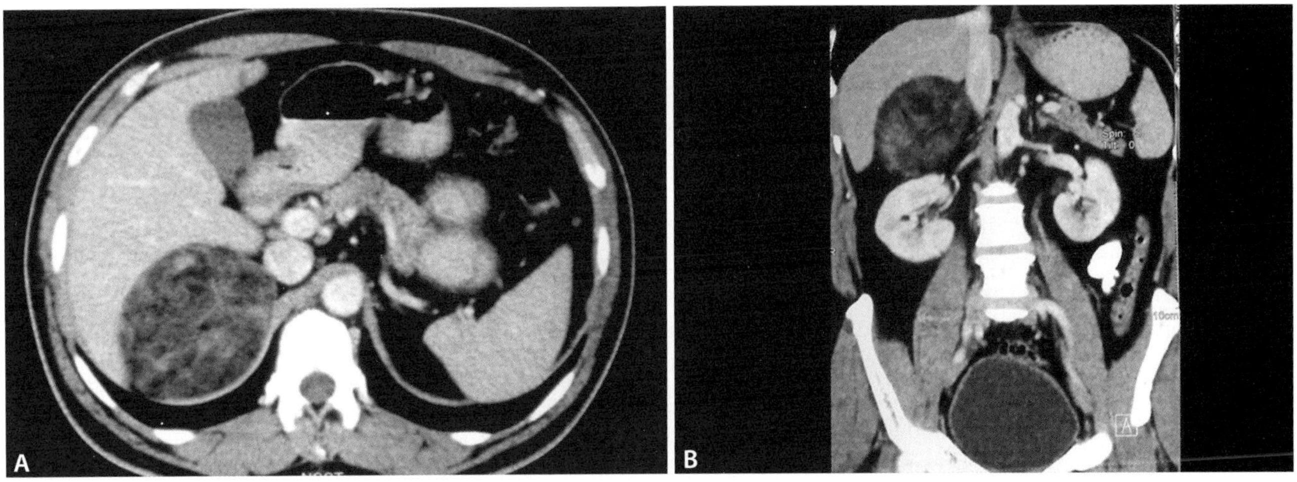

Figs. 32A and B: Adrenal myelolipoma: Axial CECT (A) and coronal MPR (B) show a mixed attenuating right adrenal mass with fat and soft tissue attenuation.

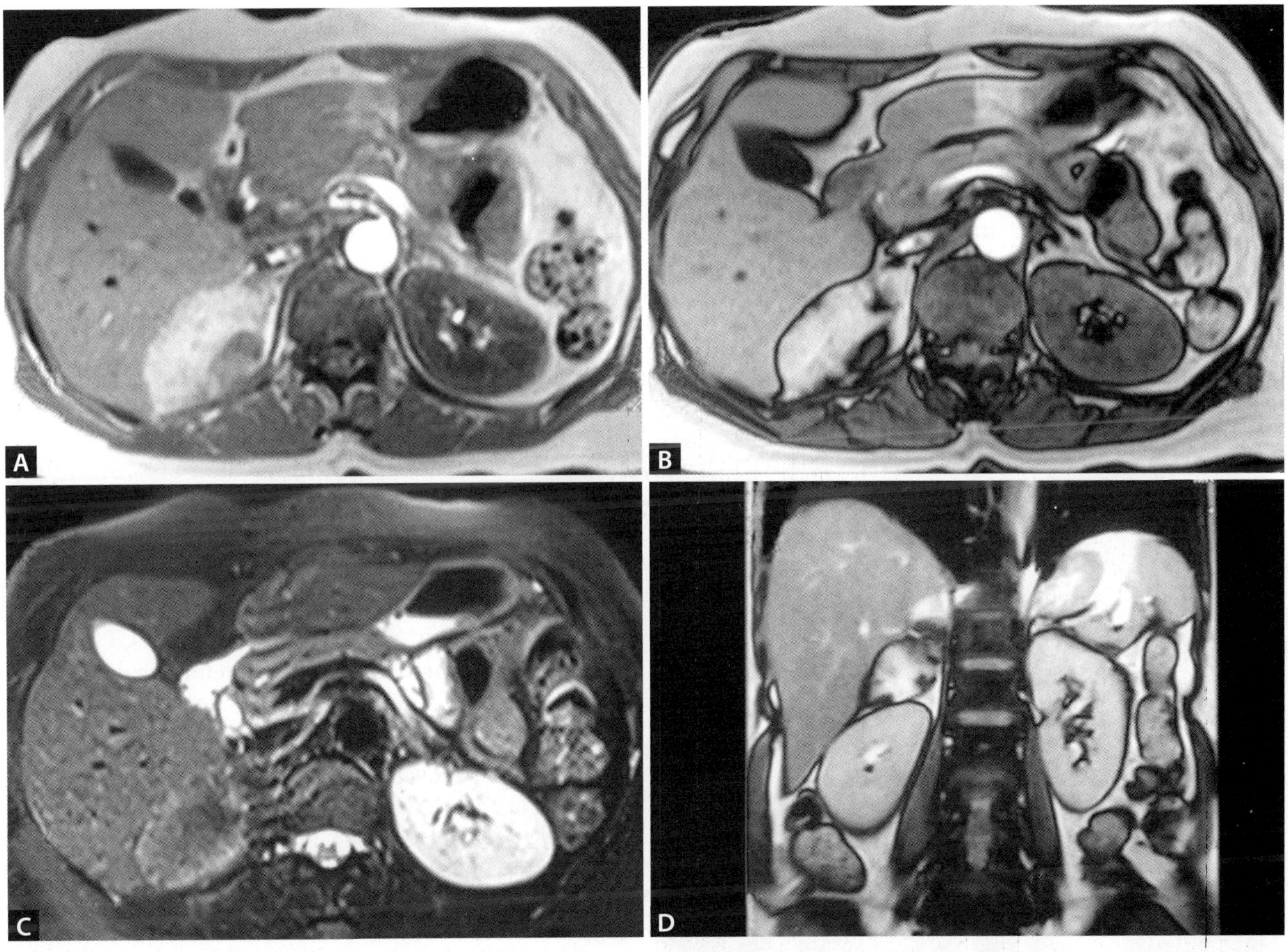

Figs. 33A to D: Adrenal myelolipoma: GRE T1W in-phase (A) and opposed phase (B) images show a hyperintense right adrenal mass which shows no drop in signal intensity but is suppressed on T2W fat suppressed image (C). Coronal true-FISP image (D) shows a hyperintense right adrenal mass.

elements show low signal on T1 and moderate signal on T2W images. Differential diagnosis includes adrenal adenoma, and large myelolipomas may mimic retroperitoneal lipoma or liposarcoma.

Neuroblastoma

Neuroblastoma is one of the most common tumor of childhood with 80% occurring below the age of 5 years. Most neuroblastomas arise from adrenal medulla but may also arise from sympathetic chain, posterior mediastinum being the second most common site. Seventy-five percent occur in the abdomen, and two-thirds of these are in the adrenal gland. Symptoms are related to the primary tumor and to metastases, which are present in more than 50% patients at the time of diagnosis. Children can present with a palpable mass, bone pain and opsomyoclonus. Common sites of metastases are lymph nodes, cortical bone, marrow, skin and liver.[4,5]

Ultrasonography almost always shows a mass which must be distinguished from nephroblastoma. Neuroblastoma is seen typically as large mass with heterogeneous echogenicity with scattered hyperechoic areas due to presence of calcification. CT shows soft tissue mass with areas of low attenuation and scattered coarse or mottled calcification, seen in almost 85% of the patients. The tumor enhances with intravenous contrast. Unlike Wilm's tumor, which usually has a well-defined pseudocapsule, neuroblastoma invades adjacent structures and encases the aorta and its branches **(Fig. 34)** early in the course of disease. On MRI, neuroblastoma shows low signal intensity on T1-weighted image and increased intensity on T2-weighted image, relative to liver intensity. Tumor heterogeneity is seen best on T2-weighted sequence and reflects calcification and necrosis.

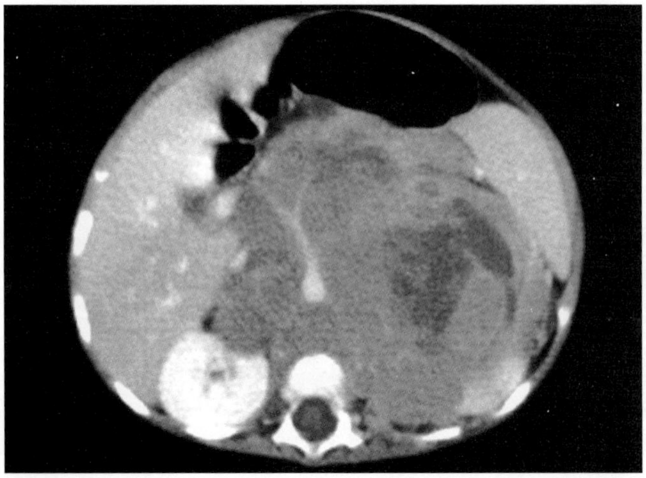

Fig. 34: Neuroblastoma: Axial CECT abdomen of a 2-year-old child shows a large left adrenal mass which is extending posterior to the aorta and inferior vena cava and encasing the celiac axis.

MRI is better than CT for defining vascular encasement, metastasis and intraspinal extension which occurs in 15% of patients. Therefore, MRI is the single best imaging modality for accurately staging the extent of the disease.[6] Neuroblastoma may also take up MIBG, which may detect bony metastasis more accurately than CT or MRI. The presence of skeletal metastasis in association with an adrenal mass in a child strongly suggests the diagnosis of neuroblastoma.

SUMMARY

With the widespread use of cross-sectional imaging techniques detection of an adrenal mass has increased over the years. However, clinical and appropriate biochemical tests in adrenal lesions, especially for functional diseases remain the most vital and initial mode of evaluation, followed by CT. The role of CT has continued to expand in both detection and characterization of an adrenal mass as benign or malignant. Based on size criteria and tumor morphology, it is not always possible to suggest benignity or malignancy. Follow-up studies are very necessary in equivocal cases. Necrosis in the tumor is related directly to prognosis. More necrosis carries worse prognosis. All attempts should be made to characterize an incidental adrenal mass as adenoma or metastasis in a patient with known malignancy. Lipid rich adenoma can be characterized with attenuation value of 10 HU or less on noncontrast CT. Lipid poor adenoma can be differentiated from metastasis on delayed enhanced CT with percentage enhancement wash out of more than 50%. If the mass remains indeterminate, chemical shift MRI is the next imaging modality for further characterization. If all these modalities still fail to characterize the lesion in a patient with known malignancy, having no other evidence of metastatic deposit, adrenal biopsy under CT guidance should be performed to establish a definitive diagnosis.

REFERENCES

1. Korobkin M. CT characterization of adrenal masses: The time has come. Radiology 2000; 217:629-32.
2. Blake MA, Holalkere NS, Boland GW. Imaging techniques for adrenal lesion characterization. Radiol Clin N Am 2008;46:65-78.
3. Gross MD, Korobkin M, Hussain H, et al. Adrenal gland imaging. In: Jameson JL, DeGroot LJ (Eds). Endocrinology, 5th edition. Philadelphia, WB Saunders; 2005.pp.2425-53.
4. Welch TJ, Sheedy PF. The adrenal glands. In: CT and MR Imaging of the Whole Body, 4th edition. Haaga, Lanzieri, Gilkeson (eds), Mosby, St Louis, USA; 2003.

5. Adrenal anatomy and imaging issues. In: Diagnostic Imaging-Abdomen. Federle MP, Jeffrey RB, Desser TS, et al (Eds). Amirsys, Salt Lake City, Utah; 2004.
6. Kelekis NL, Semelka RC, Firat RT. Zeynep. Adrenal glands. In: Abdominal-pelvic MRI. Semelka RC (Ed), 2nd edition, John Weley and Sons, New Jersey USA; 2006.pp.865-916.
7. Chung JJ, Semelka RC, Martin Dr. Adrenal adenomas. Characteristic post gadolinium capillary blush on dynamic MR imaging. J Mag Reson Imaging. 2001;13:242-8.
8. Reinig JW, Stutley JE, Leonhardt CM, Spicer KM, Margolis M, Caldwell CB. Differentiation of adrenal masses with MR imaging: Comparison of techniques. Radiology 1994;192: 41-6.
9. Lee MJ, Mayo-Smith WW, Hahn PF, et al. State-of-the-art MR imaging of the adrenal gland. Radiographics. 1994;14:1015-29, discussion 1029-32.
10. Bilbey JH, Mc Louglin RF, Kurkjian PS, et al. MR imaging of adrenal masses; value of chemical-shift imaging for distinguishing adenomas from other tumors. Am J Roentgenol. 1995;164:637-42.
11. Blake MA, Slattery JMA, Kalra MK, Halpern EF, Fischman AJ, Mueller PR, Boland GB. Adrenal lesions: Characterisation with Fused PET/CT image in patients with proved or suspected malignancy—Initial Experience. Radiology. 2006;238:970-7.
12. Shulkin BL, Thompson NW, Shapiro B, Francis IR, Sisson JC. Pheochromocytomas: Imaging with 2-[18F]fluoro-2-deoxy-D-glucose PET. Radiology 1999;212:35-41.
13. Yun M, Kim W, Alnafisi N, Lacorte L, Jang S, Alavi A. 18F-FDG PET in characterizing adrenal lesions detected on CT or MRI. J Nucl Med 2001;42:1795-9.
14. Lumachi F, Zucchetta P, Marzola MC, et al. Usefulness of CT scan, MRI and radiocholesterol scintigraphy for adrenal imaging in Cushing's syndrome. Nuclear Medicine Communications 2002;23:469-73.
15. Rockall AG, Babar SA, Sohaib SAA, et al. CT and MR imaging of the adrenal glands in ACTH-independent Cushing syndrome. Radiographics 2004;24:435-52.
16. Doppman JL, Gill JR Jr, Miller DL, et al. Distinction between hyperaldosteronism due to bilateral hyperplasia and unilateral aldosteronoma: Reliability of CT. Radiology. 1992;184:677-82.
17. Harinarayana CV, Gupta R, Ammini AC, et al. Computed tomography in untreated congenital adrenal hyperplasia. Paed Radiol. 1991;21:103-5.
18. Mayo-Smith WW, Boland GW, Noto RB, et al. State of the art adrenal imaging. Radiographics. 2001;21:995-1012.
19. Ammini AC, Gupta R, Mukhopadhya C, et al. Computed tomography morphology of adrenal gland of patients with Addison's disease. Austral Radiol. 1996;40:38-42.
20. Boland GW, Blake MA, Hahn PF, Mayosmith WW. Incidental Adrenal lesions: Principles, techniques, and algorithms for imaging characterization. Radiology. 2008;249(3):756-75.
21. Young WF Jr. The incidentally discovered adrenal mass. N Engl J Med. 2007;356:601-10.
22. Boland GW, Lee MJ, Gazelle GS, et al. Characterization of adrenal masses using unenhanced CT: An analysis of CT literature. Am J Roentgenol. 1998;171:201-4.
23. Caoili EM, Korobkin M, Francis IR, et al. Adrenal masses: characterization with combined unenhanced CT and delayed enhanced CT. Radiology. 2002;222:629-33.
24. Korobkin M, Brodeur FJ, Yutzy GG, et al. Differentiation of adrenal adenomas from nonadenomas using CT attenuation values. Am J Roengenol. 1996;166:531-6.
25. Pena CS, Boland GW, Hahn PF, Lee MJ, Mueller PR. Characterization of indeterminate (lipid-poor) adrenal masses: Use of washout characteristics at contrast enhanced CT. Radiology. 2000;217-798-802.
26. Metser U, Miller E, Lerman H, Lievshitz G, Avitla S, Even-Sapir E. 18F-FDG PET/CT the evaluation of adrenal masses. J Nucl Med. 2006;47:32-7.
27. Paling MR, Williamson BR. Adrenal involvement in non-Hodgkin lymphoma. Am J Roengenol. 1983;141:303-5.
28. Schwartz LH. Collision tumor of the adrenal gland: demonstration and characterization at MR imaging. Radiology. 1996;201(3):757-60.
29. Tung GA, Pfister RC, Papanicolaou N, Yoder IC. Adrenal cysts: Imaging and percutaneous aspiration. Radiology. 1989;173: 107-11.

CHAPTER 118

Retroperitoneum

Smriti Hari, Atin Kumar

INTRODUCTION

The retroperitoneum is the portion of the abdomen located posterior to the peritoneal cavity. It extends from the diaphragm superiorly to the pelvis inferiorly. An understanding of the complex anatomy of the retroperitoneum is imperative for calculating the distribution of inflammatory fluid collections, extravasated blood and solid masses in this region. This chapter describes the computed tomography (CT) and magnetic resonance imaging (MRI) manifestations of diseases involving the retroperitoneal spaces, aorta, inferior vena cava (IVC) and retroperitoneal lymph nodes. Disease processes confined to the retroperitoneum including, primary retroperitoneal tumors, retroperitoneal fibrosis and abnormalities related to the iliopsoas compartment are also discussed.

NORMAL ANATOMY

The retroperitoneum is divided into three main compartments: An anterior pararenal space that is continuous across the midline, a perirenal space on each side and a posterior pararenal space on each side **(Fig. 1)**. The anterior pararenal space contains the pancreas, the second, third, and fourth segments of the duodenum, the ascending and descending colon, lymph nodes and fat. This space is bordered anteriorly by the posterior parietal peritoneum, posteriorly by the anterior renal fascia (Gerota's fascia) and laterally by the lateroconal fascia, which is a continuation of the posterior renal fascia (Zuckerkandl fascia).[1] The perirenal space lies between the anterior and posterior renal fascia and contains the kidney, adrenal gland, renal pelvis, proximal ureter, renal hilar vessels, lymph nodes and fat.[2] The fascia of Gerota blends anteriorly with the connective tissue surrounding the aorta and inferior vena cava. The posterior pararenal space extends from the posterior renal fascia to the transversalis fascia and contains only a small amount of fat. Although it is located posterior to the kidneys, it continues anterolaterally as the properitoneal fat stripe.

The renal and lateroconal fascia are laminated, potentially expansile planes composed of apposed layers of embryonic mesentery: The retromesenteric plane between the leaves of the anterior pararenal fascia, the retrorenal plane formed by splitting of posterior pararenal fascia and the lateroconal plane between the leaves of the lateroconal fascia. Whereas most collections remain confined to the retroperitoneal compartment in which they originate, CT observations and cadaveric dissections suggest that rapidly accumulating collections can dissect and decompress through these retroperitoneal fascial planes themselves.[3]

Inferior to the cone of renal fat, anterior and posterior renal fascia fuse, effectively sealing the caudal perinephric space, preventing the inferior extension of perirenal fluid into the pelvis.[4] The communicating retromesenteric, retrorenal and the lateroconal fascial planes continue downwards into the true pelvis anterolateral to the psoas muscle.[5] Thus, the interfascial fluid unlike perinephric fluid can spread from the abdominal retroperitoneum into the pelvis.[6] Superiorly,

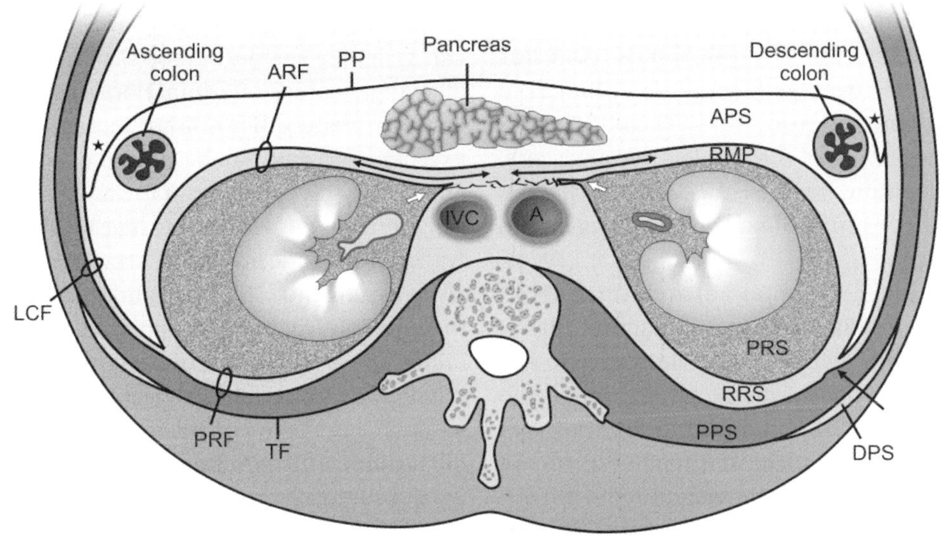

Fig. 1: Retroperitoneal and interfascial planes. Drawing at level of renal hila shows that perirenal and lateroconal fascia are laminated planes composed of apposed layers of embryonic mesentery. Note that thickness of interfascial planes is exaggerated to illustrate potentially expansile nature. Also note that perinephric spaces are closed medially (small white arrows). Retromesenteric plane is continuous across midline (bidirectional arrows). Retromesenteric plane, retrorenal space and lateroconal space communicate at fascial trifurcation (arrow). Dorsal pleural sinus may extend inferiorly to lie posterolateral to posterior pararenal space and transversalis fascia. *Abbreviations*: A: Aorta; APS: Anterior pararenal space; ARF: Anterior renal fascia; DPS: Dorsal pleural sinus; IVC: Inferior vena cava; LCF: Lateroconal fascia; PP: Parietal peritoneum; PPS: Posterior pararenal space; PRF: Posterior renal fascia; PRS: Perinephric space; RMP: Retromesenteric plane; RRS: Retrorenal space; TF: Transversalis fascia; *: Posterior peritoneal recess.

both layers of renal fascia blend with the diaphragmatic fascia to form the cephalic limit of the retroperitoneum. The normal anterior and posterior renal fascia measure 1–3 mm in thickness and are well visualized on CT scan except when abdominal fat is scanty. The posterior renal fascia is thicker and more frequently visualized than the anterior. Thickening of the retroperitoneal fascia is a sensitive but nonspecific indicator of adjacent disease and is seen in both inflammatory **(Fig. 2)** and neoplastic disorders.

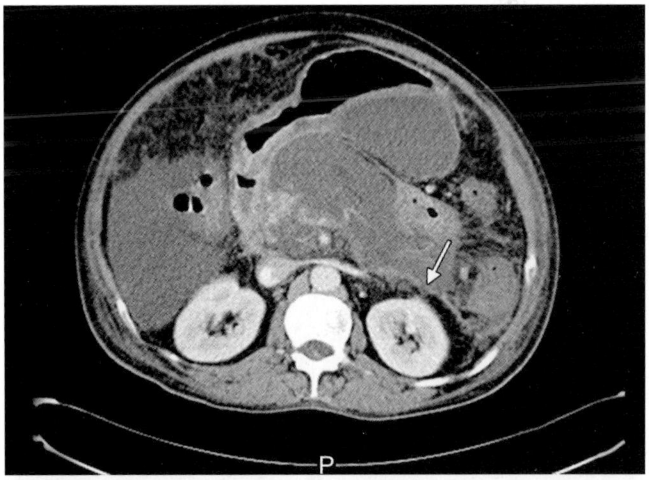

Fig. 2: Thickening of the left anterior renal fascia (arrow) in a patient of acute pancreatitis.

IMAGING MODALITIES

Multidetector CT is currently the preferred imaging modality for evaluating the retroperitoneum. It accurately displays its anatomical limits and clearly defines individual spaces separated by various fascial layers. Isotropic multiplanar reconstructions (MPRs) of thin overlapping slices in the coronal and sagittal plane provide excellent delineation of the location and extent of retroperitoneal masses. It is a useful modality for making initial diagnosis of various pathological conditions and for follow-up. The introduction of multidetector technology has substantially improved the quality and ease of performing CT angiography. The simultaneous acquisition of multiple thin collimated slices in combination with enhanced gantry rotation speed offers thin slice coverage of extended volumes without any loss in spatial resolution.

Multidetector CT angiography (MDCTA) is increasingly being used for assessing diseases affecting the vasculature of the abdominal organs, for treatment planning and post therapy follow-up.[7] CT scanners with 16 or more detectors enable full abdominal coverage from the diaphragm to the groin with high spatial resolution. These scanners permit excellent evaluation of the whole arterial visceral vasculature (e.g. hepatic vessels, mesenteric vessels, renal arteries) and the aortic–iliac axis in a single data acquisition **(Fig. 3)**.

MRI may provide additional information about retroperitoneal abnormalities because of its multiplanar capability and excellent soft tissue resolution. The MR imaging protocol should be devised to maximize the signal intensity differences between pathologies and the background tissues. Typical sequences used are precontrast T1-weighted spoiled gradient echo (SGE), fat-suppressed T2-weighted and post-gadolinium fat-suppressed T1-weighted SGE images. In the investigation of retroperitoneal hemorrhage, precontrast fat-suppressed T1-weighted SGE sequence should be obtained because it has the greatest sensitivity for subacute hemorrhage. Both T1-weighted and T2-weighted sequences are important for delineation and characterization of retroperitoneal masses, abscesses and fibrosis. Image acquisition in two orthogonal planes permits direct evaluation of the extent of retroperitoneal disease. Applications include evaluation of patients with suspected IVC thrombosis or Budd-Chiari syndrome **(Fig. 4)**, intravascular extension of renal, adrenal, or hepatic tumors and evaluation of anatomic anomalies of the IVC and systemic veins.[8]

Magnetic resonance angiography (MRA) has an important role to play in the imaging of aorta and IVC. Three-dimensional (3D) gadolinium-enhanced MRA can visualize the entire aorta with a single acquisition, allowing accurate determination of the extent of aneurysm, dissection and other abnormalities. Vascular contrast is excellent and data can be viewed in any projection, which aids in surgical planning.[9] Typically 0.1–0.2 mmol/kg body weight of gadolinium is injected intravenously as a bolus with an automatic injector at a rate of 2–4 mL/s, followed by 20 cc of saline to clear lines and veins. For aortic imaging, the time interval between initiating contrast injection and initiating the imaging sequence can be determined using a test bolus technique. 1–2 mL of contrast is injected as a test bolus and the aorta is scanned approximately once per second. The travel time can be directly observed and then used to calculate the correct scan delay. Alternatively, automated triggering may be employed in which the aorta is continuously scanned until the contrast material bolus is directly observed or the signal intensity reaches a specified level, at which time the 3D sequence is begun. The acquired dataset can be postprocessed either by MPRs or by 3D maximum intensity projection (MIP) **(Fig. 5)**. Arterial-phase MIP images demonstrate contrast material within the patent lumen and therefore may not depict the accurate diameter of an aneurysm. The walls of vessels can usually be identified on source images or axial reformatted images. In addition, axial T1-weighted spoiled gradient-echo or spin-echo MR sequences following angiography are very useful in determining the diameter of the aneurysm and the extent of intra-arterial plaque or

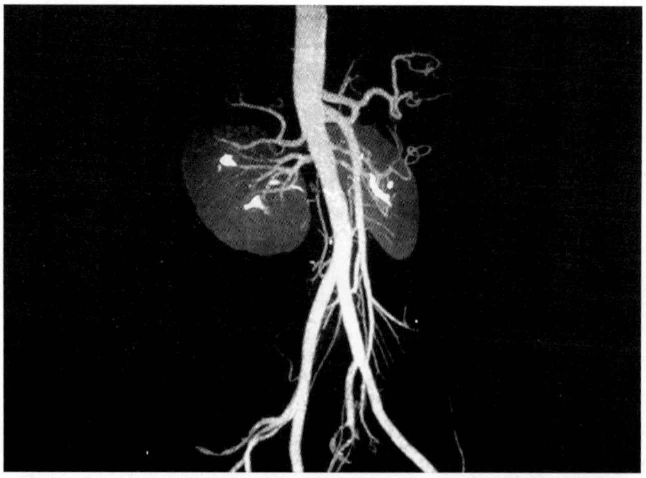

Fig. 3: Normal MDCT angiogram of the abdominal aorta. Maximum-intensity-projection (MIP) image shows good delineation of the entire abdominal aorta and its branches.The aorta has smooth walls and tapers gradually to the level of the aortic bifurcation.

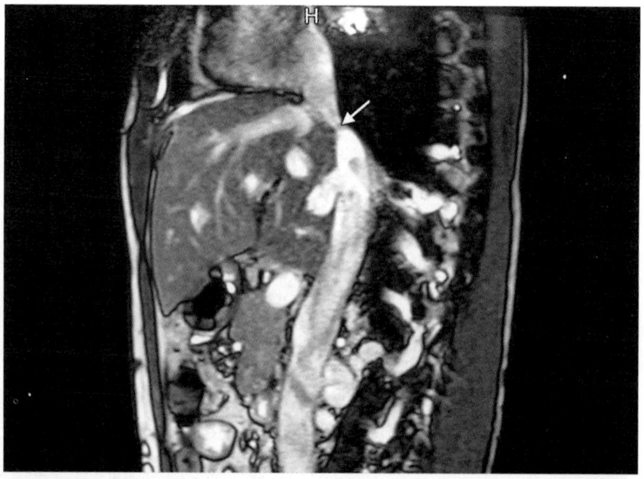

Fig. 4: Membranous obstruction of the intrahepatic IVC. Sagittal balanced steady-state (true FISP) MR image shows segmental occlusion of the IVC just below the cavoatrial junction.

thrombus. Likewise, it is important to examine the source images or thin-section reformatted images in patients who may have a dissection. An intimal flap can easily be missed if only MIP images are viewed.

Positron-emission tomography (PET) scanning has shown very high sensitivity and specificity for detection of retroperitoneal diseases. PET with 2-(fluorine-18) fluoro-2-deoxy-D-glucose (FDG) can detect small malignant nodes which are not easily identified or do not meet the size criteria for malignancy with CT **(Figs. 6A and B)** and tumor recurrences in surgical beds that are otherwise difficult to assess because of altered anatomy, surgical clip artifacts and scar issue.[10] However, evaluation of retroperitoneal malignancies or adenopathy with FDG-PET can be complicated by urinary and colonic activity or anatomic variants. Urinary artifacts are avoided with intravenous hydration, administration of furosemide and catheterization and retrograde filling of the bladder with saline solution. Colonic artifacts are avoided by cleansing the bowel with an isosmotic solution. FDG-PET is useful in assessing the retroperitoneum for adenopathy in malignancies such as testicular cancer, lymphoma, and rectal, ovarian or cervical cancer that spread along retroperitoneal lymphatics.

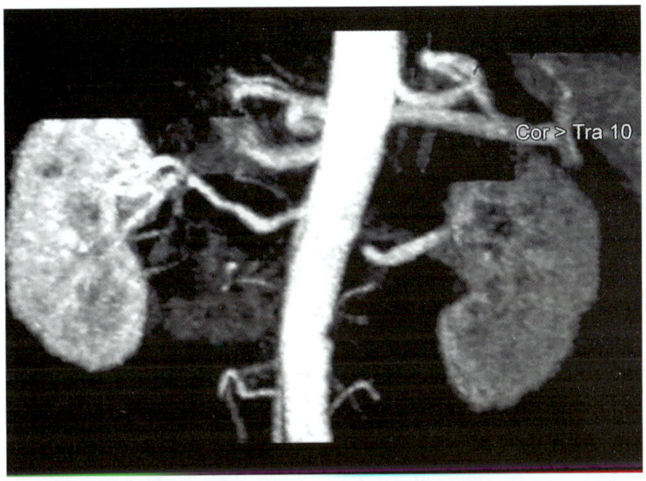

Fig. 5: Maximum intensity projection of 3D, gadolinium-enhanced MR angiogram depicting left renal artery stenosis.

RETROPERITONEAL COLLECTIONS

Fluid collection in the retroperitoneum occurs in a variety of conditions. The important conditions are acute pancreatitis, urinary tract disruption with urinoma formation, hematoma and abscess. Although the clinical presentations differ, they all share a tendency to dissect within the well-defined fascial planes in the retroperitoneal space. Most of these appear on CT as water density collections and are frequently indistin-guishable from one another.

Fluid collections in the anterior pararenal space often result from acute pancreatitis **(Fig. 7)**.[11] Fluid collections arise within or adjacent to the pancreas in about 40% and resolve spontaneously without leaving any clinical sequelae in over 50% of these patients. In others, the fluid collections persist, develop a fibrous capsule and are often associated with a variety of complications including secondary infection, perforation and erosion into the spleen, liver or vascular system. Both infected and noninfected fluid collections and pseudocysts can be treated effectively by image guided percutaneous catheter drainage.

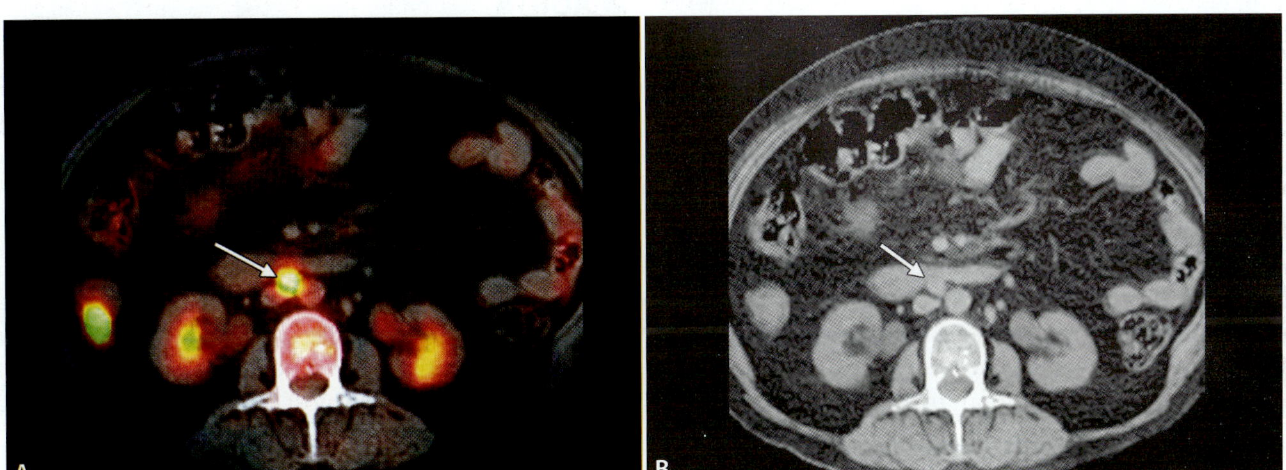

Figs. 6A and B: (A) FDG-PET image in a patient of carcinoma ovary shows increased uptake in a subcentimetric aortocaval lymph node (arrow); (B) Comparison CT image also shows the node (arrow), which was considered insignificant by the size criteria.

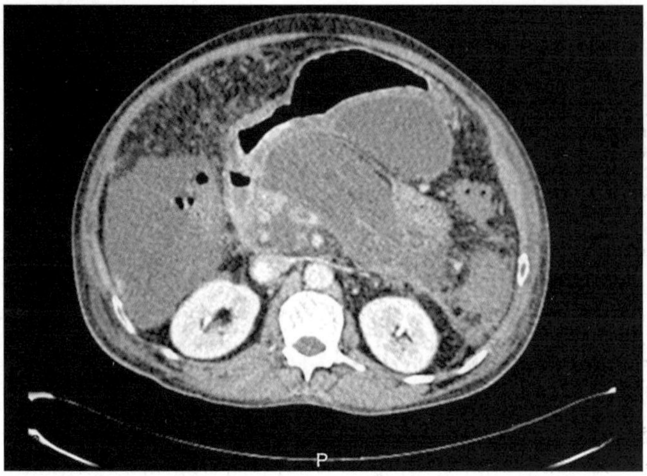

Fig. 7: Fluid collection in the anterior pararenal space. CT image in a patient with acute pancreatitis demonstrates peripancreatic fluid in the left anterior pararenal space.

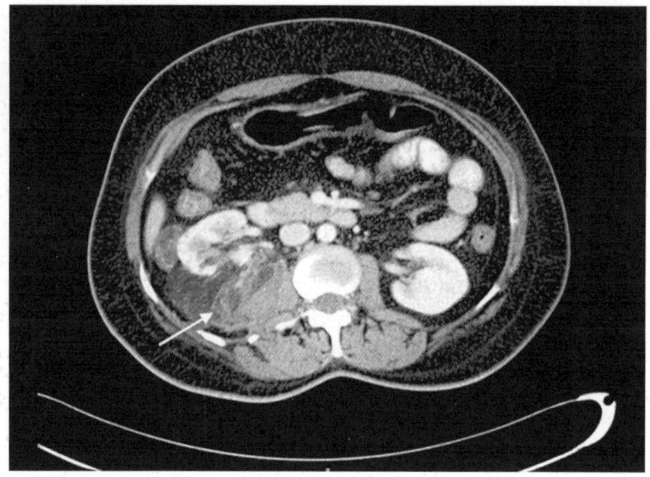

Fig. 8: Perirenal hemorrhage. Axial CT image shows right perirenal hemorrhage (arrow) that occurred spontaneously from rupture of underlying renal angiomyolipoma.

Abscesses, hematomas and urinomas can all develop in the perirenal space. Perirenal hemorrhage is usually caused by blunt trauma, rupture of an aortic aneurysm, bleeding disorders, anticoagulant therapy or spontaneous bleeding within a renal tumor **(Fig. 8)**. On CT characteristically, a hyperdense, ill-defined collection originating from the disrupted vessels and extending into the interfascial planes is seen. Loculated blood can mimic a complex cyst or neoplasm. CT attenuation of hematoma varies with time, ranging from hyperdense fresh blood, typically >50 HU to near water density within several weeks. Bleeding may be intermittent resulting in a heterogeneous appearance. MRI is more useful in determining the content of retroperitoneal fluid collections as it is more sensitive and specific for detection of blood products. An acute hematoma is isointense on T1-weighted and hyperintense on T2-weighted images. Within several days the signal gradually becomes hyperintense on T1-weighted images and a hematoma is then hyperintense on both T1- and T2-weighted images with a developing, hypointense hemosiderin rim **(Figs. 9A and B)**.

Abnormal perirenal fluid may be in either of two locations: within the renal capsule (subcapsular) or outside the capsule in the perinephric fat. Subcapsular fluid collections usually produce distortion of the renal parenchyma whereas perinephric collections do not. Urinomas result from obstructive uropathy and less frequently from abdominal trauma and surgical or diagnostic instrumentation.

Retroperitoneal abscesses are particularly difficult to diagnose, because they may not exhibit the classic clinical features, i.e. fever, chills and an elevated white blood cell count.

When an abscess is mature, its wall is thick and generally hypervascular. On contrast-enhanced CT, there is enhancement of the wall and the fluid is usually homogeneous and does not enhance. Many abscesses contain multiple septations. There may be substantial reactive inflammation in the surrounding fat.

Abnormalities in the posterior pararenal space are much less common than abnormalities in the anterior pararenal space or the perirenal space. When present, these are most commonly the result of spread of pathologic processes in the pelvis. Causes can include hematoma, infection and neoplasm.

AORTA

The most important abdominal aortic abnormalities are aneurysm formation and aortic dissection. MDCTA and MRA have gradually replaced conventional angiography as the procedures of choice for detailed evaluation of the aorta.

Aortic Aneurysm

Most abdominal aortic aneurysms result from atherosclerosis. Other causes include trauma, infection, Takayasu's arteritis, cystic medial necrosis and syphilis. The infrarenal aorta is the most common site of abdominal aortic aneurysms accounting for 95% of cases. If untreated, these aneurysms may enlarge and rupture with a mortality of 50–90%.[12]

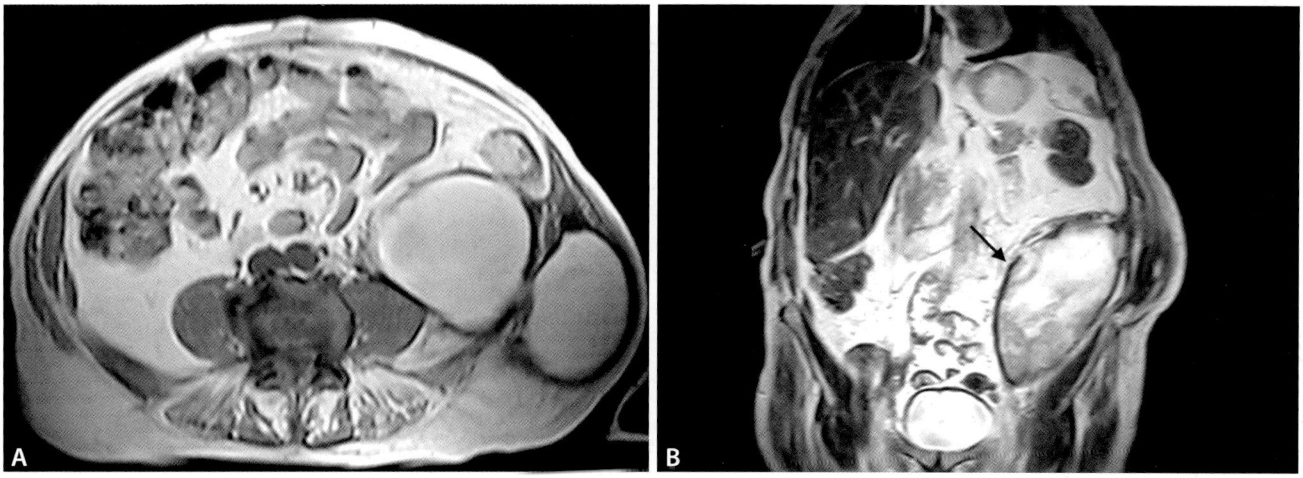

Figs. 9A and B: Spontaneous retroperitoneal hemorrhage in a patient on anticoagulant therapy. (A) Axial T1-weighted MR image shows a well-defined hyperintense lesion anterior to the left psoas. It is partially decompressing into the parietes; (B) Coronal T2-weighted image shows heterogeneous, predominantly high signal intensity within the mass. There is a markedly hypointense peripheral rim (arrow) due to hemosiderin deposition. These T1 and T2 signal intensities are diagnostic of a subacute hematoma.

The abdominal aortic aneurysm may show curvilinear calcification on plain abdominal radiography. On ultrasonography (US), CT and MRI the aneurysm is identified as focal area of dilatation exceeding 3 cm in size. Spontaneous rupture is a frequent complication of aneurysms measuring 6 cm or more in diameter. Therefore, most aneurysms larger than 6 cm require surgery. Important diagnostic information needed for management includes location, diameter of aneurysm, its longitudinal length, its relationship to the renal, common iliac and femoral arteries and assessment of the periaortic tissues for perianeurysmal fibrosis.[13] US is a good modality for initial evaluation of aortic aneurysm. It may also be used for follow-up of patients who do not undergo surgical repair. However, CT and MRI are preferred techniques for evaluating the size, extent and complications of aneurysms. At several centers, CT angiography has replaced conventional angiography because it is less invasive and can provide all the necessary information required for the management. Angiography frequently underestimates the dimensions of an aneurysm because it shows only the flowing blood in the lumen and does not show mural thrombus, which is detected on CT **(Fig. 10)**. Contrast-enhanced 3D gradient echo MRA demonstrates the full extent of the aneurysm and its relationship to aortic branches.

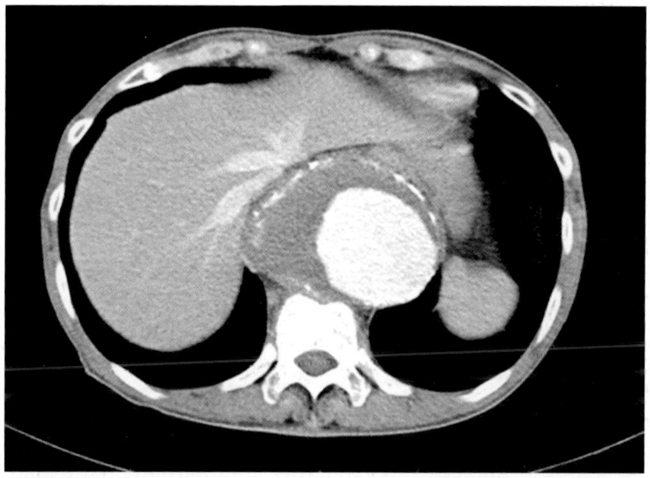

Fig. 10: Abdominal aortic aneurysm. Dynamic, contrast-enhanced axial CT image shows markedly dilated abdominal aorta with a large eccentric thrombus. A conventional angiogram on this patient would significantly underestimate the size of the aneurysm as only the patent part of the lumen containing flowing blood would be opacified.

Aneurysm rupture or leak is indicative of high morbidity and mortality if it is not promptly treated. CT findings of ruptured abdominal aortic aneurysms are often straightforward. Most ruptures are manifested as a retroperitoneal hematoma accompanied by an abdominal aortic aneurysm. Periaortic blood may extend into the perirenal space, the pararenal space, or both. Intraperitoneal extravasation may be an immediate or a delayed finding. Discontinuity of the aortic wall or a focal gap in otherwise continuous circumferential wall calcifications may point to the location of a rupture. There usually is a delay of several hours between the initial intramural hemorrhage and frank extravasation into the periaortic soft tissues. It is difficult to identify contained or impending ruptures. A small amount of periaortic blood may be confused with the duodenum, peri-aneurysmal fibrosis, or adenopathy. Imaging features suggestive of instability or impending rupture include increased aneurysm size, a low thrombus-to-lumen ratio and hemorrhage into a mural thrombus. A peripheral crescent-shaped area of hyperattenuation within an abdominal aortic aneurysm represents an acute intramural hemorrhage and is another CT sign of impending rupture. Draping of the posterior aspect of an aneurysmal aorta over the vertebrae is associated with a contained rupture.[14]

The preferred surgical treatment of abdominal aortic aneurysms is an end-to-end anastomosis with aortic graft repair. Complications of abdominal aortic surgery that can be detected on CT include graft infections, aorto-enteric fistulae, anastomotic aneurysms, graft leak or rupture.

Aortic Dissection

Aortic dissection usually originates in the thorax but sometimes extends into the abdomen. Mortality rate of untreated dissection is very high approaching 25% at 1 day, 50% at 1 week and 75% at 1 month.[15] The strategy for therapy is dependent on factors like the type and extent of dissection, the site of entry, involvement of aortic branches, patency of the false lumen and the presence of thrombus in the false lumen.

Currently, the noninvasive modalities that are most frequently used to detect aortic dissections are US, CT and MRI. US, including transthoracic echocardiography and transesophageal echocardiography, is widely available and can be performed quickly and easily at the bedside. Thus, US can be used in most patients with aortic dissections, even in relatively unstable patients. However, US has major shortcomings, namely, a limited field of view and a diagnostic accuracy that largely depends on the investigator's experience. Furthermore, US does not provide images that can be used to plan therapy. Multidetector CT has the advantages of shorter scanning times, wide availability and high diagnostic accuracy and has, therefore, classically been the modality of choice for the evaluation of aortic dissection. In the past, emergency MR imaging evaluation of aortic dissection has been impossible owing to prolonged examination times, but the advent of 3D contrast-enhanced MRA has changed this paradigm. Contrast-enhanced MR angiography has largely replaced unenhanced MR angiographic techniques and has dramatically shortened the total examination time required for confident diagnosis of aortic dissections; however, it is more suitable for stable patients. In principle, contrast-enhanced MR angiography is similar to CT angiography. Both modalities provide excellent evaluation of aortic dissections. In patients without contraindications for either modality, at most centers, the use of each modality is based on equipment availability, the personal preference of the radiologist or referring physician and patient acceptance.

Confident diagnosis and correct classification of aortic dissection is based on the detection of an intimal flap in the aorta that separates the true and false lumina **(Fig. 11)**. Such a flap manifests as a hypointense line with a linear, arc, or S shape in the axial plane. The true and false lumina can be differentiated on the basis of signal intensity, morphologic features, the relationship between the lumina and the appearance of thrombosis.

- *Signal intensity:* Similar to CT angiography, contrast-enhanced MRA shows the true lumen with higher signal intensity than the false lumen owing to a higher concentration of contrast material during the arterial phase.
- *Morphologic features:* The true lumen is usually smaller than the false lumen and would be thin or flat from being pressed, appearing oval in the axial plane. The false lumen is expanded or very large, appearing crescentic or winding around the true lumen in the axial plane.
- *Relationship between the lumina:* The lumina may be parallel to each other, the false lumen may wind around the true lumen, or the true lumen may look like a ribbon floating in the false lumen.

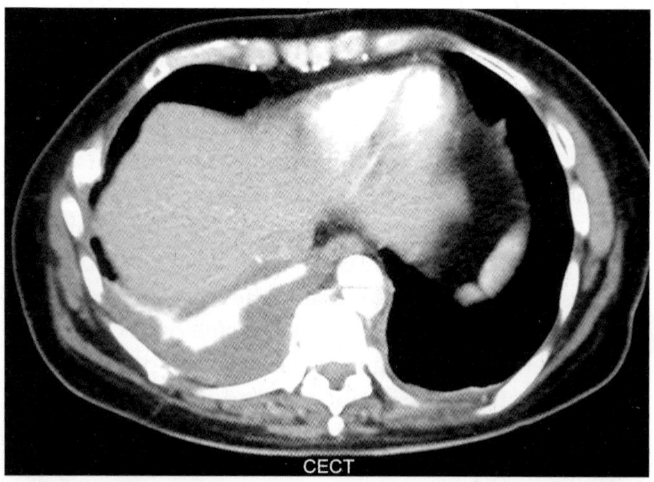

Fig. 11: Thoracoabdominal aortic dissection. Axial CT angiogram easily demonstrates the linear intimal flap between the anterior true lumen and posterior false lumen. Active extravasation into the retroperitoneum is also seen.

- *Appearance of thrombosis:* The false lumen usually contains a thrombus, especially at the retrograde end of the initial entry site, whereas the true lumen contains no thrombus in most cases.

INFERIOR VENA CAVA

Mostly a routine CT or an MR abdominal protocol employing pre- and postcontrast SGE images provides sufficient evaluation of the IVC for patient management. At least one MR sequence should be performed in the sagittal or coronal plane, because it permits direct visualization of the longitudinal extent of IVC. However, when detailed evaluation of retroperitoneal veins is required, it is prudent to obtain CT or MR venography.

Congenital Anomalies

Congenital abnormalities of the IVC and related veins are common. Preoperative knowledge of the presence of these anomalies is helpful, particularly in patients undergoing a portasystemic shunt procedure, aortic surgery or nephrectomy and reduces the risk of major venous hemorrhage associated with these anomalies.[16]

CT and MRI are well suited to determine whether rounded or tubular retroperitoneal structures are vascular in nature. Some of the developmental anomalies of inferior vena cava are: Interruption of inferior vena cava with azygos and hemiazygos vein continuation **(Fig. 12)**, left-sided inferior vena cava, duplication of the inferior vena cava, and anomalies of the left renal vein, e.g. circumaortic or retro-aortic left renal vein.[17] Retrocaval ureter is thought to be due to persistence of right posterior cardinal vein with failure of development of the infrarenal right supracardinal vein. It occurs with a frequency of 0.2 per thousand population. In retrocaval ureter the proximal right ureter courses medially behind the inferior vena cava, usually at L3 vertebral level and then courses anteriorly around the cava to partially encircle it. The anomaly is characterised by hydronephrosis and medial deviation (fish hook deformity) of the middle ureteral segment.

Venous Thrombosis

Inferior vena caval thrombus may result from proximal extension of thrombi from lower extremity, pelvis or renal veins. Intracaval tumor extension may occur via veins draining neoplasms, such as renal cell carcinoma, hepatoma or adrenal carcinoma. CT and MRI perform well in evaluating IVC thrombosis and distinguishing tumor from bland thrombus.[18] Tumor thrombus shows anatomic contiguity and an enhancement pattern identical to that of primary tumor **(Fig. 13)**. The bland thrombus does not enhance with contrast. Depiction of the supradiaphragmatic extent of the thrombus into the right atrium is important for surgical planning as it requires combined thoracoabdominal surgery, whereas thrombus that ends below the hepatic veins may require only an abdominal approach.[19]

In cases of chronic venous thrombosis, the affected vessel may not be identified if the thrombus is organized and contacted. In these cases, careful evaluation reveals the absence of a vein in the expected location in combination with the presence of collateral vessels.

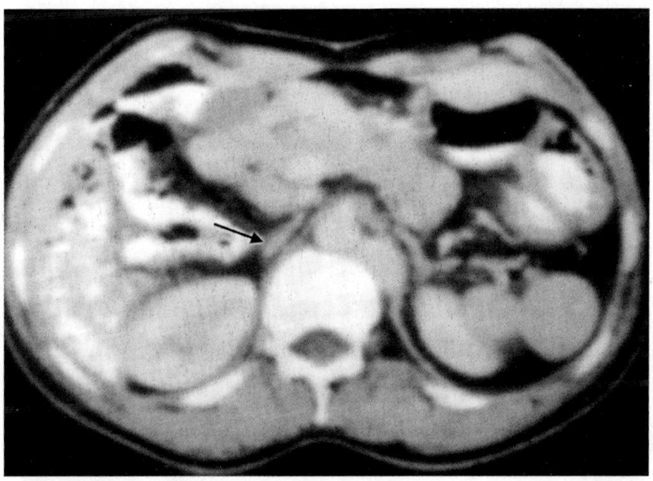

Fig. 12: Congenital polysplenia with IVC anomaly. CT scan shows multiple splenenculi and interrupted IVC with hemiazygos venous continuation. Linear density (arrow) seen lateral to the right crus is part of the right adrenal gland.

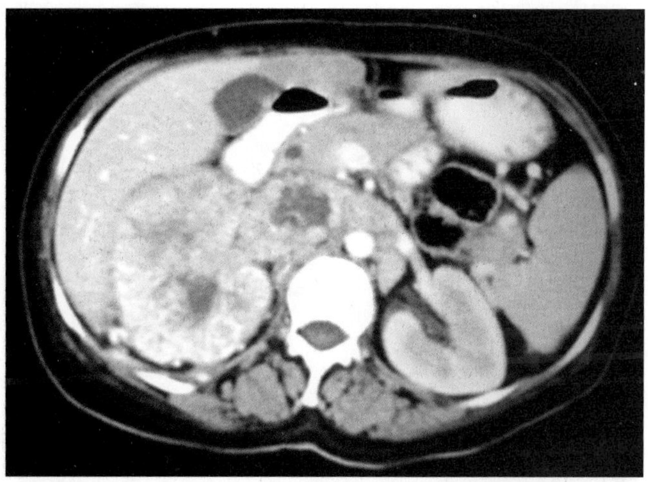

Fig. 13: IVC thrombus: Axial contrast-enhanced CT image in a 57-year-old man shows a large right renal cancer extending into the right renal vein and the IVC. The mass within the distended IVC is of the same attenuation as the primary tumor

Primary Tumors of the IVC

Primary tumors of the inferior vena cava are rare. Leiomyoma, endothelioma or leiomyosarcoma may arise as a primary neoplasm of the caval wall.[20] The tumor is usually seen as a filling defect, which may be associated with venous expansion and enhancement of the tumor wall on CT scan **(Figs. 14A and B)**. Signal intensity of these tumors is moderately low on T1-weighted images and mixed to high on T2-weighted images. Areas of intermixed tumor and blood products may show bright signal intensity on T1-weighted images. MPRs in the sagittal or coronal plane are useful for demonstrating the craniocaudal extent of the tumor. Collateral vessels such as azygous and hemiazygous veins may be enlarged.

LYMPH NODES

Normal lymph nodes appear as small, rounded soft tissue masses adjacent to the great vessels. Retrocrural, paraceliac, gastrohepatic para-aortic, aortocaval, periportal, peri-pancreatic, external and internal iliac groups together constitute the retroperitoneal nodes. Presently, CT is the most frequently used imaging technique for evaluation of enlarged retroperitoneal nodes. The diagnosis of lymph node abnormalities on CT is based on size and image morpho-logy. Size of a node is best determined by measuring its short axis diameter. The retroperitoneal lymph nodes are considered abnormal if their size is more than 10 mm, except in the retrocrural space where the upper limit is 6 mm. A variety of retroperitoneal structures can be confused with enlarged lymph nodes, including unopacified loops of bowel, vascular collaterals, dilated lymphatics and retroperitoneal fibrosis. Careful evaluation of serial CT images after oral and intravenous contrast is helpful in distinguishing between these structures.

MR sequences suited for detection of lymph nodes include precontrast T1-weighted spin-echo or SGE, fat-suppressed T2-weighted turbo spin-echo and contrast-enhanced fat-suppressed sequences. The enlarged lymph nodes appear low in signal on precontrast SGE in a background of high-signal fat and nodes are moderately high in signal on fat-suppressed T2-weighted and contrast-enhanced T1-weighted images. Fat-suppressed T2-weighted images are very sensitive for the detection of lymph nodes and perform better than CT, particularly in pediatric patients or other patients with paucity of retroperitoneal fat.

Benign Lymphadenopathy

Benign lymphadenopathy may occur secondary to inflammatory or infectious disease. Lymphadenopathy is the most common manifestation of abdominal tuberculosis.[21]

The mesenteric, omental and peripancreatic lymph nodes are most commonly involved. The nodes commonly demonstrate peripheral enhancement with central areas of low attenuation after intravenous contrast administration **(Fig. 15)**. Discrete homogeneous lymph nodes may also be seen in some cases. Calcification is frequently seen in

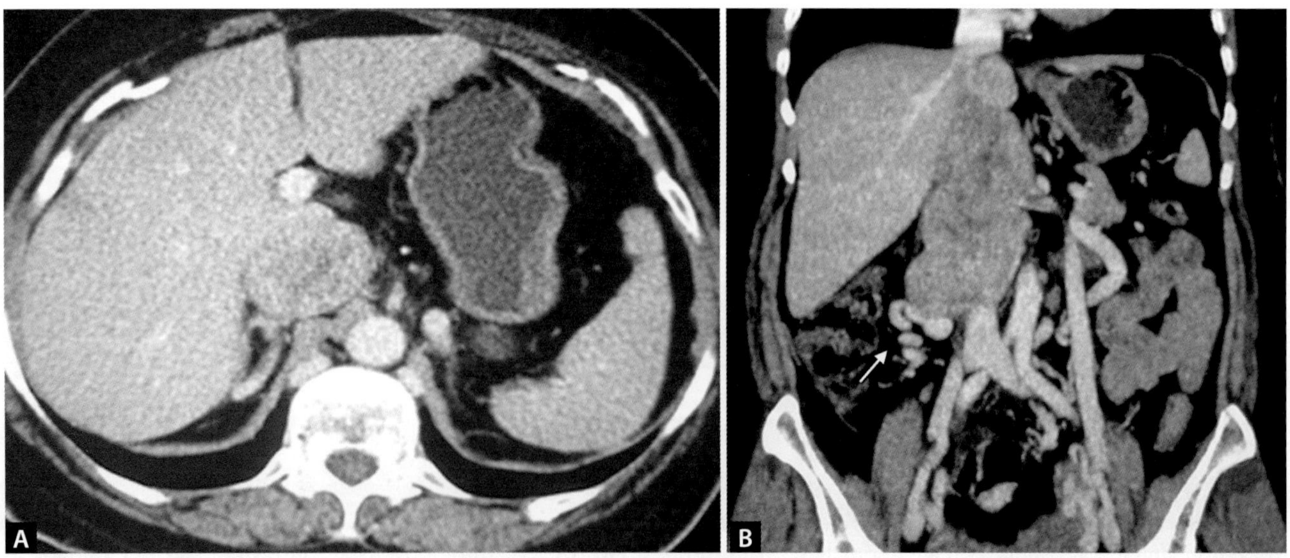

Figs. 14A and B: IVC leiomyosarcoma. (A) Contrast-enhanced CT scan of the upper abdomen shows a large, mildly enhancing mass within the hepatic portion of the IVC; (B) Coronal multiplanar image reconstructed from CT data better depicts the craniocaudal extent of the mass and the dilated venous collaterals (arrow).

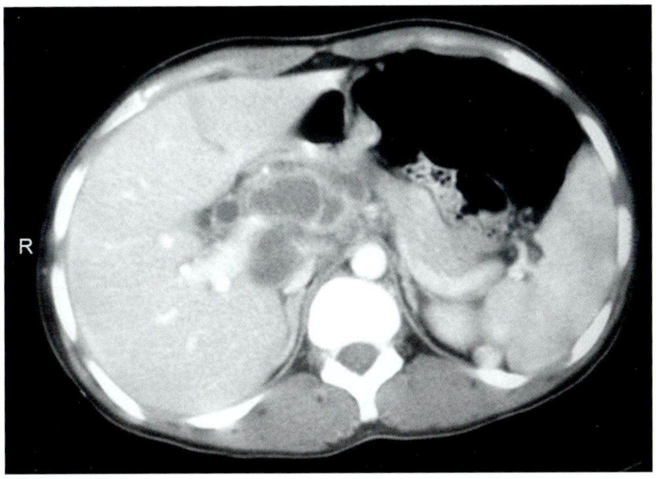

Fig. 15: Retroperitoneal tubercular lymphadenopathy. Axial CT image shows enlarged periportal and portocaval lymph nodes with characteristic central necrosis and peripheral rim enhancement.

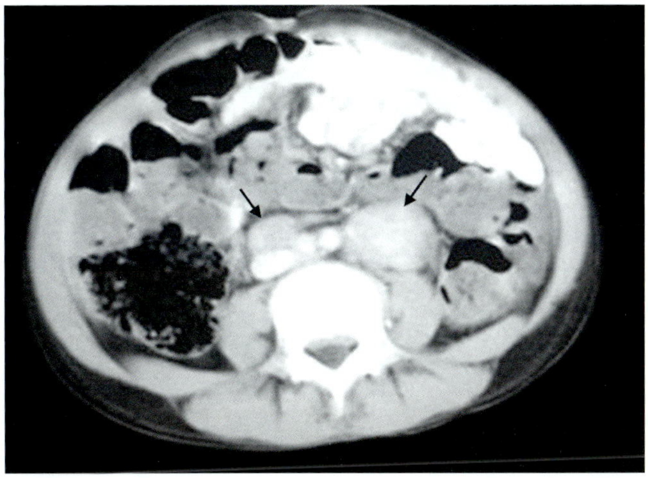

Fig. 16: Castleman disease. Contrast-enhanced axial CT image shows large, well-defined, markedly enhancing para-aortic lymph nodes (arrows) compatible with the diagnosis of Castleman disease in an 8-year-old boy.

tubercular lymph nodes. Enlarged lymph nodes with low density centers may also be seen in pyogenic infections, Whipples disease, lymphomatous or metastatic nodes following radiotherapy and chemotherapy.

Enlarged retroperitoneal nodes have also been observed in 30% of patients with sarcoidosis.[22] The periportal, paraceliac and para-aortic groups are most often involved. On CT, the nodes affected by sarcoidosis generally show homogeneous soft-tissue attenuation and remain discrete. Nodal calcification is unusual in sarcoidosis.

Castleman disease is occasionally also associated with retroperitoneal lymph node enlargement. Mostly the CT or MR appearance of these enlarged lymph nodes is not specific. However, identification of intense and uniform contrast enhancement in lymph nodes can suggest the diagnosis **(Fig. 16)**.[23]

Lymphangioleiomyomatosis is a rare cause of bulky retroperitoneal lymphadenopathy. This is a progressive disease involving the lung, lymphatic trunks and lymph nodes, typically affecting young women of child-bearing age. Sometimes, it can primarily involve retroperitoneum with or without subsequent development in the lungs.[24] On CT scans, the enlarged lymph nodes may show cystic, low-attenuation components.

Lymphoma

Abdominal lymph nodes are involved in 50% of the non-Hodgkin's lymphoma (NHL) patients as against 25% of those with Hodgkin's disease (HD) at presentation.[25] Mesenteric involvement is seen in more than half of the NHL patients (versus 5% of those with HD). The patterns of lymphadenopathy are also markedly different, slight enlargement of upper para-aortic nodes and contiguous spread being characteristic of HD. NHL on the other hand manifests with bulky lymph nodes in multiple locations.

The enlarged lymph nodes may appear as discrete masses or as confluent soft tissue mass obliterating the retroperitoneal fat **(Fig. 17)**. Lymphomas are 'soft' tumors and frequently surround the adjacent vessels (floating aorta sign) and ureters without compressing their lumina. Lymphomas are homogeneous, with minimal contrast enhancement and relatively low signal intensity at T2-weighted images representing densely packed cellular components. Nodes are rarely calcified (<1%) in untreated patients.[26]

CT is also used for follow-up of disease after treatment. Response to treatment is usually indicated by reduction in the retroperitoneal lymph node enlargement. In some patients, lymph nodes may become hypodense as an appropriate response to treatment with or without reduction in lymph node size. Occasionally, there may be post-treatment dystrophic calcification of the lymphomatous masses.

Persistent lymph nodal masses may be seen in some patients even after treatment. These may represent residual tumor, post-treatment inflammation or fibrosis. Unfortunately, there are no reliable CT characteristics that can differentiate between malignant and benign residual masses. Several studies have suggested that MRI may be helpful in distinguishing late post-therapy fibrosis (hypointense on T2-weighted images) from viable lymph

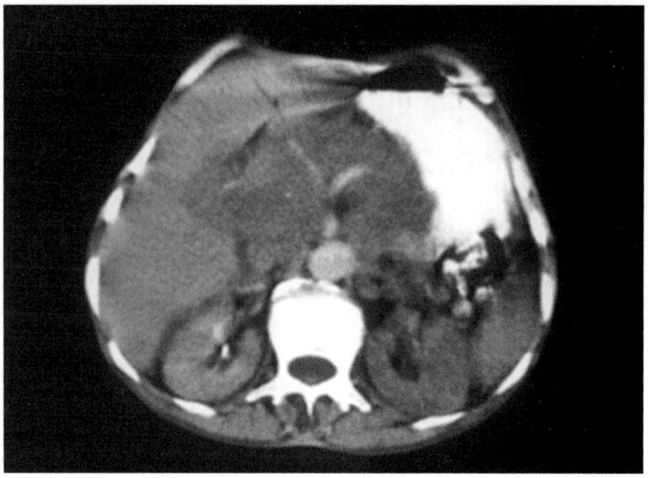

Fig. 17: Non-Hodgkin lymphoma. Contrast-enhanced axial CT image shows large, confluent lymph nodal mass in the preaortic location. The celiac axis branches are engulfed by the mass but their patency is preserved.

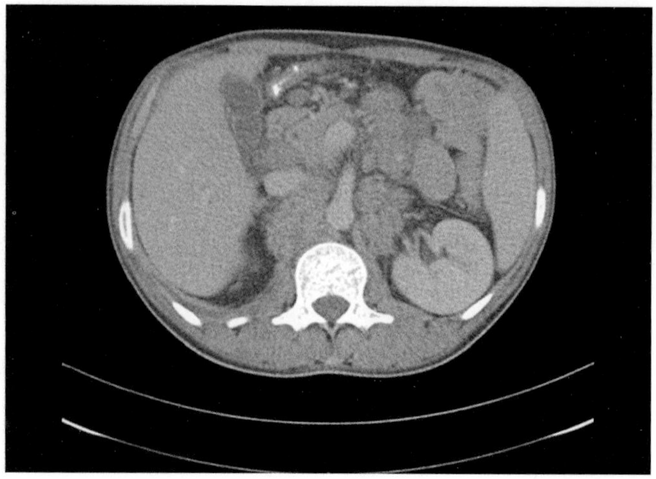

Fig. 18: *Mycobacterium tuberculosis* infection in a 35-year-old man with HIV infection. Axial CT image shows multiple, enlarged, low attenuation lymph nodes in the portocaval and paraceliac regions.

nodes (hyperintense or heterogeneous on T2-weighted images). Also chronic fibrotic tissue shows minimal MR enhancement postcontrast while recurrence generally enhances markedly.

FDG-PET has proved to be very useful in the clinical management of lymphomas. It is now considered the most accurate tool for the assessment of treatment response and prognosis in patients with Hodgkin lymphoma and aggressive non-Hodgkin lymphoma.[27] FDG-PET can detect metabolically active disease by its increased glycolysis that is proportional to the tumor mitotic activity. It can separate high from low-grade tumors and aid in prognostication. FDG-PET at the end of treatment seems to aid considerably in differentiating between residual masses with or without residual lymphoma. An early interim FDG-PET scan after 1–3 cycles of chemotherapy is a very strong predictor of outcome and trials are now in progress testing treatment modifications on this basis.[28] Like other imaging modalities, PET has its own drawbacks including inability to detect very small lesions (<5 mm) and reduced specificity due to increased uptake in metabolically active inflammatory and infective tissues.

HIV Lymphadenopathy

Enlarged lymph node are present in most (>60%) patients with HIV infection but in more than half of these patients the short-axis diameter of the largest node measures only 10–15 mm.[29] Although sometimes the nodal enlargement results only from reactive hyperplasia, many other diseases may be responsible. These include disseminated mycobacterial infections **(Fig. 18)**, histoplasmosis, lymphoma and Kaposi's sarcoma. When lymph node enlargement is massive, AIDS-related lymphoma should be suspected. Intense enhancement of lymph nodes suggest a diagnosis of Kaposi's sarcoma.

Metastatic Lymphadenopathy

Metastatic lymph nodes show varied morphological patterns, but the diagnosis is usually straightforward due to the presence of a known primary. Neoplasms of the stomach, colon, pancreas, kidney, testis, ovary, uterus, bladder and prostate may all metastasize to retroperitoneal lymph nodes. Calcification in the metastatic nodes suggest mucin producing primary from the ovary or gastrointestinal tract.

Testicular neoplasms tend to metastasize via lymphatics rather than via bloodstream. Lymphatics from the testes drain into ipsilateral lymph nodes, which follow the course of the gonadal veins. Typically, left sided neoplasms spread to involve lymph nodes in the left renal hilum, as the left gonadal vein drains into the left renal vein. Right-sided neoplasms spread to paracaval lymph nodes, an area where the right gonadal vein joins the IVC. While metastatic retroperitoneal nodes from some testicular tumors appear quite homogeneous on CT, others particularly from nonseminomatous neoplasms often appear heterogeneous containing low attenuation central areas of necrosis and rim enhancement **(Figs. 19A and B)**. Seminomas may present with bulky masses whereas non-seminomatous germ cell tumor often metastasize to normal sized nodes. On MR metastatic lymph nodes show low-intermediate signal intensity on T1-weighted images

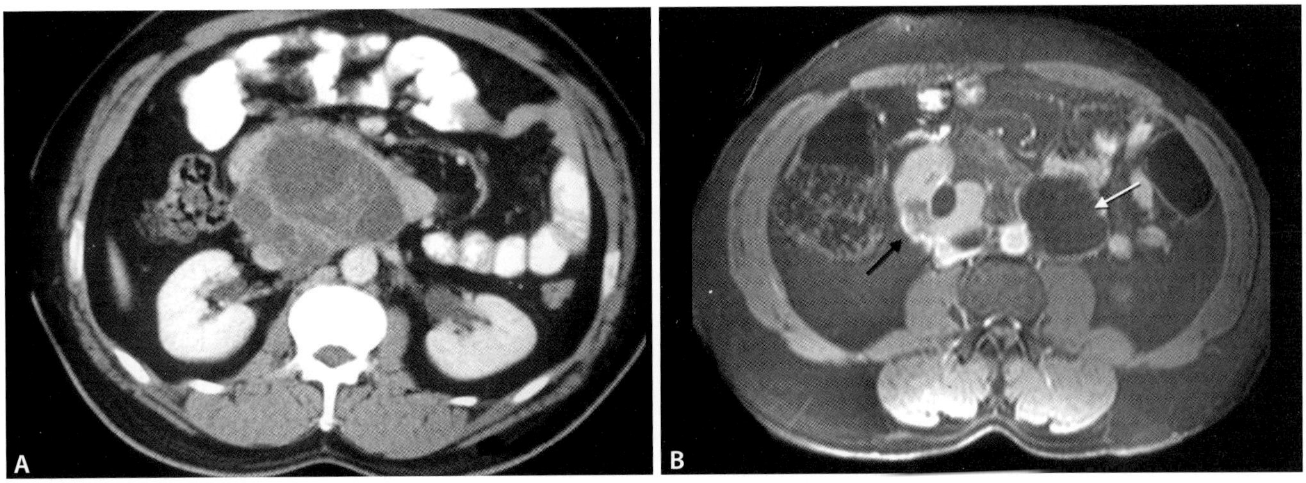

Figs. 19A and B: Metastatic testicular germ cell tumor. (A) Axial CT image shows massive, low attenuation retroperitoneal lymphadenopathy; (B) Postchemotherapy contrast-enhanced T1-weighted axial MR image in another patient shows enhancing viable tumor (black arrow) and the non-enhancing necrotic component (white arrow).

and high signal intensity on T2-weighted images. Low signal intensity masses after treatment usually represent fibrosis.

CT and MRI use the nonspecific criterion of size and are limited in their ability to differentiate benign from malignant lymph nodes. Contrast enhanced MR lymphography is a promising technique in differentiating benign from metastatic lymph nodes and providing information on lymph node morphology and function. Ultrasmall super paramagnetic iron oxide (USPIO) particles with a long plasma circulation time are suitable as MR contrast agents for MR lymphography. MR imaging is typically performed 24–36 hours after intravenous infusion of USPIO particles. Normal lymph nodes decrease in signal intensity on enhanced T2-weighted and T2-weighted gradient echo images, indicating uptake of this contrast agent. Nodes infiltrated by tumor have no appreciable USPIO uptake and thus reveal no signal change on pre- and postcontrast images.[30]

FDG-PET may be more sensitive and specific than CT for certain retroperitoneal metastases depending on the primary. Nonseminomatous germ cell tumors with well differentiated components are not very FDG-avid.

PRIMARY NEOPLASMS

Primary retroperitoneal neoplasms are rare tumors that originate in the retroperitoneal space but outside the major organs within that compartment. These neoplasms are generally derived from mesenchymal cells, neurogenic cells, or embryonic rests and may be benign or malignant. Diagnosis of these tumors is often challenging for radiologists and consists of several steps, including determining tumor location (characterizing the retroperitoneal space and identifying the organ of origin) and recognizing specific features of various retroperitoneal tumors (evaluating patterns of spread, tumor components and vascularity).

To decide whether the tumor is located within the retroperitoneal space, it is useful to observe the displacement of normal anatomic structures. Anterior displacement of retroperitoneal organs (e.g. kidneys, adrenal glands, ureters, ascending and descending colon, pancreas, portions of the duodenum) strongly suggests that the tumor arises in the retroperitoneum **(Figs. 20A and B)**. Major vessels and some of their branches are also found in the retroperitoneal cavity, so that displacement of these vessels can be helpful as well. Before a tumor can be described as primarily retroperitoneal, the possibility that the tumor originates from a retroperitoneal organ must be excluded. Some radiologic signs that are helpful in determining tumor origin include the "beak sign," the "phantom (invisible) organ sign", and the "embedded organ sign".[31] When there is no definite sign that suggests an organ of origin, the diagnosis of primary retroperitoneal tumor becomes likely.

Beak sign: When a mass deforms the edge of an adjacent organ into a "beak" shape, it is likely that the mass arises from that organ **(Figs. 21A and B)**. On the other hand, an adjacent organ with dull edges suggests that the tumor compresses the organ but does not arise from it.

Phantom (Invisible) organ sign: When a large mass arises from a small organ, the organ sometimes becomes undetectable. This is known as the phantom organ sign.

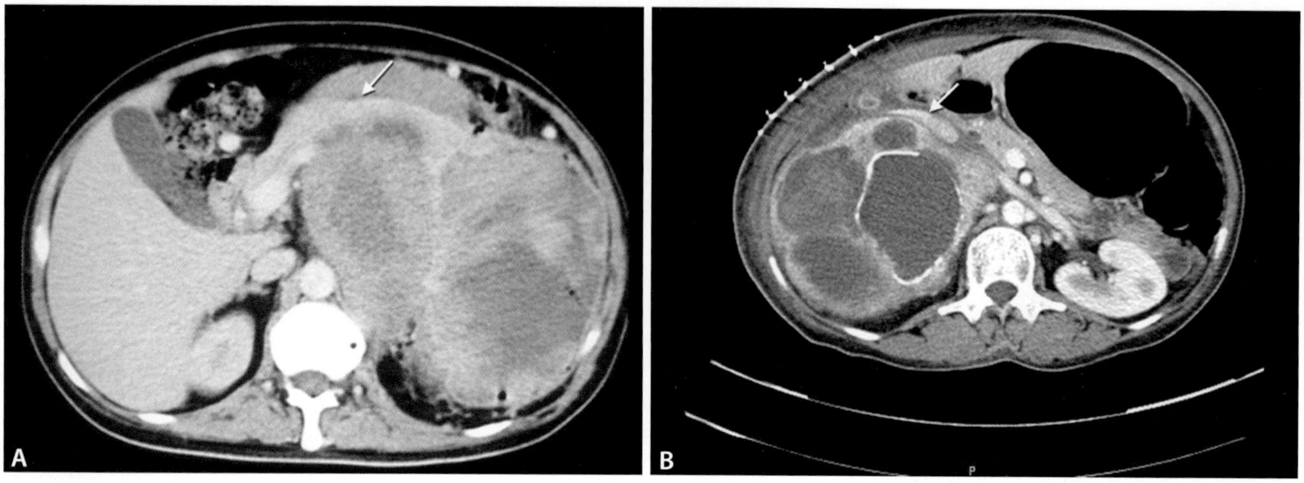

Figs. 20A and B: (A) Anterior displacement of pancreas. Axial CT image shows a large mass that is difficult to localize at first glance. However, anterior displacement of pancreas (arrow) confirms it to be in the retroperitoneal space; (B) Anterior displacement of the IVC. Axial CT image reveals a large, heterogeneous partially cystic right hypochondriac mass with septal calcification on the right. Its retroperitoneal location is suggested by the anterior displacement and stretching of the IVC (arrow). Histopathology revealed a diagnosis of paraganglioma.

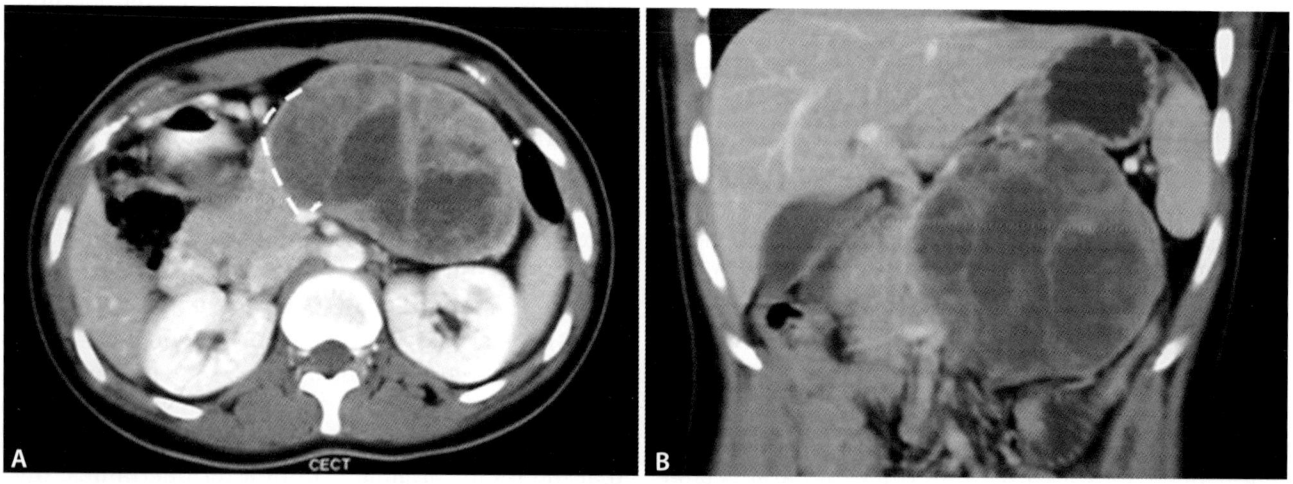

Figs. 21A and B: Beak sign. Axial CT image shows a large cystic tumor with the beak sign in its contact surface with the pancreas (broken white line). This finding represents mucinous cystadenocarcinoma of the pancreas.

However, false-positive findings do exist, as in cases of huge retroperitoneal sarcomas that involve other small organs such as the adrenal gland.

Embedded organ sign: When a tumor compresses an adjacent plastic organ (e.g. gastrointestinal tract, inferior vena cava) that is not the organ of origin, the organ is deformed into a crescent shape. In contrast, when part of an organ appears to be embedded in the tumor (positive embedded organ sign) at the contact surface, it is likely to be the organ of origin **(Fig. 22)**.

Malignant Neoplasms

Malignant tumors of the retroperitoneum are roughly four times more frequent than benign lesions, in sharp contrast to neoplasms occurring elsewhere in the body, where benign lesions predominate.[32]

Liposarcoma is the most frequent primary retroperitoneal malignant tumor followed by malignant fibrous histiocytoma.[33] Leiomyosarcomas are encountered slightly less often and a variety of other neoplasms (fibrosarcomas, malignant teratomas, rhabdomyosarcomas and

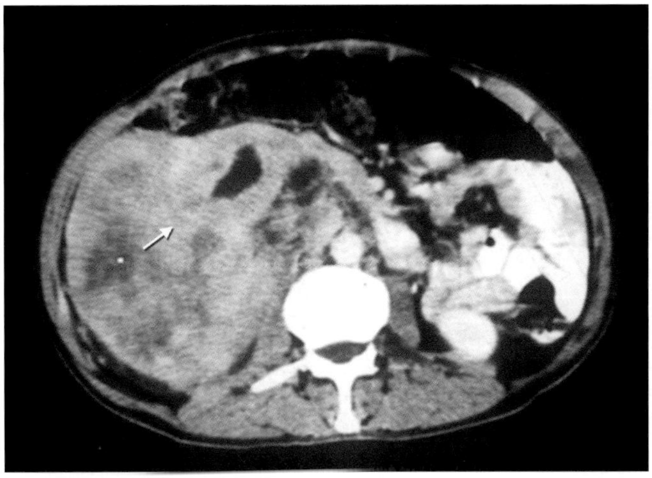

Fig. 22: Embedded organ sign. CT image shows a huge heterogeneous mass in the right side of abdomen. The lumen of the duodenum is stretched toward the mass, and the wall of the duodenum appears embedded in the mass at the contact surface (arrow). These findings represent gastrointestinal stromal tumor of the duodenum with a positive-embedded organ sign.

hemangiopericytomas) are seen only occasionally. Most primary retroperitoneal tumors arise in front of the plane of the spine and psoas muscle and despite their retroperitoneal location some may project forward as far as the anterior abdominal wall. Less commonly tumors arise in the paraspinal or posterior pararenal part of the retroperitoneal space.

Percutaneous core biopsy is often required for the complete histological analysis of these tumors and their distinction from lymphoma. Although biopsy may identify the cell type of a retroperitoneal tumor, treatment and prognosis are not affected by specific cell type. Only surgical resectability and tumor grade affect patient survival. The only consistently effective treatment for primary retroperitoneal sarcomas is operative resection. The role of imaging is to determine the tumor location and extent. It is essential to determine which organs are definitely or possibly invaded by the tumor for planning appropriate therapy.

Primary retroperitoneal sarcomas have a high rate of recurrence after local resection, even when the surgical margins are negative for tumor. Seventy five percent of recurrences typically appear within 2 years of initial surgery. The most effective treatment of recurrent retroperitoneal sarcomas is additional surgical resection. Therefore it is beneficial to have a close imaging follow-up so that recurrences can be identified when still small in size, improving the likelihood of complete resection. All patients should undergo baseline imaging CT or MRI 6 months after the initial surgical resection. Subsequently patients with grade I tumors should undergo annual imaging and patients with grade II or III tumors should undergo biannual imaging for 5 years. Thereafter, all patients should undergo annual imaging because recurrences of low- and high-grade tumors may appear late in some patients.[34]

Liposarcomas

CT or MRI can suggest a diagnosis of liposarcoma when fat is detected within a retroperitoneal mass. The amount of fat seen in liposarcomas varies widely. Three types of retroperitoneal liposarcomas are encountered, viz. well-differentiated also known as lipogenic liposarcomas, myxoid and undifferentiated.[35] On CT well-differentiated liposarcomas are predominantly of fat density and contain irregular strands of higher density **(Figs. 23A and B)**. The tumors often merge imperceptibly with adjacent normal fat and usually displace rather than invade adjacent organs. Myxoid liposarcomas have density less than muscle but greater than fat. Undifferentiated liposarcomas are indistinguishable from nonfatty soft tissue sarcomas **(Figs. 24A and B)**. It may not be possible to definitively differentiate retroperitoneal liposarcomas from benign lipomas, although some CT or MRI findings suggest that a fatty mass is more likely to be malignant than benign. These findings include identification of soft tissue septa more than 2 mm thick within a fatty retroperitoneal mass, septal irregularity or bulging and obvious enhancement.[36]

Leiomyosarcomas

Leiomyosarcomas are large, heterogeneous masses with foci of hemorrhage, necrosis and cystic degeneration **(Fig. 25)**.[37] They do not contain fat or calcification. Not infrequently, retroperitoneal leiomyosarcomas extend into the retroperitoneal veins and IVC.

Malignant Fibrous Histiocytomas

Malignant fibrous histiocytomas are high grade connective tissue tumors. They are multilobulated, infiltrative, unencapsulated but deceptively well circumscribed masses. They may contain myxoid stroma, fibrous tissue, hemorrhage and necrosis giving rise to a typical mosaic of mixed low, intermediate and high signal intensity on T2-weighted MRI images. Although both myxoid stroma and necrosis have similar T1 and T2 signal intensity, differentiation may be possible as myxoid stroma shows delayed enhancement in contrast to the nonenhancing necrotic areas. Up to 25% of malignant fibrous

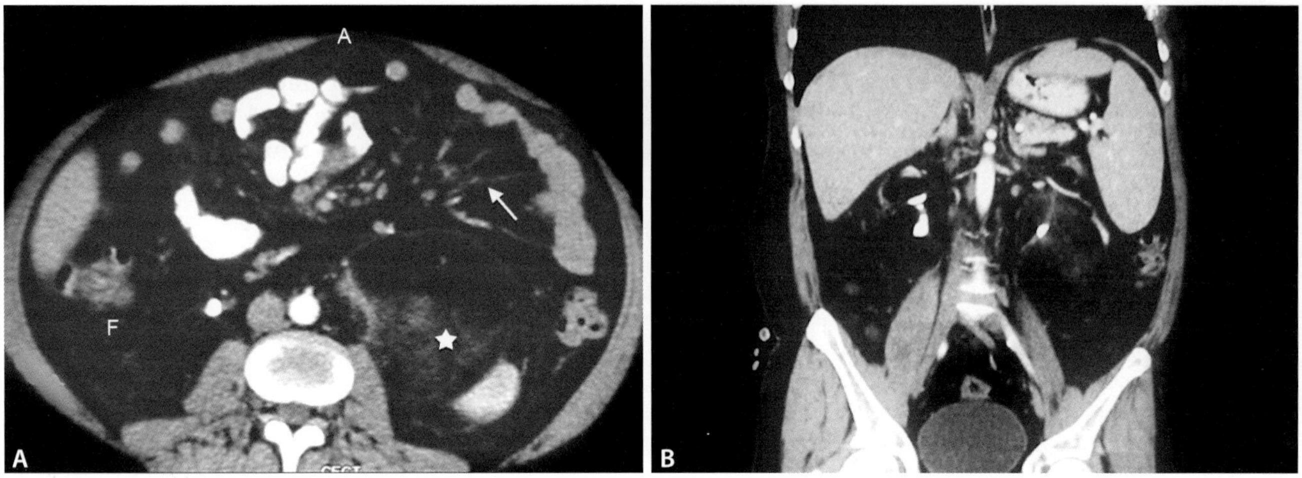

Figs. 23A and B: Retroperitoneal well-differentiated liposarcoma in a 60-year-old man with a history of increasing abdominal girth. Axial and coronal CT images show a diffusely infiltrative, retroperitoneal and abdominal mass composed of fat (F) with Hounsfield (HU) measurements of –80 to –120. There are multiple thick septa (arrow) and a posterior soft tissue component (star) with mildly higher attenuation.

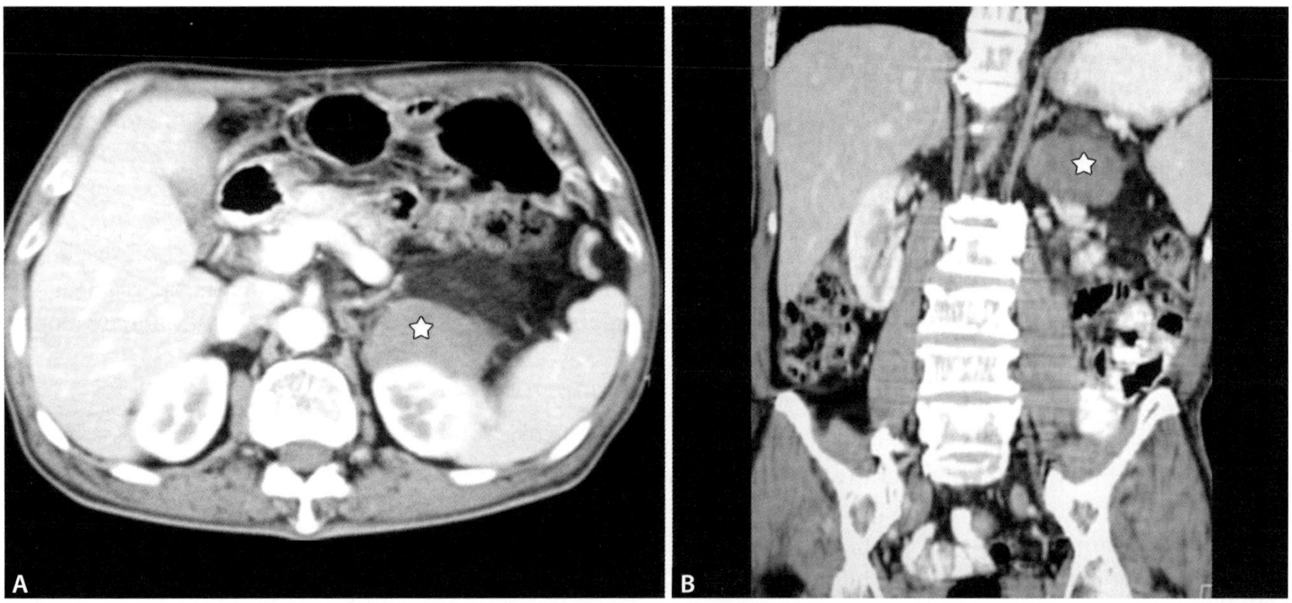

Figs. 24A and B: Poorly-differentiated retroperitoneal liposarcoma. Axial and coronal CT images show a predominantly homogeneous soft tissue density mass (star) anterior to the left kidney. The CT appearance is indistinguishable from other retroperitoneal soft tissue sarcomas. Histopathology revealed a diagnosis of poorly-differentiated liposarcoma

histiocytomas contain dystrophic calcification, a finding that is extremely uncommon in other retroperitoneal malignancies.[33]

Hemangiopericytomas

Hemangiopericytomas are highly vascular tumors thought to arise from blood vessel walls. They may demonstrate areas of intratumoral hemorrhage and multiple flow voids on MRI. Hemangiopericytomas enhance rapidly and intensely on dynamic contrast-enhanced CT or MRI.

Other Malignancies

Fibrosarcomas and neurofibrosarcomas are usually heterogeneous and thus identical in appearance to leiomyosarcomas, some liposarcomas and malignant fibrous histiocytomas. Neuroblastomas and

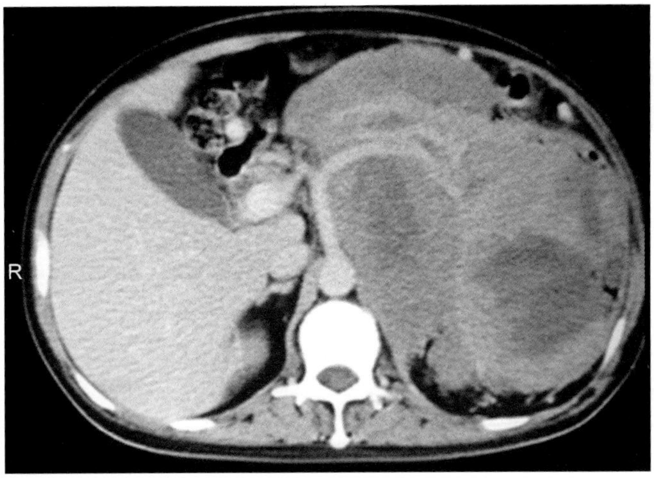

Fig. 25: Retroperitoneal leiomyosarcoma. Axial CT image shows a huge, heterogeneous, soft tissue density retroperitoneal mass on the left. Biopsy revealed it to be a leiomyosarcoma. Any non-fat containing retroperitoneal malignancy may have this appearance.

ganglioneuroblastomas often contain calcification. They are usually seen in children. Rhabdomyosarcomas are rare, heterogeneous tumors, also seen in pediatric patients.

Benign Neoplasms

Most benign lesions originate from neural tissue or neural crest remnants (neurofibroma, schwannoma, ganglioneuroma, and paraganglioma). Hemangioma, lymphangioma, lipoma, teratoma and desmoid tumors are the other benign tumors encountered in the retroperitoneum.

Paragangliomas

Majority of paragangliomas (extra-adrenal pheochromocytoma) lie in the retroperitoneum, in the immediate para-aortic region, from the level of the adrenal glands to the aortic bifurcation. Paragangliomas are well defined soft tissue masses, usually quite large at the time of diagnosis **(Figs. 26A and B)**. Paragangliomas are homogeneous when small, but become increasingly heterogeneous as they grow due to central necrosis, hemorrhage and even calcification.[38] On MR images, paragangliomas often demonstrate extremely high signal intensity on T2 weighted images. Paragangliomas are generally hypervascular and most enhance briskly after injection of IV contrast material.

Neurogenic Tumors

Neurogenic tumors are often located adjacent to the vertebral column or deep to the psoas muscles. MRI is the imaging modality of choice for imaging of these tumors as it detects tumor extension into the neural foramina, a common feature of neurogenic tumors **(Fig. 27)**. MRI also helps in the characterization of these masses, as they tend to have high signal intensity on T2 weighted, due to the myxoid stroma they contain. Central low to intermediate signal intensity may be seen corresponding to fibrous tissue and is referred to as the 'target sign'. Sometimes a whorled appearance consisting of linear or curvilinear structures of low signal intensity is seen on T2-weighted images. At histopathological analysis, this finding corresponds to bundles of Schwann cells and collagen fibres within the mass. Varying degrees of contrast enhancement in neurogenic tumors have been reported, from slight to moderate to marked with delayed heterogeneous uptake of contrast. These enhancement features are explained by the presence of abundant myxoid material in these tumors, resulting in delayed progressive accumulation of contrast material in the extracellular space.[39]

Schwannomas are the most common neurogenic soft tissue tumors occurring in the retroperitoneum. They usually appear as well-defined, heterogeneous soft tissue masses. Although they may contain cystic areas, they usually have large solid components. Retroperitoneal neurofibromas are commonly seen in patients with neurofibromatosis. On CT, neurofibromas appear as well-defined, sharply marginated, homogeneous masses that demonstrate near-water attenuation. Ganglioneuromas arise from sympathetic ganglia and are composed of mature Schwann cells, ganglion cells and nerve fibers. Predominantly children and young adults (60% of cases) are affected and the prognosis is excellent, recurrence being rare after surgical resection. At CT or MRI, ganglioneuromas appear as well-circumscribed oval, crescentic, or lobulated masses. These tumors tend to partially or completely surround major blood vessels, with little or no compromise of the lumen. At unenhanced CT, the tumors appear homogeneous, with attenuation less than that of muscle. They contain calcification in about 20% of cases. The calcifications are discrete and punctate rather than amorphous and coarse as in neuroblastomas.

Teratomas

Teratomas are congenital neoplasms containing components of all three germ layers. CT often shows calcification or even osseous elements. Fat may be seen on both CT and MRI **(Fig. 28)**. Sometimes, a dermoid plug is identifiable as a soft tissue mural nodule projecting

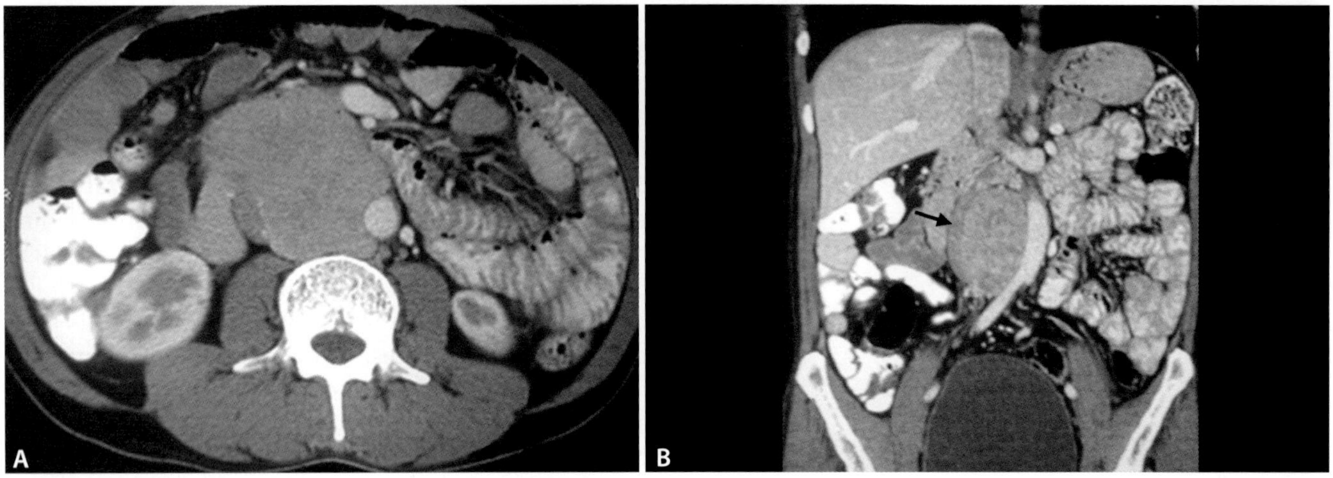

Figs. 26A and B: Retroperitoneal paraganglioma: (A) Axial CT image shows large homogeneous soft tissue density mass in the aortocaval region; (B) Coronal image shows the IVC draping around the right lateral margin of the mass (arrow).

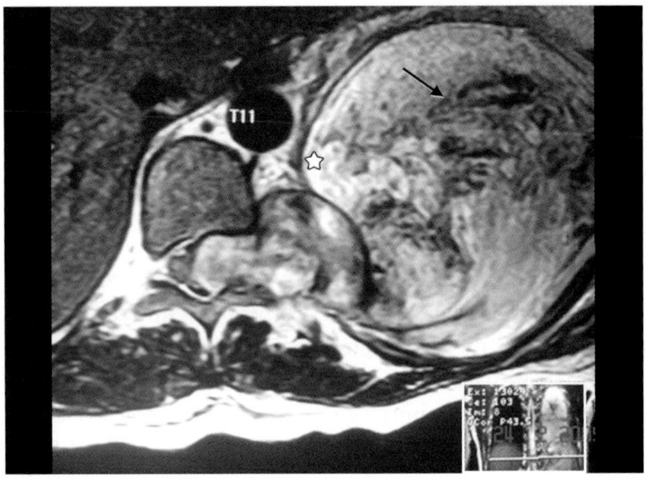

Fig. 27: Intraspinal extension of schwannoma. T2-weighted axial MR image shows a smoothly encapsulated, large heterogeneous intensity mass in the left paraspinal location. It has extended inside the extradural compartment of the spinal canal. The markedly hyperintense area (star) represents myxoid stroma. The linear, low signal intensity areas, having a somewhat whorled appearance (arrow), correspond to bundles of Schwann cells and collagen fibers within the mass.

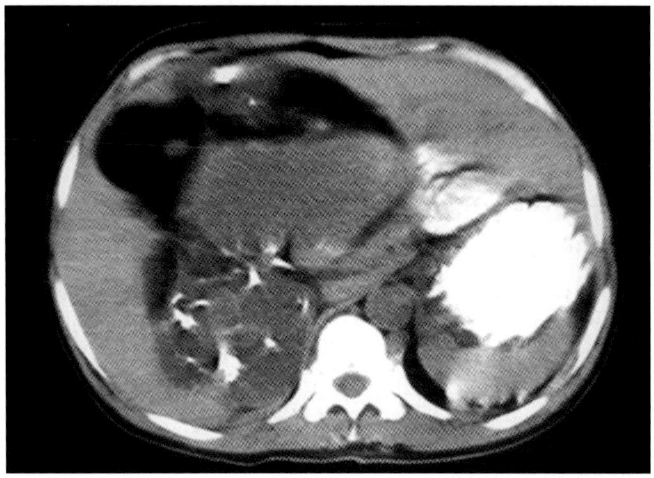

Fig. 28: Retroperitoneal teratoma. Axial CT image reveals a large heterogeneous mass containing elements that show the attenuation of fluid, fat, soft tissue and calcification.

into a cyst. The incidence of malignant degeneration is rare (<1%) and usually occurs in the dermoid plug in postmenopausal women.

Lipoma

Lipoma is a benign mesenchymal tumor that resembles normal fat. Lipomas typically demonstrate homogeneous fatty attenuation at CT and homogeneous signal intensity identical to that of fat with all MR imaging sequences. Thin fibrous septa of low signal intensity on T1- and T2-weighted images may traverse the lesion. Some lipomas have prominent fibrous septa and nodularity and may mimic well-differentiated liposarcomas at imaging.

RETROPERITONEAL FIBROSIS

Retroperitoneal fibrosis results from proliferation of fibrous tissue in the midline and para-aortic distribution. Approximately 70% cases of retroperitoneal fibrosis are idiopathic and are known as Ormond's disease. Other causes include various drugs (e.g. methysergide), previous abdominal surgery or radiation therapy, aortic hemorrhage, aortitis, aortic atherosclerosis, extravasation of urine, nonspecific gastrointestinal inflammation including appendicitis and diverticulitis, infective pathologies including tuberculosis, histoplasmosis, syphilis and actinomycosis. Retroperitoneal fibrosis may be a part of multifocal fibrosclerosis in which fibrous pseudotumor of the orbit, Riedel's thyroiditis, sclerosing cholangitis and mediastinal fibrosis may also occur. Retroperitoneal malignancy especially metastases may also produce retroperitoneal fibrosis by producing a desmoplastic reaction to the tumor cells.[40]

Idiopathic retroperitoneal fibrosis most commonly occur in patients between 40 and 60 years of age. Males are affected twice as commonly as females. Fibrous plaque typically extends from below the level of the kidneys to the bifurcation of great vessels. The fibrous tissue may involve the inferior vena cava, aorta, ureters and occasionally the iliac and renal veins in a symmetric or asymmetric distribution. Microscopically, collagen fibroblasts and inflammatory cells characterize idiopathic retroperitoneal fibrosis.

The clinical and laboratory findings of idiopathic retroperitoneal fibrosis are nonspecific and include fever, back pain and raised erythrocyte sedimentation rate. Most patients have impaired renal functions.

Excretory urography typically demonstrates bilateral hydronephrosis, which may be asymmetric and sometimes even unilateral. Retrograde studies demonstrate smooth tapering of the ureters that is most pronounced at the pelvic brim **(Fig. 29)**. The involvement may vary from focal to a long segment of ureter. Despite ureteral narrowing, there is no obstruction to retrograde passage of catheter in the ureter.

US demonstrates retroperitoneal fibrosis as a poorly demarcated periaortic mass that is typically echo-free or hypoechoic. Associated hydronephrosis may be seen. CT appearance of the fibrous plaque varies considerably: It can be midline or asymmetric, well circumscribed or poorly defined, localized or extensive **(Figs. 30A to C)**.

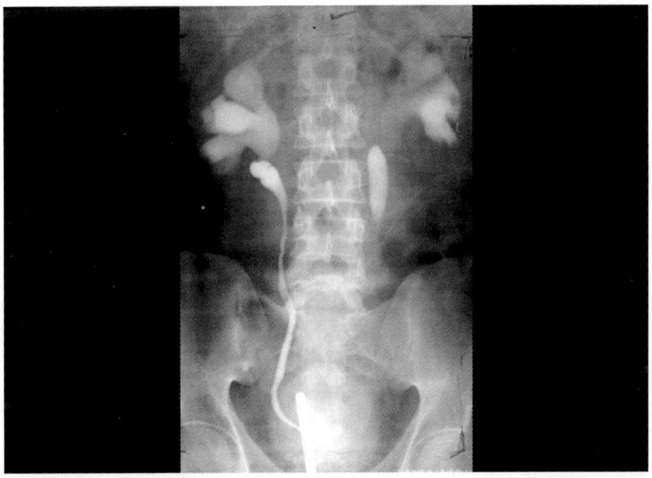

Fig. 29: Retrograde pyelography showing medial deviation of both ureters with hydroureteronephrosis in a patient with idiopathic retroperitoneal fibrosis.

Contrast enhancement varies with the age of the process, while increased enhancement is seen in early stages due to vascularity of the immature fibrosis, chronic fibrosis does not enhance appreciably. MRI may permit distinction between benign or non-neoplastic retroperitoneal fibrosis and malignant retroperitoneal fibrosis. In non-malignant retroperitoneal fibrosis low or intermediate signal intensity on T1 and T2 weighted images has been reported in contrast to higher signal intensity in most malignancies on T2W images **(Fig. 31)**. However, it has been recognized that benign retroperitoneal fibrosis also can have high signal intensity on T2-weighted images when it is in the active, inflammatory stage. MRI also demonstrates effect of the fibrotic mass on the aorta and inferior vena cava.

Iliopsoas Muscle Compartment

Diseases affecting the iliopsoas muscle more commonly originate from adjacent structures and involve the muscle by direct extension. These include hemorrhage, infections and tumors of the spine, kidneys, bowel, pancreas and retroperitoneal lymph nodes. The iliopsoas is well evaluated by both CT and MRI. Coronal or sagittal planes provide direct evaluation of the full craniocaudal extent of the muscle.

Tuberculous spondylitis and lumbar discitis are the commonest cause of an iliopsoas abscess in our country. Iliopsoas inflammatory masses display a variety of appearances, ranging from diffuse homogeneous enlargement to discrete masses containing central areas of low CT attenuation or high signal intensity on T2-weighted MR images. Postcontrast images show abscesses as expansile lesions with non-enhancing necrotic centers, intense peripheral enhancement and enhancement of the surrounding tissues **(Figs. 32A and B)**. Calcification is detected occasionally on CT in inflammatory masses, particularly in patients with tuberculosis. MRI scores over CT in detecting intraspinal extension of the inflammatory granulation tissue and cord compression.

Neoplastic involvement of psoas muscle may occur with contiguous spread from metastatic lymph nodes from primary neoplasms (of kidney, testis, bladder and cervix), lymphoma, renal cell carcinoma and retroperitoneal sarcoma. Primary neoplasms of the psoas muscle are rare. Iliopsoas malignancies often appear similar to other pathologies on imaging. The affected muscle is usually enlarged. As with abscesses, iliopsoas tumor may have enhancing peripheral rims and central necrosis **(Fig. 33)**. A specific diagnosis is possible only when a large solid enhancing component is seen.

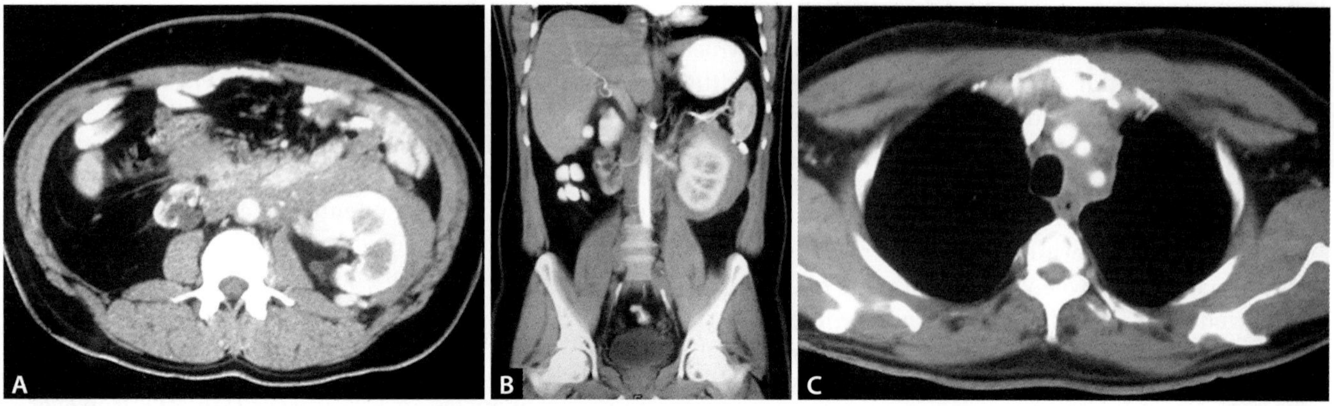

Figs. 30A to C: Retroperitoneal fibrosis. (A) Contrast-enhanced axial CT image shows hypodense, nonenhancing, infiltrating mass surrounding the aorta and IVC and extending into the left perirenal space. Right kidney is shrunken and hydronephrotic; (B) Coronal image shows the entire extent of the plaque like, perirenal soft tissue. Appearance is nonspecific and differentials include malignancy such as lymphoma. Diagnosis was confirmed by biopsy; (C) CT scan through the chest shows evidence of mediastinal fibrosis, a frequent association of retroperitoneal fibrosis.

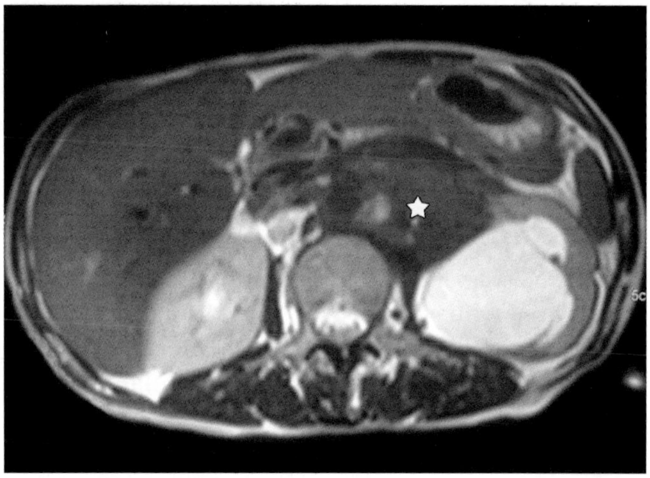

Fig. 31: Retroperitoneal fibrosis. Axial T2-weighted MR image shows a very hypointense mass (star), a finding consistent with the presence of mature fibrous tissue with little or no active inflammation.

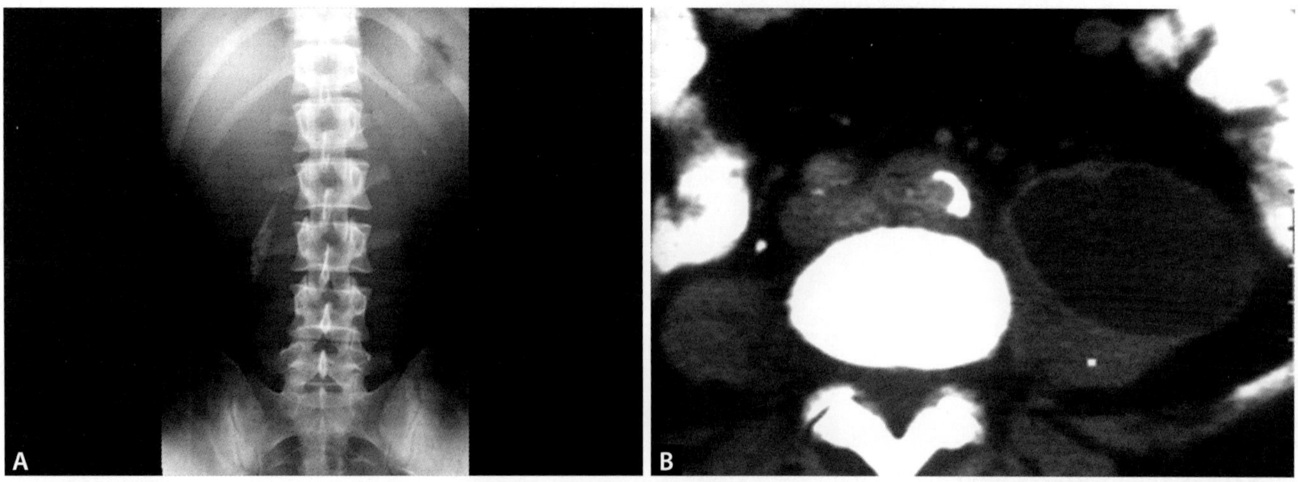

Figs. 32A and B: Psoas abscess. CT image shows a well-defined, fluid density lesion in the left psoas muscle. It has a thin, peripheral enhancing rim and large necrotic center

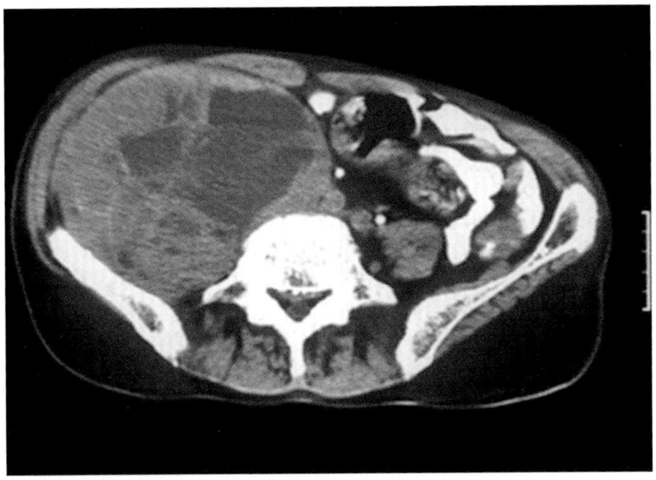

Fig. 33: Anaplastic carcinoma iliopsoas. Axial CT image shows a largest mass involving the right iliacus muscle. The large, irregular, solid component within the mass raises a possibility of malignancy.

REFERENCES

1. Korobkin M, Silverman PM, Quint LE, Francis IR. CT of the extraperitoneal space: normal anatomy and fluid collections. Am J Roentgenol. 1992;159:933-42.
2. Raptopoulos V, Kleinman PK, Marks S Jr, Snyder M, Silverman PM. Renal fascial pathway: posterior extension of pancreatic effusions within the anterior pararenal space. Radiology. 1986;158(2):367-74.
3. Molmenti EP, Balfe DM, Kanterman RY, Bennett HF. Anatomy of the retroperitoneum: observations of the distribution of pathologic fluid collections. Radiology. 1996;200(1):95-103.
4. Raptopoulos V, Lei QF, Touliopoulos P, Vrachliotis TG, Marks SC JR. Why perirenal disease does not extend into the pelvis: the importance of closure of the cone of the renal fasciae. Am J Roentgenol. 1995;164 (5):1179-84.
5. Aizensterin RL, Owens C, Sabris S, et al. The perinephric space and renal fascia. Review of normal anatomy, pathology and pathways of disease spread. Crit Rev Diagnost Imaging. 1997;38:325-67.
6. Gore RM, Balfe DM, Aizenstein RI, Silverman PM. The great escape: interfascial decompression planes of the retroperitoneum. AJR Am J Roentgenol. 2000;175(2):363-70.
7. Kang PS, Spain JW. Multidetector CT angiography of the abdomen. Radiol Clin North Am. 2005;43(6):963-76.
8. Kandpal H, Sharma R, Gamangatti S, Srivastava DN, Vashisht S. Imaging the inferior vena cava: a road less traveled. Radiographics. 2008;28(3): 669-89.
9. Glockner JF. Three-dimensional gadolinium-enhanced MR angiography: applications for abdominal imaging. Radiographics. 2001; 21(2):357-70.
10. Vesselle HJ, Miraldi FD. FDG PET of the retroperitoneum: normal anatomy, variants, pathologic conditions and strategies to avoid diagnostic pitfalls. Radiographics. 1998;18(4): 805-23.
11. Ishikawa K, Idoguchi K, Tanaka H, Tohma Y, Ukai I, Watanabe H, Matsuoka T, Yokota J, Sugimoto T. Classification of acute pancreatitis based on retroperitoneal extension: application of the concept of interfascial planes. Eur J Radiol. 2006;60(3):445-52.
12. Missiroli C, Singh AK. Nontraumatic emergencies of abdominal aorta. Semin Ultrasound CT MR. 2008;29(5):369-77.
13. Taneja K, Sharma S, Das B, et al. Aortic aneurysms and dissections: Imaging with computerised tomography. Indian Journal of Thoracic and Cardiovascular Surgery. 1994;10:52-6.
14. Rakita D, Newatia A, Hines JJ, Siegel DN, Friedman B. Spectrum of CT findings in rupture and impending rupture of abdominal aortic aneurysms. Radiographics. 2007;27(2):497-507.
15. Anagnostopolous CE, Prabhakar MJ, Kittle CF. Aortic dissections and dissecting aneurysm. Am J Cardiol. 1972;30:263-73.
16. Aljabri B, MacDonald PS, Satin R, Stein LS, Obrand DI, Steinmetz OK. Incidence of major venous and renal anomalies relevant to aortoiliac surgery as demonstrated by computed tomography. Ann Vasc Surg. 2001;15(6): 615-8.
17. Onba_ O, Kantarci M, Koplay M, Olgun H, Alper F, Aydinli B, et al. Congenital anomalies of the aorta and vena cava: 16-detector-row CT imaging findings. Diagn Interv Radiol. 2008;14(3):163-71.
18. Cuevas C, Raske M, Bush WH, Takayama T, Maki JH, Kolokythas O, Meshberg E. Imaging primary and secondary tumor thrombus of the inferior vena cava: multidetector computed tomography and magnetic resonance imaging. Curr Probl Diagn Radiol. 2006;35(3):90-101.
19. Lawrentschuk N, Gani J, Riordan R, Esler S, Bolton DM. Multidetector computed tomography vs magnetic resonance imaging for defining the upper limit of tumour thrombus in renal cell carcinoma: a study and review. BJU Int. 2005;96(3): 291-5.
20. Alfuhaid TR, Khalili K, Kirpalani A, Haider MA, Wilson SR, Daneman A. Neoplasms of the inferior vena cava—pictorial essay. Can Assoc Radiol J. 2005;56(3):140-7.
21. Hulnick D, Megibow A, Naidich D, et al. Abdominal tuberculosis: CT evaluation. Radiology. 1985;157:199-204.
22. Warshauer DM, Lee JK. Imaging manifestations of abdominal sarcoidosis. Am J Roentgenol. 2004;182(1):15-28.
23. Gossios K, Nikolaides C, Bai M, Fountzilas G. Widespread. Castleman disease: CT findings. Eur Radiol. 1996;6(1):95-8.
24. Kehagias D, Pafiti A, Vaos N, Samanidis L. Retroperitoneal lymphangioleiomyomatosis: CT appearance. Eur Radiol 1998.
25. Sheth S, Fishman EK. Non-Hodgkin lymphoma: pattern of disease at spiral CT. Crit Rev Diagn Imaging. 2001;42(6): 307-56.
26. Apter S, Avigdor A, Gayer G, Portnoy O, Zissin R, Hertz M. Calcification in lymphoma occurring before therapy: CT features and clinical correlation. Am J Roentgenol. 2002;178(4): 935-8.

27. Schöder H, Moskowitz C. PET imaging for response assessment in lymphoma: potential and limitations. Radiol Clin North Am. 2008; 46(2):225-41.
28. Specht L. 2-[18F] fluoro-2-deoxyglucose positron emission tomography in staging, response evaluation and treatment planning of lymphomas. Semin Radiat Oncol. 2007;17:190-7.
29. Radin R. HIV infection: analysis in 259 consecutive patients with abnormal abdominal CT findings. Radiology. 1995;197: 712.
30. Bellin MF, Lebleu L, Meric JB. Evaluation of retroperitoneal and pelvic lymph node metastases with MRI and MR lymphangiography. Abdom Imaging. 2003;28:155-63.
31. Minami M, Ohmoto K, Charnsangavej C, Kawauchi N, Itai Y, Sasaki S. Origin of abdominal tumors: useful findings and signs on tomographic imaging. Radiology. 1996;201:491-9.
32. Lane RH, Stephens DH, Reiman HM. Primary retroperitoneal neoplasms: CT findings in 90 cases with clinical and pathologic correlation. Am J Roentgenol. 1989;152(1):83-9.
33. Cohan RH, Baker ME, Cooper C, Moore JO, Saeed M, Dunnick NR. Computed tomography of primary retroperitoneal malignancies. J Comput Assist Tomogr. 1988;12(5):804-10.
34. Gupta AK, Cohan RH, Francis IR, Sondak VK, Korobkin M. CT of recurrent retroperitoneal sarcomas. Am J Roentgenol. 2000;174:1025-30.
35. Craig WD, Fanburg-Smith JC, Henry LR, Guerrero R, Barton JH. Fat-containing lesions of the retroperitoneum: radiologic-pathologic correlation. Radiographics. 2009;29:261-90.
36. Song T, Shen J, Liang BL, Mai WW, Li Y, Guo HC. Retroperitoneal liposarcoma: MR characteristics and pathological correlative analysis. Abdom Imaging. 2007;32:668-74.
37. Hartman DS, Hayes WS, Choyke PL, Tibbetts GP. From the archives of the AFIP. Leiomyosarcoma of the retroperitoneum and inferior vena cava: radiologic-pathologic correlation. Radiographics. 1992;12:1203-20.
38. Lee KY, Oh YW, Noh HJ, Lee YJ, Yong HS, Kang EY, et al. Extraadrenal paragangliomas of the body: imaging features. Am J Roentgenol. 2006;187:492-504.
39. Rha SE, Byun JY, Jung SE, Chun HJ, Lee HG, Lee JM. Neurogenic tumors in the abdomen: tumor types and imaging characteristics. Radiographics. 2003;23:29-43.
40. Cronin CG, Lohan DG, Blake MA, Roche C, McCarthy P, Joseph M. Murphy retroperitoneal fibrosis: A review of clinical features and imaging findings. Am J Roentgenol. 2008;191:423-31.

CHAPTER 119

Nonvascular Interventions in the Urinary Tract

Mandeep Kang, Anupam Lal, Naveen Kalra

INTRODUCTION

The past few decades have witnessed a revolution in the development of minimally invasive procedures, with interventional radiology being in the forefront of these developments. All percutaneous procedures under image guidance are based on the premise that a skinny needle (21–22 gauge) can be inserted into almost any organ part in the body with safety and accuracy. Nonvascular interventions in the urinary tract are well established procedures with the initial description of a percutaneous nephrostomy having appeared in literature more than half a century ago.[1] Propelled by technological advances, minimally invasive uroradiological interventional therapies have altered the day-to-day practice of urology.

PERCUTANEOUS NEPHROSTOMY

Percutaneous nephrostomy (PCN) is the basic technique in interventional uroradiology which provides a direct access to the urinary tract.[2] Besides urinary diversion in an obstructed system, the access can be used to create large bore tracks through which various endourological procedures can be safely performed with fewer complications than open surgical procedures.[3]

Indications

1. *Supravesical urinary tract obstruction*:
   a. Calculus disease
   b. Neoplasm
   c. Ureteral/anastomotic stricture
   d. Pyonephrosis
   e. Assessment of recoverable renal function in chronic obstruction.
2. Urinary diversion for management of a urinary leak or fistula.
3. *Access for subsequent interventions*:
   a. Antegrade ureteric stenting
   b. Nephrolithotomy/lithotripsy
   c. Stone dissolution
   d. Ureteral occlusion for urinary fistula
   e. Biopsy of urothelial lesion/fulguration
   f. Foreign body or fungal ball removal
   g. Whitaker test.

There is no absolute contraindication for PCN with the only relative contraindication being coagulopathy which should be corrected prior to the procedure.

Anatomy Relevant to Percutaneous Renal Entry

Knowledge of renal anatomy is essential for selection of a safe route through the kidney for percutaneous nephrostomy. The main renal artery divides into anterior and posterior divisions with further segmental branches. The anterior division supplies the anterior two-thirds of the renal parenchyma while the posterior division supplies the posterior third. There is a zone of relative avascularity between the two vascular territories known as the Brödel's line of bloodless incision which lies just posterior to the lateral convex border of the kidney **(Fig. 1)**. The ideal access to the collecting system should be through this

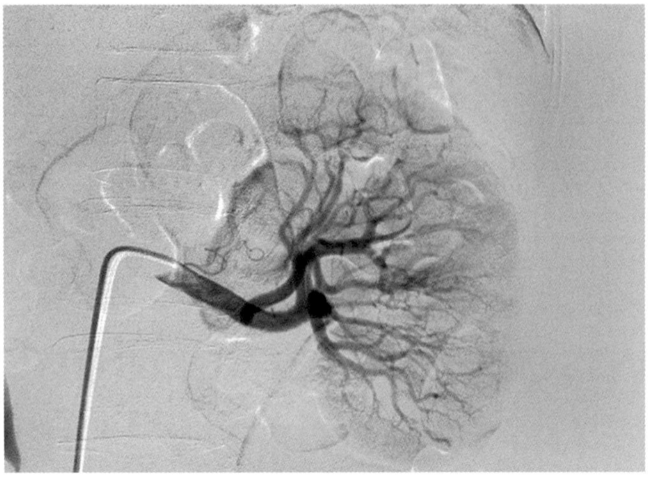

Fig. 1: Vascular anatomy of the kidney: Selective left renal arteriogram 25° left posterior oblique view shows bifurcation of the main renal artery into dorsal and ventral branches. The avascular plane of Brödel lies along the plane of division of these vascular territories.

relatively avascular plane.[4] Because of the normal rotation of the kidneys about their horizontal axis, the posterior calyces are directed posterolaterally with their long axis pointing to this avascular zone; these calyces should ideally be targeted at percutaneous nephrostomy. In the hilum of the kidney, the renal vein, artery and pelvis are located in an anteroposterior orientation. Central puncture of the collecting system should be avoided, only the calyces (which are completely surrounded by renal parenchyma) should be punctured. Central puncture can lead to two problems. Firstly, a major vessel can be injured leading to severe bleeding; secondly, there may be urinary leakage from the catheter tract due to inadequate sealing by renal tissue.[5]

The site of renal entry depends upon the indication for access. A lower pole posterior calyx can be safely accessed using a subcostal approach to avoid transgression of the pleura.[5] However, a posterior calyx of the upper pole or interpolar region provides the easiest access to the pelvi-ureteric junction for subsequent ureteral interventions. In cases of complex stone disease, entry through the posterior calyx of the upper pole allows visualization of most parts of the collecting system.[3]

Technique

An informed consent must be obtained from the patient after explaining in detail the need for the procedure, the procedure itself and the potential complications which can occur. A coagulogram must be performed and abnormalities if any, must be corrected prior to the procedure. Urine analysis to screen for possible urinary infection should also be performed. Prophylactic broad-spectrum antibiotics should be started prior to the procedure in patients with known or potential urinary infection (urinary conduit diversions, obstruction with or without fever, urinary leaks).

PCN is usually performed under fluoroscopic or ultrasound guidance. In certain cases, CT guidance may be used for example in emphysematous pyelonephritis when air in the collecting system obscures visualization on ultrasound. The use of MR guidance has also been described.[6]

The patient is placed prone on the fluoroscopy table with a bolster under the abdomen to fix the kidneys against the posterior abdominal wall and prevent their anterior displacement during the procedure. The back and flanks are cleansed and draped. The calyx to be punctured is chosen depending upon the indication and local anesthetic is infiltrated into the skin and subcutaneous tissues. This is generally adequate for pain relief during the procedure; however, conscious sedation may be required in apprehensive or noncooperative patients. Infants and young children will require general anesthesia.

The chosen calyx can be punctured with an 18 G needle under ultrasound guidance in a dilated system. After removing the stylet, a urine sample should be aspirated for culture. A small volume of iodinated contrast is injected to opacify the collecting system. A 0.035" guidewire is then passed through the needle and negotiated into the pelvis. After a stab incision along the needle tract, the needle is removed and the tract dilated using fascial dilators. For drainage of non-infected urine, catheters of 8–10 F are usually sufficient. The catheter is placed over the guidewire and coiled in the pelvis **(Figs. 2 and 3)**. A check injection of contrast should be done to confirm position of all side holes of the catheter within the collecting system. Pigtail catheters with or without locking devices may be used. The catheter is stabilized at the skin using sutures or other retention devices, connected to a urine collection bag and allowed to drain under gravity.

A variety of techniques may be used for the initial puncture. Some workers inject intravenous iodinated contrast to opacify the collecting system followed by direct puncture of the pelvis under fluoroscopic guidance with a 22 G needle. Iodinated contrast (with or without room air or carbon dioxide) is then injected under fluoroscopic control to opacify the collecting system to a degree necessary to find a suitable calyx. The selected calyx can then be punctured from the posterolateral aspect with an 18 G needle, with the subsequent steps being the same as described before. Another variation of this "two-stick"

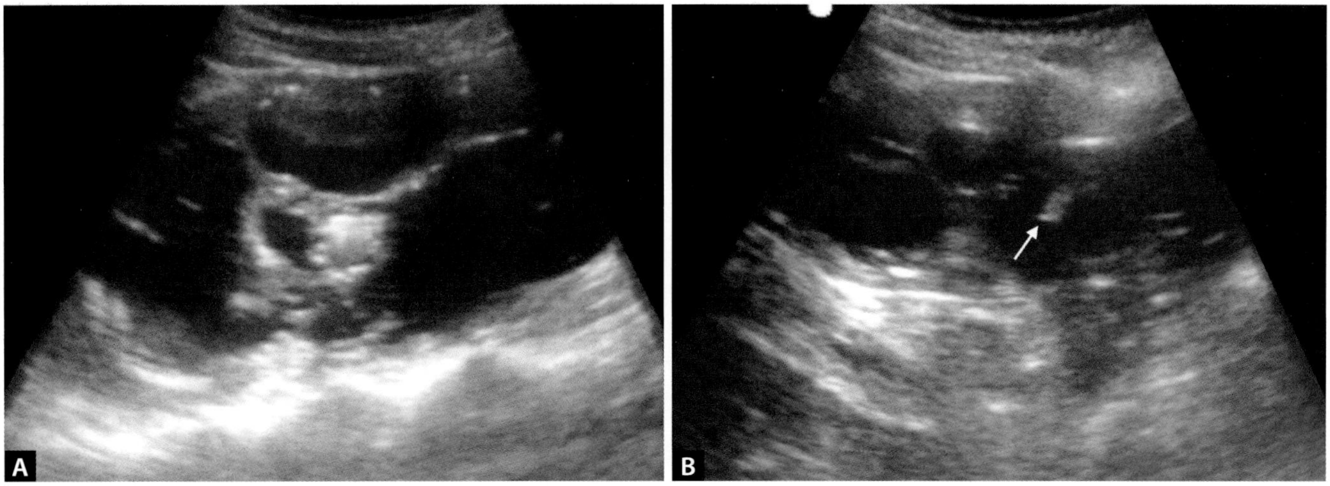

Figs. 2A and B: Percutaneous nephrostomy: (A) Longitudinal sonogram shows gross hydronephrosis with internal echoes suggestive of pyonephrosis; (B) The lower pole calyx has been punctured using an 18 G needle. Needle tip is seen *in situ* (arrow).

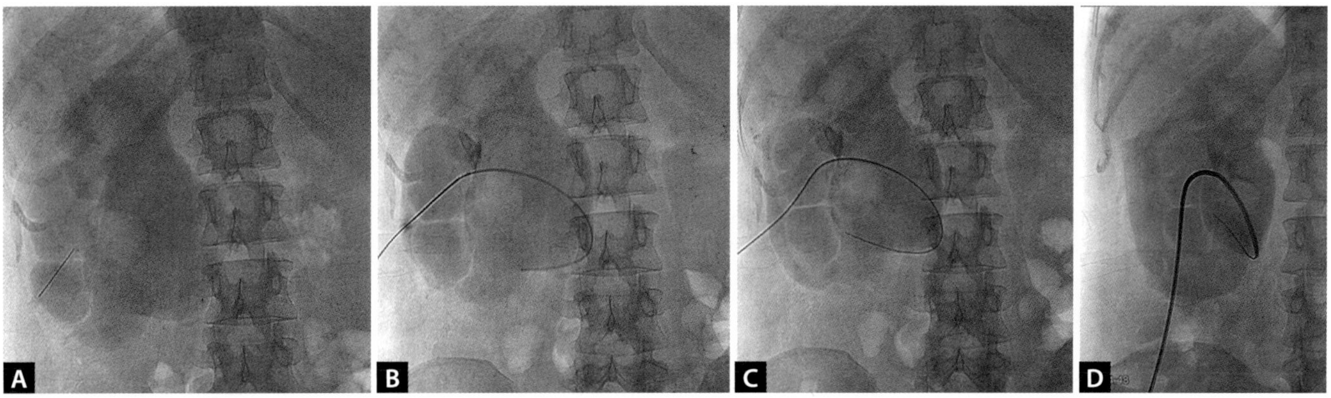

Figs. 3A to D: Percutaneous nephrostomy: (A) The grossly dilated calyces are opacified due to a CECT abdomen done the previous day. These have been directly punctured by an 18 G needle under fluoroscopic guidance; (B) A stiff guidewire has been negotiated into the pelvis; (C) The puncture needle has been withdrawn and the track is being dilated using fascial dilators; (D) An 8 F catheter is being threaded over the guide-wire to coil in the pelvis.

technique is to use a 22 G needle for the second puncture as well, a 0.014" hydrophilic guidewire is passed through this needle over which a 5F percutaneous access set is placed and the guidewire exchanged for a 0.035" stiff or super-stiff Amplatz guidewire.[3,6-8] Regardless of the technique used, care has to be taken not to over-distend the collecting system so as to avoid pyelovenous reflex, particularly in infected systems.

Occasionally, external urinary diversion is necessary in nondilated collecting systems (e.g. in urinary leak or fistulas). These kidneys can be punctured using the double stick technique with initial opacification of the collecting system with intravenous injection of iodinated contrast.[9] Alternatively, these kidneys can also be accessed using sonographic guidance after intravenous injection of frusemide. Even if the calyces do not dilate adequately to be visualized on ultrasound, the renal pelvis can be seen and punctured with a skinny needle, iodinated contrast or saline injected to distend the calyces and a definitive calyceal puncture made with fluoroscopic or US guidance.[10]

Postprocedure Care

Vital signs should be frequently monitored in the immediate post procedure period as there is a potential for ongoing blood loss or the development of septicemic shock (due to pyelovenous reflux and bacteremia) in patients at risk. Ideally, the patient should be admitted overnight for observation after the procedure, during which time the tube should be gently flushed with saline every four hours. Hematuria is initially present after percutaneous nephrostomy in virtually all patients, this usually gradually settles within 24–48 hours. The PCN tube output should be recorded to assess for adequacy of drainage. Appropriate analgesics, including narcotics if required (particularily for patients with intercostal entry) should be provided. The patients should be instructed regarding tube care, especially if long-term drainage is anticipated. The dressing around the catheter should be changed daily. The catheters need to be changed every 6–8 weeks.

Results

Placement of a nephrostomy tube is technically successful in 93–99% of cases in dilated systems. The success rate is lower in patients with nondilated systems, complex stone disease, anatomical variants and renal cysts. Use of CT guidance may improve the technical success in patients with anatomical variants or renal cysts.[11,12]

Complications

These may be divided into systemic and local complications.

Systemic Complications

The most common systemic complication which can at times be fatal is sepsis. Every obstructed system is potentially infected. Manipulation of guidewires, catheter and injection of contrast all lead to an increase in the pressure in the collecting system which can lead to pyelovenous reflux. The incidence of septic complications has been reported to be between 1% and 2.5%.[11,13,14] The incidence rises to 7% in the setting of pyonephrosis.[12] One should avoid overdistention of the system by limiting the amount of contrast injected and also keeping manipulation to a minimum in the initial procedure. Complicated or prolonged procedures should be avoided in an infected system; further imaging and manipulation should be undertaken only 48–72 hours after the initial procedure when the system is adequately decompressed.[3,5,14]

Prone position of the patient during the PCN procedure may lead to respiratory insufficiency, especially in infants or young children under sedation. Good patient monitoring is essential.[5]

Local Complications

The most common local complication is bleeding which may occur from the renal parenchymal vessels or the intercostal vessels. Transient hematuria is observed in almost every patient. Severe bleeding which requires transfusion or intervention is seen in 1–3% of patients.[11] Bleeding noticed at the time of PCN can often be controlled by tamponade of the track with a larger bore nephrostomy catheter. If bleeding persists for 2–3 days, a nephrostogram should be obtained to check for malposition of the catheter. Severe bleeding developing several days after catheter insertion requires further evaluation. A track fistulogram can be obtained by exchanging the nephrostomy catheter with an introducer sheath over a stiff guidewire. The sheath is then gradually withdrawn while injecting contrast. At times, the venous or arterial source of bleed may fill with contrast. Angiographic evaluation for identification of a renal arteriovenous fistula, pseudoaneurysm or vessel laceration should be scheduled without delay in patients with persistent or severe bleeding. Most of these vascular injuries can be managed by the endovascular route, surgical intervention is rarely necessary.[15] Bleeding can lead to a perinephric hematoma which can cause a Page kidney with subsequent deterioration in renal function. This should be drained percutaneously.

Adjacent organs may be inadvertently punctured. A retrorenal colon, an uncommon anatomic variant may be transgressed leading to a nephrocolic fistula. Treatment is conservative and consists of ensuring adequate urinary drainage by placement of an antegrade or retrograde ureteric stent, and withdrawing the nephrostomy catheter into the colon to allow the nephrocolic track to heal.[16] Pleural complications in the form of pneumothorax, pleural effusion, emphysema or hemothorax may occur in 0.1–0.2% of cases. The incidence rises with intercostal entry or complex endourologic procedures.[17]

Catheter block or dislodgement are technical complications which may occur. The blocked catheter should be cleaned with a guidewire and changed. Replacement of a dislodged catheter is usually possible through the previous tract. Many times the whole tract can be opacified by a small amount of dilute contrast injected via a sheath placed at the site of urine leak on the skin. A hydrophilic guidewire is then used to probe the tract which usually finds its way into the collecting system.

Overall, when major and minor complications are considered together, the complication rate is between 10% and 15%. The mortality rate for percutaneous nephrostomy varies from 0.046 to 0.3%.[3,5]

Extended Applications of Percutaneous Nephrostomy

Antegrade Ureteric Stenting

The most common extension of PCN is placement of a ureteric stent for obstruction or fistula. It is often much easier to negotiate areas of narrowing, fistulae or discontinuity in the ureter in an antegrade rather than retrograde manner. The stenting is usually performed under local anesthesia and conscious sedation. After the initial PCN, a safety guidewire is placed through an access sheath to avoid losing renal access during the subsequent manipulation of the working guidewire. Negotiation of an obstructed segment is often facilitated by the use of curved angiographic catheters and hydrophilic guidewires. Once the stricture has been negotiated, the guidewire–catheter combination can be coiled within the bladder and the hydrophilic guidewire exchanged for a super-stiff Amplatz wire **(Figs. 4A to D)**. Determination of the correct length of the ureteric stent required can be done by using the bent guidewire technique. Balloon dilatation of strictures, placement of ureteric stents, postprocedure drainage of the upper urinary tract and subsequent nephrostograms can all be performed via the initial PCN tract. The percutaneous external urinary catheter is left in place for 24 hours after the procedure, after which it is capped. Thereafter, if there is no hydronephrosis on sonography and contrast injection shows free flow down the double J stent, the external catheter is removed.

Balloon dilatation of benign ureteric strictures may provide durable relief in up to 50% of cases. Following the dilatation, the ureter is supported with a stent. In case repeated entry into the ureter may be required, an internal–external stent can be placed for preserving percutaneous access as well as providing mechanical support.[17] Anastomotic strictures after cystectomy and ureteric diversion to an ileal conduit can also be managed through an antegrade percutaneous approach.[18] Internal–external stents are also placed in cases of ureteric leaks or fistulas because of the anticipated need for multiple percutaneous ureteral interventions and prolonged urinary drainage to allow healing. One should ensure that a solid portion of the tube traverses the site of leak with side-holes above and below.

In patients with fistulas of the ureters or lower urinary tract associated with advanced inoperable pelvic malignancies, external drainage with a PCN catheter and urinoma drainage catheter may not provide adequate urinary diversion. Ureteral occlusion can be done using stainless steel or platinum coils deployed in the ureter above the level of leak along with a PCN to provide relief from the distressing symptoms.[19] Other materials which can be used for ureteral occlusion include gelatin sponge, n-butyl cyanoacrylate, detachable balloons or radiofrequency electrocautery.[20] The major drawback is the permanent nature of the occlusion and need for lifelong nephrostomy catheter.

Large Bore Track Creation

PCN forms the first step for creation of a large diameter track which may be necessary for percutaneous stone therapy, nephroscopy, or antegrade ureteroscopy.[21] Tracks of 30 F or larger can be created by using balloon dilatation systems, coaxial dilators or combined balloon-sheath systems. Following the procedure, a large diameter tube (24–30 F) is inserted through the sheath into the kidney to provide urinary drainage and track tamponade and the sheath is removed.

SCLEROTHERAPY FOR RENAL CYSTS

Benign renal cysts (cortical or parapelvic) are found in approximately 50% of males above the age of 50 years.

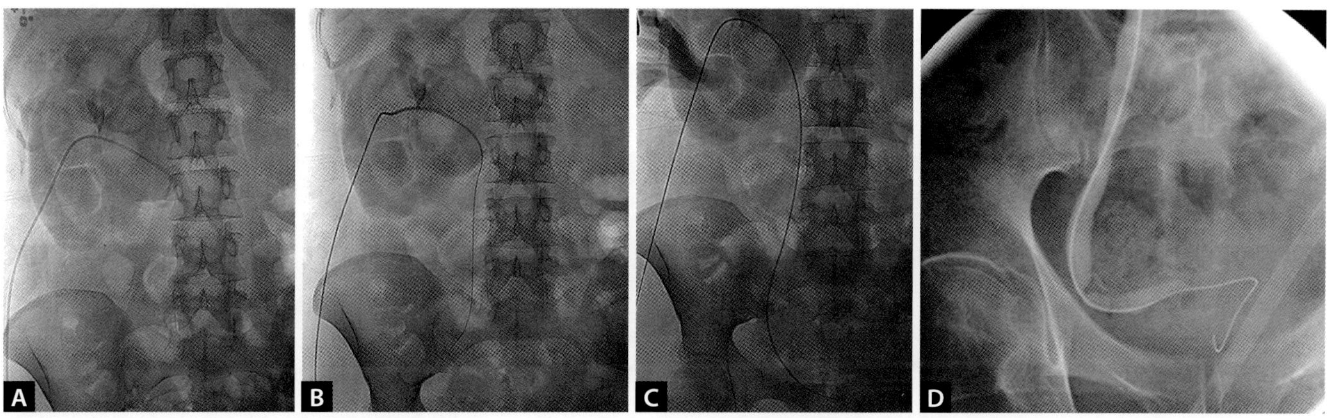

Figs. 4A to D: Antegrade stenting in a patient with carcinoma of the urinary bladder: (A) The PCN catheter has been exchanged for a curved angiographic catheter over a stiff guidewire; (B) A hydrophilic guidewire has been introduced through the catheter and is being negotiated down the ureter; (C) The catheter guidewire combination has been advanced into the urinary bladder; (D) The hydrophilic guidewire has been exchanged for a super-stiff Amplatz guidewire after negotiating a tight stricture at the ureterovesical junction. The ureteric stent is then placed over the stiff guidewire.

Renal cysts vary in size and are frequently multiple. They are usually silent, but large, infected or hemorrhagic cysts can cause symptoms. Large cysts can also cause obstruction of the pelvicalyceal system, pressure atrophy of the adjacent parenchyma and stone formation in obstructed calyces.[7,22]

A symptomatic renal cyst is managed with a combination of percutaneous drainage and sclerotherapy. Various agents which have been used to induce sclerosis of the epithelial lining of the cyst include hypertonic dextrose, hypertonic water-soluble contrast, iophandylate, absolute alcohol, tetracycline and sodium tetradecyl sulfate. The technique consists of puncture of the cyst under sonographic guidance and aspiration of the cyst contents. Contrast is then injected to demonstrate the internal appearance of the cyst and to rule out any communication of the cyst with the collecting system. If no communication is demonstrated and the cyst is small, sclerosant can be injected amounting to about one-third of the aspirated contents of the cyst. The sclerosant is left in place for 15–20 minutes with frequent postural changes of the patient to ensure contact with all the walls of the cyst and then reaspirated. If the cyst is larger, a 5 F percutaneous drainage catheter can be placed in the cyst and left to drain for 24–48 hours before sclerotherapy. Larger cysts may require multiple sessions of sclerotherapy.

If a cyst is communicating with the renal collecting system sclerosant should not be injected as it can cause strictures in the pelicalyceal system. An infected cyst is managed like an abscess with percutaneous catheter drainage. Good outcomes of sclerotherapy in renal cysts are reported with success rates of 75–100%.[7,22]

PERCUTANEOUS CATHETER DRAINAGE

Percutaneous catheter drainage (PCD) can be done to drain renal or perirenal abscesses, collections, lymphoceles or urinomas. The basic technique is similar to PCN consisting of needle puncture under imaging guidance, guidewire insertion, track dilatation and catheter placement **(Figs. 5A to C)**. The size and type of drainage catheter should be chosen according to the nature of fluid to be drained.

BIOPSIES

Core biopsy with an automated gun is more common than fine needle aspiration (FNA) in the genitourinary tract. Renal biopsy with a 16–18 G gun is used in cases of renal parenchymal disease. Biopsy or FNA can be performed for genitourinary tumors. Transrectal ultrasound guided biopsy of the prostate is useful in suspected cases of prostatic carcinoma.

COMPLICATED RENAL TRANSPLANT

Common complications in renal transplant recipients include graft rejection, perigraft or pelvic fluid collections (urinomas, lymphoceles, etc.), ureterovesical anastomotic strictures and focal parenchymal lesions. The percutaneous procedures required in this group of patients are similar to those required in native kidneys. The transplant kidney is approached from the lateral aspect with the patient supine **(Figs. 6A to D)**. These patients are usually very sick and immunocompromised, therefore, meticulous attention should be paid to antiasepsis.

RADIOFREQUENCY ABLATION OF RENAL TUMORS

The incidence of renal cell carcinoma (RCC) has been seen to rise in recent years. This is probably due to the increasing use of abdominal imaging and improvements in CT and MR technology resulting in the incidental detection of small, asymptomatic renal tumours in patients undergoing imaging for other indications. Recent

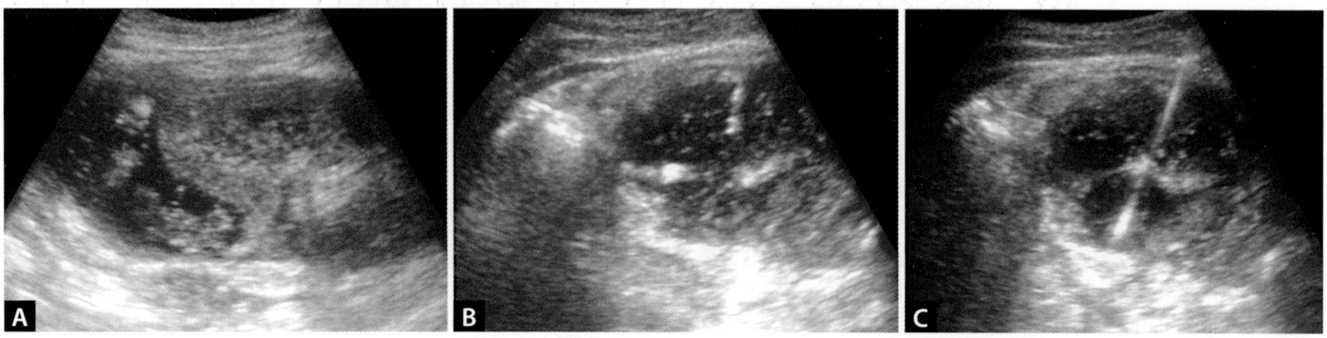

Figs. 5A to C: (A) An irregular collection with debris and internal echoes is seen in the upper pole of the kidney suggestive of renal abscess; (B) The abscess has been punctured with an 18 gauge needle; (C) Guidewire is seen coiled in the abscess.

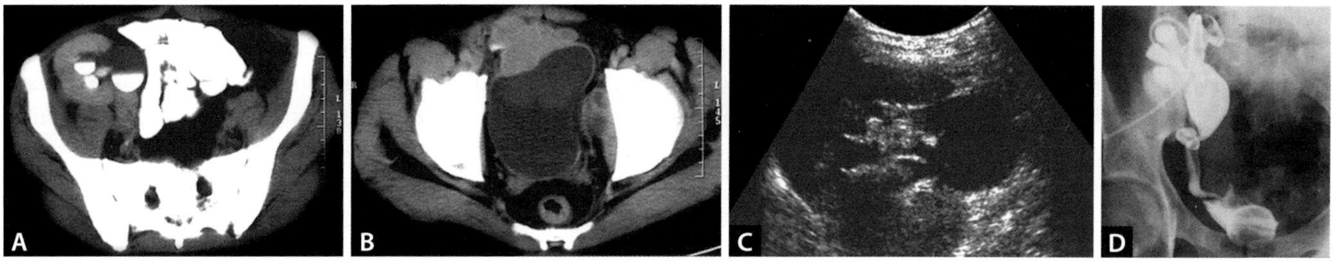

Figs. 6A to D: Anatomotic stricture in a transplant kidney: (A) CECT abdomen axial image showing hydroureteronephrosis in the transplant kidney; (B) There is a large, lobulated mass involving the ureterovesical anastomotic site engulfing the ureter; (C) Ultrasound image showing dilatation of the pelvis with minimal dilatation of the calyces; (D) Nephrostogram obtained after percutaneous nephrostomy demonstrates the stricture at the anastomotic site. This was successfully stented.

studies have indicated that RCC may be incidentally detected at cross-sectional imaging in up to 60% of patients.[23,24] Patients with RCC that have not spread outside the renal parenchyma have an excellent prognosis for cure if the RCC can be resected. In the past, radical nephrectomy has been the conventional treatment for RCC. Over the last two decades, nephron-sparing surgery has become an oncologically viable alternative in patients who would be rendered anephric by a radical nephrectomy. Nephron-sparing surgery has also been shown to be an equally effective curative treatment for patients with a single, small (<5 cm), and clearly localized RCC and a normal contralateral kidney.[23] However, nephron-sparing surgery requires more technical skills than radical nephrectomy with higher intraoperative blood loss. Many patients may be poor surgical candidates due to presence of significant comorbidities and advanced age. In addition, some patients may have multiple, bilateral tumors or poor renal function. In these patients, less invasive nephron-sparing surgical techniques have been applied, including laparoscopic partial nephrectomy, radiofrequency ablation and cryoablation. Percutaneous approaches to treatment of RCC reported include radiofrequency ablation, cryotherapy, microwave therapy and high intensity focused sonography. Radiofrequency ablation (RFA) has been successfully used for primary and metastatic hepatic tumors. The first reports on the use of RFA in the treatment of renal tumors appeared in 1997 and it is widely used as an effective curative treatment option today.[25]

Ablation Process

In RFA, a high-frequency, alternating current with a wavelength of 460–500 kHz is passed through an electrode placed within the target tumor tissue. Grounding pads placed around the patients thighs complete the electrical circuit. Deposition of radiofrequency energy results in the heating of cells near the site of energy deposition. When human tissue is heated to beyond 49°C, cell death occurs within minutes due to loss of enzymatic function, melting of cell membranes, and destruction of cytoplasm. Temperatures in excess of 60°C cause immediate cell death. When the temperature exceeds 100°C, the cells boil releasing gas vapors and causing tissue charring. These in turn inhibit the dispersion of radiofrequency energy decreasing the effectiveness of the procedure. Hence, ideal RFA devices should produce prolonged heating of target tissue between 50°C and 100°C.[25] Various modifications developed towards this purpose include: (i) pulsed energy deployment, (ii) expansion of electrode surface, (iii) intraparenchymal injection of iron compounds or saline before and during RF application, and (iv) internal cooling of the needle electrode with saline.

Equipment

All RFA devices consist of an electric generator, needle electrode and grounding pad. Among the commercially available systems, the RITA RF system (RITA Medical Systems, Inc, Fremont, CA, USA) contains a 14-gauge insulated outer needle and 4–9 internal curved prongs which deliver the RF electrical energy while affixing the needle in place. The latest RITA StarBurst Xli-Enhanced electrode, which has saline infusion capability, allows a maximum treatment volume of 7 cm. Radionics (Burlington, Mass, USA) offers the Cool-tip system which has a 17-gauge straight electrode with a beveled tip with internally circulating saline for controlling the temperature at the needle tip (<20°C), to reduce tissue charring, build-up of impedance and maximize energy deposition. A cluster of three straight electrodes arranged 0.5 cm apart in a triangular pattern is also available. The Radiotherapeutics RF 3000 system (Radiotherapeutics Corporation, Natick, MA, USA) has a 17-gauge LeVeen needle electrode consisting of an insulated metal cannula and 12 expandable wire tines which reach a diameter of 4 cm when fully deployed. Different devices use a slightly different approach to maximize energy delivery and monitor thermal destruction. The theoretical maximum size of the ablated area is twice the length of the energy emitting segment of the electrode in the long axis of the treatment zone. The maximum in the transverse axis is up to two-thirds of the long axis of the treatment zone. Practically, the ablated area is smaller than the theoretical zone. Flowing blood, large fluid containing spaces, or circulating air can decrease the effective size of the treatment zone due to the "heat-sink" effect.[26]

Patient Selection and Preprocedure Evaluation

RFA can be performed in patients with a renal tumor suggestive of RCC on the basis of the imaging findings, and who have marginal renal function, serious comorbidities that make them high-risk surgical candidates, or are at high risk for developing additional RCCs (e.g. von Hippel–Lindau disease). Contraindications are relative and include uncorrected coagulopathy and an ongoing acute illness, such as sepsis.[25,27]

All patients should undergo a contrast enhanced CT or MR of the abdomen before the procedure. The tumor should still be Robson's stage I or II to achieve curative results. Spread of the tumor beyond the renal fascia, into renal vein or lymph nodes or distant metastases are contraindications for RFA. There is no absolute size criterion for RFA; however, the likelihood of complete ablation increases in smaller tumors. Tumors larger than 7 cm are unlikely to be successfully ablated and should only be considered for cytoreduction. Peripherally located tumors are also more likely to be successfully ablated in comparison to centrally located tumors due to the heat-sink effect of the vessels in the renal hilum.[27,28] Due to the insulation offered by the perinephric fat, subcapsular or exophytic tumors can usually be completely ablated.[24]

Laboratory investigations to be performed prior to the procedure include serum creatinine, platelet count and coagulation profile. Biopsy of the tumor before ablation is usually not performed if the imaging findings are characteristic; however, some authors routinely perform a biopsy for tissue diagnosis prior to the procedure. Prophylactic antibiotics are usually administered.

Guidance

Imaging guidance for the procedure can be with the help of sonography, CT or MR. Sonography plays an important role in the guidance of both percutaneous and intraoperative procedures. It provides real-time imaging without any hazards of ionizing radiation; its easy availability and portability offer further advantages. Needle positioning can be accurately checked using 3D US. However, dissolved gases (primarily nitrogen) are released during tissue heating which form microbubbles in the tissue cause obscuration of lesion due to their hyperechogenicity.[26] This is particularly important when the tumor is more than 3 cm in size and requires multiple, overlapping ablations. In some patients, it may be difficult to visualize very small renal tumors with sonography. Air-filled bowel close to the tumor also may not be adequately visualized on US. In most cases, RFA of renal lesions is performed under CT guidance. CT offers the following advantages: (i) it can demonstrate small RCCs, (ii) there is no obscuration of the lesion after ablation, and (iii) a contrast enhanced CT can be performed after the procedure to assess adequacy of ablation before terminating the procedure.[25] MR has also been used for guidance for RFA. It provides better soft tissue contrast without need for intravenous contrast. Its multiplanar capabilities without radiation hazards and provision of MR fluoroscopy sequences makes it optimally suited for guiding RFA procedures.

Procedure

The procedure can be performed on an out patient basis. A written informed consent should be obtained. The procedure is usually performed under local anesthesia with conscious sedation. General anesthesia may be required in certain cases such as deep seated, difficult to access lesions where precise respiratory control is required.

The technique of placing the electrode is similar to that of performing an imaging-guided biopsy of a focal lesion. The goal is to ablate the target tumor tissue as well as a 0.5–1 cm circumferential rim of adjacent normal parenchyma, therefore an appropriate electrode size should be selected. The electrode is advanced to the deep margin of the tumor as there is little ablation beyond the electrode tip in some cases. The ablation is usually performed for 10–15 minutes per ablative cycle. Multiple, overlapping ablations need to be done in larger tumors. In literature, technical success rates for renal RFA range from 92 to 100% with clinical success rates for small renal tumors (mean diameter 1.7–3.5 cm) reported as between 86 and 100%.[24-28]

Postprocedure and Follow-up

All patients should be kept under observation for 4–6 hours after the procedure. Antibiotics should be continued for at least five days postprocedure. Appropriate analgesics should be prescribed for ensuring adequate analgesia.

A contrast enhanced biphasic CT should be obtained immediately after the procedure to determine adequacy of ablation. Thereafter a contrast enhanced CT or MR should be obtained at one, three, six, and twelve month intervals to look for residual or recurrent tumor. Imaging after the first year can be done at 6–9 month intervals. CT is more often used for postablation follow-up because of its lower cost and wider availability; however, MR may be used in patients with renal insufficiency **(Figs. 7A to C)**.

Immediately after ablation, the ablated tumor usually appears larger than the pre-ablation size because a peripheral margin of 0.5–1 cm of normal tissue is also ablated. On follow-up imaging, ablated tumors appear as focal, non-enhancing masses which show decrease in size with time. Soft tissue stranding may be seen in the perinephric fat. At times, a curvilinear, hyperattenuating area or halo is seen surrounding the ablated lesion.[24] Nodular enhancement in the ablated tumor or an increase in the size of lesion is considered to represent residual or recurrent tumor. On MR, the area of necrosis appears hypointense on T2-weighted images. It usually appears hyperintense relative to the renal cortex on T1 weighted images, though it may occasionally appear iso- to hypointense. Rim enhancement of the ablated lesion may be seen early after ablation but this gradually resolves over 3 months. Residual viable tumor tissue appears hyperintense on T2-weighted images and shows nodular enhancement post gadolinium on T1 images.[24]

Complications

Few complications have been reported after RFA in renal lesions. Hematuria occurs rarely, is usually self-limited and commonly resolves within 24–48 hours. Thermal necrosis of adjacent bowel has been reported. At a minimum, there should be at least 5 mm of intervening fat between the target tumor and bowel to avoid thermal injury. If bowel abuts the target, sterile water can be injected to displace the bowel and ensure safe ablation of the RCC. The RFA of lesions adjacent to the adrenal gland can cause release of vaso-active catecholamines which requires administration of alpha blockers. Perirenal hemorrhage is common but is rarely clinically significant. Needle track seeding and development of ureteric strictures are other rare complications. Overall, the rate of major complications after RFA of renal lesions is estimated to be approximately 1%.[25,29]

Other Applications of RFA

Radiofrequency ablation (RFA) has been successfully used to treat intractable hematuria in cases of unresectable RCCs. It has also been used for the treatment of recurrent RCC after surgery. The surgical resection of isolated distant metastases from RCC has been reported to be associated with prolonged survival rates. RFA has been used to successfully ablate pulmonary metastases from RCC.

To summarize, the use of RFA for the treatment of RCC is a very promising technique that should be considered as a therapeutic option for patients with early stage RCC who are poor surgical candidates.

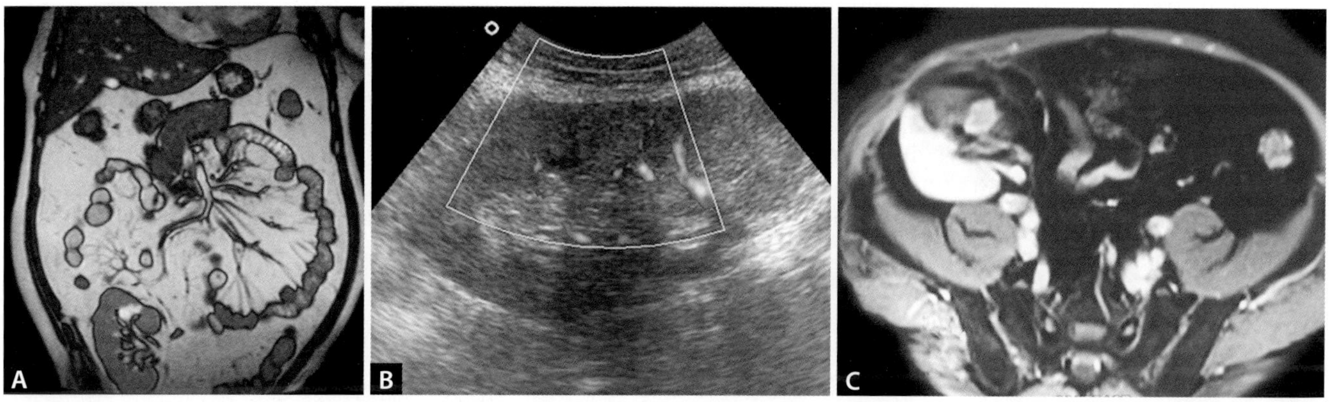

Figs. 7A to C: Radiofrequency ablation of a renal cell carcinoma in a transplant kidney: (A) Preprocedure MR coronal T2-weighted image shows a focal area of hyperintensity in the upper pole of the transplant kidney; (B) Follow-up Doppler image after six weeks shows absence of flow to the region of the ablated tumor; (C) MR axial postgadolinium T1 image one month after RFA shows absence of enhancement of the renal parenchyma in the region of ablation. Note the defect is larger than the original tumor size due to ablation of a rim of normal parenchyma around the tumor.

REFERENCES

1. Goodwin WE, Casey WL, Woolf W. Percutaneous trocar (needle) nephrostomy in hydronephrosis. JAMA. 1955;157:891-4.
2. Banner MP, Ramchandani P, Pollack HM. Interventional procedures in the upper urinary tract. Cardiovascular Intervent Radiol. 1991;14:267-84.
3. Dyer RB, Regan JD, Kavanagh PV, Khatod EG, Chen MY, Zagoria RJ. Percutaneous Nephrostomy with Extensions of the Technique: Step by Step. Radiographics. 2002;22:503-25.
4. Papanicolou N. Renal anatomy relevant to percutaneous interventions. Semin Intervent Radiol. 1995;12:163-72.
5. Hausegger KA, Portugaller HR. Percutaneous nephrostomy and antegrade ureteral stenting: technique - indications - complications. Eur Radiol. 2006;16(9):2016-30.
6. Karniemi J, Sequeiros RB, Ojala R, Tervonen O. MRI guided percutaneous nephrostomy: a feasibility study. Eur Radiol. 2008 Nov [Epub ahead of print].
7. Park BK, Kim SH, Moon MH. Nonvascular interventions of the urinary tract. J Korean Med Sci. 2002;17:727-36.
8. Funaki B, Vatakencherry G. Comparison of single-stick and double-stick techniques for percutaneous nephrostomy. Cardiovasc Intervent Radiol. 2004;27:35-7.
9. Patel U, Hussain FF. Percutaneous nephrostomy of nondilated renal collecting systems with fluoroscopic guidance: Technique and results. Radiology. 2004;233:226-33.
10. Gupta S, Gulati M, Suri S. Ultrasound guided percutaneous nephrostomy in nondilated pelvicalyceal sytem. J Clin Ultrasound. 1998;26:177-9.
11. Farrell TA, Hicks ME. A review of radiologically guided percutaneous nephrostomies in 303 patients. J Vasc Intervent Radiol. 1997;8:769-74.
12. Ramchandani P, Cardella JF, Grassi CJ, et al. Quality improvement guidelines for percutaneous nephrostomy. J Vasc Interventional Radiol. 2003;14:277-81.
13. Wah TM, Weston MJ, Irving HC. Percutaneous nephrostomy insertion: outcome data from a prospective multi-operator study at a UK training centre. Clin Radiol. 2004;59:255-61.
14. Zagoria RJ, Dyer RB. Do's and don'ts of percutaneous nephrostomy. Acad Radiol. 1999;6(6):370-77.
15. Vignali C, Lonzi S, Bargellini I, Cioni R, Petruzzi P, et al. Vascular injuries after percutaneous renal procedures: treatment by transcatheter embolization. Eur Radiol. 2004;14:723-9.
16. Gerspach JM, Bellman GC, Stoller ML, Fugelso P. Conservative management of colon injury following percutaneous renal surgery. Urology. 1997;49:831-6.
17. Seymour H, Patel U. Ureteric stenting: current status. Semin Intervent Radiol. 2000;17:351-65.
18. Tal R, Bachar GN, Baniel J, Belenky A. External Internal nephro-ureteral-ileal stents in patients with an ileal conduit: long term results. Urology. 2004;63:438-41.
19. Titton RL, Gervais DA, Hahn PF, Harisinghani MG, Arellano RS, Mueller PR. Urine leaks and urinomas: diagnosis and imaging-guided intervention. Radiographics. 2003;23:1133-47.
20. Avritscher R, Madoff DC, Ramirez PT, Wallace MJ, Ahrar K, et al. Fistulas of the lower urinary tract: Percutaneous approaches for the management of a difficult clinical entity. Radiographics. 2004;24 (Suppl 1):S217-36.
21. Bhattacharya T, Kumaradevan J, Watkinson AF. Percutaneous nephrolithotomy: State of the art. Semin Intervent Radiol. 2000;17:341-9.
22. Hanna RM, Dahniya MH. Aspiration and sclerotherapy of symptomatic simple renal cysts: value of two injections of a sclerosing agent. AJR Am J Roentgenol. 1996;167:781-3.
23. Kawamoto S, Permpongkosol S, Bluemke DA, Fishman EK, Solomon SB. Sequential changes after radiofrequency ablation and cryoablation of renal neoplasms: role of CT and MR imaging. Radiographics. 2007;27:343-55.
24. Farrell MA, Charboneau WJ, DiMarco DS, Chow GK, Zincke H, et al. Imaging-guided radiofrequency ablation of solid renal tumours. AJR Am J Roentgenol. 2003;180:1509-13.
25. Zagoria RJ. Imaging-guided radiofrequency ablation of renal masses. Radiographics. 2004;24:S59-71.
26. Chiou SY, Liu JB, Needleman L. Current status of sonographically guided radiofrequency ablation techniques. J Ultrasound Med. 2007;26:487-99.
27. Liu KW, Gervais DA, Arellano RA, Mueller PR. Radiofrequency ablation in renal cell carcinoma. Clin Radiol. 2003;58:905-13.
28. Boss A, Clasen S, Kucyzk M, Schick F, Pereira PL. Image guided radiofrequency ablation of renal cell carcinoma. Eur Radiol. 2007;17:725-33.
29. Rhim H, Dodd GD III, Chintapalli KN, et al. Radiofrequency thermal ablation of abdominal tumours: lessons learned from complications. Radiographics. 2004;24:41-52.

CHAPTER 120

Vascular Interventions in the Genitourinary Tract

Shivanand Gamanagatti, Deep Narayan Srivastava

INTRODUCTION

Interventional vascular radiology has grown over the past 2–3 decades and has placed the radiologist to play an important role in patient's management. The current technological advances have allowed more accurate and controlled deployment of embolic agents. Embolotherapy has now become the procedure of choice for the management of visceral and solid organ aneurysms and percutaneous renal revascularization has also become an accepted procedure of choice for renal artery stenosis.

Various vascular interventional procedures in genitourinary practice are directed towards vascular dilatation or vascular embolization. The commonly performed procedures include as follows:

- Renal artery angioplasty
- Renal artery stenting
- Renal artery embolization
- Uterine artery embolization
- Vaginal AVM embolization
- Scrotal AVM embolization.
- Varicocele embolization

RENAL ARTERY ANGIOPLASTY

Renal artery stenosis (RAS) is the most common cause of secondary hypertension, seen with a 14% prevalence among patients with chronic renal failure. Among the various causes of RAS, atherosclerosis is the most common etiology, others being fibromuscular dysplasia, Takayasu arteritis, neurofibromatosis, etc. Medical therapy and surgical treatment, including renal vascularization and nephrectomy are traditional methods of treatment for renovascular hypertension. These methods, however, have several disadvantages. When the blood pressure is lowered by medical therapy, it further reduces renal blood flow and further deterioration of renal function even in controlled blood pressure. The surgical revascularization methods are considerably beneficial to most patients but considering the associated morbidity and operative mortality rate of 8%, surgery should be done only on carefully selected patients. Presently, percutaneous transluminal renal angioplasty (PTRA) is the first line of treatment for renal artery stenosis due to its relatively lower morbidity and mortality compared to surgical methods. The Society of Cardiovascular and Interventional Radiology (SCVIR) has laid down guidelines for the renal artery angioplasty. Various pathological lesions are shown in **Table 1**.

According to the SCVIR guidelines, above lesions can be divided into four categories as follows:[1]

Category-I lesions: They are those for which the only procedure of choice is the balloon angioplasty. It includes

Table 1: Various pathological lesions: their causes and prevalence.

Cause	*Affected segment*	*Incidence (%)*
Atherosclerosis	Ostium and proximal 1/3	90
Fibromuscular dysplasia	Mid and distal 1/3	10
Takayasu arteritis	Ostium and proximal part	<1
NF-1	All	<1
Radiation	All	<1
Trauma	All	<1

fibromuscular dysplasia of the renal artery and unilateral short (<3 cm) and nonostial atherosclerosis **(Figs. 1 and 2)**.

Category-II lesions: They are well suited for angioplasty and are atherosclerotic bilateral nonostial stenosis, postoperative anastomotic stenosis, stenoses associated with worsening renal function **(Fig. 3)**.

Category-III lesions: They have a moderate chance of technical success or long-term benefits compared to bypass surgery and are atherosclerotic renal ostial stenosis, nonatheromatous lesions involving the proximal renal arteries.

Category-IV lesions: They have a low technical success rate. This includes renal artery stenoses in vessels that arise from an aneurysmal or severely diseased aortic segment or stenoses associated with renal artery aneurysm.

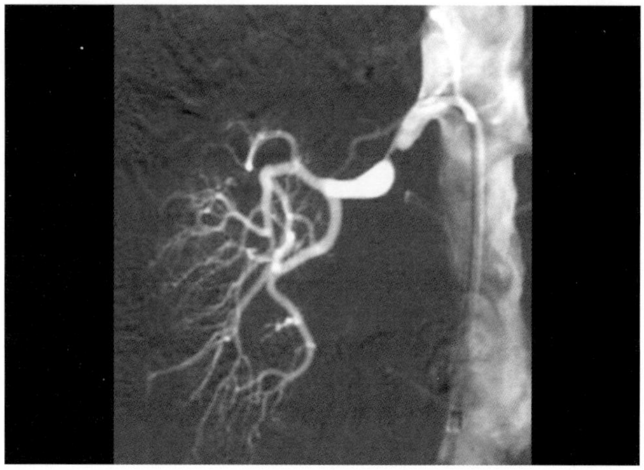

Fig. 1: Selective renal angiogram showing nonostial short segment narrowing with poststenotic dilation of right renal artery (category-I lesions).

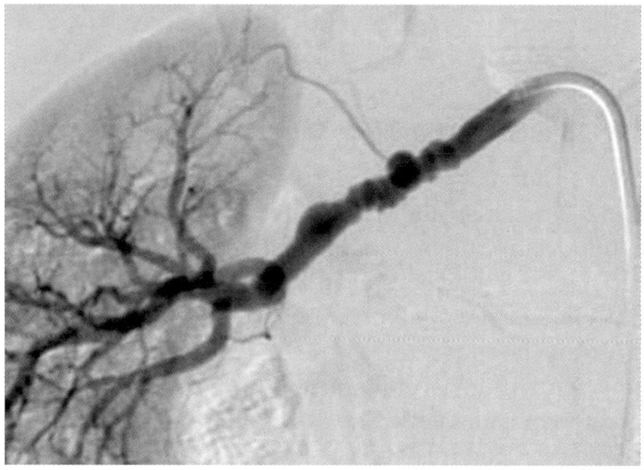

Fig. 2: Selective renal angiogram showing classic string-of-pearls appearance of right renal artery suggestive of fibromuscular dysplasia (Category-I lesions).

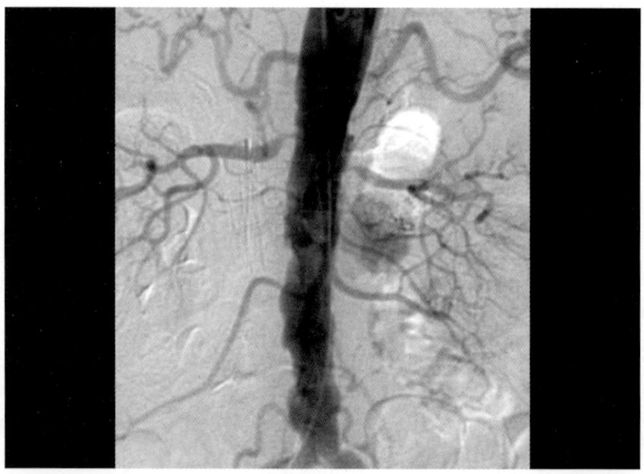

Fig. 3: Flush aortogram showing diffuse atherosclerotic abdominal aorta and ostial narrowing of bilateral renal arteries (category-II lesions).

Imaging the Renal Arteries

Conventional angiography remains to be the best anatomic study for assessing patients with renal artery stenosis. Duplex ultrasonography is very vital and should be the first imaging study in patients suspected of having renal artery stenosis. The quality of renal ultrasonography depends on the operator skill well as on other variables, such as body habitus, but even then, the sensitivity of duplex scanning has been reported to be 98%, with 98% specificity and high-positive and negative predictive values.[2]

Computed tomography angiography (CTA) is now replacing conventional angiography for the evaluation of renal arteries. The images are comparable to those of conventional angiography and vessels can be evaluated in three dimensions. CTA providess options for clarifying anatomy which may be better than with conventional angiography. Exposure of the patient to radiation from renal CTA can be compared to that of catheter angiography.[2]

Magnetic resonance angiography (MRA) is also used in evaluation of the anatomy of the renal arteries. Its resolution is lower than CTA or conventional angiography but is excellent for patients with impaired renal function because the contrast agent (gadolinium) is relatively nonnephrotoxic.[2,3]

Endovascular treatment of renal artery stenosis involves either percutaneous transluminal angioplasty or a combination of angioplasty and stent placement.

Technique[4-6]

Renal Artery Angioplasty

The procedure is mostly performed through the femoral artery approach. However, if indicated by patient's anatomy (for example presence of iliac artery occlusions or a very steeply angled renal artery), the brachial approach can also be used. A 6-F sheath is inserted into the femoral artery. It will be very effective if a long (typically 35 cm) sheath is used as guiding catheter. A preshaped catheter is then used to examine the renal artery. The catheter is used along with a guidewire for crossing the lesion. A hydrophilic guidewire, such as a Terumo can be very helpful, especially in lesions which are difficult to cross, though the soft tipped Bentson guidewire may also be used. After crossing the lesion, heparin andantispasmodic drugs are administered. The author uses 3000 units of heparin and 300 mg of isosorbide dinitrate, respectively.

With the catheter across the stenosis, the guidewire is changed to a specialist guidewire, such as the Jindo. The guidewire itself is very stiff, providing good support for the angioplasty balloon. The atraumatic nature of the tip is very important, as it can be placed in a cortical branch without any risk of causing a spasm. An angioplasty balloon is then introduced over the guidewire and then angioplasty is performed **(Figs. 4A to C)**. After confirming the proper position of balloon, it is inflated and left for 30 seconds.

Balloons are not oversized, but ideally their diameter should be the same as the artery distal to the stenosis. Typically, the diameter of balloon varies between 5 mm and 7 mm. Loin pain with balloon inflation is common, but it should not be severe. The occurrence of the latter may lead to vessel rupture, in which case the dilation should be stopped and a smaller balloon used. After dilation the balloon is removed and the guidewire is left in place. Then a check angiogram is performed through the long sheath or guiding catheter. If there has been a complication or further dilation is required, access is maintained so as to allow additional intervention. The angioplasty is considered technically successful if after the angioplasty the arterial lumen had less than 30% residual stenosis and the pressure gradient is less than 20 mm Hg. The clinical results can be evaluated through the effect on blood pressure control and improvement of renal function.

RENAL ARTERY STENTING

The renal artery stent placement is now an established method of adjunctive treatment to renal angioplasty. Several problems related with renal angioplasty, such as flow compromising dissection, residual stenosis greater than 30% with a transstenotic pressure gradient greater than 20 mm Hg or restenosis, can be successfully treated with stenting. The renal artery stenting has shown better technical results, long-term patency and a lower rate of restenosis than that of PTRA. Stents are almost exclusively placed in the renal arteries by using an angioplasty balloon (balloon-expandable rather than self-expanding stents). In many respects insertion of renal artery stents is performed in a similar way to renal angioplasty. However, stents are normally inserted at the ostium of the renal artery because they are used to treat atheromatous disease. It is therefore essential to have a clear idea of the exact location of the ostium to help in accurate placement of the stent. Before inserting the stent, it is important to predilate the stenosis with a 4 mm balloon to ease the passage of the stent across the stenosis. Although the use of a guiding catheter is highly recommended, modern long sheaths also perform very well. Use of either allows angiograms to be performed whilst finally positioning the stent prior to deployment. There have been no reports of any adverse consequences associated with leaving the stent projecting 2 mm or so into the aorta. This position of the stent ensures that the entire lesion is stented. Sometimes, it may be

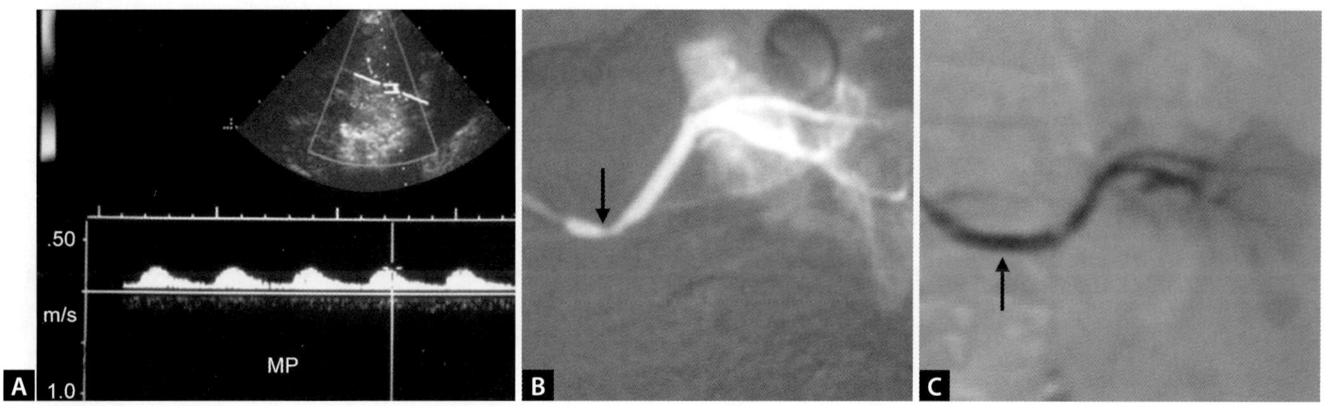

Figs. 4A to C: A case of renal artery stenosis treated by angioplasty: (A) Renal Doppler showing classic pulsus parvus et tardus wave form of renal artery stenosis; (B) Selective renal angiogram showing focal narrowing of left renal artery; (C) Postangioplasty angiogram showing successful dilatation of renal artery and 0% residual stenosis.

necessary to perform renal arterial intervention from a brachial approach, for example, when femoral access is not possible or if the renal arteries are sharply angulated inferiorly **(Figs. 5A and B)**.

Outcome

Compared with the relatively good outcomes after angioplasty for fibromuscular dysplasia, balloon angioplasty alone has not been as successful in treating atherosclerotic renal artery stenosis. This is most likely because of the high degree of elastic recoil in atherosclerotic arteries compared with that encountered in fibromuscular webs.

The restenosis rate after angioplasty alone varies widely but has been reported to be from 10 to 46%.[5] Angioplasty (without stent placement) has a higher technical success rate when applied to atherosclerotic lesions in the mid portion of the main renal artery (72–82%) than in ostial lesions (success rate ≈60%).

Stents are now almost uniformly used for all ostial lesions and almost all atherosclerotic renal artery stenosis. A recent report quotes a technical success rate for stents of 94–100% and a restenosis rate of 11–23%, with an improvement in blood pressure control in 50–80% and stabilization of renal function in 60–70%.[5,6]

Renal function at the time of stent placement strongly predicts patency and expected survival after intervention. In patients with normal renal function, 3-year survival is 94%, 74% if serum creatinine is between 1.5 mg/dL and 2.0 mg/dL, and 52% if serum creatinine is greater than 2.0 mg/dL.[6]

Renal Artery Intervention in Renal Transplants

Although technically angioplasty and stenting are similar in many ways to procedures in native kidneys, the management of transplant renal artery stenosis involves some important differences. Cadaveric transplants are generally anastomosed to the recipient external iliac artery, because it is possible to obtain the full length of renal artery and renal vein stump. These procedures are seperately described in Chapter 114 (Renal Transplant).

Complications

The complications can be divided into major (renal insufficiency, renal artery occlusion, renal artery damage, including rupture, etc.) and minor (temporary renal insufficiency, retroperitoneal hematoma, femoral artery complications, etc.).

RENAL ARTERY EMBOLIZATION

The various indications are embolization of renal neoplasms, renal pseudoaneurysms (secondary to either traumatic or iatrogenic injury), end-stage kidney, etc.

Technique

There are three different types of renal embolization: Proximal (occlusion of main/segmental renal artery), distal (occlusion of lobular or arcuate arteries) and capillary (occlusion of arterioles and glomeruli). Depending upon the type of embolization the catheter is advanced into the renal artery branches. The superselective embolization with a coaxial catheter can save part of renal parenchyma.

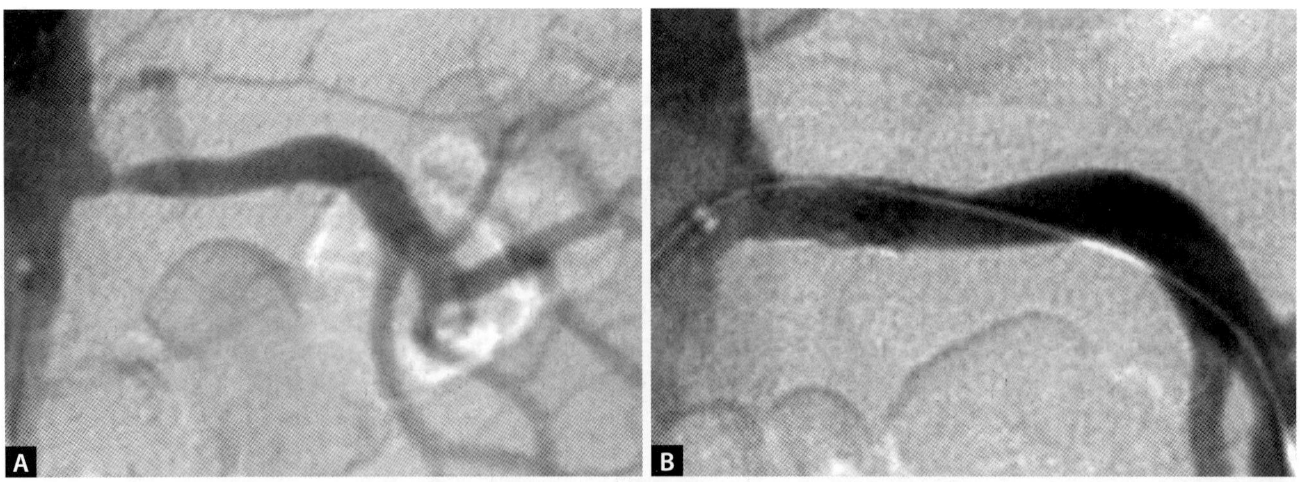

Figs. 5A and B: A case of renal artery ostial narrowing treated by stenting: (A) Renal angiogram showing ostial narrowing of left renal artery; (B) Poststenting angiogram showing 0% residual stenosis.

The selection of embolizing material also depends upon the purpose of occlusion (temporary or permanent). The various materials used for embolization are particles (gelfoam, polyvinyl alcohol), liquid agents (alcohol, sclerosants), steel coils and detachable balloons.

TRANSCATHETER EMBOLIZATION OF RENAL NEOPLASMS

The current role of renal embolization in carcinoma of the kidney is uncertain.

The most important aim of preoperative embolization of the renal artery is to prevent migration of tumor cells from being flooded out.

The various indications are as follows:

1. To relieve symptoms, such as pain, hematuria, polycythemia, congestive heart failure.
2. To facilitate surgical resection by preoperative embolization to reduce the tumor vascularity.
3. To inhibit tumor growth and to reduce tumor mass.
4. To stimulate an immune response by decreasing the tumor load.
5. Prophylactic embolotherapy in angiomyolipomas to avoid risk of hemorrhage.

The impact of the renal embolization as palliative method of treatment on the survival time is difficult to estimate but improvement in local symptoms such as hematuria and pain is evident.

Varieties of embolizing agents have been used, such as gelatin sponge, stainless steel coil, n-butyl cyanoacrylate, absolute alcohol, autologus blood clot. But the embolization material of choice is ethanol. Ethanol is widely used for permanent embolization. The optimal dose is 0.5 mL/kg of body weight with upper limit of 1 mL/kg and at the rate of 2 mL/sec. the advantage of alcohol over other permanent embolizing material are complete tissue necroses with permanent arterial occlusion, milder post infarction syndrome, less chances of infection and simple to use.

Technique for delivery of absolute alocohol to renal artery includes balloon occlusion technique and superselective technique.[7,8] Balloon occlusion technique serves several purposes like, it prevents reflux of alcohol into aorta, prolongs contact period of alcohol with endothelium.

In superselective technique, endhole catheter is advanced superselectively into lobar braches and the alcohol is injected to prevent reflux. This is then followed by large vessel embolization with coils. Mechanism of action of alcohol proposed to be combination of perivasculat necrosis, sludging of erythrocytes in small arteries and glomeruli and endothelial damage.

Rate of injection has serious impact over the success of embolization. Injection rate of 1–5 mL/sec, leads to perivascular necrosis, sludging of erythrocytes in small arteries and glomeruli indicating direct tissue toxicity. Where as at slow rate of injection 0.1 mL//sec, causes endothelial damage and less tissue toxicity. Hence, slow rate of injection is desirable in benign conditions like AVM, angiomyolipomas, where permanent arterial occlusion with minimal tissue damage is desirable.[7]

Angiographic findings of successful embolization include, all arteries smaller than major segmental arties must be occluded, stagnation of flow and extravazation of contrast material into adjacent renal parenchyma **(Figs. 6A to F)**.

Embolization with absolute ethanol should be carried out carefully due to the vigorous thrombosis it causes by denaturing proteins. Ethanol can result in seizures and intoxication if it reaches the systemic circulation. It can even permeate the tissues and causes injury to adjacent structures, such as nerves and bowel.

Transcatheter Embolization of Renal Pseudoaneurysms

Incidence

Incidence of aneurysm formation differs for the various etiologies of renal artery aneurysms. However, literature suggests that incidence ranges between 0.015% and 9.7%.[9] Poutasse have classified renal artery aneurysms into saccular, fusiform, dissecting, and pseudoaneurysms.[10] The natural history of these aneurysms has not been defined well in the literature. However, the incidence of rupture rate, ranges from 0% to 14%.[10] Renal artery aneurysms that are treated surgically are approached by nephrectomy, *ex vivo* repair and reimplntation.[9-11]

Causes

Typically, pseudoaneurysm formation in the renal artery distribution is either iatrogenic or traumatic. Other causes of aneurysm formation include fibromuscular dysplasia, polyarteritis nodosa, amphetamine abuse, angiomyolipoma (either with or without associated tuberous sclerosis) and neurofibromatosis.

Risks Posed by the Aneurysm

Risk of a rupture is rare in these aneurysms. However, pregnant women are more prone to rupture which is similar to splenic artery aneurysms rupture.

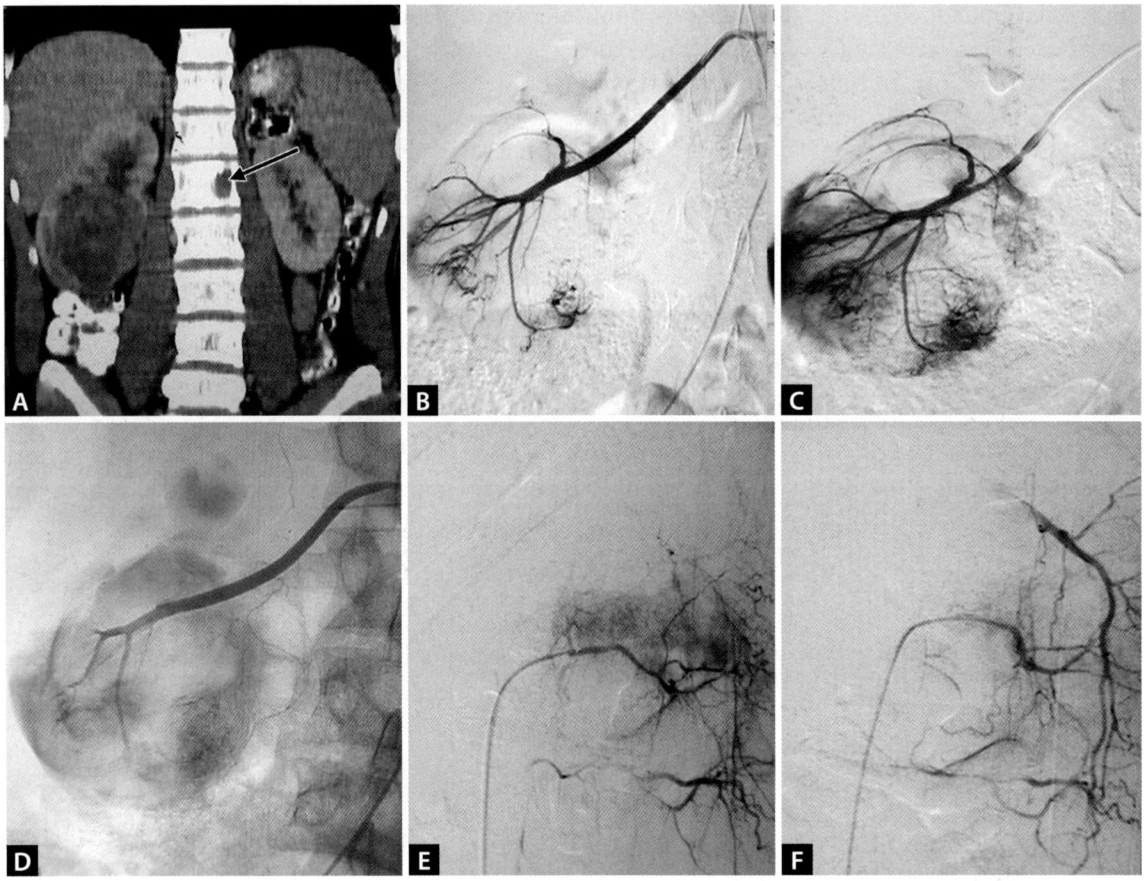

Figs. 6A to F: A case of renal cell carcinoma with vertebral metastasis treated by absolute alcohol. (A) Coronal MPR image showing large mass lesion in lower pole of right kidney. *Note*: Destructive lytic lesion in L1 vertebra (arrow); (B) Selective angiogram showing tumor neovascularity in lower polar region; (C) Delayed angiogram showing tumor blush and no arteriovenous shunting; (D) Postembolization angiogram showing stasis of contrast, persistent tumor staining and obliteration of tumor vascularity; (E) Selective angiogram of paraspinal artery showing tumor blush supplying the L1 vertebral lesion; (F) Following embolization with PVA particles (500–700 μ) showing obliteration of tumor vascularity.

Anatomic/Physiologic Considerations

The vascular supply to the kidney is considered endorgan, and hence, infarction is common after embolization. Therefore, in patients with renal insufficiency or underlying diseases, such as tuberous sclerosis or von Recklinghausen's disease, nephron-sparing procedures are vital. Superselective embolization is advisable in all cases of renal artery embolization unless partial or total nephrectomy is planned.

Technique

The renal arteries arise at the L2 level from the abdominal aorta. A LAO view during a flush injection of the aorta usually provides the best view of the origins. Careful examination for accessory renal arteries is necessary. A renal double curve or Cobra catheter will easily select the main renal ostium. A Rosen wire is an atraumatic guidewire that allows for secure exchange or upsizing to a guiding catheter or Balkin sheath. Selective injection should be performed to identify the feeding vessel or vessels. This can be done through the sheath. Many embolization techniques can be applied in this setting depending factors like the type, number, and location of the aneurysms. Commonly pseudoaneurysms are embolized superselectively by using coils **(Figs. 7A to D)**. Sometime, aneurysms of the main renal artery maybe amenable to stent graft placement, thus allowing distal perfusion to be maintained. However, until stent graft placement is perfected, surgical repair by resection, aneurysmorraphy, and autotransplantation is more commonly performed in this setting.

More peripherally located aneurysms can be selectively coil embolized using microcatheter technique **(Figs. 8A to F)**. Both distal and proximal control is not always possible, and may not be necessary due to the

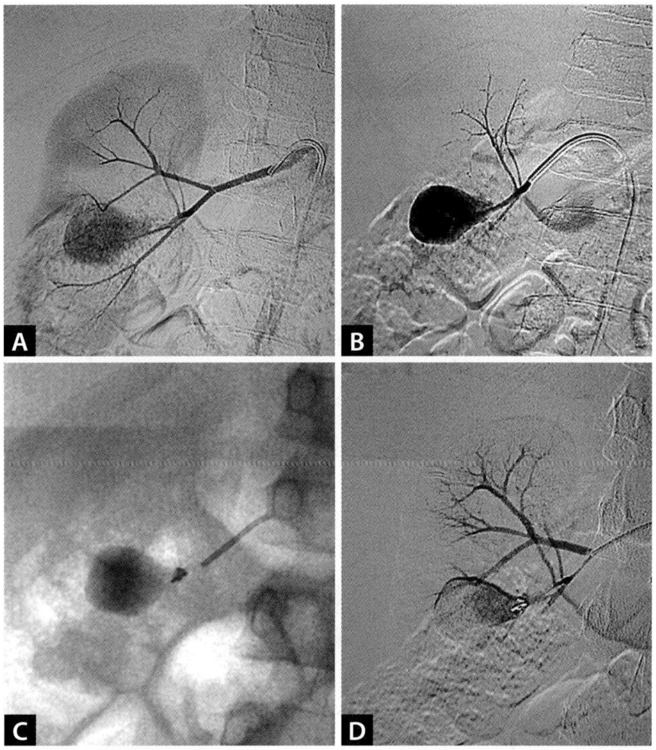

Figs. 7A to D: Post-PCNL renal artery pseudoaneurysm treated by coil embolization: (A and B) Selective renal angiogram showing large pseudoaneurysm arising from lower polar artery; (C) Spot image showing coil at the neck of pseudoaneurysm; (D) Postembolization angiogram showing nonfilling of pseudoaneurysm.

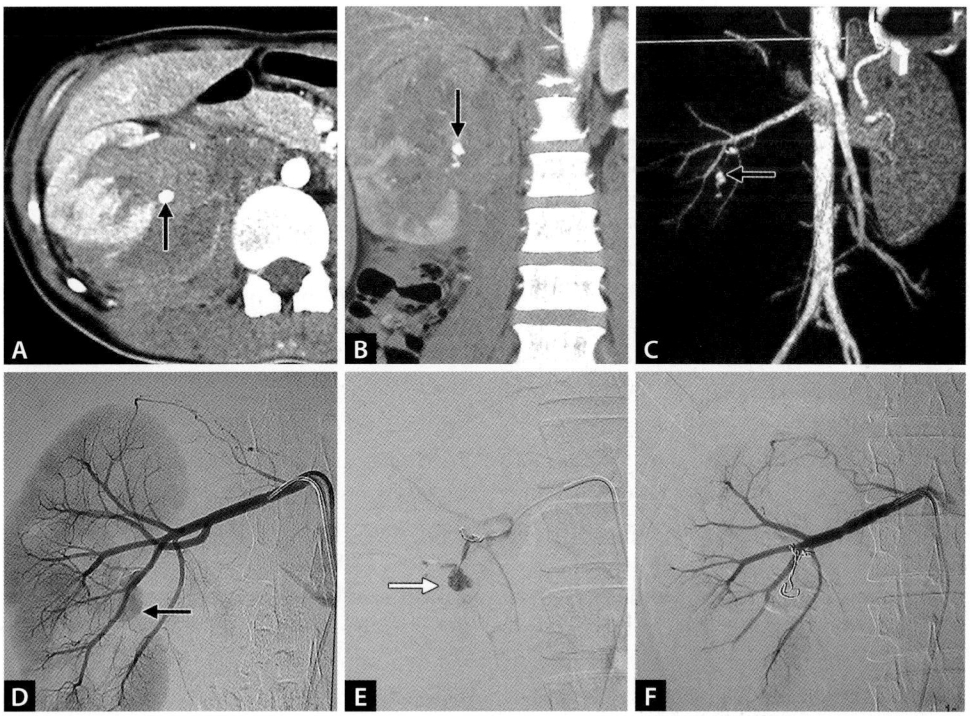

Figs. 8A to F: Post-PCNL renal artery pseudoaneurysm treated by microcoils using microcatheter coaxial technique: (A to C) Contrast-enhanced CT images showing small extrarenal pseudoaneurysm with surrounding large hematoma formation; (D) Selective renal angiogram showing filling of pseudoaneurysm supplied by lower polar branch of right renal artery; (E) Superselectively getting access into the branch supplying pseudoaneurysm using microcatheter; (F) Postembolization angiogram showing nonfilling of pseudoaneurysm.

vascular anatomy. In the presence of multiple aneurysms from a lesion, such as an angiomyolipoma, a combination of particle and coil embolization can be performed. The actively bleeding aneurysms are coiled first, followed by occlusion of the feeding vessels to the tumor with PVA or embospheres. Gelfoam can be sandwiched between coil nests to assist thrombosis.[12-15]

Results of Embolization

The success of this technique is quite high once the renal artery has securely been accessed. The use of superselective techniques results in very little ischemia, and there are minor chances of inducing renal failure.

Complications

In rare cases, dissection or perforation of the renal arteries and their branches can occur. Rupture may speed up the development of retroperitoneal hemorrhage. Both dissection flaps and rupture can be instantly controlled with balloon tamponade. Although dissection flaps can often be tacked down, rupture typically requires emergent surgery. Even perforation of smaller branch vessels can occur if a guidewire is passed too far into the periphery.

Embolization of End-stage Kidney

The nonfunctional kidney may manifest by pain, hypertension, albuminuria and other symptoms. In such cases embolization procedure can replace surgical nephrectomy **(Figs. 9A to D)**.

Technique

Absolute alcohol is a very effective 'permanent' agent for occluding capillaries. The embolization material is injected cautiously through an endhole catheter under fluoroscopic control to avoid reflux into the aorta. The embolization is considered complete when there is stasis of contrast medium in the major renal arteries without any flow of contrast material into the distal branches. There is therefore residual opacification of the parenchyma of the embolized kidney. During the embolization patients commonly experience severe flank pain on the side of the kidney being infarcted and intravenous opiate analgesia is required for pain control. This limits the procedure to embolization of a single kidney at any one sitting. Patients must be then carefully monitored for 24 hours and kept in the hospital until their pain and any associated pyrexia has settled.[7,8]

The complications are mainly postembolization syndrome in the form of flank pain for few days, fever,

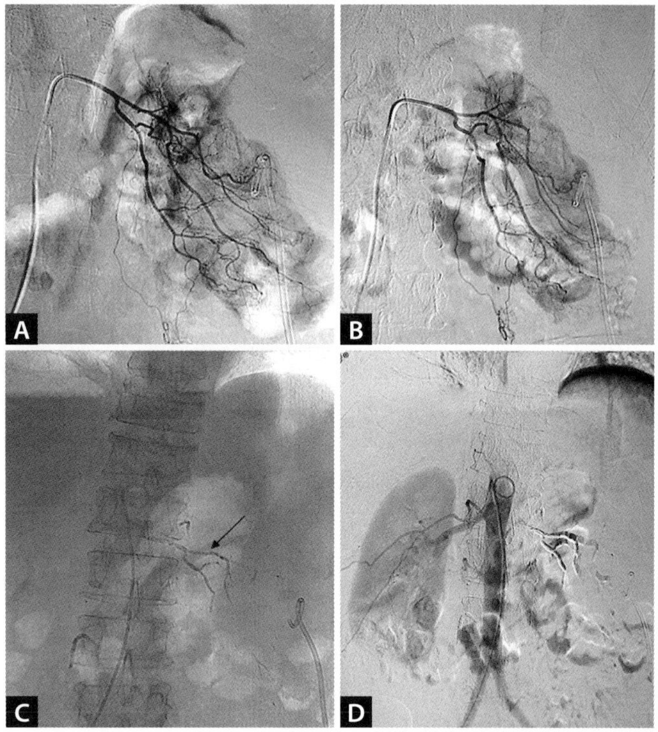

Figs. 9A to D: Glue embolization of nonfunctioning kidney. (A and B) Selective renal angiogram showing tortuous intrarenal branches; (C) Spot image showing glue cast in the intrarenal branches; (D) Postembolization flush aortogram showing complete obliteration of left renal artery and no parenchymal blush seen.

nausea, vomiting, etc. There may be hypertension in the first few hours. Majority of these symptoms are self-limited and are resolve without any specific treatment. Rarely, there may be major complications like renal failure, renal abscess and testicular infarction. The results of embolization are quite encouraging in most of the clinical situations.

Arteriovenous fistulas and malformations acquired arteriovenous fistulas in the kidney are usually the result of trauma, especially percutaneous biopsy. Massive renal arteriovenous fistulas can cause high-output heart failure. Congenital AVMs of the kidney are exceedingly rare. These lesions consist of numerous dilated, tortuous vessels within the subepithelium of the collecting system. When symptomatic, they usually present with gross hematuria and less commonly are associated with hypertension or an abdominal bruit. Color Doppler sonography, CT, and MR imaging are useful in detecting some of these lesion.

At angiography, an arteriovenous fistula produces dilatation of the feeding branch and early filling of the draining vein. Numerous segmental or interlobar arteries feed the renal AVM, which is composed of dilated, tortuous channels with rapid shunting into renal vein and IVC.

Transcatheter embolization is the first line of treatment for most of these lesions. Coils are effective for treatment of fistulas **(Figs. 10A to D)**. In AVMs, the nidus should be obliterated using a liquid agent, such as cyanoacrylate (glue).[16-19]

UTERINE ARTERY EMBOLIZATION

Indications

Uterine artery embolization (UAE) has become an extremely valuable therapy for patients with gynecological and obstetric diseases. The various indications where it can be used are uterine leiomyoma, arteriovenous malformations (AVMs) and postpartum and postoperative hemorrhage. UAE can also control bleeding following radiotherapy treatment in cases of carcinoma cervix.

Uterine Leiomyoma

Uterine artery embolization is the minimally invasive therapy in the management of uterine fibroids. The common indications for treatment are menorrhagia leading to anemia, abdominal pain, uterine enlargement with mass effect, infertility and late miscarriages. The advantages of UAE compared to operative therapies are that the patient retains the uterus, all the myomas are treated together in the same sitting and therapy is less invasive **(Figs. 11 and 12)**. The disadvantages are vaginal expulsion of necrotic fibroid if the fibroid is submucosal, postembolization syndrome and a procedure, which is not a fully curative treatment since the mean reduction of fibroid is about 40% or so.

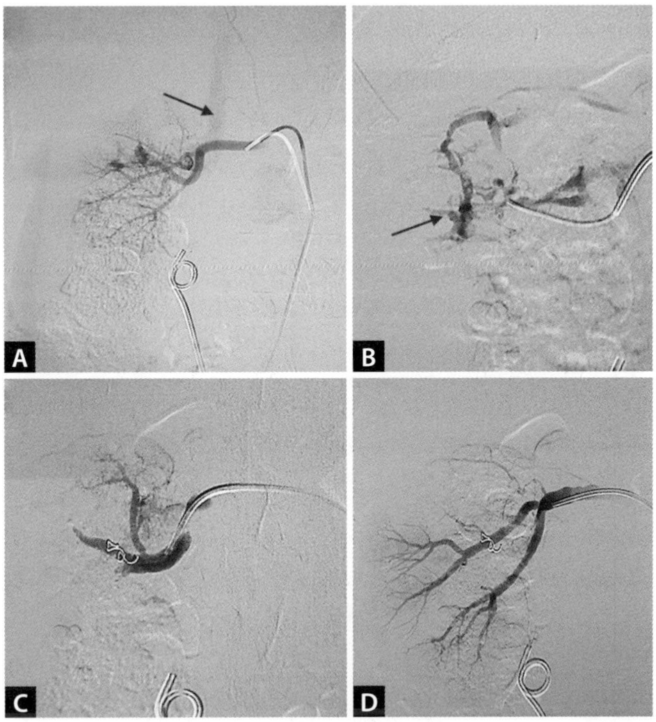

Figs. 10A to D: Post-PCNL AV fistula treated by coil embolization. (A) Selective right renal angiogram showing small contrast-filled structure supplied by upper polar artery with early draining vein; (B) Superselective angiogram showing getting close to the site of AV fistula (arrow); (C) Coil embolization of the AV fistula site; (D) Postembolization angiogram showing obliteration of the AV fistula.

Uterine Arteriovenous Malformations

The uterine arteriovenous malformations (AVMs) may either be congenital due to faulty development of arteries, veins, capillaries, lymphatics or are acquired as a result of intervillous space enlargement at the site of myometrial scar. The predisposing factors for acquired AVMs are previous uterine surgery, dilatation and curettage, intrauterine contraceptive devices, previous pregnancy, genital tuberculosis and trophoblastic disease.

Congenital AVMs are usually seen in women of child-bearing age who often present with spontaneous abortion because of bleeding. The clinical presentation in acquired AVMs is profuse, intermittent repetitive bleeding. UAE has shown good results in the treatment of these lesions with the added advantage that patient also maintains fertility **(Figs. 13A to F)**.

Postsurgical and Postpartum Hemorrhage

Role of interventional radiology in the management of PPH has gained wide acceptance in the obstetric–gynecologic community as an alternative to uterine artery ligation or hemostatic hysterectomy **(Figs. 14A to D)**.

The postsurgical hemorrhage due to vascular leak can be treated with gelfoam embolization of uterine or anterior division of internal iliac artery. The various causes of post-partum hemorrhage are abnormal placentation, retained products of conception, birth canal laceration, uterine atony or rupture of uterus. All such catastrophic bleeding conditions can be treated by angiographic embolization of uterine artery by using various embolizing materials.

Patient selection: The choice between endovascular and operative treatment should be made jointly by the patient, gynecologist, and intervention radiologist after the current status of all available treatment modalities has been considered and presented in a forthright fashion. Only symptomatic patients in whom other causes for disease have been excluded (including a recent Papanicolaou test) should undergo this treatment. The intervention

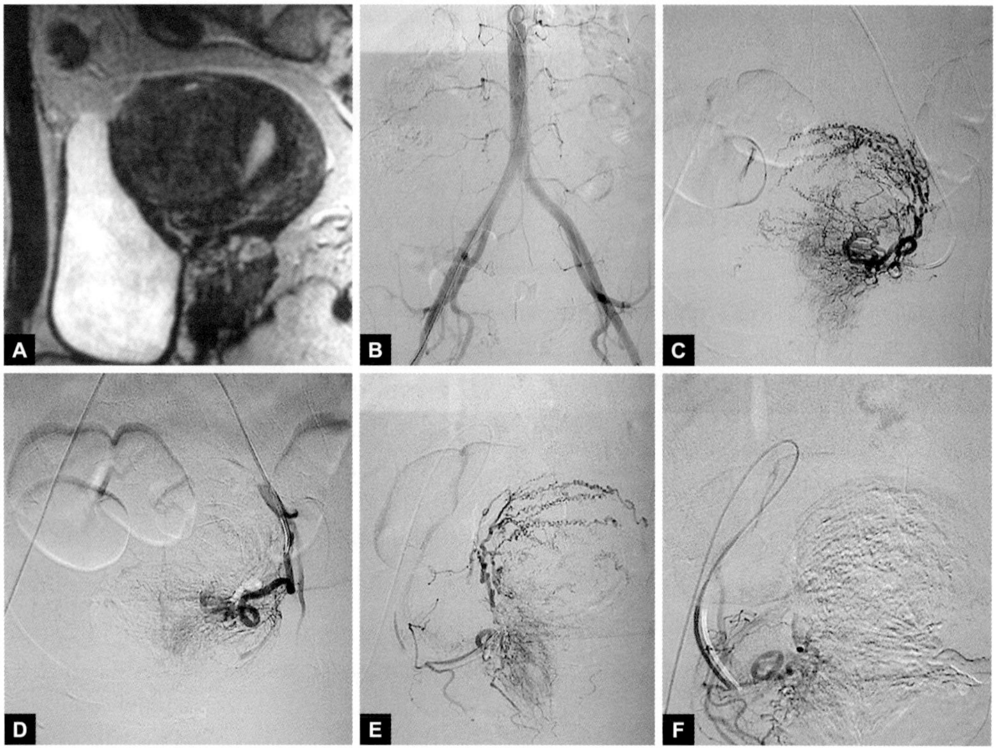

Figs. 11A to F: Uterine artery embolization of uterine fibroid. (A) Sagittal T2W MR image showing fibroid in fundal region; (B) Flush aortogram to look for any ovarian artery supply; (C) Selective left uterine artery angiogram showing increased vascularity supplying the fibroid; (D) Postembolization angiogram showing reduction in vascularity following embolization with PVA particles (500–700 μ); (E and F) Right uterine angiogram followed by embolization using PVA particles and uterine Robert's catheter.

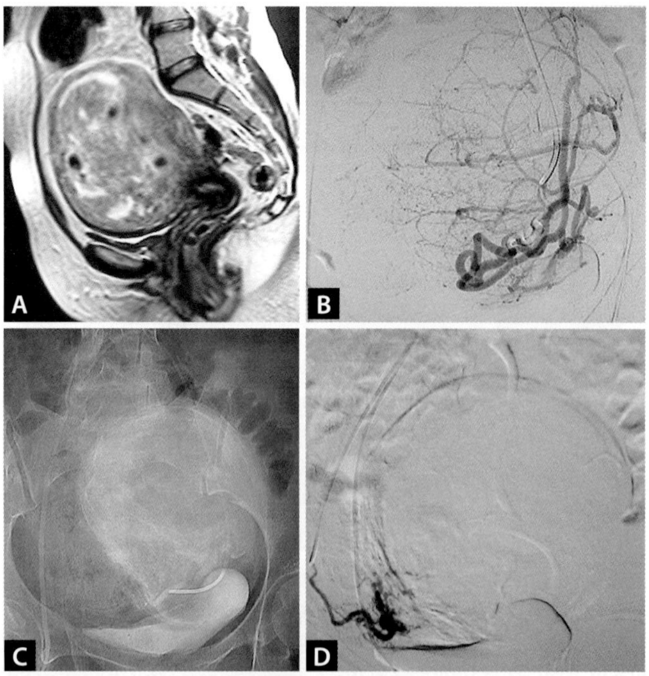

Figs. 12A to D: Uterine artery embolization of large uterine fibroid. (A) Sagittal T2W MR image showing large fibroid in fundal region; (B) Selective left uterine artery angiogram showing increased vascularity supplying the fibroid and splaying of branches by the large fibroid; (C) Postembolization angiogram showing reduction in vascularity and stasis following embolization with PVA particles (500–700 μ); (D) Right uterine angiogram after the embolization showing reduction in vascularity.

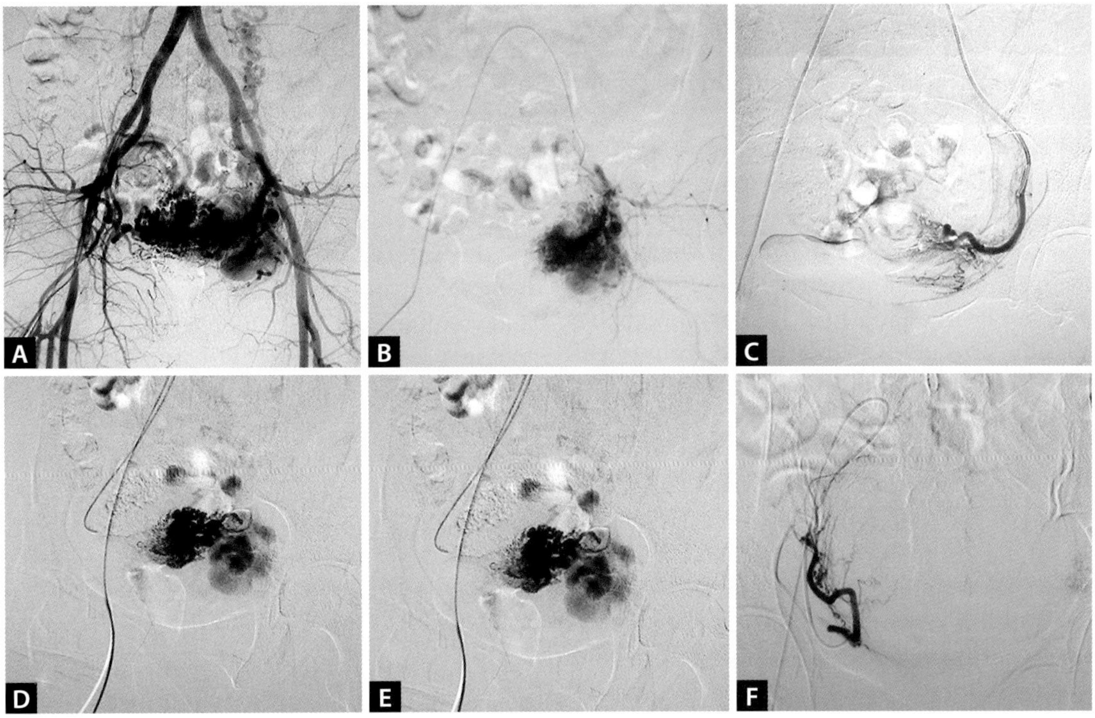

Figs. 13A to F: Uterine arteriovenous malformation treated by angioembolization. (A) Flush aortogram showing large vascular blush in the pelvis; (B) Selective angiogram of left uterine artery showing large vascular blush with nidus; (C) Postembolization angiogram following embolization with PVA particles (700–1000 μ) showing complete obliteration of the vascular blush on left side; (D to F) Selective angiogram of right uterine artery showing residual vascular blush with nidus which was obliterated with PVA particle embolization.

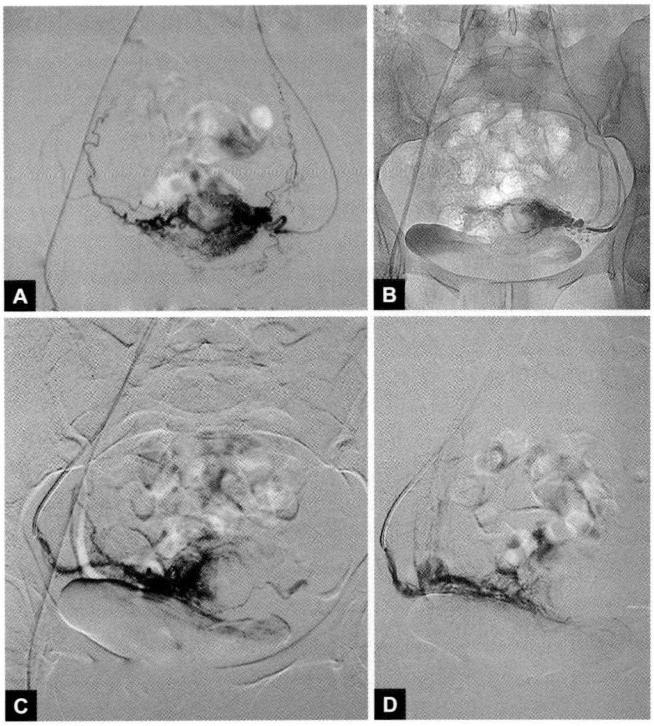

Figs. 14A to D: Post-MTP continuous uterine bleeding treated by angioembolization. (A) Selective angiogram of left uterine artery showing vascular blush; (B) Postembolization angiogram following embolization with PVA particles (700–1000 μ) showing complete obliteration of the vascular blush and stasis of contrast; (C and D) Selective angiogram of right uterine artery showing vascular blush which was obliterated with PVA particle embolization.

radiologist is obligated to become the primary physician caring for the patient in Preprocedure consultation, hospital recovery, and all outpatient management. Adenomyosis also may respond to UAE.[20,21]

Absolute or relative contraindications include pregnancy, active or chronic pelvic infection, gynecologic malignancy (unless palliative or as an adjunct to operation), uncorrectable coagulopathy, severe contrast allergy, and prior pelvic surgery or radiation therapy. The effect of UAE on fertility has not been established, although pregnancy can occur after the procedure. Pedunculated fibroids with relatively narrow stalks are prone to detachment after UAE and may require operative removal.

Technique

UAE for fibroids was first reported by Ravina et al.[22] A pelvic arteriogram with the catheter positioned in the infrarenal abdominal aorta is obtained as a road map. Selective catheterization of the anterior divisions of the internal iliac arteries is performed with a cobra or ultra-long reverse-curve (e.g. Roberts) catheter. Once the uterine artery is identified and selected, angiography shows the markedly dilated spiral arteries feeding the uterus. Tumor hypervascularity and vessel displacement is seen. In some cases, the descending portion of the uterine artery can be engaged with the 5 French diagnostic catheter. However, vasospasm may be a problem, so that coaxial placement of a microcatheter directed well into the uterine artery often is required. The preferred agents for embolization are small-caliber particulate matter, including polyvinyl alcohol (PVA) particles (350–500 or 500–700 pm), trisacryl gelatin microspheres (Embospheres, 700–900 pm), and gelfoam pieces. There does not appear to be any significant difference in clinical efficacy between the two agents. Proximal embolization (e.g. with coils) is inadvisable, because collateral vessels are very likely to develop and which will continue to feed the tumor. Embolization with particulate slurry (made with diluted contrast material) is continued until there is no flow in uterine artery branches ("pruned-tree" appearance). Regardless of the location of fibroids, bilateral embolization is necessary to prevent development of collateral vessels.[23-26]

Bilateral completion internal iliac arteriograms are obtained to identify any additional vessels feeding the tumors. The interventionalist should be observant of variant arterial anatomy and important collateral vessels. In most cases, the ovarian arteries contribute to fibroids through anastomoses with the main uterine artery. In about 10% of patients, the uterine artery is the major blood supply to the ovary, or the ovarian artery has significant direct communication with the fibroid. Embolization of these vessels theoretically increases the risk of ovarian infarction and infertility. Any other collateral vessels that feed the tumor must also be occluded. This is particularly true in women who have undergone prior pelvic surgery, had other tubal pathology, or have fundal fibroids. Postprocedure care should be directed by the interventionalist who performed the UAE. A postembolization syndrome consisting of pain, nausea and vomiting, and low-grade fever is to be expected. Most patients require overnight hospitalization. Pain must be aggressively managed with IV, and later with oral narcotic. Antiemetics are given prophylactically or as needed. Discharge medications include anti-inflammatory drugs (e.g. ketorolac) and potent oral narcotics. Follow-up is done by the interventionalist, including routine clinic evaluation at 1–3 weeks after the procedure.[27]

Results

Bilateral UAE is successful in about 95% of cases. Incomplete infarction of fibroids may be associated with the potential for continued growth. Clinical success with substantial improvement in symptoms is seen in about 80–90% of women. Submucosal lesions and small lesions seem to respond better than other tumors. Failure or recurrence is noted in about 6% of cases. If symptoms continue and leiomyomas persist or enlarge on imaging studies, repeat UAE (with aggressive search for collateral vessels, including the ovarian arteries) is often warranted.

Complications

Intra- and postprocedure pain is a common problem after UAE. Important complications after UAE are intrauterine infection, uterine ischemia and necrosis, pulmonary embolism, and expulsion of pedunculated submucosal lesions. The overall complication rate is about 5% while major complications occur in about 1%. Most patients do not have a significant change in follicle stimulating hormone level after the procedure though this is more likely to occur in women older than 45 years of age. Amenorrhea (which is often transient) occurs in less than 10% of cases, but it is much more likely in patients older than 45–50 years of age. Serious infections as complications are observed in 1% of treated women. Less than 2% require subsequent hysterectomy for any complications of UAE.[28-30]

The reasons for uterine artery embolization failure are incomplete embolization, presence of important collaterals (e.g. ovarian arteries), large fibroids and recanalization of embolized arteries.

VAGINAL AVMs EMBOLIZATION

Vaginal AVMs are rare entities and their most common presentation is vaginal hemorrhage and rarely dyspareunia. These lesions can successfully be treated by angioembolization of the supplying vessels using polyvinyl alcohol particles. Angioembolization being safe and effective should be the first treatment of choice for symptomatic vaginal vascular malformation **(Figs. 15A to C)**.

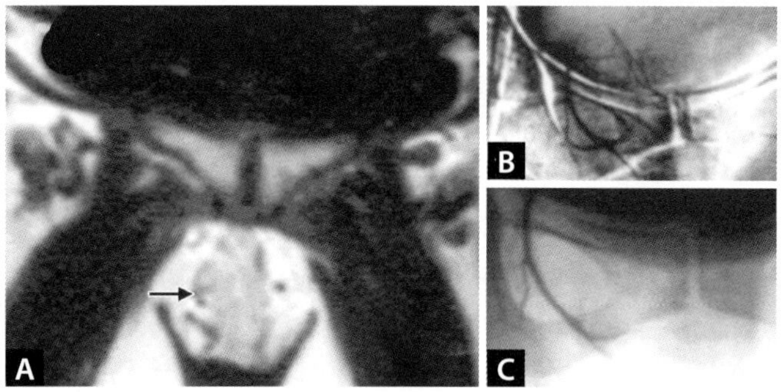

Figs. 15A to C: Vaginal AVM treated by angioembolization. (A) MR image showing abnormal vascular channels (flow voids) on right side of vagina (small arrow); (B and C) Selective angiogram of right internal pudendal artery showing vascular blush, which was obliterated using PVA particles.

SCROTAL AVMs AND TESTICULAR TUMOR EMBOLIZATION

Scrotal arteriovenous malformations are rare entity. The scrotal arteriovenous malformations and the paratesticular masses may occasionally present with uncontrollable bleeding. These lesions can be successfully treated by angioembolization of the supplying vessels using either glue or PVA particles depending upon the situations **(Figs. 16 and 17)**. Angioembolization being safe and effective should be considered as choice of treatment for the treatment of symptomatic scrotal vascular malformation.

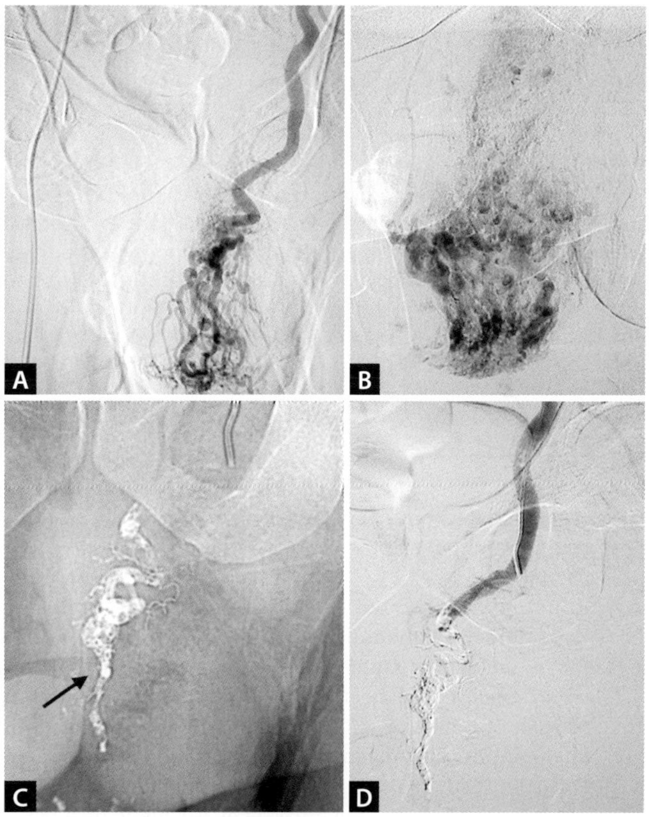

Figs. 16A to D: Scrotal AVM treated by glue embolization. (A and B) Selective left internal pudendal artery angiogram showing hypertrophied artery and large nidus; (C) Spot image showing glue cast obliterating the nidus; (D) Postembolization angiogram showing complete obliteration of the vascular nidus.

VARICOCELE EMBOLIZATION

Varicocele is an important cause of male infertility. Varicocele embolization is indicated in an individual who have been infertile for at least two years and having oligoasthenospermia without an apparent cause of infertility. The embolization is done after placing catheter deep into the internal spermatic vein. Various embolizing materials like steel coils, PVA particles, gelfoam are used.[31-33]

CONCLUSION

In conclusion, renal artery aneurysms can be life-threatening if hemorrhage occurs. Following aneurysm rupture, surgical morbidity and mortality are fairly high. Aggressive management by the interventional radiologist, therefore, is paramount, since these patients are in any case too sick for major revascularization procedures, making endovascular techniques a desirable approach. Embolization of dysfunctioning organs using various embolization techniques and regimens in the management of hypertension or protein wasting in end-stage renal disease has replaced surgical nephrectomy. The evolution of uterine fibroid embolization has established the role of embolotherapy as a viable alternative to hysterectomy, and undoubtedly revolutionized the management of postpartum bleeding. Various methods for embolization are described in the literature. The type of treatment needs to be tailored according to each individual case, since the anatomy typically dictates the therapy best suited.

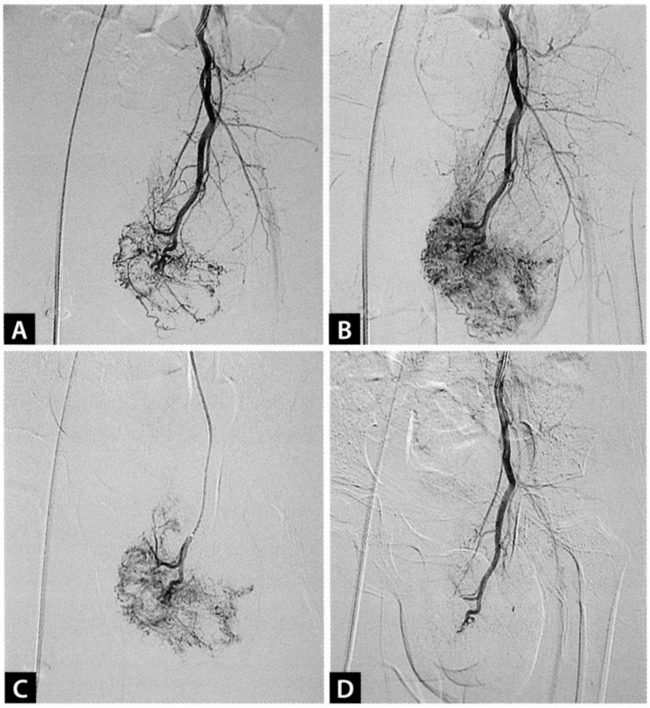

Figs. 17A to D: Left paratesticular mass in a 5-year-old child with scrotal bleeding treated by angioembolization. (A and B) Selective left internal pudendal artery angiogram showing hypertrophied artery and large tumor blush; (C) Catheter brought close to the tumor blush; (D) Postembolization angiogram following embolization using PVA particles (300–500 μ), showing complete obliteration of tumor blush.

REFERENCES

1. Cicuto KP, McLean GK, Oleaga JA, et al. Renal artery stenosis. Anatomical classification for percutaneous transluminalangioplasty. Am J Roentgenol. 1981;137: 599-601.
2. Rountas C, Vlychou M, Vassiou K, Liakopoulos V, Kapsalaki E, Koukoulis G, et al. Imaging modalities for renal artery stenosis in suspected renovascular hypertension: prospective intraindividual comparison of color Doppler US, CT angiography, GD-enhanced MR angiography, and digital substraction angiography. Ren Fail. 2007;29(3):295-302.
3. Tan KT, van Beek EJ, Brown PW, et al. Magnetic resonance angiography for the diagnosis of renal artery stenosis. A metaanalysis.Clin Radiol. 2002;57:617-24.
4. Hoffman O, Carreres T, Sapoval MR, et al. Ostial renal artery stenosis angioplasty. Immediate and mid-term angiographic and clinical results. J Vasc Interv Radiol. 1998;9:65–73.
5. Matsumoto AH, Tegtmeyer CJ, Fitzgerald EK, et al. Percutaneous transluminal angioplasty of visceral arterial stenoses: results and long-term clinical follow-up. J Vasc Interv Radiol. 1995; 6:165–74.
6. Moss JG, Hamilton G. Renal and visceral artery intervention. In: Dyet JF, Nicholson AA, Ettles DF, Wilson SE (Eds): Textbook of endovascular procedures. Churchill Livingston: Philadelphia; 2000.pp.151-73.
7. Park JH, Kim WS, Han MC, Lee CW. Renal arterial embolization with absolute ethanol. J Korean Med Sci. 1987;2(1):13-8.
8. Park JH, Kim SH, Han JK, Chung JW, Han MC. Transcatheter arterial embolization of unresectable renal cell carcinoma with a mixture of ethanol and iodized oil. Cardiovasc Intervent Radiol. 1994;17(6):323-7.
9. Martin RS 3rd, et al. Renal artery aneurysm: Selective treatment for hypertension and prevention of rupture. J Vasc Surg. 1989;9: 26-34.
10. Poutasse EF. Renal artery aneurysms: Their natural history and surgery. J Urol. 1966;95:297-306.
11. Poutasse EF. Renal artery aneurysms. J Urol. 1975;113:443-9.
12. Liguori G, et al. Percutaneous management of renal artery aneurysm with a stent-graft. J Urol. 2002;167:2518-9.
13. Pershad A, Heuser R. Renal artery aneurysm: successful exclusion with a stent graft. Catheter Cardiovasc Interv. 2004; 61:314-6.
14. Rundback JH, et al. Percutaneous stent-graft management of renal artery aneurysms. J Vasc Interv Radiol. 2000;1189-93.
15. Schneidereit NP, et al. Endovascular repair of a ruptured renal artery aneurysm. J Endovasc Ther. 2003;10:71-4.
16. Crotty KL, Orihuela E, Warren MM. Recent advances in the diagnosis and treatment of renal arteriovenous malformations and fistulas. J Urol. 1993;150:1355.
17. Takcbayashi S, Aida N, Matsui K. Arteriovenous malformations of the kidneys: diagnosis and follow-up with color Doppler sonography in six patients. Am J Roentgenol. 1991;157:991.
18. Allione A, Pomero F, Valpreda S, et al. Worsening of hypertension in a pregnant women with renal arteriovenous malformation. A successful superselective embolization after delivery. Clin Nephrol. 2003;60:211.
19. Takebayashi S, Hosaka M, Ishizuka E, et al. Arteriovenous malformations of the kidneys: ablation with alcohol. Am J Roentgenol. 1988;150:587.
20. Andrews RT, Spies JB, Sacks D, et al. Patient care and uterine artery embolization for leiomyomata. J Vasc Interv Radiol. 2004;15:115.
21. Siskin GP, Tublin ME, Stainken BF, et al. Uterine artery embolization for the treatment of adenomyosis: clinical response and evaluation with MR imaging. Am J Roentgenol. 2001;177:297.
22. Ravina JH, Herbreteau D, Ciraru-Vigneron N, et al. Arterial embolisation to treat uterine myomata. Lancet. 1995;346:671.
23. Worthington-Kirsch RL, Andrews RT, et al. Uterine fibroid embolization: technical aspects. Tech Vasc Intent Radio l. 2002;5:17.
24. Banovac F, Ascher SM, Jones DA, et al. Magnetic resonance imaging outcome after uterine artery embolization for

leiomyomata with use of trisacryl gelatin microspheres. J Vasc Interv Radiol. 2002;13:681.
25. Pelage JP, Le Dref O, Beregi JP, et al. Limited uterine artery embolization with tris-acryl gelatin microspheres for uterine fibroids. J Vasc Interv Radiol. 2003;14:15.
26. Pelage JP, Le Dref O, Soyer P, et al. Arterial anatomy of the female genital tract: variations and relevance to transcatheter embolization of the uterus. Am J Roentgenol. 1999;172:989.
27. Siskin GP, Bonn J, Worthington-Kirsch RL, et al. Uterine fibroid embolization: pain management. Tech Vasc Interv Radiol. 2002;5:35.
28. Pelage JP, Walker WJ, Dref OL. Uterine necrosis after uterine artery embolization for leiomyoma. Obstet Gynecol. 2002;99:6767.
29. Spies JB, Spector A, Roth AR, et al. Complications after uterine artery embolization for leiom-yomas. Obstet Gynecol. 2002;100:873.
30. Spies JB, Roth AR, Gonsalves SM, et al. Ovarian function after uterine artery embolization for leiomyomata. assessment with use of serum follicle stimulating hormone assay. J Vasc Interv Radiol. 2001;12:437.
31. Lima SS, Castro MP, Costa OF. A new method for the treatment of varicocele. Andrologia. 1978;10:103-6.
32. Trombetta C, Salisci E, Deriu M, Paoni A, Sanna M, Ganau A, et al. Echo-flowmetric control 6 years after percutaneous treatment of varicocele. Arch Ital Urol Androl. 1993;65:363-7.
33. Usuki N, Nakamura K, Takashima S, Takada K, Kaminoh T, Tsubakimoto M, et al. Embolization of varicocele with ethanol. Nippon Igaku Hoshasen Gakkai Zasshi. 1994;54:870-5 (Japanese).

CHAPTER 121

Imaging in Female Infertility

Rashmi Dixit

INTRODUCTION

Infertility is generally defined as one year of unprotected intercourse without conception and is one of the most prevalent chronic health disorders involving young adults.[1] Infertility is usually reported in up to 20% couples. The ability to diagnose and treat various causes of infertility is rapidly progressing and the radiologists are becoming increasingly involved in both the diagnosis and treatment of these patients.[1] Earliest evaluation and treatment of infertility is indicated in women with age above 35 years, history of oligo/amenorrhea, known or suspected uterine/tubal disease or endometriosis or a sub-fertile partner.[2] Infertility is referred to as primary when the patient has never conceived and secondary when there is a history of previous pregnancy.

CAUSES OF INFERTILITY

The statistics vary but a male factor is attributable in 40% cases, female factor 40% of the times and in about 20% cases there may be combined or unexplained causes.[3]

The initial evaluation of the infertile couple involves a complete history and examination.[4] A careful physical examination and history can identify symptoms or signs which suggest a specific cause for infertility and thereby help focus subsequent diagnostic evaluation on the most likely factor(s) responsible.[2]

The most common causes of infertility should be assessed very carefully. The most probable factors responsible are the cervical, the endometrial, uterine, the ovarian, the tubal, the peritoneal, and the male factors.[4-7]

Imaging Modalities

Imaging modalities used for evaluation of female infertility include:

1. Hysterosalpingography (HSG)
2. Sonography including transvaginal sonography (TVS) and sonohysterosalpingography.
3. Magnetic resonance imaging (MRI)

Hysterosalpingography[8,9]

Hysterosalpingography is performed during the first 7–12 days of menstural cycle and is best scheduled during the interval of 2–5 days immediately after the end of menses to reduce the risk of infection to the minimum, avoid interference from intrauterine blood clot and prevent any possibility of an Hysterosalpingography being performed in an unrecognized conception cycle. HSG does not require any specific preparation, although pretreatment with an NSAID (approximately 30 minutes before) is helpful to limit discomfort associated with the procedure. Although usually unnecessary, prophylactic antibiotic treatment may also be considered to minimize post procedure infection. HSG is best avoided altogether for at least several weeks following any episode of acute PID to minimize risk of infectious complications.

The basic technique for performing an HSG is quite standard. The study should be performed using image intensification fluoroscopy with a limited number of radiographs. The average HSG requires only 20–30 seconds of fluoroscopic time with minimal radiation exposure and has very low risk. Usually, only 3–4 basic films are required—a scout, one film during early filling, third film to document the uterine contours with the uterus fully distended and assess tubal patency and a fourth film to detect free intra peritoneal spill not seen earlier or any areas of contrast loculation **(Figs. 1 and 2)**.

Additional films may be needed when the uterus obscures the tubes or the uterine cavity appears abnormal. Contrast can be introduced using a common metal "acorn" cannula or via a balloon catheter. In general, the latter technique requires less fluoroscopic time and smaller volumes of contrast, produces less pain and is easier to perform. Slow injection of contrast (typically 3–10 mL) helps minimize the discomfort associated with HSG.

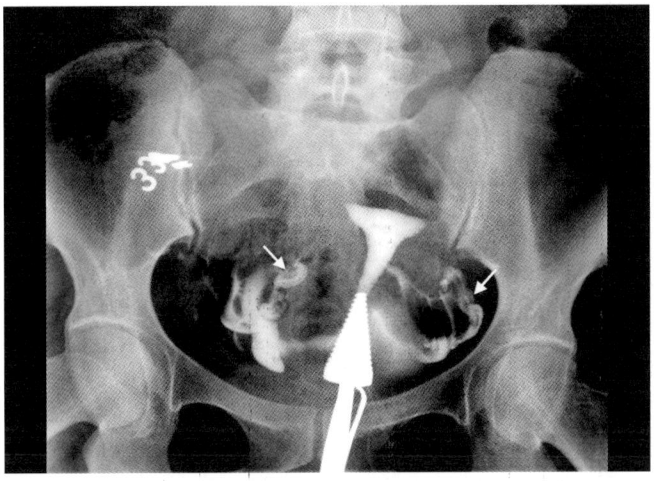

Fig. 1: Normal HSG showing an inverted triangle shaped smooth uterine outline. Both fallopian tubes are well outlined by contrast. Note the presence of longitudinal rugal folds in the ampullary portion (arrows). Free intraperitoneal spill is seen on both sides outlining the bowel loops.

Watersoluble contrast media are generally used. Oil based contrast media have also been used in the past but these are generally too viscous to reveal internal tubal architecture (having prognostic significance) disperse poorly in pelvis, so adnexal adhesions cannot be detected and are associated with significant risk of granulomatous reaction, venous intravesation and embolism. Those advocating oil soluble contrast media say that these adverse reactions are rare and numerous studies have shown that oil based contrast media increase fertility in the months immediately following HSG in women with patent tubes, however, this has been challenged by a subsequent randomized clinical trial[10-13] and these agents are generally not used.

Complications following an HSG are relatively rare but may include—light spotting after the procedure (usually lasting less than 24 hours), infection and pain. Rarely, systemic reactions to contrast media and uterine or fallopian tube perforation have been reported.[8]

Transvaginal Sonography

While evaluating patients for infertility by TVS, especially for follicular monitoring or oocyte retrieval normal condoms with spermicidal gels should be avoided.[14] Even ultrasound gels may have a detrimental effect on sperm and embryo and should not be used during oocyte retrieval or embryo transfers.[15]

Sonohysterosalpingography

Sonohysterosalpingography refers to a technique that evaluates the uterus and fallopian tubes after the uterine

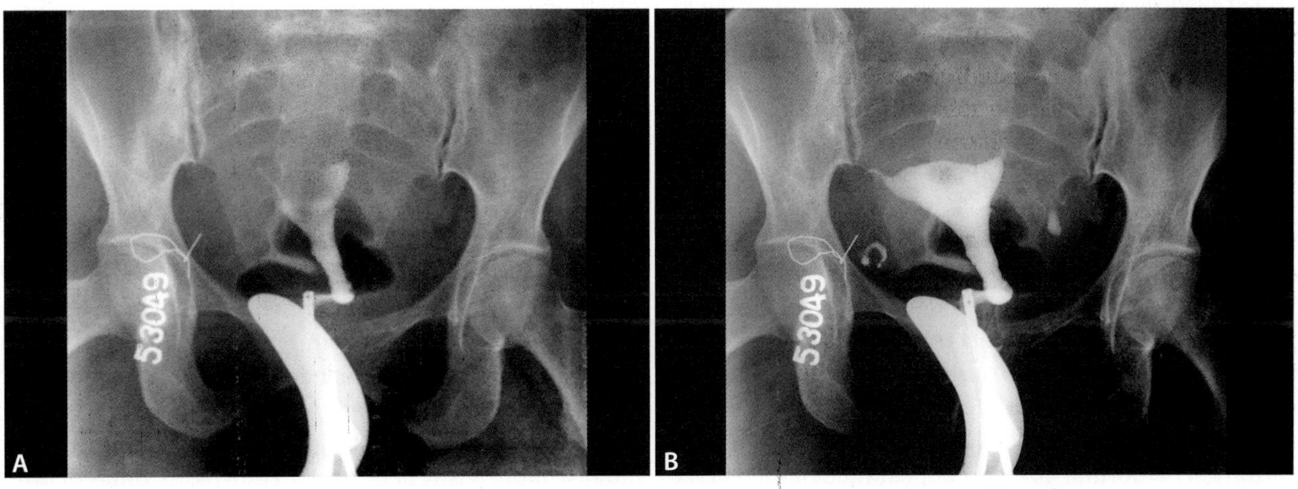

Figs. 2A and B: Uterine filling defect due to a fundal fibroid is much better appreciated on the early filling film (A) as compared with (B) where the uterine cavity is fully distended with contrast and the filling defect is much less apparent.

cavity has been distended with sonographic contrast media. Saline is the most commonly used agent, other contrast media include air and positive contrast agents such as echovist. It is a sensitive technique to detect uterine synechiae, endometrial polyps and can also be used to evaluate for tubal patency.[15,16]

Normal Menstrual Cycle[1]

A basic understanding of the normal menstrual cycle is important before trying to image female infertility.

The three stages of a normal menstrual cycle are the follicular phase, ovulation and luteal phase. The cycle is controlled by the hypothalamic-pituitary-ovarian axis. Day 1 of the average 28-day cycle initiates the menstruation. The plasma follicle stimulating hormone (FSH) level begins to rise thus stimulating the growth of the ovarian follicles and beginning the follicular phase. Usually one follicle becomes the dominant or graafian follicle. The developing follicles secrete estradiol, which stimulates endometrial proliferation; thus, the follicular phase is also called the proliferative phase. Estradiol reaches its peak about 12 hours before the luteinizing hormone (LH) ovulatory surge. This peak in estradiol causes an increase in LH/FSH levels, stimulating ovulation on or around day 14. The ovulation is followed by the luteal or secretory phase, during which the ruptured graafian follicle becomes the corpus luteum. The corpus luteum produces progesterone, which primes the endometrium for the fertilized egg. Failure of conception leads to the degeneration of corpus luteum, causing a decrease in estradiol/progesterone levels and sloughing of the endometrial lining, i.e. menstruation.

Cervical Factor

The cervical factor refers to the properties of cervical mucus and sperm transport. The hospitality of the cervix to the sperm is not evaluated by imaging the cervical anatomy but is best determined by the post coital test. Although some controversy persists about how and when to perform the post coital test, most authors suggest that it should be as close to ovulation as possible and at least 8 hours after intercourse. [1,4] The role of Imaging is limited in this evaluation except for monitoring follicle development which helps to optimize the timing of the test and avoid false positive results.[1] In recent years its utility and predictive value have been seriously questioned[2,17] but some still consider it a useful diagnostic test.[2,18]

Cervical stenosis may occasionally be the cause of infertility. The normal size and appearance of the cervix are variable and therefore diagnosis based on appearance alone is difficult. An internal os region of less than 1 mm in diameter by hysterosalpingography in a woman with painful periods may indicate cervical stenosis.[3]

Endometrial–Uterine Factor

Less than 10% of cases of infertility are caused by uterine and endometrial abnormalities.[1,4,5] Although these are a relatively uncommon cause of infertility, they should always be considered because they can adversely affect the outcome of pregnancies achieved by successful treatment of other more common factors. The abnormalities can be classified into two categories as follows: anatomic, e.g. adhesions, leiomyomas, congenital uterine malformations and physiological, i.e. lack of normal endometrial response to hormonal stimulation.

There are four basic methods for evaluating the uterine cavity, such as: HSG, Standard TVS or TVS with saline contrast (sono-hysterography) MRI and hysteroscopy. The choice of the investigation needs to be tailored to the individual patient. HSG is the traditional method and still the best initial method because it also evaluates tubal patency. However, in women with no risk for tubal disease and whose tubal status is already known (say from previous laparoscopic surgery for some other cause) TVS offers a better tolerated and simpler alternative than can also reveal suspected ovarian pathology (cyst/endometrioma) with no radiation exposure. When uterine cavity detail is critical or when congenital anomalies are suspected sonohysterography or MRI may be used. Hysteroscopy is the most definitive method but may be safely reserved for treatment of abnormalities identified by other less invasive methods.[9]

Endometrial Adhesions or Synechiae

Endometrial adhesions or synechiae cause infertility either by obstructing the cervical os or fallopian tube or by providing a sub optimal environment for embryo implantation. Synechiae are usually the sequelae of infection including tuberculosis or prior dilatation and curettage. Asherman's syndrome is the association of synechiae with hypomenorrhea or amenorrhea and infertility.

Hysterosalpingography is the imaging study of choice in the evaluation of synechiae. Synechiae appear as multiple irregular filling defects in the uterine cavity.[1] They are generally linear and irregular and extend from one uterine wall to the opposite which allows the contrast agent to flow around them only in one dimension. For this reason, they are more easily defined than polyps, myomas or other masses that generally allow contrast agent to flow around them in two dimensions.[3] Adhesions at the margins of the cavity may distort the uterine outline or obscure cornua[9] **(Fig. 3)**. It is difficult to visualize adhesions on TVS, but when seen can appear as echogenic bridges in the endometrial cavity or as irregularities of the endometrium surrounded by cystic spaces.[1,5] Synechiae are easier to identify on sonohysterography where they appear as linear echogenic bridges in the fluid filled endometrial cavity.

Leiomyoma

Leiomyoma (fibroid) is the most common neoplasm of the uterus found in up to 25% of women. Leiomyomas are rarely a primary cause of infertility and treatment should be considered only after the exclusion of other potential causes.[1,4,5] Available evidence suggests that pregnancy and implantation rates are significantly lower in women with submucous myomas but not in those with subserosal or intramural myomas that do not encroach or clearly distort the endometrial cavity, especially when modest in size (5–7 cm). Proposed mechanisms by which myomas might adversely affect fertility include cornual occlusion by myomas that involve or compress the interstitial segment of the tube, dysfunctional uterine contractility interfering with ovum or sperm transport or embryo implantation and poor regional blood flow resulting in focal endometrial attenuation or ulceration.[9]

On hysterosalpingography, leiomyomas generally appear as filling defects in the endometrial cavity with enlargement of cavity when sufficiently large **(Fig. 4)**. Care must be taken to differentiate between leiomyomas and other filling defects, including polyps, blood clots, mucus and air bubbles. Fibroids appear variable on ultrasound. They are generally hypoechoic, but can be isoechoic or hyperechoic as well. Shadowing from calcification may also be present. The reported sensitivity of ultrasound in detecting fibroid ranges from 65–93%. Ultrasound has some limitations in evaluating fibroids which include failure to detect small leiomyomas and difficulty in exact localization due to unfavorable uterine position, and poor uterine visualization because of patient body hapitus. MRI has the highest sensitivity for detection of fibroids.[1,19] Fibroids generally show low to intermediate signal intensity on T1 weighted images and low signal intensity on T2 weighted images; however, if they have degenerated, the signal characteristics may vary **(Figs. 5A and B)**. Some distinct advantages on MRI include the ability to differentiate leiomyomas from adenomyosis and improved preoperative localization for surgical planning and predicting treatment outcome. Submucosal fibroids may be resected via a hysteroscope rather than laparotomy. When submucous myomas are single and small, the benefits of hysteroscopic myomectomy generally outweigh the few associated risks. When these are multiple and large, hysteroscopic myomectomy requires much greater technical expertise and poses greater risks including severe postoperative uterine adhesions.[1,20] Leiomyomas with an intramural component may be treated by uterine artery embolization (UAE). In these patients high signal intensity on T1W images is a negative predictor of volume reduction. It is hypothesized that such leiomyomas have already undergone hemorrhagic degeneration and loss of vascular supply due to which they show poor response to UAE.[21] Gadolinium enhanced MR may be useful in predicting the outcome to hormonal (GnRH) therapy.[21]

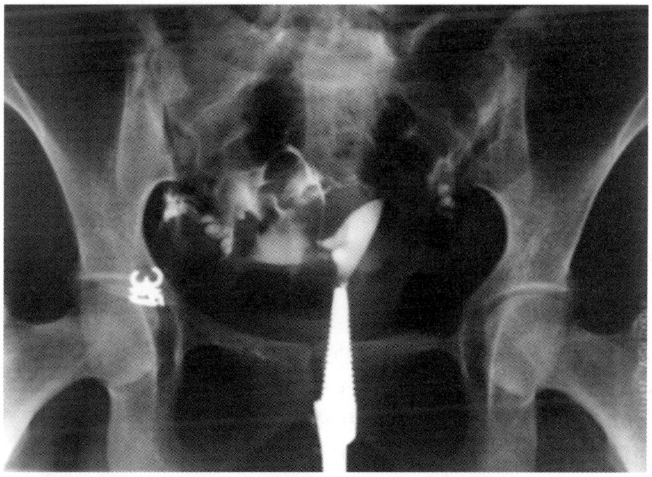

Fig. 3: HSG in a patient with secondary infertility following prior dilatation and curettage shows a distorted uterine cavity with irregular filling defects in the region of right cornu suggestive of intrauterine adhesions.

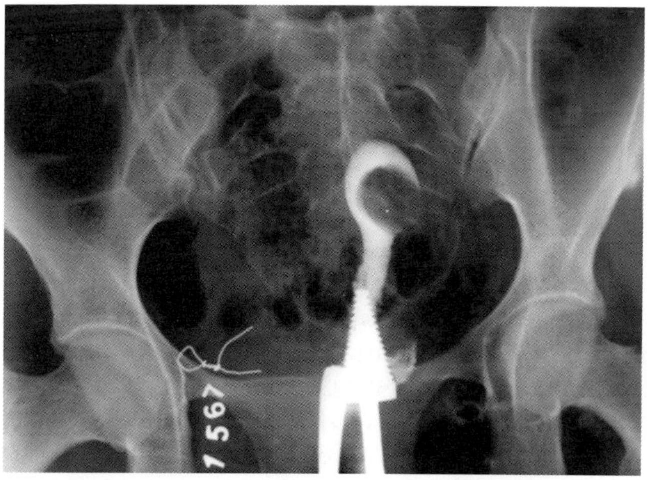

Fig. 4: A globular uterine cavity with a well-defined rounded filling defect consistent with a fibroid.

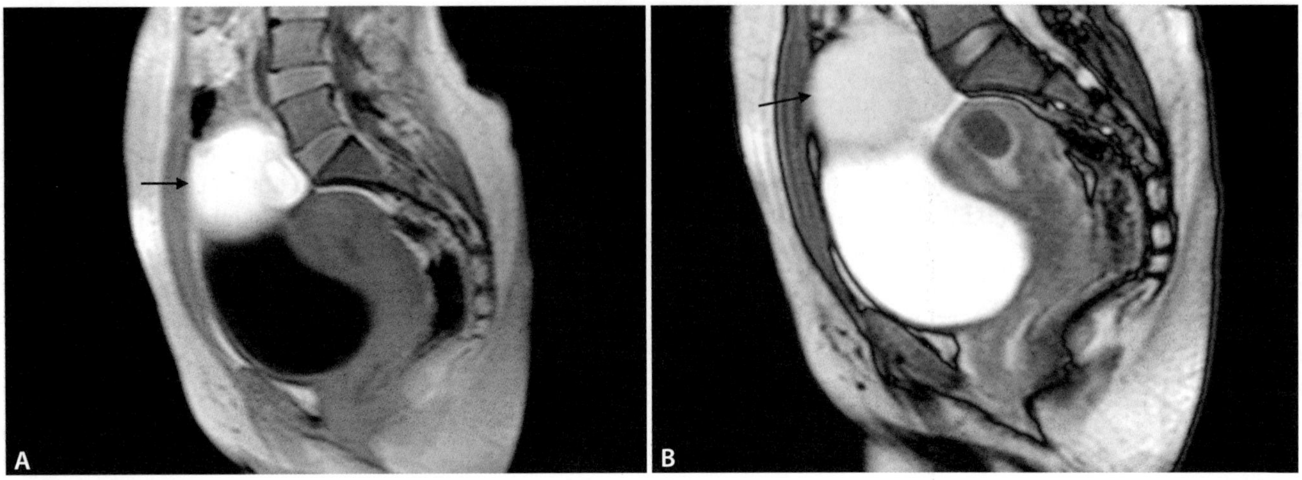

Figs. 5A and B: T1W (A) and T2W (B) weighted sagittal MR images reveal a small submucous fundal fibroid appearing iso intense on T1 and hypointense on T2W images with distortion of the endometrial cavity. Note the presence of hemorrhagic cyst in one of the ovaries lying superior to the bladder and the uterus appearing hyperintense on both T1W and T2W images (arrows).

Endometrial Polyps[9]

Endometrial polyps can be identified by HSG or TVS. The sensitivity of sonohysterography for diagnosis of endometrial polyps is greater than that of HSG and nearing hysteroscopy but false-positive results due to blood clot, mucous plug and shearing of normal endometrium are not uncommon **(Figs. 6A and B)**.

Mullerian Duct Abnormalities[1,9,21,22]

Mullerian duct abnormalities (MDAs) result from congenital non-development or fusion abnormalities of mullerian ducts, MDAs affect 1–5% of all women and although they have long been associated with pregnancy loss and complications, the ability to conceive generally remains unaffected. The anomalies have been classified into seven groups based on their prognosis for future fertility and surgical treatment. Among the MDAs septate uterus carries the highest rate of pregnancy loss (67%). Because the treatment of MDAs is dependent on the type of abnormality and because certain treatment options like IVF, super ovulation are associated with multifetal gestation which presents even greater risk to women with uterine malformations, a correct diagnosis is paramount. The most consistently accurate imaging technique for evaluation of MDAs is MRI. When transvaginal sonography is combined with hysterosalpingography, reports show that it results in diagnostic accuracy rates as high as 90%. 3D ultrasound is comparable in accuracy to MR in evaluation of congenital malformations.[23,24]

HSG evaluates mainly the internal morphology of the endometrial cavity and is less accurate. It cannot reliably distinguish a septate from a bicornuate uterus. Both these appear as two diverging endometrial cavities. A more obtuse angle ($>105^{\circ}$) favors a bicornuate uterus and an acute angle ($<75^{\circ}$) favors a septate uterus, but there is considerable overlap **(Figs. 7A to C)**. The external contour must be evaluated to make the correct diagnosis (a septate uterus has a normal contour, whereas a bicornuate uterus is heart-shaped). Using T2-weighted MR images parallel to the long axis of the uterus, both the internal and external uterine contour can be evaluated simultaneously. Not only does simultaneous internal and external visualization differentiate a bicornuate from a septate uterus, but it also helps in the planning of the treatment. On MR the bicornuate uterus has divergent uterine horns with an intercornual distance exceeding 4 cm, concavity of the fundal contour or a cleft more than 1 cm deep (heart-shaped) whereas in a septate uterus the contour is normally convex, flat or minimally indented by less than 1 cm. The septum may be a combination of fibrous tissue myometrium or both **(Figs. 8A and B)**.[21] Septoplasty via hysteroscopy is generally done for septate uterus. An incompetent cervix is often associated with bicornuate uterus and serial scanning during pregnancy may be helpful. [3] MRI is also helpful in delineating other less common MDAs, including arcuate, unicornuate uterus, uterus didelphys or uterine agenesis. Among the MDAs, uterus didelphys is associated with the highest possibility of successful pregnancy. Spontaneous abortion and premature labor may occur in pregnancies with a unicornuate uterus. Some of these patients have a rudimentary horn on the contralateral side. When this is non-communicating, endometrial tissue is

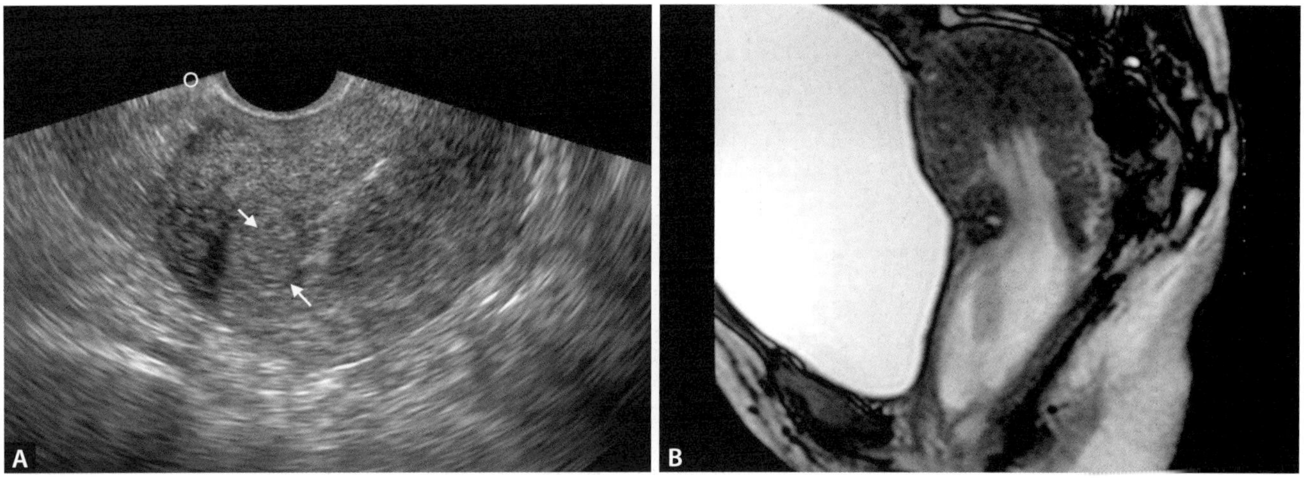

Figs. 6A and B: (A) TVS reveals a relatively well-defined hypoechoic mass within the upper endometrial cavity (arrows) due to an endometrial polyps which was hysteroscopically removed; (B) Sagittal T2W MR image (in another patient) reveals a large hyperintense endometrial polyp coming out through the cervix and bulging into the vagina.

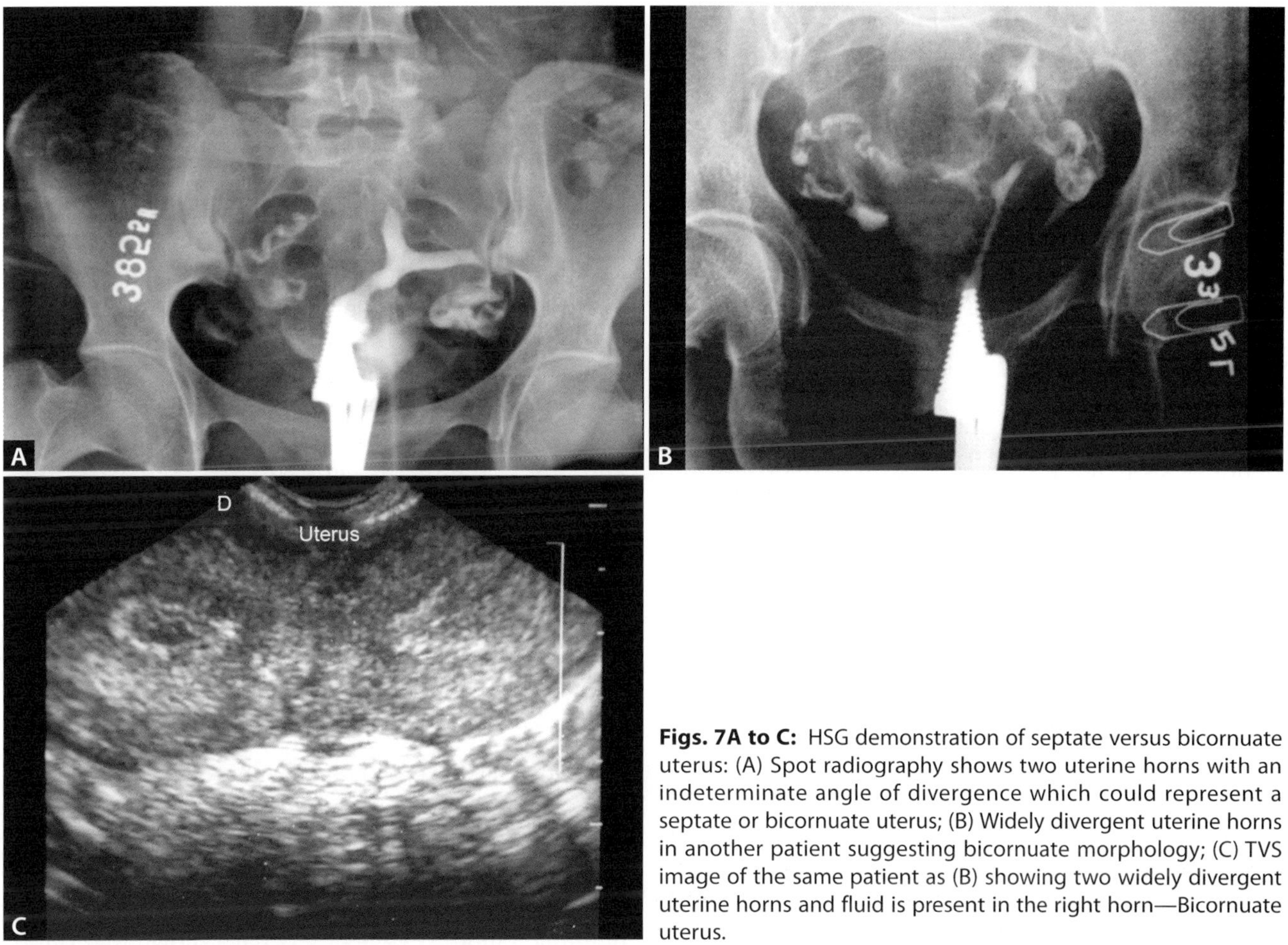

Figs. 7A to C: HSG demonstration of septate versus bicornuate uterus: (A) Spot radiography shows two uterine horns with an indeterminate angle of divergence which could represent a septate or bicornuate uterus; (B) Widely divergent uterine horns in another patient suggesting bicornuate morphology; (C) TVS image of the same patient as (B) showing two widely divergent uterine horns and fluid is present in the right horn—Bicornuate uterus.

expelled retrogradely resulting in increased frequency of endometriosis. This makes surgical resection of the horn necessary.

Arcurate uterus usually has no effect on fertility. It has been proposed that when a ratio of less than 10% between the height of fundal indentation and distance between the

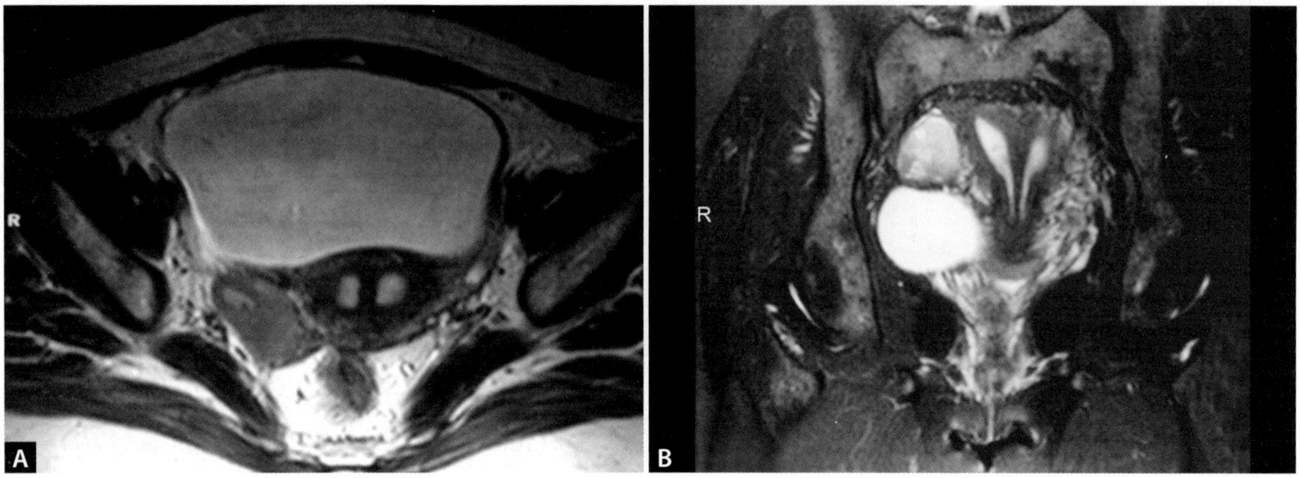

Figs. 8A and B: T2W axial and coronal MR images in a patient with complete uterine septum. Two uterine cavities are seen which are separated by a septum showing signal isointense to myometrium in its upper part and an inferior fibrous component which is T2 hypointense extending into the cervix. The external fundal contour is only mildly indented. Note the cyst in the right ovary—Septate uterus.

lateral apices of the horns is calculated on HSG, an adverse reproductive outcome is not anticipated.[22-27] However a defining depth of indentation to differentiate an arcurate configuration from a broad based septum has not been established. On MR images the normal external uterine contour is maintained with a smooth myometrial fundal indentation. The signal intensity of this is similar to normal myometrium **(Figs. 9A and B)**.

Endometrial ossification is a rare condition which acts like an IUCD. It appears as a highly reflective echo on USG.[15]

Adenomyosis

Adenomyosis is not a common cause of infertility and generally manifests as pelvic pain or bleeding. It is most commonly detected with MR imaging or ultrasound.[15] The relevant ultrasound findings are thickening and asymmetry of anterior or posterior uterine walls with a poorly defined area of increased, decreased or heterogeneous echogenicity or myometrial cysts **(Fig. 10)**. MR reveals a myometrial mass of low signal on both T1 and T2W images with indistinct margins, focal widening of the junctional zone (≥12 mm) and punctuate high signal intensity foci **(Figs. 11A and B)**.[21] Adenomyosis may occasionally be imaged with HSG when nests of endometrial tissue connect to the uterine cavity. At HSG adenomyosis appears as small diverticulae extending into the myometrium **(Fig. 12)**.[8]

The only functional uterine[9] abnormality that is of particular interest in the evaluation of infertility is chronic endometritis. Some may view defects of endometrial receptivity, including luteal phase deficiency (LPD) as another but controversies exist regarding the existence mode of diagnosis and of LPD.

Nontubercular Chronic Endometritis

Nontubercular chronic endometritis[9] is an enigmatic condition of uncertain persistence from one cycle to next and often of uncertain bacterial origin. The diagnosis is usually made histologically, but in florid cases, TVS may reveal thin echogenic endometruim that does not thicken as follicular phase advances.

Sonography has also been used to study the normal developmental response of the endometrium to try and predict implantation. In the menstrual phase the endometrium is a thin echogenic interface which thickens during the proliferative phase is relatively hypo- to isoechoic yielding a prominent trilaminar pattern. During the secretory phase the endometrim does not thicken further but becomes more echogenic. Researchers have attempted to correlate endometrial thickness and appearance and volume (using 3D ultrasound) in an effort to predict optimal implantation times, however, neither allowed a reliable prediction of subsequent implantion.[28]

Spiral and uterine artery Doppler indices have been studied to evaluate endometrial receptivity but the results have again been conflicting. Some authors have reported that a uterine artery PI to >3 correlates with poor chance of implantation[1,29] while others have shown that Doppler evaluation of the spiral or uterine arteries has little predictive value.[28] Recently, researchers have shown that presence of both endometrial and subendometrial blood flow on the day of embryo transfer (ET) indicates good endometrial

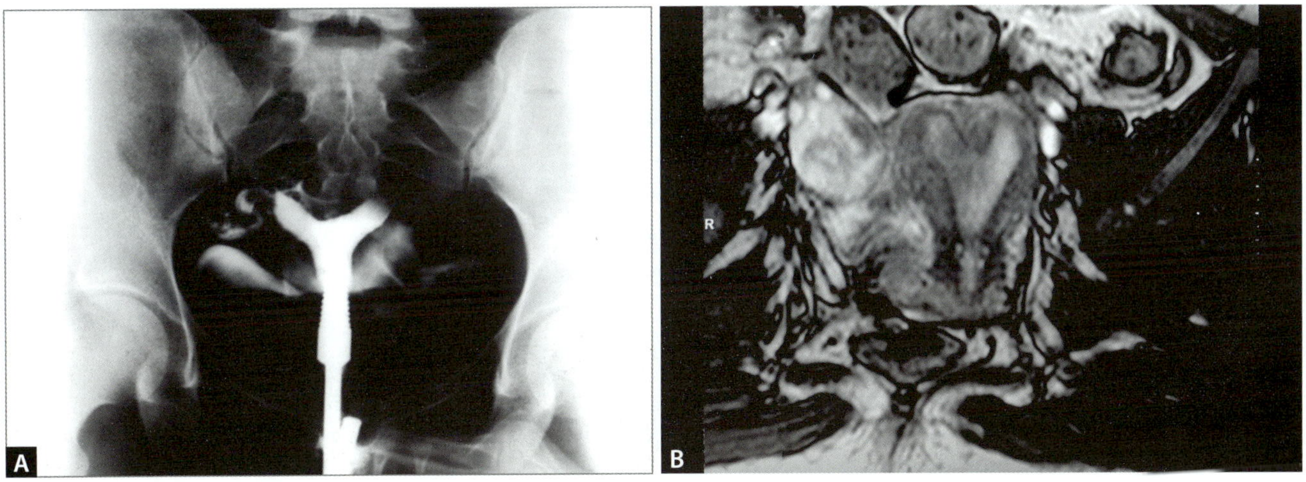

Figs. 9A and B: (A) HSG showing a broad saddle shaped indentation of fundal outline representing an arcurate deformity; (B) TSE-T2W MR image of the same patient demonstrates a normal external uterine contour with a smooth broad myometrial indentation at the fundus.

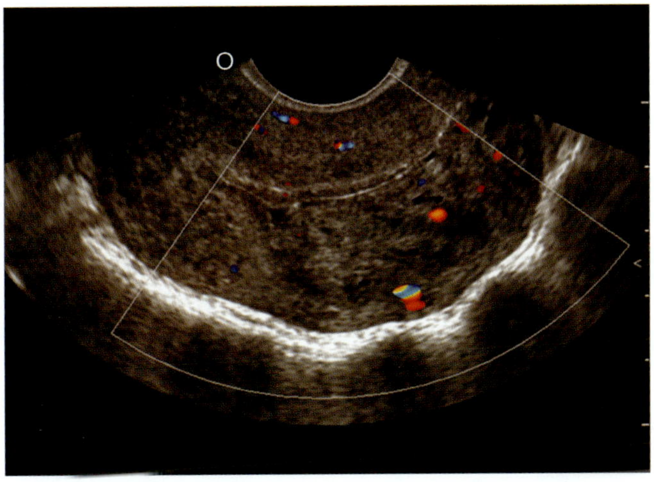

Fig. 10: TVS (CDFI) showing a poorly defined area of decreased echogenicity in the anterior myometrium with no abnormal vascularity—Adenomyosis.

receptivity whereas absence of both represents a poor uterine environment.[30] As a result of conflicting results, routine US or Doppler evaluation of the endometruim has no proven value in management of patients with infertility. According to a recent study, the relevant studies in literature differ in patient's characteristics, the day of ultrasound examination and selection of subendometrial region and further studies are required especially in the late follicular to the early luteal phase.[31]

Tubal Factor

The fallopian tubes connect the peritoneal cavity to the external environment via the uterus, cervix and vagina. Their function and their anatomy is complex and includes conduction of sperm from the uterine end towards the ampulla, conduction of ova in the other direction from the fimbriated end to the ampulla and support of the early embryo and conduction of the early embryo from the ampulla into the uterus for implantation. The normal fallopian tube ranges in length from 7 to 16 cm, with an average length of 12 cm. The tube is composed of a ciliated mucosal epithelial layer surrounded by three smooth muscle layers and is divided into four regions, which are: (i) the intramural or interstitial portion, which lies in the wall of the uterine fundus and is 1–2 cm long; (ii) the isthmic portion, which is approximately 2–3 cm long; (iii) the ampullary portion, which is 5–8 cm long; and (iv) the infundibulum, which is the trumpet-shaped distal end of the tube that terminates in the fimbria.[3]

Pathology of the fallopian tube is the cause of infertility in up to 40% women and is among the most common causes of infertility. Tubal obstruction is a common sequelae of infection or endometriosis. Another cause of tubal infertility commonly described in the western literature is salpingitis isthmica nodosa (SIN).[1,3]

Evaluation of tubal patency is an essential part of the infertility workup. The methods available to evaluate the tubes include HSG, sonohysterosalpingography and laparoscopy. HSG remains the most common initial imaging technique used to evaluate the fallopian tubes. Compared with laparoscopy (which is the gold standard test for tubal patency). HSG has only moderate sensitivity but relatively high specificity. The clinical implications are that when HSG reveals obstruction there is still a relatively high probability (approx 60%) that the tube is infact open,

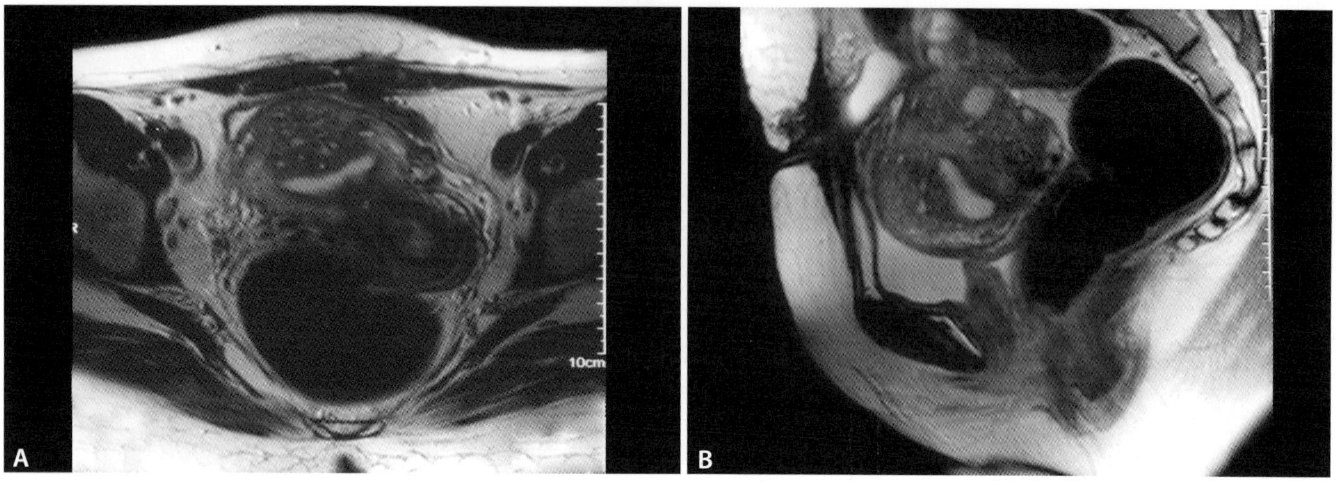

Figs. 11A and B: Axial and sagittal T2W MR images reveal ill-defined myometrial masses with indistinct margins, myometrial cysts and focal widening of junctional zone—Adenomyosis.

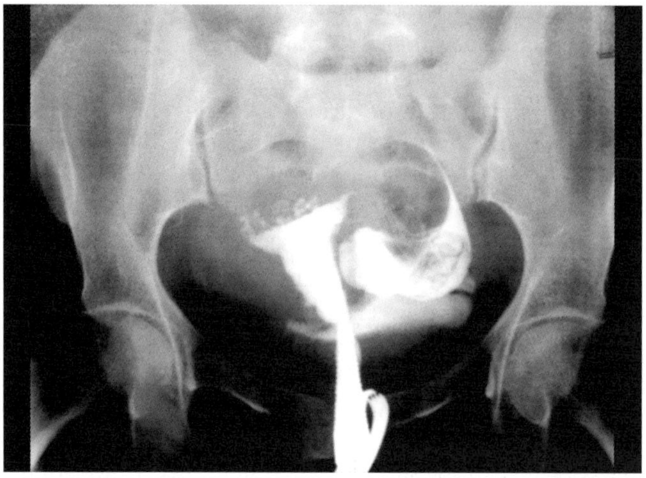

Fig. 12: HSG in a known case of adenomyosis showing multiple small irregular diverticulae in the region of fundus filling with contrast—Right-sided tube is not visualized (cornual block). Left tube is normal.

but when HSG demonstrates patency there is little chance that the tube is actually occluded (approx 5%). In these cases, contrast in a dilated tube or vaginal formix may be mistaken for peritoneal spill.[9] Sonohysterosalpingography and 3D ultrasound and Doppler techniques have been used to evaluate the tubes. However, the techniques provide no information reqarding tubal anatomy and whether one or both tubes are patent. Although 3D ultrasound and Doppler techniques have improved visualization of fluid movement through fallopian tubes but it is unlikely that they will replace traditional HSG anytime soon.[9]

On HSG, the interstitial portion of the fallopian tube may be delicate and thread-shaped or may be funnel-shaped, assuming the configuration of a small triangle or diamond. The isthmic portion is normally thread-shaped. Diameter of both these regions is approx 1 mm. Proximal tubal obstruction[1,3] is obstruction in the first 3–4 cm of the tube. Hysterosalpingography shows obstruction of the proximal end of the fallopian tube in 20% of cases. The cause of proximal tubal obstruction is frequenly unclear, but infection and subsequent inflammation are leading causes in all reported series. Histopathologic findings in resected proximal tubal segments include plugs of amorphous debris, chronic inflammation, obliterative fibrosis and salpingitis isthmica nodosa (SIN). Together these lesions account for majority of anatomic occlusions at the uterotubal junction. Other causes include granulomatous or "giant cell" salpingitis from tuberculosis, foreign bodies and some parasitic infestations. Intraluminal endometriosis occurs in approximately 10% of tubes resected for proximal occlusion and may exist without relation to visible lesions elsewhere in the pelvis. Mullerian anomalies of the fallopian tube are rare, but cornual occlusion is seen with variants of unicornuate uterus, where atresia of tubal segments, including the proximal isthmus can occur.

Another cause of proximal tubal obstruction on HSG is "tubal spasm". The cornual portion of the fallopian tube is encased by smooth muscle of the uterus. If there is spasm of the muscle during HSG, one or both tubes may not fill beyond the interstitial portion. Administration of a spasmolytic agent, such as glucagon can occasionally result in uterine muscle relaxation and consequent tube opacification. However, no reliable antispasmodic has been discovered.[32] According to some authors, however, tubal spasm is the cause of proximal tubal obstruction much less often than originally proposed. They postulate that temporary nonvisualization of the tube may be explained by some easily dislodged entity such as amorphous debris in tubal lumen.[32,33] Placing the patient prone and waiting for 5 minutes before slowly reinjecting contrast may help in some cases. If proximal tubal obstruction persists despite these maneuvers tubal catheterization with selective salpingography can be performed.

Fluoroscopically guided selective salpingography can diagnose and treat proximal tubal obstruction.[3,34-36] Selective salpingography is a minimally invasive method during which the tip of the catheter is placed in the tubal ostia and contrast is injected directly into the tube. Often the injection alone clears the obstruction. If the obstruction still persists, a guidewire can be directed into the tube fluoroscopically through the catheter. Recanalization of the tube, either by forceful injection of contrast or by clearing the obstruction with a guidewire, is possible in up to 95% of patients.[36] Pregnancy rates after one year are comparable to surgery. Complications are also similar to surgery, including a reocclusion rate 30% and an ectopic pregnancy rate of 10%.[36] Sonographic guidance has also been performed for this technique in a small number of patients.[1]

Salpingitis isthmica nodosa (SIN) is another tubal pathology commonly described in western literature. There is an association between SIN and pelvic inflammatory disease however, it is not clear whether SIN is caused by pelvic inflammation or it is congenital and predisposes to inflammation. It mostly affects the isthmic portion, occasionally interstitial and ampullary segments. On HSG it is seen as characteristic multiple small diverticule involving the proximal two thirds of the tube. In addition to causing infertility it also increases the risk of ectopic pregnancy. Tuberculous salpingitis can appear the same but may be associated with calcified lymph nodes or calcifications of the tube itself.[1] SIN associated with tubal obstruction may be treated by fluoroscopically guided tubal catheterization and recanalization.[1,3]

The ampullary portion is the longest portion of the tube. It gradually widens from 1 to 2 mm at its proximal end to approxi-mately 15 mm, where it joins the fimbriated infundibular portion. Subtle ampullary rugal folds can be demonstrated by salpingography and occasionally the fimbriae are outlined by contrast material. Abnormal rugal folds imply damage of the epithelium from infection and usually coexist with a dilated and sometimes distally obstructed tube. Abnormal rugal folds can occur in a patent tube and they indicate reduced chances for conception. The visualization of abnormal rugal folds requires optimal tubal imaging, because the normal rugal folds are subtle. Rugal folds may be best seen before the dilated tube is fully distended with contrast, i.e. during early filling.[3]

Obstruction of the fimbrial portion of the tube is characterized by dilation of the ampullary portion of the tube, which sometimes can be massive and no free spill of contrast agent into the peritoneal cavity despite adequate filling of the tubes and rolling the patient **(Fig. 13)**. It may be occasionally difficult to differentiate a dilated tube from loculated spill of contrast agent. The amount of dilation of the tube does not necessarily predict surgical results. A dilated tube may be soft and pliable with an intact epithelium and offer an opportunity for surgical correction. An obstructed but minimally dilated tube may have an indurated and thickened wall that cannot be reconstructed. The visualization of normal ampullary rugal folds probably improves the chances for successful tubal reconstruction. Dilation of the ampullary portion of the tube in the absence of complete occlusion indicates perifimbrial phimosis, or adhesions around the fimbria that impede degress of fluid. Fimbrial phimosis can be mild or severe, but generally the presence of at least a pinpoint opening in the distal tube carries a more favorable surgical prognosis than complete occlusion. It also increases the risk of post-HSG peritonitis.

Although ultrasound is unable to visualize normal fallopian tubes, blockage of the fallopian tube with fluid accumulation (hydrosalpinx) is easily seen on ultrasound **(Fig. 14)**. The distended tube coiled around the ovary with folds producing septa which do not completely cross the lumen **(Figs. 15A and B)**. A hydrosalpinx may occasionally be visible on ultrasound, distended with fluid only at midcycle, under the estrogenic influence of a preovulatory follicle.[37]

A woman with severly damaged fallopian tubes but a normal uterine cavity is a good candidate for in vitro fertilization and embryo transfer. However, presence of hydrosalpinx in a woman being treated by IVF is associated with poor embryo uptake which may be improved after treatment of hydrosalpinx. Even a unilateral hydrosalpinx is capable of disrupting natural fertility and preventing the success of IVF.[37-39] The mechanism is as follows: Estradiol produced by the preovulatory and ovulating follicle stimulates both ampullary transudation of fluid and isthmic secretion of dense mucus which along with an estrogen medicated increase in isthmic myosalpingeal tone functionally occludes the tube's communication with the cavity of the uterus. Thus the hydrosalpinx gathers fluid. With ovulation, increasing progesterone secretion from the luteinizing follicle relaxes the isthmus, allowing

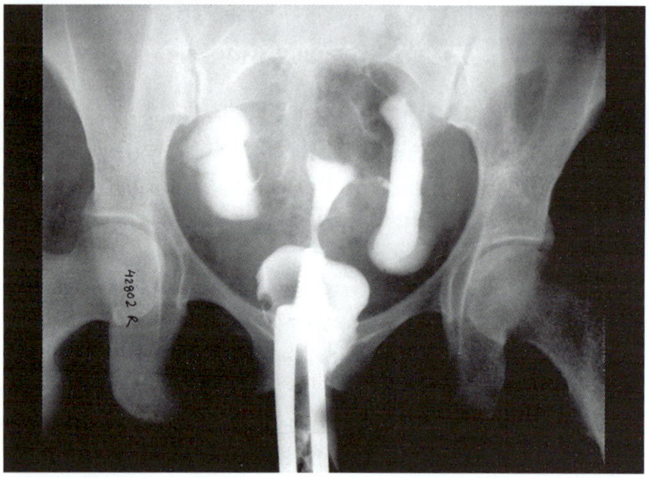

Fig. 13: HSG in a patient with bilateral fimbrial block shows markedly dilated ampullary segments (hydrosalpinx) with absence of free intraperitoneal spill.

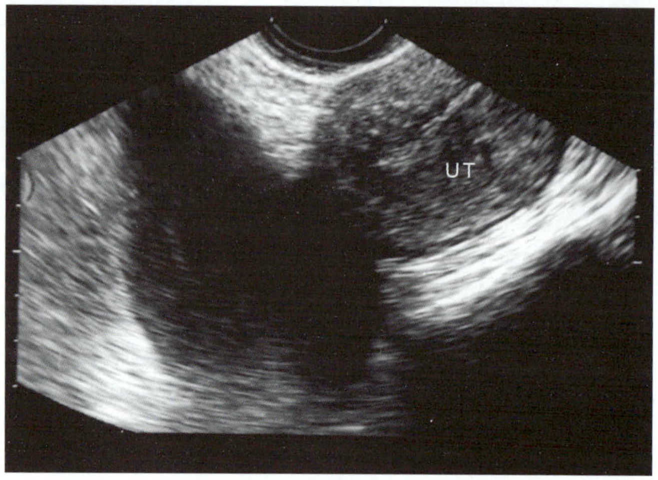

Fig. 14: USG showing a cystic hypoechoic retort shaped dilated tube with incomplete reptations—Hydrosalpinx.

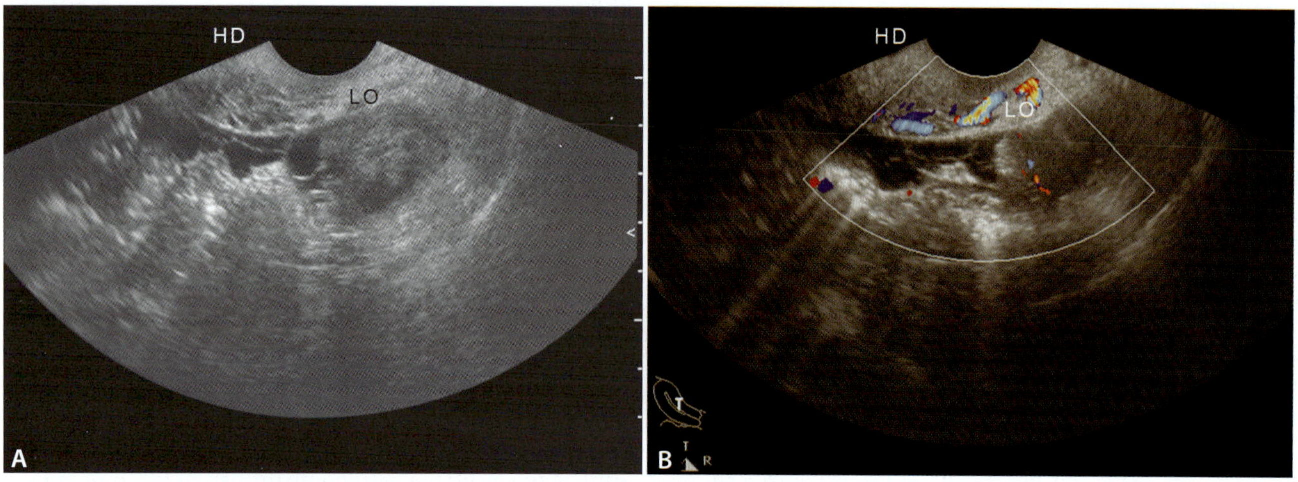

Figs. 15A and B: TVS (grayscale CDFI) showing a mildly dilated left fallopian tube seen to extend up to the left ovary.

passage of accumulated hydrosalpinx fluid down the endometrial cavity just at the time that a normal tube allows passage of pre-embryo to the uterus. This cascade from a single tube is likely to displace any pre-embryos that might have reached through the contralateral patent one or through IVF and transcervical transfer.

Conception rates following salpingostomy are less than 25% if the hydrosalpinx has a thick-wall or a diameter greater than 15 mm.[15,40]

Peritoneal Factor

The peritoneal factor responsible for infertility relates to the presence of pelvic adhesions from previous infection, endometriosis or surgery.[1,3,4] Adhesions can cause problems in oocyte pick up and transfer due to distortion of the normal anatomy, limitation of fimbrial motility and obstruction of fallopian tubes. Imaging techniques are limited in their ability to diagnose pelvic adhesions. Laparoscopy is the gold standard for visualization of pelvic adhesions and endometriosis.[1]

With HSG the presence of peritubal adhesions and endometriosis is underdiagnosed with reported sensitivities ranging from 34–75%. Peritubal adhesions can be suggested if loculated spill of contrast is seen in the peritoneal cavity, or it is seen to track along the outside of the tube producing "a halo effect" or double contour appearance to tubal wall.[41] Peritubal adhesions can also be diagnosed if a persistently convoluted, kinked, stretched or vertically oriented fallopian tube is seen **(Fig. 16)**. Delayed films or film obtained after rolling the patient may be useful to confirm loculated spill in doubtful cases.

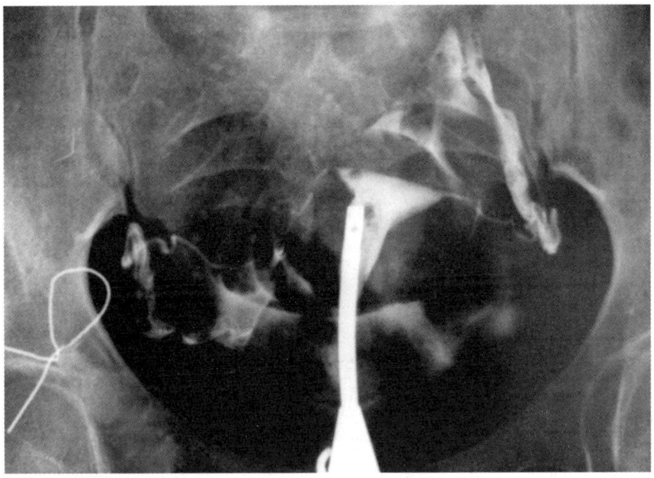

Fig. 16: HSG film reveals an irregular filling defect in the uterine body just adjacent to the cannula due to adhesions. An air bubble is seen in the right cornu. The ampullary portion of the left fallopian tube is vertically stretched with evidence of both peritubal and free spill due to peritubal adhesions.

Normally the contrast should flow freely to outline the bowel loops.[1,3,42] A tug and release maneuver has also been described to confirm the presence of adhesions. If traction is applied on the HSG system both a fixed laterodeviated uterus (due to adhesions) as well as a normal non median uterus initially follow the traction direction, however, during the releasing phase the fixed laterodeviated uterus tends to keep the original deviated position while the non median uterus keeps the pelvis midline.[41]

Ultrasound especially TVS may also allow detection of pelvic adhesions and loculated fluid collections in the adnexae. Adhesions may be suggested by enmasse movement of tethered organs when pressure is applied simultaneously by the operator's hand transabdominally and by the probe transvaginally. However, the sensitivity is low. [1,42]

Endometriosis

Endometriosis is found in 25–50% of infertile women and 30–50% of women with endometriosis are infertile.[43] Endometriosis is the result of ectopic foci of secretory endometrium located outside the uterus. It can cause adhesions, and even impair fertility through hormonally medicated mechanisms. Endometriosis occurs as diffuse peritoneal implants or focal endometriomas (chocolate cysts). Transvaginal sonography is the preferred technique to identify ovarian endometriomas which are seen as complex adnexal or cul-de-sac masses. Diffuse low level internal echoes may be seen. However, TVS has limited ability to identify generalized disease producing subtle changes, such as obliteration of margins between pelvic organs and a generalized increase in echogenicity.[21,42]

On MR imaging endometriomas may be seen as adnexal cysts with high signal on both T1W and T2W images or high signal on T1 and low signal on T2W images (shading) and indistinct margins due to adhesions. Evaluation of adhesions is limited and these may be seen as low signal intensity stranding that obscures organ interfaces, post-displacement of uterus, kissing ovaries, angulated bowel loops, elevated posterior vaginal fornix, loculated fluid collections and hydro/hematosalpinx **(Figs. 17A to C)**. Hormonal therapy, is occasionally used to treat endometriosis and shading on T2W images is the most important negative predictor for volume reduction with medical treatment, such therapy should be discontinued should low T2 signal be seen in a case on hormonal treatment.[21] It is important to remember that small implants and adhesion[6] that may cause infertility are not well visualized by any imaging technique. Laparoscopy remains the gold standard for diagnosis and staging of endometriosis and is also the mainstay for diagnosis. [2,3]

Genital Tuberculosis

About 18% of female infertility in India is attributed to genital tuberculosis (TB).[44] Tuberculosis commonly results in changes in the endometrium, the fallopian tubes and pelvic peritoneum.

Scarring in uterine TB is well demonstrated by HSG. This can take few specialized forms namely T-shaped uterus, asymmetric uterus and pseudounicornuate uterus.[45] A T-shaped uterus has been observed in a significant number of patients with uterine TB, and in the appropriate setting, it is virtually diagnostic of uterine TB. In the Western literature, a T-shaped uterus has usually been labeled as a diethylstilbestrol (DES) uterus. The DES and the tuberculous uterus both reveal irregular margins. However, tubal changes are not noted in DES uterus, whereas tubal changes are invariably seen in T-shaped uterus due to TB. The normal uterine cavity has a triangular appearance with either straight or concave lateral walls. In tuberculous endometritis, due to scarring along the long as well as the short axis of the uterus, this triangular shape is converted into a T-shape.[45]

Scarring is also recognizable by the asymmetric uterine contour it produces. An asymmetric, small sized uterine cavity is usually due to TB. Occasionally the scarring may be more unilateral which may lead to obliteration of that side of the uterine cavity leading to a unicornuate uterus-like appearance—"the pseudounicornuate uterus". Comparison with previous films, laparoscopy and

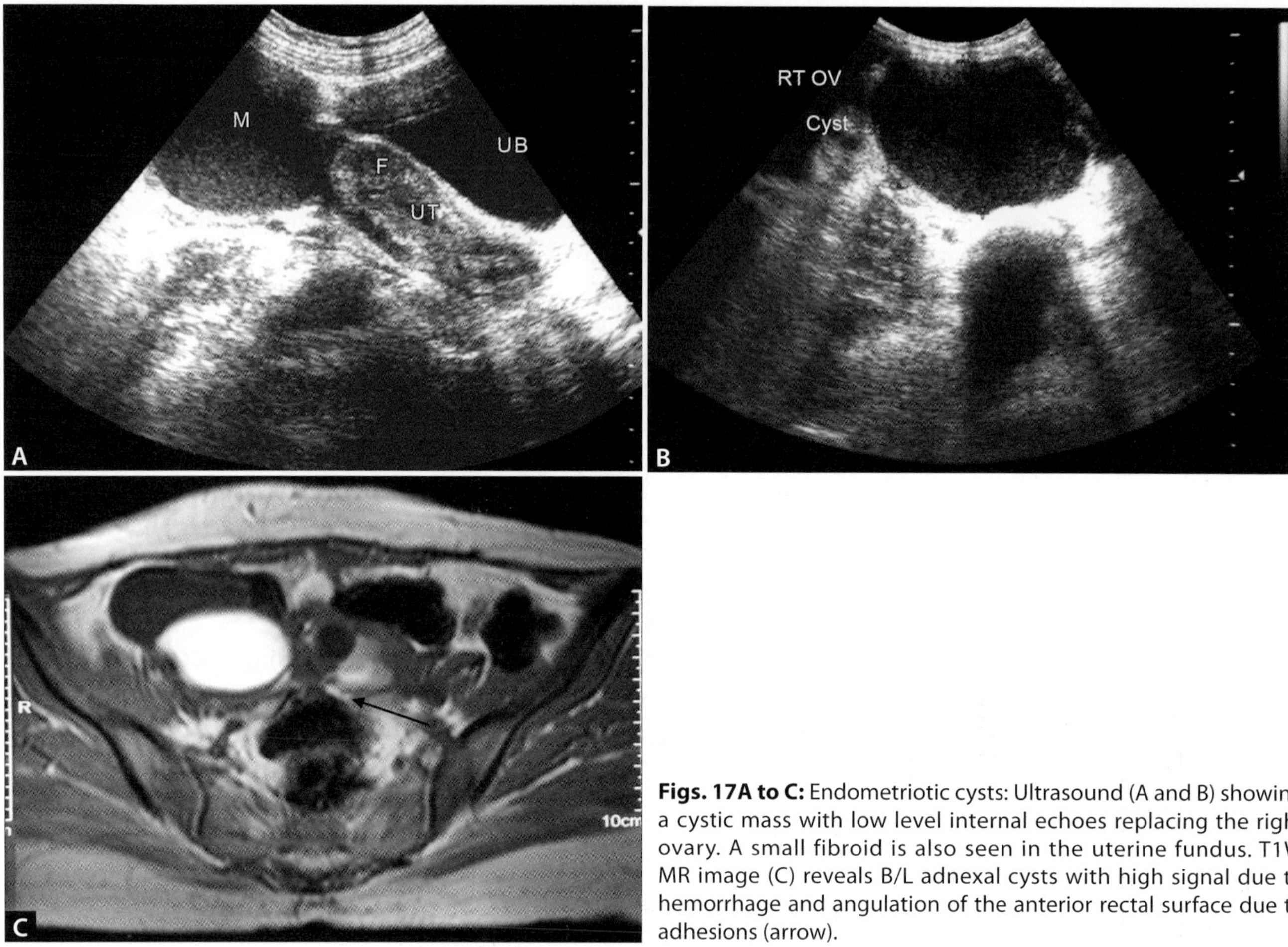

Figs. 17A to C: Endometriotic cysts: Ultrasound (A and B) showing a cystic mass with low level internal echoes replacing the right ovary. A small fibroid is also seen in the uterine fundus. T1W MR image (C) reveals B/L adnexal cysts with high signal due to hemorrhage and angulation of the anterior rectal surface due to adhesions (arrow).

awareness about this type of scarring would be essential in excluding TB in a true unicornuate uterus. A good pointer towards endometrial TB is myometrial extravasation and/or venous intravasation. This finding along with any other endometrial or tubal change **(Figs. 18 and 19)** is very suggestive of a tuberculous etiology of endometritis.[45]

Ovarian Factor

Up to 20% of infertility cases are caused by ovarian factors.[1,7,46] Normal ovarian follicular development, ovulation and formation of a functional corpus luteum are needed for adequate reproductive function, and these represent the ovulatory factors that must be evaluated in an infertility investigation. The imaging modality used to evaluate the ovaries is TVS which is used to detect both ovarian pathology and monitor ovulation. Functional ovarian cysts or other benign ovarian cysts and tumors like dermoid cysts or fibromata may occasionally interfere with ovarian function particularly when large. Endometriomas have already been discussed.

Polycystic Ovarian Syndrome

Another condition commonly found during evaluation for infertility is polycystic ovarian syndrome (POD).[1,47-51] It is a complex endocrine disorder of unknown etiology also called Stein–Leventhal syndrome. It is characterized by multiple small (<1 cm) ovarian cysts. These cysts are thought to represent graafian follicles that persist in arrested stages of development because of low levels of FSH. The classic sonographic features of polycystic ovaries are round, enlarged ovaries, with multiple 2–6 mm cysts, absence of cysts greater than 1.5 cm in diameter, smooth contours and hyperechoic ovarian stroma. The small cysts may be peripherally located or dispersed throughout the ovarian parenchyma. The presence of a thickened echogenic endometrium (due to estrogen excess) also supports the diagnosis of POD **(Figs. 20A and B)**. One third of patients with clinical manifestations of POD have normal ovaries.

Distinct from polycystic ovaries are the more chaotically distributed multiple follicles seen in what has come to be called multifollicular ovaries. The ovulatory

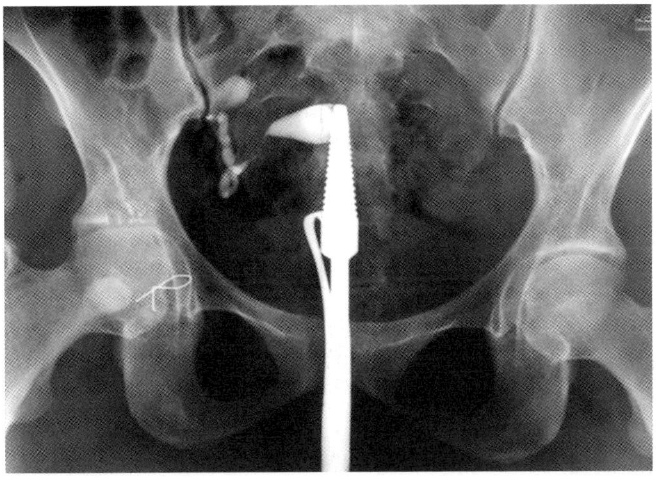

Fig. 18: A HSG showing a mildly dilated beaded right fallopian tube with evidence of loculated spill. Left tube is not visualized due to cornual block—Sequelae of tuberculosis.

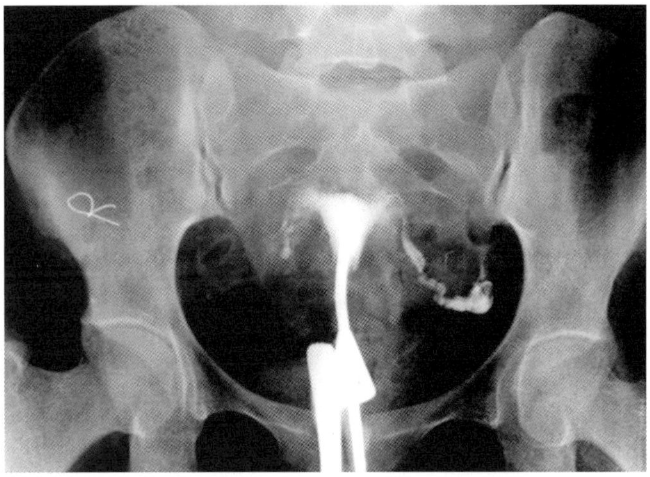

Fig. 19: HSG demonstrating a beaded left fallopian tube with no free spill. Only the proximal (isthmic and interstitial portion) of the right fallopian tube is visualized. Note the presence of myometrial extravasation suggestive of tubercular involvement.

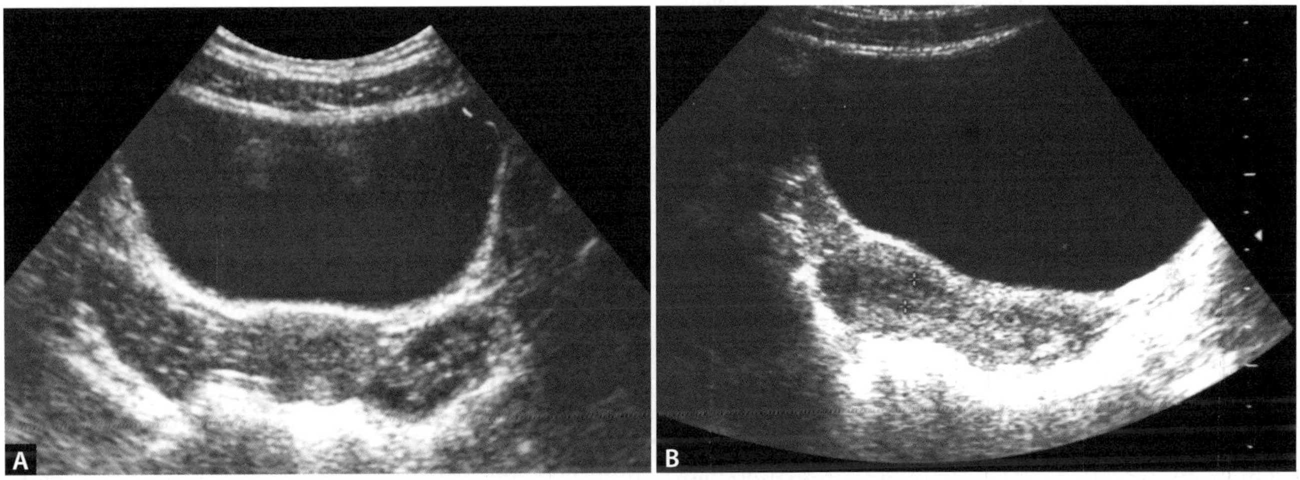

Figs. 20A and B: Transverse (A) and longitudinal (B) US images reveal markedly enlarged ovaries with multiple small diffusely scattered cysts. Note the presence of endometrial thickening in the uterus—Polycystic ovarian disease.

pattern in these patients is often irregular; reminiscent of the post-menarcheal or premenopausal states and premature menopause is common among these patients. Their response to ovarian stimulation for assisted conception can be unpredictable; many respond poorly. The ultrasound appearance of variably sized follicles, irregularly dispersed and often larger than usually seen, is not always convincingly different from normal **(Figs. 21A and B)**. A multifollicular morphology can also be seen in patients recovering from anorexia.[37]

Follicular Monitoring

Ovulation is initially monitored using simple tests like BBT mid luteal serum progesterone and urinary LH. However, when a more accurate estimation of ovulation is necessary, ultrasound is used to monitor follicular development in both natural and stimulated cysts.[9] Observation of a developing follicle, the prediction of impending ovulation allows procedure, such as postcoital testing, human chrionic gonadotropin (hCG) administration, intercourse, donor and husband insemination and egg collection to be timed optimally. Patients not shown to be ovulating may be treated by ovulation-induction agents.

Spontaneous Cycles[15,52]

Beginning with menarche, during spontaneous cycles there is usually development of one or sometimes two dominant follicles. Sonography can depict developing

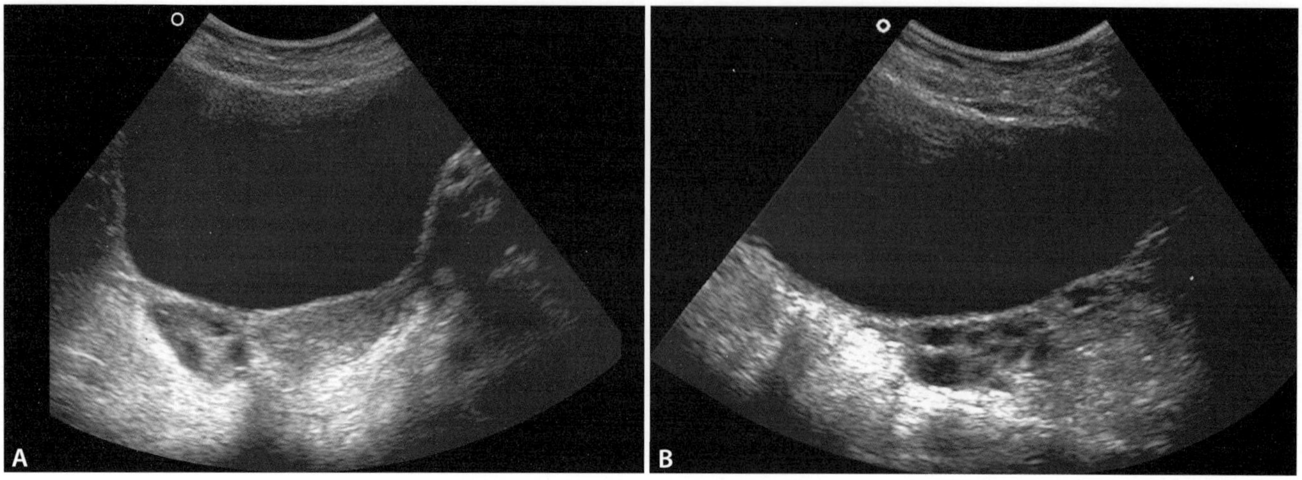

Figs. 21A and B: (A) Multifollicular ovarian morphology seen in a patient recovering from anorexia; (B) Ovaries are only mildly enlarged with multiple variably sized follicles irregularly dispersed on the left side.

follicles beginning at the time they measure 3–5 mm. In the spontaneous cycle by unknown mechanisms one or at the most two follicles that develop to approximately 10 mm. At this time (about 7 days before LH surge) a dominant follicle takes over and there is a very little further growth of other follicles. Occasionally, two dominant follicles develop. During the five days prior to ovulation the dominant follicle grows at the rate of 2–3 mm/day. As a follicle reaches maturity its inner dimensions range from 17–25 mm. However within the same individual the size of the mature follicle is relatively constant cycle to cycle.

Induced Cycles[2,15]

In patients in whom infertility can be attributed to an ovulation abnormality or anovulation, ovulation induction is indicated. Ovulation induction or superovulation therapy is also used in women with normal ovulation before assisted conception techniques such as IVF-ET or GIFT to increase the number of oocytes aspirated. This increases the number of fertilized concepti that may be transferred thereby increasing the chances of pregnancy.

Before starting treatment a baseline scanning of the pelvis should be done. Presence of one or more cysts larger than approximately 2 cm in diameter particularly if accompanied by serum estradiol concentration of more than 100 pg/mL may interfere with treatment and induction may be postponed to the next cycle or cysts treated by aspiration.

The two medications that are most commonly used for ovulation induction include clomiphere citrate and human menopausal gonadotropin (hMG). Patients undergoing ovulation induction are usually examined every other day beginning at day 10. Patients undergoing IVF-ET are examined by sonography starting earlier and usually daily in an attempt to carefully monitor their follicular development.

Clomiphene citrate is an estrogen antagonist which indirectly promotes the secretion of FSH and LH. Because the process of selection and dominance in overridden, multiple relatively synchronous follicles develop. In some women elevated serum FSH and LH results in ovulation without further therapy. In other patients, human chorionic gonadotrophin may be needed to induce ovulation.[1] Follicular development with clomiphere citrate can be quite different from that observed in natural cycles. Each follicle seems to develop at an individual rate and at times may be accelerated or slowed down. Therefore, the larger follicles on a given date may not be the same one that is the largest 2 days later and it may not even be the same one that is most mature. Furthermore correlation of estradiol levels (E2) and follicle size is poor and maximum pre ovulatory diameter can range from 19 to 24 mm. In clomiphere stimulated cycles the growth rate in the last few days preceding ovulation is higher.

Unlike clomiphene, citrate treatment with hMG does not require an intact hypothalamic-pitutary axis. This contains both FSH and LH and induces follicle development. Human chorionic gonadotropin is then given to induce ovulation of mature follicles. Although the growth of follicle can be assessed by serial measurement of serum or urinary estradiol levels, multiple, small, immature follicles may produce as much estradiol as a large mature follicle. Therefore, TVS is used to predict the optimal timing for administering a dose of hCG to induce ovulation.[1,53-55] Sonographic delineation of follicle size is critical because hCG is best administered once follicles reach 15–18 mm.[1]

Prediction of Ovulation[1,15,52]

Follicular rupture occurs at a wide range of diameters between 2 and 2.7 cm. In the unstimulated ovary follicles are approximately spherical. They may, however, be flattened in one plane by either pressure of the transducer or bladder so a mean of the maximum diameter in three planes is a better estimate of follicular size than measurements only in two planes.[15] In superovulation cycles pressure from abutting follicles distorts the follicle so exact measurements are often difficult. Serial follicular measurement is best done by the same observer using the TVS route. In a recent study assessment of follicular volume using 3D ultrasound was found to correlate better with oocyte retrieval than 2D ultrasound alone. The authors found that a follicular size of >22 mm or a volume >5 mL was correlated with poor oocyte retrieval probably due to post mature follicle.[56]

Ovulation can also be predicted by collapse of a previously seen follicle, development of internal echoes within the follicle, crenation of follicular walls, visualization of cumulus, peri follicular halo and visualization of fluid in the cul-de-sac (if not previously seen). However, fluid may commonly be seen in the pouch of Douglas in the periovulatory period and only a small percentage of women have a detectable increase with ovulation. Contrary to popular belief ovulation need not alternate between two ovaries. Unfortunately, the variable appearance of ovulation makes the use of these ultrasound signs problematic in the management of infertility.[15]

Ultrasound Doppler studies reveal an increase in blood flow to the ovary carrying the dominant follicle[57-60] (and later, the corpus luteum) – an increase that precedes other indicators of follicular dominance. With maturation of the follicle, increased flow is directed to the follicle itself within the dominant ovary. Intrafollicular neovascularization occurs over the hours preceding ovulation and becomes massive after follicular collapse as blood vessels invade the luteinizing follicular (or granulose) cells and the corpus luteum forms and impedance in intraovarian arterioles drops while velocities reach up to 40 cm/s. These changes do not occur in non ovulatory cycles. Recently, a study[61] was undertaken to investigate if corpus luteal function could be improved by increasing CL blood flow in women with LPD and high CL-RI (≥0.51). They concluded that vitamin E or L-arginine treatment improved luteal function by decreasing CL blood flow impedance.

Luteinized Unruptured Follicle (LUF)[3,15]

The corpus luteum formed after ovulation may have a variety of ultrasound appearances. It may be imperceptible from the surrounding ovarian stroma. It may show a small cystic component with echoes or may be large (>40 mm) and be hemorrhagic.[15]

Failure to detect follicular collapse but with infilling of the follicle suggests luteinization without ovulation. The LUF syndrome occurs more commonly in infertile patients than in fertile patients and may be a cause of unexplained infertility. However, ultrasound diagnosis has a 15% false positive rate. Great care should be taken in diagnosing this condition because ovulation may be associated with an increase in size of follicles and these cystic corpora lutea may indicate a conception cycle.

Ovarian Hyperstimulation Syndrome

Ovarian hyperstimulation syndrome (OHSS) is potentially the most serious complication of ovulation induction with gonadotrophins. It occurs after hCG administration to patient with a large number of immature follicles and high serum estradiol levels and is more likely to occur in those with a polycystic ovarian morphology.[1,62,63]

Two mechanisms may be responsible, which are: excessive serum levels of gonadotropins or hypersensitivity of the ovaries to these hormones. The ovarian hyperstimulation syndrome occurs when hyperstimulation of the ovaries is accompanied by an aberration of the fluid balance. This syndrome is characterized by third-space fluid accumulation and electrolyte disturbances. The syndrome may have varied severity, but it is generally more severe if pregnancy follows ovulation. The clinical features that cause concern are nausea, vomiting, ascites, pleural and pericardial effusion. These worsen hemoconcentration causing hyperviscosity and hypercoagulability which predispose to thrombosis, embolism and renal failure.[15]

Ultrasound is used to detect patients potentially likely to develop OHSS and in hyperstimulation patients to categorize the severity of the disease and to assess the size of the ovaries.[62,63] Mild cases are characterized by minimal gain in weight and enlargement of ovary to a maximum dimension of 5 cm. Moderate cases are classified as weight gain of up to 10 lb and increase in ovarian size which does not exceede 10 cm. These patients may have some ascites. In severe cases, weight gain exceeds 10 lb, the ovaries are greater than 10 cm in size, ascites is readily apparent and pleural effusions may be present. In all cases of ovarian hyperstimulation, sonographic examination shows ovarian enlargement with a myriad of cysts. The sizes of these cysts vary and are separated by thick septae. Follow-up scans show a gradual regression in size and number of cysts, as well as resolution of the ascites and pleural effusions **(Figs. 22A and B)**.

TREATING INFERTILITY

The last decade has seen a transformation in the approach to treating infertility. Increasingly assisted conception with IVF or one of its related therapeutic modalities is being used to treat infertility. These acronyms are summarized in **Table 1**. Imaging has become inseparable from all modern assisted conception practices. Besides detecting pathologies like hydrosalpinx which are likely to affect the success of IVF, imaging especially TVS is crucial for the safety of ovulation induction and is widely used in oocyte retrieval.

Follicle Aspiration[15,64,65]

In the first successful *in vitro* fertilization, oocytes were collected during laparoscopy which is an expensive procedure associated with complications like periovarian adhesions, hemorrhage infection, etc.

Ultrasound directed follicle aspiration (UDFA) has reduced costs considerably and can be done as an out patient technique. Various approaches have been used in the past for follicular aspiration including direct transabdominal, transabdominal through full bladder, transvaginal, transvaginal/ transvesical and per urethral.[15]

Oocyte collection using TVS, first described by Wikland in 1985[64] has become the technique of choice however the actual method used can be tailored according to each patient depending on where the ovaries are situated. With all these aspiration techniques, a long (30 cm) 18-gauge needle is used that is scored at the tip, which results in its enhanced sonographic visualization. The aspiration procedure is performed under local anesthesia and with supplemental intravenous or intramuscular medication.

For the transvaginal aspiration with transvaginal transducers, a needle guide is attached to the transducer/ probe. This allows the needle to transverse in the beam path of the transducer. The cursor is displayed on the scanning screen, which indicates the path of the needle. After a condom containing sterile gel is placed over the transducer and a sterile needle guide is attached, the operator manipulates the transducer to optimally delineate the ovary. The desired follicle is brought into the "line of sight" and the needle is introduced transvaginally. After the initial aspiration, the follicle may be filled with buffered medium and flushed to maximize the chances of retrieving a mature oocyte.

The technique has been associated with low complication rates which include vaginal hemorrhage and pelvic infection. When a transvesical or transurethral approach is used postoperative clot retention or occasionally urine extravasation may occur.

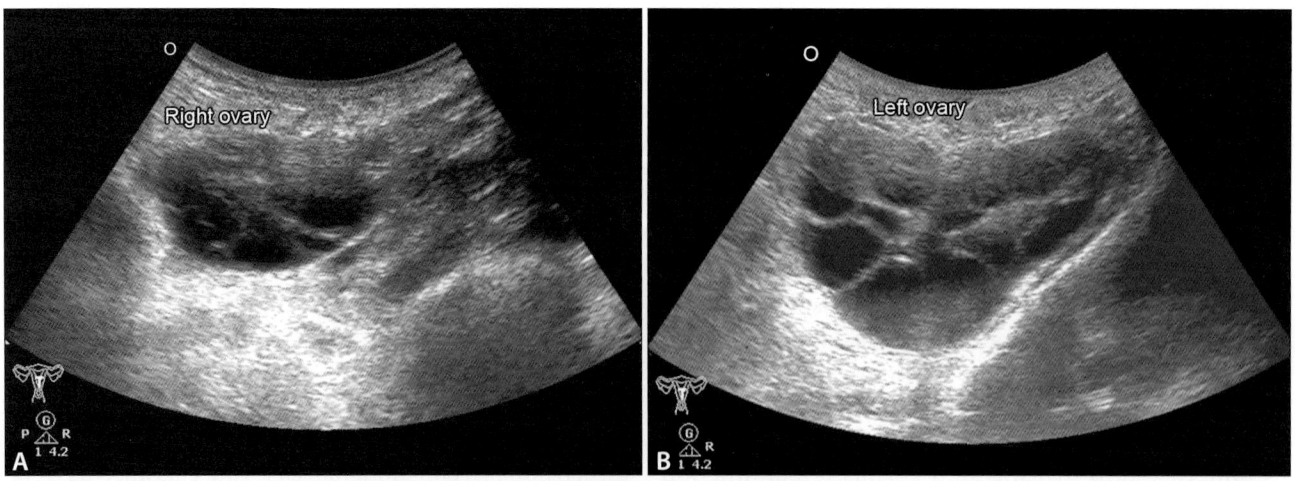

Figs. 22A and B: TVS scans of both ovaries in a patient on ovulation induction reveal enlarged ovaries with a myriad of cysts varying in size consistent with ovarian hyperstimulation syndrome (OHSS).

Table 1: Acronyms used in assisted conception.[37]

In vitro fertilization (IVF)	Recovered eggs are fertilized with prepared sperm in the laboratory and transferred back to the genital tract after usually several days' culture
Gamete intrafallopian transfer (GIFT)	Recovered eggs are almost immediately transferred, with prepared sperm, into the fallopian tubes, so that fertilization and early development occur in the normal situation; generally, a higher pregnancy rate than after IVF, provided the tube used is normal and normal sperm function can be assumed
Zygote intrafallopian transfer (ZIFT)	IVF in which 1 day fertilized eggs, or zygotes, are transferred to the fallopian tube
Uterine embryo transfer (Uterine ET)	Conventional procedure with IVF: 2-day pre-embryos are transferred through the cervix to the endometrial cavity
Frozen embryo transfer (FET, FrET)	Transfer of IVF pre-embryos previously cryostored
Tubal embryo-stage transfer (TEST)	2-day IVF pre-embryos are transferred to the tube instead of the uterus
Intracytoplasmic sperm injection (ICSI)	Laboratory refinement for IVF in cases of severely depressed sperm function, in which a single sperm is selected and microinjected into each egg
Microepididymal sperm aspiration (MESA)	A means of obtaining sperm for ICSI in men with obstructive azoospermia
Testicular sperm extraction (TESE)	A means of obtaining sperm cells from testicular tubules for ICSI in some men with nonobstructive azoospermia

Ultrasound has also been used to guide embryo transfer to the uterine cavity to assist accurate placement of the embryos in the uterine cavity rather than cervical canal.

CONCLUSION

Imaging studies have contributed greatly to the diagnosis and management of infertility in women. Hysterosalpingography remains the first-line radiologic examination for most women undergoing an infertility investigation. It can show intrauterine synechiae tubal morphology such as hydrosalpinx, myomas and congenital anomalies may also be suggested. MR imaging is the most accurate examination for detection and localization of myomata and characterization of congenital malformations. This is clinically important because the location, number, and size of myomata affect the treatment of these lesions and the correct classification of a developmental abnormality can prevent unnecessary laparoscopy and aid in appropriate surgical management. Sonography has a crucial role in monitoring ovarian follicular development in spontaneous and induced cycles and is invaluable as a guidance procedure in reproductive techniques such as oocyte collection and gamete transfer *in vitro* fertilization programs.[42]

REFERENCES

1. Collins JI, Woodward PJ. Radiological Evaluation of Infertility. Semin Ultrasound, CT and MRI. 1995;16(4): 304-16.
2. ASRM Practice Committee. Optimal evaluation of the infertile female. Fertil Steril. 2006;86(4):264-7.
3. Thurmond AS. Imaging of female infertility. Radiol Clin N Am. 2003;41:757-67.
4. Jaffe SB, Jewlewicz R. The basic infertility investigation. Fertil Steril. 1991;56:599-613.
5. Krysiewicz S. Infertility in women: Diagnostic evaluation with hysterosalpingography and other imaging techniques. Am J Roentgenol. 1992;159:253-61.
6. Winfield AC, Wentz AC. Diagnostic Imaging of Infertility. Baltimore, MD: Williams and Wilkins; 1987.
7. Moghissi K. Current concepts in infertility. Clin Obstet Gynecol. 1989;22:9-189.
8. Simpson WL, Beitia LG, Mester J. Hysterosalpingography: A reemerging study. Radiographics. 2006;26:419-31.
9. Speroff L, Fritz MA. Female Infertility. In: Clinical Gynecologic Endocrinology and Infertility, Leon Speroff, Marc A Fritz (Eds) 7th edition. 2005.pp.1013-67.
10. Grosskinsky CM, Clark RL, Wilson PA, Novotny DB. Pelvic granulomata mimicking endometriosis following the administration of oil-based contrast media for hysterosalpingo-graphy. Obstet Gynecol. 1994;83:890.
11. Nunley WC, Jr. Bateman BG, Kitchin JD, 3rd Pope TL, Jr. Intravasation during hysterosalpingography using oil-based contrast medium—a second look. Obstet Gynecol. 1987;70:309.
12. Vandekerckhove P, Watson A, Lilford R, Harada T, Hughes E. Oil-soluble versus water-soluble media for assessing tubal patency with hysterosalpingography or laparoscopy in subfertile women. Cochrane Database Syst Rev: CD000092, 2000.
13. Spring DB, Barkan HE, Pruyn SC. Potential therapeutic effects of contrast materials in hysterosalpingography: a prospective randomized clinical trail. Kaiser Permanente Infertility Work Group. Radiology. 2000:214:53.
14. Steer CV, Parsons JH. Infertility In: Dewbury K, Meire H, Cosgrove D, Farrant P (Eds.). Ultrasound in Obstetrics and Gynaecology, Churchill Livingstone; 2nd edition. 2001. pp.99-122.
15. Hill LM. Transvaginal sonography in an assisted conception program. In: Anderson JC (Ed). Gyneologic Imaging. Churchill Livingstone. 1999.pp.585-99.
16. Fleicher AC, Parsons AK, Cullinan JA. Special imaging procedures in gynecology. In: Fleischer AC (Ed). Clinical Gynecologic Imaging. Lippincott-Raven, Philadelphia; 1997.pp.315-31.

17. Oei SG, Helmerhorst FM, Bloemenkamp KW, Hollants FA, Meerpoel DE, Keirse MJ. Effectiveness of the postcoital test: randomized controlled trial. BMJ. 1998;317:502-5.
18. Glatstein IZ, Harlow BL, Hornstein MD. Practice patterns among reproductive endocrinologists: further aspects of the infertility evaluation. Fertile Steril. 1998;70:263-9.
19. Dudiak CM, Turner DA, Patel SK, et al. Uterine leiomyomas in the infertile patient: Preoperative localization with MR imaging versus US and hysterosalpingography. Radiology. 1988;167:627-30.
20. Woodward PJ. Wagner BJ, Farley TE. MR imaging in the evaluation of female infertility. Radiographics. 1993:13;293-310.
21. Imaka I, Wada A, Matsuo M, et al. MR imaging of disorders associated with female infertility: use in diagnosis, treatment and management. Radiographics. 2003;23:1401-21.
22. Troiano RN, Mc Carthy SM. Mullerian duct anomalies: imaging and clinical issues. Radiology. 2004;233:19-34.
23. Olphin JD, Heilbrum M. Imaging of Mullerian duct anomalies. Clin Obstet Gynaecol. 2007;52(1):40-56.
24. Deutch TD, Abuhamad AZ. The Role of 3D-USG and MR imaging in the diagnosis of MDA: a review of literature. J Ultrasound Med. 2008;27(3):413-23.
25. Homer HA, Li TC, Cooke ID. The septate uterus: a review of management and reproductive outcome. Fertil Steril. 2000; 73:1-14.
26. Ott DJ, Fayez JA, Zagoria RJ, (Eds). Congenital anomalies. In: Hysterosalpingography: A Text and Atlas, 2nd edition. Baltimore, Md: Williams & Wilkins; 1998.pp.59-69.
27. Stampe Sorensen S. Fundal contour of the uterine cavity in the new syndrome of minor mullerian duct anomalies and oligomenorrhea: a prospective controlled study. Am J Obstet Gynecol. 1983;145:659-67.
28. Schild RL, Knobloch C, Dorn C, et al. Endometrial receptivity in an in vitro fertilization program as assessed by spiral artery blood flow; endometrial thickness, endometrial volume and uterine artery blood flow. Fertile Stezil. 2001;75(2):361-6.
29. Steer CV, Campbell S, Tan SL, et al. The use of transvaginal colour flow imaging after in vitro fertilization to identify optimum uterine conditions before embryo transfer. Fertil Steril. 1992;576:372-6.
30. Chen LW, An HK, Chen PL, et al. Assessment of uterine receptivity by the endometrial, subendometrial blood flow distribution pattern in women undergoing in vitro fertilization—embryo transfer. Fertil Steril. 2002;78(2):245-51.
31. Alcazar JL. Three dimensional ultrasound assessment of endometrial receptivity: a review. Reprod Biol Endocrinol. 2006;4-56.
32. Thurmond AS, Novy MJ, Rosch J. Terburaline in diagnosis of interstitial fallopian tube obstruction. Invest Radiol. 1988;23:209-10.
33. Sulak PJ, Letterie GS, Coddington CC, et al. Histology of proximal tubal occlusion. Fertil Steril. 1987;48:437-40.
34. Thurmond AS. Selective salpingography and fallopian tube recanalization. Am J Roentgenol. 1991;156:33-8.
35. Rosch J, Thurmond AS, Vchida BT, et al. Selective transcervical fallopian tube catherterization—technique update. Radiology. 1988;168:1-5.
36. Thurmond AS, Rosch J. Nonsurgical fallopian tube recanalization for treatment of infertility. Radiology. 1990;174:371-4.
37. Jansen RPS, Ramsay PA. Imaging in gynecologic infertility. In: Anderson JC (Ed). Gynecologic Imaging. 1999.pp.567-80.
38. Strandell A, Waldenstrom U, Nilsson L, Hamberger L. Hydrosalpinx reduces in vitro fertilization/embryo transfer pregnancy rates. Hum Reprod. 1994;9:861-3.
39. Andersen AN, Yue Z, Meng FJ, Petersen K. Low implantation rate after in-vitro fertilization in patients with hydrosalpinges diagnosed by ultrasonography. Hum Reprod. 1994;9:1935-8.
40. Donnez J, Casanas-Roux E. Prognostic factors of fimbrial microsurgery. Fertil Steril. 1986;46:200-4.
41. Valentini AL, Muzuil L, Marana R. Improvement of hysterosalpingographic accuracy in the diagnosis of peritubal adhesions. AJR. 2000;175:1173-6.
42. Krysiewicz S. Infertility in women: Diagnostic evaluation with hysterosalpingography and other imaging techniques. AJR. 1992;158:253-61.
43. Schenken RS. Endometeriosis. In: Scott JR, Di Saia PJ, Hammona CB, Spellacy WN (Eds). Danforth's Obstetrics and Gynaecology, 8th edition. Philadelphia PA: Lippincott Williams and Wilkins; 1999.pp.669-75.
44. Das P, Ahuja A, Gupta SD. Incidence, etiopathogenesis and pathological aspects of genitourinary tuberculosis in India : A journey revisited. Indian J Urol. 2008;24:356-61.
45. Merchant SA. Tuberculosis of the genitourinary system. Ind J. Radiol Imag. 1993;3:253-74.
46. Daly DC, Reuter K, Cohen S, et al. Follicle size by ultrasound versus cervical mucus quality: Normal and abnormal patterns in spontaneous cycles. Fertil Steril. 1989;51:598-603.
47. Mendelson EB, Friedman H, Neiman HL, et al. The role of imaging in infertility management. Am J Roentgenol. 1985;144:415-20.
48. Parisi L, Tramoniti M, Derchi LE, et al. Polycystic ovarian disease: Ultrasonic evaluation and correlations with clinical and hormonal data. J Clin Ultrasound. 1984;12:21-6.
49. El Tabbakh GH, Lofty I, Azab I, et al. Correlation of sonographic ovarian disease and the clinical, hormonal and laparoscopic findings. Am J Obstet Gynecol. 1986;154:892-5.
50. Yeh H-C, Futterweit W, Thornton JC. Polycystic ovarian disease: US features in 104 patients. Radiology. 1987;163:111-6.
51. Pache TD, Wladimiroff JW, Hop WCJ, et al. How to discriminate between normal and polycystic ovaries: Transvaginal US study. Radiology. 1992;183:421-3.
52. Fleischer AC, Daniell JF, Rodein J, et al. Sonographic monitoring of ovarian follicular development. J Clin Ultrasound. 1981;9:275.
53. Fleischer AC, Herbert CM,GA, et al. Transvaginal sonography of the endometrium during induced cycles. J Ultrasound Med. 1991;10:93-5.

54. Haning RV, Zwiebel WJ. Ultrasound assistance in clinical management of infertility. Semin Ultrasound CT MR. 1983;4:226-34.
55. Hann LE, Crivello M, McArdle C, et al. In vitro fertilization: Sonographic perspective. Radiology. 1987;163:665-8.
56. Shmorgun D, Hughes E, Mohida P, Roberts R. Prospective cohort study of three- versus two-dimensional ultrasound for prediction of oocyte maturity. Fertil Steril. 2010;93(4):1337-7.
57. Campbell S, Bourne TH, Waterstone J, et al. Transvaginal colour blood flow imaging of the periovulatory follicle. Fertil Steril. 1993;60:433-8.
58. Taylor KJW, Wells PNT, Conway Pl. Ultrasound Doppler flow studies of the ovarian and uterine arteries. Br J Obstet Gynaecol. 1985;92:240-6.
59. Deutinger J, Reinthaller A, Bernaschek G. Transvaginal pulsed Doppler measurement of blood flow velocity in the ovarian arteries during cycle stimulation and after follicle puncture. Fertil Steril. 1989;51:466-70.
60. Collins W, Jurkovic D, Bourne T, et al. Ovarian morphology, endocrine function and intrafollicular blood flow during the periovulatory period. Hum Reprod. 1991;6:319-24.
61. Takasaki A, Gamura H, Taniguchi K, et al. Luteal blood flow and luteal function. J Ovarian Res. 2009;2:1.
62. Cowan BD. Ovarian hyperstimulation syndrome. Female Patient. 1991;16:37-44.
63. Ranking RN, Hutton LC. Ultrasound in the ovarian hyperstimulation syndrome. J Clin Ultrasound. 1981;9:473-6.
64. Wikland M, Lenmart E, Hamberger L. Tranvesical and transvaginal approaches for the aspiration of follicles by the use of ultrasound. NY Sci. 1985;442:182.
65. Fleishcer AC, Vasquez JM, Kepple DM. Transvaginal sonography in gynaecologic fertility disorders. In: Fleischer AC (Ed). Clinical Gynecologic Imaging. Lippincott-Raven, Philadelphia; 1997.pp.273-314.

CHAPTER 122

Benign Diseases of the Female Pelvis

Alpana Manchanda, Veena Chowdhury

INTRODUCTION

Ultrasonography is the primary modality for evaluating gynecological abnormalities as it adequately depicts normal and pathological anatomy. Ultrasound provides useful information in confirming the presence or absence of a pelvic mass, determining its site of origin and precise relationship to other pelvic organs, and evaluating the morphologic characteristics of the mass along with delineating ascites or adenopathy or other features suggesting malignancy. The diagnostic sensitivity and specificity of sonography has increased with the advent and increased use of high resolution transvaginal probes.

Color Doppler sonography (CDS) and sonohysterography (SHG) are useful adjuncts to conventional gray-scale ultrasonography in the evaluation of gynecologic disorders and can be helpful in clarifying the etiology of some of the masses with nonspecific morphological features. CT often provides diagnostic information in patients who have suspected pelvic masses in whom the initial ultrasound has proved equivocal as it is capable of detecting adenopathy, assessing fat planes and extent which are important in the staging of malignancy.

Magnetic resonance imaging (MRI) can reliably diagnose several benign lesions, such as congenital anomalies of the uterus, leiomyomas, adenomyosis, dermoid cysts and in some cases of endometriomas.

BENIGN UTERINE LESIONS

Congenital Uterine Anomalies

Congenital uterine anomalies represent a spectrum of morphological abnormalities that result from nondevelopment or varying degrees of nonfusion of the mullerian ducts and occur in 1–15% of women.[1] The clinical classification of mullerian duct anomalies follows the guidelines proposed by Buttrams and Gibbons.[2] The classification was modified by the American Fertility Society in 1988 (now the American Society of Reproductive Medicine ASRM) and is the most widely accepted scheme for classifying Mullerian duct anomalies **(Table 1)**.[3]

Classification

Congenital anomalies of the female reproductive tract are frequently associated with renal anomalies, especially renal agenesis or ectopia.[4] Renal anomalies may be present in upto 50% of patients.[5] Therefore, in individuals with suspected mullerian duct anomalies, the kidneys should be evaluated as well. Patients with uterine

Table 1: American Fertility Society (AFS) classification of congenital uterine anomalies.

Class	*Anomaly*	*% of anomalies*
Class I	Agenesis/hypoplasia	10
Class II	Unicornuate uterus	15–20
Class III	Uterus didelphys	5–7
Class IV	Bicornuate uterus	10
Class V	Septate uterus	55
Class VI	Arcuate uterus (considered a normal variant)	
Class VII	Uterine anomalies associated with DES exposure	1

anomalies may be completely asymptomatic as in uterus didelphys or they may result in infertility or spontaneous abortion. Septate uterus is associated with a higher rate of reproductive failure.[6,7] Patients may present at puberty with primary amenorrhea, pelvic mass or pain. MR is helpful in these patients of primary amenorrhea as it can determine the presence or absence of the vagina, cervix or uterus. In addition, MR can reveal the level of obstruction and whether retrograde menstruation has resulted in hematosalpinx.[3]

Hysterosalpingography (HSG) and ultrasound have been the primary imaging modalities, but each has its own-limitations. HSG permits the contour of the endometrial cavity to be defined, but its relationship to the myometrium cannot be determined. Hence, HSG cannot always differentiate between a septate and bicornuate uterus **(Fig. 3A)**. Conventional two-dimensional sonography is helpful in identifying two horns of a uterus, but the distinction between the above two conditions cannot be generally made. Before the advent of MRI, diagnosis was often possible only on laparoscopy or surgery. MRI has proved to be an accurate and noninvasive means of evaluating patients with congenital anomalies, allowing precise classification. The introduction of three-dimensional ultrasound allows identification of congenital uterine anomalies, thus replacing the use of MRI in this field.

Class I: Müllerian Agenesis or Hypoplasia

Uterine agensis or hypoplasia results from nondevelopment or rudimentary development of the mullerian ducts. A subtype of uterine agenesis is the Meyer-Rokintansky-Kuster-Hauser (MRKH) syndrome which has an incidence of approximately 1 in 5,000.[8] This syndrome results in failure of development of upper two-thirds of vagina, cervix and uterus. Ovaries are intact and are associated with variable anomalies of the urinary tract and skeletal system.[5] The T2-weighted sagittal images are most useful for identifying the presence of a uterus. Vaginal agnesis is best characterized on the axial plane with no normal vaginal zonal anatomy identified between the rectum and the urethra **(Figs. 1A to C)**. The main advantage of MRI compared with other modalities is its ability to differentiate complete from segmental uterine agenesis. Uterine hypoplasia is diagnosed when the uterus is small in size and the myometrium is of lower than normal signal intensity. In addition, the endometrial cavity is small and inter cornual diameter is less than 2 cm with poorly differentiated zonal anatomy.[9]

Class II: Unicornuate Uterus

A unicornuate uterus results from non-development or rudimentary development of one mullerian duct while the other one elongates normally. The characteristic appearance on MRI is the "banana" shaped uterine cavity with maintained zonal anatomy although the uterine volume is reduced.[2] If a rudimentary horn is present, MRI can usually distinguish it from an adnexal mass suspected on ultrasound, as well as determine if there is endometrium contained within it and if it communicates with the unicornuate uterus.

Women with a noncommunicating rudimentary horn are at a risk of endometriosis while an ectopic or ruptured pregnancy may result if the rudimentary horn communicates with the opposite normal horn. Thus, a rudimentary horn should be removed to prevent these

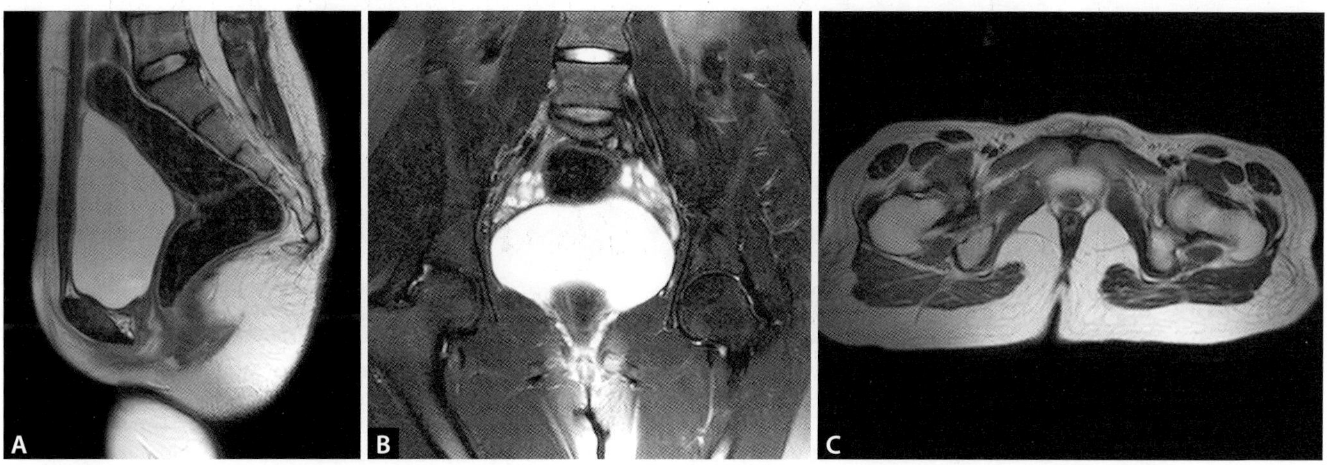

Figs. 1A to C: (A and B) T2W sagittal and coronal MR images show absence of uterus and cervix with normal morphology of both ovaries; (C) T2W axial image shows lower one-third of vagina between the bladder and rectum—Uterine agenesis.

complications.[8] Renal agenesis or other anomalies when present are generally located ipsilateral to the small or absent uterus.

Class III: Uterus Didelphys

The didelphys uterus results from non-fusion of the two mullerian ducts. Two separate normal sized uteri and cervices are demonstrated on MRI, with a septum extending upto the upper vagina. The two uteri are usually widely separated with preservation of the endometrial and myometrial widths and no communication between the endometrial cavities. While the horns in uterus didelphys are widely divergent, the cervices are often closely approximated and may show a minor degree of fusion along their medial margins. A longitudinal vaginal septum is present in 75% of cases and occasionally a transverse vaginal septum may be present causing obstruction of the hemiuterus resulting in hematometrocolpos[3] **(Figs. 2A to C).**

Class IV: Bicornuate Uterus

Partial fusion of the mullerian ducts produces the bicornuate uterus, with the resulting septum being composed of myometrium. It may be bicornuate unicollis in which the myometrial septum extends to the internal os or bicornuate bicollis where it extends as far as the external os. On T2-weighted axial MR images, two uterine horns are visualized, each containing an endometrial cavity, with the separating myometrium having a high signal intensity. In addition, MR may also document an outward fundal concavity in bicornuate uterus as opposed to the convexity seen in a normal uterus. The depth of the intervening cleft separating the uterine horns in the external fundal myometrium is greater than 1 cm **(Figs. 3A to D)**.[3] Normal zonal anatomy is seen in each horn.

Class V: Septate Uterus

Septate uterus is the most common congenital anomaly representing approximately 55% of all anomalies. Septate uterus is due to incomplete resorption of the final fibrous septum between the two mullerian ducts. It may be complete or partial. Complete septate uterus is one wherein the septum extends to the external os. While in partial septate uterus, septum extends to any level proximal to the external os. The external uterine contour is convex, flat or mildy concave, with the fundal indentation less than or equal to 1 cm.[3] The uterine septum is of low signal intensity on both T1- and T2-weighted images in contrast to the medium to high signal intensity myometrium separating the two endometrial cavities in the bicornuate uterus **(Figs. 4A and B)**. The differentiation between septate uterus and bicornuate uterus is clinically significant because of their different complications and different treatment.

Evaluation of the external fundal contour is the most important feature for distinguishing a bicornuate uterus from a septate uterus. This can be well defined by transvaginal sonography, 3D ultrasonography and magnetic resonance imaging, which show both the external contour of the fundus as well as the nature of the dividing tissue.

Table 2 lists the differentiating features between septate and bicornuate uteri.

The nature of tissues separating the two endometrial cavities has been used to distinguish between septate and bicornuate uteri but has been found to be a less reliable

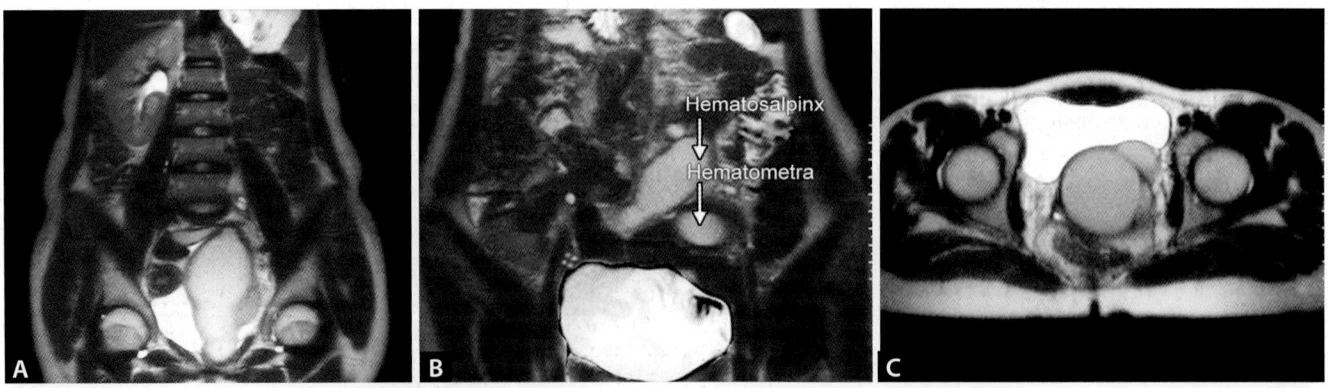

Figs. 2A to C: (A) T2W coronal MR image reveals complete duplication of uterus with normal morphology of right-sided uterus. The left uterus and vagina are distended with hyperintense contents—hematometrocolpos. Left kidney is absent; (B) T2W coronal shows a hyperintense tubular structure on the left side—hematosalpinx along with hematometra; (C) Axial T2W image shows complete duplication of vagina with hematocolpos on the left with normal vagina on the right with thin, central luminal hyperintensity: Uterus didelphys with obstructed left side system with associated developmental absence of left kidney.

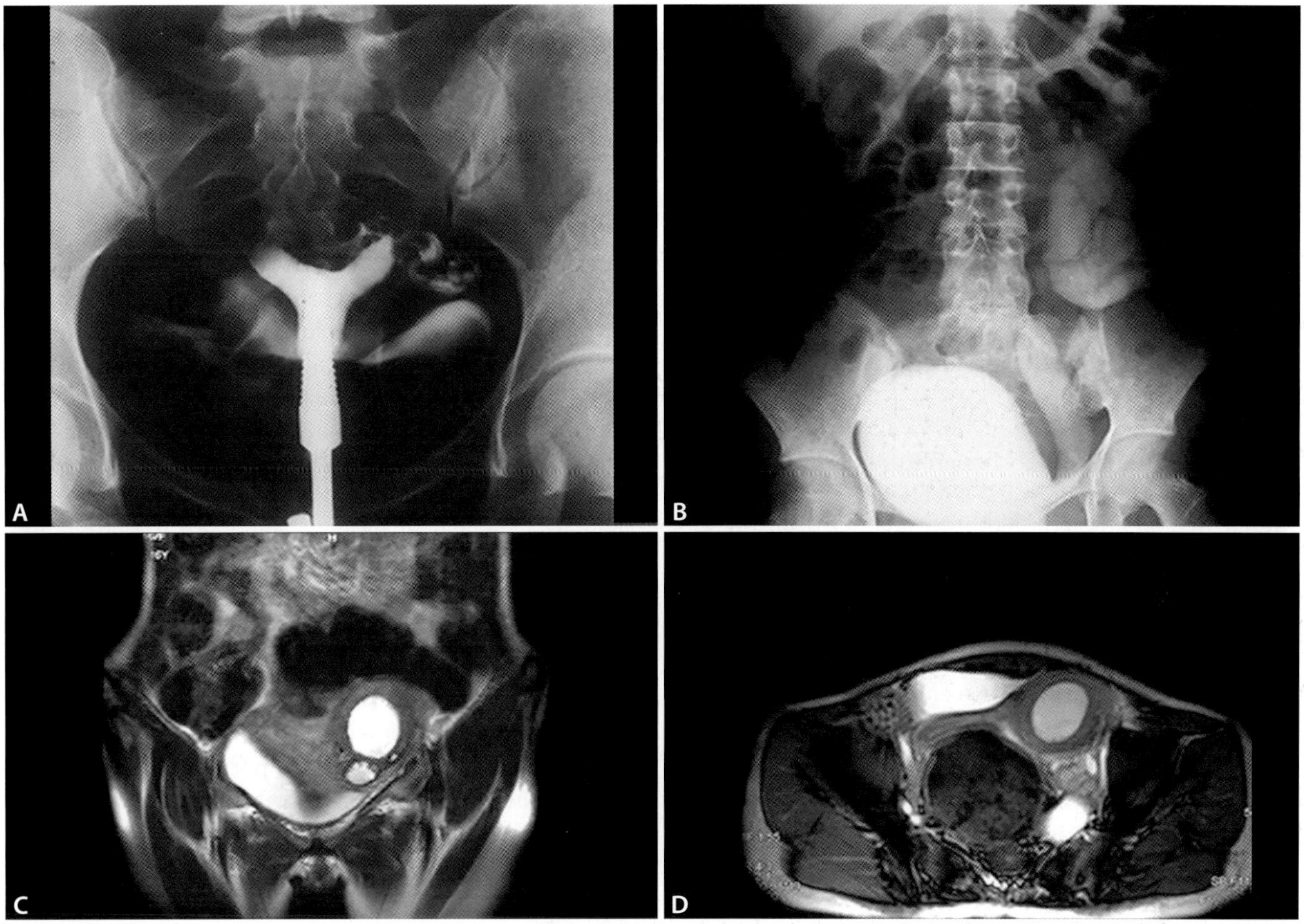

Figs. 3A to D: (A) HSG showing two separate uterine cavities: The left fallopian tube is visualized with intraperitoneal spill while the right tube is not visualized bicornuate/septate uterus; (B) IVP in another patient reveals malascended left kidney with grade IV HUN with ectopic low insertion of left ureter in retropubic region; (C and D) Coronal and axial T2W MR images of same showing two separate uterine horns with dilated and high SI endometrial collection in left horn suggestive of hematometra with small right horn with thinned endometrium. Fundal contour is concave, best appreciated on the coronal image—Bicornuate uterus.

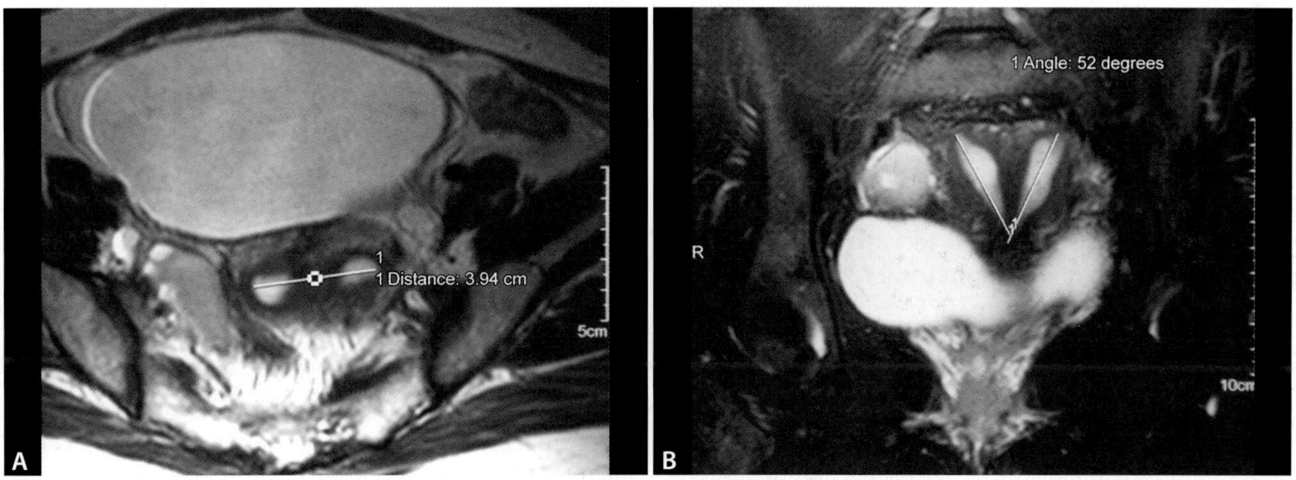

Figs. 4A and B: (A) T2W axial MR image shows two endometrial cavities with an intercornual distance <4 cm with hypointense septum separating them; (B) T2W coronal image depicts the two uterine cavities separated by a vertical septum extending from the fundus to above the internal os with an intercornual angle < 75°. Also seen is a right hemorrhagic ovarian cyst—Septate uterus.

Table 2: Distinguished features between septate and bicornuate uteri.

Features	*Septate uterus*	*Bicornuate uterus*
1. Depth of fundal cleft	≤1 cm	>1 cm
2. Fundal contour	Convex/flat	Deep fundal concavity
3. Intercornual angle	<75°	>105°
4. Intercornual distance (T2 W coronal MR image)	<4 cm	>4 cm
5. Intercornual tissue	Fibrous or myometrial	Myometrial tissue

feature than the external shape of the uterus. Typically a fibrous septum defines the septate uterus which whill appear hypoechoic compared to myometrium on TVS and hypointense on all MR pulse sequences. In contrast, a myometrial septum occurs only in a bicornuate uterus and would appear isoechoic or isointense to myometrium. However, a considerable overlap in the imaging features of the dividing tissues in these two entities have been found.[9]

Class VI: Arcuate Uterus

An arcuate configuration of the uterus is considered a normal variant and is not associated with an increase risk of infertility or pregnancy loss. It results from a near complete resorption of the uterovaginal septum, leaving a mild concave indentation at the level of the fundus. On imaging, the external uterine contour is usually flat or convex, though it may be slightly concave. There is a broad, smooth indentation of the myometrium on the endometrium in the fundal region with normal zonal anatomy being maintained. Also there is no evidence of a low signal appearing fibrous component.

Class VII: Diethylstilbestrol Exposed Uterus

Diethylstilbestrol (DES) is a synthetic estrogen that was used in the 1950s and 1960s to prevent recurrent spontaneous abortions and poor reproductive outcomes in patients. This drug has been associated with congenital anomalies of the female genital tract in the offspring of women exposed in the first trimester. Uterine malformations include narrowed, irregular endometrial cavities with constriction bands ("T" configuration), small hypoplastic uterus. Fallopain tubes can demonstrate stenosis, sacculations and shortening.[3] These anomalies of uterine shape are demonstrable by hysterosalpingography and MR imaging. They are not associated with any urinary tract abnormalities.[10]

Leiomyomas

Leiomyoma (fibroid) of the uterus is the most common gynecologic disorder occurring in 20–40% of all women during their reproductive years. It is a benign uterine tumor and consists of predominantly smooth muscle with varying amounts of fibrous and connective tissue.[11] These tumors are estrogen-dependent; hence, there is an increased prevalence of leiomyomas in patients with diseases associated with hyperestrogenism, such as endometrial hyperplasia, endometrial cancer, anovulatory states.[10] Leiomyomas may increase in size during pregnancy and decrease in size after menopause. Most women with leiomyomas are asymptomatic although some may have signs and symptoms of pelvic mass, pain, abnormal bleeding and pressure effect on adjacent pelvic organs. They are usually well circumscribed and surrounded by a pseudocapsule. Majority of the leiomyoma are found within the uterine body (90%), with a small proportion found within the cervix or broad ligament. Myoma may be solitary or multiple and occur in submucosal, intramural or subserosal locations **(Figs. 5A and B)**. It often calcifies in postmenopausal women and large tumors may develop hyaline, myxomatous, cystic or hemorrhagic degeneration.

The sonographic appearance of uterine fibroid depends on its relative composition of smooth muscle and fibrous tissue and on the presence and nature of degeneration. These masses may be difficult to detect with ultrasonography, because of variable patterns of echogenicity which may range from hypoechoic to echogenic, homogeneous to heterogeneous, with or without acoustic shadowing. It may present with uterine enlargement or distort the uterine contour. The most common appearance of a leiomyoma is that of a well-marginated, hypoechoic round or oval mass within the uterine body.[5] Intense shadowing may represent calcification.[12,13] Calcified myoma have a typical appearance on plain radiograph of the abdomen **(Fig. 6)**.

Distortion of the endometrial complex is helpful in identifying a submucosal component. Submucosal leiomyomas may mimic endometrial lesions and sonohysterosalpingography may help in differentiating the two. Submucosal fibroids are usually broad-based hypoechoic masses with an overlying layer of echogenic endometrium.[14]

The characteristic CT features of uterine leiomyoma is an enlarged uterus with solid enhancing mass **(Fig. 7)** having a lobulated contour with speckled, whorled, streaked or curvilinear calcification. The presence of dystrophic calcification is the most specific sign of leiomyoma.[15]

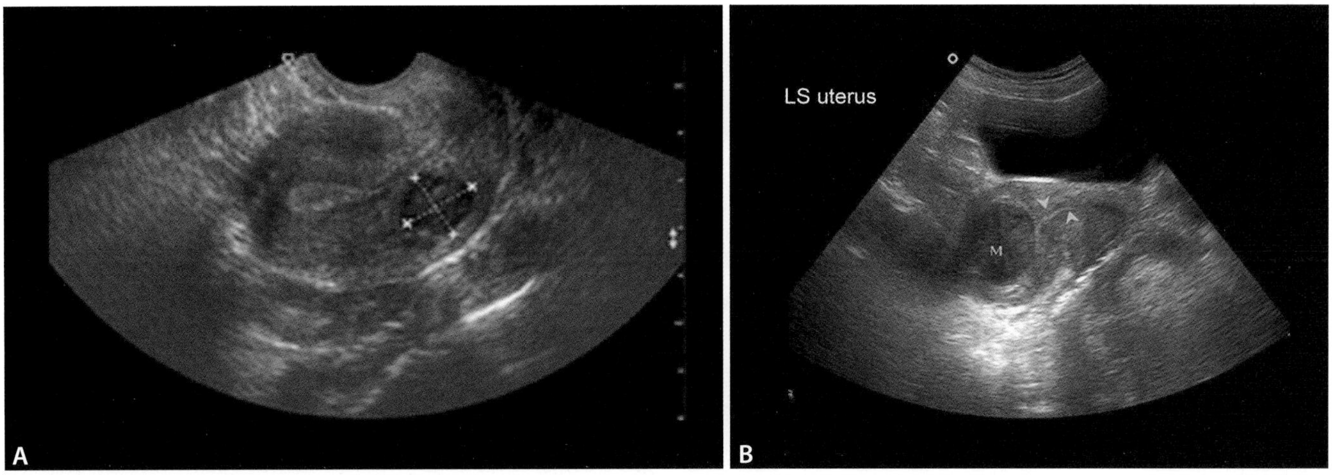

Figs. 5A and B: Uterine fibroids: TVS shows (A) Well-defined, round, hypoechoic mass in posterior myometrium—Intramural fibroid; (B) LS of the uterus reveals homogeneous, hypoechoic well marginated round to oval mass lesion in the fundus of uterus displacing the endometrium inferiorly—Submucosal fibroid.

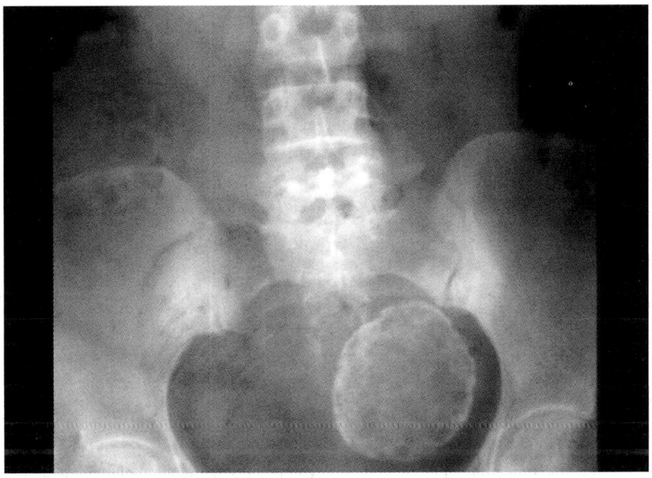

Fig. 6: Plain X-ray pelvis shows a large calcified fibroid in the pelvis.

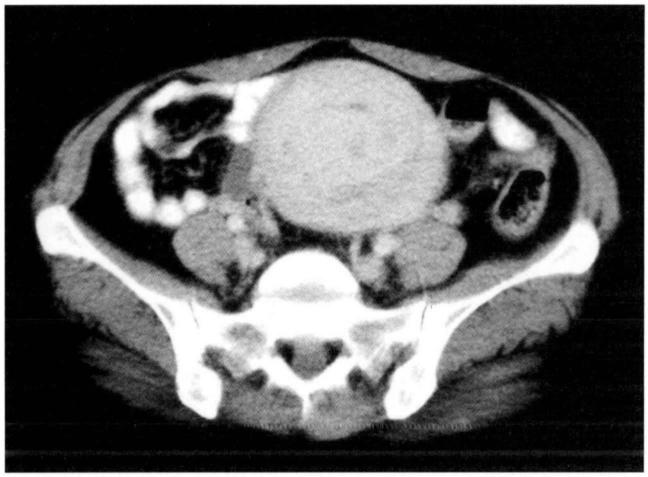

Fig. 7: CT scan through the lower abdomen shows leiomyoma as a well-defined rounded lesion with homogeneous contrast enhancement with few small hypodense areas within.

However, calcification is only seen in 10% of cases. Other CT features suggestive of a uterine leiomyoma are soft tissue masses that distort or obliterate the uterine cavity and irregular low density areas within uterine masses representing degeneration of a leiomyoma.[16] However, if there is no calcification, myoma cannot be distinguished from carcinoma on the basis of attenuation values. In the absence of calcification both ultrasound and MRI are superior to CT for demonstrating myomas.

MRI is indicated when the ultrasound examination is indeterminate or limited as in retroflexed uterus.[17]

Magnetic resonance imaging offers the most sensitive imaging of leiomyomas, being able to identify lesions as small as 0.3 cm. Leiomyoma is typically seen as sharply marginated homogeneous areas of very low signal intensity on T2-weighted sequences and isointense to myometrium on T1-weighted sequences **(Fig. 8)**. The characteristic low signal intensity on T2-W1 is due to the presence of compact, smooth muscle myoma cells and a paucity of intercellular matrix.[7] They are well circumscribed with well-defined margins. The appearance of leiomyoma after the administration of gadolinium is variable. On postcontrast T2-weighted images, leiomyoma most often appear of lower signal intensity relative to the myometrium or endometrium. The presence of calcification usually causes areas of signal void on both T1- and T2-weighted images, but unlike CT the finding is not specific. Thin, hyperintense rims are sometimes seen,

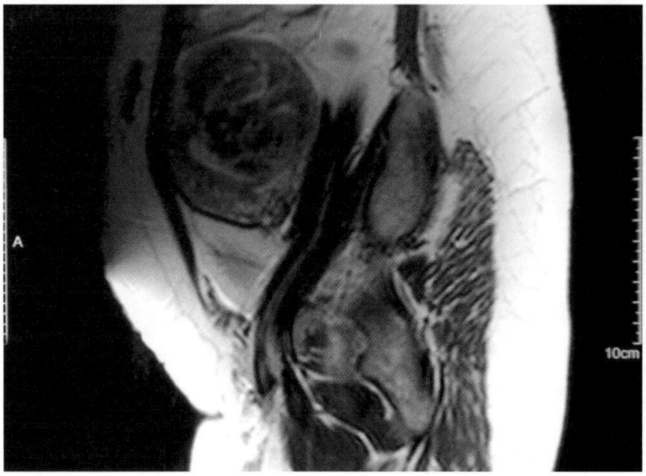

Fig. 8: T2W sagittal image of pelvis reveals a large, well-defined low signal intensity mass in the posterior myometrium with typical whorled internal appearance abutting the endometrium—Intramural fibroid.

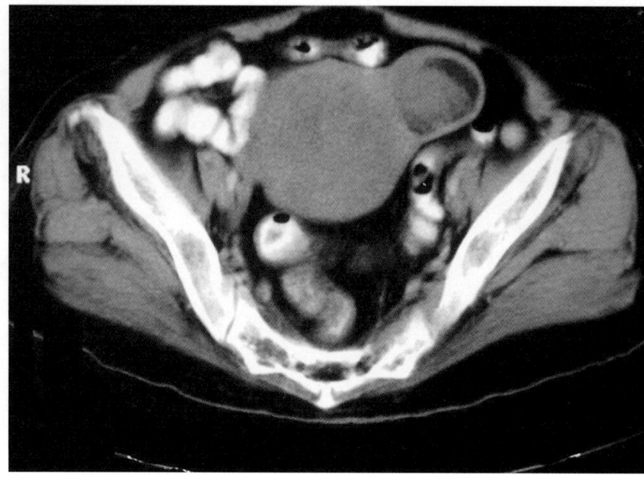

Fig. 9: CT scan of the pelvis showing a lobulated uterine mass with fatty degeneration—Lipoleiomyoma.

as well as internal signal heterogeneity due to hyaline or myxoid degeneration.[18]

MR imaging facilitates the differentiation of a pedunculated leiomyoma from an adnexal mass on basis of typical signal intensity and morphology.[19] An MR feature of exophytic leiomyomas is the "bridging vessel sign" which refers to the presence of flow voids on T1- and T2-weighted images from branches of the uterine artery that are localized between the mass and the uterus. This indicates that the tumour is supplied by branches of the uterine artery. It is the only noninvasive means available for differentiating a leiomyoma from adenomyosis and is useful in patients considered for myomectomy as it precisely determines the location and number of leiomyomas.[20]

Hemorrhagic, cystic and fatty degeneration are the three types of degeneration in fibroids that have suggestive MR features. Hemorrhagic degeneration of fibroids is uncommon and is associated with leiomyomas during pregnancy. Leiomyoma with hemorrhagic "red degeneration" often reveals peripheral or central high SI on T1-W images secondary to methemoglobin and show minimal enhancement.[8] About 5% of fibroids have foci of cystic degeneration which on MR imaging appears as very high SI on T2 W images and also do not enhance after contrast. Falty degeneration of a leiomyoma into a lipoleiomyoma is rare and has an incidence of less than 0.5%.[8] The fat tissue within the myoma can be detected and characterized using fat suppression techniques. CT is also very sensitive in identifying fat attenuation within a lipoleiomyoma **(Fig. 9)**.

Malignant degeneration is rare (0.1–0.6%) but should be suspected if a leiomyoma enlarges suddenly,[21] or if an indistinct border or irregular contour is noted on MR imaging.[22]

Treatment of Uterine Leiomyomas

Most leiomyomas are asymptomatic, and therefore, do not require any treatment. Multiple treatment options are available for women who are symptomatic. The surgical options include hystrectomy and myomectomy. Myomectomy can be via laprotomy, laproscopic or hysteroscopic route. Non surgical treatments include uterine artery embolization (UAE) and medical therapy. Hystrectomy is an effective treatment for symptomatic fibroids and routinely performed in patients with pain and abnormal bleeding. Patients with one or two sub-mucosal myomas are likely to benefit from hysteroscopic resection following which a cessation of excess bleeding and restoration of fertility may be seen.

UAE has become an alternative noninvasive treatment of symptomatic uterine fibroids. When compared with myomectomy, it has been found to be a better treatment option for fibroid related menorrhagia and equivalent method for reducing pain.[23]

MR angiography provides information to determine which patients are potential candidates for UAE therapy. MR can document the size, number, location and vascularity of uterine leiomyomas. Women with large (>10 cm) leiomyomas have been found to have equally good results after UAE as those with smaller myomas. One subtype that has shown poor response to UAE is leiomyomas with high SI on T1W images and minimal or no enhancement.[24] This is likely because the high SI myomas have already undergone ischemia/hemorrhagic necrosis and will not lose additional vascularity or volume with additional embolization.[25] Conversely, the best response to UAE therapy is seen in those myomas that show marked enhancement after contrast administration.

Contrast-enhanced MR angiography (CE-MRA) can reveal the presence of normal uterine arteries. If a separate gonadal arterial supply to the uterus is seen on CE MRA, then one should consider embolizing the gonadal artery at the time of UAE. Failure to embolize the gonadal artery that directly supplies the uterus, has been seen to be a cause of UAE failure.[26]

After UAE, MR can document a decrease in size and enhancement of fibroids, preserved enhancement of remainder of the uterus and lack of visualization of the uterine arteries on an MRA study. An MR performed immediately after UAE showing decreased enhancement of the fibroids correlates, with a subsequent successful clinical response.[25] A decrease in volume of fibroids by 40–60% and a decreased enhancement of fibroids has been documented by MR following UAE correlating with the successful necrosis.[24]

OTHER BENIGN MESENCHYMAL TUMORS

Fatty or mixed mesenchymal tumors, such as fibromyolipoma, myolipoma and lipoma of the uterus are rare benign tumors.[27] They may arise from metaplasia of connective tissue or smooth muscle cells.

Sonographically, lipoma is seen as a rounded lesion of central increased echogenicity with a hypoechoic rim.[28] On CT, the encapsulated fat density of uterine lipoma mimics the more common ovarian dermoid (benign cystic teratoma).[29] Proper diagnosis of these lesions is important because teratomas are generally managed by surgical excision, whereas lipomatous uterine tumors require no therapy unless symptomatic.

Adenomyosis

Adenomyosis is the presence of ectopic endometrial glands and stroma with surrounding smooth muscle hyperplasia within the myometrium. It occurs due to direct invasion of the basal endometrium into the myometrium and may be microscopic, focal or diffuse.[30] Diffuse form is more common and is composed of widely scattered foci of adenomyosis distributed asymmetrically within the myometrium, while the focal or nodular form is composed of circumscribed nodules called adenomyomas within the inner myometrium.[14] Adenomyosis is frequently accompanied by additional pelvic abnormalities, such as uterine myomas, and it occurs concomitantly in 6–20% patients with endometriosis.[30] It is frequently diagnosed in multiparous, premenopausal women, with clinical presentation mimicking leiomyomas or dysfunctional bleeding. Establishing the correct diagnosis is essential, as treatment of these three entities differs markedly. The definitive treatment of adenomyosis is hysterectomy, dysfunctional uterine bleeding may be controlled with dilatation and curettage and symptomatic leiomyomas may be removed via myomectomy.

Sonography shows an enlarged uterus without focal masses, more often seen to involve the posterior uterine wall.[31] The uterus has a globular configuration. On transabdominal sonography, the features suggestive of adenomyosis are a diffuse uterine enlargement with a normal contour, normal endometrial and myometrial texture. Other findings that have been described are thickening of the posterior myometrium with the involved area being slightly more anechoic than normal myometrium.[14] Transvaginal sonography (TVS) has been found to be more accurate in the diagnosis of adenomyosis.[32] On TVS the findings include (i) poorly defined hypoechoic myometrium, (ii) heterogeneous myometrial echotexture, (iii) assymmetrically thickened myometrial wall, (iv) shaggy endometrium with poor definition between endometrium and myometrium, and (v) scattered small (<5 mm) myometrial cysts.[33]

The focal and nodular involvement of the myometrium is called adenomyoma. Two sonographic features used to characterize an adenomyoma are indistinct margin and presence of hypoechoic lacunae in the hyperechoic myometrium with several cysts.[33] These two criteria have enabled correct diagnosis with TVS in 95% cases.

MR can detect and characterise adnomyosis accurately. On T2-weighted images, focal adenomyosis appears as an ill-defined poorly marginated area of low signal intensity within the myometrium but continuous with the junctional zone (JZ) (inner myometrium). The junctional zone may be evenly or irregularly thickened with a thickness of >12 mm considered abnormal.[34] Occasionally small foci (2–4 mm) of increased signal intensity in both T1- and T2-weighted images are seen within the thickened junctional zone that pathologically correspond to small foci of hemorrhagic endometrium **(Figs. 10A to C)**. MR imaging is highly accurate in diagnosing adenomyosis from leiomyomas.[35,36] MR can more accurately diagnose adenomyosis than can TVS, especially in women with coexistent leiomyomas.[8] Focal adenomyosis often has an ill-defined border and is always contiguous with the junctional zone which

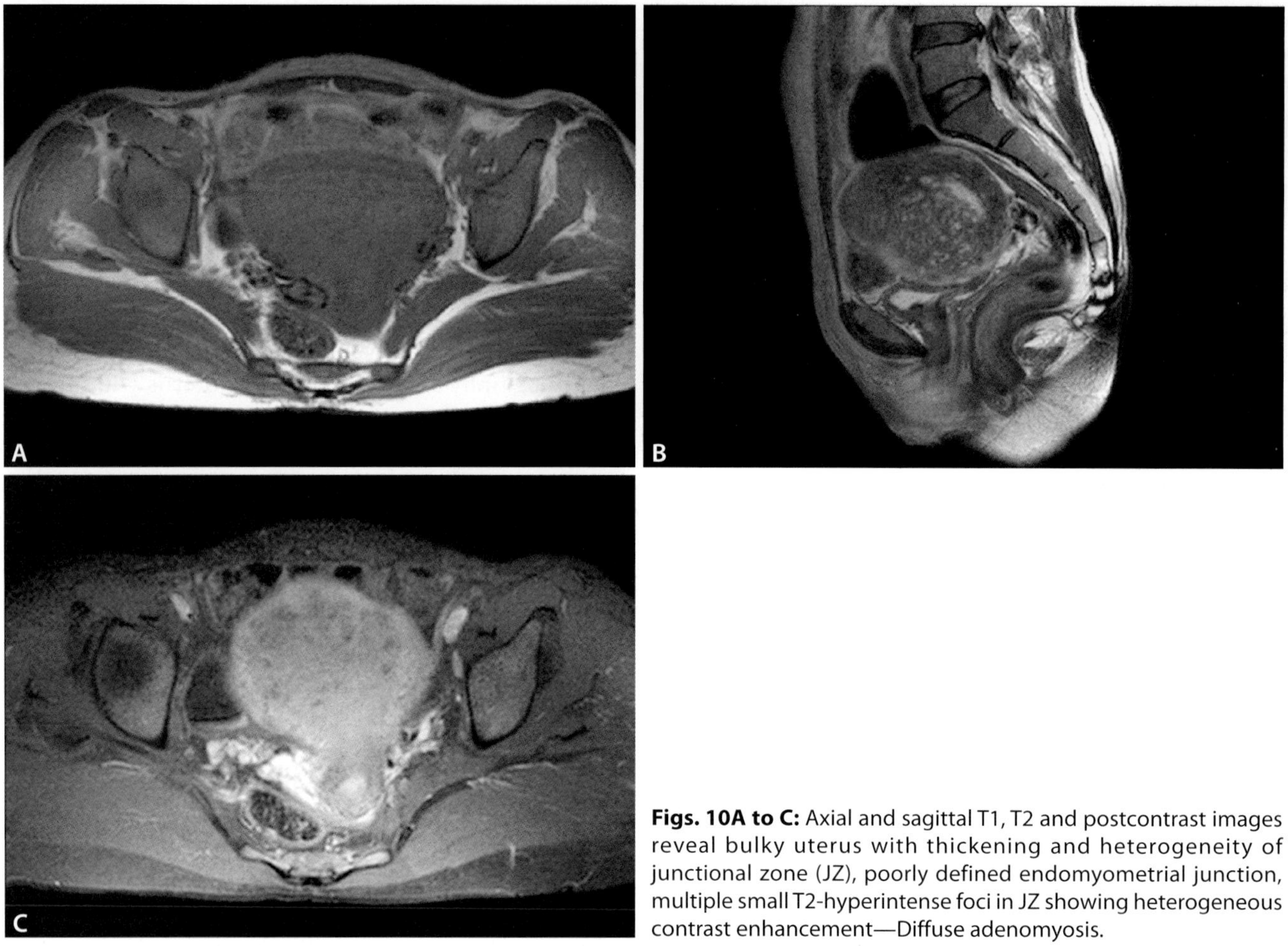

Figs. 10A to C: Axial and sagittal T1, T2 and postcontrast images reveal bulky uterus with thickening and heterogeneity of junctional zone (JZ), poorly defined endomyometrial junction, multiple small T2-hyperintense foci in JZ showing heterogeneous contrast enhancement—Diffuse adenomyosis.

is frequently thicker than 12 mm, whereas the border around leiomyomas is sharp.[35] An irregular interface between endometrium and adenomyosis is typical. T2W images will show a relatively homogeneous, low intensity mass, but the SI is not as low as that with leiomyomas.[10] Adenomyosis is often oriented parallel to the endometrial stripe and has minimal mass effect on the endometrial canal while leiomyomas do show mass effect.[37]

Table 3 shows the differentiating features between adenomyosis and leiomyomas.

Table 3: Differentiating features between adenomyosis and leiomyomas.

Features	***Adenomyosis***	***Uterine leiomyoma***
Margins	Poorly defined	Well circumscribed
Center	Junctional zone	Any layer of uterus, originates in myometrium
Appearance	Focal or diffuse	Focal
T2-signal intensity	Small hyperintense foci	Hypointense unless degeneration present
Thickened junctional zone	Yes (>12 mm)	No
Mass effect on endometrium	Minimal or none	+ if intracavitary or submucosal

Endometrial Polyps

Endometrial polyps are localized hyperplastic overgrowth of endometrial glands and stroma which are covered by endometrium and almost always benign. Endometrial polyps may be sessile or pedunculated and are usually attached to the uterine fundus. They may be small or so large as to protrude through the cervical os into the endocervical canal **(Figs. 11A and B)**. There are three types of polyps: hyperplastic (resembling glands of endometrial hyperplasia), atrophic (cystically dilated atrophic glands), and functional (undergo cyclical endometrial changes). Endometrial polyps are common, being found in perimenopausal and postmenopausal women, with 20%

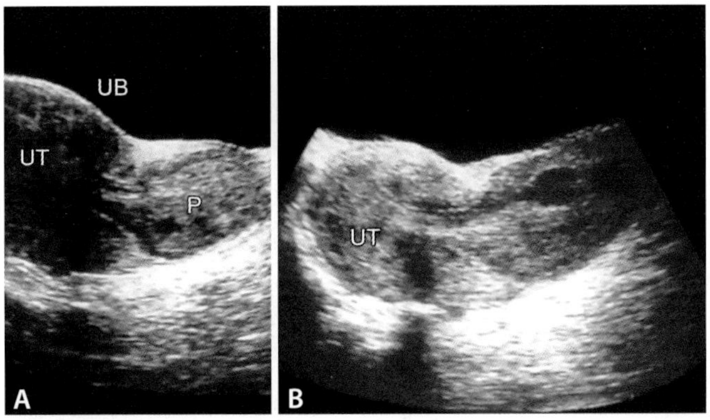

Figs. 11A and B: (A) TAS showing a well-defined oval mass in the cervix with its stalk extending into the endometrial cavity—Endometrial polyp; (B) Small cyst is seen in the lower part of the polyp with multiple myometrial fibroids.

to be multiple in the affected women. Most polyps are asymptomatic; however when symptomatic, may cause menorrhagia, intermenstrual bleeding or postmenopausal bleeding. Women on tamoxifen therapy for breast cancer treatment have an increased relative risk for developing endometrial polyps. A spectrum of endometrial abnormalities like proliferative changes, hyperplasia, polyps and cancer have been reported with tamoxifen.[3]

Ultrasound features include nonspecific thickened endometrium, a focal echogenic area in the endometrium or occasionally an endocavitary mass surrounded by fluid indistinguishable from carcinoma.[38] Sonohysterography is an ideal technique for demonstrating a polyp. This is because a polyp seen as a round echogenic mass within the endometrial cavity is much more easily identified when there is fluid in the endometrial cavity outlining the mass. A submucosal fibroid may mimic an endometrial polyp but may be differentiated by a broader base and more irregular contour of the former on sonohysterography. A normal layer of endometrium is seen overlying a submucosal fibroid while the polyp can be seen arising from the endometrium.[14] Cystic areas may be see within a polyp, representing the histologically dilated glands. With color Doppler, a feeding artery may be seen in the pedicle of the polyp.[39] On MR imaging, endometrial polyps have a variable appearance and may be seen as low/intermediate signal masses within the endometrial cavity on T2W images and appear isointense to the endometrium on T1W images. Contrast enhanced MRI has been reported to improve the sensitivity of their detection, polyps generally enhancing less than the surrounding endometrium, but more than the myometrium[40] **(Figs. 12A to C)**. Most endometrial polyps can be reliably differentiated from submucosal leiomyomas on MR imaging with leiomyomas appearing lower in signal intensity than polyps and being myometrial in origin. However, in case of a degenerated submucosal fibroid, the signal intensity of the two may overlap.[3]

Endometrial Hyperplasia

Endometrial hyperplasia is the excessive proliferation of the endometrial glands, with an increase in endometrial gland-to-stromal raito when compared with normal proliferative endometrium.[14] It may be focal or diffuse and is most often the result of unopposed estrogen stimulation (chronic anovulatory states, obesity, tamoxifen therapy) Women with endometrial hyperplasia commonly present with postmenopausal bleeding. Histologically, endometrial hyperplasia can be divided into hyperplasia without cellular atypia and hyperplasia with cellular atypia (atypical hyperplasia) with 25% of the latter subgroup progressing to endometrial cancer. Each of these types may be further subdivided into simple (cystic) or complex (adenomatous) hyperplasia depending on the glandular complexity. In simple (cystic) hyperplasia, there is cystic dilatation of the glands with surrounding abundant cellular stroma while in complex (adenomatous) hyperplasia, the glands are crowded with little intervening stroma.

The cutoff value for normal versus abnormal endometrial thickeness is controversial, but is a function of the patients hormone status [i.e. premenopausal, postmenopausal with or without hormone replacement therapy (HRT)]. On ultrasonography, a bilayer endometrial width greater than equal to 5 mm is regarded as abnormal in symptomatic postmenopausal women. In asymptomatic postmenopausal women on HRT, cut off values range from <5 to >8 mm while in premenopausal women an endometrial thickness greater than 8 mm in the proliferative phase and greater than 16 mm in the secretory phase is considered abnormal.[41]

Both TVS and sonohysterography are the modalities of choice for screening of endometrial pathology. A focal or diffuse thickening of the endometrium is seen which is usually thick and echogenic **(Fig. 13)**. Small cysts may be seen within the endometrium in cystic hyperplasia. As the sonographic appearance is nonspecific, biopsy is necessary for diagnosis.

On MR imaging, endometrial hyperplasia appears as a diffuse widening of the endometrium with the signal intensity of the hyperplastic endometrium appearing hypo to isointense relative to normal endometrium. Small, high signal intensity cystically dilated glands may be seen within it. Follwing contrast administration, the endometrial hyperplasia enhances less than the adjacent myometrium.[3]

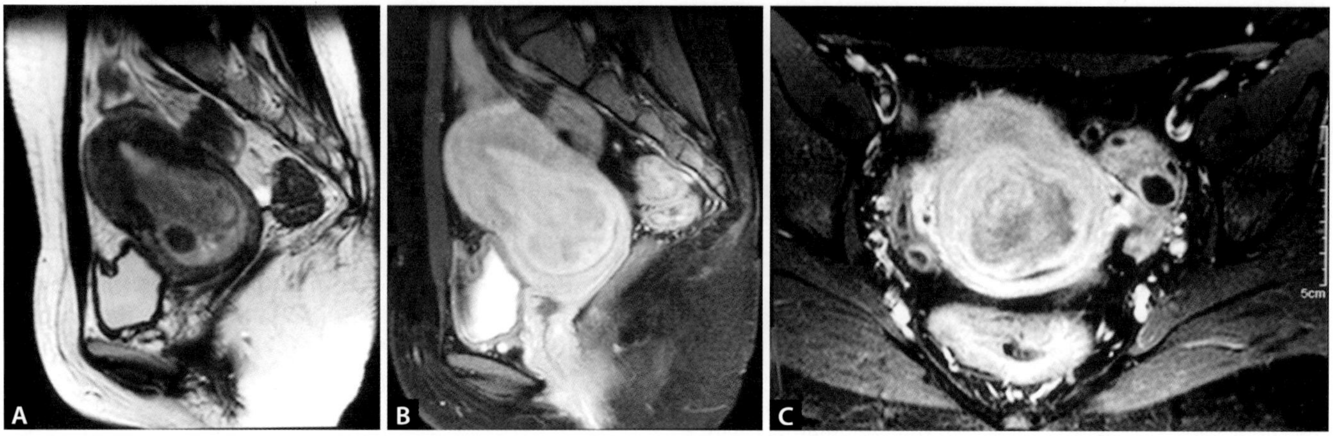

Figs. 12A to C: T2 sagittal and T1 postgadolinium images reveal a large, round to oval well-circumscribed polypoid mass hyperintense on T2W image in the endometrial cavity with widening of the cavity and extending into the lower uterine segment with heterogeneous contrast enhancement—Endometrial polyp.

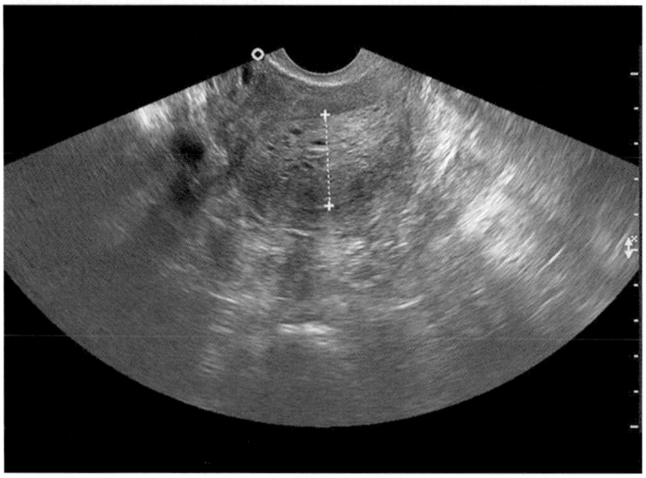

Fig. 13: TVS reveals diffuse thickened echogenic endometrium with small cysts within—Endometrial hyperplasia.

Endometrial Synechiae

Endometrial synechiae/adhesions (Asherman's syndrome) are bridging bands of tissue in the endometrial cavity which occur in response to trauma (post-curettage), infection or inflammation. They may be a cause of infertility or recurrent pregnancy loss. The sonographic diagnosis is difficult unless fluid is distending the endometrial cavity. The endometrium usually appears normal on transabdominal sonography. On TVS, adhesions may be seen as irregular, hypoechoic bridgelike bands within the endometrium which are best seen during the secretory phase when the endometrium is more hyperechoic.[42] Sonohysterography is a technique which demonstrates adhesions very well and should be performed in all cases of suspected adhesions. Adhesions appear as bridging bands of tissue that distort the cavity or as thin undulating membranes best seen on realtime sonography. Hysterosalpingography (HSG) is the other primary method for diagnosis followed by division of the adhesions under hysteroscopy. MR imaging is complementary and provides information on the etiology of synechiae.[43] On T2-weighted images, synechiae appear as low signal intensity bands that traverse the endometrial cavity and enhance after contrast administration, especially in the early phase. MR is a useful technique as it provides information of the endometrial cavity above the adhesions which is a blind spot for hysteroscopy, and has both therapeutic and prognostic significance.[44]

UTERINE ARTERIOVENOUS MALFORMATION

Uterine arteriovenous malformations (AVMs) are uncommon and may be congenital, traumatic, malignant or idiopathic in origin. Congenital AVMs are considered to be undifferentiated vascular structures resulting from the arrest of embryonic development at various stages. Acquired AVMs are usually caused by procedures such as curettage, uterine surgery or may be secondary to trauma or neoplasm.[45]

On gray-scale imaging, appearance of AVMs is nonspecific and include subtle, myometrial inhomogeneity, tubular spaces within the myometrium or prominent parametrial vessels. Doppler findings reveal a low resistance flow with high peak systolic velocities. Spectral analysis of venous flow also depict high flow velocities and systolic velocity peaks similar to arterial pattern, suggesting an arteriovenous shunting.[46]

Both CT and MR can accurately assess the size, extent, vascularity of AVMs and the degree of adjacent organ involved. On MR imaging, AVMs appear as focal uterine masses or as disruption of the junctional zones with serpiginous flow related signal voids within the myometrium, showing intense enhancement on postgadolinium imaging **(Figs. 14A to D)**. Treatment of uterine AVM consists of either surgery or transcatheter embolization. The extent of involvement of adjacent pelvic viscera is a major criteria in deciding between the two treatment options.[45]

BENIGN OVARIAN MASSES

Sonographic morphology of benign ovarian masses include either the masses being completely cystic or complex .

BENIGN CYSTIC MASSES OF PELVIS

In general, most cystic masses that arise within the pelvis are of ovarian origin. Cystic adnexal masses on sonography include physiological ovarian cysts (follicular cysts, corpus luteum cysts, and theca lutein cysts), hemorrhagic ovarian cysts, simple ovarian cysts, polycystic ovarian disease, hydrosalpinx, cystadenoma, paraovarian cysts, peritoneal inclusion cysts and endometriomas.

FUNCTIONAL CYSTS

Follicular Cysts

Follicular cysts develop when a follicle fails to ovulate or involute They occur in all age groups but are most common in women of reproductive age-group. It is a simple cyst and its diagnosis is based purely on ultrasound findings—a unilocular, round, anechoic structure with a thin and regular walls causing posterior acoustic enhancement.[47] The size of the cyst varies from 3 cm to 5 cm. CT is not the investigation of choice for evaluation of ovarian cysts, but are common incidental finding on CECT of the the pelvis wherein they are well defined, rounded, unilocular, homogeneous, water density mass with smooth thin walls and low attenuation contents.[48]

On MR imaging, they are well-circumscribed, homogeneous, intermediate to low signal intensity masses on T1-weighted images and very high signal intensity on T2-weighted images. The cyst wall is imperceptible on T1 weighted images and enhances following administration of gadolinium.[3]

Simple follicular cysts usually resolve spontaneously. Follow up ultrasound is recommended 6 weeks after initial imaging evaluation to see for cyst resolution. It should preferably be done in the first of week of the menstrual cycle in order to avoid confusion with other follicular cysts.

The differential diagnosis of follicular cysts include nonfunctional cysts and cystic neoplasm. Nonfunctional cysts include surface epithelial inclusion cysts, rete cysts and paraovarian or paratubal cysts. Paraovarian cysts are indistinguishable from functional cysts by imaging criteria except by location. A diagnosis of paraovarian cyst can be made when the ipsilateral ovary is seen close to but separate from the cyst.

Simple ovarian cysts are common in premenopausal women and with increasing use of ultrasound are also seen in upto 20% of postmenopausal women.[49] They should be followed by serial ultrasonography to see for cyst resolution and any change in cyst morphology. Earlier it was advocated that postmenopausal cysts >5 cm in size should be removed. However, studies have shown that postmenopausal simple cysts upto 10 cm in size can be followed by serial sonographic evaluation and do not warrant an immediate laprotomy as risk of malignancy is very rare (<1%).[50]

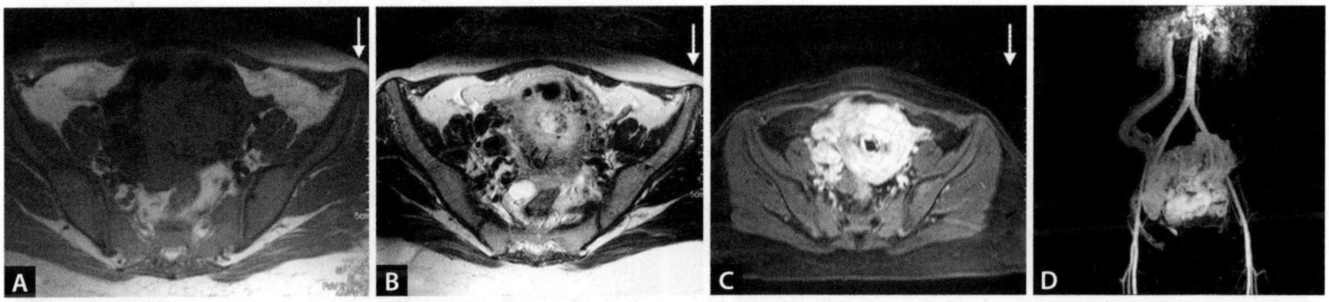

Figs. 14A to D: (A and B) T1W and T2W axial MR images reveal a bulky uterus with multiple, large tortuous flow voids within the myometrium and bilateral parametrial regions showing; (C) Intense enhancement on postgadolinium images; (D) MRA reveals prominent arterial feeder channels arising from anterior division of the internal iliac arteries. Enlarged, tortuous venous channels are seen draining into the iliac vein with early filling of the IVC—Uterine arteriovenous malformation.

Corpus Luteum Cyst

Corpus luteal cysts are normal physiological ovarian structures formed after ovulation by the dominant follicle when the follicular wall becomes vascularized, thickened and partially collapsed. The changes in the follicular wall are known as luteinization. While they are not pathological, they can cause periovulatory pain that may require radiological evaluation. Corpus luteal cysts are less common than follicular cysts but tend to be larger and symptomatic. They are usually unilateral and more prone to hemorrhage and rupture. If the ovum is fertilized, the corpus luteum continues as the corpus luteum of pregnancy. Maximum size is reached at 8–10 weeks and by 12–16 weeks the cyst usually resolves spontaneously. It represents the most common adnexal mass in pregnancy.[3]

Sonographically, corpus luteal cysts have a thicker hyperechoic and crenulated wall. The contents are usually hyperechoic and represents some bleeding into the follicle that has ovulated. A higher fat content of the cyst wall is a likely cause for the hyperechogenic wall of the corpus luteal cyst.[47] On color Doppler sonography, corpus luteal cyst shows a typical " ring of fire appearance" **(Figs. 15A and B)**.

As computed tomography (CT) is increasingly being used as a primary modality for the radiological evaluation of patients with lower abdominal or pelvic pain, therefore; recognition of CT appearance of corpus luteal cysts is desirable. They are unilocular cysts, typically less than 3 cm in diameter with thick, crenulated, hyperdense or enhancing walls. This appearance corresponds to the histopathological changes of corpus luteal cysts seen after ovulation.[48]

The characteristic appearance of corpus luteum cyst on MR allows it to be differentiated from other ovarian masses. The inner wall of the cyst wall may be seen as a line of high signal intensity on T1-weighted images and a line of low signal intensity on T2-weighted images representing hemosiderin deposited along its wall.[51] The thickened cyst wall enhances avidly following administration of gadolinium. Internal debris and hemorrhage can be present within the corpus luteum but lack of internal enhancement rules out the possibility of ovarian malignancy.[3]

The above-described characteristic appearances of corpus luteal cyst on imaging allows distinction from other ovarian masses and often obviates the need for follow-up. When in doubt, correlation with recent ultrasound and follow-up imaging is helpful as corpus luteal cysts should exhibit rapid change in size. A large amount of hemorrhage into a cyst can mimic an endometrioma, but on follow-up imaging the corpus luteum cyst will resolve whereas an endometrioma will persist.

Hemorrhagic Cyst

The most common complication of a functional cyst is hemorrhage. Hemorrhage can occur in any ovarian cyst, but most commonly seen in corpus luteal cysts. Women with hemorrhagic cysts frequently present with acute onset of pelvic pain. Hemorrhagic cysts show a spectrum of findings as a result of variable sonographic appearance of blood. The sonographic appearance depends on the amount of hemorrhage and the time of hemorrhage relative to the time of sonographic examination. Various sonographic findings include diffuse echogenic material,

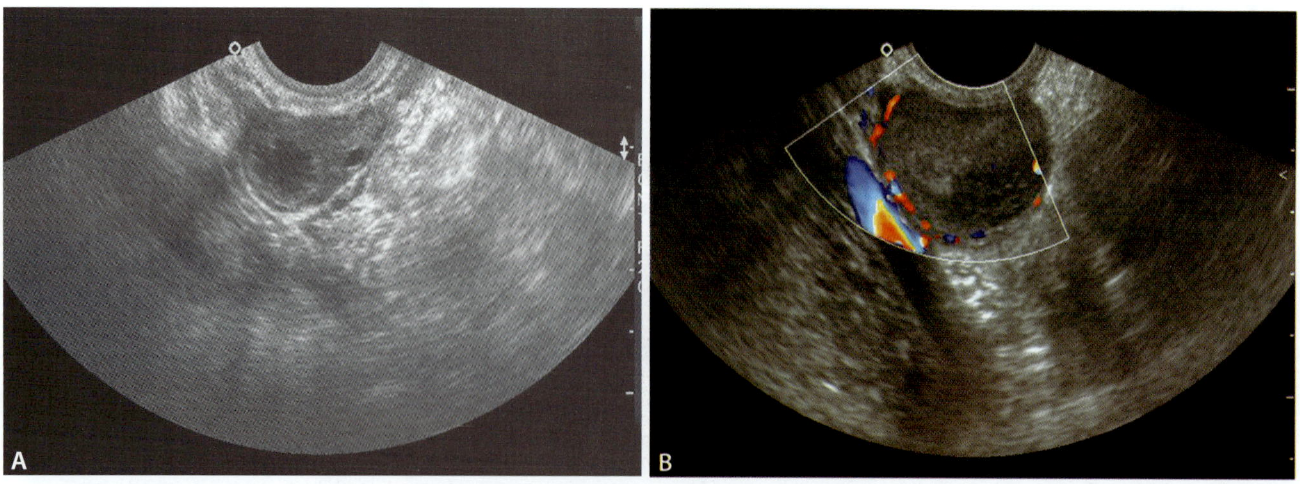

Figs. 15A and B: (A) Corpus luteum cyst showing thick wall with crenulated appearance within the ovarian parenchyma; (B) CDS showing "ring of fire" appearance around corpus luteum cyst with internal echoes due to hemorrhage.

diffuse echoes with visible fibrin strands, retracting thrombus and fluid-fluid level.

The internal characteristics of a hemorrhagic cyst are much better appreciated on TVS because of its superior resolution. Hemorrhagic ovarian cysts typically contain fine linear echoes which represent strands of fibrin. Fibrin within the internal architecture of clot is responsible for this appearance. The fibrin strands need to be differentiated from true septations which are a feature of ovarian neoplasm. Usually, fibrin strands are innumerable, discontinuous, cannot be traced on multiple frames, whereas septations are continuous, thick, linear structures seen in multiple frames on sonography.[47]

A retracting thrombus adherent to the wall of the hemorrhagic cyst is another sonographic feature. This finding may occasionally be confused with a focal mural nodule, a feature of a neoplastic ovarian mass. A retracting clot has a typically concave margin, whereas, mural nodules have a convex margin. Also, retracting clots appear to have a variable central echogenic pattern, while most mural nodules appear isoechoic in relation to the wall of the cyst. Color Doppler sonography does not reveal any blood flow within the fibrin strands or retracting thrombus thereby supporting the diagnosis of hemorrhage **(Figs. 16A and B)**.[47]

Hemorrhagic ovarian cysts have a very specific appearance in the vast majority of cases, and the presence of multiple, thin, linear fibrinous strands within the cyst has been typically described as "Fish-net" appearance[49] **(Fig. 16C)**. When a unilocular smooth walled cyst with the above mentioned appearance is identified, it is 200 times more likely to be a hemorrhagic ovarian cyst than any other possibility.[49]

On MR imaging, signal intensities vary according to the age of hemorrhage. Most frequently hemorrhagic cysts demonstrate high signal intensity on T1- and T2-weighted images due to intracellular methemoglobin in the late sub acute phase.[3] Apart from hemorrhage, fat containing lesions also appear bright on T1-weighed images. The two can be differentiated on fat suppressed T1-weighted images, wherein signal intensity of hemorrhage remains unchanged while that of fat is suppressed. This feature helps in the distinction of haemorrhagic cysts from dermoid cysts.

The cyst wall is thin and smooth and demonstrates intense enhancement after gadolinium administration. Contrast-enhanced images may help differentiate adherent clot from a mural nodule because clot will not enhance after the administration of gadolinium. Hemorrhagic cyst may be difficult to differentiate from other hemorrhagic adnexal lesions, especially endometriomas. However, hemorrhagic cyst tends to be solitary and is usually brighter on T2-weighted images than endometriomas, which typically has more profound T2 shortening, described as shading.[52]

It is important to remember that hemorrhagic cysts almost always represent non-neoplastic cysts that resolve spontaneously and gray-scale ultrasound is the investigation of choice for diagnosing the same. The main features to note are the presence of fibrin strands or retracting clot, with absence of suspected septations and wall irregularity as secondary helpful findings. Also, follow-up ultrasound should be performed 4–6 weeks after the initial sonography, preferably in the first week of menstruation to allow time for resolution of the cyst and to avoid confusion with new physiologic cysts.[52]

Theca Lutein Cysts

Theca lutein cysts are the largest of the functional cyst group. They result from overstimulation by high levels of circulating human chorionic gonadotropin (hCG) in trophoblastic disease or from iatrogenic hyperstimulation with exogenous hCG in the treatment of infertility. On ultrasonography, theca lutein cysts appear as bilateral,

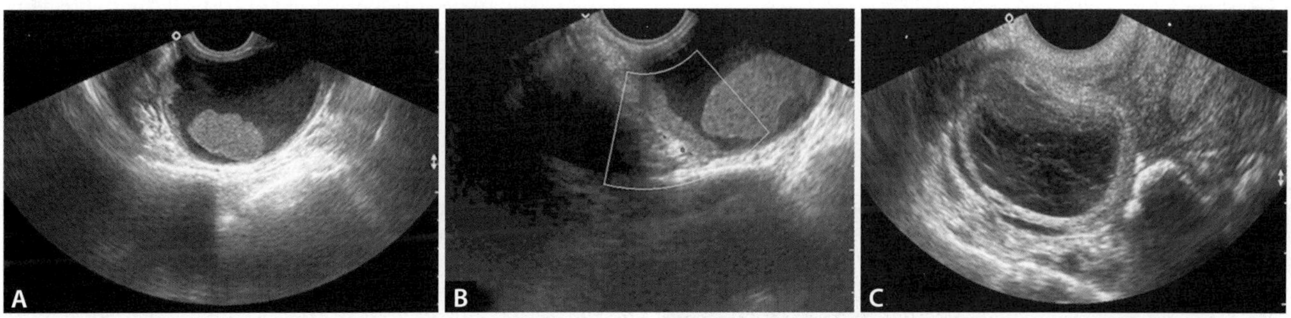

Figs. 16A to C: Hemorrhagic ovarian cysts showing (A) presence of retracting clot with wall thickness and irregularity; (B) CDS showing absence of blood flow in both; (C) "Fish-net appearance".

large multilocular cysts and may persist for days or weeks after withdrawl of the stimulus **(Figs. 17A and B)**. These cysts may undergo hemorrhage, rupture or torsion.[14]

Polycystic Ovarian Disease

Polycystic ovarian disease is a complex endocrinological disorder resulting from chronic anovulation clinically characterized by amenorrhea or oligomenorrhea, infertility, hirsuitism and obesity. The luteinising hormone to follicle-stimulating hormone (LH to FSH ratio) is more than 2 with increased androgen levels. Acylic production of estrogen results in appropriately elevated levels of LH and decreased levels of FSH. Increased LH leads to stimulation of ovarian theca and stroma and decreased FSH is responsible for chronic anovulation.

TVS has been used to distinguish the polycystic ovary from the healthy one. Classic sonographic and MR features are bilateral ovarian enlargement with multiple (10 or more) small peripheral follicles of uniform size measuring 2–8 mm in diameter **(Figs. 18A and B)**. Two patterns of cyst distribution have been described. In the peripheral cystic pattern, the cysts are present beneath the ovarian capsule, leading to a "string of pearls" appearance. In the general cystic pattern, the cysts can be seen both in the subcapsular and stromal parts of the ovary and can vary in size. In general, the polycystic ovary contains twice the number of antral follicles which are usually less than 4 mm in diameter and have twice the volume of the normal ovary.[10] The cysts show uniform high signal on T2W images. Hypertrophied ovarian stroma is depicted as broad central areas of low T1 and T2 signal intensity and appears echogenic on sonography. The ratio of ovarian stroma to ovarian area has been found to be the best predictor of polycystic ovaries by sonography.[53] However, with respect to ovarian volume and follicular number, there is considerable overlap with healthy subjects. In almost one-third of the patients with clinical and endocrinological evidence of PCOD, the ovaries show normal morphology and volume.[10]

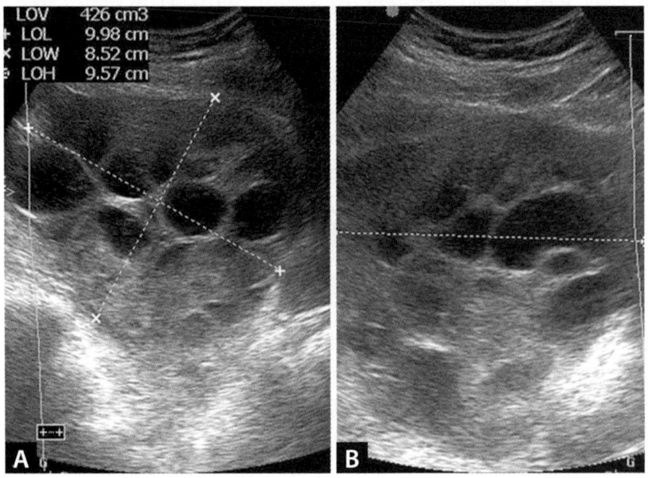

Figs. 17A and B: TAS showing a large multilocular cysts in left ovary in a patient of OHSS—Theca lutein cyst.

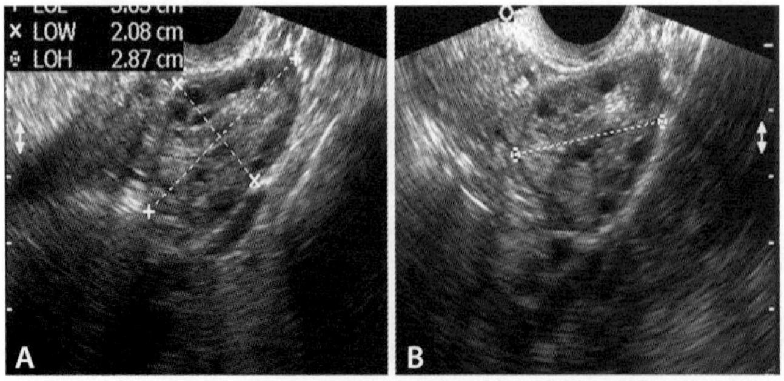

Figs. 18A and B: PCOD: Bilateral enlarged ovaries with stromal echogenicity and multiple peripheral follicles.

Peritoneal Inclusion Cyst

Peritoneal inclusion cysts occur predominantly in premenopausal women with a history of previous abdominal surgery, trauma, pelvic inflammatory disease or endometriosis. The normal peritoneum absorbs fluid produced by the ovaries. This ability is lost following inflammation or adhesions. Fluid may accumulate within adhesions and entrap the ovaries leading to a large cystic adnexal mass with multiple septations with the ovary lying centrally or in the wall of the cyst.[54] The patient may present with pain or pelvic mass. Peritoneal inclusion cysts are lined by mesothelial cysts and they are also referr to as benign cystic mesothelioma or benign encysted fluid.

On sonography, peritoneal inclusion cysts are multiloculated, cystic adnexal masses. The diagnostic finding is an intact ovary amid septations and fluid indicating the extraovarian origin of the mass.[55] The ovary may be located centrally or displaced peripherally with, margins of the cystic mass following the contour of the pelvis **(Figs. 19A to C)**.

Peritoneal inclusion cysts have a characteristic appearance on MR imaging depicting a cystic mass with thin septations, no distinct wall and bordered by the pelvic sidewall **(Figs. 19D and E)**. Usually, there is no mass effect on adjacent structures, although this can be seen in large lesions. Typically they are of low signal intensity on T1 and high signal on T2-weighted images. If protein content of the cyst is high or hemorrhage has occurred into the cyst, the cyst may be intermediate to hyperintense on T1 weighted images.[3]

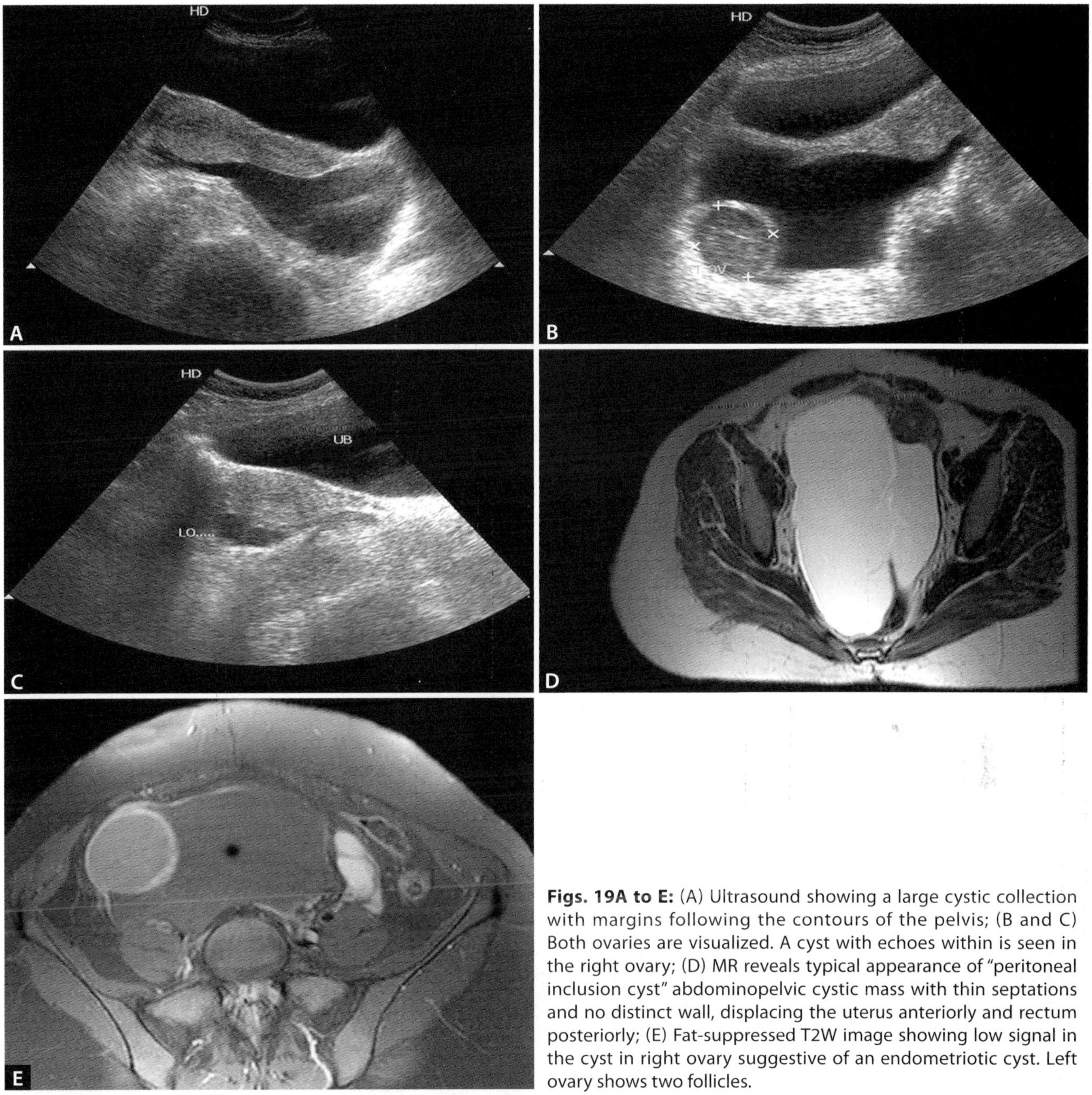

Figs. 19A to E: (A) Ultrasound showing a large cystic collection with margins following the contours of the pelvis; (B and C) Both ovaries are visualized. A cyst with echoes within is seen in the right ovary; (D) MR reveals typical appearance of "peritoneal inclusion cyst" abdominopelvic cystic mass with thin septations and no distinct wall, displacing the uterus anteriorly and rectum posteriorly; (E) Fat-suppressed T2W image showing low signal in the cyst in right ovary suggestive of an endometriotic cyst. Left ovary shows two follicles.

Peritoneal inclusion cysts need to be differentiated from paraovarian cysts and hydrosalpinx. While all these conditions are extraovarian, paraovarian cysts are separate from the ovary, whereas the ovary lies inside or in the wall of a peritoneal inclusion cyst.[56] Paraovarian cysts are usually round to ovoid and are not associated with a history of pelvic surgery, trauma or inflammation. Hydrosalpinx appears as a tubular cystic structure with visible folds and the ovary is seen to be outside the cystic structure. Peritoneal inclusion cyst may be mistaken for a cystic ovarian neoplasm and patient may undergo multiple surgeries. Accurate diagnosis of the same is essential because it is known to recur after extensive surgery in 30–50% cases.[3] Hence, treatment is conservative. Peritoneal inclusion cysts have no malignant potential.

Hydrosalpinx

Hydrosalpinx occurs when an inflammatory process produces adhesions of the fimbriated end of the fallopian tube, trapping the intraluminal secretions and dilatation of the ampullary and infundibular portions of the tube. Dilated fallopian tubes are depicted as tubular, fluid-filled structures that are folded upon themselves to form a C or S shape or, at times, a multilocular mass. The diagnosis of simple hydrosalpinx is typically made by sonography. Multiplanar imaging can be helpful in confirming the tubular nature of an adnexal mass or demonstrating incomplete septations, thus confirming it to originate from the fallopian tube.[3]

Most cases of hydrosalpinx have a typical appearance and can be easily distinguished from ovarian abnormalities. The most consistent sonographic feature described by Tessler et al. is a tubular, elongated extra-ovarian structure with folded configuration (incomplete septation) **(Figs. 20A and B)**.[57]

Recently, Patel et al. have described a combination of tubular shape and "waist sign" as being specific for the diagnosis of hydrosalpinx.[49]

Sonographically, a dilated tube is seen as a fusiform, anechoic adnexal mass with lack of peristalsis which allows differentiation from small bowel loops. Timor-Tritsch et al have described three appearances of tubal wall structure:[14] (i) cogwheel sign which is anechoic cogwheel-shaped structure visible in the cross- section of the tube with thick walls, (ii) beads on a string sign, which are hyperechoic mural nodules of 2–3 mm in size and seen on the cross-section of the fluid-filled distended tube, and (iii) incomplete septa which are hyperechoic septa that originate as a triangular protrusion from one of the walls, but do not reach the opposite wall.

In case of a complex cystic adnexal mass it may not be possible to establish the tubular nature of the process by sonography and MR can help in demonstrating incomplete septations and a separate normal ovary **(Figs. 21A and B)**. MR can also help in determining the etiology of hydrosalpinx. If hydrosalpinx is due to endometriosis, signal intensity characteristics of the tubal fluid are similar to those in endometriomas (high T1 and low T2 signal intensities). In a patient with adhesions, signal intensity of the dilated tube follows that of simple fluid (low T1 and high T2 signal intensities).[3]

Paraovarian Cysts

Paraovarian or paratubal cysts arise from mesonephric (Wolffian) or paramesonephric (Mullerian) structures. They represent 10% of all adnexal masses and most commonly occur in the 3rd and 4th decades. The hydatid of Morgagni is the most common paramesonephric cyst and is found arising from the fimbrial end of the fallopian tube.[47] They are frequently located superior to the uterine fundus.[14]

They are usually large and unilocular. Paraovarian cyst are not physiological, hence its dimensions remain constant throughout menstrual cycle. Sonographically, they are round to oval, anechoic with good sound transmission and morphologically indistinguishable from simple functional cysts. A specific diagnosis is not possible unless a normal ovary is seen separately from the cyst **(Fig. 22)**.[58] On sonography, a complicated paraovarian cyst may resemble an endometrioma, serous cystadenoma or a hemorrhagic cyst. The cyst may undergo torsion and rupture similar to other cystic masses. Malignancy is rare in cysts less than 5 cm. Benign neoplasms such as cystadenomas and cystadenofibromas of paraovarian origin are also uncommon.[14]

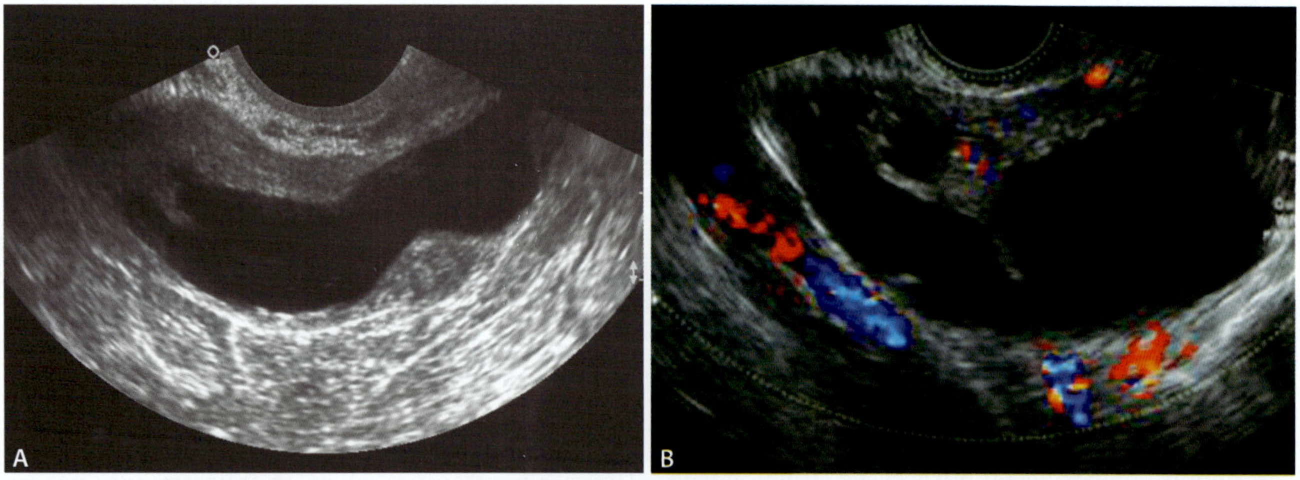

Figs. 20A and B: (A) TVS reveals tubular elongated extraovarian structure; (B) Incomplete septation and absence of vascularity on CDS—Hydrosalpinx.

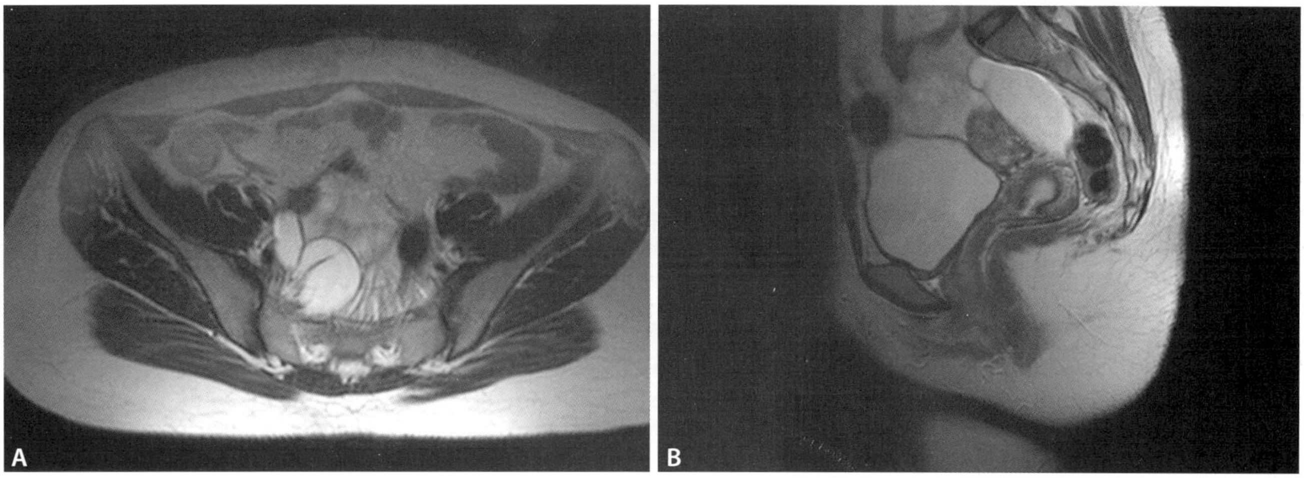

Figs. 21A and B: T2W axial and sagittal images showing a hyperintense tubular structure with folded configuration in the right adnexa—Hydrosalpinx.

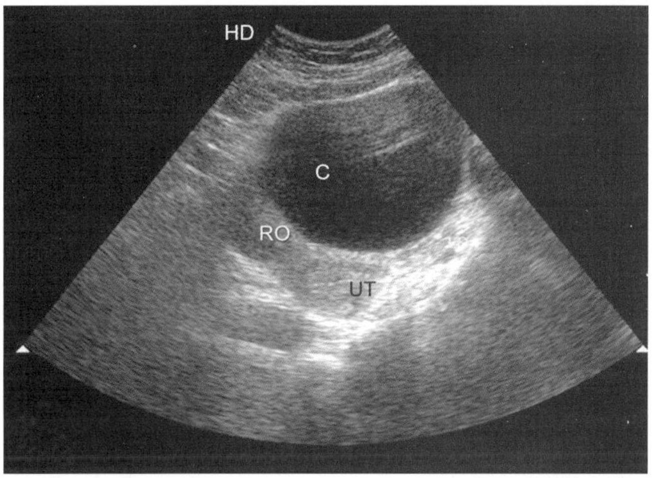

Fig. 22: Ultrasound of the right adnexa showing a unilocular smooth walled anechoic cyst with normal appearing right ovary adjacent and separate from it—Paraovarian cyst.

CYSTADENOMAS

Cystadenomas are benign epithelial tumors arising from the surface epithelium of the ovary. They are of two types: serous and mucinous.

Serous cystadenomas account for 25% of all benign ovarian neoplasms with 20% of them being bilateral. The peak incidence of presentation is in the fourth and fifth decades. Sonographically, serous cystadenomas are large, thin-walled, unilocular cystic masses with a mean size of around 10 cm. They may be multilocular in which case the septations are thin **(Fig. 23A)**. Papillary projections may be seen occasionally. Usually the cysts contain simple fluid with low signal intensity on T1 and high signal intensity on T2-weighted images. Rarely, the cyst contents may be complex due to high protein content or hemorrhage. On postcontrast T1-weighted images, the cyst wall and septa enhance with no evidence of any solid component.[3]

In contrast, mucinous cystadenomas are less common and occur most often in the 3rd to 5th decades. They are less frequently bilateral than their serous component (only 3% bilateral) Sonographically, mucinous cystadenomas are larger, measuring up to 15-30 cm having a multilocular appearance. Multiple thin septae are present and low level echoes due to mucoid material may be seen in the dependent portions of the mass. In many of the mucinous cystadenomas, the imaging appearance of the individual locules may vary as a result of difference in degree of haemorrhage or protein content. The sonographic feature of variable echogenicity in the contents of an multilocular adnexal cyst is strongly suggestive of a mucinous tumor[47] **(Fig. 23B)**. The difference in chemical composition of fluids rather than their difference in viscosity is responsible for the different sonographic echogenicities. This sign may not be seen in all mucinous tumours as some may have small differences in the chemical composition of contents. Also, some of the mucinous tumours may be unilocular and have one type of mucin.[47] Papillary projections are less frequently seen than in their serous counterpart. On MR imaging, the thick mucinous content of the cyst may result in a high signal on T1- and low signal on T2-weighted images. The loculations in these cysts vary giving a "stained glass" appearance.

Preoperative knowledge of the mucinous nature of the tumour is important because penetration of the tumor capsule or rupture may lead to intraperitoneal spread of mucin-secreting cells that may fill the peritoneal cavity

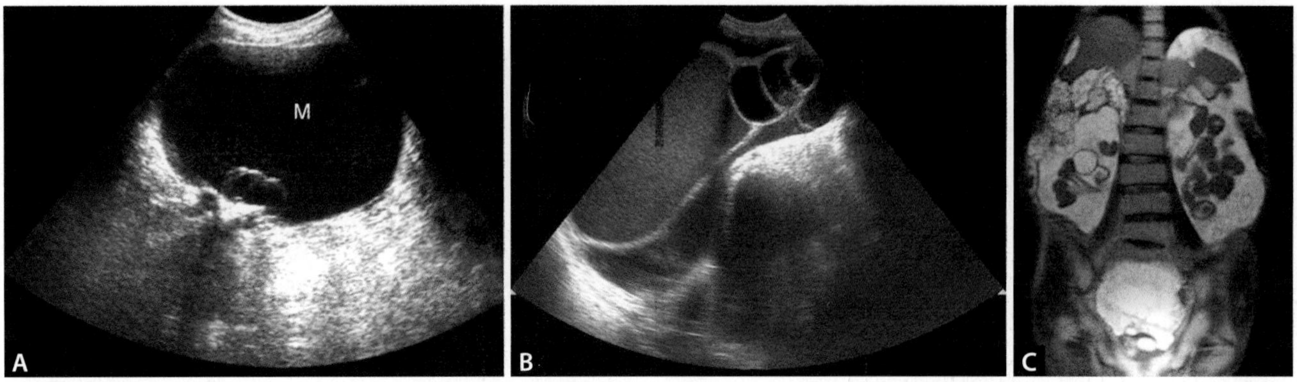

Figs. 23A to C: (A) TAS reveals a large unilocular thin walled cystic mass with thin septations within—Serous cystadenoma; (B) Characteristic appearance of mucinous cystadenoma showing "variegated echogenicity sign" in the loculi of a large multiloculated cystic mass; (C) T2W and coronal image showing mucinous implants on peritoneal surfaces with typical scalloping of liver surface secondary to ruptured mucinous tumor—Pseudomyxoma peritonei.

with a gelatinous material. This condition is known as pseudomyxoma peritonei and apart from mucinous cystadenoma and cystadenocarcinoma, can result from a ruptured mucococle of the appendix and mucinous tumours of the appendix and colon **(Fig. 23C)**.

Color Doppler sonography (CDS) has been used along with conventional unltrasound to characterise cystadenomas and other adnexal masses. CDS does not improve actual detection of a mass, but seems to improve specificity in differentiating benign from malignant masses. Presence of colour flow in echogenic portion of the cyst is indicative of malignancy while its absence indicates benignancy.[59]

Spectral Doppler analysis has been seen to be of limited value in predicting malignancy as a number of physiological (corpus luteum) and benign (inflammatory) masses have a low PI (≤1) similar to that seen in ovarian malignancy.[60]

Benign and malignant ovarian neoplasms can be differentiated by sonographic characteristics of the mass. Features suggestive of a benign ovarian mass is a cystic mass (usually <5 cm) with thin, wall defined walls and thin septations. On analysis of Doppler spectrum, a benign mass generally shows no flow or a high resistance flow. In contrast, features that suggest malignancy in an adnexal mass are a large size (>10 cm) with thick, ill-defined or irregular walls, large solid component, thick or irregular septations (>3 cm) with evidence of peritoneal, lymphatic, hematogenous spread or local invasion. Doppler features indicative of a malignancy are presence of vascular nodules within the mass with low resistance flow in them.

The diagnosis of cystadenoma is usually made by ultrasound wherein a combination of sonographic morphology and Doppler characteristics help in differentiating a benign from malignant ovarian mass. MR is helpful in the evaluation of indeterminate adnexal masses on ultrasound due to its superior tissue characterization.[3]

COMPLEX MASSES

Complex masses are those that contain both solid and cystic areas and include tubo-ovarian abscess, endometriosis, dermoid cyst, ovarian torsion and ectopic pregnancy.

Tubo-ovarian Abscess

Tubo-ovarian abscess is a result of ascending infection that spreads to involve the endometrium and fallopian tubes. The ovaries are relatively resistant to infection and are involved only in more severe cases. Bilateral adnexal involvement is the rule, and abscess formation tends to occur with late or inadequate treatment. Tubo-ovarian abscess has a variable appearance on sonography. It is typically a unilocular or multilocular complex mass with irregular borders and thickened wall.[61] Multiple internal septations may be present **(Fig. 24)**. Normal ovarian stroma with follicles is often identifiable as part of the conglomerate mass. Anechoic or hypoechoic areas represent collection of frank pus. On CT, tubo-ovarian abscess is seen as thick-walled, complex adnexal mass with centers of low attenuation and shaggy margins.[62] If air is present within the mass, a diagnosis of an abscess can be made confidently, but when no gas is present, differentiation of abscess from neoplasm is usually not possible without a percutaneous fine needle aspiration.[63] Abscess on MR imaging appears as unilocular or multilocular cystic mass with a thicker wall than that seen in functional ovarian cyst. The abscess fluid has variable signal but usually is of very high signal intensity on T2-weighted image and low signal intensity on T1-weighted image.[64] The abscess wall

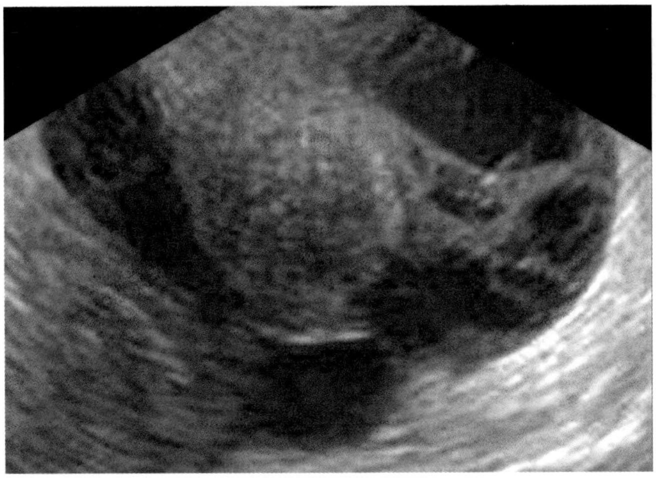

Fig. 24: TVS reveals bilateral multilocular complex adnexal masses with septations and associated free fluid—Tubo-ovarian abscesses.

and adjacent inflammatory changes enhance intensely with gadolinium showing thickened irregularly enhancing wall and septations. Infiltration of pelvic fat surrounding the mass may be evident.

Actinomycosis is an uncommon pelvic infection usually seen in the presence of an intrauterine device. The mass in actinomycosis consists predominantly of a solid lesion with low signal intensity on T2-weighted images, Cystic elements are seen less commonly. Diffuse infiltration of the uterus, adnexa and pelvic musculature with transgression of fascial planes is the hall mark of the disease. The presence of a foreign body such as an intrauterine contraceptive device (IUCD) further corroborates to the diagnosis. Following guided aspiration, indentification of sulphur granules within the aspirate is diagnostic of an actinomycotic infection.[3]

The diagnosis of tubo-ovarian abscess is typically made by clinical examination and ultrasound. Both transabdominal and TVS are useful. The transabdominal approach is helpful in assessing the extent of the disease, while TVS is superior in detecting dilated tubes, periovarian inflammatory change and internal characteristics of tubo-ovarian abscesses. Sonography is also helpful in following the response to antibiotic therapy. MR has been demonstrated to have a higher accuracy compared to TVS for making the diagnosis.[3] In chronic cases, multiple pelvic organs may be involved and inflammatory signs can be absent, making differentiation from malignancy difficult.

Endometriosis

Endometriosis is defined as the presence of functioning endometrium located outside the uterus. The sites of implantation of ectopic endometrium in decreasing order of frequency are ovary, uterosacral ligaments, cul-de-sac, posterior wall of lower uterine segment, fallopian tube, rectovaginal septum and sigmoid colon. Ectopic endometrium may be diffuse or focal, more commonly being diffuse with minute endometrial implants involving pelvic viscera and their ligamentous attachments. It is a disease of women in the reproductive age group who may present with chronic lower abdominal pain, pelvic and back pain, dysmenorrhea, irregular bleeding and infertility. However there is no direct relationship between the severity of symptoms and extent of the disease. Sonography is insensitive in evaluating diffuse endometrial implants and plaques as these lesions are too small to be imaged.[65]

Endometriomas are internal hemorrhages within an area of endometriosis resulting in endometrial cysts. 80% of pelvic endometriosis is found in the ovary. They are bilateral in 30–50% of cases and are frequently multilocular. On sonographic evaluation, endometriomas appear as ovarian cysts ranging from anechoic to solid, depending on the amount of blood and its organization.[47] They have wide range of manifestations from cystic to complex and may have a solid appearance.

The classic appearance of an endometrioma on ultrasound is a cystic mass with homogeneous low level echoes[65] **(Figs. 25A and B)**. 95% of endometriomas exhibit diffuse low level internal echoes. Though the absence of this finding does not exclude an endometrioma, it significantly decreases the likelihood of diagnosis.[49] Repeated episodes of bleeding and rebleeding may result in development of irregular walls and echogenic mural nodules. Fluid-fluid levels or fluid debris levels represent blood products. These appearances are much less specific and can be mimicked by hemorrhagic cysts, tubo-ovarian abscesses and cystadenomas. Presence of thick septations and walls, irregular mural nodules may sometimes make it difficult to differentiate from malignant ovarian neoplasms. In addition, multilocular appearance and punctate echogenicities in the wall of the endometrioma are seen less commonly but add specificity to the appearance of the lesions. These hyperechoic wall foci represent focal deposits of cholesterol secondary to degeneration and breakdown of cell membranes. A smooth walled mass with homogeneous ground glass internal echoes and coexisting hyperechoic wall foci has been described to be 32 times more likely to be an endometrioma than any other adnexal mass.[49] Doppler waveform analysis is not helpful in differentiating endometrioma from other masses. Low resistance waveform resembling malignancy

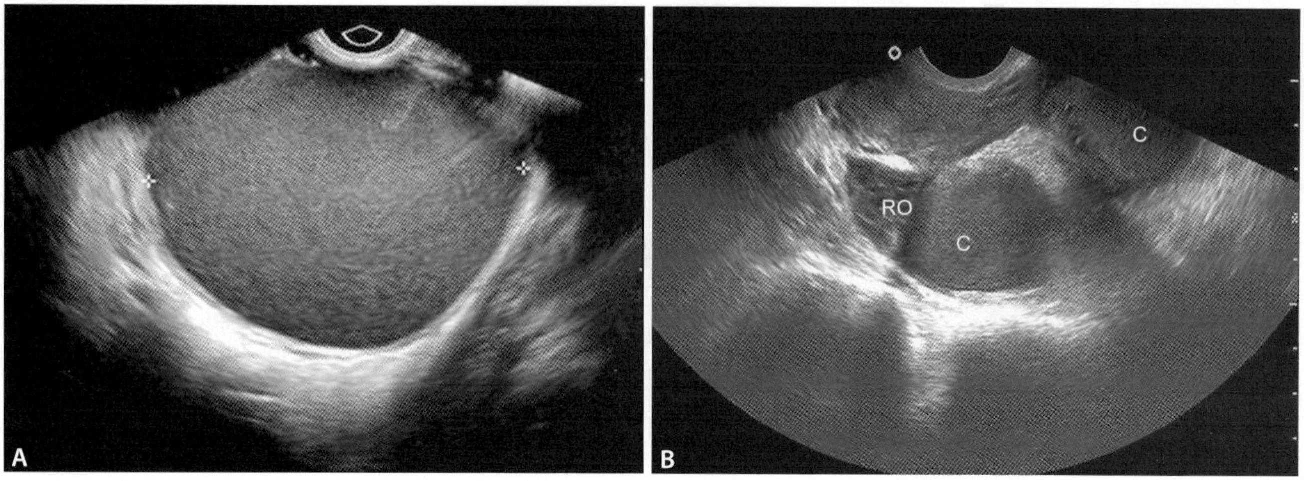

Figs. 25A and B: (A) TVS showing a unilocular ovarian cyst with low level internal echoes—characteristic of endometrioma; (B) Bilateral endometriotic cysts in another patient depicting typical ground-glass appearance.

are encountered in endometrioma. CT appearance of endometriosis and endometrioma is nonspecific and easily mimicked by PID and benign and malignant ovarian tumors.[66] MR improves diagnostic accuracy with endometrial cyst typically appearing as high signal intensity on T1-weighted sequence with shading or low signal intensity on T2-weighted sequence due to presence of blood products **(Figs. 26A to D)**.[67,68] "Shading sign" is a distinguishing feature of an endometrotic cyst at MR imaging which consists of T2 shortening in an adnexal cyst that is hyperintense on T1W images. It is most commonly manifested as a complete loss of signal intensity or dependent layering with a hypointense fluid level in an endometrioma.[69]

Its precise mechanism is complex. Endometriotic cysts are highly viscous and have a high concentration of protein and iron from recurrent hemorrhage. The concentration of iron is 10–20 times higher than in blood. The high iron and protein within the lesion leads to T2 shortening and contribute to signal intensity loss described as 'shading'. These lesions are more often multiple, with angular margins or distorted shape. Fat saturation sequence does not suppress the signal intensity of the cyst which was bright on T1-weighted sequence confirming that hemorrhage, not fat is present. This signal characteristic differentiates endometrioma from fatty adnexal masses, such as dermoids.

MR can diagnose endometriomas with 91–96% accuracy if MR features of multiple lesions with high signal intensity on T1 weighted images without fat suppression are noted and demonstrate low signal intensity on T2-weighted images.[3] The wall of an endometrioma is thick and can contain foci of low signal intensity on T1- and T2-weighted images due to a combination of fibrosis and hemosiderin—laden macrophages. On contrast enhanced T1-weighted images endometriomas show early wall enhancement.

In contrast, endometrial implants are often difficult to identify on imaging studies as they appear as small, flat lesions having variable T1 and T2 signal characteristics.[3] Implants commonly manifest as solid masses with low signal intensity on T2-weighted images due to fibrosis surrounding the glandular islands and demonstrate enhancement following contrast administration. Small hemorrhagic implants have been seen to become more conspicuous on fat-saturated T1 weighted sequences, appearing bright against the background of suppressed fat, thereby increasing the accuracy in staging the disease.

A rare complication of endometriosis is the development of clear cell carcinoma which occurs in 0.04% cases. About 25% of clear cell carcinomas arise in endometriomas and 50–70% are associated with pelvic endometriosis.[3]

As small implants and adhesions are not well-evaluated on imaging and MR may underestimate the extent of disease, therefore, laproscopy remains the standard of reference for diagnosis and staging. MR has a role in detecting lesions inaccessible to laproscopy due to dense adhesions. In addition, MR can be used for staging the disease, differentiating endometriomas from other adnexal masses and evaluating the response to treatment. Larger endometriomas with pronounced T2 shading have been reported to benefit less from medical treatment. This may be related to the more concentrated blood products in older endometriomas.[3]

The differential diagnosis of endometriomas on MR imaging include other lesions which have a high

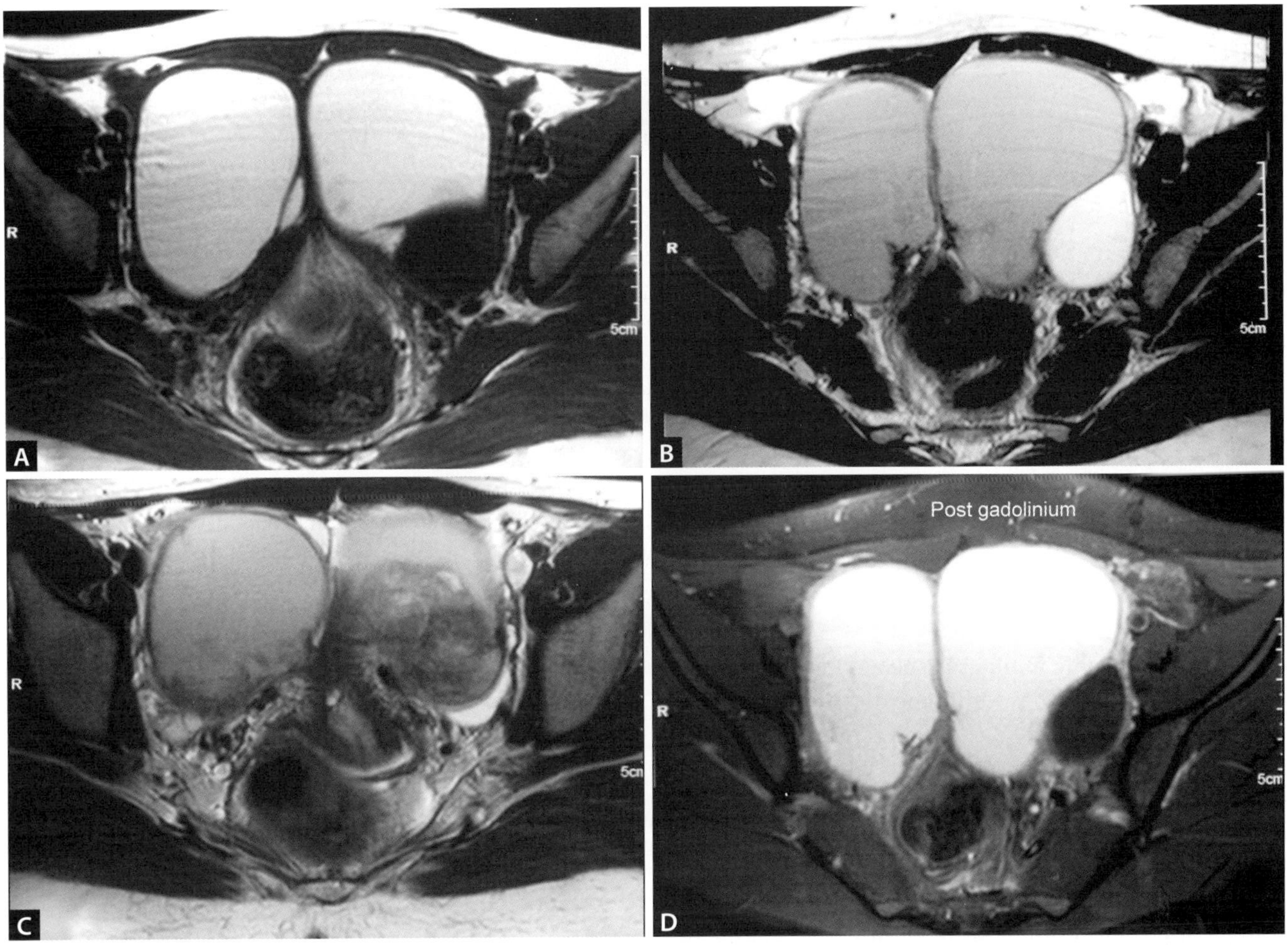

Figs. 26A to D: MR imaging in endometriomas: (A and B) Bilateral endometriotic cysts appearing as large well-defined cystic lesions in B/L adnexal regions with predominantly high SI on T1W and low SI on T2W images. One of the cysts has a low signal on T1W and high signal on T2W image; (C) T2W axial image shows hypointense debris in dependant part of cysts; (D) T1 postgadolinium fat-sat image showing early wall enhancement with lack of suppression of T1 bright signal—Confirms diagnosis of endometrioma.

signal intensity on T1 weighted sequences. These are fat containing tumors such as dermoid cysts which are reliably differentiated as they get suppressed on fat saturated sequences while the bright signal of endometriomas persist. Hemorrhagic lesions like hemorrhagic cyst and corpus luteum cyst may be difficult to differentiate from an endometrioma on imaging alone, but are generally solitary, the wall of a hemorrhagic cyst being thin while that of a corpus luteum cyst being slightly thicker and convoluted. Also, as there is no repeated hemorrhage into these lesions, marked loss of signal intensity on T2-weighted images is generally not observed.

Dermoid Cyst/Mature Cystic Teratoma

Dermoid cyst is a mature benign form of teratoma and occurs in women in their reproductive years. It is a common cause of adnexal mass accounting for approximately 20% of all ovarian neoplasms and 99% of germ cell tumors. It is bilateral in 10–15% cases.

Dermoid cyst contain all three germ layers, however the ectodermal layer predominates. Most tumors are discovered incidently on physical examination or imaging studies. If clinical symptoms are present, they are often nonspecific like pelvic mass or pain. Most common complication is ovarian torsion, seen in 16% of cases.

On plain radiograph, around 40% of ovarian teratoma shows diagnostic characteristics with presence of teeth or fat in the pelvis.[70] Variable sonographic appearances of ovarian dermoids have been described depending on the internal composition. The classic US appearance is a complex cystic mass with solid mural component called "dermoid plug" **(Fig. 27)**.[71] The dermoid plug usually contains hair, teeth or fat and is usually echogenic and frequently casts an acoustic shadow. This is seen in almost 90% of cystic teratomas.

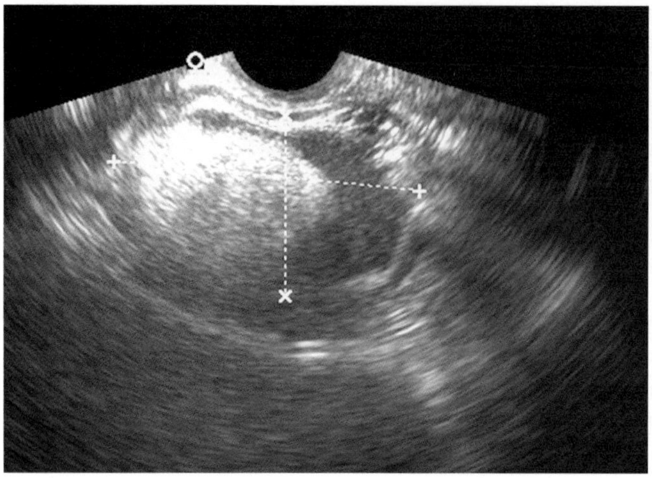

Fig. 27: Cystic ovarian mass with an echogenic mural nodule in the periphery representing "dermoid plug"—Cystic teratoma.

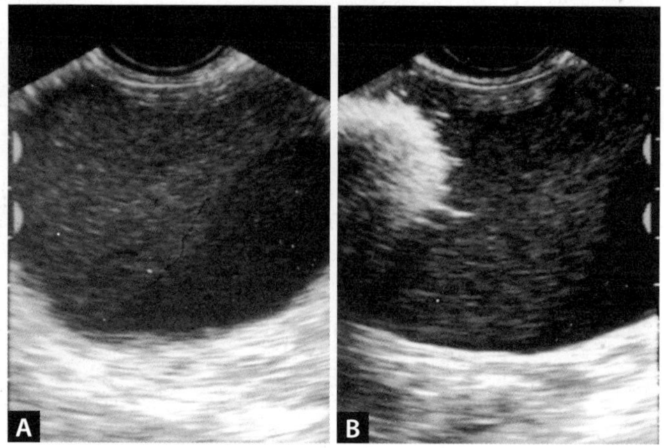

Figs. 28A and B: Transvaginal view of a dermoid with a fluid–debris level, probably produced by interface between sebum and cellular debris. Highly reflective mass in the periphery with partial shadowing represent hair in the dermoid within the ovary.

Other sonographic findings associated with dermoids are high amplitude echoes within the mass. This is seen in 60% of cystic teratomas and is due to presence of sebum. Presence of hyperechoic lines and dots within the mass, so called 'dermoid mesh' is caused by hair and also seen in 60% of cystic teratomas.[49]

A fat-fluid or hair fluid level may be seen and is considered specific **(Figs. 28A and B)**. However, these findings are seen in only one-third of cases. Echogenic dermoids may mimic bowel gas and may be missed on US. When a dermoid produces ill-defined acoustic shadowing that obscures the posterior wall of the lesion, it is termed as "Tip of the iceberg sign". This is produced by a mixture of matted hair and sebum which is highly echogenic because of multiple tissue interfaces. Often hematomas, abscesses or endometriomas cannot be distinguished ultrasonographically from teratomas. The diagnosis is commonly made on US. CT can provide a definitive diagnosis in majority of cases.[72] The characteristic CT features include detection of fat (-130 – -90 HU), hair, teeth and fat-fluid level **(Figs. 29A and B)**. Although malignant teratomas are rare, CT detection of an irregular solid component greater than 5 cm strongly suggests the diagnosis.[73]

Cystic teratomas are well-defined, heterogeneous masses and identification of fat within an adnexal mass is the key to diagnosis of a dermoid cyst on MRI.[74] On MRI, fat is identified when the signal intensity of the mass (or part of it) is isointense to subcutaneous fat on both T1- and T2-weighted sequences and internal or external chemical shift artefact indicating fat water interface is present. On fat saturation sequence, suppression of signal that was of high signal intensity on T1-weighted sequence; confirms the presence of fat within the mass[75] and thereby helps in differentiating from an endometrioma or hemorrhagic cyst **(Figs. 30A and B)**.

Ovarian Torsion

It is an acute condition requiring prompt surgical intervention caused by partial or complete rotation of the ovarian pedicle on its long axis. Ovarian torsion is most commonly associated with an adnexal mass, usually a dermoid cyst, but may also occur spontaneously. On ultrasound, the salient finding is unilateral ovarian enlargement which is edematous with multiple small cystic structures at the periphery, which is due to transudation of fluid into the follicles from circulatory impairment. Small amounts of fluid may be seen in the cul-de-sac secondary to obstructed veins and lymphatics.[76]

Color Doppler may facilitate specific diagnosis of ovarian torsion by demonstrating lack or severe restriction of arterial flow. The ovary has a dual blood supply, and torsion may effect one arterial blood supply more than the other, resulting in partial arterial flow on CDS. The arterial waveform may exhibit a lack of diastolic flow with a "spike" configuration of the systolic peak. Studies have shown that while arterial flow may be present even in nonviable ovaries, absent venous flow may be sensitive of nonviability.

MR is not a primary imaging modality but can be helpful if sonographic findings of torsion are indeterminate. The

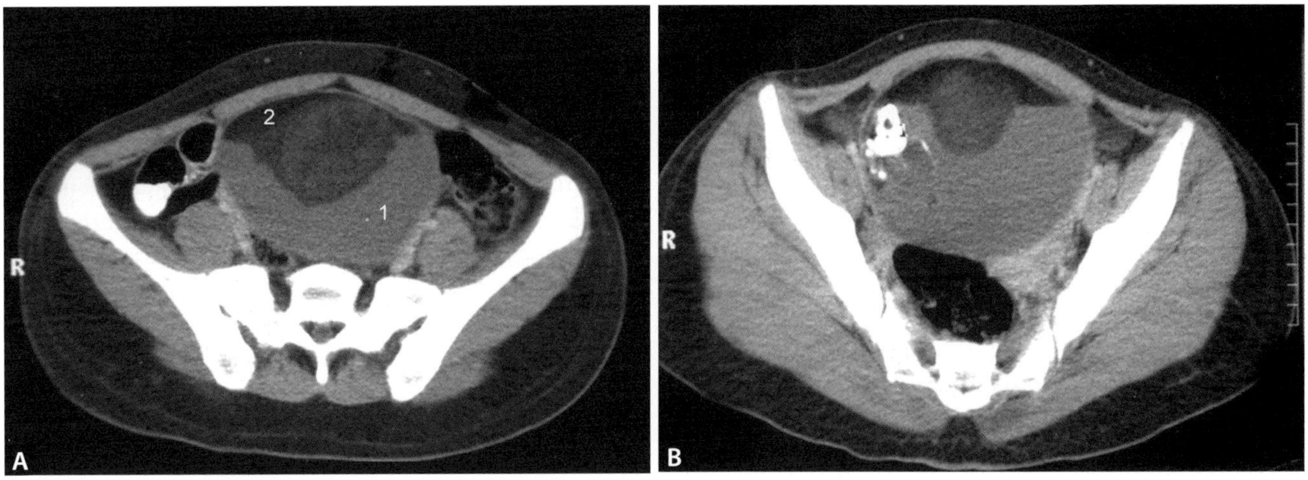

Figs. 29A and B: Right ovarian cystic teratoma: (A) CT shows a large abdominopelvic mass of fat attenuation, with fat fluid level and a central hair ball; (B) The mass shows areas of calcification.

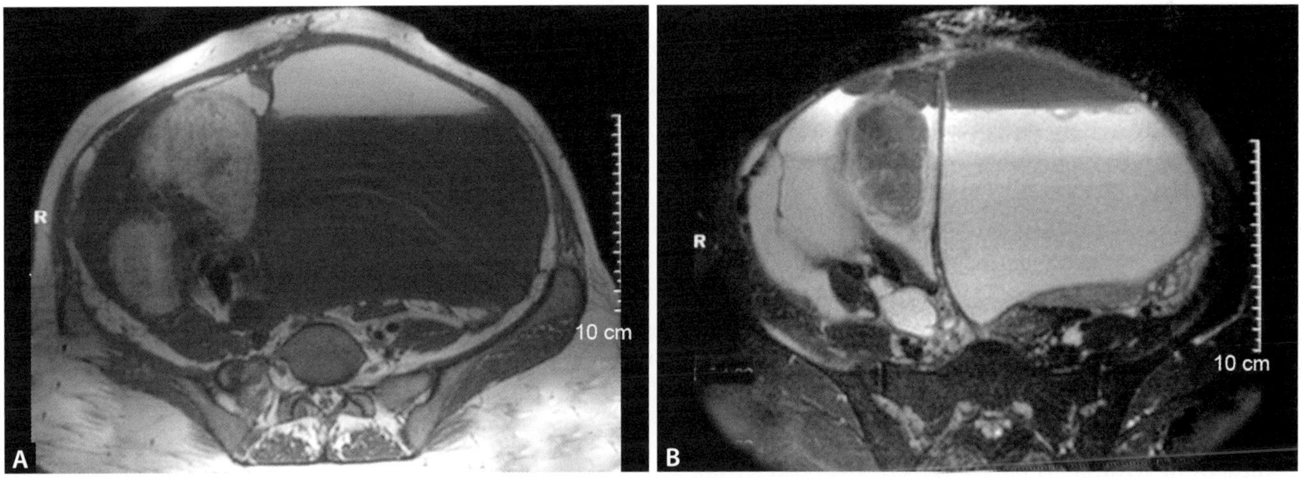

Figs. 30A and B: MR imaging in bilateral dermoid cysts: (A) B/L complex masses with bright signal of fat anteriorly on T1W image; (B) T1W fat-suppressed image showing suppression of fat signal with chemical shift artifact at fat-fluid interface.

most common finding on MR imaging is an adnexal mass with deviation of the uterus to the side of the torsion. Engorged vessels leading towards the vascular pedicle can be identified between the mass and uterus.[77] Hemorrhage in the torsed ovary can be seen as a high signal intensity ring in the periphery of the lesion, while hemorrhagic infarction is identified as low signal intensity on T1- and T2-weighted images due to interstitial hemorrhage. The most specific feature of infarction is lack of enhancement on T1-weighted contrast enhanced images.[3]

The treatment of choice for ovarian torsion is laparoscopic detwisting of the adnexa and resection of any enlarged cysts. Ovaries can remain viable up to 36 hours after twisting and thus oophorectomy can be avoided in most women.[78]

Ectopic Pregnancy

Ectopic pregnancy is one of the most common gynecological emergencies, presenting with amenorrhea followed by vaginal bleeding or pelvic pain. The diagnosis is usually reached by a combination of clinical presentation, hCG levels and findings on ultrasonography. On transabdominal and TVS, it appears as a complex cystic adnexal mass representing the ectopic gestational sac and hematoma, usually separate from the ovary.

The most common site for ectopic pregnancy is the fallopian tubes, occurring in up to 97% of cases of which 75–80% are located in the ampullary region.[79] The ovary, cervix are other less common sites of ectopic pregnancy. As most often fallopian tube is the site for an ectopic pregnancy, it is important to scan above or below the ovary and between the ovary and uterus.

The sonographic finding which is most specific for ectopic pregnancy is the presence of a live extrauterine pregnancy. However, it is positive is only 8–26% of ectopic pregnancies on TVS.[80] The next most specific sign is the presence of an extrauterine gestation sac containing a yolk sac, with or without an embryo.[81] The "tubal ring" of ectopic pregnancy is another finding which has been found to be 40–68% sensitive for ectopic pregnancy.[79] The tubal ring represents an extrauterine gestation sac with trophoblastic tissue. But the most common, but slightly less specific finding of an ectopic pregnancy is a complex adnexal mass separate from the ovary. The use of color doppler shows a "ring of fire" pattern and a high-velocity, low-impedance flow which is compatible with placental perfusion **(Figs. 31A and B)**. However, the corpus luteum is also very vascular and shows a similar appearance on color flow imaging from which it needs to be differentiated.

In a patient with suspicion of an ectopic pregnancy one should routinely screen the upper abdomen for free fluid in the Morrison's pouch or flanks. Presence of echogenic free fluid does not always signify a ruptured ectopic pregnancy, though more the fluid, greater is the possibility of finding a ruptured ectopic pregnancy.[47]

BENIGN SOLID OVARIAN MASSES

Solid ovarian masses are less common as compared to the frequency of solid masses representing uterine leiomyoma. Benign solid ovarian masses include thecomas, fibromas and fibrothecomas which arise from ovarian stroma. They are part of sex cord-stromal tumors with 80% of these tumors producing hormones, although fibromas do not. Fibromas usually arise in postmenopausal women, are mostly asymptomatic until they cause pelvic pressure or produce torsion. Ascites is seen up to 50% of patients with fibroma larger than 5 cm in diameter.[14] Meig's syndrome represents the rare triad of ovarian fibroma, ascites and pleural effusion. Sonographically, these fibrous tumors have a characteristic appearance of a hypoechoic mass with marked posterior attenuation of the sound beam seen separate from the uterus and a nonvisualized ovary.[14] MR is helpful if the sonographic appearance is nonspecific or the ovarian origin of the lesion is questionable.

On MR fibromas are usually well-defined solid tumors, with low signal intensity on both T1 and T2-weighted images. The low signal intensity results from abundant collagen content of these tumors and is relatively diagnostic of fibromas.[82] Hyalinisation and myxomatous changes in the solid masses may occasionally show irregular areas of high signal intensity on T2-weighted images. The differential diagnosis of a solid adnexal mass includes ovarian neoplasm, pedunculated uterine leiomyoma, metastasis, non-Hodgkin lymphoma.

An adnexal mass that is of low signal intensity on both T1 and T2 weighted images is most likely to be a pedunculated leiomyoma. The diagnosis is further confirmed if a stalk is seen connecting to the uterus or two normal ovaries are identified. Ovarian fibromas also present with low signal intensity on T1- and T2-weighted images, but on T1-weighted images, fibromas often have lower signal intensity than leiomyomas.[83] Fibroids have a discrete round margin and characteristic whorled internal structure and typically enhance intensely with gadolinium **(Figs. 32A to C)**. In contrast, benign ovarian stromal

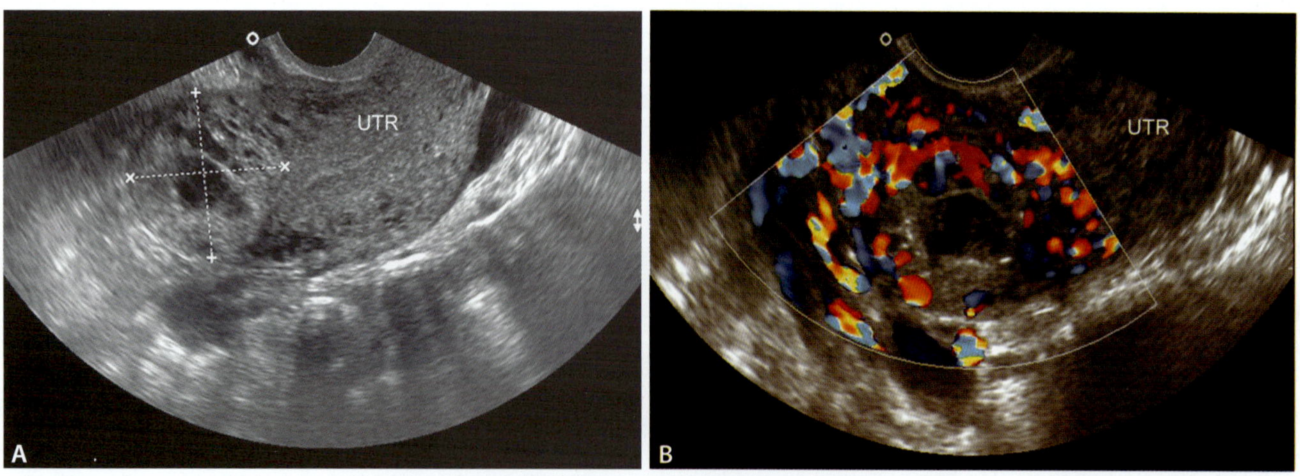

Figs. 31A and B: TVS reveals a complex cystic mass in right adnexa separate from the right ovary with increased vascularity due to vascular trophoblastic tissue—Ectopic pregnancy.

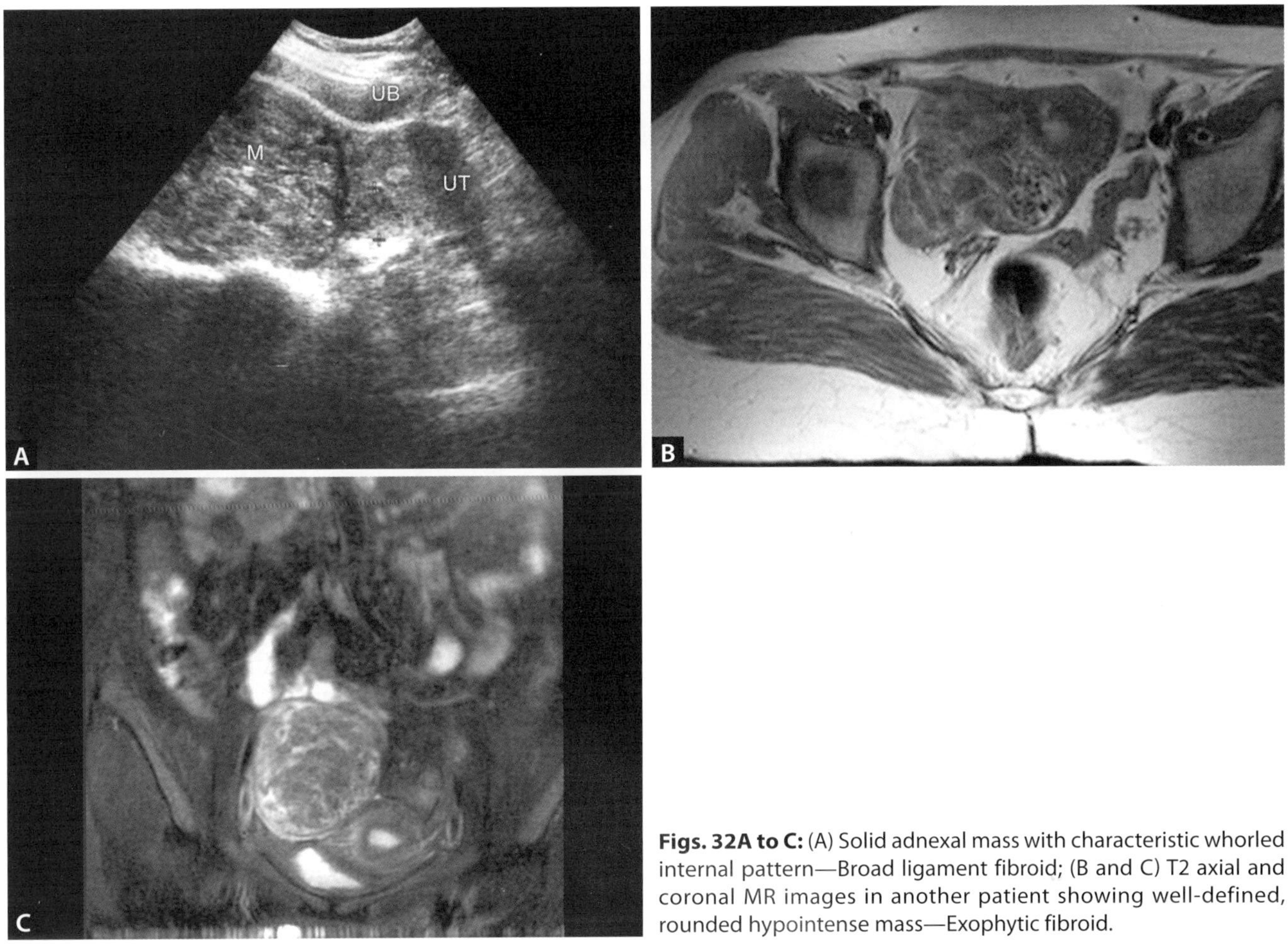

Figs. 32A to C: (A) Solid adnexal mass with characteristic whorled internal pattern—Broad ligament fibroid; (B and C) T2 axial and coronal MR images in another patient showing well-defined, rounded hypointense mass—Exophytic fibroid.

tumors have homogeneous internal structure and show a lesser degree of enhancement.[84]

A Brenner tumor is an uncommon surface epithelial stromal tumor consisting of transitional cells in prominent fibrous connective tissue. In one-third of cases they are associated with other ovarian tumors. Sonographically, they are hypoechoic solid masses usually smaller than 2 cm.[14] It is the predominantly fibrous content of Brenner tumor that results in a relatively low SI on T2-weighted images. Otherwise, ovarian fibroma and Brenner tumor may be indistinguishable by imaging.

CONCLUSION

Ultrasonography, especially transvaginal sonography is the modality of choice in detection and characterization of pelvic masses due to its superior resolution. It gives a detailed assessment of morphology of a mass on the basis of its internal contents thereby suggesting the possible etiology. Masses can be cystic, complex or solid on sonographic evaluation. It is the complex or solid masses that need a thorough evaluation. Though MR has a lower resolution than ultrasound, it has a wide range of tissue specificity and a much larger field of view.[83] MR can be used to definitely characterize simple fluid, blood, fat and fibrous tissue and the enhancement properties of solid tissues can be measured following contrast administration. The larger field of view and multiplanar capability of MR is useful for characterizing large pelvic masses and evaluating their origin (ovarian/uterine) when the adnexal anatomy is significantly distorted.

REFERENCES

1. Sorenson SS. Estimated prevalence of mullerian anomalies. Acta Obstet Gynecol Scan. 1988;67:441.
2. Buttram VC, Gibbons WF. Mullerian anomalies, a proposed classification (an analysis of 144 cases). Fertil Steril. 1979;32:40-6.
3. Ascher SM, Siewert B, Toriano R, et al. Benign conditions of the female pelvis. In: Edelman RR, Hesselink JR, Zlatkin MB (Eds): Clinical MRI, 3rd edition. Saunders, Elsiever. 2006;3:2988-3046.

4. Woolf RB, Allen WM. Concomitant malformations: The frequent simultaneous occurrence of congenital malformations of the reproductive and urinary tract. Obstet Gynecol. 1953;2:236.
5. Sala E, Allison S, Ascher S, et al. Imaging in gynaecology. In: Adam A, Dixon AK (Eds): Grainger and Allison's Diagnostic Radiology and Textbook of Medical Imaging, 5th edition. Churchill Livingstone. 2008;2:1217-41.
6. Buttram VC. Mullerian anomalies and their management. Fertil Steril. 1983;60:159.
7. Golan A, Langer R, Bukovsky I, et al. Congenital anomalies of the mullerian system. Fertil Steril. 1989;51:747.
8. Siegelman ES. MRI of the female pelvis. In: Siegelman ES (Ed): Body MRI. Elsiever Saunders; 2005.pp.269-342.
9. Carrington BM, Hricak H, Nuruddin RN, et al. Mullerian duct anomalies: MR imaging evaluation. Rad. 1990;176:715-20.
10. Zagoria RJ. The female genital tract. In: Zagoria RJ (Ed): The Requisites—Genitourinary Radiology, 2nd edition. Mosby. 2004.pp.256-311.
11. Hendrickson MR, Kempson RL (Eds). Surgical Pathology of the Uterine Corpus Philadelphia: WB Saunders; 1980.p.452.
12. Gross BH, Silver TM, Jaffe MH. Sonographic features of uterine leiomyomas: Analysis of 41 proven cases. J Ultrasound Med. 1983;2:4013.
13. Walsh JW. Grey-scale ultrasound in 204 proven gynecologic masses: Accuracy and specific diagnostic criteria. Radiology. 1979;130:391.
14. Salem S, Wilson SR. Gynaecologic ultrasound. In: Rumack CM, Wilson SR, Charbonean JW (Eds): Diagnostic Ultrasound. 3rd edition. Elsevier Mosby; 2005;1:527-87.
15. Karasick S, Lev-Toaff AS, Toaff ME. Imaging of uterine leiomyomas. AJR. 1992;158:799-805.
16. Tada S, Tsukioka M, Ishii C, et al. Computed tomographic features of uterine myoma. J Comput Assist Tomogr. 1981;5:866-9.
17. Weinreb JC, Barkoff ND, Megibow A. The value of MR imaging in distinguishing leiomyomas from other solid pelvic masses when sono-graphy is indeterminate. AJR. 1990;154:295.
18. Hricak H, Tscholakoff D, Heinrichs L. Uterine leiomyomas: Correlation of MR, histopathologic findings and symptoms. Radiology. 1986;158:385.
19. Aubel S, Wozney P, Ediwards RP. MRI of female uterine and juxtauterine masses: Clinical application in 25 pattients. Magn Reson Imaging. 1991;9:485.
20. Zwain M, McCartty S, Scoutt LM, et al. High-field MRI and US evaluation of the pelvis in women with leiomyomas. Magn Reson Imaging. 1990;8:371.
21. Muto MG, Friedman AJ. The uterine corpus. In: Ryan KJ, Berowitz RS, Barbieri RL (Eds): Kistner's Gyncology, St Louis; Mosby; 1995.
22. Pattani SJ. MRI of uterine leiomyosarcoma. Magn Reson Imaging. 1995;13(2):331-3.
23. Razavi MK, Hwang G, Jahed A, et al. Abdominal myomectomy versus uterine fibroid embolisation in the treatment of symptomatic uterine leiomyomas. AJR. 2003;180:1571-5.
24. Burn PR, Mc Call J M, Chinn RJ, et al. Uterine fibro-leiomyoma: MR imaging appearances before and after embolisation of uterine arteries. Rad. 2000;214:729-34.
25. de Souza NM, Williams AD. Uterine arterial embolisation for leiomyomas: Perfusion and volume changes at MR imaging and relation to clinical outcome. Rad. 2002;222:367-74.
26. Nikolic B, Spies JB, Abbara S, et al. Ovarian artery supply to uterine fibroids as a cause of treatment failure after uterine artery embolisation: a case report. J Vasc Interv Radiol. 1999;10:1167-70.
27. Soyer P, Harry G, Cazier A. Uterine fibromyo-lipoma: Uncommon imaging features. Eur J Radiol. 1991;13:67.
28. Houser LM, Carrasco CH, Shelhan LR. Lipomatous tumour of the uterus: Radiographic and ultrasonic appearance. BJR. 1979;52:992.
29. Lehrman BJ, Nisenbaum HL, Glasser SA. Uterine myolipoma: Magnetic resonance imaging, computed tomographic, and ultrasound appearance. J Ultrasound Med. 1990;9:665.
30. Azziz R. Adenomyosis: Current perspectives. Obstet Gynecol Clinics North Am. 1989;16:221.
31. Bohlman ME, Ensor RE, Sander RC. Sonographic findings in adenomyosis of the uterus. AJR. 1987;148:765.
32. Hulka CA, Hall DA, Mc Carthy K, et al. Sonographic findings in patients with adenomyosis: Can sonography assist in predicting extent of disease? AJR. 2002;179:379-83.
33. Dimitrios Botsis, Dimitrios Kassasnos, George Antomou. Adenomyoma and leiomyoma: Differential diagnosis with transvaginal sonography. J Clin Ultrasound. 1998;26:21-5.
34. Kido A, Togashi K, Koyama T, et al. Diffusely enlarged uterus: evaluation with MR imaging. Radiographics. 2003;23:1423-39.
35. Mark AS, Hricak H. Adenomyosis and leiomyoma: Differential diagnosis by means of magnetic resonance imaging. Radiology. 1987;163:527.
36. Togashi K, Ozasa H, Konishi I. Enlarged uterus: Differentiation between adenomyosis and leiomyoma with MRI. Radiology. 1989;171:531.
37. Ascher SM, Jha RC, Reinhold C. Benign myometrial conditions: Leiomyomas and adenomyosis. Top Magn Reson Imaging. 2003;14:281-304.
38. Johnson MA, Graham MF, Cooperberg PL. Abnormal endometrial echoes: Sonographic spectrum of endometrial pathology. J Ultrasound Med. 1982;1:161-6.
39. Sheth S, Hamper UM, Kurman RJ. Thickened endometrium in the post-menopausal woman: Sonographic pathologic correlation. Rad. 1993;187:135-9.
40. Hricak H, Frick S, Honda G. MR imaging in the evaluation of benign uterine masses. Am J Roent. 1992;158:1043.
41. SmithBindman R, Kerlikowske K, Feldstein VA, et al. Endovaginal ultrasound to exclude endometrial cancer and other endometrial abnormalities. JAMA. 1998;280:1510-617.
42. Fedele L, Bianchi S, Dorta M, et al. Intrauterine adhesions: Detection with transvaginal US. Rad. 1996;199:757-9.
43. Letterie GS, Haggerty MF. Magnetic resonance imaging of intrauterine synechiae. Gynecol Obstet Invest. 1994;37:66-8.

44. Bacclar AC, Wilcock D, Powell M, et al. The value of MRI in the assessment of traumatic intra-uterine adhesions (Asherman's syndrome). Clin Radiol. 1995;50:80-3.
45. Dixit R, Prakash A, Chowdhury V, et al. Pelvic Arterio-venous Malfaormation. Radiological quiz - GU Imaging IJRI. 2000;10:177-9.
46. Huang MW, Muradali D, Thurston WA, et al. Uterine arterio-venous malformation. Grey-scale and Doppler US features with MR imaging correlation. Radiology. 1998;206(1):115.
47. Joshi M, Ganeshan K, Munshi HN. Ultrasound of adnexal masses. Semin Ultrasound CT MRI. 2008;29:72-97.
48. Siddall KA, Rubens DJ. Multi-detector CT of the female pelvis. RCNA. 2005;43:1097-118.
49. Patel MD. Practical approach to the adnexal mass. RCNA. 2006;44:879-99.
50. Giede KC. Ovarian cysts in postmenopausal women: When to worry. The Canadian Journal of CME; 2007.pp.21-4.
51. Togashi K. MR imaging of the ovaries: Normal appearance and benign disease. RCNA. 2003;41:799-811.
52. Scoutt LM, Mc Carthy SM, Lange R. MR evaluation of clinically suspected adnexal masses. J Comput Assist Tomogr. 1994;18(4):609.
53. Fulgheshu AM, Ciampelli M, Belosi C, et al. A new ultrasound criteria for the diagnosis of polycystic ovary syndrome: The ovarian stroma/total area ratio. Fertil Steril. 2001;76:326-31.
54. Hoffer FA, Kozakewich H, Colodny A, et al. Peritoneal inclusion cysts: Ovarian fluid in peritoneal adhesions. Rad. 1988;169:189-91.
55. Jain KA. Imaging of Peritoneal inclusion cysts. AJR. 2000;174:1559-63.
56. Sohaey R, Gardner TL, Woodward PJ, et al. Sonographic diagnosis of peritoneal inclusion cyst. J Ultrasound Med. 1995;14:913-7.
57. Tessler FN, Perrella RR, Fleischer AC, et al. Endovaginal sonographic diagnosis of dilated fallopian tubes. AJR. 1989;153:523-5.
58. Athey PA, Cooper NB. Sonographic feature of parovarian cysts. AJR. 1985;144:83-6.
59. Fleischer AC, Cullinan JC. Pelvic masses. In: Copel JA, Reed KL (Eds): Doppler Ultrasound in Obstetrics and Gynecology. Raven Press Ltd; 1995;6:61-70.
60. Buy JN, Ghossain MA, Hugol D. Characterisation of adnexal masses: Combination of colour Doppler and conventional sonography compared with spectral Doppler analysis alone and conventional sonography alone. AJR. 1996;166:385-93.
61. Coleman BG. Transvaginal sonography of adnexal masses. In The Female Pelvis. RCNA. 1992;30(4):677-91.
62. Wilbur A. Computed tomography of tubovarian abscesses. J Comput Assist Tomogr. 1990;14(4):625-8.
63. Shamam OM, Bennel WF, Teteris NJ, et al. Primary fallopian tube adenocarcinoma presenting as a hydrosalpinx. CT appearance. J Comput Assist Tomogr. 1988;12(4):674-5.
64. Mitchell DG, Mintz MC, Spritzer CE. Adnexal masses: MR imaging observations at 1.5 T, with US and CT correlation. Radiology. 1987;162:319.
65. Friedman H, Vogelzang RL, Mendelson EB. Endometriosis detection by US with laparo-scopic correlation. Radiology. 1985;157:217-20.
66. Fishman EK. Computed tomography of endometriosis. J Comput Assist Tomogr. 1983;7:257-64.
67. Togashi K, Nishimura K, Kimura I. Endometrial cysts: Diagnosis with MR imaging. Radiology. 1991;180:73.
68. Outwater EK, Dunton CJ. Imaging of the ovary and adnexa: clinical issues and applications of MR imaging. Radiology. 1995;194:1-18.
69. Glastonbury CM. The shading sign. Rad. 2002;224:199-201.
70. Sloan RD. Cystic teratomas (dermoid) of the ovary. Radiology. 1963;81:847.
71. Quinn SF, Erickson S, Black WC. Cystic ovarian teratomas: The sonographic appearance of the dermoid plug. Radiology. 1985;155:477-8.
72. Friedman AC, Pyatt RS, Hartman DS. CT of benign cystic teratomas. AJR. 1982;138:659.
73. Buy JN. Cystic teratoma of the ovary: CT detection. Radiology. 1989;171:697-701.
74. Togashi K, Nishimura K, Itoh K. Ovarian cystic teratomas. MR imaging. Radiology. 1987;162:669.
75. Mitchell DG. Chemical shift magnetic resonance imaging: Applications in the abdomen and pelvis. Top Magn Reson Imaging. 1992;4(3):46.
76. Graif H, Shalev J, Strauss S. Torsion of the ovary: Sonographic features. Am J Roentgenol. 1984;143:1331.
77. Rha SE, Byun JY, Tung SE, et al. CT and MRI imaging findings of adnexal torsion. Radiographics. 2002;22:283-94.
78. Argenta PA, Yeagley TJ, Ott G, et al. Torsion of the uterine adnexa: pathological correlations and current management trends. J Reprod Med. 2000;45:831-6.
79. Eyvazzadeh AD, Levine D. Imaging of pelvic pain in the first trimester of pregnancy. RCNA. 2006;44:863-77.
80. Nuberg DA, Mack LA, Jeffrey RBJr, et al. Endovaginal sonographic evaluation of ectopic pregnancy: a prospective study. AJR. 1987;149:1181-6.
81. Russel SA, Filly RA, Damato N. Sonographic diagnosis of ectopic pregnancy with endovaginal probes. What really has changed? Ultrasound Med. 1993;12:145-51.
82. Jeong YY, Outwater EK, Kang HK. Imaging Evaluation of Ovarian Masses: Radiographics. 2000;20:1445-70.
83. Funt SA, Hann LE. Detection and characterisation of adnexal masses. RCNA. 2002;40:591-608.
84. Lee SI. Radiological Reasoning: Imaging characterisation of bilateral adnexal masses. AJR. 2006;187:S460-66.

CHAPTER 123

Imaging in Gynecological Malignancies

Sanjay Thulkar, Smriti Hari

GYNECOLOGICAL MALIGNANCIES IN INDIA

The incidence of various gynecological cancers in India is different from that of the developed countries. The incidence of cervical cancer is high in India and that of the endometrial cancer and ovarian cancer is low as compared with the western population. Socioeconomic and environmental factors are mainly responsible for this phenomena.[1] Annual age adjusted incidence (AAR) of cervical cancer in India ranges from 13 (Mumbai) to 24.8 (Chennai) per 100,000 women per year.[2] It used to be the most common cancer in females in India, however, now the breast cancer has taken over this position in most population based cancer registries of India. The incidence of ovarian cancer is 2.2–8 and that of endometrial cancer is 0.7–9.5 per 100,000 women per year.

CARCINOMA OF CERVIX

Peak incidence of carcinoma of cervix occurs between 30 and 50 years of age. Main risk factors for the cervical cancer include early age at first coitus, multiple sexual partners and sexually transmitted human papilloma virus (HPV) infection.[3] Widespread screening and early detection of cervical cancer has been made possible with Papanicolaou (PAP) smear examinations.

Approximately, 90% of cervical cancers are squamous cell carcinomas, others include adenocarcinomas and sarcomas.[3] Cervical carcinoma develops through various stages of dysplasia of cervical epithelium. It is designated as cervical intraepithelial neoplasia (CIN). Highest grade of CIN is called carcinoma *in situ* which is still limited by basement membrane. Breach of the basement membrane leads to invasive carcinoma. Clinically, patients present with vaginal bleeding and discharge. Patients with advanced disease may complain of pelvic pain and other symptoms related to lower urinary tract.

Spread of cervical cancer occurs through direct extension into parametrium and the pelvic lymph nodes. Direct invasion of uterus and upper vagina also occurs. Involvement of urinary bladder, rectum and pelvic side-walls occurs late. Hematogenous spread to lungs, bone, liver and brain is uncommon and late feature in the course of the cervical cancer. Invasive cervical cancers are staged according to International Federation of Gynecologists and Obstetricians (FIGO) staging system into four stages **(Table 1)**. The staging is clinical and may include findings of hysteroscopy, cystoscopy, proctoscopy, curettage, biopsy, IVP and X-rays. Prognosis depends on patient's age, tumor size and lymph node status as well histopathological type and grade of the tumor. Lymph node status is an important prognostic factor; the 5 years survival rates are 90% for node-negative and 50% for node-positive diseases.[4,5]

Imaging Modalities

Conventional Radiography

International Federation of Gynecologists and Obstetricians (FIGO) staging system uses the findings on chest radiography, IVP and barium enema. The

Table 1: Staging of the carcinoma of cervix.

Stage 0	**Carcinoma *in situ***
Stage I	**Invasive tumor confined to cervix** *IA:* Preclinical (subdivided into IA1 when stromal invasion is < 3 mm deep and 7 mm wide and IA2 when it is greater) *IB:* Clinically detectable (subdivided into IB1, if <4 cm and IB2, if >4 cm)
Stage II	**Spread beyond uterus** *IIA:* Involvement of upper third of vagina *IIB:* Involvement of parametrium not extending to side wall
Stage III	**Extension to the pelvic side wall/lower 3rd of vagina/hydronephrosis** *IIIA:* Involvement of lower third of vagina *IIIB:* Involvement of pelvic side wall and/or hydronephrosis
Stage IV	**Pelvic visceral involvement or distant metastases** *IVA:* Involvement of bladder or rectum *IVB:* Distant metastases

demonstration of urinary obstruction on IVU is classified as stage IIIB. The findings on IVU include delayed nephrogram, hydroureteronephrosis or extrinsic compression or deviation of ureters. Involvement of rectum and sigmoid colon can be seen on barium enema as irregularity of outline, ulceration and fistula formation. Presently, IVU and barium enema are not routinely performed, instead cross-sectional imaging modalities such as US, computed tomography (CT) and magnetic resonance imaging (MRI) are preferred.[4] These may be supplemented with sigmoidoscopy and cystoscopy.

Ultrasonography

Cervical tumors are usually isoechoic to normal cervix and hence are not readily identified on ultrasonography.[4] Transvaginal and transrectal ultrasonography may show nonspecific enlargement of the cervix.[6] Transvaginal color Doppler imaging does not offer any improvement in detection and characterization of cervical cancer.[7] Large necrotic tumors are hypoechoic and hence these can be identified on ultrasonography. Presence of hydro/pyometra suggests obstruction of endocervical canal by the tumor. Ultrasonography readily detects hydronephrosis.

Computed Tomography

Cervical cancer is poorly depicted on CT. The mass may not be seen or seen as nonspecific enlargement of the cervix. When mass is demonstrated, it is hypodense and heterogeneous, often with peripheral enhancement[4,8] **(Fig. 1)** CT does not accurately detect early parametrial invasion. Features suggestive of early parametrial invasion include irregular margins of the cervix and stranding in parametrium. However, these findings can also be caused by reactive or inflammatory changes without tumor extension. Advanced parametrial invasion on CT is suggested by soft tissue mass in parametrial fat, encasement of ureter or thickening and nodularity of uterosacral ligament[9] **(Figs. 2 and 3)**. CT findings suggestive of pelvic sidewall invasion include extension of the tumor within 3 mm of lateral wall of pelvis, encasement of iliac vessels, invasion of obturator internus or pyriformis muscles or bone destruction.[4]

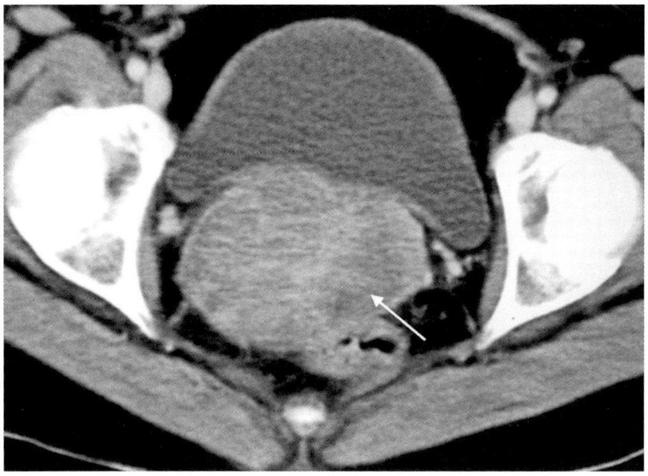

Fig. 1: Carcinoma of cervix. CECT of pelvis shows a bulky heterogeneously enhancing mass (arrow). It is confined to cervix as there is smooth interphase with the myometrium.

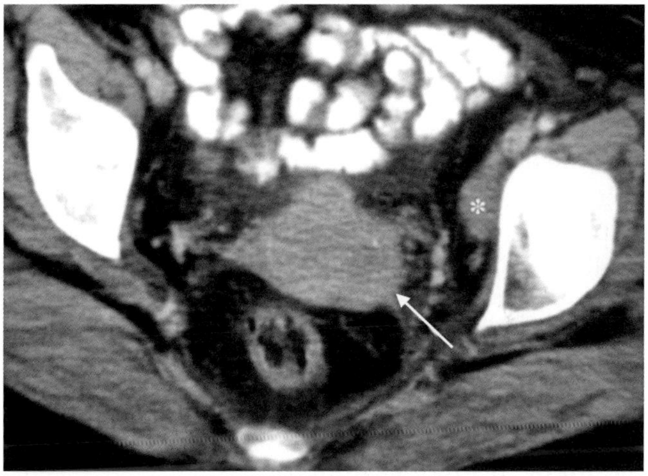

Fig. 2: Carcinoma of cervix: CECT shows isodense cervical mass with irregularity of the outline and extension of soft tissue (arrow) in left parametrium suggestive of parametrial invasion. Enlarged left obturator lymph node (asterisk) is also seen.

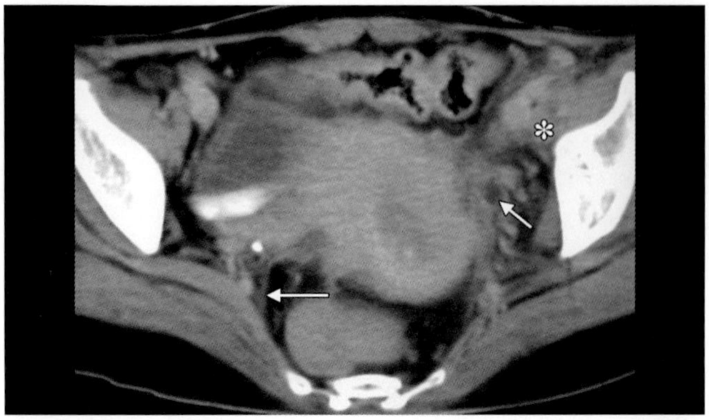

Fig. 3: Carcinoma of cervix: Delayed pelvic image of the CECT shows large cervical mass with soft tissue stranding involving the right pyriformis muscle (arrow) suggestive of pelvic wall invasion. Urinary bladder and right ureter is opacified, however, left ureter is dilated and unopacified (small arrow) suggestive of poorly functioning left kidney. Enlarged left external iliac lymph node (asterisk) is also seen.

Ureteric obstruction is reliably detected by CT, thereby obviating the need for IVU **(Fig. 3)**. Invasion of urinary bladder or rectum occurs late in course of the disease. On CT, this may be seen as loss of fat plane and irregular wall thickening.

CT is fairly accurate in evaluation of lymph nodal metastases **(Figs. 2 and 3)**. Presence of central necrosis in the lymph nodes is highly specific for metastatic involvement.[10] Distant metastases may be seen in lungs, liver and bones. Peritoneal metastases may also occur in carcinoma of cervix. These are seen as peritoneal nodules, thickening and ascites.

Magnetic Resonance Imaging

Superior contrast resolution has made MRI the imaging modality of choice for evaluation of cervical cancer. Indications of MRI include pre-treatment evaluation of local tumor extent and nodal involvement, assessment of treatment response and detection of recurrent disease.[9]

T1, T2 and contrast-enhanced T1-weighted images are normally obtained in axial and sagittal planes. Excellent contrast between tumor and the cervical tissue allows accurate delineation and measurement of tumor size on these images.[11] On T2W image, the tumor is seen as a hyperintense mass surrounded by hypointense cervical stroma. On contrast-enhanced T1W image, small tumors enhance homogeneously **(Figs. 4A and B)**. Large tumors may be necrotic and do not enhance, however, they often have enhancing rim surrounding them. Demonstration of intact peripheral fibrous layer of the cervix, which is normally seen as a hypointense ring on T2W images **(Fig. 4A)**, has 95% negative predictive value for parametrial invasion.[5,12] Disruption of stromal ring suggests full thickness stromal invasion but not necessarily parametrial invasion. Various MRI features of parametrial invasion include nodular or irregular tumor signal intensity extending into the parametrium **(Figs. 5A and B)**, focal tumor bulge into the parametrium, encasement of ureter or periuterine vessels and thickening and nodularity of uterosacral ligament.[4,9] Parametrial invasion may be overestimated on T2W images in large size tumors because of stromal edema caused by tumor compression.[5]

Lateral pelvic wall involvement is suggested by tumor proximity (less than 3 mm) or hyperintensity of muscles on T2W images, encasement of iliac vessels or bony destruction. MRI is highly accurate for detection of the invasion of urinary bladder, vagina and rectum.[9,11] Bladder invasion is suggested by disruption of low signal intensity bladder wall, irregularity of bladder wall or mass protruding into the lumen. Rectal invasion is rare and seen as segmental thickening or loss of anterior rectal wall.[13]

Imaging Strategies in Cervical Cancer

Imaging has no role in the diagnosis of cervical cancer. Routine pretreatment work up includes clinical examination, laboratory studies and chest radiography. FIGO staging system is clinical, and it has several limitations. Estimation of tumor size and spread may not be always accurate on clinical examination. Lymph node status is not included in staging. Findings on chest X-ray, IVP or barium enema are included in staging but not the USG, CT or MRI. Even though cross-sectional imaging findings have been shown to improve the accuracy of staging.[14,15] FIGO guidelines prohibits the use of US, CT or MR imaging findings for staging purpose.[3] In practice, however, cross-sectional imaging findings are often used to choose most appropriate treatment options without changing the clinical stage.

In early cervical cancers (clinically stage IA) with tumor size less than 2 cm, chances of local or lymphatic spread are minimal and hence no cross-sectional imaging is necessary. MRI is the investigation of choice when clinical stage is 1B or higher.[13] In advanced disease (stage II or more), both MRI and CT can be used for evaluation, MRI being the preferred modality.[16] MRI is also recommended when clinical examination and staging is equivocal. Imaging assessment of the tumor and its spread assist in correct therapeutic decisions. Patients with clinically occult bulky tumors (>4 cm) or lymphadenopathy may receive chemoradiation instead of upfront surgery.

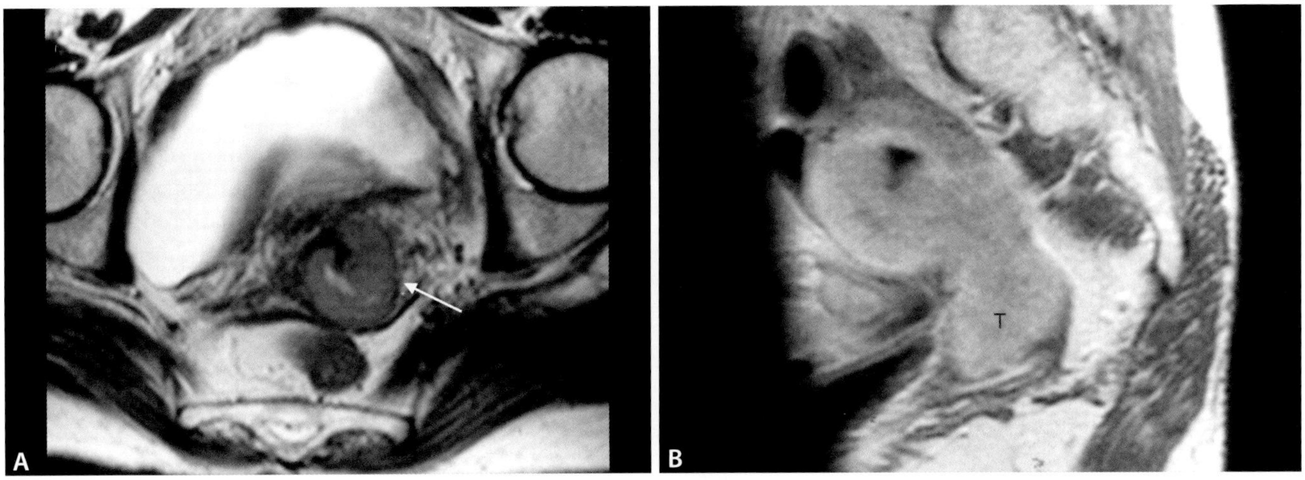

Figs. 4A and B: Carcinoma of cervix: (A) T2W axial MR image shows hyperintense mass in the cervic surrounded by the hypointense rim of cervical stroma (arrow); (B) Contrast-enhanced sagittal T1 W image shows extension of the tumor (T) in lower part of the body of the uterus.

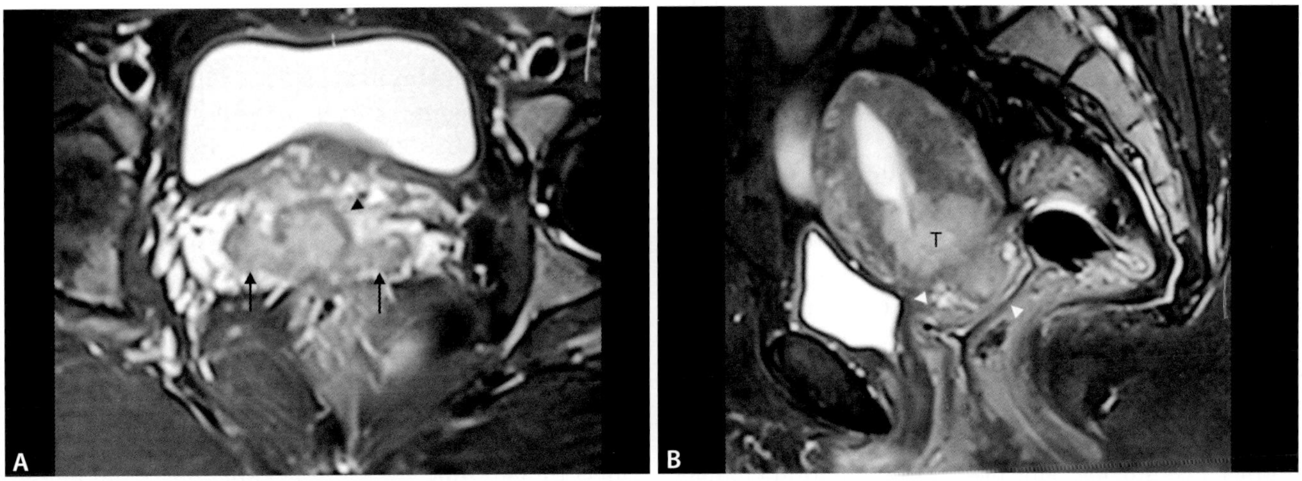

Figs. 5A and B: Carcinoma of cervix: (A) T2W axial MR image shows hyperintense mass in the cervix. It is surrounded by hypointense stromal ring anteriorly (black arrowhead); however, this ring is disrupted posterolaterally with tumor sensitivity soft tissue extension in bilateral parametrium (arrows); (B) Contrast-enhanced sagittal T1W images shows enhancing tumor (T) in the cervix. Preserved hypointense walls of urinary bladder and rectum (white arrowheads) exclude their invasion by the tumor.

For parametrial invasion, overall sensitivity of CT is 55% and that of MRI is 74%.[17] Early parametrial invasion, however, is better assessed clinically.[18] IVP and barium enema have now become obsolete in staging work-up as same information can also be obtained with CT or MRI. Absence of rectal and bladder involvement on MRI has 100% negative predictive value and this can obviate the cystoscopy and sigmoidoscopy in patients with cervical cancer **(Fig. 5B)**.[19]

Accuracy of MRI in detection of lymph nodal metastases is similar to CT. It is up to 85% for CT and 89% for MRI.[9] The sensitivity is poor as metastases in normal sized lymph nodes cannot be identified using size criteria. Use of lymph node specific contrast agent, such as ultra-small superparamagnetic iron oxide (USPIO) can significantly improve the sensitivity of MRI in detection of lymph node involvement.[20]

Positron Emission Tomography

Positron emission tomography (PET) imaging is not routinely obtained in cervical cancer; however, it is a useful adjunct to CT and MRI for the evaluation of lymph nodes, detection of distant metastases and assessment of treatment response.[9] PET has sensitivity and specificity of 84% and 95% for para-aortic lymph nodes and 79% and 99% for pelvic lymph nodes.[21] It is more sensitive than MRI for this purpose.[22] FDG uptake in primary tumor is also an independent predictor of the disease free survival.[23] Hence, PET is useful imaging modality in patients with advanced cervical cancer for making treatment decisions and determining the prognosis.

Treatment and Follow-up

Early cervical cancers (up to stage IIA) can be treated with both surgery and radiotherapy, surgery being the preferred modality for younger women. Those with positive margin or nodes on surgery also receive postoperative chemoradiotherapy. Radiotherapy is the primary treatment modality for most patients with advanced (stage IIB or more) disease.[3]

After radiation treatment, the tumor and uterus normally decrease in size and the cervix shows low signal intensity on T2W images.[9] However, sometimes edema or necrosis may appear hyperintense mimicking residual tumor. Patients are normally followed up for five years with clinical examinations, lab studies, PAP smear and chest radiography.

Recurrence of carcinoma of cervix is most commonly detected within first two years after the treatment.[3] It is uncommon after five years. Vaginal vault and lymph nodes are the most common sites of the local recurrence. These may invade, pelvic sidewall, bladder or rectum. Recurrence at distant metastatic sites includes metastases in liver, lung, bone adrenals and peritoneal carcinomatosis.[13] Both CT and MRI demonstrate the recurrences but it is better assessed with MRI. Recurrence is seen on T2W images as heterogeneous mass and enhancement on post-contrast T1W images. However, early radiation changes and infection may also show similar findings.[13] MRI has high sensitivity (90–91%) but low specificity (22–38%) for detection of recurrence.[9] PET is a better investigation for detection of recurrence with sensitivity and specificity of more than 80% and its use may improve the management of recurrent cervical cancer in many patients.[24,25]

CARCINOMA OF ENDOMETRIUM

Prolonged estrogen stimulation is the main risk factor for endometrial cancer.[4] An increased incidence of endometrial carcinoma is seen in women taking estrogen, such as for oral contraception or postmenopausal hormone replacement therapy. Increased incidence is also noted in postmenopausal women taking tamoxifen as a part of hormonal therapy for breast cancer. Other risk factors include nulliparity, obesity, diabetes. The peak incidence of endometrial carcinoma is between the ages of 55 and 65 years.

Most patients present with postmenopausal vaginal bleeding or discharge; however, it can also occur in premenopausal women. In less than 5% of patients, the tumor is detected incidentally on cervical cytology or histopathology of uterus removed for benign causes.[3] The diagnosis of endometrial carcinoma in suspected patients is made by histopathological examination of endometrial biopsy and curettage. Up to 90% of the endometrial cancers are adenocarcinoma, the rest include adenosquamous carcinoma, clear cell carcinoma and papillary serous carcinoma.[13]

Spread and Staging

Endometrial carcinoma typically arises from body of uterus (upper uterine corpus). The early growth is exophytic into the endometrial cavity followed by progressive invasion of myometrium. This pattern causes uterine enlargement. The tumor spreads caudally to involve cervix and vagina and axially to involve adnexa, parametrium and other pelvic organs. Lymphatic spread of the endometrial carcinoma is complex in nature and hence any group of pelvic lymph nodes or retroperitoneal para-aortic lymph nodes may be involved.[4] Hematogenous spread to lungs, liver, bones and brain occurs late in the course of the disease. Endometrial cancer is staged according FIGO staging system **(Table 2)**. It is a surgicopathological staging system.

Imaging Modalities

Conventional Radiography

Chest radiographs are routinely obtained in all patients diagnosed to have endometrial carcinoma. Skeletal radiography or scintigraphy can be performed if bone metastases are suspected. Similar to the carcinoma of cervix, IVU and barium studies are obsolete in evaluation of endometrial carcinoma.[4]

Ultrasonography

Ultrasonography is an important modality for screening, diagnosis as well as staging of endometrial carcinoma. Transvaginal sonography is more accurate than trans-abdominal sonography for this purpose. Normal endometrium is seen as an echogenic stripe in the uterine cavity. It is surrounded by inner myometrium, which is seen as hypoechoic layer around the echogenic endo-metrium (endometrial halo).

Early endometrial cancers typically appear as widening of endometrial layer **(Fig. 6)**. Double layer endometrial thickness of greater than 5 mm in postmenopausal women

Table 2: Staging of the carcinoma of endometrium.

Stage I	**Tumor confined to the body of uterus** *IA:* Limited to endometrium *IB:* Invade less than half of myometrium *IC:* Invade half or more of myometrium
Stage II	**Tumor involving cervix** *IIA:* Endocervical invasion only *IIB:* Cervical stromal invasion
Stage III	**Tumor extending outside uterus but not outside true pelvis** *IIIA:* Involement of serosa, adnexa or malignant ascites *IIIB:* Vaginal involvement *IIIC:* Pelvic or para-aortic lymph nodes
Stage IV	**Bladder/rectum invasion or distant metastases** *IVA:* Bladder or bowel involvement *IVB:* Distant metastases

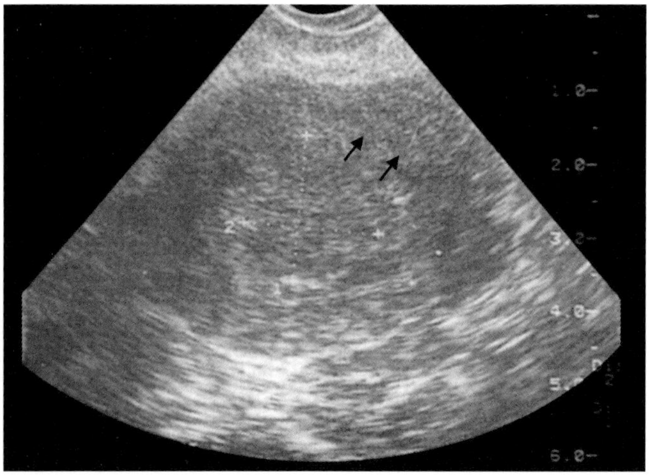

Fig. 6: Carcinoma of endometrium: Transvaginal sonogram shows thickened endometrium with loss of subendometrial halo (arrows) by endometrial carcinoma

is considered abnormal.[26] Exception to this is women on estrogen therapy in whom endometrial stripe thickness up to 7 mm is considered normal.[4] In premenopausal women, the upper limit of endometrial thickness is 15 mm. Thickening of endometrium can also be seen in endometrial hyperplasia or polyps. Saline infusion sonohysterography improves the accuracy of the diagnosis.[27] Color Doppler shows diffusely increased vascularity in multivessel pattern in endometrial cancer, in contrast to the pedicle artery sign seen in polyps.[28] Transvaginal sonography along with endometrial aspiration samplings can be used for screening of endometrial cancer in high-risk women.

Obliteration of endometrial halo (produced by inner myometrium) or irregularity of endometrium-myometrium interphase on transvaginal sonography is suggestive of myometrial invasion.[9] Larger tumors cause enlargement and distortion of the echotexture of the uterus **(Fig. 7A)**. Sonography is not suitable to detect extrauterine spread of the tumor and lymph nodal metastases.

Computed Tomography

Endometrial cancer appears as diffuse or focal enlargement of endometrium. The tumor enhances less than the adjacent myometrium **(Fig. 7B)**. Irregularity of uterine outline and stranding of parametrium is suggestive of an extrauterine spread. CT readily demonstrates lymph nodal enlargement, peritoneal deposits and distant metastases.[9] Myometrial invasion of the tumor is difficult to assess on the CT. Both false positive and false negative errors are common with CT.

Magnetic Resonance Imaging

This imaging modality is the technique of choice for evaluation of endometrial carcinoma. It provides an excellent morphological display of uterus and adjacent structures. T2W and gadolinium enhanced T1W axial and sagittal images are mostly used. The zonal anatomy is best demonstrated on T2W image. Endometrium appears hyperintense and is surrounded by hypointense rim of junctional zone representing inner myometrium. The outer myometrium shows medium signal intensity.

Endometrial cancer appears isointense on T1W and hyperintense on T2W images when compared with myometrium **(Figs. 8A and B)**. Large tumors are often seen as polypoidal masses expanding the endometrial cavity. Presence of normal hypointense junctional zone seen on T2W images excludes myometrial invasion. Obliteration of junctional zone or irregularity of endometrium–myometrium interphase suggests myometrial invasion[9] **(Fig. 9)**. After intravenous gadolinium, endometrial carcinoma shows less enhancement compared to myometrium **(Fig. 8C)**. Dynamic contrast-enhanced studies are more useful in detection of small tumors and to assess myometrial invasion. Early phase (0–1 minute) shows better contrast between inner and outer myometrium, the former enhances earlier. Deep myometrial invasion is best assessed at equilibrium (2–3 minutes) as tumor myometrium contrast is highest at this time. Presence of low signal intensity tumor in outer myometrium suggests deep invasion (stage 1C) disease. Cervical invasion (stage II) is better assessed at delayed (4–5 minutes) phase.[13] Spread to parametrium (stage IIIA) is seen as disruption of serosal

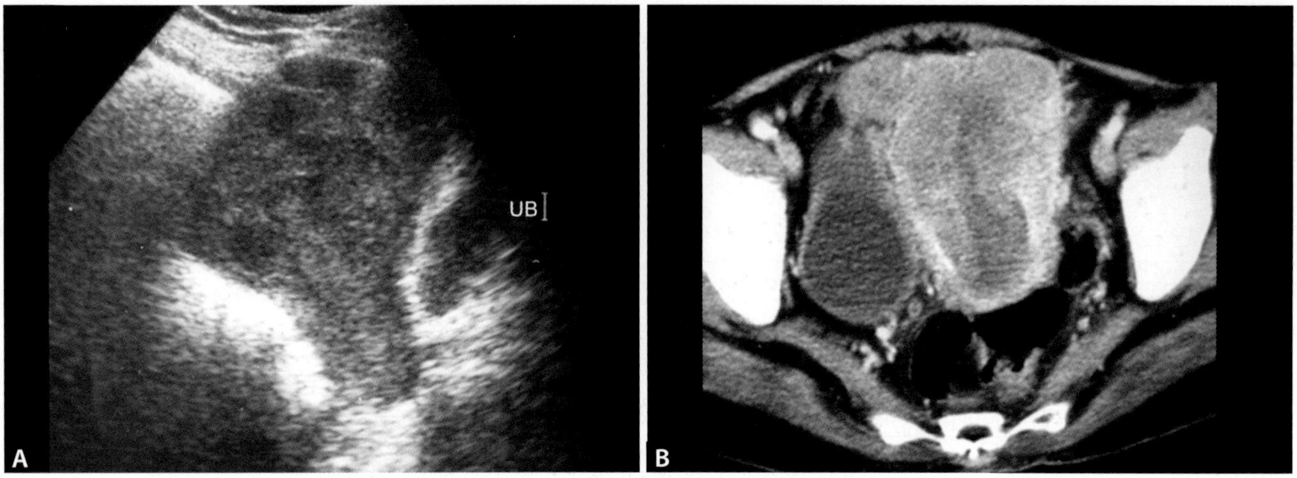

Figs. 7A and B: Carcinoma of the endometrium: (A) Sonography shows enlarged, distorted and heterogeneous uterus; (B) CECT also shows the similar findings. The tumor enhancement is lesser than that of the myometrium.

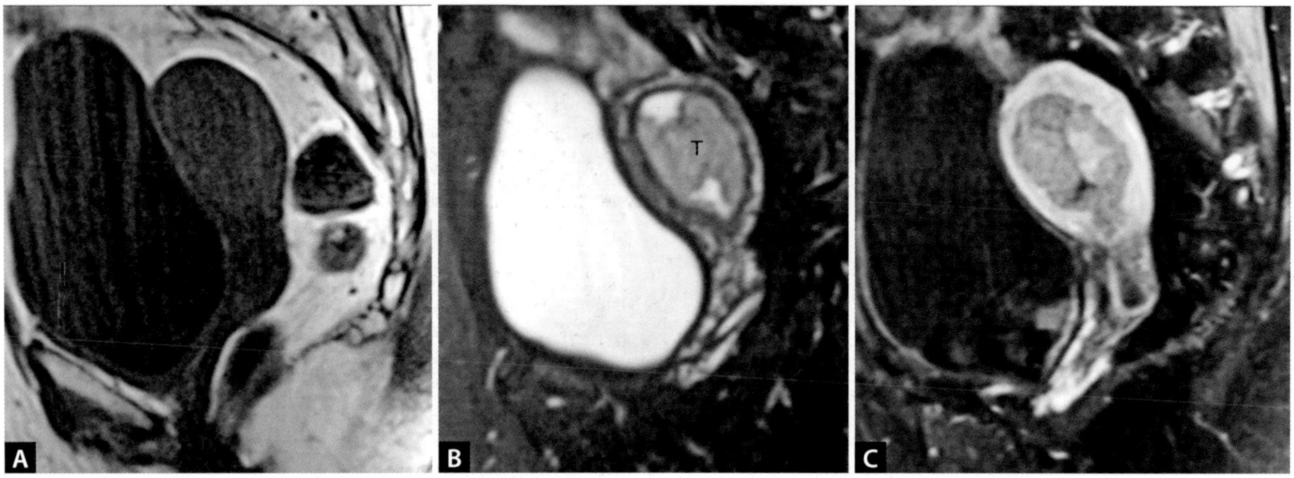

Figs. 8A to C: Carcinoma of endometrium: Sagittal T1W MRI shows nonspecific enlargement of the uterus as the tumor is isointense; (B) Sagittal fat suppressed T2W-MR image shows large tumor (T) distending the uterine cavity. It is moderately hyperintense as compared with surrounding myometrium. The junctional zone is indistinct in this atrophic uterus; (C) On contrast-enhanced T1W MR image, the tumor enhances less than the myometrium.

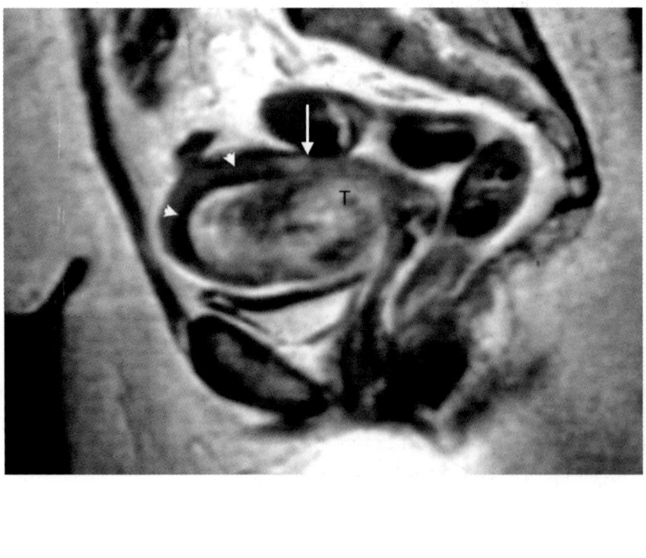

Fig. 9: Carcinoma of endometrium: T2W sagittal MR images shows hyperintense endometrial tumor (T). The junctional zone, seen as hypointense rim, is intact in fundus (arrowheads); however, it is obliterated in lower part with tumor extension into deep myometrium (arrow).

outline and direct toumor extension into the parametrium. Vaginal involvement (stage IIIB) is seen as segmental loss of the low intensity vaginal wall.

Imaging Strategies in Endometrial Cancer

Transvaginal sonography is the most useful modality for detection of endometrial cancer. Patients with abnormal findings on sonography then undergo dilatation and curettage or endometrial biopsy for definitive diagnosis. Transvaginal sonography is also useful to determine the extent of myometrial invasion; however, MRI provides more accurate information about the degree of invasion and locoregional extent of the disease.

Determining the presence and depth of myometrial invasion on MRI is important. There is six–sevenfold increased prevalence of lymphadenopathy if depth myometrial invasion is more than 50% (stage 1C) when compared with patients with less than 50% (stage 1B) or absent (stage 1A) myometrial invasion. The preoperative assessment of myometrial invasion helps to plan the extent of lymph node sampling.[9] MR evaluation of endometrial cancer may be difficult in elderly women with atrophic uterus as junctional zone may be indistinct **(Fig. 8B)**. The junctional zone is also difficult to evaluate when it is irregular and thickened in women with adenomyosis and in presence of myometrial distortion by large tumor or fibroid. MRI has 87% sensitivity and 91% specificity in assessment of myometrial invasion; however, sensitivity for detection of lymph node involvement is only 50%.[29]

Treatment and Follow-up

Carcinoma of the endometrium is surgically stagzed and treated tumor. All patients with early (stages I and II) endometrial cancers are treated with hysterectomy and bilateral salpingo-oophorectomy. After surgery, those with high risk of recurrence receive adjuvant radiotherapy. Tumor grade and stage, depth of myometrial invasion, cervical stromal invasion and lymph node status are important prognostic indicators in this regard. Advanced (stages III and IV) tumors are treated with pelvic radiotherapy. After radiotherapy, patients with resectable tumors are operated for removal of residual tumor. Rests of the patients are subjected to extended field radiotherapy or chemotherapy.[4]

Patients are followed with clinical examination. Recurrence can be local or at distant metastatic sites. Almost all recurrences occur within three years.[30] Local recurrences usually develop in vaginal vault and these are detected on follow-up clinical examinations. Hence, routine imaging for follow-up is not required. CT and MRI are performed only when pelvic examination is abnormal or distant metastases are suspected.[4]

OVARIAN MALIGNANCIES

Carcinoma of the ovary is the second most common gynecological malignancy. This is classified according to tissue of origin. Majority are epithelial tumors. Others include germ cell tumors, stromal-sex cord tumors and metastatic cancers from extraovarian primary sites. Incidence of these types varies widely. As per ten years data at author's institute, epithelial tumors constitute 83% while germ cell tumors constitute 9.5% of ovarian tumors. 3.2% each are stromal tumors and metastatic carcinomas of the ovary.[31]

Epithelial Ovarian Carcinoma

These account for up to 90% of all malignant ovarian cancers. These are separated into two major categories: invasive (80%) and noninvasive or borderline (20%) tumors. Epithelial invasive cancers are further classified into serous cystadenocarcinoma, mucinous cystadenocarcinoma, endometroid carcinoma, clear cell carcinoma and undifferentiated tumor.[32] Ovarian carcinoma predominantly occurs in postmenopausal women and up to 85% of them present with peritoneal spread[33] (stage III). About 10% of epithelial ovarian cancers are hereditary. These include women with breast ovarian cancer syndrome (with BRCA1 and BRCA2 mutations) and hereditary nonpolyposis colorectal cancer syndrome. These women have up to 60% lifetime risk of developing ovarian cancers and the risk can be reduced with prophylactic bilateral salpingo-oophorectomy after childbearing.[34]

Patients usually present with abdominal pain, distention or symptoms related to gastrointestinal tract/ or and genitourinary tract compression or nonspecific constitutional symptoms. A pelvic mass may be evident on abdominal palpation or pelvic examination but it is usually detected or confirmed on initial sonographic examination.

Spread of the tumor is transcoelomic and follows the pathways of peritoneal fluid circulation. Accordingly, deposits in right subdiaphragmatic region and paracolic gutters occur early along with ascites. Eventually all peritoneal surfaces, omentum and mesentery may be involved. Metastases to the para-aortic and pelvic lymph nodes also occur.

Ultrasonography

Ultrasonography is the first imaging modality to diagnose or confirm the clinically suspected adnexal mass. It is also used to characterize the adnexal masses based on their morphological features. Transvaginal sonography is better than transabdominal approach for characterization of adnexal masses. Large, bilateral, complex solid-cystic masses are usually malignant. Cysts with thick walls, irregular thick septation (more than 3 mm), papillary projections or mural nodules favor malignancy **(Fig. 10A)**. Ovaries enlarged for the age are also suspicious for malignancy. Presence of ascites, peritoneal deposits and lymph node enlargement are other supportive evidences. Physiological hemorrhagic cysts may sometimes have suspicious appearances on ultrasound and hence it is important to follow these with ultrasound and only persistent lesions should be considered abnormal.[32]

Doppler studies are important in evaluation of adnexal masses. Nonhyperechoic mass with central vascularity on color Doppler is suggestive of malignancy.[35,36] On pulsed Doppler, malignant tumors have abnormal neovascularity and low resistance flow pattern. Low pulsatility index (1.4 or less) and low resistive index (0.4 or less) suggest malignancy. Positive predictive value of 98% has been reported for the diagnosis of ovarian malignancy using these features.[37] However, subsequent studies found that characterization of the adnexal masses based on Doppler studies only is unreliable as similar findings may also be seen in inflammatory diseases and physiological cysts.[38,39] A large meta-analysis of the studies concluded that combined morphological and Doppler transvaginal sonographic evaluation provides the best results in detection of ovarian cancer.[40]

Screening for Ovarian Cancer

The five-year survival rates up to 90% for stage I cancers as compared to 15–20% in stage III or IV cancers and the fact that most patients present with advanced disease make screening important option.[41] Transvaginal ultrasound, Doppler studies and serum CA-125 measurement can be used in combination for screening of the ovarian cancer.

There are several difficulties for screening of ovarian cancer. Ultrasound features are nonspecific. This leads to several false-positive results and unnecessary surgeries. CA 125 is elevated in only 50% of stage 1 epithelial cancers and it is relatively insensitive for mucinous tumors.[34] Also, there is low incidence of ovarian cancer in general population and the cost of screening is high. Currently, a large screening trial is going on in USA (PLCO or prostate, lung, colorectal and ovary) but the results and recommendations will be available only after a decade.[34] At present, there is no evidence that screening reduces the mortality from ovarian cancer and hence not recommended for women with or without family history of ovarian cancer.[42] The exception may be women with BRCA mutations in whom screening may be performed until prophylactic bilateral oophorectomy after childbearing.[43]

Computed Tomography

CT is the main stay of preoperative evaluation of ovarian cancer. The CT features of ovarian cancer show varied morphological patterns: A multilocular cyst, thick wall or internal septations, solid mural nodules, complex cystic-solid mass or lobulated papillary mass **(Figs. 10 to 12)**. Solid looking areas that do not enhance may represent blood or mucinous fluid with high protein content.[32,33] Normal size ovaries which are large for the age, especially when these show papillary excrescences are also suspicious for malignancy **(Fig. 13)**. Calcification is occasionally seen in papillary serous adenocarcinoma and Brenner

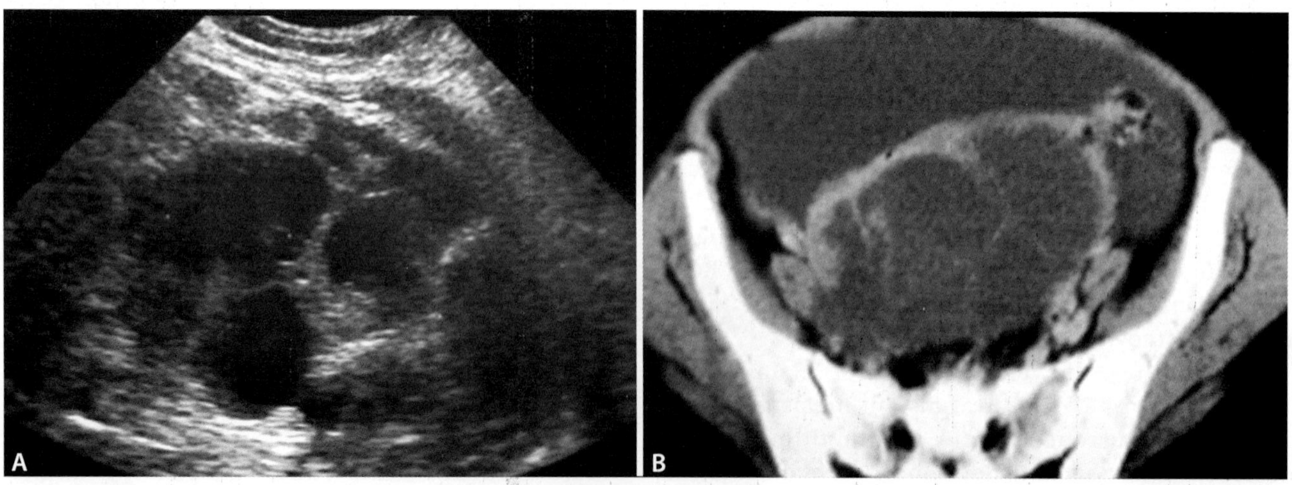

Figs. 10A and B: Carcinoma of ovary: (A) Ultrasonography shows complex cystic pelvic mass with irregular thick septations and solid component; (B) CECT of pelvis shows similar findings.

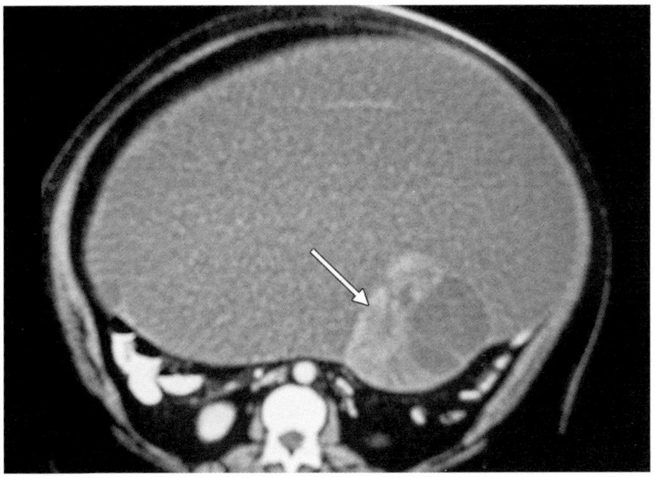

Fig. 11: Carcinoma of ovary: CECT of pelvis shows clear cell carcinoma of ovary as a large cyst with solid mural nodule (arrow).

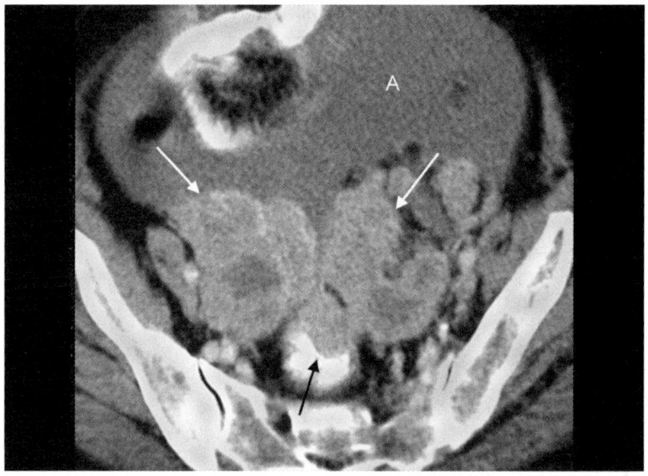

Fig. 12: Carcinoma of ovary: CECT shows bilateral complex solid cystic adnexal masses (white arrows) with invasion of the rectum (black arrow) seen as wall thickening and luminal bulge. Ascites (A) is also seen.

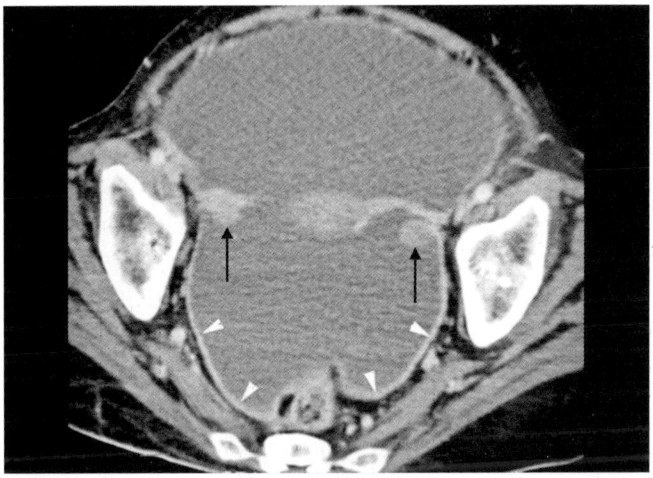

Fig. 13: Carcinoma of ovary: Bilateral normal sized but irregular ovaries (arrows) are definitely abnormal for this elderly woman with atrophic uterus. Gross ascites as well as peritoneal deposits are present. The latter is seen as enhancing and thickened peritoneum in pouch of Douglas (arrowheads).

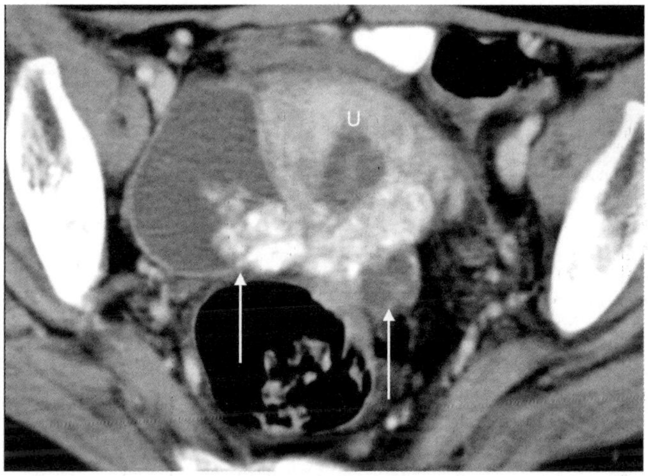

Fig. 14: Carcinoma of ovary: CECT shows bilateral complex cystic masses (arrows) with calcifications in solid component are seen. Invasion of the uterus (U) and the rectum is also seen.

tumor **(Fig. 14)**. Ancillary findings of malignancy, such as ascites, peritoneal deposits, lymphadenopathy and pleural effusion may also be present. Although CT is not normally used for differentiation of benign and malignant adnexal masses, it is equivalent to ultrasonography for this purpose.[44]

Involvement of uterus, rectum, colon and small bowel by the tumor is well demonstrated on CT **(Figs. 12 and 14)**. It can also detect deposits on peritoneum, liver or bowel surfaces. Peritoneal deposits are seen as soft tissue nodules or plaque like thickening and enhancement of the peritoneum **(Figs. 15 and 16)**. These may coalesce to form large masses. Peritoneal deposits are more commonly seen at the peritoneal reflections where the peritoneal fluid tends to accumulate. Accordingly, common sites are pouch of Doglous, paracolic gutters, right subdiaphragmatic space and liver surface.[45] The sensitivity of CT in detection of peritoneal deposits is moderate, conventional CT scanners detected only up to 50% of peritoneal deposits that are 5 mm or less in size. The multidetector CT scanners have improved sensitivity in detection of small peritoneal deposits, especially in upper

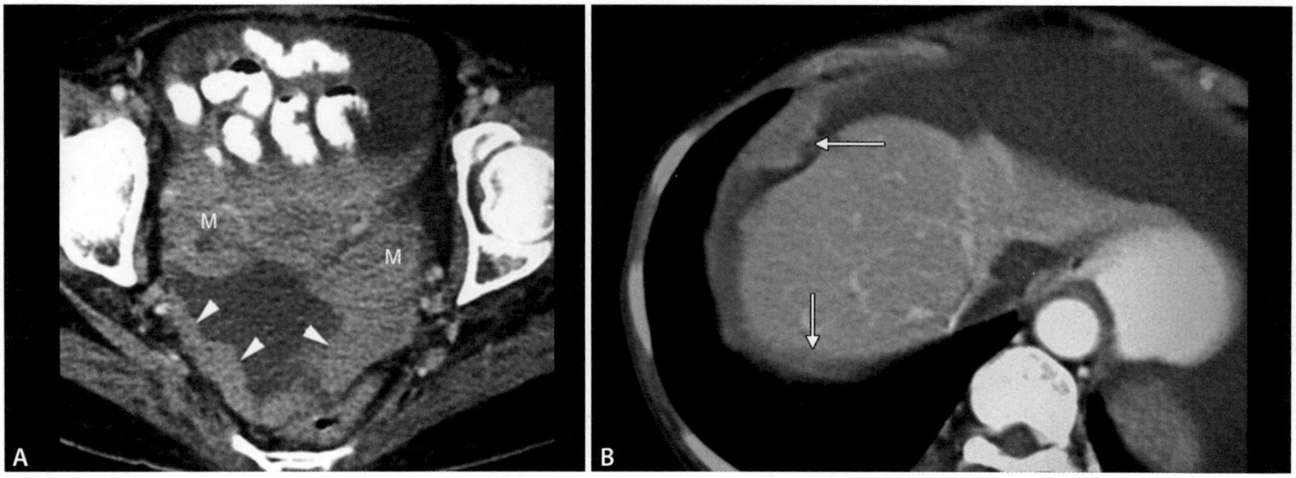

Figs. 15A and B: Carcinoma of ovary with peritoneal deposits: (A) CECT of the pelvis shows bilateral adnexal masses (M) and ascites with plaque-like peritoneal deposits (arrowheads) in pouch of Douglas; (B) Peritoneal deposits are also seen of the surfaces of liver and diaphragm (arrows).

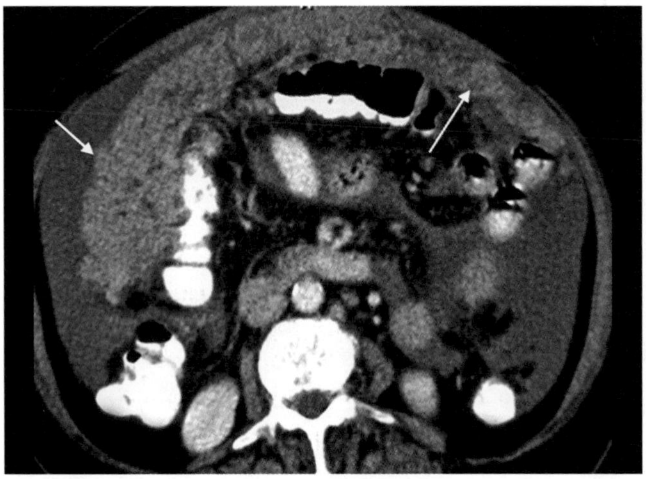

Fig. 16: Carcinoma of ovary: Multiple omental deposits coalesce to form a characteristic solid omental cake (arrows).

abdomen.[46] CT detection of peritoneal or liver surface deposits is facilitated by presence of ascites **(Fig. 15B)**. Small foci of peritoneal calcifications may also represent deposits, especially, if it is a new finding.

Omental deposits are initially seen as multiple nodular lesions in omental fat. Later, they coalesce to form a solid 'omental cake', which is seen along the greater curvature of stomach or anterior to transverse colon or small bowel **(Fig. 16)**. It may be seen beneath the anterior abdominal wall located anywhere from upper abdomen to pelvis and at times, mistaken for unopacified bowel loops. Mesenteric metastases are seen as rounded, ill-defined soft tissue masses surrounded by small bowel loops or as thickening along the mesenteric vessels and lymphatics.[33]

CT accurately detects para-aortic and pelvic lymph node enlargement. Superior diaphragmatic (paracardiac) lymphadenopathy is a characteristic finding some advanced ovarian cancers and these are associated with poor prognosis.[47] Intrahepatic metastases are rare and occur late in the course of the disease. Ovarian cancer is one of the few primary cancers to have splenic metastases.

Although it is not possible to suggest specific histological diagnosis on CT, some features are considered typical for various types.[32] Seorus cystadenocarcinoma, endometroid carcinoma and undifferentiated carcinoma are frequently bilateral. Serous cystadenocarcinomas are usually seen as bilateral complex masses of irregular shape with papillary excrescences on the surface **(*see* Fig. 13)**. Endometroid cancers are usually bilateral masses which can be both cystic as well as completely solid **(Fig. 17)**. Concomitant endometrial hyperplasia, endometriosis or endometrial carcinoma may be associated. Undifferentiated tumors are usually solid masses with areas of necrosis. Mucinous adenocarcinomas and clear cell carcinomas are more commonly unilateral and seen in comparatively younger age group. The mucinous tumor typically manifests as multiloculated cystic solid mass with variable densities in different locules. Clear cell carcinoma is characterisitically seen as unilateral cystic lesion with solid mural nodule in relatively younger women **(*see* Fig. 11)**. Unlike endometrial counterpart of this tumor, ovarian clear cell carcinoma has a better prognosis.

Magnetic Resonance Imaging

The morphological features of ovarian cancer on MRI are similar to those seen on sonography or CT, but because

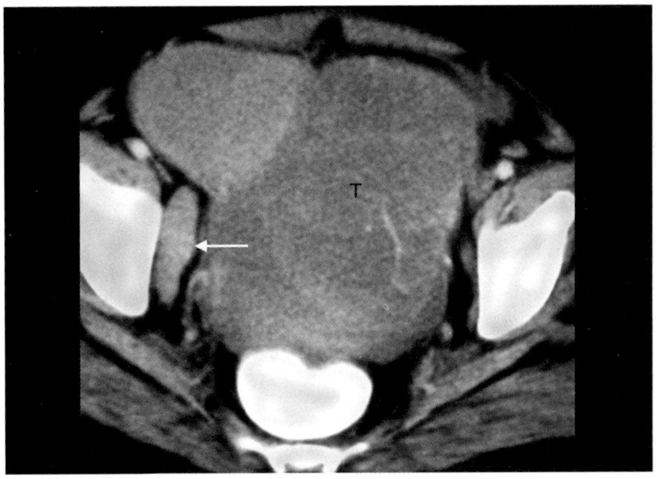

Fig. 17: Endometroid carcinoma of the ovary: CECT of the pelvis shows solid well-defined adnexal mass (T) with minimal contrast enhancement. Enlarged right obturator lymph node (arrow) is also seen.

of excellent soft tissue contrast, the details are better demonstrated. T1W fat suppressed, T2W and gadolinium enhanced T1W sequences are important in ovarian cancer. Most tumors are low or intermediate in signal intensity on T1W and high in signal intensity on T2W images **(Figs. 18A and B)**. Contrast enhancement helps to differentiate solid component of the tumor from blood clot or debris which do not enhance. MRI is better than other modalities in determining the origin of a pelvic mass as well as its characterization into benign and malignant.[33,48] Hence, it is used as a problem solving tool in the settings of indeterminate mass on sonography.[32] MR signal characteristic do not help in differentiation of benign versus malignant lesions, instead, morphological features are used for this purpose. MR features favoring malignancy are same as those for ultrasonography and CT: Size more than 4 cm, large, wall or septal thickness of more than 3 mm, solid component or nodularity and presence of necrosis.[32,49] Ancillary features supporting the diagnosis of malignancy include invasion of other pelvic structures, peritoneal deposits, ascites and lymphadenopathy. These features have accuracy of 91% in characterization of malignant ovarian tumors. Necrosis in a solid mass and vegetations in cystic masses are most reliable predictors of malignancy on MR imaging of adnexal masses.[50] MR is also accurate in demonstration of direct involvement of other pelvic structures by the ovarian tumor.

Positron Emission Tomography

PET scanning is of limited use in characterization of ovarian masses. Physiological uptake in ovaries in different phases of menstruation is a limitation in detection and characterization of ovarian cancer on PET.[51] Various benign conditions like corpus luteum cysts, dermoid and benign cystadenomas may also show FDG uptake leading to false positive result.[52] On the other hand, mucinous cystadenocarcinomas may not show uptake on PET. Hence, PET is not useful for detection and characterization of the adnexal masses.

Staging and Treatment

The prognosis and management depends on type and stage of the disease. Staging is surgical and it is done according to FIGO guidelines into four stages **(Table 3)**.

In standard surgical procedure both staging as well as therapeutic resection of the tumor are combined. The complete surgical procedure includes total abdominal hysterectomy with bilateral salpingo-oophorectomy, omentectomy, retroperitoneal lymph node sampling, peritoneal biopsies and cytology of peritoneal washings. The aim of the surgery is to stage the disease as well to achieve optimal debulking of the tumor, because adjuvant therapy is effective only if the residual tumor is less than 1 cm in size. If residual tumor is more than 1 cm, the survival of patients is poor and similar regardless of the size of the residual tumor.[34,53]

Although only 10–15% patients present with early stage (Stages I and II) diseases, high cure rate is achieved with surgery and adjuvant (postoperative) chemotherapy. Platinum and taxane based chemotherapy is normally used in combination. Patients with advanced diseases (stages III and IV) are also treated with surgery and adjuvant (postoperative) chemotherapy; however, relapses are common and most patients eventually develop resistance to the treatment.[34] Neoadjuvant (preoperative chemotherapy) is given to the patients in whom optimal cytoreductive surgery may not be possible. Many of these patients can then undergo optimal surgery.[31]

Imaging Strategies in Carcinoma of Ovary

Role of imaging in ovarian cancer is to detect and characterize adnexal masses, recognize unusual findings that may suggest atypical or alternative diagnosis, demonstrate metastases in order to prevent surgical understaging and detect specific sites of the disease that may be unresectable.[45]

Ultrasound is the primary modality is important to detect and characterize the adnexal masses in patients who are clinically suspected to have ovarian cancer. MRI may be used in equivocal cases.[32,33]

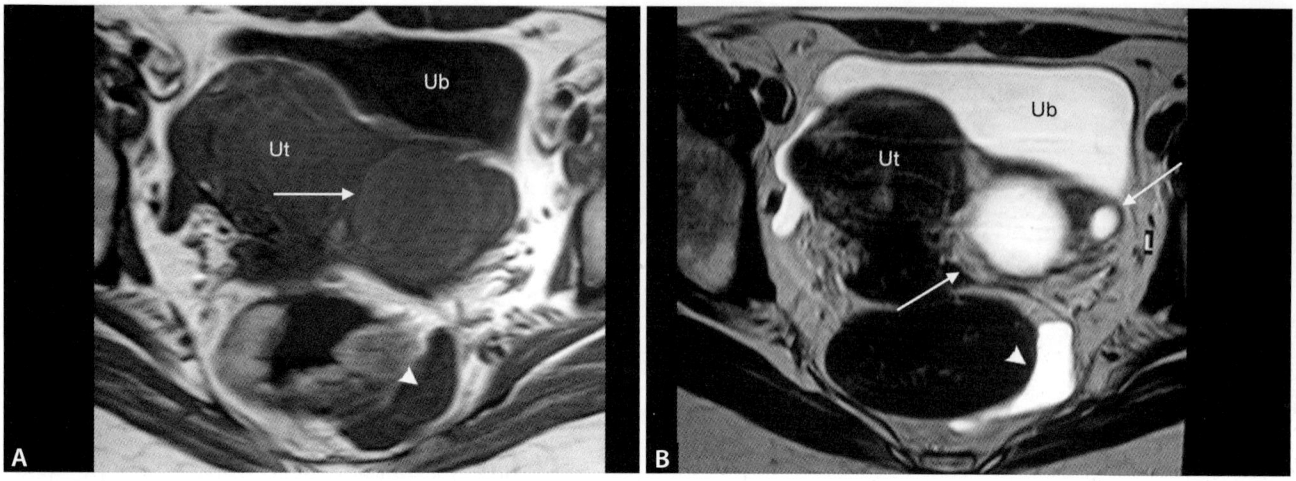

Figs. 18A and B: Carcinoma of ovary: (A) T1W and (B) T2W MR images show left adnexal mass which is homogeneously isointense on T1W image and heterogeneously hyperintense on T2W image (arrows); A large uterosacral ligament deposit is seen on left side (arrowhead) with signal intensity similar to the primary tumor.

Table 3: Staging of carcinoma of the ovary.

Stage I	**Tumor limited to ovaries** *IA:* Limited to one ovary *IB:* Limited to both ovaries *IC:* IA or IB with malignant ascites
Stage II	**Pelvic extension** *IIA:* Involvement of uterus and/or fallopian tubes *IIB:* Involvement of other pelvic organs *IIC:* IIA or IIB with malignant ascites
Stage III	**Peritoneal deposits/lymphadenopathy** *IIIA:* Microscopic deposits *IIIB:* Macroscopic (<2 cm) deposits *IIIC:* Large (>2 cm) deposits and/or lymphadenopathy
Stage IV	**Distant metastases**

Although staging of the ovarian cancer is always surgical, preoperative CT is recommended and it is now routinely obtained. Preoperative estimation of the gross extent of the disease on imaging may guide the referral to appropriate specialty. Demonstration of GIT and urinary tract involvement helps to modify the surgical plan.[45] Preoperative CT can also accurately predict the surgical outcome and hence has important role in deciding the management of ovarian cancer. Findings that suggest unresectable disease include greater than 1–2 cm deposits at porta hepatis, fissure for falciform ligament or ligamentum teres, GB fossa, diaphragm, gastrohepatic ligament, lesser sac and root of the mesentery **(Figs. 15B, 19 and 20)**. Invasion of pelvic sidewall and ureters as well as presence of retroperitoneal lymphadenopathy encasing aorta or lymphadenopathy located above the renal hilum also suggest unresectable disease. Such patients can be spared of surgery and put on neo-adjuvant chemotherapy, as optimal debulking of the disease is unlikely to be achieved in these patients.[45,54,55] Detection of distant metastases on imaging help to prevent surgical under staging, although it does not necessarily makes the patient inoperable.

In few patients with clinically diagnosed carcinoma of ovary, imaging may suggest alternative diagnosis and hence, change the management. Metastatic ovarian cancer is often similar to primary ovarian cancer in clinical presentation as well as imaging features, hence, careful search to exclude other primary site should be made on CT. The identification of different primary with metastases to ovary on imaging may change the treatment from surgery to chemotherapy. Similarly, identification of benign or less aggressive tumors like germ cell tumors on CT also change the management as these are treated with more conservative surgery.[45]

Although CT is the primary imaging modality for preoperative staging, MRI may be equal to CT.[56] At present, use of MRI in ovarian cancer limited primarily because of long imaging time required for MRI evaluation of entire abdomen and pelvis, high cost and limited availability.[32]

Borderline Epithelial Carcinoma

About 20% of all epithelial ovarian cancers are borderline tumors, also known as tumors of low malignant potential. Histologically these can be serous or mucinous and characterized by absence of stromal invasion.[34] Most patients present with stage I disease and have good

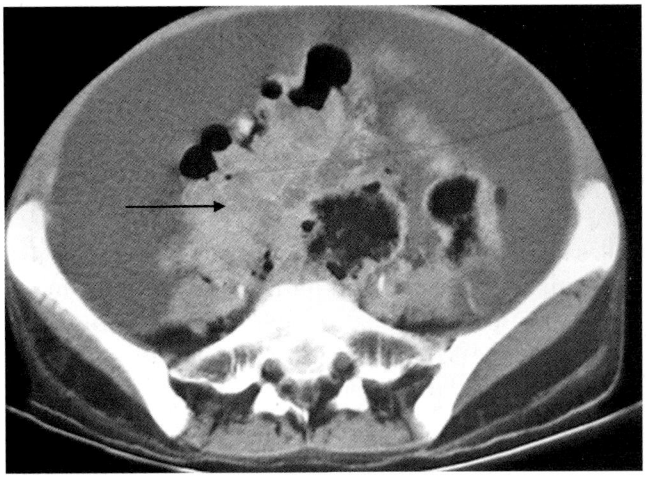

Fig. 19: Carcinoma of ovary: Large conglomerate mesenteric deposits (arrow) are seen in the mesentery involving multiple bowel loops.

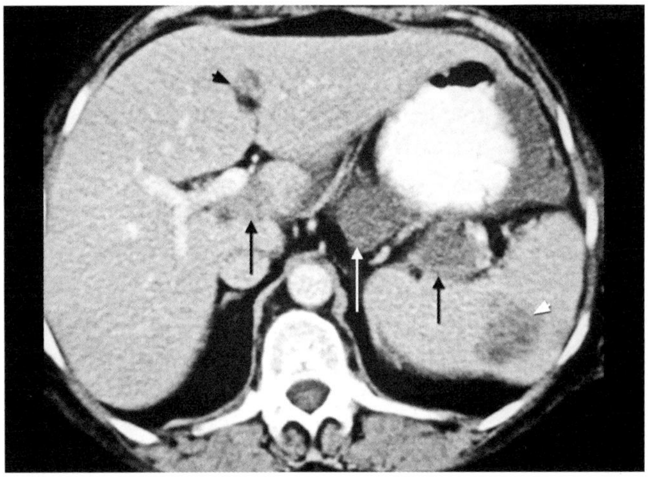

Fig. 20: Carcinoma of ovary with multiple unresectable deposits: CECT shows multiple deposits at falciform ligament (black arrowhead), porta hepatis (black arrows), lesser sac and splenic hilum (white arrow). A parenchymal deposit is also seen in the spleen (white arrowhead).

prognosis. Imaging features are similar to invasive epithelial cancers and hence imaging cannot differentiate between stage I invasive cancers and borderline cancers. Borderline tumors are treated with surgical excision and staging. Fertility preserving unilateral oophorectomy or cystectomy can also be performed. Such patients require prolonged imaging follow-up to detect recurrences.[32]

Pseudomyxoma Peritonei

Pseudomyxoma peritonei occurs due to rupture of mucinous adenocarcinoma into the peritoneal cavity leading to gelatinous deposits throughout the peritoneum.[33] Primary is often unclear and may be located in ovary, appendix or elsewhere.[57] On CT, it resembles high density ascites. Mass effect of the gelatinous material may result in characteristic scalloping of liver, spleen and bowel surfaces and septations within the fluid[45,57] **(Fig. 21)**. Prognosis is generally poor.

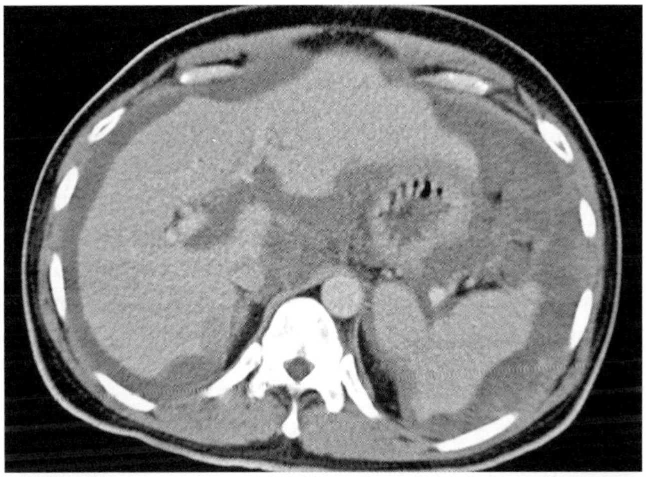

Fig. 21: Pseudomyxoma peritonei: CECT shows presence of high density ascites with indentations and scalloping on the surfaces of liver and spleen.

Primary Papillary Serous Carcinoma of the Peritoneum

Some cases of serous adenocarcinoma in women with raised serum CA-125 may demonstrate extensive peritoneal carcinomatosis but no adnexal masses. Ovaries may be normal or not visualized. Calcifications may also be present. These tumors are considered to have arisen from extraovarian peritoneum and the condition is called primary papillary serous carcinoma of the peritoneum.[58] The management however, is same as that of ovarian cancer.[34] Peritoneal tuberculosis may also mimic peritoneal carcinomatosis and the differentiation from malignancy is possible only on histopathology.[59]

Follow-up Imaging

Recurrence rate is high in ovarian cancer even after complete remission. The patients are followed up with pelvic examination, serum tumor markers (CA-125), and CT of abdomen and pelvis every 3–4 months for 2 years.[33] Less frequent follow-up is required after that. After completion of the treatment, a surgical exploration of the asymptomatic patient (second look laparotomy—SLL) was the standard procedure to document pathological complete remission. This procedure is now uncommonly performed, as CT with tumor markers is adequate for majority of the patients.

Both CT and MRI are useful in detection of macroscopic recurrences. On CT and MRI, recurrences can be seen in various forms; pelvic or vault masses, peritoneal deposits, ascites, lymphadenopathy or rarely, hematogenous metastases to various distant organs. Peritoneal deposits may be cystic or solid **(Fig. 22)**. These can be easily mistaken for unopacified bowel loops, and hence, careful search on CT is essential. The recurrences are also common at the sites of previous lesions, and hence, review of preoperative CT scans is desirable while evaluating the follow-up CT scans. Careful search for the recurrences should be made at these sites. PET CT is also useful to detect recurrences, especially in patients with rising tumor markers and normal CT scan.[60] Recurrent disease may be treated with surgery and/or chemotherapy. The CT criteria suggesting unresectability of recurrent disease are same as those for primary disease. In addition, presence of pelvic sidewall invasion, hydronephrosis and bowel obstruction are important findings which preclude the pelvic exenteration.[61]

Germ Cell Tumors of the Ovary

Germ cell tumors (GCT) of the ovary are rare. These constitute only 2–3% of ovarian cancers in west but up to 15% of ovarian cancers in Asia.[34] These affect young women below 30 years of age. GCT is the most common ovarian tumor in pediatric age group. The most common of these tumors is dysgerminoma, which is a histological counterpart of seminoma in males. Others include immature teratoma, embryonal tumor, endodermal sinus (yolk sac) tumor, choriocarcinoma and mixed germ cell tumors, which is any combination of the other tumors.

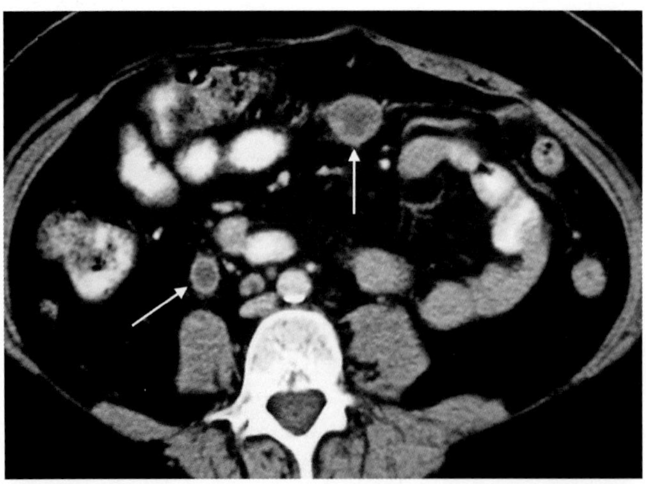

Fig. 22: Recurrent carcinoma of ovary: Multiple small cystic peritoneal deposits with enhancing nodular walls are seen (arrows). These resemble unopacified bowel loops and hence, can get overlooked.

Patients often present early when the tumor is sill confined to the ovary. Most present with abdominal pain, mass or with acute abdomen because of torsion, rupture or hemorrhage in the tumor mass. Tumor markers, such as AFP, hCG and LDH are elevated. These help diagnose yolk sac tumor (AFP only), choriocarcinoma (hCG only) and embryonal cell carcinoma (both AFP and hCG). Patients with pure immature teratoma have normal AFP and hCG levels.[34] FIGO staging of the GCT is same as that of epithelial ovarian cancer.

On cross-sectional imaging, germ cell tumors are unilateral, solid and well-defined, however cystic, necrotic or hemorrhagic areas may also be seen **(*see* Fig. 10)**. These tumors are often quite large but well defined at presentation. Spread of most germ cell tumors occur by direct extension into adjacent organs and/or by lymphatic or hematogenous dissemination. Ascites and peritoneal deposits may also be seen with germ cell tumors. Metastases to the lymph nodes, liver and lungs are more common with germ cell tumors than with epithelial carcinomas.

Dysgerminoma is the most common ovarian malignancy in children and young adults with 80% of patient under 30 years of age.[33] It is seen as large, unilateral, well-defined solid mass **(Figs. 23A and B)**. It is usually homogeneous; however, varying degree of necrosis or hemorrhage may be present. Numerous fibrovascular septa are present within the mass. Prominent arterial flow may be demonstrated in these septa on color Doppler.[62] On MRI, these septa are hypointense on T2W images and show strong enhancement.[63]

Immature teratoma is usually a unilateral solid mass with coarse calcifications and rarely intratumoral fat **(Fig. 24)**. Mature teratoma element may coexist in same or contralateral ovary.[32] Peritoneal spread is common. Gliomatosis peritonei is a condition when multiple benign or low grade malignant deposits of immature teratoma are seen throughout the peritoneal cavity. After chemotherapy, some of the immature teratoma disappear while other may transform into mature (benign) teratoma.

Yolk sac or endodermal sinus tumor is a highly malignant ovarian tumor characterized by rapid growth and early metastases. On CT and MRI, these are seen as complex cystic or solid tumors with heterogeneous and intense contrast enhancement **(Fig. 25)**. Areas of necrosis and hemorrhages are often present.

Pure embryonal cell carcinomas and choriocarcinomas (nongestational) are rare and most often these are part

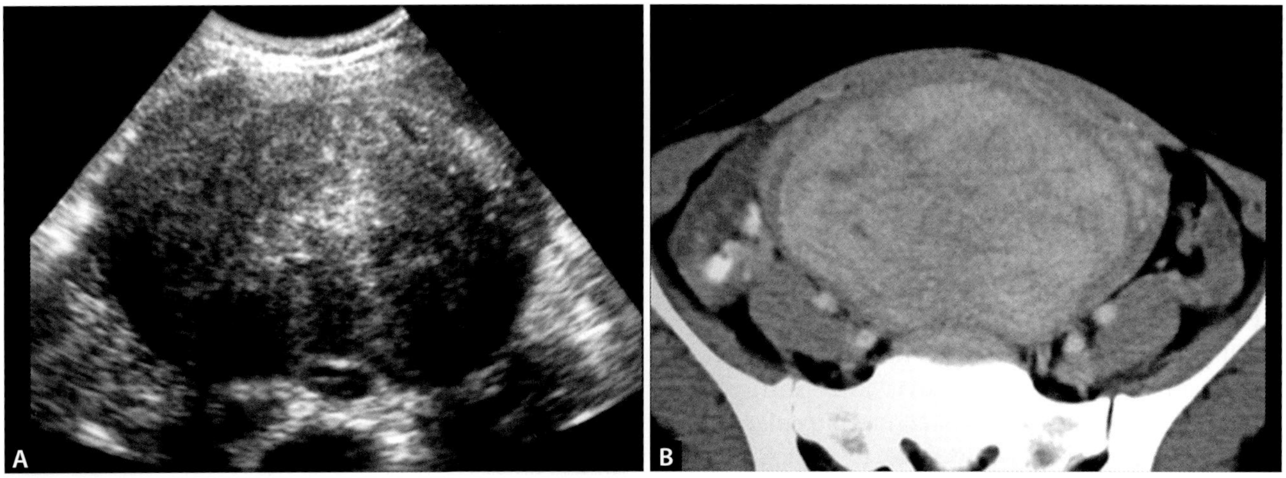

Figs. 23A and B: Dysgerminoma: (A) Ultrasonography of pelvis in a young woman shows a large, well-defined, homogeneous mass; (B) CECT shows moderately enhancing mass with same morphological features.

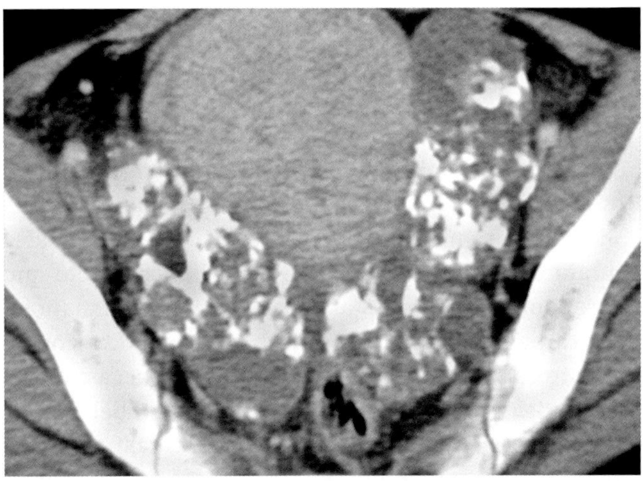

Fig. 24: Immature teratoma: CECT shows bilateral solid adnexal masses with coarse calcifications.

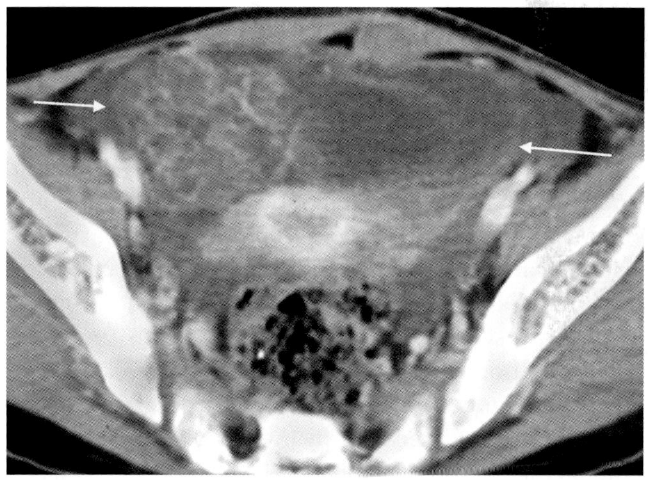

Fig. 25: Yolk sac tumor: CECT of pelvis of a female child shows large heterogeneous pelvic mass (bounded by arrows) with areas of necrosis and invasion of the uterus.

of other germ cell tumors, i.e. mixed germ cell tumors. Imaging features are nonspecific.

Most patients with germ cell tumors present with early stage disease, and hence, prognosis is usually good. Surgery with unilateral salpingo-oophorectomy and preservation of uterus and contralateral ovary can be performed in most patients, thus preserving the fertility. Advanced diseases are treated with surgery and chemotherapy. Dysgerminoma like seminoma, are radiosensitive and can be treated with radiotherapy, if preservation of fertility is not the main concern.[64] Patients are followed with periodic physical examination, serum tumor markers and sonography. CT is performed if sonographic examination is equivocal or tumor markers are rising. Functional ovarian cyst are often seen in normal ovary after fertility preserving surgery and these evoke anxiety and fear of recurrent disease; however, these can be safely followed up.[64] Recurrences after complete remission of GCTs are uncommon and occur in 10–20% of patients. Most of these occur in first two years and late relapses are extremely rare.

Stromal Sex Cord Tumors

Neoplasms arising from sex cord or stromal cells constitute 1–2% of ovarian malignancies.[32] The most common of these is granulosa cell tumor, which is almost always malignant, while fibromas, thecomas and Sertoli–Leydig cell tumors, which usually behave in benign fashion. Histology of stromal-sex cord tumors cannot accurately predict the clinical behavior and actual grade of malignancy cannot be defined. These tumors occur either in postmenopausal women or in prepubertal girls. Majority of these tumors secret estrogen and hence cause sexual precocity in girls or resumption of menses in postmenopausal women. These tumors are usually diagnosed at early stage, treated surgically and have good prognosis.

On imaging, granulosa cell tumor is usually seen as predominantly solid and multilobulated adnexal mass. MRI may show characteristic sponge like appearance as well as extensive intratumoral hemorrhages.[65] These tumors enhance heterogeneously after intravenous contrast on CT or MRI. Associated uterine enlargement and endometrial hyperplasia may also be seen. Granulosa cell tumors also have high propensity for local invasion and sacral involvement is may be present.[33] Fibrothecomas solid benign tumors but rarely, these can be malignant. Because of the high fibrous content, these show low signal intensity in T2W MRI.[65]

Metastatic Ovarian Tumors

Up to 15% of ovarian malignancies are metastatic in nature.

Common primary sites are stomach, colon and breast. Uncommon primary sites include lung, gallbladder and pancreas. 'Krukenberg tumor' is the term used for specific histological pattern of mucin-secreting signet cells with sarcomatous stroma, usually from a gastric primary.[66] Clinical presentation in metastatic ovarian tumors is variable. About one-third of the patients present with pelvic mass and not with the symptoms of primary site. Melanoma usually secondarily involves ovaries; however, primary malignant melanoma of the ovary also occurs.[67]

On cross-sectional imaging, ovarian metastases are usually seen as bilateral, large, lobulated solid or complex cystic masses **(Fig. 26)**. These are indistinguishable from primary ovarian carcinoma, although multilocularity on ultrasound or MRI is uncommon with metastases.[33,68] Ascites, peritoneal nodules and omental deposits are also seen both in primary as well as metastatic ovarian tumors. Hematogenous spread to liver is rare with primary ovarian carcinoma but common with metastatic ovarian disease. Hence, presence of intrahepatic metastases should warrant a search for primary tumor in stomach or colon. Possibility of metastatic ovarian tumor must be considered in any patient with ovarian mass if there is a known extraovarian primary cancer or liver metastases.

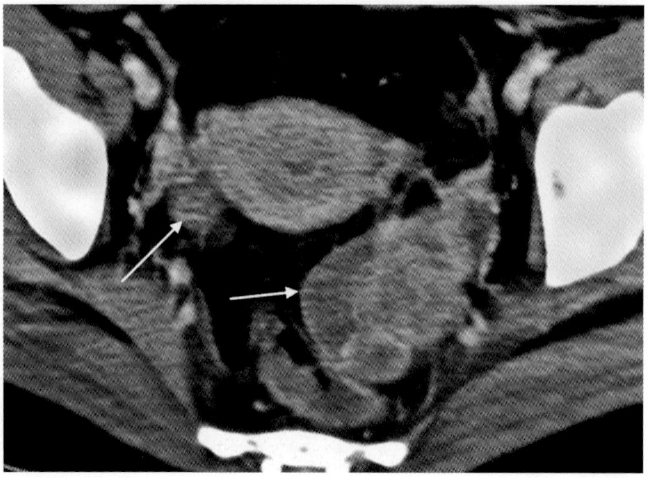

Fig. 26: Metastases to ovary: CECT of a pelvis in a woman with metastatic breast cancer shows bilateral cystic solid adnexal metastases (arrows). The appearance is indistinguishable from that of primary ovarian carcinoma.

Rare Ovarian Tumors

Brenner tumors are epithelial tumors of ovary. These are usually benign; however, some of them can be borderline or frankly malignant. Malignant Brenner tumors are also known as transitional cell carcinoma of the ovary. An imaging benign Brenner tumors are seen as homogenously solid or unilocular cystic lesions. Malignant Brenner tumor however, is indistinguishable from other epithelial carcinomas on imaging.[65,69] These may also contain calcifications.[45] Primary ovarian carcinoid and neuroendocrine tumors are rare ovarian malignancies which are related to teratoma. Hepatoid adenocarcinoma is a rare tumor which involves ovary and occasionally, the uterus. These are aggressive tumors and believed to be type of yolk sac tumors. These histologically resemble hepatocellular carcinoma and serum AFP may also be elevated. Imaging findings are nonspecific and range from solid to complex cystic-solid masses.

MISCELLANEOUS GYNECOLOGICAL MALIGNANCIES

Carcinoma of Vagina and Vulva

Secondary involvement of vagina and vulva by adjacent tumors like rectum, cervix or urinary bladder is more common than the primary carcinoma.[70] Vaginal and vulval carcinomas are rare and seen in old women. Majority of these are squamous cell carcinomas. Others include clear cell adenocarcinoma, melanoma and leiomyosarcoma.[71]

Vaginal carcinomas usually occur in upper third of the vagina. They may spread to involve adjacent structures like urinary bladder and rectum **(Fig. 27)**. Involvement of pelvic lymph nodes and hematogenous metastases

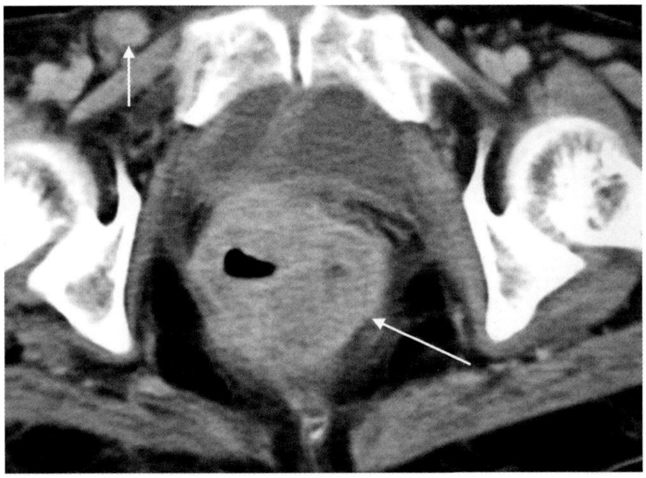

Fig. 27: Carcinoma of vagina: CECT shows enhancing pelvic floor mass involving vagina and rectum (large arrow). Enlarged right inguinal lymph node is also seen (small arrow).

may also be seen. Vulval tumors commonly involve labia majora and uncommonly, labia minora, clitoris and perineum.

These tumors are diagnosed and staged using FIGO staging similar to that of carcinoma of cervix. MRI is the preferred modality to determine the site of origin as well as extent of the tumor when this is difficult to assess clinically. Most tumors are seen as hyperintense masses on T2W and contrast-enhanced T1W images. As majority of these tumors are treated with radiotherapy, MRI facilitates the treatment planning by defining the extent of the tumor.[71]

Sarcoma of the Uterus

Uterine sarcoma are highly malignant tumors and account for 1–3% of all gynecological malignancies. These include endometrial stromal sarcoma, malignant mixed mullerian tumor (carcinosarcoma) and leiomyosarcoma. These can also arise from ovaries. Prior pelvic irradiation is associated with increased risk for the development of uterine sarcomas. Imaging features of uterine sarcomas are nonspecific and may be similar to the endometrial carcinoma or fibroids. However, these are often large at presentation and it may be difficult to determine the organ of origin on imaging. Areas of necrosis and hemorrhage, myometrial invasion and peritoneal deposits are usually seen on imaging.[13]

Rhabdomyosarcoma of uterus, cervix or vagina occurs in children and have nonspecific imaging features. Clear cell adenocarcinoma of vagina is associated with diethyl stilbesterol exposure. The characteristic imaging finding is multicystic, expansile mass in the vagina.

Fallopian Tube Carcinoma

Fallopian tube carcinoma is extremely rare. On imaging, it is seen as solid or cystic adnexal masses similar to ovarian tumors.[72] Serum CA-125 may also be elevated in cases of fallopian tube carcinoma. Hence, preoperative diagnosis of fallopian tube carcinoma is rarely made.

Gestational Trophoblastic Neoplasms

Gestational trophoblastic disease includes hydatidiform mole, invasive mole, placental site trophoblastic tumor and choriocarcinoma. These are associated with elevated serum hCG. Hydatidiform mole or molar pregnancy is not a neoplasm. Gestational trophoblastic neoplasms include placental site trophoblastic tumor and choriocarcinoma. Placental site trophoblastic tumor is a slow growing tumor and remains localized in uterus for long before metastasizing while choriocarcinoma is an aggressive variant characterized by rapid growth, widespread dissemination and propensity for hemorrhage.

Choriocarcinoma may evolve from a molar pregnancy or a full-term pregnancy. Patients usually present with vaginal bleeding, and there is elevated serum hCG. On sonography, uterus is enlarged. Endometrial cavity contains echogenic solid mass with numerous small cystic spaces and the placenta **(Fig. 28)**. Associated theca lutin cysts of the ovaries are seen in 20–50% cases.[73] Myometrial invasion in choriocarcinoma is seen as hyperechoic nodules, thickening and hypervascularity of the myometrium. CECT may show enlarged uterus with heterogeneous mass in endometrial cavity **(Fig. 29A)**. On T2W-MR images, distention of the uterus by high signal intensity mass is seen. Myometrial invasion is also better appreciated on MRI. If myometrial invasion is not seen on imaging, appearance is same as that of hydatidiform mole. Purpose of imaging however, is to establish the presence of gestational trophoblastic disease in appropriate clinical setting and to determine its extent and spread.

Choriocarcinoma spreads hematogenously. The metastases can be seen in lungs **(Fig. 29B)**, vagina, liver, spleen, GIT or brain. Few patients present with metastases from occult primary. Treatment with surgery and chemotherapy results in rapid improvement, even with widespread metastases. Choriocarcinoma should be considered in any women in reproductive age, even without a history of sexual activity, who present with abnormal bleeding, enlarged uterine cavity or metastases with occult primary. Imaging evaluation and serum hCG estimation are essential part of diagnostic work up in these patients. Nongestational choriocarcinoma are part of germ cell tumors of the ovary and usually seen as part of mixed germ cell tumors rather than pure choriocarcinoma.

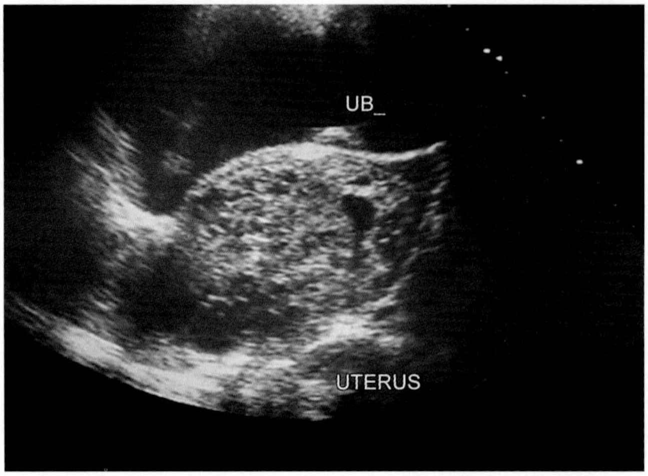

Fig. 28: Choriocarcinoma: Ultrasonography shows enlarged uterus distended with echogenic mass containing numerous tiny cystic spaces. The appearance is similar to hydatidiform mole.

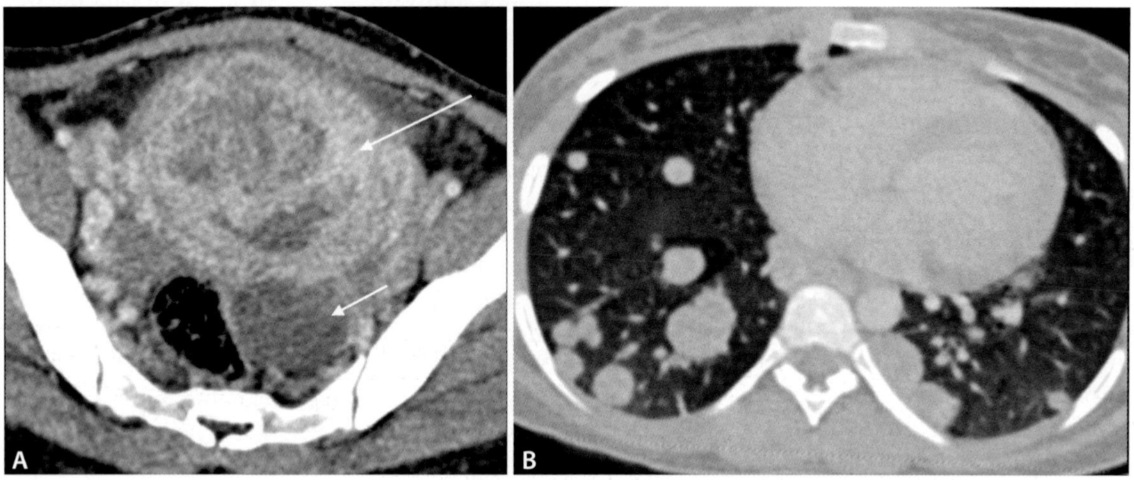

Figs. 29A and B: Choriocarcinoma: (A) CECT shows enlarged uterus distended with heterogeneously enhancing mass (large arrow), associated theca lutein cyst is also seen (small arrow); (B) Lung window of the chest CT shows characteristic cannonball metastases

Lymphoma of the Female Genital Tract

Secondary involvement of the female genital tract as a part of disseminated non-Hodgkin's lymphoma is more common than primary involvement. Infiltration of the uterus causes its diffuse enlargement **(Fig. 30)**. On MRI, the signal intesity is homogeneous with preserved normal junctional zone.[74] Lymphoma of the ovary is usually seen as bilateral, solid, large adnexal masses with little contrast enhancement.[32] On MRI, it is homogeneously hypointense on T1W images with only minimal increase in signal intensity on T2W images.[75] Ovary is the most common organ of female genital tract to be involved in leukemia, in the form of granulocytic sarcoma.[76] On imaging, these are seen as lobulated solid or complex cystic solid adnexal masses with variable contrast enhancement, similar to the primary ovarian carcinoma.[77]

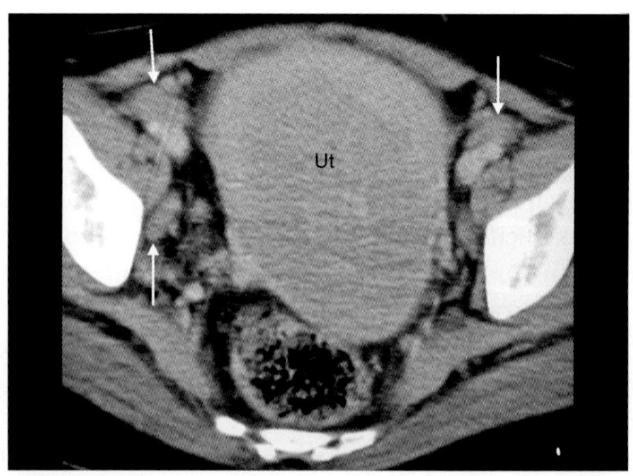

Fig. 30: Lymphoma of the uterus: CECT of the pelvis of a woman with disseminated non-Hodgkin lymphoma shows diffuse homogeneous enlargement of the uterus (Ut). Multiple enlarged pelvic lymph nodes are also seen (arrows).

REFERENCES

1. Shanta V. Perspectives in gynecological oncology. In: Lalit Kumar (Ed). Current trends in gynecologic oncology. 1st edition, Mumbai, Himalaya Publishing House; 1999. pp.1-15.
2. Indian Council of Medical Research: Consolidated report of population based cancer registries 2001-2004. At: http://icmr.nic.in/ncrp/report.pop_2001-04.
3. Eifel PJ, Berek JS, Markman MA. Cancer of the cervix, vagina and vulva. In: Devita VT, Lawrence TS, Rosenberg SA (Eds). Cancer: Principles and practice of oncology (8th edition). Lippincot, Wiliams and Wilkins, Philadelphia; 2008.pp.1496-543.
4. Boles SM, Hricak H, Rubin P. Carcinoma of the cervix and endometrium. In: Bragg DG, Rubin P, Hricak H (Eds): Oncologic Imaging, 2nd edn. Philadelphia: WB Saunders; 2002.pp.523-48.
5. Kaur H, Silverman M, Iyer RB, et al. Diagnosis, staging and surveillance of cervical carcinoma. AJR. 2003;180:1621-31.
6. Innocenti P, Pulli F, Sarini L. Staging of cervical cancer: Reliability of trans-rectal US. Radiology. 1992;185:201-05.
7. Carter JR. Cervical tumor characterization by transvaginal colour flow Doppler ultrasound. Int J Gyn Ca. 1999;9:279-84.
8. Pannu HK, Corl FM, Fishman EK. CT evaluation of cervical cancer: Spectrum of disease. Radiographics. 2001;21:1155-68.
9. Akin O, Mironav S, Taskar NP, et al. Imaging of uterinecancer. Radiol Clin N Am. 2007;45:167-82.
10. Yang WT, Lam WW, Yu MY, et al. Comparison of dynamic helical CT and Dynamic MR imaging in evaluation of pelvic lymph nodes in cervical carcinoma. AJR. 2000;175:759-66.
11. Sheu MH, Chang CY, Wang JH, et al. Preoperative staging of cervical carcinoma with MR imaging: A reappraisal of diagnostic accuracy and pitfalls. Eur Radiol. 2001;1:1828-33.
12. Lien HH, Blomlie V, Iverson T, Clinical stage 1 carcinoma of cervix: value of MR imaging in determining parametrial invasion. Acta Radiol. 1993;34:130-32.
13. Sala E, Wakely S, Senior E, et al. MRI of malignant neoplasms of the uterine corpus and cervix. AJR. 2007;188:1577-87.
14. Hricak H, Lacey CG, Sandles LG, et al. Invasive cervical carcinoma: comparison of MR imaging and surgical findings. Radiology. 1998;166:623-31.
15. Ozsarlak O, Tjalma W, Schepens E, et al. The correlation of preoperative CT, MR imaging and clinical staging with histopathology in primary cervical carcinoma. Eur Radiol. 2003;13:2338-45.
16. Hricak H, Powel GB, Yu KK. Invasive cervical carcinoma: Role of MR imaging in pretreatment work up: Cost minimization and diagnostic efficacy analysis. Radiology. 1996;198:403-9.
17. Bipat S, Glas AS, Van Der Valden J, et al. Computed tomography and magnetic resonance imaging in staging of uterine cervical carcinoma: A systematic review. Gynecol Oncol. 2003;91:59-66.
18. Hanke K, Heilman V, Straka P, et al. Pretreatment staging of cervical cancer: Is imaging better than palpation? Role of CT and MRI in preoperative staging of cervical cancer: Single institution results for 255 patients. Ann Surg Oncol. 2008:15:2856-61.
19. Rockall AG, Ghosh S, Alexander SF, et al. Can MRI rule out bladder and rectal invasion in cervical cancer to help select patients for limited EUA? Gynecol Oncol. 2006;101:244-9.
20. Rockall AG, Sohaib SA, Harsinghani MG, et al. Diagnostic performance of nanoparticle enhanced magnetic resonance imaging in the diagnosis of lymph node metastases in patients with endometrial and cervical cancer. J Clin Oncol. 2005;23:2813-21.
21. Havrilesky LJ, Kulasingam SL, Matchar DB, et al. FDG-PET for management of cervical and ovarian cancer. Gynecol Oncol. 2005:97;183-91.
22. Choi HJ, Roh JW, Seo SS, et al. Comparison of accuracy of magnetic resonance imaging and positron emission tomography/computed tomography in presurgical detection of lymph node metastases in patients with uterine cervical carcinoma: A prospective study. Cancer. 2006;106:914-22.
23. Xue F, Lin LL, Dehdashti F, et al. F-18 fluorodeoxyglucose uptake in primary cervical cancer as an indicator of prognosis after radiation therapy. Gynecol Oncol. 2006;101: 147-51.
24. Chung HH, Jo H, Kang WJ, et al. Clinical impact of integrated PET/CT on the management of suspected cervical cancer recurrence. Gynecol Oncol. 2007;104:529-34.
25. van der Veldt AA, Buist MR, van Baal MW, et al. Clarifying the diagnosis of clinically suspected recurrences of cervical cancer: Impact of 18FDG PET. J Nucl Med. 2008;49:1936-43.
26. Smith-bindman R, Kerlikoweske K, Feldstien VA, et al. Endovaginal ultrasound to exclude endometrial cancer and other endometrial abnormalities. JAMA. 1998;280:1510-17.
27. Bree RL, Bowerman RA, Bohm-Velez M, et al. US evaluation of the uterus in patients with postmenopausal bleeding: A positive effect on diagnostic decision-making. Radiology. 2000;216:260-64.
28. Alcazar JA, Ajossa S, Floris S, et al. Reproducibility of endometrial vascular patterns in endometrial diseased as assessed by transvaginal power Doppler sonography in women with post-menopausal bleeding. J Ultrasound Med. 2006;25:159-63.
29. Manfredi R, Mirk P, Maresca G, et al. Local-regional staging of endometrial carcinoma: Role of MR imaging in surgical planning. Radiology. 2004;231:372-8.
30. Shumskey AG, Stuart GC, Brasher PN, et al. An evaluation of routine follow ups of the patients treated for endometrial carcinoma. Gynecol Oncol. 2004;55:231-5.
31. Kumar L, Janga D, Berge S, et al. chemotherapy for advanced epithelial ovarian cancer. Ind J Med Pediatr Oncol. 2004;25:21-5.
32. Mironov S, Akin O, Taskar NP, et al. Ovarian cancer. Radiol Clin N Am. 2007;45:149-66.
33. Ascher SM, Imauka I, Jha RC. Tumors of adnexa. In: Bragg DG, Rubin P, Hricak H (Eds). Oncologic Imaging, (2nd edn). Philadelphia: WB Saunders; 2002.pp.549-74.

34. Cannistra SA, Gershenson DM, Recht A. Ovarian cancer, fallopian tube carcinoma and peritoneal carcinoma. In: Devita VT, Lawrence TS, Rosenberg SA (Eds). Cancer: Principles and practice of oncology, 8th edition. Lippincot, Wiliams and Wilkins, Philadelphia; 2008.pp.1568-94.
35. Brown DL, Doubilet PM, Miller FH, et al. Benign and malignant ovarian masses: Selection of the most distinguishing grey scale Doppler sonographic feature. Radiology. 1998;208:103-08.
36. Guerriero S, Alcozar JL, Coccia ME, et al. Complex pelvic masses: A target of evaluation of vessel distribution by color Doppler sonography for the diagnosis of adnexal malignancies: Results of a multicenter European study. J Ultrasound Med. 2002;21:1105-11.
37. Kurjak A, Zalud I, Alfirec Z. Evaluation of adnexal masses with transvaginal color Doppler ultrasound. J Ultrasound Med. 1991;10:295-97.
38. Levine D, Feldstein VA, Babcock CJ, et al. Sonography of ovarian masses: Poor sensitivity of resistive index for identifying malignant lesions. AJR. 1994;162:1355-9.
39. Liu J, Xu Y, Wang J. Ultrasonography, computed tomography and magnetic resonance imaging for the diagnosis of ovarian carcinoma. Eur J Radiol. 2007;62:328-34.
40. Kinkel K, Hricak H, Ying L, et al. US characterization of ovarian masses: A meta-analysis. Radiology. 2000;217: 803-11.
41. Neelam, Banerjee S, Kriplani A. Screening for ovarian cancer. In : Kumar L (Ed). Current trends in gynecologic oncology. 1st edition, Mumbai: Himalaya Publishing House; 1999.pp.80-7.
42. Sterling D, Evans GR, Pichert GR, et al. Screening for familial ovarian cancer: Failure of current protocols to detect ovarian cancer at an early stage according to the international federation of gynecology and oncology system. J Clin Oncol. 2005;23:5588-96.
43. Kauf NT, Satagopan JM, Robson ME, et al. Risk reducing salpingo-oophorectomy in women with BRCA1 or BRCA2 mutations. N Engl J Med. 2002;346:1609-15.
44. Zhang J, Mironov S, Hricak H, et al. Characterization of adnexal masses using feature analysis at contrast enhanced helical computed tomography. J Comput Assist Tomogr. 2008;32:533-40.
45. Cookley FV. Staging ovarian cancer: Role of imaging. Radiol Cin N Am. 2002;40:609-36.
46. Pannu HK, Horton KM, Fishman EK, et al. Thin section dual phase multidetector row computed tomography detection of peritoneal metastases in gynecologic cancers. J Comput Assist Tomogr. 2003;27:333-40.
47. Holloway BJ, Gore PH, Hern RP, et al. The significance of paracardiac lymph nodes enlargement in ovarian cancer. Clin Radiol. 1997;52:692-7.
48. Kurtz AB, Tsimikas JV, Tempany CM, et al. Diagnosis and staging of ovarian cancer: Comparative values of Doppler and conventional US, CT and MR imaging correlated with surgery and histopathologic analysis-report of the Radiology Diagnostic Oncology group. Radiology. 1999;212:19-27.
49. Sohaib SA, Sahdev A, Van Trappen P, et al. Characterization of adnexal mass lesions on MR imaging. AJR. 2003;180:1297-304.
50. Hricak H, Chen M, Coakely FV, et al. Complex adnexal masses: Detection and characterization with MR imaging-multivariate analysis. Radiology. 2000;214:39-46.
51. Subhas N, Patel PV, Pannu HK, et al. Imaging of pelvic malignancies with in-line FDG PET-CT: Case examples and common pitfalls of FDG-PET. Radiographics. 2005;25:1031-43.
52. Frenchel S, Grab D, Nuesle K, et al. Asymptomatic adnexal masses: Correlation of FDG-PET and histologic findings. Radiology. 2002;223:780-8.
53. Hoskins WJ. Epithelial ovarian carcinoma: Principle of primary surgery. Gynecol Oncol. 1994;55:S91-6.
54. Nelson BE, Rosenfield AT, Schwartz PE. Preoperative abdominopelvic computed tomography prediction of optimal cytoreduction in epithelial ovarian carcinoma. J Clin Oncol. 1993;11:166-72.
55. Qayyum A, Coakley FV, Westphalen AC, et al. Role of CT and MR imaging in predicting optimal cytoreduction of newly diagnosed primary epithelial ovarian cancer. Gynecol Oncol. 2005;96:301-6.
56. Tempany CM, Zou KH, Silverman SG, et al. Staging of advanced ovarian cancer: Comparison of imaging modalities-report from Radiological Diagnostic Oncology Group. Radiology. 2000;215:761-7.
57. Zissin R, Gayer G, Fishman A, et al. Synchronous mucinous tumors of the ovary and appendix associated with pseudomyxoma peritonei: CT findings. Abdom Imaging. 2000;25:311-6.
58. Chopra S, Laurie LR, Chintapally KN, et al. Primary papillary serous carcinoma of the peritoneum: CT–pathologic correlation. J Comput Assist Tomogr. 2000;24:395-9.
59. Ha HK, Jung JL, Lee MS, et al. CT differentiation of tubercular peritonitis and peritoneal carcinomatosis. AJR. 1996;167: 743-78.
60. Murakami M, Miyamato T, Lida T, et al. Whole body positron emission tomography and tumor marker CA 125 for detection of recurrence in epithelial ovarian cancer. Int J Gynecol Cancer. 2006;16:99-107.
61. Funt FA, Hricak H, Abu Rustum N, et al. Role of CT in the management of recurrent ovarian cancer. AJR. 2004;182:393-8.
62. Kim SH, Kang SB. Ovarian dysgerminomas: Colour Doppler ultrasonographic findings and comparison with CT and MR findings. J Ultrasound Med. 1995;14:843-8.
63. Tanaka YO, Kurosaki Y, Nishida M, et al. Ovarian dysgerminoma: MR and CT appearance. J Comput Assist Tomogr. 1994;18:443-8.
64. Kumar L, Kumar S, Kriplani A, et al. Malignant germ cell tumors of ovary In: Kumar L (Ed). Current trends in gynecologic oncology. (1st ed); Himalaya Publishing House Mumbai; 1999.pp.100-17.
65. Imaoka I, Wada A, Kaji Y, et al. Developing and MR imaging strategy for diagnosis of ovarian masses. Radiographics. 2006;26:1431-48.

66. Ha HK, Back SY, Kim SH, et al. Krukenbergs's tumor of the ovary: MR imaging features. AJR. 1995;164:1435-9.
67. Vimla N, Kumar L, Thulkar S. Primary malignant melanoma in ovarian cystic teratoma. Gynecol Oncology. 2001;82:380-83.
68. Brown DL, Zou KH, Tempany CM, et al. Primary versus secondary ovarian malignancy: Imaging findings of adnexal masses in radiology diagnostic oncology group study. Radiology. 2001;219:213-8.
69. Oh SN, Rha SE, Jung SE, et al. Transitional cell tumor of the ovary: Computed tomographic and magnetic resonance imaging features with pathologic correlation. J Comput Assist Tomogr. 2009;33:106-12.
70. Parikh JH, Barton DP, Ind TE, et al. MR imaging features of vaginal malignancies. Radiographics. 2008;28:49-63.
71. Chang SD. Imaging of vagina and vulva. Radiol Clin N Am. 2002;40:637-58.
72. Slanetz PJ, Whitman GJ, Halpern EF, et al. Imaging of fallopian tube tumors. AJR. 1997;169:1321-4.
73. Green CL, Angtuaco TL, Shah HR. Gestational trophoblastic disease: A spectrum of radiologic diagnosis. Radiographics. 1996;16:1371-84.
74. Kim YS, Cho O, Song S, et al. MR imaging of primary uterine lymphoma. Abdom Imaging. 1997;22:441-4.
75. Ferrozzi F, Tognini G, Bova D, et al. Non-Hodgkin lymphomas of the ovaries: MR findings. J Comput Assist Tomogr. 2000;24: 416-20.
76. Kamble R, Sharma A, Thulkar S, et al. Granulocytic sarcoma of uterine cervix as presentation of acute myeloid leukemia: A case report and review of literature. J Obstet Gynecol Res. 1997;23:261-6.
77. Jung SE, Chun KA, Park SH, et al. MR findings in ovarian granulocytic sarcoma. Br J Radiol. 1997;72:301-3.

CHAPTER 124

Imaging of Scrotum

Anupam Lal, Manphool Singhal

ANATOMY

The scrotum is a cutaneous pouch which contains the testes and parts of the spermatic cords. It is formed by the fusion of two scrotal sacs separated by an inner septum that corresponds to a midline ridge or raphé on the surface, which continues on the ventral surface anteriorly and in the midline of the perineum up to the anus. The left half of the scrotum hangs lower than the right to correspond with the greater length of the left spermatic cord. The wall of the scrotum is made of the following structures from the deep to the superficial layers: internal spermatic fascia, cremasteric fascia, external spermatic fascia, dartos muscle, superficial fascia and rugated skin. The testes are suspended in the scrotal sac by the spermatic cord and are anchored to scrotal wall caudally by gubernaculum testis. It is a cord-like structure located caudal to the testis and guides the testicular descent.

Each testis is ovoid in shape and is placed obliquely in the scrotal sac; the superior and inferior poles are directed anteriorly and slightly laterally, posteriorly and slightly medially, respectively; the anterior border is convex and is oriented in anteroinferior direction, and posterosuperiorly the cord is attached to the posterior or straight border. The anterior border, lateral surfaces and poles are smooth, free, convex, and covered by the visceral layer of the tunica vaginalis all around except the posterior border which is only partially covered. The body of the epididymis is located on the posterior border in its lateral edge. Visceral and parietal layers of tunica vaginalis surround the testis and epididymis with presence of cavity in between containing little serous fluid secreted by the peritoneal lining 'saccus vaginalis' which descends from the abdomen into the scrotum before the decent of testis. The testicular capsule is formed by tunica albuginea and is covered by tunica vaginalis, except at the sites where epididymis is attached to testis and at the entry of spermatic vessels along its posterior border. An incomplete vertical septum is formed at the posterior border due to interior reflection of tunica vasculosa over the testicular glandular septum called the mediastinum testis. The testis is divided into 250–400 lobules by multiple fibrous septae entering the mediastinum testis. Seminiferous tubules are seen with in these lobules which supports the Sertoli cells and spermatocytes forming the sperm. Testosterone-secreting Leydig cells are also seen within the loose connective tissue within these tubules.

All tubules drain into larger ducts called tubuli recti. These tubuli recti converge to form the rete testis, an anastomosing network of draining tubules, and enter into mediastinum testis, which caries the sperms from testis to the epididymis. The mediastinum testis consists of invagination of tunica albuginea and the rete testis. It also contains branches of testicular arteries, centripetal veins and lymphatics of the testis and hence is the anatomical hilum of the testis.

Size of the testes is dependent on stage of sexual development and age. Approximate dimension of the testis at birth is 1.5 cm in length and 1 cm in width. The volume of testis is around 1–2 cm^3 before the age 12 years. Clinical consideration for a male individual to have reached puberty is testicular volume of 4 cm^3. Postpubertal testis measures 4–5 cm in length, 2.5 cm in breadth, and 3 cm in the antero-posterior diameter and weighs 10.5–14 g.

Parts of epididymis are the head, an enlarged upper extremity (globus major), body or the central portion, and the tail, a pointed lower extremity (globus minor). The head of the epididymis consists of 8–12 efferent ducts converging into a single larger duct in the body and tail and it lies cephalad to the testis. The vas deferens is derived from this single larger duct and continues in the spermatic cord.

Remnants of embryonic ducts give rise to various testicular appendages like the appendix epididymis, the appendix testis, the vas aberrans, and the paradidymis.[1] The appendix testis (hydatid of Morgagni) is the remnant of the upper part of the Müllerian duct and is seen on ultrasound as a small oval sessile body near superior pole of the testis beneath the epididymis head. The appendix of the epididymis (pedunculated hydatid) lying on the head of the epididymis as a small stalked appendage (sometimes duplication is regarded as detached part of efferent duct). The spermatic cord consists of the internal and external spermatic arteries, the artery to the ductus deferens, veins, lymphatics, nerves, and the excretory duct of the testis. They are anchored together by areolar tissue and covered by the layers of peritoneal lining brought down during the descent of the testis.

Testicular covering is supplied by the external pudendal branches of the femoral (superficial and deep), the superficial perineal branch of the internal pudendal, and the cremasteric branch from the inferior epigastric artery and veins of the corresponding arteries. The lymphatics drain into the inguinal lymph glands. Nerve supply is by lumboinguinal and ilioinguinal branches of the lumbar plexus, the two superficial perineal branches of the internal pudendal nerve, and the pudendal branch of the posterior femoral cutaneous nerve.

IMAGING MODALITIES

Ultrasonography (USG) with a high-frequency transducer (7.5–10 MHz) has been considered the best imaging modality for the scrotum. Sonography combined with color Doppler and power Doppler has evolved into an all-encompassing scrotal imaging technique as both structural and perfusion abnormalities can be detected. The ability to detect testicular perfusion in acute scrotal pain using color and power Doppler USG helps making specific diagnosis. MRI and nuclear scan are other important complementary modalities. CT scan and MRI have important role in staging of testicular cancer and for the localization of testis in patients with cryptorchidism.

Technique of Sonography

The patient is placed in the supine position and the scrotal support given by placing a towel between the thighs. Optimal images can be obtained with a high-frequency linear-array transducer (7–10 MHz). Superficial lesions can be evaluated using a stand-off pad. The examination of the testes should be carried out in least two planes, i.e. longitudinal and transverse axes. Comparison made between the size and echogenicity of each testis and the epididymis with contralateral side. In patients with an acute scrotum, the examination should start with the asymptomatic side to adjust the gain settings of grayscale and color Doppler for comparing comparison with the diseased side. Small palpable nodules can be imaged effectively by directly placing the transducer over the nodule after placing the finger beneath the nodule. Scrotal skin thickness should be evaluated, and it depends on the state of the cremasteric muscle contraction (normal 2–8 mm). Extratesticular masses and other abnormalities are detected by examining the scrotal sac structures. Venous structures are evaluated using additional techniques like Valsalva maneuver or erect posture.

Echogenicity of testes during prepubertal age is low to medium, while pubertal and postpubertal testes is medium and the reason being maturation of tubules and the development of germ cell elements.[2] An echogenic band of variable thickness and length is seen oriented in craniocaudal direction called the mediastinum testis **(Fig. 1)**. Minimal fluid is seen normally between the

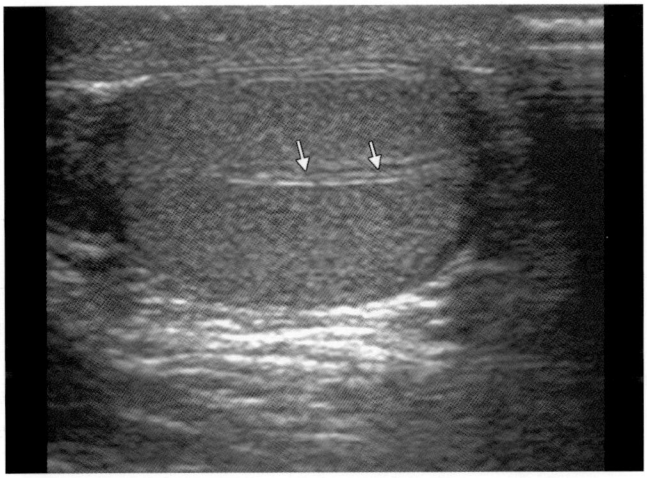

Fig. 1: USG of the testis in its long axis showing echogenic line of mediastinum testes (arrows).

two leaves of the tunica vaginalis that appear as thin echolucent area adjacent to epididymis head, and it should not be misinterpreted as hydrocele. Longitudinal view best shows the epididymis, and its head appears as a pyramidal structure 5–12 mm in maximum length seen over the superior pole of the testis with same echogenicity as that of testis with coarser echotexture as compared to the testis.[3] The body of epididymis is narrower (2–4 mm in diameter) and is difficult to distinguish from the adjacent peritesticular tissue. The tail of the epididymis (approximately 2–5 mm in diameter) is a curved structure and becomes the proximal portion of the ductus deferens near the inferior pole of the testis.

Doppler shows characteristic low-resistance spectral pattern,[4] with a mean resistive index of 0.62 (range, 0.48–0.75);[2] however, diastolic flow may not be detectable when the testicular volume is less than 4 cm,[3] often found in prepubertal boys.[5]

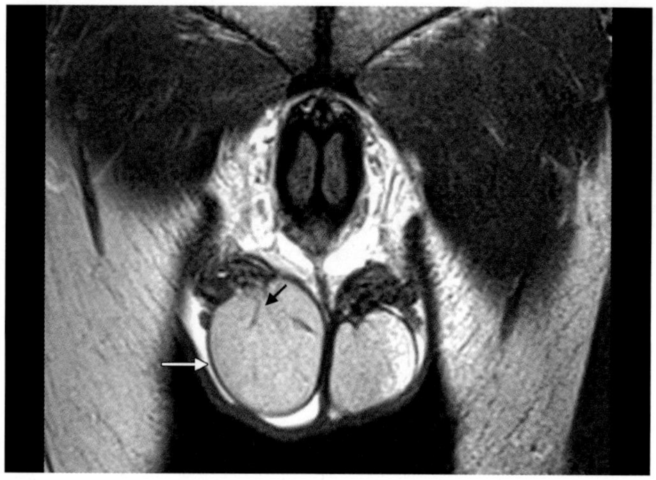

Fig. 2: T2 coronal MR image of the scrotum showing testes as high-signal intensity structures within the scrotum. Note the hypointense rim of tunica albuginea (white arrow) around the testes and the mediastinum testis (black arrow) within it.

MRI of Scrotum

MRI of the scrotum is extremely valuable as a problem solving modality. The MR examination is performed in supine position with scrotum supported by towel. Symmetric placement of testis is important for optimal coronal scans. The scrotum is then covered by small cloth or gauze and the surface coil is placed over it in a flat position. T1- and T2-weighted spin echo images are acquired in coronal and axial planes. Contrast-enhancement or fat-suppression sequences are also obtained when further tissue characterization is required. Optimum coverage is provided by thin (4–5 mm) slices with 1–2 mm interslice gaps and 8–20 cm field of view. The scan area must be extended to lower pole of kidneys when looking for undescended testis and up to the diaphragm when MRI is performed for staging of testicular cancer.

On MRI, the testis appears as an oval, well-defined structure with uniform intermediate signal intensity on T1W images and high-signal intensity on T2W images **(Fig. 2)**. The tunica albuginea appears as a thin hypointense rim around the testis.

The mediastinum testis is also hypointense, and it is seen as a dark stripe invaginating into the testis. The epididymis appears similar to testis on T1W images and much lower on T2W images. The pampiniform plexus is seen as a tortuous tubular structure extending from upper pole of testis up to the inguinal canal. Vas deferens can sometimes be seen as a low intensity tubular structure that can be traced from tail of the epididymis to the inguinal canal.

CONGENITAL ANOMALIES OF THE TESTIS

Cryptorchidism

Cryptorchidism is defined as failure of migration of one or both testes to scrotal base. It is more common in premature males (9–30%) than full-term (4–5%). The testis is positioned anywhere along its usual path of descent (the position can be abdominal, inguinal, prescrotal, or gliding); however, about 80% of nonpalpable undescended testis are located in inguinal canal and remaining 20% are intra-abdominal.[6] Current advice is early correction at 3–6 months of age. Normal complete descent is necessary for full maturation of the testis. Complications of undescended testis include infertility, malignant degeneration, torsion and inguinal hernia. Orchiopexy can be performed even after puberty for better surveillance of the testis. If orchiopexy is not feasible, orchidectomy is considered in patients after puberty. Recent epidemiologic studies indicate a 2.5–8 times greater risk of developing malignancy in cryptorchid testis.[7] The most common malignancy in the undescended testis is seminoma. Orchiopexy does not reduce the risk of malignant degeneration of the undescended testis; however, it allows better surveillance. Seminoma occurrence in one testis may prompt unilateral orchiectomy; however, the remaining testis also pose higher risk for development of malignancy.

Ultrasound examination is indicated for the localization of undescended testis and also for the follow-up after orchiopexy. The undescended testis is often smaller and iso- or hypoechoic in echogenicity. Identification of mediastinum testis helps in differentiating this with other similar appearing structures like lymph nodes. The most common location of undescended testis is distal to external inguinal ring anterior to the pubic tubercle. Even small rudimentary testis can be identified if it is located here, and hence, sonography is the primary imaging modality used for the localization of undescended testis **(Fig. 3)**. Suprapubic, perineal and femoral regions should also be examined if testis is not detected in the inguinal canal or base of the scrotum. Intra-abdominal testis is difficult to locate on sonography.

MRI is an excellent modality for demonstration of penoscrotal or intracanalicular testis but is not very satisfactory for demonstration of high intra-abdominal testis. Bladder should be emptied before the scanning. Fast T1W and T2W axial and coronal images are obtained from scrotum to above the seminal vesicles. The examination is extended up to lower pole of the kidneys if testis is not located in the pelvis. The undescended testis can be easily identified with its characteristic signal intensity pattern. It tends to be oval in inguinal canal and round in intra-abdominal position. Sometimes, the gubernaculum testis may be misdiagnosed as the undescended testis. While testis typically is hypointense on T1W and hyperintense on T2W images, the guber-naculum testis is hypointense on both T1W and T2W images. Hypertrophied inguinal lymph nodes may also have the signal characteristics similar to the testis; however, typical location of the nodes (adjacent to vessels or below the inguinal ligament) and demonstration of mediastinum in undescended testis help differentiate testis from the lymph nodes. CT, like MRI, also allows accurate identification of the cryptorchid testis.

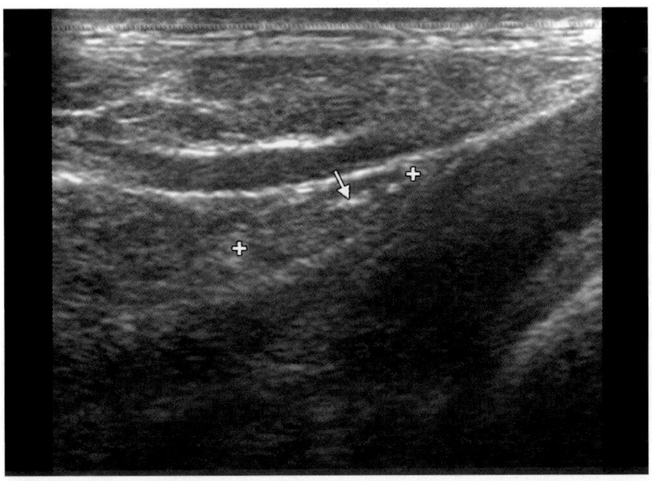

Fig. 3: USG of left undescended testis in a 24-year-male. The testis is atrophic and located distal to external inguinal ring anterior to the pubic tubercle. Mediastinum testes is identified within the testis (arrow).

Miscellaneous Congenital Anomalies

Retractile or migratory testis is common in boys 5–6 years old and is due to a hyperactive cremaster muscle reflex. The testis slides back and forth between scrotum and external inguinal ring. These usually take normal intrascrotal position by puberty and no treatment is required. The ectopic testis, i.e. location outside the descent path, is rare and the usual sites of testicular ectopia are perineum, femoral canal, superficial inguinal pouch (lateral to external inguinal ring), suprapubic area, and contralateral scrotal pouch.[8] The etiology is believed to be misdirected attachment to the scrotum. Unilateral absence of testis (monorchia) is usually left sided.[9] Unlike cryptorchidism, the testis in the patients with monorchia is not at increased risk of malignancy. Polyorchidism or testicular duplication is very rare and only few cases have been reported.[8]

ACUTE SCROTUM

Acute scrotum is a clinical condition characterized by sudden onset of pain, swelling and redness of the scrotum that may occur alone or in any combination. It is essential to differentiate as early as possible from the conditions, such as testicular torsion or rupture that require immediate surgery from those that are managed conservatively, such as epididymitis. Clinical examination alone may not be helpful or it may be difficult to perform in patients with acute tender scrotum. Acute inflammation and testicular torsion are most important causes of acute scrotal pain. Other causes include torsion of appendix of testis or epididymis, trauma, tumor, incarcerated inguinal hernia and thrombophlebitis of the pampiniform plexus.

Epididymitis and Orchitis

The most common cause of acute scrotum in postpubertal adults is epididymitis. It is almost always caused by descending lower urinary tract infection. In children and older men *E. coli, Proteus* and *Pseudomonas* are the usual causative organisms. In young men, sexually transmitted organisms, such as gonococci and *Chlamydia* are responsible. Rare causes of epididymitis and orchitis include tuberculosis, sarcoidosis,[10] mumps, brucellosis,[11] and cryptococosis. Drugs causing epididymitis is amiodarone hydrochloride (chemical epididymitis).[12] Direct extension of the inflammation in testis, resulting in epididymo-orchitis occurs in about 20% of patients with epididymitis.[13] Isolated orchitis is rare except when caused by viral infections, such as mumps and AIDS.[14] Infarction, abscess, gangrene, chronic pain, infertility, atrophy, and pyocele are various complications of acute epididymitis.

Patients present with insidious pain and scrotal swelling. Fever, dysuria and urethral discharge may also be present. Clinically, epididymitis is identified using the Prehn sign where epididymitis-associated scrotal pain is usually relieved on elevation of the testes over the symphysis pubis.[15] Findings on grayscale USG include a bulky hypoechoic or hyper-echoic (likely secondary to hemorrhage) epididymis[2] **(Fig. 4)**. Reactive hydrocele or pyocele with scrotal wall thickening represents indirect signs of inflammation.

The presence of testicular enlargement and heterogeneous echotexture indicates diffuse testicular involvement. Testicular edema from orchitis results heterogeneous echogenicity on ultrasound.[16] Involvement could be either focal or diffuse, with the former presenting as multiple hypoechoic lesions within the parenchyma of testis **(Fig. 5)**. Similar appearance can also be seen in lymphoma and leukemia of the testis; however, they are often (but not always) bilateral, whereas infection is usually unilateral (except mumps).

The color Doppler USG has got sensitivity of nearly 100% in identifying scrotal inflammation.[17] There is increase in number and density of vessels due to hyperemia causing high-flow, low-resistance pattern in acute epididymitis.[18] Spectral waveform and resistive index assessment provide useful information, and the resistive index is rarely less than 0.5 in a normal person and is less than 0.5 in more than 50% patients with epididymo-orchitis.[19] Use of a peak systolic velocity threshold of 15 cm/sec results in a diagnostic accuracy of 90% for orchitis and 93% for epididymitis.[20] Reversal of flow during diastole in acute epididymo-orchitis is suggestive of venous infarction.[21] Follow-up sonography is necessary in patients who do not respond to therapy. However, it is not required in patients with uncomplicated epididymitis.

In acute epididymitis, enlarged epididymis with high-signal intensity on T2W images is seen on MRI. Areas of hemorrhages and hypervascularity (in the form of engorged vessels with signal void) can also be demonstrated. The inflamed epididymis shows marked enhancement on postcontrast images. Associated orchitis, if present, is seen as homogeneous or heterogeneous hypointense areas in testis on T2W images.

The sonographic findings in chronic epididymitis are nonspecific and diagnosis is usually made on the basis of clinical findings. Patients presents with persistent pain in the scrotum. An enlarged epididymis with increased echogenicity is seen at grayscale USG.[22] Calcifications may be seen in the epididymis. Granulomatous epididymo-orchitis can be caused by tuberculosis, brucellosis, sarcoidosis, leprosy, and syphilis **(Fig. 6)**.

Torsion

Testicular torsion occurs due to rotation of testis on the longitudinal axis of spermatic cord. Initially, venous drainage is stopped resulting in edema and hemorrhages. Subsequently, arterial flow is also impaired resulting in ischemia and hemorrhagic necrosis of the gonad. It is a surgical emergency, as delay in diagnosis and intervention leads to irreversible damage to the testis. There may be varying degrees of testicular torsion from 180 to 720° or greater. The salvage rate depends on the duration of ischemia and the degree of torsion. Almost 100%

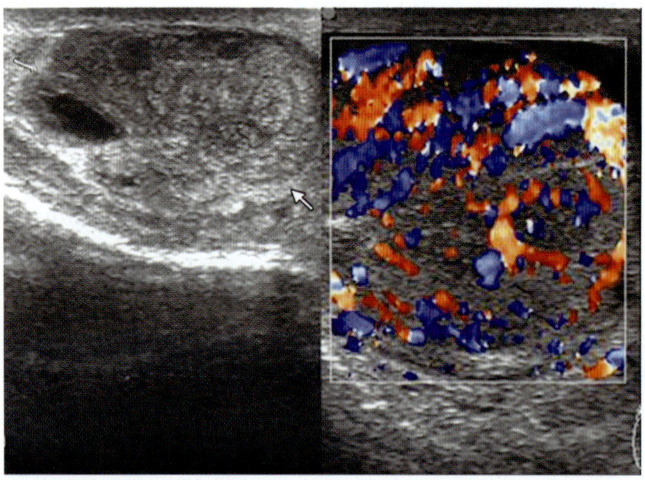

Fig. 4: USG and color Doppler of acute epididymitis showing enlarged heterogeneous epididymal head with increased vascularity.

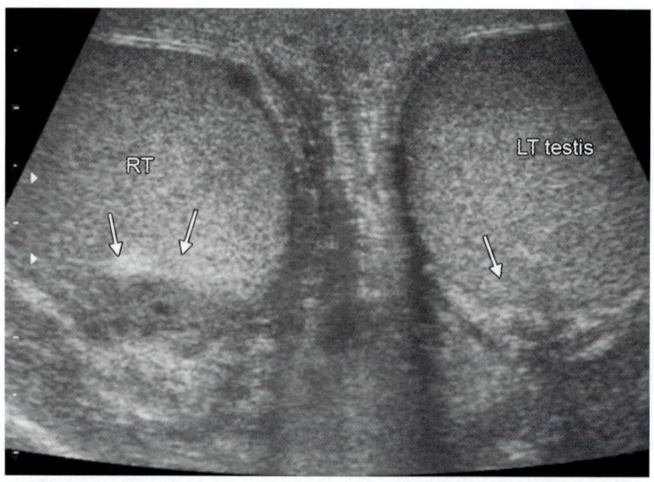

Fig. 5: Bilateral epididymorchitis: USG showing enlarged heterogeneous epididymis posterior to both testes and hypoechoic areas within the testes (arrows).

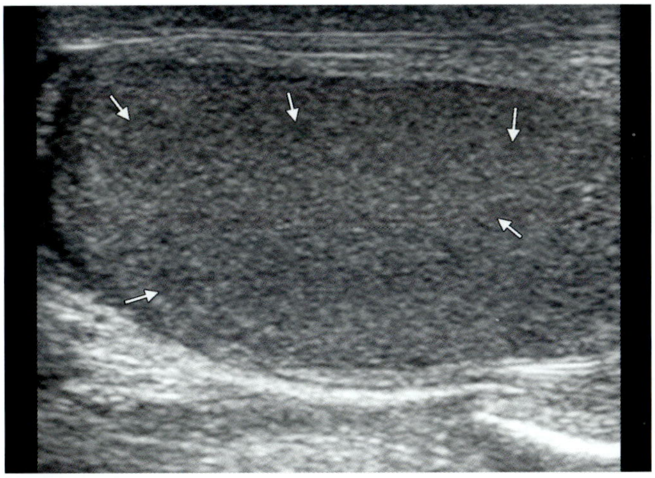

Fig. 6: Granulomatous orchitis in a case of syphilis: USG showing multiple ill-defined hypoechoic lesions (arrows) within the testis.

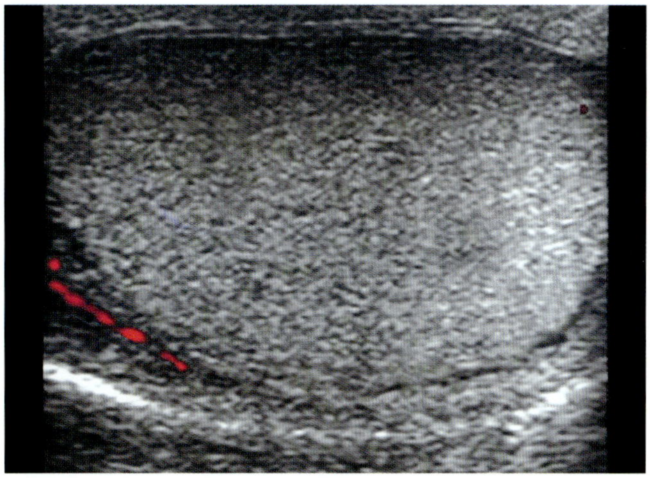

Fig. 7: Power Doppler USG showing heterogeneous appearing testis with reduced intratesticular flow in a case of torsion of testis.

successful salvage rate is seen in the first 6 hours after the onset of symptoms which decreases to 70% in 6–12 hours and 20% in 12–24 hours.[23]

Two types of testicular torsion are extravaginal and intravaginal. Extravaginal torsion is rare and occurs almost exclusively in neonates. It occurs when testis and gubernaculum are freely rotating in the scrotum and not fixed. The entire vaginal sac, including testis rotates at the level of external inguinal ring. It often presents as a mass in the groin in newborns. Intravaginal torsion occurs within the vaginal sac. It results from anomalous suspension of testis by a long stalk of spermatic cord and most commonly occurs in boys around the puberty. There is tenfold increased incidence of torsion in undescended testis after orchiopexy.[24]

Approximately two-third cases of torsion occur between 12 and 18 years of age. Clinically, patients present with sudden onset of pain in scrotal region with associated low-grade fever, nausea and vomiting. On local examination inflamed hemiscrotum is tender and swollen. USG is considered the first step in evaluation. Findings depend on the degree and duration of rotation of the spermatic cord. The testis may show normal appearance during the early stage of torsion, so grayscale images are nonspecific. The most commonly encountered findings seen around 4–6 hours after the onset of torsion are increased bulk of the testis and decreased echogenicity **(Fig. 7)**. Heterogeneous appearance of testis due to congestion of vessels, hemorrhage, and infarction (late or missed torsion) occurs after 24 hours of onset of pain. Epididymal head appears enlarged and hypoechoic due to involvement of deferential artery supplying the epididymis.[25] A strong predictor of testicular viability is presence of normal testicular echogenicity in a case of torsion. Presence of thickening of scrotal wall and reactive hydrocele are other indicators.

Torsion may be complete, incomplete, or transient. Diagnostic dilemma is seen in cases of partial or transient torsion. The accuracy of color Doppler USG imaging to diagnose incomplete torsion remains elusive. The detection of color or power Doppler signal does not exclude torsion in a patient with the clinical findings of torsion.[26]

For accurate diagnosis the scanner should be optimized for detection of slow flow and be adjusted for the low threshold setting with the lowest repetition frequency. The threshold setting is set just above the level for detection of color noise. Absent intratesticular color flow on Doppler US has sensitivity of 86%, specificity of 100%, and accuracy of 97% in diagnosing torsion and ischemia in patients of acute scrotum.[17] The accuracy of diagnosing torsion in adolescents and adults is similar among both scintigraphy and color Doppler US.[17] When the sensitivity of detecting low-velocity, low-volume testicular blood flow is insufficient in color Doppler US, scintigraphy can be used as an alternative for diagnosing torsion **(Fig. 8)**.

Torsion of the appendix testis and appendix epididymis mimics torsion testis; however no other physical symptoms is present in these cases. On local examination, "blue dot" sign can be seen which is palpation of a small firm nodule on the superior aspect of the testis exhibiting bluish discoloration through the overlying skin.[27] Approximately 91–95% of twisted testicular appendices involve the appendix testis and occur most often in boys in the age group of 7–14 years. A hyperechoic mass with a central hypoechoic area is seen near the epididymis or

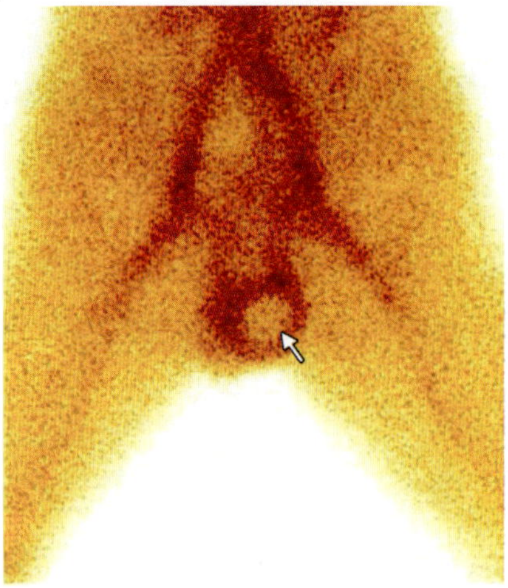

Fig. 8: Tc-99m pertechnetate scan showing photopenic area (arrow) in scrotum due to torsion of left testis.

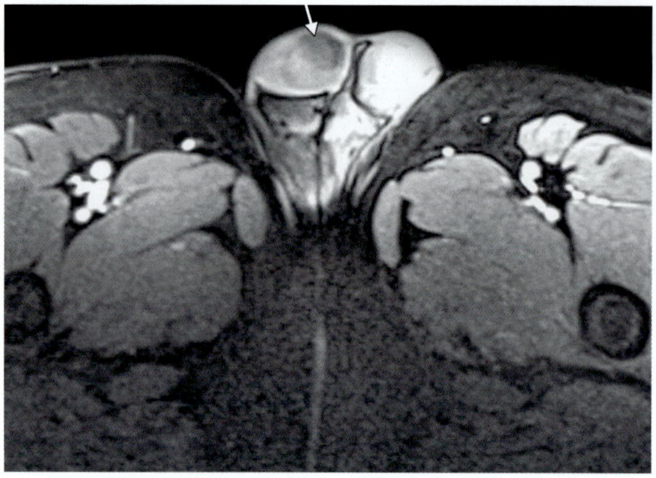

Fig. 9: Intermittent torsion: CEMR axial image showing hypoenhancing area within the right testis (arrow).

testis on ultrasound with associated skin thickening and reactive hydrocele. Color Doppler US shows increased color flow in the periphery of the twisted testicular appendage.[17] Conservative management of pain is adequate in these cases. Resolution of pain is seen in 2–3 days, with calcification of atrophied appendix. Exclusion of testicular torsion and acute epididymo-orchitis remains important while evaluating torsion of testicular appendages.

MRI in testicular torsion can show twisted cord as curvilinear structure with multiple radiating low intensity areas in a 'whirlpool' pattern. The torsion knot appears an area of signal void. In patients with intermittent torsion, the testis is enlarged and hyperintense on both T1- and T2-weighted images owing to subacute hemorrhages **(Fig. 9)**. Phosphorus MR spectroscopy has been reported to be helpful in evaluation of acute torsion. It demonstrates decreased levels of beta-ATP and phosphomonoester and increased levels of inorganic phosphorus.[13]

Scrotal Trauma

Scrotal trauma usually occurs due to direct injury or from straddle injuries. History is very helpful in the diagnosis; however, marked scrotal swelling, pain and open injuries limit adequate clinical examination. Patients with open and penetrating scrotal injuries undergo immediate surgery and are not candidates for scrotal sonography.

In cases of blunt trauma, sonography is used to confirm or exclude testicular rupture, differentiate a hematoma from hematocele and for follow-up of patients undergoing conservative management. Testicular rupture is a surgical emergency and such patients are taken up for immediate surgery whereas patients with small hematomas or hematocele are managed conservatively. Hence, scrotal sonography has a decisive influence on clinical management.[28]

On sonography, intratesticular hematoma is seen as sharply defined hypoechoic space-occupying lesion (SOL). Irregularities of testicular contour and hypo- or hyperechoic heterogeneous areas suggest testicular rupture. These parenchymal areas correspond to hemorrhages and infarction. Visualization of solid and cystic intrascrotal mass and absence of testis like structure is a characteristic feature of testicular fragmentation. Sometimes, a distinct fracture line may also be identified. Hematocele usually accompanies testicular rupture, but its absence does not exclude the possibility of rupture.[14] Scrotal hematoma between the layers of scrotal wall is seen as nonspecific soft tissue thickening. If the urethra is injured, extravasation of urine between the layers of scrotal wall produces 'onion peel' thickening of scrotal wall.

Acute hematocele or accumulation of blood in vaginal sac contains numerous small internal echoes. In chronic hematocele, thick septae and wall-thickening is demonstrated.

MRI may be required in patients with scrotal injury when satisfactory sonographic examination is not possible. It is also indicated if testicular rupture cannot be confidently excluded on the sonography. The diagnosis of testicular rupture is facilitated by unequivocal depiction of tunica albuginea on MRI.

The integrity of tunica albuginea is best assessed on T2W or contrast-enhanced T1W images. Intratesticular injuries demonstrate decreased contrast enhancement. MRI is also valuable in demonstration of hematomas.

TESTICULAR TUMORS

Testicular cancer represents 1% of all cancers in men. It is the most common malignancy affecting young men of 20–34 years of age. However, developments in diagnostic and therapeutic modalities during past decade have led to improved outcomes even in patients with advanced disease.[16] Various risk factors for development of testicular cancer are undescended testis, testicular atrophy (e.g. mumps), testicular microlithiasis, Klinefelter's syndrome, Down syndrome and maternal use of diethyl stilbesterol.[29]

Common presentation of testicular cancer is a vague discomfort or painless mass in the scrotum. US examination is very useful as it differentiates intratesticular and extratesticular lesions as the majority of intratesticular lesions are malignant whereas the extratesticular lesions are usually benign.[30] The sensitivity of grayscale US for detection of testicular tumors is nearly 100%.[31] Various mimics of testicular malignancy are benign intratesticular processes, such as hematoma, orchitis, abscess, infarction, and granuloma which must therefore be considered in the differential diagnosis. Color Doppler and power Doppler US show increased color flow in malignant testicular masses.

Testicular tumors are divided in germ-cell and nongerm-cell tumors.

Germ-cell Tumors

Germ-cell tumors account for 90–95% of testicular cancer. The rest are accounted for by those of stromal or lymphoid origin, leukemic infiltration and metastases. Two groups of germ-cell tumors are seminomatous and nonseminomatous germ-cell tumor (NSGCT). The later includes embryonal cell carcinoma, teratoma, choriocarcinoma, endodermal sinus tumor or any combination of these tumors. This distinction determines treatment and prognosis.

In the initial diagnosis, staging and follow-up tumor markers are important. These include lactose dehydrogenase (LDH), alpha-fetoprotein (AFP) and human chorionic gonadotrophin (hCG). LDH may increase in any type of tumor and it correlates well with the extent of the disease. Pure seminoma never shows elevated AFP level. In other words even a histological seminoma with elevated AFP level is treated as non-semino-matous.[32] hCG is elevated in all patients of choriocarcinoma, majority of NSGCT and only in few patients with seminomas.[29]

Seminomas

Seminomas are the most common type of testicular tumor and constitute 50% of all germ-cell tumors. They most commonly occur in the fourth decade, almost unheard in infancy.[33] Due to their sensitivity to chemoradiation, it carries best prognosis among all the germ-cell tumors.[7] The subtypes of seminomas include typical, anaplastic and spermatocytic seminomas with incidence of 85%, 5–10% and 4–6%, respectively. The incidence of spermatocytic seminomas is in men in 60s and 70s and carries excellent prognosis. Gross pathology demonstrates a uniform appearance appearing as a hypoechoic lesion on grayscale, homogeneous in echotexture **(Fig. 10)**. Replacement of the entire testis by tumor is seen in more than 50% of the cases. In one prospective study,[34] cystic components noted in 10% of seminomas. Seminomas rarely involves peritesticular structures as the tumor is usually confined by the tunica albuginea. Lymphogenous spread to retroperitoneal lymph nodes and hematogenous distant metastases to brain, lung or both are seen in about 25% of presenting population.

Nonseminomatous Germ-cell Tumors

Nonseminomatous germ-cell tumors (NSGCTs) occur most often in men aged in their 30s, have multiple histologic patterns in 40–60% of cases.[30] Various patterns are (a) teratoma and embryonal carcinoma (teratocarcinoma), (b) teratoma, embryonal carcinoma, yolk sac tumor, and human chorionic gonadotrophic hormone-containing syncytiotrophoblast, (c) seminoma and embryonal carcinoma. Both the gross and grayscale appearance of these tumors depends on the proportion of individual components often showing infiltrative/ill-defined margins (45%) inhomogeneous echotexture (71%), echogenic foci (35%), and cystic areas (61%).[34] Hemorrhage, fibrosis or calcific foci can appear echogenic. Most of the NSGCTs (~60%) are quite advanced at presentation.[30]

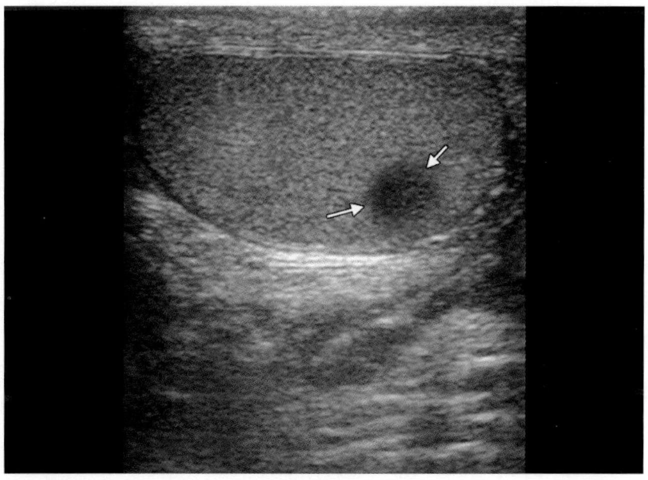

Fig. 10: USG showing a nonpalpable seminoma (arrows) of testis.

Embryonal carcinoma: It is more aggressive than seminomas and seen in men in their 30s. Only 3% NSGCTs are pure embryonal; a large percentage of the tumours with mixed histology however contain embryonal components (45%). No scrotal enlargement is seen in pure embryonal carcinoma as it is small. On grayscale, they are heterogeneously hypoechoic with indistinct margins with echogenic foci representing either calcificstion/ hemorrhage or fibrosis. Hemorrhage, calcification, or fibrosis commonly appear as echogenic foci. Cystic components are seen in 20% of embryonal carcinomas and 89% of teratocarcinomas. Contour abnormality of the testis due to tumor invasion of the tunica albuginea is quite common.[7]

Yolk sac tumor: synonymous with endodermal sinus/ infantile embryonal carcinomas. Most common age group affected are children less than 5 years of age. Exclusive tumor marker is an AFP.[33]

When present as a component of mixed tumors, they are a marker for poor prognosis. On USG, they are heterogeneous in echotexture often with hemorrhagic (echogenic) foci.

Choriocarcinoma: Pure choriocarcinomas are a rarity constituting only 0.3% of the testicular tumors. However microscopic foci are seen in up to 16% of mixed germ-cell tumors. Vascular invasion is quite common, with consequent tendency for early blood borne metastasis, particularly to the lungs, even with a very small primary lesion.[30] Central tumoral hemorrhagic necrosis with a mixed solid-cystic morphology at ultrasound is seen in many cases.[35]

Teratoma: Unique in its embryological derivation from all the three germ-cell layers: endo, meso and ectoderm. Pure teratomas are more common in children—second MC tumor in prepubertal age group (male sex), with the tumors more commonly being of a benign nature. Pure teratomas are rarer in adults (2–3%), and regardless of age should be considered malignant. In addition, 50% of mixed tumors contain teratomatous elements. They have an inhomogeneous appearance with a large tumor size with numerous foci of increased echogenicity representing calcification/cartilage/immature bone or fibrosis. Cystic component is very common in this tumor **(Fig. 11)**.

Burned-out germ-cell tumor often a teratocarcinoma or choriocarcinoma to begin with, which outgrow their blood supply due to rapid division of tumor cells with resultant tumor necrosis, fibrosis and scar tissue formation.

These appear as echogenic or hypoechoic foci depending on stage of fibrosis.[36]

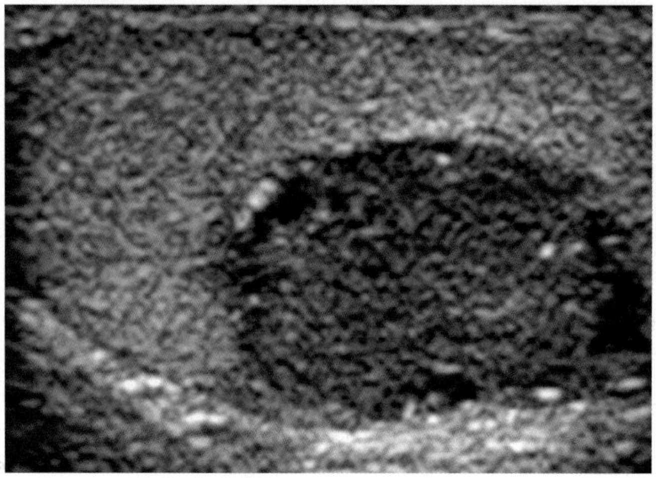

Fig. 11: USG showing teratoma of testis. Note small cystic areas and foci of calcification within the lesion.

Non-germ Cell Testicular Tumors

These include tumors of gonadal stroma (Leydig cell tumors, Sertoli cell tumors and gonadoblastoma), lymphoma, leukemia, metastases and other rare tumors. Majority of stromal tumors are benign. These may be endocrinally active and hence patients may present with precocious puberty, gynecomastia or other endocrinopathies. They are usually benign with Leydig cell subtype being the most common. Any age group can be affected with interesting symptomatology. In children often there is precocious puberty due to androgen secretion by the tumor cells, whereas enlargement of scrotum (42.5%) and gynecomastia (30%) is common presentation in adults, with the latter usually preceding the former.[37] Malignant transformation is not very common.

Gonadoblastoma (contains both germ-cell and stromal cell elements) is rare and is almost exclusively seen in intersex problems and gonadal dysgenesis. Eighty percent are phenotypically female.

Sonographically stromal tumors are seen as small, smoothly demarcated, homogeneous hypoechoic intra-testicular masses **(Fig. 12)**.[29]

Lymphomas constitute only 5% of testicular tumors. Histologically, they are usually non-Hodgkin's lymphoma: B-cell subtype **(Fig. 13)**. In the 6th decade, it is the MC testicular tumor, accounting for about half of the cases.[38] Sonographically, these tumors resemble seminomas but asynchronous involvement of the contralateral testis and spermatic cord/epididymal involvement gives a clue towards the diagnosis. 40 to 65% of patients with acute leukemia and 20 to 35% of patients with chronic leukemia have testicular infiltration at autopsy.[39] Testicular

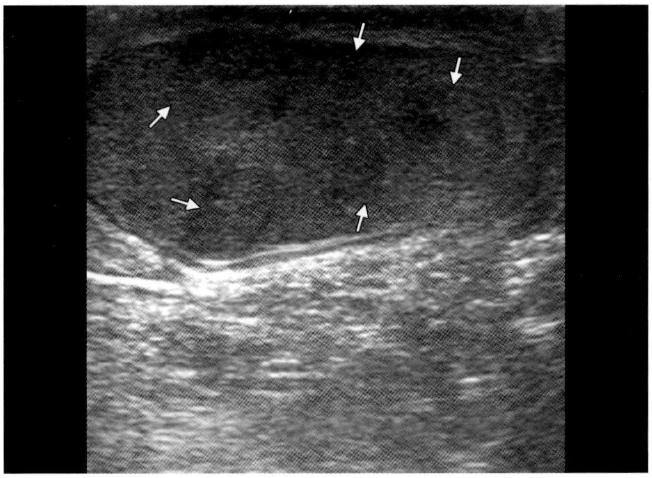

Fig. 12: US image showing multicentric rhabdomyosarcoma of testis.

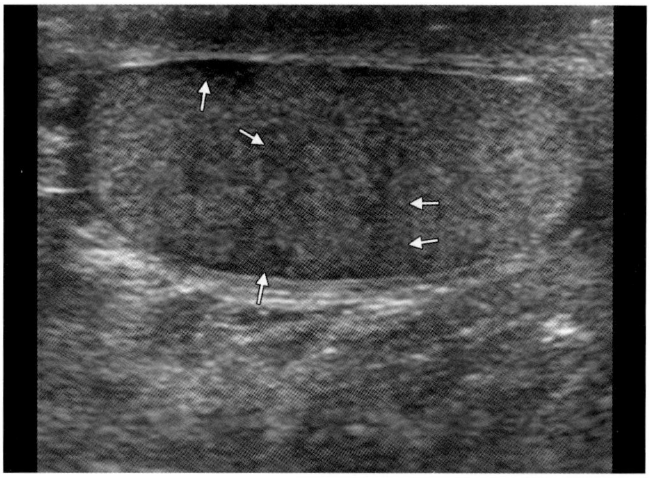

Fig. 13: US image showing sheet-like hypoechoic areas within the testis (arrows) due to lymphoma (NHL).

involvement is seen in 5–10% of boys during clinical remission of acute lymphoblastic leukemia. Bilateral testicular involvement is seen in about 50% of the patients. Sonographically, lymphoma/leukemia deposits are seen as focal or diffuse hypoechoic areas. The testis is usually enlarged. In leukemia patients after remission due to the blood–testis barrier the testes are a favorable site for persistence of leukemic cells.

Intrascrotal metastases from tumors of other organs are rare and are usually found in older patients. Most frequent primaries are from lung, kidney, prostate and melanoma.[14] Sonographic appearances are nonspecific.

Staging or Testicular Cancer

Testicular cancer is staged using the TNM system created by the American Joint Committee on Cancer (AJCC) **(Tables 1 to 3)**.

Primary Tumor (T)

TX: The primary tumor cannot be assessed.

T0: There is no evidence of primary tumor.

Tis: Carcinoma in situ (noninvasive cancer cells).

T1: The tumor has not spread beyond the testicle and the narrow tubules next to the testicles where sperm undergo final maturation (epididymis). Cancer cells are not found inside blood vessels or lymph vessels next to the tumor. The cancer may have grown through the inner layer surrounding the testicle (tunica albuginea) but not the outer layer covering the testicle (tunica vaginalis).

T2: Similar to T1 except that the cancer has spread to blood vessels, lymphatic vessels, or the tunica vaginalis.

T3: The tumor invades the spermatic cord (which contains blood vessels, lymphatic vessels, nerves, and the vas deferens).

T4: The tumor invades the skin surrounding the testicles (scrotum).

Regional Lymph Nodes (N)

NX: Regional (nearby) lymph nodes cannot be assessed.

N0: No metastasis (spread) to regional lymph nodes is seen on X-rays.

N1: There is metastasis in at least one lymph node, but no lymph node is larger than 2 cm (about 3/4 inch) in any dimension.

N2: There is metastasis in at least one lymph node that is larger than 2 cm but is not bigger than 5 cm (2 inches) in any dimension.

N3: There is metastasis to at least 1 lymph node that is larger than 5 cm in any dimension.

If the lymph nodes were taken out during surgery, there is a slightly different classification:

pNX: Regional (nearby) lymph nodes cannot be assessed.

pN0: There is no metastasis to regional lymph nodes.

pN1: There is metastasis (spread) to 1–5 lymph nodes, with no lymph node larger than 2 cm (about 3/4 inch) across in greatest dimension.

pN2: There is metastasis in at least one lymph node that is bigger than 2 cm but not larger than 5 cm; or metastasis to more than 5 lymph nodes that are not bigger than 5 cm (one inch) across (in greatest dimension), or the cancer is growing out the side of the lymph node.

pN3: There is metastasis to at least one lymph node that is bigger than 5 cm.

Table 1: Serum tumor markers (S).

	LDH (U/liter)	*hCG (mIU/mL)*	*AFP (ng/mL)*
SX	Marker studies not available or not performed		
S0	Normal	Normal	Normal
S1	<1.5X Normal	<5,000	<1,000
S2	1.5–10X Normal	5,000–50,000	1,000–10,000
S3	>10X Normal	>50,000	>10,000

Abbreviations: LDH: Lactate dehydrogenase (measured in units per liter); hCG: Human chorionic gonadotropin [measured in milli-International units per milliliter (mL)]; AFP: Alpha-fetoprotein [measured in nanograms per milliliter (mL)].

Table 2: Stage grouping.

Stage	*T*	*N*	*M*	*S*
Stage 0	Tis (*in situ*)	N0	M0	S0
Stage I	T1–4	N0	M0	SX
Stage IA	T1	N0	M0	S0
Stage IB	T2–T4	N0	M0	S0
Stage IS	Any T	N0	M0	S1–3
Stage II	Any T	N1–3	M0	SX
Stage IIA	Any T	N1	M0	S0–1
Stage IIB	Any T	N2	M0	S0–1
Stage IIC	Any T	N3	M0	S0–1
Stage III	Any T	Any N	M1	SX
Stage IIIA	Any T	Any N	M1a	S0–1
	Any T	Any N	M1a	S1
Stage IIIB	Any T	N1–3	M0	S2
	Any T	Any N	M1a	S2
Stage IIIC	Any T	N1–3	M0	S3
	Any T	Any N	M1a	S3
	Any T	Any N	M1b	Any S

Table 3: Tumor markers and stage grouping of nonseminoma and seminoma.

Risk status	*Nonseminoma*	*Stages*	*Seminoma*	*Stages*
Good outlook	No nonlung spread	IS (S1)		
	Good markers	IIA (S1)	No nonlung spread	IIC
	AFP < 1,000	IIB (S1)	AFP normal	IIIA
	hCG < 5,000	IIC (S1)	hCG and LDH can be any level	IIIB
				IIIC
	LDH < 1.5	IIIA		
	No nonlung spread			
	Intermediate markers	IS (S2)	Nonlung spread	IIIC with nonlung spread
Intermediate outlook	AFP 1,000–10,000	IIC (S2)	AFP normal	
	hCG 5,000–50,000	IIIB	hCG and LDH can be any level	
	LDH 1.5–10			
	Nonlung spread			
	High markers	IS (S3)		
Poor outlook	AFP > 10,000	IIC (S3)	None (seminoma is never classified as poor outlook)	
	hCG > 50,000	All IIIC		
	LDH > 10			

Distant Metastasis (M)

MX: Distant metastasis cannot be assessed. M0: There is no distant metastasis (no spread to lymph nodes outside the area of the tumor or other organs, such as the lungs).

M1: Distant metastasis is present.

M1a: The tumor has metastasized to distant lymph nodes or to the lung.

M1b: The tumor has metastasized to organs, such as liver, brain, bone, and others.

Another application of the TNM system used for advanced disease takes into account the markers and classifies the cancer as low, medium, and poor outlook.

Imaging in Evaluation of Testicular Cancer

MRI

MRI is used as a problem solving modality. MRI of scrotum is more sensitive than sonography for detection of testicular tumors; however, the findings are variable and nonspecific. Most testicular tumors are isointense to testis on T1W images and hypo-intense on T2W images. On dynamic gadolinium enhanced MRI, the tumor enhancement is often earlier and greater than the normal testicular parenchyma. Similar to their sonographic appearances, seminomas tend to be homogeneous, whereas NSGCTs are heterogeneous on MRI. Lymphoma and leukemia show testicular enlargement with decreased T2 signal, in a homogeneous and diffuse pattern. MRI is also useful in staging work-up of testicular tumors when CT is inconclusive or contraindicated. It is also useful for follow-up after the treatment.

CT

CT is most commonly used for evaluation of tumor spread, staging and follow-up. CT is useful for detection of enlarged retroperitoneal or mediastinal lymph nodes as well as extranodal metastases in lungs and liver. In testicular carcinoma, even subcentimetric nodes are suspicious especially when seen in the regional nodal drainage site (e.g. aortocaval location on right side or renal hilum on the left) **(Fig. 14)**. 7 mm as a cutoff has been suggested as more useful for nodal involvement in testicular cancer.[29] The enlarged lymph nodes may demonstrate necrotic center or heterogeneous contrast enhancement, particularly in NSGCTs. After completion of the treatment, some lymph nodes may not decrease in size and instead, develop more necrosis and fibrotic strands. Majority of such lymph nodal masses do not contain viable tumor; however, it cannot be ruled out on the basis of CT alone.

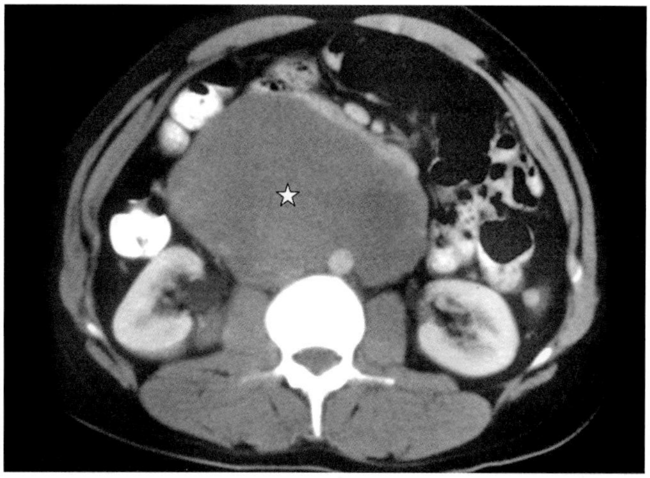

Fig. 14: Axial CECT image at the level of renal hilum showing a large metastatic homogeneous lymph nodal mass (star) in a case of seminomas testis.

PET

The role of fluoro-D-deoxyglucose positron-emission tomography (FDG-PET) in testicular tumors include three specific settings:

1. After chemotherapy in distinguishing active disease from fibrosis/mature teratoma.
2. After orchidectomy in primary disease staging and assessment and when there is elevation of tumor markers; looking for recurrence.
3. Predicting response to treatment.

PET is more sensitive and specific for disgnosing recurrent disease at local and remote sites especially in patients with residual tumor masses or increasing tumor marker following treatment.[40]

Further investigation is needed to determine its eventual place as an imaging modality for staging at diagnosis. The exact role of PET in determining the prognosis of disease is not clearly defined in testicular malignancy but the initial results appear promising.

BENIGN INTRATESTICULAR LESIONS

Cysts

Testicular cysts are incidentally detected on sonography. These need to be differentiated from cystic tumors. Symptomatic or palpable testicular cysts or those with suspicious solid component need further evaluation and/or exploration. Others can be followed-up. Two types of simple benign cysts can be identified—cysts of tunica albuginea and simple testicular cysts. Tunica albuginea cysts are typically small (<5 mm) and are usually palpated as firm nodular masses. These are located at the periphery.

Simple testicular cysts are usually located near the mediastinum testis and are not palpable.

Tubular ectasia of rete testis may be mistaken for tumors. These are typically located at the mediastinum testis and consist of areas of multiple tiny cystic spaces with no flow on CDFI **(Fig. 15)**. It is usually associated with epididymal obstruction. Epidermoid and dermoid cysts of the testis are rare and these are also seen as palpable simple cysts with characteristic echogenic margins. They do not have malignant potential.

Adrenal Rests

Aberrant adrenal tissue rests may be found in testis in about 8% of patients with congenital adrenal hyperplasia. Pathogenesis may be related to the common embryonic origin of adrenals and gonads. On sonography, they are seen as multifocal and often bilateral hypoechoic lesions.

Calcifications

Testicular microlithiasis (TM) is an uncommon condition in which multiple, fine calcifications are present within seminiferous tubules. Sonography demonstrates innumerable, small, hyperechoic foci scattered throughout the testicular parenchyma, which rarely show acoustic shadowing **(Fig. 16)**. Abnormal finding is presence of 5 or more foci per transducer field.[13] Testicular malignancy has been reported in 18–75% of testicular microlithiasis.[41] TM is neither a premalignant condition nor a causative factor in testicular malignancy and exact prevalence of neoplasia is unknown; however, due to reported association with neoplasia, one US follow-up on an yearly basis is recommended for several years after the diagnosis.[41]

Extratesticular scrotal calculi or scrotoliths (scrotal pearls) represent loose bodies and occur due to torsion of the appendix testis or epididymis.[16] Ultrasound diagnosis of scrotoliths is easy due to presence of small amount of fluid usually around the testis **(Fig. 17)**. Other considerations for Intratesticular macrocalcifications are calcifying large cell Sertoli-cell tumor, burned-out germ-cell tumor, or post-traumatic change.

EXTRATESTICULAR PATHOLOGIES

Fluid Collections

Hydrocele is an abnormal accumulation of serous fluid in vaginal cavity. The congenital type is seen in infants, and it is due to persistent communication between scrotal sac and the peritoneum. Acquired hydrocele is idiopathic or secondary to inflammation, torsion, trauma or tumor. Sonographically, a clear fluid is seen surrounding the testis. However, fine mobile echogenic concretions or a few thin septations can be seen in any long-standing hydrocele, and it does not necessarily suggests complicated collection. Rarely, the concretion may be fairly large when it gives a 'bull's eye' appearance with central calcification surrounded by the hypoechoic layer.

Hematocele and pyocele result from hemorrhage and abscess formation respectively. Both contain multiple septations and echogenic debris. Thickening of scrotal skin and calcifications may be seen in both of these conditions **(Fig. 18)**.[13]

Inguinoscrotal hernia is usually diagnosed on the basis of clinical examination. Hernia may contain small bowel, large bowel and/or omentum. Sonographically, hernia is seen as echogenic structure of varying shapes, which

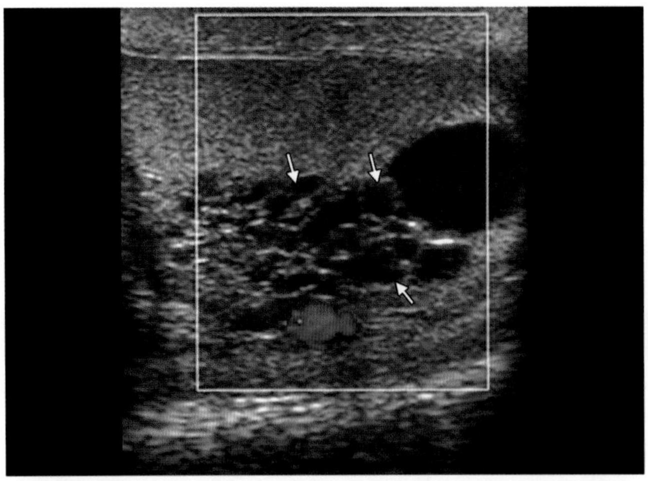

Fig. 15: US showing tubular ectasia of rete testis (arrows). Note absence of flow of color Doppler.

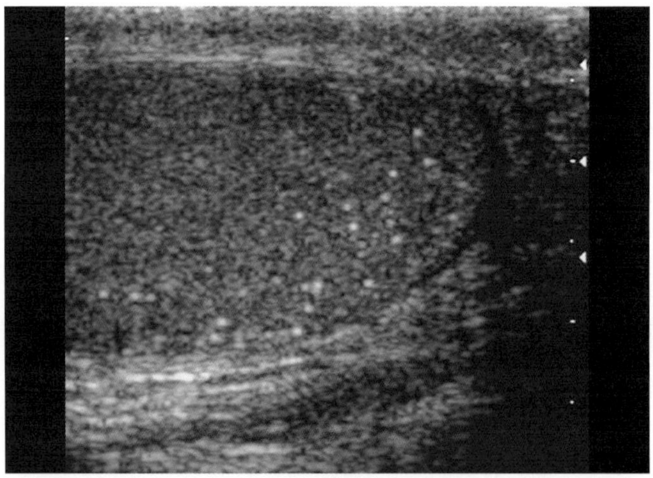

Fig. 16: US image showing multiple punctate hyperechoic nonshadowing foci of testicular microlithiasis.

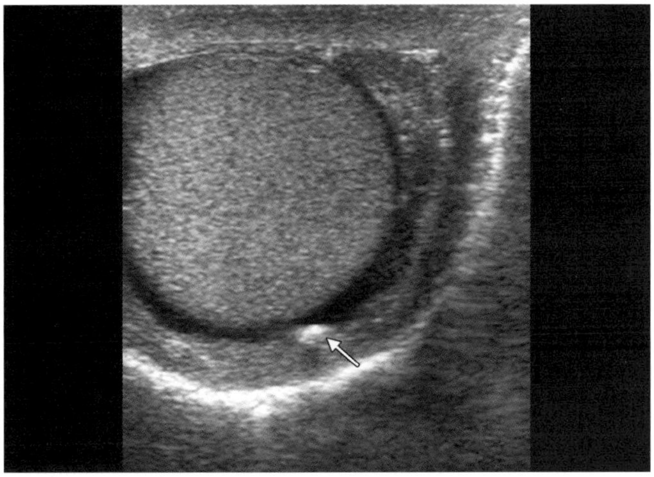

Fig. 17: US image showing a scrotal pearl (arrow).

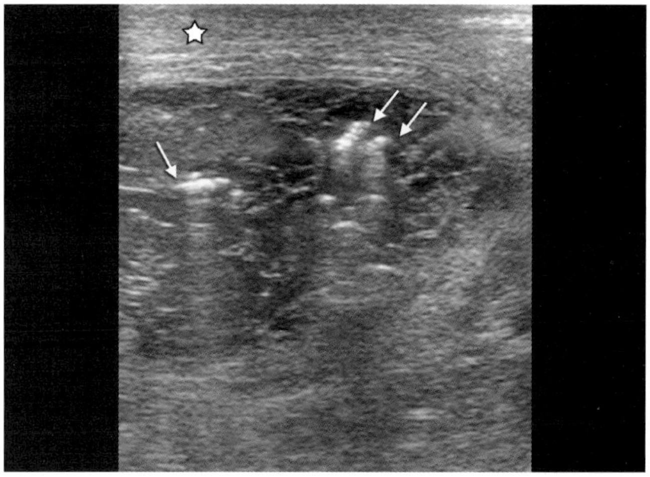

Fig. 18: Pyocele of scrotum: US image showing echogenic fluid collection within the scrotum and air foci (arrows) trapped within thin septations. Note the thickened skin of scrotum (star).

moves in the inguinal canal with breathing. Sometimes, bowel loops with their mucosal folds and peristalsis can also be identified. The presence of real-time peristalsis is very suggestive of bowel. Indirect inguinal hernia is more commonly associated with strangulation of bowel than direct inguinal hernia. Features of strangulation on ultrasound are an akinetic dilated bowel loop in the hernial sac or hyperemic scrotal soft tissue and bowel wall.[2] The testis and epididymis are separately seen and they retain their normal appearance.

Epididymal Cysts

The most common scrotal pathologies are spermatoceles and epididymal cysts and these may be encountered in up to 70% of all patients subjected to scrotal sonography.[12] Spermatoceles contains debris and sperms in addition to serous fluid and occur secondary to the obstruction of spermatic pathway. Head of epididymis is the most common location. Cysts are more common than spermatoceles and they do not contain sperms. These are usually smaller in size and are located anywhere in the epididymis. Spermatoceles and epididymal cysts are identical on sonography and are seen as anechoic, well-circumscribed cysts with no or few internal echoes **(Fig. 19)**. Sperm granulomas may be found in patients with epididymal obstruction or after vasectomy.[12] On sonography, these are seen as hypoechoic epididymal lesions, sometimes with focal calcification.

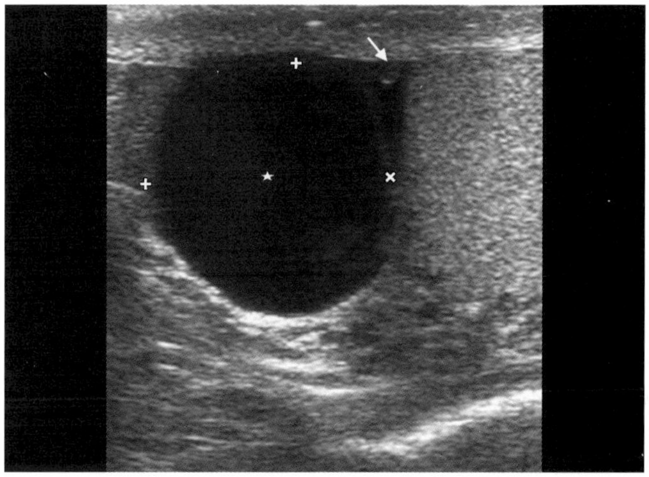

Fig. 19: US image showing an epididymal cyst. Appendix of testis (arrow) is seen between the cyst and the testis.

Postorchidectomy Scrotum

After orchidectomy, small amount of clear fluid is usually seen in the empty hemiscrotal sac, which resolves gradually. The scrotal wall appears thickened because of contraction. Hematomas are common in early postoperative period. Fresh hematomas are echogenic. These become hypoechoic or cystic as these resolve after 5–6 weeks. Tumor recurrence may be suspected if the mass develops several months after the orchidectomy. On sonography, the recurrence is seen as a poorly defined hypoechoic lesion. Color Doppler, MRI or sonography guided biopsies are useful to differentiate recurrent tumor from hematoma.[42]

Testicular prosthesis is usually made up of silicone. On sonography, it is seen as a sharply defined, anechoic structure, frequently with excessive reverberations.[42]

Extratesticular Tumors

Extratesticular scrotal tumors are mostly benign and usually involve the epididymis. The most common is adenomatoid tumor constituting 30% of these tumors. It arises in epididymis or spermatic cord. On sonography, it is generally seen as solitary, well-defined, round-to-oval, small mass with variable echogenicity.[14] It may occasionally invade adjacent testicular parenchyma. Other benign paratesticular tumors include hemangioma, lipoma, neurofibroma and leiomyoma. Malignant paratesticular tumors include liposarcoma, fibrosarcoma and lymphoma in adults and rhabdomyosarcoma in children. The sonographic appearances of these tumors are nonspecific.[13]

Varicocele

Varicocele is an abnormal dilatation and tortuosity of the veins of the pampiniform plexus. It is described in detail in Chapter 125: Male Infertility and Erectile Dysfunction.

REFERENCES

1. Trainer TD. Testis and the excretory duct system. In Sternberg S, (Eds). Histology for pathologists. New York, NY: Raven; 1992.pp.744-6.
2. Siegel MJ. The acute scrotum. Radiol Clin North Am. 1997;35:959-76.
3. Bree RL, Hoang DT. Scrotal ultrasound. Radiol Clin North Am. 1996;34:1183-205.
4. Middleton WD, Thorne DA, Melson GL. Color Doppler ultrasound of the normal testis. AJR. 1989;152:293-7.
5. Paltiel HJ, Rupich RC, Babcock DS. Maturational changes in arterial impedance of the normal testis in boys: Doppler sonographic study. AJR Am J Roentgenol. 1994;163:1189-93.
6. Friedland GW, Chang P. The role of imaging in the management of the impalpable undescen-ded testis. AJR. 1988;151:1107-11.
7. Heiken JP. Tumors of the testis and testicular adnexa. In: Pollack HM, McClennan BL, (Eds). Clinical Urography. Philadelphia, Pa: Saunders. 2000;1716-41.
8. Hricak H: Congenital anomalies of the testis. In: Hricak H, Hamn B, Kim B (Eds). Imaging of Scrotum. New York: Raven press. 1995;1:37-48.
9. Levitt SB, Konyan SJ, Engel RM. The impalp-able testis: A rational approach to management. J Urol. 1978;120:515-20.
10. Toyoshima M, Chida K, Masuda M. Testicular sarcoidosis. Nihon Kokyuki Gakkai Zasshi. 2000;38:63-6.
11. Bayram MM, Kervancioglu R. Scrotal gray-scale and color Doppler sonographic findings in genitourinary brucellosis. J Clin Ultrasound. 1997;25:443-7.
12. Cook JL, Dewbury K. The changes seen on high-resolution ultrasound in orchitis. Clin Radiol. 2000;55:13-8.
13. Gorman B, Carroll BA. The scrotum. In Rummak CM, Wilson SR, Charhoneau JW (Eds). Diagnostic Ultrasound. Mosby: St Louis. 2005;3:849-88.
14. Oyen RH. Scrotal ultrasound. Eur Radiol. 2002;12:19-34.
15. Noske HD, Kraus SW, Altinkilic BM, Weidner W. Historical milestones regarding torsion of the scrotal organs. J Urol. 1998;159:13-6.
16. Dewbury KC. Scrotal ultrasonography: An update. BJU Int. 2000;86:143-52.
17. Burks DD, Markey BJ, Burkhard TK, Balsara ZN, Haluszka MM, Canning DA. Suspected testicular torsion and ischemia: evaluation with color Doppler sonography. Radiology. 1990; 175:815-21.
18. Horstman WG. Scrotal imaging. Urol Clin North Am. 1997;24:653-71.
19. Jee WH, Choe BY, Byun JY, Shinn KS, Hwang TK. Resistive index of the intrascrotal artery in scrotal inflammatory disease. Acta Radiol. 1997;38:1026-30.
20. Brown JM, Hammers LW, Barton JW, et al. Quantitative Doppler assessment of acute scrotal inflammation. Radiology. 1995;197:427-31.
21. Sanders LM, Haber S, Dembner A, Aquino A. Significance of reversal of diastolic flow in the acute scrotum. J Ultrasound Med. 1994;13:137-9.
22. Rifkin MD. Inflammation of the lower genito-urinary tract: The prostate, seminal vesicles, and scrotum. In: Pollack HM, McClennan BL (Eds): Clinical Urography 2nd ed. Philadelphia, Pa: Saunders; 2000.pp.1058-87.
23. Patriquin HB, Yazbeck S, Trinh B, et al. Testicular torsion in infants and children: Diagnosis with Doppler sonography. Radiology. 1993;188:781-5.
24. Williamson RCN. Torsion of the testis and allied conditions. Br J Surg. 1976;63:465-76.
25. Berman JM, Beidle TR, Kunberger LE, Letourneau JG. Sonographic evaluation of acute intrascrotal pathology. AJR Am J Roentgenol. 1996;166:857-61.
26. Dogra VS, Sessions A, Mevorach A, Rubens DJ. Reversal of diastolic plateau in partial testicular torsion. J Clin Ultrasound. 2001;29:105-8.
27. Skoglund RW, McRoberts JW, Ragde H. Torsion of testicular appendages: Presentation of 43 new cases and a collective review. J Urol. 1970;104:598-600.
28. Kratzik C, Hainz A, Kuber W. Has ultrasound influenced the therapy concept of blunt scrotal trauma. J Urol. 1989;142:1243-6.
29. Hari A, Grossfeld G, Hricak A. Tumors of the scrotum. In Bragg DG, Rubin P, Hricak H (Eds): Oncologic Imaging. Philadelphia: WB Saunders Co. 2002;2:603-28.
30. Geraghty MJ, Lee FT, Jr, Bernsten SA, Gilchrist K, Pozniak MA, Yandow DJ. Sonography of testicular tumors and tumor-like conditions: a radiologic-pathologic correlation. Crit Rev Diagn Imaging. 1998;39:1-63.
31. Rifkin MD, Kurtz AB, Pasto ME, Goldberg BB. Diagnostic capabilities of high-resolution scrotal ultrasonography: Prospective evaluation. J Ultrasound Med. 1985;4:13-9.
32. Guthrie JA, Fowler RC. Ultrasound diagnosis of testicular tumours presenting as epididymal disease. Clin Radiol. 1992;46:397-400.

33. Cotran RS, Kumar P, Collins T. The male genital tract In: Robbins Pathologic Basis of Disease. 6th ed. Philadelphia, Pa: Saunders. 1999.pp.1011-34.
34. Schwerk WB, Schwerk WN, Rodeck G. Testicular tumors: Prospective analysis of real-time US patterns and abdominal staging. Radiology. 1987;164:369-74.
35. Comiter CV, Renshaw AA, Benson CB, Loughlin KR. Burned-out primary testicular cancer: sonographic and pathological charac-teristics. J Urol. 1996;156:85-8.
36. Hamm B. Differential diagnosis of scrotal masses by ultrasound. Eur Radiol. 1997;7:668-79.
37. Kim I, Young RH, Scully RE. Leydig cell tumors of the testis: A clinicopathological analysis of 40 cases and review of the literature. Am J Surg Pathol. 1985;9:177-92.
38. Nonomura N, Aozasa K, Ueda T, et al. Malignant lymphoma of the testis: histological and immunohistological study of 28 cases. J Urol. 1989;141:1368-71.
39. Richie JP. Neoplasms of the testis. In Walch PC, Retik AB, Vaughan ED, Wein AJ, (Eds). Campbell's urology. (7th edn) Philadelphia, Pa: Saunders; 1998.pp.2411-52.
40. Basu S, Rubello D. PET imaging in the management of tumors of testis and ovary: current thinking and future directions. Minerva Endocrinol. 2008;33:229-56.
41. Ganem JP, Workman KR, Shaban SF. Testicular microlithiasis is associated with testicular pathology. Urology. 1999;53:209-13.
42. Eftekhari F, Smith JK. Sonography of scrotum after orchiectomy: normal and abnormal findings. AJR. 1993;160;543-7.

CHAPTER 125

Male Infertility and Erectile Dysfunction

Deep Narayan Srivastava, Sanjay Thulkar

MALE INFERTILITY

Defects in male partner may be responsible for infertility in up to 50% of the infertile couples.[1] These defects account for a reduction in the quantity and quality of the semen. The evaluation of infertile male begins with a careful history and physical examination of the patient. This is followed by semen analysis in which ejaculate volume and its pH, sperms count, their motility and morphology are studied. Average sperm count in normal fertile man is 70–80 million sperms per mL and it contains more than 60% motile sperms. Sperm count of less than 20 million per mL is termed as oligospermia, however, significant decrease in pregnancy rates occur only at sperm concentration of less than 5 million per mL. Oligospermia is present in 80% and azoospermia is present in another 15–20% of the infertile men.[1]

Etiology

Male infertility results from many diverse conditions. Congenital anomalies include cryptorchidism, Klinefelter's syndrome, agenesis of vas deferens and/or seminal vesicles and congenital ejaculatory duct cyst. Endocrinal abnormalities are uncommon causes of the male infertility and these are diagnosed primarily on the basis of clinical examination and laboratory findings. Luiteinizing hormone secreted by the pituitary gland regulates the *testosterone* secretion by Leydig cells of the testis. Low testosterone affects spermatogensis, growth of the prostate and seminal vesicle secretion.[2]

Acquired testicular abnormalities such as trauma, tumor, infection and paratesticular abnormalities such as varicocele and epididymitis are responsible for infertility in significant number of patients. Tuberculosis and gonorrhea cause inflammation and obstruction of the ductal transport system. Other diseases, such as mumps and syphilis may affect seminiferous tubules in the testicular parenchyma.

Primary or secondary neoplastic infiltration of testes, as occurs in lymphoma and leukemia, may affect fertility. Chemotherapy; especially with cisplatin or alkylating agents can produce irreversible damage to germinal epithelium. Radiotherapy of more than 15 Gy also produces testicular damage. Testicular tumors and hematological malignancies are common neoplasms in young males and infertility counseling before treatment is mandatory in these patients. Cryopreservation of sperms is a preferred option.[3]

Imaging Approach in Male Infertility

Normal volume (more than 1 mL), fructose positive ejaculate with azoospermia or oligospermia is usually caused by lesions of the testis or of paratesticular structures, such as varicocele and epididymal diseases.[4] These lesions can be satisfactorily evaluated with scrotal ultrasonography, supplemented with color Doppler flow imaging. Although clinical examination is an integral part of diagnostic work-up in these patients, upto 67% of scrotal pathologies detected on sonography and responsible for infertility are not apparent clinically.[5]

Low volume ejaculate (less than 1 mL) is caused by stenosis, obstruction or congenital anomalies of distal sperm transport system, which include vas deferens, seminal vesicles, ejaculatory duct and prostate. Abnormalities in these structures result in decreased semen volume and blockage of flow of sperms into the ejaculate leading to azoospermia or oligospermia. These abnormalities include agenesis of vas deferens or seminal vesicles or both, inflammatory strictures and obstruction of seminal vesicles and vas deferens, ejaculatory duct cysts and obstruction. Vasography is the traditional modality for evaluation of distal ductal system. It is an invasive technique and requires surgical exploration of the vas deferens in scrotum. The procedure itself may cause iatrogenic scarring and obstruction of the vas.[6] Transrectal ultrasonogrpahy (TRUS) has now replaced vasography as the primary imaging modality for distal ductal system.[1,7] It is now widely used to diagnose congenital and other obstructive lesions that produce low volume ejaculate and azoospermia. MRI is indicated only if TRUS findings are inconclusive.[8]

Varicocele

Varicocele is the most common surgically correctable cause of male infertility. There is abnormal dilatation of veins of the pampiniform plexus, which is due to venous reflux in these veins. The incidence of varicocele is 15% in general population and 35–40% in men presenting with infertility.[9,10] Primary varicocele is seen in young men and is due to incompetent testicular vein. It is mostly left-sided or bilateral. Left testicular vein is maximally predisposed to develop varicocele. Various factors responsible include right-angled entry of left testicular vein into left renal vein, the intermittent compression of left renal vein between aorta and the superior mesenteric artery (nutcracker syndrome) and pressure of the left colon.[11] Secondary varicocele results from compression of testicular veins by adjacent masses such as tumor, lymph nodes or hydronephrosis.[12] Cross communications exist between veins of the pampiniform plexus and cremasteric veins as well as external spermatic veins and veins of vas deferens. In patients, subjected to high ligation, these communications may lead to recurrence.

Although most men with varicocele are not infertile, varicocele is present in up to 40% of infertile men. Repair of varicocele improves quality of semen in majority of patients.[13] Proposed mechanisms by which varicocele causes testicular dysfunction include hormonal imbalance, hypoxia secondary to venous stasis, reflux of adrenal and renal metabolites and elevated testicular temperature.[14] During adolescence, when the testis is growing rapidly, it may be very susceptible to harmful effects of varicocele.

The simplest and most widely used method for diagnosis of varicocele is physical examination; however, subclinical varicocele cannot be diagnosed with physical examination alone. Ultrasonography with color duplex flow imaging is the preferred imaging modality for evaluation of varicocele. Thermogrpahy and venography are rarely performed for diagnostic purpose.[13] The patient is examined in supine and erect position during quite breathing, deep breathing and Valsalva maneuver before interpreting the examination as normal.[9] Vessels are scanned on each side from the scrotal neck to the lower pole of testis. As the flow in pampiniform plexus is very slow, Doppler parameters must be adjusted to detect very slow flow during color Doppler examination. On grey scale ultrasonography, visualization of three or more dilated veins with at least one of them having a diameter of 3 mm or more is suggestive of varicocele.[13] These tortuous venous channels are easily compressible as opposed to other cystic abnormalities in this region. On color Doppler study, continuous retrograde flow towards testis during Valsalva maneuver, is taken as a positive sign for varicocele[13,15] **(Figs. 1A and B)**. A brief reflux in veins of pampiniform plexus followed by cessation of flow is physiological. Pulsed Doppler is not required for the diagnosis of varicocele.[13] Some varicoceles can be demonstrated in erect position of the patient only and hence scanning in erect position is mandatory before the study is interpreted as normal.[13] Intratesticular varicocele is rare and always associated with paratesticular varicocele. It is usually located in subcapsular location or in the mediastinum testis.[16]

Size of the varicocele does not correlate with degree of impairment of spermatogenesis. Thus a small varicocele detected only on radiological assessment may have a profound effect on spermatogenesis.[17] The treatment of subclinical varicocele in infertility is still controversial, however, it has been demonstrated that sperm motility improvement after varicocele surgery is comparable in patients with both clinical and subclinical varicocele.[18]

Spermatic venography is the gold standard for diagnosis of varicocele. When compared with venography, color Doppler ultrasonography had a sensitivity of 93% and specificity of 80% in a group of infertile patients with normal physical examinations.[19] In addition to the diagnosis, spermatic venography has therapeutic application for embolization of varicocele. In this technique, an angiographic catheter is placed into the testicular vein via transfemoral venous route. About 5–10 mL of contrast is injected during Valsalva maneuver and radiographs of

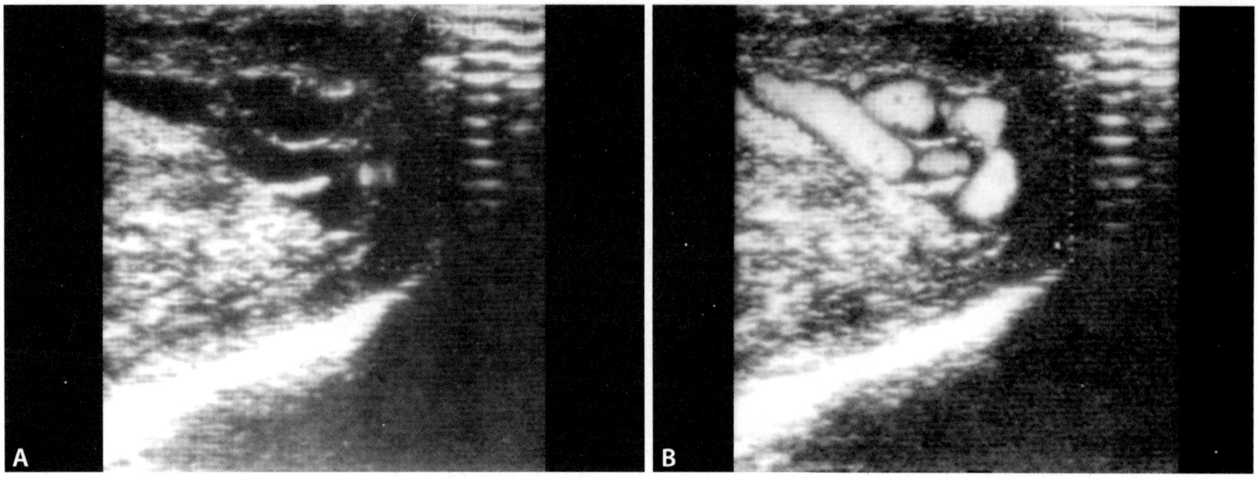

Figs. 1A and B: Varicocele: (A) Multiple dilated vascular channels with minimal detectable flow is seen at the lower pole of testes on this black and white image of color Doppler scan; (B) Significant increase in flow is seen during Valsalva maneuver.

abdomen and pelvis are taken. The venography can be followed by embolization performed using coils or sclerosants such as sodium tetradecyl sulfate foam.[13] Correct identification of all venous collaterals with their selective embolization is necessary. High technical success rate with significant improvement in semen quality can be achieved with this technique.[20] This technique is especially suitable for post-surgical recurrent varicocele.[21]

Testis

Sonographic examination of the testis is important in the evaluation of infertile male, specifically for measurement of testicular size for atrophy or for tumor identification. Normal adult testis is homogenous with low to medium echogenicity and measures 3–5 cm in length, 2–3 cm in width and 2–3 cm in antero-posterior thickness. Testicular volume in cc can be calculated using the formula of length × width × thickness × 0.53. The normal volume of adult testis is 15–20 cc and testis is symmetrical on both sides.[21]

Cryptorchidism occurs in approximately 0.8% of all one-year-old boys and if left untreated can represent a congenital cause of male infertility.[22] Progressive germ cell damage occurs in the cryptorchoid testis secondary to the increased temperature at its extra scrotal location. Significant germ cell damage occurs by two years of age and untreated postpubertal undescended testis may be completely devoid of germ cells. It also has a deleterious effect on contral-ateral normal descended testis. Pregnancy rates in men who have undergone pre pubertal treatment of unilateral cryptorchoidism ranges between 65% and 80%.[22] In addition to infertility, undescended testis is highly susceptible for malignant transformation.

Most of the undescended testes are located at or close to the inguinal canal and ultrasonography is very sensitive to identify their location. Ultrasonography is less accurate in detection of undescended testis when it is located in the retroperitoneum. CT or MRI scans of abdomen and pelvis from the level of inguinal rings to lower poles of the kidney are required for testicular localization in such situations. MRI is more accurate because of its high soft tissue contrast and multi planner capabilities. The characteristic high signal intensity of testis on T2-weighted sequences aid in easy recognition of undescended testis. MRI scores over ultrasonography and CT in localization of atrophic undescended testis.

Testicular tumors are most common in the same age group in which fertility disorders of male are most prevalent. Testicular tumors may be identified in-patients presenting with oligospermia or azoospermia.[23] Seminomas are the most common testicular tumours and are usually homogeneously hypoechoic on sonography. Nonseminomatous tumors are complex and heterogeneous in echotexture. Testicular tumors are described in details in Chapter 124: Imaging of Scrotum.

Testicular torsion occurs most frequently during adolescence and therefore has the potential impact on fertility of affected young males. Acute testicular torsion is an emergency and torsed testis must be salvaged at the earliest. The degree of ischemic damage due to torsion depends on the duration of testicular torsion. There are good chances of salvage when patients are operated within seven hours. If it is delayed for more than 24 hours, virtually all testicular function is lost. On sonography, the affected testis is hypoechoic and may be enlarged. Color Doppler shows decreased vascularity, which is best appreciated when compared with contralateral normal testis.

Testicular trauma has less impact on male fertility than the other testicular factors such as torsion or cryptorchoidism.[22] Spermatogenic dysfunction may develop in testicular trauma patients, secondary to direct cell injury and the formation of anti sperm antibodies from disruption of blood–testis barrier in them. Ultrasonography with color Doppler is most suitable investigation to determine the extent of testicular trauma; however, satisfactory ultrasonography examination may not be possible in acutely traumatized and painful scrotum. In such situations, MRI is more accurate to detect disruption of the testicular capsule; however, most of these patients will need surgical exploration.

Higher incidence of testicular microlithiasis is found on scrotal ultrasonography in infertile men; however, its relationship with infertility is not known.[10]

Epididymis

The epididymis is located along the postero-lateral aspect of testis and runs parallel and posterior to the mediastinum testis. The head of the epididymis is pyramidal in shape and it is larger than rest of the epididymis. The head measures 5–12 mm in thickness.

Infertile man may have infection or inflammation of the epididymis. The normal epididymis has the echogenicity similar to the testis. In acute epididymitis, epididymis is enlarged and hypoechoic with increased vascularity on color Doppler. Chronic inflammation results in an enlarged and heterogeneously hyperechoic epididymis, sometimes with foci of calcification.[12] Scarring in chronically inflamed epididymis may result in epididymal obstruction, which can be avoided with early and aggressive treatment of epididymitis.

Epididymal cysts and spermatoceles are usually located at the head of the epididymis and these can be easily detected on sonography. Most epididymal cysts do not cause obstruction, however, rarely, these may compress the epididymal tubules and cause epididymal obstruction, especially if large, and produce oligo or azoospermia, Very large epididymal cysts may occasionally be difficult to differentiate from hydrocele on sonography, however, compression of epididymis and adjacent testicular margin and presence of the fluid at one end of the testis instead of surrounding the testis help to differentiate large epididymal cyst from hydrocele **(Fig. 2)**.

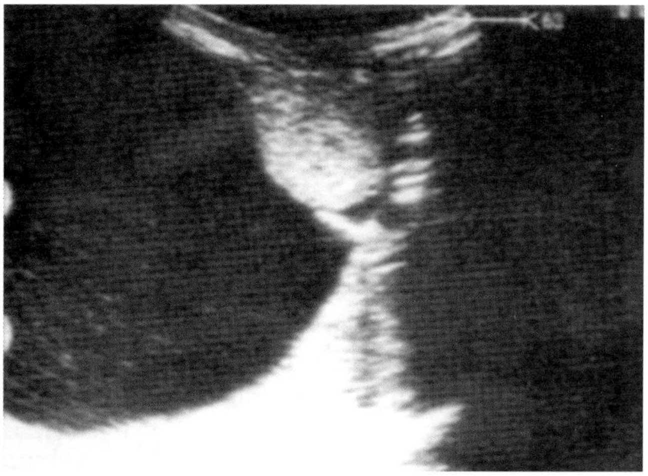

Fig. 2: Large epididymal cyst at the upper pole of testis seen on scrotal ultrasonography. Nonvisualization of normal epididymal head and eccentric displacement of testis instead of being surrounded by fluid helps differentiate this condition from hydrocele.

TRUS Evaluation of Distal Genital Ductal System

TRUS is indicated in infertile men with suspicion of obstructive pathology in distal sperm transport system. This is suggested by low volume ejaculate with oligo- or azoospermia and palpable abnormality on digital rectal examination. The conditions that produce low volume ejaculate with oligo- or azoospermia include agenesis of vas deferens and seminal vesicle, ejaculatory duct obstruction and urethral strictures.[1,7] Other indications of TRUS include hematospermia, painful ejaculation, severe sperm motility defects and azoospermia in normal volume ejaculate without testicular atrophy.[24]

On TRUS, normal prostate is a symmetric, triangular and ellipsoid structure with homogeneous echogenicity surrounded by a thin layer of echogenic capsule. Normal seminal vesicles are paired, well defined, sacular, elongated hypoechoic organs, situated cranial to the prostate and posterior to urinary bladder with 'bow-tie' appearance on axial images. These may vary in size, shape and degree of distention; however, usually these are symmetrical. On axial plane, ampulla of vasa deferentia are seen as round or oval tubular structures that are just cranial to prostate and medial to seminal vesicles. In sagittal plane, these can be seen behind prostate projecting medially towards seminal vesicles. Ejaculatory ducts are difficult to visualize on TRUS in normal men. These may sometimes be seen as tubular structures obliquely traversing the prostate and entering the urethra at verumontanum.[1]

Seminal Vesicles and Vas Deferens

Seminal vesicle secretions contribute about 80–90% of sperm volume. They also secrete fructose and maintain an acidic pH of semen. Congenital anomalies and obstructive lesions of seminal vesicles result in decreased semen volume, low pH and low fructose levels.

Wolffian duct anomalies include renal agenesis, agenesis of vas deferens, agenesis or atrophy of seminal vesicles and cysts of seminal vesicles. Seminal vesicle atrophy or agenesis may be unilateral or bilateral.[2] It occurs in all patients with agenesis of vas deferens. Bilateral absence of seminal vesicles may be seen in up to 40% of patients with low volume azoospermia.[4] It can be diagnosed with semen analysis and clinical examination in most patients.[25] Large number of these patients also has associated renal anomalies. Another strong association is with cystic fibrosis in which 98% of men have agenesis of seminal vesicles and vas deferens.[4] On TRUS or MRI, seminal vesicle is considered atrophic if it measures less than 7 mm in width and dilated (as in ejaculatory duct obstruction) when it measures more than 15 mm.[2,8] Diagnosis of seminal vesicle and vas agenesis is made when these are not visualized **(Fig. 3)**.

Cysts of seminal vesicles may be congenital or acquired. Congenital cyst of seminal vesicle results from an ectopic ureter insertion into the seminal vesicle and is associated with a hypoplastic kidney on the same side. This cyst may compress ejaculatory duct and produce obstruction. Acquired cysts of seminal vesicles are secondary to infection. Chronic inflammation produces cystic dilatation with scarring and obstruction of the lumen of the seminal vesicles and causes infertility **(Fig. 4)**. Stone formation in dilated seminal vesicles can be readily demonstrated on TRUS **(Figs. 5A and B)**, however, this appears to be secondary to stasis rather than cause of the obstruction.[8,26]

Ejaculatory Ducts

These are formed by confluence of seminal vesicles and terminal ampullary portion of the vas deferens, and hence, ejaculatory duct obstruction results in decreased semen volume with absence of seminal fructose. TRUS may demonstrate ejaculatory duct cysts, dilatation of ejaculatory ducts **(Fig. 6)** or calcification in ejaculatory ducts along with dilated seminal vesicles 4.[27] Any of these findings strongly suggest ejaculatory duct obstruction.

Many of these conditions can be treated with transurethral resection of the ejaculatory duct (TURED).[27] Specificity of TRUS in the diagnosis of ejaculatory duct obstruction is unsatisfactory, hence, TRUS-guided seminal vesicle aspiration followed by vesiculography is useful before TURED.[28,29] TRUS-guided seminal vesicle aspiration is performed with a 21G needle introduced transrectally. Presence of motile sperms in seminal vesicle fluid strongly suggests ejaculatory duct obstruction because sperms are not normally seen in seminal vesicles. The aspiration is followed by injection of 5–20 mL of dilute noniodinated contrast under fluoroscopic guidance and images are obtained to study the seminal vesicles and ejaculatory ducts. Pelvic and inguinal portions of vas deferens may also be visualized with this technique.[24]

Prostate

Müllerian duct cyst and utricle cyst are congenital prostatic cysts which may be indistinguishable from each other. When large, these may compress and produce ejaculatory duct obstruction.[2] On imaging, both are seen as midline cyst in

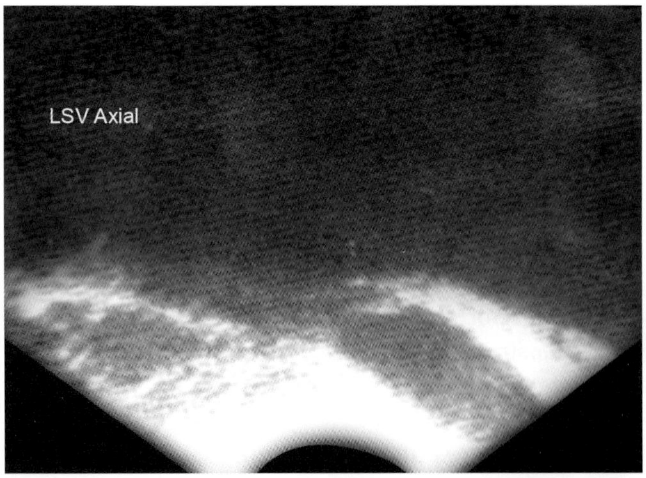

Fig. 3: Agenesis of seminal vesicle: TRUS shows absence of seminal vesicle on right side on axial scan. Normal left seminal vesicle (LSV) is seen as hypoechoic elongated structure behind the urinary bladder.

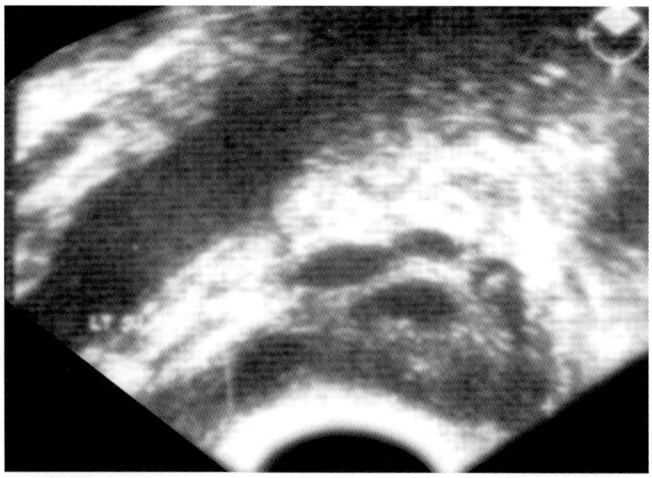

Fig. 4: Multiple postinflammatory seminal vesicle cysts are seen on axial TRUS scan.

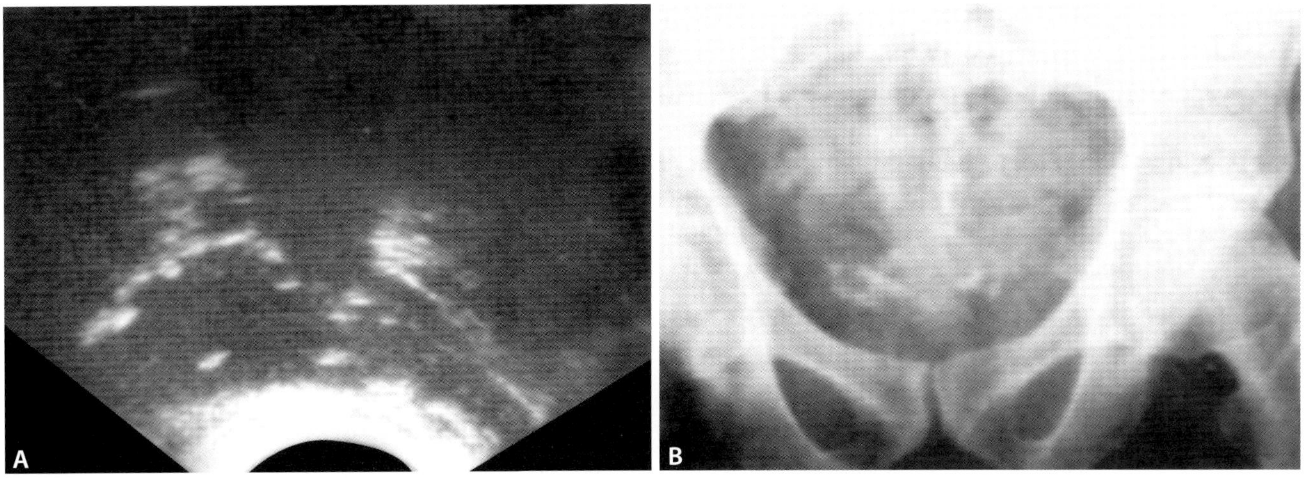

Figs. 5A and B: Seminal vesicle calculi: (A) Axial TRUS scan; (B) AP radiograph of pelvis.

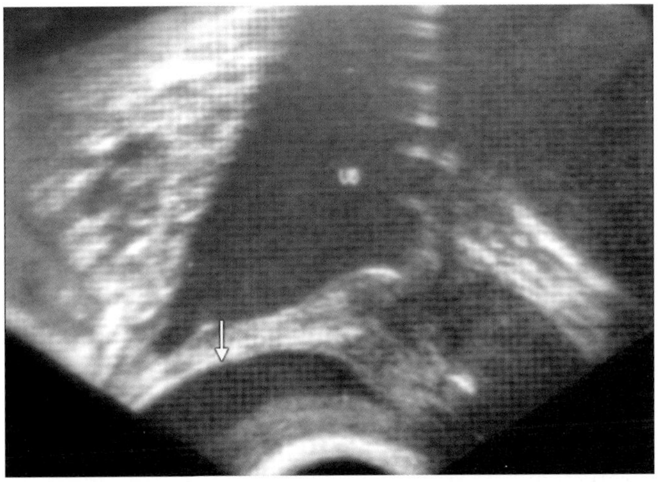

Fig. 6: Ejaculatory duct obstruction: Cystic dilatation of ejaculatory duct (arrow) is seen on sagittal TRUS image.

prostate. Müllerian duct cysts do not communicate with urethra and when large, may extend above the prostate. Utricle cysts communicate with urethra and do not extend above prostate. Acquired prostatic cysts like parasitic and prostatic retention cysts are usually located peripherally. These may produce obstruction to semen flow within the prostate and subsequent infertility. Chronic prostatitis may produce scarring, atrophy of seminal vesicles and strictures of ejaculatory duct which may lead to infertility.[2] These can be identified on TRUS as disorganization of normal anatomy produced by scarring of prostatic tissue and occasional stone formation.[4]

MRI in Infertility

Scrotal MRI is the most important adjunct to ultrasonography in evaluation of testicular and paratesticular abnormalities. It is highly accurate in cryptorchidism, testicular tumors, trauma and infection. Scrotal MRI is described in details in Chapter 124: Imaging of Scrotum.

MRI is recommended for the evaluation of distal genital tract when TRUS findings are equivocal.[8,26] Various abnormalities of prostate and seminal vesicles, such as cysts of seminal vesicles and ejaculatory duct, dilatation of vas deferens and seminal vesicles secondary to ejaculatory duct obstruction can be satisfactorily demonstrated. On MRI, absence or atrophy of seminal vesicles with very small size and loss of normal high-signal intensity is seen in up to 40% of patients.[26] Agenesis of vas may be demonstrated. MRI is particularly advantageous in suspected case of ejaculatory duct obstruction as demonstration of normal ejaculatory ducts rules out presence of ejaculatory duct obstruction.[30]

Imaging in Assisted Fertilization

Scrotal sonography is also useful in the work up of assisted fertilization. Testicular volume as calculated on sonography can predict the outcome of testicular biopsies for sperm retrieval. Chances of successful sperm retrieval are significantly higher in patients with testicular volume more than 12 cc.[31] Similarly, sonography guided testicular sperm aspiration is more accurate and it has less complications when compared with the blind aspiration as sonography allows good visualization of testicular parenchyma, easy sampling and avoidance of prominent vessels.[32] In patients with ejaculatory duct obstruction, sperms can also be aspirated from seminal vesicles under TRUS guidance. Intra operative use of TRUS is helpful in identification of obstructing cyst and determining the depth of resection during trans urethral resection of ejaculatory duct for the treatment of ejaculatory duct obstruction.[33]

ERECTILE DYSFUNCTION

Erectile dysfunction (ED) or impotence is defined as inability to achieve and/or maintain an erection for satisfactory sexual intercourse.[34] Its prevalence increases with age and affects up to 52% men between age group of 40 and 69 years.[35] ED is broadly classified into two categories: organic and psychologic. Vasculogenic impotence is the most common cause of organic impotence and may be a marker for occult cardiovascular disease.[36] Vascular ED does not rule out the presence of contributing psychological factors, but merely means that vascular factors are predominant cause of ED. Vascular ED has two different mechanisms: obstruction in penile inflow tract, termed as arterial ED and the inability to trap the incoming blood in the cavernosa, termed as veno-occlusive ED.

Anatomy and Physiology of Penile Erection

The paired internal pudendal arteries give rise to common penile arteries which divide into four branches, one each to spongiosa, cavernosa, proximal urethra and the dorsum of the penis (deep dorsal artery). The cavernosal artery provides blood to cavernosa through multiple helicine arteries that open directly into the cavernosal sinusoids. Venules located within the subtunical space between the periphery of erectile tissue and the tunica albugenia provide venous outflow channel from corpora cavernosa via peripheral lacunae. These vein pierce tunica albuginea and drain into cavernosal and then into deep dorsal vein.

Penile erection is a neurovascular phenomenon in which neurological stimulus via parasympathetic nerves from sacral 2–4 leads to arterial response. It is initiated by relaxation of smooth muscles of helicine arteries leading to vasodilatation. The phase of arterial response is followed by the phase of tumescence, in which relaxation of trabecular smooth muscles and increased arterial flow lead to increase in size and length of the penis. The phase of erectile response follows when subtunical venules are compressed against tunica albuginea due to dilatation of sinusoids and increase in intracavernosal pressure. If this veno-occlusive mechanism is intact, the arterial inflow leads to increase in intracavernosal pressure to the levels of mean arterial blood pressure. Perineal muscles contractions generate further increase in pressure, which leads erectile response to rigidity.

Parameters of quality of the arterial response are peak systolic velocity and acceleration time as measured by pharmacopenile duplex ultrasonography (PPDU) and cavernosal artery occlusion pressure as measured by cavernosometry. Parameters to assess the quality of veno-occlusive mechanism are end diastolic velocity and resistive index on PPDU and maintenance flow and pressure loss on cavernosometry.

Evaluation of Erectile Dysfunction

Psychologic factors or systemic illnesses are responsible for erectile dysfunction in majority of patients. Careful history, clinical examination and routine laboratory tests are extremely important for the evaluation of ED as these can identify the underlying cause in up to 80% of patients.[37] Such work-up may detect reversible cause of ED or unmask the systemic illness responsible for ED. With advent of effective oral pharmacotherapy, the diagnostic approach has significantly changed over past decade. A good erectile response to these drugs excludes significant arterial or vascular disease as a cause of ED. Hence, most patients are first given a therapeutic trial and only those with failure are referred for invasive diagnostic tests like PPDU, cavernosography or angiography.[34]

Pharmacopenile Duplex Ultrasonography

Pharmacopenile duplex ultrasonography (PPDU) is most widely used investigation to define vascular ED and to differentiate between arterial insufficiency and defective veno-occlusive mechanism.

The different vasoactive agents used for PPDU are papaverine, combination of papaverine and phentolamine and prostaglandin PGE_1 (Trimix).[34] Papaverine may lead to false negative erectile response in some patients and persistent painful erection (priapism) may occur in other. Prostaglandin PGE_1 has better erection rate and less incidence of priapism.[38] Genital self-stimulation, visual erotic stimulus or application of penoscrotal tourniquet may augment the erectile response. Gadgets like virtual glasses with facility for audio-visual erotic stimulus improve the erectile response and Doppler waveform, thereby eliminating the false positive results of PPDU examination.[39]

Technique of PPDU: The examination must be conducted in an atmosphere of privacy. The ultrasonographic evaluation begins with scanning of flaccid penile shaft in transverse plane to measure the diameter of cavernosal artery. It ranges from 0.2 to 1 mm.[34] Although the arterial flow in the flaccid penis is difficult to demonstrate, Doppler flowmetry of flaccid penis has the potential to detect arteriogenic ED. Peak systolic velocity of less than 10 cm/sec in the cavernosal artery of flaccid penis is suggestive of arteriogenic ED.[40] Later, intracavernosal injection of 60 mg of papaverine is made with 30 G needle in either of the cavernosa as cross communications exist between both sides. Care must be taken not to inject into a vessel or urethra. The erectile response is graded visually from E0 to E5 as suggested by Broderick et al.[41] **(Table 1)**. Grade E4 and E5 are sufficient for penetration.

After evaluating the erectile response, scanning is started from the base at the penoscrotal junction to distal part, both in transverse and longitudinal planes. Dorsal scanning in saggital plane is necessary to identify cavernosal collaterals and penile deformities such as Peyronie's disease. The post-injection diameter of both cavernosal arteries is measured. Angle corrected flow velocities are measured as proximal as possible in cavernosal arteries. Most accurate flowmetry values are obtained at the time of peak rigidity, however, this time is highly variable. Hence, flowmetry values are normally obtained at 0, 5,10 and 20 minutes after the injection.

Post-papaverine injection normal spectral waveform has been described to have five phases **(Figs. 7A to D)**.[42]

Table 1: Visual grading of penile erection during PPDU.

E0	No response
E1	Elongation of shaft only
E2	Moderate tumescence, no rigidity
E3	Full tumescence, no rigidity, easily bendable
E4	Full erection, partial rigidity
E5	Full rigidity for at least 20 minutes

Phase 1 is characterized by increase in both systolic and diastolic velocities. In phase 2, there is progressive decrease in end diastolic velocity and appearance of a diachrotic notch. Patients with severe venous leakage do not progress beyond phase 2. In phase 3, diastolic flow approximates zero and it is reversed in phase 4. Phase 5 is characterized by eventual loss of both systolic and diastolic signals.

Various parameters studied on flowmetry are peak systolic velocity (PSV), end diastolic velocity (EDV), acceleration time (AT), and resistive index (RI). Mild variations are seen in cutoff values described in different studies. PSV of more than 35 cm/sec rules out arterial insufficiency and PSV of 25 cm/sec is highly suggestive of the same. Lot of overlap is seen between these two values in normal and abnormal individuals.[2] Currently acceptable reference values to interpret the examination as normal are given in **Table 2.**[34,38]

In a study of 32 men without evidence of vascular ED conducted at AIIMS, the mean PSV was 61.3 cm/sec, the mean EDV was –1.2 cm (minus sign denotes flow reversal) and the mean AT was 0.06 sec.[43] Mean RI was 0.93 in whom diastolic flow reversal was not achieved. Another interesting observation was the linear relationship between PSV and ages of the individuals, which implies that use of single cut-off value for all ages may be debatable.

Abnormal PSV (less than 25 cm/sec) and AT (more than 0.11 sec) are suggestive of arterial disease. Similarly,

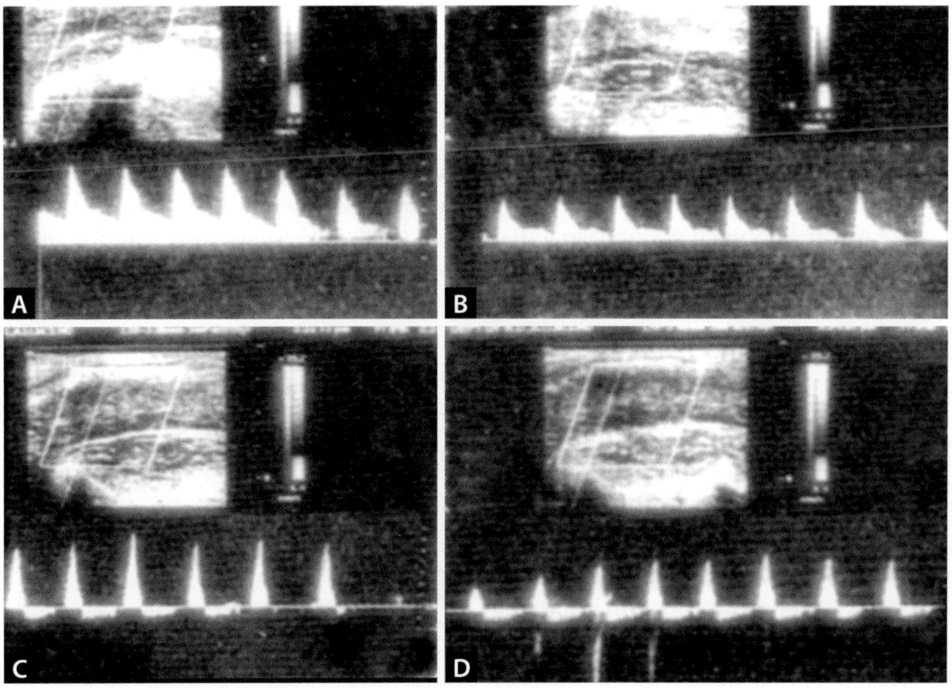

Figs. 7A to D: Normal spectral waveform progression of PPDU: (A) Early tumescence; (B) Late tumescence; (C) Early rigidity; (D) Peak rigidity.

Table 2: Normal reference values for PPDU.

PSV	25 cm/sec or more
EDV	5 cm/sec or less
AT	0.11 sec or less
RI	0.85 or more

Abbreviations: PSV: Peak systolic velocity; EDV: End diastolic velocity; AT: Acceleration time; RI: Resistive index.

any increase in the cavernosal artery diameter by less than 75% of the baseline diameter also indicates possibility of arterial disease. Abnormal EDV (more than 5 cm/ sec) and RI (less than 0.85) denote venous leakage. RI is considered more reliable than EDV for assessment of veno occlusive mechanism.[43] If arterial disease is present, intracavernosal pressure remains below systemic pressure and veno-occlusion cannot occur, even if this mechanism is intact, and diastolic flow will continue to persist. Therefore, veno-occlusive mechanism cannot be assessed with EDV and RI in presence of arterial disease.

PPDU with oral sidenafil: Sidenafil citrate (Viagra) has been studied as an alternative to intracavernosal injection of vasoactive drugs for PPDU, in order to make the examination noninvasive. However, the results are inconsistent.[44,45] Oral dose of 50 or 100 mg is normally used. Unlike intracavernosal agents, sidenafil alone cannot achieve erection and it must be supplemented with audiovisual sexual stimulation. Effect of sidenafil is also slow and peak erection is usually achieved between 60–75 minutes after its oral administration. The quality of erection and the PSV achieved with sidenafil is lower than the same parameters achieved after intracavernosal injection. This may lead to false-positive PPDU results in some patients.[45] With these limitations, oral sidenafil has failed to replace intracavernosal injections of vasoactive drugs for PPDU. A recent study has suggested that best results are obtained with combination of oral sidenafil and intracavernosal injection of trimix during PPDU.[46]

Peyronie's Disease

This is a benign condition resulting from inelastic scar of tunica albuginea, which produces curvature deformities of penis and the ED. It is traumatic in origin in majority of the patients and the ED in these patients is primarily because of penile deformities, painful erection or associated vascular disorders.[47] On sonography, the penile plaques are seen as echogenic focal thickenings of tunica, which may displace or encase dorsal vasculature. Dense plaques may contain calcifications and cause acoustic shadowing **(Fig. 8)**; however, shadowing can be seen even without

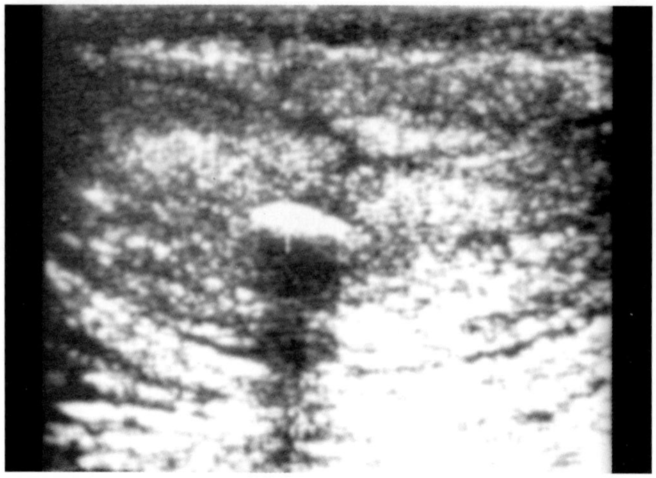

Fig. 8: Peyronie's disease: Dense echogenic plaque of tunica albuginea with distal shadowing is seen on PPDU.

evidence of calcification on plain radiographs. Most plaques are located in the middle third of the shaft of the penis.[38]

Cavernosometry

Cavernosometry is a primary modality available for quantifying and mapping of veno-occlusive dysfunction. However, because of its invasive nature, it is reserved for patients with suggestion of venous leakage on PPDU if surgical repair is being considered for them. In cavernosometry, venous outflow resistance is assessed by determining the intracavernosal flow rate required to sustain an erection in a state of complete sinusoidal relaxation.

In this technique, two 19G needles are introduced, one in each cavernosa. One needle is connected to the infusion pump and the other needle to a pressure monitor. A mixture of 30 mg of papaverine and 1 mg of phentolamine is infused. The intracavernosal pressure rises gradually and then remains steady. After this, the infusion flow rate is gradually increased to demonstrate linearly proportional increase in intracavernosal pressure. Linear relationship between cavernosal pressure and infusion rate is suggestive of a state of complete sinusoidal relaxation. If a nonlinear relationship is observed, a second dose of papaverine may be given to achieve complete sinusoidal relaxation.

Maintenance flow rate is considered as the most important parameter of cavernosometry and it involves recording of minimum flow rate, which is required to maintain intra cavernous pressure at 150 mm Hg. Maintenance flow rate of more than 3 mL/min is suggestive of venous leakage. After this, the infusion is stopped and the rate of fall of cavernosal pressure is observed for

30 seconds. The rate of fall, termed as 'pressure loss', of more than 1.5 mm Hg per second is considered abnormal.[38]

Gravity cavernosometry is a simple and cost effective modification of the above technique in which the inflow needle is connected to heparinized normal saline kept at the height of 160 cm. The infusion produces increase in cavernosal pressure which subsequently reaches at a pleatuea, termed as 'steady state pressure'. Steady state pressure of less than 97 mm Hg is considered abnormal.[48]

Cavernosography

Patient can be taken up for cavernosography after cavernosometry in the same sitting. About 40 mL of iodinated contrast is injected in infusion line while keeping intra cavernosal pressure just above mean arterial pressure. Spot films of penis and pelvis are obtained under fluoroscopic guidance in AP and both oblique projections **(Figs. 9A and B)**. Normally draining veins are not opacified. In case of venous leakage, veins are visualized draining from the veins of corpus spongiosum, the deep dorsal, cavernosal and crural veins **(Figs. 10A and B)**. More than one site is present in most patients, with deep dorsal and cavernosal veins being the most common combination.[49]

Penile Angiography

Internal pudendal angiography is indicated in younger patients with suspected isolated arterial disease, such as post-traumatic narrowing, who may benefit from

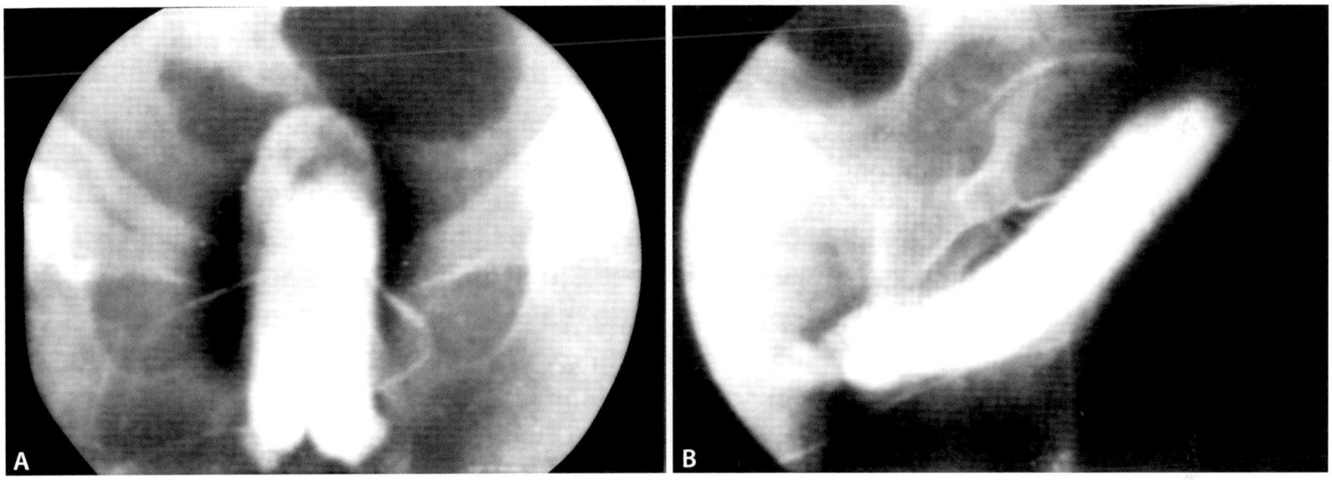

Figs. 9A and B: Normal cavernosogram: (A) AP and (B) oblique views show homogeneous opacification of bilateral cavernosa without visualization of any vein in victinity.

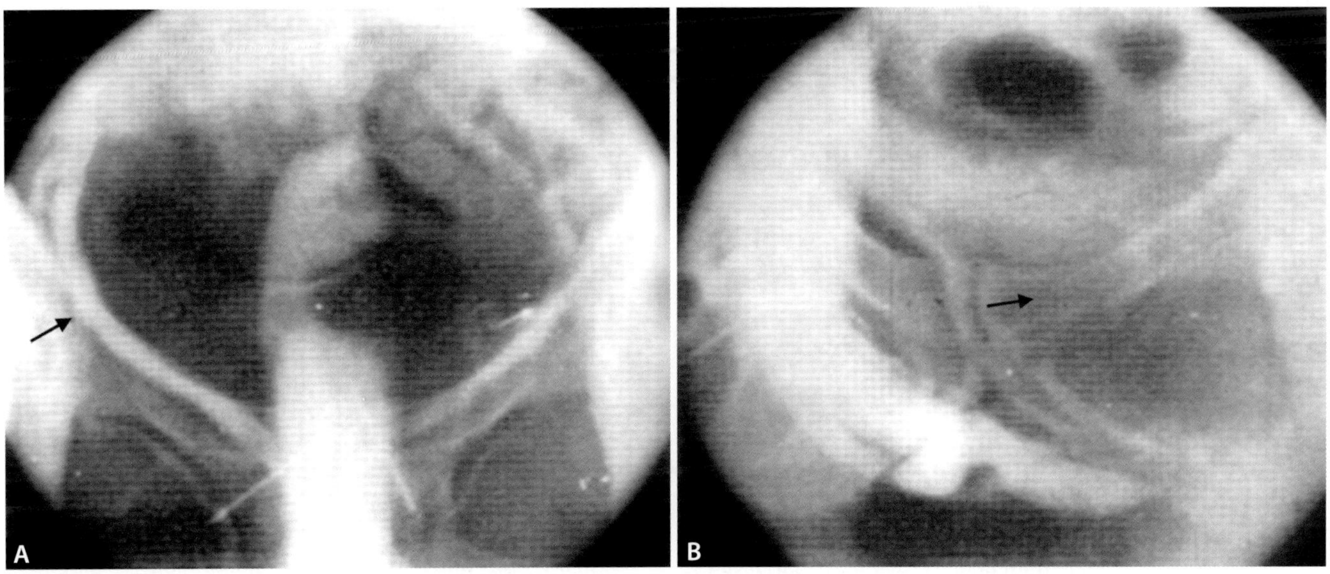

Figs. 10A and B: Cavernosogram: Veno-occlusive ED: (A) AP view shows venous leak into internal pudendal vein (arrow); (B) Oblique view shows venous leak into deep dorsal vein in the cavernosogram of another patient.

surgical repair rather than in elderly patients with diffuse atheromatous involvement. Patency of common iliac, internal iliac and internal pudendal arteries is established on initial angiographic films. Later, 60 mg of papaverine is injected in cavernosa followed by selective angiography of anterior division of internal pudendal artery. Contrast is injected at the rate of 3–4 mL per second and images are obtained in posterior oblique projection. In majority of the patients, anatomy of the penile arterial supply and the precise location of the arterial lesion is demonstrated which allows planning of appropriate surgical approach **(Figs. 11A and B)**.

Priapism

The most common complication during the diagnostic work-up and especially during PPDU and cavernosometry is papaverine induced prolonged and painful erection or priapism. The incidence can be as high as 11%.[34] Chances of priapism are high if PSV of more than 66 cm/s or RI of more than 1 (diastolic flow reversal) is observed.[50] It is prudent to observe the patient for at least 2 hours after the procedure. Not all priapism cases require specific treatment as penis detumescence generally occurs within few hours. In case the duration of erection exceeds six hours, the corpora cavernosa are drained to decrease the pressure and 10 micrograms of adrenaline is injected intracavernosally to induce cavernosal smooth muscle contraction, effective venous drainage and restriction of arterial flow. Compression bandage is also applied for few minutes. In case of recurrence of erection, the procedure is repeated.

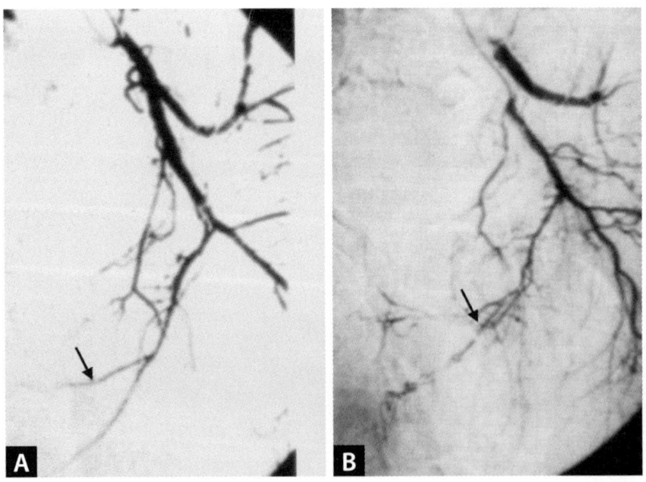

Figs. 11A and B: Internal pudendal angiogram: (A) Normal internal pudendal and common penile (arrow) arteries; (B) Internal pudendal angiogram of another patient shows post-traumatic narrowing of common penile artery (arrow) as a cause of arteriogenic ED.

Broadly, priapism is divided into high flow and low flow priapism. High flow priapism is usually associated with trauma. The patients have painless erection and venous outflow is usually maintained. The diagnosis of high flow priapism is usually clinical but color Doppler US may provide useful information. No cavernosal injection is required for the study. A hypoechoic area may be seen in cavernosa on gray-scale US which suggest laceration. Color Doppler study may demonstrate the cavernosal artery tear and arterial–lacunar fistula. Selective embolization of the torn artery with blood clots, coils or PVA is the treatment of choice to treat these lesions.[51]

Low flow or ischemic priapism is seen as complication of intracavernosal injection of drugs or leukostasis in leukemic patients. The diagnosis is clinical and imaging is not required before surgical intervention. The condition is considered as an urologic emergency. US and color Doppler findings are same as that of normal rigid erection.

REFERENCES

1. Kuligowska E. Transrectal ultrasonography in diagnosis and management of male infertility: In Jaffe R, Pierson RA, Abramowics JS (Eds): Imaging in Infertility and Reproductive Endocrinology, JB Lippincot Co. Philadelphia; 1994.pp.217-29.
2. Parsons RB, Fisher AM, Bar-Chama N, et al. MR imaging in male infertility. Radiographics. 1997;17:627-37.
3. Colpi GM, Contalbi GF, Nerva F, et al. Testicular function following chemoradiotherpay. Eur J Obstet Gynecol Reprod Biol. 2004;113 Suppl: S2-6.
4. Cornund E, Amar E, Hamida K, et al. Ultrasound findings in male hypofertility and impotence. Eur Radiol. 2001;11:2126-36.
5. Pierik FH, Dohle GR, Muiswinkel JM, et al. Is routine scrotal ultrasonography advantageous in infertile men? J Urol. 1999;162:1618-20.
6. Jarrow JP. Transrectal ultrasonography of infertile men. Fertil Steril. 1993;60:1035-39.
7. Raviv G, Mor Y, Levron J, et al. Role of transrectal ultrasonography in the evaluation of azoospermic men with low volume ejaculate. J Ultrasound Med. 2006;25:825-9.
8. Engin G, Kadioglu A, Orhan I, et al. Transrectal US and endorectal MR imaging in partial and complete obstruction of the seminal duct system: a comparative study. Acta Radiol. 2000;41:288-95.
9. Dhabuwala CB, Parulkar BG. Doppler flow analysis and conventional ultrasonography for evaluation of the infertile male: In Jafe R, Pierson RA, Abramowics JS (Eds): Imaging in Infertility and Reproductive Endocrinology, JB Lippincot Co. Philadelphia; 1994.pp.207-16.

10. Qublan HS, Al-Okoor K, Al-Ghoweri AS, et al. Sonographic spectrum of scrotal abnormalities in infertile men. J Clin Ultrasound. 2007;35:437-41.
11. Howards SS. Varicocele. Infertil Reprod Med Clin N Am 1992;3:429-41.
12. Dambro TJ, Stewart RR, Carroll BA, et al. The scrotum. In: Rumack CM, Wilson SR, Charboneau JW (Eds). Diagnostic ultrasound, 2nd edition, St Louis, Mosby; 1998.pp.719-822.
13. Beddy P, Geoghegan T, Browne RF, et al. Testicular varicocele. Clin Radiol. 2005;60:1248-55.
14. McLure RD, Hrickak H. Scrotal ultrasound in infertile man: detection of subclinical unilateral and bilateral varicocele. J Urol. 1986;135:711-4.
15. Kokacok E, Serhatlioglu S, Kiris S, et al. Colour Doppler sonographic evaluation of interrelations between diameter, reflux and flow volume of testicular veins in varicocele. Eur J Radiol. 2003;47:251-6.
16. Kessler A, Meirsdorf S, Graif M, et al. Intratesticular varicocele: grey scale and color Doppler sonographic appearance. J Ultrasound Med. 2005;24:1711-6.
17. Dubin L, Amelar R. Varicocele size and results of varicocelectomy in selected infertile men with a varicocele. Fertil Steril. 1970;21:606-9.
18. McLure R, Kho D, Dale R, et al. Subclinical varicocele- the effectiveness of varicocelectomy. J Urol. 1991;145:786-90.
19. Gonda RL Jr, Kaw JJ, Forte KA et al. Diagnosis of subclinical varicocele in infertility. AJR 1987;148:71-5.
20. Gandini R, Konda D, Reale CA, et al. Male varicocele: transcatheter foam sclerotherapy with sodium tetradecyl sulfate- outcome in 244 patients. Radiology. 2008;246:612-8.
21. Halden W, White RI. Outpatient embolotherapy of varicocele. Urol Clin N Am. 1987;14:137-40.
22. Thompson ST. Prevention of male infertility - an update. Urol Clin N Am. 1994;21:365-76.
23. Simon SD, Lee RD, Mulhall PP. Should all infertile males undergo urologic evaluation before assisted reproductive technologies? Fertil Steril. 2001;75:1226-7.
24. Kim Ed, Lipshultz LI: Role of ultrasound in assessment of male infertility. J Clin Ultrasound. 1996;24:437-53.
25. Kumar R, Thulkar S, Kumar V, et al. Contributions of investigations to the diagnosis of bilateral vas aplasia. ANZ J Surg. 2005;75:807-9.
26. Kim MJ, Lee JT, Lee MS, et al. MR imaging of male infertility with an endo rectal surface coil. Abdom Imaging. 1997;22:348-53.
27. Fisch H, Lambert SM, Goluboff ET. Management of ejaculatory duct obstruction: etiology, diagnosis and treatment. World J Urol. 2006;24:604-10.
28. Colpi GM, Negri L, Nappi RE, et al. Is transrectal ultrasonography a reliable diagnostic approach in ejaculatory duct sub obstruction? Hum Reprod. 1997;12: 2186-91.
29. Purohit RS, Wu DS, Shinohara K, et al. A prospective comparison of three diagnostic methods to evaluate ejaculatory duct obstruction. J Urol. 2004;171:232-5.
30. Schnall MD, Pollack HM, Arsdalen KV, et al. The seminal tract in patients with ejaculatory dysfunction: MR imaging with an endorectal surface coil. AJR. 1992;159:337-41.
31. Toov JH, Fait G, Houser R, et al. Can Doppler ultrasonographic measurements of the testis predict spermatozoa retrieval in azoospermic patients undergoing testicular biopsy? Fertil Steril. 2001;76:1276-7.
32. Belenky A, Avrech CM, Bacher GN, et al. Ultrasound guided testicular sperm aspiration in azospermic patient: a new sperm retrieval method for intra cytoplasmic sperm injection. J Clin Ultrasound. 2001;6:339-43.
33. Belker AM, Steinbock GS. Transrectal prostate ultrasonography as a diagnostic and therapeutic aid for ejaculatory duct obstruction. J Urol. 1990;144:356-8.
34. Mihmanli I, Kantarci F. Erectile dysfunction. Semin Ultrasound CT MRI. 2007;28:274-86.
35. Araujo AB, Mohr BA, McKinley JB. Changes in sexual function in middle aged and older men: longitudinal data from the Massachusetts male aging study. J Am Geriatr Soc. 2004;52:1502-9.
36. Montorsi F, Briganti A, Salonia A, et al. Erectile dysfunction prevalence, time of onset, and association with risk factors in 300 consecutive patients with acute chest pain, and angiographically documented coronary artery disease. Eur Urol. 2003;44:360-4.
37. Hatzichristan D, Hatzimouratidis K, Bekas M, et al. Diagnostic steps in evaluation of patients with erectile dysfunction. J Urol. 2002;168:615-20.
38. Meuleman E, Diemont WL. Investigation of erectile dysfunction. Urol Clin N Am. 1995;22:803-19.
39. Park K, Kwon DD, Oh BR, et al. Efficacy of virtual glasses in audio-visual sexual stimulation during penile colour duplex Doppler ultrasonography. Eur Urol. 2002;41:62-5.
40. Roy C, Saussine C, Tuchman C, et al. Duplex Doppler sonography of flaccid penis: potential role in the evaluation of impotence. J Clin Ultrasound. 2000;28:290-4.
41. Broderick GA, Arger P. Duplex Doppler ultrasonography: noninvasive assessment of penile anatomy and function. Semin Roentgen. 1993;28:43-56.
42. Shwartz AM, Lawe M, Berger RE, et al: Assessment of normal and abnormal erectile function-color Doppler sonography versus conventional techniques. Radiology. 1991; 180:105-9.
43. Bhargava R, Srivastava DN, Thulkar S, et al. Colour duplex Doppler ultrasonography evaluation of non-vasculogenic male erectile dysfunction: an Indian perspective. Australas Radiol. 2002;44:170-73.
44. Arslan D, Esen AA, Secil M. A new method for evaluation of ED: Sidenafil plus Doppler ultrasonography. J Urol. 2001;166:181-4.
45. Copel L, Ktz R, Blacher A, et al. Clinical and duplex US assessment of effects of sidenafil on cavernosal arteries of the penis: comparison with intracavernosal injection of vasoactive agents- initial experience. Radiology. 2005;237:986-91.

46. Park JK, Park JS, Jeon SB, et al. Why a combined intracavernosal injection with trimix and oral sidenafil is reliable therapy in ultrasonic evaluation of erectile dysfunction. BJU Int. 2008;102:993-7.
47. Gholami SS, Lue TF. Peyronie's disease. Urol Clin N Am. 2001;28:377-90.
48. Meulman EJ, Wijkstra H, Doesbury WH, et al: Comparison of diagnostic values of pump and gravity cavernosometry in the evaluation of cavernous veno-occlusive mechanism. J Urol. 1991;146:1266-70.
49. Shabsingh R, Fishman IJ, Toombs BD et al. Venous leaks: Anatomical and physiological observations. J Urol. 1991;146: 1260-4.
50. Metawea B, El-Nashar AR, Gad-Allah A, et al. Intracavernos papaverine phentolamine induced priapism can be accurately predicted with colour Doppler ultrasonography. Urology. 2005;66:858-60.
51. Campliani S, Savoca G, Buttazi L, et al. High flow priapism: treatment and long term follow-up. Urology. 2002;59: 110-3.

Section 5

Pediatric Imaging

CHAPTER 126

Technical Considerations in Pediatric Imaging

Ashu Seith Bhalla, Arun Kumar Gupta, Amar Mukund

INTRODUCTION

Technical factors such as the ability to position the patient and expose the radiograph with the patient immobile, which are often taken for granted in adult radiography, may appear as crippling problems in pediatric radiography. For this reason and because of the importance of minimizing radiation to the child, special attention must be paid to certain technical points. These will be discussed under the following five broad groups:

1. Minimizing heat loss
2. Immobilization
3. Sedation
4. Reduction of radiation dosage
5. Use of contrast media

MINIMIZING HEAT LOSS

Neonates and infants lose body heat rapidly, the risk of hypothermia being greatest in the premature baby with little subcutaneous fat. Local warmth may be obtained by special tabletop heating cradles, but the most convenient way of avoiding heat loss is to maintain a room temperature of about 27°C in room. A room thermometer is an important piece of equipment. Enhanced humidity is not normally required for the duration of an X-ray examination.[1]

IMMOBILIZATION

Atraumatic immobilization is essential in order to ensure proper positioning and to minimize patient motion. Newborn babies and small infants need only soft sandbags and adhesive tape to stop movement. Towels and sheets can also be used to tightly wrap babies. Older, stronger children require wrapping on immobilization boards in addition to tape and sandbags. Special X-ray equipment is available which is designed specifically for the examination of infants and children. The essential factors for an immobilization device are: (1) Absence of artifacts; (2) Safety; (3) No disturbance of the patient's sedation, and (4) Ease of handling. It is not always possible to accommodate older children on such apparatus. Cradle-holding devices are provided which enable the infant to be rotated in relation to the tabletop. When this type of equipment is not available, views such as the prone shoot through swallow for tracheoesophageal fistula may be obtained by using a device such as the Charteris baby holder inverted on the step of an up-right adult screening table.[1-3]

SEDATION

One fundamental technical component for imaging is the need for the child to remain motionless during the duration of imaging. Babies and infants under 6 months of age will often sleep after a feed and may not need sedation unless they are known to be restless, or the procedure is painful. Adjunctive measures such as sleep deprivation can also be useful. In older children, verbal reassurance may be sufficient. Venous access produces less disturbance, if a cannula is put in place after the area has been treated with a topical gel. Two possible areas can be prepared about 30 minutes before injection. Small gauge needles are used, often 22 to 25 gauge.

Warming of contrast medium makes injection through fine needles easier and less painful.[1,4,5]

Sedation, however, is often necessary, especially for procedures such as MRI due to its long duration, and for interventions due to the pain involved. Once it is deemed that both the procedure and sedation are necessary, every effort must be made to provide safety for the child. Even if the radiologist is not directly responsible for the sedation procedure, he or she must expedite the procedure in order to minimize the length of sedation. The timing of sedation and of the procedure need careful coordination.[1,5]

Monitoring the patient in the radiology suite is not an easy task for the clinicians. Observing children from the CT or MRI control room through a glass window is much more difficult for the clinician than direct observation at the bedside and increases their reliance on monitoring devices. Hence, adequate monitoring devices should be available. Pulse oximetry is commonly used during sedation. Monitoring is further complicated during MRI because the scanner generates strong static, radiofrequency and time varied magnetic fields which interfere with the monitoring devices. New nonferromagnetic monitors and cables have been deviced which are safe and reliable within the scanning suite. Standard ferromagnetic monitors, if used, need to be placed outside the magnetic field or carefully shielded.[4,5]

The radiology suite is less than ideal environment for dealing with respiratory arrest or cardiovascular collapse. Hence, the most important prerequisite to sedation is the availability of adequate equipment for resuscitation and personnel experienced in managing sedation complications. If the radiology suite is not equipped with wall outlets for oxygen and suction, portable oxygen cylinders and suction apparatus should be available. Also, a cart with resuscitation drugs, defibrillator, and age and size appropriate equipment for different age groups and body sizes for purpose of oxygen administration and intubation are absolutely essential.[4,5]

Risk factors must be taken into consideration before planning sedation. If the child's condition is tenuous enough for sedation to be a significant risk, precautionary measures like securing the airway should be taken before the child arrives in the radiology department. Knowledge of both the past and the present medical history is equally important.

Nil Per Orally Status

Aspiration is a significant concern in sedated children and nil per orally (NPO) guidelines should be as stringent as those in children undergoing general anesthesia. Guidelines recommended by American Academy of Pediatrics Committee on Drugs (AAPCOD) are as follows: clear liquids are allowable up to 2 hours before the procedure for any age; semisolid liquid (including breast milk) and solid foods are acceptable for up to 4 hours for children less than 6 months, 6 hours for children 6–36 months old and 8 hours for older children. Whenever possible, these recommendations must be followed. Bowel obstruction or ileus are other factors that increase the risk of aspiration because they delay gastric emptying. In these patients, nasogastric suction of gastric contents should be performed and agents given that promote gastric emptying, such as metoclopramide. The actual risk of aspiration in children undergoing diagnostic imaging is unknown, but it is probably quite low. In one recent report, aspiration of gastric contrast was present in no more than 4% of children undergoing CT scan examination in a setting of trauma.[4,6]

The practice of administering oral contrast material in children before sedation for abdominal CT is controversial. At some institutions, the practice of administering an enteric contrast material before sedation is being discouraged, because it violates the "nothing by mouth" status that is otherwise strictly enforced before sedation. However, recent studies have indicated that oral contrast appears to be safe when using the sedation drugs such as chloral hydrate and propofol. Further study of the safety of this practice is required.[7]

Pharmacological Agents

Several different agents have been successfully used for sedation of children for imaging studies. The choice of the agent depends on availability, local expertise and patient risk factors. The route of administration could be oral or parenteral. Intravenous route has the advantage of faster onset and reliable titration of dose. Other non-parenteral routes include the intranasal or rectal route.

The most commonly used sedative agents belong to one of the three classes of drugs:

1. Barbiturates,
2. Benzodiazepines, or
3. Narcotics.

Most often used *barbiturate* is pentobarbital. Others being methohexital and thiopental sodium. Pentobarbital and quinalbar-bitone are safe, effective oral agents in children under the age of 5 years. The *benzodiazepines* include diazepam and midazolam. Diazepam is not used routinely as a sedative for diagnostic imaging in children.

Respiratory depression is the most important concern with barbiturates while vomiting is often seen with midazolam. *Narcotics* are commonly used as an adjunct to other sedative agents in situations where pain control is desirable in addition to sedation.[4,5]

Besides these three groups of drugs, other commonly used agents include triclofos, chloral hydrate, propofol, ketamine and a combination of meperidine (Demerol), chlorpromazine (Phenargan) and promethazine (Thorazine) [also known as DPT, or the "lytic" cocktail], injected intramuscularly. Triclofos (pedicloryl) is a good sedative agent which can be used orally to sedate infants and children under 5 years undergoing procedure or imaging. Maximum dose of 70-100 mg/kg body weight may be given.[8] Years of experience, ease of administration, and an excellent safety record have made chloral hydrate the most widely used sedative for children undergoing radiologic imaging. It is most effective in children under 2 years of age. Use of propofol by radiologists is not widespread due to its anesthetic properties. Ketamine is a safe and effective agent for pediatric outpatient sedation and analgesia. Ketamine can be given by multiple routes and is one of only a few agents that are extremely predictable when administered intramuscularly. Furthermore, unlike benzodiazepines, barbiturates, and sedative/hypnotic agents; ketamine seldom causes respiratory depression. Ketamine, however, may cause raised intracranial pressure and should not be used when this is an issue. DPT has been popular as an analgesic and sedative to facilitate a variety of painful or anxiety-provoking procedures in children, but prolonged sedation times and the possibility of respiratory depression argue against the use of DPT in any setting. **Table 1** enlists the routes and doses of frequently used sedatives.[4,9]

REDUCTION OF RADIATION DOSAGE

It is essential to limit the dose of ionizing radiation to children as much as possible. Based on information concerning the effects of low-dose radiation to atomic bomb survivors who were irradiated as children with doses that are comparable to those received by children in helical CT, it is now known that there is a statistically significant, albeit, small individual risk for excess cancer in patients with doses used in CT. Children are more sensitive than adults by a factor of 10 because firstly, they have more time to express cancers than do adults and also because they have more dividing cells. Also, girls are more sensitive than boys. Hence, applying the ALARA principle in imaging becomes especially important in children. Gonad protection especially is essential.[10-12] Reduction of dose during an examination can be done at several levels, i.e. rational use of referral criteria, modification of equipment and technique. The most important prerequisite is the evaluation of need for an examination and the choice of most suitable modality accordingly. Specific pediatric adaptation of equipment such as restriction devices, tubes for immobilization and a removable grid are very useful for dose saving. Besides modification of equipment, operator-dependent factors, i.e. the technique is equally important.[12,13] Two major areas where reduction of radiation dose are critical are:

1. Radiography and fluoroscopy
2. Computed tomography

Table 1: Sedative agents and antagonists for pediatric imaging[4,8]

Agent	*Class and route**	*Effect and onset*	*Dose*	*Duration*
Chloral hydrate	PO (PR)	Sedative	50–100 mg/kg; up to 120 mg/kg reported. Maximum single dose 2 g	30–90 minutes
Pentobarbital sodium	Barbiturate IV (PO, IM)	Sedative 5–10 minutes	2–3 mg/kg dose titrated over 5–7 min until sedated, maximum cumulative dose of 8 mg/kg or 150–200 mg	40–60 minutes
Fentanyl citrate	Narcotic IV	Analgesic with sedative properties 1–2 minutes	1 mg/kg slowly IV over 5 minutes; adult-size patients 25–50 mg/dose; maximum cumulative dose 4 mg/kg	30–60 minutes
Midazolam	Benzodiazepine IV (PO)	Sedative, anxiolytic, Amnestic 1-5 minutes (IV)	0.02–0.05 mg/kg; titrate using half of original dose (over 2–4 minutes) based on effect and oxygen saturation; maximum of 1 mg	20–30 minutes

Abbreviations: IV: Intravenous; IM: Intramuscular; PO: Per os; PR: Per rectum.
*Preferred route listed first with alternate routes in brackets.

Radiography and Fluoroscopy

In procedures involving radiography and fluoroscopy, radiation dose reduction can be achieved at two broad levels:

1. Radiographic equipment factors
2. Operator dependent techniques.

Radiographic Equipment Factors

- Use of increased film-screen sensitivity
- Use of digital radiography
- Addition of filtration
- Use of carbon fiber materials
- In fluoroscopy
  - Modern image intensifiers
  - Pulsed fluoroscopy
  - Last image hold up system

Dynamic recording on videotape for screening procedures. Potential reduction using these changes have been studied by many investigators like Gozalez et al. (1995), Martin et al. (1994), Mooney et al. (1998), etc. who found dose reduction ranging from 30–85%.[14-16]

Screen-Film Combinations

The choice of the optimal screen-film combination has the greatest impact on dose reduction. The higher the sensitivity of the screen-film combination, the lower the patient dose. A dose reduction by a factor of 8–10 in comparison to universal screens is possible when rare earth screens with a high speed are used. Generally speaking, for routine examinations (with the exception of some bone disease like osteomyelitis, battered child), screens with a speed of at least 400 should be used. Some authors recommend systems with a speed of 600 because the radiation doses are minimum and their use permits very short exposure times, which also prevents motion blurring artifacts. These advantages outweigh the slightly lower resolution.[12,17]

Digital Radiography

Phosphor plates are now frequently used for intensive care radiography and even portable DR systems are available. Most modern CR and DR systems now effectively offer substantial patient dose reduction compared to screen-film radiography, however, in pediatric radiography this may not be true due to lack of standardization in exposure factors due to lack of understanding of fundamentals of CR and DR technology.[18,19] Moreover, other advantages of digital radiography are the fact that images can be stored and transferred electronically. Repeated exposures are no longer necessary because the contrast resolution is sufficient over a wider range than with conventional screen-film combinations; in particular, fine catheters and tubes are clearly seen. Also modern equipment have integrated "diagnostic reference dose levels". This is defined as dose levels for typical examinations for groups of standard sized patients. Using these presets, exposure can be adjusted as per the patient's size and hence dose may be reduced. Despite these advantages, these may be counterbalanced by dose increases due to the radiographer's unawareness of possible overexposure, since the visible film blackening is standardized by the reading mechanism of the laser imaging device. So, in order to reduce the radiation dose all guidelines implemented for conventional radiography, including appropriate collimation, appropriate source-to-image distance (SID), focal spot size, and patient positioning should be practiced in digital techniques as well.[18,19] It should be emphasized that while doing various portable examinations and pediatric applications requiring manual tube settings, special care should be taken as there may be unnoticed increase in exposure.

Additional Filtration

Additional filtration can reduce the entrance surface dose considerably up to about 50%, depending on the material used. Its use has the disadvantage that the image contrast is deteriorated and the tube load is increased. Adjustable additional filtration should be available for all X-ray tubes, which are used for pediatric exposures (Bucky tables, fluoroscopic equipment and mobile X-ray units). The recommended materials for additional filtration are 1.0 mm aluminum and 0.1–0.2 mm copper. Steel filtration (0.7 mm) can also be used.[12,20,21]

Use of Carbon Materials

The use of carbon materials for patient support, in anti-scatter grids and for the radiographic cassette face, allows transmission of a larger portion of the X-ray beam. The overall reduction in the absorbed dose due to this measure is in the range of about 30% to more than 50%.[13]

Fluoroscopy

Image intensifiers: Direct dark room fluoroscopy delivers higher radiation dose to the patient than fluoroscopy with image intensification, and produces images of lower quality. The use of direct fluoroscopy should hence be discontinued.

Also, the size of the image intensifier determines the receptor dose rate. The rule is that because of the need for constancy of brightness at the image intensifier input, smaller sizes of the image intensifier require higher dose rates. A similar increase in dose occurs, if electronic magnification is used. Two different dose rates should be available in order to select the lower dose for simple follow-through contrast studies, such as the barium enema, and to switch to the higher dose rate, if a high-contrast examine is needed, such as the tracheoesophageal fistula. Electronic magnification during fluoroscopy should be restricted to rare cases.[12,13]

Pulsed fluoroscopy: Pulsed fluoroscopy with and without grid controlled tubes reduces the effective screening time and hence, the dose can be dramatically reduced.[12,13]

Last image hold up system, Dynamic recording on videotape for screening procedures: Use of these techniques essentially contributes to a decrease in screening time by the operator and thus the dose.[12,13]

Flat-panel detector units: Recently, flat-panel detector units have been introduced for fluoroscopic and angiographic use. These units offer high quality images. However, the available studies do not show these units to be superior to conventional units with image intensifiers in reducing the radiation dose.[22,23] Hence, the guidelines implemented for conventional fluoroscopy should be followed to reduce patients dose.

Operator-dependent Techniques

- Field size
- Focus film distance
- Use of high voltage
- Shielding of sensitive organs
- Beam direction
- Avoid use of anti-scatter grid
- Minimizing fluoroscopic time
- Decrease in number of films.

Studies in the previous decade have shown that operator-dependent changes could lead to dose reductions of about 30–50% with no increase in the cost.

Field Size

This is the most important and most variable factor in the amount of radiation dose imparted to the patient and hence accurate field collimation should be meticulously followed. This is especially important in children because an increase in the field size in pediatric patients will cause a proportionally greater increase in individual exposure as compared to adults. This relatively higher increase is due to the smaller anatomical size of young patients. Compared to adults a similar edge length increase in pediatric patients will lead to a larger percentage of the body surface area being irradiated. Also because, up to 35% of the red bone marrow of infants is in the long bones of the arms and the legs, correct patient positioning and collimation in the transverse axis is also important when chest and/or abdominal films are taken.[12,13]

The actual field size also depends on a correctly functioning collimating system. In most machines, an automatic setting prevents collimation of radiographic exposure even if fluoroscopic field is collimated. This can be identified and switched off[12,24] **(Figs. 1A and B)**.

Five frequent reasons for bad collimation in daily practice, and consequently for oversized field areas, are:

1. Lack of knowledge of age-dependent anatomy
2. No information on pathology
3. Difficulty in patient positioning
4. Difficulty in patient immobilization
5. Difficulty in handling of the X-ray equipment.

Permanent training and supervision of the technicians and young radiologists is needed to optimize collimation, especially in neonates. In a European survey on neonatal chest radiography only 15% of the films had an acceptable field size.[25] In chest X-ray, inadvertent exposure of both the

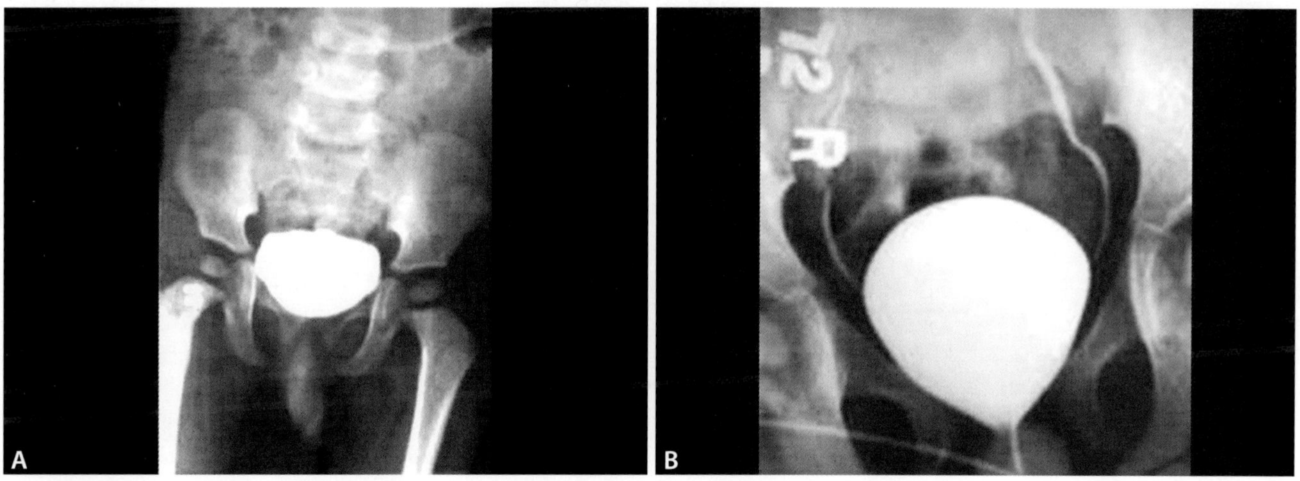

Figs. 1A and B: MCU, AP view bladder area: (A) Without automatic setting switched off showing unsatisfactory collimation; (B) With the setting is switched off, desired collimation is achieved.

skull and the abdomen, and in abdominal films of both the chest and the legs is too high, thereby increasing the red bone marrow dose. Up to 40% of the red bone marrow of infants and toddlers is in the skull, and 25% in the femora of premature babies.[12]

Focus Film Distance

The radiographer should always try to select the largest possible focus-patient distance during radiography. For example the longest distances are used for the upright anteroposterior (AP) spine for scoliosis (up to 300 cm). On the other hand, the focus-film distances (FFD) for X-rays performed with mobile units in neonatal wards (mainly chest and abdominal films) are often too short (less than 80 cm, sometimes even less than 60 cm). Ideally, the focus-film distance should be at least 100 cm. Incorrect and varying focus-film distances are the most important factor responsible for over-exposure of patients in the intensive care units.[12,13]

Use of High Voltage

In terms of radiation protection, there is an important relationship between the absorbed dose and the voltage used. A reduction in the kV causes a steep increase in the relative dose. A basic rule of radiation protection is that voltage values below 60 kV should not be used for X-rays of the body, trunk and head. The highest possible kV should be used. An increase in the voltage up to 120 kV can diminish the dose slightly, further, but is not at all useful in infants and young children because the image contrast is significantly degraded. Many generators cannot cope with the short switching times needed for high kV exposures. When voltage settings above 50 kV are used for small patients, one should use additional filtration to counterbalance the very small mAs-product, and thus allow for longer switching times.[12,13,24]

An increase in patient thickness causes an enormous increase in the required dose. The AP diameter in children up to one year of age is only 10–12 cm and is about 15 cm in older children up to five. In patients with a body diameter above 15 cm the dose increase is very steep. In order to deal with these relatively higher doses in school children, one should at first increase the kV-setting to avoid an undesirable concomitant increase in exposure time. This simple relationship is also important for fluoroscopy when lateral views have to be performed during voiding cystourethrography. Increasing the kV not only reduces the dose but also shortens the exposure time and thereby reduces motion blurring artifacts. However, the scatter will be increased with the use of higher kV. Scattered radiation can be diminished if the irradiated volume can be kept small by good collimation.[12]

In a study in our department at AIIMS, the use of high kV and low mA in radiographic exposures was studied during micturating cystourethrograms, under fluoroscopic guidance. The kV used was about 25% higher and mA about 50% lower than the routinely used parameters. It was found that the resultant dose area product (DAP) value per radiograph during an exposure was 25–28% lower than the DAP value per radiograph at the routinely used parameters when the same degree of collimation was used, and comparable image quality was obtained[23] **(Figs. 2A and B)**.

Low kV settings for the bones are only rarely needed for special indications, i.e. mostly for special skeletal disorders (osteogenesis imperfecta, etc).[12]

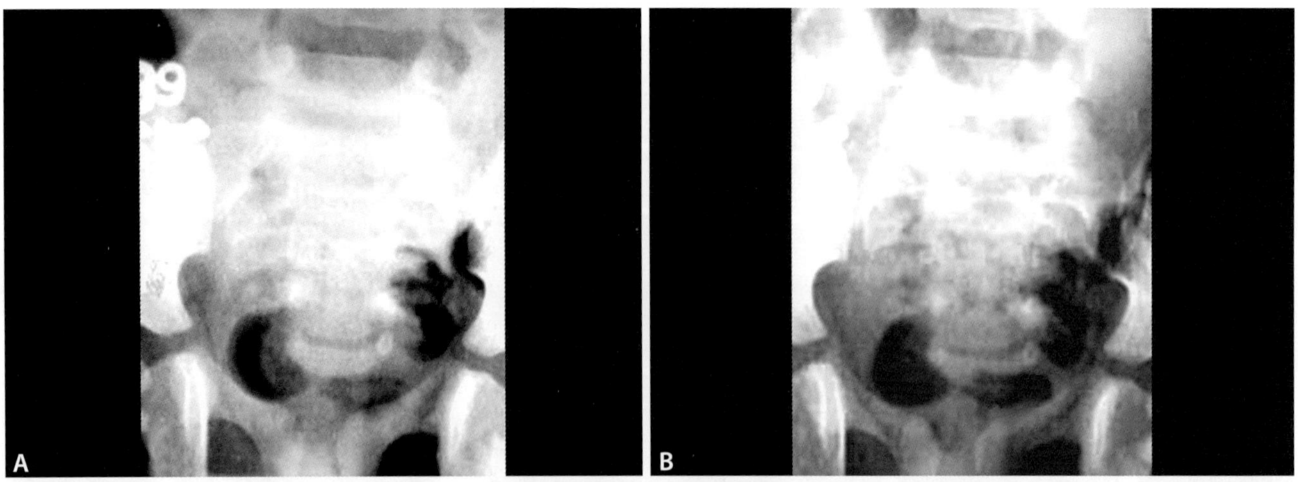

Figs. 2A and B: Pelvis anteroposterior view: (A) Taken at 48 kV and 8 mA; (B) Taken at 58.5 kV and 3.6 mA. No significant difference in image quality, dose reduction by 28% in high kV technique.

Shielding of Sensitive Organs

The best gonadal protection is tight collimation to exclude the gonads from direct exposure. If this is not possible, gonadal shielding should be used. It is recommended that the gonads should be shielded when they are directly in the X-ray beam or within 5 cm of it, unless such shielding excludes or degrades important diagnostic information. Various gonadal shields are available. Every pediatric radiology department must have different size shields for the various age groups. Contrary to general opinion, it has been shown that shields like lead capsules, can be used in over 90% of cases for a voiding micturition cystourethrography without overshadowing the urethra, and even for pelvic examinations.

Effective protection of the ovaries is more difficult because these generally lie within the pelvis.[13] Ovarial masks (fixation of the shadowing material at the collimator) should be preferred over contact shielding which can be easily displaced during the examination, thereby possibly shadowing the hip joints causing a need for retakes.[3,25-27]

Beam Direction

Another important aspect for patient exposure is the beam direction [anteroposterior (AP)/posteroanterior (PA)].[28] The standard AP projection can be replaced by prone positions for a large number of examinations **(Table 2)**. For example, the gonadal and breast tissue dose in gastrointestinal or urographic examinations can greatly be decreased using PA instead of AP projection. In addition patient thickness is decreased by compression of the belly in prone positioning, thereby decreasing the scattered dose.[12]

Anti-scatter Grid

Scattered radiation plays no major role in pediatric patients. Use of anti-scatter grid increases patient dose by a factor of 3 to 5. No grid is needed if the object thickness is less than 12 cm. No anti-scatter grid is needed for chest X-ray in patients up to 8 years of age, for the infant hip, for abdominal films in infants or for most of the fluoroscopic examinations (with the exception of double-contrast examinations of the gastrointestinal tract studies in older children). However, a grid is needed for imaging of fat patients (diameter over 15 cm) and for high kV exposures (over 90 kV). A grid ratio of 8:1 is sufficient for all pediatric examinations.[12,13,29]

In nearly all pediatric fluoroscopic examinations, grids are not needed, because no significant scatter is produced, especially when collimation is good. A removable grid is essential for pediatric fluoroscopy equipment. Gridless screening may reduce the radiation dose by as much as 50%. Infants under 1 year of age are always examined with the explorator grid removed since there is little scatter and no appreciable loss of detail. When fine detail such as mucosal pattern is not required, gridless screening may be used in children up to 5 years of age.[1,12,13,29]

Table 2: The possible use of posterior-anterior beam projection for radiographic examinations in pediatric patients.[11]

Radiographic examinations	***Clinical setting***	***Critical organ***
Skull	Trauma, ventriculo-peritoneal shunt	Lens
Chest in lateral decubitus	Foreign body aspiration, empyema	Breast
Abdomen in lateral decubitus	Bowel perforation, ileus	Breast
Spine	Scoliosis	Breast, gonads
Abdomen postcontrast films	Intravenous urography	Breast
Abdomen	Enteroclysis	Breast

Minimizing Fluoroscopic Time

The most important factor for dose reduction in fluoroscopy is the limitation of screening time. This depends mostly on the clear definition of the clinical questions, on the patient's disease and on the radiologist's experience. Reduction of fluoroscopic time can be achieved by modifying some practices as a habit. Techniques like collimating fluoroscopic field before placing the child on the table and use of fluoroscopy only after satisfactory positioning of the child and the explorator are useful.[1,13,24]

Decrease in Number of Films

Tailoring an examination based on clinical problem and minimizing the number of films can significantly reduce the radiation dose.[13,24]

Computed Tomography

Various studies have established that CT scans performed in children result in a significantly increased life time radiation risk over adult CT, both because of the increased dose per milliampere second as well as the increased life time unit dose. This underlines the importance of dose reduction in pediatric CT examinations. In older helical CT scanners, parameters were not adjusted on the basis of examination type or age of the child so that most pediatric CT scans were performed using the same parameters as for adult CT. Donnelly et al. suggested a number of techniques for minimizing radiation dose in pediatric helical CT. Most important of these include reduction in mA and increase in pitch **(Table 3)**.[30,31]

Table 3: Suggested tube current (mA) by weight of pediatric patients for single-detector helical CT.[38]

	mA	
Weight (kg)	***Chest***	***Abdomen or pelvis***
4.5–8.9	40	60
9.0–17.9	50	70
18.0–26.9	60	80
27.0–35.9	70	100
36.0–45.0	80	120
45.1–70.0	100–120	140–150
>70	≥140	≥170

Dose is directly proportional to the product of scan time and tube current. Hence, keeping other parameters constant, absorbed dose shows a linear relationship with mA. This has been shown by numerous investigators including Fearon et al. and Donnelly et al. in phantom studies.[30,31] Selection of the most appropriate mA is a compromise between image quality and radiation dose. Phantom experiments have shown that an increase in mAs will always result in a decrease in image noise and thus an improvement in image quality. But at high tube current settings the gain in image quality will not be significant. Tube current should be adjusted to provide the lowest dose consistent with adequate diagnostic quality. A technique chart that relates current to patient's weight is appropriate. Scan time can be shortened by more rapid gantry rotation or by decreasing beam rotation to less than a full 360°. In general, the fastest scan time that uses full rotation should be used.[31-33]

Similarly, it has been seen that radiation dose in helical CT is inversely proportional to the pitch used. When pitch is doubled, radiation dose gets halved.[31]

The dose increase caused by increasing kilovoltage is not linear, and is greater than often appreciated. An increase from 120–140 kVp increase dose by approximately 40%. Pediatric patients are rarely large enough to warrant the use of increased kVp.[33]

Newer multidetector CT scanners are equipped with automatic exposure control system (AEC) under different names (Care dose 4D, Dose right, AutomA, etc.). These dose modulation systems work in various ways, so as to adjust the radiation dose according to the patient's body size and attenuation. AEC reduces the patient's dose without compromising image quality.[34,35] The radiation dose is essentially reduced by controlling the tube current which is performed by three methods. These methods are based on: (a) patient size, (b) z-axis, and (c) angular or rotational AEC. Most of the scanners use combination of all these methods.[35] The scanner uses the projection radiograph data (topogram/scanogram) to assess size and attenuation of patient and accordingly dose is modulated using patient size and z-axis. In angular AEC, the dose is modulated so as to equalize the photon flux to the detector while the tube is rotating. This is needed because the human body is noncircular, and hence the attenuation of the beam varies at different projections. Generally, lateral projections are more attenuating than AP projections. By using AEC, there is considerable reduction in the magnitude exposure dose, in the range of 35–60%.[36] AEC thus is helpful in reducing the patient's dose, especially in pediatric cases.

Despite these developments, following facts should always be taken into account while performing a CT in pediatric cases. In a neonate approximately 30% of the marrow is contained in the skull and the marrow absorbed dose for a CT brain examination in a 6 years old patient phantom has been reported to be even higher than that for a CT chest or abdomen examination. Therefore, high priority should be given to dose reduction measures for head scans in children. Results of a study in our department at AIIMS also showed that a reduction of mAs from 115 or 141 mAs to 77 or 94 mA, which represents a 53–65% reduction in dose did not result in any significant difference in diagnostic accuracy although there was a slight reduction in image quality which was also not statistically significant,[37] **(Figs. 3A and B)**. Chest is a naturally high contrast area because of large attenuation differences that result from the presence of air in lungs and fat in mediastinum. Scans of objects with large differences in attenuation values such as lungs are less likely to be sensitive to image noise as image noise mainly affects low-contrast resolution. So, low doses may be used. Low radiation dose technique was used by Rogalla et al. in their study of chest CT. Rogalla et al. had found that although there is no consensus regarding which mA setting may be regarded as ideal low dose technique for spiral CT scanning of pediatric chest, 25–75 mAs is sufficient for lung window and 50–75 mAs for mediastinal window. A mA of 77 (57.5 mAs) time represents a nearly 67% reduction in dose as compared to mA of 240 (180 mAs) with no significant loss of diagnostic information.[38] Our departmental study also showed similar results[37] **(Figs. 4A and B)**. Now-a-days, most of the modern scanners provide CT dose index (CTDI) which is the most commonly used dose indicator. It does not provide the precise dose, rather it is an index of dose measured using a phantom. However, CTDI may greatly help in comparing radiation dose at different scanning parameters.[35]

Various manufacturers provide multiple protocols for different examination and as per the age of patient.

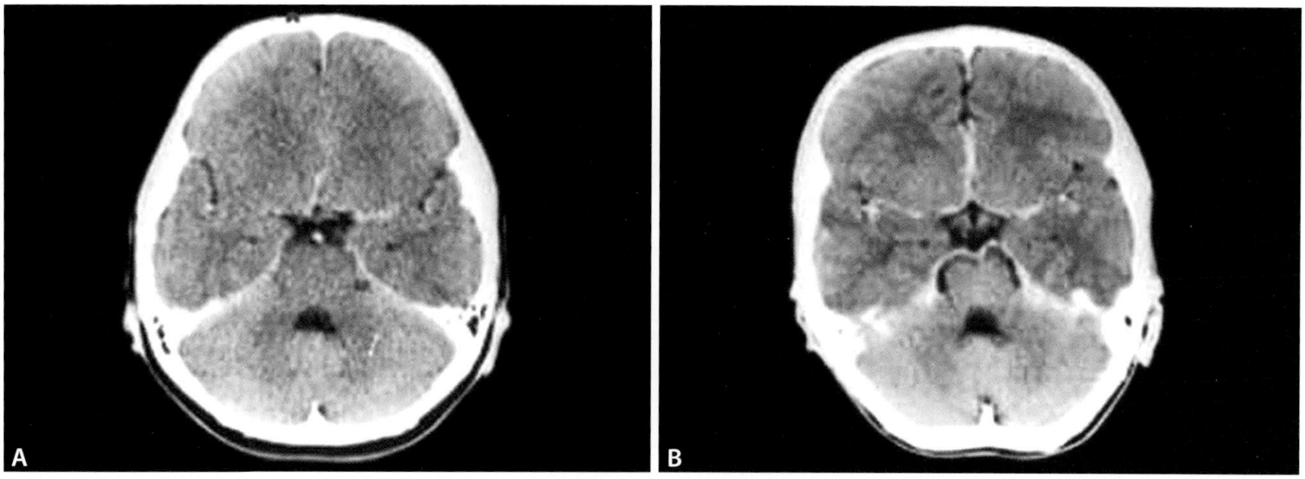

Figs. 3A and B: CT head: (A) At 94 mA and (B) at 206 mA. No significant difference in overall image quality. Radiation dose in A is 50% of B.

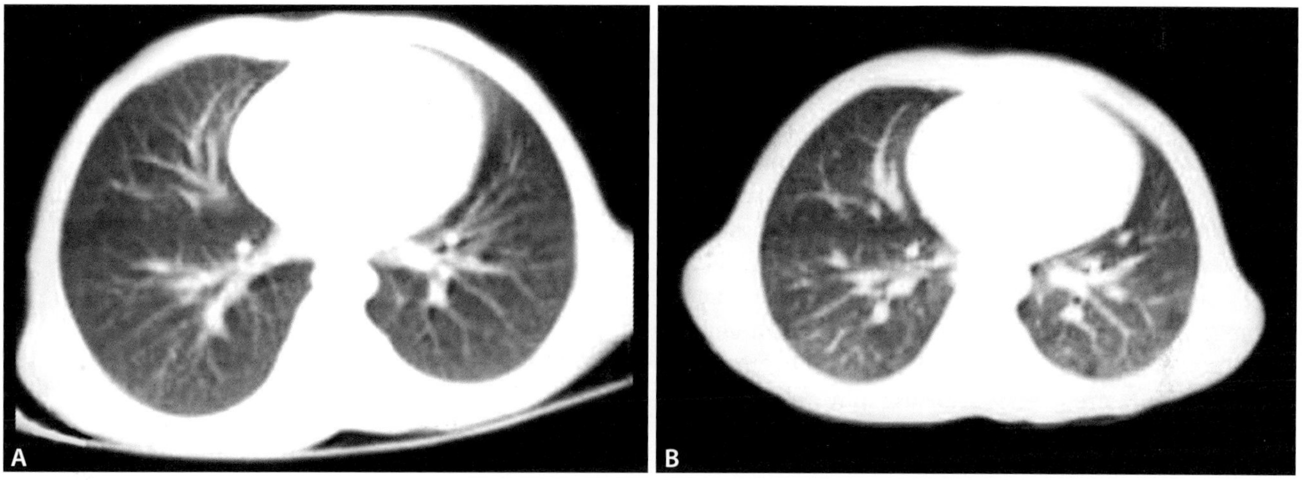

Figs. 4A and B: Chest CT: (A) At 240 mA and (B) at 77 mA. Image quality is comparable while radiation dose in B is less than one-third of that in A.

Hence when imaging for children, pediatric protocols should be followed. Ideally, all institutions must set their own scanning protocol, involving various parameters (tube voltage, tube current, slice thickness, collimation and pitch) optimized as per the use. The important point to remember is that different manufacturers use different techniques for dose modulation so the user should know about the system's characteristics before trying to attempt any change in scanning parameters.[39] Any changes should be performed using appropriate (weight range) phantoms.

Recently dual energy CT scanners have been introduced which are faster and have ability to provide greater information about tissue composition than obtained by single energy scanners. Although not much is known about its use in pediatric cases, however, with dual energy scanners noncontrast CT scans are not needed as contrast media can be subtracted, and the patient is spared the radiation dose of a second scan.

USE OF CONTRAST MEDIA

Contrast media available for intravenous (IV) use in radiography are categorized as high-osmolality contrast media (HOCM), low-osmolality contrast media (LOCM) and isosmolar contrast media (IOCM). Considerations in choice amongst these are the concentration of iodine achieved within plasma and urine, economic factors, and safety factors.

High Osmolality Contrast Media

High osmolality contrast media (HOCM) have an iodine content ranging from 280 to 480 mg/mL and an osmolality range from 1,400 to 2,500 mOsm/kg. Dosage of contrast material is based upon grams of iodine administered in relation to body mass. It is appropriate to use a dosage of approximately 300 mg of iodine per kilogram. This represents approximately 1.0 mL/kg in the most commonly used forms of diatrizoate or iothalamate. The total dose for excretory urography or for CT is usually 2.0 mL/kg in children or 3.0 mL/kg in the newborn.

Speed of injection is important for the resultant plasma concentration of contrast material. After rapid injection, there is an increase in serum osmolality within 3 minutes, a decrease in serum sodium concentration, and an increase in heart rate. The osmotic effect is particularly significant in young infants. A mean increase of 3% in serum osmolality is observed in adults. Excretion occurs rapidly by renal glomerular filtration. Because of a high osmotic load, these contrast media also produce diuresis, opposing tubular resorption.[38]

Low Osmolality Contrast Agents

Low osmolality contrast agents have an iodine content ranging from 128–320 mg/mL and an osmolality range from 290–702 mOsm/kg. Agents with low iodine content are most suitable for intra-arterial digital subtraction arteriography. Those with iodine content of 240–300 mg/mL are used for excretory urography, venography, venous injection digital subtraction arteriography, and bolus IV enhancement for CT scans. The contrast media with high iodine content, 320–370 mg/mL, are used for aortography and selective arteriography.

Iso-osmolar Contrast Agents

Iso-osmolar contrast media (IOCM) has an iodine content ranging from 270–320 mg/mL and an osmolality of 290 mOsm/kg.

Initial-reports showed that the IOCM reduces the risk of contrast-induced nephropathy (CIN) in patients with deranged renal parameters. However, recently various meta-analysis of randomized control trials have shown that there is no statistically significant reduction in CIN-associated with iodixanol as compared to LOCM.[39,40] Hence, with this equivocal kind of reports IOCM offers no significant advantage over LOCM.

Unlike HOCM, LOCM and IOCM have little or no effect on serum osmolality, serum sodium, vasodilation, hemodilution, red blood cell morphology, or vascular permeability. There is little or no effect on the blood-brain barrier, fewer electrocardiographic changes, and fewer alterations in myocardial contractility, cardiac output, and left ventricular, pulmonary artery, and aortic pressures. There is less endothelial damage, and lower release or activation of vasoactive substances including complement activation, histamine release, and acetylcholinesterase inhibition. Diminished effects on coagulation pathways have been demonstrated. These effects are attributed to the lower osmolality and the reduced chemotactic effect of the molecules. Of importance is reduction in the nephrotoxic effect noted with HOCM. Hence, there are definite advantages to adoption of LOCM. A major consideration is degradation of the resulting examination resulting from pain, heat or vomiting with HOCM.[38]

Performing a multiphasic CT scans in neonate and infants may be challenging, as the IV cannula is of smaller gauge limiting the injection rate of power injector, moreover only small amount of IV contrast can be used depending on the weight of the child. These situations may be handled by: (1) Using bolus tracking and saline chasing technique and, (2) Large bore cannula.[41,42] An injection rate of 2–3 mL/sec is safe and provides good results.[40] Although there is no consensus, but contrast may be administered using central venous line with a maximum injection rate of 2 mL/sec.[41]

MR Contrast Agents

The most commonly used contrast agents are paramagnetic substances and amongst these gadolinium diethylenetriamine penta-acetic acid (Gd-DTPA) dimeglumine is most frequently used. Gd-DTPA is excreted by glomerular filtration with 90% excreted within 24 hours. Rapid renal clearance, and low toxicity are important features of this contrast material. The clinical dose of Gd-DTPA is 0.1 mmol/kg. It has an osmolality of 1,900 mOsm/kg. However, the high osmolality is of little importance because of the small volume administered.[38,43]

Although, gadolinium-enhanced MRI was once considered one of the safer imaging procedures, but recently there has been a significant concern regarding nephrogenic systemic fibrosis (NSF) associated with gadolinium-based contrast agents. The identified risk factors associated with development of NSF include—administration of a high dose of gadolinium-based contrast agent, acute or chronic renal failure, venous thrombosis and coagulopathy and vascular surgery.[44,45]

Some additional guiding principles for use of contrast in the neonates are:

- Use warm contrast for maintenance of body temperature.
- Use iso-osmolar positive, non-ionic contrast in most instances.

- When giving oral or rectal contrast, use low-osmolar, nonionic agents instead of barium to avoid barium contamination of the peritoneal cavity.
- Do not give contrast blindly; oral contrast may be aspirated, and rectal contrast may get into peritoneal cavity via a perforation. Even in the intact bowel, the contrast may not progress distally as quickly as predicted and therefore may lead to unnecessary radiographs.
- Be judicious in the volume of contrast administered. Renal function in neonates is less than in babies over 1 month of age, therefore excretion of contrast may be delayed.
- Gadolinium is the preferred contrast agent for magnetic resonance imaging. However, it should be used with a caution.[43-47]

In conclusion the aim of all departments and radiologists dealing with pediatric imaging should be to achieve a diagnostically adequate radiograph or examination, with minimum radiation exposure and discomfort to the child. This goal can only be achieved, if the radiologists and technicians in charge are committed to quality control programs, and are aware of the necessity for radiation protection in children.

REFERENCES

1. Levick RK, Spriqq A. In: Whitehouse GH, Worthington BS (Eds): Pediatric Radiology in Techniques in Diagnostic Imaging, 3rd edition. 1996. pp. 389-404.
2. Tani S, Mizuno N, Abe S. Availability and improvement of a vacuum-type immobilization device in pediatric CT. Abstract in English on pubmed. Nippon Hoshasen Gijutsu Gakkai Zasshi. 2002;58(8):1073-79.
3. Bontrages KL. Pediatric Radiography in Textbook of Radiographic Positioning and Related Anatomy, 5th edition. St Louis: Mosby; 2001. pp. 629-64.
4. Frush DP, Bisset GS. Sedation of children for emergency imaging. RCNA. 1997;35(4):789-97.
5. Chudnofsky C, Krauss B, Brustowic Z (Eds). Sedation for Radiologic Imaging in Pediatric Procedural Sedation and Analgesia Maryland, USA: Lippincott Williams and Wilkins; 2001. pp. 169-78.
6. Lim-Dunham JE, Narra J, Benya EC, et al. Aspiration following oral contrast administration for pediatric trauma CT scans [abstract 46]. In 82nd Scientific Assembly and Annual Meeting, Radiological Society of North America. Chicago, Radiological Society of North America. 1996. p. 137.
7. Ziegler MA, Fricke BL, Donnelly LF. Is administration of enteric contrast matrial safe before abdominal CT in children who require sedation? Experience with chloral hydrate and pentobarbital. AJR. 2003;180(1):13-5.
8. Iwata S, Okumura A, Kato T, et al. Efficacy and adverse effects of rectal thiamylal with oral triclofos for children undergoing magnetic resonance imaging. Brain Dev. 2006;28(3):175-7.
9. Frush DP, Bisset GS, Hal SC. Pediatric sedation in radiology: The practice of safe sleep. AJR. 1996;167:1381.
10. Pierce DA, Preston DL. Radiation-related cancer risks at low doses among atomic bomb survivors. Radiat Res. 2000;154:178-86.
11. Slovis TL. Executive summary, ALARA Conference: Pediatr Radiol. 2002;32:221.
12. Schneider K. Radiation Protection in pediatric radiology: How important is what? In syllabus of 20th Postgraduate Course European Society of Pediatric Radiology. 1997; 95-101.
13. Protection of the patient in diagnostic radiology: Summary of the current ICRP principles, by Atomic Energy Regulatory Board: Mumbai. 1987;3-16.
14. Gonzalez L, Vano E, Ruiz MJ. Radiation dose to pediatric patients undergoing micturating cystourethography examinations and potential reduction by radiation protection optimization. Br J Radiol. 1993;68:291-5.
15. Martin CJ, Darragh CL, Mc Kenzie GA, et al. Implementation of a program for reduction of radiographic doses and result achieved through increase in tube potential. Br J Radiol. 1993;66:228-33.
16. Mooney R, Thomas PS. Dose reduction in a pediatric X-ray department following optimization of radiographic technique. Br J Radiol. 1998;71:852-60.
17. Kohn MM, et al. Guidelines on Quality Criteria for Diagnostic Radiographic Images in Pediatrics. CEC Directorate General XII/D/3, Brussels, 1996.
18. Uffmann M, Schaefer-Prokop C. Digital radiography: The balance between image quality and required radiation dose. Eur J Radiol. 2009;72(2):202-8.
19. Willis CE. Optimizing digital radiography of children. Eur J Radiol. 2009;72(2):266-73.
20. Fearon T, Vucich J. Normalized pediatric organ absorbed doses from CT examinations. AJR. 1987;148:171-74.
21. Nicholson RA, Thornton A, Akpan M. Radiation dose reduction in pediatric fluoroscopy using added filtration. Br J Radiol. 1995;68(807):296-300.
22. Bogaert E, Bacher K, Lapere R, et al. Does digital flat detector technology tip the scale towards better image quality or reduced patient dose in interventional cardiology? Eur J Radiol. 2009;72(2):348-53.
23. Chida K, Inaba Y, Saito H, et al. Radiation dose of interventional radiology system using a flat-panel detector. AJR. 2009;193(6):1680-5.
24. Shah R, Gupta AK, Rehani M. Evaluation of radiation dose to children undergoing radiological examinations and reduction of dose by protective methods. (Unpublished data) Department of Radiodiagnosis, AIIMS, 2002.
25. Schneider K. Evolution of Quality assurance in pediatric radiology. Radiation Protection Dosimetry. 1995;57:119-23.

26. Fendel H, Schineider K, Bakowski C, et al. Specific principles for optimization of image quality and patient exposure in pediatric diagnostic imaging. BJR. 1990;20:91-110.
27. Fendel H. Die zehn Gebote des Strahlenshutzes bei der Rontgendiagnostikim Kindesalter. Pediatric Prax. 1976;17:339-46.
28. Fendel H, Schneider K, Schofer H, et al. Optimization in pediatric radiology: Are there specific problems for quality-assurance in pediatric radiology. Brit J Radiol. 1985;18:159-65.
29. Drury P, Robinson A. Fluoroscopy without the grid: A method of reducing the radiation dose. Br J Radiol. 1980;53(626):93-9.
30. Brenner DJ, Ellison CD. Estimated risks of radiation induced fatal cancer from pediatric CT. AJR. 2001;176:289-96.
31. Frush DP, Donnelly LF. Helical CT in children technical considerations and body applications: Radiology. 1998;209:37-48.
32. Fearon T, Vucich J. Normalized pediatric organ absorbed doses from CT examinations. AJR. 1987;148:171-4.
33. Kuhn JP, Brody AS. High resolution of CT pediatric lung disease. RCNA. 2002;40(1):89-110.
34. McCollough CH, Bruesewitz MR, Kofler JM. CT dose reduction and dose management tools: Overview of available options. Radiographics. 2006;26(2):503-12.
35. Lee CH, Goo JM, Ye HJ, et al. Radiation dose modulation techniques in the multidetector CT era: From basics to practice. Radiographics. 2008;28(5):1451-9.
36. Söderberg M, Gunnarsson M. Automatic exposure control in computed tomography: An evaluation of systems from different manufacturers. Acta Radiol. 2010;51(6):625-34.
37. Shah R, Gupta AK, Rehani MM, et al. Effect of reduction in tube current on reader confidence in pediatric computed tomography. Clinical Radiology. 2005;60(2):224-31.
38. Rogalla P, Stöver B, Scheer I, et al. Low dose spiral CT applicability to pediatric chest imaging. Pediatr Radiol. 1999;29:565-9.
39. Gudjónsdóttir J, Ween B, Olsen DR. Optimal use of AEC in CT: A literature review. Radiol Technol. 2010;81(4):309-17.
40. Currarino G, Wood B, Mayd. In: Silverman FN, Kuhn JP (Eds). Diagnostic Procedures: The Genitourinary Tract and Retroperitoneum in Caffey's Pediatric X-Ray Diagnosis, 9th edition. St Louis: Mosby; 1993. pp. 1148-71.
41. From AM, Al Badarin FJ, McDonald FS, et al. Iodixanol versus low-osmolar contrast media for prevention of contrast-induced nephropathy: meta-analysis of randomized, controlled trials. Circ Cardiovasc Interv. 2010;3(4):351-8.
42. Heinrich MC, Häberle L, Müller V, et al. Nephrotoxicity of iso-osmolar iodixanol compared with nonionic low-osmolar contrast media: Meta-analysis of randomized controlled trials. Radiology. 2009;250(1):68-86.
43. Nievelstein RA, van Dam IM, van der Molen AJ. Multidetector CT in children: Current concepts and dose reduction strategies. Pediatr Radiol. 2010;40(8):1324-44.
44. Fleishmann D, Kamaya A. Optimal vascular and parenchymal contrast enhancement: The current state of the art. Radiol Clin North Am. 2009;47:13-26.
45. Slovin TL. In: Kuhn JP, Slovin TL, Halles JO (Eds). Neonatal Imaging: Overview in Caffey's Paediatric Diagnostic Imaging, 10th edition. Penn Sylvania: Mosby; 2004. pp. 15-8.
46. Prince MR, Zhang HL, Prowda JC, et al. Nephrogenic systemic fibrosis and its impact on abdominal imaging. Radiographics. 2009;29(6):1565-74.
47. Juluru K, Vogel-Claussen J, Macura KJ, et al. MR imaging in patients at risk for developing nephrogenic systemic fibrosis: Protocols, practices, and imaging techniques to maximize patient safety. Radiographics. 2009;29(1):9-22.

CHAPTER 127

Recent Advances in Pediatric Radiology

Akshay Kumar Saxena, Kushaljit Singh Sodhi

INTRODUCTION

The articles dwelling upon pediatric radiology are published not only in the radiology journals, but also in journals in the fields of allied specialties, like pediatrics and pediatric surgery. There is no strict definition of recent advances. For an avid reader, recent advances mean the literature published in last few months (say 1 year); for a research worker dedicated to a particular topic, only the articles published in that context would constitute recent advances while for a general radiologist, changing trends over last few years would qualify for recent advances. Given the vast plethora of articles available in medical literature and differing needs of radiologists, it is impossible to cater to the need of all. This chapter dwells upon some of the recent trends in speciality of pediatric radiology as applicable to Indian scenario. Readers are encouraged to update their knowledge by reading the recent journals.

RADIATION PROTECTION

The children are known to be at high-risk for developing radiation-induced malignancies. This is because the growing tissues are more radiosensitive. In addition, children have long lifespan available to manifest the ill effects of radiation. Hence, there is a need to keep the radiation dose to the minimum possible level in children. An Alliance for Radiation Safety in Pediatric Imaging (Image Gently campaign)[1] has recently taken shape with the objective of making the imaging community aware of the need to adjust the dose of radiation when they are imaging the children. In late 2006, it was started as a Committee within the Society for Pediatric Radiology and currently encompasses 56 professional associations globally. This alliance aims at changing the practice. The initial focus of the alliance has been computed tomography (CT) scan as there has been dramatic global increase in number of CT scans being performed for children. The alliance website *(www.imagegently.org)* provides information for radiologists, parents, pediatricians, medical physicists and radiology technologists. The alliance has evoked widespread interest. The website has already been visited over 300,000 times, the CT protocol has been downloaded more than 20,000 times and the pledge has been taken by 4,528 medical professionals. Recently, the alliance has started targeting radiation safety pediatric interventional radiology. It has been labeled "Image Gently, Step Lightly". It encourages the radiologists to "Step Lightly" on the fluoroscopy pedal during the pediatric interventional procedures. It also encourages the radiologists to use ultrasound or magnetic resonance imaging (MRI) for guidance during interventional procedures. The image gently campaign has been named to the 2009 Associations Advance America Honor Roll. Sponsored by the American Society of Association Executives, this award recognizes the ways in which nonprofit associations contribute towards improving the quality of life in America. Detailed guidelines are now available for reducing radiation dose during fluoroscopy, CT scan and interventional procedures in children.[2-4]

NEURORADIOLOGY

Computed tomography scan of head is commonly performed for head trauma in children. However, very few of these patients show CT evidence of intracranial injury. Since CT scan imparts high-radiation dose, it is desirable to minimize number of children who do not require CT scan after head trauma. Palchak and colleagues[5] conducted a prospective observational study to derive a decision rule for identifying those children who were at low risk for traumatic brain injuries. They enrolled 2,043 children and evaluated clinical predictors of traumatic brain injury on CT scan and traumatic brain injury requiring acute intervention, defined by: (1) a neurosurgical procedure (2) antiepileptic medications for more than 1 week (3) persistent neurologic deficits or (4) hospitalization for at least two nights. CT scan was performed in 1,271 (62%) patients of which 98 (7.7%) had traumatic brain injuries on CT scan. 105 (5.1% of 2,043 enrolled patients) had traumatic brain injuries which requires acute intervention. Abnormal mental status, clinical signs of skull fracture, history of vomiting, scalp hematoma (in children ≤ 2 years of age), or headache identified 97/98 (99%) of those with traumatic brain injuries on CT scan and 105/105 (100%) of those with traumatic brain injuries requiring acute intervention. Amongst the 304 (24%) children undergoing CT with none of these predictors, only 1 (0.3%) patient had traumatic brain injury on CT. This patient was discharged from the emergency department without complications. The authors concluded that absence of abnormal mental status, clinical signs of skull fracture, history of vomiting, scalp hematoma (in children ≤ 2 years of age), and headache were important factors for identifying children at low risk for traumatic brain injuries after blunt head trauma.

Magnetic resonance imaging, diffusion tensor imaging (DTI) and MR spectroscopy are important constituents of evaluation of neonatal encephalopathy. Barkovich and colleagues[6] performed serial MRI in 10 neonates to describe the time course of changes in various regions of the brain during the first 2 weeks of life. DTI and MR spectroscopy of most patients revealed a characteristic pattern of evolution during the first 2 weeks after birth. Although, the anatomic images were normal or nearly normal on the first 2 days after birth in most patients, some abnormalities were observed on DTI and spectroscopy. The parameters would worsen until about day 5 and then become normal, though there was persistence of abnormal metabolite ratios on spectroscopy in several cases. During the serial scans, the areas of reduced diffusion pseudonormalized in some parts, while new abnormal areas developed in other parts. Thus, the pattern of injury looked very different on serial scans.

Liauw and colleagues[7] evaluated the predictive value of diffusion-weighted imaging (DWI) and apparent diffusion coefficient (ADC) measurements for outcome in children with perinatal asphyxia. MRI was performed in term neonates within 10 days of life because of birth asphyxia. In survivors, developmental outcome until early school age was graded as: I (normal), II (mildly abnormal) and III (definitely abnormal). For analysis, category III and death (category IV) were labeled "adverse", I and II were "favorable" and II-III and death were "abnormal" outcome. The study demonstrated that ADC values in normal-appearing basal ganglia and brainstem correlated with outcome independent of all MRI findings. However, ADC values in visibly abnormal brain tissue on DWI did not show a predictive value for outcome. Another study (by Vermeulen and colleagues), which evaluated DWI and conventional MRI in neonatal hypoxic ischemia reported DWI to be a useful additional MR tool to predict the motor outcome at 2 years. In this study, local ADC values had a limited value. Recognition of the patterns of brain damage with DWI and conventional MRI appeared useful as a diagnostic tool.

Although, ultrasound and MRI are frequently utilized for evaluation of neonatal hypoxic ischemic injury, there is striking paucity of prospective studies comparing these two modalities. Epelman and colleagues[8] prospectively performed ultrasound and MRI of 76 neonates and young infants (age range: 1–44 days; means age 9.8 days). Both the studies were done within 2 hours of each other. The diagnostic accuracy of ultrasound was found to be 95.7%. The authors recommended the use of ultrasound as screening modality with emphasis on correct technique. They also recommended early MRI for mapping delineating extent of injury.

Tovar-Moll and colleagues[9] utilized magnetic resonance DTI and tractography in patients of callosal dysgenesis to reveal the aberrant circuit. The study group consisted of 11 patients 9 of which belonged to pediatric age-group. Four main findings were reported:

1. In the presence of a callosal remnant or a hypoplastic corpus callosum (CC), fibers therein largely connect the expected neocortical regions.
2. Callosal remnants and hypoplastic CC display a fiber topography similar to normal.
3. At least two long abnormal tracts are formed in patients with defective CC: Probst bundle (PB) and a sigmoid, asymmetrical aberrant bundle connecting the frontal lobe with the contralateral occipito-parietal cortex.

4. Whereas the PB is topographically organized and has an ipsilateral U-connectivity, the sigmoid bundle is a long, heterotopic commissural tract.

These observations revealed that when the process of CC fibers to cross the midline is obstructed, some properties of the miswired fibers are maintained (such as side-by-side topography), whereas others change dramatically, leading to the formation of grossly abnormal white matter tracts.

Magnetic resonance imaging is considered inferior to CT scan in detecting calcification. However, susceptibility-weighted imaging (SWI) technique can identify calcification by using phase images. Using this technique, Wu and colleagues[10] were able to detect a partially calcified oligodendroglioma, multiple calcified cysticercosis lesions and multiple physiologic calcifications in a single patient. The authors concluded that SWI-filtered phase images can identify calcifications as well as CT scan.

Wang and colleagues[11] evaluated serial MRI changes compared to clinical outcome and evaluated their impact on clinical outcome in the follow-up of pyogenic spinal infection in children. In this study, 17 patients (age 2 months to 16 years) underwent 51 follow-up MRI scans done 2 weeks to 4.75 years after baseline scan. Follow-up scans done at short-term revealed epidural and/or paraspinal soft-tissue changes which correlated with the clinical status and laboratory findings in all patients. However, in some cases progression of bone and disk abnormalities was noted in spite of clinical improvement. Long-term follow-up scans revealed soft tissue, bone and disk changes 1–3 years after initial scan in spite of these children being symptom free. The authors concluded that management should be based on the clinical response and that long-term or serial routine follow-ups are not necessary.

THORACIC IMAGING

Lung pathologies have traditionally been evaluated using radiography and CT scan. A few recent studies have explored utility of ultrasound and MRI in lung pathologies. Bober and Swietliński[12] investigated the possible role of chest ultrasound in the diagnosis of the respiratory distress syndrome in newborn. Using transabdominal approach, they performed ultrasound examination in 131 consecutive newborns (admitted to the neonatal intensive care unit) in their 1st day of life with symptoms of respiratory failure. Retrohepatic or retrosplenic hyperechogenicity was shown in 109/131 newborns examined and the diagnosis of respiratory distress syndrome was confirmed by radiography in 101 cases. Respiratory distress syndrome was diagnosed in any patient without retrohepatic or retrosplenic hyperechogenicity. In 8 patients with positive ultrasound images unconfirmed by chest X-ray (i.e. false-positive sonographic examination), congenital pneumonia was diagnosed in 4 cases and pneumothorax in 1 case while in 3 cases no pathology was found. The authors reported 100% sensitivity and 92% specificity of ultrasound in diagnosis of respiratory distress syndrome.

Copetti and Cattarossi[13] evaluated sonographic appearance of transient tachypnea of newborn (TTN) and its clinical relevance. They performed sonographic examination of 32 neonates with clinical suspicion of TTN and compared the findings with 60 normal infants, 29 with respiratory distress syndrome, 6 with pneumonia and 5 each with pulmonary hemorrhage and atelectasis. They noted that in TTN the echogenicity of upper lung fields was different from lower lung fields. Specifically, the lower lung fields showed very compact comet tail artifacts while these were rare in superior lung fields. The authors labeled this as "double lung point" which had 100% sensitivity and specificity for diagnosis of TTN.

In another study, Copetti and colleagues[14] attempted to define the sonographic appearance of neonatal respiratory distress syndrome and evaluate its clinical relevance. They enrolled 40 neonates with respiratory distress syndrome and performed transthoracic ultrasound. In all the patients, sonography revealed echographic "white lung", pleural line abnormalities (small subpleural consolidations, thickening, irregularity and coarse appearance) and an absence of areas with a normal pattern (i.e. spared areas). When presented simultaneously, these signs had 100% sensitivity and specificity for diagnosis of respiratory distress syndrome.

Kurian and colleagues[15] compared the findings of sonography and CT in pediatric patients suffering from pneumonia complicated by parapneumonic effusion. In this retrospective study of 19 patients (age range: 8 months to 17 years), images were assessed for traces of effusion, loculation, fibrin strands, parenchymal consolidation, necrosis and abscess. In this study, CT of the thorax could not provide any added clinically useful information that was unavailable on chest ultrasound. The authors suggested that the imaging workup of complicated pediatric pneumonia be done with chest radiography and chest ultrasound and CT be reserved for cases where the chest ultrasound is technically limited or discrepant with the clinical findings.

Montella and colleagues[16] compared the efficacy of high-field MRI and high-resolution CT (HRCT) in children and adults with non-cystic fibrosis (CF) chronic lung disease with the aims of assessing whether chest high-field

MRI is as efficient as chest HRCT in identifying pulmonary abnormalities; and to investigate the relationships between the severity and extent of lung disease, and functional data in patients with nonCF chronic lung disease. There were 30 children and 11 adults in this study (age range: 5.9–29.3 years; median age 13.8 years). The 14 patients each had primary ciliary dyskinesia and primary immunodeficiency while another 13 had recurrent pneumonia. All the patients underwent pulmonary function tests, chest HRCT (120 kV, dose-modulated mAs) and high-field 3.0 Tesla MRI (HASTE; transversal orientation; repetition time/echo time/flip angle/acquisition time, infinite/92 ms/150°/approximately 90 seconds). The images of both HRCT and MRI were scored in consensus by two observers using a modified version of the Helbich scoring system. The maximal score was 25. HRCT and high-field MRI total scores were 11 (range: 1–20) and 11 (range: 1–17), respectively. There was good agreement between the two techniques for all scores ($r > 0.8$). HRCT and MRI total scores, and extent of bronchiectasis scores were significantly related to pulmonary function tests ($r = -0.4$, $p < 0.05$). Similarly, the MRI mucus plugging score was also notably related to pulmonary function tests ($r = -0.4$, $p < 0.05$). The authors concluded that high-field 3.0 Tesla MRI of chest surfaces to be as efficient as HRCT in determining the extent and severity of lung abnormalities in nonCF chronic lung diseases, and it might be a more dependable radiation-free option as compared to HRCT.

Bannier and colleagues[17] evaluated the sensitivity of hyperpolarized helium-3 (^{3}He) MRI for the detection of peripheral airway obstruction in younger CF patients showing normal spirometric results and the immediate effects of a single chest physical therapy (CPT) session. The study involved 10 children with ages varying from 8 years to 16 years. Spirometry followed by proton and hyperpolarized ^{3}He three-dimensional lung imaging were performed on a 1.5 Tesla MRI unit before and after 20 minutes of CPT. The number of ventilation defects per image (VDI) and the ventilated lung fraction (VF) were quantified. Despite the normality of Spirometry in all the patients, ventilation defects were discovered in all the patients (mean VDI: 5.1 ± 1.9; mean global VF: 78.5% ± 12.3; and mean peripheral VF: 75.5% ± 17.1). This was well above the VDI in healthy subjects (1.6) as reported in literature. Although disparate changes in the distribution of ventilation defects were observed after CPT there was no significant change in the average VDI and VF.

Tracheomalacia is characterized by excessive collapsibility of trachea in expiration. Lee and colleagues[18] evaluated air trapping in pediatric patients with and without tracheomalacia. In this retrospective study, the study group and comparison group had 15 patients each. Tracheomalacia was diagnosed if the cross-sectional luminal area of trachea decreased by more than or equal to 50% during expiration as seen on CT scan and confirmed by bronchoscopy. The authors graded the severity of air trapping visually on a 5-point score. All the patients with tracheomalacia and 10/15 children without tracheomalacia showed air trapping. The median air trapping score was significantly higher ($p = 0.002$) in the study group. However, the patterns of air trapping were not significantly different. These findings have potential implications for diagnosis and management of children with tracheomalacia.

Chest radiography, catheter angiography and echocardiography (ECG) have remained the mainstay of evaluation of patients with heart disease. With the recent availability of advanced multidetector scanners, it has now become possible to evaluate congenital heart diseases using CT scan. Cheng and colleagues[19] evaluated the clinical value of low-dose prospective ECG-triggered dual-source CT angiography (DSCT) in infants and children with complex congenital cardiac diseases. They compared DSCT findings with transthoracic echocardiography (TTE). The study includes 35 patients with the age range of 2 months to 6 years. They demonstrated high sensitivity (97.3%) and specificity (99.8%) with mean effective dose of 0.38 ± 0.09 mSv. In this study, the subjective mean image quality score was 4.3 ± 0.7 using a 5-point scale. Another study evaluated step-and-shoot DSCT for evaluation of heart coronary artery and other thoracic structures in young children (age < 6 years) with congenital heart disease.[20] They utilized prospective gating with end-systolic reconstruction. The image quality was evaluated using a 5-point scoring system. They reported mean image quality score of 4.7 ± 0.6 and mean effective radiation dose of 0.26 ± 1.6 mSv.

GASTROINTESTINAL IMAGING

Necrotizing enterocolitis (NEC) refers almost exclusively to an idiopathic, often severe, enterocolitis that occurs in neonates with premature babies being more at risk.[21] The radiological evaluation is traditionally dependent upon radiography. Although there are sporadic reports of use of ultrasound in NEC, the first comprehensive evaluation of NEC with abdominal sonography was reported by Faingold and colleagues.[22] They enrolled 30 controlled and 32 neonate of proven or suspected NEC. They performed color Doppler of the bowel wall and described the normal and abnormal flow patterns. In this study, the sensitivity of absent flow in bowel wall on color Doppler, as marker for severe NEC, was 100%. This was significantly superior to 40% sensitivity of abdominal radiography which relied upon free air as sign of severe NEC.

A recent study[23] reported the findings of ultrasonography in early NEC. The authors evaluated 40 neonates with clinically diagnosed NEC and 10 controls. They evaluated the echogenicity of the bowel wall, involved region, ascites, and portal venous gas at initial and follow-up examinations. Echogenic dots were seen in bowel wall in 16 patients (40%) and dense granular echogenicities in 24 patients (60%). Portal venous gas was not visualized in any of the patients. None of the neonates in control group had echogenic foci in bowel wall. Follow-up examinations revealed decrease in the echogenicity of the bowel wall and ascites in 37 patients (93%).

Silva and colleagues,[24] in a retrospective study, correlated the sonographic findings with clinical outcome in 40 neonates. They divided the patients into two groups based on outcome: group A included neonates who had been treated medically and had fully recovered, while group B included neonates who required surgery for perforation in the acute setting (laparotomy or placement of a peritoneal drain), surgery for late strictures or those who died as a result of NEC. They calculated the risk ratios and 95% confidence intervals (CI) for those features for different sonographic patterns. The reports showed an adverse outcome associated with the sonographic findings of free gas, focal fluid collections or three or more of the following: increased bowel wall echogenicity, absent bowel perfusion, portal venous gas, bowel wall thinning, bowel wall thickening, free fluid with echoes and intramural gas. Interestingly, in this study, two babies in group A revealed absent flow in bowel wall suggesting that absent flow in bowel wall need not always be associated with adverse outcome.

Dilli and colleagues[25] also reported sonographic findings in NEC. They stated that sonography had high specificity but low sensitivity for detection of portal venous gas. In addition, sonography provided valuable information regarding intra-abdominal collections.

Bora and colleagues[26] evaluated the role of postnatal superior mesenteric artery (SMA) flow in predicting feed intolerance and NEC in the babies of mothers showing absent end-diastolic flow in umbilical arteries during antenatal sonography. There were three groups in this study: group 1 (n = 23) was small for gestational age with mothers having absent end-diastolic flow; group 2 was small-for-gestational age (n = 20) while the group 3 was appropriate for gestational age (n = 19). Antenatal color Doppler revealed normal umbilical artery blood flow in group 2 and 3. In all the patients, postnatal SMA color Doppler was performed before test feed (0.5 mL) and repeated every 15 minutes till 1 hour after administration of test feed. The study revealed higher incidence of NEC and feed intolerance in group 1. The study also suggested that serial SMA flow evaluation, especially the 60 minutes postfeed study may help in identifying babies likely to develop feed intolerance.

Extrahepatic biliary atresia (EHBA) and neonatal hepatitis are two important causes of neonatal conjugated hyperbilirubinemia. Together, they account for 60–90% of patients.[27,28] It is essential to differentiate between these two entities as the treatment is completely different. Some of the recent articles have utilized ultrasound and/or color Doppler for evaluation of babies suspected of having EHBA. Humphrey and Stringer[29] performed sonographic evaluation of 90 infants with conjugated hyperbilirubinemia for gallbladder morphology, triangular cord sign, presence of a common bile duct, liver size and echotexture, splenic appearance and vascular anatomy. Using all of the above mentioned features, they were able to correctly classify 88/90 infants as having or not having EHBA (98% accuracy). The features with the greatest individual sensitivity and specificity, respectively, in the diagnosis of biliary atresia (BA) were triangular cord sign had sensitivity of 73% and specificity of 100% for diagnosis of EHBA. Corresponding figures were 91% and 95% for abnormal gallbladder wall; 70% and 100% for gallbladder shape, and 93% and 92% for absent common bile duct. The hepatic artery had statistically significant ($p < 0.001$) larger diameter in infants with EHBA than in those without EHBA. However, portal vein diameters were not significantly different between the two groups.

Kim and colleagues[30] prospectively evaluated the accuracy of hepatic artery diameter and hepatic artery diameter-to-portal vein diameter ratio for ultrasonographic diagnosis of BA. The diameter of right hepatic artery and the ratio of hepatic artery diameter-to-portal vein diameter were larger in the EHBA group. The authors suggested right hepatic arterial diameter of 1.5 mm and hepatic artery diameter-to-portal vein diameter ratio of 0.45 as optimal cut-off values for diagnosis of EHBA.

Lee and colleagues[31] described the color Doppler ultrasonographic findings in livers of neonates with EHBA and compared them with US findings in livers of neonates with nonBA and control subjects. The study included 64 patients of neonatal cholestasis of which 29 had EHBA. In additional, they enrolled 19 control subjects. The authors evaluated the triangular cord sign and hepatic subcapsular flow. The images were interpreted by three pediatric radiologists independently and discrepancies were resolved by consensus. The triangular cord sign had sensitivity of 62% and specificity of 100% for diagnosis of EHBA.

Hepatic subcapsular flow on color Doppler had sensitivity and specificity of 100% and 86% respectively for diagnosis EHBA on the basis of consensus reading.

The gold standard for diagnosis of EHBA is intraoperative cholangiogram.[32] Unfortunately, some infants are found not to have EHBA on peroperative cholangiogram. In a retrospective study, Nwomeh and colleagues[33] evaluated the contribution of percutaneous cholecystocholangiography in preventing unnecessary laparotomy in infants with cholestatic jaundice. The study included 35 infants of which 9 had sonographically visible gallbladder. In these patients ultrasound-guided percutaneous cholecystocholangiography was performed and diagnosis of EHBA excluded. This obviated the need of laparotomy in these patients.

Rectal bleeding is commonly evaluated using CT colonoscopy (CTC) in adult population. However, this modality has not been extensively used in pediatric population. Anupindi and colleagues[34] evaluated eight (3–17 years of age) children with noncontrast CTC and reported it to be a well tolerated, safe and useful investigation. The estimated mean effective dose in this study for CTC was 2.17 mSv as compared to 5–6 mSv for a standard air-contrast barium enema in a small child. Capuñay and colleagues[35] performed 100 CTC studies in children with rectal bleeding. No complications were encountered. They reported sensitivity and specificity of 89% and 80% of CTC in diagnosis of elevated colonic lesions. The authors concluded that virtual colonoscopy is an alternative method for the evaluating the children with elevated lesions. It has fast speed without complications, and uses a low dose of radiation. The postulated advantages of using CTC included diagnosis of the exact location of the polyp, faster and easier polypectomy by conventional colonoscopist, reduction in the time of anesthesia and less complications in relation to the conventional procedure of colonoscopy.

Sugiyama and colleagues[36] evaluated the feasibility of single scan CTC using polyethylene glycol electrolytes solution with contrast medium (PEG-C) bowel preparation in children. Seven patients suspected of colorectal-elevated lesions were subjected to CTC. All patients underwent bowel preparation using PEG at a dose of 32 ± 3 mL/kg body weight (BW) during the evening before the day of CTC. The water-soluble contrast agent (Gastrografin, Nihon Schering, Osaka, Japan) was given to the patients orally or through a nasogastric tube at a dose of 0.6 ± 0.1 mL/kg BW, the next morning. The water-soluble contrast agent was diluted 1:9 with PEG. The contrast agent was used for residual fluid tagging. Air was insufflated into the colon in the left decubitus position. The patient was scanned axially with a single run from the colonic flexures to the pelvis in the supine position. CTCs were negative for polyps in 2 patients and positive in 5 patients. The endoscopic findings were similar to the CTC images. In two cases which did not reveal polyps on CTC, no symptoms were noticed on follow-up for a period of more than 6 months. The authors concluded that the single scan CTC using PEG-C preparation was safe and less invasive compared to conventional colonoscopy due to the shorter examination time and lower radiation dose. Radiation exposure in this study was between 6.5 mGy and 15.0 mGy (mean dose: 9.1 mGy).

Intussusception is a common emergency in infants and young children. Ultrasound or fluoroscopy guided reduction is frequently attempted to avoid surgery. However, many a times the reduction is incomplete. Curtis and colleagues[37] retrospectively reviewed whether a failed reduction of ileocolic intussusception at a referring hospital is predictor of failure of repeat attempt at a children's hospital. The children with pathological lead point, these with age more than 10 years, those having successful reduction at referring hospital and those who did not undergo an enema reduction at the authors' institute were excluded. 152 patients met the enrollment criteria. The authors did not find any significant difference in the rate of successful reduction for the patients who initially presented to author's institute (60.5% as compared to those who had failed reduction at a referring hospital 60.7%). They concluded that children referred to a children's hospital after failed enema reduction at a referring hospital should undergo repeat enema reduction provided there are no other contraindications.

In another retrospective study, Pazo and Losek[38] evaluated the demographic and clinical characteristics of children with intussusception and failed initial air enema reduction who were managed by delayed repeat enema attempts. They attempted to identify predictors associated with successful reduction. In this study, there were 21 intussusception events in 20 patients which were managed by delayed repeat air enemas. 9/21 repeat enemas were successful. 4 of the patients who had unsuccessful reduction at first repeat enema underwent a second repeat enema with successful reduction in 3 patients. Thus, 12/25 (48%) repeat enemas were successful. The success rate of delayed repeat enemas was found to be greatest when the intussusception was initially reduced to the ileocecal valve. Demographic characteristics, clinical characteristics, or time from initial enema to first repeat enema were not significant determinant of success at repeat enema.

Cystic fibrosis frequently involves liver early in evolution. Liver steatosis is the most common manifestation while focal biliary cirrhosis is the pathognomonic manifestation. Menten and colleagues[39] evaluated the role of transient elastography of liver in patients of CF. In this prospective study, the authors evaluated 134 patients of CF of which 75 were children. In addition, 31 children without CF were enrolled as controls. Liver morphology was classified on a scale of 1–5 representing increasingly severe liver disease. 10 measurements were recorded for tissue elastography for each subject and median value was considered the elastic modulus of liver. The authors found elasticity values of controls, pancreatic sufficient CF and pancreatic insufficient CF patients with ultrasound score less than 3 to be comparable and significantly lower than compared to CF patients with ultrasound score of more than or equal to 3. In addition, male patients with CF had significantly higher median elasticity (4.7 kilopascals) as compared to female patients with CF (3.9 kilopascals). This preliminary study suggests that transient elastography may be an attractive noninvasive technique to assess and follow-up hepatic disease in CF patients.

UROR ADIOLOGY

Intravenous urography and micturating cystourethrography are important radiological investigations in pediatric uroradiology. However, both of these investigations impart ionizing radiation to the children. Magnetic resonance urography (MRU) and voiding ultrasonography are being evaluated as radiation-free alternatives.

Hydronephrosis is common urological problem in pediatric population which is evaluated using a combination of several modalities. Perez-Brayfield and colleagues[40] conducted a prospective study to compare ultrasound, nuclear scintigraphy and dynamic contrast-enhanced MRI for the estimation of hydronephrosis. 96 children with mean age of 4 years (range: 1 month to 17 years) were enrolled in the study. Patient sedation, an important issue in pediatric MRI, was administered without complications. The split renal function as calculated by nuclear and MRI scans were comparable in 71 cases ($r = 0.93$) evaluated. In 50/64 (78%) cases, the final diagnosis at MRU was similar to that on a combination of ultrasound and nuclear scintigraphy. The authors concluded that dynamic contrast-enhanced MRI provided the same information about renal function but superior information regarding morphology in a single study without ionizing radiation.

Akgun and colleagues[41] conducted a retrospective study to assess whether diuretic agent administration in MRU affects the renal length and to clarify whether the increase in length can be useful in assessing renal function. The study group consisted of 20 children of age group 10 months to 13 years. All these children had ureteropelvic junction stenosis. All had technetium-99m (^{99m}Tc)-mercaptoacetyltriglycine (MAG-3) and ^{99m}Tc-diethylene triamine pentaacetic acid (DTPA) diuretic renography performed within 1 month of MRU. The authors reported that the mean renal lengths measured before and after diuretic administration were 79.02 ± 16.84 mm and 85.61 ± 18.49 mm, respectively. This increase in renal length after diuretic administration was found to be statistically significant ($p < 0.001$; $t = 8.082$). In addition, a positive correlation was observed between the increase in renal length after diuretic injection and functional status of kidneys ($p < 0.001$; $r = 0.547$). The better functioning kidneys had higher increase in renal length after diuretic administration.

Availability of sonographic-contrast agents and harmonic imaging has contributed significantly to the sonographic evaluation of vesicoureteric reflux. In a recent study, Papadopoulo and colleagues[42] prospectively evaluated sensitivity of voiding urosonography harmonic imaging (VUS HI) using a second-generation contrast agent (sulfur-hexafluoride gas microbubbles, SonoVue, Bracco, Italy) for the diagnosis of vesicoureteral reflux. The study group included 228 children with 463 kidney-ureter units (KUUs). The patients underwent two cycles of VUS HI and two cycles of voiding cystourethrography (VCUG) at the same session. The findings of two modalities were compared. Vesicoureteric reflux was demonstrated in 161/463 (34.7%) KUUs, 57 by both methods, 90 only by VUS HI, and 14 only by micturating cystourethrogram. There was (77.5%) ($k = 0.40$) concordance (359/463 KUUs) in findings regarding the presence or absence of vesicoureteric reflux. There was a significant difference in the detection rate of reflux between the two methods ($p < 0.01$). Apart from showing inferior sensitivity, micturating cystourethrography also missed reflux of higher grade (2 grade I, 65 grade II, 19 grade III, 4 grade IV) as compared to VUS HI (8 grade I, 5 grade II, 1 grade III). The authors suggested that VUS HI and a second-generation contrast agent can be used as an alternative radiation-free imaging method for evaluation of vesicoureteric reflux.

Another radiation-free approach to evaluation of vesicoureteric reflux involves utilization of MR fluoroscopy.

Vasanwala and colleagues[43] have attempted to develop an MRI voiding cystography protocol with continuous real-time MR fluoroscopy and validate it against micturating cystourethrography. In this study, eight follow-up patients of vesicoureteric reflux were evaluated in a specially designed machine capable of performing MRI as well as fluoroscopic VCUG. In this study, MRI had sensitivity of 88% when the grade of reflux differed by less than 1 on two modalities. MRI detected reflux in one patient which was not detected by fluoroscopic VCUG.

MUSCULOSKELETAL IMAGING

Magni-Manzoni and colleagues[44] conducted a study to compare clinical evaluation and ultrasound in the assessment of joint synovitis in children with juvenile idiopathic arthritis. 52 joints in 32 children were evaluated by two pediatric rheumatologists for swelling, tenderness/pain on motion, and restricted motion. The same joints were evaluated by an experienced sonographer for synovial hyperplasia, joint effusion and power Doppler signal. Overall, 1,664 joints were assessed both clinically and sonographically. On clinical examination joint swelling, tenderness and restricted motion were noticed in 98 (5.9%), 59 (3.5%) and 40 (2.4%) of joints, respectively. Sonographic evaluation revealed synovial hyperplasia in 125 (7.5%), joint effusion in 153 (9.2%) and power Doppler signal in 53 (3.2%) joints. A total of 104 (6.3%) and 167 (10%) joints had clinical and sonographic evidence of synovitis, respectively. 86 (5.5%) of the clinically "normal" joints had sonographic features of synovitis. 5 patients were classified as having polyarthritis who were classified as having oligoarthritis or no synovitis on clinical evaluation. In this study, sonographic features moderately correlated with clinical measures of joint swelling, but poorly correlated with those of joint tenderness/pain on motion and restricted motion. The authors concluded that subclinical synovitis is common in juvenile idiopathic arthritis which may have important implications for patient classification and may affect the therapeutic strategy in individual patients.

Rooney and colleagues[45] prevalence of synovitis and tenosynovitis in children with juvenile idiopathic arthritis who were felt clinically to have active inflammatory disease of the ankle. Forty-nine clinically swollen ankle joints in 34 patients were included in this study. There were 19 patients with polyarticular disease and 13 with oligoarticular disease. One patient had systemic juvenile idiopathic arthritis. The authors found that 71% of ankles had tenosynovitis and 39% had tenosynovitis alone. Only 29% of clinically swollen ankles had tibiotalar joint effusion alone while 33% had both tenosynovitis and tibiotalar joint effusion. There was statistically significant difference between different subgroups for the frequency of occurrence of medial ankle tenosynovitis ($p = 0.048$) and lateral ankle tenosynovitis ($p = 0.001$).

SUMMARY

Several good articles have been published in recent years contributing to improved patient care. The current trends stress on the need of keeping the radiation dose to the minimum possible level when investigating the pediatric patients. Readers are encouraged to stay in touch with recent developments. Use of electronic resources is recommended as quick and inexpensive means for maintaining up to date knowledge.

REFERENCES

1. Image Gently: The Alliance for Radiation Safety in Pediatric Imaging. (2014). Campaign Overview. [online] Available from: *www.imagegently.org/FAQsMore/CampaignOverview.aspx*. [Accessed July, 2015].
2. Strauss KJ, Kaste SC. The ALARA concept in pediatric interventional and fluoroscopic imaging: striving to keep radiation doses as low as possible during fluoroscopy of pediatric patients—a white paper executive summary. Am J Roentgenol. 2006;187(3):818-9.
3. Strauss KJ, Goske MJ, Kaste SC, et al. Image gently: ten steps you can take to optimize image quality and lower CT dose for pediatric patients. Am J Roentgenol. 2010;194(4):868-73.
4. Sidhu M, Strauss KJ, Connolly B, ct al. Radiation safety in pediatric interventional radiology. Tech Vasc Interv Radiol. 2010;13(3):158-66.
5. Palchak MJ, Holmes JF, Vance CW, et al. A decision rule for identifying children at low risk for brain injuries after blunt head trauma. Ann Emerg Med. 2003;42(4):492-506.
6. Barkovich AJ, Miller SP, Bartha A, et al. MR imaging, MR spectroscopy, and diffusion tensor imaging of sequential studies in neonates with encephalopathy. Am J Neuroradiol. 2006;27(3):533-47.
7. Liauw L, van Wezel-Meijler G, Veen S, et al. Do apparent diffusion coefficient measurements predict outcome in children with neonatal hypoxic-ischemic encephalopathy? Am J Neuroradiol. 2009;30(2):264-70.
8. Epelman M, Daneman A, Kellenberger CJ, et al. Neonatal encephalopathy: a prospective comparison of head US and MRI. Pediatr Radiol. 2010;40(10):1640-50.
9. Tovar-Moll F, Moll J, de Oliveira-Souza R, et al. Neuroplasticity in human callosal dysgenesis: a diffusion tensor imaging study. Cereb Cortex. 2007;17(3):531-41.
10. Wu Z, Mittal S, Kish K, et al. Identification of calcification with MRI using susceptibility-weighted imaging: a case study. J Magn Reson Imaging. 2009;29(1):177-82.
11. Wang Q, Babyn P, Branson H, et al. Utility of MRI in the follow-up of pyogenic spinal infection in children. Pediatr Radiol. 2010;40(1):118-30.

12. Bober K, Swietliñski J. Diagnostic utility of ultrasonography for respiratory distress syndrome in neonates. Med Sci Monit. 2006;12(10):CR440-6.
13. Copetti R, Cattarossi L. The 'double lung point': an ultrasound sign diagnostic of transient tachypnea of the newborn. Neonatology. 2007;91(3):203-9.
14. Copetti R, Cattarossi L, Macagno F, et al. Lung ultrasound in respiratory distress syndrome: a useful tool for early diagnosis. Neonatology. 2008;94(1):52-9.
15. Kurian J, Levin TL, Han BK, et al. Comparison of ultrasound and CT in the evaluation of pneumonia complicated by parapneumonic effusion in children. Am J Roentgenol. 2009;193(6):1648-54.
16. Montella S, Santamaria F, Salvatore M, et al. Assessment of chest high-field magnetic resonance imaging in children and young adults with noncystic fibrosis chronic lung disease: comparison to high-resolution computed tomography and correlation with pulmonary function. Invest Radiol. 2009;44(9):532-8.
17. Bannier E, Cieslar K, Mosbah K, et al. Hyperpolarized 3He MR for sensitive imaging of ventilation function and treatment efficiency in young cystic fibrosis patients with normal lung function. Radiology. 2010;255(1):225-32.
18. Lee EY, Tracy DA, Bastos M, et al. Expiratory volumetric MDCT evaluation of air trapping in pediatric patients with and without tracheomalacia. Am J Roentgenol. 2010;194(5):1210-5.
19. Cheng Z, Wang X, Duan Y, et al. Low-dose prospective ECG-triggering dual-source CT angiography in infants and children with complex congenital heart disease: first experience. Eur Radiol. 2010;20(10):2503-11.
20. Paul JF, Rohnean A, Elfassy E, et al. Radiation dose for thoracic and coronary step-and-shoot CT using a 128-slice dual-source machine in infants and small children with congenital heart disease. Pediatr Radiol. 2010;41(2):244-9.
21. Buonomo C. The radiology of necrotizing enterocolitis. Radiol Clin North Am. 1999;37(6):1187-98.
22. Faingold R, Daneman A, Tomlinson G, et al. Necrotizing enterocolitis: assessment of bowel viability with color Doppler US. Radiology. 2005;235(2):587-94.
23. Kim WY, Kim WS, Kim IO, et al. Sonographic evaluation of neonates with early-stage necrotizing enterocolitis. Pediatr Radiol. 2005;35(11):1056-61.
24. Silva CT, Daneman A, Navarro OM, et al. Correlation of sonographic findings and outcome in necrotizing enterocolitis. Pediatr Radiol. 2007;37(3):274-82.
25. Dilli D, Oguz SS, Ulu HO, et al. Sonographic findings in premature infants with necrotising enterocolitis. Arch Dis Child Fetal Neonatal Ed. 2009;94(3):F232-3.
26. Bora R, Mukhopadhyay K, Saxena AK, et al. Prediction of feed intolerance and necrotizing enterocolitis in neonates with absent end diastolic flow in umbilical artery and the correlation of feed intolerance with postnatal superior mesenteric artery flow. J Matern Fetal Neonatal Med. 2009;22(11):1092-6.
27. Jonas MM, Perez-Atayde AR. Liver disease in infancy and childhood. In: Schiff ER, Sorell MF, Maddrey WC (Eds). Schiff's diseases of liver, 10th edition. Philadelphia, PA, USA: Lippincott Williams & Wilkins. 2007. pp. 1307-31.
28. Nicotra JJ, Kramer SS, Bellah RD, et al. Congenital and acquired biliary disorders in children. Semin Roentgenol. 1997;32(3):215-27.
29. Humphrey TM, Stringer MD. Biliary atresia: US diagnosis. Radiology. 2007;244(3):845-51.
30. Kim WS, Cheon JE, Youn BJ, et al. Hepatic arterial diameter measured with US: adjunct for US diagnosis of biliary atresia. Radiology. 2007;245(2):549-55.
31. Lee MS, Kim MJ, Lee MJ, et al. Biliary atresia: color Doppler US findings in neonates and infants. Radiology. 2009;252(1):282-9.
32. de Carvalho E, Ivantes CA, Bezerra JA. Extrahepatic biliary atresia: current concepts and future directions. J Pediatr (Rio J). 2007;83(2):105-20.
33. Nwomeh BC, Caniano DA, Hogan M. Definitive exclusion of biliary atresia in infants with cholestatic jaundice: the role of percutaneous cholecysto-cholangiography. Pediatr Surg Int. 2007;23(9):845-9.
34. Anupindi S, Perumpillichira J, Jaramillo D, et al. Low-dose CT colonography in children: initial experience, technical feasibility, and utility. Pediatr Radiol. 2005;35(5):518-24.
35. Capuñay CM, Carrascosa PM, Bou-Khair A, et al. Low radiation dose multislice CT colonography in children: Experience after 100 studies. Eur J Radiol. 2005;56(3):398-402.
36. Sugiyama A, Ohashi Y, Gomi A, et al. Colorectal screening with single scan CT colonography in children. Pediatr Sur Int. 2007;23(10):987-90.
37. Curtis JL, Gutierrez IM, Kirk SR, et al. Failure of enema reduction for ileocolic intussusception at a referring hospital does not preclude repeat attempts at a children's hospital. J Pediatr Surg. 2010;45(6):1178-81.
38. Pazo A, Hill J, Losek JD. Delayed repeat enema in the management of intussusception. Pediatr Emerg Care. 2010;26(9):640-5.
39. Menten R, Leonard A, Clapuyt P, et al. Transient elastography in patients with cystic fibrosis. Pediatr Radiol. 2010;40(7):1231-5.
40. Perez-Brayfield MR, Kirsch AJ, Jones RA, et al. A prospective study comparing ultrasound, nuclear scintigraphy and dynamic contrast enhanced magnetic resonance imaging in the evaluation of hydronephrosis. J Urol. 2003;170(4 Pt 1):1330-4.
41. Akgun V, Kocaoglu M, Ilgan S, et al. Diuretic-induced renal length changes in the estimation of renal function with MR urography. Am J Roentgenol. 2010;194(2):W218-20.
42. Papadopoulou F, Anthopoulou A, Siomou E, et al. Harmonic voiding urosonography with a second-generation contrast agent for the diagnosis of vesicoureteral reflux. Pediatr Radiol. 2009;39(3):239-44.
43. Vasanawala SS, Kennedy WA, Ganguly A, et al. MR voiding cystography for evaluation of vesicoureteral reflux. Am J Roentgenol. 2009;192(5):W206-11.
44. Magni-Manzoni S, Epis O, Ravelli A, et al. Comparison of clinical versus ultrasound-determined synovitis in juvenile idiopathic arthritis. Arthritis Rheum. 2009;61(11):1497-504.
45. Rooney ME, McAllister C, Burns JF. Ankle disease in juvenile idiopathic arthritis: ultrasound findings in clinically swollen ankles. J Rheumatol. 2009;36(8):1725-9.

CHAPTER 128

Interventions in Children

Gurpreet Singh Gulati, Sanjiv Sharma, Amar Mukund, Ashu Seith Bhalla, Shivanand Gamanagatti

VASCULAR INTERVENTIONS

Gurpreet Singh Gulati, Sanjiv Sharma

INTRODUCTION

Interventional procedures in the pediatric age group have a long history. Probably the first intervention performed in a pediatric patient was the reduction of intussusception. The earliest cardio-vascular intervention in children performed with angiographic guidance was balloon atrial septostomy. Over the years, although vascular interventional techniques as applied to the adult population have undergone dramatic and continuous innovation, their application to pediatric patients has been delayed, due to a conservative attitude of pediatric medicine practitioners, lack of adequately trained physicians and staff in this subspecialty, and need for special equipment appropriate for pediatric use.

Children are not merely "little adults", nor are the diseases to which they are particularly susceptible, variants of diseases in adult life. Excessive crying, unwillingness for examination, and their inability to describe complaints make a child the most difficult patient. However, it is a challenge to the pediatric interventionist to master the art of "talking" and achieve a successful examination. A friendly environment, affectionate attitude of the medical staff, and a carefully and rapidly performed study, go a long way in conducting a successful procedure.

SPECIAL CONSIDERATIONS FOR THE PEDIATRIC PATIENT

The interventional radiologist and referring physician hold a detailed discussion to decide the appropriate procedure to be performed. The risks for the particular patient are appreciated, and the likely benefit to accrue to the patient is understood. It is particularly imperative to pay special attention to the following details while conducting a pediatric angiography or intervention. These are:

- Choice of sedation or anesthesia
- Maintenance of temperature control
- Fluid balance
- Radiation safety
- Equipment selection.

A dedicated team consisting of the operating radiologist, the radiation and hemodynamic technologists, and the nursing attendant are needed to prepare the catheterization laboratory, prepare and handle the patient, and assist during the procedure. A high-resolution digital angiography system is required to obtain reliable diagnostic images quickly and to monitor the interventional procedure.

Table 1: Pre-procedure clinical evaluation of the patient.

1.	History of the current problem
2.	Pertinent medical and surgical history
3.	Review of the organ systems • Cardiac • Pulmonary • Renal • Hepatic • Hematologic (e.g. coagulopathy, hypercoagulable state) • Endocrine (diabetes)
4.	History of allergies
5.	Current medications
6.	Directed physical examination

PATIENT PREPARATION

History and Physical Examination

A detailed discussion on the patient's history taking and examination relevant to general as well as specific angiographic interventional procedures is outside the scope of this chapter. **Table 1** lists the several components that need to be assessed while evaluating the patient.

Informed Consent

The parent or guardian of a minor child, and when possible, the patient himself, should understand the reasons for undergoing the procedure. The risks and benefits should be clarified along with the consequences of refusing the procedure, and the alternative therapies available should be discussed. He/she should then give consent for the procedure.

Coagulation

Whenever there is a bleeding diathesis, risk of hemorrhage, or a plan to perform systemic thrombolysis, coagulation studies are obtained. Blood is sent for grouping and cross-matching whenever there is ongoing or expected blood loss. Heparin is administered for arterial catheterization procedures in a dose of 50 units/kg for diagnostic and 100 units/kg for revascularization procedures.

Anesthesia

Most diagnostic studies are carried out with intravenous sedation. Difficult interventions such as device implantation or particularly painful procedures are conducted under general anesthesia.

In most children, conscious sedation is used, in which the child is conscious, drowsy, and may even close his eyes, but is responsive to verbal commands and able to protect his reflexes and airway. *Midazolam* is a commonly used, short-acting benzodiazepine that is metabolized by the liver. Its dose is 0.2–1 mg/KBW IV. The onset of action is 3–5 minutes and the duration of action is 60 minutes. The major side effects are respiratory depression and apnea. A combination of three drugs namely, *demerol* (50 mg), *promethazine* (12.5 mg) and *triclofos* (12.5 mg), known as *DPT,* is the other agent used for conscious sedation. A mixture of the three is made into a 2 mL solution, to be given in a dose of 0.06–0.1 mL/KBW IM. For deeper sedation, a combination of *diazepam* (0.1 mg/KBW) and *morphine* (0.1 mg/KBW) may be given IV. Respiratory depression may occur with higher doses.

Patient Immobilization

Smaller children are immobilized on a restraining board. Older children will have hand and leg restraints but, if uncooperative, will need to be anesthetized.

Temperature Control

Neonates and especially premature babies may become hypo-thermic if a warm operating environment is not maintained. The room temperature should be increased, radiation heaters are required, and the child should be covered quickly while preparing the groin and draping.

Diet and Medications

Small children need not be kept fasting for more than 3–4 hours prior to the procedure. Routine antibiotics are not prescribed except for high-risk procedures, e.g. splenic embolization.

Dose of Radiation and Fluids

Isky Gordon et al.[1] calculated and published the ratio of radiation dose to the skin (in rads) for various procedures as follows:

Age (years)	*1*	*5*	*10*	*15*
Angiography – 20 films	1.4	3.0	4.8	7.5
Fluoroscopy – 4 minutes	3.2	4.8	6.8	8.8

One must try and minimize the radiation exposure to children who are believed to be more sensitive to the effects of radiation and likely to live for many years with these effects. Digital systems probably do not reduce radiation exposure. However, several precautions may be taken by the operator to reduce the dose. Fluoroscopy at the lowest dose possible (reduce the mAS), pulsed fluoroscopy, removing the scatter grids, and addition of rare earth filters in the X-ray tubes help to reduce radiation doses to the patient.

All fluids and medication must be scaled to the patient size. One may easily administer excessive amounts of fluids and contrast without realizing it. Digital systems (more so with biplane angiography systems) help to bring down the volume of contrast material and speeding up procedures. Most infants can tolerate 4 mL/kg of contrast, whereas children over 6 months can tolerate 6 mL/kg, if it is delivered as several injections spread over a period of time. It is important to maintain patient hydration if such large doses are employed.

TECHNIQUES

The vascular procedures used in pediatric patients require a substantially different approach than that of the adult population. An account must be kept of a few considerations when treating the pediatric population, including the small size of the caliber vessel, anticipation of spasm, the risk for infection, the tendency of children to rapidly form collateral circulation, the inevitability of growth, and the strong tendency for restenosis and growth arrest to occur.

Access

Introducer sheaths should be used to preserve vascular access, since multiple catheter/guidewire insertions or exchanges may be needed. Special pediatric access sheaths are available in 4–6 F sizes. These are usually introduced by using a cannula (18–21 G) and a 0.021" guidewire. The angle of entry of the needle should be less perpendicular to the skin, and a small nick in the skin with the blade should be given before introducing the sheath, to prevent pain and a possible vasovagal reaction. Care should be taken to prevent an inadvertent incision in the anterior vessel wall while using the blade.

PROCEDURES

The major vascular interventional procedures performed in children can be grouped into:

- Embolization
- Angioplasty
- Thrombolysis
- Foreign body removal.

EMBOLIZATION

Percutaneous transcatheter embolization has replaced surgery for many pediatric vascular problems, and is a treatment alternative in patients where surgery has little to offer. Microcatheter systems, which were initially developed for adult neurovascular interventions, are ideal for pediatric applications. They permit access to small vessels and territories that were previously inaccessible. Hydrophilic coated steerable guidewires permit negotiation of complex vascular loops without provoking spasm or causing dissection.

Embolization procedures should only be performed by experienced physicians familiar with the equipment and technical aspects of the procedure. Discussion with the pediatric physicians or surgeons, their support and backup is essential for a safe and successful procedure.

The various pediatric vascular conditions treated by using embolotherapy can be grouped as follows:

- Vascular anomalies, e.g. arteriovenous malformation (AVM), arteriovenous fistula (AVF), venous malformation (VM), lymphatic malformation (LM), and hemangioma.
- Hemorrhage from bleeding vessels (due to pseudoaneurysms or vascular involvement in trauma, tumor or inflammation) in various organ systems.
- Other conditions, e.g. tumors and organ ablation.

Goals of embolotherapy include: (1) an adjunctive goal, e.g. preoperative, adjunct to chemotherapy or radiation therapy; (2) a curative goal, e.g. definitive treatment such as that performed in cases of aneurysms, AVFs, AVMs, and traumatic bleeding; and (3) a palliative goal, e.g. relieving symptoms, such as of a large AVM, which cannot be cured by using embolotherapy alone.

Embolization Materials and Substances

Materials required in embolization include coils, sodium tetradecyl sulfate, ethanol, n-butyl cyanoacrylate (NBCA) glue, polyvinyl alcohol (PVA) particles, gelatin sponge (Gelfoam) and microspheres.

Vascular Anomalies

Vascular anomalies can be grouped into two categories: Hemangiomas and vascular malformations. Vascular malformations are categorized further as high-flow lesions (AVM, AVF), low-flow lesions (capillary malformation, VM, LM), or combined vascular malformations. Embolotherapy with a variety of embolic materials is commonly used in the treatment of vascular anomalies.

Hemangioma

Hemangiomas are very benign tumors which do not require treatment in most patients. In some of the rare cases, embolization may be essential (particularly in patients with urgent need of therapy) because of spontaneous hemorrhage or functional abnormality caused by the extreme size of the lesion or the particular anatomic location or because of significant congestive heart failure.[2] Additionly, embolotherapy is deemed useful prior to surgical resection in select patients, and in patients in whom a hemangio-endothelioma causes Kasabach-Merritt phenomenon (platelet trapping).[2] Embolotherapy of a hemangioma or hemangioendothelioma can be performed with the use of PVA particles. Coils are not used frequently as they cause more proximal occlusion with potential for recruitment of supply from other arteries and they block future access to the lesion if the need arises.

Embolotherapy aims at blocking a large percentage of the tumoral vessels, thus preventing further trapping and destruction of the platelets and hastening involution of the lesion. Several sessions of embolotherapy may be required for some tumors because of revascularization of the tumor or to prevent exceeding the limits of radiation and contrast burden in one session. Infantile hepatic hemangioendotheliomas, a variant of infantile hemangioma, usually are multiple and are frequently complicated by congestive heart failure. In the clinical setting, embolotherapy aims at reducing the hepatic arterial flow, which sufficiently relieves high-output cardiac failure. A variety of embolic materials have been used. In some patients, embolization of other nearby arteries (e.g. intercostals) may also be necessary.[3] Arterial portography should be performed to exclude the possibility of feeders from the portal system.

A rare entity called noninvoluting hemangioma, which is found in the adult population, may also respond to transcatheter embolization (usually with particles such as PVA or micro-spheres). This procedure is usually performed to improve the cosmetic appearance.

Arteriovenous Malformation

Arteriovenous malformations are typically characterized by a nidus of abnormal vessels in which shunting of arterial blood to veins occurs. These vascular anomalies are usually present during childhood but often demonstrate a sudden increase in size in response to trauma, hormones or other stimuli. Although, a clinical grading system has been used among surgeons, no grading system has yet been developed for imaging. Most AVMs can be managed by transcatheter embolization and/or sclerotherapy. Surgical excision can treat some focal AVMs. Proximal embolization or ligation of the feeding arteries usually has adverse effects because of subsequent recruitment of collaterals, and transluminal embolization of the nidus which cannot be performed afterwards. The collaterals that develop are more problematic in terms of transcatheter treatment; however, proximal embolization of the feeding arteries may be performed if it is indicated prior to surgical excision.

During primary embolotherapy, the nidus should be embolized when possible.[2] Absolute alcohol is the most effective agent in the treatment of AVMs. If the nidus is not reachable through the feeding arteries, then an attempt can be made for direct percutaneous cannulation of the nidus. In selected patients with AVMs, another therapeutic approach is embolic occlusion of the venous outflow.

Cervicofacial AVMs

For dental arcade AVMs, spontaneous or catastrophic hemorrhage during tooth extraction is a common presentation. Embolization of an AVM in this region requires superselective catheterization of the involved branches of external carotid artery and other regional arterial branches (e.g. thyrocervical trunk) using microcatheters and the coaxial technique.[4]

Embolotherapy can be performed with NBCA, alcohol, particles, and/or microcoils, depending on the nature and extent of the malformation. Gelfoam can also be used for preoperative embolization. In cases of patients with dental AVMs associated with acute bleeding and loose teeth embolization should be performed immediately prior to tooth extraction. Some complications related to embolotherapy of cervicofacial AVMs include stroke, nerve paralysis, skin necrosis, infection, blindness, and pulmonary embolism.

Extremity AVMs

In the extremities, AVMs can be diffuse and may involve the entire extremity (Parkes-Weber syndrome). Extremity AVMs typically present with extremity-length discrepancy, high cardiac output, pain, and ulceration. Extremity lesions can be treated with multiple embolizations[5] and/or surgical resections or amputation of the extremity **(Figs. 1A and B)**.

A detailed pre-embolization angiographic examination is important for mapping the feeders and draining veins. During the injection of contrast material, the injection rate and duration should be adjusted so that there is accurate identification of arteriovenous connections. A high injection rate in a short period is appropriate for AVMs.

Selective catheterization with microcatheters is required to reach the nidus of the AVM. Some possible complications of embolotherapy include skin necrosis (blisters), nontarget embolization (which also includes

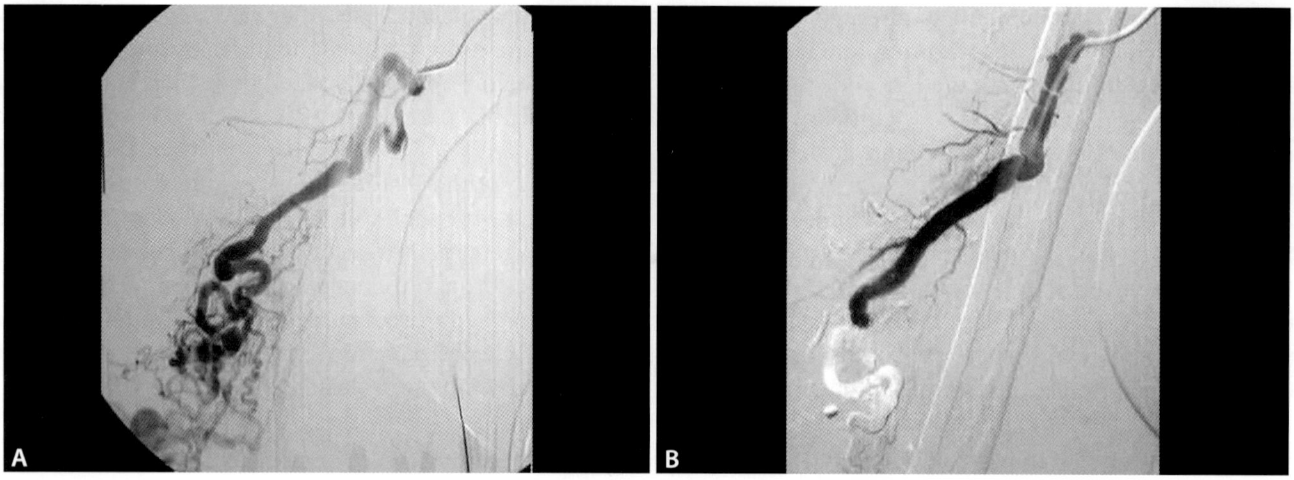

Figs. 1A and B: An arteriovenous malformation of the right arm, with feeders from the profunda brachii artery. (A) Pre-embolization; (B) Postembolization (polyvinyl alcohol particles) angiograms.

pulmonary emboli), and systemic sclerosant toxicity if a liquid agent (e.g. alcohol) is used.

Pulmonary AVMs

Pulmonary AVMs are also termed as pulmonary AVFs. They have a high association with Osler-Weber-Rendu syndrome (also called hereditary hemorrhagic telangiectasia syndrome). Symptoms of which may include dyspnea, cyanosis, and clubbing. Paradoxical embolization may cause stroke or brain abscess. This anomaly can be classified as simple or complex on the basis of the number of feeders and draining veins. In simple lesions, a single artery and vein are involved; in complex lesions, 2 or more supplying arteries and 1 or more draining veins are involved.

Most pulmonary AVMs (80%) are simple. Although a surgical approach (thoracotomy and resection) is the traditional mode of therapy, currently, transcatheter embolization is a preferred alternative.[6] Transcatheter embolization offers significantly reduced morbidity and mortality rates, particularly in hereditary hemorrhagic telangiectasia syndrome.

Embolotherapy for AVMs can be performed with coils, vascular plugs or detachable balloons. Possible complications of embolotherapy include nontarget embolization in the systemic circulation (through the AVM shunt) or in other noninvolved pulmonary arteries. Therefore, it is vital to properly measure the size of the coil to the feeding (afferent) artery. A preliminary detailed angiography is essential for mapping the feeders and draining veins, while paying particular attention to the size of the feeders. Basically, a successful embolization is achieved by nesting 1 or more coils in the feeding artery, which occludes flow through the AVM shunt **(Figs. 2A and B)**.

Generally, feeding arteries larger than 3 mm should be embolized. Feeders smaller than 3 mm have low risk of paradoxic embolization and should be left alone unless they are simple and straightforward technically. A coil that is 2–3 mm larger than the feeding artery is usually selected. For vascular plug, a 30–50% oversizing is recommended. If the feeding artery is large in caliber (>12 mm), a balloon occlusion of the proximal artery via a second groin puncture can be used for a more controlled coil deployment. Postembolization syndrome can occur and is characterized by pleuritic chest pain, pleural fluid, atelectasis, fever and leukocytosis.

Arteriovenous Fistula

Arteriovenous fistulas are relatively large arteriovenous connections and may be congenital or secondary to trauma, surgery, or underlying vascular abnormality (e.g. neurofibromatosis). AVFs may be seen in any part of the body. A patient may present with cardiac failure, localized growth disturbances, neurologic deficits, and ischemic changes. Unlike AVMs, AVFs can be cured with embolotherapy. The embolotherapy technique used depends on the size, location, and hemodynamics of individual lesions. The goal of embolotherapy is to occlude the fistula and the immediate draining vein.

Embolization can be achieved by using detachable coils or balloons, or tissue adhesives (glue or onyx). It is not appropriate to use Gelfoam or particles in AVF embolization. Detachable coils[7] or balloons are ideal

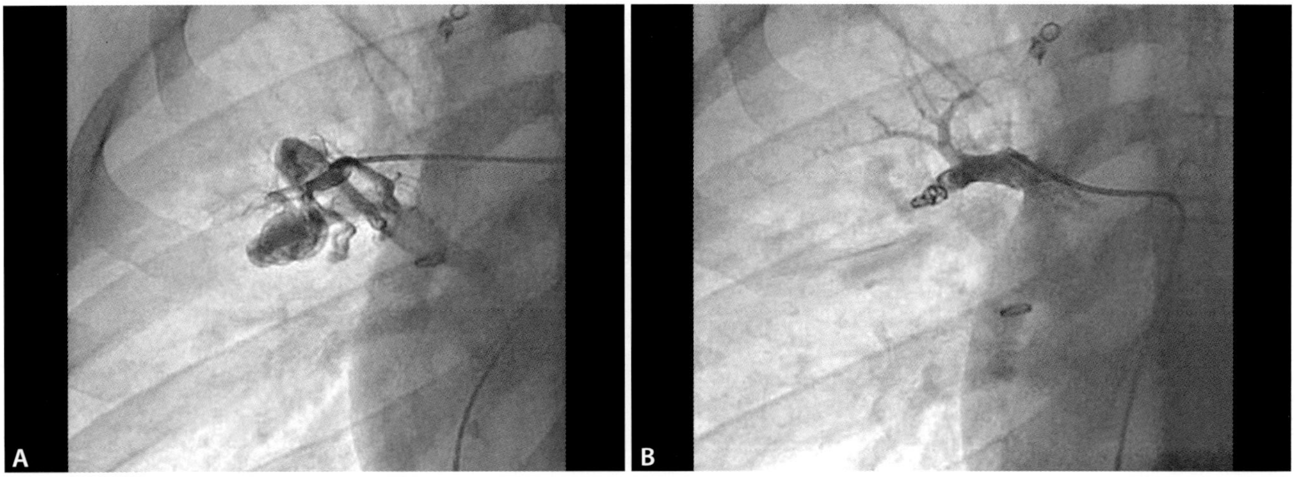

Figs. 2A and B: Right upper lobe pulmonary arteriovenous malformation: (A) Pre-embolization; (B) Postembolization (fibered platinum coils) angiograms. Coils elsewhere are from embolization carried out for other PAVMs in the right lung.

because these embolic materials can be positioned optimally before they are detached. Balloons also have the advantage of conforming to the size and shape of the abnormal vessels. Microcoils can be dislodged; however, this complication can be minimized by performing flow-control techniques (e.g. balloon occlusion, tourniquet, or blood pressure cuff control). The other disadvantage of coil embolization is that the clot that forms around the coil may dissolve, leading to recanalization. Appropriate nesting of several coils (packing) can minimize recanalization. Also, thrombosis can be augmented by soaking the coils in thrombin before deployment or by injecting sclerosants around the coils. If adequate coil packing cannot be accomplished, tissue adhesive can be effectively used in combination with coils. Covered stents can also be particularly useful for acquired AVFs (single communications). They have the advantage of maintaining patency of the parent artery. Often, combining strategies by using different techniques becomes necessary.

Vascular Malformation

The most common type of vascular malformations are VMs and can have significant variations in size and clinical presentation. These lesions (usually distinguished by a bluish discoloration with swelling and pain) may also be associated with systemic syndromes such as blue rubber-bleb nevus syndrome or Maffucci syndrome. Sinus pericranii (communication between intracranial and extracranial venous drainage) is also commonly associated with craniofacial VMs. These lesions can be treated with embolotherapy (sclerotherapy) and/or surgical excision.[8,9] The type of treatment used depends on the morphology, size, and location of the malformation.

A preliminary venogram is usually obtained to evaluate the deep venous system and to determine if any communication exists between the VM and the extremity veins. In particular, a venogram is performed on extremity VMs. The lesion is localized by using ultrasonography, and the largest-appearing cystic portion of the lesion is selected. Then, the lesion is accessed by using real-time ultrasonographic guidance and a small Angiocath needle [typically, 20–22 gauge (G)]. The lesion is studied with contrast agent injections under fluoroscopy as well as digital subtraction angiography. Subsequently, sclerotherapy is performed by using ethanol (absolute alcohol) or sodium tetradecyl sulfate mixed with a contrast medium (Ethiodol or iodinated contrast) under real-time fluoroscopic control **(Figs. 3A and B)**. Foam sclerotherapy is a technique where a mixture of room air and sclerosant is injected and potentially results in greater agent-malformation contact and lowers volume of sclerosant required.

If draining veins are present (as they commonly are), manual compression or a tourniquet should be used to reduce washout of the sclerosant material from the malformation. If large draining veins are present, these veins can be embolized with coils via a percutaneous approach before sclerotherapy. For large head and neck VMs, airway involvement can be a challenging component of the condition in terms of treating the patients. Because alcohol and sodium tetradecyl cause significant edema after sclerotherapy, airway patency should be carefully monitored during and after the sclerotherapy procedure. In patients with large head and neck VMs requiring surgical debulking, presurgical sclerotherapy with NBCA glue can be performed because NBCA causes no significant edema.

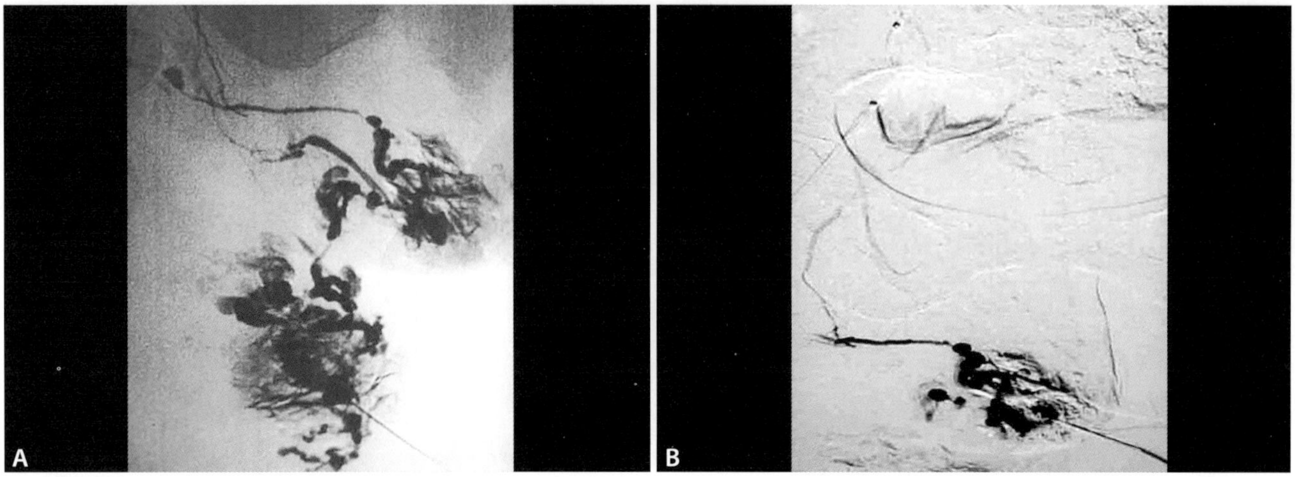

Figs. 3A and B: A diffuse venous malformation in the right thigh: (A) Direct puncture venogram showed minimal flow into deep veins. Sodium tetradecyl sulphate was slowly injected under fluoroscopic control; (B) Successful occlusion of the malformation was achieved.

Two common problems associated with sclerotherapy include skin necrosis (blisters) and/or nerve damage or paralysis. Nerve damage or paralysis can result from the direct toxic effect of the sclerosant agent and/or compression of the nerve by focal compartmental tissue edema (compartment syndrome). In addition, hemoglobulinuria is a relatively common complication; this is treated by aggressive hydration and alkalinization. A less common but more severe complication is cardiac toxicity resulting from the systemic effect of absolute alcohol.

Lymphatic Malformation

Lymphatic malformations (LM) can be grouped as microcystic, macrocystic, and mixed. The mixed form of anomaly is probably the most common form of LM.

Lymphatic cysts contain lymphatic fluid. When a single cystic mass (previously termed cystic hygroma when found in the neck) or a conglomerate mass containing a few macrocysts is encountered, surgical excision is considered the most effective treatment. However, some lesions respond really well to sclerotherapy without any complications after 1 or several sclerotherapy sessions.

When a mixed form of LM is encountered, the best therapeutic approach may be sclerotherapy for cystic masses, followed by surgical debulking. The microcystic LM, or the microcystic component of the mixed form, does not contain cystic spaces on radiologic studies (including MRI). It demonstrates a characteristic contrast-enhanced pattern of rings and arcs. The sclerosant agents most commonly used are antibiotics (doxycycline), ethanol, sodium tetradecyl sulfate and, most recently, OK-432 (a derivative of group A streptococci). For patients older than 8 years of age, doxycycline is the most commonly used sclerosant agent. But if the patient is younger than 8 years, the options are alcohol, sodium tetradecyl, or OK-432. The amount of alcohol used depends on the weight of the patient, which proves to be a limiting factor in most procedures which involve alcohol.

The interventional therapeutic approach used for LMs is similar to the sclerotherapy technique used for VMs; however, an initial venogram is usually unnecessary.

Hemorrhage

Embolization can treat several types of hemorrhage. Examples of these include hemoptysis; epistaxis; and gastrointestinal (GI) tract, post-traumatic, and iatrogenic hemorrhage (e.g. postbiopsy or nephrostomy tube insertion).

Gastrointestinal Hemorrhage

Major causes of upper GI tract hemorrhage are ulcer disease, varices and gastritis. The most common causes of a lower GI tract hemorrhage are vascular malformations and bleeding after endoscopic biopsy. If the bleeding source is identified on arterial angiogram, the patient is treated by using either intra-arterial vasopressin infusion (Pitressin) or embolization of the bleeding mesenteric artery. Embolization is usually the first line of treatment in patients with upper GI tract bleeding and is used as the second line of treatment in patients with lower GI tract bleeding (usually used if vasopressin treatment fails).[10]

Embolization in the arcades proximal to the bleeding vasa recta is recommended to minimize the risk of bowel necrosis. The most commonly used embolic agents are coils (macrocoils or microcoils) and Gelfoam pieces (torpedoes). Coil embolization is particularly helpful if the bleeding is caused by focal vascular abnormalities such as a false aneurysm. Some interventional radiologists have also used PVA, although the use of PVA or other particles should be avoided because of the risk of bowel infarction. After embolization, control angiography is performed to determine if bleeding (contrast material extra-vasation) continues via any collaterals. The primary advantage of embolotherapy is the immediate cessation of bleeding without need for prolonged catheterization (unlike vasopressin infusion therapy).

Pelvic Hemorrhage

Intractable pelvic hemorrhage, usually post-traumatic, should be approached in a similar interventional fashion. It is usually not favorable to employ a surgical approach to control active bleeding in acute trauma setting. It is mandatory to hold a detailed angiographic examination with super selective injections in the branches of the internal iliac artery. Embolization can be performed by using an autologous blood clot, Gelfoam torpedoes, PVA particles, NBCA, coils, or detachable balloons.[11] At the capillary level, embolization with small particles or Gelfoam powder is contraindicated (because of the elimination of collateral flow, which results in massive tissue necrosis).

A specific anatomic relationship between the fracture site and the affected vessel often allows embolization of the branch (frequently the obturator artery) even when no obvious bleeding site is detected.[12] In particular, liquid or particle embolization of the inferior gluteal branch of the anterior division should be avoided to minimize the possibility of sciatic nerve injury (this branch supplies muscles of the thigh and buttocks and the sciatic nerve). In addition, embolization of the posterior division of the internal iliac artery should be avoided because of the risk of gluteal necrosis.

Hemoptysis

Hemoptysis is considered massive when at least 300 mL of blood is lost in less than 24 hours, and it may be life-threatening. Common causes of massive hemoptysis are cystic fibrosis, bronchiectasis, tuberculosis, and aspergillosis. Malignancy is rarely a cause. Surgical intervention is usually not feasible because of severe pulmonary disease; therefore, embolization of the bleeding bronchial arteries can be lifesaving.[13]

Bronchial arteries are variable. They usually arise from the descending thoracic aorta between thoracic vertebrae T4 and T7. The right bronchial artery arises from the intercostobronchial trunk in most patients (>90%). The left bronchial artery usually arises directly from the aorta and is multiple in most patients. Occasionally, the right and left bronchial arteries arise from a common trunk.

Although some bronchial branches may supply the spinal cord, the most important of these branches is the artery of Adamkiewicz. This artery usually arises from an intercostal or lumbar artery on the left. Other spinal branches from the right intercostobronchial artery, thyrocervical, or costocervical arteries may be identified. A preliminary thoracic aortogram may be performed, which usually shows abnormal bronchial arteries. An aortogram helps in outlining the bronchial anatomy.

Because of potential source of collaterals, a subclavian arteriogram also is obtained, particularly if the upper lung field is involved. Then, the bronchial arteries are catheterized and studied with selective injections. The most common appearance of the abnormal bronchial artery (the bleeding source) is increased caliber of the bronchial artery with some hypervascularity over the lung field. Contrast agent extravasation, shunting from bronchial to pulmonary arteries, or aneurysmal changes in the involved bronchial artery rarely are identified.

Embolotherapy is usually performed with particles (PVA or embospheres) and Gelfoam pledgets **(Figs. 4A and B)**. When the decision is made to use particles, appropriately sized particles should be used. Sizes are usually 500–710 μm for PVA and 500–800 μm for embospheres. Use of coils is inappropriate, and absolute alcohol or cyanoacrylate is no longer used for bronchial artery embolization because of the risk of tissue necrosis (bronchial and/or esophageal).

Embolization is performed as selectively as possible (when necessary, by using a microcatheter and coaxial technique) to minimize tissue necrosis and nontarget embolization (e.g. spinal artery). Special care should be taken to prevent reflux by injecting the embolic material slowly under continuous fluoroscopic control. Gelfoam pledgets/torpedoes usually are used to occlude the abnormal artery more proximally after particle embolization.

Epistaxis

Intractable epistaxis is a nosebleed that does not respond to conservative treatment (nasal spraying of vasoconstrictors, nasal packing, blood transfusion). Etiologies include

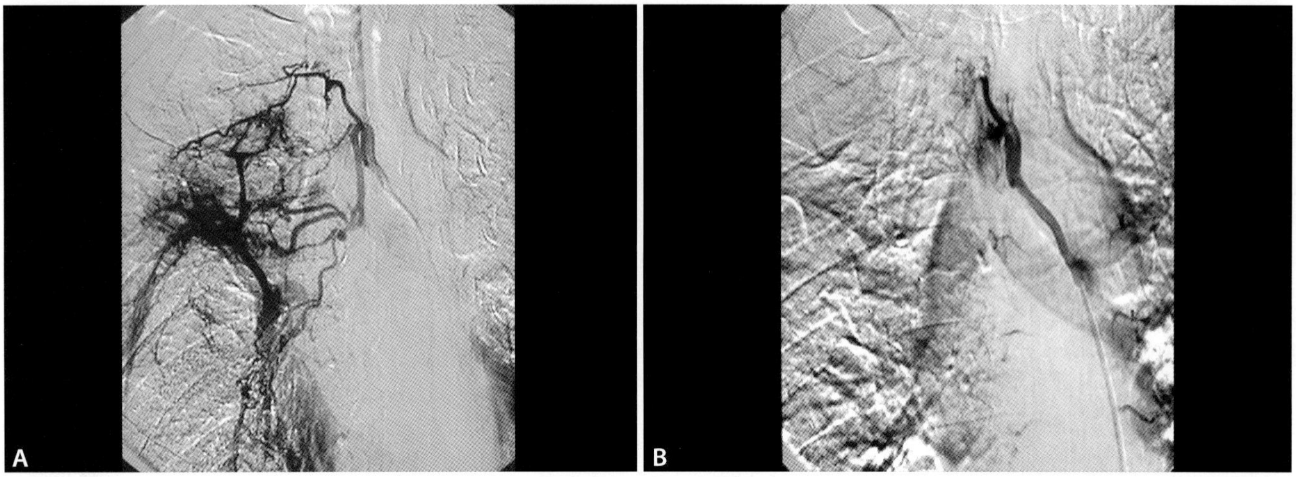

Figs. 4A and B: A patient with hemoptysis due to bronchiectasis in the right upper and middle lobe. Selective injection of the hypertrophied right intercostobronchial trunk: (A) Revealed multiple feeders with parenchymal blush; (B) After embolization with PVA particles and gelfoam, the culprit vessel is completely occluded.

uncontrolled hypertension with or without superficial mucosal abnormality (e.g. Osler-Weber-Rendu syndrome).

Epistaxis can be treated by either surgical means (e.g. cautery, vascular ligation) or endovascular embolotherapy. Internal carotid arteriograms are obtained to exclude aneurysms. Then, the external carotid artery is catheterized and control angiography is performed initially to map the vascular anatomy and to check for the presence of a collateral supply to the intracranial circulation.

During catheterization of the external carotid artery and its branches, vasospasm is a common problem. Nitroglycerin can be used to treat this. The target branch is usually the pterygopalatine division of the internal maxillary artery, which is distal to the origin of the meningeal and temporal arteries. By using a microcatheter, the pterygopalatine division is catheterized and embolized with particles (most commonly PVA). If bleeding is not caused by a neoplastic entity, embolotherapy can be performed in the 250–500 μm range. If a neoplastic entity is the cause, the capillary bed needs to be embolized. This embolization can be accomplished by using smaller particles (150–250 μm).

Although the procedure is considered safe if performed by an experienced physician, possible complications can occur. These include ischemia, pain, cranial nerve damage, blindness, and stroke.

Post-traumatic Hemorrhage

Post-traumatic hemorrhage can be due to either a blunt or penetrating injury to a vessel, typically arteries in the extremities with penetrating injuries or associated fractures or arteries to the organs (e.g. renal arteries, after blunt trauma). Some patients may present after an orthopedic procedure, such as total hip replacement. An angiographic study is mandatory, not only to aid selecting in the appropriate subsequent embolization procedure but also in planning for possible future surgical interventions.

Coil embolization is appropriate in extremity branch arteries responsible for the bleeding because it offers a fast and permanent occlusion of the vessel. The bleeding vessel should be embolized proximal and distal to the site of arterial injury. Avoid embolization of arteries that endangers limb viability. Hemorrhage or AVF formation after organ biopsy (particularly renal biopsy), or iatrogenic traumatic hemorrhage, is a common complication (i.e. iatrogenic traumatic hemorrhage) that can be treated with embolization **(Figs. 5A and B)**.

Pseudoaneurysm

Pseudoaneurysms occur secondary to trauma or infection and consist of leakage of blood into the confined perivascular space at the site of a vessel wall disruption. Embolization is a good alternative to surgical repair, and is often the treatment of choice, especially when pseudoaneurysms are not accessible or when the patient is not a surgical candidate because of sepsis or other medical conditions.[14,15]

Embolic materials used for pseudoaneurysms include coils, detachable balloons, thrombin, gelfoam, and NBCA. In large-neck pseudoaneurysms, a stent placement combined with coil embolization has been described. If the involved vessel cannot be catheterized

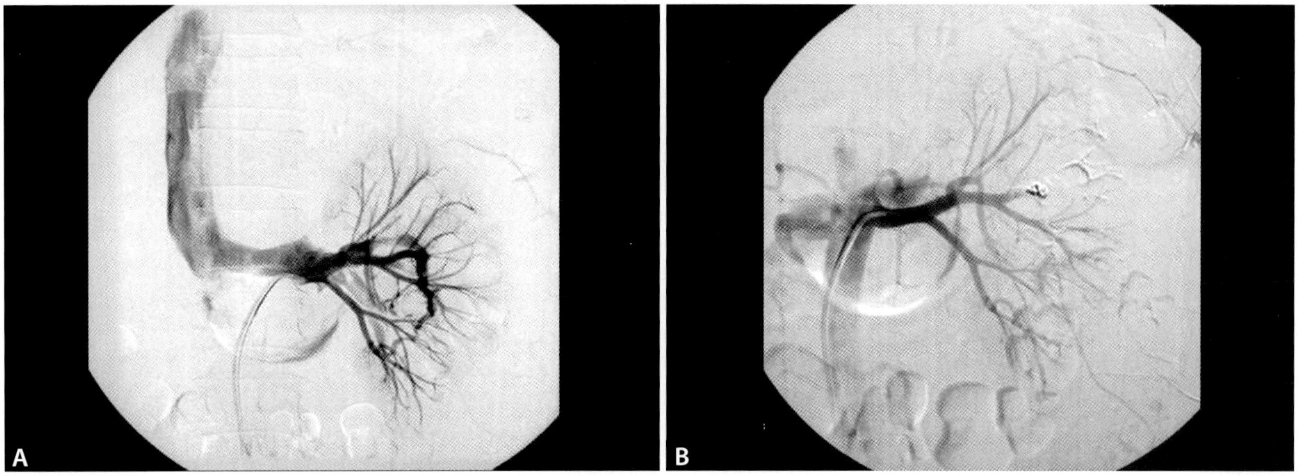

Figs. 5A and B: A patient with postrenal biopsy hematuria: (A) Selective left renal angiogram shows an arteriovenous fistula from an interlobar artery in the midpole with early filling of the inferior vena cava; (B) Complete occlusion of the branch was achieved with coils.

or if a pseudoaneurysm is close to the skin surface (typically a pseudoaneurysm in the groin after cardiac catheterization), the pseudoaneurysm can be directly punctured with a fine needle (e.g. 22 G), and thrombin or NBCA can be injected **(Figs. 6A to D)**. When the involved artery is embolized with coils, the artery also should be embolized distal to the origin of the pseudoaneurysm so that collaterals do not fill the aneurysm

Malignant Tumors

Indications for embolotherapy in neoplastic conditions include preoperative embolization and palliative embolization. Embolization helps to alleviate symptoms, reduces further dissemination, and increases the response to other treatment modalities (e.g. radiation therapy). Embolotherapy can be used for many types of malignant tumors.[16] Renal malignancy is the most common type of tumor treated with embolotherapy. In particular, tumors extending into the hilum or other adjacent structures for which surgical removal is difficult are treated by using embolotherapy. In these patients, prior embolization of the tumor shrinks the mass and minimizes blood loss during surgical removal.

Unresectable tumors can be made operable by means of embolotherapy. If the entity is in its end-stage (disseminated metastatic deposits), the technique can be used for palliation to control pain and hematuria. Other reported malignancies in which embolotherapy has been used include pelvic malignancies and bone tumors. Hemorrhage resulting from malignancy or radiotherapy (e.g. due to radiation cystitis) can be controlled by using embolotherapy.

Chemoembolization

Chemoembolization is commonly performed in hepatic malig-nancies.[17] The technique is used in patients with unresectable liver tumors and metastatic liver disease. An essential prerequisite for chemoinfusion/chemoembolization is the presence of a patent portal vein with hepatopetal flow. The bilirubin level should be less than 3 mg/dL to perform chemoinfusion/chemoembolization safely.

Vigorous intravenous hydration is required before the procedure for at least 24 hours. Initially, a superior mesenteric arteriogram is usually obtained to demonstrate a variant origin of hepatic artery (accessory or replaced, originating from the superior mesenteric artery) and to demonstrate patency of the portal vein. Then, the celiac trunk and, subsequently, the common hepatic artery are catheterized and studied to outline the vascular anatomy.

The involved lobar hepatic artery or, more commonly, the first- or second-order branches of this artery is subsequently catheterized by using a microcatheter and the chemoinfusion material is injected under fluoroscopic guidance. The tip of the catheter must be placed distal to the cystic and gastroduodenal arteries. The most commonly used chemoinfusion mixture consists of 10 mL of iopamidol (Isovue), 20 mL of Ethiodol, and 60 mg of doxorubicin. The chemoinfusion is usually followed by embolization with slurry of gelatin sponge powder (Gelfoam).

Lidocaine is intra-arterially administered to reduce pain after the chemoinfusion/chemoembolization treatment.

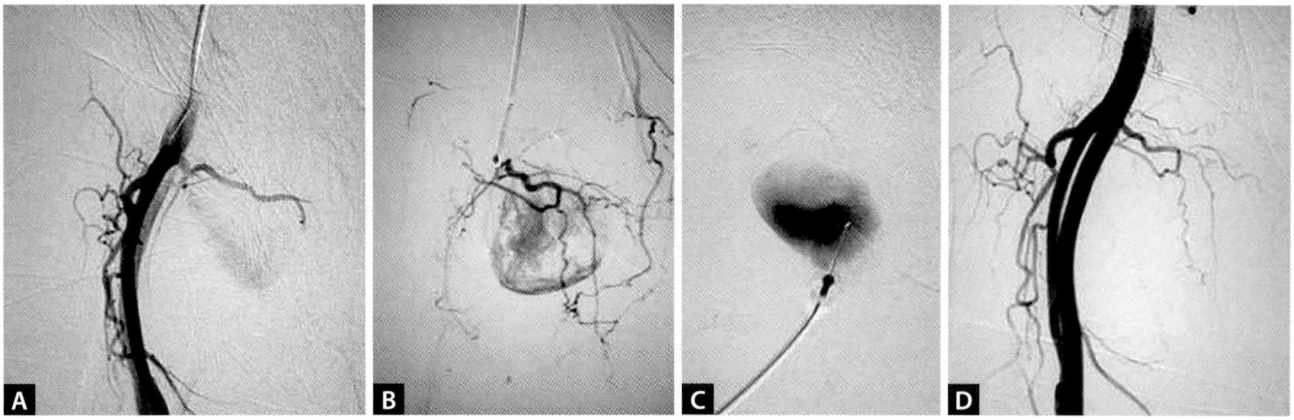

Figs. 6A to D: A postcatheterization pseudoaneurysm in the right groin: (A) Selective injections into the right common femoral artery; (B) A branch of the profunda femoris artery show the jet and the lesion; (C) The lesion was percutaneously punctured and 800 U thrombin was injected; (D) Though the pseudoaneurysm occluded immediately, it recanalized a few days later and needed surgical repair.

Organ Ablation

Splenic embolization can be used as a preoperative therapy or as an alternative to surgical removal of the spleen. Indications include post-traumatic bleeding, variceal bleeding secondary to portal hypertension or splenic vein thrombosis, hypersplenism, thalassemia major, thrombocytopenia, idiopathic thrombocytopenic purpura, Gaucher's disease, and Hodgkin's disease. Embolotherapy is performed with superselective catheterization/embolization of the splenic artery by using embolic particles while the tip of the catheter is beyond the caudal pancreatic artery. Careful fluoroscopic control of the splenic area is required to limit the total infarction to approximately 60% of the spleen.

Renal embolization is an alternative to surgical removal of the kidney, and indications include end-stage renal disease or renovascular hypertension requiring unilateral or bilateral nephrectomy and renal transplant with native kidneys *in situ*. The procedure requires selective catheterization of the renal artery with further advancement of the catheter so that the catheter is wedged or with the use of a balloon occlusion catheter to minimize the possibility of embolic material spillage into the aorta. The preferred embolic agents are particles (e.g. PVA) and/or liquid agents such as ethanol or NBCA. Postinfarction syndrome is relatively common and characterized by pain, which can be managed with narcotics. This pain usually subsides within 48–72 hours.

ANGIOPLASTY

The techniques for balloon dilatation of vascular stenosis are the same for children as for adults. Balloon dilatation can be carried out safely even in small children and can permit access to peripheral stenoses. Small balloon catheters (2 mm) and small shaft catheters (3.8 F) can be used with 4 F delivery systems. Small steerable guidewires (e.g. 0.018" or 0.014" PTCA wires) can be used to cross small distal stenosis. For the renal arteries, low profile balloons in diameters of 3–4 mm are employed. Larger balloons up to 20 mm in size are used to treat recurrent coarctation or peripheral pulmonary stenosis. High pressure balloons (up to 17 atm burst pressure) are available with smaller sizes for fibrous stenosis or restenotic lesions.

The major indications for angioplasty in children are:

- Renal artery stenosis (RAS)
- Aortic stenosis
- Coarctation of aorta
- Transplant renal artery stenosis
- Peripheral pulmonary stenosis
- Systemic-to-pulmonary artery shunt stenosis
- Budd-Chiari syndrome due to hepatic vein/inferior vena cava (IVC) stenosis.

Percutaneous transluminal renal angioplasty (PTRA) is the treatment of choice for RAS. Nonspecific aortoarteritis (NSAA) is responsible for 61% of RAS in our country. Other causes include fibromuscular dysplasia (28%), atherosclerosis (8%), polyarteritis nodosa (2.5%) and renal artery aneurysm of indeterminate etiology (0.5%). NSAA is a chronic and progressive panarteritis of unknown cause that commonly affects the aorta, its major branches and the pulmonary arteries, and results in stenosis, occlusion, dilatation or formation of aneurysms in the involved blood vessels.[18,19] Stenosis or obstruction is the most common angiographic abnormality, frequently involving the aorta and the renal arteries, and resulting in systemic hypertension. The complexity of pathological changes in the wall of the aorta and widespread nature of involvement make surgical revascularization a very difficult option. There is also a high prevalence of graft occlusion. Due to these reasons, nonsurgical revascularization techniques have been increasingly used in the treatment of this group of patients.[20-22]

The therapy in RVH aims at controlling the blood pressure (BP) and restoration of renal blood flow. We accept the patients for treatment by nonsurgical revascularization if they have hypertension uncontrolled by single-drug therapy, angiographic evidence of at least 70% stenosis in the renal artery or the aorta with a pressure gradient of more than 20 mm Hg and a normal erythtrocyte sedimentation rate (ESR). Patients with an elevated ESR and/or a positive C-reactive protein test are considered to have an active arteritis and are not generally accepted for this treatment except in certain situations (uncontrolled hypertension, severe ventricular dysfunction, flash pulmonary edema and deteriorating renal function).

Antihypertensive medication is stopped 24 hours before angioplasty, except for sublingual administration of 5–10 mg nifedipine if the blood pressure is more than 170/110 mm Hg. The patients are treated with aspirin (175–330 mg) daily for 3 days before angioplasty, and this treatment is continued for 6 months after treatment. Heparin (100 IU/kg body weight) is given IV during the procedure and is not reversed afterwards. Blood pressure medication is withheld for 24 hours after the procedure, except for sublingual administration of nifedipine (5–10 mg) if the blood pressure is above 160/100 mm Hg. If there is severe, uncontrolled hypertension before renal angioplasty, the BP is controlled with nitroprusside drip infusion.

For renal angioplasty **(Figs. 7A to C)**, a pigtail catheter is positioned in the abdominal aorta above the origin of renal arteries for continuous pressure measurement and diagnostic DSA. The diseased renal artery is selectively catheterized through another arterial sheath in the opposite groin and transstenotic pressure gradient is measured. The angiographic catheter is replaced by a commercially available, appropriate sized balloon catheter by using standard exchange technique. The diameter of the involved vessel is measured and a balloon catheter of same size is used for angioplasty. Three to five inflations, for up to 45 seconds each, are performed until the balloon "waist" is no longer present or has decreased substantially. We do not use oversized balloon catheters in patients with mild residual stenosis or transstenotic pressure gradients in order to avoid the risk of arterial rupture. Immediately after the procedure, transstenotic pressure is measured and an angiogram is obtained to assess the adequacy of angioplasty.

Alternatively, the procedure can be completed through a single groin approach too. After crossing the stenosis with the angiographic catheter, an 0.014" or 0.018" exchange guidewire is placed in a distal intrarenal branch, and a 6F or 7F (depending upon the patient size) guiding (right coronary or renal double curve configuration) catheter is placed at the ostium of the diseased artery. The appropriately compatible balloon catheters (sometimes, PTCA balloons in monorail configuration may also be used) are then used to dilate the lesion. The advantage of this approach is the avoidance of a second puncture, although the cost of hardware increases.

If there is an obstructive dissection or a recurrent ostial stenosis, renal artery stent placement is considered. Pretreatment with ticlopidine (250 mg twice daily)

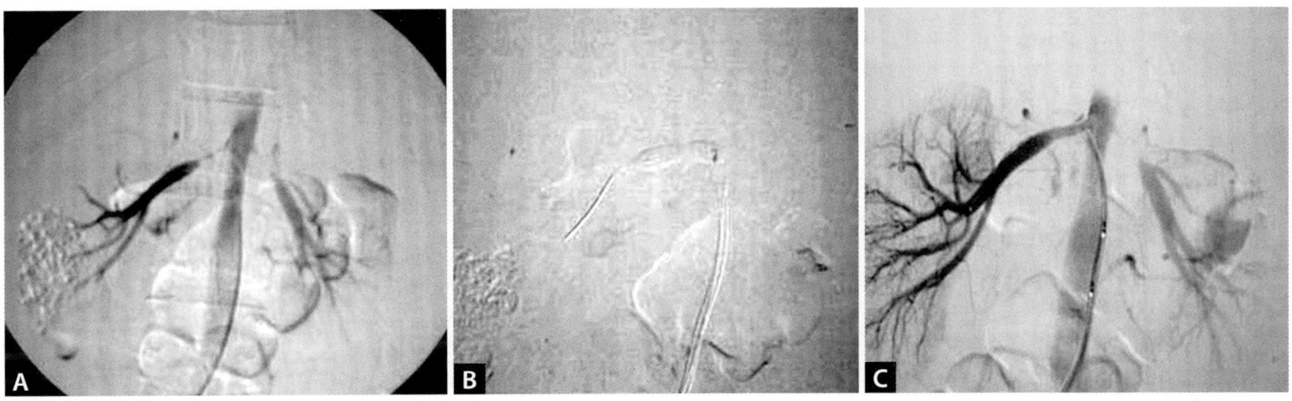

Figs. 7A to C: A 12-year-old female with hypertension: (A) Tight bilateral ostial renal artery stenosis due to aortoarteritis; (B) The right stenosis was treated with balloon angioplasty with a mild residual waist; (C) The lesion opened up well with mild residual disease. The left stenosis was then subjected to angioplasty with a similar result.

beginning three days before angioplasty is then advisable. This should be continued for at least 6 weeks after the procedure. A preshaped renal guiding catheter is positioned at the ostium of the diseased renal artery over an exchange guidewire positioned in a secure distal location in the artery. The selection of the diameter and length of the stent is based on the angiographic morphology of the involved artery. It is advisable to give sublingual nifedipine (5–10 mg) or an intra-arterial bolus of trinitroglycerine (100–200 mg) in the renal artery before stent placement. The stent is positioned across the lesion and released by inflating the balloon at the desired inflation pressure for up to 30 seconds. Various stent designs are available for use in this location. Balloon-mounted stents are generally preferred for an ostial stenosis. A check angiogram is obtained at the end of the procedure to assess the adequacy of stent release. Intravascular ultrasound is a useful technique to define the endpoint of intervention. Angioplasty or stent placement in the aorta is performed by a similar technique.

Angioplasty is considered technically successful if: (1) the aortic or renal artery lumen after angioplasty has less than 30% residual stenosis (2) the arterial lumen is at least 50% larger than its pretreatment diameter, and (3) the pressure gradient is less than 20 mm Hg and has decreased at least 15 mm Hg from the pretreatment gradient.

The clinical results of the angioplasty are judged as follows: (1) cure (normal BP after the procedure without antihypertensive drug therapy), (2) improved (at least 15% reduction in diastolic pressure or a diastolic pressure less than 90 mm Hg with the patient taking less antihypertensive medication than before the procedure), and (3) failed (no change in BP after the procedure). All patients cured or improved are considered to have benefited from angioplasty. Follow-up is performed by BP and medication evaluation 1 day, 1 week, and 4–6 weeks after treatment and then at 6-month intervals. Follow-up angiograms are performed in patients with recurrence of hypertension, in whom contralateral nephrectomy of poorly or nonfunctioning kidney for residual hypertension is planned and in those patients who consent for the procedure. Angioplasty is repeated if restenosis is detected.

Percutaneous transluminal angioplasty (PTA) of the aortic stenosis in NSAA can also be carried out by a similar technique **(Figs. 8A and B)**. The angiographic features, including eccentricity of the stenosis and presence of diffuse adjacent disease, location of the stenosis in juxtadiaphrag-matic segment of the aorta and presence of calcification adversely affect the outcome of PTA, most of whom develop large intimal flaps. Stents have been

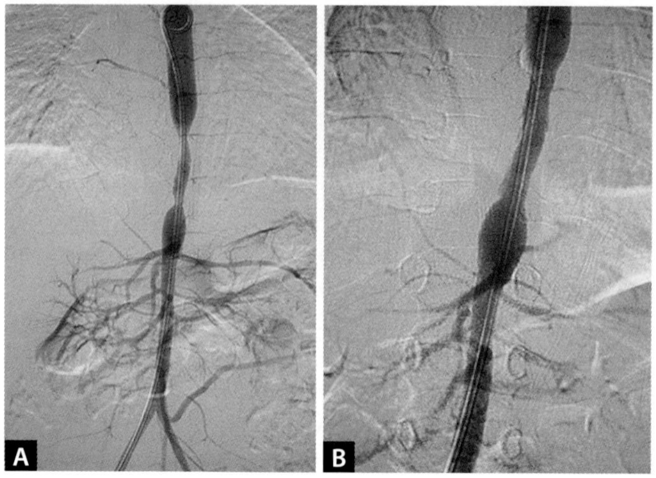

Figs. 8A and B: (A) Juxtadiaphgramatic aortic stenosis (due to aortoarteritis) in an 18-year-old girl with resistant hypertension; (B) The stenosis responded well to balloon angioplasty alone with a small dissection flap. The systolic pressure gradient across the lesion was significantly reduced and the patient did well on clinical follow-up.

occasionally used as a "bail-out" measure in salvaging an obstructive dissection in such situations and rarely electively in the treatment of native stenosis. Stents provide an immediate relief of symptomatic obstructive dissection and are also useful in the treatment of recurrent stenosis after successful angioplasty. We do not advocate elective use of stents due to young age of the patients, the cost involved and lack of knowledge about the long-term behavior of stents in the aorta at a growing age. Until recently, it was felt that this diesease is characterized by skip areas of involvement. The findings of recent studies, using cross-sectional imaging techniques, suggest that nonspecific aortitis involves a continuous length of the aorta, producing mural and luminal changes in some areas, and only mural changes in the intervening segments. This observation has therapeutic implications. The site of surgical reconstruction or balloon positioning in PTA is based on the demonstration of angiographically normal adjacent segments. The results of cross-sectional imaging suggest that there are extensive wall changes even in angiographically normal areas. The unpredictable outcome of PTA and surgical revascularization in nonspecific aortitis, in our opinion, is caused by the placement of a bypass graft or the balloon catheter within the diseased segments and not from normal to normal aortic segment. In this regard, intravascular ultrasound may be useful in guiding the interventional procedures. Overall, aortic PTA has specific technical problems but has a high technical and clinical success rate. The complication rate is low. Late remodeling occurs in most patients and is responsible for delayed clinical benefit despite poor technical success in some patients.

Arterial stenosis associated with renal transplantation can often be improved. These obstructions may be at or beyond the suture line. It is important to evaluate the hemodynamic significance of proximal stenosis because in some of these patients extensive peripheral disease due to rejection nullifies the benefit of dilating the proximal lesions.

Peripheral pulmonary artery stenosis can sometimes be treated effectively but at moderate risk. Because of the elasticity of pulmonary arteries, these lesions require large balloons for small increases in artery size. Arterial rupture can occur, resulting in death. Because there are no surgical options to treat these lesions, balloon dilatation is the procedure of choice when treatment is clinically indicated. Stenting is a safer and more effective approach to these lesions.

After the modified Blalock-Taussig (BT shunt) is placed, stenosis can develop in the subclavian artery, the proximal or distal anastomosis, the graft, or the pulmonary artery. All of these may be treated except the graft stenosis. The best results are obtained in those patients with a traditional BT shunt where the subclavian artery has been directly connected to the pulmonary artery, but this surgery is rarely performed nowadays. Most BT shunts are performed with Goretex grafts, which limit the amount of stretching of the stenosis. Narrowing within the graft is probably caused by kinking, thrombosis, or fibrointimal proliferation.

Complications of Angioplasty Procedures

Vascular spasm can occur, particularly in PTRA, and may in turn provoke thrombosis and segmental infarction. 100 Units/kg of heparin is usually given to prevent this, and more may be required for prolonged procedures. Monitoring of heparinization with measurements of activated clotting time (ACT) should be done. Spasm may be treated with direct intra-arterial injection of nitroglycerin (0.25–1.00 μg/kg/minute).

Thrombosis may occur at the PTA site or at the groin. If it does, then thrombolytic therapy is indicated. Intimal dissection is part of any PTA procedure, and usually does not cause flow obstruction. If an obstructive dissection develops, stents may be used. Vascular rupture is always a concern but can be avoided by appropriate balloon selection.

THROMBOLYSIS

Experience with thrombolysis in children is limited but has increased because of the need to treat complications of cardiac or peripheral angiography or intervention. Procedures requiring insertion of devices mounted on large shafts are more likely to result in femoral artery thrombosis. The other indications include thrombosis of BT shunts, dialysis fistula, pulmonary artery thrombosis, iliofemoral thrombophlebitis, aortic thrombosis in neonates, and brachial artery occlusion after supracondylar fracture. Contraindications for the procedure include recent surgery or trauma (within the past 6 weeks), any intracranial or gastrointestinal bleed within the past 3 months, renal failure, gangrene or significant pregangrenous changes in the affected organ system or extremity.

Thrombolytic agents include streptokinase, urokinase, or r-tpa. Urokinase is the most commonly employed agent. Local low-dose therapy is unlikely to produce systemic changes in coagulation, whereas systemic therapy may cause undesirable bleeding. The dose of urokinase for local low dose infusion is 300–500 IU/kg/hour. High-dose, short-duration treatment given locally often produces clearing of thrombus **(Figs. 9A to D)**. Treatment failures usually relate to delays in implementing therapy, resulting in maturation of thrombus. The fibrinogen level, thrombin time, prothrombin time, and activated partial thromboplastin time are monitored at regular intervals, and the children are observed in an intensive care unit or neonatal nursery.

Complications of intra-arterial thrombolysis include systemic bleeding (<5% cases), compartment syndrome due to extremity edema, tissue breakdown products entering systemic circulation causing renal shut down, hyperkalemia causing cardiac arrhythmias, etc. Appropriate patient selection and preprocedure evaluation may help prevent these complications.

FOREIGN BODY REMOVAL

Intravascular foreign bodies may result from the complex interventional hardware, monitoring systems, and indwelling catheters that are increasingly being used these days. These may be catheter fragments, pieces of guidewires, metallic coils, stents, electrodes, or ventriculoatrial shunt tubing. Large fragments are believed to pose a risk of thrombosis, spasm, hemorrhage, and arrhythmia. Snares, deflectable guidewires, wire baskets, and intravascular forceps (bioptomes) may be used to retrieve these objects.

CONCLUSION

The future is indeed bright for the practice and practitioners of pediatric vascular interventions. As more and more of the procedures that are currently being

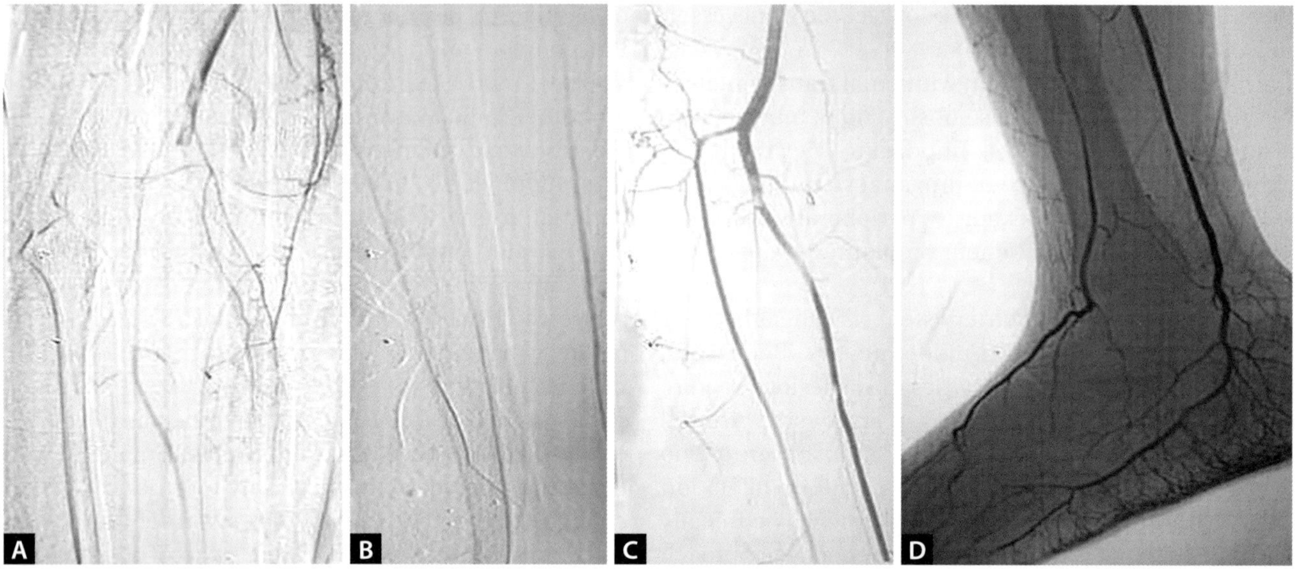

Figs. 9A to D: (A) Acute thrombotic occlusion of the right popliteal artery; (B) The infrapopliteal arteries are not visualized; (C and D) After intra-arterial mechanical and pharmacological thrombolysis with urokinase antegrade flow has been re-established.

performed in adults get gradually adapted for use in the pediatric population, it may be possible to perform safe and successful interventions in many of the pediatric vascular lesions that are otherwise being referred for surgery. These include use of atherectomy devices or lasers that may be used for fibrointimal proliferation that develops in bypass grafts or stents, or in cases of coarctation and recoarctation of the aorta once the vessel wall structure is better understood. Endovascular stenting of the neonatal ductus may replace the surgical creation of aortopulmonary shunts. Percutaneous insertion of central lines and creation of portocaval anastomosis may increasingly get applied to the pediatric patients as well.

However, a note of caution may be made at this point. Risk of radiation damage and the long lasting impact of its after effects may be a serious problem in this age-group, particularly in interventional procedures that require increased fluoroscopic times or multiple sessions. Newer devices or materials or those with uncertain safety should be used with caution in children, and only in situations where other more suitable and safer alternatives do not exist.

REFERENCES

1. Gordon I, Evans K, Peters AM, et al. The quantitation of 99Tcm-DMSA in paediatrics. Nucl Med Commun. 1987;8:661-70.
2. Castaneda-Zuniga WR. Vascular embolotherapy. In Interventional Radiology. Lippincott William and Wilkins; 1997.
3. Tadavarthy SM, Knight L, Ovitt TW, et al. Therapeutic transcatheter arterial embolization. Radiology. 1974;112(1):13-6.
4. Yakes WF, Rossi P, Odink H. How I do it. Arteriovenous malformation management. Cardiovasc Intervent Radiol. 1996;19(2):65-71.
5. Yoshimoto T, Takahashi A, Kinouchi H, et al. Role of embolization in the management of arteriovenous malformations. Clin Neurosurg. 1995;42:313-27.
6. White RI, Pollak JS, Wirth JA. Pulmonary arteriovenous malformations: Diagnosis and transcatheter embolotherapy. J Vasc Interv Radiol. 1996;7(6):787-804.
7. Kaufman SL, Martin LG, Zuckerman AM, et al. Peripheral transcatheter embolization with platinum microcoils. Radiology. 1992;184(2):369-72.
8. Berenguer B, Burrows PE, Zurakowski D, et al. Sclerotherapy of craniofacial venous malformations: Complications and results. Plast Reconstr Surg. 1999;104(1):1-11; discussion 12-5.
9. Dubois JM, Sebag GH, De Prost Y, et al. Soft-tissue venous malformations in children: Percutaneous sclerotherapy with Ethibloc. Radiology. 1991;180(1):195-8.
10. Goldman ML, Land WC, Bradley EL, et al. Transcatheter therapeutic embolization in the management of massive upper gastrointestinal bleeding. Radiology. 1976;120(3):513-21.
11. Moore HM, List A, Holden A, et al. Therapeutic embolization for acute hemorrhage in the abdomen and pelvis. Australas Radiol. 2000;44(2):161-8.
12. Agolini SF, Shah K, Jaffe J, et al. Arterial embolization is a rapid and effective technique for controlling pelvic fracture hemorrhage. J Trauma. 1997;43(3):395-9.

13. Fellows KE, Khaw KT, Schuster S, et al. Bronchial artery embolization in cystic fibrosis; technique and long-term results. J Pediatr. 1979;95(6):959-63.
14. Mazer MJ, Baltaxe HA, Wolf GL. Therapeutic embolization of the renal artery with Gianturco coils: Limitations and technical pitfalls. Radiology. 1981;138(1):37-46.
15. Stambo GW, Hallisey MJ, Gallagher JJ. Arteriographic embolization of visceral artery pseudoaneurysms. Ann Vasc Surg. 1996;10(5):476-80.
16. Chuang VP, Soo CS, Wallace S. Ivalon embolization in abdominal neoplasms. AJR Am J Roentgenol. 1981;136(4): 729-33.
17. Gates J, Hartnell GG, Stuart KE, et al. Chemoembolization of hepatic neoplasms: Safety, complications, and when to worry. Radiographics. 1999;19(2):399-414.
18. Liu YQ. Radiology of aortoarteritis. Radiol Clin North Am. 1985;23:671-88.
19. Sharma S, Rajani M, Talwar KK. Angiographic morphology in nonspecific Aortoarteritis (Takayasu's arteritis): A study of 126 patients from North India. Cardiovasc Intervent Radiol. 1992;15:160-5.
20. Sharma S, Saxena A, Talwar KK, et al. Renal artery stenosis caused by nonspecific arteritis (Takayasu disease): Results of treatment with percutaneous transluminal angioplasty. AJR. 1992;157:417-22.
21. Sharma S, Bahl VK, Saxena A, et al. Stenosis in the aorta caused by nonspecific aortitis: Results of treatment by percutaneous stent placement. Clin Radiol. 1999;54: 46-50.
22. Sharma S, Gupta H, Saxena A, et al. Results of renal angioplasty in nonspecific aortoarteritis (Takayasu's disease). JVIR. 1998;9:429-35.

NONVASCULAR INTERVENTIONS

Amar Mukund, Ashu Seith Bhalla, Shivanand Gamanagatti

Pediatric interventional radiology has emerged as an essential adjunct to management of various surgical and medical conditions of children. The interventional procedure may be categorized into: (1) Vascular interventions and (2) Nonvascular interventions. Vascular interventions have been described in the previous section of this chapter, and in this section nonvascular procedures will be addressed. Prior to any intervention the most important step consists of patient evaluation and preprocedure care. Every intervention should have a proper and valid referral. If necessary, a direct discussion with the referring physician is appropriate.

PATIENT EVALUATION

This includes reviewing of the medical records as well as the available imaging. Patient/guardian counseling with proper explanation about the procedure should be done and then an informed consent obtained. Other prerequisite prior to the procedure is evaluation of the various necessary laboratory reports. The coagulation parameters should be within normal limits or else these should be rectified prior to intervention. Renal function parameters should be evaluated prior to any intervention needing administration of intravenous (IV) contrast media; however IV contrast is seldom needed in nonvascular procedures.

SEDATION AND ANESTHESIA

Sedation is one of the most important factors determining the technical success of a procedure and it also decrease the actual time of procedure. Children may be unable to cooperate for the procedure and crying and body movements can significantly impair the procedure. Hence, anesthetic agents are required to perform a successful intervention. Choice of anesthetic agent depends upon the estimated duration and the degree of pain associated with the procedure. Longer and painful procedure may need general anesthesia (GA) while shorter and less painful procedure may be performed under conscious sedation. Moreover, all procedures should be done in a room well equipped with pulse oximeter monitor, resuscitation devices and emergency drugs needed to handle any adverse situation.

BASIC PROCEDURES

Fine Needle Aspiration/Biopsy

The most common image guided nonvascular procedures requested are fine needle aspiration (FNA) and biopsy. Common indications for these procedures are diagnosis of underlying inflammatory/malignant pathology, metastatic disease and tumor staging. The few contraindications, although relative, include—uncorrectable coagulation abnormalities and nonavailability of safe percutaneous pathway to reach the desired lesion. For abdominal biopsies ascites is also considered a contraindication.

The basic prerequisite for FNA and biopsies are the same as described earlier. Special care should be taken for correcting the coagulopathies, if any, prior to the procedure. A 22-23 G spinal (LP) needle is the most preferred needle for FNA. For deep seated lesions 22 G chiba needle may be needed. Most of the FNAs may be performed under sedation and local anesthesia (LA).

Image-guided biopsies although, safe still carry a risk of bleeding and hence, should always be performed with all precautions. Nowadays most of the procedures are performed using either automated or semiautomated biopsy guns. In certain situations coaxial system may prove to be very helpful in cases where multiple passes are required like FNAs and biopsies from lung lesions. Generally, 18-20 G biopsy gun suffices for most of the true cut biopsies but the throw length of the cutting needle should be chosen depending upon the size of the lesion. US guidance is preferred over CT guidance for most of the pediatric FNAs and biopsies barring few procedures related to lung lesions, where CT may be needed.[1] Also US guidance prevents the child from unnecessary radiation.

Sampling Technique

Patient should be kept in a comfortable position preferably supine for most of the procedures, but other positions like prone, oblique and even sitting position may be opted for, if deemed necessary. For all FNAs and biopsies the shortest and safest path should be chosen and any vital structure lying in the path between the target and skin should be avoided **(Fig. 1)**. Lesions situated on the surface of the liver should be approached by a path having a sizable amount of normal liver parenchyma between the lesion and site of capsular puncture to reduce hemorrhagic complications. FNAs and biopsies should not be attempted if the child is crying or restless as patient movement may cause inadvertent needle movement resulting in organ injury and bleeding. Also the needle tip should always be monitored throughout the procedure.

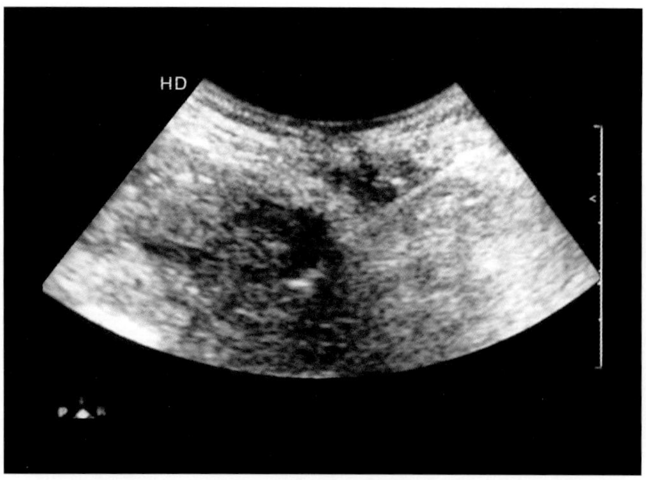

Fig. 1: USG image showing FNA being performed with needle tip in retroperitoneal lymph node.

For FNA, once the needle tip reaches the target organ the stylet should be removed and small to and fro as well as rotating movement should be done with the tip placed in the lesion. Sample for FNA may be obtained using either slight suction technique with a 10-mL syringe or nonsuction technique to prevent contamination of sample by red blood cells.

Various needles and biopsy guns are commercially available, and prior to any biopsy proper knowledge of the device is mandatory. The performing radiologist should know about the functioning of device (automated or semiautomated gun) and throw length of the cutting needle. While performing biopsy special care is to be taken (more than FNA) to avoid any vital structure as slight negligence leading to vital structure injury may be catastrophic.

Abscess Drainage

Percutaneous drainage is the preferred treatment for various abdominal/pleural collections and abscesses. This may be performed using either of the two basic techniques. For large and superficial collections one step procedure (*Trochar technique*) may be used; whereas relatively small and deeper collections or collections adjoining vital structures are suitable for *Seldinger technique*. In trochar technique, the catheter is mounted over a stiff cannula with a stylet; and this assembly is directly inserted into the collection under image guidance as a one-step procedure. In Seldinger technique 18/17.5 G needle is used for the initial puncture and a guidewire is introduced into the collection via this needle. Further serial dilatation of the track is done and then a catheter is placed. Choice of catheter depends upon the consistency of the collection. For thick collections wide bore catheters (10–14 F) with large holes like Malecot's may be required whereas for clear or less viscous collections 8–10 F pigtail catheter may suffice.

THORACIC INTERVENTIONS

Guided aspiration of pleural fluid is the most commonly requested nonvascular intervention of the thorax. Other interventions include guided insertion of percutaneous drainage catheters for large/thick/septated pleural/mediastinal collections and FNA/biopsy of lung/mediastinal lesions.

Pleural fluid aspiration may be requested either for diagnostic purpose or sometimes it may be a therapeutic

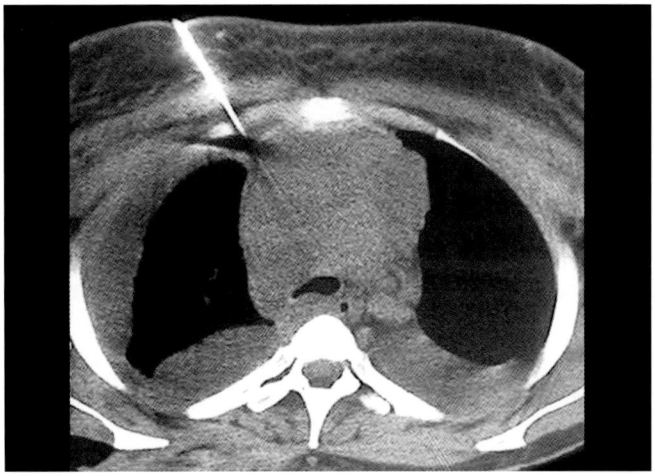

Fig. 2: Anterior mediastinal mass being sampled through right parasternal approach under CT guidance.

tap. Single time aspiration using a small gauge needle is performed for small and clear pleural effusions, however thick/septated and nonresolving effusions require continuous drainage via a percutaneous drainage catheter. For large collections *trochar technique* may be used but for smaller collections *Seldinger technique* is preferable. Special care should be taken to prevent pneumothorax while attempting these procedures, for instance in single time aspiration a three way stop cock along with tubing should be attached to the hub of the needle to prevent entry of air into the pleural cavity. Similarly, if a drainage catheter is placed it should be connected to an underwater seal bag rather than a routine urobag. Fibrinolytic therapy may be needed for thick and septated collections and various agents like streptokinase, urokinase and tPA (tissue type plasminogen activator) are available. Studies have shown urokinase and tPA to be safer options.[2,3]

Thoracic lesions in contact with the chest wall and hence, visible on US should be sampled under US guidance; however, lung/mediastinal lesions not visible on US will require CT guidance **(Fig. 2)**. The basic technique remains the same as described above except for few modifications and precautions. Multiple pleural punctures should be avoided to prevent pneumothorax and for this purpose coaxial devices are useful. Facility for oxygen administration, suction and chest tube insertion should be available.

GASTROINTESTINAL INTERVENTIONS

Salivary Gland Interventions

These include US guided injection of botulinum toxin in submandibular and sometimes parotid glands. Botulinum injection is performed for treatment of drooling in children with neurological impairment.[4] While injecting botulinum, care should be taken so as to provide uniform distribution of drug throughout the gland. This may be achieved by placing the needle at deeper level and withdrawing it while drug is being injected. FNAs and biopsy of salivary gland lesions may be safely done under US guidance; however the risk of needle track seeding exists in cases of epithelial malignancy.

Esophageal Interventions

One of the common childhood problems is *esophageal stricture*, which may be secondary to corrosive ingestion or anstomosis.[5,6] Balloon dilatation for esophageal strictures is a well-recognized radiological treatment **(Figs. 3A to D)**.[5,6] It should be done under sedation/GA and fluoroscopic guidance. Curved/straight tip angiographic catheter with (0.035") hydrophilic, floppy J tip guidewire may be used to cross the stricture. Size of balloon depends upon the size of patient and ranges from 8 mm to 18 mm. A rough guide may be obtained from the width of the thumb of the child, which should be the upper limit of the size of the balloon to be used. [5] Complete dilatation should be attempted progressively in two or more sessions.[7] There is no consensus regarding the time to keep balloon inflated, however authors have suggested balloon inflation for 10–30 seconds.[8]

Gastric Interventions

Percutaneous gastrostomy is one of the radiological interventions which may be requested in patients requiring long term (>6 weeks) nutritional supplementation such as patients having neurodisability, craniofacial anomalies, severe gastroesophageal reflux disease, etc. This is done under fluoroscopic guidance and initially the stomach is distended with air and punctured by a thin gauge needle. An anchor device is then inserted and pulled to fix the anterior wall of stomach to the abdominal wall.[9] Thereafter, again the stomach is punctured and the tract is dilated in order to insert a pigtail catheter. This may be further converted to gastrojejunostomy by passing the guidewire into the jejunum through the same track and inserting the catheter over it **(Fig. 4)**. Care should be taken during the procedure to prevent colonic puncture/injury, which may lead to formation of gastrocolic fistula.

Hepatic Interventions

Common hepatic interventions requested in pediatric patients are percutaneous FNA, biopsy and drainage of

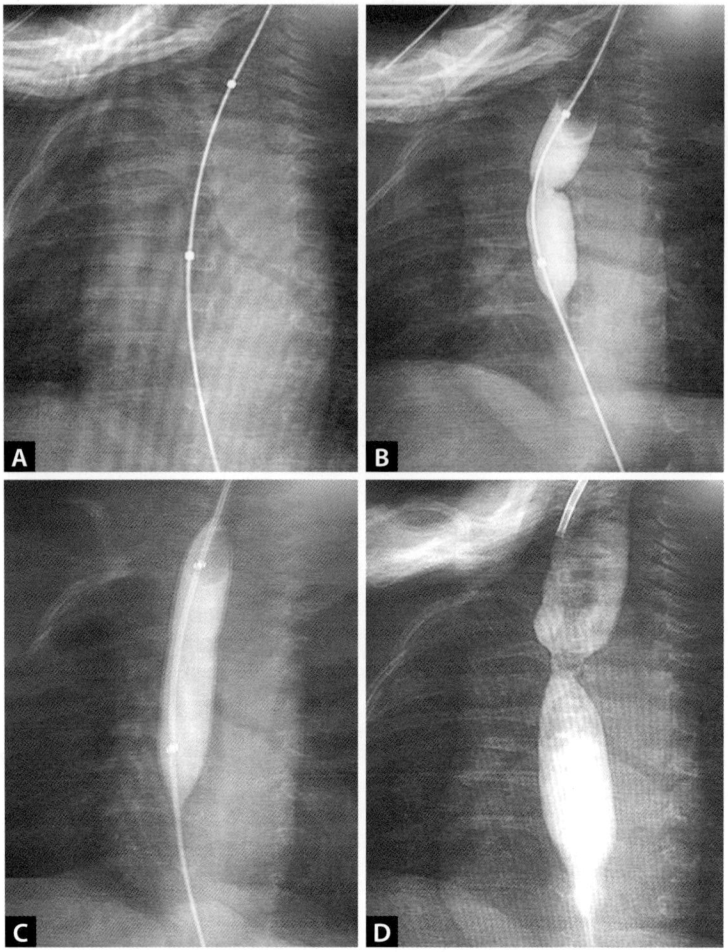

Figs. 3A to D: (A) Image showing balloon catheter placed across the stricture; (B) Balloon catheter being inflated with formation of waist at the site of stricture; (C) The waist within the balloon was removed; (D) Postdilatation contrast study showing free flow of contrast, however, residual stricture seen, which requires another session.

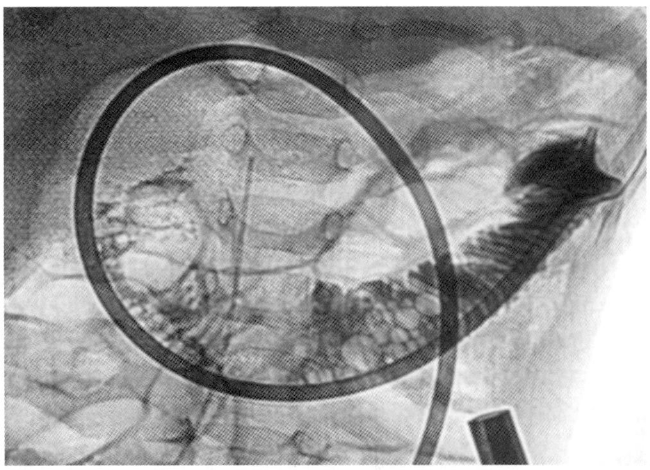

Fig. 4: Gastrojejunostomy image with tip of malecots in proximal jejunum.

liver abscess. The technique remains the same for FNA and biopsy as described previously. However, the coagulation profile should be within normal limits for any patient undergoing hepatic intervention, especially biopsy. Also the lesion should be approached via substantial normal liver parenchyma.

Percutaneous insertion of the drainage catheter may be required in selected cases of liver abscess.[10,11] Depending upon the size and location of the abscess either trochar or seldinger technique may be used.

Biliary Intervention

Percutaneous biliary drainage may be required in children having malignant obstructive jaundice as in patients with metastatic lymph nodes encasing the common bile duct, primary pancreatic tumors or metastatic involvement of pancreas.[12] Prior to the procedure, status of biliary confluence (patent/blocked) should be ascertained and accordingly procedure should be performed. In case of a patent primary confluence the catheter may either be placed in the right or the left ductal system. Left sided drainage is generally better tolerated by the children because of less inconvenience caused; and also it is easy to perform under US guidance. In case of a blocked primary confluence the duct which is draining the maximum part of liver should be targeted and at least one-third of liver should be drained.

Sedation is a must with coagulation profile under normal limits. For patients with a deranged prothrombin time FFP (fresh frozen plasma) may be required. Ideally, the puncture should be performed using a micropuncture set containing a 21G needle and 018" guidewire which can be further dilated to accommodate 035" guidewire. After initial puncture performed under US guidance the procedure should be carried under fluoroscopic guidance and efforts should be made to cross the strictured segment and place an internal-external drainage catheter across the stricture reaching up to the duodenum **(Fig. 5A)**. However at times, it may not be possible to negotiate the stricture in the first attempt when the system is grossly dilated. In these cases patient may be scheduled for a second session to attempt internalization while the external drain is left in place **(Fig. 5B)**. Once the system collapses the internalization of the biliary drainage becomes easier. If internalization fails and the patient is on an external drainage then adequate care should be taken to maintain hydration and electrolyte balance caused by bile loss.

Pancreatic Interventions

Pancreatic interventions include FNA/biopsy of pancreatic mass and drainage of peripancreatic collections. While attempting pancreatic FNA/biopsy, care should be taken to avoid traversing through spleen, colon and normal pancreatic parenchyma.

Pancreatitis is relatively rare in children and is generally seen secondary to trauma. Sometimes, a pseudocyst may form and drainage may be required. While planning drainage the smallest and safest pathway without any intervening abdominal viscera should be chosen for catheter placement, however, if no safe pathway is available transgastric approach may be taken.[13] US guidance is preferred for drainage of various abdominal collections, however if proper acoustic window is not available then the drainage should be performed under CT guidance.

GENITOURINARY INTERVENTIONS

Common interventions of genitourinary system include renal biopsies, drainage procedures, percutaneous nephrostomy and ureteric dilatation and stenting.

Renal Biopsy

Renal biopsy is required for the diagnosis of renal parenchymal disease or renal masses for tissue diagnosis. Being a painful procedure sedation/GA may be needed for a successful biopsy. All renal biopsies are done under US guidance and retroperitoneal approach is preferred especially in cases with renal masses to prevent intraperitoneal seeding. While sampling renal masses a coaxial technique is preferred.[14] Sampling of renal capsule should be avoided as it may increase the

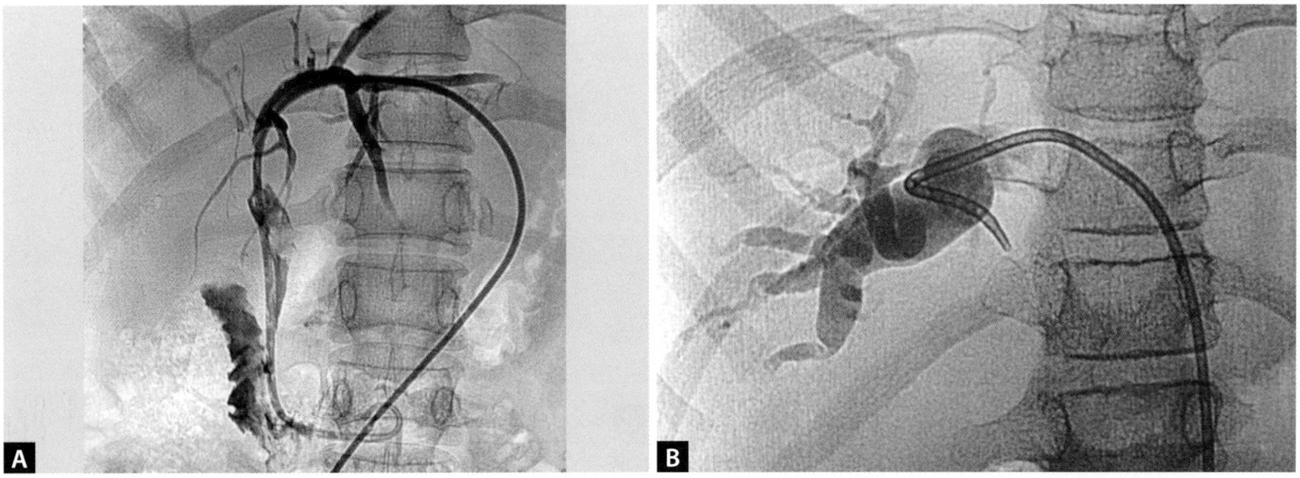

Figs. 5A and B: (A) Image showing internal external drainage catheter (Ring biliary catheter) placed across the stricture with collapsed biliary system; (B) Grossly dilated biliary system with external drainage catheter *in situ*.

chances of bleeding/hematoma. Postbiopsy hematuria though common is minimal and self-limiting. In cases of continuous significant hematuria, patient should be worked up to rule out pseudoaneurysm/AVF, which if present, may need angiographic embolization for treatment.

Percutaneous Nephrostomy

Common indications for percutaneous nephrostomy (PCN)are obstructive renal disease, urinary diversion, for removal of renal stones or placement of antegrade ureteric stent. In cases of obstructive disease or when simply urinary diversion is needed lower polar calyx puncture is preferred. However, if PCN is performed as an initial step for ureteric stenting or percutaneous nephrolithotomy then upper/interpolar calyx should be punctured **(Figs. 6A and B)**. Intercostal approach may be needed to access the upper pole calyx.[15]

Commonly, the patient is placed in a prone or semiprone position. The initial puncture of selected calyx (upper or lower) is done under USG guidance. It is preferable to puncture the selected calyx via an oblique posterolateral approach (at 25° from the median plane, with the hub towards patient's flank) to avoid renal hilar vessels.[16] Once the needle tip is inside the calyceal system, urine is seen coming out of the needle as soon as the stylet is removed. At this point, a small amount of diluted contrast may be injected to map the anatomy of pelvicalyceal system and ureter. Further, a floppy-tip wire is inserted and directed toward the ureter and using Seldinger technique drainage catheter is positioned in the renal pelvis. The catheter should be properly secured by using various commercially available devices or may be sutured to the skin and dressing should be applied.

Ureteric Dilatation and Stenting

Common indication of ureteric dilatation and stenting in pediatric patients is post-transplant ureteral stricture. Upper pole calyx or interpolar calyx puncture is required for all ureteric interventions **(Fig. 7A)**. Dilatation and stenting may be done via a pre-existing PCN catheter or through a new antegrade puncture. Initially, a 0.035" hydrophilic floppy J tip guidewire is placed in the ureter **(Fig. 7B)**. Then an angled 5F angiographic catheter is advanced over it to reach the stricture site and using the combination of guidewire and catheter the stricture is negotiated **(Fig. 7C)**. Sometimes, floppy straight tip guidewire may be needed to cross the stricture. After crossing the stricture hydrophilic floppy guidewire is exchanged for a stiff metallic (0.035' Amplatz extra stiff) guidewire, over which the balloon dilatation of stricture is done. Thereafter, a double J ureteric stent is inserted over the same guidewire using the stent pusher **(Fig. 7D)**. The proximal end of the stent may be secured using a suture anchored in one of the side hole so as to position the proximal end of the stent in the renal pelvis while the wire is being withdrawn. A PCN tube should also be placed in the renal pelvis with external end capped for next 24 hours so as to perform antegrade nephrostogram to ensure proper functioning of the stent. Later these stents are removed cystoscopically.

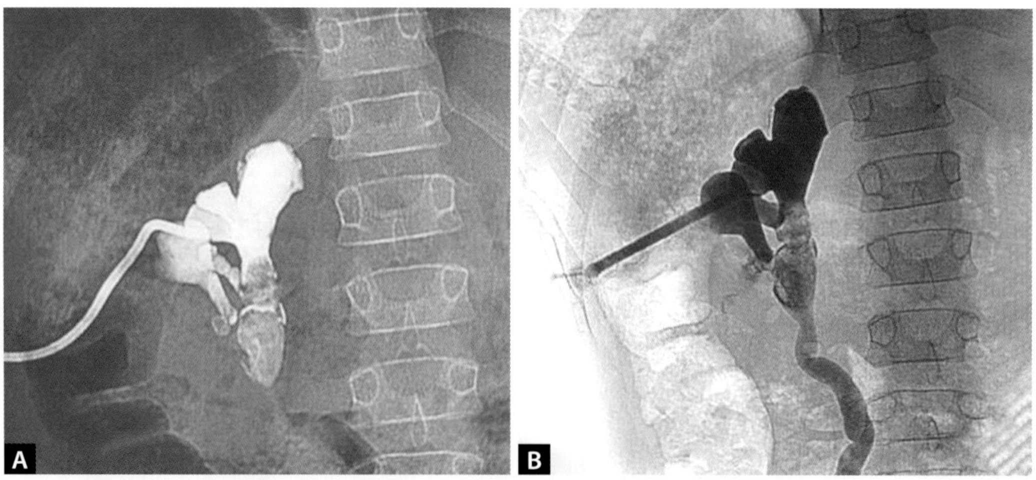

Figs. 6A and B: (A) Pigtail drainage catheter (PCN) through upper pole calyx, as patient planned for PCNL; (B) Pigtail catheter replaced with a 12F sheath in upper pole calyx for PCNL.

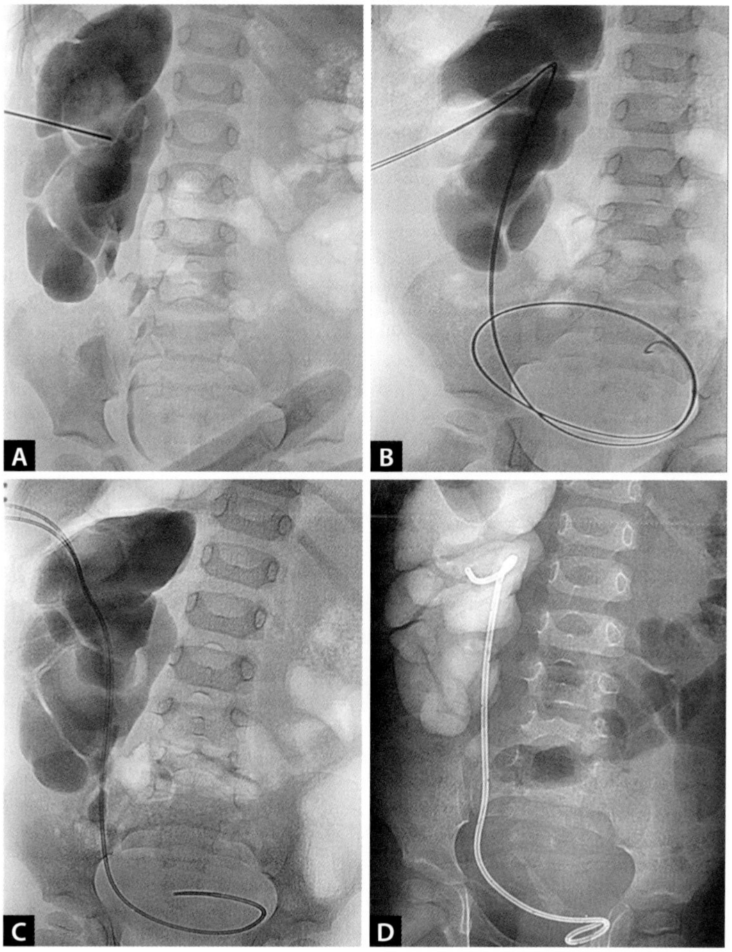

Figs. 7A to D: (A) Contrast study following interpolar calyx puncture; (B) Guidewire was negotiated across the stricture with tip lying within the urinary bladder lumen; (C) Further catheter was advanced into the bladder; (D) Double J stent was placed over the stiff metallic guidewire.

CONCLUSION

Barring a few, most interventions performed in children are similar to adults; but interventions in children are more challenging due to their small size and uncooperative nature due to the associated pain. It is thus essential to have an experienced team consisting of interventional radiologists, anesthetists and nurses for successful pediatric interventions. Also critical is the availability of size appropriate hardware. Concern regarding radiation may be addressed by performing most of the interventions under US guidance, with judicious use of fluoroscopy/CT.

REFERENCES

1. Roebuck DJ. Pediatric interventional radiology. Imaging. 2001;13:302-20.
2. Haaga JR, Nakamoto D, Stellato T, et al. Intracavitary urokinase for enhancement of percutaneous abscess drainage: Phase II trial. AJR Am J Roentgenol. 2000; 174(6):1681-5.
3. Beland MD, Gervais DA, Levis DA, et al. Complex abdominal and pelvic abscesses: Efficacy of adjunctive tissue-type plasminogen activator for drainage. Radiology. 2008; 247(2):567-73.
4. Pena AH, Cahill AM, Gonzalez L, et al. Botulinum toxin A injection of salivary glands in children with drooling and chronic aspiration. J Vasc Interv Radiol. 2009;20:368-73.
5. Hamza AF, Abdelhay S, Sherif H, et al. Caustic esophageal strictures in children: 30 years' experience. J Pediatr Surg. 2003;38:828-33.
6. Ko HK, Shin JH, Song HY, et al. Balloon dilation of anastomotic strictures secondary to surgical repair of esophageal atresia in a pediatric population: Long-term results. J Vasc Interv Radiol. 2006;17:1327-33.
7. Gercek A, Ay B, Dogan V, et al. Esophageal balloon dilation in children: Prospective analysis of hemodynamic changes

and complications during general anesthesia. J Clin Anesth. 2007;19:286-9.
8. Roebuck DJ, McLaren CA. Gastrointestinal intervention in children. Pediatr Radiol. 2011;41(1):27-41.
9. Amaral J, Connolly B. Pediatric interventional radiology. In: Geary DF, Schefer F (Eds) Comprehensive pediatric nephrology. Philadelphia; Elsevier: 2008. pp. 1053-78.
10. Simeunovic E, Arnold M, Sidler D, et al. Liver abscess in neonates. Pediatr Surg Int. 2009;25:153-6.
11. Lee SH, Tomlinson C, Temple M, et al. Imaging-guided percutaneous needle aspiration or catheter drainage of neonatal liver abscesses: 14-year experience. AJR. 2008;190: 616-22.
12. Roebuck DJ, Stanley P. External and internal-external biliary drainage in children with malignant obstructive jaundice. Pediatr Radiol. 2000;30:659-64.
13. Curry L, Sookur P, Low D, et al. Percutaneous cystgastrostomy as a single-step procedure. Cardiovasc Intervent Radiol. 2009;32:289-95.
14. Roebuck D, Michalski AJ. Core biopsy of renal tumors in childhood [abstract]. Med Pediatr Oncol. 2003;41:283.
15. El-Nahas AR, Shokeir AA, El-Kenawy MR, et al. Safety and efficacy of supracostal percutaneous nephrolithotomy in pediatric patients. J Urol. 2008;180:676-80.
16. Roebuck D. Pediatric interventional radiology: An overview. In: Spitz L, Coran A (Eds) Operative pediatric surgery. London; Hodder Arnold: 2006. pp. 1025-37.

CHAPTER 129

Imaging of Pediatric Trauma

Shivanand Gamanagatti, Atin Kumar

Nearly 50% of all deaths in children from 1 to 14 years are the result of trauma.[1] The estimates of mortality for children hospitalized after injury are uniformly low because most fatalities occur prior to arrival at a healthcare facility.[1,2]

The most common single organ system injury which is associated with highest mortality in pediatric age group is head trauma and nearly 80% of patients with head injuries have associated other organ injuries such as thoracoabdominal injuries. Children are not simple mini adults. Pediatric patients have major anatomic, physiologic, and psychological differences in comparison to adult patients, which play a significant role in the evaluation and management of pediatric trauma patient.

List of anatomic differences in adults and children: Implications for pediatric trauma management.[3]

- Pediatric body size allows a greater distribution of traumatic injuries, hence multiple injuries are common.
- Relatively greater body surface area of children contributes to greater heat loss.
- More anterior position of liver and spleen with less protective musculature and subcutaneous tissue mass, makes them more susceptible to injury.
- Relatively large size of the kidneys compared to their body size, more mobility and less protection from rib cage makes them very susceptible to deceleration injury.
- The child's growth plates are not yet closed, leading to Salter-type fractures with possible limb-length abnormalities following healing.
- Children have larger head-to-body ratio and thinner cranial bones (< age of 4 years, the calvarium is unilaminar and lacks dipole) due to which injuries to the head are more serious.

Imaging differences in children from adults:[3-5] Imaging differences in children is based on following aspects:

- In children, periosteum is stronger, thicker, highly vascularized, loosely attached to the underlying bone, biologically more active, and often remains intact even in the presence of significant trauma. The bones have more elasticity and plasticity and therefore sometimes may lead to reversible deformities, without manifesting a typical fracture.
- Because of increased elasticity of the pediatric bones, we may come across significant organ injuries without any osseous injuries. The child's cortical bone is also relatively thicker.
- The growth zone, (consists of transition zone between the elastic metaphysis, with a thinner cortical layer and more spongiosa that is prone to bulge fractures, and the initially purely cartilaginous epiphysis) is the most vulnerable part of the growing bone.
- In children, the bones and also other injuries heal quicker. Growth potentially corrects axial deviations, hence an anatomically exact repositioning of a fracture may not always be necessary as in adults, and even severe parenchymal injuries may be completely compensated by organ growth. On the other hand, even slight injuries of the growth zone may cause

severe growth retardation, osseous deformities and joint problems.

- Abdominal parenchymal organs are more mobile in childhood, and less protected by the osseous thoracic skeleton. This exposes them to a higher risk of injury.
- In children, circulation remains stable for very long time but can deteriorate dramatically at any point. Hence, reliable initial assessment as well as effective continuous monitoring and precautionary measures have to be taken to either preventively stabilize the patient or to ensure prompt treatment, particularly important in the era of conservative treatment approach.
- Children are smaller, have higher breathing and heart rates, and have less fatty tissue or not yet ossified skeletal parts, hence their imaging demands a higher spatial and temporal resolution. Some conditions can be assessed by ultrasound (US) in infants and children that in adults could only be reliably assessed by computed tomography (CT), e.g. injuries of abdominal parenchymal organs and neonatal cerebral hemorrhage.
- Children are more sensitive to radiation, and have a higher probability to develop radiation-induced cancer. Therefore, utmost radiation protection is compulsory, one should use dedicated imaging algorithms, alternative imaging modality, and radiation reduction imaging protocols (e.g. reduce X-rays and adapt CT protocols).
- Finally, non-accidental injuries comprise an important aspect of pediatric trauma imaging. It is the duty of any radiologist to pick up potential victims as early as possible to prevent future harm or even life-threatening events.

IMAGING METHODS[6]

The initial assessment of any child should focus on the following questions:

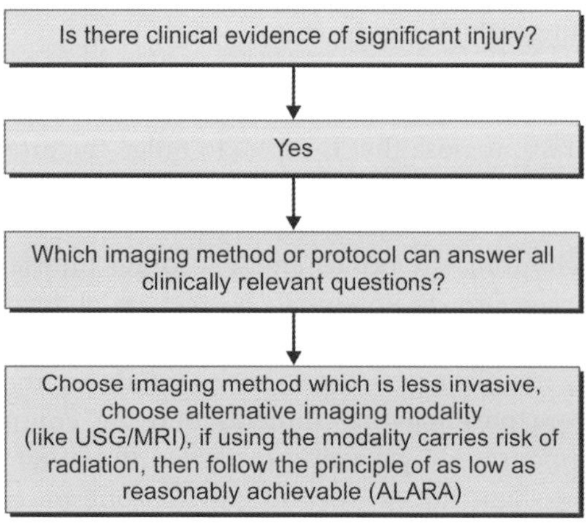

Radiographs: Radiographs are the first imaging method used following trauma. Radiographs will be obtained based on the physical examination. For patients sustaining minor trauma, radiographs may not be needed. Plain film radiography is the method most often relied upon in the assessment of suspected non-accidental injury of children. Children younger than 2 years of age with injuries consistent with child abuse will need a skeletal survey including skull, chest, abdomen, and long bone radiographs. It is important that good quality radiographs are obtained in all circumstances and that quality should not be compromised just because of the age and lack of cooperation of the child. It is important that all individuals interpreting radiographs in the acute trauma situation should have an understanding of the normal anatomy and basic radiographic projections used. In majority of the cases, X-ray films are taken because of medicolegal considerations rather than clinical necessity.[7]

Ultrasound: High frequency transducers (7–5 MHz) and ultrasound machines with high spatial and temporal resolution having color Doppler ability are mandatory for a thorough investigation, particularly for imaging neonates and infants. However, in the emergency room just for checking free fluid can be performed using normal equipment using 3–5 MHz transducer. An important use of ultrasound in the acutely traumatized pediatric patient is the 'Focused Abdominal Sonography for Trauma (FAST)' examination. When used by a trained radiologist, the FAST evaluation has the potential to provide sensitive and specific identification of intraperitoneal hemorrhage without invasive measures. The FAST examination does not have the ability to reliably detect specific organ injuries.

Potential Uses of the FAST Examination[8]

- Rapidly identify the source of hypotension in the hemodynamically unstable patient
- Assist in decision making in the child with head and abdominal trauma (head and abdominal CT versus laparotomy and/or craniotomy)
- Evaluate a stable and alert trauma patient with negative physical examination who otherwise would not routinely undergo radiology imaging
- Help prioritize imaging studies in the multiple-trauma patient
- Help avoid additional imaging in a child with an already low likelihood of intra-abdominal injury.

Computed Tomography

Computed tomography (CT) is still and will remain (at least for the near future) the modality of choice for a quick, reliable and comprehensive assessment of any polytraumatized child. The current generation CT scanners are very fast, have extremely short rotation time, improved Z-axis resolution and offer multiplanar reconstruction facilities. Contrast media is essential just as in adults, using weight adapted contrast media dose and age adapted delay. The modern CT scanners have automated radiation dose reduction techniques such as *automatic tube current modulation* that can substantially reduce patient dose. Currently, there are two methods used in the CT systems: Z-axis modulation and angular (X- and Y-axis) modulation. The aim of this dose reduction or low dose CT strategy is to still achieve a diagnostically reliable image quality at lowest possible radiation dose, by accepting some noise and speckle with consecutive image degradation. In pediatric patients, however, a more critical approach should be adopted with the CT examination being tailored to the specific clinical question being asked, to avoid unnecessary radiation dose.[9]

The specific indications for chest CT in blunt trauma should be guided by the findings of the initial clinical examination and chest radiograph.

- A spinal fracture or fractures of the upper ribs, shoulder girdle, and sternum will often necessitate a contrast-enhanced CT to look for vascular injury
- If there is persistent hemorrhagic output from these tubes or progressive pneumomediastinum, to look for bronchial or vascular injury
- In the presence of an abnormal mediastinum on plain radiographs, to evaluate for thoracic aortic injury.

The most common indications for abdominal CT include lap-belt ecchymosis, gross hematuria, positive FAST scan, all patients with penetrating injury and signs of peritonitis to look for bowel injury.

There are three arguments against the routine use of total-body CT in pediatric trauma imaging:[9]

1. An important issue of radiation dose in the pediatric age group
2. Consideration of cost effectiveness in the use of expensive imaging resources
3. There is the risk of the possible demonstration of pseudo-disease and clinically unimportant findings by over-interpretation of CT findings

Hence, there is a critical need for developing clinical appropriateness criteria for the application of CT in pediatric trauma patients.

Given these controversies, the initial imaging evaluation of pediatric trauma should consist of the conventional trauma series (lateral radiograph of the cervical spine, AP radiograph of the pelvis and chest radiograph), in conjunction with a careful and rapid triage by an experienced clinician after taking the mechanism and force of injury into account. This approach will determine the need for additional imaging with cross-sectional techniques, such as ultrasound and spiral or multidetector-row CT.

Magnetic Resonance Imaging

Magnetic resonance imaging (MRI) is rarely used for the initial assessment of acute severe trauma except in some rare situations, most commonly related to the central nervous system and spinal cord. However, MRI is also widely used for assessment of traumatic musculoskeletal changes at multiple body areas, particularly the joints. Diagnostic MRI needs appropriate sequence selection and good quality images. Sequence selection is dependent on the clinical question being asked and the possible pathological processes that may be encountered. Image quality is dependent on the signal to noise ratio, spatial resolution, image contrast and any associated artifacts.[10]

Abdominal Trauma[11-13]

The management of pediatric blunt abdominal trauma has become increasingly nonoperative over the past several decades. Blunt trauma accounts for nearly 90% of injuries in children. Although skeletal, thoracic, and central nervous system injuries are often clinically evident but intra-abdominal injuries in children are difficult to detect on physical examination, especially in an unconscious child. Hence, imaging plays an important role in diagnosis and management.

Contrast-enhanced CT is the preferred imaging modality in the evaluation of intra-abdominal injury. The radiologist's job is not simply to recognize injuries but also to actively seek imaging signs that indicate the need for surgery. Imaging signs that indicate need of either surgical or endovascular intervention include presence of pneumoperitoneum, intraperitoneal bladder rupture, grade V renovascular injury and active contrast extravasation.[14]

Nonoperative management is typical for uncomplicated spleen and liver injuries and is gaining popularity for uncomplicated pancreatic and renal injuries. The injuries detected at CT help in determining the appropriate degree of patient monitoring in the hospital (i.e. intensive care unit versus regular ward), length of hospitalization, and amount of activity restriction after discharge. In children, following blunt abdominal trauma, solid-organ injuries predominate, with the spleen being the most commonly injured organ, followed by the liver and kidney.

Spleen and Liver

Injury to the liver and spleen occurs in 6–9% of pediatric patients after blunt abdominal trauma. Although these injuries occur with nearly equal frequency, mortality is greater in patients with hepatic injuries. Patterns of hepatic and splenic injury includes laceration, fracture, hematoma, and rupture **(Figs. 1 and 2)**. Complications of splenic and liver injury include arterial pseudoaneurysm, active intra-abdominal hemorrhage, delayed hemorrhage, and biloma.

Pancreas

Pancreatic injuries occur in approximately 1–2% of children undergoing CT for blunt abdominal trauma. Bicycle handlebar injuries are the most common mechanism of pancreatic injury in children. Pediatric pancreatic injuries are most often isolated, whereas in adults they commonly accompany other abdominal injuries.

Direct signs of pancreatic injury include pancreatic laceration, transection, and comminution **(Figs. 3A to D)**. Peri-pancreatic fat stranding, hemorrhage, and fluid between the splenic vein and pancreas are useful secondary signs of pancreatic injury. Presence of peri-pancreatic fluid in the absence of other abdominal visceral injury should strongly suggest pancreatic injury.

CT is useful in delineating the location of pancreatic injury in relation to superior mesenteric artery and vein, as well as the status of main pancreatic duct.

Common complications of pancreatic injury in children include pancreatitis and pseudocyst formation. In contrast to adults, trauma is the most common cause of pancreatitis in children.

Nonoperative management is preferred in children with blunt pancreatic trauma in contrast to adult patients who undergo surgery in most cases.

Kidney

Injury to kidney occurs in 4–14% of children presenting with blunt abdominal trauma. Children are more susceptible to renal injury after trauma than adults due to

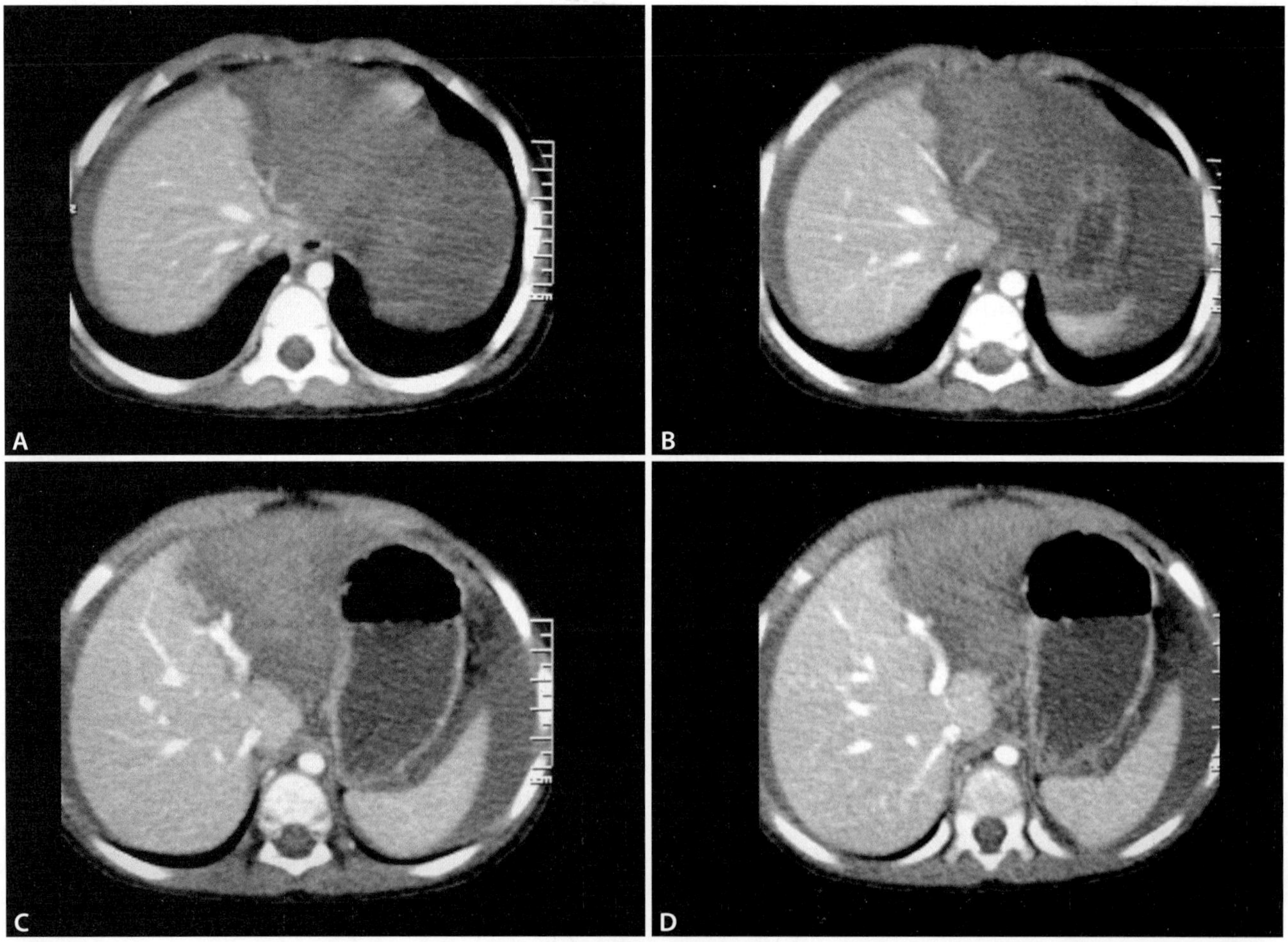

Figs. 1A to D: Axial CT sections of liver showing large contusion involving lateral segment of left lobe of liver with hemoperitoneum.

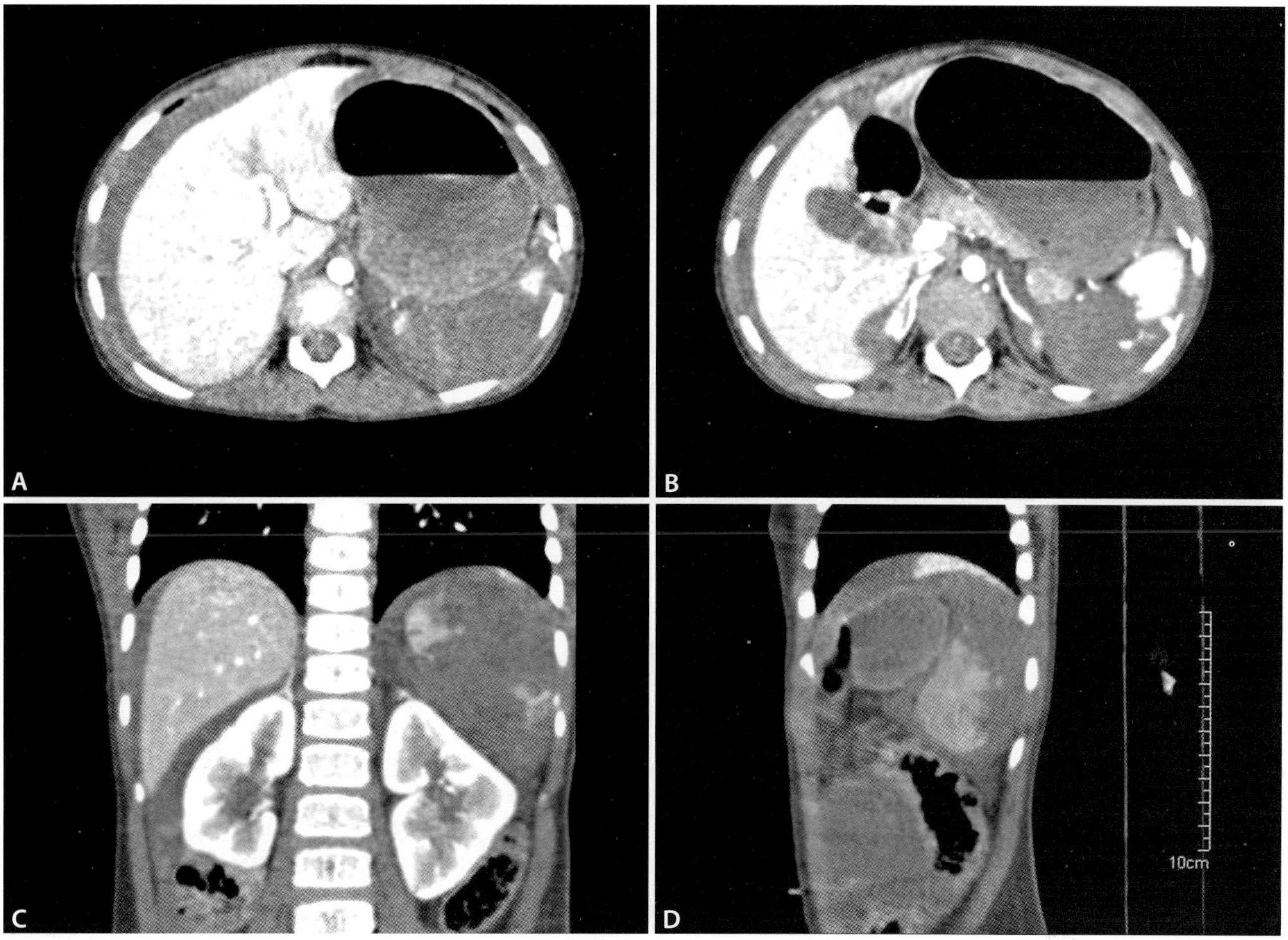

Figs. 2A to D: Axial CT (A and B), coronal (C) and sagittal MPR (D) images of upper abdomen showing large contusion involving more than 50% of splenic parenchyma suggesting Grade 3 lesion with hemoperitoneum.

the relatively increased renal size and mobility, decreased amount of perinephric fat, and decreased chest wall protection. Presence of an underlying abnormality such as a mass, horse-shoe kidney, hydronephrosis, or multiple cysts may increase that susceptibility by causing the kidney to become bulky and oversized. Most patients with significant renal injury present with hematuria. In some cases, significant renal injuries are present in children with only microscopic hematuria or a normal urinalysis.

Majority (64-96%) of renal injuries is mild (grade 1-2) **(Figs. 4A to D)**. Just as with other solid organ injuries in children, nonoperative management is preferred in the management of renal trauma.

Complications of nonoperative management include delayed hemorrhage, renal pseudoaneurysm, delayed hematuria, renal scarring, renal cysts, hypertension, infections, and persistent urinoma.

Bowel and Mesentery

A specific history of lap-belt or handle-bar injury should heighten suspicion for bowel injury. Bowel injury occurs in 1 to 8.5% of children after blunt abdominal trauma.

Although bowel perforation is one of the few indications for surgery after abdominal trauma, the diagnosis is difficult to establish at CT. Differentiating perforating from nonperforating bowel injury remains a challenge even for an experienced radiologist.

Most common CT findings in children with bowel rupture are free peritoneal fluid and bowel wall enhancement **(Figs. 5A and B)**. Other CT findings include extraluminal gas, bowel wall thickening, bowel dilation, bowel wall defect, mesenteric stranding, fluid at the mesenteric root, focal hematoma, active hemorrhage, and mesenteric pseudoaneurysm.

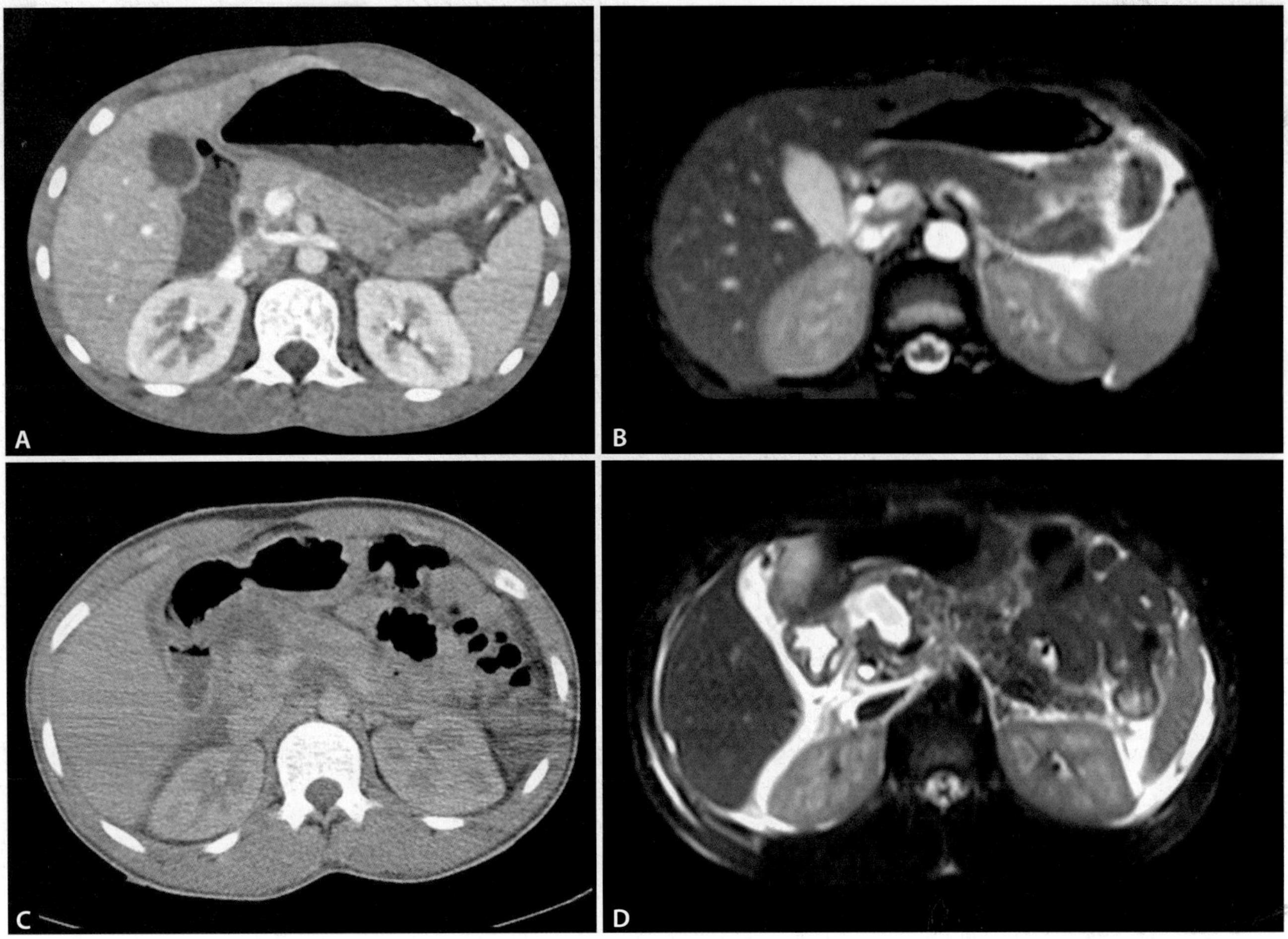

Figs. 3A to D: Axial CT and TRUE FISP MR images showing linear complete laceration involving tail of pancreas with peripancreatic minimal free fluid collection (A and B). Axial CT and T2W-FS images showing complete laceration with fluid collection in the region of head of pancreas (C and D).

Unexplained peritoneal fluid (free fluid without any solid parenchymal injury, pelvic fracture, or hypoperfusion complex) is another useful indicator of bowel or mesenteric injury.

Duodenal injury is rare, occurring in less than 1% of children after blunt abdominal trauma. CT findings that are strongly suggestive of a nonperforating duodenal injury include a thickened duodenum, mural hematoma, retroperitoneal fluid, and intraperitoneal fluid. Presence of retroperitoneal air has a strong association with duodenal perforation. The distinction is critical, as perforating injuries require surgery, while duodenal hematomas can be managed nonoperatively.

Complications of bowel injury include abscess, fistula formation, bowel obstruction, and wound infection.

One common mimicker of bowel injury at CT is overhydration, or increased central venous pressure that occurs during aggressive resuscitation. This can lead to bowel wall or mesenteric edema that can obscure or simulate bowel injury.

Chest Trauma

Blunt Trauma Chest[9]

Thoracic injury is a leading cause of death resulting from trauma in children, second only to head injury. Blunt chest injuries are more common than penetrating injury. Physical evaluation of chest is limited in children with polytrauma either because of loss of consciousness due to head injury, or because of lack of co-operation; imaging plays an important role in diagnosis.

The supine anteroposterior (AP) chest radiograph performed in emergency room may be limited because of technical factors and artifact from overlying immobi-

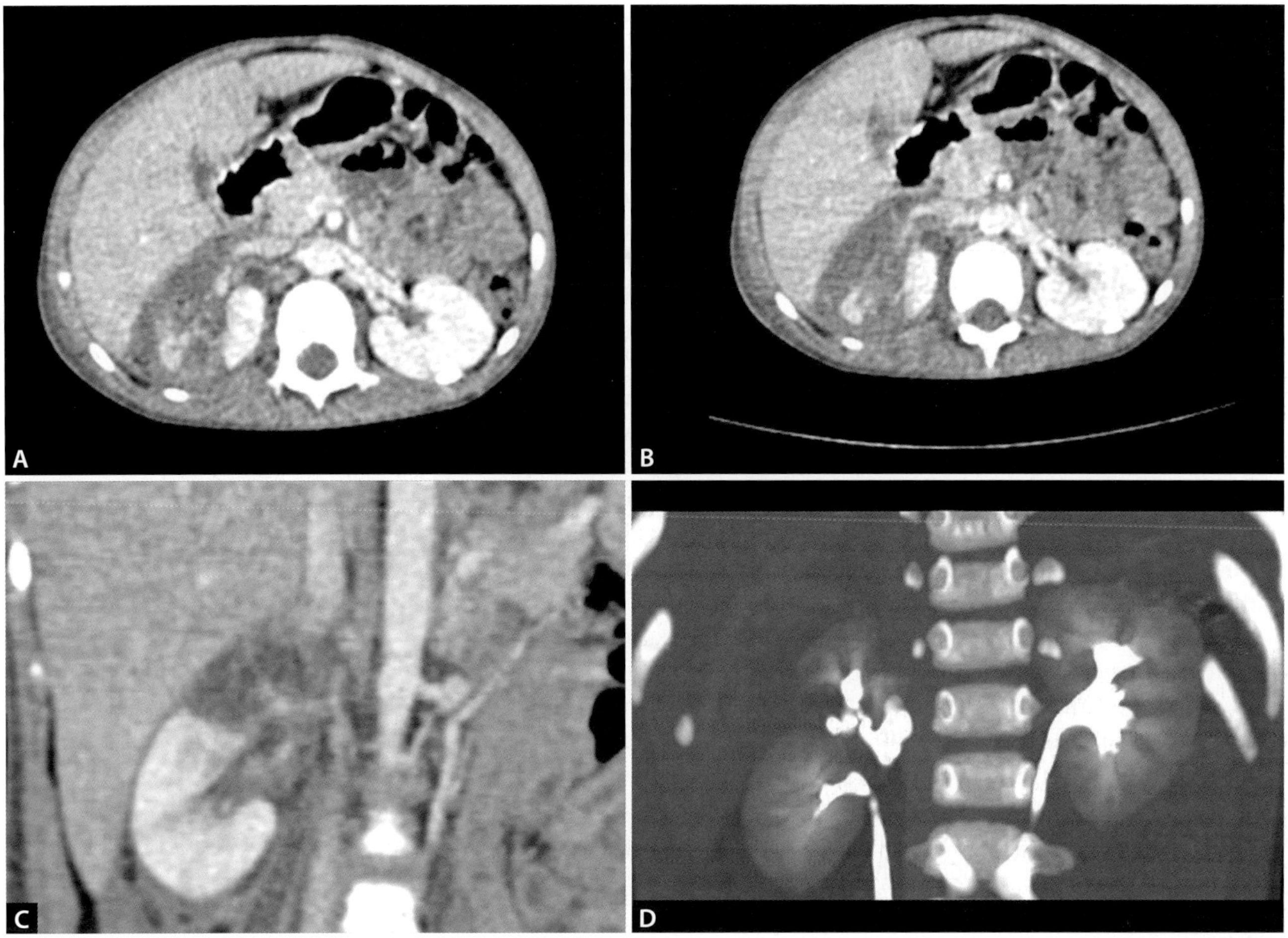

Figs. 4A to D: Axial CT (A and B) and Coronal MPR (C) images of upper abdomen showing laceration involving upper pole of right kidney with perinephric hematoma and there is evidence of contrast leakage from the upper pole calyx in delayed scan (D).

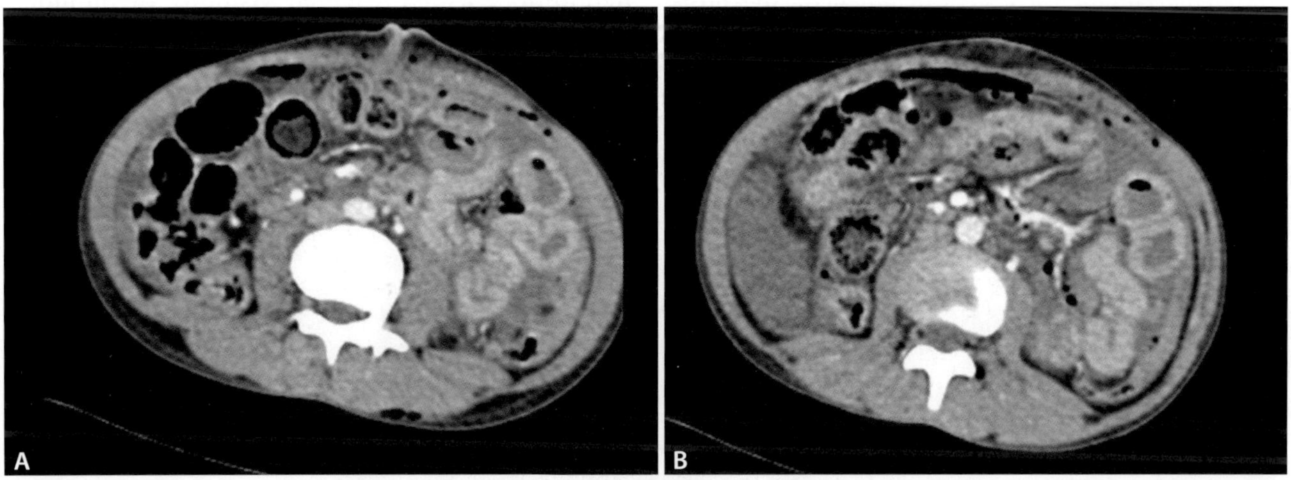

Figs. 5A and B: Axial CT sections (A and B) of mid abdomen showing presence of pneumoperitoneum and abnormal enhancement of walls of small bowel loops with hemoperitoneum suggestive of bowel injury.

lization hardware; however, it remains an important tool for the prompt diagnosis of life-threatening conditions such as a tension pneumothorax.

Focused sonography of the lower chest and pericardial space may be very helpful in identifying presence of significant hemo-thorax or hemopericardium, which may require urgent drainage.

Once a severely injured child is stabilized hemodynamically, further imaging tests need to be undertaken to identify internal injury such as contusion, laceration, pneumothorax, hemothorax, pericardial effusion or any vascular injury.

Currently, CT is the imaging modality of choice to evaluate chest injury in multitrauma patients, not only in adults, but increasingly in the pediatric population.

Chest wall injuries: Rib fractures are less common in children than in adults because of the compliance/ elasticity of the anterior chest wall in children, hence, major internal injuries can occur without rib fractures. Dislocated rib fractures/ unstable flail chest are rarely seen in smaller children. Fractures of the upper ribs and clavicle are often combined with either vascular or esophago-tracheo-bronchial injuries.

Lower rib fractures are often combined with lacerations of the upper abdominal organs. The fractures of the upper ribs, clavicles, sternum, scapulae, and vertebral bodies or processes are all better assessed with CT than with plain films.

Fracture of the trachea or of a bronchus gives following radiological findings:

- Misplaced endotracheal tube, but a deformed bronchial contour can also be helpful in the diagnosis.
- In the most advanced cases fallen lung sign with collapse of the lung *not to* the hilum *but towards* the diaphragm can be seen.

Pleura

Pneumothorax can result from penetrating injury to the chest wall, from air leak into the pleural space from an injured lung (laceration), or in association with central air leak from the tracheobronchial tree (pneumomediastinum).

Diagnosis of pneumothorax is straightforward on upright chest radiographs, with demonstration of the visceral pleural line outlined by free pleural air in the apex of the chest. Expiratory films may enhance the visibility of pneumothoraces. In the multitrauma situation, patient is typically in the supine position hence pneumothorax is more difficult to detect and often can be diagnosed only by indirect signs such as deep sulcus sign and double diaphragm sign.

CT is more sensitive than chest radiography for small pneumothoraces **(Fig. 6A)**, but it is of no clinical significance unless the patient is receiving positive-pressure ventilation support.

Presence of a tension pneumothorax **(Fig. 6B)**, as evidenced by midline shift on chest radiograph, requires urgent chest tube insertion and therefore this information should be communicated to the treatment team.

Hemothorax: Hemothorax is a result of venous or arterial bleeding into the pleural cavity.

On supine chest radiography, pleural effusions manifest as a veil-like increased density over the involved hemithorax with preserved visibility of pulmonary

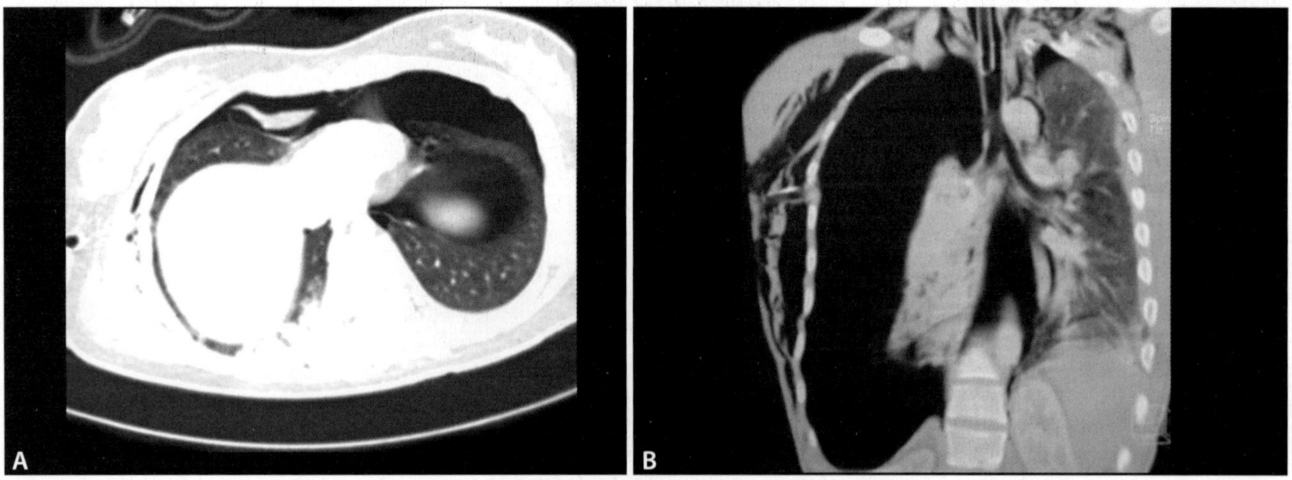

Figs. 6A and B: Axial and coronal MPR images of lungs showing bilateral minimal pneumothorax (A) and tension pneumothorax on right side with collapse of underlying lung (B).

vascular markings and, in the case of larger amounts of fluid, thickening of the lateral pleural line. CT is more sensitive than radiography for demonstrating small effusions, and Hounsfield density measurements may help confirm their hemorrhagic nature **(Figs. 7A and B)**. CT is also superior for accurate assessment of chest tube placement and related complications.

Pulmonary parenchyma: The radiological findings in pulmonary contusion can vary considerably from patient to patient. There is no air bronchogram but the pattern and extent varies. There are many different radiological appearances. They can be patchy or extensive and confluent, they can be solitary or multifocal, and they can be unilateral or bilateral. Simultaneous aspiration can sometimes confuse the radiological assessment and complicate the outcome. Lung laceration initially may be indistinguishable from the surrounding contusion **(Figs. 8A to D)**. Because of the disruption of lung tissue, one or more air cavities develop over time and may contain a central density or fluid level because of intrapulmonary hematoma. In the case of large lacerations involving the pleural surface, a bronchopleural fistula may develop. Cavitation of contusions or hematomas, sometimes with air-blood levels on upright chest films or on CT occurs earlier in time in children than in adults. They can be seen as residual infiltrates for months.

Mediastinum: The momentary chest compression and re-expansion of the chest at the time of incident may lead to mediastinal injury and a pneumomediastinum with air tracking and sometimes extending into the neck as subcutaneous emphysema. Pneumo-mediastinum is recognized by streaky air collections outlining mediastinal structures such as thymus. Another sign of pneumo-mediastinum is the so called continuous diaphragm sign which is due to air beneath the heart.

Perforation/rupture of the esophagus may be caused by blunt trauma of chest or by penetrating injury. Unexplained pneumomediastinum and pleural effusions are the most important radiologic signs. If the injury is suspected, an esophagogram should be performed, initially with water-soluble contrast material, followed by dilute barium **(Figs. 9A and B)**.

Detection of a *mediastinal hematoma* is extremely important, because it may be a clue to an occult traumatic aortic injury (TAI), which is often clinically silent. Mediastinal measurement criteria published in the adult, i.e. mediastinal width greater than 8 cm, mediastinum-to-chest ratio greater than 0.25 have been proven to lack a sufficient predictive value for TAI and do not necessarily apply to children. Multidetector-row CT angiography has emerged in recent years as a test that is helpful to rule out or demonstrate TAI in patients with an abnormal mediastinum on chest radiography.[9]

Cardiac injuries are rare but may include both myocardial laceration with ventricular shunting or pericardial hemorrhage **(*see* Figs. 7A and B)** and possibly a cardiac tamponade. Chest radiographs can demonstrate enlargement of cardiac silhouette, but they are generally more accurately assessed by CT.

Traumatic ruptures of the diaphragm are more common on the left side but are generally very rare.

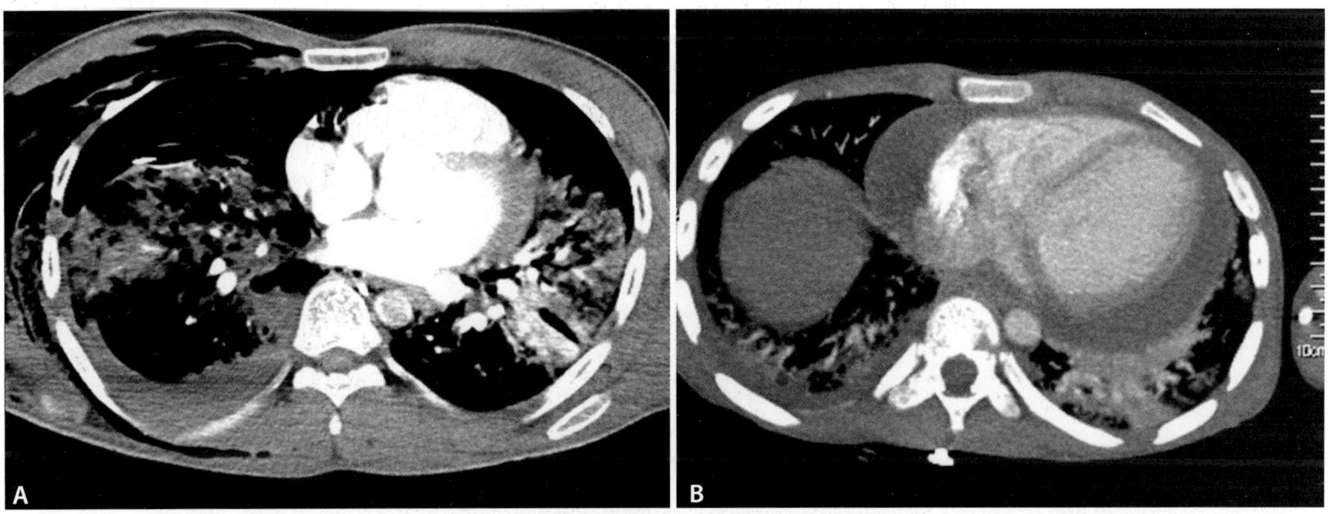

Figs. 7A and B: Axial CT section of thorax showing right side hemothorax with contusion in bilateral lungs (A) and hemopericardium with minimal right side hemothorax (B).

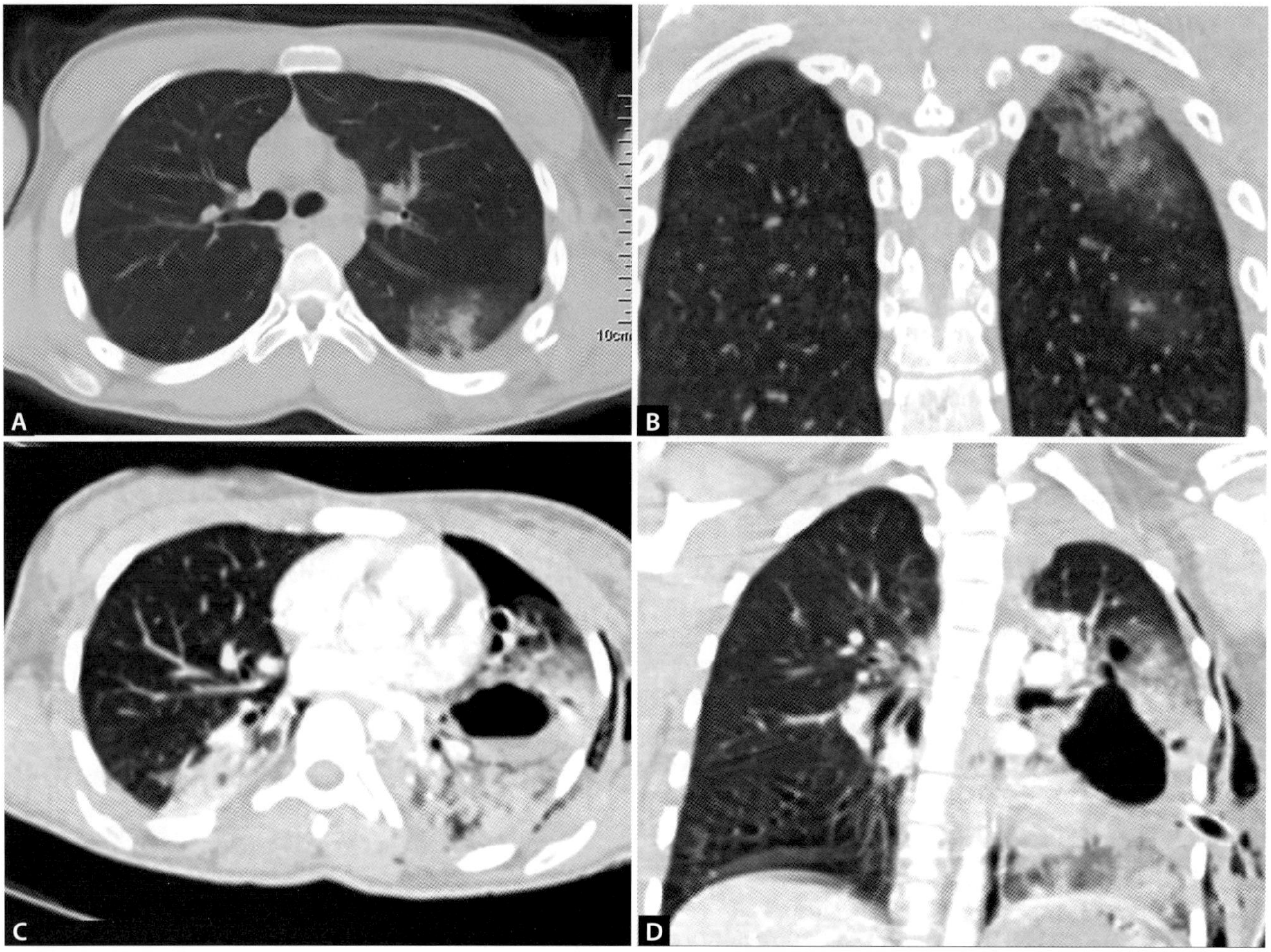

Figs. 8A to D: Axial and coronal MIP images (A and B) of lung showing ground-glass attenuation lesion in left upper lobe close to the chest wall suggestive of lung contusion. Axial and coronal MIP (C and D) images of lung showing large air-filled cavity in left upper lobe with surrounding consolidation suggestive of laceration with surrounding contusion. Note the minimal pneumothorax on left side.

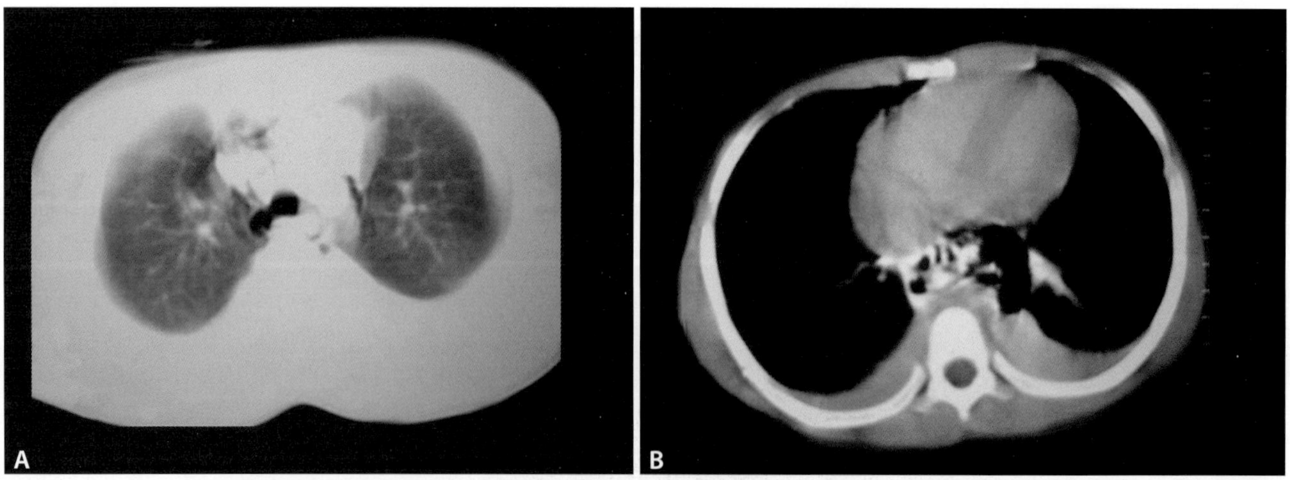

Figs. 9A and B: Axial CT sections of thorax showing pneumomediastinum (A) and contrast leakage from the esophagus (B) given orally suggestive of esophageal rupture.

Penetrating Chest Trauma

When they involve the lungs, heart or great vessels they produce similar findings to those that occur with blunt chest trauma. Gunshot wounds are relatively common and the pellet is most often accompanied by a pulmonary consolidation. Even if the pellet has passed through the body a circular tube-like consolidation around the track of the bullet can be seen. Specifically, penetrating pediatric chest trauma tends to produce air within the pleural space, heart, mediastinum or great vessels. Metallic and sometimes other foreign bodies may be seen.

Musculoskeletal Injuries[7,10]

Many unique features of the growing skeleton pose specific challenges in imaging skeletal trauma (Vide supra). Differences in the composition and development of the pediatric skeleton (as compared with adults) result in characteristic injuries and fractures. Imaging of these injuries typically begin with plain films, and in the majority no further radiologic evaluation is required. However, Computed tomography (CT) and magnetic resonance imaging (MRI) are used as supplementary imaging studies in pediatric patients with suspected skeletal trauma.

Imaging[15]

Plain radiographs: In most cases, imaging of pediatric skeletal trauma begins with radiographs, and very few patients require imaging beyond plain films, this is particularly true in cases of common fractures.

At least, two perpendicular views should be performed. Occasionally, oblique or other views may be needed to diagnose a fracture.

CT Scan: Multidetector CT (MDCT) with multiplanar and 3-D reconstruction may help in the identification or exclusion of fractures in anatomically complex areas such as the pelvis, spine, elbow and ankle that are not definite on plain radiography. MDCT is also excellent for the evaluation of fracture healing and complications such as pseudoarthrosis formation, post-traumatic physeal closure and growth arrest.

MRI: With acute pediatric trauma, although plain radiography is still the primary imaging tool, MR imaging has evolved into an essential adjunct diagnostic tool for the prompt identification of occult musculoskeletal injuries. Growth plate injuries and their complications, osteochondritis dissecans **(Figs. 10A to C)**, avulsion, stress fractures, and soft tissue injuries can be diagnosed early and confidently with MR imaging when other imaging modalities are equivocal. MR imaging, therefore, offers invaluable aid in clinical decisions regarding the timely institution of necessary management to help alleviate symptoms, promote healing, and, more importantly, prevent further complications, such as fractures, degenerative changes, malunion, and growth arrest. MRI is able to accurately evaluate occult and physeal fractures. MRI has been shown to change the classification of physeal fractures significantly, thus affecting surgical management of these patients. Complications such as physeal growth arrest are also well demonstrated on MRI. In other circumstances it is of limited value, being relatively insensitive in detecting small ossific fragments within a joint and when there is a considerable amount of metallic hardware within the bone. While protocols are important, each examination should be tailored to the

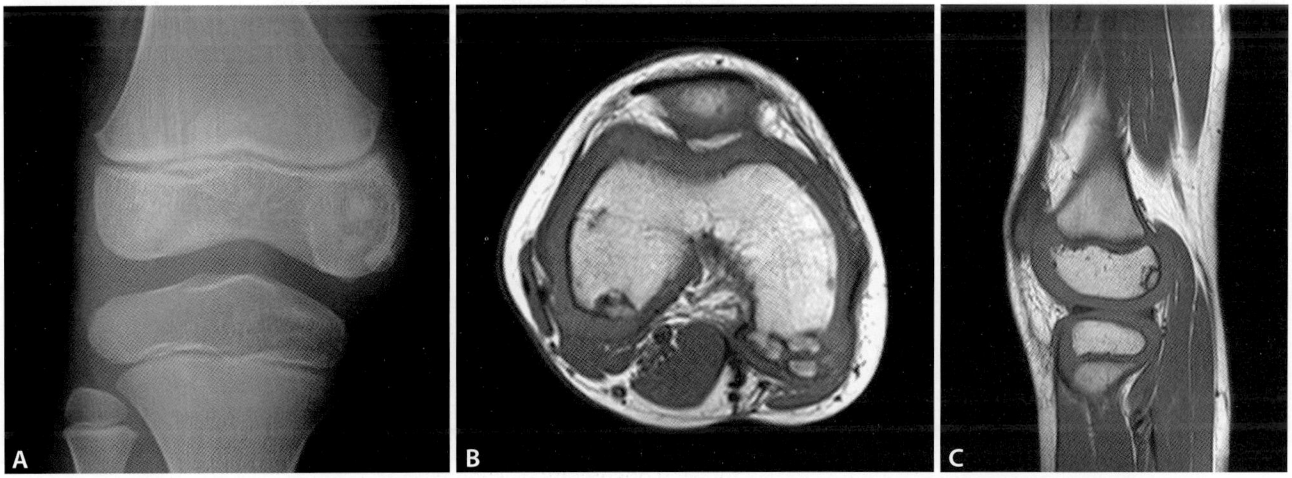

Figs. 10A to C: Anteroposterior radiograph of left knee (A) showing multiple loose bodies overlying the medial condyle of left femur. Axial and sagittal MR (B and C) images showing osteochondral lesions involving both condyles of left femur with multiple loose bodies in relation to medial condyle.

individual patient and address the specific area of clinical concern. Drawbacks of MRI include longer imaging times, dependence on patient cooperation, and frequent need for sedation.

Musculoskeletal injuries account for 12% of pediatric visits to the emergency department, with fractures making up a large proportion of these numbers. Pediatric bone is more elastic than adult bone and can bend without breaking. This results in unique childhood fractures such as the plastic deformation, torus and greenstick fractures.[7,10]

Fractures extending into the physeal plate may cause growth arrest, and angular deformity may result. Fractures involving the physis have been classified and described by Salter and Harris.

Types of Pediatric Fractures

- Plastic deformation of bone
- Torus
- Greenstick
- Complete diaphyseal fractures
  - Plastic deformation occurs as a result of longitudinal compression of a long bone. With increasing force, microfractures occur and the bone then loses its capacity to regain its original shape and remains bowed. This fracture occurs most commonly in the radius and ulna.
  - Torus fractures are also known as buckle fractures and are incomplete fractures occurring on the concave side of the bone with outward buckling of the cortical margin. These fractures occur most commonly in the metaphyseal regions of long bones **(Fig. 11)**.
  - A greenstick fracture is an incomplete fracture occurring only on the convex side of the long bone **(Figs. 12A and B)**.
  - A complete fracture occurs when the fracture line propagates completely through the bone and most commonly involve the diaphyseal region.

Physeal Fractures

The Salter-Harris classification of physeal fractures is the most widely accepted classification and it relates the radiological appearance of physeal fractures with treatment and morbidity.

Salter-Harris Classification

I : Transverse through physis.
II : Through physis but with a metaphyseal fragment.
III : Through physis and epiphysis and therefore intra-articular.
IV : Through epiphysis, across physis and through metaphysis (II and III).
V : Physeal crush injury **(Figs. 13A to C)**.

A useful rule of thumb is that the higher the grades of injuries, the greater likelihood that the growth plate will be damaged, which can result in long-term complications. Types I, II and III have a relatively good prognosis, whereas type V has a poorer prognosis due to damage to the growth plate. Complications of growth plate injuries include malunion, premature fusion resulting in growth impairment and avascular necrosis.

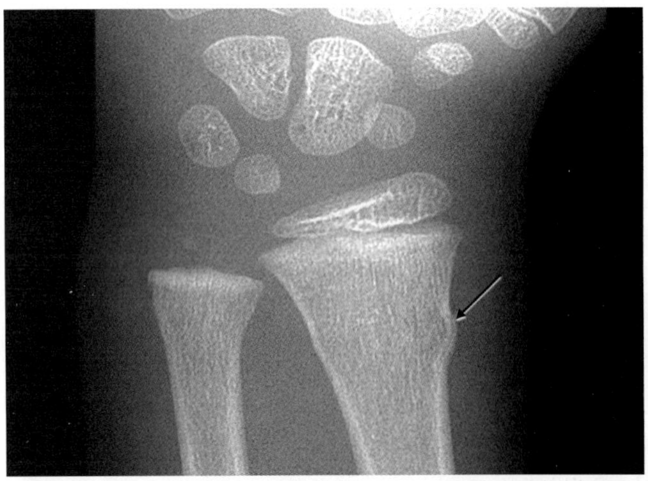

Fig. 11: Anteroposterior radiograph of wrist showing torus fracture with outward buckling of the cortical margin of lower end of radius in the metaphyseal region (arrow).

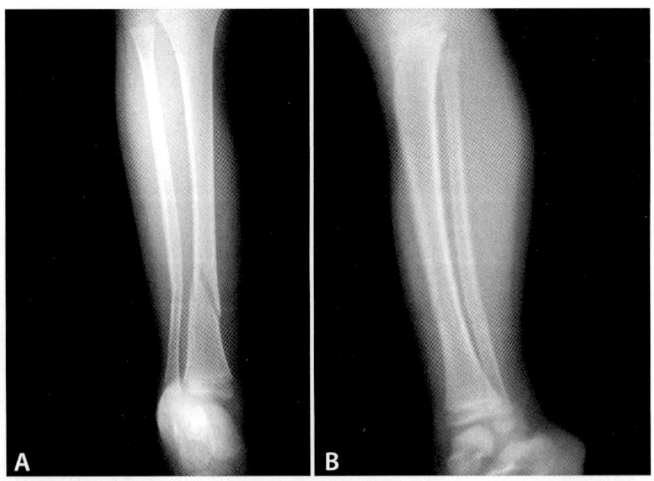

Figs. 12A and B: Anteroposterior (A) and lateral (B) radiographs of right leg showing a green-stick fracture of fibula and oblique fracture of tibia.

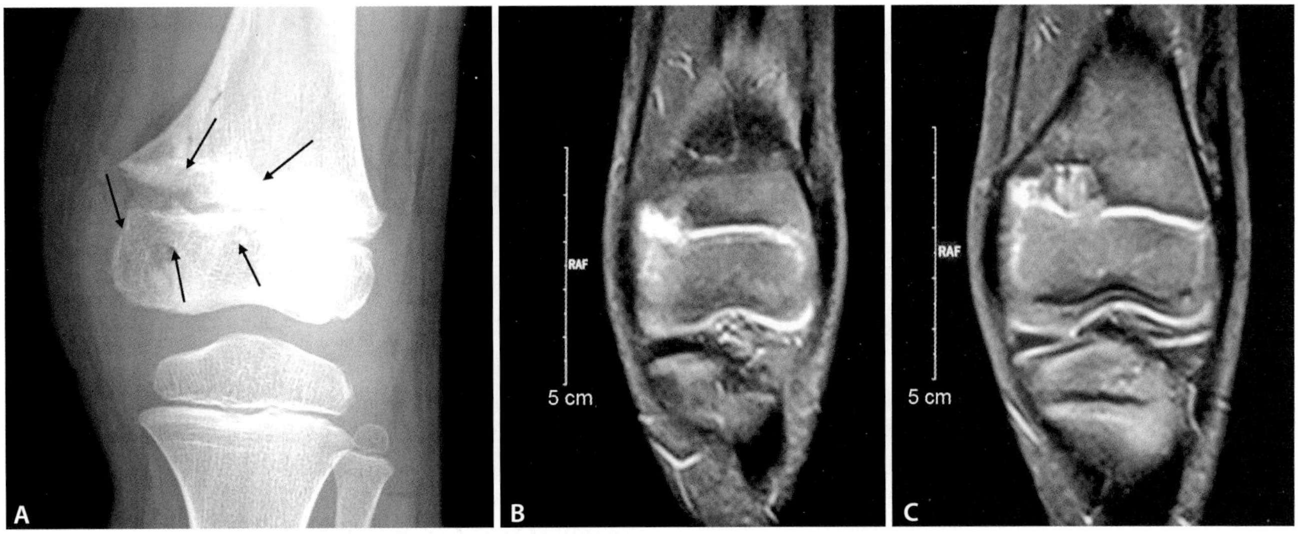

Figs. 13A to C: Anteroposterior radiograph (A) and coronal STIR MR images (B and C) of right knee showing type V fracture of Salter-Harris classification involving the medial aspect of growth plate.

Head Trauma[16]

Pediatric head trauma is one of the primary causes of injury, mortality and morbidity in childhood. Imaging supports the diagnosis and treatment of intracranial injuries.

The mechanisms of injury in children vary depending on age. The younger the child, the higher the risk of injury, and the risk for asymptomatic intracranial injury is highest for infants younger than 6 months, because of their large heads, weak neck musculature, and relatively thin calvarium. As the child gets older, falls become a less frequent cause of accidental trauma, whereas bicycle injuries and motor vehicle accidents become more common.

Broad Classification

- *Primary lesions:* Are the direct result of trauma (Already occurred at the time of presentation)
- *Secondary lesions:* As complications of primary lesions (preventable)
  - *Acute and subacute:* Include cerebral edema, ischemia, and brain herniation.
  - *Chronic:* Hydrocephalus, the cerebrospinal fluid (CSF) leak, leptomeningeal cyst, and encephalomalacia.

According to Location of Lesions

- *Intra-axial:* Cortical contusions, intracerebral hematoma, axonal shearing injuries, gray matter injury, and vascular injury
- *Extra-axial:* Epidural, subdural, subarachnoid, and intraventricular hemorrhage.

Skull Fractures[17]

Skull fractures in neonates may be of the following types: Linear, diastatic, depressed, compound or buckled. Skull fractures may be diagnosed by CT or plain radiography. Complications from depressed skull fractures include dural tear, cerebral contusion, retained osseous fragments, and cosmetic deformity.

Imaging findings of these abnormalities in children are similar to those in adults.

However, there are few differences as compared to adults[18]

- Skull fractures from minor trauma are more common in children than adults, especially in children younger than 2 years of age.
  The calvarium in a child is softer and thinner than an adult' and is, therefore, susceptible to fracture.
- The calvarium is unilaminar without diploe till the age of 4 years. Therefore, skull offers less protection to the child's brain than it does in the adult, and children with skull fractures are at an increased risk of having intracranial injury.

Extra-axial Injury

- Epidural hematoma (EDH) **(Figs. 14A and B)**
- Subdural hematoma (SDH) **(Figs. 15A and B)**
- Subarachnoid hemorrhage
- Intraventricular hemorrhage

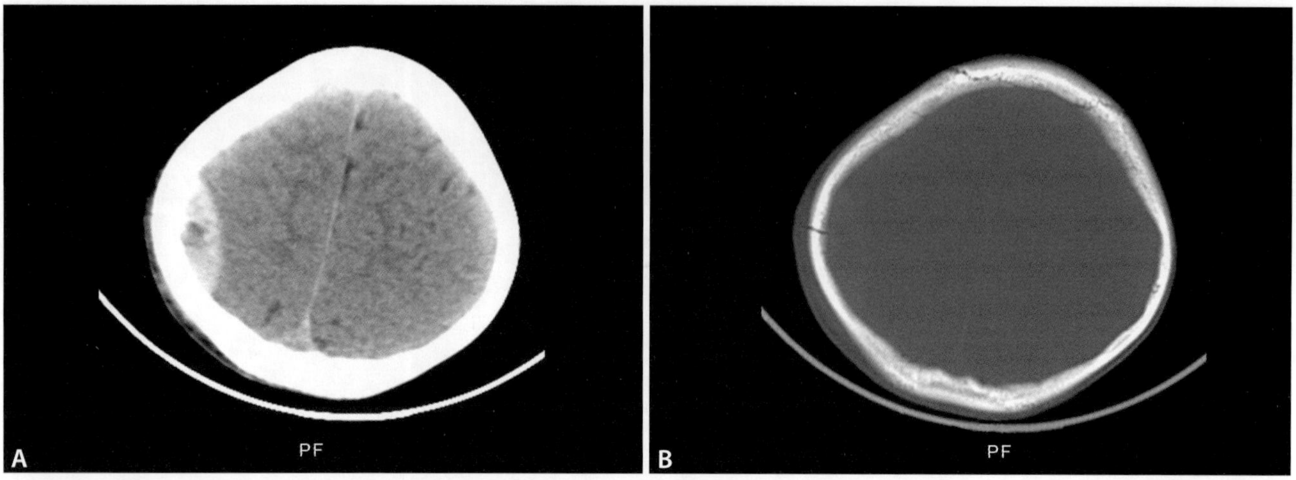

Figs. 14A and B: Axial CT sections in brain window (A) and bone window (B) showing small biconvex epidural hematoma in parietal region with linear non-depressed fracture of overlying parietal bone.

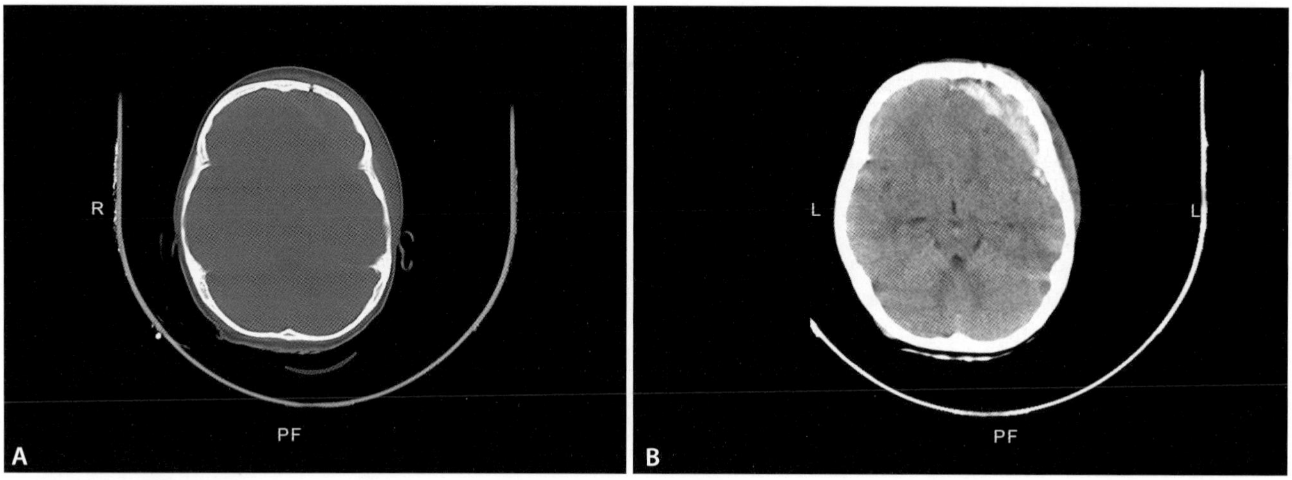

Figs. 15A and B: Axial CT sections in bone window (A) and brain window (B) showing small subdural hematoma in left frontal region with linear non-depressed fracture of overlying frontal bone.

Imaging findings of these abnormalities in children are similar to those in adults.

However, there are few differences as compared to adults:

- SDH are more common than EDH
- In children, the dura is more firmly adherent to the inner table of the skull and the groove for the middle meningeal artery is shallow, allowing for more mobility of the vessel. For these reasons EDH is less common, and when it does occur, is more often from venous bleeding than arterial.
- Skull fractures are less commonly associated with EDH in children because of the increased plasticity of the child' skull.
- Since the bleeding is often venous, these hematomas evolve slowly, and the clinical presentation of acute EDH in the young child can be less dramatic than in an adult.
- Unlike in adults, where the SDH is often unilateral, SDH in children is bilateral in up to 80% of cases.
- Often SDH in the pediatric age group is extensive, with involvement of the temporal, frontal and parietal regions. This results from the lack of adhesions in the subdural space that are present in the adult.

Intra-axial injuries include contusions **(Figs. 16A and B)**, diffuse axonal injury (DAI) **(Figs. 17 and 18)** and intracerebral hematomas. The imaging appearances of these abnormalities are similar to those in adults. However, skull is relatively smooth in children compared with adults, contusions are less common in the former.

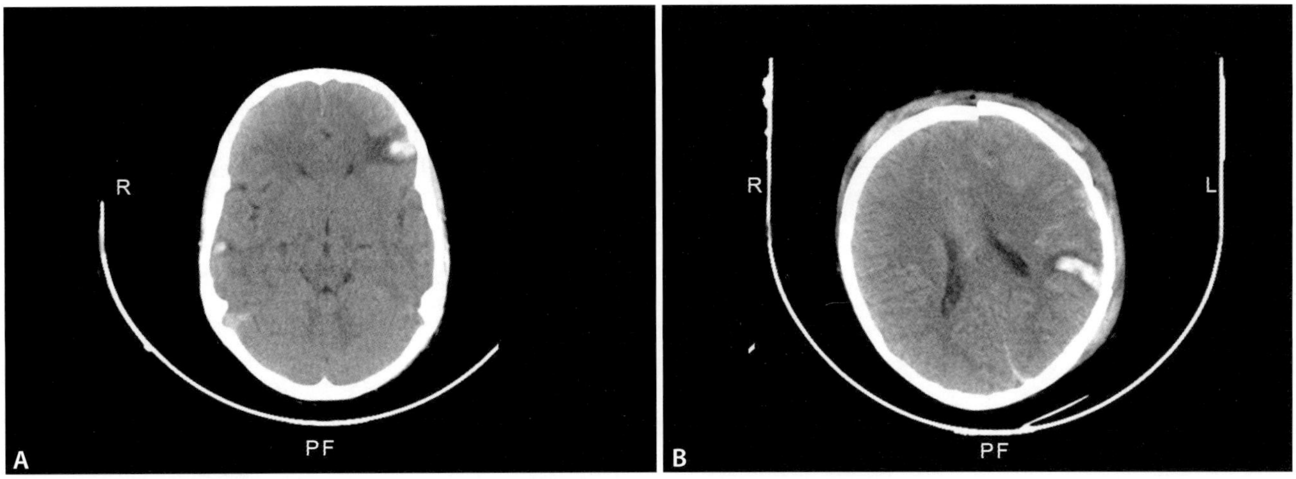

Figs. 16A and B: Axial CT sections of brain showing multiple contusions in left frontal, parietal and right temporal lobes associated with mild perilesional edema. Note the depressed fracture of frontal bone.

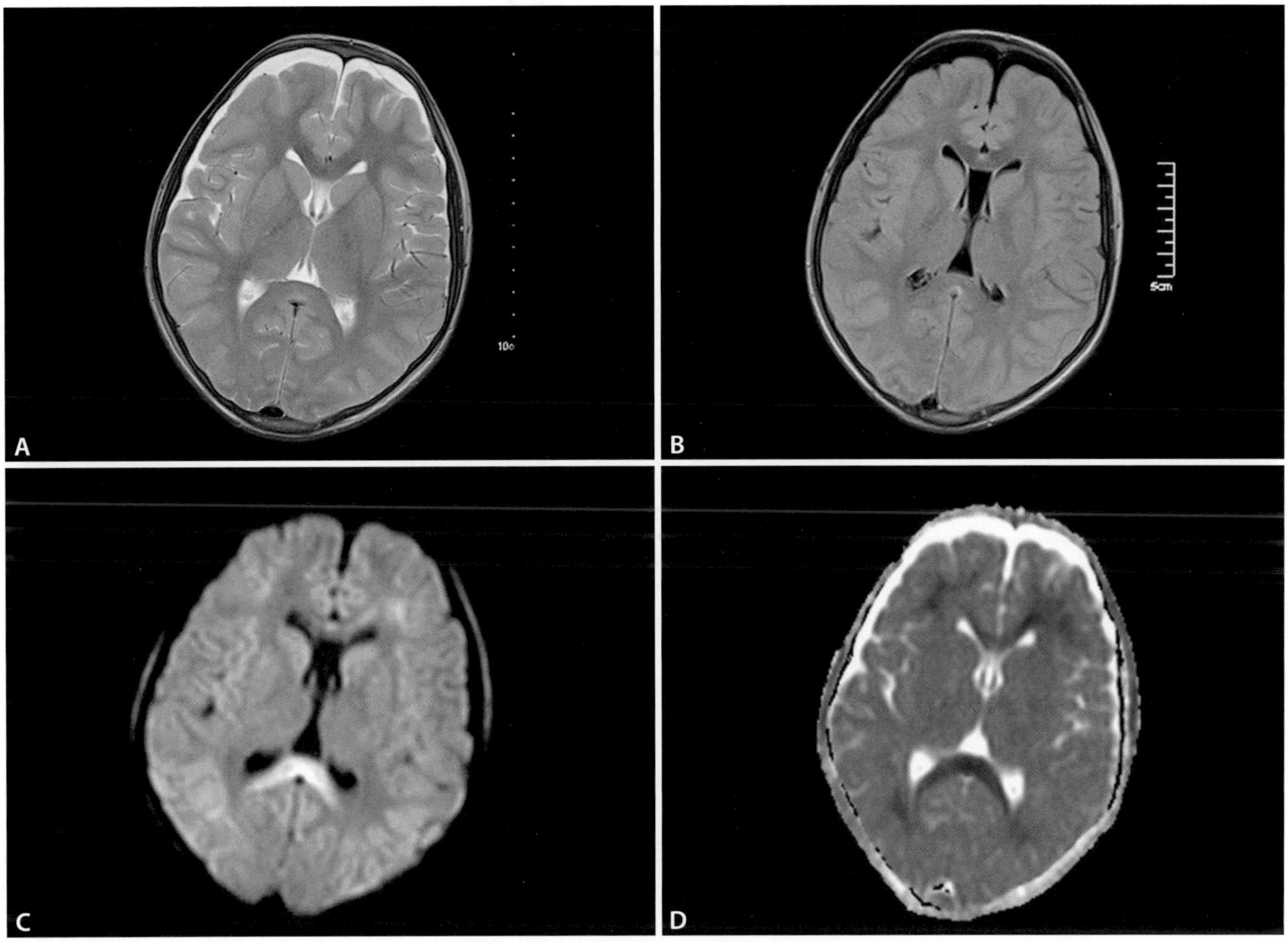

Figs. 17A to D: Axial T2W (A), FLAIR (B), DWI (C) and ADC map (D) showing diffuse axonal injury involving the splenium of corpus callosum.

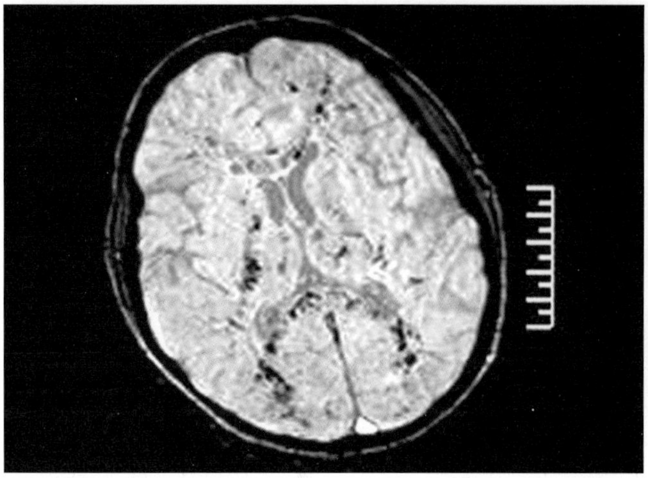

Fig. 18: FLASH MR image showing multiple foci of hemorrhages involving gray-white matter junctions and corpus callosum with blooming effect suggestive of diffuse axonal injury.

Secondary Head Injury

Diffuse cerebral swelling (edema) results from:

- Increase in cerebral blood volume (hyperemia),
- Vasogenic edema, or
- An increase in tissue fluid (cytotoxic edema).

Imaging features of cerebral edema include effacement of the cerebral sulci and cisterns, compression of the ventricles and loss of gray-white differentiation. The cerebellum and brainstem are usually spared in cerebral edema and may appear hyperdense (On CT) relative to the affected cerebral hemispheres.

Brain herniation occurs secondary to mass effect produced by other causes.

There are three types of herniation:

1. Subfalcine
2. Uncal
3. *Transtentorial*:
   - Descending
   - Ascending

All types of herniation are a serious sign of cerebral injury accompanied by displacement of blood vessels and nerves.

Traumatic Ischmemia–infarction

Infarctions may occur when cerebral swelling leads to transfalcine or transtentorial herniation that compresses the anterior or posterior cerebral arteries respectively. Cerebral ischemia can occur due to regional or global cerebral blood flow changes **(Figs. 19A and B)**.

Spinal Injuries

Spinal injuries in children are rare compared with similar injuries in adults. The prevalence of spinal injuries in children has been reported at less than 10% of all spinal injuries in several studies; however, the mortality rate of craniospinal injury in children is significantly higher than in adults. The cervical spine of young children is fundamentally different from that of adults and the type and outcome of spinal injuries in children also differs from adults.[16]

Anatomic differences in the pediatric cervical spine:[3]

- Relatively larger head size, resulting in greater flexion and extension injuries
- Smaller neck muscle mass with ligamentous injuries more common than fractures
- Increased flexibility of interspinous ligaments
- Infantile bony column can lengthen significantly without rupture
- Flatter facet joints with a more horizontal orientation
- Incomplete ossification making interpretation of bony alignment difficult
- Basilar odontoid synchondrosis fuse at 3 to 7 years of age
- Apical odontoid epiphysis fuse at 5–7 years of age
- Posterior arch of C1 fuses at 4 years of age
- Anterior arch fuses at 7–10 years of age
- Epiphyses of spinous process tips may mimic fractures
- Increased preodontoid space up to 4–5 mm (3 mm in an adult)
- Pseudosubluxation of C2 on C3 seen in 40% of children
- Prevertebral space size may change because of variations with respiration.

Indications for imaging cervical spine:[19,20]

- Midline cervical tenderness
- Altered level of alertness
- Evidence of intoxication
- Focal neurologic deficits
- Presence of a painful distracting injury
- Significant head or facial injury

Indications for thoracolumbar CT:[20]

- Motor vehicle crash at greater than 35 mph
- Falls of greater than 15 feet
- Automobile hitting pedestrian with pedestrian thrown more than 10 feet
- Assaulted with a depressed level of consciousness
- Known cervical injury
- Rigid spine disease

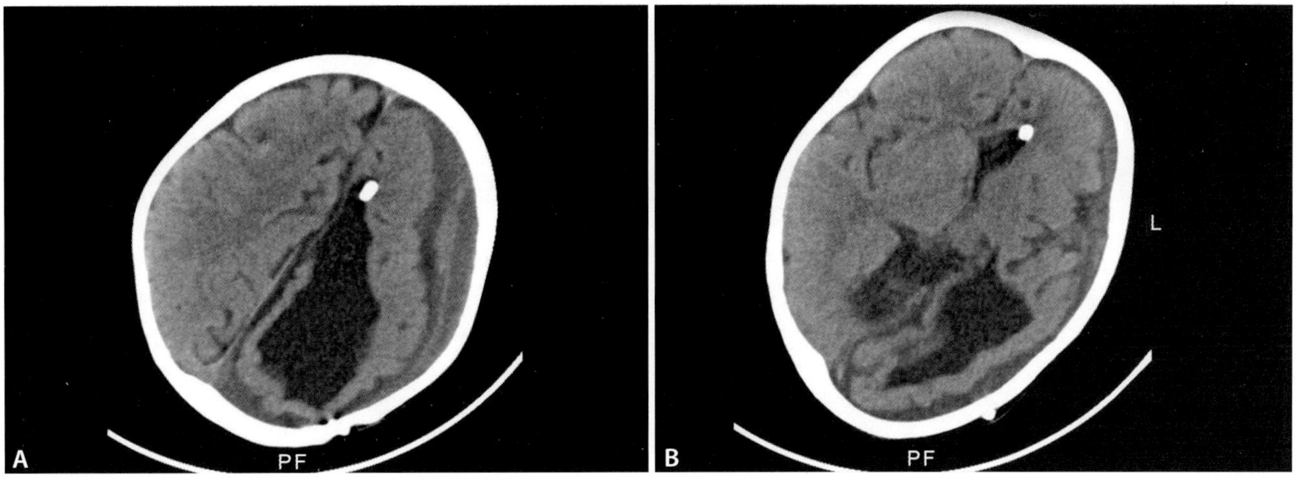

Figs. 19A and B: Axial CT sections of brain showing atrophic changes in left cerebral hemisphere with ex-vacuo ventriculomegaly with VP shunt *in situ* and subdural hygroma, sequelae of post-traumatic brain injury.

One should be very cautious in using these criteria in children younger than 2 years old, and also in children with congenital or acquired abnormalities (e.g. Down syndrome, juvenile rheumatoid arthritis, prior fracture).

When indicated, radiographic evaluation should routinely consist of three views: a cross-table lateral view, an anteroposterior view, and an open-mouth view to help visualize the odontoid process of C1. With these three plain film views of the cervical region, the sensitivity for detecting cervical fractures is 89% and the negative predictive value of these three views adequately done is nearly 100%.

CT with multiplanar reformatting has a crucial role in the assessment of cervical spine injury (CSI). MRI is the investigation of choice in the presence of neurological deficit, or if there is concern for ligamentous injury as it provides direct evaluation of soft tissue abnormalities such as cord compression/contusion, hematoma, disk herniation and ligament disruption.

Types of cervical spine injuries:[16]

- Spinal cord injury without radiographic abnormality (SCIWORA), **(Figs. 20A and B)**
- Occiput–C1 injury
- Atlantoaxial injuries **(Figs. 21A and B)**
- Traumatic spondylolisthesis of C2 (Hangman fracture)
- Subaxial injuries (C3–C7)
- Posterior ligamentous injuries
- Wedge compression fractures
- Facet dislocations

Spinal Cord Injury Without Radiological Abnormality (SCIWORA) is almost unique to the pediatric population and occurs as a consequence of a stretch or distraction injury to the relatively flexible spinal column that exceeds the tensile limits of the spinal cord. Because of increased musculoskeletal elasticity which serves to dissipate the kinetic energy transferred to the child's body during trauma thus preventing fracture or dislocation is not shared by the spinal cord, which may lead to the occurrence of spinal cord injury without radiological abnormality. There is another hypothesis that SCIWORA results from ischemia due to direct vessel injury or due to hypoperfusion of the spinal cord parenchyma.[16]

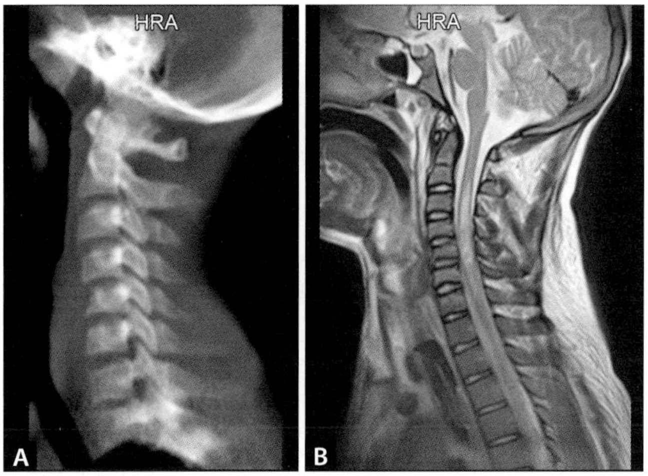

Figs. 20A and B: Lateral radiograph of cervical spine (A) and sagittal T2W MR image (B) showing evidence of cord contusion without any obvious visible radiographic abnormality suggestive of SCIWORA.

MRI can demonstrate a variety of neural and extraneural findings. The neural findings vary from cord

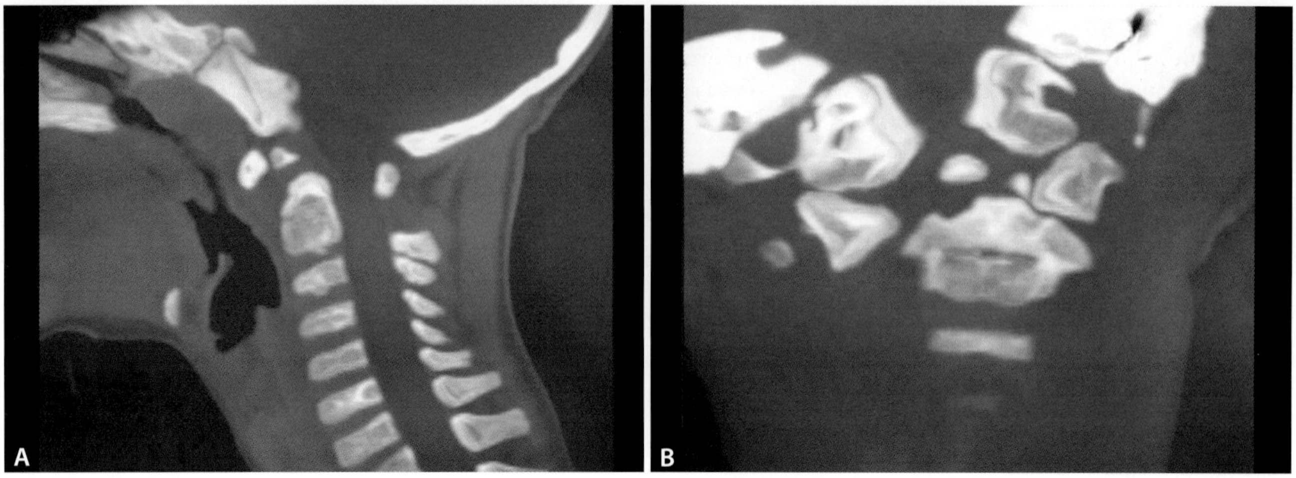

Figs. 21A and B: Sagittal MPR (A) and coronal thick MIP (B) images showing type1 fracture of dense of C2 vertebra and atlanto-occipital subluxation.

edema, minor or major hemorrhage, to complete cord transection. The extraneural findings are more useful for assessing the stability of the spinal column and include ligamentous disruption, edema or hemorrhage in the paraspinal muscles, disk edema or herniation, or epidural/subdural hematomas.

Thoracic and Lumbar Spine Trauma

Approximately, 30% of all spinal injury in children occurs in the thoracic region and 17–28% of spinal injury is seen in lumbar vertebrae. The most frequent fracture in the thoracolumbar spine is vertebral body compression fracture **(Figs. 22A and B)**, almost invariably due to a fall. Anterior wedging is seen on a radiograph. CT is essential to fully demonstrate the fracture extent.[16]

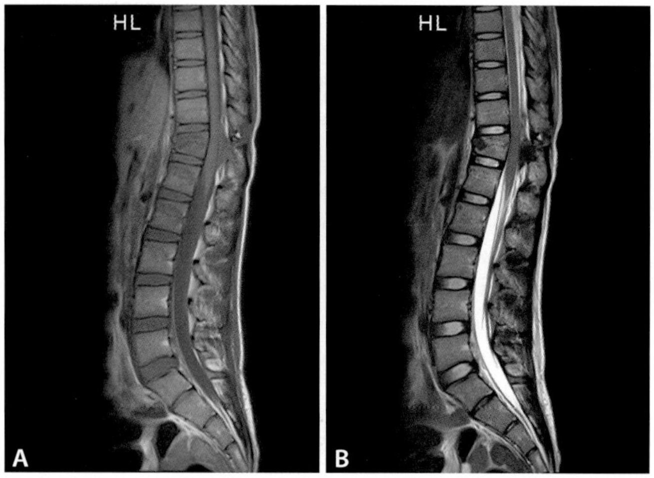

Figs. 22A and B: Sagittal T1W (A) and T2W MR (B) images showing wedge compression fracture of D12 vertebral body with epidural hematoma. Cord shows normal signal intensity.

Normal radiographic parameters and variants: There are several normal anatomical variants that may be encountered during imaging of the pediatric cervical spine[16]

- The atlanto-dens interval (ADI) is defined as the distance between the anterior aspect of the dens and the posterior aspect of the anterior ring of the atlas. This distance should be 5 mm or less in children. An ADI that exceeds 5 mm in lateral flexion and 4 mm in lateral extension indicates instability and is suspicious for ligamentous disruption.
- Pseudospread of the atlas on the axis (pseudo-Jefferson fracture) can be seen on anterior open-mouth radiographs. Up to 6 mm of displacement of the lateral masses relative to the dens is common in patients up to 4 years old and may be seen in patients up to 7 years old.
- *Pseudosubluxation:* In children, it is seen most commonly at the C2–3 level, but can also be seen at the C3–4 level. This can be differentiated from true subluxation by the posterior cervical line described by Swischuk. The posterior cervical line is drawn along the posterior arches of C1 and C3, and in normal children the posterior arch of C2 lies within 1.5 mm of the posterior cervical line. An abnormal posterior cervical line measurement often indicates the presence of a bilateral pars interarticularis ('Hangman fracture') of C2.
- The absence of lordosis, although potentially pathologic in an adult, can be seen in children up to 16 years of age, when the neck is in a neutral position.

- *Posterior interspinous distance:* It is a good indicator of ligamentous integrity and should not be more than 1.5 times greater than the interspinous distance one level either above or below the level in question.
- *Vertebral body wedging:* In early infancy, cervical vertebral bodies have an oval appearance. These vertebrae take on a more rectangular appearance with advancing age. Anterior wedging of up to 3 mm of the vertebral bodies should not be confused with compression fracture.
- *Retropharyngeal soft tissue buckling:* In pediatric patients, widening of the prevertebral soft tissues can be a normal finding that is related to expiration. When lateral radiography of the cervical spine in an infant with possible spinal injury shows wide prevertebral soft tissues, repeat lateral radiography in mild extension and in inspiration should be performed to determine, if the apparent soft-tissue abnormality is real.

CONCLUSION

Imaging in pediatric trauma must use specific techniques with adapted protocols and algorithms taking the child's specific conditions into consideration. These differ from standard adult imaging strategies and protocols.

REFERENCES

1. Jaffe D. Emergency management of blunt trauma in children. N Engl J Med 1991; 324:1477–82.
2. Miniño A, Heron M, Smith B, et al. Deaths: final data for 2004. National vital statistics reports. Hyattsville (MD). National Center for Health Statistics, 2007.
3. Marx JA, Holberger RS. Rosen's emergency medicine: Concepts and clinical practice, 5th edition. Mosby. 2002. pp.267–81.
4. Kao SC, Smith WL. Skeletal injuries in the pediatric patient. Radiol Clin North Am. 1997;35:727-46.
5. Resnik CS. Diagnostic imaging of pediatric skeletal trauma. Radiol Clin North Am. 1989;27:1013-22.
6. Kellenberger CJ. Imaging children: What is special? Ther Umsch. 2009;66(1):55-9. Review.
7. AL Baert, et al. Imaging in Pediatric Skeletal Trauma: Techniques and Applications, 1st edition. Springer. 2008. pp.1-11
8. Soudack M, Epelman M, Maor R, et al. Experience with Focused Abdominal Sonography for Trauma (FAST) in 313 pediatric patients. Journal of Clinical Ultrasound. 2004;32:53–61.
9. Westra SJ, Wallace EC. Imaging evaluation of pediatric chest trauma. Radiol Clin North Am. 2005; 43(2):267-81. Review.
10. Sanchez TR, Jadhav SP, Swischuk LE. MR imaging of pediatric trauma. Magn Reson Imaging Clin N Am. 2009;17(3):439-50.Review.
11. Stanescu LA, Gross JA, Bittle M, et al. Imaging of blunt abdominal trauma. Semin Roentgenol. 2006;41(3):196–208.
12. Saladino RA, Lund DP. Abdominal trauma. In: Fleisher GR, Ludwig S, Henretig FM, et al. Textbook of Pediatric Emergency medicine, 5th edition. Philadelphia: Lippincott. Williams & Wilkins. 2006.pp.1339-48.
13. Rose JS. Ultrasound in abdominal trauma. Emerg Med Clin North Am. 2004; 22(3):581-9.
14. Bixby SD, Callahan MJ, Taylor GA. Imaging in pediatric blunt abdominal trauma. Semin Roentgenol. 2008; 43(1):72-82.
15. Hussain, Barnes. Pediatric Skeletal Trauma—Plain Film to MRI: Imaging Techniques. Applied Radiology. 2007; 36(8):24-33.
16. Cakmakci H. Essentials of trauma: Head and spine. Pediatr Radiol. 2009; 39 (Suppl 3):391-405.
17. Zimmerman RA, Bilaniuk LT. Pediatric head trauma. Neuroimaging Clin N Am. 1994;4:349-66.
18. Schutzman SA, Greenes DS. Pediatric minor head trauma. Ann Emerg Med. 2001;37:65-74.
19. Daffner RH. Controversies in cervical spine imaging in trauma patients. Semin Musculoskelet Radiol. 2005; 9(2):105-15.
20. Daffner RH, Hackney DB. ACR Appropriateness criteria on suspected spine trauma. J Am Coll Radiol. 2007;4(11):762-75.

CHAPTER 130

Neonatal Respiratory Distress

Akshay Kumar Saxena, Kushaljit Singh Sodhi

INTRODUCTION

A newborn is considered neonate till the age of 28 postnatal days. Respiratory distress constitutes the most common morbidity requiring admission of a neonate in an intensive care unit (ICU). Respiratory distress is defined by presence of at least two of the following three features:[1]

1. Tachypnea (respiratory rate > 60 per minute)
2. Retractions (intercostal, subcostal, sternal or suprasternal)
3. Noisy respiration (grunt, stridor or wheeze).

Respiratory distress occurs in 11–14% of all live births.[2] Gestational age has pronounced effect on incidence of neonatal respiratory distress with incidence of respiratory distress on first day of life being higher in babies born at lesser gestation. Kumar et al. reported 60% incidence of respiratory distress in babies less than 30 weeks of gestational age which reduced to 5–6% in babies with gestational age more than 34 weeks.[2] There are several causes which can give rise to respiratory distress during the neonatal period. They can broadly be classified as follows:[3]

- *Causes affecting respiration at alveolar level:* Hyaline membrane disease (HMD), pneumonia, meconium aspiration syndrome, pneumothorax, pulmonary hemorrhage, primary pulmonary hypertension, transient tachypnea of newborn (TTNB), etc.
- *Structural anomalies of the respiratory tract:* Congenital lobar emphysema (CLE), congenital caustic adenomatoid malformation (CCAM), congenital diaphragmatic hernia (CDH), choanal atresia, tracheoesophageal fistula (TEF), etc.
- *Extrapulmonary causes:* Chest wall abnormalities, congenital heart disease, metabolic acidosis, etc.

The management of neonatal respiratory distress depends upon clinical history, examination, radiology and laboratory data. The radiology of important causes of respiratory distress in neonatal period is discussed in this chapter.

MEDICAL CAUSES OF NEONATAL RESPIRATORY DISTRESS

Hyaline Membrane Disease

Hyaline membrane disease, also known as respiratory distress syndrome (RDS), constitutes the most common cause of respiratory distress in the premature newborn infant accounting for up to 60% incidence in babies born at or before 29 weeks of gestation.[4] It is a manifestation of pulmonary immaturity and results from impaired surfactant production by type 2 pneumocytes leading to formation of hyaline membranes within alveoli and terminal airways, hence the name. Oxygen therapy along with surfactant supplementation currently forms the cornerstone of treatment for HMD. Persistent barotraumas and oxygen toxicity in these neonates, due to intensive oxygen and ventilation therapy, can lead to bronchopulmonary dysplasia (BPD).[5]

The radiological evaluation of HMD has traditionally relied upon chest radiography. The radiographic findings in untreated HMD reflect the generalized acinar collapse that results from surfactant deficiency. Chest radiograph features in these neonates demonstrate decreased expansion of lungs, symmetric generalized consolidation of variable severity, effacement of normal pulmonary vessels and air bronchograms **(Figs. 1A and B)**.[6] The commonly seen "reticulogranular" pattern of lung opacities in HMD represents the summation of collapsed alveoli, transudation of fluid into the interstitium from capillary leak and distension by air of innumerable bronchioles that are more compliant than surfactant deficient lung. This radiographic picture reaches maximum severity around 12–24 hours of life. In severe cases, there may be complete bilateral "whiteout" of lungs due to extensive consolidation.[7]

The radiographic findings of HMD also depend on the timing of the administration of surfactant. Early on, despite prevention with surfactant, the lungs are hypoaerated and have a reticulogranular pattern due to interstitial fluid and atelectatic alveoli. The administration of surfactant usually produces some clearing **(Figs. 2A and B)**, which may be symmetrical or asymmetrical; the asymmetry usually disappears in 2–5 days. Since the surfactant is not evenly distributed throughout the lungs, areas of improving lung alternating with areas of unchanged RDS are common findings.[8]

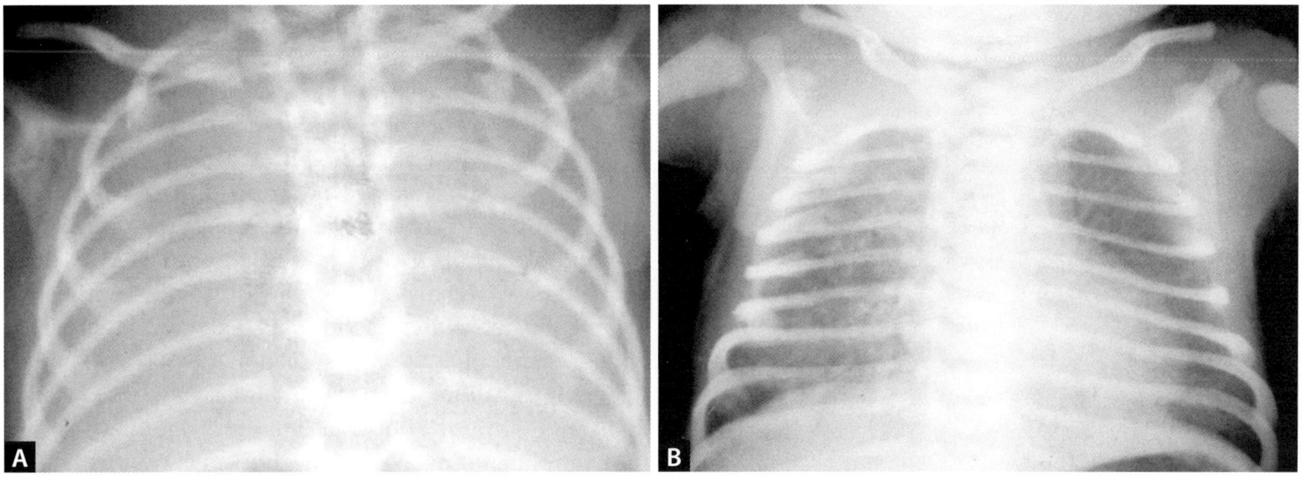

Figs. 1A and B: (A) Chest X-ray AP view of a preterm neonate with respiratory distress soon after birth reveals low volume lungs with bilateral consolidation with "whiteout" of lungs suggestive of hyaline membrane disease (HMD); (B) In another preterm neonate with respiratory distress soon after birth, consolidation is less extensive.

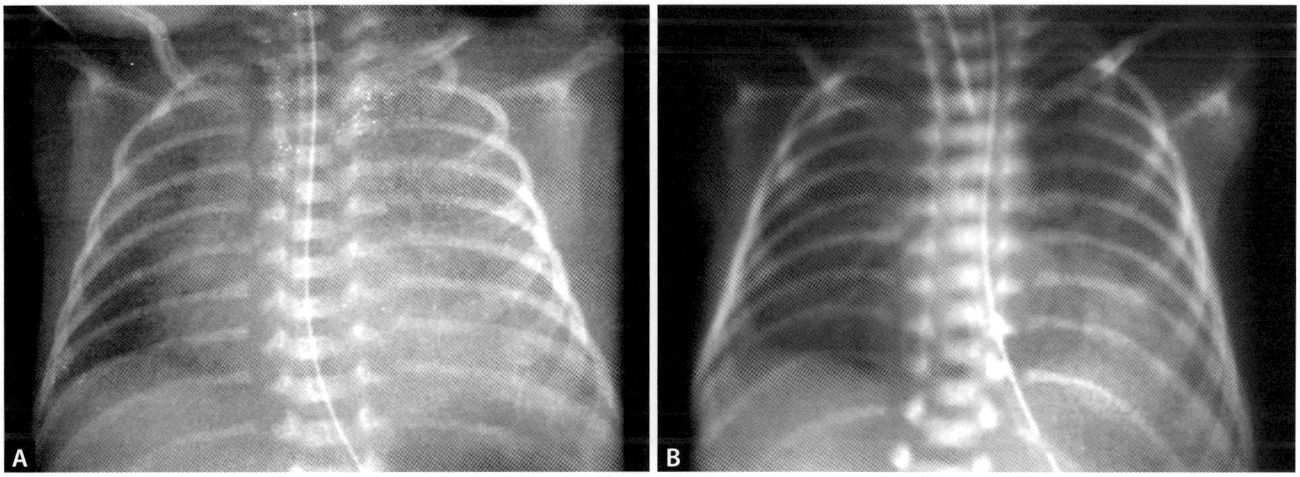

Figs. 2A and B: (A) Chest X-ray AP view of a preterm neonate with respiratory distress soon after birth reveals low volume lungs with bilateral consolidation with "whiteout" of lungs suggestive of hyaline membrane disease (HMD); (B) 18 hours after surfactant administration, there is asymmetric clearing of upper zones.

With positive-pressure ventilation usually given in these infants, the lung opacity decreases, and they appear radiographically improved. However, the positive pressure required to aerate the lungs can disrupt the epithelium, producing interstitial and alveolar edema. It can also cause the dissection of air into the interlobar septae and their lymphatics, producing pulmonary interstitial emphysema (PIE) **(Fig. 3)**. Radiographically, PIE appears as tortuous, 1–4 mm linear lucencies that are relatively uniform in size and radiate outwards from the pulmonary hilum. The lucencies do not empty on expiration and extend to the periphery of the lungs.[9] PIE can be symmetrical, asymmetrical, or localized to one portion of a lung. Peripheral PIE can produce subpleural blebs which can rupture into pleural space to produce pneumothorax or can extend centrally to produce pneumomediastinum or pneumopericardium.

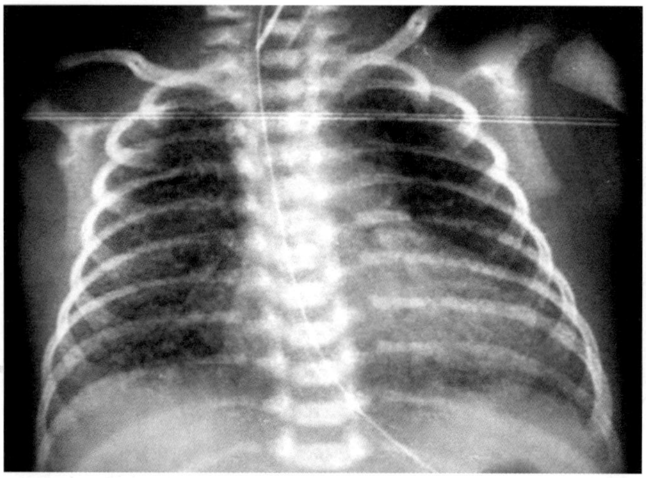

Fig. 3: Follow-up chest X-ray of a patient of hyaline membrane disease (HMD) reveals lucent lesions suggestive of pulmonary interstitial emphysema (PIE).

Since, portable chest radiography imparts ionizing radiation and involves delay in availability of information to the clinician, alternative strategies in evaluation of HMD are desirable. A few studies have evaluated use of sonography in diagnosis of HMD.[10,11] Using the transabdominal approach for visualization of lung bases, these studies reported a typical pattern of increased retrodiaphragmatic hyperechogenicity which has high sensitivity and specificity for diagnosis of HMD **(Figs. 4A and B)**. Another study by Copetti et al.[12] tried transthoracic approach for evaluation of HMD. They suggested that a combination of whiteout lung, absence of areas of sparing and pleural line abnormalities to be 100% sensitive and specific for diagnosis of RDS.

Sonography has also been used for follow-up of HMD and early prediction of BPD in neonates suffering from HMD.[13,14] In these studies, the incomplete clearance of retrodiaphragmatic hyperechogenicity was found to be a good predictor of later development of BPD. Avni and colleagues[13] suggested that day 18 was the earliest day where the persistence of the abnormal retrodiaphragmatic hyperechogenicity was observed in 100% of the patients developing BPD at day 28. At that time, 95.2% of the patients without abnormal hyperechogenicity showed uncomplicated evolution and no BPD. They concluded that sonography can be a useful diagnostic tool to determine the occurrence of BPD and to predict as

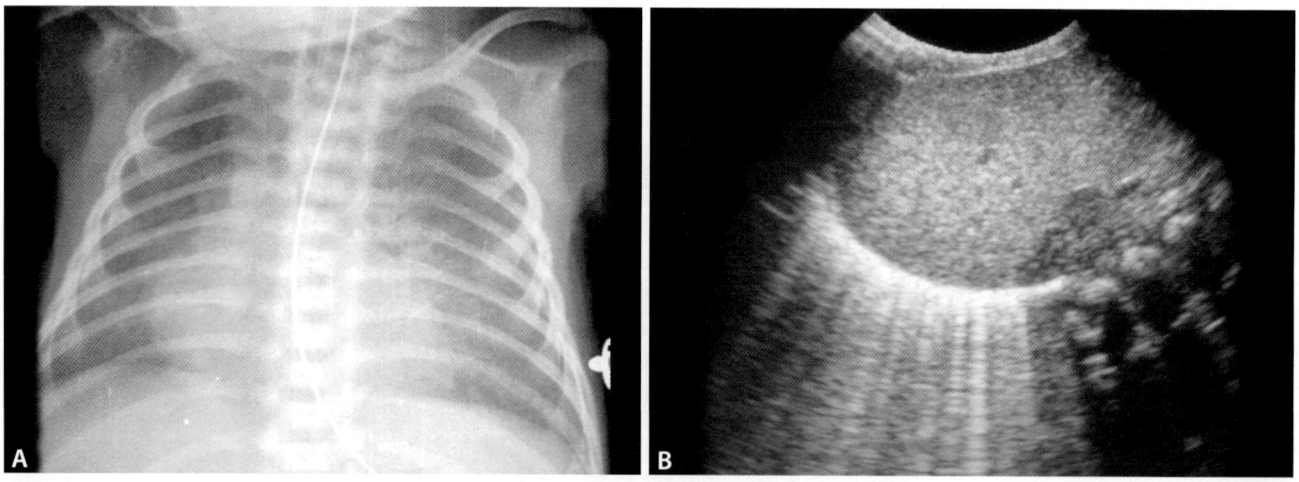

Figs. 4A and B: (A) Chest X-ray AP view of a preterm neonate with respiratory distress soon after birth reveals low volume lungs with bilateral consolidation with "whiteout" of lungs suggestive of hyaline membrane disease (HMD); (B) Coronal transabdominal sonography reveals diffuse retrodiaphragmatic hyperechogenicity suggestive of HMD.

early as day 18 the premature at risk for the disease. In another similar study, Pieper et al.[14] reported that day 9 was the earliest day where persistence of abnormal retrodiaphragmatic hyperechogenicity was observed with the highest predictor values for the development of BPD. These preliminary studies suggest that sonography has a role in early identification of neonates who are at risk of developing BPD in future. However, there is some discrepancy regarding the exact postnatal age at which this can be achieved.

Transient Tachypnea of Newborn

Whereas HMD is a disease of premature neonates, transient tachypnea of newborn (TTNB) affects term babies. In the fetal life, the lungs are distended with fluid. This fluid is cleared from the lungs during the squeeze through the birth canal while additional fluid is removed by pulmonary capillaries and lymphatics. The delay in clearance of pulmonary fluid leads to TTNB which is also known as "wet lung disease". The risk factors include delivery by cesarean section; precipitous delivery; and very small, hypotonic or sedated babies. The babies present with mild or moderate respiratory distress soon after birth.[15] Typically, the disease is self-limiting with resolution of symptoms in 6–24 hours. Uncommonly, the symptoms may last 2–5 days when it becomes necessary to exclude alternative causes of respiratory distress.[3]

The radiographic features of TTNB include mild overaeration, mild cardiomegaly, small pulmonary effusion and prominent perihilar interstitial markings **(Fig. 5)**. TTNB may mimic reticulogranular pattern of HMD but lacks the underaeration seen in HMD. The radiographic features may occasionally look similar to pulmonary edema or meconium aspiration syndrome.[15]

Copetti and Cattarossi[16] have recently evaluated the lung sonographic findings in TTNB and its clinical relevance. They reported that in neonates with TTNB, lung sonography revealed difference in lung echogenicity between the upper and lower lung areas. There were very compact comet-tail artifacts in the inferior lung fields which were rare in the superior lung fields. They designated this finding the "double lung point". In this study, "double lung point" was not seen in healthy infants, infants with RDS, atelectasis, pneumothorax, pneumonia, or pulmonary hemorrhage. Thus, the sensitivity and specificity of the "double lung point" was 100% for the diagnosis of TTNB. However, a recent report suggests that "double lung point" may be seen in pneumothorax as well.[17]

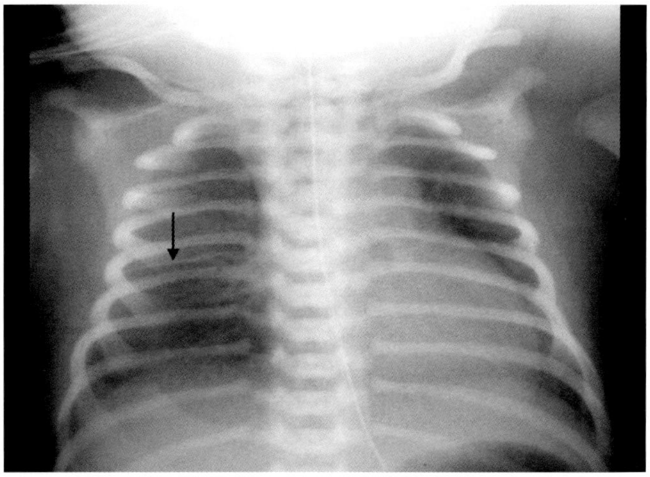

Fig. 5: Transient tachypnea of newborn: Chest X-ray of a term neonate born by cesarean section and respiratory distress soon after birth reveals normal volume lungs with perihilar infiltrates, prominent cardiac silhouette and pleural fluid in minor fissure (arrow).

Neonatal Pneumonia

Pneumonia is an important cause of neonatal respiratory distress in India with all cases of neonatal respiratory distress being treated as pneumonia at the first referral unit.[18] In a recent study which evaluated the causes of respiratory distress in outborn neonates brought to a referral unit, Mathur et al.[18] reported pneumonia to be the cause of respiratory distress in more than two-thirds of cases. However, this study did not include patients having surgical causes of respiratory distress. The pneumonia may set in due to transplacental spread, lack of asepsis during delivery, aspiration of amniotic fluid or be acquired during hospital stay for other ailments. Ventilator associated pneumonia is the second most common hospital-acquired infection among pediatric and neonatal ICU patients,[19,20] and is responsible for a very high mortality in neonatal ICU patients. The majority of cases are of bacterial etiology.

Radiographically, pneumonia is characterized by pulmonary opacities **(Fig. 6)**. However, similar appearance may be seen in hyaline membrane disease, transient tachypnea of newborn and meconium aspiration syndrome. Presence of pleural effusion is a helpful pointer towards pneumonia. Furthermore, some of these conditions may coexist with pneumonia.[15] The patients with positive radiograph who do not grow causative organism from blood culture are considered "probable pneumonia".[21] It is important to note that in some of the patients with pneumonia, chest X-ray may be normal and diagnosis is made on isolation of organism from blood culture.[18] Rarely, pneumonia may mimic mass lesion **(Figs. 7A to D)**.

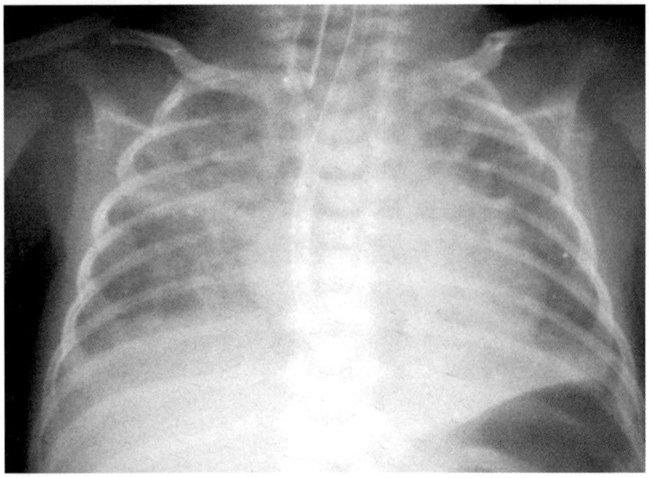

Fig. 6: Chest X-ray AP view of a neonate on ventilator with respiratory distress reveals patchy consolidation in right lung suggestive of pneumonia.

Meconium Aspiration Syndrome

Meconium aspiration is a disease predominantly affecting term and postmature neonates. While, 10–15% of neonates pass meconium in utero, it is rare before 37 weeks.[21] Fetus manifests normal shallow regular respiratory movements during intrauterine life. Fetal hypoxia stimulates deep gasping respirations. In addition, it also leads to premature passage of meconium in utero. Meconium is sterile but locally irritant. It can cause obstruction of medium and small airways. In addition, it is a good medium for bacterial growth. The severity of meconium aspiration syndrome depends on several factors including consistency of meconium, adequacy of oropharyngeal suction, associated asphyxia, resuscitative measures, etc.

The radiographic appearance in meconium aspiration is variable **(Figs. 8A and B)**. Incomplete bronchial

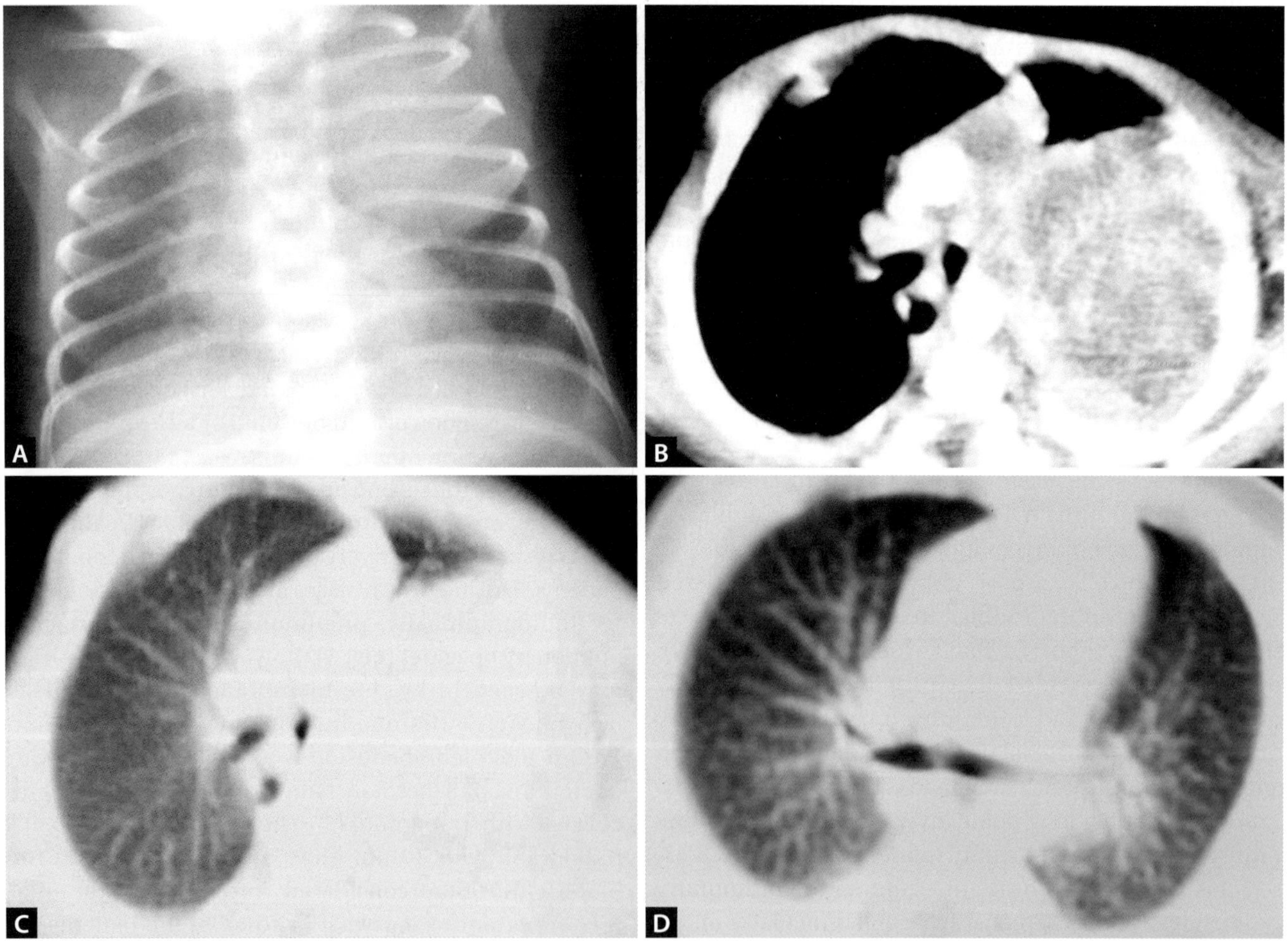

Figs. 7A to D: Pneumonia mimicking mass lesion: (A) Chest X-ray AP view of a 3-week-old male child with fever and respiratory distress reveals mass like opacity in left upper zone; (B) Mediastinal; and (C) Lung window of contrast-enhanced computed tomography (CECT) scan confirm mass-like consolidation in left upper lobe; (D) Lung window of repeat CECT scan after 4 weeks of antibiotics reveals resolution of opacity.

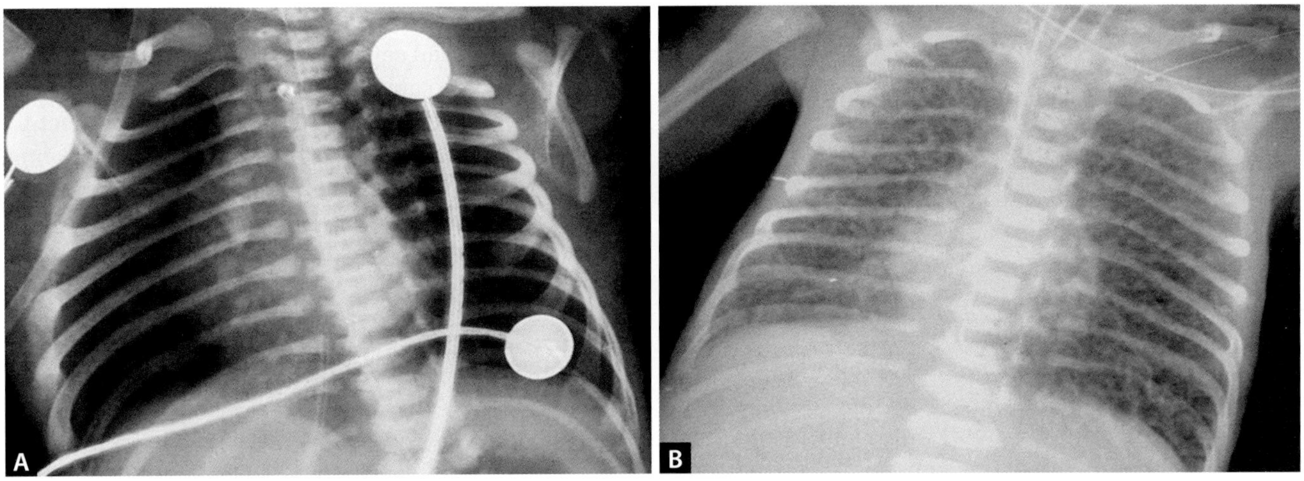

Figs. 8A and B: (A) Term neonate with meconium aspiration. Chest X-ray AP view reveals bilateral hyperinflation; (B) In another neonate with respiratory distress and suspected meconium aspiration, chest X-ray AP view reveals bilateral pulmonary opacities. Pulmonary opacities in meconium aspiration may be due to atelectasis, chemical pneumonitis or super added pneumonia.

obstruction leads to generalized overaeration along with patchy areas of atelectasis secondary to complete bronchial obstruction. There may be subsequent development of pneumothorax and pneumomediastinum. The radiographic appearance may be further complicated by pulmonary edema (because of cerebral, myocardial or renal dysfunction secondary to ischemia), pulmonary hemorrhage, RDS or pneumonia.[15] Some of the babies with meconium aspiration may eventually develop persistent pulmonary hypertension of newborn.[3]

Pneumothorax

Pneumothorax, defined as presence of air in the pleural cavity, is an uncommon but significant cause of neonatal respiratory distress.[18,22] Timely identification can be lifesaving. It can occur spontaneously or be secondary to infection, meconium aspiration, ventilation barotraumas **(Fig. 9)** or lung deformity. The incidence of spontaneous pneumothorax is more in premature babies (about 6%) as compared to term babies (1–2%). The radiographic diagnosis of pneumothorax, although of great clinical significance, can be missed on the X-rays as apicolateral accumulation of air is rather uncommon in the supine films. In the supine position, air preferentially accumulates in anteromedial and subpulmonic recesses.[23] The position of air collection is also modified by underlying lung disease. Subpulmonic pneumothorax presents as a relatively lucent region in the left or right upper abdominal quadrant. Sometimes, the only radiographic sign of subpulmonic pneumothorax is deep lateral costophrenic angle (deep sulcus sign).[24]

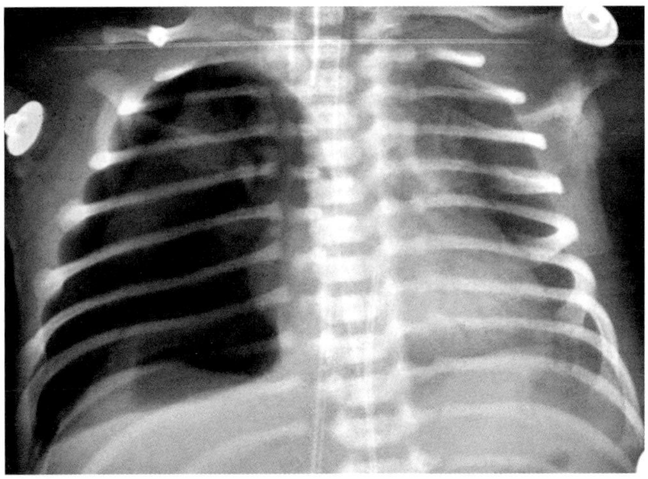

Fig. 9: Neonate on ventilator developed respiratory distress. Chest X-ray AP view revealed gross right pneumothorax.

SURGICAL CAUSES OF NEONATAL RESPIRATORY DISTRESS

Several conditions of neonatal chest require surgical procedure for management. Although listed here as causes of neonatal respiratory distress, it is to be remembered that they may present beyond the neonatal period. In addition, even if discovered during neonatal period, they may be managed conservatively initially. Some of these conditions, like diaphragmatic hernia, can be diagnosed antenatally. Conversely, some of these pathologies may be discovered accidentally in later life and pose dilemma regarding the need for surgery.

Congenital Lobar Emphysema

Congenital lobar emphysema or congenital lobar hyperinflation is a disease of multifactorial origin characterized by focal abnormality of a large airway. Unfortunately, the exact abnormality of large airway frequently remains a mystery as it is left inside the body of the patient proximal to the ligated bronchial stump. However, potential culprits include bronchomalacia, kinks, webs, mucosal webs and crossing vessels. Whatever the etiology may be, the result is impairment of bronchial function and hyperinflation of a pulmonary lobe.[25] Left upper lobe is the most common site of involvement (40–50%) followed by right middle lobe (28–34%) and right upper lobe (20%).[26] The hyperinflated lobe causes mediastinal shift and atelectasis of the adjacent lobes.

Prenatal diagnosis is unusual in congenital lobar emphysema. Postnatally, the age of onset of symptoms and degree of respiratory distress may be variable. However, more than 50% become symptomatic within first week. Not all the symptomatic patients may require immediate surgery.[25,27] The postnatal chest radiograph, if acquired early in life, may reveal overdistended fluid filled lobe. Later on, the radiograph shows characteristic hyperinflation of a lobe with splayed pulmonary vessels, atelectasis of adjacent lobes and contralateral mediastinal shift **(Fig. 10)**. The differential diagnosis is pneumothorax wherein the hyperlucent region will be devoid of pulmonary vascular markings. If required, computed tomography (CT) scan can be performed to resolve the diagnosis. The findings seen on chest X-ray can all be seen on CT scan. CT scan can also reveal treatable extrinsic and intrinsic treatable cause of partial bronchial obstruction.[26]

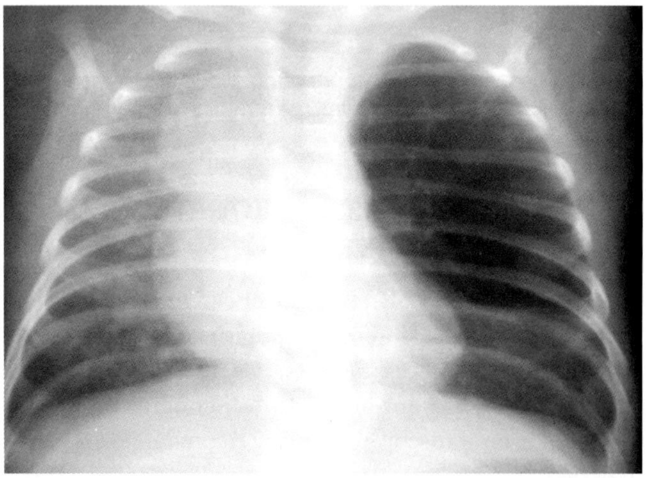

Fig. 10: Chest X-ray AP view of a neonate with respiratory distress reveals emphysematous left upper lobe with contralateral mediastinal shift suggestive of congenital lobar emphysema. Presence of vascular markings differentiate congenital lobar emphysema from pneumothorax.

Uncommonly, the lobar emphysema may affect two lobes. Either the lobes may be affected simultaneously or the second hyperinflated lobe may be detected after first thoracotomy. The bilobectomy procedure may be performed as one stage or two stage procedure.[27]

Congenital Cystic Adenomatoid Malformation

Congenital caustic adenomatoid malformation (CCAM), also called congenital pulmonary airway malformations (CPAM), is a hamartomatous lesion believed to occur because of the failure of pulmonary mesenchyme into normal bronchoalveolar tissue.[15,26] On the basis of pathological findings, Stocker,[28] classified the CCAM into five types. However, radiological classification consists of three types:[26]

1. *Type I:* It constitutes 50% of CCAM patients and shows multiple or single large cysts which communicate with the bronchial tree of the affected lobe.
2. *Type II:* It constitutes 40% of CCAM and shows multiple cysts that rarely exceed 1.2 cm in diameter and communicate with the bronchial tree of the affected lobe. About one-third of these patients have associated congenital anomalies.
3. *Type III:* It is least common type (10% of patients). It consists of multiple small (<0.5 cm) cysts and may appear solid on imaging. It usually causes mass effect on mediastinum.

Antenatal ultrasound may depict CCAM as a pulmonary mass with associated polyhydramnios or fetal anasarca. The disease is usually unilateral with single lobe involvement seen in 95% of patients. Bilateral disease is rare (2%). Neonatal respiratory distress occurs if the CCAM is large and causes mediastinal shift. The cysts may be detected radiographically in 90% of patients[26] and better characterized with CT **(Figs. 11A to D)** which also helps in excluding congenital lobar emphysema as differential diagnosis. It is to be noted that radiological classification of CCAM may not corroborate with pathological classification.[29] When the lesion abuts diaphragm, CDH needs to be excluded. This can be done through contrast study of the gastrointestinal tract. CCAM also needs to be differentiated from pneumatoceles. The diagnosis of pneumatoceles can be made if an earlier normal chest radiograph is available or when subsequent radiographs (or CT scan) show complete resolution of disease. Mesenchymal cystic hamartoma can mimic CCAM

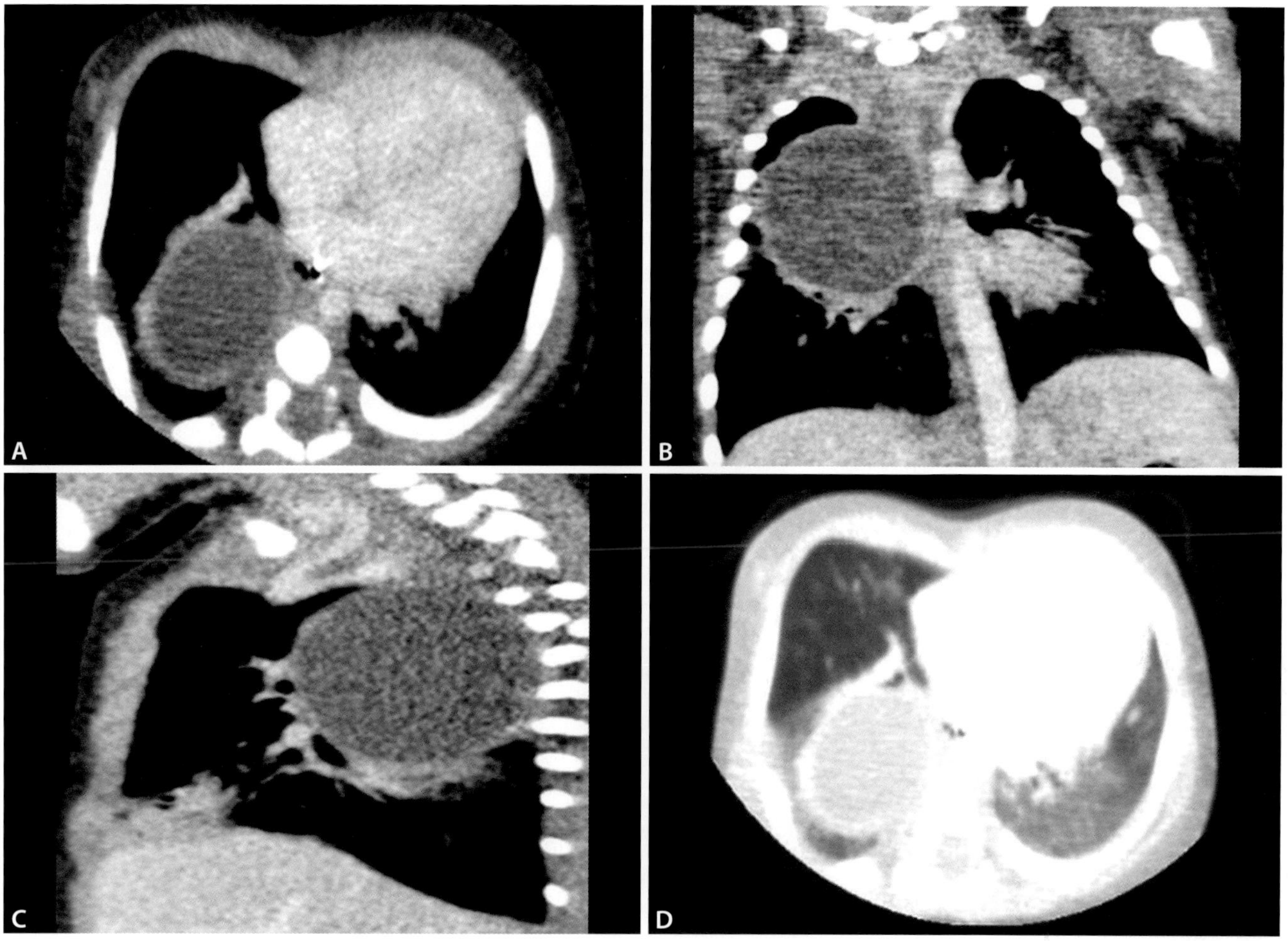

Figs. 11A to D: A 3-day-old neonate with respiratory distress. Mediastinal window of contrast-enhanced computed tomography (CECT) scan—(A) Axial; (B) Coronal reconstruction; and (C) Right parasagittal reconstruction reveal a cystic mass lesion in right upper lobe; (D) Lung window additionally reveals bilateral pneumonia. This lesion can be congenital caustic adenomatoid malformation (CCAM) or bronchogenic cyst. The patient was managed conservatively and is awaiting surgery.

radiographically. Malignant masses may occasionally be seen within CCAM.[30,31]

Congenital Diaphragmatic Hernia

Congenital diaphragmatic hernia signifies intrathoracic herniation of abdominal contents through a defect in the diaphragm. Its incidence varies from 1:2,000 to 1:5,000 in live births. Many fetuses with the diaphragmatic hernia are stillborn. Among the live born, 28–50% may have associated anomalies. The diaphragmatic defect may be located anteromedially (Morgagni hernia) **(Figs. 12A to C)**; posterolaterally (Bochdalek hernia) **(Figs. 13A to C)** or in the central tendon of diaphragm.[26] The condition is being diagnosed increasingly during antenatal ultrasound which facilitates supervised institutional delivery. Bag and mask therapy during neonatal resuscitation may worsen the respiratory distress. Diaphragmatic hernia is accompanied by pulmonary hypoplasia, pulmonary immaturity, hypoplastic left heart and persistent pulmonary artery hypertension of the newborn.[32]

The radiographic appearance depends on the contents of hernia sac and distension of bowel. If radiograph is acquired early, the bowel may be fluid filled or collapse resulting is opacity of variable size in lower hemithorax with contralateral mediastinal shift. Subsequently, air can be identified in the herniated bowel loops making the diagnosis straight forward. However, in some cases, it may need to be differentiated from congenital cystic adenomatoid malformation. This may require a contrast study of the gastrointestinal tract to establish the diagnosis.

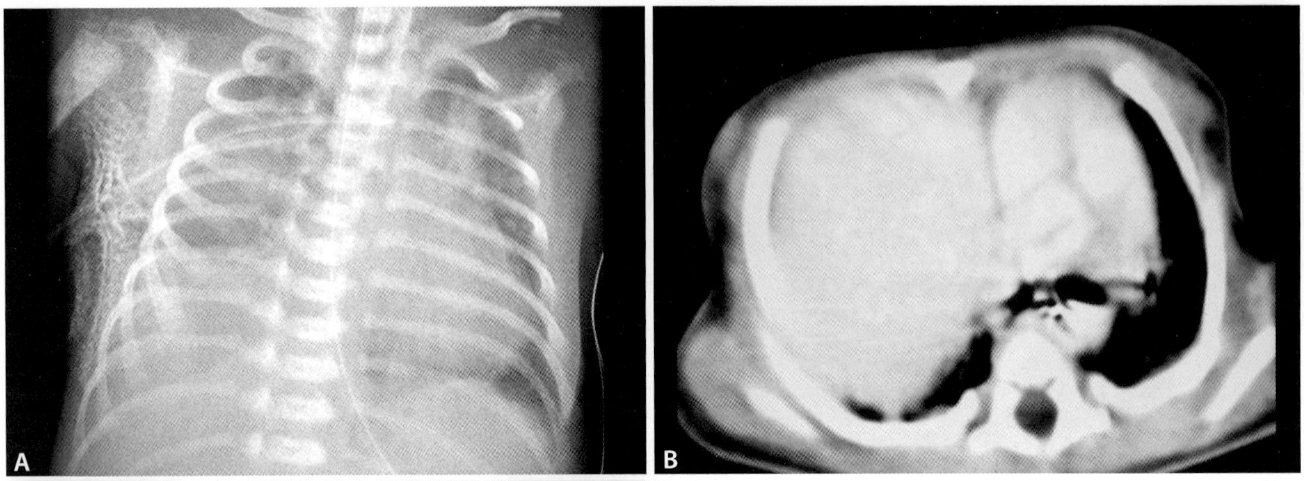

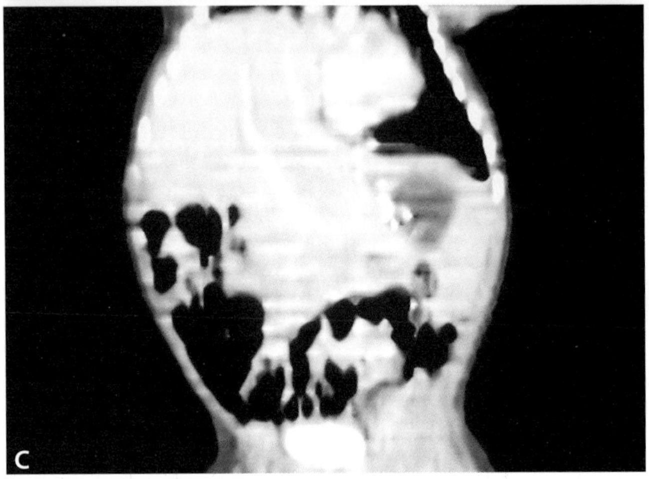

Figs. 12A to C: One-day-old neonate with respiratory distress: (A) Chest X-ray AP view reveals high placed liver, right sided pneumonia and contralateral mediastinal shift. Contrast-enhanced computed tomography (CECT) scan axial (B); and Reconstructed coronal (C) images confirm herniation of liver through foramen of Morgagni.

After the diagnosis of diaphragmatic hernia is established, search should be made for associated congenital malformations using sonography (abdomen and head) and echocardiography.

Esophageal Atresia with Tracheoesophageal Fistula

Although western literature does not consider esophageal atresia with TEF a common cause of neonatal respiratory distress,[22] but a recent Indian study reported it to be the most common cause of neonatal respiratory distress which required admission in neonatal surgical ICU.[33] Esophageal atresia can be diagnosed at birth with the baby pouring out oral secretions. The baby can develop respiratory distress due to aspiration pneumonia as also due to distended stomach. Antenatal sonography may reveal polyhydramnios. Postnatal diagnosis can be made by localizing the "gastric" tube coiled in the upper esophageal pouch **(Fig. 14)**. Small volume of nonionic contrast can be injected through the tube before acquiring the radiograph for better localization.[3,26] However, spillage of contrast may make the situation worse.[33]

MISCELLANEOUS CAUSES

Bronchogenic and esophageal duplication cysts[34] **(Figs. 15A to C)** are congenital lesions which can cause neonatal respiratory distress by virtue of mass effect on surrounding structures or because of superadded pneumonia. If located in mediastinum, CT is required to characterize the lesion and demarcate its size and extent. Careful scrutiny is required to exclude intraspinal communication to exclude neuroenteric cyst. Intrapulmonary bronchogenic cyst is difficult to differentiate radiologically from other congenital cystic lesions.

Some of the congenital cardiac anomalies (e.g. transposition of great arteries) can cause neonatal respiratory distress. Echocardiography and catheter angiography are the mainstay of diagnostic work-up.

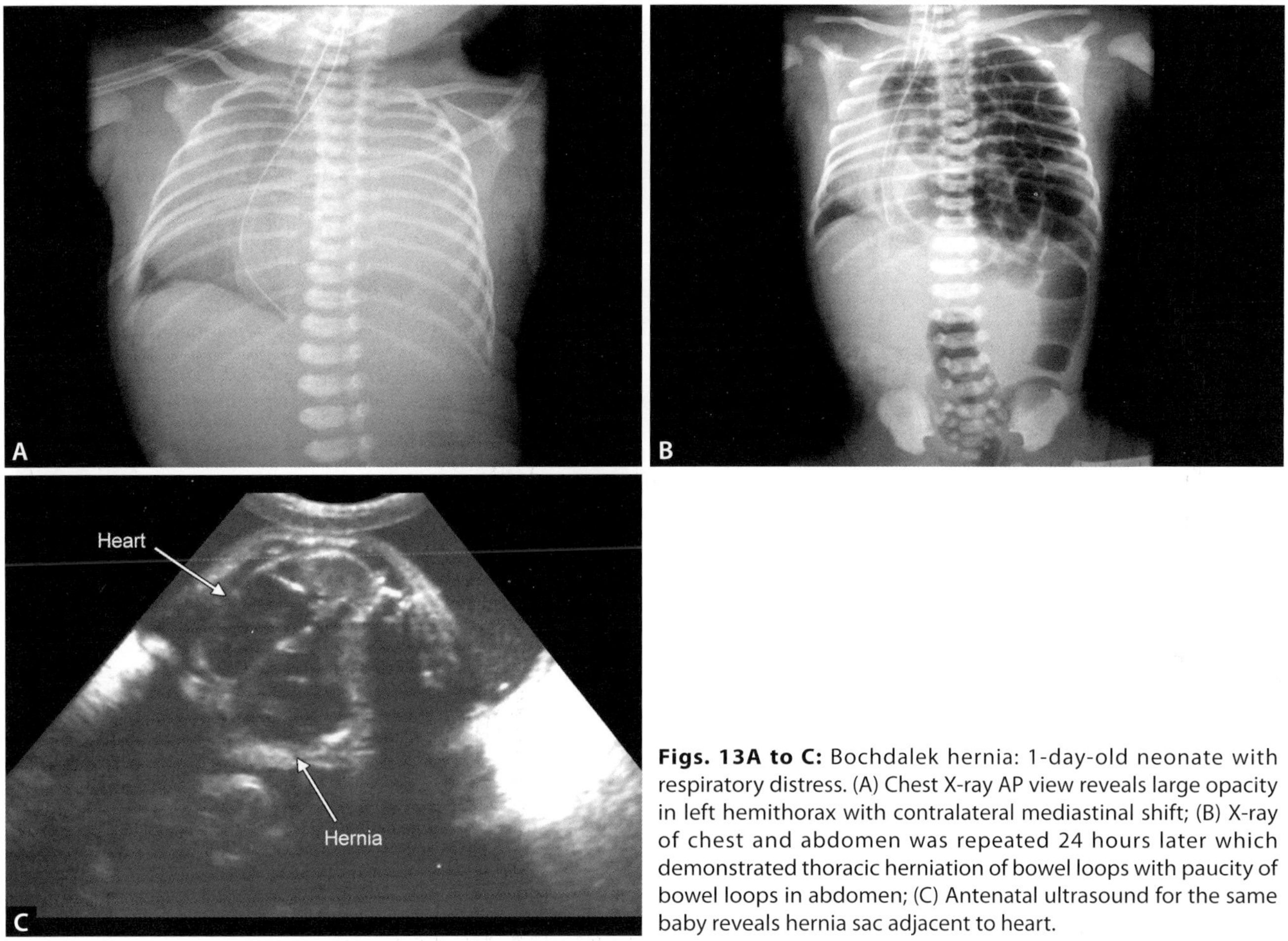

Figs. 13A to C: Bochdalek hernia: 1-day-old neonate with respiratory distress. (A) Chest X-ray AP view reveals large opacity in left hemithorax with contralateral mediastinal shift; (B) X-ray of chest and abdomen was repeated 24 hours later which demonstrated thoracic herniation of bowel loops with paucity of bowel loops in abdomen; (C) Antenatal ultrasound for the same baby reveals hernia sac adjacent to heart.

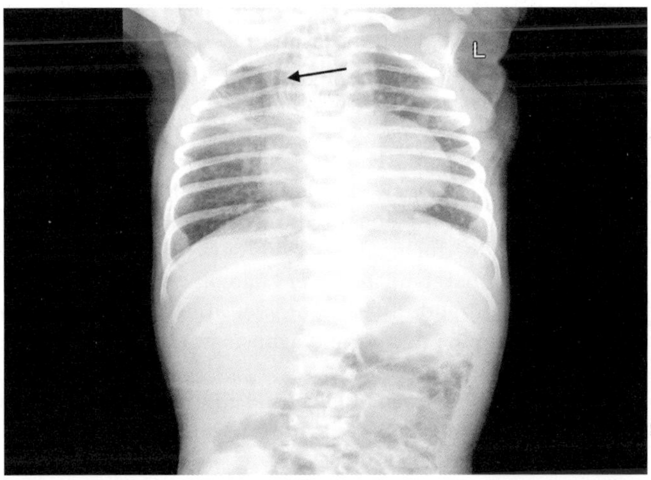

Fig. 14: A 1-day-old neonate with respiratory distress and pooling of saliva. Chest X-ray AP view reveals coiling of nasogastric tube in upper esophageal pouch (arrow) suggestive of esophageal atresia. Presence of air in abdomen confirms the presence of tracheoesophageal fistula.

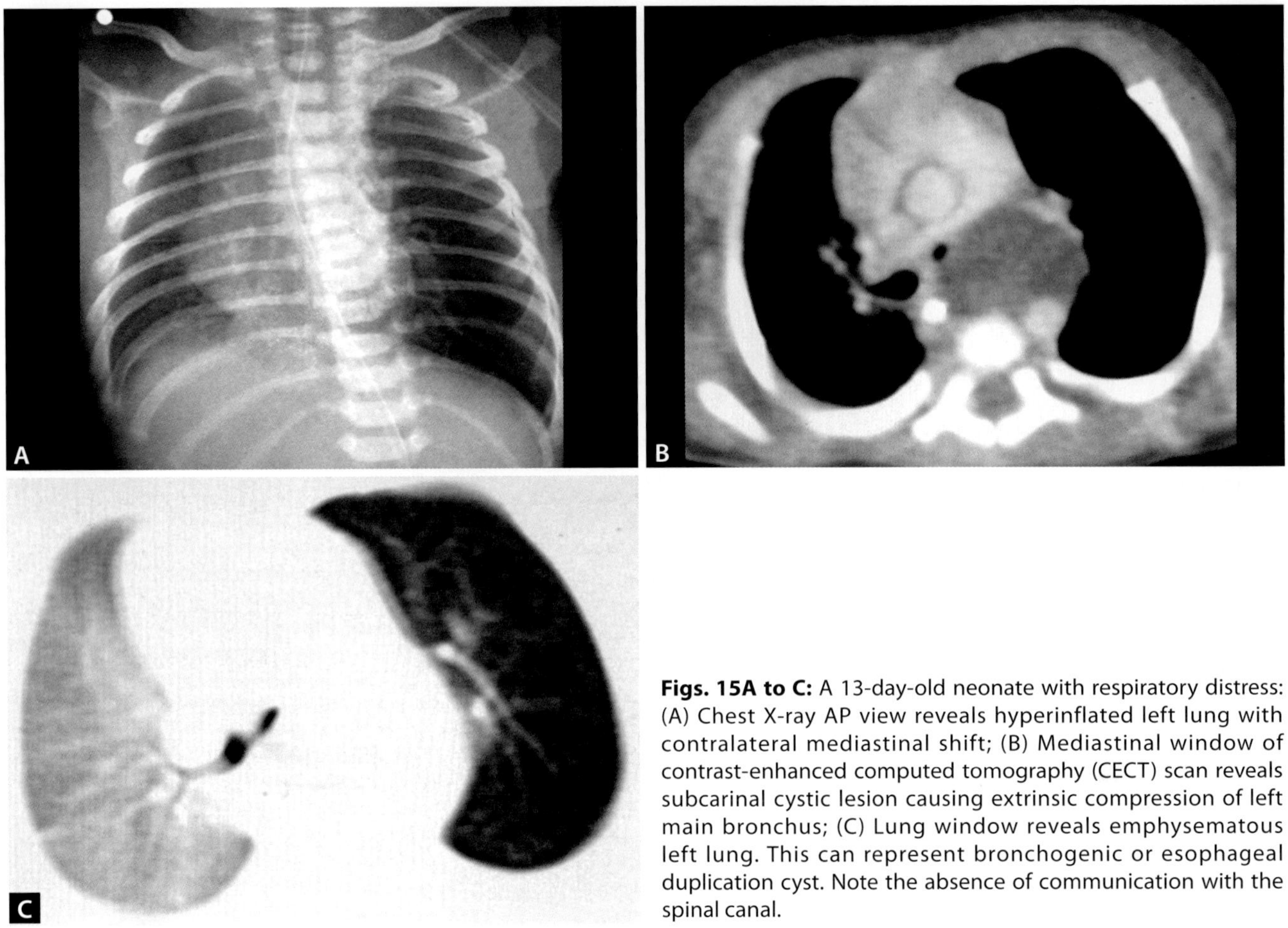

Figs. 15A to C: A 13-day-old neonate with respiratory distress: (A) Chest X-ray AP view reveals hyperinflated left lung with contralateral mediastinal shift; (B) Mediastinal window of contrast-enhanced computed tomography (CECT) scan reveals subcarinal cystic lesion causing extrinsic compression of left main bronchus; (C) Lung window reveals emphysematous left lung. This can represent bronchogenic or esophageal duplication cyst. Note the absence of communication with the spinal canal.

Several other conditions can cause respiratory distress in neonates. These include bony defects of the chest wall, metabolic acidosis, anemia, polycythemia, primary pulmonary artery hypertension, hyperthermia, choanal atresia, etc.[3,18,22]

REFERENCES

1. NNF recommended basic perinatal-neonatal nomenclature. In: DK Guha (Ed). Neonatology—Principles and Practice, 1st edition. New Delhi: Jaypee Brothers Medical Publishers (P) Ltd. 1998. pp. 131-2.
2. Kumar P, Kumar R, Narang A. Spectrum of neonatal respiratory distress at PGI. Bulletin NNF. 2000;14:8-12.
3. Diwakar KK. Clinical approach to respiratory distress in newborn. Indian J Pediatr. 2003;70:S53-9.
4. Guyer B, Hoyert DL, Martin JA, et al. Annual summary of vital statistics—1998. Pediatrics. 1999;104:1229-46.
5. Northway WH, Rosan RC, Porter DY. Pulmonary disease following respirator therapy of hyaline-membrane disease. Bronchopulmonary dysplasia. N Engl J Med. 1967;276:357-68.
6. Marini C, Bulleri A, Cambi L, et al. The neonatal respiratory insufficiency syndrome: the role of the chest radiogram. Radiol Med (Torino). 1997;94:463-7.
7. Kurl S, Heinonen KM, Kiekara O. The first chest radiograph in neonates exhibiting respiratory distress at birth. Clin Pediatr. 1997;36:285-9.
8. Dinger J, Schwarze R, Rupprecht E. Radiological changes after therapeutic use of surfactant in infants with respiratory distress syndrome. Pediatr Radiol. 1997;27:26-31.
9. Helbich TH, Popow C, Dobner M, et al. Newborn infants with severe hyaline membrane disease: radiological evaluation during high frequency oscillatory versus conventional ventilation. Eur J Radiol. 1998;28:243-9.
10. Avni EF, Braude P, Pardou A, et al. Hyaline membrane disease in the newborn: diagnosis by ultrasound. Pediatr Radiol. 1990;20:143-6.
11. Bober K, Swietliński J. Diagnostic utility of ultrasonography for respiratory distress syndrome in neonates. Med Sci Monit. 2006;12:440-6.
12. Copetti R, Cattarossi L, Macagno F, et al. Lung ultrasound in respiratory distress syndrome: a useful tool for early diagnosis. Neonatology. 2008;94:52-9.

13. Avni EF, Cassart M, de Maertelaer V, et al. Sonographic prediction of chronic lung disease in the premature undergoing mechanical ventilation. Pediatr Radiol. 1996;26:463-9.
14. Pieper CH, Smith J, Brand EJ. The value of ultrasound examination of the lungs in predicting BPD. Pediatr Radiol. 2004;34:227-31.
15. Newman B. Imaging of medical disease of the newborn lung. RCNA. 1999;37:1049-65.
16. Copetti R, Cattarossi L. The "double lung point": an ultrasound sign diagnostic of transient tachypnea of the newborn. Neonatology. 2007;91:203-9.
17. Volpicelli G, Audino B. The "double lung point": an unusual sonographic sign of juvenile spontaneous pneumothorax. Am J Emerg Med. 2011;29(3):355.e1-2.
18. Mathur NB, Garg K, Kumar S. Respiratory distress in neonates with special reference to pneumonia. Indian Pediatr. 2002;39:529-37.
19. Garner JS, Jarvis WR, Emori TG, et al. CDC definitions for nosocomial infections. In: Olmsted RN (Ed). APIC Infection Control and Applied Epidemiology: Principles and Practice. St. Louis, MO: Mosby. 1996. pp. A1-19.
20. Gaynes RP, Edwards JR, Jarvis WR, et al. National Nosocomial Infection Surveillance System. Nosocomial infections among neonates in high-risk nurseries in the United States. Pediatrics. 1996;98:357-61.
21. Wiswell TE, Bent RC. Meconium staining and meconium aspiration syndrome. Pediatr Clinics North Am. 1993;40:955-81.
22. Hermansen CL, Lorah KN. Respiratory distress in the newborn. Am Fam Physician. 2007;76:987-94.
23. Tocino IM, Miller MH, Fairfax WR. Distribution of pneumothorax in the supine and semirecumbent critically ill adult. Am J Roentgenol. 1985;144:901-5.
24. Gordon R. The deep sulcus sign. Radiology. 1980;136:25-7.
25. Schwartz DS, Reyes-Mugica M, Keller MS. Imaging of surgical diseases of the newborn chest. Intrapleural mass lesions. Radiol Clin North Am. 1999;37:1067-78.
26. Slovis TL. Congenital and acquired lesions (Most causing respiratory distress). In: Kuhn JP, Slovis TL, Haller JO (Eds). Caffey's Pediatric Diagnostic imaging, 10th edition. USA: Mosby. 2004. pp. 58-101.
27. Ghribi A, Mekki M, Krichene I, et al. Congenital bilobar emphysema. J Pediatr Surg. 2008;43:e5-7.
28. Stocker JT. Congenital and developmental diseases. In: Dail OH, Hammar SP (Eds). Pulmonary Pathology, 2nd edition. Heidelberg: Springer-Verlag. 1994. pp. 155-90.
29. Shimohira M, Hara M, Kitase M, et al. Congenital pulmonary airway malformation: CT-pathologic correlation. J Thorac Imaging. 2007;22:149-53.
30. d'Agostino S, Bonoldi E, Dante S, et al. Embryonal rhabdomyosarcoma of the lung arising in cystic adenomatoid malformation: case report and review of the literature. J Pediatr Surg. 1997;32:1381-3.
31. West D, Nicholson AG, Colquhoun I, et al. Bronchioloalveolar carcinoma in congenital cystic adenomatoid malformation of lung. Ann Thorac Surg. 2007;83:687-9.
32. Thébaud B, Mercier JC, Dinh-Xuan AT. Congenital diaphragmatic hernia. A cause of persistent pulmonary hypertension of the newborn which lacks an effective therapy. Biol Neonate. 1998;74:323-36.
33. Kumar A, Bhatnagar V. Respiratory distress in neonates. Indian J Pediatr. 2005;72:425-8.
34. Sodhi KS, Saxena AK, Narasimha Rao KL, et al. Esophageal duplication cyst: an unusual cause of respiratory distress in infants. Pediatr Emerg Care. 2005;21:854-6.

CHAPTER 131

Childhood Pulmonary Infections

Jyoti Kumar

INTRODUCTION

Respiratory tract infections are the most common cause of illness in children and one of the most common indications for imaging. It should be remembered that children are not small adults and the spectrum of disorders that affect the pediatric population can be quite different from that seen in adults. Clinical evaluation is difficult and the history is inevitably difficult to elicit, no matter how observant the parents are. There is extra emotional concern when children fall sick and all together; these issues are of great importance to a radiologist, especially in thoracic disorders where imaging of the chest is frequently one of the first tools after clinical assessment.[1]

PNEUMONIA

Epidemiology

In preschool-aged infants and children (4 months to 5 years old), viruses cause 95% of all respiratory infections. In the school-aged children, although viral agents remain the most common cause of lower respiratory infections, the incidence of bacterial infection increases and *Mycoplasma pneumoniae* is the cause in approximately 30%.[2]

The factors that increase the risk for childhood pneumonia are large families, siblings of school-aged children, congenital heart disease, congenital immune disorders and neuromuscular disorders that depress the patient's ability to clear infected secretions or to suppress aspiration.[3]

Infections reach the lower respiratory tract via three routes: (1) The airways, (2) Vasculature and (3) Direct spread from extrapulmonary sites. Inhalation or aspiration of airborne organisms or infected secretions is the most common route for infection. Infection via pulmonary vasculature may be a result of diffuse sepsis or septic emboli as in cases of endocarditis. Nodules may be miliary and diffuse or fewer and random in distribution. These may or may not cavitate and vessels may be seen reaching up to the nodules. Direct spread of infection from mediastinum, chest wall, abdomen or neck is an uncommon occurrence.[3]

Imaging

Although clinical symptoms and signs are helpful indicators of the presence of disease, radiographic investigation is often required to confirm the clinical diagnosis and to help sort out whether or not antibiotics or more extensive work-up is necessary.[4] The various roles of imaging in children with pneumonia are: evaluation of possible pneumonia, determination of specific etiologic agent, exclusion of other pathology, evaluation of the child with failure of pneumonia to clear, and evaluation of complications related to pneumonia.[5]

In infants and young children, the signs and symptoms of pneumonia may be more nonspecific than in adults. Although fever and respiratory symptoms like cough, wheezing, tachypnea or retractions are the presenting symptoms in most cases, nonrespiratory symptoms like malaise and irritability, headaches, chest pain, or abdominal pain are also a common mode of presentation in children. Lower lobe pneumonia may be recognized on the superior aspect of abdominal radiographs being obtained for abdominal pain. Physical examination may be less reliable in children. Also, laboratory tests including elevated erythrocyte sedimentation rate, C-reactive protein and leukocytosis are neither sensitive nor specific.[2] Chest radiography is a technique which is heavily relied upon to determine the likelihood of underlying bacterial illness in children and has been shown to alter the management decisions in children with pneumonia.[5]

Most chest infection imaging is carried out using radiographs. It is generally agreed that chest radiographs should be obtained when fever is present in conjunction with respiratory symptoms.[2] Although cost, radiation dose and procedure time increase, when both frontal and lateral radiographs are used, certain radiographic findings like hyperinflation are better evaluated on a lateral radiograph, especially in infants.[2]

The etiological agent cannot be characterized from radiographs alone.[4] The main objective of imaging in pneumonia is whether the patient is likely to have viral or bacterial pneumonia. The specific bacterial agent is usually not the clinical question expected to be resolved by radiography.

Computed tomography (CT) has a very limited role in primary assessment of uncomplicated pneumonia. In pediatric lower respiratory infection, CT is indicated:[6,7]

- When complications of bacterial pneumonia are suspected. One of the goals of CT in cases of persistent illness is to separate suppurative pleural from parenchymal pathology as most of the former require interventional procedures while lung parenchymal complications are managed conservatively.
- To exclude underlying abnormality in recurrent infection
- To evaluate immunocompromised children with normal radiograph but with clinical suspicion of respiratory infection
- To guide the type and site of tissue sampling
- To assess the sequelae of respiratory infection (e.g. post-viral bronchiolitis obliterans).

Viral Pneumonia

Viral infection predominantly affects the mucosa of the airways resulting in bronchiolitis. The process may remain confined to the medium and small airways or may extend into the adjacent lung tissue resulting in peribronchiolar opacities. Respiratory syncytial virus (RSV) is the most common cause, others being parainfluenza and adenovirus.[4] Most of these are acquired by inhalational route. Edema, increased mucosal secretions and necrotic debris in the lumen result in blockade of airways, more marked at the level of the bronchioles and cause air trapping. Children are more predisposed to air trapping and collapse in viral infection than adults due to the following reasons: (1) Bronchi and bronchioles are smaller in diameter; (2) Collateral pathways of ventilation, including pores of Kahn and channels of Lambert are not well developed; these do not mature until about 8 years of age; and (3) Mucus secretion is more in children.[2]

Radiographic signs of diffuse hyperinflation are hyperlucency, depression of the hemidiaphragm to more than 10 posterior ribs, flattening of the diaphragms, widening of intercostal spaces and increased retrosternal space. On the lateral view, findings of flattening of the hemidiaphragms and increased anteroposterior diameter, which often becomes more than the superior to inferior diameter, are often better evaluated **(Figs. 1 and 2)**. When thick mucus inspissates resulting in complete plugging of the airway, there is segmental atelectasis. This is seen as wedge-shaped areas of density, more common in the middle and lower lung **(Fig. 3)**. Inflammation extending into the adjacent lung tissue can cause peribronchial edema and result in bronchopneumonia which manifests as bilateral, usually symmetrical peribronchial cuffing and thickening in the central perihilar location. On the lateral view, increased hilar size and density may be used as a marker for perihilar peribronchial thickening. Doughnut-like appearance on cross-section and tram-track line appearance of bronchi are seen radiating from the hilum.[2,4,5]

Although the central peribronchial thickening, hyperinflation and areas of segmental atelectasis are typical of viral infection in infants and small children, there

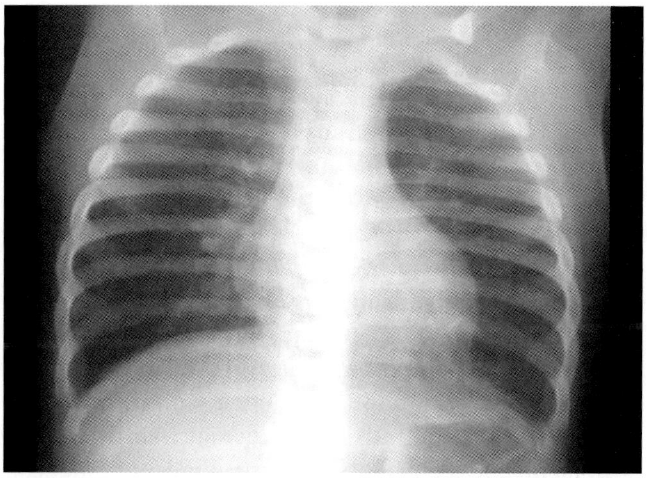

Fig. 1: Viral pneumonia: Frontal radiograph in a 4-month-old boy shows hyperinflation with increased peribronchial markings.

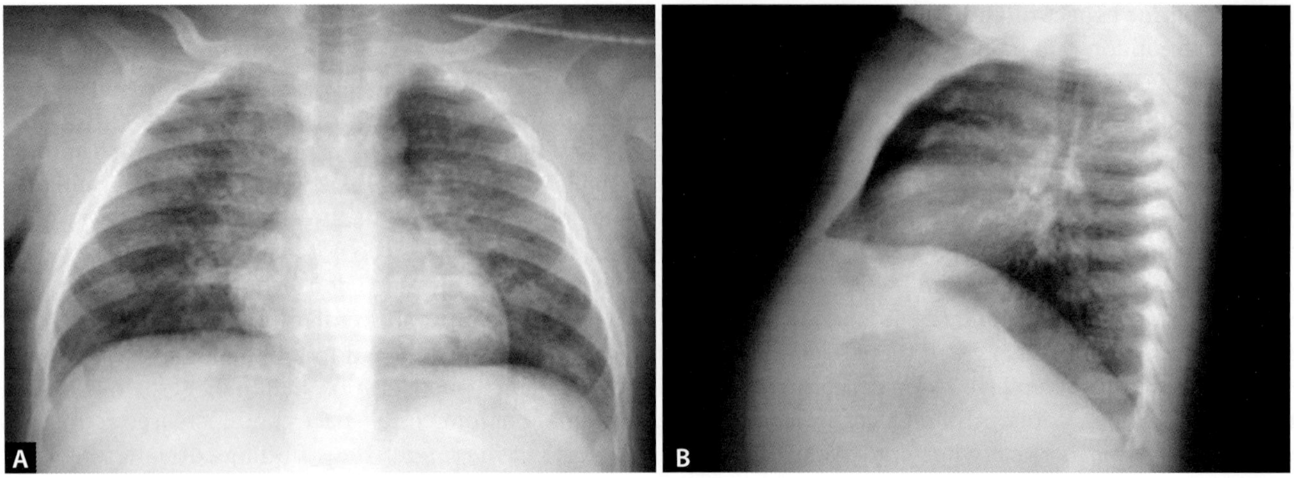

Figs. 2A and B: Viral pneumonia: (A) Frontal radiograph in a 5-month-old child shows increased peribronchial markings, and (B) Lateral radiograph shows prominent density and size of the hila, a supportive finding of increased peribronchial markings.

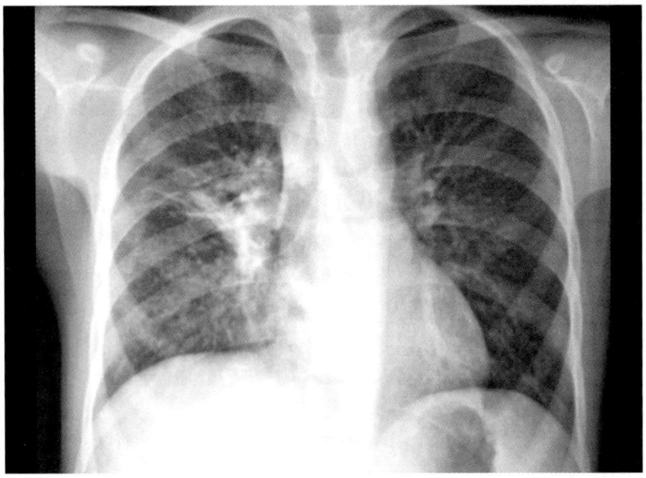

Fig. 3: Viral pneumonia: Frontal radiograph in a 4-year-old girl depicts prominent bronchovascular markings with triangular right perihilar area of atelectasis.

are various pitfalls. Perivascular edema and reactive airway disease may simulate the appearance of peribronchial thickening. Expiratory films may give the erroneous impression of peribronchial thickening. Sometimes, bacterial pneumonia like pertussis pneumonia (rare due to widespread immunization) mimics the appearance of viral pneumonia. Segmental atelectasis in viral pneumonia may be overinterpreted as consolidation in bacterial pneumonia. Secondary bacterial infection may develop in few cases of viral infection, related to altered immunity and ubiquitous pathogen, confounding the radiological picture.[4] Also, if bronchial wall thickening is present between bouts of acute illness, it suggests chronic airway disease such as asthma or cystic fibrosis, immunodeficiency or chronic aspiration.[3]

Although most infants recover uneventfully, viral pneumonias may result in long-standing complications of bronchiolitis obliterans and Swyer-James syndrome (unilateral hyperlucent lung) discussed later.[4]

Bacterial Pneumonia

Bacterial pneumonia is usually a result of *Streptococcus pneumoniae*, other common agents being *Haemophilus influenzae* and *Staphylococcus pneumoniae*. The usual route of spread is via the inhalational route. Airspace pneumonia is classically the result of *S. pneumoniae* and *Klebsiella pneumonia*e. Inflammatory exudates and edema within the acini result in segmental or lobar consolidation **(Fig. 4)**. This is usually unilateral in contrast to viral pneumonias. Air bronchograms, when seen, are typical. There is usually little or no volume loss as the airways are not primarily affected. *Staphylococcus aureus*, Gram-negative bacteria and *Mycoplasma* usually result in bronchopneumonia that begins in terminal and respiratory bronchioles rather than alveoli. The disease then spreads to peribronchiolar alveoli that produce acinar filling and lobular consolidations. This results in patchy consolidation, loss of volume with absence of air bronchograms. When affected areas coalesce, the shadowing may become more uniform and resemble lobar pneumonia. There may be accompanying pleural effusions, which are rarely associated with viral disease.

Sometimes, lobar consolidation may be difficult to distinguish from atelectasis seen in viral pneumonias (in fact, these may coexist as superadded infection is common secondary to obstructed airway). It may be remembered that accompanying signs of volume loss like fissural distortion, mediastinal shift and compensatory hyperinflation, seen with atelectasis are unusual in consolidated lung.[4]

Although more gradual, the pneumonia generally resolves completely. Radiological improvement may lag behind clinical improvement by days or weeks, usually taking 1–2 weeks **(Figs. 5A and B)**. However, severity of the disease agent and underlying host factors may result in complications like cavitatory necrosis, empyema and abscess formation.[4,5] Increase in antibiotic usage has led to increase in the incidence of complications.[4] Lung abscess is uncommon in children and suggests underlying aspiration and infection with Gram-negative bacilli or *Staphylococcus*. Multilobar consolidation with mixed flora in debilitated patients suggests aspiration as the underlying mechanism. Aspiration of gastric contents can also result in chemical pneumonitis.[4]

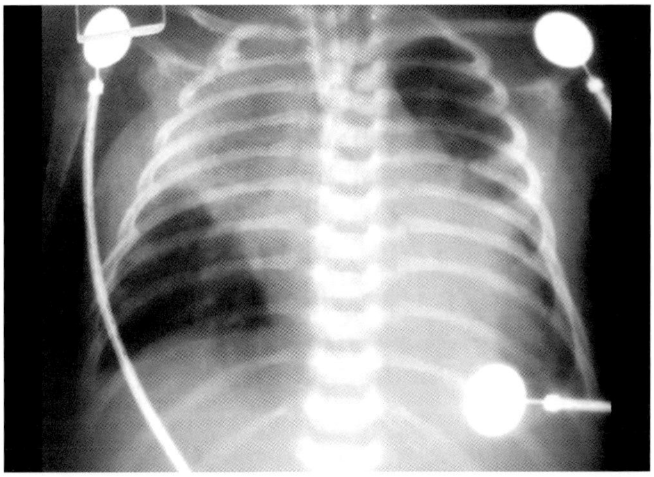

Fig. 4: Lobar pneumonia: Frontal radiograph in a 3-month-old infant shows consolidation of the right upper lobe suggesting a bacterial pneumonia.

Round pneumonia is also common in young children, less than 8 years of age. This is due to paucity of collateral channels of ventilation as described earlier. This is most often due to *S. pneumoniae* and simulates a mass lesion.[2,5] These often involve the lower lobes, especially the superior segments. In a child with fever, diagnosis of round pneumonia should always be considered when a round mass-like lesion is encountered **(Figs. 6A and B)**. Round pneumonia may contain air bronchograms and show ill-defined margins in at least a part of the border, suggesting the diagnosis. Follow-up radiography after antibiotic therapy is essential to rule out an underlying mass lesion, like bronchogenic cyst.[2]

M. pneumoniae, which is an atypical cause of pneumonia, is a common cause of pneumonia in school-aged children. It is uncommon in children less than 3 years of age. It can have a broad-spectrum of appearances which may simulate viral or bacterial pneumoniae. The radiographic changes are more severe than the clinical symptoms. Hilar lymph nodes and pleural effusions can be associated.[2,6]

In most children with pulmonary infections, specific etiological agent is never documented. Invasive diagnostic procedures are usually not warranted and even when done, specific etiological agent is still not identifiable because of ongoing treatment with antibiotics.[5]

In a study by Bettenay et al.[8] it was suggested that both clinical and radiographic criteria overestimate the number of children with bacterial pneumonia by a significant proportion, owing to low-positive predictive value.

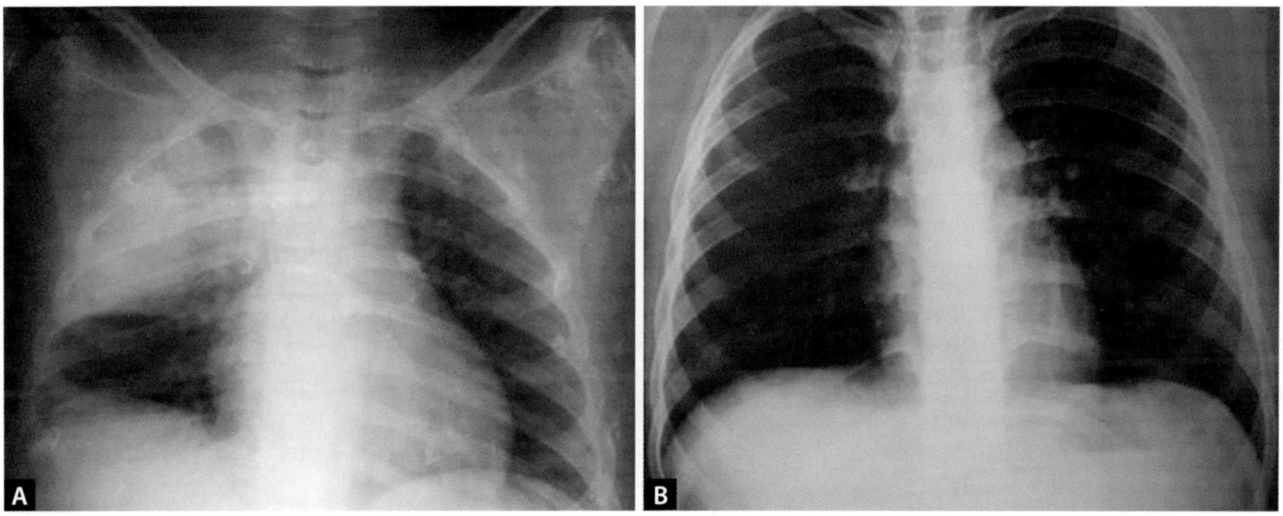

Figs. 5A and B: Lobar pneumonia: (A) Frontal radiograph in a 2-year-old child shows consolidation of the right upper lobe, and (B) Patient was put on antibiotics and radiograph obtained 2 weeks later shows complete radiological clearance.

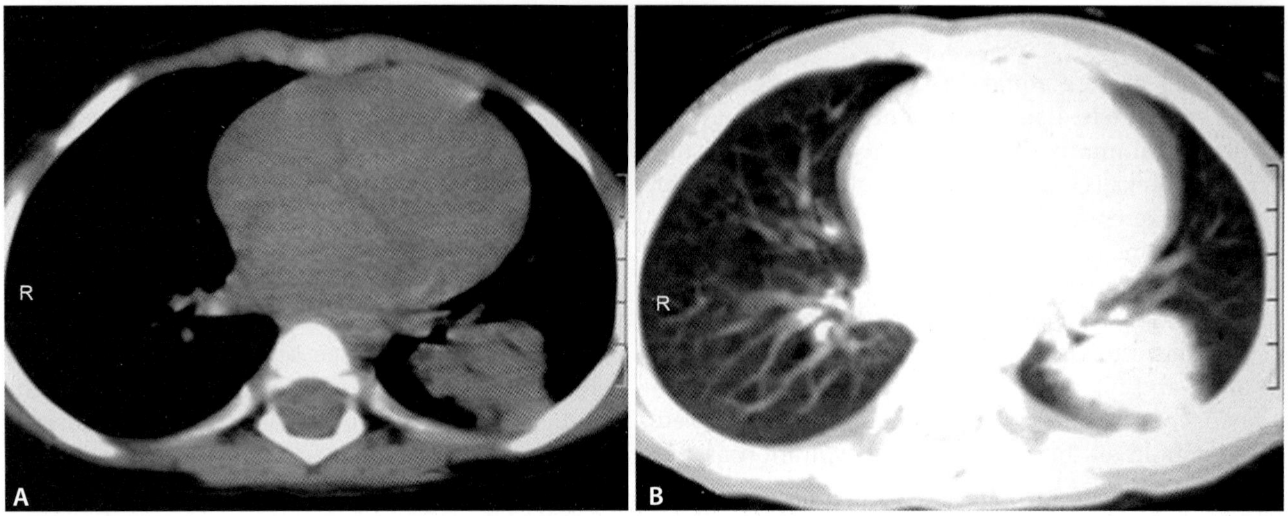

Figs. 6A and B: Round pneumonia: Axial computed tomography (CT) images in a 2-year-old child with fever shows a round mass-like lesion with air bronchogram. This was a case of round pneumonia.

However, it was the high-negative predictive value in the range of 80–90% of the clinical and radiographic findings that were useful in excluding bacterial pneumonia and affected the management decisions.

Few specific appearances pertaining to different bacterial agents may be mentioned here. *Staphylococcal pneumonia* presents with lobar or multilobar consolidation. Complications are most common with this organism. Pleural effusion is common which may develop into empyema. A frequent feature of *S. pneumonia* is pneumatocele formation, which is otherwise rare. It is seen as a round thin-walled lucency due to collection of air in the interstitium. This may result in pneumothorax secondary to rupture. Although they generally disappear in days or weeks, few may persist for months.[6] Septicemic staphylococcal infection may result in multiple nodules which may also cavitate **(Figs. 7A and B)**.

In cases of infection with *K. pneumoniae,* a Gram-negative bacillus, there is homogeneous opacification with copious inflammatory exudate which may result in an increase in the lung volume resulting in expansile pneumonia **(Fig. 8)**. Empyema and abscess are common complications.[6]

Exclusion of Other Pathologies

Since the clinical symptoms of pneumonia in children are fairly nonspecific, other pathologies that may simulate pneumonia must be excluded. It is essential to look at the ribs and the airways to exclude other potential causes of respiratory distress in children, e.g. rib erosions in cases of neuroblastoma **(Figs. 9A and B)** and fractures in cases of child abuse are pointers to the correct diagnosis. Also, stridor due to vascular rings around the airway is common in children, compared to adults and warrants a careful look at the airways. Evaluation of the diameter of the airways should be stressed as a routine part of evaluation of pediatric chest radiographs.[2]

Nonresolving Pneumonia

In children, follow-up radiographs are usually reserved for those children who have persistent or recurrent symptoms or who have an underlying condition such as immunodeficiency, cystic fibrosis, or sickle-cell anemia. These should also be considered in children with round pneumonia. When obtained, they should be done after at least 2–3 weeks.[2] In patients with nonresolving pneumonia on antibiotic and other therapy, with noncontributory chest radiograph, contrast-enhanced CT (CECT) is the modality of choice.

The various causes of recurrent or nonresolving pneumonia are enumerated here:[5,9-11]

- *Aspiration syndromes:* Swallowing disorders due to neuromuscular disorders or immaturity, gastroesophageal reflux, H-type fistula, esophageal obstruction (foreign body, vascular ring)
- *Underlying developmental lesions:* Like congenital cystic adenomatoid malformation (CCAM) **(Fig. 10)**, bronchogenic cyst, sequestration
- *Bronchial obstruction:* Foreign body, neoplasm
- *Underlying systemic disorders:* Immunodeficiency (congenital and acquired), asthma, cystic fibrosis, immotile cilia disease.

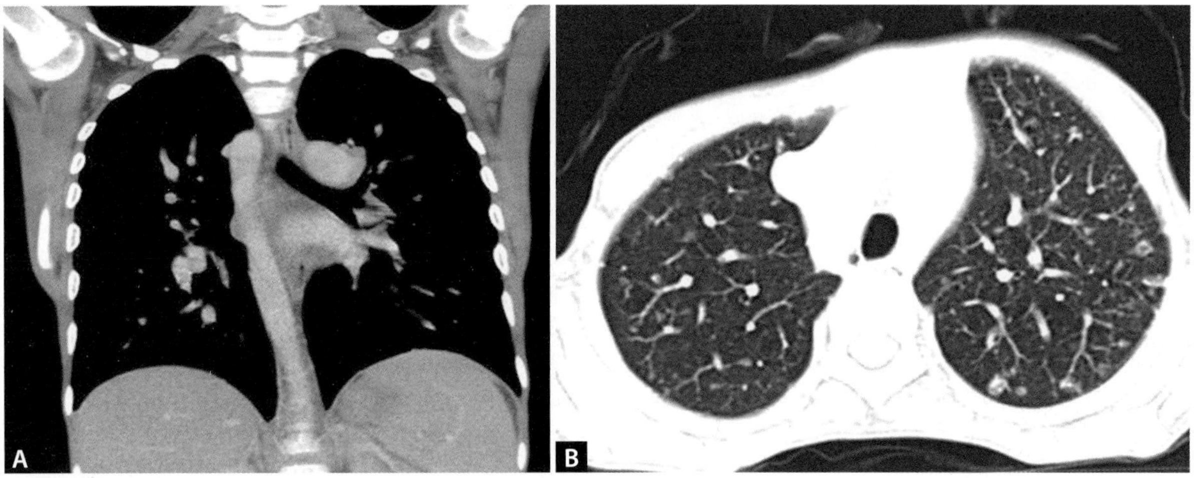

Figs. 7A and B: Infective endocarditis with septic emboli: (A) Coronal reformatted computed tomography (CT) image on mediastinal window settings shows right-sided aortic arch in a case of ventricular septal defect with infective endocarditis, and (B) Multiple nodular lesions, few showing feeding vessel sign, are seen on axial contrast-enhanced CT (CECT) at lung window settings.

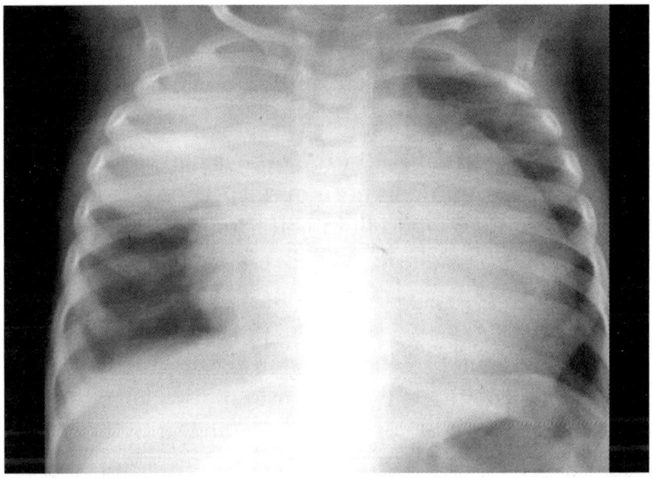

Fig. 8: Expansile pneumonia: Frontal radiograph in a 4-month-old infant shows lobar consolidation with bulging of the fissure suggesting expansile pneumonia.

Foreign bodies usually lodge in the bronchial tree and affect the lower lobes or the right middle lobe. Only large ones may lodge in the trachea. Children usually do not remember the episode or are too young to do so, hence present with pneumonia. This is usually chronic and develops slowly. Although the child may be very ill at presentation, but without the toxicity of acute infection. Very small foreign bodies such as grass may migrate to the peripheral bronchi. Inorganic foreign bodies are usually inert and only result in mechanical obstruction, whereas organic foreign bodies such as peanuts also incite an inflammatory reaction in addition to the mechanical obstruction. Also, they may be fragmented and then spread into peripheral bronchi or bronchi of other lobes. Up to 85% are nonopaque on chest radiographs. When a foreign body is suspected, radiographic assessment should start with paired inspiratory and expiratory films or fluoroscopy. Decubitus film may be obtained, if fluoroscopy is not available and expiratory film is difficult to obtain. Fluoroscopy can depict air trapping, mediastinal shift to affected side on inspiration and reduced diaphragmatic movement on the affected side. Distal atelectasis, especially in the lower lobes, pulmonary abscess, bronchiectasis and bronchiolitis obliterans are the complications that may be encountered. Stenosis of the bronchus can also result which predisposes to further infections.[6]

For assessment of swallowing mechanism, swallow should be done using solid food coated with barium, followed by thickened barium mixture and finally thin liquid barium. In case, H-type tracheoesophageal fistula is suspected, tube esophagogram should be done, with patient in the prone position and using a horizontal beam. Combined bronchoscopy and endoscopy is the investigation of choice.[6]

EVALUATION OF ASSOCIATED COMPLICATIONS

Suppurative complications of pneumonia may involve the pleura, lung parenchyma and rarely the pericardium.

Pleural Complications

A parapneumonic effusion (PPE) is a pleural fluid collection adjacent to infected lung. It may be simple or complicated depending on whether the infective organism

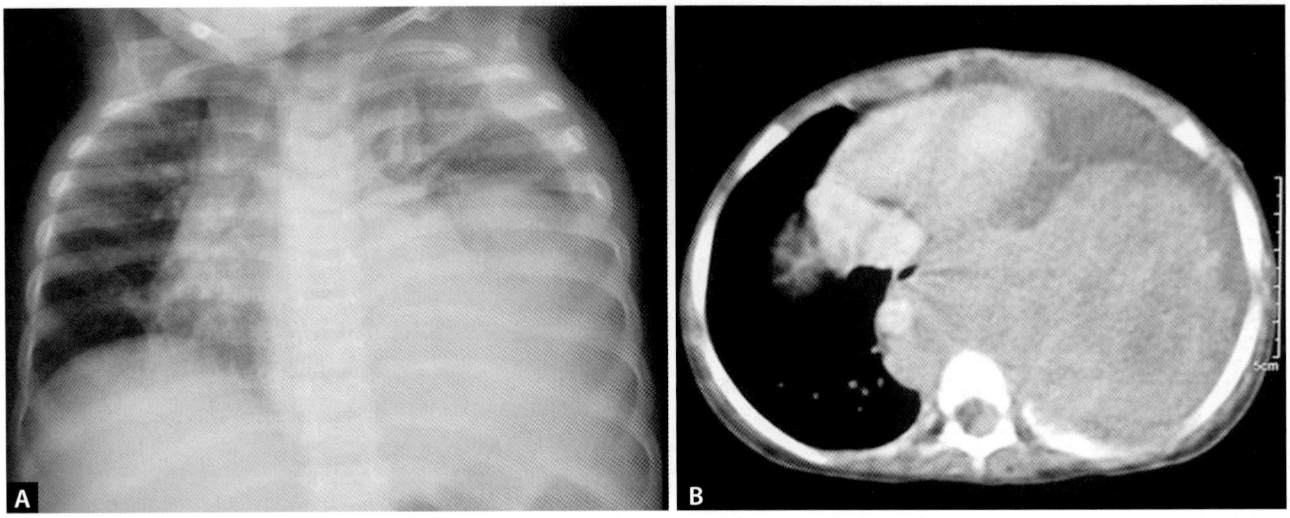

Figs. 9A and B: Neuroblastoma: (A) Chest radiograph in a 2-year-old girl shows opacity in the left mid and lower zone with accompanying left pleural effusion. Note erosion and splaying of the left posterior 7th to 10th ribs differentiating neuroblastoma from pneumonia, and (B) Computed tomography (CT) scan shows a posterior mediastinal mass displacing heart and aorta with extension into spinal canal.

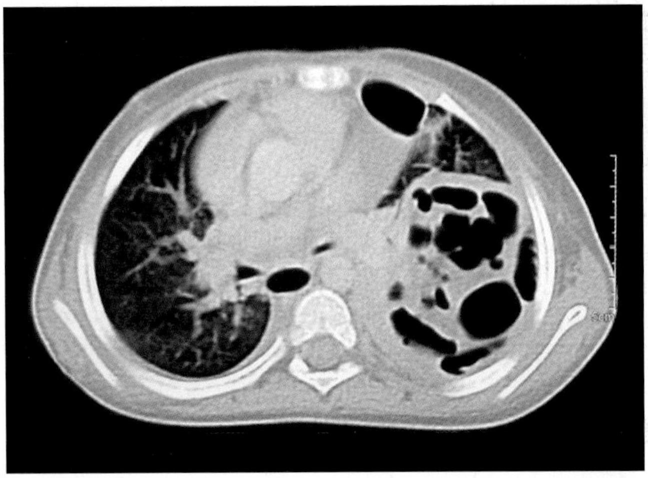

Fig. 10: Congenital cystic adenomatoid malformation (CCAM). Computed tomography (CT) in a 3-year-old child with recurrent pneumonia shows multiseptated cystic mass with thickened walls in the left lower lobe. The diagnosis of CCAM was confirmed at surgery.

is present or not within the collection. The term *empyema* is used when there is frank pus within the collection.[12]

Empyema in children is a different condition from that in adults. Although associated with significant morbidity, it is almost never fatal in contrast to adults, where mortality is nearly 20%, probably due to the higher incidence of premorbid conditions.[12] The most common agents involved are *S. pneumoniae, S. aureus*, other *Streptococci* (including *S. pyogenes*), *H. influenzae, M. pneumoniae, Pseudomonas spp.* and *Mycobacterium tuberculosis (MTB).*[12]

Initially, there is pleural inflammation secondary to involvement of the subpleural lung. This leads to increase in pleural fluid production with influx of inflammatory cells resulting in simple PPE. There is consequent fibrin production, resulting in fibrinous septations, resulting in complicated PPE when fluid is thickened. Later, there is pus formation, resulting in frank empyema. Eventually, a thick fibrous peel may trap the lung and may result in long-term restriction of lung function.[12]

Chest radiography and ultrasound (US) are the imaging modalities of choice to detect effusions and guide drainage of complicated effusions. Chest radiography is usually the first investigation. The signs vary from obliteration of the costophrenic angle, meniscus of fluid tracking along the lateral chest wall in small effusions to complete opacification of the hemithorax with contralateral mediastinal shift in larger effusions **(Figs. 11 and 12)**. Pleural cap may be visualized. Loculated effusions tend to have a lenticular shape **(Fig. 13)**. In cases of empyema, there may be scoliosis concave to the side of the collection, due to pain. On supine films, there may be homogeneous haze of the affected hemithorax.

Ultrasound is used to confirm the presence of effusion, characterize it, and guide drainage. Effusions may be anechoic, or show fine internal echoes and fibrinous septations **(Figs. 14A to C)**. US may also be used to characterize nonshifting nature of loculated fluid by scanning the patient in supine and sitting positions. In cases of fibrous rind formation, pleural thickening is seen with lack of mobility of the underlying lung, suggesting

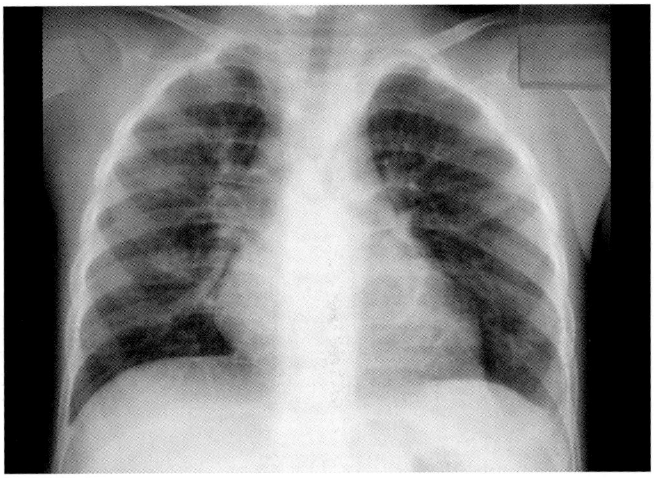

Fig. 11: Pleural effusion. Frontal radiograph of a child shows blunting of the left costophrenic angle suggesting effusion. This was confirmed on ultrasound (US)

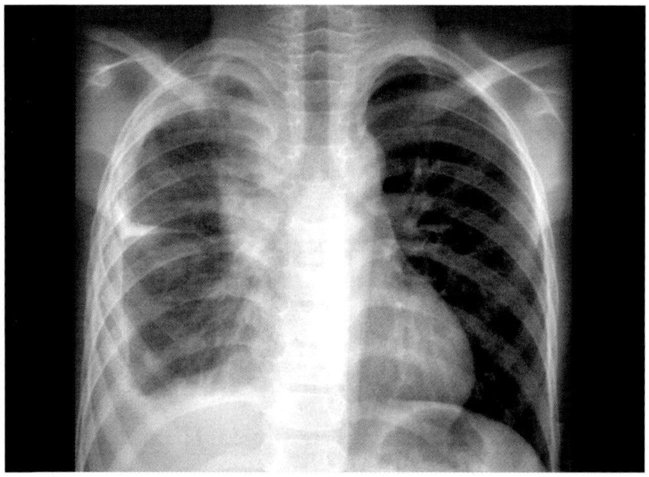

Fig. 12: Pleural effusion. Frontal radiograph of a 10-year-old child shows blunting of the right costophrenic angle with fluid tracking along the lateral chest wall and the horizontal fissure in addition to the opacities in the right lung.

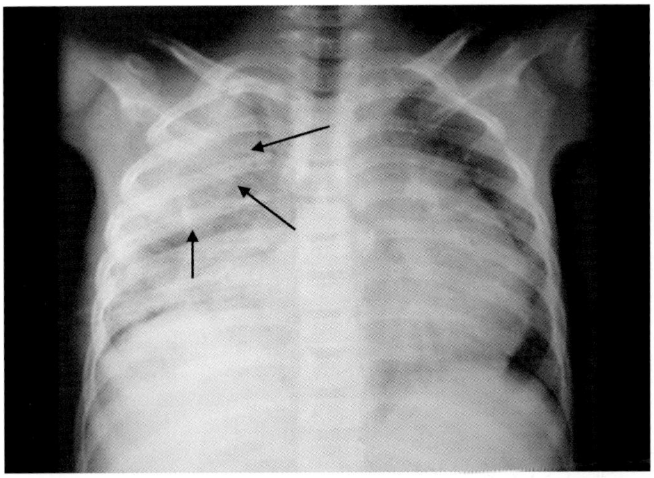

Fig. 13: Loculated pleural effusion. Frontal radiograph of a 10-year-old child shows lenticular shaped soft-tissue opacity along the right upper lateral chest wall suggesting loculated pleural effusion (arrows). The underlying lung shows areas of consolidation and atelectasis.

entrapment. When a very organized collection is difficult to distinguish from the underlying consolidated lung, color Doppler may be used to demonstrate vessels in the consolidated lung in contrast to the avascular pleural collection.[12]

Computed tomography is reserved for special circumstances. As per the British Thoracic Society guidelines, CT should be reserved for failing tube drainage, and in immunocompromised individuals to detect associated parenchymal and mediastinal abnormalities. On CT, features of empyema include pleural thickening and enhancement, increased density and thickening of extrapleural fat, increased density of extrathoracic fat and lenticular shape suggesting loculation. Pleural thickening and enhancement is better appreciated in the parietal pleura, as the visceral pleura are difficult to differentiate from the underlying consolidated lung. Although septations are not readily appreciable on CT, their presence may be inferred from air loculi within the pleural collection. This is due to air separating into tiny bubbles due to septations rather than forming an air-fluid level **(Fig. 15)**.[12] CT can also be helpful in depicting malpositioned chest tubes **(Figs. 16A and B)**.

We have to remember that even an anechoic collection may contain frank pus. Therefore, imaging is not the basis for deciding whether the patient requires drainage. This decision is dependent on whether the collection is increasing in size or the patient is having respiratory embarrassment due to the collection.[12]

Another clinical problem which may arise is whether we are dealing with empyema or a lung abscess. This is important because the treatment of abscess is primarily medical, and insertion of drainage tube increases the risk for bronchopleural fistula formation. While irregular thick wall and acute angle with chest wall favor the diagnosis of lung abscess, split pleura sign and compression of the adjacent lung favor the diagnosis of empyema.[12]

Lung Parenchymal Complications

The various complications include cavitatory necrosis, pulmonary abscess, pulmonary gangrene, pneumatocele and bronchopleural fistulae. The names given to the suppurative process depends on several factors including

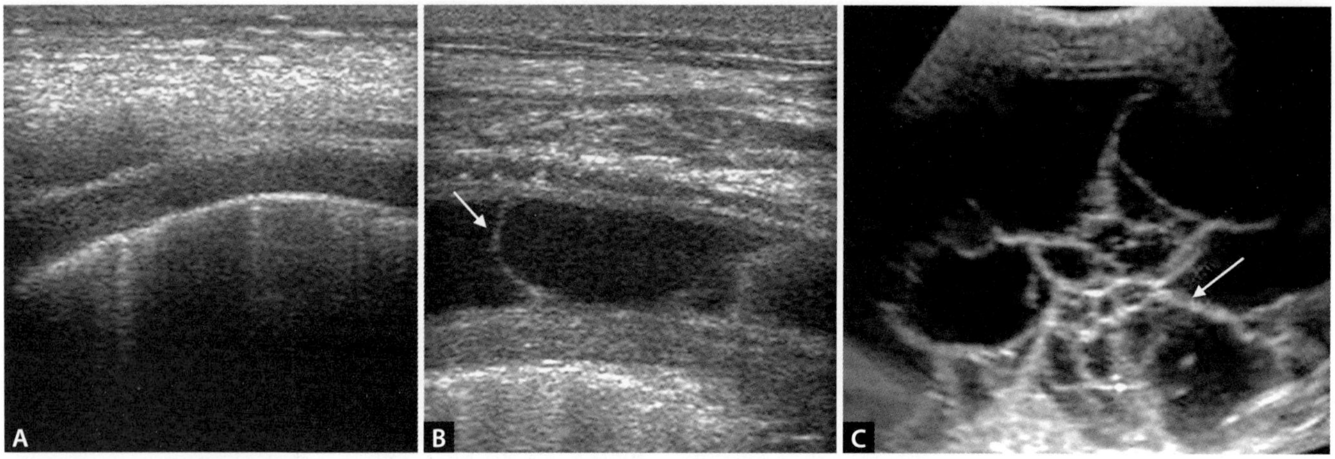

Figs. 14A to C: Ultrasound (US) in cases of pleural effusion may depict the clear nature of fluid (A) or show fine fibrinous septations (B and C).

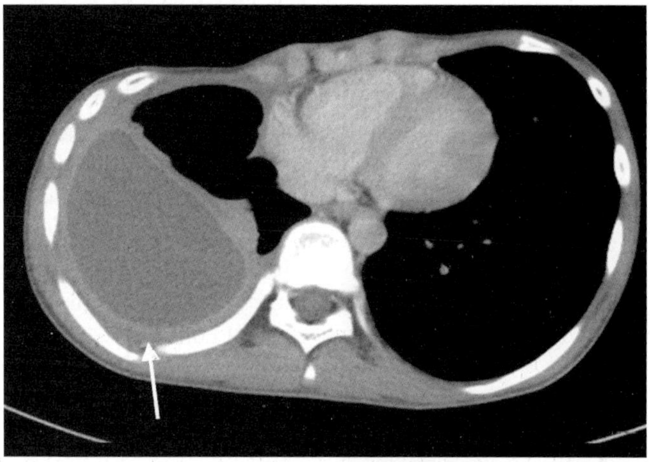

Fig. 15: Empyema: Axial contrast-enhanced computed tomography (CECT) shows lenticular shape of the collection with pleural thickening and enhancement with increased thickness and density of extrapleural fat (arrow).

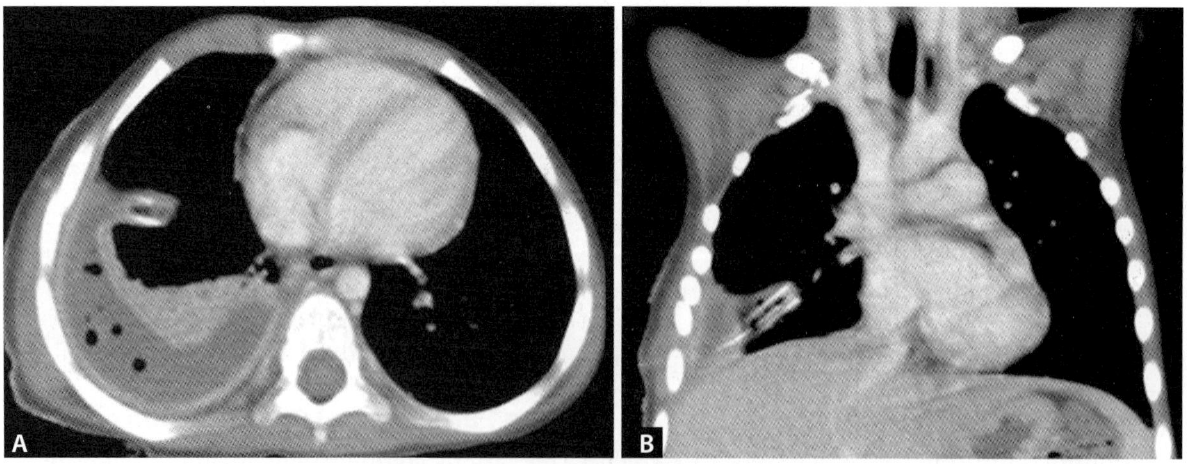

Figs. 16A and B: Empyema: Axial and coronal reformatted contrast-enhanced computed tomography (CECT) images depict the loculated right pleural collection with foci of air within.
Note: It is made of split pleura sign and underlying atelectasis. It is important to note the position of the chest tube which appears malpositioned.

the severity, distribution, and condition of the adjacent lung parenchyma and temporal relationship with disease resolution.[2,5,13-15]

Cavitatory necrosis is the most common complication encountered in children. *S. pneumoniae* and *S. aureus* are the frequent associated organisms. It is defined as a dominant area of necrosis with associated variable number of thin-walled cysts. On CT, it appears as decreased contrast enhancement, lack of normal lung architecture, loss of lung pleura margin, multiple thin-walled cavities filled with air or fluid with no peripheral enhancement **(Figs. 17A and B)**. The finding of decreased enhancement is indicative of pulmonary parenchymal ischemia, or impending cavitatory necrosis **(Figs. 18A and B)**. This is visualized on chest radiographs when air enters the cavities due to bronchial communication. Although associated with a protracted course, most patients are managed conservatively in contrast to adults.[5,15]

Lung abscess is fairly uncommon in immunocompetent children and is defined as collection of fluid or air within the lung parenchyma with a well-defined enhancing rim **(Figs. 19A and B)**.[5,13-15] In early stages, pulmonary consolidation may show a low-density center with no definite cavity formation.[7]

Pneumatoceles are seen as thin-walled cysts on imaging and may represent a later or less severe stage of resolving or healing necrosis.[2] Although pneumatoceles are most characteristic of *S. pneumonia*, other causes are *Pneumococcus, H. influenza, Streptococcus, MTB* and *Escherichia coli*. They are also known after hydrocarbon

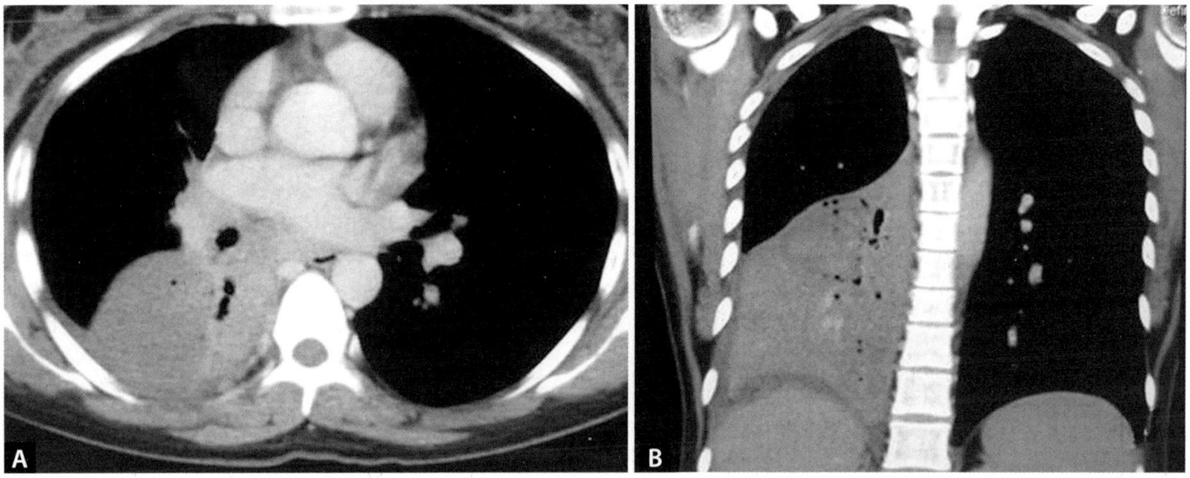

Figs. 17A and B: Cavitatory necrosis: Computed tomography (CT) findings in a 7-year-old boy shows multiloculated cavity within consolidated lung.

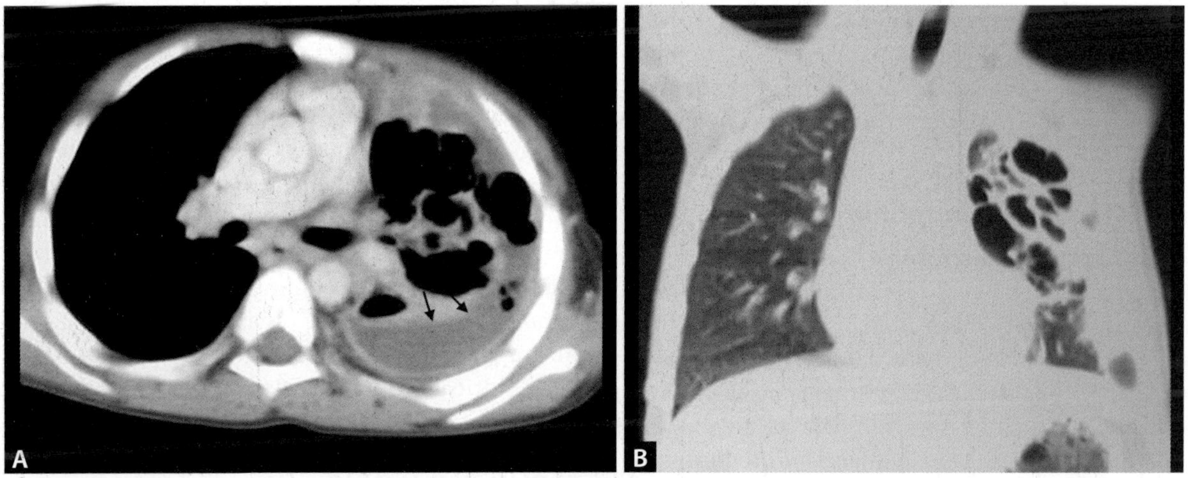

Figs. 18A and B: Axial (A) and coronal reformatted (B) computed tomography (CT) images of an adolescent with severe pneumonia shows consolidation of the right lower lobe with bulging of the lobe and areas of decreased parenchymal enhancement within (arrows), probably reflecting areas of ischemia and impending gangrene.

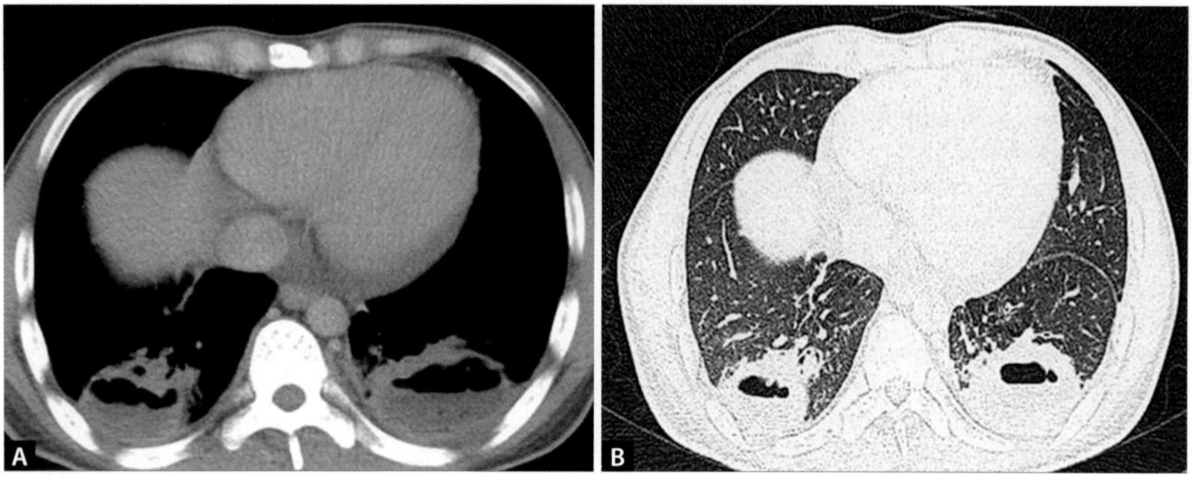

Figs. 19A and B: Lung abscesses: Axial contrast-enhanced computed tomography (CECT) images show abscesses with air-fluid levels in bilateral posterior dependent lungs suggesting aspiration as the probable cause

ingestion. When pneumatoceles develop in infected areas, inflammatory exudate may seep into them and produce air-fluid levels that simulate lung abscesses. However, true lung abscesses have a thicker and often somewhat shaggy wall.

Bronchopleural fistula is a communication between a bronchus and the pleural cavity. While it most commonly follows pneumonectomy, it may follow lung abscess, bacterial or fungal pneumonias and TB. Diagnosis is based upon increasing amount of sputum production, air in the pleural cavity which may be loculated.[6] CT may demonstrate direct communication between the pleural space and the bronchial tree in these cases.

Purulent Pericarditis

Pericardial fluid is not uncommonly encountered during US and CT of children with pneumonia. This may also result in cardiac tamponade when there is rapid accumulation. When the clinical features go unrecognized, the radiologist may be the first one to suggest the diagnosis **(Figs. 20A and B)**.[12]

Chronic Effects of Pneumonia

Most cases of pneumonia resolve completely. However, a few children may develop chronic complications. Increased susceptibility to infection in the same area of the lung may be a result of underlying damage to the airways in this area. Focal bronchiectasis is another complication that may occur in cases of infection with persistent collapse or foreign body aspiration. It usually affects the medium-sized bronchi, as the proximal bronchi have more cartilage in their walls. Only allergic bronchopulmonary aspergillosis shows a tendency to attack the proximal bronchi. Diffuse bronchiectasis may also occur due to chronic recurrent pulmonary infection, particularly in cases of cystic fibrosis and primary ciliary dyskinesia syndromes.[3]

Bronchiolitis obliterans may result from a severe viral pneumonia. Swyer-James/McLeod syndrome is a form of postinfectious obliterative bronchiolitis that has special features. It occurs following an insult to the developing lung (before the age of 8 years). The most frequently encountered scenario is post-viral infection, in particular adenoviral and post-mycoplasma infection. Noninfectious causes include hydrocarbon ingestion. The lung served by the affected bronchi and bronchioles remains inflated due to collateral air drift. Pulmonary tissue as well as pulmonary artery and its branches are hypoplastic. Patients are typically asymptomatic, presenting in adulthood or less commonly, may present with progressive exertional dyspnea or repeated respiratory infections. Disease on chest radiography is predominantly unilateral, giving rise to the key finding of unilateral transradiancy. This reflects hypoplasia of pulmonary vasculature as well as obliterative bronchiolitis. The hilum of the affected lung is small. The affected lung is small or normal in volume in contrast to congenital lobar emphysema. Ipsilateral air trapping is the key finding. CT changes are more complex than chest radiographs. It more commonly shows areas of bilateral abnormalities depicting areas of decreased attenuation. Air trapping can be confirmed on expiratory scans. Areas of cylindrical bronchiectasis may also be seen. There may be areas of collapse and scarring.[16]

TUBERCULOSIS

The pathological form is dependent on sensitivity of the infected host and is classified as primary or postprimary.[17]

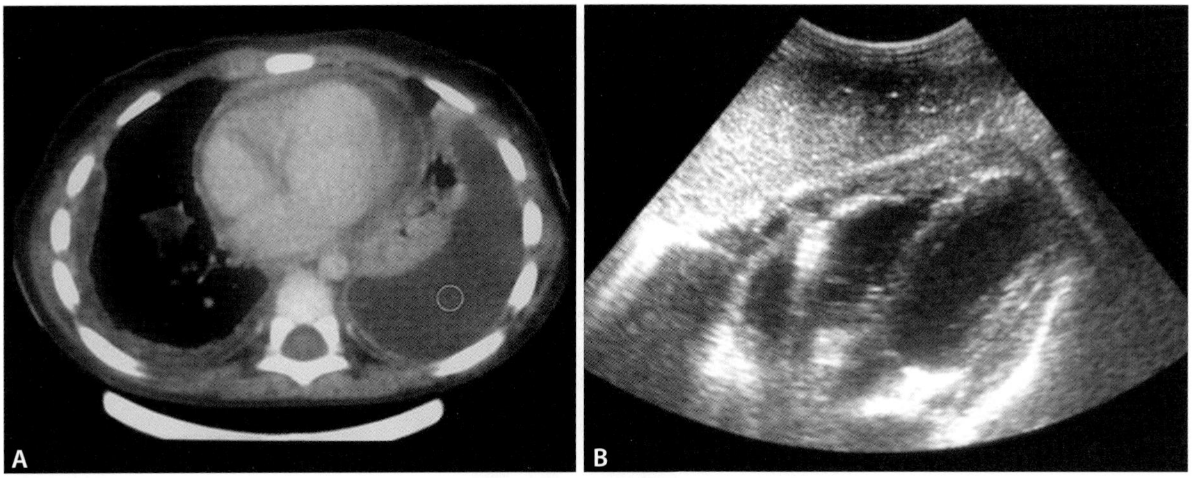

Figs. 20A and B: Pericarditis: (A) Axial contrast-enhanced computed tomography (CECT) image shows pericardial as well as pleural fluid in a case of pneumonia; (B) Correlative ultrasound (US) image shows thick pericardial fluid with septations.

Primary TB, the most common form in childhood, is radiologically distinct from postprimary TB, the most common form occurring in adults. Due to difficulty in obtaining suitable sputum samples and low sensitivity of gastric washings, chest radiography plays an important role in evaluation for TB in pediatric cases.[18]

Primary Pulmonary Tuberculosis

Primary TB represents the reaction to first exposure and is often a subclinical condition. Incubation period varies from 2–10 weeks and ends when the patient becomes sensitized (i.e. has a positive skin test). As the infecting bacteria are inhaled, it incites a local inflammatory reaction in the bronchiole/alveolus, usually peripherally in a subpleural focus, called the Ghon's focus. From this focus, lymphatic spread to the local hilar or mediastinal lymph nodes may occur.[17] The combination of a peripheral granuloma, involved lymphatics and lymph nodes is known as Ghon's or Ranke's complex. In most cases, the immune response is usually enough to limit the infection, which heals as a small granuloma. Primary focus is usually quite small as compared to the large lymph nodes. In young infants, or in cases with underlying illness or impaired nutrition resulting in impaired defenses, progressive primary disease may occur. Enlarging pulmonary focus of consolidation and caseation followed by liquefaction occurs. This leads to cavitation and rupture into a bronchus, may result in acute tuberculous bronchopneumonia.[18] These children are usually quite ill with weight loss and failure to thrive.

Primary TB may be asymptomatic when the child is well and the disease is detected during a routine skin test. It may otherwise present in four major ways in childhood, in addition to a normal chest radiograph:

1. Lymphadenopathy
2. Lobar or segmental parenchymal disease
3. Pleural effusion
4. Miliary involvement.

Lymphadenopathy with or without parenchymal abnormality is the radiological hallmark of primary TB in childhood. The favored lymph nodal sites are right paratracheal, hilar, subcarinal and aortopulmonary window region. Children less than 3 years of age have shown a higher prevalence of lymphadenopathy than parenchymal changes as compared to older children. The reverse, however, does not hold true.[18,19] CECT may depict characteristic low-attenuation nodes with rim enhancement **(Figs. 21A and B)**.

There is a tendency towards right sided parenchymal involvement, likely due to increased probability of inhalation of particles into the straighter right bronchus. No consensus has been reached regarding zonal predilection in primary TB.[18] The parenchymal involvement patterns described vary from ill-defined parenchymal opacities to segmental or lobar consolidation.[18] Homogeneous, dense and well-defined air space consolidation is a typical appearance of primary TB **(Fig. 22)**. Lymph nodes obstructing the adjacent bronchi can result in obstructive hyperinflation and atelectasis **(Figs. 23A to C)**. They may open into adjacent bronchi resulting in bronchopneumonia. There may be multifocal air space consolidation or diffuse nodularity. Bronchiectasis may be seen in areas of previous collapse. Evolution to cavitatory TB is uncommon in children. Cavitation may raise the possibility of previously unsuspected underlying immune disorder. Calcification occurs after caseation of the primary lesion and is seen earlier in infants (6

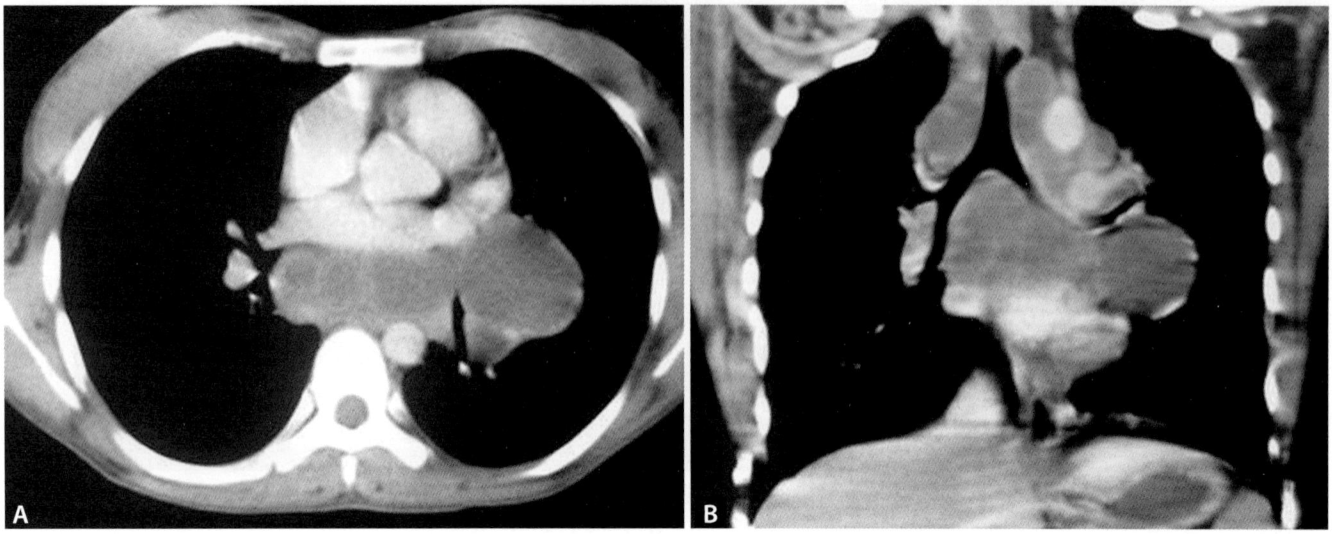

Figs. 21A and B: Tuberculosis (TB): Axial and coronal reformatted contrast-enhanced computed tomography (CECT) images at mediastinal window settings depict large necrotic rim enhancing lymph nodes in a case of TB in a 5-year-old girl.

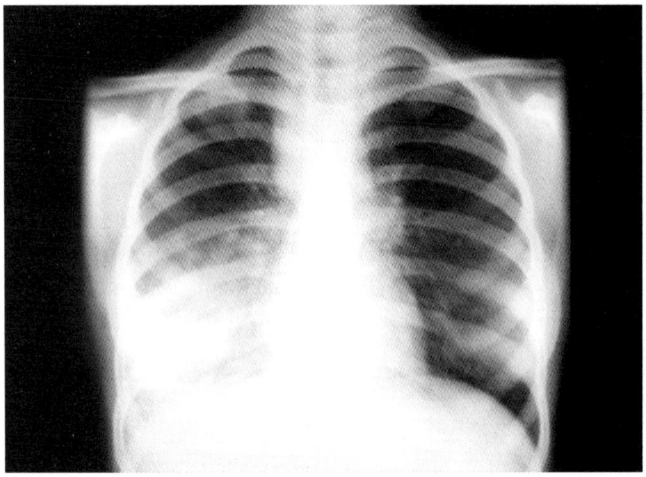

Fig. 22: Tuberculosis (TB): Frontal radiograph in an 8-year-old child with proven TB shows right paratracheal lymphadenopathy with homogeneous consolidation in the right lower lobe.

months after infection) than in older children (2–3 years after infection). Fibrotic and calcified lesions may persist. Single or multiple tuberculomas may develop in primary TB, but they are seen less frequently than in reactivation TB **(Figs. 24A and B)**.[3,7,20]

Pleural effusions usually occur due to direct extension from the parenchymal focus in cases of primary tuberculosis (TB). Effusions are not a common feature of primary TB in young children and are more commonly encountered in adolescents and adults.[18]

Hematogenous spread occurs as a rule but is self-limited in primary TB. However, when an overwhelming number of mycobacteria are discharged into the bloodstream, it can cause miliary infection of the lungs.[6,17] Infants are more susceptible to miliary TB, possibly due to low immunity at this age. CT can detect miliary disease earlier than chest radiographs **(Figs. 25A to C)**.[18]

Postprimary Tuberculosis

This is unusual in children and when seen in the pediatric age-group, it is usually seen in adolescents. It results from reactivation of dormant residual foci. Reactivation TB is rarer in children who were infected with primary disease before the age of 2 years. It is much more frequent in children who were afflicted by the primary disease after the age of 7 years, especially near puberty.[3] It is characterized by parenchymal disease with an anatomic bias for the upper lung zones. Typically the lesions are located in the apical and posterior segments of the upper lobes and superior segments of the lower lobes, probably due to relatively higher oxygen tension and impaired lymphatic drainage.[18] However, no portion of the lungs has immunity. Bilateral and multilobar involvement is fairly frequent. Cavitation is a characteristic radiographic finding. Necrotic rim enhancing lymph nodes or calcified lymph nodes may be encountered **(Figs. 26 to 28)**. Fluid levels may be seen within cavities. Heavy seeding of the bronchial tree is likely, particularly in the presence of cavitation and widespread bronchopneumonia may result. Cicatrization atelectasis is a common finding after postprimary TB. Bronchiectasis may be seen, either as a result of cicatricial broncho-stenosis after local infection, or more commonly due to

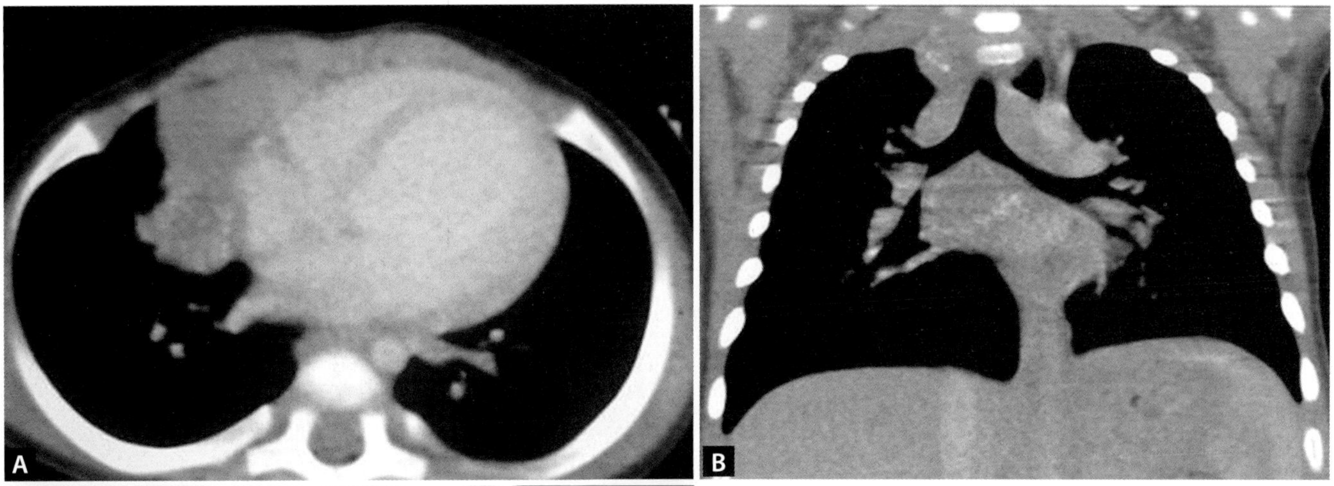

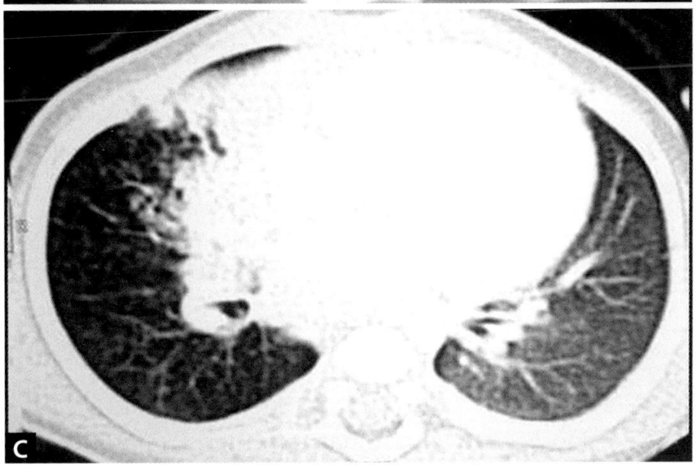

Figs. 23A to C: Tuberculosis (TB) in a 1-year-old child: Computed tomography (CT) images show right paratracheal, hilar and subcarinal node enlargement with foci of calcification. There is also collapse of the right middle lobe. This was probably due to the bronchial compression by enlarged lymph nodes.

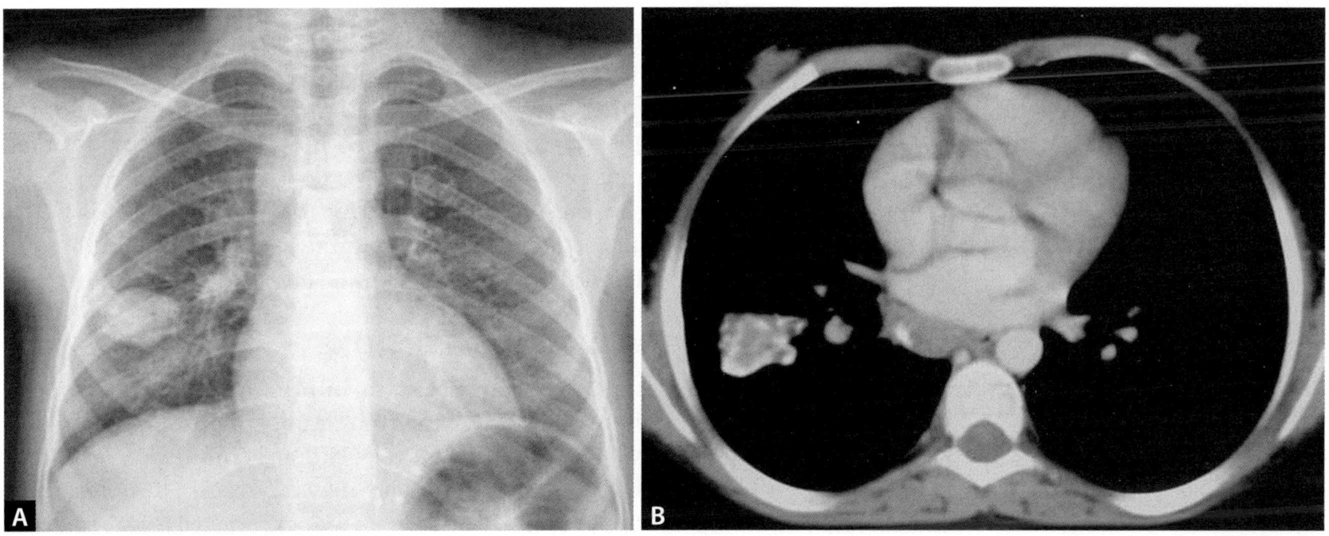

Figs. 24A and B: Tuberculoma (A): Frontal radiograph of an 11-year-old child reveals prominence of the right paratracheal stripe and hilum with nodule in the right lung field. (B) Axial contrast-enhanced computed tomography (CECT) image shows the calcified lymph nodes with granuloma in the right lung with foci of calcification.

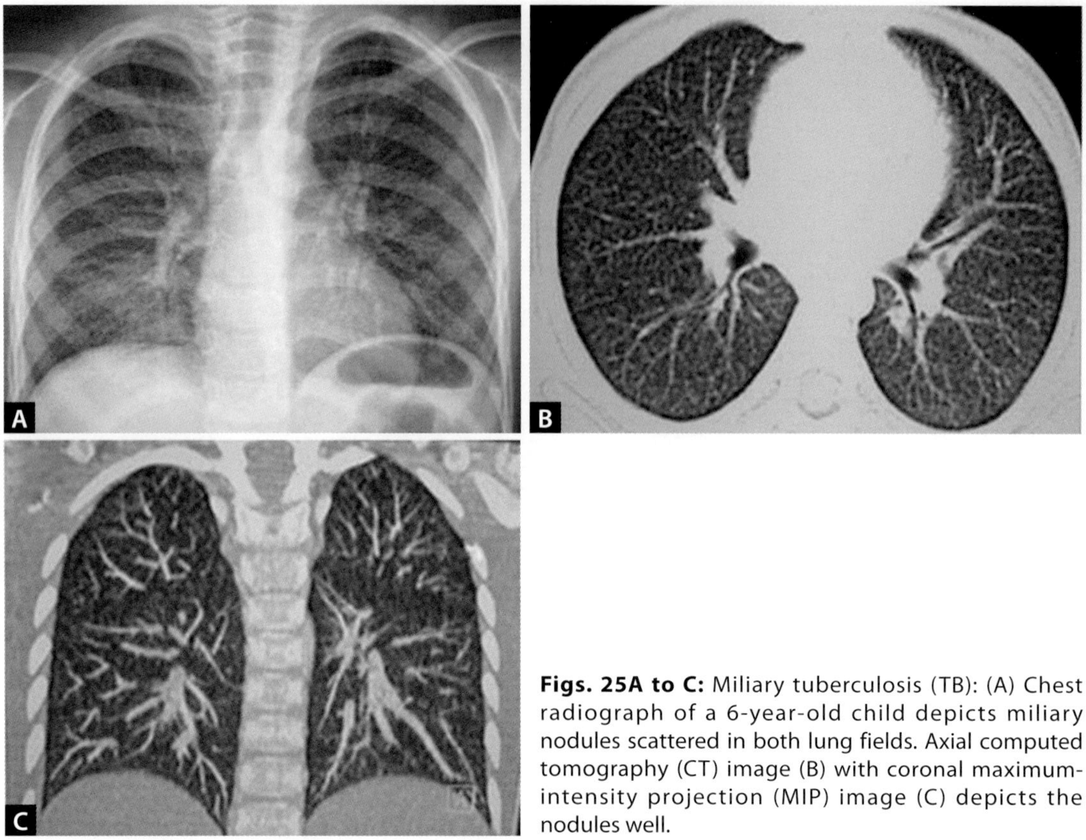

Figs. 25A to C: Miliary tuberculosis (TB): (A) Chest radiograph of a 6-year-old child depicts miliary nodules scattered in both lung fields. Axial computed tomography (CT) image (B) with coronal maximum-intensity projection (MIP) image (C) depicts the nodules well.

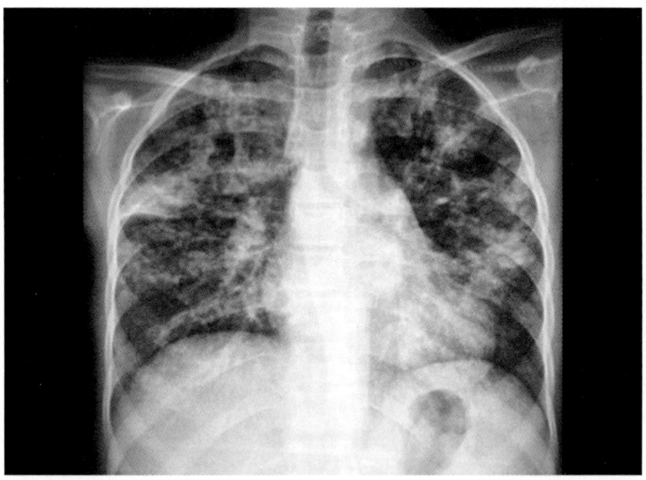

Fig. 26: Tuberculosis (TB): In an adolescent with TB, frontal radiograph depicts multifocal area of consolidation in both lungs with an area of cavitation in the right upper lobe.

fibrosis of lung parenchyma with secondary bronchial dilatation **(Figs. 29A to C)**. Calcification is often seen coincident with increasing fibrosis.[6,17]

Miliary TB, due to hematogenous spread can be seen with both primary and postprimary TB. Both well-defined and poorly-defined nodular opacities, 2–3 mm in size are seen scattered randomly in both lungs. Coalescence of small nodules may form larger nodules or even consolidation. There may be reticulonodular opacities with thickening of the interlobular septa. Ground-glass opacities may also be seen on high-resolution CT (HRCT) when small granulomas below the resolution of the scan are superimposed on exudative changes of the lung.[6,17]

Computed tomography may be done when TB is suspected in children, but the radiographic findings are inconclusive or when complications are suspected.[21]

FUNGAL INFECTIONS

Although may occur in immunocompetent patients, these are mostly seen in immunocompromised patients. Necrosis, cavitation, calcifications, chronic inflammatory reaction, pleural disease may all occur. These resemble tuberculous lesions. There are no conclusive radiographic criteria that can distinguish mycosis from TB or one mycosis from another. Few common radiographic patterns are enumerated in **Table 1**. Other important features are highlighted in the following discussion.

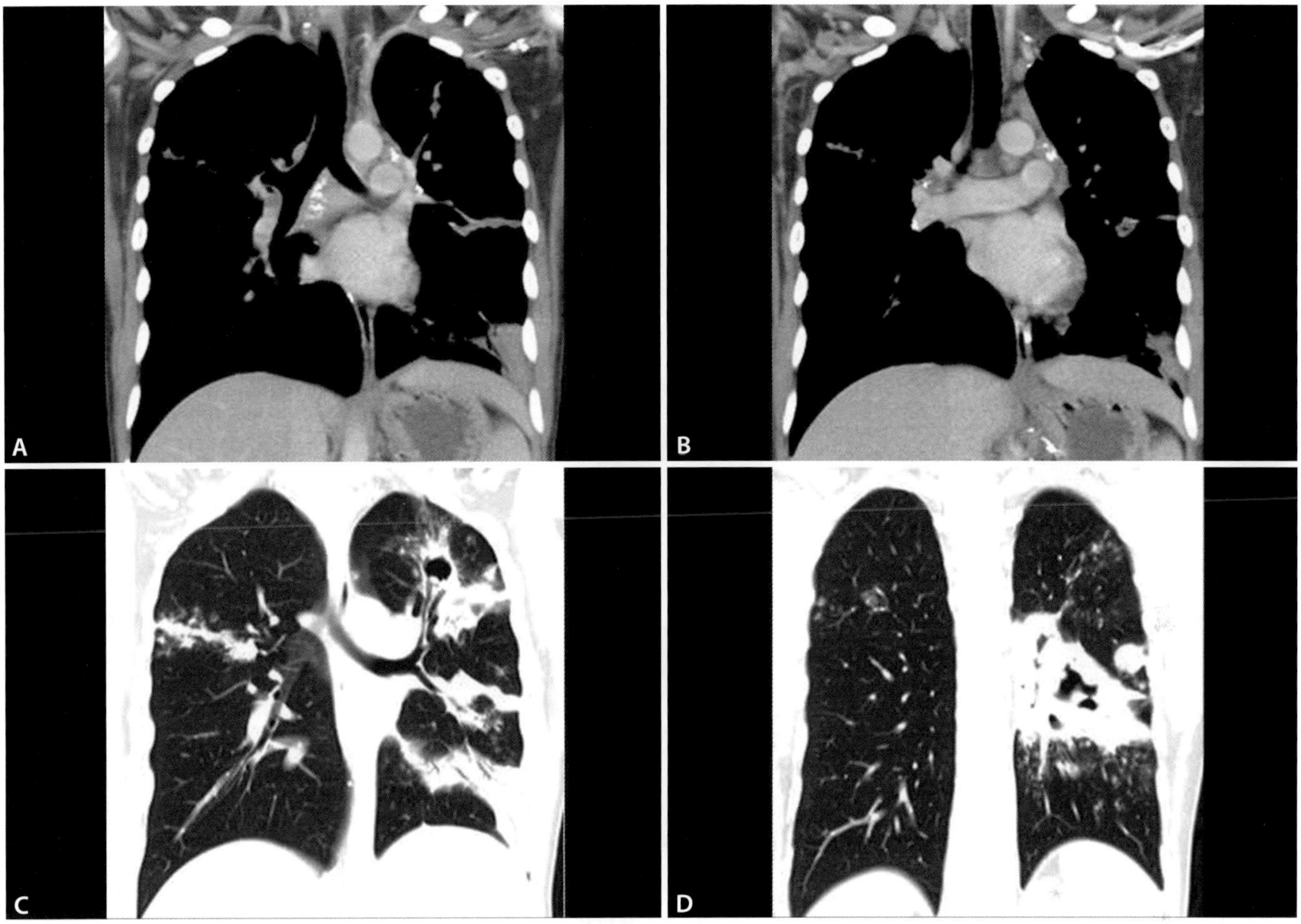

Figs. 27A to D: Tuberculosis (TB): In a 12-year-old girl, coronal reformatted computed tomography (CT) images at mediastinal and lung window settings show mediastinal nodes with foci of calcification and multifocal patches of consolidation bilaterally with areas of cavitation and other centrilobular nodules.

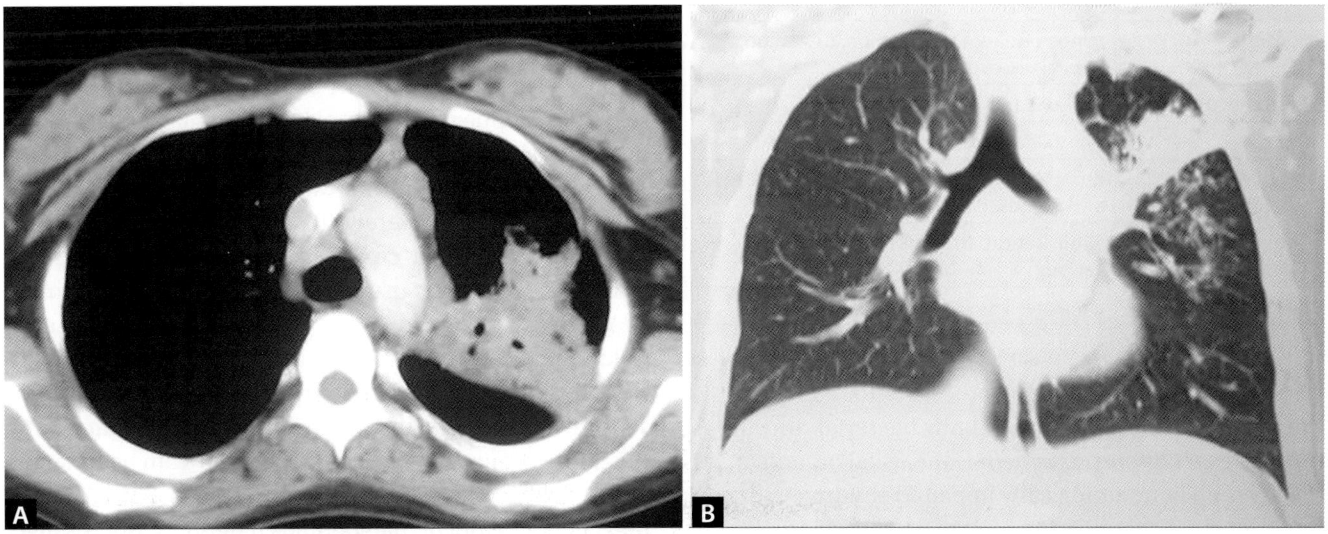

Figs. 28A and B: Tuberculosis (TB): In an adolescent, axial contrast-enhanced computed tomography (CECT) image at mediastinal window (A) shows evidence of mediastinal lymph nodes with left upper lobe consolidation. Coronal reformatted CT image (B) at lung window depicts consolidation in the left upper lobe with few adjacent centrilobular nodules.

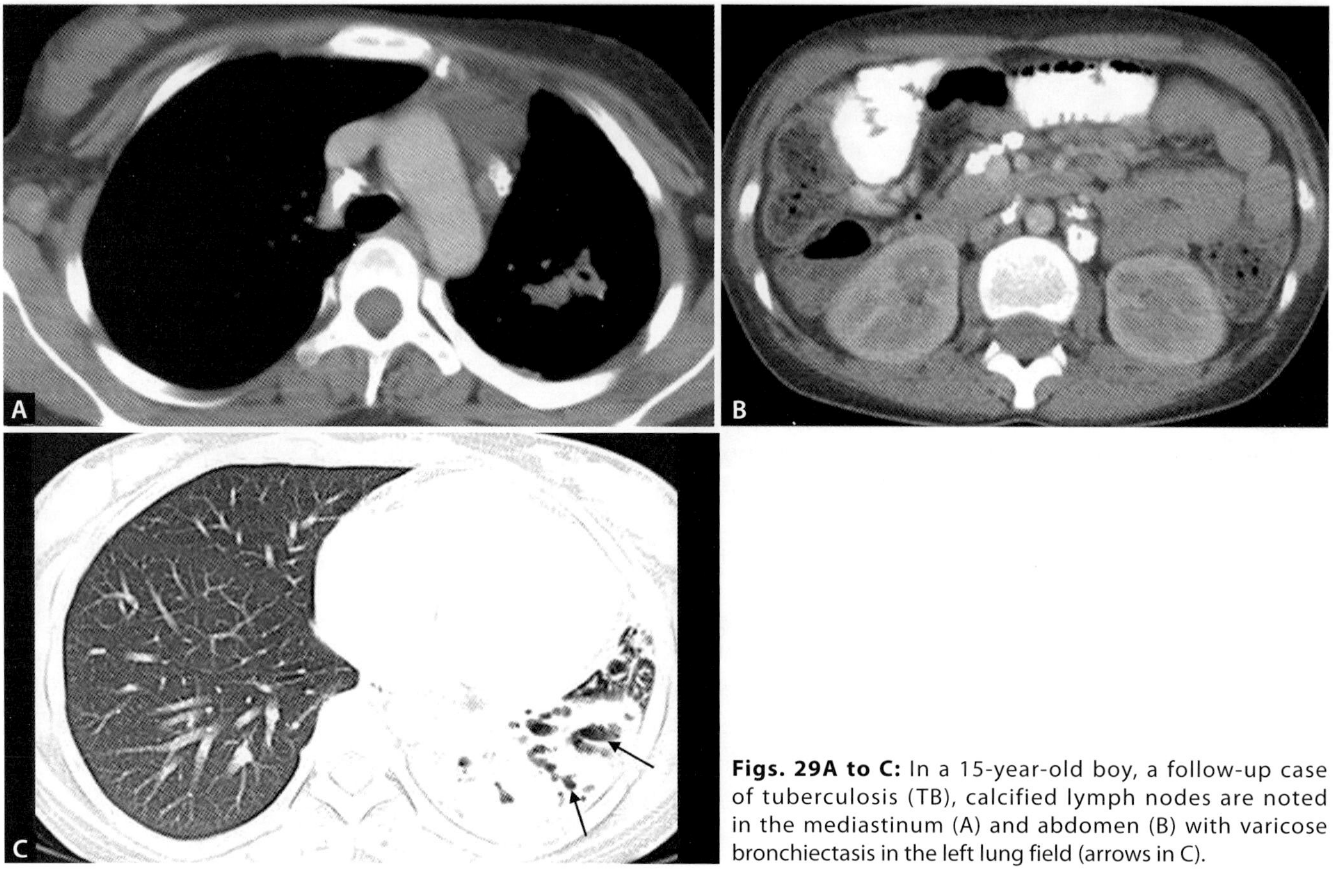

Figs. 29A to C: In a 15-year-old boy, a follow-up case of tuberculosis (TB), calcified lymph nodes are noted in the mediastinum (A) and abdomen (B) with varicose bronchiectasis in the left lung field (arrows in C).

Table 1: Radiographic characteristics of fungal and actinomyces infection.[3]

Infection	*Common radiographic patterns*
Actinomyces	Lung, nodal, pleural disease, chest wall involvement
Nocardia	Lung nodules, consolidation, cavitation, pleural disease
Blastomycosis	Consolidation, cavitation
Cryptococcosis	Consolidation, nodules
Invasive aspergillosis	Bronchocentric or angiocentric lesions, halo and air-crescent signs
Coccidioidomycosis	Simulates tuberculosis (TB), thin-walled cavities
Histoplasmosis	Simulates TB

Actinomyces

This anaerobic organism has both bacterial and fungal properties. *Actinomyces israelii* is the usual organism. It is mostly seen in neurologically impaired children with poor oral hygiene. Aggressive invasion of the thoracic wall when present is characteristic and often distinguishes this from fungal infections other than mucormycosis.[3]

Aspergillosis

Aspergillus can produce four distinct patterns in children depending on immune status and patient's pre-existing disease.

Fungal balls can form in pre-existing cavities formed by tuberculous infection, bronchiectasis or fibrotic lung disease and are unusual in children. These are usually seen in the upper lobes or apical segments of lower lobes, because most of the cavities are caused by previous TB. Mobility can be demonstrated in most cases except when it nearly completely fills the cavity with no space to move around. In contrast, the air-crescent sign of invasive aspergillosis usually does not have a background of fibrocavitatory disease. Pronounced associated inflammatory reaction may result in hemoptysis.[16]

Allergic bronchopulmonary aspergillosis is a hypersensitivity reaction to the presence of *Aspergillus fumigatus*. It is most commonly seen in association with asthma and cystic fibrosis. The immune reaction results in thick mucin plugging the bronchi. Radiographs may show gloved-finger appearance due to mucin-filled bronchi outlined because of collateral air drift. There may be patchy areas of atelectasis and emphysema. Central bronchiectasis may be seen. Aspergillus infection may be suggested in children with cystic fibrosis, when there are large patches of consolidation, often disproportionate to the magnitude of disease.

Invasive aspergillosis is invariably noted in immunocompromised neutropenic patients with leukemia or after bone marrow or solid organ transplantation. It may be airway invasive or angioinvasive. The two forms may coexist and it is not always possible to distinguish between the two types. Multifocal bronchocentric or angiocentric air-space opacities may be seen. Peribronchiolar nodules, centrilobular micronodules (<5 mm), ground-glass opacities and consolidation may be seen. In the angioinvasive form, wedge-shaped opacities can result from infarction as a consequence of hyphal invasion of blood vessels. Few nonspecific but distinctive features are halo sign and air crescent sign. The halo sign represents hemorrhage surrounding the nodule due to vascular invasion. It is seen earlier and with greater frequency than the air-crescent sign. The air-crescent sign is seen in the recovery phase when neutrophillic count rises; retraction of the necrotic lung from the viable lung parenchyma results in a crescent of air collection, partially outlining the necrotic lung.[16] Semi-invasive aspergillosis is a less aggressive form seen in patients with underlying lung disease or with mild immunosuppression.[3] This is also known as chronic airway invasive aspergillosis and may mimic reactivation TB. It usually starts as a focus of consolidation in the upper lobes, which may have cavitation and pleural thickening.

Histoplasmosis

This is endemic in many parts of the United States of America (USA), especially in Ohio and Mississippi river valleys. The initial exudative phase simulates primary complex of TB; only the pulmonary foci are mostly multifocal. 95% of patients are asymptomatic in the initial phase. The disease resembles TB in all phases.

Disseminated histoplasmosis may occur in an infant in the exudative phase, and resembles miliary TB. Massive hepatosplenomegaly may be seen with granulomatous or calcific foci.

A rare but serious complication is fibrosing mediastinitis, which may result in compression of the pulmonary artery, superior vena cava, airway and esophagus. In the west, chronic histoplasmosis is a frequent cause of mediastinal fibrosis in children.[3]

Coccidioidomycosis

Coccidioidomycosis, caused by *Coccidioides immitis*, is endemic in south-western deserts of USA. The radiographic manifestations are similar to TB in all phases, including consolidation, lymph nodes and pleural effusions. The primary complex lasts only a few weeks, duration being shorter than in TB. Residual calcifications may occur. Small thin-walled cavities, commonly seen in adults, are less common in children.[3]

PARASITIC INFESTATIONS

Hydatid Disease of the Lung

Hydatidosis, caused by larval stage of *Echinococcus granulosus*, is the most frequently encountered type of hydatid disease in humans. While in adults, hepatic involvement is more common than lungs, in children, the lungs are the most common site of involvement. The lung facilitates the growth of cyst due to compressible nature and the presence of negative pressure. Intact cysts are seen as sharply defined round to oval masses of variable size **(Figs. 30A and B)**. Lung cysts rarely calcify. Rupture or superimposed infection may result in varied appearances giving rise to air-crescent sign, air-bubble sign, water-lily sign, mass within cavity sign and ring enhancement sign amongst others.[22]

Others

Few parasites including *Ascaris lumbricoides, Necator americanus, Ancylostoma duodenale, Strongyloides stercoralis* may pass through lungs as a part of their life cycle. These may result in transient migratory pulmonary opacities without recognizable segmental distribution. Blood and sputum eosinophilia may be present along with pulmonary opacities (Löffler's syndrome).[16]

Paragonimiasis is endemic in the Orient and is a common cause of necrosis and calcification in lungs and is difficult to distinguish from TB radiologically.

PULMONARY INFECTIONS IN HIV-POSITIVE CHILDREN

Most children are infected after vertical transmission from their mother, and majorities develop acquired immunodeficiency syndrome (AIDS) early in life. Majority of perinatally infected children develop symptoms during the first 24 months of life. Children who develop human immunodeficiency virus (HIV) infection as a result of blood transfusion frequently are asymptomatic for long periods of time, although immunological abnormalities may be seen. Respiratory infection is very common in children and more than 70% of patients with AIDS will suffer from at least one episode of respiratory infection in the course of their illness. In pediatric age-group,

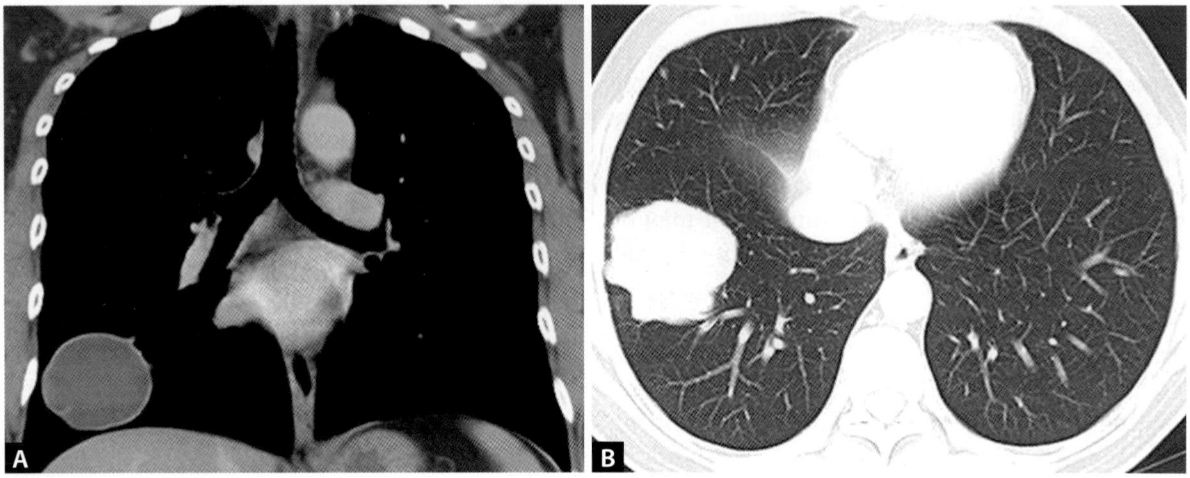

Figs. 30A and B: Hydatid cyst: Homogeneous well-defined rounded fluid attenuation mass lesion noted in the right lower lobe.

lungs are often the site of life-threatening illness in these patients. As the radiographic appearance is not specific, the aim of imaging is to narrow the differential diagnosis based upon pattern recognition, clinical presentation, level of immunocompromise and current drug therapy such as highly active antiretroviral therapy (HAART) and *Pneumocystis jiroveci* pneumonia (PJP) prophylaxis.[23,24]

Bacterial Pneumonias

Typical pneumonias (*S. pneumoniae, S. aureus*) occur as in immunocompetent children, but with increased frequency and severity. The radiological appearance is that of bronchopneumonia and lobar pneumonia as in immunocompetent children but with an increased incidence of empyema and lung abscesses. Other uncommon pathogens include *Salmonella spp., Klebsiella spp., Pseudomonas spp., E. coli* and other atypical organisms such as *Mycoplasma*. These can produce a wide variety of appearances, including bilateral patchy reticulonodular infiltrates and patchy or confluent air-space opacification. Also common are polymicrobial infections.[23]

Pyogenic infectious airway disease has been increasingly recognized in recent years in HIV population, including bronchitis, bronchiolitis and bronchiectasis.

Mycobacterial Pneumonias

As CD4 lymphocytes, which play an important role in cellular immunity against mycobacterial infections, are the primary target of HIV infection, the risk of TB increases. Tuberculin test is less useful and treatment response is poorer in this subset of patients. Primary TB usually manifests as massive adenopathy, and pattern of consolidation similar to that in primary TB in immunocompetent children. Miliary pattern may also be encountered. Subcarinal group of lymph nodes are the most common. On magnetic resonance imaging (MRI), lymph nodes have a strikingly low signal on T_2 and short tau inversion recovery (STIR) images. Pleural effusion is uncommon.[23,25]

Mycobacterium avium-intracellulare has also been observed in pediatric AIDS patients. Children tend to be older with lower CD4 lymphocyte counts (< 50 cells/mm^3) than the general pediatric HIV population. Children have nonspecific features of air-space opacification, nodular opacities, cavitation, bronchiectasis and mediastinal nodes.[23,25]

Fungal Pneumonias

Pneumocystis jiroveci pneumonia remains the most common pulmonary pathogen in children with AIDS, although the incidence appears to decrease because of prophylactic treatment.[25] Children with PJP are usually younger than those with other pulmonary conditions, with a peak age incidence at 4–5 months. PJP can be fulminant, with a mortality rate as high as 40–50%. Most patients have a CD4 count less than 100 cells/mm^3. Radiographic findings include a normal radiograph, hyperinflation with prominent perihilar bronchovascular markings or air-space opacities. PJP needs to be included in the differential diagnosis of any infant with rapidly progressive pneumonia, even in those not known to have HIV infection as approximately 45% of children with PJP are not known to have HIV at the time of presentation. The use of PJP prophylaxis does not exclude the diagnosis. CT is the imaging modality of choice. CT features include patchy areas of ground glassing, especially in the perihilar location **(Figs. 31A and B)**. Interlobular septal thickening

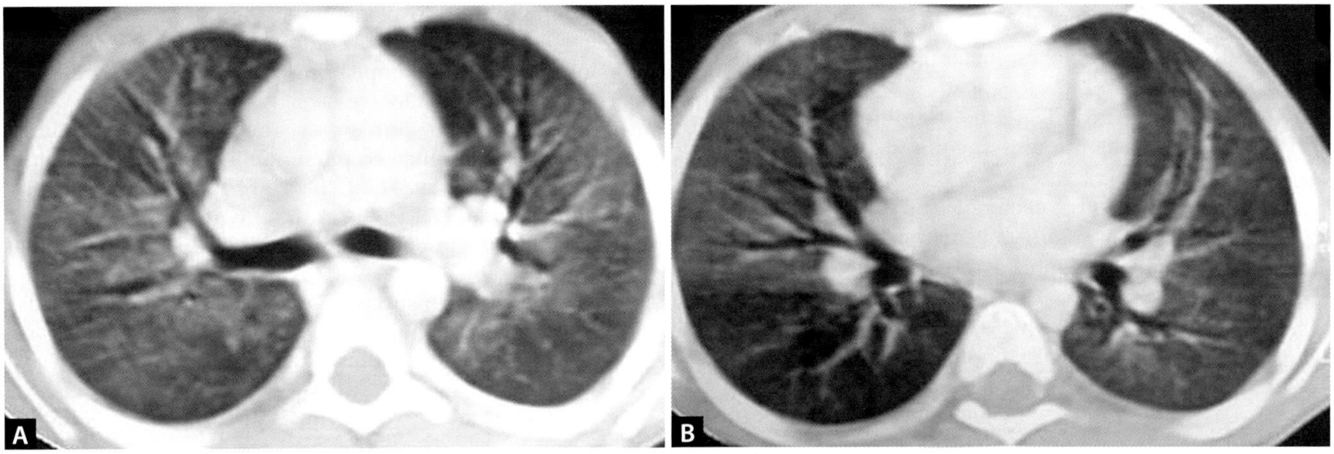

Figs. 31A and B: *Pneumocystis jiroveci* pneumonia (PJP): Areas of ground-glass opacification are seen in bilateral lungs in a proven case of PJP in a 6-year-old human immunodeficiency virus (HIV) positive boy.

may be present. Other findings include lymphadenopathy, nodules and mass lesions. Pulmonary air cysts may be seen. Pneumothorax and pneumomediastinum may occur. Pleural effusion is uncommon and suggests other pathology.[23,25]

Infection with *Cryptococcus neoformans, Histoplasmosis, Mucormycosis* and *Invasive aspergillosis* are the other fungal infections that may be encountered.

Viral Pneumonias

Viral pathogens include RSV, parainfluenza, influenza, adenovirus, cytomegalovirus (CMV), measles, varicella and herpes simplex virus. Signs of consolidation are more common than wheezing in immunocompromised children.

Transmission of RSV is primarily via the hands contaminated with secretions from the mouth or nose. The radiographic findings are diffuse, patchy or nodular air-space opacities rather than interstitial infiltrates. Secondary bacterial infections are more common.[23]

Cytomegalovirus pneumonia usually presents when the CD4 counts fall below the level of 50 cells/mm^3. Chest radiographs may be normal, may show reticulonodular or air-space pattern of disease. CT features include ground-glass attenuation, nodules, consolidation and masses. Other features may be cavitation, bronchiectasis, lymphadenopathy and pleural effusions.

Lymphocytic Interstitial Pneumonitis

Lymphocytic interstitial pneumonitis (LIP) is seen in 30–40% of patients with HIV infection. It is believed to be a response of the lymphoid system to circulating antigens of infectious agents (Epstein-Barr virus) or to HIV itself. Patients tend to be a little older at diagnosis than those with opportunistic infections. It is most frequently diagnosed in children over 2 years of age. The course of the disease is relatively indolent compared to PJP. It presents with insidious development of respiratory distress and mild cough. Associated findings include generalized lymphadenopathy, salivary gland enlargement, hepatosplenomegaly and clubbing of fingers. It has a relatively good prognosis with resolution indicating severe immunosuppression and impending opportunistic infections.[26]

Clinical features and radiographic appearances are usually sufficient to make the diagnosis. Chest radiographs range from mild prominence of bronchovascular markings to the more classical description of adenopathy and reticulonodular markings. Nodules may measure up to 2–3 mm in diameter. Lymphadenopathy may be massive, but with no airway compression, in contradistinction to tuberculous adenopathy. On CT, diffuse ground-glass opacity, poorly-defined centrilobular nodules, interlobular septal thickening and thickening of the bronchovascular interstitium may be seen. Bronchiectasis and cyst formation may complicate the disease. LIP responds successfully to steroid treatment.[24,16]

CONCLUSION

Because of the high frequency of lower respiratory tract infections in children, it is important to be familiar with the role of imaging in the diagnosis and management of various pediatric pulmonary infections.

REFERENCES

1. Frush DP. Pediatric chest imaging. Radiol Clinics N Am. 2005;43:xi-xii.
2. Donnelly LF. Maximizing the usefulness of imaging in children with community-acquired pneumonia. AJR. 1999;172(2):505-12.
3. Adler B, Effmann EL. Pneumonia and pulmonary infection. In: Slovis TL (Eds). Caffey's Pediatric Diagnostic Imaging, 11th edition. Philadelphia, PA, USA: Mosby-Elsevier; 2008. pp. 1184-7.
4. Markowitz RI, Ruchelli E. Pneumonia in infants and children: Radiological-pathological correlation. Semin Roentgenol. 1998;33(2):151-62.
5. Donnelly LF. Imaging in immunocompetent children who have pneumonia. Radiol Clinics North Am. 2005;43(2):253-65.
6. McPhillips M. Infection. In: Carty H, Brunelle F, Stringer DA, Kao SC (Eds). Imaging in Children, 2nd edition. Philadelphia, PA, USA: Elsevier Churchill Livingstone; 2005. pp. 1075-118.
7. Copley SJ. Application of computed tomography in childhood respiratory infections. Br Med Bull. 2002;61:263-79.
8. Bettenay FA, de Campo JF, McCrossin DB. Differentiating bacterial from viral pneumonias in children. Pediatr Radiol. 1988;18(6):453-4.
9. Burko H. Considerations in the roentgen diagnosis of pneumonia in children. Am J Roentgenol Radium Ther Nucl Med. 1962;88:555-65.
10. Kirkpatrick JA. Pneumonia in children as it differs from adult pneumonia. Semin Roentgenol. 1980;15(1): 96-103.
11. Griscom NT, Wohl MB, Kirkpatrick JA. Lower respiratory infections: How infants differ from adults. Radiol Clin North Am. 1978;16(3):367-87.
12. Calder A, Owens CM. Imaging of parapneumonic pleural effusions and empyema in children. Pediatr Radiol. 2009;39(6):527-37.
13. Donnelly LF, Klosterman LA. Pneumonia in children: decreased parenchymal contrast enhancement: CT sign of intense illness and impending cavitary necrosis. Radiology. 1997;205(3):817-20.
14. Donnelly LF, Klosterman LA. The yield of CT of children who have complicated pneumonia and noncontributory chest radiography. AJR. 1998;170(6):1627-31.
15. Donnelly LF, Klosterman LA. Cavitary necrosis complicating pneumonia in children: Sequential findings on chest radiography. AJR. 1998;171(1):253-6.
16. Hansell DM, Armstrong P, Lynch DA, McAdams HP (Eds). Infections of the lungs and pleura. In: Imaging of Diseases of the Chest, 4th edition. Philadelphia, PA, USA: Mosby-Elsevier; 2005. pp. 183-276.
17. Fonseca-Santos J. Tuberculosis in children. Eur J Radiol. 2005;55(2):202-8.
18. Agrons GA, Markowitz RI, Kramer SS. Pulmonary tuberculosis in children. Semin Roentgenol. 1993;28(2):158-72.
19. Leung AN, Müller NL, Pineda PR, et al. Primary tuberculosis in childhood: Radiographic manifestations. Radiology. 1992;182(1):87-91.
20. Lamont AC, Cremin BJ, Pelteret RM. Radiological patterns of pulmonary tuberculosis in the pediatric age group. Pediatr Radiol. 1986;16(1):2-7.
21. Kim WS, Moon WK, Kim IO, et al. Pulmonary tuberculosis in children: Evaluation with CT. AJR. 1997;168(4):1005-9.
22. Turgut AT, Altinok T, Topçu S, et al. Local complications of hydatid disease involving thoracic cavity: imaging findings. Eur J Radiol. 2009;70(1):49-56.
23. George R, Andronikou S, Theron S, et al. Pulmonary infection in HIV-positive children. Pediatr Radiol. 2009;39(6):545-54.
24. Harty MP, Markowitz RI, Rutstein RM, et al. Imaging features of human immunodeficiency virus infection in infants and children. Seminars Roentgenol. 1994;29(3):303-14.
25. Marks MJ, Haney PJ, McDermott MP, et al. Thoracic disease in children with AIDS. Radiographics. 1996;16(6):1349-62.
26. Theron S, Andronikou S, George R, et al. Non-infective pulmonary disease in HIV-positive children. Pediatr Radiol. 2009;39(6):555-64.

CHAPTER 132

Chest Masses

Sanjay Thulkar, Arun Kumar Gupta

INTRODUCTION

Thoracic masses in children may be located in mediastinum, lung or the chest wall. Majority of these are surgical conditions. The spectrum ranges from incidentally detected developmental lesions to aggressive malignant tumors. Chest radiography is the initial modality for their detection; however, most require further evaluation with CT or MRI. While obtaining the CT, special attention must be given radiation issues in children and dedicated pediatric CT protocols should be followed. Although MRI has the limitations of long imaging time often-requiring general anesthesia as well as poor lung evaluation, it should be substituted for CT whenever possible.

LUNG MASSES

These can be classified as:

- *Congenital*
  - *Abnormal lung bud development*: Congenital lobar emphysema, unilateral pulmonary agenesis/aplasia, pulmonary hypoplasia and hypogenetic lung syndrome (The conditions are described separately in this book)
  - *Abnormality of separation of lung bud*: Sequestration
  - *Hamartomatous lesions*: Congenital cystic adenomatoid malformation (CCAM); lung cysts, hamartoma
  - *Vascular anomalies*: Congenital arteriovenous malformation (AVM)
- *Inflammatory*: Lung abscess, hydatid cyst
- *Neoplastic*: Metastases, pulmonary sarcoma/blastoma.

Congenital Cystic Adenomatoid Malformation

This relatively rare entity is considered a focal pulmonary dysplasia and is defined as "a multicystic mass of pulmonary tissue in which there is proliferation of immature bronchial structures at the expense of alveolar development". Pathologically, the affected lobe is increased in volume and weight. The cysts are lined by cuboidal or columnar epithelium and the walls contain smooth muscle and elastic tissue. Type I is most common and contains one to four, varying sized air-filled large cysts over 2.0 cm in diameter. It may resemble congenital lobar emphysema especially if unilocular. Type II is characterized by numerous small to medium sized thin walled cysts of up to 2 cm in diameter, and prognosis is bad when associated with other congenital malformations. Type III is the least common. It is seen as a large solid lesion with multiple tiny fluid-filled cysts.[1]

Congenital cystic adenomatoid malformation may be seen in stillborn infant with a classical triad of hydramnios, fetal ascites and cystic or solid mass in the fetal chest. The intrathoracic mass causes venous obstruction, which in turn is responsible for fetal ascites. On antenatal ultrasound, CCAM is seen as an echogenic intrathoracic mass, which may or may not have cysts. After birth, it presents with neonatal respiratory distress. In the older infant, it may cause pulmonary infection. The lesion is usually unilateral and occurs with equal frequency in both lungs with slight predilection for the upper lobes. CCAM usually involves an entire lobe or lung and produces mediastinal shift. The prognosis is usually poor due to large size and early *in utero* cardiovascular compromise.

Type I appears as a multicystic lesion with a tendency for recurrent infection in older children. Types II and III are usually associated with respiratory distress in the newborn, often with other congenital anomalies. Radiographically, types I and II demonstrate a multilocular air-filled bubbly mass. At this stage the differential diagnosis includes congenital diaphragmatic hernia (in which the abdomen will be gasless) and staphylococcal pneumatoceles (uncommon in the neonatal period). If one of the cysts becomes extremely large with very thin walls, it may resemble a pneumothorax or congenital lobar emphysema. Prenatal diagnosis may be made on ultrasound. Ultrasound is also helpful in the evaluation of fluid-filled or solid-appearing lesions. The solid lesions demonstrate highly reflective interfaces within due to the walls of the minute cysts. In uninfected CCAM, CT shows multilocular cystic mass with thin walls **(Fig. 1)** while in infected lesion, CT shows a complex mass with a mixture of solid and cystic lesions with variable definition and thick walls. The treatment is surgical excision even if the patient is asymptomatic. Type III lesion is seen as a solid pulmonary mass may be seen in the neonatal period.[2]

Pulmonary Sequestration

A bronchopulmonary sequestration is defined as a congenital mass of nonfunctioning lung tissue, which contains both bronchial and alveolar elements but lacks communication with tracheobronchial tree and receives blood supply from an anomalous systemic artery. Its venous drainage may be via the pulmonary veins, inferior vena cava or the azygos system. Sequestration occurs when a supernumerary lung bud develops caudal to the normal lung bud. If arrest occurs early in development, its communication with the foregut remains, sharing its blood supply. If arrest occurs later, sequestrated segment is connected with foregut through a fibrous band. This malformation has been further classified as intralobar in which the abnormal tissue is contained within the normal lung and its pleural covering and extralobar in which the sequestration is separate from the lung parenchyma and has its own pleural covering.

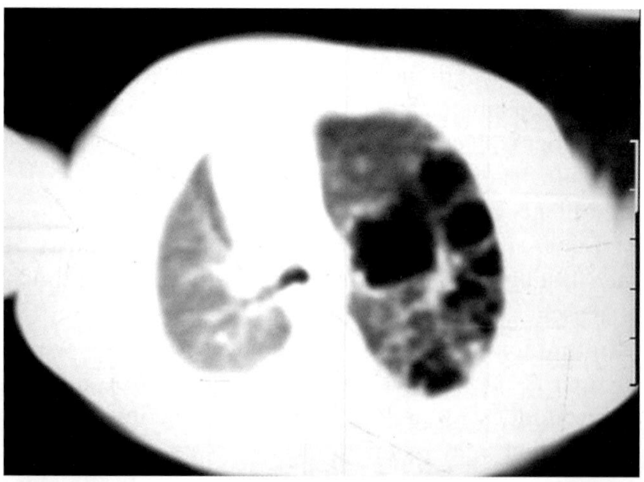

Fig. 1: Congenital cystic adenomatoid malformation. CT of chest shows a thin-walled multicystic left lung mass.

Intralobar sequestration predominantly occurs in lower lobes, usually on the left side. It tends to present later in life as an incidental finding on chest radiograph or because of recurrent infections. Patients may also present with hemoptysis if there is communication with bronchial tree. The sequestrated segment may communicate with the adjacent lung as a result of infection or occasionally cystic spaces in the lesion may communicate directly with bronchial tree.

On a chest radiograph and CT, the lesion appears as an oval, spherical or triangular basal opacity **(Figs. 2A to C)**. It is ill-defined and often contains multiple cysts of variable sizes, simulating CCAM. Indeed pulmonary sequestration may coexist with CCAM and then it is called as hybrid lesion of the lung. Other differential diagnosis includes pneumonia, bronchogenic cyst or pulmonary neoplasm. Most often, the abnormal vascular supply is a large vessel arising from the aorta either above or below the diaphragm. It is important to demonstrate the abnormal vascular channel on CT or MR angiography not only for diagnosis but also to avoid potential hemorrhage if surgery is contemplated.[3]

Extralobar sequestration occurs in contiguity with the left hemidiaphragm in 90% of the patients and is often seen incidentally as a basal soft tissue mass at or below the diaphragm with associated diaphragmatic hernia in almost 30% of patients. These masses enhance on contrast-enhanced CT. Sometimes aeration may occur in this opacity. As it is completely separated from lung, there is less chance of secondary infection.

Bronchogenic Cyst

This congenital lesion presents after the newborn period. It arises as a result of anomalous supernumerary budding of the tracheal diverticulum of the ventral foregut. The cyst has a fibrous wall containing cartilage, and is lined by respiratory epithelium and may be filled with air, mucoid or

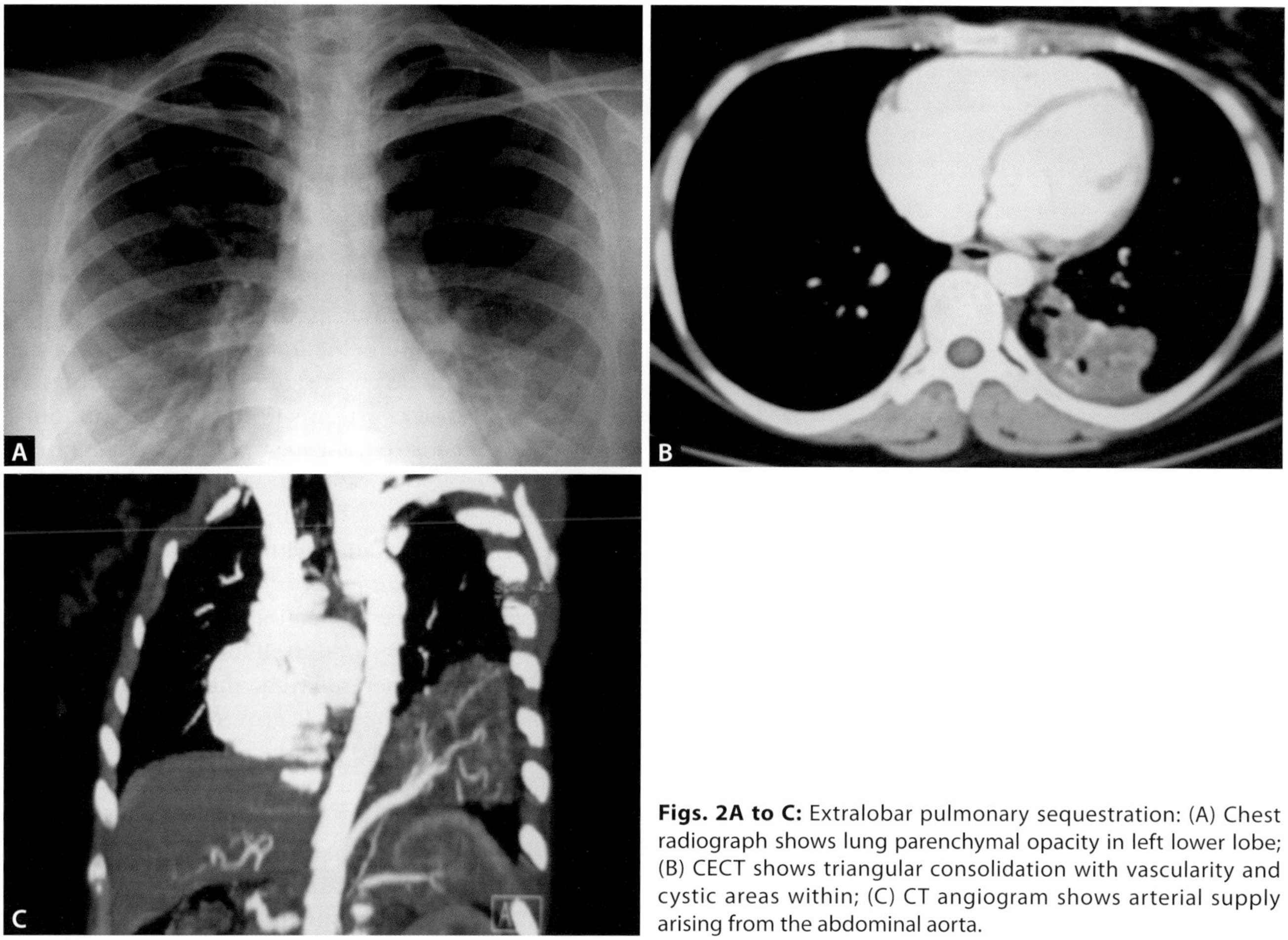

Figs. 2A to C: Extralobar pulmonary sequestration: (A) Chest radiograph shows lung parenchymal opacity in left lower lobe; (B) CECT shows triangular consolidation with vascularity and cystic areas within; (C) CT angiogram shows arterial supply arising from the abdominal aorta.

serous fluid or combination of these. The location of the cyst may be central (near hilum or mediastinum) or peripheral in the lung. Mediastinal bronchogenic cysts are more common and the usual locations are subcarinal, paratracheal and along the bronchi. Intrapulmonary cysts can be perihilar or peripheral. The central cyst is usually solitary and asymptomatic until infection occurs that produces hemoptysis, fever, cough or purulent expectoration. There is no direct communication of mediastinal bronchogenic cysts with the tracheobronchial tree. However, the mediastinal bronchogenic cysts may be attached to major airways through a stalk. Rapid enlargement may be seen in infected cysts and respiratory distress may be profound. When peripheral, the cysts may be multiple and extensive. With multiple cysts, respiratory distress and even death may occur shortly after birth. Bronchial communication is common with peripheral cysts with air-fluid levels and more rapid development of infection.

Chest radiograph shows round or oval, smooth, sharply marginated, thin walled, homogeneous water density mass or air-filled cyst in the mediastinal or perihilar location. Mass effect over the adjacent trachea, bronchus or esophagus may be demonstrable. An air-fluid level and thick wall may be seen in infected cysts. On CT, a hypodense, isodense or hyperdense mass lesion may be seen depending on the nature of fluid contents[4] **(Fig. 3)**. The differential diagnosis on chest radiograph of a fluid-filled intrapulmonary bronchogenic cyst includes round pneumonia, primary or metastatic pulmonary neoplasm, interlobar effusion. Air or air fluid-filled cyst should be differentiated from small congenital cystic adenomatoid malformation, pneumatocele and pulmonary abscess. Complications of bronchogenic cysts include infection, hemorrhage, spontaneous pneumothorax and rarely, development of malignancy.[5]

Vascular Lesions

Vascular malformations may be isolated or part of a congenital syndrome like hereditary telangiectasia. When multiple or large, they may cause high output cardiac failure

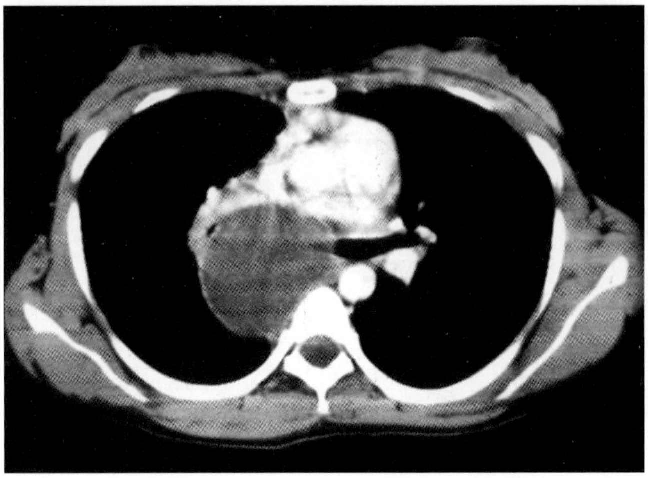

Fig. 3: Bronchogenic cyst: CT of chest shows a subcarinal fluid-filled cyst.

and cyanosis from right to left shunting. A pulmonary AVM or varix may be seen on a radiograph as a well-defined serpiginous or lobulated opacity. Calcification is rare.[6] Associated linear density representing a feeding vessel may be seen. If the feeding vessel is not apparent, the lesion may simulate a granuloma or metastasis. A thin-section CT pulmonary angiogram would demonstrate an arterial malformation to best advantage. Pulmonary angiography with and embolization is the treatment of choice.[7]

Lung Abscess

A lung abscess develops when necrosis, suppuration and cavitation occur in a localized infection of lung parenchyma. The necrotic cavity filled with purulent material may develop an air-fluid level if erosion into the airway has occurred. Staphylococci, alpha and beta hemolytic streptococci, *Pseudomonas, Klebsiella* and aspirated anaerobic mouth flora are the common organisms for the lung abscesses. With advent of antibiotics and prompt therapy, incidence of primary lung abscess has markedly reduced. However, secondary abscess in an immunocompromised and severely ill patient has become more frequent.

The radiological appearance depends on the relative amount of necrosis, consolidation and presence of gas in the necrosis. In early stages, discrete pneumonic consolidation is seen on chest radiograph. CT at this stage may show low-density center in the area of consolidation. There is absence of air bronchogram within the abscess. When the cavity attains sufficient size and is filled with air after a bronchial communication, an air-fluid level will be seen. The abscess wall is enhancing, thick and shaggy **(Fig. 4)**. Ultrasound is also useful to demonstrate lung abscess and to perform ultrasound-guided aspiration.[8]

Cavitary necrosis is a more common complication of chest infection in children. It is seen as well-demarcated area of necrosis filled with multiple small irregular cysts **(Fig. 5)**. Affected part of the lung parenchyma does not enhance.[9] Round pneumonia is a localized infective pneumonia which appears as a rounded lung mass. This occurs in young children in whom collateral air circulation through pores of Kohn is not well developed. The consolidation remains localized and forms a mass like round opacity on chest radiographs. In children with clinical features of chest infection, round pneumonia is the most likely cause of lung mass on chest radiographs.[10]

Hydatid Cysts

This is caused by infestation with *Echinococcus granulosus* and *Echinococcus multilocularis*. As hydatid cyst grows, it compresses the adjacent lung tissue into a fibrotic capsule known as pericyst. The cyst itself has a thin smooth wall, consisting of two adherent layers, the laminated ectocyst and thin lining endocyst. It grows rapidly and nearly two-thirds may rupture in either the surrounding lung, bronchial tree or pleura.

Chest radiograph shows spherical or oval well-defined homogeneous opacity **(Fig. 6)**. It may be single, multiple, unilateral or bilateral. Lung hydatids rarely calcify. When the pericyst ruptures into an airway and air dissects between pericyst and ectocyst, this gives rise to the characteristic meniscus or crescent sign. When the cyst ruptures into an airway, an air-fluid level results. Sometimes the cyst wall is seen crumpled up and floating in fluid, which lies within the noncollapsed pericyst. This is described as water-lily sign or camalote sign. Fluid content is demonstrated on CT or MRI. With secondary infection, the membranes may disintegrate, walls thicken and the appearance is indistinguishable from bacterial lung abscess on chest radiograph. Sometimes all contents of the cyst may be expelled through the bronchial tree and resultant dry cyst is seen as air-filled cavity.[11] Lesions abutting the chest wall or diaphragm can also be diagnosed on ultrasound, which shows the characteristic cystic mass, with floating membranes.

Pulmonary Metastasis

Metastases are the most common malignant lesion of the lung in children. The common primary tumors that metastasize to lung include Wilms' tumor, osteosarcoma, Ewing's sarcoma, rhabdomyosarcoma, lymphoma, leukemia, germ cell tumors and neuroblastoma. The

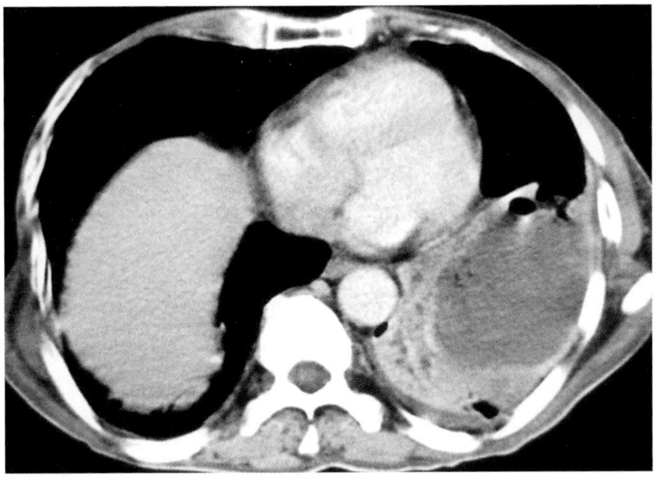

Fig. 4: Lung abscess: CECT shows a fluid-filled rounded lesion with air lucencies within and thick enhancing wall.

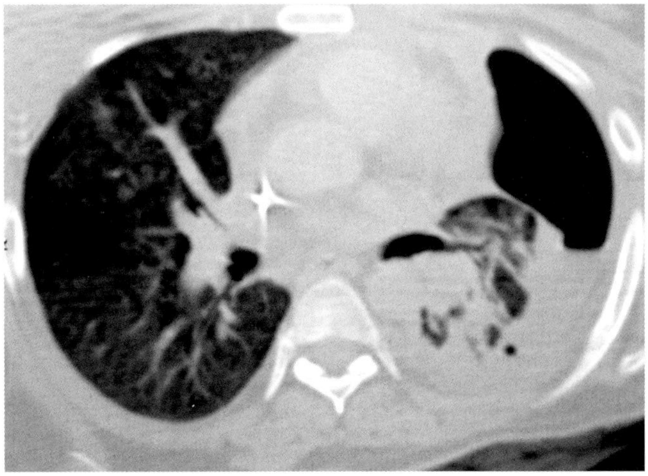

Fig. 5: Cavitary necrosis: CECT of chest of a leukemic man shows left lung consolidation with irregular cavities within. Variable sizes of the cavities help to distinguish it from air bronchogram. Associated hydropneumothorax is also seen.

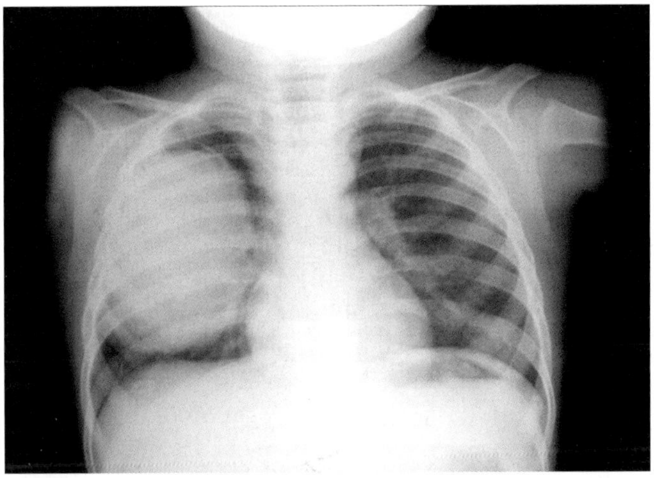

Fig. 6: Hydatid cyst: Chest radiograph shows a well-defined homogeneous oval mass in right lung.

metastasis may be single or multiple, vary in size from a small nodule to large mass or a lymphangitis pattern may be seen. With a known primary malignancy, chest radiograph is always necessary to look for metastasis, and if present, further imaging studies may not be indicated. However, CT is routinely indicated in patients with normal chest radiographs in cancers with high incidence of lung metastases and whom the management would alter. Such cancers include most sarcomas, choriocarcinoma, and germ cell tumors. CT is also required if metastasectomy is considered. On CT, the metastases are seen as a round sharply defined nodules or masses with homogeneous attenuation. Deposits from Wilms' tumor, Hodgkin's disease and osteosarcoma may cavitate and when peripheral, these may cause a pneumothorax.

Osteosarcoma is the most common cause of calcified metastases; it may also be associated with calcified mediastinal lymph nodes and calcified pleural deposits[12] **(Figs. 7A and B)**. Thyroid carcinoma causes miliary deposits with 2–5 mm nodules. Lymphoma and leukemia may also cause lung deposits. An air bronchogram within a lung nodule is a characteristic feature of the lymphomatous nodule. Hilar adenopathy and interstitial disease may be associated. Lymphangitic spread on chest radiograph is seen as reticular or reticulonodular pattern. On high resolution CT, nodules are seen in continuity with a vessel. Also, there is beading and thickening of interlobular and interlobar septa and irregular thickening of bronchovascular bundles. It is important to note that in patients with known extrathoracic malignancies, large number of the lung nodules detected on CT as metastases are actually benign and may represent granulomas.[13] This is especially common in areas with high incidence of tuberculosis or histoplasmosis.

Primary Lung Tumors

Primary pulmonary neoplasms in children are uncommon. The largest group of malignant tumors in childhood is grouped under the name *pleuropulmonary blastoma*. These occur in children as well as in adults; however, both are considered distinct entities. Pleuropulmonary blastoma of the childhood arises from primitive blastomatous tissues and develops in pre-existing congenital lung lesions like cystic adenomatoid malformation, sequestration or bronchogenic cysts.[14]

This tumor may be small and present as a solitary pulmonary nodule, or large and occupy the entire thorax.

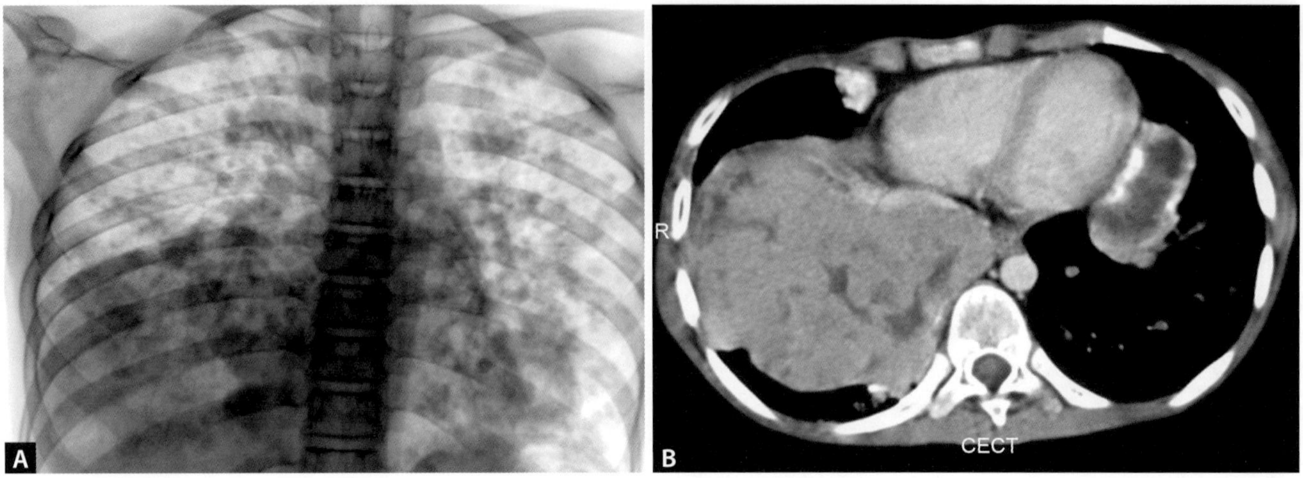

Figs. 7A and B: Lung metastases from osteosarcoma: (A) Chest radiograph shows bilateral extensive nodules and masses; (B) CT shows a right lower lobe mass with multiple smaller bilateral nodules and masses with calcifications.

The lesion may be multicystic, cystic solid or entirely solid; with malignancy rate increasing in that order. The chest radiograph shows a large mass, which may have features of local invasion **(Figs. 8A and B)**. CT and MR features are variable and ranges from fluid-filled cysts with solid nodule, solid mass causing mediastinal shift, and lung collapse shows areas of necrosis within a heterogeneously enhancing mass. Pleural effusion may be present; however, chest wall invasion is uncommon.[15] Metastases may occur in liver and central nervous system. Prognosis is poor.

Mesenchymal sarcomas of childhood may be associated with developmental cystic lesions like bronchogenic cyst, cystic adenomatoid malformation or congenital pulmonary cyst. These include leiomyosarcoma, rhabdomyosarcoma and fibrosarcoma. Bronchogenic carcinoma is extremely rare but can occur in older children. Usual histologies include carcinoid tumor, adenocarcinoma, basaloid carcinoma and mucoepidermoid carcinoma. Initial diagnostic consideration is usually pneumonia in these children; resulting in delayed diagnosis.[16] Other rare primary lung tumors include hemangiopericytoma and Askin tumor.

Plasma cell granuloma, also called inflammatory pseudotumor, is a proliferation of plasma cells, histiocytes and granulocytes and could represent a reparative response to infection. On radiographs, a well-circumscribed mass, mostly uncalcified and of a large size is seen. On CT, central necrosis and peripheral contrast enhancement may be seen.

MEDIASTINAL MASSES

The primary thoracic masses in children are most commonly located in the mediastinum. The mediastinal masses represent a wide variety of congenital anomalies and cysts in addition to neoplasms. Children with mediastinal masses are frequently asymptomatic and most often chest X-ray is done for nonspecific symptoms like fever, malaise, cough, airway compression, particularly before the age of one year is an important presentation. Respiratory distress results from easily compressible rings of the infant's trachea and bronchi. The risk of airway compression and high incidence of malignancy require prompt diagnosis and treatment for a child with mediastinal tumor.

Mediastinal masses can be classified as per their location into anterior, middle and posterior mediastinal masses. Since these compartments are not anatomical spaces, masses may often involve more than one compartment. In this situation, location of the center of the mass direction of displacement of adjacent structures, such as trachea and great vessels, is useful to suggest the likely region of origin.

Anterior Mediastinal Masses

Approximately 30% of mediastinal masses occur in anterior mediastinum. These include the four 'T's: teratoma (and other germ cell tumors), thymic tumor, thyroid tumor or cysts and 'terrible' lymphoma/leukemia. As thymus or thyroid tumors are rare in pediatric age group, important differential diagnosis of anterior mediastinal mass consists of germ cell tumor and lymphoma.

Germ Cell Tumors

These include dermoid, teratoma, teratocarcinoma, choriocarcinoma, embryonal carcinoma, seminoma, endodermal sinus tumors and mixed germ cell tumors. Most germ cell tumors arise in anterior mediastinum near thymus and few arise in other mediastinal compartments.

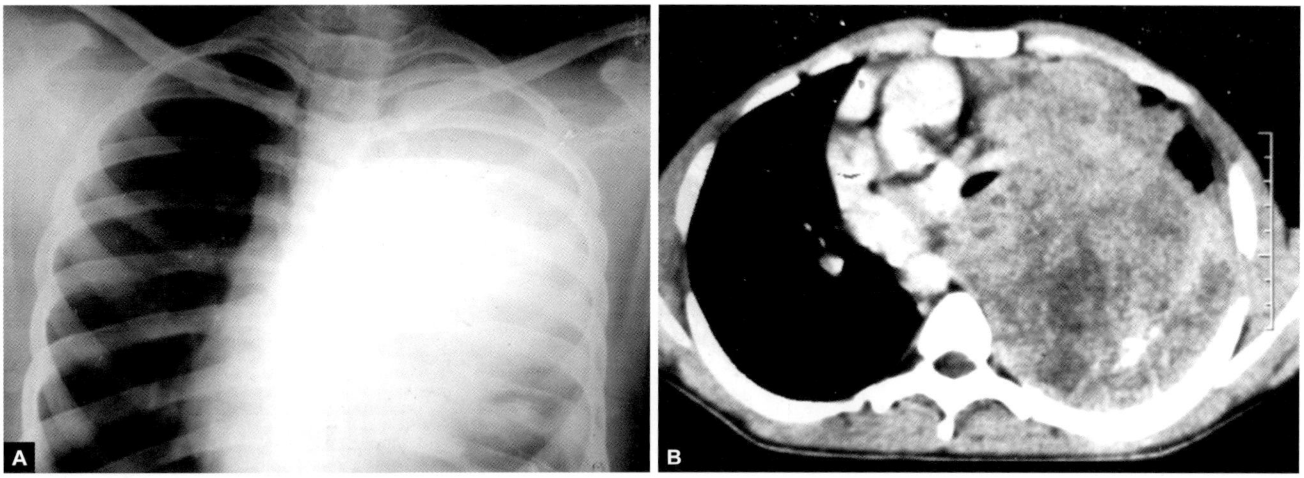

Figs. 8A and B: Pulmonary blastoma: (A) Chest radiograph shows a large left lung mass with mediastinal shift to right side; (B) CT shows a large solid mass with areas of necrosis and calcifications with mediastinal and pleural invasion.

Teratomas may be benign (mature) or malignant (immature). Mature teratomas usually attain a large size before they present with symptoms. Both mature and immature teratomas are seen as lobulated anterior mediastinal soft tissue masses. Calcifications are common. On CT, teratomas are seen as complex solid or cystic solid masses with variable wall thickness. Calcification, teeth and fat densities are more readily visualized on CT[17] **(Fig. 9)**. However, macroscopically demonstrable fat is unusual in malignant teratoma.

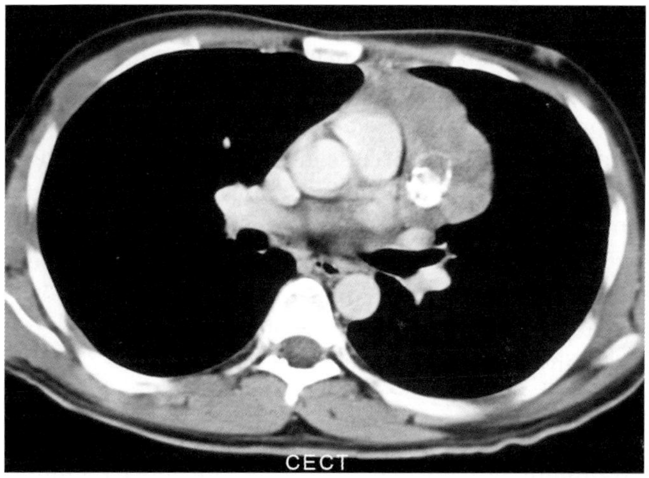

Fig. 9: Mediastinal germ cell tumor: CT shows an anterior mediastinal mass containing coarse calcification.

Seminoma arising in mediastinum is rare and metastatic seminoma in the mediastinum from occult gonadal lesion should always be excluded with USG of scrotum. Seminoma is seen as a bulky, homogenous anterior mediastinal mass on CT and may simulate lymphoma. Rarely, calcifications may be present. Involvement of adjacent structures is uncommon however; metastases to lymph nodes, lung or bone may be present. *Endodermal sinus tumor* (yolk sac tumor) is a poorly differentiated embryonal carcinoma, occurs often in males and patients usually have systemic symptoms and elevated serum alpha-fetoprotein. These tumors as well as most other nonseminomatous malignant germ cell tumors have nonspecific imaging features. On CT, these are seen as large irregular, heterogeneous mediastinal masses with areas of necrosis, cystic degeneration and hemorrhages.[18]

Lymphoma

Lymphomas are the most common cause of mediastinal masses in children. Both Hodgkin and non-Hodgkin (especially lymphoblastic lymphoma) can present with large anterior mediastinal masses. However, the lymphadenopathy may be present anywhere in the mediastinum or the hila. CT is the modality of choice for evaluation and staging of lymphoma. On CT, mediastinal lymphadenopathy in lymphoma may be discrete, however, more often it produces conglomerate homogenous lymph node masses **(Figs. 10A and B)**. Mass effect such as vascular displacement, compression of trachea or obstruction of superior vena cava is common with large masses.[19] Necrosis and hemorrhages are rare but it may be seen in large masses of lymphoma. Calcification is also rare in lymphoma.

In Hodgkin's lymphoma, if transverse diameter of mediastinal lymph nodal mass measured on chest radiograph at T4–5 level exceeds transverse thoracic diameter, it is called as bulky disease.

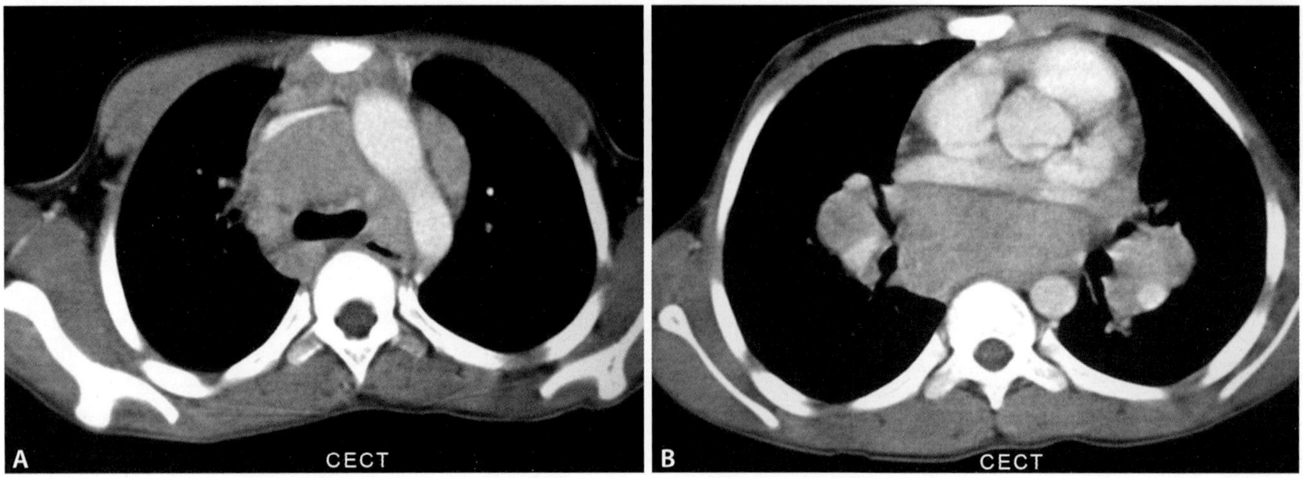

Figs. 10A and B: Hodgkin's lymphoma: CT images at (A) carinal and (B) subcarinal levels show bilateral conglomerate homogeneous lymph node enlargement.

It is denoted as suffix X to the stage and associated with inferior prognosis. It is uncommon for non-Hodgkin's lymphoma (NHL) to be limited to mediastinum only at the presentation. However, some NHL primarily involves anterior mediastinum. These include primary mediastinal large B-cell lymphoma and lymphoblastic lymphoma, the latter is a T-cell NHL. Both these are aggressive lymphomas seen in children and young adults. Patients usually present with dyspnea, stridor and superior vena cava (SVC) syndrome.[20] On imaging, large, often heterogeneous and infiltrative anterior mediastinal mass is seen.

Thymic Masses

Prominent but normal thymus is the most common pseudotumor of anterior mediastinum. On imaging, anterior mediastinal tumors displace the trachea and esophagus posteriorly and laterally in contradistinction to a normal enlarged thymus, which does not displace adjacent structures.

Hyperplasia of thymus is uncommon and may occur in Graves' disease, lymphoma, leukemia and Langerhans' cell histiocytosis. It may also occur as a rebound thymic enlargement after chemotherapy.

Thymic cyst is of developmental origin, representing persistent tubular remnants of the third pharyngeal pouch. The cyst is usually asymptomatic and incidentally seen on chest radiograph. It is unilocular or multilocular and varies is size. CT is helpful in diagnosis.

Thymoma is rare in childhood. The association of thymoma and myasthenia gravis is also much less in children than in adults. On radiographs, thymoma is seen a variable sized lobulated soft tissue mass in anterior mediastinum. On CT, thymomas are generally seen as lobulated, homogeneously enhancing masses with smooth contour. They tend to grow asymmetrically to one side of the mediastinum. Calcifications may be present and this helps to differentiate thymoma from lymphoma. Rarely, thymoma may have pleural effusion with nodular pleural deposits or diffuse pleural thickening mimicking mesothelioma or pleural metastases.[21] On MRI, thymomas are homogenously isointense on T1-weighted images and heterogeneously hyperintense on T2-weighted images.[22]

Lymphangioma

Lymphangioma, also known as cystic hygroma, results from failure of primary lymphatic sac to establish drainage into the venous system. It is an uncommon cause of mediastinal masses in children. Most are caused by extension from other sites, such as neck or axilla, into the mediastinum.[23] Most are located in anterior or middle mediastinum but few may be seen in posterior mediastinum. It often presents as a large soft consistency mass and rarely causes airway obstruction. Pathologically these are lymphatic malformations macrocystic, microcystic or combined morphology. Chest radiograph shows well-demarcated mass, which may have a lobulated outline. On USG, macrocystic component is seen as cystic masses with internal echoes and septations. Mild vascularity may be seen on color Doppler. Microcystic component is highly echogenic. MRI is required to assess the entire extent of lymphangioma. CT and MRI demonstrate a well-circumscribed avascular cystic mass with septations and mild wall enhancement **(Fig. 11)**. Areas of fat density may be demonstrated. Fluid-fluid levels may also be seen due

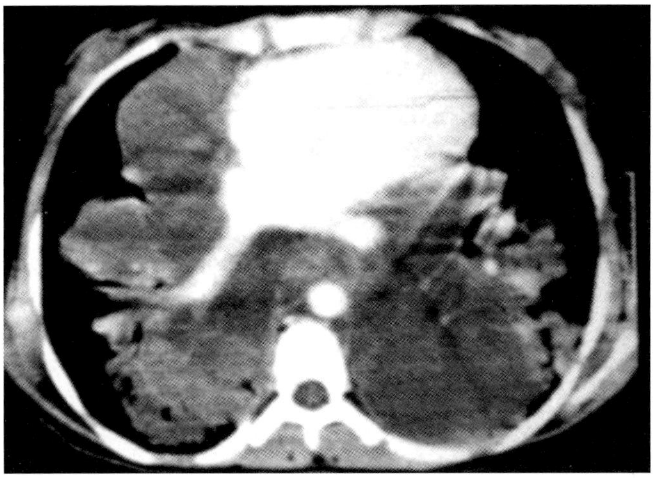

Fig. 11: Mediastinal lymphangioma: CT shows a multiseptated, lobulated bilateral cystic mediastinal mass.

to hemorrhages or protein contents. The septations show enhancement on contrast-enhanced MRI. The mass tends to envelop or mould to adjacent structures. The microcystic type may be seen as highly enhancing soft tissue mass on contrast-enhanced MRI.[24]

Pericardial Cysts

These are rare benign unilocular anterior mediastinal cyst containing clear fluid. Most are developmental in origin. On radiographs, these are seen as well defined, rounded or teardrop shaped mass in cardiophrenic angles abutting the heart. Most are seen on right side. On CT or MRI, these are seen as well-demarcated nonenhancing cysts.

Middle and Posterior Mediastinal Masses

Common masses in middle mediastinum are enlarged lymph nodes or bronchogenic cyst. Lymph node enlargement may be in the paratracheal or hilar locations are mostly due to viral, tubercular or fungal infections, leukemia, lymphoma and histiocytosis. Massive adenopathy is seen in lymphoma and leukemia in which the nodes are confluent. Aneurysms of aorta, pulmonary artery or coronary artery are also rare causes of middle mediastinal masses. Bronchogenic cyst is discussed under congenital lung conditions. Almost 40% of mediastinal masses in children are located in the posterior mediastinum and majority of these are neurogenic tumors or cystic duplications.[25] Rare causes of posterior mediastinal tumors include hemangiomas and vascular malformations, extramedullary hematopoiesis, germ cell tumors, Ewing's sarcoma and rhabdomyosarcoma.

Neurogenic Tumors

These include ganglion tumors (ganglioneuroma, ganglioneuroblastoma and neuroblastoma), nerve sheath tumors (neurofibroma and schwannoma) and paraganglioma.

Neuroblastoma and Other Ganglion Tumors

Ganglion tumors are derived from the sympathetic ganglia and include neuroblastoma (malignant), ganglioneuroma (benign) and ganglioneuroblastoma (having both components). They usually occur in the superior half of the posterior mediastinum and cannot be differentiated on the basis of imaging alone.

Neuroblastoma is the second most common solid tumor in children after brain tumors and represent 10% of all childhood cancers.[26] Thorax is the second most common site for neuroblastoma after the abdomen. It usually occurs in children less than two years of age but may rarely occur up to the age of 10 years. These may also be diagnosed on prenatal USG. Neuroblastoma is malignant but has a better prognosis in mediastinum when diagnosed less than one year of age.

Patients with thoracic neuroblastoma have symptoms due to primary mass or the metastases. They present with respiratory distress or cord compression. Those with metastatic disease have pain, fever and weight loss. Rarely, neuroblastoma may be detected as an asymptomatic mass on chest radiograph. Usual appearance of neuroblastoma on chest radiograph is of a smooth elongated paraspinal mass with rib or vertebral erosion and characteristic splaying of ribs. Calcifications are seen in up to 30% cases.[27] On CT, a soft tissue mass with speckled, irregular and granular calcification is seen in the posterior mediastinum **(Fig. 12)**. It shows mild contrast enhancement, occasionally with areas of necrosis and hemorrhages. Rib erosion and widened intervertebral foramina may be seen. Other bony changes include pedicular flattening, spinal canal enlargement, posterior vertebral scalloping and localized kyphoscoliosis. Intraspinal extension is frequent even in absence of neurologic signs and symptoms. Vascular encasement and mediastinal lymphadenopathy may also be seen, though uncommonly. MRI is the modality of choice for staging because the intraspinal spread and spread along nerves and bone marrow involvement are better demonstrated by MRI. As bone metastases are common, radiographic skeletal survey and a bone scan using ^{99m}TC-MDP or ^{123}I-MIBG is usually obtained as a part of imaging work-up. Bony metastases are lytic or lytic sclerotic and have characteristic appearances.[28]

Median age for the diagnosis of ganglioneuroblastoma is 5 years and that for the ganglioneuroma is 10 years.[26] *Ganglioneuroblastoma* is more differentiated malignancy and has a good prognosis. These tumors are usually asymptomatic until they invade or compress adjacent structures, metastasize to distant sites or produce unusual paraneoplastic syndromes. Nonspecific symptoms include fever, malaise, back pain or anemia. Lower limb weakness is present in lesions involving the spinal canal. The imaging features of ganglioneuroblastoma are similar to neuroblastoma. Twenty percent of ganglioneuroblastomas have calcification and show low homogeneous attenuation with minimal contrast enhancement **(Figs. 13A and B)**. *Ganglioneuroma* is a benign tumor, which occurs in older children is seen as a large smooth spherical mass or small elongated sausage-shaped mass, which shows low homogeneous attenuation with minimal contrast enhancement. Differential diagnosis of neurogenic tumors includes malignant sarcoma arising from chest wall or inflammatory lesion such as actinomycosis.

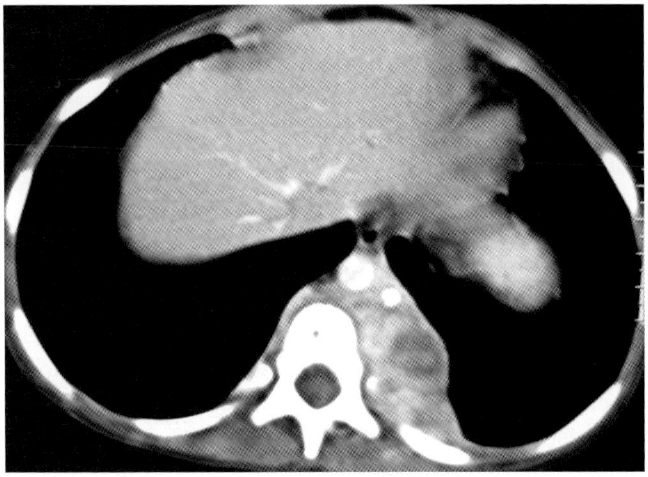

Fig. 12: Mediastinal neuroblastoma: CT shows enhancing left paravertebral mass with areas of necrosis and calcification.

Neurofibroma and Schwannoma

Neurofibroma and schwannomas are nerve sheath tumors. Schwannoma is encapsulated and does not contain nerve fibers while neurofibroma is uncapsulated and hence have nerve fiber within it. In thorax, these tumors arise from intercostals or sympathetic nerves. These tumors are mostly benign, asymptomatic and seen under 20 years of age. On imaging, neurofibroma and schwannoma are similar in appearance and seen as solid, well-defined round or oval masses.[29] Neurofibroma usually occurs in patients with systemic neurofibromatosis rather than a solitary lesion. It is more often bilaterally located in posterior mediastinum. Chest radiograph in addition to this lesion shows 'ribbon-like' rib deformities or scoliosis. On CT, the soft tissue mass is homogeneous with low attenuation and mildly enhances with contrast. It may extend to spinal canal, showing characteristic dumb-bell shape. In the plexiform variety, the mass may be confluent.

Paraganglioma

These are rare neurogenic tumors of the posterior mediastinum and actually represent extra-adrenal pheochromocytoma. These are derived from chromaffin cells of the sympathetic nervous system. Imaging features are nonspecific, but the diagnosis is usually established on the basis of excessive catecholamine secretions.

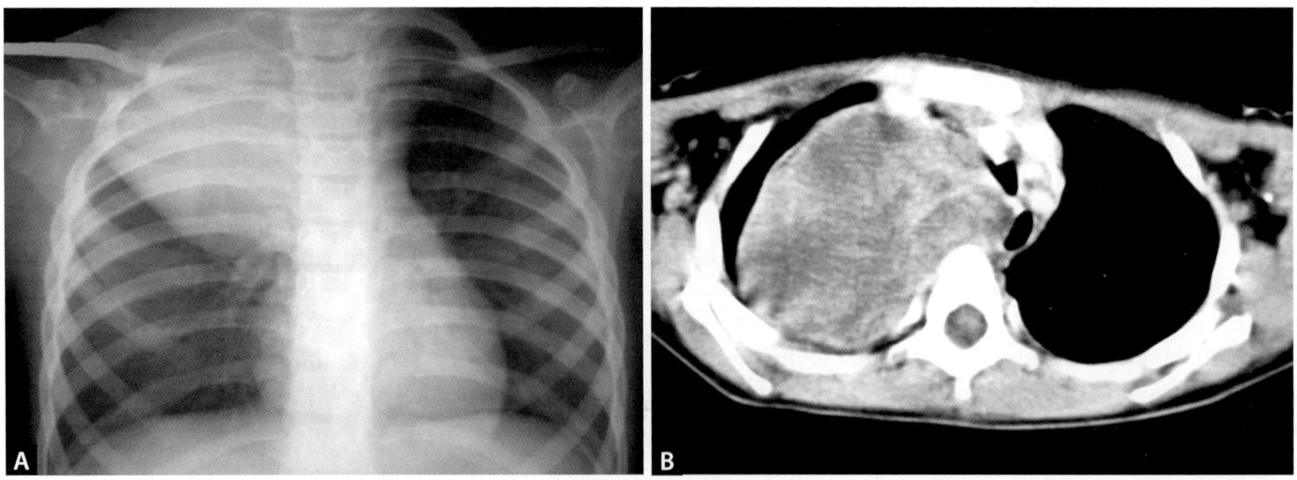

Figs. 13A and B: Ganglioneuroblastoma: (A) Chest radiograph shows a large right mediastinal mass; (B) CT shows a large posterior mediastinal mass with displacement and compression of mediastinal structures.

Duplication Cysts

Abnormal closure of ventral foregut results in formation of *bronchogenic cyst*. These are described above in congenital lung conditions. Abnormal closure of dorsal foregut results in enterogenic duplication cysts and these include esophageal duplication cyst and neuroenteric cyst. *Esophageal duplication cyst* constitutes almost 10–15% of all duplications of the gastrointestinal tract. In contrast to bronchogenic cyst, which occurs in early age, the majority of children with esophageal duplications are over 10 years of age at the onset of symptoms. The lesion is smooth in outline, varies in size and usually impinges on a barium-filled esophagus but rarely communicates with esophageal lumen. CT and MRI demonstrate the cystic and avascular nature of the lesion. These modalities clearly demonstrate precise size, location, its relation to adjacent organs and transdiaphragmatic extension. Technetium^{99}m-pertechnetate scintigraphy demonstrates gastric mucosa in the cyst, thereby confirms the preoperative diagnosis.

The *neurenteric cyst* results from incomplete separation of the foregut from notochord. These have a vertebral body cleft communicating with the spinal canal. It contains both neural and gastrointestinal element. It may be limited to the chest as a blind sac or may extend below the diaphragm where it either ends blindly or communicates with the intestinal tract. Most neurenteric cysts are discovered in infancy because of esophageal and tracheobronchial compression.[30]

Anterior Thoracic Meningocele

Though rare, this entity is to be considered in the differential diagnosis of posterior mediastinal masses. It occurs due to spinal canal anomalies in which the leptomeninges herniate through the neural foramina. It is seen usually in patients of neurofibromatosis with kyphoscoliosis where the meningocele is at the apex of the convexity. MRI confirms the diagnosis.

Extramedullary Hematopoiesis

It is rarely seen in hematological disorders, most commonly in thalassemia. It is usually asymptomatic but may rarely cause cord compression. On imaging, it is seen as bilaterally symmetrical, well-defined, lobulated lower thoracic paraspinal soft tissue mass.

CHEST WALL MASSES

Chest Wall Infections

Chest wall is the uncommon site for infections and abscesses as compared to the lungs. These are easily diagnosed clinically however; imaging is required to assess the deeper extent. Ultrasound is useful to detect and localize chest wall abscess. It is seen as cystic mass with debris. On CT, the abscess is seen as cystic area with wall enhancement. CT is especially useful to detect associated osteomyelitis of the rib and deeper extent of the abscess. Chest wall infection without the well-formed abscess is seen as a heterogeneous, ill-defined mass on CT.

Lymphangioma

These are focal or diffuse masses that tend to involve subcutaneous tissues of neck, chest wall or axilla. These may extend into mediastinum. Imaging features are similar to those described above for mediastinal lymphangiomas.

Hemangioma

Hemangiomas are the most common soft tissue tumors in children. The usual sites are head and neck, chest and extremities. These are usually present at birth, however, after initial proliferation, majority of these disappear spontaneously. Small superficial hemangiomas have characteristic appearance and of no clinical significance. Large and extensive lesions may have mass effect. On color Doppler USG, large vascular channels with both arterial as well as venous flow are seen.[31] On MRI, hemangiomas are seen as lobulated masses iso and high-signal intensity on T1- and T2-weighted images respectively, with areas of flow voids representing vascular channels. Diffuse enhancement following contrast administration. During involution, high T1 signal intensity is seen due to fatty replacement.

Venous malformations may have similar appearance; however, unlike hemangiomas, these are not tumors. On imaging, venous malformations tend to be solid without dilated vascular channels and on color Doppler, there is minimal or no detectable flow at all. Phleboliths are frequently seen as calcified focal lesions within the mass.

Neurofibroma

Neurofibroma and *schwannoma* may also involve chest wall. Extensive chest wall involvement by plexiform neurofibromatosis may be seen in children with NF1. These tumors may cause secondary bony abnormalities in the form of ribbon appearance of the ribs, scalloping of the vertebral bodies and kyphoscoliosis.

Benign Osseous Masses

Fibrous dysplasia of the rib is the most common osseous lesion of the chest wall. These are frequently seen as incidental findings on imaging. Radiographically, it is seen as a focal, well-defined, expansile lytic lesion of the rib. Alternatively, there may be diffuse fusiform enlargement of the rib with ground glass matrix. *Osteochondromas* (or exostosis) are benign bony outgrowths with cartilage cap on the surface. These usually occur in long bones; however, ribs, sternum, scapula, clavicle or spine may also be involved. Most are asymptomatic and detected incidentally while others may be symptomatic due to mass effect on adjacent structures. Malignant transformation is rare. On radiography, osteochondroma is seen as a bony outgrowth with both cortex and medulla that are continuous with the host bone. CT and MRI show similar features and cartilage cap is better evaluated on these modalities. Irregularity or thickening of the cartilage cap more than 2 cm is suspicious for malignant transformation into chondrosarcoma.[32] *Enchondroma* of the rib usually occurs in adults and uncommon in children. It is seen as a well-defined, expansile lytic lesion of the rib with endosteal scalloping. Calcifications may also be present.

Mesenchymal hamartoma of the chest wall is a rare benign tumor of the infancy. It is a mature mesenchymal tumor containing bone, cartilages, fat and fibrous tissues. On imaging, it is seen as a large complex cystic solid soft issue mass along with destruction of one or several contiguous ribs. Intense enhancement is seen in solid parts of the mass.[33]

Primitive Neuroectodermal Tumor

These include Ewing's sarcoma of the bone and primitive neuroectodermal tumor (PNET) of the chest wall (Askin's tumor). Clinically, these present a large painful soft tissue masses, often associated with cough and dyspnea. On chest radiographs, large thoracic soft tissue mass with or without associated rib destruction is seen **(Figs. 14A and B)**.

CT demonstrates large extrapleural mass with heterogeneous contrast enhancement and rib destruction. The extraosseous soft-tissue mass component is disproportionately larger than the bone lesion. Very large tumors may occupy most part of the hemithorax and cause lung collapse and mediastinal shift to the contralateral side. Pleural effusion may be present but it is usually not massive. Incidence of lung metastases is high and hence, careful lung evaluation should also be done on CT. MRI appearance is similar to CT. These tumors may also have skip lesions along the intercostal nerves. These tumors are usually treated with chemoradiotherapy followed by surgery; however, the prognosis is poor.[34]

Rhabdomyosarcoma

It is the second most common malignancy of the chest wall in children.[35] Chest wall rhabdomyosarcomas are more aggressive than those occurring in head and neck or genitourinary tract. On radiographs, soft tissue mass is seen with or without rib destruction. CT and MR features are nonspecific and similar to those of PNET.

Miscellaneous Malignant Chest Wall Masses

Both Hodgkin and non-Hodgkin's lymphoma may secondarily involve the chest wall by direct extension from mediastinal or pleural disease. Most common pattern is of homogeneous parasternal chest wall mass contiguous with anterior mediastinal lymphadenopathy. Rib or sternum

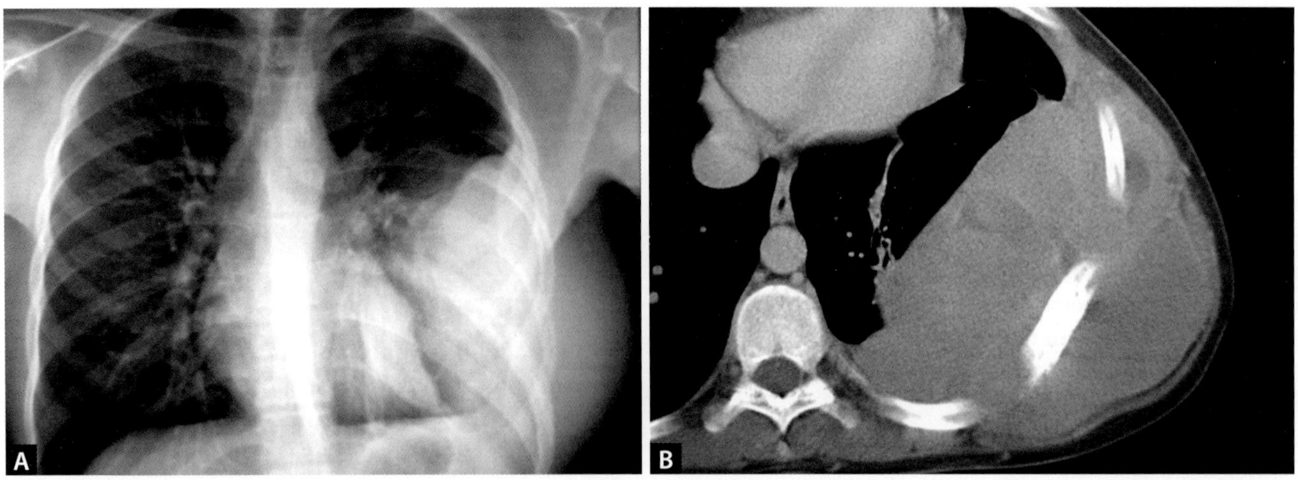

Figs. 14A and B: Primitive neuroectodermal tumor of chest wall: (A) Chest radiograph shows a large left-sided chest wall mass with both intra- and extrathoracic components; (B) CT shows lytic sclerotic rib within the mass.

may be eroded or appear normal in spite of large chest wall mass. Uncommonly, discrete and isolated chest wall may also be seen with lymphoma. Neuroblastoma may involve the chest wall as a direct extension from posterior mediastinal tumor.[36] MRI is most useful to evaluate the extent of chest wall as well as spinal involvement by neuroblastoma. Osteosarcoma of the rib is uncommon in children. It is seen as destructive lesion of the rib with new bone formation. Associated soft tissue component is also present although not as massive as PNET.

Other rare malignant chest wall tumors in children include congenital fibrosarcoma, mesenchymal chondrosarcoma and malignant peripheral nerve sheath tumor (MPNST). Their imaging features are nonspecific.

REFERENCES

1. Stocker JT, Madewell JE, Drake RM. Congenital cystic adenomatoid malformation of the lung: classification and morphologic spectrum. Hum Pathol. 1977;8:155-71.
2. Winters WD, Effaman EL. Congenital masses of the lung: prenatal and postnatal imaging evaluation. J Thorac Imaging. 2001;16:196-206.
3. Lee EY, Siegel MJ, Sierra LM, et al. Evaluation of architecture of pulmonary sequestration in pediatric patients using 3D MDCT angiography. Am J Roentgenol. 2004;183:183-8.
4. Reed JC, Sobonya RE. Morphologic analysis of foregut cysts in the thorax. Am J Roentgenol Radium Ther Nucl Med. 1974;120:851-60.
5. McAdams HP, Kitejczyk WM, Rosado-de-Christensen ML, et al. Bronchogenic cysts: imaging features with clinical and histopathologic correlation. Radiology. 2000;217:441-6.
6. Paterson A. Imaging evaluation of congenital lung abnormalities in infant and children. Radiol Clin N Am. 2005;43:303-23.
7. Abushaban L, Uthaman B, Endrys J. Transcatheter coil closure of pulmonary arteriovenous malformations in children. J Interven Cardiol. 2004;17:23-6.
8. Yang P, Lih K, Lee Y, et al. Lung abscesses: ultrasonography and ultrasound guided transthoracic aspiration. Radiology. 1991;180:171-5.
9. Donnely LF. Practical issues concerning imaging of pulmonary infections in children. J Thorac Imaging. 2001;16:238-50.
10. Rose RE, Ward BH. Spherical pneumonias in children simulating pulmonary and mediastinal masses. Radiology. 1973;106:179-82.
11. Erdem CZ, Erdem LO. Radiological characteristics of pulmonary hydatid disease in children: less common radiological appearances. Eur Radiol. 2003;45:123-8.
12. Rastogi R, Garg R, Thulkar S, et al. Unusual thoracic CT manifestations of osteosarcoma: review of 16 cases. Pediatr Radiol. 2008;38:551-8.
13. Aquino SL. Imaging of metastatic disease to the thorax. Radio Clin N Am. 2005;43:481-95.
14. Maniwell JC, Priest JR, Watterson J, et al. Pleuropulmonary blastoma: the so called pulmonary blastoma of childhood. Cancer. 1988;62:1516-26.
15. Orazi C, Inserra A, Schingo PM, et al. Pleuropulmonary blastoma, a distinct neoplasm of childhood: report of three cases. Pediatr Radiol. 2007;37:337-44.
16. Lal DR, Clark I, Shalkow J, et al. Primary epithelial lung malignancies in pediatric population. Pediatr Blood Cancer. 2005;45:683-6.
17. Brown LR, Muhm JR, Aughenbaugh GL, et al. Computed tomography of benign mature teratomas of the mediastinum. J Thorac Imaging. 1987;2:66-71.
18. Lee KS, IM JG, Han CH, et al. Malignant primary germ cell tumors of the mediastinum: CT features. Am J Roentgenol. 1989;153:947-51.
19. Arya LS, Narain S, Tomar S, et al. Superior vena cava syndrome. Indian J Pediatr. 2001;69:293-7.
20. Shukla NN, Trippett TM. Non-Hodgkin lymphoma in children and adolescents. Curr Oncol Rep. 2006;8:387-94.
21. Thomas CR, Wright CD, Loeherer PJ. Thymoma: state of art. J Clin Oncol. 1999;17:2280-9.
22. Santana L, Givica A, Camacho C. Best cases from AFIP: thymoma. Radiographics. 2002;22:95-102.
23. Sumner TE, Volberg FM, Kiser PE, et al. Mediastinal cystic hygroma in children. Pediatr Radiol. 1981;11:160-2.
24. Konez O, Borrows PE. Magnetic resonance of vascular anomalies. Magn Reson Imaging Clin N Am. 2002;10:363-88.
25. Mea MP, Benson M, Slovis TL. Imaging of mediastinal masses in children. Radiol Clin N Am. 1993;31:583-604.
26. Lonergan CJ, Schwab CJ, Suarez ES, et al. Neuroblastoma, ganglioneuroblastoma and ganglioneuroma: radiologic-pathologic correlation. Radiographics. 2002;22:911-34.
27. Softka CM, Semelka RC, Kelekis NL, et al. Magnetic resonance imaging of neuroblastoma using current techniques. Magn Reson Imaging. 1999;17:193-8.
28. Hiorns MP, Owens CM. Radiology of neuroblastoma in children. Eur Radiol. 2001;11:2071-81.
29. Laurent F, Latrabe V, Lecesne R, et al. Mediastinal masses: diagnostic approach. Eur Radiol. 1998;8:1149-59.
30. Strollo DC, Rosado-de-Christenson ML, Jett JR. Primary mediastinal tumours. Part II: tumors of the middle and posterior mediastinum. Chest. 1997;112:1344-57.
31. Paltiel HJ, Burrows PE, Kozakewich HPW, et al. Soft tissue vascular anomalies: utility of US for diagnosis. Radiology. 2000;214:747-54.
32. Lee KC, Davis AM, Cassar-Pullicino VN. Imaging the complications of osteochondromas. Clin Radiol. 2001;57:18-28.
33. Groom KR, Murphy MD, Howard LM. Mesenchymal hamartoma of the chest wall: radiologic manifestations with emphasis on cross-sectional imaging and histopathological comparison. Radiology. 2002;222:205-11.
34. Fefferman NR, Pinkney LP. Imaging evaluation of chest wall disorders in children. Radiol Clin N Am. 2005;43:355-70.
35. Shamberger RC, Grier HE. Chest wall tumours in infants and children. Semin Pediatr Surg. 1994;3:267-76.
36. Wyttenbach R, Vock P, Tschappeler H. Cross-sectional imaging with CT and/or MRI of pediatric chest tumours. Eur Radiol. 1998;8:1040-9.

CHAPTER 133

Pediatric Airway

Ashu Seith Bhalla

Diseases affecting the airway, extrinsic or intrinsic, are much more common in children than in adults. Also, the smaller airway caliber coupled with the greater collapsibility of the airway in infants and young children, leads to early and more symptomatic airflow disturbances, even with minor amounts of airway edema and mucus. Clinically, the presentation of these disorders may be acute or chronic. In their acute form, the airway disorders can be life threatening. "Always look at the airway" is a lesson that must be emphasized in pediatric radiology.[1-4]

The airway is referred to as the upper airway (above the thoracic inlet) or lower airway being below it. While the predominant presentation of upper airway obstruction is inspiratory stridor, that of lower airway obstruction is expiratory wheeze.[1-4] Other clinical presentations include feeding difficulty, respiratory distress, tachypnea, nasal flaring, chest wall retractions, hemoptysis, fever, failure to thrive and even no symptoms.[4] Diseases affecting the pediatric airway are broadly classified in **Table 1**.

IMAGING MODALITIES

The purpose of imaging is to delineate: location of the abnormality, if the involvement diffuse or focal and extrinsic or intrinsic. If the lesion is an intrinsic process, is it mural or intraluminal and is the obstruction fixed or dynamic.[4] The radiographic evaluation of airways in infants and young children is challenging due to inability to obtain motionless end-inspiratory and end-expiratory images. The resultant artifacts are especially noticeable in HRCT images. Also the caliber of airways of young children is small and difficult to detail in infants and small children.

Plain Radiographs

Plain radiographs are the primary and often only imaging modality used in evaluation of children with airway obstruction. The evaluation should include frontal and lateral high kV radiographs of the upper airways, and frontal and lateral views of the chest. When an endobronchial foreign body is a consideration, decubitus chest views may be helpful. Expiratory radiographs aid in demonstrating air trapping.

Fluoroscopy

Fluoroscopy of the airway demonstrates dynamic airway collapse during expiration in children with tracheobronchomalacia.[4] Decubitus fluoroscopy may be performed in cases of suspected foreign body in infants and young children.

Barium Swallow

A barium swallow may be useful for demonstrating gastroesophageal reflux in patients with chronic aspiration simulating asthma. This study is also helpful for establishing the diagnosis of vascular rings and slings, although cross-sectional imaging is eventually required for better anatomic delineation.

Table 1: Diseases affecting the pediatric airway.

Upper Airway Obstruction		
Acute		
• Croup		
• Epiglottitis		
• Retropharyngeal cellulitis and abscess		
• Exudative tracheitis		
• Foreign body		
Chronic		
Space-occupying lesions		- Adenoidal enlargement
		- Enlarged pharyngeal tonsils
		- Juvenile nasopharyngeal angiofibroma
Fixed airway narrowing		- Stenosis/stricture
Congenital		- Micrognathia
		- Macroglossia
		- Laryngeal malacia
		- Laryngeal cysts
Lower Airway Obstruction		
Central airways		
Extrinsic:	Congenital	- Vascular compression, vascular malformations
		- Bronchopulmonary foregut malformations—Bronchogenic cyst
		- Thoracic deformity
	Inflammatory	- Lymph nodes
		- Mediastinal abscess/cellulitis
	Masses	- Hemangioma
		- Lymphoma
		- Germ cell tumor
Intrinsic:		
Wall abnormality:		
	Congenital	- Tracheobronchomalacia
		- Tracheal stenosis
		- Bronchopulmonary foregut malformations—Bronchial atresia, tracheoesophageal fistula
		- Tracheobronchial branching anomalies
	Inflammatory	- Exudative tracheitis, tuberculosis
		- Fibrotic stricture
	Postintubation stricture	
Intraluminal:		- Foreign body
		- Masses: hemangioma, carcinoid
Peripheral Airway Abnormalities		
• Asthma		
• Bronchiectasis		
• Bronchiolitis/Small airway disease		

Multidetector Computed Tomography

Relative to MRI, CT has the advantage of rapid scan times enabling performance of the examination without sedation, it has the disadvantage of radiation exposure and need for using contrast. *Dynamic CT* can be obtained as a paired inspiratory-expiratory scan in older cooperative children.

In uncooperative children, some authors have reported a controlled ventilation CT (CVCT). CVCT uses positive pressure feedback ventilation. The child is sedated but otherwise breathing on his/her own; and images are acquired during hyperventilation-induced transient respiratory pause. The technique does not require intubation or general anesthesia and provides motionless inspiratory and expiratory phase images. In this technique, several sequential inspirations are augmented by face-mask ventilation which induces hypocarbia. Hypocarbia (through Hering-Breuer reflex) results in brief apneic periods during which images can be acquired.[3,4] CT images can be acquired at desired degrees of airway distention.

In those uncooperative children in whom even the controlled-ventilation technique is not feasible or not available, cine CT can be used. *Cine-CT* involves rapid acquisition of images of the airway throughout the respiratory cycle during free breathing. Once the site of suspected airway stenosis or malacia is localized, CT images are rapidly and sequentially acquired at the same axial level. Cine CT technique can provide multiple images of the airway during inspiration and expiration, even in tachypneic patients.

Multiplanar and 3D volume-rendered image reconstructions further enhance the accuracy of multidetector computed tomography (MDCT) in delineating the level of narrowing, degree of obstruction, segment length and distal airway.[5]

Magnetic Resonance Imaging

Magnetic resonance imaging (MRI) can demonstrate abnormal airway motion in addition to anatomic causes of obstruction. The protocol includes axial and sagittal T1-weighted as well as STIR images.

Dynamic (cine) MRI studies can be used to evaluate airway motion in real time. Sagittal midline MR cine (fast gradient echo imaging) is performed. Axial MR Cine images are obtained craniocaudally at the level of mid-tongue in those with obstructive sleep apnea.[2] The use of cine MR imaging during coughing for evaluation of tracheal collapsibility in patients with suspected tracheomalacia has been described.[6]

UPPER AIRWAY OBSTRUCTION

Normal Anatomy (Plain Radiographs) (Figs. 1A and B)

Epiglottis: The normal epiglottis has very thin borders. Epiglottis may appear artefactually thickened if imaged

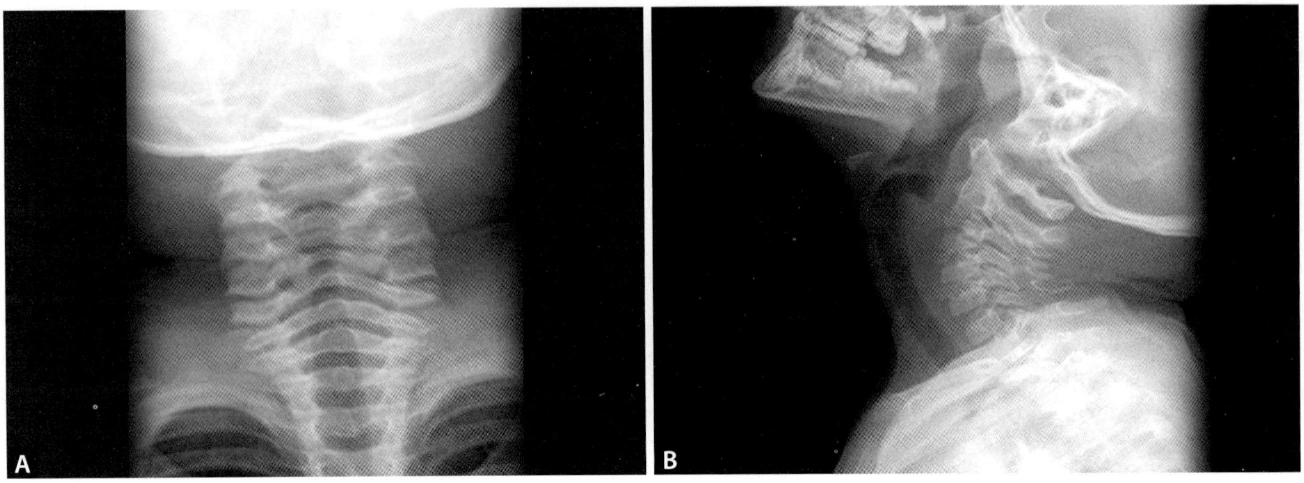

Figs. 1A and B: Normal frontal (A) and lateral (B) radiographs neck of a 5-year-old child.

obliquely—this is due both the left and right sides being imaged next to each other. This is referred to as the "omega" appearance.[1,2]

Aryepiglottic folds: Aryepiglottic folds are mucosal folds which extend from the epiglottis superiorly to the arytenoids cartilages, posteroinferiorly. On a lateral radiograph, these appear thin and convex inferiorly.

Subglottic trachea: On frontal views subglottic trachea appears rounded with lateral convexities or "shoulders". On the lateral view, it should not be narrower than the airway above or below it.

Retropharyngeal soft tissues: Normally, the soft tissues between the posterior aspect of the aerated pharynx and anterior aspect of the vertebral column, should not be more than the anteroposterior diameter of the vertebral bodies. However, "pseudothickening" of the retropharyngeal soft tissues may be seen if the radiographs are obtained in a flexed position of the neck, especially in infants with short necks. The radiographs should hence be performed with adequate neck extension. The thickness of soft tissues is measured transversely somewhere between the level of adenoids superiorly to base of epiglottis inferiorly, below which these are normally thicker due to the presence of esophagus.

Tonsils/Adenoids: At less than 6 months of age, the adenoids are rarely visible on radiography. There is rapid proliferation during infancy with peak size reaching between 2 years and 10 years. A size up to 12 mm is considered normal. Subsequently, during the second decade there is reduction in size.

ACUTE OBSTRUCTION

The most common causes of acute upper airway obstruction are inflammatory, followed by foreign body. Ingestion of corrosive/caustic substances is another cause.[1,2]

Croup (Acute Laryngotracheobronchitis)

Croup is a benign, self-limiting acute inflammatory condition of the upper airways. It results from viral infection, and is the most common cause of upper airway obstruction in young children and infants[1,2] (6 months–3 years of age). Affected children present with "croupy" (barky) cough and inspiratory stridor.

The purpose of obtaining radiographs in a suspected case of croup is to exclude secondary causes such as foreign body. It, however, has characteristic findings–on frontal radiographs there is loss of the normal shoulders (lateral convexities) of the subglottic trachea due to subglottic edema. The subglottic trachea becomes elongated, extending below the level of the pyriform sinuses. The appearance is referred to as a "church steeple" or "inverted V" appearance. Lateral radiographs may reveal similar narrowing of the subglottic trachea with loss of its wall definition.[1]

Epiglottitis

Unlike croup, epiglottitis is a life-threatening condition requiring emergency intubation. The most common organism responsible is *Haemophilus influenzae*. Affected children present with abrupt onset fever, dysphagia, stridor and worsening of respiratory distress in recumbent

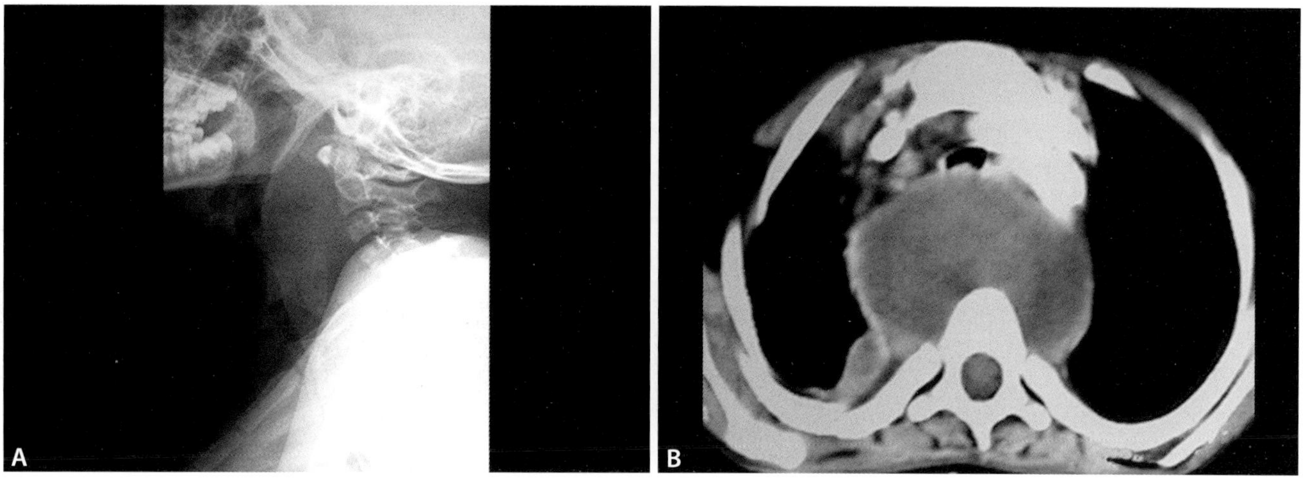

Figs. 2A and B: Retropharyngeal and mediastinal abscess: (A) Lateral radiograph neck of an 8-year-old boy with low-grade fever, respiratory distress and dysphagia reveals widening of the retropharyngeal soft tissues; (B) Contrast-enhanced CT scan at the level of the thoracic inlet shows a large prevertebral abscess compressing the trachea.

position. The 'classic' mean age of presentation is 3–5 years (older than croup). Now with availability of vaccination the incidence of this entity has significantly declined, and patients may present at a later age (13–14 years).[1,2]

Diagnosis is made on basis of presentation and physical examination. If not, a single lateral radiograph of neck may be obtained. This reveals markedly thickened epiglottis ("thumb" appearance). The pathological thickening of epiglottis can be differentiated from "omega" appearance, due to associated thickening of aryepiglottic folds in the former. The thickened aryepiglottic folds appear convex superiorly.

Retropharyngeal Cellulitis and Abscess

Retropharyngeal space inflammation is usually of pyogenic origin, following upper respiratory tract infection. Patients present with fever, dysphagia, a stiff neck and occasional stridor. It is most common between 6 months and 12 months of age.

Lateral radiographs reveal thickening of the retropharyngeal soft tissues. On radiographs, the only conclusive finding differentiating cellulitis from abscess is the presence of gas within the latter. Contrast-enhanced CT scans can aid in the distinction of cellulitis from a drainable fluid collection. An abscess appears as a well-defined, low-attenuation area with an enhancing rim[1] **(Figs. 2A and B)**.

Exudative Tracheitis

Exudative tracheitis is also referred to as membranous laryngotracheobronchitis or membranous croup. It is a purulent infection of the trachea characterized by formation of exudative plaques along the tracheal walls. Patients are older than croup, typically 6–10 years of age, and are also more ill. The causative organism may be *Staphylococcus aureus*, or the infections may be multimicrobial.

The characteristic finding on radiographs is a linear soft tissue filling defect (membrane) seen within the airway. A plaque-like irregularity of the tracheal wall is also suggestive. Other findings include narrowing of subglottic trachea (symmetric or asymmetric) with loss of its wall definition. The older age of the patient (> 3 years) aid distinction from croup.

Foreign Body

Post aspiration most foreign bodies lodge in the lower airway. Foreign bodies in the larynx or trachea are much less common, and the patients present with sudden onset stridor and respiratory distress. Foreign bodies if lodged in the esophagus may also present with respiratory symptoms. Radiographs reveal either a radiopaque foreign body or soft tissue density within the airway or loss of definition of the airway wall[1] **(Figs. 3A to C)**.

CHRONIC OBSTRUCTION

Obstructive Sleep Apnea (OSA)

The clinical presentation in children with chronic upper airway obstruction differs from that of acute obstruction. While these children may present with stridor, symptoms of sleep apnea or snoring are more common.[1,2] Sleep apnea

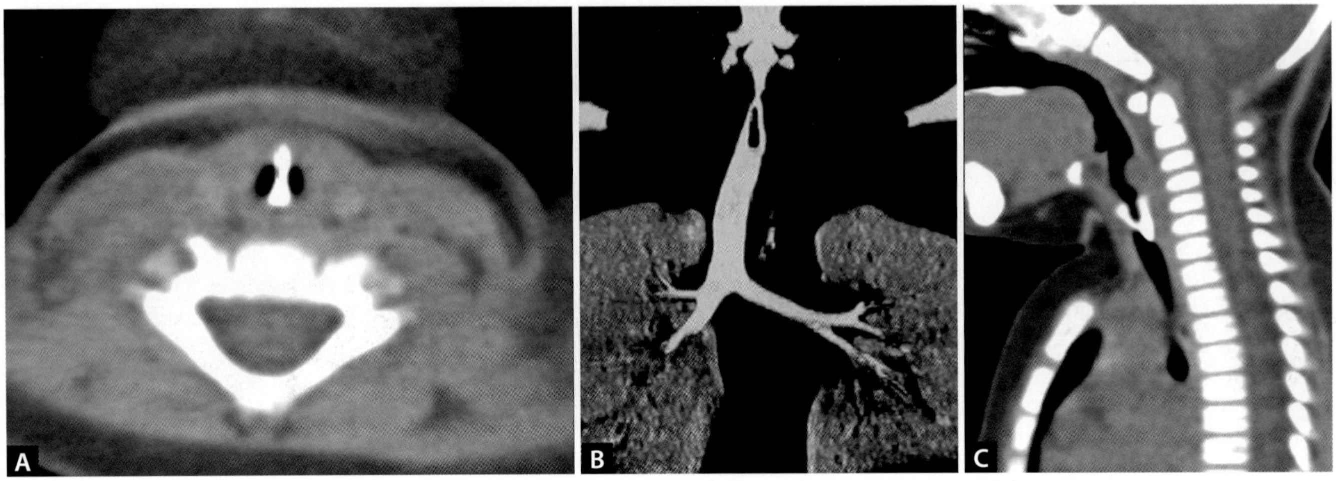

Figs. 3A to C: Foreign body: Axial CT scan (A) of a 7-month-old infant with sudden onset stridor reveals a radiopaque foreign body lodged in the trachea. Coronal minIP (B) and sagittal MPR (C) demonstrate the object well.

may be seen in up to 3% of children.[3] The various causes include any space occupying lesion or fixed narrowing, which maybe congenital, inflammatory or neoplastic in etiology.

At various levels the causes are:

Nasal cavity/Nasopharynx: Adenoidal enlargement, choanal atresia, juvenile angiofibroma.

Oropharynx: Micrognathia with posterior displacement of tongue, macroglossia, glossoptosis.

Hypopharynx: Hypopharyngeal collapse.

Larynx: Laryngomalacia, congenital cysts.

Large hemangiomas/vascular malformations can cause airway obstruction at any level.

MRI is useful in evaluation of patients with OSA. Indications for dynamic MR sleep imaging include persistence of OSA despite tonsillectomy and adenoidectomy, OSA with predisposition to obstruction at multiple sites (craniofacial anomalies, Down syndrome), evaluation of OSA before any complex airway surgery and obesity.

Enlarged Tonsils/Adenoids

The most common cause of chronic upper airway obstruction is enlargement of adenoids and palatine tonsils. Enlargement of lingual tonsils results in OSA only uncommonly. On a lateral radiograph, enlarged adenoids appear as convex soft tissue mass (>2 cm) in the posterior nasopharyx narrowing or obliterating the nasopharyngeal air lucency. CT also demonstrates tonsillar adenoidal enlargements well **(Figs. 4A to C)**. Enlarged palatine tonsils appear as soft tissue mass projecting on the posterior aspect of soft palate.[1] On T2W and STIR images adenoids and tonsils appear hyperintense.

Glossoptosis

Glossoptosis means abnormal posterior motion of the tongue during sleep and is associated with underlying hypotonia, macroglossia or micrognathia. Macroglossia and micrognathia may be diagnosed on lateral radiograph. However, glossoptosis can be demonstrated on dynamic sleep fluoroscopy or cine MRI.

Hypopharyngeal Collapse

Hypopharyngeal collapse refers to cylindrical collapse of the hypopharynx; with its anterior, posterior and lateral walls all moving centrally. It is associated with disorders of decreased muscular tone. This can be diagnosed on cine fluoroscopy or MRI.

Subglottic Obstruction

Subglottic Stenosis

Short segment subglottic stenosis is often congenital in origin **(Figs. 5A and B)**.

Postintubation Stenosis

Prolonged intubation can lead to either tracheomalacia or airway stenosis, particularly with oversized endotracheal tubes or balloon cuffs. Airway stenosis consequent to prolonged intubation usually occurs at the level of cricoid cartilage, which is the narrowest part of the upper airway[7] **(Figs. 6A to C)**.

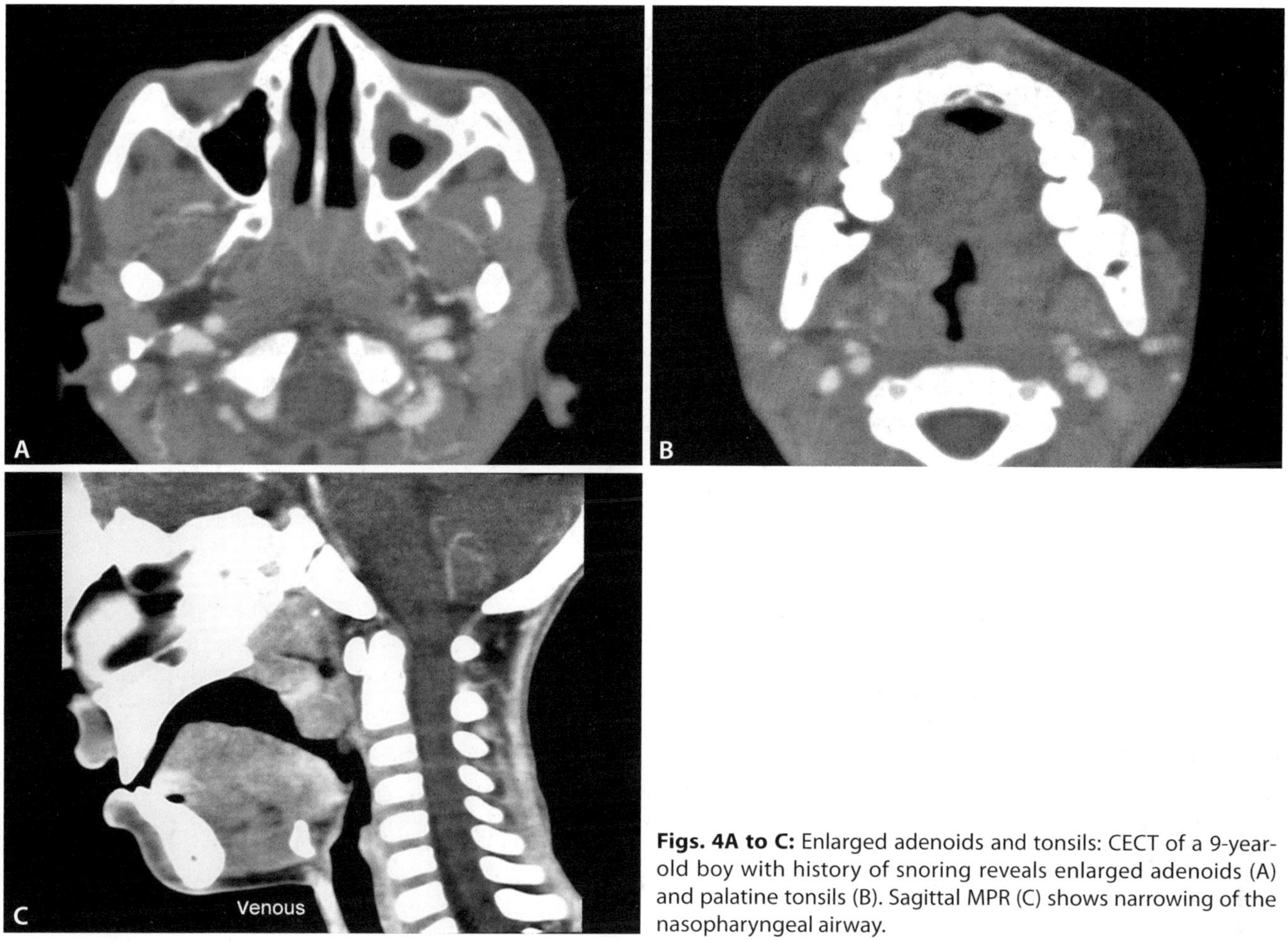

Figs. 4A to C: Enlarged adenoids and tonsils: CECT of a 9-year-old boy with history of snoring reveals enlarged adenoids (A) and palatine tonsils (B). Sagittal MPR (C) shows narrowing of the nasopharyngeal airway.

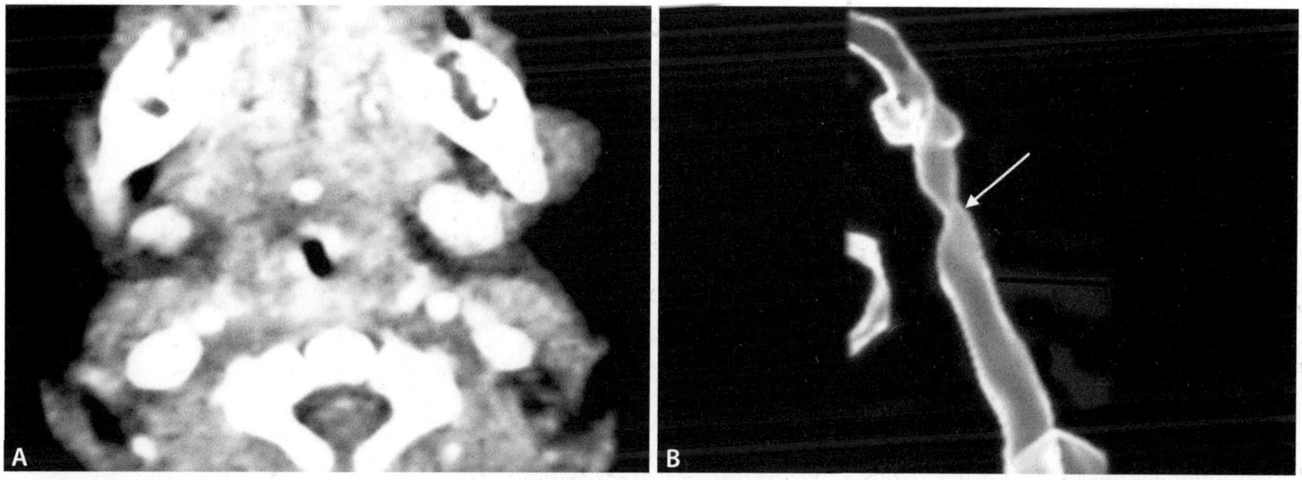

Figs. 5A and B: Subglottic stenosis: CECT of a newborn with stridor. Axial (A), sagittal VRT (B) images show a short segment, smooth subglottic stenosis (arrow).

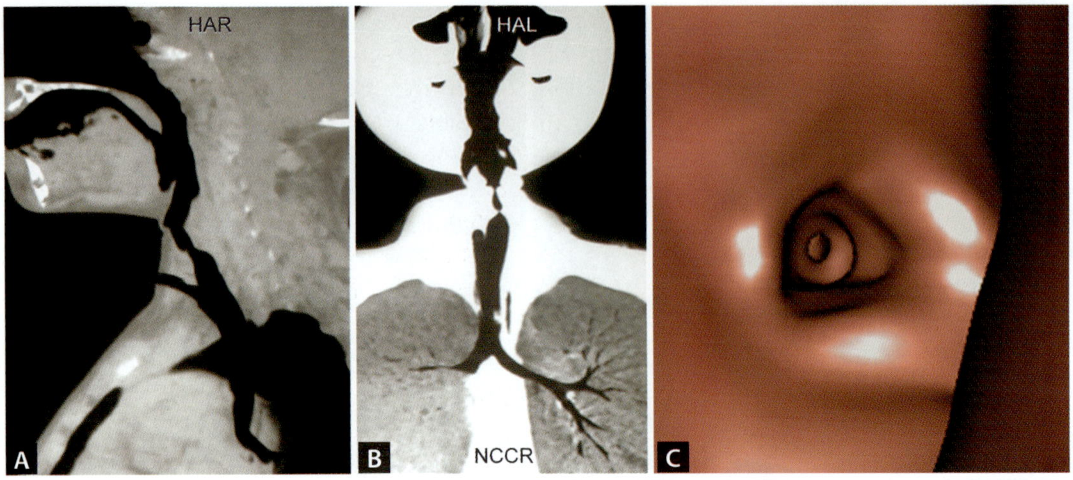

Figs. 6A to C: Postintubation stenosis: A short segment, smooth subglottic stenosis is seen on sagittal MPR (A), coronal minIP (B) and VB (C) CT images of a child with history of prolonged intubation.

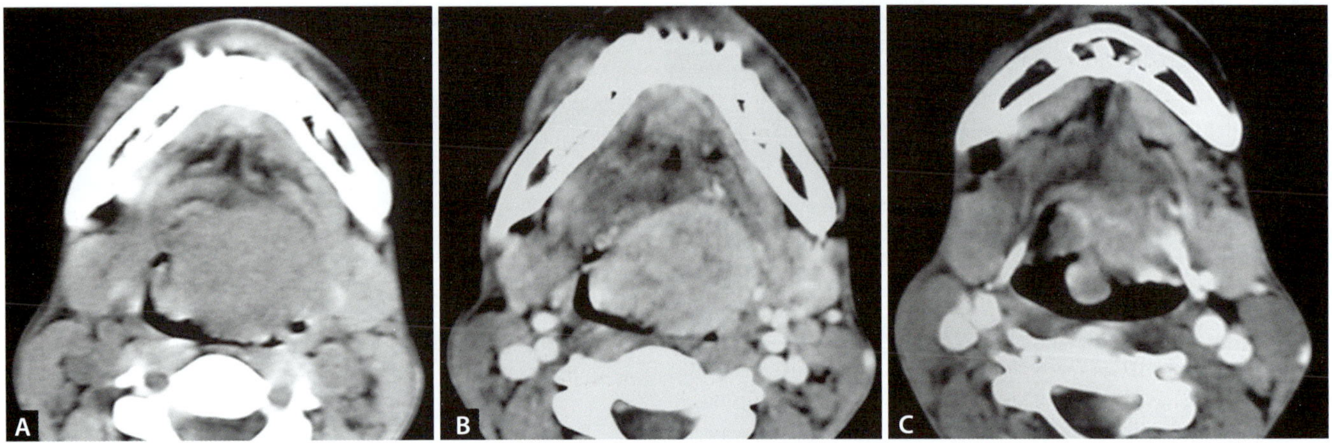

Figs. 7A to C: Hemangioma: NCCT (A) and CECT (B, C) image reveal an enhancing, well-defined soft tissue mass significantly narrowing the oropharyngeal and subglottic airway.

Subglottic Hemangioma

Hemangiomas located in the soft tissues of the neck may extend into the subglottic airway. Large hemangiomas or vascular malformations can cause obstruction at any level **(Figs. 7 and 8)**. These present in infancy, often at less than 6 months of age; and may be associated with hemangiomas of the face or trunk.

Plain radiographs reveal asymmetric subglottic narrowing with associated soft tissue. On cross-sectional imaging, the lesions show intense contrast enhancement which may be nodular. These lesions are unilateral or bilateral, but often asymmetric and occasionally circumferential. On T2W images, as elsewhere hemangiomas appear hyperintense.[2] Although a benign lesion with a natural history of proliferation and involution,

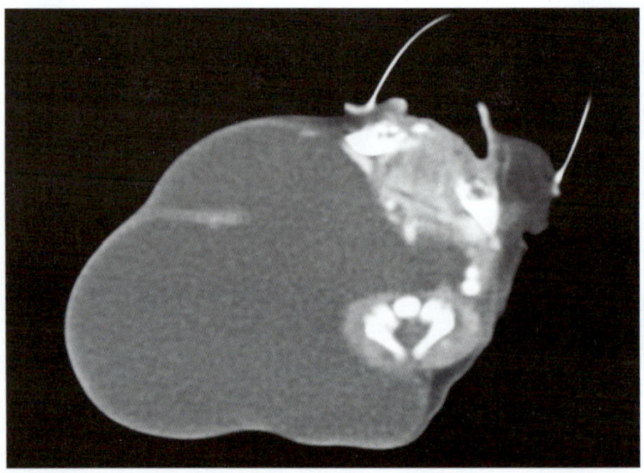

Fig. 8: Lymphangioma: CECT neck of a neonate showing a large multiseptated, multicompartmental cystic lesion obliterating the oropharyngeal airway.

complications of bleeding and airway obstruction can be life threatening. Spontaneous regression is typical. Endoscopy confirms the diagnosis. When the presentation demands active management, as in patients with symptomatic airway compromise, treatment options include systemic or intralesional corticosteroids, laser ablation, interferon therapy or surgical excision.[4,8]

LOWER AIRWAY OBSTRUCTION

Central Airways

Small airway diseases such as asthma and bronchiolitis are more common than central causes of obstruction. The central causes may be extrinisic or intrinsic (involving either the wall or lumen).

Investigations include frontal and lateral radiographs of the airway and chest. The neck radiographs help to exclude upper airway obstruction. Chest radiographs should be evaluated for tracheal caliber, cardiac size, position of the aortic arch, mediastinal widening, asymmetric lung aeration, lung collapse or consolidation and radiopaque foreign body. The length of tracheal narrowing and involvement of anterior/posterior walls should be noted. If the radiographs are suggestive of an intrinsic cause of obstruction, then one can proceed with fiberoptic bronchoscopy. If the suspected cause is extrinsic then further cross-sectional imaging is indicated.

The choice between CT and MRI is not clearly defined. While MRI has the advantage of being radiation free and not dependent on intravenous contrast, its main drawback is the long scanning times. The need for sedation especially in a child with airway compromise often negates the advantages of MRI, making CT the preferred modality. Both modalities offer good contrast between the central airway and surrounding structures, while the lungs are better visualized on CT.

Extrinsic Causes

Any mass lesion of the mediastinum such as nodes and cysts include the nonvascular causes of airway compression. Chest wall deformities may similarly result in airway compromise.

The classical vascular causes include double aortic arch, anomalous left pulmonary artery (pulmonary sling) and innominate artery compression syndrome. However, several other vascular causes such as dilatation of pulmonary artery **(Figs. 9A to C)**, enlargement of ascending aorta, midline descending aorta and right arch with aberrant left subclavian artery can also result in airway compression. A vascular ring encircling the airway occurs as a result of the failure of primitive vascular structures to fuse and regress normally during the development of the aortic arch, pulmonary arteries, and/or ductus arteriosus. Patients with vascular rings may have wheezing, stridor, feeding difficulties, choking episodes, or even aspiration pneumonia; depending on the degree of tracheal and esophageal narrowing.[4]

Plain radiographs and barium swallow cannot reliably distinguish among the types of vascular ring. Cross-sectional imaging, either with CT or MR, is helpful in delineating the anatomy and aiding in presurgical planning and postsurgical assessment.[4,9,10]

Vascular Causes

Vascular Rings

Double aortic arch: Double aortic arch is a congenital arch anomaly, and is the most common vascular ring to cause airway compression. It is usually an isolated anomaly. Both right and left arches are seen to arise from the ascending aorta and join to form the descending aorta. Right arch is commonly larger and posterosuperior.[1,2]

The two arches surround and compress the trachea anteriorly, and esophagus posteriorly. The level of compression is mid to lower thirds of intrathoracic trachea.[1,2]

On radiography, lateral tracheal indentations are seen. On cross-sectional imaging, it is important to determine the dominant arch (side), as the surgical approach differs accordingly.

Pulmonary sling: Pulmonary sling refers to a pulmonary artery anomaly wherein the left pulmonary artery arises from the proximal right pulmonary artery, forming a "sling" around the trachea. It subsequently passes between the trachea and esophagus as it courses towards the left lung. It may be associated with congenital heart disease and complete tracheal rings, worsening the airway compromise.[1,2]

Frontal radiograph reveals asymmetric lung inflation. On lateral radiograph, there is posterior compression of the trachea with anterior esophageal impression. It is the only vascular ring to course between the trachea and esophagus, to be associated with asymmetric lung inflation and also the only one to cause anterior indentation on the esophagus.[1,2]

Innominate artery compression syndrome: Innominate artery (Brachiocephalic) crosses the trachea anteriorly, just below the thoracic inlet. In infants, it arises more to the left than adults. In addition the presence of a large thymus in the mediastinum and lack of rigidity of infantile

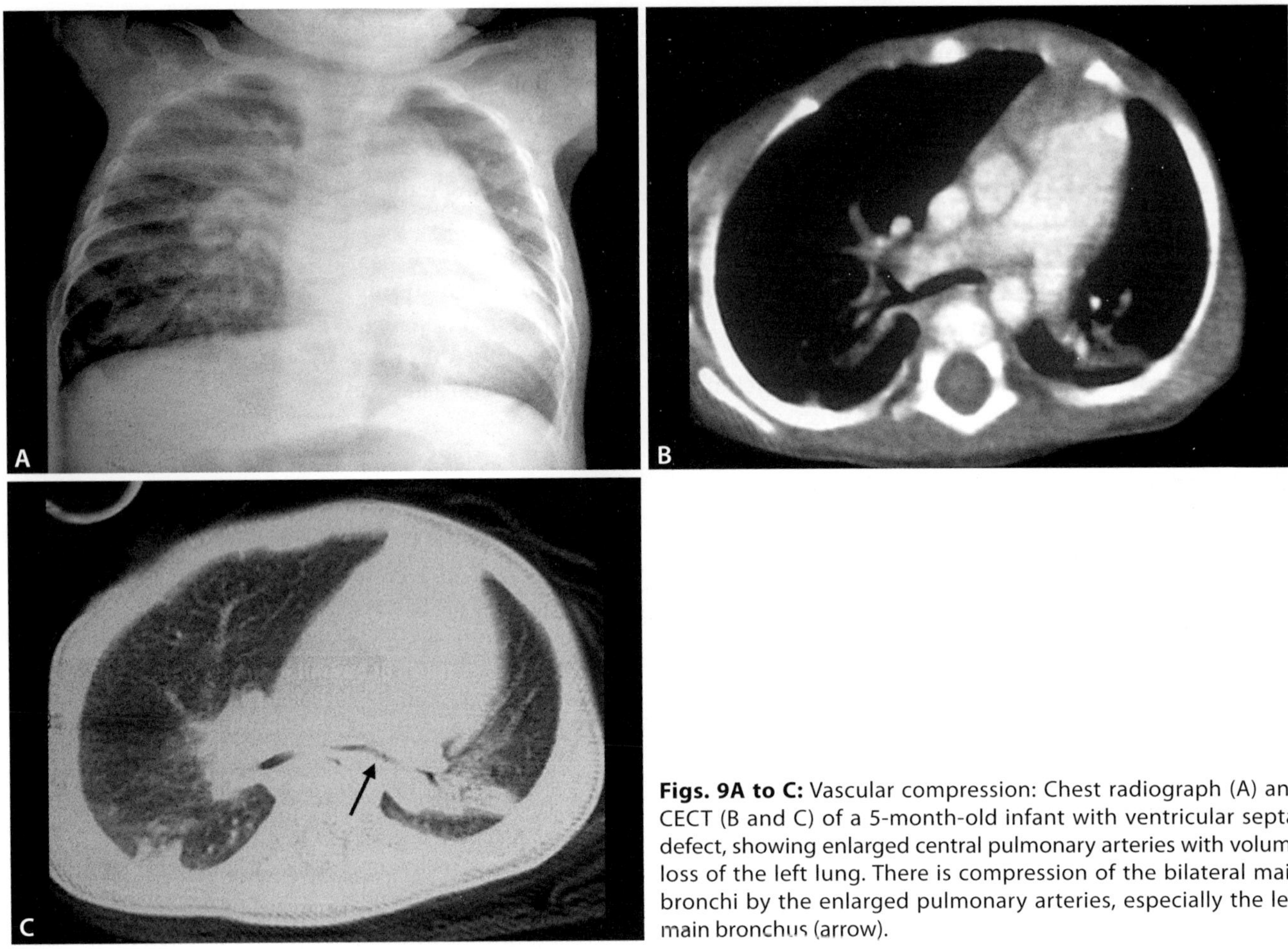

Figs. 9A to C: Vascular compression: Chest radiograph (A) and CECT (B and C) of a 5-month-old infant with ventricular septal defect, showing enlarged central pulmonary arteries with volume loss of the left lung. There is compression of the bilateral main bronchi by the enlarged pulmonary arteries, especially the left main bronchus (arrow).

trachea results in tracheal compression. The range of symptoms vary from none to stridor and dyspnea resulting from severe compression. Most children outgrow the disease and surgery is reserved only for those with severe compression.

Lateral radiographs reveal focal anterior indentation of the trachea. CT and MRI detail the severity of the compression and exclude other causes.[1,2]

Right arch with aberrant left subclavian artery: This is an arch anomaly wherein the aortic arch is located to the right of trachea. The left subclavian artery (LSA) originates from the proximal descending aorta and courses to the left behind the esophagus. In 60% cases, there is dilatation of origin of the LSA (aortic diverticulum of Kommerell). It is commonly an asymptomatic finding with only 5% patients having symptoms.[2] However, this anomaly may be associated with a constricting left ligamentum arteriosum, forming a vascular ring and causing airway compression. If the ligamentum arteriosum connects to LSA it forms a loose vascular ring, while if it extends to the aortic diverticulum of Kommerell, a tight ring is formed.

On frontal radiograph, there is aortic arch indentation on the right wall of the trachea with tracheal deviation to the left **(Figs. 10A to C)**. Right sided descending aorta may also be seen. Lateral view reveals indentation on the posterior aspect of trachea. On barium swallow, frontal views show a filling defect coursing from right inferior to left superior. On lateral view, there is posterior esophageal indentation. Cross-sectional imaging is indicated when there is clinical or radiographic evidence of airway compression.

Midline descending aorta: In this anomaly, the descending aorta is positioned immediately anterior to the vertebral body, instead of the normal left paravertebral location. It may be an isolated lesion or be associated with hypoplastic right lung and hence mediastinal shift; or aortic arch anomalies.

Malposition may result in airway compression due to crowding of structures. Radiographs are often normal, cross-sectional imaging reveals the diagnosis.

Vascular Malformations

Vascular malformations may be venous, lymphatic, or mixed venolymphatic. Although these lesions are usually

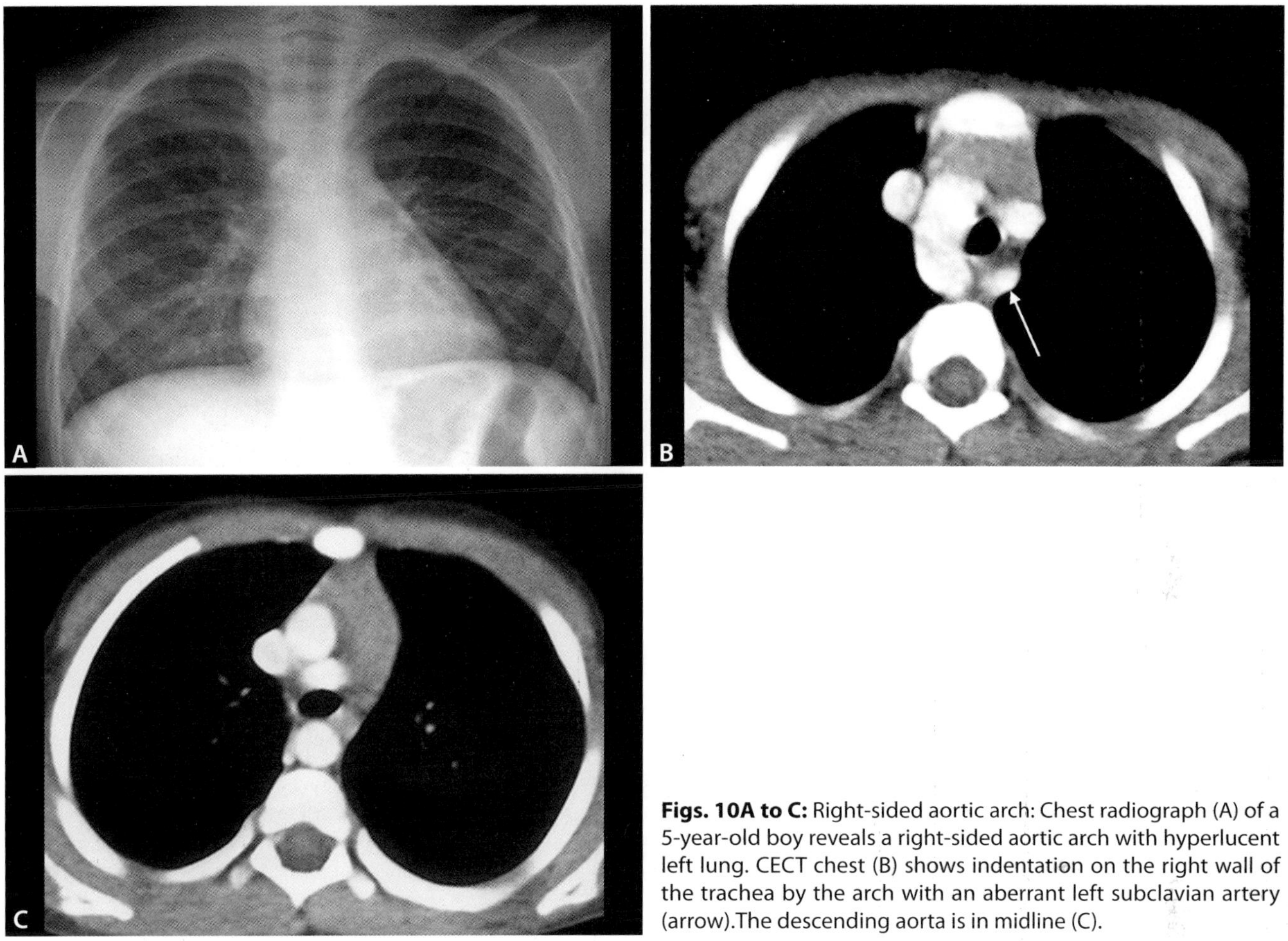

Figs. 10A to C: Right-sided aortic arch: Chest radiograph (A) of a 5-year-old boy reveals a right-sided aortic arch with hyperlucent left lung. CECT chest (B) shows indentation on the right wall of the trachea by the arch with an aberrant left subclavian artery (arrow).The descending aorta is in midline (C).

soft and compressible, giant malformations of the neck and/or chest can compress airway.

Bronchopulmonary foregut malformations: Bronchogenic cysts are among the most common cystic lesions in the pediatric chest. The most common location is around the carina. Hence, when large, these result in compression of the proximal bronchi. They can occur anywhere along the respiratory tract.[4]

The dilated proximal esophageal pouch in patients of esophageal atresia can also exert a mass effect on the adjoining airway[4] **(Fig. 11)**.

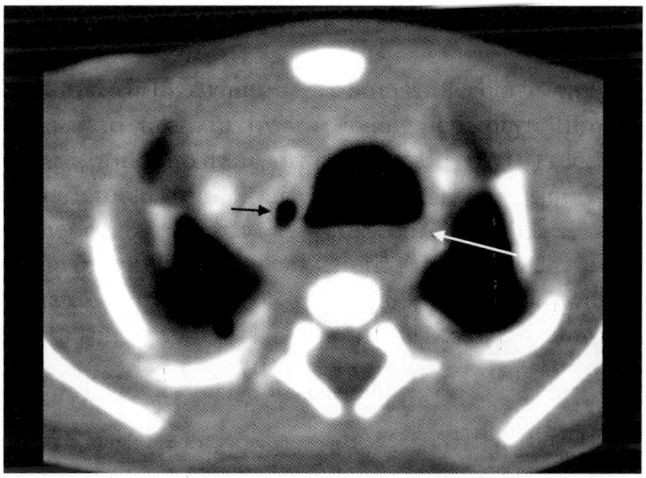

Fig. 11: Esophageal atresia: CECT of a neonate with esophageal atresia, performed to evaluate respiratory distress shows the dilated proximal esophageal pouch (white arrow) causing significant compression of the trachea (black arrow).

Inflammatory causes: Deep neck space infections, when they spread into the mediastinum, can compress the airway. Large paravertebral abscesses, even tubercular may result in significant airway compression **(Fig. 2)**.

Mediastinal lymphadenopathy, tubercular or fungal infections can also narrow the airway by mass effect **(Figs. 12A to D)**.

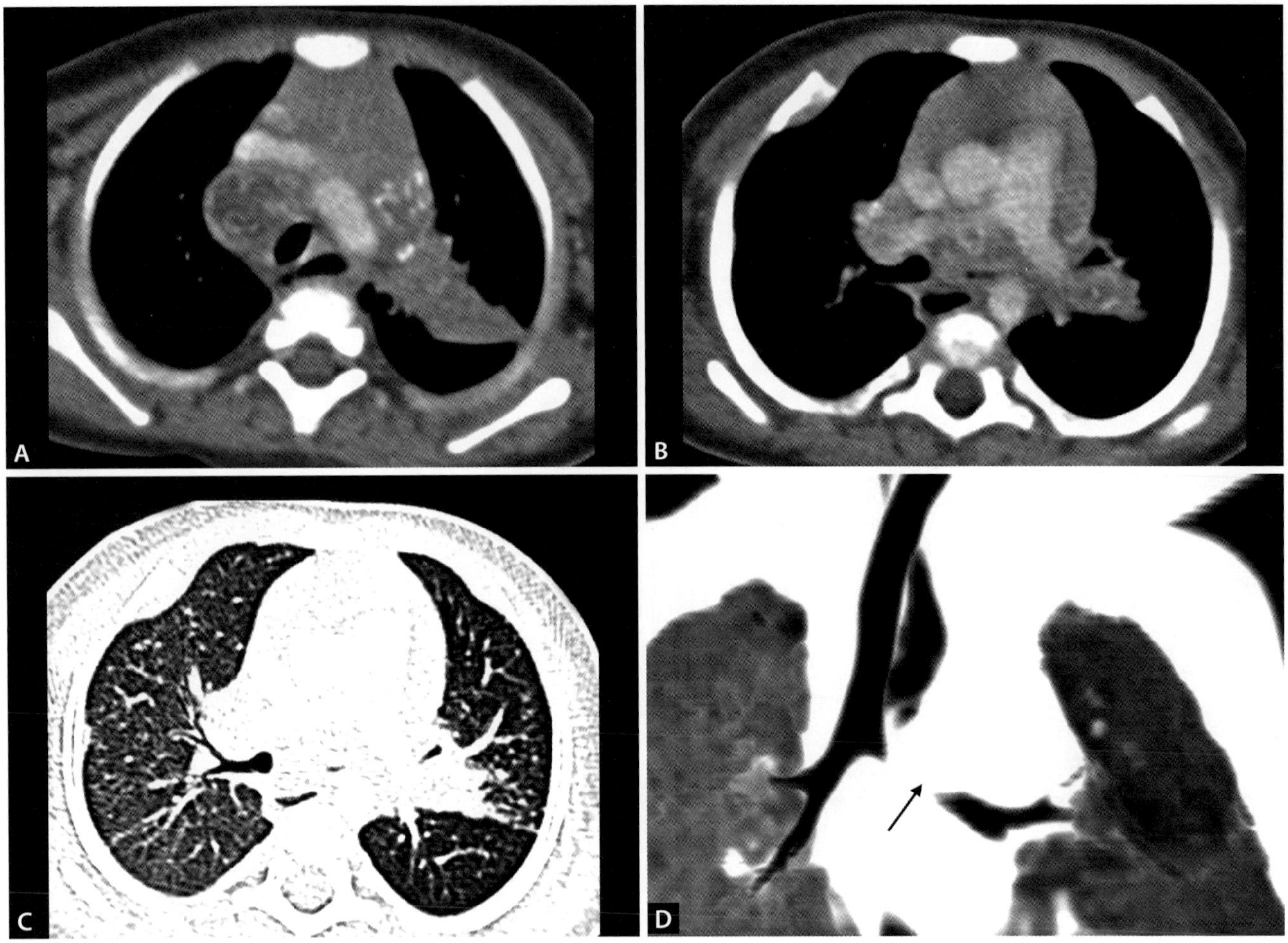

Figs. 12A to D: Tubercular lymphadenopathy: CECT of a 6-year-old boy reveals conglomerate, necrotic, calcific mediastinal lymphadenopathy with left upper lobe consolidation (A). A more caudal section mediastinal window (B), and lung window (C) and minIP (D) show narrowing of the left main (arrow) and upper lobe bronchii.

Masses: Lymphoma is the most common childhood neoplasm to cause symptomatic airway compromise in children.[11] Other neoplasms that tend to narrow the airway by extrinsic mass effect include infantile hemangiomas, germ cell tumors, rhabdomyosarcomas and neurogenic tumors **(Figs. 13A and B)**.

Intrinsic Causes

Intrinsic causes include those involving the wall which may be dynamic (tracheomalacia) or fixed (stenosis) and intraluminal lesions.

Wall Abnormalities

Tracheomalacia: Tracheomalacia refers to abnormal softening of the trachea due to abnormality of the cartilaginous rings. This results in intermittent (expiratory) collapse of the trachea. The narrowing of the tracheal lumen is most marked during forced expiration, coughing, or the Valsalva maneuver.[4] It may be primary or secondary to compression by masses or vascular structures. Similar condition may involve the proximal bronchi. It may be congenital associated with syndromes such as cystic fibrosis, or even result from chronic inflammation, chronic extrinsic compression or prior intubation. The characteristic clinical presentation is of an expiratory wheeze.

The diagnosis cannot be made on the basis of a single radiograph. Fluoroscopy, and typically fiberoptic bronchoscopy can demonstrate the characteristic dynamic collapse of the trachea. Airway fluoroscopy done in a lateral projection is the traditional radiographic method of diagnosing tracheomalacia. However, bronchomalacia is difficult to diagnose on fluoroscopy,

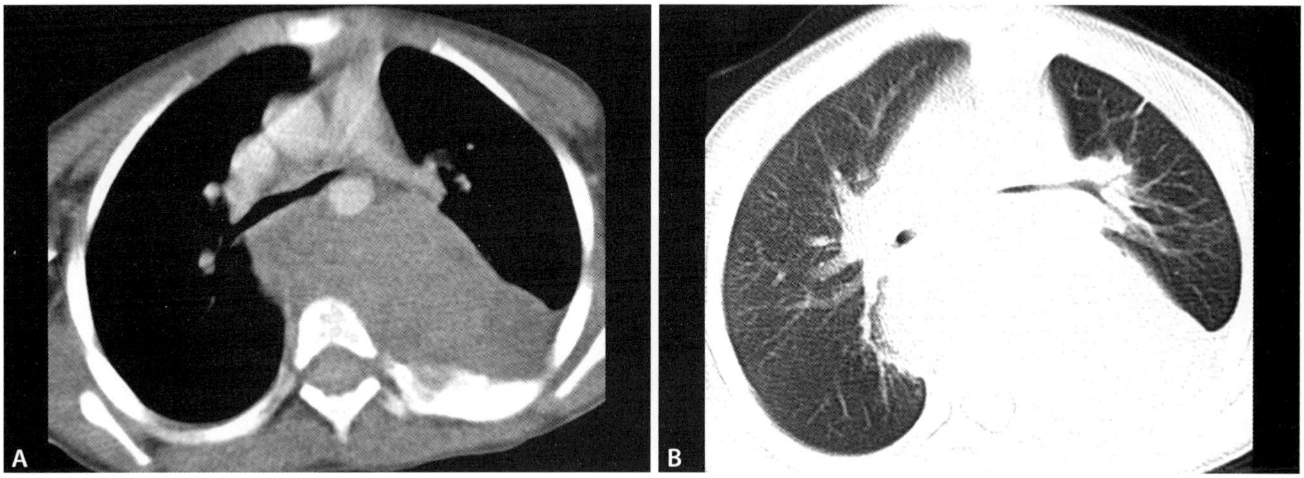

Figs. 13A and B: Neuroblastoma: CECT (A) showing a large posterior mediastinal mass lesion causing displacement and compression of the major bronchi, especially the left main bronchus. Lung window (B) reveals a hyperlucent left lung.

and controlled-ventilation CT, cine CT, or cine MR imaging are preferred methods for this entity.[4] On a single phase inspiratory CT the diagnosis is difficult, although the trachea may demonstrate an abnormal shape being flattened slightly posteriorly in the membranous part[1,2] **(Figs. 14A to C)**. Paired inspiratory-expiratory MDCT/cine MDCT is more sensitive to demonstrate the expiratory collapse, and require the measurement of the area of trachea in both the phases.[12]

Stenosis: Fixed trachea stenosis may be congenital or acquired. Congenital tracheal stenosis results from absence of the membranous portion of the trachea resulting in complete or near complete cartilaginous tracheal rings. The various patterns of tracheal stenosis include generalized stenosis, carrot- or funnel-shaped segmental stenosis, and focal stenosis. Focal stenosis usually involves the lower trachea. A tight focal stenosis causes more severe symptoms than a long, mild stenosis. It may be associated with congenital heart disease, pulmonary sling, TEF, or skeletal abnormalities.[2,4] On axial imaging, trachea appears as a round or complete circle (O-shaped). Other findings include: circumferential narrowing of the entire length of the trachea and fusion of the cartilaginous tracheal rings posteriorly.[4, 13]

Congenital tracheal web is a rare entity. The web is usually not associated with deformity of the tracheal cartilage or the tracheal wall. CT reveals a weblike structure traversing and narrowing the tracheal lumen,[14] which is well demonstrated on coronal reformatted images and virtual bronchoscopy.[4]

Bronchopulmonary foregut malformations: Bronchopulmonary foregut malformations include a wide spectrum of disorders such as: tracheal agenesis, tracheal stenosis, tracheal fistula, branching anomalies, bronchial stenosis, or lung agenesis and hypoplasia; as well as bronchogenic cysts are also included in this group.[3] These anomalies may present with respiratory distress in the newborn, recurrent pulmonary infections or mass lesions later in life. This chapter deals with anomalies affecting the major bronchi.

Bronchial atresia and sequestration: Bronchial atresia most often involves the left upper lobe. On CT, a mucocele is identified as a hypo- or fluid-attenuating branching structure distal to the atretic bronchus near the hilum. The pulmonary parenchyma distal to the atretic segment is often lucent and demonstrates air trapping. The affected region may even be outlined by pseudofissures.[4]

Bronchial atresia may be isolated or associated with a retained systemic vascular connection, when it is referred to as intralobar sequestration. The imaging appearance is virtually identical to that of isolated bronchial atresia, except that the atretic bronchus is ectopically located at the margin of the lung. Rarely, such ectopic bronchi may not be atretic but have a connection with the gastrointestinal tract, usually the esophagus. Such cases are usually accompanied by bronchiectasis and accumulated secretions from impaired clearance of lung parenchyma. It is hence important to look for airway abnormalities, pulmonary parenchymal abnormalities, retained systemic vascular connections, anomalous pulmonary venous drainage, and airway communication with the gastrointestinal tract in patients with suspected bronchopulmonary foregut malformations.[4, 15,16]

Tracheoesophageal fistula (TEF): Esophageal atresia with or without TEF is believed to result from a faulty separation

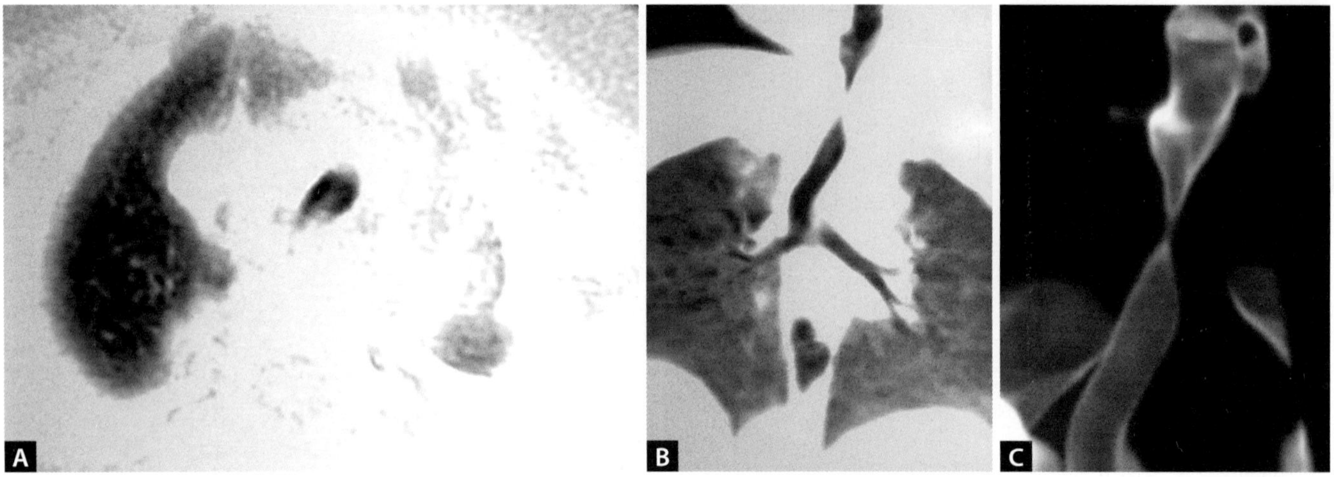

Figs. 14A to C: Tracheomalacia: Axial CT (A) of a neonate with stridor showing slight posterior flattening of the trachea; min IP (B) and VRT images (C) show narrowing of subglottic trachea. On bronchoscopy, this narrowing was found to be dynamic.

of the embryonic trachea and esophageal remnants. The most common type of these is proximal esophageal atresia with distal TEF (up to 80–90%). H-shaped TEFs with no atresia constitute up to 5–8%.[4] Typical clinical presentation includes failure to pass a feeding tube in a newborn with a history of polyhydramnios at prenatal US, excessive secretions from the mouth, and respiratory distress.[4] Chest radiograph demonstrates the feeding tube catheter ending/coiling in the proximal thoracic esophagus. The presence of air in the distal gastrointestinal tract confirms the presence of a distal TEF. In such patients, it is important to observe the airway as there is frequently associated tracheomalacia.[17] Also, a dilated proximal esophageal pouch can result in airway compression. Patients with H type fistula may present with recurrent aspiration or small airway disease. While contrast esophagogram is the investigation of choice, CT scan may demonstrate the fistula **(Figs. 15A and B)**.

Tracheobronchial branching anomalies: Tracheobronchial branching anomalies may be seen as an isolated finding or accompanying heterotaxy syndromes, pulmonary sling, and conditions associated with pulmonary underdevelopment (agenesis, aplasia or hypoplasia). The most common amongst these is the tracheal bronchus or "pig bronchus" **(Figs. 16A and B)**. A tracheal bronchus arises from the trachea or mainstem bronchus and aerates either the entire upper lobe or a segment.[4,18] An accessory cardiac bronchus or tracheal diverticulum are also relatively common anomalies. An accessory cardiac bronchus arises from the medial wall of the right mainstem bronchus or bronchus intermedius, grows toward the pericardium terminating as a blind-ending stump or branching further.[19] Tracheal diverticula is seen arising with a narrow stalk from the right posterolateral wall of the trachea near the thoracic inlet.[4] Other abnormal branching patterns include tracheal trifurcation, bilateral right-sided isomerism or bilateral left-sided isomerism. A detailed classification of tracheobronchial branching anomalies has been given in "Imaging of the tracheobronchial tree" in AIIMS-MAMC-PGI Imaging Course Series, Diagnostic Radiology-Chest and Cardiovascular Imaging 3rd edition.[20]

Metabolic conditions: Hunter syndrome (a muco-polysac-charidosis) may cause the deposition of mucopolysaccharides in the walls of the major airways results in progressive airway narrowing due to wall thickening and anteroposterior collapse.[4,21]

Acquired: Acquired tracheal or bronchial strictures usually result from *chronic inflammation*, often tubercular **(Figs. 17A to E)**. Another cause of acquired airway strictures is *post-traumatic* sequelae.

Intraluminal Causes

A foreign body (FB) is the most common cause of bronchial obstruction. Soft tissue masses of the trachea and bronchi are rare.

Foreign body: Foreign body aspiration is most often seen in infants and toddlers (8 months–3 years). The bronchi are the most common site of lodgement (76%), while laryngeal (6%) or tracheal (4%) lodgement is far less common. Right bronchus is more common (58%), than the left (42%).[2] The clinical presentation may be acute, while more often the symptoms remain indolent. The symptoms and signs can mimic asthma, upper

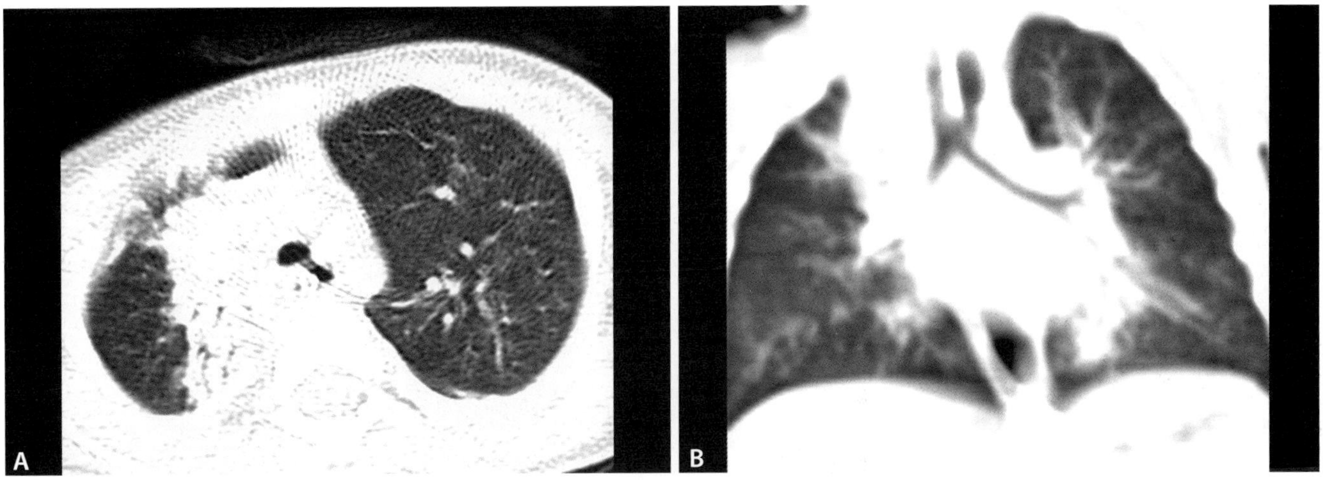

Figs. 15A and B: Tracheoesophageal fistula (TEF): Axial CT (A) of an infant reveals a communication between the trachea and esophagus with right upper lobe consolidation. Coronal MPR (B) also demonstrates the fistula.

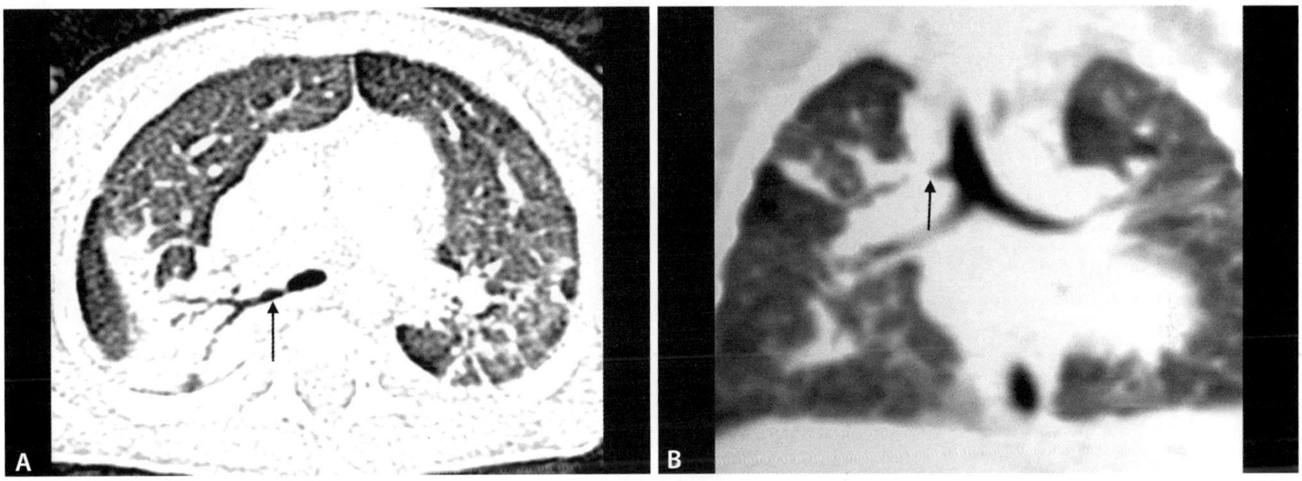

Figs. 16A and B: Tracheal bronchus: Axial lung window (A), coronal MPR (B) reveal an accessory bronchus arising from the trachea and aerating the posterior segment of right upper lobe (arrows).

respiratory infection, or pneumonia. The history of aspiration is often not elicited. Foreign body may lead to partial ("ball-valve" effect) or complete obstruction, resulting in hyperinflation or collapse respectively. Chest radiograph findings include asymmetric lung aeration, lung consolidation or atelectasis, and even pneumothorax or pneumomediastinum[1] **(Figs. 18 and 19)**. Metallic foreign bodies can be identified on plain radiographs **(Fig. 18)**. However, commonly aspirated airway foreign bodies are food products, particularly nuts, and seeds, which are not radiopaque enough to be identified at conventional radiography **(Figs. 20A to D)**. These organic materials can swell following absorption of water and then rapidly change a partial airway obstruction to a complete obstruction.[4]

Inspiratory radiographs alone may be normal in up to a third of patients (14–35%) with foreign bodies.[1,2] The lung volume of the affected lung/segment may be normal, increased or decreased.[1,2] Majority (up to 97%) of the foreign bodies are nonradiopaque.[1] The characteristic radiographic finding is that the lung volume remains static with no change in different phases of respiration. This can be demonstrated by obtaining paired inspiratory-expiratory radiographs in cooperative children. In infants and uncooperative children bilateral decubitus radiographs of the chest or fluoroscopy can demonstrate the same finding.[1,2] The differential diagnosis of an asymmetric, lucent lung include Swyer-James syndrome and pulmonary hypoplasia.[1,2] However, air trapping may be seen in partial obstruction.

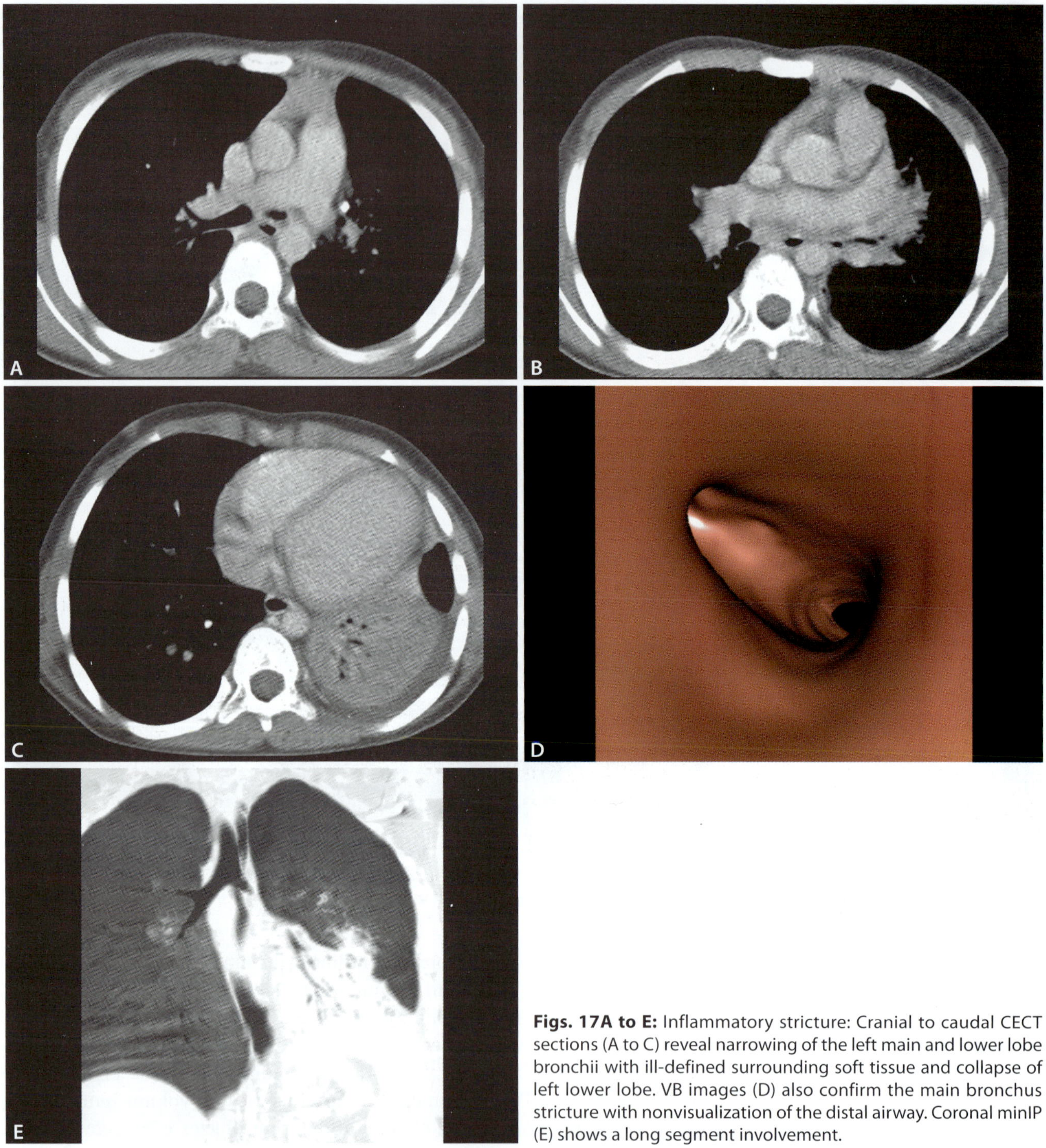

Figs. 17A to E: Inflammatory stricture: Cranial to caudal CECT sections (A to C) reveal narrowing of the left main and lower lobe bronchii with ill-defined surrounding soft tissue and collapse of left lower lobe. VB images (D) also confirm the main bronchus stricture with nonvisualization of the distal airway. Coronal minIP (E) shows a long segment involvement.

CT is not routinely advocated in evaluation of a bronchial foreign body. It may, however, be performed as work-up for nonresolving pneumonia or collapse, or even stridor **(Fig. 20)**. CT is also a good option when the clinical setting does not strongly warrant bronchoscopy or if bronchoscopy is not readily available.[4] On CT, foreign bodies are well demonstrated as filling defects in the bronchus, besides detailing the changes in the distal lung. It can identify both opaque and nonopaque foreign bodies. Kosucu et al reported a 100% sensitivity and specificity of CT in the evaluation of endobronchial foreign bodies.[22] Applegate et al while evaluating low-dose helical CT found

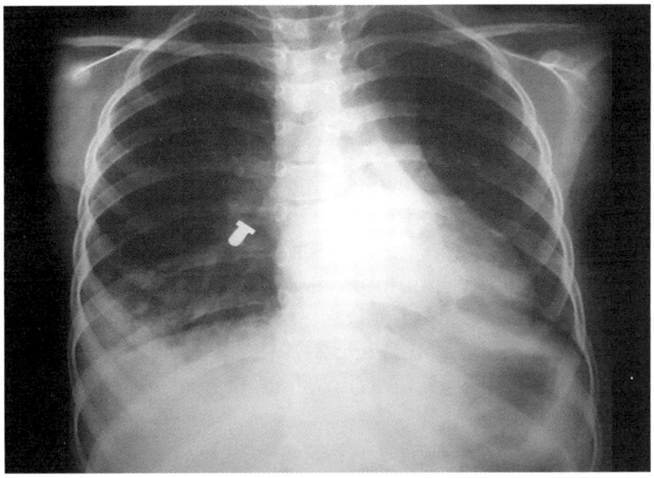

Fig. 18: Foreign body. Chest radiograph demonstrates a radiopaque foreign body in the right lower lobe bronchus with consolidation in the distal lung,

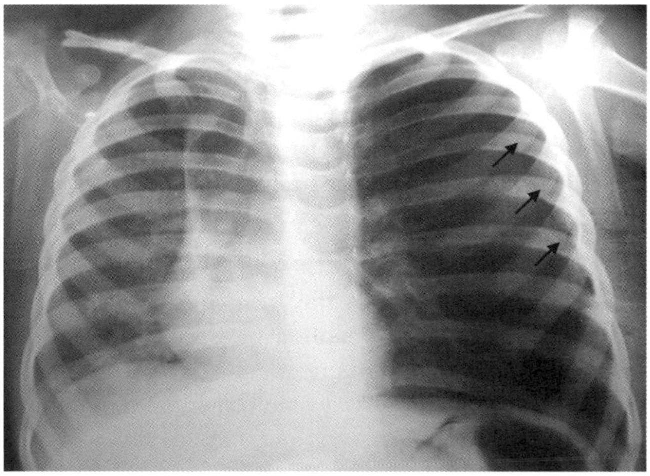

Fig. 19: Foreign body. Chest radiograph of a 2-year-old boy with history of foreign body aspiration and sudden onset respiratory distress reveals a hyperinflated left lung with spontaneous pneumothorax (arrows) and extensive subcutaneous emphysema.

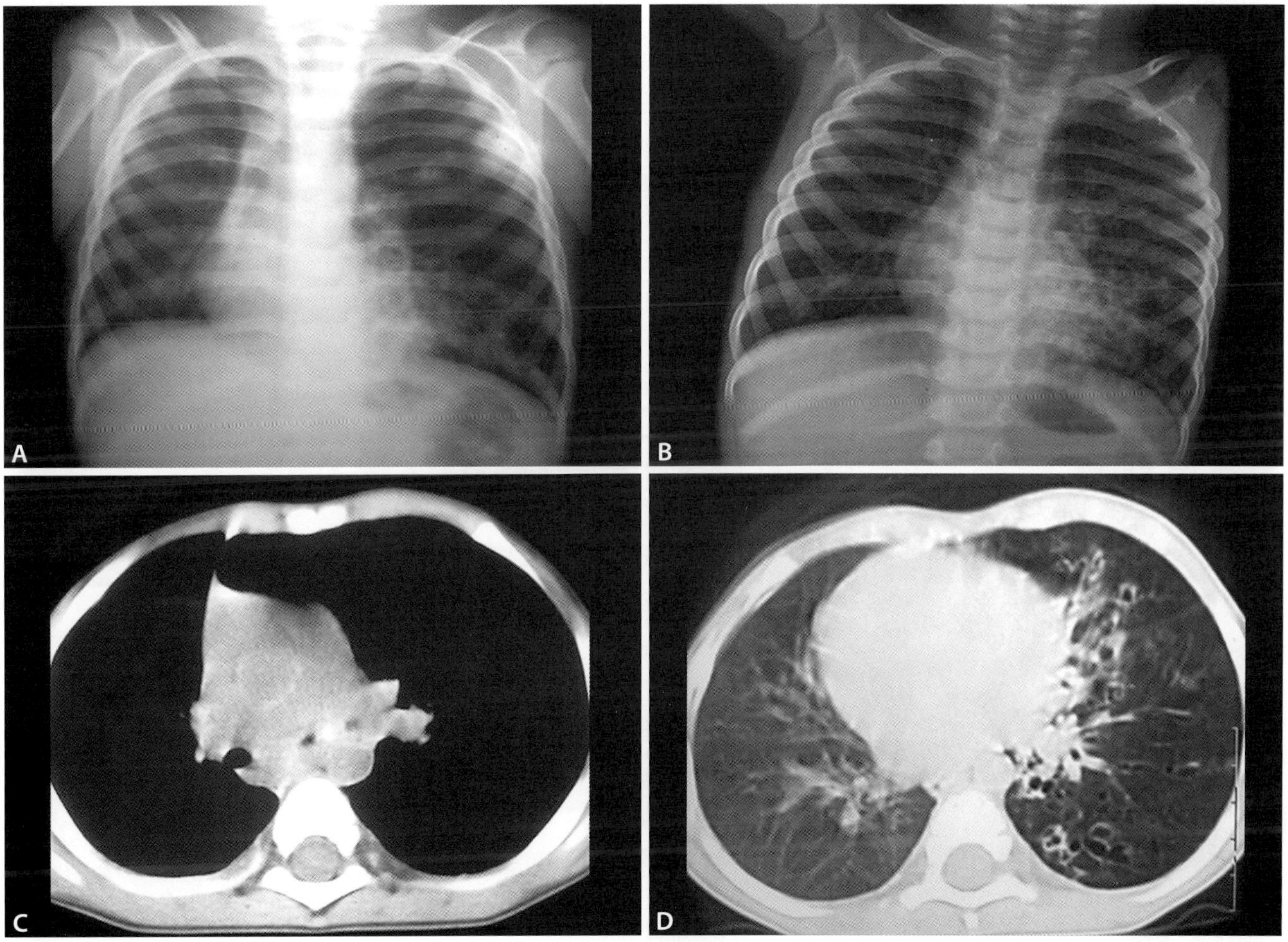

Figs. 20A to D: Foreign body: Chest radiograph (A) of a toddler with history of recurrent high-grade fever reveals a hyperinflated left lung with tram-track lesions in the left lower zone. A subsequent chest radiograph (B) shows progression in the lung parenchymal lesions with decrease in the hyperinflation. CT scans (C and D) reveals abrupt cut-off of the left main bronchus with intraluminal contents, and distal bronchiectasis. A "neem fruit ball" was removed from the left main bronchus on bronchoscopy.

a sensitivity of 83% and specificity of 89% for visualizing plastic pieces in the airway. Peanuts however were not well visualized in the same study.[23]

Even esophageal foreign bodies can present acutely with symptoms related to airway compression or with complications consequent to perforation and neck and/or mediastinal infection.[4]

Inflammatory: Tuberculosis—Occasionally, enlarged lymph nodes erode into the bronchus and result in endobronchial fibrosis or luminal occlusion. Intraluminal granulomas may occur in the trachea or bronchi.[4,24] In a series by Weber et al., airway involvement in tuberculosis was seen in up to 30% cases.[25]

Tumors: Tracheal soft tissue masses include tracheal papilloma; while bronchial masses may be carcinoid tumors.[1] Carcinoid tumor is the most common amongst these. Rare lesions include adenoid cystic carcinoma, mucoepidermoid carcinoma, inflammatory myofibroblastic tumor, juvenile xanthogranuloma, and metastasis.[4]

Carcinoid tumors comprise about 80% of endobronchial neoplasms in children and adolescents. These present in children or young adults and may be associated with neuroendocrine secretion.[3,26] Most carcinoid tumors occur in the mainstem or lobar bronchi, and patients present with dyspnea, wheezing, cough or hemoptysis. CT reveals typically intensely enhancing, ovoid lesions with a long axis parallel to the bronchovascular bundle.[4] These lesions may have intraluminal, mural, and extrabronchial components. Associated collapse, consolidation, or air trapping is often seen **(Figs. 21A to C)**. They are relatively slow growing masses, and complete surgical resection offers the best chance of cure.[27,28]

Peripheral Airways

Bronchiolitis/Small Airway Disease

Acute: Acute inflammation of the bronchi and bronchioles is common in children, and is most often infective in etiology. Plain radiographs reveal hyperinflation with increased perihilar markings. This entity is covered in detail in the chapter on Pulmonary Infections.

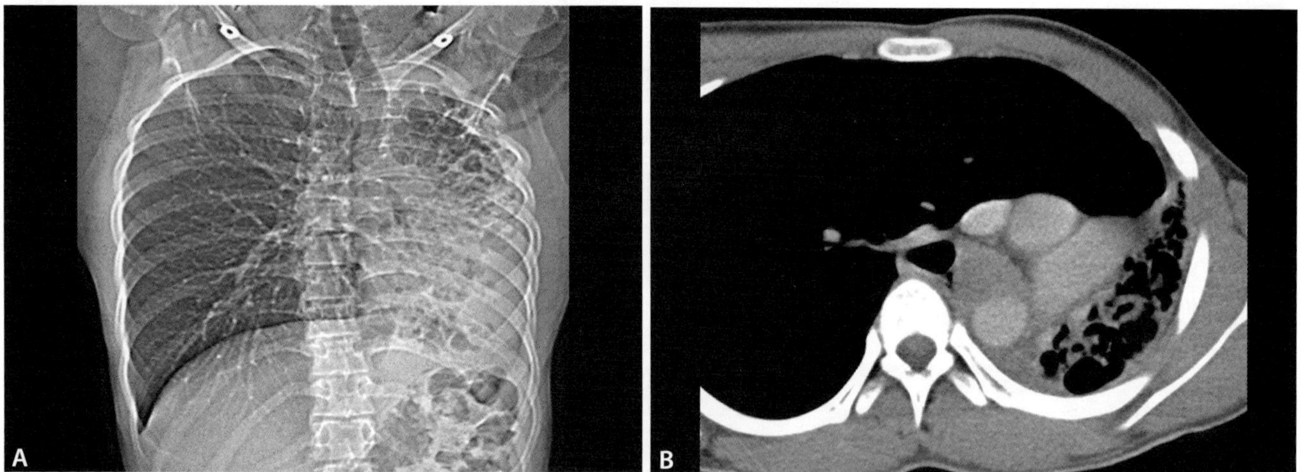

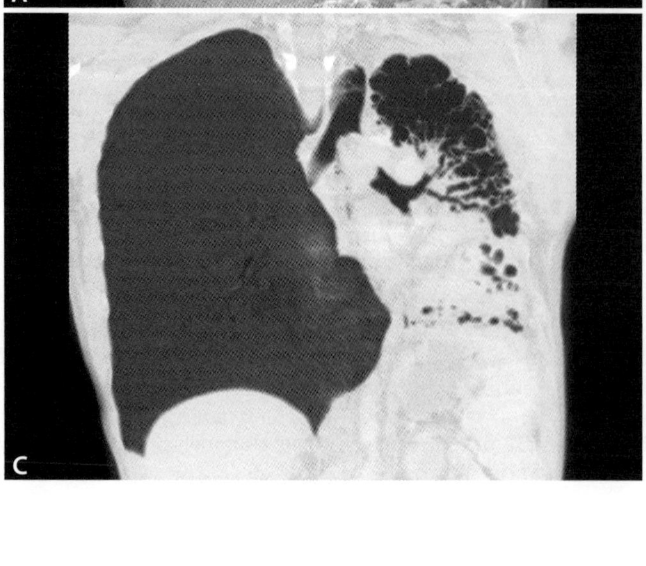

Figs. 21A to C: Carcinoid tumor: CT scout (A) of a 16-year-old boy with history of recurrent pulmonary infections reveals volume loss of left lung with extensive consolidation and bronchiectasis. Axial CECT (B) shows a homogeneous mass in the left main bronchus with mediastinal shift to left. minIP (C) demonstrates the entire extent of the mass with distal lung changes. Histopathology revealed a carcinoid tumor.

Chronic: The causes of chronic, small airway disease in children include: constrictive bronchiolitis, extrinsic allergic bronchiolitis, diffuse panbronchiolitis, follicular bronchiolitis and lung disease of prematurity.[3]

The chest radiograph and even CT findings are often nonspecific though the underlying etiologies may be quite variable. CT scan reveals ground glass opacities with mosaic attenuation and air trapping. Mild bronchiectasis with bronchial wall thickening may be seen **(Figs. 22 and 23)**.

Constrictive bronchiolitis or bronchiolitis obliterans: Although constrictive bronchiolitis may present as a unilateral hyperlucent lung (Swyer James syndrome), it is more often bilateral. There are several causes of this entity including infection (viral or mycoplasma), toxic and fume exposure, collagen vascular diseases such as Rheumatoid arthritis; and complication of bone-marrow or heart-lung transplant.[3,29]

HRCT reveals a prominent mosaic attenuation with bronchial abnormalities including bronchiectasis; and air-trapping[3,30] **(Figs. 22A and B)**. The pattern is similar to severe asthma or cystic fibrosis.

Extrinsic allergic alveolitis: Extrinsic allergic alveolitis or hypersensitivity pneumonitis is a form of cellular bronchilitis. In the acute stage CT reveals multiple, ill-defined centriliobular nodules; while in the subacute or chronic stage mosaic alternation with expiratory air trapping are seen[3,29] **(Figs. 23A and B)**. Areas of fibrosis may also be present.

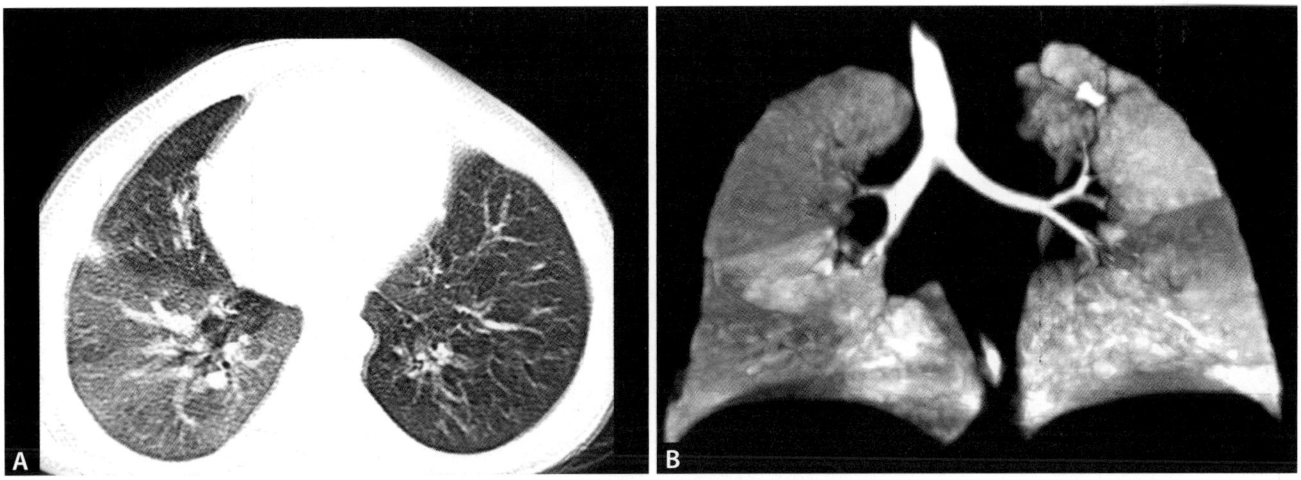

Figs. 22A and B: Chronic bronchiolitis: Axial CT lung window (A) and minIP (B) of a 3-year-old girl with history of dyspnea reveals prominent mosaic attenuation with air-trapping and mild bronchiectasis.

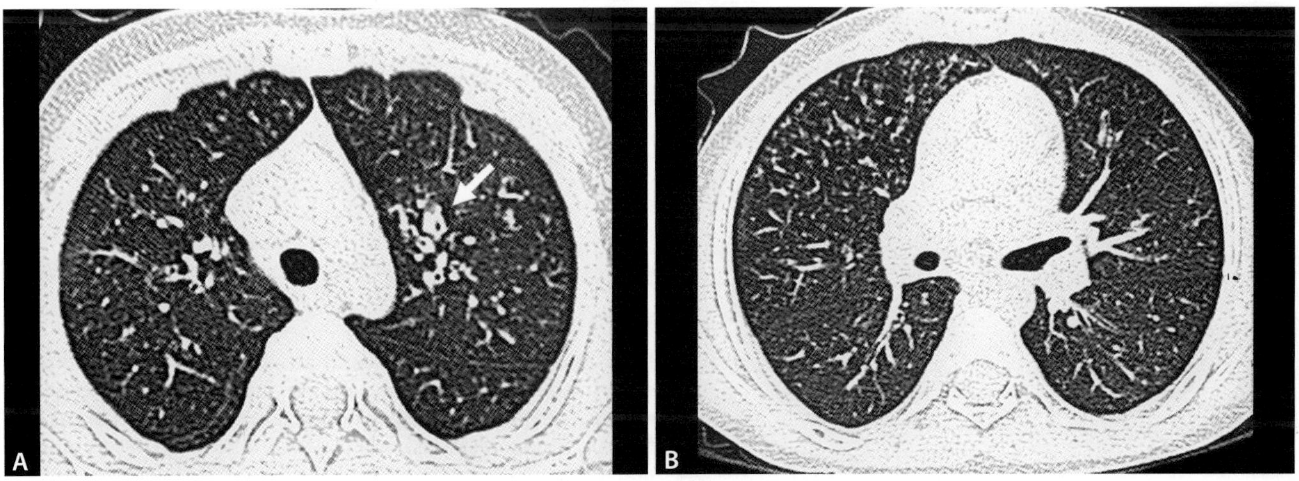

Figs. 23A and B: Chronic bronchiolitis: HRCT (A and B) of 8-year-old child reveals multiple, ill-defined centriliobular nodules and bronchial wall thickening (arrow).

Diffuse panbronchiolitis: Diffuse panbronchiolitis is an exudative form of bronchiolitis seen in Eastern and South-Eastern Asia. CT reveals multiple small centrilobular nodules and linear opacities diffusely distributed in both the lungs.[3]

Follicular bronchiolitis: Follicular bronchiolitis or lung hyperplasia of the bronchus associated lymphoid tissue is also a cause chronic obstructive diffuse lung disease. In addition to expiratory air trapping, CT reveals areas of ground glass opacity.[3, 31]

Lung Disease of Prematurity

This is a unique form of airway disease seen in premature infants with bronchopulmonary dysplasia. It is a destructive diffuse lung disease occurring in a background of rapid alveolar growth. CT helps in excluding other causes of chronic respiratory distress such as central airway lesions.[3]

Bronchiectasis

Bronchiectasis is a common cause of respiratory symptoms in children.[28] It is often the result of chronic inflammation causing damage to the supporting structure of the airways. Also, chronic or recurrent inflammation due to immunodeficiency states may cause bronchiectasis. Other etiologies include, abnormal mucus as in cystic fibrosis and abnormal mucociliary clearance in children with ciliary dyskinesias **(Figs. 24A to C)**. Proximal bronchial obstruction due to an intrinsic or extrinsic cause may also lead to bronchiectasis in the distal lung. Aspiration secondary to gastroesophageal reflux due to its chronic, recurrent nature has also been postulated as a cause of bronchiectasis.[3,32]

Patients typically present with recurrent infections. Chest radiographs are relatively insensitive in detecting early changes, with HRCT being the imaging modality

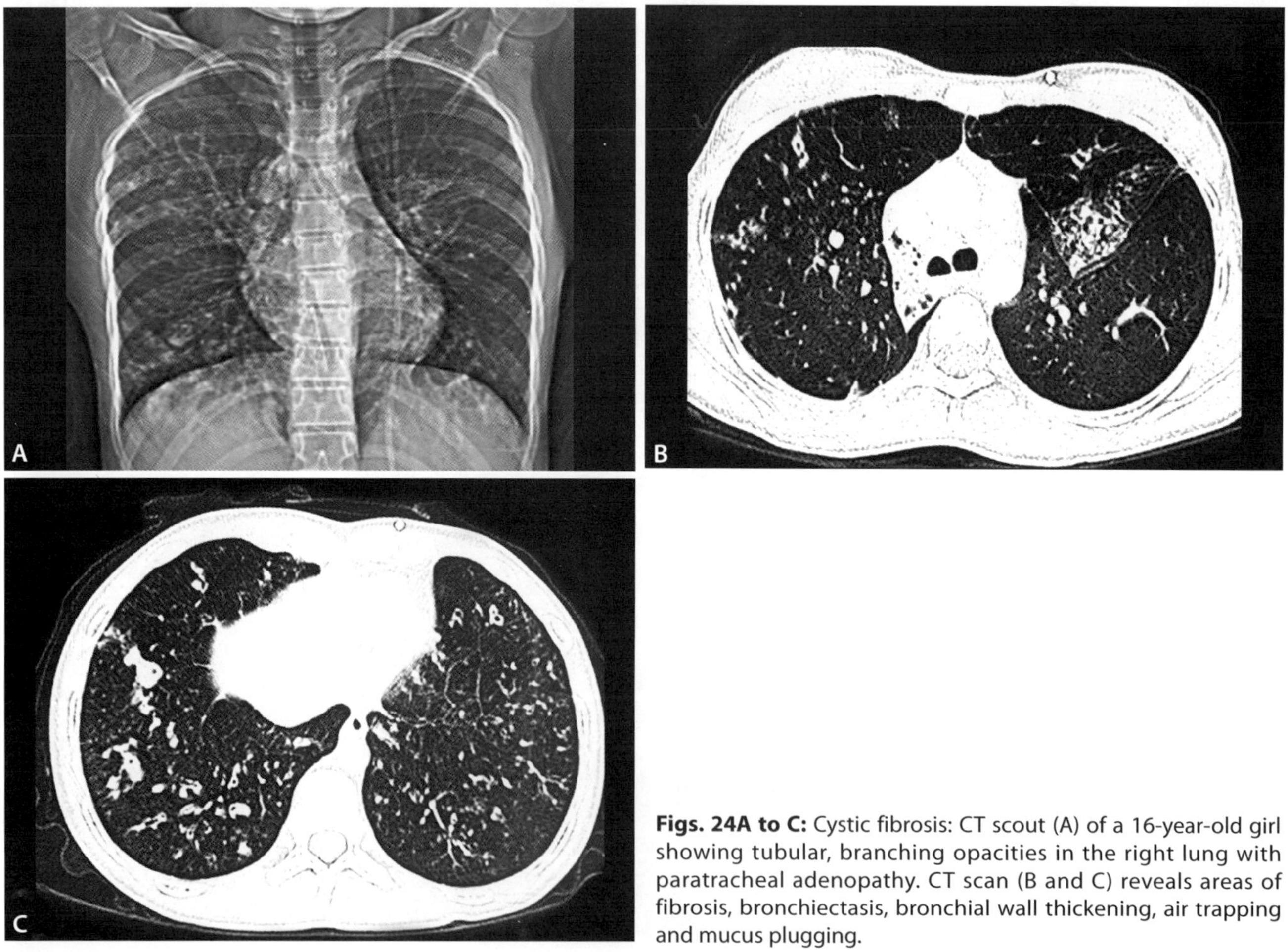

Figs. 24A to C: Cystic fibrosis: CT scout (A) of a 16-year-old girl showing tubular, branching opacities in the right lung with paratracheal adenopathy. CT scan (B and C) reveals areas of fibrosis, bronchiectasis, bronchial wall thickening, air trapping and mucus plugging.

of choice.[3] Chest radiographs reveal multiple cystic, ring or tram-track lucencies with bronchial wall thickening. In case of secondary infection mucous plugging, air-fluid levels, bronchial wall thickening and even enlarged draining nodes may be seen **(Figs. 24 and 25)**.

Asthma

The peak age of prevalence of asthma in children is 6–11 years, with a male predominance. 30% of these persist into adulthood.[2] Chest radiographs are usually normal and are indicated in case of poor response to therapy, suspected complications or suspicion of an alternate diagnosis.[2]

Radiographs reveal hyperlucency of lungs or foci of atelectasis. The differential diagnosis includes viral bronchiolitis. CT is seldom indicated in asthma and reveals nonspecific findings of small airway disease **(Figs. 26A and B)**. Findings of secondary allergic bronchopulmonary aspergillosis (ABPA) may be seen **(Figs. 27A and B)**.

Complications are more frequent in younger children as their bronchi are smaller and more easily occluded in an exacerbation. Complications include: lobar collapse, segmental or subsegmental atelectasis, pneumonia, air leaks (pneumomediastinum), subcutaneous emphysema and rarely pneumothorax or pulmonary interstitial emphysema (PIE).

In conclusion, it is critical to evaluate the airway in all children presenting with acute, chronic or recurrent respiratory symptoms. Multiphasic imaging is essential. Plain radiographs and fluoroscopy form the initial methods of evaluation, with CT being required often for a complete diagnosis.

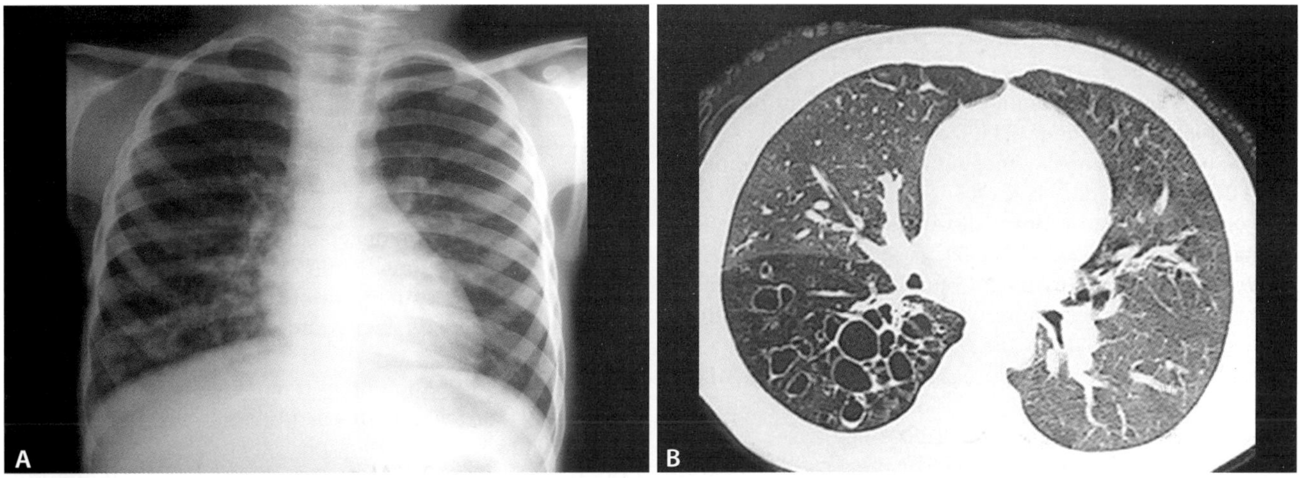

Figs. 25A and B: Bronchiectasis: Chest radiograph (A) showing cystic lucencies with air-space nodules in the right lower zone suggesting secondary infection. CT scan (B) at a different date shows tubular and cystic bronchiectasis in right lower lobe with air trapping.

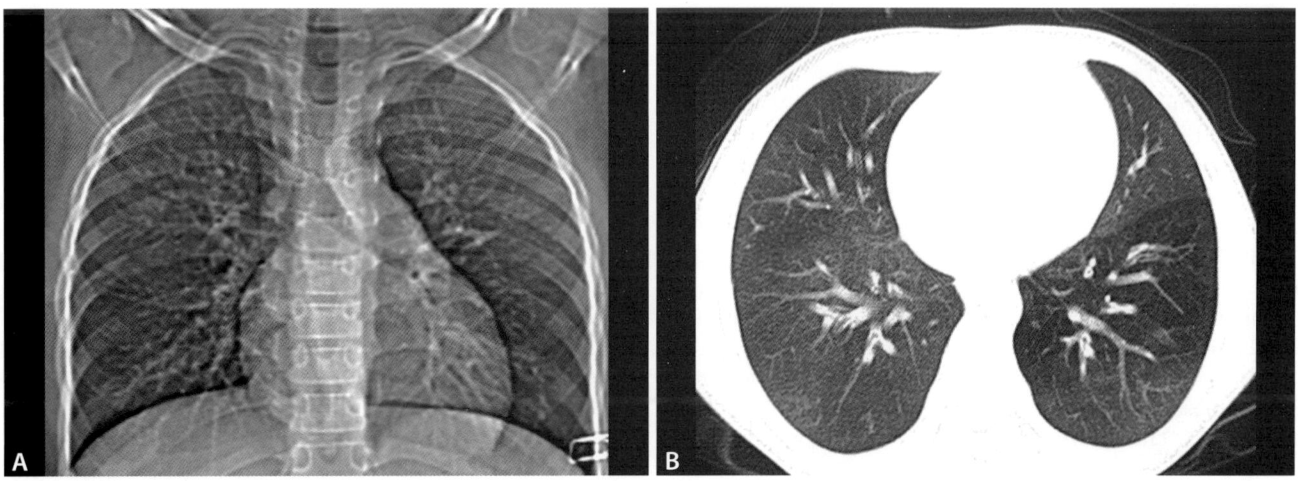

Figs. 26A and B: Asthma: CT scout (A) showing relative hyperlucency of left lower zone. CT scan (B) shows multiple areas of air trapping.

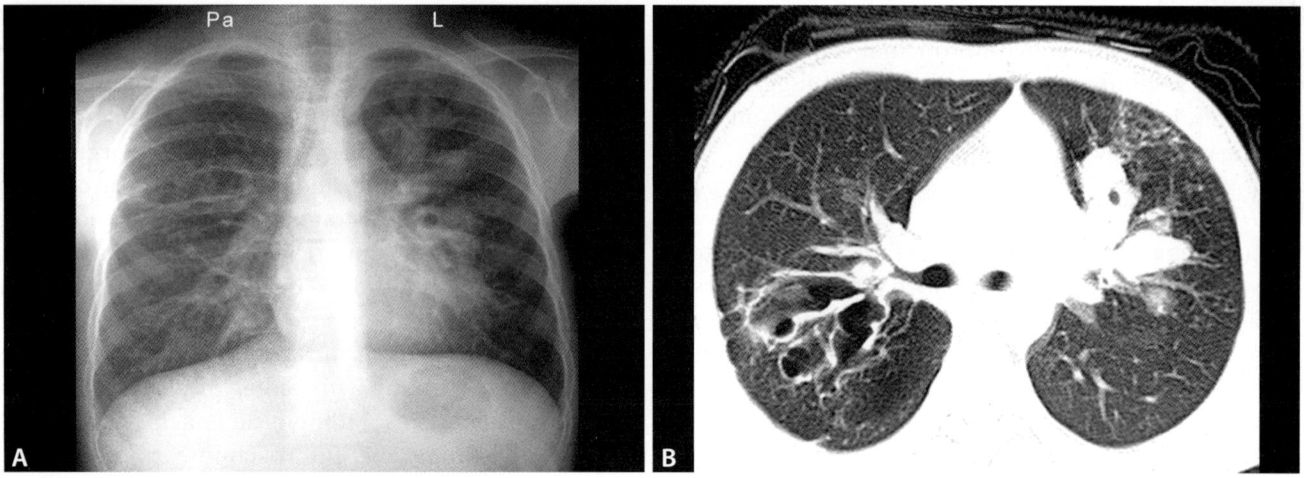

Figs. 27A and B: Allergic bronchopulmonary aspergillosis (ABPA): Chest radiograph (A) of a 16-year-old asthmatic boy showing multiple tubular, branching opacities in bilateral lung fields giving a "finger-in-glove" appearance. CT scan (B) confirms the presence of bilateral tubular bronchiectasis with bronchoceles.

REFERENCES

1. 'Airway' in Fundamentals of Paediatric Radiology LF Donnelly. 2001 Saunders, Philadelphia, USA.
2. 'Airway' in Diagnostic imaging Paediatrics. LF Donnelly (Ed). Amirsys, Utah, USA, 2005.
3. Long FR. Paediatric airway disorders: Imaging evaluation. Radiol Cl N Am. 2005;43:371-89.
4. Yedururi S, Guillerman RP, Chung T, et al. Multimodality Imaging of Tracheobronchial Disorders in Children Radiographics. 2008;28(3):e29.
5. Kumar D, Seith A, Sharma R, et al. Unpublished data AIIMS, Postgraduate Thesis: Evaluation of tracheobronchial lesions by multi-detector row CT. 2003-06.
6. Suto Y, Tanable Y. Evaluation of tracheal collapsibility in patients with tracheomalacia using dynamic MR imaging during coughing. Am J Roentgenol. 1998;171:393-4.
7. John SD, Swischuk LE. Stridor and upper airway obstruction in infants and children. Radiographics. 1992;12:625-43.
8. Bitar MA, Moukarbel RV, Zalzal GH. Management of congenital subglottic hemangioma: trends and success over the past 17 years. Otolaryngol Head Neck Surg. 2005;132:226-31.
9. Choo KS, Lee HD, Ban JE, et al. Evaluation of obstructive airway lesions in complex congenital heart disease using composite volume-rendered images from multislice CT. Pediatr Radiol. 2006;36:219-23.
10. Swischuk LE. Cardiovascular system: imaging of the newborn, infant and child. 5th edn. Philadelphia, Pa: Lippincott Williams & Wilkins. 2003. pp. 303-17.
11. Glick RD, La Quaglia MP. Lymphomas of the anterior mediastinum. Semin Pediatr Surg. 1999;8:69-77.
12. Lee EY, Litmanovich D, Boiselle PM. Multidetector CT evaluation of tracheobronchomalacia Radiol Clin N Am. 2009;47(2):261-9.
13. Berrocal T, Madrid C, Novo S, Gutierrez J, Arjonilla A, Gomez-Leon N. Congenital anomalies of the tracheobronchial tree, lung, and mediastinum: embryology, radiology, and pathology. Radiographics. 2004;24:e17.
14. Legasto AC, Haller JO, Giusti RJ. Tracheal web. Pediatr Radiol. 2004;34:256-8.
15. Langston C. New concepts in the pathology of congenital lung malformations. Semin Pediatr Surg. 2003;12:17-37.
16. Newman B. Congenital bronchopulmonary foregut malformations: concepts and controversies. Pediatr Radiol. 2006;36:773-91.
17. Swischuk LE. Alimentary tract, imaging of the newborn, infant and child. 5th ed. Philadelphia, Pa: Lippincott Williams &Wilkins. 2003. pp. 350-6.
18. Ghaye B, Szapiro D, Fanchamps JM, Dondelinger RF. Congenital bronchial abnormalities revisited. Radiographics. 2001;21:105-19.
19. McGuinness G, Naidich DP, Garay SM, Davis AL, Boyd AD, Mizrachi HH. Accessory cardiac bronchus: CT features and clinical significance. Radiology. 1993;189:562-6.
20. Bhalla AS, Sharma R. Imaging of the tracheobronchial tree in AIIMS-MAMC-PGI Imaging Course Series, Diagnostic Radiology-Chest and Cardiovascular Imaging, 3rd edn, Jaypee Publishers, New Delhi. 2009. pp. 90-116.
21. Davitt SM, Hatrick A, Sabharwal T, Pearce A, Gleeson M, Adam A. Tracheobronchial stent insertions in the management of major airway obstruction in a patient with Hunter's syndrome (type-II mucopolysaccharidosis). Eur Radiol. 2002;12:458-62.
22. Kosucu P, Ahmetoglu A, Koramaz I, et al. Low-dose MDCT and virtual bronchoscopy in pediatric patients with foreign body aspiration. Am J Roentgenol. 2004;183:1771-7.
23. Applegate KE, Dardinger JT, Lieber ML, et al. Spiral CT scanning technique in the detection of aspiration of LEGO foreign bodies. Pediatr Radiol. 2001;31:836-40.

24. Mukhopadhyay S, Gupta AK, Seith A. Imaging of tuberculosis in children in essentials of tuberculosis in children 3rd edn, Vimlesh Seth, SK Kabra (Eds) Jaypee Brothers, New Delhi. 2006. pp. 375-404.
25. Weber AL, Bird KT, Janower ML. Primary tuberculosis of childhood with particular emphasis on changes affecting the tracheobronchial tree. Am J Roentgenol. 1968;103:123-32.
26. Ferretti GR, Thony F, Bosson JL, et al. Benign abnormalities and carcinoid tumors of the central airways: diagnostic impact of CT bronchography. Am J Roentgenol. 2000;174: 1307-13.
27. Curtis JM, Lacey D, Smyth R, Carty H. Endobronchial tumours in childhood. Eur J Radiol. 1998;29:11-20.
28. Kothari NA, Kramer SS. Bronchial diseases and lung aeration in children. J Thorac Imaging. 2001;16:207-23.
29. Hansell DM. Small airways disease: detection and insights with computed tomography. Eur Respir J. 2001;17: 1294-313.
30. Lau DM, Siegel MJ, Hildebolt CF, et al. Bronchiolitis obliterans syndrome: thin section CT diagnosis of obstructive changes in infants and young children after lung transplantation. Radiology. 1998;208:783-8.
31. Kinane BT, Mansell AL, Zwerdling RG, et al. Follicular bronchitis in the paediatric population. Chest. 1993;104:1183-6.
32. Patterson PE, Harding SM. Gastroesophageal reflux disorders and asthma. Curr Opin Pulm Med. 1999;5:63-7.

CHAPTER 134

Developmental Anomalies of Gastrointestinal Tract

Alpana Manchanda, Sumedha Pawa

Derangement of embryological development can lead to malformations at any point along the gastrointestinal tract (GIT) from the oropharynx to the anorectum. Most of these abnormalities manifest clinically with GIT obstruction and present with vomiting and abdominal distention. Bile-stained vomiting occurs when the obstruction is below the ampulla of Vater, whereas vomiting of clear gastric contents indicates obstruction above the second part of the duodenum. Abdominal distention indicates a low level of obstruction. However, one must remember that both vomiting and abdominal distention may occur in conditions like sepsis, increased intracranial pressure, etc. in the absence of anatomic abnormality of the GI tract.[1] Infants who have undergone resuscitative efforts, or infants on continuous positive airway pressure, may swallow an excessive amount of air, leading to clinically significant abdominal distention. Since the distention is by air only, the walls of the distended loops on the abdominal radiograph are razor-sharp. Pathological conditions, involving the gut, such as ileus and obstruction, are characterized by dilatation with both air and fluid.[2] Developmental lesions of the neonatal gastrointestinal tract can be grouped as follows:[1]

ANATOMICAL

Attributed to embryological maldevelopment:

- Esophageal atresia with or without fistula
- Antropyloric atresia
- Antral diaphragm
- Duodenal atresia
- Duodenal stenosis
  - *Intrinsic:* Windsock duodenum
  - *Extrinsic:* Annular pancreas
  - Midgut malrotation with peritoneal bands
- Anorectal atresia.

Attributed to in utero catastrophic (ischemic) complication:

- Jejunoileal atresia
- Colonic atresia or stenosis
- Complicated meconium ileus.

FUNCTIONAL

- Meconium plug syndrome and its variants
- Megacystis-microcolon-intestinal hypoperistalsis.

COMBINED ANATOMICAL: FUNCTIONAL

- Hypertrophic pyloric stenosis
- Midgut volvulus (complicating midgut malrotation)
- Uncomplicated meconium ileus
- Colonic aganglionosis (Hirschsprung's disease).

IMAGING MODALITIES

The imaging methods available to investigate the gastrointestinal tract in the neonate include, plain film radiography, ultrasonography and contrast studies of the GI tract. Nuclear scintigraphy, computed tomography and magnetic resonance imaging are uncommonly required in infants.[1]

Plain Film Radiography

It is the simplest, usually the first and sometimes the only examination performed. An anteroposterior supine radiograph may be sufficient, only if the purpose is to evaluate a palpable mass or the presence of calcification. If obstruction is suspected, additional films are required. A cross-table lateral projection with the infant in supine position is best in terms of leaving the patient virtually undisturbed. However, a left-lateral decubitus view with a horizontal beam has the advantage of better identification of free gas over the liver and better anatomical definition of bowel loops in a frontal projection. If only one film is desired, a prone radiograph will give the most information regarding free gas as well as defining the level of obstruction. Occasionally, a prone lateral film is valuable for detection of gas in the rectum.[1]

Within seconds after birth, air enters the gastrointestinal tract and it can be seen radiographically in the stomach. Air is seen in the small bowel within the first hour, it reaches the cecum within 3–4 hours, and appears in the sigmoid colon by 11 hours. Gas-fluid levels are generally absent except in the stomach and occasionally in the right colon. The normal bowel gas pattern in neonates is quite different from that seen in older children and adults. It is characterized by gas throughout the small and large bowel and little fluid with respect to air, so that bowel-air interfaces are thin and sharp, with few, if any loops identified; rather, the gas distribution is one of multiple, closely apposed, rounded or polyhedral structures. Small and large bowels cannot be distinguished.[2]

A gasless abdomen after the first few hours of life is occasionally seen in normal infants as well as in those with uncontrollable vomiting, continuous gastric aspiration, severe dehydration, esophageal atresia without a fistula and deficient air swallowing, secondary to CNS depression. Obstruction is manifested by distention of portion of the GI tract proximal to the obstruction, with little or no gas below. By observing the number and distribution of distended bowel loops and air-fluid levels, one can estimate the approximate level of obstruction **(Figs. 1A and B)**.

Contrast Studies

Air is the cheapest, easiest and most commonly available contrast medium. The presence of gas within the bowel can be very useful in delineating abnormalities, particularly, a proximal high atresia. Occasionally, one may require to inject air to delineate the bowel better and it can be instilled by nasogastric tube or per rectum.[3]

Barium is not used in the following circumstances: (i) Suspected perforation, where preferably a non-ionic contrast medium should be used; (ii) Instances of lower small-bowel obstruction when retained fluid proximally is likely to cause oral barium suspension to precipitate and degrade the images; (iii) When a cleansing effect is also desired, as in attempted reduction of meconium ileus or meconium plug.

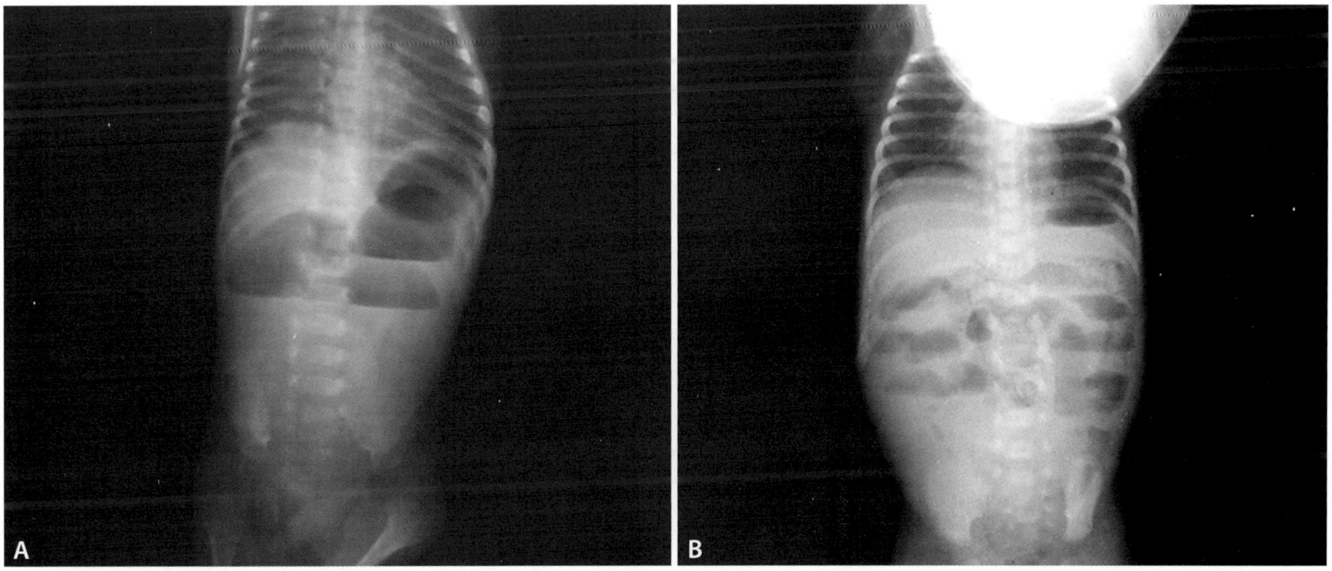

Figs. 1A and B: Plain X-ray abdomen erect view reveals (A) few (three) air-fluid levels in proximal small bowel with absence of distal air diagnostic of a high small bowel (jejunal) obstruction in a newborn presenting with bilious vomiting; (B) In contrast, multiple air-fluid levels seen in another neonate with abdominal distention, is indicative of a low small bowel (ileal) obstruction.

Ionic water-soluble contrast media are ideal for stimulating evacuation of retained thick tenacious intestinal contents by virtue of their high osmolarity, which increases the intraluminal fluid and bulk. This, however, may cause water and electrolyte imbalance and appropriate patient hydration and electrolyte homeostasis should be carefully maintained. Ionic contrast media are contraindicated when investigating esophageal problems because aspiration may cause pulmonary edema. Non-ionic contrast media are ideal for most of the circumstances. In suspected Hirschsprung's disease, in which the rate of evacuation has some potential diagnostic value, barium should be preferred. The radiologist should modify the routine use of contrast as needed in a particular case.

Ultrasonography

Ultrasonography (US) has been found to be highly accurate in the diagnosis of hypertrophic pyloric stenosis. It is useful in the diagnosis of gastric and duodenal duplications and in the detection of duodenal dilatation accompanying intrinsic or extrinsic duodenal obstruction, such as duodenal atresia and stenosis. Although duodenal dilatation is non-specific and additional contrast studies may be required to identify the specific cause, US is an excellent screening technique for localization of the site of obstruction. Ultrasound is valuable in the investigation of abdominal distention or palpable mass lesions because of easy and accurate detection of ascites as well as meconium peritonitis and intraperitoneal cystic lesions such as intestinal duplications and mesenteric or omental cysts.[1]

ESOPHAGUS

Esophageal Atresia and Tracheoesophageal Fistula

Esophageal atresia with or without tracheoesophageal fistula (TEF) is the most common congenital abnormality of the esophagus, manifesting itself during the neonatal period, occurring in about 1 in 2,500 to 4,000 livebirths.[4] It is usually sporadic and its etiology is uncertain.[3] No definite familial tendency has been documented in esophageal artesia, but more than one case in the same family has been noted.

Embryology

The trachea and esophagus develop from the common foregut during the early first trimester. During the 5th and 6th weeks of gestation, the common foregut divides into trachea and esophagus. Incomplete separation results in esophageal atresia with or without associated tracheoesophageal fistula. Because separation of the trachea and esophagus occurs cranial to tracheal branching of the carina, Tracheoesophageal fistulas generally present above the carina.[5]

Clinical Features

The presentation is usually in the first few hours of life, with the newborn having excessive oral secretions, choking and sometimes even cyanosis. Typically, symptoms become more pronounced during the first feed. The abdomen may be distended due to air passing through the distal fistula into the stomach or may be scaphoid or gasless in patients who have atresia without a fistula or atresia with a proximal fistula. Patients with an H-fistula usually present later with history of choking while feeding, cough, cyanosis, recurrent or chronic pneumonias and a distended abdomen from tracheal gas passing through the fistula into the esophagus and stomach.[5]

Esophageal atresia may be diagnosed by antenatal ultrasound. It is suspected on the basis of maternal polyhydroamnios with an absent fluid-filled stomach, the proximal esophageal pouch seen as a central anechoic area in the fetal neck or upper chest. The presence and size of the tracheoesophageal fistula determines the amount of fluid in the stomach and gastrointestinal tract. Associated anomalies in the other systems may be identified. The atresias may be multiple and involve the esophagus, duodenum and anus.

Classification

Esophageal atresia and tracheoesophageal fistula have been classified based on their anatomical and radiographic appearance, i.e. on the basis of presence (and location) or absence of a tracheoesophageal fistula **(Figs. 2A to E)**. They have been variously designated as types A to E (or 1 to 5) as follows:[3]

Type A: Esophageal atresia without fistula (7.8%)

Type B: Esophageal atresia with proximal fistula (0.8%)

Type C: Esophageal atresia with distal fistula (85.8%)

Type D: Esophageal atresia with fistula in both the pouches (1.4%)

Type E: H-type fistula without atresia (4.2%)

In the majority of patients, the atresia occurs between the proximal and middle thirds of the esophagus with a gap of varying length between the atretic pouches.[3]

Most commonly, there is a proximal esophageal atresia with a distal tracheoesophageal fistula. This occurs in approximately 85.8% of cases. Next most common, occurring approximately in 7.8% cases, is isolated

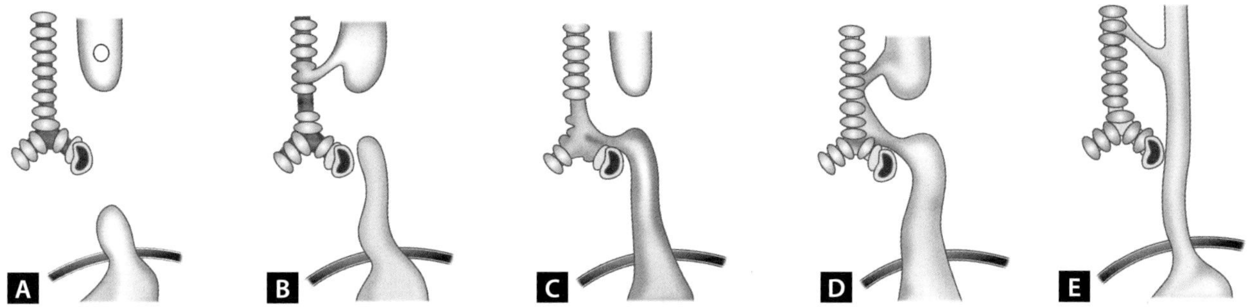

Figs. 2A to E: Types of esophageal atresia/tracheoesophageal fistula. The plain radiographs for Types A and B are similar as in case for Types C and D.

esophageal atresia. H-type fistula occurs in approximately 4.2% of cases. Esophageal atresia with proximal tracheoesophageal fistula or with both proximal and distal tracheoesophageal fistulas are quite rare.[6]

Approximately 50–70% of patients with esophageal atresia have additional anomalies. The VACTERL syndrome is seen in 15–30% of patients. "V" is for vertebral and vascular abnormalities. Of these, a right-sided aortic arch is seen in 5% cases. "A" is for anal and auricular malformations. "C" is for cardiac abnormalities like ventricular septal defects, patent ductus arteriosus and complex cyanotic heart disease. "TE" is for tracheoesophageal fistula and esophageal atresia. "R" represents renal abnormalities. "L" is for limb malformations.[7]

Imaging Features

Plain film of the chest taken soon after birth reveals proximal esophageal pouch distended with air, thereby indicating the diagnosis on plain radiographs. In unequivocal cases, a thin soft rubber nasogastric tube is passed into the proximal pouch and about 5 cc of air is injected. A frontal radiograph of the chest showing dilated proximal esophageal pouch with round distal margin and coiled nasogastric tube within is diagnostic. The distended air filled proximal esophageal pouch may make visualization of the lower cervical and upper dorsal spine more clear. A lateral radiograph though not routinely indicated, if obtained, shows considerable anterior bowing and narrowing of the trachea by the dilated blind esophageal pouch.[3] Plain radiograph of the chest should include the abdomen to evaluate the presence of air in the gastrointestinal tract. The presence of air in the stomach and the small bowel indicates esophageal atresia with a distal tracheoesophageal fistula. Absence of air in the stomach eliminates the possibility of a distal fistula. The possibility of proximal tracheoesophageal fistula, however, cannot be eliminated **(Figs. 3 and 4)**.

Air confined to the stomach raises the possibility of associated duodenal atresia and necessitates a follow-up plain film examination.

Routine contrast examinations are not required in the neonate with esophageal atresia and TEF.[3] Use of radiopaque contrast in the proximal pouch should be avoided, owing to the possibility of aspiration. Swallowed air or air through nasogastric tube is usually adequate for the diagnosis and to demonstrate the extent of the proximal pouch. If positive contrast examination is needed then isotonic nonionic contrast medium should be used in minimal amount under fluoroscopic monitoring. Immediately after the study, contrast should be aspirated out.

Through H-type fistulas can be at any level, most are at the thoracic inlet, between C_7 and T_2 vertebral bodies. The connection is angulated superiorly from the esophagus to the trachea, thus accounting for the more precise but less popular appellation of the N-type fistula **(Fig. 5)**. The best way to demonstrate H-type tracheoesophageal fistula is with careful injection of contrast medium via a nasogastric tube, first placed at GE junction and then gradually withdrawing the nasogastric tube with simultaneous injection of contrast under fluoroscopic guidance at various levels of the esophagus. The main reason that the H-type TEF is inconstantaly patent is that the normal esophageal mucosa is quite redundant and usually occludes the esophageal side of the fistula. Normal active swallowing may not distend the esophagus sufficiently to allow passage of contrast into the fistula.[8] The patient should be viewed in the lateral or steep prone oblique projection with the right side down. Care should be taken to separate tracheal and esophageal lumens during the study so that fistula is readily identified between them. If the contrast appears in the trachea or lungs, it is very important to be certain, if the contrast went through a fistula or was aspirated. If in doubt, then the investigation

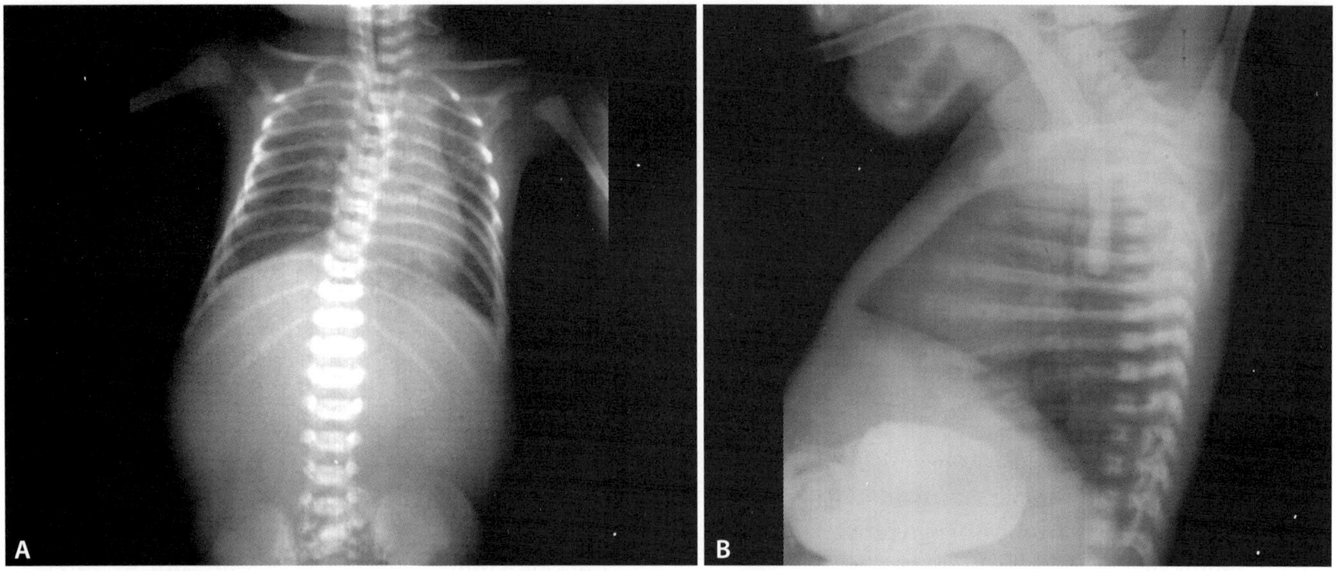

Figs. 3A and B: Esophageal atresia. (A) Frontal radiograph of chest and abdomen showing a catheter in the proximal pouch. The abdomen is gasless; (B) Lateral film shows the tip of the nasogastric tube at the level of 4th dorsal vertebra.

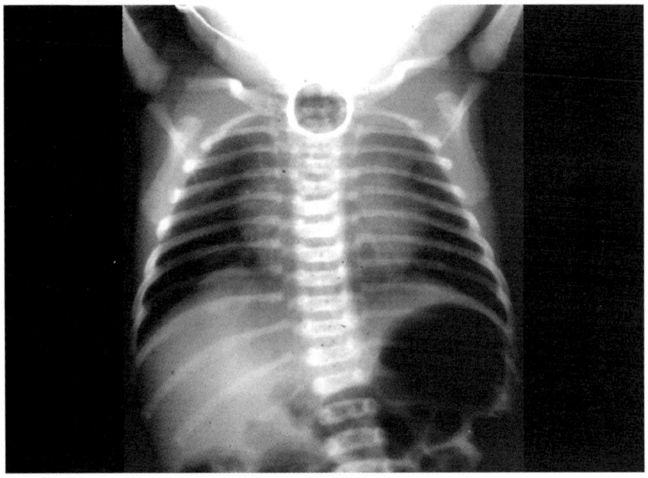

Fig. 4: Esophageal atresia with distal tracheoesophageal fistula. Coiled nasogastric tube is seen in the proximal esophageal pouch. Air is seen in the stomach and bowel.

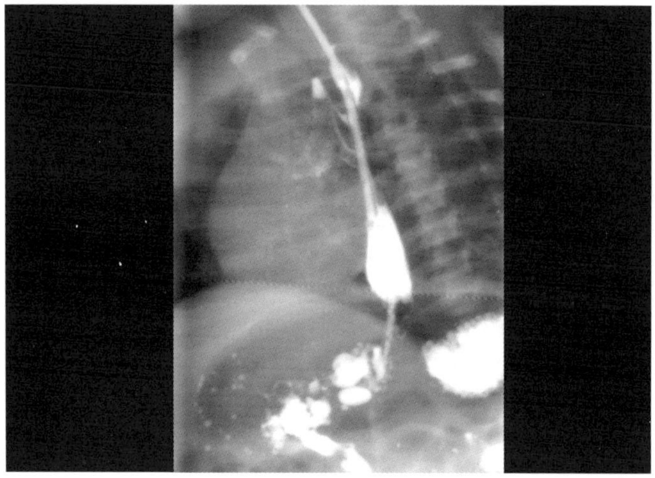

Fig. 5: Contrast esophagogram demonstrating an oblique tract of an H-type tracheoesophageal fistula arising from the anterior wall of the esophagus and passing cephalad to the posterior tracheal wall, with contrast filling the tracheobronchial tree.

must be repeated once the trachea is cleared of the contrast.

The side of the aortic arch should be determined. This information is important to the surgeon because the surgical approach to the mediastinum for repair of esophageal atresia with a distal TEF is from the side opposite to the aortic arch. When plain radiograph fails to indicate the side of the arch, computed tomography or a cardiac ultrasound can localize the arch.

H-type fistulas are commonly demonstrated by contrast studies.[3] However, bronchoscopy and endoscopy are more sensitive methods and may be indicated to confirm the diagnosis, especially in a symptomatic older child where the contrast esophagogram is normal.

Computed tomography (CT) is occasionally used in the preoperative evaluation of neonates with TEF and has proved to be a noninvasive and quick investigation. As compared with conventional bronchoscopy or catheterization, CT does not require any general anesthesia. The improved spatial and temporal resolution of new generation of scanners facilitates assessment of such small defects such as TEF. Either direct sagittal acquisition or axial acquisition with multiplanar reconstruction may help in demonstrating the precise location of fistula and the length of the gap between esophageal segments. Alternatively, length of the atretic segment can be assessed by passing a feeding tube from above and a metal bougie from below, via a gastrostomy.

The knowledge of the origin of the fistula is helpful to the surgeon not only in deciding the side of the thoracotomy (right or left), but also in anticipating the gap to be bridged. The most important advantage of CT is that both esophagus and trachea are seen in their natural (unstretched) positions, and the interpouch gap can be measured accurately.[9]

High resolution CT scan on a 64-slice CT scanner has shown to provide definitive diagnosis and help in surgical planning in a critically ill neonate with H-Type TEF by distending the esophagus with air (by means of nasogastric feeding tube) during CT acquisition. Such a maneuver has proved to be very useful in optimizing the visualization of the fistula which may be totally or partially closed by a valve like mucosal flap or by a spasm of the muscular layer of the esophagus.[10]

When there is a proximal fistula, then it is located in the anterior wall of the esophagus. In esophageal atresia with a distal fistula, primary repair is possible as the length of the gap between the esophageal segments is usually short. When there is atresia with no distal fistula, there is usually a long gap (of the order of about five vertebral bodies) between the proximal and distal esophageal segments. The growth of the esophageal segments during the first few months of life tends to lessen the gap, thereby making a delayed primary repair feasible. A gastrostomy is established for feeding in the meantime.

Radiological Evaluation of Postoperative Complications

Most patients of isolated esophageal atresia and tracheoesophageal fistula do well following surgical repair. Nevertheless, complications following surgery do occur and can be grouped under early and late complications. The early complications include: (i) Leakage at the anastomotic site (14–16%), (ii) Esophageal stricture, and (iii) Recurrent fistula. Oral feeding is not started for 1–2 weeks following surgery, till the edema subsides. A contrast study of the esophagus should be performed prior to the institution of oral feeds. A low-osmolal nonionic contrast should be used as leakage at the anastomotic site and is the most commonly identified early complication of surgical repair. Anastomotic leak increases the risk of esophageal stricture in the future. Donnelly et al. found that the appearance of an extrapleural fluid collection after esophageal atresia repair performed via an extrapleural approach was associated with a high incidence of anastomotic leakage.[8] If an anastomotic leak is left untreated, it may eventually lead to diverticulum formation. Most anastomotic leaks have been seen to close spontaneously.

Stricture is another common complication which can occur following esophageal atresia repair. Most often, the stricture or narrowing is slight at the site of anastomotic repair and may persist for years, even though the patient has no functional problem **(Figs. 6A and B)**. Those with true stricture at anastomotic site are symptomatic and generally respond to bougie dilatation, with reoperation generally not required. However, if a stricture is associated with gastroesophageal reflux, the stricture may not respond to dilatation if it continues to be exposed to the acidic gastric contents. Hence, patients with postoperative strictures should be evaluated for reflux by upper gastrointestinal series or pH monitoring.

A tracheoesophageal fistula can recur (3–14% cases) again at the anastomotic site, following surgery and is believed to be related to anastomotic leakage with erosion into trachea caused by local inflammation.

The late complications which can occur following repair of an esophageal atresia are dysmotitily, gastroesophageal reflux, tracheomalacia, rib fusion and scolosis. Dysmotility is present in nearly all patients who have had esophageal atresia.

Gastroesophageal reflux is also commonly associated and has been reported in 40–70% of cases. Reflux is thought to be related to the shortening of the intra-abdominal portion of the esophagus, or occur secondary to the surgical repair. Reflux may lead to peptic esophagitis and is likely to be the cause of more distal strictures in those who have had a history of repaired esophageal atresia.

Tracheomalacia is thought to occur due to chronic intrauterine compression of trachea by a distended upper esophageal pouch.

STOMACH

Microgastria

Congenital microgastria is an extremely rare anomaly in which fetal rotation of the stomach fails to occur. There is no differentiation into fundus, body, antrum and pyloric canal and the lesser and greater curvatures also do not develop.[8] It is believed to occur as a result of atresia of normal foregut development in the 5th week of embryonal development.

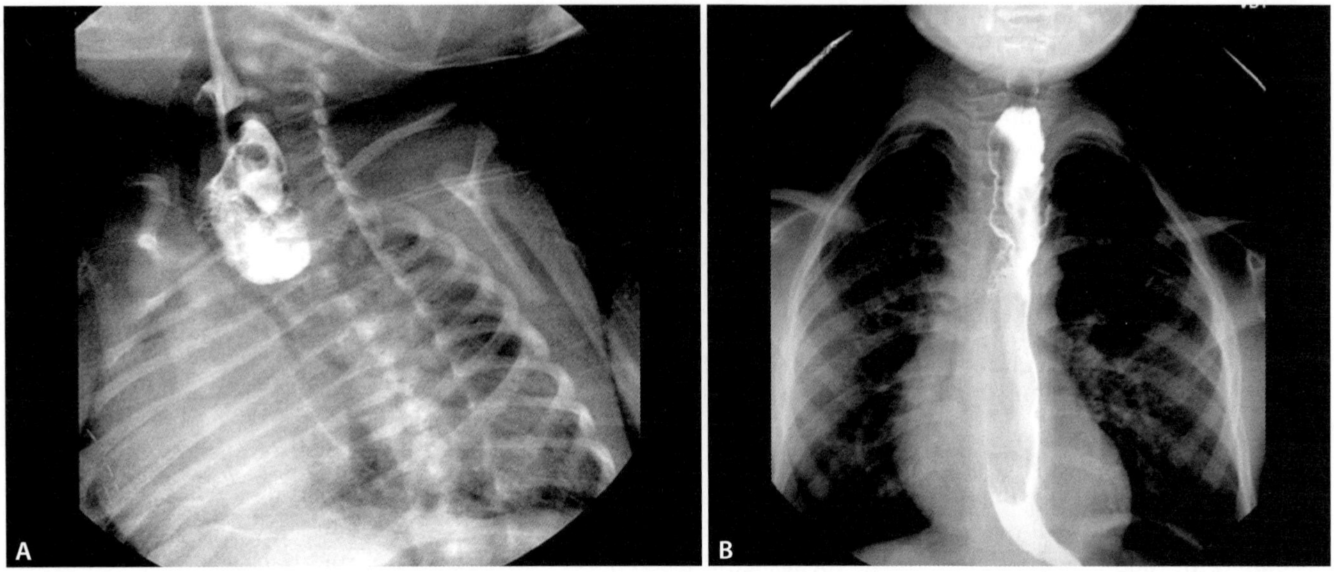

Figs. 6A and B: (A) Esophageal atresia with distal TEF in a neonate. Lateral radiograph shows contrast-filled dilated proximal esophageal pouch bowing the trachea anteriorly; (B) Barium swallow following primary anastomosis of esophageal atresia demonstrates slight narrowing at the anastomotic site (D4 vertebral level). The child had mild respiratory distress with dysphagia.

Microgastria is often accompanied by other congenital anomalies such as malrotation, asplenia, renal, limb, vertebral and cardiac anomalies (VACTERL syndrome).[4] The common association between microgastria and upper extremity limb reduction defects, has led to the term microgastria-limb reduction complex.[8]

The clinical presentation of microgastria depends on the stage at which gastric development has been arrested. On prenatal ultrasound it may mimic esophageal atresia due to failure to visualize a distended stomach. Postnatally, microgastria presents with postprandial vomiting, failure to thrive, developmental delay, growth retardation, malnutrition and aspiration pneumonia. Most of the symptoms are due to secondary gastroesophageal reflux (GER).[4]

An upper GI study shows a small tubular stomach in the midline. The esophagus is dilated and appears to take over the storage function of the small capacity stomach. The gastroesophageal junction is incompetent and GER is present. There is associated esophageal dysmotility, secondary to its massive dilatation.[4]

The treatment of microgastria depends on its severity. The less severe forms may be treated conservatively, with surgery reserved as the first line of treatment in severe cases. The surgical treatment consists of creation of a Hunt-Lawrence pouch as a gastric reservoir, which allows for the secondary esophageal changes to resolve.[4]

DEVELOPMENTAL OBSTRUCTIVE DEFECTS

Congenital gastric obstruction is rare, as unlike the esophagus, the stomach undergoes little alteration in form during development. Gastric obstruction in the newborn may be due to:

1. Gastric atresia
2. Pyloric stenosis
3. Pyloric/prepyloric membrane/Antral web.

Gastric Atresia

Isolated gastric atresia is very rare and accounts for less than 1% of all congenital obstructions.[11] Almost all gastric atresias occur at the pylorus or antrum. They are thought to be due to localized vascular occlusion in fetal life and not to failure of recanalization of the intestinal tract.[3] Gastric atresia is classified into three types:[12]

1. Complete atresia with no connection between the stomach and duodenum
2. Complete atresia with the fibrous band connecting the stomach and duodenum, and
3. A gastric membrane or diaphragm producing atresia. Gastric atresia may be familial or associated with epidermolysis bullosa. The newborn presents mainly with regurgitation of non-bilious vomitus within the first few hours after birth. As obstruction is complete, a plain radiograph of the abdomen reveals a "single bubble appearance" with marked dilatation of the

stomach, proximal to the obstruction and absence of gas in the small bowel and colon. This appearance is diagnostic and most patients are taken directly to surgery without any contrast imaging.[11]

Pyloric Stenosis or Prepyloric Membrane or Antral Web

A pyloric stenosis or prepyloric membrane or antral web is a rare cause of symptomatic gastric obstruction in the newborn.[2] Patients with webs or stenosis of the pylorus, rather than complete atresia may present later in life or even in adulthood because the obstruction is incomplete.[8] The most common presenting symptoms are cyclic postprandial vomiting and episodes of transient vomiting.[9] Radiographically, the stomach is dilated with varying degrees of distal air, the extent of which depends on the degree of obstruction. In patients with incomplete obstruction, webs are more common than stenosis.[4]

It is difficult to diagnose an antral web on imaging studies. On UGI barium studies, a web is seen as a thin, 2–3 mm, linear circumferential filling defect traversing the barium column producing a reduction in the antral lumen, with a normal pyloric canal.[11] On ultrasound, the membrane may be visible, if the stomach is filled with clear fluid and appears as echogenic band extending centrally from the lesser and greater curvatures in the prepyloric region. A mucus strand may be mistaken for an antral membrane. On the basis of clinical and radiographical findings, the definitive diagnosis of antral web can be made endoscopically.[2]

Ectopic Pancreas

Ectopic pancreas is an uncommon anomaly in which pancreatic tissue is found in the antropyloric region, less commonly in the duodenum. It is seen as an incidental finding. Less commonly, it can cause symptoms of pain, GI bleeding or obstruction.[8] An upper GI study shows a smooth, dome shaped filling defect, 1–3 cm in diameter on the greater curvature of stomach, with central umbilication at times. Ectopic pancreatic tissue may produce intermittent obstruction, if it prolapses into the pylorus.[11]

Hypertrophic Pyloric Stenosis

Hypertrophic pyloric stenosis (HPS) is a common developmental condition affecting young infants. The incidence of HPS is approximately 3 in 1000 livebirths and boys are affected four to five times more commonly than girls. There is a familial disposition. Affected patients usually present between 2 and 6 weeks of age, with projectile non-bilious vomiting. Other conditions that can manifest with non-bilious vomiting include pylorospasm, hiatus hernia and preampullary duodenal stenosis.[13] HPS is never seen beyond 3 months of age, except reported in premature infants, in whom, enteral feeding has been started late.[14]

Diagnosis can be made on appropriate history and palpation of an 'olive' mass in the subhepatic region of an infant. The mass is reported to be seen in up to 80% of cases. Antral peristaltic waves can also be observed.[3]

HPS is characterized by hypertrophy of pyloric circular muscle and redundancy of the pyloric mucosa. However, its etiology is unknown. Possible causes include hypersecretion with resulting duodenal irritation and pylorospasm. There is a constant association with hyperplasia of the antral mucosa.[3] Recent work has confirmed that the pylorus is abnormally innervated, and suggested that a lack of nitric oxide synthetase may be responsible for the pylorospasm that leads to gastric outlet obstruction and muscular hypertrophy.[5]

In most cases, a clinical diagnosis can be confidently made. However, further investigation may be required when the diagnosis remains in doubt. The diagnosis of HPS can be established by either barium studies or US. Ultrasonography has replaced barium examination being noninvasive and its ability to visualize the pyloric muscle directly to obtain measurements of muscle thickness.[15,16]

Ultrasonography

Ultrasonography (US) is the imaging modality of choice in an infant suspected of having pyloric stenosis, with a reported accuracy approaching 100%.[13] The examination is typically performed with a high frequency linear transducer (>5 MHz) as the stomach, pylorus and duodenum are very superficial in an infant.[17] The gallbladder which is adjacent to the pylorus, serves as a good landmark.[3] Longitudinal and transverse images through the pylorus are obtained with the infant in the right posterior oblique position while scanning the right upper quadrant just off the midline. In this position, any fluid in the fundus of the stomach moves into the antrum and pyloric region, distending these regions. The stomach should not be emptied prior to the examination as this makes identification of antropyloric area difficult. If there is inadequate distention of the antrum, the infant may be given a glucose solution or water, orally or via a nasogastric tube. If fluid is administered, then it should be removed at the end of the examination to prevent further vomiting and the risk of aspiration. In addition, if there is lot of gas, scanning the baby in the prone position may help in visualization of the pyloric region.[17]

The US evaluation of HPS includes assessment of both morphological and quantitative features. The classic findings are of a thickened echo-poor pyloric muscle and an elongated pyloric canal.[15,16,18] The thickened muscle is seen as two curved bundles of mixed but generally low reflectivity bulging into the base of the duodenal cap and gastric antrum. The mucosal echoes are seen as one or two central bright lines. On transverse images, the hypertrophic pylorus has a doughnut appearance, representing the reflective central mucosa and submucosa surrounded by echo-poor muscle. The hypertrophic muscle may look non-uniform on transverse scanning of the pylorus. This is related to the sonographic artifact of anisotropic effect because of the orientation of the muscle fibers.[3] Other signs include exaggerated peristaltic waves that terminate at the pylorus, esophageal reflux and little, if any gastric emptying.

An experienced examiner can frequently make the diagnosis just by qualitative assessment of the thickness of the pyloric wall. The exact measurements that separate a normal pylorus from a hypertrophic one, are controversial.[16,18-20] However, as a general guide, a pyloric canal length greater than 15 mm, muscle thickness greater than 3.0 mm, and transverse serosa-to-serosa diameter greater than 15 mm is consistent with HPS **(Figs. 7A and B)**. At least two values should be positive. A muscle thickness less than 2.0 mm is unequivocally normal. A muscle thickness between 2 and 2.9 mm is abnormal but nonspecific, and can be seen in gastritis and pylorospasm as well as in HPS. Though pylorospasm may mimic HPS on sonography as there is some pyloric muscle thickening and/or slight elongation of the pyloric canal, pylorospasm is transient and generally resolves in 30 minutes. An important pointer for diagnosing pylorospasm is that there is considerable variation in measurement or image appearance with time during the study.[21] Borderline muscle thickness measurements are more likely to occur in premature than in term infants.

A number of ancillary sonographic signs of HPS have been described.[17]

- Shoulder sign—refers to an indentation upon the gastric antrum produced by hypertrophy of the pyloric muscle
- Double tract sign—this refers to fluid, trapped in the mucosal folds in the center of an elongated pyloric canal seen as two sonolucent streaks in the center
- Nipple sign is produced due to the evagination of redundant pyloric mucosa into the distended portion of the antrum. Color Doppler evaluation of the pylorus may reveal hyperemia within the muscle and mucosal layers.

False negative diagnosis may be made, if the stomach is overdistended, because it can displace the pylorus posteriorly, making it difficult to visualize the pyloric canal. If the scan is not in the midline, or is tangential

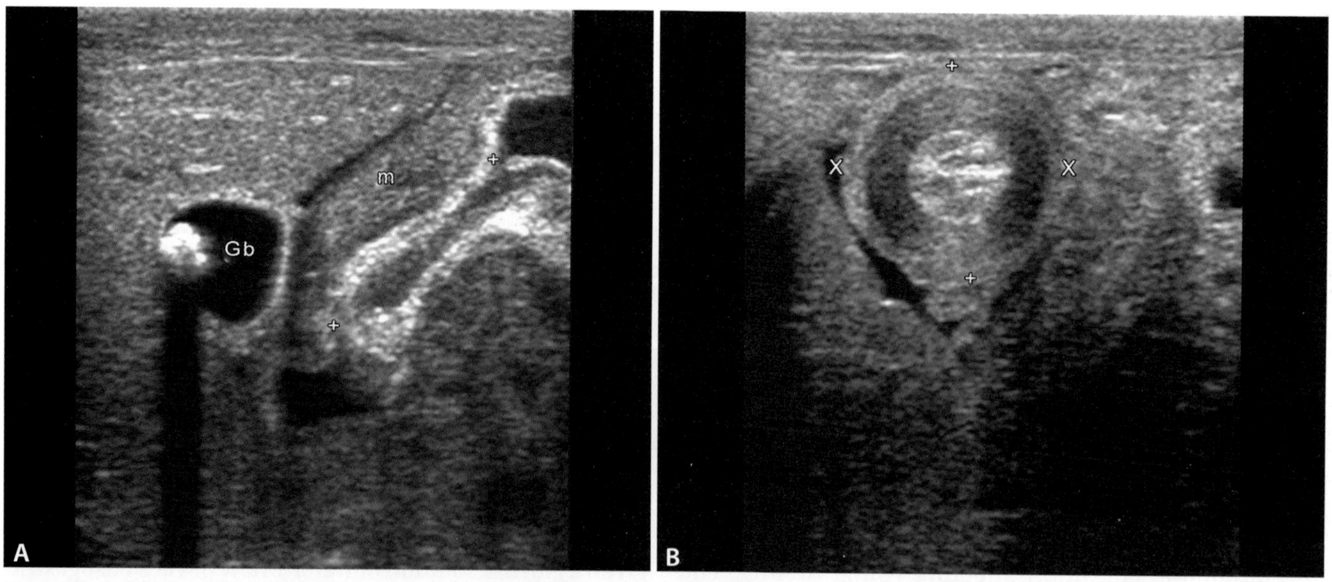

Figs. 7A and B: Hypertrophic pyloric stenosis: (A) Longitudinal ultrasound image showing an elongated thickened pylorus seen as two curved bundles of low reflectivity (m). The mucosal echoes are seen as central bright lines. Gallbladder (Gb) shows sludge within. Minimal fluid is present around the stomach; (B) Transverse section shows the muscle thickness as an echo poor rim—Bull's eye sign. Serosa to serosa measures 15 mm (cursors).

to the antrum, the antral wall can simulate a thickened pyloric muscle, leading to a false positive diagnosis.

Barium Study

A barium study should be performed, if ultrasound is inconclusive or gastroesophageal reflux is suspected.[21] If gastric distention is severe, a nasogastric tube should be passed and the stomach emptied. With the patient in the prone oblique position, the tube is placed in the antrum and adequate barium is injected via the tube under fluoroscopic control and spot films are taken.

Most of the infants, with and without HPS, show some degree of pylorospasm. In HPS, generally barium will pass through the antropyloric region within 1–10 minutes, but may be delayed as long as 20–25 minutes. The pyloric canal is narrowed (the "string sign") and elongated and almost always curved upward posteriorly **(Fig. 8)**. Combination of narrowing and elongation is the hallmark of HPS on barium study. Barium may be caught between folds overlying the hypertrophied muscle and parallel lines (the "double string sign") may be seen **(Fig. 9)**. The enlarged muscle mass looks much like an "apple-core lesion", with undercutting of the distal antrum and proximal duodenal bulb. The "beak sign" is noted as the thick muscle narrows the barium column as it enters the pyloric canal. Virtually all of the above signs can be seen transiently in infants especially those with some degree of spasm. The study should be continued sufficiently long to document the persistence of the findings in order to assure the diagnosis of pyloric stenosis. Occasionally, an associated antral web or diaphragm may be identified.

Adult Idiopathic Hypertrophic Pyloric Stenosis (AIHPS)

It is a mild form of hypertrophic pyloric stenosis (HPS) which may rarely present later in adult life. Its exact incidence is not known, as majority of these patients are asymptomatic for years. Around 80% of patients with the adult form of the disease are men which is in concordance with the male preponderance of congenital HPS. The primary form of AIHPS should be differentiated from the secondary form which is caused by diseases such as peptic ulcer disease, hypertrophic gastritis or malignancy.[23]

In AIHPS, the pylorus is bulbous or fusiform with its thickest portion at the pyloroduodenal junction. Patients present with symptoms of delayed gastric emptying not associated with any pain.

The radiologic and endoscopic studies may be nonspecific. However, the diagnosis should be suspected, if there is elongation of the pyloric canal and is accompanied by marked dilatation of the stomach.

In AIHPS, the "string sign" may be seen as an extremely thin line of barium on an upper GI study. A marked thickening of the pyloric muscle may produce a convex indentation at the base of the duodenal bulb, causing a mushroom-like deformity ("Kirklin's sign"). The presence of a barium-filled cleft between the hypertrophied muscle and the fibers of the pylorus can project into either one or both sides of the pylorus, proximal to the base of the bulb ("Twining's sign"). However, none of these signs are pathognomic and presence of two or more of them strengthens the radiologic diagnosis. Endoscopy may be useful and the classic finding that has been described is

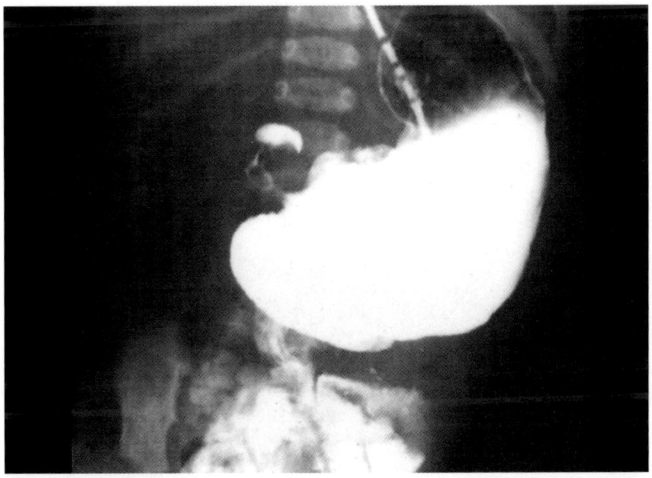

Fig. 8: Upper GI barium study in a child with pyloric stenosis. The markedly narrowed pylorus curves upward and posteriorly to the duodenal bulb which shows an impression of the hypertrophied muscle in the base.

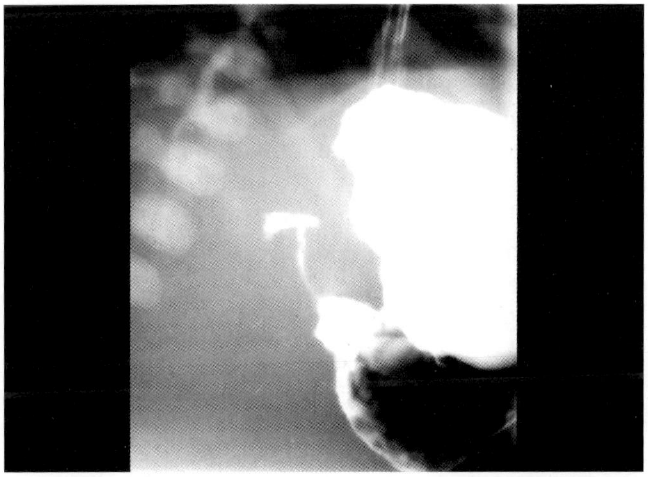

Fig. 9: Characteristic findings of HPS in a 6-week-old boy with history of vomiting. The pyloric canal is narrowed and elongated and the base of the duodenal bulb is stretched by the pyloric mass.

the "donut" or the cervix sign which consists of a fixed narrow pylorus with a smooth border.

In the congenital type of HPS, pyloromyotomy is the preferred treatment. Normal emptying of the stomach occurs within 2–3 days after the procedure. However, muscle thickness gradually regresses to normal and may even take 6–8 weeks.[3] In contrast, in AIHPS, pyloroplasty and recently, laparoscopic pyloromyotomy have been tried with successful results.[22]

An increased incidence of renal anomalies like pelviureteric junction obstruction, primary megaureter, duplex kidney, renal agenesis or ectopia and horse-shoe kidney have been reported in patients with HPS.[23]

DUODENUM

Duodenal obstruction is a relatively common form of intestinal obstruction in the newborn **(Table 1)**. It may be complete (duodenal atresia) or incomplete. Complete duodenal obstruction is seen more frequently than congenital gastric obstruction.[11] Incomplete obstruction may be intrinsic, such as duodenal stenosis caused by a web or "windsock" membrane; or it is more often extrinsic, e.g. duodenal compression from bands, annular pancreas, etc. Intrinsic and extrinsic obstructions may coexist.

Duodenal Atresia and Stenosis

Atresia is much more common than stenosis, but the etiology is the same. Atresia or stenosis occurs when the duodenum, which is a solid tube till about 3–6 weeks' gestation, fails to recanalize partially or completely. Unlike jejunal and ileal atresia, it does not appear to be related to intrauterine ischemia.[11] Atresia and stenosis almost always occur in the region of the ampulla of Vater (about 80% are just distal to the ampulla); thus they are frequently accompanied by abnormalities of the bile duct and pancreas. Annular pancreas occurs in 20% of patients with duodenal atresia or stenosis. It may contribute to the duodenal obstruction but is seldom or never found without intrinsic obstruction of the duodenum.

Duodenal atresia and stenosis may be associated with other congenital anomalies, like intestinal atresia and congenital heart disease and may be part of VACTERL association. About 30% of the patients have Down's syndrome.[24-26]

Duodenal atresia and stenosis occur with equal frequency in boys and girls. Prematurity and maternal polyhydramnios are common. Bilious vomiting in the first few hours of life is the cardinal symptom but those with duodenal stensois can present at variable times, because the clinical findings depend on the degree of stenosis. Bilious vomiting is a feature in 80% of neonates with duodenal atresia as the atresia is present distal to the ampulla of Vater. In the remaining 20%, the vomitus is non-bilious.[3]

Table 1: Causes of duodenal obstruction in the newborn.

Intrinsic	*Extrinsic*
Duodenal atresia	Ladd's bands
Duodenal stenosis	Midgut volvulus with malrotation
Duodenal web or diaphragm	Annular pancreas Duplication Preduodenal portal vein

Imaging Features

In newborns with duodenal atresia, the abdominal radiograph is usually diagnostic. Air is present in the stomach and proximal duodenum, but there is no air distally in the gastrointestinal tract. Erect film shows two gas-fluid levels in which the higher, larger bubble to the left is the stomach and the other bubble is the dilated proximal duodenum which is seen above the region of obstruction.[11] Thus, the typical appearance of a "double-bubble sign" represents air, or air and fluid-filled distended stomach and duodenal bulb **(Fig. 10)**.

In duodenal stenosis, the stomach and duodenal bulb usually are distended, but air is present in the distal bowel.

In newborns with evidence of complete duodenal obstruction on abdominal radiograph, there is mostly no need for further radiologic investigation. If enough air is not present to adequately demonstrate the obstruction, one can introduce through a nasogastric tube.[12] However, a contrast enema in patients with complete duodenal obstruction

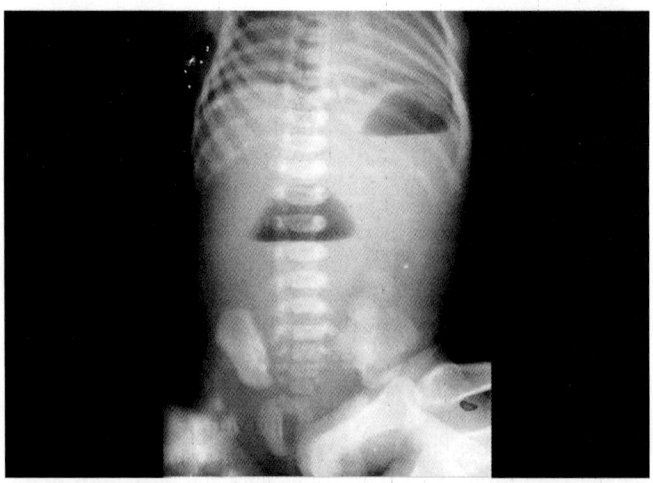

Fig. 10: Duondenal atresia. Erect film of the abdomen demonstrating the "double bubble" sign.

may be done to exclude additional, more distal atresia.[7] A microcolon implies that there is a distal atresia or atresias.

The newborn with congenital duodenal obstruction, complete or partial, requires surgery and is frequently taken to surgery without any more radiological investigation other than the plain film. However, further radiological study is required for making a preoperative diagnosis, specifically to distinguish between a cause of partial obstruction for which operation may be delayed, such as duodenal stenosis, from midgut volvulus, which requires emergent surgery. In these cases, when the infant is clinically stable, an upper gastrointestinal (UGI) series may be very useful. On UGI study, duodenal stenosis appears as dilatation of the duodenum proximal to the point of obstruction with abrupt caliber change.[3]

Duodenal Web

In patients with duodenal webs, the findings on UGI vary. In some, the appearance is of complete obstruction, in others there is narrowing of the duodenum. In the latter, a web is indistinguishable from simple duodenal stenosis. The most diagnostic appearance of a web is that of a thin, convex, curvilinear defect extending for a variable distance across the lumen of the duodenum. The "windsock" appearance that a duodenal web may have in an adult or older child, the so called intraluminal duodenal diverticulum, is not seen in newborns. This appearance is probably due to stretching and redundancy of the web caused by years of peristalsis, proximal to an incomplete obstruction.[27]

Annular Pancreas

Annular pancreas is due to anomalous pancreatic tissue encircling the second part of duodenum. It is believed to result from the failure of normal pancreatic tissue to rotate around the duodenum. The duodenal obstruction may be total at the time of birth, if a complete ring is formed. If the ring is incomplete, the obstruction may occur later in life or may never produce symptoms.[11] With severe obstruction, patient presents as a neonate. Presenting symptoms with delayed presentation are usually pain and vomiting. Radiographs are normal. On upper GI studies, a persistent waist is seen, partially obstructing the second part of duodenum.[3]

Preduodenal Portal Vein

Preduodenal portal vein is rarely the sole cause of duodenal obstruction and is rarely diagnosed preoperatively. It is thus important for the surgeon to be aware of the association of this anomaly with the other congenital lesions causing duodenal obstruction.[3]

A preduodenal portal vein (persistent left vitelline vein) results from normal situs asymmetry and is commonly seen in patients with heterotaxy. The resultant portal vein courses anterior to the pancreas and duodenum. The condition is diagnosed by identifying the prepancreatic course of the portal vein on sonography, CT and MR imaging. It is now believed that in most cases of duodenal obstruction associated with a preduodenal portal vein, the obstruction is due to a primary, obstructing duodenal lesion such as intraluminal membrane or web and such a lesion should be suspected in these patients, if duodenal obstruction is present.[21]

SMALL BOWEL

Anomalies of Rotation and Fixation

Embryology

At approximately sixth week of gestation, the primitive midgut herniates into the extraembryonic celom in the umbilical cord. The proximal and distal portions of the midgut elongate and rotate 270° anticlockwise around the axis of the superior mesenteric artery. By the end of the third month of gestation, the bowel loops return to their final position in the abdominal cavity. Fixation of the duodenojejunal junction or the ligament of Treitz in left upper quadrant occurs. The cecum is the last part of the GIT to be fixed and it normally comes to lie in the right lower quadrant. When all or part of the physiological rotation of bowel fails to occur, a wide variety of anomalies of intestinal rotation and mesenteric fixation occurs which consist of nonrotation, malrotation or reversed rotation.[12]

1. *Nonrotation:* It is an asymptomatic condition in which the small bowel lies entirely on the right side and the colon on the left side. It is demonstrated incidentally on barium studies in older children or adults **(Figs. 11A and B)**. The bowel is not very mobile and volvulus is not a common complication of nonrotation of the bowel.
2. *Malrotation:* In malrotation of the bowel, final position of the GI tract is somewhere between normal and complete nonrotation.[12] Malrotation is a general term that includes a wide spectrum of anomalies that occur when this intestinal rotation and fixation occurs in an abnormal fashion. It can also be referred to as "malfixation". Most commonly, there is incomplete rotation, which leads to a shortened mesenteric root which may have a narrow rather than a broad base that

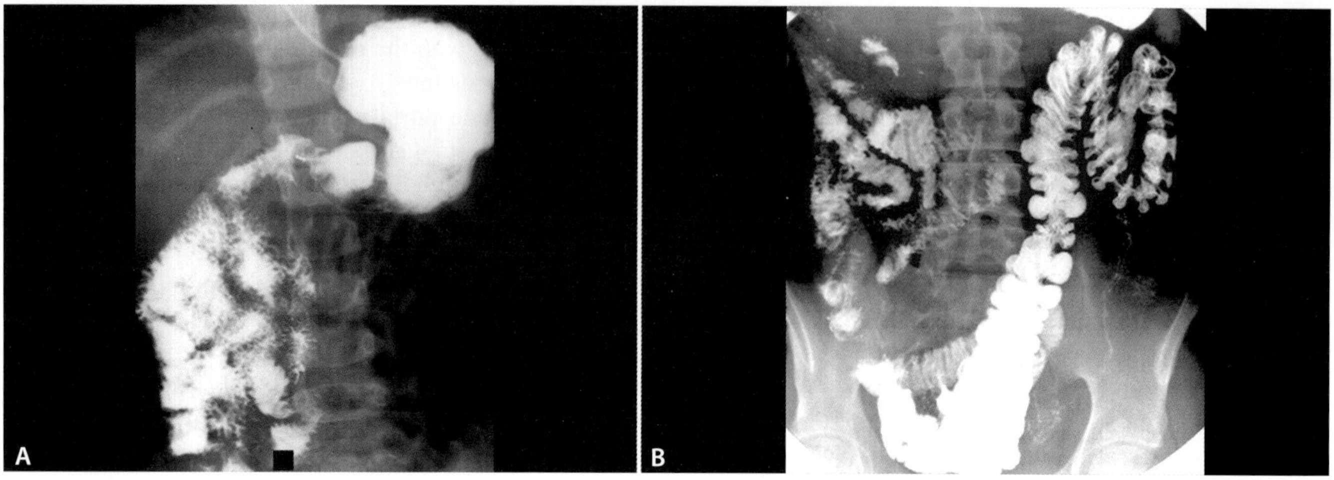

Figs. 11A and B: Barium meal follow through study shows (A) jejunal loops on the right side of the abdomen and (B) colon and cecum on the left side, with the ileum seen crossing the midline from right to left—Nonrotation.

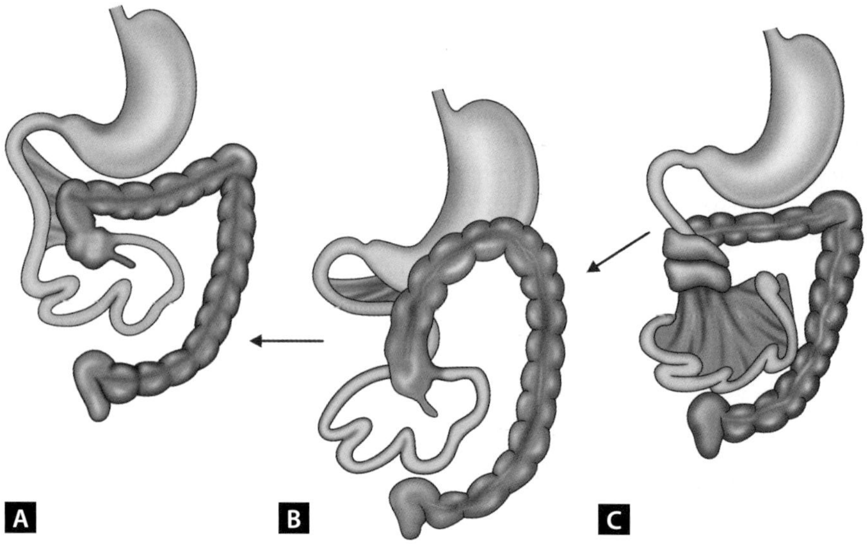

Figs. 12A to C: Illustration of midgut volvulus. Narrow mesenteric attachment of nonrotation (A) or incomplete rotation (B) may lead to midgut volvulus (C).

has a tendency to twist on its axis. This leads to extrinsic compression of the bowel, causing bowel obstruction, and if the twist persists, it may lead to occlusion of the mesenteric vessels. This twist of malfixed intestines around the short mesentery is called a midgut volvulus **(Figs. 12A to C)**. In patients with malfixation of the bowel, in addition to the absence of a normal mesentery, frequently there are aberrant peritoneal bands (**Ladd's bands**). These bands extend from the malpositioned cecum across the duodenum and attach to the hilum of the liver, posterior peritoneum or abdominal wall and can cause extrinsic duodenal obstruction **(Figs. 13 and 14)**.[24]

3. *Reversed intestinal rotation:* It is a rare rotational anomaly which renders the hepatic flexure and left transverse colon posterior in position. These portions of the colon lie behind the descending duodenum and the superior mesenteric artery. The cecum is usually malrotated and medially placed and the small bowel is more right-sided than normal. Obstructing bands and midgut volvulus can occur.[12]

Clinical Features

Two-thirds of patients who are symptomatic present with an acute onset of bilious vomiting in the first month of life with many of them presenting in the first week of life.

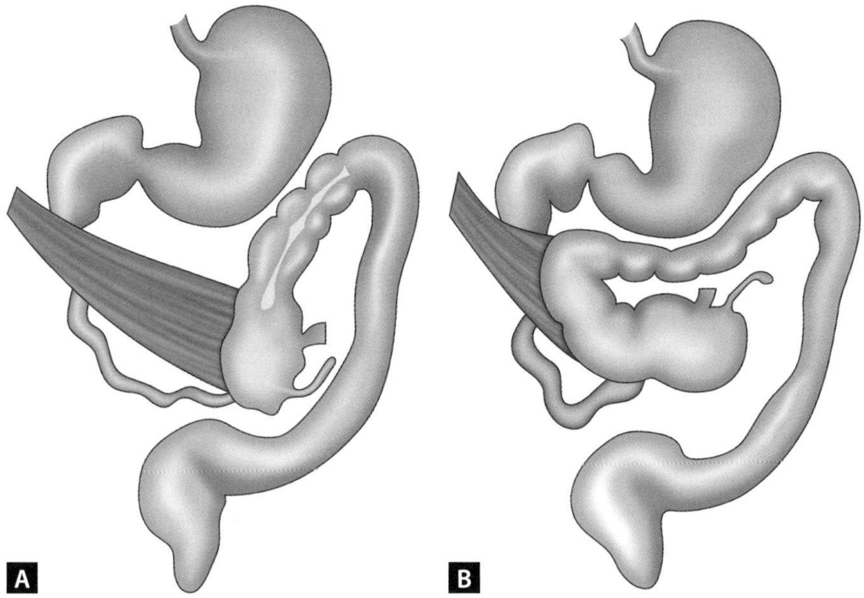

Figs. 13A and B: Diagrammatic representation of Ladd's bands causing duodenal compression in patients with malrotation. The cecum is left sided (A) and midline (B) in position and has dense peritoneal bands crossing over the duodenum.

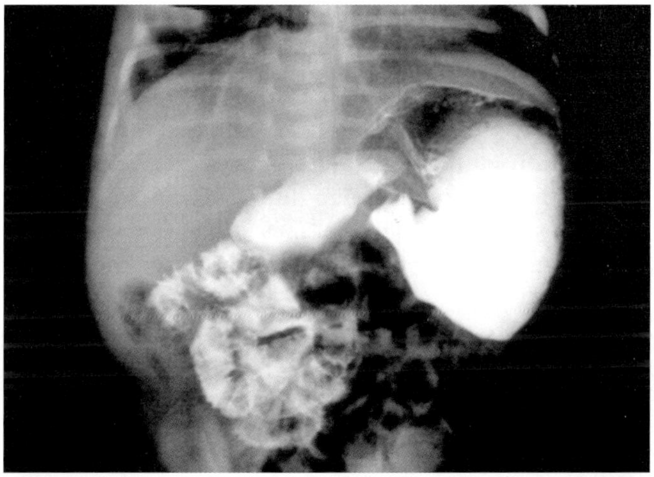

Fig. 14: Midgut malrotation with Ladd's bands: Barium study shows distended proximal duodenum with tapering at the level of obstruction indicative of extrinsic compression. The small intestine, distal to the usual site of the ligament of Treitz lies below the duodenum and to the right.

About 15–20% of patients present in late infancy or early childhood. In the remaining patients, malrotation is seen as an incidental finding.

The bowel obstruction may be caused by the volvulus, by Ladd's bands, or both. The sudden onset of bilious vomiting in a newborn who has been normal for the first few days of life should be considered to be due to a midgut volvulus until proved otherwise.

Imaging Features

Plain radiographs may show feature of duodenal obstruction due to partially obstructing Ladd's bands. The duodenal bulb dilatation is less than that seen with duodenal atresia. There may be little distal bowel gas. When there is a volvulus, the plain films may show features of distal bowel obstruction. Bowel-wall thickening and pneumatosis may be present due to volvulus-induced ischemia. The fluid-filled bowel loops associated with volvulus can simulate an abdominal mass. The abdomen may be gasless, which may be due either to proximal obstruction or to diffuse bowel necrosis in midgut volvulus. Of all the congenital anomalies that result in bilious emesis, only malrotation is likely to produce a normal abdominal film.[24]

Upper gastrointestinal barium examination is performed to document the location of ligament of Treitz and to evaluate for duodenal obstruction. Normally, the duodenojejunal junction lies to the left of the body of the first or second lumbar vertebra at the level of the duodenal bulb. In malrotation, it is located lower and to the right of normal. It is important to remember that the duodenojejunal junction is mobile in children and may be pushed inferomedially by an overdistended stomach, chronic bowel dilatation, enlarged spleen or in the presence of a nasojejunal tube.[3] A lateral view of the contrast-filled duodenum is an important additional view in the upper GI study when evaluating for malrotation.

Normal duodenum being a retroperitoneal structure, on lateral views is seen to lie behind the level of the stomach, with the fourth part of the duodenum superimposed on the second part of duodenum. This superimposed relationship is lost in case of malrotation of duodenum as it is seen to course anteriorly. An abnormal position of the duodenojejunal flexure may be the only indication of malrotation, as in 16% of cases cecum occupies its normal position.

In addition, in malrotation the jejunum is usually on the right side of the abdomen. However, this should not be taken as an indication of malrotation as the jejunum in a normal child is relatively mobile and may be seen to the right of the spine.[3]

When volvulus occurs, there may be complete or partial duodenal obstruction. With complete obstruction, a beaked tapering of the obstructed duodenum may be seen. More commonly, the volvulus is intermittent with incomplete bowel obstruction with contrast filling the proximal small bowel. Occasionally, the pathognomonic corkscrew pattern of the twisted duodenum and jejunum is seen due to their clockwise twisting around the superior mesenteric artery **(Figs. 15A and B)**. In malrotation, the cecum and right colon may have abnormal mobility. The cecum is in the right upper quadrant or in midline in malrotation. A colonic beak may be present in the right colon on barium enema in the presence of volvulus.[24] In the past, a contrast enema was the first investigation performed to evaluate for malrotation.[3] This has been replaced by an upper GI study due to its greater sensitivity and specificity for malrotation. The cecum may be mobile in neonates and may be seen in the right upper quadrant in the absence of malrotation.

A barium meal upper GI study should be done for suspected malrotation since a normal barium enema does not exclude malrotation. The position of the cecum may be normal in a significant number of patients with malrotation.[21] Hence, the upper GI study is the investigation of choice for the diagnosis of malrotation.

Ultrasound may be useful in the early detection of midgut malrotation as well as complicating midgut volvulus. A distended proximal duodenum with a tapered end in front of the spine is consistent with malrotation in the proper clinical set-up. If in addition, one finds peritoneal fluid and edematous bowel loops on the right, the diagnosis of volvulus can be made. A normal anatomical relationship, however, in no way excludes the possibility of malrotation. A UGI series is mandatory, if this diagnosis must be confirmed or excluded prior to surgery.

Ultrasound and CT scan may be helpful in suggesting the diagnosis of malrotation owing to abnormal superior mesenteric artery (SMA) or superior mesenteric vein (SMV) anatomy. The SMV normally rests to the right and anterior to the SMA. When the SMV is to the left of the SMA, this is highly suggestive of volvulus. When the SMV is anterior to the SMA, this is suggestive of malrotation with possible volvulus. Color Doppler US demonstrates **whirlpool sign** due to clockwise spiralling of the mesentery and superior mesenteric vein around the superior mesenteric artery. Inversion of the mesenteric

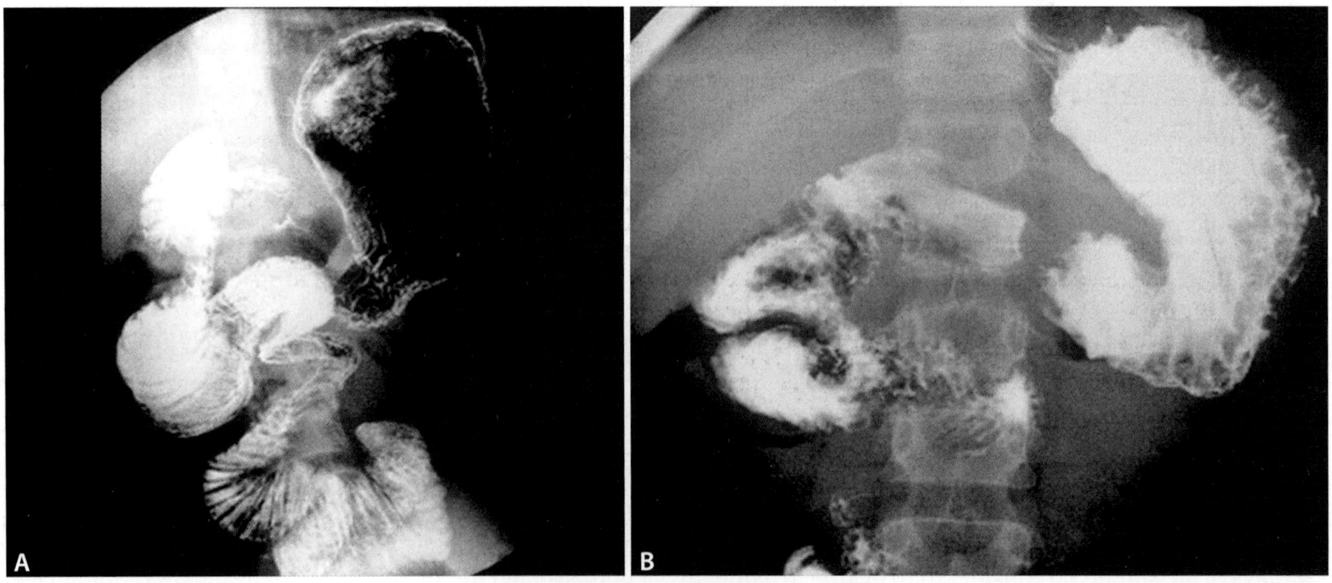

Figs. 15A and B: Upper GI barium study in two different patients showing classic "corkscrew" appearance of the duodenum in midgut volvulus.

vessels or the SMV rotation sign is not a sensitive screening test, because it may be present in normal population, patients with situs inversus and patients with abdominal masses. Other CT findings of midgut malrotation complicated by midgut volvulus are: (1) The 'whirl' sign of small-bowel loops revolved around the SMA; **(Fig. 16)** (2) A dilated, fluid-filled, obstructed stomach and proximal duodenum; (3) Thick-walled loops of ischemic right-sided small bowel loops with potential pneumatosis intestinalis and mesenteric edema; and (4) free intraperitoneal fluid.

Jejunoileal Atresia and Stenosis

Small bowel atresias (i.e. jejunal, jejunoileal or ileal) are more common than duodenal or colonic atresia. They are more common in the proximal jejunum and distal ileum than in the intervening small intestine.[24] Jejunal atresias comprise around 50% of small bowel atresias and may be associated with other jejunal and ileal atresias.[2]

Embryology

Most jejunal and ileal atresias and stenoses, except those that are familial, are thought to be secondary to ischemic injury to the developing gut. The ischemia may be due to primary vascular accident, usually in the mid second trimester or secondarily to a mechanical obstruction, as may occur in case of an in utero volvulus.[24] There is no solid core phase in the development of jejunum and ileum, so recanalization is not thought to be involved. Jejunoileal atresia may involve the bowel anywhere from the ligament of Treitz to the ileocecal valve with the majority of cases of atresia occurring at the extremes of the small bowel. The devascularized bowel becomes necrotic and is resorbed leaving an atretic area of varying length with its attached mesentery. Several forms of atresia have been described surgically, but it is not possible to differentiate them by imaging studies.[4]

Clinical Features

Antenatal diagnosis of small bowel atresia may be suggested on ultrasound by the presence of polyhydramnios and dilated fluid-filled bowel loops. These findings are non-specific and the diagnosis is usually not confirmed until after birth.[3] Proximal atresia may present with bilious vomiting; whereas more distal atresias present with abdominal distention. There may be failure to pass meconium. It is commonly associated with prematurity. Meconium may be passed, if atresia is located in the jejunum or occurred later in intrauterine life.

Classification

Small bowel atresia usually occurs as an isolated anomaly of the gastrointestinal tract. There are four types of small bowel atresia[3] **(Figs. 17A to D)**:

Type 1: Membranous or web-like atresia, composed of mucosal and submucosal elements with no interruption of the muscularis.

Type 2: Atresia with a solid fibrous cord connecting the atretic bowel ends, but the mesentery is intact. All the three layers of the intestinal wall are interrupted.

Type 3: Complete absence of a segment of bowel (total atresia) as well as a portion of the mesentery (V-shaped defect in the mesentry).

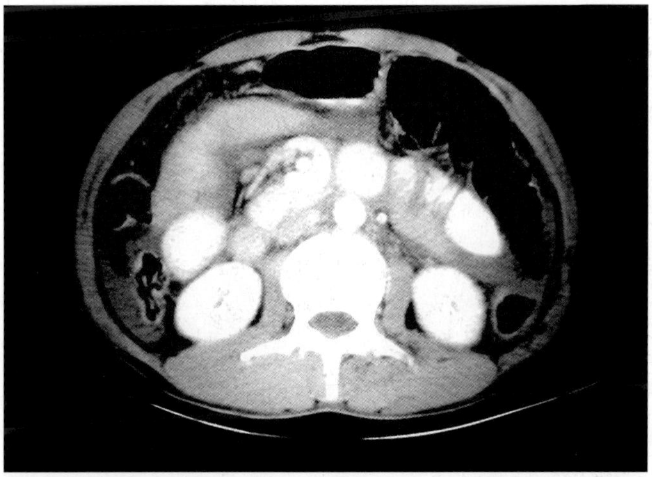

Fig. 16: Axial CECT of the abdomen showing characteristic "whirlpool" sign of clockwise twisting of the SMV and mesentery around the SMA.

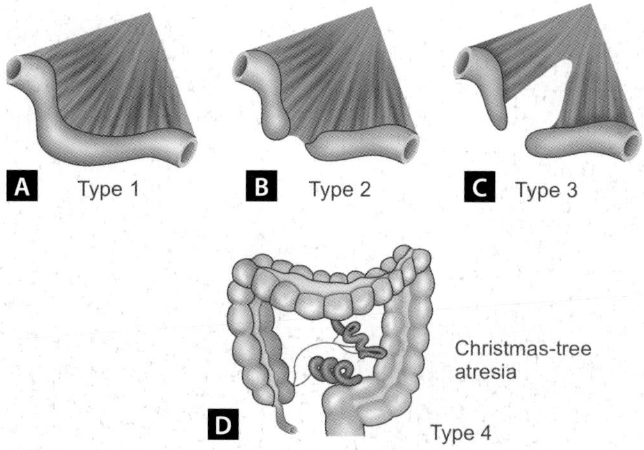

Figs. 17A to D: Types of small bowel atresia.

Type 4: The familial form of multiple atresias.

There are two unusual forms of atresia that are inherited:[24]

1. "Apple peel" or "Christmas tree" atresia
2. A syndrome of multiple intestinal atresias

Apple peel or *Christmas tree* atresia is a rare variant of Type 3 atresia which consists of proximal jejunal atresia with absence of the distal superior mesenteric artery, shortening of the small bowel distal to the atresia and absence of the dorsal mesentery. This type of atresia is probably caused by prenatal occlusion of the SMA, distal to the origin of the midcolic artery. The distal small intestine spirals around its vascular supply giving the characteristic apple peel appearance **(Fig. 17D)**. The result is a very short intestine with a propensity towards necrotizing enterocolitis.[28]

The syndrome of multiple intestinal atresias with intraluminal calcification is transmitted as an autosomal recessive pattern. There are multiple atresias from stomach to rectum. The radiological hallmark of this syndrome is extensive calcification of intraluminal contents between the areas of atresia. Nonhereditary bowel atresias may also demonstrate intraluminal calcification.[24]

Imaging Features

Plain radiograph of the abdomen demonstrates typical findings of small-bowel obstruction. The site (jejunal or distal ileal) of the atresia can be suspected by the number and location of gas-filled loops of bowel **(Fig. 18)**.[3] Proximal jejunal atresia may have a few markedly dilated loops, the so-called triple bubble sign, more distal atresia typically has a more uniform dilatation of small bowel with associated air-fluid levels. The loop just proximal to the site of atresia is frequently disproportionately distended, with a bulbous end. If the ischemic event that produced the atresia caused a perforation, there may be evidence of meconium peritonitis which is a chemical peritonitis occurring as a result of extruded bowel contents producing an intense peritoneal inflammatory reaction. It leads to the formation of dense fibrotic tissue which often calcifies, resulting in characteristic intraperitoneal calcifications. Peritoneal calcifications may be identified on plain films as a consequence of meconium peritonitis, wherein they are seen as linear or flocculent areas of calcification within the peritoneal cavity **(Fig. 19)**. The most frequent finding is a linear calcification under the free edge of the liver, though any or all portions of the peritoneum may be involved.[4] The calcification may extend into the scrotum through a patent vaginal process to produce a calcified mass in the scrotum.[28] The association of meconium peritonitis with small bowel obstruction is virtually diagnostic of small bowel atresia.[4]

Ultrasound depicts the calcifications of meconium peritonitis as highly echogenic linear or clumped foci in the abdomen or pelvis. The appearance of meconium peritonitis on US may be either generalized or cystic. In the generalized condition, highly echogenic material spreads throughout the abdomen and around the bowel loops to produce a characteristic "snowstorm" appearance. Encysted collections of meconium show a variable appearance from homogeneous to heterogeneous echogenicity and may be ill-defined or well defined.

Sonography may also be useful in differentiating ileal atresia from meconium ileus. In ileal atresia, the bowel

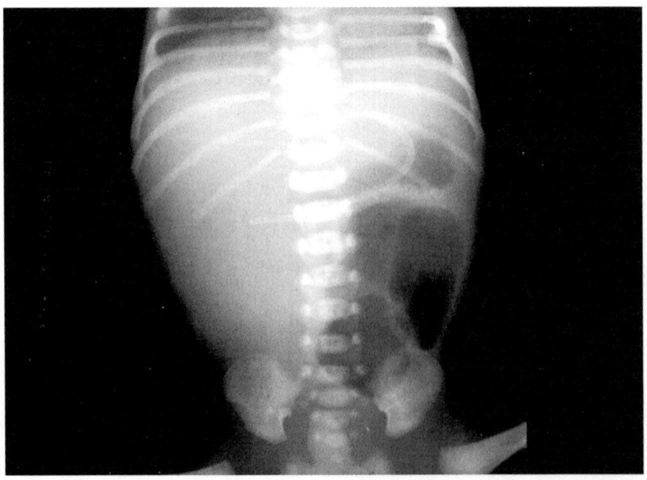

Fig. 18: Small bowel atresia: Air is seen in the stomach and dilated part of the jejunum proximal to the atresia.

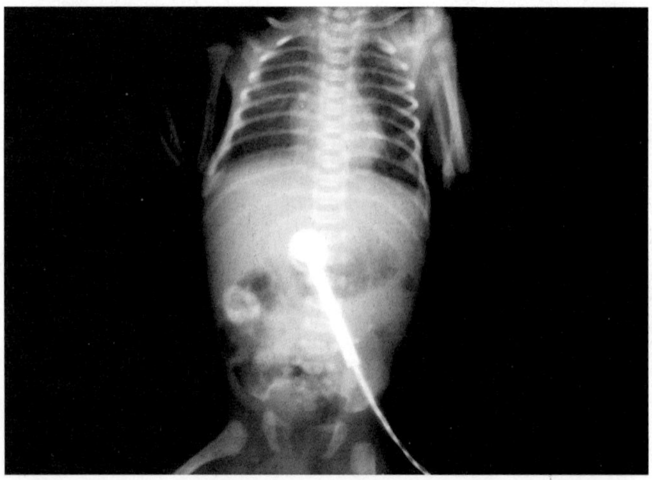

Fig. 19: Plain radiograph of the abdomen in a case of meconium peritonitis shows curvilinear calcification in the right flank.

contents are echopoor while in meconium ileus, the dilated bowel loops are filled with echogenic material.[21]

Additional imaging is not required in the presence of a high intestinal obstruction. A contrast enema is required for further evaluation for low bowel obstruction to distinguish between a large or distal small bowel obstruction, as the differentiation of the two on plain radiographs may be difficult or impossible. The most common causes of neonatal distal small bowel obstruction are ileal atresia and meconium ileus.[3]

Contrast enema should be performed with water soluble low osmolar contrast media introduced via a soft rectal catheter. Care must be taken to perform the enema as the distal blind pouch is prone to perforation. The one diagnostic finding to be looked for in the contrast enema performed in a setting of low bowel obstruction, is the presence or absence of a microcolon **(Fig. 20)**. A microcolon is a colon of very small caliber, generally less than 1 cm diameter, and the entire colon must be involved (i.e. not a portion as in small left colon syndrome). Normally, colonic measurements are not needed for diagnosing microcolon as it is usually obvious on inspection. The colon is small owing to lack of use rather than anatomic or functional abnormality. The more distal the small bowel obstruction, the smaller the colon. A microcolon or unused colon occurs when no or little intestinal juices (succus entericus) reaches the colon and is highly suggestive of a distal small bowel obstruction (meconium ileus or ileal atresia). A normal sized colon almost always excludes these diagnoses.[24]

It is important to remember that the presence of microcolon is diagnostic of long standing distal small bowel obstruction, but a normal colon does not exclude it in all cases. Also, microcolon on contrast enemas may be seen in premature infants and occasionally, in total colonic aganglionosis (long segment Hirschsprung's disease). The rectum is distensible in distal ileal atresia, thereby distinguishing it from the microcolon of long segment Hirschsprung's disease.[3]

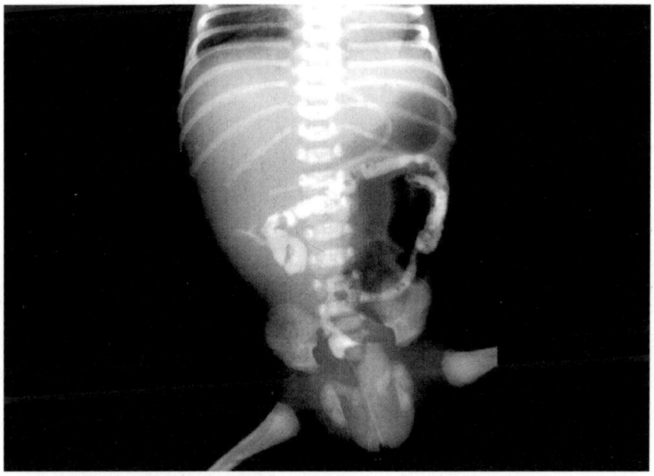

Fig. 20: Small bowel atresia: Contrast enema demonstrates a microcolon.

Jejunal atresia does not lead to a microcolon because the remaining small bowel, distal to the atresia produces sufficient succus entericus to give a colon of normal caliber. Hence, a microcolon in the presence of a high bowel obstruction indicates a second, more distal atresia.[3]

Surgical treatment involves resection of the atretic portion of the intestine with reanastomosis. The proximal dilated bowel may remain dilated for sometime in the postoperative period, showing delayed motility with delayed passage of contrast across a widely patent anastomosis.

Meconium Ileus

Meconium ileus is a low intestinal obstruction caused by inspissation of abnormal meconium in the distal ileum.[24] It is almost always associated with cystic fibrosis and is a presenting feature of cystic fibrosis in 5–10% of these patients.[24] The lack of normal pancreatic enzymes leads to thick, tenacious meconium that collects in the distal ileum and cecum, occluding its lumen and resulting in high-grade distal small bowel obstruction.

Meconium ileus can be complicated or uncomplicated, with complicated meconium ileus being seen in up to half of the patients which include intestinal atresia, volvulus of the distal intestinal loop and perforation with meconium or pseudocyst formation.[3]

Imaging Features

Meconium ileus is the most common mimic of small bowel atresia clinically and on plain films.[4] Plain radiograph may demonstrate a distal bowel obstructive pattern with air-fluid levels. Bowel loops may vary in size, a finding seen less often in atresia. The dilated small-bowel loops that contain air can mimic colon loops in size and course. In addition, some air mixes with the viscid meconium and results in a bubbly appearance in the right lower quadrant. This "soap-bubble appearance" is not specific and a similar fecal pattern can be seen with any cause of distal intestinal obstruction like ileal atresia, colonic atresia, aganglionosis of the terminal ileum and meconium plug syndrome.[28] Patients with meconium ileus have fewer air-fluid levels than patients with small-bowel atresias.

Meconium peritonitis may occur and be associated with peritoneal calcifications. However, this differential point is not specific in all cases. A localized perforation forms a meconium pseudocyst which may have peripheral curvilinear calcifications seen on plain radiographs. The term pseudocyst is also used to refer for a mass of necrotic, fluid-filled bowel loops with a fibrous wall which may be seen as a mass on radiographs.[3]

Ultrasound can detect abnormal bowel dilatation and echogenic bowel contents in infants with meconium ileus. Ultrasound can also pick-up complications of meconium peritonitis or pseudocyst which is seen as echogenic material lying outside the bowel loops, with or without associated calcification.

The colon of babies with meconium ileus is often said to be the smallest of all colons, and is empty except for a few occasional pellets of meconium. The distal 10–30 cm of ileum appears dilated due to meconium within and may even displace the right colon to the left.[24]

Definitive diagnosis is made with a low osmolal water soluble contrast enema which demonstrates a microcolon with inspissated meconium pellets identified in the collapsed distal ileum with dilated small bowel proximal to the obstruction **(Fig. 21)**.

Uncomplicated cases of meconium ileus may be treated with multiple contrast enemas, i.e. one or two enemas per day. The aim is to introduce the contrast into the dilated small bowel, proximal to the obstructing inspissated meconium. But care must be taken not to overdistend the meconium. This leads to mechanical loosening of the meconium pellets. The patient should be well hydrated, if high osmolarity agents are used because of fluid shifts. The therapy is largely mechanical and the osmotic load probably plays little role. Repeated enemas may be used only, if progress is seen in decreasing the obstructing pellets. In premature infants, isotonic non-ionic contrast medium is used. Enema has a success rate of about 50 to 60% in treating meconium ileus.[3] If signs of obstruction are not relieved or perforation/perintornitis develop, further attempts at therapeutic enema should be abandoned. Surgery in such patients often reveals complicated meconium ileus.

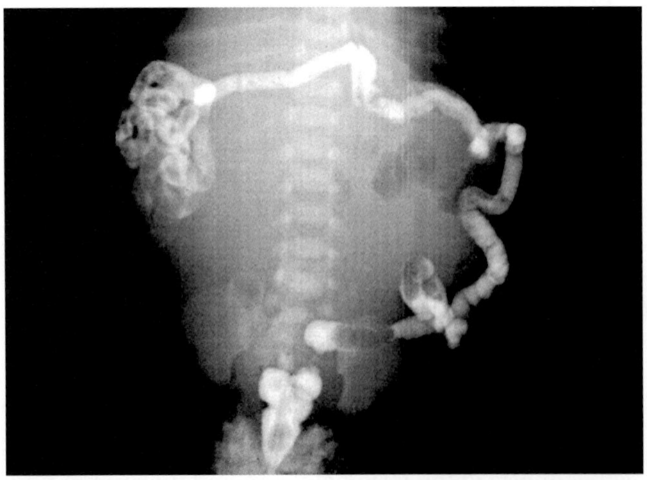

Fig. 21: Meconium ileus: Water-soluble contrast enema showing a microcolon. Filling defects due to meconium are seen in colon and distal ileum.

Megacystis-microcolon-intestinal Hypoperistalsis Syndrome (Berdon's Syndrome)

Megacystis-microcolon-intestinal hypoperistalsis syndrome is a pseudoatresia. There is a functional small bowel obstruction with a microcolon, malrotation and a large unobstructed bladder. There is four-to-one female predominance with associated genitourinary and congenital heart malformation in up to 14% cases.

Upper GI contrast study shows hypomotility of small bowel with retrograde peristalsis. Ultrasound reveals a dilated bladder with bilateral hydroureteronephrosis.[21] The prognosis is poor for long-term survival.

Meckel's Diverticulum

Meckel's diverticulum is a congenital blind pouch in the small bowel which results from an incomplete obliteration of the proximal part of the vitelline duct (omphalomesenteric duct) during the fifth week of gestation. It results in a true diverticulum arising from the antimesenteric border of the distal ileum.[29] For Meckel's diverticulum, the common rule by which it is known is the "rule of twos", i.e. it is found in 2% of the population, twice as common in males, most frequently found in those less than 2 years of age and usually 2 feet from the ileocecal valve. It may contain ectopic mucosa, usually gastric mucosa which is responsible for the adjacent ulceration in the ileum.

Meckel's diverticulum usually does not give rise to symptoms. Bleeding is the most common complication in children reported in over 50% of cases, while it is seen in only around 12% cases in adults. Bleeding is usually minor, resulting in chronic anemia.[22] It may present with malena due to ulceration of ectopic gastric mucosa in its wall. In 20–30% of patients, it may give rise to symptoms such as inflammation, and or perforation which may often be indistinguishable from acute appendicitis.

Obstructive symptoms have been seen to occur more frequently than hemorrhage in patients with Meckel's diverticulum presenting in adulthood. The obstruction may occur due to intussusception, volvulus, inflammatory adhesions. The diverticulum may get obstructed with resulting diverticulitis, may present as a mass and initiate intussusception in childhood.

Preoperative evaluation of a Meckel's diverticulum is difficult, and routine and special radiological studies such as plain abdominal radiograph, barium meal follow through, arteriography and computed tomography are often nondiagnostic and often of limited diagnostic value. The diverticulum is seldom recognized on a small bowel follow-through study because there is no significant hold-up, and the barium residue remaining in it is very small because of its wide neck.[29,30] In suspected symptomatic Meckel's diverticulum, preoperative evaluation includes ^{99m}Tc (technetium-99m pertechnetate) scanning which relies on the presence of ectopic gastric mucosa. In this study, ^{99m}Tc is injected intravenously, and over time it accumulates in the gastric mucosa.

As symptoms such as bleeding is caused by the ectopic gastric issue, ^{99m}Tc scanning may help in the diagnosis in symptomatic cases. In children, the scan has a sensitivity of 85% and specificity of 95%, but in adults the sensitivity is 62.5% and the specificity 9%. The accuracy of the scan can be improved with the use of pentagastrin or cimetidine. In patients with nondiagnostic scan or with nonbleeding presentation, ultrasonography could prove to be useful in achieving a diagnosis.

Enteric Duplication

Gastrointestinal duplications are uncommon congenital abnormalities that may occur anywhere in the gastrointestinal tract. But the most common locations are the distal ileum (35%), distal esophagus (20%) and stomach (9%) followed by duodenum and jejunum. Colonic and rectal duplications are rare. Multiple duplications may be present in 15–20% cases.[21] Enteric duplication occurs in the late first or early second trimester owing to abnormal canalization of the bowel. The duplication has smooth muscle in its wall with gastrointestinal mucosal lining. The wall thickness is 3–5 mm as seen in normal bowel. It is usually adjacent to and in most instances, does not communicate with the gastrointestinal tract. In most cases of hemorrhage or ulceration, gastric mucosa is present. Esophageal duplications are located at the posterior aspect of the esophagus. Gastric duplication is found along the greater curvature of the stomach interposed between the stomach and the transverse colon. Duplications may be spherical or tubular. Tubular duplication is more likely to communicate with the adjacent bowel. They typically occur along the mesenteric border of the intestine and share a common blood supply. Thus the tubular type of duplication may complicate bowel-sparing surgery because of difficulty in preserving the enteric blood supply. Unlike neurenteric cysts, duplication cysts are usually not associated with vertebral segmental anomalies.[29]

Clinical Features

Duplications can present with a variety of symptoms and signs depending on the site of duplication and its size. Upper esophageal duplications present with symptoms due to tracheal compression. Other symptoms include nausea and vomiting. In the presence of heterotopic gastric mucosa, patients may present with gastrointestinal hemorrhage or even perforation. Patient may also present with distention, ulceration, volvulus, an abdominal mass lesion or with obstruction, particularly when the duplication is in the region of the ileocecal valve or duodenum.

About 40% of patients with enteric duplication present by one month of age, with 85% diagnosed during the first year of life.

Malrotation, genitourinary anomalies and jejunal or ileal atresias are also seen. Duplications are more common in boys except for gastric ones, which occur without gender predominance.

Imaging Features

Plain radiographs may demonstrate a mass lesion, especially in the chest in the case of esophageal duplication, **(Figs. 22A and B)**. The bowel gas pattern may suggest an obstruction, particularly with duodenal or ileal duplications. Enteric duplication cysts may reveal mural calcifications.

Occasionally, duplication may get filled with barium suspension during gastrointestinal examinations. In most cases, however, the duplications are not demonstrated in this manner. Barium study usually reveals extrinsic compression **(Figs. 23A and B)** of the bowel or an obstruction.

On ultrasonography, a duplication cyst appears as a well-defined, unilocular anechoic mass with good through transmission **(Fig. 24)**. Rarely, the contents are reflective or contain septations secondary to hemorrhage or inspissated material within the lumen. A highly reflective mucosa and a surrounding echo poor muscular wall may be seen as the duplication is of gastrointestinal origin.[31,32] This is most easily identified in the dependent portion of the cyst.[21] The presence of this double-layered appearance

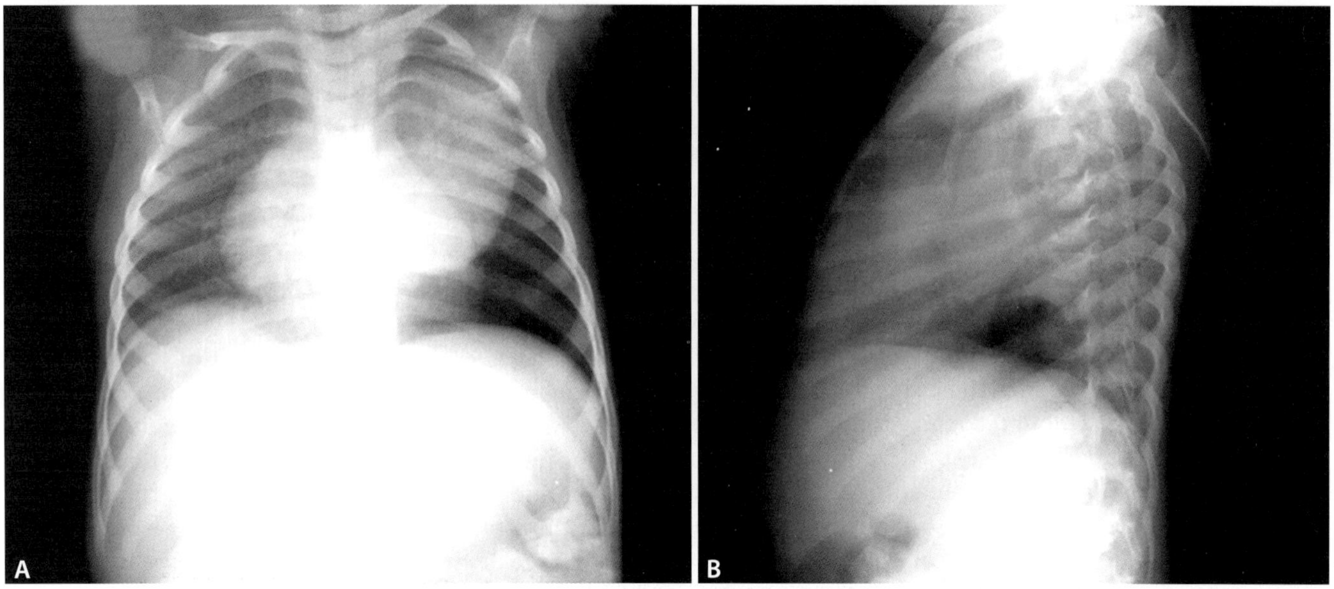

Figs. 22A and B: Esophageal duplication: Chest PA showing a well-defined soft tissue mass in the left hemithorax (A) lying posterior in the lateral film (B). There is associated hyperinflation of the left lung. The vertebral bodies appear normal.

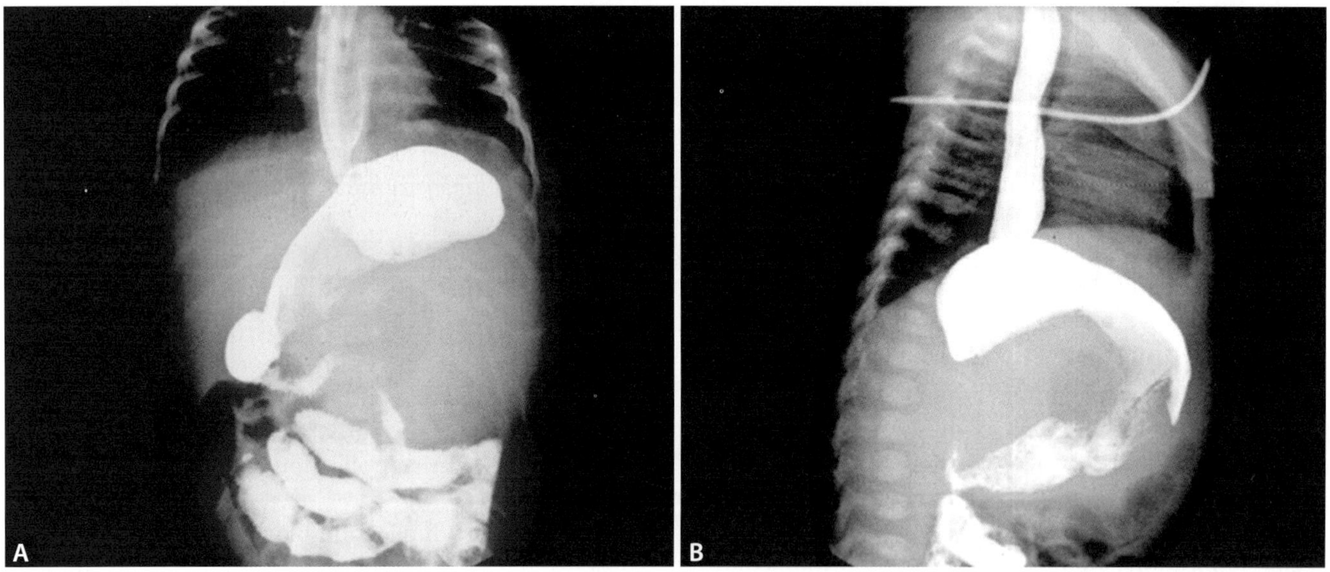

Figs. 23A and B: Barium study shows extrinsic impression on the body of the stomach with effacement of the mucosa in AP and lateral views in a case of gastric duplication.

("gut wall signature") is relatively specific for the diagnosis of duplication cyst and is useful to exclude other cystic masses, such as mesenteric or omental cyst, choledochal cyst, ovarian cyst, pancreatic pseudocyst or abscess. The reflective lining may be absent as a result of extensive mucosal ulceration by gastric enzymes.

Radionuclide studies may be useful in 30% of patients, where the enteric duplications have gastric mucosa. Free pertechnetate is taken up and secreted by gastric mucosa, thus localizing the enteric duplication.[5]

CT or MRI may be useful in further characterizing the nature of enteric duplication cysts when the diagnosis is unclear, wherein they are seen as well-marginated, smooth-walled masses of fluid attenuation/signal not showing any contrast enhancement **(Figs. 25A and B)**.

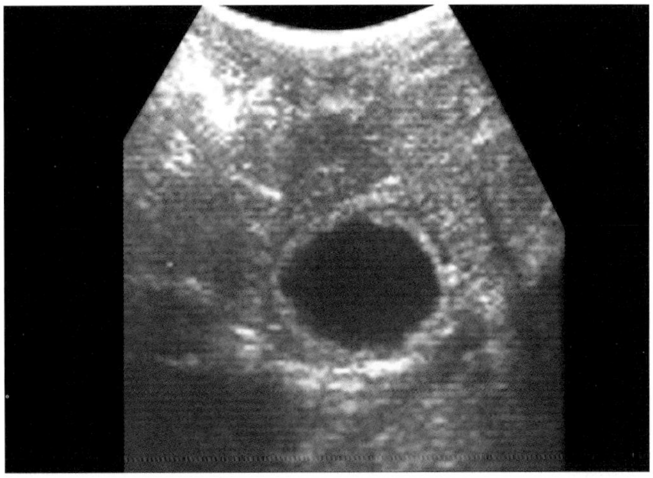

Fig. 24: Ultrasound abdomen reveals a well-defined, smooth rounded cystic lesion with inner echogenic mucosal stripe and outer hypoechoic muscle layer—enteric duplication.

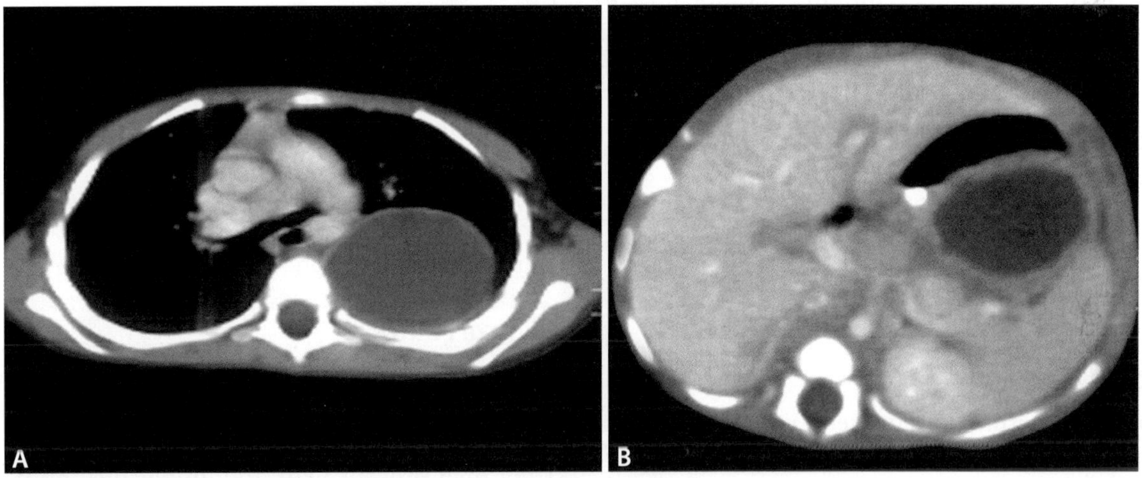

Figs. 25A and B: CECT images of esophageal and gastric duplications of the two patients of the same case as in Figures 22 and 23 show sharply marginated, non-enhancing, homogeneous mass of water attenuation in the (A) posterior mediastinum and (B) along the greater curvature of stomach.

LARGE BOWEL

Colonic Obstruction

Obstruction of the colon in the newborn may be either anatomical or functional. The first type includes atresia of the colon, anorectal atresia, and with a functional element, aganglionosis or Hirschsprung's disease. A group of poorly understood disorders like meconium plug, neonatal small left colon syndrome, etc. cause transient self-limited functional obstruction.

Colonic Atresia

Colonic atresia is quite rare as compared to atresias of the small bowel.[24] It is thought to be secondary to vascular insult. Multiple atresia syndromes may involve the colon in addition to small bowel. Proximal location is more common than distal, with atresias beyond the splenic flexure being unusual. If atresia is located in the ascending colon, it may often be indistinguishable from obstruction of the distal ileum.[28] The classification system based on the anatomic appearance is same as with jejunoileal atresia. Type 1 represents a diaphragmatic occlusion; type 2 represents a complete atresia with a blind, solid cord extending between the two ends of atretic segment; and type 3 represents a complete atresia with complete separation and an associated V-shaped mesenteric defect.

Clinical Features

Patients present with distension and failure to pass meconium. Presentation may be delayed up to 48 hours, if the atresia is proximal.

Imaging Features

Prenatal sonography may demonstrate dilatation of the colon proximal to the atresia.

Plain radiograph may demonstrate a distal obstruction with multiple air-fluid levels and may be nonspecific. Occasionally, a hugely and disproportionately dilated loop of bowel may be present and render the plain film evaluation highly suggestive of the diagnosis.[2] A "soap-bubble" appearance of retained meconium may be seen. There is dilatation of the proximal colon up to the level of the atresia, unless multiple atresias are present.

Contrast enema shows a microcolon, distal to the atresia with obstruction to the retrograde flow of barium at the site of atresia. The colon may have a hook or question-mark appearance at the site of atresia. The colon is often non-fixed or malpositioned in the midline. The distal colon segment may perforate into the peritoneal cavity during a contrast enema because often the blind end is covered with only mucosa.

Hirschsprung's Disease (Aganglionosis of the Colon)

Hirschsprung's disease is a condition caused by absence of normal ganglion cells in a segment of the colon, leading to a form of low intestinal obstruction. It accounts for around 15–20% of cases of neonatal bowel obstruction.[28]

Embryology

In normal intrauterine development, neuroenteric cells migrate from the neural crest to the upper end of the gastrointestinal tract by 5 weeks and then proceeds in a caudal direction. These cells reach the rectum by 12 weeks and commence the intramural migration from Auerbach's (myenteric) plexus to the submucosal plexus. Hirschsprung's disease is caused by abnormal neural crest cell migration, resulting in arrested distal migration of these cells.[3] As the normal migration is continuous from proximal to distal, the part of the GI tract distal to the site of arrest is aganglionic.[8]

In the majority of cases (75–80%), the aganglionic segment is limited to the rectosigmoid region (short segment aganglionosis). The aganglionosis always involves the anus and internal sphincter and extends proximally for a variable distance. The transition from innervated to aganglionic bowel is found in the rectosigmoid region in 73% of patients, the descending colon in 14%, and more proximal colon in 10%, according to Swenson et al.[8] Total colon aganglionosis involves the entire colon and part of the terminal ileum. It can very rarely involve the large as well as whole of the small bowel, which is incompatible with life. At the other end of the spectrum is ultrashort segment Hirschsprung's disease which is also rare. In this type, the aganglionosis is limited to the region of the internal sphincter.[3] The ultrashort segment can only be diagnosed by manometry (not biopsy or imaging) and is usually not diagnosed in the neonatal period.[4] Skip lesions in Hirschsprung's disease are believed to be unlikely to exist if one accepts the concept of neuronal migration down the GI tract. It is likely that such areas represent areas of intrauterine ischemic insult leading to destruction of ganglion cells.[12]

However, according to recently published literature, skip lesions in Hirschsprung's disease, though a controvertial condition, is a definite entity, with 24 cases reported till date. Skip lesions have been found to occur predominantly in patients with total colonic aganglionosis (92%). The presence of a skip area of normally innervated colon in total colonic aganglionosis may influence the surgical management, enabling the surgeons to preserve and use the ganglionated skip area during pull through operations.[33]

Hirschsprung's disease may be associated with certain congenital anomalies like intestinal atresia, malrotation. Down's syndrome is present in 2–3% cases.

Clinical Features

The absence of ganglion cells interrupts the normal propagation of colonic peristalsis. Patients with Hirschsprung's disease fail to pass meconium in the first 48 hours of life. They may present with abdominal distention, bilious vomiting, or enterocolitis. Over 80% of patients present within the first 6 weeks in life. Hirschsprung's disease is about three to four times as common in boys as in girls. Older children may present with chronic constipation. Hirschsprung's disease can be complicated by life-threatening enterocolitis which presents with diarrhea, abdominal distention and fever and may progress to perforation with peritonitis.[3]

Imaging Features

Plain films may demonstrate features of distal bowel obstruction. However, a dilated colon proximal to the distal and smaller aganglionic segment is the more typical finding **(Fig. 26)**. A small gas-filled rectum can be seen, especially on prone films and may help in the diagnosis. The absence of rectal gas is not specific for Hirschsprung's disease as it is commonly seen in infants with sepsis and necrotizing enterocolitis.[21] At times, the bowel pattern may

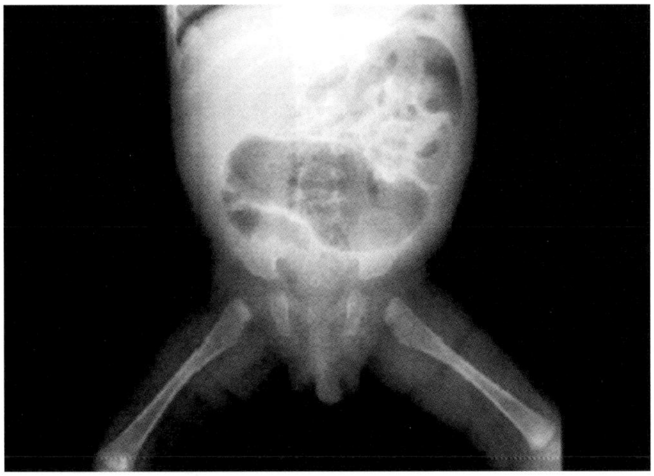

Fig. 26: Plain X-ray abdomen showing a dilated proximal sigmoid colon with a smaller distal sigmoid with relatively little rectal gas in a neonate with Hirschsprung's disease.

appear normal. Less commonly (4%), pneumoperitoneum may be seen in patients with long segment or total colonic disease secondary to colonic perforation.

The radiographic diagnosis is made by contrast enema and is directed towards identifying the transition zone which is the most specific sign of Hirschsprung's disease. This is where the normal-sized, distal aganglionic bowel changes in caliber to join the proximal ganglionic bowel.[3] This findings may not be obvious in the newborn, hence, careful attention should be given to the technique of performing barium enema.

Barium enema is performed on an unprepared patient by inserting a straight-tipped catheter to a point just beyond the anal sphincter. Balloon catheters are not used to avoid expanding a narrow segment of aganglionic colon, and may thus obscure the diagnosis. There is also risk of perforation of the stiff aganglionic rectum.[24] Barium contrast should be prepared with normal saline to avoid possibility of water absorption from the large surface area of dilated colon.[29] With the patient in the lateral position, barium suspension is introduced slowly by gravity drip infusion, under fluoroscopic monitoring. The infusion is stopped and restarted as serial spot radiographs are obtained. As filling progresses into the descending colon, the patient is rolled into the supine position. If the examination is positive, the diagnosis in most cases is made by the time the barium fills the proximal descending colon. Rapid infusion of barium suspension can distend and mask the transition zone. When the transition zone is observed, the examination should be discontinued because filling of the more proximal dialated bowel beyond the transition zone may lead to impaction. However, the distention of the bowel, proximal to the aganglionic segent is gradual, and a transition zone is seen in only 50% of neonates during the first week of life.[28]

The transition zone generally is funnel-shaped and it is an important diagnostic feature. In some instances, the transformation from dilated bowel to narrowed bowel is abrupt **(Fig. 27)**. In other cases, the funneling of the bowel occurs incrementally over a long segment of bowel to appear almost imperceptible because of the gradual change in caliber. In long segment Hirschsprung's disease, a variable portion of the colon proximal to the sigmoid colon is aganglionic **(Fig. 28)**. The pathological transition zone is usually somewhat more proximal than the radiographical one. Under fluoroscopic visualization, irregular saw-toothed mucosal pattern may be seen due to disordered contractions in the aganglionic colon **(Fig. 29)**. Another radiographic appearance of Hirschsprung's disease that has been described in neonates and young infants in whom the rectosigmoid region appears normal, is the presence of straight transverse bands in the involved segment of colon. These bands are thought to represent areas of persistent spasm.[12]

The rectosigmoid index can be used in the diagnosis of Hirschsprung's disease confined to the rectum. This compares the ratio of the rectal diameter to the sigmoid diameter and is considered abnormal, if the sigmoid colon is more dilated than the rectum (R/S index <1).[3]

The immediate postevacuation film may be useful in identifying the collapsed distal aganglionic segment. Delayed radiographs taken after 24 hours may show prolonged retention of barium, which is a strong indicator of Hirschsprung's disease when enema findings have been inconclusive **(Figs. 30A and B)**. Other signs observed in Hirschsprung's disease are contrast media mixed with stool or a more obvious transition zone than seen on immediate films.[3]

In total colonic Hirschsprung's disease, barium enema may be non-diagnostic with no discordant sizes in the distal large bowel. A useful sign is a colon that is shortened with flexures pulled down and rounded in appearance (question mark colon) A true microcolon appearance similar to that seen in distal ileal atresia is rare.[5]

Confirmation of Hirschsprung's disease is by means of a suction biopsy which should be taken 2 cm above the dentate line, as below this line the normal anus shows relative hypoganglionosis. Contrast enema can be safely performed 24 hours after a suction biopsy, though ideally the enema should precede a biopsy.[3]

In equivocal cases, further investigation which may help is anorectal manometry. This relies on anal sphincter

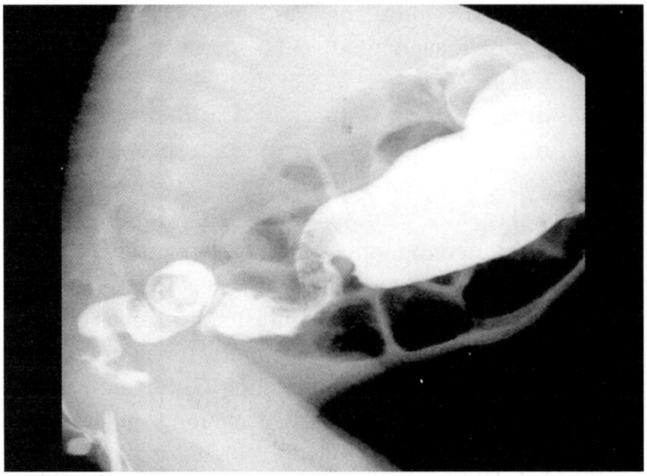

Fig. 27: *Hirschsprung's disease:* Barium enema shows an abrupt transition from the narrow caliber rectosigmoid (aganglionic) to the larger caliber more proximal sigmoid colon.

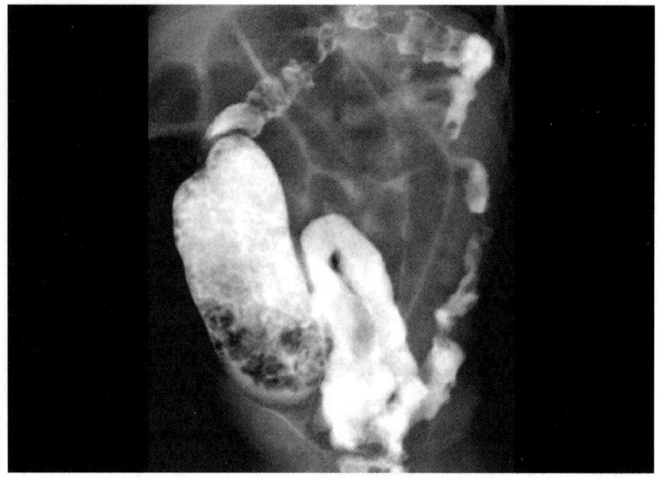

Fig. 28: Barium enema reveals a colon of reduced caliber from rectum to hepatic flexure with markedly dilated colon (cecum and ascending colon) proximal to it—long segment aganglionosis.

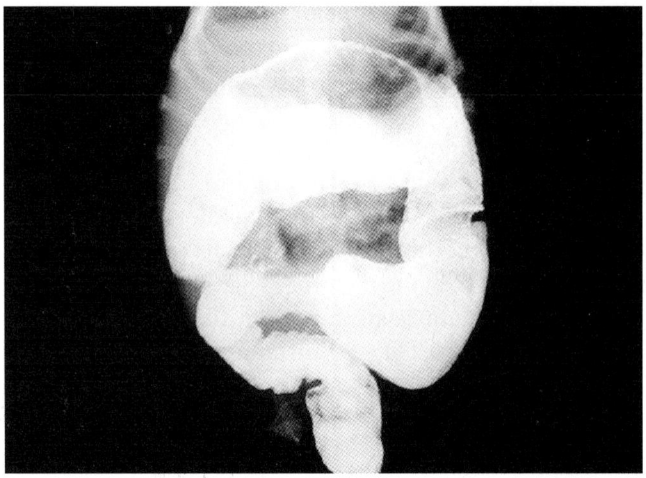

Fig. 29: Colonic aganglionosis with transition zone in sigmoid colon showing irregular mucosal outline/contractions.

reflex relaxation in response to distention of the rectum and is absent in patients with Hirschsprung's disease.

Enterecolitis is a major cause of death in patients with Hirschsprung's disease, with enema contraindicated in these patients.

Surgical treatment of Hirschsprung's disease consists of resection of the aganglionic segment, confirmation of ganglia in the proximal bowel and reanastomosis of the bowel.

Functional Immaturity of the Colon/Neonatal Functional Colonic Obstruction

Functional immaturity of the colon is a common cause of neonatal obstruction, especially in premature babies. It comprises of several entities, most common being *small left colon syndrome* and *meconium plug syndrome.*[28] Its exact etiology is not known and it is thought to be associated with functional immaturity of the ganglion cells of the colon. The babies are frequently infants of diabetic mothers or mothers who have received magnesium sulfate for eclampsia.

Clinical Features

In general, babies with functional immaturity of the colon are not sick as compared to other babies presenting with low intestinal obstruction.[24]

Most infants present within the first 24–36 hours of life with abdominal distention, biliary emesis and failure to initiate the normal passage of meconium. This is due to transient colonic inertia with failure of normal peristalsis in a normally innervated colon.[12]

Plain radiography findings are nonspecific, showing distal bowel obstruction with no gas seen in the distal colon or rectum.[3] Both the conditions causing neonatal functional colonic obstruction will be dealt separately.

Meconium Plug Syndrome

This is the most frequent cause of delayed passage of meconium in infants. Contrast enema performed is both diagnostic and therapeutic in such infants. Low osmolal contrast should be used with careful attention of hydration of the neonate.

The colon is usually of normal caliber. The meconium plug occupies the rectosigmoid region, but may extend throughout the colon. A normal evacuation pattern is

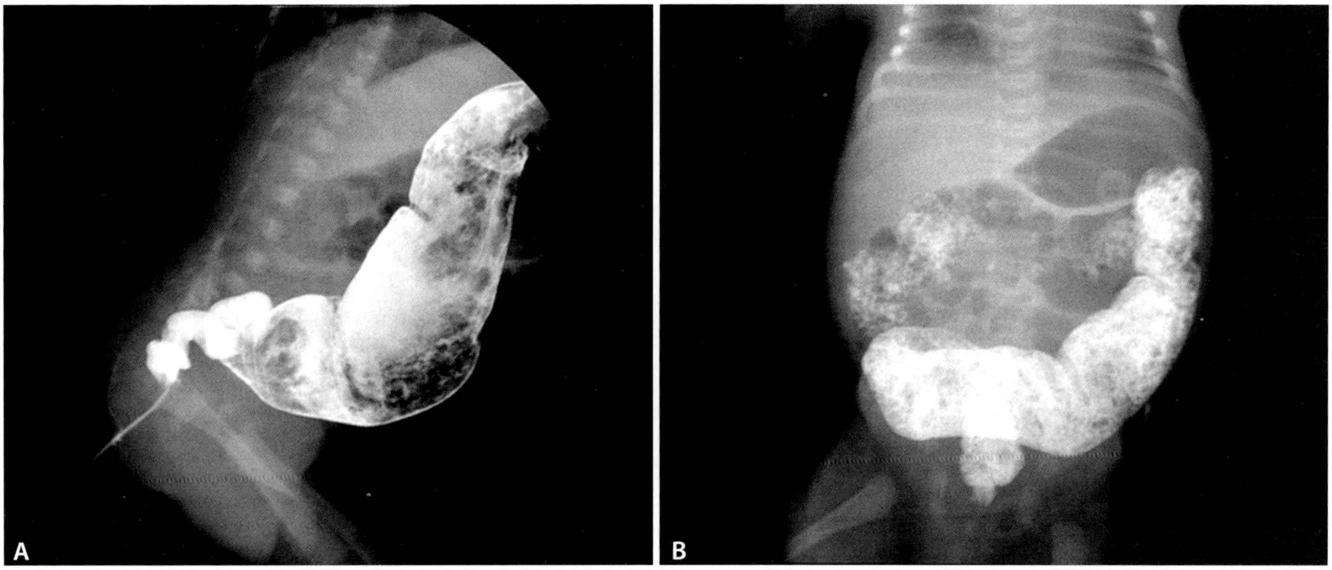

Figs. 30A and B: (A) Short segment Hirschsprung's disease with aganglionosis of rectum and distal sigmoid and marked dilatation proximal to it; (B) 24 hours film showing significant retention of barium.

Table 2: Differentiating features between small left colon syndrome and Hirschsprung's disease.

Points of difference	*Small left colon syndrome*	*Hirschsprung's disease*
1. Change in caliber/transition	Usually at splenic flexure, with proximal distended right colon and transverse colon	Transition usually more distal, most commonly at rectosigmoid
2. Type of transition	Abrupt change in caliber	Cone-shaped and gradual change
3. Caliber of involved segment	Left colon is usually smaller in caliber than normal colon	Near normal caliber of aganglionic colon
4. Rectum	In most patients, rectum is quite distensible	The aganglionic colon is of uniform caliber to the anus

established following stimulation of rectum by enema or occasionally digital examination.[3]

Meconium plug syndrome needs to be differentiated from meconium ileus. The term meconium ileus is reserved for bowel obstruction secondary to inspissated meconium in the distal small bowel and proximal colon, most often seen in patients of cystic fibrosis.[3]

Small Left Colon Syndrome

In this, the contrast enema demonstrates a distended right and transverse colon with transition to a very small diameter descending and rectosigmoid colon, occurring near the splenic flexure, with the rectum being quite distensible. Typically, there is improvement in the clinical and radiological finding over the next few hours or days. The condition may mimic Hirschsprung's disease, but there are several findings which help in differentiating the two **(Table 2)**.[2]

It is important to follow the patients closely, because if they have Hirschsprung's disease, they will return with intestinal problems like constipation or diarrhea.[12] At times, distinction between the two is not possible and a rectal biopsy should be performed in those children in whom the symptoms do not resolve.[24]

CONCLUSION

Imaging plays an important role in most neonatal as well as childhood developmental lesions of the gastrointestinal tract, which usually present with obstruction. The role of imaging may vary from establishment of diagnosis, evaluation of associated abnormalities, surgical planning or therapy for some conditions. Plain radiographs and contrast examinations serve as primary imaging modalities. CT and MR imaging help in more complex cases as they provide excellent anatomical detail.

Plain radiographs are often diagnostic in neonates with complete gastric and duodenal atresia and generally do not require any further radiological investigation. An upper GI contrast study should be performed in all patients presenting with incomplete intestinal obstruction.

Ultrasound is useful in evaluating developmental lesions such as hypertrophic pyloric stenosis, entertic duplication cysts, midgut malrotation, meconium ileus and meconium peritonitis.[21]

It is important to be familiar with the role and usefulness of various imaging modalities so that they can be used judiciously. The aim of every radiological study is to obtain maximum possible information while avoiding unnecessary radiation exposure and minimizing patient discomfort.

REFERENCES

1. Silverman FN, Kuhn (Eds). The gastrointestinal tract. Caffey's Pediatric X-ray Diagnosis: An Integrated Imaging Approach Mosby, 1993.
2. Hernanz-Schulman M. Imaging of neonatal gastrointestinal obstruction. Radiol Clin North Am. 1999;37:1163.
3. Donohue V, Twomey EL. The neonatal and non-neonatal gastrointestinal tract. Carty H, Brunelle F, Stringer DA Kazo Simon CS (Eds). Imaging Children, 2nd edition. Elsevier Churchill Livingstone. 2005;2:1305-528.
4. Leonidas JC, Singh SP, Slovis TL. Congenital anomalies of the gastrointestinal tract. In: Kuhn Jerald P, Slovis Thomas L, Haller Jack O (Eds): Caffey's Pediatric Diagnostic Imaging, 10th edition, Mosby. 2004;1:113-62.
5. McAlister WH, Kronemer KA. Emergency gastrointestinal radiology of the newborn. Radiol Clin North Am. 1996;34:819.
6. Ein SH, Shandling B. Pure esophageal atresia: A 50-year review. J Pediatr Surg. 1994;29:1208.
7. Iuchtman M, Brereton RJ, Spitz L, et al. Morbidity and mortality in 46 patients with the VACTERL association. Isr J Med Sci. 1992;28:281.
8. Schlesinger AE, Parker BR. Abdomen and gastrointestinal tract. In: Kuhn JP Slovis TL, Haller JO (Eds). Caffey's Pediatric Diagnostic Imaging volume 2, 10th edition, Mosby. Section VI 2004.pp.1421-690.
9. Ratan SK, Varshney A, Mullick S, Saxena NC. Evaluation of neonates with esophageal atresia using chest CT Scan. Pediatr Surg Int. 2004;20:757-61.
10. Ou P, Seror E, Layouss W, Revillon Y, Brunelle F. Definitive diagnosis and surgical planning of H-type tracheoesophageal fistula in a critically ill neonate: First experience using air distension of the esophagus during high-resolution computed tomography acquisition. J Thorac Cardiovasc Surg. 2007; 133:1116-7.
11. Berrocal T, Torres I, Gutierrez J, Prietio C, del Hoyo ML, Lamas M. Congential anomalies of the upper gastrointestinal tract. Radiographics. 1999;19(4):855-72.
12. Swischuk, LE. Alimentary tract. In: Swischurk LE (Ed). Imaging of the Newborn, Infant and Young Child, 5th edition Lippincott Williams and Wilkims. 2004.pp.341-482.
13. Schulman MH. Infantile hypertrophic pyloric stenosis. Radiology. 2003;227:319-31.
14. Chung E. Infantile hypertrophic pylotic stenosis: Genes and environment. Arch Dis Child. 2008;93:1003-4.
15. Haller JO, Cohen HL. Hypertrophic pyloric stenosis: Diagnosis using ultrasound. Radiology. 1986;161:335.
16. Hayden CK Jr, Swischuk LE, Lobe TE, et al. Ultrasound: The definitive imaging modality in pyloric stenosis. Radiographics. 1984;4:517.
17. Amodio J, Fefferman N. Ultrasound of pediatric abdominal and scrotal emergencies. Applied Radiology. 2007;36(12): 22-9.
18. Blumhagen JD, Maclin L, Krauter D, et al. Sonographic diagnosis of hypertrophic pyloric stenosis. Am J Roentgenol. 1988;150:1367.
19. Hernanz-Schulman M, Sells LL, Ambrosino MM, et al. Hypertrophic pyloric stenosis in the infant without a palpable olive: Accuracy of sonographic diagnosis. Radiology. 1994;193:771.
20. O'Keeffe FN, Stansberry SD, Swischuk LE, et al. Antropyloric muscle thickness at US in infants: what is normal? Radiology. 1991;178:827.
21. Gupta AK, Guglani B. Imaging of congenital anomalies of the gastrointestinal tract. Indian J Pediatr. 2005;72(5):403-14.
22. Vaos G, Misiakos EP. Congenital anomalies of the gastro-inestinal tract diagnosed in adulthood: Diagnosis and management. J Gastrointest Surg. 2010;14:916-25.
23. Atwell JD, Levick P. Congenital hypertrophic pyloric stenosis and associated anomalies in the genitourinary tract. J Pediatr Surg. 1981;16:1029.
24. Buonomo C. Neonatal gastrointestinal emergencies. Radiol Clin North Am. 1997;35:845.
25. Bailey PV, Tracy TF, Connors RH, et al. Congenital duodenal obstruction: A 32-year review. J Pediatr Surg. 1993; 28:92.
26. Fonkalsrud E, de Lorimier A, Hays D. Congenital atresia and stenosis of the duodenum: A review compiled from the members of the surgical section of the American Academy of Pediatrics. Pediatrics. 1969.pp.43:79.
27. Pratt A. Current concepts of the obstructing duodenal diaphragm. Radiology. 1971;100:637.
28. Berrocal T, Lamas M, Gutierrez J, Torres I, Prieto C, del Hoyo ML. Congenital anomalies of the small intestine, colon and rectum. Radiographics. 1999;19(5):1219-36.
29. Thomas KE Owens CM. The pediatric abdomen. In: Sutton D (Ed). Textbook of Radiology and Imaging Volume 1, 7th edition. Churchill Livingstone. 2002.pp.849-84.
30. Macari M, Balthazar EJ. The acute right lower quadrant: CT evaluation. Radiol Clin North Am. 2003;41:1117-36.
31. Macpherson RI. Gastrointestinal tract duplications: Clinical, pathologic, etiologic and radiologic considerations. Radiographics. 1993;13:1063.
32. Barr LL, Hayden CK Jr, Stansberry SD, et al. Enteric duplication cysts in children: Are their ultrasonographic wall characteristics diagnostic? Pediatr Radiol. 1990;20:326.
33. O' Donnell AM, Puri. Skip segment Hirschsprung's disease: A systematic review. Pediatr Surg Int. Published online 17th Aug. 2010.

CHAPTER 135

Imaging of Anorectal Anomalies

Arun Kumar Gupta

Anorectal anomalies (ARA) are rare with an incidence of approximately 1 in 5,000 births. They have a male preponderance.

EMBRYOLOGY OF THE CLOACA RELATED TO ARA

Embryology of the cloaca can be described under internal and external cloaca.

Internal Cloaca

It is an endodermal reservoir which is in contact with the surface ectoderm at the cloacal membrane. At present, there is a general agreement that the division of internal cloaca occurs in two stages (Tourneux's method), i.e. a combination of craniocaudal extension of the urorectal septum and lateral ingrowths of the mesenchyma. Most of the ARA can be explained by this mechanism of combined division.

External Cloaca

On the other hand, external cloaca refers to the partitioning of the proctodeal pit, the perineum and the genital folds. Essentially, the rectal group of ARA consists of those abnormalities which are intrinsic in the partitioning of the internal cloaca, whereas aberrations in the external cloacal division results in the anal group of malformations.

CLASSIFICATION

Two major classifications presently in use are the following:

1. International classification, 1970 **(Table 1)**
2. Wingspread classification, 1984 **(Table 2)**

International classification was considered by some to be too detailed and too complex. A simplified version of it was, therefore, considered and is known by the name of Wingspread classification (so called because the meeting to decide it was held at the Wingspread convention center in Racine, Wisconsin).

In the author's experience, if one is dealing with a large number of ARA in a major hospital, then use of international classification is essential. On the other hand for general teaching and occasional encounter with these patients, Wingspread classification should be adequate.

INFORMATION REQUIRED IN A PATIENT OF ARA

Four major answers, one is looking for, are the following:

1. Level of the blind terminal bowel and of any fistula, if present.
2. Levator muscle mass status.
3. Associated congenital anomalies.
4. Nerve supply status to the levator muscle group.

The last one is assessed by clinical tests while the rest are evaluated by imaging.

Table 1: Anorectal anomalies: International classification (1970).

Level	*Male*	*Female*
High anomalies	1. *Anorectal agenesis:* a. Without fistula b. *With fistula:* i. Rectovesical ii. Rectoprostatic urethral (including H or N type) 2. Rectal atresia	1. *Anorectal agenesis:* a. Without fistula b. *With fistula:* i. Rectovesical ii. Cloacal anomalies iii. Rectovaginal (high) 2. Rectal atresia
Intermediate anomalies	1. *Anal agenesis:* a. Without fistula b. *With fistula:* i. Rectobulbar 2. Anorectal stenosis	1. *Anal agenesis:* a. Without fistula b. *With fistula:* i. Rectovaginal (low) ii. Rectovestibular 2. Anorectal stenosis
Low anomalies	1. *At normal anal site:* a. Covered anus, complete b. Anal stenosis 2. *At perineal site:* a. Anterior perineal anus b. Anocutaneous fistula	1. *At normal anal site:* a. Covered anus, complete b. Anal stenosis 2. *At perineal site:* a. Anterior perineal anus b. Anocutaneous fistula 3. *At vulvar site:* a. Anovestibular fistula b. Vulvar anus c. Anovulvar anus

Table 2: Anorectal anomalies: Wingspread classification.

Level	*Male*	*Female*
High anomalies	1. *Anorectal agenesis:* a. Without fistula b. With rectoprostatic urethral fistula 2. Rectal atresia	1. *Anorectal agenesis:* a. Without fistula b. With rectovaginal fistula 2. Rectal atresia
Intermediate anomalies	1. Anal agenesis without fistula 2. Rectobulbar urethral fistula	1. Anal agenesis without fistula 2. Rectovaginal fistula 3. Rectovestibular fistula
Low anomalies	1. Anocutaneous fistula 2. Anal stenosis	1. Anovestibular fistula 2. Anocutaneous fistula 3. Anal stenosis
Cloacal malformations	Rare	Rare

CLINICAL CLUES

Males

Perineum should be carefully scrutinized for any orifice. Visible orifice suggests an anal translevator anomaly (exception—rectal atresia). External orifice may be located anywhere from the normal anal site to the tip of penis.

In the absence of a perineal orifice, level of the anomaly is difficult to predict although the majority will be rectal lesions. In these patients, urine may be examined next (after collection and not catheterization) for meconium or squamous epithelial cells. In the absence of meconium an invertogram should be done while presence of meconium in urine requires a defunctioning colostomy.

Females

Noncommunicating anomalies occur rarely in females. Careful examination for the site and number of orifices must be made.

If only one orifice is present, then it indicates a cloacal anomaly with a common cloaca for the urethra, vagina and rectum. Colostomy is required.

If two orifices are visible in the vulva with no anal orifice, then one of them is of the urethral, while the other one is of the vaginal orifice. Meconiun would come from the latter due to the associated rectovaginal fistula. Colostomy is again indicated.

If three orifices are visible, then two of them are respectively, of the urethra and the vagina, both at their normal site, while the third one is the bowel which could be at the normal anal site, or it might open as a fistulous track anteriorly at an abnormal site—either in the perineum or in the vestibule.

IMAGING WORK-UP

During the imaging of a case with ARA, one or more of a number of investigations can be carried out—invertography; contrast opacification of the urinary tract, fistula or colon; ultrasound; CT and MRI scan. All these investigations are complementary, providing information regarding different facets of the complex problem of ARA.

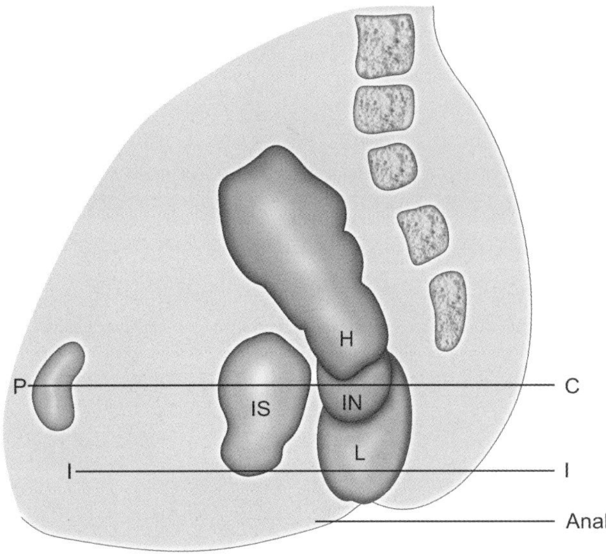

Fig. 1: Line drawing showing high (H), intermediate (IN) and low (L) anomalies and their relationship to pubococcygeal (PC) and ischial (I) lines.

Invertography

Invertography was first described by Wangensteen and Rice in 1930.[1]

Technique: Six to eight hours after the birth, a newborn baby with ARA should be held upside down for at least 3 minutes, and then a strict lateral view (in this upside down position) is taken with the thighs of the baby flexed at hip, and beam accurately centered on the greater trochanter. Anal dimple and the natal cleft should be outlined by barium paste. In a correctly taken radiograph: (i) both the ischial bones would accurately superimpose, and (ii) the terminal blind bowel will be rounded and well-distended. Interpretation of an invertogram should be attempted only, if both these features are present otherwise it may be fallacious.

Interpretation: Basic purpose of invertography is to identify the relationship of the gas bubble in the blind pouch to the bony pelvis, which in turn indicates the relation to the levator ani muscle complex. Information contained in an invertogram can be interpreted in two ways:

1. By using three lines, a concept which was first put forward by Stephens and Smith (1971).[2] The three lines are: (i) PC (pubococcygeal) line, (ii) the I (ischial) line or I point, and (iii) the anal pit line **(Fig. 1)**. A gas bubble situated above the PC line is designated "high" anomaly, one located between the PC and I line or point "Intermediate" anomaly, and if it extends below the I line (point), then it is called "low" anomaly **(Figs. 2A to C)**.
2. However, Cremin (1971)[3] did not find PC line very accurate. They proposed a "M line" or "M point", which is located at the junction of upper two-third and lower one-third of the ischium **(Figs. 2A to C)**. Anomalies are then divided into "high" and "low" types with no intermediate category.

Accuracy of invertography to differentiate supralevator (gas bubble above the I line or point) and infralevator lesions (gas bubble below the I line or point) has been reported to range from 60 to 87%. One must be aware of the potential pitfalls of this technique in order to avoid misdiagnosis. Some of the common reasons are listed here:

- Insufficient time for the gas to reach the terminal bowel.
- Meconium blocking the terminal segment.
- In a crying child, puborectalis sling may move significantly up or down giving erroneous results.
- Gas may escape through a fistula.
- Improper technique—in positioning, centering or marker placement.

Besides the conventional upside down invertography described earlier, two more methods have been described to obtain the same information. They are as follows:

- Prone cross table lateral view (Narasimharao et al, 1983).[4]
- CT invertography (Leighton and de Campo, 1989).[5]

During the reading of an invertogram, besides evaluating the level of bowel gas, one should also look for the following:

- Spine congenital anomalies of the spine are common.
- Presence of gas in the region of urinary bladder and vagina, which would indicate an underlying fistula.

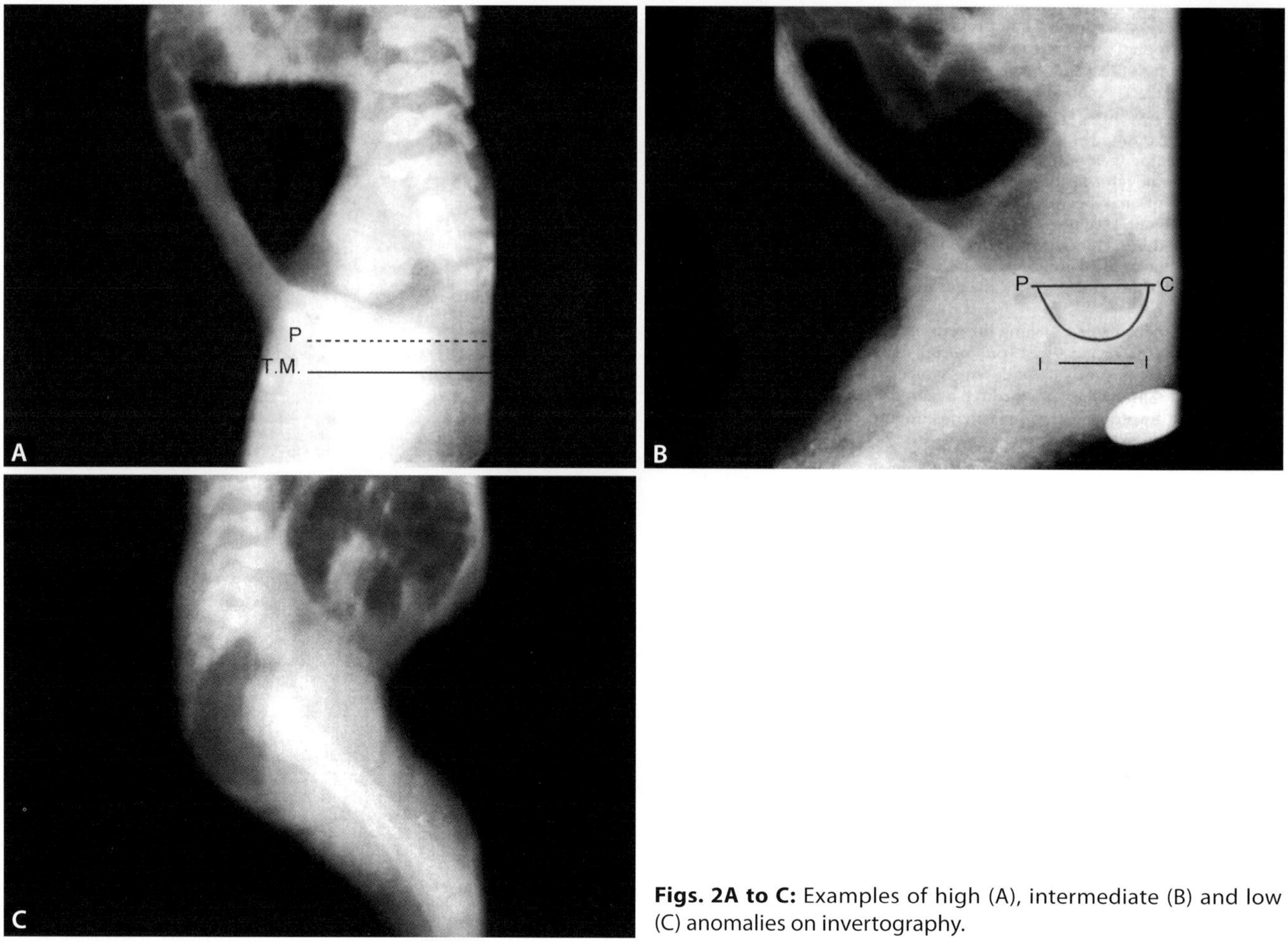

Figs. 2A to C: Examples of high (A), intermediate (B) and low (C) anomalies on invertography.

Contrast Studies

Purpose of any contrast study is:

- To confirm the level of blind bowel pouch, and
- To document the presence (or absence) and level of the fistula between the GI (gastrointestinal) and the GU (genitourinary) system.

Contrast Studies in Males

1. *Retrograde urethrography (RGU)/micturating cysto-urethrography (MCU):* Prior to or even after the colostomy, RGU is a good technique to demonstrate the fistula. If negative, then RGU is followed by MCU in the same sitting to demonstrate the possible fistula.
2. *Distal cologram:* Once colostomy has already been done, then distal cologram, in the author's experience, is a reliable technique to demonstrate the fistula. Fluoroscopy with image intensifier, use of water-soluble contrast media and raising the intraluminal pressure in the distal colon to fill the fistula more consistently are some of the pre-requisites in this technique. In a case with colostomy, distal cologram should be done first, and only if it is negative in demonstrating the fistula, then RGU/MCU should be done in the same sitting.

   Sometimes the fistula is not documented inpite of all the efforts but on RGU, an acute backward angulation of the posterior urethra and on colography an anteroinferior "beaking" of the blind rectal pouch is seen **(Figs. 3A and B)**—these findings suggest the presence of fistula or adhesion.
3. *Direct catheterization:* If a patient has a cutaneous fistula, then direct catheterization and retrograde injection of contrast into the fistula should be carried out. However, urethra and bladder should be first outlined with a catheter (filled with radiopaque contrast) in situ.

ANORECTAL ANOMALIES IN MALES

These are discussed under high, intermediate and low anomalies.

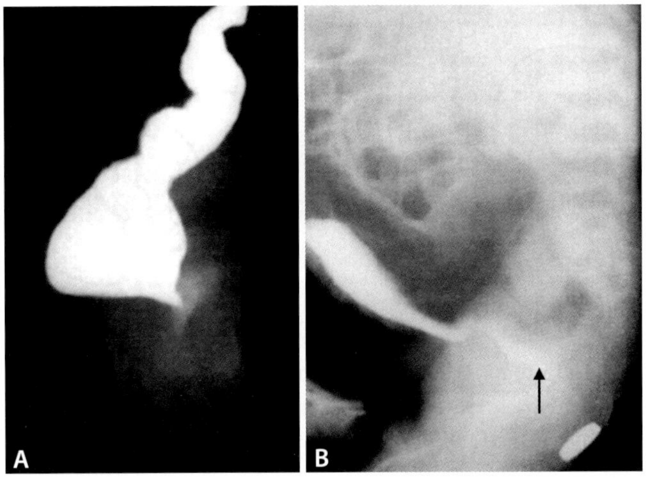

Figs. 3A and B: "Beaking" from anteroinferior angle of blind rectal pouch on colography (A) and "acute backward angulation" (arrow) of posterior urethra on RGU (retrograde urethrography) (B) without actually filling the fistula, indicating presence of underlying fistula or adhesion.

High Anomalies

In these patients, the imperforate bowel or its fistulous connection lies above the puborectalis sling of the levator ani muscle. Various types described under this group are the following:

Anorectal Agenesis without Fistula

Anorectal agenesis without fistula is uncommon. Invertography and contrast studies would show the blind rectal pouch lying at or cranial to the PC line with no suggestion or demonstration of a fistula.

Anorectal Agenesis with Rectoprostatic Urethral Fistula

Anorectal agenesis with rectoprostatic urethral fistula is the most common type in this group. Most common site of fistulous opening is at the level of the verumontanum, but rarely it may open either more cranially closer to the bladder neck or more distally just above the bulb **(Figs. 4A and B)**.

H or N Type of Rectoprostatic Urethral Fistula

H or N type of rectoprostatic urethral fistula is extremely rare. This entity was not even described in the original International classification. There is a H or N-shaped fistulous connection between the prostatic urethra and the anterior wall of the rectum just cranial to the valves. Characteristically, urethra distal to the site of fistula is usually stenotic **(Figs. 5A and B)**.

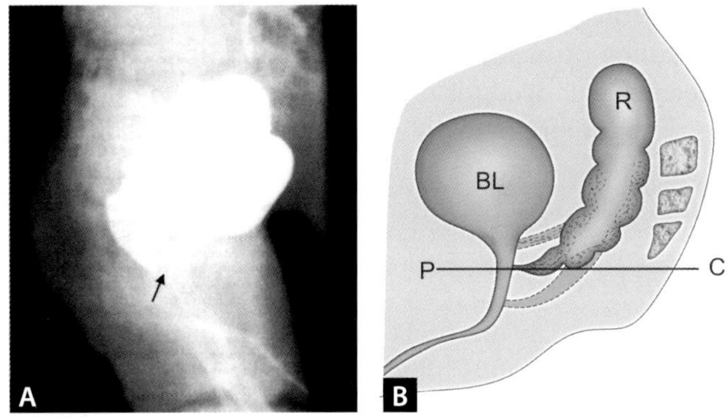

Figs. 4A and B: Rectoprostatic urethral fistula—schematic drawing (A) and a case (B). As indicated by dotted lines fistula may enter either more cranial or distal to verumontanum (arrow—fistula).

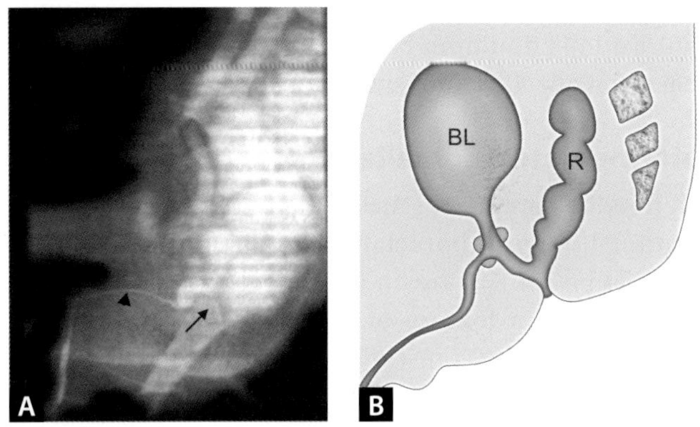

Figs. 5A and B: H or N fistula is extremely rare—note the patent anal canal and the microcaliber of the penile urethra (arrowhead—fistula, arrow—narrow penile urethra).

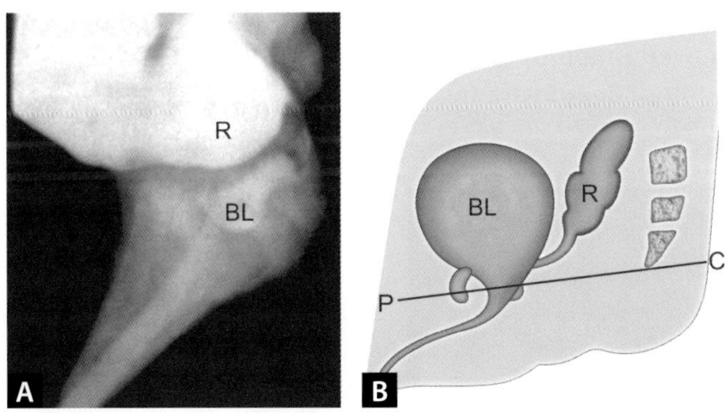

Figs. 6A and B: Rectovesical fistula—another rare type filling on distal colography—note the filling of urinary bladder immediately after opacification of the rectum (arrowhead—fistula).

Rectovesical Fistula

Rectovesical fistula is also rare. Fistulous tract usually enters close to the bladder base. During contrast injection into the distal colon via colostomy site, urinary bladder would fill first **(Figs. 6A and B)** without opacifying the urethra, thereby, excluding a urethral fistula. This sequence of events must be carefully monitored and specifically looked for real time on the image intensifier. It is very important to differentiate this type of fistula from the rare more cranially located rectoprostatic urethral fistula by the observations described earlier.

Rectal Atresia

It is a rare and an unusual condition. In these patients, the terminal bowel ends blindly at varying levels. Anus and the anal canal are normal and the bowel in between these two segments is deficient (either a short membranous or a long, string-like) **(Fig. 7A)**. Its etiopathogenesis is believed to be a vascular insult after the formation of a normal rectum. Complete documentation in such cases require contrast injection from both ends (i.e. distal cologram + anal canal opacification) simultaneously **(Fig. 7B)**.

Intermediate Anomalies

Intermediate anomalies are termed so due to a complex relationship to puborectalis muscle. Thus, the blind terminal bowel is lying on (i.e. above) the puborectalis sling muscle, a feature of "high" anomalies, but the fistulous track when present is within or through the sling, a criterion for diagnosing "low" anomalies. Thus, features of both the "high" and the "low" anomalies are present in this group of anomalies.

Anal Agenesis without Fistula

Invertography and distal cologram would reveal the blind bowel pouch to lie between the PC line and the I point without demonstrating a fistula.

Anal Agenesis with Rectobulbar Urethral Fistula

Two types are described **(Fig. 8A)**—either the fistula is short, wide and enters the posterior surface of the bulb directly **(Fig. 8B)**, or it is long, thin, passing distally within the cavernous tissues of the penis in midline to enter on the undersurface of the urethra.

Anorectal Stenosis

Anorectal stenosis is rare. It is generally agreed that "anal stenosis" should be classified under the low anomalies while stenosis occurring up to 4 cm within the anus are more appropriate to be termed "anorectal stenosis". Mechanism of its formation is postulated to be ischemic and is thus similar to rectal atresia described earlier.

Low Anomalies

These are essentially "anal deformities". Various types are listed here:

1. Anocutaneous fistula (covered anus, incomplete)
2. Anterior perineal anus
3. Covered anal stenosis
4. Anal membrane stenosis
5. Covered anus, complete
6. Imperforate anal membrane

The entire group of low anomalies can be readily appreciated on the clinical examination itself, and imaging is usually not indicated. First two subtypes are briefly described below.

Anocutaneous Fistula

In this condition, the anal canal is of normal caliber till the level of anal valves beyond which it is suddenly

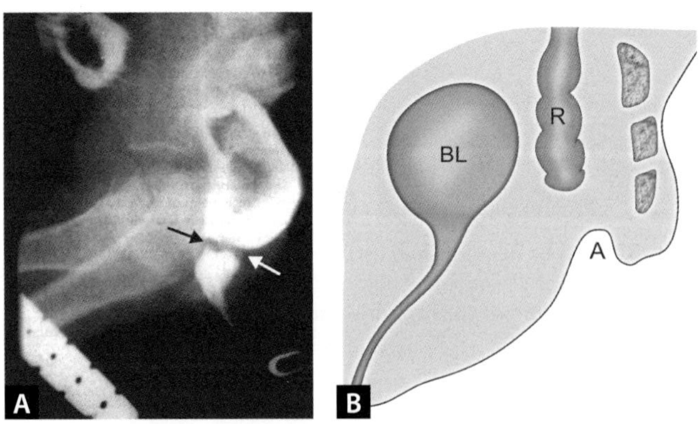

Figs. 7A and B: Rectal atresia—opacification was done from both ends of the site of atresia. One cm metallic scale helps in accurately measuring the distance of atretic bowel (arrows—atretic segment).

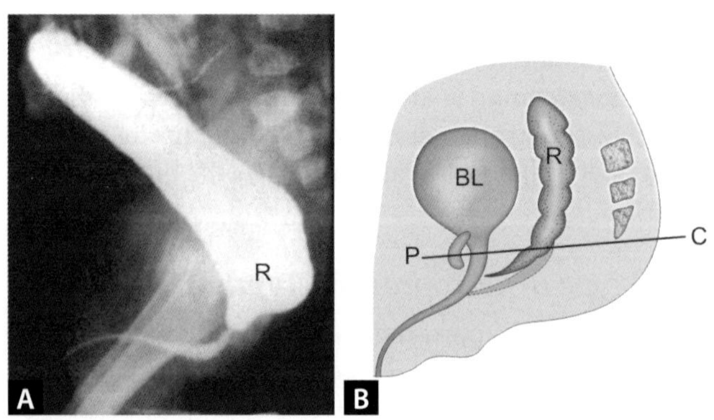

Figs. 8A and B: Rectobulbar urethral fistula—note short, wide fistula entering directly into the posterior wall of bulb of urethra. Other variety is long and narrow which enters into the under surface of penile urethra.

reduced to a tube of small caliber and runs forward covered by skin to open anywhere from the ventral surface of the penile shaft to an area adjacent to the anal site **(Figs. 9A and B)**. Although fistulogram is not necessary, but if required it can be readily carried out.

Anterior Perineal Anus

In this condition, anus is normal in appearance but is located more anteriorly than the normal site close to the posterior or membranous urethra. This is an important differential in the list of causes of constipation in children. On per rectal examination, "posterior shelf"—a characteristic finding of this condition might be felt which can also be demonstrated on barium enema examination **(Fig. 10)**. Cannula may distort the anal anatomy due to sheer mechanical pressure. Therefore, the catheter/cannula should be removed before the film is taken in strict lateral view at the time of barium defecation.

ANORECTAL ANOMALIES IN FEMALES

Anorectal anomalies are divided into high, intermediate and low types.

High Anomalies

Anorectal Agenesis without Fistula

Anorectal agenesis without fistula is rare and is similar to that seen in males, i.e. the blind terminal bowel lies above the PC line without any fistula.

Anorectal Agenesis with High Rectovaginal Fistula (Without a Urogenital Sinus Defect)

The vagina, urinary bladder and urethra are normal. Rectal fistula enters the posterior (dorsal) wall of the vagina **(Fig. 11A)**. Rectovaginal fistulae have been classified as "high" or "low" depending on the level of the terminal bowel, and these terms do not refer to the level of entry of fistula into the vagina.

Vaginogram or distal cologram following colostomy would readily demonstrate these fistulae **(Fig. 11B)**.

Cloacal Anomalies

This is a very large and one of the the most complex group of anomalies which is beyond the scope of this text. In these anomalies, there is only a single orifice for the urethra, vagina and rectum. A large number of subtypes based on the internal anatomy have been described. Retrograde injection of contrast through the external orifice as well as colography would delineate the internal

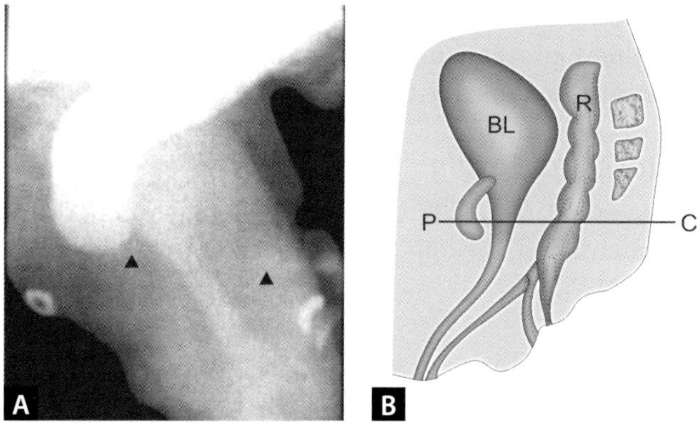

Figs. 9A and B: Rectocutaneous fistula (arrowheads)—fistula, as shown in schematic drawing, can open anywhere from near the anal opening to the tip of penis.

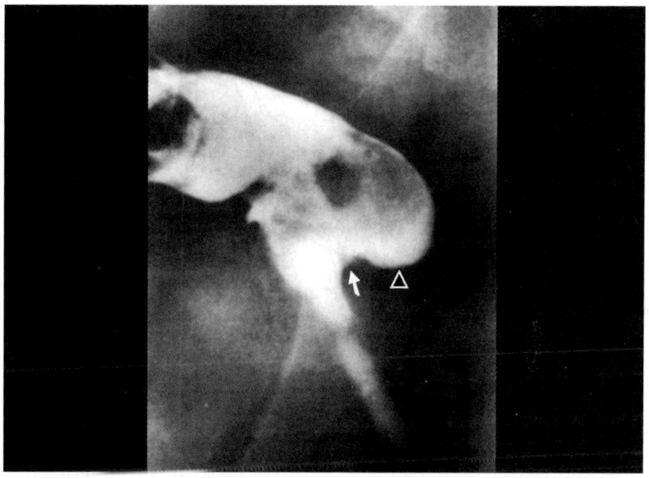

Fig. 10: Anterior perineal anus demonstrated on barium enema. Note the removal of cannula and posterior shelf (arrowhead).

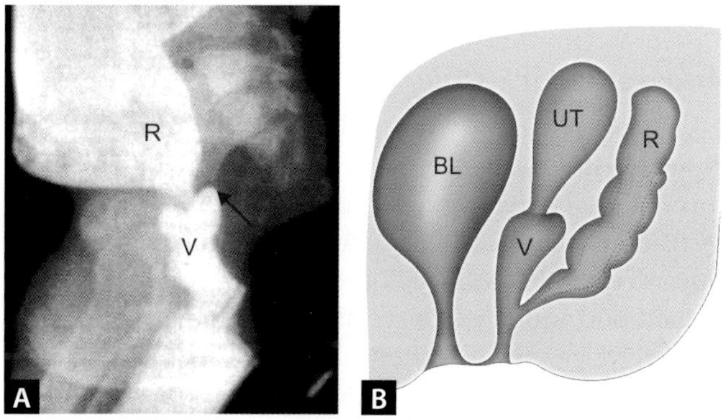

Figs. 11A and B: Rectovaginal fistula demonstrated on vaginogram. Difference in "high" and "low" rectovaginal fistulae lies in the level of blind bowel pouch and not on the site of entry of fistula into the vagina (R—rectum, V—vagina, BL—bladder, UT—Uterus).

anatomy **(Figs. 12A and B)**. Some of the most severe forms may present immediately after birth with acute respiratory distress due to a hugely dilated vagina.

Rectovesical Fistula

Rectovesical fistula is extremely rare in females. On documentation, the appearance is similar to that seen in males.

Rectal Atresia

Rectal atresia is similar to the lesions seen in males.

Intermediate Anomalies

Anal Agenesis without Fistula

Anal agenesis without fistula is easy to diagnose by inverted plain films of the abdomen especially taken in lateral views.

Rectovestibular Fistula

From the anterior wall of the rectum arises a fistula which opens in the vestibule. Usually, it is thin and long (more than 1 cm) **(Fig. 13A)**. Diagnosis is evident on clinical examination by noting three orifices in the vestibule and combining it with a gentle probe test. Retrograde injection of contrast would readily opacify the fistula and the rectum **(Fig. 13B)**.

Low Rectovaginal Fistula

Low rectovaginal fistula is very rare. Its difference from the high type has already been discussed earlier.

Low Anomalies

These are again designated as "anal deformities".

Anovestibular Fistula

Like rectovestibular fistula, it opens in the vestibule. However, its length is very short (less than 1 cm) and well-formed anal canal extends quite low down close to the skin at the anal site **(Fig. 14)**. A probe would pass not only upwards parallel to the vagina, but to some extent, it can be turned posteriorly just beneath the perineum. The latter maneuver cannot be achieved in rectovestibular fistula. Contrast study, if at all done, demonstrates the anatomy clearly.

Anocutaneous Fistula/Anterior Perineal Anus

Anocutaneous fistula/anterior perineal anus is similar to those observed in males.

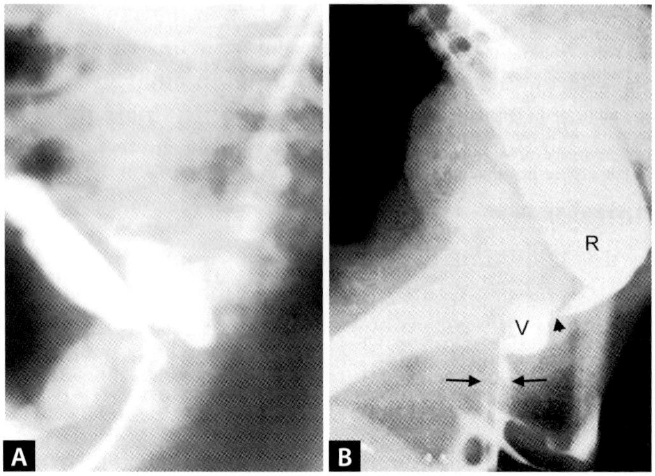

Figs. 12A and B: Cloacal anomalies—two different cases: (A) retrograde injection showing urethra and rectum only with absent vagina, and (B) One of the variants in which common channel leading into urethra and vagina (arrows) while rectum opening into the vagina (arrowhead).

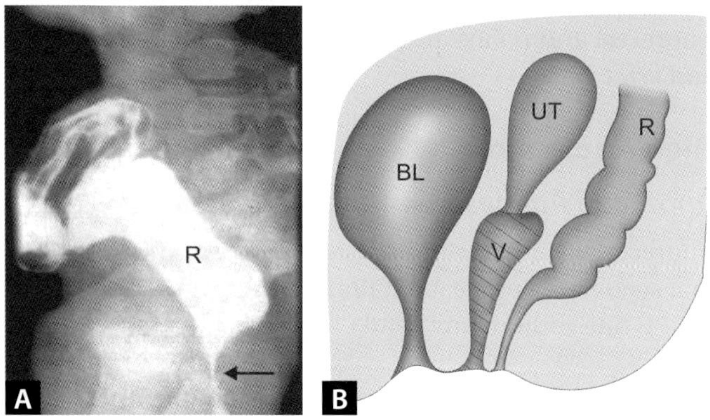

Figs. 13A and B: Rectovestibular fistula—demonstrated on retrograde contrast injection. Note the long, narrow fistulous track (arrow).

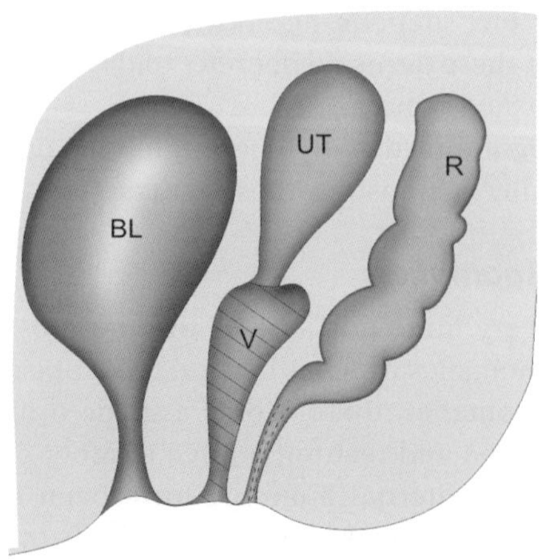

Fig. 14: Schematic drawing of anovestibular fistula.

Anal Stenosis

Anal stenosis is similar to the lesions in males.

INVESTIGATIONS

As the first step, a careful and detailed clinical examination is absolutely essential. This may provide a number of clues pointing to a specific type of the anomaly. This has been discussed earlier.

Invertography: Its role is similar to that described earlier in males.

Contrast studies: Noncommunicating anomalies are rare in females. Communication of the bowel may be either to the exterior and, therefore, visible as an abnormal orifice or internally into one of the pelvic viscus. Contrast studies can be carried out to demonstrate both the types.

OTHER INVESTIGATIONS

Besides the invertography and the conventional contrast studies, other newer imaging modalities have also an important role to play prior to as well as after the surgery.

Ultrasound

In spite of being an ideal imaging modality in the pediatric age group, i.e. its painless, requires no, contrast or sedation and without ionizing radiation, yet ultrasound has still not been established as a reliable technique. Reason is obvious—high incidence of fallacies and operator dependence. However, probably ultrasound still has potential in this clinical problem, and one should explore it before deciding its fate. It is, however, routinely used in screening the abdomen for the detection of congenital malformations, especially of the upper urinary tracts.

CT Scan

Computed tomography has established an important place in the work-up of ARA. It is used preoperatively to demonstrate the thickness of muscles (puborectalis sling and external anal sphincter) **(Figs. 15A and B)**.

In the postoperative period, it demonstrates the relationship of the pulled-through bowel (neorectum) to the above muscles (i.e. whether neorectum is central, eccentric or even outside the sling) and any evidence of fat drawn into the sling **(Fig. 16)**—all of these may be the reason for the incontinence in the postoperative period.

MRI Scan

With the introduction of MRI, not only has the visualization of the sphincter muscles become easy and better, but they can also be seen in multiple planes (axial, coronal and sagittal)—thereby allowing better understanding of the relationship of the bowel with the muscles. MRI has a tremendous potential in demonstrating the pelvic muscle anatomy with a very high degree of sensitivity and is used for obtaining the same information for which CT is otherwise used.

Relationship of Sacral Development and Levator Muscle Development

In order to determine the levator muscle mass prior to surgery, CT and MRI are routinely used. However, if these modalities are not available, then a good indicator is the development of the sacrum as seen on plain radiographs. It has been observed that:

- If sacrum is normal, then muscle mass and innervation are also normal;

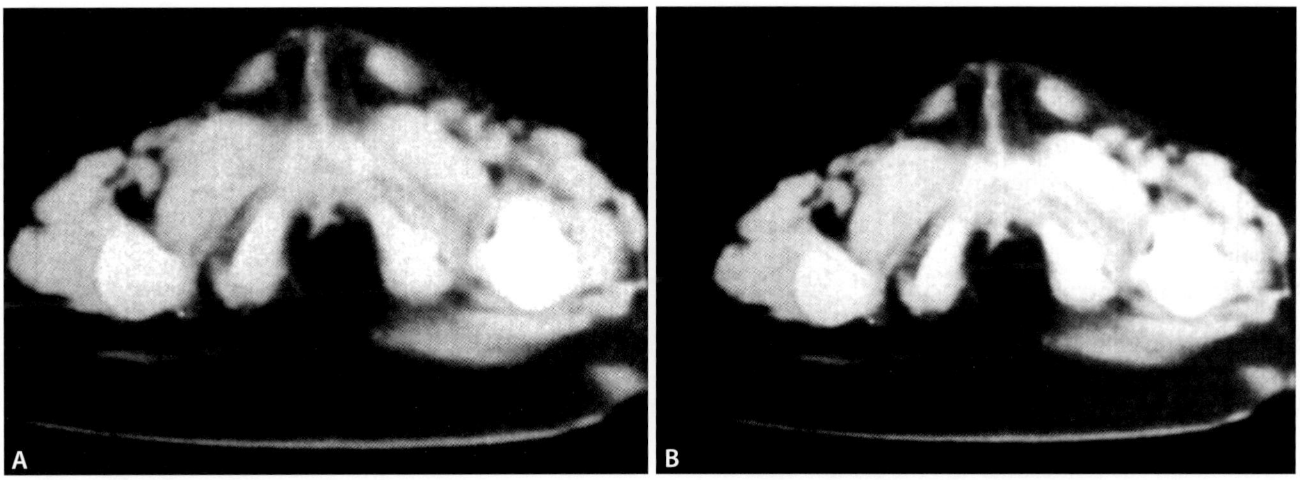

Figs. 15A and B: Pelvic CT, preoperative—puborectalis sling and external anal sphincter are very poorly formed.

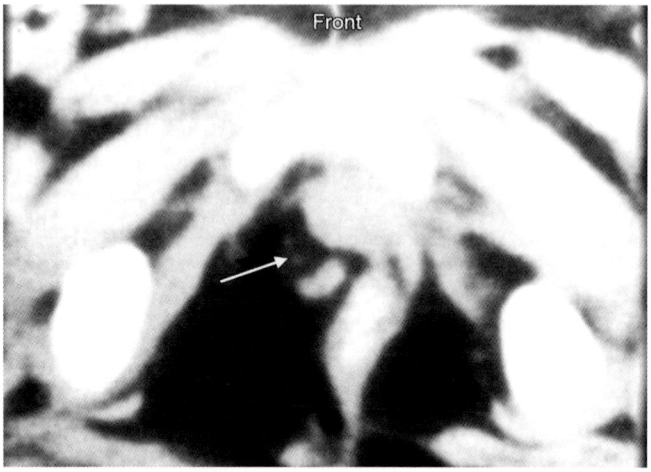

Fig. 16: Pelvic CT, postoperative—fat has been drawn along with the neorectum (arrow) which was the cause of incontinence.

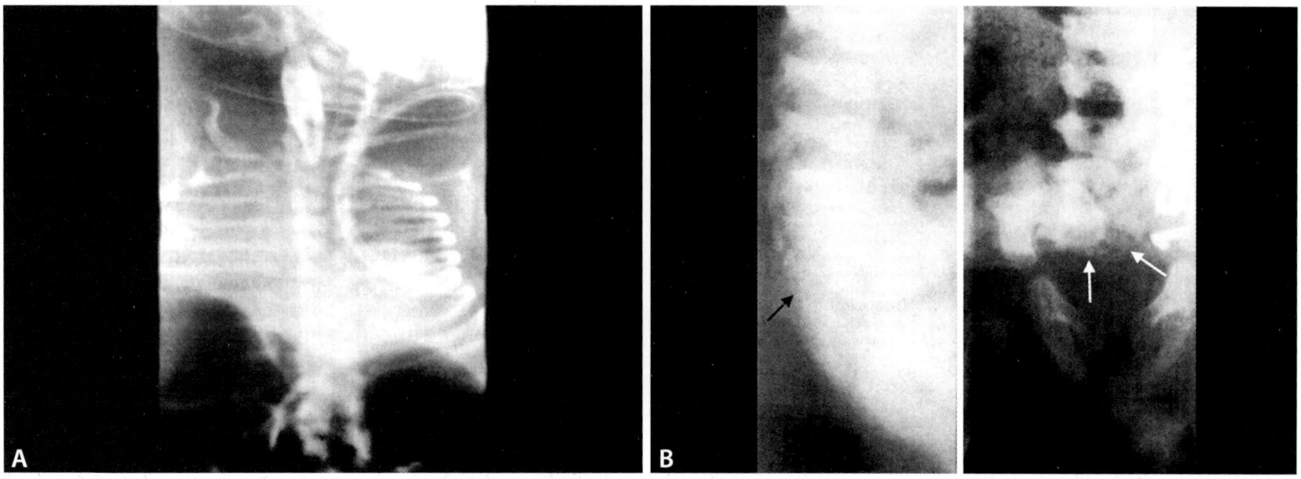

Figs. 17A and B: (A) Associated anomalies—esophageal atresia; (B) Associated anomalies—gross spinal abnormalities (Partial agenesis of sacrum, arrows).

- If S4, S5 are absent, then muscle and innervation are usually still normal;
- If S3–S5 are absent, then there is variable degree of deficiency of the muscle mass, and patient is usually incontinent;
- If S1–S5 are absent, then muscles are markedly hypoplastic, and all the patients are incontinent.

Associated Anomalies

Anorectal anomalies are frequently associated with other congenital anomalies. Its incidence varies from 20 to 70% depending upon the efforts put into find the anomalies. Almost any system may be affected, but the spine, genitourinary, gastrointestinal and the cardiac systems are more frequently affected **(Figs. 17A and B)**. Supralevator, i.e. high and intermediate anomalies are much more likely to have the associated anomalies than the infralevator lesions.

Diagnostic Algorithm

Diagnostic algorithms in a new case of ARA are shown in **(Flowcharts 1 and 2)** for male and female respectively. A combination of the clinical findings and the information provided by invertography are used to make the crucial decision on day 1.

Anorectal anomalies are rare complex congenital malformations which need a teamwork between the pediatrician, pediatric surgeon and the pediatric radiologist with an aim to deliver the best possible management, utilizing the available investigations and resources in a planned and judicious manner.

Flowchart 1: Diagnostic algorithm in a male anorectal anomalies (ARA).

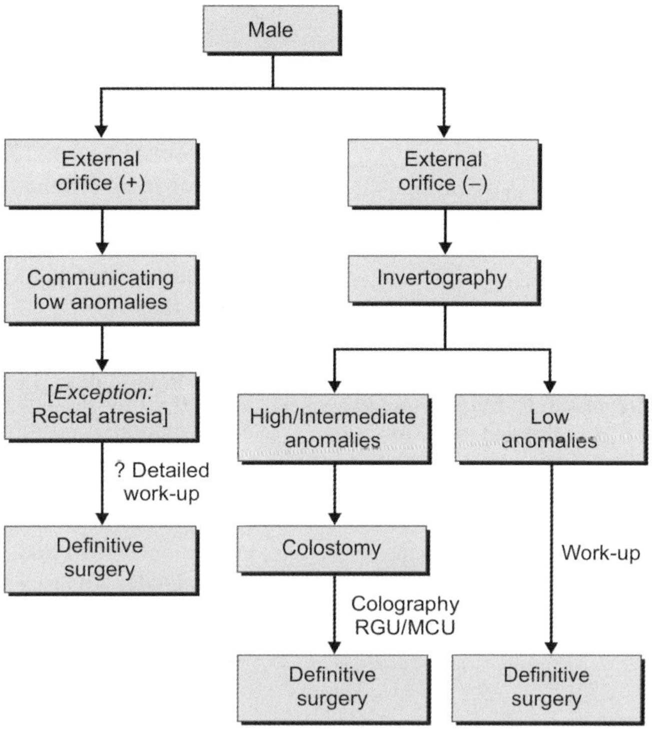

Flowchart 2: Diagnostic algorithm in a female ARA.

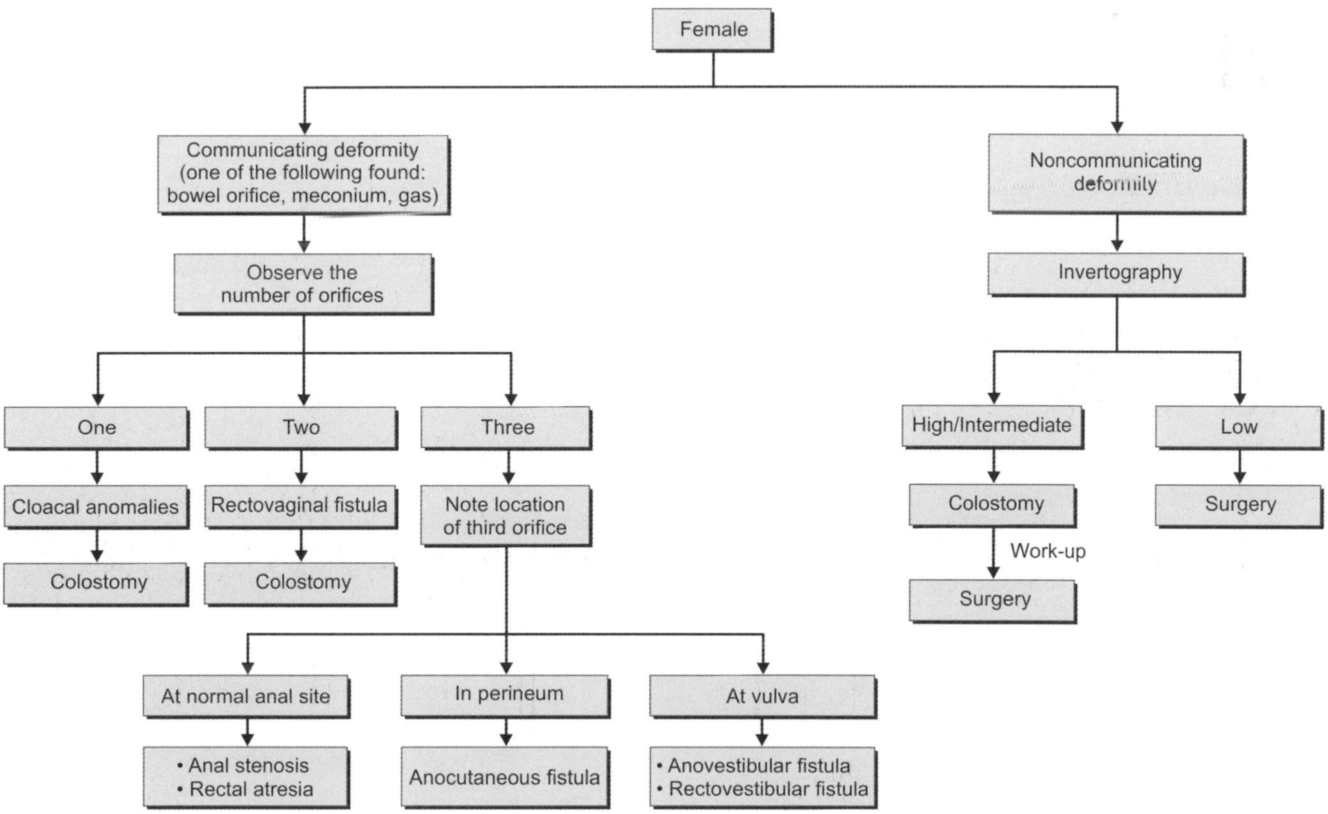

REFERENCES

1. Wangensteen OH, Rice CO. Imperforate anus: A method of determining the surgical approach. Ann surg. 1930;92:77.
2. Stephens FD, Smith ED. Anorectal Malformations in Children Chicago: Year Book Medical Publishers, 1971.
3. Cremin BJ. The radiological assessment of anorectal anomalies. Clin Radiol. 1971;22:239.
4. Narasimharao K, Prasad G, Katariya S, et al. Prone cross table lateral view: An alternative to the invertogram in imperforate anus. AJR. 1983;140:227-9.
5. Leighton DM, de Campo M. CT invertograms. Pediatr Radiol. 1989;19:176-8.

BIBLIOGRAPHY

1. Arnbjornsson E, Laurin S, Mikaelssan C. CT of anorectal anomalies: Correlation between radiologic findings and clinical evaluation of fecal incontinence. Acta Radiol. 1989;30:25-8.
2. Harris RD, Nyberg DA, Mack LA, et al. Anorectal atresia: Prenatal sonographic diagnosis. AJR. 1987;149:395-400.
3. Ikawa H, Yokoyama J, Sanbonmatsu T. The use of computerized tomography to evaluate anorectal anomalies. JPS. 1985; 20:640-4.
4. Kohda E, Fujioka M, Ikawa H et al. Congenital anorectal anomaly: CT evaluation. Radiology. 1985;157:349-52.
5. Oppenheimer DA, Carroll BA, Schuchat SJ. Sonography of imperforate anus. Radiology. 1983;148:127-8.
6. Sato Y, Pringle KC, Bergman RA et al. Congenital anorectal anomalies: MR imaging. Radiology. 1988;168:157.
7. Schuster SR, Teele RL. An analysis of ultrasound scanning as guide in determination of "high" or "low" imperforate anus. JPS. 1979;14:798-800.
8. Silverman F (Ed). Caffey's Pediatric X-ray Diagnosis, 8th edition Chicago: Year Book Medical Publishers 1985;2:1863-73.
9. Stephens FD, Smith ED, Paul NW. Anorectal malformations in children: Update 1988. Birth Defects. 1988;24(4).
10. Taccone A, Martucciello G, Fondelli P et al. CT of anorectal malformation: A postoperative evaluation. Pediatr Radiol. 1989;19:375-8.
11. Vade A, Reyes H, Wilbur A, et al. Anorectal sphincter after rectal pull-through surgery for anorectal anomalies: MRI evaluation. Pediatr Radiol. 1989;19:179-83.
12. Willital GH. Advances in the diagnosis of anal and rectal atresia by ultrasonic echo examination. JPS. 1971;6: 454-7.

CHAPTER 136

Gastrointestinal Masses in Children

Arun Kumar Gupta

The diagnostic evaluation of a gastrointestinal tract (GIT) mass in an infant or child is a challenging problem. The role of diagnostic imaging is to identify the precise location, the organ of origin and the extent of pathologic process with a minimal number of imaging procedures.

GIT masses in children include:

- Masses arising from the GIT, i.e. esophagus to rectum
- Mesenteric and omental masses.

Clinically, the patient may present with either a **palpable** abdominal lump as in hypertrophic pyloric stenosis, large GIT tumors, mesenteric masses or the mass may be clinically **non-palpable**, e.g. gastrointestinal polyps and these latter group of patients may present with other abdominal symptoms like abdominal pain, distension, bleeding or occasionally with the symptoms related to the mass effect on other organs.

Imaging modalities available for the evaluation of GIT masses in children are:

- Plain radiographs
- Contrast studies
- Ultrasonography (US)
- Computed tomography (CT)
- Magnetic resonance imaging (MRI)
- Angiography

The presenting symptoms of a patient govern to a large extent, the type of initial investigation performed. Thus, in a child with an abdominal lump, US is the initial investigation of choice whereas in patients presenting with nonspecific abdominal symptoms without a palpable abdominal mass, an abdominal radiograph or contrast study may be done initially.

PLAIN RADIOGRAPHS

Plain radiographs do not have any significant role in the diagnostic evaluation of patients with GIT masses. However, in certain clinical situations, where a patient presents with atypical features, plain radiographs may be obtained to exclude an acute process such as small bowel obstruction and bowel perforation. Also in masses with calcification, e.g. teratoma, plain radiographs are diagnostic.[1]

CONTRAST STUDIES

Clinical circumstances of the patient determine which contrast study to be performed and in what fashion. Over the years, with advancements in the imaging technology and increasing experience with newer modalities, the diagnostic algorithms have changed dramatically in most diseases. The role of barium studies in the evaluation of GIT masses in children has declined significantly in most situations except for conditions like polyposis where they continue to be the initial investigation of choice.

ULTRASONOGRAPHY

US is the screening modality of choice in a child suspected to have an intra-abdominal mass.[2] It is quick, easy to perform, rarely requires sedation, requires no patient preparation and is non-ionizing. Lack of intra-abdominal fat in infants and children allows better visualization of intra-abdominal structures when compared with adults. It can yield information about intraperitoneal fluid, presence and location of mass, nature of mass, i.e. whether cystic or solid, presence or absence of adenopathy, etc.

COMPUTED TOMOGRAPHY

CT is an extremely accurate and fast imaging modality, and is playing an increasing role in the radiological evaluation of GIT masses in children. It can provide information about the bowel wall, mesentery, lymph node status, peritoneum, omentum and solid organs. It is useful in assessing the extent of mass lesion. Optimal and uniform opacification of bowel loops is required along with intravenous contrast in a dose of 2 ml/kg. Short sedation may be required especially in children between 4 months to 4 years of age. Relative disadvantage of CT is the radiation exposure. Spiral CT further decreases the scan time and allows the use of 3D reconstruction algorithms.

MAGNETIC RESONANCE IMAGING

MR imaging offers exquisite soft tissue resolution, excellent delineation of vascular structures, multiplanar ability, absence of ionizing radiation but because of expense, limited availability, motion artifacts from bowel peristalsis and frequent need for sedation, it is usually reserved only for equivocal cases. Also the total scan time is considerably longer than in CT and claustrophobia is a real issue in paediatric patients. MR compatible anesthesia equipment is another important requirement.

ESOPHAGEAL MASSES IN CHILDREN

In general, the appearance of the normal esophagus in infants and children is similar to that in adults, except for the following variations:

- Air is more often noted in the esophagus in neonates and children than in adults and is a normal finding due to aerophagia from feeding or crying.
- In children <5 years of age, thoracic esophagus may lie slightly to the right of the spine. This variation must be borne in mind in these young patients so that the esophagus is not mistaken for adenopathy.

Masses arising from the esophagus are very rare in children. They can be broadly classified into:

- Congenital
- Neoplastic

Congenital Masses

Esophageal duplication cysts[3] occur most commonly in the distal third of esophagus. Duplication cyst (DC) is a spherical/tubular structure that is lined by alimentary tract epithelium, has smooth muscle in its wall, and is usually attached to the GI tract. They share a common muscular wall and blood supply with the adjacent bowel. Ectopic gastric mucosa can be seen in all locations of enteric duplication cysts but is most common in esophageal duplications where autodigestion of pulmonary tissue can lead to massive hemoptysis.

Clinical Presentation

- Patient may be asymptomatic and DC is diagnosed incidentally on a chest radiograph
- Dysphagia or dyspnea may be present due to compression of the esophagus or tracheobronchial tree, respectively, especially, if located in upper 2/3rd of esophagus.
- Rarely, *pain* from peptic ulceration or *hemoptysis,* if the cyst ruptures into the tracheobronchial tree, may be the presenting features.

Associated anomalies include gastric duplication and partial pericardial absence.

Imaging Features

Plain radiograph: A well-defined posterior mediastinal mass with displacement of the trachea/bronchus may be seen depending upon the site and size of mass.

Barium swallow: Extrinsic compression of the esophagus by the mass may be appreciated.

US: Using a high frequency transducer through posterior chest wall an esophageal DC located in the posterior mediastinum and abutting the posterior chest wall can be diagnosed based on the wall characteristics.

The cyst is typically anechoic, but the presence of echogenic contents represents either hemorrhage or inspissated secretions.

CT and MRI are helpful in demonstrating the relationship of the cyst to the surrounding structures. DC appears as a homogeneous, round, sharply outlined, fluid-filled mass located adjacent to the esophagus. If mucoid material or calcium is present within, then higher attenuation values of the fluid will be noted.

Technetium 99m pertechnetate scan confirms the presence of ectopic gastric mucosa within the DC.

Neuroenteric cysts arise due to incomplete separation of foregut from the notochord. They can have residual communication with the spinal canal either via a sinus tract or a fibrous band. They contain both the GI and neural elements in the wall. Radiographic appearance is similar to that of enteric duplication cyst except for the presence of associated vertebral anomalies.

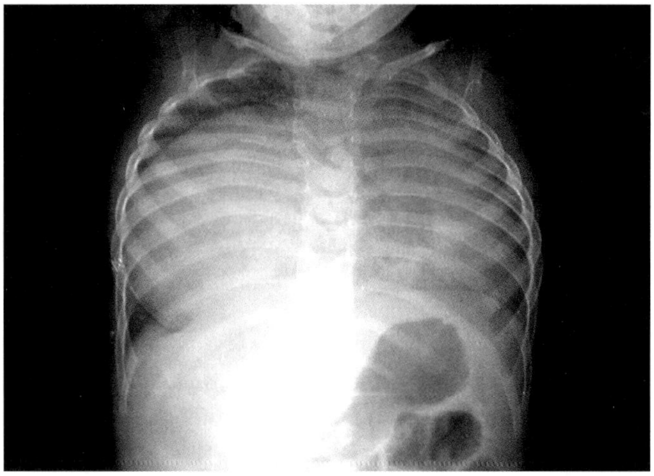

Fig. 1: Neuroenteric cyst, frontal chest radiograph: Large right posterior mediastinal mass with congenital dorsal vertebral anomalies.

Presence of dorsal vertebral anomalies in association with a posterior mediastinal mass on a frontal chest radiograph **(Fig. 1)** in a child suggests the diagnosis of neuroenteric cyst.[3,4] MRI can help to delineate the associated intraspinal anomalies.

Neoplasms

Primary esophageal tumors are extremely rare in children. Most of those that do occur are benign tumors like leiomyoma, neurofibroma, fibroma, hemangiomas and polyps. Of the malignant esophageal tumors, secondary tumors, especially lymphomas and rarely metastasis are more likely to affect children than a primary neoplasm.

Esophageal lymphomas account for <1% of total GIT lymphomas in children.

GASTRIC MASSES IN CHILDREN

Gastric masses can be broadly classified into:

- *Congenital:* Duplication cyst
- *Acquired outlet obstruction of stomach:* Hypertrophic pyloric stenosis
- *Neoplasms:* Both benign and malignant.
- *Miscellaneous:* Bezoars

Significant differences occur in the radiographic appearance and investigation of gastric masses in younger children as compared with adults:

- Distended, air-filled stomach is commonly seen in normal infants because they swallow a large amount of air while crying/feeding.
- Because ulcers and mucosal diseases are relatively rare in children, single contrast barium studies are usually more helpful than double contrast studies.
- In single contrast studies, gastric emptying may normally be slow in infancy, and this should not be confused as indicative of hypertrophic pyloric stenosis.

Congenital

Gastric duplication cysts are rare accounting for only 3.8% of all gastrointestinal duplications. A female preponderance has been noted. Duplication cysts usually occur in the antral region along its greater curvature.[4,5] Gastric DC may have associated multiple duplications in the bowel.

Clinical Presentation

Gastric DC usually presents in early infancy with one or more of the following:

- Vomiting, fever, pain, anemia. Vomiting may be related to partial or complete small bowel or pyloric obstruction. Larger cysts may also be palpable clinically.
- Complications such as perforation, hemorrhage, fistula from ulceration due to aberrant pancreatic or gastric tissue may be present.

Imaging Features

Barium studies: In its typical location along the greater curvature, gastric DC impinges on the stomach causing its upward displacement while in the late films of the same follow through study transverse colon is displaced downwards. This combination of gastric and colonic displacements in the same study is reported to be a specific finding in an appropriate clinical setting.

Ultrasonography: Gastric DC are typically anechoic on US but the presence of echogenic contents represents either hemorrhage or inspissated secretions.

Due to its location, gastric DC may simulate pseudopancreatic cyst on US but a more specific diagnosis can usually be made using a high frequency, usually linear, transducer probe by observing the characteristic appearance of bowel wall, i.e. echogenic mucosal stripe surrounded by hypoechoic line of muscle wall.

US is usually more than sufficient to diagnose cystic duplication.

Computed tomography: On CT scan, DC is seen as a fluid filled mass with an enhancing well-defined rim or wall.

Acquired Outlet Obstruction of Stomach

Hypertrophic pyloric stenosis (HPS) is the most common cause of gastric outlet obstruction in infants. There is hypertrophy and hyperplasia of the circular muscle of pylorus with thickening and lengthening of pylorus gradually progressing to gastric outlet obstruction.[4]

Etiology

Etiology is unknown but several mechanisms have been postulated, two important ones are:

1. Abnormal nerve cells of myenteric plexus. Electron microscope studies have disproved this hypothesis.
2. Hyperacidity causing prolonged pylorospasm leading to muscle hypertrophy.

Clinical Presentation

Typically, the child presents at 3 weeks of age with nonbilious, projectile vomiting. There is a male predominance with a ratio of 4:1. Usually, the baby is well at birth and vomiting begins at 2nd to 3rd week of life with progression from regurgitation to projectile vomiting after every feed. On clinical examination, a lump (olive) may be palpable in the epigastrium in about 80% of cases. Exaggerated peristaltic wave may be seen travelling from LUQ across the epigastrium. Presentation before 1st week and after 3 months of age is rare.

Diagnosis of classical HPS is based on clinical history and finding of a hypertrophied mass on abdominal palpation.

For confirmation of clinical findings, nowadays ultrasonography is the modality of choice. Only in equivocal cases barium study should be done.

Imaging Features

Plain radiograph if done, may show increased gastric distention with air and little amount of small bowel or colonic air.

Ultrasound[6-12]

Technique

- A high frequency linear transducer probe (7–10 MHz) should be used.
- Child is positioned in supine or RPO position.
- Adequate amount of gastric fluid is essential to provide the ultrasonic window and identification of anatomical structures. By placing a nasogastric tube and filling of saline through it keeps the whole procedure under control.
- On transverse section, the upper pole of right kidney is identified and the transducer is moved towards the xiphoid process. When pyloric canal is located, then transducer is angled to align it to the long axis of pyloric canal. *The lumen of pylorus is always a straight line in HPS in the longitudinal plane.* This is important because scanning in tangential plane can produce false positive results.

Findings on US

- Thickness of muscle is the most sensitive and specific measurement. It is measured from the outer edge of echogenic mucosa to the outer edge of muscle on both longitudinal and transverse scan and these measurements should be in close agreement. Normal wall thickness of pyloric canal is <2 mm. Earlier workers had proposed that thickness >4 mm is abnormal but recently it has been agreed that the critical value should be decreased, and presently if pyloric wall thickness is >3 mm, then it is considered abnormal **(Fig. 2A)**.
- Total pyloric canal length (TPL) is more variable than muscle thickness. Length >17 mm is considered abnormal, whereas <14 mm is felt to be unequivocally normal. However, diagnosis should not be made on pyloric canal length alone.

Increase in wall thickness and TPL are the two main diagnostic features.

Other findings which may be present are:

- *Empty cervix sign:* Hypertrophic muscle mass indents the duodenal bulb and bulges into the antrum, an appearance resembling that of empty cervix.
- *Mucosal nipple sign:* Redundant pyloric mucosa may protrude into the antrum.
- Hyperperistalsis of stomach with failure of gastric contents to pass into the duodenum.
- Overdistended, fluid-filled stomach and also the squared off rather than rounded configuration of the end of stomach can provide indirect clues to the diagnosis of HPS.

Barium Study[4]

It is always advisable to put a nasogastric tube so that gastric filling with barium is better. Findings could be:

- Delayed gastric emptying.
- Elongated and narrowed pyloric canal—string sign. This is one of the most important finding for diagnosis of HPS on barium study **(Fig. 2B)**.
- "Double track" of barium may be seen, if the hypertrophied muscle squeezes the lumen into separate compartments.
- Indentation of the gastric antrum and duodenal bulb producing "shoulder sign"
- "Beak sign" is produced as the barium column enters the narrowed pylorus.
- Hyperperistaltic waves seen stopping at the pylorus.

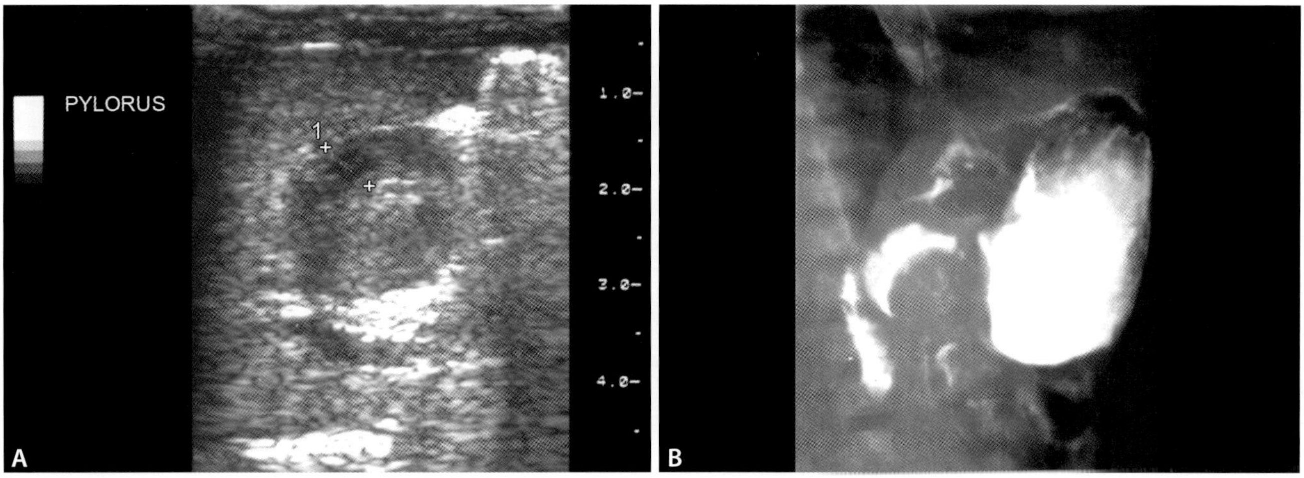

Figs. 2A and B: Hypertrophic pyloric stenosis (HPS): (A) Ultrasonography, transverse view shows significant wall thickening of the pyloric canal; (B) *Barium UGI study:* Pyloric canal is narrow and elongated. Note the indentations on the duodenal cap and the antrum by the hypertrophied muscle. Gastric emptying is delayed.

Diagnosis of HPS cannot be based only on delayed gastric emptying because delay could be due to pylorospasm and gastritis as well.

After the completion of the barium study, residual barium should be drained via the nasogastric tube before tube removal in order to prevent aspiration of barium into the lungs.

Treatment

Ramstedt pyloromyotomy: Postoperatively, the normal gastric emptying is usually resumed within 2–3 days. Muscle thickness may remain abnormal on US for up to 6 weeks. Most important is to assess the gastric emptying in postoperative period preferably with barium.

HPS is not an emergency. *False positive diagnosis must be avoided. Since HPS is a progressive disease* borderline cases must be re-examined in a day or two to avoid unnecessary surgeries.

Neoplastic Masses

These could be **benign** or **malignant.**

Benign Masses[4,13]

Polyps may be present in isolation or may be associated with several polyposis syndromes like Peutz-Jeghers, juvenile polyposis syndromes as well as familial polyposis coli. They are commonly hamartomatous polyps. Barium upper gastrointestinal study readily detects these as well circumscribed filling defects that interrupt the normal mucosal pattern.

Benign gastric tumors are rare in children. They are usually derived from mesenchymal tissue. Two relatively common masses are teratoma and leiomyoma.

Gastric Teratoma[1,4,14,15]

Stomach is a rare site for development of teratoma. They have a benign clinical course. These usually occur in infants <1 year of age. A strong male preponderance is observed. Most common site is along the greater curvature.

Clinical presentation: They are often large in size and presents as a palpable abdominal mass. GI bleeding and proximal GIT obstruction may be the other presenting features.

Imaging features: On both US and CT, a large solid mass with areas of cystic component is seen in the epigastric region, usually along the greater curvature. Calcification is seen in nearly half the cases **(Fig. 3)**. Abdominal radiographs would show an epigastric soft tissue mass with areas of calcification.

Gastric Leiomyoma[4,16-19]

Gastric leiomyomas are extremely rare in children.

Imaging features: Barium is a smooth, rounded, well-circumscribed filling defect in the stomach with or without central ulceration may be seen on barium study.

CT: A homogeneous soft tissue mass with uniform contrast enhancement is seen on CT. Very large myomas may contain necrotic areas. CT provides excellent delineation of exophytic component of the mass which is otherwise

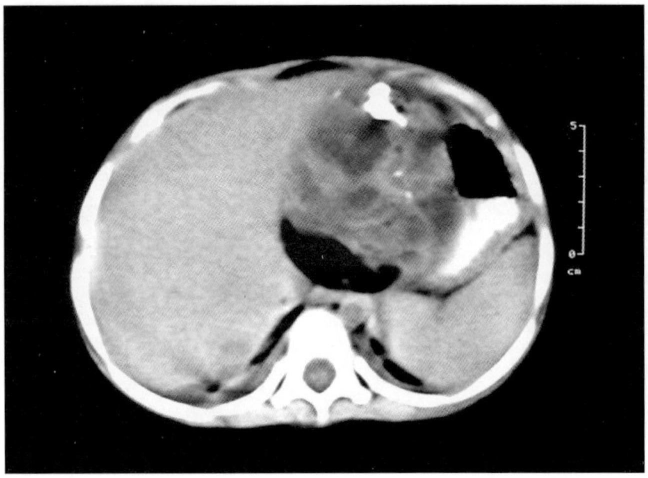

Fig. 3: Gastric teratoma, *CT abdomen:* A heterogeneous mass with areas of calcification is seen in the lesser omentum displacing the stomach down and outwards.

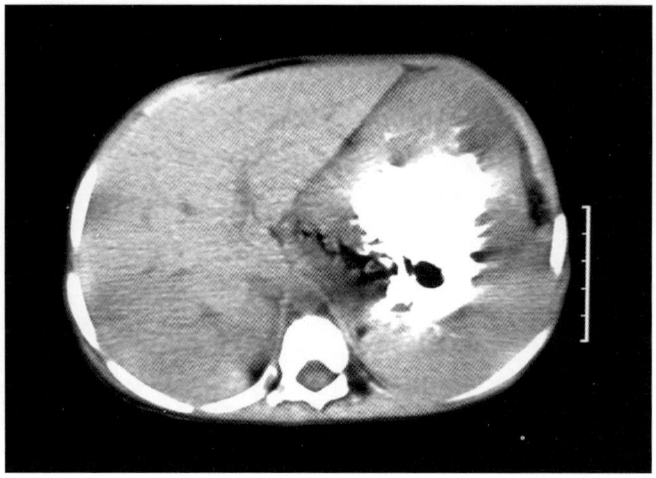

Fig. 4: Ossified gastric leiomyoma: NCCT abdomen shows a densely ossified mass in the epigastrium. Note the extension of gas into the center of the mass from its medial side. Tumor had communication with the gastric lumen.

difficult to assess on barium studies. Calcification is uncommon. A rare case of ossified leiomyoma (**Fig. 4**) has also been reported.[16]

Other benign tumors are teratoma, leiomyoma, lipoma,[20] fibroma, neurogenic tumor, hemangiomas.

Malignant Gastric Tumors

Adenocarcinoma of Stomach

Adenocarcinoma of stomach is a disease of adults but cases have occasionally been reported in children.[21] Clinical presentation is as a chronic gastric ulcer. Detection is usually late **(Fig. 5)** and is associated with a poor prognosis. Endoscopy should therefore be undertaken in any patient with persistent chronic gastric ulcer symptoms.

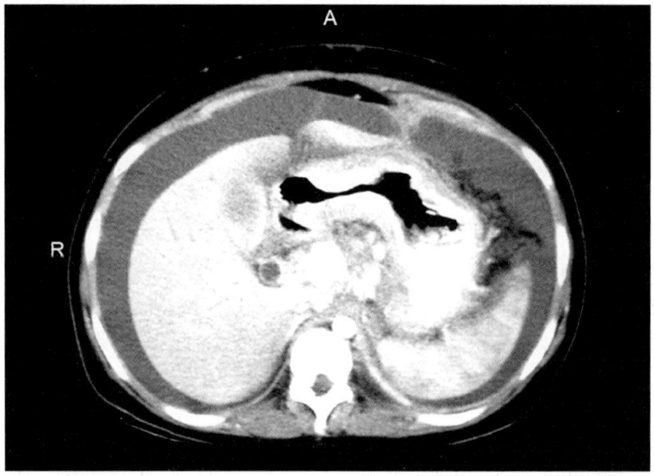

Fig. 5: Gastric adenocarcinoma: CT shows significant thickening of gastric walls with luminal narrowing and ascites.

Gastric Lymphoma

Gastric lymphoma is the most common malignancy of stomach in children.[4,22-24] Stomach is the second most common site of primary GIT lymphomas in children after ileum. This is in contrast with adults where stomach is the commonest site of primary GIT lymphomas and accounts for approximately 80% of all cases.

Clinical presentation: Patient may present with abdominal pain, abdominal mass, weight loss.

Imaging features: Barium studies may show an intraluminal mass with ulceration, fold thickening, or narrowing of lumen.

CT usually demonstrates gastric wall thickening with smoothly lobulated outer border. CT is particularly valuable in the diagnosis of gastric lymphoma since the disease originates in the submucosa and endoscopic biopsy may yield limited information especially in early stages.

Gastric Leiomyosarcoma

Gastric leiomyosarcoma is an exceedingly rare condition.[17] It is usually seen in children <1 year of age but can occur at any age. *Carney's triad* has been described, i.e. gastric leiomyosarcoma, pulmonary chondromas and extra-adrenal paraganglioma. It usually affects young females with an average age of 19 years. Mortality rate is almost 20% mostly due to paraganglioma.

Gastrointestinal Stromal Tumors

Gastrointestinal stromal tumors (GIST) are a subset of GI mesenchymal tumors. About 60-70% of total GIST occur in the stomach.[27] Histologically and on imaging, they resemble leiomyoma group. However, for definitive diagnosis, presence of CD34 and CD117 is essential.[25-27] About 10–30% are malignant but majority are benign.[27] Factors indicating higher probability of malignancy are: extraintestinal location, size more than 5 cm, central necrosis, extension into adjacent organs and presence of metastases.[27]

BEZOARS[4,28]

A bezoar is a mass of ingested, non-opaque foreign material in the stomach. At one time, they were mainly a problem of older children and for most part were trichobezoars (hair) and phytobezoars (vegetable matter). Recently, lactobezoars have become common especially in premature infants, due to the formation of dense milk coagulum when powdered milk is mixed with inadequate quantities of water.

Trichobezoars is the most common and is due to chronic hair swallowing by mentally disturbed children especially young females. Over a period of time, an intraluminal mass develops representing matted hair, trapped food particles and air taking the shape of stomach. It may extend into the duodenum and even small bowel.

Clinical Presentation

Patient may present with a mass or with history of gastric outlet obstruction. A palpable mass in the LUQ or epigastrium is common. Limited mobility is typically seen in smaller masses. Complications like gastric outlet obstruction, perforation, hemorrhage and ulceration may also be cause for presentation.

Imaging Features

Plain abdominal radiograph may show a mottled epigastric mass often rimmed by gas. This can mimic food residue. Therefore, it is important to know when the child ate last and a delayed fasting film can sort out problem cases.

Barium studies: Bezoar produces a filling defect. After the free barium has been expelled from the stomach, barium that has adhered to the surface of the bezoar forms a mottled shadow of increased density. Delayed films may show extension of the bezoar into the duodenum or jejunum.

On US, a curved broadband of increased echogenicity is seen with distal acoustic shadowing produced by air inside and around the bezoar. No details of the mass can be appreciated.

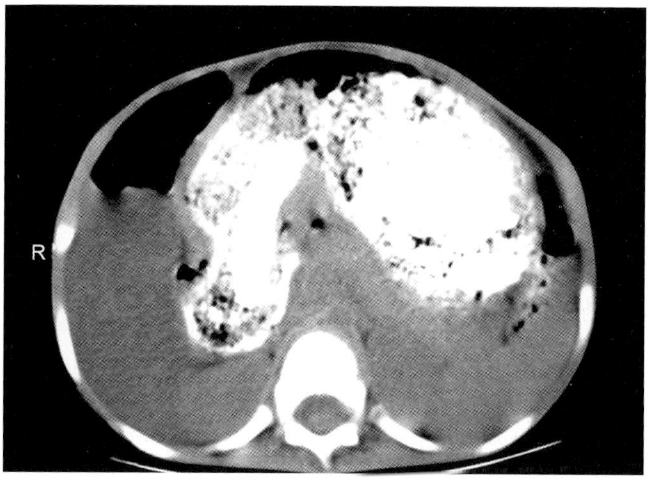

Fig. 6: Gastric bezoar: CT with oral contrast demonstrates a heterogeneous mass filling and distending the gastric and duodenal lumens (also jejunal in lower sections). Pockets of air and positive contrast are trapped within the mass.

On CT, an intragastric mass with entrapped air, debris and contrast is seen **(Fig. 6)**.

Lactobezoars usually disappear after formula adjustment and increased water intake.

Tricho- and phytobezoars require surgical removal to prevent complications.

SMALL BOWEL MASSES IN CHILDREN

Masses can be classified into:
- *Congenital:* Enteric duplication cysts.
- *Infectious:* Abdominal Koch's
- *Neoplastic:* Both benign and malignant
- *Miscellaneous:* Intussusception, intramural hematoma.

Congenital Masses

Enteric Duplication Cyst[4,29-32]

Embryologically DC arise from abnormalities of development, separation and recanalization of primitive foregut during the late first or early second trimester. Spherical duplications usually do not communicate with the GIT while the much less common tubular type frequently does communicate. Although they can occur anywhere in the GI tract, the most common site is the distal ileum followed by esophagus. Approximately 40% of the patients present by first month of age while 85% present during the first year of life.

Duodenal duplication cysts are rare. They may present with gastric outlet obstruction and on imaging can mimic pseudopancreatic cyst. Ileal DC lie on the mesenteric border of normal small bowel and their muscular wall is often intimately attached to the muscular wall of the normal bowel. Therefore, surgical removal is often impossible without resecting the adjacent loop of bowel. Very rarely, persistent fibrous connection to the spinal cord can exist. In such cases anterior vertebral body segmentation anomalies can be seen. Most are solitary, but they can be multiple. Transdiaphragmatic extension into chest has been reported.

Clinical presentation: Patient may present with abdominal pain, abdominal mass, vomiting or abdominal distention secondary to intestinal obstruction. Presence of ectopic gastric or pancreatic mucosa may result in complications such as bleeding or perforation.

Imaging features: US is the modality of choice in the initial examination of any child suspected to have DC. It shows a well-defined, usually unilocular, cystic anechoic mass. The characteristic appearance of bowel wall showing "rim-sign" with echogenic inner-rim of mucosa surrounded by a relatively hypoechoic layer representing gut muscle is diagnostic **(Fig. 7)**. Unfortunately, not all duplication cysts have this sign either because the mucosal layer has been enzymatically destroyed or the duplication is tubular and communicating type and so is not always fluid filled. Also, rimming may be seen in any cyst where bleeding occurs and fibrin is deposited along the cyst wall, most often in the ovarian cyst. ^{99m}Tc pertechnetate scan then becomes useful since ectopic gut mucosa usually takes up ^{99m}Tc pertechnetate. Another interesting finding of duplication cyst is the presence of peristalsis in the cyst wall, which may be appreciated in real-time scanning.

CT would show a cystic mass with sharp, enhancing wall.

Differential diagnosis includes mesenteric cyst, omental cyst, ovarian cyst, choledochal cyst and pancreatic pseudocyst.

Infectious Masses

Abdominal tuberculosis, particularly involving the *ileocecal* region and *tubercular peritonitis* can present as an abdominal mass in children.[4,33-35]

In ileocecal TB, the ileocecal (IC) valve may be so thick that it mimics a mass in the RIF. The patient may present with nonspecific complaints and a RIF mass and both CT and US would demonstrate adherent bowel loops, gross bowel wall thickening, thickened mesentery and large regional nodes producing a soft tissue mass centered around the IC junction. Barium may demonstrate contracted, coned, irregular cecum; gaping, incontinent IC valve; narrowed, rigid terminal ileum; matted, fixed bowel loops with or without strictures.

Loculated ascites, as may be seen with tuberculous peritonitis (*wet form*), may present as an abdominal mass in children. It may contain septations, debris. US appearance of loculated ascites can mimic mesenteric or omental cyst.

In the d*ry form of* tuberculous peritonitis, bowel, omentum or mesentery may be clumped together **(Fig. 8)** due to multiple caseous nodules on the surface and adhesions, often becoming palpable and may present as a mass. On US, a very characteristic "Swiss-Cheese" appearance is noted.

Neoplastic Masses

Neoplastic masses could be benign or malignant.

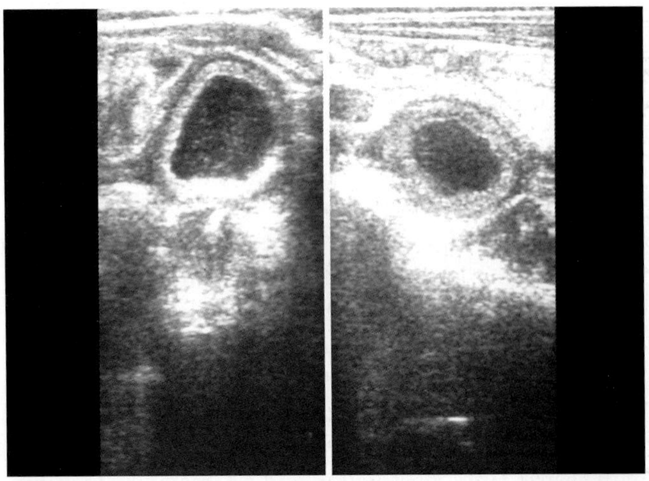

Fig. 7: Duplication cyst: Ultrasonography shows the typical wall characteristics of duplication cyst.

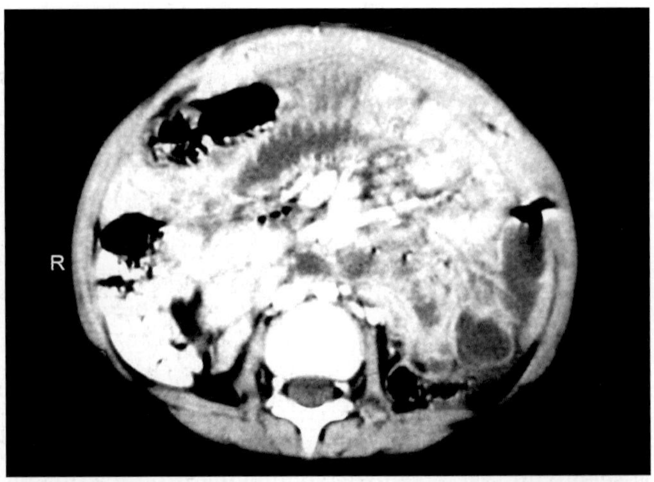

Fig. 8: Abdominal tuberculosis: On CECT abdomen matted bowel loops, mesenteric nodes and small pockets of fluid are seen.

Benign

Benign small bowel tumors,[4,36] which include hemangiomas,[37] lipomas, leiomyomas **(Fig. 9)**, neurofibromas and fibromas are rare in children.

Polyps of small bowel are usually seen in association with polyposis syndromes especially Peutz-Jeghers and juvenile gastrointestinal polyposis.

Clinical presentation: Patient may be asymptomatic and detection is incidental. Most common clinical presentation is crampy abdominal pain and bloody stools due to recurrent entero-enteric intussusception.

Imaging features: If the presentation is not acute, the polypoidal mass or masses are readily identified in most cases as filling defects on barium follow through. If the condition presents as intussusception, the lead point may be seen as a polypoidal mass on barium meal follow through studies.

Malignant Small Bowel Masses

Malignant masses of the small bowel include lymphoma, adenocarcinoma, leiomyosarcomas and carcinoid. Of these, lymphoma is the commonest tumor. All the benign tumors have their malignant counterparts. Also patients with polyposis syndromes can develop GI malignancies.

Small Bowel Lymphoma[4,17,23,38]

Although relatively rare in childhood *lymphomas constitute the most common small bowel malignancy in children.* Those under 8 years of age are at greatest risk. Burkitt lymphomas, which has a strong male predominance, is the most common type of lymphoma.

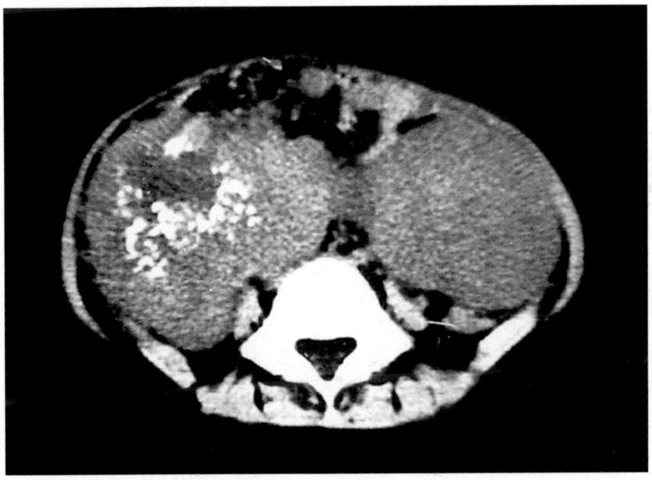

Fig. 9: Small bowel leiomyoma: NCCT abdomen shows a large bilobed soft tissue mass with areas of calcification.

In children, GI lymphomas account for 19% of total lymphomas and *majority occur in ileum* followed by stomach and jejunum. This is in contrast with adults in whom primary GI lymphomas occur in only 4–12% cases and the most common site is stomach.

Clinical presentation: Nausea, vomiting, abdominal pain, altered bowel habits, GI bleeding, small bowel obstruction, a palpable abdominal mass or features of intussusception are some of the features with which a patient may present. Approximately, *25% patients present with intussusception. Burkitt lymphoma is the most common lead point in children of >4 years of age presenting with ileocolic intussusception.*

Imaging features: The investigations performed would depend upon the clinical presentation. Plain abdominal radiograph is usually nonspecific and may be normal, show a soft tissue mass or may show features of intussusception with small bowel obstruction.

Barium meal follow through (BaMFT) may be the initial investigation performed, if the patient presents with unusual abdominal pain or features of subacute intestinal obstruction. BaMFT may demonstrate a stricture, mass or features of intussusception. Findings are similar to that seen in adult lymphomas and six radiological patterns have been described on barium: Aneurysmal **(Fig. 10A)**, nodular, ulcerative, constrictive, mesenteric and sprue patterns.

The appearance on BaMFT may mimic Crohn's disease or tuberculosis and differentiation may be difficult based only on imaging.

If there is a suspicion of an abdominal mass, then US is the most appropriate initial imaging study. On US, an atypical target is seen, i.e. a hypoechoic mass due to bowel wall thickening, usually in the RIF, with a central irregular echogenic area due to the bowel lumen **(Fig. 10B)**. Also, enlarged nodes and ascites may be frequently seen.

CT is crucial to demonstrate the full extent of the mass and any associated lesions.

CT findings include one or more of the following:

- Marked bowel wall thickening
- Luminal narrowing
- Aneurysmal dilatation **(Fig. 10C)**
- Bulky mesenteric and RP nodal masses with loop separation
- Intussusception
- Small bowel obstruction.
- Omental, mesenteric, peritoneal dissemination.
- Ascites and pleural effusion
- Renal, hepatic, splenic and pancreatic lesions
- Calcification, uncommon in untreated cases.

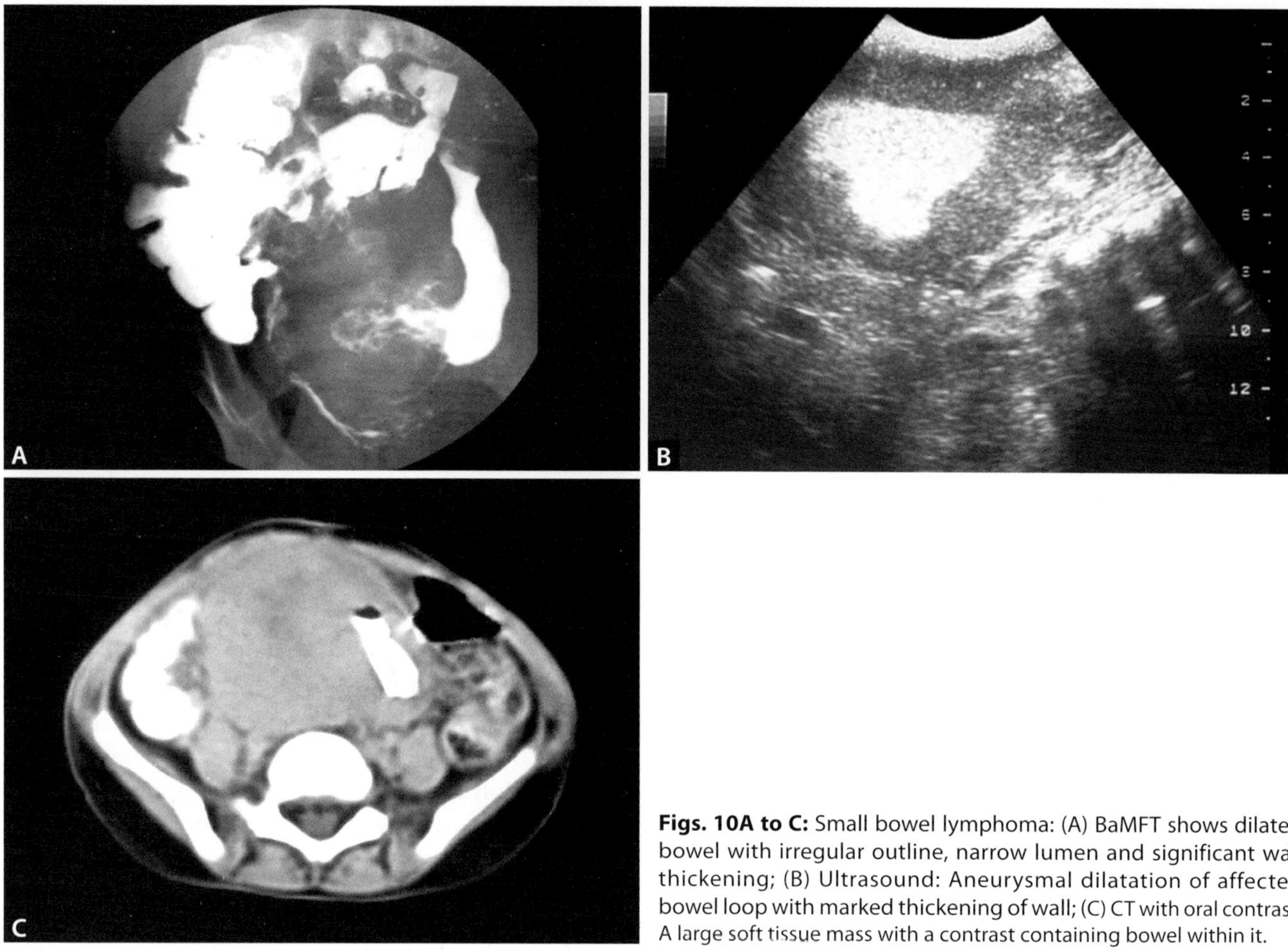

Figs. 10A to C: Small bowel lymphoma: (A) BaMFT shows dilated bowel with irregular outline, narrow lumen and significant wall thickening; (B) Ultrasound: Aneurysmal dilatation of affected bowel loop with marked thickening of wall; (C) CT with oral contrast: A large soft tissue mass with a contrast containing bowel within it.

Leiomyosarcomas[36]

Leiomyosarcomas can also rarely occur in small bowel especially in <1 year age group. Most commonly, they present with small bowel obstruction, perforation, intussusception, bleeding, and anemia. Obstruction in a newborn can cause meconium peritonitis. On CT, they resemble leiomyomas, i.e. soft tissue mass with areas of necrosis **(Fig. 11)** and may be even calcification. Intestinal leiomyosarcomas in children are smaller at diagnosis than in adults and majority are resectable and have a slightly better prognosis. Metastases have been reported in regional lymph nodes, lung, liver, bone.

Gastrointestinal Stromal Tumor (GIST)[27]

These tumors are similar to those in stomach. Small bowel GIST account for 20–30% of total cases.[27] Large mass with areas of necrosis are common CT findings.

Adenocarcinoma

Adenocarcinoma of the small bowel is extremely rare in children. Most cases occur in the second decade. *Clinical presentation* may be nonspecific and includes nausea, vomiting, small bowel obstruction. On *barium follow through* study tumor is seen as a short segment narrowing **(Fig. 12)**, an appearance which may simulate tubercular stricture of small bowel.

Generally, the prognosis is poorer than in adults because of late diagnosis since symptoms are nonspecific and there is a low index of suspicion.

Intussusception

Intussusception is the prolapse of one portion of bowel into the other. The segment of intestine that prolapses is called the *intussusceptum* while the receiving segment is the *intussuscipiens*.[4] Ileocolic intussusception is most commonly seen (90%) in children. Ileoileocolic, colocolic

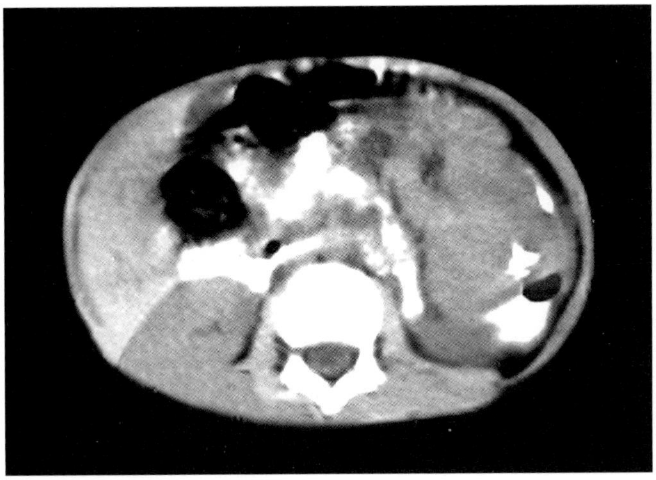

Fig. 11: Small bowel leiomyosarcoma: On CT, a soft tissue mass on the left side of abdomen with a contrast opacified bowel loop located eccentrically.

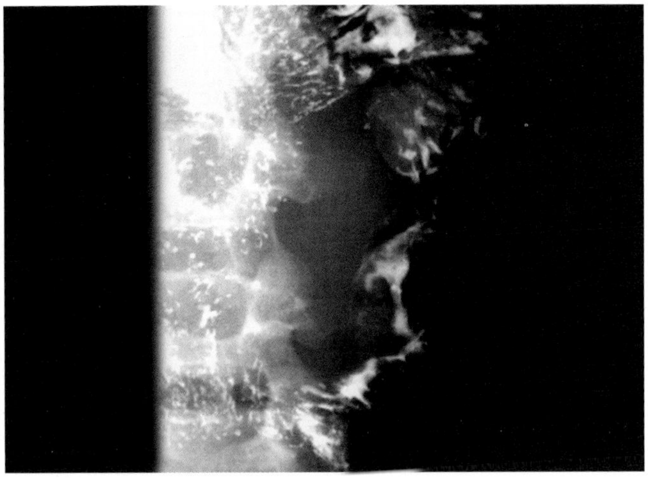

Fig. 12: Small bowel adenocarcinoma: BaMFT shows marked degree of narrowing, irregularity and loss of normal fold pattern in a segment of small bowel.

and ileoileal intussusceptions are rarer. It commonly affects children < 2 years of age and is more frequent in boys.

Unlike in adults where majority of intussusception are due to pedunculated polypoidal tumor (80%, mostly lipoma), in children only 5% cases are due to identifiable lead points such as Meckel's diverticulum, duplication cysts, lymphoma, polyps, hematoma. Lead points are more frequent in children less than 1 month or more than 4 years of age where approximately 50% of cases may be caused by lead points.

Clinical Presentation

The classical triad of abdominal pain, currant jelly stools and palpable abdominal mass is seen in <50% cases. Diagnosis may be difficult and delay may be life-threatening due to bowel necrosis and complications. Therefore, imaging modalities play a vital role in diagnosing or excluding intussusception.

Imaging Features

Although US is the initial investigation of choice, plain abdominal radiograph[39] and barium enema may be done in equivocal cases during the course of evaluation.

Ultrasound features are:[40-42]

- A mass with either an atypical target or a concentric ring appearance in transverse section **(Fig. 13A)** and sandwich/pseudokidney appearance in sagittal plane.
- Since any condition causing bowel wall thickening, e.g. inflammation, edema, hematoma, etc. may mimic intussusception on US, an extremely useful differentiating sonographic feature is the characteristic appearance of *eccentric, semilunar, echogenic mesenteric fat* on transverse section that is pulled along with the vessels and lymph nodes into the intussusception.
- US may be able to depict lead point and detect other intra-abdominal lesions unrelated to intussusception.
- On color Doppler imaging, absence of blood flow might indicate the presence of ischemia or necrosis and that vigorous attempts at reduction in such patients should be avoided.

Plain radiographs: If done might show:[39]

- Soft-tissue mass in the region of cecum or transverse colon with meniscus sign (due to the presence of rim of gas around the intussusceptum).
- Absence of caecal gas or stool.
- Features of small bowel obstruction.

The sensitivity of plain abdominal radiographs in diagnosing intussusception is low. *The best positive predictor is the presence of a soft tissue mass in the abdomen and the absence of cecal gas even in prone position. The only way to exclude intussusception is the presence of cecal gas.* However, misidentification of air can lead to false negative results.

Diagnostic barium enema had been the gold standard for the diagnosis till mid-80s when it was realized that sonography could be highly accurate in the diagnosis of intussusception. Since about 50% of patients with clinical suspicion of intussusception turn out to be normal on barium enema, US rather than barium enema should be done initially in all patients with suspected

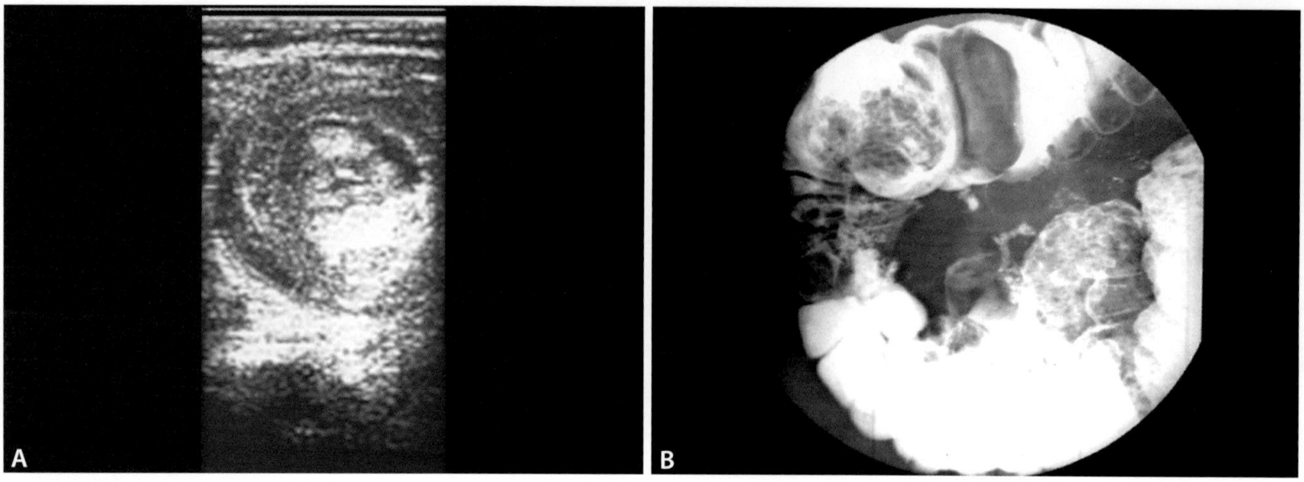

Figs. 13A and B: Intussusception: (A) US transverse view demonstrates concentric ring pattern. Note the characteristic eccentric echogenic mesenteric fat and (B) Barium enema shows a filling defect due to intussusceptum head in the proximal transverse colon.

intussusception. When used appropriately, a negative US obviates unnecessary diagnostic enemas and the use of enema can be limited to therapeutic purpose only. On a diagnostic barium enema study, an intussusception is seen as a convex intraluminal filling defect **(Fig. 13B)**. Coiled spring appearance may be produced as the contrast insinuates between the intussusceptum and the intussuscipiens.

Reduction can be attempted using either dilute barium/ water-soluble contrast (hydrostatic) or more recently using air (pneumatic) each under either fluoroscopic or US guidance.[43-46]

Procedure for reduction using barium enema:

- Hydration status and vitals should be checked, an intravenous line should be established, procedure is explained to the parents and their written consent is obtained.
- Anal opening is occluded using an appropriate sized Foley's catheter.
- 25% weight/volume (w/v) barium or a diluted (1:3 or 1:4) water soluble contrast is used, latter is preferred in young infants with long duration of symptoms.
- Rule of three is followed, i.e.
  - Reservoir is kept at 3 ft high from the table (5 ft in case of water soluble contrast)
  - Reduction attempt is maintained for 3 minutes
  - A maximum of 3 attempts are made.

For air-enema reduction pressure between 85 and 120 mm Hg is safe.

Successful reduction is marked by free flow of contrast into the terminal ileum with disappearance of soft tissue mass.

Some workers prefer air enema under fluoroscopy than barium reduction because it is quicker, easy, less messy and exposes patient to lower amount of radiation. Recent studies have shown that US with saline reduction is safe with comparable results. Pneumatic reduction under US guidance has been tried and might have fewer complications but is much more cumbersome.

The only contraindications to enema reduction are clinical features of *peritonitis, shock*[43] and radiological features *of perforation.*

Relatively lower rates of successful reduction are obtained in the following situations:

- Symptoms for >24 hours
- Presence of associated small bowel obstruction or rectal bleeding
- Presence of lead points
- Position of intussusceptum, e.g. those located distally are more difficult to reduce
- Ileoileal and ileoileocolic types are more difficult to reduce.
- US appearance of an atypical target indicating more tight intussusception is less likely to be reduced than one with concentric ring appearance suggesting a more loose type of intussusception, though this criteria is not considered reliable now.

Major complication of enema reduction is perforation. Perforation rates in both hydrostatic and pneumatic reduction are comparable and is <1%, provided air pressures are not exceeded and proper technique is followed.

Increased risk of perforation is noted in infants <6 months of age, >36 hours duration of onset and absent flow on color Doppler imaging.

There is 5–10% recurrence rate after successful hydrostatic or pneumatic reduction. Most recur within 72 hours. Children with recurrent intussusception appear to be *no more* likely to have a lead point than those with single episode.

MESENTERIC MASSES IN CHILDREN

Mesenteric masses[47-49] may be classified as:
- Cystic
- Neoplastic

Mesenteric cysts, omental cysts and lymphangiomas are believed to be different manifestations of a common problem, i.e. malformation of lymphatic system in which the lymphatic vessels of the mesentery fail to establish communication with the central lymphatic system resulting in the formation of large masses with dilated fluid-filled lymphatic spaces. They may adhere to the adjacent organs but do not invade them. Rarely, they may be associated with lymphatic malformation elsewhere.

Clinical Presentation

Most of these patients present in the first few years of life but rarely in the newborn period. Presenting features include:
- Abdominal distension, pain, abdominal mass or features of small bowel obstruction.
- Rarely, diffuse lymphangiomas may extend via patent processus vaginalis and present as an inguinal hernia
- Diffuse lymphangiomas can produce protein losing enteropathy.

Imaging Features

Plain radiograph may show a soft tissue mass displacing the gas filled bowel loops. Mesenteric mass would displace the bowel loops around it while an omental mass would displace the bowel loops posteriorly **(Fig. 14)**. Features of small bowel obstruction may also be seen.

US features include:
- Cystic anechoic mass which is usually unilocular but may show fine septations. Presence of echoes within suggest blood, chyle or purulent material.
- Mesenteric and omental cysts are solitary and occasionally multiloculated, whereas abdominal lymphangiomas are more widespread and multicystic.
- Mesenteric cysts are usually mobile and changes shape.

CT: On CT a large, thin walled cystic, sometimes multiseptate, mass is seen which displaces the bowel loops posteriorly **(Fig. 15)**. Mural calcification is rare.

MRI: Cyst may have signal intensity ranging from fluid (low on T1W and high on T2W) to fat (high on T1W) depending upon the content of fluid.

Differential Diagnosis

Includes loculated ascites, fluid-filled viscus (pseudo-ascites), ovarian cyst, cystic teratoma and duplication cyst.

Mesenteric and Omental Tumors

Most common neoplasms involving the mesentery are *lymphomas* (usually in the disseminated form) and *metastasis.*

Lymphoma: NHL is more common than Hodgkin's disease. It is usually associated with retroperitoneal lymphadenopathy.

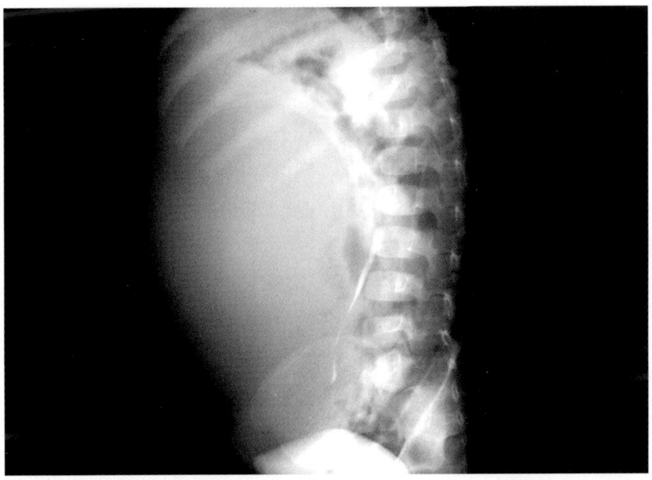

Fig. 14: Lateral view of an excretory urography shows a large omental mass displacing the bowel loops posteriorly.

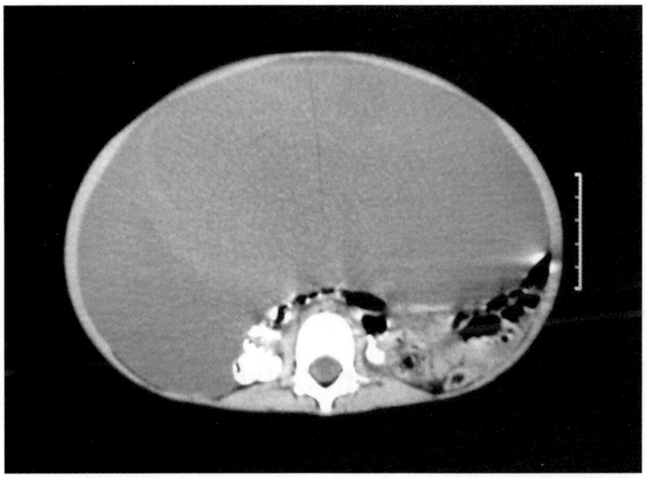

Fig. 15: Omental cyst on a CT displaces the bowel loops posteriorly around the spine.

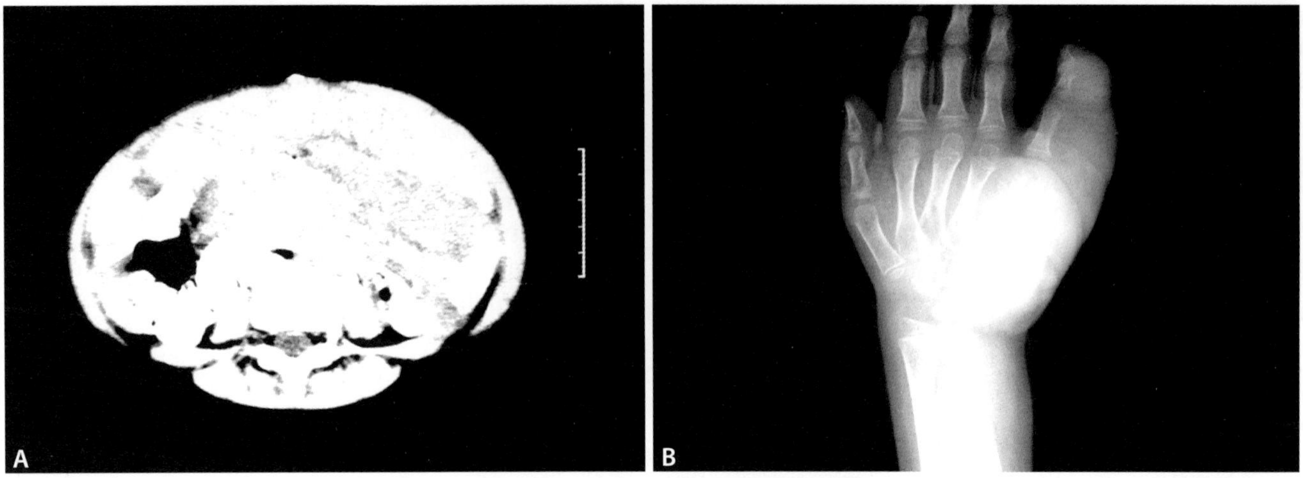

Figs. 16A and B: Mesenteric neurofibroma: (A) CT shows a diffuse relatively homogeneous soft tissue mass in the mesentery; (B) Right hand radiograph: A large neurofibromatosis mass on the ulnar side.

Metastasis may appear on CT as discrete rounded or cake like masses, ill-defined masses or simply as mesenteric fat streakiness.

Primary omental and mesenteric neoplasms are rare and include fibromas, neurofibromas **(Figs. 16A and B)**, lipomas, lipoblastomas, desmoid, yolk sac tumor.

Fibroma: It is the most common primary mesenteric neoplasm. It appears solid, homogeneous on CT.

Lipomas are well-defined homogeneous mass of fat attenuation **(Fig. 17)**.

Lipoblastoma is a heterogeneous mass with soft tissue attenuation areas within a focal fatty mass.

Desmoid tumor occurs typically in post colectomy patients with Gardener's syndrome.

Yolk sac tumor is highly malignant. It is the most common gonadal tumor occurring in childhood. Occasionally, however, they can arise in mesentery and can appear on CT as well-defined heterogeneous solid mass with low attenuation areas within.

Intraperitoneal teratoma are usually cystic. Identification of multi-tissue origin, especially, when fat and calcification are seen, can lead to the correct diagnosis.

Cystic mesothelioma is a rare primary neoplasm of peritoneal cavity, seen most commonly in adult females but may occasionally be seen in children. It has a predilection for surface of pelvic viscera.

COLONIC MASSES IN CHILDREN

Colonic masses can also be classified as:

- Congenital
- Inflammatory
- Neoplastic

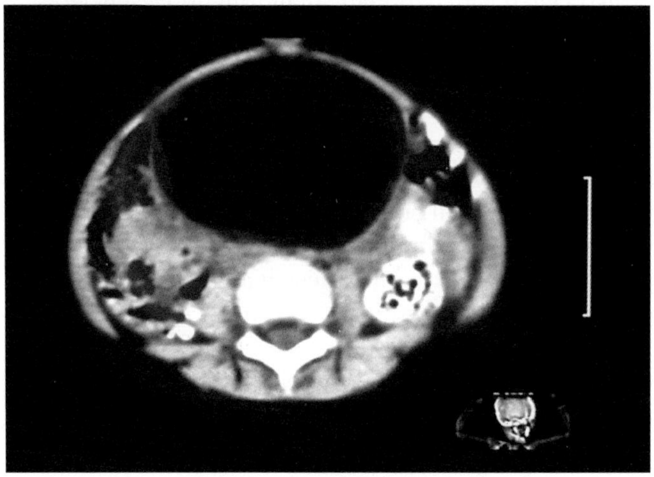

Fig. 17: Mesenteric lipoma: On CT a large fat attenuating mesenteric mass is seen.

Congenital Mass

Duplication Cysts[50]

Colonic duplication cysts are much less frequent than in small bowel, but if they are large, then they can produce mass effect or obstruction of the bowel. Urinary tract obstruction due to pressure on the urinary bladder by rectal duplication cyst has been observed. Ectopic gastric or pancreatic mucosa can cause ulceration, bleeding and perforation. They may be spherical but in about 50% of cases it is tubular.

Inflammatory Mass

Appendicular Lump[51]

Appendicitis is reported to be a common cause for abdominal surgery in children in the west. Early diagnosis is important because morbidity increases after appendix perforation. History and examination are often atypical. Up to approximately 25% of patients are found to have normal appendix at surgery. Therefore, imaging plays an important role to eliminate negative surgery.

Perforation can lead to generalized peritonitis but a local abscess adjacent to appendix is more likely because perforation is usually contained by the omentum. And in such cases, patient may present with lump in RLQ. The ultrasound is the investigation of choice.

US: It may show variable findings:

- A mass of mixed echogenicity in RLQ with periappendiceal fluid or intraperitoneal fluid
- Inflamed appendix may be seen as a tubular aperistaltic, noncompressible, blind-ending structure with total diameter > 6 mm
- Appendicolith may be seen as an echogenic lesion with an acoustic shadowing **(Fig. 18A)**
- Appendiceal abscess is seen as a hypoechoic mass in the RLQ **(Fig. 18B)** and its extension into the cul-de-sac occurs frequently forming a hypoechoic mass between the bladder and the rectum.

Plain abdominal radiograph: A number of findings may be seen:

- Mass effect on the cecum
- Thickened cecal wall
- Air-fluid level in the terminal ileum and cecum.
- Loss of obturator internus fat plane.
- *Appendicolith:* Calcified concretions in the appendix are seen in about 5–10% of cases on plain radiograph.

Identification of appendicolith in a child with acute abdominal pain is diagnostic of appendicitis and atleast 50% of such patients have perforation, abscess or both.

CT due to its superior soft tissue contrast is more sensitive than US for diagnosis of abscess **(Fig. 18C)**.

Neoplastic Mass

Most large bowel tumors in children are benign, i.e. juvenile polyps.[4] Less common causes include hereditary polyposis syndrome and primary colonic malignancy.

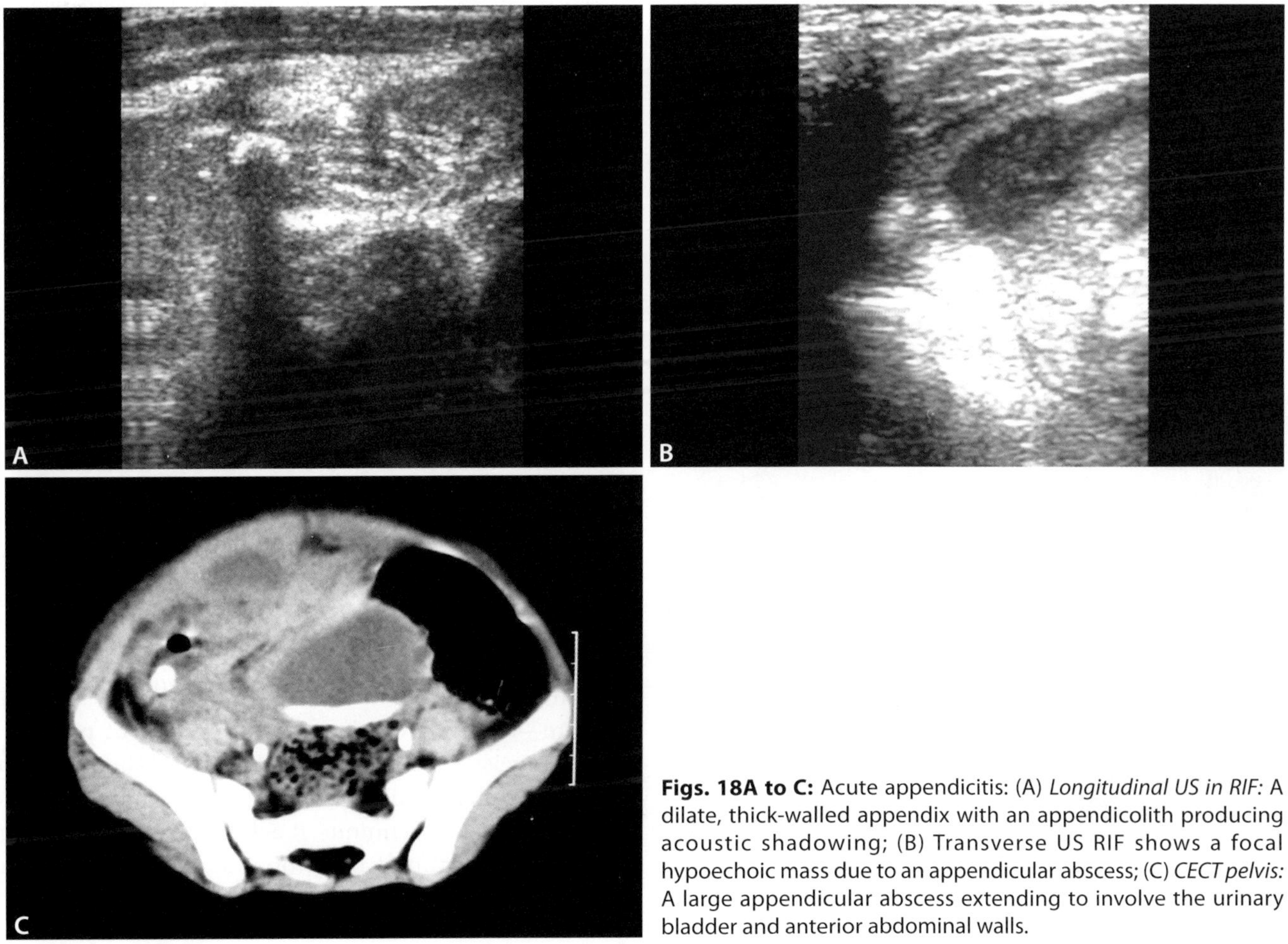

Figs. 18A to C: Acute appendicitis: (A) *Longitudinal US in RIF:* A dilate, thick-walled appendix with an appendicolith producing acoustic shadowing; (B) Transverse US RIF shows a focal hypoechoic mass due to an appendicular abscess; (C) *CECT pelvis:* A large appendicular abscess extending to involve the urinary bladder and anterior abdominal walls.

Benign Colonic Neoplasms

Isolated juvenile polyp: This is the most common tumor of colon in children between 4 and 6 years of age. Some consider it inflammatory, others describe them as hamartomatous. These are not true neoplasms. They can be single or multiple and are most commonly (75–85%) located in the rectum or sigmoid region but they can occur anywhere in the colon. They are rarely seen in neonates.

They usually present with bleeding per rectum. Occasionally, there may be anemia, mucoid diarrhea or colocolic intussusception.

Polyposis syndromes: A number of syndromes have been described with multiple colonic polyps **(Fig. 19)**. Peutz-Jeghers, Gardner's, Generalized juvenile polyposis syndrome, familial adenomatous colonic polyposis syndrome and Turcot syndrome.

Malignant Colonic Neoplasm[52,53]

Adenocarcinoma of colon are uncommon in childhood. Most occur in the colon and rectum, usually in the second decade. No sex predilection is observed. In young infants, a colonic tumor is more likely to be leiomyoma, leiomyosarcoma and other sarcomas than adenocarcinoma. Predisposing conditions are seen in only about 9–12% of cases and includes FAP, Gardner's syndrome, ulcerative colitis, cystic fibrosis.

Clinical features include abdominal pain, nausea, vomiting, diarrhea, weight loss, gastrointestinal bleed and obstructive symptoms. In children, the diagnosis of colorectal carcinoma has a much poorer prognosis than in adults for several reasons:

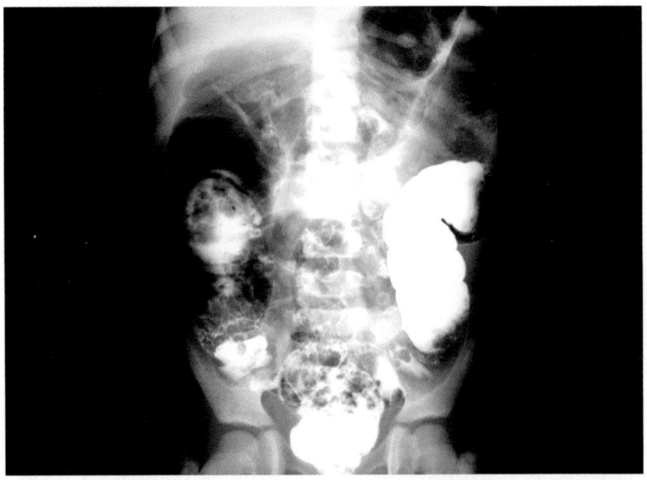

Fig. 19: Multiple polyps involving the entire colon in a double contrast barium enema.

- Because of nonspecific clinical features and a low index of suspicion patients usually present at an advanced stage at the time of diagnosis. About 70–90% already have local, nodal or metastatic spread at the time of diagnosis compared with 40% in adults.
- *Aggressive histological subtype:* Approximately, 50% are aggressive mucinous adenocarcinomas as compared to 5% in adults.

Imaging: Appearance is similar to that in adults **(Figs. 20 and 21)**.

Plain films are either normal or show features of intestinal obstruction. Mucinous tumors may show areas of punctate calcification at the primary site and also in the metastatic deposits.

Barium enema is used as a screening modality. Intraluminal filling defect or apple core lesion may be seen.

US is not performed for suspected colorectal carcinoma, but when used for evaluation of nonspecific abdominal pain, may demonstrate a mass lesion involving the bowel.

CT is very valuable for diagnosis and staging of disease. The bowel wall thickness, relation of mass to surrounding structures, adenopathy and distant metastasis can be evaluated.

MRI improved soft tissue contrast, but because of expense, low availability, motion artifacts and need for sedation CT is preferred.

GIST: Colonic GIST accounts for only about 5% of cases.[27] Features are similar to GIST anywhere in the intestine.[54]

Colon is a much less frequent site for the development of *lymphoma* than the small bowel.

CONCLUSION

- GI masses in children are significantly different when compared with GI masses in adults. In children, primary malignant tumors of GIT hollow viscera are very rare. Masses in intestinal tract are much more likely to be benign developmental lesions like duplication cysts. Benign neoplastic processes are also more common than malignant lesions.
- The ultimate goal of imaging—better patient care—depends on coordinated efforts of pediatric radiologists, pediatricians and pediatric surgeons. The age of patient and the clinical presentation guides the initial imaging technique. Precise diagnostic evaluation allows selection of the proper surgical and medical treatment.

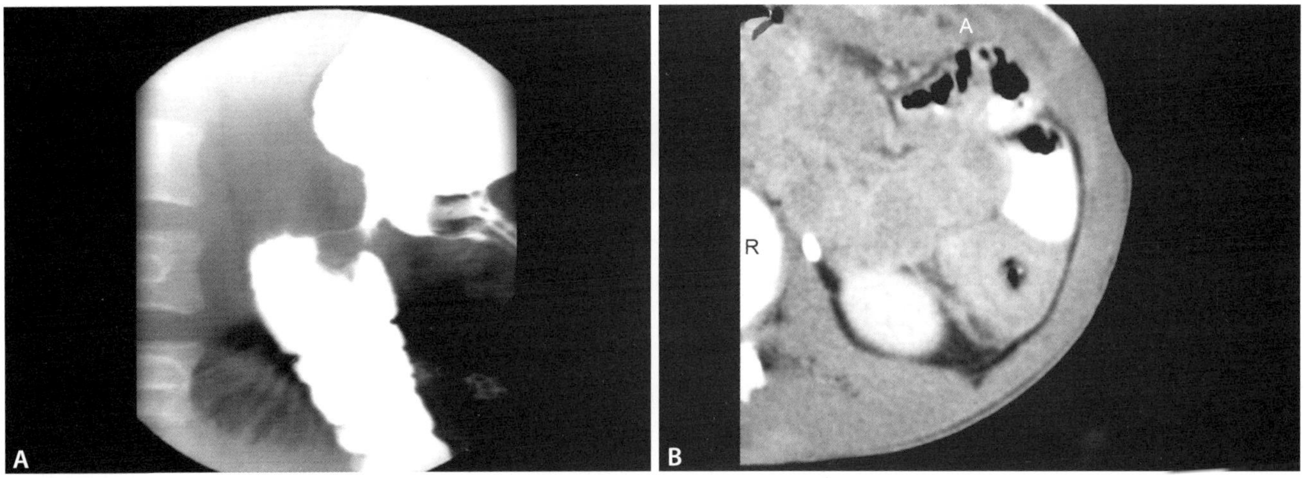

Figs. 20A and B: Adenocarcinoma descending colon: (A) On barium enema, short significant narrowing in mid descending colon seen; (B) CT at the same level shows concentric wall thickening with luminal narrowing of the affected colon.

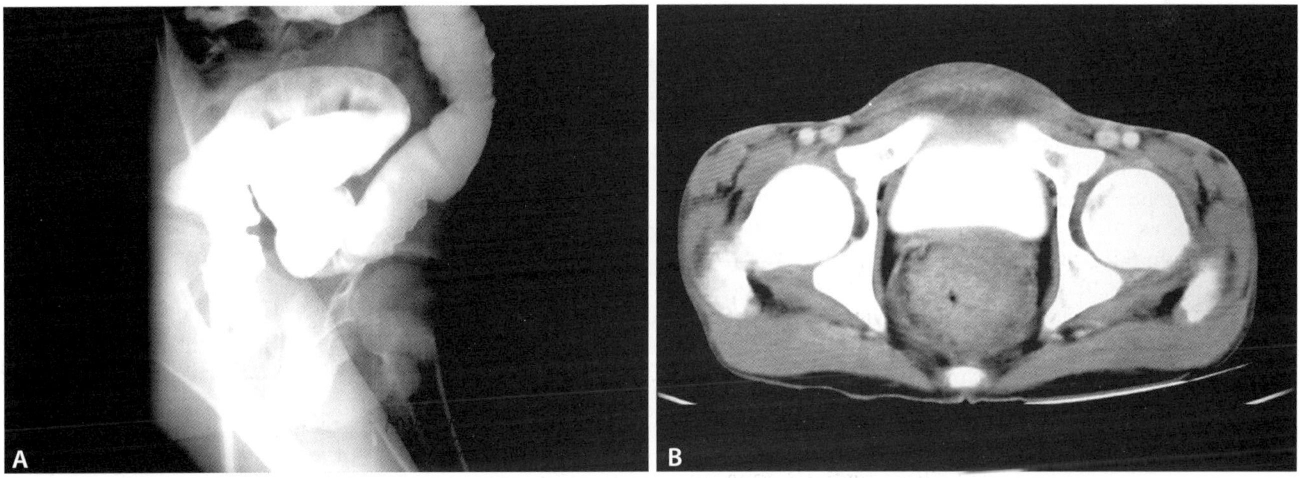

Figs. 21A and B: Carcinoma rectum: (A) Barium enema—marked narrowing and irregularity of the rectum; (B) CT pelvis shows diffuse thickening of rectal wall with early infiltration of adjacent tissues.

REFERENCES

1. Cairo MS, Grosfeld JL, Weetman RM. Gastric teratoma: Unusual cause for bleeding of the upper gastrointestinal tract in the newborn. Pediatrics 1981;67:721-4.
2. Golden CB, Feusner JH. Malignant abdominal masses in children: Quick guide to evaluation and diagnosis. Pediatr Clin North Am. 2002;49(6):1369-92.
3. Superina RA, Ein SH. Cystic duplications of the esophagus and neuroenteric cysts. J Pediatr Surg. 1984;19:517-30.
4. Parker BR. The abdomen and gastrointestinal tract. In Silverman FN, Kuhn JP (Eds): Caffey's Pediatric X-Ray Diagnosis, 9th edition. Mosby, 1993.
5. Gupta AK, Berry M, Mitra DK. Gastric duplication cyst in children: Report of two cases. Pediatr Radiol. 1994;24:346-7.
6. Teele RL, Smith EH. Ultrasound in the diagnosis of idiopathic hypertrophic pyloric stenosis. N Engl J Med. 1977;296:1149-50.
7. Hayden CK, Swischuk LE. Ultrasound: The definite imaging modality in pyloric stenosis. Radiographics. 1984;4:517-30.
8. Hallam D, Hansen B, Bodker B, et al. Pyloric size in normal infants and in infants suspected of having hypertrophic pyloric stenosis. Acta Radiol. 1995;36(3):261-64.
9. Neilson D, Hollman AS. The ultrasonic diagnosis of infantile hypertrophic pyloric stenosis: Technique and accuracy. Clin Radiol. 1994;49(4):246-7.
10. Hernanz-Schulman M, Sells LL, Ambrosino MM, et al. Hypertrophic pyloric stenosis in the infant without a palpable olive: Accuracy of sonographic diagnosis. Radiology. 1994;193(3):771-6.
11. Blumhagen JD, Noble HGS. Muscle thickness in hypertrophic pyloric stenosis: Sonographic determination. AJR. 1983;140: 221-3.
12. Daniel AB. Pyloric stenosis, hypertrophic. *http://www.emedicine.com/ped/topic1103.htm.*

13. Murphy S, Shaw K, Blanchard H. Report of three gastric tumors in children. J Pediatr Surg. 1994;29(9):1202-24.
14. Mirbagheri SA, Nahidi AR, Mohammod SP. Report of an 8 years old boy presenting with repeated GIT bleeding. *http://pearl.sums.ac.ir/AIM/9923/mirbagheri9923.html*
15. Mathew M, Gupta A, Narula MK, et al. Gastric teratoma: A report of three cases. Ind J Radiol Imag. 2002;12(4):507-10.
16. Gupta AK, Berry M, Mitra DK. Ossified gastric leiomyoma in a child: A case report. Pediatr Radiol. 1995;25:48-9.
17. Navaro O, Dugougeat F, Daneman A. Sonographic signs that characterize the gastrointestinal origin of abdominal neoplasms in children: 4 case reports. Can Assoc Radiol J. 2000;51(4):250-53.
18. Bluth EI, Merritt CRB, Sullvian MA. Ultrasonic evaluation of the stomach, small bowel and colon. Radiology. 1979;133:677-80.
19. Golden T, Stout AP. Smooth muscle tumours of GIT and retroperitoneal tissue. Surg Gynecol Obstet. 1941;73:784.
20. Thompson WM, Kende AI, Levy AD. Imaging characteristics of gastric lipomas in 16 adults and pediatric patients. AJR. 2003;181:981-5.
21. Dixon WL, Fazzari PJ. Carcinoma of stomach in a child. JAMA. 1976;235:2414-5.
22. Dunnick NR, Harell GS, Parker BR. Multiple "bull's eye" lesions in gastric lymphoma. AJR. 1976;126:965.
23. Ng YY, Healy JC. The radiology of non-Hodgkin's lymphoma in childhood: A review of 80 cases. Clin Radiol. 1994;49(9): 594-600.
24. Kurugoglu S, Mihmanli I, Celkan T, et al. Radiological features in pediatric primary gastric MALT lymphoma and association with *Helicobacter Pylori*. Pediatr Radiol. 2002;32:82-7.
25. Li P, Wei J, West AB, et al. Epithelial GI stromal tumours of stomach with liver metastases in a 12 years old girl: Aspiration cytology and molecular study. Pediatr Dev Pathol. 2003;6(3):278-9.
26. Oguzkurt P, Akcoren Z, Senocak ME, et al. A huge gastric stromal tumour in a 13 years old girl. Turk J Pediatr. 2002;44(1):65-8.
27. Nguyen VU, Taylor A. Gastric stromal tumours: Leiomyoma, leiomyosarcoma. *http://www.emedicine.com/radio/topic338.htm.*
28. Newman B, Girdany BR. Gastric trichobezoars: Sonographic and CT appearance. Pediatr Radiol. 1990;20:526-7.
29. Barr LL, Hyden CK, Stansberry SD, et al. Enteric duplication cysts in childen: Are their ultrasonographic wall characteristics diagnostic? Pediatr Radiol. 1990;20:326-8.
30. Macpherson RI. Gastrointestinal duplications: Clinical, pathologic, etiologic and radiologic considerations. Radiographics. 1993;13:1063-80.
31. Lister J, Rickham PP. Duplication of the alimentary tract. In: Rickham PP, Lister J, Irving T (Eds). Neonatal Surgery, 2nd edition. London: Butterworth. 1990;474-84.
32. Spottswood SE. Peristalsis in duplication cyst: A new diagnostic sonographic finding. Pediatr Radiol. 1994;24:344-5.
33. Andronikou S, Welman CJ, Kader E. The CT features of abdominal tuberculosis in children. Pediatr Radiol. 2002;32(2): 75-81.
34. Denath FM. Abdominal tuberculosis in children: CT findings. Gastrointestinal Radiology. 1990;15(4):303-06.
35. Ozbey H, Tireli GA. Abdominal tuberculosis in children. Eur J Pediatr Surg. 2003;13(2):116-9.
36. Gupta AK, Berry M, Mitra DK. Gastrointestinal smooth muscle tumours in children: Report of three cases. Pediatr Radiol. 1994;24:498-9.
37. Chattopadhyay A, Kumar A, Maruliah M, et al. Duodenojejunal obstruction by a haemangioma. Pediatr Surg Int. 2002;18(5-6):501-2.
38. Vade A, Blane CE. Imaging of Burkitt lymphoma in paediatric patients. Pediatr Radiol. 1985;15:123-6.
39. Sargent MA, Babyn P, Alton DJ. Plain abdominal radiography in suspected intussusception: A reassessment. Pediatr Radiol. 1994;24:17-20.
40. Bowerman RA, Silver TM, Jaffe MH. Real time ultrasound diagnosis of intussusception in children. Radiology. 1982;143:527-9.
41. Harrington L, et al. Ultrasonographic and clinical predictors of intussusception. J Pediatrics. 1998;132(5):836-9.
42. Stanley A, Logan H, Bate TW, et al. Ultrasound in the diagnosis and exclusion of intussuception. Ir Med J. 1997;90(2):64-5.
43. Intussusception reduction. British Society of Paediatric Radiology draft guidelines for suggested safe practice. *http://www.bspr.org.uk/intus.doc*
44. Del-Pozo G, et al. Intussuception in children: Current concepts in diagnosis and enema reduction. Radiographics. 1999;19(2):299.
45. Chan KL, Saing H, Peh WC, et al. Childhood intussusception: Ultrasound guide Hartmann's solution hydrostatic reduction or barium enema reduction? J Pediatr Surg. 1997;32(1):3-6.
46. Swischuk LE. The current radiology management of intussusception: A survey and review. Pediatr Radiol. 1992;2:317.
47. Haney PJ, Whitley NO. CT of benign cystic abdominal masses in children. AJR. 1984;142:1279-81.
48. Konen O, Rathaus V, Dlugy E, et al. Childhood abdominal cystic lymphangioma. Pediatr Radiol. 2002;32:88-94.
49. Zarewych ZM, Donnelly LF, Frush DP, et al. Imaging of pediatric mesenteric abnormalities. Pediatr Radiol. 1999;29(9):711-9.
50. Jewell CT, Miller ID, Ehrlich FE. Rectal duplication: An unusual cause for an abdominal mass. Surgery. 1973;74:783-5.
51. Sivit CJ, Newman KD. Appendicitis: Usefulness of ultrasound in diagnosis in a pediatric population. Radiology. 1992;185:549-52.
52. Karnak I. Colorectal cancers in children. J Pediatr Surg. 1999;34(10):1499-504.
53. Radha Krishnan CN, Bruce J. Colorectal cancers in children without any predisposing factors: A report of eight cases and review of literature. Eur J Pediatr Surg. 2003;13(1):66-8.
54. Karnak I, Kale G, Tanyel FC, et al. Malignant stromal tumour of the colon in an infant: Diagnostic difficulties and differential diagnosis. J Pediatr Surg. 2003;38(2):245-7.

CHAPTER 137

Hepatic and Pancreatic Masses in Children

Akshay Kumar Saxena, Kushaljit Singh Sodhi, Naveen Kalra

Focal hepatic masses in children include benign lesions such as cysts (congenital, i.e. simple or acquired like hydatid cysts), abscesses, granulomas and neoplasms (benign and malignant tumors, primary and metastatic lesions). Malignant neoplasms and abscesses are more common than simple cysts and benign tumors.

Pancreatic tumors are rare in infants and children. They can be cystic or solid, benign or malignant and endocrine or exocrine in origin. Pancreatoblastoma, islet cell tumors and solid and papillary epithelial neoplasms (SPEN) are the most important tumors of childhood. Pseudocysts of pancreas secondary to pancreatitis are more common than cystic tumors of the pancreas.

IMAGING

Ultrasonography (US) and computed tomography (CT) remain the primary imaging modalities for investigating hepatic and pancreatic masses. Majority of the lesions, particularly tumors, require more than one modality to reach at a definitive diagnosis. Ultrasonography is the initial investigation of choice as the location, nature of the lesion (cystic or solid), relationship to adjacent organs, associated lymphadenopathy and invasion of the vascular structures by the mass can all be well seen on US. In children, ultrasonography has the ability to visualize the entire pancreas well because of the relatively large left lobe of liver as an acoustic window during scanning. Color Doppler flow imaging and intra-operative ultrasonography further help in the diagnosis and patient's management.[1]

Once a mass is suspected to be a tumor, dynamic contrast enhanced CT scan should be performed as it is more accurate than US in distinguishing various neoplastic lesions and it has the best capability to assess extrahepatic spread of the disease such as lymphadenopathy and omental or peritoneal spread.[1] However, it is important to note a few technical considerations while performing the CT scan. Many of the patients require sedation for performing a technically satisfactory study. Generally, the sedation is provided by the anesthetists. The radiologist should ensure that the patient undergoes pre-anesthetic check up prior to the date of appointment. In addition, need for keeping the child nil orally on the day of appointment should be carefully impressed upon. Failure to adhere to these precautions may lead to postponement of study. The nil per oral guidelines are less stringent for smaller children and for clear fluids **(Table 1)**.[2]

With the advent of multidetector spiral CT, it is now possible to image the abdomen during the arterial

Table 1: Nil per oral guidelines for CT scan.[2]

Age	*Solids and milk/formula*	*Clear liquids*
> 3 years	Stop 6–8 hours before sedation	Stop 2–3 hours before sedation
6 months to 3 years	Stop 6 hours before sedation	Stop 2–3 hours before sedation
< 6 months	Stop 4–6 hours before sedation	Stop 2 hours before sedation

and portal venous phases. Lu et al.[3] however have advocated that imaging of the pancreas should be done in the 'pancreatic phase' only. This phase occurs in the interval between the arterial and portal venous phase at 40–70 seconds after the bolus injection of contrast at a rate of 3 mL/second. During this phase there is maximum pancreatic parenchymal enhancement with accentuation of the lesion-to-pancreas contrast. The use of this phase alone has the benefit of reducing the radiation exposure to the patient. Single phase evaluation of focal hepatic lesions is also recommended by "Image gently" campaign.[4] Apart from doing the single phase studies, it is important to carefully adjust the KV and mAs according to the weight of the child.[2] This will avoid unnecessary high radiation to these children. Most of the vendors now provide for children specific scanning protocols and radiologists should ensure that technologists are adhering to these protocols.

Magnetic resonance imaging (MRI) is superior to both US and CT in characterizing the lesion and showing its extent, particularly vascular invasion,[5,6] but it is reserved as a problem solving modality because of its inherent limitations namely high cost, lack of easy availability and compulsory sedation in nearly all infants and children which makes its routine use impractical. However due to the lack of ionizing radiation and multiplanar imaging capabilities, MR and MRCP are especially useful in the pediatric population.

Radionuclide scanning of the liver using ^{99m}Tc-Sulphur colloid has a sensitivity and specificity of 80-85% each. It can be supplemented with single photon emission computed tomography (SPECT) which can detect lesions as small as 1 cm diameter (sensitivity and specificity of 90–95% each). Regarding characterization of a known hepatic mass, ^{99m}Tc-labeled red blood cell (RBC) scanning has the greatest utility in diagnosing cavernous hemangiomas by achieving a specificity of nearly 100% (barring occasional false positives due to small hepatocellular carcinomas or hypervascular metastasis).[7]

Angiography has limited role except for the vascular road-mapping of tumors when surgery or therapeutic embolization is considered.

Plain radiography is of limited diagnostic value in the evaluation of pediatric masses. Calcification in tumors like hepatoblastoma and pancreatoblastoma may be detected on abdominal radiographs. Pulmonary complications like basal pneumonitis, pleural effusions in hepatic abscesses and pulmonary metastasis may be seen on chest radiographs.

Imaging, usually ultrasonography, may also be required for providing guidance for interventional procedures like fine needle aspiration cytology (FNAC).

HEPATIC MASSES

Malignant Hepatic Tumors

Primary malignant hepatic tumors constitute nearly 1.5% of all pediatric tumors and 15% of all abdominal masses in children.[8] About 2/3rd of these are malignant, of which hepatoblastoma, hepatocellular carcinoma and rarely sarcomas constitute the majority.[5,9]

HEPATOBLASTOMA

The term hepatoblastoma was coined by Willis in 1962 for hepatic tumors of embryonal origin which were histologically different from hepatocellular carcinoma.[10] Hepatoblastoma is the most frequent malignancy of liver in children and is seen at less than 5 years of age.[2,11] The peak incidence occurs between 18 and 24 months of age. The patient usually presents with an abdominal mass but less frequently anorexia, weight loss, jaundice and pain due to hemorrhage or rupture may be the presenting features. A number of conditions such as Beckwith-Wiedemann syndrome, hemihypertrophy, familial adenomatous polyposis (FAP), Gardner's syndrome, Wilms' tumor, sexual precocity and osteopenia can be associated with hepatoblastoma. Serum alpha-fetoprotein is elevated in about 80% of these patients.[9]

Pathologically, hepatoblastoma contains small, primitive, epithelial cells resembling those in fetal liver tissue. When mesenchymal elements like osteoid are also present in addition to epithelial elements, the hepatoblastoma is classified as mixed variant. There is no significant survival difference between the epithelial and mixed forms of hepatoblastoma. Vascular invasion is less frequent compared to hepatocellular carcinoma. Calcification may be present. The tumor metastasizes most commonly to the lungs followed by lymph nodes, brain, peritoneum and diaphragm.

Several methods are available for staging of hepatoblastoma.[12] The most commonly used is PRETEXT system. This system is predominantly dependent on radiological findings. The liver, in this system, is divided into right anterior (Couniad's segments V and VIII), right posterior (Couniad's segments VI and VII), left medial (Couniad's segments IVa and IVb) and left lateral (Couniad's segments II and III) sections (also called sectors). The caudate lobe and the caudate process, i.e. segments I and IX are currently considered not to have any independent significance in PRETEXT system. The PRETEXT group number reflects the maximum number of contiguous liver sections that are free of tumor **(Table 2)**.[12] Extrahepatic spread is classified separately **(Table 3)**.[12] In contrast, Children's Oncology

Group (widely used in North America) is based on postoperative evaluation **(Table 4)**[12] and, therefore, relies much less on the imaging findings. TNM classification is not widely used for hepatoblastoma.

On imaging, hepatoblastoma is generally seen as a single, well-defined lesion with lobulated outline, mostly located in the right lobe. Less commonly the lesion may involve the left lobe or even be multicentric. On US, the lesion has generally inhomogeneous echotexture, may be hyperechoic[13] with anechoic areas corres-ponding to necrosis or hemorrhage. Calcifications in the lesion appear as echogenic foci with distal shadowing. A rare cystic form of hepatoblastoma has also been described which is completely anechoic on US but may reveal mural nodule.[11] Hepatoblastoma may also appear as diffuse parenchymal inhomogeneity with multiple cystic lesions.[14] In case of vascular invasion, portal vein may show intraluminal thrombus. On Doppler studies, peak systolic Doppler frequency shifts in the hepatic artery are usually greater than 4 KHz.[9] If available, noncontrast CT **(Fig. 1A)** scan generally reveals hypodense or isodense and calcification may be detected in as many as 50% of cases.[15] Calcification is typically coarse and dense in contrast to fine calcification seen in hemangioendothelioma. Other features which differentiate hepatoblastoma from hemangioendothelioma include predominantly hyperechoic pattern, absence of congestive heart failure and markedly elevated level of alpha-fetoproteins in hepatoblastoma. On CECT hepatoblastoma appears as low attenuating mass which may show inhomogeneous enhancement **(Fig. 1B)**. In the early phase of dynamic

Table 2: PRETEXT staging of hepatic tumors.[12]

PRETEXT-I	One section is involved and three adjoining sections are free
PRETEXT-II	One or two sections are involved, but two adjoining sections are free
PRETEXT–III	Two or three sections are involved and no two adjoining sections are free
PRETEXT-IV	All four sections are involved

Table 3: PRETEXT staging of extrahepatic disease.[12]

V +	Involvement of the inferior vena cava and/or all three hepatic veins
P +	Involvement of the main portal vein and/or both left and right branches of the portal vein
E +	Extrahepatic disease in the abdomen
M +	Distant metastases

Table 4: Children's oncology group staging of liver cancer.[12]

Stage I	Tumor completely resected
Stage II	Tumor grossly resected with microscopic residual disease
Stage III	• Tumor unresectable or resected with gross residual disease • Nodal involvement • Tumor spill • Gross residual intrahepatic disease
Stage IV	Distant metastases

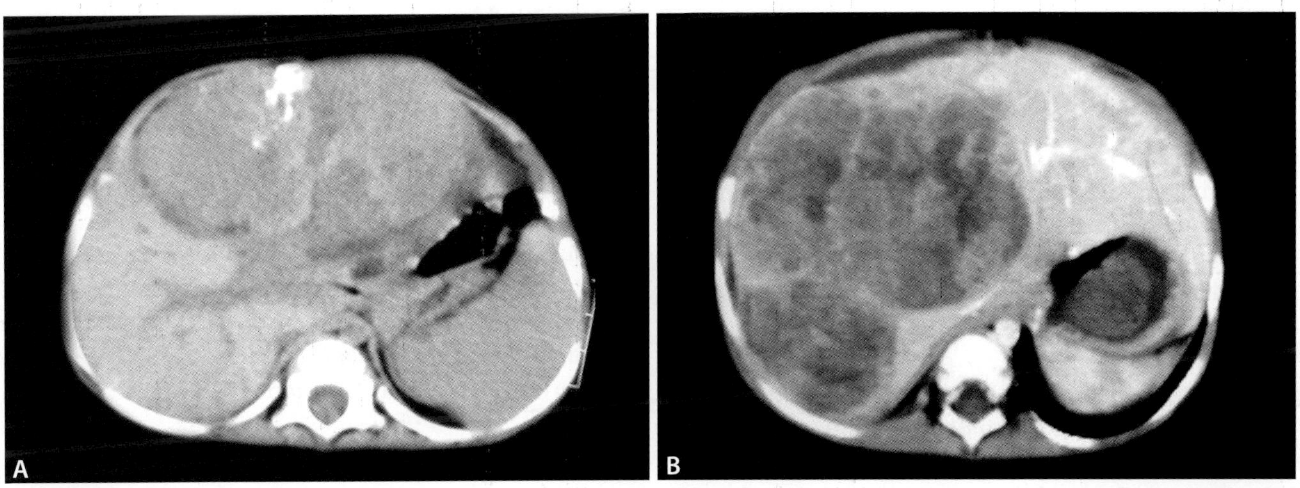

Figs. 1A and B: (A) NCCT scan in a 14-month-old male patient with hepatoblastoma shows a large well defined hypodense mass replacing the left lobe of liver. Coarse calcification is seen within the mass; (B) CECT in another patient of hepatoblastoma shows heterogeneously enhancing mass lesion in right lobe.

CT, the tumor may appear hyperdense and show rim enhancement indicating increased vascularity. The septations within the tumor are best seen after contrast enhancement **(Fig. 2)**.

On MRI, hepatoblastoma appears as low intensity mass on T1WI and increased signal intensity mass on T2WI. Hypointense bands (corresponding to fibrotic areas) may be seen on both T1W and T2W images. Tumor thrombus in the hepatic or portal vein appears as an area of increased signal intensity in the normal flow of vessels. MRI is better than CT and US for demonstration of tumor margins and vascular invasion. However, CT is superior for detecting calcification.

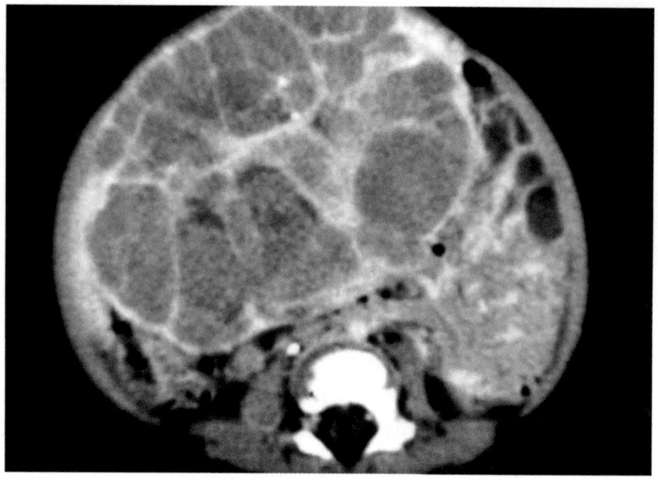

Fig. 2: CT in a case of hepatoblastoma shows inhomogeneous enhancement and multiple enhancing septae.

HEPATOCELLULAR CARCINOMA

This tumor generally occurs in children older than 5 years. There are two age peaks in childhood, the first is between 2 and 4 years and the second one occurs between 12 to 14 years.[16] Childhood hepatocellular carcinoma (HCC) is associated with diseases like glycogen storage disease (Type I), cystinosis, hereditary tyrosinemia, Wilson's disease, alpha 1-antitrypsin deficiency, extrahepatic biliary atresia and giant cell hepatitis. Association with cirrhosis is less common than in adults. Serum alpha-fetoprotein is elevated in 40–50% of patients.[6]

HCC can appear as focal, multinodular or diffuse form with variable and nonspecific appearances. When solitary, the lesion is common in the right lobe. On sonography, HCC is characterized by variable echogenicity pattern with predominantly hypo-, iso- or hyperechoic echotexture. Calcification may be seen in 10% of patients but is less common than in hepatoblastoma. US appearances may be indistinguishable from hepatoblastoma.

On noncontrast CT scan, lesion is of low attenuation and generally reveals inhomogeneous enhancement after contrast. On dynamic CT, majority are hypervascular and may reveal areas of peripheral enhancement in the early vascular phase and later become hypodense to liver parenchyma **(Figs. 3A and B)**. On MRI, these tumors are usually hypointense on T1WI and hyperintense on T2WI. The vascular invasion is demonstrated as loss of normal flow void in the vessels.

Fibrolamellar HCC

It is a rare subtype of HCC but it has a better prognosis if resected. This tumor is usually seen in young females (mean age 23 years); but it can occur in children. Alpha-fetoprotein level is usually not elevated.[17] CT reveals a well-defined hypodense mass which shows variable enhancement after contrast injection. A central fibrotic scar and calcification are more commonly seen (30% and 50% of cases respectively)[18] in fibrolamellar subtype of HCC **(Figs. 4A and B)**. MRI can be used to distinguish fibrolamellar HCC from focal nodular hyperplasia (FNH). The fibrous central scar of fibrolamellar HCC is hypointense on both T1WI and T2WI. On the other hand, the central scar of FNH is hyperintense on T2WI.[19]

RHABDOMYOSARCOMA

This is the most common tumor of the biliary tree in children and accounts for 0.04% of all cancers in children. It occurs at a median age of 3 years and is rare after the first decade.[20] There is a male preponderance. The tumor may arise in the liver, intrahepatic ducts, intrahepatic cyst, gallbladder, cystic duct, extrahepatic duct, ampulla or choledochal cyst. Patient usually presents with jaundice and abdominal distention. Ultrasonography **(Fig. 5A)** shows biliary dilatation with a hyperechoic intraductal mass. The portal vein may be displaced but is not thrombosed. Larger lesions have areas of necrosis. CT **(Figs. 5B and C)** shows an intraductal mass with or without biliary dilatation. The mass is heterogeneous in attenuation with variable contrast enhancement. On MRI, the mass is of low signal intensity on T1W images and hyperintense on T2W images. MRCP shows dilated ducts and the entire extent of the lesion **(Fig. 6)**.

HEPATIC METASTASES

The common primary malignancy to metastasize to liver in children are neuroblastoma, Wilms' tumor, GI tumors, Ewing's sarcoma, rhabdomyosarcoma, lymphomas and

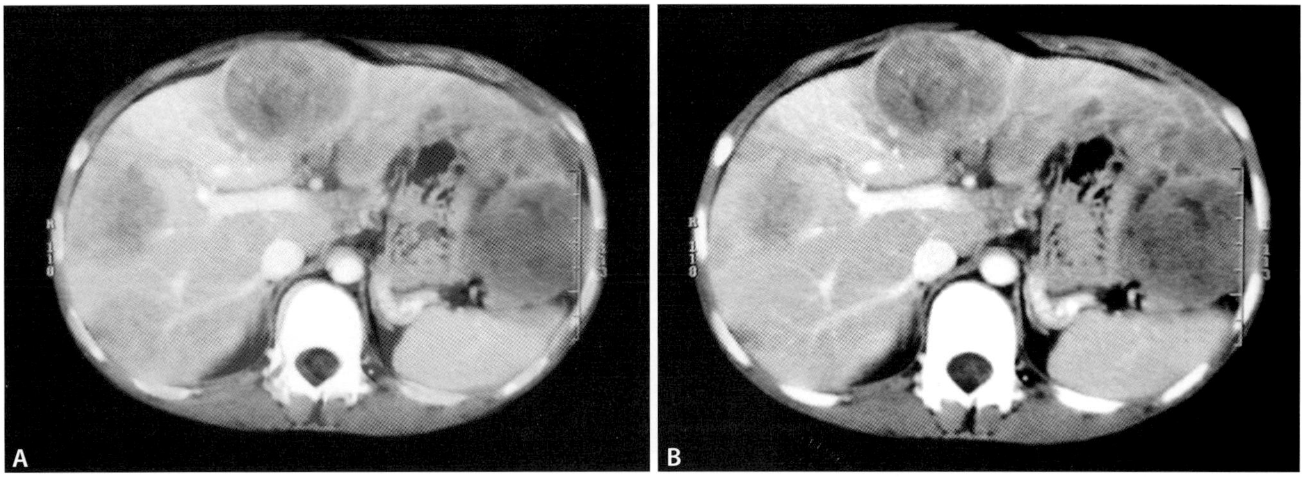

Figs. 3A and B: CT scan in an 11-year-old male patient with multicentric HCC. There are multiple lesions seen in both lobes of liver which show peripheral enhancement. The left branch of portal vein is not opacified suggestive of invasion.

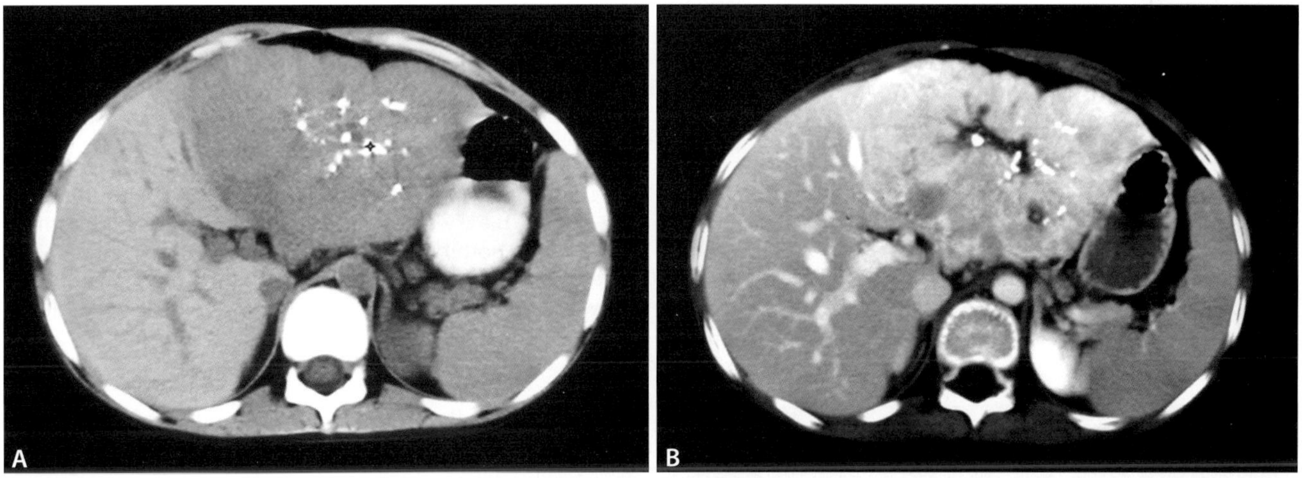

Figs. 4A and B: CT scan in a 16-year-old female patient with fibrolamellar HCC: (A) NCCT shows a well-defined hypodense mass in the left lobe of liver with central calcification and lobulated border; (B) CECT shows inhomogeneous enhancement with central hypodense scar.

leukemias.[2,11] The metastases may be single or multiple **(Figs. 7 and 8)**. These are usually nonspecific lesions appearing hypoechoic on ultrasonography, hypodense on contrast enhance CT scan, hypointense on T1 and hyperintense on T2W MR images. If required, diagnosis can be clinched by fine needle aspiration cytology under sonographic guidance.

Benign Hepatic Neoplasms

These account for one-third of all primary hepatic tumors. Most of these tumors are of vascular origin, viz. infantile hemangioendothelioma and cavernous hemangioma.[9] Less common tumors are mesenchymal hamartoma, focal nodular hyperplasia (FNH) and hepatic adenoma.

INFANTILE HEMANGIOENDOTHELIOMA

Infantile hemangioendothelioma is the most common benign tumor in children less than one year of age.[2,21] It commonly presents before 6 months of age in more than 85% of patients and is more common in females. Hemangioendothelioma may present with high output cardiac failure, asymptomatic hepatomegaly or an abdominal mass. Heart failure occurs in nearly 50% of infants with this tumor.[22] Occasionally, thrombocytopenia due to platelet sequestration or massive intraperitoneal bleeding and shock due to spontaneous tumor rupture can be the presenting features. Cutaneous hemangiomata are reported in 40% of patients.[23] Spontaneous regression

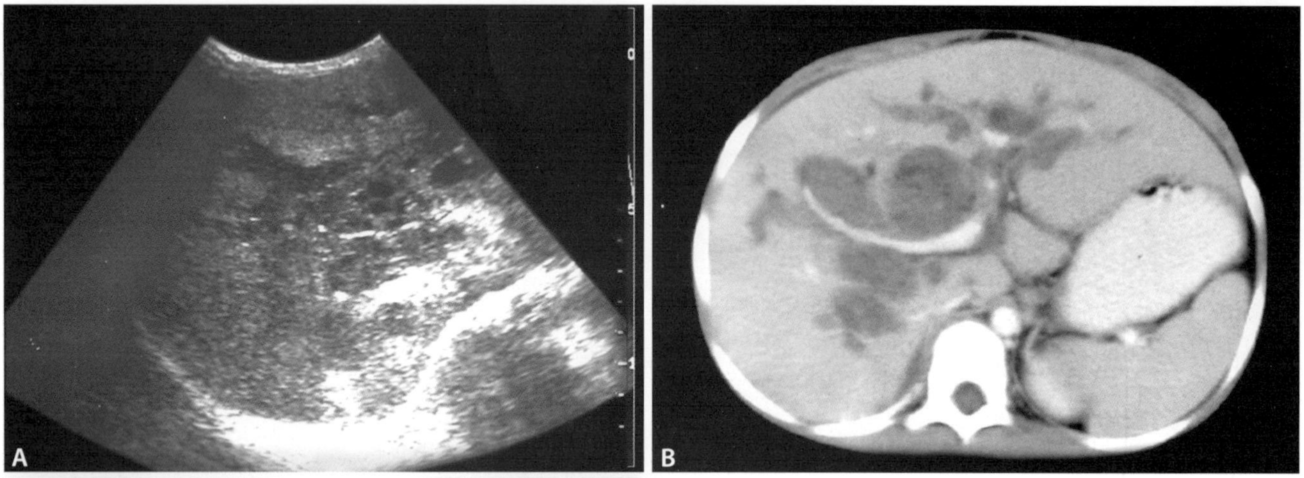

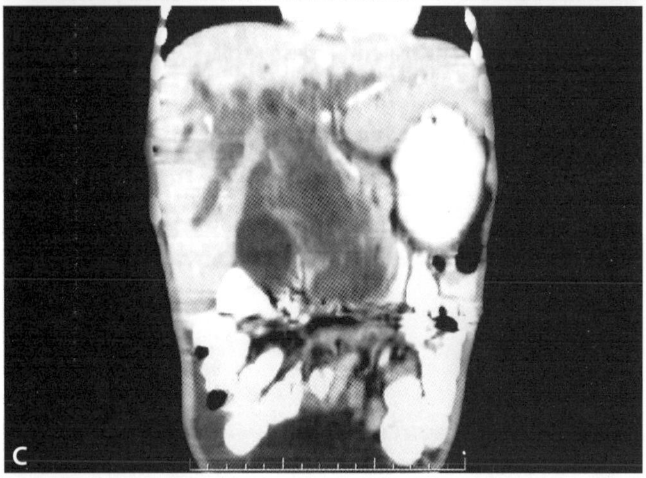

Figs. 5A to C: An 8-year-old female child with jaundice: (A) Ultrasound scan reveals echogenic soft tissue filling the dilated biliary channels; (B) CECT shows biliary radicle dilatation in both lobes of liver with presence of intraluminal heterogeneous attenuation mass; (C) Coronal reconstruction shows the entire extent of the lesion. FNAC revealed biliary rhabdomyosarcoma.

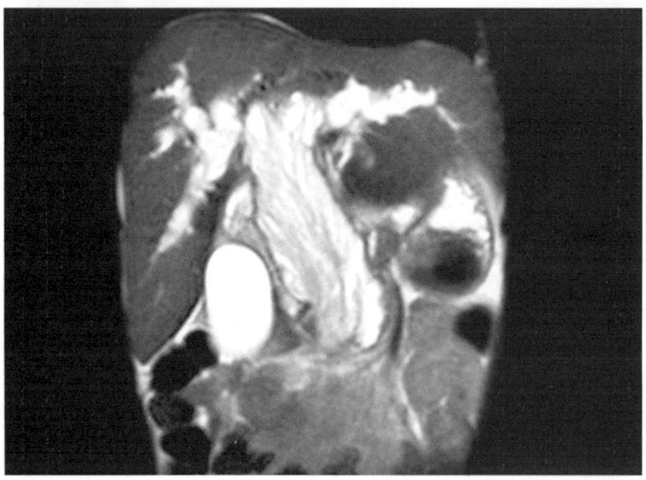

Fig. 6: T2W coronal image in a case of biliary rhabdomyosarcoma shows the dilatation of the biliary tree with heterogeneous hyperintensity of the intraductal tumor.

has also been described. The clinical as well as radiological features depend on the rate of blood flow and the extent of arteriovenous shunting.

Pathologically, hemangioendothelioma is composed of multiple, round, discrete nodules ranging from 2–15 cm in size. Microscopically, the tumor is quite vascular. There are two histological subtypes.[24] Type I consists of variable sized vascular spaces lined by relatively immature plump endothelial cells. Type II has more immature pleomorphic cells with hyperchromatic nuclei and reflects more aggressive form. They may mimic hemangioendothelial sarcoma and rare cases of metastasis have also been described.[25] Uncommonly, these tumors may be solitary with a slight predilection for the posterior segment of right lobe.

On sonography the lesion shows multiple well-defined hypoechoic masses throughout the liver **(Figs. 9A and B)**. Enlargement of the celiac and hepatic arteries along with decreased caliber of the aorta distal to the origin of the celiac artery strongly suggests the diagnosis. Large draining hepatic veins are also seen. Ultrasonography can also be used to monitor the response of hemangioendothelioma to steroid therapy.

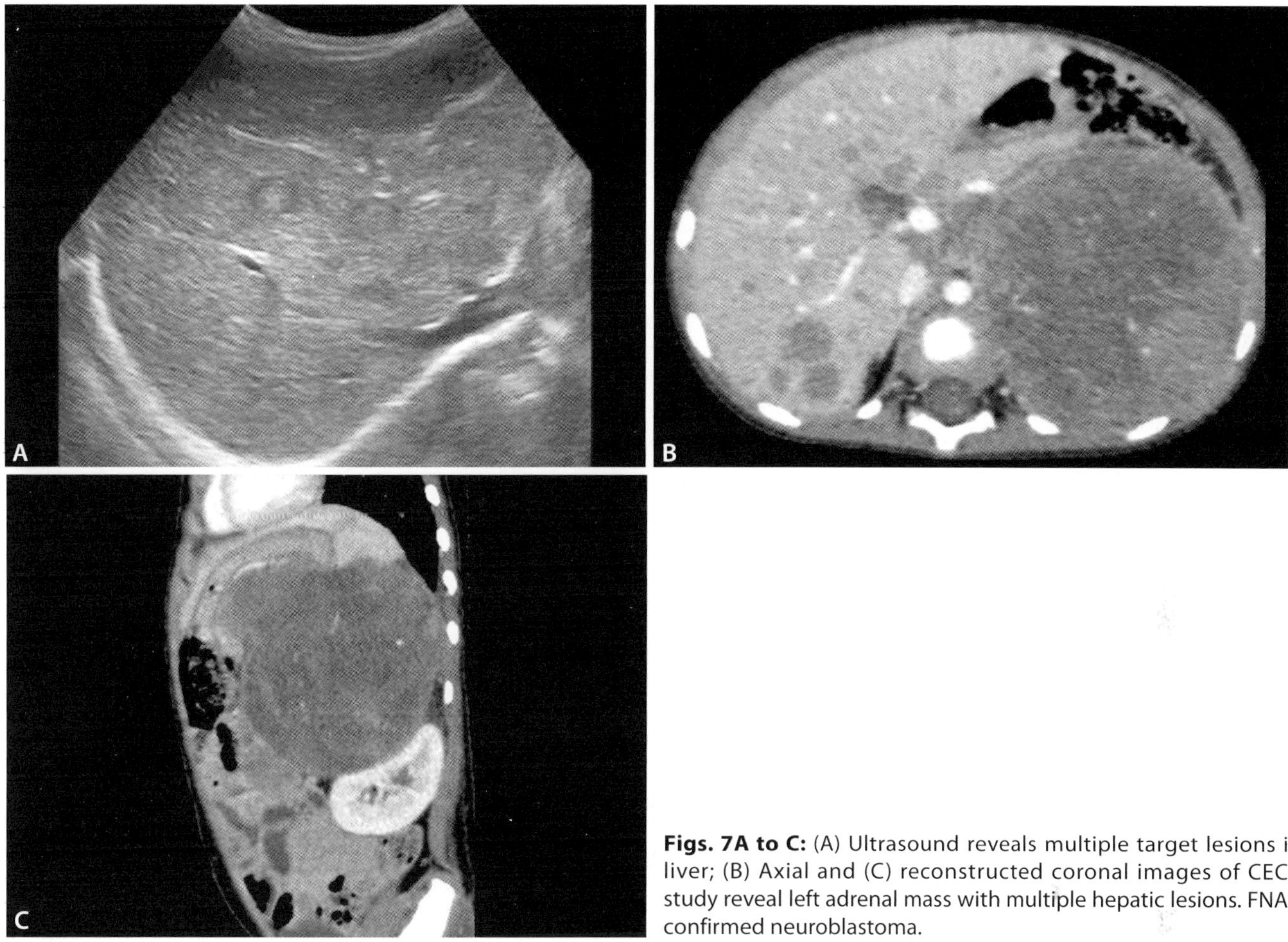

Figs. 7A to C: (A) Ultrasound reveals multiple target lesions in liver; (B) Axial and (C) reconstructed coronal images of CECT study reveal left adrenal mass with multiple hepatic lesions. FNAC confirmed neuroblastoma.

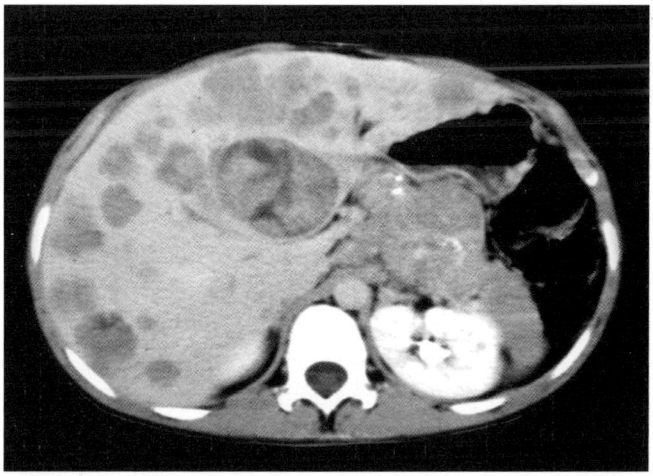

Fig. 8: Multiple well-defined hypodense lesions are seen in liver on CECT in a case of pancreatoblastoma metastasizing to liver.

On noncontrast CT, these tumors appear as well-defined, homogeneous hypodense masses. Calcification is seen in 40% of patients.[16] Early peripheral, nodular enhancement with gradual central filling is seen on dynamic CT scanning similar to hemangioma in adults. Larger lesions usually show incomplete filling with central hypodense areas representing fibrosis and thrombus **(Figs. 9C and D)**.[26]

When CT or US findings are equivocal, radionuclide or MRI studies can be helpful. Tc-labeled red blood cell scan shows increased activity in the blood pool phase and on delayed scanning. Radionuclide study has nearly 100% specificity for the diagnosis and should be used whenever diagnosis is in doubt.[17,27] On MRI, tumor is hypointense on T1WI and hyperintense or heterogeneous on T2WI.

HEMANGIOMA

Hemangiomas may be single or multiple; the latter being associated with hemangiomatosis syndrome of childhood.

Pathologically it is very vascular and shows multiple, dilated, blood filled spaces lined by mature, flat endothelium and separated by fibrous stroma. This lesion does not have any malignant potential.

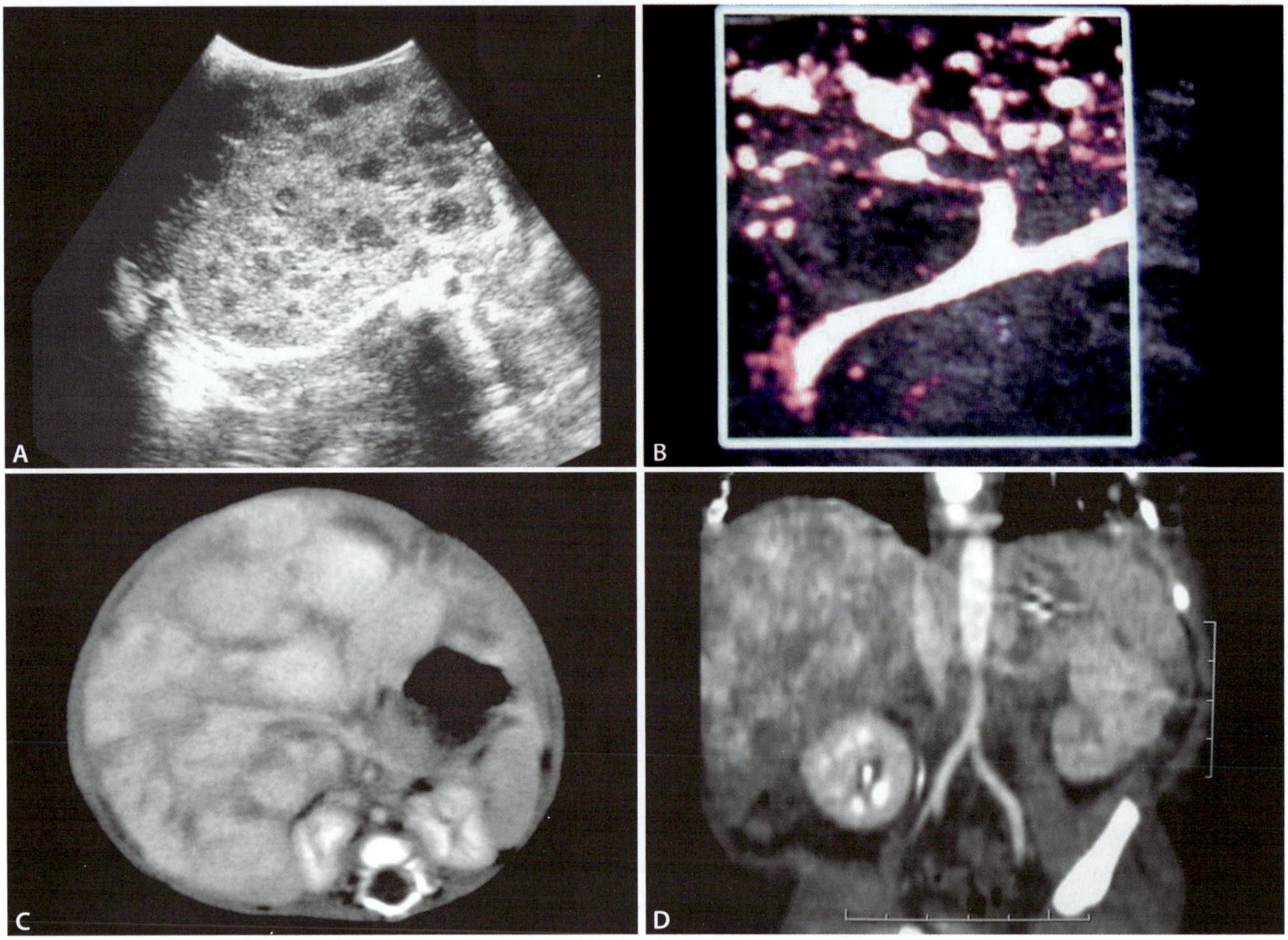

Figs. 9A to D: Imaging finding in infantile hemangioendothelioma: (A) Grayscale ultrasound reveals multiple well-defined hypo- to anechoic lesions in both lobes of liver; (B) Power Doppler revealed markedly increased vascularity in these lesions; (C) In another patient axial CECT scan demonstrates multiple enhancing hypervascular lesions diffusedly distributed in both lobes of liver while coronal reformatted image (D) shows sudden change in aortic caliber, distal to celiac artery, which is a characteristic feature of infantile hemangioendothelioma.

On sonography, hemangioma is typically small (<3 cm in diameter), homogeneous, well-defined and hyperechoic with distal acoustic enhancement. Larger lesion can be heterogeneous.[28] On noncontrast CT, it is hypo-to isodense and well-defined. On dynamic contrast studies, early, peripheral, dense nodular enhancement with later centripetal fill in is noted **(Figs. 10A and B)**. Complete isodense filling occurs in not less than 3 minutes and not more than 30 minutes after injection in 2/3rd of these lesions. When above features can be demonstrated, no further investigation is required. But the lesion can show variable contrast enhancement and variable fill in. In this equivocal state, MRI and scintigraphy are helpful.

On MRI, hemangioma appears hypo-or isointense to liver on T1WI. On T2WI, it shows marked hyperintensity which is maintained even on heavily T2WI.[2] After Gd-DTPA injection, the appearance is similar to CT, i.e. peripheral enhancement with centripetal fill in.

On Tc-labeled red blood cell scanning, it shows increased activity in blood pool phase and on delayed scanning. This study has 100% specificity for the diagnosis of hemangioma. For lesion larger than 2 cm, both MRI and ^{99m}Tc RBC imaging have similar accuracy (95%) but for lesion smaller than 2 cm, MRI is more sensitive. However, SPECT ^{99m}Tc RBC imaging is more specific than MRI.

Hepatic angiography is rarely required in establishing the diagnosis of hemangioma. Rarely when surgery is contemplated in symptomatic hemangioma, angiography can be helpful in defining the vascular anatomy.

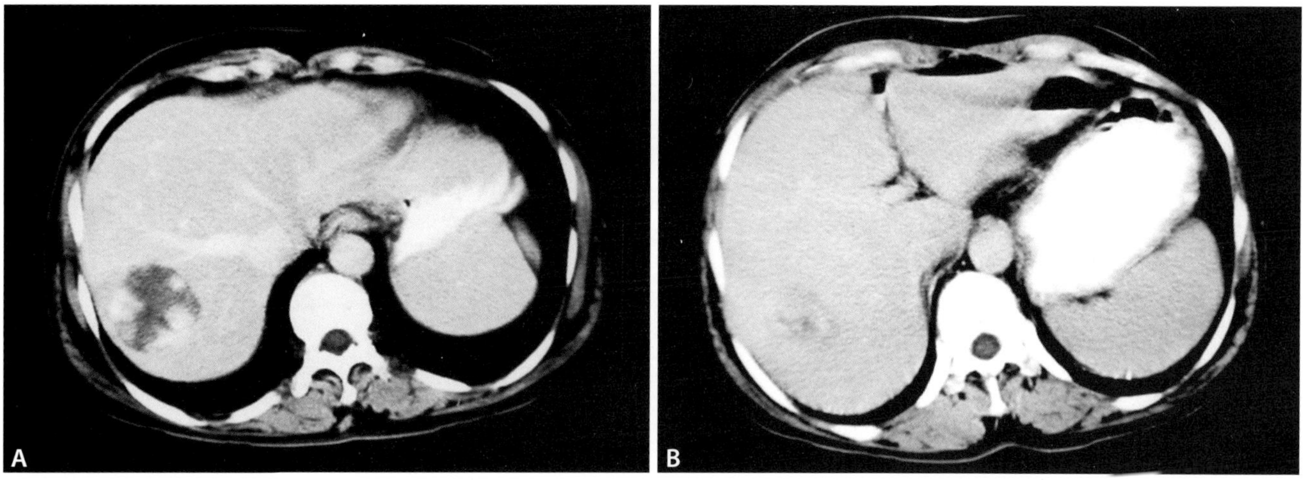

Figs. 10A and B: (A) Venous phase CECT image in a case of cavenous hemangioma showing dense nodular enhancement in a peripherally located hepatic mass; (B) Delayed phase reveals lesion to be almost isodense to liver.

MESENCHYMAL HAMARTOMA

Mesenchymal hamartoma is the second most common benign hepatic tumor next to vascular lesions.[29] This tumor usually presents as an asymptomatic abdominal mass in children less than 2 years of age and is twice as common in boys than girls. Rarely children may present with cardiac failure due to presence of large shunt in the lesion.

Pathologically, this tumor is seen as a well-circumscribed mass with multiple cystic areas.[29] On sonography,[30] the tumor appears as a well-defined, multilocular mass with anechoic spaces separated by echogenic septae **(Figs. 11A and B)**. This has been described as 'swiss cheese' appearance.[29] On CT scanning, the tumor is seen as a complex mass containing areas of low attenuation separated by solid septae and stroma which enhance with intravenous contrast administration[31] **(Figs. 12A and B)**. On MRI, the cystic spaces show high signal on T2WI and low signal on T1WI. The signal intensity however depends on the protein content and presence of hemorrhage within the cysts.

FOCAL NODULAR HYPERPLASIA (FNH) AND HEPATIC ADENOMA

This benign lesion is uncommon and constitutes less than 2% of pediatric hepatic tumors.[7] Childhood hepatic adenoma is associated with glycogen storage disease, Fanconi's anemia and galactosemia. Both these tumors are well-circumscribed masses with variable echogenicity and enhancement patterns. However, presence of a central low attenuation scar favors the diagnosis of FNH. When the distinction based on these imaging modalities is uncertain, radionuclide sulphur colloid scintigraphic study is very helpful. As high as 60% of FNH accumulate colloid while hepatic adenoma appears as focal defects.[7,9,32] Focal hepatic mass which is seen as hot area on sulphur colloid scan is diagnostic of FNH.

PELIOSIS HEPATIS

This is a rare entity characterized by small blood filled spaces in the liver. It is found in association with type I glycogen storage disease, HIV infection and intake of androgens.[10,16] On US, there are scattered areas of heterogeneous echogenicity of liver along with cystic lesions. CT demonstrates areas of low attenuation which show variable contrast enhancement. MRI shows increased signal intensity on T2WI and variable signal on T1WI depending upon the contents of the cysts.[11]

INFLAMMATORY LESIONS

Pyogenic Hepatic Abscess

These are usually associated with various predisposing conditions like systemic sepsis, appendicitis, inflammatory bowel disease, omphalitis, trauma or chronic granulomatous disease of childhood.[33] In neonates gram-negative, and in older children *Staphylococcus aureus* are the most common organisms. When the abscesses are multiple, they usually are the result of ascending biliary infection. When solitary, right lobe is affected more often. Children often present with fever, upper abdominal pain, tender hepatomegaly and leukocytosis.

The abscesses pass through three stages viz. the stage of suppuration, the stage of liquefaction and the stage of

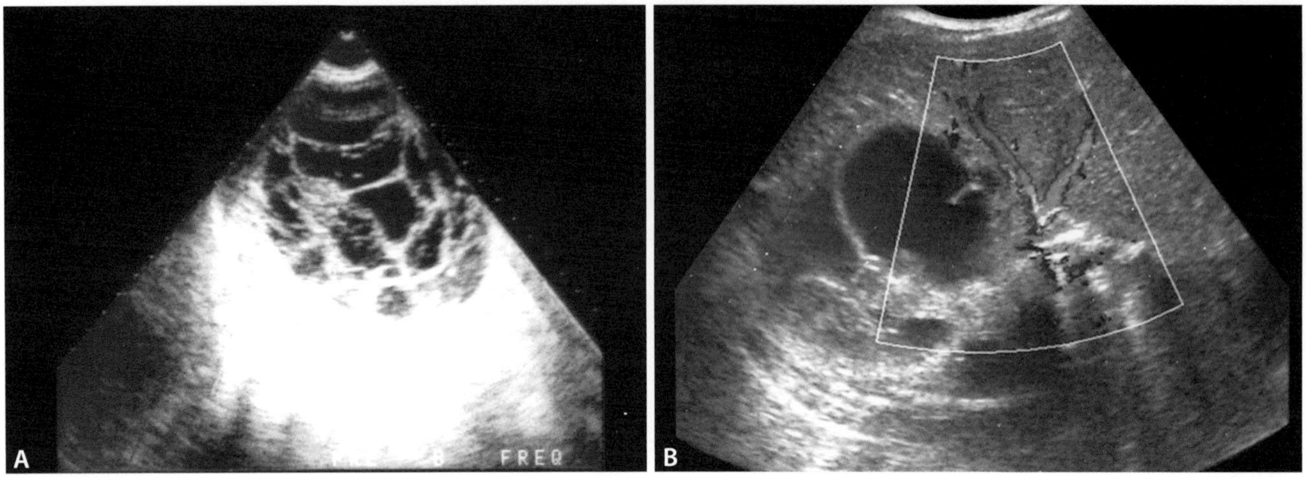

Figs. 11A and B: (A) US scan in a 7-month-old boy reveals a large multilocular cystic mass with septae in the right lobe of liver in a case of mesenchymal hamartoma; (B) Doppler reveals absence of intralesional blood flow.

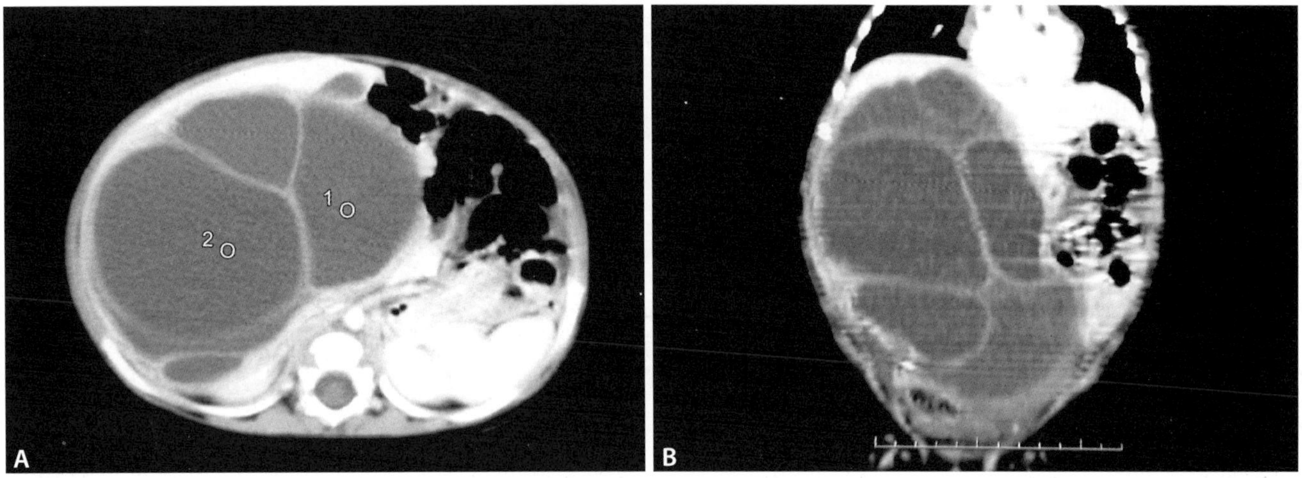

Figs. 12A and B: CT scan (A) axial and (B) coronal reconstruction in a 7-month-old male patient with mesenchymal hamartoma reveals a multiloculated cystic mass with enhancing septae.

resolution including fibrosis, cystic residual lesion and calcification. These stages influence imaging appearance of the abscesses.

Sonography is the initial and usually the only investigation required in patients suspected to have hepatic abscesses. Abscess may appear anechoic, hypoechoic, hyperechoic or as a complex mass with thick irregular walls and through-transmission **(Fig. 13)**. Early lesions tend to be echogenic and ill-defined. If gas is detected it clinches the diagnosis. Occasionally septations, fluid-fluid levels and echogenic debris may be noted.[34]

On CT, most abscesses are sharply defined, hypodense masses which may show rim enhancement on contrast administration.[9] Intralesional gas, although highly suggestive of the diagnosis, is seen in only 20% of patients. Double-target sign, consisting of a low density central area surrounded by hyperdense zone and then a peripheral hypodense zone may also be noted.

On scintigraphy examination using either Ga-67 or In-111, the lesions are "hot". In-111 scanning provides increased specificity because it is not taken up by benign or malignant lesions. Chest radiographs show elevated hemidiaphragm, pleural effusion, basal atelectasis or infiltrates.

When the diagnosis cannot be established based on clinical or CT findings, percutaneous needle aspiration performed under sonographic or CT guidance can be helpful in diagnosis and also for providing percutaneous aspiration or catheter drainage.[35,36]

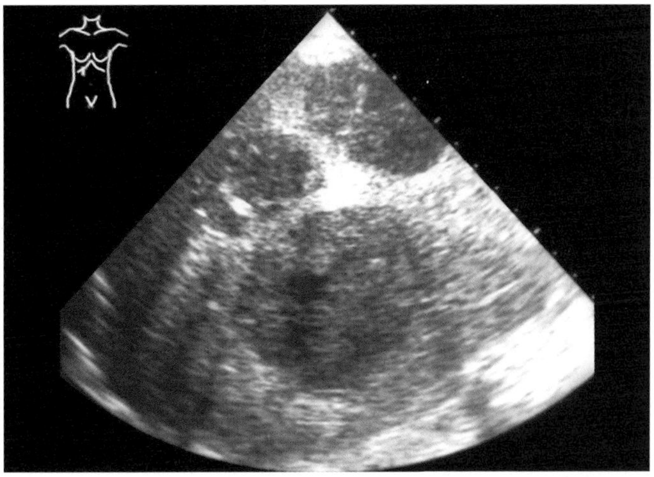

Fig. 13: US liver showing multiple pyogenic liver abscesses as multiple hypoechoic lesions with thick irregular wall and coarse internal echoes.

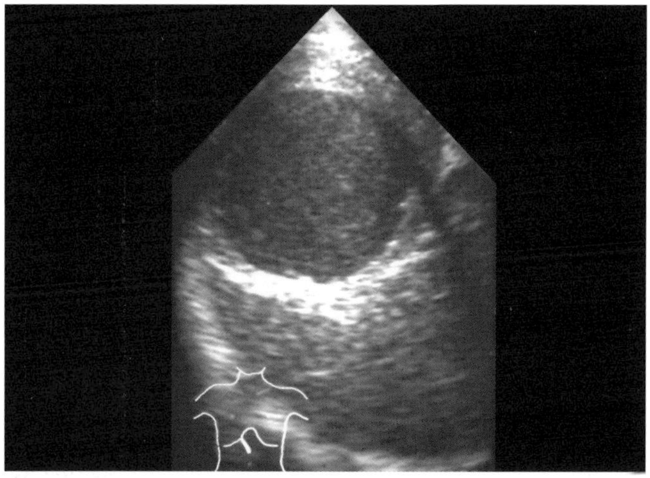

Fig. 14: US liver in a case of amebic liver abscess shows a well-defined rounded hypoehoic lesion with fine low level internal echoes and an almost imperceptible wall.

Amebic Hepatic Abscess

It is caused by *E. histolytica* and approximately 3–9% of cases of intestinal amoebiasis are complicated by hepatic abscesses. Liver is invaded by one of the three routes viz. (i) portal vein (most common), (ii) lymphatics, or (iii) via direct extension through colonic wall.

Amebic abscess is most often solitary (85%) and affects the right lobe more (72%) than left lobe (13%). Chest radiograph is abnormal in approximately 50–78% of cases which includes elevation of right hemidiaphragm, basal pulmonary infiltrates or pleural effusion. On sulphur colloid scans and gallium scans, the abscess appears as cold center with a hot rim. On ultrasound, the lesion is usually round or oval, hypoechoic mass with homogeneous low level internal echoes and distal acoustic enhancement **(Fig. 14)**. Compared to pyogenic abscess, amoebic abscess is more likely to be round or oval in shape (82% vs. 60%), sonographically hypoechoic with fine low level echoes (58% vs. 36%) and show absence of a definite wall.[37]

CT appearance of amoebic abscess is variable and nonspecific. Lesion is usually low attenuating (10–20 HU) with an enhancing rim **(Fig. 15)**. It may appear uni- or multiocular and may demonstrate nodularity of the margin. On MRI, amoebic abscess appears as a round or oval area showing low signal intensity on T1WI and hyperintensity on T2WI.

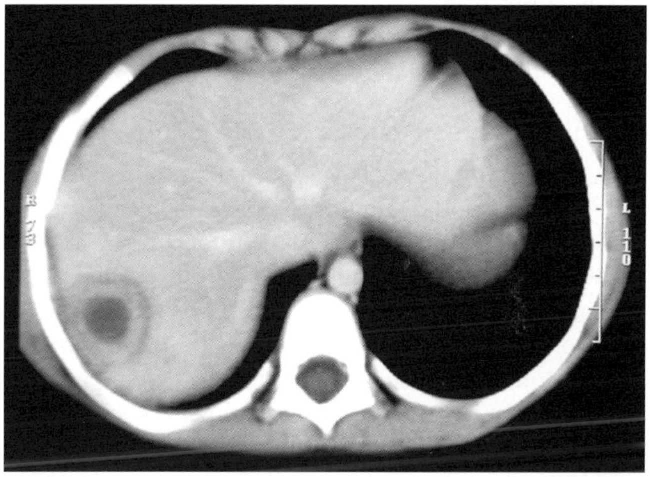

Fig. 15: CT scan in a case of liver abscess shows a hypodense lesion with thick wall in the right lobe of liver. A thin rim of perilesional fluid is seen.

Fungal Abscess

This is more commonly seen in immunocompromised patients like those receiving chemotherapy, AIDS, lymphoma or acute leukemia. Liver is frequently involved secondary to hematogeneous spread of mycotic infection from other organs, most commonly the lungs. Of the various fungi, candida is the most common agent.[38]

Sonographically four major types are seen: (i) "Wheel within a wheel" appearance where a peripheral hypoechoic zone surrounds an inner echogenic wheel which, in turn surrounds a central hypoechoic nidus, (ii) "Bull's eye" lesion where a hyperechoic center is surrounded by hypoechoic rim, (iii) "Uniformly hypoechoic"—the most common appearance **(Fig. 16)**, and (iv) "Echogenic" lesion, caused by scar formation.

On CT scan, most common pattern is multiple, small, rounded lesions of low-attenuation. The lesion may show

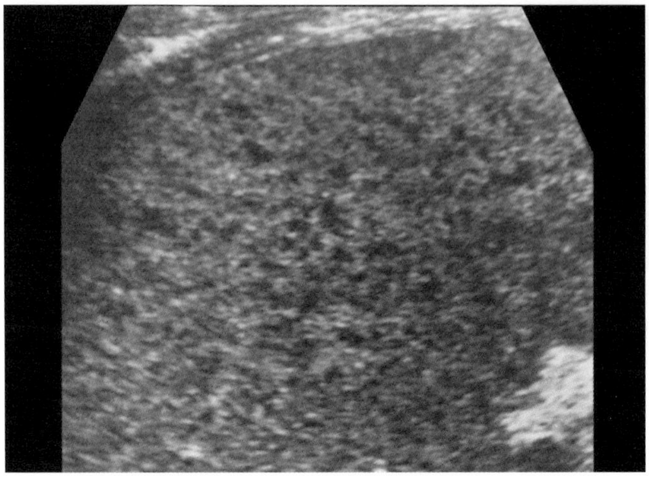

Fig. 16: Ultrasound reveals multiple tiny hypoechoic lesions diffusedly scattered in both lobes of liver in a case of candidiasis.

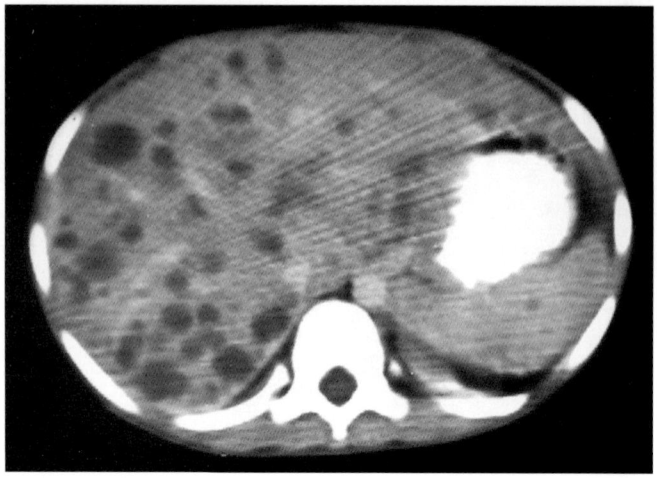

Fig. 17: CECT abdomen shows multiple well-defined hypodense lesions in both lobes of liver and spleen. FNAC confirmed tuberculosis.

calcification. It is cold on sulphur colloid and gallium scans. MR shows increased signal intensity on T1WI and STIR (short T1 inversion recovery) sequences.

Granulomatous Lesions

Various granulomatous diseases which may affect liver include tuberculosis, histiocytosis and sarcoidosis.

Tuberculosis of the liver usually occurs in miliary form with nodules ranging in size from 0.5 to 2 mm which are too small to be seen on US or CT. The most common finding in such cases is hepatomegaly without focal lesions. A diffusely heterogeneous echotexture on US has also been reported. Macronodular involvement is uncommon[39] and usually manifests as single or multiple focal lesions of varying sizes which are hypoechoic on US and hypodense on CT **(Fig. 17)**. These lesions may show peripheral rim enhancement and a central hypodensity due to caseation.[39,40]

Echinococcal Disease (Hydatid Cyst)

The disease is worldwide and is most often caused by *Echinococcus granulosus. E. multilocularis* is less common but is more aggressive pathogen and rarely encountered in our country.

Hydatid cyst has three layers. The outer pericyst is formed by the compressed, modified host tissue which is a rigid protective zone. The two inner layers (ectocyst and endocyst) are parasitic in origin. The ectocyst is approximately 1 mm thick and may calcify. Innermost germinal layer (endocyst) is the living parasite which produces laminated membrane and scolices. Up to 60% of the cysts are multiple.

Plain radiograph shows calcification of the cyst wall in 20–30% of cases. Calcification, however, does not indicate death of the parasite.[41] On sulphur colloid scans they are cold and may show a rim of increased activity on gallium scans.

Sonographic appearance depends on the maturity of the cyst. It can be (i) completely anechoic, well encapsulated cyst, (ii) anechoic cyst with hydatid sand, (iii) multiseptated cyst, with daughter cysts and echogenic material within cysts - the characteristic "Water-lily" sign, and (iv) a densely calcified mass. When infected, the hydatid cysts lose their characteristic appearance and are indistinguishable from liver abscess.

On CT **(Figs. 18A to D)**, hydatid cyst is usually uni- or multilocular, well-defined with either thick or thin wall. Daughter cysts are usually located at the periphery and can be floating freely and altering the patient's position may change the position of these cysts thereby confirming the diagnosis. Curvilinear wall calcification may be seen.

On MR, hydatid cyst has low intensity on T1WI and high signal intensity on T2WI. Pericyst usually has low intensity signal on both TI and T2WI. Calcification is not detected on MR.

Hydatid cyst may rupture into the biliary tree, and pleural, pericardial or the peritoneal cavity, thereby increasing the mortality to 50%.[42,43] Presence of undulating membrane on either US or CT suggests contained rupture.

SIMPLE HEPATIC CYST

This arises from bile duct epithelium and is seen in about 5–14% of the general population. It is usually asymptomatic and rarely causes pain, biliary obstruction or hepatomegaly.

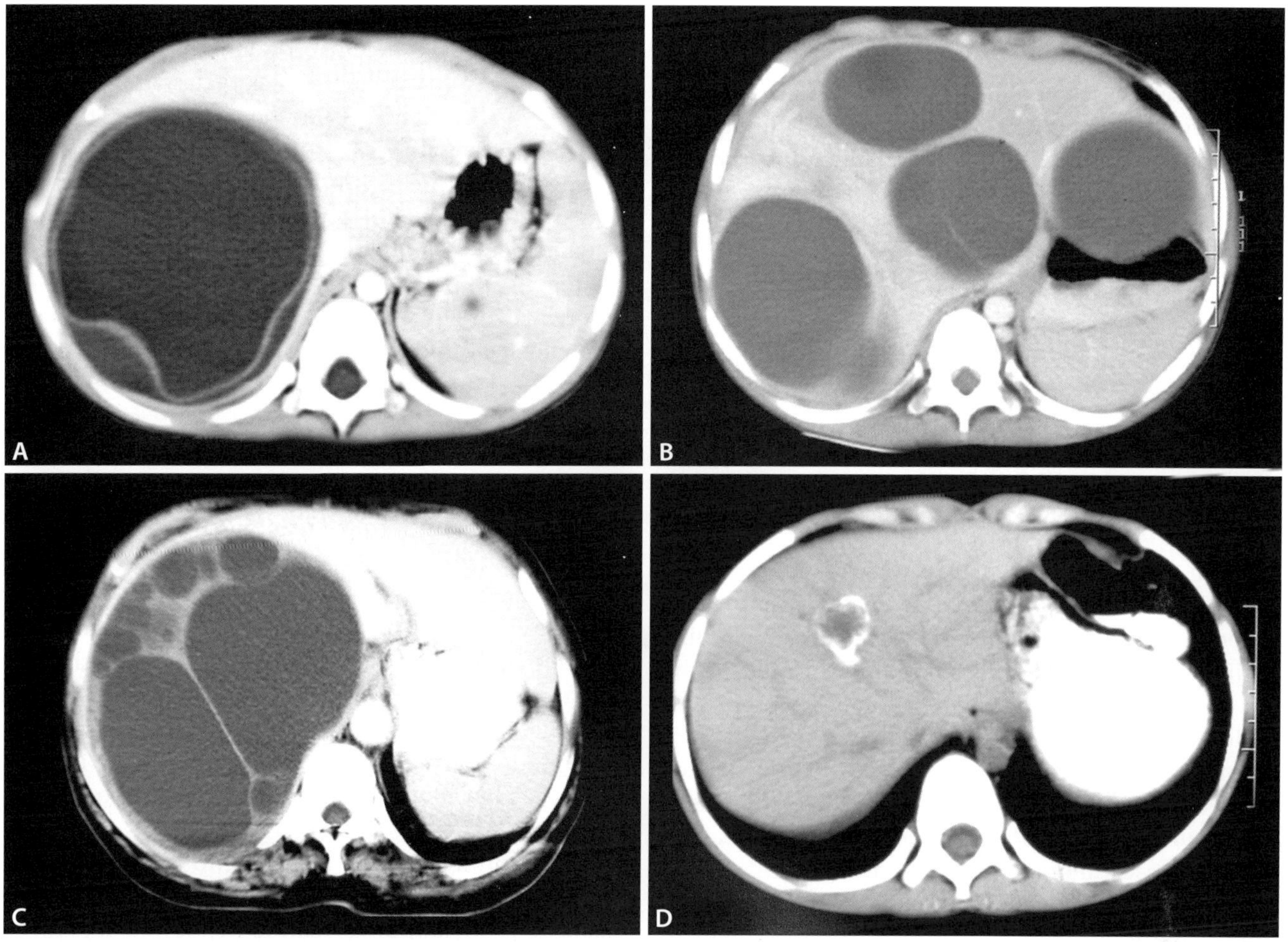

Figs. 18A to D: CT scan findings in hydatid cysts: (A) Unilocular cyst with undulating membrane; (B) Multiple cysts with one of them showing septation; (C) Multiseptated cyst in right lobe of liver with multiple peripheral daughter cysts; (D) Partially calcified cyst.

On sonography **(Fig. 19)**, this lesion is usually solitary, well-defined, anechoic and reveals enhanced through transmission. CT features of simple cyst include low attenuating (0-15 HU) lesion with imperceptible or thin smooth walls, homogeneous appearance and total lack of contrast enhancement. On MR, they are sharply demarcated hypointense lesion on T1WI and hyperintense on T2WI.[9]

POLYCYSTIC LIVER DISEASE

This is characterized by multiple liver cysts of varying sizes. Approximately 57–74% of patients with adult polycystic kidney disease will show liver cysts. Extent of liver involvement is not proportional to the renal disease. In typical congenital hepatic fibrosis, cysts are not grossly visible. However, in the polycystic variant, numerous large and small cysts coexist with hepatic fibrosis.[44]

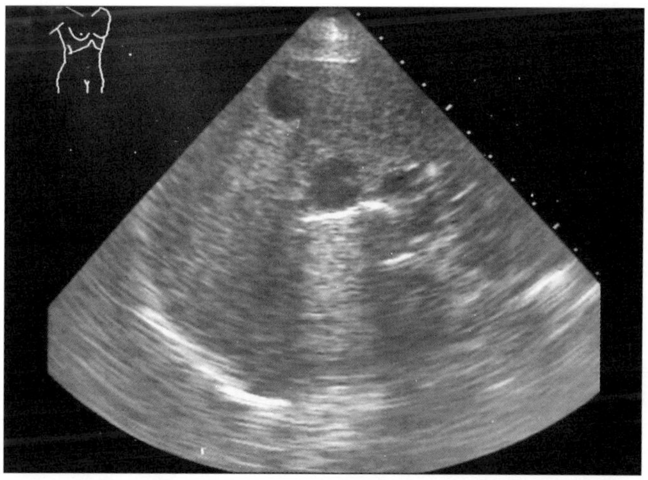

Fig. 19: Ultrasound of liver in a 4-year-old child reveals two anechoic lesions with imperceptible wall and distal acoustic enhancement suggestive of simple cysts.

CAROLI'S DISEASE

This represents type V (Todani) choledochal cyst and is characterized by segmental nonobstructive dilatation of the intrahepatic bile ducts. It is associated with hepatic fibrosis, medullary sponge kidney and infantile polycystic renal disease. Patient presents with abdominal pain secondary to cholangitis or to biliary calculi. US typically shows ectatic ducts surrounding portal vein radicles ('intraluminal portal vein sign').[45] The counterpart of this intraluminal portal vein sign is the 'central dot' sign seen on CT. The common duct and gallbladder are dilated. MRCP is indicated to define the anatomy of the biliary tree in Caroli's disease.

PANCREATIC MASSES

Pancreatoblastoma

The term pancreatoblastoma was first coined by Horie et al for infantile tumors of the pancreas.[46] This tumor is located in the body or tail region of pancreas. According to some authors it is more commonly located in the pancreatic head.[46,47] It usually occurs in newborns and children less than 8 years of age. The mean age at presentation is 6 years. The congenital form is associated with Beckwith-Wiedemann syndrome.[48] Patient presents with an abdominal mass, weight loss, pain, nausea and diarrhea. These tumors secrete alpha-fetoprotein, alpha1-antitrypsin and lactate dehydrogenase. These tumors are usually large at presentation (7–12 cm) and show areas of necrosis.

Microscopically pancreatoblastoma consists of acinar cells. Small areas of squamous differentiation ('squamoid corpuscles') are typically present. The tumor is well-encapsulated and has a good prognosis after surgery. If metastases are seen at the time of diagnosis, the prognosis is poor.

Barium studies may reveal features of mass effect **(Fig. 20A)**. Ultrasound shows a heterogeneous or predominantly hypoechoic mass. Sometimes cystic areas and foci of calcification are seen within the mass **(Fig. 20B)**. Even when these tumors are present in the head of pancreas they do not cause biliary obstruction despite their large size **(Fig. 20C)**. This is due to the soft and gelatinous consistency of these tumors.[49] The tumor may directly spread into the portal vein.[50] Vascular encasement commonly involves the mesenteric vessels and inferior vena cava. Aortic encasement, however, has not been described.

On CT, the tumor is hypodense and shows mild enhancement. Sometimes it is seen as a multiloculated mass with enhancing septae. Central necrosis may be seen **(Figs. 21A and B)**. The most common metastases seen in pancreatoblastoma are to the liver. Metastatic spread may also occur to lymph nodes, peritoneal cavity and the lungs. Bony metastases are very rare.

MR shows these tumors as hypointense on T1W images and iso—or hyperintense on T2W images. Contrast enhancement is variable.

Imaging in pancreatoblastoma is required to localize the organ of origin of the mass and to determine the extent of spread. It is important to distinguish pancreatoblastoma from other pediatric masses like neuroblastoma, lymphoma or Wilms' tumor.

ISLET CELL TUMORS

Islet cell tumors are rare pancreatic neoplasms that produce and secrete hormones to a variable degree. Insulinoma, glucagonoma, gastrinoma, vasoactive intestinal polypeptide producing tumor and somatostatinoma have been reported in childhood.[11] Insulinomas are the most common islet cell tumors. The majority of these lesions are solitary (80%) and benign (90%). The usual age of presentation is over 4 years of age although islet cell adenomas have been reported to occur in the neonatal period.

Functional tumors are diagnosed due to the hormonal activity and imaging is needed for preoperative localization. Insulinomas lead to hypoglycemia and the affected children show seizure activity and erratic behavior which is relieved by the administration of glucose. The diagnosis is confirmed by reproducible hypoglycemia in a controlled environment (fasting) and by showing concomitant hyperinsulinemia. **Table 5** shows the clinical and laboratory features of patients with functional islet cell tumors.

Nonfunctioning tumors are usually large at time of presentation and contain necrotic and calcified areas. They are easily detected due to the mass effect that they produce.

With the availability of helical CT and MRI, invasive imaging techniques like selective celiac and mesenteric angiography and venography with venous sampling are rarely being used for the diagnosis of islet cell tumors. Selective arteriography is diagnostic in 60–70% of cases while transhepatic portal venous sampling has been reported to have an 86% success rate for tumor localization.[51]

Endoscopic ultrasound is an excellent imaging technique with sensitivity and specificity of 93% and 95% respectively.[52] On US, these tumors are usually seen as

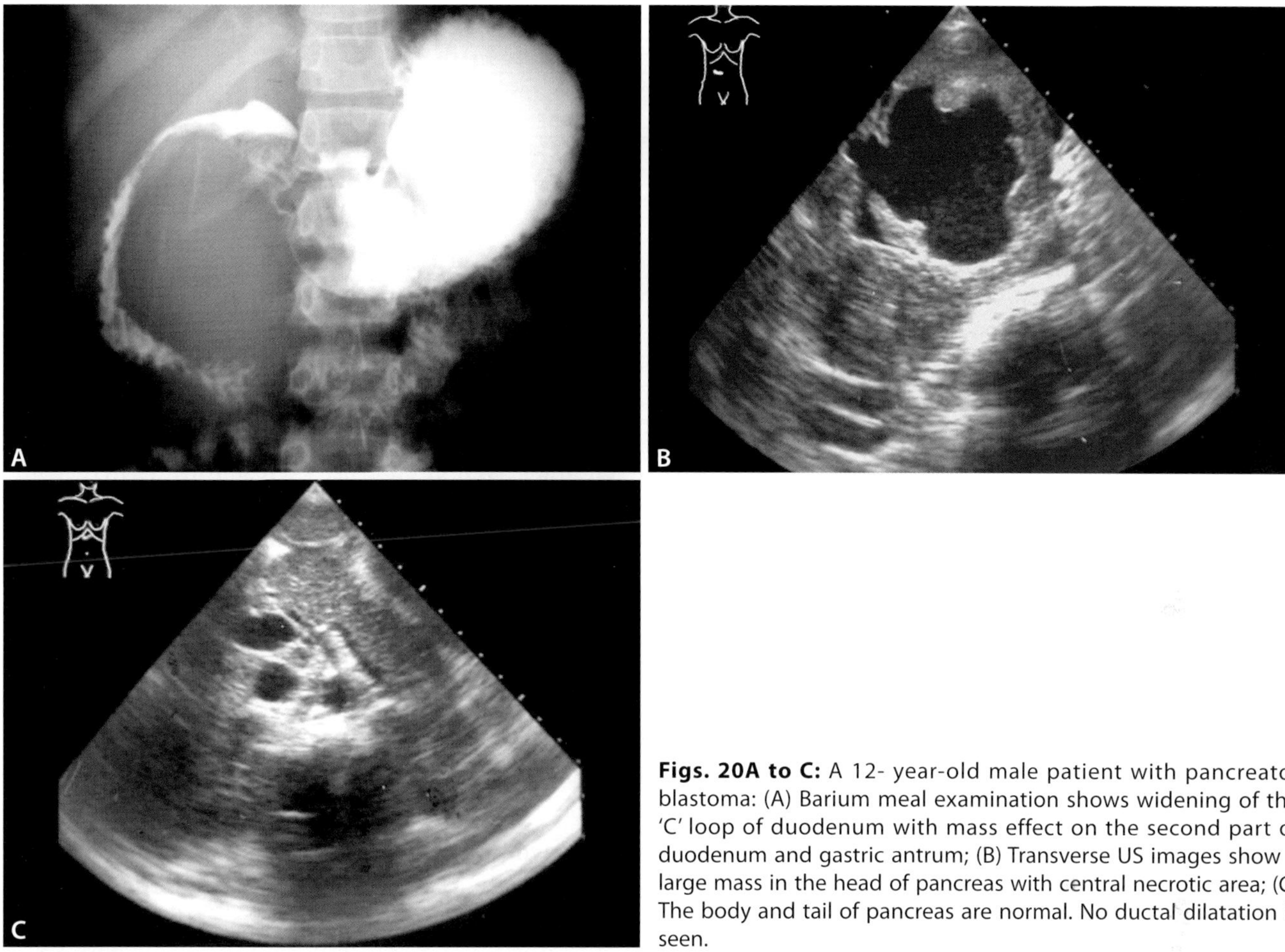

Figs. 20A to C: A 12- year-old male patient with pancreatoblastoma: (A) Barium meal examination shows widening of the 'C' loop of duodenum with mass effect on the second part of duodenum and gastric antrum; (B) Transverse US images show a large mass in the head of pancreas with central necrotic area; (C) The body and tail of pancreas are normal. No ductal dilatation is seen.

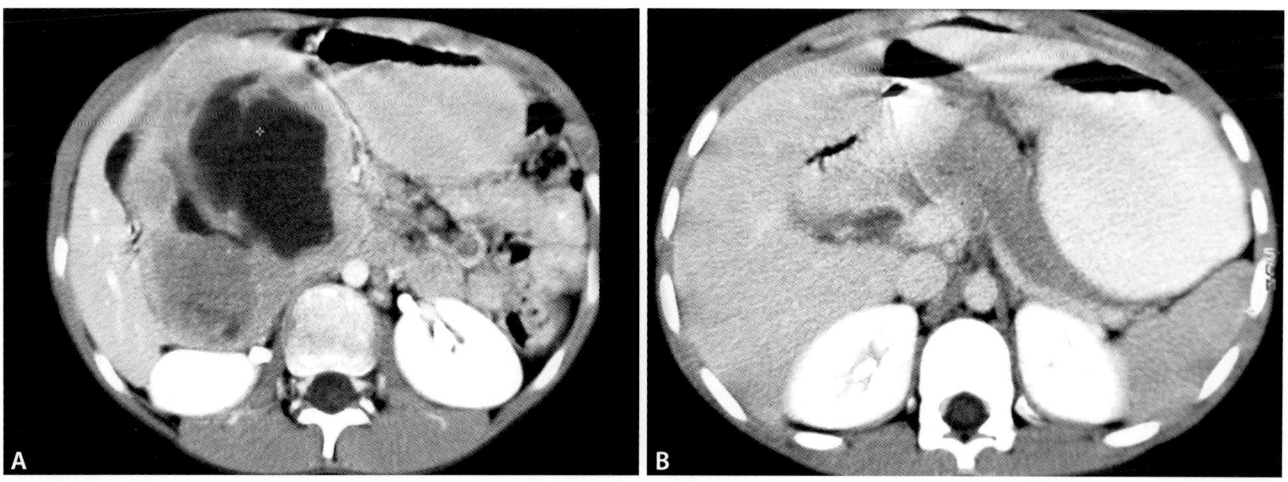

Figs. 21A and B: (A) CECT in the case of pancreatoblastoma shows a large heterogeneous mass in the head of pancreas with central necrosis; (B) There is no dilatation of biliary radicles or pancreatic duct.

well-defined hypoechoic lesions. A hyperechoic rim may sometimes be seen. Isoechoic and hyperechoic lesions have also been described.

On dual phase helical CT, small islet cell tumors are seen as homogeneous hyperattenuating lesions on the arterial as well as portal venous phase. However,

Table 5: Clinical and laboratory features of islet cell tumors.

Functioning islet cell tumor	***Clinical presentation***	***Laboratory findings***
Insulinoma	Hypoglycemic attacks, atypical seizures	Low fasting plasma glucose, hyperinsulinemia
Gastrinoma	Peptic ulcers, diarrhea, malabsorption	Elevated serum gastrin
Glucagonoma	Necrolytic migratory erythema	Hyperglycemia
VIPoma	Watery diarrhea, flushing	Hypokalemia, achlorhydria, elevated plasma peptide

these tumors are hypervascular and the attenuation difference between the lesion and the normal pancreatic parenchyma is more in the arterial phase than in the portal venous phase. Nonfunctioning islet cell tumors also have similar characteristics. Larger lesions show heterogeneous enhancement **(Figs. 22A and B)**. There is no precise data about the sensitivity of biphasic CT for islet cell tumor diagnosis because of the rarity of such studies. The reported sensitivity of CT for localizing functional islet cell tumors is 71–82%.[53]

Fat suppressed T1WI shows islet cell tumors as low signal intensity lesions compared to the normal pancreas. These lesions are hyperintense on T2WI. Some islet cell tumors may be hypointense on T2WI also due to the presence of fibrous tissue. The sensitivity of MR imaging ranges from 24 to 100%.[54] This conflicting data is due to the small reported patient series and the variations in the imaging sequences used.

SOLID AND PAPILLARY EPITHELIAL NEOPLASM (SPEN) (FRANTZ TUMOR)

This tumor was first described by Frantz in 1959. SPEN is an uncommon low grade malignant pancreatic tumor which occurs in young women. The usual age of presentation ranges from 10 to 74 years with the mean age at diagnosis being 25 years.[55] However it also occurs in the pediatric population. It is common in blacks and East Asian patients.

Patients present with an abdominal mass, pain, nausea and early satiety. The tumor is usually large at presentation and shows areas of necrosis and hemorrhage resulting in cystic cavities. Peripheral calcification is seen in one third of cases.

Microscopically SPEN has characteristic histological features. The solid areas in the lesion are traversed by numerous delicate blood vessels. The disruption of this delicate vascular network leads to intralesional hemorrhage. Acellular spaces form subsequently, which fill with myxoid connective tissue.

On US, the tumor shows variable echotexture. Hyperechoic areas are seen due to hemorrhage. The tumor shows heterogeneous attenuation on CT. On MRI **(Figs. 23A to C)**, areas of high signal intensity may be seen on T1WI due to presence of hemorrhagic debris within the tumor. A fluid-debris level may be seen on imaging.

SPEN needs to be distinguished from other cystic lesions of the pancreas like microcystic adenoma, mucinous cystadenoma and cystadenocarcinoma, nonfunctioning islet cell tumor and hemorrhagic pseudocysts. Microcystic adenoma is well-circumscribed lesion with microscopic cystic spaces. This lesion is seen in older women and has no malignant potential. Mucinous cystadenoma may have large cystic spaces and shows fluid-debris levels like SPEN. This can be differentiated from SPEN due to the presence of multiple loculi and septations. Mucinous cystadenoma is a premalignant lesion and can transform into cystadenocarcinoma.

MESENCHYMAL TUMORS

These account for 1–2% of all pancreatic tumors.[49] These include lymphangioma, lipoma, teratoma, schwannoma and lymphoma. Their exact prevalence in the pediatric population is unknown.

Lymphangioma is a multicystic lesion with cysts of varying sizes separated by thin septa. CT shows a uni- or multilocular cystic mass with enhancing septa. Calcification is rarely seen within the lesion. Pancreatic lymphangioma may be intraglandular or may be connected to the gland by a pedicle. These lymphangiomas are liable to undergo torsion.

Lipoma is seen as homogeneous well-defined nonenhancing lesion with attenuation value of –30 to –120 HU.

Pancreatic teratoma originates from pluripotential cells and contains both cystic and solid elements like hair, teeth, cartilage and dermal appendages. On CT, a complex solid cystic mass with calcifications and fatty component is seen.

Pancreas is an unusual site for visceral Schwannomas. In tumors with Antoni type A tissue (organized cellular component), a solid enhancing mass with central necrosis or an in homogeneous hypodense lesion is seen on CT. In tumors with Antoni type B tissue (loose hypocellular component), CT shows a homogeneous fluid attenuation lesion without any significant contrast enhancement.

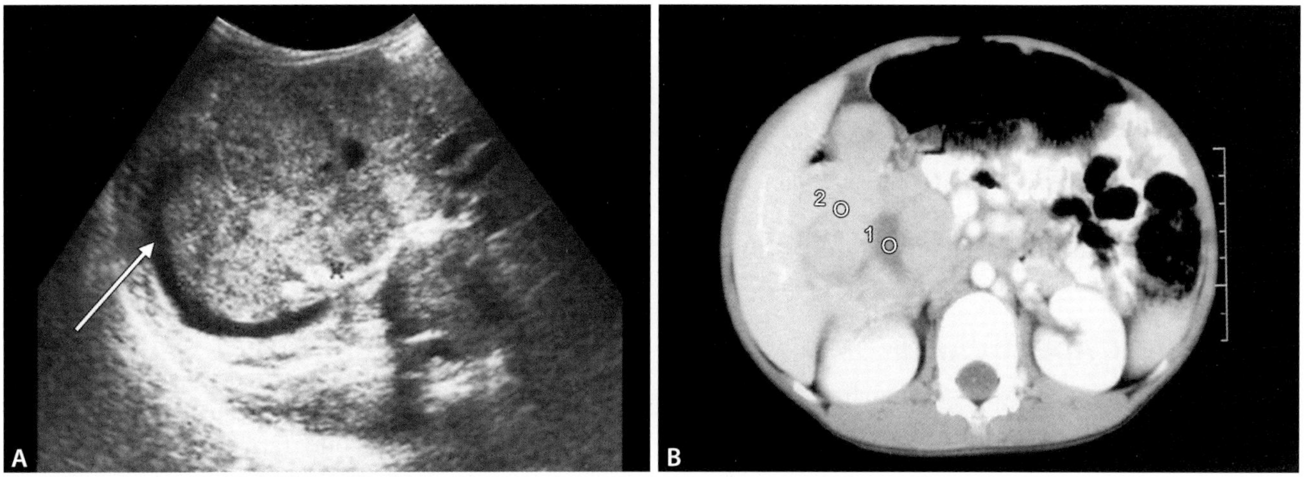

Figs. 22A and B: An 8-year-old boy with abdominal mass: (A) US reveals a solid mass lesion with duodenum (arrow) draped around it; (B) CECT confirms a large heterogeneous mass with central necrosis in the head of pancreas. Histopathological examination of surgical specimen revealed nonfunctioning neuroendocrine tumor of the pancreas.

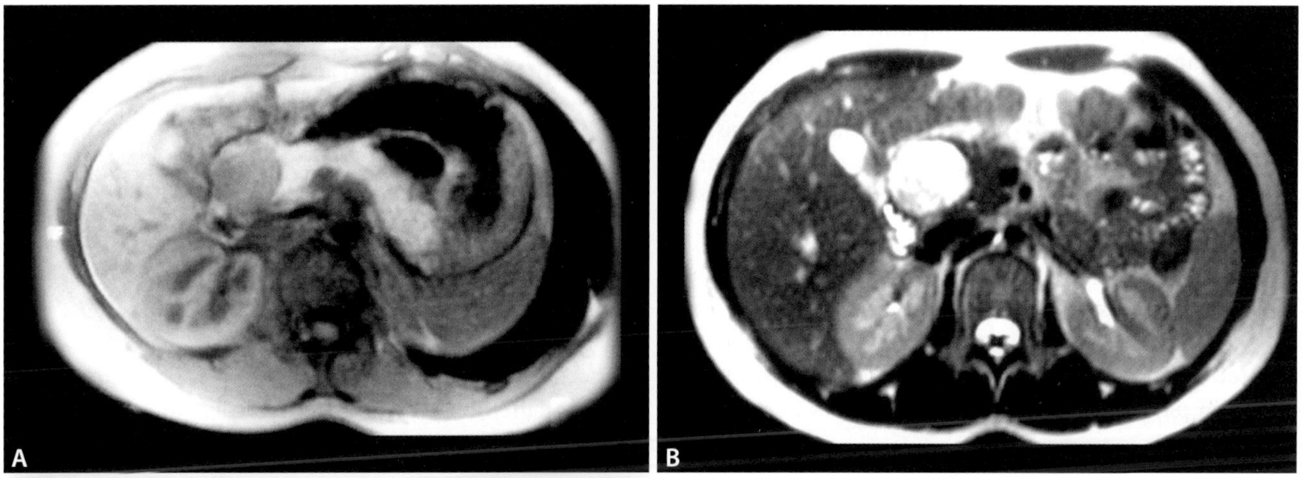

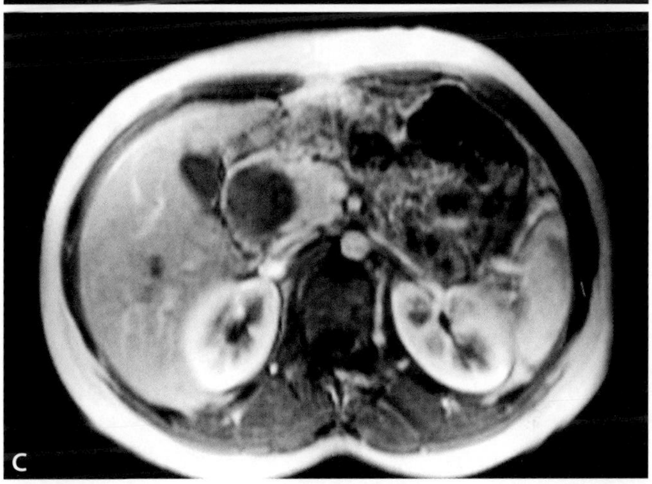

Figs. 23A to C: Biopsy proven SPEN: (A) Fat-saturated T1W; (B) T2W MRI images show the lesion to be hypointense on T1W image and hyperintense on T2W image. The lesion does not show any significant contrast enhancement (C).

Less than one percent of non-Hodgkin's lymphoma can be seen in the pancreas. AIDS-related NHL may also involve the pancreas. Pancreatic lymphoma can present as diffuse infiltrating lesion in the pancreas or as focal well-defined mass.

Primary pancreatic sarcoma accounts for 0.6% of pancreatic malignancies. CT shows a heterogeneous solid mass with inhomogeneous enhancement.[56] Imaging findings cannot distinguish sarcoma from adenocarcinoma.

PANCREATIC ADENOCARCINOMA

It is the most common pancreatic malignancy occurring in the sixth decade of life but is relatively rare in children. The incidence of pancreatic carcinoma in children is not known. Welch[57] reviewed 38 patients of pancreatic carcinoma in children and found that the age at time of diagnosis ranged from 3 months to 18 years with a mean age of 9.2 years. Abdominal pain and epigastric mass were the common presentations. Unlike in adult patient, jaundice was found to be less common presenting symptom in children.

The imaging features are similar to those seen in adults. Ultrasound shows a poorly defined, homogeneous or inhomogeneous hypoechoic mass in the pancreas. CT assesses the local extension of the tumor and determines the resectability of the lesion.

PSEUDOCYSTS

These are frequent complications of pancreatitis regardless of its etiology. An overall incidence of 10–12% has been reported in pancreatitis with a 30% incidence in case of traumatic pancreatitis.[58] Thus, pseudocysts occur more often in children with traumatic pancreatitis compared with those with nontraumatic pancreatitis.

Acute pancreatitis is uncommon in childhood. The most common etiology is multisystem disease (Reye's syndrome, sepsis, shock, viral infections, hemolyticuremic syndrome).[59] Other common causes include blunt trauma, congenital anatomic abnormalities, drug toxicity and metabolic diseases. Children with pancreatitis present with abdominal pain, nausea and vomiting.

Ultrasonography is the initial imaging modality for detecting pseudocysts in children with pancreatitis. Pseudocyst is seen as a well-defined anechoic lesion with or without debris. CT is indicated when the pancreas is not well-visualized on ultrasonography. On CT, pseudocyst is seen as a low attenuating lesion with enhancing walls **(Figs. 24A and B)**. High attenuation in the pseudocyst occurs due to hemorrhage or infection. In case of complicated or recurrent pancreatitis, MRCP is done to evaluate the pancreatic ductal system for congenital ductal anomalies. However for pancreatic duct injury in patients with traumatic pancreatitis, ERCP is required to delineate the site of disruption.

Pancreatic pseudocysts may resolve spontaneously. In the past nonresolving or infected pseudocyst was drained surgically. Percutaneous drainage is an alternative mode of treatment. Its advantages over surgical drainage include early treatment prior to cyst wall maturation and reduction of length and cost of hospital stay.[60]

PANCREATIC TUBERCULOSIS

Abdominal tuberculosis is uncommon in children with a reported incidence of 10% under the age of 10 years.[61] Only

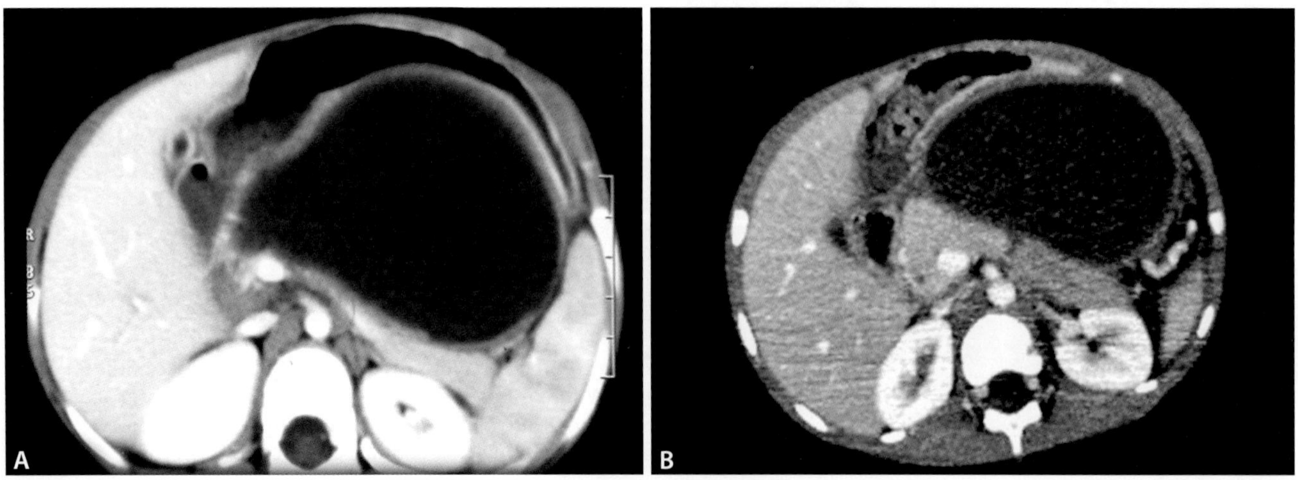

Figs. 24A and B: (A) CECT in a 3-year-old female patient with pancreatitis and pseudocyst shows a large well-defined fluid attenuation lesion with enhancing wall in the lesser sac; (B) CECT section in another patient with traumatic pancreatitis shows laceration of the pancreas with a fluid collection in the lesser sac.

1–5% of cases of pulmonary tuberculosis are complicated by abdominal tuberculosis. Tuberculosis infrequently involves the pancreas. Pancreatic involvement in children was first reported by Andronikou et al in 2002.[62]

The common presenting features are pain, fever, anorexia and weight loss. Obstructive jaundice, vomiting and anemia are less common symptoms.

Ultrasound shows an enlarged pancreas with focal hypoechoic lesions especially in the head region. A cystic lesion may sometimes be seen. CT shows multiple hypodense lesions. The imaging findings are nonspecific and may be mimicked by pancreatic carcinoma or focal pancreatitis. Associated ancillary findings such as hypodense peripancreatic or mesenteric lymph nodes, ascites, mural thickening of the ileocaecal region can help in prospectively diagnosing tuberculosis.[63] The diagnosis should however be confirmed on US or CT guided biopsy.

SUMMARY

Hepatic and pancreatic masses in children are a common clinical problem in pediatric population. Judicious use of various imaging modalities can help to reach at a correct preoperative diagnosis in the majority. Awareness of the imaging characteristics, advantages and limitations of different imaging techniques are crucial for diagnosis and management.

REFERENCES

1. Kane RA. Liver imaging update. Seminars in ultrasound, CT and MRI. 1992;13:311-2.
2. Takano H, Smith WL. Gastrointestinal tumors of childhood. Radiol Clin North Am. 1997;35:1367-89.
3. Lu DS, Vedantham S, Krasny RM, Kadell B, Berger WL, Reber HA. Two-phase helical CT for pancreatic tumors: Pancreatic versus hepatic phase enhancement of tumor, pancreas, and vascular structures. Radiology. 1996;199:697-701.
4. www.imagegently.org last accessed on 15.10.10.
5. Boechat MI, Kangarloo H, Ortega J, et al. Primary liver tumors in children: Comparison of CT and MR imaging. Radiology. 1988;169:727-32.
6. Weinreb JC, Cohen JM, Armstrong E, Smith T. Imaging the pediatric liver: MRI and CT. AJR. 1986;147:785-90.
7. Drane WE. Nuclear medicine techniques for the liver and biliary system. Update for the 1990s. Radiol Clin North Am. 1991;29:1129-50.
8. Weinberg AG, Finegold MJ. Primary hepatic tumors of childhood. Hum Pathol. 1983;14:512-37.
9. Siegel MJ. Pediatric liver and biliary tract. In Margulis, Burhennes (Eds): Alimentary Tract Radiology, 5th edition. Mosby-Year Book Inc., USA, 1994.
10. Willis RA. The pathology of the tumors of children. In Cameron R, Wright GP (Eds): Pathological Monographs. Oliver and Boyd, London. 1962. pp.57-61.
11. Miller JH, Greenspan BS. Integrated imaging of hepatic tumors in childhood. Part I: Malignant lesions (primary and metastatic). Radiology. 1985;154:83-90.
12. Roebuck DJ, Olsen Ø, Pariente D. Radiological staging in children with hepatoblastoma. Pediatr Radiol. 2006;36:176-82.
13. Dachman AH, Pakter RL, Ros PR, Fishman EK, Goodman ZD, Lichtenstein JE. Hepatoblastoma: Radiologic-pathologic correlation in 50 cases. Radiology. 1987;164:15-9.
14. Men S, Hekimoðlu B, Tüzün M, Arda IS, Pinar A. Unusual US and CT findings in hepatoblastoma: a case report. Pediatr Radiol. 1995;25:507-8.
15. Amendola MA, Blane CE, Amendola BE, Glazer GM. CT findings in hepatoblastoma. J Comput Assist Tomogr. 1984;8:1105-9.
16. Schlesinger AE, Parker BR. Tumors and tumor-like conditions. In Kuhn JP, Slovis TL, Haller JO (Eds): Caffey's Pediatric Diagnostic imaging, 10th edition. Mosby, USA. 2004.pp.1493-1508.
17. Blickman JG , Connolly SA. Pediatric imaging: Liver, biliary tree, and pancreas. In Gazelle GS, Saini S, Mueller PR (Eds): Hepatobiliary and Pancreatic Radiology, Imaging and Intervention, 1st edition. Thieme, Germany. 1998.pp.240-70.
18. Brandt DJ, Johnson CD, Stephens DH, Weiland LH. Imaging of fibrolamellar hepatocellular carcinoma. AJR. 1988;151:295-9.
19. Horton KM, Bluemke DA, Hruban RH, Soyer P, Fishman EK. CT and MR imaging of benign hepatic and biliary tumors. Radiographics. 1999;19:431-51.
20. Ruymann FB, Raney RB Jr, Crist WM, Lawrence W Jr, Lindberg RD, Soule EH. Rhabdomyosarcoma of the biliary tree in childhood. A report from the Intergroup Rhabdomyosarcoma Study. Cancer. 1985;56:575-81.
21. Craig JR, Peters RL, Edmondson HA. Tumors of the liver and intrahepatic bile ducts. In Craig JR, Peters RL, Edmondson HA (Eds). Atlas of tumor pathology, fasc 26, ser 2, Wasnigton DC, Armed forces Istitute of Pathology. 1989. pp.1-280.
22. Smith WL, Franken EA, Mitros FA. Liver tumors in children. Semin Roentgenol. 1983;18:136-48.
23. Dachman AH, Lichtenstein JE, Friedman AC, Hartman DS. Infantile hemangioendothelioma of the liver: A radiologic-pathologic-clinical correlation. AJR. 1983;140:1091-6.
24. Dehner LP, Ishak KG. Vascular tumors of the liver in infants and children. A study of 30 cases and review of the literature. Arch Pathol. 1971;92:101-11.
25. Connolly B. The paediatric liver, biliary tree and spleen. In Grainger RG, Allison DJ, Adam A, Dixon AK (Eds): *Diagnostic Radiology,* 4th edition. Churchill Livingstone, USA. 2001. pp.1447-65.
26. Thapa BR, Yaccha S, Narsimharao KL, Gupta HL, Kataryia S, Mehta S. Multinodular infantile hemangioendothelioma of liver. Indian Pediatr. 1988;25:199-203.
27. Bar-Sever Z, Horev G, Lubin E, Kornreich L, Naor N, Ziv N, Shimoni A, Grunebaum M. A rare coexistence of a multicentric hepatic hemangioendothelioma with a large brain hemangioma in a preterm infant. Pediatr Radiol. 1994;24:141-2.

28. Abramson SJ, Lack EE, Teele RL. Benign vascular tumors of the liver in infants: Sonographic appearance. AJR. 1982;138:629-32.
29. Ros PR, Goodman ZD, Ishak KG, et al. Mesenchymal hamartoma of the liver: Radiologic-pathologic correlation. Radiology. 1986;158:619-24.
30. Narasimharao KL, Narasimhan KL, Katariya S, Suri S, Kaushik S, Mitra SK. Giant hamartoma of liver mimicking malignancy. Postgrad Med J. 1988;64:398-400.
31. Stanley P, Hall TR, Woolley MM, Diament MJ, Gilsanz V, Miller JH. Mesenchymal hamartomas of the liver in childhood: sonographic and CT findings. AJR. 1986;147:1035-9.
32. Rogers JV, Mack LA, Freeny PC, Johnson ML, Sones PJ. Hepatic focal nodular hyperplasia: Angiography, CT, sonography, and scintigraphy. AJR. 1981;137:983-90.
33. Chusid MJ. Pyogenic hepatic abscess in infancy and childhood. Pediatrics. 1978;62:554-9.
34. Newlin N, Silver TM, Stuck KJ, Sandler MA. Ultrasonic features of pyogenic liver abscesses. Radiology. 1981;139:155-9.
35. Towbin RB, Strife JL. Percutaneous aspiration, drainage, and biopsies in children. Radiology. 1985;157:81-5.
36. Rajak CL, Gupta S, Jain S, Chawla Y, Gulati M, Suri S. Percutaneous treatment of liver abscesses: needle aspiration versus catheter drainage. AJR. 1998;170:1035-9.
37. Ralls PW, Colletti PM, Quinn MF, Halls J. Sonographic findings in hepatic amebic abscess. Radiology. 1982;145:123-6.
38. Miller JH, Greenfield LD, Wald BR. Candidiasis of the liver and spleen in childhood. Radiology. 1982;142:375-80.
39. Brauner M, Buffard MD, Jeantils V, Legrand I, Gotheil C. Sonography and computed tomography of macroscopic tuberculosis of the liver. J Clin Ultrasound. 1989;17:563-8.
40. Denton T, Hossain J. A radiological study of abdominal tuberculosis in a Saudi population, with special reference to ultrasound and computed tomography. Clin Radiol. 1993;47:409-14.
41. Beggs I. The radiology of hydatid disease. AJR. 1985;145:639-48.
42. Lewall DB, McCorkell SJ. Rupture of echinococcal cysts: Diagnosis, classification, and clinical implications. AJR. 1986;146:391-4.
43. Jain R, Sawhney S, Berry M. Hydatid disease: CT demonstration and follow-up of a cystogastric fistula. Am J Roentgenol. 1992;158:212.
44. Wan SK, Cochlin DL. Sonographic and computed tomographic features of polycystic disease of the liver. Gastrointest Radiol. 1990;15:310-2.
45. Tomà P, Lucigrai G, Pelizza A. Sonographic patterns of Caroli's disease: Report of 5 new cases. J Clin Ultrasound. 1991; 19:155-61.
46. Horie A, Yano Y, Kotoo Y, Miwa A. Morphogenesis of pancreatoblastoma, infantile carcinoma of the pancreas: Report of two cases. Cancer. 197;39:247-54.
47. Willnow U, Willberg B, Schwamborn D, Körholz D, Göbel U. Pancreatoblastoma in children. Case report and review of the literature. Eur J Pediatr Surg. 1996;6:369-72.
48. Drut R, Jones MC. Congenital pancreatoblastoma in Beckwith-Wiedemann syndrome: An emerging association. Pediatr Pathol. 1988;8:331-9.
49. Klöppel G, Maillet B. Classification and staging of pancreatic nonendocrine tumors. Radiol Clin North Am. 1989;27:105-19.
50. Gupta AK, Mitra DK, Berry M, Dinda AK, Bhatnagar V. Sonography and CT of pancreatoblastoma in children. AJR. 2000;174:1639-41.
51. Grosfeld JL, Vane DW, Rescorla FJ, McGuire W, West KW. Pancreatic tumors in childhood: analysis of 13 cases. J Pediatr Surg. 1990;25:1057-62.
52. Anderson MA, Carpenter S, Thompson NW, Nostrant TT, Elta GH, Scheiman JM. Endoscopic ultrasound is highly accurate and directs management in patients with neuroendocrine tumors of the pancreas. Am J Gastroenterol. 2000;95:2271-7.
53. Sheth S, Fishman EK. Imaging of uncommon tumors of the pancreas. Radiol Clin North Am. 2002;40:1273-87.
54. Ichikawa T, Peterson MS, Federle MP, Baron RL, Haradome H, Kawamori Y, Nawano S, Araki T. Islet cell tumor of the pancreas: Biphasic CT versus MR imaging in tumor detection. Radiology. 2000;216:163-71.
55. Buetow PC, Buck JL, Pantongrag-Brown L, Beck KG, Ros PR, Adair CF. Solid and papillary epithelial neoplasm of the pancreas: Imaging-pathologic correlation on 56 cases. Radiology. 1996;199:707-11.
56. Ferrozzi F, Zuccoli G, Bova D, Calculli L. Mesenchymal tumors of the pancreas: CT findings. J Comput Assist Tomogr. 2000;24:622-7.
57. Welch KJ. The pancreas. In Ravitch MM, Randolph JG, Rowe MI, et al (Eds): Pediatric Surgery, 3rd edition. Chicago, IL:Year book. 1984. pp.1090-6.
58. Eichelberger MR, Hoelzer DJ, Koop CE. Acute pancreatitis: The difficulties of diagnosis and therapy. J Pediatr Surg. 1982;17:244-54.
59. Weizman Z, Durie PR. Acute pancreatitis in childhood. J Pediatr. 1988;113:24-9.
60. Amundson GM, Towbin RB, Mueller DL, Seagram CG. Percutaneous transgastric drainage of the lesser sac in children. Pediatr Radiol. 1990;20:590-3.
61. Aston NO. Abdominal tuberculosis. World J Surg. 1997;21:492-9.
62. Andronikou S, Welman CJ, Kader E. The CT features of abdominal tuberculosis in children. Pediatr Radiol. 2002;32:75-81.
63. Takhtani D, Gupta S, Suman K, et al. Radiology of pancreatic tuberculosis: a report of three cases. Am J Gastroenterol. 1996;91:1832-4.

CHAPTER 138

Childhood Biliopathies

Veena Chowdhury

Cholestasis is the principal manifestation of hepatobiliary disease and jaundice is the most common clinical problem which necessitates examination of biliary tract in childhood. There are few disorders which can manifest within the first year of life and these present an important challenge because, not only is hepatic structure and function disturbed but also normal development may be retarded or altered by the disease process.

DEFINITION AND PATHOPHYSIOLOGY OF CHOLESTASIS

Cholestasis is defined as a pathological state of reduced bile formation or flow. The clinical state of jaundice occurs in any condition in which substances normally excreted into the bile are retained in varying proportion.[1]

PHYSIOLOGICAL NEONATAL JAUNDICE

Jaundice is the most common problem in the neonatal period, occurring in approximately 60% of term infants and 80% of preterm infants.[2,3] Metabolism of bilirubin in the neonate is in transition from the fetal stage, when the placenta eliminates bilirubin, to the adult stage, during which bilirubin is excreted from the hepatocytes into the biliary system and then into the gastrointestinal tract. Jaundice occurs when the liver is unable to clear sufficient bilirubin from the plasma. Excessive bilirubin formation or limited uptake and conjugation leads to excess unconjugated bilirubin in the blood. Impaired bile flow and bilirubin excretion result in excess conjugated bilirubin in the blood and urine causing cholestatic jaundice.

During the first 24 hours of life, jaundice may be due to erythroblastosis fetalis, hemorrhage, sepsis and intrauterine infections. Jaundice that appears in the second or third day is usually physiologic but may represent a more severe form of hyperbilirubinemia of the newborn.[3]

Physiologic jaundice is the most common cause of neonatal jaundice. It has its onset by the third day of life and usually resolves by 7 days of life. The bilirubin levels usually do not exceed 12 mg/dL in full-term infants and 14 mg/dL in preterm infants. The cause of neonatal jaundice should be investigated, if:

- The onset of jaundice is within the first 24 hours of life or if jaundice persists beyond 7 days of life.
- The bilirubin level is above 12 mg/dL in full-term infants and 14 mg/dL in preterm infants and a direct-reacting bilirubin component exceeds 1 mg/dL at any time.

Breastfed term infants (1 in 200) may have non-cholestatic jaundice that persists into the second week of life and if nursing is discontinued, the serum bilirubin falls to normal levels within a few days. This is due to substances in the breast milk of some mothers that impair conjugation of bilirubin.

Nonobstructive jaundice in the neonate and infant is due to sepsis, Rh/ABO incompatibility, red blood cell defects, drug effects, congenital enzyme deficiencies, systemic metabolic disorders, gastrointestinal obstruction and cystic fibrosis.[4,5]

ETIOLOGY OF JAUNDICE IN THE NEONATE AND INFANT

Hepatocellular cholestasis results from impairment of mechanisms of bile formation. The reduction in bile flow with retention of substances normally excreted in the bile is due to an anatomic or functional obstruction in the biliary system resulting in obstructive jaundice. The obstruction may be either at the level of larger extrahepatic bile ducts or at the smaller intrahepatic bile ducts.

Major causes of jaundice in neonates are:

Transient Causes

- Hepatic infection
- Sepsis
- Metabolic disease
- Bile plug syndrome
- Adrenal hemorrhage
- Drug related

Persistent Causes

- Neonatal hepatitis
- Biliary atresia
- Choledochal cyst
- Alagille syndrome
- Spontaneous perforation of the common bile duct

Major causes of obstructive jaundice in infancy are:

Common

- Biliary atresia
- Congenital bile duct anomalies (Choledochal cysts)

Uncommon

- Infectious cholangitis
- Primary sclerosing cholangitis
- Langerhans' cell histiocytosis
- Cholelithiasis
- Tumor-Sarcoma botryoides

Biliary atresia accounts for more than 90% of cases with obstructive jaundice in infancy.

Other Causes of Cholestasis

Cholestasis may also occur in conditions associated with paucity of ducts. These are:

- Syndromatic paucity: Alagille's syndrome[6]
- Nonsyndromatic ductal paucity

Rare causes of bile duct disease in children are idiopathic congenital stricture of the bile duct, obstruction of bile duct due to pancreatic disease, post-traumatic or spontaneous perforation of the common bile duct, biliary helminthiasis and cystic fibrosis.

DIAGNOSIS OF JAUNDICE IN INFANCY AND CHILDHOOD

The differential diagnosis of cholestasis in neonates and infants is much broader than in children and adults.[7,8] This is because the immature liver is sensitive to injury and the response of immature liver is more limited. The so called "physiologic stasis" results from functional immaturity. The sensitivity of the infant to insults that would not produce cholestasis in the adults, such as gram negative sepsis, heart failure, metabolic disease and exposure to minimally toxic substances alerts the clinician to look beyond the liver for the causes of cholestasis present in the newborn or young infant. A more focussed investigation can be undertaken if these causes are excluded.

The differential diagnosis of hepatobiliary diseases resulting in jaundice in infants is limited, and major concern is to differentiate hepatocellular from obstructive cholestasis because it represents the differential between the disorders of physiology and anatomy or medical versus surgical jaundice. Laboratory tests are often not diagnostic as the biochemical differences between hepatocellular and obstructive cholestasis are few and there is an overlap in values. The diagnosis is usually made with the help of imaging and biopsy.

The imaging modalities routinely used are:

- Ultrasonography (US)
- Computed tomography (CT)
- MRI and MRCP
- Biliary scintigraphy (99mTc HIDA scan)
- Cholangiography—percutaneous transhepatic cholangiography (PTC), and Endoscopic retrograde cholangiopancreatography (ERCP).

Sonography is the preferred screening method for detection of intrahepatic ductal dilatation and to exclude anatomic anomalies of the extrahepatic biliary system, the most common being choledochal cyst. Sonography may identify other anatomic causes for the patient's jaundice, such as stones or inspissated bile in the bile plug syndrome. Bile plug syndrome is a rare cause of perinatal jaundice of unclear etiology that may be related to total parenteral nutrition or cystic fibrosis in which sludge (echogenic or hypoechoic) in the bile ducts and gallbladder forms plugs and may cause transient gallbladder hydrops and duct dilatation.

Computed tomography can be used to identify associated congenital and acquired abnormalities such as polysplenia and portal hypertension.

Magnetic resonance cholangiopancreatography is an effective noninvasive imaging technique for the evaluation of pancreaticobiliary disease in children.[9,10]

Pediatric MR cholangiopancreatography needs to be optimized and tailored to the different body sizes intrinsic to children of various ages. For visualization of small caliber ducts, spatial resolution and SNR needs to be improved. The first step toward such improvement is proper coil selection.[11] Either a phased-array or a surface coil that fits the child well should be used for signal reception. Poor signal in children can be compensated for to some extent by increasing the number of signals averaged to between four and eight. However, this needs to be balanced with the ETL, since increasing the number of signals averaged increases scanning time. Proper slab thickness in 2D FSE and SSFSE imaging is the next step towards obtaining optimal-quality images. Smaller children such as neonates and infants do not need a slab thickness of more than 2 cm. Thin-section (3–5 mm) images in the axial and coronal planes, as well as thick slabs in radiating coronal planes, should be acquired. A 3D FSE sequence should be performed whenever breathing is regular. It provides better SNR and spatial resolution than 2D FSE imaging. Moreover, anomalies can be better understood by rotating 3D images. Because neonates and infants usually have irregular breathing with varying respiratory amplitude, 3D FSE imaging with respiratory triggering may not be possible in many of these patients. SSFSE imaging with varying section thickness can be useful in this situation providing adequate image quality even with free shallow breathing.

Hepatobiliary scintigraphy (99mTc HIDA scan) **is usually required to differentiate between neonatal hepatitis and biliary atresia.**

Operative cholangiograms are performed to evaluate the intrahepatic and extrahepatic portions of the biliary system as biliary atresia may affect only portions of the biliary tree.

NEONATAL HEPATITIS

Neonatal hepatitis (giant cell neonatal hepatitis) represents a morphologic alteration of the liver that occurs as a nonspecific reaction to various insults. The disease is idiopathic (55%), familial (10%), infectious (20%), and metabolic in 15% of cases.[12] Idiopathic neonatal hepatitis is the most common cause of neonatal cholestasis accounting for one third to two third of cases. The incidence ranges from 1 in 4800 to 1 in 9000 live births. Male preterm infants are more commonly affected.

More than half of neonates with this disorder have jaundice of varying degree within the first week of life, about one-third show failure to thrive and have a fulminant course leading to extensive hepatocellular damage. On clinical examination, hepatosplenomegaly is found and a bleeding diathesis may be present. Laboratory tests reveal abnormal elevation of liver enzyme levels.

Pathology

Liver biopsy is helpful in confirming the diagnosis of idiopathic neonatal hepatitis and in excluding other causes of neonatal cholestasis. Histologic examination demonstrates hepatocellular swelling with marked variation in cell size, portal inflammatory exudate, regeneration and individual cell necrosis, multinucleated giant cells throughout the lobules, and increased extramedullary hematopoiesis.

Imaging Features

Ultrasonography and radionuclide scintigraphy are the most widely used imaging modalities used in this disorder. US findings are, however, nonspecific. The liver may be normal or increased in size with increased periportal echogenicity. Intrahepatic and extrahepatic bile ducts are normal in caliber while the gallbladder may be normal, small, large, or not visualized **(Figs. 1A and B)**. The normal common bile duct should measure less than 1 mm in neonates, less than 2 mm in infants up to 1-year-old, less than 4 mm in older children and less than 7 mm in adolescents and adults. In infants the normal gallbladder length is 1.5–3 cm.[13,14] Ikeda et al. have reported that serial ultrasound may be useful in the differentiation of neonatal hepatitis and biliary atresia when the gallbladder is visualized. According to these authors, postprandial gallbladder contraction can be seen in patients with neonatal hepatitis but not in patients with biliary atresia.[15]

A radionuclide hepatobiliary study demonstrates the radiopharmaceutical agent in the bowel, thereby excluding biliary atresia. Nuclear medicine studies of the biliary tree have been the traditional definitive imaging method for the differentiation of biliary atresia from neonatal hepatitis and are typically performed after US. Evaluation of the blood pool and hepatic phases and determination of the presence or absence of radioisotope in the gastrointestinal tract on delayed images are all necessary for the proper investigation of biliary atresia. Patients should be pretreated with phenobarbital. The oral administration of phenobarbital for 5 days before the study is said to enhance

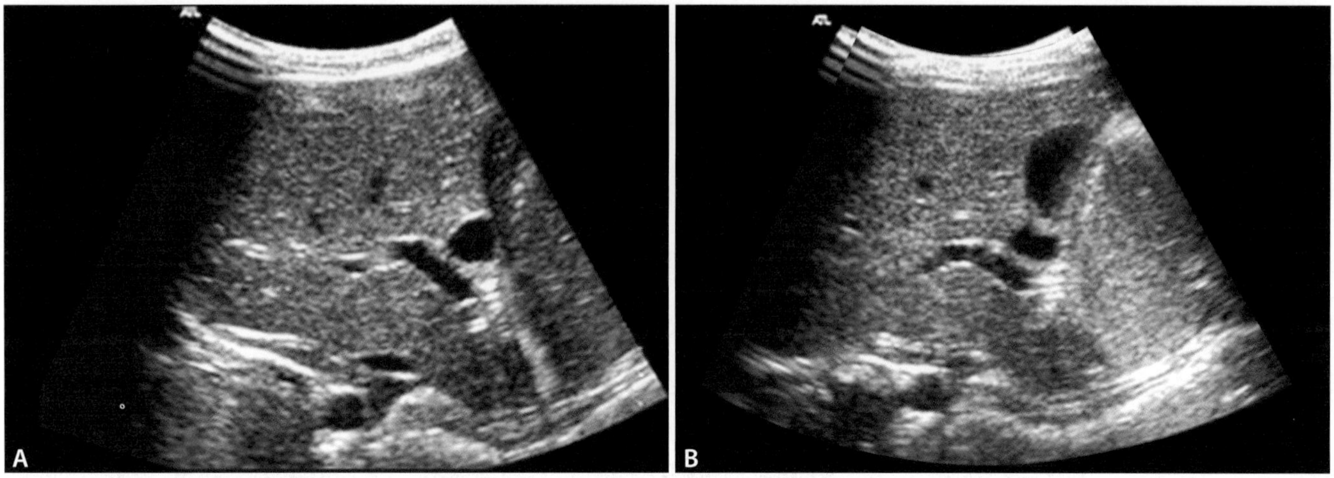

Figs. 1A and B: Grayscale sonograms of a jaundiced neonate showing increased periportal echogenicity with a normal sized gallbladder—neonatal hepatitis.

the biliary excretion of the isotope. If the early scans do not demonstrate isotopic activity in the gastrointestinal tract, delayed scans, up to 24 hours, should be obtained. The presence of radioisotope in the gastrointestinal tract essentially excludes biliary atresia. Scintigraphy has an excellent sensitivity of 96–97% in differentiating biliary atresia from neonatal hepatitis.[16] Although, most patients with neonatal hepatitis have excretion of the radionuclide into the gut, patients with severe hepatic injury may not have sufficient liver function to excrete detectable amounts of radiotracer into the gastrointestinal tract. Thus, if there is lack of demonstration of the radionuclide in the bowel, the distinction between severe hepatocellular disease and biliary atresia cannot be made with certainty.[17]

On MR imaging, T2 weighted images reveal a collar of high signal intensity surrounding portal vein branches due to periportal edema, however, this finding is nonspecific **(Figs. 2A to E)**. Overall, if the gallbladder is normal or near normal in size and hepatic bile duct filling occurs, even if it is minimal, the preferred diagnosis should be neonatal hepatitis.

BILIARY ATRESIA

Extrahepatic biliary atresia (EHBA) accounts for approximately one-third of the cases of neonatal cholestasis, the incidence varying from 1 in 8000 to 1 in 25,000 live births, with females being more commonly affected.[18]

This disorder has a 15–30% incidence of associated anomalies such as polysplenia, malrotation, trisomy 17-18 and cardiovascular abnormalities, suggesting a congenital etiology.[19] The exact etiology of biliary atresia is unknown, although proposed mechanisms include viral infections, immune-mediated bile duct injury, and autoimmune disease of the biliary tree.[20]

In terms of infection, it is theorized that a viral infection in an infant, first induces a cholangiohepatitis and in response an immune response is invoked. This entails the production of α-fetoprotein, an immune response regulator that attempts to control the disease process. Characteristically, it is elevated in infants with neonatal hepatitis but not in infants with biliary atresia. This is of considerable importance because it has also been demonstrated that those patients with elevated α-fetoprotein generally do not go on to develop biliary atresia, while those with low levels do. This would suggest that some infants are able to control the initial viral infection better than others and that those who are not able to, develop biliary atresia. Based on this concept, different degrees of biliary duct obliteration will be seen, infants with reasonably well-preserved ducts, infants with ducts that appear hypoplastic and are visible only on microscopic examination and infants with no remaining bile ducts at all and finally a few with cystic transformation of the intrahepatic bile ducts. Thus, main interlobar ducts are present in their entire course in the early stages of the disease, but they diminish in number and size with time (The "disappearing bile duct syndrome").

Pathology

In the first month of life histologic findings in the liver may be indistinguishable from those of neonatal hepatitis, and the two diseases may, in fact be different final processes of a single initial disease state.

Liver biopsy after the first month of life will help differentiate the two diseases. While biliary atresia shows many of the same histologic features as neonatal hepatitis,

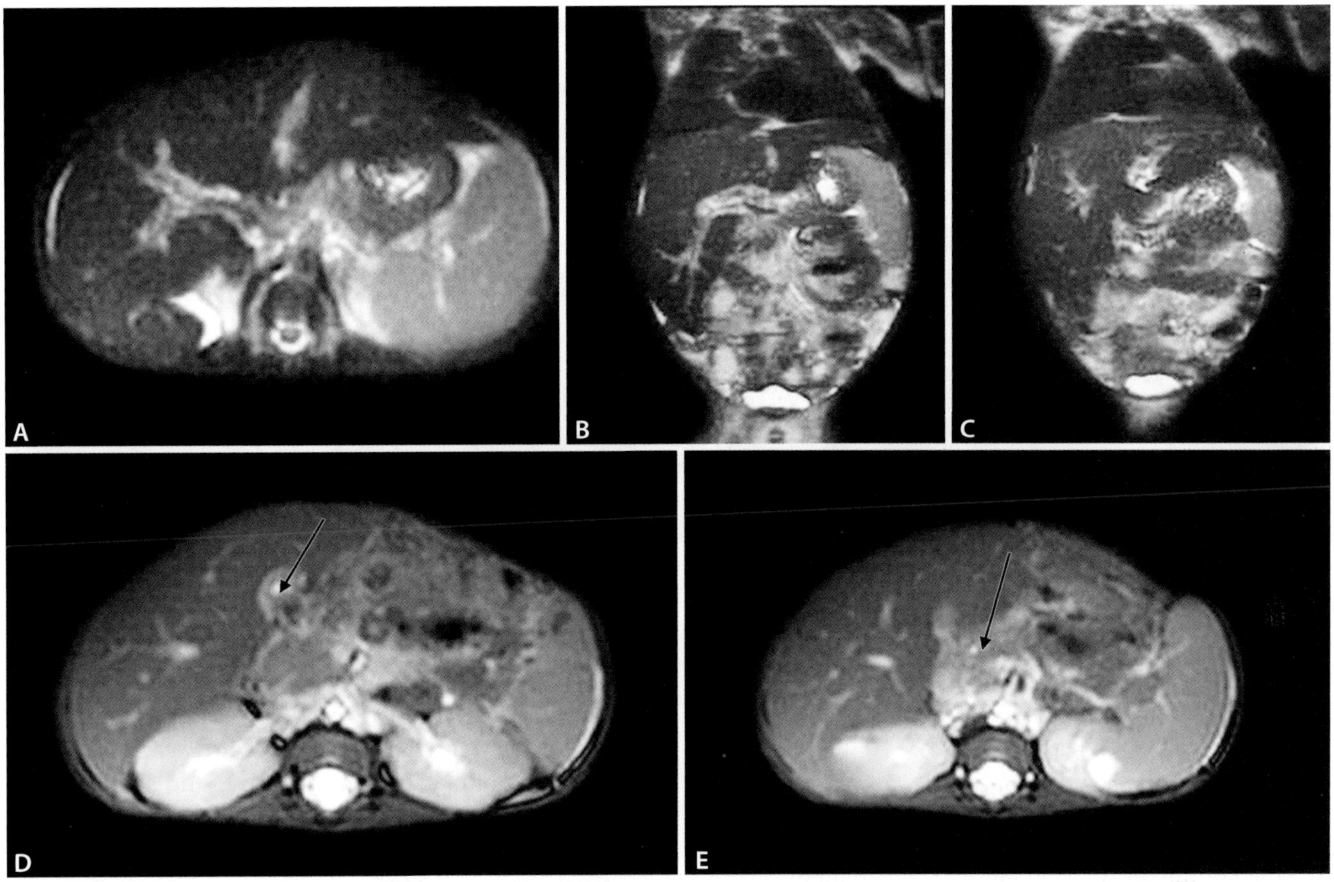

Figs. 2A to E: HASTE axial (A) HASTE coronal (B and C) revealing a collar of high signal intensity surrounding the portal vein branches due to periportal edema. TRUFISP axial (D and E) MR images reveal a near normal gallbladder (D) and the intrapancreatic CBD is visualized shown by an arrow (E) Neonatal hepatitis.

proliferation of bile ducts in all the portal tracts is an additional cardinal feature.

Based on the predominant site of atresia the following classification of anatomical variants has been evolved:[21,22]

- *Type I:* Obliteration of the common bile duct but proximal ducts are patent.
- *Type II:* Common hepatic duct is obliterated but dilated bile ducts are found at porta hepatitis.
- *Type IIA:* Both cystic and common bile ducts are patent.
- *Type IIB:* Obliteration of both cystic and common bile duct.
- *Type III:* No patent hepatic or hilar ducts.

If untreated, the vast majority of cases of EHBA progress to irreversible biliary cirrhosis and death. Because the treatment for biliary atresia and neonatal hepatitis are very different (surgical in the former and medical in the latter), definitive diagnosis is mandatory. Diagnostic imaging tests with or without liver biopsy are utilized to help facilitate a rapid diagnosis because the likelihood of re-establishing bile flow after Kasai hepatoportoenterostomy is greater if the procedure is performed within the first 2 months after birth.[22,23]

Imaging Features

Ultrasonography

A spectrum of changes may be seen sonographically in cases of biliary atresia, depending on the type and severity. Both the liver size and the echogenicity of hepatic parenchyma, may be normal or increased. There may be decreased visualization of the peripheral portal venous vasculature, indicative of fibrosis.[24]

Gallbladder Length and Gallbladder Contraction

On US, an atretic gallbladder that appears small, has an irregular contour and lacks echogenic mucosal lining is the characteristic imaging finding of biliary atresia **(Figs. 3A to C)**. A combination of three gallbladder features, i.e. (i) The length of the gallbladder less than 19 mm, (ii) an irregular wall, (iii) indistinct mucosal lining—the so called

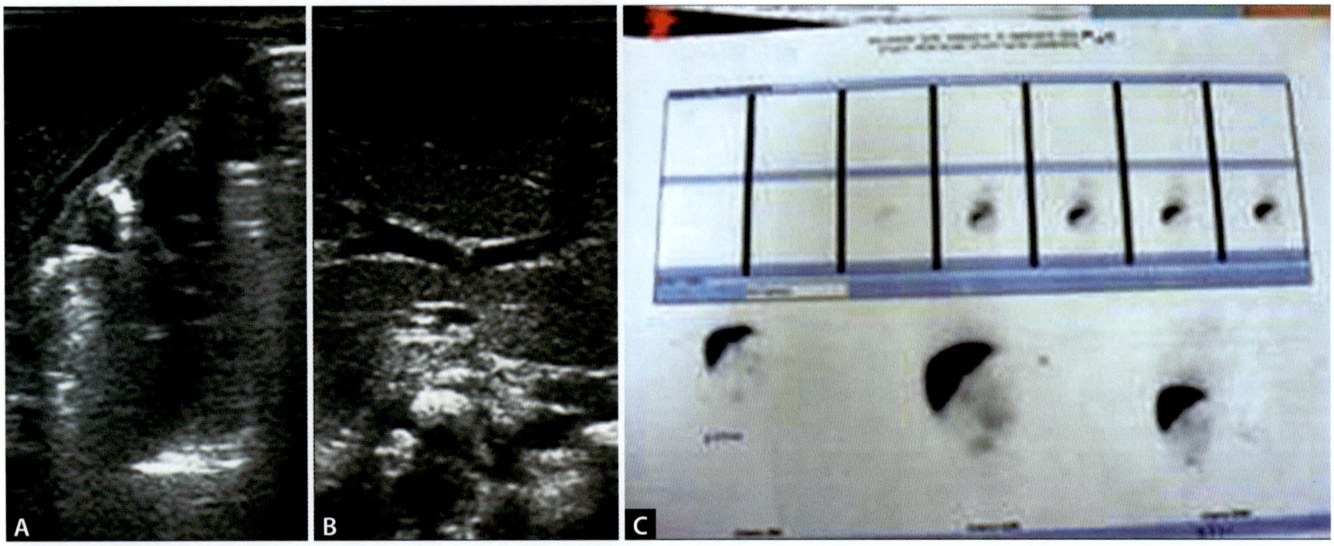

Figs. 3A to C: Sonography reveals an atretic gallbladder. The length of the gallbladder is less than 19 mm with an irregular wall and an indistinct mucosal lining. (A) Bile duct is not identified anterior to the portal vein; (B) HIDA scan reveals no bowel opacification; (C) Biliary atresia.

"gallbladder ghost triad" is diagnostic of biliary atresia.[25] Gallbladder contraction is evaluated by calculating the contraction index (CI) as follows:[26]

$$\text{CI (\%)} = \frac{\text{Fasting volume–Postprandial volume} \times 100}{\text{Fasting volume}}$$

The volume of the gallbladder is calculated as 0.52 × length × width × height. A normal contraction index has been reported to be 86 ± 18% (mean ± SD) in a 6-week-old infant and 67 ± 42% in a 4-months-old infant. If the contraction index was less than mean ± SD, the gallbladder was described as uncontracted. An uncontracted gallbladder is more suggestive of biliary atresia than of neonatal hepatitis or other causes of infantile cholestasis.[26]

Although, the finding of a normal sized gallbladder usually implies neonatal hepatitis, it may also be seen when the atretic common bile duct is distal to the insertion of the cystic duct. About 10% of infants with biliary atresia are found to have a normal gallbladder with a diameter greater than 1.5 cm. Change in gallbladder size after a milk feeding suggests patency of the common hepatic and common bile ducts and is seen only with neonatal hepatitis.

Biliary Atresia Splenic Malformation Syndrome

This syndrome has been reported by Davenport et al.[27] Biliary atresia can be associated with polysplenia, situs inversus, an interrupted inferior vena cava and other cardiovascular anomalies. Furthermore, infants with BA have a degree of hepatic fibrosis or cirrhosis and the majority have some evidence of portal hypertension as early as 8 weeks. Biliary atresia is associated with polysplenia in 10–12% of cases. The abdomen should be examined for signs of end-stage liver disease including ascites, hepatofugal flow in the portal and splenic veins and collateral venous channels.

Triangular Cord Sign

Several investigators have recently reported the importance of assessing for the presence or absence of an echogenic triangular cord seen just cranial to the bifurcation of the portal vein on US. This echogenic region corresponds to fibrous tissue found adjacent to the portal vein bifurcation in cases of biliary atresia **(Fig. 4)**. In their series of 61 infants with neonatal cholestasis, Park et al. found that US had a diagnostic accuracy of 95%, a sensitivity of 85%, and a specificity of 100% when using the presence of the triangular cord sign to identify infants with biliary atresia.[28-30]

Objective Criteria of Triangular Cord Sign in Biliary Atresia on US

Biliary atresia is characterized by fibrous obliteration of the extrahepatic bile duct with fibrous ductal remnant in the porta hepatis. The hepatic ducts transform into a fibrous ductal remnant that is usually anterior and slightly cranial to the hepatic artery and the portal vein. The fibrous ductal remnant takes the same course as the common hepatic duct and smoothly tapers proximally along both sides of the intrahepatic ducts. Thus, the location of the fibrous ductal remnant in the porta hepatis should be the same as

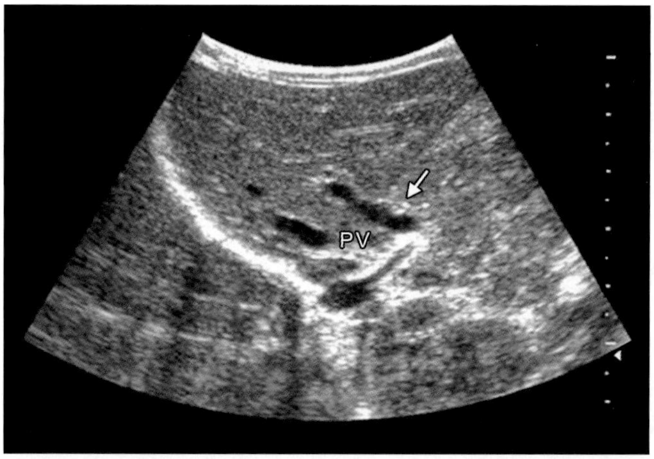

Fig. 4: US of a neonate with biliary atresia showing an echogenic triangular cord anterior to the portal vein—"Triangular cord" sign.

that of the common hepatic duct. The original definition of the TC sign was based on the idea that this fibrous ductal remnant could be seen as a thick tubular or triangular echogenic density along the anterior aspect of the portal vein.

The normal possible structures positioned along the anterior aspect of the portal vein, include the anterior wall of the right portal vein, the anterior wall of the right hepatic artery and the common hepatic duct. Lee et al, therefore, took the thickness of the echogenic anterior wall of the right portal vein which they called as EARPV.[31] The triangular cord sign was defined as thickness of the EARPV of more than 4 mm on a longitudinal scan. They stated that the triangular echogenic density was hard to measure exactly on a transverse scan because of errors related to its tapering structure into the liver. Also, the fibrous ductal remnant may not be in the pattern of a triangular, cone-shaped fibrous mass. Other patterns of the fibrous ductal remnant do not appear as triangular echogenic density on a transverse scan, hence they used a longitudinal scan rather than a transverse scan for measurement. These authors, thus proposed that the TC sign be defined as a thickness of the EARPV or the echogenic anterior wall of the right portal vein of more than 4 mm on a longitudinal scan as an objective criterion of diagnosing biliary atresia **(Figs. 5A to C)**. The use of this criterion for the diagnosis of biliary atresia resulted in a sensitivity of 80%, specificity of 98%, a positive predictive value of 94%, a negative predictive value of 94% and an accuracy of 94%.[31]

Color Doppler US in Biliary Atresia

The triangular cord sign cannot always be found in every patient. The detection of this sign is largely operator dependent. This sign can also be masked in the presence of diffuse periportal echogenicity due to nonspecific inflammation or cirrhosis. A few authors have described enlargement of the hepatic artery as a useful sign in the diagnosis of biliary atresia. In an angiographic study of biliary atresia, all patients with biliary atresia had hepatic artery enlargement and the branches of the intrahepatic peripheral hepatic artery manifested with irregular contrs suggestive of peripheral occlusion.[32] It has been stated that enlargement may be a compensatory change to improve the blood supply for the biliary trees or a secondary change of liver cirrhosis or a vascular malformation **(Figs. 6A and B)**. Enlargement of the hepatic artery diameter (> 1.5 mm at the level of the proximal right hepatic artery) or a value of 0.45 for the hepatic artery diameter to portal vein diameter ratio is highly suggestive of biliary atresia.[33] Color Doppler US can also be used to detect hepatic subcapsular flow in patients with biliary atresia. Uflaker and Pariente reported the presence of angiographically demonstrable perivascular arterial tufts in the periphery of the hepatic arterial circulations in patients with biliary atresia and suggested that these findings may be useful in the diagnosis.[34] Hepatic subcapsular flow has been reported to have sensitivity, specificity, positive and negative predictive values of 100%, 86%, 88% and 100% respectively for the diagnosis of biliary atresia.[34]

Hepatobiliary scintigraphy definitively excludes biliary atresia if gut excretion of radiotracer is observed. But this test demonstrates poor accuracy (56%) and specificity (35%), with a sensitivity of 96% **(Fig. 7)**.[28]

More recently, investigators have evaluated the ability of MRI and MR cholangiography to diagnose biliary atresia. Jaw et al found that the common hepatic ducts and common bile duct could be readily visualized in control subjects and infants with neonatal hepatitis, whereas infants with surgically confirmed biliary atresia failed to demonstrate a visible common bile or hepatic duct on MRCP.[35] In their study, Giubaud et al found that failure to visualize the extrahepatic bile ducts on MRCP and presence of high signal intensity periportal thickening has a strong association with the presence of biliary atresia.[36,37]

Contrast-enhanced MR Cholangiography for Evaluation of Biliary Atresia

Mangafodipir trisodium (Mn-DPDP) is a non radio-isotopic liver specific contrast medium that is taken up mainly by the liver cells and excreted into the biliary system. The active ingredient in Mn-DPDP is manganese dipryidoxyl diphosphate, a metal chelate of manganese that is essentially a paramagnetic T1 enhancer.[38] After

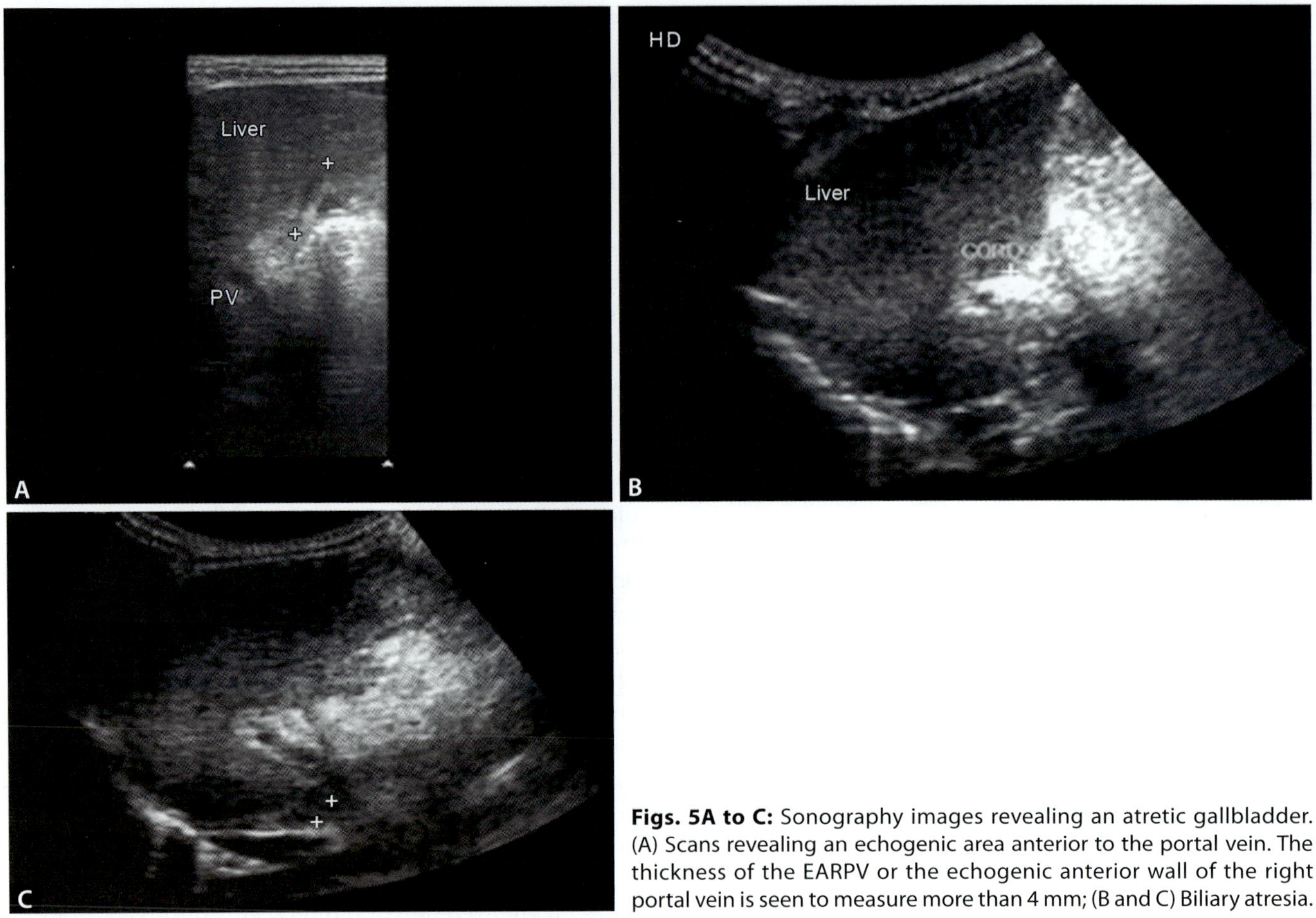

Figs. 5A to C: Sonography images revealing an atretic gallbladder. (A) Scans revealing an echogenic area anterior to the portal vein. The thickness of the EARPV or the echogenic anterior wall of the right portal vein is seen to measure more than 4 mm; (B and C) Biliary atresia.

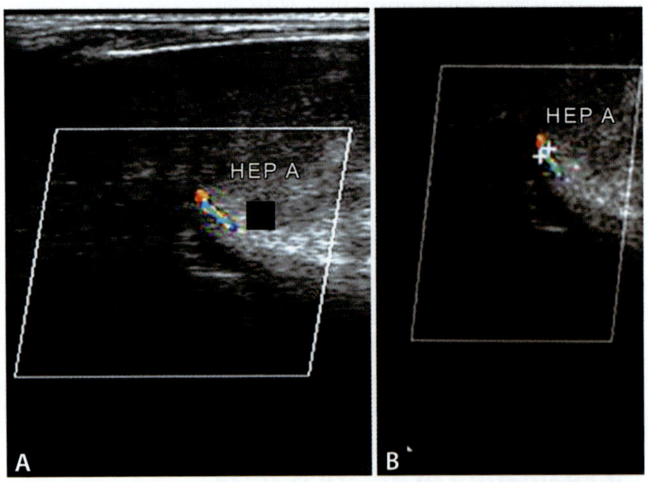

Figs. 6A and B: Color Doppler showing color fill in of the hepatic artery which is enlarged. The diameter of the artery >1.5 mm—Biliary atresia.

intravenous administration, a proportion of manganese is slowly released from the chelate and binds to the blood/protein and the main uptake of manganese occurs in the liver. Enhancement of the liver parenchyma peaks after 5–10 minutes and plateaus over several hours.[39] Most of the manganese is then eliminated through the biliary route with about 20% excreted in the urine. Precontrast images are compared with the postcontrast and contrast material filling of the gallbladder, extrahepatic bile duct, duodenum or small bowel loops is observed. Contrast enhanced MR cholangiography can also yield functional information similar to that obtained with hepatic scintigraphy, anatomic information similar to that yielded by conventional contrast-enhanced cholangiography and cross-sectional information similar to that obtained at computed tomography and US. Thus, a prominent gallbladder and extrahepatic bile duct filling, together with duodenal excretion of Mn-DPDP within 1 hour are definite exclusion criteria of biliary atresia.

Kasai Operation

In the Kasai operation, the porta hepatis is dissected and a loop of small intestine is brought up and anastomosed

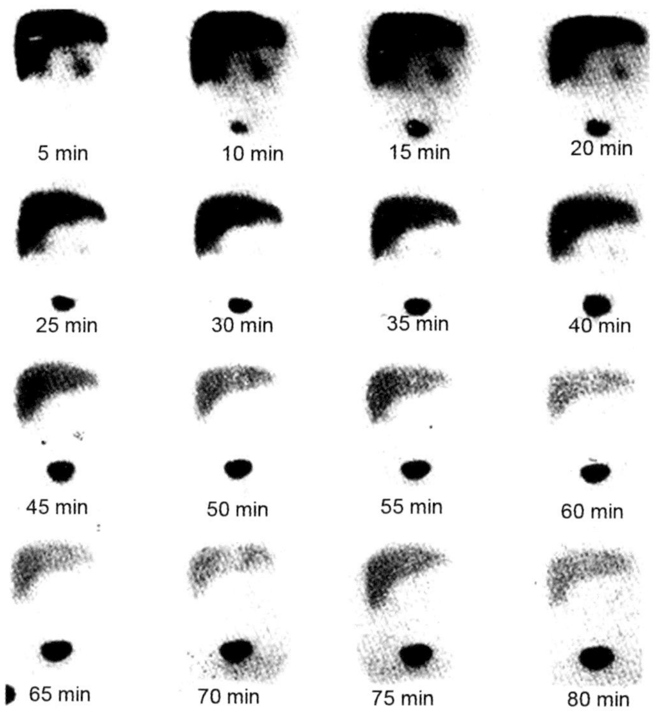

Fig. 7: Scintigraphy using ^{99m}TC IDA scan in a neonate with cholestasis shows good hepatocyte extraction of the radiotracer but no bowel opacification due to biliary atresia.

to the exposed draining biliary radicles.[40] This bowel loop, if it is fluid filled, may be seen in the region of the porta hepatis on postoperative US scans. Biliary scintigraphy can be used to evaluate the patency of the portoenterostomy. Isotopic activity should appear in the bowel by 1 hour after administration. Patients may develop ascending cholangitis with cystic dilatation of the intrahepatic bile ducts and subsequent "bile lakes" secondary to stasis.[41] These accumulations of bile are easily seen on US, CT and magnetic resonance imaging (MRI) and can be drained percutaneously with variable results. Though the operation is successful in more than 50% of patients when performed under the age of 2–3 months, but, because of progressive obliteration of the bile ducts, survival rates drop rapidly when surgery is performed after this age. At times, even with good short-term to mid-term results, cholangitis, cirrhosis and portal hypertension may develop. These patients ultimately need to undergo liver transplantation.

HEPATOBILIARY CYSTIC MALFORMATIONS

Choledochal Cyst

Choledochal cysts are uncommon anomalies of the biliary system with dilatation of the extrahepatic and/or intrahepatic bile ducts. Their incidence in Western countries is approximately 1 in 15,000 live births.[42] About 60% of cases are diagnosed before the age of 10, with about 20% of patients remaining asymptomatic until adulthood and 75% occur in females. Choledochal cysts are generally considered congenital in origin, since they are seen even in fetuses and neonates.

Etiopathogenesis

Yotsuyanagi theorized that unequal proliferation of epithelial cells occurred within the primitive solid bile ducts, with cyst formation occurring at these more "active" locations on subsequent recanalization. Alonso-Lej postulated that cystic dilatation was a result of a primary weakness in the bile duct wall. Subsequently, Babbitt (1969) theorized that an anomalous insertion of the common bile duct into the pancreatic duct with a long common channel caused chronic reflux of digestive pancreatic enzymes into the biliary tree, leading to inflammation, dilation, and scarring. This theory of choledochal cyst development is currently the most popular and is supported by the occurrence of an anomalous pancreaticobiliary junction in 10.5–58% of cases.[43]

The following classification system to describe the various types of choledochal cysts was initially developed by Alonso-Lej et al [44] and subsequently revised by Todani et al:[45]

- *Type IA:* Cystic choledochal dilatation
- *Type IB:* Focal segmental dilatation
- *Type IC:* Fusiform choledochal dilatation
- *Type II:* Eccentric dilatation of CBD referred to as choledochal diverticulum
- *Type III:* Focal dilatation of the intraduodenal portion of CBD—choledochocele
- *Type IVA:* Intrahepatic and extrahepatic cysts
- *Type IVB:* Multiple extrahepatic cysts (may overlap with Type I)
- *Type V:* Single or multiple dilatations of the intrahepatic ducts (Caroli's disease).

Choledochal cysts may manifest clinically with the classic triad of jaundice, abdominal pain and palpable mass. They may be discovered during prenatal sonography. Laboratory abnormalities are often consistent with obstructive jaundice. Surgical resection is the treatment of choice for choledochal cysts to avoid the potential complications of cholelithiasis, choledocholithiasis, cystolithiasis, cholangitis, cirrhosis, pancreatitis, portal hypertension, cyst rupture with bile peritonitis and malignant degeneration with development of cholangiocarcinoma. Malignancy arising within the cyst is reported to occur in 2.5–15% of cases.[46]

Hepatobiliary anomalies associated with choledochal cysts include single or multiple intrahepatic and extrahepatic biliary duct strictures, pancreatic duct strictures, ectopic pancreas, malrotation, double common bile duct, double gallbladder, gallbladder atresia, congenital hepatic fibrosis and sclerosing cholangitis.

Anomalous Junction of the Pancreaticobiliary Duct

In general, the main pancreatic duct and the common bile duct open into the second part of the duodenum separately or by a common channel. A common channel is present in 60–80% of people and 20–40% of the population have separate openings for the two ducts.[47] The length of the normal common channel ranges from 1 to 12 mm, with a mean of 4.5 mm.[48] AJPB is defined as the presence of a common channel longer than 15 mm with or without dilatation of the common channel (>5 mm). Many patients with AJPB have associated choledochal cysts. The pathogenesis of choledochal cyst is complex. Babbitt et al. proposed that AJPB predisposes to the reflux of pancreatic juice into the bile duct because pressure is higher in the pancreatic duct. High amylase levels in the bile aspirated from choldedochal cysts confirm the presence of reflux and this finding supports this theory. However, AJPB is not associated with all cases of choledochal cyst. Wiedmeyer et al. identified ectasia of the common channel, larger than 5 mm in diameter, in addition to a long common channel as important radiographic findings in the diagnosis of choledochal cyst.[49]

The anomalous junction of the pancreaticobiliary duct (AJPB) was classified according to the system of Kimura et al. as type BP when the common bile duct joins the pancreatic duct at a right angle and as type PB when the pancreatic duct joins the common bile duct at an acute angle.[50] Komi proposed a new classification of AJPB into types I, II, and III **(Figs. 8A to C)**. Type I, or type BP, is divided further into type Ia or Ib according to whether the common channel is or is not dilated.[51] The normal caliber of the common channel is 3–5 mm. Similarly, type II is divided into type IIa or IIb. Type III is subclassified as types IIIa, IIIb,and IIIc, which is equivalent to Warshaw's types of pancreas divisum with biliary dilatation. Recently, Guelrud et al. added a Y type AJPB to describe a long common channel without common bile duct dilatation.[52]

The most common complications of choledochal cyst is ascending cholangitis. Eventually, cirrhosis of the liver can occur with subsequent portal hypertension. Spontaneous cyst rupture has also been reported. There is a 20 fold increased incidence of carcinoma of the biliary

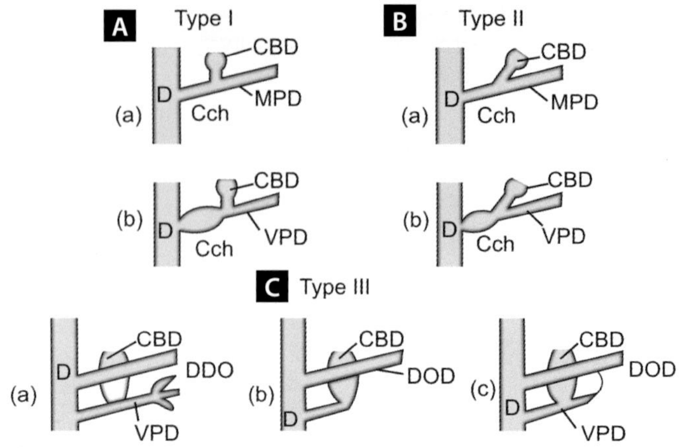

Figs. 8A to C: Komi's classification of the anomalous junction of pancreatic duct and biliary duct—Types I, II, and III.
Abbreviations: D: Duodenum; Cch: Common channel; CBD: Common bile duct; DDD: Dominant dorsal duct; MPD: Main pancreatic duct; VPD: Ventral pancreatic duct.

tree in a patient with choledochal cyst. The risk is low in the first decade of life but increases with advancing age. AJPB has also been implicated as a cause of bile duct and gallbladder carcinoma and pancreatitis. Carcinoma is a recognized complication of choledochal cyst, with a reported frequency of 3–28%.There is a 12–16 times higher incidence of carcinoma in choledochal cyst, and the risk is especially high in patients with cystolithiasis.[53] Bile duct carcinoma appears to be related to long standing ulceration and inflammation and the formation of carcinogens in the bile. Cystolithiasis and cholelithiasis reflect the effects of prolonged stasis and infection. It has been postulated that, in AJPB, pancreatic juice refluxes freely into the biliary tree, leading to chronic inflammation and metaplasia. When pancreatic juice mixes with bile, lysolecithin and phospholipase A2 are produced, which may also be irritants. In patients with choledochal cyst, irritation occurs in the cyst rather than in the gallbladder, so there is a high incidence of choledochus carcinoma.[54] The incidence of carcinoma of the gallbladder is 73% in patients with AJPB without a choledochal cyst and only 10% in patients with AJPB with a choledochal cyst. AJPB not only predisposes to biliary tract anomalies but also causes pancreatic duct abnormalities. Guelrud et al. found that dysfunction of the sphincter of Oddi associated with AJPB is responsible for episodes of recurrent pancreatitis.[52] They associated AJPB with 28% of patients with recurrent pancreatitis. The combination of AJPB and choledochal cyst is responsible for protein plugs and pancreatolithiasis. Kaneko et al. proposed that increased mucin production from the bile duct caused by pancreaticobiliary malfunction is responsible for protein plug formation.[55] These protein plugs are usually seen in the common channel but may be seen distal to the common channel as reported by Yamataka et al.[56] Pancreatolithiasis in patients with choledochal cyst ranges from 0.2% to 33%, as noted by various investigators.[55,56]

Imaging Features

On plain radiograph, a soft tissue mass may be appreciated in the right upper quadrant adjacent to the liver. The cyst wall rarely demonstrates calcification, but opaque calculi may be visible.

An upper GI series demonstrates anterior displacement of the first and second portions of duodenum and gastric antrum, widening of the duodenal sweep. On barium enema, there is inferior displacement of the hepatic flexure.

Choledochal cysts of types I, II or III are detected at sonography as anechoic or hypoechoic cystic lesions in the region of the porta hepatis ventral to the portal vein with communication to the biliary tree **(Figs. 9A to C)**. The gallbladder is seen separate from the cystic lesion. The rapid, almost focal transition between a grossly dilated and nondilated biliary system is further indication of the presence of a choledochal cyst. US is the recommended initial imaging study in the newborn infant with persistent jaundice in whom the differential diagnostic consideration include choledochal cyst, biliary atresia, neonatal hepatitis, etc. Choledochal cyst and biliary atresia might occur together in neonates[57] **(Fig. 10)**. Depending on the type of choledochal cyst, other intrahepatic cysts may or may not be demonstrated. The pancreas and pancreatic duct should be examined for evidence of pancreatitis or ductal dilatation.

Hepatobiliary scintigraphy confirms excretion of radiotracer into the choledochal cyst, but yields limited anatomic delineation and is insufficient for determining cyst type or planning surgical reconstruction. At times, the choledochal cyst does not fill with the radionuclide and the diagnosis can be missed.

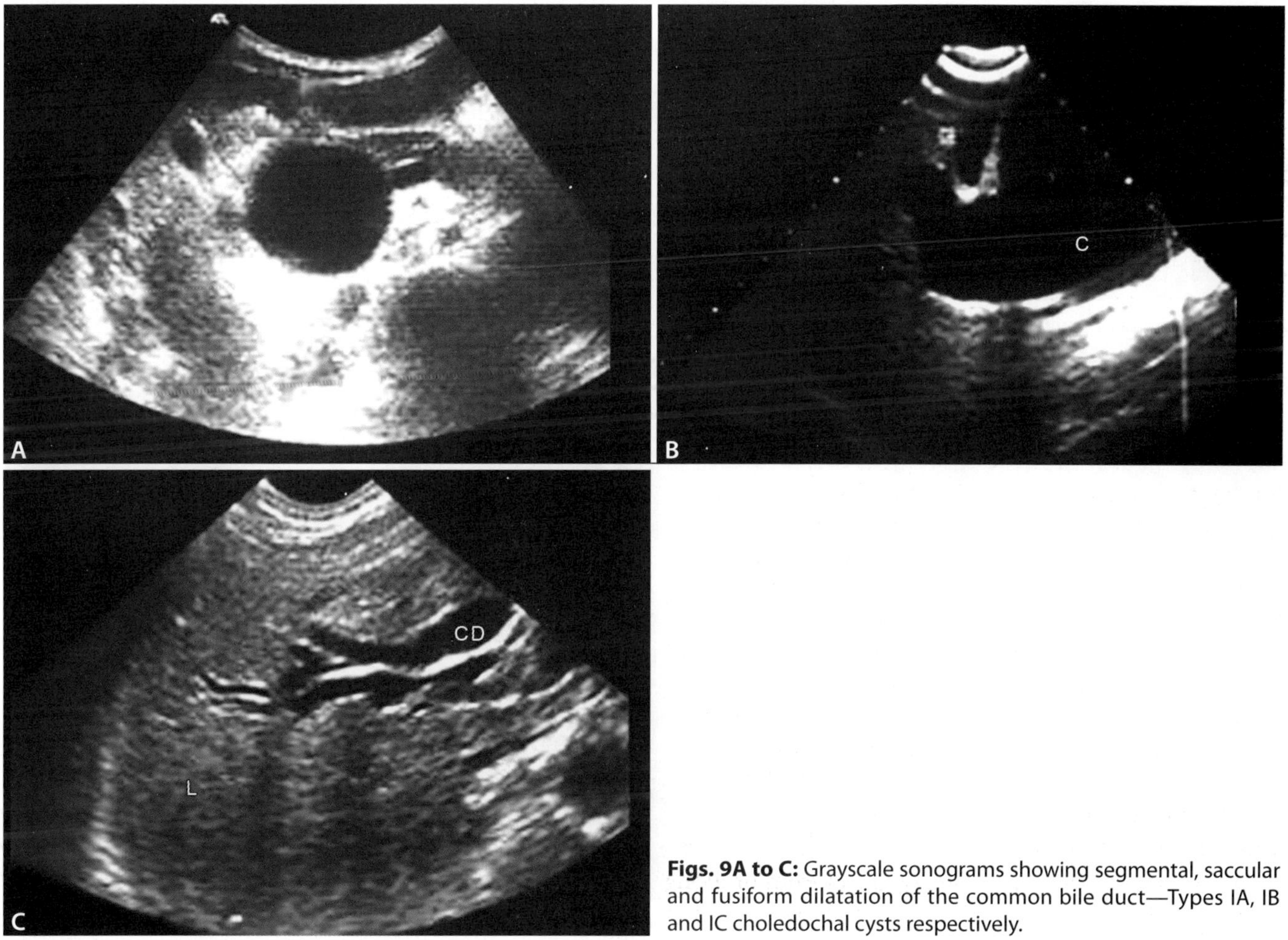

Figs. 9A to C: Grayscale sonograms showing segmental, saccular and fusiform dilatation of the common bile duct—Types IA, IB and IC choledochal cysts respectively.

CT is helpful in demonstrating the size and extent of both extrahepatic and intrahepatic choledochal cysts. It can globally delineate the relationship of the cystic mass to adjacent intraperitoneal and extraperitoneal structures, allowing a thorough evaluation of the abdominal cavity and retroperitoneum. Mural irregularities or focal nodularity within the choledochal cyst, suggesting malignant changes, may be identified by CT and US.

On MRI, long T1 and T2 relaxation times characteristic of fluid can confirm the cystic nature of the lesion when US yields inconclusive results because of internal echoes within the cyst **(Figs. 11 and 12)**. MRI can also yield detailed information on surrounding abdominal anatomy.

For preoperative planning, MR cholangiopancreatography (MRCP) may be performed **(Figs. 13A to D)**. MRCP is a noninvasive procedure and provides the best available projection image for revealing the extent of choledochal cyst in children and adults **(Figs. 14A and B)**. Thin slice and thick slab MR images enable visualization of the accessory pancreatic duct and the common channel. The global quality of images obtained with single-slab images is better than that of maximum-intensity-projection images in adults with suspected biliary or pancreatic abnormalities **(Figs. 15 and 16)**. In a study by Chan et al. anomalous pancreaticobiliary ductal union was not visualized on MRCP using a two-dimensional turbo spin-echo sequence with the MIP technique. However, in pediatric patients, MRCP with a half-Fourier acquisition of a single shot fast spin-echo or a turbo spin-echo sequence might increase the sensitivity of anomalous pancreaticobiliary ductal union detection.[58,59] The main drawback of using MRCP for the determination of anomalous pancreaticobiliary ductal union seems to be that large choledochal cysts obscure the common channel. ERCP is regarded as the most definitive and reliable diagnostic method of revealing choledochal cysts and anomalous pancreaticobiliary ductal union **(Figs. 17A and B)**.[60]

Surgeons need an exact anatomic map of the pancreaticobiliary ductal union because it is essential that the choledochal cyst be completely resected without pancreatic ductal injury. Surgical excision with Roux-en-Y anastomosis gives excellent results and reduces bile stasis, risk of cholangitis and malignancy. When the anatomy is more complicated, a simple drainage is carried out but these patients have risk of recurrent cholangitis, lithiasis, pancreatitis and cancer **(Figs. 18 to 20)**.

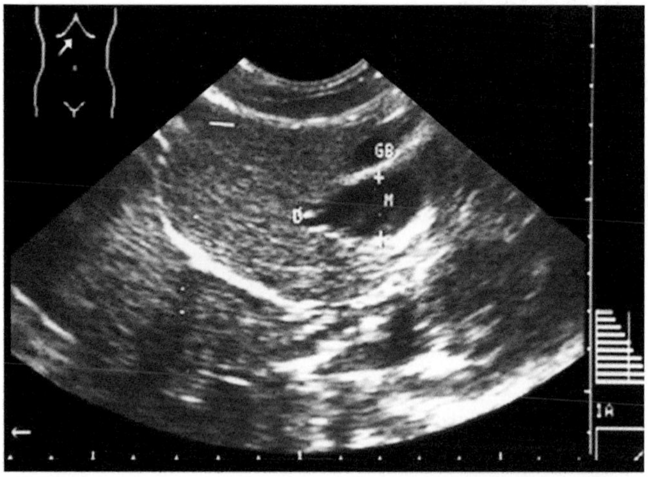

Fig. 10: Sonogram showing a diffuse increase in liver echogenicity with saccular dilatation of distal CBD—biliary atresia with associated choledochal cyst.

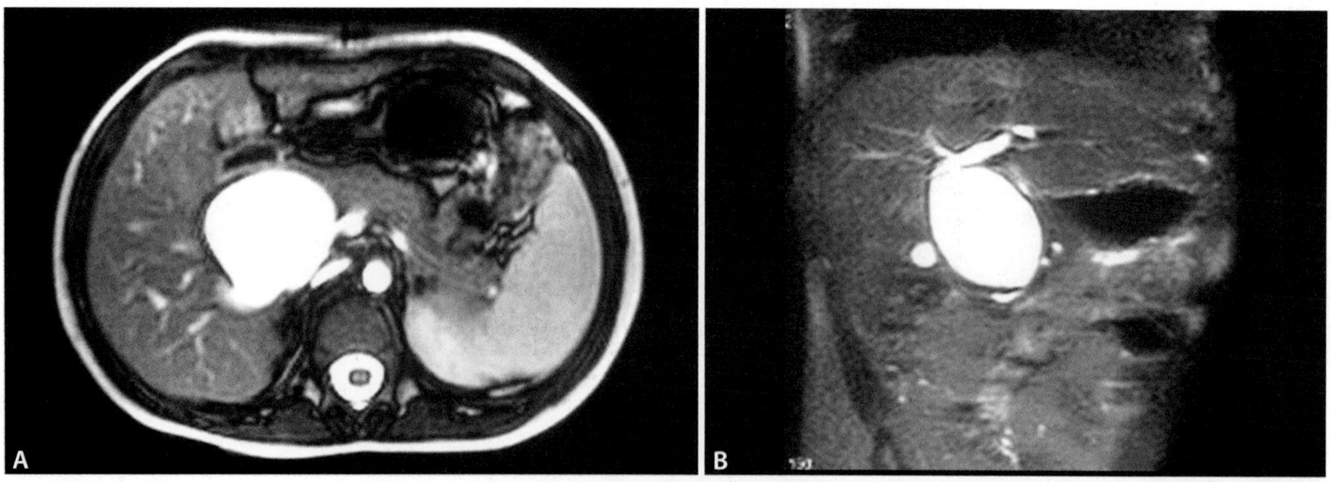

Figs. 11A and B: TRUE FISP axial and HASTE coronal MR images showing cystically dilated common bile duct due to Type I choledochal cyst.

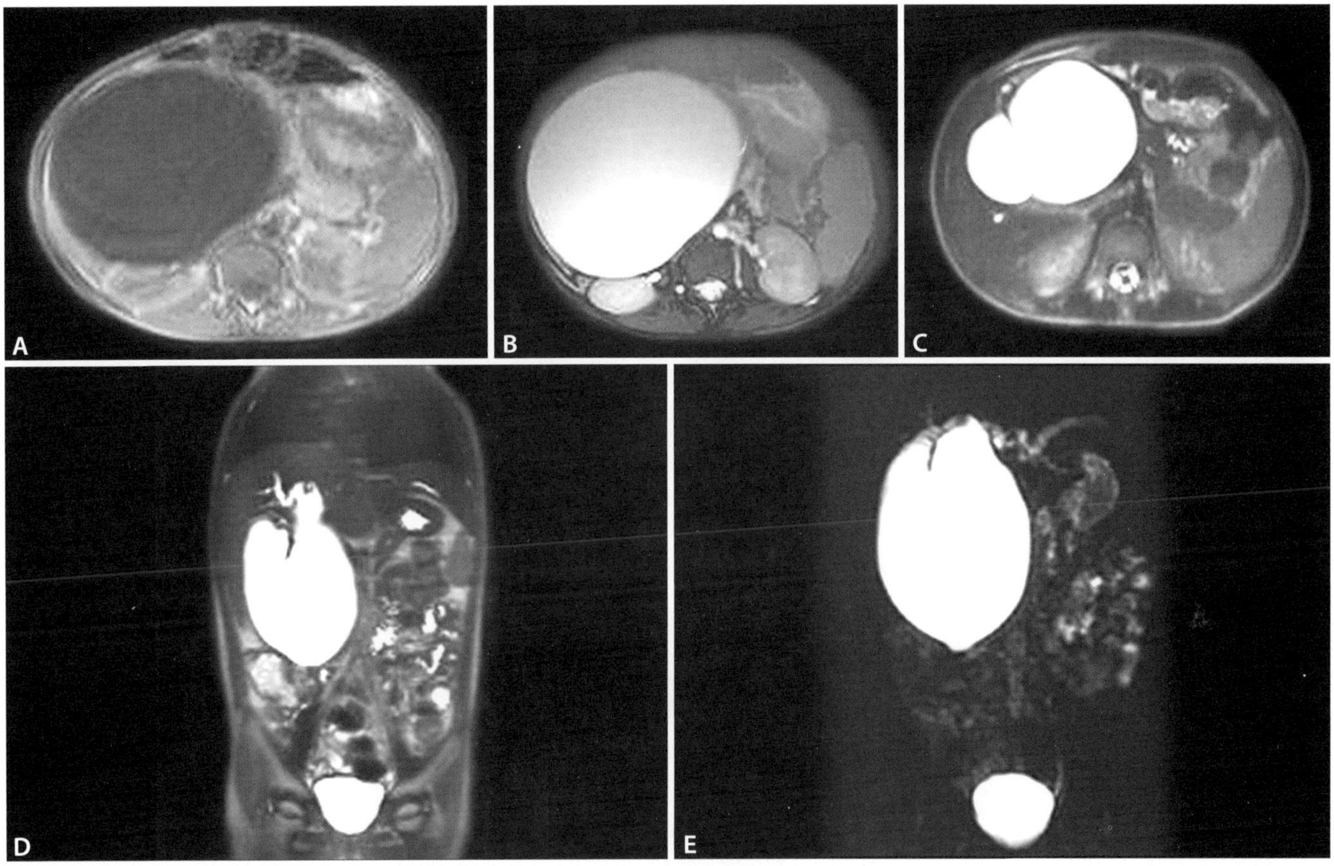

Figs. 12A to E: Axial T1W (A), axial T2W (B and C) and HASTE coronal (D) images revealing the cystic nature of the choledochal cyst seen as hypointense signal on T1 and hyperintense on T2W MR images. A small septation is seen within the cyst. RARE sequence showing the cyst to a saccular dilatation of the common bile duct Type I A choledochal cyst.

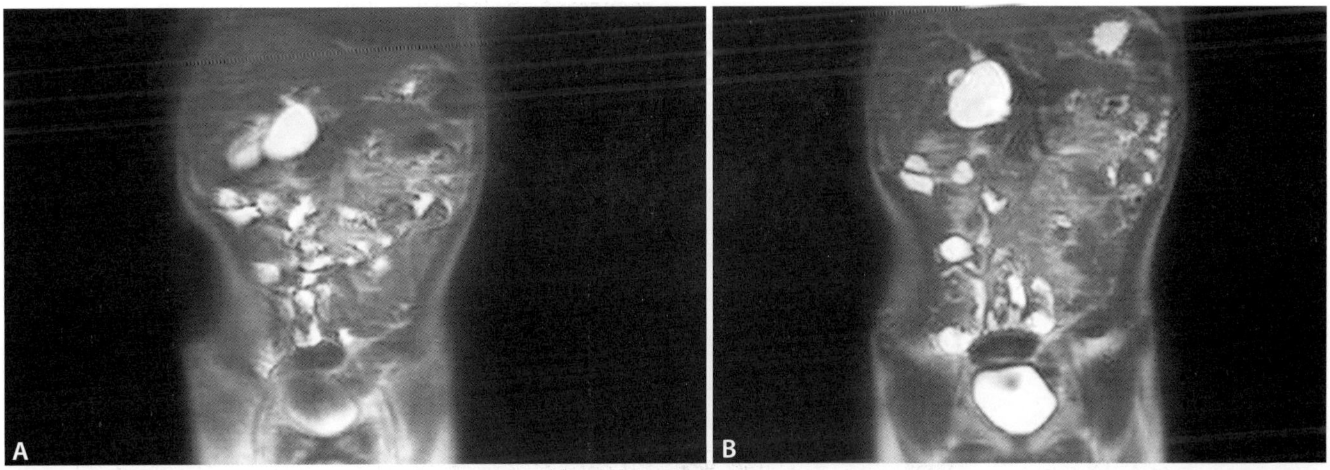

Figs. 13A and B

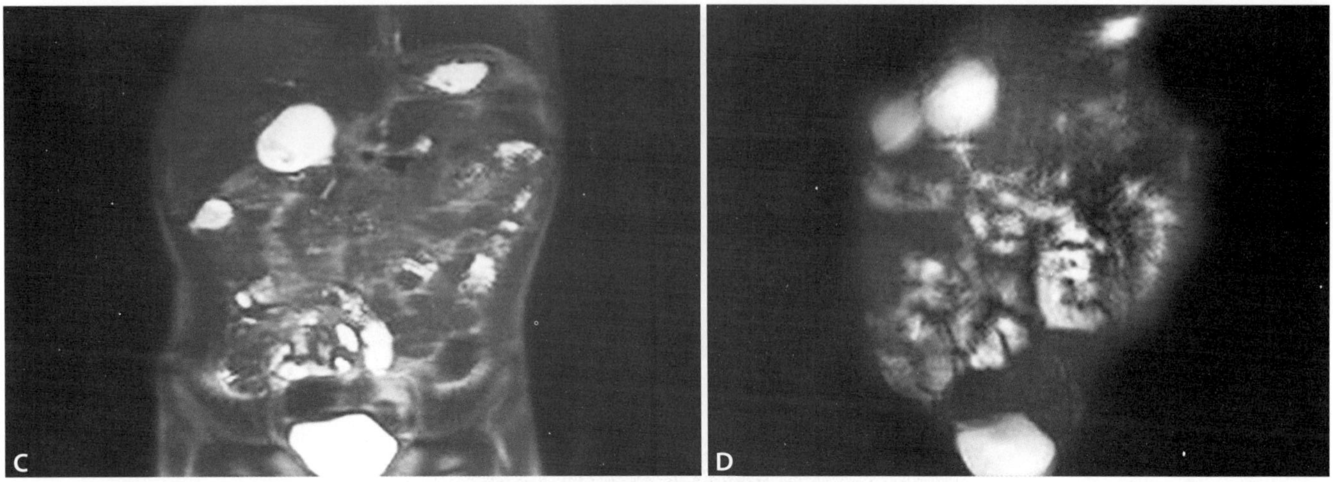

Figs. 13C and D

Figs. 13A to D: HASTE coronal (A to C) and RARE sequence (D) MR images showing a focal segmental dilatation of the common bile duct. The normal caliber duct proximal and distal to the dilatation is visualized—Type IB choledochal cyst.

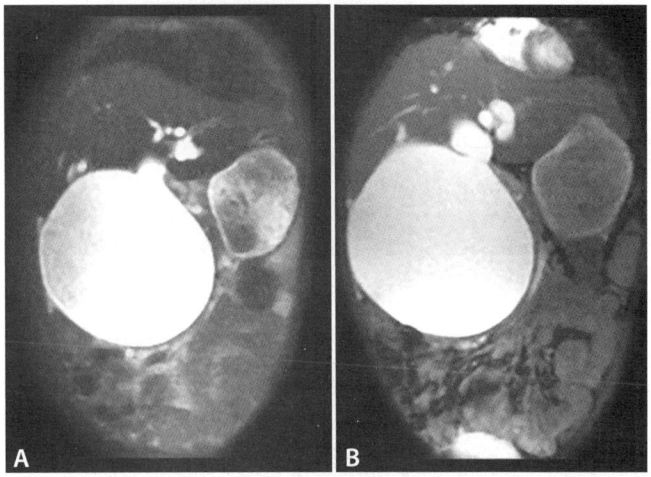

Figs. 14A and B: HASTE coronal MR images revealing a large eccentric dilatation of the CBD seen as a large outpouching from the CBD—Type II choledochal cyst/choledochal diverticulum.

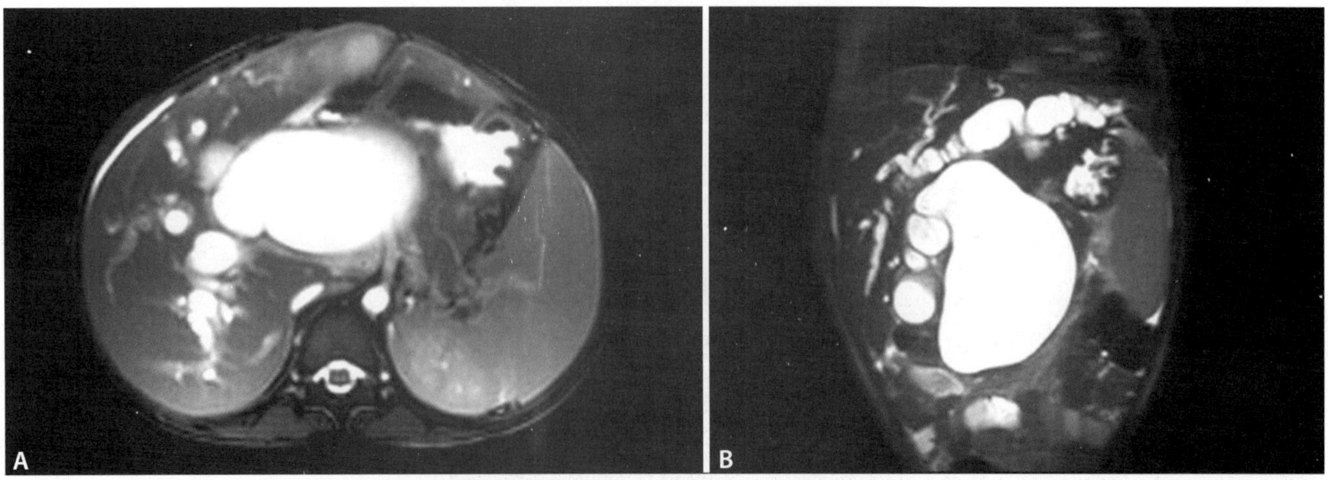

Figs. 15A and B: Type IVA choledochal cyst seen on TrueFISP axial and HASTE coronal MR images as cystically dilated intra- and extrahepatic bite ducts.

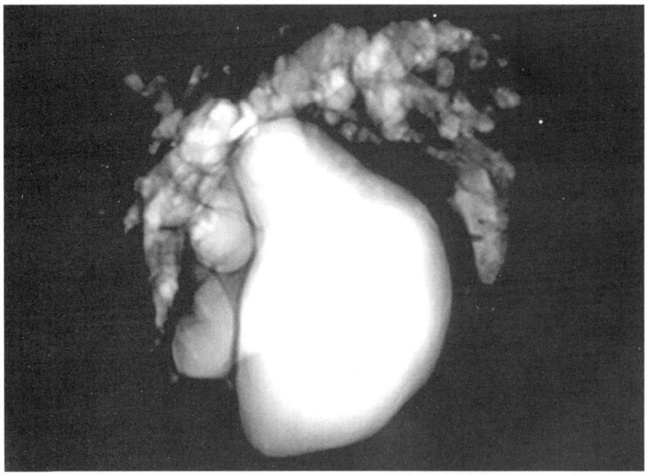

Fig. 16: SSFSE (RARE) image showing Type IVA choledochal cyst.

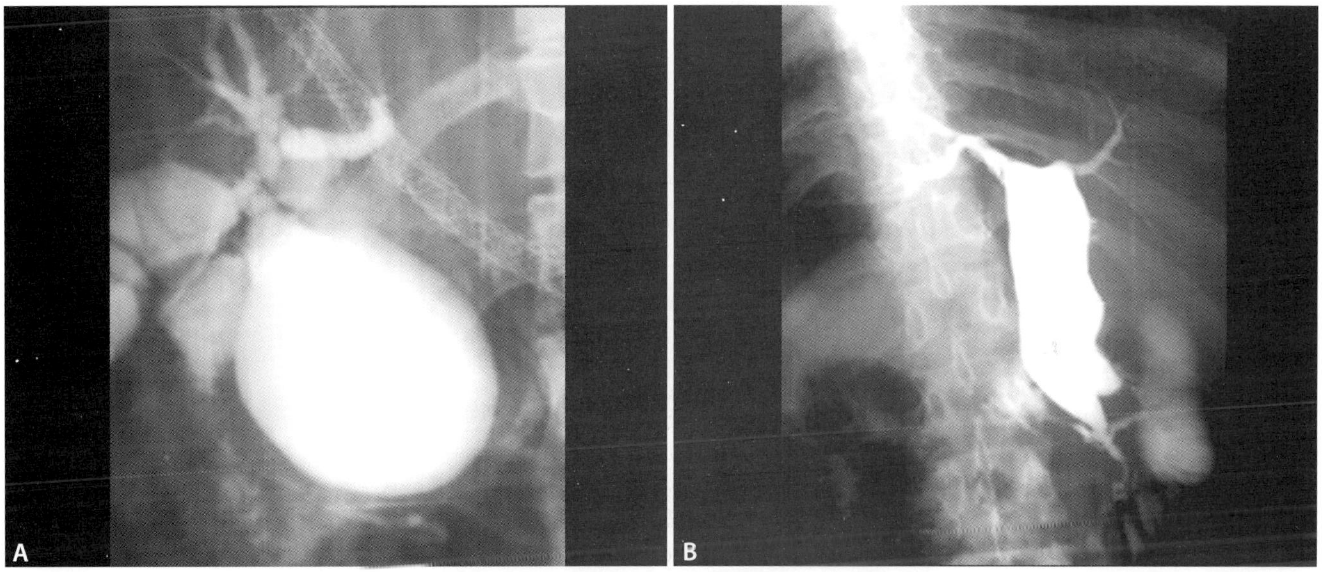

Figs. 17A and B: ERCP images illustrating saccular and fusiform dilatation of common duct with nondilated intrahepatic biliary radicles—Type I choledochal cysts.

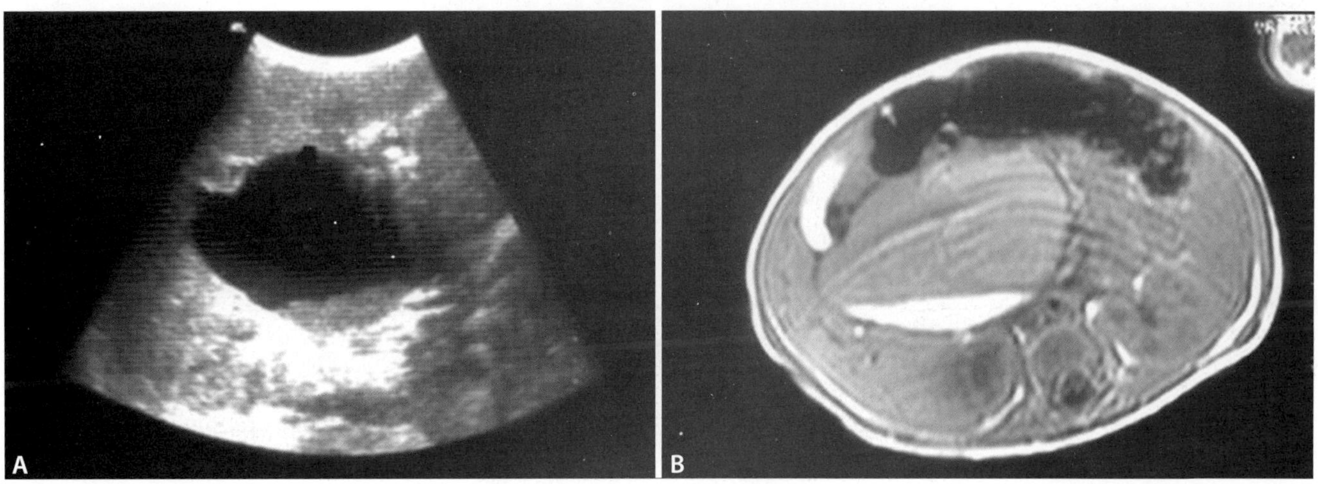

Figs. 18A and B: US(A) and T1W axial (B) MR image showing fluid–sludge level within a huge Type I choledochal cyst.

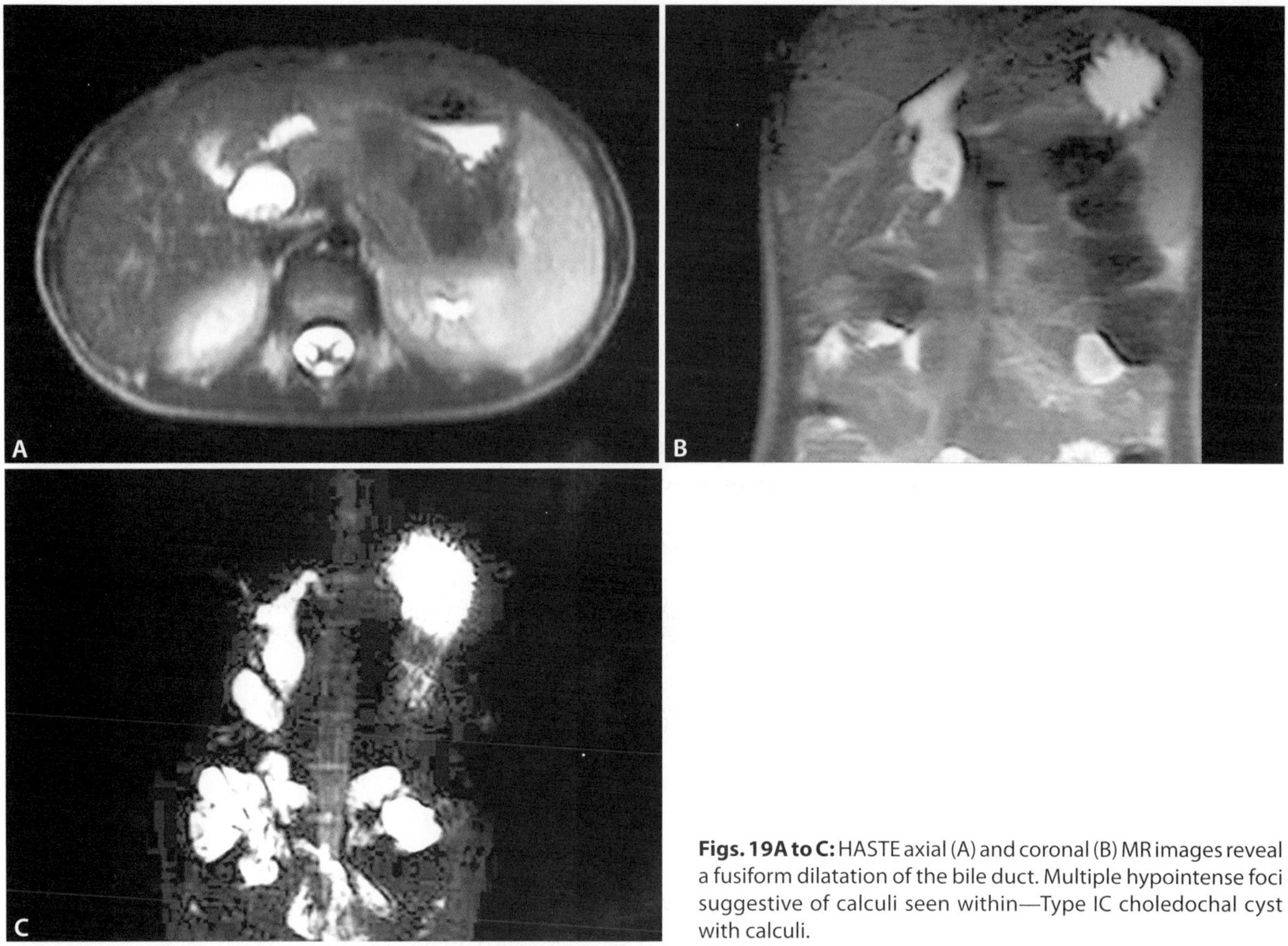

Figs. 19A to C: HASTE axial (A) and coronal (B) MR images reveal a fusiform dilatation of the bile duct. Multiple hypointense foci suggestive of calculi seen within—Type IC choledochal cyst with calculi.

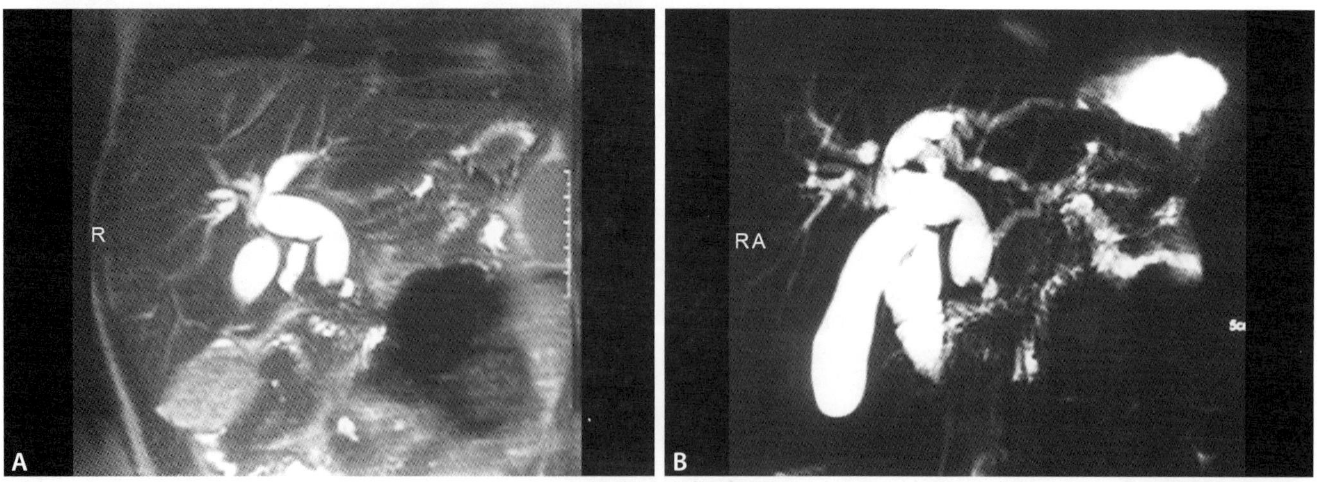

Figs. 20A and B: HASTE coronal and SSFSE MR images illustrate fusiform dilatation of common duct with an irregular polypoid filling defect at its lower end—Malignant transformation in a Type I choledochal cyst.

The differential diagnosis of choledochal cyst includes several other cystic lesions including hepatic cyst, enteric duplication cyst, pancreatic pseudocyst, hepatic artery aneurysm and spontaneous perforation of the common bile duct. Use of careful 2D imaging combined with CDFI can readily differentiate these conditions.

CAROLI'S DISEASE

Caroli's disease is Type IV (Alonson-Lej) or type V (Todani) Choledochal cyst.

Caroli's disease or communicating cavernous ectasia of the intrahepatic bile ducts is a rare congenital disorder with segmental, saccular dilatation of the intrahepatic bile ducts. Although, congenital cystic dilation of the intrahepatic bile ducts was first described by Vachell and Stevens in 1906, Caroli first clearly defined this disease entity in 1958.[61]

It is an autosomal recessive disorder and is among the ductal plate malformations that occur at different levels in the developing biliary tree. The disease results from the arrest of or a derangement in the normal embryologic remodeling of ducts and causes varying degrees of destructive inflammation and segmental dilatation. When the large intrahepatic bile ducts are affected, the result is Caroli's disease. Abnormal development of the small interlobular bile ducts results in congenital hepatic fibrosis. Features of both congenital hepatic fibrosis and Caroli's disease are present if all levels of the biliary tree are involved and this condition has been termed "Caroli's syndrome". Two primary types of the disease have been identified:

- Nonhereditary form (Type I), also known as the "sporadic pure type" is often limited to one hepatic lobe (usually the left lobe). Multifocal saccular dilatations of segmental bile ducts are frequently accompanied with calculi formation and recurrent bacterial cholangitis.
- Hereditary form (Type II) involves the entire liver. The bile duct dilatation is usually less prominent than in Type I, and the patients present with abnormalities related to hepatic fibrosis and portal hypertension.

Associated conditions, including choledochal cysts and cystic lesions of the kidney known as autosomal—recessive polycystic kidney disease (ARPKD) occur mainly in the hereditary form.[62] Hepatic fibrosis, medullary sponge kidney, nephronophthisis are other associated conditions.

Although, the Todani classification of choledochal cysts includes Caroli's disease as a type V choledochal cyst, the current understanding of the pathogenesis of Caroli's disease makes it unlikely that these entities are related. The cause of Caroli's disease is unknown. Postulated mechanisms include occlusion of the hepatic artery in the neonatal period with associated ischemia of the bile ducts. Abnormal growth rate of the biliary epithelium and lack of the normal involution of the ductal plates surrounding the portal tracts, leads to biliary cysts surrounding the portal tracts.

Caroli's disease has an autosomal recessive inheritance and is often associated with renal disorders whereas choledochal cysts are congenital and not associated with renal disorders.[63]

Caroli's disease typically develops during childhood or early adulthood with recurrent episodes of right upper quadrant or epigastric pain, fever, and sometimes jaundice (typical triad).

Liver function tests may be normal or demonstrate mild elevations in serum alkaline phosphatase and transaminase levels.

Complications of the "simple form" of Caroli's disease include cholelithiasis, choledocholithiasis, intrahepatic calculi, intrahepatic abscesses, subphrenic abscesses, and cholangiocarcinomas.

Bloustein reported a 7% incidence of malignancy in Caroli's disease.[64] Portal hypertension, although less common, does occur with the fibroangioadenomatous form of Caroli's disease and the patient may have episodes of hematemesis secondary to variceal bleeding.

Pathology

Pathologically, two forms of the disease have been recognized:

1. The "simple" form, which is more common, is characterized by dilatation of the intrahepatic bile ducts and is most often manifested as repeated episodes of ascending cholangitis.
2. The "fibroangioadenomatic" form is characterized by congenital hepatic fibrosis, portal hypertension and bleeding esophageal varices.[63]

Imaging Features

The spectrum of radiologic appearances of Caroli's disease ranges from segmental to diffuse biliary dilatation, from saccular to fusiform dilatation, and from isolated intrahepatic involvement to intra- and extrahepatic involvement.[65-67]

Plain films occasionally show gallstones, intrahepatic calculi, or medullary nephrocalcinosis. Excretory urography may demonstrate the renal tubular ectasia of medullary sponge kidney or the corticomedullary cystic changes of renal cystic disease.

US demonstrates sonolucent intrahepatic tubular structures converging on the porta hepatis, representing the grossly dilated intrahepatic biliary tree. The dilated ducts may give the appearance of surrounding the portal vein radicles ("the intra-aluminal portal vein sign") Toma et al believed this sign to be pathognomonic Caroli's disease.[68] On color Doppler they show lack of color fill-in *the dilated ducts and color flow can be seen in portal vein branches*. It is important to demonstrate a communication between these multiple dilated structures in order to distinguish Caroli's disease from polycystic liver disease or multiple hepatic abscesses. Additional, findings include intrahepatic calculi, bulbar protrusions into the ductal lumina, bridge formation across dilated ductal lumina, and portal radicles surrounded by dilated bile ducts ("central dot" sign).

Intrahepatic dilatation of the bile ducts with multiple cysts can also be seen in Byler's disease but the large cysts do not communicate with the biliary system. Renal sonography may show medullary cysts, loss of corticomedullary differentiation, or increased medullary or parenchymal echogenicity.[65]

CT depicts low-density, irregular, dilated cystic structures communicating with the biliary tree[66] **(Figs. 21A and B)**. CT is an excellent modality to show the extent of the disease especially the intrahepatic ductal ectasia. A central dot may be seen that corresponds to the intraluminal portal vein seen sonographically. These will enhance on administration of contrast. If the ducts are only minimally dilated the connections will be better seen on CT than US[69] **(Figs. 22 to 24)**.

CT cholangiography has also been described as a noninvasive method of confirming the biliary nature of the disease process.

Hepatic scintigraphy may show multiple filling defects if the ducts are sufficiently dilated. Biliary imaging with, ^{99}Tc iminodiacetic acid compounds show focal defects during

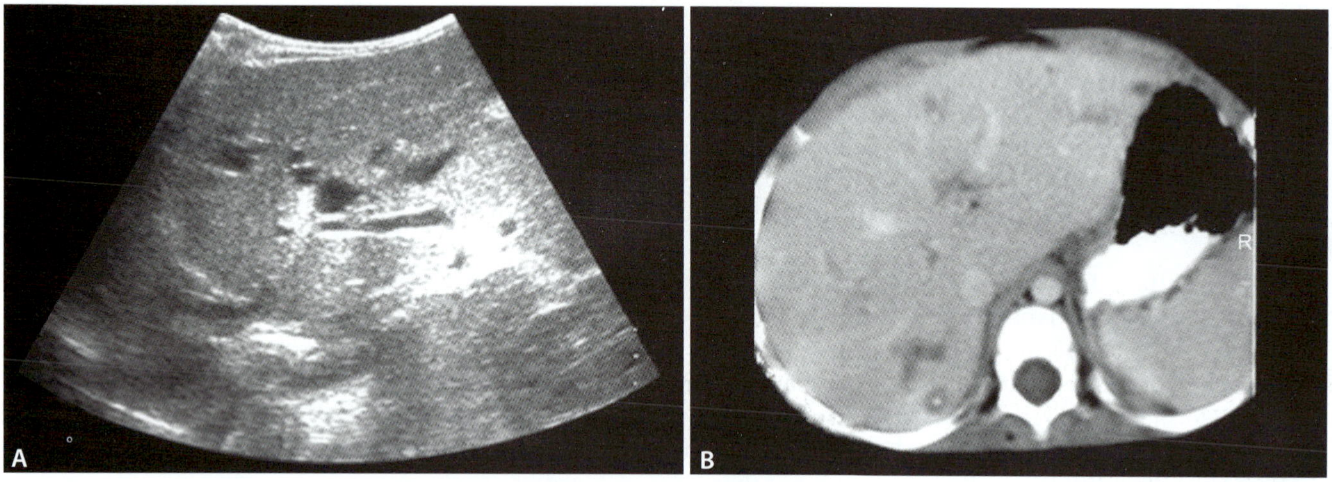

Figs. 21A and B: Transverse sonogram (A) showing multiple intrahepatic cysts communicating with the biliary tree. CECT (B) in another patient showing segmental intrahepatic duct dilatation with the "central dot" sign—Caroli's disease.

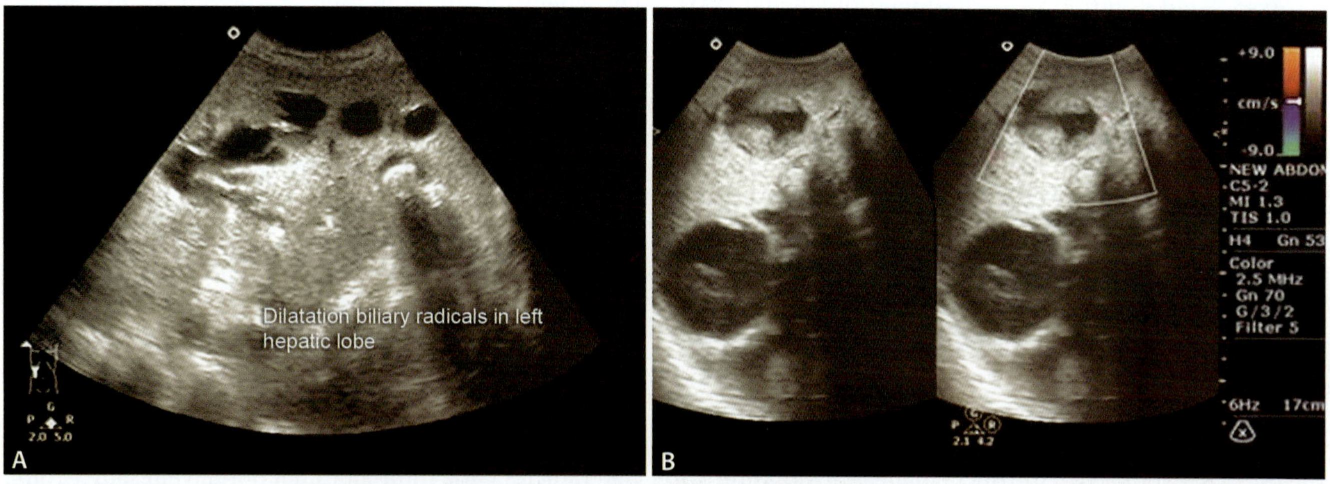

Figs. 22A and B: Ultrasound images in an adolescent male showing multiple saccular areas of biliary dilatation within the liver parenchyma. Echogenic foci with distal acoustic shadowing seen in one of the cysts s/o intraductal calculi. One of the larger cysts shows presence of soft tissue along the walls.

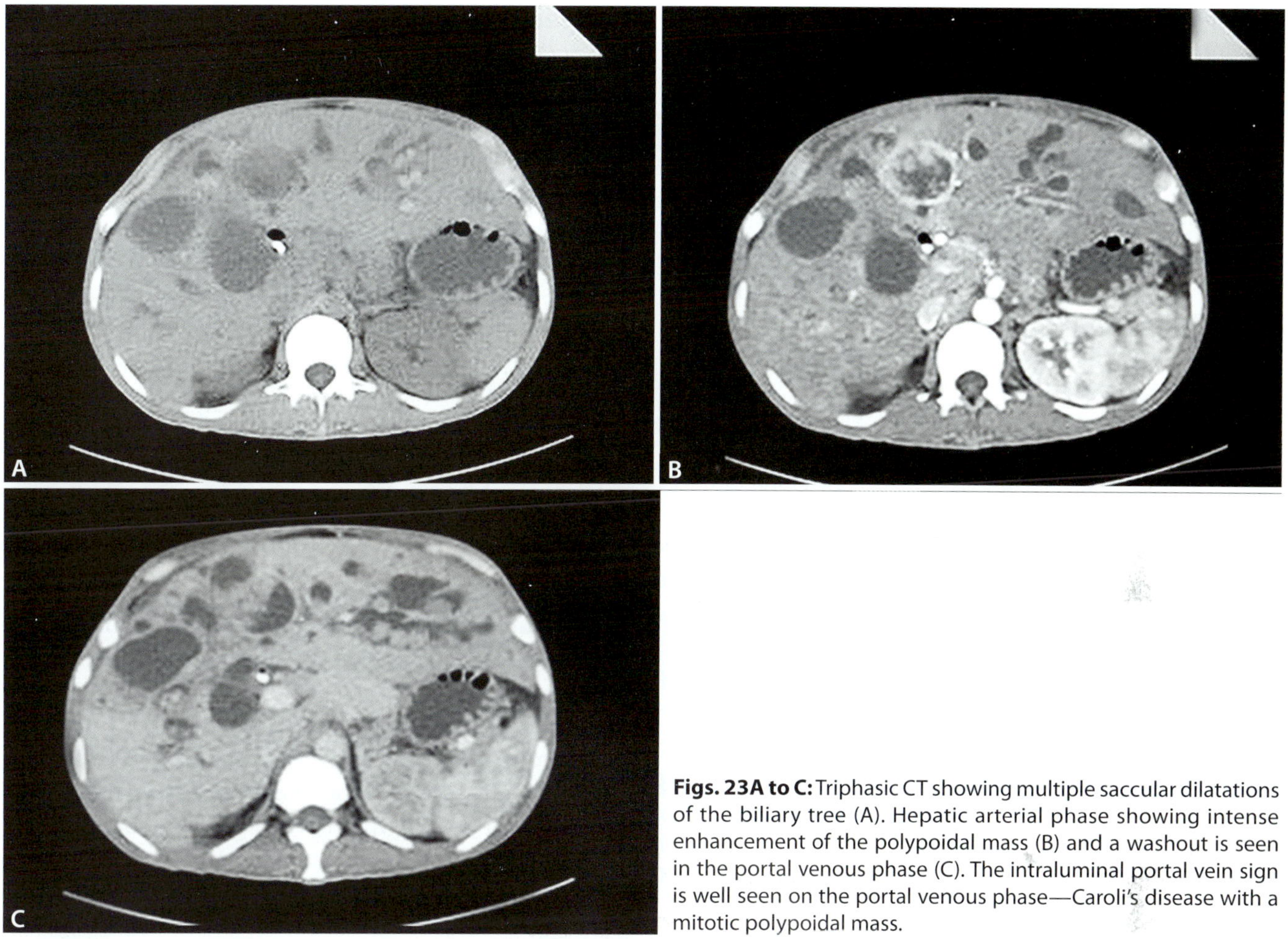

Figs. 23A to C: Triphasic CT showing multiple saccular dilatations of the biliary tree (A). Hepatic arterial phase showing intense enhancement of the polypoidal mass (B) and a washout is seen in the portal venous phase (C). The intraluminal portal vein sign is well seen on the portal venous phase—Caroli's disease with a mitotic polypoidal mass.

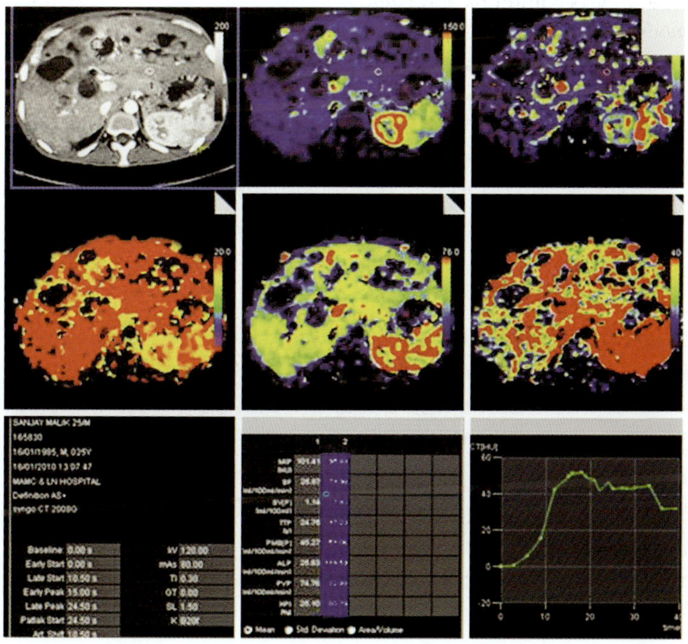

Fig. 24: Perfusion study with ROI placed over the intraductal lesion and normal liver reveals increased HPI values 80.79% for the lesion. Higher BF BV PMB HPI are observed. Biopsy revealed it to be a intraductal cholangiocarcinoma.

the hepatic phase that gradually increases in activity as the radiopharmaceutical collects in the dilated ducts while the remainder of the liver shows decreased activity with time. Radiotracer activity in the gastrointestinal tract will be seen but is frequently delayed because of the stasis.[70]

The cholangiographic features of Caroli's disease are well established as saccular or fusiform dilatation of the intrahepatic bile ducts, irregular bile duct walls, strictures, and stones. Segmental ductal dilatation is more common (82%) than diffuse ductal dilatation with alternating areas of stricture and dilation. The presence of diffuse fusiform dilatation of the extrahepatic duct measuring 3 cm or less in diameter combined with the characteristic intrahepatic ductal findings may be helpful in differentiating patients with Caroli's disease from patients with choledochal cyst and intrahepatic biliary dilatation.

Direct bile duct opacification by ERCP or PTC is the most sensitive method for investigating bile duct abnormalities, and, more specifically, for demonstrating communications between cystic dilatations and bile ducts, however, both techniques are invasive and carry a risk of complications including sepsis and bleeding.[65]

Advantages of MRCP consist of depiction of the entire biliary tree in a noninvasive fashion and a spatial resolution as high as 1.5 mm.[67] Guy et al (2002) reported three main patterns of Caroli's disease using an MR imaging protocol which included MRCP and a dynamic contrast-enhanced study.[71]

- The first pattern was characterized by multiple cystic ectasias connected with fusiform dilatations of the intrahepatic bile ducts throughout the liver. On gadolinium-enhanced scans, the 'dot sign' was seen as a tiny dot or an internal septum showing strong contrast enhancement due to a portal radicle surrounded by a dilated bile duct.
- The second pattern was characterized by isolated fusiform dilatation of the intrahepatic bile ducts.
- The third pattern was characterized by a monoliform dilatation of the left intrahepatic bile ducts with hepatic cystic lesions. MRCP may be useful in the evaluation of a suspected malignancy. The modality has the added benefit of revealing both intraluminal and extraluminal disease and has recently been reported as an aid in the diagnosis of malignancy in Caroli's disease.

The differential diagnosis of Caroli's disease includes primary sclerosing cholangitis, recurrent pyogenic cholangitis, polycystic liver disease, a choledochal cyst, biliary papillomatosis, and (occasionally) obstructive biliary dilatation.[63]

Congenital Hepatic Fibrosis

Congenital hepatic fibrosis, with or without associated biliary duct ectasia, is an autosomal recessive inherited abnormality. The associated renal abnormalities are infantile and adult polycystic disease, renal dysplasia, and medullary cystic disease.[72] Those patients who present as newborns or infants do so because of the severity of their renal disease which usually dictates their course and prognosis. Those patients who present later in childhood or in adulthood have less renal involvement and frequently come to attention because of hepatomegaly or portal hypertension.

US characteristics of congenital hepatic fibrosis described by Alvarez et al is a large liver with or without splenomegaly depending on the presence or absence of portal hypertension.[72] The hepatic echogenicity is homogeneously or heterogeneously increased. With associated Caroli's disease there will be intrahepatic biliary duct ectasia and dilatation of the gallbladder. If portal hypertension is present, its characteristic imaging findings will be seen.[73] Associated renal lesions can also be identified and should always be sought. CT does not have a routine role in this disease but may be performed if complications are suspected or in the evaluation of patients with portal hypertension.[74] MR angiography can demonstrate vascular sequelae of portal hypertension and MR cholangiopancreatography may reveal biliary cysts or intra- or extrahepatic biliary duct dilatation or ectasia.[75]

PRIMARY SCLEROSING CHOLANGITIS

Primary sclerosing cholangitis (PSC) is an uncommon, progressive idiopathic chronic cholestatic disorder characterized by inflammation of bile ducts leading to their fibrosis and destruction. It can involve both intrahepatic and extrahepatic ducts, gallbladder and small bile ducts down to the interlobular ducts in any combination. There may be focal or diffuse liver involvement.

Pathology

Pathologically, the extrahepatic ducts are thickened with small lumen, described as cord-like or rope-like ducts and the intrahepatic ducts are almost always affected. Histologically, the constellation of reduced numbers of small bile ducts, surrounded by cuff of fibrous tissue, ductular proliferation, copper deposition, and piecemeal necrosis is very suggestive of PSC.

PSC is an uncommon condition in infants and children. It can present either alone or in association with ulcerative colitis, histiocytosis X and immune deficiency. In children many cases are idiopathic with a subset of it presenting in the neonatal period.[76] The neonatal form presents with jaundice within the first two weeks of age which resolves by one year. These children develop cirrhosis between 1 and 10 years of age.

No definite test is available for the diagnosis of primary sclerosing cholangitis and diagnosis is based on the combination of biochemical, histological and imaging data.

Radiological visualization of biliary tree is essential for its diagnosis and cholangiographic techniques are the gold standard.

Imaging Features

On sonography, extensive thickening of intrahepatic and extrahepatic ducts is depicted as brightly echogenic tissue surrounding the portal venules and common duct. Intraluminal debris consisting of nonshadowing, mobile echogenic particles may be present, consistent with pus, biliary sludge or desquamated bile duct epithelium. Irregular, multisegmental intrahepatic biliary dilatation on sonography can suggest PSC **(Figs. 25A and B)**.

CT may show a spectrum of findings including intrahepatic duct pruning, beading, and skip dilatation. Most commonly, multifocal discontinuous areas of minimal intrahepatic biliary dilatation without a mass are seen **(Figs. 25C and D)**. As benign reactive lymphadenopathy may occur in PSC, it should not be taken as a strong indicator of malignancy without other supportive signs.

Cholangiography is the gold standard for diagnosis of PSC and ERCP is preferable to PTC for demonstrating the intrahepatic and extrahepatic ductal narrowing and dilatations with "skip" lesions.

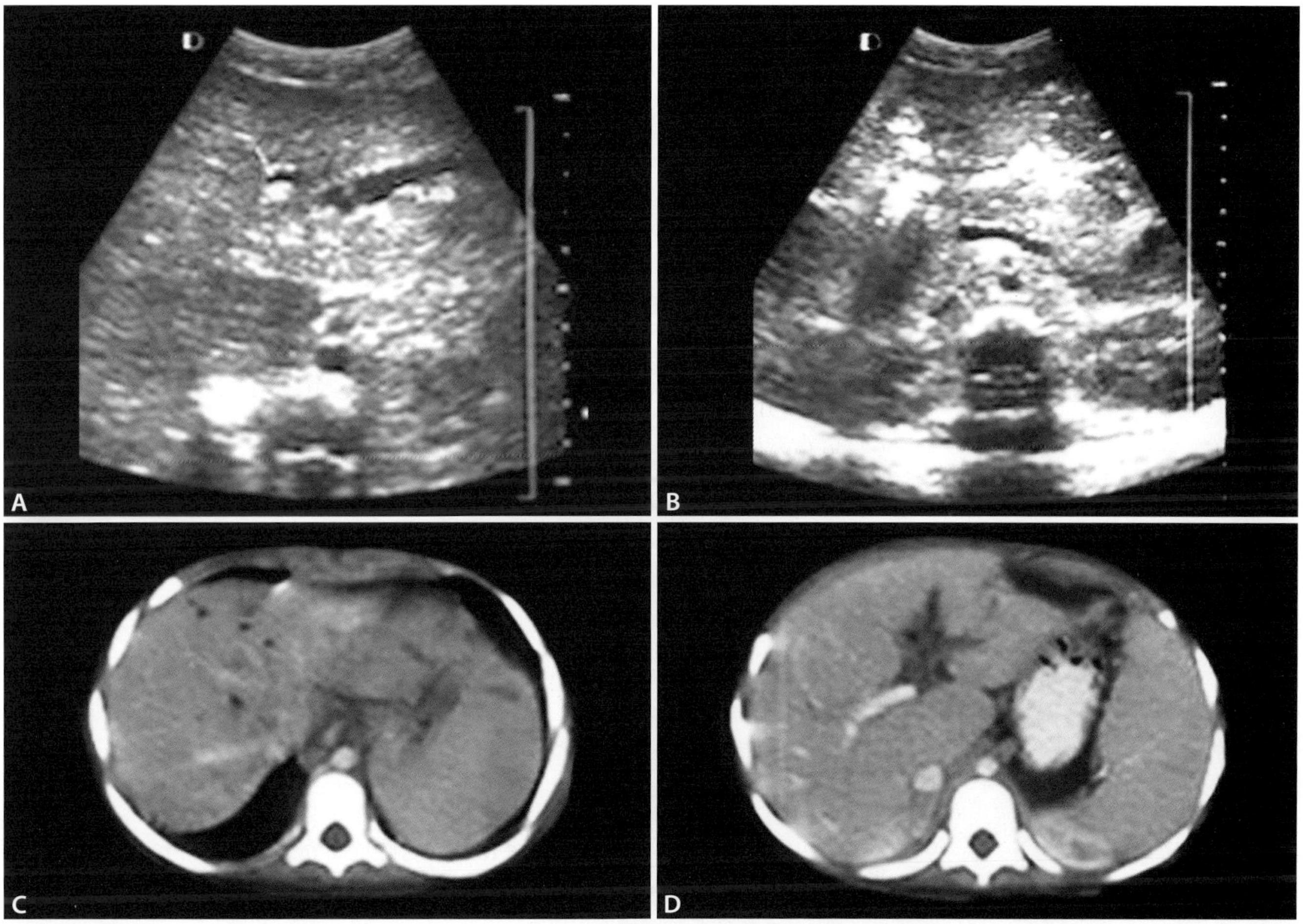

Figs. 25A to D: (A and B) Transverse sonograms of liver showing irregular intrahepatic biliary dilatation with shadowing and nonshadowing intraluminal echogenic debris—primary sclerosing cholangitis; (C and D) CECT scans of the same patient show tubular structures in left lobe with "skip" areas of biliary dilatation.

Magnetic resonance imaging has been used to evaluate children with sclerosing cholangitis and has demonstrated peripheral wedge shaped areas of high signal in association with dilated bile duct.[10]

The biliary tree is markedly irregular with areas of stricture and focal dilatation proximal to the stricture **(Figs. 26A to C)**.

The prognosis of PSC in children is variable and hepatocellular carcinoma, as a complication of PSC seen in adults, has not been reported in children.[77]

CYSTIC FIBROSIS

Symptomatic liver disease is seen in 2–18% patients of cystic fibrosis and can be the presenting feature of this disorder.[78] Rarely the patient may present in the neonatal period with cholestatic jaundice. Focal or multilobular biliary cirrhosis can be attributed to intrahepatic bile plugging causing ductular obstruction, with common and intrahepatic bile duct strictures.

Initially the liver function tests may be normal but later there is mild to moderate elevation of liver enzymes and as the disease advances, conjugated bilirubin levels are also elevated.

Imaging Features

Sonography and CT can demonstrate intrahepatic ductal dilatation which is often focal or multifocal with intraductal echogenic foci with or without shadowing due to inspissated bile and stones **(Fig. 27)**.

Hepatobiliary scintigraphy shows intraparenchymal and intrahepatic ductal retention of activity with delayed clearance of isotope and a nonvisualized or poorly visualized gallbladder.

Cholangiography reveals features similar to PSC including variable dilatation, narrowing and beading of the intrahepatic ducts with occasional strictures of the common bile duct.[78]

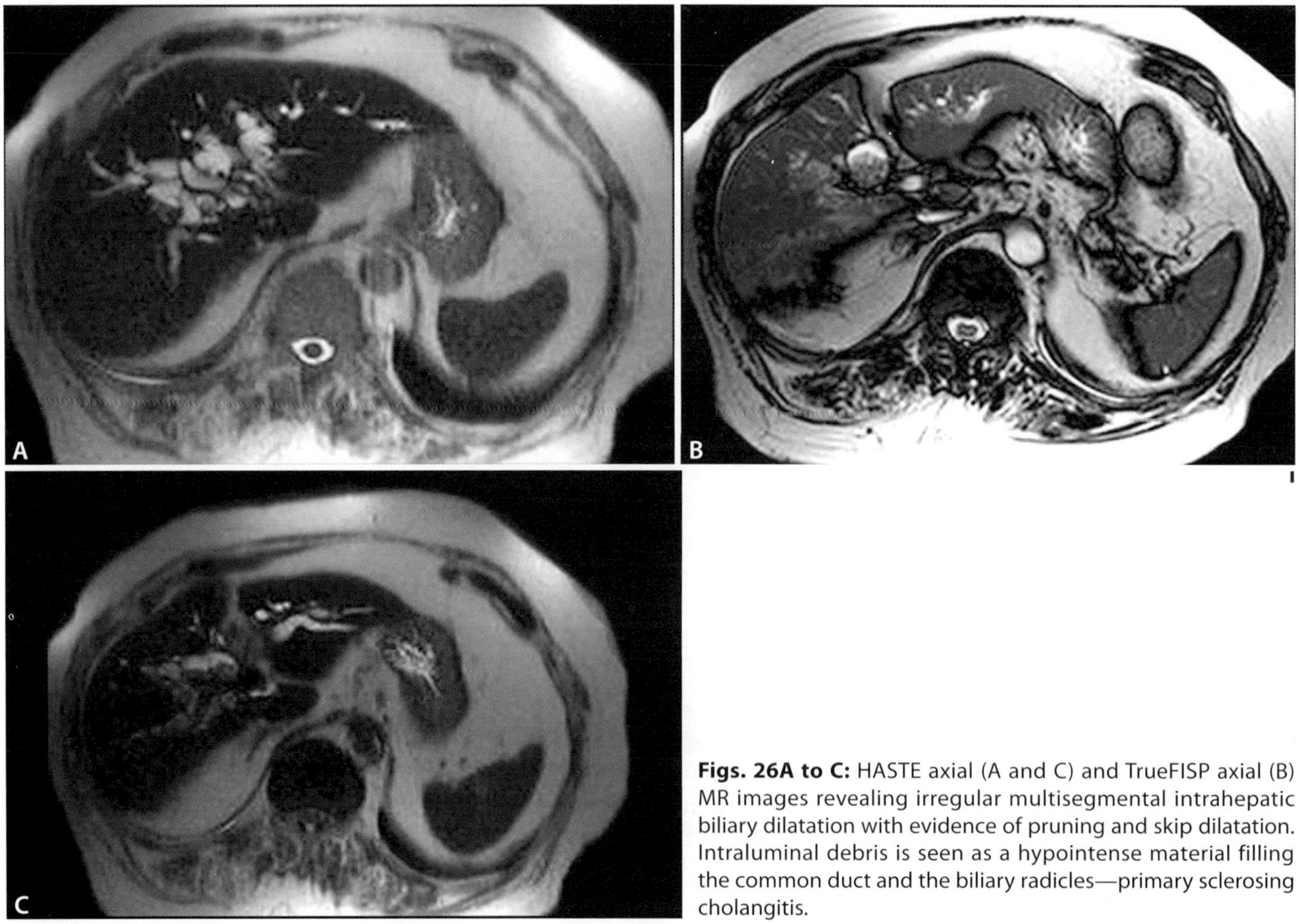

Figs. 26A to C: HASTE axial (A and C) and TrueFISP axial (B) MR images revealing irregular multisegmental intrahepatic biliary dilatation with evidence of pruning and skip dilatation. Intraluminal debris is seen as a hypointense material filling the common duct and the biliary radicles—primary sclerosing cholangitis.

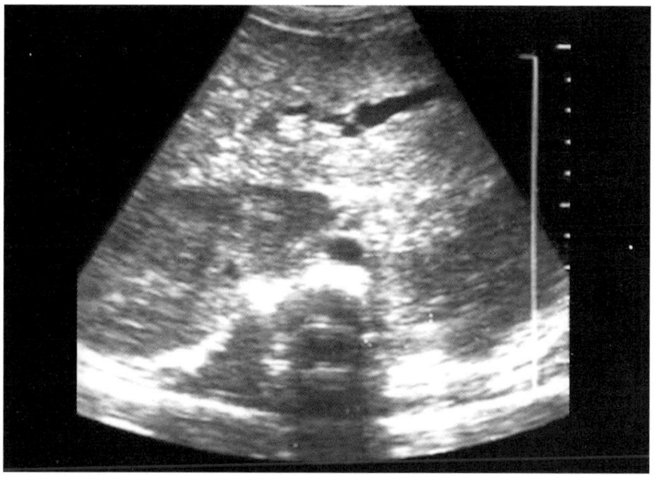

Fig. 27: US of a child with cystic fibrosis reveals irregular left hepatic duct dilatation with nonshadowing intraluminal echogenic foci.

DESTRUCTIVE CHOLANGITIS ASSOCIATED WITH LANGERHANS' CELL HISTIOCYTOSIS

Some infants develop an acute hepatitis like picture while others develop severe progressive cholestasis with duct lesions.[79]

Pathology

There is marked destruction of intrahepatic bile ducts and their walls show intense necrosis, inflammation and fibrosis. Periductal bile lakes are seen due to extrusion of bile into the surrounding parenchyma.

Imaging Features

Cholangiography shows "puff of smoke" appearance in the parenchyma around major bile ducts due to the leakage of bile and contrast.

BILE DUCT PAUCITY

Bile duct paucity is present when histologic examination demonstrates that the ratio of intralobular ducts to portal tracts is less than 0.9.[80] Disorders with bile duct paucity have been divided into two major groups: nonsyndromic and syndromic bile duct paucity (SBDP), or Alagille's syndrome.

Nonsyndromic bile duct paucity refers to many conditions associated with bile duct paucity including idiopathic, metabolic (a-IAT deficiency, hypopituitarism, cystic fibrosis), infectious (rubella, congenital syphilis, CMV, hepatitis B), immunologic, chromosomal (Down's syndrome) and miscellaneous disorders (Zeilweger's syndrome, Ivemark's syndrome).[81]

Alagille's syndrome (SBDP, Watson-Alagille syndrome, arteriohepatic dysplasia) is recognized as an important and relatively common cause of neonatal jaundice and cholestasis in older children with an estimated incidence of 1 in 100,000 births. The syndrome, which is inherited in an autosomal dominant pattern, is characterized by a typical facies, hepatic abnormalities, cardiovascular abnormalities, musculoskeletal, vertebral, ocular and genitourinary abnormalities, marked mental retardation, and growth failure.[6] The abnormal facies include a large forehead, small pointed chin, hypertelorism and a poorly developed nasal bridge. Ocular abnormalities are most typically posterior embryotoxon and pigmentary retinopathy. The cardiovascular abnormalities include pulmonary artery hypoplasia or stenosis.

Imaging Features

On US, the liver shows increased echogenicity and may demonstrate evidence of regenerating cirrhotic nodules. In addition, US helps to exclude any surgically correctable cause of jaundice. There is progressive decrease in ducts after three months of age and extrahepatic ducts are narrowed or hypoplastic. Presence of a patent biliary tract on HIDA distinguishes bile duct paucity from biliary atresia.

SPONTANEOUS PERFORATION OF CBD

Perforation usually occurs at the junction of the cystic and common hepatic duct and rarely it occurs in the common hepatic or common bile duct or the gallbladder. The etiology is uncertain but several causes have been postulated including developmental weakness of the bile duct wall, wall weakness resulting from the reflux of pancreatic secretions, calculi or inspissated bile.

It is seen in infants within the first three months of life who present with jaundice and ascites. The liver function tests are essentially normal.

Diagnosis is established based on clinical, sonographic and scintigraphic findings.

Imaging Features

Sonography reveals normal ducts with fluid in the peritoneal cavity. The fluid may be septated and is located in subhepatic region.

Hepatobiliary scintigraphy depicts the leak.

INSPISSATED BILE SYNDROME

The inspissated syndrome (IBS) is an uncommon cause of jaundice in neonates. Sludge may be seen within the gallbladder as low-level echoes without distal shadowing. It may also be seen within the biliary ducts associated with partial or complete ductal obstruction. IBS may be associated with massive hemolysis (Rh incompatibility), hemorrhage (intra-abdominal, intracranial or retroperitoneal), and increased enterohepatic circulation in various intestinal diseases (Hirschsprung disease, intestinal atresias and stenoses).[82]

JAUNDICE IN OLDER CHILDREN

The causes of jaundice in older children can be divided into primary diseases of the hepatocytes and obstructive causes.

Hepatocellular Causes

Hepatocellular disease can be subdivided into hepatitis (both acute and chronic) and metabolic.

HEPATITIS

Acute hepatitis may be caused by infection, toxic agents or drugs.

Imaging Features

On US, the liver size may be normal or enlarged with diffuse decrease in parenchymal echogenicity and brightly echogenic portal venous walls due to edema in the hepatocytes. The gallbladder wall may be diffusely thickened with intraluminal sludge[83] **(Figs. 28A and B)**.

CHRONIC ACTIVE HEPATITIS

Imaging Features

Sonograms generally show increased hepatic parenchymal echogenicity with a coarsened echotexture and decreased visualization of the peripheral portal venous vasculature **(Fig. 29)**.

On T2W MR images of patients with acute or chronic active hepatitis, a periportal cuff of high signal intensity can often be seen, corresponding to inflammation. However, this finding is nonspecific. In some patients with focal inflammatory changes or fibrosis, diffuse or regional high signal intensity can be identified on T2W images. Enlarged periportal lymph nodes are common in patients with hepatitis.[84]

METABOLIC

Metabolic causes of jaundice include Wilson's disease, cystic fibrosis, glycogen storage disease, tyrosinuria and α1-AT deficiency. The sonographic findings are nonspecific with the liver often appearing hyperechoic with decreased visualization of the peripheral portal venous vasculature. Liver biopsy may be necessary to confirm the diagnosis.

CIRRHOSIS

Cirrhosis is rare in neonates but may occur in older children as a cause of jaundice. Various etiological factors that cause childhood cirrhosis include chronic hepatitis, congenital hepatic fibrosis, biliary atresia, cystic fibrosis, metabolic disease, Budd-Chiari syndrome and total parenteral nutrition.

Duplex and color Doppler evaluation of biliary vessels is important in pediatric patients with chronic liver disease to establish whether the flow is hepatopedal or hepatofugal; presence of varices and collateral venous channels, evidence of spontaneous portosystemic shunts,

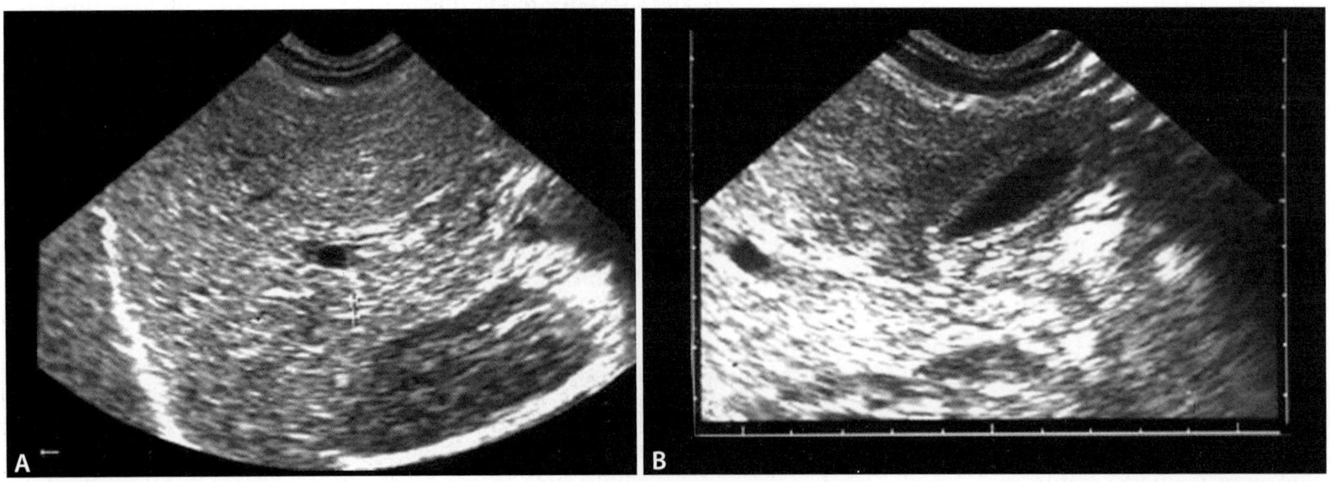

Figs. 28A and B: Grayscale sonograms of a child with acute hepatitis reveal hepatomegaly with bright portal radicles (A) and a diffusely thickened gallbladder wall (B).

if "portalization" of the hepatic veins is evident and if satisfactory flow is seen in the hepatic artery and IVC **(Figs. 30A and B)**.[85]

Portal Hypertensive Biliopathy

It is a rare cause of childhood cholestasis. Portal hypertensive biliopathy (PHB) is defined as abnormal biliary changes that take place most likely secondary to extrahepatic portal vein obstruction (EHPVO) with portal hypertension.[86] This condition may be asymptomatic or could lead to a cholestatic state which is rare in children. The term "portal biliopathy" actually describes an intra-or extrahepatic biliary stricture in patients with portal cavernoma.[87] Portal cavernomas are usually associated with portal hypertension, which frequently causes bleeding from esophageal or gastric varices. Cavernomatous transformation of the portal vein may also lead to biliary obstruction **(Figs. 31A and B)**. In fact, portal cavernous transformation gives rise to many dilated pericholedochal and periportal collaterals that bypass the portal vein obstruction. Extrinsic compression of the common duct by dilated venous collaterals together with pericholedochal fibrosis from the inflammatory process causing portal thrombosis may lead to biliary stricture and dilatation of the proximal biliary tree.[88] This condition sometimes causes the formation of secondary biliary stones and cholangitis. There are two types of clinical features in portal biliopathy: (1) those related to chronic cholestasis, probably explained by strictures caused by either compression of the biliary lumen by enlarged collaterals or by ischemia and (2) those related to biliary stones, which are probably responsible for biliary pain and cholangitis.

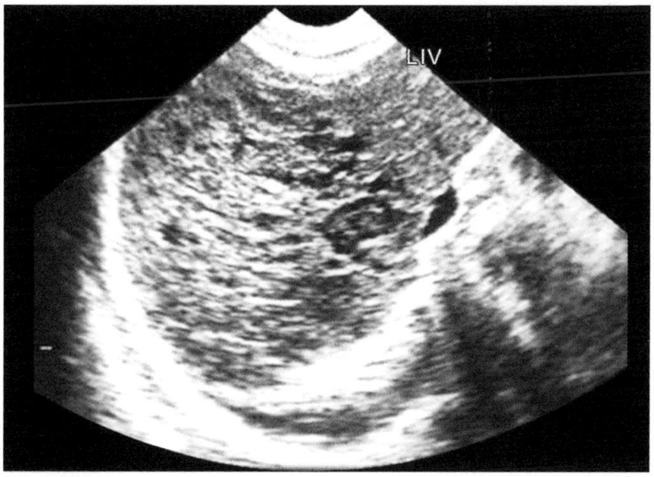

Fig. 29: US in a case of chronic active hepatitis shows coarsened liver echotexture with multiple ill-defined hypoechoic nodules.

The diagnosis of PB is mostly made by ERCP. The typical changes are irregularities in the CBD and hepatic ducts (smooth tapering strictures) and localized saccular dilatations. Filling defects suggestive of CBD stones may be seen. Abdominal ultrasound provides additional information regarding the presence of gallbladder varices (tortuous vessels in and around the gallbladder) and is helpful to provide the complete spectrum of PB.

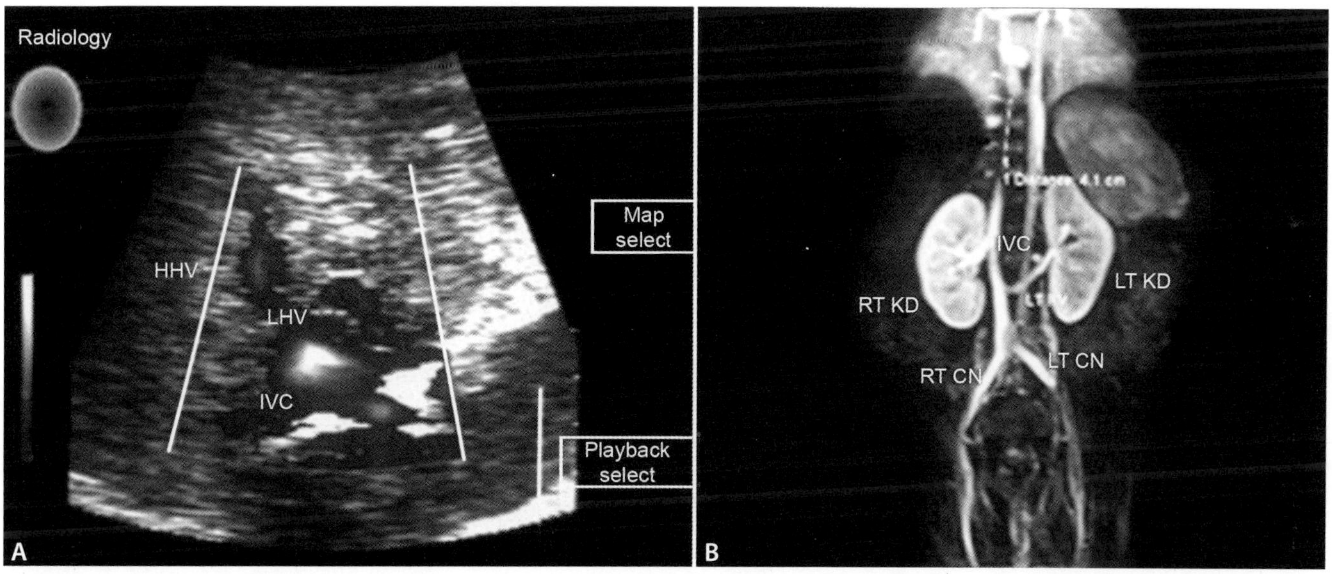

Figs. 30A and B: (A) Doppler image of a child with Budd-Chiari syndrome showing attenuated hepatic veins and intrahepatic IVC. MIP MR venogram (B) of the same patient well depicts the long segment of IVC attenuation.

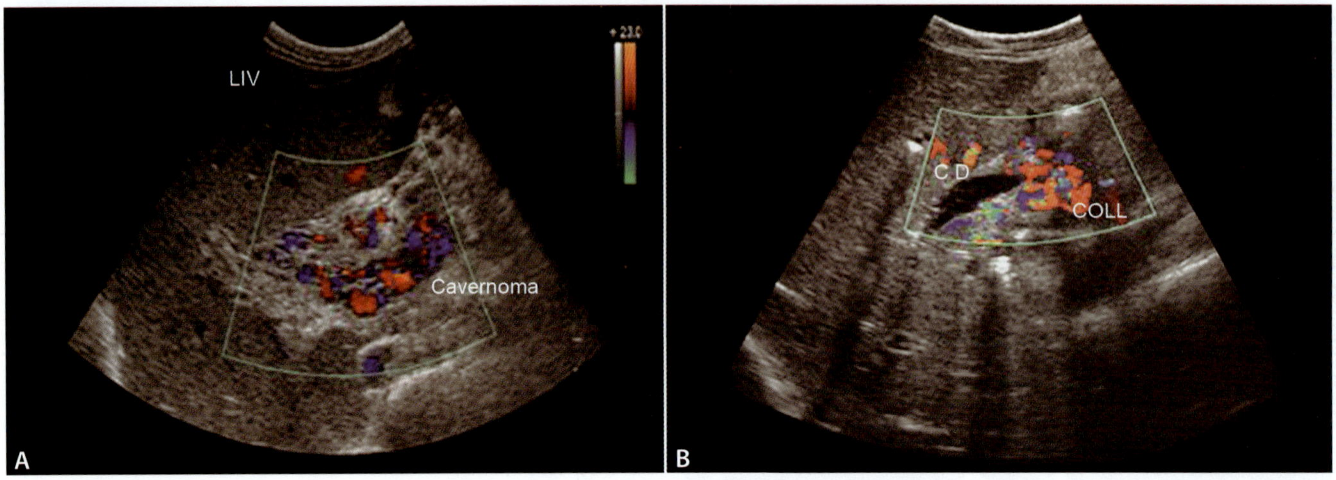

Figs. 31A and B: Doppler images revealing multiple anechoic tubular structures replacing the portal vein with color fill in s/o portal cavernoma formation.There is extrinsic compression with resultant dilatation of the common bile duct—Portal hypertensive biliopathy.

Chandra et al. have graded the severity of biliopathy changes as follows:[89]

- *Type I:* Involvement of extrahepatic bile duct
- *Type II:* Involvement of intrahepatic bile duct
- *Type IIIa:* Involvement of extrahepatic bile duct and unilateral intrahepatic bile duct (left or right)
- *Type IIIb*: Involvement of extrahepatic bile duct and bilateral intrahepatic bile duct.

Treatment is focussed on the management of portal hypertension and relief of obstructive jaundice due to the portal cavernoma is managed endoscopically. Stenting with or without balloon dilatation of CBD is recommended and the stent needs to be replaced regularly. Portosystemic shunt surgery can be done in cases which cannot be managed endoscopically.

BILIARY TRACT NEOPLASMS

Embryonal Rhabdomyosarcoma (Sarcoma Botryoides)

Sarcoma botryoides is a variant of embryonal rhabdomyosarcoma that arises in proximity to the mucosal surface of a hollow viscus or body cavity. After choledochal cyst, sarcoma botryoides is the most common cause of obstructive jaundice in children post infancy.[90,91] Average age at onset is four years with a 2:1 female preponderance. Children present with malaise, fever, jaundice and death is usually from local invasion of contiguous structures.

Pathology

Biliary sarcoma botryoides usually grows from or along the wall of the common bile duct beneath the lining mucosa, with polypoid projections into the lumen. The projecting polyps often undergo hemorrhage and necrosis and are covered by biliary epithelium overlying a dense zone of neoplastic cells (cambium layer) resembling rhabdomyoblasts.[90]

Imaging Features

Sonography and CT show intrahepatic duct dilatation and a soft tissue mass in the region of the common bile duct or porta hepatis. MRCP and direct cholangiography reveal grapelike intraluminal filling defects, usually in extrahepatic ducts, that obstruct the duct only after the tumor has reached a considerable size. Ducts proximal to the obstruction are usually not as dilated as ducts containing the tumor.[91]

DISEASES OF THE GALLBLADDER

Cholelithiasis

Cholelithiasis is uncommon in otherwise healthy children but certain conditions are associated with increased risk of cholelithiasis.

Pathogenesis of Gallstones in Infancy and Childhood

Pigmented gallstones predominate in infants and children. Cholecystitis occurs in premature infants on prolonged parenteral nutrition, following bouts of sepsis, repeated blood transfusions and use of diuretics. An enlarged distended gallbladder filled with sludge may develop before the evolution of cholelithiasis.

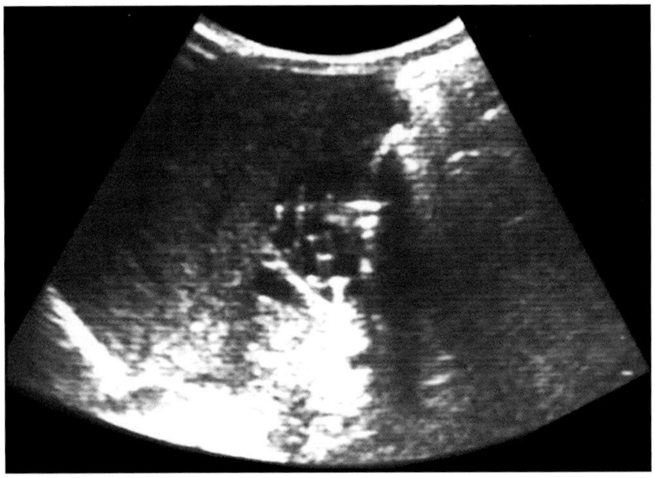

Fig. 32: US showing multiple echogenic foci within the gallbladder lumen causing distal shadowing—gallstones in a neonate.

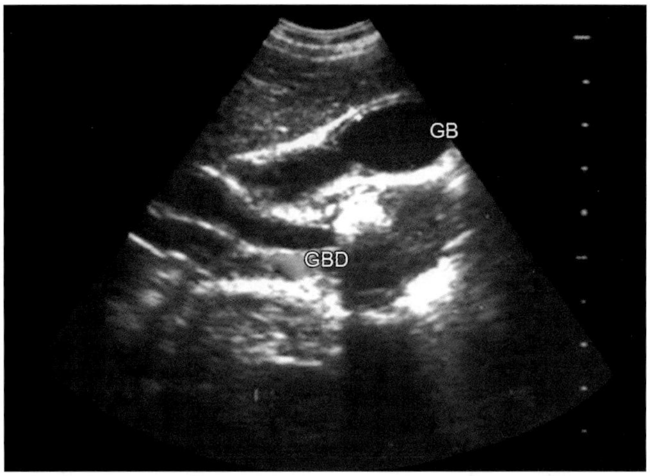

Fig. 33: Grayscale sonogram of a 9-year-old child showing choledocholithiasis with proximal CBD dilatation.

Chronic hemolytic disorders are also associated with gallstones. The 30–60% of patients with sickle cell disease develop pigment stones. Older children and adolescents without an identifiable cause of cholelithiasis are more likely to be obese females.

Other predisposing causes include pancreatic abnormalities and intestinal problems that interfere with the normal enterohepatic circulation such as inflammatory bowel disease, cystic fibrosis and the short gut syndrome. Cystic fibrosis can also produce cholelithiasis.

Imaging Features

Ultrasonography is the most sensitive, specific and the only imaging technique required for demonstrating gallstones and any associated dilatation of the intrahepatic or extrahepatic bile ducts[92,93] **(Figs. 32 and 33)**.

Acute Acalculus Cholecystitis and Acute Hydrops of the Gallbladder

Acute acalculus cholecystitis is an acute inflammation of the gallbladder without gallstones which is associated with infection or systemic illness. Infections due to streptococcal group, gram-negative organisms including *Salmonella, Shigella, E.coli* and parasitic infestation with ascariasis or giardia lamblia may be the cause of acute acalculus cholecystitis. Systemic vasculitis from periarteritis nodosa and Kawasaki disease are more often associated with acute hydrops of the gallbladder. Sometimes congenital narrowing or inflammation of the cystic duct or compression by lymph nodes may be the cause of acalculus cholecystitis. The diagnosis is based on the clinical findings of right upper quadrant or epigastric pain, nausea, vomiting, fever and jaundice. An enlarged gallbladder may be palpable. Laboratory investigations reveal elevated alkaline phosphatase and bilirubin with leukocytosis.

Sonography reveals a distended gallbladder without calculi. The gallbladder appears biconvex on longitudinal scan instead of its normal ovoid shape. The gallbladder wall is edematous and measures more than 3 mm. US findings in cholecystitis include thickened gallbladder wall, distention of the gallbladder, pericholecystic fluid, biliary sludge gallbladder wall edema, irregularity of the gallbladder wall (may suggest gangrene) and echogenic nonshadowing foci in gallbladder wall (may suggest emphysematous change).[94]

Serial imaging of the gallbladder is useful in following the course of the illness.[95]

To conclude hepatobiliary cholestasis in childhood is both a diagnostic and therapeutic challenge. New diagnostic tools, experience in endoscopy, better imaging and understanding of the molecular mechanisms underlying childhood cholestasis have contributed to an early diagnosis with improved management and better outcome for these children. A multimodality imaging approach is required for the diagnosis of obstructive biliopathies.[96]

REFERENCES

1. Elias E, Boyer JL. Mechanism of intrahepatic cholestasis. In Popper H, Schaffer F (Eds): Progress in Liver Diseases. New York: Crune and Stratton. 1979;4:457-70.
2. Maisels MG. Neonatal jaundice. In Avery GB (Ed): Neonatology, Pathophysiology and Management of the Newborn. Philadelphia: JB Lippincott. 1987.

3. Kliegman RM, Behrman RE. Jaundice and hyperbilirubinaemia in the newborn. In Behrman RE, Vaughan VC III (Eds): Nelson Textbook of Pediatrics, 13th edn. Philadelphia: WB Saunders. 1987.
4. Ferry GD, Selbi ML, Udall J, et al. Guide to early diagnosis of biliary obstruction in infancy. Clin Pediatrics. 1985;24:305-11.
5. Markle BM, Potter BM, Majd M. The jaundiced infant and child. Semin Ultrasound. 1980;1:123-33.
6. Alagille D, Estrada A, Hadchovel M. Syndromatic paucity of interlobular bile ducts (Allagille syndrome or arteriohepatic dysplasia); Review of 80 cases. J Pediatrics. 1987;110:195-200.
7. Balistreri WF. Neonatal cholestasis. J Pediatrics. 1985;106:171-84.
8. Fitzgerald JF. Cholestatic disorders of infancy. Pediatric Clinics of North America. 1988;35:357-73.
9. Delaney L, Applegate KE, Karmazyn B, Akisik MF, Jennigs SR. MR Chlangiopancreatography in children: Feasibility, safety an initial experience. Paediatr Radiol. 2008;38:64-75.
10. Tipnis NA, Dua KS, Werlin SA. A retrospective assessment of magnetic resonance chlangiopancreatography in children. J Paediat Gastroentrol. 2008;46:59-64.
11. Chavhan GB, Babyn PS, Manson D, Vidarsson L. Paediatric MR Cholangiopancreatography: Principles, Technique and Clinical Applications. Radiographics. 2008;28:1951-62.
12. Moyer MS, Balisteri WF. Prolonged neonatal obstructive jaundice. In Walker WA, Durie PR, Hamilton JR, et al (Eds): Pediaric Gastrointestinal Disease. Philadelphia: BC Decker. 1991.
13. Carroll BA, Oppenheimer DA, Muller HH. High frequency real time ultrasound of the neonatal biliary system. Radiology. 1982;145:437-40.
14. McGahan JP, Phillips HE, Cox KL. Sonography of the normal pediatric gallbladder and the biliary tract. Radiology. 1982;144:873-5.
15. Ikeda S, Sera Y, Akagi M. Serial ultrasonic examination to differentiate biliary atresia from neonatal hepatitis—special reference to changes in size of the gallbladder. Eur J Pediatr. 1989;148:396.
16. Nadel HR. Hepatobiliary scintigraphy in children. Seminar Nucl Med. 1996;26:25-42.
17. Majd M. Nuclear Medicine. In Franken EA Jr, Smith WL (Eds): Gastrointestinal Imaging in Pediatrics. (2nd edn). New York: Harper and Row. 1982.pp.530-79.
18. Lilly JR. Biliary atresia: The jaundiced infant. In Welch KJ, Randolph JG, Ravitch MM (Eds): Pediatric Surgery Chicago: Year Book,l. 1985.
19. Abramson SJ, Berdon WE, Altman RP, et al. Biliary atresia and non-cardiac polysplenia syndrome: US and surgical considerations. Radiology. 1987;163:377-9.
20. Sokol RJ, Mack C. Etiopathogenesis of biliary atresia. Semin Liv Dis. 2001;21:517-24.
21. Miyano T, Fujimoto T, Ohya T. Current concept of treatment of biliary atresia. World Journal Surgery. 1993;17:332-36.
22. Kasai M. Treatment of biliary atresia with special reference to hepatic portoenterostomy and its modifications. Prog Pediatric Surgery. 1974;6:5.
23. Balisterie WF, Grand R, Hoofnagal JH, et al. Biliary atresia: Current concepts and research directions. Hepatology. 1996;23:1682-92.
24. Kirks DR, Coleman RE, Filson HC, et al. An imaging approach to persistent neonatal jaundice. AJR. 1984;142:461-5.
25. Tan Kendrick AP, Phua OB, Ooi Bc, Tan CE. Biliary atresia making the diagnosis by gallbladder ghost triad. Pediatr Radiol. 2003;33:311-5.
26. Kanegawa K, Akasaka Y, et al. Sonographic diagnosis of biliary atresia in pediatric patients using the "Triangular Cord" Sign Versus gallbladder Length and Contraction. AJR. 2003;181:1387-90.
27. Davenport M, Savage M, Mowat AP, Howard ER. The biliary atresia splenic malformation syndrome. Surgery. 1993;113:662-8.
28. Park WH, Choi SO, Lee HJ, et al. A new diagnostic approach to biliary atresia with emphasis on the ultrasonographic triangular cord sign: Comparison of ultrasonography, hepatobiliary scintigraphy and liver needle biopsy on the evaluation of infantile cholestasis. J Pediatric Surgery. 1997;32: 1555-9.
29. Kotb MA, Kotb A, Sheba MF, et al. Evaluation of the triangular cord sign in the diagnosis of biliary atresia. Pediatrics. 2001;108:416-20.
30. Brun P, Gauthier F, Bouchar D, et al. Ultrasound findings in biliary atresia in children. Ann Radiol. 1985;28:259.
31. Lee HJ, Lee SM, Park WH, Choi SO. Objective criteria of Triangular cord sign in biliary atresia on US scans. Radiology. 2003;229:395-400.
32. dos Santos JL, da Silveira TR, da Silva VD, Cerski CT, Wagner MB. Medial thickening of hepatic artery branches in biliary atresia: A morphometric study. J Pediatr Surg. 2005;40:637-42.
33. Kim WS, Cheon JE, Youn BJ, et al. Hepatic arterial diameter measured with US: Adjunct for US diagnosis of biliary atresia. Radiology. 2007;245:549-55.
34. Uflacker R, Pariente DM. Angiographic findings in biliary atresia. Cardiovasc Intervent Radiol. 2004;27:486-90.
35. Jaw TS, Kuo YT, Liu GC, et al. MR cholangiography in the evaluation of neonatal cholestasis. Radiology. 1999;212:249-56.
36. Arcement CM, Meza MP, Arunmanla S, et al. MRCP in the evaluation of pancreatobiliary disease in children. Pediatr Radiol. 2001;31:92-7.
37. Giubaud L, Lachaud A, Touraine R, et al. MR cholangiography in neonates and infants: Feasibility and preliminary applications. AJR. 1998;170:27-31.
38. Mitchell DG, Alam F. Mangafodipir trisodium: Effects on T1 and T2 weighted MR cholangiography. J Magn Reson Imaging. 1999;9:366-8.
39. Ryeom HK, Choe BH, et al. Biliary atresia: Feasibility of Mangafodipir Trisodium Enhanced MR cholangiography for Evaluation. Radiology. 2005;235:250-8.
40. Kasai M, Kimura S, Asakura Y, et al. Surgical treatment of biliary atresia. J Pediatr Surg. 1968;3:665.
41. Takahashi A. Tsuchida Y, Suzuki N, et al. Incidence of intrahepatic biliary cysts in biliary atresia after hepatic

portoenterostomy and histopathologic findings in the liver and porta hepatis at diagnosis. J Pediatr Surg. 1999;34:1364.
42. Sela-Herman S, Scharschmidt BF. Choledochal cyst: a disease for all ages. Lancet. 1996;347:779.
43. Babbitt DP. Congenital choledochal cyst: New etiologic concept based on anomalous relationships of common bile duct and pancreatic bulb. Ann Radiol. 1969;12:231-40.
44. Alonso-Lej F, Rever Jr WB, Pessagno DJ. Congenital choledochal cysts, with a report of 2, and an analysis of 94 cases. Surg Gynecol Obstet. 1959;108:1-30.
45. Todani T, Watanabe Y, Narusue M, et al. Congenital bile duct cysts. Am J Surg. 1977;134:263-9.
46. Todani T, Tabuchi K, Watanabi Y, et al. Carcinoma arising in the walls of congenital bile duct cysts. Cancer. 1979;44:1134-41.
47. DiMagno EP, Shorter RG, Taylor WG, Go LW. Relationship between pancreaticobiliary ductal anatomy and parenchymal histology. Cancer. 1982;49:361-8.
48. Misra SP, Gulati P, Thorat VK, et al. Pancreaticobiliary ductal union in biliary diseases. An endoscopic retrograde cholangiopancreatico-graphic study. Gastroenterology. 1989;96:907-12.
49. Wiedmeyer DA, Stewart ET, Dodds WJ, et al. Choledochal cyst: findings on cholangiopancreatography with emphasis on ectasia of the common channel. AJR. 1989;153:969-72.
50. Kimura K, Ohto M, Saisho H, et al. Association of gallbladder carcinoma and anomalous pancreaticobiliary duct union. Gastroenterology. 1985;89:1258-65.
51. Komi N. New classification of anomalous arrangement of the pancreaticobiliary ductal (APBD) in choledochal cyst: A proposal of new Komi classification of APBD. J Jpn Pancr Soci. 1991;6:234-43.
52. Guelrud M, Morera C, Rodrigues H, et al. Sphincter of Oddi dysfunction in children with recurrent pancreatitis and anomalous pancreaticobiliary union: An etiologic concept. Gastrointest Endoscopy. 1999;50:194-9.
53. Voyles CR, Smajda C, Shands WC, et al. Carcinoma in choledochal cysts. Arch Surg. 1983;118;969.
54. Nagi B, Kochhar R, Bhasin D, Singh K. Endoscopic retrograde cholangiopancreatography in the evaluation of anomalous junction of the pancreaticobiliary duct and related disorders. Abdom Imaging. 2003;28:847-52.
55. Kaneko K, Ando M, Ito T, et al. Protein plug causes symptoms in patients with choledochal cysts. Am J Gastroenterol. 1997;92:1018-21.
56. Yamtaka A, Segawa O, Kobayashi H, et al. Intraoperative pancreatoscopy for pancreatic stone debris distal to the common channel in choledochal cysts. J Pediatr Surg. 2000;35:1-4.
57. Torrisi JM, Haller JO, Velcek FT. Choledochal cyst and biliary atresia in the neonate: Imaging findings in five cases. AJR. 1990;155:1273-6.
58. Chan Y, Yeung C, Fork T, et al. Magnetic resonance cholangiography: Feasibility and application in the pediatric population. Pediatr Radiol. 1998;28:307-11.
59. Dinsmore JE, Murphy JJ, Jamieson D. MRCP evaluation of choledochal cysts. J Pediatric Surgery. 2001;36:829-30.
60. Lamb WWN, Lamb TPW, Saing H, et al. MR cholangiography and CT cholangiography of pediatric patients with choledochal cysts. AJR. 1999;173:401-5.
61. Caroli J, Soupault R, Kossakowsky J, et al. La Dilatation Polycystique congenitale des voies biliairis intrahepatiques. Semin Hop Paris. 1958;14:128-35.
62. Lonergan GJ, Rice RR, Suarez ES. Autosomal recessive polycystic kidney disease: Radiologic-pathologic correlation. Radiographics. 2000;20:837-55.
63. Levy AD, Rohrmann CA, Murakata LA, et al. Caroli's disease: Radiologic spectrum with pathologic correlation. AJR. 2002;179:1053-7.
64. Bloustein PA. Association of carcinoma with congenital cystic conditions of the liver and bile ducts. Am J Gastroenterol. 1977;67:40-6.
65. Miller WJ, Sechtin AG, Campbell WL. Imaging findings in Caroli's disease. AJR. 1995;165:333-7.
66. Choi BI, Yeon KM, Kim SH, et al. Caroli disease: Central dot sign in CT. Radiology. 1990;174:161-3.
67. Pavone P, Laghi A, Basso N, et al. Caroli's disease: Evaluation with MRCP. Abdom Imaging. 1996;21:117-9.
68. Toma P, Lucigraj G, Pelizza A. Sonographic patterns of Caroli's disease report of 5 new cases. J Clin Ultrasound. 1999;19:155.
69. Sood GK, Mahaptra JR, Khurana, et al. Caroli disease: Computed tomographic diagnosis. Gastrointest Radiol. 1991;16:243.
70. Sty JR, Hubbard AM, Starshak RJ. Radionuclide hepatobiliary imaging in congenital tract ectasia (Caroli disease) Pediatr Radiol. 1982;12:111.
71. Guy F, Cognet F, Dranssart M, et al. Caroli's disease: magnetic resonance imaging features. Am Radiol. 2002;12:2730-6.
72. Alvarez A, Bernard O, Brunelle F, et al. Congenital hepatic fibrosis in children. J Paediatr. 1981;99:370.
73. Premkumar A, Berdon WE, Levy J, et al. The emergence of hepatic fibrosis and portal hypertension in infants and children with autosomal recessive polycystic kidney disease: Initial and follow up sonographic findings. Pediatr Radiol. 1988;18:123.
74. Summerfield JA, Nagaguchi Y, Sherlock S, et al. Hepatobiliary fibropolycystic diseases clinical and histological review of 51 patients. J Hepatol. 1986;2:141.
75. Brancatelli G, Federle MP, et al. Fibropolycystic liver disease: CT and MR Imaging findings. Radiographics. 2005;25:659-70.
76. Debray D, Pariente D, Uryoas E. Sclerosing cholangitis in children. J Pediatrics. 1994;124:49.
77. Sisto A, Feldman P, Garel L. Primary sclerosing cholangitis in children: Study of five cases and review of the literature. Pediatrics. 1987;80:918-23.
78. Oppenheimer EH, Esterly JR. Hepatic changes in young infants with cystic fibrosis. Possible relation to focal biliary cirrhosis. J Pediatrics. 1975;86:683.
79. Leblanc A, Hadchouel M, Jehan P. Obstructive jaundice in children with Histiocytosis X. Gastroenterology. 1981;80:143.
80. Piccoli DA, Witzleben CL. Disorders of intrahepatic bile ducts. In Walker WA, Hamilton JR, Walker-Smith JA, et al

(Eds): Pediatric Gastrointestinal Disease, Philadelphia: BC Decker. 1991.
81. Altman RP. Personal communication, 1992.
82. Pfeiffer WR, Robbinson LH, Balsara VJ. Sonographic features of bile plug syndrome. J Ultrasound Med. 1986;5:161-3.
83. Kurtz AB, Rubin CS, Cooper HS, et al. Ultrasound findings in hepatitis. Radiology. 1980;136:717-23.
84. Donnelly LF, Bisset GS III. Pediatric hepatic imaging. Radiol Clin North Am. 1998;36:413-27.
85. Subramanyam BR, Balthazar EY, Horri SC, et al. Sonography of portosystemic venous collaterals in portal hypertension. Radiology. 1983;146:161-6.
86. Matary WZ, Roberts EA, Kim P, et al. Portal hypertensive biliopathy: A rare cause of childhood cholestasis. Eur J Pediatr. 2008;167:1339-42.
87. Perego P, Cozzi G, Bertolini A. Portal bioliopathy. Surgical Endoscopy. 2002 (online publication).
88. Malkan GH, Bathia SJ, Bashir K. Cholangiopathy associated with portal hypertension. Gastroint Endos. 1999;49:344-8.
89. Chandra R, Kapoor D, Tharakan A, et al. Portal biliopathy. J Gastro Hepatol. 2001;16:1086-92.
90. Orloff MJ, Charters AC. Tumours of the gallbladder and bile ducts. In Bockus HL (Ed): Gastroenterology. Philadelphia: WB Saunders. 1976.
91. Davis GL, Kissane JM, Ishak KG. Embryonal rhabdomyosarcoma (Sarcoma botryoides) of the biliary tree: A report of five cases and review of the literature. Lancet. 1969;24:333-42.
92. Debray D, Pariente D, Gauthier F. Cholelithiasis in infancy: A study of 40 cases. J Pediatrics. 1993;122:385-91.
93. Greenberg M, Kangarloo H, Cochran ST, et al. The ultrasonographic diagnosis of cholecystitis and cholelithiasis in children. Radiology. 1980;137:745-9.
94. Coughlin JR, Mann DA. Detection of acute cholecystitis in children. J Can Assoc Radiol. 1990;41:213.
95. Gubernick JA, Rosenberg HK, Kessler A, et al. US approach to jaundice in infants and children. Radiographics. 2000;20:173-95.
96. Mortele KJ, Rocha TC, et al. Multimodality imaging of pancreatic and biliary congenital anomalies. Radiographics. 2006;26:715-31.

CHAPTER 139

Congenital Anomalies of the Urinary Tract

Smriti Hari, Arun Kumar Gupta

INTRODUCTION

Anomalies of the urogenital tract are among the most common organ system anomalies found in the neonate. With use of real-time ultrasound (US) as a screening test in healthy infants, Steinhardt et al. found that 3.2% of infants had an abnormality of the genitourinary tract and one-half of these patients required surgical intervention.[1] Prompt and accurate imaging analysis of these anomalies is important so that correctible abnormalities can be treated in a timely manner. Correct diagnosis can also help in genetic workup that may aid in future pregnancy planning.

IMAGING MODALITIES

Diagnostic imaging of pediatric urologic disorders is continuously changing as technological advances are made. Although, the backbone of pediatric urologic imaging has been US, voiding cystourethrography (VCUG), and radionuclide scintigraphy, newer and advanced modalities are increasingly becoming important. The small physical habitus of infants and children and absence of abdominal fat make US an ideal imaging method for providing excellent anatomic images of the urinary system. US has replaced intravenous urography (IVU) as the initial examination, and the results of US usually determine what further examination is required. The role of IVU is to answer specific questions (e.g. to show the calyceal anatomy which may be helpful in establishing the cause of a small kidney), and to differentiate some unusual causes of ureteral obstruction (ureteral valve, ureteral polyp, retrocaval ureter) from the usual pelviureteric junction (PUJ) obstruction.[2] VCUG is essential for the evaluation of the anatomy and abnormalities of the bladder and urethra. Diuretic renography is used to differentiate obstructive from nonobstructive hydronephrosis or hydroureter. It is performed by the intravenous injection of a radiopharmaceutical Tc-diethylene triamine pentaacetic acid (DTPA) or Tc-mercaptoacetyl glycyl3 (MAG3) that is extracted rapidly from the bloodstream and excreted by the kidney. US is the preferred modality when anatomic detail is required, whereas diuretic renography is better for quantitative functional information, such as differential renal function.

Antenatal Sonography

It is estimated that a structural fetal anomaly is detected by antenatal sonography in 1% of all screened pregnancies. Of these anomalies, a fifth are believed to be manifestations of genitourinary origin, second only to those found within the central nervous system.[3] Fetal sonography allows for early detection of renal lesions, especially those characterized by hydronephrosis. Because it has been shown that renal growth and development are affected adversely by prenatal urinary tract obstruction, antenatal hydronephrosis has become a common indication for postnatal renal and bladder sonography. Once postnatal hydronephrosis or hydroureteronephrosis is detected, the radiologic workup should include evaluation for vesicoureteral reflux (VUR) and posterior urethral valve (PUV), evaluation of individual renal function, and determination of whether the lesion is obstructive or nonobstructive. The most common causes of nonobstructive hydronephrosis are VUR and nonobstructive primary megaureter; "prune-belly syndrome" is a much less common cause. Obstructive causes include PUJ obstruction, ureterovesical junction (UVJ) obstruction, ureteral ectopia with or without ureterocele, and PUV (in boys).[4]

Magnetic Resonance Urography

Magnetic resonance urography (MRU) has become a useful adjuvant in evaluating urogenital anomalies when the results of conventional imaging modalities are inconclusive.[5] MRU is a powerful examination that has the distinct advantage of providing both anatomic and functional information in one examination. MRU allows a one-stop-shop evaluation of the renal parenchyma, collecting system, vasculature, bladder, and surrounding structures. MRU has intrinsic high soft tissue contrast resolution and multiplanar 3D reconstruction capabilities, without the use of radiation. Additionally, MRU allows quantification of numerous renal functional parameters including transit times, an index of glomerular filtration rate (GFR), and differential renal functions. A comprehensive MRU protocol is a 2-part imaging technique composed of precontrast sequences (static MRU) and postcontrast sequences (dynamic or excretory MRU).

Static MR Urography (Precontrast Imaging)

Static MRU uses heavily T2-weighted fluid-sensitive sequences in which urine-containing structures are bright. These T2-weighted images serve to delineate the anatomy of the renal collecting systems and ureters. 3D respiratory triggered T2 sequences can be reconstructed to create maximum intensity projections (MIPs) and volume rendered images of the entire collecting system. Additional, high-quality axial T2 sequences are also obtained to provide a high-resolution view of the renal parenchyma. MRU has been shown to be superior to US both in the detection of occult upper pole moieties and in demonstrating ureteral ectopy.[6] In this instance, excretory function of the kidney is not a limiting factor in diagnosing an ectopic ureter because the static-fluid MRU images are sufficient. This is also true for the detection of dysplastic ectopic kidneys that are very difficult to see with other imaging modalities **(Figs. 1A and B)**. MRU can also clarify the anatomy and complications related to complex urinary tract anomalies, such as crossed fused renal ectopia and horseshoe kidney.

Dynamic MR Urography (Postcontrast Imaging)

Dynamic MRU not only provides anatomic information including that of the vascular system, it also offers functional information, which is in many ways analogous to a nuclear medicine study. Intravenous gadolinium is administered and sequential 3D dynamic sequences of the whole urinary tract are acquired. These images can be presented as a MIP and a cine loop. The former provides morphologic information. The dynamic sequences are the basis of the functional calculation, assess renal perfusion, evaluate renal transit and excretion, and allow generation of signal intensity versus time curves. MRU has been shown to be superior to renal scintigraphy in many regards.[7] MRU

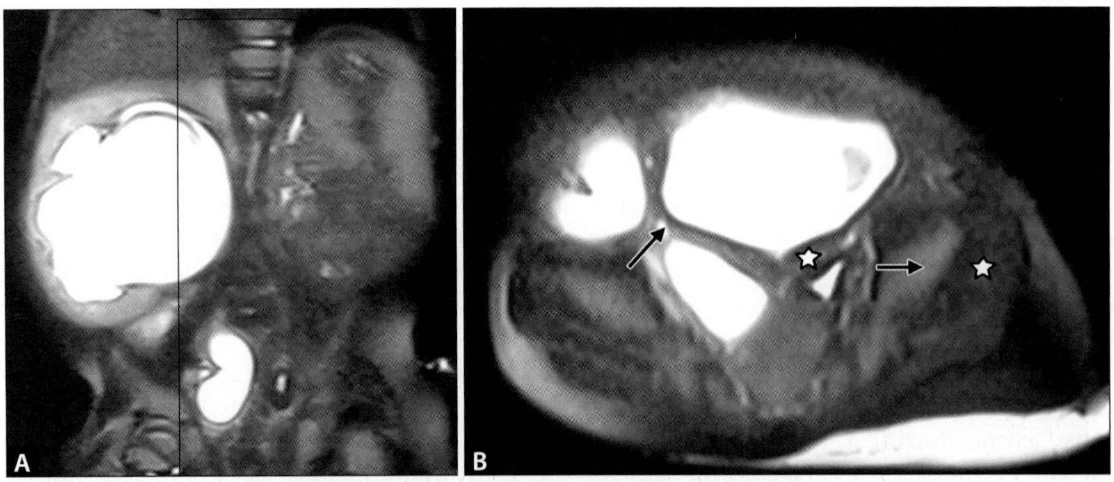

Figs. 1A and B: MR Urogram: (A) Coronal HASTE image shows gross right hydroureteronephrosis and empty left renal fossa in a one-year-old child; (B) Axial HASTE image demonstrates the dysplastic, small left pelvic kidney (stars) and the right lower ureteric stricture (arrows), the cause of proximal gross hydroureteronephrosis.

has superior contrast and temporal and spatial resolution, and MRU has been shown to be superior to renal scintigraphy in many regards.[10] MRU has superior contrast and temporal and spatial resolution, and can provide precise anatomic information, which radionuclide studies cannot. MRU has also been shown to be superior to renal scintigraphy in distinguishing between pyelonephritis and scar.[8]

Limitations

Although MRU is a powerful study with numerous advantages, few limitations do exist. MRU can have relatively long imaging times and is sensitive to motion artifact, which necessitates sedation for young children. An important limitation of the dynamic postcontrast part of the MRU is that it can be contraindicated in patients with moderate renal insufficiency. As stated, excretory MRU involves the administration of intravenous gadolinium and requires excretion into the collecting systems. Although, it was previously thought that gadolinium could be safely administered in patients with renal insufficiency/failure in an effort to avoid iodinated contrast material, relatively recent reports have linked the disorder nephrogenic systemic fibrosis (NSF) to gadolinium administration.[9] New recommendations are to make every effort to avoid administering gadolinium-based contrast material in patients with moderate-to-severe renal insufficiency (GFR <30 mL/min).

Voiding Urosonography

Voiding urosonography (VUS) is a relatively new modality in the detection of VUR in children. Although, VCUG and radionuclide cystography are currently the two methods most commonly used to evaluate for VUR, recent developments of commercially available echoenhancing agents have significantly improved the sonographic detection of fluid movement within the urinary tract. The most commonly used echoenhancing agent is Levovist (Bayer-Schering, Berlin, Germany). This introduces stabilized microbubbles, which allow improved visualization of fluid movement. More recently, a newer-generation US contrast agent, namely SonoVue (Bracco, Milan, Italy), is starting to be used. These US contrast agents have made VUS a reliable alternative to VCUG and radionuclide cystography with the distinct advantage of avoiding ionizing radiation and, at the same time, increasing the detection rate of VUR. Overall, the VUS examination consists of scanning the patient before, during, and after the intravesical administration of US contrast agent, as well as during voiding. The kidneys, ureter, and bladder are then imaged to assess for possible VUR, which is diagnosed by the presence of echogenic microbubbles in either the ureters or the renal pelves. VUS can be used in workup of urinary tract infections, follow-up of known VUR, and in the evaluation of reflux in renal transplant patients.

CT Angiography and CT Urography

State-of-the-art CT technology offers two advanced imaging protocols for pediatric urological applications: CT angiography (CTA) and CT urography (CTU). Among many technical factors, CTA and CTU require precise synchronization between contrast medium delivery and the scan acquisition. For CTA, synchronization is to the arterial or venous phase, whereas for CTU, synchronization is to the delayed excretory renal phase. Although inherently dependent on radiation and iodinated contrast medium, CTA and CTU can be performed safely in pediatric patients using low radiation and contrast medium dose strategies. Current state-of-the-art scanners offer 64- to 320-channel multidetector-row CT (MDCT) technology. Both isotropic (0.50–0.75 mm thick images) and high-resolution (1.25–1.50 mm thick images) datasets can be generated. In most instances, however, a high-resolution acquisition provides sufficient detail for accurate CTA and CTU diagnoses. In selecting this mode, patients are exposed to less radiation, as MDCT collimation will not be submillimeter. Additional, strategies and acquisition parameters to control radiation exposure include restricting coverage to the anatomy of interest and using the lowest possible voltage (kVp) and amperage (mA). Coverage, voltage, and amperage all have direct relationships with the amount of patient radiation exposure. Voltage options include 80, 100, 120, and 140 kVp; 80 kVp is recommended until 50 kg, 100 kVp from 50 to 90 kg, and 120 kVp greater than 90 kg. Amperage is typically prescribed using an automated dose algorithm, which delivers a variable range of amperage over the length of the coverage, based on prescan determined body density and a targeted threshold value for acceptable noise. Using a 64-channel MDCT scanner for abdominal CTA and abdominopelvic CTU in neonates to adolescent patients, average radiation exposures are approximately 1 to 2 mSv with scan times of 1.5 to 4.0 seconds.[10] This radiation dose is equivalent to that of approximately 50 to 100 chest radiographs. As with 3D MRI-MRA and 3D US, CTA, and CTU, datasets are transferred to a workstation for real-time display and review using a combination of multiplanar and curved planar reconstructions, 3D volume rendering, and maximum intensity projections. Pediatric CTA and CTU are considered only after US and MRI have been exhausted or when CT is considered superior for clinical imaging objectives. Emphasizing the advantages of CT, appropriate primary indications for CTA or CTU include the presence of metallic hardware and implantable devices; the requirement for higher spatial resolution; and the need for rapid scan time, such as in emergent imaging or in the high-risk sedation/anesthesia patient. Once there is a decision to proceed forward with CT, the pediatric urology patient should be screened to confirm normal renal function and an absence of contrast allergies. CTA applications for the pediatric urology patient include evaluation of suspected or known renovascular hypertension, crossing renal hilar vessels (in the setting of PUJ obstruction), renal aneurysms, small-vessel vasculitis, renal venous occlusive disease (i.e. tumour invasion), vascular malformations (in the setting of hematuria), and traumatic renovascular injury. Additional, indications include preoperative vascular mapping (i.e. before resection of vascular renal and adrenal tumors) and if involved with hemodialysis access care, assessment of upper or lower extremity dysfunctional grafts and fistulas. Diagnostic quality pediatric renal CT arteriograms are motion free, achieving robust enhancement of extraparenchymal renal arteries through to at least the third to fourth order intraparenchymal segments. CTU applications include the evaluation of suspected or known congenital anomalies, obstructive uropathy, trauma, reflux nephropathy, and papillary necrosis. Acquisitions may be performed as a single dedicated urographic 8 to 10 minutes delay acquisition or as a second series following a routine CT or CTA acquisition. Diagnostic quality CT urograms, achieve dense enhancement of the upper and lower collecting systems and the bladder, while maintaining enhancement in the renal parenchyma. As with MRU or conventional IVU, evaluation addresses the number, caliber, contour, course, and patency of native and anomalous upper and lower collecting systems.

Neonatal Kidney

The normal US appearance of the neonatal kidney **(Fig. 2)** is markedly different from that of an older child or an adult, i.e. the cortex is thinner and more reflective than the liver, the pyramids are large and relatively hypoechoic compared with the cortex, the capsule is not well-defined and the sinus fat is much less noticeable.[11] The age of transition from the neonatal to an adult pattern is very variable and may occur at 2 to 3 months after birth, but can persist for up to 6 months of age.

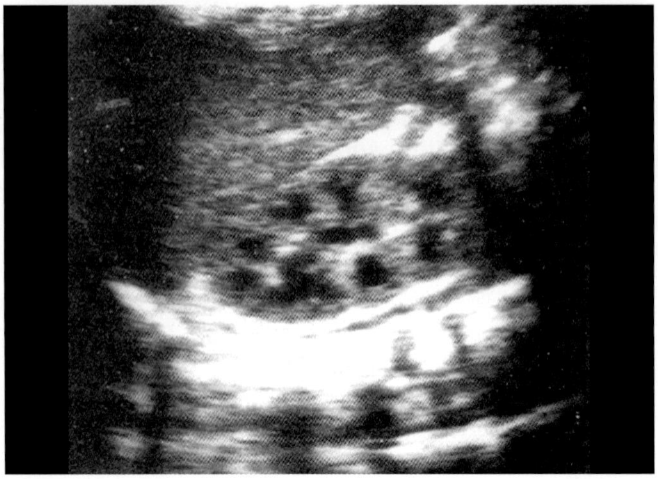

Fig. 2: Normal neonatal kidney: The cortex is relatively thin and echogenic, the medullary pyramids appear large and relatively hypoechoic and minimal sinus structures are seen.

The large pyramids have been mistaken for renal cysts. The important diagnostic features of the neonatal renal medulla are the pyramids with their regular triangular shape, with the base on the cortex and the highly reflective foci of the arcuate vessels on the triangular base. The infant kidney is often lobulated in outline because of residual fetal lobulations, and this should not be mistaken for scarring.

Dynamic radionuclide scans are generally best obtained after 4 weeks of age when some renal maturity has occurred. The neonatal DTPA scan is characterized by poor visualization of the kidneys. Relatively poor function as seen on nuclear scanning does not imply irreversible damage, and no long-term management decisions should be taken on the basis of these results; rather the scan should be repeated either when the infant is older (around 3 months) or following a drainage procedure.[12]

IVU requiring administration of an osmotically active contrast medium may be detrimental to the immature kidney of a neonate; it may also aggravate renal vein thrombosis or medullary necrosis. Even in normal neonates, an IVU may fail to outline the kidneys, especially in the first 48 hours of life. These considerations suggest that there is generally no place for an IVU in the first 2–3 days of life. US is the imaging modality of choice for the kidneys in the first week of life. If an IVU is undertaken, delayed images at 6, 12 and 18 hours may be necessary to visualize the kidneys. IVU should be done with a nonionic contrast medium at a concentration of 30% iodine up to a maximum dose of 3 mL/kg.

Embryologic Development of the Urinary Tract

The following brief review of the embryologic development of the urinary tract is very helpful in understanding these congenital genitourinary malformations. The renal parenchyma is derived from the primitive metanephros, which arises from mesenchymal tissue in the presacral area.[13] This primitive tissue is referred to as the nephrogenic blastema. As the primitive metanephros migrates upwards and matures, it takes the form of normal kidney. A specific rotation also occurs so that whereas the renal pelvis originally points anteriorly, a gradual inward and medial turning takes place. Any arrest along this line results in an abnormal orientation of the kidney and some degree of malrotation.

The ureteric bud develops as an outpouching from the metanephric or Wolffian duct at a site near the cloaca. It soon separates from the Wolffian duct and opens into the portion of the cloaca destined to become the urinary bladder. Then the ureteric bud grows upwards and eventually meets the primitive renal parenchymal tissue. At its upper end it forms the renal pelvis and then divides to form the calyces and the collecting tubules. The cloaca forms the larger portion of the bladder and urethra. The Wolffian duct descends and forms the epididymis, ejaculatory duct and vas deferens in the male. In the female, the Wolffian duct disappears and the Mullerian ducts give rise to the female internal genitalia.

ABNORMALITIES OF KIDNEY

Renal Agenesis

Renal agenesis, the complete congenital absence of renal tissue results from the failure of the ipsilateral ureteric bud to contact the nephrogenic blastema. The ipsilateral ureter and renal artery are absent. There is ipsilateral absence of the trigone and ureteral orifice of the bladder when evaluated by cystoscopy.

Bilateral renal agenesis is the most severe anomaly of the genitourinary system and occurs in 1 to 3 per 10,000 live births. It is noted predominantly in males and is incompatible with life. On prenatal US, severe oligohydramnios, absence of fetal bladder and both kidneys are highly suggestive of bilateral renal agenesis. Early neonatal death is usually because of pulmonary hypoplasia resulting from a lack of transmitted pulsations from amniotic fluid necessary for tracheobronchial tree development. Affected fetuses develop a Potter facies (flattened nose, recession of chin, epicanthic folds, low set ears and hypertelorism) as well as brachycephaly and clubfoot as a result of markedly restricted space for growth.

Unilateral agenesis occurs in about 1 in 1000 of the general population, predominantly in males and on the left side. Sonographically, fetuses with unilateral renal agenesis have a normal amount of amniotic fluid and a readily visualized urinary bladder. The contralateral kidney may be large secondary to compensatory hypertrophy. The most common associated genitourinary anomalies include uterovaginal atresia (or duplication) in females and absent seminal vesicle or seminal vesicle cyst in males.[14]

A number of syndromes are associated with unilateral renal agenesis, such as the VACTERL association, Fanconi pancytopenia, Kallman syndrome, and Fraser syndrome. Abnormalities of the remaining kidney have been described in up to 90% of patients. The most common abnormality is VUR followed by renal ectopia and malrotation, PUJ obstruction and multicystic dysplasia.

Imaging Features

In clinical practice it is quite difficult to be certain that one is dealing with true unilateral agenesis since a very small nonfunctioning kidney may be either ectopic or located medially in the renal bed overlying the transverse processes of the lumbar vertebra. A combination of US and ^{99m}tc dimercaptosuccinic acid (DMSA) scan is needed to make the diagnosis. US might show that a nonexcreting kidney on scintigraphy is actually present but abnormal. Conversely, scintigraphy might reveal a small unilateral dysplastic/hypoplastic kidney that was difficult to be evaluated on US, but which is nonetheless present and retains some function. If the US and nuclear studies fail to show a small kidney, then contrast enhanced CT should be done before RGP. RGP can exclude renal agenesis if it shows pelvicalyceal system and ureter on the suspected side.

Rotational Anomalies

As the kidney ascends in fetal life from its origin in the pelvis to its final position opposite the second lumbar vertebra, it undergoes a 90° inward rotation along its longitudinal axis so that finally the renal hilum is directed medially and slightly forward. Any anomaly in this process, results in deficient, excessive, or reversed rotation. In incomplete rotation, or nonrotation, the hilum continues to face anteriorly, the calices project out from either side of the pelvis on a standard frontal radiograph, and the proximal ureter is displaced laterally. In excessive rotation, the normal inward rotation is prolonged beyond 90° so that the hilum faces posteriorly or posteromedially and the renal vessels lie posterior to the kidney. In reversed rotation, the kidney rotates outward with the renal hilum facing laterally, the proximal ureter is displaced laterally, and the renal vessels lie anterior to the kidney **(Fig. 3)**. Nonrotation and incomplete rotations are most common rotational anomalies. They may be unilateral or bilateral and often accompany ectopia or fusion anomalies. In an IVU, oblique views are of great help in establishing that the malrotated kidney is otherwise normal.[15]

Anomalies of Renal Position

Normally, the kidneys are located opposite 1st–3rd lumbar vertebrae. Anomalies of renal position range from minor degrees of unilateral malposition to totally abnormal positioning of both kidneys. The clinical significance of this finding lies in the fact that these ectopic kidneys are more susceptible to trauma, iatrogenic injury, obstruction, calculi, reflux and infection. There is a high incidence of aberrant and multiple renal arteries and veins.

Ipsilateral/Uncrossed Ectopia

In this anomaly, the ectopic kidney is on the same side as the vesical opening of its ureter. It can be further divided into cranial or caudal ectopias according to whether they are above or below the normal position. In cranial renal ectopia, the affected kidney, usually the left, is within the lower thorax posteriorly, either below a localized diaphragmatic eventration or within a diaphragmatic hernia (intrathoracic kidney).[16] In caudal renal ectopia the abnormal kidney lies below normal position; it may be abdominal (above iliac crest, below L3), iliac (iliac fossa) or pelvic (true pelvis).

Imaging Features

Chest X-ray shows a thoracic kidney as a well-defined, posteroinferior mediastinal mass. IVU confirms the thoracic location of the kidney. CT may show the diaphragmatic defect through which the kidney passes and the adrenal gland is seen lying above, behind or below the kidney. Blood supply is from an elongated renal artery from aorta at normal level **(Figs. 4A and B)**, or occasionally from an accessory renal artery from thoracic aorta. In cases of caudal renal ectopia, renal outline is not visible in expected position on an abdominal X-ray. Bowel gas can be seen to occupy the renal fossa; typically the hepatic and splenic flexures are repositioned. IVU shows the malrotated, ectopic kidney with a bizarre pattern of calyces draining into the bladder via a short ureter. Tightly coned views can miss early nephrogram as the ectopic kidney may not be included in the field of view. Fluoroscopic spot views may be required to delineate the course of ureters. Adrenal gland remains in normal location; appears linear on CT and the colonic flexures, spleen and tail of pancreas are seen occupying the empty renal fossa. CT can easily distinguish the ectopic kidney from various abdominal and pelvic masses **(Fig. 5A)**. Delayed imaging is helpful in hydronephrosis and to delineate distal ureters. CT angiography can be used for mapping of renal vasculature. Renal arteries are seen to arise lower than normal and may be multiple. When the kidney is pelvic, the arterial supply usually arises from the aortic bifurcation **(Fig. 5B)**. These aberrant arteries may cross and obstruct the ureter. It is important to recognize these vessels prior to aortic surgery as they

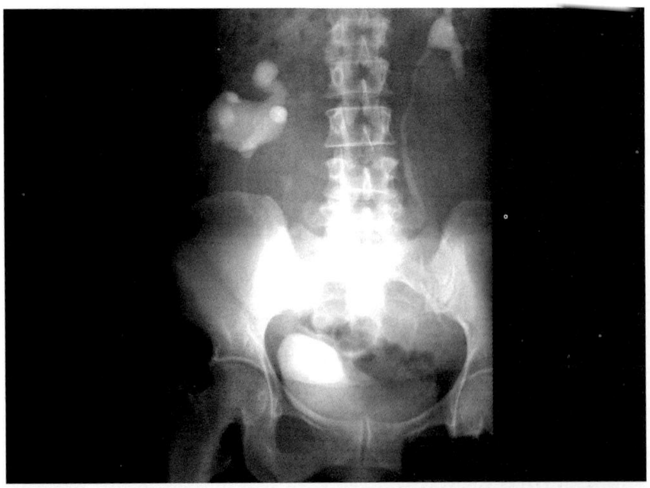

Fig. 3: Rotational anomaly of the kidney: IVU showing right caudal ectopia with a rotational anomaly. Note that the calyces are facing medially while the pelvis is facing laterally.

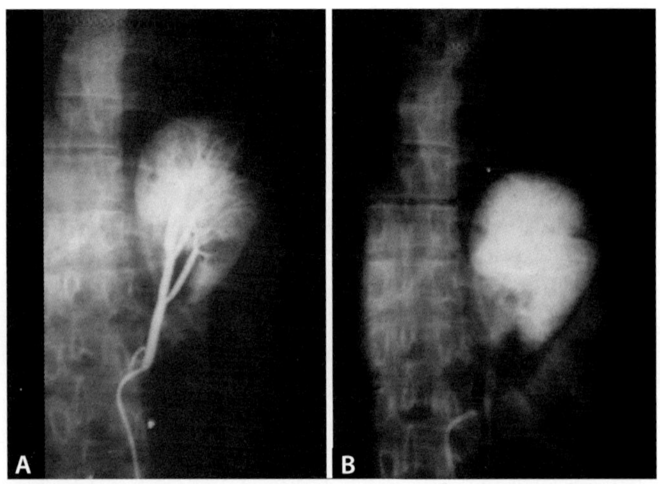

Figs. 4A and B: Thoracic kidney: Conventional angiogram showing intrathoracic left kidney being supplied by an abnormally long renal artery.

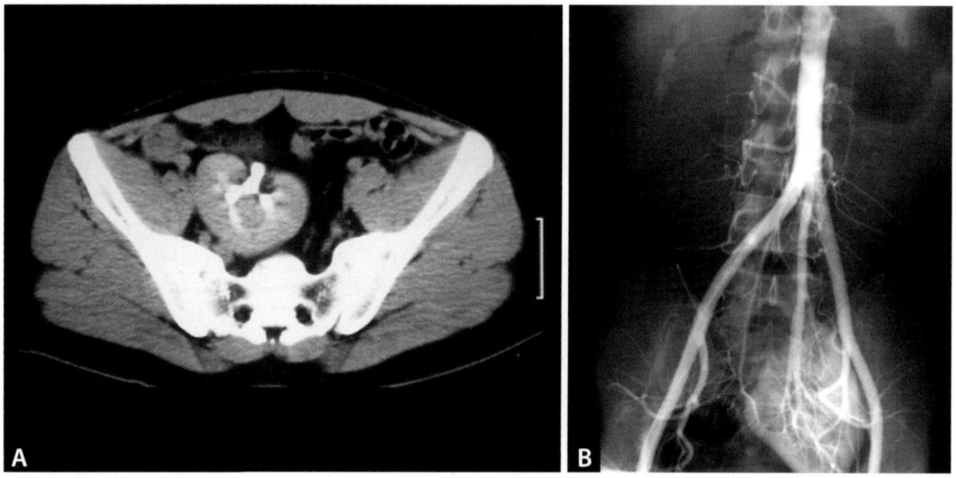

Figs. 5A and B: Pelvic kidney: (A) Contrast enhanced CT axial image showing ectopic right kidney lying in the right iliac fossa; (B) Aortogram showing an ectopic left pelvic kidney drawing its blood supply from the aortic bifurcation.

may be inadvertently injured. DMSA scan detects ectopic kidney by outlining the kidney shape. A ptotic kidney has to be differentiated from a caudal renal ectopia. In ptosis of kidney the renal artery arises from normal site and the ureter is redundant.[17]

Crossed Renal Ectopia

In crossed renal ectopia the kidney is located in opposite side of midline from its ureteral orifice. It may occur with fusion (most common), without fusion (15%), or in a solitary kidney (least common).[18] In fused crossed ectopia (unilateral fused kidney), the kidney crosses the midline to the opposite side of the body and fuses with the kidney on that side. Crossed, fused renal ectopia is more common in males and on the right side. The anomalous kidney usually lies below the orthotopic kidney, and the fusion is between the lower pole of the orthotopic kidney and the upper pole of the ectopic kidney. Malrotation, particularly in the ectopic kidney, is the rule. Occasionally, the pelvis of the lower, ectopic kidney faces laterally (sigmoid or S-shaped kidney) or is horizontal (L-shaped kidney). In rare cases, the two fused kidneys are at the same level and are fused completely (unilateral lump kidney). Instances of bilateral crossed renal ectopia and of crossed ectopia of a solitary kidney have been reported.[19] The importance of these conditions is that it may present as an abdominal mass or as an obstructive uropathy with PUJ obstruction. There is an increased incidence of VUR into the crossed kidney.

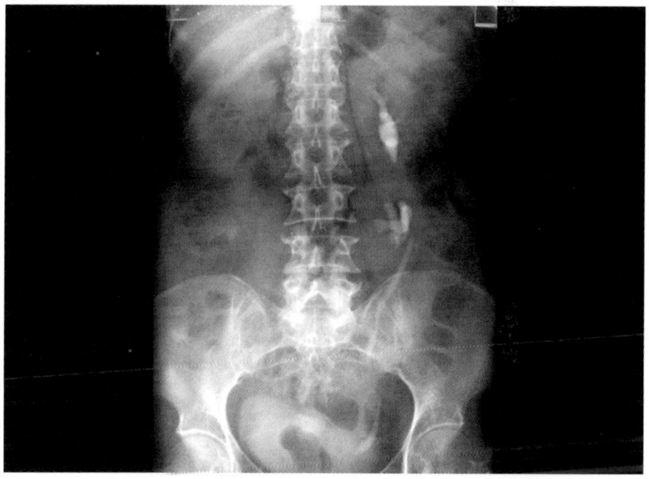

Fig. 6: Crossed fused ectopia: IVU showing the right kidney crossing over and fusing with the lower pole of left kidney.

Imaging Features

The US reveals an unusually large kidney on the affected side with an absent kidney on the opposite side. If the kidneys are not fused, they may be seen to move separately from each other during respiration. In cases of fused ectopia, the renal sinuses lie in different planes, run in different directions and the fused kidneys are inseparable. The diagnosis of renal ectopia is generally established from the IVU or CT. IVU delineates the morphology of the crossed kidneys and shows the insertion of ureter into the trigone on the side of origin **(Fig. 6)**. CT with thin slices is helpful in showing the degree of separation of the kidneys. CT angiography can show the anomalous vascular supply arising from the vessels in the vicinity.

Horseshoe Kidney

The horseshoe kidney is the most frequent renal fusion anomaly, occurring in 1 in 400 people. It is characterized by fusion of the lower poles across the midline. The kidney is lower in position than a normal kidney and lies anterior to the aorta and inferior vena cava. The horseshoe kidney's polar fusion results in an isthmus of tissue (parenchymal or fibrous) between the two. The usual position of the isthmus is at the junction of the aorta with the inferior mesenteric artery. The isthmus prevents normal renal rotation. The ureters exit the anteriorly positioned renal pelves to descend inferiorly. Most (90%) cases are asymptomatic. Horseshoe kidneys are at greater risk than normal kidneys for PUJ obstruction as well as VUR, infection, urolithiasis and malignancy. Carcinoma of the renal pelvis and Wilms' tumor are more likely to occur in the horseshoe kidney.[20] The abnormal position also leaves the kidney more susceptible to trauma. Many anomalies are associated with horseshoe kidney. Urinary tract anomalies include PUJ obstruction, duplicated collecting systems, ureterocele, megaureter, and renal dysplasia. Horseshoe kidney may be associated with Turner's syndrome, trisomy 18, Fanconi's anemia, and Laurence-Moon-Biedl syndrome, or as a part of VACTERL association.

Imaging Features

On X-ray the lower poles of the kidneys are seen to lie too close to the spine and sometimes the isthmus may be seen. US shows the curved configuration of the horseshoe kidney with elongated, poorly defined lower poles.[21] IVU reveals that the nephrogram is U-shaped and the lower calyces descend towards the midline near the isthmus, resulting in the "hand-holding calyces" appearance **(Fig. 7A)**. The lower calyces are often medial to the ureter on the same side. As each ureter crosses the isthmus, it curves laterally and then assumes a normal medial course giving rise to the "flower-vase" appearance. The renal pelvis is usually large and extrarenal with an abnormally high insertion of the ureter. PUJ (more common) or UVJ obstruction may lead to delayed clearing of the contrast. VCUG often demonstrates VUR. CT is especially useful in showing the degree and site of fusion, and whether the isthmus is composed of functioning renal parenchyma or of fibrous tissue **(Fig. 7B)**. Renal parenchymal changes (scarring, cystic disease) and collecting system abnormalities (duplex system, hydronephrosis, calculi) are also picked up on CT.[22] Angiographic images show renal arterial supply from aorta, common iliac, internal iliac, external iliac or inferior mesenteric arteries.

Ureteropelvic Duplication (Duplex Kidney)

A duplex kidney shows two separate pelvicaliceal systems. The two draining ureters may join before emptying into the bladder (partial duplication/bifid ureters) or insert separately into the bladder (complete duplication). 85% of completely duplicated ureters follow the Weigert-Meyer rule according to which the upper ureter inserts into the bladder in a position more inferior and medial to the orifice of the lower moiety ureter. In these cases, the ectopic ureter draining the upper pole moiety frequently ends in a ureterocele and is obstructed, whereas reflux typically occurs into the lower moiety. The duplication process may involve the entire urinary tract: from the renal parenchyma to urethra.

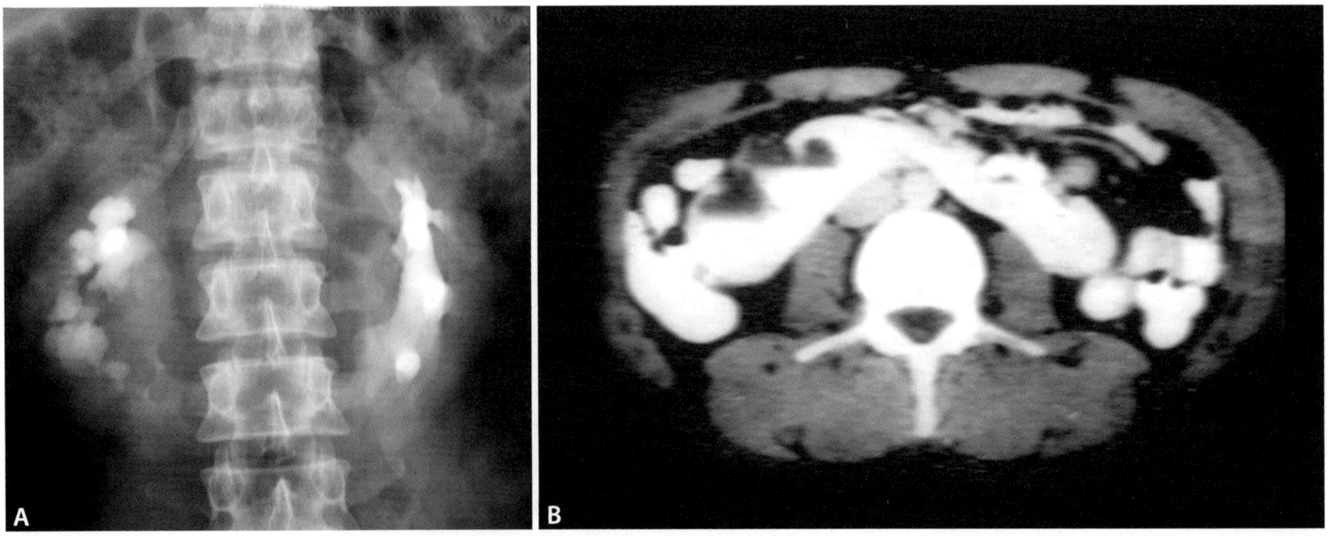

Figs. 7A and B: Horseshoe kidney: (A) IVU shows the typical U-shape of the horseshoe kidney. The calyces are pointing medially and the pelvis faces laterally; (B) CECT showing a horseshoe kidney with hydronephrosis on the right side and an isthmus of functioning renal parenchyma.

Imaging Features

The US diagnosis of a duplex kidney is usually straightforward, the calyces forming two distinct echo complexes with intervening renal parenchyma. Separate renal pelves are often visible along with separate proximal ureters. Distal nondilated ureters are more difficult to image because of bowel gas. One should carefully look for associated ureterocele and assess for the presence and location of ureteral jets in the bladder. Concomitant genital anomalies, especially uterine should also be looked for.

On IVU or CT Urography, duplex kidney is well seen with double ureters leading to two jets of contrast. There is poor or no excretion by the upper pole moiety. Nonfilling of the obstructed upper pole moiety results in the downward displacement of the lower pole calyces, called the "drooping lily" sign **(Fig. 8)**. Lower pole may also show calyceal clubbing with thinning and scarring of overlying renal parenchyma. VCUG demonstrates reflux into the lower pole ureter and the frequently present ureterocele at the distal end of upper pole ureter. Saddle reflux or yo-yo reflux is unique to partial duplications which have a single distal ureter. It refers to the refluxed contrast first entering one moiety, draining and then entering the other moiety of the duplicated pelvicaliceal system. Occasionally, nuclear scan is the first to suggest a renal duplication. Renal scan is helpful in estimating differential function, drainage and scarring. MR urography is often the best modality when an ectopic ureter can not be shown by any other imaging modality.[23] Coronal thick slab sequences are most useful in this regard.

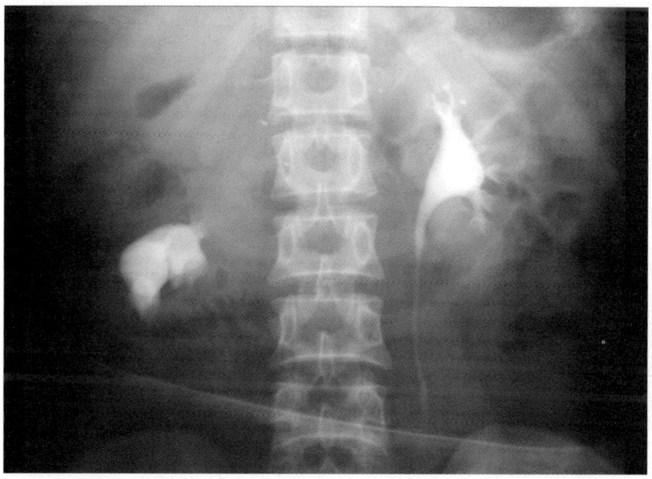

Fig. 8: Duplex right kidney. IVU shows that the upper moiety is non-functioning and displaces the lower pelvicaliceal system downwards, producing the "drooping lily sign".

Renal Hypoplasia

In simple renal hypoplasia, also called miniature or dwarf kidney, the affected kidney is significantly smaller than normal, but is otherwise well formed both grossly and histologically, and functions normally in proportion to its mass. The main renal artery and its branches are uniformly small. On IVU, it is small, usually excretes contrast material well, smooth in outline, has normal appearance but has fewer than normal (less than 7) calyces, and a normal ureter. The opposite kidney is usually large owing to compensatory hypertrophy. It does not affect total kidney function unless the opposite kidney is diseased or absent, but rarely it may cause severe hypertension in the neonate.[24]

Cystic Renal Dysplasia

Renal dysplasia is a congenital renal parenchymal malformation in which abnormal nephrons and mesenchymal stroma are found in absence of either neoplasm or infection. It occurs in 2 to 4 in every 1,000 births. Cystic renal dysplasia has been classified into 4 types.[25] Type I is infantile or Autosomal Recessive Polycystic Kidney Disease (ARPKD); II, Multicystic Dysplastic Kidney Disease (MDK); III, Autosomal Dominant (Adult Type) Polycystic Kidney Disease (ADPKD); and IV, cystic renal dysplasia due to early urinary tract obstruction (at any level).

Autosomal Recessive Polycystic Kidney Disease

Autosomal recessive polycystic kidney disease (ARPKD) is a single gene disorder characterized by bilateral, symmetrical renal cystic disease involving distal convoluting tubules and collecting ducts. There is 25% likelihood of recurrence in a future pregnancy. Pathologically, there is saccular dilatation of renal collecting tubules noted as hundreds of tiny 1–2 mm cysts on gross examination. In ARPKD the liver is always involved by hepatic cysts, bile duct ectasia and periportal fibrosis. Clinically, it is characterized by a variable mixture of renal failure and portal hypertension. ARPKD is divided into four categories: Perinatal, neonatal, infantile and juvenile, depending upon the age at the time of presentation. It is generally accepted that the abnormality is expressed within a spectrum that varies from predominant renal and minimal hepatic involvement in the infant, to predominant hepatic and minimal renal involvement in the late childhood.[26]

Imaging Features

Plain radiograph shows bilateral large flank masses (enlarged kidneys) that displace the bowel gas centrally.

Dilated renal collecting tubules are, too small to be imaged on US as separate cysts and because of the numerous acoustic interfaces provided by the cyst walls the kidney appears solid and homogeneously hyperechoic **(Fig. 9A)**. The size of kidneys is 2–4 standard deviations more than the mean size, in majority of patients. The enlarged kidneys maintain their reniform shape and show absent or poor corticomedullary differentiation. Dilated renal collecting tubules are seen radially arranged from the hilum to the periphery in two-third patients when high frequency linear transducer is used.[27] Cysts are only occasionally visible and they are small (0.5–1 cm). A characteristic perirenal halo may be seen, representing the peripherally compressed hypoechic normal cortex around the hyperechoic medulla. Tiny, punctuate, echogenic foci develop with time due to calcium deposition and correlate with renal failure. These foci do not show posterior acoustic shadowing, but may cause ring-down artifacts.

IVU is seldom performed today. Decreased renal function leads to poor visualization of the pelvicaliceal system. Classic urographic appearance, best seen on delayed films taken 6–24 hours after the administration of IV contrast medium, was persistence of contrast in the dilated tubules leading to a streaked nephrogram **(Fig. 9B)**.

CT shows bilateral symmetrically enlarged kidneys with multiple punctuate calcific foci. Contrast enhanced CT shows a prolonged striated nephrogram **(Fig. 9C)**, due to trapping of contrast in the medulla. There is minimal excretion of contrast and the bladder is typically empty or small. Few small cysts (2 cm) may be identifiable within the kidneys.

Nuclear scan shows loss of kidney outline with patchy, tracer uptake with focal defects throughout the renal parenchyma.

Antenatal US diagnosis of ARPKD can be made when oligohydramnios with markedly enlarged, echogenic kidneys is noted. In general, earlier the diagnosis is made, worse is the prognosis. These infants are at risk for pulmonary hypoplasia and often die in the neonatal period due to pulmonary complications.

Multicystic Dysplastic Kidney

Multicystic dysplastic kidney (MDK) is the second most common abdominal mass in a neonate after hydronephrosis, with an incidence of 1 in 4300 live births. The affected kidney is nonfunctioning, replaced by numerous cysts and dysplastic tissue. It varies in size from 10–15 cm to only 1–2 cm. Classically, two forms are recognized on imaging:

- *Pelvi-infundibular* MDK, the more common type results from atresia of renal pelvis and proximal ureter in early fetal life. The cysts represent the dilated calyces.
- *Hydronephrotic* MDK, the less frequent type results from atresia of the proximal segment of the ureter (sometimes the entire ureter). In this form cysts represent the entire pelvicaliceal system.

The abnormality is usually unilateral with a normal contralateral kidney allowing for a good prognosis. Bilateral disease, including bilateral MDK (19%) or MDK with contralateral kidney agenesis (11%), is lethal. There is a 3–5% familial recurrence of the disease suggesting a genetic influence.[28] The importance of recognizing MDK

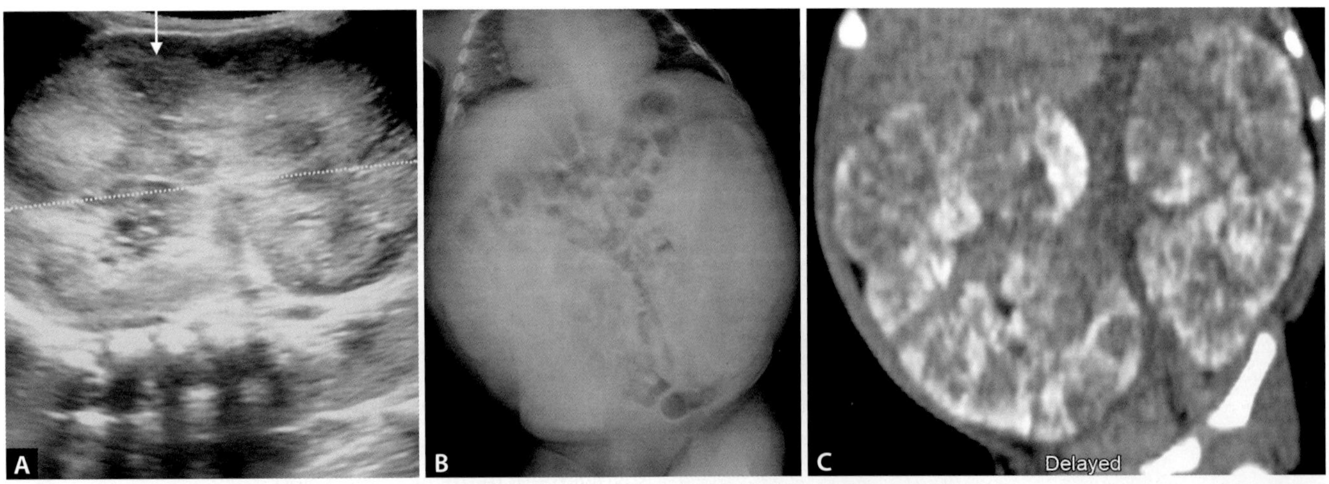

Figs. 9A to C: Autosomal recessive polycystic kidney: (A) US shows markedly enlarged, homogeneously hyperechoic, kidney with absent corticomedullary differentiation. A characteristic perirenal halo is also seen (arrow), representing the peripherally compressed hypoechoic normal cortex around the hyperechoic medulla; (B) Radiograph taken postcontrast enhanced CT shows classic persistence of contrast in the dilated tubules leading to a streaked nephrogram; (C) Contrast-enhanced CT shows bilateral symmetrically enlarged kidneys showing a prolonged striated nephrogram, due to trapping of contrast in the medulla.

lies in the knowledge that, approximately 30–50% of affected patients have contralateral renal abnormalities including vesicoureteral reflux, PUJ obstruction, and ureterovesical junction obstruction.[29] Postnatally, the natural history of MDK is one of progressive involution of the cystic spaces within the first two years of life.

Imaging Features

MDK is often discovered on routine prenatal US or during an US investigation of a flank mass in the neonate.[30] The findings include the presence of variably-sized cysts separated by echogenic areas throughout the kidney. Outer contour is often lobulated with outer cyst walls forming the margins of the mass. There is no demonstrable communication between these cysts, and no normal renal parenchyma is seen **(Fig. 10)**. The kidney may lose its reniform contour. Microscopically, connective tissue, thick walled cysts, small groups of tubules and poorly formed glomeruli are seen between cysts. Color Doppler shows minimal flow in the parenchyma and the central hilar vessels tend to be small. In the majority of cases US allows a definitive diagnosis to be made, however in a small percentage of cases in the neonate it may be difficult to distinguish between a multicystic dysplastic kidney and a large PUJ obstruction. In the multicystic kidney there is usually one 'cyst' which is larger than the others and lies laterally, whereas in PUJ obstruction the dilated renal pelvis is centrally located and the peripheral calyces are seen to extend from it **(Figs. 11A and B)**. The kidney maintains a reniform shape and its parenchyma surrounds the dilated calyces. In such situations dynamic nuclear imaging may be useful since the demonstration of function indicates PUJ obstruction. In MDK, initial blood flow images show perfusion but sequential images demonstrate lack of any excretory function. CECT also shows multiple low attenuation cysts (debris may lead to higher attenuation in some cysts) replacing normal renal parenchyma. There is minimal or no contrast enhancement and no excretion on delayed images.

Autosomal Dominant (Adult Type) Polycystic Kidney Disease (ADPKD)

ADPKD is a hereditary disease characterized by the presence of multiple bilateral renal macrocysts. There is

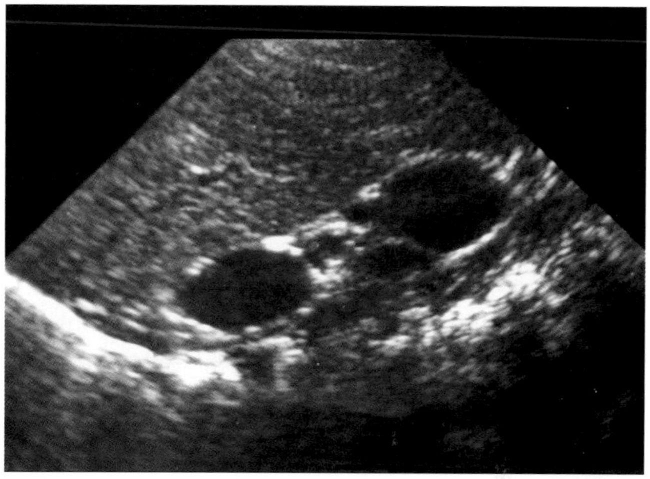

Fig. 10: Multicystic dysplastic kidney US shows variably-sized cysts separated by echogenic areas throughout the kidney. There is no demonstrable communication between these cysts, and no normal renal parenchyma is seen.

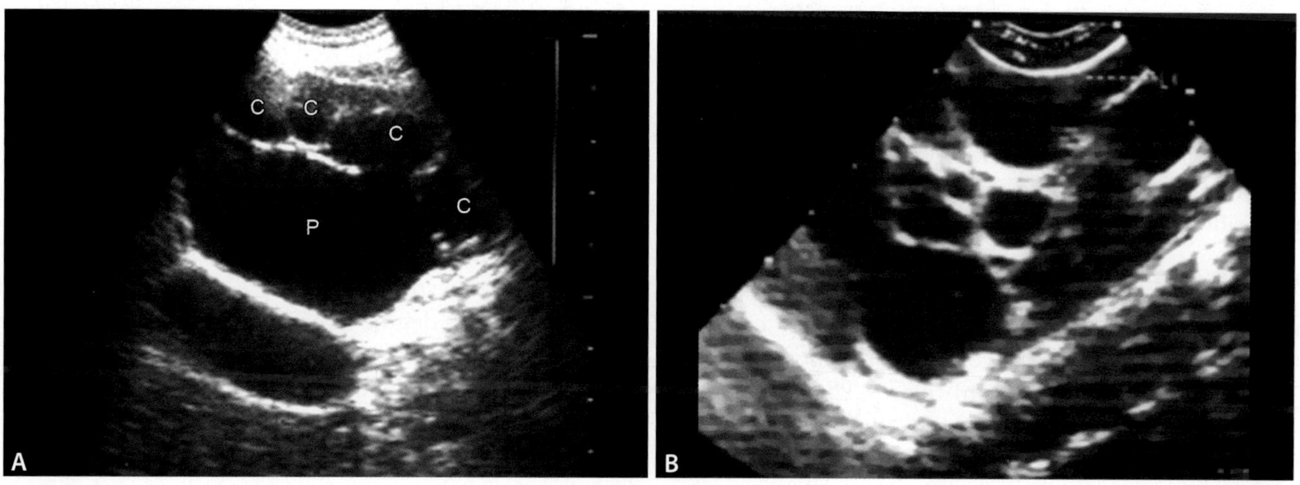

Figs. 11A and B: (A) PUJ obstruction: Longitudinal US scan of the kidney showing a central distended pelvis (P) and communicating dilated calyces (C); (B) Multicystic dysplastic kidney: The kidney is replaced by multiple simple appearing cysts, which are not connected to each other, the largest ones are peripherally situated.

cystic involvement of liver (50%), pancreas (9%), spleen, brain, ovaries or testes (1%). It has autosomal dominant inheritance with a high degree of penetrance. This disorder most frequently manifests after the third decade of life but now is frequently being diagnosed in infants and children. Children with ADPKD may have hypertension, proteinuria or hyperlipidemia. ADPKD is rarely seen in utero because less than 5% of nephrons are cystic antenatally.

Imaging Features

Renal cysts are rarely seen in normal children; hence, when imaged, although at times part of some syndromes, one must consider the possibility of ADPKD. Analysis of the US or medical history of older family members can help make the diagnosis. Cysts are readily seen in the affected adults, with a reported US sensitivity of 100% in those more than 30 years of age. Renal contor is typically normal early in life, becoming bosselated as more cysts develop.[31] Renal size and echotexture is normal in young patients, aside from the few small cysts.

IVU shows mildly to markedly enlarged kidneys. Dystrophic calcification of cyst walls and renal calculi are typically only seen in adult patients. Smoothly marginated rounded, radiolucent defects may be seen in the nephrographic phase, leading to a "Swiss-cheese" pattern. The pelvicaliceal system is splayed around the renal cysts.

Contrast enhanced CT can readily show the nonenhancing hypodense cysts with intervening normally enhancing renal parenchyma and the associated cysts in the liver, pancreas or spleen. Cysts complicated by hemorrhage appear hyperdense (60–90 HU) and may be associated with perinephric hematoma due to rupture. Cyst wall calcification and secondary calculi are easily identified. Infected cysts are hypodense with thick walls showing variable contrast enhancement. Adjacent renal fascia is also thickened with stranding of the perinephric fat. MRI is useful in equivocal cases as it can reliably demonstrate hemorrhage within the cysts as T1 hyperintensity, fluid-fluid levels or T2 hypointense hemosiderin deposition.

PUJ Obstruction

Idiopathic obstruction at the PUJ is a major cause of obstructive uropathy at all ages and is the most common cause of neonatal hydronephrosis.[32] The etiology of obstruction is varied and in more than half the cases obstruction is functional rather than anatomical. Histologically, the PUJ shows a deficiency of muscle fibers with an increase in collagen tissue. This results in an impaired transmission of the peristaltic waves and urine from the renal pelvis to the ureter (segmental dysfunction, adynamic segment).[33] Obstruction may also be due to an intrinsic stenosis of the PUJ, an infolding of the local mucosa and musculature or local kink and angulation of the ureter associated with adhesions and overlying fibrous bands. An aberrant renal artery to the lower pole of the kidney crossing the PUJ is seen in about one-third of patients.[34]

PUJ obstruction may occur in a duplex system where it almost always affects the lower moiety. Malrotated, horseshoe and ectopic kidneys are prone to PUJ obstruction, mainly due to aberrant and multiple arterial vasculature. PUJ obstruction has also been reported to be associated with primary megaureter and VUR. In unilateral PUJ obstruction, the opposite kidney is sometimes absent, duplicated or cystic dysplastic. There is a definite relationship between fetal urinary obstruction and cystic renal dysplasia. The location and timing of obstruction in utero appear to determine whether dysplasia, cystic dysplasia or ordinary hydronephrosis will result.[35] Whatever the cause, the renal pelvis and calyces fail to empty leading to various degrees of dilatation with corresponding degree of atrophy of the renal parenchyma.

PUJ obstruction occurs more commonly in males than females and the left side is more commonly affected. There can be bilateral involvement in 10–30% of patients. Newborns and infants (if not diagnosed antenatally) present with a palpable abdominal lump. Older children may present with intermittent abdominal pain with vomiting, hematuria or urinary tract infection.

Imaging Features

In infants with known or suspected hydronephrosis from a prenatal US, a re-evaluation by abdominal US should be done soon after birth followed by a diuretic DTPA nuclear scan and, if still indicated, by a conventional urogram. In other patients, both infants and older children, the diagnosis is often suggested on sonography. On US, the hydronephrotic kidney is often enlarged and contains a central cystic structure, representing the renal pelvis, around which and communicating with it are multiple cystic areas corresponding to the dilated calyces. US can also evaluate the degree of cortical atrophy. As the ureter is not dilated, it is not visualized.

Duplex Doppler can be used to differentiate obstructive from nonobstructive dilatation of the renal collecting system. A resistive index (RI) of more than 0.7 in the peripheral intrarenal arteries indicates obstructive dilatation. However, the RI value is age-dependent and in children less than 4 years of age the RI is normally greater than 0.7. In these cases the RI of the affected system can be compared with the opposite side.[36] Measurements of the resting RI and after a diuretic challenge, i.e. 10 minutes following intravenous frusemide, can give better results in the pediatric population. The post-frusemide study shows an increase in RI in both the obstructed and nonobstructed kidneys, but the obstructed kidney shows a significant increase of greater than 0.1.[37]

On IVU, the classical PUJ obstruction presents with delayed opacification of the collecting system, marked pyelocaliectasis, narrowing at PUJ, incomplete visualization of a normal sized ureter, and retention of contrast material in the collecting system on delayed films **(Fig. 12)**. In severe cases the nephrographic phase of the urogram may show an opaque rim of functioning parenchyma of variable thickness peripherally with multiple centrally placed round radiolucencies representing dilated calyces (rim sign).[38] Contrast in the compressed and realigned or dilated collecting tubules of Bellini may be visible in the early phase of the study as dense curved bands (calyceal crescents)[39] or as a row of dense dots located around the outer border of the calyces. The markedly dilated pelvis and calyces fill only on delayed films and absence of function is uncommon.

The urographic appearance of PUJ obstruction varies depending upon the cause. Obstructing vessels may produce a linear or band like oblique crossing defect in the proximal ureter.[40] Both intrinsic stenosis and functional obstruction cause a focal, smooth narrowing. In most PUJ obstructions the extrarenal pelvis enlarges out of proportion to the degree of caliectasis. Rarely, PUJ obstruction occurs with an intrarenal pelvis, in which case caliectasis may be in proportion with or relatively more severe than the pyelectasis.

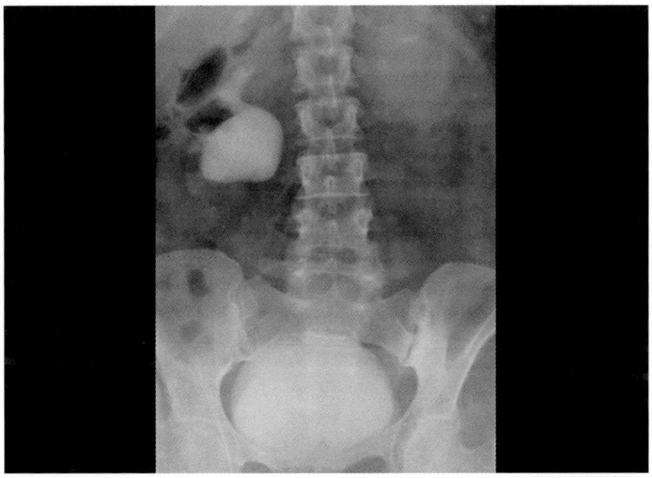

Fig. 12: PUJ obstruction: IVU showing dilatation of right renal pelvis out of proportion to the calyces, with abrupt narrowing at the junction of pelvis with ureter.

Diuresis renography can help in two circumstances: (i) to confirm that a prominent renal pelvis is not obstructed and (ii) to bring out a suspected intermittent PUJ obstruction. It is an adjunct to the basic IVU. Furosemide, 0.5 mg/kg is injected intravenously, 15–20 minutes after the injection of contrast. Films are taken at 5, 10 and 15 minutes after the diuretic injection. In nonobstructive PUJ, all contrast material should clear by 10 minutes. Delayed clearance, appearance of pyelocaliectasis and/or flank pain is the classic signs of a flow related PUJ obstruction.[41]

Radionuclide studies give the best objective assessment of renal function. Diuresis renography effectively separates obstructive from nonobstructive dilatation in many patients and can also localize the probable site of obstruction. Even in patients with equivocal test results, serial renograms are useful to assess whether urine transport is stable or deteriorating.

VCUG is done in infants with PUJ obstruction to exclude coincidental reflux.[42] Older children need VCUG only if a dilated ureter has been demonstrated on IVU or US or if urinary infection is present.

CT is needed in very few circumstances. CT is the best method for assessing isthmus anatomy when PUJ obstruction involves a horseshoe kidney. It may also be used to determine the level of obstruction in nonfunctioning kidneys. Hydronephrosis without ureterectasis places the obstruction near or at the PUJ.

The Prominent Normal Extrarenal Pelvis

Rounded extrarenal pelvis is seen in approximately 10% of normal individuals. It tends to be flabby, distensible, often narrow or closed at outlet and may appear turgid during some phases of IVU **(Fig. 13)**. The features which caution against diagnosing this as PUJ obstruction are: The absence of symptoms, prompt appearance of contrast material in the calyces, normal sized calyces with sharp fornices and prompt drainage on films made with the patient prone/erect.

Postoperative Evaluation

Postsurgical edema at the anastomosis frequently causes partial obstruction in the early postoperative period and gradual resolution takes place over days to weeks. Routine imaging studies during this interval are likely to be confusing and misleading.

Serial diuretic radionuclide renography is probably the most informative way to monitor urodynamics

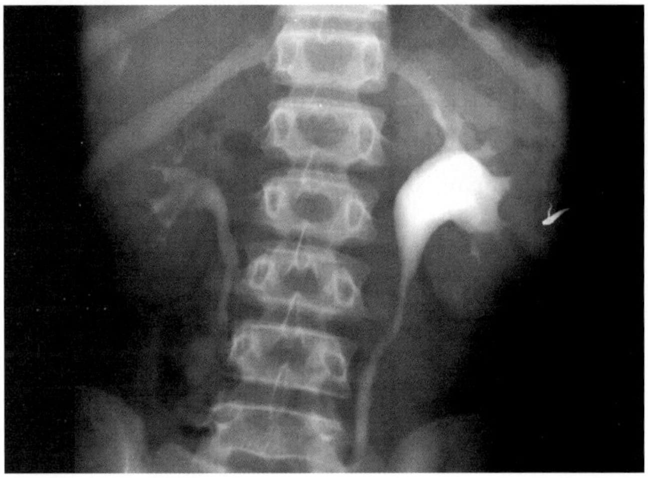

Fig. 13: Left extrarenal pelvis without obstruction. Though the pelvis appears distended it tapers smoothly into the ureter with no evidence of hold up of contrast.

postsurgically as long as renal function is satisfactory. Improvement in function and/or drainage has been shown by renography in approximately 90% of patients.[43]

IVU or renography should be done 3–6 months postoperatively. Following successful PUJ repair the contour of the renal pelvis will be altered according to the type of surgery performed. Reduction in size of the renal pelvis reflects the extent of the plastic repair and is not, per se, an indication that obstruction is gone.

Improvement in the emptying rate should result in earlier appearance of contrast material in the upper ureter compared with preoperative studies. Although, drainage may still be delayed in comparison with the normal, contralateral kidney, this should not be taken as evidence for persistent obstruction. Calyces that were minimally dilated preoperatively may return completely to normal after surgery, but if moderate or severe caliectasis was well established, little or no change is common. Maximum improvement is attained by 6 months. Increased caliectasis or further delay in appearance of contrast material in the ureter at 6 months always indicates a poor clinical result.

In view of the unpredictability of pyelocaliectasis following PUJ repair, US has limited usefulness for postsurgical evaluation. Moreover, different states of hydration and bladder filling affect the caliber of the collecting system and make interpretation difficult. A decrease in both renal size and pelvic dilatation has been observed by US immediately following PUJ surgery in uncomplicated cases. The comparison of renal RI as measured by duplex Doppler in pre- and post-pyeloplasty cases can be used as an index to assess the post-surgical status.

ANOMALIES OF THE URETER

Ectopic Ureter

An ectopic ureter is one that does not insert at its normal position at the superolateral aspect of the bladder trigone. Intravesical ectopia is not so common and is manifested by the ureter opening either lateral or caudal to the normal opening.

Extravesical ectopia is more common and also more clinically important. It is more common in girls than in boys and is associated with a duplicated system in at least 85% of cases. It is the upper pole ureter that opens ectopically. In girls the ectopic ureter may open in the urethra, vestibule or vagina and a common presenting feature is continuous leakage of urine with a normal voiding pattern. In boys, the anomalous ureter may insert in the prostatic urethra, near the bladder neck or sometimes in the genital ducts. Urinary incontinence is not a problem with boys since the ectopic opening is above the strongly developed external sphincter but urinary tract infection is a common clinical manifestation.

Imaging Features

The renal parenchyma drained by the ectopic ureter is often dysplastic and its function is usually decreased or absent. The corresponding pelvicalyceal system and ureter draining ectopically may be visualized on delayed films of an IVU **(Fig. 14A)**. A nonfunctioning second system can be suspected when the visualized pelvicalyceal system is displaced downward and laterally. When the aberrant ureter empties in the urethra, reflux into the ectopic ureter is occasionally demonstrated in the voiding study. In girls, a vaginogram may show reflux in the affected ureter if this terminates in the vagina. US is helpful if the anomalous ureter is dilated, in which case it can be followed down to and beyond the bladder **(Fig. 14B)**. Renal scan can demonstrate function not apparent in the urogram. Recently, MR urography has proved capable of displaying dilated collecting systems, ectopic ureters, and ureteroceles. It has an advantage over US and IVU in that it is capable of demonstrating ectopic extravesical ureteric insertions, thereby providing a global view of the malformation.

Ureterocele

Ureterocele is a cystic dilatation of the intravesical segment of the ureter projecting into the lumen of the bladder. It is of two types: (1) Simple ureterocele and (2) Ectopic ureterocele.

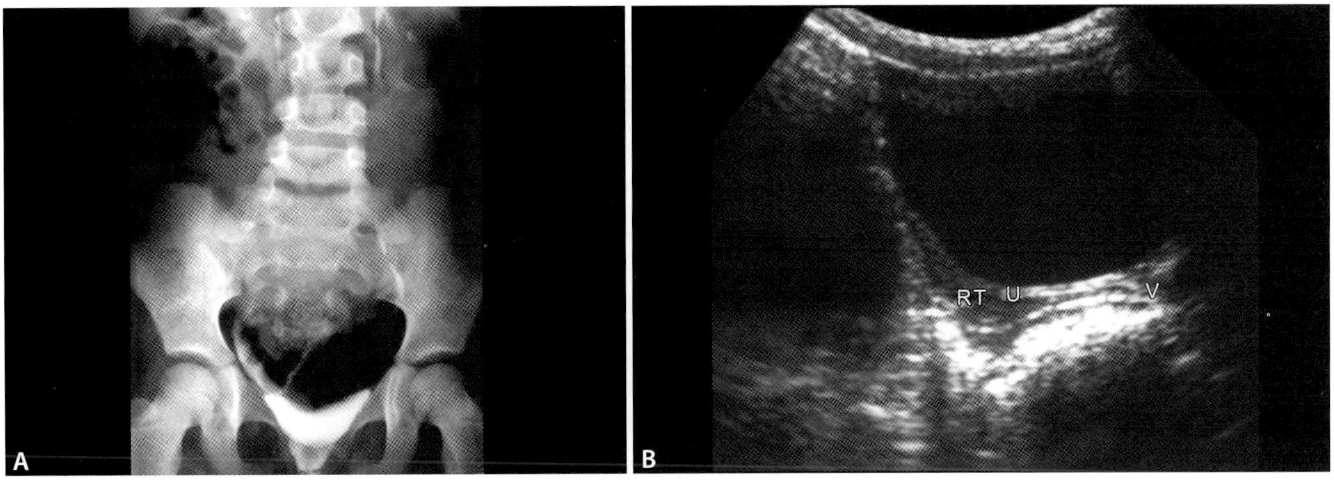

Figs. 14A and B: Ectopic ureter: (A) Delayed IVU fim showing the low-lying ectopic insertion of the right ureter into the vagina which has been opacified by contrast; (B) US showing mildly dilated right ureter draining into the vagina in a 6-year-old girl with complaints of continuous dribbling of urine.

Simple Ureterocele

In simple ureterocele, stenosis of the distal end of the normally positioned ureteral orifice leads to ballooning of the segment immediately above it, forming the ureterocele which presents as a rounded cystic mass. It is more commonly bilateral and is seen in nonduplicated systems. Complications include stone formation and urinary tract infection.

Imaging Features

A simple ureterocele may be demonstrated on US, VCUG or IVU. The ureterocele is located at the lateral angle of the trigone, and is entirely within the bladder. The findings on excretory urography are characteristic. In the early films, the ureterocele is seen as a round, radiolucent defect at the trigone. As contrast collects within the bladder and in the ureterocele a radiolucent halo representing the nonopacified wall of the ureterocele is seen. This is the well known "Cobra head" appearance **(Fig. 15)**. On US, ureterocele may be seen as a cystic mass projecting into the lumen of the bladder. On real time US scanning the ureterocele may show distension and collapse with ureteric peristalsis **(Figs. 16A and B)**. On VCUG the negative defect of the ureterocele is best seen during early filling of the bladder before the contrast becomes too dense and before the intravesical pressure compresses the ureterocele.

Ectopic Ureterocele

Ectopic ureterocele is more common than the simple type and is unilateral in 90% of patients. It differs from simple ureterocele in several respects.[44]

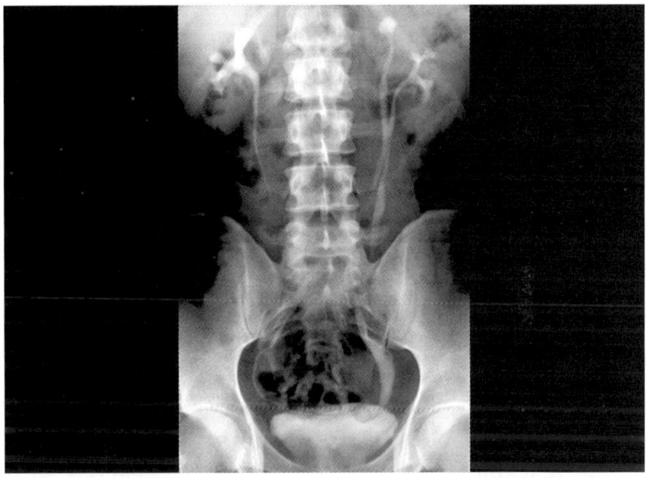

Fig. 15: Simple Ureterocele: IVU showing duplex left kidney. The ureter draining the lower moiety inserts into the lateral trigone of the bladder ending into a ureterocele. A radiolucent halo representing the nonopacified wall of the ureterocele is seen producing the "Cobra head" appearance.

- Ectopic ureterocele commonly occurs in a duplicated system and is almost always connected with the upper moiety ureter.
- The ureter connected with the ureterocele enters the bladder wall at the normal site, descends towards the bladder neck submucosally, passes through the internal urethral sphincter and terminates ectopically in the proximal urethra. In contrast to the simple ureterocele in which the cyst is formed by herniation of distal end of the ureter, the ectopic ureterocele represents the dilatation and protrusion of the entire submucosal

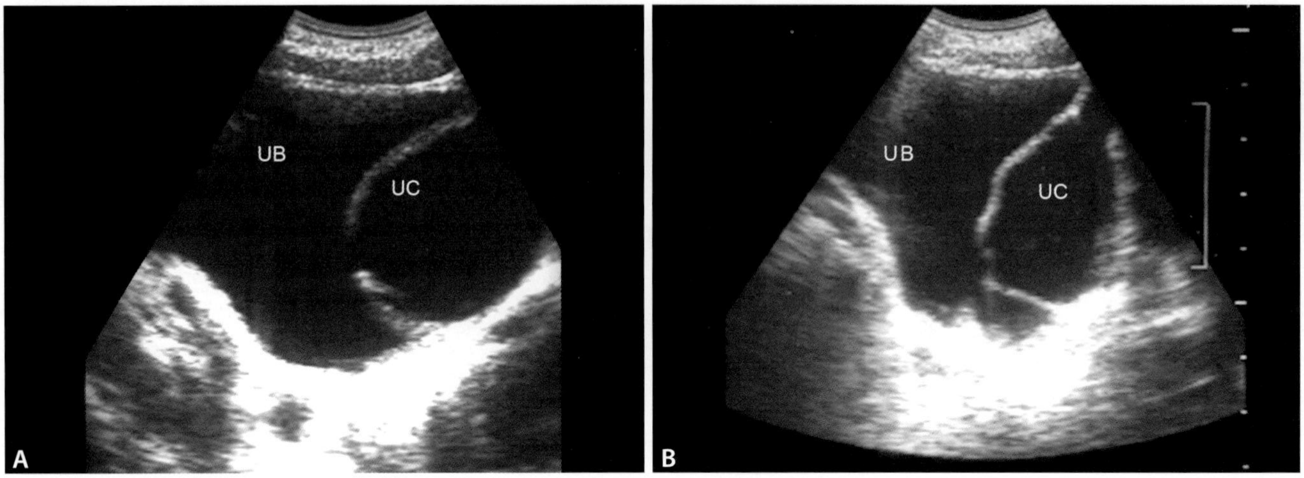

Figs. 16A and B: Ectopic ureterocele: (A) US shows the ureterocele as an intravesical cyst attached to the posterolateral wall of the bladder (cyst within a cyst appearance); (B) Dynamic scanning shows a collapsing ureterocele.

segment of the ureter into the lumen of the bladder and at the bladder neck.

- Ectopic ureterocele has a broad base and is usually larger than the simple intravesical type. It is located more inferiorly in the bladder and extends to the bladder neck area or urethra. The ureter connected with ureterocele is often dilated and tortuous.

Imaging Features

US is the single, most important investigation to diagnose ectopic ureterocele. It shows not only the ureterocele but also the upper pole collecting system of a duplex kidney which is typically dilated and is continuous with the dilated tortuous ureter entering the ureterocele (The upper pole kidney may not be seen on IVU). The ureterocele is seen as an intravesical cystic lesion of variable size attached to the posterolateral wall of the urinary bladder (cyst within cyst).

Renal scintigraphy has an important role in evaluation of functional status of kidneys in these patients.

On IVU the ectopic ureter and its insertion point may be visualized, although IVU is now performed less frequently because the dilated upper pole often shows reduced function and is rarely opacified. The visualized pelvicalyceal system of the lower moiety is displaced downwards and laterally by the dilated nonvisualized upper moiety. Ureterocele is usually seen as a rounded and eccentric filling defect at the base of the urinary bladder **(Fig. 17)**. The outline of the ureterocele is usually clearly defined by the contrast material except for its lower margin which is confluent with the bladder base and bladder neck. This is in contrast to the simple ureterocele which is intravesical and therefore completely outlined.

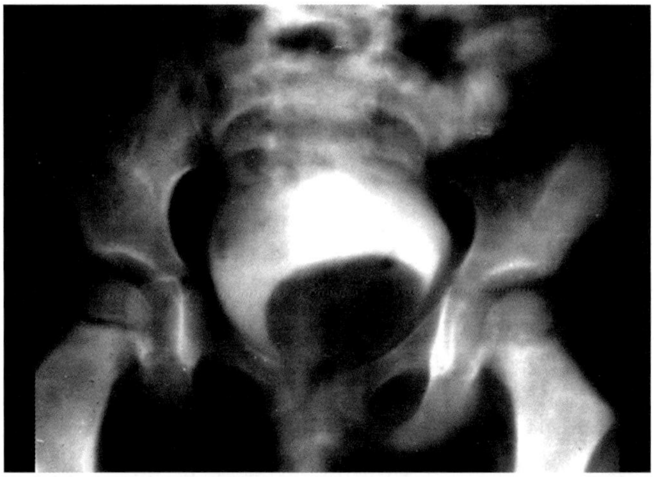

Fig. 17: Ectopic ureterocele: Contrast filled bladder on an IVU shows the ureterocele as a well-defined eccentrically placed filling defect confluent with the bladder base.

Primary Megaureter

Primary megaureter, is an uncommon, nonhereditary lesion caused by an adynamic distal segment that prevents normal, caudal progression of ureteral peristalsis.

The diagnosis of primary megaureter is usually made from the IVU. Typically the dilated ureter tapers smoothly but abruptly just above the ureterovesical junction. The terminal aperistaltic segment varies between 0.5 cm to 4 cm in length. Mild forms are common, resulting only in fusiform dilatation of the lower ureter. Even when the entire ureter is affected, the lower third shows greatest dilatation.

At its extreme, primary megaureter causes severe obstructive hydronephrosis with parenchymal thinning and loss of renal function. In bilateral cases, dilatation is often asymmetrical. Calculi may form or trap proximal to the adynamic segment and often remain long enough to become very large **(Figs. 18A and B)**.

Real time US shows ureterectasis, disproportionately greater dilatation of the lower ureter, hyperperistalsis with to and fro movement of urine, and the relatively narrowed adynamic distal segment.

VCUG should always be performed to make sure VUR is not the major cause of a wide ureter. Although, the strict definition of primary megaureter excludes patients with reflux, ipsilateral reflux has been seen in a significant number of children with otherwise classical findings of primary megaureter. Clues to the diagnosis of primary megaureter being primary rather than secondary to reflux are:

- The distal ureteral segment is normal in caliber
- The opacity of refluxed contrast material in the ureter and collecting system is less than that in the bladder, indicating dilution by stagnant urine trapped above the aperistaltic segment, and
- There is delayed drainage of contrast-laden urine back into the bladder.[45]

ANOMALIES OF THE URINARY BLADDER

Agenesis

Agenesis of the bladder is a rare anomaly that is more commonly seen in females. When seen, it is mostly part of a complex anomaly in a stillborn fetus. On antenatal US, bladder absence may be simulated by recent emptying, requiring follow-up imaging. An axial US image of the umbilical arteries as they course lateral to the bladder can help point out where the bladder should be imaged in the fetus.

Complete Duplication

Complete duplication of the urinary bladder and related anomalies are also extremely rare.[46] Two bladders lie side by side separated by peritoneal fold. Each bladder has a separate urethra **(Fig. 19)**. Bladder may be compartmentalized into two parts by a septum in the sagittal or coronal plane. The complete septum results in a ureter draining into the closed portion resulting in a dysplastic or nonfunctional kidney. IVU shows one kidney with an associated hemibladder.

Bladder Exstrophy

Exstrophy of the bladder **(Fig. 20)** occurs as a result of defect in the formation of anterior abdominal wall. Exstrophy is the most common anomaly of the urinary bladder.[47] In its most severe manifestation, the rectus abdominus muscle is widely separated and bladder lies open and everted on the anterior abdominal wall. The bladder mucosa is continuous with the skin. The exposed transitional cell mucosa often undergoes metaplasia, creating an increased risk for adenocarcinoma of the bladder. With an associated epispadias the urethral mucosa covers the dorsum of a short penis and the urethra opens on the dorsal surface of the penis. Plain radiograph of abdomen and pelvis demonstrates diastasis of the symphysis pubis. On intravenous urography there is a wide lateral curve of the pelvic portion of the distal ureters,

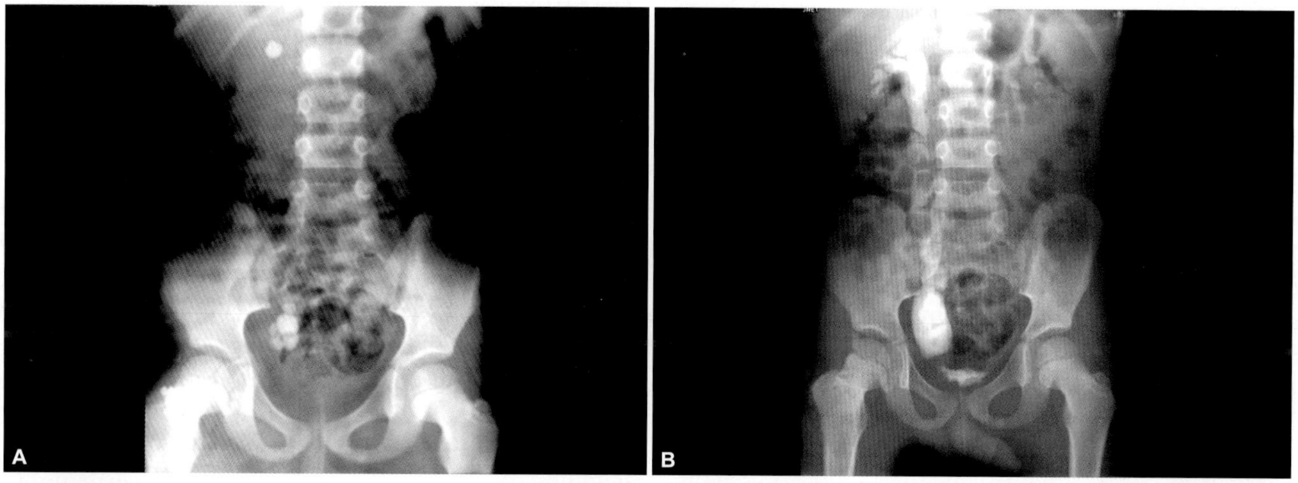

Figs. 18A and B: Calculi complicating primary obstructive megaureter: (A) Plain radiograph of the pelvis shows large, faceted stones in the right hemipelvis, and a single right renal calculus; (B) IVU shows grossly dilated juxtavesical segment of the primary megaureter in which the faceted stones are located.

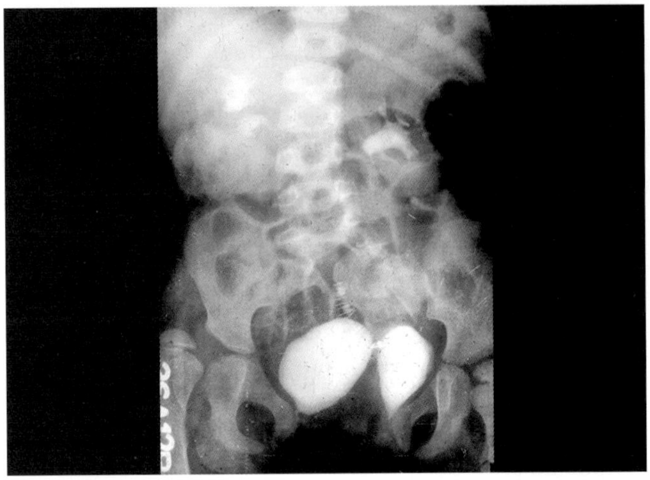

Fig. 19: Bladder duplication: IVU showing duplication of the urinary bladder in the sagittal plane.

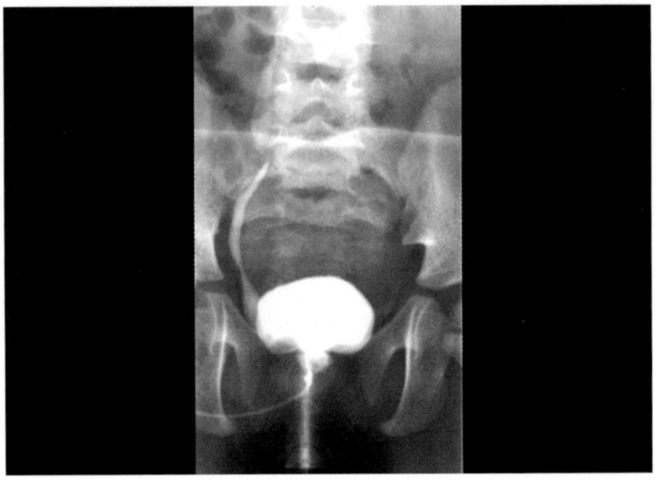

Fig. 20: Exstrophy of the bladder (Postoperative patient): Evidence of diastasis of symphysis pubis with reconstructed bladder seen. Also bilateral VUR seen.

which then turn slightly medially and upwards and pass through the bladder wall in a perpendicular direction.

Bladder Diverticulae

Congenital bladder diverticulae occur almost exclusively in boys. Most bladder diverticulae are localized outpouchings of the bladder mucosa between fibers of the detrussor muscles (pseudo-diverticulae) resulting from a congenital or acquired defect in the bladder wall. Bladder diverticulae may be primary (idiopathic), secondary or iatrogenic (postoperative).

Primary or idiopathic diverticulae are the most common, occur anywhere but most frequently in the trigonal areas. A common type of bladder diverticulum, referred to as paraureteral diverticulum or "Hutch diverticulum", is located laterally and cephalad to the ureteral orifice **(Fig. 21)**. Associated VUR is present in about half of the patients. This is because the presence of the diverticulum alters the normal slanted insertion of the ureter into the bladder. A large diverticulum may cause bladder outlet obstruction. Bladder diverticulae may be seen in several syndromes, e.g. Cutix Laxa, Ehlers-Danlos syndrome, Fetal alcohol syndrome. In male infants, bladder diverticulum must be distinguished from bilateral protrusion of the urinary bladder into the inguinal rings anteriorly. These outpouchings also called "bladder ears" are transient and disappear with growth. Lateral VCUG usually helps differentiate between the two conditions.

Secondary diverticulae develop as a result of chronically increased intravesical pressure and are seen mostly in patients with posterior urethral valves or other causes of severe lower urinary tract obstruction and in patients with neurogenic bladder disease.

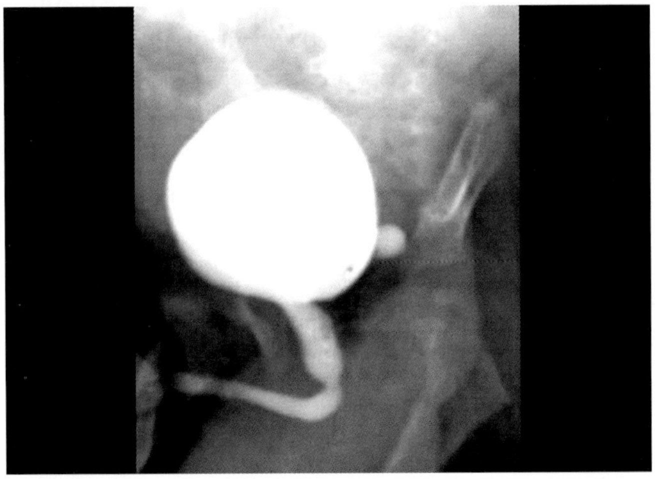

Fig. 21: Hutch diverticulum: MCU showing a paraureteric (Hutch) diverticulum.

Iatrogenic diverticulae are most often seen in the anterior wall of the bladder at the site of previous vesicostomy or suprapubic drainage catheter and at VUJ following ureteral reimplantation.

Bladder diverticulae are best imaged by contrast cystography, US and CT. The appearance of diverticulae varies with location, size and pressure effect due to adjacent structures and the presence of complicating stone or tumor. A wide neck diverticulum fills and empties readily with the bladder, if the neck of diverticulum is narrow with poor emptying, the diverticulum may be better appreciated on post void film.

Neurogenic Bladder

In contrast to adult patient in whom neurogenic bladder is most often due to an acquired, usually traumatic spinal cord lesion, the vast majority of children affected with this disorder have a myelomeningocele or a related myelodysplastic anomaly (occult spinal dysraphism, sacral agenesis).

Myelomeningocele can occur at any level of the spine but is most often located in the lumbosacral area. The radiographs of the affected area show widening of the neural canal, defective posterior neural arches, absence of the posterior spinous processes, and widened interpedicular distance involving several segments, with elongated and flattened or defective pedicles.

Occult myelodysplasia is a group of congenital anomalies of the spinal cord in which the overlying skin is intact although cutaneous stigmata of the disorder may be present such as local hair overgrowth, hyperpigmentation, hemangioma, a skin dimple, or an ill-defined soft tissue mass due to a lipoma. These anomalies include tethered cord, diastematomyelia, intraspinal lipoma, dermoid cyst, and hamartoma. Radiographs of the spine may show osseous changes similar to those seen in myelomeningocele, and sometimes scoliosis or broad vertebral bodies.

Children with this disorder commonly have inappropriate detrusor muscle contraction and external sphincter relaxation, resulting in uncontrolled voiding pattern with incomplete bladder emptying.[48] Initially, the upper tracts are normal but due to poor bladder emptying secondary changes of reflux and infection result.

Complete evaluation of patients suspected of having neurogenic bladder requires VCUG for assessment of lower urinary tract, US and one of the functional studies of IVU or scintigraphy for upper tract. However, for the diagnosis of primary cause, examination with plain radiographs and MRI is essential.

On VCUG, bladder is usually elongated, pointing upwards (Christmas tree shape) with varying degrees of trabeculation and sacculation **(Fig. 22)**. Rarely bladder may be large, smooth, atonic type. During voiding, bladder neck and proximal posterior urethra are dilated forming a funnel shape with the point of the funnel directed caudally at mid posterior urethra level. Distal urinary stream is usually poor with significant post void residual urine. Associated VUR is common. Urodynamic techniques have assumed a major role in the evaluation of neurogenic bladder and contributed significantly to the management.

Megacystis

Megacystis is a descriptive term for a large, smooth walled bladder. It may be a normal variation or a congenital anomaly of little clinical significance. A large smooth walled bladder is a common finding in Prune Belly syndrome. It may be seen in patients with excessive urine formation, e.g. diabetes insipidus. Uncommonly it may be seen in neurogenic disease.

Prune Belly Syndrome

Prune belly syndrome is a rare congenital syndrome usually affecting the males. The term prune belly refers to a lax, wrinkled abdominal wall, which is frequently associated with other anomalies.[49] The syndrome comprises of deficiency of abdominal muscles, undescended testis and urinary tract anomalies. On voiding cystourethrography, bladder is enlarged and elongated but lacks trabeculations and dilated high placed posterior urethra is a characteristic finding **(Fig. 23)**. Upper tract findings include renal dysmorphism or marked hydroureteronephrosis. Nonfunctioning kidney may also be seen.

Urachal Anomalies

In early fetal life the bladder extends to the umbilicus where it is in continuity with the allantois. As the fetus grows the cephalad part of bladder narrows to form a channel, the urachus, which obliterates into a fibrous cord called the medial umbilical ligament. Failure of the urachus to regress may result in one of the following four types of congential anomalies.[50]

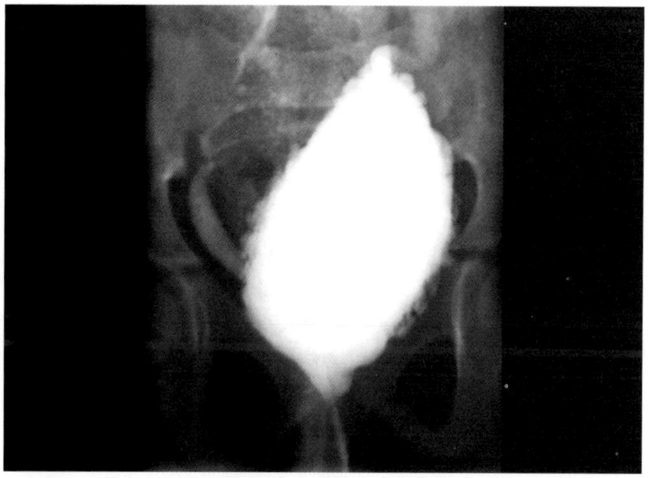

Fig. 22: Neurogenic bladder: Bladder is elongated upwards with trabeculations and sacculations.

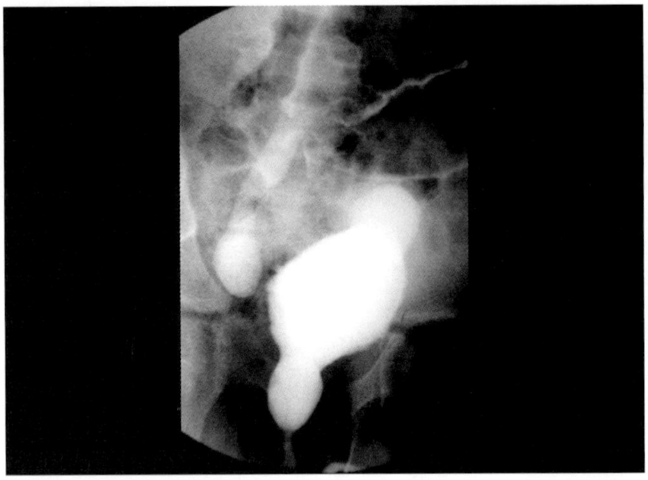

Fig. 23: Prune belly syndrome. VCUG showing enlarged and elongated bladder that lacks trabeculations, dilated high placed posterior urethra and dilated right ureter.

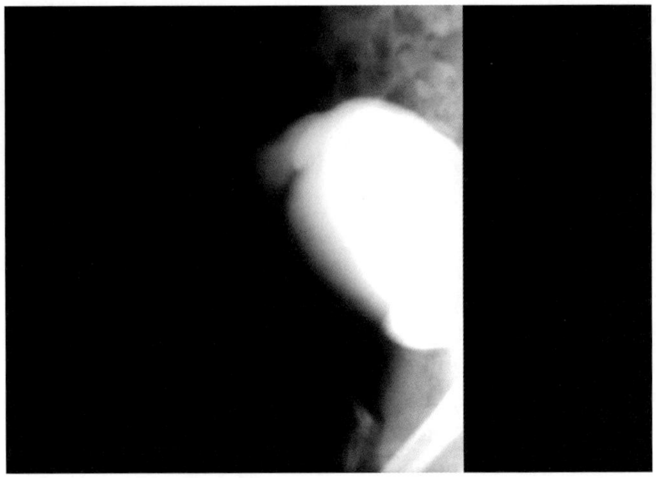

Fig. 24: Urachal diverticulum: Blind ending dilated urachus seen at the anterior superior aspect of the bladder.

Types of Anomalies

1. Patent urachus
2. Urachal cyst
3. Urachal sinus
4. Urachal diverticulum

Patent urachus: The failure of the entire course of the urachus to close results in an open channel between the bladder and the umbilicus. A patent urachus is diagnosed in a newborn when urine is seen leaking from the umbilicus.

Urachal cyst: It results from obliteration of both the umbilical and the vesical ends of the urachal lumen with an intervening portion remaining patent and fluid filled. Generally, it occurs in that part of the urachus which is closer to the bladder. It usually remains clinically obscure till complicated by either infection or rarely a tumor.

Urachal sinus: Urachal sinus is a blind ending dilatation of the urachus at the umbilical end.

Urachal diverticulum: Urachal diverticulum is a blind ending dilatation of the urachus at the anterosuperior aspect of the bladder as a result of failure of closure of the urachus at the bladder end **(Fig. 24)**.

The diagnosis of patent urachus can be made either by catheterization of the bladder through the umbilicus or by VCUG with films taken in lateral projection. Diagnosis of urachal sinus is made by catheterization and opacification of the umbilical fistula. Urachal diverticulum is demonstrated by VCUG with films in lateral projection. Diagnosis of urachal cysts is more difficult. The cystogram may show only an extrinsic compression on the dome of the bladder in the mid line or slightly to one side. US, CT or MRI may demonstrate the lesion better.

ABNORMALITIES OF THE URETHRA

Posterior Urethral Valve

Posterior urethral valve is the most common congenital obstructive lesion of the urethra and the most important cause of end stage renal disease in boys. Three types of posterior urethral valves (PUV) have been recognized based on urethroscopic findings.[51]

Type I: Two fibroepithelial valve like folds originate from the lower pole of the verumontanum and course obliquely to the most distal portion of the prostatic urethra. The two folds fuse anteriorly, leaving a cleft as the only passage for urine. This is the most common form of PUV.

Type II: PUV related to superior urethral crest and its fins, is believed to be very rare or nonexistent.

Type III: This type of PUV is also relatively less common as compared to Type I. In patients with this type of valve a transverse membrane is seen in the posterior urethra just below the verumontanum sometimes near the urogenital diaphragm.

Imaging Features

VCUG is the gold standard for imaging PUV. On voiding films, the posterior urethra is markedly dilated and elongated down to the level of PUV. The transition between the dilated posterior and anterior normal urethra is abrupt with a thin stream **(Fig. 25)**. The valves may be seen as two

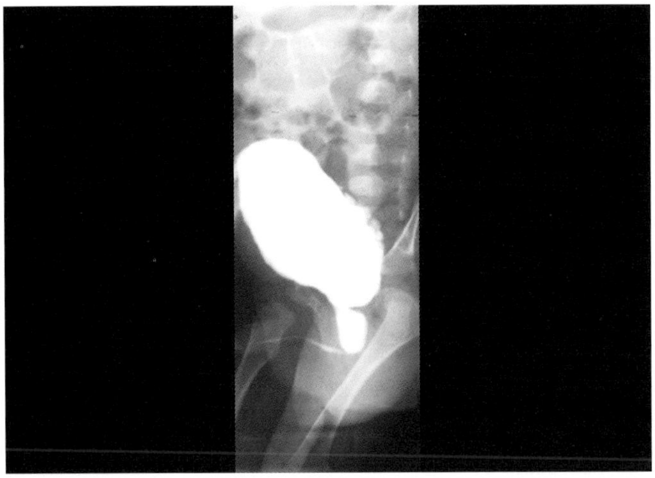

Fig. 25: Posterior urethral valve: MCU showing markedly dilated posterior urethra and thin stream of contrast in anterior urethra. Bladder shows back pressure changes of multiple saccules and diverticulae.

radiolucent lines. A posterior indentation or posterior lip is often present at the level of bladder neck due to bladder neck hypertrophy. Reflux of contrast into the prostatic or ejaculatory ducts may occur and a prominent utricle may be seen. Classic PUV is not visible on a retrograde urethrogam since the valves are displaced and flattened against the urethral wall by the retrograde flow of contrast.

Secondary, obstructive changes of varying severity develop in the bladder, ureters and kidneys. The bladder becomes hypertrophied and trabeculated and develops saccules and diverticulae. In approximately 50% of patients VUR may be present.[52] The ureters are often dilated, elongated and tortuous, along with hydronephrosis. Associated renal dysplasia of varying degree is common and the affected kidney may be small.

Apart from VCUG, US is a valuable modality for evaluation of PUV. US evaluates size of the kidneys, thickness of renal parenchyma, degree of hydronephrosis, dilatation of the ureters, and bladder wall thickness. Mid line sagittal scans of the base of the bladder through suprapubic approach or through perineum may show dilatation of the proximal posterior urethra.[53] Evaluation of kidneys may be carried out by nuclear scan.

The newborns with PUV and severe degree of obstructive changes may be associated with Potter facies and pulmonary hypoplasia. Abdominal distension and palpable abdominal masses due to an enlarged bladder and kidneys may be noted. A localized perirenal urinoma or urinary ascites due to a rent in the caliceal fornix or in the bladder may also contribute to the abdominal enlargement. The prenatal US may reveal bilateral hydronephrosis, hydroureters, a thickened bladder wall and a dilated posterior urethra in sagittal scans (Keyhole sign).[54] Fetal MRI is the best imaging test for antenatal diagnosis in late gestation when ossifying pelvic bones interfere with the visualization of bladder outlet on sonography.

Posterior Urethral Polyp

This is a relatively uncommon lesion of the male posterior urethra and is usually diagnosed in children between 3 to 6 years of age but may be seen even in infants or adults.The lesion is also called congenital polyp of the verumontanum which consists of an elongated, freely mobile polypoid mass on a long stalk originating from the verumontanum. It is a benign hamartomatous lesion. The symptoms are those of intermittent urethral obstruction. On VCUG urethral polyp is seen as a rounded/oval filling defect in the distal posterior urethra. At the end of voiding the polyp is displaced upwards at the level of bladder outlet.[55]

Prostatic Utricle and Müllerian Duct Cyst

Prostatic utricle is a small diverticulum of the prostatic urethra located in verumontanum between the two openings of the ejaculatory ducts and extends backwards and slightly upwards for a short distance within the medial lobe of the prostate. The utricle is occasionally seen on routine VCUG as a tiny diverticulum of few millimeters length. Large size prostatic utricle occasionally may be seen in normal males and in other conditions, e.g. Male hypospadias, Prune Belly syndrome and anorectal anomalies.

Müllerian duct cyst or cyst of the prostatic utricle is a cystic dilatation of an obstructed utricle occurring in patients with otherwise normal lower urinary tract. The obstruction could be due to congenital valves, mucosal folds, or local infection. The cysts vary in size from a few cm in diameter to a large pelvic mass, displacing the bladder upwards and forwards and sometimes obstructing the urethra. Stones may form in these cysts. The cysts may communicate with urethra by a minute tract. The cystic nature and location of the pelvic mass is readily determined by US, CT or MRI.

Cowper's Duct Cyst

Cowper's glands are paired structures located on either side of the membranous urethra within the urogenital diaphragm. Their ducts are directed forward through the bulb of the corpus spongiosum to end in the ventral aspect of the bulbar urethra. The ducts and the glands may sometimes be opacified during VCUG. Abnormalities of the Cowper's duct are uncommon. Syringoceles or cystic dilatation occurs most commonly in infants and young children secondary to narrowing of the duct orifice. Clinical findings include recurrent urinary tract infection and obstructive voiding symptoms. Rarely Cowper's duct cyst appears as a perineal mass. The dilated duct is seen on VCUG as a filling defect on the ventral surface of the bulbar urethra. Reflux of contrast material into a patulous or perforated syringocele opacifies the dilated duct.

Male Hypospadias/Epispadias

Hypospadias is a condition in which the urethral meatus opens on the ventral surface of the penis at a point proximal to the glans. In epispadias, in contradistinction, the urethral orifice is located on the dorsal aspect of the penis. Epispadias is usually seen in association with various forms of exstrophy. Epispadias in female is associated with a short patulous urethra, widely separated labia and a bifid clitoris. In either, hypospadias or epispadias, VCUG demonstrates a foreshortened urethra.

Anterior Urethral Diverticulum and Anterior Urethral Valve

Anterior urethral diverticulum, although uncommon, is the second most common cause of congenital urethral obstruction in boys. Anterior urethral diverticulum is a saccular outpouching of the ventral aspect of the anterior urethra commonly near penoscrotal junction. The diverticulum has a well defined valve like anterior lip and a less well defined posterior lip. The diverticulum fills during voiding, thereby narrowing and obstructing the true urethra. Complications resulting from the presence of diverticulum are incomplete bladder emptying and infection. On VCUG, the typical saccular diverticulum of the anterior urethra fills with contrast material and appears as an oval shaped structure on the ventral aspect of anterior urethra **(Fig. 26)**. At times RGU may be required to demonstrate the neck of the diverticulum.

Anterior urethral valve is a semilunar fold similar to anterior lip of a urethral diverticulum with absence of posterior lip. 40% of the anterior urethral valves are located in the bulbar urethra, 30% at the penoscrotal junction, and 30% in the pendulous urethra. VCUG is the diagnostic modality of choice for anterior urethral valves. Typically, the urethra appears dilated proximal to the valve and narrowed distal to it. A valve may appear as a linear filling defect along the ventral wall, or it may be indicated by an abrupt change in the caliber of the dilated urethra.

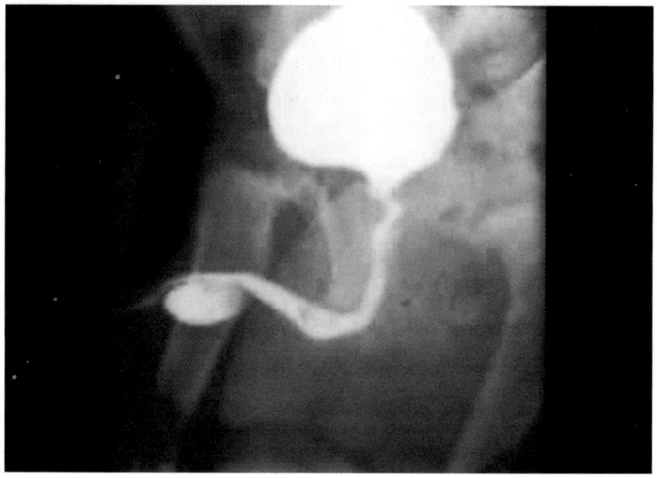

Fig. 26: Anterior urethral diverticulum: A large diverticulum is seen on the ventral aspect of the anterior urethra.

Urethral Duplication

Urethral duplication may be complete or incomplete and may take several forms. Two separate structures may originate from the bladder and persist with separate external drainage; a common urethra may originate from the bladder and duplicate distally; or a duplicated origin may unite distally into a single external orifice.[56] According, to the location of the accessory urethral opening on the dorsal or ventral aspect of the penis, urethral duplications are divided into epispadiac (more common) and hypospadiac types. The diagnosis is made by VCUG or catheterization and opacification of both the urethras.

Megalourethra

Megalourethra is a rare anomaly in which abnormal development of the corpus spongiosum and corpus cavernosum results in congenital dilatation of penile urethra without obstruction. On VCUG the penile urethra is seen markedly dilated and fusiform, with tapering both distally and proximally into a relatively normal urethra. Sometimes, the anomaly affects a small portion of the urethra. The anomaly may occur as an isolated lesion but is seen more commonly in prune belly syndrome.

Scaphoid megalourethra is more common than fusiform type. It consists of a localized saccular dilatation of the penile urethra caused by a localized absence of the corpus spongiosum. During voiding the affected part of urethra balloons markedly causing a large smooth bulge on the ventral surface of the urethra assuming a scaphoid configuration.[57]

Congenital Meatal Stenosis

Congenital meatal stenosis is a pin point narrowing of the urethral orifice and is seen in patients with hypospadias. Acquired meatal stenosis is more common than congenital stenosis. VCUG demonstrates dilatation of the urethra proximal to a narrowed meatal orifice. Radiologic evaluation of meatal stenosis, however, is usually not required.

REFERENCES

1. Steinhardt JM, Kuhn LP, Eisenberg B. Ultrasound screening of healthy infants for urinary tract abnormalities. Pediatrics. 1988;82:609-12.
2. Kraus SJ. Genitourinary Imaging in children in pediatric urology. Pediatr Clin North Am. 2001;48:1381-424.
3. Johnson CE, Elder JS, Judge NE, et al. The accuracy of antenatal ultrasonography in identifying renal abnormalities. Am J Dis Child. 1992;146(10):1181-4.
4. Harvie S, McLeod L, Acott P, Walsh E, Abdolell M, Macken MB. Abnormal antenatal sonogram: An indicator of disease severity in children with posterior urethral valves. Can Assoc Radiol J. 2009;60(4):185-9.
5. Payabvash S, Kajbafzadeh AM, Saeedi P, Sadeghi Z, Elmi A, Mehdizadeh M. Application of magnetic resonance urography in diagnosis of congenital urogenital anomalies in children. Pediatr Surg Int. 2008;24(9):979-86.
6. Staatz G, Rohrmann D, Nolte-Ernsting CC, et al. Magnetic resonance urography in children: Evaluation of suspected ureteral ectopia in duplex systems. J Urol. 2001;166:2346-50.
7. Perez-Brayfield MR, Kirsch AJ, Jones RA, et al. A prospective study comparing ultrasound, nuclear scintigraphy and dynamic contrast enhanced magnetic resonance imaging in the evaluation of hydronephrosis. J Urol. 2003;170:1330-4.
8. Grattan-Smith JD, Jones RA. MR urography in children. Pediatr Radiol. 2006;36:1119-32.
9. Grobner T. Gadolinium—a specific trigger for the development of nephrogenic fibrosing dermopathy and nephrogenic systemic fibrosis? Nephrol Dial Transplant. 2006;21:1104-8.
10. Brody AS, Frush DP, Huda W, et al. Radiation risk to children from computed tomography. Pediatrics. 2007;120:677-82.
11. Han BK, Babcock DS. Sonographic measurements and appearances of normal kidneys in children. AJR. 1985;145:611-6.
12. De Brugn R, Gordon I, Mc Hugh K. Pediatric Uroradiology. In Grainger RG, Allison D (Eds): Diagnostic Radiology: A Textbook of Medical Imaging. New York: Churchill Livingstone; 2001.pp.1717-64.
13. Sadler TW (Ed). Langman's Medical Embryology, 9th edition. Philadelphia, PA, Lippincott Williams and Wilkins; 2004.
14. Trigaux JP, Van Beers B, Delchambre F. Male genital tract malformations associated with ipsilateral renal agenesis: Sonographic findings. J Clin Ultrasound. 1991;19:3-10.
15. Shalaby-Rana E, Lowe LH, Blask AN, et al. Imaging in pediatric urology. Pediatr Clin North Am. 1997;44:1065-89.
16. Jefferson KP, et al. Thoracic kidney; a rare form of renal ectopia. J Urol. 2001;165(2):502.
17. Pennington DJ, Zerin JM. Imaging of the urinary tract in children. Pediatr Ann. 1999;28:678-86.
18. Glodny B, Petersen J, Hofmann KJ, Schenk C, Herwig R, Trieb T, Koppelstaetter C, Steingruber I, Rehder P. Kidney fusion anomalies revisited: Clinical and radiological analysis of. 209 cases of crossed fused ectopia and horseshoe kidney. BJU Int. 2009;103(2):224-35.
19. Gu LL, et al. Crossed solitary renal ectopia. Urology. 1991;38(6):556-8.
20. Begin LR, Guy L, Jacobson SA, et al. Renal carcinoid and horseshoe kidney: A frequent association of the two rare entities—a case report and review of the literature. J Surg Oncol. 1998;68:113-9.
21. Strauss S. Sonographic features of horseshoe kidney. J Ultrasound Med. 2000;19(1):27-31.
22. Pozniak MA, Nakada SY. Three-dimensional computed tomographic angiography of a horseshoe kidney with ureteropelvic junction obstruction. Urology. 1997;49(2):267-8.
23. El-Nahas AR, Abou El-Ghar ME, Refae HF, Gad HM, El-Diasty TA. Magnetic resonance imaging in the evaluation of pelvi-ureteric junction obstruction: An all-in-one approach. BJU Int. 2007;99(3):641-5.
24. Tokunaka S, Osanai H, Hashimoto H, et al. Severe hypertension in infant with unilateral hypoplastic kidney. Urology. 1987;29:618-20.
25. Osathanondh V, Potter EL. Pathogenesis of polycystic kidneys. Survey of results of microdissection. Arch Pathol. 1964;77:510-2.
26. Turkbey B, Ocak I, Daryanani K, Font-Montgomery E, Lukose L, Bryant J, Tuchman M, Mohan P, Heller T, Gahl WA, Choyke PL, Gunay-Aygun M. Autosomal recessive polycystic kidney disease and congenital hepatic fibrosis (ARPKD/CHF). Pediatr Radiol. 2009;39(2):100-11.
27. Traubici J, Daneman A. High-resolution renal sonography in children with autosomal recessive polycystic kidney disease. Am J Roentgenol. 2005;184(5):1630-3.
28. Srivastava T, Garola RE, Hellerstein S. Autosomal dominant inheritance of multicystic dysplastic kidney. Pediatr Nephrol. 1999;13(6):481-3.
29. Kaneyama K, Yamataka A, Satake S, Yanai T, Lane GJ, Kaneko K, Yamashiro Y, Miyano T. Associated urologic anomalies in children with solitary kidney. J Pediatr Surg. 2004;39(1):85-7.
30. Eckoldt F, Woderich R, Smith RD, Heling KS. Antenatal diagnostic aspects of unilateral multicystic kidney dysplasia—sensitivity, specificity, predictive values, differential diagnoses, associated malformations and consequences. Fetal Diagn Ther. 2004;19(2):163-9.
31. Avni FE, Guissard G, Hall M, Janssen F, DeMaertelaer V, Rypens F. Hereditary polycystic kidney diseases in children: Changing sonographic patterns through childhood. Pediatr Radiol. 2002;32(3):169-74.
32. Talner LB. "Specific causes of obstruction". In Pollack HM (Ed): Clinical Urography. Philadelphia: WB Saunders Co. 1990;2:1629-751.

33. Park JM, Bloom DA. The pathophysiology of UPJ obstruction. Current concepts. Urol Clin North Am. 1998; 25(2):161-9.
34. Khaira HS, Platt JF, Cohan RH, Wolf JS, Faerber GJ. Helical computed tomography for identification of crossing vessels in ureteropelvic junction obstruction-comparison with operative findings. Urology. 2003;62(1):35-9.
35. Beck AD. The effect of intrauterine urinary obstruction upon the development of fetal kidney. J Urol. 1971;105:784.
36. Platt JF, Rubin JM, Ellis JH, et al. Duplex Doppler US of the kidney-differentiation of obstructive from non-obstructive dilatation. Radiology. 1989;171:515-7.
37. Malleck R, Bankiee AA, Hainz E, et al. Distinction between obstructive and non-obstructive hydronephrosis: Value of diuresis duplex Doppler sonography. AJR. 1996;166:113.
38. Ramsey PG. Opacification of the renal parenchyma in obstruction and reflux. Paediatr Radiol. 1976;4:226.
39. Dunbar JS, Nogardy MB. The calyceal crescent—a roentgenographic sign of obstructive hydronephrosis. AJR. 1970;110:520.
40. Stephens FD. Ureterovascular hydronephrosis and the "aberrant" renal vessels. J Urol. 1982;128:984.
41. Whitfield HN, Britton KE, Hendry WF, et al. Furosemide intravenous urography in the diagnosis of PUJ obstruction. Br J Urol. 1985;57:351.
42. Lebowitz RL, Blickman JG. The coexistence of ureteropelvic junction obstruction and reflux. AJR. 1983;140:231.
43. Lupton EW, Testa HJ, Lawsan RS, et al. Diuresis renography and the results of pyelplasty for idopathic hydronephrosis. Br J Urol. 1979;51:449.
44. Nussbaum AR, Dort JP, Jeffs RD, et al. Ectopic ureter and uroterocoele: Their varied radiographic manifestations. Radiology. 1986;159:227-35.
45. Blickman JG, Lebowitz RL. The coexistence of primary megaureter and reflux. AJR. 1984;143:1053.
46. Dunetz GN, Bauer SB. Complete duplication of bladder and urethra. Urology. 1985;25:179-82.
47. Cohen HL, Kravets F, Zucconi W, Ratani R, Shah S, Dougherty D. Congenital abnormalities of the genitourinary system. Semin Roentgenol. 2004;39(2):282-303.
48. Bauer SB. Neurogenic bladder dysfunction. Pediatr Cli North America. 1987;34:1121-40.
49. Jennings RW. Prune Belly syndrome. Semin Pediatr Surg. 2000;9:115-20.
50. Suita S, Nagasaki A. Urachal remnants. Semin Pediatr Surg. 1996;5:107-15.
51. Wendelin SH. The urinary bladder. In Davidson AJ, Hartman DS (Eds): Radiology of the Kidney and Urinary Tract Philadelphia: WB Saunders Co. 1994. pp.607-48.
52. Chatterjee SK, Banerjee S, Basak D, et al. Posterior urethral valves: The scenario in a developing center. Pediatr Surg Int. 2001;17:2-7.
53. Cohen HL, Susman M, Haller JO, et al. Posterior urethral valve: Transperineal US for imaging and diagnosis in male infants. Radiology. 1994;192:261-4.
54. Eckoldt F, Heling KS, Woderich R, Wolke S. Posterior urethral valves: Prenatal diagnostic signs and outcome. Urol Int. 2004;73(4):296-301.
55. Silverman FN, Kuhn JP. Abnormalities of the lower urinary tract. Caffey's Paediatric X-ray Diagnosis: An Integrated Imaging Approach, 9th edition. Mosby. 1993. pp.1278-98.
56. Effman EL, Lebowitz RL, Colodny AH. Duplication of urethra. Radiology. 1976;119:179-85.
57. Kester RR, Woopan UM, Ohm HK. Congenital megalo-urethra. J Urol. 1990;4:1213-5.

CHAPTER 140

Urinary Tract Infections (Including VUR and Neurogenic Bladder)

Kushaljit Singh Sodhi, Akshay Kumar Saxena

Urinary tract infection (UTI) is a common febrile illness in children. Although, most of these children recover with an excellent prognosis, a minority will still have long-term complications and sequelae, such as hypertension, chronic renal insufficiency, and end-stage renal failure. These potential complications are the basis for rapid appropriate investigations, prompt treatment, and subsequent customized follow-up of UTI in children.[1,2] Interventions, such as follow-up imaging, antibiotic prophylaxis, and surgical correction, are thought to reduce the incidence of the long-term complications.[3-5]

The urine culture is a critical component of the workup for a presumed UTI. The culture identifies the organism causing the infection and helps guide treatment with right antibiotics. The traditional definition for a clinically significant UTI is more than 100,000 cfu/mL.[3,4] However, lower numbers can also constitute a UTI because of additional factors (e.g. hydrational dilution and frequent voiding).[3,4]

INCIDENCE

It has been estimated that 7% of girls and 2% of boys have a UTI prior to 6 years of age.[3,6] During the first year of life more boys than girls are diagnosed with a UTI, with uncircumcized boys having a 10-fold greater risk than those circumcized.[3,6] This trend reverses after the first year of life, with more girls than boys being diagnosed with a UTI.

Of children who have UTI, between 25% and 40% are found to have vesicoureteral reflux (VUR).[5,7] Of children who have febrile UTI, 50–91% are found to have defects on renal cortical scintigraphy, indicating acute pyelonephritis (APN).[5,8] However, when VUR is present, renal cortical abnormalities are shown by scintigraphy in 79–86% of the kidneys.[8]

Although, these statistics show that VUR is a precipitating factor in APN, studies[5,9] have also found that 61% of kidneys with evidence of APN on scintigraphy did not have VUR, and 53% of refluxing kidneys did not have any defect on scintigraphy to suggest APN. Therefore, VUR and APN frequently also occur independently of one another.[9,10]

Of children with APN diagnosed by scintigraphy, 38–57% will develop permanent renal scarring.[5,11,12] A recent study by Oh et al.[13] found a correlation between the severity VUR grade and frequency of APN on renal scintigraphy; however, the likelihood of APN becoming permanent renal scarring was independent of the VUR grade.

RADIOLOGICAL MODALITIES FOR IMAGING OF UTI

Imaging may entail renal ultrasound (US) for the detection of congenital abnormalities, obstruction, and scarring; micturating cystourethrography (MCU) for the identification of vesicoureteric reflux; and ^{99m}Tc-labeled dimer captosuccinic acid (DMSA) renal scintigraphy for the determination of scarring. Depending on the clinical scenario, one or more of these examinations may be performed after a child's first episode of UTI; indeed, in many cases, all three investigations are performed.[1]

ROLE OF ULTRASOUND IN FIRST TIME UTI

Ultrasound has always been a part of the routine evaluation of first time UTI because it is very useful in depicting structural abnormalities such as asymmetric renal size, hydronephrosis, and duplex kidneys. Ultrasound is a noninvasive study which requires no sedation or ionizing radiation.

However, due to its low yield for additional clinical information, its role has been questioned in many recent articles. Zamir et al.[14] found that ultrasound failed to alter clinical management in any of 255 first uncomplicated UTI patients. Many other studies raise concern that routine ultrasound for UTI may not be justifiable, given its somewhat negligible effect on patient management.

On the contrary, in a more recent study, Huang et al.[15] found ultrasound abnormalities in 112 (28.7%) of 390 children with UTI residing in a country in which antenatal ultrasound is routinely performed. The abnormalities detected included asymmetric renal size, intermittent hydronephrosis, and duplicated collecting system. The presence of these findings correlated to a higher prevalence and grade of VUR. The authors concluded that routine ultrasound for UTI is worth performing.

Vesicoureteral Reflux

Vesicoureteral reflux (VUR) refers to the retrograde passage of urine from the bladder into the ureter and often to the calices. VUR can occur due to one of the following causes:[16,17]

- Abnormality of ureterovesical junction (UVJ).
- Marginally competent UVJ becoming incompetent due to urinary tract infection.
- Lateral ureteral ectopia.
- Abnormal bladder wall, e.g. Prune belly syndrome.
- Bladder outlet obstruction and neurogenic bladder.
- Reflux following interference of UVJ (iatrogenic).

As it is generally believed that VUR correlates to risk of renal scar development, pediatric patients with UTI undergo various imaging tests to detect vesicoureteral reflux.

PATHOPHYSIOLOGY OF VUR AND PYELONEPHRITIS

The distal most part of ureter traverses obliquely through the bladder wall into the ureteral orifice. Over a period of time, as the bladder distends with urine, increasing compression of the intramural and submucosal segment of ureter prevents retrograde flow of urine into the distal most ureter. However, the effectiveness of this particular valvular function is dependent on the length of the distal ureteral segment that lies within the bladder wall: A shorter intramural-submucosal segment increases the likelihood of VUR.[5] The normal length of the intramural-submucosal segment varies with age in children, is reported to range from 7 to 12 mm.[18] The objective of ureteral reimplantation surgery for VUR is to construct a more oblique ureteral course through the bladder wall, thus lengthening the intramural-submucosal segment.[5]

Pyelonephritis on the other hand, is usually caused by ascending bacterial infection in the urinary tract. VUR and urinary stasis predispose urine in the renal pelvis to infection. Bacteria are thus able to enter the renal parenchyma, leading to inflammation and edema. Subsequently, the parenchymal microvasculature becomes compressed, which can lead to ischemia, microabscess formation, and necrosis.[5] If the renal parenchyma is unable to recover from these injuries, permanent renal scarring with loss of parenchymal volume and function can also result. Renal cortical scintigraphy with ^{99m}Tc-dimercaptosuccinic acid (DMSA) is considered to be the imaging technique of choice to detect acute pyelonephritis and renal scarring because of its high sensitivity,[5,19] both entities appear as photopenic defects on DMSA scans, and the radiologist/nuclear physician has to rely on the clinical time course to distinguish between the two entities.

IMAGING FINDINGS IN ACUTE PYELONEPHRITIS

Urographic (Intravenous Urography-(IVU)) findings consist of diffuse renal enlargement, decreased patchy or striated nephrogram, delayed calyceal opacification and attenuation or effacement of the PCS. Renal US may be entirely normal or may show generalized or patchy decrease (rarely increase) in parenchymal echogenicity with decreased vascularity **(Fig. 1)**. Ultrasound is mainly performed for detection of associated abnormalities, e.g. calculi, obstructive uropathy or nephrocalcinosis.[20]

Renal cortical scintigraphy with ^{99m}Tc glucoheptonate (GH) or DMSA with a sensitivity of 91% and specificity of 99.9%, is the imaging procedure of choice for acute pyelonephritis.[21] Cortical scintigraphy demonstrates a pattern of focally reduced or absent cortical accumulation of the radio-pharmaceutical with no evidence of volume loss; the defects may be solitary, multiple, or involve the entire kidney giving rise to a mottled tracer distribution **(Figs. 2 and 3)**. On contrast-enhanced computed tomography (CECT) and contrast-enhanced magnetic resonance (CEMR), the affected kidney may show a

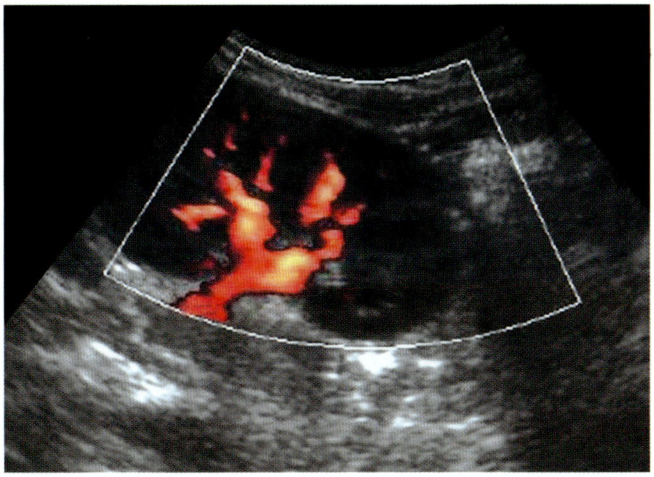

Fig. 1: Power Doppler ultrasound of kidney reveals a well-defined area of altered echogenicity at lower pole, which demonstrates decreased flow and perfusion, corresponding to acute pyelonephritis.

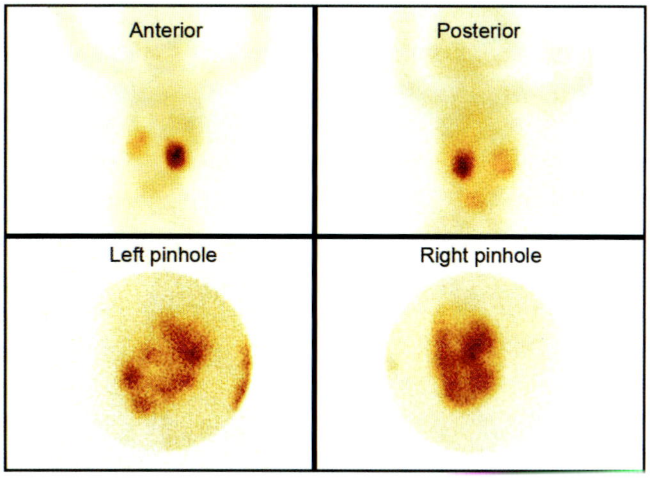

Fig. 2: ^{99m}Tc DMSA scan showing multiple photopenic areas in both kidneys, suggestive of pyelonephritis.

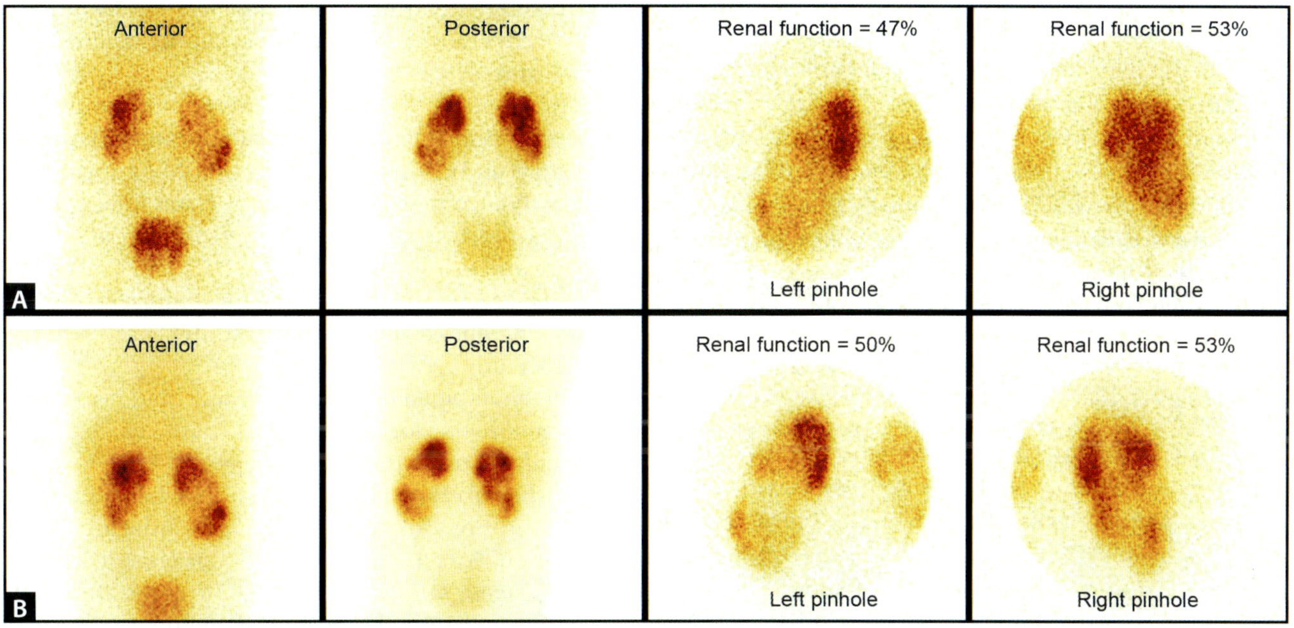

Figs. 3A and B: Consecutive ^{99m}Tc DMSA scans in 2008 (A) and 2010 (B) showing persistent photopenic defects in both kidney cortices, indicative of renal scarring.

striated nephrogram with multiple, poorly enhancing wedge-shaped (rarely round and irregular) areas fanning out from the calyces, and reaching upto the cortex of the kidney **(Fig. 4)**.

All children with acute pyelonephritis require US and DMSA scans in the acute phase; if the US is normal but the isotope scan is abnormal, follow-up scanning 3–6 months later is suggested, to detect whether the kidney has healed or scarred.[20,22]

ACUTE FOCAL BACTERIAL NEPHRITIS

In this form of acute pyelonephritis, which is also called acute lobar nephronia, the inflammatory process is localized or segmental, often affecting a renal pole or one moiety of a duplex kidney. On renal ultrasound, the swollen part of the kidney appears as a hypoechoic poorly marginated mass with low-level echoes scattered throughout. Acute infection produces wedge-shaped areas with decreased perfusion on Doppler US.[23]

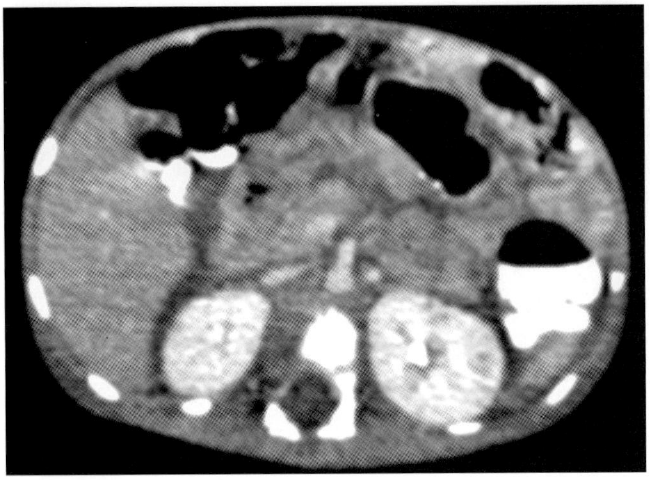

Fig. 4: CECT abdomen demonstrates well-defined poorly enhancing areas of acute pyelonephritis in left kidney.

These are better shown with power Doppler.[20] However, Power Doppler US is not as sensitive for pyelonephritis as renal scintigraphy performed with DMSA. CECT shows poor and mottled enhancement of the area sometimes associated with wedge-shaped hypodense zones. In general, the renal mass is not sharply defined from rest of the kidney and lacks a well-defined wall in contrast with a renal abscess which shows a relatively well-defined wall which enhances on CECT. A decreased uptake of the tracer is seen on nuclear scintigraphy. IVU shows localized enlargement of part of the kidney with focally reduced nephrographic density and is non-specific for pyelonephritis.

Grading of VUR

The accepted technique for reporting and grading VUR is the International Reflux Study Committee's classification for radiographic grades of reflux, which was suggested as a system to provide standardization of reporting technique.[24] The classification is shown below and should be used in radiology reports, wherever possible so that effective communication between clinicians and radiologists takes place.

Grade I: Reflux to the ureter but not to the kidney.

Grade II: Reflux to the ureter, pelvis and calyces without dilatation.

Grade III: Reflux to the calyces with mild dilatation or tortuosity of the ureter, mild dilatation of renal pelvis and calyces, with normal or slightly blunted calyceal fornices.

Grade IV: Reflux into moderately dilated ureter and pelvicalyceal system with blunting of the fornices but preservation of papillary indentation.

Grade V: Reflux into grossly dilated ureter and pelvicalyceal system with loss of papillary indentation.

Imaging of VUR

- Micturating cystourethrogram (MCU)
- Radionuclide cystography (RNC)
- Voiding urosonography (VUS)
- MRI

MICTURATING CYSTOURETHROGRAM

Micturating cystourethrogram (MCU), also known as voiding cystourethrogram (VCUG) is one of the most commonly performed fluoroscopic investigations in pediatric radiology departments.[25] It is currently the investigation of choice for delineating the anatomy and determining the function of the lower urogenital tract.[25] It is the primary diagnostic procedure for evaluation of VUR in children. MCU should be used to document the presence of VUR and to determine the grade of reflux and whether reflux occurs during micturation or during bladder filling **(Figs. 5 and 6)**.

A proper technique is essential for performing MCU. Catheterization should be performed using strict aseptic technique and contrast medium should be instilled via the gravity drip method and not by hand injection. This prevents the introduction of contrast medium under pressure and is less likely to cause transmucosal contrast medium absorption and consequent contrast reactions.[26]

Recommended views for MCU study[25] are:

- Early filling view of bladder.
- *Full bladder view:* The expected bladder capacity (in milliliters) for children less than 2 years of age is calculated using the formula (age + 2) × 30.[25,27]
- *Voiding urethra view:* This should be obtained by turning boys in the right or left anterior oblique position. For girls, supine position is obtained.
- *Renal view following voiding:* To determine, if any contrast medium has reached the kidneys (reflux).
- *Bladder view following voiding:* This assesses the degree of bladder emptying. The majority of children under 1 year of age do not empty their bladder completely during a VCUG,[28] but a complete bladder emptying episode does help, exclude bladder neuropathy.

The last three images should be repeated as part of a cyclical voiding study.

PRACTICE AND CONCEPT OF CYCLICAL VOIDING

It has been recommended that in order to increase the diagnostic yield of VUR in MCU examinations,

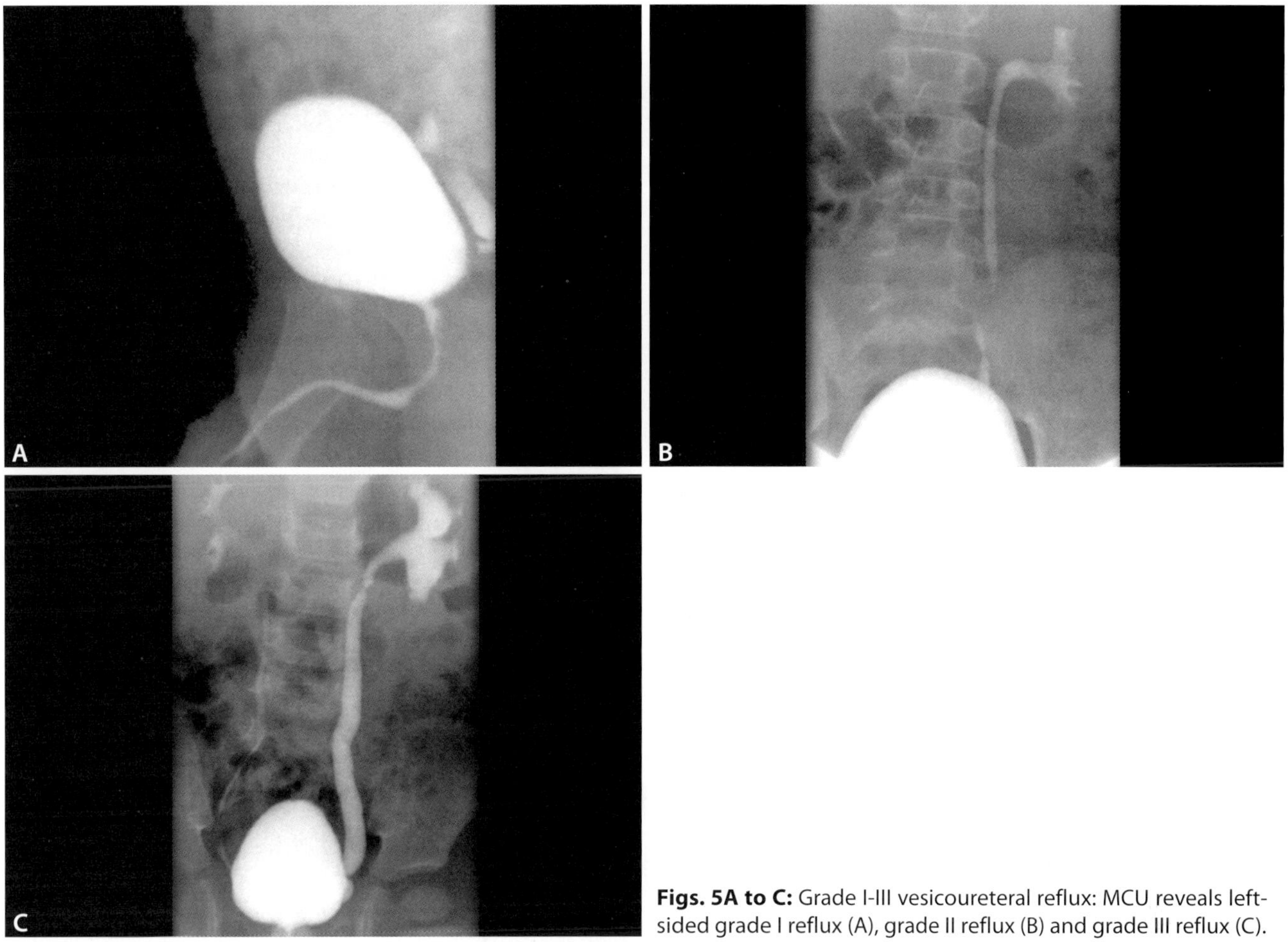

Figs. 5A to C: Grade I-III vesicoureteral reflux: MCU reveals left-sided grade I reflux (A), grade II reflux (B) and grade III reflux (C).

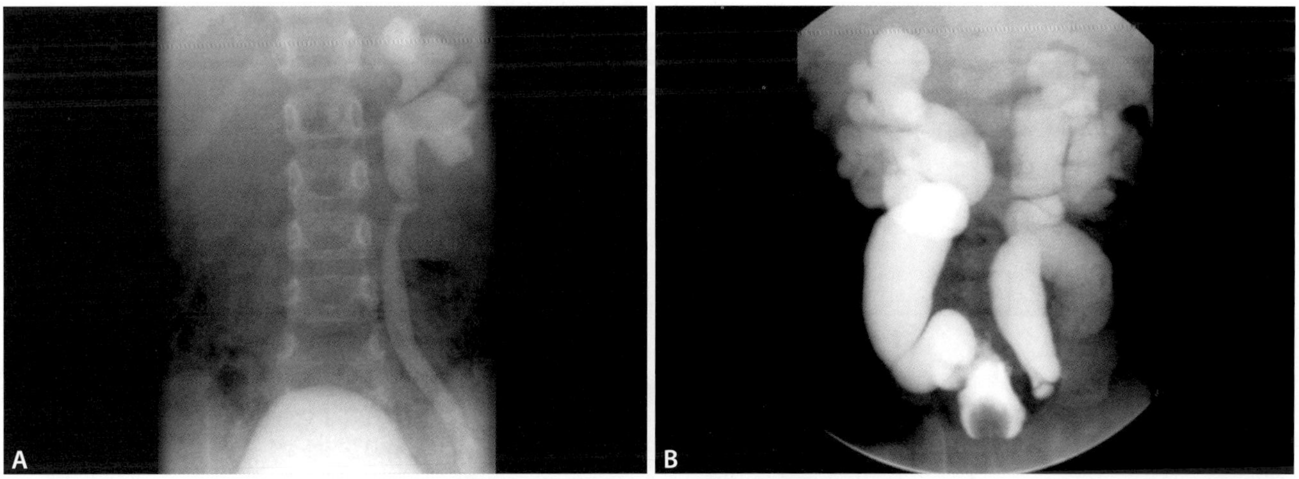

Figs 6A and B: Left grade IV (A) and bilateral grade V reflux (B) seen on MCU.

cyclical voiding is required. Obtaining a second voiding cycle has been shown to increase the detection of VUR significantly.[25,29,30] The increased detection rate using cyclical voiding can be as high as 19.5%.[29] Grade 5 reflux has been detected on a second repeat cycle, where no VUR was seen on the first void.[29] Second-cycle voids can also increase the grade of reflux that was detected on the first void.[29,30] This is most important when grade 1 reflux is upgraded to grade 2 or above, since many clinicians will not treat grade 1 reflux alone.

With recent advances in fluoroscopy, dose reduction can be easily achieved without any perceived loss of image quality.[31-34] Using high-quality image-capture technology can also reduce radiation dose.[35,36]

In a comparison between spot films and image-capture acquisition, the latter provided diagnostically comparable images with a 57% reduction in skin radiation dose.[25] Per se, low magnification, low-pulse-per-second fluoroscopy and image-grab acquisition should be used as much as possible within locally formulated MCU protocols.

RADIONUCLIDE CYSTOGRAPHY

Reflux can also be graded, with radionuclide cystography **(Fig. 7)**. There are two types of radionuclide cystography: Direct and indirect.

Indirect radionuclide cystography is performed by IV injection of a radiopharmaceutical such as ^{99m}Tc mercaptoacetyltriglycine (^{99m}Tc-MAG3) or ^{99m}Tc-diethylenetriaminepenta-acetic acid (^{99m}Tc-DTPA) followed by dynamic imaging of the kidneys.[5] A time-activity curve will show a sudden rise in activity in the renal pelvis when VUR occurs. The main advantage of indirect RNC is that bladder catheterization is not required, although an IV catheter is needed.

The reported sensitivity of indirect RNC, is less than direct RNC, and ranges between 22% and 51%.[5,37] If indirect RNC is to be performed, it should be restricted to patients in whom bladder catheterization is impossible. To maximize sensitivity, patients should be toilet-trained.

The radionuclide cystogram has traditionally had approximately 1/100th of the radiation exposure of a standard MCU.[3] Further, because imaging is continuous with a direct radionuclide cystogram (versus intermittent with fluoroscopy), it seems to be more sensitive in determining reflux than a traditional contrast VCUG.[3,38,39] Fluoroscopic MCU is more accurate at grading reflux,

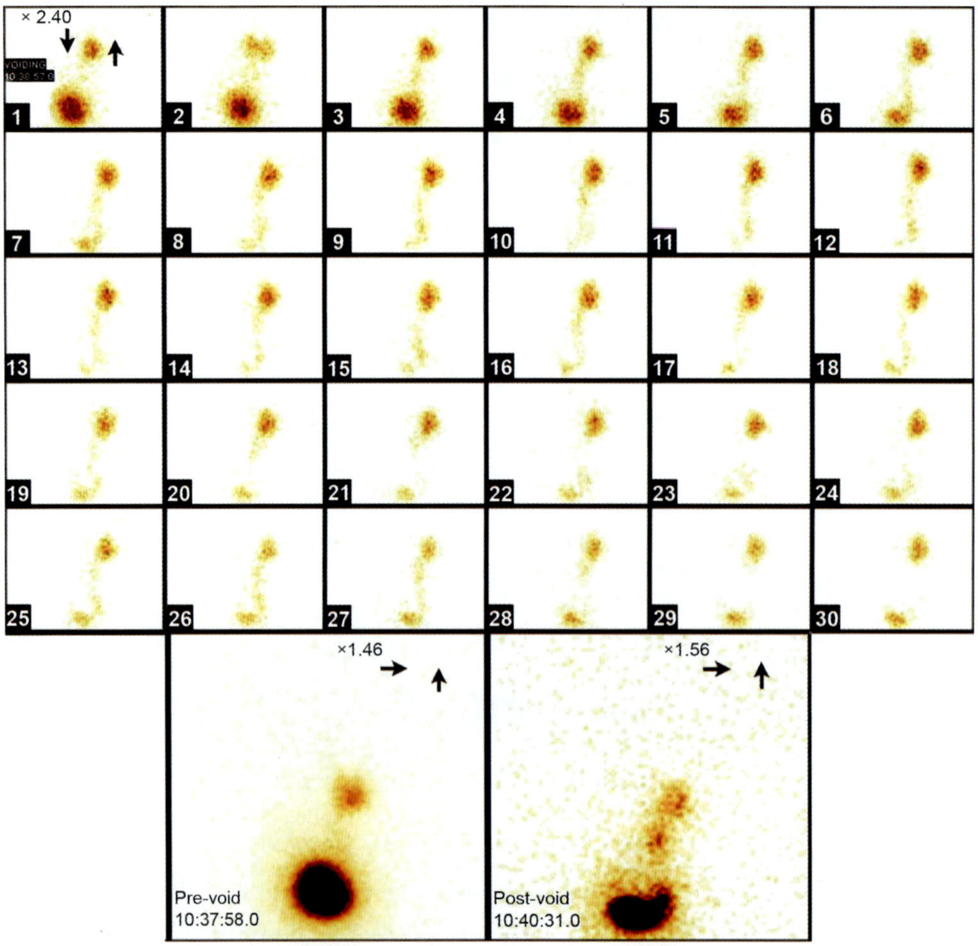

Fig. 7: *^{99m}Tc sulphur colloid DRCG:* Retrograde movement of tracer is seen from the right kidney into the upper ureter, indicative of high grade right-sided VU reflux.

however, and can show spinal abnormalities, bladder and urethral anatomy, periureteral diverticula, and other upper tract detail that cannot be identified with radionuclide cystography.[3,4]

The commonly accepted practice is to perform MCU as the initial test for the presence and severity of VUR as well as any anatomic abnormalities. RNC is typically used at follow-up to determine, if VUR subsequently persists or resolves, especially after antireflux surgery and in girls with first-time UTI because urethral pathology is far less common in girls or when there is a low clinical suspicion of VUR.[40] The sensitivity of RNC has been found to be equal to or slightly higher than that of MCU.[38,41,42] Some studies have found that VCUG is more likely to miss reflux due to its noncontinuous imaging and that RNC is more likely to miss grade I reflux because of its poor anatomic detail.[39,42]

The gonadal radiation dose in RNC has been reported in the range of 10–20 μGy.[5,43] A tailored, low-dose fluoroscopy technique using "last-frame grabber" technology can potentially result in a VCUG gonadal dose as low as 17–52 μGy.[5,44] As stated above, the use of modern variable-rate pulsed fluoroscopy reduces effective radiation dose by eight-fold compared with older continuous fluoroscopy machines; however, the effective dose of VCUG performed with this technique is still ten-fold higher than that received during RNC.[45]

To summarize, nuclear cystography has an advantage due to the lower radiation dosage, which makes it an excellent tool for screening female patients and for follow-up of patients of both sexes. The disadvantages are difficulty in recognizing important anatomical details, i.e. associated bladder disease, e.g. bladder diverticula and male urethra.

ULTRASOUND IN VUR

Echo-enhanced cystosonography has now emerged as a promising new method for detecting and grading VUR without exposing patients to ionizing radiation.

Recent studies[46] have shown that ureteral dilatation has the best diagnostic accuracy for the ultrasound based diagnosis of both all-grade and high-grade VUR (compared with pelvic dilatation, renal length, urinary tract dilatation, and corticomedulary differentiation) with 73% sensitivity and 88% specificity for the detection of high grade VUR.

In voiding urosonography (VUS) intravesical administration of US contrast agent (USCA) is performed for the diagnosis of vesicoureteric reflux (VUR).[47] Many institutions now recognize VUS as a practical, safe, radiation-free modality with comparable or higher sensitivity than direct radionuclide cystography (DRNC) and voiding cystourethrography (VCUG), respectively.

The basic procedural steps of VUS are:

- Ultrasound of the kidneys and bladder.
- Bladder catheterization and intravesical administration of normal saline and USCA.
- Repeat scan of the bladder and kidneys during and after bladder filling and finally all through voiding.[47,48]

Reflux is ranked in grades I–V similar to that for VCUG. The most commonly used USCAs are first generation ultrasound contrast agent, Levovist (Bayer-Schering Pharma, Berlin, Germany) and second generation ultrasound contrast agent SonoVue (Bracco, Milan, Italy).[47,48] Harmonic Imaging (HI) improves the detection of microbubbles and increases the sensitivity of VUS.[47]

MICTURATING CYSTOURETHROGRAM VERSUS VOIDING UROSONOGRAPHY

The largest comparative study between VCUG and VUS with the intravesical administration of the second generation USCA SonoVue, published to date, is by Papadopoulou et al.[49] It comprises a total of 228 children, 123 boys and 105 girls, 6 days to 13 years old, with a total of 463 pelvi-ureteral-units (PUUs). SonoVue was administered at a dose of 1 mL/bladder filling. In 161 (35%), PUUs reflux was detected by one or both methods. In 90 (56%), PUUs reflux was detected only by VUS and in 14 (9%), PUUs only by VCUG. This implies a 47% higher reflux detection rate for SonoVue-enhanced VUS compared to VCUG, which is almost 1.5-times higher than the highest reported rate for Levovist-enhanced VUS.[48] Concordance of VUS and VCUG was 78%. More importantly refluxes missed by VCUG were of higher grades (2 grade 1, 65 grade II, 19 grade III, 4 grade IV) compared to those missed by VUS (8 grade I, 5 grade II, 1 grade III). When VCUG was used as the reference method, the sensitivity of VUS was 80%. When all refluxing PUUs in either method were considered as true positive, sensitivity of VUS and VCUG was 92% and 64%, respectively. These results emphasize that as VUS with a second generation USCA is a safe modality with a much higher sensitivity, it has the potential to become the study of choice in future.

Eva K et al.[50] also evaluated the sensitivity of VUS using a second generation ultrasound (US) contrast agent and compared it with standard fluoroscopic voiding cystourethrography (VCUG) in a study group comprising 183 children.VUR was detected in 140 out of 366 cases (38%); in 89 (24.3%) by both methods, in 37 (10.1%) by VUS only, and in 14 (3.8%) by VCUG only. Although, there was considerable agreement in the diagnosis of VUR by VUS and VCUG ($\kappa = 0.68$, standard error $[\kappa] = 0.04$), the difference in the detection rate of reflux between VUS and VCUG was significant ($p<0.00001$).Their findings also suggest that contrast-enhanced harmonic VUS using a second generation contrast agent is superior to VCUG in the detection and grading of VUR, and it should be the method of choice in UTI.

Most of the publications on VUS are from Europe.[47,48] Limited availability of these contrast agents, however limits its wider use. However, this is a very promising investigation and has the potential to change the conventional management algorithm of VUR.

ROLE OF MRI IN UTI IMAGING

Although, MR urography has yielded very promising results in obstructive uropathy, its role in MR cystography is yet to be established. Few recently published articles on direct and indirect MR cystography techniques have shown technical feasibility details,[51,52] however, there have been no studies comparing it with VCUG.

MRI with its great anatomical detail can help in detection of pyelonephritis and scarring. Many studies have established superior or atleast similar sensitivity of MRI to DMSA scintigraphy, in acute pyelonephritis and scarring. It also offers additional advantage of being a radiation free modality and provides structural detail even in children with poor renal function.

GUIDELINES FOR IMAGING IN UTI: FROM HISTORY TO CURRENT PERSPECTIVE

First set of guidelines were published by Royal College of Physicians (RCP) in 1991 for imaging of UTI in children.[53,54] It was recommended that every child between 0 and 7 years of age with first UTI should have an ultrasound and DMSA scan. Children who are in first year of life should also have a Micturating Cystourography (MCU). These guidelines obviously led to huge burden on radiology departments.

Subsequent to this, practice parameters were established by the American Academy of Pediatrics (AAP) in 1999,which guided physicians in the evaluation of UTI in infants and children.[55,56] Their recommendations for imaging workup were broad, advocating ultrasound and voiding cystourethrography (VCUG) or radionuclide cystography (RNC) in all infants and young children (< 2 years old) with UTI. The American Academy of Family Physicians suggested performing DMSA scanning after treatment of UTI to evaluate for permanent renal scarring.[56] This imaging algorithm and its variants have been described as the "bottom-up" approach because the initial diagnostic concern is detection of VUR. Once VUR is diagnosed, the patient is presumed to be at increased risk for renal scarring, and DMSA scanning is performed several months later to detect any permanent renal scarring.

Since, the 1999 recommendations, physician's experience in managing pediatric UTI and published scientific data has expanded. As a result, there has been a gradual drift away from the AAP guidelines, resulting in several imaging algorithms that can differ among various physicians, practice groups, cities, countries, and continents. One recent survey by Shah et al.[57] showed only a 61% adherence rate to the AAP imaging guidelines.

Another evolution in practice guidelines is now seen in the 2007 European Society of Pediatric Radiology recommendations.[58] This algorithm advocates ultrasound examination of all pediatric UTI patients, and if the ultrasound is normal and there is clinical suspicion for APN, early DMSA scanning is performed at the time of the acute infection. If the DMSA scan shows evidence of APN, then VCUG or RNC is performed later to evaluate for VUR.[5] Normal findings on DMSA scanning obviate subsequent VCUG or RNC.[59,60]

This reversal in the sequence of DMSA scanning and cystography has been referred to as the "top-down" approach by Lim et al. because the initial diagnostic concern is now that of APN, not VUR.[5] The rationale behind most of these recent guidelines is that only 47% of VUR is severe enough to cause APN.[5,9] Therefore, it may not be worthwhile to diagnose and treat all cases of mild VUR. Conversely, 61% of APN occurs in children who do not have reflux;[5,9] using the presence of VUR as the criterion to decide which patients will undergo continued follow-up results in great potential to underdiagnose APN in children without reflux.

To prevent serious long-term sequelae such as hypertension and renal failure, it is now believed that the critical clinical goal is the early recognition of infants and children who are at risk of permanent renal scarring. Detection of APN using DMSA renal scintigraphy may be a more sensitive and appropriate screening tool than VCUG or RNC to determine who is at risk for renal scarring.[5]

DMSA for Renal Scar: When is the Best Time to Scan?

There is no consensus amongst the physicians and radiologists on what is the best time to perform DMSA scan for renal scarring.It is vital as the affected patients would need appropriate urinanalysis,interval renal imaging, hypertensive check ups and follow-ups. In their consensus report, Piepsz et al.[61] found that there is no consensus: 42% of experts perform DMSA scanning at 3 months, 33% at 6 months, and 15% at 12 months after the acute UTI. Agras et al.,[62] have demonstrated in a group of 37 children with DMSA scintigraphic defects, 13 (38.2%) had persistent defects at 6 months but only six (17.6%) showed defects at 12-months after acute UTI. This study suggests a high rate of continuing resolution of pyelonephritis even beyond 6 months after infection and that a 12-month time interval is more reliable for determining the presence of permanent renal scarring.

TREATMENT GUIDELINES FOR REFLUX

The significance of reflux deals with the issue of recurrent pyelonephritis and potentially renal scarring. A common dilemma has been the decision to treat or not to treat a particular child. Traditional therapy has included long-term prophylactic antibiotic treatment, to prevent infections alongside observation, in anticipation of the child outgrowing the reflux.[3]

High spontaneous resolution rates have been obtained, especially for lower grades of reflux, but admittedly with the cost of long-term use of antimicrobials and repeated imaging with MCUs. Surgical intervention has traditionally been reserved for those children who have noncompliance with medical therapy, or nonresolution of VUR, febrile breakthrough UTIs, and progression of renal scarring, after prolonged follow-up.[3]

Bauer et al. in their review article on UTI,[3] have described results of a recent meta-analysis of 10 trials, involving 964 children, which compared long-term antibiotics and surgical correction of VUR with antibiotics (seven trials); antibiotics with no treatment (one trial);and different materials for endoscopic correction of VUR (two trials). Risk of UTI by 1 to 2 and 5 years was not significantly different between surgical and medical groups. Surgical treatment did result in a 60% reduction in febrile UTI by 5 years but no concomitant significant reduction in risk of new or progressive renal damage at 5 years.

American Urological Association has convened the Pediatric Vesicoureteral Reflux Guidelines Panel to make a set of guidelines to determine when to treat reflux medically versus surgically.[63] As is evident from the recommendations, surgery is recommended for higher grades of reflux. Different surgical treatment options are available to these children. The standard surgical care has always been open surgical repair (e.g. ureteral reimplantation). After various attempts made to minimize the morbidity, extravesical approach has been proposed. Success rates for surgical techniques are 98% for curing reflux. These surgical developments, combined with a new general tendency to avoid overuse of antibiotics, have resulted in a drift toward earlier surgery. This has been emphasized even more by the use of laparoscopic techniques in many centers.[64] In endoscopic treatment of reflux, however, success rates of 70–90% for curing reflux have been reported and VCUGs remain essential for endoscopic treatment. It is important to remember that not all VUR needs intervention, and treatment does not always prevent complications.[65]

NEUROGENIC BLADDER

In contrast to adult patient in whom neurogenic bladder is most often due to an acquired, usually traumatic spinal cord lesion, the vast majority of children affected with this disorder have a myelomeningocele or a related myelodysplastic anomaly (occult spinal dysraphism, sacral agenesis).

Myelomeningocele can occur at any level of the spine but is most often located in the lumbosacral area. The radiographs of the affected area show widening of the neural canal, defective posterior neural arches, absence of the posterior spinous processes, and widened interpedicular distance involving several segments, with elongated and flattened or defective pedicles.[16]

Occult myelodysplasia is a group of congenital anomalies of the spinal cord in which the overlying skin is intact although cutaneous stigmata of the disorder may be present such as, local hair overgrowth, hyperpigmentation, hemangioma, a skin dimple, or an ill-defined soft tissue mass due to a lipoma. These anomalies include tethered cord, diastematomyelia, intraspinal lipoma, dermoid cyst, and hamartoma. Radiographs of the spine may show osseous changes similar to those seen in myelomeningocele, and sometimes scoliosis or broad vertebral bodies.

Children with this disorder commonly have inappropriate detrusor muscle contraction and external sphincter relaxation, resulting in uncontrolled voiding pattern with incomplete bladder emptying.[16,66] Initially, the upper tracts are normal but due to poor bladder emptying secondary changes of reflux and infection result.

Complete evaluation of patients suspected of having neurogenic bladder requires MCU for assessment of lower urinary tract, US and one of the functional studies of IVU or scintigraphy for upper tract. However, for the diagnosis of primary cause, examination with plain radiographs and MRI is essential. In case of nonavailability of MRI, myelography with nonionic contrast followed by CT is mandatory.

On MCU, bladder is usually elongated, pointing upwards (Christmas-tree shape) with varying degrees of trabeculation and sacculation **(Figs. 8A and B)**. Rarely, bladder may be large, smooth, atonic type. During voiding, bladder neck and proximal posterior urethra

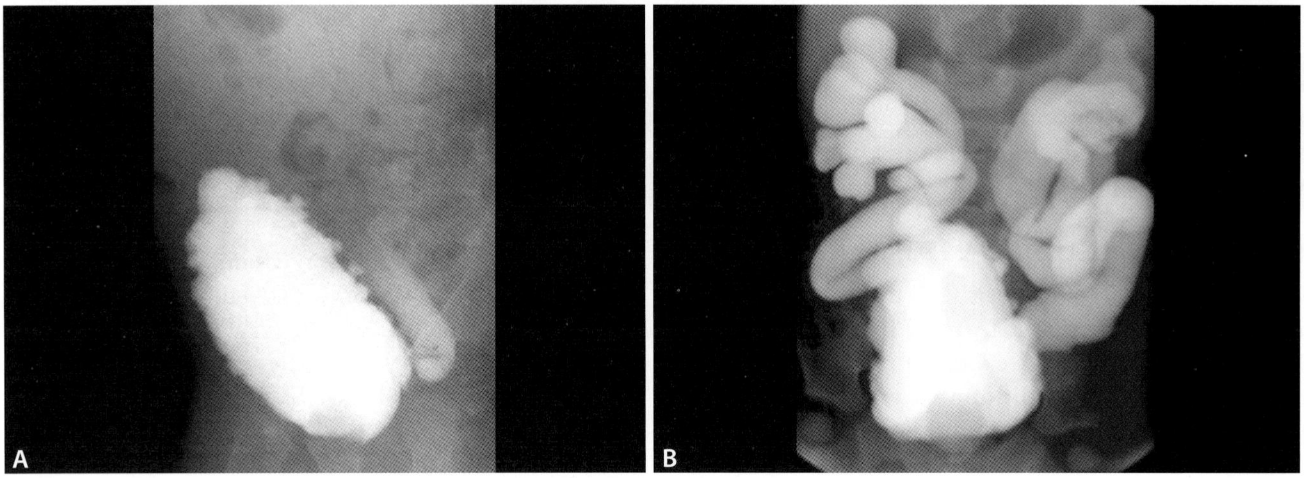

Figs. 8A and B: Neurogenic bladder: MCU shows an elongated bladder with trabeculations and sacculations with grade I VUR (A); MCU in another patient showing neurogenic bladder with grade V VUR (B).

are dilated forming a funnel shape with the point of the funnel directed caudally at midposterior urethra level. Distal urinary stream is usually poor with significant post void residual urine. Associated vesicoureteral reflux is common.[16] Urodynamic techniques have assumed a major role in the evaluation of neurogenic bladder and contributed significantly to the management.

ACKNOWLEDGMENTS

We wish to thank Dr Anish Bhattacharya, Associate Professor, and Dr BR Mittal, Proffessor and Head, Department of Nuclear Medicine, for their kind help and support in providing images of ^{99m}Tc DMSA scans and ^{99m}Tc sulphur-colloid DRCG scans.

REFERENCES

1. Luk WH, Woo YH, San Au-Yeung AW, Chan JCS. Imaging in Pediatric Urinary Tract Infection: A 9-Year Local Experience. AJR. 2009;192:1253-60.
2. Larcombe J. Urinary tract infection in children: Clinical evidence. BMJ. 1999;319:1173-5.
3. Bauer R, Kogan BA. New Developments in the Diagnosis and Management of Pediatric UTIs. Urol Clin N Am. 2008;35:47-58.
4. Linda S. Urinary tract infections in infants and children. In: Walsh P (Ed), 8th edition. Campbell's Urology, Vol. 3. Baltimore (MD): Saunders 2002; pp. 1846-84.
5. Lim R. Vesicoureteral reflux and urinary tract infection: Evolving Practices and Current Controversies in Pediatric Imaging. AJR. 2009;192:1197-208.
6. Marild S, Jodal U. Incidence rate of first-time symptomatic urinary tract infection in children under 6 years of age. Acta Pediatr. 1998;87:549–52.
7. Cleper R, Krause I, Eisenstein B, Davidovits M. Prevalence of vesicoureteral reflux in neonatal urinary tract infection. Clin Pediatr (Phila). 2004;43:619-25.
8. Rushton HG, Majd M. Dimercaptosuccinic acid renal scintigraphy for the evaluation of pyelonephritis and scarring: A review of experimental and clinical studies. J Urol. 1992;148:1726-32.
9. Ditchfield MR, De Campo JF, Cook DJ, et al. Vesicoureteral reflux: An accurate predictor of acute pyelonephritis in childhood urinary tract infection? Radiology. 1994;190:413-5.
10. Sastre JB, Aparicio AR, Cotallo GD, Colomer BF, Hernandez MC. Urinary tract infection in the newborn: Clinical and radio imaging studies. Pediatr Nephrol. 2007;22:1735-41.
11. Lin KY, Chiu NT, Chen MJ, et al. Acute pyelonephritis and sequelae of renal scar in pediatric first febrile urinary tract infection. Pediatr Nephrol 2003;18:362-5.
12. Zaki M, Badawi M, Al Mutari G, Ramadan D, Adul Rahman M. Acute pyelonephritis and renal scarring in Kuwaiti children: A follow-up study using ^{99m}Tc DMSA renal scintigraphy. Pediatr Nephrol. 2005;20:1116-9.
13. Oh MM, Jin MH, Bae JH, Park HS, Lee JG. Moon du G. The role of vesicoureteral reflux in acute renal cortical scintigraphic lesion and ultimate scar formation. J Urol. 2008;180:2167-70.
14. Zamir G, Sakran W, Horowitz Y, Koren A, Miron D. Urinary tract infection: Is there a need for routine renal ultrasonography? Arch Dis Child. 2004;89:466-8.
15. Huang HP, Lai YC, Tsai IJ, Chen SY, Tsau YK. Renal ultrasonography should be done routinely in children with first urinary tract infections. Urology. 2008;71:439-43.
16. Vashist S. Radiology of lower Urinary tract;In Diagnostic Radiology. Pediatric Imaging, 2nd edition. Jaypee Brothers Medical Publishers. 2004;11:208-22.
17. Alon U, Berant M, Pery M. Intravenous pyelography in children with urinary tract infection and vesicoureteral reflux. Pediatrics. 1989;83:332-7.

18. Cussen LJ. Dimensions of the normal ureter in infancy and childhood. Invest Urol. 1967;5:164-78.
19. Ataei N, Madani A, Habibi R, Khorasani M. Evaluation of acute pyelonephritis with DMSA scans in children presenting after the age of 5 years. Pediatr Nephrol. 2005;20:1439-44.
20. Sandhu MS, Lal A. Pediatric Kidney: Medical Conditions. Radiology of lower urinary tract in Diagnostic Radiology, 2nd edition. Pediatric Imaging. Jaypee Brothers Medical Publisher. 2004;9;160-181.
21. Jakobson B, Soderlungh S, Berg U. Diagnostic significance of ^{99m}Tc-DMSA scintigraphy in urinary tract infection. Arch Dis Child. 1992;67:1338-42.
22. Lebowitz RL, Mandell J. Urinary tract infection in children: Putting radiology in its place. Radiology. 1987;165:1-9.
23. Dubbins PA. The kidney. In: Allen PL, Dubbins PA, Pozniak MA and McDicken WN (Eds). Clinical Doppler ultrasound. New York: Churchil Livingstone. 2000.pp.169-90.
24. International Reflux Study Committee. Medical versus surgical treatment of primary vesicoureteral reflux: A prospective international reflux study in children. J Urol. 1981;125:277-83.
25. Agrawalla S, Pearce R, Goodman TR. How to perform the perfect voiding cystourethrogram? Pediatr Radiol. 2004;34:114-9.
26. Weese DL, Greenberg HM, Zimmern PE. Contrast media reactions during voiding cystourethrography or retrograde pyelography. Urology. 1993;41:81-3.
27. Kaefer M, Zurakowski D, Bauer SB, et al. Estimating normal bladdercapacity in children. J Urol. 1997;158:2261-4.
28. Sillen U. Bladder function inhealthy neonates and its development during infancy. Urology. 2001;166:2376-81.
29. Papadopoulou F, Efremidis SC, Economou A, et al. Cyclic voiding cystourethrography: Is vesicoureteral reflux missed with standard voiding cystourethrography? Eur Radiol. 2002;12:666-70.
30. Paltiel HJ, Rupich RC, Kiruluta HC. Enhanced detection of vesicoureteral reflux in infants and children with use of cyclic voiding cystourethrography. Radiology. 1992;184:753-5.
31. Boland GW, Murphy B, Arellano R, et al. Dose reduction in Gastrointestinal and genitourinary fluoroscopy: Use of grid-controlled pulsedfluoroscopy. AJR. 2000;175:1453-7.
32. Hernandez RJ, Goodsitt MM. Reduction of radiation dose in pediatric patients using pulsed fluoroscopy. AJR. 1996;167:1247-53.
33. Lederman HM, Khademian ZP, Felice M, et al. Dose reduction fluoroscopy in pediatrics. Pediatr Radiol. 2002;32:844-8.
34. Brown PH, Silberberg PJ, Thomas RD, et al. A multihospital survey of radiation exposure and image quality in pediatric fluoroscopy. Pediatr Radiol. 2000;30:236-42.
35. Bazopoulos EV, Prassopoulos PK, DamilakisJE, et al. A comparison between digital fluoroscopic hard copiesand 105 mm spot films in evaluating vesicoureteric reflux in children. Pediatr Radiol. 1998;28:162-6.
36. Diamond DA, Kleinman PK, Spevak M, et al. The tailored low dosefluoroscopic voiding cystogram for familial reflux screening. J Urol. 1996;155:681-2.
37. De Sadeleer C, De Boe V, Keuppens F, Desprechins B, Verboven M, Piepsz A. How good is technetium-99m mercaptoacetyltriglycine indirect cystography? Eur J Nucl Med. 1994;21:223-7.
38. Unver T, Alpay H, Biyikli NK, Ones T. Comparison of direct radionuclide cystography and voiding cystourethrography in detecting vesicoureteral reflux. Pediatr Int. 2006;48:287-91.
39. McLaren CJ, Simpson ET. Direct comparison of radiology and nuclear medicine cystograms in young infants with vesico-ureteric reflux. BJU Int. 2001;87:93-7.
40. Lebowitz RL. The detection and characterization of vesicoureteral reflux in the child. J Urol. 1992;148:1640-2.
41. Sukan A, Bayazit AK, Kibar M, et al. Comparison of direct radionuclide cystography and voiding direct cystography in the detection of vesicoureteral reflux. Ann Nucl Med. 2003;17:549-53.
42. Saraga M, Stanicic A, Markovic V. The role of direct radionuclide cystography in evaluation of vesicoureteral reflux. Scand J Urol Nephrol. 1996;30:367-71.
43. Van den Abbeele AD, Treves ST, Lebowitz RL, et al. Vesicoureteral reflux in asymptomatic siblings of patients with known reflux: Radionuclide cystography. Pediatrics. 1987;79:147-53.
44. Kleinman PK, Diamond DA, Karellas A, Spevak MR, Nimkin K, Belanger P. Tailored low-dose fluoroscopic voiding cystourethrography for the reevaluation of vesicoureteral reflux in girls. AJR. 1994;162:1151-4;discussion 1155-6.
45. Ward VL, Strauss KJ, Barnewolt CE, et al. Pediatric radiation exposure and effective dose reduction during voiding cystourethrography. Radiology. 2008;249:1002-9.
46. Leroy S,Vantalon S, Larakeb A, Ducou-Le-Pointe H, Bensman A. Vesicoutertral reflux in children with urinary tarct infection: Comparison of diagnostic accuracy of renal US criteria. Radiology. 2010;255:890-8.
47. Darge K. Voiding urosonography with US contrast agent for the diagnosis of vesicoureteric reflux in children: An update. Pediatr Radiol. 2010;40:956-62.
48. Darge K. Voiding urosonography with ultrasound contrast agents for the diagnosis of vesicoureteric reflux in children. Pediatr Radiol. 2008;38:40-53.
49. Papadopoulou F, Anthopoulou A, Siomou E, et al. Harmonic voiding urosonography with a second generation contrast agent for the diagnosis of vesicoureteral reflux. Pediatr Radiol. 2009;39:239-44.
50. Éva K, Nyitrai A,Várkonyi I, et al. Voiding urosonography with second generation contrast agent versus voiding cystourethrography. Pediatr Nephrol. 2010;25:2289-93.
51. Teh HS, Gan JS, Ng FC. Magnetic resonance cystography: Novel imaging technique for evaluation of vesicoureteral reflux. Urology. 2005;65:793-4.
52. Takazakura R, Johnin K, Furukawa A, et al. Magnetic resonance voiding cystourethrography for vesicoureteral reflux. J Magn Reson Imaging. 2007;25:170-4.

53. [No authors listed]. Guidelines for the management of acute urinary tract infection in childhood. Report of a Working Group of the Research Unit, Royal College of Physicians. JR Coll Physicians Lond. 1991;25:36-42.
54. Biassoni L, Chippington S. Imaging in urinary tract Infections: Current strategies and new trends. Seminars in Nucl Medicine. 2008;38:56-66.
55. [No authors listed]. Practice parameter: The diagnosis, treatment, and evaluation of the initial urinary tract infection in febrile infants and young children. American Academy of Pediatrics. Committee on Quality Improvement. Subcommittee on Urinary Tract Infection. Pediatrics. 1999;103: 843-52.
56. Ross JH, Kay R. Pediatric urinary tract infection and reflux. Am Fam Physician. 1999;59:1472-8, 1485-6.
57. Shah L, Mandlik N, Kumar P, Andaya S, Patamasucon P. Adherence to AAP Practice Guidelines for Urinary Tract Infections at Our Teaching Institution. Clin Pediatr (Phila). 2008;47:861-4.
58. Riccabona M, Avni FE, Blickman JG, et al. Imaging recommendations in pediatric uroradiology: Minutes of the ESPR workgroup session on urinary tract infection, fetal hydronephrosis, urinary tract ultrasonography and voiding cystourethrography. Barcelona, Spain, June 2007. Pediatr Radiol. 2008;38:138-45.
59. Preda I, Jodal U, Sixt R, Stokland E, Hansson S. Normal dimercaptosuccinic acid scintigraphy makes voiding cystourethrography unnecessary after urinary tract infection. J Pediatr. 2007;151:581-4.
60. Tseng MH, Lin WJ, Lo WT, Wang SR, Chu ML, Wang CC. Does a normal DMSA obviate the performance of voiding cystourethrography in evaluation of young children after their first urinary tract infection? J Pediatr. 2007;150:96-9.
61. Piepsz A, Blaufox MD, Gordon I, et al. Consensus on renal cortical scintigraphy in children with urinary tract infection: Scientific Committee of Radionuclides in Nephrourology. Semin Nucl Med. 1999;29:160-74.
62. Agras K, Ortapamuk H, Naldoken S, Tuncel A, Atan A. Resolution of cortical lesions on serial renal scans in children with acute pyelonephritis. Pediatr Radiol. 2007;37:153-8.
63. Elder JS, Peters CA, Arant B Jr, et al. Pediatric vesicoureteral reflux guidelines panel summary reporton the management of primary vesicoureteral reflux in children. J Urol. 1997;157: 1846-51.
64. Yeung CK, Sihoe JD, Tam YH, et al. Laparoscopic excision of prostatic utricles in children. BJU Int. 2001;87:505-8.
65. Lorenzo AJ, Khoury AE. Endoscopic treatment of reflux: Management pros and cons. Curr Opin Urol. 2006;16:299-304.
66. Bauer SB. Neurogenic Bladder dysfunction. Pediatr Cli North America. 1987;34:1121-40.

CHAPTER 141

Renal and Retroperitoneal Masses

Anju Garg

The retroperitoneum is a potential space that extends along the posterior most aspect of the abdominal cavity from the level of the diaphragm to the pelvic brim. Masses in this space can arise from the kidneys, adrenal glands, lymph nodes, lymphatic channels, sympathetic ganglia or other neural tissue and iliopsoas muscle. As symptoms of retroperitoneal disease are non-specific and physical examination is difficult, retroperitoneal masses grow quite large before they are detected.

IMAGING

The multitude of diagnostic imaging modalities available for evaluation of abdominal masses in infants and children requires a logical and analytical approach to avoid unnecessary expense, radiation and potential morbidity. Ultrasound (US) is the most frequently selected first imaging modality on the basis of availability, ease of performance (as there is no need for intravenous contrast or patient sedation), low cost and absence of radiation exposure. The highest possible frequency probes should be used to maximize resolution. Color Doppler enables characterization of tumor vascularization and assessment of vascular invasion. US has a high diagnostic efficacy for common pediatric abdominal masses and in many cases, it may give a complete diagnosis obviating the need for any further investigation. If the US examination is technically limited because of excessive bowel gas or body habitus, or if the mass is incompletely evaluated by US or thought to be neoplastic, computed tomography or magnetic resonance imaging can be done. In the case of a suspected neoplasm, these modalities further refine the differential diagnosis, define the local and regional extent of the mass and detect metastases.

Computed tomography (CT) is an extremely accurate and fast imaging modality, displaying high quality cross-sectional images. Multidetector CT allows excellent reconstructions in planes other than the original scanning plane. Isotropic multiplanar reconstructions (MPRs) of thin overlapping slices in the coronal and sagittal plane provide excellent delineation of the location and extent of retroperitoneal masses. The use of pre- and post-contrast scanning should be minimized in children; the use of oral contrast is helpful in distinguishing bowel from nodal disease. Short sedation may be required, especially in younger children. A relative disadvantage of CT is the radiation exposure. Chest CT may be required in cases of suspected neoplasms to evaluate presence of lung metastases.

The advantages of *magnetic resonance imaging (MRI)* include its unique ability to directly acquire multiplanar images, superior contrast resolution and lack of ionizing radiation. Its major disadvantages are cost, limited availability and need for sedation. Faster scanners and newer imaging sequences currently allow accurate lesion characterization in a reasonably short scanning time. Typical sequences used are pre-contrast T1- and T2-weighted gradient echo sequences and post-contrast fat suppressed T1-weighted images. Images should be obtained in at least two orthogonal planes to permit direct evaluation of extent of retroperitoneal disease.

Conventional abdominal radiographs infrequently provide a definite diagnosis for a suspected abdominal mass but can suggest a mimicking process such as constipation and fecal retention or a distended urinary bladder. The nature of an abdominal mass can sometimes be inferred on abdominal radiographs by the presence or absence of calcification in the mass and the location of the mass as indicated by the pattern of bowel displacement and other signs of mass effect.

With the availability of cross-sectional imaging modalities like US, CT and MRI, *intravenous urography* has a very limited role to play in the evaluation of suspected cases of retroperitoneal or even renal masses as it provides only indirect evidence of the mass.

The first step in evaluating these masses is to decide whether the mass is located in the retroperitoneal space. Anterior displacement of retroperitoneal organs and major abdominal vessels strongly suggest that the mass arises in the retroperitoneum. After confirming the retroperitoneal location, the next step is to decide whether it is arising from a retroperitoneal organ or is a primary retroperitoneal tumor arising outside the major retroperitoneal organs. Certain radiologic signs have been described to determine the origin of a mass.[1] When a tumor arises from an organ, then the organ appears to be embedded in the tumor. This is called the *positive embedded organ sign.* When a tumor compresses an adjacent pliable organ (such as the hollow viscera or IVC), it deforms the organ into a crescent shape. This is the *negative embedded organ sign* and is seen in primary retroperitoneal tumors. When the edge of an adjacent organ is distorted into a "beak", it indicates that the tumor probably arises from the organ. This is called the *positive beak sign.* On the other hand, when an adjacent organ has rounded edges, it indicates that the retroperitoneal mass does not arise from that organ, this finding is called a *negative beak sign* **(Figs. 1A to D)**. When a large mass arises from a small organ, the organ sometimes becomes undetectable—the *phantom (invisible) organ sign.*

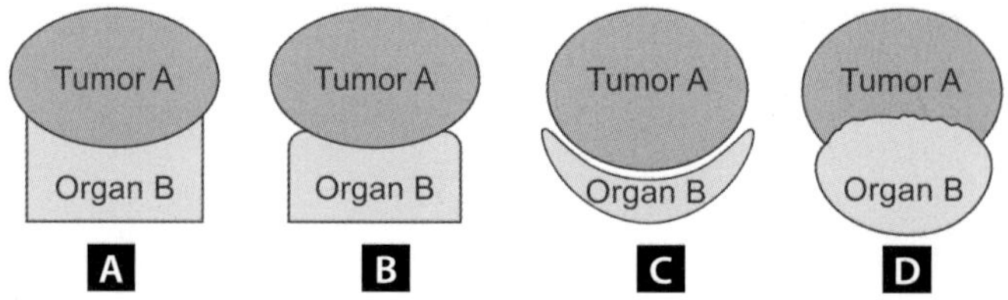

Figs. 1A to D: Possible relationships of retroperitoneal masses to retroperitoneal organs.[1] (A and B) Beak sign: Drawings illustrate the positive beak sign (A), in which Tumor A arises from Organ B, and the negative beak sign (B), in which Tumor A does not arise from Organ B. (C and D) Embedded organ sign: Drawings illustrate the negative embedded organ sign (C), in which Tumor A simply compresses Organ B, and the positive embedded organ sign (D), in which Tumor A arises from Organ B so that the organ appears to be embedded in the tumor.

RENAL MASSES

Renal masses can be congenital, infective, inflammatory or neoplastic in nature. Non-neoplastic masses have been discussed elsewhere in the book and this chapter will deal with the renal neoplasms in children.

An abdominal mass in a child in the first year of life is usually of renal origin. Benign renal masses (mainly developmental, only 20% being true neoplasms)[2] predominate in early infancy, but beyond the first year of life and during the first decade, primary tumors of the kidney become more common. The various pediatric renal neoplasms, their frequency and age of presentation are given in **Table 1**.[3]

WILMS' TUMOR (NEPHROBLASTOMA)

Wilms' tumor was first described by a German surgeon named Max Wilms in 1899. It is the most common renal malignancy in childhood accounting for 80–90% of pediatric renal tumors and 12% of childhood cancers. It is rare during the first year of life and is commonly seen between 1 and 5 years of age with a peak at 3 years.[4] Occasionally, Wilms' tumor has been described in teenagers and adults.

Etiopathogenesis

Wilms' tumors can arise sporadically, can develop in association with genetic syndromes, or can be familial. Upto 12% of children with Wilms' tumor have associated congenital anomalies. The incidence of co-existent genitourinary anomalies—cryptorchidism, hypospadias, ambiguous genitalia, horseshoe kidney is the highest (5%) followed by hemihypertrophy (2.5%), and aniridia (1%). About 33% of children with sporadic aniridia develop Wilms' tumor and these tumors are frequently bilateral. Certain syndromes have a predisposition to Wilms' tumor. These include the Beckwith-Wiedeman syndrome (macroglossia, exomphalos, gigantism), Denys-Drash (pseudohermaphroditism, glomerulonephritis), Sotos (cerebral gigantism), Bloom (immunodeficiency and facial telangiectasia) and Perlman syndromes.[2] Wilms' tumor has also been reported in children with neurofibromatosis, with imperforate anus and rectourethral fistula.

Two loci on chromosome 11 have been implicated in the genesis of a minority of Wilms' tumors. Locus 11p13 is known as the WT1 gene, and locus 11p15 is known

Table 1: Most common age at presentation for renal neoplasms.[3]

Renal neoplasm (Prevalence)	*Age range*	*Peak age*
• *Wilms' tumor (80%)*:		
– Unilateral form	1–11 years	3½ years
– Bilateral form	2 months–2 years	15 months
• Nephroblastomatosis	Any age	6–18 months
• Mesoblastic nephroma (3%)	0–1 year	1–3 months
• Clear cell sarcoma (4–5%)	1–4 years	2 years
• Rhabdoid tumor (2%)	6 months–9 years	6–12 months
• *Miscellaneous tumors (7%)*:		
– Renal cell carcinoma	6 months–60 years	10–20 years*
– Multilocular cystic renal tumor (Cystic nephroma)	3 months–4 years	1–2 years
– Angiomyolipoma	6–41 years	10 years†
– Ossifying renal tumor of infancy	6 days–14 months	1–3 months
• *Metanephric adenoma*:		
– Renal medullary carcinoma	15 months–83 years	None
– Lymphoma	10–39 years	20 years
♦ Hodgkin	>10 years	Late teens
♦ Non-Hodgkin	Any age child	<10 years

*von Hippel–Lindau syndrome
†Tuberous sclerosis, neurofibromatosis, von Hippel–Lindau syndrome.

as the WT2 gene. An abnormal WT1 gene is present in patients with WAGR syndrome (Wilms' tumor, aniridia, genitourinary abnormalities, mental retardation) or Drash syndrome; an abnormal WT2 gene is present in patients with Beckwith-Wiedeman syndrome or hemihypertrophy. However, the genetics of Wilms' tumor appear to be multifactorial, and abnormalities at other sites, including chromosomes 1, 12, and 8, are also recognized. Familial Wilms' tumor is rare, occurring in approximately 1% of cases, and is not associated with mutations in chromosome 11.[5]

Clinical Features

Most children present with a painless abdominal mass often discovered accidentally by the parents or by the physician on a routine examination. The mass is hard rather than firm, non-tender and commonly unilateral. Wilms' tumor can be bilateral in 4–13% of children of which two-thirds are synchronous and one-third metachronous.[6] Bilateral tumors occur earlier, have a higher incidence of associated congenital anomalies and a higher incidence of nephroblastomatosis than seen in unilateral tumors.[7]

If the tumor ruptures, or if hemorrhage occurs, there may be rapid enlargement of the mass with development of acute symptoms. Fever, leukocytosis, malaise, anorexia and gross or microscopic hematuria may occur. Hypertension can occur due to disruption of blood flow to and from the kidney, compression of renal tissues by tumor or rarely production of renin by the tumor itself.[8] Rarely, some tumors may become hormonally active and can cause Cushing's syndrome or hypoglycemia.

Pathology

Wilms' tumor is characterized by an abnormal proliferation of the metanephric blastema cells, which are believed to be primitive embryologic cells of the kidney. The gross appearance of a Wilms' tumor is that of a large, bulky, solid mass with a well-defined pseudocapsule of compressed renal parenchyma that separates it from the rest of the kidney, with distortion of the renal parenchyma and collecting system. The tumor typically spreads by direct extension and displaces adjacent structures but does not usually encase or elevate the aorta. Foci of hemorrhage, necrosis and cyst formation are commonly found, specially if the tumor is large or has previously been treated with radiation or chemotherapy. There may be vascular invasion of the renal vein and inferior vena cava with occasional extension into the right atrium. Metastases are most commonly found in the lungs (85% of cases), liver, and regional lymph nodes.

Histologically, the classic Wilms' tumor is "triphasic": it contains epithelial (tubular, glomerular), blastemal (small round cells), and stromal (spindle, myxoid) cell lines. Not all tumors, however, contain all cell lines and the proportion as well of degree of differentiation of cell lines is highly variable from one tumor to the next.[9] Apart from the predominant cell lines, the prognosis of children with Wilms' tumor is heavily dependent on the presence of anaplasia. Its presence has been found to be more significant than tumor staging when assigning prognosis. A 'favorable' histology lacks anaplastic changes, whereas one with "unfavorable" histology demonstrates extreme nuclear and mitotic atypia characteristic of anaplasia. Approximately 90% of Wilms' tumors are of 'favorable" histology.

Staging

The current staging according to the North American National Wilms' Tumor Study Group (NWTSG) is based on surgical, pathological and radiological findings and is given in **Table 2.**[10]

Table 2: Staging system for National Wilms' tumor study.[10]

Stage I	The tumor is limited to the kidney and is excised completely
Stage II	The tumor extends beyond the kidney but is excised completely. Capsular penetration, renal vein involvement, and renal sinus involvement may also be found. No residual tumor apparent at or beyond margins of excision
Stage III	Residual intra-abdominal tumor (nonhematogenous) exists after the completion of surgery. Lymph node findings are positive, or peritoneal implants are found. Tumor extends beyond surgical margins either microscopically or macroscopically
Stage IV	Hematogenous or lymph node metastasis has occurred outside the abdomen or pelvis
Stage V	Synchronous bilateral involvement has occurred. Each side is assigned a stage from I to III, and histology is based on biopsy findings

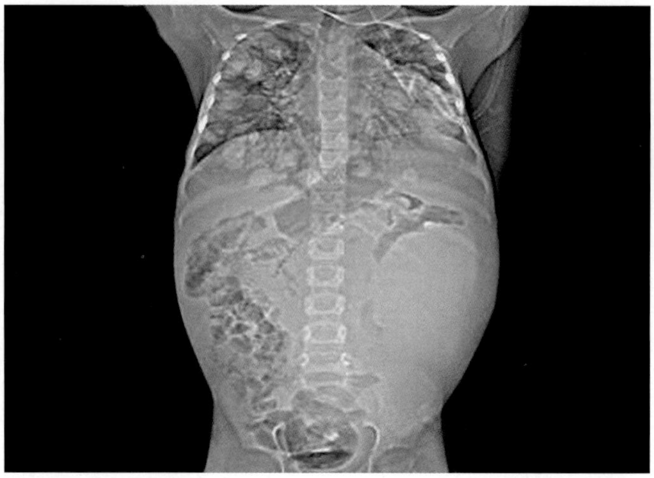

Fig. 2: Plain radiograph of the chest and abdomen shows evidence of a soft tissue mass in the left lumbar and iliac fossa with displaced bowel loops. Multiple rounded opacities seen scattered through both lung fields—pulmonary metastasis.

Imaging

Plain abdominal radiographs show evidence of a large flank mass. Calcification is seen in less than 10% of cases.[2] *Chest radiographs* are routinely done in all cases to look for evidence of lung metastases which indicate advanced stage disease **(Fig. 2)**.

On *ultrasound*, the tumor is visualized as a predominantly solid, slightly hyperechoic mass causing gross renal enlargement. A clear margination of the tumor from the rest of the kidney is often possible due to the pseudocapsule which may be hypo- or hyperechoic **(Figs. 3A and B)**. Normal native renal tissue can be difficult to detect and is typically stretched at the periphery of the lesion. It may show hydronephrotic changes. Cystic areas are often seen within the mass which correlate with presence of hemorrhage or cystic degeneration. Invasion of the IVC and extension into the right atrium can be readily detected on US **(Figs. 4A and B)**. Intrahepatic IVC can be assessed relatively easily but differentiation of invasion from displacement and compression may be difficult. A clue to the presence of obstruction is the dilatation of the hepatic veins. Doppler can also confirm the presence of a thrombus and show its extent. Thrombus confined to the renal vein is less easy to detect because of distortion. US is excellent for detecting the tumor itself and its vascular extension but is limited in its ability to assess extracapsular extension of tumor, lymph node involvement and small contralateral tumors.

Abdominal *CT scan* is more sensitive than ultrasound in identifying tumor extent, nodal, liver and contralateral kidney involvement.[11] CT has the advantage of detecting the precursor condition, nephroblastomatosis.[12] On CT, Wilms' tumor is seen as a large, well-defined mass of heterogeneous attenuation, which enhances to a lesser degree than the normal renal parenchyma. The normal renal parenchyma can be seen stretched and splayed at the periphery of the mass—the "positive beak sign". Areas of low attenuation coincide with tumor necrosis and/or fat deposition. Calcification may be seen in a few cases **(Figs. 3C, 5 and 6A and B)**. Capsular invasion may be suggested by a pattern of exophytic growth and contour irregularity. Contrast-enhanced CT scan allows evaluation of the renal veins and inferior vena cava for tumor thrombus though sensitivity is less than sonography **(Fig. 6C)**.[13] CT scan may identify regional adenopathy, although it cannot differentiate tumor replacement from reactive adenopathy. Nodal involvement differentiates between stage II and III, but neither CT nor surgical exploration is accurate and its distinction remains histological at present. Peritoneal, omental and mesenteric involvement of Wilms' tumor can be depicted accurately by CT.

On *MR imaging* the tumor appears as a well-defined mass with signal intensity similar to that of the spleen and slightly lower than that of the normal renal cortex on T1W images. On T2W images, the tumor appears isointense to normal renal cortex. Areas of high-signal intensity correspond to the presence of hemorrhage or necrosis. The pseudocapsule is seen as a hypointense rim surrounding the tumor on both T1 and T2 pulse sequences **(Figs. 3D and E)**. On contrast administration, the tumor enhances heterogeneously and characteristically less than the normal renal parenchyma.

MR imaging can accurately assess tumor size, gross composition, and regional spread, although, as with all

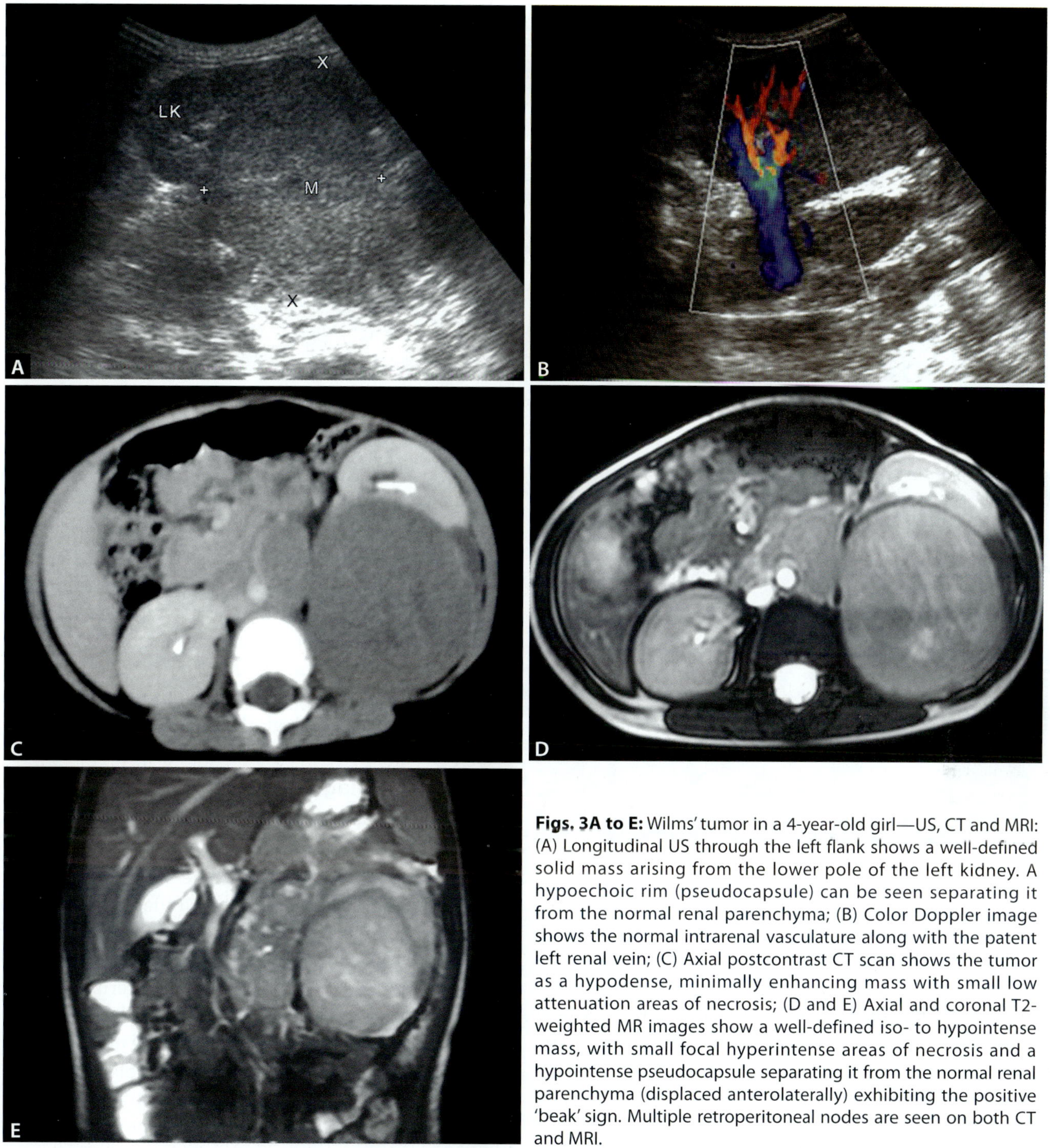

Figs. 3A to E: Wilms' tumor in a 4-year-old girl—US, CT and MRI: (A) Longitudinal US through the left flank shows a well-defined solid mass arising from the lower pole of the left kidney. A hypoechoic rim (pseudocapsule) can be seen separating it from the normal renal parenchyma; (B) Color Doppler image shows the normal intrarenal vasculature along with the patent left renal vein; (C) Axial postcontrast CT scan shows the tumor as a hypodense, minimally enhancing mass with small low attenuation areas of necrosis; (D and E) Axial and coronal T2-weighted MR images show a well-defined iso- to hypointense mass, with small focal hyperintense areas of necrosis and a hypointense pseudocapsule separating it from the normal renal parenchyma (displaced anterolaterally) exhibiting the positive 'beak' sign. Multiple retroperitoneal nodes are seen on both CT and MRI.

other imaging modalities, it cannot define subtle capsular invasion.[2] It can also accurately identify the presence of liver metastases and caval thrombus. Advantages over US and CT scan include the use of specific flow sequences in the search for tumor thrombus and multiplanar imaging in evaluating caval displacement by tumor.

With the diagnostic information provided by US, CT/MRI, the role of intravenous urography (IVU) has significantly reduced in the present day imaging work-up of Wilms' tumor. On IVU, both frontal and lateral views are required for a proper three-dimensional concept of the mass. The appearance of the tumor on the IVU depends on

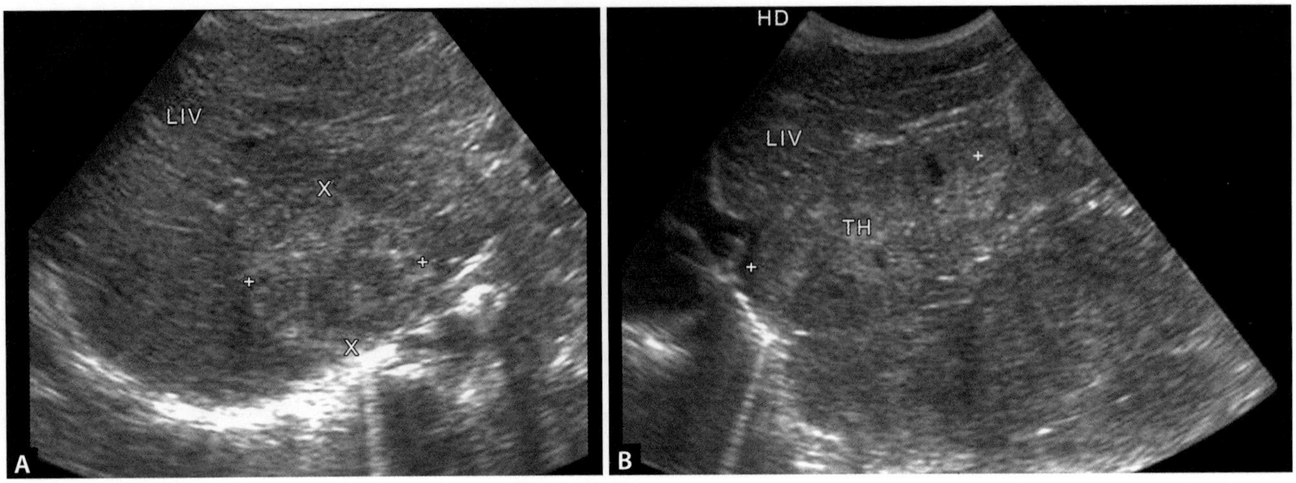

Figs. 4A and B: Transverse and longitudinal US images in a case of Wilms' tumor showing an isoechoic thrombus (TH) filling the IVC.

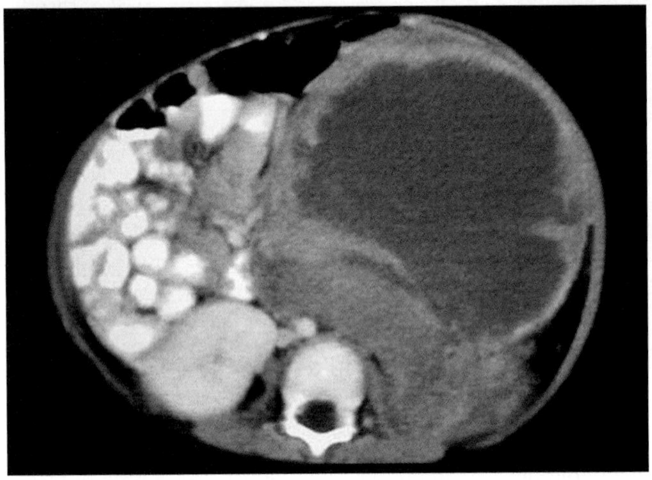

Fig. 5: Cystic Wilm's tumor: Contrast-enhanced axial CT shows a Wilms' tumor of the left kidney with a large cystic component within. The tumor mass extends across the midline, displacing the aorta and IVC to the right, but not elevating or encasing these vessels (unlike neuroblastoma).

the location of the tumor within the kidney. An intrarenal mass can be seen to cause splaying and distortion of the calyces. Tumors in the upper pole and posterior location cause more calyceal distortion than lower pole or anterior tumors, which can readily grow exophytically. A centrally located tumor may cause a hydronephrotic appearance associated with calyceal distortion.

Chest CT and pulmonary metastases: The role of CT scan of the chest in the evaluation and subsequent management of pulmonary lesions found only on CT is controversial and its prognostic importance is equivocal.[14,15] Chest CT, currently required by the NWTSG-5 imaging protocol, is a highly sensitive technique in the evaluation of parenchymal lung disease and enables the identification of lesions not visible on chest radiographs. It is also more sensitive in the detection of calcified nodules. Controversy arises in staging the disease when chest CT identifies lesions (CT-only lesions) not seen on chest radiographs. The results of many studies have shown that treating according to chest CT findings does not change the final outcome of children with Wilms' tumor.[14] Also, it has been shown that CT-only lesions are not invariably tumor, demonstrating the need for histopathological confirmation.[16]

Differential Diagnosis

The most important differential diagnosis of a Wilms' tumor is *neuroblastoma*. Although Wilms' tumor characteristically arises from the kidney, whereas a neuroblastoma displaces the kidney, differentiation may be difficult in the presence of a large exophytic Wilms' tumor or with renal invasion of neuroblastoma. Features favoring Wilms' tumor are non-homogeneous internal structure of tumor with hemorrhage and necrosis, round or oval-shaped with regular margins and absence of calcification. Classical features of an abdominal neuroblastoma are ill-defined margins, tumor calcifications, tumor extension across midline, displacement and encasement of vascular structures. Encasement of aorta, paravertebral extension and invasion of spinal canal, if seen, are highly predictive of neuroblastoma whereas tumor invasion of IVC suggests Wilms' tumor.

Other differentials are mesoblastic nephroma (seen in children younger than 6 months), renal cell carcinoma (peak age 10–20 years), clear cell sarcoma and rhabdoid tumor of the kidney.

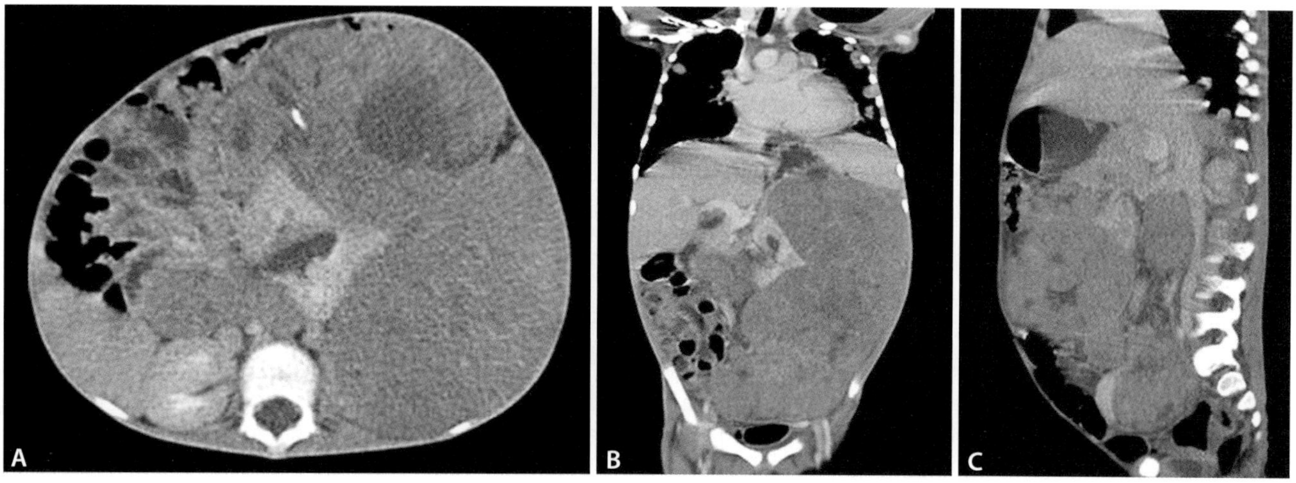

Figs. 6A to C: MDCT of a large left Wilms' tumor: (A and B) Axial CT and coronal MPR shows a large heterogeneous left renal mass with areas of low attenuation due to necrosis. Small focus of calcification is also seen. Residual renal parenchyma is displaced anteromedially by the mass and shows the positive "embedded organ" sign. The mass enhances less than the normal renal parenchyma. Note the ill-defined nodular hypoattenuating area anterior to the right kidney, aorta and IVC representing adenopathy. Vessels are not encased or elevated. Multiple metastases can be seen in the lung fields; (C) Parasagittal MPR image shows the entire IVC which is compressed by the mass but there is no invasion or thrombus formation.

Treatment and Prognosis

The treatment strategy of Wilms' tumors has become a model for the successful multidisciplinary approach to pediatric solid tumors. North American practice is initial surgical removal of the tumor followed by adjuvant chemotherapy dictated by the staging found at surgery. European oncologists favor initial chemotherapy (after biopsy confirmation in the UK) with later resection. The optimal surgery includes a transperitoneal approach with biopsy of adjacent regional lymph nodes, whether enlarged or not. Nephrectomy is usually carried out except in the setting of bilateral Wilms' tumors where partial nephrectomies, when possible, are indicated to preserve as much normal kidney tissue with the hope of avoiding or delaying the subsequent onset of chronic renal failure. The prognosis for Wilms' tumor patients is excellent and there is little evidence to suggest that the overall relapse-free survival is adversely affected by either approach. The 4-year overall survival rate, and presumed cure, ranges between 86% and 96% for stages I–III disease, is up to 83% for stage IV and 70% for stage V disease. Patients with the much less common diffuse anaplastic Wilms' tumors have a much poorer outcome, however. Their 4-year survival figures are 45% for stage III and only 7% for stage IV disease.[17]

Follow-up and Screening

Follow-up care after treatment must be long (if possible, lifelong) because Wilms' tumor may recur after several years. Most relapses occur within the chest and abdomen, and 94% of relapses occur within the first 2 years following diagnosis. Follow-up consists of chest radiography, abdominal ultrasonography and CT scan or MRI every 3 months for the first 2 years, every 6 months for another 2 years, and once every 2 years thereafter.[2]

Screening for Wilms' tumor in patients with associated syndromes should begin at 6 months of age with initial computed tomography (CT) followed by serial ultrasonography (US) every 3 months up to 7 years of age. After the age of 7 years, screening can be discontinued because the risk of developing Wilms' tumor decreases significantly.[6,18]

NEPHROBLASTOMATOSIS

The nephrons of the kidney develop from the metanephric blastema. This development is normally complete by the 36th week of intrauterine life. The term "nephrogenic rests" implies persistence of the metanephric blastema beyond 36 weeks of gestation. Nephroblastomatosis is the presence of multiple nephrogenic rests. These abnormal foci of persistent nephrogenic cells are regarded as precursor lesions and have the potential for malignant transformation into Wilms' tumor. They are found incidentally in 1% of infants. It is currently believed that nephrogenic rests give rise to approximately 30–40% of unilateral Wilms' tumors,[6] and they are found in up to 99% of bilateral Wilms' tumors.[19]

Pathology

Nephrogenic rests are classified histologically as *dormant, sclerosing, hyperplastic*, or *neoplastic*. Dormant and sclerosing rests are usually microscopic and not considered to have malignant potential. *Hyperplastic* and *neoplastic* rests are grossly visible as small nodules surrounded by normal parenchyma. Nephrogenic rests can also be classified into *perilobar* and *intralobar* on the basis of location and the syndromes with which they are associated. Perilobar rests lie in the peripheral cortex or columns of Bertin. They are associated with Beckwith-Wiedemann syndrome and hemihypertrophy, Perlman syndrome, and trisomy 18. Malignant degeneration into Wilms' tumor is most common in patients with Beckwith-Wiedemann syndrome and hemihypertrophy, occurring in 3% of cases.[6] Intralobar rests are considerably less common than the perilobar type but have a higher association with Wilms' tumor development. These rests are found in 78% of patients with Drash syndrome and nearly 100% of patients with sporadic aniridia and are also seen in patients with WAGR syndrome.

Imaging Features

Nephroblastomatosis may either be *diffuse* or *multifocal*. In the more common *multifocal* type, the nephrogenic rests resemble normal renal cortex on all modalities and can be scattered throughout the kidneys; US shows large, irregularly lobulated kidneys with hypoechoic to isoechoic homogeneous mass like regions within the renal parenchyma. These masses are often asymmetric and peripheral and the corticomedullary differentiation is poor. They are better defined on Contrast-enhanced CT and MRI as focal non-enhancing masses **(Fig. 7)**.[20] In general, these nodules appear fairly homogeneous in contrast to a Wilms' tumor which is always heterogeneous in appearance.

The *diffuse* form typically manifests as reniform enlargement with a thick hypoechoic rim on US. This abnormal tissue surrounds the renal periphery and compresses the centrally located residual parenchyma. At CT, the peripheral rim of nephroblastomatosis is homogeneously hypodense and non-enhancing, and causes distortion of the pelvicalyceal system. The remaining functional parenchyma may characteristically exhibit a pattern resembling Stag's antlers. On MRI, the nephroblastomatosis is homogeneously hypointense on T1W images and varies from iso- to hyperintensity on T2W images. It is best seen after contrast administration becoming sharply demarcated from the highly enhancing normal renal parenchyma.

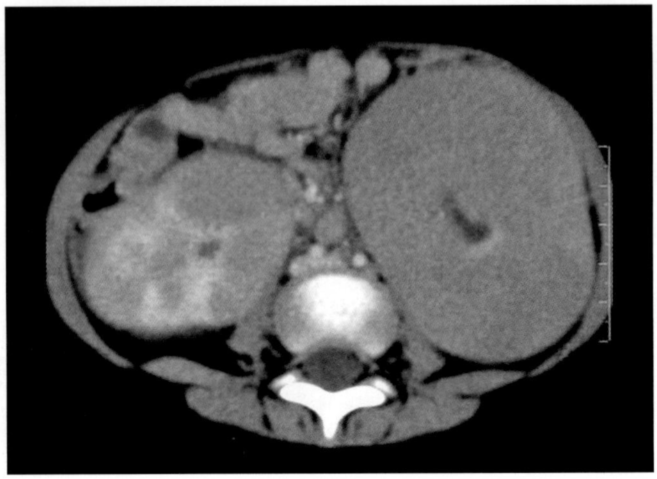

Fig. 7: Nephroblastomatosis in a 1-year-old child: Contrast-enhanced axial CT scan shows large nonenhancing hypodense masses in both the kidneys, larger on the left. Histological examination showed Wilms' tumor on the left.

MRI may be able to distinguish a sclerotic from a hyperplastic nephrogenic rest.[21] Sclerotic rests are thought to be in a regressive phase and to thus lack the potential to develop into a Wilms' tumor. Sclerotic rests typically appear dark on T2-weighted images, whilst hyperplastic rests are usually hyperintense, similar to Wilms' tumor. In the setting of bilateral nephroblastomatosis or bilateral Wilms' tumors on treatment, it is thought that hypointense lesions on T2-weighted images (sclerotic rests) may simply be observed, whereas hyperintense lesions may require further chemotherapy or local resection.[21] CT is unable to make this distinction.

The *differential diagnosis* of nephroblastomatosis includes renal lymphoma, leukemia or even polycystic kidneys.

MESOBLASTIC NEPHROMA (BOLANDE'S TUMOR)

Mesoblastic nephroma is the most common solid renal tumor identified in the first 3–6 months of life. It is a non-familial, benign tumor arising from the renal connective tissue. Originally thought to represent congenital Wilms' tumor, it was first described as a separate entity by Bolande et al. in 1967.[22]

Clinical Presentation

A large, palpable abdominal mass in a neonate is the most common presentation. The peak age at presentation is approximately 3 months. Additional signs and symptoms include hematuria, hypertension, vomiting, and hypercalcemia, seen in a minority of cases. Increased renin levels are often present. Some cases are detected at prenatal sonography and may be associated with polyhydramnios, hydrops, and premature delivery.

Pathology

Grossly, mesoblastic nephroma has a yellow, homogeneous, rubbery appearance likened to a *uterine leiomyoma* with no capsule and poorly defined margins. Unlike Wilms' tumor, foci of hemorrhage and necrosis are uncommon in this entity. The tumor has 2 morphologic variants—namely, the classic and cellular type. Microscopically, the classic type shows sheets of benign connective tissue and mature spindle cells arranged in bundles and fascicles with entrapped dysplastic tubules and glomeruli. The cellular variant is highly cellular, with immature mesenchymal cells and a high number of active mitotic figures, but no significant pleomorphism. Tumor *necrosis* and hemorrhage are more frequently seen with the cellular variant. These tend to have a poorer prognosis and are mainly seen in infants and children older than 3 months.[20]

Imaging

On US imaging, a mesoblastic nephroma appears typically as a well-defined, solid, homogeneous lesion **(Fig. 8A)**. There may be some heterogeneity due to hypoechoic areas of hemorrhage or necrosis. A distinctive "ring sign" may be seen in typical intrarenal CMN. This vascular ring sign, as described by Chan et al.[23] is an anechoic or hypoechoic vascular ring surrounding the tumor on ultrasound and is considered a feature of the typical or nonaggressive mesoblastic nephroma. On color Doppler examination, this vascular ring demonstrates significant vascularity, and on spectral Doppler examination, it demonstrates both arterial and venous waveforms.

CT and MRI demonstrate the presence of a large solid, mostly homogeneous intrarenal mass typically involving the renal sinus. On contrast administration, the tumor shows no or minimal enhancement **(Fig. 8B)**. Entrapment of urine or collecting system may lead to the excretion of contrast material within the mass. Areas of necrosis may be seen with the aggressive variant. On MRI, the mass shows intermediate signal intensity, similar to the renal cortex and the skeletal muscle on the T1- and increased signal on the T2-weighted images. The benign or the classic mesoblastic nephroma may demonstrate a peripheral, markedly enhancing ring on the postcontrast T1-weighted images, corresponding to the vascular ring seen on US.

On prenatal sonography, a mesoblastic nephroma may be first diagnosed when the detailed fetal anomaly scan is performed at 18–20 weeks' gestation, as a unilateral, solid paravertebral mass with low level echoes. Differentiation between a solid and a cystic mass can easily be made on ultrasound to differentiate between a mass and hydronephrosis. Associated polyhydramnios is common and is thought to occur due to increased renal blood flow and impaired renal concentrating ability leading to fetal polyuria and subsequent polyhydramnios. If the mass is very large, it may be difficult to determine the organ of origin in some cases. Fetal MRI may be helpful in determining the organ of origin.

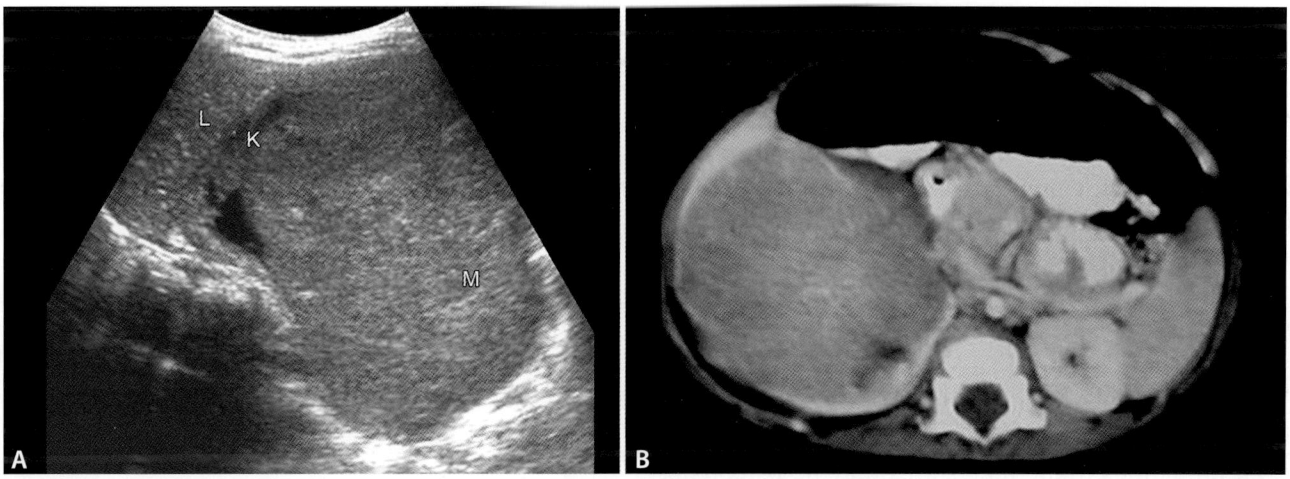

Figs. 8A and B: Mesoblastic nephroma: (A) Longitudinal US and (B) contrast-enhanced axial CT in a 6-month-old infant with a palpable abdominal mass show a large, central, solid homogeneous mass arising from the right kidney. The enhancing normal renal tissue is seen along the periphery in (B).
Abbreviations: M: Mass; K: Hydronephrotic kidney; L: Liver.

Differential Diagnosis

Imaging cannot definitively differentiate a mesoblastic nephroma from a congenital Wilms' tumor. Histologic examination is the only definitive test. The younger age of presentation, lack of well-defined margins, absence of tumor capsule, and central intrarenal location with involvement of renal sinus favor the diagnosis of mesoblastic nephroma. Other differential diagnoses include multicystic dysplastic kidney and congenital adrenal neuroblastoma.

Treatment and Prognosis

Mesoblastic nephroma generally exhibits benign behavior and is successfully treated with nephrectomy alone. Rarely, the lesion may recur locally, if incompletely resected or metastasize to the lungs, brain, or bones. Therefore, it is currently recommended that patients be closely followed-up for 1 year after surgical resection.[3] The prognosis is best, if the tumor is diagnosed and resected before 6 months of age.

CLEAR CELL SARCOMA

Clear cell sarcoma of the kidney once thought to be a variant of Wilms' tumor, accounts for 4–5% of primary renal tumors in childhood.[2] The peak incidence is at 1–4 years of age, and a male predominance has been reported.[3] It has a nonspecific presentation, most often manifesting as an abdominal mass. The tumor is characterized by its aggressive behavior and is associated with a higher rate of relapse and mortality than Wilms' tumor. It may metastasize to the bones, lymph nodes, brain, liver, and lungs; in some cases long after nephrectomy.

Pathology

At gross analysis, the tumor is soft and well circumscribed. At histologic analysis, small cells with inconspicuous nucleoli and ill-defined cell membranes and a prominent capillary network commonly characterize this tumor. However, there is a spectrum of appearances, in which only 20% have clear cells.[3]

Imaging

Imaging studies do not allow differentiation of clear cell sarcoma from Wilms' tumor. A sharply demarcated solid intrarenal mass without intravascular extension is seen on all modalities. Bone metastases may be osteolytic, osteoblastic or mixed. The discovery of a metastatic lesion in the skeleton in a child with a presumed diagnosis of Wilms' tumor should suggest that the tumor is likely to be a clear cell sarcoma. Once diagnosed, a ^{99m}Tc-MDP bone scintigraphy is indicated for staging purposes.

Treatment consists of nephrectomy and chemotherapy with current survival rates of 60–70%.[3] The most common site of recurrence is bone and current recommendations of the NWTSG-5 include periodic screening with bone scintigraphy and skeletal survey.

RHABDOID TUMOR

Rhabdoid tumor of the kidney (RTK) is a rare, highly aggressive malignancy of early childhood comprising 2% of all pediatric renal malignancies.[3] It was formerly considered a Wilms' tumor variant with unfavorable histology, but is now recognized as a separate entity. Rhabdoid tumor is seen early in life: 80% of cases occur in patients less than 2 years and 60% before 1 year of age. The median age at presentation is 11 months with a slight male predominance.[24]

Clinical Presentation

Most patients present with advanced stage disease and symptoms may be referable to metastatic disease. Concomitant brain tumor or other soft tissue tumors are distinctive features of this entity.

Pathology

The macroscopic appearance of rhabdoid tumor is nonspecific. It arises centrally (unlike Wilms' tumor) and has an infiltrative growth pattern. Local invasion of renal parenchyma and renal vein are common. Distant metastases to the lung and liver are also common and association with synchronous and metachronous brain metastases is a distinctive feature. Association with synchronous primary brain tumors has been reported in 10–15% of patients. Primitive neuroectodermal tumor, ependymoma, and cerebellar and brainstem astrocytoma have all been documented.[24] Soft tissue and thymic tumors may also occur in association with malignant rhabdoid tumor.

At histologic analysis, the tumor is characterized by monomorphic cells with prominent eosinophilic nucleoli and characteristic filamentous intracytoplasmic inclusions.[25] Some areas of the tumor may superficially resemble the blastemal pattern of Wilms' tumor.

Imaging

In most instances, RTK cannot be differentiated from Wilms' tumor based on imaging alone. US, CT and MRI show a large heterogeneous mass, characteristically involving the renal hilum with associated vascular invasion. If present, a number of features may suggest the diagnosis of RTK: subcapsular fluid collections, tumor lobules separated by dark areas of necrosis or hemorrhage, and linear calcifications outlining tumor lobules.[26] Vascular and local invasion is common. Radiological investigation should also include cross-sectional imaging for the common sites of metastases (lung, liver, brain), bone scintigraphy and skeletal survey (bone metastases).

Treatment and Prognosis

Of all the pediatric renal tumors, the prognosis of children with RTK is the poorest. Despite aggressive surgery and chemotherapy, RTK has the poorest prognosis amongst all pediatric renal tumors. There is a high rate of local tumor recurrence following surgical resection. Survival is poor, with an 18-month survival rate of only 20%.[26]

RENAL CELL CARCINOMA

Renal cell carcinoma (RCC) is primarily a tumor of the adult population and less than 2% of all cases occur in the pediatric age range. The mean age of presentation is 9 years. Although Wilms' tumor is much more common than any other malignancy in the first decade of life, Wilms' tumor and RCC have an almost equal incidence in the second decade.[27]

Renal cell carcinoma is associated with von Hippel-Lindau syndrome, in which the tumors tend to be multiple and manifest at a younger age. This syndrome must be ruled out in pediatric patients diagnosed with renal cell carcinoma, especially when the tumor is bilateral.[27]

Clinical Presentation

Clinical manifestations are similar to those in adults. Gross painless hematuria, flank pain, and a palpable mass are the most common presenting symptoms. Hematuria is more frequent in patients with renal cell carcinoma than in patients with Wilms' tumor.

Pathology

The tumor forms an infiltrative solid mass with variable necrosis, hemorrhage, calcification, and cystic degeneration. There is distortion of the normal renal architecture and formation of a pseudocapsule. The tumor invades locally with spread to adjacent retroperitoneal lymph nodes. Metastases to the lungs, bones, liver, or brain are found in 20% of patients at diagnosis. Compared with Wilms' tumor, renal cell carcinoma is more likely to manifest bilaterally and more likely to metastasize to bone.[2]

Imaging

RCC and Wilms' tumor may be indistinguishable based on imaging features alone. RCC tends to be smaller and exhibits calcifications more frequently (25% of RCC versus 9% of Wilms' tumor).[6] On CT and MRI, RCC appears as a heterogeneous intrarenal mass, due to the presence of necrosis and/or hemorrhage. Ring like calcifications may be present. On contrast administration, the mass shows little or no enhancement.

MULTILOCULAR CYSTIC RENAL TUMOR

The term multilocular cystic renal tumor (MCRT) refers to two distinct entities: Cystic nephroma (CN) and cystic partially differentiated nephroblastoma (CPDN). Both are benign renal tumors that have well-defined margins and consist entirely of cystic lesions with multiple thin-walled septations. In CN, the septa are composed entirely of differentiated tissues. If immature or blastemal cells are present in the septa, the lesion is termed CPDN.[20]

Multilocular cystic renal tumors have a biphasic age and sex distribution—two-thirds occur in a predominately male pediatric population between 3 months and 2-years-old; approximately one-third occur in a mostly female population, with a peak in the 5th and 6th decades of life.[28] There is no association with cysts in other organs and only sporadic association with other congenital anomalies.

Clinical Presentation

Presenting symptoms vary with patient age. Children typically present with a painless, progressively enlarging, palpable abdominal or flank mass that has a variable growth rate and may be discovered incidentally. Adults can present with a variety of nonspecific signs and symptoms, including abdominal and flank pain, urinary tract infection, and hypertension.[28]

Pathology

Cystic nephroma (CN) and cystic partially differentiated nephroblastoma (CPDN) are indistinguishable from each other on gross examination and consist of a well-defined multiloculated mass of non-communicating cysts that is surrounded by a thick fibrous capsule and compressed renal parenchyma. The mass is typically large and commonly arises from the lower pole of the kidney. Calcification is rare. Necrosis and hemorrhage are uncommon but are usually seen in association with herniation of the tumor into the renal pelvis or ureter, which damages the thin layer of transitional epithelium.[28]

At microscopic examination, however, CN is clearly distinct from CPDN. In CN, the septa consist of fibrous tissue, which may contain well-differentiated epithelial cells. The presence of poorly differentiated tissues or blastemal cells in the septa characterize CPDN. It is essential to distinguish between cystic nephroma and CPDN because the blastemal component theoretically portends the risk of Wilms' tumor development.

Imaging

Abdominal radiography may demonstrate a soft-tissue mass. Curvilinear and peripheral calcification may be seen, although it is uncommon. On US, CT and MRI, a MCRT typically appears as an intrarenal multicystic mass with no solid or nodular elements **(Figs. 9A and B)**. The loculi can range in size from microscopic to 4 cm in diameter and very small loculi may mimic solid components because of their innumerable, closely packed acoustic interfaces.[29,30] On CT, the cystic spaces have an attenuation value similar to or slightly greater than water. On MR T1-weighted images the cyst contents show variable signal intensities, depending on the concentration of old hemorrhage or protein and a high signal intensity on T2-weighted images. Septal enhancement is seen on contrast administration on both CT and MRI. Associated urinary tract obstruction may be evident.

Differential Diagnosis

The main differential diagnosis is cystic Wilms' tumor. Identification of solid nodular elements in the septa should suggest the diagnosis of WT and not MCRT. Other lesions that may mimic MCRT include multicystic dysplastic kidney, cellular variety of mesoblastic nephroma, clear cell carcinoma and renal cell carcinoma.[20]

Treatment and Follow-up

Because neither the clinical nor the imaging features of multilocular cystic renal tumor (MCRT) can predict its histologic characteristics, surgery—either nephrectomy or nephron-sparing surgery—is required for both diagnosis and treatment.[29] If pathologic analysis proves that the tumor is a CPDN, regular noninvasive monitoring is suggested because the presence of blastemal cells in the septa of a CPDN implies the potential for more aggressive behavior, despite the usually benign course of the tumor.

ANGIOMYOLIPOMA

Angiomyolipomas (AML) are benign hamartomatous masses in the kidney containing fat, smooth muscle and blood vessels in varying proportions. Up to 80% of all patients with tuberous sclerosis (both adults and children) have angiomyolipomas.[2] When associated with tuberous sclerosis, these tumors are more likely to be multifocal, bilateral and of greater size. Association with neurofibromatosis and von Hippel-Lindau syndrome has also been described.

Clinical Presentation

Most commonly AMLs are found incidentally in asymptomatic children. Clinical symptoms are related to the occurrence of tumor bleeding which correlates with the size of tumor. AMLs smaller than 4 cm are usually asymptomatic. Those larger than 4 cm are more likely to

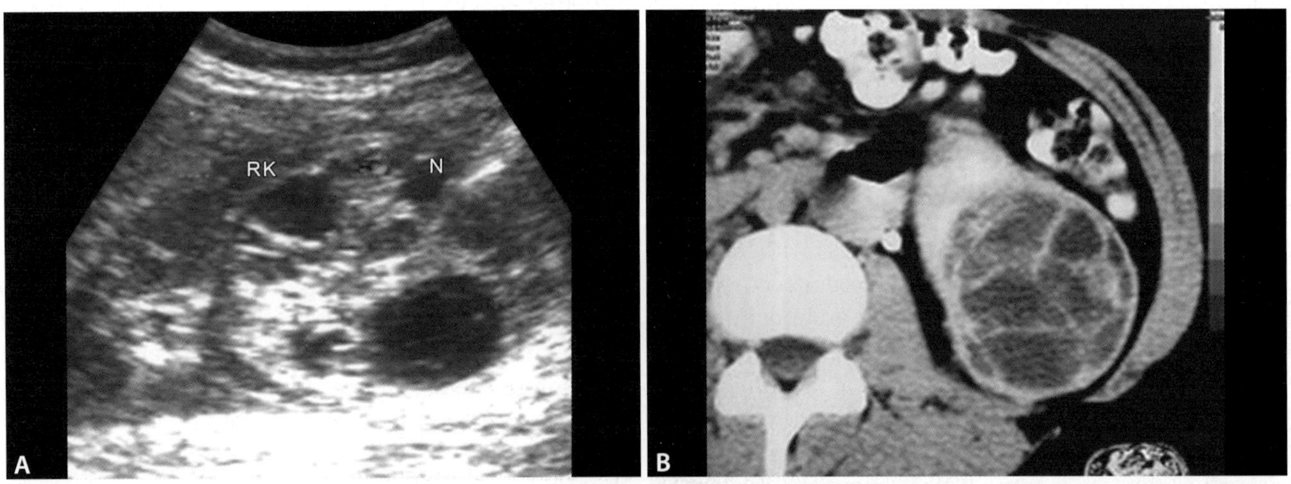

Figs. 9A and B: Multilocular cystic nephroma: (A) Longitudinal US and (B) contrast-enhanced axial CT demonstrate an intrarenal sharply circumscribed, multiloculated mass with enhancing septae on CECT.

bleed spontaneously and manifest clinically as pain and hematuria or even severe life- threatening hemorrhage.[2,31]

Pathology

On gross examination, angiomyolipoma appears as an intrarenal mass, varying in diameter from 3–20 cm. It is well demarcated from surrounding compressed renal parenchyma but it has no capsule. Rarely, it may behave aggressively and invade the collecting system, renal vein, IVC and retroperitoneal lymph nodes. Microscopically, a mixture of lipomatous tissue, blood vessels and smooth muscle characterizes angiomyolipoma.

Imaging

Imaging studies are diagnostic, if a characteristic fatty component is identified. On US, AML is seen as a heterogeneous mass, predominantly echogenic, without through transmission **(Fig. 10A)**. CT is the most reliable imaging modality and shows the presence of a renal mass with significant fat attenuation within it **(Figs. 10B and C)**. However, in the case of small lesions thin sections and single voxel measurements may be needed to confirm the diagnosis.[32] MRI can also detect fat within an AML which gives high signal intensity signal on both T1- and T2-weighted images. The signal intensity decreases on out of phase T1W and fat-suppressed pulse sequences. Angiography which may be performed for embolization of a focal lesion prior to surgery, shows a hypervascular lesion with tortuous, somewhat aneurysmal arteries, venous puddling, but no vascular encasement or arteriovenous shunting.[33]

Screening, Follow-up and Treatment

Conservative management is recommended for patients with known masses smaller than 4 cm. In children with tuberous sclerosis, it is expected that by 10 years of age, 80% will have developed angiomyolipomas if monitored. The intensity of monitoring varies between centres. Serial US examinations every 2–3 years before 10 years of age and every 8–12 months thereafter are recommended, with

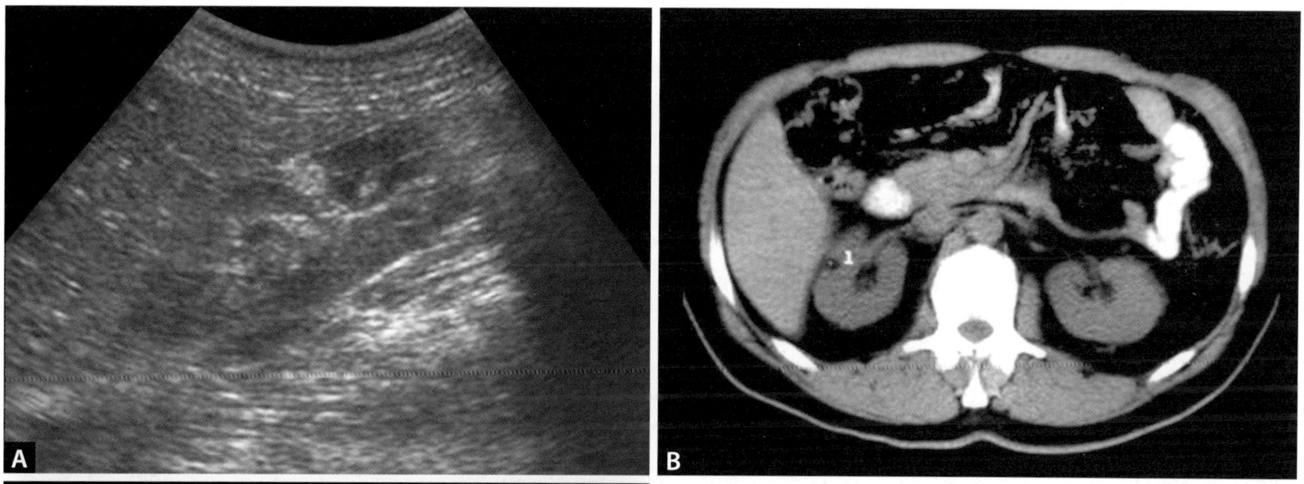

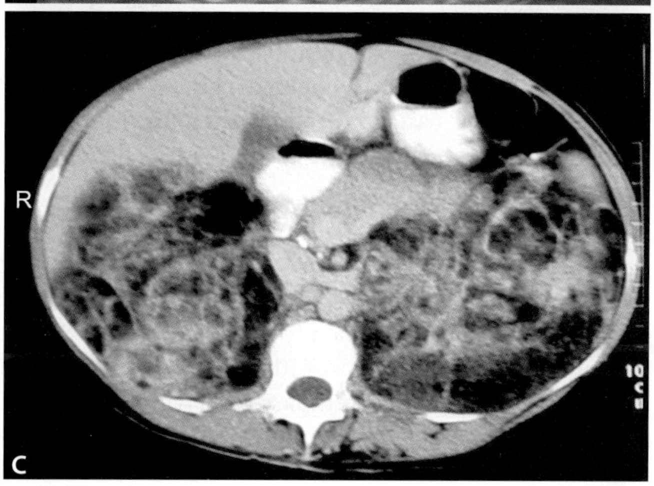

Figs. 10A to C: Angiomyolipoma: (A) Longitudinal US of the right kidney shows a small well-defined hyperechoic mass in peripheral cortex; (B) Contrast-enhanced axial CT shows fatty attenuation (–50 HU) in the mass; (C) Contrast-enhanced CT shows large heterogeneous masses in both kidneys with multiple fat density areas in a child with tuberous sclerosis.

the aim of identifying and monitoring growing lesions.[3] Lesions that have bled or lesions larger than 4 cm may require renal-sparing surgery or selective transcatheter embolization in an attempt to spare as much renal parenchyma as possible.[2]

OSSIFYING RENAL TUMOR OF INFANCY

Ossifying renal tumor of infancy is a rare benign renal mass and is reported only in young children ranging from 6 days to 14 months, Boys are more commonly affected than girls.[34,35] The tumor is relatively small (2–3 cm) and resembles renal calculi, except that it is attached to the renal parenchyma. The mass is centrally located at or near the renal papilla from where it extends in a polypoid fashion into the collecting system. Microscopically, ossifying tumors are composed of an osteoid core, osteoblasts and proliferating spindle cells.

Imaging

The renal outline is usually maintained; however, filling defects with partial obstruction of the collecting system are often seen. Because of its location within the collecting system and its characteristic ossification, ossifying renal tumor of infancy may mimic a staghorn calculus, which would be exceedingly rare in the age group in which this lesion occurs. At US, the mass is echogenic with shadowing, and hydronephrosis may be present. CT shows a well-defined mass, often calcified, with poor enhancement.[3]

METANEPHRIC ADENOMA (NEPHROGENIC ADENOFIBROMA, EMBRYONAL ADENOMA)

Metanephric adenoma is a benign renal tumor that can occur at any age and has been reported in patients as young as 15 months and as old as 83 years. It is more common in female patients.[3] Presenting features include pain, hypertension, hematoma, a flank mass, hypercalcemia, and polycythemia.

Imaging

At US, the mass is well-defined and solid. It can be hypoechoic or hyperechoic or even cystic with a mural nodule. Doppler evaluation shows the lesion to be hypovascular. CT shows an iso- to hyperattenuating mass which enhances less than normal renal parenchyma. Small calcifications may be present.[36]

LYMPHOMA

Lymphoma either involves the kidney secondarily from direct retroperitoneal extension or by hematogenous metastases. In children, non-Hodgkin lymphoma—especially Burkitt lymphoma—is more likely to involve the kidney. As many as 62% of patients with lymphoma have renal involvement at autopsy although only 3–8% of these patients demonstrate renal involvement at CT.[3,37] The existence of primary renal lymphoma without evidence of systemic disease is still debatable.

Clinical Presentation

Lymphomatous involvement of the kidney typically does not produce symptoms until late in the disease. Flank or abdominal pain, hematuria, anemia, weight loss, and a palpable mass are the most common clinical findings. Hypertension is rare.[3]

Imaging

Imaging findings are variable and include solitary or multiple renal masses or nodules, diffuse infiltration, direct invasion from contiguous retroperitoneal extension, and least commonly isolated perinephric disease. The most common radiologic pattern is multiple parenchymal masses or nodules that occasionally distort the renal contour and displace the collecting system. Lymphomatous masses have a nonspecific CT appearance. They are usually homogeneous, hypodense on non-enhanced and contrast-enhanced images, and may mimic multiple renal cysts. At US, they are hypoechoic and may demonstrate increased through transmission **(Fig. 11A)**. On MRI, lymphomatous nodules exhibit signal intensity slightly higher than that of muscle on T1- and higher than fat on T2-weighted images.

Diffuse infiltration of the kidney may result in reniform enlargement. Retroperitoneal disease occasionally leads to vascular and ureteric encasement. Perinephric involvement can arise from retroperitoneal disease (most commonly) or transcapsular spread of parenchymal involvement. The CT findings of perinephric disease are variable and include small curvilinear areas of high attenuation, soft-tissue attenuation nodules, thickening of the Gerota fascia, or a mass contiguous with retroperitoneal disease.

LEUKEMIA

Renal involvement by leukemia is rare at presentation but may occur at relapse. Renal involvement generally occurs along with involvement of other extramedullary sites such as mediastinum, liver, pancreas, lymph nodes, etc. Renal symptoms such as hypertension or renal failure are rare. Leukemic infiltration of the kidneys most commonly

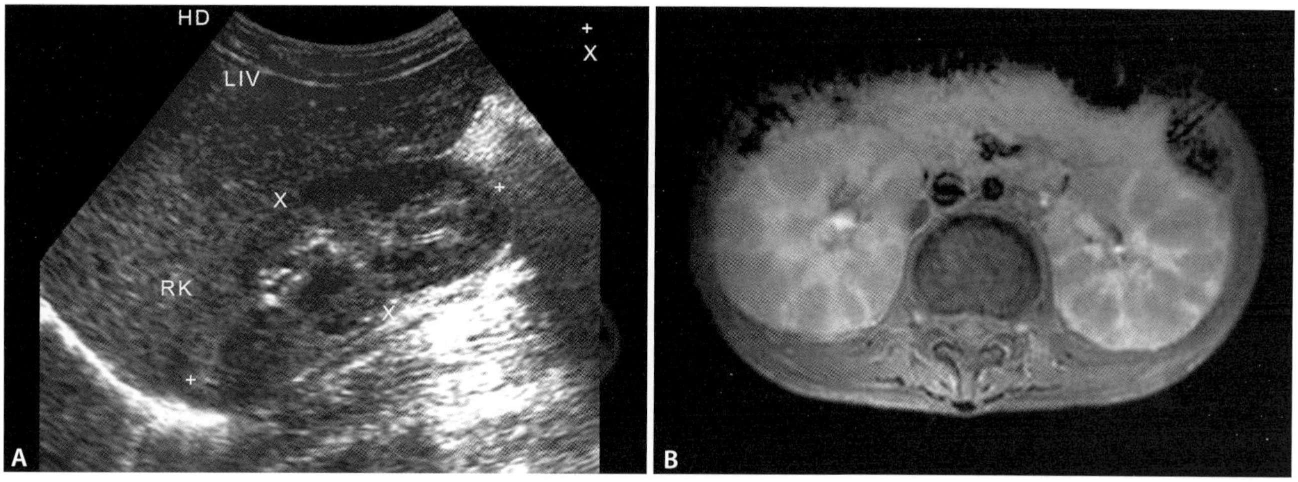

Figs. 11A and B: (A) Renal lymphoma: Longitudinal US through the kidney shows multiple focal hypoechoic masses in the kidney; (B) Renal Leukemia: Postcontrast T1-weighted axial image shows leukemic infiltration of the kidneys in a 12-year-old boy as multiple nonenhancing nodular lesions in the renal parenchyma. This appearance is indistinguishable from that of lymphoma.

causes bilateral, diffuse renal enlargement with distortion of the calyceal system. solitary or multiple focal nodular deposits may be seen in the renal parenchyma. On imaging, the kidneys are enlarged but maintain their shape. There is loss of corticomedullary differentiation on US with a heterogeneouses echotexture. CT and MRI show the same findings, i.e. bilaterally enlarged kidneys with loss of corticomedullary differentiation, altered parenchymal attenuation and decreased cortical enhancement.[2] Nodular deposits are seen as hypoechoic on US which are non-enhancing on CT and MRI **(Fig. 11B)**. The differential diagnosis includes nephroblastomatosis, lymphomatous deposits and simple cysts.

PRIMARY NEUROGENIC TUMORS OF THE KIDNEY

Primitive Neuroectodermal Tumor

Primitive Neuroectodermal Tumors (PNETs) are rare malignant lesions most commonly occurring in the chest and extremities but have been reported to occur in the kidney. At histological examination, the tumor features small round cells and areas of extensive necrosis. On imaging, these lesions resemble Wilms' tumors. A large heterogeneous mass with areas of necrosis and minimal or no enhancement are found. Calcifications may be present.[20]

Neuroblastoma

Primary renal neuroblastomas have been reported but are rare. Imaging appearances resemble those of Wilms' tumor. Secondary renal involvement from contiguous adrenal and retroperitoneal neuroblastoma is more common and an incidence of 20% of cases has been reported.[38] Renal invasion occurs more frequently in undifferentiated histology and high stage (3 or 4) tumors. Extension may occur by tumor spread along vessels or by direct infiltration of the renal capsule, especially the upper pole contiguous with the adrenal gland.

Other rare primary tumors of the kidney are *renal medullary carcinoma,*[3] *metanephric stromal tumor and hemangiopericytoma* or reninoma.[2] *Metastases* to the kidney are extremely rare in children. Osteosarcoma metastases have been reported.[39]

CYSTIC DISEASES OF THE KIDNEY

Although simple cysts of the kidneys are more common in adults, they are more frequent in childhood than was previously appreciated and may even be seen *in utero*. The routine use of US nowadays and its high sensitivity in the diagnosis of cystic lesions, account for the increased number of cysts reported.

It is believed that if a cyst is small, asymptomatic and meets all the standard US criteria for a simple cyst (no internal echoes or septations, good through transmission, smooth wall) then no further evaluation is required. Follow-up sonography is recommended to detect changes in the size or appearance of the cyst that might indicate the need for surgical treatment. If a cyst is symptomatic (producing hypertension or dangerously attenuating the overlying cortex), surgery may be indicated despite a benign appearance at US.

If a cystic lesion fails to meet the criteria for a simple renal cyst, then additional imaging studies, e.g. CT or MRI, are indicated, to exclude developmental lesions (e.g. multicystic dysplastic kidney) or cystic neoplasms (cystic Wilms' tumor, clear cell sarcoma and multilocular cystic renal tumor).

ADRENAL MASSES

Adrenal masses in children may be due to neoplasms, hemorrhage, abscess and cysts. Neoplasms of the adrenal gland may arise from the medulla or the cortex. Medullary neoplasms are of neural crest origin and so may arise not only from the adrenal medulla but also from the sympathetic chain and include neuroblastoma, ganglioneuroblastoma, ganglioneuroma and pheochromocytoma. Adrenal cortical neoplasms are the carcinoma and adenoma. Rarely, other neoplasms like smooth muscle tumors can occur in children.

NEUROBLASTOMA

Neuroblastoma (NBL) is by far the most frequent adrenal neoplasm, being the third most common pediatric malignancy, after leukemia and central nervous system tumors.[40] It is also the most common malignancy encountered in the first month of life. The median age of diagnosis is 2 years and 90% of the diagnoses are made in children under the age of 5 years.[41] The tumor is congenital and cases have been identified on in utero ultrasound examination. There is a genetic predisposition to neuroblastoma and the tumor has occurred in siblings and in identical twins.[42]

Site

Neuroblastomas arise from primordial neural crest cells, which are the precursors of the sympathetic nervous system. As a result, they can be found anywhere along the sympathetic chain or in the adrenal medulla. Two thirds of NBLs are located in the abdomen and of these approximately two-thirds arise in the adrenal gland and the rest from the retropritoneal sympathetic ganglia, followed by the posterior mediastinum (20%).[43] Less common sites are the pelvis (2–3%) and the neck (1–5%). Occasionally, in the presence of metastatic disease, no definite primary tumor can be found.

Clinical Features

NBL has overall a wide spectrum of clinical symptoms which depend on the site, extent and the biological features of the primary tumor, and the presence of distant metastatic disease. The majority of children with NBL present with a palpable abdominal mass. This may be an incidental finding in an otherwise healthy child or in a child clearly unwell with lethargy, anemia, weight loss and failure to thrive from widespread dissemination of tumor. In half of the patients with intraspinal tumor extension, peripheral neurologic deficits and neurological symptoms from compression of the nerve roots or the cord may be present.[42] Metastatic involvement of the periorbital bones and soft tissues results in ecchymosed orbital proptosis, which is also described as "raccoon eyes" and may be misinterpreted as non-accidental injury. Compression of the optic nerves by metastases may cause blindness. Massive hepatic metastases can cause increased intra-abdominal pressure and death from respiratory insufficiency. Encephalopathic symptoms may be encountered. In less than 2% of cases, NBLs can present with paraneoplastic syndromes: opsoclonus-myoclonus-ataxia syndrome or watery diarrhea.[44] NBLs may also be discovered incidentally during scanning for other reasons, e.g. antenatal ultrasound, chest radiograph for pneumonia or screening protocols.

Urinary excretion of high levels of catecholamine metabolites occurs in 85–90% of patients. These metabolites are identified as vanillylmandelic acid (VMA) and homovanillic acid (HVA). The VMA/HVA ratio in patients with disseminated disease correlates with prognosis. Vanillacetic acid (VLA) in urine indicates a poor prognosis.[45]

Pathology

The tumors arise from the primitive neuroectodermal cells. Histologically, NBLs are composed of small round and rosette- forming cells which may be difficult to distinguish from similar round cells seen in Ewing's sarcoma, rhabdomyosarcoma, and even leukemia. Classically, three different types of neural crest tumors are described based on the degree of differentiation of these primitive cells and subsequent variable malignancy. Neuroblastoma is considered the most malignant, ganglioneuroma a benign and ganglioneuroblastoma with a mixed mature and undifferentiated histology as a "semi malignant" or intermediate manifestation of this neoplastic disease. Within a given tumor, the state of maturation may change: especially in an infant, the degree of malignancy may decrease and the neoplastic process may disappear.

Staging

The age of the patient and the stage of disease at diagnosis are the two most important predictors of survival in neuroblastoma. The International Neuroblastoma Staging System (INSS)[46] is based on radiological findings, surgical resectability, lymph node involvement and bone marrow involvement **(Table 3)**. Patients with stage 1 have greater than 90% 5-year survival. The survival rate falls with increasing stage of disease, the exception being stage 4S in which the survival can be between 60–90%. Spontaneous regression has been demonstrated in a small group of stage 4S patients. The overall survival of patients less than 1 year of age is almost 75%. As the age of the patient at diagnosis increases the survival rate falls.[42]

A more recently introduced recognized variant of NBL, stage 4N (N = nodes) has been described which is not included in the INSS classification. This has been added for children with distant nodal spread, but no bony cortical involvement on account of better prognosis.[44]

Imaging

Imaging of neuroblastoma requires evaluation of the primary tumor and the metastatic extent of disease.

Plain radiographs: Abdominal radiographs may show the presence of an abdominal mass. One of the characteristic findings in neuroblastoma is calcification, which can be demonstrated in about one half of abdominal neuroblastomas (compared with only less than 10% in Wilms' tumor). The calcification is usually finely stippled but may also be linear or ring shaped and can sometimes be seen in areas of metastases such as lymph nodes or liver. Evidence of erosion of vertebral body or widened interpedicular distance suggests intraspinal extension.

If the child has presented with bone pain, it is likely that initial imaging will include skeletal radiographs. Discrete lytic areas or metaphyseal lucencies are typical of metastatic involvement and plain film appearances can simulate leukemic infiltration. However, the bones may appear normal even in the presence of metastases. Skull radiographs may also show lytic areas or sutural widening due to underlying dural involvement **(Fig. 12)**.

Ultrasound: The mass is seen as a predominantly solid, poorly defined, heterogeneous, echogenic mass with few echopoor areas. Calcification is commonly seen **(Fig. 13A)**. The displaced kidney can be identified, most often inferolateral to the mass, with a well-defined plane between the mass and the kidney. In rare cases, a neuroblastoma may invade the kidney and then it is impossible to differentiate from Wilms' tumor. The tumor often extends across the midline and can be seen to encase and anteriorly displace the aorta, IVC and other vascular structures rather than invade them. The opposite kidney may also be displaced by large masses. US is useful in detecting differential movements of the tumor relative to the adjacent organs, i.e. liver and ipsilateral kidney. If there is no differential movement, involvement is likely. Nodal and focal hepatic metastases can be identified.

Antenatal and perinatal US examination has resulted in an apparent increase in the incidence of fetal or congenital neuroblastoma. The US appearance is variable and ranges from cystic through solid to mixed with foci of calcification.[46] The differential diagnosis of this appearance is adrenal hemorrhage, extralobar pulmonary sequestration and congenital mesoblastic nephroma.

Table 3: International Neuroblastoma Staging System.[46]

Stage 1	Localized tumor confined to the area of origin; complete gross resection with or without microscopic residual disease; identifiable ipsilateral and contralateral lymph nodes negative macroscopically
Stage 2A	Localized tumor with incomplete gross excision, identifiable ipsilateral and contralateral lymph nodes negative microscopically
Stage 2B	Unilateral tumor with complete or incomplete gross resection with positive ipsilateral regional lymph nodes contralateral lymph nodes negative microscopically
Stage 3	Tumor infiltrating across the midline with or without regional lymph node involvement; unilateral tumor with contralateral regional lymph node involvement; or midline tumor with bilateral regional lymph node involvement
Stage 4	Dissemination of tumor to distant lymph nodes, bone, bone marrow, liver, or other organs (except as defined in stage 4S)
Stage 4S	Localized primary tumor (as defined for stage 1 or 2) with dissemination limited to skin, liver, or bone marrow (<10% tumor cells, and MIBG scan negative in the marrow) limited to infants <1 year of age

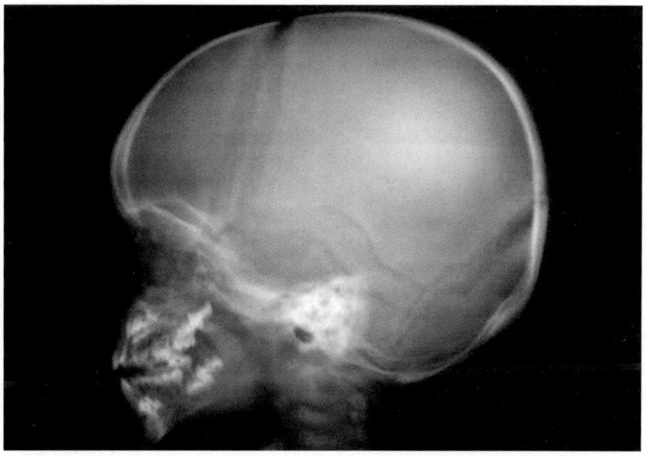

Fig. 12: Lateral film of the skull shows sutural widening due to underlying dural involvement.

CT and MRI: Further axial imaging for staging of a newly discovered NBL can be performed with either CT or MRI of the primary site. Both modalities can accurately assess the location and the size of the primary tumor, the vascular encasement and tumor resectability, but may sometimes be equivocal in the evaluation of invasive growth and lymphadenopathy. MRI is superior to CT in determining marrow infiltration and intraspinal extension of tumor.

On CT, a NBL is seen as a large, heterogeneous, lobulated soft-tissue mass that shows mild heterogeneous enhancement. Coarse, finely stippled or curvilinear calcifications are seen in more than 90% of the abdominal **(Figs. 13B and 14)** and 50% of the thoracic NBLs on CT.[44] Low attenuation areas seen within the tumor represent necrosis or hemorrhage. On MRI, the tumor is typically heterogeneous, with low signal on T1- and high signal intensity on T2-weighted images, and shows little or no enhancement **(Figs. 15A and B)**. Cystic and hemorrhagic areas within the tumor can be well identified but not calcification. On diffusion-weighted images, NBLs show increased tumor signal which is attributed to restricted diffusion of water protons within the dense tumor matrix.[47]

The tumor is usually lobulated and lacks an identifiable capsule. Involved nodes at the renal hila, porta, and in the retroperitoneum are often large. Distinguishing between the primary tumor and the adjacent nodal disease is often difficult. Adrenal tumors frequently displace the ipsilateral kidney inferiorly while paravertebral tumors may push the kidney anteriorly.

Both CT and MRI can demonstrate retrocrural and paravertebral extension and encasement and compression of the major abdominal vessels. Spinal canal extension is more common with thoracic than with abdominal tumors and the extent of extension, spinal cord displacement and compression are better seen on MRI.

Hepatic metastases have two distinct patterns—either diffuse infiltration seen in 4S infants, which maybe indiscernible on CT, but is clearly seen on MRI as characteristically bright signal on T2-weighted images; or focal nodular lesions seen in older children with stage 4 disease which can be readily identified on both CT and MRI. Lung metastases are rare, occurring in approximately 3% cases.[48] MRI plays an important role is assessing disseminated disease in the bone marrow. Bone marrow disease is usually seen as diffuse infiltration but it may also present a nodular pattern with areas of low and high signal intensity on T1- and T2-weighted images, respectively. Both CT and MRI may be needed for detection and follow-up of cranial disease particularly with recurrent disease. Bony erosion is identified on CT **(Fig. 16)**, both CT and MRI can demonstrate soft tissue deposits and focal dural involvement whereas diffuse leptomeningeal disease is best seen on contrast-enhanced MRI.

Some studies suggest that MRI with whole body short- time inversion recovery (STIR) imaging can replace the combination of CT and bone scintigraphy for overall assessment of stage 4 disease in children with NBL, reducing the radiation exposure and the number of sedation procedures required.[49]

Nuclear scanning: Two-thirds of patients with neuroblastoma have metastatic bone disease at diagnosis. *^{99m}Technetium methylene diphosphonate (^{99m}Tc MDP) whole-body bone scintigraphy* should be performed

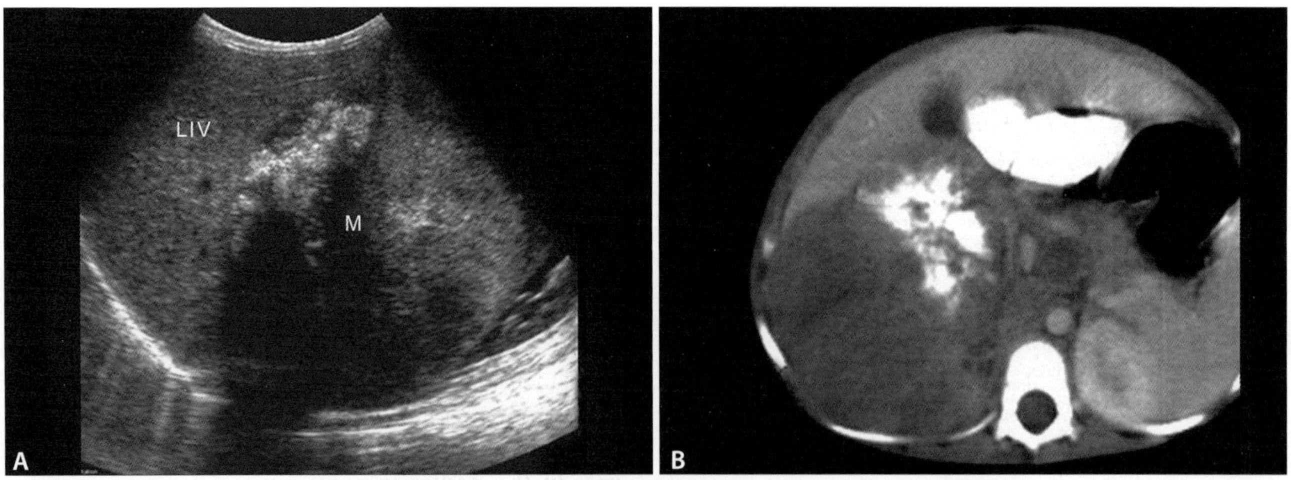

Figs. 13A and B: Neuroblastoma: (A) US and (B) contrast-enhanced axial CT show a solid, right adrenal mass with a large area of calcification within. Multiple retroperitoneal nodes are also seen on CT.

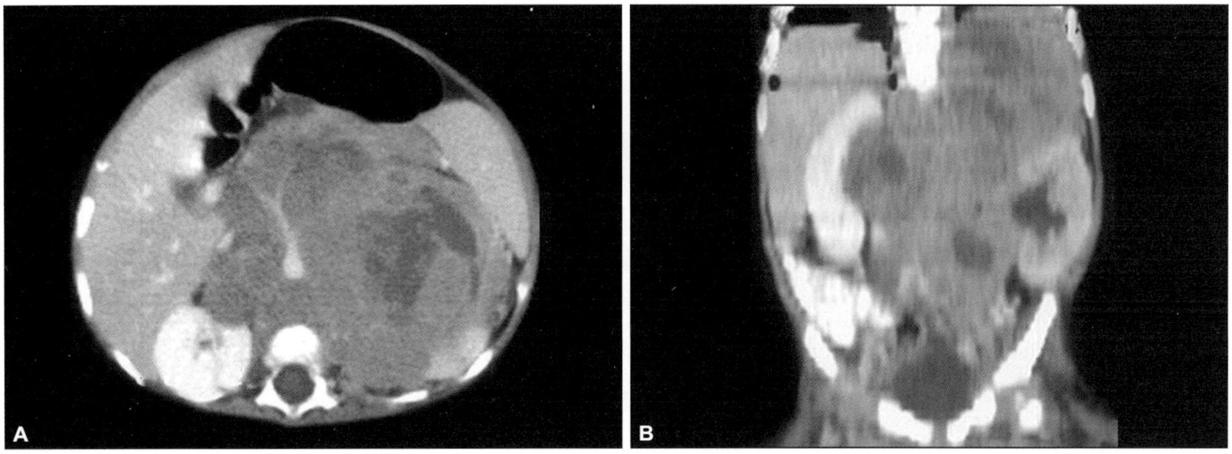

Figs. 14A and B: Neuroblastoma: CECT (A) axial and (B) coronal reconstruction in a 2-year-old child show a large lobulated left abdominal mass with few hypodense necrotic areas within. The mass elevates and encases the aorta and its branches. The IVC is displaced anteriorly and to the right. The left kidney is displaced inferolaterally and shows the negative beak sign suggesting an extra-renal origin.

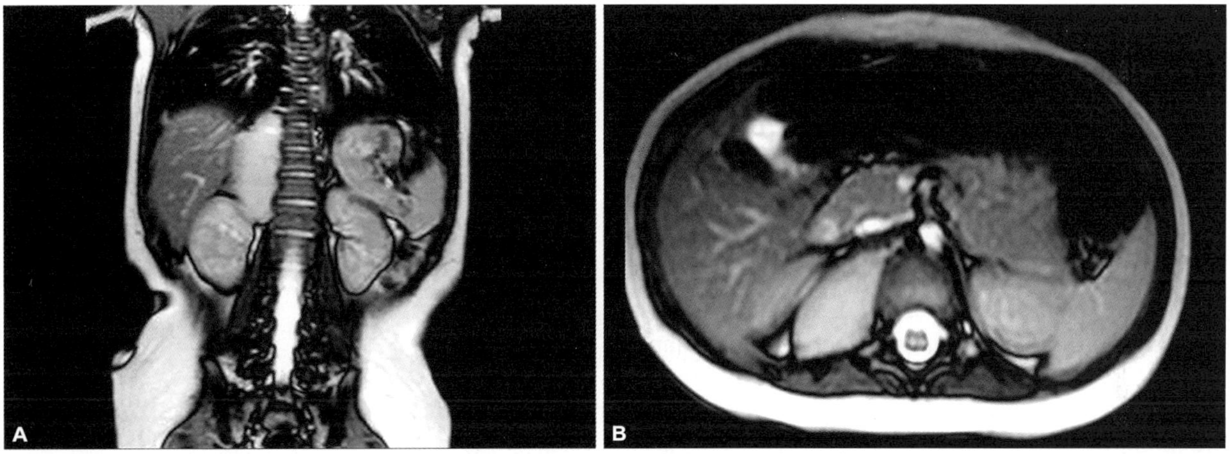

Figs. 15A and B: Paravertebral neuroblastoma: (A) Coronal and (B) axial T2-weighted MR images in a child presenting with opsoclonus-myoclonus syndrome show a well-defined hyperintense solid mass seen in the right paravertebral region superior to the right kidney. There is no evidence of intraspinal extension of the tumor.

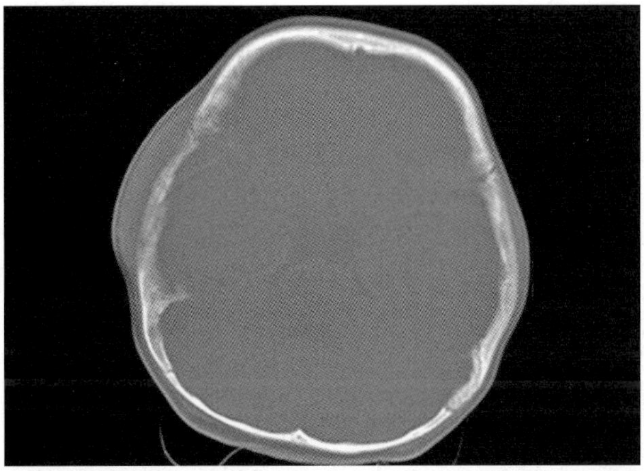

Fig. 16: Cranial metastasis in neuroblastoma: CT cranium shows bony erosion of the right parietal bone with overlying soft tissue thickening.

on all patients at diagnosis. It is more sensitive than a radiographic skeletal survey. Plain radiographs should be performed on suspicious areas of abnormal increased tracer uptake. The primary tumor frequently takes up ^{99m}Tc MDP and is consequently seen on bone data acquisition.[50]

Metaiodobenzylguanidine (MIBG) imaging plays an important role in diagnosis and follow-up of patients with NBL. MIBG labeled with either I^{123} or I^{131} should be done in all patients. MIBG is an analog of catecholamine precursors and is taken up by catecholamine-producing cells and although other neuroendocrine tumors such as pheochromocytoma, medullary carcinoma of thyroid and carcinoid tumors also take up MIBG, these are extremely rare in the pediatric population. Therefore, uptake of MIBG is considered specific for neuroblastoma.

MIBG is taken up by both—the primary tumor and metastases and shows high sensitivity (88%) and specificity (99%) in detecting primary tumor and metastatic involvement (cortical bone, bone marrow and lymph nodes) in more than 90% of patients.[49] MIBG scanning is less sensitive than MDP at detecting bone involvement, and using only MIBG may result in an underestimate of bone metastases. False negative MIBG scans do occur and therefore many centers combine MIBG and MDP in the diagnostic work-up of children with NBL to minimize the incidence of false-positive or false-negative results.

Positron Emission Tomography (PET), using ^{18}fluoro-2-deoxy-glucose, has emerged as a promising modality for revealing NBL in both soft-tissue and skeleton. FDG uptake is directly proportional to tumor burden and to tumor-cell proliferation. Primary tumor and metastatic spread concentrate FDG avidly before therapy, whereas after therapy variable patterns of accumulation have been observed. PET scanning can be useful in MIBG-negative cases and during follow-up when assessing response to treatment.[51]

Differential Diagnosis

The differential diagnosis encompasses all pediatric abdominal masses, particularly Wilms' tumor (discussed in earlier section), teratoma, lymphoma, metastatic retroperitoneal lymhadenopathy and rhabdoid tumor. A congenital neuroblastoma diagnosed in the neonatal period needs to be differentiated from neonatal adrenal hemorrhage. The diagnosis of adrenal hemorrhage is usually made by ultrasound, which identifies the mass and shows, in sequential examinations, decreasing size and cystic evolution. Color Doppler is useful to show avascularity of adrenal hemorrhage. MRI may show the classic signal intensity pattern of aging blood products, but diagnostic difficulties can occur because of bleeds of different ages. Other pediatric adrenal tumors, such as pheochromocytoma and adrenal carcinoma, are much less common.

Management and Follow-up

Treatment depends on several factors, including stage of the disease at the time of presentation and response to initial therapy. Surgery, chemotherapy and radiation therapy all have a role to play. Primary surgical resection is done for localized tumors and initial chemotherapy for those that are unresectable, followed by delayed surgery once, they decrease in size.

The imaging strategy in the follow-up period depends largely on the imaging protocols followed by various pediatric oncology set-ups. Regular follow-up is required after surgery to assess the tumor bed for local recurrence. Follow-up is also essential in non operable tumors to assess response to chemotherapy and to determine the most appropriate time for delayed surgery. Imaging includes chest radiographs, abdominal US, and CT/MRI of the primary site. ^{99m}Tc MDP and I^{123} MIBG scanning are performed until they have returned to normal or until the end of treatment.[51]

GANGLIONEUROBLASTOMA

A ganglioneuroblastoma is intermediate in aggressiveness in the spectrum of neural crest tumors between the frankly malignant neuroblastoma and the benign ganglioneuroma. Most occur in the abdomen and thorax. Clinically, they present with effects of a mass lesion, hormonal manifestations being rare. Occasionally, they can be discovered incidentally on radiographs performed for some other purpose.

Imaging and investigation are the same as described for neuroblastomas **(Figs. 17A to C)**. Catecholamine excretion is usually increased. Biopsy is required for diagnosis but sampling errors may occur due to variable tumor composition.[51]

GANGLIONEUROMA

This tumor is benign and is formed of nerve fibers and mature ganglion cells. Most ganglioneuromas occur in the posterior mediastinum. Only one-third occur in the abdomen, and most are paravertebral, rarely from adrenal medulla. These tumors generally occur in older children or adolescents, who are often asymptomatic. Hormonally active lesions are rare. They may be discovered incidentally on radiographs or present with mass effect.

The imaging appearances are similar to those of neuroblastoma but unlike NBLs, they are well encapsulated masses. The abdominal lesions may even encase the aorta and the inferior vena cava and their branches or invade the spinal canal. The definitive diagnosis depends on histological examination of tumor tissue. Surgical removal may be difficult particularly when the mass is encasing vital structures or with intraspinal extension. In these cases, conservative management is advocated with regular clinical and imaging follow-up.[51,52]

PHEOCHROMOCYTOMA

Pheochromocytoma is an uncommon neoplasm in children.[42] Like neuroblastoma, pheochromocytoma is of neural crest origin, secretes catecholamines, and

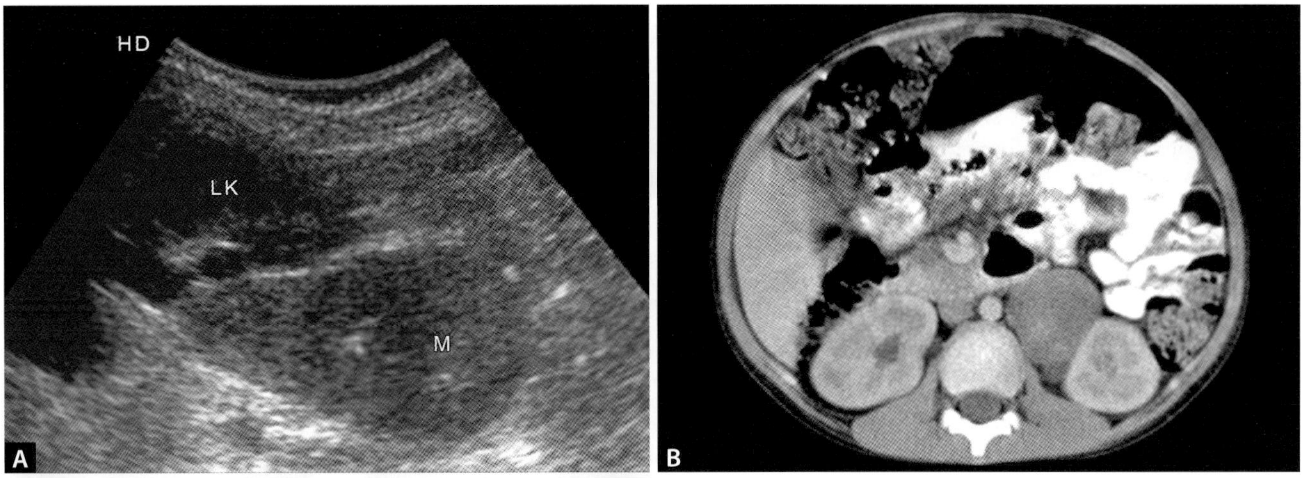

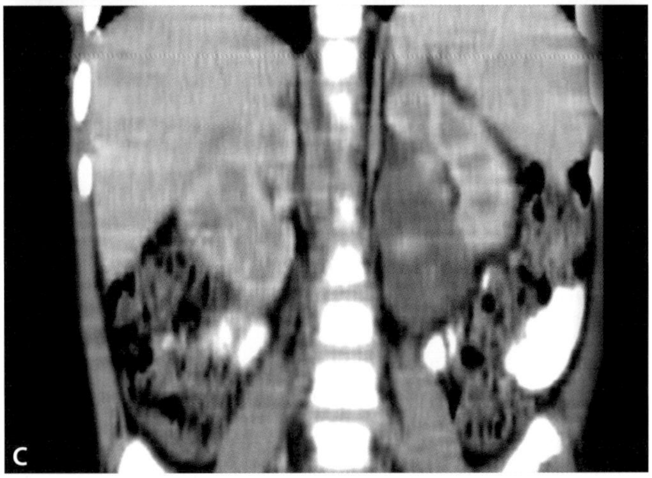

Figs. 17A to C: Paravertebral ganglioneuroblastoma in a 10-month-old infant: (A) Longitudinal US and (B and C) Contrast-enhanced CT (axial and coronal reformation) show a well-defined, oval, solid mass medial and inferior to lower pole of left kidney displacing it laterally. The imaging features cannot differentiate it from a paravertebral neuroblastoma. The diagnosis was made on histopathology.

may be located in the adrenal medulla or anywhere along the sympathetic chain. In children, 70% of pheochromocytomas occur in the adrenal gland and 20% have bilateral involvement. 30% have extra adrenal involvement, and most of these occur in the upper abdomen. Other less common extra-adrenal sites include the sympathetic chain anywhere from base of skull to pelvis, urinary bladder, spermatic cord and vagina. Multiple lesions are present in 30–70% of children. Malignancy occurs in less than 10%.[53]

Pheochromocytoma usually presents in older children and a familial occurrence is well documented. It has been seen as a part of multiple endocrine neoplasia syndrome (MEN 2). It has also been associated with a number of diseases, including neurofibro-matosis, von Hippel-Lindau disease and Sturge-Weber syndrome.

Clinical Presentation

Clinical presentation is usually related to the secretion of catecholamines. Patients may present with hypertension, sweating, headaches, visual blurring, flushing, tachycardia, hypertensive encephalopathy, weight loss and diarrhea. Urinary catecholamines are usually markedly elevated, much more so than with neuroblastoma.[42]

Imaging

On ultrasound, a pheochromocytoma may be seen as a well-defined hypoechoic mass which may be homogeneous or heterogeneous due to hemorrhage and necrosis **(Fig. 18A)**. Calcification is uncommon. Sonography easily detects lesions in and adjacent to adrenal glands but is less sensitive than CT and MRI for lesions in mid and lower abdomen.[52] On CT, the lesions have a soft tissue attenuation with diffuse, mottled or rim-like enhancement **(Fig. 18B)**. Adrenergic blockade, to prevent a hypertensive crisis, is not required prior to nonionic contrast administration during CT scanning.[17] On MRI, pheochromocytomas have a low signal on T1-weighted images and high signal on T2-weighted images, with intense enhancement and slow wash-out after

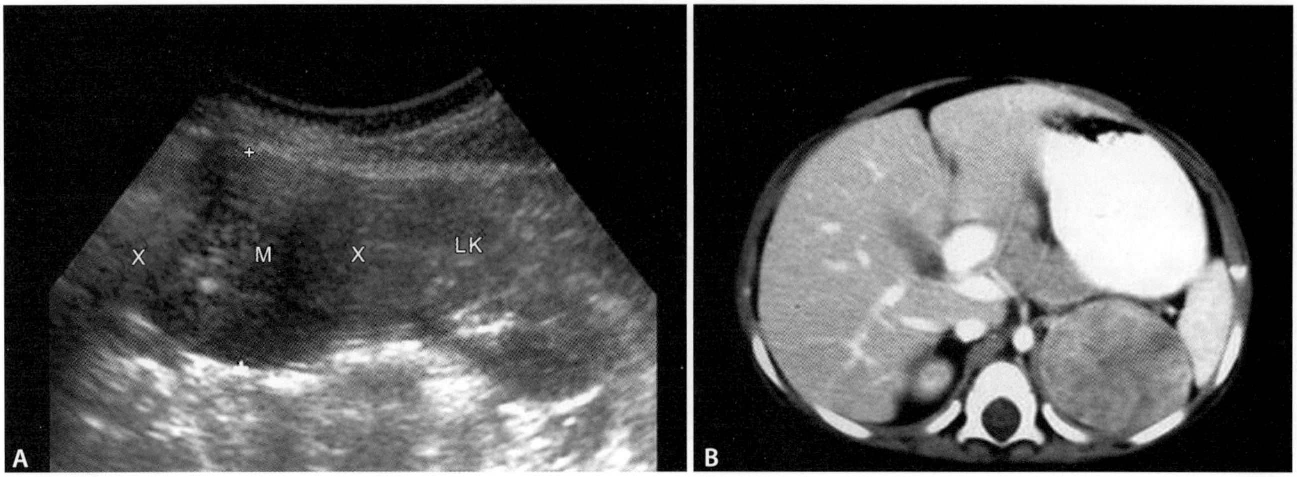

Figs. 18A and B: Pheochromocytoma: (A) Longitudinal sonogram in a 2-year-old girl shows a well-defined, solid, hypoechoic mass with few small hyperechoic foci in the left suprarenal region; (B) Contrast-enhanced CT shows the tumor as a well-defined solid mass which shows mottled enhancement.
Abbreviations: M: Mass; LK: Left kidney.

contrast administration. Malignancy is best determined by identifying distant metastases to nonchromaffin tissues like lung, liver, bone and lymph nodes.[53] I^{131} MIBG can accurately localize a pheochromocytoma, but does not show the anatomy as well as CT or MRI. It is particularly helpful in detecting nonadrenal tumors (paragangliomas). MIBG may be positive in the abdomen even when an US is negative and MIBG should always be done prior to surgery to detect or exclude multiple sites of disease.

ADRENAL CORTICAL TUMORS

Adrenocortical tumors (ACT) are very rare in children with a worldwide annual incidence of 0.3 per million children below the age of 15 years. About 75% of children who develop adrenocortical tumors are less than 5 years old at the time of diagnosis. The incidence is higher in young girls with a female/male ratio of 2:1, whereas in adolescence the sex ratio is equal. Two syndromes have a clear association with this tumor: Li-Fraumeni syndrome is associated with mutations of the *p53* gene, and Beckwith-Wiedemann syndrome which has mutations in the 11p15 region.[54]

Clinical Features

More than 75% of adrenocortical tumors are functional, secreting one or more hormones (androgens, cortisol, aldosterone, or estrogens). Virilization, with early onset of pubic hair, hypertrophy of the clitoris or penis, accelerated growth, gynecomastia or acne, is the most common presentation. The second most common manifestation is with hypercortisolism (Cushing's syndrome), whilst presentation with a palpable abdominal mass is unusual. Hypertension may be seen in up to 43% at diagnosis.[55] This may be due to either mineralocorticoid or glucocorticoid excess, increased aldosterone production or simply renal artery compression by the tumor, and the hypertension usually resolves after tumor resection. Diagnosis of an ACT is supported by raised levels of androstenedione, dehydroepiandrosterone sulfate (DHEAS), testosterone, and urinary steroids. These hormones are also useful markers for the detection of tumor recurrence during follow-up. The combination of hormone production and adrenal mass is diagnostic of an adrenocortical tumor.

Imaging Features

On all 3 modalities (US, CT and MRI), the smaller lesions tend to have a fairly homogeneous appearance **(Figs. 19A and B)** and areas of hemorrhage, necrosis and calcification are seen in the larger lesions. A characteristic central scar with radiating linear bands representing areas of necrosis and calcification is often seen in the large lesion.[53]

The tumor tends to be locally aggressive and frequently invades the IVC and may extend into the right atrium.[56] The tumor may also metastasize to lung, nodes, bone, and liver. MR imaging is the modality of choice and demonstrates the primary tumor, caval extension, and liver metastases.[57] Chest CT to exclude or detect pulmonary metastases should be performed at first diagnosis.

The classification of benign from malignant ACTs is not clear cut and is the subject of much debate.[17] Even established histopathological criteria and algorithms

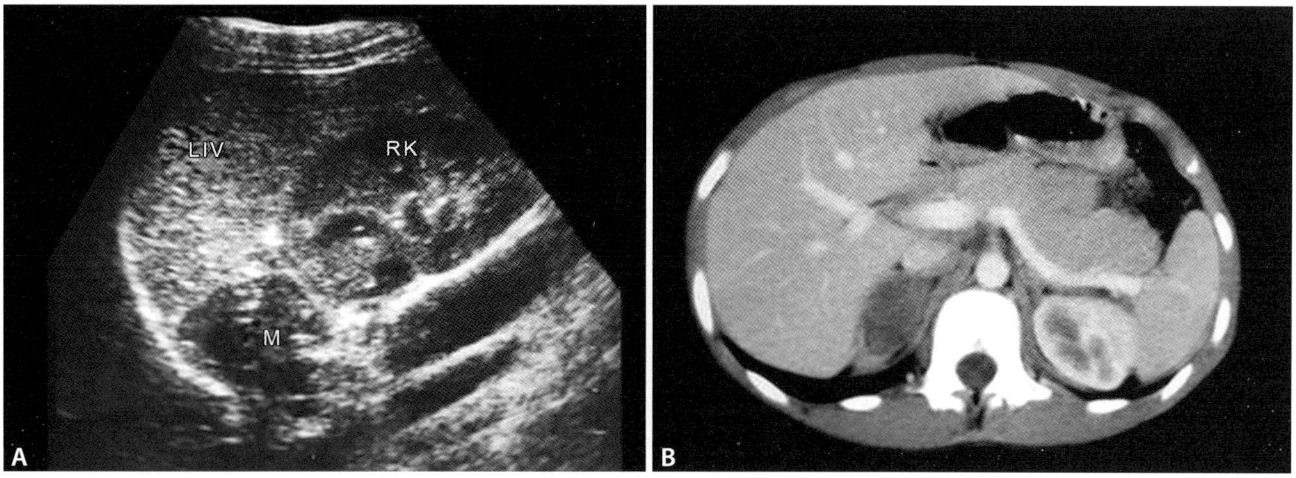

Figs. 19A and B: Adrenal adenoma: US and contrast-enhanced axial CT scans show a small well-defined mass in the right suprarenal region in a 12-year-old boy, hypodense on CT with no evidence of calcification.

adapted from tumors in adults do not allow a clear classification in children. Differentiation between adenoma and carcinoma is in practice somewhat arbitrary, and all patients (even those with a seemingly benign adenoma completely resected) require close follow-up initially. The majority of ACTs in children are interpreted pathologically as malignant in most studies. Factors favoring malignancy include size over 5–10 cm, weight over 200 g, invasion into the periadrenal soft tissues or IVC.[17]

Surgical resection is the mainstay of treatment. Younger children, particularly those less than 5 years, with pathologically malignant ACTs, have a significantly better prognosis than older children and adolescents.[17]

ADRENAL HEMORRHAGE

Adrenal hemorrhage occurs almost exclusively in newborns in association with perinatal asphyxia, trauma or bacterial (typically meningococcal) septicemia. The precise cause is unknown but is thought to be stress related or due to birth trauma, as there is an increased frequency in larger babies or babies of diabetic mothers. The hemorrhagic process may involve the whole gland or part of one, or both adrenal glands in about 10% of cases.

Clinical Features

In a moderate or massive degree of adrenal hemorrhage, there is clinically a palpable flank mass due to the caudal displacement of the ipsilateral kidney from the hemorrhagic mass. The mass is usually not palpable at birth and develops over the following 24 hours. The child will often become jaundiced and present with vomiting. The mass typically regresses within days to a few weeks with resorption of the clot. Acute or late adrenal insufficiency is uncommon, even in bilateral adrenal hemorrhage.

Imaging Features

Ultrasound demonstrates a suprarenal mass that is variable in echogenicity.[57] In the acute phase, the hemorrhage is usually echogenic, representing clot formation **(Fig. 20)**. Over several weeks, the hemorrhage becomes echofree as the clot lyses and becomes liquefied. The hemorrhage gradually decreases in size and may result in adrenal calcification. If there is no evidence of ultrasonographic resolution after several days, other diagnoses, including

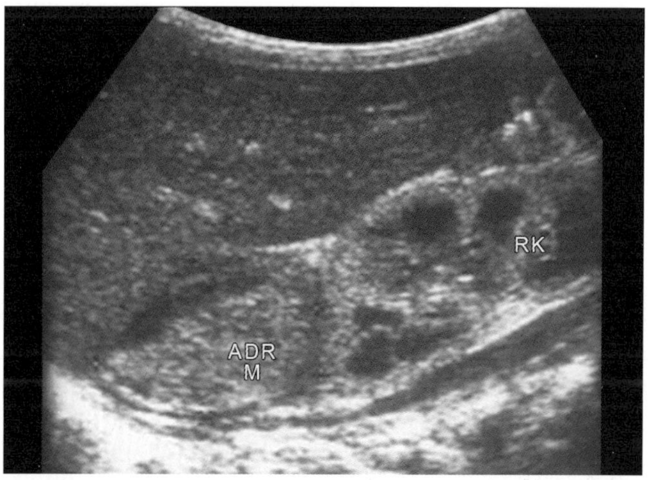

Fig. 20: Adrenal hemorrhage: Longitudinal US scan through the right flank in a 9-day-old infant shows a well-defined cystic mass in the right suprarenal regional with a fluid-fluid level.

neuroblastoma and its variants, but also benign conditions such as an adrenal cyst or extraadrenal abnormality from a surrounding structure including an enteric duplication cyst, need to be considered.

In older children, post traumatic adrenal hemorrhage has been described to occur in some 3% of blunt abdominal injury and often associated with ipsilateral lesions of the liver, kidney or spleen. It seems more likely to occur on the right side, is usually asymptomatic and, also, without evidence of subsequent adrenal insufficiency.[52]

ADRENAL CYSTS

Large adrenal cysts may be found in older children. These are usually endothelial lined and found incidentally. Their importance lies in their being mistaken for adrenal neoplasms. If cross sectional imaging shows a smooth thin-walled cyst without any evidence of solid components, and there is no endocrine dysfunction, hypertension, infection or metastatic disease, they can be managed conservatively because adrenal neoplasms seldom have large cystic components and never present as thin smooth-walled cystic structures without solid components.

PRIMARY RETROPERITONEAL TUMORS

Primary tumors of retroperitoneum are rare tumors that originate in the retroperitoneal space but outside the major organs in that space. These neoplasms are generally derived from neurogenic cells, embryonic rests or mesenchymal cells and may be benign or malignant.

NEUROGENIC TUMORS

Neurogenic tumors may arise from tissue of the sympathetic (autonomic) nervous system and include extra-adrenal neuroblastoma **(*see* Figs. 15A and B)**, ganglio-neuroblastoma **(*see* Figs. 17A and B)** and ganglioneuroma, or from neuroectoderm as in the case of a primitive peripheral neuroectodermal tumor. Extra-adrenal pheochromocytoma also arises in the retroperitoneum. The site of origin of all these tumors is in the paravertebral gutter with resultant anterior and lateral displacement of other retroperitoneal structures including kidneys, ureters and the inferior vena cava. Their imaging and investigations are similar to that of their adrenal counterparts and have been discussed earlier. Uncommon neuro-ectodermal tumors are paraganglioma, neurofibroma, neurofibrosarcoma, neurolemmoma, or schwannoma. Although occasionally isolated tumors, they are often seen as multiple tumors in patients with neurofibromatosis.[58]

GERM CELL TUMORS

Germ cell tumors are derived from the primordial germinal epithelial layer cells and two-thirds of these tumors are extragonadal in location. These include germinomas, embryonal carcinoma, endodermal sinus tumor, choriocarcinoma, gonadoblastoma and teratoma. *Teratomas*, the most common of germ cell tumor, account for 3.5–4% of all germ cell tumors in children. They contain all three embryonal layers—ectoderm, mesoderm and endoderm. They are the third most common tumors of the retroperitoneum in children following neuroblastoma and Wilms' tumor. The ratio of girls to boys is 2:1. Malignancy is seen in 10–15% cases.[59] Increase in abdominal girth is the most common presenting symptom, frequently accompanied by pain, nausea, vomiting and weight loss. The presence of a palpable abdominal mass is an almost universal finding. Occasionally, the tumor is present antenatally and diagnosed at birth, these neonatal teratomas have a higher incidence of malignancy than those in older children. Malignant teratomas can produce alpha-fetoprotein and its serum levels can be used to monitor response to therapy/recurrence.[60]

Imaging

Plain radiographs may demonstrate calcification or formed bony components such as teeth and phalanges, which are pathognomic. The tumor may be cystic, solid, or mixed. Although US demonstrates the solid or cystic nature of the tumor, CT defines the true location and character of the mass better and is useful to delineate the extent of the disease in retroperitoneum and its relationship to major vessels **(Figs. 21A and B)**. Fat may be identified in about half the cases and fat-fluid levels may sometimes be seen. Internal homogeneity, fat density, cyst formation, and calcification are important predictors of a benign retroperitoneal tumor on CT.[61]

MESENCHYMAL TUMORS

Lipomatous Tumors

These are often quite large at the time of diagnosis and are usually benign. They include lipoma, lipoblastoma and liposarcoma-like lipoblastomatosis. These tumors are best visualized on CT and MRI, showing homogeneous fatty attenuation at CT and homogeneous signal identical to that of fat on all MR imaging sequences. The boundaries of the mass are clearly delineated because of marked contrast in signal intensity with surrounding structures. Lipoblastoma

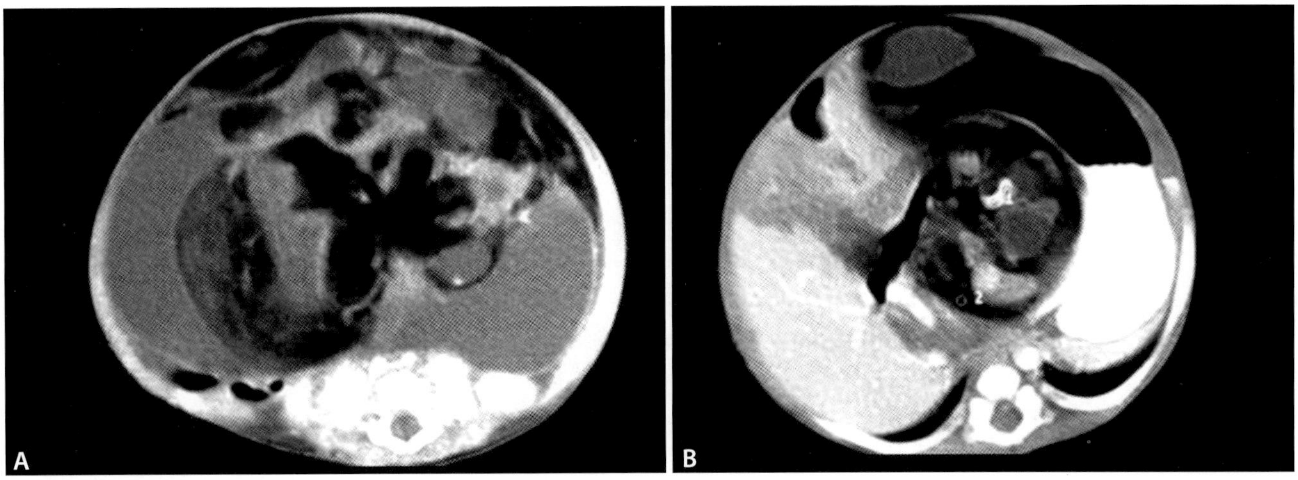

Figs. 21A and B: Teratoma: (A) Contrast-enhanced axial CT section shows a large well-defined heterogeneous mass with cystic, solid and fat attenuation components in a 3-month-old child; (B) A higher section shows the presence of a tooth within the mass, clinching the diagnosis.

is extensive and locally invasive, and difficult or impossible to remove completely. Its appearance on imaging studies may be similar to lipoma but some cases have shown areas of relatively increased attenuation on CT, which on pathologic examination have been shown to be regions of myxoid material. Liposarcoma is extremely rare in children, but is locally invasive and also metastatic to distant sites.

Rhabdomyosarcoma and Undifferentiated Sarcomas

Rhabdomyosarcoma (RMS) accounts for 5 to 8% of childhood cancer and presents in a wide variety of histologic types and patterns of spread of tumor. Retroperitoneal rhabdo-myosarcomas are rare tumors. The tumors infiltrate locally, invade lymphatics and blood vessels, and frequently present with distant hematogenous metastases to the lungs, bone marrow, and bone. Retroperitoneal lymph nodes, bone marrow metastases, and distant hematogenous metastases to the lungs are common at presentation. Other sarcomas occasionally seen in children and adolescents include fibrosarcoma, neurofibrosarcoma, malignant fibrous histiocytoma, hemangiopericytoma and leiomyosarcoma.[62]

RETROPERITONEAL LYMPHANGIOMA

Retroperitoneal lymphangioma is a benign tumor of congenital lymphatic origin. Cystic lymphangioma or hygroma consist of multiple dilated, poorly developed lymphatic channels. The cystic spaces are lined with endothelium and contain multiple thin septa and chylous fluid. Although it may present early as a palpable abdominal mass, the soft nature of this lesion, makes it difficult to identify on physical examination. The mass may compress adjacent structures, particularly displacing and obstructing the ureters. On US, a lymphangioma is seen as a cystic mass with multiple, apparently non-communicating, fluid-containing cystic regions, separated by thin septae. CT also shows the cystic nature of the mass, although the septae are not well seen **(Fig. 22)**. Rarely, hemorrhage or infection may complicate a lymphangioma.

LYMPH NODE MASSES

Isolated retroperitoneal lymph node enlargement in children is unusual and associated findings help to clarify the diagnosis. Retroperitoneal lymphadenopathy can be benign, most often infective—tubercular, or it can occur with a variety of malignant processes including metastatic lymph node enlargement or lymphoma.

Metastasis to retroperitoneal nodes in children occur by spread from primary retroperitoneal malignancies such as Wilms' tumor, neuroblastoma, or spread from testicular or ovarian malignancies **(Fig. 23)**. Intra-abdominal lymphoma in children is nearly always non-Hodgkin's lymphoma, most commonly Burkitt's lymphoma. Retroperitoneal lymphadenopathy generally occurs along with bowel, hepatic or spleen involvement. Initial presentation with retroperitoneal masses is uncommon and more likely to be associated with lymphomas related to pharmacologic immunosuppression.[63]

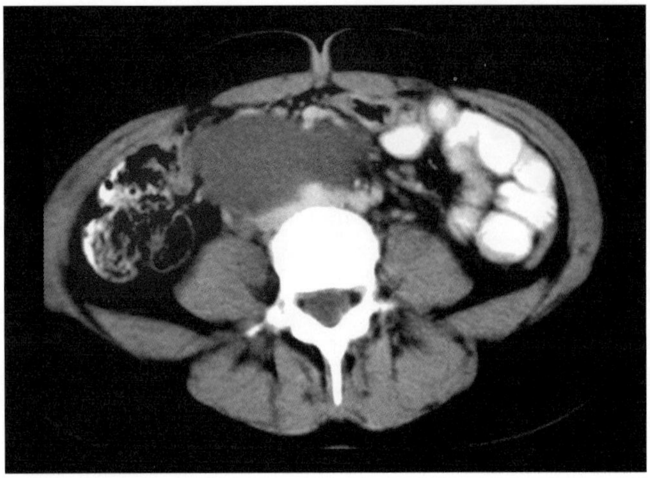

Fig. 22: Lymphangioma: Contrast-enhanced axial CT shows a cystic mass in midline with thin imperceptible walls, just anterior to the major abdominal vessels, displacing the mesenteric vessels anteriorly.

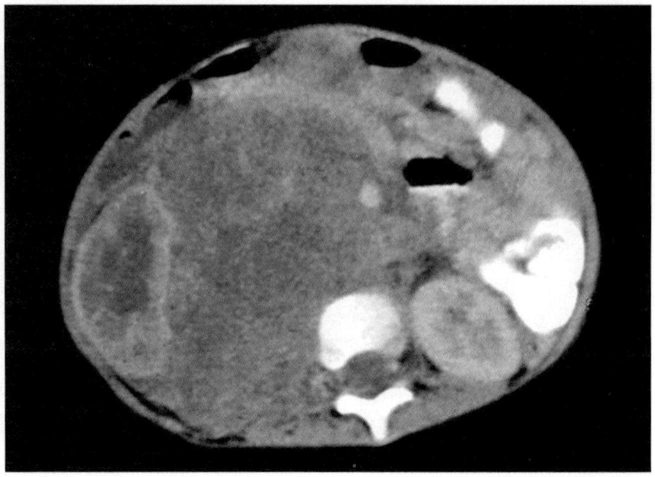

Fig. 23: Metastatic testicular germ cell tumor: Contrast-enhanced CT shows massive, low attenuation retroperitoneal lymphadenopathy displacing the right kidney laterally (negative beak sign seen) in a diagnosed case of testicular germ cell tumor in a 2-year-old boy.

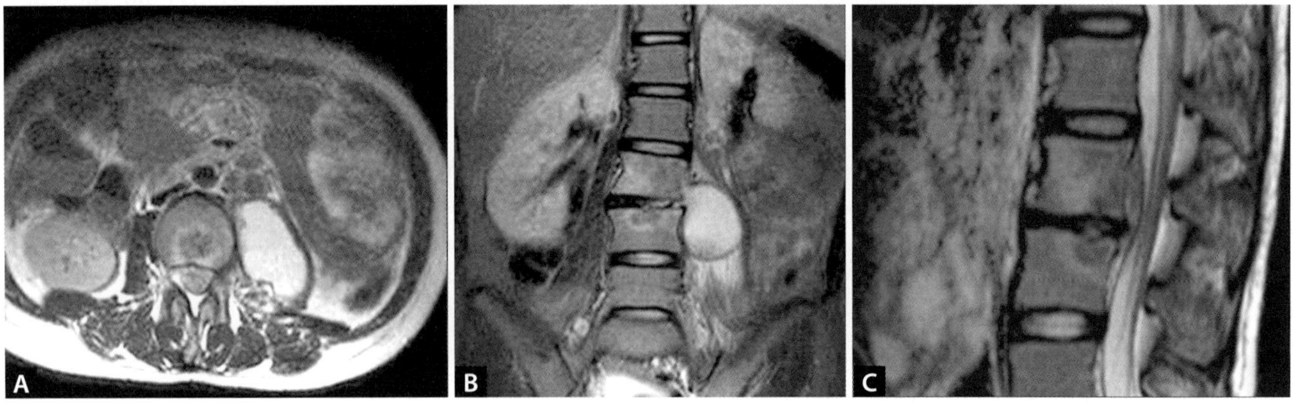

Figs. 24A to C: Psoas abscess: (A) Axial T2W, (B) coronal STIR and (C) sagittal T2-weighted MR images show the abscess as a well-defined hyperintense lesion with a smooth hypointense rim in the left psoas muscle. The whole muscle appears hyperintense. Vertebral and discal involvement is well seen. A small epidural extension of the abscess can be seen in the sagittal section.

CT is the most frequently used modality for evaluation of enlarged nodes. However, MRI, especially fat suppressed T2-weighted images are very sensitive for the detection of lymph nodes and performs better than CT particularly in children who have a paucity of fat. CT and MRI use nonspecific criterion of size and are limited in their ability to differentiate benign from malignant nodes. Contrast-enhanced MR lympho-graphy using ultrasmall supermagnetic iron oxide (USPIO) particles is a promising technique in differentiating benign from metastatic nodes and providing information on lymph node morphology and function.[64] FDG-PET may be more sensitive and specific for evaluation of lymphomas and certain retroperitoneal metastases depending on the primary.

RETROPERITONEAL ABSCESS AND HEMATOMA

Tuberculous spondylitis is the most common cause of an iliopsoas abscess in our country. The inflammatory mass shows a variety of appearances ranging from diffuse homogeneous enlargement of the iliopsoas muscle to discrete masses containing central areas of low CT attenuation or high signal intensity on T2-weighted MR images **(Figs. 24A to C)**. Post-contrast images show abscesses as expansile lesions with nonenhancing necrotic centers, intense peripheral enhancement and enhancement of the surrounding tissue. Calcification may occasionally be seen on CT and plain radiographs. Although vertebral involvement can be well appreciated on both CT and MRI, MRI scores over CT in detecting intraspinal extension of the inflammatory granulation tissue/abscess and cord compression. US can detect the psoas abscess as a sonolucent region within the psoas muscle with associated fluid along the margins of the psoas and can serve as a guide for diagnostic and therapeutic drainage of these abscesses.

Hematomas of the retroperitoneum are most commonly the result of severe blunt trauma or a surgical procedure. Spontaneous retroperitoneal hematomas, usually within the iliopsoas muscle, can be seen in patients with hemophilia or other bleeding diathesis. On US, CT and MRI, the muscle is seen to be enlarged with characteristic changing pattern of a evolving hemorrhage within it.

CONCLUSION

About 70–80% of abdominal masses in infants and children are retroperitoneal in origin, renal being the most common. Imaging aims to diagnose the site, nature, extent and stage of the disease, so as to determine the appropriate management. The various imaging modalities available need to be used in a logical sequence as governed by the findings in an individual case and availability of facilities.

REFERENCES

1. Minami M, Ohmoto K, Chansangavej C, et al. Origin of abdominal tumors: Useful findings and signs on tomographic imaging. Radiology. 1996;201:491-9.
2. Geller E, Smergel EM, Lowry PA. Renal neoplasms of childhood. RCNA. 1997;35(6):1391-413.
3. Lowe HL, Isuani BH, Heller RM, et al. Paediatric renal masses: Wilms' tumor and beyond. Radiographics. 2000;20(6):1585-603.
4. Breslow NE, Beckwith JB, Ciol M, et al. Age distribution of Wilms' tumor. Report from the National Wilms' Tumor Study. Cancer Res. 1988;48:1653-7.
5. Charles AK, Vujanic GM, Berry PJ. Renal tumors of childhood. Histopathology. 1998;32:293-309.
6. LoneganGJ,Martinez-LeonMI,AgronsGA,MontemaranoH, Suarez ES. Nephrogenic rests, nephroblastomatosis, and associated lesions of the kidney. Radiographics. 1998;18: 947-68.
7. Bond JV. Bilateral Wilms' tumor: Age at diagnosis, associated congenital anomalies and possible patterns of inheritance. Lancet. 1975;2:482-4.
8. Yokomori K, Hori T, Takemura T, et al. Demonstration of both primary and secondary remission in renal tumors in children. J Paediatr Surg. 1988;23:403-9.
9. R White KS, Grossman H: Wilms' and associated renal tumors of childhood. Paedr Radiol. 1990;21:81-8.
10. D'Angio GJ, Evans AE, Breslow N, et al. The treatment of Wilms' tumor: Results of the second National Wilms' Tumor Study. Cancer. 1981;47:2302-11.
11. Fernbach SK, Feinstein KA, Donaldson JS, et al. Nephroblastomatosis: Comparison of CT with US and urography. Radiology. 1988;166:153.
12. Remain TAH, Siegel MJ, Shackeyord GD. Wilms' tumor in children: Abdominal CT and US evaluation. Radiology. 1986;160:501-5.
13. Ritchey ML, Kelalis P, Breslow NE, et al. Intracaval and atrial involvement with nephroblastoma: Review of National Wilms' Tumor Study-3. J Urol. 1988;140:1113.
14. Tongaonkar HB, Qureshi SS, Kurkure PA, Muckaden MA, Arora B, Yuvaraja TB. Wilms' tumor: an update. Indian J Urol. 2007;23:458-66.
15. Owens CM, Veys PA, Pritchard J, Levitt G, Imeson J, Dicks-Mireaux C. Role of chest computed tomography at diagnosis in the management of Wilms' tumor: A study by the United Kingdom Children's Cancer Study Group. J Clin Oncol. 2002;20:2768-73.
16. Ehrlich PF, Hamilton TE, Grundy P, Ritchey M, Haase G, Shamberger RC, et al. The value of surgery in directing therapy for patients with Wilms' tumor with pulmonary disease: A Report from the National Wilms' Tumor Study Group (National Wilms' Tumor Study 5). J Pediatr Surg. 2006;41:162-7.
17. McHugh K. Renal and adrenal tumors in children. Cancer Imaging. 2007;7(1):41-51.
18. Beckwith JB. Children at increased risk for Wilms' tumor: Monitoring issues. J Pediatr. 1998;132:377-9.
19. White KS, Grossman H. Wilms' and associated renal tumors of childhood. Pediatr Radiol. 1991;21:81-8.
20. Carneiro RC, Fordham LA. Tumors of the Urinary Tract in Carty H, Brunelle F, Stringer DA, et al (Eds). Imaging Children, 2nd edition. Churchill Livingstone Publications. 2005;1:777-804.
21. Grundy P, Perlman E, Rosen NS, et al. Current issues in Wilms' tumor management. Curr Probl Cancer. 2005;29:221-60 [PubMed].
22. Bolande RP, Brough AJ, Izant RJ Jr. Congenital mesoblastic nephroma of infancy: A report of eight cases and the relationship to Wilms' tumor. Paediatrics. 1967;40:272-8.
23. Chan HS, Cheng MY, Mancer K, et al. Congenital mesoblastic nephroma: clinicoradiological study of 17 cases representing the pathological spectrum of the disease. J Paediatrics. 1987;111(1): 64-70.
24. Agrons GA, Kingsman KD, Wagner BJ, Sotelo-Avila C. Rhabdoid tumor of the kidney in children: a comparative study. AJR. 1997;168:447-51.
25. Charles AK, Vujanic GM, Berry PJ. Renal tumors of childhood. Histopathology. 1998;32:293-309.
26. Chung CJ, Lorenzo R, Rayder S, et al. Rhabdoid tumors of the kidney in children: CT findings. AJR. 1995;164:697-700.
27. Hartman DS, Davis CJ, Jr, Madewell JE, Friedman AC. Primary malignant renal tumors in the second decade of life: Wilms' tumor versus renal cell carcinoma. J Urol. 1982;127:888-91.
28. Madewell JE, Goldman SM, Davis CJ, Hartman DS, Feigin DS, Lichtenstein JE. Multilocular cystic nephroma: a radiologic-pathologic correlation of 58 patients. Radiology. 1983;146:309-21.

29. Agrons GA, Wagner BJ, Davidson AJ, Suarez ES. Multilocular cystic renal tumor in children: Radiologic-pathologic correlation. Radiographics. 1995;15:653-69.
30. Wood BP, Muurahainen N, Anderson VM, et al. Multicystic nephroblastoma: Ultrasound diagnosis (with a pathologic-anatomic commentary). Pediatr Radiol. 1982;12:43-7.
31. Lemaitre L, Robert Y, Dubrulle F, et al. Renal angiomyolipoma: Growth followed-up with CT and/or US. Radiology. 1995;197:598-602.
32. Kurosaki Y, Tanaka Y, Kuramoto K, et al. Improved CT fat detection in small kidney angiomyolipomas using thin sections and single voxel measurements. JCAT. 1993;17:745-8.
33. Strouse PJ. Paediatric Renal Neoplasms. RCNA. 1996;34(6): 1081-100.
34. Vazquez JL, Barnewolt CE, Shamberger RC, Chung T, Perez-Atayde AR. Ossifying renal tumor of infancy presenting as a palpable abdominal mass. Pediatr Radiol. 1998;28:454-7.
35. Ito J, Shinohara N, Koyanagi T, Hanioka K. Ossifying renal tumor of infancy: the first Japanese case with long-term follow-up. Pathol Int. 1998;48:151-9.
36. Navarro O, Conolly B, Taylor G, Bagli DJ. Metanephric adenoma of the kidney: a case report. Pediatr Radiol. 1999;29:100-3.
37. Hartman DS, Davis CJ, Jr, Goldman SM, Friedman AC, Fritzsche P. Renal lymphoma: Radiologic-pathologic correlation of 21 cases. Radiology. 1982;144:759-66.
38. Albregts AE, Cohen MD, Gallani CA. Neuroblastoma invading the kidney. J Paediatric Surgery. 1994;29:930-3.
39. Raby WN, Kopplin P, Weitzman S. Metastatic osteosarcoma of the kidney presenting as renal haemorrhage. Journal of Paediatric Haematology/Oncology. 1996;18:321-2.
40. Kushner BH. Neuroblastoma: A disease requiring a multitude of imaging studies. J Nucl Med. 2004;45:1172-88 [PubMed].
41. Kushner B, Cheung NK: Neuroblastoma: an overview. Haem/Onc Annals. 1993;1:189-201.
42. Abramson SJ. Adrenal Neoplasms in children. RCNA. 1997;35(6):1415-51.
43. Rha SE, Byun JY, Jung SE, Chun HJ, Lee HG, Lee JM. Neurogenic tumors in the abdomen: Tumor types and imaging characteristics. Radiographics. 2003;23:29-43 [PubMed].
44. Hirons MP, Owens CM. Radiology of neuroblastoma in children. Eur Radiol. 2001;11:2071-81 [PubMed].
45. Currarino G, Wood B, Massond M: The genitourinary tract and Retroperitoneum. In: Silverman FN, Kuhn JP (Eds). Caffey's Paediatric X-ray Diagnosis: An Integrated Imaging Approach. Mosby. 1993;2:1145-375.
46. Brodeur GM, Pritchard J, Berthold F, et al. Revisions of the international criteria for neuroblastoma diagnosis, staging and response to treatment. J Clin Oncol. 1993;11:1466.
47. Ferraro EM, Fakhry J, Aruny JE, et al. Prenatal adrenal neuroblastoma. Case report with review of the literature. J Ultrasound Medicine. 1988;7:275-8.
48. Uhl M, Altehoefer C, Kontny U, et al. MRI diffusion imaging of neuroblastomas: first results and correlation to histology. Eur Radiol. 2002;12:2335-8.
49. Lonergan GJ, Schwab CM, Suarez ES, et al. Neuroblastoma, ganglioneuroblastoma, and ganglioneuroma: radiologic-pathologic correlation. Radiograhics. 2002;22:911-34.
50. Laffan EE, O' Connor R, Ryan SP, et al. Whole body magnetic resonance imaging: a useful additional sequence in paediatric imaging. Paediatr Radiol. 2004;34:472-80.
51. Chaya SA. Neuroblastoma. In: Grainger and Allison (Eds). Diagnostic Radiology: A Textbook of Medical Imaging, 4th edition. 2001;2:1483-6.
52. Willi UV. The adrenal glands. In: Carty H, Brunelle F, Stringer DA, et al (Eds). Imaging Children. 2nd edition. Churchill Livingstone Publications. 2005;1:975-96.
53. Daneman A. Adrenal Gland. In: Kuhn JP, Slovis TL, Haller JO (Eds). Caffey's Pediatric Diagnostic Imaging, Vol 2, 10th edition. Mosby Publications. 2004. pp. 1894-908.
54. Ein S, Wertzman S, Thorner P, et al. Paediatric malignant phaeochromocytoma. J Paediatr Surg. 1994;29:1197-201.
55. Bonfig W, Bittman I, Bechtold S, et al. Virilizing adrenocortical tumors in children. Eur J Paediatr. 2003;162:623-8.
56. Michalkiewicz E, Sandrini R, Figueiredo B, et al. Clinical and outcome characteristics of children with adrenocortical tumors: A report from the International Pediatric Adrenocortical Tumor Registry. J Clin Oncol. 2004;22:838-45 [PubMed].
57. Godine L, Bordon W, Brasch R, et al. Adrenocortical carcinoma with extension into IVC and right atrium: Report of 3 cases in children. Pediatric Radiology. 1990;20:166-8.
58. Mittelstaedt CA, Volberg FM, Merten D, et al. The sonographic diagnosis of neonatal adrenal haemorrhage. Radiology. 1979;131:453-7.
59. Grosfield JL, Billimere DF. Teratomas in infancy and childhood. Curr Prob Cancer. 1985;9:1-53.
60. Rattan KN, Kadian YS, Nair VJ, et al. Primary retroperitoneal tumors in children: a single institution experience. African J of Paed Surg. 2010;7(1):5-8.
61. Hayasaka K, Yamada T, Saitoh Y, et al. CT evaluation of primary benign retroperitoneal tumor. Radiat Med. 1994;12:115-20.
62. Haller J. Retroperitoneal masses. In: Kuhn JP, Slovis TL, Haller JO (Eds). Caffey's Pediatric Diagnostic Imaging, Vol 2, 10th edition. Mosby Publications. 2004; pp. 1909-14.
63. Parker BR. Leukemia and lymphoma in childhood. Radiol Clin North Am. 1997;35:1495.
64. Bellin MF, Lebleu L, Meric JB. Evaluation of retroperitoneal and pelvic node metastases with MRI lymphangiography. Abdominal Imaging. 2003;28:155-63.

CHAPTER 142

Evaluation of Female Pelvis and Testicular Abnormalities

Kushaljit Singh Sodhi, Akshay Kumar Saxena

INTRODUCTION

Ultrasonography (USG) is the most useful modality for imaging genital organs in infants and children, because it is a noninvasive and painless study which does not require sedation for the baby (in contrast to computed tomography (CT) and magnetic resonance (MR) examinations). The lack of ionizing radiation makes ultrasound very attractive as a pediatric imaging modality.[1,2]

Knowledge of simple embryology and basic physiology is necessary in investigating cases of precocious puberty, amenorrhea, pelvic pain, pelvic masses, or ambiguous genitalia in children, which are key reasons for imaging of female pelvis in children.

CT remains useful for tumor staging, follow-up and in acute abdomen. Magnetic resonance imaging provides precise demonstration of anatomic features in multiple planes in cases of complex anomalies, when US findings are inconclusive.[3]

NORMAL US ANATOMY OF GENITAL ORGANS IN INFANTS AND CHILDREN

The size and shape of the ovaries and of uterus vary during childhood, are age dependent, and under hormonal influence. The maternal and placental hormones produce a relatively larger size of the neonatal uterus and ovaries. The uterus has a prominent, echogenic endometrial lining.[1,2]

During infancy, the size, shape, and echotexture of the uterus and ovaries remain relatively stable. However, the ovaries are never dormant and follicles or cysts can be seen at every age. Two to three years before the onset of puberty, the uterine volume gradually increases with accelerated growth occurring during puberty.[2]

UTERUS

Uterine anatomy changes with age of the child **(Figs. 1A to C)**. The neonatal uterus is prominent under the influence of maternal and placental hormones.[4,5] The cervix is larger than the fundus (fundus-to-cervix ratio= 1/2), the uterine length is approximately 3.5 cm, and the maximum thickness is approximately 1.4 cm. The endometrial lining is often echogenic. Some fluid can also be seen within the endometrial cavity. During infancy the proportion of cervix to uterine body changes to 1:1. This tubular shape is stable until 2 to 3 years before the onset of puberty.[2]

The prepubertal uterus has a tubular configuration (anteroposterior cervix equal to anteroposterior fundus) or sometimes a spade shape (anteroposterior cervix larger than anteroposterior fundus).[6-9] The endometrium is normally not apparent; however, high-frequency transducers can demonstrate the central lining in some cases. The length is 2.5–4 cm; the thickness does not exceed 10 mm.

During puberty the greatest growth occurs in the fundus and corpus, altering to a pear-shaped uterus (~25 mL). The pubertal uterus has the adult pear configuration (fundus larger than cervix) (fundus-to-cervix ratio = 2/1

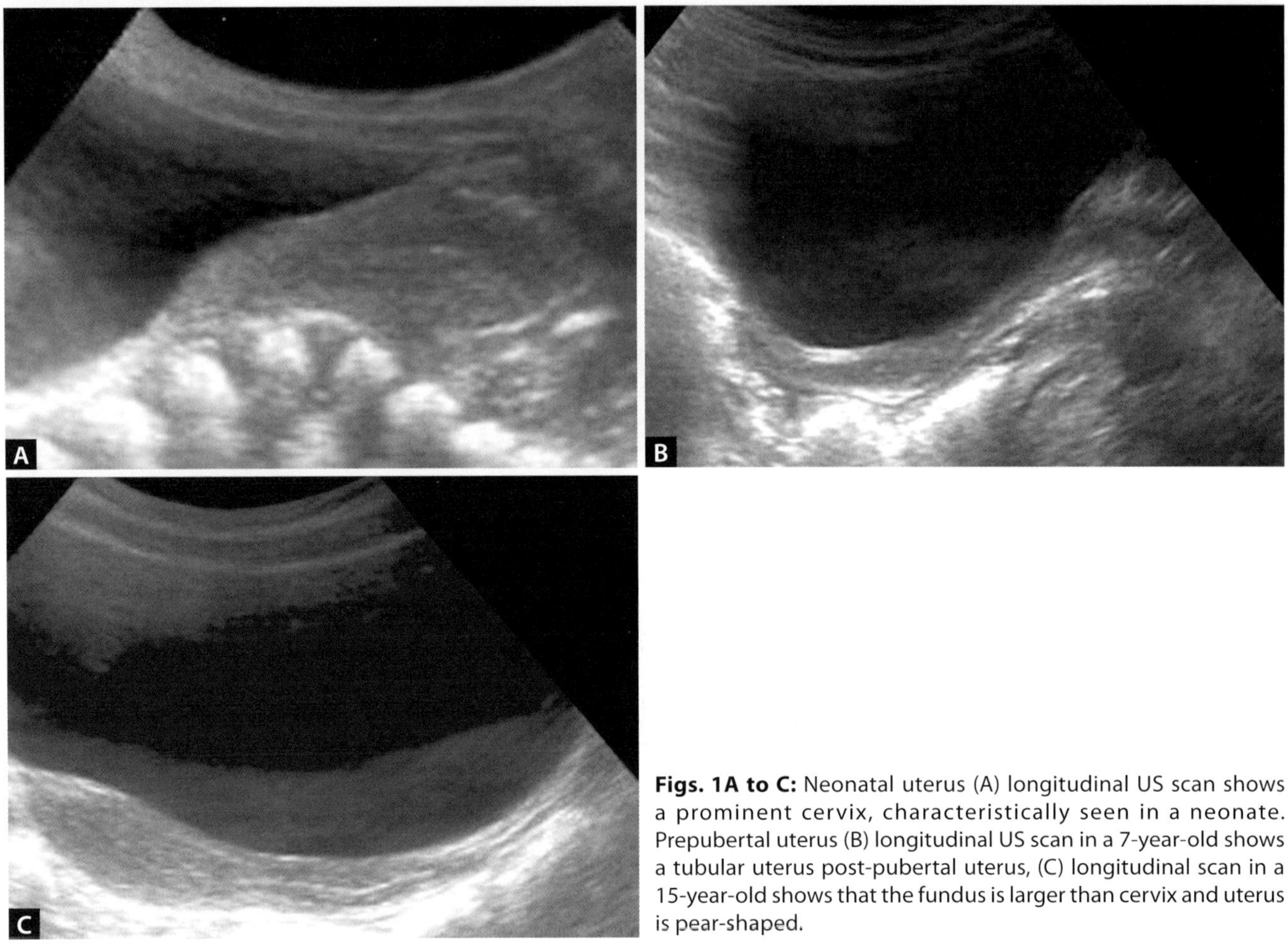

Figs. 1A to C: Neonatal uterus (A) longitudinal US scan shows a prominent cervix, characteristically seen in a neonate. Prepubertal uterus (B) longitudinal US scan in a 7-year-old shows a tubular uterus post-pubertal uterus, (C) longitudinal scan in a 15-year-old shows that the fundus is larger than cervix and uterus is pear-shaped.

to 3/1)[6-9] **(Fig. 1C)** and is 5–8 cm long, 3 cm wide, and 1.5 cm thick. The endometrial lining is seen and varies with the phases of the menstrual cycle. The endometrial canal is seen as a thin echogenic interface and the endometrium demonstrates cyclical changes every cycle. The measurement of the endometrial thickness includes both endometrial lines.

Doppler ultrasound of the uterine artery can be used to confirm the onset of puberty. In prepubertal girls, the pulsed Doppler demonstrates a narrow systolic waveform without positive diastolic flow. In postpubertal girls, a broad systolic waveform is seen with positive diastolic flow.[6]

OVARIES

Ovarian size is usually described by assessment of the ovarian volume: Neonatal ovaries measure 1 to 3.6 mL.[2,6] In infants, measurements are average of slightly greater than 1 cm^3 for the first year of life and 0.67 cm^3 for the second year.[10,11]

Multiple follicles in the ovaries are normal in a neonatal ovary. After birth, follicle stimulating hormone (FSH) rises in the newborn period due to the abrupt lack of the placental and maternal hormones. During the second year of life, the FSH level decreases, but a pulsatile secretion of FSH persists at a low level. The ovary thus contains mature follicles at all ages. Antral follicles (tertiary follicles) are fluid-filled follicles, which are round in shape and usually <9 mm in size in the prepubertal girl.[1,2]

The mean ovarian volume in girls less than 6 years of age is less than or equal to 1 cm^3. The increase in ovarian volume begins after 6 years of age.

In prepubertal girls (6–10 years old), ovarian volumes range from 1.2 to 2.3 cm^3. In Premenarchal girls (11–12 years old), ovarian volumes range from 2 to 4 cm^3 **(Table 1)**. In post-menarchal girls, the ovarian volume averages 8 cm^3.

Normal microcystic follicles are routinely imaged (in 84% of cases) from birth to 24 months of age and in 68% of cases between 2 and 12 years of age).[12] Practically, the following

Table 1: Pediatric ovarian volumes.[10,11]

Age (year)	Mean volume (cm^3)	Standard deviation
1	1.05	0.7
2	0.67	0.35
3	0.7	0.2
4	0.8	0.4
5	0.9	0.02
6	1.2	0.4
7	1.3	0.6
8	1.1	0.5
9	2.0	0.8
10	2.2	0.7
11	2.5	1.3
12	3.8	1.4
13	4.2	2.3

measurements can be considered as upper values for prepubertal girls: Uterine length = 4.5 cm, uterine thickness = 1 cm (the single most useful criterion), and ovarian volume = 4–5 cm^3.[1,2]

OVARIAN CYSTS

Ovarian cysts can be classified as physiological, functional, or neoplastic.[13] When a normal mature follicle fails to involute and continues to enlarge, secondary to hormonal imbalance, a functional or retention cyst results. These cysts may develop from preovulatory follicles (follicular cysts) or from postovulatory follicles (corpus luteum cysts) and usually range from 1 to 10 cm in size.[13-15]

Cysts up to 2 cm are usually follicles. Larger cysts (>2 cm) may be pathologic, particularly if persistent.[2] Follow-up ultrasound of ovarian cysts is recommended to ensure resolution after 6 weeks or after one and a half menstrual cycles.[16-18] Maternal hormones may cause large neonatal ovarian cysts.[19] Although, retention cysts are usually asymptomatic and detected incidentally on sonograms, they may cause pain related to pressure or hemorrhage.

Follicular and corpus luteum retention cysts cannot be differentiated with imaging studies. However, corpus luteum cysts tend to be more symptomatic. Diagnosis requires correlation with the date of the last menstrual period or tissue sampling. Serial sonography is suggested, since the majority of functional cysts demonstrate cyclic changes or regress spontaneously.

On sonograms, a non-hemorrhagic functional cyst appears as a smooth, unilocular cystic mass. The sonographic features that suggest hemorrhage within a simple cystare variable and depend on the age of the blood. Most hemorrhagic ovarian cysts are seen as complex masses with septations, low-level echoes, a fluid-debris level, or coagulated blood. Hemorrhagic cysts are a avascular on Doppler sonography. Clot lysis and resolution is an important diagnostic feature. With time, the cyst becomes more sonolucent or anechoic.[2,13]

ANOMALIES OF THE FEMALE PELVIS

Müllerian Anomalies

Müllerian anomalies are classified into: (a) Müllerian agenesis, (b) Disorders of lateral fusion (duplication defects) with or without obstruction, and (c) Disorders of vertical fusion (canalization defects) with or without obstruction.[1]

Because of the frequent association between anomalies of lateral fusion and anomalies of vertical fusion, it is helpful to consider these anomalies according to the presence or absence of obstruction.

Müllerian agenesis: Müllerian agenesis (Mayer-Rokitansky-Kuster-Hauser syndrome) is the second most common cause of primary infertility/primary amenorrhea, after gonadal dysgenesis.[20,21] Müllerian agenesis is characterized by vaginal atresia associated with an absent or rudimentary uterus (unicornuate or bicornuate) and normal ovaries. The karyotype is normal (46, XX). Renal anomalies (agenesis, ectopia) occur in 50% of cases; skeletal or spinal anomalies occur in 12% of cases. In 6–10% of patients, functioning endometrium may be present within the rudimentary uterus, resulting in unilateral hematometra.

Obstructive Müllerian Anomalies

Failure of vertical fusion or canalization of the urogenital sinus or the Müllerian duct system may result in cervical stenosis or atresia, vaginal atresia, or transverse vaginal septa. A transverse vaginal septum can occur at many levels of the vagina and creates a blockage of the vagina and uterus. In addition, hymenal tissue may be imperforate. Imperforate hymen is the most common genital outflow tract anomaly.

Most of the cases of hydrometrocolpos in the neonatal group are associated with a urogenital sinus or cloacal malformation.[22,23] Hematometrocolpos presenting in adolescent girls is secondary to vaginal obstruction by an imperforate hymen. The patient presents at puberty with primary amenorrhea and cyclic lower abdominal or pelvic pain.[24] Ultrasound typically shows a fluid-filled mass posterior to the bladder, which represents the dilated vagina **(Figs. 2 and 3)**. The uterus may also be dilated. The dilated uterus can be differentiated from the vagina by the cervical margin and thicker wall. Not infrequently, hematometrocolpos is present with duplication anomalies.[25] In the newborn period, a bulging mass (hydrocolpos) may be noted at the introitus.

Hematometrocolpos is cured by relieving the obstruction, whereas, hematometra usually requires a hysterectomy. Approximately, 45% of vaginal septa occur in the upper vagina, 40% in the middle vagina, and 15% in the lower vagina. An obstructed hemivagina with a double uterus is almost always associated with ipsilateral renal agenesis. At clinical examination, cyclic abdominal pain (due to the obstruction) coexists with normal menses (through the unobstructed system).[1,2]

Nonobstructive Müllerian Anomalies

These include septate, bicornuate, didelphys, and unicornuate uterus. A longitudinal vaginal septum can be associated with uterine duplication defects (e.g. uterus didelphys, uterus bicollis with a complete vaginal septum).

Primary Amenorrhea

Primary amenorrhea is defined as: (a) no menarche by 16 years of age, (b) no thelarche or adrenarche by 14 years of age, or (c) no menarche more than 3 years after adrenarche and thelarche.[1]

The presence or absence of secondary sexual development at clinical examination and müllerian structures at US is the basis for further laboratory tests.

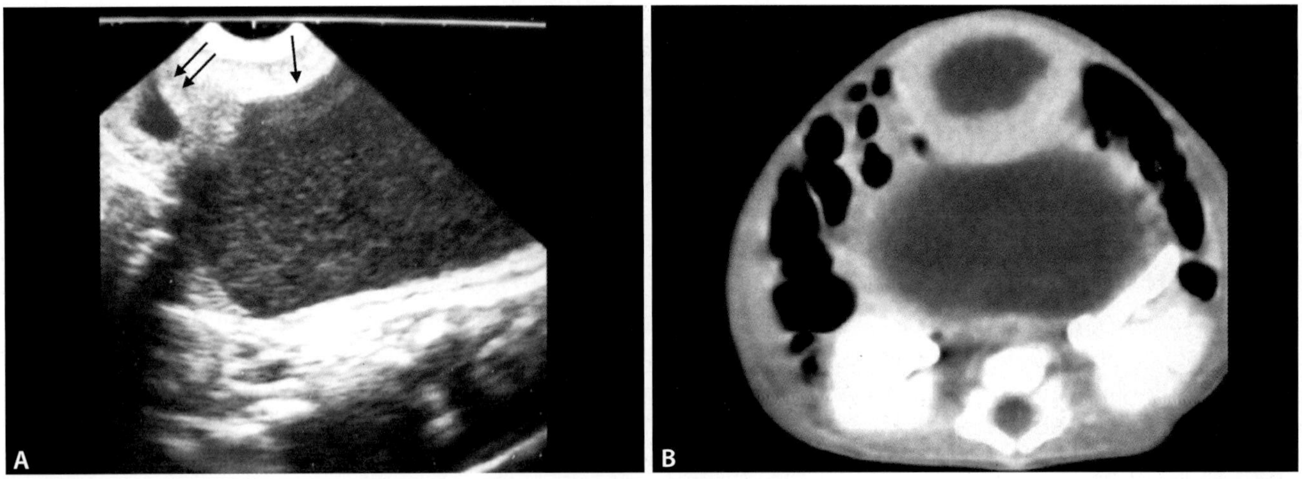

Figs. 2A and B: Hydrometrocolpos in a 1-year-old female child with palpable midline pelvic lump. Ultrasound (A) shows a fluid-filled distended vagina (arrow) and the uterine cavity with its thick myometrium (double arrow). CT scan (B) reveals two fluid-filled structures separate from the displaced small urinary bladder, consistent with distended uterine cavity and vagina.

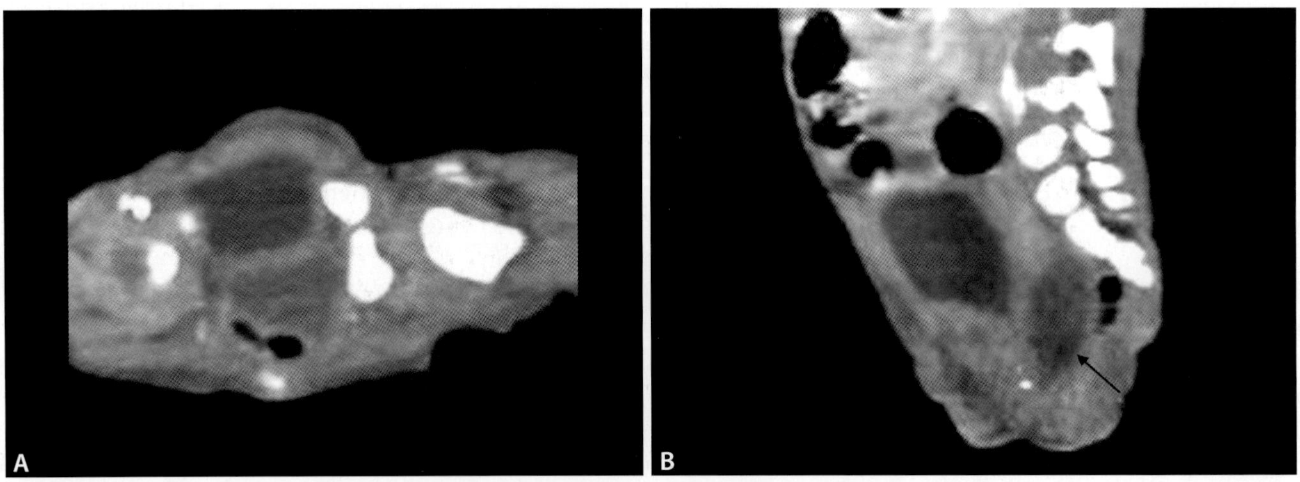

Figs. 3A and B: CT scan: Axial (A) and sagittal (B) images of hydrocolpos in a 4-month-old IUGR child showing cystic structure (arrow) behind urinary bladder, anterior to rectum, and inferior to uterus, consistent with hydrocolpos.

Common causes include gonadal dysgenesis (Turner syndrome) (33% of cases), müllerian (uterovaginal) anomalies (20%), hypothalamic-pituitary causes (15%), constitutional delay (often familial) (10%), and other causes (e.g. systemic, psychiatric) (22%).

Multiple syndromes result in primary amenorrhea including Turner syndrome, MRKH syndrome, Kallmann syndrome, Prader-Willi syndrome, Androgen Insensitivity syndrome, and Swyer syndrome.[26-28]

In Swyer syndrome (XY gonadal dysgenesis), no functional gonads are present to induce puberty, in an otherwise normal girl whose karyotype is found to be XY. The gonads are found to be nonfunctional streaks. Estrogen and progesterone therapy is commenced. The nonfunctioning gonads are removed because of their risk of developing gonadoblastoma.[2]

Turner syndrome: Patients with XO karyotype (approximately 70% of those with Turner syndrome) have a pre-pubertal uterus and non visualized or streaky ovaries.[29] In rare instances, especially in mosaic karyotypes, the ovaries can be normal in appearance.[29] Spontaneous puberty occurs in 5–15% of patients with Turner syndrome.[30]

Polycystic Ovary Syndrome

Polycystic ovary syndrome (PCOS) is an endocrine disorder resulting in chronic anovulation. PCOS is a common cause of infertility and amenorrhea. It is associated with Stein-Leventhal syndrome, which includes obesity and hirsutism. On ultrasound, multiple, small follicles (over 10) may be noted with increased echogenicity of the stroma. The ovaries are often 1.5–3 times larger than normal; however, the ovarian volume may be normal in 30% of cases.[2] The diagnosis of PCOS is confirmed biochemically.

PELVIC MASSES IN CHILDREN

Benign Ovarian Neoplasms

Ovarian teratomas are the most common benign ovarian neoplasm in pediatric patients.[2] Mature teratomas or dermoid cysts constitute for two-thirds of pediatric ovarian tumors.[13]

Typically, they are found in adolescents. Dermoids contains two cell layers: Mesoderm and Ectoderm. Teratomas are made up of elements from all three layers, including the endoderm. Two-thirds of patients present with an abdominal mass and the rest with pain due to torsion or hemorrhage. 25% of teratomas are bilateral. Malignancy is found in 2–10%. Teratomas may have cystic, solid, or mixed appearance on ultrasound due to its contents. They appear echogenic due to contained fat, hair, sebum, or calcium (teeth, bone). Anechoic components are due to serous fluid or sebum.[31] Approximately, 10–15% of benign teratomas are purely anechoic masses at sonography. Another 10–15% of teratomas are predominantly echogenic.

Peripheral nodules and shadowing each occur in 70% of teratomas in postpubertal girls. In contrast, mural nodules occur in only 40% of prepubertal girls and shadowing in only 15%.[13] Other features of teratomas include fat- or hair-fluid levels and central soft-tissue masses.[31,32]

CT and MR imaging are useful in further characterization. The most characteristic CT appearance of a benign teratoma is that of a predominantly fluid-filled lesion containing a mixture of fat, hair, debris, and calcifications **(Figs. 4A to C)**. Calcifications (either teeth or bone) often are localized to the solid globular protuberance (i.e. mural nodule or dermoid plug) arising from the cyst wall. Rarely, a teratoma appears on CT scans as a primarily fatty mass without calcification. If fat or a combination of fat and calcium is identified within a cystic mass, a specific diagnosis of teratoma can be made. In general, two thirds of teratomas display characteristic CT features. On MR images also, cystic teratomas vary in signal intensity depending on their tissue composition.[19] On T1-weighted images, fat appears as an area of high signal intensity, while serous fluid has low signal intensity. On T2-weighted images, fat and serous fluid have high signal intensity. Calcifications, bone, and hair have low signal intensity on MR images.[13]

Malignant Neoplasms

Malignant pelvic lesions in the female pelvis are rare and can arise from bone (Ewing sarcoma, coccygeal teratomas), soft tissue of muscles, uterus, or bladder (rhabdomyosarcoma) or have neurogenic origin (neuroblastoma). Some cystic and solid masses have particular diagnostic features (teratomas), but often additional imaging modalities (MR/CT) and/or histology are necessary to confirm a specific diagnosis.

Sacrococcygeal teratoma is one of the most common presacral tumors which contains derivates of three germinal layers. These tumors occur more frequently in girls and are classified into four types, according to the location. Type I is predominantly external, while type IV is presacral with no external component in it. CT and MRI are useful for depiction of location, its differentiation and extent of this tumor **(Figs. 5 and 6)**.

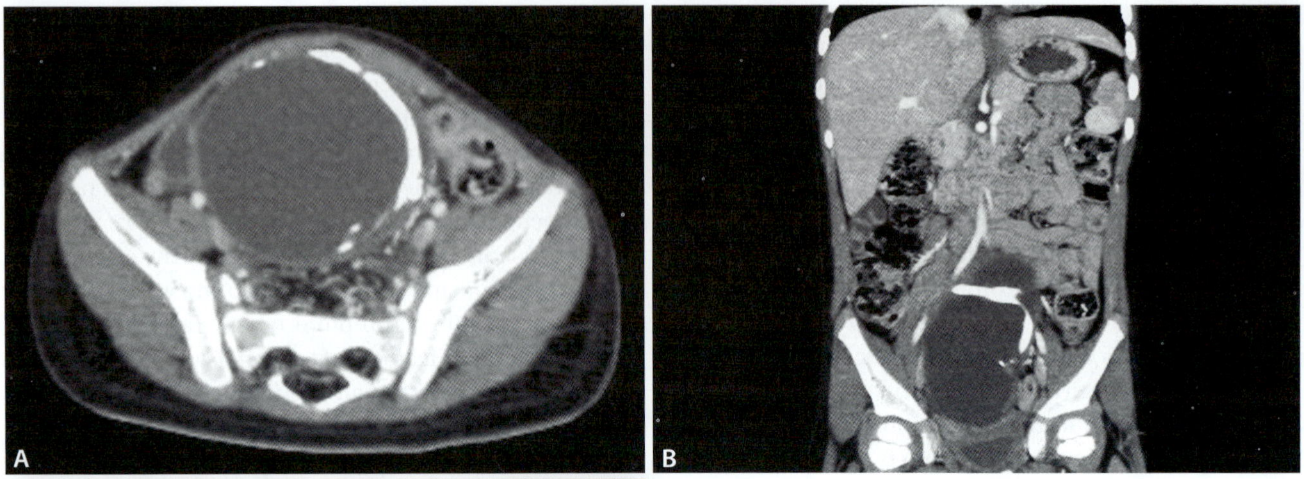

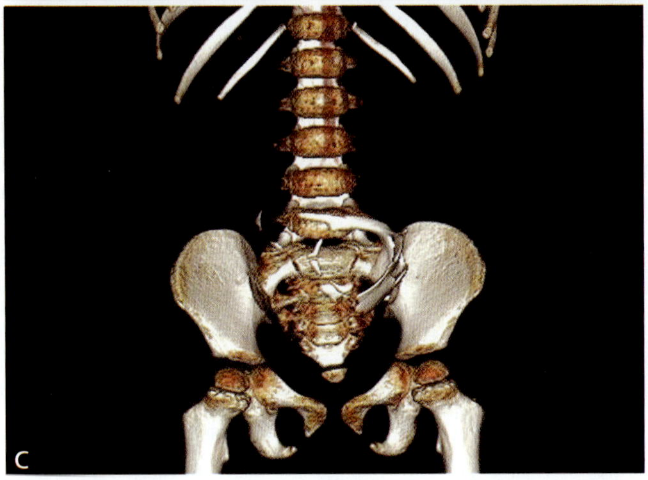

Figs. 4A to C: CT abdomen demonstrates a pelvic cystic tumor with bony elements in axial (A), coronal (B) and volume-rendered images (C) in a case of mature teratoma in a 3-year-old girl.

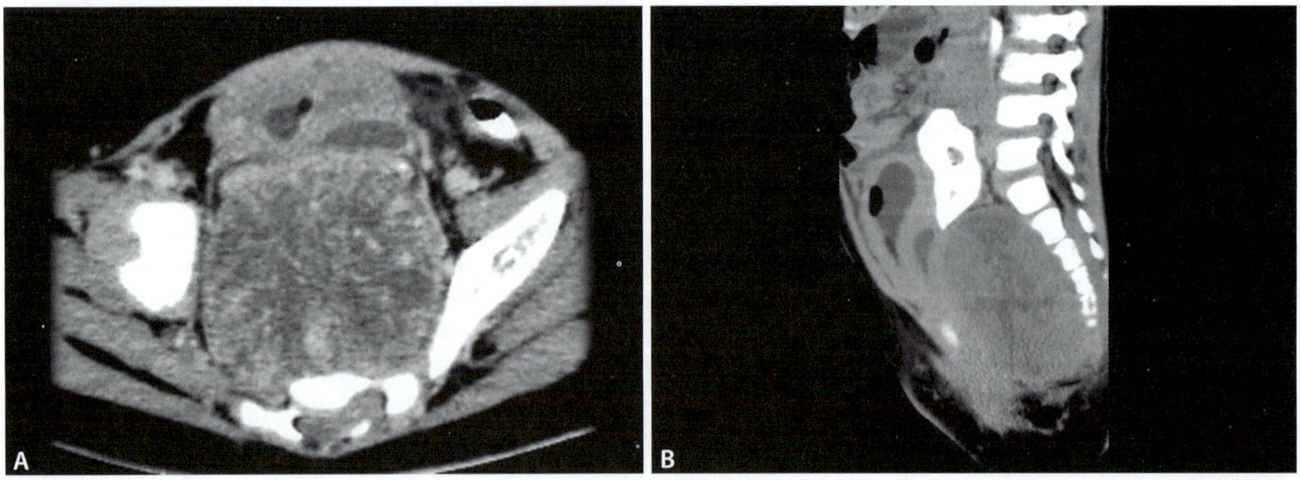

Figs. 5A and B: CT scan: Axial (A) and sagittal (B) images of malignant sacrococcygeal teratoma in a 2-year-old female child which also demonstrated bony involvement along with markedly raised AFP levels.

Rhabdomyosarcoma is the most common soft-tissue sarcoma in children. Peak incidence is between 2 and 6 years. The genitourinary tract is a common site of origin.

In girls, rhabdomyosarcoma can arise from the bladder, or vagina and surrounding tissues. 6% are sarcoma botryoides, which is an embryonal rhabdomyosarcoma

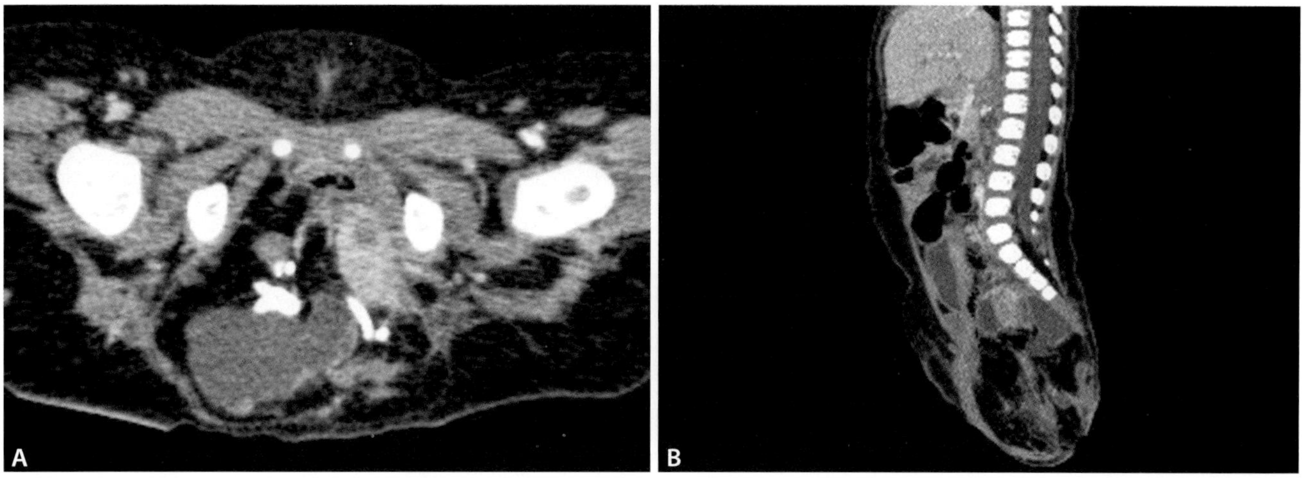

Figs. 6A and B: Axial (A) and sagittal (B) CT scans in another patient of sacrococcygeal teratoma which demonstrate areas of fat, calcification, and cystic components within this tumor.

originating from the vagina, cervix, or bladder of young girls. The tumor characteristically resembles a bunch of grapes.

Vaginal rhabdomyosarcomas are commonly botryoid and are almost exclusively found in very young children. At US, a vaginal rhabdomyosarcoma appears as a large, solid, heterogeneous or hypoechoic mass posterior to the bladder.

Malignant Ovarian Neoplasm

Malignant pelvic neoplasms with gynecologic origin are rare in children and include sex cord stromal tumors (granulosa cell, theca cell, fibroblast, Leydig and Sertoli cells) and germ cell tumors (dysgerminoma, malignant teratoma, endodermal sinus tumor, embryonal carcinoma, choriocarcinoma) **(Figs. 7 and 8)**. Sex cord stromal tumors represent 8% of ovarian neoplasm and affect all age groups. The more common type is granulosa cell tumors. Due to the estrogenic effects of these tumors, females present with pseudoprecocious puberty, endometrial bleeding, and sonographic findings of enlargement of the uterus and thickening of the endometrium. The appearance of sex cord tumors vary and range from large multicystic masses to small solid masses.[33]

Children with germ-cell tumors present often with asymptomatic pelvic or abdominal masses. With imaging, solid masses are found, which are echogenic on ultrasound and have soft-tissue attenuation on CT **(Figs. 7A and B)**. Other findings include calcifications, central necrosis, irregular walls, thick septations, papillary projections, and free abdominal and pelvic fluid. Metastasis occurs in lungs, liver, and peritoneum. Yolk sac tumor is a germ-cell tumor and is a rare, malignant tumor composed of cells that line the yolk sac of the embryo. The tumor is most often found in children before the age of 2 years. As with most other pelvic masses, ovarian yolk sac tumors grow very large before being noticed clinically.[2]

Ovarian Torsion

Ovarian torsion is the twisting of an ovary on its ligamentous supports, which can lead to a compromised blood supply.[23] Adnexal torsion is a term that includes either ovary, fallopian tube, or both. Concomitant ovarian and tubal torsion has been shown to occur in up to 67% of cases of adnexal torsion.[34,35]

Symptoms of ovarian torsion are often nonspecific, making it difficult to differentiate from other causes of acute abdominal pain. Ovarian torsion is frequently associated with a cyst or tumor, which is typically benign; the most common is mature cystic teratoma. Ultrasonography (US) is the primary imaging modality for evaluation of ovarian torsion.[36]

With US, the typical findings of ovarian torsion can be visualized in patients of all ages, although they are not always present. One series studying the effectiveness of US in diagnosing ovarian torsion yielded a positive predictive value of 87.5% and specificity of 93.3%.[37] The most constant finding in ovarian torsion is a large ovary.[35] Early in the disease, even before infarction has occurred, unilateral ovarian enlargement (>4 cm) is most commonly detected. In up to 74% of cases, US may demonstrate multiple small (up to 25 mm), uniform cysts aligned in the periphery of the engorged ovary. This appearance is likely secondary to follicles that have been displaced to the periphery

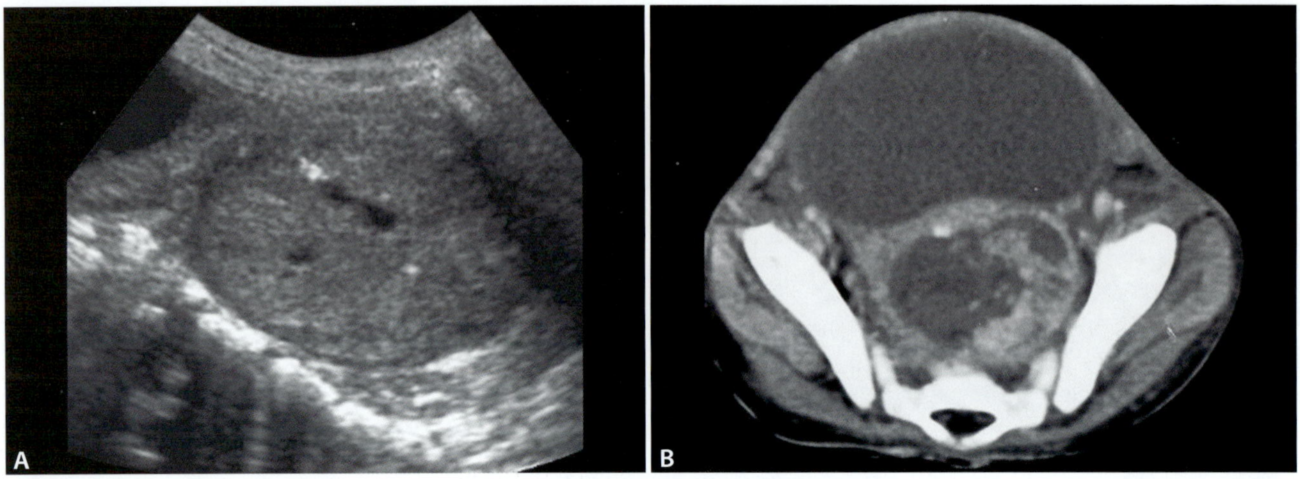

Figs. 7A and B: Ultrasound (A) shows a well-encapsulated predominantly solid adnexal mass with calcific foci and few cystic areas. Biopsy revealed malignant germ cell tumor; CT scan (B) reveals a large heterogeneous solid cystic pelvic mass, with a calcific foci.

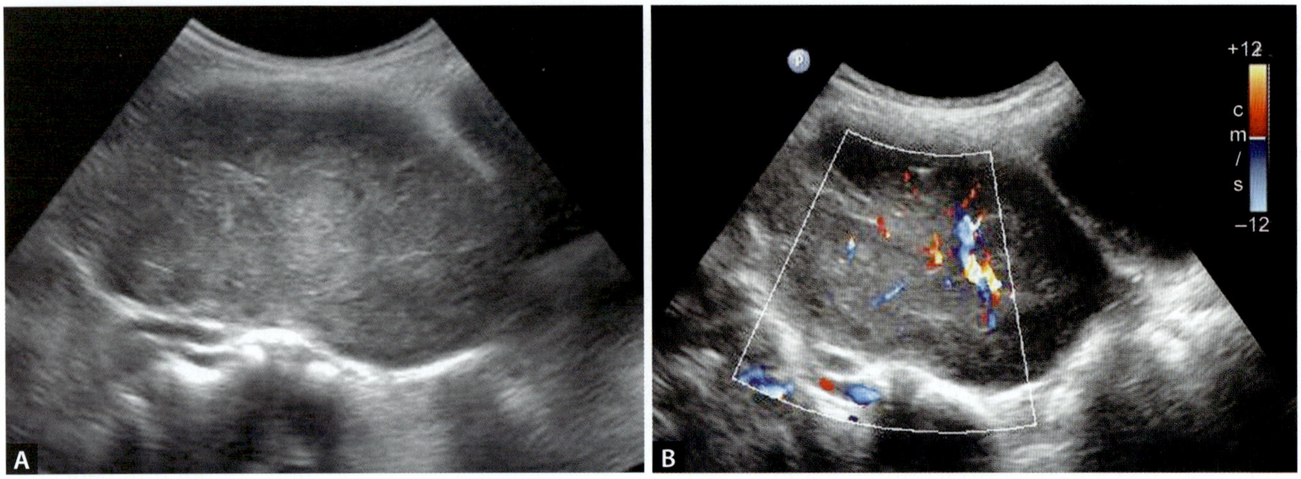

Figs. 8A and B: Dysgerminoma right ovary: Ultrasound pelvis reveals a solid pelvic mass in the right adnexa (A), which on color Doppler (B) demonstrates mild increased central vascularity.

due to the marked edema and venous congestion.[34,37] Peripherally arranged follicles is also an non-specific sign and may be seen in normal ovaries of fertile women and in patients with polycystic ovary disease and are not solely diagnostic of ovarian torsion. Multiple peripheral cysts in the setting of pain with a unilaterally enlarged ovary are helpful in diagnosing ovarian torsion.[34]

Color Doppler Imaging in Ovarian Torsion

The color Doppler flow manifestations of ovarian torsion are variable and are based, in part, on the degree of vascular compromise. The typical color Doppler sonographic finding in ovarian torsion is the absence of arterial flow. However, in one study involving patients with confirmed ovarian torsion, the absence of arterial flow was found in only 73% of cases.[35] In yet another study, 60% had normal color Doppler flow findings.[10,38] However, the most frequent finding is either decrease or absence of venous flow (93%),which may reflect the early collapse of the compliant venous walls.[35] The most promising findings incorporating both grayscale and color Doppler sonography are a twisted vascular pedicle and the whirlpool sign.[38,39] In a study by Lee et al.[39] a twisted vascular pedicle was detected in 88% of cases of ovarian torsion.

To summarize, US features of ovarian torsion include a unilateral enlarged ovary, uniform peripheral cystic structures, a coexistent mass within the affected ovary, free pelvic fluid, lack of arterial or venous flow, and a twisted vascular pedicle. It is important to remember that the presence of flow at color Doppler imaging does not allow exclusion of torsion but instead suggests that the ovary may be viable, especially if flow is present centrally. Absence of flow in the twisted vascular pedicle may indicate that the ovary is not viable.[34]

The role of computed tomography (CT) has expanded, and it is increasingly being used in evaluation of abdominal pain. Common CT features of ovarian torsion include an enlarged ovary, uterine deviation to the twisted side, smooth wall thickening of the twisted adnexal cystic mass, fallopian tube thickening, peripheral cystic structures, and ascites.[1,2,23] Understanding the imaging appearance of ovarian torsion will lead to conservative, ovary-sparing treatment.

Tubo-ovarian Abscess

Pelvic inflammatory disease more commonly affects postpubertal girls. The inflammatory process usually begins in the cervix, ascending to the endometrium; fallopian tubes; and, rarely, to the ovaries, parametrium, and peritoneal cavity. The diagnosis is made clinically, based on symptoms of pain, vaginal discharge, and fever. US, CT or MRI are useful for detecting complications such as pyosalpinx, tubo-ovarian abscess.[13]

Pyosalpinx appears as a hypoechoic tubular mass with internal debris, whereas tubo-ovarian abscess is seen as a complex mass, often with debris, septations, and irregular thick walls. After antibiotics, pelvic inflammatory disease may resolve completely or lead to sequelae such as hydrosalpinx or adhesions. CT can complement US. At CT, a tuboovarian abscess often appears as a soft-tissue mass with central areas of lower attenuation and thick walls. Occasionally, air or an air-fluid level may be seen.

Ectopic Pregnancy

Ectopic pregnancy is a known but infrequent cause of pelvic mass in postpubertal girls.

The most specific US finding for diagnosing an ectopic pregnancy is the visualization of an extrauterine embryo. More often, ectopic pregnancy is manifested as a nonspecific echogenic or complex adnexal mass, often associated with cul-de-sac fluid and an enlarged uterus with a pseudogestational sac.[40,41] A pseudogestational sac has only a single echogenic ring representing parietal decidua, whereas an early intrauterine pregnancy has a double-ring appearance resulting from visualization of the inner capsulari decidua and outer parietal decidua. Because of the non-specficity of the adnexal masses, it is vital to correlate the US appearance with the level of the β subunit of human chorionic gonadotropin (hCG).

NONGYNECOLOGIC PELVIC MASSES

Pelvic masses of non-gynecologic origin include appendiceal abscesses, fluid collections, and fluid-filled bowel ,which can be confounded with primary adnexal lesions.[13,42]

On sonograms, periappendiceal abscess appears as a complex mass in the right lower quadrant. If an appendicolith or gas is present, bright echoes with shadowing may be noted. Positive ultrasound findings of appendicitis are diameter over 6 mm, lack of compressibility, increased vascularity of the appendical wall, appendicolith, adjacent abdominal free fluid, increased echogenicity of adjacent mesenteric fat, and enlarged lymph nodes.

Cerebrospinal fluid pseudocysts are infrequent complications of ventriculoperitoneal shunting, resulting from loculation of draining cerebrospinalfluid. On sonograms, uninfected pseudocysts appear as hypoechoic masses. When infected, pseudocysts become more complex, containing internal echoes or septations.

Fluid-filled bowel may potentially be confused with an adnexal cyst at US. In most cases, bowel can be identified due to peristalsis detected with real-time imaging. In addition, complicated fluid collections resulting from bleeding or ascites due to peritoneal metastases may be confused with ovarian masses. These collections may change with changes in patient position.

Other non-gynecological cystic masses which can be seen in the pelvis include mesenteric cysts, duplication cysts, urachal remnants, Meckel's diverticulum, ureteroceles, dilated ureters, hydronephrosis in ectopic kidneys, vascular and lymphatic malformations, abscess, and hematoma. The larger the size of the lesion, the more difficult it is to determine its origin.

Role of MRI in Imaging of Female Pelvis

Magnetic resonance imaging (MRI) also plays a crucial role in diagnosis, treatment selection, treatment planning, and follow-up of both benign and malignant gynecological conditions. Advantages of MRI include superb spatial and tissue contrast resolution, lack of ionizing radiation, multiplanar capability, and fast techniques. However, optimization of MRI sequences and clinical protocols is crucial to ensure best results.[43] In pediatrics, MRI is mainly used for congenital anomalies and in evaluation of indeterminate adenexal masses.

Congenital Uterine Anomalies

Müllerian duct anomalies result from nondevelopment or varying degrees of nonfusion or nonresorption of the Müllerian ducts. The role of MRI is to provide both precise classification and demonstration of associated complications.[44] (Classification of Müllerian anomalies has been discussed at the start of this chapter).

In Mayer–Rokitansky–Kuster–Hauser syndrome, there is absence or anomalies of the uterus and upper vagina, with varying degrees of development of the lower vagina.[43]

The unicornuate uterus appears as a curved, elongated uterus with tapering of the fundal segment off midline (the"banana-like" configuration) on T2-weighted MR images.

Normal uterine zonal anatomy is maintained. The rudimentary horn, when present, usually demonstrates lower signal intensity on T2-weighted images. Communication with rudimentary horn can be easily demonstrated on MRI.

Partial fusion of the Müllerian ducts results in the bicornuate uterus. MRI shows uterine horns separated by an interveningcleft in the external fundal myometrium of longer than 1 cm. Normal zonal anatomy is seen in each horn and there is a dividing septum which is composed of myometrium.

The uterus didelphys results from nonfusion of the two Müllerian ducts. Two separate normal-sized uterine horns and cervices are demonstrated on T2-weighted MR images.

A longitudinal vaginal septum is present in 75% of cases, occasionally complicated by transverse septa causing obstruction. The two uterine horns are usually widely separated, with preservation of the endometrial and myometrial widths.

A septate uterus is seen when there is incomplete resorption of the final fibrous septum between the two uterine horns. The septum may be partial, or it may be complete and extend to the external cervical os. The differentiation between the septate and the bicornuate uterus is clinically important as the septate uterus is associated with a higher rate of reproductive complications. T2-weighted MR images taken parallel to the long axis of the uterus demonstrate a convex, flat, or concave (less than 1 cm) external uterine contor and the presence of the fibrous septa.[43]

Role of MRI in Characterization of Adnexal Lesions

The strength of MRI is its ability to characterize ovarian lesions, especially in the case of masses that are indeterminate on ultrasound. The signal intensity characteristics of ovarian masses can lead to a systematic approach to diagnosis. The signal intensity of a specific tumor depends on the presence, type, and extent of cystic and solid components within a lesion. Lesions that have a homogeneous low signal intensity on T1-weighted images and high signal intensity on T2-weighted images are simple fluid-filled structures and are considered benign. In general, benign epithelial ovarian neoplasms are predominantly cystic. Fat, hemorrhage, and mucin-containing lesions have high signal intensity on T1-weighted images. Fat-saturated T1-weighted images help distinguish between hemorrhage and fat within a lesion (e.g. endometriosis versus mature cystic teratoma). An adnexal mass of low or intermediate signal intensity on T1-weighted images and low signal intensity on T2-weighted images contain fibrosis and smooth muscle components. Such lesions include pedunculated leiomyoma, fibroma, fibrothecoma, cystadenofibroma, and Brenner tumors. The absence of a normal ipsilateral ovary or the presence of small follicles surrounding the mass helps identify the ovarian origin of fibromas.[43-45]

It is imperative to note that as there are no MRI signal intensity characteristics, that are specific for malignant epithelial tumor, such tumors must be distinguished based on morphologic criteria. The MRI features which are most predictive of malignancy are an enhancing solid component or vegetations within a cystic lesion, presence of necrosis within a solid lesion, as well as presence of ascites and peritoneal deposits.[46,47]

Although, both ultrasound and contrast-enhanced MRI have high sensitivity (97 and 100%, respectively) in the identification of solid components within an adnexal mass. MRI, however, is reported to demonstrate higher accuracy (93%).[46,47]

CONCLUSION

Ultrasound has proven to be a powerful imaging tool for most clinical indications, related to the pediatric female pelvis. Knowledge of the normal physiologic and age varying appearance of the pelvic organs during childhood is essential. Most pathology within the pediatric pelvis is well delineated with ultrasound. MRI is useful in depicting congenital anomalies and in evaluation of indeterminate adenexal masses.

IMAGING OF TESTICULAR ABNORMALITIES

The clinical manifestations in testicular abnormalities include pain, swelling, redness, or a palpable mass. These include undescended testes, hydrocoele, varicocele, acute scrotum, scrotal tumors, benign testicular cysts, testicular microlithiasis, scrotal trauma, scrotal hernia and systemic diseases with testicular involvement.

Gray-scale ultrasonography (US) in combination with color or power Doppler imaging, is a well accepted technique for assessing testicular abnormalities.[48] US permits differentiation between lesions that require urgent surgery (testicular torsion, malignant tumors, and traumatic rupture) and those that can be managed conservatively (e.g. epididymo-orchitis, torsion of the testicular appendages).

Undescended Testes

Various terms such as maldescended, undescended, retractile and ectopic testes have been used in the literature. Hormann M, have illustrated the entity of 'undescended testes' in their review on scrotal imaging in children.[49] The term "undescended testes" summarizes all conditions, in which the testes are absent from the scrotal sac:[50]

1. *Maldescended:* Testis not descended into the normal position 4 cm below the inguinal ligament.
2. *Cryptorchidism:* A maldescended, abdominally positioned testis.
3. *Incompletely descended:* Testis lying in the inguinal canal between the external and internal ring (most common site 75–80%).[51]
4. *Obstructed testis:* Testis lying in the superficial pouch.
5. *Prescrotal retention:* Testis lying within the scrotal sac, at a high position less than 4 cm below the inguinal ligament.
6. *Retractile testis:* Testis lies in normal position, retracts in cases of patent processus vaginalis and cremasteric muscle contraction.
7. *Ectopic testis:* Testis lying outside the normal path of descent—groin, perineum, penile root, femoral triangle, opposite scrotum (crossed ectopia).
8. *Absent testis:* No viable testicular tissue can be found.

Approximately, 3.5% of all male term infants, 20% of premature, and 100% of infants with a birth weight of less than 800 g have undescended testis. In 80% of these male infants, the testes are descended by the age of 1 year.[49] After 1 year of age, the descent of the undescended testis is almost not observed. Initial strategy, therefore, is to wait and reevaluate the child at age of 9–12 months and operate within this time.

Untreated undescended testes may lead to infertility when lying in the abdominal cavity. Also, undescended testes carry a significantly higher risk for development of malignancy. It is reported that 10% of all testicular malignancies occur in undescended testes or in testes treated for cryptorchidism.[51,52] Intra-abdominal testes carry a four times greater risk for development of malignancy than an inguinal testis.[53] The most frequent tumors in undescended testes are seminoma and embryonal cell carcinoma. The majority of undescended testes can be detected with the ultrasound, as 75–80% are located between the internal and external inguinal ring.[51]

Higher intra-abdominal locations make detection with ultrasound more difficult. MR imaging has been recommended in such cases. MR imaging offers excellent images of the testes, although, it has the disadvantage of a relative high cost and the need for sedation or anaesthesia in small children.[49] The location of the testis influences the optimal section orientation. In the lower abdomen and inguinal canal, coronal orientation offers the best results, while intra-abdominal testes are best depicted in axial and sagittal orientations. Surgeons in many institutions prefer laparoscopy as a diagnostic and at the same time a therapeutic tool in small children in cases in which ultrasound findings are inconclusive.

Inguinal-Scrotal Hernia

Inguinal-scrotal hernia is defined as the passage of intestinal loops and/or omentum into the scrotum.[48] The prevalence of inguinal hernia is higher in preterm neonates.[26] The hernia is more frequently located on the right side, as the right processus vaginalis closes later than the left.[54] Physical examination is usually sufficient to allow diagnosis in most cases. US examination is indicated in patients with inconclusive physical findings, in patients with acute scrotum, and also to investigate contralateral involvement in patients in whom only a unilateral hernia is clinically evident.[55]

The diagnosis of hernia is achieved by visualization of air bubble movement and/or intestinal peristalsis during the real-time examination. The herniated omentum is seen as a highly echogenic structure on US. Inguinal rings larger than 4 mm are an indication for prophylactic herniorrhaphy.[55] Color or power Doppler imaging is useful in inguinal-scrotal hernia to investigate intestinal and testicular perfusion. Urgent surgery is indicated in patients with an aperistaltic akinetic dilated bowel loop (a sign of strangulation).[56]

Varicoceles

Varicoceles are seldom seen in early childhood, but occur in adolescents and adults, and are a leading cause of male infertility. A varicocele is abnormal dilatation of the veins of the spermatic cord, which is usually caused by incompetent valves of the internal spermatic vein, and results in impaired drainage into the spermatic cord veins. Varicoceles can be visible, palpable or subclinical at clinical examination. Palpable and subclinical varicoceles are diagnosed with ultrasound: On grayscale imaging, they appear as multiple, serpiginous, tubular structures of varying sizes, larger than 2 mm in diameter.[49] On color and pulsed-wave Doppler images, venous flow is better demonstrated during the Valsalva maneuver **(Fig. 9)**. Varicocele may affect testicular growth;[57] hence, testicular volumes should be systematically measured and any asymmetry evaluated with US.[48]

Hydrocele

Hydrocele, is collection of fluid between the visceral and parietal layers of the tunica vaginalis and/or along the spermatic cord. It is one of the most common cause of painless scrotal swelling in children. In the normal scrotum, 1–2 mL of serous fluid may be observed in the potential tunica vaginalis cavity and should not be mistaken for hydrocele. Virtually, all hydroceles are congenital in neonates and infants and associated with a patent processus vaginalis, which allows peritoneal fluid to enter the scrotal sac.[48,58] In older children and adolescents, hydroceles are usually acquired and are often result of an inflammatory process, testicular torsion, trauma, or a tumor.

At USG, congenital hydrocele appears as an anechoic fluid collection surrounding the anterolateral aspects of the testis, which may sometimes extend to the inguinal canal or as a fluid collection with low-level swirling echoes[58] **(Fig. 10)**.

Spermatic cord cyst, a less common type of hydrocele, which more commonly appears as a fluid collection in the spermatic cord and results from closure of the processus vaginalis above the testis and below the internal inguinal ring **(Figs. 11A and B)**. Two types of spermatic cord hydrocole are known. The first type is encysted hydrocele of the cord, where the fluid collection does not communicate with the peritoneum or the tunica vaginalis. The second type is the funicular hydrocele, where there is a fluid collection along the cord, communicating with the peritoneum at the internal ring.

Most congenital hydroceles (80%) resolve spontaneously before the age of 2 years. However, surgical treatment is usually applied in spermatic cord and abdominoscrotal hydroceles.[48]

Cystic Dysplasia of the Testis

Cystic dysplasia of the testis is primarily incidentally found when evaluating children with renal dysplasia. It involves cystic dilatation of the rete testes. It is associated with dysplasia or agenesis of the ipsilateral kidney.[49]

Testicular Calcification (Microcalcification)

Testicular microcalcification is usually an incidental finding. Testicular microlithiasis is defined as multiple calcifications that are smaller than 2 mm and appear as hyperechoic structures throughout or in a large area of the testis.[49] They are associated with congenital syndromes (Klinefelter syndrome, pseudohermaphroditism), with congenital anomalies (undescended testes) or they could be idiopathic; they are also seen in tumors and are of unknown cause.

The calcifications are seen as fine, bright, non-shadowing hyperechoic foci (five or more on any single

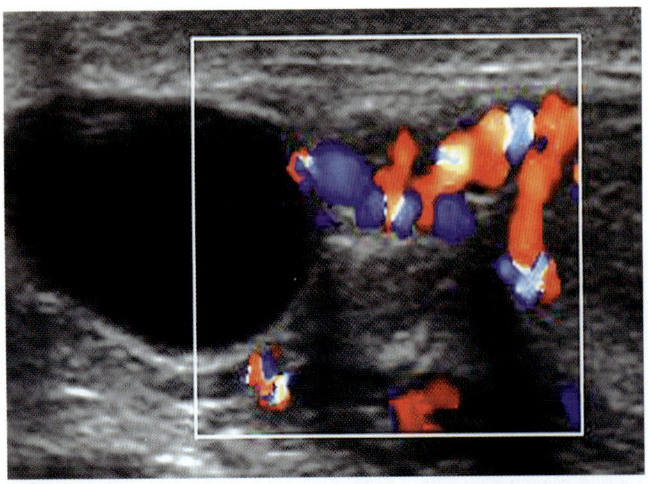

Fig. 9: Color Doppler ultrasound demonstrates typical dilated veins of spermatic cord, seen in child with varicocele along with encysted cord hydrocele.

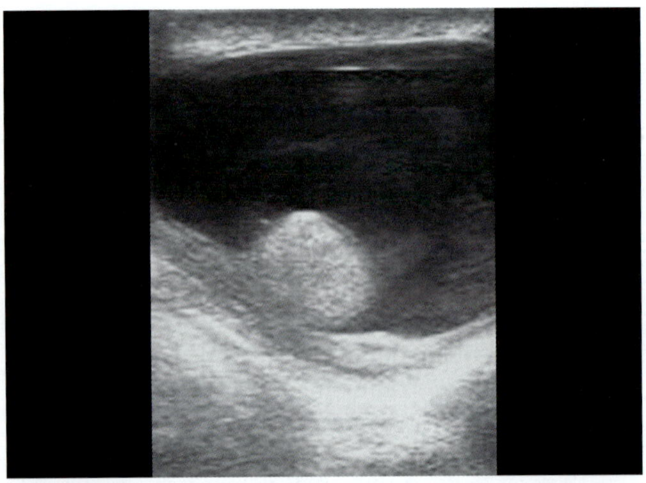

Fig. 10: Hydrocele: Longitudinal ultrasound of the right hemiscrotum shows a fluid collection surrounding the testes.

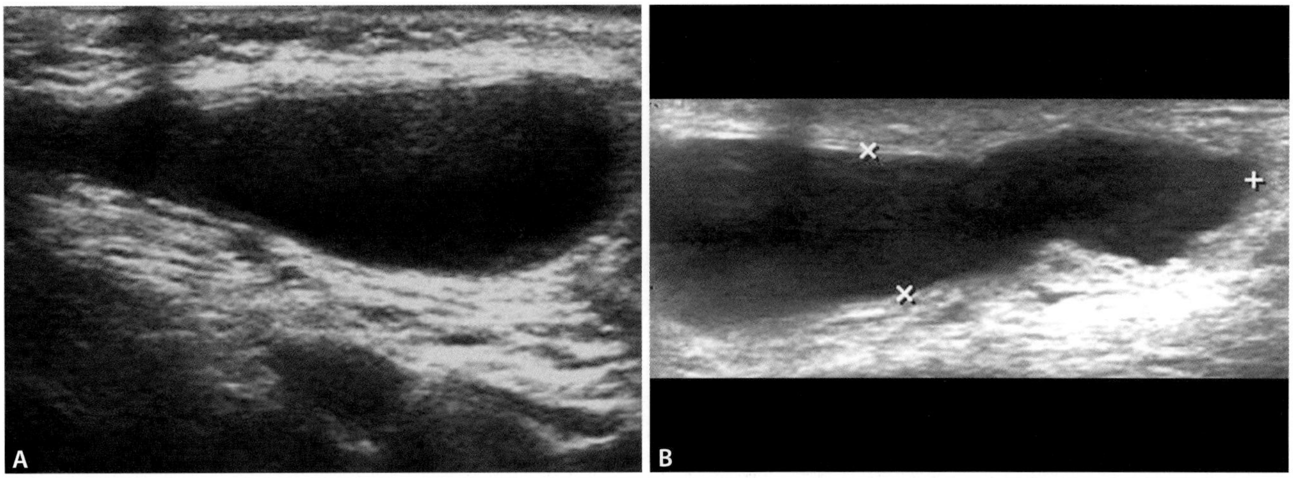

Figs. 11A and B: Spermatic cord hydrocele (funicular hydrocele). Longitudinal scan of the right spermatic cord of a 2-year-old child, shows a fluid collection along the cord, communicating with the peritoneum at the internal ring (A). Ultrasound in another patient (B) with spermatic cord hydrocele

view) that are uniform in size and are distributed in a diffuse pattern or in peripheral clusters.[48] As testicular microlithiasis is considered to be a premalignant condition; thus, serial scrotal US monitoring (once per year) is recommended.[59]

Acute Scrotum

Acute scrotum refers to a clinical setting of sudden-onset scrotal pain, redness, and swelling, which is most frequently caused by acute epididymo-orchitis, torsion of the testicular appendages, or testicular torsion.[48] Since scrotal involvement is usually unilateral, one should start the examination on the asymptomatic side first to have a basis for comparison. Color Doppler imaging, or power Doppler imaging should be added to grey-scale ultrasound.

Epididymo-orchitis

Epididymo-orchitis, is a common cause of acute scrotum in children.[48] It is mainly of infectious origin. The infection usually originates in the bladder or prostate gland, spreads through the vas deferens and the lymphatics of the spermatic cord to the epididymis, and finally reaches the testis, causing epididymo-orchitis. Isolated orchitis can also occur, but is rare.

There are two reported peaks of prevalence: under 2 years of age and over 6 years of age. Many conditions predispose to epididymo-orchitis, which include Imperforate anus, ureteral ectopia to the seminal vesicle, bladder exstrophy, neurogenic bladder, posterior urethral valves, and dysfunctional voiding. Chronic mild trauma can also lead to mild non-infective epididymo-orchitis.[49]

Children present with pain of acute onset, which is typically not as rapid as in torsion, and with reddening of the skin and edema. Clinical examination may be difficult because of pain, and elevating the scrotum beyond the symphysis pubis (Prehn's sign) relieves pain.[49]

The epididymal head is the most affected region, and reactive hydrocele and wall thickening are also frequently present. Increased size and, decreased, increased, or heterogeneous echogenicity of the affected organ are usually observed. On color Doppler imaging, there is increased blood flow within the epididymis, testis, or both **(Figs. 12 and 13)**.[48]

Occasionally, the entire epididymis is affected. Malignancies such as leukemia and lymphoma, that diffusely infiltrate the testicular parenchyma, may have a US appearance similar to that of diffuse orchitis. In such cases, the clinical history is extremely important.

In cases with accompanying orchitis, the testis is also enlarged and shows a heterogeneous echotexture.[60] Color Doppler studies show hyperemia in all cases in the affected regions, and ideally should help to distinguish from torsion. However, hyperemia disappears rapidly with improvement of symptoms under therapy.[61] With spectral Doppler studies, a low-resistance waveform with decreased resistance index (RI < 0.5) is observed.[62] Hyperemia of the testis also may be the result of vasculitis in Henoch–Schönlein purpura. In these cases, different presentations of vasculitis can be observed and therefore can be differentiated from inflammation of other cause.[49]

Granulomatous epididymo-orchitis is a chronic inflammation occurring in postpubertal boys.[48] The affected part of the epididymis, mainly the tail, is

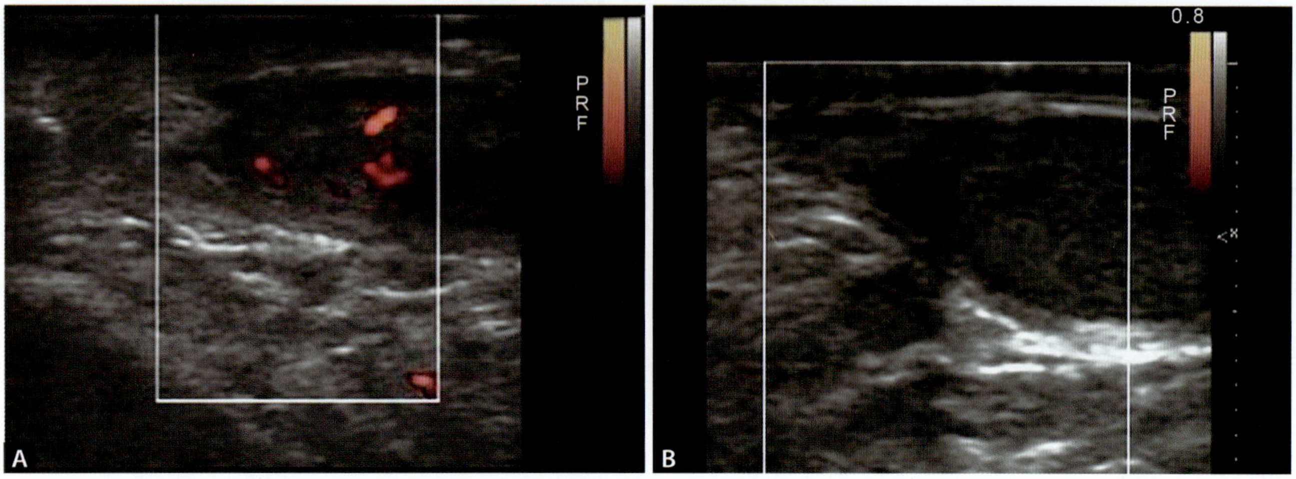

Figs. 12A and B: Epididymitis: Epididymis is enlarged, heterogeneous and demonstrates increased flow on color Doppler (A). Normal opposite epididymis is shown for comparison (B).

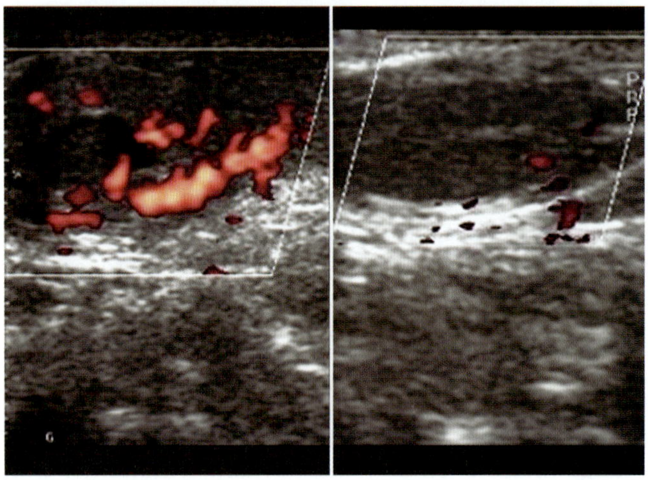

Fig. 13: Epididymo-orchitis in a 9-year-old boy. Ultrasound revealed enlarged epididymal head with heterogeneous echotexture of epididymus and testes, which demonstrated increased vascularity on power Doppler. Oppisite normal left testis is shown for comparison.

enlarged with heterogeneous echogenicity.[63] At color Doppler imaging, chronic epididymo-orchitis does not demonstrate the increased blood flow, typical of acute epididymitis. The sonographic features can be similar to those of epididymal adenomatoid tumor; however, patients with chronic epididymitis present with a painful mass, whereas the tumor is usually painless.

Torsion of the Testicular Appendages

The appendages are sessile structures, which thus predisposes them to torsion, and the appendix testis is most often affected.[48] Torsion of the appendix testis occurs mainly in prepubertal boys (aged 7–14 years), is more frequent on the left side, and is a common cause of acute scrotum in this age group.[64]

Affected patients typically present with gradual or sudden intense pain, usually localized in the upper pole of the testis. At physical examination, the classic finding in these children is a small palpable nodule on the superior aspect of the testis, which is called the "blue dot" sign. This is seen in nearly one third of patients, and this is a pathognomonic feature of this entity.

At US, the twisted appendage is seen as a round extra-testicular mass with high or mixed echogenicity depending on the evolution time.[65] Associated findings include an enlarged epididymal head, reactive hydrocele, and scrotal skin thickening. There is no Doppler signal in the twisted appendage, and the epididymis and scrotal tunics are hypervascularized. Management is conservative, in contrast to torsion of the spermatic cord, and the pain resolves after 2–3 days. The appendix becomes atrophic and finally calcifies.

Testicular Torsion

Testicular torsion, entails first venous and later arterial flow obstruction. The extent of testicular ischemia in these patients depends on the degree of twisting (180°–720°) and the duration of the torsion. Testicular salvage is more likely in patients treated within 6 hours after the onset of torsion, hence the need for an urgent, immediate diagnosis.[48]

Testicular torsion are of two types: Extravaginal and intravaginal.

Extravaginal torsion or supravaginal torsion, can only occur before the tunica vaginalis and the gubernaculum become fixed to the scrotal wall, and therefore can only occur in the perinatal period.[66] At birth, the testis is infarcted and necrotic, and clinically, children present with a painless mass, swelling and discoloration of the scrotal sac. Ultrasound, typically demonstrates an enlarged heterogeneous testis, ipsilateral hydrocoele, thickening, and absent flow in the spermatic cord and testis.

Intravaginal torsion can occur at any age but is more common in adolescents. A known predisposing factor is the "bellclapper" deformity, in which the tunica vaginalis joins high on the spermatic cord, leaving the testis free to rotate.[49]

Differentiation between testicular torsion and epididymo-orchitis is important, since scrotal pain, swelling, and redness are clinical symptoms common to these two entities. Generally, pain in testicular torsion has a sudden onset, whereas in orchitis, it is more gradual. However, 5% of children with orchitis have sudden onset of pain, and only 50% of patients with testicular torsion have an acute attack.[44]

The pain is constant and does not increase with palpation or movement and is not relieved when the scrotum is elevated above the symphysis, in contrast to inflammatory conditions.

In the early phases of torsion (1–3 hours), testicular echogenicity appears normal. With progression, enlargement of the affected testis and increased or heterogeneous echogenicity are common findings. Sonographic evaluation of the spermatic cord is an essential part of the examination. The point of cord twisting can be identified at the external inguinal orifice. More than 24 hours after the onset of symptoms, there is reversion to normal echogenicity and after 10 days the testis becomes atrophic.[49] A definitive diagnosis of complete testicular torsion is made when blood flow is visualized on the normal side but is absent on the affected side.[48]

Two kinds of torsion can be differentiated: Complete torsion (>360°) and incomplete torsion (<360°).[49] In complete torsion, initially the epididymis is the first organ without flow, but after about 6 hour a collateral arterial supply from the inferior epigastric artery is opened, which can mislead the examiner. Incomplete torsion refers to cord twisting of less than 360°, in which some arterial flow persists in the affected testis (seen in 20% cases in one series). The venous flow is obstructed. Therefore, it is important to study the testicular perforating arteries to avoid false-negative ultrasound results.[49]

Additional, information can be obtained from pulsed-wave Doppler imaging, with which decreased or reversed diastolic flow may be evident on the affected side, and from scintigraphy and MR imaging.[67,68]

Normal echogenicity with mild testicular enlargement has been reported as a good sign of viability, whereas marked enlargement, heterogeneous echotexture, and scrotal wall hypervascularity are signs of testicular infarction and necrosis.

Acute Idiopathic Scrotal Edema

Acute idiopathic scrotal edema is a self-limiting disease which is characterized by edema and erythema of the scrotum.[69] It is the fourth most common cause of acute scrotum in patients aged below 20 years, following epididymitis, testicular torsion, and torsion of appendages.[69,70] Since clinically it manifests similar to those of other surgically correctable acute scrotal disease, it is important to confirm diagnosis, using US and Doppler to avoid unnecessary surgery.

Exact etiology of this entity remains unclear, however, it is considered a variant of angioneurotic edema.[70] Patients with idiopathic scrotal edema may also show eosinophilia, which may be the result of allergic reaction. In most reported cases, all source of infection was excluded from surrounding structures. It is also known that as mostly unilateral, and perineal or inguinal erythema is coexistent in half the cases.[70-72] However, bilateral involvement was more common in one study by Lee et al. (75%) compared with previous studies.[69] The most common characteristic of is scrotal wall edema **(Fig. 14)**, which is easily visualized on US, which has also been confirmed by surgical findings.[72]

Several studies have described the following US and Doppler findings:

1. Marked thickening of the scrotal wall, with heterogeneous striated and edematous appearance, with increased flow.

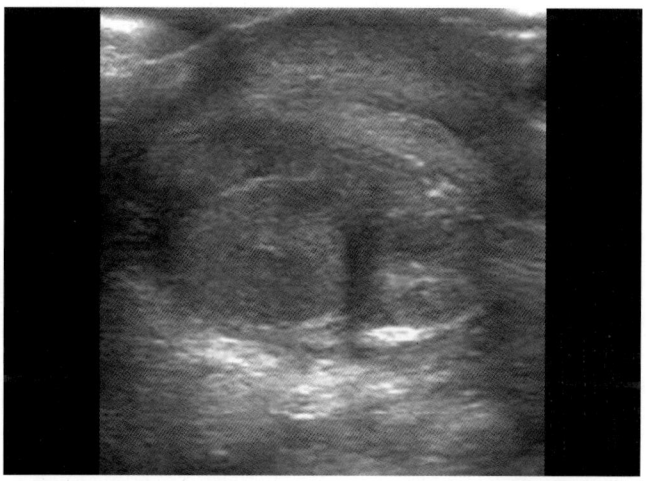

Fig. 14: Acute idiopathic scrotal edema. Transverse ultrasound scan of both hemiscrota shows marked thickening of scrotal walls.

2. Increased peritesticular blood flow.
3. Mildly reactive hydrocele.[71,72]
4. The testes and epididymis are normal in appearance and do not show increased vascularity.[73]
5. Enlargement and increased vascularity of the inguinal lymph nodes.

As, it is an self-limiting disease, surgical intervention should be avoided. US examination along with Doppler is very useful to differentiate between other acute scrotal diseases and acute idiopathic scrotal edema.

Scrotal Tumors

The incidence of scrotal tumors is estimated at 0.5–2.0 cases per 100,000 boys.[74] Scrotal tumors typically manifest as painless scrotal swelling. Owing to its excellent spatial resolution, US is highly sensitive for identifying scrotal masses.[75] This technique allows differentiation between cystic and solid tumors and classification as intra- or extratesticular. The term *paratesticular* refers to a group of extratesticular lesions that are not easily identified as originating from a particular tissue. Computed tomography (CT) is reserved for detecting spread in malignant tumors, while MR imaging is useful for characterizing the tumor content or better delineation of extratesticular solid masses.[76] Certain tumor markers (α-fetoprotein and human chorionic gonadotropin) also help to make a more precise diagnosis.

Testicular Tumors

Testicular tumors account for 1% of all pediatric solid tumors.[48] They have two peaks of prevalence, first before 3 years of age and secondly, in the postpubertal period. They usually manifest as a painless scrotal mass. However, in approximately 10% of patients, testicular tumor is associated with pain due to hemorrhage or infarction, mimicking torsion or epididymitis. Testicular tumors are subdivided into two groups: Germ cell tumors and nongerm cell tumors.

Germ cell tumors: Germ cell tumors result from the transformation of primitive germ cells. These pluripotential cells can remain nondifferentiated (seminomas), become slightly differentiated (embryonal carcinoma), or transform into differentiated embryonal (mature or immature teratomas) or extraembryonal (choriocarcinoma) structures.[77]

For clinical purposes, germ cell tumors are also divided into two groups: seminomatous and nonseminomatous germ cell tumors.[78]

Seminomas, in comparison with nonseminomatous tumors, occur in older population,with an average patient age of 40.5 years. Seminoma is extremely radiosensitive, and radiotherapy for low-stage tumors is very effective, resulting in a 5-year survival rate of 95%.[78]

Nonseminomatous Germ Cell Tumors

Yolk sac tumor, also known as endodermal sinus tumor, is the most common germ cell tumor, accounts for 80% of childhood testicular tumors, with most cases occurring before the age of 2 years. In its pure form, yolk sac tumor is rare in adults; however, it is present in 44% of adult cases of mixed germ cell tumor.[79]

α-fetoprotein is normally produced by the embryonic yolk sac, and thus serum α-fetoprotein levels are elevated in greater than 90% of patients with yolk sac tumor.[78] These markers are also useful in follow-up to check for regression or recurrence of the tumor.

The US findings are nonspecific, usually showing a solid mass replacing the entire testis.The presence of hypoechoic areas within the tumor, which indicates areas of necrosis, is a frequent finding **(Figs. 15A to C)**. As with all germ cell tumors, spread is predominantly via the lymphatic system; hence, the lymphatic pathway should be included in the initial work-up.

The second most common germ cell tumor is *teratoma*, which is classified as mature, immature and those with malignant areas. Generally, teratomas occur in children less than 4 years of age.[78]

The sonographic appearance depends on the components of the three germinal layers (endodermal, mesodermal, and ectodermal). Cysts are a common feature and may be an echoic or complex, depending on the cyst contents (i.e. serous, mucoid, or keratinous fluid). Teratoma may appear as a complex mass with cystic components, or a cystic lesion with peripheral solid components or calcifications, and echogenic intratumor fat.[78] These tumors are usually benign in prepubertal children, so tissue sparing surgery may be possible; however, in adolescents they are often malignant and require orchidectomy.

Testicular epidermoid cyst is the most common benign testicular tumor with no malignant potential. Epidermoid cysts are composed of keratinizing, stratified, squamous epithelium with a well-defined fibrous wall. The cyst contains cheesy material and may resemble a solid tumor at US. Several sonographic patterns have been described: An echogenic lesion surrounded by a hypoechoic or echogenic rim, a target appearance, and an "onionring" configuration with alternating echogenic and anechoic areas within the lesion.[80] The presence of well-delineated borders and a vascularity at color Doppler imaging favors

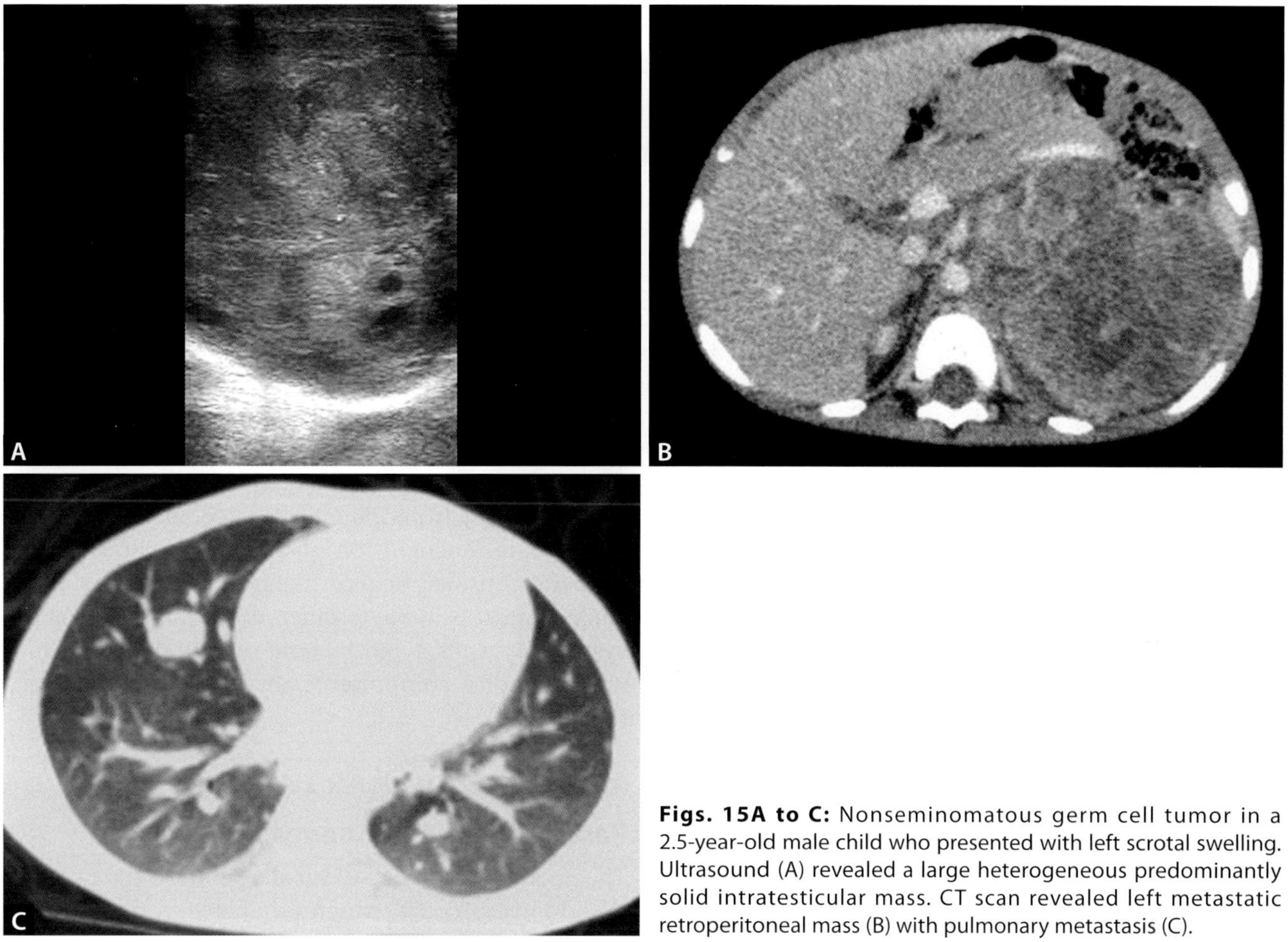

Figs. 15A to C: Nonseminomatous germ cell tumor in a 2.5-year-old male child who presented with left scrotal swelling. Ultrasound (A) revealed a large heterogeneous predominantly solid intratesticular mass. CT scan revealed left metastatic retroperitoneal mass (B) with pulmonary metastasis (C).

the diagnosis. In inconclusive cases, MR imaging can aid in identification. On contrast-enhanced images, they are seen as sharply demarcated, low signal-intensity, non-enhancing lesions.[81]

Although, the radiologic appearance of epidermoid cyst is quite characteristic, it is not however, pathognomonic. Teratomas and other malignant tumors may also have a similar appearance, and mass should be carefully evaluated for any irregular borders, which might suggest a malignant lesion. Because carcinoma cannot be completely excluded, orchiectomy is usually performed. However, if the lesion has been thoroughly evaluated, and if there is a strong possibility that it is an epidermoid cyst, it is recommended to perform a testis sparing enucleation rather than orchiectomy.[78]

Non-germ cell tumors: Non-germ cell tumors, are less frequent than germ cell tumors, and can develop from the gonadal stroma (Leydig cell tumor), sex cord cells (Sertoli cell tumor), or sex cord cells plus stroma (gonadoblastoma).[48]

These account for nearly 4% of all testicular tumors.[78] The prevalence is higher in the pediatric age group, for which non-germ cell tumors constitute 10–30% of all testicular neoplasms.[78] 90% of all non-germ cell tumors are benign. Unfortunately, no radiologic criteria allows definite differentiation of benign from malignant disease, and orchiectomy is usually performed in all cases. Even with histologic analysis, it is difficult at times, to determine the biologic behavior of these tumors.

Leydig cell tumors are the most common in this group, accounting for 1–3% of all testicular tumors. They can be seen in any age group, with 20% of cases reported to occur in patients younger than 10 years, 25% in patients aged 10–30 years, 30% in patients aged 30–50 years, and 25% in patients older than 50 years.[82] Nearly 30% of patients will have an endocrinopathy secondary to secretion of androgens or estrogens by the tumor. Leydig cell tumors are generally small solid masses, but they may show cystic areas, hemorrhage, or necrosis **(Fig. 16)**.[82] Their sonographic appearance is also variable and is indistinguishable from that of germ cell tumors.

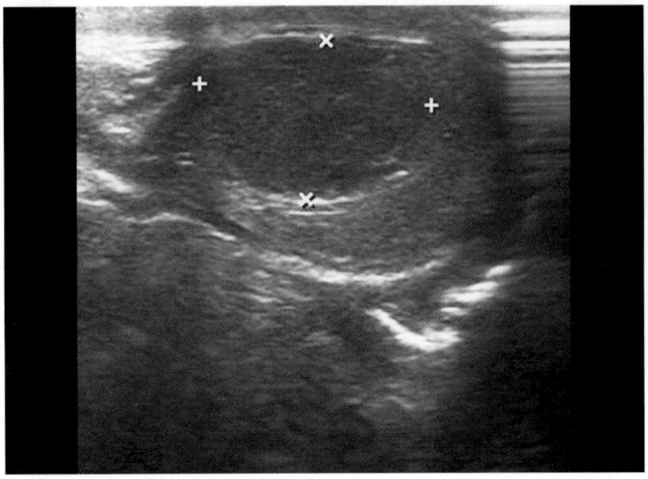

Fig. 16: Testicular ultrasound showing a hypoechoic intratesticular lesion in a child with Leydig cell tumor of testes.

Sertoli cell tumors are less common than leydig cell tumors, and constitute less than 1% of testicular tumors. They are less hormonally active, but gynecomastia can occur.[82] Sertoli cell tumors are typically well-circumscribed, unilateral, round to lobulated masses. An subtype is the large-cell calcifying Sertoli cell tumor, which is most often seen in the pediatric age group. This subtype commonly manifests as multiple and bilateral masses, which, as the name implies, are distinguished by large areas of calcification that are readily seen with US.[83] This subgroup has been associated with Peutz-Jeghers syndrome and Carney syndrome (pituitary adenomas, mucocutaneous pigmentation, and myxomas of the heart, skin, eyelids, and breast).[78,83]

Gonadoblastoma is a dysgenetic lesion occurring in the setting of gonadal dysgenesis and intersex syndromes. Approximately, 80% of the patients are phenotypically female.[82,83]

Other Testicular Tumors

Primary follicular lymphoma of the testes is an infrequent tumor, with only few reported cases.[84] However, secondary involvement is common in patients with acute lymphoblastic leukemia and non-Hodgkin B-cell lymphoma.[85] At US, there are two relatively more common patterns of involvement, which are seen in both leukemia and lymphoma: the more common diffuse type, in which the testis is enlarged and hypoechoic, and the focal type, which demonstrates multiple hypoechoic nodules. Increased blood flow may be seen on color Doppler images, which may simulate an inflammatory lesion.

Primary leukemia of the testis is rare. However, the testis is a common site of leukemia recurrence in children, with 80% of patients being in bone marrow remission.[86,87] It is believed that the blood testis barrier allows leukemic cells to be "hidden" during chemotherapy. The clinical characteristics and sonographic appearance of leukemia of the testis can be quite varied, as the tumors may be unilateral or bilateral, diffuse or focal, hypoechoic or hyperechoic **(Figs. 17A and B)**.[86,87]

Metastasis of other solid tumors, such as Wilms' tumor, neuroblastoma, and retinoblastoma, that may affect the testis have also been reported.[48]

Benign testicular cysts can be located either within the tunica albuginea or the parenchyma.[78] Tunica albuginea cysts are typically peripherally located and may be single or multiple. Recognition of their classic location and appearance usually helps in making this diagnosis. Careful analysis must be done to differentiate these lesions from cystic neoplasms, typically teratomas. If the cystic lesion has any solid components, it should be considered malignant.

EXTRATESTICULAR TUMORS

Paratesticular Rhabdomyosarcoma

The most common extratesticular tumor is paratesticular rhabdomyosarcoma, which originates in the spermatic cord or scrotal tunics.[48] The majority of these tumors occur in the first two decades of life and belong to the embryonal histopathologic subtype. At US, paratesticular rhabdomyosarcoma is seen as a hypo- or hyperechoic solid mass that may envelop or invade the epididymis and testis, which demonstrates hypervascularity at color Doppler imaging.[88]

CT is often recommended in the initial work-up to determine tumor spread, and MR imaging can be performed, if required,to delimit the borders of the mass relative to the epididymis and testis.[89] Long-term survival is expected in patients under 10 years of age with disease confined to the scrotum.

Adenomatoid Tumor

Adenomatoid tumors are benign, solid extratesticular lesions that can originate from the epididymis, tunica vaginalis, or spermatic cord. They are the most common tumor of the epididymis and occur more often in the lower pole than in the upper pole by a ratio of 4:1.[90] Usually, an incidental finding, adenomatoid tumors manifest

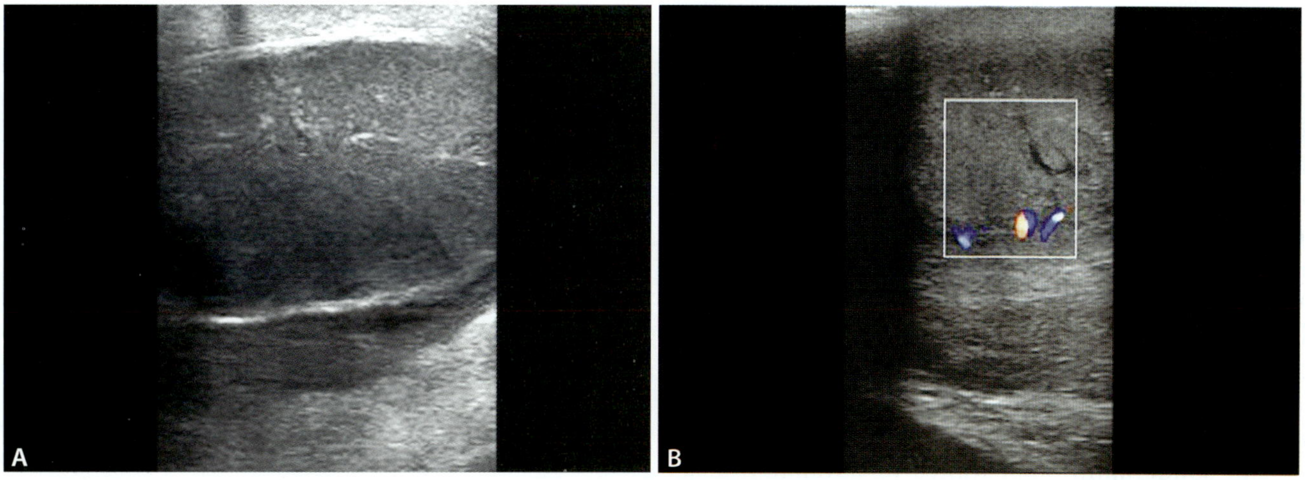

Figs. 17A and B: Ultrasound (A and B) reveals diffuse leukemic infiltration of testes in a child with lymphoblastic leukemia.

as a painless scrotal mass, with the majority diagnosed inpatients aged 20–50 years.[91] They are typically unilateral and occur more frequently on the left side. When they grow noninvasively into the testicular parenchyma, they can simulate intratesticular disease.

At US, they appear as a solid extratesticular mass with variable echogenicity.[91,92] Commonly, MR imaging demonstrates low signal intensity relative to the testicular parenchyma on T2-weighted images. However, the appearance is not specific and should be differentiated from granulomatous epididymitis, a chronic form of epididymitis that manifests as a painful palpable mass. At color Doppler imaging, vessels are observed within the adenomatous tumor, whereas usually no vessels are seen in granulomatous epididymitis.[48,60]

Epididymal cysts, although not true tumors, typically manifest as a palpable mass and are of lymphatic origin. Because they contain clear serous fluid, they are seen as an anechoic, well-defined mass with increased through transmission. Epididymal cysts cannot be differentiated from spermatoceles, which are secondary to obstruction and dilatation of the efferent ductal system. However, the latter occur exclusively in postpubertal boys.[91]

Primary malignant tumors of the epididymis are rare in children; epididymal involvement is largely due to metastatic spread from B-cell acute lymphoblastic leukemia and B-cell non-Hodgkin lymphoma.[91]

Epididymal Cystadenoma

Papillary cystadenoma of the epididymis is a benign epithelial neoplasm. It is seen in up to 60% of men with von Hippel–Lindau disease.[91] Although, the sporadic variety is usually seen in middle-aged men, it is seen earlier in patients with von Hippel–Lindau disease. The sonographic appearance is variable. It can appear as a solid appearance with few cystic spaces or can appear as multiloculated cystic lesion with small papillary projections.[90-92] In patients with von Hippel–Lindau disease, sonographic criteria for diagnosis of epididymal cystadenoma consist of (a) A predominantly solid epididymal mass larger than 10 × 14 mm and (b) Slow growth. At MR imaging, a cystic mass with septations or mural nodules can be seen.

Lipoma

Lipoma is the most common benign tumor of the spermatic cord and can occur at any age.[91] At US, it is a well-defined, homogeneous, hyperechoic paratesticular lesion.[92] At MR imaging, lipoma appears uniform and follows fat signal intensity with all sequences, including fat-suppressed sequences, which confirms the diagnosis.[93]

Fibrous Pseudotumor

Fibrous pseudotumor is considered as a benign, reactive fibrous paratesticular tissue. As it can grow up to large sizes, therefore, it can mimic a neoplasm. It commonly arises from the tunica vaginalis. The sonographic appearance is nonspecific,[90,92] and calcification is commonly seen. The lesion can dislodge and become freely mobile within the scrotal sac; such a lesion is known as a "scrotal pearl". At MR imaging, owing to the presence of fibrosis, the lesion has low signal intensity on both T1- and T2-weighted images with variable enhancement.

ADRENAL RESTS

These are a rare cause of testicular masses, which can be seen in patients with congenital adrenal hyperplasia and rarely in those with Cushing syndrome. These rests are usually less than 5 mm and can be found in the testis and surrounding tissues in 7.5–15% of newborns and 1.6% of adults.[94] If these cells are exposed to elevated levels of adrenocorticotropic hormone, they can enlarge to form masses.

These were present in 11 of 20 patients (55%) with CAH, in one series reported by Aso C et al.[48] As potential malignancy is extremely rare, testicular biopsy is not required, even when the mass increases in size.

The sonographic appearance of adrenal rests is variable, with some series describing predominantly hypoechoic masses and others reporting heterogeneously hyperechoic masses with shadowing.[94,95] On MR imaging, these have been reported to have low signal intensity on both T1- and T2-weighted images.[96] It is important to recognize these as benign lesions to avoid unnecessary orchiectomy.[78]

Sarcoidosis is a multisystem, chronic granulomatous disease that rarely affects the genital tract. Although, it more commonly affects the epididymis but can, in some cases, also involve the testis. Testicular lesions can be solitary, but they are more commonly multiple, small, bilateral masses.[97] Testicular sarcoidosis is more common in African-Americans than in other racial groups.[82]

Scrotal Involvement in Systemic Diseases

Scrotal involvement can be seen in many systemic diseases.[48] The testes are affected in 15–37% of patients with Henoch-Schönlein purpura.[98,99] In this disease, scrotal symptoms may even precede other manifestations. US findings include scrotal wall thickening, epididymal enlargement, and reactive hydrocele. Involvement is bilateral in the majority of cases; hence, this entity should be considered when bilateral US findings similar to those of inflammatory epididymitis are visualized.

Scrotal Trauma

Scrotal trauma, in children can result from a trivial fall, sports or motor vehicle and straddle accidents. Since physical examination is limited by swelling and pain, US is an good modality for its detection. Lesions range from extratesticular hematoma to testicular rupture. Extratesticular hematomas may be quite large and their echogenicity changes over time, being echogenic in the acute state and anechoic during follow-up **(Fig. 18)**.

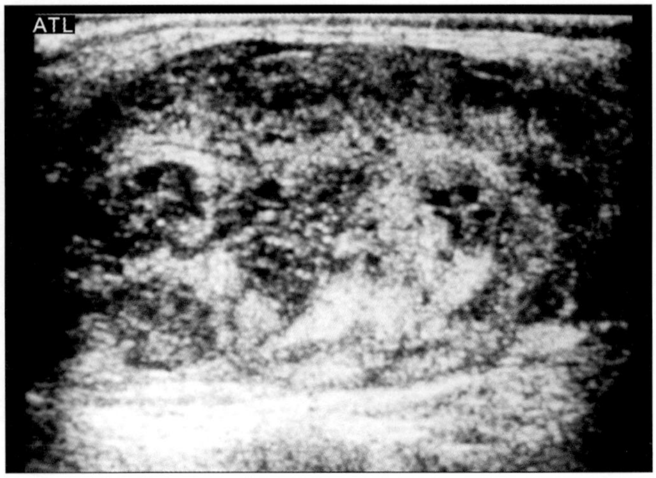

Fig. 18: Longitudinal ultrasonogram in a 12-year-old child (with history of scrotal injury while playing football) shows a large heterogeneous soft tissue mass in the left scrotal sac, suggestive of testicular hematoma.

Conservative treatment is recommended except in cases of impaired testicular flow testicular rupture is rare, but should be suspected when the margins of the testis are poorly defined or disruption of the capsular blood flow is observed.[48,60] MR imaging increases the diagnostic confidence and is useful in preoperative work-up of testicular rupture.[100] MRI is extremely helpful for evaluation of scrotal blunt trauma owing to its high tissue contrast, multiplanar imaging, and ability to depict hemorrhage at different stages. The low signal from the albuginea is a remarkable sign, ensuring testicular integrity.

Role of MRI in Testicular Abnormalities

MR imaging is useful as a problem-solving tool when sonographic findings are equivocal.[90] Magnetic resonance imaging (MRI) has been tested, with good results in different scrotal diseases because of its superb anatomic details, and great tissue contrast.[100-102] MRI dramatically improves the diagnostic reliability in certain given conditions, such as scrotal blunt trauma, nonpalpable lesions with an inconclusive sonographic appearance, patients with chronic scrotal pain with nonspecific sonograms, and when the US and clinical findings are discrepant.

MR imaging accurately allows characterization of scrotal masses as intratesticular or extratesticular and can demonstrate various types of lesions and tissue, including cysts or fluid, solid masses, fat, and fibrosis. MR imaging can be of additional value when the location of a scrotal mass is uncertain or when US does not allow differentiation between a solid mass and an inflammatory or vascular abnormality. Gadolinium-enhanced MR imaging can further help differentiate between a benign cystic lesion and a cystic neoplasm. Contrast-enhanced MRI can also be used to demonstrate areas of absent or reduced testicular perfusion, such as in segmental testicular infarct. MR imaging can demonstrate an intra-abdominal undescended testis, which can be difficult to detect with US, and is superior to US in differentiation between an undescended testis and testicular agenesis.[90]

CONCLUSION

A wide spectrum of diseases can involve the scrotum in children. Ultrasonography (US) performed by using a high-frequency transducer, with color Doppler, is the initial imaging modality of choice when evaluating testicular abnormalities. US can suggest a specific diagnosis for a wide variety of intrascrotal diseases, appropriately guiding treatment. Magnetic resonance imaging can be useful as a problem-solving tool when sonographic findings are equivocal or suboptimal. CT scan has no current role in evaluation of scrotal disorders in children, however, it is useful in staging of malignancy.

REFERENCES

1. Gare L, Dubois J, Grignon A, Filiatrault D, Vliet GV. US of the Pediatric Female Pelvis: A Clinical Perspective. Radiographics. 2001;21:1393-407.
2. Stranzinger E, Strouse PJ. Ultrasound of the Pediatric Female Pelvis Seminars in US, CT. MRI. 2008;29:98-113.
3. Lang IM, Babyn P, Oliver GD. MR imaging of pediatric uterovaginal anomalies. Pediatr Radiol. 1999;29:163-70.
4. Nussbaum AR, Sanders RC, Jones MD. Neonatal uterine morphology as seen on real-time US. Radiology. 1986; 160:641-3.
5. Hata K, Nishigaki A, Makihara K, Takamiya O, Hata T, Kitao M. Ultrasonic evaluation of the normal uterus in the neonate. J Perinat Med. 1989;17:313-7.
6. Haber HP, Mayer EI. Ultrasound evaluation of uterine and ovarian size from birth to puberty. Pediatr Radiol. 1994;24:11-3.
7. Holm K, Laursen EM, Brocks V, Muller J. Pubertal maturation of the internal genitalia: An ultrasound evaluation of 166 healthy girls. Ultrasound Obstet Gynecol. 1995;6:175-81.
8. Buzi F, Pilotta A, Dordoni D, Lombardi A, Zaglio S, Adlard P. Pelvic ultrasonography in normal girls and in girls with pubertal precocity. Acta Paediatr. 1998;87:1138-45.
9. Orbak Z, Sagsoz N, Alp H, Tan H, Yildirim H, Kaya D. Pelvic ultrasound measurements in normal girls: Relation to puberty and sex hormone concentration. J Pediatr Endocrinol Metab. 1998;11:525-30.
10. Cohen HL, Shapiro MA, Mandel FS, Shapiro ML. Normal ovaries in neonates and infants: A sonographic study of 77 patients 1 day to 24 months old. AJR. 1993;160:583-6.
11. Orsini LF, Salardi S, Pilu G, Bovicelli L, Cacciari E. Pelvic organs in premenarcheal girls: Real-time ultrasonography. Radiology. 1984;153:113-6.
12. Cohen HL, Eisenberg P, Mandel F, Haller JO. Ovarian cysts are common in premenarchal girls: A sonographic study of 101 children 2–12 years old. AJR. 1992;159:89-91.
13. Surratt, JT, Siegel MJ. Imaging of pediatric ovarian masses. Radiographics. 1991;11:533-48.
14. Fleischer AC, Daniel JF, Rodier J, Lindsay AM, James AE Jr. Sonographic monitoring of ovarian follicular development. JCU. 1981;9:275-80.
15. Ritchie WGM. Sonographic evaluation of normal and induced ovulation. Radiology. 1986;161:1-10.
16. Templeman C, Fallat ME, Blinchevsky A, et al. Non inflammatory ovarian masses in girls and young women. Obstet Gynecol. 2000;96:229-33.
17. De Silva KS, Kanumakala S, Grover SR, et al. Ovarian lesions in children and adolescents: An 11-year review. J Pediatr Endocrinol Metab. 2004;17:951-7.
18. Brandt ML, Helmrath MA. Ovarian cysts in infants and children. Semin Pediatr Surg. 2005;14:78-85.
19. Nussbaum AR, Sanders RC, Hartman DS, et al. Neonatal ovarian cysts: Sonographic-pathologic correlation. Radiology. 1988;168:817-21.
20. Rosenberg HK, Sherman NH, Tarry WF, Duckett JW, Snyder HM. Mayer-Rokitansky-Kuster-Hauser syndrome: US AID to diagnosis. Radiology. 1986;161:815-9.
21. Carranza-Lira S, Forbin K, Martinez-Chequer JC. Rokitansky syndrome and MURCS association: Clinical features and basis for diagnosis. Int J Fertil Womens Med. 1999;44:250-5.
22. Blask AR, Sanders RC, Gearhart JP. Obstructed uterovaginal anomalies: Demonstration with sonography. I. Neonates and infants. Radiology. 1991;179:79-83.
23. Banerjee AK, Clarke O, MacDonald LM. Sonographic detection of neonatal hydrometrocolpos. Br J Radiol. 1992;65:268-71.
24. Sugar NF, Graham EA. Common gynecologic problems in prepubertal girls. Pediatr Rev. 2006;27:213-23.
25. Strouse PJ. Sonographic evaluation of the child with lower abdominal or pelvic pain. Radiol Clin North Am. 2006;44:911-23.
26. Ziereisen F, Guissard G, Damry N, et al. Sonographic imaging of the pediatric female pelvis. Eur Radiol. 2005;15:1296-309.
27. Robert Y, Mestdagh P, Ziereisen F, et al. Imaging of the female pelvis in adolescence. J Radiol. 2001;82:1765-80.
28. Haber HP, Ranke MB. Pelvic ultrasonography in Turner syndrome: Standards for uterine and ovarian volume. J Ultrasound Med. 1999;18:271-6.
29. Mazzanti L, Nizzoli G, Tassinari D, et al. Spontaneous growth and pubertal development in Turner's syndrome with different karyotypes. Acta Paediatr. 1994;83:299-304.
30. Matarazzo P, Lala R, Artesani L, Franceshini PG, De Sanctis C. Sonographic appearance of ovaries and gonadotropin secretions as prognostic tools of spontaneous puberty in girls with Turner's syndrome. J Pediatr Endocrinol Metab. 1995;8:267-74.

31. Sheth S, Fishman EK, Buck JL, et al. The variable sonographic appearances of ovarian teratomas: Correlation with CT. AJR. 1988;151:331-4.
32. Sisler CL, Siegel MJ. Ovarian teratomas: A comparison of the sonographic appearance in prepubertal and postpubertal girls. AJR. 1990;154:139-41.
33. Outwater EK, Wagner BJ, Mannion C, et al. Sex cord-stromal and steroid cell tumors of the ovary. Radiographics. 1998;18:1523-46.
34. Chang HC, Bhatt S, Dogra VS. Pearls and Pitfalls in diagnosis of Ovarian Torsion. Radiographics. 2008;28:1355-68.
35. Albayram F, Hamper UM. Ovarian and adnexal torsion: Spectrum of sonographic findings with pathologic correlation. J Ultrasound Med. 2001;20(10):1083-9.
36. Breech LL, Hillard PJ. Adnexal torsion in pediatric and adolescent girls. Curr Opin Obstet Gynecol. 2005;17(5):483-9.
37. Graif M, Itzchak Y. Sonographic evaluation of ovarian torsion in childhood and adolescence. AJR. 1988;150(3): 647-9.
38. Lee EJ, Kwon HC, Joo HJ, Suh JH, Fleischer AC. Diagnosis of ovarian torsion with color Doppler sonography: Depiction of twisted vascular pedicle. J Ultrasound Med. 1998;17(2):83-9.
39. Vijayaraghavan SB. Sonographic whirlpool sign in ovarian torsion. J Ultrasound Med. 2004;23(12):1643-9.
40. Dashefsky SM, Lyons EA, Levi CS, Lindsay DJ. Suspected ectopic pregnancy: Endovaginal and transvesical US. Radiology. 1988;169:181-4.
41. Filly RA. Ectopic pregnancy: The role of sonography. Radiology. 1987;162:661-8.
42. Strouse PJ, DiPietro MA, Saez F. Transient small-bowel intussusceptions in children on CT. Pediatr Radiol. 2003;33: 316-20.
43. Sala E. Magnetic Resonance Imaging of the Female Pelvis. Seminars in Roentogenology. 2008;290-302.
44. Carrington BM, Hricak H, Nuruddin RN, et al. Mullerian duct anomalies: MR imaging evaluation. Radiology. 1990;176:715-20.
45. Jeong YY, Outwater EK, Kang HK. Imaging evaluation of ovarian masses. Radiographics. 2000;20:1445-70.
46. Hricak H, Chen M, Coakley FV, et al. Complex adnexal masses: Detection and characterization with MR imaging–multivariate analysis. Radiology. 2000;214:39-46.
47. Tempany CM, Zou KH, Silverman SG, et al. Staging of advanced ovarian cancer: Comparison of imaging modalities. Report from the Radiological Diagnostic Oncology Group. Radiology. 2000;215:761-7.
48. Aso C, Enrl´quez G, Fite M´, Tora´n N, Piro´C, Piqueras J, Lucaya J. Gray-scale and color Doppler sonography of scrotal disorders in children: An update. Radiographics. 2005;25:1197-214.
49. Hormann M, Balassy C, Marcel O, Philipp MO, Pumberger W. Imaging of the scrotum in children. Eur Radiol. 2004;14: 974-83.
50. Whitaker RH. Undescended testes: The need for a standard classification. Br J Urol. 1992;70:1-6.
51. Oyen RH. Scrotal ultrasound. Eur Radiol. 2002;12:19-34.
52. Nguyen HT, Coakely F, Hricak H. Cryptorchidism: Strategies in detection. Eur Radiol. 1999;9:336-43.
53. Campbell HE. The incidence of malignant growth in the undescended testicle: A reply and re-evaluation. J Urol. 1959;81:663-8.
54. Siegel MJ. The acute scrotum. Radiol Clin North Am. 1997;35:959-76.
55. Chou TY, Chu CC, Diau GY, Wu CJ, Gueng MK. Inguinal hernia in children: US versus exploratory surgery and intraoperative contralateral laparoscopy. Radiology. 1996;201:385-8.
56. Ogata M, Imai S, Hosotani R, Aoyama H, Hayashi M, Ishikawa T. Abdominal ultrasonography for the diagnosis of strangulation in small bowel obstruction. Br J Surg. 1994;81:421-4.
57. Thomas JC, Elder JS. Testicular growth arrest and adolescent varicocele: Does varicocele size make a difference? J Urol. 2002;168:1689-91.
58. Gooding GA, Leonhardt WC, Marshall G, Seltzer MA, Presti JC Jr. Cholesterol crystals in hydroceles: Sonographic detection and possible significance. AJR. 1997;169:527-9.
59. Drut R. Yolk sac tumor and testicular microlithiasis. Pediatr Pathol Mol Med. 2003;22:343-7.
60. Dogra VS, Gottlieb RH, Mayumi O, Rubens DJ. Sonography of the scrotum. Radiology. 2003;227:18-36.
61. Rifkin MD, Cochlin DLI. Scrotal masses (and scrotal enlargement). In: Rifkin MD, Cochlin DLI (Eds). Imaging of the Scrotum and Penis. Martin Dunitz Ltd, London. 2002; pp.33-95.
62. Jee WH, Choe BY, Byun JY, Shinn KS, Hwang TK. Resistive index of the intrascrotal artery in scrotal inflammatory disease. Acta Radiol. 1997;38:1026-30.
63. Salmeron I, Ramirez-Escobar M, Puertas F, Marcos R, Garcia-Marcos F, Sanchez R. Granulomatous epididymo-orchitis: Sonographic features and clinical outcome in brucellosis, tuberculosis and idiopathic granulomatous epididymo-orchitis. J Urol. 1998;159:1954-7.
64. Monga M, Scarpero HM, Ortenberg J. Metachronous bilateral torsion of the testicular appendices. Int J Urol. 1999;6:589-91.
65. Hesser U, Rosenborg M, Gierup J, Karpe B, Nystrom A, Hedenborg L. Gray-scale sonography in torsion of the testicular appendages. Pediatr Radiol. 1993;23:529-32.
66. Brown Casillas VJ, Montalvo AM, Albores-Saavedra J. Intrauterine spermatic cord torsion in the newborn: Sonographic and pathologic correlation. Radiology. 1990;177:755-7.
67. Paltiel HJ, Connolly LP, Atala A, Paltiel AD, Zurakowski D, Treves ST. Acute scrotal symptoms in boys with an indeterminate clinical presentation: Comparison of color Doppler sonography and scintigraphy. Radiology. 1998;207:223-31.
68. Watanabe Y, Dohke M, Ohkubo K, et al. Scrotal disorders: Evaluation of testicular enhancement patterns at dynamic contrast-enhanced subtraction MR imaging. Radiology. 2000;217:219-27.

69. Lee A, Park SJ, Lee HK, Hong HS, Lee BH, Kim DH. Acute idiopathic scrotal edema: Ultrasonographic findings at an emergency unit. Eur Radiol. 2009;19:2075-80.
70. Klin B, Lotan G, Efrati Y, Zlotkevich L, Strauss S. Acute idiopathic scrotal edema in childred-revisited. J Pediatr Surg. 2002;37:1200-2.
71. Van Langen AM, Gal S, Hulsmann AR, De Nef JJ. Acute idiopathic scrotal oedema: Four cases and a short review. Eur J Pediatr. 2001;160:455-6.
72. Kaplan GW. Acute idiopathic scrotal edema. J Pediatr Surg. 1977;12:647-9.
73. Varga J, Zivkovic D, Grebeldinger S, Somer D. Acute scrotal pain. In children—ten years' experience. Urol Int. 2007;78:73-7.
74. Kay R. Prepubertal Testicular Tumor Registry. J Urol. 1993. 150:671-4.
75. Woodward PJ, Schwab CM, Sesterhenn IA. Extratesticular scrotal masses: Radiologic-pathologic correlation. Radiographics. 2003;23:215-40.
76. Cramer BM, Schlegel EA, Thueroff JW. MR imaging in the differential diagnosis of scrotal and testicular disease. Radiographics. 1991;11:9-21.
77. Martelli H, Patte C. Gonadal tumours in children. Arch Pediatr. 2003;10:246-50.
78. Paula J, Woodward PJ, Sohaey R, O'Donoghue MJ, Green DE. Tumors and tumor-like lesions of the testis: Radiologic-pathologic correlation. Radiographics. 2002;22:189-216.
79. Frush DP, Sheldon CA. Diagnostic imaging for pediatric scrotal disorders. Radiographics. 1998;18:969-85.
80. Schwerk WB, Schwerk WN, Rodeck G. Testicular tumors: Prospective analysis of real-time US patterns and abdominal staging. Radiology. 1987;164:369-74.
81. Cho JH, Chang JC, Park BH, Lee JG, Son CH. Sonographic and MR imaging findings of testicular epidermoid cysts. AJR. 2002;178:743-8.
82. Ulbright TM, Amin MB, Young RH. Tumors of the testis, adnexa, spermatic cord, and scrotum. In: Atlas of Tumor Pathology, FASC 25, SER 3. Washington, DC: Armed Forces Institute of Pathology. 1999.pp.1-290.
83. Chang B, Borer JG, Tan PE, Diamond DA. Large-cell calcifying Sertoli cell tumor of the testis: Case report and review of the literature. Urology. 1998;52:520-2.
84. Pileri SA, Sabattini E, Rosito P, et al. Primary follicular lymphoma of the testis in childhood: Anentity with peculiar clinical and molecular characteristics. J Clin Pathol. 2002;55: 684-8.
85. Dalle JH, Mechinaud F, Michon J, et al. Testicular disease in childhood B-cell non-Hodgkin's lymphoma: The French Society of Pediatric Oncology experience. J Clin Oncol. 2001;19:2397-403.
86. Mazzu D, Jeffrey RB Jr, Ralls PW. Lymphoma and leukemia involving the testicles: Findings on gray-scale and color Doppler sonography. AJR. 1995;164:645-7.
87. Heaney JA, Klauber GT, Conley GR. Acute leukemia: Diagnosis and management of testicular involvement. Urology. 1983;21:573-7.
88. Mask CW, Chou CK, Su CC, Huan SK, Chang JM. Ultrasound diagnosis of paratesticular rhabdomyosarcoma. Br J Radiol. 2004;77:250-2.
89. Mason BJ, Kier R. Sonographic and MR imaging appearances of paratesticular rhabdomyosarcoma. AJR. 1998;171: 523-4.
90. Kim W, Rosen MA, Langer JE, Banner MP, Siegelman ES, Ramchandani P. US–MR imaging correlation in pathologic conditions of the scrotum. Radiographics. 2007;27:1239-53.
91. Yang DM, Kim SH, Kim HN, et al. Differential diagnosis of focal epididymal lesions with gray scale sonographic, color Doppler sonographic, and clinical features. J Ultrasound Med. 2003;22:135-42.
92. Akbar SA, Sayyed TA, Jafri SZ, Hasteh F, Neill JS. Multimodality imaging of paratesticular neoplasms and their rare mimics. Radiographics. 2003;23:1461-76.
93. Pretorius E. MRI of the male pelvis and bladder. In: Siegelman ES (Ed). Body MRI. Philadelphia, Pa: Elsevier Saunders. 2005.pp.372-86.
94. Vanzulli A, DelMaschio A, Paesano P, et al. Testicular masses in association with adrenogenital syndrome: US findings. Radiology. 1992;183:425-9.
95. Seidenwurm D, Smathers RL, Kan P, Hoffman A. Intratesticular adrenal rests diagnosed by ultrasound. Radiology. 1985;155:479-81.
96. Berg NB, Schenkman NS, Skoog SJ, Davis CJ. Testicular masses associated with congenital adrenal hyperplasia: MRI findings. Urology. 1996;47:252-3.
97. Burke BJ, Parker SH, Parker KD, Pienkos EJ. The ultrasonographic appearance of coexistent epididymal and testicular sarcoidosis. J Clin Ultrasound. 1990;18:522-6.
98. Ben-Sira L, Laor T. Severe scrotal pain in boys with Henoch-Schönlein purpura: Incidence and sonography. Pediatr Radiol. 2000;30:125-8.
99. Laor T, Atala A, Teele RL. Scrotal ultrasonography in Henoch-Schönlein purpura. Pediatr Radiol. 1992;22:505-6.
100. Muglia V, Tucci S, Elias J, Trad CVS, Bilbey J, Cooperberg PL. Magnetic resonance imaging of scrotal diseases: When it makes the difference. Urology. 2002;59:419-23.
101. Schultz-Lampel D, Bogaert G, Thuroff JW, et al. MRI for evaluation of scrotal pathology. Urol Res. 1991;19:289-92.
102. Sica GT, Teeger S. MR imaging of scrotal, testicular and penile diseases. MRI Clin North Am. 1996;4:545-62.

CHAPTER 143

Imaging of Intersex Disorders

Sanjay Sharma, Arun Kumar Gupta

INTRODUCTION

Intersex disorders presenting with ambiguous genitalia are complex and uncommon conditions that involve intermingling of characteristics of each sex to varying degrees due to a defect in embryological development. The incidence is approximately one per 1,000 live births. Although most are not medical emergencies, they are considered psychologic emergencies. Prompt diagnosis of ambiguous genitalia is necessary to help the family and later the child adjust psychologically. Most cases of ambiguous genitalia are discovered at birth. Knowledge of internal genital anatomy is crucial in the overall management of these patients. The role of a radiologist is to demonstrate this anatomy using different imaging techniques. An understanding of the normal sexual differentiation is essential before interpreting the pathological state.

NORMAL SEXUAL DIFFERENTIATION[1]

Genital primordia of a fetus are intrinsically programmed to differentiate into female sex. However, in the presence of a Y chromosome the undifferentiated gonads differentiate into testes. Anti-Müllerian hormone (AMH), which is secreted by the Sertoli cells of the testes inhibits the development of Müllerian ducts (i.e. female structures), while testosterone secreted from Leydig cells of the testes maintain and differentiate Wolffian ducts (i.e. male structures). Thus, presence of Y chromosome differentiates the genital primordia into a male. On the other hand, in the absence of Y chromosome, testicular tissue and its two hormones are absent due to which there is no inhibition of Müllerian ducts by AMH. Wolffian ducts regress because of lack of testosterone. End result is a normal female child.

IMAGING OF AN INTERSEX CHILD[2-6]

Intersex disorders presenting with ambiguous genitalia form a challenging clinical problem. Biochemical and chromosomal assays, besides the radiological evaluation are required in order to completely address its different aspects. Genitography, ultrasound, and MR imaging, are routinely employed. Judicious use of minimum investigations to obtain maximum information should be the goal.

Genitography[2,7]

As most of these children have a urogenital sinus, the anatomy displayed using genitography becomes essential in treatment planning as regards the corrective surgery for gender assignment. In this technique, water soluble contrast is injected retrogradely, via the external genital opening so as to outline the genital anatomy. Contrast is injected, either by placing the nozzle of a syringe (flush technique) or the tip of an end hole catheter (catheter technique), within the external genital opening **(Figs. 1A and B)**. It aims to address the following:

a. Degree of masculinization of the urogenital sinus and the urethra.
b. Vaginal status, i.e. its presence, size and any cervical indentation by the uterus.

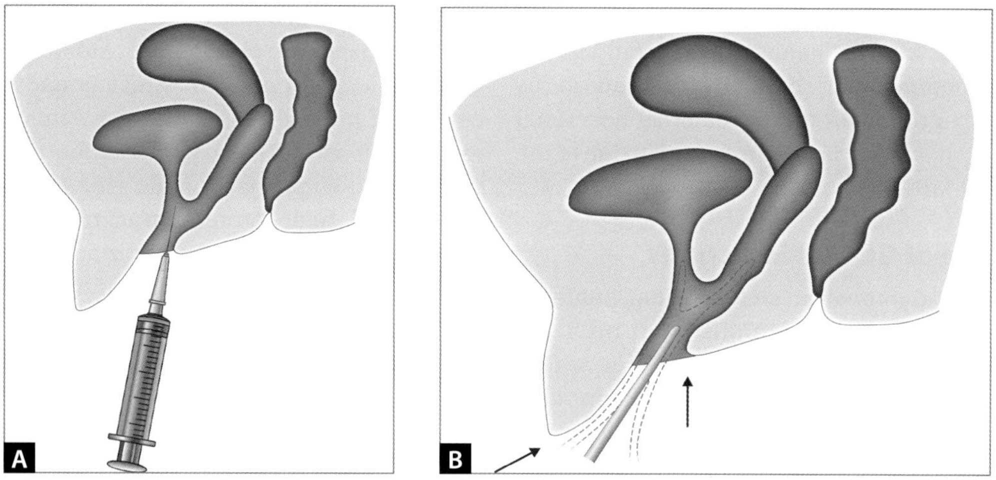

Figs. 1A and B: Techniques of genitography: (A) Flush technique; (B) Catheter technique. In (A), tip of the syringe nozzle is within the external opening and barrel is pressed against the perineum. In (B), single hole catheter should be used and its tip should be in the common urogenital sinus. Dotted lines in (B) show the potential pitfall if the tip enters either channel selectively. Arrows in (B) indicate compression of perineal skin around the catheter to prevent reflux of contrast.

c. Junctional site of vagina with the urethra, i.e. whether low, middle or high junction **(Figs. 2A to C)**. Low, middle or high vaginal insertion determines the morphological female, indeterminate or the male urethral type, respectively.
d. Presence of uterus/fallopian tubes, either by their direct opacification or indirectly by visualization of cervical indentation at the cranial end of the contrast filled vagina.

It must be realized that no genitographic appearance is specific for one particular type of intersex disorder. It only depicts the degree of virilization of genitalia. Genitography only provides information about the status of the derivatives of Müllerian and Wolffian ducts. Gonadal evaluation is not possible. The technique is 'invasive' and it uses ionizing radiation.

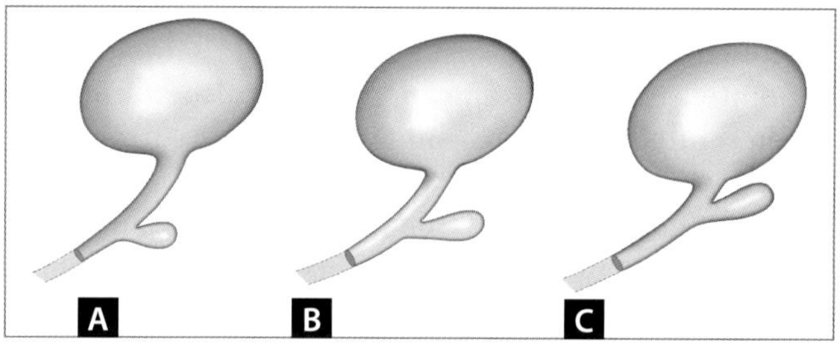

Figs. 2A to C: Schematic drawing of possible junctional sites of vagina (or its remnant) with the urethra: Low (A), middle (B) and high (C). Generally higher the junctional site, more degree of masculinization will be present.

Other Imaging Modalities

Ultrasound and MRI are two noninvasive cross-sectional imaging techniques available for examination of the pelvicstructures. Asstatedearlier, roleofimagingistoidentify (a) structures derived from Müllerian or Wolffian ducts and (b) status of gonads. Therefore, image analysis should include evaluation for the presence or absence of uterus, vagina, clitoris/penis, ovaries, prostate and testes. Addition of pelvic ultrasonography has been a valuable supplement to genitography and karyotyping in the work-up of an intersex child for assessing not only gonads but also the presence of uterus and cervix, but has its limitations of small field of view, poor demonstration of complex anomalies and inability to keep the child's urinary bladder adequately distended to provide a sonographic window.

Recent reports on the use of MRI in these disorders have been promising.[8,9] Strength of MRI lies in its multiplanar capability, excellent soft tissue characterization, large field of view, and nonionizing nature. It contributes to the accurate morphological evaluation of Müllerian and Wolffian duct structures, gonads and the development of phallus, all of which are essential for appropriate gender assignment and planning surgical reconstruction. Axial, sagittal and coronal T1- and T2W images are obtained using fast/turbo spin echo sequences. Suggested section thickness is 5 mm in patients older than 5 years and 3 mm in patients under 5 years. Secaf et al.[8] have suggested use of an image matrix of 256 × 192 with two to four signal averages. Image analysis includes the assessment of uterus, vagina, ovaries, testes, penis and clitoris. MRI is now considered to be more valuable than ultrasound in the evaluation of internal genitalia, especially in the newborn. In the neonatal period, the ovaries and uterus are physiologically prominent due to maternal hormonal influence. CT now has a very limited role to play due to the widespread use of MRI.

MR Appearance of Genital Structures

The normal *uterus* demonstrates clear zonal anatomy on T2W images. Three zones demonstrated on T2WI **(Fig. 3)**, i.e. innermost hyperintense linear area within the uterus corresponds to endometrium, the surrounding hypointense band represents the junctional zone (inner myometrium) and the outer intermediate signal intensity zone corresponds to outer myometrium.[10] However, a hypoplastic uterus is not only small but demonstrates low signal intensity of the entire myometrium on T2W images. For complete evaluation of the uterus, both axial and sagittal T2W images are most useful. The *vagina* is best visualized on axial T2W images. Sagittal images are complementary to the axial images. On T2W images, the hypointense vaginal wall can be distinguished from the bright central canal representing mucosa and surrounding adipose tissue. Demonstration of *urogenital sinus* on MRI is difficult. Normal *testes and ovaries* have medium to low signal intensity on T1W images and high signal intensity on T2W images. Gonadal tissue characterization is not always possible, unless follicles are seen in case of ovary. Ectopic gonads frequently demonstrate an outer rim of medium signal intensity on T2W images, which differentiates it from lymph nodes. Axial T1W and T2W images are useful in the evaluation of gonads. Sagittal and coronal images are also helpful. Although signal intensity of atrophic, dysgenetic, or streak gonads are not as high as that of normal gonads on T2W images, histological evaluation is necessary for differentiation between normal and abnormal gonads. Gonads are sought in the intrascrotal, high scrotal, intracanalicular or intrapelvic location. The normal *penis* is composed of paired corpora cavernosa, corpus spongiosum, and supporting muscular structures, such as bulbocavernosus, ischiocavernosus and transverse perineal muscles. Paired corpora cavernosa and corpus spongiosum have medium signal intensity on T1W images and high signal intensity on T2W images. On T2W images, these structures are easily differentiated from the supporting muscles and urethra. Presence of normal *clitoris* is established when on a T2W image, high signal intensity tissue is seen adjacent to ischium in the anatomical location of crura of corpora cavernosa **(Fig. 4)**. When full length of the clitoris extends for greater than 1 cm anterior to the pubic ramus, it is considered hypertrophied.[8]

CLASSIFICATION OF INTERSEX

Over the years, a number of workers have put forth contradictory views regarding classification of intersex states. Paquin et al.[11] based on a study of 7 patients concluded that presence and appearance of urogenital sinus on imaging itself is not diagnostic of any specific type of hermaphroditism. Shopfner[12] studied 66 intersex children and classified them into six types, demonstrating progressive masculinization from type I to type VI. He

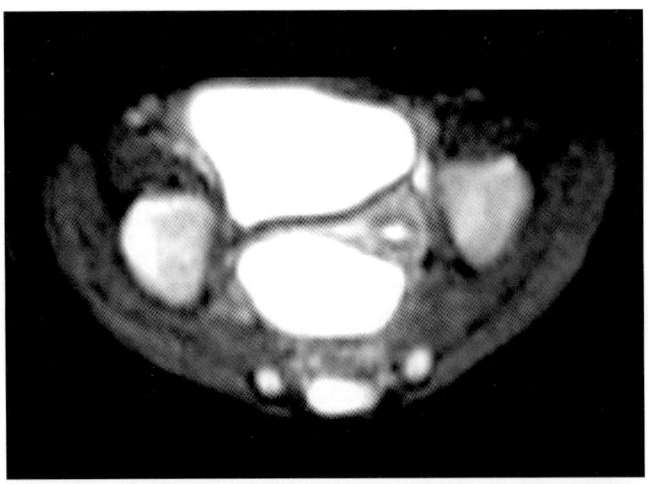

Fig. 3: Axial T2W MRI shows the normal zonal anatomy of uterus, i.e. central hyper, outer hypo and outermost intermediate signal uterine tissues.

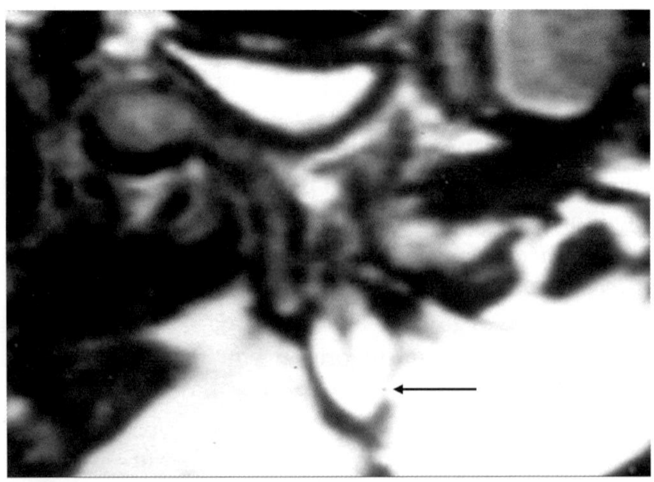

Fig. 4: Coronal T2W MRI shows the normal clitoral appearance. Compare this with Figure 11.

believed that each genitographic type represented a specific type of intersexuality, an observation in direct contradiction to Paquin et al.[11] and other subsequent workers. A French team of endocrinologists and radiologists[1,13] carried out studies in more than 120 patients and concluded, unlike Shopfner,[12] that no genitographic pattern is specific for any particular type of intersexual state. At AIIMS, our conclusion is similar to that of Paquin et al.[11] and the French team.[1]

Presently, intersex patients are assigned to one of the following types:

- Female pseudohermaphroditism (FPH)
- Male pseudohermaphroditism (MPH)
- True hermaphroditism (TH)
- Mixed gonadal dysgenesis (MGD)
- Dysgenetic male pseudohermaphroditism (DMP).

Female Pseudohermaphroditism[1,2,7,14]

The female pseudohermaphroditism (FPH) denotes a female karyotype 46XX with presence of normal ovaries, uterus and tubes. Although the external genitalia are ambiguous, the testes or internal Wolffian duct derivatives like vas deferens and seminal vesicles are absent.

Etiology

It results from the action of an extragonadal testosterone on a normal female fetus resulting in virilization of genitalia to varying degrees. A number of mechanisms may be responsible but the most common one is congenital adrenal hyperplasia, resulting from an enzymatic defect (21 hydroxylase deficiency being the most common) in adrenal steroidogenesis.

Types

Degree of virilization of the urogenital sinus and the external genitalia vary, depending upon the time of onset of the insult and the amount of androgen. Prader[14] had classified them into 5 types based on clinical and genitographic findings. Some surgeons, however, are not fully satisfied with this classification from surgical point of view. Based on the degree of virilization FPH can be classified either as complete or incomplete.

Complete virilization is equivalent to Prader type V and results from massive amounts of androgens in the early phase of embryonic development. Clinically the external genitalia, i.e. the penis and the scrotum are like that of a normal male except that the scrotum is empty. Genitography reveals a male type urethra **(Fig. 5A)**, which at times may be associated with an underdeveloped vagina opening high on the vertical portion (high junction). Cervical impression is absent or difficult to appreciate. MRI or pelvic sonography would demonstrate presence of uterus and gonads **(Fig. 5B)**. MRI or CT shows bilateral adrenal hyperplasia **(Fig. 5C)**. Bone age is accelerated **(Fig. 5D)**. It is advisable to rear these children as male.

Incomplete virilization type is equivalent to Prader types I–IV and occurs as a result of exposure to lesser amounts of androgens later during the embryonic development. Clinically, external genital appearance varies from simple clitoral hypertrophy (Prader type I) to perineal hypospadias (Prader type IV). Genitography reveals a well-developed vagina with cervical impression **(Figs. 6A and B)**, uterus and tubes **(Figs. 6C and D)**. These patients should be reared as female.

MR images demonstrate masculinized external genitalia with normal ovaries **(Fig. 7A)** and uterus **(Fig. 7B)**. It may show enlarged adrenal glands due to adrenal hyperplasia. Although external genitalia of complete virilization type of FPH are similar to those of males, there are no testes at any site. In patients of incomplete virilization type of FPH, the hypertrophied clitoris mimics penis due to prominent corpora cavernosa and corpus spongiosum **(Fig. 7C)**. The uterus and the vagina may be filled with clear urine due to reflux into them through the urogenital sinus.[15]

Male Pseudohermaphroditism[1,2,7]

The male pseudohermaphroditism (MPH) represents a genetic male having 46XY karyotype with normal or mildly defective testes.

Cause

Five well-recognized types based on etiology are:

- Combined anti-Müllerian hormone (AMH) and testosterone deficiency
- AMH deficiency alone
- Androgen receptor insensitivity (testicular feminization syndrome: complete and incomplete types)
- Defective testosterone biosynthesis
- 5 α-reductase deficiency resulting in decreased dihydro-testosterone production.

Final definitive diagnosis would require sophisticated laboratory facilities for estimation of these hormones.

Without going into the details of each subtypes of MPH listed above, it would suffice to state that the clinical (i.e., external genitalia) and genitographic appearance (i.e. internal genitalia) of three of these MPH, i.e. incomplete testicular feminization syndrome; defective testosterone biosynthesis and steroid 5 alpha reductase deficiency, are similar, i.e. externally they all show ambiguous

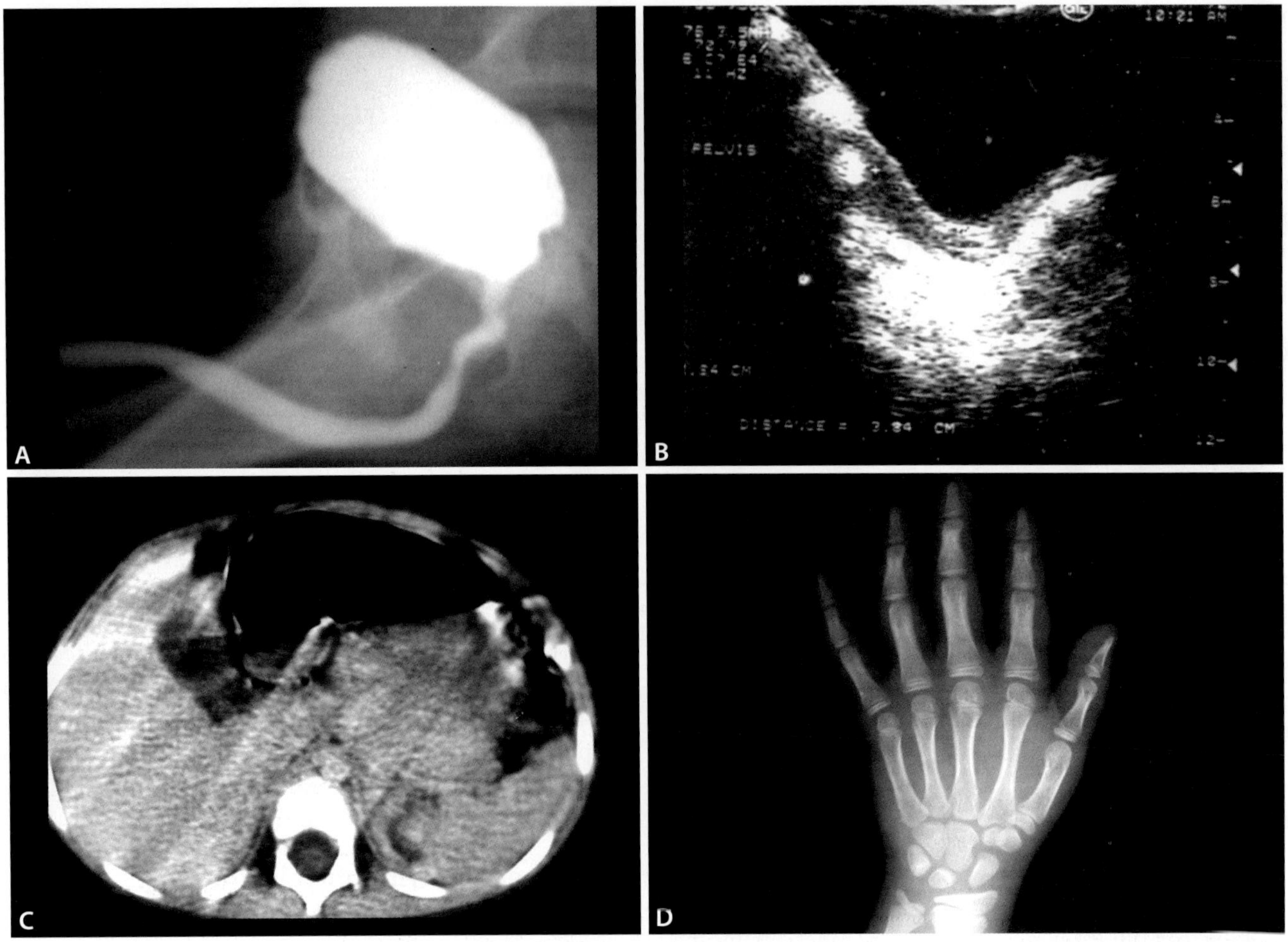

Figs. 5A to D: A 4-year-old child with FPH, complete virilization type: Genitography (A) did not show any Müllerian duct derivative in a boy with normal external genitalia with cryptorchidism. Pelvic sonography (B) revealed presence of a well-formed uterus. CT (C) demonstrated bilateral adrenal hyperplasia, (D) bone age is accelerated.

genitalia with perineal hypospadias while internally, on genitographic study, they show variable sized urogenital sinus and a small sized vagina without cervical impression **(Figs. 8A to C)**.

MRI demonstrates bilateral testes (commonly undescended) **(Figs. 9A and B)** and incompletely musculinized or frankly feminized external genitalia. There is no uterus **(Fig. 10)** or ovaries. Both testes are of normal size and signal intensity and are located in the scrotum or in the inguinal canals. The corpora cavernosa and, corpus spongiosum, and the supporting muscular structures are well-demonstrated **(Fig. 11)** and the prostatic tissue appears to be present. Hypospadias is well-visualized on sagittal images. Pseudovagina may be seen on MR images.[15]

Patient with AMH deficiency is also called 'male with uterus' because on clinical examination of the external genitalia, these patients appear as normal male with the urethra opening at the tip of a normally formed penis. They also have cryptorchidism (or inguinal hernia) and internally fully developed Müllerian duct derivatives, i.e. well-formed vagina and uterus **(Figs. 12A and B)** are present.

In complete testicular feminization syndrome, on the other hand, externally there is no sexual ambiguity and the external genitalia appears as that of a normal female but genitography would demonstrate a short, blind ending vagina without any evidence of cervix and a separate urethral opening **(Fig. 13)**.

If a newborn has perineal hypospadias and 46XY karyotype, it is important to assume that the child is a male with congenital urogenital malformation. In these patients, one must keep MPH in the differential diagnosis. Genitography and, if facilities are available, d-hydroxy

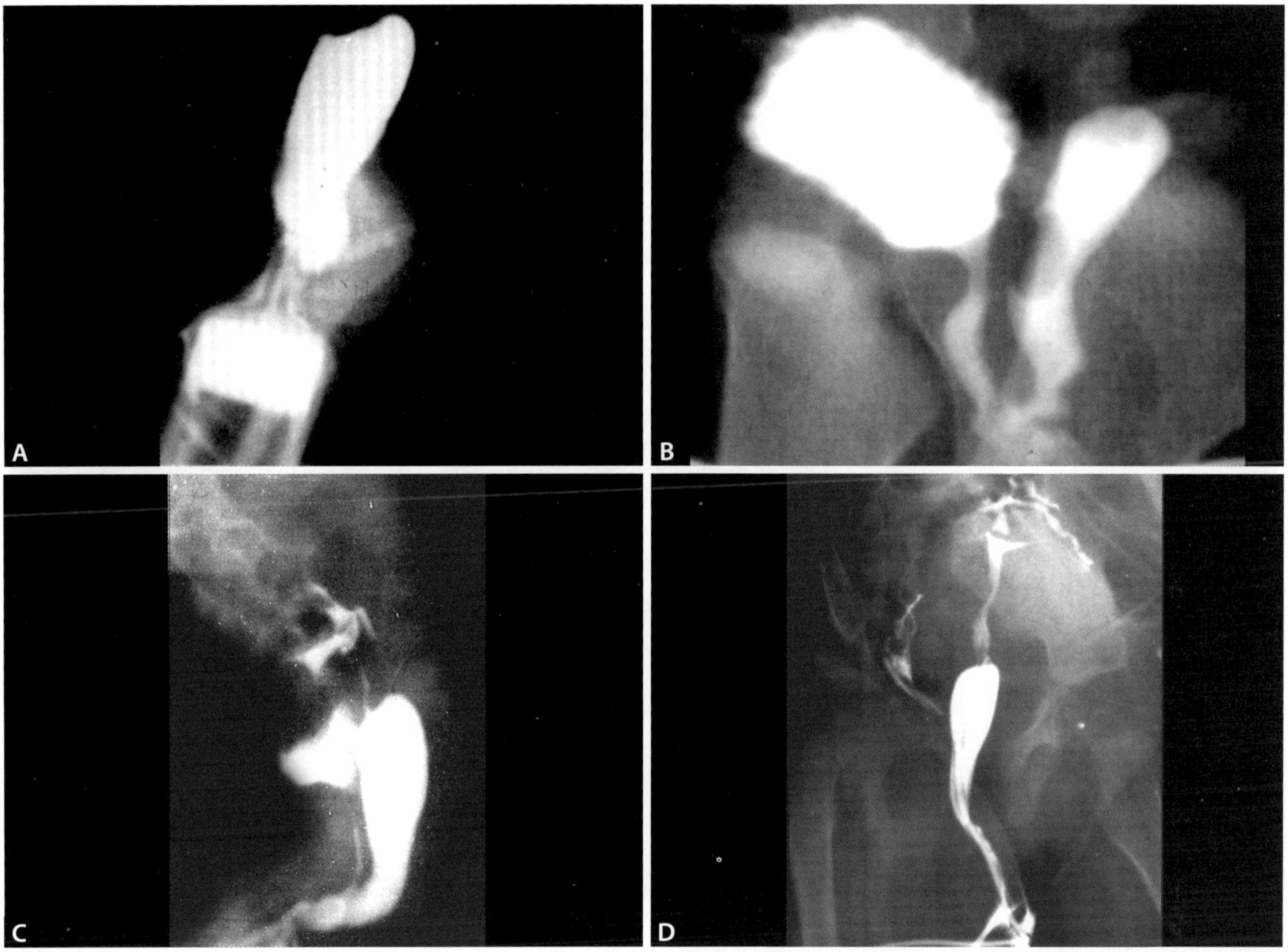

Figs. 6A to D: (A) Female pseudohermaphroditism (FPH) incomplete virilization types (different cases): (A) Flush technique genitography filled only a well-formed vagina. Note a concave upward filling defect on top of the vagina, the cervical identification, presence of which indirectly denotes a well-formed uterus; (B) Both urethra and vagina, open together very low, close to the surface of perineum. Again note negative filling defect, the cervical indentation. Uterus and tubes are not opacified in both Figures 6A and B; (C and D) Picture is similar to Figure 6B except that contrast has entered the uterine cavity and tubes with spill over into the peritoneal cavity.

testosterone therapeutic test, are mandatory prior to reaching at the final diagnosis and assigning a particular sex to the child.

Rarely, MPH also forms part of a syndrome called Drash's syndrome which has three components, i.e. MPH, progressive mesangial sclerosis with nephrotic syndrome and Wilms' tumor.

True Hermaphroditism[1,7]

Majority (50–80%) of true hermaphrodites (TH) are have a 46XX karyotype with both the ovary and the testicular tissue present in the same patient or even same gonad. Various possible combinations in which these tissues may occur in TH are shown in **Figure 14**.

Clinically, before puberty, patients with TH present with an ambiguous external genitalia but later presentation may be varying such as cryptorchidism, breast development in a patient reared up as a male, hematuria (actually menstruation through the urogenital sinus opening) in those reared up as a male, amenorrhea in those reared up as female, inguinal hernia, etc.

Genitography shows a urogenital sinus of variable size with a relatively well-developed vagina which may open at varying level into the urethra. Contrast might also enter into the uterus and tubes **(Fig. 15)**.

MRI demonstrates both an ovary and a testis (one or both of which may be replaced by an ovotestis) and variable internal and external genitalia.

Final diagnosis is made only after laparotomy, identification of the Müllerian and Wolffian duct derivatives and gonadal biopsy and histopathological examination of the gonads.

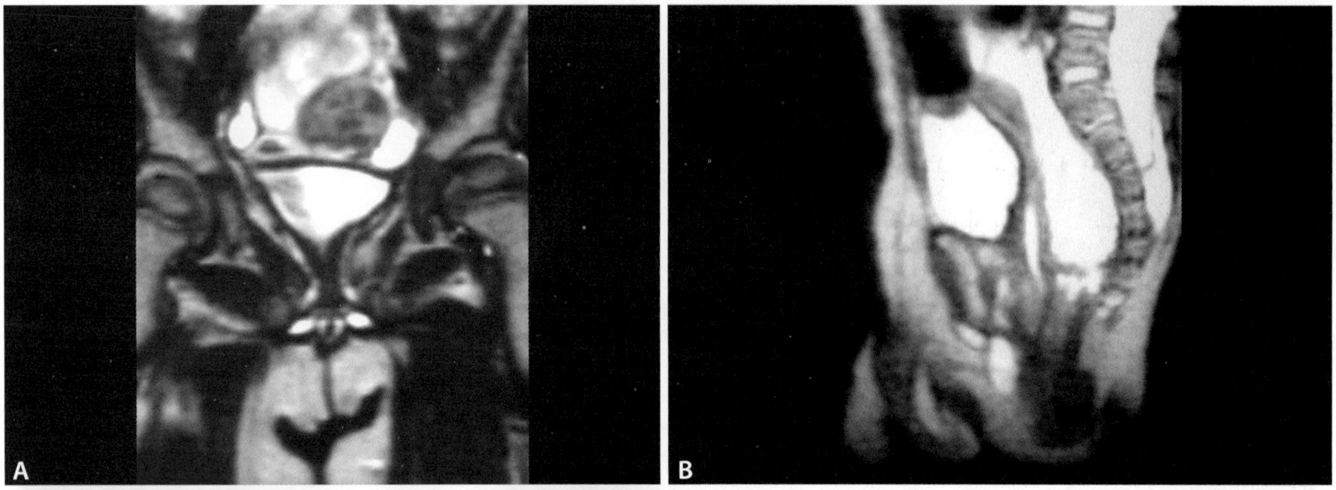

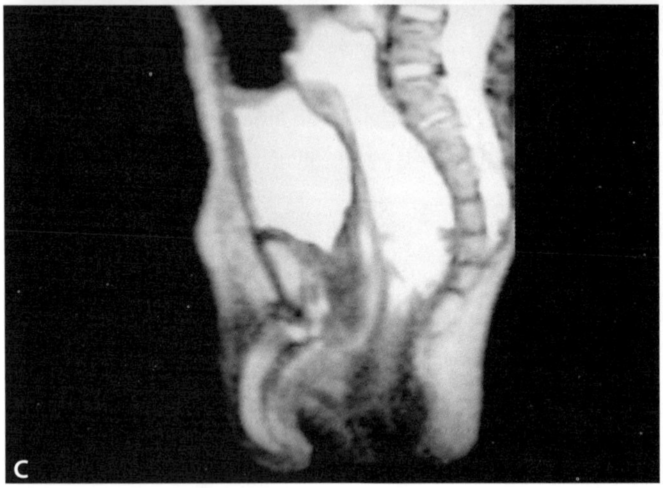

Figs. 7A to C: MRI in female pseudohermaphroditism (FPH): (A) Coronal T2WI shows bilateral normal ovaries with high signal intensity; (B) Midline sagittal MRI: Normal uterus well seen. (C) Externally, hypertrophied clitoris seen.

Surgical management consists of excision of inappropriate gonadal tissues followed by appropriate genitoplasty of external genitalia.

Mixed Gonadal Dysgenesis and Dysgenetic Male Pseudohermaphroditism[1,2,7]

It is believed that mixed gonadal dysgenesis (MGD) and dysgenetic male pseudohermaphroditism (DMP) represent different spectra of the same condition. In both MGD and DMP, karyotypes are similar, i.e. XY; internally Müllerian ducts are always present **(Fig. 16)** and externally hypospadias is almost always found. The only difference between the two is in the histology of the gonads **(Fig. 17)**, i.e. MGD **(Figs. 18A to F)** has a normal testis on one side and dysgenetic testis on the contralateral side, while DMP has dysgenetic testes on both the sides. On MRI, dysgenetic gonads have a spectrum of appearances ranging from normal size to streak gonads. Although dysgenetic gonads have intermediate signal intensity on T1W and T2W images, histological confirmation is essential for definitive diagnosis. In any case, prophylactic early gonadectomy must be performed because of a high incidence of testicular tumors developing in both these disorders. The small, hypoplastic uterus and vagina are well demonstrated on MRI.

There are only few MRI studies in the literature regarding imaging of patients with intersex disorders.[15] Role of MRI in patients with intersex patients seems to be two folds: (a) to delineate internal genital anatomy, including gonads, and (b) to characterize the external genital structures, especially to differentiate hypertrophied phallus from normal penis. In a study by Secaf et al.[8] MRI depiction of uterus was possible in 93%, vagina in 95%, penis in 10%, testes in 88%, and ovary in 74% patients. At AIIMS, genitography, ultrasound and MRI were performed in 33 children of intersex disorder (13 days to 17 years of age) after appropriate clinical work-up, karyotyping and hormonal analysis.[15] The ability to detect common

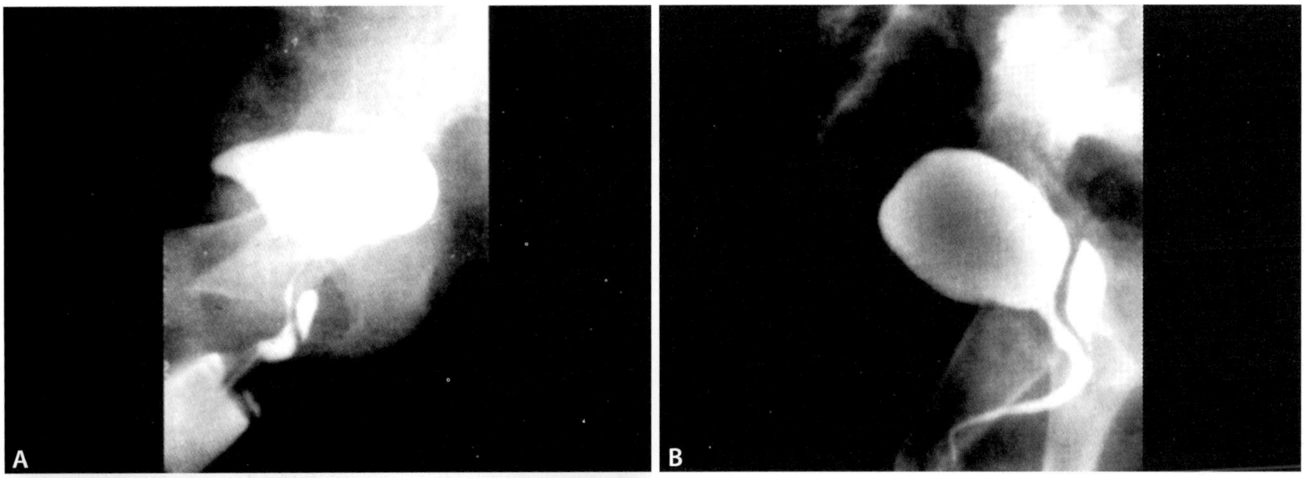

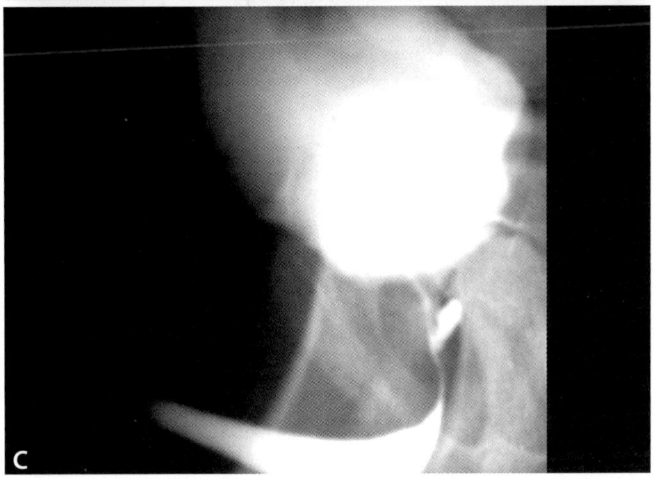

Figs. 8A to C: Male pseudohermaphroditism (MPH) (different cases): Note that the junctional site is low (A), middle (B) and high (C). As the junctional site moves up, the degree of masculinization also increases which is evident by longer, male type urethra. In (C), small vaginal remnant, also called utriculus is arising from the vertical portion of the urethra. Also note absence of cervical indentation and the top of the vaginal remnants remaining round.

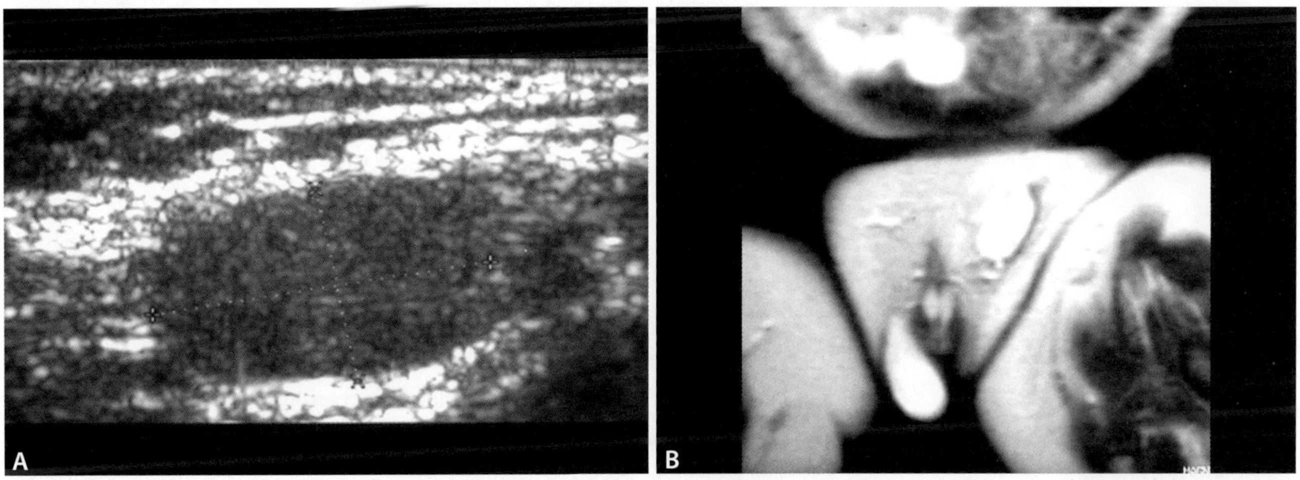

Figs. 9A and B: Male pseudohermaphroditism (MPH)—Undescended testes: (A) Ultrasonography detects a gonad at inguinal canal; (B) T2W coronal MRI demonstrates bilateral undescended testes as high signal masses.

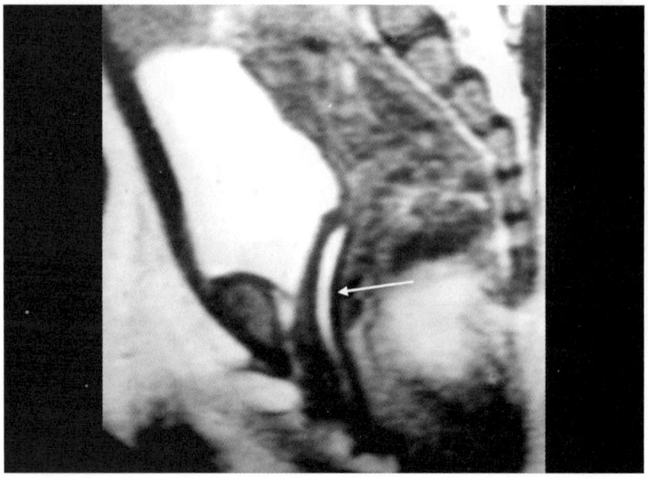

Fig. 10: Male pseudohermaphroditism (MPH): Midline sagittal T2W MRI shows fluid-filled vagina but absent uterus.

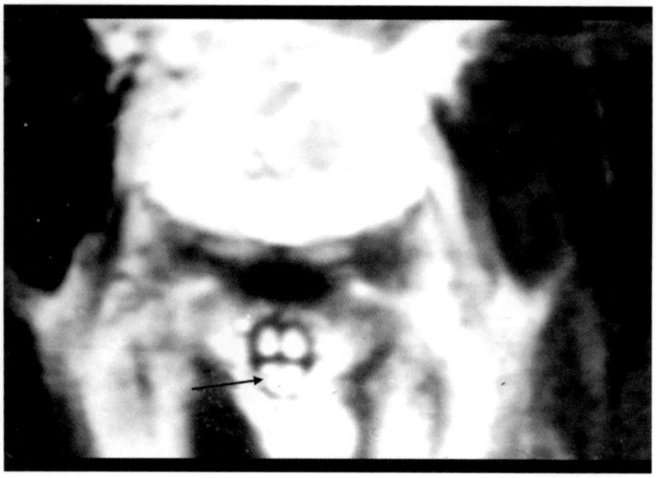

Fig. 11: Male pseudohermaphroditism (MPH): Corpora cavernosa and spongiosum are well-demonstrated, presence of these suggest male type of anatomy.

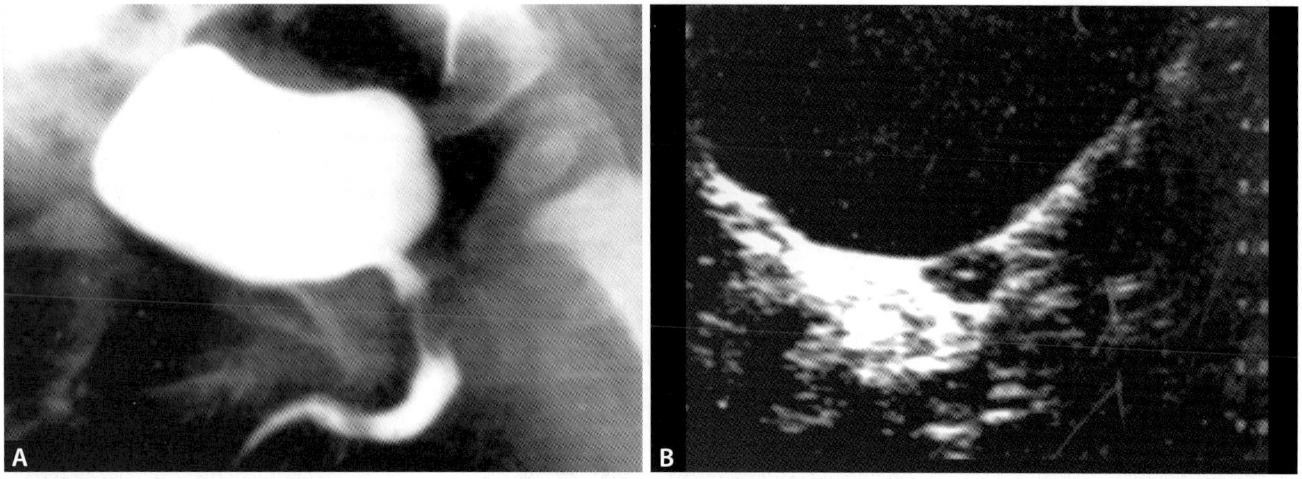

Figs. 12A and B: MPH, AMH deficiency type: Genitography (A) documents a male type urethra only. On sonography (B), however, a good sized uterus and cervix was detected. Example of 'male with uterus'.

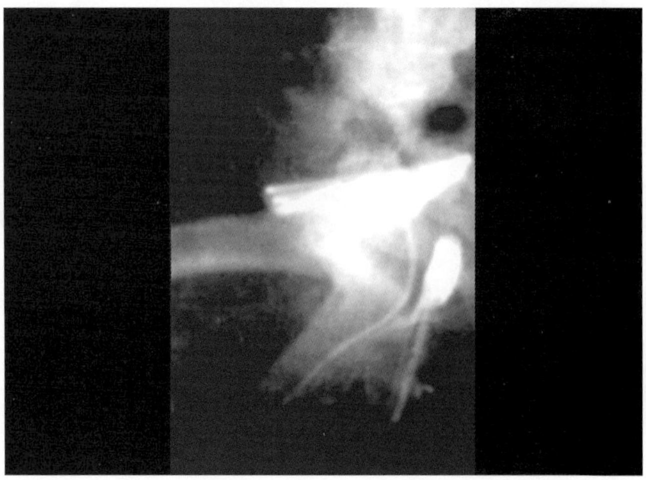

Fig. 13: Male pseudohermaphroditism (MPH), complete testicular feminization syndrome type: Clinically, no ambiguity in the external genitalia which was female type, i.e. two separate openings, one each for urethra and vagina present. Simultaneous, separate catheterization of both the openings with retrograde contrast injection demonstrates a small, hypoplastic, blind ending vagina with rounded top and absence of cervical indentation. Sonography or MRI would show absence of uterus or cervix.

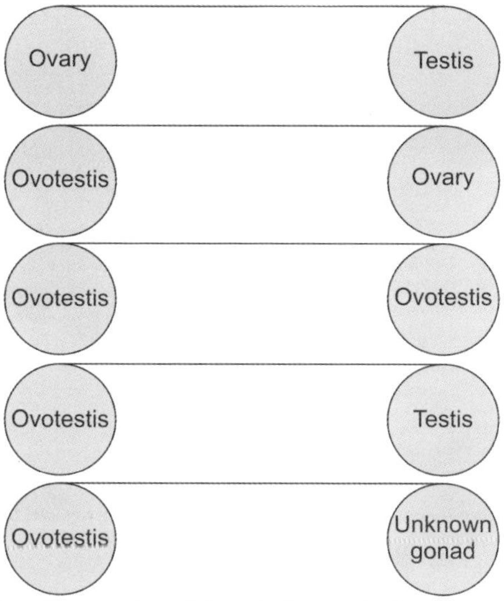

Fig. 14: True hermaphroditism: Schematic drawing to show all possible combinations of testicular and an ovarian tissue, on the two sides.

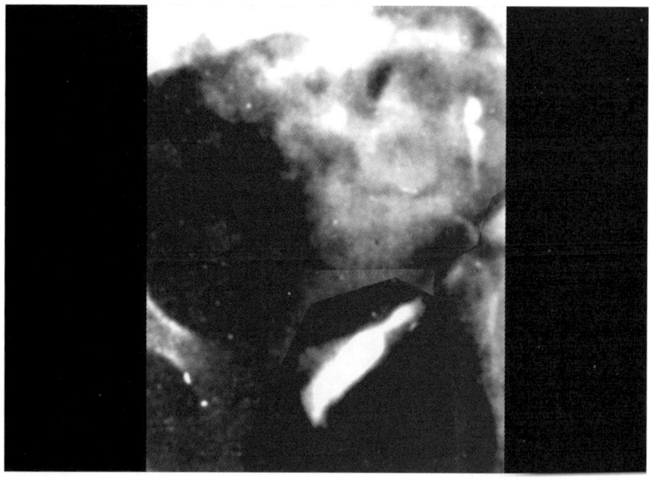

Fig. 15: True hermaphroditism, genitography demonstrates presence of Müllerian duct derivative only on the left side. Due to the presence of testicular tissue on the contralateral side, Müllerian duct structures do not differentiate on that side.

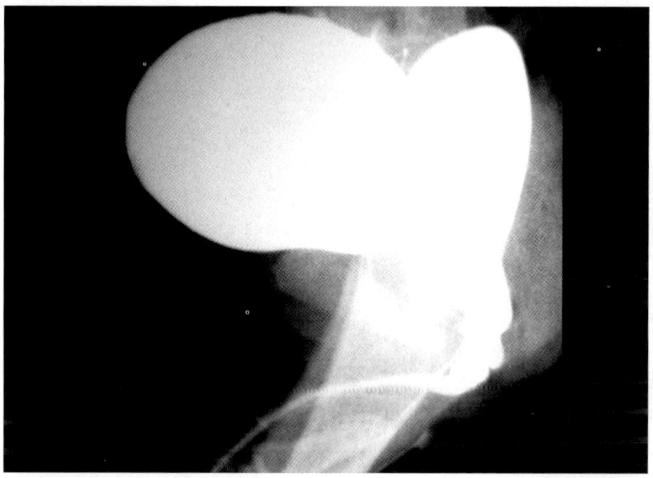

Fig. 16: DMP, genitography demonstrates well-formed Müllerian duct derivatives internally.

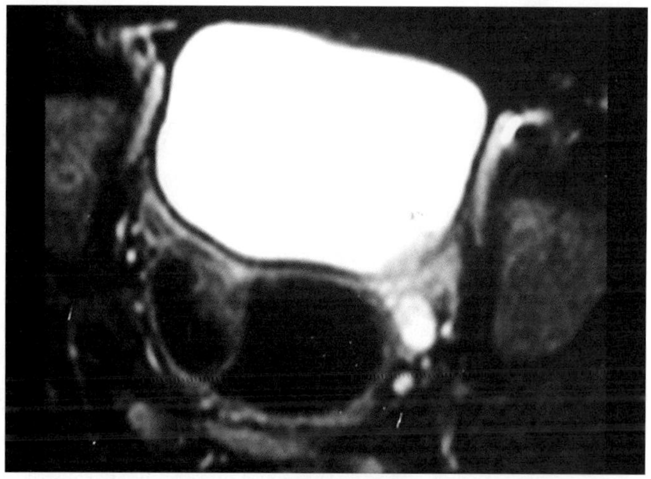

Fig. 17: DMP, T2W axial MRI shows left-sided gonad with high signal. Histopathologically, it was a dysgenetic gonad.

urogenital sinus (UGS), vagina and gonads by each modality was assessed. Surgical follow-up was available in 17 cases whereas karyotype, hormonal assay and biochemical profile was taken as a proof of diagnosis in the remaining 16 cases. Common UGS was properly evaluated in 48% cases by genitography, and none by ultrasound or MRI. Vagina was detected by genitography, US and MRI in 100%, 39.4% and 78% respectively. Uterus was detected by genitography, US and MRI in 69%, 75% and 100% cases respectively. US detected 21 inguinal and 8 intra-abdominal gonads (total 44%), whereas MRI detected 40 inguinal and 11 intra-abdominal gonads (total 77.3%).[16]

Relatively hypointense (even hyperintense) gonad on T2W images could be atrophic or dysgenetic gonads and requires histological analysis.

Supporting muscles of phallus, viz. bulbospongiosus (BS), ischiocavernosus (IC) and superficial transverse perinii (STP) have been stated to help differentiate enlarged clitoris from penis on MRI.[8] In the study at AIIMS, it was found that well-developed BS and IC muscles are a better indicator of chromosomal (karyotype) than hormonal (urethral type) sex. Well-developed supporting muscles suggest a likely male karyotype. However, when these muscles are indeterminate or nonvisualized, it

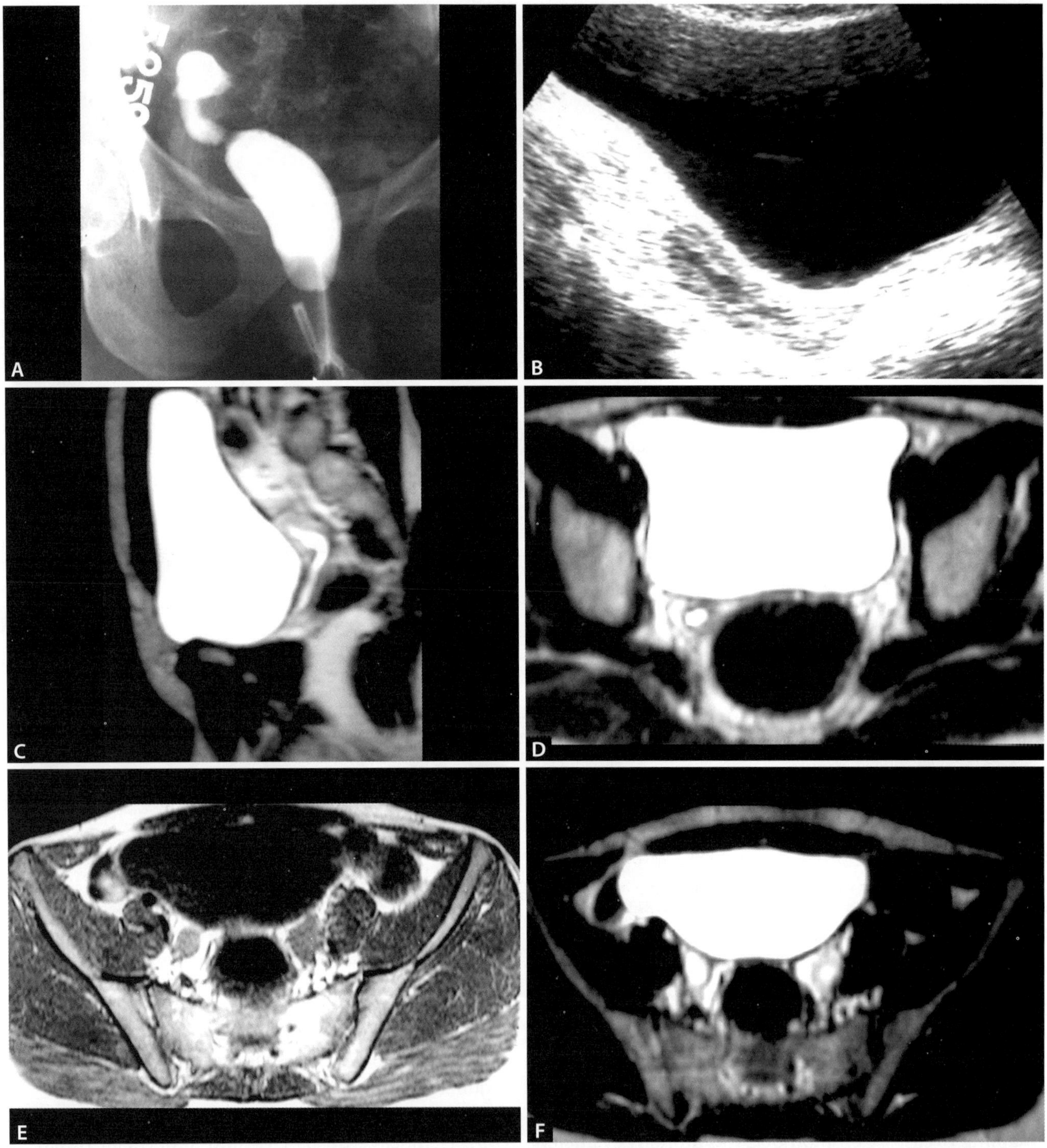

Figs. 18A to F: Mixed gonadal dysgenesis (MGD): (A) Genitography documents a right sided Müllerian duct structures; (B) On US, longitudinal section uterus is seen; (C) Sagittal T2W MRI demonstrates well-formed uterus; (D) Axial T2W MRI localizes the uterus to right side only; Axial T1W (E) and T2W MRI (F) demonstrate bilateral gonads. Histologically, both were dysgenetic.

cannot predict the chromosomal (karyotype) sex, but may suggest a female or indeterminate urethral type. STP muscle is not visualized in a large majority but when seen, it suggests a likely male karyotype. Poor or nonvisualization of this muscle gives no clue about the chromosomal sex or urethral type.[17] Literature is silent on MRI findings of these muscles in different types of intersex patients.

Table 1: Diagnostic algorithm in an intersex child. Criteria used: Karyotyping + genitographic anatomy.

Genitographic anatomy → ***karyotyping*** ↓	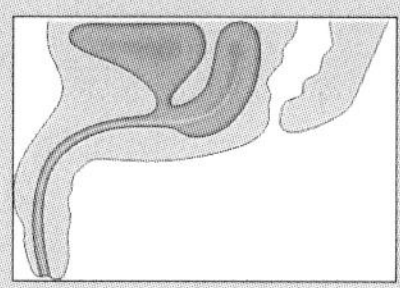	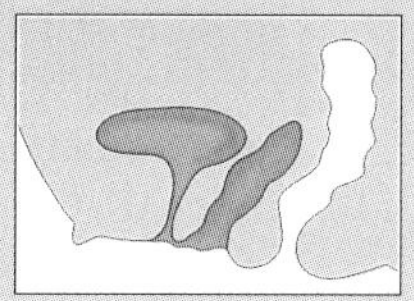	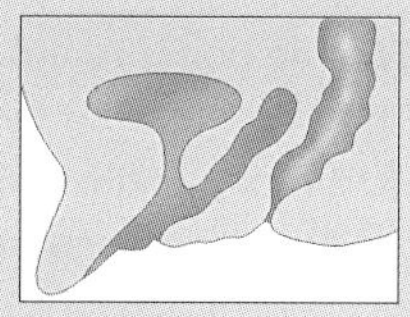	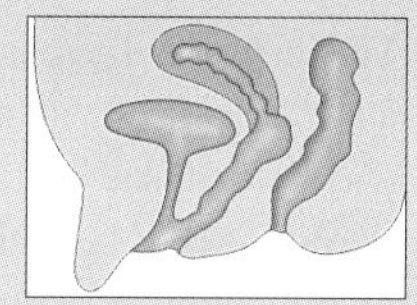
Chromatin positive (XX)	FPH (Total virilization type)	—	—	• FPH (Partial virilization type) • TH
Chromatin negative (XY)	MPH (AMH deficiency only)	MPH (Androgen receptor insensitivity type: complete testicular feminization syndrome)	MPH *Causes*: • Deficiency of 5 alpha reductase • Defective biosynthesis of testosterone • Incomplete testicular feminization syndrome	• MGD • DMP • MPH with combined AMH and testosterone deficiency

Abbreviations: MPH: Male pseudohermaphroditism; FPH: Female pseudohermaphroditism; TH: True hermaphroditism; MGD: Mixed gonadal dysgenesis; DMP: Dysgenetic male pseudohermaphroditism; AMH: Anti-Müllerian hormone.

More work in this field comparing MRI with ultrasound, genitography and correlation with surgical findings is required before a final algorithmic approach can be decided.

CLUES TO THE DIAGNOSIS

At most centers especially in India, laboratory facilities for a detailed investigation of a case of intersex child are lacking. Under these circumstances, by combining the information of karyotyping genitographic anatomy and MRI, one can reach at a reasonably correct "working diagnosis" within a short period of time and thus the sex of rearing can be assigned to the child at an early age. The diagnostic approach is shown in **Table 1**. MRI is now more widely used. With increasing experience in interpreting the complex anatomy of intersex disorders, it is necessary that MRI should form an essential component in the diagnostic work-up of these patients for reaching definitive diagnosis.

CONCLUSION

Intersex disorders are complex clinical problems. Genitography, ultrasonography and more recently MRI are important imaging tools. Except perhaps for the evaluation of urogenital sinus, most of the other information required in an intersex child can now be obtained noninvasively and reliably by MRI without use of ionizing radiation. Role of the radiologist is not to arrive at a diagnosis, but to accurately demonstrate the genital anatomy. This is often difficult as the conditions encountered are diverse in aetiology and often incompletely expressed. The final diagnosis is established by putting clinical findings with a combination of cytogenetic, biochemical and radiological studies. An early decision regarding the phenotypic sex, lessens the psychological impact on the child and is crucial in parent counselling. A close cooperation between a pediatric endocrinologist, pediatric surgeon and pediatric radiologist is vital for comprehensive management of these challenging disorders.

REFERENCES

1. Nihoul-Fekete C. Feminising genitoplasty in the intersex child. In: Josso N, Karger S, Basel (Eds): The Intersex Child. Pediatric and Adolescent Endocrinology. 1981;8:240-60.
2. Silverman F (Ed). Caffey's Pediatric X-ray Diagnosis (9th ed). Chicago: Year Book Medical Publishers Inc. 1993;2.
3. Cohen HL, Bober SE. Imaging the pediatric pelvis: The normal and abnormal genital tract and simulators in its diseases. Urol Radiol. 1992;14:273-83.
4. Cremin BJ. Intersex states in young children: The importance of radiology in making a correct diagnosis. Clin Radiol. 1974;25:63-73.
5. Gambino J, Coldwell B, Dietrich R, et al. Congenital disorders of sexual differentiation: MR findings. Pictorial Essay AJR. 1992;158:363-7.
6. Horowity M, Glassberg KI. Ambiguous genitalia: Diagnosis, evaluation, and treatment. Urol Radiol. 1992;14:306-18.
7. Gupta AK. Imaging of intersex. In: Subbarao K, Banerjee S, Aggarwal SK, et al (Eds): Diagnostic Radiology and Imaging. 1997;1:860-9.
8. Secaf E, Hricak H, Gooding CA, et al. Role of MRI in the evaluation of ambiguous genitalia. Pediatric Radiology. 1994;24:231-5.

9. Wright NB, Smith C, Rickwood AMK, et al. Review: Imaging children with ambiguous genitalia and intersex states. Clini Radio. 1995;50:823-9.
10. McCarthy S, Tauber C, Gore J. Female pelvic anatomy: MR assessment of variations during the menstrual cycle and with use of oral contraceptives. Radiology. 1986;160:119-23.
11. Paquin AJ, Baker DH, Finby N, et al. The urogenital sinus: Its demonstration and significance. J Urol. 1957;78:796-807.
12. S Karger, Basel (Eds). Genitography in Intersex Problems. Progr Pediat Radiol. 1970;3:97-115.
13. Josso N, Fortier B, Faure C. Genitography in intersexual states: a review of 86 cases with new criteria for the study of the urogenital sinus. Acuta Endocrinologica. 1969;62:165-80.
14. Prader A. Helv Paediat 9: 231-48 (Quoted in reference number 8) 1954.
15. Choi HK, Cho KS, Lee HW, Kim KS. MR imaging of intersexuality. Radiographics. 1998;18:83-96.
16. Haloi AK, Gupta AK, Sharma S, et al. Radiological evaluation of children with intersex disorders with ambiguous genitalia using genitography, ultrasonography and MR imaging. AJR 2001;178:50, Abstract (Suppl).
17. Sharma S, Gupta AK, Haloi AK. MR imaging of muscles supporting the phallus: A clue to the true sex in an intersex child. Radiology. 2002;225:669, Abstract (Suppl).

CHAPTER 144

Skeletal Dysplasias

Gaurav S Pradhan

INTRODUCTION

The skeletal dysplasias are a large heterogeneous group of genetic conditions characterized by abnormal shape, growth, number or integrity of bones. In the broadest sense, skeletal dysplasias may be divided into the osteodysplasias and the chondrodysplasias depending on the fact that the dysplasias are due to disturbance in osteoid production or in chondroid formation, respectively. The dysplasias may result from the following:

- Abnormal growth—affecting shape and size of skeleton.
- Abnormal number of bones—either decreased or increased.
- Abnormal texture—decreased or increased activity of remodelling process and mineral deposition.

The birth prevalence of skeletal dysplasias recognizable in the neonatal period has been estimated to be 2.4/10,000 births.[1] The lack of understanding of etiology of skeletal dysplasias resulted in classifications that were mainly descriptive and the technique most likely to identify the findings was predominantly used to categorize the anomalies.[2,3] Therefore, many definitions are based on radiological criteria with a few based on histological or clinical criteria.

TERMINOLOGY

Most skeletal dysplasias are forms of disproportionate short stature. To date about 220 well-established skeletal dysplasias are known to exist. Despite recent breakthroughs in the areas of collagen biochemistry and gene localization, the diagnosis still lies primarily in the hands of the radiologist.[4-6]

For the evaluation of skeletal dysplasias, certain basic definitions are important. Skeletal dysplasias can involve either the spine or the long bones. When the spine or any of its parts are shortened, the prefix "spondylo" is used. Involvement of the long bones on the other hand is subclassified into rhizomelia (proximal shortening involving the humerus and/or femur), mesomelic when, there is shortening of distal limb (radius and tibia) and micromelic when there is shortening of proximal and distal limbs. Dysostosis are skeletal abnormalities caused by embryonic developmental errors as opposed to dysplasias, which exert their effect during the entire period of skeletal growth.

These definitions are important because the terminologies of many disorders were created based on radiologic findings, although they may be confusing at times. The skeletal dysplasias are often classified according to whether the epiphysis, the metaphysis or the diaphysis is involved. Thus, it is important that the tubular bones are viewed before closure of the epiphyseal plate.

Another important consideration in dealing with skeletal dysplasia is the concept of lethality. About 25 disorders are included in the group of lethal dysplasias.

By far the most common lethal dysplasia, at or before birth, is thanatophoric dysplasia. Other relatively common lethal skeletal dysplasias include homozygous achondroplasia, osteogenesis imperfecta type II and achondrogenesis type II/hypochondrogenesis.

Usually, these conditions are lethal because the infant possesses a small chest cage as a direct result of having short ribs, leading to respiratory insufficiency and death in most cases. The chest circumference to abdominal circumference ratio in most of these cases is usually less than 0.85 and reflects the reduction of chest size. No children of asphyxiating thoracic dysplasia who have managed to live beyond 2 years have been reported to die of respiratory insufficiency. The reason for this appears to be growth of thoracic cage, resulting in adequate respiratory function. It is therefore very critical when dealing with a newborn with skeletal dysplasia to establish the diagnosis quickly and then to decide if the child should receive ventilator care.[7, 8]

The nonlethal skeletal dysplasias are a much larger group. They are considered according to the time of appearance, at birth or early infancy, or others after 2 years of age. Heterozygous achondroplasia is the most common condition that appears close to birth. The radiographic findings are specific to this disorder, which is differentiated from pseudoachondroplasia where the head is normal sized.

Most patients of nonlethal dysplasias if managed properly, could live relatively normal and productive lives.

Skeletal survey for the diagnosis of skeletal dysplasia should include the following radiographs:

- Skull—AP, lateral and Towne's
- Spine—AP and lateral
- Chest—AP view
- Pelvis—AP view
- Upper and lower extremities—AP view
- Hands and feet—AP view
- Lateral view of foot in neonatal disorders and a full body AP and lateral radiograph in postmortem examination of newborn.

Newer Imaging Modalities

Computed tomography and magnetic resonance imaging have an important role to play in the evaluation of intracranial and spinal cord anomalies in skeletal dysplasias. They are also helpful in assessing abnormalities of the cranium and the bony spinal canal. This is important in prognosticating the outcome of the dysplasia. 3-dimensional CT scan is used to evaluate craniofacial anomalies prior to reconstructive surgery while MR imaging of the spine is helpful in the presurgical planning prior to surgical treatment of spinal abnormalities.[7,8]

Despite recent advances in imaging, fetal skeletal dysplasias are difficult to diagnose in utero. This is especially so, as there are large number of skeletal dysplasias with overlapping phenotypic features, lack of systemic approach and due to variable time of presentation of the dysplasia. The dysplasia may be suspected during routine ultrasound, if an abnormal or short bone or some other abnormal skeletal finding is detected. It is also important to evaluate chest circumference, femur length-abdominal circumference ratio to assess the possibility of lethality, besides evaluating for other craniofacial and skeletal anomalies. The bones should be evaluated for presence, curvature, degree of mineralization and fractures. The femur length-abdominal circumference ratio of less than 0.16 suggests lung hypoplasia, while femur length-foot length ratio of less than 1, suggests skeletal dysplasias. If there is disproportionate limb shortening, then the segment (rhizo, meso or acromelic) involved should be assessed.[9,10]

The dysplasias and dysostoses group of skeletal abnormalities have been broadly classified into five major groups **(Table 1)**.[11]

OSTEOCHONDRODYSPLASIAS

Defects of Growth of Tubular Bones, Spine or Both

Dysplasias Manifested at Birth

Achondrogenesis:

1. *Clinicopathologic features:* Achondrogenesis is a phenotypically diverse group of chondrodysplasias characterized by a short trunk and micromelia. Achondrogenesis is classified into two types: type I and type II. In achondrogenesis I, the child is usually stillborn or dies soon after birth. Achondrogenesis II is not lethal and usually appears in children of consanguinous parents.
2. *Imaging features:* The radiologic findings in achondrogenesis I include severe lack of ossification of vertebral bodies, small deformed iliac bones, absent or poor ossification of pubic and ischial bones. There is severe micromelia involving the tubular bones, which are markedly shortened and malformed with wide cupped ends. The ribs are short and show cupped and flared ends. Rib fractures are present in some patients. The skull and other membranous bones are involved.

   Imaging features in achondrogenesis II include shortening of bones in distal extremities. The bones are curved and distal segments may be absent. The ossification of bones of hand and feet is delayed.

Table 1: Classification of skeletal abnormalities.

1. ***Osteochondrodysplasias (Abnormalities of Cartilage or Bone Growth and Development)***
   - **i. Defects of growth of tubular bones, spine or both**
     - *Manifested at birth*:
       - Achondrogenesis
       - Thanatophoric dysplasia
       - Achondroplasia
       - Chondrodysplasia punctata
       - Metatrophic dwarfism
       - Diastophic dwarfism
       - Chondroectodermal dysplasia
       - Asphyxiating thoracic dysplasia (Jeune syndrome)
       - Spondyloepiphyseal dysplasia congenita
       - Cleidocranial dysplasia
       - Mesomelic dwarfism
     - *Manifested in later life*:
       - Hypochondroplasia
       - Metaphyseal chondrodysplasia
       - Spondylometaphyseal dysplasia
       - Multiple epiphyseal dysplasia
       - X-linked Spondyloepiphyseal dysplasia tarda
       - Acrodysplasia
   - **ii. Disorganized development of cartilage and fibrous components of the skeleton**
     - Dysplasia epiphysealis hemimelica
     - Multiple cartilaginous exostoses
     - Enchondromatosis (Ollier's disease)
     - Enchondromatosis with hemangiomas (Maffucci syndrome)
     - Fibrous dysplasia
   - **iii. Abnormalities in the density of cortical diaphyseal structure or metaphyseal modeling, or both**
     - Osteogenesis imperfecta congenita
     - Osteogenesis imperfecta tarda
     - Osteopetrosis
     - Pycnodysostosis
     - Osteopoikilosis
     - Osteopathia striata
     - Melorheostosis
     - Diaphyseal dysplasia

Contd...

Contd...

     - Metaphyseal dysplasia
     - Craniodiaphyseal dysplasia
     - Craniometaphyseal dysplasia
     - Frontometaphyseal dysplasia
2. ***Dysostoses (Malformation of Individual Bone, Singly or in Combination)***
   - **i. Dysostoses with cranial and facial involvement**
     - Craniosynostosis
     - Craniofacial synostosis
   - **ii. Dysostosis with predominantly axial involvement**
     - Vertebral segmentation defects
     - Sprengel's deformity
     - Osteo-onychodysostosis
   - **iii. Dysostosis with predominant involvement of extremities**
     - Amelia
     - Hemimelia
     - Phocomelia
     - Radioulnar synostosis
     - Polysyndactyly
     - Clinodactyly
3. ***Idiopathic Osteolysis***
   - Acro-osteolysis (phalangeal type, tarsocarpal type)
   - Multicentric osteolysis
4. ***Primary Disturbances of Growth***
   - Cornelia de Lange syndrome
   - Progeria
5. ***Constitutional Diseases of Bone with Known Pathogenesis***
   - **i. Chromosomal aberrations**
   - **ii. Primary metabolic abnormalities**
     - Calcium phosphorous metabolism (Hypophosphatasia)
     - Mucopolysaccharidosis
     - Mucolipidosis and lipidosis
   - **iii. Bone abnormalities secondary to disturbances of extra-skeleton systems**
     - Endocrine
     - Hematologic
     - Neurologic
     - Renal
     - Gastrointestinal
     - Cardiopulmonary

Polydactyly of the hands and feet is common. The skull and other membranous bones are not involved, distinguishing it from type I.

Thanatophoric Dysplasia:

1. *Clinical features:* As the name implies, thanatophoric dysplasia meaning "death bearing", is the most common lethal bony dysplasia. Clinically the disease is so severe that it may be recognized in utero, with a family history of polyhydramnios and spontaneous abortions. The thorax is markedly narrow with resultant inability of the infant to inflate the lung. Prenatal diagnosis by sonography is possible. Polyhydraminos, poor foetal activity and presence of extra ossification pelvic centres can help in the diagnosis of the dysplasia in utero.[12]
2. *Imaging features:* The radiological features include marked rhizomelic shortening of tubular bones with presence of metaphyseal flaring, osseous widening and bowing. Bowed femora are characteristic and appear like telephone receivers **(Fig. 1)**. Skull changes include frontal bossing, macrocephaly, small skull base and small foramen magnum and cloverleaf skull. Thorax is slender with short ribs with flared anterior ends. There is marked flattening of vertebral bodies with constriction of their mid portions, prominent intervertebral disk spaces against a back drop of well formed neural arches giving a typical H or inverted U appearance on AP view. Narrowing of spinal canal is most marked in lumbar region. Changes in pelvis include small rectangular iliac bones, small sacrosciatic notches with short and wide pubic and ischial bones.

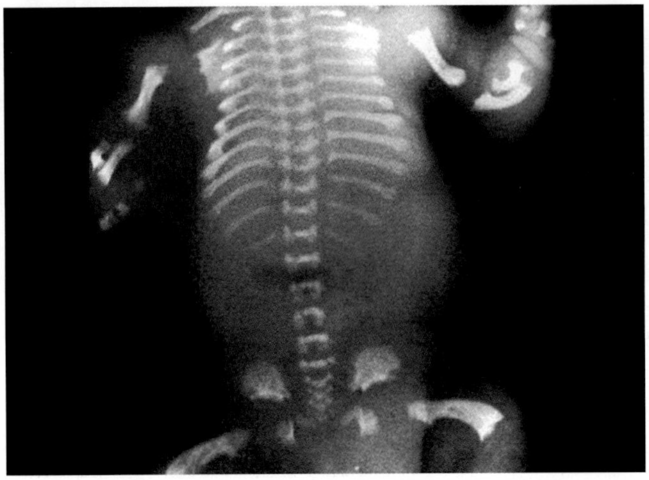

Fig. 1: AP projection of a thanatophoric dwarf showing short and curved tubular bones with telephone receiver configuration of the femora. There is deficient ossification of the vertebral bodies producing an H-shaped appearance. The ribs are short with undercut scapulae.

The features distinguishing this dysplasia from achondroplasia are severe universal vertebra plana in spine and short tubular bowed bones of limbs.

Achondroplasia:

1. *Clinicopathological features:* Achondroplasia is the most common type of nonlethal dysplasia presenting with dwarfism. It is a hereditary condition with an autosomal dominant mode of transmission, though now most cases may be due to mutation of gene in older fathers, in 85% of cases. It presents at birth and is characterized clinically by a large head with brachycephaly, prominent frontal bones with nasal bridge recession, rhizomelic dwarfism, constricted thorax and trident hands due to separation of second and third digits. There is generalized defect in enchondral bone formation. The apophyseal growth is deficient towards the metaphysis, resulting in a V-shaped defect in which the epiphysis is incorporated. A fibrous band growing from periosteum can interpose between epiphysis and the ossifying cartilage, with resultant stunting of longitudinal growth.
2. *Imaging features:* The radiographic findings include a large cranium with respect to size of face with defective growth of base of skull giving a pinched appearance. The foramen magnum is small and funnel shaped. CT and MRI of craniocervical region show associated abnormalities of the cervicomedullary junction. Anteroposterior diameter of chest is decreased due to short ribs. Spinal abnormalities include reduction in interpedicular distances in lumbar region with short pedicles, narrow spinal canal and posterior vertebral scalloping **(Fig. 2A)**. Vertebral bodies are flattened and can appear bullet-shaped in infancy and early childhood. Changes in pelvis include square iliac bones with posteriorly set horizontal acetabular roof and small sacrosciatic notches giving classical "tombstone appearance" **(Fig. 2B)**. Rhizomelic shortening of proximal bones, with deepseated epiphysis in flared metaphysis gives a V-shaped appearance **(Fig. 2C)**. Shortening and widening of tubular bones of hand and feet, with typical involvement of proximal and middle phalanges can also be seen.

   With advancing age, severe spinal cord compromise and disk protrusions become especially important and are best evaluated by MRI **(Figs. 2D and E)**.

   In hypochondroplasia, the radiologic findings are similar but less severe than those of achondroplasia and the skull is never affected.

   Achondroplasia needs to be differentiated from thanatophoric dysplasia, spondyloepiphyseal dysplasia, diastrophic dwarfism, metatrophic dwarfism, asphyxiating thoracic dysplasia, Ellis-van-Creveld syndrome, cartilage hair hypoplasia and metaphyseal dysostosis.

Chondrodysplasia Punctata (CDP) Group:

1. *Clinicopathological features:* It is transmitted as an autosomal recessive trait, with a female preponderance. Most of the cases are manifest clinically before two years of age. There is craniofacial dysmorphism, ocular abnormalities, severe mental retardation, spastic tetraplegia and joint contractures with shortening of one or more limbs. There is a benign non-rhizomelic group with good prognosis with little residual deformity, and a potentially lethal rhizomelic group. Death occurs in the rhizomelic group due to tracheal stenosis or spinal cord compression usually within the first decade. Mucoid degeneration in epiphyseal center has been seen histologically which leads to fragmentation of the epiphysis. This becomes a nidus for calcareous deposits or punctate ossification.
2. *Imaging features:* Radiologic findings include stippled calcification of the cartilage at the end of bones. There is symmetric rhizomelic or mesomelic limb shortening with metaphyseal splaying.[13] There can be delayed ossification of carpal bones. There is hypoplasia of bones of mid-face with nasal

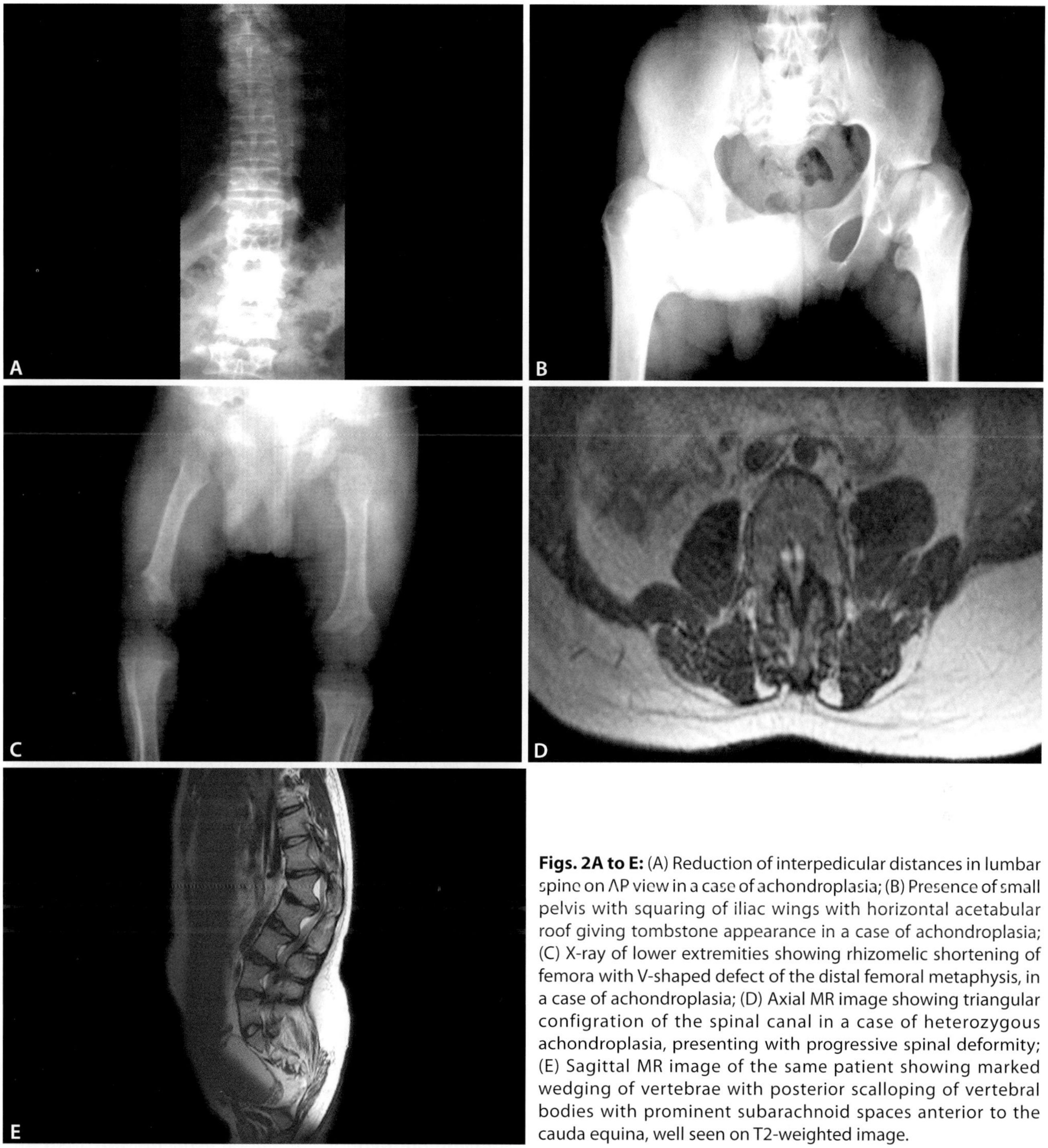

Figs. 2A to E: (A) Reduction of interpedicular distances in lumbar spine on AP view in a case of achondroplasia; (B) Presence of small pelvis with squaring of iliac wings with horizontal acetabular roof giving tombstone appearance in a case of achondroplasia; (C) X-ray of lower extremities showing rhizomelic shortening of femora with V-shaped defect of the distal femoral metaphysis, in a case of achondroplasia; (D) Axial MR image showing triangular configration of the spinal canal in a case of heterozygous achondroplasia, presenting with progressive spinal deformity; (E) Sagittal MR image of the same patient showing marked wedging of vertebrae with posterior scalloping of vertebral bodies with prominent subarachnoid spaces anterior to the cauda equina, well seen on T2-weighted image.

flattening. Changes in spine include defective vertebral ossification, flattening of vertebral column, transient lucent vertebral defect, and abnormalities of segmentation, kyphosis and scoliosis. Neurologic abnormalities, such as Dandy-Walker frequently coexist. Iliac blades lack normal flaring. Calcifications in and around epiphysis are frequently seen in region of acetabulum, femur, spine and carpal and tarsal bones in Conradi-Hünermann type.

The radiologic appearance is characteristic and should not be confused with other conditions **(Fig. 3)**. In cretins, there can be epiphyseal fragmentation which is however, larger and conforms to the expected shadow of the epiphysis.

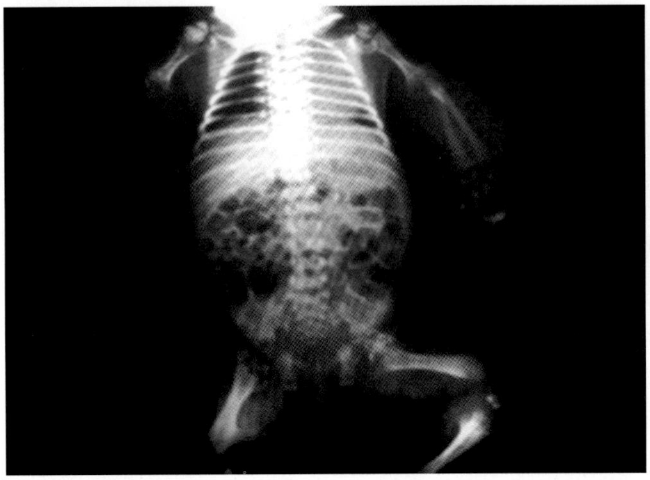

Fig. 3: Rhizomelic dwarfism with stippled epiphyseal calcification in a newborn, in a case of chondrodysplasia punctata.

Metatrophic Dysplasia:

1. *Clinical features:* Metatrophic dysplasia is characterized by short extremities and a normal trunk at birth, and short trunk with kyphoscoliosis later in life.
2. *Imaging features:* The radiologic findings include marked metaphyseal widening with short bones of extremity giving a dumbbell appearance. The trochanters are large, typically the lesser trochanter with the appearance simulating a battle-axe. The epiphyses show delayed appearance and are small and deformed. The vertebral bodies are markedly reduced in height and appear rectangular or diamond shaped and can show anterior wedging. The intervertebral disk spaces consequently appear large. The neural arches are well developed. There may be hypoplasia of the dens with resultant atlantoaxial instability. The thorax is elongated with decreased AP diameter due to short ribs in infancy. There is severe anterior bowing of sternum with development of kyphoscoliosis in childhood. Changes in pelvis include short ilia with curved lateral margins, flat acetabular roof, wide Y-shaped triradiate cartilage and small sacrosciatic notches.

Diastrophic Dysplasia Group:

1. *Clinical features:* The term diastrophic meaning twisted or crooked has been used to highlight the phenotype resulting from this autosomal recessive disorder. This dysplasia group has a mutation in the sulfate transporter gene. It is characterized by short stature, progressive scoliosis, kyphosis, clubfeet, Hitchiker's thumb, multiple contractures, dislocations, deformed ears and cleft palate.
2. *Imaging features:* There is micromelic dwarfism with marked shortening of tubular bones with metaphyseal widening and rounding. The first metacarpal is oval and usually hypoplastic. There is delayed appearance of the epiphysis with flattening and deformity, seen characteristically in proximal and distal femora. Epiphysis in hand and foot bones may be irregular, distorted and deformed. A disproportionate shortening of ulna and fibula can be present. Narrowing of joint spaces especially of hip and elbows can be seen. Femora may have broad inter trochanteric regions with short femoral necks. Scoliosis is progressive leading to spinal abnormalities, instability, cord compression, and death.

Diastrophic dysplasia needs to be differentiated from achondroplasia and Morquio's syndrome. The oval metacarpal of diastrophic dwarfism is the most distinguishing feature. The presence of a basal segment of innominate bone and the lack of narrowing of the interpedicular distances in the lumbar region distinguish it from achondroplasia. The characteristic spinal changes in form of anterior beaking of lumbar vertebrae and "simian-shaped" pelvis in Morquio's syndrome help in differentiating it from diastrophic dysplasia.

Chondroectodermal Dysplasia:

1. *Clinical features:* This is a short-limbed dwarfism characterized by ectodermal dysplasia, polydactyly and congenital heart disease. There is distal shortening of limbs, absent or hypoplastic nails, abnormal hair, dysplastic teeth and upper lip abnormalities. It is inherited as an autosomal recessive trait and is evident at birth. Death is common in childhood due to cardiac and pulmonary complications.
2. *Imaging features:* In addition to changes in asphyxiating thoracic dysplasia, there is presence of carpal fusion, post-axial poly- and syndactyly, enlargement of proximal end of ulna and distal end of radius giving drumstick appearance with anterior dislocation of radial heads. Medial tibial exostoses, wide but hypoplastic lateral aspect of proximal tibia, genu valgum and fibular shortening are other typical features. Atrial septal defect is a commonly associated cardiac abnormality.
   The spine and skull are normal.

Asphyxiating Thoracic Dysplasia (Jeune Syndrome):

1. *Clinical features:* This is an autosomal recessive condition, which is evident at birth. The infants have

characteristically constricted chests with shortening of the extremities. There is in addition, marked pulmonary hypoplasia. Most infants die due to respiratory distress while renal failure is frequent in those that survive.

2. *Imaging features:* The significant radiological features include high handle bar appearance of clavicles along with narrow thorax, short horizontal ribs and wide irregular costochondral junctions. Changes in pelvis include short ilia with flat acetabular roof and downward spike like projections giving trident appearance to the acetabulum. Premature ossification of capital femoral epiphysis is fairly common with presence of metaphyseal irregularity. Epiphysis in hand bones can be cone shaped and fuse prematurely, producing shortening of middle and distal phalanges. Skull and spine are normal. It is not associated with congenital heart disease.[14]

   It can be differentiated from chondroectodermal dysplasia by the presence of short ribs, hepatic fibrosis and higher incidence of progressive renal disease. In addition, there is less frequent polydactyly and less frequent nail changes.

Spondyloepiphyseal Dysplasia Congenita:

1. *Clinical features:* Spondyloepiphyseal dysplasia congenita is a hereditary dysplasia transmitted as an autosomal dominant trait that affects the spine and proximal epiphysis of long bones at birth. This short limb dwarfism is characterized by mild shortening of the limbs, cleft palate, flat face, short neck and increased anteroposterior chest diameter. Progressive kyphoscoliosis occurs as the child grows. Knock-knees and bowleg deformities are common. The hands and feet are normal.
2. *Imaging features:* The height of vertebral bodies is decreased with pear-shaped vertebrae seen in infancy due to lack of development of the posterior portion of vertebral bodies. Anterior wedging, irregularity and generalised flattening can be present in childhood with development of kyphoscoliosis and lumbar lordosis. The interpedicular distances are narrowed in lumbar region. Atlantoaxial dislocation due to hypoplasia of dens can also be present. The chest is broad and bell shaped and of decreased height. There is in addition, short squared scapulae with flared anterior ends of ribs, delay in sternal ossification and pectus carinatum. There is marked delay in ossification of the pubic bones and proximal portion of femora. The femoral heads often ossify from multiple centers and progressive coxa vara develops with premature osteoarthritis. Prominent shortening of neck of femora with small femoral heads well below the level of greater trochanter can be seen. The epiphyses are irregular and the metaphyses show flaring and irregularity in long tubular bones. The ossification may be delayed **(Fig. 4)**.

   Spondyloepiphyseal dysplasia congenita needs to be differentiated from Morquio's disease, diastrophic dwarfism, metatrophic dwarfism and multiple epiphyseal dysplasias.

Cleidocranial Dysplasia:

1. *Clinical features:* It is an uncommon autosomal dominant condition characterized by delayed or incomplete calvarial ossification and clavicular hypoplasia or aplasia. Midline structures are primarily affected in this dysplasia and the disease manifests in infancy. Mild shortening of the stature may also be present in cleidocranial dysplasia.
2. *Imaging features:* Radiologic findings include poor ossification of skull bones with presence of multiple wormian bones and wide sutures. The parietal bone ossification may be absent at birth. The foramen magnum is large and deformed, basilar invagination may occur. The clavicle is deficient in its outer or middle parts, though rarely it may be totally absent **(Fig. 5A)**. The thorax is narrow and bell shaped with a small hypoplastic scapula.[14,15] Pelvic abnormalities are common and include delayed ossification of pubic bones, narrow iliac wings and wide pubic symphysis giving a 'see-through' appearance **(Fig. 5B)**. Coxa valga deformity is frequently present. The changes

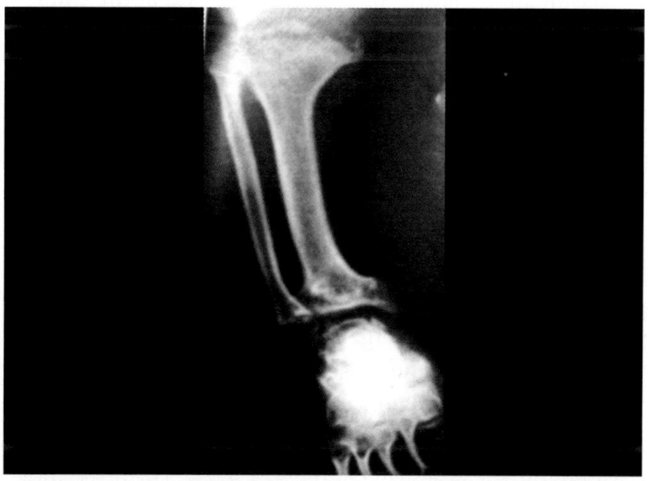

Fig. 4: Epiphyseal and metaphyseal irregularities with metaphyseal widening involving both tibia and fibula with angular deformity at the ankle joint, in a case of spondyloepiphyseal dysplasia congenita.

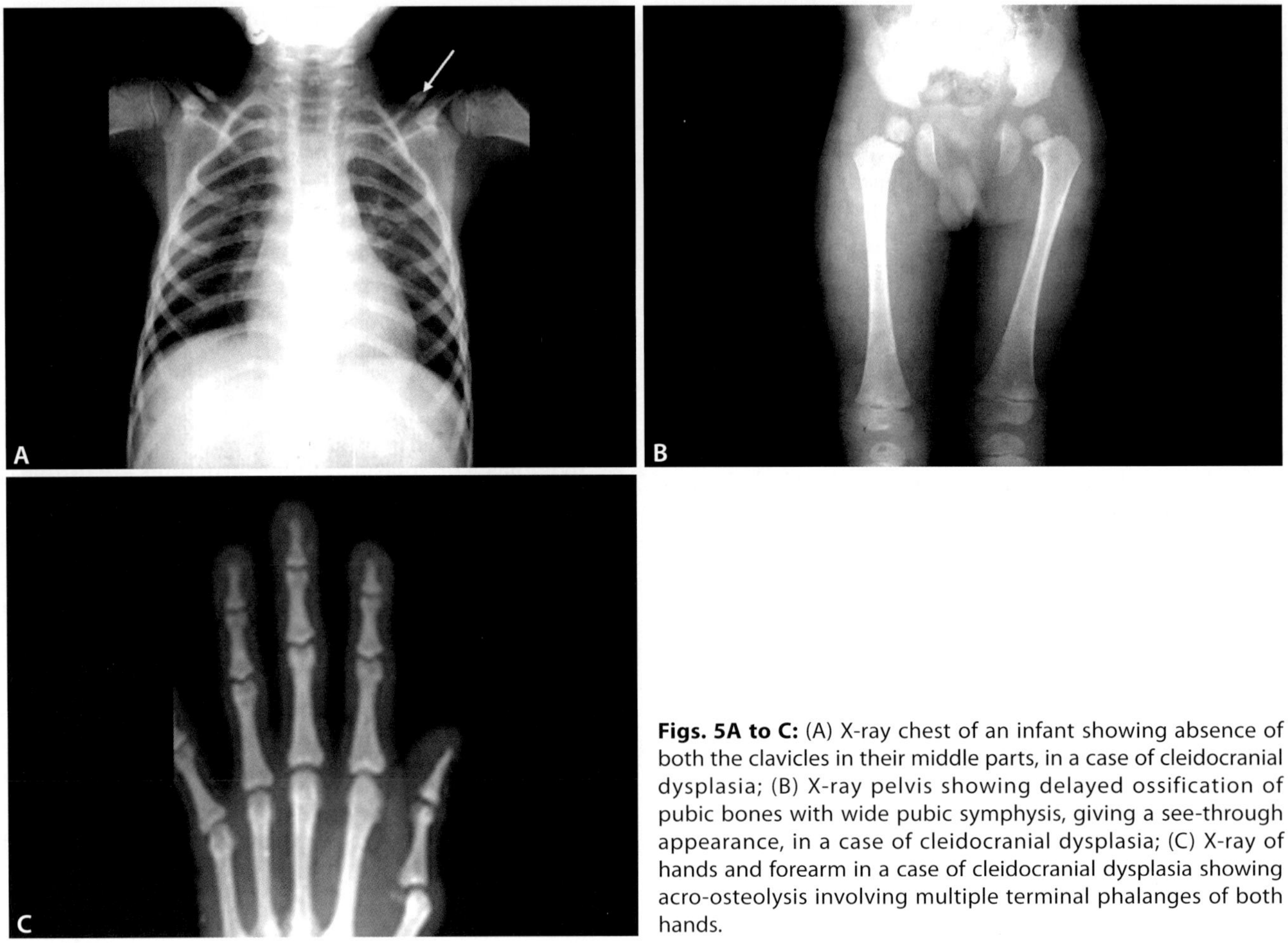

Figs. 5A to C: (A) X-ray chest of an infant showing absence of both the clavicles in their middle parts, in a case of cleidocranial dysplasia; (B) X-ray pelvis showing delayed ossification of pubic bones with wide pubic symphysis, giving a see-through appearance, in a case of cleidocranial dysplasia; (C) X-ray of hands and forearm in a case of cleidocranial dysplasia showing acro-osteolysis involving multiple terminal phalanges of both hands.

in spine include failure of fusion of neural arches, wedging of vertebral bodies with scoliosis, multiple ossification centres of thoracic vertebral bodies, defect in pars interarticularis in lumbar spine and spina bifida occulta in cervical and thoracic vertebrae.[16] There can be mild widening of the metaphysis and narrowing of the diaphysis of tubular bones. Hand changes include long 2nd and 5th metacarpals with supernumerary ossification centers and short 2nd and 5th phalanges, small middle and small tapered distal phalanges, pseudoepiphysis in metacarpal bones, and cone-shaped epiphysis and retarded ossification of the carpal bones **(Fig. 5C)**. Tibiotalar slant and short fibulae may also be present.

Yunis-Varon syndrome comprises cleidocranial dysostosis, micrognathia, absence of thumbs and first metatarsals and distal aphalangia.

Mesomelic Dysplasias:

Dyschondrosteosis is the most common mesomelic dysplasia.

It is transmitted as an autosomal dominant trait with a female predominance. Dorsal dislocation of distal ulna is present with limited elbow and wrist movement.

1. *Radiological features:* It is characterized by mesomelic limb shortening with Madelung deformity of the forearm. It is also called as Léri-Weill syndrome. There is shortening of radius with bowing deformity and subluxated distal end of ulna. The lack of development of distal radial epiphysis results in tilting of the distal end of radius in a volar and ulnar direction. The radial head can also dislocate. Similar changes in lower leg can result in deformity of ankle mortice.

   Nievergelt type is the most severe type of mesomelic dysplasia, which is also accompanied by bony prominences in the lower legs. Hypoplasia of bones of forearm and leg is common **(Fig. 6)**. Dysplasia of tibia may result in triangular or rhomboid configuration of tibia and slanting of the growth plate of tibia. Proximal radioulnar synostosis with elbow dislocation and fusion of carpal bones may also be seen.

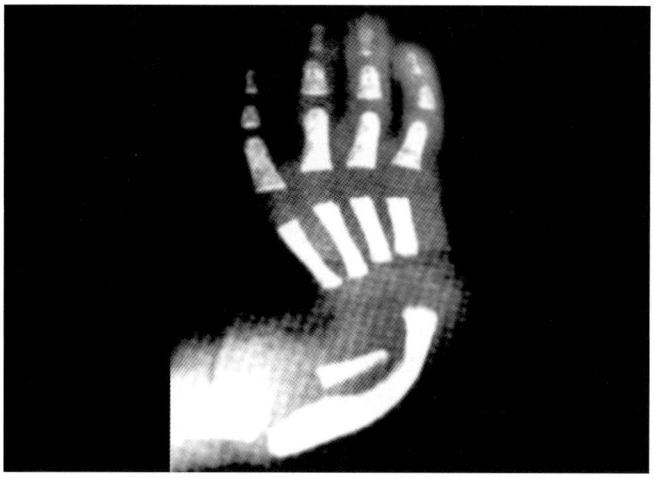

Fig. 6: Newborn infant with hypoplastic radius, curved ulna with absent thumb in a case of mesomelic dysplasia.

Dysplasias Manifested in Later Life

Hypochondroplasia:

1. *Clinical features:* This dysplasia is transmitted in an autosomal dominant mode. The clinical features include short stature with relatively long trunk and disproportionate short limbs. The head is normal, which distinguishes it from achondroplasia.
2. *Imaging features:* The radiologic features include rhizomelia with metaphyseal flaring, spinal stenosis due to reduced interpedicular distances, small pelvis and lordotic sacrum. There is broadening of femoral neck and the distal fibula is overgrown as compared to proximal fibula.The differential diagnosis includes achondroplasia, diastrophic dwarfism, spondyloepiphyseal dysplasia and chondroectodermal dysplasia.

Metaphyseal Chondrodysplasia:

Metaphyseal chondrodysplasias are a large heterogeneous groups of disorders.

1. *Jansen type*

   Clinical features: This is a rare severe dysplasia due to excessive proliferating hypertrophic cartilage in the metaphysis. There is marked dwarfism, swelling of joints and bowed legs and forearms detectable at birth.

   Imaging features: In infancy there is marked irregularity of the metaphysis, widened growth plate and bowing of tubular bones with diffuse osteopenia. Subperiosteal resorption of bones and fractures also occur in childhood. There is cupping of the metaphysis with a wide zone of irregular calcification. There is resultant dwarfism with metaphyseal flaring and bowed bones. Spine shows minimal platyspondyly. There is basilar and supraorbital ridge sclerosis with osteopenia of the skull vault.

   In the early cases, differential diagnosis includes renal osteodystrophy and hypophosphatasia, however the radiological features are diagnostic.
2. *Schmid type*

   Clinical features: Presents in early childhood, and this is often misdiagnosed as rickets because of metaphyseal changes.

   It is transmitted as an autosomal dominant trait and manifests as mild dwarfism. The skeletal abnormalities are not evident at birth but appear in third and fourth year of life. Radiological findings include growth plate widening, metaphyseal irregularity, and flaring especially in knee and hip joints. Coxa vara is common due to involvement of metaphyses of proximal femora. The spine and hands are not involved.

   Patients with cartilage hair hypoplasia also show irregular metaphyses with bowing and dwarfism, but the brittle, short hair accompanying the syndrome help in differentiating the two conditions.

Spondylometaphyseal Dysplasia (SMD)

1. *Clinical features:* This dysplasia is characterized by abnormalities in the vertebrae and metaphyses of tubular bones. In Kozlowski type there is short stature, kyphosis and scoliosis, diminutive hands, and feet with bowing of bones.
2. *Imaging features:* Radiological findings include markedly retarded skeletal maturation with degenerative changes in joints. There is flattening of vertebral bodies with pedicles located medially and altered spinal curvatures **(Fig. 7A)**. Metaphyseal irregularity is most evident at the ends of long bones **(Fig. 7B)**. Proximal femora are commonly involved with resultant coxa vara. The iliac bones are shortened with small sacrosciatic notches and horizontal acetabular roof. In Sutcliffe type, there are small triangular bony fragments at the periphery of metaphysis adjacent to growth plate (corner fracture appearance) and severe coxa vara. In spine, the findings include exaggerated end plate convexity, anterior wedging of vertebral bodies and square or ovoid vertebral bodies.[17]

Multiple Epiphyseal Dysplasia (MED)

1. *Clinical features:* It is transmitted in an autosomal dominant manner in most of the cases. Mild dwarfism with flexion deformities and degenerative arthritis are frequently present.
2. *Imaging features:* Radiographic findings are especially prominent in hip, knee, wrist and ankles.

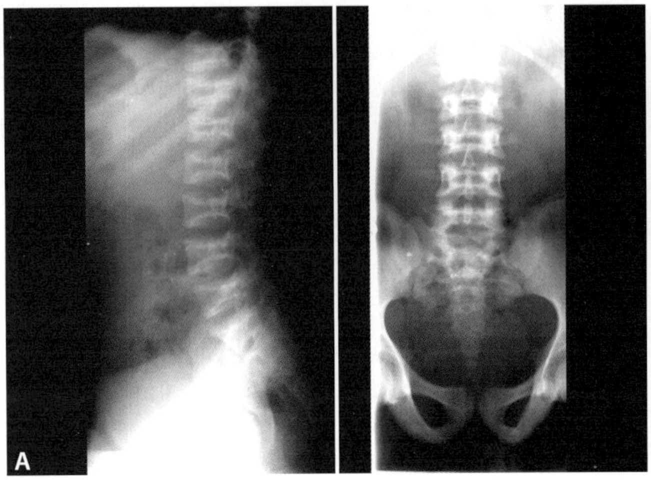

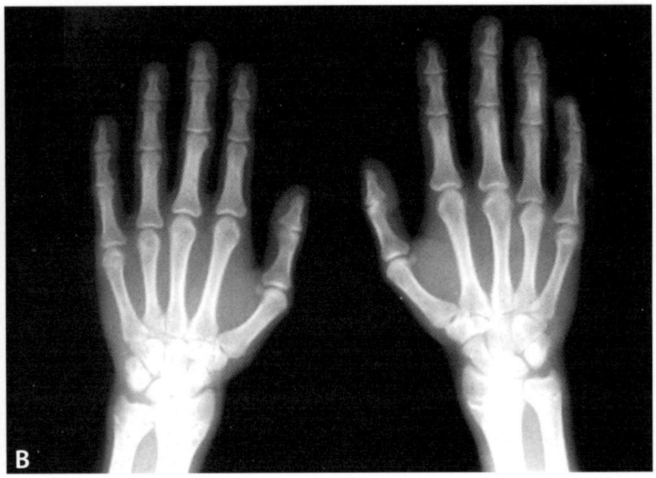

Figs. 7A and B: (A) X-ray lumbar spine AP and lateral views showing platyspondyly with end-plate irregularity and sclerosis; (B) X-ray of both hands AP view showing metaphyseal cupping and irregularity involving distal metaphysis of radius and ulna, in a case of spondylometaphyseal dysplasia.

The ossification centers appear late, show delayed mineralisation and are fragmented. They ossify from multiple centers and can have a "mulberry appearance". The secondary centers are small and flattened. Fusion of ossification centers is also delayed, and a fragmented piece of the center may result in the formation of loose body. In older patients slipped epiphysis may result with resultant deformities of joint, such as tibiotalar slant, genu valgum and premature osteoarthritis **(Fig. 8)**. The metaphyseal changes are especially noticeable in metacarpal and metatarsal bones. There are short broad phalanges with irregularity of epiphyseal ends of bones. The spine is affected in two-thirds of patients and changes include mild platyspondyly, anterior wedging with irregularity of anterior aspect of end plates associated with scoliosis, typically in mid thoracic spine.

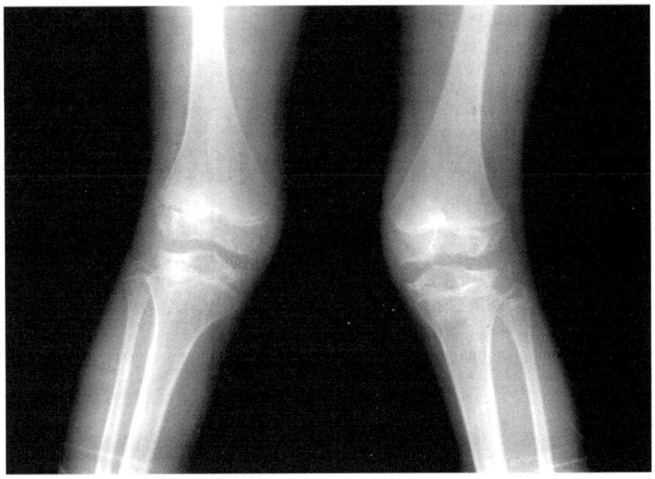

Fig. 8: X-ray of both knees AP view showing epiphyseal flattening with irregularity of both distal femora and proximal tibia with mild fibular flattening and resultant genu valgum, in a case of multiple epiphyseal dysplasia.

The involvement of multiple epiphyses with lack of metaphyseal change helps in differentiating this condition from Perthes' disease.

In cretins, the bone age is severely retarded, which is a helpful differentiating feature.

X-linked Spondyloepiphyseal Dysplasia Tarda:

1. *Clinical features:* This condition is seen exclusively in males as it is transmitted as a sex-linked trait. It becomes evident after five years of age due to impaired growth of spine. The dwarfism is of the short limb type. Premature hip osteoarthritis with pain and limited motion is noticed around puberty.
2. *Imaging features:* Radiologically, platyspondyly is prominently present in the spine **(Figs. 9A and B)**. Other features include hump-shaped area of dense bone on the central and posterior portion of the end plates. The disk spaces consequently appear wide anteriorly and narrow posteriorly. The odontoid process may be deformed. There may be disk protrusions in the thoracic region. There is relative increase in the anteroposterior diameter of chest. Degenerative changes in spine develop in early adult life. Pelvic bones and femoral necks may be small with presence of coxa vara. Osteoarthritis involving hip can be disabling **(Fig. 9C)**.

Morquio's disease can be excluded by the absence of severe platyspondyly and severe dysplasia of the peripheral epiphyses.

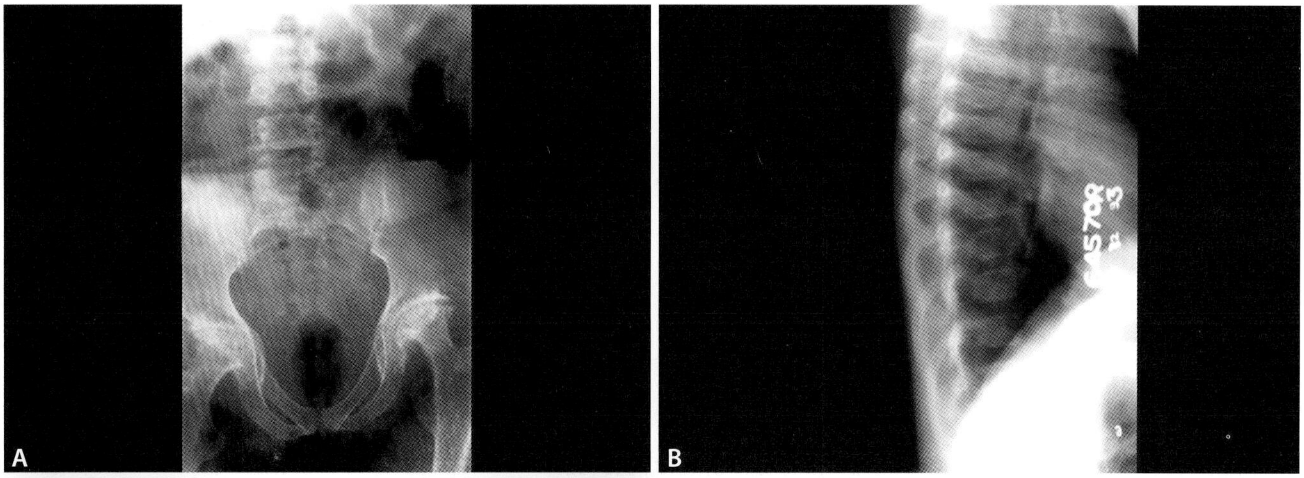

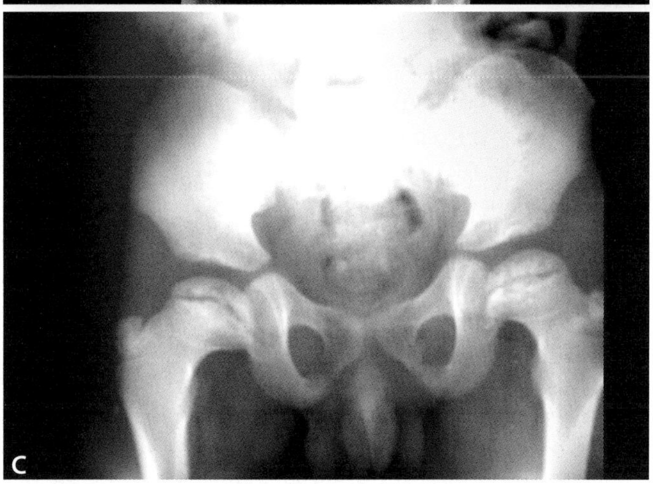

Figs. 9A to C: X-ray spine (A) AP and (B) lateral views showing generalized platyspondyly; (C) X-ray pelvis AP view-rounded flared ilia with distal tapering and bilateral symmetrical capital femoral epiphyseal flattening, sclerosis and fissuring, in a case of spondyloepiphyseal dysplasia tarda.

Acrodysplasia—Trichorhinophalangeal Dysplasia:

1. *Clinical features:* It is transmitted as an autosomal dominant trait. Clinical features include sparse scalp hair, pear shaped nose, short stature, joint laxity and deformity of proximal interphalangeal joints. Three types of dysplasias have been described.
2. *Imaging features:* The characteristic radiologic findings in type I dysplasia include cone-shaped epiphysis in hands producing a U-shaped pattern with osseous shortening, especially in middle phalanges of second and third digit with ivory epiphysis being common in the distal phalanges. The proximal femoral epiphyses are small and often demonstrate changes resembling Perthes' disease. Pectus carinatum, scoliosis and kyphosis can also be seen. In type II dysplasia, there are cone shaped epiphyses in thumb and other digits with presence of multiple exostoses, which distort and expand the bone. There is asymmetric limb growth, tibiofibular synostosis, short fibula, wide femoral neck and changes similar to Perthes' disease. Segmentation errors in spine and macrocephaly may occasionally be present. In type III dysplasia, there is severe generalized shortening of all the phalanges and metacarpals without the presence of exostosis.[18]

Disorganized Development of Cartilage and Fibrous Components of the Skeleton

Dysplasia Epiphysealis Hemimelica

1. *Clinical features:* The clinical features consist of pain, deformity, and restricted motion of affected joints.
2. *Imaging features:* The radiological features of this dysplasia include early appearance and excessive growth of epiphysis with irregularly calcified mass projecting from the epiphysis. The irregular mass may initially appear distinct from the surrounding bone, though eventually, it fuses with the adjacent epiphysis. Distal femur and distal tibia are among the common sites of involvement. Epiphyseal involvement on one side of body may be associated with hemihypertrophy. Spinal abnormalities, including scoliosis can occur.

Multiple Cartilaginous Exostoses

1. *Clinical features:* This condition also called diaphyseal aclasis is characterized by cartilage capped exostosis. It occurs more commonly in boys, who develop painless lumps near ends of long bones. They have mild shortness of stature.
2. *Imaging features:* The radiological appearance and size of exostosis is variable. They arise on metaphyseal side of growth plate and point away from the epiphyses with associated metaphyseal expansion and deformity **(Fig. 10)**. In hands, however, the origin can be in the epiphysis. The forearms are frequently deformed as a consequence of bowing of radius, dislocation of radial head, ulnar angulation of distal end of radius and shortening of ulna. The long tubular bones are frequently involved, however ribs, scapula and pelvis can also be affected. Vertebral involvement though uncommon, can lead to compression of spinal cord or nerve roots. Complications related to osteochondroma include interference with growth, compression of adjacent structures and malignant transformation. Malignant transformation may be indicated by continued growth of osteochondroma even after cessation of normal growth, changing appearance of calcification in cartilage cap and irregular outline or bony destruction of exostosis.

Enchondromatosis (Ollier's Disease)

1. *Clinical features:* Clinically there is asymmetrical limb shortening with expansion of affected bone and occasionally pathological fracture.
2. *Imaging features:* The radiological features include radiolucent masses, which may be round or triangular in the tubular bones of hand, which may show considerable expansion and pathological fracture. Focal area of calcification can be present in the mass **(Fig. 11)**. Cartilaginous areas extending from physis lead to interference with growth and resultant shortening and deformity. The femur and tibia are most commonly involved. In pelvis V-shaped radiolucent areas are seen in iliac bones. The enchondromas typically stabilise or even regress in adulthood. Malignant transformation to chondrosarcoma in one-fourth of patients can occur.

Enchondromatosis with Hemangiomas (Maffucci Syndrome)

The radiological features are similar to Ollier's disease with the additional presence of phleboliths and soft tissue masses due to hemangiomas, more commonly in hands and feet **(Fig. 12)**. The hemangiomas can disappear, and they need not overlie the bone lesions. A higher incidence of malignant transformation is seen compared to Ollier's disease.

Fibrous Dysplasia

1. *Clinical features:* This dysplasia is seen in the first three decades with a female preponderance. There is deformity and pain related to involved bones, with pathological fracture at times. The lesions tend to be unilateral. Histologically, medullary bone is seen to be replaced by fibrous tissue and cysts. This dysplasia can be monostotic or polyostotic. The

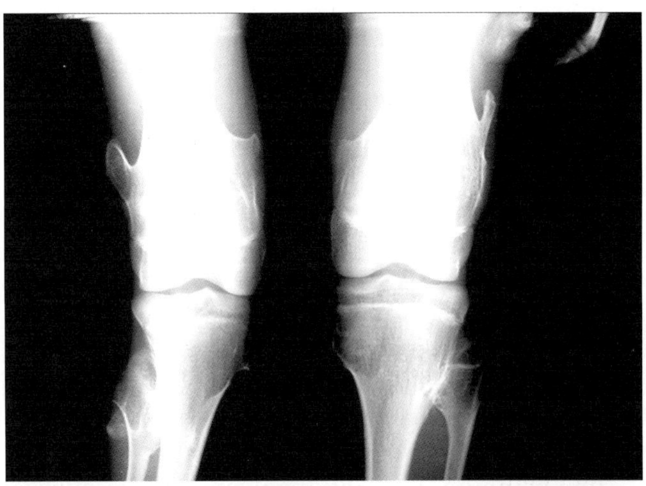

Fig. 10: Multiple bony exostosis seen involving both lower femora and upper ends of tibia and fibulae with metaphyseal modeling deformity.

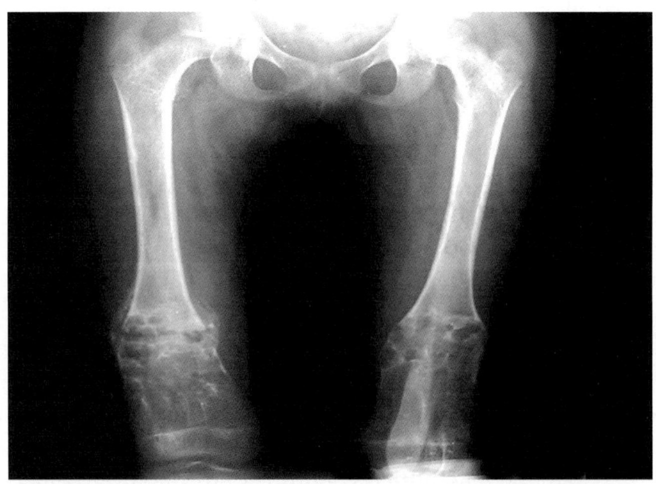

Fig. 11: X-ray of both knees AP view showing marked bony expansion with loss of cortical integrity of the distal femoral metaphysis with intramedullary calcification and lucencies, in a case of Ollier's disease.

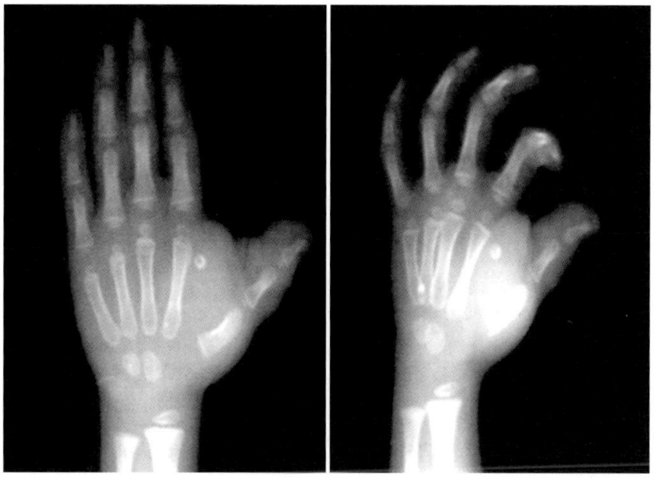

Fig. 12: X-ray of right hand AP view showing soft tissue swelling with presence of calcified phleboliths suggestive of hemangioma between the metacarpal bones, in a case of Maffucci syndrome. Enchondromatosis may not be present in the region of hemangioma, as in this case.

association of polyostotic fibrous dysplasia, sexual precocity, café-au-lait pigmentation in females, constitutes the McCune-Albright syndrome. Sarcomatous degeneration can occur in about 1% cases.

2. *Imaging features:* The radiological features include "ground-glass" appearance or radiolucent areas of altered trabeculae in the ribs and long bones with associated patchy sclerosis and expansion **(Fig. 13A)**. There is endosteal scalloping and cortical thinning. Localized or asymmetrical overgrowth of bones may be seen. Pathological fractures and deformities due to bone softening, such as 'Shepherd's crook deformity' can occur. The skull shows asymmetrical thickening of the vault with sclerosis of the base with obliteration of the paranasal sinuses **(Fig. 13B)** and marked facial deformity giving a "leontiasis ossea" appearance.[19]

Abnormalities of the Density of Cortical Diaphyseal Structure or Metaphyseal Modeling or Both

Dysplasias with Decreased Bone Density

Osteogenesis Imperfecta

1. *Clinical features:* Clinically there is thin skin with ligamentous laxity and easy bruising, blue sclerae, dentinogenesis imperfecta, premature otosclerosis, with presence of hydrocephalus. The dysplasia is seen to result from abnormality of type I collagen. Osteogenesis imperfecta congenita occurs early in life while osteogenesis imperfecta tarda is less severe and occurs later in life. Clinical features in osteogenesis imperfecta congenita include paper thin soft skull with short broad extremities with deformities due to multiple fractures.
2. *Imaging features:* There is diffuse decrease in bone density in both axial and appendicular skeleton. Based on radiographic appearance of the extremities, Fairbank classified osteogenesis imperfecta into three groups. The first group includes patients with thin gracile bones **(Fig. 14A)**. This is the most common expression of the disease. The bone cortices and shafts are thin with poorly defined trabeculae. The second group includes those patients with short thick limbs. The term thick bone type is a misnomer, as the cortices are thin with reduced bony density. In this group, there is severe micromelia with an increase in the width of the bones **(Fig. 14B)**. This group has a poor prognosis. Third and least common, is a group of cases with cystic changes in the extremities with altered modelling of the bone. These occur in severely affected patients and other features include flared hyperlucent metaphyses traversed by coarse trabeculae giving a honeycomb appearance. Patients who survive infancy often undergo change from the thick limb type to the cystic or gracile type.[17]

Fractures in osteogenesis imperfecta occur most commonly in the lower limbs. Microfractures can occur at the junction of metaphysis and epiphysis. These fractures are asymmetrical and are seen as dense lines due to repeated trauma. Avulsion injury due to normal muscle pull can occur. Multiple telescoping fractures, which begin to occur in utero, lead to micromelia and bowing deformities. Fracture healing is usually normal, but tumoral callus and pseudoarthoses can occur. Hyperplastic callus usually occurs after trauma or surgical intervention. Multiple radiolucent scalloped areas with sclerotic margins referred to as popcorn calcifications can occur in metaphysis or epiphysis in severely affected patients. This is thought to result from traumatic fragmentation of cartilage growth plate. Laxity, tendon ruptures, fractures deformities and premature degenerative processes all contribute to wide scale deformities.

In the skull, changes include enlargement of mastoid and frontal sinuses. Wormian bones are commonly seen, arranged in mosaic pattern, along the lambdoid suture. Platybasia with or without basilar impression is a frequent deformity. Basilar impression with platybasia is referred to as "Tam-o-Shanter"

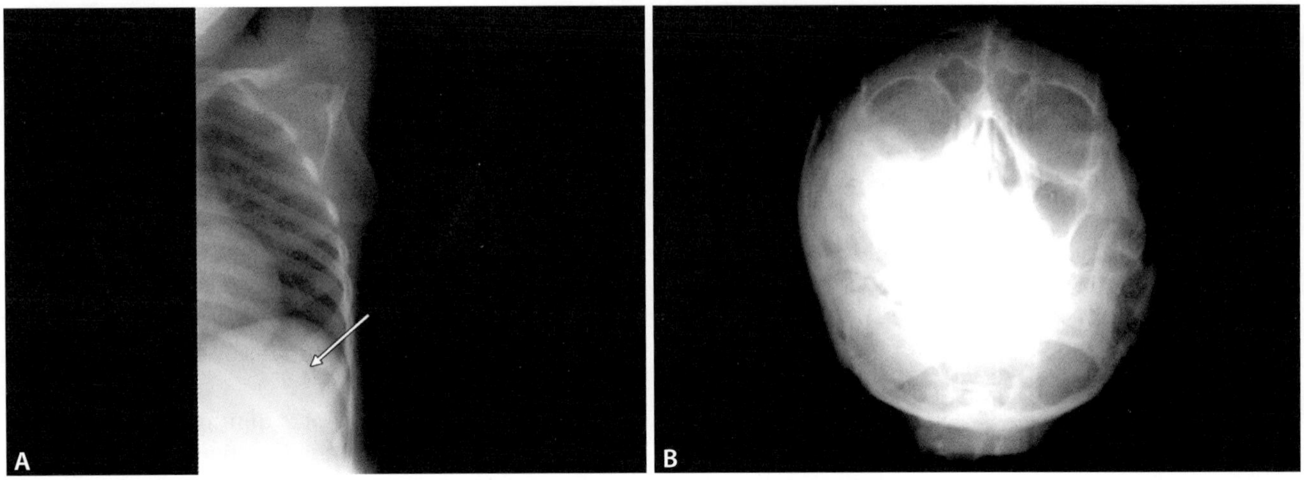

Figs. 13A and B: (A) Bony expansion with lysis and ground-glass haze in a case of fibrous dysplasia involving the 10th rib posteriorly (arrow); (B) Bony expansion with ground-glass haze and uniformily increased density seen involving the right maxillay sinus, right zygoma and right hemimandible on Water's view.

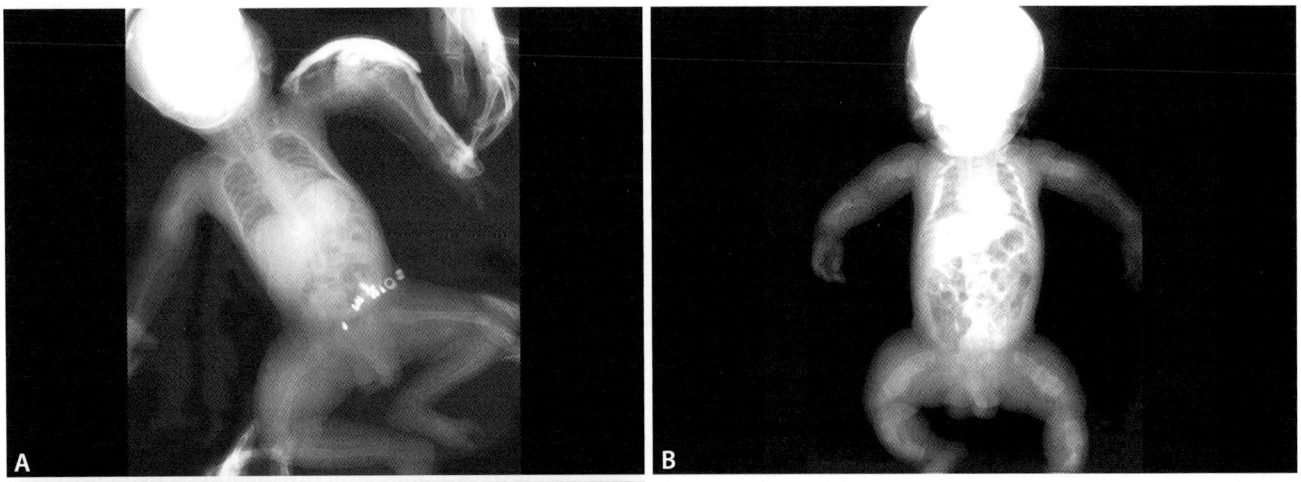

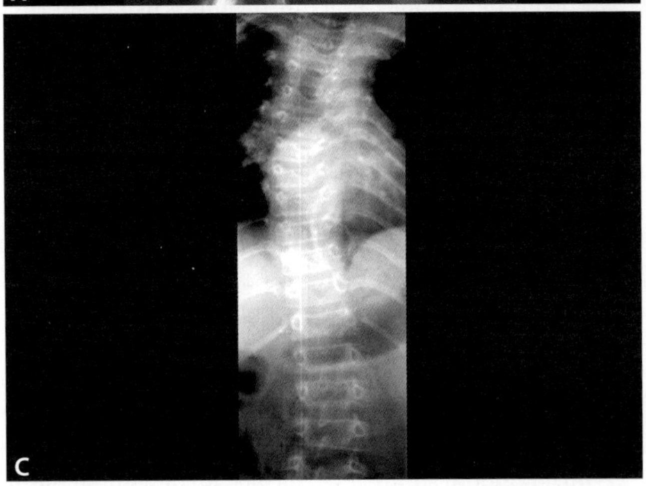

Figs. 14A to C: (A) Infantogram showing a case of osteogenesis imperfecta congenita (thin bone type) with bone with thin cortices and decreased bone density with presence of fractures in diaphysis of both humeri and right femora with exuberant callous formation; (B) Infantogram showing a classical case of osteogenesis imperfecta congenita (thick bone type) with short and broad bones and decreased bony density, platyspondyly, multiple diaphyseal fractures in all the long bones of the extremities and ribs with callous formation; (C) Radiograph of the lumbar spine (AP view) showing generalized decrease in bone density with platyspondyly, in a case of osteogenesis imperfecta tarda.

skull. Premature otosclerosis can also result, due to thickening of stapes footplate, stapedial crural fractures, obliteration of oval window and flattening of cochlea, which can be well depicted by computed tomography. Dental abnormalities include teeth with absent pulp chambers and root canals, deformed and twisted roots and absence of enamel. Jaw fractures with excessive callus can follow dental extraction.

Spinal changes include flattened vertebral bodies, which can be biconcave or wedged anteriorly, with severe kyphoscoliosis, which is progressive **(Fig. 14C)**. Pelvis is frequently triradiate with presence of compression fractures and protrusio acetabulae. Shepherd's crook deformity can also be present. Sonographic detection of disease is possible in utero by using three diagnostic criteria described by Münoz et al. i.e.:

1. Detection of crumpled or wrinkled appearance due to fractures of long bones.
2. Detection of severe demineralization of calvaria, which is associated with excellent visualization of intracranial contents, and
3. Shortening of femur to more than three standard deviations below mean value. Other features can also be detected which include platyspondyly, beaded ribs, small thoracic circumference and Wormian bones. Serial scans are important, as they can help in determining prognosis and in planning type of delivery.[20]

Increased Bone Density without Modification of Bone Shape

Osteopetrosis:

1. *Clinicopathological features:* The primary defect is the failure of osteoclastic activity. There is enlargement of liver and spleen, anaemia and cranial nerve palsies. There can be variable modes of inheritance, both autosomal recessive and dominant types have been described.

   Four different types can be commonly recognised, which include the precocious type, the delayed type, the intermediate type and the tubular acidosis type.
2. *Imaging features:* The radiological findings in precocious type include generalized osteosclerosis, failure of corticomedullary differentiation and defective modelling of bones. This defective modeling of distal femora leads to the deformity called as "Erlenmeyer flask deformity".[21] A club-like appearance due to defective modeling frequently results, with presence of transverse striations **(Fig. 15A)**. Alternating areas of mature bone and sclerotic osseous tissue can give a "bone within bone" appearance.

   The entire skull is involved with the cartilaginous portion of the base being most severely involved. Calvaria is thick with dense inner and outer tables, broad diploic spaces with hair-on-end appearance and small cranial foramina. The skull base shows appreciable marrow activity, well shown by MR imaging. Osteomyelitis of the mandible is fairly common. The changes in spine include radiodense vertebral bodies with end plate sclerosis.

   In the delayed type, the findings are less severe compared to the precocious type. Osteosclerosis, defective undertubulation with thick cortex and a bone within bone appearance, characterize this type of osteopetrosis **(Figs. 15B and C)**.

   In intermediate type, there is bone sclerosis, primarily of the skull base with involvement of facial bones. Interference with normal bone modeling, bone within bone appearance and ischemic necrosis of femoral head an also be present.

   In the tubular acidosis type, there is osteopetrosis with renal tubular acidosis and intracerebral calcifications, primarily in basal ganglia and periventricular region. Other radiologic findings include obliteration of medullary cavity and pathologic fractures. A significant aspect of this type is progressive improvement of the abnormalities.

Pycnodysostosis:

1. *Clinical features:* It is transmitted as an autosomal recessive trait. Clinically, there are short limbs with tendency to fracture, irregular dentition and respiratory problems. Patients are usually short and less than 150 cm in height.
2. *Imaging features:* The radiologic findings include generalized osteosclerosis with thick sclerotic skull base. There is marked delay in closure of sutures with presence of wormian bones. The mandible is frequently hypoplastic with loss of normal angulation **(Fig. 16A)**. Changes in spine include sclerosis of vertebral bodies, segmentation anomalies and spondylolisthesis **(Fig. 16B)**. The bones of hand are short with hypoplasia or osteolysis of the distal phalanges **(Fig. 16C)**. The medullary cavity of tubular bones may be mildly narrow.

Osteopoikilosis:

1. *Clinical features:* This condition is asymptomatic and does not produce physical deformity. Male

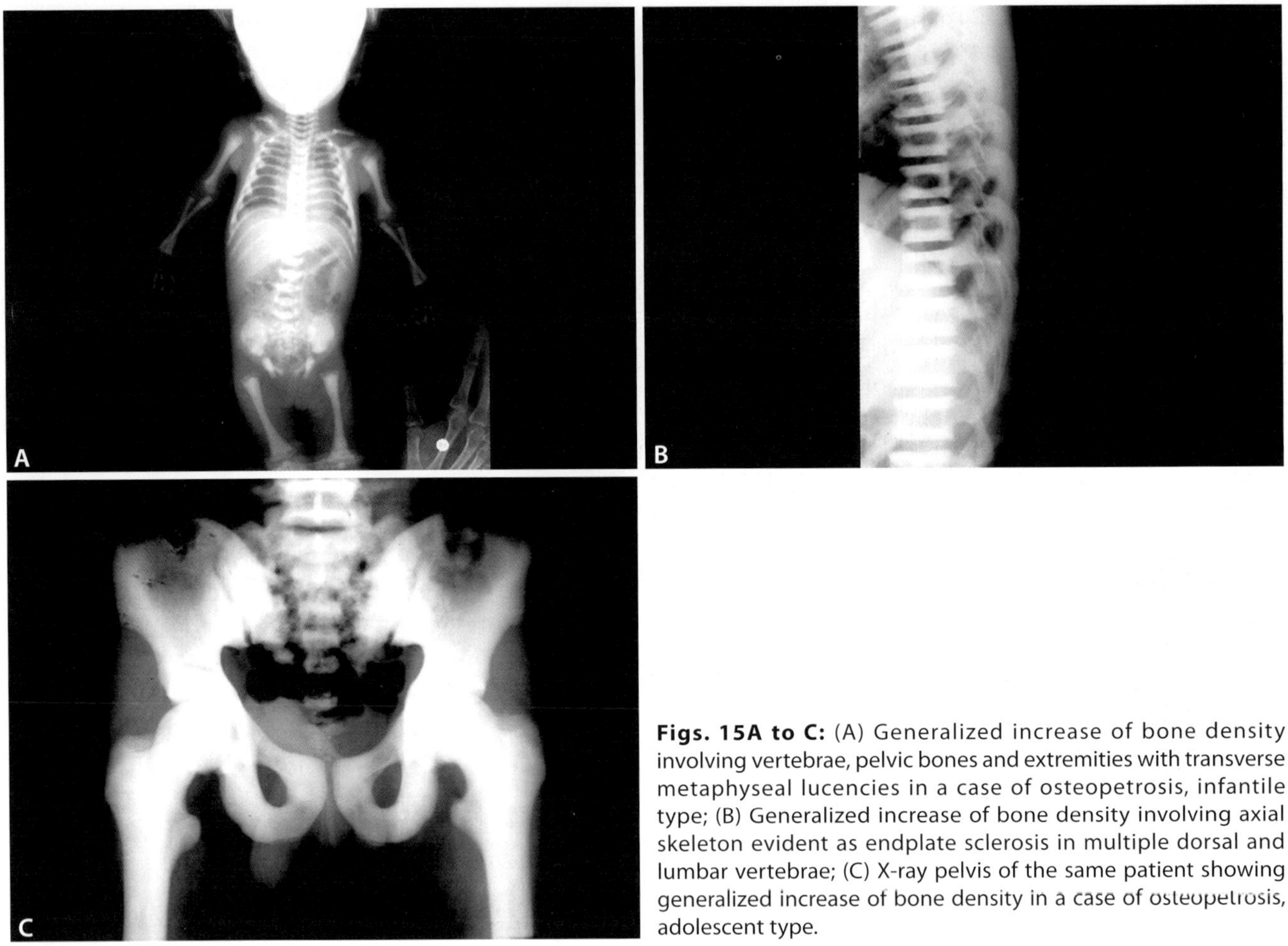

Figs. 15A to C: (A) Generalized increase of bone density involving vertebrae, pelvic bones and extremities with transverse metaphyseal lucencies in a case of osteopetrosis, infantile type; (B) Generalized increase of bone density involving axial skeleton evident as endplate sclerosis in multiple dorsal and lumbar vertebrae; (C) X-ray pelvis of the same patient showing generalized increase of bone density in a case of osteopetrosis, adolescent type.

preponderance is seen. The condition has been found to be associated with linear scleroderma. The disease is of little clinical consequence.

2. *Imaging features:* Punctate, rounded, and sometimes linear sclerotic densities of one to ten millimeters are seen in medullary cavities of compact bone. These densities predominate towards ends of long bones. The pelvis is affected frequently **(Fig. 17)**. The skull, ribs and spine are usually spared in this condition.

Osteopathia Striata:

1. *Clinical features:* The condition is usually asymptomatic, although sometimes it may be associated with vague joint pains.
2. *Imaging features:* There are multiple linear densities of varying width having an axial distribution, prominently seen in the ends of long bones. They usually extend into the epiphysis, where punctate and confluent opacities can occur **(Fig. 18)**. Except for skull and clavicles, the remaining skeleton can all be involved. It is a disease of little clinical consequence.

Melorheostosis:

1. *Clinical features:* It is also called Leri's disease. It is usually observed after three years of age. Severe pain is often the presenting symptom. Thickness and fibrosis of overlying skin is present. Tumors or malformations of blood vessels and lymphatics can be other cutaneous associations.
2. *Imaging features:* Multiple areas of dense hyperostosis are observed with a linear and segmental distribution corresponding to one or more dermatomes in this condition. Superficial cortical deposits are the rule, though the disease may also encroach the medullary cavity **(Fig. 19)**. The resulting contour has been likened to candle wax flowing down the margin of the bone. The disease is usually monomelic and involves bones in one limb. Bony overgrowth can occur. Soft tissue ossification commonly occurs in the periarticular region between two affected bones of a limb.

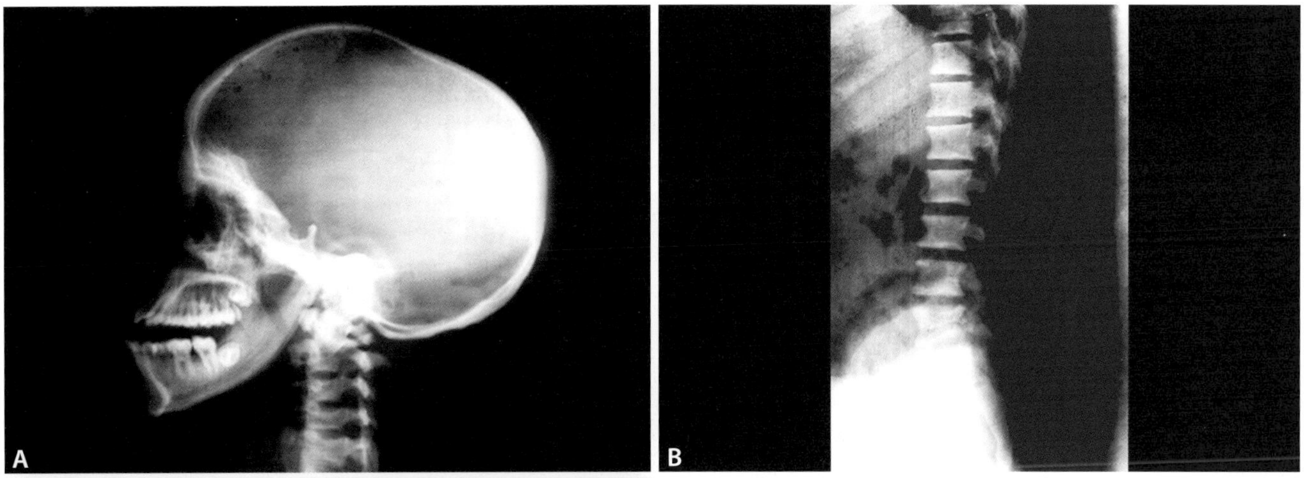

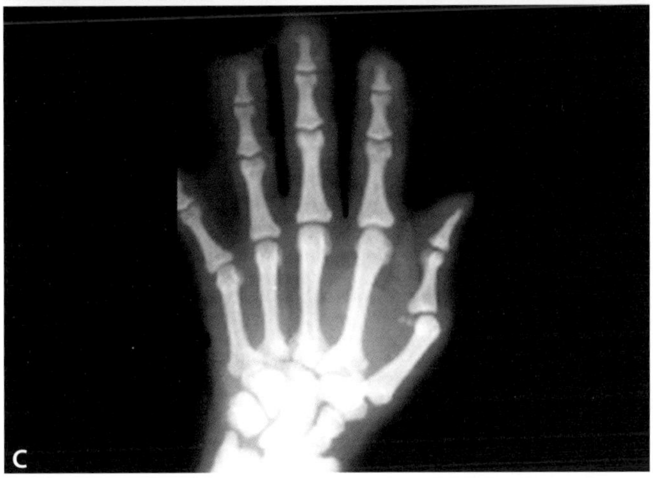

Figs. 16A to C: Skull lateral view showing widely open sutures, open anterior and posterior fontanelles with absent angle of mandible in a case of pyknodysostosis; (B) Increased bone density with spool-shaped lumbar vertebral bodies along with fractures involving pars interarticularis at multiple levels; (C) Increased bone density with acro-osteolysis, in a case of pyknodysostosis.

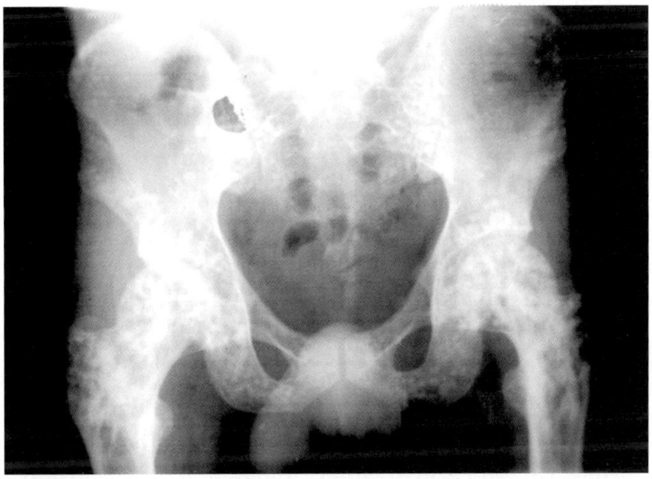

Fig. 17: Numerous small dense rounded opacities symmetrically involving the pubic bones and both femora, in a case of osteopoikilosis.

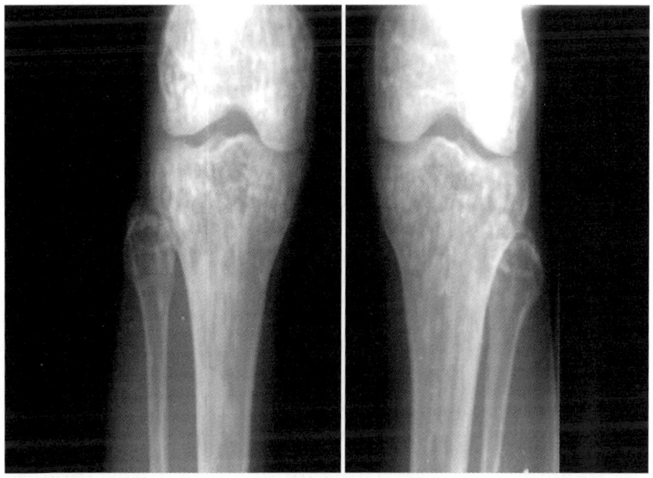

Fig. 18: Multiple linear opacities running vertically through the metadiaphysis and epiphysis with punctate opacities, in a case of osteopathia striata.

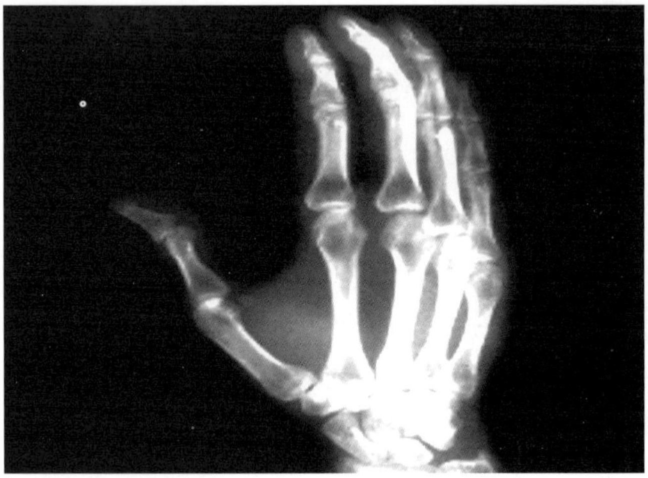

Fig. 19: Hyperostosis encroaching on the medulla of the proximal phalanges of the ring and middle fingers, in a case of melorheostosis.

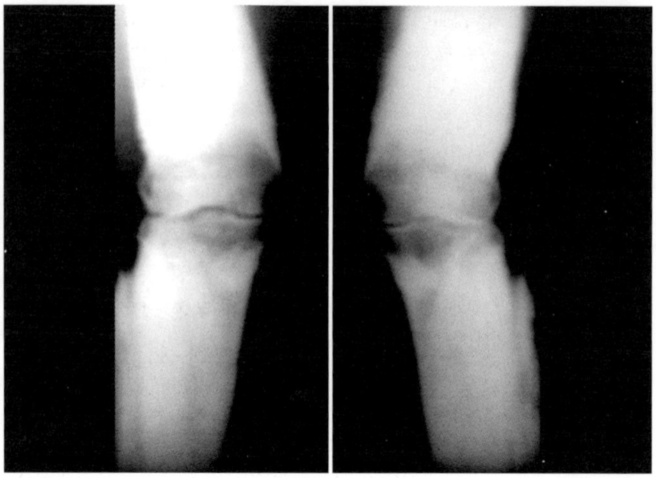

Fig. 20: Symmetrical (both periosteal and endosteal) new bone formation, obliterating the medullary cavity, sparing only the ends of the bones, in a case of diastrophic dysplasia.

Increased Bone Density with Diaphyseal Involvement

Diaphyseal dysplasia:

1. *Clinical features:* It is an autosomal dominant disorder with variability of expression with symptoms usually occurring in or after second decade, such as bone enlargement, abnormal gait, leg pain and muscle weakness. It is a generalized, bilaterally symmetric dysplasia of bone primarily involving the diaphysis and sparing the epiphysis. It is also called Camurati Engelmann disease.
2. *Imaging features:* The radiologic features include cortical thickening and diaphyseal sclerosis. The endosteal involvement is more than the periosteal involvement **(Fig. 20)**. Tibia, femur and humerus are commonly involved in decreasing order of frequency, while any bone can be involved. Sclerosis of skull base is common with encroachment of cranial nerves with associated complications. Changes in the spine include vertebral sclerosis, especially in the posterior parts of vertebral bodies and neural arches.

Craniodiaphyseal Dysplasia:

1. *Clinical features:* It is autosomal recessive disorder characterized by deformity of face, nasal and lacrimal obstruction and cranial nerve palsies.
2. *Imaging features:* The radiologic features include massive and progressive hyperostosis of the skull and facial bones with obliteration of the paranasal sinuses. Involvement of the long bones varies in severity, although cortical thickening and lack of normal modeling are typical. The ribs, clavicles and ilia are wide and sclerotic, whereas the changes in spine are mild and preferentially located in the vertebral arches.

Increased Bone Density with Metaphyseal Involvement

Pyle's Dysplasia:

It is a rare disorder with variable modes of transmission, and mild clinical symptoms, such as joint pain, muscular weakness, bone fragility and dental malocclusion.

The radiologic features of Pyle's dysplasia include marked expansion of the metaphyseal segments of the tubular bones leading to an Erlenmeyer flask appearance, especially in the distal portions of femur and proximal portions of the tibia and fibula. The changes in upper limb are milder. There is an abrupt transition between the cylindrical and flared portions of the bone. Minor involvement of skull can occur and includes mild sclerosis of vault and prominence of supraorbital region. The spine may show platyspondyly or biconcave vertebrae. The bones of pelvis, medial portions of the clavicles, and sternal ends of ribs are frequently expanded.

Craniometaphyseal Dysplasia:

1. *Clinical features:* It is clinically characterized by facial deformity, hypertelorism, broad mass at base of nose, nasal obstruction, deafness and dental malocclusion.
2. *Imaging features:* There is progressive sclerosis around the sutures with sclerosis of the skull base. In addition, there is obliteration of paranasal sinuses and loss of lamina dura of teeth. Osteosclerosis in

diaphysis of tubular bones is noted in infancy, which later disappears and is replaced by modelling defects. There is an addition metaphyseal expansion and club shaped epiphysis. Ribs and medial part of clavicles can be widened. Spine is rarely affected.

Frontometaphyseal Dysplasia:

1. *Clinical features:* Clinical manifestations include childhood onset, short trunk with long extremities, prominent supraorbital ridges, micrognathia and joint contractures.
2. *Imaging features:* The radiologic features of this dysplasia include calvarial hyperostosis, prominent supraorbital ridge, absent frontal sinuses, hypoplasia of angle and condylar processes of mandible, antegonial notching of body of mandible, flaring of the iliac wings with widening of ischial bones. Changes in tubular bones include fibular waviness and bowing, tibia recurvatum, elongation of metacarpal bones and phalanges with erosion and fusion of carpal and tarsal bones.

DYSOSTOSES

Dysostoses with Cranial and Facial Involvement

Craniosynostosis

1. *Clinical features:* There is local cessation of growth and distortion of calvarial configuration due to premature fusion of one or more cranial sutures.
2. *Imaging features:* Isolated closure of sagittal suture is encountered most frequently. Unilateral closure of lambdoid suture leads to flattening of back of head or plagiocephaly. Cloverleaf skull is associated with premature synostosis of multiple sutures.

Craniofacial Synostosis

Clinical features: Crouzon's syndrome is characterized by craniosynostosis, exophthalmos and midface recession. The disorder is caused by mutation in the gene for fibroblast growth factor. The skull is brachycephalic, with fusion of coronal, sagittal and lambdoid sutures, usually seen by three years of age. Hypertelorism, hypoplastic maxilla, hydrocephalus and spinal anomalies can also occur.

Dysostoses with Predominant Axial Involvement

Vertebral segmentation defects, Sprengel's deformity: Various vertebral segmentation defects can occur. Multiple block vertebrae are seen in cervico-oculo-acoustic syndrome or Wildervanck syndrome. Sprengel's deformity can occur as an isolated abnormality of the scapula, which is small, triangular, elevated and rotated, so that its medial border faces spine, or as a part of Klippel–Feil syndrome.

Osteo-onychodysostosis

Nail-patella dysplasia (Hereditary osteo-onychodysostosis) The radiological features include dysplastic abnormalities of knee, iliac bone, and elbow. Hypoplasia or absence of one or both patellae and asymmetry of condyles of the femur, tibia and humerus are characteristic. Flaring of the iliac crests associated with iliac horns is pathognomonic of this syndrome. The medial femoral condyle is enlarged while the lateral condyle is hypoplastic resulting in patellar instability and genu valgum. The elbow characteristically shows hypoplasia of the radial head, which is frequently subluxated with narrow neck of radius. The abnormalities in knee and elbow are more common than the abnormality of iliac bone. However, the iliac horns arising from posterior aspect of iliac bones near sacroiliac joint are generally bilateral and pathognomonic of this condition. The iliac bones by themselves are hypoplastic. Hypoplasia of scapula, carpal bones, presence of eleven pair of ribs and Madelung's deformity are less common findings.

Dysostosis with Predominant Involvement of Extremities

Dysostosis with predominant involvement of extremities can occur alone, or as a part of a widespread dysplasia. There can be various deformities affecting the limbs, for example, there can be partial or complete absence of limbs or fingers, radioulnar synostosis, polysyndactyly, clinodactyly.

Certain neonatal anomalies in hand, foot and arm can be a pointer to the presence of skeletal dysplasia. For instance, clinodactyly (finger curvature in medial or lateral plane) can be seen in Cornelia de Lange syndrome, Down syndrome, Nail-patella syndrome, radial hypoplasia or aplasia can be seen in Cornelia de Lange syndrome, Trisomy 18 **(Fig. 21)**, metacarpal hypoplasia can be seen in chondrodystrophia calcificans congenita, polydactyly in chondrodystrophia calcificans congenita, Ellis-van Creveld syndrome, syndactyly in acrocephalosyndactyly (Apert's syndrome), chondrodystrophia calcificans congenita, Cornelia de Lange syndrome, broad thumb in acrocephalosyndactyly camptodactyly (permanent finger flexion at the proximal interphalangeal joint due to contractures or fascial abnormality) in Morquio's syndrome and nail-patella syndrome.

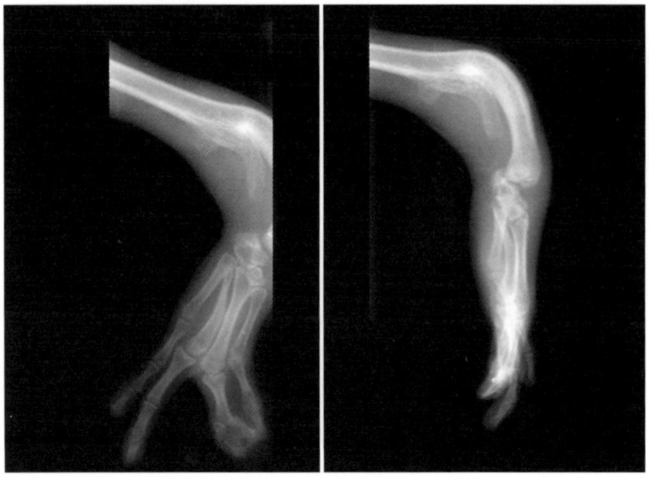

Fig. 21: Radial aplasia with curved ulna and absent thumb in a case of trisomy 18.

IDIOPATHIC MULTICENTRIC OSTEOLYSIS

1. *Clinical features:* The carpotarsal osteolysis syndromes include multicentric osteolysis with nephropathy, hereditary multicentric osteolysis and miscellaneous conditions characterized by localized osteolysis involving carpal and tarsal bones. Histologically, there is proliferation and hyperplasia of smooth muscle cells of synovial arterioles suggesting underlying vascular abnormity. The articular cartilage is replaced by fibrous tissue.
2. *Imaging features:* Radiologically, it is seen as progressive dissolution and disappearance of carpal and tarsal bones. Multicentric osteolysis with nephropathy is characteristically associated with tapering of adjacent tubular bones.

PRIMARY DISTURBANCE OF GROWTH

Cornelia de Lange Syndrome

1. *Clinical features:* Clinical features include bushy eyebrows meeting in midline, high forehead, depressed nasal bridge, excessive distance between nose and lips and antimongoloid slant.
2. *Imaging features:* Radiologic findings include small brachycephalic skull, small cervical spine, short proximally placed thumbs, clinodactyly involving fifth finger, small distal phalanges, hypoplasia of long bones, absent forearm bones with resultant elbow dislocation and retarded skeletal maturation.

Progeria

Progeria or premature aging is a rare disorder characterized by absence of hair, atrophic skin and failure to grow at normal rate. In first two years of life, the child develops degeneration of hair follicles, loss of subcutaneous fat, joint stiffness and poor growth. Skeletal hypoplasia is most evident in facial bones, mandible and hands. Fontanelle ossification is delayed. The tubular bones, ribs and calvaria are thin. The distal phalanges and clavicles are hypoplastic.

CONSTITUTIONAL DISEASES OF BONE WITH KNOWN PATHOGENESIS

Chromosomal Aberrations

Chromosomal aberrations due to morphologic change in the individual chromosomes with addition or deletion have been associated with diseases having effect on bony skeleton but have been kept out of definition of bony dysplasias, which in contrast continue to exert their effect throughout life. Failure of proper disjunction of sex chromosomes is seen in Turner and Klinefelter syndrome. Autosomal trisomy defects are usually result of nondisjunction or due to translocation involving autosomal chromosomes, as is seen in mongolism.

In Turner's syndrome clinically there is agenesis of the gonads, webbing of the neck and cubitus valgus. Radiological features include decreased density of bones, maldeveloped clavicles and slender ribs, depressed medial tibial condyle and shortening of the fourth metacarpal.

Down syndrome occurs due to chromosomal aberration involving 21 chromosome. The radiological features include brachycephalic skull with decreased interorbital distance, hypoplasia of nasal bones, eleven pairs of ribs, clinodactyly involving middle phalanx of fifth digit besides widespread defects including cardiac and gastrointestinal defects.

Primary Metabolic Abnormalities

Calcium Phosphorus Metabolism (Hypophosphatasia)

Four clinical groups are recognized, although distinction between them is not always possible due to the variability in presentation due to variable deficiency of alkaline phosphatase. These include the neonatal, infantile, childhood and adult form. The neonatal form presents soon after birth, the infants dying within six months of age, while most infants usually survive in infantile form of hypophosphatasia. The childhood form presents between six months and two years of age and is clinically less severe. Bone fragility and dental abnormalities are frequent in adult form of hypophosphatasia.

Imaging features: The radiological features in neonatal form include diffuse profound defective ossification with broad, irregular metaphyses, seen prominently at the wrists, knee and costochondral junctions. The cranial sutures also appear wide due to defective ossification. Fractures are common.

Infantile form is characterized by widening of cartilaginous growth plate and frayed and cupped metaphysis with the epiphysis showing spotty demineralisation. Mild irregularity of the diaphysis can also be evident due to defective mineralisation. The skull shows premature fusion with subsequent craniosynostosis, often with a brachycephalic configuration.[18]

The characteristic features in childhood form include bowed legs or knock knees, mild rachitic changes, premature loss of deciduous teeth and dental caries. Craniosynostosis is usually not present.

The adult form is characterized by presence of osteopaenia, Looser's zones and actual fractures.

The differential diagnosis of the neonatal form includes other fatal short limb dwarfism, osteogenesis imperfecta and severe rickets.

Mucopolysaccharidoses and Mucolipidoses

They are complex carbohydrate metabolism abnormalities. They can be diagnosed by means of specific metabolic test such as fibroblast culture and assay. The role of radiologist in this group of disorders is limited but important.

Mucopolysaccharidosis-I (Hurler's Syndrome):

1. *Clinical features:* It is a rare disorder of mucopolysaccharide metabolism and is transmitted as an autosomal dominant trait. Clinical features manifest in early infancy and include large head with eyes wide apart, shrunken bridge of the nose, everted lips, protruding tongue, poorly formed teeth, hepatosplenomegaly and dorsolumbar kyphosis. Progressive mental retardation and corneal opacities are invariably present with death occurring at a younger age compared to other mucopolysaccharidoses.
2. *Imaging features:* The radiological features of this disorder include macrocephaly, craniostenosis, J-shaped sella, atlantoaxial subluxation, ovoid vertebral bodies, hypoplasia of vertebra around thoracolumbar region **(Fig. 22)**. The changes in pelvis include hypoplasia of base of ilia, pseudoenlargement of acetabula and coxa valga. In the hands changes include pointing of proximal ends of metacarpal bones and shortening and widening of short tubular bones. Progressive hydrocephalus and deficient myelination can often be present. Hurler's syndrome may be confused with Morquio's syndrome, but changes in the spine, skull and long bones help in differentiating between the two conditions.

Mucopolysaccharidosis-IV (Morquio's Syndrome)

1. *Clinical features:* Clinical features include dwarfism with low dorsal kyphosis, flexion deformities of both hips and knees, knock knees and flat feet. The head is thrust forward and appears shrunken between high shoulders. Deformities become noticeable after one year of age.
2. *Imaging features:* The radiological features of this disorder are characteristic and include slightly rounded vertebral bodies in infancy with small anterior beak. In childhood, a central tongue or projection appears from the anterior aspect of vertebral bodies **(Fig. 23)**. In adults, the vertebrae are flat and rectangular with irregular margins. Hypoplasia of the dens is often present. There is anterior bowing of sternum with increased diameter of chest. Changes in pelvis include flaring of iliac wings with increased obliquity of acetabular roofs. The femoral capital epiphysis is dysplastic with resultant coxa valga. There is widening of metacarpals with pointed anterior ends and small and irregular carpals with slanting of distal articular surfaces of radius and ulna at the wrist. The long tubular bones show diminished growth, epiphyseal deformity and metaphyseal flaring.

   Differential diagnosis of Morquio's syndrome includes Hurler's syndrome, spondyloepiphyseal dysplasia and diastrophic dwarfism.

Mucolipidosis:

These are inherited as autosomal recessive trait and this group exhibits clinical features depending on the

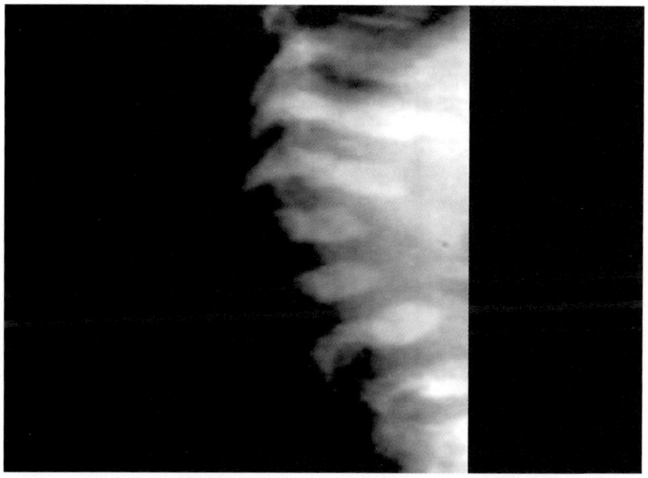

Fig. 22: Case of MPS-1 (Hurler's syndrome): Spine lateral view showing characteristic anteroinferior beaking in lumbar vertebrae.

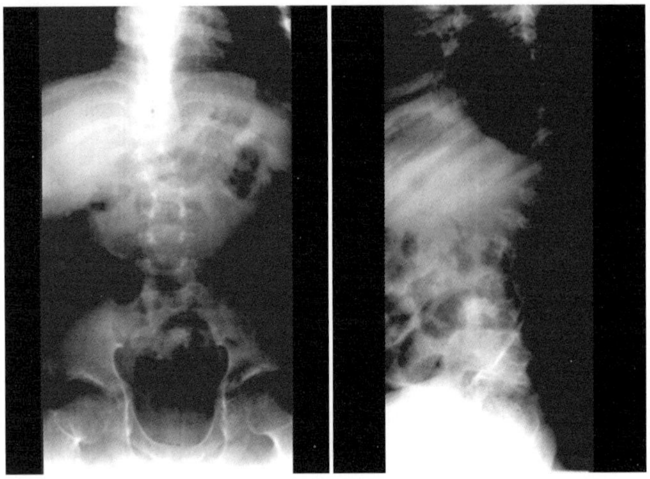

Fig. 23: Case of MPS-1V (Morquio's syndrome): Spine AP and lateral views showing generalized platyspondyly and characteristic central anterior tongue-like beak in multiple lumbar vertebrae with ape shaped pelvis.

deficiency of the enzyme involved. The radiologic features resemble those of mucopolysaccharidosis except that urinary excretion of mucopolysaccharides is not increased.

Bone Abnormalities Secondary to Disturbances of Extraskeleton Systems

Bone abnormalities can result secondary to endocrine, hematologic, neurologic, renal, gastrointestinal and cardiopulmonary diseases. These diseases of bone classified under "constitutional diseases of bone" are secondary abnormalities and not classified under skeletal dysplasias.

CONCLUSION

Methodical evaluation in some and pathognomonic features in others can lead to a specific diagnosis of skeletal dysplasia.

The establishment of a precise diagnosis is important for numerous reasons, such as genetic counseling, accurate recurrence risk, prenatal diagnosis in future pregnancies, prediction of adult height and most importantly, clinical management, including prevention of complications and disabilities.

REFERENCES

1. Camera G, Mastroiacovo P. Birth prevalence of skeletal dysplasias in the Italian multi-centric monitoring system for birth defects. In: Papadatos CJ, Bartsocas CS (Eds). Skeletal Dysplasias. New York: Alan R Liss; 1982.pp.441-9.
2. Spranger J. International classification of osteochondrodysplasias. Eur Pediatr. 1992;151:407-15.
3. Lachman Ralph S. International nomenclature and classification of the osteochondrodysplasias. Pediatr Radiol. 1998;28:737-44.
4. Frézal Jean, Le Merrer M, Chauvet ML. Osteochondrodysplasias, dysostosis, disorders of calcium metabolism, congenital malformations syndromes and other disorders. Pediatr Radiol. 1997;27:366-87.
5. Horton W. Advances in the genetics of human chondrodysplasias. Pediatr Radiol. 1997;27:422-27.
6. Superti-Furga Andrea, Bonafé Luisa, Rimoin David L. Molecular pathogenetic classification of genetic disorders of the skeleton. Am J Med Gene (Semin Med Genet). 2001; 106:282-93.
7. Behrman Richard E, Kliegman Robert M, Jenson Hal B. Nelson Textbook of Pediatrics, 16th edition. India reprint. Noida Harcourt Asia Pte Ltd, Thompson press (I) Ltd; 2000. pp.2113-36.
8. Kirks Donald R, Thorne Griscom N. Practical Pediatric Imaging-Diagnostic Radiology of Infants and Children. 3rd edition. Philadelphia, New York: Lippincott-Raven Publishers; 1999.
9. Deborah Krakow, Yasemin Alanay, Lauren P. Rimoin, et al. Evaluation of prenatal onset osteochondrodysplasias by ultrasonography; A retrospective and prospective analysis. Am J Med Genet A. 2008;1;146A[15]:1917-24.
10. Deborah Krakow, Ralph S Lachman, David L. Rimoin. Guidelines for prenatal diagnosis of fetal skeletal dysplasias. Genet Med. 2009;11[2]:127-33.
11. Edeiken's Roentgen Diagnosis of Diseases of Bone, 4th edition. Williams and Wilkins; 1990.p.2.
12. Kitoch Hiroshi, Lachman Ralph S, Brodie Steven G, et al. Extrapelvic ossification centers in thanatophoric dysplasia and platyspondylic lethal skeletal dysplasia. Pediatr Radiol. 1998;28:759-63.
13. Pozanski AK. Punctate epiphysis: a radiological sign not a disease. Pediatr Radiol. 1994;24:418-24.
14. Taybi H, Lachman RS. Radiology of syndromes, metabolic disorders and skeletal dysplasias. St Louis: Mosby Year Book Publications; 1996.
15. Sutton David. Textbook of Radiology and Imaging, 7th edition. Churchill Livingstone; 2003.p.2.
16. Lachman Ralph S. The cervical spine in the skeletal dysplasias and associated disorders. Pediatr Radiol. 1997;27:402-8.
17. Resnick Donald. Diagnosis of Bone and Joint Disorders, 4th edition. WB Saunders Company. An imprint of Elsevier Science; 2002.p.5.
18. Gledion Andres. Phalangeal cone shaped epiphyses of the hand: Their history, diagnostic sensitivity and specificity in cartilage hair dysplasia and the trichorhinophalangeal syndrome I and II. Pediatr Radiol. 1998;28:751-8.
19. Arabella I Leet, Mchael T Collins. Current approach to fibrous Dysplasia and McCune Albright syndrome J Child Orthop. 2007;1(1):3-17.
20. Murray Ronald O, Jacobson Harold G, Stoker Dennis J. The Radiology of Skeletal Disorders, Exercises in Diagnosis, 3rd edition. Churchill Livingstone; 1990.p.2.
21. Maha A Faden, Deborah Krakow, et al. Erlenmeyer Flask bone deformity in the skeletal dysplasias. Am J Med Genet A. 2009;149A(6):1334-45.

CHAPTER 145

Skeletal Maturity Assessment

Arun Kumar Gupta

INTRODUCTION

From the moment one is born until the time one has grown up, the bones go through a set of characteristic changes—the skeletal maturity or sometimes also referred to as bone age. Therefore, skeletal maturity is the only indicator of development that is available from birth to full maturity.[1] Skeletal maturity in pathological terms denotes consolidation of new tissues by calcification of the fibrous and cartilaginous elements. It is distinct from growth. In clinical terms one may describe each individual passing from a stage of "wholly immature" to a stage of "wholly mature" through a normal growth process. At any particular stage, one individual might be more or less mature than another individual.

MEASUREMENT OF MATURITY

Maturity can be measured by observing certain events which occur in all individuals along the "Road to full maturity". These are called developmental milestones,[2] which could be dental, skeletal or pubertal development (secondary sexual characters, i.e. pubic hair, breast development, penis development).

In an ideal situation, the developmental milestones should occur in all the individuals, invariably in the same order and should cover the entire developmental span evenly and completely. Only skeletal maturity provides developmental milestones closest to such an ideal situation. It is, therefore, the most commonly used parameter of maturity in clinical practice.

In addition, the method employed to assess 'skeletal maturity' is noninvasive, inexpensive and independent of body size, weight and chronological age. All these advantages make assessment of maturity by 'skeletal maturity' method an ideal clinical tool.

Skeletal Maturity Assessment: Why is it Necessary?

Skeletal maturity assessment is required in clinical practice for two major reasons: (i) in pediatric endocrinological problems and growth disorders; (ii) for medicolegal reasons.

- In the field of pediatric endocrinology, skeletal maturity assessment is not only essential but highly crucial for a number of reasons:[2]
  - For diagnosing underlying cause in short stature children with growth delay **(Fig. 1)**
  - For reassuring young people with nonpathological but unusual growth delay
  - Monitoring growth hormone and anabolic steroid therapy
  - Monitoring treatment in various endocrinopathies, e.g. hypothyroidism, congenital adrenal hyperplasia
  - In the differential diagnosis of sexual precocity
  - For prediction of adult height
  - For selection of children in sports
  - Public health reasons—Comparison of environmental, dietary and other factors between different populations.

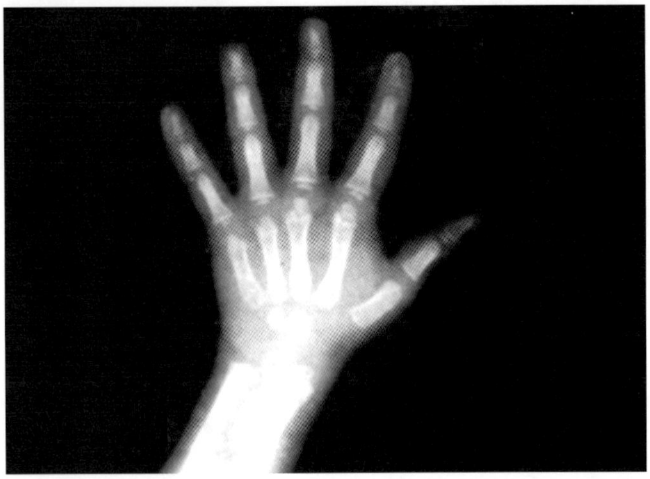

Fig. 1: Radiograph of left hand and wrist of a male child. Chronological age: 9 years and 9 months. Bone age, TW2 method: RUS-2.9 years, CS-2.3 years, 20 bones, Bone age-2.7 years (RUS, radius, ulna and short bones; CS, carpal score).

- For medicolegal reasons, estimation of age of an individual is important both for the medical jurist and lawyers. The gravity of offence is dependent upon particular age and also certain rights are given to the persons only at certain age.[3] Estimation of age, is therefore, of considerable importance from the point of view of administration of justice. This is important in a number of situations: identification, employment, criminal responsibility, judicial punishment, consent for marriage, rape, criminal abortion, prostitution, etc.[3]

Most difficult problem arises in estimation of age of adolescent girls. Period of adolescence extends from puberty to full maturity.

Factors to be taken into consideration for estimation of age are:[3]

- Dentition, i.e. number of teeth in each jaw
- Appearance of hair in the armpits and on pubis
- Development of breasts
- Appearance of first menstrual period
- Height, weight, general configuration and development of body
- Radiological examination of joints.

Methods to Assess Skeletal Maturity

Skeletal maturity in an individual child is assessed by comparing his or her state of bone development with the standards that have already been evolved from examination of radiographs of normal children.[2-4] Different methods use different standards for determining skeletal maturity. The three important methods are as follows:

1. Appearance and fusion of ossification centers.
2. Greulich and Pyle atlas method (G–P method).
3. Tanner and Whitehouse II method (TW2 method).

Appearance and Fusion of Ossification Centers

The earliest method for assessing skeletal maturity was by observing the time of appearance and fusion of various ossification centers.

Although this method has the advantage of being simple, quick and easy to calculate, it has significant drawbacks[5-7] and the two major ones are as follows: First, ossification centers especially those of carpal bones may have extremely variable appearance and fusion time **(Fig. 2)** even on the two sides of the same individual, and secondly the bone age calculated by this method usually has a wide range, thereby, diminishing its clinical usefulness in pediatric endocrine diseases.

For these reasons, it became apparent that this method was neither valid nor reliable and hence inadequate and unsatisfactory for estimating skeletal maturity in children with pediatric endocrine diseases where crucial decisions for treatment are based to a large extent on this information.[7]

However, this method still has its utility in medicolegal cases.[3,8] This is more so in adolescent girls involved in rape, kidnapping and prostitution where courts directive will change depending on age. Also, whether to try a boy or girl involved in some offence under juvenile act or not will depend on his/her age.

Radiology plays a crucial role in all these cases.[3] However, it is important to remember that radiological bone age must be interpreted along with other clinical parameters of growth before final decision.

For Indian children, standards have been established by a number of workers.[3,7-11] Using prepared charts the degree of skeletal development or 'bone age' can be calculated readily. Different sets of radiographs are required for bone age estimation depending upon the chronological age, e.g.

- PA radiograph of wrist and hand
- Elbow, knee, shoulder—either one or both ends depending upon expected age
- Pelvis AP for iliac crest appearance and fusion.

At AIIMS two published data for children from Delhi are followed[8,9] for calculating bone age by this method.

Greulich and Pyle (G–P) Method

In 1940, Greulich and Pyle published an atlas of standards of skeletal maturity based on longitudinal studies in 1930s of a relatively small number of Euro-American children living in Cleveland who were above average in economic and educational status.[12] This atlas was the turning point in establishing scientific standards of skeletal maturity. It is still the most widely used method in the Western countries due to its relative simplicity to use.

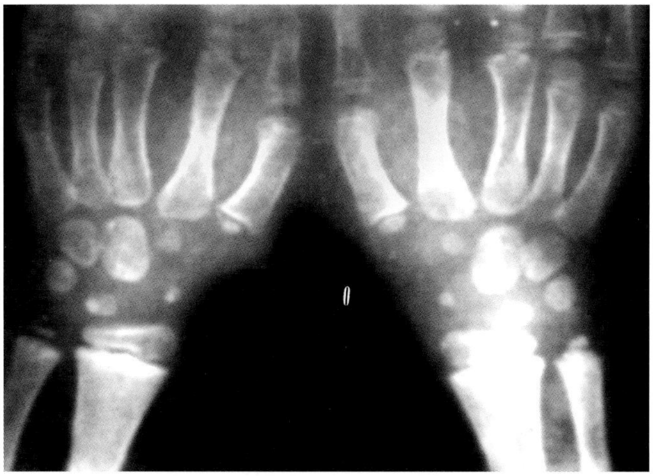

Fig. 2: Posteroanterior radiograph of both wrists of a 14 years male. Note asymmetrical appearance of carpal centers on the two sides, a major drawback of the technique using 'appearance-fusion' of centers as the basis.

The atlas consists of a set of standard (typical) radiographs of the wrist and hand representing a particular bone age at some 30 points along the maturity scale. Standards for boys and girls are separate since girls mature earlier than boys. In order to determine the skeletal maturity of a child, the user should match the radiograph under question "as close as possible" to one of the plates in the atlas and the closest match represents that child's bone age. Thus a bone age of "12" means the child is as mature as the 'average 12 years old'.

Although the atlas for G–P method is most commonly used as described above but the same atlas also describes 'maturity indicators' for individual bones which forms the basis for the Tanner and Whitehouse method.

Popularity of G–P method is due to its simple methodology providing accurate information and similar reproducibility.[13] However, two important drawbacks are[2] subjectivity of matching process and the scale used for expressing maturity, i.e. maturity is expressed by 'most likely' chronological age after the matching process and this 'most likely' age is then designated as 'bone age'. Some studies found G-P method to be inaccurate.[14]

Tanner and Whitehouse Method

Tanner et al. in 1962 revolutionized skeletal maturity assessment by introducing the bone specific scoring system.[2] The study was carried out in an average socioeconomic level British (Scottish) children in 1950s. It was later modified to TW2 method in 1975. The conclusion drawn from the greatest drawback of G–P method was that the maturity scale should be defined in a manner which does not refer directly to age. In TW2 method this disadvantage was eliminated.[2] Till date this is the most accurate and reliable method for skeletal maturity assessment.

TW2 method is based on the principle that each bone develops to a reasonable, constant final shape and a sequence of recognizable state can be defined right from the appearance to the final shape all along the developmental journey. Each bone is thus classified into eight or nine stages (A to H or I) to which weighted scores are assigned. Boys and girls have different scores for the same stage of a bone. Each stage differs from the next by 'maturity indicators', i.e. slight change in shape which is presented both in visual form as well as written descriptions by the side of each stage in the atlas. While calculating skeletal maturity, both the visual and the descriptive information are used for assigning the stage but in case of any doubt, latter, i.e. descriptive information is used for making the final decision.

Technique

For TW2 method a posteroanterior radiograph of the left hand and wrist is used. During positioning, it is important to keep the long axis of the middle finger, forearm and arm in direct line and also upper arm and forearm in the same horizontal plane. Centering is done on the third metacarpal head at a film focus distance of 30 inches (75 cm).

X-ray plate is put up for viewing with fingers pointing upwards and thumb on the right side of the viewer **(Fig. 3)**.

In this method, 20 bones are assessed and score is assigned to them. The scores are summed up. Three separate maturity scoring systems are derived, i.e. carpal score (CS) for the 7 carpals (out of the eight carpals pisiform is not considered for calculations), the Radius-Ulna-Short bone (RUS) score for 13 bones comprising the radius, ulna and short bones of hand (I, III and V fingers only) and finally the TW2-20 bone score which combines both the carpal and the RUS components. For each of these three scoring systems, different 'weighted scores' are assigned. At the end of the atlas a series of tables as well as centile standard curves are given for each of these three bone age scores from which 'bone age' can be directly read for a given total score **(Figs. 4 to 6)**.

Finally, three bone ages are thus obtained:

1. RUS bone age.
2. Carpal bone age.
3. 20 bone-bone age.

TW2 method is useful till the age of 18 years (RUS and 20 bone-bone age) in boys and till 16 years in girls (RUS and 20 bone-bone age). However, upper limit for carpal bone age is 15 years in boys and 13 years in girls.

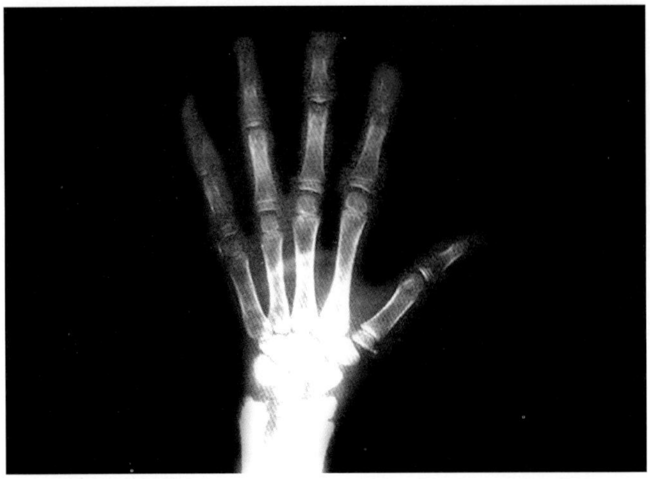

Fig. 3: While reviewing the radiograph of left hand and wrist by TW2 method, X-ray plate is put up with fingers pointing upwards and thumb directed to viewer's right side.

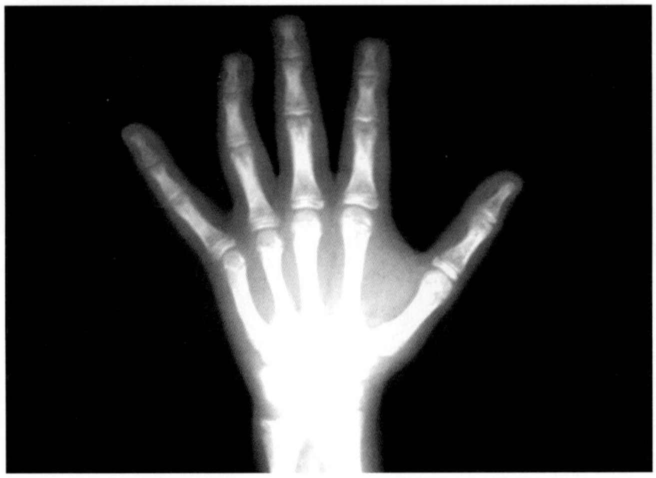

Fig. 4: *Female*: Chronological age is 11 years. RUS bone age is 11.9 years. Both matching.

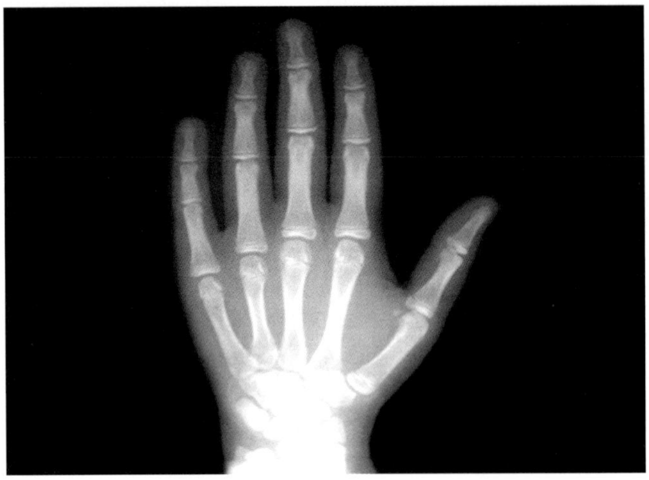

Fig. 5: An 8-year-old female. RUS bone age is 13.2 years. Accelerated bone age.

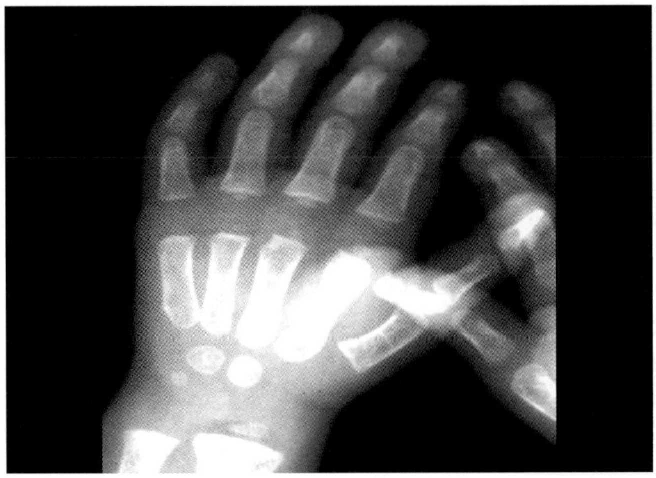

Fig. 6: Advantage of TW2 over conventional. By conventional method age is 3.7 +/–1.5 years. RUS age is 1.8 years. Chronological age 1.6 matches with RUS.

Comparison of G–P and TW2 Methods

A number of studies have compared the two standard methods. G–P method is easy and faster to do while TW2 is a more laborious, time consuming technique and requires more training. Bone age was found to be closer to chronological age by TW2 method.[15] However, TW2 was less reproducible between observers in this study.[15] The conclusion of most studies[13-17] is to use one method, preferably TW2 method, when performing serial measurements on an individual patient.

Computer-assisted Skeletal Age Scores

To eliminate the various sources of inter- and intraobserver errors associated with TW2 method (as well as for G–P method and even for carpal bone maturation) a number of studies[18-22] have reported use of computer systems. Almost all of them found computer-aided systems to be reliable with results close to that with experts interpretation. With time, TW2 method may become easy and a routine procedure with the help of these computer programs.

Ultrasound-based Bone Age Calculation

In November 2003, a German company called Sunlight introduced an ultrasound-based device to test skeletal age in children and adolescents.[23] In this method of bone age estimation, the child need not be referred to some specialized center but can be performed at the pediatrician's clinic with results in years and months available on the spot. Results are reported to be closely related to those produced by traditional method of Greulich and Pyle atlas.

But this needs larger studies at various centers by independent workers before finally it can be accepted as a routine technique.

INDIAN SCENE

Skeletal maturation is dependent not only on intrinsic factors such as genetic, racial, familial and hormonal but also on extrinsic factors like socioeconomic status, nutrition, chronic illness and climate. When there is interplay of so many factors then the standards for one population may not be applicable to another population. Ideally each country, even within each country different regions, should establish their own standards through longitudinal (or at least cross-sectional) studies of normal children. However, due to an ethical issue of exposing normal children to radiation hazard such studies have not been carried out in large numbers. The next best thing is to apply well-established methods to our own population and compare the results. From India few studies[7,24] have been carried out using both G–P and TW2 methods to assess skeletal maturity. Maniar[7] assessed Indian children with G–P method but found progressively increasing delay after second year of life. This method was therefore not found applicable to Indian children by the author.[7]

On the other hand, Maniar[7] applied the same set of radiographs as above to TW2 method. At any age between one to seven years, the difference was found to be less than 0.8 years. Hence, TW2 method was found to be by far the best method applicable to Indian children. Our experience at AIIMS[25] in 100 normal healthy children is similar (unpublished data) and we concluded that TW2 method can be directly applied to Indian children. TW2 has been a standard method used in all pediatric endocrinology OPD patients at AIIMS for the last two decades.

CONCLUSION

To conclude, despite the difficulties of assessing bone age, and the assumptions on which various methods are based, skeletal maturity assessment is clinically relevant in that it provides the only means of assessing rates of maturational change throughout the growing period.[1] Of the various methods available, TW2 is the most accurate method, and it can be applied directly to Indian population. However, this method requires correct positioning, precise radiographic technique and skilled interpretation. Awareness amongst the pediatricians and radiologists of India about TW2 method and its advantages is essential before it can become part of routine workup in every department all over the country. For medicolegal purposes however method of appearance and fusion of ossification centers continues to be in use because age groups covered under MLC problems cannot be evaluated by other two methods.

REFERENCES

1. Cox LA. The biology of bone maturation and ageing. Acta Paediatr Suppl. 1997;423:107-8.
2. Tanner JM, Whitehouse RH, Cameron N, et al. Assessment of Skeletal Maturity and Prediction of Adult Height (TW2 method) (2nd edn). London: Academic Press; 1983.
3. Kangne RN, Sami SA, Deshpande VL. Age estimation of adolescent girls by radiography. JFMT 1999;16(1):20-6.
4. How is skeletal age measured? http://vms.cc.wmich.edu/~Anemone/anth354/tsld091.htm.
5. Kovi R, Korner A, Varkony J, et al. Bone age discrepancy on hand radiographs. Pediatr Radiol. 2000;30(7):500.
6. Marshall WA. Individual variations in rate of skeletal maturation. Nature. 1969; 221(195):91.
7. Maniar B. Skeletal maturity in Indian children. Indian J Pediatr. 1987;54:295-302.
8. Modi's Medical Jurisprudence and Toxicology; 1999.
9. Jain S. Estimation of age from 13 to 21 years. JFMT. 1999; 16(1): 27-30.
10. Bajaj ID, Bhardwaj OP, Bhardwaj S. Appearance and fusion of important ossification centers. A study in Delhi population. Indian J Med Res. 1967;55:1064-7.
11. Sharat S, Khanduja PC, Agarwal KN, et al. Skeletal growth in school children. Indian Pediatric 1970;7:98-108.
12. Greulich WW, Pyle SI. Radiographic atlas of skeletal development of hand and wrist. Stanford: Stanford University Press; 1950.
13. King DG, Steventon DM, O'Sullivan MP, et al. Reproducibility of bone ages when performed by radiology registrars: An audit of Tanner and Whitehouse II versus Greulich and Pyle methods. BJR. 1994;801(67):848-51.
14. Gilli G. The assessment of skeletal maturation. Horm Res. 1996; 45(2):49-52.
15. Cole AJ, Webb L, Cole TJ. Bone age estimation: A comparison of methods. BJR. 1988;728(61):683-6.
16. Benso L, Vannelli S, et al. Main problems associated with bone age and maturity evaluation. Horm Res. 1996; 45(2):42-8.
17. Bull RK, Edwards PD, Kemp PM, et al. Bone age assessment: A large scale comparison of the Greulich and Pyle, and Tanner and Whitehouse (TW2) methods. Arch Dis Child. 1999; 81:172-3.

18. Canovas F, Banegas C, Cyteval M, et al. Carpal bone maturation assessment by image analysis from computed tomography scans. Horm Res. 2000;54:6-13.
19. Drayer NM, Cox LA. Assessment of bone age by Tanner and Whitehouse method using a computer-aided system. Acta Paediatr Suppl. 1994;406:77-80.
20. Frisch H, Riedl S, Wadhor T. Computer-aided estimation of skeletal age and comparison with bone age evaluation by the method of Greulich-Pyle and Tanner-Whitehouse. Pediatr Radiol. 1996;26(3):226-31.
21. Sato A, Ashizawa K, et al. Setting up an automated system for evaluation of bone age. Endocr J. 1999;46:597-600.
22. Tanner JM, Gibbons RD. A computerized image analysis system for estimating Tanner-Whitehouse 2 bone age. Horm Res. 1994;42(6):282-7.
23. Sunlight introduces Ultrasound-based bone age testing. http://www9.medica.de/cgi-bin/md.../content.cgi?lang=2 and ticket=g_u_e_s_t and oid= 11275 and print= 1/1/99.
24. Prakash S, Cameron N. Skeletal maturity of well-off children in Chandigarh, North India. Ann Hum Biol. 1981;8:175-80.
25. Gupta AK, Menon PSN, Seth V. Skeletal maturity by TW2 method in normal, healthy children at AIIMS (unpublished data).

CHAPTER 146

Spinal Dysraphism

Raju Sharma, Ankur Gadodia

INTRODUCTION

Spinal dysraphism is one of the most common congenital disorders associated with significant morbidity and mortality with estimated incidence of approximately 0.05–0.25 per 1000 births.[1] It can be defined as an incomplete fusion of midline mesenchymal, bony and neural structures.[2]

Spinal dysraphism is broadly classified into open and closed type. Most of the open spinal dysraphic states can be detected prenatally using ultrasound or fetal MRI. Postnatal imaging is usually performed to look for associated CNS anomalies (hydrocephalus, Chiari malformation), and in postoperative patients presenting with progressive neurological deficit to look for any treatable cause. Most of the closed spinal dysraphic states remain asymptomatic at birth and are suspected in the presence of high risk cutaneous markers, or when these children present with neurological deficit later in life.[3]

MRI is the modality of choice for evaluating spinal dysraphism.[4-6] It is helpful in the classification, diagnosis and treatment planning of these disorders.

CLASSIFICATION

Most of the dysraphic spinal states can be explained on the basis of specific abnormality in early embryonic development which spans over the period of 3rd–8th weeks of intrauterine life, and classification based on embryology has been proposed **(Table 1)**. Since, our understanding of human embryology is likely to evolve, this classification is also likely to change over a period of time. Recently, Paolo Tortori-Donati et al.[5,6] proposed a classification system based on clinicoradiological features **(Fig. 1)**, which is now widely accepted and followed. Spinal dysraphism is classified into two categories: Open spinal dysraphism

Table 1: Embryological classification of spinal dysraphism

• Anomalies of gastrulation • *Disorders of notochordal integration*: – Dorsal enteric fistula – Neurenteric cysts – Split cord malformations (diastematomyelia) – Dermal sinus • *Disorders of notochord formation*: – Caudal regression syndrome – Segmental spinal dysgenesis
• *Anomalies of primary neurulation*: – Myelomeningocele – Myeloschisis • *Lipomas with dural defect*: – Lipomyelomeningocele – Lipomyeloschisis • Intradural lipoma
• *Anomalies of secondary neurulation and retrogressive differentiation*: – Filar lipoma – Tight filum terminale – Abnormally elongated spinal cord – Persistent terminal ventricle – Terminal myelocystocele
• *Anomalies of unknown origin*: – Cervical myelocystocele – Meningocele

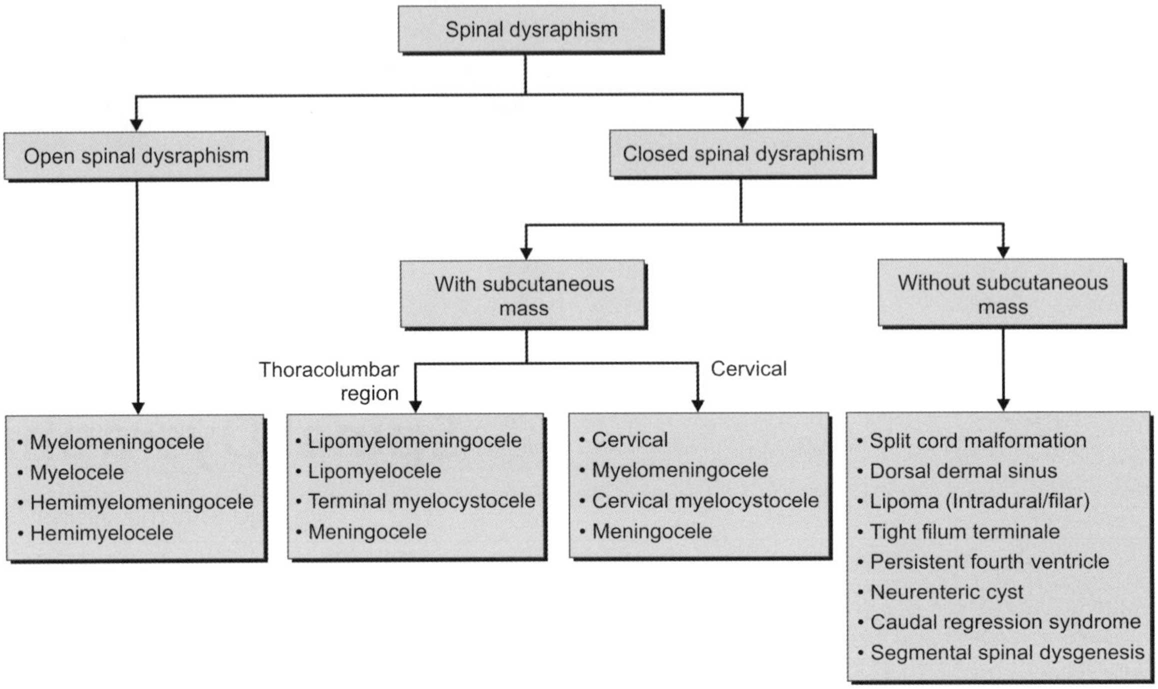

Fig. 1: Clinicoradiological classification proposed by Tortori–Donati et al.

(OSD) and closed spinal dysraphism (CSD). Neural tissue is exposed to the environment in OSDs, whereas CSDs are covered by skin, with cutaneous markers present in up to 50% of cases.

First step in the evaluation of patient with dysraphism is thorough clinical assessment. The child's back should be evaluated to look for presence/absence of skin covering, back mass and cutaneous stigmata of dysraphism **(Table 2)** **(Figs. 2A to C)**.[3,5,6]

EMBRYOLOGY

It is vital to know the development of the spinal cord to understand the different types of spinal dysraphism. The development of the bony spine and intraspinal contents begins in the first month of gestation.[7,8] The spinal cord develops from ectoderm, and the development occurs during three stages: neurulation, canalization and retrogressive differentiation. During the first week of gestation, there is a proliferation of ectodermal cells along the surface of the embryo to form the primitive streak. This is the neural plate which forms a groove in the midline and during the third week of gestation it begins to fold laterally. The folds begin to approach each other dorsally near the midline at the neural groove and the neural plate thus closes to form the neural tube. This is referred to as the stage of neurulation.

Table 2: Cutaneous lesions associated with spinal dysraphism.

• *High index of suspicion*: – Hypertrichosis – Atypical dimples – Acrochordons/pseudo-tails/true tails – Lipomas – Hemangiomas – Aplasia cutis or scar – Dermoid cyst or sinus
• *Low index of suspicion*: – Telangiectasia – Capillary malformation (port-wine stain) – Hyperpigmentation – Melanocytic nevi – Teratomas

Simultaneous with the stage of neurulation, the overlying ectoderm of the skin separates from the neural tube and fuses in the midline. The perineural mesenchyme grows around the neural tube to form the meninges, bone and muscle. Majority of the dysraphic states including myelomeningocele, myelocele and lipomyelomeningocele are thought to occur at this stage of development of the spine and spinal cord.

During the next stage called canalization, the caudal end of the neural tube elongates into a caudal cell mass and ependyma lines a central tubular structure. It is believed that persistence of portions or abnormal development of

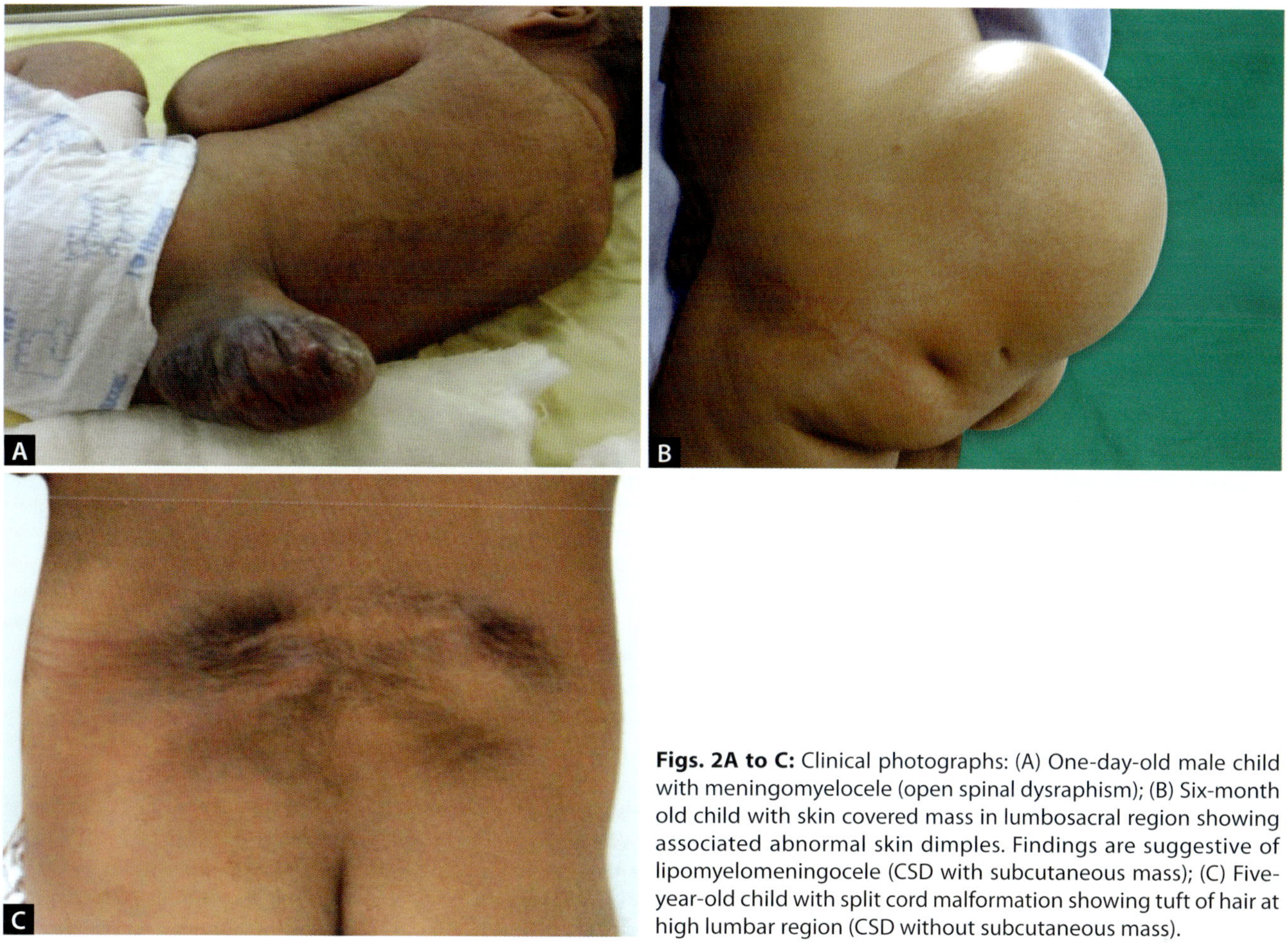

Figs. 2A to C: Clinical photographs: (A) One-day-old male child with meningomyelocele (open spinal dysraphism); (B) Six-month old child with skin covered mass in lumbosacral region showing associated abnormal skin dimples. Findings are suggestive of lipomyelomeningocele (CSD with subcutaneous mass); (C) Five-year-old child with split cord malformation showing tuft of hair at high lumbar region (CSD without subcutaneous mass).

the caudal cell mass may give rise to intradural lipoma, sacral teratoma and tethered low lying spinal cord.

Finally, during the stage of retrogressive differentiation (between 5 and 6 weeks), there is a decrease in the size of the central lumen and in the caudal cell mass and formation of the spinal cord, conus medullaris and filum terminale. The underlying cause for different types of spinal dysraphism is thought to be an insult—either genetic or acquired, that interferes with the normal process of neurulation, canalization or retrogressive differentiation.

IMAGING MODALITIES

Magnetic resonance imaging (MRI) is the imaging modality of choice in the diagnosis and characterization of spinal dysraphism. Other modalities play a supplemental role.

Plain radiographs (anteroposterior and lateral views) are mandatory for evaluation of the vertebral column.[5,9] The findings seen on plain radiographs include focal spina bifida, widened spinal canal, scoliosis, segmentation anomalies like block vertebrae, butterfly vertebrae and other congenital abnormalities. Bony spur may be seen in cases of diastematomyelia. Radiographs are used as preliminary screening examination that can help to guide the further imaging work up.

Ultrasonography is primarily useful in the antenatal diagnosis of spinal dysraphism **(Figs. 3 to 5)** and is also of some use in the neonate and infant.[4] It becomes progressively less useful as ossification of posterior elements proceeds during the first year of life. Prenatal sonography can detect the open widened neural arch with flared laminae, can show the meningomyelocele sac and detect hydrocephalus and other associated cranial anomalies. Direct sonography of the sac in children using high frequency transducers can provide information regarding the contents of the sac. However, for complete and more detailed information, an MR scan is usually required.

CT is useful in demonstration of the bony spur in cases of split cord malformation. Myelography and postmyelogram CT were used prior to the advent of MRI.

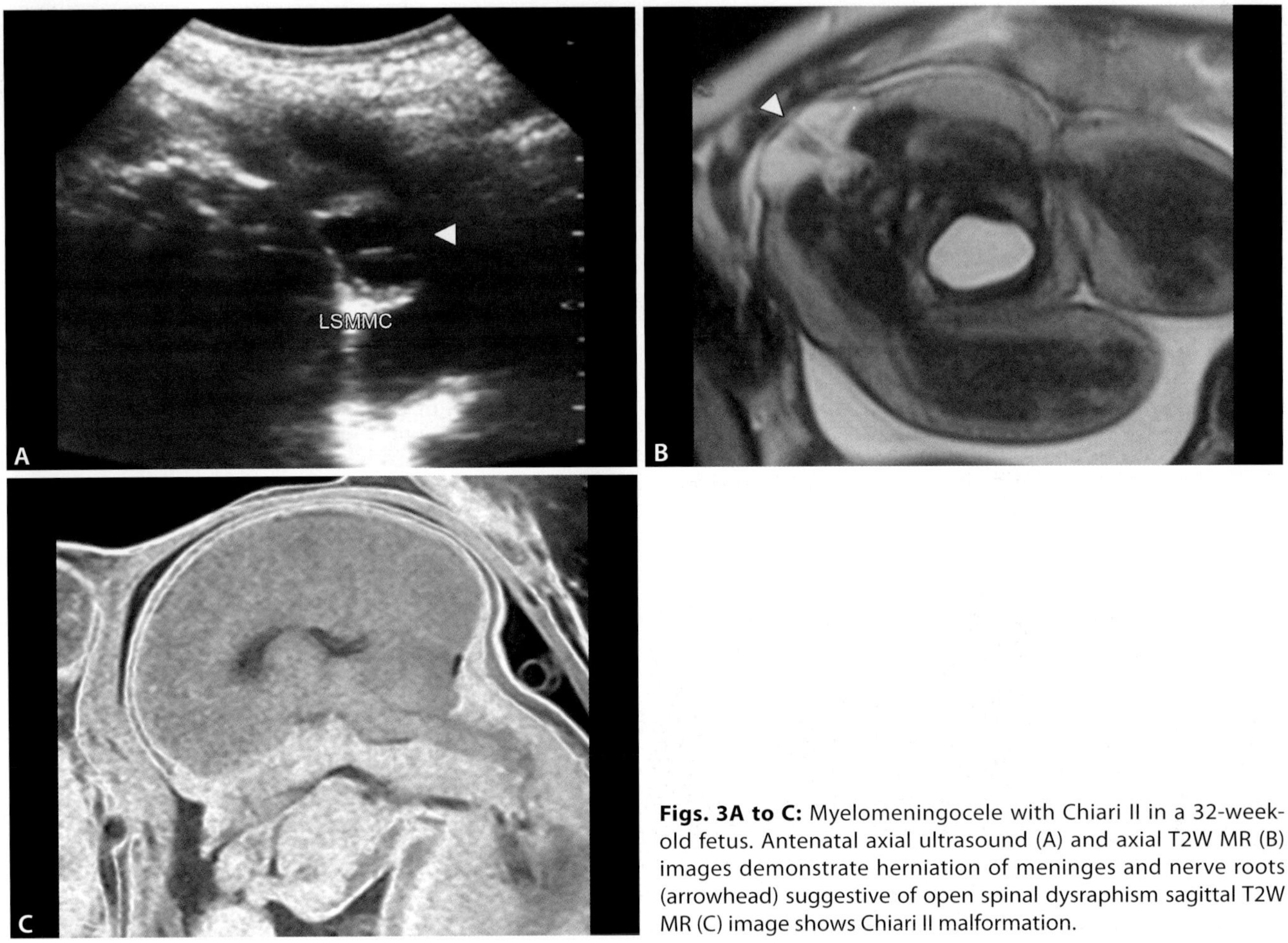

Figs. 3A to C: Myelomeningocele with Chiari II in a 32-week-old fetus. Antenatal axial ultrasound (A) and axial T2W MR (B) images demonstrate herniation of meninges and nerve roots (arrowhead) suggestive of open spinal dysraphism sagittal T2W MR (C) image shows Chiari II malformation.

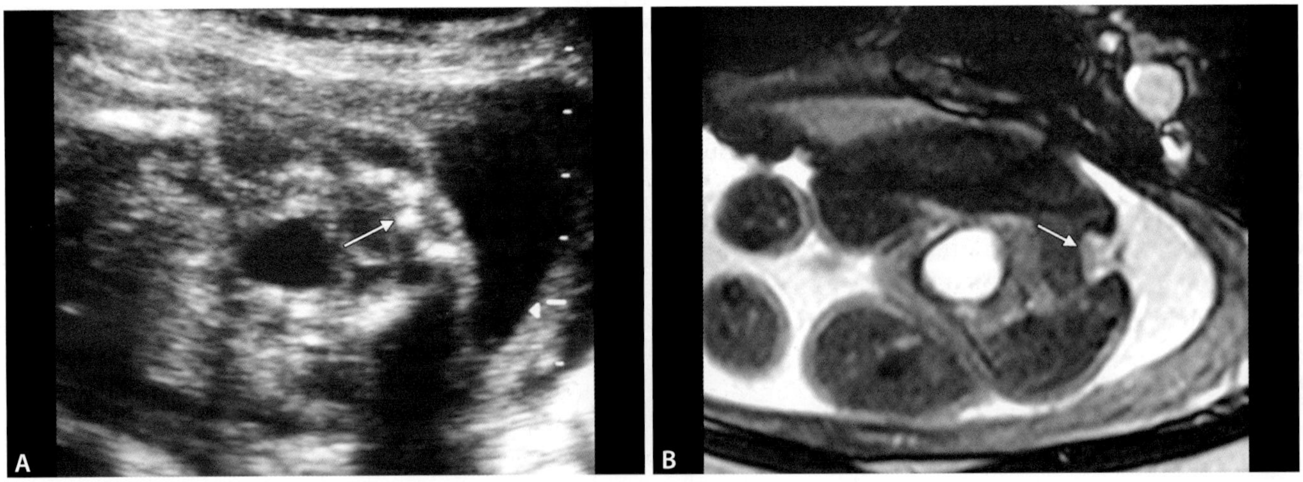

Figs. 4A and B: Meningocele with Chiari II in a 26-week-old fetus. Antenatal axial ultrasound (A) axial T2W (B) images demonstrate widening of the spinal canal with absence of posterior elements. Neural placode is flushed with the skin surface (arrows).

MRI provides an accurate and noninvasive method for evaluating spinal dysraphism, making it the modality of choice. The excellent contrast resolution, wide field of view and multiplanar images allow evaluation of the entire spinal cord, contents of the back mass; detect cord tethering, associated syringomyelia, Chiari malformation

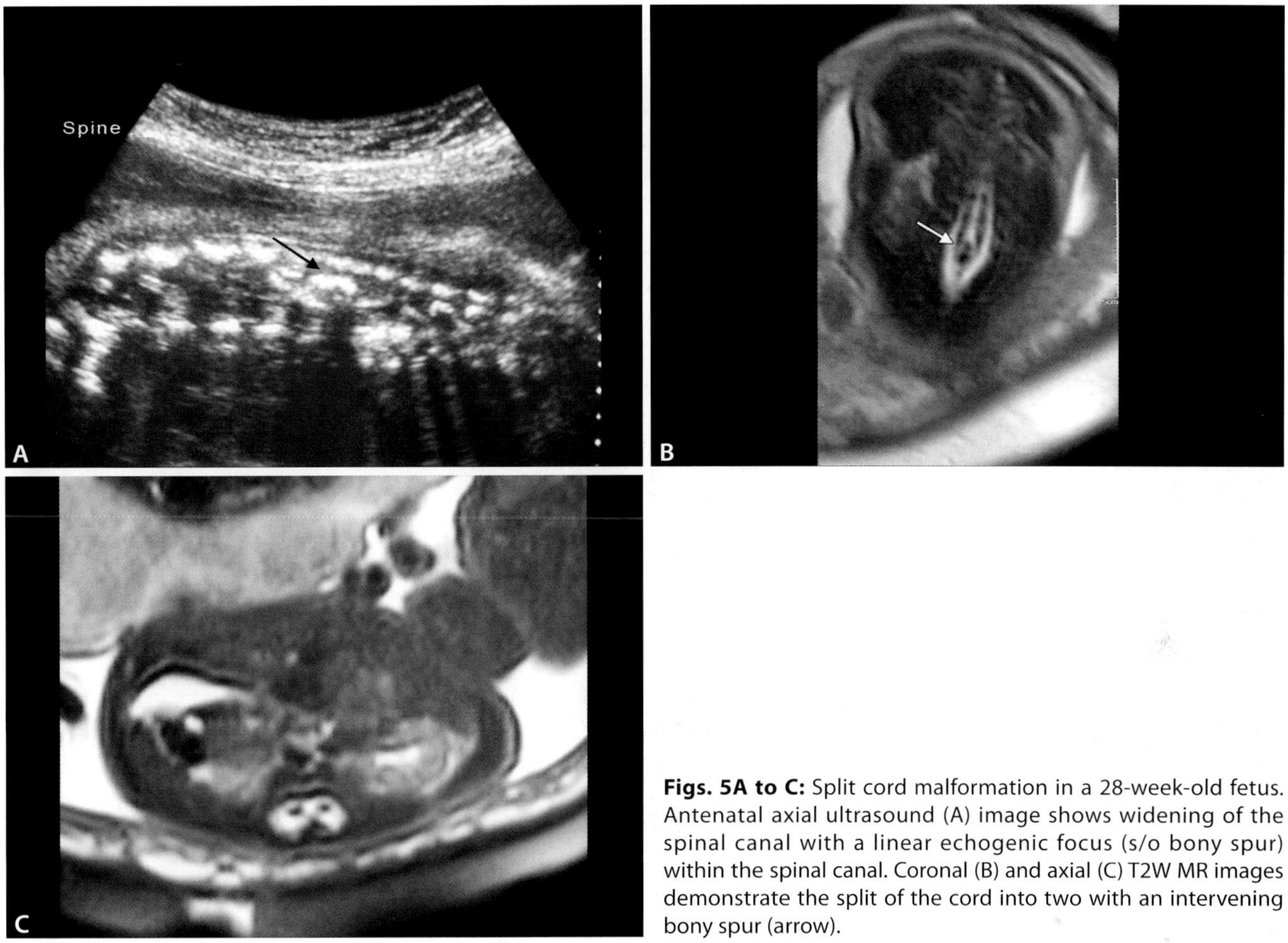

Figs. 5A to C: Split cord malformation in a 28-week-old fetus. Antenatal axial ultrasound (A) image shows widening of the spinal canal with a linear echogenic focus (s/o bony spur) within the spinal canal. Coronal (B) and axial (C) T2W MR images demonstrate the split of the cord into two with an intervening bony spur (arrow).

and other associated abnormalities. T1W images (sagittal, axial and coronal plane) demonstrate the malformation in the majority of the cases. T2W images are helpful in the demonstration of syrinx and associated pathologies like dermoid and epidermoid cyst.[6,9] Patients with spinal dysraphism may have multiple spinal anomalies. For instance, a patient with myelomeningocele may have associated syringohydromyelia and Chiari malformation. Therefore, it cannot be overemphasised that the entire spine needs to be imaged if a cutaneous or vertebral anomaly suggests the presence of a malformation. Fetal MRI is used as complementary modality to USG **(Figs. 3 to 5)**, for the antenatal diagnosis of spinal anomalies and associated hydrocephalus.[10,11]

OPEN SPINAL DYSRAPHISM

Open spinal dysraphism (OSD) implies exposure of neural tissue or its covering meninges to external environment without any cutaneous covering. Exposed non-neurulated neural tissue is called placode.[5] This category includes myelomeningocele, myelocele, hemimeningocele and hemimyelomeningocele. Myelomeningocele accounts for approximately 99% cases of OSD while myelocele, hemimeningocele and hemimyelomeningocele are distinctively rare.

Myelocele and Myelomeningocele

Myelomeningocele and myelocele are the most common form of OSD, occurring in up to 2 per 1000 live births and females are affected slightly more than males.[5] The incidence has decreased in the last two decades because of the use of folate supplementation in pregnant mothers in the period before conception to six weeks after conception.[4,12] The mechanism of preventive action of folate is not fully understood.

Superficial ectoderm does not disjoin from the neuroectoderm, thereby producing a midline defect. The neural tube remains open and the neural folds remain in continuity with the cutaneous ectoderm at the skin surface.[5,6] The affected newborn is identified by the presence of a placode of reddish neural tissue in the middle of the back that is exposed to air because of the absence of overlying skin. Most common location of OSDs is lumbosacral region (44%) followed by thoracolumbar region (32%). In contrast to lumbar meningomyelocele, cervical meningomyelocele is a classified as a closed spinal dysraphism. Imaging is usually not done as the diagnosis is clinically obvious and is a neurosurgical emergency.

Some authors suggest that MRI should be performed whenever possible as it can characterize the various components of the malformation, evaluate associated abnormalities (hydromyelia, Chiari II malformation, and hydrocephalus) and identify hemimyelomeningocele and hemimyeloceles.[13] Imaging of untreated OSDs demonstrates dehiscense of skin, subcutaneous fat, muscle and bone at the level of spina bifida **(Figs. 6 and 7)**. In a meningomyelocele the ventral subarachnoid space is distended displacing the neural placode posteriorly **(Figs. 6A to C)**, while myelocele lies flush with the skin surface without CSF space expansion **(Figs. 7A to C)**.

After surgery the infants have a neurological defect that is stable. Imaging is indicated if the patient deteriorates neurologically despite adequate treatment of associated hydrocephalus or if the neurological examination findings are unusual.[14,15] MRI done in the postoperative setting may show the cord to be low lying and covered by skin graft; the

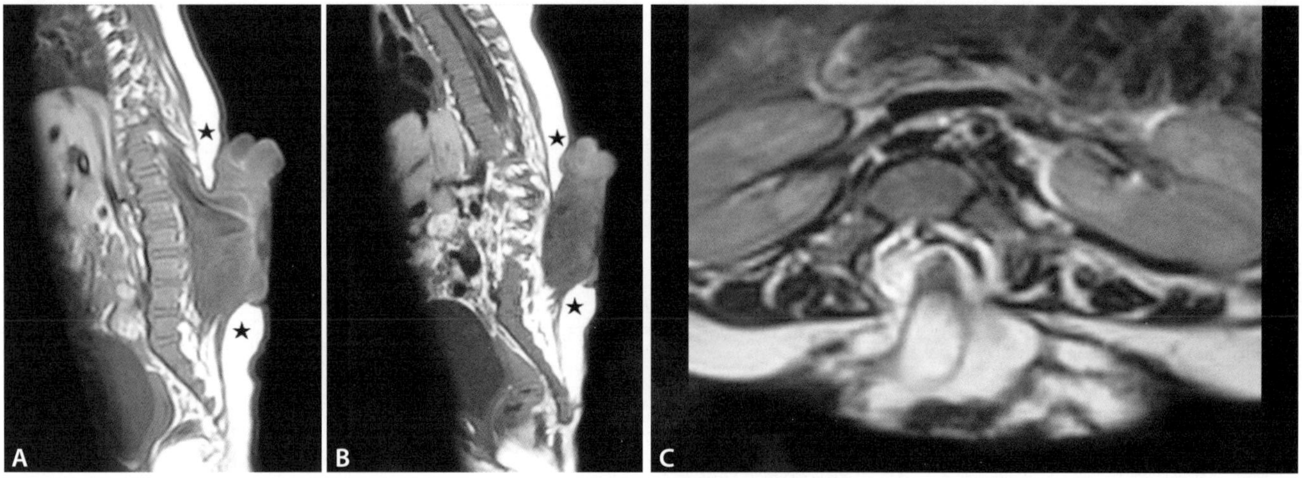

Figs. 6A to C: Lumbosacral meningomyelocele in a 2-day-old female. Sagittal T1W (A and B) images show a large mass in lower lumbar region without skin covering. Axial T2W image (C) shows exposed neural placode with traversing dorsal and ventral nerve roots. Notice dehiscent subcutaneous fat (stars). Ventral subarachnoid space is distended in contrast to myelocele which lies flush with the skin surface without CSF space expansion. Also note small syrinx in the cord at thoracic level.

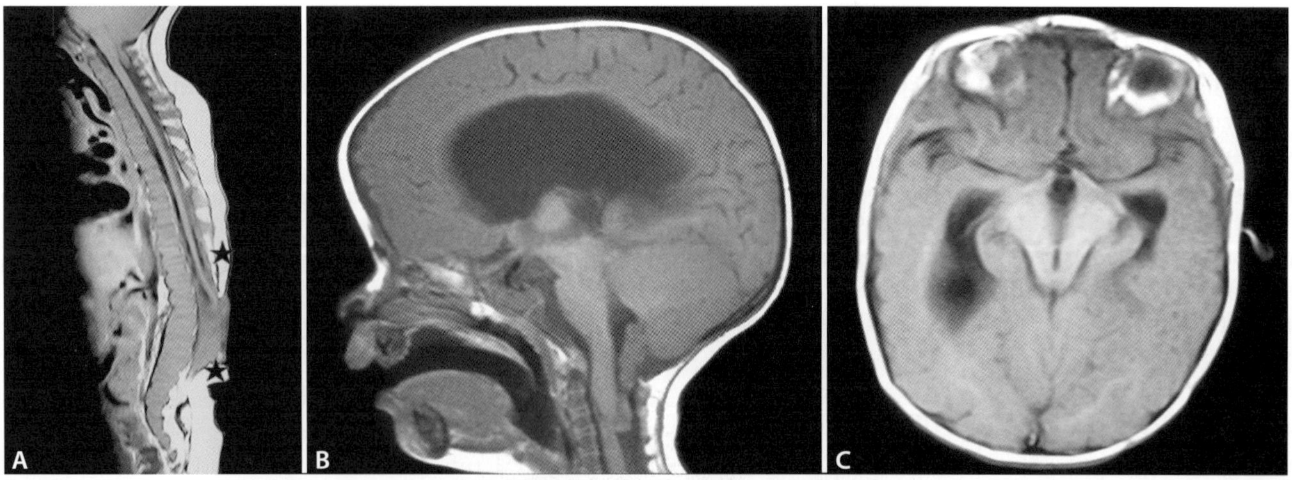

Figs. 7A to C: Myelocele with Chiari II malformation in a 1-day-old newborn. Sagittal T1W (A) image shows dehiscence of the subcutaneous fat (stars). Neural placode is exposed and flush with the skin surface without expansion of the subarachnoid space. Sagittal T1W image (B) of brain shows small posterior fossa with herniation of cerebellar tonsil behind cervical cord. Axial T1W image (C) at mid brain level shows abnormal posterior tectal beaking with dilated temporal horns.

stretched spinal cord may be tethered at this level **(Figs. 8 and 9)**. The spinal cord may be thinned out and may show cavitation at any level **(Figs. 8A and B)**. Intraspinal mass (epidermoid or dermoid cyst) may be associated.[15] Dermoid differs from epidermoid by the presence of appendages of skin. On imaging both conditions appear similar. These lesions usually appear hypointense on T1W images, and hyperintense on T2W images similar to CSF **(Figs. 10A to D)**. They may have complex signal intensity when there is hemorrhage or when the cyst becomes infected.

Causes of postoperative neurological deterioration include retethering **(Figs. 8 and 9)**, cord ischemia, spinal cord cysts and cavitation **(Figs. 8A and B)**, diastematomyelia and hydrocephalus. All these are easily amenable to detection by MR.[14] Surgical release of the adherent cord is effective and leads to improved motor function in almost 80% patients. Up to 85% of OSD patients have a concurrent hydrocephalus, and nearly all patients have an associated Chiari II malformation.[5,16]

Chiari II Malformation

Various theories have been put forward to explain this entity, but the recent theory by McLone and Knepper[17] best explains this association which is shown in **Figure 11**, and it has also been shown that most of these CNS anomalies

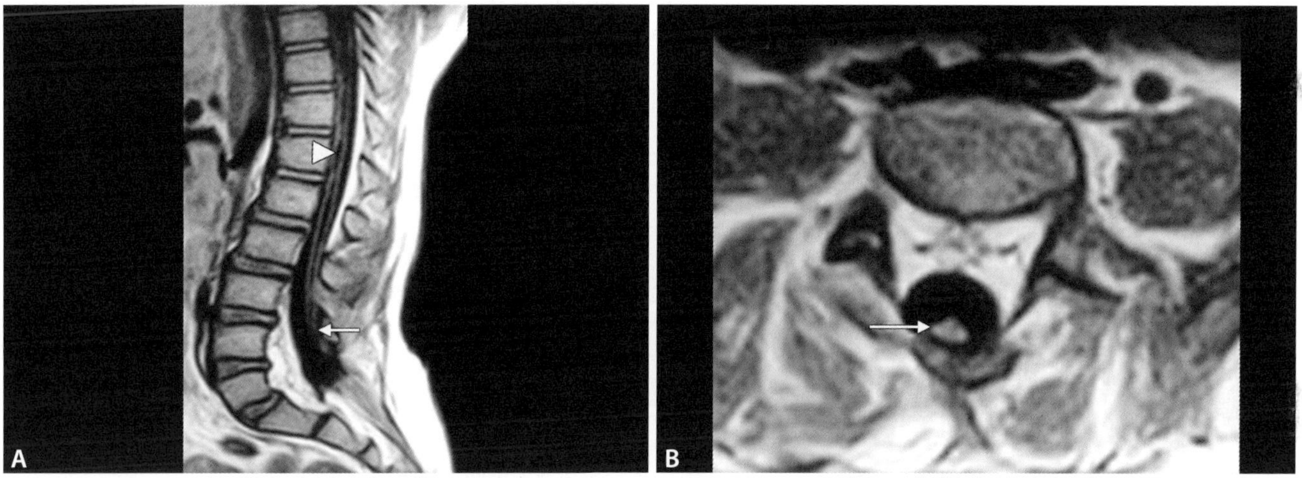

Figs. 8A and B: Tethered cord with hydromyelia in a 2-year-old male after surgery for lumbosacral meningocele. Sagittal T1W (A) and axial T1W (B) images show low lying tethered cord reaching up to L4–L5 disk level with thinning (arrow) and hydromelia (arrowhead) with abnormal eccentric location of cord indicating adhesion.

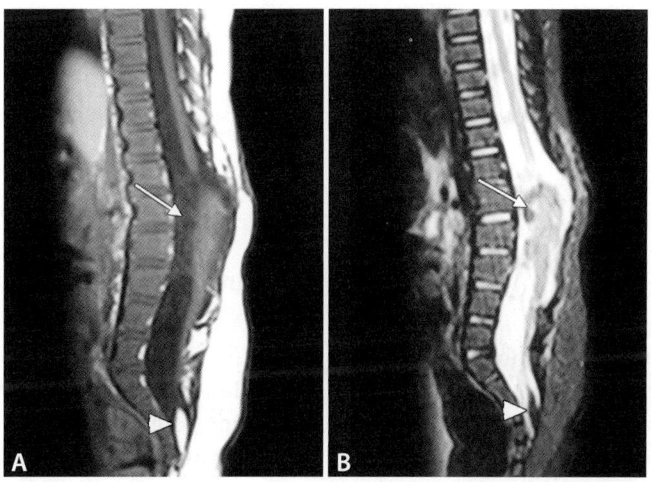

Figs. 9A and B: Postoperative fibrosis following meningomyelocele closure in a 5-year-old female. Sagittal T1W (A) and T2W (B) images demonstrate low-lying cord tethered by fibrotic tissue, hypointense on T1W and T2W images (arrows). Also note presence of filar lipoma (arrowheads) showing hyperintensity on T1W and hypointensity on T2W fat suppressed images.

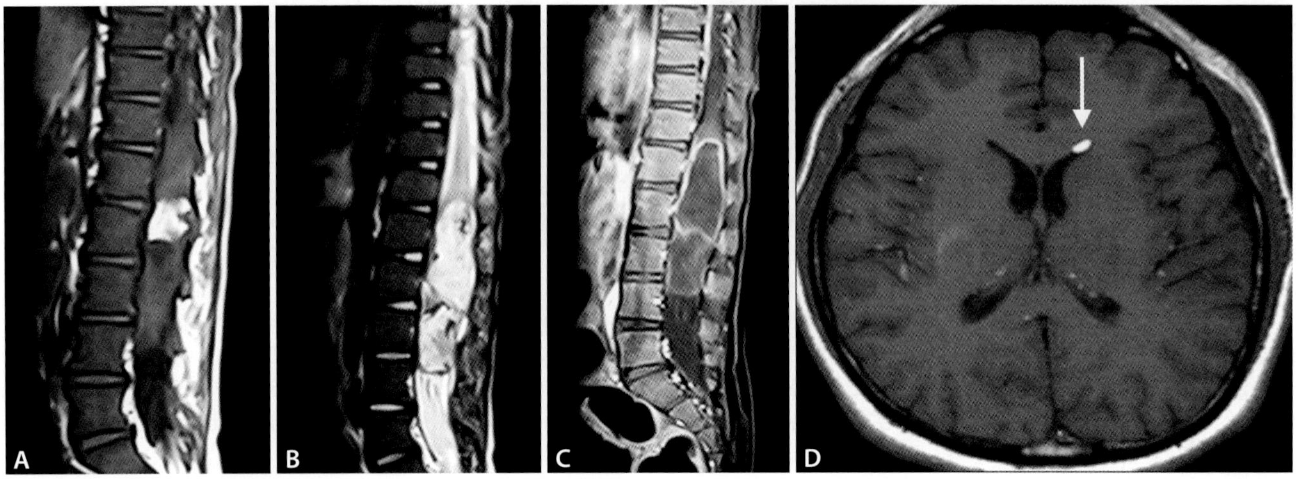

Figs. 10A to D: Infected dermoid cyst in a 12-year-old child with history of meningomyelocele repair. Sagittal T1W (A), T2W (B) and post-gadolinium (C) images show focal expansion of spinal cord at level of conus by a hyperintense (on T2W) mass with foci of T1 hyperintensity suggesting fat. Note peripheral rim enhancement following gadolinium indicating infected cyst. Axial T1W image of brain (D) demonstrates a hyperintense focus in left frontal horn (arrow). Findings are suggestive of infected dermoid cyst with rupture.

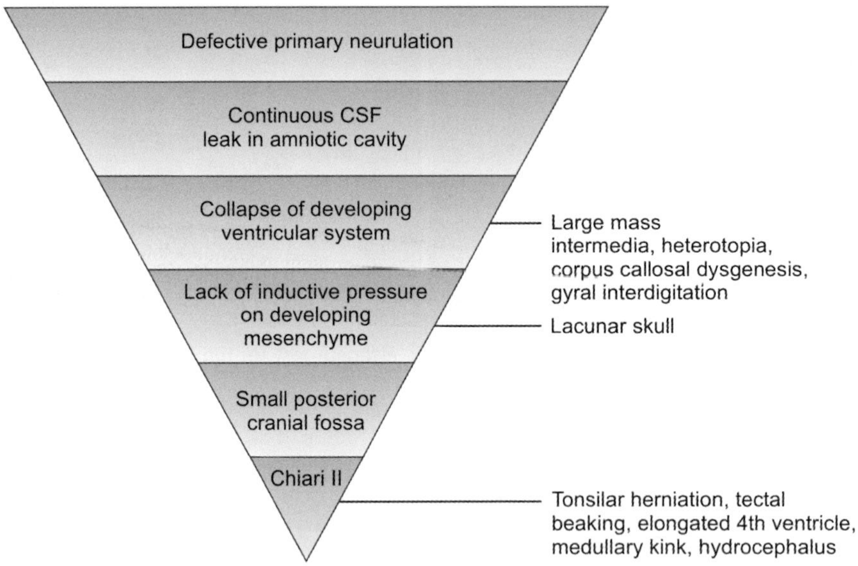

Fig. 11: McLone and Knepper theory explaining the pathogenesis of Chiari II malformation.

can be reversed or even prevented by early intrauterine repair of the defect which highlights the importance of early diagnosis of this condition.[18,19] As against less pronounced tonsilar herniation seen with Chiari I, in Chiari II there is marked tonsilar herniation **(Figs. 4 and 7)**. Tectal beaking, low lying torcular herophile, and hydrocephalus are usual associations with this malformation. Tonsilar herniation should be assessed on mid-sagittal non-fat suppressed T1W image. Anatomical landmark followed is a line connecting basion with opisthion.[20] While drawing the line signal intensity of bone, not marrow should be used. Since there is gradual ascent of cerebellar tonsil with age, criteria for tonsilar ectopia changes with age (≥6 mm 0–10 years; ≥5 mm 10–30 years; ≥4 mm 30–80 years; ≥3 mm >80 years).

Hemimyelocele/Hemimyelomeningocele

This is the rarest form of OSD and results when split cord malformation is associated with defective primary neurulation of one of the hemicord which forms part of myelomeningocele. Hemimyelocele/myelomeningocele **(Figs. 12 and 13)**, also has associated chiari malformation in up to 40% of cases.[21,22] Clinical clues to the diagnosis include asymmetrical neurological deficit and presence of hirsutism along one side of the exposed neural defect.[23]

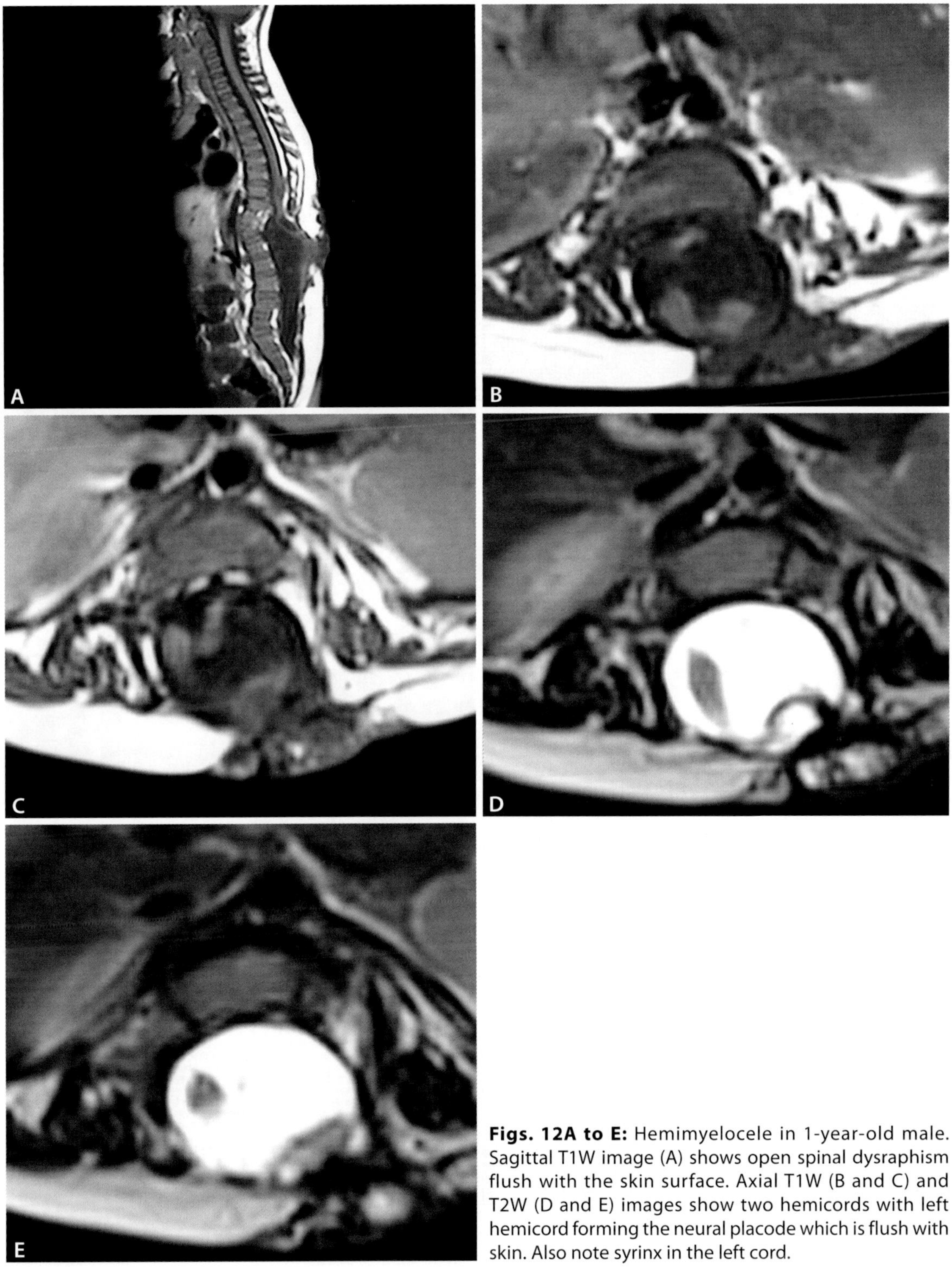

Figs. 12A to E: Hemimyelocele in 1-year-old male. Sagittal T1W image (A) shows open spinal dysraphism flush with the skin surface. Axial T1W (B and C) and T2W (D and E) images show two hemicords with left hemicord forming the neural placode which is flush with skin. Also note syrinx in the left cord.

CLOSED SPINAL DYSRAPHISM

Closed spinal dysraphism (CSD) is a heterogenous group of disorders. In patients with CSD, early diagnosis may be useful, as SD may lead to distortion of the nerve roots with growth, resulting in neurological sequelae in the lower extremities. Early diagnosis is necessary to prevent neurological sequelae by performing early surgical procedures.

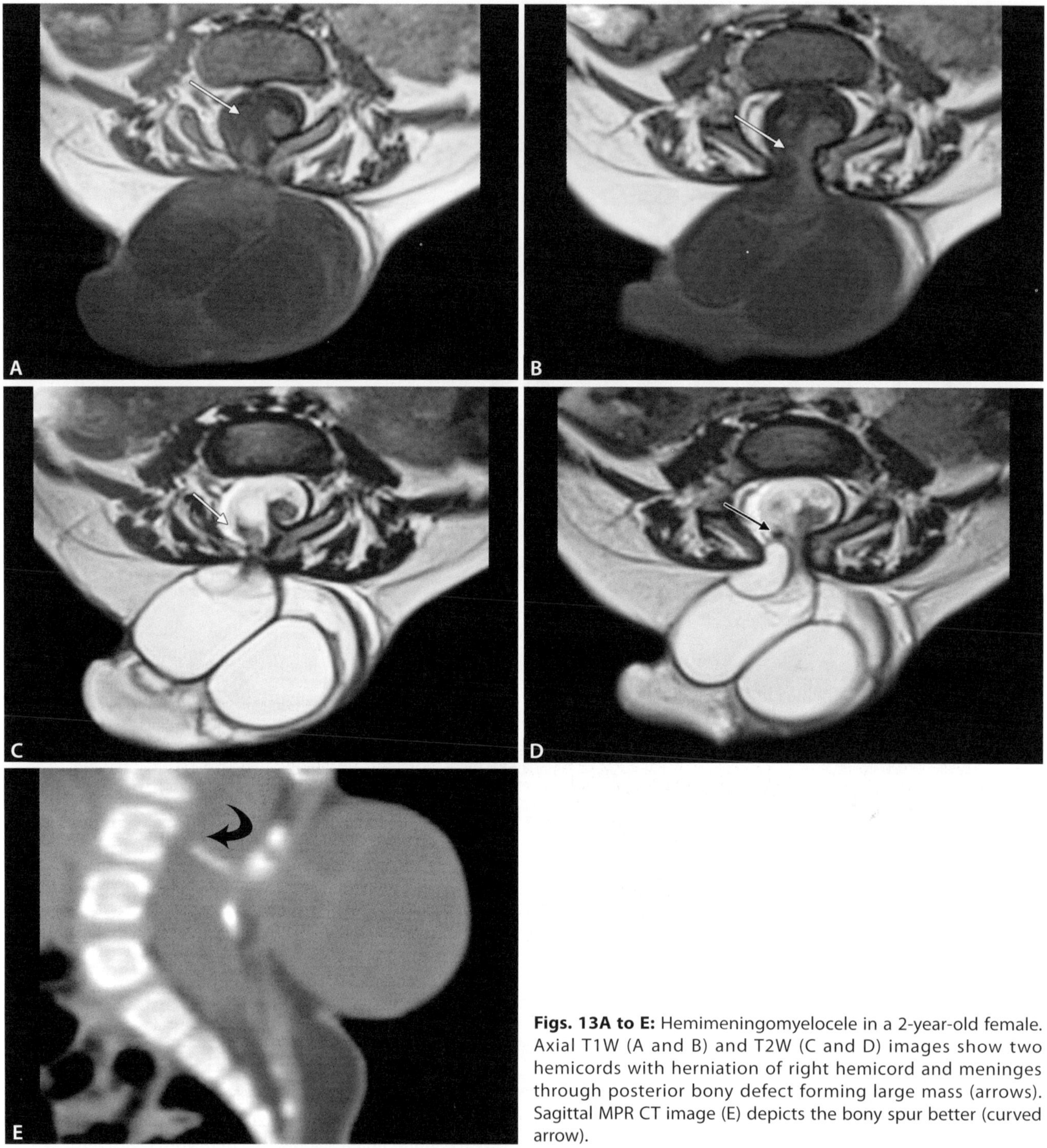

Figs. 13A to E: Hemimeningomyelocele in a 2-year-old female. Axial T1W (A and B) and T2W (C and D) images show two hemicords with herniation of right hemicord and meninges through posterior bony defect forming large mass (arrows). Sagittal MPR CT image (E) depicts the bony spur better (curved arrow).

CSD with Subcutaneous Mass

CSDs with subcutaneous mass at lumbosacral region include lipomyelocele, lipomeningomyelocele, meningocele, myelocystocele. Among these lipomyelocele and lipomyelomeningocele are common entities, and lipomyelocele is twice as common as lipomyelomeningocele. At cervical level differential diagnosis of CSD with subcutaneous mass includes cervical meningomyelocele, meningocele and myelocystocele.[5,6]

Lipoma with Dural Defect (Lipomyelocele and Lipomyelomeningocele)

Lipomyelomeningocele consists of a large subcutaneous skin covered mass in lumbosacral region that contains fat, neural tissue, CSF and meninges.[24] This results from premature separation of surface ectoderm from neural ectoderm prior to formation of proper neural tube which allows ingress of intervening mesoderm into neural tube which in turn prevents further neurulation.[8] These mesodermal components specifically differentiate towards adipose tissue and form fatty component of these disorders. Clinically there is a mid-line soft non-tender mass above level of the intergluteal crease which extends asymmetrically into one buttock. Associated cutaneous malformation is seen in 50% cases. Differentiation of lipomyelocele from lipomyelomeningocele is by position of lipoma-placode interface. In lipomyelomeningocele the lipoma-placode interface is outside the confines of spinal canal **(Figs. 14A to C)**, whereas in lipomyelocele interface is either inside or at the edge of spinal canal **(Figs. 15A to C)**. In lipomyelocele, size of the subarachnoid space ventral to the cord is normal; however, the size of the canal may be increased depending on size of the lipoma. On the other hand, in the lipomyelomeningocele, there is ballooning of subarachnoid space ventral to the cord. This condition is associated with tethered cord, hydromyelia and Chiari I malformation.[9]

Meningocele

Meningocele is characterized by herniation of meninges through bony defect covered externally by the skin. The embryological basis remains unexplained.[8] As per definition the mass should not contain any of spinal cord segments or nerve root as content **(Figs. 16A and B)**. Rarely, filum terminale may remain tethered within the sac. On imaging, CSF filled dural outpouching is seen to herniate via the spina bifida, intervertebral foramen or sacral foramen. More than 80% meningoceles are

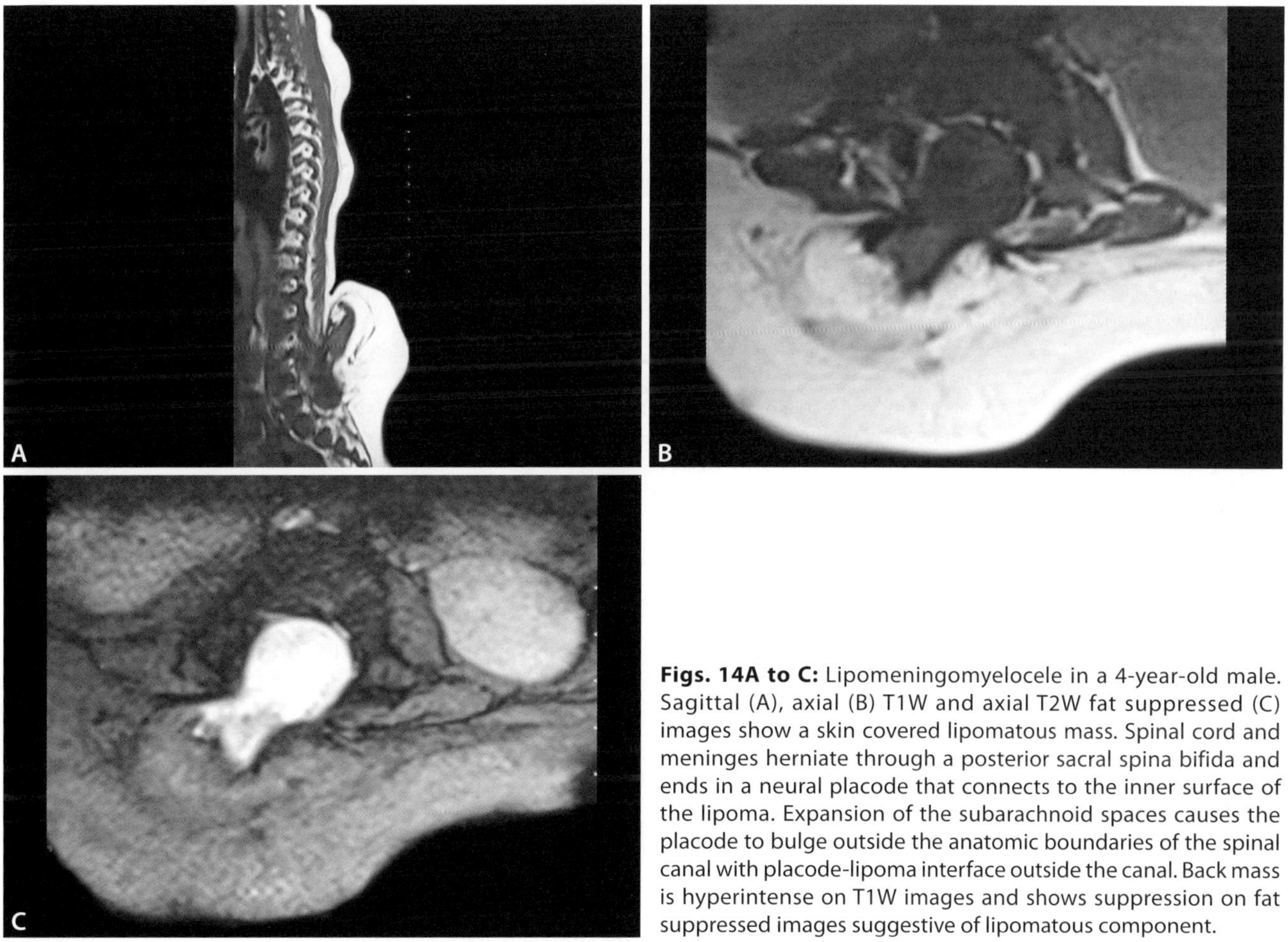

Figs. 14A to C: Lipomeningomyelocele in a 4-year-old male. Sagittal (A), axial (B) T1W and axial T2W fat suppressed (C) images show a skin covered lipomatous mass. Spinal cord and meninges herniate through a posterior sacral spina bifida and ends in a neural placode that connects to the inner surface of the lipoma. Expansion of the subarachnoid spaces causes the placode to bulge outside the anatomic boundaries of the spinal canal with placode-lipoma interface outside the canal. Back mass is hyperintense on T1W images and shows suppression on fat suppressed images suggestive of lipomatous component.

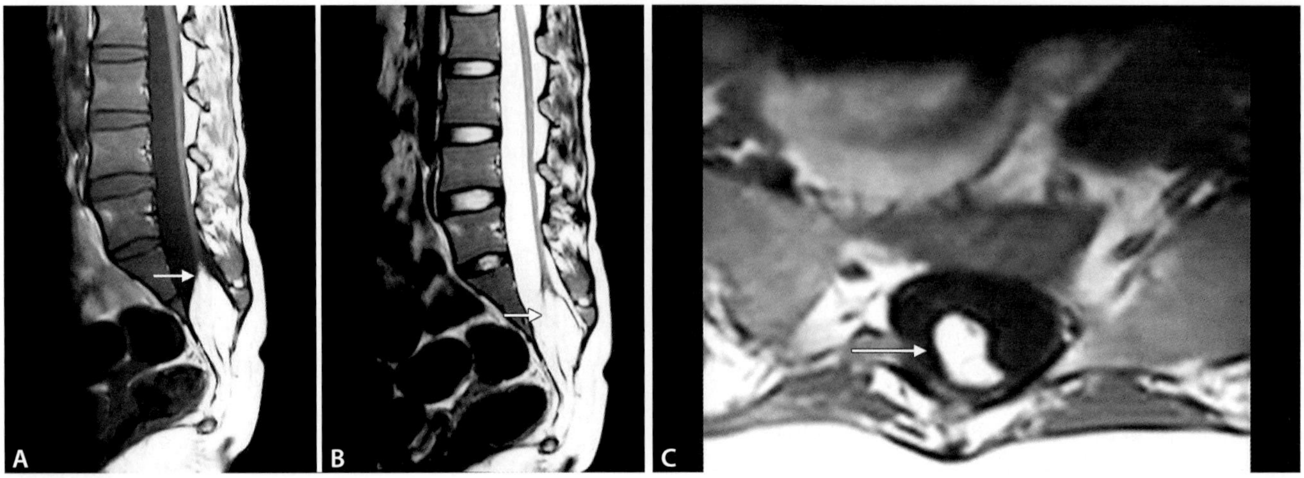

Figs. 15A to C: Lipomyelocele in a 2-year-old male. Sagittal T1W (A) and T2W (B) images show T1 hyperintense intraspinal mass adherent to cord continuous with subcutaneous fat through wide spina bifida. Axial (C) T1W image better depicts intraspinal fatty component. Note lipoma–placode interface within confines of the spinal canal (arrow).

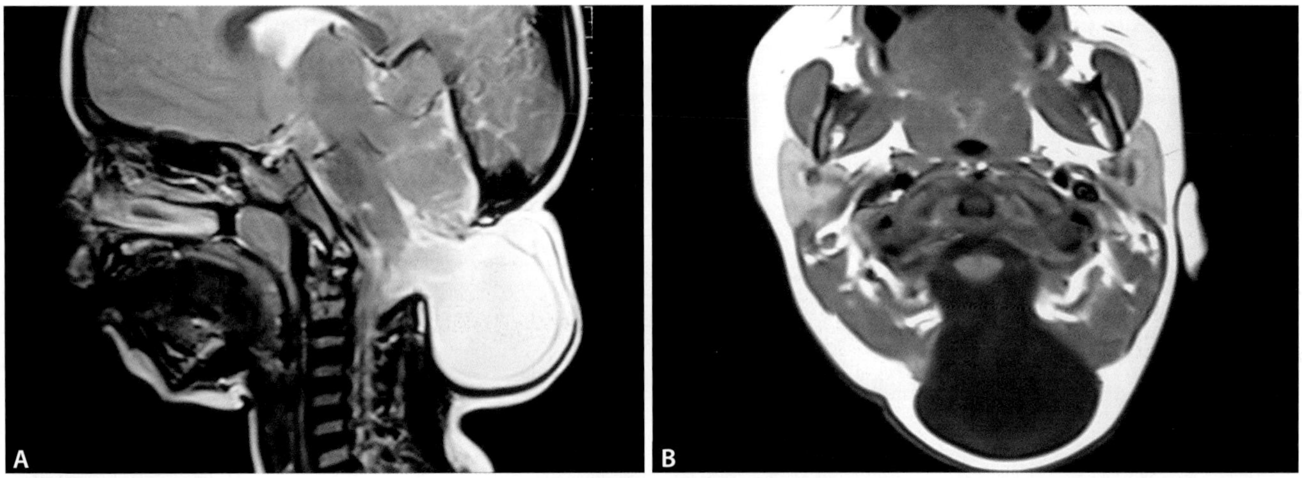

Figs. 16A and B: Posterior cervical meningocele in a 6-month-old male. Sagittal T2W (A) and axial T1W (B) images show herniation of the meninges in the upper cervical region. Note associated skin covering and lack of herniation of neural elements.

located in the lumbosacral spine. The bony defect may involve the posterior elements, anterior aspect of sacrum, lateral aspect of spine or distal sacrum (intrasacral meningocele).

Anterior Sacral Meningocele

Anterior sacral meningocele is characterized by herniation of meninges through anterior sacral defect, forming cyst like structure filled with CSF continuous with subarachnoid space of spinal cord. When this condition is associated with anorectal anomaly, it is called Currarino's triad. Majority of cases remains asymptomatic and are detected incidentally either on pelvic examination or imaging.[25] Differential diagnosis includes cystic sacrococcygeal teratoma, large ovarian cyst and neurenteric cyst. Demonstration of continuity of cyst with thecal sac ensures diagnosis of anterior sacral meningocele **(Figs. 17A to C)**.

Myelocystocele

This rare entity constitutes about 5% cases of CSD and its embryological basis is not fully understood.[5,8] It could represent severe disruptive form of terminal ventricle, a defect in secondary neurulation. It has three components: skin covered posterior meningocele, hydromelic terminal cord into meningocele and posterior spina bifida. Myelocystocele may be terminal or segmental (cervical). Differential diagnosis includes simple dorsal meningocele and myelomeningocele. Continuity of the dilated central canal with the caudal cyst is diagnostic of myelocystocele and helps differentiate it from other entities.[26]

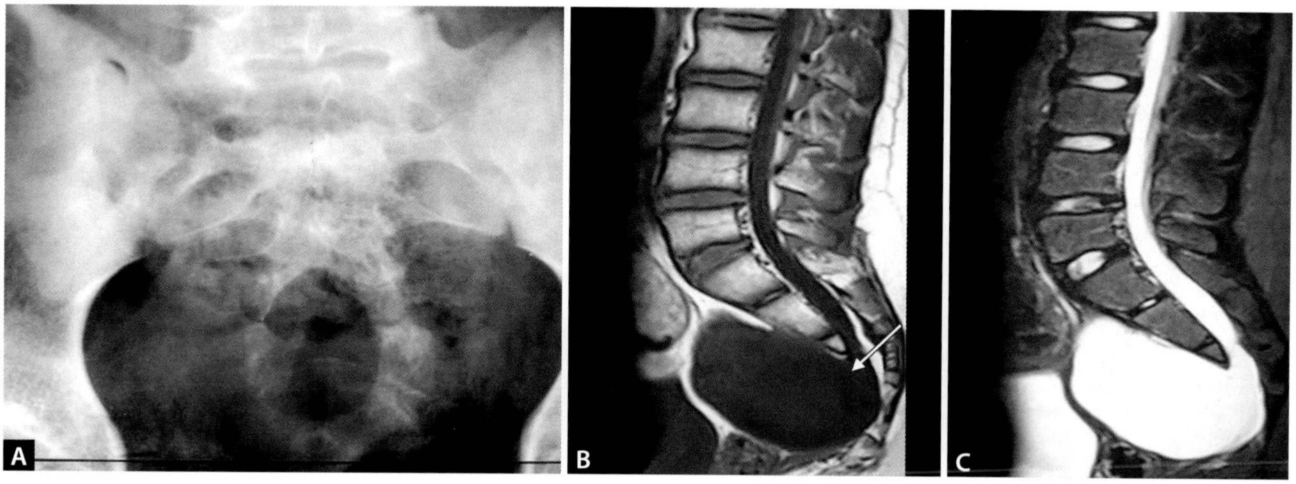

Figs. 17A to C: Anterior sacral meningocele in a 15-year-old female. Radiograph sacrum AP view (A) shows scimitar sacrum. Sagittal T1W (B) and T2W (C) images show a large presacral cyst contiguous with the spinal canal (arrow). Also note sacral hypogenesis.

CLOSED SPINAL DYSRAPHISM WITHOUT SUBCUTANEOUS MASS

This group includes wide variety of abnormalities in which imaging plays a crucial role in making the diagnosis.

Posterior Bony Spina Bifida

This is the simplest form of CSD and is characterized by defective fusion of posterior bony element. Isolated posterior spina bifida is seen in up to 5% of the general population. Usually, insignificant, further imaging is not indicated unless there is neurological deficit or high risk cutaneous markers are present **(Table 2)**. Defect is commonly seen at L5–S1 level **(Fig. 18)**. Care should be taken not to diagnose this entity in children less than 6 years since it is physiological to see unfused posterior elements in lumbosacral region up to 6 years of age.[9]

Lipoma (Intradural and Intramedullary)

Lipoma results from early disjunction between neuroectoderm and ectoderm.[8] Lipoma is most commonly seen at lumbosacral level and is usually subpial in location. They occur more commonly in females, peak in the first five years of life and usually present with tethered cord syndrome. Lipomas are contained within intact dural sac and are located in midline dorsally. On MR, lipoma appears as a mass which follows signal intensity of subcutaneous fat on all pulse sequences (high signal intensity on T1W and FSE T2W images, hypointense on fat saturated images).

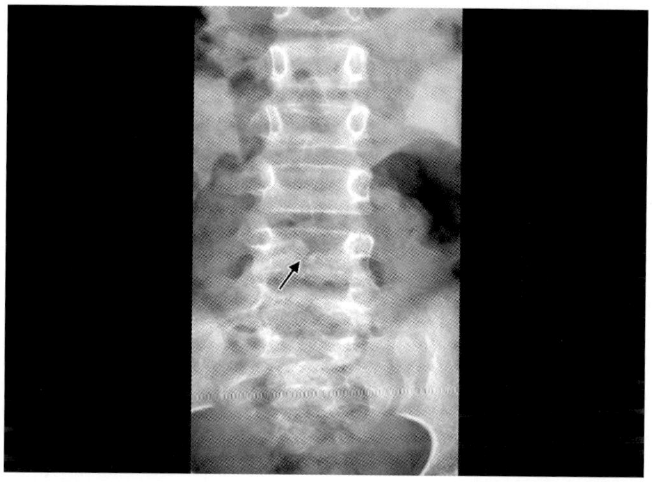

Fig. 18: Isolated spina bifida in an 8-year-old male. Radiograph lumbosacral spine AP view shows absence of fusion of posterior elements of L4–L5 (arrow).

Filum Terminale Lipoma

Filum terminale lipoma probably results from defective secondary neurulation which leads to persistence of mesodermal elements within filum terminale which later differentiate towards adipose tissue.[5,8] Incidental detection of fatty signal (hyperintense on T1W) in the filum is a normal finding seen in upto 5% of general population and is referred as fatty filum.[27] Diagnosis of filum terminale lipoma should be made when the fatty filum measures more than 2 mm **(Figs. 9 and 19A and B)**. This condition may or may not be associated with cord tethering.

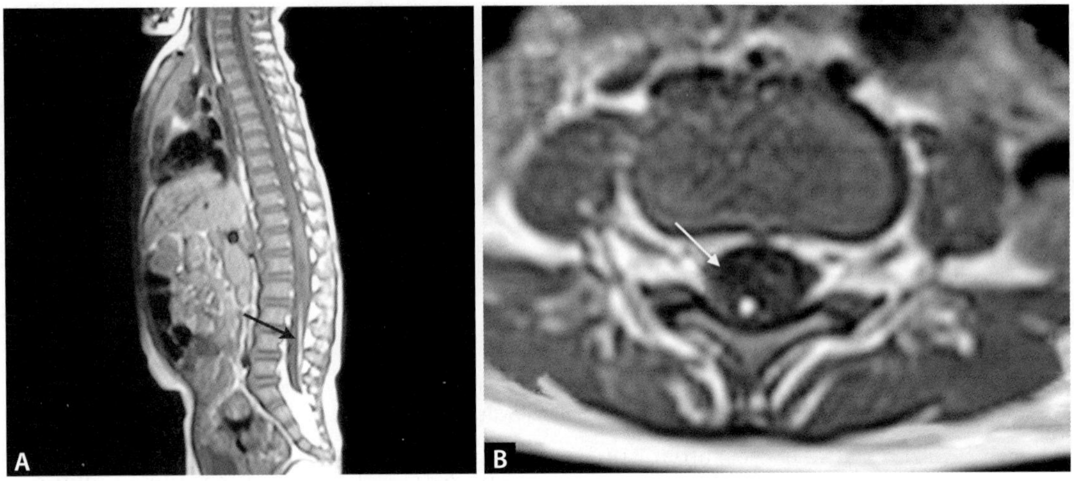

Figs. 19A and B: Filum terminale lipoma in a 10-month-old female. Sagittal T1W (A) and axial T2W (B) images show thickened filum terminale with T1 hyperintensity indicating fat in filum terminale (arrow).

Tight Filum Terminale Syndrome

Tight filum terminale syndrome occurs due to defective retrogressive differentiation of neural tube formed by the process of secondary neurulation resulting in short and thick filum terminale (>2 mm) which causes abnormal stretching of spinal cord with secondary neurological deficit.[5,6,9] Associated anomalies include posterior spina bifida, scoliosis and kyphoscoliosis. According to some authors tight filum terminale is a clinical syndrome and not an imaging diagnosis. It can be seen with anomalous filum terminale, split cord malformation and in postoperative period after surgery for open spinal dysraphism **(Figs. 20A and B)**. The treatment is surgical section of the filum terminale.

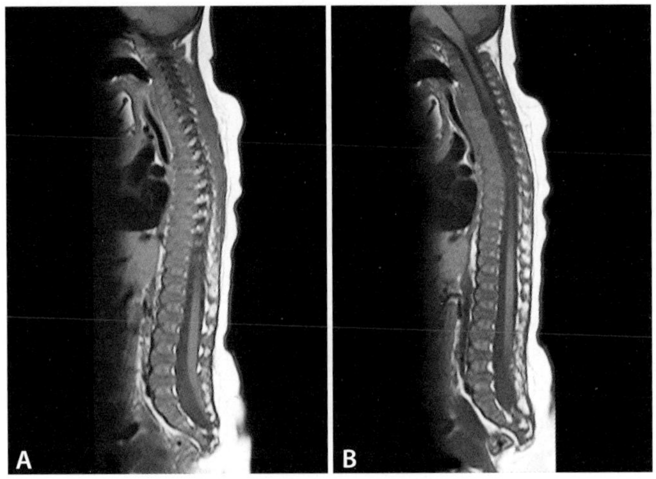

Figs. 20A and B: Tight filum terminale (tethered cord syndrome) in an 8-month-old female. Sagittal T1W images (A and B) show thickened filum terminale with tethered, low conus medullaris.

Persistent Terminal Ventricle

Persistent terminal ventricle results from defect in the process of secondary neurulation, resulting in the formation of small ependymal lined cavity with in conus medullaris. Usually, asymptomatic but may present with low backache and bladder dysfunction. There is dilatation of ependymal canal immediately above the filum terminale with slight expansion of conus. This condition needs to be differentiated from intramedullary tumor which can be done by its central location, CSF isointense signal intensity, and by noting lack of contrast enhancement following gadolinium and on follow up imaging.[6,9]

Neurenteric Cyst

Neurenteric cyst results from incomplete regression of neuroenteric canal. Complete failure of regression manifest as dorsal enteric fistula which is very rare.[8] They are enteric lined cysts that present within the spinal canal and exhibit a definite connection with the spinal cord and/or vertebra. They may communicate with an extraspinal component of cyst in the mediastinum or mesentery through a dysraphic vertebra or they may attach by a fibrous stalk to the vertebra or gut.[5,28] The peak incidence is during the first two decades of life, and the most common location is thoracic spine followed by cervical spine. Vertebral anomalies are common though not invariable. Most cysts lie in the cervicothoracic junction or close to the conus medullaris.

Typically neurenteric cysts are located ventral to the cervicothoracic cord. Diagnosis should be thought, whenever a posterior mediastinal mass is seen along with congenital vertebral anomalies **(Figs. 21A to C)**. Neurenteric cysts are isointense to CSF on T1W images and hyperintense on T2W images.[28] No enhancement occurs after contrast administration. Usually, the child is asymptomatic, but can present with symptoms related to compression of airways, oesophagus, or atrium. Neurological deficit occurs secondary to intraspinal component of cyst and demonstration of this component and associated vertebral segmentation anomaly is critical in establishing the diagnosis.

SPLIT CORD MALFORMATION

In split cord malformation (SCM), the spinal cord is partially or completely spilt into two hemicords by either an osteocartilaginous septum or by a fibrous septum. Usually, these hemicord unite distally after splitting into two. Each segment has a central canal, and dorsal and ventral nerve roots. Over 90% of the cases occur in female patients. SCM most commonly occurs in the thoraco-lumbar region (between D9 and S1 vertebral levels) and approximately 50–75% of patients have cutaneous stigmata at the site of cord split.[4-6]

SCM is classified as type 1 and type 2 based on state of the dural tube and nature of the medial septum.[21] In Pang type 1 **(Figs. 22A to F)**, each hemicord has a separate dural and arachnoid covering separated by a bony spur or septum (osteocartilaginous). In type 2 **(Figs. 23A to F)**, the hemicord are contained in a single dural sac and arachnoid covering without a rigid median septum (60% cases). Medial septum may be complete or incomplete and may course obliquely dividing the cord asymmetrically. Cleft is located at caudal end of splitting in majority of cases. SCM may be difficult to appreciate on sagittal MR images. Axial and coronal images show cord splitting as well as septum. However, fibrous septum may be very thin and is best demonstrated using thin axial/coronal T2W images.[9] SCM is suspected clinically in the presence of asymmetric neurological deficit and in presence of hairy tuft high along the back. It is important to look for this abnormality in all cases of dysraphic spine because of its frequent association. If not recognized prior to repair, it may be responsible for neurological deficit secondary to cord tethering. Commonly associated anomalies include cord tethering seen in around 75% of patients and syringohydromyelia (50% patients). It may affect the normal cord above or below the cleft and extend into one or both hemicords. Intramedullary tumors **(Figs. 24A to C)** have also been reported in the hemicord.[29] Vertebral anomalies are a rule and include spina bifida, widened interpedicular distance, hemivertebrae and fused vertebrae.

DORSAL DERMAL SINUS

Dorsal dermal sinus (DDS) is an epithelium lined tract beginning at the skin surface which can communicate with the CNS and its meningeal coating. This results from defective disjunction of surface ectoderm from developing neural tube which leads to persistence of ectodermal connection between spinal cord and external skin.[8] Sinus tract usually ends at a level above the external opening because of the ascent of the spinal cord. The points of attachment of skin and spinal cord remain segmental or

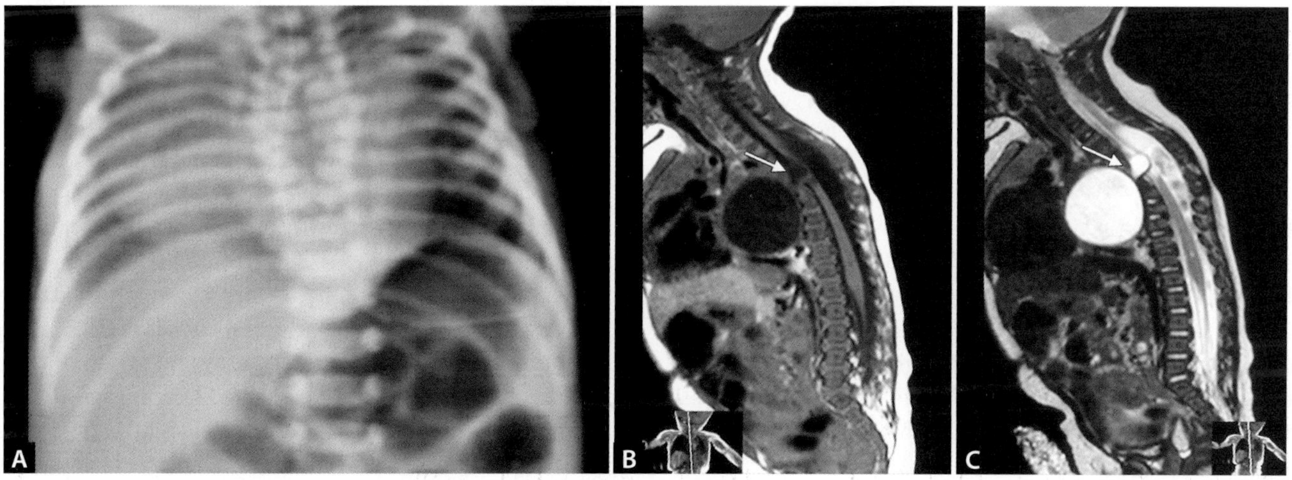

Figs. 21A to C: Neurenteric cyst in a 1-month-old male. Chest radiograph AP view (A) shows vertebral segmentation anomalies with large posterior mediastinal mass. Sagittal T1W (B) and T2W (C) images demonstrate a dumb-bell shaped mass extending from mediastinum into the spinal canal. Posterior subarachnoid space is dilated.

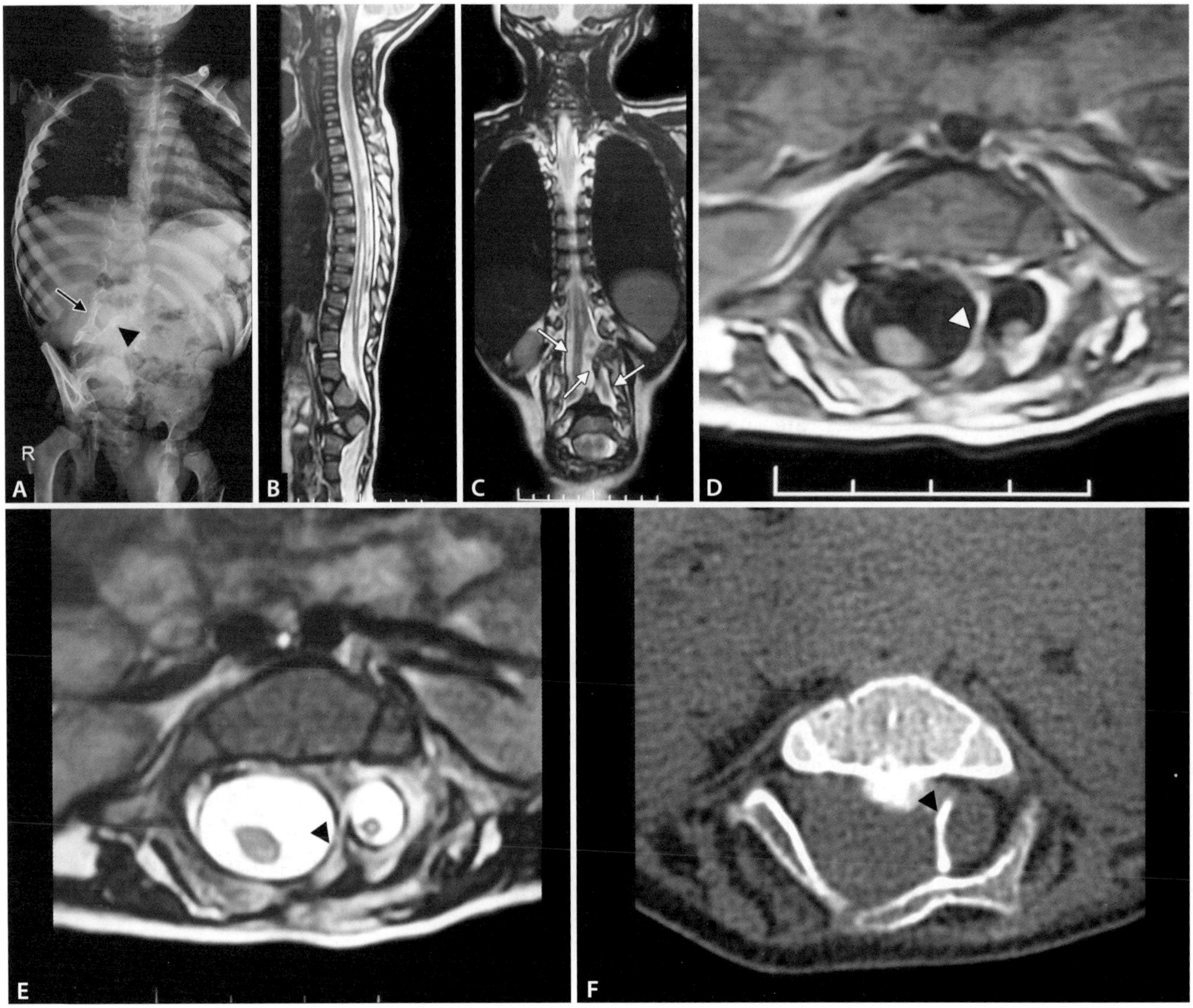

Figs. 22A to F: Type 1 split cord malformation in an 8-year-old boy. (A) Radiograph whole spine demonstrates vertebral segmentation anomalies with intersegmental bar (arrow). Presence of vertical intersegmental bar strongly suggests split cord malformation. Also, note presence of bony spur (arrowhead); (B) Sagittal T2W image demonstrates thinning of cord with hydromyelia. Cord is also low-lying and tethered; Coronal T2W image (C), axial T1W (D) and T2W (E) images show asymmetric split of cord (arrows) into two hemicords with bony spur (arrowhead) in between. Axial CT (F) shows bony spur better.

metameric, so the dermatome of involvement predicts the site of neural abnormality. Males and females are affected equally. The sinus ostium is typically midline and small hemangiomas may surround the ostium. The sinus tract extends deeply through the subcutaneous layer and between the bifid laminae toward the dura. It may end superficial to the dura, at the dura or deep to the dura.

Clinically dimples below top of the intergluteal crease end blindly whereas dimples above the level of intergluteal crease are highly suspicious. Patients become symptomatic either by infection or due to associated dermoid and epidermoid tumours.[30] Dorsal dermal sinus will be seen as hypointense tract in both T1- and T2-weighted images extending from skin surface to spinal canal **(Figs. 25A and B)**. Sagittal and axial MR sequences are good to demonstrate the extraspinal portion of the dermal sinus tract, though the intraspinal portion is hard to identify. In such cases 3D MR myelography can better delineate the tract and its intraspinal component. The differential diagnosis of DDS includes low sacrococcygeal midline dimple and pilonidal sinus, both of which do not enter spinal canal.

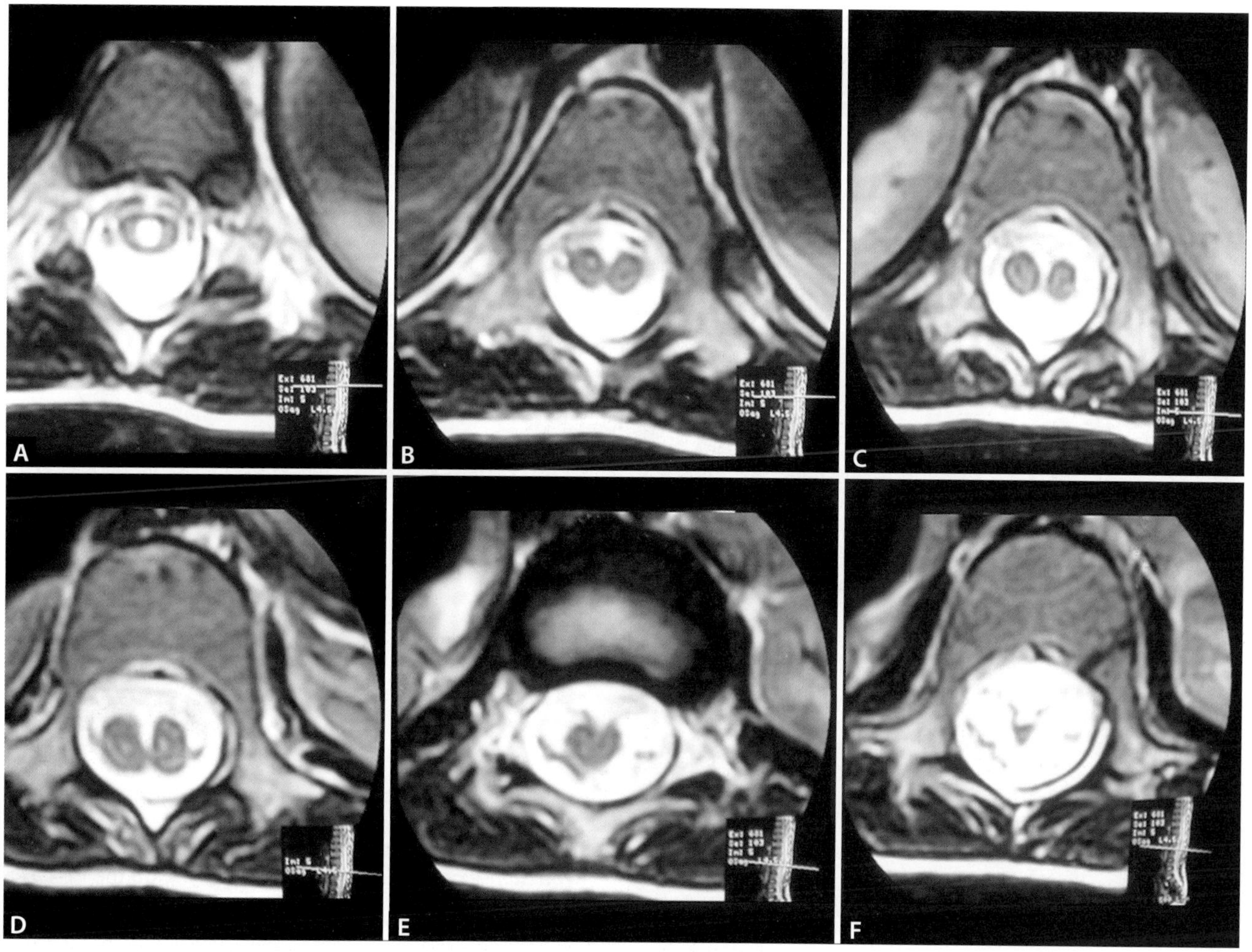

Figs. 23A to F: Type 2 split cord malformation in a 10-year-old male. (A to F) Axial T2W images show two hemicords spur contained within a single dural sac. Syrinx is seen in the cord proximal to split and there is no bony/fibrous spur.

CAUDAL AGENESIS (CAUDAL REGRESSION SYNDROME, CRS)

This is an uncommon malformation seen in 0.1–0.25:10,000 of normal pregnancies. However, it occurs in about one in 350 infants of diabetic mothers, representing an increase of about 200 times.[31] This syndrome is characterized by partial agenesis of lumbosacral spine, imperforate anus, malformed external genitalia, renal aplasia, extrophy bladder, etc. Plain films are adequate for demonstrating bony hypogenesis but do not show associated cord abnormalities. Sagittal T1W MR images are excellent for evaluating caudal vertebral agenesis, level and shape of conus and cord tethering.[6,31]

The anatomy and position of the conus defines two distinct types of abnormalities.[32] In type 1 **(Fig. 26)**, the conus ends above the level of L1, is typically deformed and terminates abruptly at D11 or D12, as if the normal distal tip were absent (nearly always club or wedge shaped). In this type with high conus, the sacral deficit is typically large and the sacrum typically ends at or above S1. More severe the malformation, greater the number of absent vertebra and more cephalic is cord termination. In type 2 **(Fig. 27)**, the conus ends lower (below L1) and is elongated, stretched caudally and tethered by a thick filum or transitional lipoma. In these patients the sacrum tends to be relatively well-preserved, with identifiable portions of S2 or lower vertebral segments. Type 1 is associated with significant neurological deficit when compared to type 2 caudal agenesis.

Lumbosacral agenesis has also been classified into five different types depending on the nature and severity of agenesis. Type 1 is total sacral agenesis with some lumbar vertebra also missing. Type 2 is total sacral agenesis but

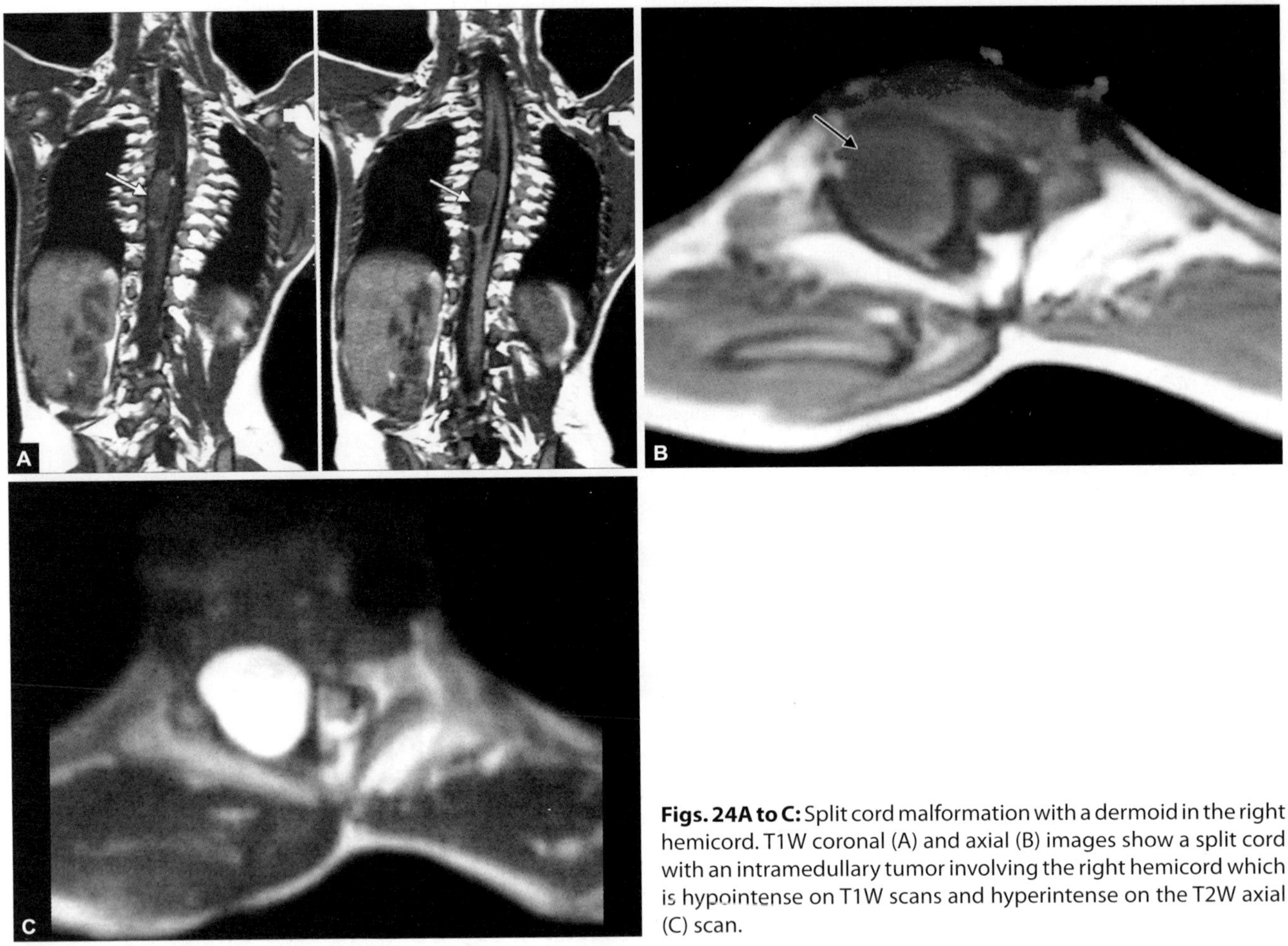

Figs. 24A to C: Split cord malformation with a dermoid in the right hemicord. T1W coronal (A) and axial (B) images show a split cord with an intramedullary tumor involving the right hemicord which is hypointense on T1W scans and hyperintense on the T2W axial (C) scan.

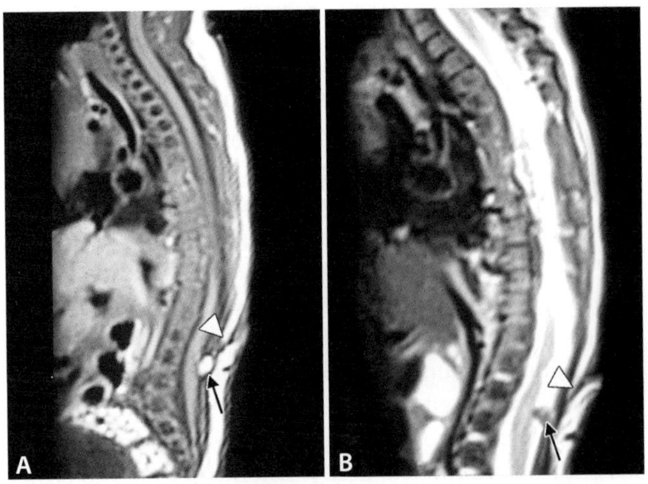

Figs. 25A and B: Dorsal dermal sinus in a 9-day-old child with skin dimple at back. Sagittal T1W (A) and T2W (B) images show a hypointense linear tract (arrowhead) extending from skin till dura and terminates in a well-defined T1 hyperintense oval lesion (arrows) suggestive of dermoid cyst.

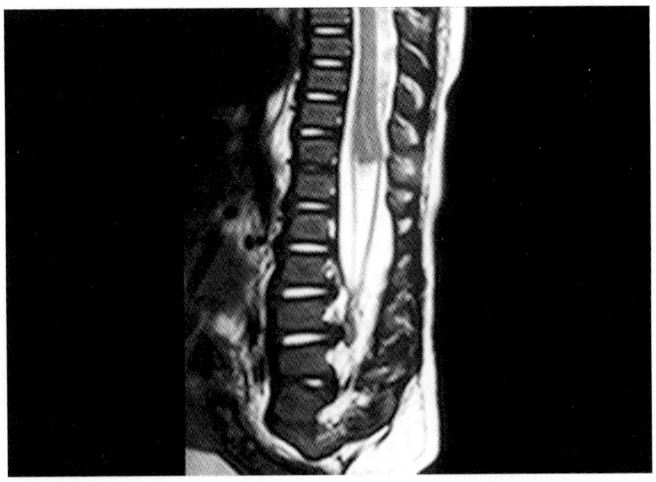

Fig. 26: Caudal agenesis type 1 in an 8-month-old male. Sagittal T2W image shows absence of the sacral segments below S1 with abrupt bulbous termination of cord at D12–L1 disk level with abnormal distal nerve roots.

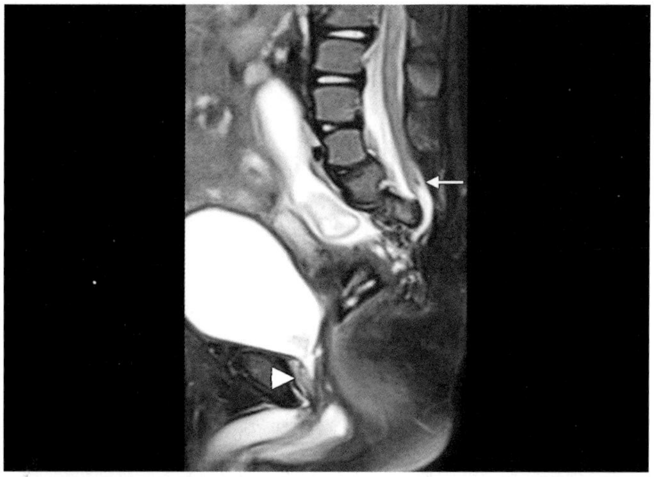

Fig. 27: Caudal agenesis type 2 in a 2-year-old male: Sagittal T2W image demonstrates abnormal low lying cord reaching up to S1 (arrow) with agenesis of distal sacral segments. Bladder neck is patulous (arrowhead) suggestive of neurogenic bladder.

the lumbar vertebra are not involved, while type 3 is subtotal sacral agenesis and atleast S1 is present. Type 4 is a hemisacrum whereas type 5 is coccygeal agenesis.[4]

SEGMENTAL SPINAL DYSGENESIS

Segmental spinal dysgenesis (SSD) is a rare form of dysraphic spinal state resulting from defective development of segment of notochord during preneurulation stage. This is characterized by segmental agenesis of spine with dysgenesis of spinal cord at the level of bony abnormality. Severity of this anomaly varies from minimal segmental thinning of cord to complete loss of segment of spinal cord.[33]

CONCLUSION

Spinal dysraphism is a heterogeneous group of developmental abnormalities in which there is a defective closure of the neural tube. MRI is a single stop-shop imaging modality in majority of cases and also helps to classify them based on the commonly followed clinicoradiological classification proposed by Torotti et al. It is important for the radiologist and clinicians to be familiar with normal embryologic development of spine and MR findings of spinal dysraphism. Various other congenital anomalies are frequently associated and should be meticulously looked for when dysraphism is detected.

REFERENCES

1. Warder DE. Tethered cord syndrome and occult spinal dysraphism. Neurosurg Focus. 2001;15:10:e1.
2. Byrd SR, Darling CP, Mclone DG. Developmental disorders of the pediatric spine. Radiol Cl North Am. 1991;29:9-21.
3. Drolet B. Birthmarks to worry about. Cutaneous markers of dysraphism. Dermatol Clin. 1998;16:447-53.
4. Silverman FN, et al. Spinal dysraphism. In Silverman FN, Kuhn JP (Eds): Caffey's Pediatric X-ray Diagnosis (9th edn). Lippincott Williams and Wilkins; 1993. Vol. 1.pp.312-24.
5. Tortori-Donati P, Rossi A, Cama A. Spinal dysraphism: A review of neuroradiological features with embryological correlations and proposal for a new classification. Neuroradiology. 2000;42:471-91.
6. Tortori-Donati P, Rossi A, Biancheri R, Cama A. Magnetic resonance imaging of spinal dysraphism. Top Magn Reson Imaging. 2001;12:375-409.
7. Nievelstein RAJ, Hartwig NG, Vermeji-Keers C, Valk J. Embryonic development of the mammalian caudal neural tube. Teratology. 1993;48:21-31.
8. French BN. The embryology of spinal dysraphism. Clin. Neurosurg. 1983;30:295-340.
9. Rossi A, Biancheri R, Cama A, Piatelli G, Ravegnani M, Tortori-Donati P. Imaging in spine and spinal cord malformations. Eur J Radiol. 2004;50(2):177-200.
10. Bulas D. Fetal evaluation of spine dysraphism. Pediatr Radiol. 2010;40(6):1029-37.
11. Von Koch CS, Glenn OA, Goldstein RB, Barkovich AJ. Fetal magnetic resonance imaging enhances detection of spinal cord anomalies in patients with sonographically detected bony anomalies of the spine. J Ultrasound Med. 2005;24(6):781-9.
12. Hahn YS. Open myelomeningocele. Neurosurg Cl North Am 1995;6:231-41.
13. Tortori-Donati P, Cama A, Fondelli MP, Rossi A. Le malformazioni di Chiari. In: Tortori-Donati P, Taccone A, Longo M. (Eds.), Malformazioni cranio-encefaliche. Neuroradiologia. Turin: Minerva Medica; 1996.pp.209-36.
14. McLone DG, Dias MS. Complications of myelomeningocele closure. Pediatr. Neurosurg. 1991;17:267-73.
15. Scott RM, Wolpert SM, Bartoshesky LF, Zimbler S, Klauber GT. Dermoid tumors occurring at the site of previous myelomeningocele repair. J Neurosurg. 1986;65:779-83.
16. Cama A, Tortori-Donati P, Piatelli GL, Fondelli MP, Andreussi L. Chiari complex in children. Neuroradiological diagnosis, neurosurgical treatment and proposal of a new classification (312 cases). Eur. J Pediatr Surg. 1995; 5 Suppl 1:35-8.
17. McLone DG, Knepper PA. The cause of Chiari II malformation: A unified theory. Pediatr Neurosci. 1989;15(1):1-12.
18. Fichter MA, Dornseifer U, Henke J, Schneider KT, Kovacs L, Biemer E, Bruner J, Adzick NS, Harrison MR, Papadopulos NA. Fetal spina bifida repair—current trends and prospects of intrauterine neurosurgery. Fetal Diagn Ther. 2008;23(4):271-86.
19. Hirose S, Farmer DL. Fetal surgery for myelomeningocele. Clin Perinatol. 2009;36(2):431-8.

20. Naidich TP, McLone DG, Fulling F. The Chiari II malformation. Part IV. The hindbrain deformity. Neuroradiology. 1983;25:179-97.
21. Pang D, Dias MS, Ahab-Barmada M. Split cord malformation, Part I: A unified theory of embryogenesis for double spinal cord malformations. Neurosurgery. 1992;31:451-80.
22. D Pang. Split cord malformation. Part II: Clinical syndrome. Neurosurgery. 1992;31:481-500.
23. Breningstall GN, Marker SM, Tubman DE. Hydrosyringomyelia and diastematomyelia detected by MRI in myelomeningocele. Pediatr. Neurol. 1992;8:267-71.
24. Naidich TP, McLone DG, Mutleur S. A new understanding of dorsal dysraphism with lipoma (lipomyeloschisis): Radiological evaluation and surgical correction. AJNR Am. J Neuroradiol. 1983;4:103-16.
25. Lee KS, Gower DJ, McWhorter JM, Albertson DA. The role of MR imaging in the diagnosis and treatment of anterior sacral meningocele. Report of 2 cases. J Neurosurg. 1988;69:628-31.
26. Byrd SE, Darling CF, McLone DG, Tomita T. MR imaging of the pediatric spine. Magn Reson Imaging Clin N Am. 1996; 4:797-833.
27. Brown E, Matthes JC, Bazan C, III, Jinkins JR. Prevalence of incidental intraspinal lipoma of the lumbosacral spine as determined by MRI. Spine. 1994;19:833-6.
28. Gadodia A, Sharma R, Jeyaseelan N, Aggarwala S, Gupta P. Prenatal diagnosis of mediastinal neurentric cyst with an intraspinal component. J Pediatr Surg. 2010;45(6):1377-9.
29. Sharma A, Sharma R, Goyal M, Vashisht S, Berry M. Diastemato-myelia associated with intramedullary tumour in a hemicord: A report of two cases. Australas Radiol. 1997; 41(2):185-7.
30. Barkovich AJ, Edwards MSB, Cogen PH. MR evaluation of spinal dermal sinus tracts in children. AJNR Am J Neuroradiol. 1991;12:123-9.
31. Nievelstein RAJ, Valk J, Smit LME, Vermeji-Keers C. MR of the caudal regression syndrome: Embryologic implications. AJNR Am J Neuroradiol. 1994;15:1021-9.
32. Pang D. Sacral agenesis and caudal spinal cord malformations. Neurosurg. 1993; 32:755-79.
33. Tortori-Donati P, Fondelli MP, Rossi A, Raybaud CA, Cama A, Capra V. Segmental spinal dysgenesis. Neuroradiologic findings with clinical and embryologic correlation. AJNR Am J Neuroradiol. 1999;20:445-56.

CHAPTER 147

Imaging of Pediatric Hip

Anjali Prakash

INTRODUCTION

The hip joint is a large and complex ball and socket joint consisting of a cup like acetabulum and a spherical femoral head.

Normal hip growth occurs as a result of genetically determined balanced growth of the acetabular and triradiate cartilages and the presence of a properly located femoral head. Absence of normal femoral head within the acetabulum during acetabular growth results in a flat shape of both the femoral head and acetabulum. The concave shape of the normal acetabulum is attributed to the presence of a spherical femoral head in close apposition to the acetabulum. Most acetabular development occurs by 8 years of age. The head, neck and greater trochanter of the infant hip is cartilaginous with early ossification of the femoral head seen between 3 and 6 months in girls and 6 and 9 months in boys.

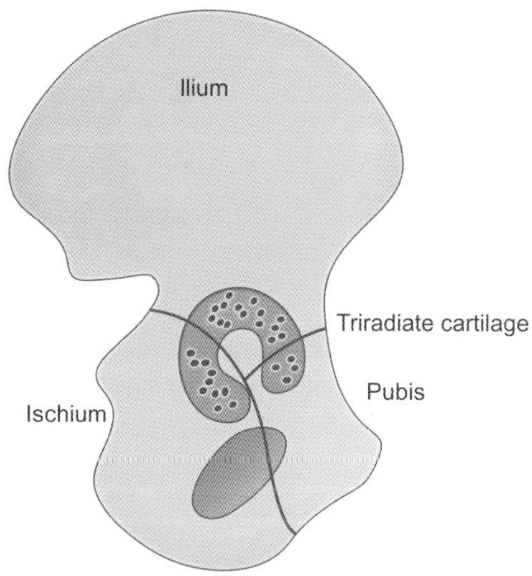

Fig. 1: Anatomy of the acetabulum.

Normal Anatomy

The acetabulum is formed of two fifths ischium, two fifths ilium and one fifth pubis joined by the triradiate cartilage **(Fig. 1)**. Acetabulum at birth has a rim of hyaline cartilage. A fibrocartilaginous rim, the labrum that forms lateral extension of the acetabular roof, extends the acetabulum peripherally. The strong transverse ligament completes the inferior gap in the labrum. The ligamentum teres connects the acetabulum to the femoral head. A dense capsule encloses the joint and attaches superiorly to labrum on the ilium and distally along the intertrochanteric line of the femur. The joint surfaces are lined by a synovial membrane containing synovial fluid. The entire joint is surrounded and stabilized by large (extensor, flexor and adductor) muscle groups arising from the pelvis.

METHODS OF INVESTIGATION

Conventional Radiography

Hip radiography should include an anteroposterior view of the pelvis which allows quick comparison with the normal hip for subtle changes. The frog lateral view is X-ray lateral view of both hips taken together in abduction and external rotation **(Fig. 2)**. Additional views may include oblique or a weight bearing view for dynamic evaluation of the joint space.

Various measurements are made on conventional radiography to assess alignment across the hip joint. Hilgenreiner line[1,2] is a YY line drawn through the center of the triradiate cartilage on both sides. Perkin's line is drawn through the superior lateral aspect of the acetabulum perpendicular to the YY line. The position of the femoral head can be surmised by evaluating the intersection of the Hilgenreiner line with the Perkin's line. In a normally positioned hip the femoral capital epiphysis primarily occupies the medial inferior quadrant **(Fig. 3)**. The acetabular angle is the angle subtended between the Hilgenreiner line and a line parallel to the acetabular roof with the normal acetabular angle,[1] being less than 30° **(Fig. 4)**.

The Shenton's line is a smooth unbroken curved line bridging the medial femoral metaphysis and the inferior margin of the superior pubic ramus. Disruption of this normally curved line suggests hip dislocation **(Fig. 5)**.

Andren and von Rosen,[3] described an anteroposterior projection in which the child is supine with knees extended, hip extended and abducted to 45° from the midline and the femora fully internally rotated. A line drawn through the midshaft of an undislocated femur will pass within the acetabulum and will, if extended, cross the spine at the level of lumbosacral junction **(Fig. 6)**. Andren and von

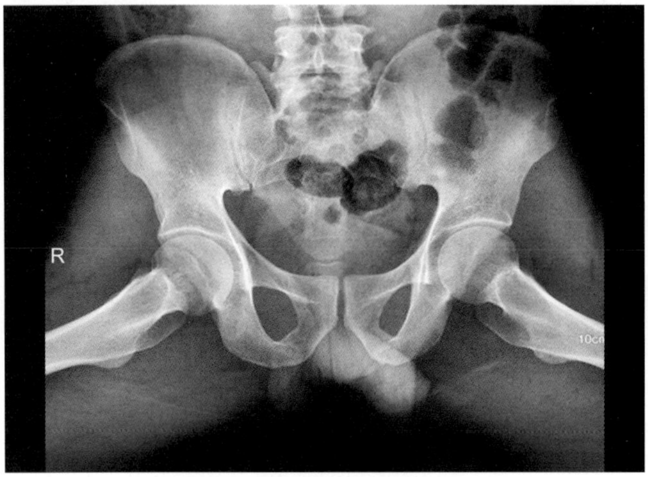

Fig. 2: X-ray both hips—frog-leg view.

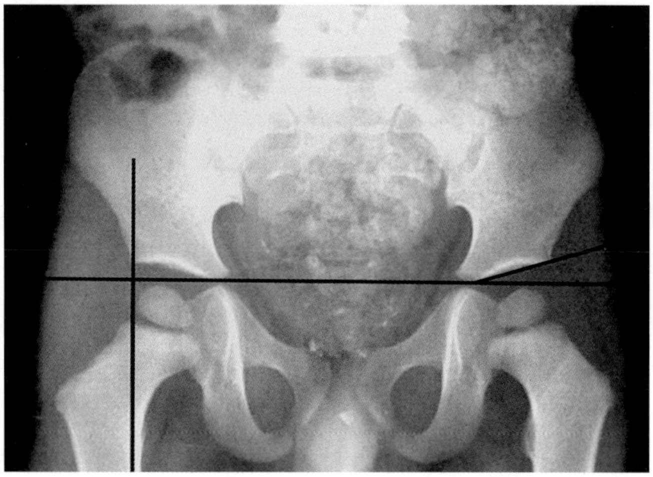

Fig. 3: X-ray pelvis depicting Hilgenreiner's line and Perkin's line, femoral epiphysis lies in the medial inferior quadrant.

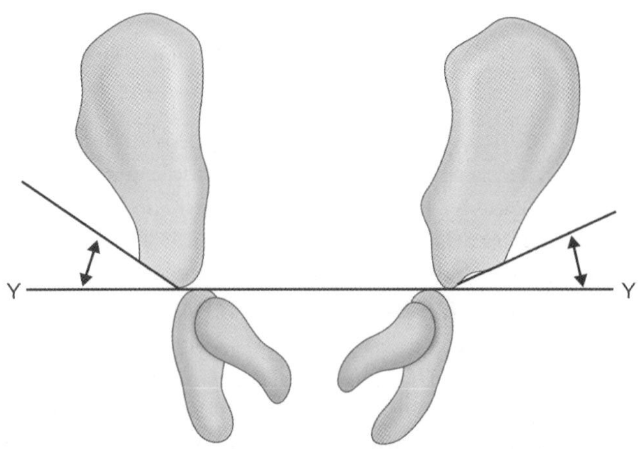

Fig. 4: Schematic diagram showing method for measurement of acetabular angle .

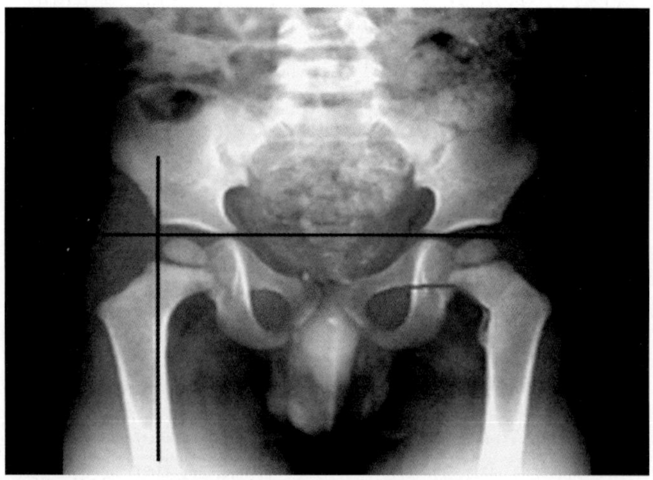

Fig. 5: X-ray pelvis showing acetabular angle and smooth unbroken Shenton's line.

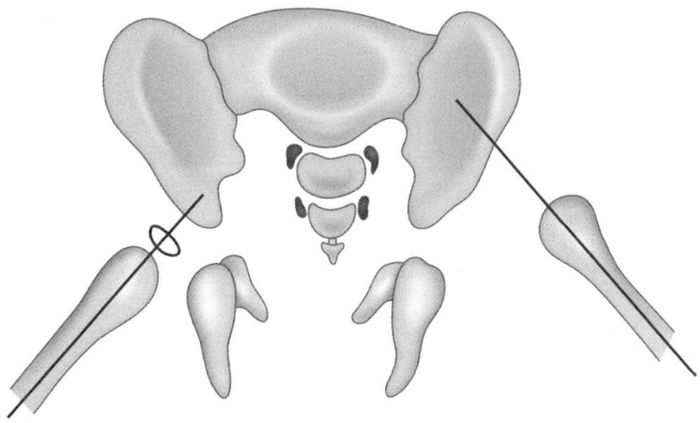

Fig. 6: Andren and von Rosen's method for detection of congenital dislocation of the hip before appearance of the capital femoral epiphysis.

Rosen view may have false negative results because of the inability to image the cartilaginous portions of the infant hip joint. False positive results may occur due to improper positioning and rotation of the pelvis.

These classical landmarks, lines and measurements were established as criteria for plain radiographic depiction of dislocation of the hip.

Ultrasonography

Real time sonography has gained wide acceptance as the method of choice for imaging the infant hip. Sonography is particularly appropriate as it can image the cartilaginous femoral head and acetabulum without the use of radiation. Cartilage forms the major part of the femoral head and acetabulum in the first 6 months of life and this is not visible on plain radiograph. Not only can the detailed anatomy be demonstrated but the hip can be observed by the dynamic technique of hip sonography which incorporates motion and stress maneuvers that are based on accepted clinical examination technique. Ultrasonography is also valuable to assess the hip in older children presenting with hip pain or limp. The procedure is noninvasive, involves no radiation, is easily available, inexpensive and in most patients sedation is not required.

Normal Sonoanatomy of the Hip

A linear array transducer with good near field resolution should be used. For infants, less than 7 months of age a 7.5 MHz transducer is appropriate and a 5 MHz transducer is used for infants between 7 and 12 months of age.

Sonographically, the normal cartilaginous femoral head is spherical measuring 1.2 to 2.1 cm in diameter in the neonatal age group. It is echopoor with finely stippled echoes, due to vascular channels **(Fig. 7)**. The greater trochanter is of the same echogenicity and sonographically continuous with the femoral head. The femoral ossific nucleus is highly echogenic and becomes visible by 2–8 months of age **(Fig. 8)**.[4]

The femoral head should be seated within the bony acetabulum formed by the ossification centers of ilium, ischium and pubis which are separated by the triradiate cartilage. The triangular cartilaginous roof of the acetabulum extends laterally beyond the bony acetabulum. This is echopoor except for a small fibrocartilaginous tip that is echogenic—labrum. The labrum appears as an echogenic triangle, caudal and lateral to the hypoechoic hyaline cartilage. The synovial membrane, fibrous capsule and supportive ligaments cover the limbus externally **(Fig. 9)**.

In transverse images acetabulum appears as a V shaped structure with shadowing from bony anterior (pubic) and posterior (ischial) parts and echoes penetrating the vertical part of the triradiate cartilage **(Fig. 10)**. The ischial component is larger than pubic part and femoral head is bisected by line continuous with the echoes penetrating the mid acetabulum.

The ligamentum teres is seen as a broad echogenic structure attached to the medial aspect of the femoral head in infants. In older children, it is obscured by the ossified femoral head. In neonates, the two layers of the synovial membrane are not distinct while in older children; some synovial fluid is normally present.

The joint capsule and ligaments are visualized as echogenic fibrous structures, which are closely approximated and cannot be separated on sonography. The hip is studied in two planes from the lateral approach, coronal and transverse with respect to the bony pelvis. The anterior approach in the parasagittal plane parallel to the femoral neck is used for evaluation of joint effusion. On anterior approach, the capsule ligament complex has a concave shape paralleling the underlying femoral neck **(Figs. 11 and 12)**.

Arthrography

Arthrography, although ideal for visualization of joint anatomy has limited use in infants due to high morbidity and risks of general anesthesia and infection. Intraoperative arthrography in conjunction with arthroscopic procedures provides precise direct visualization of anatomy and biopsy specimens but is impractical for children who require serial or frequent investigation.

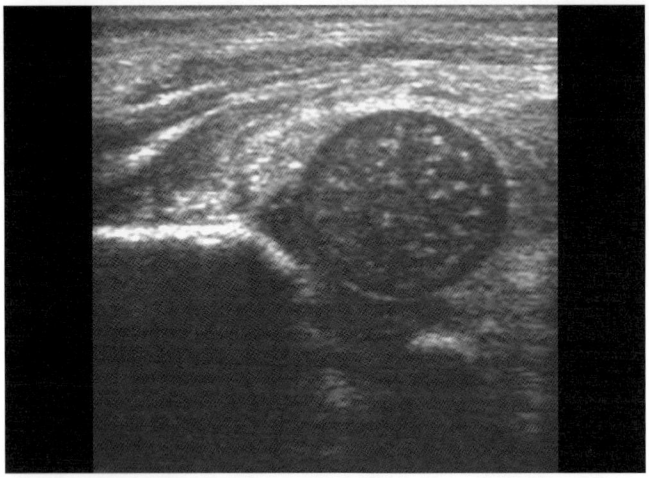

Fig. 7: USG (Coronal view): Femoral epiphysis shows low echogenicity with fine stippled echoes.

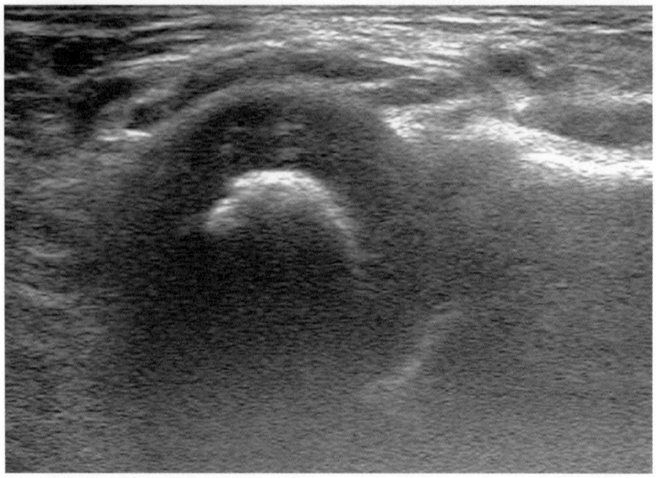

Fig. 8: USG: Beginning of ossification of femoral epiphysis from center.

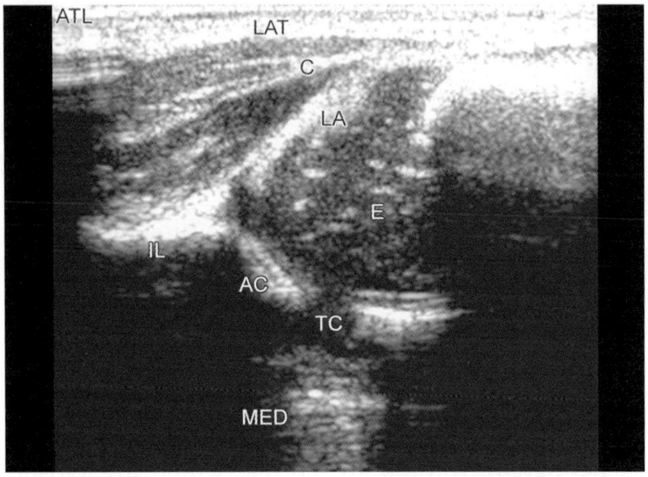

Fig. 9: USG (Coronal) depicting normal structures.
Abbreviations: IL: Ilium; AC: Acetabulum; LA: Labrum; C: Capsule; TC: Triradiate cartilage.

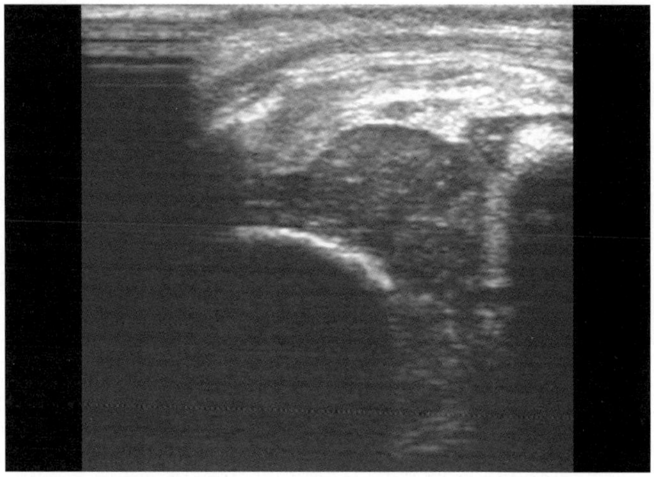

Fig. 10: USG transverse image: Triradiate cartilage is seen between pubis anteriorly and ischium posteriorly.

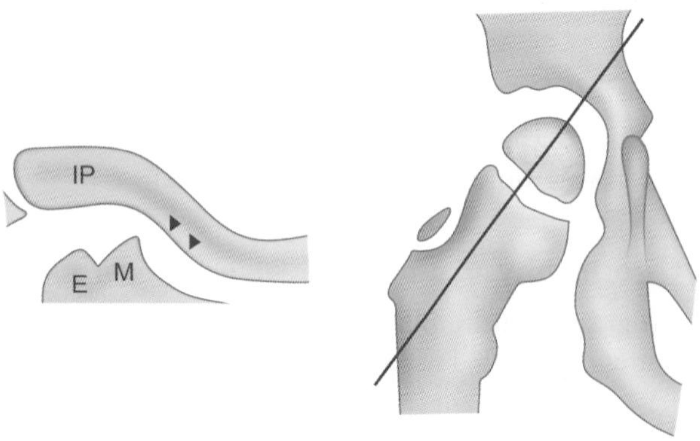

Fig. 11: Plane of section obtained when the transducer is positioned parallel to the femoral neck and anatomy of the hip for detection of joint effusion in the anterior approach.
Abbreviations: E: Femoral epiphysis; M: Metaphysis; IP: Iliopsoas; Arrowheads: Joint capsule/Iliofemoral ligament.

Scintigraphy

Radionuclide bone scintigraphy is a sensitive, but relatively nonspecific modality for detection and characterization of articular diseases. ^{99m}Technetium-labeled polyphosphate is the most commonly used radionuclide which shows increased uptake in areas of bone turnover regardless of etiology, i.e. the growth plate in children and at abnormal sites, such as in tumor, infection, fracture, arthritis and periostitis. In osteonecrosis of the hip, it can demonstrate infarctive, reparative and inactive stages.

Computed Tomography

The use of helical computed tomography (CT) has made three-dimensional reconstructions possible which optimizes visualization of hip articulations. CT

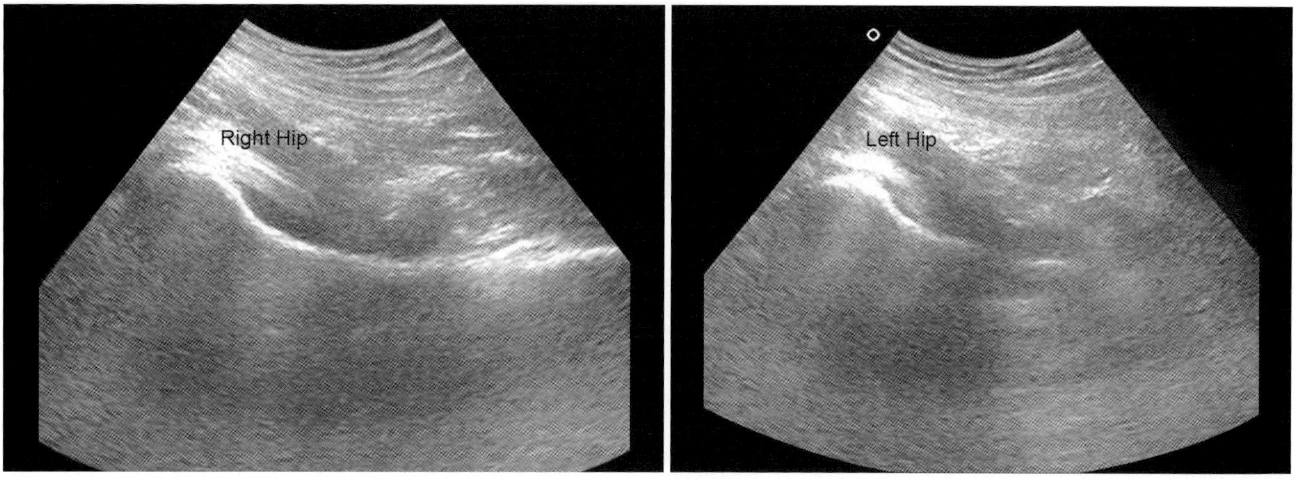

Fig. 12: USG anterior approach shows right hip effusion.

allows accurate evaluation regarding reduction of hip in complicated cases, in the postoperative period and in presence of a spica cast.[5] Pediatric protocols that involve reduced doses can be used and study can be tailored for individual cases. A CT examination is, however, unnecessary for the treatment of the neonate or young infant with easily reducible dislocation of the hip.

Magnetic Resonance Imaging

Magnetic resonance imaging (MRI) has become increasingly important in the evaluation of pediatric musculoskeletal diseases. The advantages being no known deleterious biological effect, no radiation, contrast resolution of soft tissue and muscle is superior to any other modality and fatty as well as cellular marrow components can be imaged.

Cortical bone produces a thin sharply defined black line surrounding the medullary cavity. The nonossified epiphyseal cartilage of the child is homogeneous and moderately high in signal intensity. Maturation replaces the cartilage with fatty marrow resulting in high signal of the femoral head on T1W images. The immature metaphysis contains hematopoietic marrow and has an intermediate signal on all sequences **(Figs. 13A to C)**.

Axial, coronal and sagittal MRI, using body or surface coils are useful in evaluation of hip joint. Coronal images allow assessment of shape of the acetabulum and femoral head coverage. MR images improve visualization of surrounding soft tissue structures—labrum, iliopsoas tendon, capsular tissue, ligamentum teres, transverse acetabular ligament and associated fibrofatty pulvinar. Ligaments and labrum have a low signal on all pulse sequences.

Fat saturation techniques and sequences like STIR (short tau inversion recovery) may be used to decrease the high signal intensity of the fat and enhance visualization of abnormal tissue and oedema within the marrow.

Dynamic multipositional (neutral and 2° flexion and abduction) MR in an open magnet configuration is being used to assess femoral head containment and joint congruency. This can also be used to position the femoral head, under direct visualization.[6]

MR arthrography, with direct intra-articular injection of dilute Gd-DTPA is a combination of joint distension and multiplanar imaging which provides detailed assessment of intra-articular structures especially acetabular labrum. This creates an arthrographic effect by delineating the synovial space.[7]

MR is particularly useful in cases of failed reduction of a dislocated hip to ascertain exact cause.

PEDIATRIC HIP DISORDERS

The most frequently encountered pediatric hip disorders are:

- *Dislocation*:
  - Developmental dysplasia of the hip
  - Traumatic hip dislocation
- *Hip disorders causing effusion-painful hip*:
  - Septic arthritis
  - Tubercular arthritis
  - Transient synovitis
- *Miscellaneous*:
  - Legg-Calve-Perthes disease
  - Slipped capital femoral epiphysis
  - Proximal focal femoral deficiency
  - Rotational deformities.

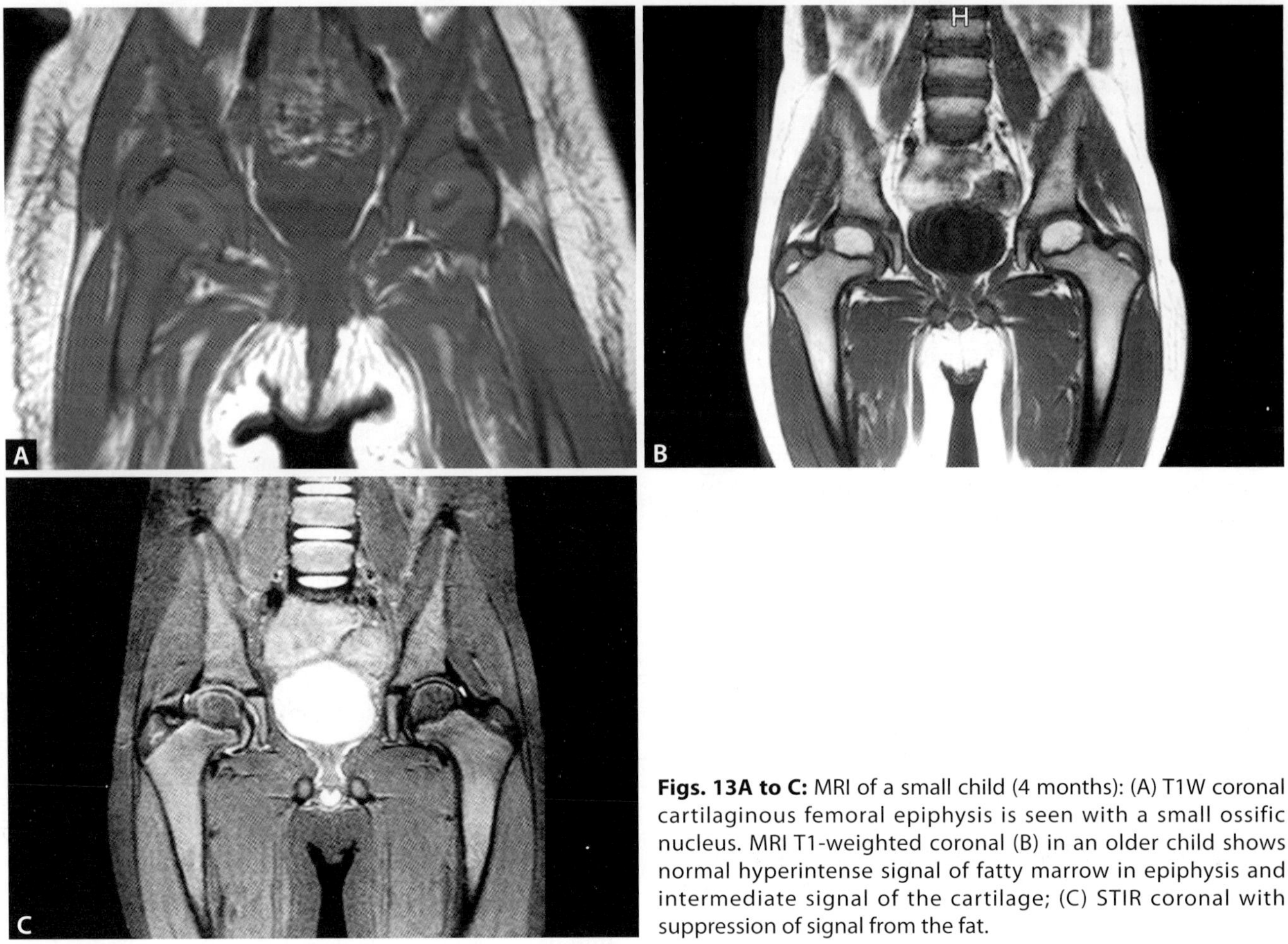

Figs. 13A to C: MRI of a small child (4 months): (A) T1W coronal cartilaginous femoral epiphysis is seen with a small ossific nucleus. MRI T1-weighted coronal (B) in an older child shows normal hyperintense signal of fatty marrow in epiphysis and intermediate signal of the cartilage; (C) STIR coronal with suppression of signal from the fat.

DEVELOPMENTAL DYSPLASIA OF THE HIP

The terminology congenital dislocation of the hip is now referred to as developmental dysplasia of the hip (DDH).[8] This broader term includes all the variants of the disorder during embryologic, foetal and infantile growth. DDH implies a dynamic disorder, that maybe unstable, subluxated or dislocated. DDH is composed of two elements—(1) Instability and (2) Abnormal morphology. Some authors observed that instability resulting in displacement of the femoral head prevents the acetabulum from developing properly, while other authors found that a primary deficiency in development of acetabulum allows the hip to become displaced, creating instability.

The hip is at risk for dislocation at several critical periods in utero,including shortly after its formation is complete at 12 weeks and at 18 weeks, when the hip muscles develop. The early in utero dislocations are often associated with other anomalies and are termed teratologic dislocations. These are fixed and secondary to paralysis from myelodysplasia, arthrogryposis or other neuromuscular disorders. The vast majority of cases of DDH result from forces acting on vulnerable, unstable, but otherwise normal hip in the immediate prenatal or postnatal period. These forces alter the relative proportion of ossified to cartilaginous portions of the acetabular roof in favor of structurally weaker cartilage, predisposing to dislocation.

Natural History and Pathology

The hip joint is entirely cartilaginous at birth, the proximal femur has growth areas including the physeal plate, growth plate of the greater trochanter and along the isthmus of the femoral neck. The normal concave cup shaped acetabulum develops in response to the presence of a spheric femoral head. In DDH, there is a shallow saucer shaped acetabulum that is not congruent with the femoral head and there is persistent femoral anteversion. Secondary changes can be observed in the surrounding soft tissue, with contractures, thickening of the ligamentum teres, increased pulvinar fat, interposition of iliopsoas tendon and hip joint capsule. Soft tissue adaptations can develop at the acetabulum labrum with the formation of a neolimbus with superior migration of the femoral head; there is gradual eversion of the labrum with capsular tissue interposed between it and the outer wall of the acetabulum. In the older infants with DDH, the labrum may be deformed, elongated, inverted and may impede reduction. With abnormal pressure on the labrum there is formation of fibrous tissue that merges with the hyaline cartilage of the acetabulum to form the neolimbus.[9]

The reported incidence of fixed dislocation is 1 in 1000, whereas it is 0.4 to 0.6 in 1000 for late dislocation, subluxation and dysplasia. DDH is more common in girls (M:F = 1:6). The condition is usually unilateral (left > right 11:1), but both hips may be involved. Causes of DDH are multifactorial, with a combination of hormonal, familial and mechanical factors. The hormonal factor may explain the 6:1 female–male incidence and 20% familial incidence. The mechanical factor involves *in utero* spatial constraint and compression of the foetus as can be seen in oligohydramnios and breech position. Other risk factors include, talipes, arthrogryposis and spinal dysraphism and generalized ligamentous laxity.

Early detection of DDH results in an excellent outcome, failing which the condition can cause significant long-term morbidity.

Clinical Examination

DDH may be suspected clinically in the newborn, when a physical examination reveals asymmetrical skin folds, shortened thigh and irritability of the hip.

A "click" during the Ortolani reduction test performed by flexing the hip 90° with gentle abduction or an abnormal Barlow dislocation test performed by grasping the thigh in abduction with downward pressure on the hip indicates instability.

Radiological Diagnosis and Screening of DDH

The maximum potential for acetabular maturation is within the first 3 months of life; hence DDH should be diagnosed and treated before this time. It is important to be aware that a certain amount of instability in the hips of newborns, representing capsular laxity is normal in both boys and girls. This resolves spontaneously by 4 weeks. Delaying hip ultrasound till 6 weeks of age allows resolution of the same and hence ultrasound of clinically normal hips should be done at 4-6 weeks of age, while a clinically unstable hip should be scanned at approximately 2 weeks.[10]

The absolute indications for hip imaging include: (a) Family history of DDH, (b) Neonatal hip instability, (c) Limb shortening and (d) Limitation of hip abduction in flexion.

The relative indications, if more than two are present, imaging for to be done are: (a) Breech presentation, (b) First born child, (c) Cesarean section, (d) Other congenital anomalies, and (e) Excessive fetal moulding.

IMAGING IN DEVELOPMENTAL DYSPLASIA OF THE HIP

Conventional Radiography

As the neonatal hip is composed entirely of cartilage radiographs of the hip are frequently normal, especially if instability alone is present. An AP projection is obtained; the infant must be placed so that the pelvis is in neutral position and not rotated with hips slightly flexed. By 4–6 months, once the femoral head ossifies, radiographs become more reliable.

The site of non-ossified epiphysis may be inferred as lying superior to the femoral epiphyseal plate. The superoinferior and lateral displacement of the femur can be determined by Perkin's line. The Shenton's line is disrupted in cases of dislocation. In dislocated hip, a line through the femoral shaft will point outside the acetabulum and will cross the spine at a higher level than normal as described in the Andrew and von Rosen method **(Figs. 14A and B)**.

From the age of six months onwards, radiological diagnosis is usually easy. The femoral head is displaced upwards and outwards with delayed ossification of its epiphysis. The acetabulum is shallow with its roof sloping upwards and outwards with an increased acetabular angle **(Fig. 15)**. A false acetabulum can develop in a frankly dislocated hip and is a pathognomonic sign of dislocated hip **(Fig. 16)**.

In older children, other radiographic measurements may be useful. In children older than 5 years center edge angle is used. This is obtained by drawing a vertical line through the center of femoral head and perpendicular to the Hilgenreiner's line. A second line is drawn obliquely from the outer edge of the acetabulum through the center of the femoral head **(Fig. 17)**. The resulting angle reflects the degree of acetabulum coverage in dysplasia and the degree of femoral head displacement in an unstable hip. The center edge angle less than 20° is abnormal.

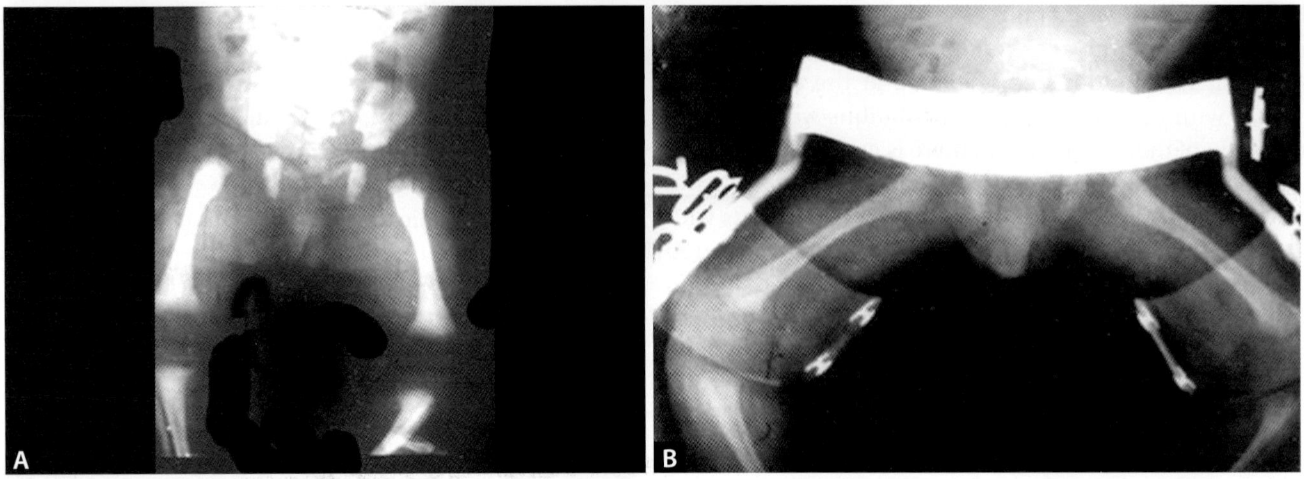

Fig. 14A and B: X-ray pelvis: Congenital dislocation of the right hip in a newborn (A) before reduction; (B) after reduction.

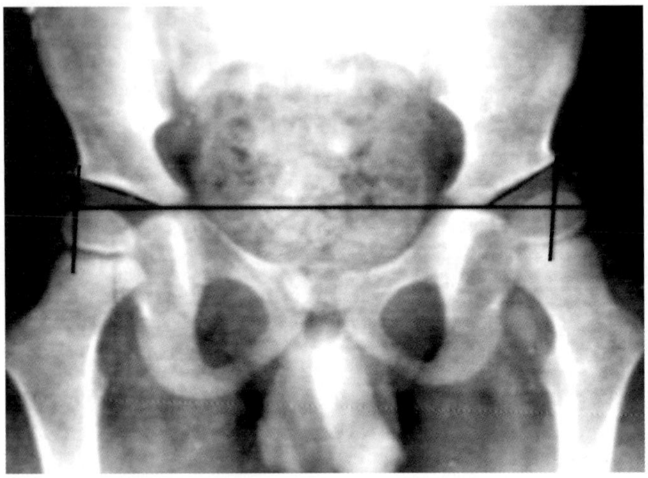

Fig. 15: X-ray pelvis: Subluxation of the left hip.

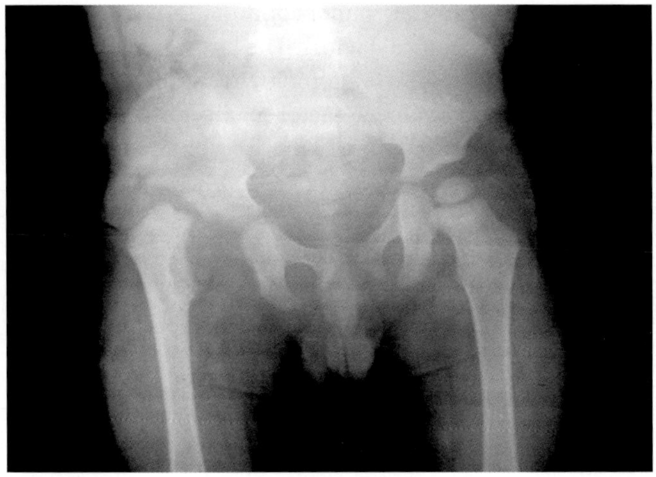

Fig. 16: X-ray pelvis with both hips: Anteroposterior view shows a neglected DDH on the right side, with pseudoacetabulum formation.

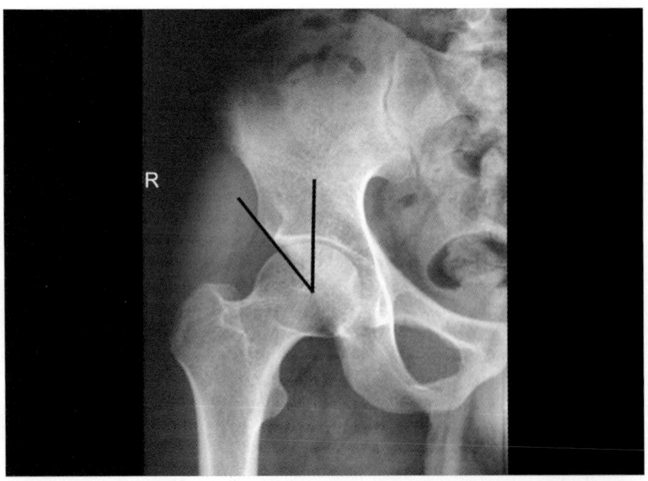

Fig. 17: X-ray of right hip: Measurement of center–edge angle.

Conventional radiography suffers from the following drawbacks—the cartilage is not directly visualized and its position has to be inferred from the bony landmarks, the standard radiographs are taken in a position in which subluxation is least likely to occur and the examination is static.

Ultrasonography in DDH

Sonography is now the primary imaging technique in the diagnosis and follow-up of DDH and has been shown to be more accurate than either clinical or radiographic assessment with a sensitivity of 100% and a specificity of 98%.[11] Ultrasound examination has the following advantages—it visualizes the nonossified cartilage of the femoral epiphyses and the cartilaginous labrum and permits dynamic assessment of stability. It cannot be used over the age of 12 months due to acoustic shadowing from the developing ossification center of the epiphysis.

The sonographic features to be noted in an infant hip include the following:

- Position of femoral head, its coverage and change in position with stress.
- Assessment of acetabular dysplasia.
- Acetabular roof–horizontal or inclined.
- Acetabular edge—sharp, rounded or flattened.
- Labrum everted or inverted.
- Acetabular fossa for presence of interposed soft tissues such as excessive fat or hypertrophied ligamentum teres.

The use of ultrasound in evaluation of DDH was first described by Graf[12] in 1978 and Harcke[13] et al soon after. Modifications of these methods- by Rosendahl, Morin have been suggested and are used at some centers.

Graf assessed acetabular morphology and devised a classification system based on angles of inclination of the bony and cartilaginous roof.

A static coronal image of the hip is obtained for interpretation. The baby is supported in a lateral decubitus position, knees slightly flexed. The hip is positioned in approximately 20° of flexion and slight internal rotation; this represents the neutral position for an infant. The transducer is positioned over the greater trochanter and held perpendicular to the skin and parallel to the table in order to obtain a coronal image of the acetabulum showing its maximum depth.

The cardinal landmarks are the inferior edge of the ilium, the lateral margin of the ilium projected as a horizontal line and the acetabular labrum. The appearance of this standard plane has been likened to a "Ball on Spoon" appearance, with the femoral head representing the ball, the acetabulum, the bowl of the spoon and the ilium, the handle of the spoon **(Fig. 18)**.

The proper coronal view contains three elements (a) the echoes from the bony ilium should be in a straight line parallel to the transducer (b) the transition between the os ilium and the triradiate cartilage should be seen definitively (c) the echogenic tip of the labrum should be in the same plane as the other two. Minor anterior or posterior adjustment may be required until the standard plane is obtained. False positive diagnosis of dysplasia may be made when the transducer is not in mid plane and is rotated anteriorly. Conversely a dysplastic acetabulum may appear normal if the transducer is rotated posteriorly.

Graf demonstrated that in normal hips the round, hypoechoic, speckled femoral head lies centered in

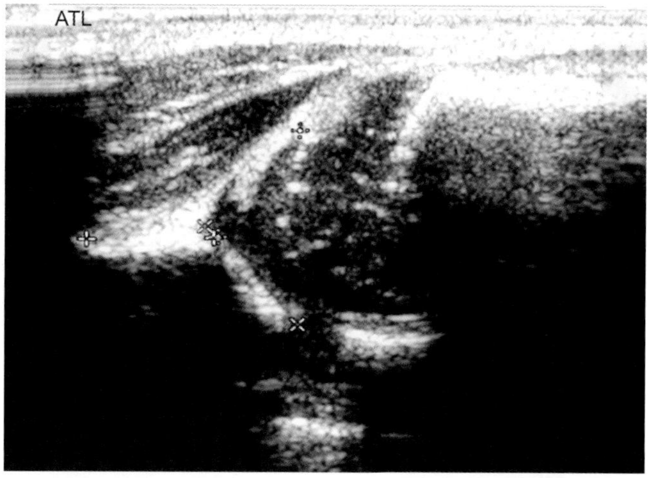

Fig. 18: USG: Coronal view 'Ball on Spoon' appearance.

the acetabulum. His protocol had 3 lines drawn on the coronal view about the acetabulum from which the α and β angles could be measured. The first baseline A is drawn along the straight lateral margin of the ilium, where the perichondrium meets the ilium. A second inclination line B connects osseous convexity to labrum and the third roof line C connects lower edge of acetabular roof medially to osseous convexity. One between acetabular roofline and baseline measures the α angle, which denotes inclination of the acetabular. A small alpha indicates a shallow bony acetabulum **(Figs. 19A and B)**.

The β angle is measured between the baseline and the line of inclination, giving an indication of coverage of femoral head by cartilaginous acetabular rim. A large β angle indicates lateral migration of femoral head. Classification of hip types on ultrasound studies is given in **Table 1**.

Calculation of α and β angles is not possible if the femoral head is dislocated in anterior or posterior direction. Graf described type I and II a/b as inherently stable and types II d, III and IV as inherently unstable and found that it is only necessary to test for stability with type IIc **(Figs. 20 and 21)**.

Coronal images are also used to evaluate the position of the femoral head within the acetabulum. If the acetabular cup accommodates less than one-third of the femoral head, then acetabular dysplasia is definitely present and must be suspected, if only half to one-third is accommodated **(Fig. 22)**.

Harcke and Grisson[14] advocate the use of dynamic sonography of the infant hip, based on the premise that the position and stability of the femoral head are key factors in the diagnosis and management of DDH. If the femoral

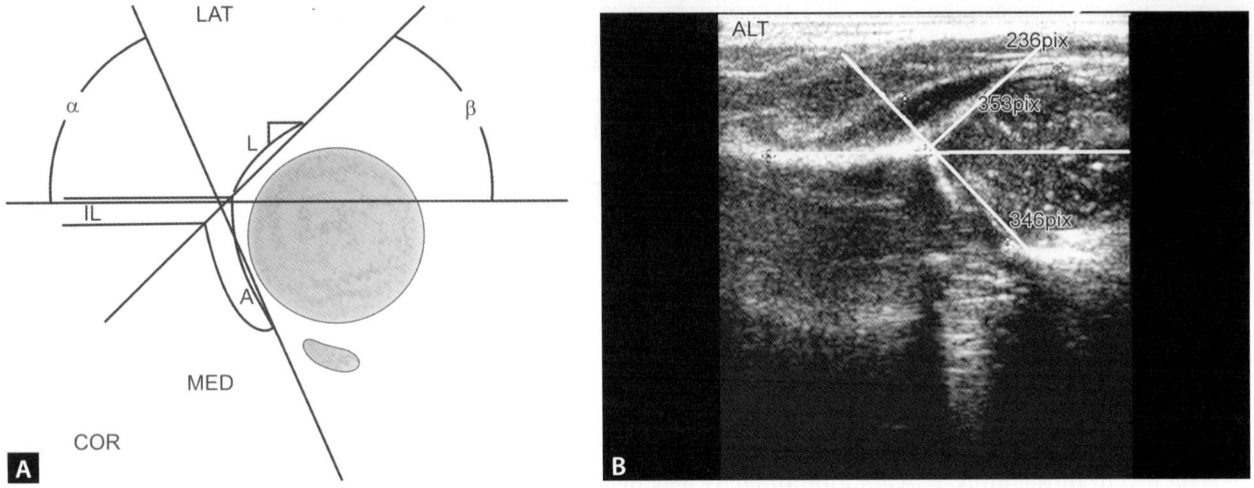

Figs. 19A and B: (A) Straight bony iliac interface (IL), bony acetabulum (A) and echogenic labrum (L), the α and β angles are shown; (B) Sonogram depicting base line, inclination line and acetabular roof lines—normal hip type I.

Table 1: Graf hip types.

Type	*Description*	*α*	*β*	*Comments*	*Treatment*
I	Normal hip	>60°	< 55°	Stable	None
II	• *Concentric position*:				
	– Physiological immaturity (age < 3 months)	50°–60°	<77°	—	Observed till change to type 1
	– Delayed ossification (age > 3 months)	50°–60°	55°–77°	—	Evaluation by orthopedic surgeon
	– Concentric position	43°–49°	—	—	Evaluation by orthopedic surgeon
	– Subluxation	43°–49°	> 77°	Labrum everted	Required
III	Low dislocation	<43°	>70°	Bony roof deficient labrum everted	Required
IV	High dislocation	Not measurable		Flat bony acetabulum, interposed labrum	Required

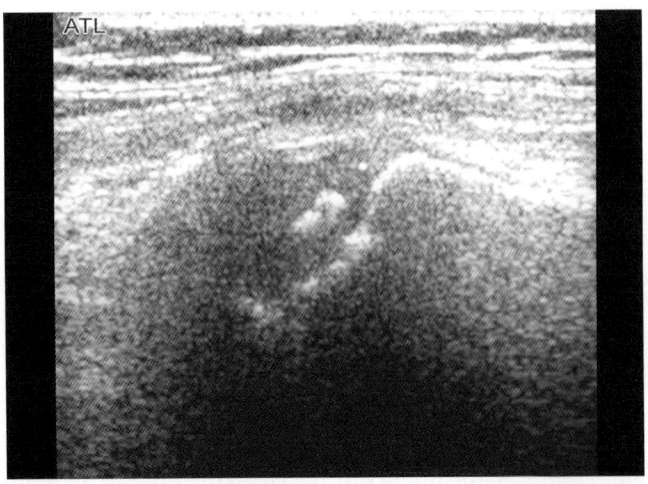

Fig. 20: USG: Gross superolateral hip dislocation with complete disruption in alignment with the acetabulum (Type IV CDH).

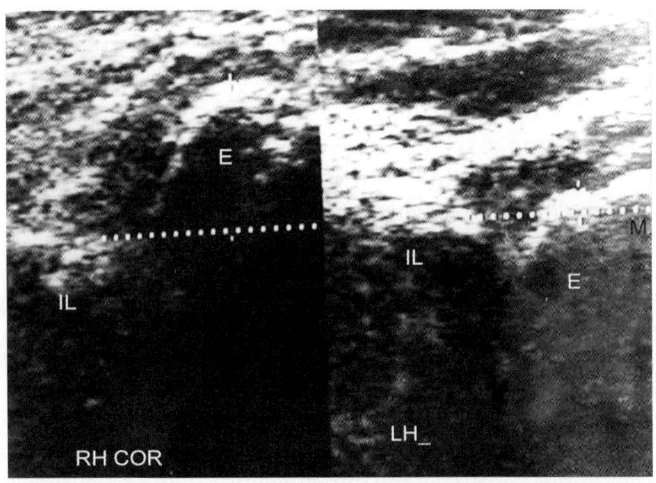

Fig. 21: USG old neglected CDH on the right with normal left hip.

head is properly positioned and stability is achieved, then acetabular development will proceed.

The US examination is modeled after clinical examination and based on provocative tests for dislocating the unstable hip and the reduction of the dislocated hip. The standard US examination should consist of two particular views: Transverse neutral and coronal-flexion **(Figs. 23A to D)**. The value of the coronal flexion view is that it reflects the position in which the physician places the hips during the dynamic physical examination. The ossific nucleus is graded for size (0 = no center present, 1 = center size ≤ 0.5 cm; 2 = center size of > 0.5 cm but acetabulum visible; 3 = center size large enough to prevent visualization) **(Figs. 23A to D)**.

In the transverse plane, with the infant's hip flexed, the hypoechoic cartilaginous femoral head is viewed between two echogenic limbs of a 'V' (in adduction) or U (in abduction). Stability can also be assessed in the coronal plane while pistoning the hip anteroposteriorly (knees flexed), **(Fig. 24)**.

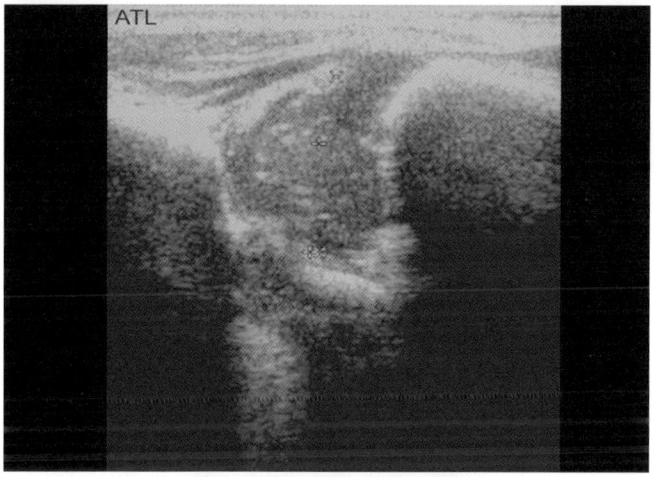

Fig. 22: USG: 62% coverage of the femoral head within the acetabular cup.

Rosendahl and coworkers in 1992 described a modified Graf's method classifying hip morphology and hip stability separately. Hip morphology (alpha angle) was assessed using the standard coronal view with the femoral head centered. In cases of decentered or dislocated hips-Graf type 2c, D, 3, 4a, the femoral head was relocated by mild traction on the thigh before morphology could be studied. A Barlow maneuver was applied to assess a coexisting instability. A technique for assessing the degree of lateralization of the femoral head on the basis of Harcke's coronal flexion view was proposed by Morin et al. in 1985. Based on two lines paralleling Graf's baseline, one tangent to the lateral part of the femoral head and one tangent to the medial junction of the head and acetabular fossa were drawn, they measured distance between medial and iliac lines (d) and between the medial and lateral lines (D). The ratio of d to D multiplied by 100 indicated the percentage of the femoral head covered by the bony acetabulum.[15]

Pediatric radiologists are relying increasingly on the use of dynamic sonography as this allows real time observation of maneuvers allowing a more accurate depiction of the femoral head in relation to the acetabulum as the hip position is changed. Hence, it allows not only depiction of DDH but is also able to assess whether a particular closed reduction is appropriate.

Sonography can also be used to monitor treatment of patients with DDH in a spica cast, brace or Pavlik harness. The long axis anterior approach may be useful in a patient with a spica cast in which a window cannot be cut for lateral scanning. The window should be repositioned and the cast repaired to avoid posterior hip dislocation. The sonographic follow-up of patients being treated in a Pavlik harness is however easy as it permits movement within a safe zone while the degree of restriction prevents subluxation or dislocation. Improvement should be seen within 3 weeks of treatment. Duplex Doppler US has been used to assess vascularity of the femoral head in an infant

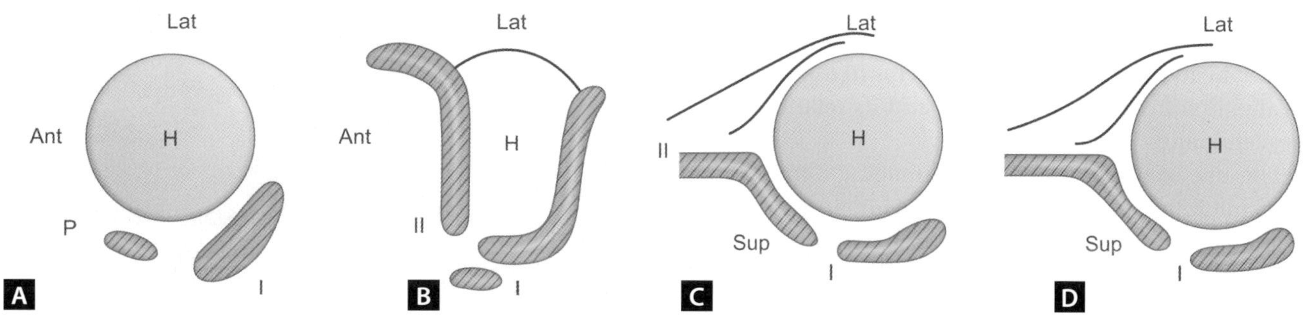

Figs. 23A to D: Harcke's dynamic four step method: (A) Transverse neutral view; (B) Transverse flexion view; (C) Coronal flexion view; (D) Coronal neutral view.
Abbreviations: Ant: Anterior; Lat: Lateral; P: Pubis; I: Ischium; Il: Ilium.

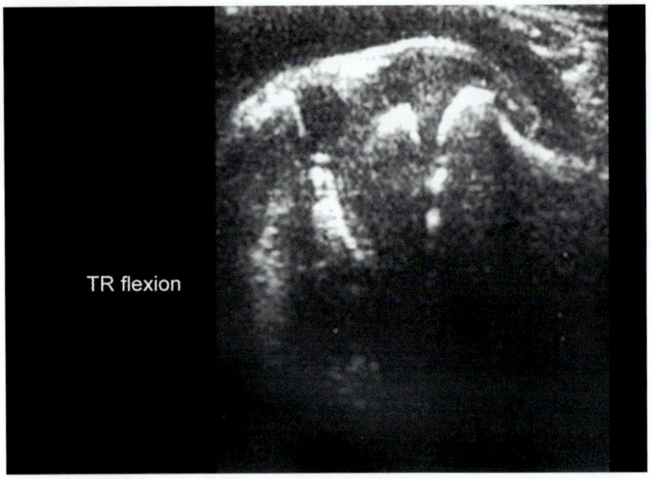

Fig. 24: USG—hip flexed transverse plane: Femoral head viewed between two echogenic limbs of pubis and ischium in adduction ('V').

undergoing abduction treatment. The normal spectral waveform of arterioles in the femoral head of an infant is a slow flow, low resistance arterial pattern with resistive indices ranging from 0.2 to 0.68 (mean 0.48 ± 0.11).[16] Power Doppler can be used to visualize blood flow in the cartilaginous femoral head to ensure that flow is not compromised during treatment.

COMPUTED TOMOGRAPHY

Computed tomography is useful for the evaluation of concentricity of closed reduction, detection of iliopsoas muscle deformity or intra-articular soft tissue obstacles such as hypertrophied fibrofatty pulvinar which can make it difficult to achieve concentric reduction by the closed method, for detection when the surgical procedures are to be performed and for the determination of femoral torsion and acetabular configuration. It can be performed even when the patient is casted **(Figs. 25 and 26)**. CT is most useful in postoperative assessment of reduction. Injection of contrast medium into joint is often performed during intraoperative reduction. CT done soon after allows the contrast medium surrounding the nonossified femoral head to be identified. This helps in assessment of the alignment of the femoral head and its relationship to the acetabulum.

The use of three-dimensional imaging allows direct assessment of the amount of anterior and posterior acetabular coverage. Standard CT protocols allow images to be obtained in the standard frog leg position. Even though the femoral head may not be ossified the position of the femoral metaphysis relative to the midportion of acetabulum can be evaluated.

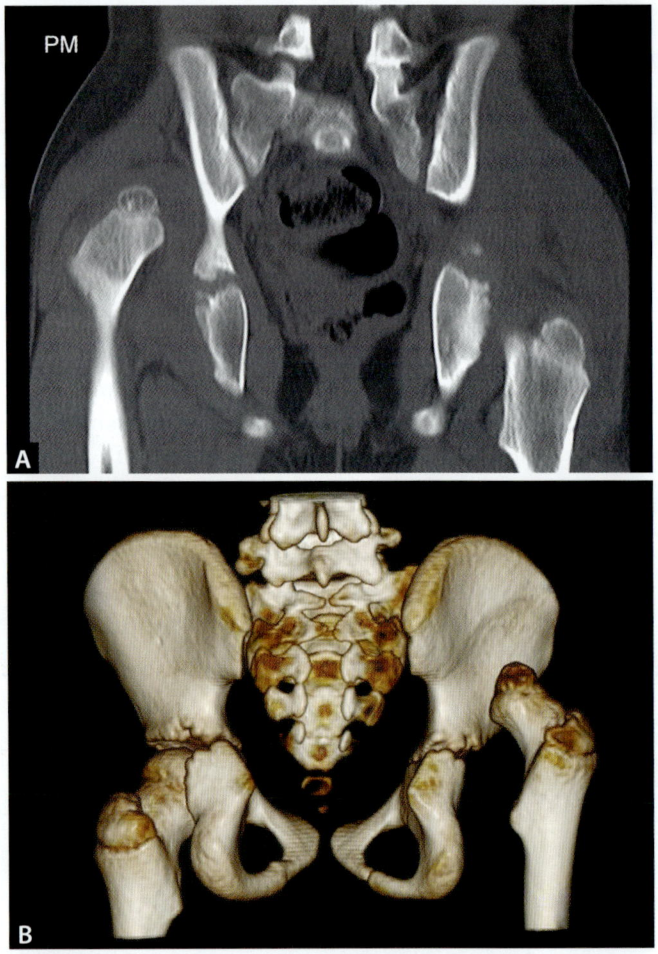

Figs. 25A and B: CT-MPR (A) and VRT (B) show right femoral epiphysis dislocated superiorly and posteriorly.

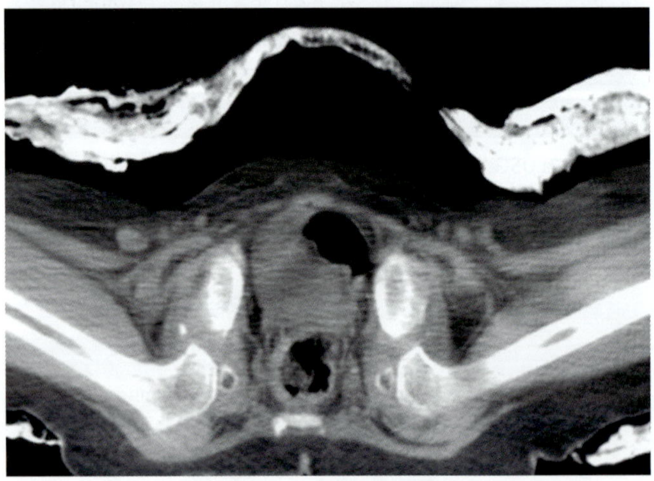

Fig. 26: CT case of DDH with hip spica.

CT scanning allows differentiation of lateral from posterior hip dislocations. Lateral displacement shows the labrum and capsule unfolded secondary to a tight iliopsoas tendon. In posterior dislocation approximation of the femoral metaphysis and acetabulum, projection of a mass behind the ischium and posterior displacement of pregluteal fat plane is seen. Acetabular anteversion is measured by determining the angle of the anterior and posterior rim relative to the vertical axis of the pelvis **(Figs. 27A and B)**. Increased acetabular anteversion has been noted in dysplastic hips and also in some healthy volunteers. Acetabular sector angles are more specific to the presence of hip dysplasia **(Figs. 28A and B)**. Anterior and posterior sector angles reflect the degree of anterior and posterior acetabular support.[17] The sector angles are determined by measurement of the angle drawn between the center of the femoral head and the anterior and posterior acetabular rim relative to the horizontal axis of the pelvis. A normal anterior angle is greater than 50° and a normal posterior angle is greater than 90°. These angles are reduced in developmental dysplasia, which reflects acetabular support. Measurements of acetabular angles, have however not been found predictive of the outcome of DDH.[18]

MAGNETIC RESONANCE

Magnetic resonance is used in the evaluation of dysplasia of the hip when there is (i) a complex dysplasia, (ii) there has been inadequate response to treatment, (iii) in late

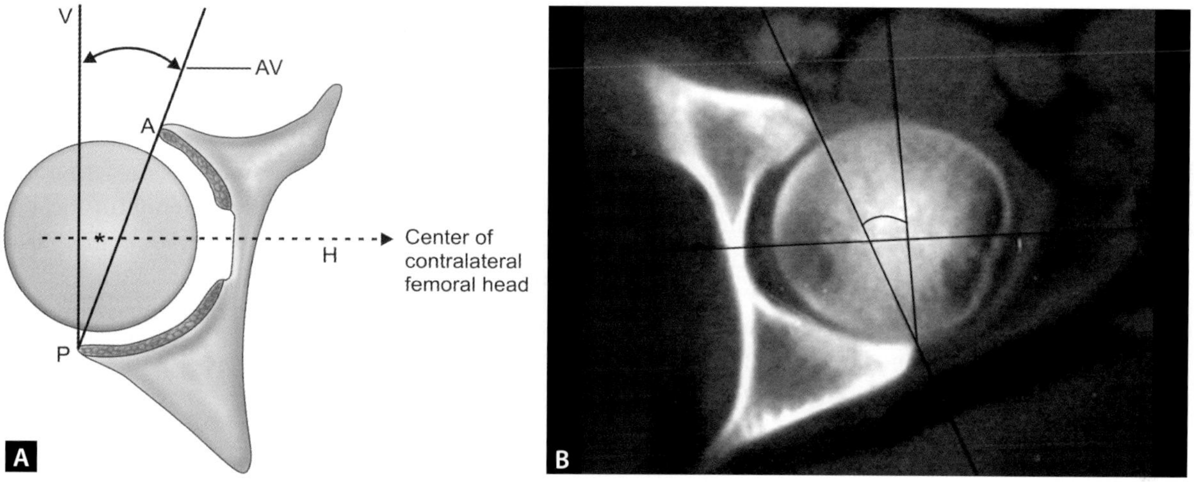

Figs. 27A and B: Schematic diagram (A) and CT (B). Measurement of femoral anteversion from an axial CT slice.
Abbreviations: H: Horizontal line through femoral head center; P: Posterior margin of acetabulum; A: Anterior margin of acetabulum; V: Line perpendicular to line H through point PAC; AV: Angle of anteversion.

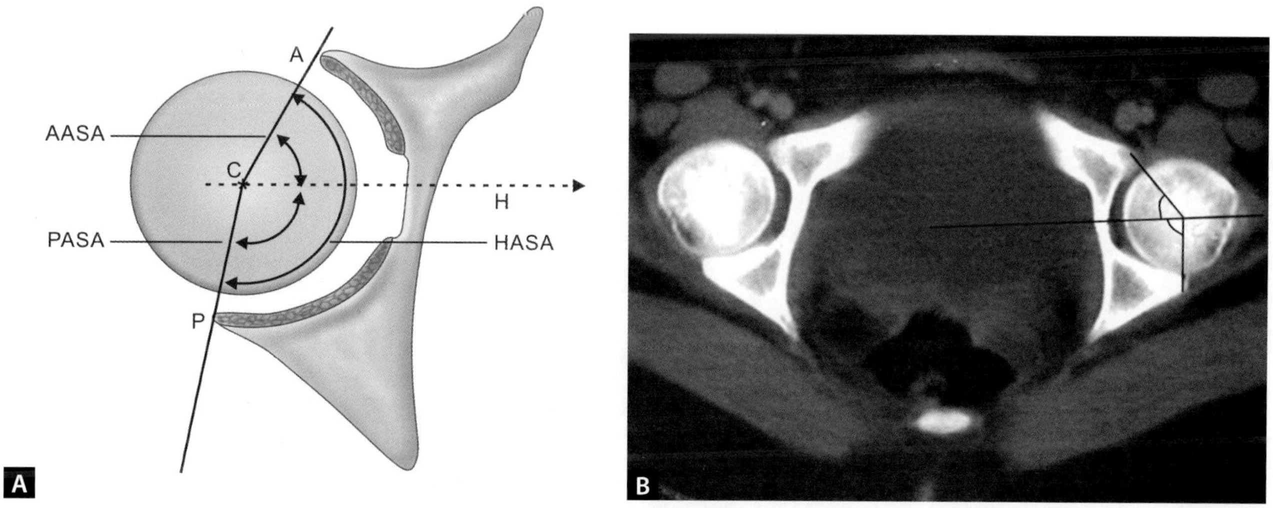

Figs. 28A and B: Schematic diagram (A) and CT (B). Measurement of acetabular sector angles.
Abbreviations: H: Horizontal line through femoral head center; P: Posterior margin of acetabulum; A: Anterior margin of acetabulum; C: Center of femoral head; HASA: Horizontal sector angle; AASA: Anterior sector angle; PASA: Posterior sector angle.

presentation and (iv) teratological dislocation. Axial and coronal MR images are most useful and small surface coils with high spatial resolution are necessary to evaluate DDH.

The value of MR imaging in preoperative planning is due to its ability to portray the cartilaginous part of the pelvis and also analyze the relationship of the femoral head to the acetabulum and labrum. The femoral head is variably laterally displaced in DDH, with posterior and superior reduction. MR shows femoral head coverage in both coronal and axial planes without need for complex radiographic projections or magnification correction. The degree of coverage by the cartilaginous acetabulum and labrum can be evaluated by MR. MR imaging can show changes in the shape of the acetabulum, not demonstrated on CT sonography or radiography. In DDH, the acetabulum becomes elongated posteriorly or superiorly. The rim of the acetabulum becomes oval and the acetabular cartilage becomes thickened and may become displaced.[19]

Any obstruction to the reduction can be visualized, especially in cases where there is a history of failed closed reduction. These include a flipped labrum, prominent pulvinar and a redundant ligamentum teres; capsule or illiopsoas tendon or transverse acetabular ligament, which may be interposed into the joint **(Figs. 29A and B)**. Prominent pulvinar is visualized as fibro fatty material in the joint, which does not allow normal seating of the femoral head within the joint. There can be a small amount of pulvinar normally present with the head being slightly laterally displaced. If the head is encompassed by the confines of the acetabulum and pointing at the triradiate cartilage, the pulvinar usually atrophies. Gadolinium enhanced magnetic resonance arthrography visualizes the labrum, ligamentum teres, transverse acetabular ligament and the pulvinar.[20]

In the immediate postoperative period, MR imaging is useful in evaluation of proper reduction of the dislocated femoral head and its vascular health.

Recently dynamic interventional MRI in an open configuration scanner has been used in the management of developmental dysplasia. The hip can be visualized during reduction and spica can be applied within the scanner itself.[21]

Differential Diagnosis of DDH

Radiographic features such as shallow acetabulam with high angled roof lateral and cephalad displacement of the upper end of the femur and small ossification center for the head can be seen in congenital hypothyroidism. Following appropriate therapy, spontaneous resolution may occur.

Traumatic epiphyseal separation of the femoral neck in very young infants may simulate congenital dislocation. The possibility of trauma may be considered if there is history of an abnormal presentation/difficult labor. Acquired non traumatic dislocation may develop in pyoarthrosis of hip. In such a case clinical sign of infection will be present.

The Painful Hip

Hip pain in a child is always potentially serious and presents a diagnostic challenge since clinical differentiation between septic arthritis; transient synovitis and Perthes' disease may be difficult. The principle concern is to distinguish sepsis of the hip joint from an irritable hip,

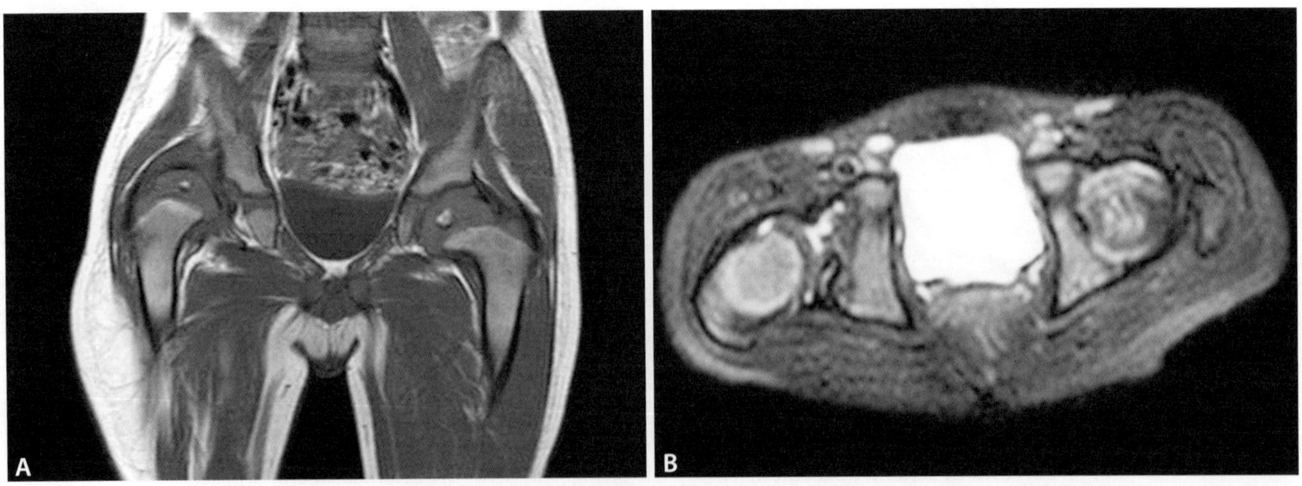

Figs. 29A and B: MRI T1 coronal (A) and T2 axial (B) show dislocated femoral epiphysis with hypertrophied ligamentum teres preventing relocation.

as untreated sepsis can destroy the hip within days. The presentation may be mild and atypical and therefore imaging plays an important role in the management of such cases.

Septic Arthritis

Acute purulent infection of the joints is more common in infancy and early childhood because of greater blood flow to the joints during active growth. Hematogenous seeding is the most common cause related to an upper respiratory tract infection or pyoderma. Infection may also spread from adjacent osteomyelitis in metaphysis (specially in hip, where metaphysis is intra-articular) or from cellulitis, abscess, etc. During infancy, septic arthritis frequently complicates osteomyelitis because capillaries from the metaphysis traverses the physis into the epiphysis. Infants with immune dysfunction, indwelling cathetars, vascular lines are at increased risk. Over 90% of cases of septic arthritis are monoarticular with hip being one of the most commonly affected joints.

Staphylococcus aureus is the most common cause of bacterial arthritis, with group B *Streptococcus* seen in neonates. *H. influenzae* in the 1–4 years age group. Children with chickenpox are at increased risk of developing septic arthritis and other musculoskeletal infections secondary to group A Streptococcus. Pneumococcal joint infection may be seen in children with splenic dysfunction. Over 90% of cases of septic arthritis are monoarticular with the hip being most commonly involved.

Clinically there is fever, joint pain and swelling. Boys are affected twice as frequently as girls. It is a medical emergency as it may lead to joint destruction and impairment, if not immediately and adequately treated.

Pathology

The joint cartilage is vascular and the synovial fluid cushions, lubricates and nourishes the joint cartilage. Bacteria may seed into the synovial space through the highly vascular synovial membrane. Initially, there is edema and hypertrophy of the synovial membrane with joint effusion, which distends the joint. Hyperemia and immobilization leads to demineralization and osteoporosis. The ensuing inflammatory reaction results in destruction of the cartilage matrix leading to reduction of the joint space. Inflammatory pannus destroys the articular cortex, which is eroded. Severe cases are characterized by massive destruction, separation of bone ends, subluxation and dislocation. During recovery bones recalcify and bony and fibrous ankylosis may occur.

Imaging

Imaging evaluation is initially by **conventional radiography**. Plain films may be normal or demonstrate joint space widening with adjacent soft tissue swelling and disruption of normal tissue planes. It may show joint space loss and erosions with relative preservation of mineralization **(Fig. 30)**.

Radionuclide imaging is more sensitive than radiographs. A bone scan localizes the site of infection and is positive as early as 2 days after the onset of symptoms. In septic arthritis there is increased articular activity in the blood flow and blood pool phases. Reduced uptake within the epiphysis may be as a result of ischemia.

Ultrasonography can clearly delineate presence and nature of joint fluid by direct visualization[22] and can be used to guide needle aspiration. The anterior approach along the plane of the neck is used as this is the most easily distensible part of the joint and fluid first accumulates in this area. In normal hip, the joint capsule is seen as a continuous concave reflective line paralleling the anterior aspect of the femoral neck and capital femoral epiphysis. Synovial thickening or an effusion causes the joint capsule to become convex and bulge anteriorly. A difference of 2 mm in the Anterior Capsule Distance (ACD) is indicative of effusion. Asymmetry is an unreliable parameter as effusion may be bilateral. The normal ACD increases with age and the upper limit of normal are 5 mm (<4 years) 6 mm (4–7 years) and 7 mm (8 years or over).[4]

Ultrasound can detect as little as 1 mm of fluid and all cases of septic arthritis have effusion **(Figs. 31 and 32)**. Neither the size nor the relative echogenicity of fluid can be used to distinguish an infected from a simple effusion.

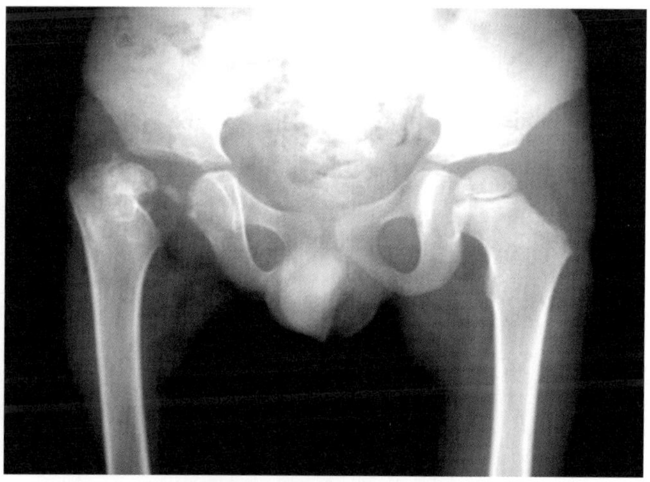

Fig. 30: X-ray pelvis erosions in right femoral head with dislocation and widening of joint space septic arthritis.

Power Doppler ultrasound has been used to differentiate septic arthritis from sterile synovitis. Strouse et al found that though increased flow in the hip suggested infection, findings of normal flow do not exclude infection and should not preclude hip joint aspiration.[23]

MRI is extremely sensitive for detection of even a very minimal effusion with sensitivity and specificity of Gd-DTPA enhanced MR imaging of 100% and 77% in detection of septic arthritis.[24,25] Patients with both septic arthritis and transient synovitis may show joint effusion, intense enhancement and hypertrophy of the synovial membrane. Patients with septic arthritis, however, also show signal abnormalities in adjacent bone marrow on fat suppressed CE MRI, a finding not seen in patients with transient synovitis. The joint space becomes an abscess cavity. Pyogenic abscess in a joint space can be differentiated from reactive fluid based on diffusion MR. A pyogenic abscess shows an increased signal intensity on diffusion weighted imaging whereas a reactive effusion shows a low signal.[26]

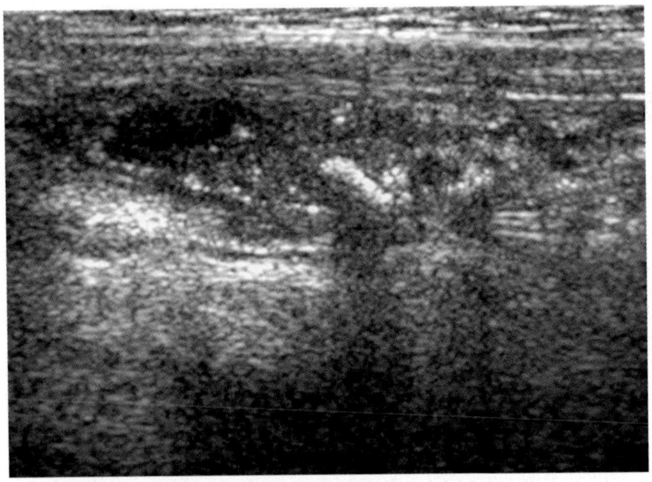

Fig. 31: USG: Collection with echogenic debris following infection.

The earliest MR finding of acute osteomyelitis is marrow edema with decreased signal on T1 and increased signal on T2 and STIR images.[27] As infection progresses, periosteal soft tissue inflammation and cortical abnormalities may be seen **(Fig. 33)**. Differentiation of pyogenic from tubercular joint infection is important as treatment is different in both. Serology and joint fluid analysis form the basis of diagnosis. MR imaging may offer some clues to the diagnosis.[28] The presence of bone erosions, absence of subchondral marrow signal intensity abnormality favors a diagnosis of tubercular arthritis.A thin and smooth abscess rim favors tubercular arthritis, where as a thick and irregularly enhancing rim is indicative of pyogenic arthritis.

Septic arthritis is a surgical emergency and a delay in diagnosis and therapy may lead to femoral head destruction, arthritis and deformity **(Fig. 34)**. Once an effusion has been detected, prompt arthrocentesis should be carried out. A needle with a central stylet such as spinal needle is recommended to avoid the theoretical risk of creating an implantation dermoid.

Tuberculosis of the Hip Joint

Tuberculosis of the skeletal system is widespread in our country and accounts for 15% of all (adults and children) patients of osteoarticular TB,[29] hip involvement, being second to spine. The patient may present with a limp,

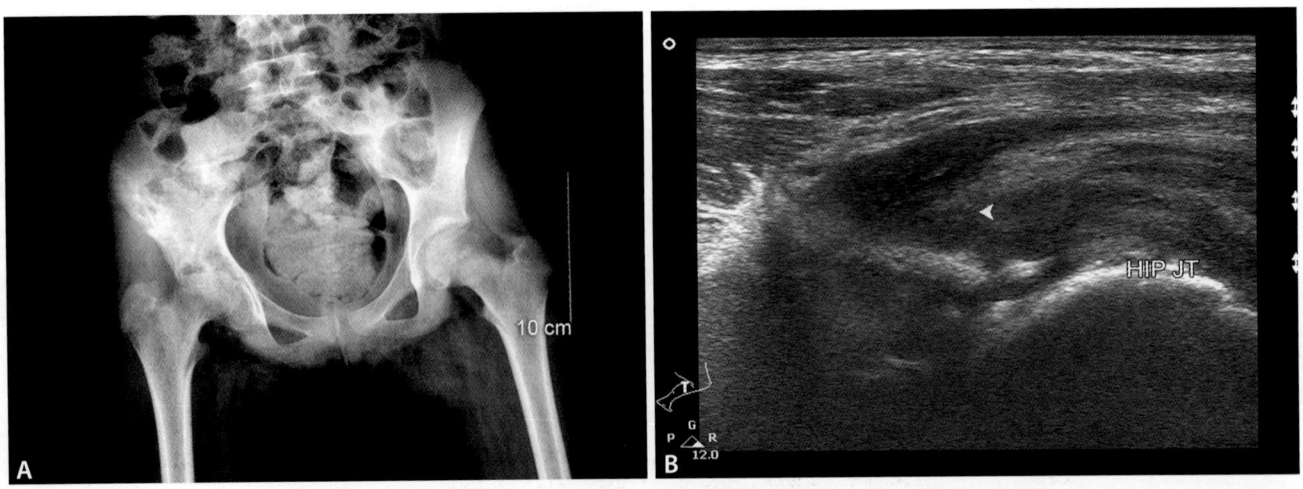

Figs. 32A and B: X-ray (A) reduced right hip joint space with irregularity of articular outline. Ultrasound hip (B) of the same patient shows disorganized joint with effusion that shows debris—A case of septic arthritis.

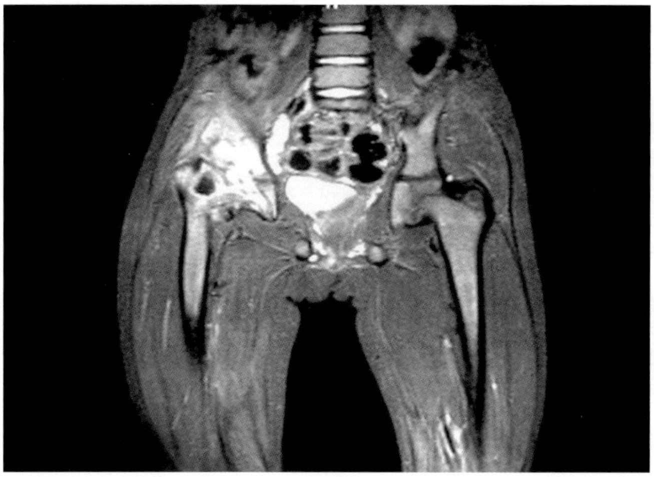
Fig. 33: MRI-STIR coronal: Hyperintensity within femoral head and acetabulum with joint effusion—septic arthritis.

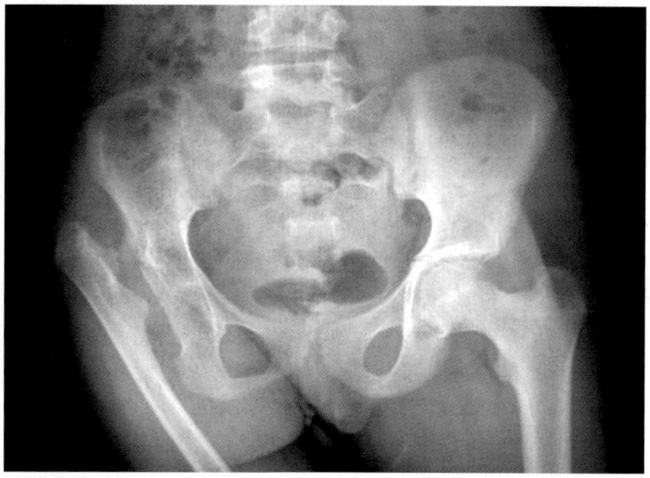
Fig. 34: X-ray pelvis: Completely destroyed right femoral head with dislocation—Sequelae of septic arthritis.

pain, or fullness around the hip with referred pain to the knee. The initial focus of tuberculous lesion may start in the acetabular roof, epiphysis, metaphysis, greater trochanter or synovial membrane. The destruction of articular cartilage is characteristically slow; consequently the cartilage space is preserved for long joint involvement and the patient may then present with extensive bony destruction.

Pathology and Imaging

The different stages of tuberculosis are:[30,31]

Stage I—Tubercular Synovitis

Synovial edema and outpouring of a large fibrinous exudate results in joint effusion and soft tissue swelling **(Fig. 35)**. Osteopenia may be noted 12–18 months after onset of symptoms. Flexion deformity of the hip may be seen.

Stage II—Tubercular Arthritis with Damage to Articular Cartilage

There is destruction of the articular cartilage and erosion of the acetabular margins and femoral head. Periarticular osteopenia may be seen with reduction of the joint space multiple lesions, involving the epiphysis of the neck and acetabulum may be noted due to common blood supply **(Figs. 36 to 38)**.

Stage III—Advanced Arthritis

There is gross destruction of the articular cartilage, bone of femoral head and the acetabulum. Subluxation and dislocation of the joint may be seen. This leads to a broken Shenton's line with bird beak appearance of the femoral head and a mortar and pestle appearance of the joint. There may be 'wandering acetabulum'. In this there is a lesion in the acetabular roof which may result in subluxation with the femur being displaced upwards and dorsally with clinical features of limb shortening.

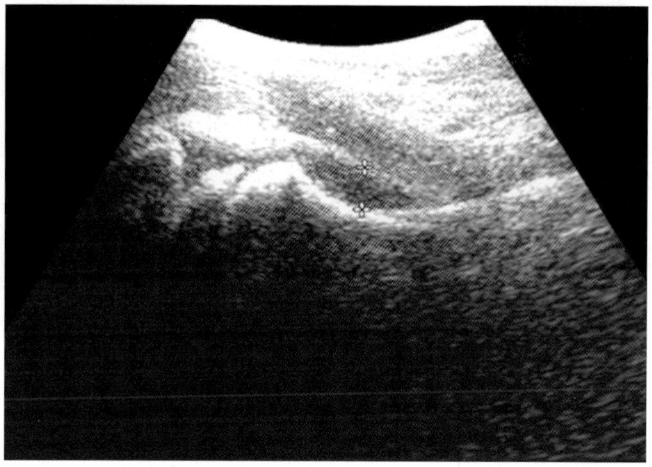
Fig. 35: Hip joint effusion—a case of early tubercular arthritis.

Ultrasound can be used to guide aspiration and evaluate femoral head destruction and joint congruency. Erosive changes are better delineated on CT. MRI can detect early tubercular involvement as it is highly sensitive to marrow pathology **(Figs. 39 to 41)**.

TRANSIENT SYNOVITIS OF HIP

Transient synovitis is a self limited inflammatory condition specific to the hip. It affects boys more commonly than girls

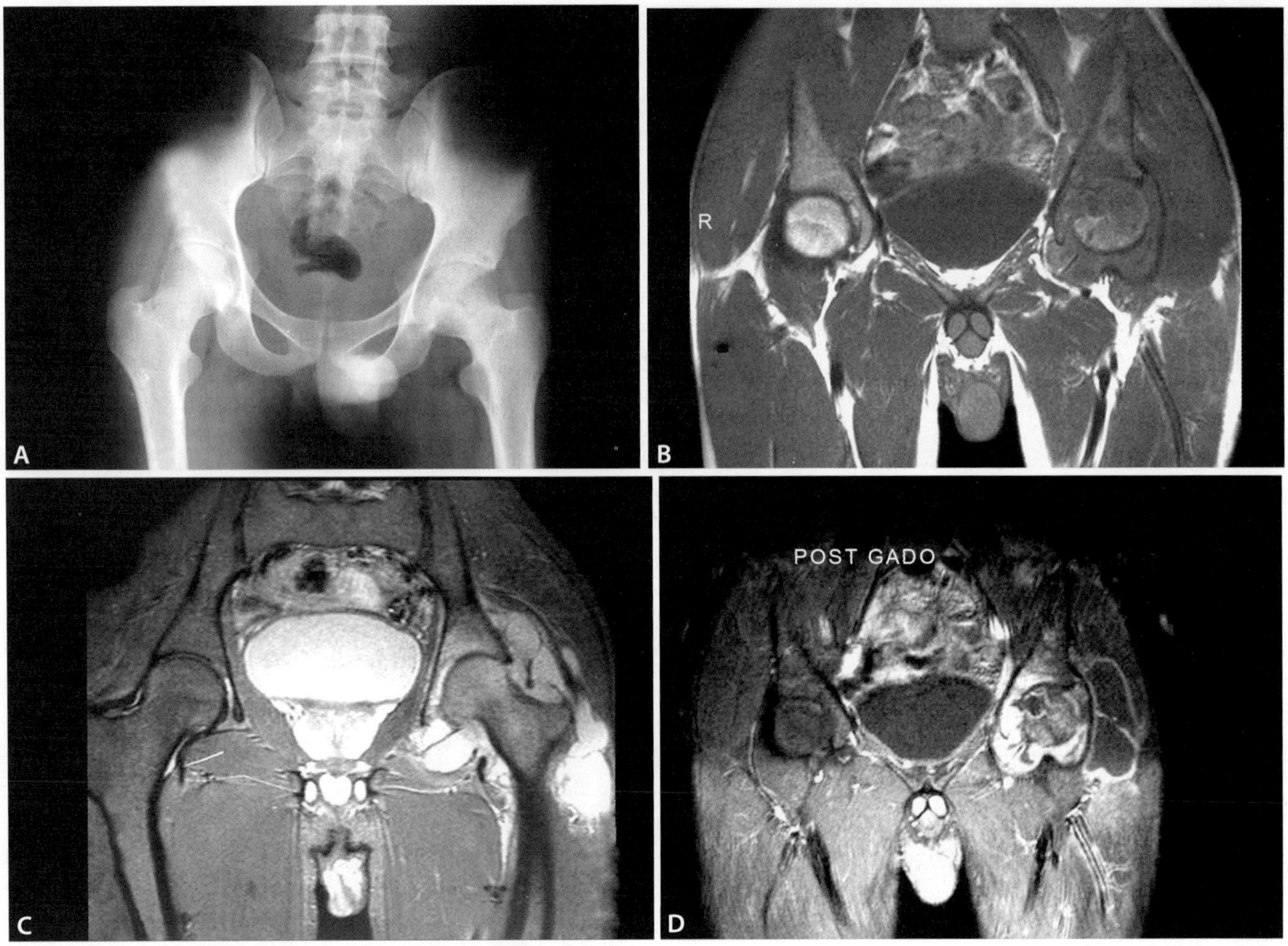

Figs. 36A to D: X-ray pelvis: (A) Mild osteopenia on the left side with decrease in joint space. MRI T1 Coronal (B) STIR Coronal (C), and T1 Coronal post-gadolinium (D). Marrow signal alteration with lytic lesion in left femoral head and acetabular margin, hypointense on T1, hyperintense on T2, with cortical irregularity. Heterogeneous enhancement is noted. There is a large multilocular, peripherally enhancing collection in the adjacent muscles—TB hip.

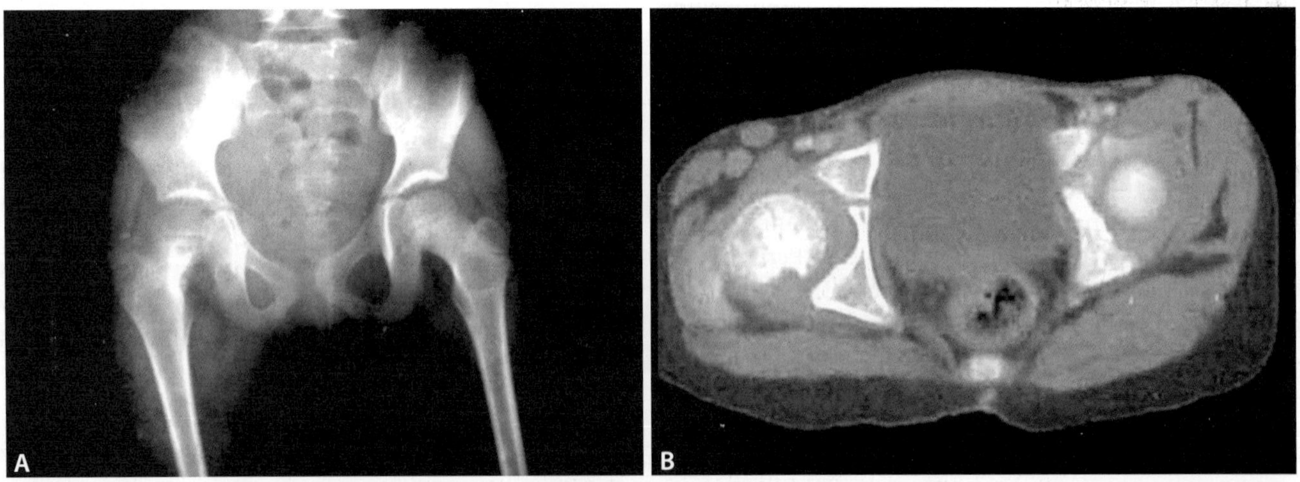

Figs. 37A and B: (A) X-ray pelvis: Erosion of head and medial aspect of femoral neck; (B) CT pelvis: Cortical erosion of femoral head-TB.

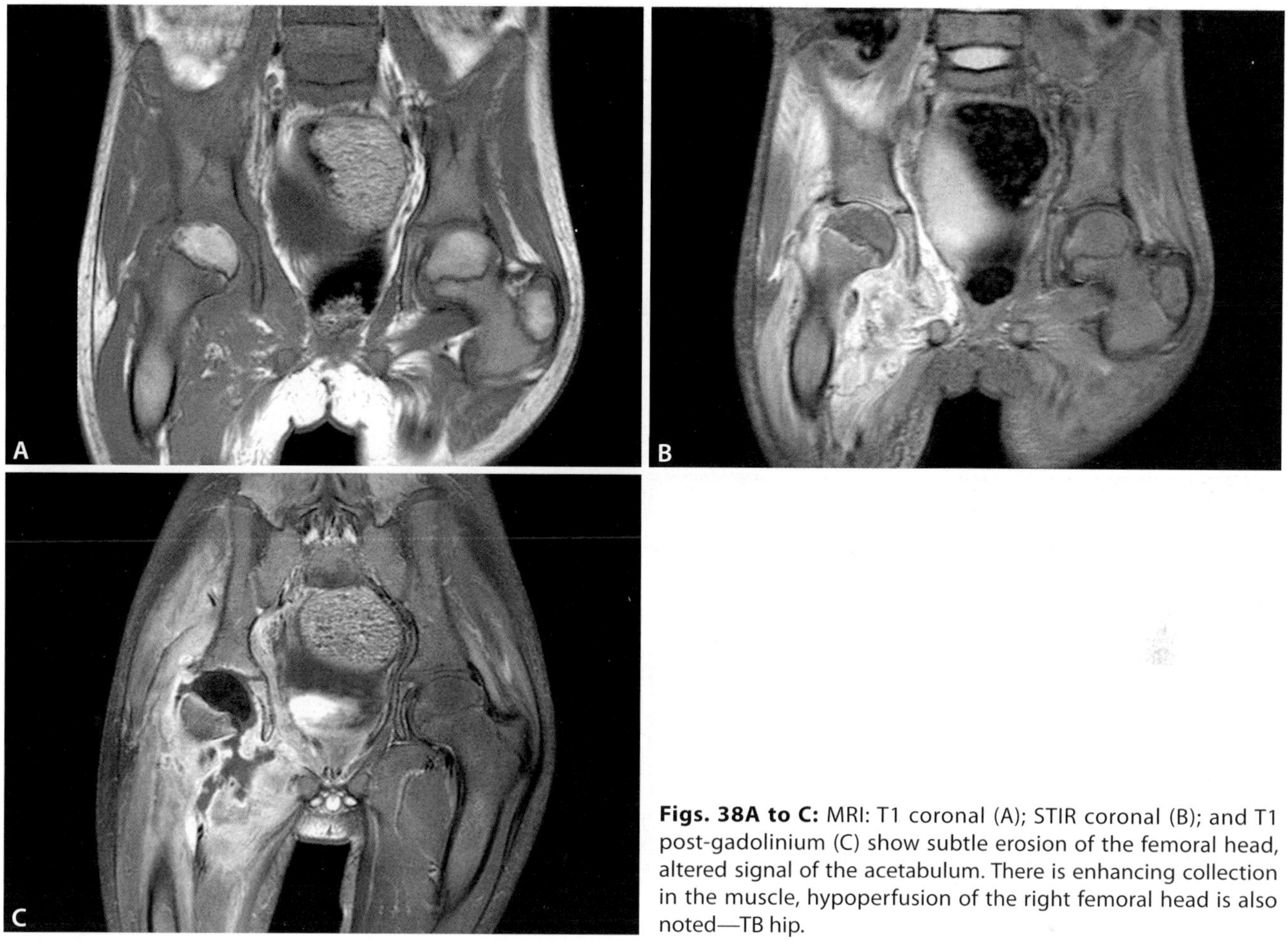

Figs. 38A to C: MRI: T1 coronal (A); STIR coronal (B); and T1 post-gadolinium (C) show subtle erosion of the femoral head, altered signal of the acetabulum. There is enhancing collection in the muscle, hypoperfusion of the right femoral head is also noted—TB hip.

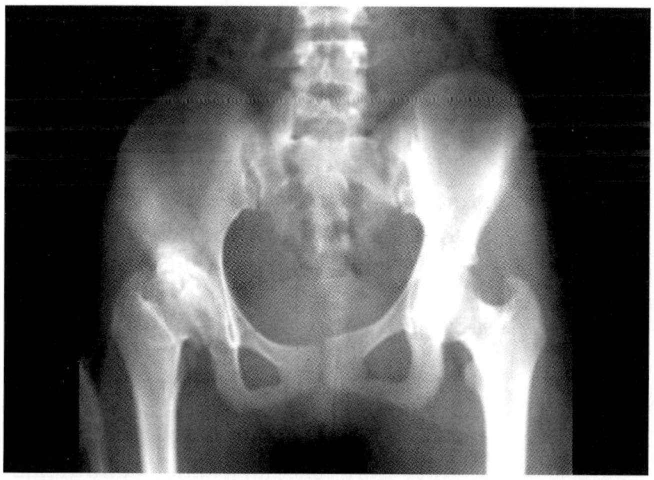

Fig. 39: X-ray pelvis: Advanced TB arthritis—Erosion and sclerosis of femoral head with partial collapse and decreased joint space.

in all age ranges, but is more common between 3 and 6 years. The etiology is unknown; some children have a preceding history of upper respiratory infection or trauma. Patients present with acute onset of pain, limp, refusal to bear weight. None of the symptoms or laboratory investigation is pathgnomic. ESR may be raised and symptoms usually regress within ten days with simple bed rest, prolonged immobilization and traction are very rarely needed.

Only 1% have bilateral disease. Transient synovitis is a diagnosis of exclusion with the most common differentials being traumatic synovitis, JRA and perthes disease. Treatment consists of rest and NSAIDs. Long term sequlae are rare.

Radiographs are usually normal but may show joint effusion with mild widening of joint space. Sonography is sensitive to the presence of effusion.[19] Joint effusion is not a specific finding and aspiration is required to rule out infection. On MRI, there is evidence of joint effusion, but there is no concomitant bony abnormality **(Figs. 42A and B)**.[27] Scintigraphy may demonstrate a transient decrease in isotope uptake for the first week followed by rebound hyperemia within a month. Biopsies performed

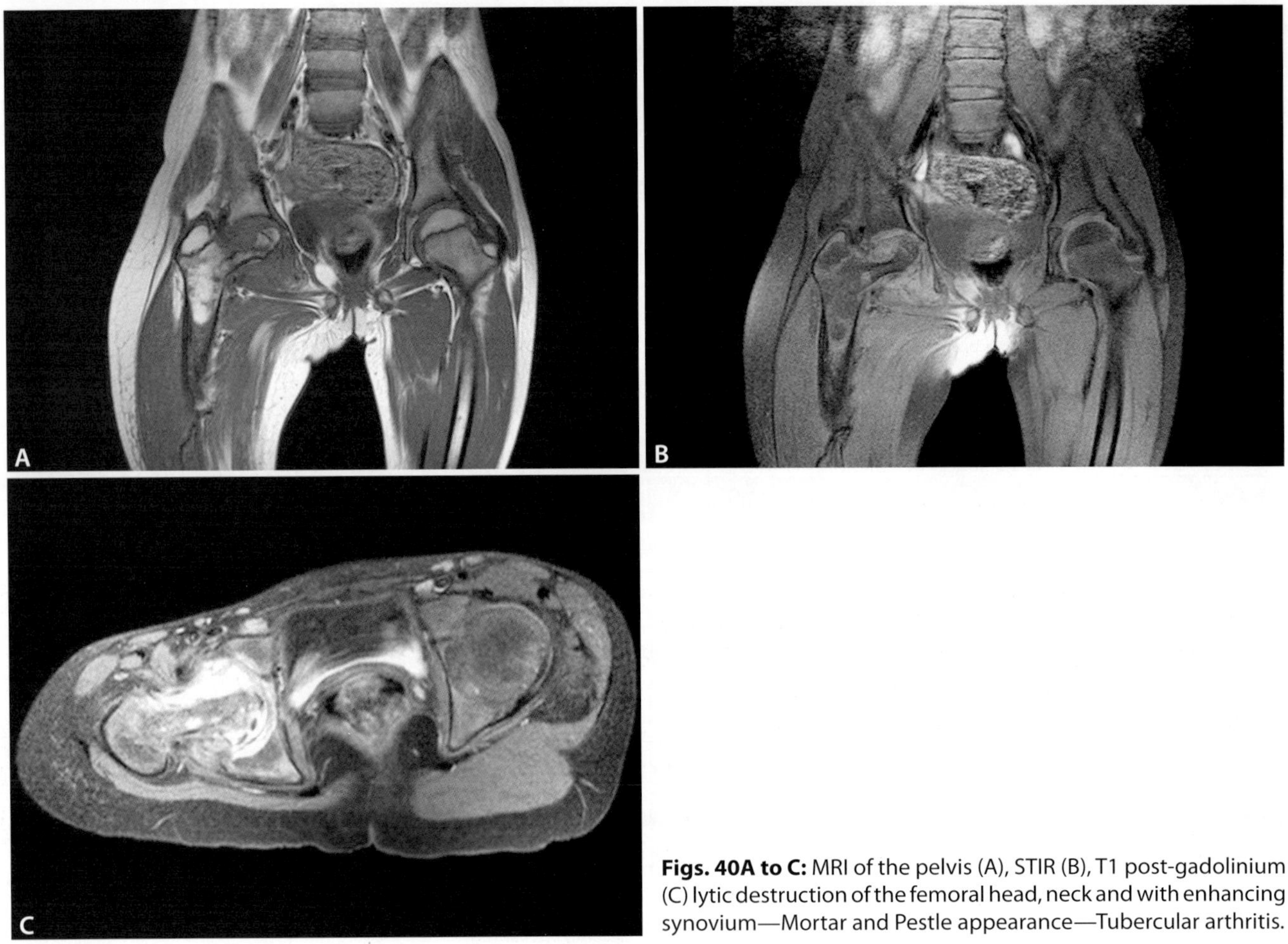

Figs. 40A to C: MRI of the pelvis (A), STIR (B), T1 post-gadolinium (C) lytic destruction of the femoral head, neck and with enhancing synovium—Mortar and Pestle appearance—Tubercular arthritis.

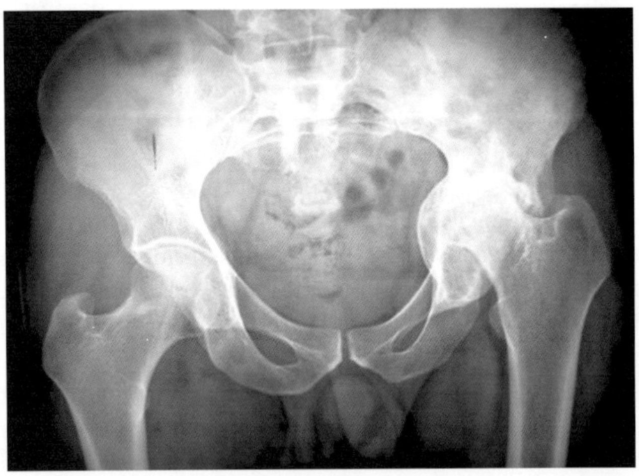

Fig. 41: X-ray pelvis: Protusio acetabuli seen on the left in a case of tubercular hip arthritis.

on these joints reveals nonspecific synovial inflammation and hypertrophy with joint effusion and normal articular cartilage and joint capsule.

LEGG-CALVE-PERTHES' DISEASE

Legg-Calve-Perthes' disease is a self-limiting osteonecrosis of the femoral head epiphysis which typically occurs between the ages of 3 and 12 years, more common in boys (M:F = 5:1). Both hips are involved in 15% of patients, with involvement being asymmetric. If there is a symmetric involvement, hypothyroidism or multiple epiphyseal dysplasias should be excluded. The first symptom is a limp sometimes painless, but usually associated with pain in groin, lateral hip or knee.

The origin of LCP remains unknown. It is believed to represent multiple vascular occlusive episodes that involve the femoral head, causing changes of AVN with a long ongoing process of vascular changes and repair. This differs from AVN seen in adults, because in most cases, there is remodeling and healing with little residual deformity of the femoral head. If the age of the patient at the onset of disease is more than 9 years and the shape of femoral head at skeletal maturity is non-spherical a worse outcome can be expected.

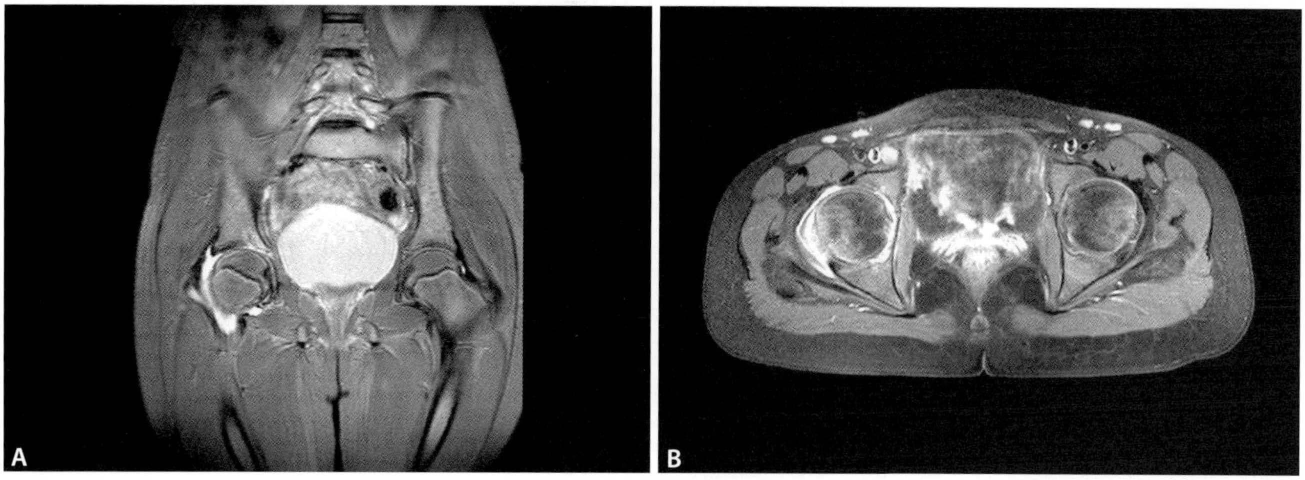

Figs. 42A and B: MRI: T2 coronal (A) and T1 post-gadolinium (B) show minimal joint effusion and enhancing synovim—Transient synovitis.

Following ischemia, the ossific nucleus of the epiphysis undergoes necrosis, causing growth arrest. The overlying cartilage, supplied by synovial fluid, survives and thickens medially and laterally in the non-weight bearing regions. Creeping substitution eventually occurs in the ossific nucleus, which becomes dense.[32]

Imaging

The goal of imaging in Perthes's is early diagnosis, assessment of the extent and location of epiphyseal involvement and of the femoral head coverage. Imaging is also required to follow healing of the disease and measure sphericity of the femoral head at completion of healing.

Radiographs remain the mainstay of diagnosis, classification and follow-up of the disease. Most children of LCP present with an abnormal radiograph. The earliest radiographic abnormality includes asymmetry of the intergluteal fat planes, growth retardation and reduced size of the capital femoral epiphysis. Subchondral fractures are noted and best seen in the frog lateral view. Increased radiographic density of the femoral ossific nucleus occurs due to trabecular compression, dystrophic calcification in the debris and creeping substitution. The classical triad comprises of condensation, collapse and fragmentation. The amount of subchondral fissuring of the femoral head on the radiograph during the initial stages, is thought to be predictive of later involvement of the femoral head. A poor prognosis is associated with subchondral fissuring of more than 50% of the head **(Figs. 43 to 45)**.

There is a radiographic staging described by Waldenstrom which is as follows:

- *Initial stage*: Increased head socket distance, subchondal plate thinning, dense epiphysis.

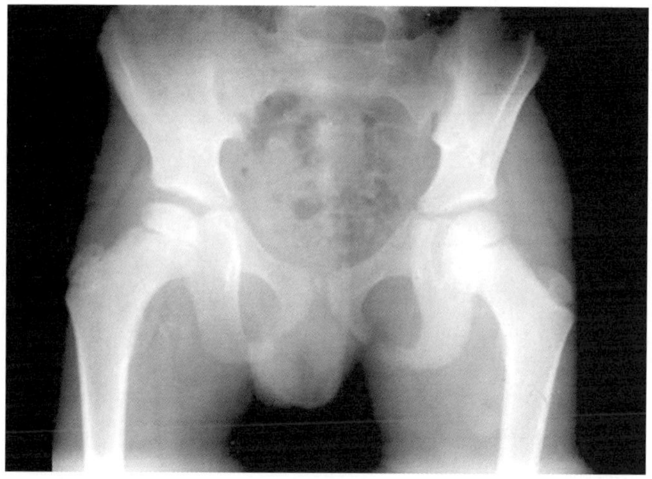

Fig. 43: X-ray pelvis: Subtle flattening of the right femoral epiphysis. No subchondral fracture appreciated.

- *Fragmentation stage*: Subchondral fracture in homogeneous dense epiphysis, metaphyseal cysts/ pseudocysts.
- *Reparative stage*: Removal of sclerotic bone and replacement with normal bone, epiphysis more homogeneous.
- *Growth stage*: Approach the final stage.
- *Definative stage*: Final shape—Congruent or incongruent hip joint.

To classify the extent of ischemic process for purpose of prognostication, based on plain X-rays. Catterall[33] has described four groups, estimating the extent of involvement of the head by ischemia, deformity of the head by lateral displacement, collapse and resorption of bone in the head.

Group I—Only the anterior part of the epiphysis is involved. Collapse does not occur and healing begins from the periphery of the defect.

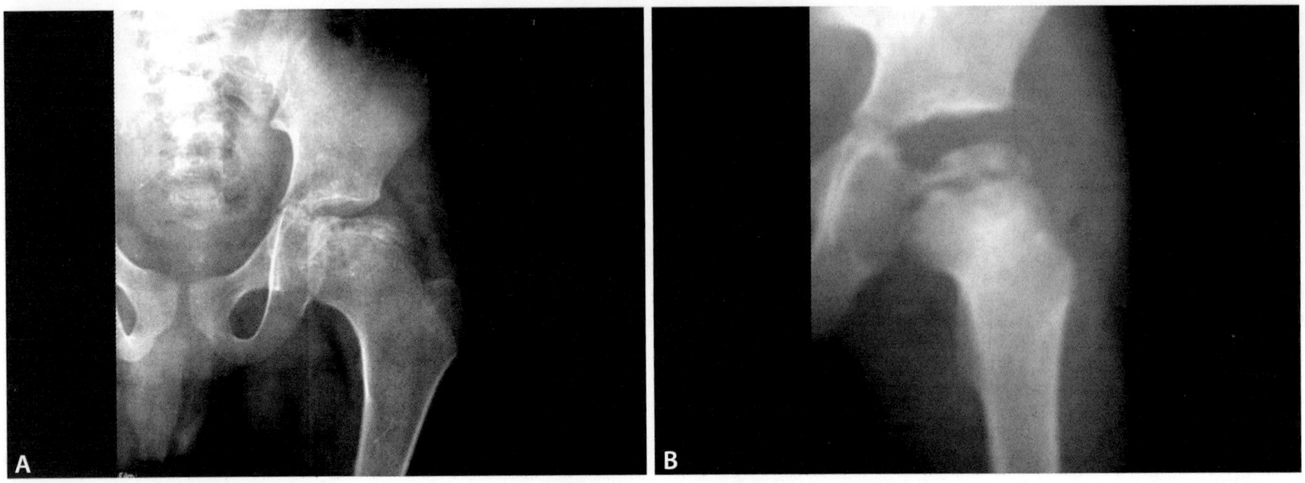

Figs. 44A and B: X-ray pelvis: Flattening and sclerosis with fissuring of femoral head and metaphyseal changes—Perthes' disease.

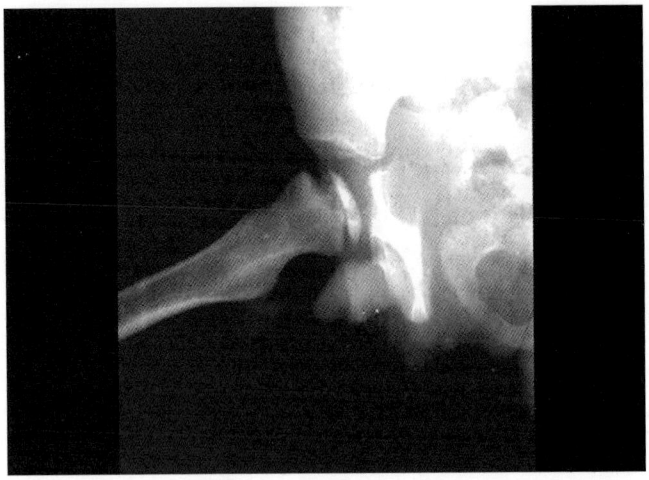

Fig. 45: X-ray left hip: Severe flattening of femoral head involving the entire epiphysis and sclerosis—Perthes' disease.

Group II—More of the anterior epiphysis is involved which collapses and a dense sequestrum form. The unaffected segment retains its height and reaches epiphyseal plate normally. Metaphyseal changes are minor and the involved segment heals by ossification from the periphery.

Group III—Only a small uninvolved part remains posteriorly. Subchondral fissuring is prominent. Speckled ossification occurs in cartilage around the nucleus. Metaphyseal changes are more, collapse and deformity is present.

Group IV—The whole epiphysis is involved and flattened to a thin dense line. All quadrants are flattened and a mushroom deformity remains.

Herring system[34] is based on lateral pillar involvement (Lateral pillar is defined as the lateral 5-30% of epiphysis).

A—LP uninvolved

B < 50% LP loss of height

B/C Border group—Narrow LP 75% original height, poorly ossified LP with at least 50% original height or exactly 50% that is depressed relative to the central pillar.

C—75% LP loss of height

Sonography can be used as an adjuvant to other imaging modalities. The following parameters are assessed ultrasonographically: (i) medial joint space, (ii) epiphyseal changes and flattening, condensation and fragmentation, (iii) metaphyseal changes such as fissures, widening and sclerosis. The earliest ultrasound appearance is of hip joint effusion. Although this is a nonspecific finding, persistence of a hip joint effusion for more than 2 weeks should raise the possibility of Perthes' disease.[5] Synovial thickening is often more marked than is seen in transient synovitis and thickening of the articular cartilage may be seen at an earlier stage. Ultrasound may demonstrate irregularity, flattening and fragmentation of the capital femoral epiphysis, osteoid new bone, and recalcification in the healing phase. The articular cartilage thickens. Contrast-enhanced Power Doppler has been used to demonstrate changes of the revascularization process in LCP, particularly within the physis.[35]

In very early stages of disease, the plain films may be normal and **scintigraphy** is helpful in making the diagnosis. A focal area of decreased uptake of the isotope is seen within the femoral head, the size of the scintigraphic defect is believed to correlate with the eventual amount of involvement of the femoral head.

CT and MRI in Perthes' Disease

CT depicts changes of Perthes' disease. The area of femoral head necrosis is usually located in the superior anterior aspect with characteristic marginal sclerosis.[36]

MR imaging is a sensitive and specific imaging technique for the evaluation of LCP. This condition can be diagnosed even in the setting of normal or equivocal radiographs. In a suspected case of LCP, MR should include imaging in all the three planes. The coronal plane allows comparative analysis of both hips; sagittal plane is the most accurate in estimating the volume of necrotic bone as well as the angular span of involvement.[37] Axial plane is limited in the evaluation of LCP because the superior portion of the head is often inadequately visualized because of partial volume averaging. MR imaging can be used during manual positioning of the hip or multipositional MR imaging, in an open magnet configuration to study femoral head containment, articular congruency and femoral head deformity.[38] It is comparable to arthrography for demonstration of femoral head containment and congruency of articular surface of the hip.

The typical MR appearance in the **avascular phase** is loss of the normally bright signal intensity of the femoral epiphysis on T1 weighted images **(Figs. 46A and B)**. Loss of signal may be subtle and needs to be compared to the contralateral hip **(Figs. 47A and B)**. T2 weighted/STIR imaging shows variable signal intensity, including hyperintensity representing bone marrow edema. Curvilinear subchondral T2 hyperintensity and T1 hypointensity may be observed in the anterosuperior aspect of the femoral head. This finding, referred to as the **crescent or Caffey sign,** suggests presence of a subchondral fracture. The normal hip shows rapid enhancement after IV gadolinium. In Perthes disease, there may be partial or complete nonenhancement of the proximal femoral epiphysis in the avascular phase. This is best depicted approximately 2 minutes after injection using subtraction techniques. Asymmeteric involvement is noted with the anterior portion frequently and most prominently. There may also be flattening of the head. This is due to combination of necrotic trabecular bone collapse and resorption. Articular cartilage and labrum hypertrophy as they continue to derive nutrition from synovium. Periarticular T2/STIR hyperintensity and contrast enhancement may be seen due to associated synovitis.

In the **revascularization and reparative phase** of the disease, MRI reveals heterogeneous proximal femoral epiphyseal signal. Revascularized areas show T2/STIR hyperintensity and contrast enhancement.[39,40] Areas of revascularized epiphysis may hyperenhance after the IV administration of contrast when compared with areas that were never avascular. Revascularized areas may also show persistent enhancement on delayed imaging.

Dynamic gadolinium-enhanced subtraction MR allows early detection of epiphyseal ischemia and accurate analysis of revascularization patterns which can aid therapeutic decision-making.[41] Nonionic gadoteriol is the preferred contrast agent.[42] Acquisition is usually obtained in coronal plane. The acquisition should be early as the enhancement of the early vascular phase decreases after 2–5 minutes post injection. The disparity between normal and abnormal side becomes less clear. The lack of perfusion, in an acute setting, does not necessarily mean that necrosis has occurred, or will occur as therapeutic intervention may interrupt the ischemic pathway.[43] Dynamic postcontrast imaging accurately quantifies the viable bone which enhances brightly. Early enhancement of the lateral pillar (the lateral one-third of the femoral head) is associated with better prognosis.

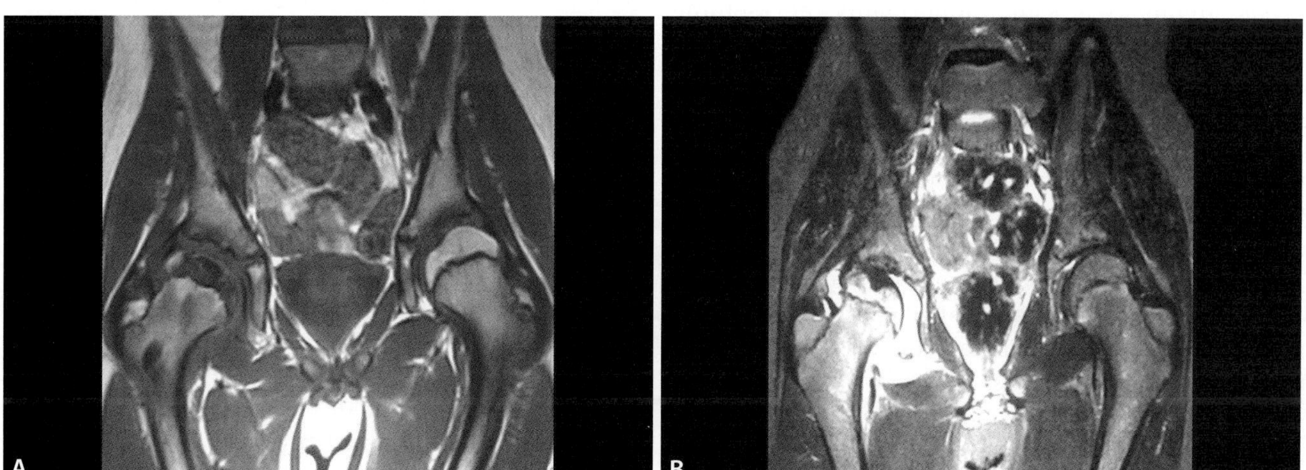

Figs. 46A and B: MRI: T1 coronal (A) and STIR coronal (B) Flattening of femoral head with loss of normal hyperintense signal of femoral epiphysis—Perthes' disease.

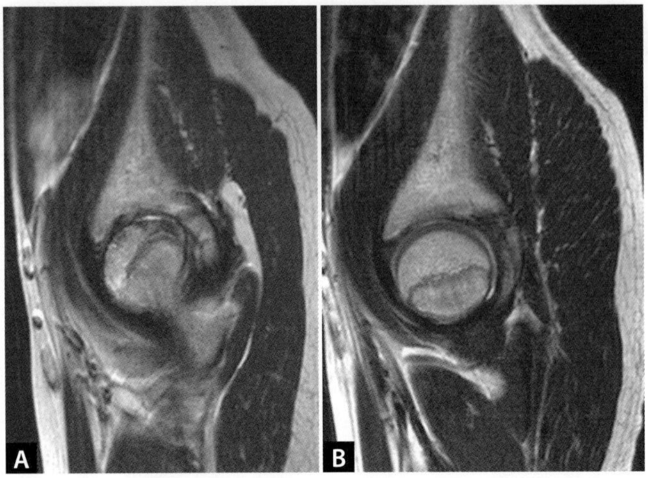

Figs. 47A and B: T1-saggital of the affected (A) and normal (B) hip in a case of Perthes seen as decrease in size of the femoral epiphysis on the affected side.

Morphological changes related to epiphyseal necrosis may include articular surface flattening (coxa plana) and fragmentation. There may be lateral subluxation of the femoral head or loss of containment. This finding is due to cartilage thickening, joint effusion and synovial thickening.

Abnormality of the proximal femoral physis is also seen. This may be due to the primary ischemic insult or secondary to abnormal mechanical loads. Physeal abnormalities include increased undulation of the growth plate (W or M shaped, deepening of the growth plate, epiphyseal-metaphyseal osseus fusion or physeal cystic changes. This may lead to premature growth arrest of the femur). Metaphyseal lesions can be a cystic fluid collection in the metaphysis adjacent to the physis. Metaphyseal signal abnormality representing cartilaginous metaphyseal ingrowth indicates higher possibility of growth abnormalities.

Subsequently, in the fragmentation stage, the involved area takes on speckled appearance, an indication of non-homogeneous revascularization of necrotic zone. As revascularization and reossification progresses, the epiphysis regains a more uniform signal.

With healing, proximal femoral epiphyseal height is slowly restored,ossific fragments coalesce and mature trabecular bone again constitutes the entire ossific nucleus. After approximately six years, the epiphysis shows normal MR signal.

The extent and distribution of epiphyseal necrosis has prognostic implications. As the extent of femoral head necrosis increases, overall prognosis worsens. Prognosis is also adversly affected by the involvement of the lateral pillar, the lateral most one-third of the femoral head. Disturbance of the physis is the single most important predictor of growth disturbance. Extensive epiphyseal necrosis can sometimes be predicted by MRI in very early Perthes disease. The two features predicting the same are (a) decreased signal intensity on both T1 and T2W images covering over two thirds of the epiphysis and (b) diffuse bone marrow edema of the femoral neck and metaphysis.[44] Factors that predict early degeneration of the hip joint include later age of disease onset and abnormal shape of the femoral head at the time of skeletal maturity.

Prognostic evaluation of Legg-Calve-Perthes's disease by MRI has been proposed and takes into account the predictive value of four MRI indices—extension of necrosis, lateral extrusion, physeal involvement and metaphyseal changes. The extent of necrosis (up to or >50%) separates the two main groups A and B.[45]

DWI may be a noninvasive means of distinguishing between Perthes disease with favorable and unfavorable prognosis. Femoral epiphysis showed increased diffusivity in the affected hip. Increased metaphyseal diffusivity was found in all cases with absent lateral pillar enhancement at dynamic post contrast MR,[46] signifying poor prognosis.

The main differential diagnosis of LCP are toxic synovitis, septic hip, juvenile chronic arthritis and juvenile osteonecrosis (AVN due to a known cause-sickle cell anemia, thalassemia).

Proximal Femoral Focal Deficiency

Proximal femoral focal deficiency (PFFD) is a malformation in which complete growth and development of upper femur fails to occur. It encompasses spectrum ranging from mild shortening of an otherwise normal femur to severe handicap of absent femur, except for condyles accompanied by acetabular aplasia and thigh muscular dysplasia.

Imaging

The radiographic findings consist of failure of development and delayed ossification of a lesser or greater part of the proximal femur. Hence, a short femur that is laterally situated and proximally displaced is demonstrated at birth. The distal femur is by definition always present **(Figs. 48 and 49)**, there is a misshapen femoral head and neck, upper end of disconnected distal femur—either bulbous or pointed. The femoral head is situated low in the acetabulum with a woolly outline. Secondary deformity of the acetabulum may result. In later cases, the greater trochanter will be found to curve like a beak and it may articulate with the ilium. Pelvis may show

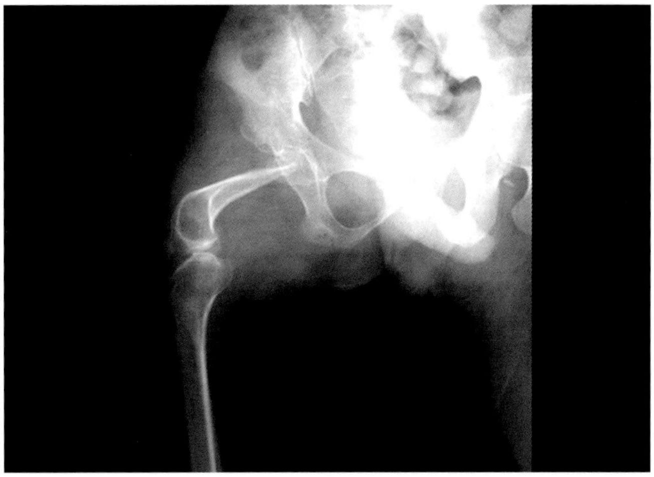

Fig. 48: X-ray pelvis: Focal femoral deficiency in the right side.

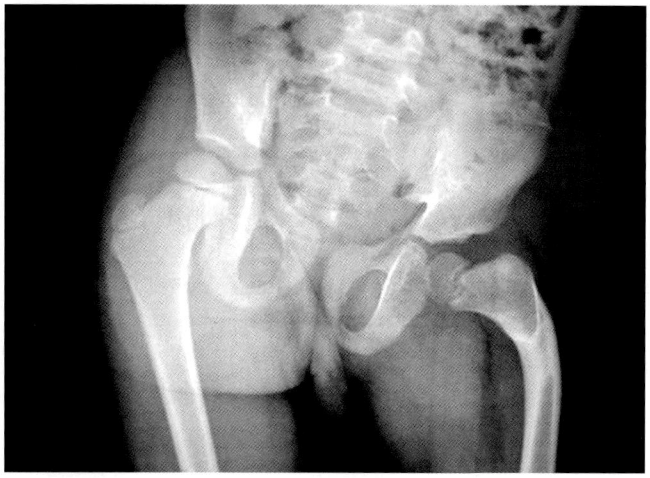

Fig. 49: Aitken class A PFFD: Femoral head is present and connected to the shaft of femur.

enlarged obturator foramen with a supra acetabular bump or horizontal/dysplastic roof of the acetabulum. If radiographs show a normal acetabulam at birth, presence of normal cartilaginous femoral head is likely.

Hip sonography plays a role in the classification of PFFD and in confirming the location of the femoral head with respect to the acetabulum, especially when no proximal femur is seen on radiography. US may reveal a cartilaginous head and neck.[47] Ultrasonography may be useful in prenatal diagnosis and in infants to identify the femoral head. Mobility of the femoral head within the acetabulum may also be assessed.[48]

Magnetic resonance imaging can identify correctly the size and position of the femoral head present. Thin section coronal and axial imaging is of use in locating a small femur head. Continuity to the rest of the femur may also be assessed. Presurgical evaluation is important to guide the orthopedic surgeon in reconstruction. There may be a wide variation in the gap between femoral head and subtrochanteric femur. The gap may be small with pseudoarthrosis or be filled with fibro-osseous tissue. It can also be devoid of any connective tissue. This and the resultant coxa vara deformity cannot be adequately seen on a radiograph as the gap is radiolucent. On CT, the nonossified areas have soft tissue attenuation. On MRI, the femoral head, if present exhibits the intensity of yellow marrow, whereas fibrous tissue is low in signal intensity on all pulse sequence.

The prognosis and treatment options depend on grading of the abnormalities. The most commonly used system is the Aitken classification which assigns types A to D to the abnormality depending in the presence or absence of the femoral head and the acetabulum and osseous integrity of the remainder of the femoral shaft. In patients with type A PFFD, the femoral is short. The femoral head and acetabulum are present. In type D the femur is very short and head and acetabulum are absent. Acetabular deformity is correlated with the presence or absence of the femur which can be inferred from the relative development of the acetabulum.

The **differential diagnosis** can be a congenital short femur (no specific abnormalities of head, neck and shaft):
- Congenital coxa vara-Head, neck normal
- Developmental dysplasia of hip-Graf type 4

Traumatic femoral capital epiphysiolysis in newborn—Pain plus edema of inguinal crease and upper thigh is noted.

Slipped Capital Femoral Epiphysis

Slipped capital femoral epiphysis (SCFE) is an uncommon skeletal disorder of adolescence often overlooked because of its non-specific presentation. It is a unique disorder because no other bone shows similar changes. It is usually seen during adolescent growth spurt in overweight children, with the incidence of bilaterality being 25%. There is a morphological change in the relationship of the femoral head to the femoral neck centered at the physeal level probably caused by obesity. The femoral head becomes relatively retroverted at the physeal level placing the head and physis at a mechanical disadvantage when subjected to stress.

It is Salter 1 fracture through the proximal femoral physis with displacement of the capital femoral epiphysis. In most cases, the displacement of the head is usually medial and posterior relative to the metaphysis. In a few cases, there may be a valgus slip with the head rotating superiorly and posteriorly relative to the neck. This term does not include traumatic Salter-harris 1 as the etiology and management are different.

The most common sign/symptom is limp, painful limitation of hip motion while walking/running. It coincides with adolescent growth and is related to endocrine disorders like hypothyroidism, pituitary dysfunction.

The slip is classified as stable or unstable with the criterion being the ability to bear weight with or without crutches. The incidence of complications is higher with unstable variety.

Imaging

Radiographs remain the prime method of diagnosing SCFE, though it may be difficult to diagnose on anterior projection alone. Medial displacement of the capital epiphysis is seen on the antero posterior projection. A line drawn along the lateral border of the femoral neck (Klein's line) in a normal individual intercepts the epiphyseal ossification center so that a small portion of the head remains lateral to this line **(Figs. 50A and B)**. With SCFE, no part of femoral head ossification center is seen lateral to the line. On the anterior projection, there may be mild widening, lucency and irregularity of the physis. The femoral head may appear foreshortened and there may be apparent sclerosis in the regional femoral neck as the femoral head rotates posteriorly. In the frogleg or true lateral position, the anterior and posterior corners of the epiphysis and metaphysis line up closely in a normal patient, whereas they are displaced in SCFE **(Figs. 51 and 52)**. Posterior displacement is seen on frog lateral radiograph as medial displacement of epiphysis relative to metaphysis. Approximately 90° external rotation of femur on frog-lateral means what is actually a posterior displacement of epiphysis looks like medial displacement on radiograph. On the cross table lateral radiograph with 25 flexion, it is seen as true posterior displacement of epiphysis. Metaphysis shows scalloping, irregularity, sclerosis and posterior beaking. One needs to be careful when using opposite asymptomatic hip as control for radiographic evaluation of painful one as the opposite side may have unrecognized SCFE.

Staging of radiographic findings is mild-moderate-severe based on the displacement of ossification center by <1/3 - 1/3-2/3 - >2/3 metaphyseal diameter.

Ultrasound may suggest malalignment of the capital femoral epiphysis relative to the metaphysis.[4] The alignment of the epiphysis relative to the metaphysis should be assessed as part of hip ultrasound study. Joint effusion, which may accompany SCFE, is recognized by US. US can be used as follow-up of SCFE due to risk of slippage in the contralateral hip.[49]

CT demonstrates the slip and the reduced femoral anteversion, which may be quantified. CT head/neck angles range from 4 to 57 degrees in symptomatic and 0 to 14 degrees in asymptomatic patient.[50] It may also demonstrate metaphyseal scalloping and beaking **(Figs. 53A to C)**.

Magnetic resonance imaging relies on identification of the morphological change at head/neck function and the abnormal signal intensity centered on the physis, indicating stress and edema. Physeal widening is a constant feature and can be seen on MR before being apparent

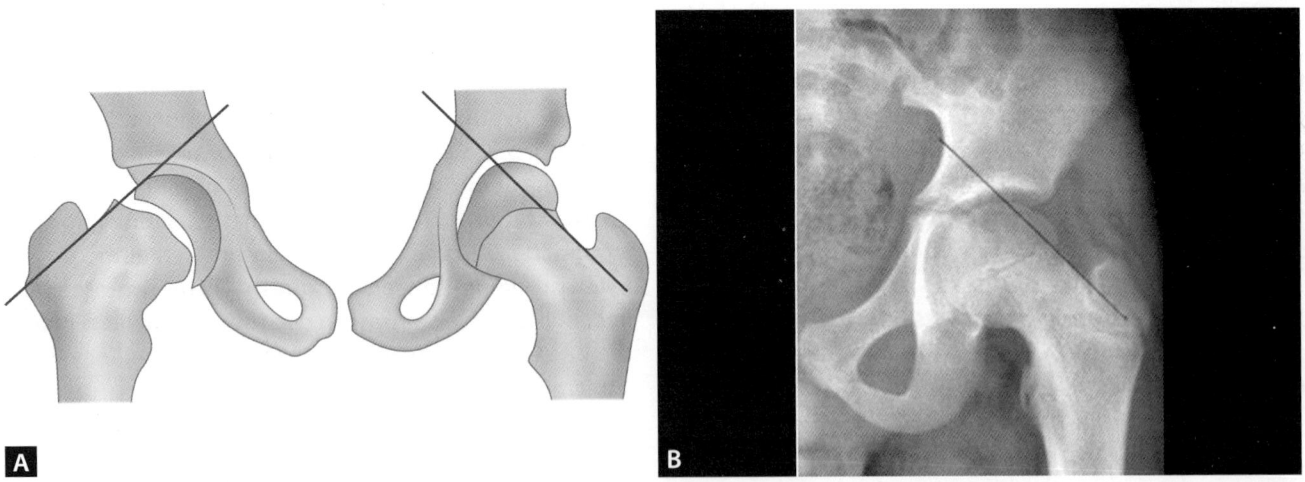

Figs. 50A and B: Schematic representation (A) of hip shows Klein's line that normally intersects lateral 1/3rd of the femoral epiphysis on the left, whereas in slipped epiphysis, no part of the epiphysis is lateral to it as seen on the right; X-ray pelvis (B) depicting the normal position of the femoral head in relation to the Klein's line.

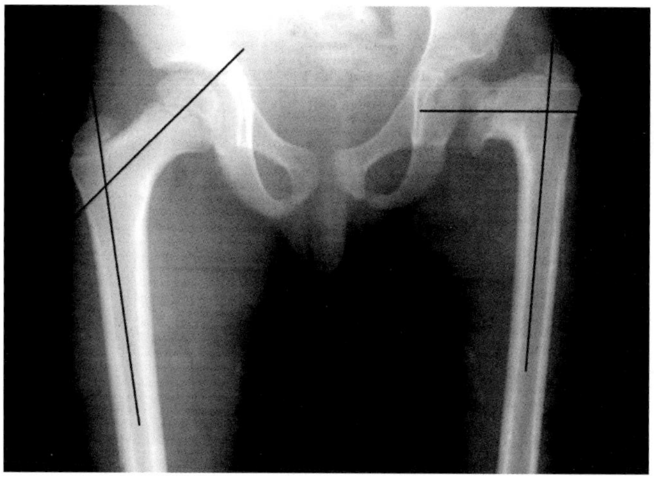

Fig. 51: X-ray pelvis: Slipped capital epiphysis left side.

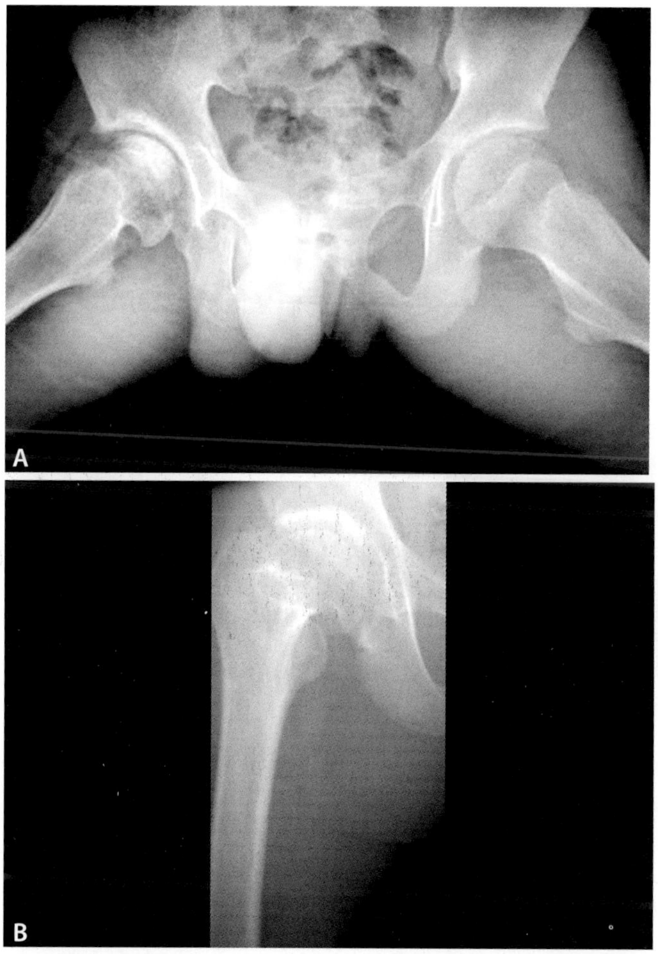

Figs. 52A and B: X-ray frog's leg view (A) and AP view (B) show medial and inferior displacement of the right capital epiphysis with widening of the physis.

on radiographs. 3D volume acquisition can be used to reconstruct sagittal oblique images along the axis of the femoral neck to identify any retroversion. MR image can be oriented to a plane orthogonal to the plane of the physis to assess the width of the same. Physeal widening is seen on T1 weighted MRI, whereas synovitis and marrow oedema are appreciated on T2 weighted images **(Figs. 54A and B)**. MRI can also demonstrate physeal widening in the center or posteromedial origin of the physis in a contralateral asymptomatic hip, providing for prophylactic treatment of the same.[51] Hyperintensity on fluid sensitive images at the physis is indicative of a chronic slip condition. Subtle abnormalities include edema on the metaphyseal side, usually at the extreme medial end of the physis.

The complications of SCFE are avascular necrosis, occurring in 20–45% of cases and chondrolysis. Treatment consists of preventing further displacement and to cause closure of the physis. Chondrolysis is less common than AVN and is recognized by progressive thinning of the medial joint space on the radiographs. Premature closure of the physis of the greater trochanter is considered as predictive sign for chondrolysis. Premature osteo arthritis may develop in 1/4–1/3 of patient with SCFE. Prognosis is poorer with unstable variety.

Differential Diagnosis

- Legg-Calve-Perthes's disease—the patient is younger with irritable hip progressing to sclerosis and collapse of epiphysis, there is a hairline fracture with marrow edema:
  - Hip joint inflammation
  - Osteoid osteoma
  - Traumatic SCFE

Developmental Coxa Vara

The normal femoral neck shaft angle changes from about 150 degrees in the infant decreasing to 120 degrees in the adult. The femoral neck is valgus in infants because of relatively increased growth in the medial portion of the physis in the perinatal period. During childhood there is a greater amount of growth in the lateral portion of the femoral physis that is influenced by weight bearing. Coxa vara is defined as femoral neck shaft angle of less than 120 degrees.[52]

True coxa vara may be secondary to congenital anomalies, osteomalacia, or syndromes. Functional coxa vara occurs as a result of overgrowth of the greater trochanter secondary to AVN, infection or trauma. Developmental coxa vara, bilateral in 40% of cases, presents

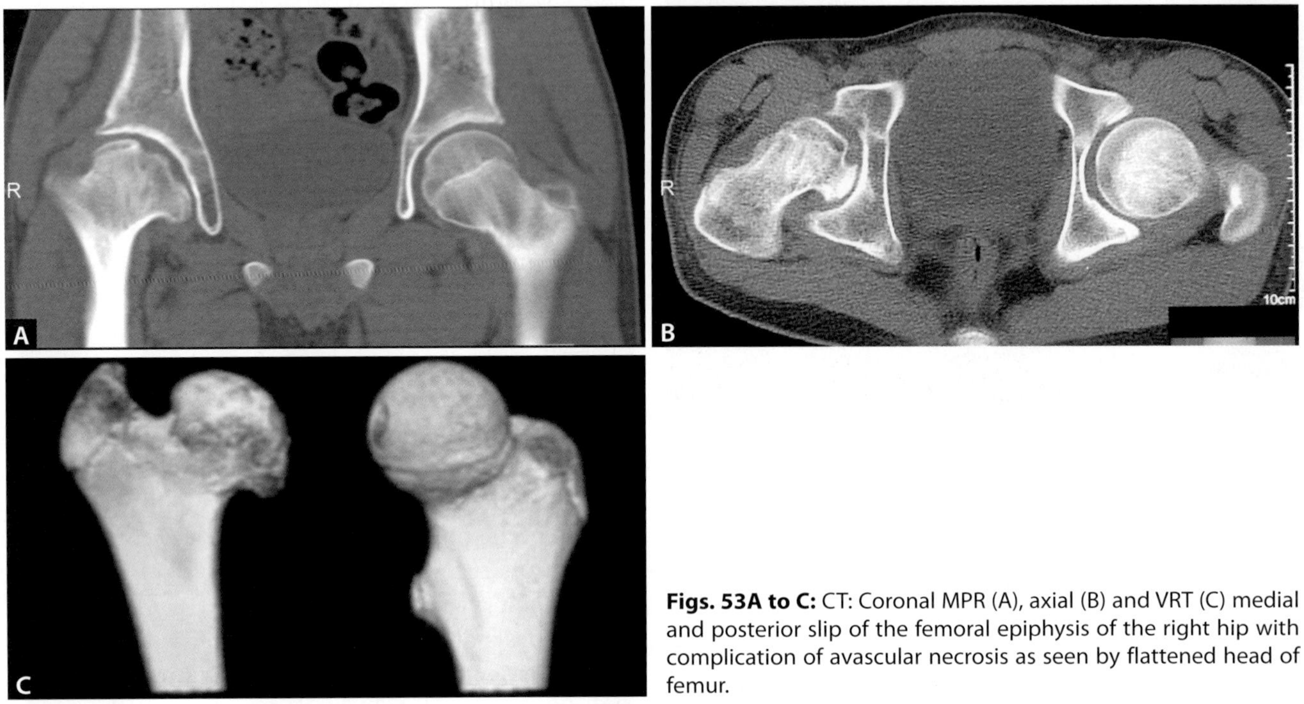

Figs. 53A to C: CT: Coronal MPR (A), axial (B) and VRT (C) medial and posterior slip of the femoral epiphysis of the right hip with complication of avascular necrosis as seen by flattened head of femur.

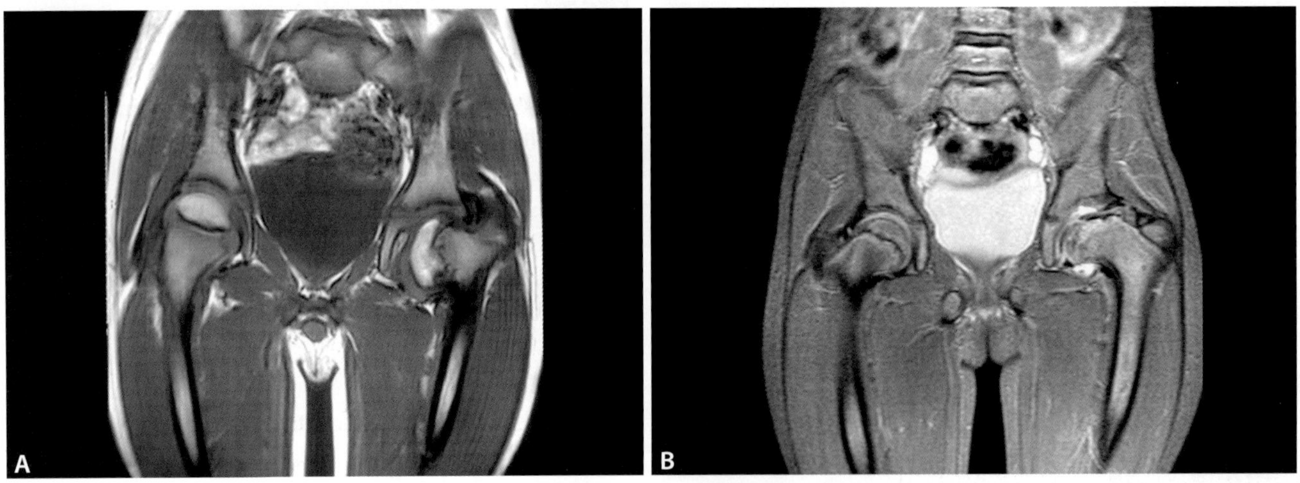

Figs. 54A and B: (A) MRI: T1-weighted coronal and (B) STIR coronal depicting widening and irregularity of the physis on the left side with physeal slip—Slipped capital femoral epiphysis.

at 2 years of age with an abnormal gait. It is caused by an abnormality of bone growth at the physis with a greater rate of growth of the lateral aspect of the physis causing the physis to be more vertical than usual. Radiographs show a widened and an abnormally oriented physis **(Fig. 55)**. As stress occurs along the physis multiple small steps occurs and small triangular corner fractures develop along the medial aspect of the physis. MR imaging demonstrates widening of the physis with expansion of the cartilage.

Pediatric Hip Trauma

Traumatic hip dislocations rarely occur in childhood. Posterior hip dislocations comprise majority of such dislocations.[53] A soft pliable acetabulum and ligamentous laxity may predispose the immature hip joint to a dislocation secondary to minimal trauma. Potential associated injuries include fracture and neurovascular injury while avascular necrosis and degenerative joint disease are potential sequelae. Osteochondral fractures

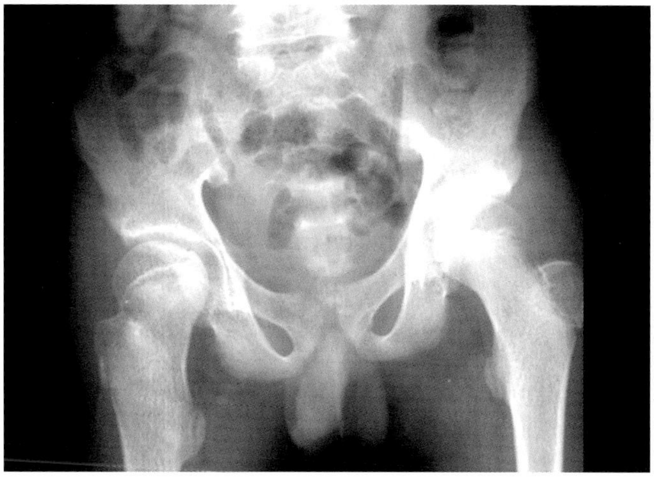

Fig. 55: Right coxa vara.

may be difficult to recognize on plain radiography. CT is useful in the definition of the extent and displacement of complex and impacted fractures around the hip joint.

Growth plate injuries are important to recognize as they have potential implications for growth arrest. Growth disturbance of the proximal femur can be post-traumatic or may be secondary to ischaemia following hyperabduction for DDH, Legg-Calve-Perthes' disease and rapidly developing effusions. The proximal femur physis is particularly vulnerable because the epiphyseal artery is intraarticular. Physeal widening or narrowing may be seen on radiographs. MR imaging is the modality of choice. T1 weighted images demonstrate low signal intensity growth recovery line and variable signal intensity bony bridge on GRE sequences, a bridge appears as a low signal intensity interruption in high signal physeal cartilage. Physeal widening on GRE and T2 weighted images implies physeal dysfunction. Medial physeal impairment leads to a short wide femoral neck and coxa vara deformity whereas vertex arrest causes Coxa valga[54] **(Figs. 56 and 57)**.

Neuromuscular Hip Dysplasia

Children who suffer from cerebral palsy or other neuromuscular disorders, who are unable to walk have a 58% incidence of hip dislocations. With muscle imbalance and lack of weight bearing, there is a coxa valga deformity with persistence of a straight neck shaft angle, which leads to hip dislocation.

Simulated standing radiographs show pelvic tilt, valgus deformity of the femoral neck, abnormal shape and placement of the femoral head. CT is helpful for evaluation of the shape of the acetabulum and the degree of femoral articulation.

Childhood Idiopathic Chondrolysis of the Hip

This is a rare disorder, which causes progressive destruction of the articular cartilage of the hip joint with associated bone remodeling. Cartilage loss, bone remodeling, and small joint effusions along with muscle wasting are seen.[55]

Calcification of Cartilage and Joints

Idiopathic calcification of the cartilages of the hips, i.e. acetabular rims and femoral hands has been reported in children and the patients may be asymptomatic or have a limp with restricted hip movements. This is believed to be an acquired pathology due to local chemical trauma from partial extravasation of an intravenous injection via the femoral route. On serial studies, calcification may remain unchanged, increase, or show gradual resorption with early fusion of the femoral head and neck.

The hip joint may also be involved as part of a large number of skeletal dysplasias or systemic disorders as in nutritional disorders, neoplasia like leukemia, metastatic neuroblastoma.

Developmental and acquired abnormalities of the hip are relatively common in childhood. Radiographs, ultrasonography, MR imaging, computed tomography and nuclear medicine play an important role in the diagnosis and management of these disorders.

Femoroacetabular Impingement

The geometry of femoral neck and acetabulum plays a role in the etiology of degenerative disease.[56,57]

Normally, the femoral neck has a definite narrowing or waist which allows the femur to abduct fully without impingement on the lateral aspect of the acetabulum. In patients with FAI, the femoral neck is not tabulated normally. Instead of having an identifiable constriction, a pistol grip deformity is seen in which tabulation is lacking. A small bump or protuberance may be identified on the anterior femoral neck. Slipped capital femoral epiphysis may be a contributing factor **(Fig. 58)**.

Axial oblique images prescribed along the axis of the femoral neck or reconstruction of 3D volume acquisition into axial oblique plane allows for measurement of α angle. First the center of the femoral head is identified using the contour of the head to fit a circle to outline and define the position of the center of the head. Two lines are extended from the center point of the head, one down the axis of the femoral neck and the second to the intersection point between the head and the neck, when the convexity of the femoral head becomes the concavity of the femoral neck. Angles less than 55 degrees are abnormal or if the

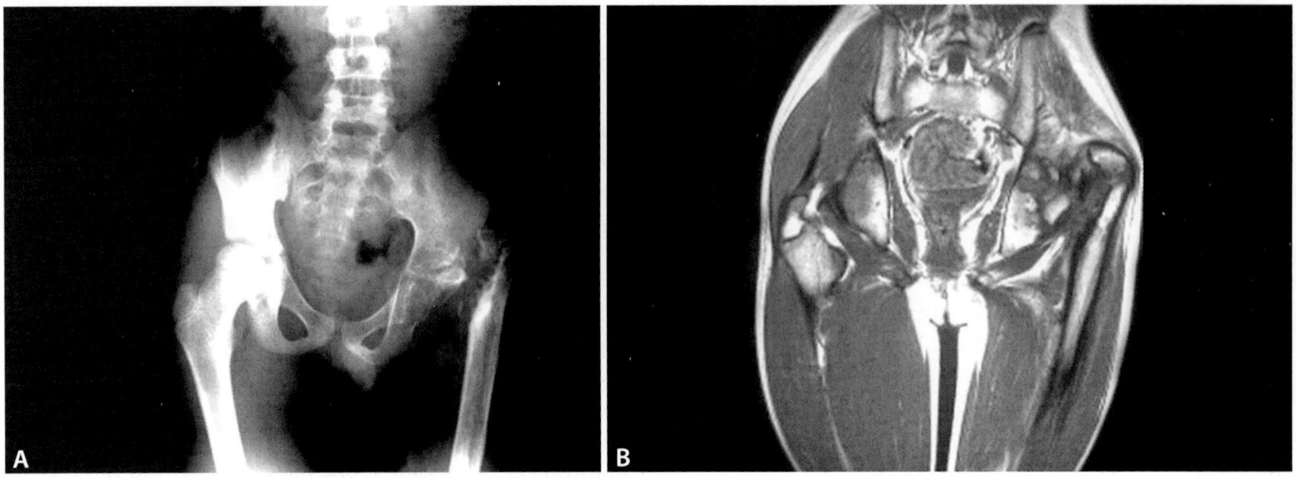

Figs. 56A and B: X-ray pelvis (A) traumatic posterosuperior dislocation of the left femur; MRI-T1 coronal (B) depicting the superior and posterior dislocation.

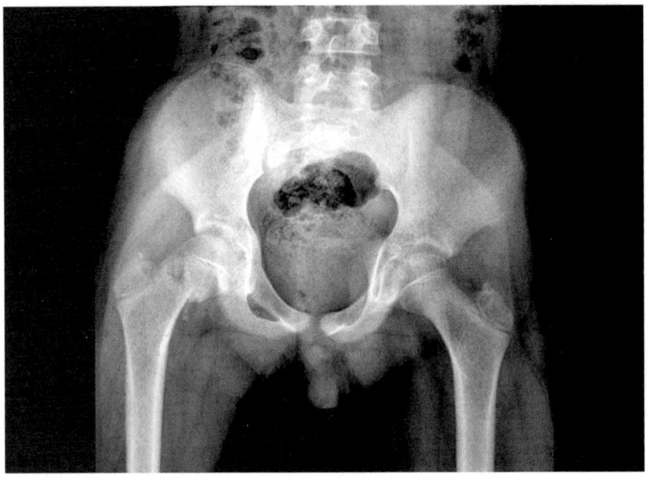

Fig. 57: X-ray pelvis: Fracture right femoral neck.

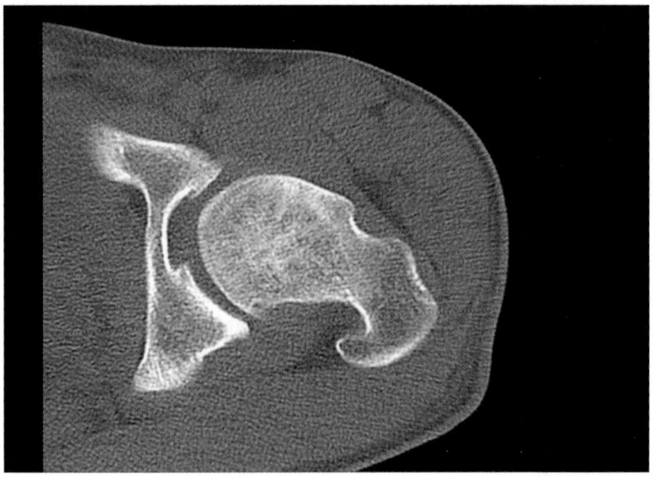

Fig. 58: CT: Oblique axial image shows evidence of CAM impingement with a bump at the femoral neck.

head-neck line measures greater than the radius of the circle defining the femoral head, then a femoral waist deficiency is present.

FAI may also be caused by over coverage of the femoral head and neck. This may be caused by acetabular retroversion. Normally the acetabulum has its lateral opening directed slightly anteriorly. In abnormal cases, the anterolateral edge of the acetabulum extends further laterally than the posterolateral edge so that the acetabular opening is directed posteriorly. On radiographs,this is visualized as the cross over sign. This is present when the anterior lip of the acetabulum crosses over the posterior lip on a standard frontal film. This limits the ability to flex at the hip as the femoral neck impinges on the anterior acetabulum.

Abnormal morphology in the pediatric age group may not reflect the pathological abnormalities seen in adulthood, however subtle osseous abnormalities can help guide prognosis.

REFERENCES

1. Jacobs P, Renton P. Congenital anomalies: Skeletal dysplasias; chromosomal disorders. In Sutton D (Ed): Textbook of Radiology and Imaging (4th edn). Churchill Livingstone. 1987;1:2-50.
2. Hilgenreiner H. Zur Fruhdiagnose and Fruhbehandlung derangegorenen Huftgelenkrerrenkueg Med Klink. 1925; 21:1385-88,1425-9.
3. Andren L, von Rosen S. The diagnosis of dislocation of hip in newborns and the preliminary results of immediate treatment. Acta Radiol. 1958;49:89-95.

4. Gibbon Wayne W, Long G. In Meire H, Cosgrove D, Dewbury K, et al (Eds). Musculoskeletal System: Abdominal and General Ultrasound (2nd edn). London: Churchill Livingstone. 2000.p.2.
5. Fayed LM, Johnson P, Fishman EK. Multidetector CT of musculoskeletal disease in pediatric patient; principles, techniques and clinical applications. Radiographics. 2005; 25:603-61.
6. Jaramillo D, Galen TA, Winalski CS, et al. Legg-Calve-Perthes disease: MR imaging evaluation during manual positioning of the hip-comparison with conventional arthrography. Radiology. 1999;212(2):519-25.
7. Aubry S, Belanger D, Giguere C. Magnetic resonance arthrography of the hip: Insights Imaging. 2010;1:72-82.
8. Klisie PJ. Congenital dislocation of the hip: A misleading term. J Bone Joint Surg Br. 1981;63:38-42.
9. Kuhn JP, et al. Caffey's Pediatric Diagnostic Imaging. 10th edn 2277-9,2004: Mosby. The joints BabynPS, RansOm MD 2435-93.
10. Havije HT, Waller RS. Ultrasound screening for dysplasia of the hip (Letter). Pediatrics. 1995; 95:799-800.
11. Zieger M. Ultrasound of the infant hip Part 2 validity of the method. Pediatric Radiol. 1986;16:488-92.
12. Graf R. Classification of hip joint dysplasia by means of sonography. Arch Orthop Trauma Surg. 1984;102:248.
13. Harcke HT, Lee MS, Born P, et al. Examination of the infant hip with real time ultrasonography. J Ultrasound Med. 1984;3:131.
14. Harcke HT, Grissom LE. Performing dynamic sonography of the infant hip. Am J Roentgenol. 1990;155:837.
15. Rosendahl K, Toma P. Ultrasound in the diagnosis of developmental dysplasia of the new borns. The European approach. A review of methods, accuracy and clinical validity: Eur Radiol. 2007;17:1960-7.
16. Schwartz DS, Kellar MS, Fields JM, et al. Arterial waveforms of the femoral heads of healthy neonates. Am J Roentgenol. 1998;170:465-6.
17. Browing WH, Rosenkrantz II, Tarquinio T. Computed Tomography in congenital hip dislocation. J Bone Joint Surgery (AM). 1982;64:27-31.
18. Hubbard AM. Imaging of pediatric hip disorders. Rad Clin North Am. 2001;39(4).
19. Dwek JR. The Hip: MR Imaging of Uniquely Pediatric Disorders: Radiol Clin North Am. 2009;47:997-1008.
20. Kawaguchi AT, Otsuka NY, Deigado ED, et al. Magnetic resonance arthrography in children with developmental hip dysplasia. Clin Orthop. 2000;374:235-46.
21. Tennant S, Kinmant C, Lamb G, et al. The use of dynamic interventional MRI in developmental dysplasia of the hip. J Bone Joint Surg B. 1999;81(3):392-7.
22. Jawin J, Hoffer F, Rand F, et al. Joint effusion in children with an irritable hip: Ultrasound diagnosis and aspiration. Radiology. 1993;1987:459.
23. Strouse PJ, Di Pietro MA, Adler RS. Hip Effusions: Evaluation with Power Doppler Sonography. Radiology. 1998;206:731-5.
24. Hopkins K, Li K, Bergmon G. Gadolinium DTPA enhanced magnetic resonance imaging of musculoskeletal infections processes. Skeletal Radiol. 1995;24:325.
25. Lee SK, Suh KJ, Kim YW, et al. Septic arthritis, versus transient synovitis at MR imaging preliminary assessment with signal intensity alterations in bone marrow. Radiology. 1999;211:459.
26. Park JK, Kim BS, Choi G, et al. Distinction of reactive joint fluid from pyogenic abscess by diffusion-weighted imaging. J Magn Reson Imaging. 2007;25(4):859-61.
27. Daldrup-Link HE, Steinbach L. MR imaging of Pediatric arthritis. Radiol Clin N Am. 2009;47:939-55.
28. Hong SH, Kim SM, Ahn JM, et al. Tuberculous versus pyogenic arthritis: MR imaging evaluation. Radiology. 2001;218:843-53.
29. Sawhney S, Jain R. Tuberculosis of the bones and joints. In Berry, Chowdhury, Suri (Eds): Diagnostic Radiology-Musculoskeletal and Breast imaging (1st edn). Jaypee Brothers Medical Publishers 1998.
30. Chapman H, Murray RD, Stoken OJ. Tuberculosis of the bone and joints. Semin Roentgenol. 1979;19:26-282.
31. Murray RO, Jacobson HG. Infections: Radiology of Skeletal Disorders (2nd edn). Churchill Livingstone. 1997.p.1.
32. Jacobs P, Renton P. Avascular necrosis of bone: Osteochondritis: Miscellaneous bone lesions. In Sutton D (Ed): Textbook of Radiology and Imaging (4th edn). Churchill Livingstone. 1987;1:77-94.
33. Caterall A. Legg-Calve-Perthes disease. New York, Churchill Livingston 1982.
34. O'hara SM. Benton C-abnormalities of hip in Diagnostic Imaging-Donelly. Amirsys 2005.
35. Doria AS, Guarniero R, Gunha FG, et al. Contrast enhanced power Doppler Sonography: Assessment of revascularization flow in Legg-Calve-Perthes' disease. Ultrasound Med Biol. 2002;28(2):171-82.
36. Strouse PJ. Musculoskeletal system. In Haaga JR, Lanzieri, Gilkeson (Eds): CT and MR Imaging of the Whole Body (4th edn). 2002;2:2095-122.
37. Ha As, Wells J, Jaramillo D. Importance of sagittal MR imaging in nontraumatic femoral head osteonecrosis in children. Pediatr Radiol. 2008;38(ii):1195-200.
38. Jaramillo D, Galen TA, Winalski CS, et al. Legg-Calve-Perthes' disease: MR imaging evaluation during manual positioning of the hip. Comparison with conventional arthrography. Radiology. 1999;212(2):519-25.
39. Dillman JR, Hernandez RJ. MRI of Legg-Calve-Perthes disease. AJR. 2009;193:1394-1407.
40. Mahnken AH, Staatz G, Ihme IV, et al. MR signal intensity characteristics in Legg-Calve-Perthes' disease value of fat suppressed (STIR) images and contrast enhanced T1 weighted images. Acta Radiol. 2002;43(3):329-35.
41. Lamer S, Dogeret S, Khairouni A, et al. Femoral head vascularization in Legg-Calve-Perthes' disease Comparison of dynamic gadolinium enhanced substraction MRI with bone scintigraphy. Pediatric Radiol. 2002;32(8):580-85.

42. Menezes NM, Olear EA, Li X, et al. Gadolinium enhanced MR images of the growing piglet skeleton: Ionic versus. Nonionic contrast agent. Radiology. 2006;239(2):406-14.
43. Menezes NM, Connolly SA, Shapiro P, et al. Early ischemia in growing piglet skeleton. MR diffusion and perfusion imaging. Radiology. 2007;242(1):129-36.
44. Lahdes-Vasama T, Lamminen A, Merikanto J, et al. The Value of MRI in early Perthes' disease: An MRI study with a 2 year follow up. Pediatric Radiol. 1997;27(6):517-22.
45. De Sanctis N, Rega AN, Rondinella F. Prognostic evaluation of Legg-Calve-Perthes' disease by MRI—Pathomorphogenesis and new classification. J Pediatr Orthop. 2000;20(4):403-70.
46. Merlinic L, Combescure C, De Rosa V, et al. Diffusion—weighted imaging findings in perthes disease with dynamic gadolinuim-enhanced subtracted (DGS) with MR correlation—a preliminary study. Pediatr Radiol. 2010;40(3):31.
47. Grissom LE, Harcke HT. Sonography in congenital deficiency of the femur. J Paediatr Orthop. 1994;14:29-33.
48. Kayser R, et al. Proximalfocal femoral deficiency—rare entity in the sonographic differential diagnosis of developmental dysplasia of the hip. J Pediatr. 2005;146(1):141.
49. Castriota-Scandfrberg A, Orsi E. Slipped capital femoral epiphysis ultrasonographic findings skeletal. Radiol. 1993; 22(3):191-93.
50. Umans H, Liebling MS, Moy L, et al. Slipped capital femoral epiphysis: A physeal lesion diagnosed by MRI with radiographic and CT correlation. Skeletal Radiol. 1998;27(3):139-44.
51. Futami T, Suzuki S, Seto Y, et al. Sequential magnetic resonance imaging in slipped capital femoral epiphysis, assessment of prestep in the contralateral hip. J Paediatr Orthop B. 2001;10(4):298-303.
52. Ozonof MB. Pediatric Orthopaedic. Radiology Philadelphia: WB Saunders 1992.
53. Petrie SG, Harris MB, Willis RB. Traumatic hip dislocation during childhood. A case report and review of the literature. Am J Ortho. 1996;25(a):645-9.
54. Ecklund K, Jaramillo D. Imaging of growth disturbance in children. Radiol Clin North Am. 2001;39(4):823-42.
55. Johnson K, Haigh SF, Ehtisham S, et al. Childhood Idiopathic Chondrolysis of the hip: MRI features. Paediatr Radiol. 2003; 33(3):194-9.
56. Pfirrmann CW, Mengiardi B, Dara C, et al. Ca M and pincer femora acetabular impingement: Characteristic MR authrographic findings in 50 patients. Radiology. 2006;240(3):778-85.
57. Gam R, Parvizi J, Beck M, et al. Femoracetabular impingement: a cause of osteo arthritis of the hip. Clin Orthop Relat Res. 2003;417:112-20.

CHAPTER 148

Benign Bone and Soft Tissue Tumors and Conditions

Mahesh Prakash, Kushaljit Singh Sodhi

INTRODUCTION

Benign bone tumor and tumor-like lesions are very common in children. More than half of all childhood bone neoplasms are benign.[1] It is important that radiologists recognize the typical imaging features of benign tumors so that patient can avoid unnecessary diagnostic and surgical procedures.

The differential diagnosis of bone tumors can be narrowed, based on knowledge of age of the patient, gender, constitutional complaints, location of the lesion in body and bone and general radiographic characteristics.[2] Plain film radiographs remain the primary tool for evaluating bone tumors. However, other imaging methods, particularly magnetic resonance imaging (MRI) and in some cases computed tomography (CT) and nuclear studies, provide support for initial diagnosis by demonstrating specific features.[1,2] Common benign bone lesions in children are osteochondroma, nonossifying fibroma, Langerhans' cell histiocytosis, unicameral bone cyst and aneurysmal bone cyst. Benign bone tumors and tumor like lesions in children may be classified as follows:[1]

- *Cartilaginous tumors*:
  - Osteochondroma
  - Enchondroma
  - Chondroblastoma
  - Chondromyxoid fibroma
- *Osseous tumors*:
  - Osteoid osteoma
  - Osteoblastoma
- *Fibrous tumors*:
  - Nonossifying fibroma
  - Fibrous dysplasia
  - Osteofibrous dysplasia
- Langerhans cell histiocytosis:
- Giant cell tumor
- *Tumor-like lesions*:
  - Simple bone cyst
  - Aneurysmal bone cyst
  - Pseudotumor of hemophilia

CARTILAGINOUS TUMORS

Osteochondroma

Osteochondromas are common lesions of the growing skeleton, occurring in approximately 1% of the general population. It is the most common benign neoplasm and constitutes 20–50% of all benign tumors.[3] They arise from bony metaphysis with cartilage cap covering **(Fig. 1)**. These tumors are either pedunculated or sessile. The long axis of the osteochondroma pedicle or stalk is almost always directed away from the adjacent joint. The direct communication between the osteochondroma and the cortex and marrow cavity of the bone from which it arises is a distinctive feature, that is particularly well demonstrated on computed tomography and magnetic resonance imaging. T2-weighted MR images is useful to demonstrate an cartilaginous cap **(Fig. 2)**. The cap can be quite thick in early childhood and like the normal physis, becomes thinner with age. After epiphyseal closure, growth of the

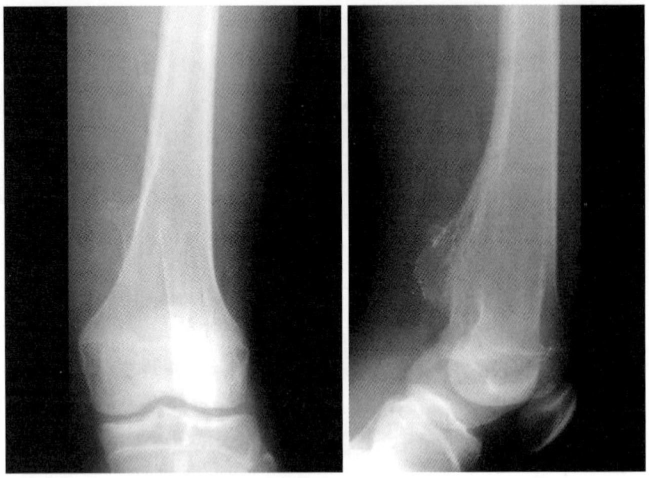

Fig. 1: Osteochondroma: Radiographs of lower end of femur (AP and lateral view) show large well-defined bony outgrowth, with broad-based attachment to femur.

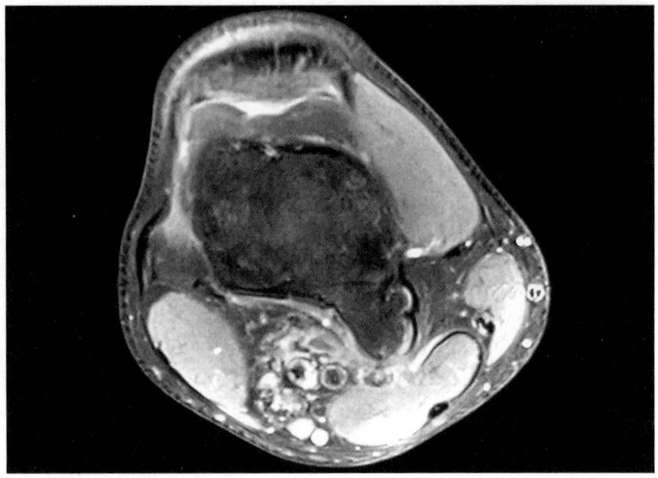

Fig. 2: MRI (T1W fat sat): Axial section of the same patient shows clear demonstration of continuity of marrow and cortex of host bone into osteochondroma with covering cartilage cap.

osteochondroma ceases. Multiple osteochondroma occur as a manifestation of diaphyseal aclasia, an inherited disorder with autosomal dominance **(Fig. 3)**. Because most osteochondromas are asymptomatic, they are usually discovered incidentally. However, mechanical irritation of adjacent soft tissues or nerves, vascular injuries, fracture of the stalk, or malignant transformation can produce symptoms.

Malignant transformation into low-grade chondrosarcoma occurs in 1% of osteochondromas, however, the risk is 10–30% in cases of multiple osteochondromatosis.[3,4] Malignant transformation should be considered when the osteochondroma grows after epiphyseal closure. Malignancy occurs in the cartilaginous cap, which becomes thickened. The cap of an osteochondroma usually measures less than 1 cm in thickness, whereas that of a chondrosarcoma often exceeds 2 cm.

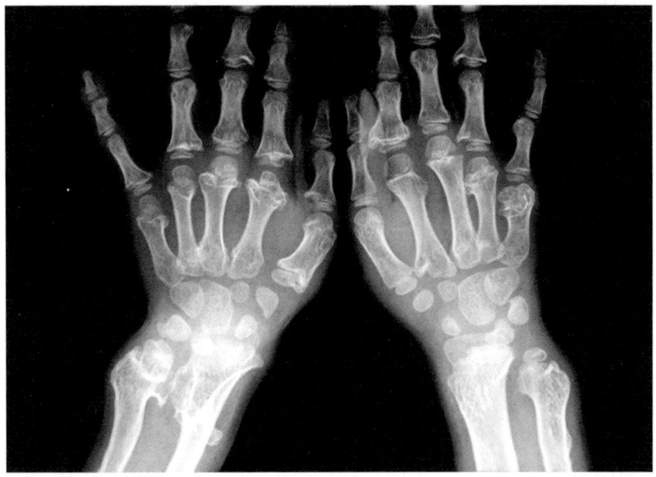

Fig. 3: Diaphyseal aclasia: PA radiograph of bilateral hands show multiple pedunculated osteochondromas, involving multiple bones of hands and forearm.

Enchondroma

Enchondromas accounts for 12% of benign bone tumors.[3] These are most frequently located in the large and small tubular bones of the limbs, particularly those of the hand **(Fig. 4)**. Like other cartilaginous tumors, enchondromas exhibit a lobulated growth pattern, that results in asymmetric expansion of the medullary cavity and endosteal scalloping. Tumor matrix may be radiolucent or show calcification. Characteristic cartilaginous ring and arc pattern of calcifications is seen on radiographs and CT images. On MR imaging, the tumor is isointense to muscle on T1-weighted and exhibits a heterogeneous, predominantly high T2-weighted signal.[5] Contrast enhanced MRI may demonstrate a pattern of thin arcs and rings.

Ollier's disease is a nonheritable disorder of cartilage proliferation in which enchondromas involve multiple bones, especially those of the hands and may result in severe skeletal deformity. Enchondromatosis accompanied by multiple hemangiomas is known as Maffucci's syndrome. Calcified phleboliths may be demonstrated radiographically in the hemangiomatous soft tissue masses. Lesions associated with both Ollier's disease and Maffucci's syndrome carry a significant risk of malignant degeneration (30–70%).[6]

Chondroblastoma

It is less common than enchondroma. Chondroblastoma is composed of primitive cartilage cells, usually occurs

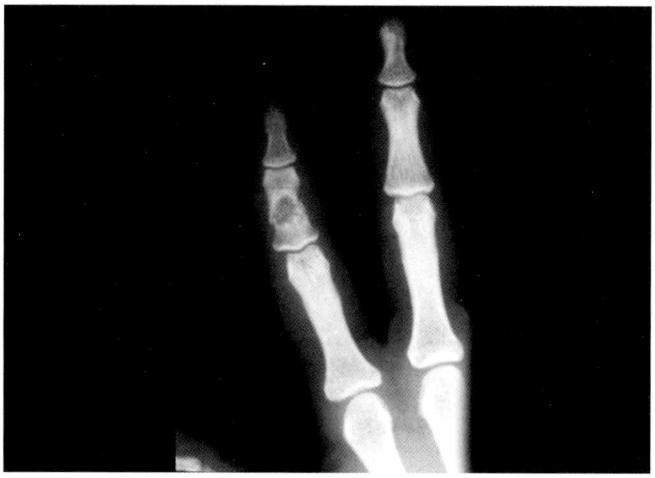

Fig. 4: Enchondroma: Radiograph shows a sharply demarcated expansile lytic lesion with pathological fracture in the middle phalanx of index finger.

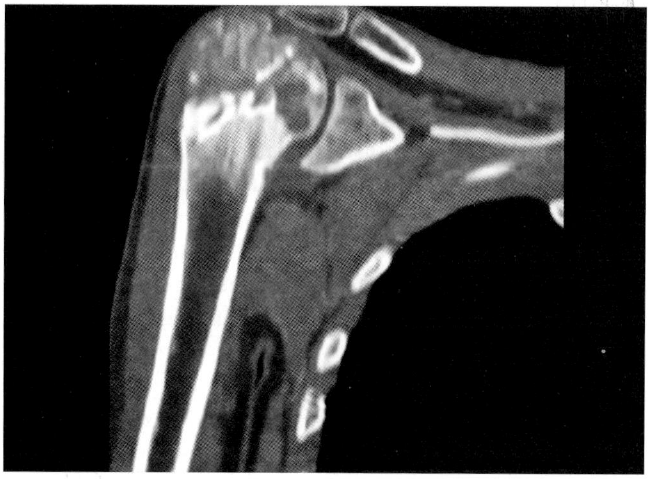

Fig. 5: Chondroblastoma: CT (coronal reformation) shows lytic lesion in epiphysis of upper humerus with matrix calcification.

in the age group of 10–20 years. It is typically located in epiphysis and apophysis of bone, most often the proximal humerus, distal femur, or proximal tibia. On plain X-ray, chondroblastoma is an eccentric, lucent, well-defined lesion with sclerotic borders. Periosteal reaction, far from the lesion is another common feature suggesting an accompanying inflammatory process. Approximately one third of chondrobastoma have a calcified matrix which can be better seen on CT scan **(Fig. 5)**.

The tumor shows signal intensity similar to that of muscle on MR imaging; however, the rim of the tumor has lower signal intensity. On T2-weighted images, the signal intensity of the tumor is low to intermediate. This tumor also shows extensive surrounding inflammation which may be confused with more aggressive lesion. Malignant transformation of chondroblastoma is extremely uncommon.[7]

Chondromyxoid Fibroma

Chondromyxoid fibroma is less common than chondroblastoma, affecting predominantly males in the age group of 15–35 years.[8] Histologically, it is composed of chondroid, myxoid and fibrous tissue in varying amounts. The common locations of tumor are ilium and the bones of the knee and foot. These tumors are located characteristically in metadiaphyseal location unlike chondroblastoma and do not cross an open growth plate. On plain radiograph, it appears as a well-marginated central or eccentric lucent lesion, with sclerotic margins and cortical expansion **(Fig. 6)**. Half of the lesions may show parallel orientation to the long axis of the involved bone. Matrix calcification and periosteal new bone formation usually do not occur.

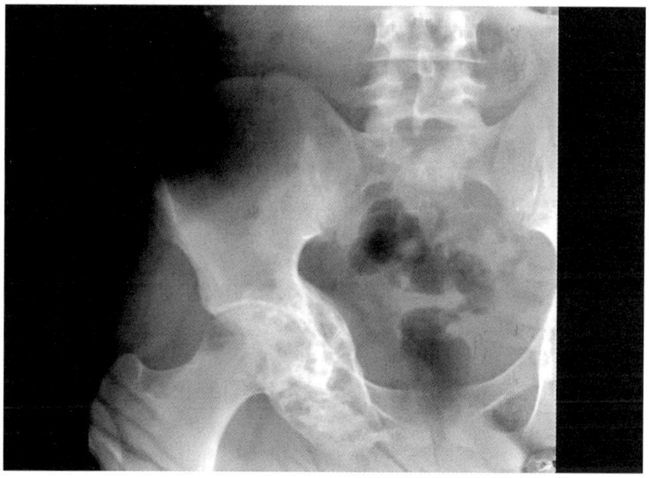

Fig. 6: Chondromyxoid fibroma: Radiograph of right hip shows large expansile lesion with sclerotic border involving right acetabulum.

OSSEOUS TUMORS

Osteoid Osteoma

Osteoid osteoma is a fairly common tumor, accounting for approximately 10–12% of all benign tumors.[9] These tumors usually affect boys in the second decade of life. Clinically most patients presents with pain that is especially severe at night and relieved by aspirin or other nonsteroidal antiinflammatory agents.

More than half of tumors are located in proximal femur and tibia. They occur less frequently in the upper extremities than in the lower extremities. Osteoid osteomas also frequently affect the tubular bones of the hands and feet. They are however less common in the spine, where they affect the posterior arches of the vertebra. Histologically, the lesion consists of a nidus which is usually surrounded by dense sclerotic bone. The nidus contains interlacing trabeculae at various stages of ossification within a stroma of loose, vascular connective tissue. Osteoid osteoma can be cortical (the most common type), cancellous or medullary, and subperiosteal. The latter two types produce less sclerotic bone than those in the cortex do, making radiologic diagnosis difficult.

Radiographically, the lesion appears as well-defined lytic lesion, surrounded by reactive sclerosis **(Figs. 7A and B)**. Solid or lamellated periosteal reaction is seen in 60% of patients. Nidus may be purely radiolucent or contain a dense center. Intra-articular osteoid osteomas may be either cancellous or periosteal and have little reactive bone or periosteal new bone formation.

CT is very useful in showing the nidus, which can vary in its degree of ossification. CT appears to display the nidus better than MRI. The tumor nidus typically shows hypo to intermediate signal on T1W images and low-to-high signal on T2W images. The nidus shows enhancement with gadolinium.[10] Intra-articular osteoid osteomas produce joint effusions and synovial proliferation. Radionuclide bone scans have been used for many years to help in diagnosis of osteoid osteomas. Bone scintigraphy, which is a highly sensitive method of detecting osteoid osteoma typically shows increased flow to the lesion on immediate images and a focus of increased activity on skeletal equilibrium images with double density sign. Many times, osteomyelitis can mimick osteoid osteoma clinically as well radiographically; however, presence of soft tissue extension favors the diagnosis of osteomyelitis. The traditional treatment of choice has been surgical excision; however, it can also be successfully treated by radiofrequency ablation under image guidance.[11]

Osteoblastoma

Osteoblastoma constitutes 2–6% of all bone tumors and most commonly occurs in patients in the second and third decade of life.[12] This tumor is more common in males than in females. Histologically, the osteoblastoma is closely related to osteoid osteomas except that bony trabeculae are broader and longer with absence of surrounding sclerotic halo. Size is an important consideration in distinguishing between these two types of tumors. If the size of lesion is less than 1.5 cm in diameter than it is likely to be osteoid osteomas, whereas tumors larger than 1.5 cm are usually osteoblastoma.

The most common location of osteoblastoma is spine where it classically affects posterior elements (33%) **(Figs. 8A and B)**. [12] The other common locations are proximal femur and talus. On plain X-ray, spinal osteoblastoma is osteolytic lesion with destruction of overlying cortex and may extend to in the spinal canal. In the long bones, osteoblastoma appear radiologically as round or oval lucent tumors in the medulla. Periosteal reaction is common. Edema in the soft tissues or marrow appears hyperintense on T2-weighted images but the signal characteristics are not specific. Treatment is by surgical excision or curettage, but there is a moderate recurrence rate after these procedures.

FIBROUS TUMORS

Nonossifying Fibroma

Nonossifying fibroma is a benign fibroblastic mass that occurs in long bones of children and represents

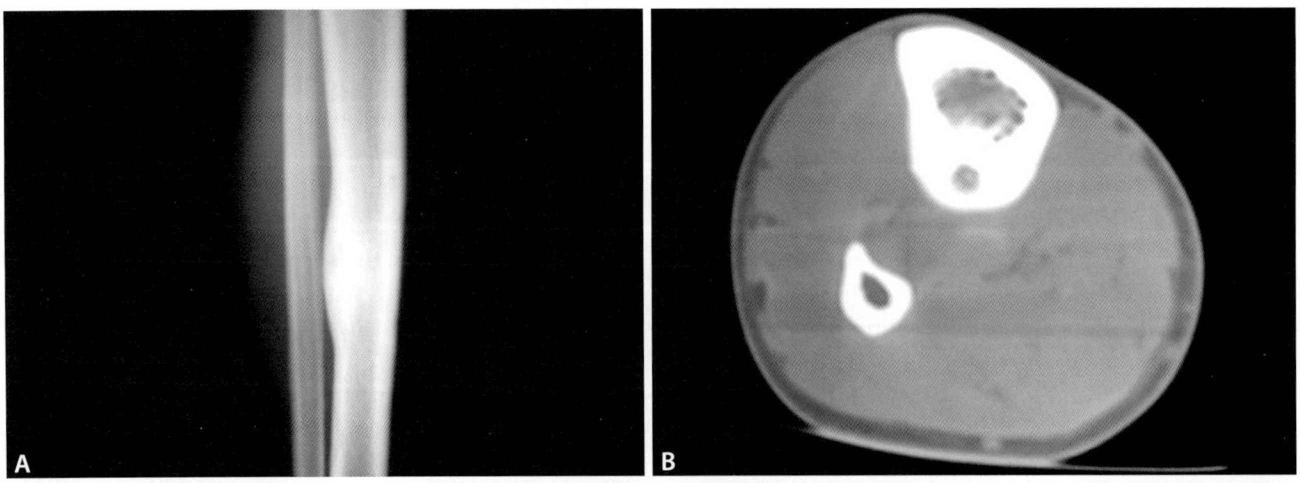

Figs. 7A and B: Osteoid osteoma: (A) Radiograph of leg shows dense sclerosis and solid periosteal reaction in the diaphysis of tibia; (B) CT scan axial sections reveals well-defined lytic lesion with calcified nidus with gross adjacent sclerosis

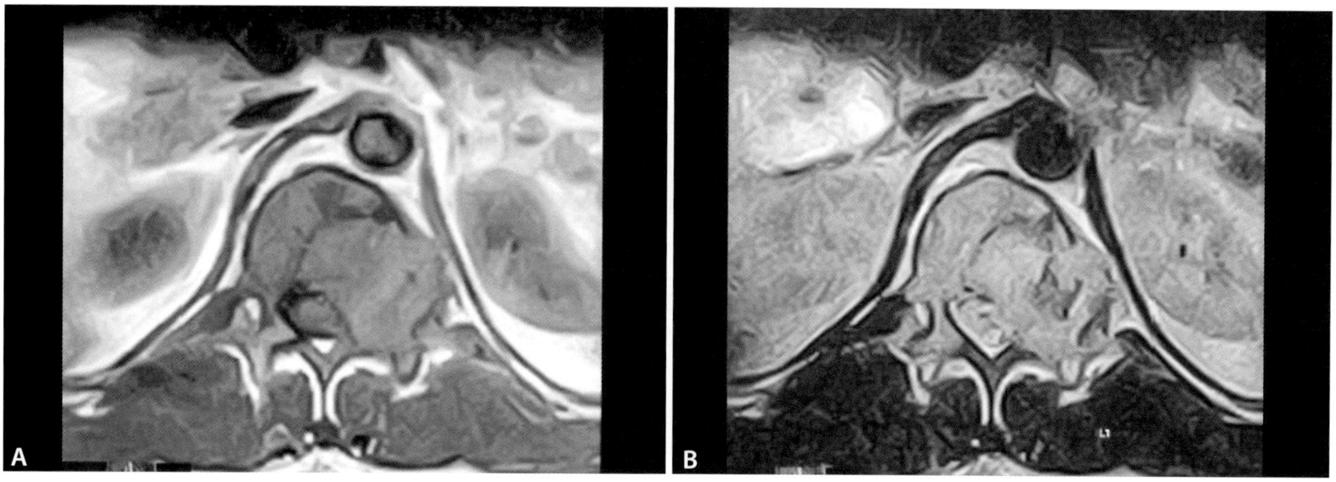

Figs. 8A and B: Osteoblastoma (A and B): MRI axial section, T1 and T2WI images reveal heterogeneous signal lesion, predominantly involving posterior elements of vertebra with extension into spinal canal and left paravertebral location

continuation of growth of fibrous cortical defect. It occurs eccentrically in the medullary cavity. The common location of lesion is in the bones around the knee joints. These lesions are usually asymptomatic and do not require specific treatment. On plain radiography, the lesion appears as well-marginated eccentric lytic lesion with scalloped margin **(Fig. 9)**. Its inner border is often sclerotic and may appear multilocular due to corrugations. Differential diagnosis includes unicameral bone cyst, aneurysmal bone cyst, fibrous dysplasia, and chondromyxoid fibroma. The signal intensity of nonossifying fibroma is equal to or less than muscle on T1-weighted MR images and hypointense to fat on T2-weighted images. Postcontrast images usually show heterogeneous enhancement.

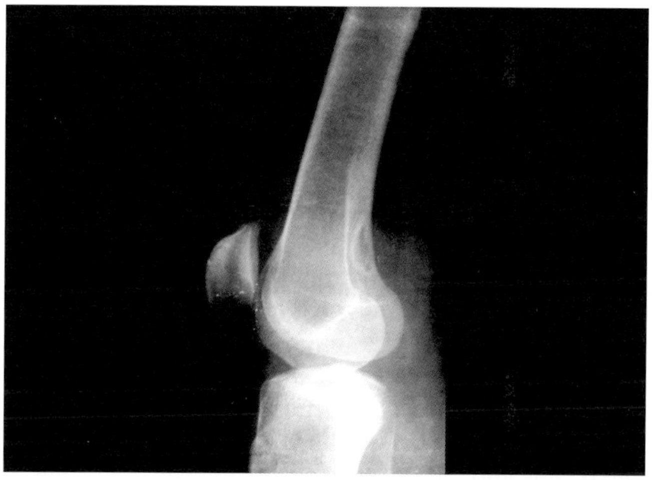

Fig. 9: Nonossifying fibroma: Radiograph of knee joint (Lateral view) shows well-defined lytic lesion with sclerotic margin in characteristic location of lower end of femur.

Fibrous Dysplasia

Fibrous dysplasia is disorders where bone is replaced by abnormal fibrous tissue. Fibrous dysplasia can be monostotic, polyostotic, monomelic, or polymelic. It is more common in young females. It is occasionally seen in the first decade of life. In a small percentage of cases (2–3%), fibrous dysplasia is associated with endocrine disorders, especially precocious puberty in girls (McCune–Albright syndrome).[13] Although it is not a true neoplasm, fibrous dysplasia involving a long bone may mimic a bone tumor or cyst. This type of fibrous dysplasia causes expansion of the medullary cavity of tubular bones, endosteal scalloping and trabeculation. The margin is sclerotic. The lesion may appear as ground glass or radiolucent, and this depends upon amount of fibrous tissue within the lesion. Bowing of the affected long bone may occur; when the affected bone is femur, the resulting deformity is called a "Shepherd's crook" **(Fig. 10)**. Thinning and destruction of the bony cortex may be seen on CT or MR images. Soft tissue extension of the lesion is unusual. On T1-weighted MR images, the signal intensity of fibrous dysplasia is similar to that of skeletal muscle. Although, the signal of pure fibrous tissue is hypointense on T2-weighted images, the signal of fibrous dysplasia is variable.

Osteofibrous Dysplasia

It is a rare lesion that is usually confined to the tibia but can also involve the fibula. Most cases occur during the first decade of life. On plain X-ray, the lesion appears as an eccentric, lucent, solitary or multiloculated, lesion involving the anterior aspect of tibia. CT is very helpful

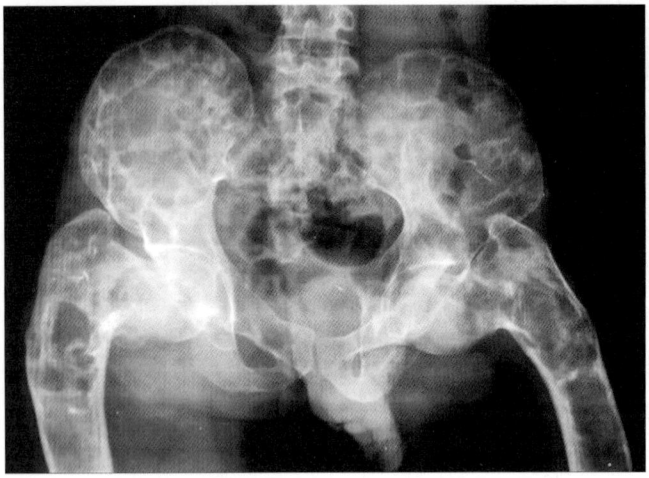

Fig. 10: Fibrous dysplasia: Radiograph of pelvis shows multiple lytic lesions involving all the visualized bones with characteristic Shepherd's crook deformity.

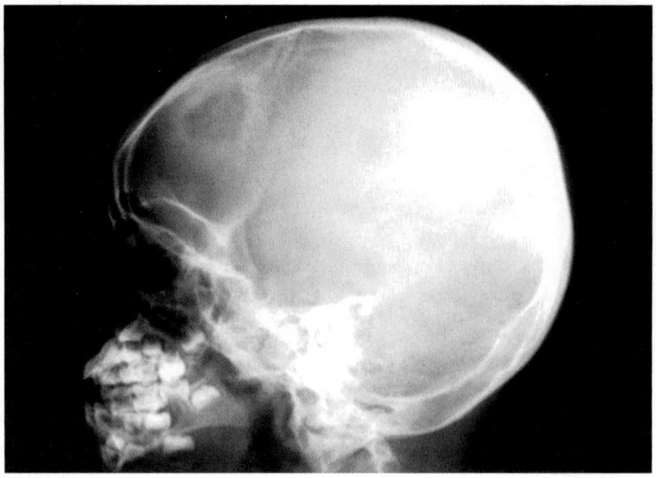

Fig. 11: Histiocytosis: Radiograph of skull (Lateral view) shows well-defined lytic lesion with beveled margins in frontal lobe.

in determining its intracortical location, an important feature in distinguishing osteofibrous dysplasia from fibrous dysplasia.[14]

HISTIOCYTOSIS X (LANGERHANS CELL HISTIOCYTOSIS)

Histiocytosis X is a syndrome that consists of group of clinical pathological entities: eosinophilic granuloma, Hand-Schüler-Christian disease and Letterer-Siwe disease. Eosinophilic granuloma is localized skeletal disease and is one of the commonly occurring bone tumors of boys in the first decade of life.[15] The skull is the most frequent location, followed by the femur, mandible, pelvis, ribs and spine. The lesions are usually located in the medulla of the diaphysis and metaphysis and rarely involves the cortex and epiphysis. Multiple lesions occur in about 25% of cases.[15] Pain is most common presenting problem with local tenderness and palpable mass. Histologically, the tumors are composed of Langerhans histiocytes containing their characteristic cleaved nuclei, and electron microscopy reveals Birbeck granules in the cytoplasm adjacent to the cell membrane. Radiographic appearance is variable. The lesion in calvarium typically appears as well defined lytic lesion with scalloped/beveled borders **(Fig. 11)**. Sometimes, a button sequestrum may be seen in the lesion. Most of the lesions in long bones appear as lytic lesion with well-defined borders; however some of the lesions are permeative and associated with periosteal new bone formation **(Fig. 12)**. The later findings suggest aggressive behavior. MRI is a very sensitive but nonspecific method of detecting eosinophilic granuloma. The lesion can be hypointense or hyperintense on T1 and

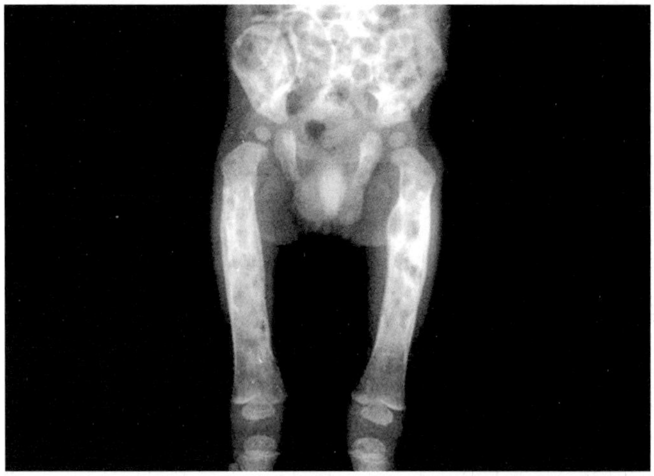

Fig. 12: Histiocytosis: Radiograph of the pelvis and upper femora shows multiple well-defined and ill-defined lesions with associated periosteal reaction in both femora.

hyperintense on T2W images, associated with extensive marrow and soft tissue edema. Occasionally, there is cortical disruption with adjacent soft tissue seen on MRI **(Fig. 13)**. The natural history of isolated lesion is gradual healing.[16] Treatment depends upon the site, location and multiplicity of lesion.

GIANT CELL TUMOR

Giant cell tumors are very rare in children under 15 years of age, and commonly seen in girls.[17] Radiographically, these tumors are well defined, eccentric lytic lesions usually located around the knee. The lesion usually shows nonsclerotic margin, cortical thinning without matrix calcification **(Fig. 14)**. GCT is located in the metaphysis

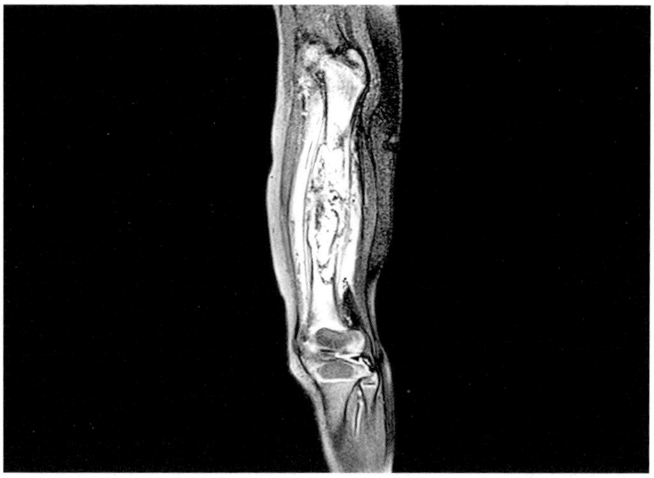

Fig. 13: Histiocytosis: MRI of femur shows large heterogeneous signal intensity lesion in diaphysis with cortical destruction, soft tissue and periosteal reaction.

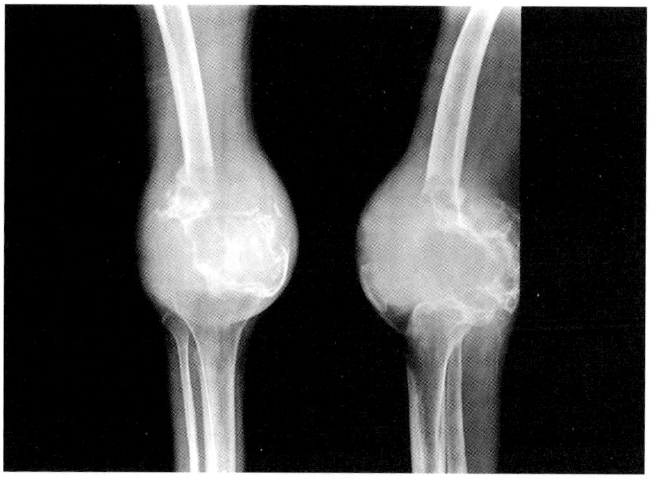

Fig. 14: Giant cell tumor: Radiograph of knee (AP and Lateral view) show large grossly expansile lytic lesion in lower end of femur, extending up to subchondral region.

and do not cross the open physis, but may extend to the subchondral bone if the physis is closed. On MRI, the lesion shows generalized hypointensity on T2-weighted images. This T2 hypointensity may result from the tumor cellularity, or from recurrent hemorrhage within the lesion. The solid portions of GCT enhance diffusely after gadolinium administration. Secondary, ABC formation can be seen in about 14% of GCT.[17]

TUMOR-LIKE LESIONS

Simple Bone Cyst

A bone cyst is a fluid filled lesion with fibrous lining. It occurs in metaphysis of long bones and adjacent to physis in children and young adults. Common locations are proximal humerus and femur.[18] Calcaneum and ileum are less common sites. On plain radiograph, the lesion appears as moderately expansile, well marginated with or without sclerosis **(Fig. 15)**. The cortex may be thinned out and may lead to pathological fracture. "Fallen fragment" sign may be seen, when there is piece of bone which migrates into the cavity and settles at the base. CT and MRI can confirm the cystic nature of the lesion. The fluid contents are usually of low intensity on T1-weighted images and hyperintensity on T2-weighted images. However, hemorrhage into the cyst can alter the signal characteristics of the lesion.[5,18]

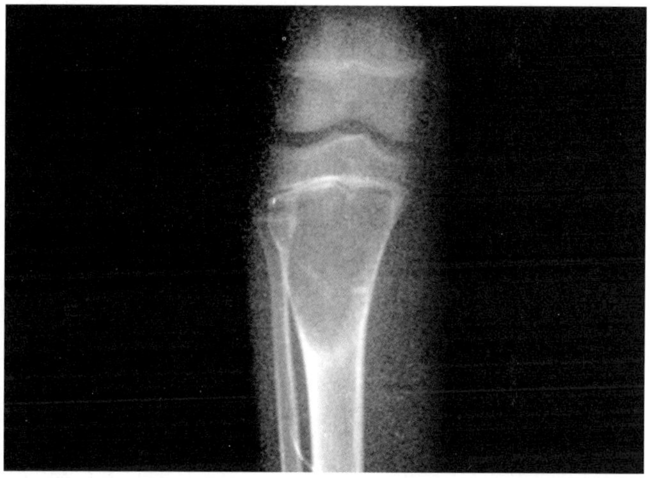

Fig. 15: Bone cyst: Radiograph of knee joint show mildly expansile lytic lesion in metaphysis of tibia with thinning of cortex.

Aneurysmal Bone Cyst

Aneurysmal bone cyst is solitary, expansile radiolucent lesion and generally located in metaphysis of long bones. Other sites are dorsolumbar spine, small bones of hand, feet and pelvis. Pathologically, the lesion contains multiples cystic spaces containing various stages of blood. Radiologically, the lesion appears as expansile, lytic sharply circumscribed with thin cortex. The characteristic features are its ballooned out appearance and trabeculated appearance **(Fig. 16)**. CT may demonstrate fluid-fluid level and thin rim of bone overlying the lesion. MRI shows the various stages of blood products which appear as layers of different signal intensity on both T1 and T2W images[18] **(Figs. 17A and B)**. The differential diagnosis includes giant cell tumor, osteoblastoma, chondroblastoma, osteosarcoma and simple bone cyst.

Pseudotumor of Hemophilia

Hemophilia is a bleeding disorder that occurs in males. Repetitive hemorrhage occurs close to muscle

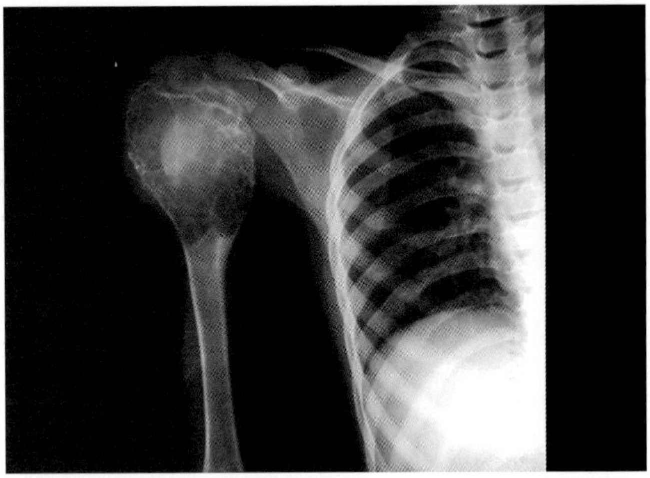

Fig. 16: Aneurysmal bone cyst: Radiograph of shoulder joint shows multiloculated expansile lytic lesion, involving upper end of humerus.

attachments without significant history of trauma. The common locations are iliopsoas and gastrocnemius muscles. Sometimes, there is intraosseous or subperiosteal hemorrhage, which can cause pressure erosion of bone. Plain X-ray shows pressure erosion/destruction of bone associated with large soft tissue component **(Fig. 18A)**. Calcification within soft tissue hematoma may be seen. MRI shows variable heterogeneous signal, in form of various stages of blood products **(Fig. 18B)**.

SOFT TISSUE TUMORS

The diagnosis of soft tissue tumors in children can be challenging due to broad spectrum of developmental anomalies, neoplasms, inflammatory conditions and pseudotumors. Ultrasonography (USG) and magnetic resonance imaging (MRI) are extremely useful in the

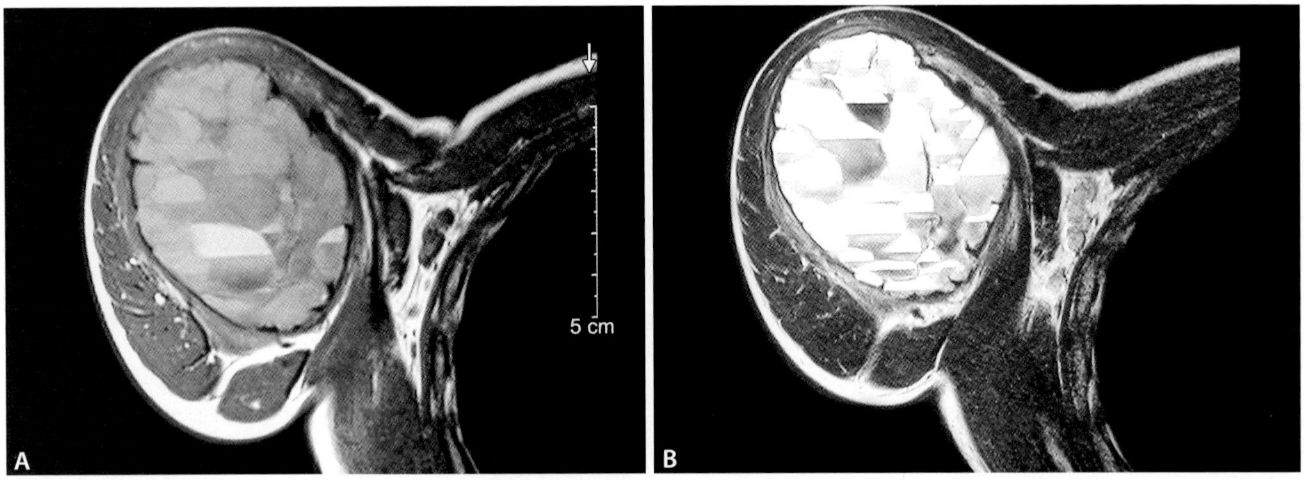

Figs. 17A and B: Aneurysmal bone cyst: MRI of the same patient, axial T1 and T2W images (A and B) show well-defined multiloculated expansile lesion with fluid-fluid/hemorrhage levels.

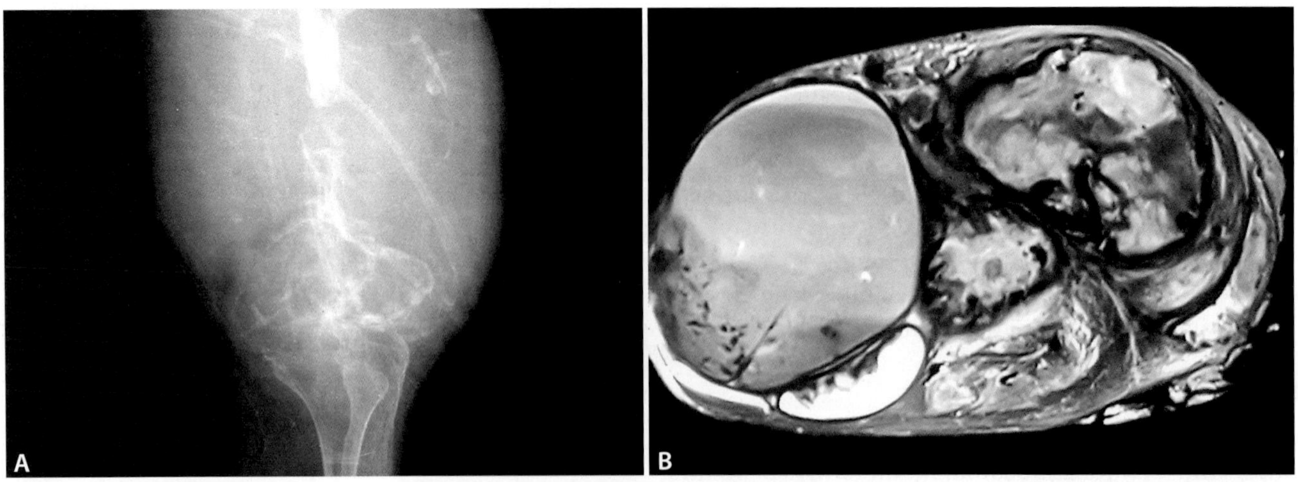

Figs. 18A and B: Pseudotumor of hemophilia: Radiograph of lower end of femur: (A) Shows lytic destruction of femur associated with large soft tissue component and bony spicules. MRI of the same patient, fat sat T2WI image; (B) Shows large soft tissue with various stages of blood components.

characterization of these tumors. However, an accurate diagnosis can only be made by correlating with the patient's age, clinical history and physical examination. Ultrasound is usually the modality of choice for the small and superficial soft tissue masses. It has the advantages of relatively low cost, portability, lack of radiation, no need for sedation, and widespread availability. Grayscale imaging should be performed with the highest frequency transducer available. Color Doppler should be performed to demonstrate the presence of vessels within the lesion.

Due to its multiplanar imaging capabilities, high tissue contrast resolution, and lack of radiation, MR imaging is the modality of choice for the evaluation of large and deep masses or for those cases in which US is not adequate. Magnetic resonance imaging (MRI) should include the entire tumor so as to demonstrate its margins. MR images of soft tissue tumors have low specificity, are only occasionally helpful in differentiating between benign and malignant masses with certainty. Some MR imaging criteria have been postulated as indicators of malignancy, particularly in adults. These include size (>5–6 cm), absence of low signal on T2-weighted images, signal heterogeneity on T1-weighted images, early contrast enhancement, peripheral or heterogeneous enhancement, rapid initial enhancement followed by a plateau or a washout phase, and invasion of adjacent bone, neurovascular bundles, or both.[19]

Vascular Lesions

Vascular lesions are the most common cause of soft tissue masses in children. Mulliken and Glowacki,[20] divided them in two groups based on the findings on physical examination, clinical evolution, histology, and cellular kinetics: hemangiomas and vascular malformations. Hemangiomas are neoplastic lesions, whereas vascular malformations are errors of vascular morphogenesis. Categorization of a lesion into one of these two groups has significant implications for a patient's management and prognosis.

Hemangioma

Hemangiomas are considered to be true neoplasms and they account for 7–10% of all benign soft tissue tumors.[20] Hemangiomas may be localized or diffuse and are histogically benign. Capillary (usually cutaneous), cavernous, venous and mixed types of hemangiomas have been described and classified according to the apparent origin of their vascular channels. Hemangiomas also contain variable amounts of nonvascular tissue and other elements, including fat, smooth muscle, fibrous tissue, myxoid stroma and hemosiderin.

USG, CT, MRI and radiolabeled red cell scintigraphy, can facilitate preoperative diagnosis. Radiographs are important for detecting associated osseous abnormality, and the finding of calcified phelebolìths on radiographs or CT images is an indication of a hemangioma **(Figs. 19A and B)**. Ultrasound shows hemangioma as a well-defined mass of variable echogenicity.[21] Color Doppler may show high flow pattern in proliferative phase; however, vascularity decreases in involuting phase. On T1-weighted MRI images, hemangiomas are either isointense or when they contain sufficient fat, hyperintense to muscle. On T2-weighted images, the lesions are well defined and markedly hyperintense with serpiginous high signal zones,

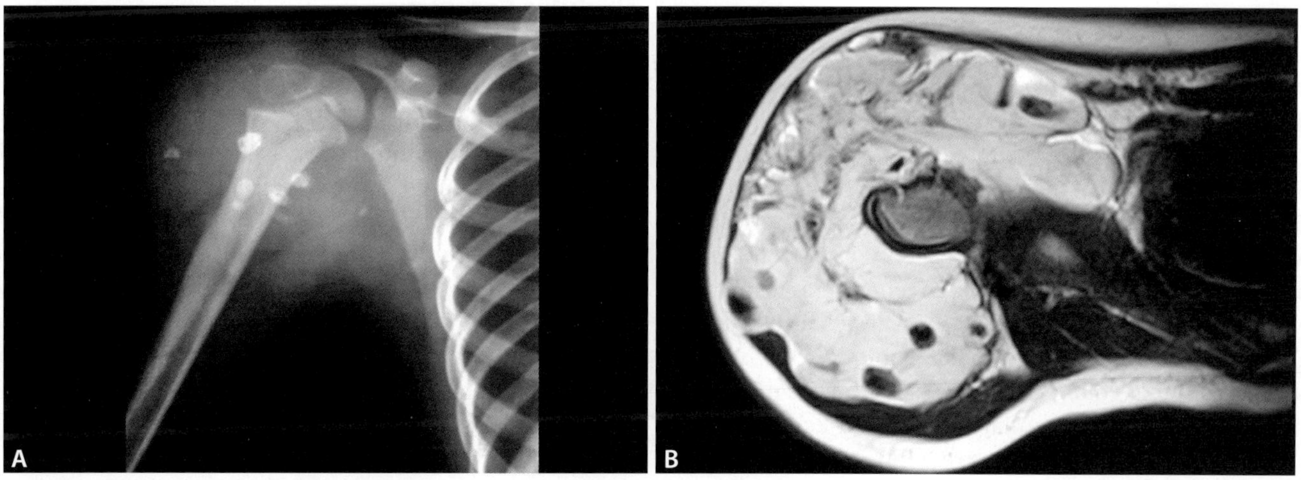

Figs. 19A and B: Hemangioma: (A) Radiograph of shoulder joint shows large soft tissue around the joint with phleboliths; (B) MRI of same patient shows large lobulated soft tissue with multiple phleboliths.

that correlate with torturous vascular channels interlaced with lower intensity fibrous or fatty tissue. Phleboliths are hypointense on both T1 and T2-weighted sequences.

Hemangiopericytoma is a rare soft tissue tumor of low but unpredictable malignant potential that is believed to arise from vascular endothelial pericytes. These tumors are usually located in the thigh or the pelvic retroperitoneum but can arise in any part of the body. Approximately 10% of hemangiopericytomas occur during childhood, and about one-third of these are congenital.[22] Congenital hemangiopericytoma can exhibit rapid initial growth, but spontaneous regression has also been reported. Microscopically, these tumors show endothelial proliferation with some similarity to hemangioma. Calcifications may be detected radiographically or by CT, and the tumors are well circumscribed. There may be partial destruction of adjacent bone. Hemangiopericytomas are very vascular lesions and show marked enhancement and frequently, central necrosis on contrast enhanced CT images.

Like most soft tissue sarcomas, hemangiopericytomas are isointense to muscle on T1-weighted images and exhibit high signal intensity on T2-weighted and STIR images, and they enhance moderately with gadolinium.

Vascular Malformations

Vascular malformations occur due to errors in vascular development that are always present at birth. Based on the main vascular channel present within the lesion, they are classified as arteriovenous, venous, lymphatic, capillary, or mixed. Arteriovenous malformations are high-flow vascular malformations characterized by direct communication between the arterial and venous systems without an intervening capillary bed. These lesions may be detected at birth (40% of cases) and grow commensurately with the child.[23] On US, they appear as multiple dilated tortuous channels diffusely involving subcutaneous soft tissues, which may not be apparent on grayscale but are easily demonstrated with color Doppler evaluation. These lesions have a high vascular density, and spectral Doppler analysis reveals high velocity in the arteries, but well-defined mass is usually not seen.[21] On MR imaging, they appear as enlarged vascular channels associated with dilated feeding and draining vessels and without an associated well-defined mass. The high-flow vessels appear as signal void foci on spin echo images or as high signal intensity on flow-enhanced gradient-echo images.

Venous malformations are characterized by the presence of anomalous ectatic venous channels. They may be small and localized or extensive. On US, venous malformations are usually of heterogeneous echogenicity, more commonly hypoechoic in comparison with the adjacent subcutaneous tissues phleboliths, may be present in 16% of cases. Doppler US usually detects slow venous flow within these lesions, although absence of flow is not uncommon which may reflect very slow flow or thrombosis. On MR imaging, they may appear as dilated tortuous veins or more often as lobulated masses, comprised of multiple locules reflecting dilated venous spaces separated by thin interstitial septa. They are iso- to hypointense to muscle on T1-weighted images, hyperintense on T2-weighted images, and show patchy enhancement after the administration of intravenous gadolinium.[24]

Lymphangioma usually visible at birth, is more frequent in the head and neck but also seen in the trunk, extremities, and in viscera. It may present clinically as, soft, smooth, translucent masses. On US, the macrocystic lymphatic malformations appear as well-defined, multicystic lesions. On MR imaging, the macrocystic lymphatic malformations appear as clearly defined cysts usually of low signal intensity on T1-weighted images and high signal intensity on T2-weighted images, often with fluid-fluid levels. Postcontrast images show only septal enhancement without enhancement of the cystic spaces. This is a helpful feature in the differentiation from venous malformations.[24]

FIBROBLASTIC/MYOFIBROBLASTIC TUMORS

Fibroblastic/myofibroblastic tumors comprise a large number of mesenchymal tumors with both fibroblastic and myofibroblastic features. Common lesions of this group are described here.

Nodular Fasciitis

Nodular fasciitis is an idiopathic, self-limited focal fibrous proliferation, usually confined to the subcutaneous tissues. Common locations include the upper extremities and trunk. On US, nodular fasciitis is a well-defined lesion with, homogeneous/heterogeneous echotexture. The MR imaging appearance is variable, although more commonly, it appears as a fascia-based lesion of homogeneous isointense or slightly hyperintense to muscle on T1-weighted images, hyperintense on T2-weighted images, and homogeneous enhancement after gadolinium administration.[25]

Myositis Ossificans

Myositis ossificans is a localized, self-limited, reparative hypercellular lesion, composed of reactive hypercellular fibrous tissue and bone. In most cases, a clear history of trauma is obtained. It often occurs in an area exposed to trauma, more commonly in the thighs and arms. Plain X-ray can show heterogeneous calcification, adjacent to bony attachment **(Fig. 20)**. CT is the modality of choice for the evaluation of myositis ossificans. The appearance of the lesion changes with time. In the first 2 weeks after trauma, it appears as a noncalcified hypodense mass, with edema of surrounding soft tissues. Curvilinear peripheral calcification becomes evident after 4–6 weeks, with progressive internal ossification over the next several weeks and months.[26]

Myofibroma/Myofibromatosis

Solitary myofibroma is a common, benign fibrous tumor commonly seen in children <2 years of age. It may present as a solitary nodule in the subcutaneous tissues or muscle or as multiple nodules involving soft tissues and bone. The multicentric presentation is known as myofibromatosis. The natural history of myofibromatosis is spontaneous regression; however, a high mortality is reported in multicentric cases with visceral involvement. On US, myofibromas have varied appearances but are often well marginated with an anechoic center, reflecting central necrosis, which can be traversed by thick septa.[27] On MR imaging; myofibromas appear as nodules of low signal intensity on T1-weighted images and a more variable appearance on T2-weighted images.

Fibromatosis

Fibromatosis is a benign proliferation of fibroblasts and myofibroblasts with a marked production of collagen. It is characterized by infiltrative growth and a propensity for local recurrence. These tumors are variably echogenic on ultrasound and their borders may be smooth or irregular. CT scan is useful to show extent of soft tissue and bony erosion **(Figs. 21A and B)**. On MR images, their appearance is also variable with a signal that is isointense or slightly hyperintense when compared with that of muscle on T1-weighted images and either intermediate between muscles and fat or high signal on T2-weighted images.[28]

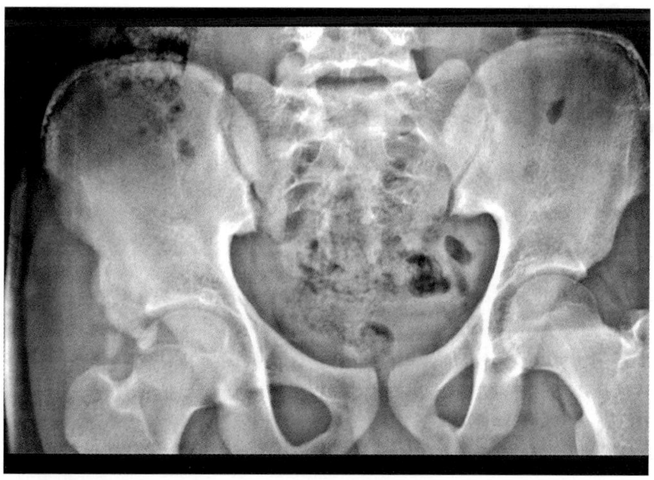

Fig. 20: Myositis ossificans: Radiograph of pelvis shows soft tissue ossification adjacent to superior aspect of right acetabulum.

Neurogenic Tumor

Most common neurogenic tumor arising from peripheral nerves in children is neurofibroma. Three types of neurofibroma has been described, localized, diffuse and plexiform type.[29] Localized neurofibroma are usually well defined, encapsulated soft tissue masses less than 5 cm in diameter. They are isointense to muscle on T1 and heterogeneous signal on T2-weighted images and may show target pattern.[29] Plexiform neurofibroma is a diffuse mass involving multiple fascicles of nerve. These lesions can be deep, superficial or combination of both, depending upon the location of tumor. Superficial types of lesions are more common, diffuse and asymmetric in distribution and extend to skin surface **(Fig. 22)**.

Adipocytic Tumor

Common adipocytic tumors are lipoma, lipoblastoma, and lipomatosis of nerve in the pediatric age group. Liposarcoma, which is the most common type of soft tissue sarcoma in adults is rare in children.

Lipoma

Lipoma is the most common adipocytic tumor in children, it is often found in the upper back, neck, proximal extremities, and abdomen. Lipomas are usually subcutaneous, although deep ones are not rare, and these will more often require imaging. On US, lipomas have a variable appearance, with about two thirds of cases demonstrating homogeneous echogenicity and 60% with well-defined margins. The echogenicity is varied with hypoechoic, isoechoic, hyperechoic, and mixed echogenicity patterns reported.[30] On MR imaging, lipomas have similar signal characteristics compared with subcutaneous fat, characterized by high signal intensity on T1-weighted images and low signal intensity on fat-suppressed images **(Fig. 23)**.

Lipoblastoma

Lipoblastoma is a tumor composed of mature adipocytes and lipoblasts in various stages of development. It represents up to 30% of adipocytic tumors in children.[31] It occurs primarily in children <3 years of age and commonly

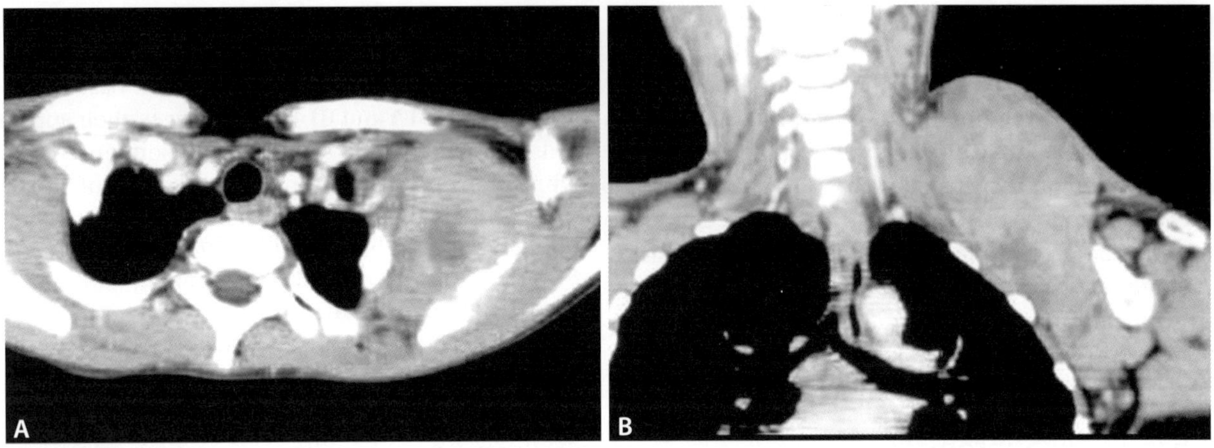

Figs. 21A and B: Fibromatosis: (A) CT scan axial section and (B) coronal reformation show large soft tissue mass in the lower part of neck extending into axilla with erosion of adjacent scapula.

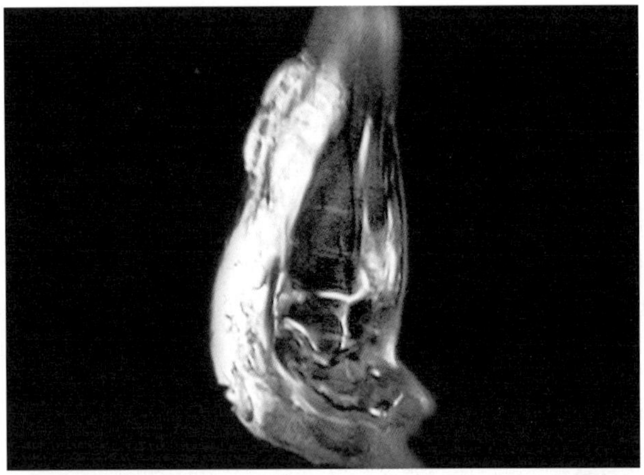

Fig. 22: Plexiform neurofibroma: MRI of leg shows large lobulated heterogeneous signal intensity lesion involving skin and deep soft tissue of leg.

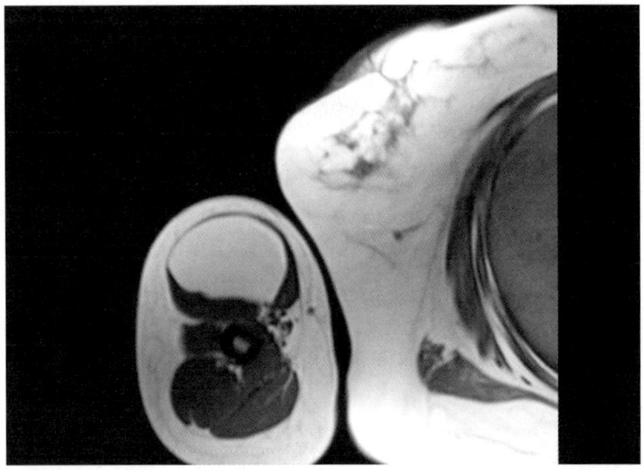

Fig. 23: Lipoma: MRI, axial section (T1W image) of shows well-defined lesion in anterior compartment of arm with similar signal intensity of subcutaneous fat.

manifests as a painless, progressively growing mass. On US, lipoblastoma usually appears as a homogeneous, hyperechoic mass, although mixed echogenicity and fluid-filled spaces have also been reported. On MR imaging, the appearance reflects the amount of mature adipose tissue relative to lipoblasts and myxocollagenous stromal tissue. They can appear similar to lipoma. When the myxoid component is large the MR signal is heterogeneous and shows contrast enhancement. This imaging appearance is indistinguishable from liposarcoma **(Fig. 24)**.[32]

Pseudotumors

Pseudotumors are non-neoplastic lesions and can present as soft tissue mass. These include hematoma, fat necrosis, inflammatory lesions and periarticular cysts.

Fat Necrosis

It is self-limiting entity and presents as small nontender subcutaneous nodule. The causes of fat necrosis include cold exposure, trauma, injection, autoimmune disorders and vasculitis. Common locations include the soft tissues overlying bone prominences in the shoulders, back, buttocks, thighs, and cheeks. Imaging findings on ultrasound is quite variable; however, predominantly it is a hyperechoic nodule with fuzzy margins. Fat necrosis appears as linear shaped abnormal signal in subcutaneous tissue which is usually hypointense on T1 and hypo/hyperintense on T2-weighted images.[33]

Hematoma

Imaging of hematoma is usually not required; however, it may be indicated in very symptomatic cases, in children without clear history of trauma and in bleeding disorders to know extent of involvement. The imaging appearance of hematoma depends on the age of blood. Ultrasound is the initial investigation of choice. In acute stage, hematoma is hyperechoic; however, it becomes anechoic/ heterogeneous in few days **(Fig. 25)**. MRI is useful and it can show hyperintensity on T1-weighted images, hypointense on T2-weighted images and blooming on GRE sequences.[34]

Inflammatory Lesions

Cellulitis occasionally presents as soft tissue mass. Ultrasound shows increased echogenecity of subcutaneous fat. On MRI, cellulitis appears as illdefined T1 hypointense and T2 hyperintense area seen in subcutaneous tissue. Sometimes, aggressive infection leads to abscess formation in soft tissue. On ultrasound, abscess appears as hypoechoic fluid collection **(Fig. 26)**. MRI shows, well defined T1 hypointense and T2 hyperintense lesion with peripheral enhancement on postcontrast images.[35]

Periarticular Cysts

These include ganglion, synovial cyst and meniscal cyst. Ganglion is cystic lesion which has fibrous capsule and composed of mucoid material. Imaging (USG and MRI) shows typical features of cyst; however, sometimes, internal echoes and septae can be seen.[36] Synovial cyst is lined by synovial cells. Synovial cyst may communicate with joint space. Typical example of synovial cyst is popliteal cyst. Collection of fluid in the meniscus or parameniscal tissue is called meniscal cyst **(Fig. 27)**. It is associated with meniscus tear. MR imaging shows well defined cyst/fluid collection in continuity with meniscus tear.[37]

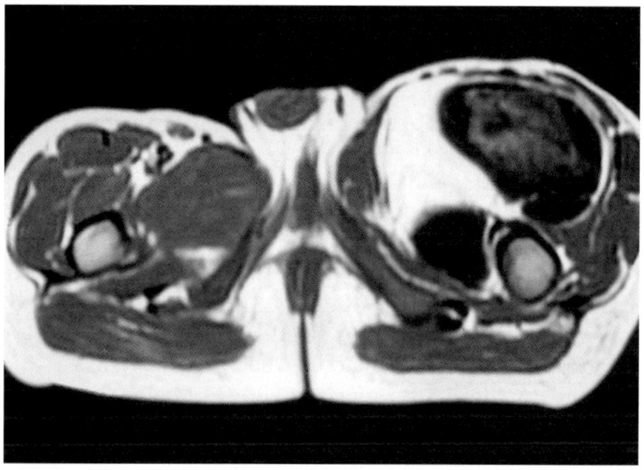

Fig. 24: Lipoblastoma: MRI, axial section (T1 W images) of upper thigh, shows large soft tissue mass in left upper thigh with signal intensity of fat as well as soft tissue

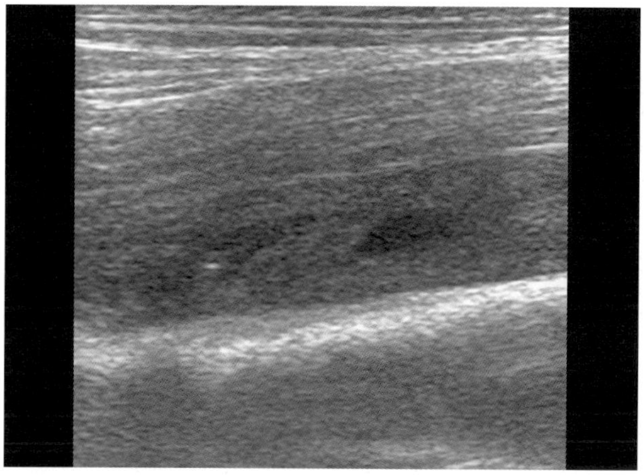

Fig. 25: Hematoma: Ultrasound image shows ill-defined heterogeneous echotexture lesion with in the deep muscles of thigh, suggestive of hematoma.

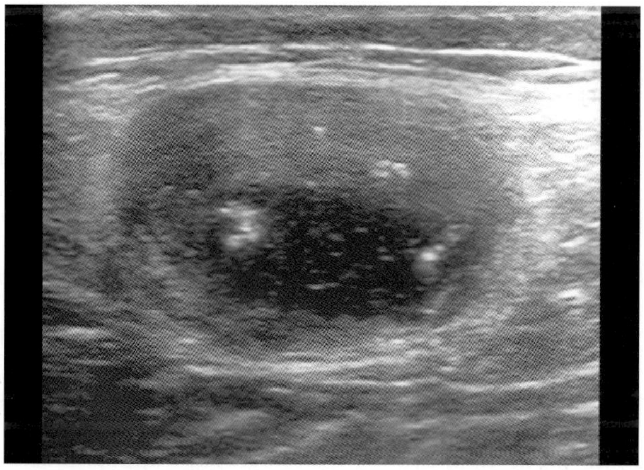

Fig. 26: Abscess: Ultrasound image shows well-defined collection in subcutaneous soft tissue with internal echoes suggestive of abscess.

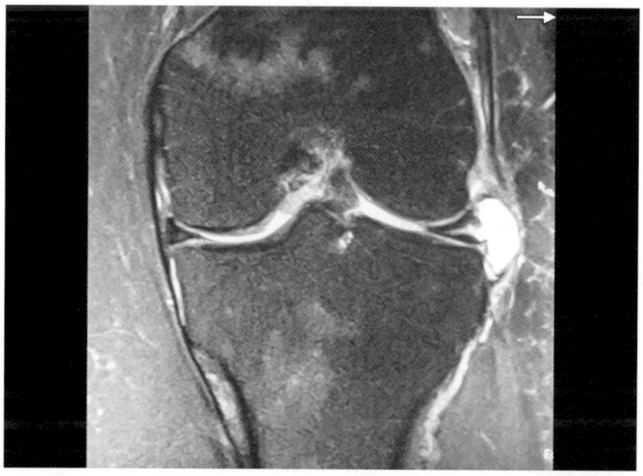

Fig. 27: Meniscal cyst: MRI, coronal section of knee shows tear of meniscus with large adjacent fluid collection communicating with tear suggestive of meniscal cyst.

CONCLUSION

A wide spectrum of benign bone and soft tissue tumor and conditions is seen in children. It is imperative for the radiologist to be aware of entire gamut of imaging findings, so as to avoid unwarranted biopsies and surgeries in these children. Plain radiograph continue to be first line imaging modality of choice and is the cornerstone in diagnosis of pediatric benign bone tumors. MR imaging has emerged to become an integral part of diagnostic algorithm of these lesions, owing to its excellent soft tissue resolution, multiplanar capabilities and nonionizing nature.

REFERENCES

1. Fletcher BD. Benign and malignant bone tumor. In Caffey's Pediatric Diagnostic Imaging Volume 2, Mosby, Elsevier, Philadelphia; 2004.
2. Biermann JS. Musculoskeletal neoplasms in children. In: Orthopaedic knowledge update. Sponseller PD, Shaughnessy JW (Eds): Rosemont, IL: American Academy of Orthopaedic Surgeons. 2002.pp.51-61.
3. Giudici MA, Moser RP, Kransdorf MJ. Cartilaginous bone tumor. Radiol Clin of North Am. 1993;31:237-59.
4. Mirra JM, Picci P, Gold RH. Bone tumors: Clinical, radiologic and pathologic correlation. Philadelphia; Lea and Fabiger; 1989.
5. Steven S, Srinivas K, Javicr B. MR imaging of tumors and tumor like lesions of upper extremity. Magn Reson imaging Clin of N America. 2004;12:349-59.
6. Holtz P, Sundaram M. Enchondroma. Orthopedics. 1995;18: 509-10.
7. Mermelstein LE, Friedlaender GE, Katz LD. Chondroblastoma. Orthopedics. 1997;20:67-71.
8. McGrory BJ, Inwards CY, Mcleod RA, et al. Chondromyxoid fibroma. Orthopadedics. 1995;18(3):307-10.
9. Bloem JL, Kroon HM. Osseous lesions. Radiol Clin of North America. 1993;31(2):261-5.
10. Assoun J, Riichardi G, Railhac JJ, et al. Osteoid osteoma: MR Imaging versus CT Radiology. 1994;191:217-36.
11. Bruners P, Penzkofer T, Günther RW, Mahnken A. Percutaneous radiofrequency ablation of osteoid osteomas: Technique and results. Rofo. 2009;181(8):740-7.
12. Moulton JS, Bvaley SE, Biedel JS. Bone and soft tissue tumors. In clinical Magnetic resonance imaging (2nd edn), 1996.pp.2042-77.
13. Lucas E, Sundaram M, Boccini T. Polyostotic fibrous dysplasia. Orthopaedics. 1995;18(3):311-3.
14. Zeanah WR, Hudson TM. Springfield DS. Computed tomography of ossifying fibroma of the tibia. J Comput Assist Tomogr. 1983;7:688-91.
15. Marin C, Warrier RP. Langerhan's cell histiocytosis. Orthop Clin of North Am. 1996;27(3):615-23.
16. Copley L, Dormans JP. Benign pediatric bone tumors. Evaluation and treatment. Pediatr Clin North Am. 1996;43:949-66.
17. Murphey MD, Nomikos GC, Flemming DJ, et al. Imaging of giant cell tumor and giant cell reparative granuloma of bone: Radiologic-pathologic correlation. Radiographics. 2001;21:1283–309.
18. Conway WF, Hayes CW. Miscellaneous lesions of bone. Radiol Clin of North Am. 1993;31(2):339-58.
19. Brisse H, Orbach D, Klijanienko J, Fréneaux P, Neuenschwander S. Imaging and diagnostic strategy of soft tissue tumors in children. Eur Radiol. 2006;16(5):1147-64.
20. Mulliken JB, Glowacki J. Hemangiomas and vascular malformations in infants and children: A classification based on endothelial characteristics. Plast Reconstr Surg. 1982;69(3):412-22.
21. Paltiel HJ, Burrows PE, Kozakewich HPW, Zurakowski D, Mulliken JB. Soft-tissue vascular anomalies: Utility of US for diagnosis. Radiology. 2000;214(3):747-54.
22. Auguste LJ. Razack MS, Sako K. Hemangiopericytoma. J Surg Oncol. 1982;20:260-4.
23. Frieden I, Enjolras O, Esterly N. Vascular birthmarks, other abnormalities of blood vessels and lymphatics. In: Schachner LA, Hansen RC (Eds). Pediatric Dermatology, 3rd edn. New York, NY: Mosby. 2003. pp. 833-62.
24. Konez O, Burrows PE. Magnetic resonance of vascular anomalies. Magn Reson Imaging Clin N Am. 2002;10(2):363-88.
25. Leung LYJ, Shu SJ, Chan ACL, Chan MK, Chan CHS. Nodular fasciitis: MRI appearance and literature review. Skeletal Radiol. 2002;31(1):9-13.
26. Siegel MJ. Magnetic resonance imaging of musculoskeletal soft tissue masses. Radiol Clin North Am. 2001;39(4):701-20.
27. Koujok K, Ruiz RE, Hernandez RJ. Myofibromatosis: Imaging characteristics. Pediatr Radiol. 2005;35(4):374-80.
28. Lee JC, Thomas JM, Phillips S, Fisher C, Moskovic E. Aggressive fibromatosis: MRI features with pathologic correlation. Am J Roentgenol. 2006;186(1):247-54.
29. Stull MA, Moser RP, Kransdorf MJ, et al. Magnetic resonance appearance of peripheral nerve sheath tumors. Skeletal Radiol. 1991;20:9-14.
30. Fornage BD, Tassin GB. Sonographic appearances of superficial soft tissue lipomas. J Clin Ultrasound. 1991;19(4):215-20.
31. Miller GG, Yanchar NL, Magee JF, Blair GK. Lipoblastoma and liposarcoma in children: An analysis of 9 cases and a review of the literature. Can J Surg. 1998;41(6):455-8.
32. Murphey MD, Carroll JF, Flemming DJ, Pope TL, Gannon FH, Kransdorf MJ. From the archives of the AFIP: Benign musculo-skeletal lipomatous lesions. Radiographics. 2004;24(5):1433-66.
33. Tsai TS, Evans HA, Donnelly LF, Bisset GS III, Emery KH. Fat necrosis after trauma: A benign cause of palpable lumps in children. Am J Roentgenol. 1997;169(6):1623-6.
34. Bush CH. The magnetic resonance imaging of musculoskeletal hemorrhage. Skeletal Radiol. 2000;29(1):1-9.
35. Faingold R, Oudjhane K, Armstrong DC, Albuquerque PAB. Magnetic resonance imaging of congenital, inflammatory, and infectious soft-tissue lesions in children. Top Magn Reson Imaging. 2002;13(4):241-61.
36. Seymour R, Lloyd DCF. Sonographic appearances of meniscal cysts. J Clin Ultrasound. 1998;26(1):15-20.
37. McCarthy CL, McNally EG. The MRI appearance of cystic lesions around the knee. Skeletal Radiol. 2004;33(4):187-209.

CHAPTER 149

Pediatric Malignant Bone and Soft Tissue Tumors

Manisha Jana, Ashu Seith Bhalla, Deep Narayan Srivastava

INTRODUCTION

Malignant bone tumors account for about 6% of all childhood malignancies,[1,2] though malignant soft tissue tumors are rare in childhood. The most common malignant bone tumors include osteosarcoma and Ewing's sarcoma, while rhabdomyosarcoma is the most common pediatric malignant soft tissue tumor.[3,4] Most of the tumors affect the appendicular skeleton and result in significant morbidity and mortality. **Table 1** shows age distribution of these tumors.

Table 1: Age distribution of pediatric bone and soft tissue tumors.

Age	*Bone tumor*	*Soft tissue tumor*
Less than 5 years	• Osteosarcoma • Ewing's sarcoma • Lymphoma	• Rhabdomyosarcoma • Infantile fibrosarcoma • Hemangiopericytoma • Granulocytic sarcoma
More than 5 years	• Osteosarcoma • Ewing's sarcoma • Lymphoma • Malignant fibrous histiocytoma (rare) • Chondrosarcoma (rare)	• Rhabdomyosarcoma • Synovial sarcoma • Granulocytic sarcoma • Hemangiopericytoma

IMAGING MODALITIES

Plain Radiographs

Radiographs are the primary imaging modality in cases of bone tumors, and often a specific diagnosis can be made on plain radiographs alone depending on location of the lesion **(Table 2)**. The appearance of the lesion and the patient age remain important considerations for diagnosis. Most of the pediatric malignant bone tumors involve the metaphysis; however, Ewing's sarcoma and lymphoma have a propensity to involve diaphysis. The pattern of bone destruction is a pointer towards the aggressiveness of the lesion. Most malignant bone tumors present radiographically with a permeative lytic or moth-eaten pattern of bone destruction **(Fig. 1)**.

Table 2: Common locations of primary malignant bone tumors.

Location	*Tumors*
Metaphysis	• Osteosarcoma • Metastases • Ewing's sarcoma • Lymphoma • Malignant fibrous histiocytoma
Diaphysis	• Ewing's sarcoma • Lymphoma
Epiphysis	• Aggressive giant cell tumor (rare)

In cases of pediatric soft tissue tumors, plain radiographs are often of limited importance. Clinical examination can often prove useful in evaluating small superficial lesions (e.g. lipoma), but for proper assessment of extent of most soft tissue tumors, radiologic evaluation is imperative.

Sonography

Ultrasonography is useful for characterization of some lesions, especially for superficial lesions.[5] Doppler can

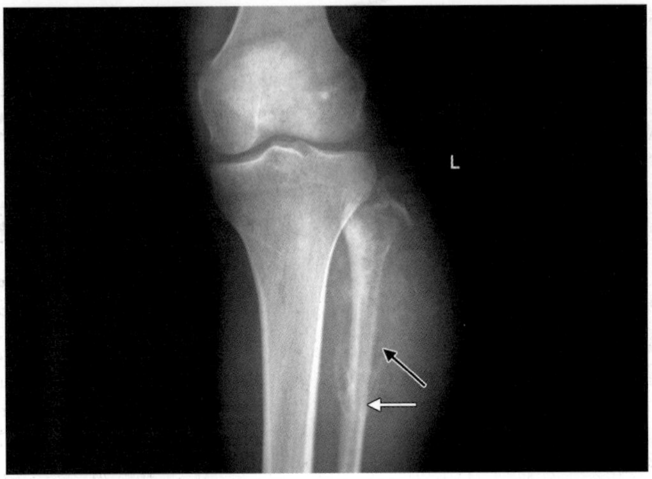

Fig. 1: Plain radiograph of the left leg shows permeative lytic destruction, periosteal reaction (white arrow) and Codman triangle (black arrow), typical imaging features of a malignant bone tumor. *Histopathology*: Osteosarcoma.

help in the assessment of vascularity of lesion and also for guided biopsies and in monitoring tumor response to chemotherapy.

Computed Tomography

Among the cross-sectional imaging, role of CT has considerably reduced after the introduction of MRI. However, CT is superior to MRI in the detection and characterization of matrix mineralization, bone trabeculation and periosteal reaction. CT is also used in the detection of pulmonary metastases.

Magnetic Resonance Imaging

The roles of magnetic resonance imaging (MRI) in pediatric bone tumors include accurate assessment of the extent of the lesion, evaluation of skip lesions, neurovascular and articular involvement. T1W spin echo images remain the most important sequence to assess the tumor extent, owing to the contrast between normal hyperintense fatty marrow and hypointense tumor.[6] Inversion recovery sequence (short tau inversion recovery—STIR) sequence makes the tumor more conspicuous by suppressing normal marrow fat as the hyperintense tumor stands bright. Postcontrast images (after Gadolinium administration) can define the exact extent of the tumor, define viable tumor and the necrotic areas[7] and help in tumor edema differentiation.[8] Peritumoral edema can either be intraosseous or extraosseous and often show high signal on T2 weighted or STIR images. In the bones, edema has poorly defined margin and often difficult to differentiate from the tumor mass. In the soft tissues, edema does not have mass effect and follows muscle and fascial planes.

Most of the malignant bone and soft tissue tumors share common similar imaging features, e.g. they are hypointense on T1W and hyperintense on T2W images.[9-12] However, few lesions show characteristic signal intensities, e.g. fat containing lesions are bright on T1W as well as T2W sequences and fibrous tumors may show hypointense signal on both T1 as well as T2W images. The differentiation of benign from malignant nature of a mass is not possible in most cases on MR imaging; but the useful role of MRI is in tumor staging.

MRI Techniques for Bone and Soft Tissue Tumors

The sequences should include T1W images in coronal or sagittal plane for accurate delineation of tumor extent **(Fig. 2A)** and articular involvement, if any. T2W fat saturated or STIR images is useful for better demonstration of relationship with adjacent muscles, nerves and vascular structures **(Fig. 2B)**.

Role of Contrast-enhanced MRI

In primary bone and soft tissue tumors, contrast administration is often not required. However, T1W fat saturated images are helpful in follow-up imaging for detection of recurrence. Dynamic contrast-enhanced MRI is specifically helpful in detecting tumor recurrence,[13] which often shows early contrast enhancement and washout.

Newer MR Imaging Techniques

Diffusion-weighted MRI: Diffusion-weighted MRI has been used to predict the tumor viability after treatment, and hence, to reflect the response to treatment. After treatment, many a times the tumor bulk may not reduce significantly but the apparent diffusion coefficient (ADC) value increases[14] indicating response to treatment.

Dynamic Contrast-enhanced MRI: Dynamic contrast-enhanced MRI is a new addition in the imaging of malignant bone tumors, especially osteosarcoma. It measures the tumor viability by determining the contrast accumulation within the tumor. Dynamic contrast-enhanced MRI assessment of dynamic vector magnitude (based on contrast accumulation rate over time and maximal intensity of the tumor) and Kep (measure of the gadolinium exchange between the vascular and the interstitial space) tend to predict the outcome after treatment.[15]

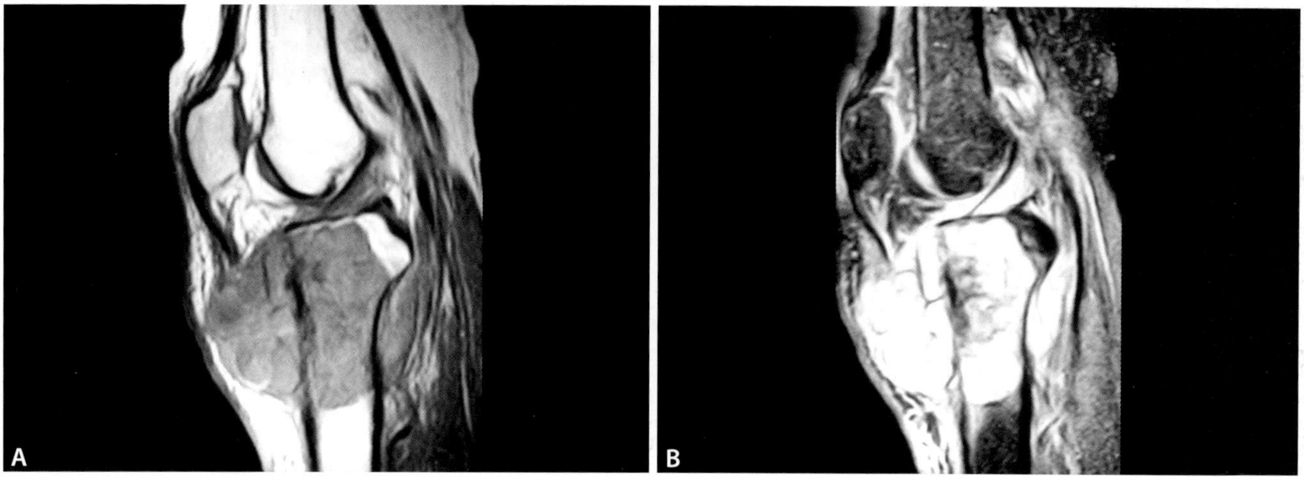

Figs. 2A and B: Sagittal T1W (A) and T2W (B) MR of a case of osteosarcoma. The tumor is hypointense in contrast to hyperintense fatty marrow on T1W and hyperintense on T2W sequences. The tumor has an extracompartmental extension into the muscle plane (stage T2).

MR spectroscopy: In vivo proton MR spectroscopy is a promising modality in the evaluation of malignant bone and soft tissue tumors. On MR spectroscopy, these tumors show choline peak (resonance at 3.2 ppm);[16] which is highly sensitive and specific.

Staging of Malignant Bone and Soft Tissue Tumors

The Enneking system of staging malignant bone and soft tissue tumors[17] **(Table 3)** was based on three criteria: extent of tumor (T1 suggests an intracompartmental tumor, T2 an extracompartmental spread **(Figs. 2A and B)**), presence or absence of metastases (M0 and M1 respectively) and histologic grade of the tumor (low grade G1, high grade G2). Low grade tumors (stage IA or IB; T1G1M0 or T2G1M0) are candidates for wide local excision or limb salvage surgeries. High grade tumor (G2) without metastases are treated with radical surgeries like amputation.

In 1983, AJCC developed another system of staging of bone and soft tissue tumors depending on four criteria: extent of tumor (confined by bone cortex T1; with transcortical extension T2), nodal disease (N0 no nodal disease; N1 regional nodal spread), metastases (absence of metastases M0; presence of metastases M1) and histologic grade of tumor (G1-well differentiated tumor, G2-moderately differentiated, G3-poorly differentiated and G4 undifferentiated). The recent revision in this staging is based on the size of the tumor rather than transcortical extension (T1 tumors being less than 8 cm and T2 more than 8 cm).[18] A new stage T3 has been added to indicate skip matastases. These classification system did not include bone lymphoma or myeloma.

Table 3: Enneking staging for primary malignant bone tumors.

Stage	*Tumor*	*Metastases*	*Histologic grade*
IA	T1 (intracompartmental tumor)	M0	G1
IB	T2 (extracompartmental tumor)	M0	G1
IIA	T1	M0	G2
IIB	T2	M0	G2
III	T1 or T2	M1	G1 or G2

MALIGNANT BONE TUMORS

Osteosarcoma

Osteosarcoma is the most common pediatric malignant bone tumor,[19] usually affecting children in the second decade. Patients with retinoblastoma, Li-fraumeni syndrome, prior radiation therapy are more prone to develop osteosarcoma. The usual clinical presentation is with a painful mass.

Histologic subgroups in osteosarcoma include osteoblastic, chondroblastic, fibroblastic, giant cell rich, telangiectatic or small cell type.[20]

Plain radiographs are usually the first investigation performed. Osteosarcoma in pediatric age groups predominantly involve the metaphyses. On radiographs they present with a permeative lytic destruction with wide zone of transition **(Fig. 1)**, blastic lesion **(Fig. 3)** or a mixed pattern. Often there is an associated soft tissue component, 'sunburst' type of periosteal reaction, 'Codman triangle' formation **(Fig. 1)**; and an osteoid tumor matrix mineralization **(Fig. 3)**. Pathological fractures are more common in a telangiectatic variety.

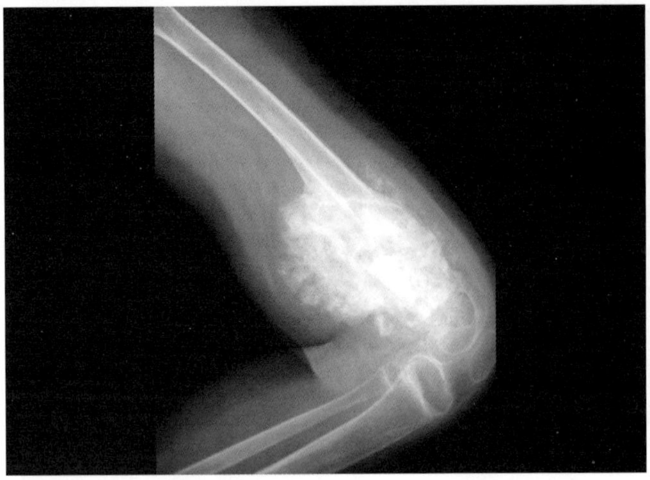

Fig. 3: Lateral radiograph of the knee in a child with osteosarcoma of the tibia. The tumor shows dense osteoid matrix mineralization.

The workup of a child with osteosarcoma include computed tomography (CT) of chest **(Figs. 4A to C)**, ^{99m}Tc MDP bone scan (to detect metastases as it spreads via the bloodstream and about 20% may have metastases at presentation)[6] and MRI for the local tumor extent.

MRI tends to show accurate intramedullary extent of the tumor. Tumor mass is usually hypointense on T1W and hyperintense on T2W and STIR images **(Fig. 5)**. The rare telangiectatic variety shows blood-fluid levels secondary to intratumoral hemorrhage **(Fig. 6)**.[3] Skip lesions within the same bone, may be seen in 15% of cases.

Survival and response to chemotherapy depends on the tumor burden which can be measured by tumor size. Histologic response to preoperative neoadjuvant chemotherapy (percent of necrosis) is the strongest predictor of survival.[21-23] Often the tumor size remains unchanged after treatment and it is difficult to determine response based on the size criteria.[15] Newer MR imaging techniques which help in predicting tumor response include diffusion weighted images and dynamic contrast-enhanced MRI. With treatment, the apparent diffusion coefficient (ADC) of the tumor mass increases.[14] Dynamic contrast-enhanced MRI assessment of dymanic vector magnitude (based on contrast accumulation rate overtime and maximal intensity of the tumor) and Kep (measure of the gadolinium exchange between the vascular and the interstitial space) tend to predict the outcome after treatment.[15]

Ewing's Sarcoma

Ewing's family of tumors include classic Ewing's sarcoma, primitive neuroectodermal tumor (PNET), Askin tumor (PNET of the chest wall), extraosseous Ewing's tumor and peripheral neuroepithelioma. All these tumors have a common neuroectodermal origin and frequently seen in children.

Classic Ewing's sarcoma: It is the second most common bone malignancy in children, predominantly seen in the second decade of life. Males and females have equal incidence. Usual clinical presentation is with local pain and swelling; often with constitutional symptoms. Laboratory investigations may show elevated erythrocyte sedimentation rate and leukocytosis; hence the picture often mimics osteomyelitis.

Metadiaphyses of the long bones are the most common site for Ewing's sarcoma. On plain radiographs, the tumor presents as a permeative lytic bone destruction with a wide zone of transition; cortical destruction; onion-peel type of periosteal reaction and often extensive noncalcified soft tissue mass.[24] Saucerization of the outer cortex may occur due to erosions by tumor growth in the subperiosteal region. In cases of flat bone involvement, the soft tissue component is larger than osseous destruction. CT scan, though not commonly indicated, can define the bony destruction **(Fig. 7)**. However, chest CT is done to detect pulmonary metastasis. Radionuclide study is useful in the detection of bone metastasis. The differential diagnosis includes osteomyelitis.

On T1W MRI the mass is isointense to mildly hypointense; on T2W or STIR images it is hyperintense **(Figs. 8A and B)** and shows variable contrast enhancement. Skip lesions may be present in 14% cases.[24] The soft tissue mass tends to decrease in size and undergo necrosis with treatment. As with osteosarcoma, diffusion weighted MRI and dynamic CE-MRI can predict the response to neoadjuvant chemotherapy or radiotherapy.[23] Positron emission tomography (PET) is also used in monitoring response to therapy and metastatic disease.

PNET of the chest wall (Askin tumor) **(Fig. 9)**: It usually presents with an intrathoracic extrapulmonary mass having rib involvement and extrathoracic component. They are hypointense on T1W and hyperintense on T2W images, showing moderate contrast enhancement. Multiplanar imaging using MRI or CT is helpful in determining the extent of the soft tissue mass.

Chondrosarcoma

Chondrosarcoma is rare in pediatric age group, and should be differentiated from the chondroblastic variety of osteosarcoma. It predominantly involving the long bones of pelvis and shoulder girdle followed by metaphyses

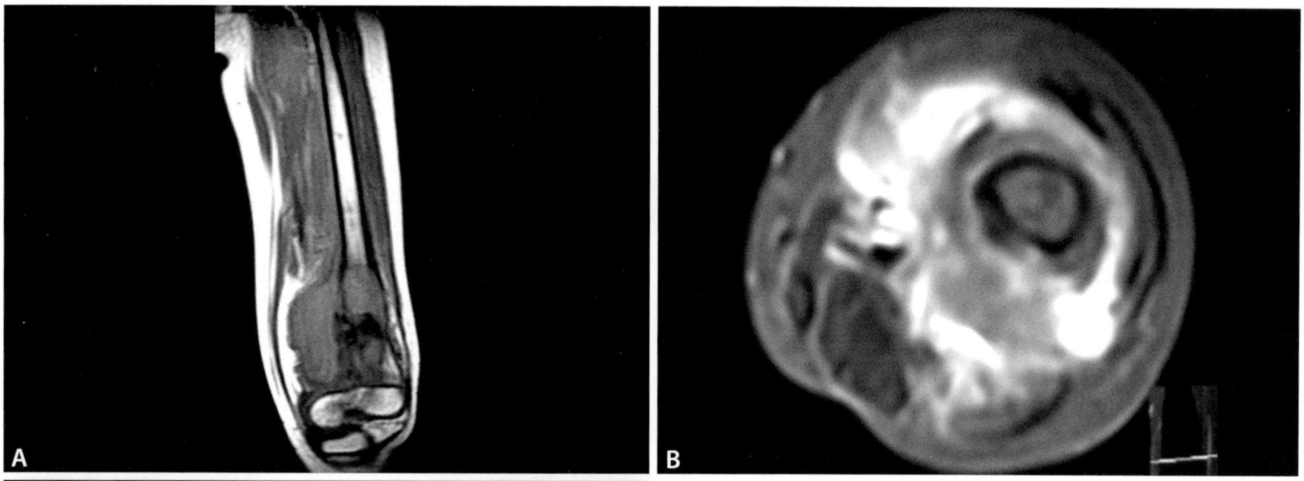

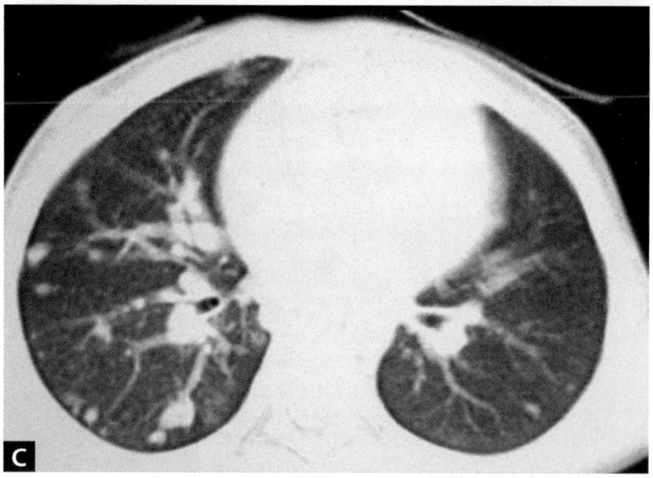

Figs 4A to C: Coronal T1W (A) and axial T2W fat saturated (B) MR of a case of osteosarcoma showing the craniocaudal and axial extent of the marrow involvement. The tumor has extracompartmental extension into the muscle plane (stage T2). Axial CT thorax (lung window) (C) of the same patient show multiple lung metastases.

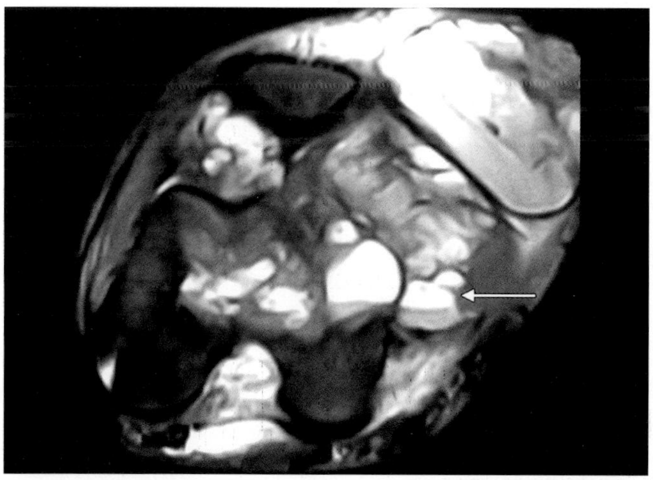

Fig. 5: Axial T2W fat saturated MR image in a case of telangiectatic osteosarcoma showing multiple areas of blood-fluid levels (white arrow) suggesting intratumoral hemorrhage.

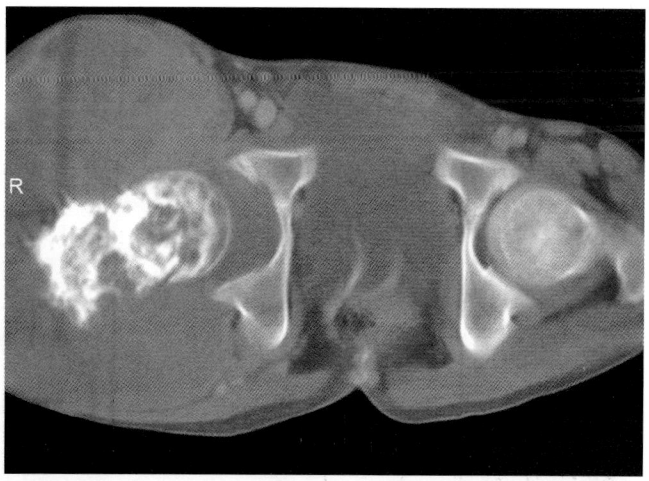

Fig. 6: PNET of the right femur: Axial CT scan bone window reconstruction reveals mixed lytic–sclerotic destruction of the right femoral head and neck with adjacent large soft tissue.

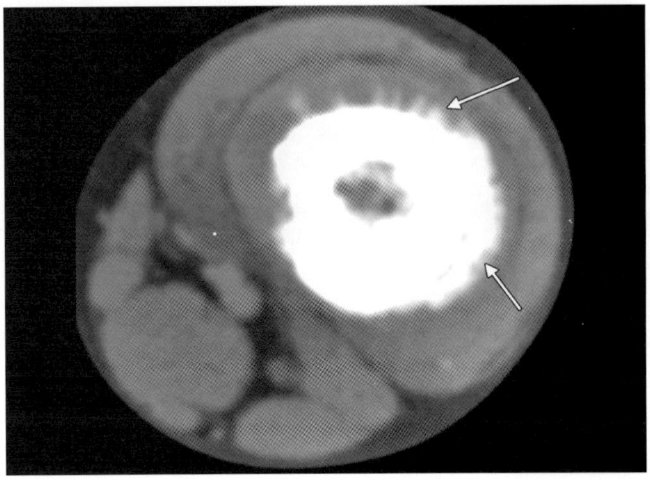

Fig. 7: Ewing's sarcoma: Axial CT bone window reconstruction reveals permeative lytic destruction of the femoral diaphysis, with spiculated periosteal reaction (arrows) and associated soft tissue.

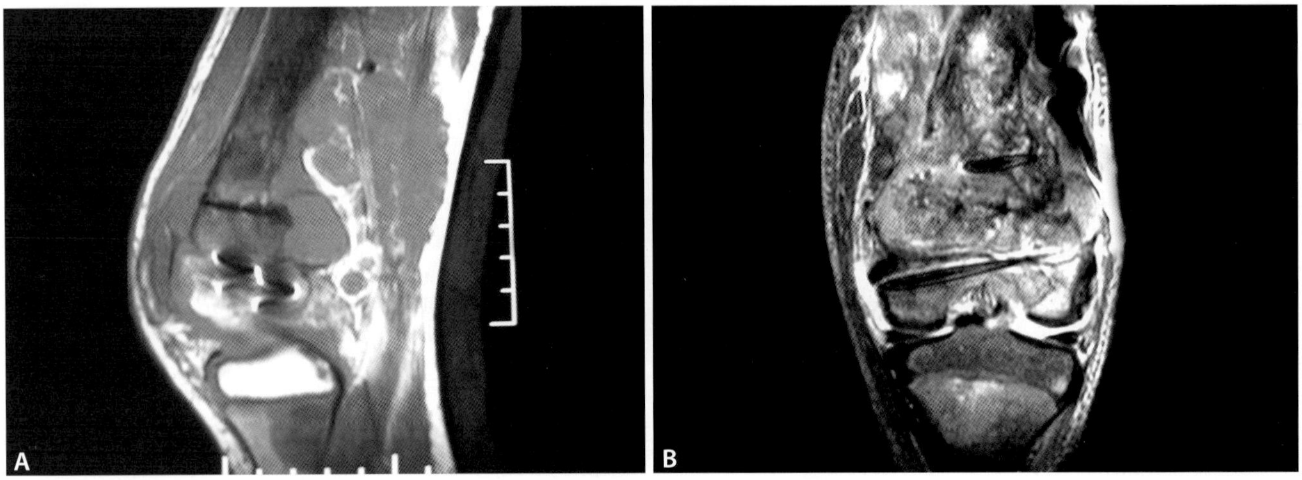

Figs. 8A and B: Sagittal T1W (A) and coronal T2W (B) MR of a case of Ewing's sarcoma. The tumor is hypointense on T1 and heterogeneously hyperintense on T2 with diffuse marrow infiltration and extraosseous spread.

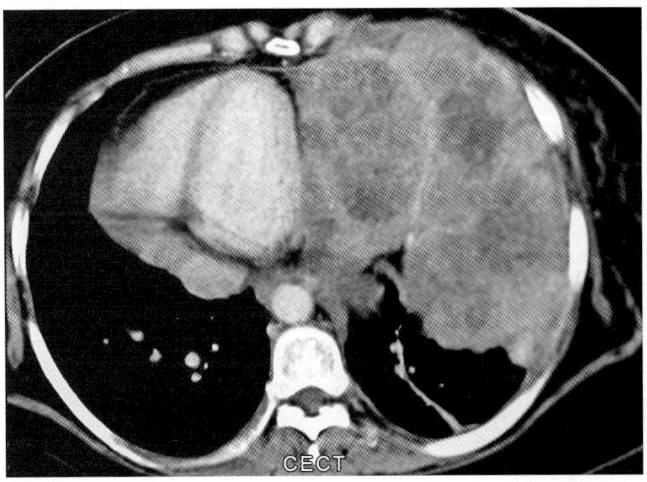

Fig. 9: PNET of the left thoracic wall (Askin tumor): Axial image of CECT thorax mediastinal window shows a large heterogeneous mass lesion in the left hemithorax with a small extrathoracic component.

of long bones, ribs and spine. The tumors can either be primary or secondary. On radiographs they are usually expansile lytic lesions with variable matrix mineralization (chondroid type). On MR imaging they show low signal intensity on T1W images. The signal on T2W images are variable, depending on the matrix. Cartilaginous matrix is bright on T2WI whereas areas of calcification and hemorrhage are hypointense.[25]

Lymphoma

Primary bone lymphoma: It comprises of 5% of all children with lymphoma and most of them are high grade B-cell NHL.[20] Usual locations include the spine and the long bones. On imaging, they commonly show permeative lytic destruction, sometimes with periosteal reaction and commonly associated with soft tissue component. Frank cortical destruction is often not evident, and the lesions are easily missed on radiographs.[26] Hodgkin's disease can cause sclerotic bony lesions and 'ivory' vertebra. MRI reveals the marrow of the affected bone to be hypointense on T1W and hyperintense on T2W images, enhancing after contrast **(Figs. 10A and B)**.

Secondary bone lymphoma: It is more common than primary bone lymphoma, especially in children. The incidence can be as high as 25% in children. Secondary skeletal involvement in Hodgkin's disease is usually from contiguous lymph nodal spread, and the lesions are more commonly sclerotic. In secondary involvement by non-Hodgkin's lymphoma, most commonly affected sites are pelvis, spine and skull. The usual presentation is with permeative lytic destruction of bone with cortical destruction.

Metastases

Metastases to bone in pediatric age group commonly occurs from primary tumors like neuroblastoma, Ewing's sarcoma or neuroblastoma. Osseous metastases in osteosarcoma are usually blastic. Metastases from neuroblastoma show a 'sunburst' type of periosteal reaction. When occurring in the calvarium, they often give rise to sutural diastasis secondary to dural deposits.

Malignant Fibrous Histiocytoma

Malignant fibrous histiocytoma occurs very rarely in pediatric age group, and usually affects the adolescents. Most common location includes metaphysis of a long bone. The radiographic findings range from geographic to permeative lytic destruction. Periosteal reaction is uncommon,[27] unlike other malignant tumors. MRI features are nonspecific.

SOFT TISSUE TUMORS

In the pediatric age group, most of the soft tissue masses are benign; only 1–6% being malignant.[28] Rhabdomyosarcoma alone comprises more than half of the pediatric soft tissue sarcomas.[3,4] In the 0–5 years age group, fibrosarcoma is the most common and in 6–15 years age group, malignant fibrous histiocytoma, synovial sarcoma and rhabdomyosarcoma are common.[29] MR imaging often cannot accurately determine the benignity or malignant nature of a soft tissue mass, but some indicators which favor a benign etiology include younger age group, smaller size of the mass, well-circumscribed lesion, subcutaneous or fascial location, homogeneous signal on T2W imaging and no

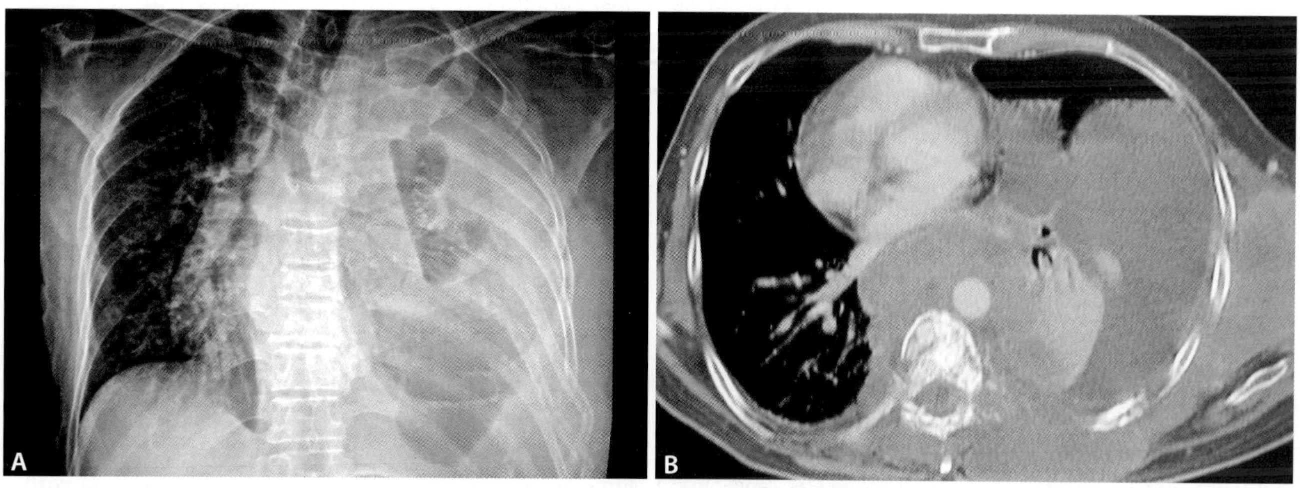

Figs. 10A and B: (A) NHL of the left thoracic wall. Chest radiograph reveals opaque left hemithorax with lytic–sclerotic destruction of left 7th and 8th ribs as well as the 8th dorsal vertebral body; (B) Axial CECT bone window of the same patient shows permeative lytic–sclerotic bone destruction involving the vertebral body, posterior element and the posterior ribs having a large soft tissue component in the paraspinal locations and along posterolateral thoracic wall.

surrounding edema.[30] Sometimes, a malignant soft tissue tumor may have well-defined margins with a pseudocapsule and homogeneous in signal intensity on MRI.

The prime important role of imaging in soft tissue tumor is not to provide an accurate diagnosis but to provide information regarding the extent of tumor, extension beyond fascial planes, adjacent bone and neurovascular bundle involvement. Other important role of imaging include response assessment after treatment. Differentiating a residual or recurrent tumor from post-treatment changes is the most challenging part in follow-up imaging. Both can present with high T2W signal intensity. Tumor recurrence is often associated with mass effect and contrast enhancement; whereas post-treatment changes lack these features.[31]

Rhabdomyosarcoma

Rhabdomyosarcoma **(Figs. 11 and 12)** accounts for 4–5% of all childhood cancers and 10–15% of solid tumors in the extremities.[32] The most common locations are the head and neck region, genitourinary tract, the retroperitoneum and the extremities. The histologic subtypes include embryonal, alveolar and the undifferentiated types. The alveolar subtype, which is relatively aggressive, is seen in the extremities. The prognosis of this tumor depends on the size, local invasion, nodal spread and distant metastases. Tumors with a diameter less than 5 cm has better overall prognosis. Extremity tumors, which are usually of alveolar subtype, have a poorer prognosis. Prognosis is better in case of proximal extremity tumors than distal tumors.[33] Complete resection is the treatment of choice and survival in unresectable tumors is poor.

On MR imaging, the tumor is isointense to muscle on T1W and hyperintense on T2W images and shows strong contrast enhancement.[30]

Synovial Sarcoma

Synovial sarcoma **(Figs. 13A and B)** is the most common non-rhabdomyosarcomatous soft tissue sarcoma in the children. It is a high grade tumor showing differentiation of tumor cells into spindle cells resembling synoviocytes; and not derived from synovial cells. The usual location of this tumor is in periarticular regions, though it can occur in other places. These tumors commonly present as a painless extremity mass, most commonly around the knee joints. On imaging, they are well defined, lobulated in outline, isointense to muscle on T1W and heterogeneously hyperintense on T2W images, with areas of hemorrhage.[34] Scattered calcification is seen in as high as one-third of the lesions.[35] Sometimes, the lesions are cystic, mimicking a ganglion cyst or Baker's cyst.[28]

Other Non-rhabdomyosarcomatous Tumors

Other non-rhabdomyosarcomatous tumors are rare in childhood and include fibrosarcoma, hemangio-pericytoma, granulocytic sarcoma, malignant fibrous histiocytoma, epithelioid sarcoma and clear cell sarcoma.

The peak age group affected by infantile fibrosarcoma is below 5 years, specifically in infants or neonates. These are usually large disfiguring masses, but biologic

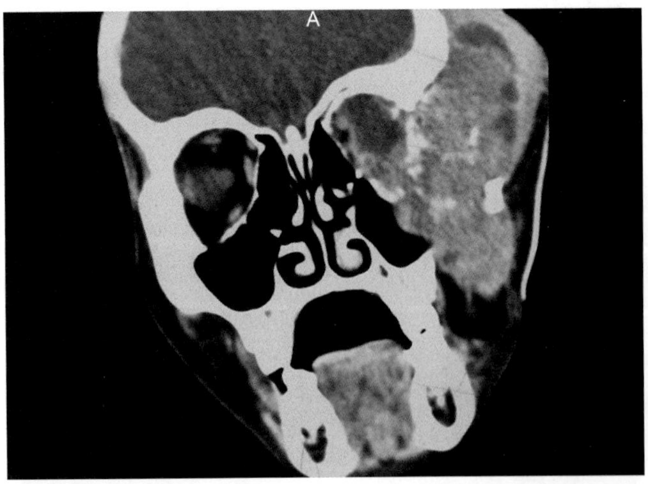

Fig. 11: Rhabdomyosarcoma in a child presenting with rapid onset proptosis and facial swelling. CECT orbit coronal reformatted image shows a large heterogeneously enhancing mass lesion causing destruction of the left zygoma and lateral maxillary and orbital wall.

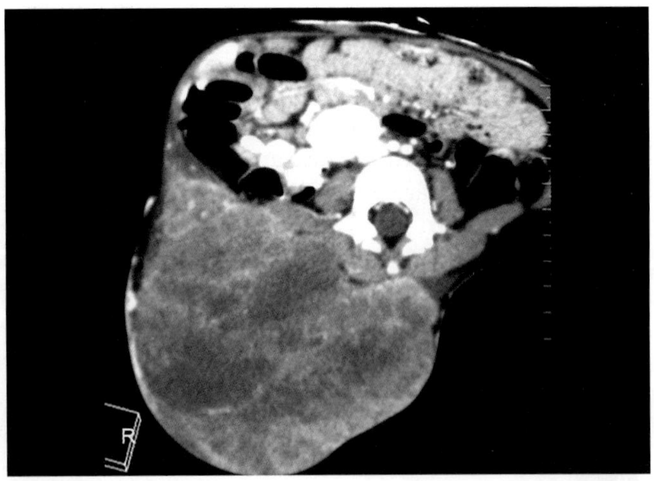

Fig. 12: Rhabdomyosarcoma in a child presenting with an enlarging back mass. Axial CECT abdomen shows infiltration of the mass into the paraspinal and posterior abdominal muscles on right side.

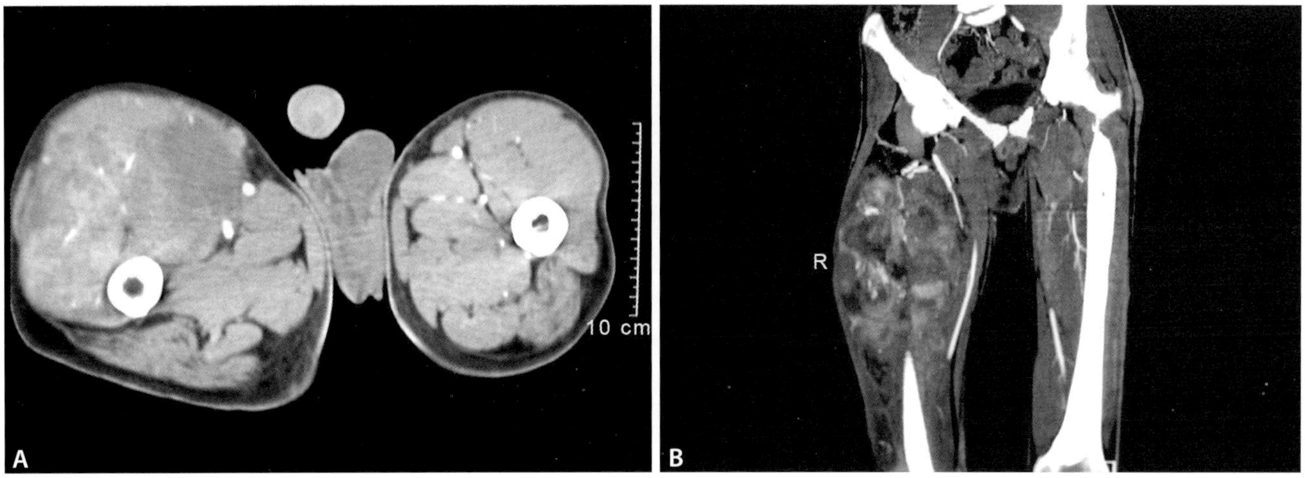

Figs. 13A and B: Synovial sarcoma in a 15-year-old. CECT thigh axial soft tissue window and (A) and (B) coronal maximum intensity projection (MIP) images show a heterogeneous mass lesion in the extensor compartment, abutting and displacing the right superficial femoral artery.

behavior is favorable than their adult counterparts. They rarely metastasize. They are isointense to muscles on T1W images and heterogeneously hyperintense on T2W images.[36] Contrast enhancement is usually heterogeneous. In older children the tumor behaves like those in adults, with a more aggressive course.[4]

Granulocytic sarcoma (also called chloroma): It is seen in 5% cases of acute myeloid leukemia and contains primitive precursors of granulocytes. To begin with, they arise in bone marrow and traverses the haversian canals to extraosseous locations. The most common site in head and neck region **(Fig. 14)**. They are isointense to muscle one as well as T2W images, showing homogeneous enhancement.[37]

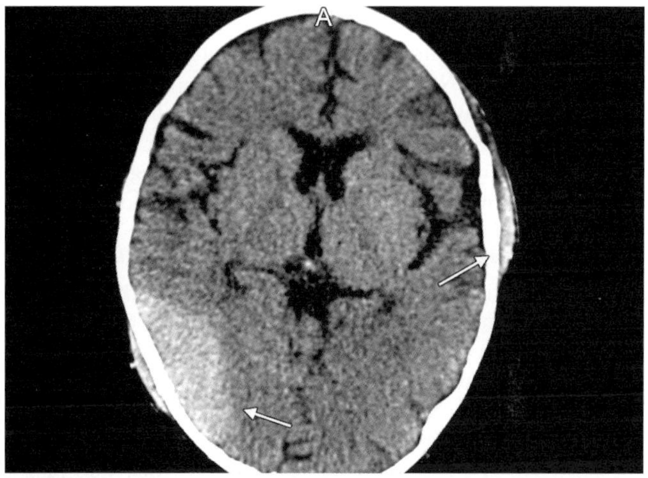

Fig. 14: Granulocytic sarcoma in a case of acute myeloid leukemia. CECT of head reveals multiple enhancing soft tissue masses (arrows) involving the calvarium.

CONCLUSION

Though the pediatric malignant bone tumors account for about 6% of all childhood malignancies, malignant soft tissue tumors are rare in childhood. The role of imaging is to assess the extent of the lesion, thus establishing the accurate stage and determining resectability. Plain radiographs are the most important tool in evaluating bone tumors. MRI offers better assessment of the bony and extraosseous extent and neurovascular involvement, the knowledge of which is crucial for surgery. CT scan of thorax and bone scans are required to determine the presence or absence of metastases.

Soft tissue lesions in childhood are usually benign. The primary role of imaging is to assess the extent in a soft tissue lesion, thus establishing the accurate stage and determining resectability.

REFERENCES

1. Wootton-Gorges SL. MR imaging of primary bone tumors and tumor-like conditions in children. Radiol Clin N Am. 2009;47:957-75.
2. Caudill JSC, Arndt CAS. Diagnosis and management of bone malignancy in adolescence. Adolesc Med. 2007;18: 62-78.
3. Arndt CA, Crist WM. Common musculoskeletal tumors of childhood and adolescence. N Engl J Med. 1999; 341(5): 342-52.
4. Miser JS, Pizzo PA. Soft tissue sarcomas in childhood. Pediatr Clin North Am. 1985;32(3):779-800.
5. Stein-Wexler R. MR imaging of soft tissue masses in children. Radiol Clin N Am. 2009;47:977-95.

6. Hoffer FA. Primary skeletal neoplasms: Osteosarcoma and Ewing sarcoma. Top Magn Reson Imaging. 2002;13: 231-400.
7. Meyer JS, Nadel HR, Marina N, et al. Imaging guidelines for children with Ewing sarcoma and osteosarcoma: A report from the children's oncology group bone tumor committee. Pediatr Blood Cancer. 2008;51:63-70.
8. Alyas F, James SL, Davies AM, et al. The role of MR imaging in the diagnostic characterization of appendicular bone tumors and tumor-like conditiond. Eur Radiol. 2007;17:2675-86.
9. Berquist TH, Ehman RL, King BF, et al. Value of MR imaging in differentiating benign from malignant soft-tissue masses: Study of 95 lesions. Am J Roentgenol. 1990;155(6):1251-5.
10. Kransdorf MJ, Murphy MD. Radiologic evaluation of soft-tissue masses: A current perspective. Am J Roentgenol. 2000; 175(3):575-87.
11. Soler R, Castro JM, Rodriguez E. Value of MR findings in predicting the nature of soft tissue lesions: Benign, malignant or undetermined lesion? Comput Med Imaging Graph. 1996;20(3):163-9.
12. Jelinek J, Kransdorf MJ. MR imaging of soft-tissue masses. Mass like lesions that simulate neoplasma. Magn Reson Imaging Clin N Am. 1995;3(4):727-41.
13. Woude HJ, Bloem JL, Verstraete KL, Taminiau AH, et al. Osteosarcoma and Ewing's sarcoma after neoadjuvant chemotherapy: Value of dynamic MR imaging in detecting viable tumor before surgery. Am J Roentgenol. 1995;165: 593-8.
14. Hayashida Y, Yakushiji T, Awai K, et al. Monitoring therapeutic responses of primary bone tumors by diffusion-weighted image: initial results. Eur Radiol. 2006;16:2637-43.
15. McCarville MB. New frontiers in pediatric oncologic imaging. Cancer Imaging. 2008;8:87-92.
16. Wang C-K, Li C-W, Hsieh T-J, Chien S-H, Liu G-C, Tsai K-B. Characterization of bone and soft-tissue tumors with in vivo ^{1}H MR spectroscopy: Initial results. Radiology. 2004;232:599-605.
17. Enneking WF, Spanier SS, Goodman MA. A system for surgical staging of musculoskeletal sarcoma. Clin Orthop. 1980;153:106-20.
18. American Joint Committee on Cancer, Bone. In: Greene FL, Page DL, Fleming ID, et al, (Eds): AJCC Cancer Staging Manual. New York, NY. Springer-Verlag. 2002;213-9.
19. Longhi A, Errani C, De Paolis M, et al. Primary bone osteosarcoma in the pediatric age: State of the art. Cancer Treat Rev. 2006;32:423-36.
20. Vlychou M, Athanasou N. Radiological and pathological diagnosis of pediatric bone tumours and tumour-like lesions. Pathology. 2008;40(2):196-216.
21. Reddick WE, Wang S, Xiong X, et al. Dynamic magnetic resonance imaging of regional contrast access as an additional prognostic factor in pediatric osteosarcoma. Cancer. 2001;91: 2230-7.
22. Bacci G, Ferrari S, Bertoni F, et al. Histologic response of high-grade nonmetastatic osteosarcoma of the extremity to chemotherapy. Clin Orthop Relat Res. 2001;386:186-96.
23. Provisor AJ, Ettinger LJ, Nachman JB, et al. Treatment of nonmetastatic osteosarcoma of the extremity with preoperative and postoperative chemotherapy: A report from the Children's cancer Group. J Clin Oncol. 1997;15:76-84.
24. Peersman B, Vanhoenakcker FM, Heyman S, et al. Ewing's sarcoma: Imaging features. JBR-BTR. 2007;90:368-76.
25. KaimAH,HugliR,BonelHM,etal.Chondroblastomaandclear cell chondrosarcoma: radiological and MRI characteristics with histopathological correlation. Skeletal Radiol. 2002;31: 88-95.
26. Krishnan A, Shirkhoda A, Tehrznzadeh J, et al. Primary bone lymphoma: Radiographic-MR imaging correlation. Radiographics. 2003;23:1371-87.
27. Murphey MD, Gross TM, Rosenthal HG. Musculoskeletal malignant fibrous histiocytoma: Radiologic-pathologic correlation. Radiographics. 1994;14:807-26.
28. Bissett GS 3rd. MR imaging of soft-tissue masses in children. Magn Reson Imaging Clin N Am. 1996;4(4):696-719.
29. Kransdorf MJ. Malignant soft-tissue tumors in a large referral population: Distribution of diagnoses by age, sex and location. AJR Am J Roentgenol. 1995;164(1):129-34.
30. Moulton JS, Blebea JS, Dunco DM, et al. MR imaging of soft tissue masses: Diagnostic efficacy and value of distinguishing between benign and malignant lesions. Am J Roentgenol. 1995;164(5):1191-9.
31. Siegel MJ. Magnetic resonance imaging of musculoskeletal soft tissue masses. Radiol Clin North Am. 2001;39(4): 701-20.
32. Kim EE, Valenzuela RF, Kumar AJ, et al. Imaging and clinical spectrum of rhabdomyosarcoma in children. Clin Imaning. 2000;24(5):257-62.
33. Tabrizi P, Letts M. Childhood rhabdomyosarcoma of the trunk and extremities. Am J Orthp. 1999;28(8):440-6.
34. Jones BC, Sundaram M, Kransdorf MJ. Synovial sarcoma: MR imaging findings in 34 patients. Am J Roentgenol. 1993; 161(4):827-30.
35. Frassica FJ, Khanna JA, McCarthy EF. The role of MR imaging in soft tissue tumor evaluation: Perspective of the orthopaedic oncologist and musculoskeletal pathologist. Magn Reson Imaging Clin N Am. 2000;8(4):915-27.
36. Eich GF, Hoeffel JC, Tschappeler H, et al. Fibrous tumors in children: Imaging features of a heterogeneous group of disorders. Pediatr Radiol. 1998;28(7):500-09.
37. Stein-Wexler R, Wootton-Gorges SL, West DC. Orbital granulocytic sarcoma: An unusual presentation of acute myelocytic leukemia. Pediatr Radiol. 2003;33(2):136-9.

CHAPTER 150

Congenital Brain Anomalies

Niranjan Khandelwal

INTRODUCTION

Congenital malformations of the brain are numerous with over 2000 malformations described so far. Its incidence is reported to be about 1% of all live births. About 60% of cases have no known etiology while 40% may have chromosomal inheritance or acquired cause. Approximately 75% of fetal deaths are attributed to these malformations.[1]

Congenital malformations result from abnormal formation of the brain structure during intrauterine development.[2,3] Various classifications have been proposed. **Table 1** shows the broad subgroups.

Table 1: Classification of congenital brain anomalies.

- ***Disorders of organization*:**
  (Due to arrest of brain development and with normal histogenesis)
  - *Supratentorial*:
    - *Migrational disorders*:
      - Lissencephaly
      - Hemimegalencephaly
      - Heterotopias
      - Schizencephaly
      - Polymicrogyria
    - Holoprosencephaly
    - Syndrome of septo-optic dysplasia
    - Dysgenesis of corpus callosum
    - Hydranencephaly
  - *Infratentorial anomalies*:
    - Dandy–Walker complex
    - Cerebellar aplasia/ hypoplasia
    - Chiari malformation
  - *Both intratentorial and supratentorial anomalies*:
    - Cephalocele
    - Arachnoid cyst
- ***Disorders of histogenesis*:**
  (Result from persistent development of abnormal cells in the otherwise normally structured brain)
  - Neurofibromatosis
  - Tuberous sclerosis
  - Sturge–Weber syndrome
  - Von Hippel–Lindau disease
  - Ataxia–telangiectasia

Source: Adapted from Byrd and Charles[2]

DISORDERS OF ORGANIZATION

Supratentorial Malformations

Migrational Disorders

Lissencephaly or smooth brain: In this condition, there is complete or partial absence of sulcation. Complete lack of gyri is termed as agyria and the presence of few, broad and flat gyri is termed as pachygyria. Patient of lissencephaly presents with dysmorphic facies, seizures, mental retardation and microcephaly. Sonographic findings include a smooth surfaced cortex without sulcal or gyral formation. Sonography can only suggest the diagnosis of lissencephaly but the characteristic findings are more readily identifiable on CT or MRI. Based on CT and MRI, three types of lissencephaly have been described:

- Classic (type I) lissencephaly (4-layer lissencephaly)
- Cobblestone (type II) lissencephaly (congenital muscular dystrophy), and
- Lissencephaly not otherwise classified.

Classic lissencephaly is further divided into three subcategories based on associated genetic abnormalities, namely:

1. Deletion of the LIS 1 gene on chromosome 17
2. An X-linked lissencephaly, and
3. An indeterminate subset with neither of the above chromosomal abnormalities.

In classical lissencephaly,[4] the MRI features are that of an abnormal contour and surface of the brain. The cerebral surface is smooth, devoid of sulci (agyric) or with few areas of pachygyria or with equal areas of pachygyria and agyria. The brain assumes a figure of 8 appearance due to the bilateral shallow sylvian fissures. There is marked reduction in the white matter, the gray white matter interface is smooth with loss of cortical white matter distribution **(Figs. 1A and B)**.[5]

Hemimegalencephaly or unilateral megalencephaly: This condition may be idiopathic or may be associated with contralateral somatic hemihypertrophy, linear sebaceous nevus syndrome, neurofibromatosis NF1.[4] The affected cortex is typically dysplastic with broad gyri, shallow sulci and cortical thickening. Gyral pattern may appear grossly normal. It may be associated with lissencephaly or polymicrogyria. There is an indistinct differentiation between the cortex and subcortical white matter. The ipsilateral lateral ventricle is enlarged with the frontal horn directed anterosuperiorly **(Figs. 2A to C)**. Rarely, brain has a bizarre, hamartomatous appearance.

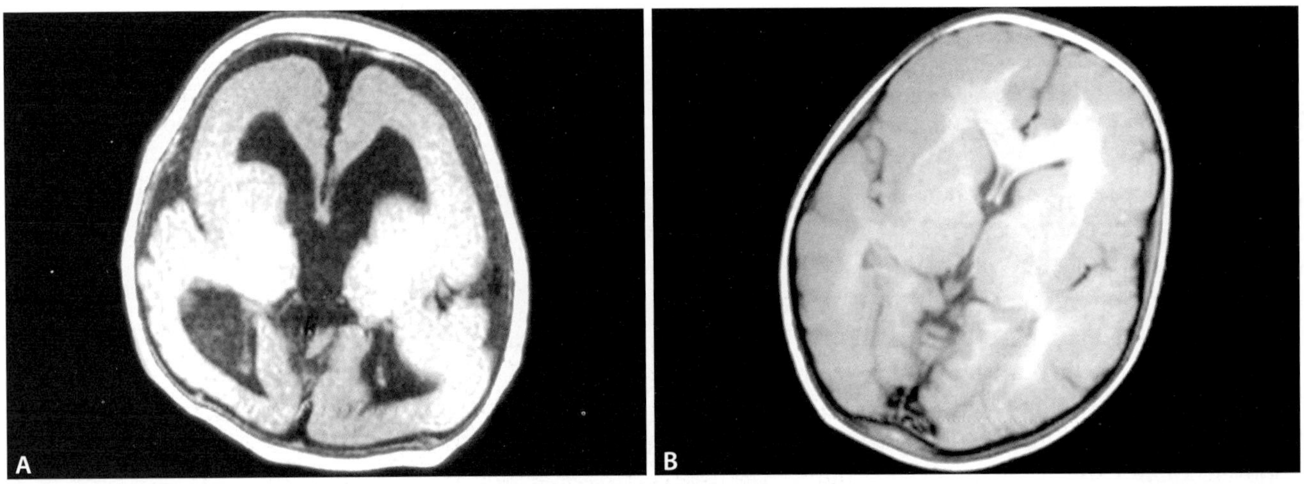

Figs. 1A and B: Lissencephaly: Short TR axial MR sections in two patients showing the shallow sylvian fissures giving a figure of eight configuration of the cerebral hemispheres. Note the thickened cortex better delineated in (B).

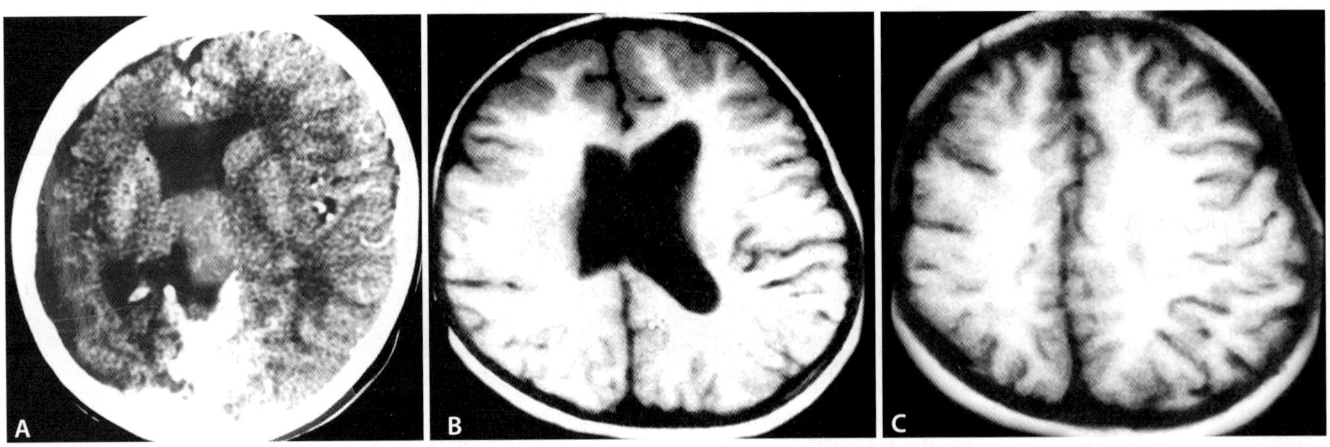

Figs. 2A to C: Hemimegalencephaly: (A) Axial CT scan shows overgrowth of the left hemisphere giving asymmetrical appearance of the brain; (B and C) T1W1 shows unilateral megalencephaly with a larger left hemisphere. Note the larger left lateral ventricle (B) and the prominent sulcation of that hemisphere (C).

Heterotopias: Heterotopias are the least severe of all the migrational disorders. The term denotes presence of normal neural tissue at an abnormal location secondary to arrest of neuronal migration along the radial glial fibers.[4] The abnormally located gray matter is isointense with cortical gray matter in all MR imaging sequences and this is a diagnostic feature. Heterotopias are of two types: the common, nodular type **(Figs. 3A and B)** is characterized by multiple masses of gray matter which are of variable size. They are commonly located in the subependymal region of the lateral ventricles or in the subcortical white matter. The second type is the uncommon band or lamellar heterotopia (double cortex) **(Figs. 3C and D)** which appears as a homogeneous gray matter band between the cerebral cortex and the lateral ventricle. It is characteristically surrounded by a zone of white matter. The cortex overlying the heterotopia is nearly always abnormal with pachygyria or polymicrogyria.

Schizencephaly or split brain: It is a form of migrational disorder characterized by abnormal columns of gray matter across the cerebral hemisphere. The basic abnormality is a pial-ependymal seam (gray matter lined cleft) which extends across full thickness of cerebral hemisphere from the ventricular system (ependyma) to the periphery (pial surface) of the brain. These clefts are usually perisylvian but can occur anywhere in the brain. Two types have been described:

- Type I or closed lip schizencephaly is characterized by a gray matter lined pial ependymal seam with both the lips apposed to each other. There is no intervening CSF cavity. The common site of involvement is the roof or lateral borders of lateral ventricle. MR or CT scan

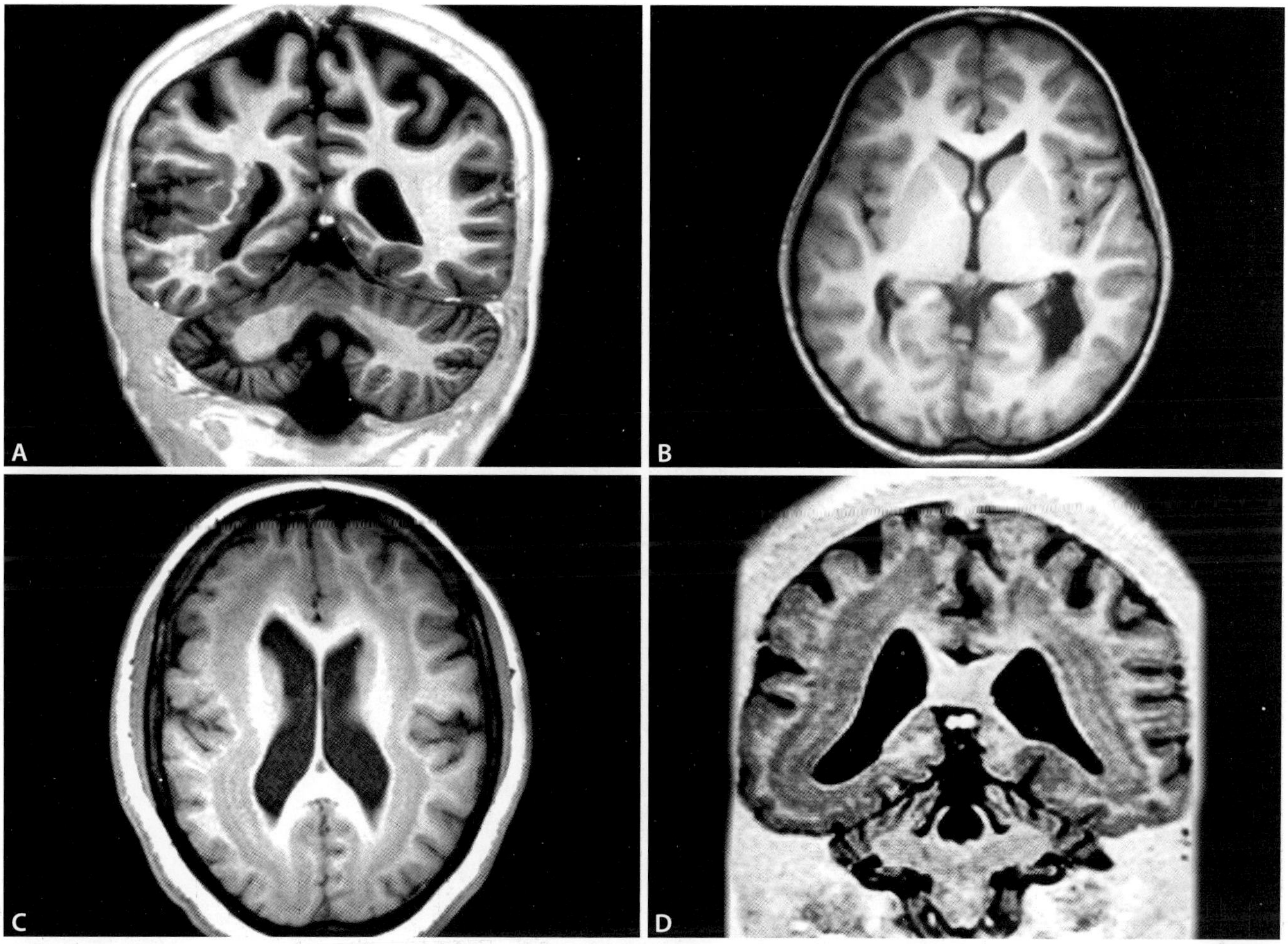

Figs. 3A to D: Nodular heterotopia: Coronal IR (A) and axial T1W (B) images showing undulating layer of gray matter lining the lateral ventricles; (C and D) Lamellar heterotopia: Axial T1W (A) and coronal IR images (B) show a band of gray matter in the periventricular region which is isointense with the cortex.

will show an outpouching or nipple at the ependymal surface of the cleft in closed lip schizencephaly. MRI demonstrates the full thickness of cleft and the pial-ependymal seam of gray matter **(Figs. 4A and B)**.

- Type II or open lip schizencephaly in which the pial ependymal seam is widened by a CSF cleft. CT and MRI shows the CSF cleft extending from the ventricular system to the pial surface of brain. The CSF cavity is usually bilateral and symmetric. However, it may be asymmetric or even unilateral. Severe form of open lip schizencephaly presents with massive CSF cavities which communicate with the ventricular system and has an appearance which is a called "basket brain". This congenital malformation has a high association with absence of septum pellucidum, polymicrogyria, septo-optic dysplasia, heterotopia **(Figs. 4C and D)**.[4]

Holoprosencephaly

Holoprosencephaly is a congenital malformation characterized by incomplete cleavage and differentiation of the prosencephalon (forebrain) into cerebral hemispheres. Mutation of at least 4 different genetic loci have been identified to be associated with this condition and these are on chromosome 21, 2, 7 and 18. Syndromic association of this condition are encountered in trisomy 13 (Patau's syndrome) and trisomy 18 (Edwards' syndrome). Embryogenesis of holoprosencephaly is postulated to be the lack of mesenchyme in the developing rostral neural tube, as a result of which the telencephalon does not separate from the diencephalon. The telencephalon does not develop in the two hemispheres and there is lack of cortical organization.[6]

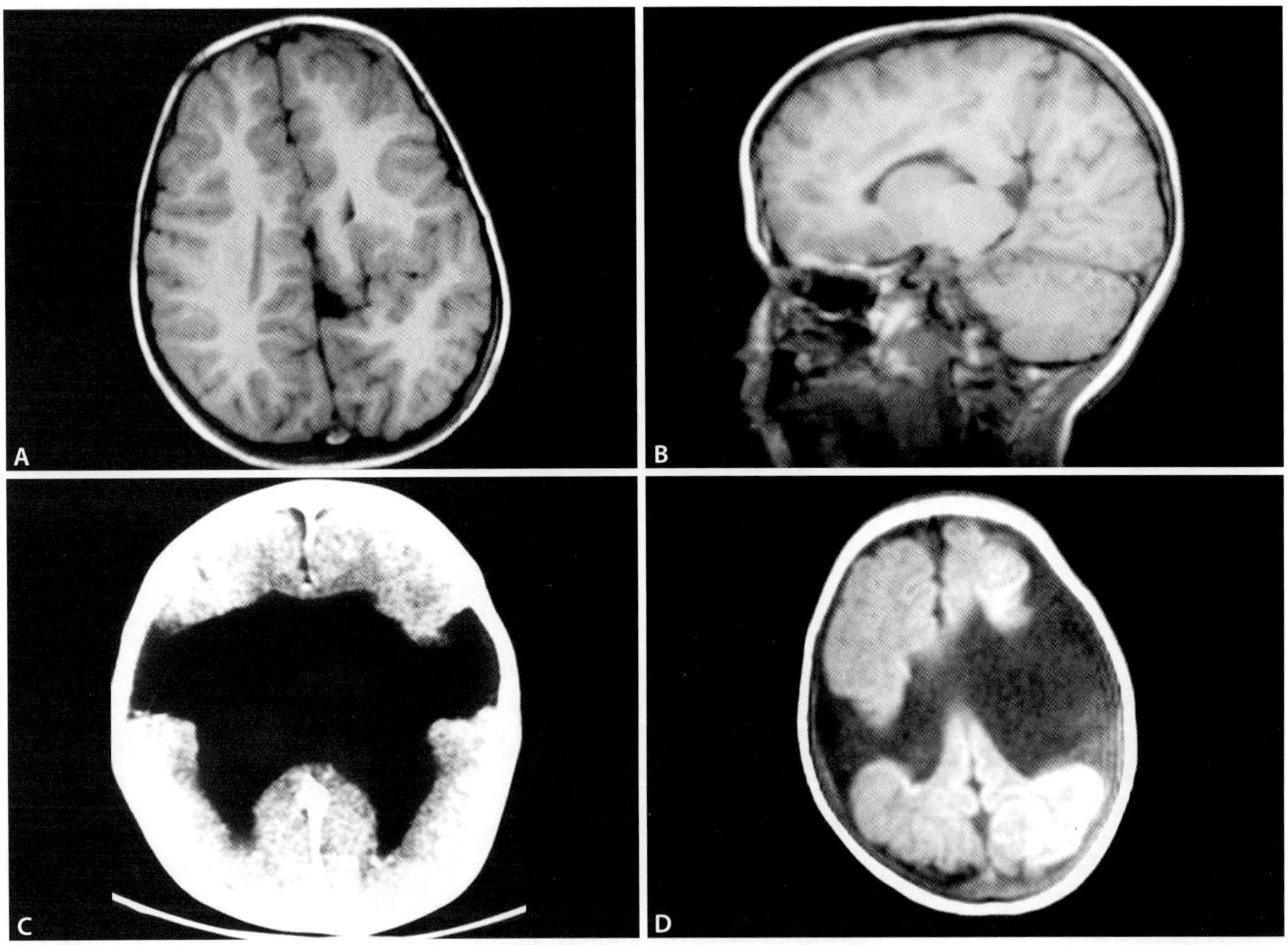

Figs. 4A to D: Schizencephaly: *Closed lip*: Axial (A) and sagittal (B) T1 W MR sections show deep extension of cerebral sulci reaching uptil the ventricle with gray matter lining; *Open lip*: Axial CT (C) and T1 MR (D) sections show bilateral CSF clefts communicating with the lateral ventricles.

There are three types of holoprosencephaly: (i) alobar, (ii) semilobar and (iii) lobar. Prenatal ultrasound, and postnatal CT or MRI can image the confluent ventricles and thalami adequately:

- *Alobar holoprosencephaly* is the most severe form of holoprosencephaly. There is no differentiation of the frontal, occipital or temporal lobes. The cerebral hemispheres are fused to form a small flat mass of tissue containing single crescent shaped holoventricle. The flattened cerebrum occupies a small rostral segment of the calvarium. The calvarium is occupied with the large dorsal cyst which communicates with the holoventricle. Thalami may be fused with absence of interhemispheric fissure, falx cerebri and septum pellucidum. The cerebellum and brainstem are relatively normal. This condition is associated with a severely dysmorphic facies, abnormal reflexes and increased tone at birth.
- *Semilobar holoprosencephaly* **(Fig. 5A)** is a less severe form of holoprosencephaly. There is partial separation of the cerebral hemispheres with rudimentary temporal and occipital lobes. The frontal lobes are fused. There is a monoventricle with presence of the falx cerebri which is only partially seen posteriorly and suggestion of presence of an interhemispheric fissure. Septum pellucidum is absent and thalami are partially separated. The splenium of the corpus callosum is formed without the genu or body **(Fig. 5A)**.
- *Lobar holoprosencephaly* **(Fig. 5B)** is the least severe form. Brain appears normal but the frontal horns remain fused with absence of septum pellucidum. Appearance of the frontal horns with angular corners is termed "box-like". Temporal and occipital horns are separated and are of normal size and shape. However, the bodies of the lateral ventricles may be closely apposed. Interhemispheric fissure is formed but is shallow anteriorly. The thalami are separated.

Septo-optic Dysplasia

Septo-optic dysplasia is believed to be a mild form of lobar holoprosencephaly and consists of absence of septum pellucidum with hypoplasia of the optic nerve and optic chiasma and hypoplasia of the hypothalamus. MRI shows these findings with clarity. In addition abnormally squared or flattened frontal horns of the lateral ventricles and an enlarged anterior recess of the third ventricle may be seen. It may be associated with aqueductal stenosis, Chiari II malformation, schizencephaly, and corpus callosum agenesis. In addition, an association of hypothalamus pituitary dysfunction is seen in two-thirds of the patients with this condition.[7]

Dysgenesis of Corpus Callosum

The corpus callosum is a midline commissure that crosses from one cerebral hemisphere to the other. The corpus callosum develops in the cephalocaudal direction with the genu developing at 2.5 months of gestation followed by the body and splenium. The rostrum is the last to develop. Adult configuration is achieved by 5th month of gestation.[8] In corpus callosum agenesis, genu is usually present but body and splenium are dysgenic.

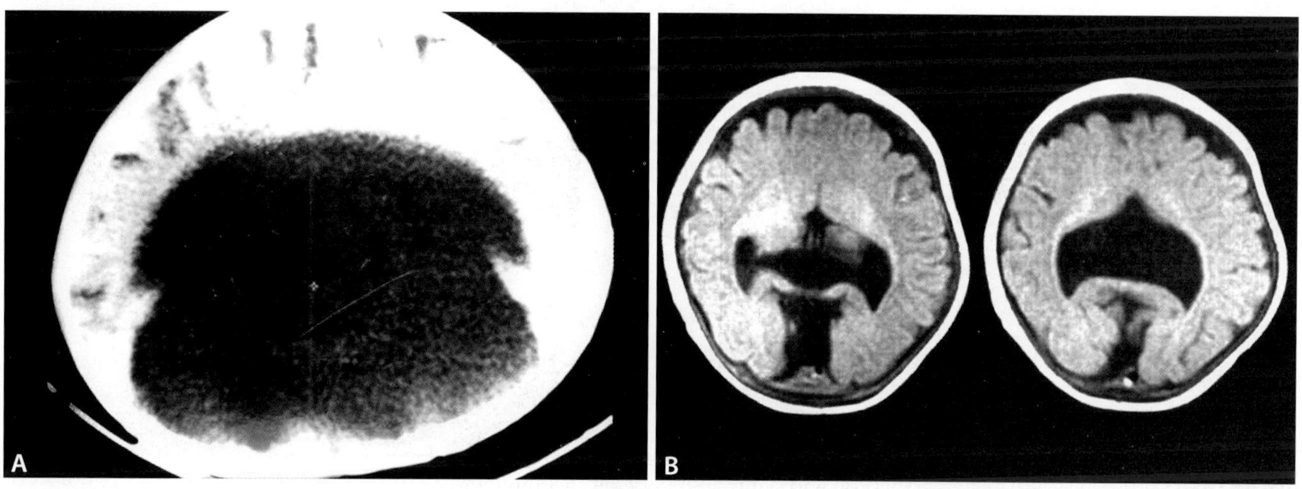

Figs. 5A and B: (A) Semilobar holoprosencephaly: Axial CT section shows a monoventricle with a dorsal cyst and partially formed temporal lobes; (B) Lobar holoprocencephaly: Axial short TR sequence MR section shows fused frontal horns of the lateral ventricles. The cerebral hemisphere are well formed; however, the anterior interhemispheric fissure is partially delineated.

Diagnostic features on imaging are parallel nonconverging lateral ventricles, dilated occipital horns (colpocephaly) **(Fig. 6A)**. The third ventricle is widended and is placed between the lateral ventricles. If the dilated third ventricle reaches the interhemispheric fissure it is referred to as dorsal interhemispheric cyst **(Fig. 6B)**. Midsagittal MR scan readily demonstrates absence of the corpus callosum. Cingulate sulcus is absent and the gyri appear to radiate from a high riding third ventricle **(Figs. 6C and D)**. Presence of Probst bundle (longitudinally oriented tracts) cause indentation on the medial aspect of the lateral ventricles which appear concave medially on coronal MR sections.[2]

Coexisting congenital malformations are common which include Dandy-Walker complex, arachnoid cyst, cephalocele and colobomas. Aicardi syndrome is association of corpus callosum agenesis, infantile spasms and ocular abnormalities and is especially seen in females.[2,5]

Hydranencephaly

Hydranencephaly is an encephaloclastic porencephaly which results presumably secondary to *in utero* occlusion of either of the internal carotid arteries, or infection, such as CMV or due to a genetic cause. This results in infarction, necrosis and destruction of the cerebral cortex. The cerebral hemispheres are replaced by a thin-walled membranous sac which is lined by glial tissue on the inside and leptomeninges on the outside. Diagnosis on ultrasound is easy as the falx cerebri, thalami and cerebellar hemispheres are identified in the presence of the two large fluid-filled sacs.[2]

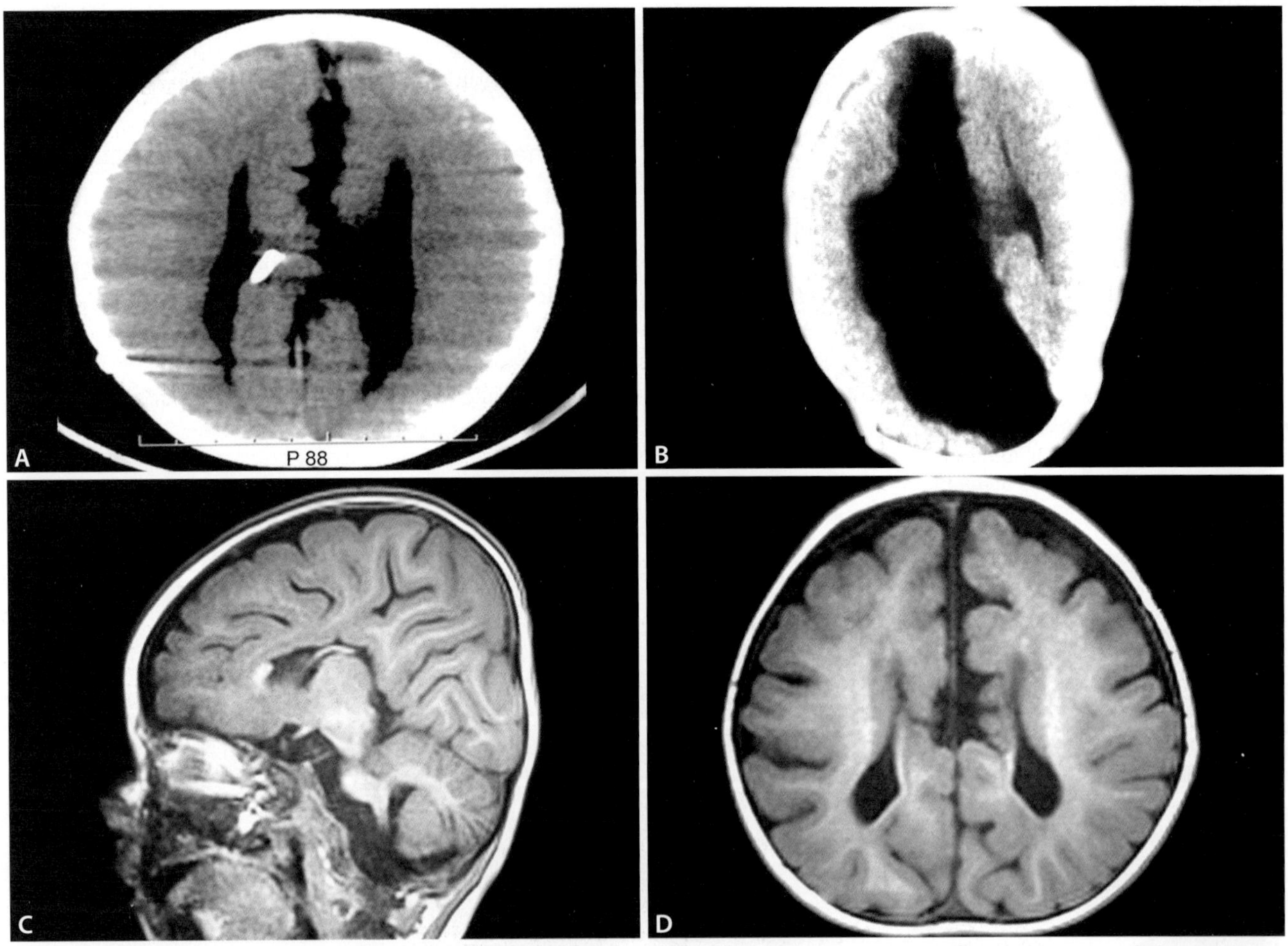

Figs. 6A to D: Corpus callosum agenesis: (A) Axial CT section shows parallel configuration of the lateral ventricles. Absence of the corpus callosum leads to separation of the interhemispheric fissure. A shunt has been placed in the right lateral ventricle; (B) Corpus callosum agenesis associated with an interhemispheric cyst which extends across the midline; (C and D) T1W sagittal and axial images depicting partial corpus callosum agenesis with parallel alignment of lateral ventricles (colpocephaly) and radiating pattern of cerebral gyri.

Differential diagnosis includes severe hydrocephalus, in which a rind of remaining cortical mantle can be identified, and alobar holoprosencephaly where absence of falx and presence of fused thalami clinches the diagnosis. CT or MRI may be done when US findings are equivocal **(Figs. 7A and B)**.

Infratentorial Malformations

Dandy-Walker (DW) complex: This includes Dandy-Walker malformation, Dandy-Walker variant and the mega cisterna magna.[9]

This represents the morphological spectrum of fundamental anomalous cerebellar vermis and adjacent cerebellar hemispheres. The cerebellar vermis is usually hypoplastic with atresia of the outlet of fourth ventricle, resulting in abnormal dilatation of 4th ventricle with expansion of posterior fossa **(Figs. 8A and B)**. There is consequently superior displacement of the tentorium and dural sinuses.

Skull radiographs show expansion of posterior cranial fossa, thinning and ballooning of occipital bone and upward displacement of lateral sinus groove which indicates elevation of tentorium.

Sonographic features of Dandy-Walker complex include anechoic posterior fossa cyst, small cerebellar hemispheres, elevated tentorium and hydrocephalus.

CT and MRI are helpful to show the structures in their proper perspective. Multiplanar imaging of MRI is superior

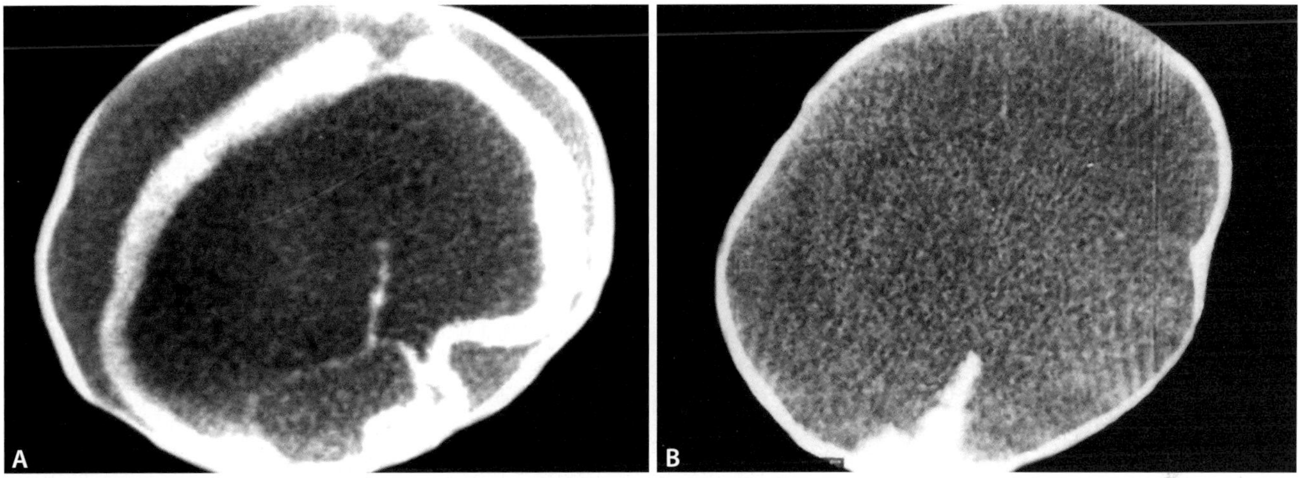

Figs. 7A and B: Hydranencephaly vs congenital hydrocephalus: Axial CT section (A) shows presence of a preserved cortical mantle with interhemispheric fissure. Bilateral subdural collection favor the diagnosis of hydrocephalus. In hydranencephaly the brain is replaced by a fluid-filled sac (B). No cortical mantle is identified.

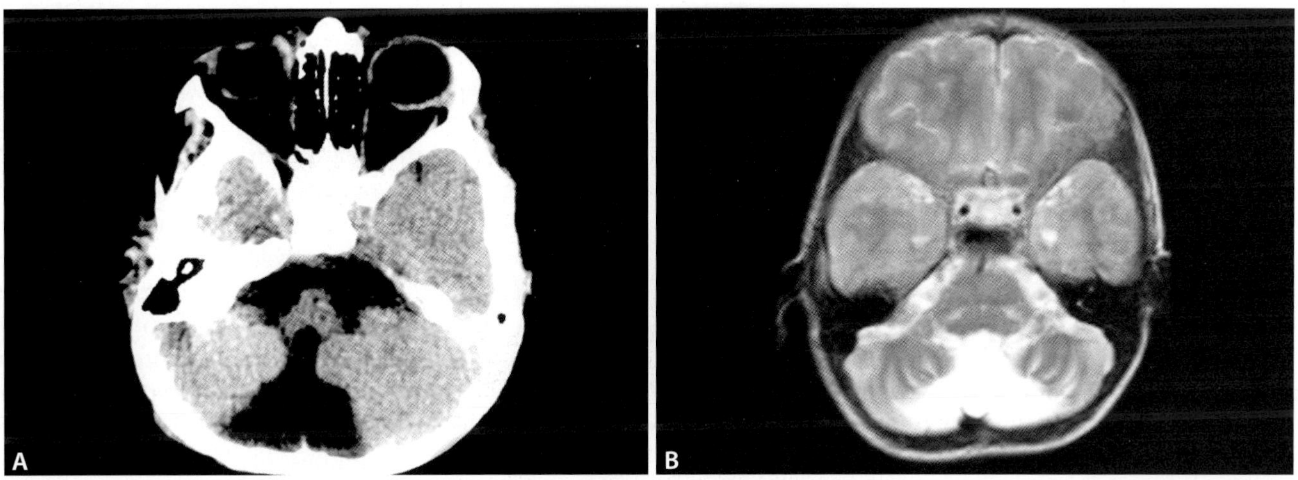

Figs. 8A and B: Dandy-Walker malformation: Absent vermis with the fourth ventricle communicating directly with a posterior fossa cyst; winged cerebellar hemispheres are characteristic of this malformation.

to CT for demonstrating the anatomy. Diagnostic criteria of DW complex on CT/MR are as follows:

- Dandy-Walker malformation is characterized by absence of or hypoplasia of the cerebellar vermis. There is associated hypoplasia of the cerebellar hemispheres giving a characteristic winged appearance to these hemispheres. The fourth ventricle is enlarged and opens dorsally into a CSF containing cyst. The posterior fossa is enlarged with a high insertion of the tentorium consequently the transverse sinuses are higher in position than normal. 80% of patients have associated hydrocephalus. Associated anomalies include corpus callosum agenesis (20–25%), heterotopias, polymicrogyria, occipital cephaloceles and schizencephaly.[9]
- In Dandy-Walker variant, there is varying degree of inferior vermian and cerebellar hypoplasia. The retrocerebellar CSF collection communicates with normal or mildly enlarged 4th ventricle via a prominent vallecula. The tentorial position and size of posterior fossa are normal. Coronal images through posterior fossa may show absence of the vermis. The brainstem is usually normal and hydrocephalus is an uncommon association.[7,8]
- Mega cisterna magna is a large subarachnoid cistern lying posterior to the vermis and can extend all the way up to the straight sinus superiorly and the C1–C2 level inferiorly. It may cause scalloping of the inner table of occipital squama, without any compression of the fourth ventricle. One of the differential diagnoses is a retrocerebellar arachnoid cyst, which is a CSF collection within the layers of arachnoid membrane and does not communicate fully with the subarachnoid or ventricular spaces. The posterior fossa and ventricular system are normal. The fourth ventricle and vermis may be displaced by the cyst.

Chiari Malformations

There are four Chiari malformations[10] which represent a spectrum of anomalies of primary neurulation, i.e. those which occur when the brain and upper spine are developing at about 3–4 weeks of gestation.

Chiari I malformation (caudal-cerebellar-tonsillar ectopia) consists of herniation of elongated peg like cerebellar tonsils through the foramen magnum into the upper cervical spinal canal.

Chiari's original description of this anomaly included associated hydrocephalus, though it is not mandatory for the diagnosis to be made.[11] Tonsillar descent has been described in four categories of Chiari I malformation:[4]

1. This malformation can be associated with abnormal intracranial pressure. Intracranial hypotension due to chronic CSF leaks or associated with CSF shunts can result in 'sagging brain'. Raised intracranial tension due to cerebral edema or intracranial masses can push the tonsils downwards.
2. Chiari I malformation can be seen with platybasia or basilar invagination or craniovertebral anomalies such as persistence of proatlas remnants, shortened clivus and C-1 assimilation.
3. Prenatal or postnatal hydrocephalus can result in Chiari 1 malformation, this subset was included in the original description of the malformation.
4. Asymptomatic tonsillar ectopia with no obvious abnormality has been described and may be congenital. The degree of tonsillar descent is of some importance. Descent less than 5 mm below a line from the basion to the opisthion is considered to be of no clinical significance whereas tonsillary descent more than 6 mm can be associated with clinical symptoms. Correlation between age of the patient and tonsillar descent is also important. Between the age of 5 years and 15 years descent of up to 6 mm is not considered pathologic. In older individuals protrusion more than 5 mm below the foramen magnum is invariably associated with an increasing incidence of symptoms. Association of syringomyelia is another important aspect of Chiari I malformation.[12] The incidence reported varies between 25% and 65%. The focus on MR studies which is the mainstay of diagnosis of this condition is to show the degree of tonsillar herniation in midsagittal section, evaluation of the craniovertebral junction, assessment of the lateral ventricles for hydrocephalus and to detect presence of syrinx in the upper cervical spine. MR CSF flow studies show increased motion of the tonsil and brainstem and decreased CSF flow to the vallecula **(Figs. 9A and B)**.[13]

Chiari II malformation is characterized by caudal displacement of the brainstem and inferior part of cerebellum into the upper cervical spinal canal. All patients of Chiari II malformations have a lumbar meningomyelocele. They nearly always develop hydrocephalus after closure of the meningomyelocele for which they are initially imaged when the lesions of the Chiari II malformation are detected.[1] These patients can present with epilepsy (17%), dysphagia, apnoeic spells, shoulder or arm weakness, weak cry or stridor. The hind brain malformations have been best explained in a theory by McLone and Knepper[14] who have postulated that the basic anomaly is a small posterior fossa into which a

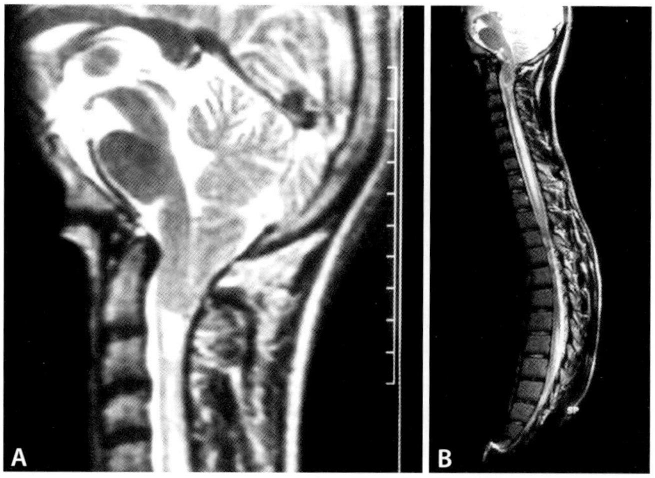

Figs. 9A and B: Chiari I malformation: (A) Midline sagittal long TR MR section showing herniation of the cerebellar tonsil below the foramen magnum; (B) Sagittal MR section of the whole spine shows presence of the associated syrinx of the cervical and dorsal segments of the spinal cord.

normal sized cerebellum develops. Lack of space within the posterior fossa together with a low lying tentorium forces the brainstem and cerebellum through the enlarged foramen magnum.

Sagittal MR scan shows stretching of the pons inferiorly. It is compressed anteroposteriorly. The medulla is pushed inferiorly through the widened foramen. The cervical spinal cord is in turn stretched inferiorly as well. Caudal displacement of the cervical cord is restricted by the dentate ligaments. Therefore, there is kink at the junction of the displaced medulla at the cervicomedullary junction. In severe cases, the cerebellum may wrap around the brainstem. The fourth ventricle is vertically oriented, compressed and displaced inferiorly. The vermis herniates and may be compressed by the superior arch of the C1. The herniated and compressed vermis may degenerate. In severe cases the whole of the cerebellum may atrophy. Beaking of the quadrigeminal plate is probably secondary to the compression by the expanded temporal lobes due to hydrocephalus. Isolation of the fourth ventricle may occur due to aqueductal narrowing and diminished flow through the fourth ventricular outflow foramina. Paradoxically, the fourth ventricle is not dilated, however, the supratentorial ventricles will dilate. In these patients, attempt should be made to look for the presence of syringohydromyelia. Chiari II malformation can be associated with corpus callosum agenesis, enlarged massa intermedia, fenestrated falx cerebri, an abnormal gyral pattern on the medial aspect of the occipital lobe termed as stenogyria.[4]

The Chiari III malformation includes the feature of the Chiari II malformation with a low occipital or high cervical encephalocele. The encephalocele contains occipital lobes, part of the cerebellum and occasionally medulla and pons.

The Chiari IV malformation includes severe cerebellar hypoplasia or absent cerebellum. There is a large posterior fossa CSF space. There is no obstructive hydrocephalus.

Detailed evaluations using current imaging methods have introduced more subtle forms of the malformation, currently named as Chiari 0 and Chiari 1.5 which are characterized by altered CSF flow dynamics.[8]

Supra- and Infratentorial Malformations

Cephalocele is a term given to herniation of intracranial contents through defects in the skull.[15] If the herniated contents are leptomeninges and CSF, the cephalocele is termed as a meningocele. When one contains brain tissue, leptomeninges and CSF, it is called a meningoencephalocele. Herniation of meninges, brain and ventricles is termed encephalocystomeningocele. Herniation of intracranial contents occurring through fracture (growing fracture) or through surgical defect is an acquired cephalocele.

In South-east Asia the most common cephaloceles encountered in clinical practice are nasal encephaloceles. Occipital (70%), parietal (10%) frontal (9%) and nasopharyngeal (1%) are the most common types of encephaloceles encountered in North America and Europe.[2]

On plain radiograph defects in the calvarium associated with cephaloceles appear well defined with sclerotic margins. If the protrusion of the brain content is large, there is a reduction in the craniofacial ratio.

Cross-sectional imaging is necessary to define the contents of the cephalocele. Sonography is a valuable mode of investigation in the prenatal diagnosis of cephaloceles. It can also differentiate whether the cephalocele contains CFS alone or CSF with brain matter. The former appears anechoic and the latter as a complex mass. CT demonstrates the extent of bony defect as well as contents of the cephalocele. MR is the most sensitive and accurate modality to detect and characterise the cephalocele. In addition multiplanar acquisition helps in the assessment of location of the cephelocele. MR venography is useful to assess the position of superior sagittal sinus and torcular herophili as they may herniate into parietal or occipital encephocele.

Frontoethmoidal cephaloceles lie between the nasal and ethmoid bones. They are not associated with neural tube defects.

Nasal encephalocele is formed when there is failure of closure of the dural diverticulum in the prenasal space.

This diverticulum connects the superficial ectoderm of the developing nose to the developing brain with the cranium. Thus, there can be a large patent opening through which brain matter can herniate or there can be a sinus tract, i.e. dermal sinus or sequestration of heterotopic or dysplastic glial tissue resulting in the so-called nasal glioma. Thus, these lesions appear as soft tissue masses and CSF collections which appear in continuum with intracranial structures. Absence of the crista galli is a constant feature of a cephalocele, alternatively, it can be split by the presence of a dermal sinus or dermoid in this location. Coronal CT scaning is partially useful in demonstrating the bony defects within location.

Occipital encephalocele originates between foramen magnum and lambda. It contains variable amount of brain matter which is usually gliotic and non-functional. Association with Chiari II and III malformation is common **(Fig. 10A)**.

Parietal cephalocele arises between bregma and lambda. Associated anomalies include corpus callosum agenesis, Chiari II malformation and Dandy–Walker complex **(Fig. 10B)**. Encephaloceles involving the sphenoid bone are further classified as transsphenoid, transsellar sphenoidal, sphenoethmoidal, sphenomaxillary, spheno-orbital and transethmoidal encehaloceles. These are occult cephalocele with patients presenting with hypertelorism, endocrine dysfunction and mental retardation. They are associated with true clefts of the lip and nose. These cephaloceles protrude through the body of the sphenoid into the nasal cavity or in severe cases, through the palate into the oral cavity. They invariably contain parts of the hypothalamus, pituitary gland and the third ventricle.[16]

DISORDERS OF HISTOGENESIS

"Neurocutaneous syndromes" or "phakomatoses" constitute a group of congenital malformations which are characterized by cutaneous lesions associated with CNS anomalies.[17]

Prominent amongst these are as follows:
- Neurofibromatosis/von Recklinghausen's disease.
- Tuberous sclerosis/Bourneville disease
- Sturge–Weber syndrome.
- von Hippel–Lindau disease
- Ataxia telangiectasia.

Neuroimaging studies are important in the diagnosis of these conditions because based on clinical presentations there are specific diagnostic imaging features in many of the conditions. The diagnosis can almost always be made on MRI because it can differentiate gray and white matter, characterize tumors from hamartomas, show extent of soft tissue lesions through bony defect and to some extent differentiate various vascular anomalies associated with these conditions.[15,16]

Neurofibromatosis

Neurofibromatosis comprises of a group of heterogeneous diseases which have been classified into two groups: Neurofibromatosis 1 (NF1) and neurofibromatosis 2 (NF2).

Neurofibromatosis type 1 (NF1) accounts for 90% of cases of neurofibromatosis with an incidence of 1: 2000–3000 live births. This autosomal dominant condition occurs due to mutation on the long arm of chromosome 17. The condition is of variable expression and high penetrance. Inactivation of the tumor repressor gene or *NF1* gene is

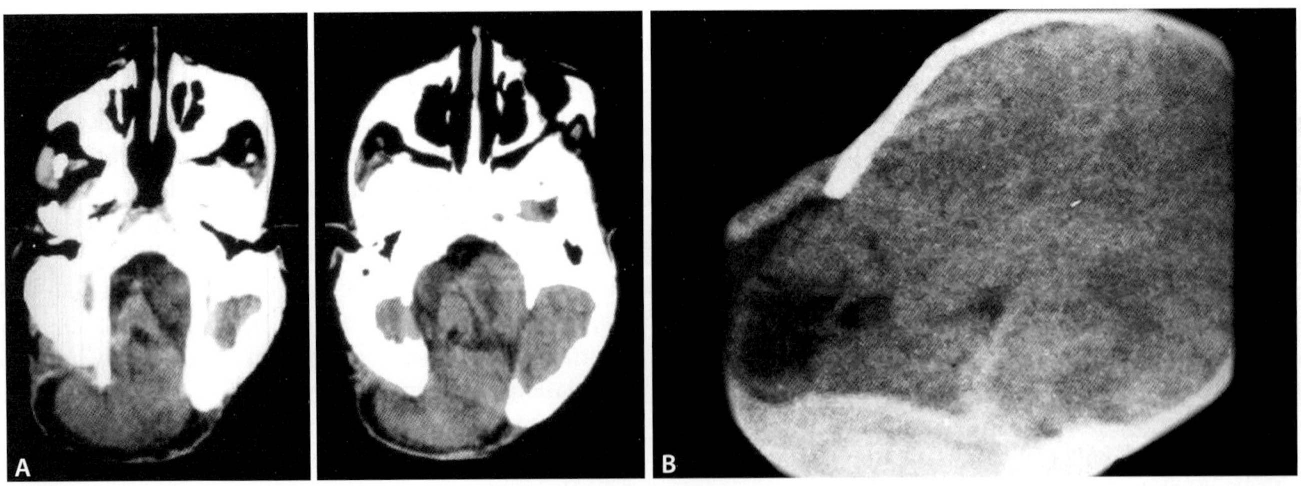

Figs. 10A and B: (A) Occipital encephocele: Axial CT section shows a defect in the occipital bone with protrusion of the right cerebellar hemisphere through the defect; (B) Parietal cephalocele: A large right parietal cephalocele containing brain matter, CSF and ectatic enhanced dura.

thought to be the genetic basis of the disease. Diagnosis of NF1 is made when two or more of the following findings are present:[18,19]

- Six or more café-au-lait spots measuring 5 mm or more in largest diameter in prepubertal children or 15 mm or more in the postpubertal period.
- One plexiform neurofibroma or two or more neurofibromas of any type.
- Two or more pigmented hamartomas (Lisch nodules) of the iris.
- Optic nerve glioma
- A distinctive osseous lesion, such as dysplasia of the sphenoidal wing.
- Axillary or inguinal freckling
- A first degree relative with NF1.

Optic pathway glioma is the most common CNS lesion in NF1. It is best imaged by MRI which delineates the entire extent of the lesion from the optic nerve, chiasma, optic tract, optic radiation and the lateral geniculate bodies although latter three structures are rarely involved. It is a low-grade pilocytic astrocytoma. On MR scan it appears a fusiform lesion which is hypo- to isointense on T1WI with variable contrast enhancement. The optic canal is enlarged. Other gliomas associated with NF1 involve the brainstem, tectum and periaqueductal white matter.

Plexiform neurofibroma is a hallmark of NF1. It is an unencapsulated neurofibroma along the path of a major cutaneous nerve, of the scalp and neck. The commonly involved nerve is the first division of the trigeminal nerve. It is invariably associated with dysplasia of the sphenoid bone and bony orbit **(Fig. 11)**. On CT scan this lesion appears as low attenuating lesion which generally do not enhance. On MR T1WI they are isointense to muscle and show variable enhancement after contrast administration.

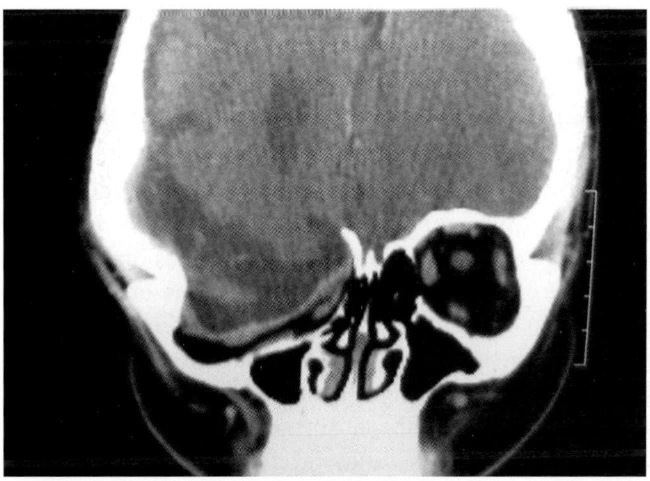

Fig. 11: Neurofibromatosis type 1: Noncontrast coronal CT showing sphenoid wing dysplasia with intraorbital herniation of the dura.

Other intracranial lesions include hamartoma, astrocytic proliferation of the retina, intracranial aneurysms, non-aneurysmal vascular ectasias and a progressive cerebral arterial occlusive disease akin to moya moya pattern.[2]

Skeletal dysplasias that may occur include calvarial defects, hypoplasia of the sphenoid wing, scoliosis, scalloping the posterior aspects of the vertebral bodies with hypoplasia of the pedicles, spinous and transverse processes. Dural dysplasia and lateral/anterior intrathoracic meningoceles are other associated anomalies.[2,16]

Neurofibromatosis type 2 (NF2) is an autosomal dominant entity which is associated with defect in the chromosome 22. Bilateral acoustic nerve schwannomas are the most consistent and hence diagnostic feature of this condition **(Figs. 11 and 12)**.

Cutaneous manifestations include neurofibroma and pale café au lait spots. Skin lesions appear in the first decade of life which are followed by development of acoustic neuromas between the age of 10 years and 15 years. Presence of cataracts and skin lesions in a child are valuable clinical indicators of NF2.

The diagnostic criteria[20] for NF2 include:

- Bilateral eighth nerve schwannoma
- A first degree relative with NF2 and
  - A unilateral eighth nerve acoustic schwannoma or
  - *Two of the following*:
    - Neurofibroma
    - Meningioma
    - Glioma
    - Schwannoma
    - Juvenile posterior subcapsular opacity or
    - Cerebral calcification
- *Two of the following*:
  - Unilateral vestibular schwannoma
  - Multiple meningiomas
  - Features listed under 2b above (Except for meningiomas).

Apart from VIIIth nerve schwannoma, the trigeminal nerve, oculomotor nerve, trochlear or the abducens nerve schwannoma are also seen in NF2. These tend to be isodense to hypodense on CT and shows patchy but significant enhancement after contrast administration.

On MR studies schwannoma appear as well delineated masses which are isohyperintense on T2WI. Intense patchy enhancement occurs after gadolinium administration. Other forms of neurofibromatosis have been described.

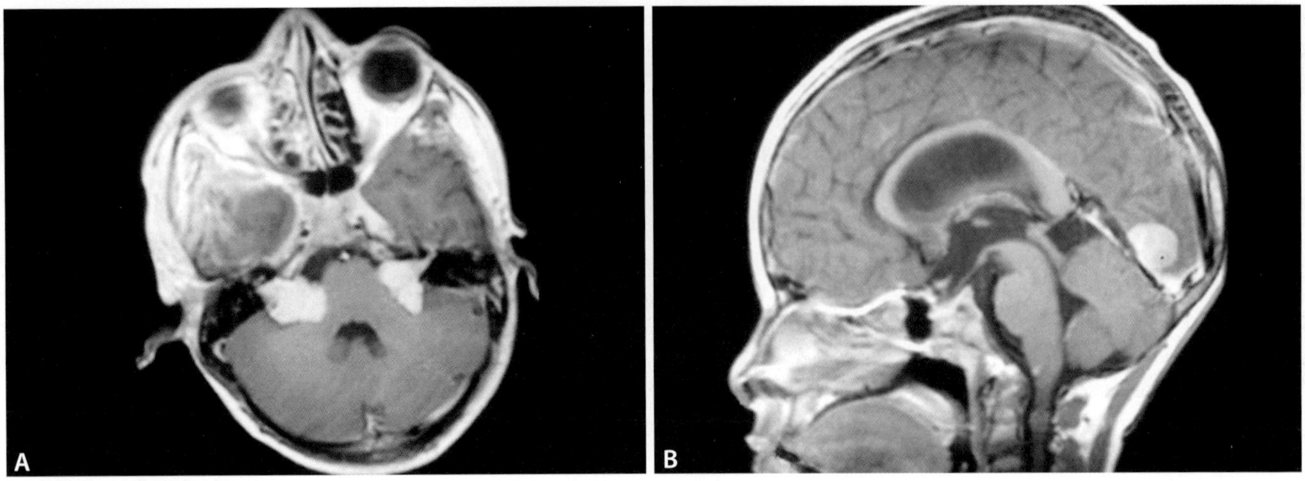

Figs. 12A and B: Neurofibromatosis type 2: Contrast-enhanced axial T1 section (A) shows enhancing CP angle masses with intracanalicular extension consistent with B/L acoustic schwannomas. The enhancing tentorial based lesion is a meningioma (B).

They have been labelled as NF3 to NF7. An eighth category NF-NOS includes cases which are atypical and do not fit into the labelled categories.[19,20] Details of these form of neurofibromatosis are beyond the scope of this chapter.

Tuberous Sclerosis

Tuberous sclerosis (TS) is an inherited autosomal dominant condition with a low penetrance. The locus of this condition is identified on two chromosomes. The TSC1 gene is localized to chromosome 9q34 and the TSC2 gene is localized to chromosome 6p13.3 which are associated with hamartoma formations in multiple organ systems.[21] The classical triad of papular facial lesions (adenoma sebaceum), seizure disorder and mental retardation are the hallmark of this disease.[16]

Subependymal hamartomas are the hallmark of tuberous sclerosis. They are located on the ventricular surface of caudate nucleus, immediately posterior to the foramen of Monro and along the frontal and temporal horns of the lateral ventricles. On MR they protrude into the adjacent ventricle. They are hyperintense on T1WI they appear hyper- and hypointense on T2 WI relation to gray and white matter. They show minimal contrast enhancement **(Figs. 13A to C)**.

Subependymal giant cell astrocytoma (SGCA) are benign tumors associated with TS usually located at the foramen of Monro in about 15%. They are hypo to isointense on T1WI and hyperintense on T2WI and enhance uniformly after contrast administration. Cerebral hamartomas are most characteristic. They are low attenuating on CT and with age become calcified. White matter low attenuating, well-defined lesions are highly characteristic lesions of TS. Like NF2, retinal hamartoma, aneurysm and vascular dysplasia have also been described with tuberous sclerosis.[2,16]

Sturge–Weber Syndrome

Sturge–Weber syndrome (encephalotrigeminal angiomatosis) is a congenital noninherited entity. It is a syndrome characterized by angiomatous malformation affecting the skin, eye and brain. The typical lesion is a facial angioma (port wine stain) in the distribution of all the divisions of the trigeminal nerve. It is usually unilateral and there is concomitant involvement of the ipsilateral occipital lobe, parietal lobes, and choroid plexus. Ocular findings of buphthalmos, optic atrophy, iris heterochromia and strabismus may be encountered. Patients may present with hemiparesis, homonymous hemianopia and seizures.

The vascular malformations are low pressure, slowly-flowing leptomeningeal angiomata. There is a congenital absence of cortical veins, therefore the blood is shunted towards the hypertrophied deep medullary veins and thence to the choroid plexus. The relatively static venous flow leads to hypoxia of the affected cortex which inturn leads to cortical atrophy and dystrophic calcification **(Fig. 14)** which can be demonstrated on plain X-ray and CT. The resulting curvilinear calcification is diagnostic of the syndrome. It is commonly seen in the occipital and posterior parietal lobe on the side of the facial angioma. If there is extensive atrophy, there is marked dilatation of the ipsiventricle, thickening of the calvarium and prominence of the ipsilateral paranasal sinuses which are obvious on plain radiograph. The ipsilateral choroid plexus is enlarged and may contain cysts and enhance intensely. The pial angiomas can show enhancement on both MR and CT **(Figs. 15A and B)**.[22] The abnormal venous channels of the

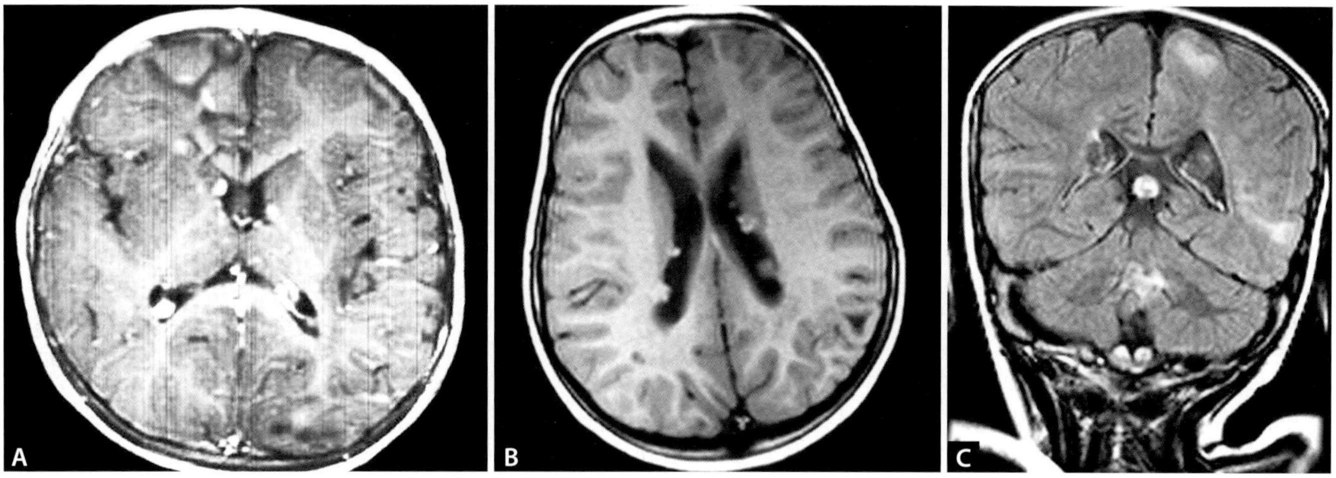

Figs. 13A to C: Tuberous sclerosis: Contrast-enhanced T1 axial MR sections showing subependymal nodules in two patients (A and B) along with cortical tubers on FLAIR coronal sections (C).

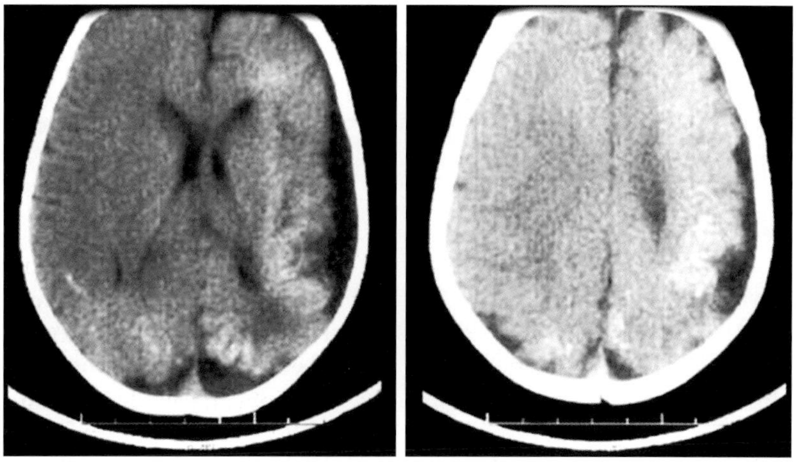

Fig. 14: Sturge–Weber syndrome: Noncontrast CT scan shows subcortical calcification with atrophy of the affected left parietal and occipital lobes. Calcification is also present in the right occipital lobe.

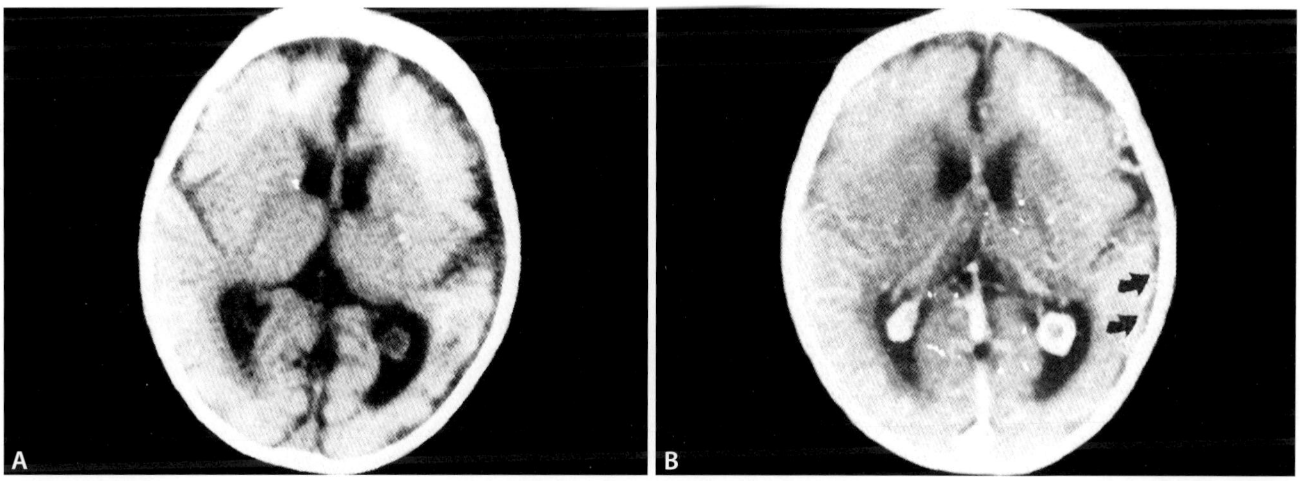

Figs. 15A and B: Sturge–Weber syndrome: A 4-year-old presented with a nevus flammeus on the left half of face. (A) Contrast-enhanced CT shows diffuse cortical calcification on both frontal lobes and atrophy of left temporal and occipital lobe; (B) Enhancement of prominent choroid plexus and temporal angioma (curved arrows) can be appreciated.

cortex and subependymal location can be identified on angiograms or MRI.

Thus, congenital malformations of the CNS includes a large number of diverse conditions. CT and especially MRI has a very important role to play in characterizing the lesions which help in establishing the diagnosis. MR imaging has been used extensively in recent years to investigate the neuroanatomical basis of congenital brain malformations. Newer techniques like diffusion imaging including diffusion tensor imaging (DTI) and high angular resolution diffusion imaging (HARDI) have helped in fiber tractography and have elucidated the aberrant connectivity underlying a number of congenital brain malformations.[23] They however still remain in the research arena and will take time to come to the clinical field.

REFERENCES

1. Osborn AG. Brain development and congenital malformation. In: Osborn AG (Ed): Diagnostic Neuroradiology St Louis: Mosby Year Book; 1994.pp.3-116.
2. ByrdSE, CharlesRF. Congenitalbrainmalformations. In: Khun JP, Slovis TL, Haller JO (Eds): Caffey's Pediatric Diagnostic Imaging, 10th edition. St. louis: Mosby Year Book; 2004. pp. 506-29.
3. Barkovich AJ, Kuzhiecky RI, Dobyns WB, et al. A classification scheme for malformations and cortical development. Neuropediatrics. 1996;27:59-63.
4. Abdel Razek AA, Kandell AY, Elsorogy LG, Elmongy A, Basett AA. Disorders of cortical formation: MR imaging features. Am J Neuroradiol. 2009;30:4-11.
5. Robertson R, Casuso PA, Truwit CL. Disorders of brain development. In: Atlas SW (Ed): Magnetic Resonance Imaging of the Brain. Philadelphia: Lippincott Williams and Wilkins; 2002.pp.279-369.
6. Hahn JS, Barnes PD. Neuroimaging advances in holoprosencephaly: Refining the spectrum of the midline malformation. Am J Med Genet C Semin Med Genet. 2010;15:120-32.
7. Morishima A, Aranoff G. Syndrome of septo-optic pituitary dysplasia: The clinical spectrum brain dev. 1986;8:233-5.
8. Paul LK, Brown WS, Adolphs R, Tyszka JM, Richards LJ, Mukherjee P, Sherr EH. Agenesis of the corpus callosum: genetic, developmental and functional aspects of connectivity. Nat Rev Neurosci. 2007;8:287-99.
9. Altman N, Naidich T, Braffman B. Posterior fossa malformation Am J Neuroradiology. 1992;13:691-724.
10. Vannemreddy P, Nourbakhsh A, Willis B, Guthikonda B. Congenital Chiari malformations. Neurol India. 2010;58(1): 6-14.
11. Kollias S, Ball W, Prenger E. Cystic malformations of the posterior fossa, differential diagnosis classified through embryologic analysis. Radiographics. 1993;13:1211-31.
12. Chiari H, Uber Veranderungen des Kleinhirns, des Pons unde der. Medulla oblongata infolge von congenitaler hydrocephalie des Gross hirns Denkschr Kais Akad Wiss Mathnaturew. 1896;63:71-116.
13. Bhaddelia RA, Bogdan AR, Wolpert SM. Analysis of cerebrospinal fluid flow waveforms with gated phase contrast MR velocity measurements. AM J Neurorad. 1995;10:389-400.
14. McLone DG, Knepper PA. The cause of Chiari II malformaiton. A unified theory. Pediatr Neuroscience. 1989;15:1-12.
15. Naidich T, Altman N, Braffman B, et al. Cephaloceles and related malformations. Am J Neuroradiology. 1992;13: 655-90.
16. Smirniotopoulous JG, Murphy FM. Central nervous system manifestations of the phakomatoses and other inherited syndromes. In: Atlas SW (Ed): Magnetic Resonance Imaging of Brain and Spine, 3rd edition. Philadelphia: Lippincott Williams and Wilkins. 2002;371-413.
17. Barkovich AJ. The phakomatoses. In: Barkovich AJ. Pediatric Neuroimaging, 4th edition. Philadelphia: Lippincott Williams and Wilkins; 2005.pp.476–81.
18. Neurofibromatosis, conference statement. National Institutes of Health Consensus Development Conference. Arch Neurol. 1988;45:575-8.
19. Mulvihill JJ. (moderator) Neurofibromatosis I (Recklinghausen's disease) and neurofibromatosis 2 (bilateral acoustic neurofibromatosis) an update. Ann Inter Med. 1990;113:39-52.
20. Ricardi VM. Neurofibromatosis. Neurol Clin. 1987;5:337-49.
21. Orlova KA, Crino PB. The tuberous sclerosis complex. Ann N Y Acad Sci. 2010;1184:87-105.
22. Stimac GK, Solomon MA, Newton TH. CT and MR of angiomatous malformations of the choroids plexus in patients with Sturge-Weber disease. Am J Neuroradiology. 1986;7:623-7.
23. Wahl M, Barkovich AJ, Mukherjee P. Diffusion imaging and tractography of congenital brain malformations. Pediatr Radiol. 2010;40:59-67.

CHAPTER 151

Hypoxic–Ischemic Encephalopathy

Atin Kumar, Arun Kumar Gupta

INTRODUCTION

Neonatal encephalopathy following birth asphyxia or perinatal hypoxia is referred to as hypoxic–ischemic encephalopathy (HIE).[1]

An HIE is a common clinical problem with far-reaching consequences. It, therefore, becomes mandatory for the pediatrician and the pediatric radiologist to understand its etiology, pathology, pathophysiological mechanism and imaging features with awareness of the limitations and advantages of each imaging modality.

Exact incidence of HIE is not known but at most centers incidence of perinatal hypoxic–ischemia is between 1% and 1.5%.[2] Clinically, HIE has been graded into mild, moderate and severe grades with prognosis directly related to the severity.[3] Approximately, 15–20% of neonates with hypoxic ischemia would die within the newborn period.[4]

NEUROIMAGING IN INFANTS WITH HIE

Role of neuroimaging in the work-up of infants with HIE is twofolds:

1. Imaging of the pathologic lesions and their follow-up.
2. Prediction of clinical outcome based on pathologic lesions observed on imaging.

Three important imaging techniques used for examination of the newborn brain are sonography, computed tomography (CT) and magnetic resonance imaging (MRI). Although maturity of the neonatal brain and suspected pathology should dictate the choice of imaging but expertise in conducting and interpreting the images on a particular diagnostic technique, may decide the final selection of an investigation. Sonography, being widely available, possible even at cribside for sick babies, non-ionizing, painless, not requiring sedation or intravenous contrast makes it an ideal screening modality in children. Depending upon the sonographic findings and the clinical status, further imaging protocol may be decided later.

It is a well-established fact that the pattern of cerebral injury in a newborn infant depends, to a great extent, on the maturity of the brain at the time of insult. It is generally agreed that the dividing line between the immature and the mature brain is around 34 weeks.[5,6]

Therefore, two broad groups, i.e. 'below 34 weeks group–the premature neonate' and 'above 34 weeks group–the term neonate' are discussed separately.

BELOW 34 WEEKS GROUP: THE PREMATURE NEONATE

Preterm neonates are much more prone to HIE than term neonates. It occurs because of increased chances of hypoxic insult due to very low birth weight (<1500 g),[7,8] hyaline membrane disease, antepartum placental abruption, hypocapnia, twin pregnancy, septicemia, patent ductus arteriosus and also due to poor autoregulatory capacity of the premature brain.[6,9-15]

Imaging features can be subdivided based on severity (and to some extent duration) of injury into two types—severe hypoxia versus mild-to-moderate or partial asphyxia. It must be remembered that features of both severe and partial asphyxia may be seen together in any given patient.

Severe, Total Hypoxia

The most metabolically active regions within the brain in this period, i.e. the deep gray matter, including thalami, basal ganglia, hippocampus, cerebellum, dorsal brainstem and corticospinal tracts are the areas of involvement. The thalami, anterior vermis and the dorsal brainstem are the most frequently affected. The basal ganglia and perirolandic cortex myelinate at around 35–36 weeks of gestational age and therefore are less severely and less frequently involved than the thalami.[16]

Cranial ultrasound is the first modality performed in the preterm neonates for screening and diagnosis for HIE. It may be normal in the first 48 hours but may show hyperechogenicity in the basal ganglia and thalami by the third day.[6] CT will similarly show hypodensity within the basal ganglia and thalami with their attenuation values close to that of white matter.

MRI is a sensitive modality to detect the changes of HIE. Diffusion weighted images may show restriction of diffusion within the involved areas, most commonly the thalami, in the first 24 hours. The abnormalities on conventional MRI start appearing in the form of T1 and T2 hyperintensity in the thalami and basal ganglia from 3rd day onwards. The restriction of diffusion reaches peak at around 3–5 days and then starts to 'pseudonormalize' after a week. T2 shortening starts to occur after 1 week in the affected areas. The T1 hyperintense signal may persist into the chronic stage **(Figs. 1A and B)**.

Mild-to-Moderate Hypoxia

This is by far the most common pattern of insult to the premature neonatal brain. The two major pathological lesions observed in this setting are hemorrhage and periventricular leukomalacia (PVL).[5,6]

Hemorrhage

Intracranial hemorrhage (ICH) in premature neonates is directly related to the degree of gestational immaturity. Germinal matrix (GM), the site of initial bleed, is a highly vascular area within the ventricular wall. GM is most prominent and active between 8 and 28 weeks of gestation.[6,17,18] Hemorrhage could be at germinal matrix (GMH), intraventricular (IVH), or parenchymal.[17-21]

Germinal Matrix Hemorrhage (GMH)

Prematurity coupled with respiratory distress syndrome are the two main factors presumed to be responsible for hemorrhage in the immature brain. Following ischemic insult when the ischemic tissue is reperfused, damaged cerebral autoregulation[22-24] associated with sudden rapid rise in cerebral blood flow or perfusion pressure as with handling, suction, artificial ventilation; leads to rupture of fragile weakened blood vessels in the germinal matrix bed.[6,17,18] The germinal matrix involutes by 34 weeks of gestation. The last portion of germinal matrix to involute is the ganglionic eminence located deep to the ependyma in the caudothalamic notch in the groove between the head of caudate nucleus and the thalamus. Hence, it is the most common site for germinal matrix hemorrhage **(Figs. 2 and 3)**. It may also occur in the cerebellum from the

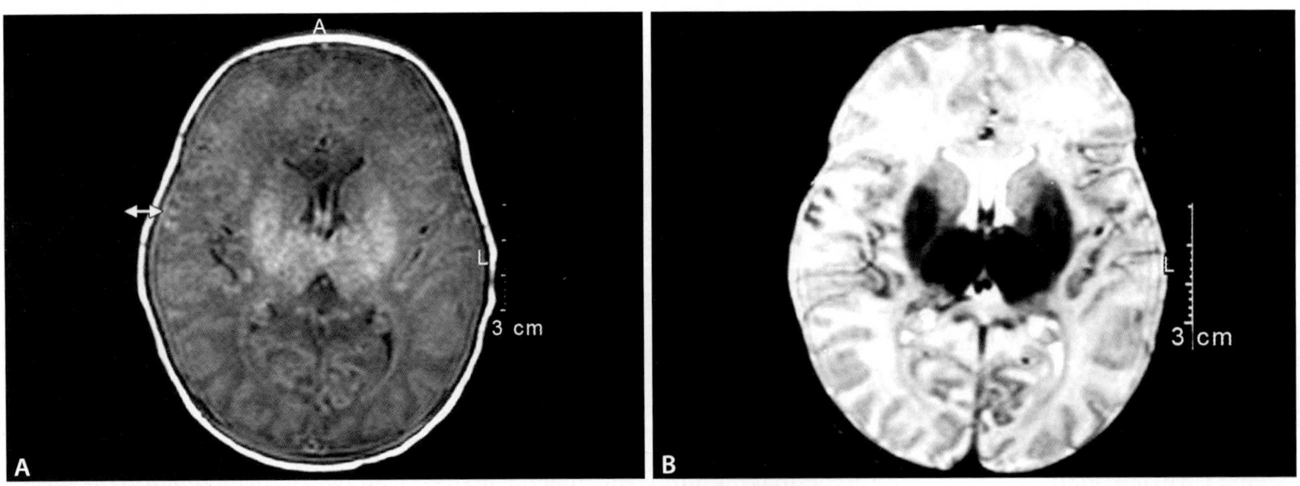

Figs. 1A and B: Axial MR images of a 9-day-old premature neonate show the thalami and basal ganglia appearing hyperintense on T1-weighted image (A) and hypointense signal on T2-weighted image (B).

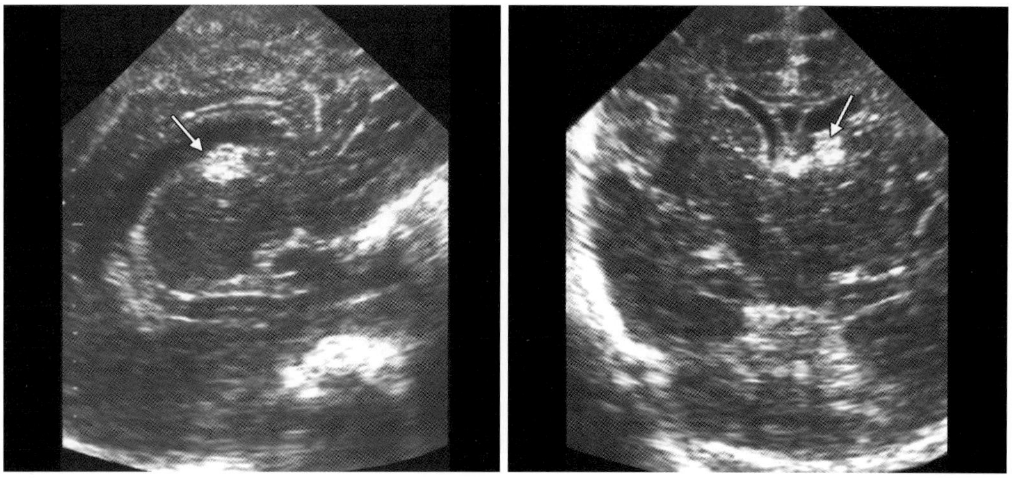

Fig. 2: US: Grade II bleed (SEH) on left side (arrow). Note location of bleed at caudothalamic junction in sagittal view

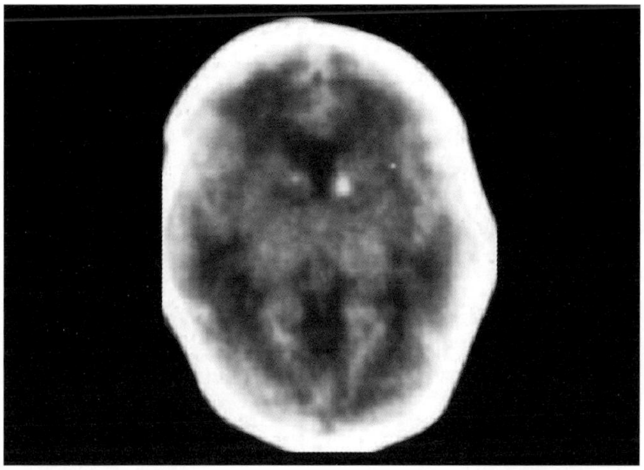

Fig. 3: Bilateral grade II bleed (subependymal hemorrhage, SEH) on NCCT.

germinal zones within the cerebellum and subependymal layer of roof of fourth ventricle.

Intraventricular Hemorrhage (IVH)

An IVH results either from rupture of a GMH into the ventricle or from choroid plexus bleeding. Depending upon the amount of bleeding and alteration in the CSF dynamics, ventricles may or may not show dilatation **(Figs. 4 and 5)**.

Parenchymal Hemorrhage (Periventricular Hemorrhagic Infarction)

It is typically unilateral, extensive and always associated with intraventricular hemorrhage. Unlike hemorrhage

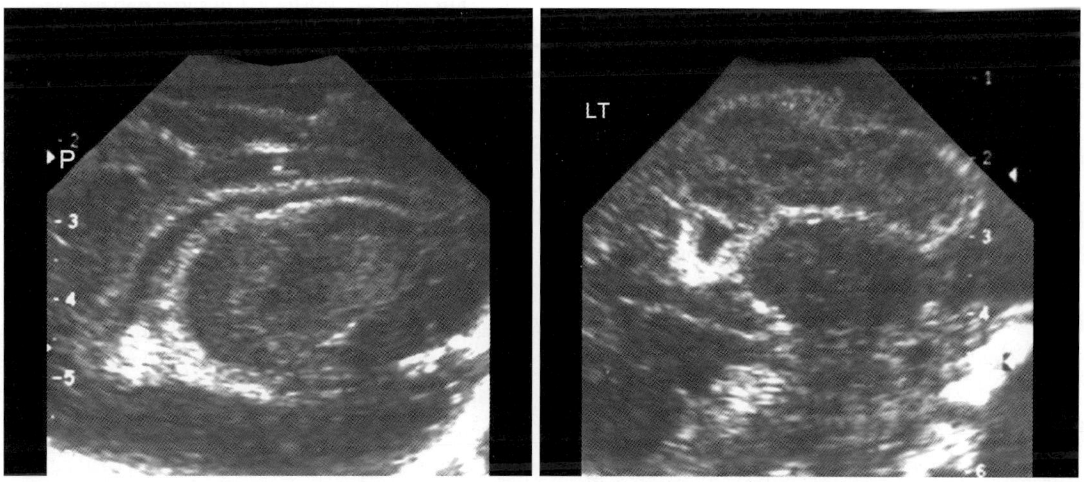

Fig. 4: US—Sagittal views: Grade III bleed, IVH with ventriculomegaly. Compare with normal ventricle on opposite side.

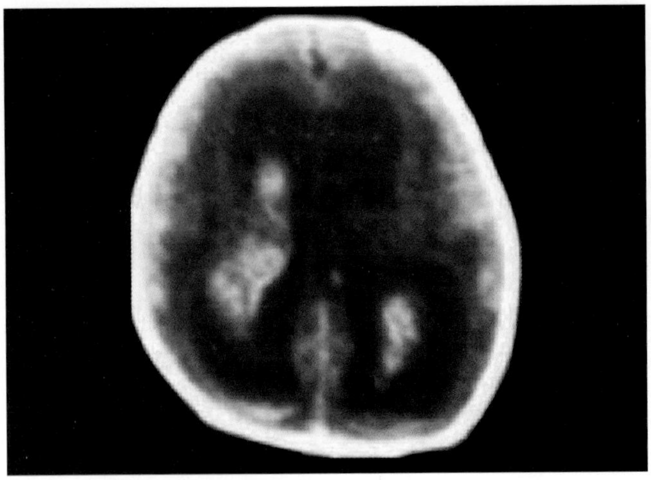

Fig. 5: NCCT: Grade III bleed. Note CSF-blood level in dependent parts.

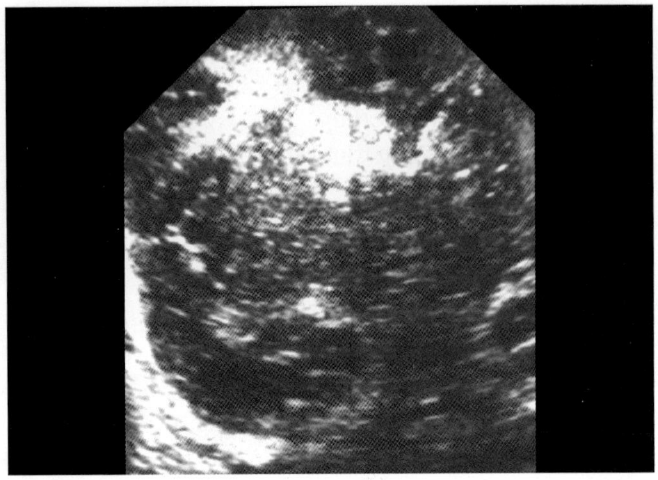

Fig. 6: US—PVHI on right side. Note typical appearance of a triangular echodensity extending from apex of frontal horn and associated IVH on same side.

occurring in an area of ischemia, periventricular hemorrhagic infarction (PVHI) occurs more anteriorly, roughly triangular in shape with apex of the triangle in the midline **(Figs. 6 and 7)**. Germinal matrix and intraventricular hemorrhage causes compromise of terminal veins underlying germinal matrix leading on to congestion, thrombosis and rupture of medullary veins draining the deep white matter. This leads to a hemorrhagic venous infarct in the periventricular parenchyma.[25] PVHI occurs about 24–48 hours after the onset of GMH and IVH. About 15% of patients with IVH develop PVHI.[21] On follow-up, such a hemorrhage results in the development of a porencephalic cyst on imaging and hemiplegia on clinical examination.

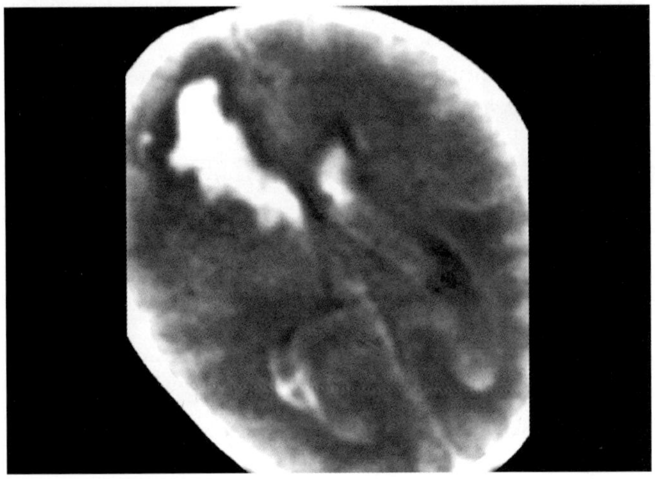

Fig. 7: NCCT: PVHI—CT of same patient as in Figure 6.

Grading of Intracranial Hemorrhage

Papile et al.[19] proposed four grades of severity: Grade (I) hemorrhage confined to germinal matrix in the subependymal region (SEH or GMH); Grade (II) is associated with IVH but without ventricular dilatation; Grade (III) IVH is associated with ventricular dilatation, and Grade (IV) bleeding occurs into the brain parenchyma (PVHI). A number of other classifications followed but none has been universally accepted so far due to their limitations.

Imaging of Intracranial Hemorrhage

Transfontanel sonography is the most sensitive modality to detect SEH and IVH in the acute stage.[26] SEH is seen as a focal echogenic area at the head of caudate nucleus in the most anterior end of caudothalamic groove.[5,6,26] It is important to document the abnormality in two planes, since normal choroid plexus in the same area may be mistaken for SEH. Normal choroid plexus tapers as it extends anteriorly and disappears beyond foramen of Monro. On the other hand, in a GM bleed, there is prominent, bulbous enlargement of choroid density which also extends beyond foramen of Monro **(Fig. 2)**. On NCCT head **(Fig. 3)** SEH is visible as a focal, high attenuating area. IVH is echogenic on sonography **(Fig. 4)** and the organized clot takes the shape of the ventricle which later shows dilatation. With time the clot becomes iso and then hypoechoic. On NCCT IVH is high attenuating initially **(Fig. 5)** becoming iso- and finally hypoattenuating. Periventricular hemorrhagic infarction (PVHI) in the acute stage is brightly echogenic, unilateral, clearly defined echodensity **(Fig. 6)** on sonography[6] with the apex of the triangle pointing towards the ventricle in the midline. Associated IVH is almost always present **(Fig. 7)**.

Subarachnoid hemorrhage (SAH) and hemorrhage in the posterior fossa and parieto-occipital area can be easily missed on the sonography. Noncontrast CT (NCCT) head is more sensitive in depicting these bleeds in the acute phase. On MRI both T1WI and even T2WI may miss these bleeds in the acute stage.

On follow-up, initially SEH becomes a subependymal cyst **(Figs. 8A and B)** which may later disappear completely. IVH cast also resolves with time **(Fig. 9)**. Ventriculomegaly may be the only clue of an earlier episode of bleed. Periventricular hemorrhagic infarction evolves into a porencephalic cyst which is usually in communication with the ventricle. With time, visibility of the hemorrhage, both on sonography and CT, decreases but on MRI visibility increases due to the formation of methemoglobin **(Fig. 10)**. Also, MRI is more specific for assessing the time of hemorrhage.

Optimum time for sonographic detection of intracranial hemorrhage secondary to HIE is from 4th to 7th day, by end of which 97% of hemorrhages will be visible.[26] In order to monitor for the development of hydrocephalus as a complication of IVH, sonography is recommended on the 14th day, and if negative, then at 3rd month.[26]

White Matter Injury of Prematurity/ Periventricular Leukomalacia

The term periventricular leukomalacia (PVL) in literal terms means "white matter softening". A number of theories have been proposed for its pathogenesis. Unlike ICH where prematurity is a clear risk factor; for the development of PVL, a large number of ante or perinatal events have been identified which may result in hypoperfusion to fetal cerebral tissue or injury to oligodendroglial cells, and are thus important causative factors.[27-29] However, besides hypoxic-ischemic insult, other causes like infection, metabolic diseases and hydrocephalus also can cause similar injury to the white matter. Also the whole white matter may be involved, not just the periventricular white matter. Therefore, these insults are better termed as 'White Matter Injury of Prematurity' rather than PVL.

In a premature neonatal brain, the periventricular area is almost totally perfused by penetrating arteries that extend inward from the surface of the brain (ventriculopetal vessels). Junction of ventriculopetal and the ventriculofugal vessels (watershed area) exists in the periventricular region. In the event of any hypoxic ischemic insult, therefore, this periventricular (watershed) area is at the highest risk. This combined with relative hypovascularity of the periventricular white matter plays a role in the development of PVL. Recently it has been believed that presence of oligodendrocyte lineage cells prooligodendrocytes within this area makes them most susceptible to changes of hypoxia–ischemia. These cells mature into oligodendrocytes which are less prone to insult by around 32 weeks of age and hence, there is decreased frequency of PVL after this gestational age.[30,31] Also toxins and excitatory amino acids, especially maternal chorioamnionitis,[32] may play a role in reducing local blood and energy supply and subsequent development of PVL.

Exact incidence of PVL is not clear and would vary depending upon the imaging modality used. Autopsy

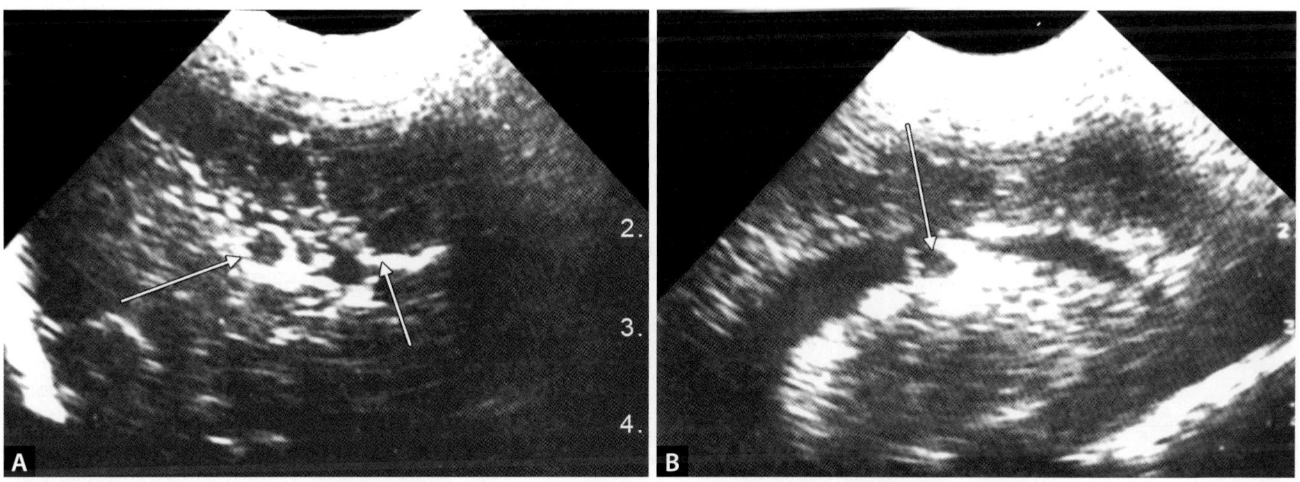

Figs. 8A and B: Coronal (A) and sagittal (B) transfontanel sonography. Subependymal hemorrhage (SEH) (arrow) in the anterior end of right caudothalamic groove with cystic changes. Note that in (A) the normal choroid plexus on the left side (long arrow) may mimick SEH. However, bleed (arrow) is slightly more laterally located in the coronal plane and US examination in sagittal plane (B) confirms the echodensity to be bleed.

series report an incidence ranging from 25% to 75%. On sonography incidence of PVL is reported to vary from 15% to 35%.[6,33,34]

Pathologically, the temporal sequence of events in the development of PVL are coagulation necrosis in the first 24–48 hours followed by cavitation evolving over the next 2–4 weeks (when these cysts can be detected on ultrasound) and after several weeks the cysts collapse and disappear completely with residual white matter atrophy and ventri culomegaly as the only evidence.[6,24] The ventricles have irregular lateral walls and cerebral cortex reaches upto the lateral ventricle wall. PVL may be purely ischemic or at times complicated by blood. Imaging features will therefore vary depending upon the time of imaging in relation to the ischemic insult and whether it is purely ischemic or complicated by hemorrhage.

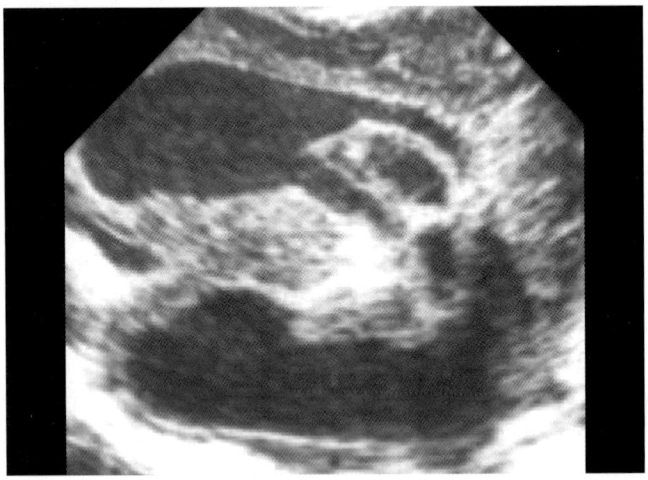

Fig. 9: Follow-up of grade III bleed shows a resolving clot and echogenic debris

PVL lesions could be focal or diffuse.[21] Classically, focal PVL lesions are distributed bilaterally, symmetrically, primarily around the trigone areas but may extend also to involve the frontal lobes adjacent to the foramen of Monro.[12,14,35,36] However, lesions may be visible only on one side on imaging and that should not exclude the diagnosis of PVL. Diffuse lesions involve the entire periventricular region.

Clinically, the characteristic neurological abnormality due to PVL is spastic diplegia[26,36] in about 5–15%. This is because the site of pathological lesions of PVL are located in the periventricular region from where also the corticospinal tracts descend. Tracts of lower limbs are located in the most medial region, i.e. closest to the PVL lesion and are thus first to be affected resulting in diplegia.[24,37] Visual impairment[38,39] and cognitive impairment[40] may occur without spastic diplegia.

Imaging of Early PVL

Ultrasound

Due to hemodynamically unstable state of most of these neonates, a cribside ultrasound (US) in the ICU/nursery is usually the first investigation. Besides portability the other advantages of US are nonionizing, no IV contrast or sedation is required and can be repeated frequently without harmful effects. Addition of color Doppler and quantitative analysis[41] to 2 D imaging may improve information content. PVL should be suspected on US studies when increased echogenicity is present in the periventricular regions. On ultrasound **(Figs. 11A and B)**, periventricular areas of increased echogenicity is visible within 24–48 hours of ischemic insult. However, there are two major potential pitfalls: Firstly, in normal newborns also there is a periventricular increased echogenicity, so

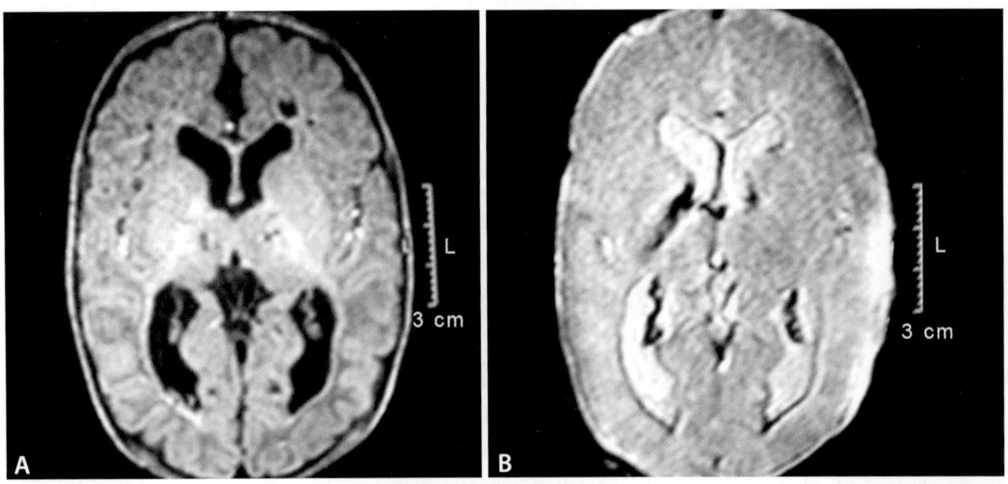

Figs. 10A and B: Axial T1 weighted MR image (A) in a premature neonate shows IVH appearing hyperintense in the occipital horns (dependent part). The gradient T2 weighted image (B) is more sensitive in detecting the bleed which is evident as hypointense signal lining the ventricular margins, choroid plexus and right caudothalamic groove.

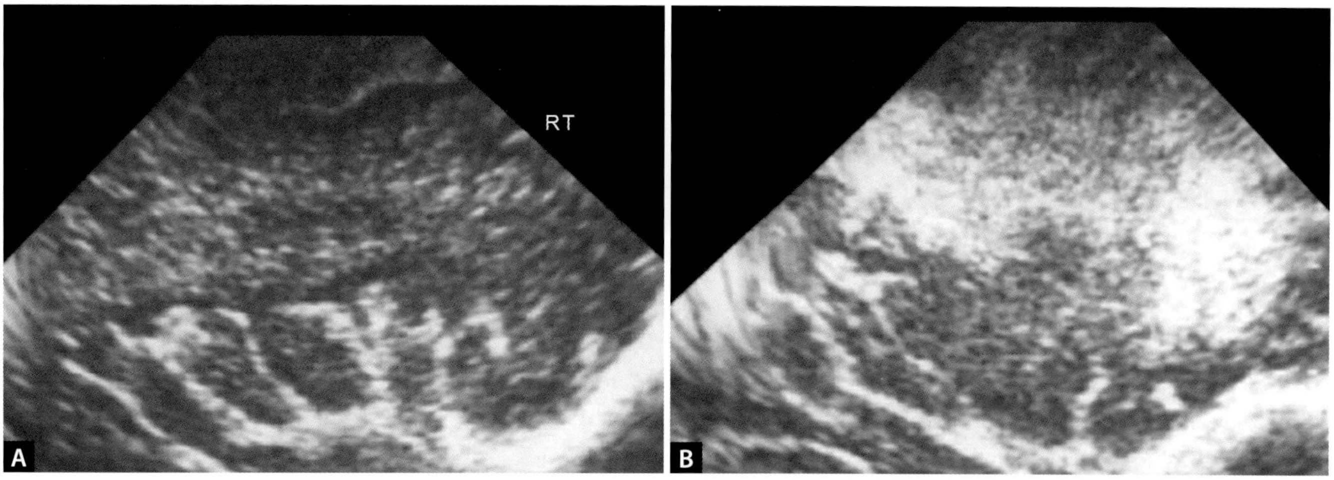

Figs. 11A and B: Periventricular leukomalacia (PVL)—early: Sagittal US both sides show marked degree of increased echogenicity on right. *Note*: Loss of normal brain architecture on the affected side.

called 'periventricular blush'.[5,6] Secondly, brain edema also appears bright on US.[42,43] Therefore, presence of increased echogenicity in itself is not enough to diagnose PVL. Reliable sign of PVL is the presence of periventricular "flares". The brightness of echogenicity due to PVL 'flare' is more than the normal periventricular echogenicity and approaches or becomes equal to that of adjacent choroid plexus. Also the normal tissue architechture is lost.[6,44,45] However, this limits the capability of US[46-48] since a certain degree of subjective element creeps in, especially in milder degrees of abnormality. 'Periventricular flare' should be confirmed and documented in both the coronal and the parasagittal views.

If ischemic PVL is complicated by hemorrhage, then the abnormalities are readily detected by sonography. It is important to recognize that both, the edema **(Fig. 12)** as well as the hemorrhage **(Figs. 13A and B)**, in the brain parenchyma will produce increased echogenicity on ultrasound. Differentiation is possible by observing the *degree of brightness*. In these situations, CT and MRI help differentiate between the two.

On follow-up, the flares may completely disappear, usually in about half of the patients, within 7–10 days. If however the flares persist beyond 1 week then the term "persistent flares" is used and are considered as grade I PVL.[44] In about 10%, the flares may progress to the next pathological stage, i.e. of cavitation, usually within 2–4 weeks. Development of few, small cysts represent milder end of the spectrum of PVL but multiple cysts **(Figs. 14 and 15)** is an indicator of a poor neurological prognosis with development of cerebral palsy.[26] Not only the size but also the distribution of cysts is important for predicting the severity of clinical outcome.[49]

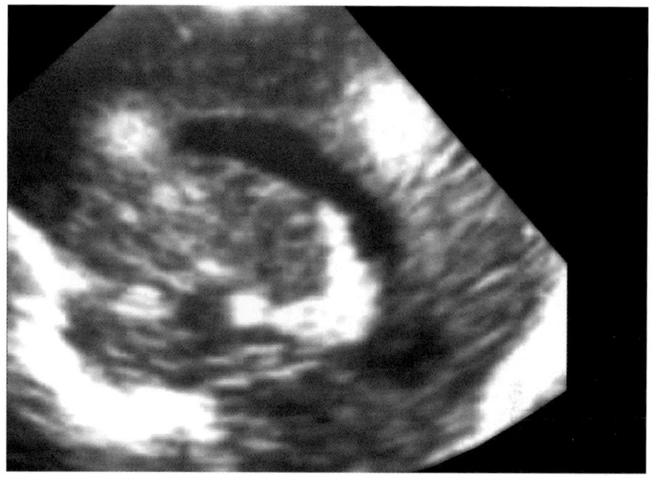

Fig. 12: Sagittal US: Focal edema mimicking PVL.

Thus, cysts in the frontoparietal area have a better prognosis as compared to those in the posterior parieto-occipital region. Again ultrasound is superior to CT **(Fig. 16)** for the detection of small cysts of PVL. However, MRI is a superior modality for detection of these cysts **(Figs. 17 and 18)**.

Ultrasound also has been used to grade the PVL. The classification suggested by De Vries[44] is simple to use **(Table 1)**. The grading increases with extent and the severity of pathological lesions and is, therefore, directly related to the severity of neurological abnormality.

CT

CT has no added advantage over ultrasound and should be avoided because of the associated ionizing radiation exposure. The only exception where CT scores over ultrasound is differentiation of bleed from edema.

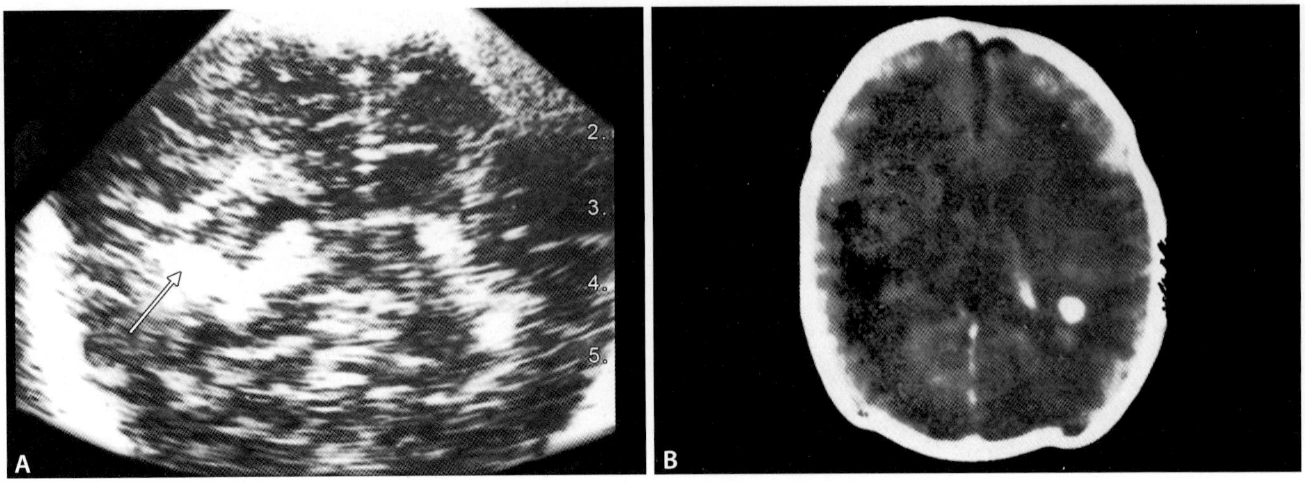

Figs. 13A and B: Focal parenchymal bleed: On sonography (A) bleed (arrow) is again echogenic but "more bright" than edema. CT (B) focal bleed readily diagnosed.

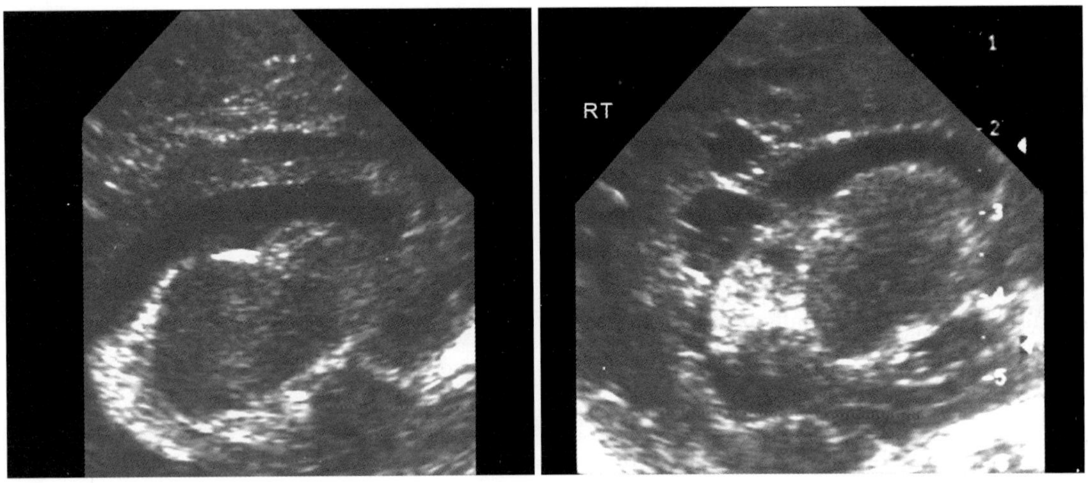

Fig. 14: Sagittal US: Large cystic PVL in posterior parieto-occipital region on right side.

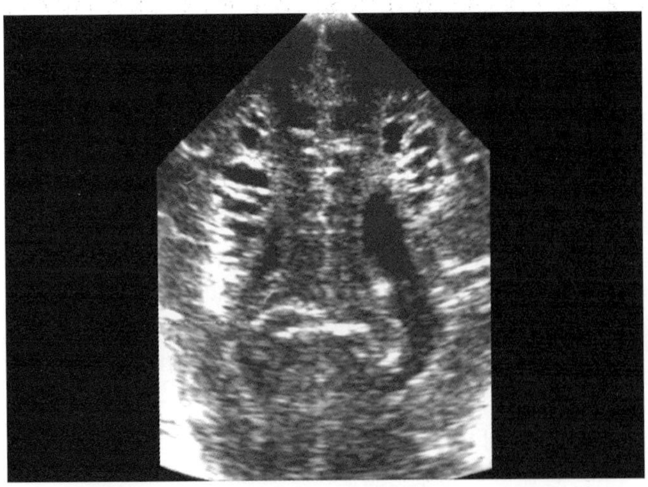

Fig. 15: Coronal US: Bilateral extensive cystic PVL.

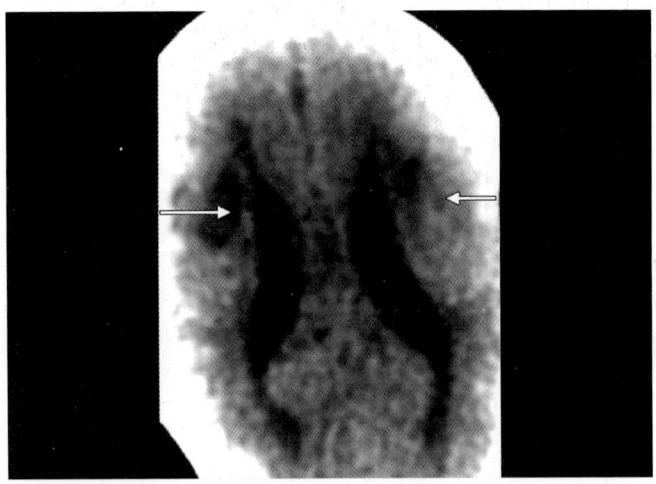

Fig. 16: Cystic PVL (arrows) on a NCCT: Same patient as in Figure 15. Demonstration on US is easier and better than on CT.

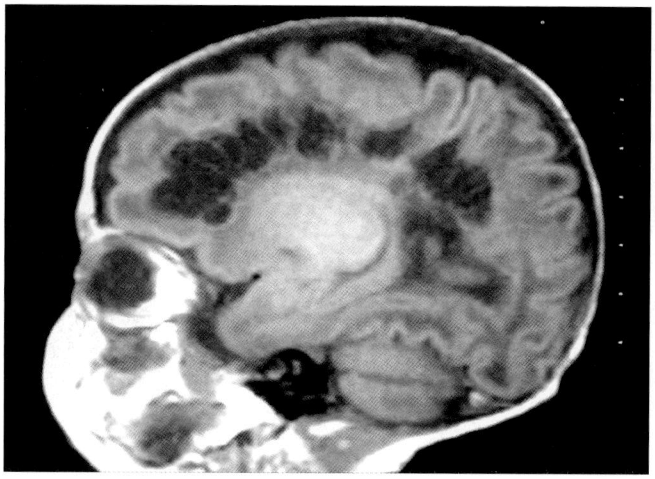

Fig. 17: Sagittal T1W MRI shows extensive large cystic PVL.

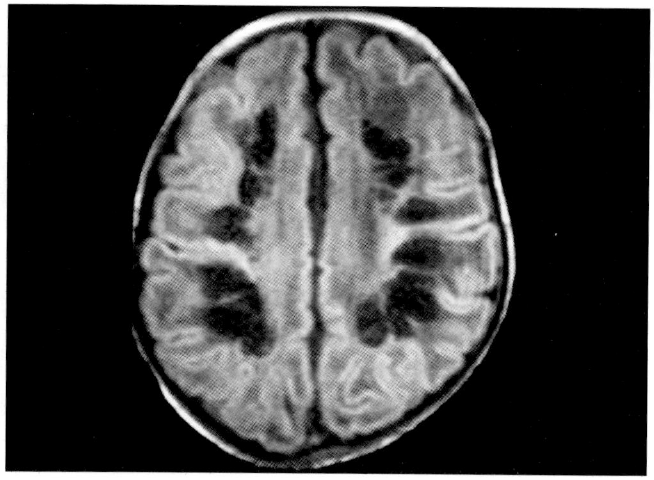

Fig. 18: Axial T1W MRI: Extensive bilateral large cystic PVL.

Table 1: Grading of periventricular leukomalacia (PVL).

Grade of PVL	*Description*
Grade I	Periventricular echogenic area, persistent for more than seven days
Grade II	Periventricular echogenic areas, evolving into localized small frontoparietal cysts
Grade III	Periventricular echogenic areas evolving into multiple cysts in the parieto-occipital white matter
Grade IV	Echogenic areas in the deep white matter evolving into multiple subcortical cysts (multicystic encephalopathy)

However, since MRI can also differentiate the two and is generally more sensitive for other findings, it is the next preferred modality after ultrasound.

MRI

The capability of MRI to detect subtle injuries, its superior contrast resolution and its multiplanar potential makes it a far superior technique to ultrasound for detection of white matter abnormalities. With recent advances in MRI, ventilators and anesthesia equipment hardware, the problems of feasibility of MRI in very sick and premature neonates have been largely overcome.[50]

Early white matter injury appears as foci of T1 hyperintensity in the periventricular white matter by 3–4 days postinsult. These lesions are not evident on T2 weighted images at this time. Instead T2 weighted images show diffuse hyperintense signal within the periventricular white matter. The T1 hyperintense foci subsequently become hypointense on T2 weighted images by 5–6 days. Hemorrhage also gives rise to T2 hypointense lesions but in this case the hypointensity is more marked.

Advances in MRI have made it possible to diagnose early white matter injury. Diffusion weighted imaging (DWI) in a number of studies has been found to be much more accurate than conventional MRI in the acute phase of PVL.[6,46,51,52] Recently further advances have been made and studies using serial quantitative diffusion tensor MRI[53,54] have reported very high degree of accuracy in diagnosing early white matter injuries. In this technique, two parameters are assessed: apparent diffusion coefficient (ADC) mapping and relative anisotropy of cerebral water. This method has been found so accurate that it is being nowadays used for white matter tractography.[55,56]

Imaging of End-stage PVL

After several weeks, usually 3 months onwards, the cysts collapse and completely disappear. Diagnosis on US at this stage is very difficult, if not impossible. A characteristic triad of findings due to white matter collapse is seen both on CT and MRI **(Figs. 19A and B)**.[5,6,12,14,57] The triad consists of the following:

- Abnormally increased bilateral periventricular white matter signal intensity on a T2W sequence, most commonly in the trigone regions of lateral ventricles. This increased signal intensity corresponds to gliosis and demyelination observed pathologically in late PVL. Important differential diagnosis of similar increased signal intensity includes normal, unmyelinated white matter; myelinoclastic disorders and postradiation or chemotherapeutic administration. However, by careful interpretation of the images in the proper clinical background, one can differentiate each of these conditions from one another and from PVL.

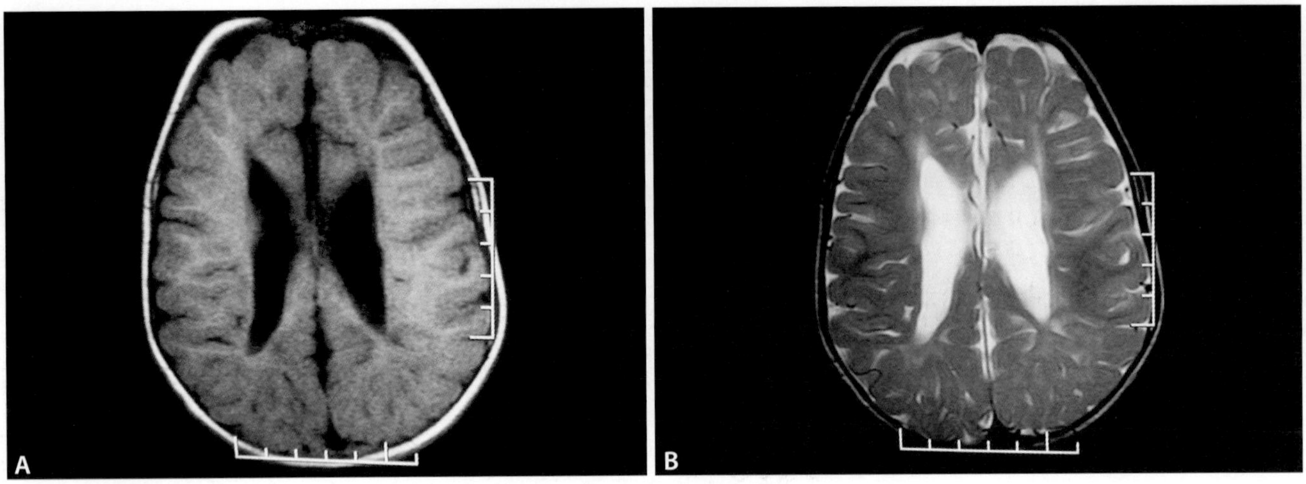

Figs. 19A and B: End-stage PVL: T1 (A) and T2 (B) weighted axial MR images show loss of volume with signal changes in the deep periventricular white matter and ventricular dilatation with irregular margins.

- Marked loss of periventricular white matter in the regions of abnormal high signal intensity results in close approximation of the cortical sulci to the ventricles. Many a times, this may be the only clue of an end-stage PVL.
- Compensatory focal enlargement of the ventricle adjacent to the regions of abnormal high-signal intensity with irregular outlines.

On MRI, two other findings may also be seen,[6] i.e. observation of delayed myelination and thin, atrophic corpus callosum particularly in the posterior body and splenium. However, it should always be remembered that all these above late stage signs on imaging may be caused by many different disorders, such as ventriculitis (a common sequel of meningitis in infants), inborn errors of metabolism, hydrocephalus and in utero events.[6] The diagnosis is best made in conjunction with a thorough past medical history.

In addition to PVL, two other distinct type of white matter abnormalities have been described in the premature neonates—punctuate lesions and diffuse excessive high signal (DEHSI).[25,50] These are much better seen on MRI as compared to ultrasound. The punctate lesions, though more common in premature neonates, may also be seen in term neonates. They are most frequently seen in the corona radiata, posterior periventricular white matter and the optic radiation and rarely in deep gray matter. In some cases, they may represent the early and mild end of PVL spectrum. They are seen as T1 hyperintense and T2 hypointense lesions which occasionally show evidence of bleed on gradient sequences and restricted diffusion on DWI. These may regress with time. In contrast, DEHSI refers to diffuse signal changes in deep white matter appearing hypointense on T1 and hyperintense on T2 weighted images. These signal changes are more profound than the normal appearances of unmyelinated white matter in the premature neonatal brain. It may be noted here that even in the normal developing brain there are more distinct zones of high signal intensity on T2 and low on T1 weighted images. These appear in the shape of caps anteriorly in the frontal white matter and arrowheads posteriorly in the peritrigonal white matter.[50] The DEHSI can be differentiated from these by being diffuse. Neonates with DEHSI have been shown to have impaired development in about 50% of the cases with rest leading on to develop normally.[25]

ABOVE 34 WEEKS GROUP: THE TERM NEONATE

Incidence of HIE in term neonates has decreased over the years and is reported to be about 1–2 per 1000 live births.[6,58] Affected neonates may have significant neurologic abnormalities,[24] mental retardation[24] or visual impairment.[59] Hypoxic–ischemic injury in the term neonate usually occurs in association with antepartum risk factors either alone or in combination with intrapartum risk factors. Remaining few cases are associated with intrapartum factors alone or secondary to postnatal complications, such as sepsis, shock and respiratory distress.

With the maturity of the infant three important anatomic changes occur:[5,6] (i) involution and regression of the germinal matrix resulting in decreased incidence of intracranial hemorrhage in term neonates in contrast to preterm neonates, (ii) the site susceptible for hypoxic–ischemic injury changes. The watershed zone shifts from the earlier periventricular location in a preterm to a more peripheral location in the subcortical region, and (iii) while earlier the response of the preterm brain to trauma was by liquefaction and resorption of the damaged brain, the mature brain responds to the same trauma by reactive astrogliosis.[6,60]

The pathological lesions and imaging characteristics due to HIE in infants beyond 34 weeks gestation are again dependent on severity and duration of hypoxia and is divided into severe and mild-to-moderate groups.

Severe Total Hypoxia

Severe hypoxia refers to sudden total loss of oxygenation as may be seen in abruption placenta, prolapsed cord or ruptured uterus. As seen in the preterm neonates, the deep gray matter, including putamen, ventrolateral thalamus, hippocampus, dorsal brainstem and lateral geniculate nuclei, are the areas of involvement.[6] In contrast to preterm neonates, the basal ganglia involvement is more severe compared to thalami. The perirolandic cortex may also be affected. The remaining cortex is involved only with more prolonged insults. In this type of injury hypoxia is the predominant component of insult rather than hypotension.

Cranial ultrasound done within the first week has low sensitivity. It may show pattern of diffuse cerebral edema seen as diffuse increased echogenicity of brain with obliterated CSF spaces **(Fig. 20)**. Ultrasound done after a week may show increased echogenicity of involved areas of basal ganglia, thalami and brainstem. Follow-up ultrasound shows diffuse cerebral atrophy.

CT is much less sensitive and specific than MRI. CT findings include decrease in the density of basal ganglia, cortex with subsequent loss of gray white matter differentiation **(Fig. 21)**. CT may also show evidence of diffuse cerebral edema evident as effacement of sylvian fissures and basal cisterns **(Fig. 22)**. It may be seen about 8 hours after insult and peak by 3–4 days.

MRI is the most sensitive modality for evaluation of HIE in the term neonate. Conventional T1 and T2 weighted images in combination with diffusion-weighted images (DWI) depict the extent of damage. The conventional images may start showing findings from second day onwards but the abnormalities on these images are best visualized after a week.[6] DWI usually shows the abnormality within the first 24 hours when the conventional images are normal. However the DWI done on the first day, though sensitive, underestimates the extent of injury which is seen to progress on these images to a peak on 3–5 days. The findings then subsequently 'pseudonormalize' by the end of first week. DWI, however, can objectively categorize tissue injury based on values of ADC and subsequently predict outcome to a certain extent.[61,62] MR spectroscopy has been shown to be sensitive modality for detecting hypoxic damage in the early period within first 24 hours even when the DWI images are normal. Elevated choline, decreased NAA, increased lacatate and increased glutamine-glutamate are seen. Lactate elevation seen as a lactate doublet (2 sharp peaks) centerd at 1.33 ppm is typically seen due to anaerobic glycosis secondary to mitochondrial dysfunction. It can be detected as early as 4–8 hours after birth but peaks at around 5 days of life.[63] Increased lactate/NAA ratio observed on first day of life has been shown to be a very sensitive parameter for injury and may be considered as gold standard. It may be useful in identification of infants who may benefit

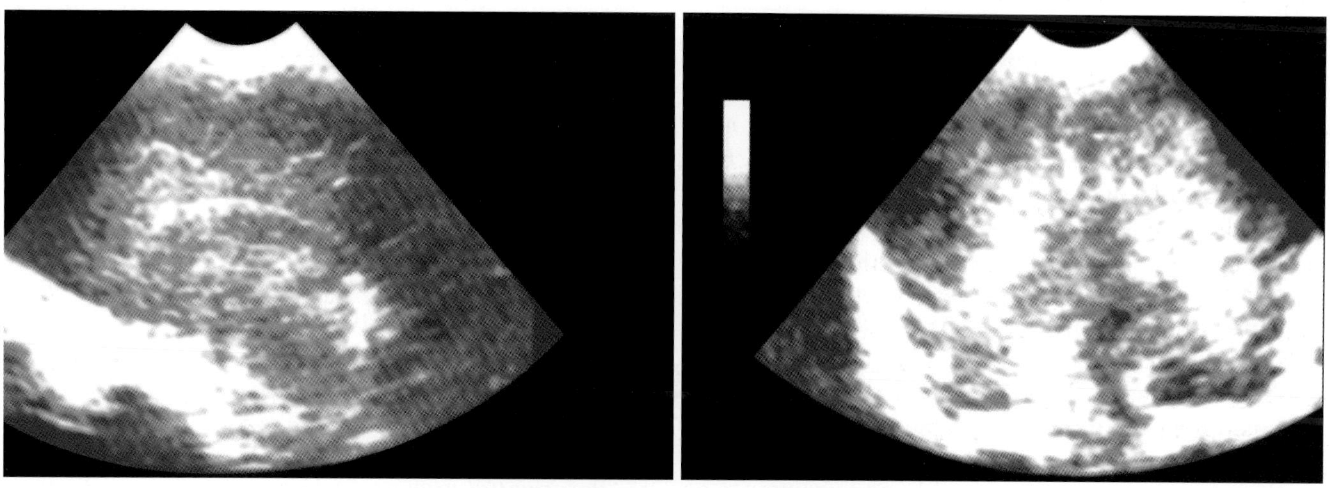

Fig. 20: Cerebral edema: On sonography 'a bright brain' with diffuse increase in echogenicity is seen. Lateral ventricles and other landmarks are obliterated.

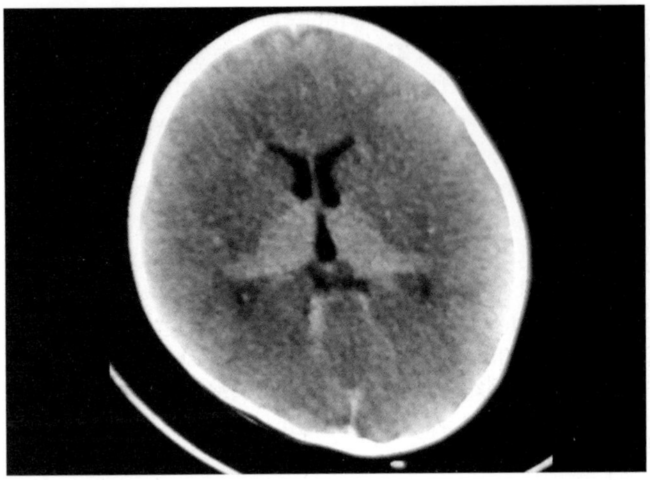

Fig. 21: Axial CT image in a term neonate with severe hypoxia shows diffuse hypodensity involving the cortical gray matter and basal ganglia with loss of gray-white matter differentiation

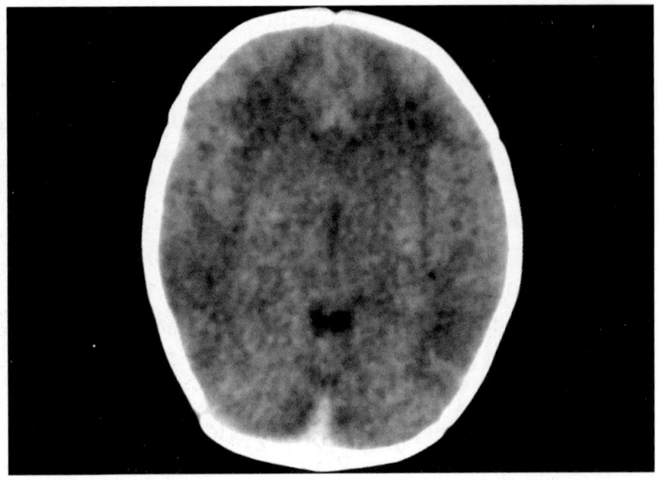

Fig. 22: Axial CT image in another term neonate with severe hypoxic injury shows diffuse cerebral edema with effacement of sulci, cisterns and ventricles.

from early therapeutic intervention.[63-67] Diffusion tensor imaging has also recently shown promise in detecting and timing these lesions by showing decreased FA values in the affected parts of brain which may be seen even after 'pseudonormalization' on DWI.[61]

MRI findings include as follows:

- *T1 hyperintense basal ganglia:* They seen in the first 3 days of life. The posterior putamina are the most commonly involved. It should be remembered that mild T1 hyperintensity of the basal ganglia may be seen in normal infants also. Hence, it is important to see for associated findings of HIE.
- *T1 hyperintense thalami:* The signal change is subtle compared to that of the basal ganglia. When abnormal, the thalami show diffuse hyperintense signal on T1 weighted images **(Figs. 23A and B)**. This should be differentiated from the focal hyperintense signal seen within the posterolateral part of thalami in normal neonates corresponding to the myelination of ventrolateral thalamic nuclei just medial to the terminal portion of the posterior limb of internal capsule. Both the putamina and thalami appear hyperintense on T2 weighted images in the early period but then progress to develop T2 hypointensity by the 2nd week **(Figs. 23A and B)**. The T1 hyperintense signal within the basal ganglia, thalami and also in the perirolandic cortex has been shown to persist for several months.
- *'Absent posterior limb' sign:* The posterior 50% of the posterior limb of internal capsule (PLIC) normally gets myelinated by 37 weeks of gestational age and is then seen as hyperintense on T1 and hypointense on T2 weighted images. Absence of this normal signal characteristics of the PLIC is a sensitive marker of hypoxia in a term infant (beyond 37 weeks of age). Although, it may be seen on the first day of life, it is usually best evident after 3–4 days. In doubtful cases the signal characteristics of PLIC may be compared with the adjacent posterolateral putamen. In normal neonates, the PLIC appears more hyperintense than the posterolateral putamen on T1 weighted images. Reversal of this pattern is considered very sensitive for hypoxic damage. T2 weighted images showing loss of normal hypointensity in the PLIC may be useful in case of doubt on T1 images especially in the setting of abnormal hyperintense signal within the adjacent basal ganglia and thalami secondary to HII **(Figs. 24A and B)**.
- *Abnormal DWI:* Restriction of diffusion may be seen in the basal ganglia, PLIC and thalami in the affected neonates. As stated above, the abnormality may be seen within the first day but usually peaks by about 4–5 days and starts to 'pseudonormalize' by 7–10 days. Initial findings on DWI may underestimate the true extent of injury. Hence, a 'normal' appearing DWI does not exclude insult.
- *Profound global injury*: It involves both the cortical gray and subcortical white matter. It is seen much less commonly than the above 4 patterns. On DWI it is seen as the 'white cerebrum' contrast from normal appearing cerebellum. It is usually fatal. Survivors show multicystic encephalomalacia on follow-up imaging **(Figs. 25A and B)**.
- *Parasagittal gray and white matter injury*: Bilateral cortical and subcortical white matter necrosis in the

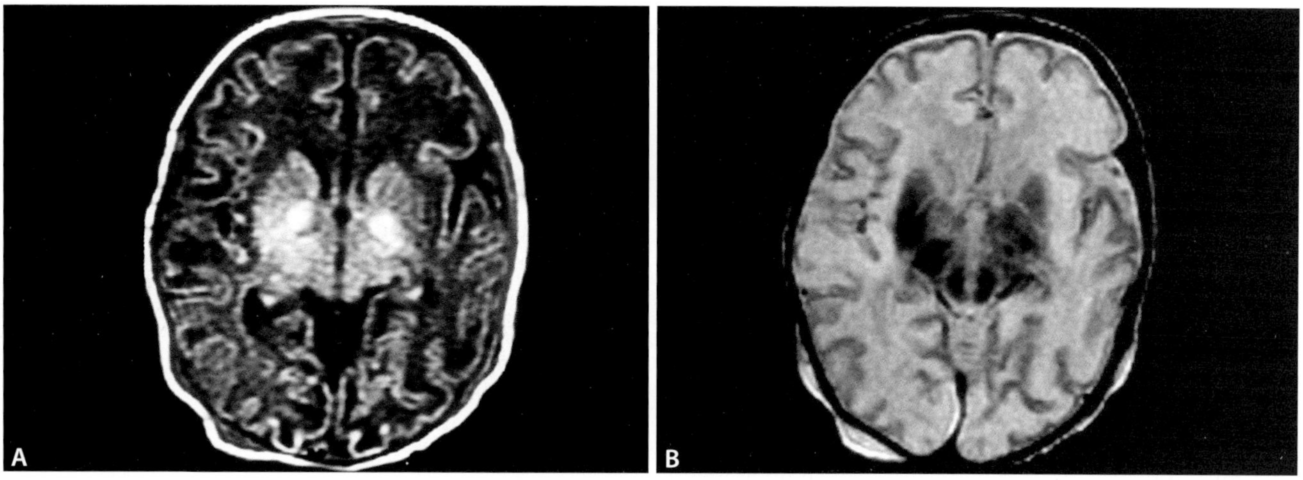

Figs. 23A and B: Axial T1 (A) and T2 (B) weighted MR images in a 6-day-old term neonate with severe hypoxic injury shows the thalami and basal ganglia appearing hyperintense on T1 and hypointense on T2. Also note the loss of normal T1 hyperintense and T2 hypointense signal within the posterior limb of internal capsule.

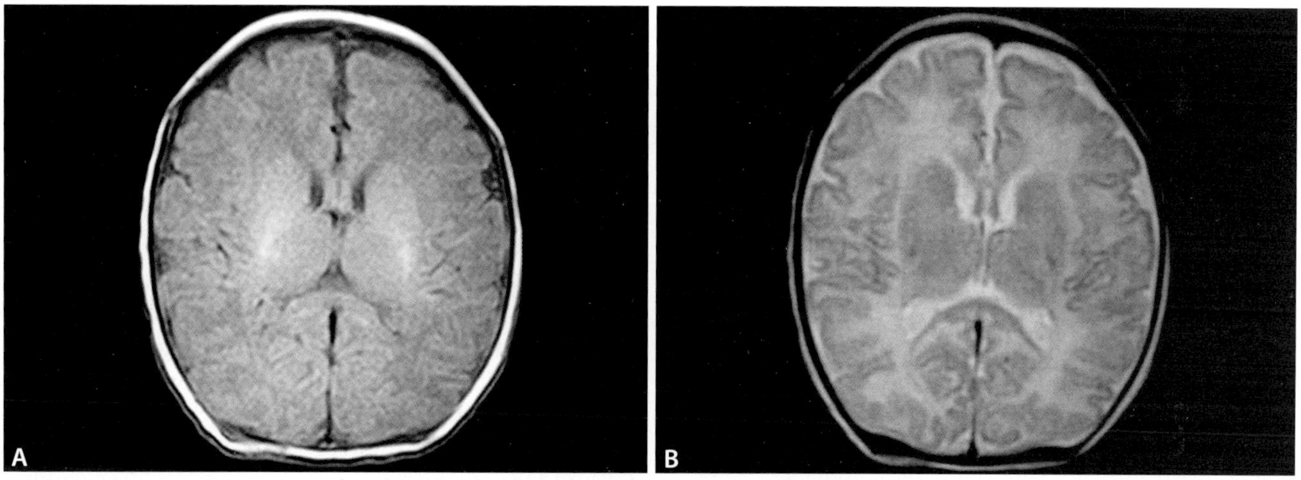

Figs. 24A and B: A 9-day-old term neonate with severe hypoxic injury shows lack of myelination of posterior limb of internal capsule on T1-weighted (A) and T2-weighted (B) axial MR images.

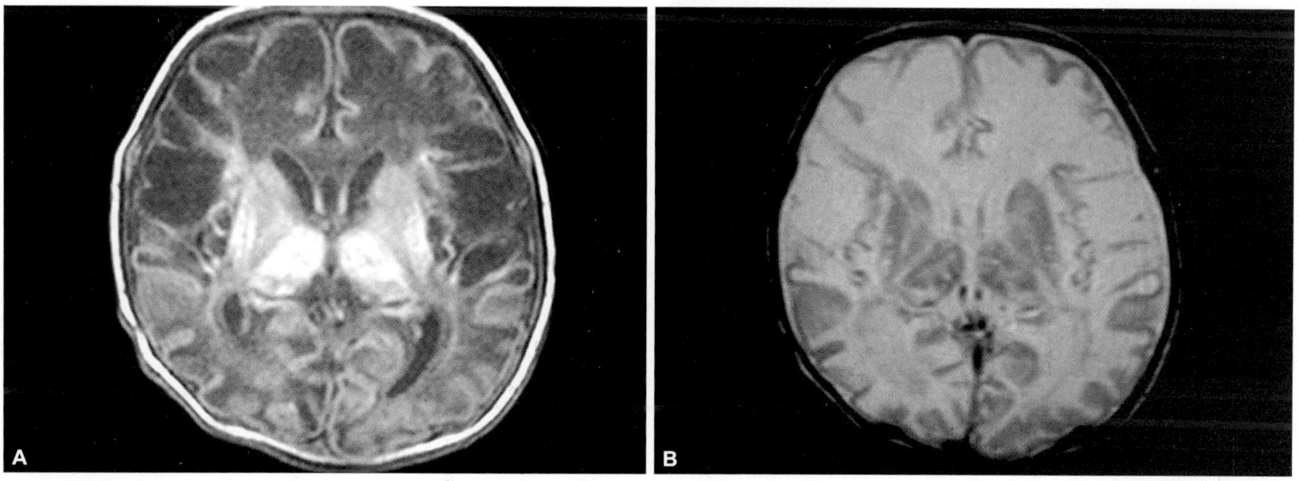

Figs. 25A and B: T1 (A) and T2 (B) weighted axial MR images of an 18-day-old term neonate with severe hypoxic injury show diffuse multicystic encephalomalacia involving cortex and subcortical white matter. Also note the persistent signal changes in the basal ganglia and thalami.

parasagittal areas extending to involve the parieto-occipital areas of the brain.

Follow-up imaging in these neonates show atrophy of the involved structures with T2 hyperintense signal especially in the posterior putamina, ventrolateral thalami and cortcospinal tracts. Also appreciated is thinning of the corpus callosum in the region of the middle or posterior body, secondary to degeneration of the transcallosal fibers.

Prolonged Partial Hypoxia

Prolonged partial asphyxia refers to a more sustained but incomplete loss of oxygenation as seen in prolonged difficult labor with fetal bradycardia. It is also more common after hypotension, hypoglycemia and infection. Hypotension plays a more major role in this type of insult rather than hypoxia. It results in shunting of blood to the vital brain structures, including brainstem, basal ganglia, thalami, hippocampi and cerebellum from the cerebral cortex and white matter which are not so metabolically active. Hence, these above vital brain structures are spared from injury whereas the watershed zones in cortical and subcortical areas get affected. Abnormalities are earliest seen on DWI (best evident as hypointensity on ADC maps) followed by findings on conventional T1 and T2 weighted images. T2 weighted images show cortical swelling and hyperintense signal within the gray and subcortical white matter with loss of gray-white matter differentiation. The parasaggital watershed zones are the most favored site of involvement but the findings may be diffusely seen in the cerebral hemispheres **(Fig. 26)**. Follow-up imaging may show leukomalacia especially in the subcortical areas. This pattern is different from that of a premature neonate where there occurs periventricular leukomalacia.

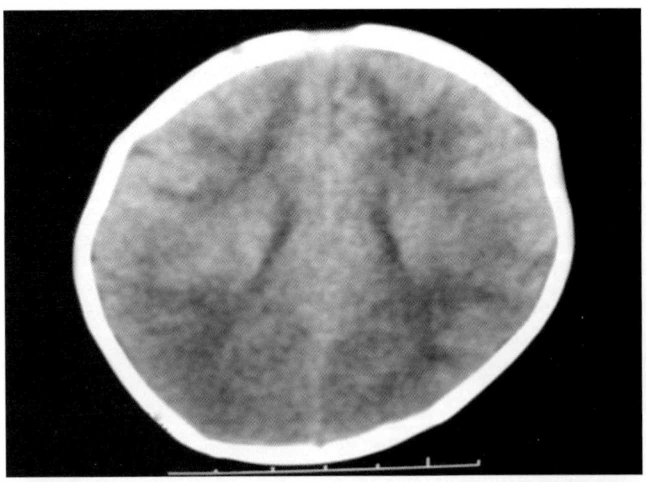

Fig. 26: Axial CT image of a 10-day-old term neonate with prolonged partial asphyxia shows hypodensity involving the watershed zones in the frontal and parieto-occipital regions.

It is important to remember that any given patient may show imaging features suggestive of both severe and partial prolonged hypoxic insult.

HYPOXIC–ISCHEMIC INJURY IN POSTNATAL AGE GROUP

Rapid brain maturation is observed in the postnatal period and the brain becomes almost completed myelinated by 2 years of age. So after 2 years of age the hypoxic injury patterns are similar to those seen in adults. The usual causes for injury in this period are non-accidental trauma, choking, drowning and asphyxiation.

Severe, Total Hypoxia

Profound hypoxic ischemic injury in children between 1 year and 2 years of age affects the basal ganglia, hippocampi, lateral geniculate body and cerebral cortex in the anterior frontal and parieto-occipital region. The perirolandic cortex and thalami are typically spared in contrast to their involvement seen in the perinatal period.[68] Infants below 1 year of age, however, may show an overlap between these categories and therefore may show involvement of thalami and perirolandic cortex along with involvement of basal ganglia, brainstem and other cortical areas. Children above 2 years behave same as adults and basal ganglia, thalami, hippocampi, cerebellum and cortical gray matter gets affected **(Figs. 27A and B)**. Cortex may be diffusely involved or may be limited to perirolandic and parieto-occipital regions. Since cranial ultrasound is not feasible after the closure of anterior fontanelle which occurs by about 4 months of age, CT and MRI are the mainstay of imaging in these children.

CT shows features of basal ganglia hypodensity with features of diffuse cerebral edema with relative sparing of perirolandic regions. Few affected children may also show 'reversal sign' defined as white matter appearing hyperdense compared to the gray matter on CT. This results when diffuse edema in the brain leads to elevated intracranial pressure which causes partial venous obstruction and distension of deep medullary veins within the white matter. The 'white cerebellum sign' may also be noted when the supratentorial brain parenchyma shows diffuse hypodensity and the brainstem and cerebellum are spared. This occurs due to redistribution of blood flow to the posterior circulation.

MRI is more sensitive in showing abnormalities in the affected regions which are seen as hyperintense signal changes in the affected regions on T2-weighted images. DWI are most sensitive with abnormal signal detected within 24 hours.

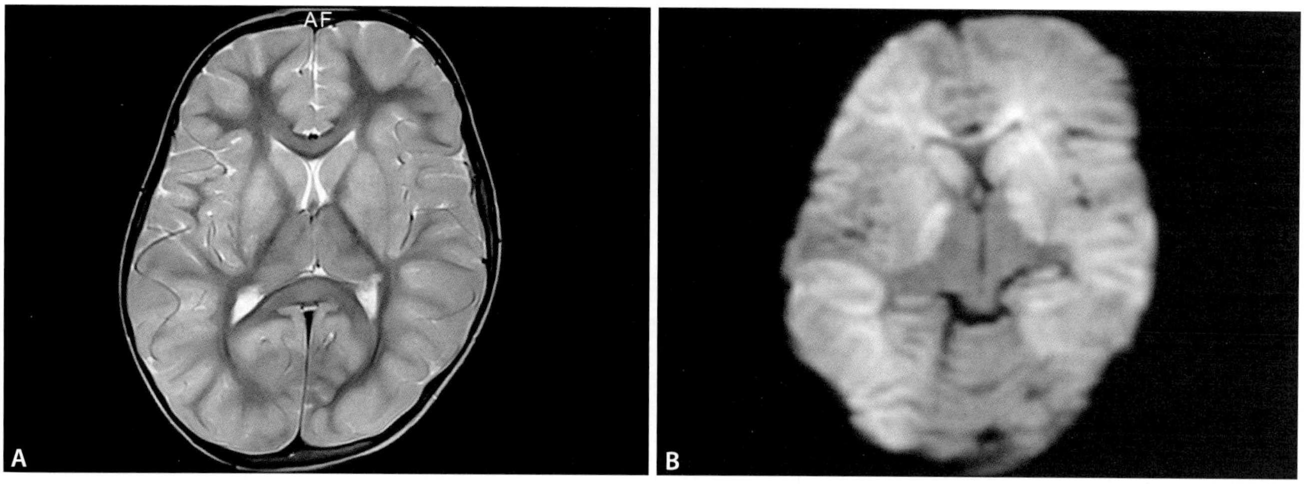

Figs. 27A and B: A 3-year-old girl with hypoxic injury. Axial T2-weighted (A) MR images show hyperintense signal changes within the basal ganglia, thalami and the cortical gray matter which show restricted diffusion on the DWI image (B).

Mild-to-Moderate Hypoxia

The older infants and children below 2 years of age who suffer from mild-to-moderate hypoxia show involvement of cortex and subcortical white matter similar to the pattern seen in the neonates with partial prolonged hypoxia. The watershed zone infarcts are seen with relative sparing of the deep periventricular white matter. The CT and MR features are similar to those described above. On follow-up imaging, T2-weighted MR images may show residual persisting hyperintensity within the involved regions especially within the basal ganglia. T1-weighted images may show gyriform pattern of hyperintensity within the affected cortex representing cortical laminar necrosis.

IMAGING CHOICE FOR EVALUATION OF HYPOXIC–ISCHEMIC INJURY

Neonates with suspected HIE are usually hemodynamically unstable and very sick and therefore a cribside ultrasound in the ICU/nursery is usually the first investigation for screening. Besides portability, the other advantages of US are nonionizing, no IV contrast or sedation is required and can be repeated frequently without harmful effects. Addition of color Doppler and quantitative analysis to 2D imaging may improve information content. However, limitations include low sensitivity and operator dependence. It has good positive predictive value but a negative scan does not rule out injury and in a high-risk scenario the neonate should be evaluated with MRI. CT because of radiation exposure and low sensitivity in presence of unmyelinated white matter is not preferred in the neonatal age group. MRI with conventional T1 and T2 weighted images along with DWI is the modality of choice for further evaluation. It is also more sensitive than ultrasound for early detection and mild changes specially myelination abnormalities. If MR is negative in the early period, MR spectroscopy may be performed or the MRI can be repeated after 3–4 days.[68]

In postnatal age group especially after 4 months of age when anterior fontanelle closes, cranial ultrasound is no longer feasible. In these children, noncontrast CT can be performed as the first investigation. MR may be required for negative scans with high suspicion or for better extent of the injury where CT is positive.

PREDICTION OF CLINICAL OUTCOME

After imaging, the second most important role of a pediatric radiologist in the workup of infants with HIE is to predict, if possible, the clinical outcome based on imaging findings at an early stage. This is a crucial but difficult situation. A number of workers have used different imaging modalities and have reported various parameters to predict the clinical outcome.

Clinically, it has been observed that decreased rate of head growth during early months in a term neonate correlates closely with the neurological dysfunction and cerebral atrophy at a later stage.

Various studies based on imaging to predict the clinical outcome are as follows:

Ultrasound

Echogenic Thalamus

Normal thalamus and basal ganglia region have medium level echoes on ultrasound. In infants with HIE, characteristic increase in the echogenicity of these tissue has been reported,[69] usually in the second week after the episode of asphyxia. Visualization of this sign predicts poor prognosis and has been reported to be associated with mortality in 1% and long-term morbidity in 56%.

Cerebral Artery Doppler

Duplex scanning of the cerebral arteries has been studied, both in normal neonates as well as in those affected by perinatal asphyxia.[70,71] Resistive Index (RI), the single most important Doppler parameter, has been used to measure the flow abnormality. Mean RI in normal healthy neonates is 75 and is inversely related to gestational age. With an RI of 60 as the critical level and all cases with values below 60 taken as abnormal, it has been observed that clinical outcome is poor even though 2D sonogram may appear normal. Thus, Doppler scanning of cerebral arteries may provide an easy and a reliable parameter on day 1 of life to predict the clinical outcome in a neonate with HIE.

CT

Reversal Sign

Presence of reversal sign, i.e. diffuse decreased attenuation of the cerebral cortex **(Figs. 24A and B)** with a relative preservation of density in the thalami, brainstem and cerebellum, has been observed to be associated with poor prognosis **(Fig. 21)**.[72] Exact mechanism of this sign is not clear although a number of theories have been put forward, e.g. mechanical factor, postischemic hypervascularity, distension of deep medullary veins and high serum glucose level. The sonographic counterpart of reversal sign of CT is echogenic thalamus discussed earlier.

Diffuse Decreased Density

Diffuse low attenuation is a common finding, both in the preterm and term neonates,[6] affected by perinatal asphyxia. However, diffuse low attenuation in preterm (below 34 weeks gestation) has no predictive value because there is very poor correlation with late neurologic sequelae. Reason for it is obvious, i.e. difficulty in differentiating pathological low attenuation from normal immature myelin tissue at this age. On the other hand, diffuse low attenuation in a term neonate is a very important prognostic predictor because it has a good correlation with poor clinical outcome.

MR Imaging

Conventional Sequences

Delayed myelination is one of the hallmark of HIE which can be detected only on MRI. Studies have shown that delayed myelination in a term neonate in the first few days of life suggests significant perinatal asphyxia and hence poor prognosis. With the introduction of serial quantitative tensor MRI technique, assessment for white matter injury has become more reliable and at an early stage.[53-56] Delayed myelination on MRI may, therefore, be used as an early predictor of clinical outcome.

In mature term neonates, abnormal signal intensity within the PLIC has been found to be an excellent predictor of abnormal motor outcome. Asymmetrical involvement predicts hemiplegia and bilateral symmetrical involvement correlates with subsequent development of spastic diplegia or quadriplegia.[73] The severity of basal ganglia and thalamic lesions detected on MRI also has good correlate with severity and nature of cerebral palsy. The involvement of white matter exacerbates cognitive impairment and poor head growth.[74]

In premature neonates, finding of PVHI correlates well with development of hemiplegia in survivors whereas PVL correlates more with spastic diplegia. It has also been observed that most of the neonates with documented PVL on US/CT alongwith DEHSI had neurologic abnormality.[75-77] Also, a general correlation between the neurological impairment and the severity of MR abnormalities was demonstrated. Abnormalities on MRI scan, therefore, can be used not only to predict the neurological deficit but also its severity.

MR Spectroscopy

MR spectroscopy has proved invaluable to detect early brain injury with good correlation between the degree of abnormality and the clinical outcome. Therefore, MRS may be used as a predictor of prognosis.

CONCLUSION

Hypoxic–ischemic encephalopathy is a relatively common clinical problem in the neonatal period. Pathological changes depend upon the gestational age. Imaging features, therefore, also differ in the preterm and term infants. Depending upon the gestational age and the abnormality suspected, a particular imaging modality is chosen.

Cranial ultrasound remains the first screening modality specially in the premature neonate. However, MRI has a vast potential not only to detect subtle, early, specific abnormalities, but also to predict clinical outcome based on imaging features in the first few days of life. MR spectroscopy has also shown good promise in early detection of changes.

A close cooperation and teamwork is, therefore, required between the neonatologist and the pediatric radiologist to decide the imaging approach appropriate for the gestational age, suspected pathology, imaging facilities available and the expertise, both in performing and interpreting the images, without duplicating the information and keeping the cost-benefit in view.

REFERENCES

1. Singh M. Hypoxic ischemic encephalopathy. In: Talukdar B (Ed): Essentials of Pediatric Neurology, New Age International (P) Ltd Publishers. 1997;95-107.
2. Legido A, Katoseos CD, Mishra OP, et al. Perinatal hypoxic ischemic encephalopathy: Current and future treatments. International Pediatrics. 2000;15:143-51.
3. Teaching files. Perinatal asphyxia (Hypoxic ischaemic encephalopathy). By: Division of Neonatology, Cedars-Sinai Medical Center, Los Angeles, California, Webmaster@ neonatology.org.
4. Vannucci RC, Perlman JM. Interventions for perinatal hypoxic ischaemic encephalopathy. Pediatrics. 1997;100:1004-114.
5. Flodmark O. The neonatal brain-imaging for prognosis. In: Harwood-Nash DC, Pettersson H (Eds): Paediatric Radiology. NICER series on Diagnostic Imaging, Merit Communications; 1992.pp.16-25.
6. Barkovich AJ. Brain and spine injuries. In Barkovich AJ (Ed). Pediatric Neuroimaging, 4th edition. Lippincott Williams & Wilkins; 2005.pp.190-290.
7. Horwood LJ, Mogridge N, Darlow BA. Cognitive, educational and behavioral outcomes at 7 to 8 years in a national very low birthweight cohort. Arch Dis Child Fetal Neonatal. 1998;79:12-20.
8. Emslie HC, Wardle SP, Sims DG, et al. Increased survival and deteriorating developmental outcome in 23–25 weeks gestation infants. 1990–1994 compared with 1984–1989. Arch Dis Child Fetal Neonatal. 1998;78:99-104.
9. Keeney SE, Adecock EW, McArdle CB. Prospective observations of 100 high risk neonates by high field (1.5 Tesla) magnetic resonance imaging of the central nervous system: I. Intraventricular and extracerebral lesions. Pediatrics. 1991;87:421-30.
10. Keeney SE, Adecock EW, McArdle CB. Prospective observations of 100 high risk neonates by high field (1.5 Tesla) magnetic resonance imaging of the central nervous system:II. Lesions associated with hypoxic-ischemic encephalopathy. Pediatrics. 1991;87:431-8.
11. Koeda T, Suganuma I, Kohno Y, et al. MR imaging of spastic diplegia: Comparative study between preterm and term infants. Neuroradiology. 1990;32:187-90.
12. Flodmark O, Roland EH, Hill A, et al. Periventricular leukomalacia: Radiologic diagnosis. Radiology. 1987;162: 119-24.
13. Barkovich AJ, Westmark K, Partridge C, et al. Perinatal asphyxia: MR findings in the first 10 days. AJNR. 1995;16:427-38.
14. Flodmark O, Lupton B, Li D, et al. MR imaging of periventricular leukomalacia in childhood. Am J Neuroradiol. 1989;10:111-8.
15. Huppi PS. MR in HIE. Clinical Perinatol. 2002;29(4):827-56.
16. Barkovich AJ, Sargent SK. Profound asphyxia in the premature infant: Imaging findings. Am J Neuroradiol. 1995;16:1837-46.
17. Hambleton G, Wigglesworth JS. Origin of intraventricular hemorrhage in preterm infant. Arch Dis Child. 1976;51:651-60.
18. Wigglesworth JS, Pape KE. An integrated model for hemorrhage and ischemic lesions in the newborn brain. Early Hum Dev. 1978;2:179-99.
19. Papile LA, Brustein J, Koffer H. Incidence and evolution of subependymal and intraventricular hemorrhage: A study of infants with birth weight less than 1500 gm. J Pediatr. 1978;92:529-34.
20. Gould SJ, Howard S, Hope PL, et al. Periventricular intraparenchymal cerebral hemorrhage in preterm infants: Role of venous infarction. J Pathol. 1987;151:197-202.
21. Volpe JJ: Brain injury in premature infant. Neuropathology, clinical aspects and pathogenesis. MRDD Res Rev. 1997;3:3-12.
22. Del Toro J, Louis PT, Goddard–Finegold J. Cerebrovascular regulation and neonatal brain injury. Pediatr Neurol. 1991;7:3-12.
23. Hill A. Current concepts of hypoxic-ischemic cerebral injury in the term newborn. Pediatr Neurol. 1991;7:317-25.
24. Volpe JJ. Hypoxic-ischemic encephalopathy: Neuropathology and pathogenesis. In: Volpe JJ (Ed): Neurology of the Newborn, 3rd edition. Philadelphia: Saunders. 1995;279-313.
25. Rutherford MA, Supramaniam V, Ederies A, Chew A, Bassi L, Groppo M, et al. Magnetic resonance imaging of white matter diseases of prematurity. Neuroradiology. 2010;52:505-21.
26. Maria A, Gupta AK, Paul VK, et al. Germinal matrix-Intraventricular hemorrhage of the premature infants and PVL. In: Kalra V (Ed): Practical Paediatric Neurology, Arya Publications 36-38. 2002. [From DM Dissertation of Maria A at AIIMS: Periventricular leukomalacia among the very low birth weight neonates, August. 2003].
27. Zupan V, Gonzalez P, Lacaze-Masmonteil T, et al. Periventricular leukomalacia: Risk factors revisited. Dev Med Child Neurol. 1996;38:1061-7.
28. Verma U, Tehani N, Klein S, et al. Obstetric antecedents of intraventricular haemorrhage and periventricular leukomalacia in the low birth weight neonate. Am J Obstet Gynecol. 1997;176:275-81.
29. Nelson K, Ellenberg J. Antecedents of cerebral palsy: Multivariate analysis of risk. N Engl J Med. 1986;315:81-6.
30. Back SA, Luo NL, Borenstein NS, Levine JM, Volpe JJ, Kinney HC. Late oligodendrocyte progenitors coincide with the developmental window of vulnerability for human perinatal white matter injury. J Neurosci. 2001;21:1302-12.

31. Back SA, Han BH, Luo NL, et al. Selective vulnerability of late oligodendrocyte progenitors to hypoxia-ischemia. J Neurosci. 2002;22:455-63.
32. Perlman JM, et al. Bilateral cystic PVL in the premature infants: Associated risk factors. Pediatrics. 1996;97:822-7.
33. Hesser U, Katz-Salamon M, Mortensson W, et al. Diagnosis of intracranial lesions in very low birth weight infants by ultrasound: Incidence and association with potential risk factors. Acta Pediatr Suppl. 1997;419:16-26.
34. Claris O, Besnier S, Lapillonne A, et al. Incidence of ischemic hemorrhagic cerebral lesions in premature infants of gestational age 28 weeks: A prospective ultrasound study. Biol Neonate. 1996;70:29-34.
35. McArdle CB, Richardson CJ, Hayden CK, et al. Abnormalities of the neonatal brain: MR Imaging Part II. Hypoxic-Ischemic brain injury. Radiology. 1987;163:395-403.
36. Banker BQ, Larroche JC. Periventricular leukomalacia in infancy: A form of neonatal anoxic encephalopathy. Arch Neurol. 1962;7:386-410.
37. Weisglas-Kuperus N, Baerts W, Fetter W, et al. Minor neurological dysfunction and quality of movement in relation to neonatal cerebral damage and subsequent development. Dev Med Child Neurol. 1994;36:727-35.
38. Pinto-Martin JA, Dobson V, Cnaan A, et al. Vision outcome at age 2 years in a low birth weight population. Pediatr Neurol. 1996;14:281-87.
39. Uggetti C, Egitto ME, Fazzi E, et al. Cerebral visual impairment in periventricular leukomalacia: MR correlation. AJNR. 1996;17:979-85.
40. Roth SC, Baudin J, McCormick DC, et al. Relation between ultrasound appearance of the brain of very preterm infants and neurodevelopmental impairment at eight years. Dev Med Child Neurol. 1993;35:755-68.
41. Barr LL, McCullough PJ, Ball WS, et al. Quantitative sonographic feature analysis of clinical infant hypoxia: A pilot study. AJNR. 1996;17:1025-31.
42. Vannucci RC, Christensen MA, Yager JY. Nature, time course and extent of cerebral edema in perinatal hypoxic ischaemic brain damage. Pediatr Neurol. 1993;9:29-34.
43. Grant EG, Schellinger D, Richardson JD, et al. Echogenic periventricular halo: Normal sonographic finding or neonatal cerebral hemorrhage? AJNR. 1983;4:43-6.
44. de Vries LS, Eken P, Dubowitz LMS. The spectrum of leukomalacia using cranial ultrasound. Behav Brain Res. 1992;49:1-6.
45. Perlman JM. Guidelines for cranial ultrasounds in premature infants. In *http://neonatal.peds.washington.edu/NICU-WEB/ultrasound.pdf.*
46. Debillon, et al. Limitations of ultrasound for diagnosing white matter damage in preterm infants. Archives of Diseases in Childhood Fetal & Neonatal. 2003;88:275.
47. Miller, et al. Comparing the diagnosis of white matter injury in premature newborns with serial MR imaging and transfontanel ultrasonography findings. AJNR. 2003;24:1661-9.
48. Inder TE, et al. White matter injury in the premature infants: A comparison between serial cranial sonographic and MR findings at term. AJNR. 2003;24(5):805-9.
49. Graham, et al. Prediction of cerebral palsy in very low birth weight infants: Prospective ultrasound study. Lancet. 1987;2(8559):593-6.
50. Arthur R. Magnetic resonance imaging in preterm infants. Pediatr Radiol. 2006;36:593-607.
51. Bozzao, et al. Diffusion weighted MR imaging in the early diagnosis of PVL. Eur Radiol. 2003;13(7):1571-6.
52. Roelants-van Rijn, et al. Neonatal diffusion weighted MRI: Relation with histopathology or follow-up MR examination. Neuropediatrics. 2001;32(6):286-94.
53. Arzoumanian Y, et al. Diffusion Tensor Brain imaging findings at term equivalent age may predict neurologic abnormalities in low birth weight preterm infants. AJNR. 2003;24:1646-53.
54. Miller, et al. Serial quantitative diffusion tensor MRI of the premature brain—development in newborns with and without injury. J Magn Reson Imaging. 2002;16(6):621-32.
55. Hoon, et al. Diffusion Tensor imaging of PVL shows affected sensory cortex white matter pathways. Neurology. 2002;59(5):752-6.
56. Melhelm ER, et al. Diffusion Tensor MR imaging of the brain and white matter tractography. AJR. 2002;178:3-16.
57. Baker LL, Stevenson DK, Enzmann DR. End stage periventricular leukomalacia: MR evaluation. Radiology. 1988;168:809-15.
58. Hull J, Dodd KL. Falling incidence of hypoxic ischemic encephalopathy in term infants. Br J Obstet Gynecol. 1992;99: 386-91.
59. Truwit CL, Barkovich AJ, Koch TK, et al. Cerebral palsy: MR findings in 40 patients. AJNR. 1992;13:67-78.
60. Raybaud C. Destructive lesions of the brain. Neuroradiology. 1983;25:265-91.
61. Rutherford M, Srinivasan L, Dyet L, Ward P, Allsop J, Counsell S, Cowan F. Magnetic resonance imaging in perinatal brain injury: Clinical presentation, lesions and outcome. Pediatr Radiol. 2006;36:582-92.
62. Hunt RW, Neil JJ, Coleman LT, Kean MJ, Inder TE. Apparent diffusion coefficient in the posterior limb of the internal capsule predicts outcome after perinatal asphyxia. Pediatrics. 2004;114(4):999-1003.
63. De Vries LS, Groenendaal F. Patterns of neonatal hypoxic-ischemic brain injury. Neuroradiology. 2010;52:555-66.
64. Hanrahan JD, Sargentoni J, Azzopardi D, et al. Cerebral metabolism within 18 hours of birth asphyxia: A proton magnetic resonance spectroscopy study. Pediatr Res. 1996;39:584-90.
65. Peden CJ, Cowan FM, Bryant DJ, et al. Proton MR spectroscopy of the brain in infants. J Comput Assist Tomogr. 1990;14:886-94.
66. Holshouser BA, Ashwal S, Luh GY, et al. Proton MR spectroscopy after acute central nervous system injury: Outcome prediction in neonates, infants and children. Radiology. 1997;202:487-96.

67. Penrice J, Cady EB, Lorek A, et al. Proton MR spectroscopy of the brain in normal preterm and term infants and early changes after perinatal hypoxic ischemia. Pediatr Res. 1996;40:6-14.
68. Huang BY, Castillo M. Hypoxic-ischemic brain injury: Imaging findings from birth to adulthood. Radiographics. 2008;28:417-39.
69. Connolly B, Kelehan P, Brien NO, et al. The echogenic thalamus in hypoxic-ischemic encephalopathy. Pediatr Radiol. 1994;24:268-71.
70. Seibert JJ, McCowan TC, Chadduck WM, et al. Duplex pulsed Doppler US vs intracranial pressure in the neonate. Clinical and experimental studies. Radiology. 1989;171:155-9.
71. Stark JE, Seibert JJ. Cerebral artery Doppler ultrasonography for prediction of outcome after perinatal asphyxia. J Ultrasound Med. 1994;13:595-600.
72. KimHan B, Towbin RB, DeCourten-Meyers G, et al. Reversal sign on CT: Effect of anoxic/ischaemic cerebral injury in children. AJR. 1990;154:361-8.
73. Rutherford MA, Pennock JM, Counsell SJ, et al. Abnormal magnetic resonance signal in the internal capsule predicts poor neurodevelopmental outcome in infants with hypoxic-ischemic encephalopathy. Pediatrics. 1998;102:323-8.
74. Rutherford M, Biarge MM, Allsop J, Counsell S, Cowan F. MRI of perinatal brain injury. Pediatr Radiol. 2010;40:819-33.
75. Cordes I, Roland EH, Lupton BA, et al. Early prediction of the development of microcephaly after HIE in full term newborn. Pediatrics. 1994;93:703-7.
76. Han, et al. Risk factors for cerebral palsy in preterm. Am J Phy Med Rehab. 2002;81:297-303.
77. van de Bor, et al. Value of cranial ultrasound and MRI in predicting neurodevelopmental outcome in preterm infants. Pediatrics. 1992;90:196-9.

CHAPTER 152

Cranial Sonography

Rashmi Dixit, Veena Chowdhury

INTRODUCTION

Neurosonography is an integral part of neonatal and infant brain imaging while the fontanels remain open. Current ultrasound equipment allows rapid evaluation of infants in the intensive care nursery with excellent visualization of normal structures and a wide range of pathologies.[1] The advantages of sonography over computed tomography or magnetic resonance imaging include portability, lower cost, lack of ionizing radiation and no need for sedation.[2]

TECHNIQUE AND NORMAL ANATOMY

Neurosonography is most successfully performed in a warm environment, when the baby is quiet or after feeding. For neonates, a 5–7.5 MHz sector transducer and for older infants, a 3–5 MHz transducer provides adequate visualization of the whole brain.[3,4] High frequency (7–10 MHz) sector or curvilinear array probes are excellent for demonstrating the superficial extracerebral spaces and to delineate the sulcal pattern as well as corticomedullary regions in the near field.[5] 3D ultrasound has also been used to evaluate the infant brain.

The anterior fontanel is the primary acoustic window and remains open for the first 6–12 months of life.[6] Images are obtained in the coronal and sagittal planes. Additional views may be obtained through the posterior fontanel, mastoid fontanel and by transaxial scanning through the squamous temporal bone.[4] The posterior fontanel and mastoid fontanel approach can significantly improve the diagnostic utility of neurosonography. The mastoid fontanel approach improves visualization of the brainstem, cerebellum and subarachnoid cisterns which are suboptimally seen through the anterior fontanel. Also, small intraventricular hemorrhages may be better visualized through posterior fontanel. The midline post-fontanel usually closes by about 3 months of age, whereas mastoid (posterolateral) fontanel may not fuse until 2 years of age.[7] Important intracranial structures seen on coronal and sagittal sonograms are shown in **Figures 1 and 2**.

Cranial Doppler US

The anterior fontanel approach for Doppler US provides the most easily accessible view and reveals the best anatomic detail. A combination of coronal scans allows consistent identification of the major intracranial vessels, including anterior cerebral artery (A1 segment and distal segment), internal carotid artery and basilar artery. The M1 segment of the middle cerebral artery is not well demonstrated as the direction of blood flow is nearly perpendicular to the Doppler beam. The internal cerebral veins and the vein of Galen are easily seen on the midsagittal view. The superior sagittal sinus and straight sinus can also be identified.[2]

The temporal approach through the thin squamous portion of the temporal bone provides detailed images of the midbrain and the vessels forming the circle of Willis. The proximal segments of the anterior and middle cerebral arteries and the M1 portion is well seen due to the more favorable Doppler angle. This approach can also be used in older children when the anterior fontanel is closed.[2,4]

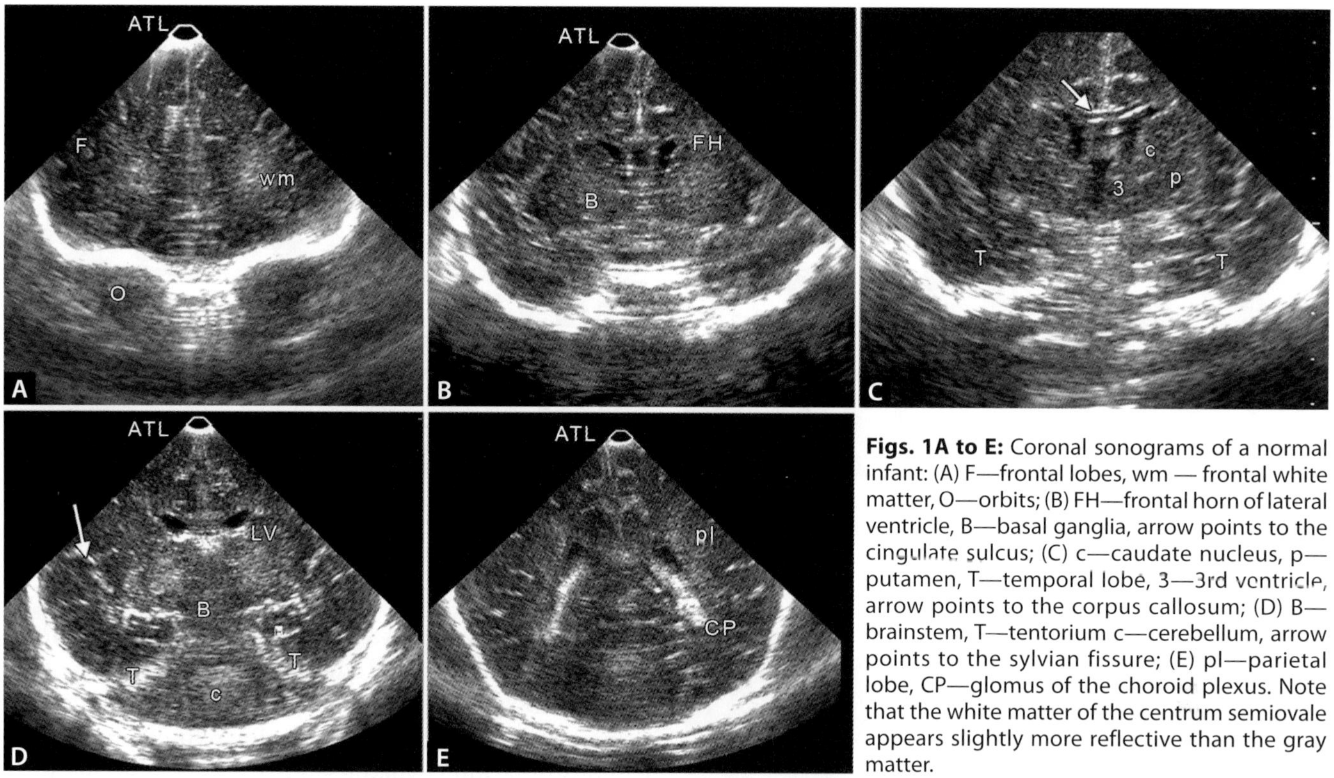

Figs. 1A to E: Coronal sonograms of a normal infant: (A) F—frontal lobes, wm — frontal white matter, O—orbits; (B) FH—frontal horn of lateral ventricle, B—basal ganglia, arrow points to the cingulate sulcus; (C) c—caudate nucleus, p—putamen, T—temporal lobe, 3—3rd ventricle, arrow points to the corpus callosum; (D) B—brainstem, T—tentorium c—cerebellum, arrow points to the sylvian fissure; (E) pl—parietal lobe, CP—glomus of the choroid plexus. Note that the white matter of the centrum semiovale appears slightly more reflective than the gray matter.

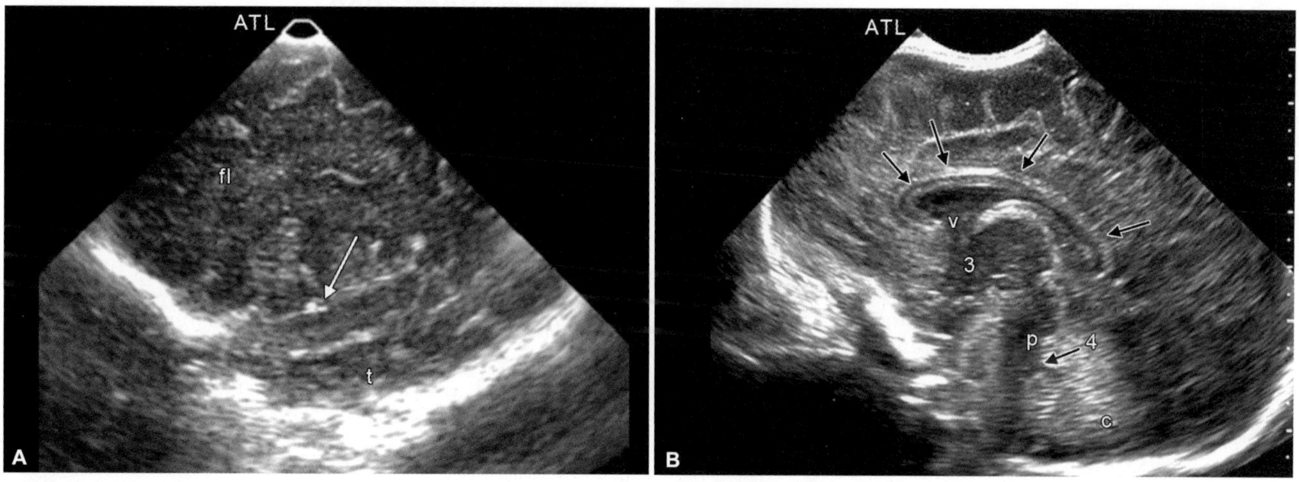

Figs. 2A and B: (A) Parasagittal and (B) midline sagittal scans of a normal infant: (A) fl—frontal lobe, t—temporal lobe, arrow points to the sylvian fissure; (B) v—cavum septum pellucidum and cavum vergae, 3—3rd ventricle, p—pons, 4—4th ventricle.

The brain is a low-resistance vascular bed and continuous forward flow should be seen throughout the arteries in systole and diastole. In term infant, RI ranges from 60 to 78%.[8,9] It is slightly higher (68–88%) in infants less than 34 weeks gestational age.[8] Besides pathological conditions, elevated RI may be seen with increased scanning pressure, high pass filter settings and in the presence of a patent ductus arteriosus. Continued refinement of ultrasound contrast agents allows quantitative cerebral perfusion mapping.[10]

The normal vascular anatomy as seen by CDFI is depicted in **Figures 3 to 5**.

CONGENITAL BRAIN ANOMALIES

These may occur at any stage of brain development. Sonography is often the first modality used for an infant

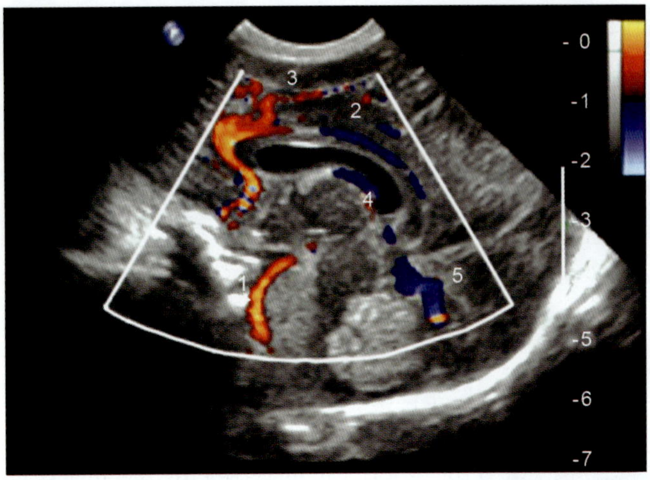

Fig. 3: Midline sagittal color Doppler scan showing internal cerebral artery (1), pericallosal artery (2), callosomarginal artery (3), internal cerebral vein (4), straight sinus (5).

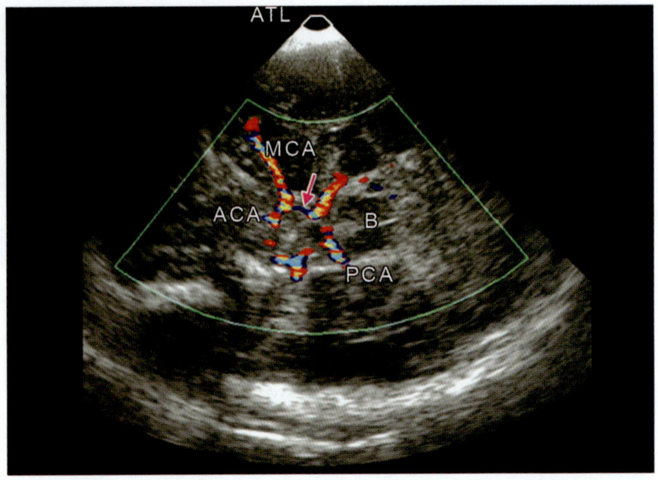

Fig. 4: Axial section through the squamous temporal bone showing the vessels of the circle of Willis, arrow points to the posterior communicating artery.

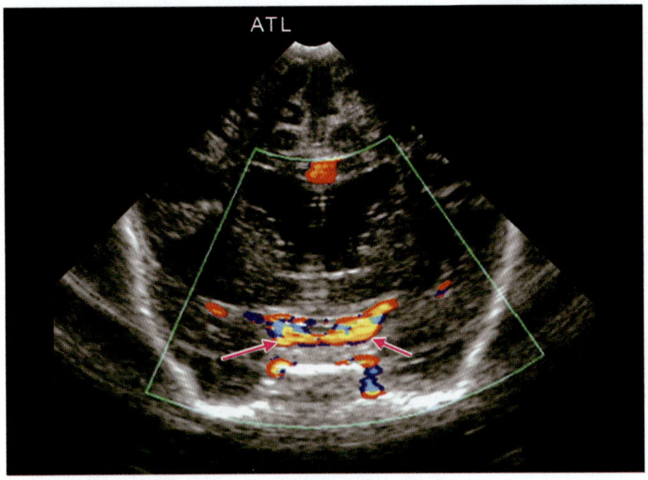

Fig. 5: Coronal CDFI scan showing ICA on both sides, arrows point to their bifurcation on both sides.

with a congenital brain malformation. Many anomalies will be diagnozed, while in others, it is useful in directing the patient to MR imaging which is the current standard of reference.

Failure of Neural Tube Closure

The first stage in brain development is neural tube closure in the 1st month of gestation, failure of which caudally causes myelomeningocele and cranially causes anencephaly or encephalocele. A myelomeningocele is very often associated with a Chiari II malformation. Aqueductal stenosis may also develop during neural tube closure in the first trimester. It often causes obstructive hydrocephalus and may lead to severe brain damage.

Infants born with a myelomeningocele require a cranial examination to establish the baseline status of the ventricular system, which frequently enlarges following primary repair of the spinal lesion, due to change in cerebrospinal fluid dynamics.

Chiari II Malformation

Sonographic Appearance

Sagittal sonograms demonstrate a small posterior fossa resulting in displacement of the cerebellar vermis, fourth ventricle and medulla into the cervical canal with a medullary kink. The fourth ventricle is often poorly visualized as it is thin, elongated, compressed and displaced into the upper spinal canal.

The degree of ventricular dilatation is variable at presentation but is usually progressive. The occipital horns and atria are disproportionately dilated compared to the frontal and temporal horns (colpocephaly). On coronal images, there is anterior and inferior pointing of the frontal horns referred to as 'batwing configuration'. The septum pellucidum may be partially or completely absent. The massa intermedia is enlarged and fills a dilated third ventricle. The interhemispheric fissure is often prominent in these patients.[2] Sonography has been a reliable method for follow-up of shunting procedures and evaluation of hydrocephalus in the first year of life,[2] although abnormalities of the Chiari malformation are best appreciated on MRI.

Agenesis of the Corpus Callosum

Corpus callosum forms during the first 8–12 weeks of gestation. Depending on the timing of intrauterine insult, the development can be partially arrested or complete agenesis may occur and is frequently associated with major malformations. The bundles of Probst that failed to fuse will persist as rounded masses on each side of the midline. The key sonographic findings are widely spaced lateral ventricles which are tiny anteriorly and enlarged posteriorly. The frontal horns are slit like, widely separated with concave medial margins and superolateral peaks. The third ventricle is dilated and high placed and often associated with a dorsal cyst **(Fig. 6)**. On midline sagittal images, the sulci are arranged radially above the third ventricle.[2,4] It is difficult to diagnose partial agenesis on sonography.

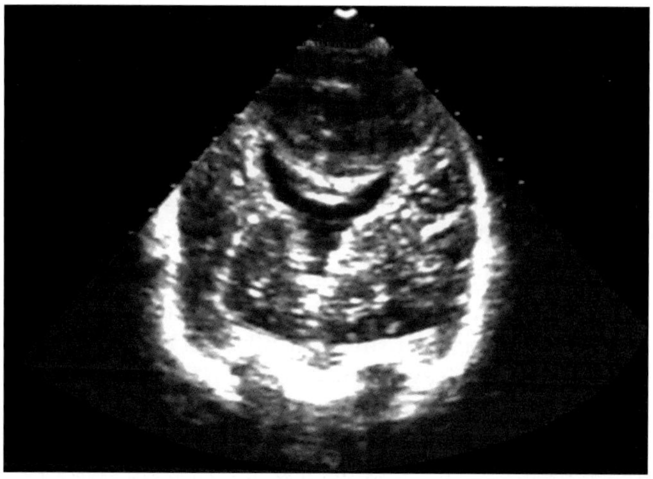

Fig. 6: Coronal sonogram showing frontal horns with concave medial borders and sharply angled lateral peaks. The third ventricle is also mildly dilated and slightly high placed, consistent with agenesis of corpus callosum.

Dandy–Walker Complex

This includes the Dandy-Walker syndrome and Dandy-Walker variant.

The Dandy-Walker (DW) syndrome may be caused by obstruction of the outlet of the fourth ventricle. The fourth ventricle is enlarged and communicates with a large posterior fossa cyst. There is hypoplasia of the cerebellar vermis and cerebellar hemispheres which are displaced anterolaterally. The posterior fossa is large with elevation of tentorium cerebelli, straight sinus and torcular herophili. The brainstem may be compressed or hypoplastic. The cerebral aqueduct may be narrowed or occluded. Generalized obstructive hydrocephalus occurs in 80% of patients **(Figs. 7A and B)**. If corpus callosum is hypogenetic, colpocephaly is present. In patients with aqueductal stenosis, separate shunts may be required for the supratentorial ventricles and post fossa cyst.

In the DW variant, the posterior fossa is normal in size and although the vermis is small, the cerebellar hemispheres are normal. The fourth ventricle is slightly to moderately enlarged and communicates with the cisterna magna. The differential diagnosis includes a giant cisterna magna and posterior fossa arachnoid cyst **(Fig. 8)**. In these conditions, the cerebellar vermis and hemispheres are not hypoplastic and the cyst does not communicate with the fourth ventricle.[11-14]

Disorders of Diverticulation

The second stage of brain development during the 2nd month of gestation is diverticulation into two hemispheres, development of the pineal and pituitary glands as well

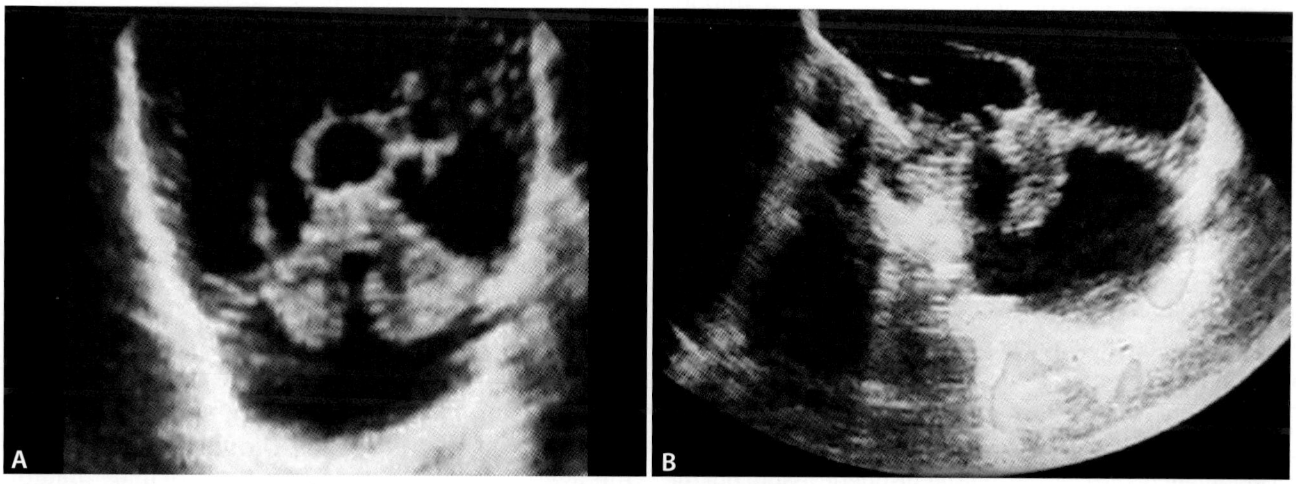

Figs. 7A and B: Coronal and sagittal sonograms showing a large posterior fossa cyst communicating with the fourth ventricle with hypoplastic vermis and cerebellar hemispheres which are displaced anterolaterally. Marked generalized hydrocephalus is present.

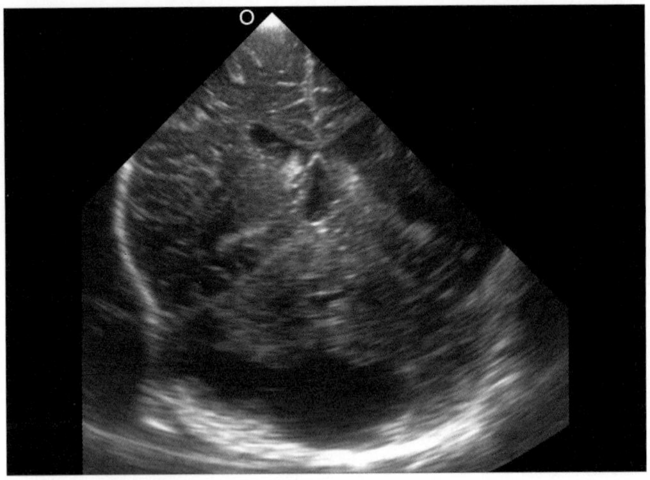

Fig. 8: Coronal sonogram through the anterior fontanel shows a large cyst in the posterior fossa not communicating with the fourth ventricle with normal cerebellum—Giant cisterna magna.

as optic and olfactory tracts. Malformations include the spectrum from simple absence of the septum pellucidum to alobar holoprosencephaly. Since the face is formed at the same time, severe midline facial abnormalities are often present.[13]

Holoprosencephaly

A failure of midline cleavage of the prosencephalon causes failure of formation of separate cerebral hemispheres.

The most severe form of holoprosencephaly is **alobar holoprosencephaly**. On sonography, there is a single horseshoe or crescent-shaped monoventricle which communicates with a large dorsal cyst. The thalami are fused and the third ventricle is absent, as are the corpus callosum and interhemispheric fissure. The cortex is thin with sparse convolutional markings and a smooth appearance to the brain surface. The cerebellum and brainstem are often spared. If Doppler is applied, absence of anterior cerebral arteries or occurrence of only a single vessel may be noted. There is absence of internal cerebral veins, the superior sagittal sinus and straight sinus.[3,15]

Semilobar holoprosencephaly is the less severe, variant. The single ventricle persists, but there may be separate occipital and temporal horns. Portions of the septum pellucidum and corpus callosum may be present posteriorly. The thalami are partially fused along the floor of the malformed third ventricle.

Lobar holoprosencephaly is the least severe form. There is nearly complete separation of the hemispheres with development of the falx and interhemispheric fissure but the anteroinferior portion is incomplete and the frontal lobes are fused. The septum pellucidum is absent. The anterior horns of the lateral ventricles are fused and square shaped but occipital horns are separated. The third ventricle is usually present, separating the thalami and the splenium and body of corpus callosum are often present with absence of the genu and rostrum.

Pellucidal Agenesis and Dysgenesis

Absence of septum pellucidum is often associated with other malformations, such as holoprosencephaly, septo-optic dysplasia, callosal agenesis, Chiari II malformation, etc. Secondary destruction is more common than primary agenesis and may occur following trauma, inflammation or ventricular obstruction **(Fig. 9)**.[16]

Disorders of sulcation and migration occur during the 3rd to 6th month of gestation. These result when the neuronal cells fail to migrate to the cortex such that the cortex becomes too thick and/or too smooth or heterotopic nodules of grey matter are left in unusual places. Neuronal migration anomalies are best evaluated by MR imaging.

Schizencephaly

Schizencephaly is a developmental defect resulting in a brain cleft lined by gray matter, which is an asymmetric process resulting in a single or bilateral cleft extending from the surface of the brain to the ventricular system. The asymmetry suggests that in some patients, schizencephaly may represent an early insult during brain development. The lesions have been divided into two groups based on fused or separated lips of the clefts.[16] Type I represents the closed lip schizencephaly and type II represents the open lip schizencephaly. The open lipped type may be easily diagnosed by ultrasound where an echofree cavity extends from the surface of the brain to fuse with the lateral wall of the lateral ventricle.[4]

Lissencephaly

In lissencephaly, the cerebral sulci and gyri fail to develop fully with a thick smooth four cell layered cortex resembling an hourglass in the coronal plane. In type I lissencephaly, microcephaly, facial dysmorphism and severe mental retardation are the rule. On ultrasound, the cerebral cortex resembles that of a 24-week fetus with no cerebral sulci, nearly absent operculization of the insula giving a figure-of-8 appearance. Type II lissencephaly typically presents with macrocephaly, secondary to obstructive hydrocephalus. Ultrasound may help identify the agyric cortex despite severe ventricular dilatation which may be difficult to identify on CT scanning.[4]

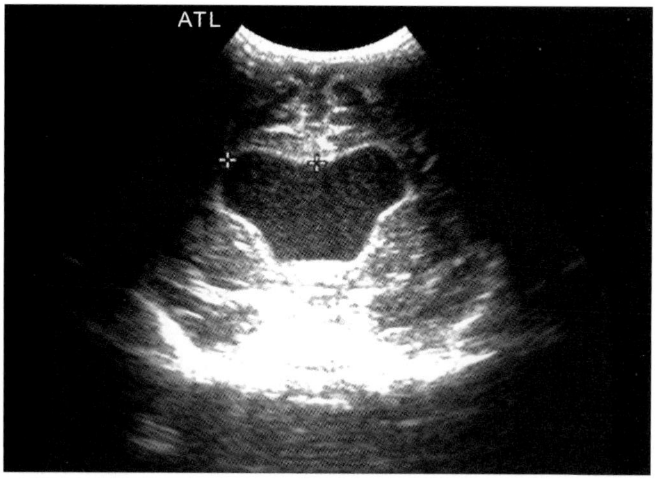

Fig. 9: Coronal sonogram showing hydrocephalus with low-level echoes within the ventricular system due to ventriculitis. Note the absence of septum pellucidum due to secondary destruction.

Disorders of histogenesis may result in tumors, arteriovenous malformations or cysts, but they are uncommon in infancy.

Tuberous Sclerosis

CNS manifestations of tuberous sclerosis include hamartomas of the periphery of the brain parenchyma and benign subependymal tubers. Subependymal nodules are seen on sonography as small focal highly reflective nodules in the wall of the lateral ventricle. Echogenic lesions in the brain parenchyma represent peripheral hamartomas.[16]

Sturge–Weber Syndrome

Serpiginous echodensities due to leptomeningeal angiomatosis may be identified in the brain periphery associated with decreased cortical volume of the involved hemisphere, i.e. cortical hemiatrophy. Usually the choroid plexus is enlarged due to the presence of angiomas within the structure.

Vascular Malformations

The most common intracranial vascular malformation presenting in the neonatal period is the vein of Galen malformation. Sonographic hallmark of the lesion is a midline echofree or mixed echogenicity, pulsatile mass that blooms with color when Doppler modalities are applied. CDFI may be helpful in distinguishing the two most common types.[17] The choroidal type is characterized by multiple abnormal feeding vessels arising in the midbrain with venous drainage via the aneurysmally dilated vein of Galen and straight sinus. The infundibular type consists of an arteriovenous fistula with one or few arterial feeders draining directly into the vein of Galen.

Spectral Doppler imaging typically shows arterialization of venous flow and increased flow velocities with reduced pulsatility of arterial feeders. Whether embolization or surgery is planned, intraprocedural neurosonography is useful in evaluating completeness of therapy. Patients are generally monitored post treatment with Doppler sonography.[16]

DESTRUCTIVE BRAIN LESIONS

Porencephalic Cyst

A porencephalic cyst is an area of normally developed brain that has been damaged and heals with a lining of gliotic white matter. The resultant lesion usually communicates with the ventricles. On sonography, an anechoic cavity communicating with the ventricular system is seen. The term should ideally be restricted to true *in utero* causes of cystic brain damage[4] **(Fig. 10)**.

Focal or diffuse brain damage in neonates can result in areas of cystic encephalomalacia. These typically do not communicate with the ventricular system[2,4] **(Fig. 11)**.

Hydranencephaly

Occlusion of the supraclinoid internal carotid arteries between the 12th and 26th weeks of gestation, results in destruction of the formed cerebral hemispheres. A fluid filled membranous sac fills the calvarium but the falx is present, differentiating this condition from holoprosencephaly. Variable amounts of frontal and occipital lobes may be preserved. The thalami, basal ganglia, midbrain and posterior fossa contents are essentially normal. On CDFI flow in the internal carotid arteries is absent.[2,4] It can be difficult to differentiate hydranencephaly from severe hydrocephalus but a thin rim of cortex should be visualized by sonography in hydrocephalus.[18-20] Macrocephaly is usual although the head may be normal or even small in size.

HYDROCEPHALUS

Hydrocephalus is an excessive accumulation of CSF in the ventricular system, subarachnoid spaces overlying the brain or a combination of both. It results when there is an imbalance between its production and absorption or an obstruction to the free flow of CSF.[21] Hydrocephalus may be considered to be communicating, i.e. extraventricular obstruction to CSF flow or noncommunicating, i.e. intraventricular obstruction to CSF flow, up to the level

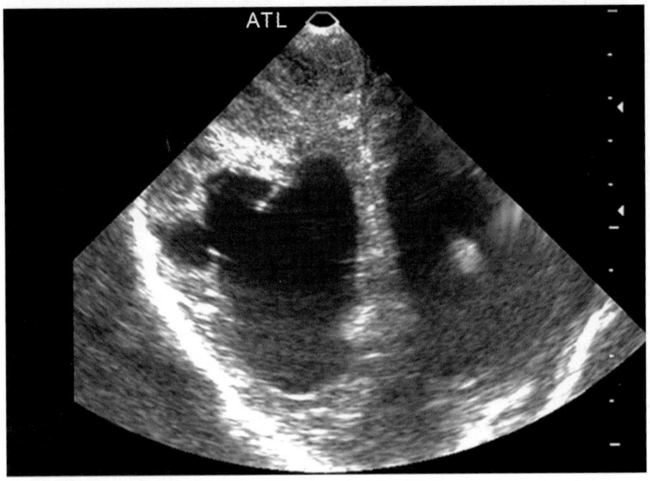

Fig. 10: Coronal sonogram showing dilated lateral ventricles with a porencephalic cyst communicating with the left lateral ventricle.

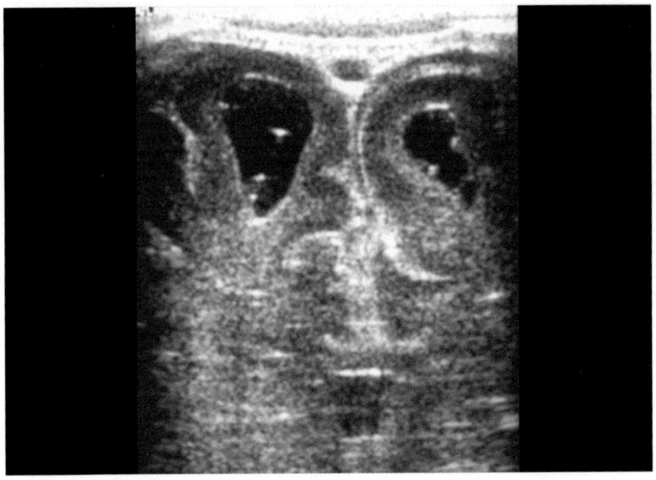

Fig. 11: Coronal sonogram showing well-defined anechoic areas representing cystic encephalomalacia in both frontal lobes.

of the outlet foramina of the fourth ventricle. Rarely, excessive production of CSF may result in hydrocephalus.

Sonography is the preferred modality for the initial evaluation of an infant with suspected hydrocephalus. Often, hydrocephalus can be diagnosed *in utero* by 15 weeks of gestation. The size of the atrium and glomus remain constant in second and third trimester. *In utero*, an upper limit of 10 mm for the ventricular atrium has been established. On neonatal sonography, the ventricular system is well defined with separation of the walls in preterm infants, whereas in the full term and older infant the ventricles are less distended and ventricular walls are often apposed. Measurements taken in the coronal section at the level of foramen of Monro are the most reproducible[4] **(Fig. 12)**. Reported values range from 9 to 13 mm for term infants.[4] In preterm infants, lateral ventricular width varies from 6 to 12 mm while lateral ventricular ratio ranges from 20.9 to 26.4% with a steady decline with increasing age.[22-24]

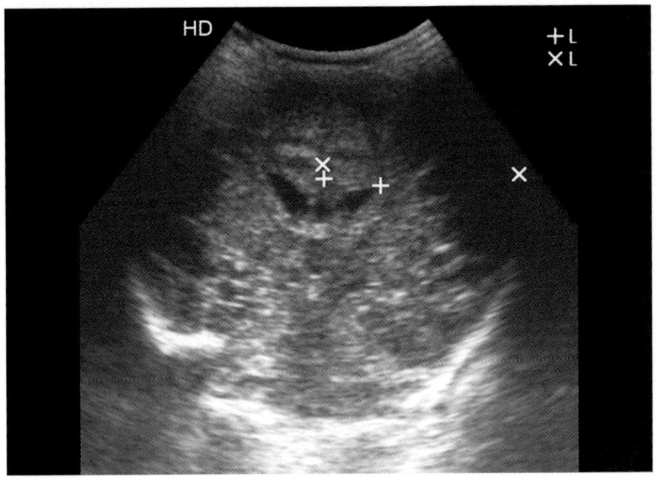

Fig. 12: Coronal section at the level of foramen of Monro. The calipers show the points for measurement of lateral ventricles and hemispheric measurement for VH ratio.

Some authors have described measurement of anterior horn width—measured between the medial wall and floor of the frontal horn at the widest point in coronal section **(Fig. 13)**. In normal preterm and term infants, anterior horn width of <3 mm has been described.[25,26] Qualitative assessment of ventricular size is often used in practice. The most useful signs are progressive rounding and bulging of the superolateral angles of the frontal horns and dilatation of occipital horns.

Sonographic criteria for the enlargement of third and fourth ventricles on transfontanel scans are not well established. Third ventricular width of 0–2.6 mm on axial scans **(Fig. 14)** and fourth ventricle width of 3.3–7.4 mm and length of 2.6–6.9 mm on scans through the asterion **(Fig. 15)** have been described in preterm neonates <33 weeks GA.[25] The presence of rounded fourth ventricle with no recognized cisterna is suggestive of noncommunicating dilation, whereas a triangular fourth ventricle with wide cisterna magna indicates a communicating dilatation.

CDFI techniques may also be helpful in evaluating CSF flow dynamics in these infants. Particulate matter and microbubble formation in CSF passing through the aqueduct, results in flow related color encoded jets. CSF flow produces a highly characteristic sinusoidal spectral Doppler waveform, indicative of cyclical to and fro motion of CSF within the ventricular system.[4] Examination of the ventricular system during cranial and abdominal compression may induce movement of CSF detectable with color flow or Doppler scanning.[27]

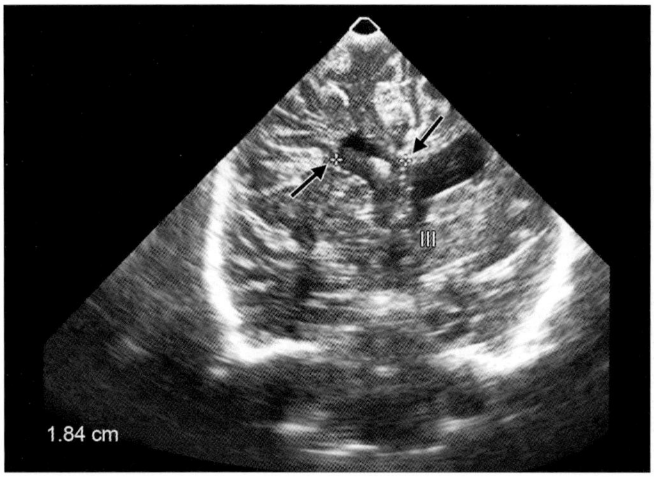

Fig. 13: Coronal section at the level of foramen of Monro. Arrows mark the points for measurement of anterior horn width.

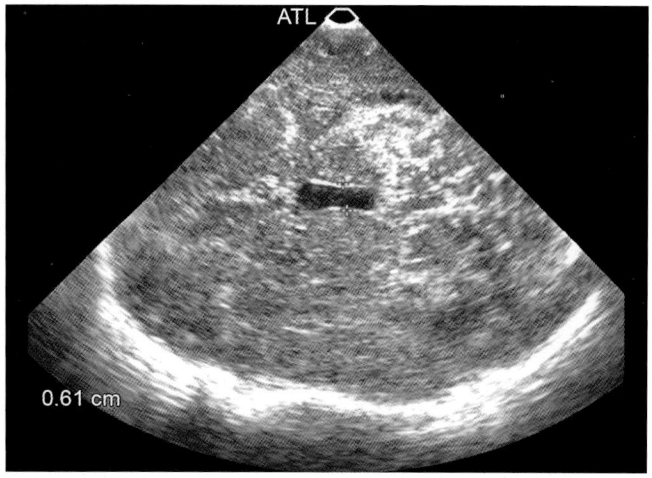

Fig. 14: Axial section through the squamous temporal bone demonstrating the third ventricle.

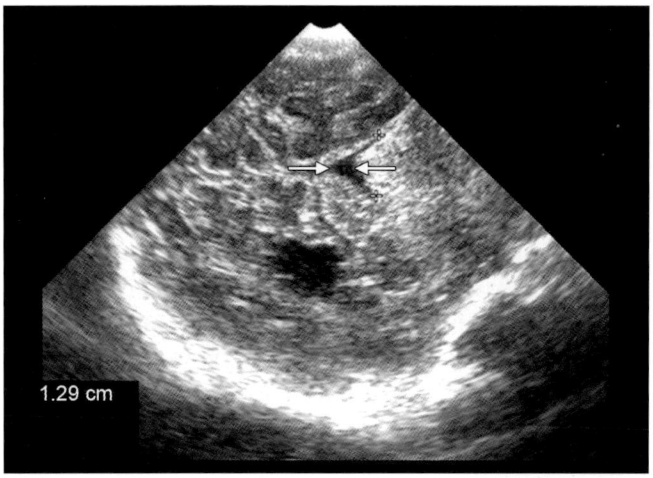

Fig. 15: Sonogram through the posterolateral fontanel showing the triangular fourth ventricle. Calipers mark the position for measurement of width and arrows mark the position for the length.

The effect of hydrocephalus on cerebral circulation can be evaluated and the resistive index correlated linearly with the intracranial pressure (ICP) in hydrocephalus, which is more important than the anatomic assessment of ventricular size alone. As the intracranial pressure rises, arterial flow tends to be more affected during diastole than during systole resulting in an increased pulsatility of flow. Increasing RI correlates well with elevation in ICP **(Figs. 16A and B)**. The resistive index decreases after ventriculoperitoneal shunting or tapping.[28,29] Doppler examination of the anterior or middle cerebral artery during fontanel compression may be useful in the early identification of infants with abnormal intracranial compliance prior to the development of increased ICP as shown by elevated base line RI.[30] In normal infants, CSF or blood flow can be readily displaced compensating for the small increase in volume caused by compression of anterior fontanel resulting in no increase in ICP. In infants with hydrocephalus, however, this maneuver results in transient increased intracranial pressure and an acute increase in arterial pulsatility.[30,31]

Sonography is also useful in determining the level of obstruction. Evaluation of the entire ventricular system should be done so that the level at which there is a transition from a large to small ventricle can be identified.[25] Dilatation of the lateral and third ventricles indicates an obstruction at the aqueductal level, most often secondary to intraventricular hemorrhage or infection or sometimes congenital, often an X-linked recessive trait. Regional flow imaging with color Doppler has been investigated as a method to exclude obstructive hydrocephalus.[27] Free passage of CSF through the ventricles and out into the basal cistern confirms the diagnosis of communicating hydrocephalus.[4]

Sonography is ideal for following ventricular size in infants who are on treatment for hydrocephalus, displaying the position of the shunt tube and size of the ventricles. Following successful shunting, a fall in the arterial RI has also been demonstrated.

Another important type of hydrocephalus in infancy is the so called **benign communicating hydrocephalus** which has also been described as **benign external hydrocephalus** of infancy or chronic subdural hygromas of infancy. It is characterized by an enlargement of the subarachnoid spaces greater than 5 mm overlying the cerebral hemispheres,

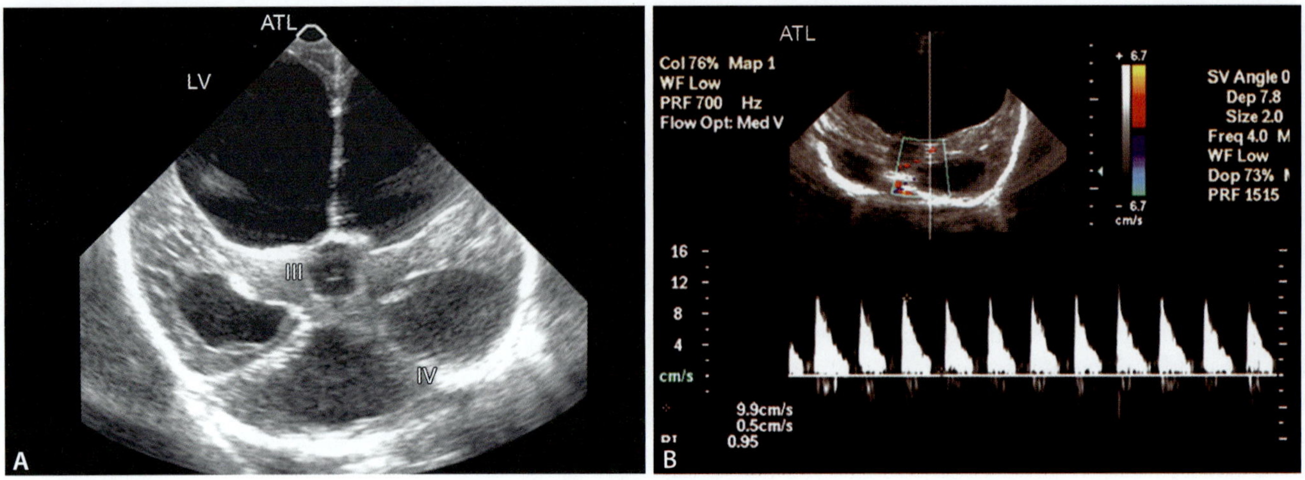

Figs. 16A and B: (A) Coronal sonogram showing generalized dilatation of the ventricular system; (B) CDFI of the same patient showing markedly elevated RI in the MCA s/o increased ICP.

particularly over the frontal and temporal convexities. There is associated mild-or-moderate ventricular dilatation. The condition usually presents in the first year of life, the infant presenting with a large head. It is generally a self limiting process that resolves without treatment by two years of age. The etiology is probably transient immaturity of the arachnoid granulations or villi.[32] In the past, excess fluid overlying the hemispheres has been misconstrued as being subdural hygromas of indeterminate etiology. However, both ultrasound and MRI can demonstrate that the excess fluid is actually in the subarachnoid space dipping into the sulci. This condition is also termed as benign enlargement of subarachnoid space **(BESS) syndrome**. Follow-up imaging is not required but serial head circumference measurements should be obtained. The condition is not entirely benign, as it predisposes to extra-axial hemorrhage after minor head trauma, and transient minor developmental delay occurs in a minority of cases during the period of most rapid head growth at 5–12 months of age.

The differential diagnosis of benign enlargement of the extra-axial fluid spaces includes cerebral atrophy (widened sulci, small or normal head circumference, proportionate ventricular enlargement), subdural collections (arachnoid neomembranes, echogenic fluid, displacement of bridging cortical veins within the subarachnoid space away from skull toward the brain), meningitis (thickened leptomeninges, echogenic fluid), communicating hydrocephalus (larger ventricles), etc.

INTRACRANIAL HEMORRHAGE

One of the most important roles of cranial ultrasound in infancy is the investigation of intracranial hemorrhage in the newborn. The patterns and etiology of hemorrhage are different in premature and term infants.

The germinal matrix is the most common site of origin of intracranial hemorrhage in the **preterm infant**. It occurs in 20–45% of preterm low birth weight neonates.[33-35] The aetiological factors associated with hemorrhage and hypoxic/ischemic encephalopathy overlap to a considerable degree. Hemorrhage probably arises due to varying cerebral blood flow in the delicate and immature vessels of the highly vascular germinal matrix.[36] These vessels are particularly vulnerable between 25 and 28 weeks of gestation and become less vulnerable as blood flow is shifted towards the cortex by 32–34 weeks.[37] Veins of the germinal matrix are the likely source of hemorrhage.

The classification/grading[38] of germinal matrix hemorrhage (GMH) most widely used is as follows:

- *Grade I*: Subependymal hemorrhage.
- *Grade II*: Intraventricular extension without hydrocephalus.
- *Grade III*: Intraventricular hemorrhage with hydrocephalus
- *Grade IV*: Intraventricular hemorrhage with deep intraparenchymal hemorrhage with or without hydrocephalus.

Sonography is the most effective method for detecting this hemorrhage in the newborn period and for follow-up in subsequent weeks. Most hemorrhages (90%) occur in the first 7 days of life, only one-third occur in the first 24 hours. The recommended time for US screening in preterm infants (<33 weeks) is around 7–10 days to detect GMH and evolving hemorrhage followed by a late scan at one month to detect cystic changes of PVL and hydrocephalus.[35]

Grade I

These are small hemorrhages confined to the subependymal or germinal matrix area between the lateral ventricle and head of caudate nucleus or the caudothalamic groove[39] **(Fig. 17)**. They may be unilateral or bilateral. In the acute stage, this appears as a moderately or highly reflective area in the inferolateral wall of the frontal horn superficially resembling the choroid plexus but in a site where the choroid is absent, i.e. anterior to foramen of Monro. As the hematoma ages, it liquefies, becomes sonolucent, and subsequently may resolve completely or persist as a subependymal cyst or as a linear echo[2,4] **(Fig. 18)**. The neurological outcome of these children does not differ significantly from preterm infants with normal cranial ultrasound.

Abnormal hyperechogenicity of the subependymal germinal matrix is not always hemorrhagic. Nonhemorrhagic germinal matrix hyperechogenicity has been reported as an isolated finding or in association with cerebral infection CMV, rubella), extracerebral infection (especially rotavirus gastroenteritis), etc. The location is the same as with germinal matrix hemorrhage but the timing, appearance, and evolution are different.

Nonhemorrhagic germinal matrix hyperechogenicity is seen primarily in near-term and term neonates, is teardrop-shaped and bilaterally symmetric, whereas germinal matrix hemorrhage occurs in premature infants predominantly in the first 2 weeks of life and tends to be round and asymmetric or unilateral. Also, nonhemorrhagic germinal matrix hyperechogenicity persists or evolves by germinolysis into subependymal pseudocysts with gliotic walls lacking hemosiderin, whereas germinal matrix hemorrhage liquefies and resolves by resorption, occasionally with hemosiderin-lined subependymal pseudocysts as residua.[40]

Grade II

This is an intraventricular hemorrhage with minimal or no significant ventriculomegaly at presentation. Before the blood has clotted it is difficult to visualize in the ventricles, but subsequently it can be seen as hyperechoic material that fills a portion or whole of the ventricular system.[2,4] The clots may just produce an echogenic irregular outline/thickening of the choroid plexus **(Fig. 19)**. Small clots tend to settle in the dependent occipital horns in the supine infant and are difficult to detect through the anterior fontanel approach. Use of posterior fontanel or axial views may improve detection of IVH in normal sized ventricles.[41] If blood extends into the cisterna magna, there is an increased risk of post hemorrhagic hydrocephalus.[35] The incidence of neurological deficits is marginally higher in this group.[42,43]

Grade III

Large intraventricular hemorrhages result in significant ventricular dilatation at presentation. Large highly reflective areas fill the ventricular system producing a 'cast like' appearance. A chemical ventriculitis as a response to blood in the CSF typically produces thickening of the ependymal lining of the ventricle. Hydrocephalus occurs due to expansion of the ventricle by the blood along with impairment of CSF resorption at the level of arachnoid

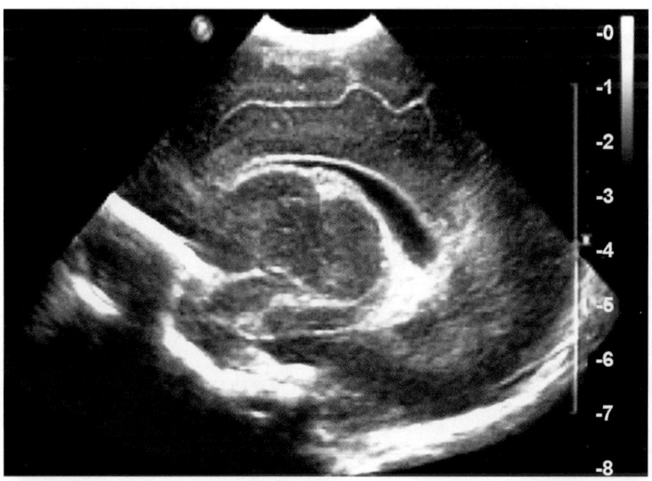

Fig. 17: Sagittal sonogram showing a small hyperechoic area in the caudothalamic groove with no evidence of hydrocephalus consistent with grade I periventricular hemorrhage.

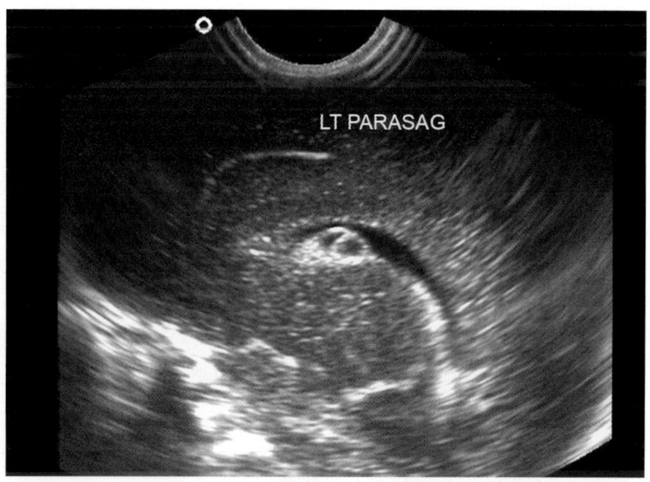

Fig. 18: Sagittal scan (of the same patient as in Figure 17) after a week shows liquefaction of the hematoma with formation of subependymal cysts.

granulations **(Figs. 20A and B)**. Hydrocephalus should be monitored by serial ultrasound scans. In most cases the hydrocephalus may resolve and approximately 34% of very low-birth infants require shunting.[35,39] The clinical outcome with varying degrees of permanent neurological impairment is significantly worse in this group.[44]

Grade IV

This consists of simultaneous intraventricular and intraparenchymal cerebral hemorrhage **(Fig. 21)**. It is usually located in the frontal or parietal lobes, because it often extends from the germinal matrix. It has been suggested that the culprit may be venous ischemia complicated by hemorrhage. CDFI may be used to show initial displacement and gradual encasement and obstruction of the terminal veins by an enlarging germinal matrix hemorrhage. This finding may be useful for early prediction of infants at risk for worsening intracranial hemorrhage.[45,46] The neurological sequelae in this group are usually severe and tend to be developmental delay and poor tone as opposed to spastic diplegia or quadriplegia in patient with ischemia in the same region.

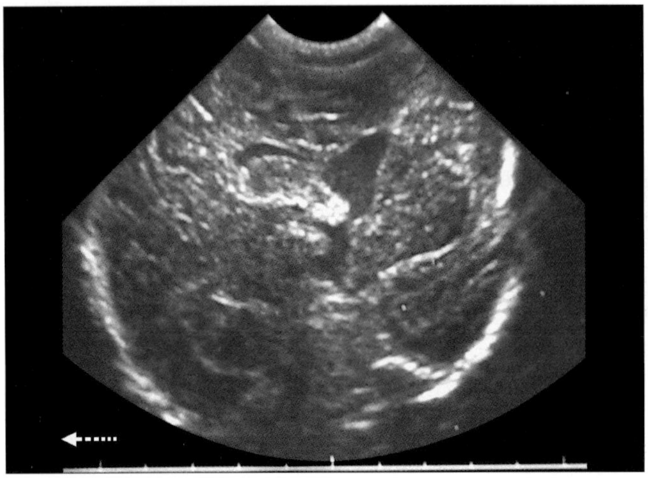

Fig. 19: Intraventricular clot in the left lateral ventricle extending to the 3rd ventricle with only minimal prominence of the ventricular system—well seen on this coronal scan, suggesting grade 2 hemorrhage.

Subarachnoid hemorrhage may also occur in preterm newborns and is usually difficult to identify on ultrasound due to normal variation in the appearance of subarachnoid cisterns. It may be seen as widening of sylvian fissures with increased reflectivity.

Hemorrhage in the **term newborn** may occur due to birth trauma and subdural hemorrhage is the most commonly encountered lesion due to falcine or tentorial laceration, while extradural hemorrhage is uncommon. Acute SDH appears as a highly reflective linear or elliptical collection that compresses the brain parenchyma. Transcranial scanning may be useful to demonstrate this lesion. Cerebellar hemorrhage is a reported complication of traumatic delivery in full term neonates, in ECMO or with coagulopathy. Posterior fossa hemorrhages are more difficult to demonstrate by the anterior fontanel approach and the mastoid fontanel scanning is now routinely used. Subarachnoid hemorrhage may occur in neonates who have experienced asphyxia or trauma and may be the only hemorrhage in full term infants not at risk for GMH.[2,4] Intraventricular hemorrhage has also been reported in term infants probably arising from the choroid plexus or germinal matrix.[35,47,48]

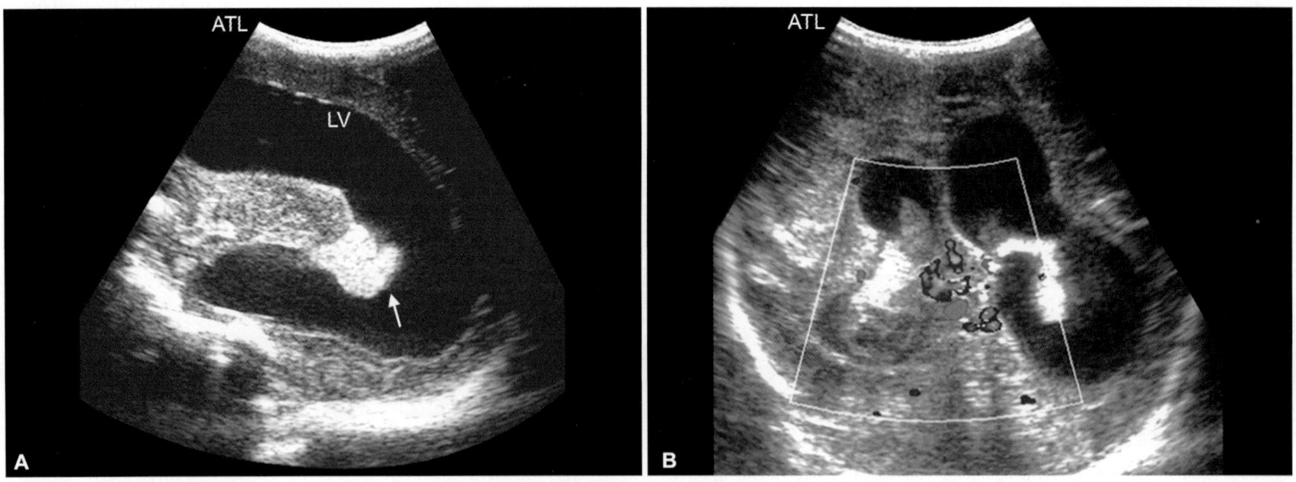

Figs. 20A and B: Sagittal and coronal sonograms showing a grossly dilated lateral ventricles with enlarged and echogenic choroid plexus appearing avascular on CDFI consistent with hemorrhage.

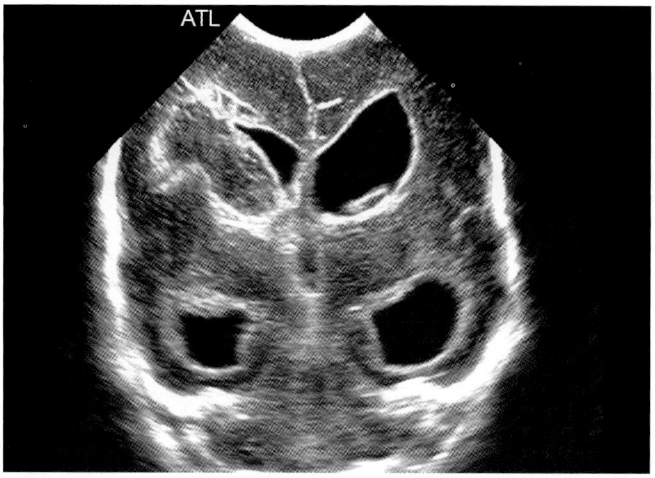

Fig. 21: Coronal sonogram showing marked dilatation of both lateral ventricles with intraventricular hemorrhage and deep parenchymal hemorrhage (grade IV) on the left side and intraventricular hemorrhage (grade III) on the right. The ependyma appears echogenic due to chemical ventriculitis.

HYPOXIC OR ISCHEMIC ENCEPHALOPATHY

The pattern of involvement differs in the preterm and term neonate and also varies with the degree of hypoxia.

Mild-to-moderate Hypotension in the Preterm Neonate

The most common location for injury to the premature brain is the periventricular white matter the periventricular white matter, since this is the water shed area in the preterm infant, resulting in periventricular leukomalacia or **PVL**.

PVL is an ischemic lesion, that occurs in the periventricular white matter and centrum semiovale in the preterm infant. In the premature infant, these areas are the most vulnerable to hypoperfusion and ischemia. The areas of infarction vary in size and severity.[2,4] There may be mild involvement with resulting gliosis or more severe involvement with resulting cystic changes. Areas of necrosis and infarction may be complicated by superimposed hemorrhage. The white matter in the region of the posterior trigone and adjacent to the frontal horns of the lateral ventricles is most commonly affected.[49]

Diagnosis of PVL may be made during the neonatal period with sonography, although the diagnosis is easier to miss than subependymal hemorrhage because there may be only subtle increase in echogenicity in the first week of life. These areas are more echogenic than the choroid in the acute phase but when they resolve, they may be mistaken for the normal periventricular echogenic blush. Cystic changes may develop later, usually between day 8 and day 28 **(Figs. 22A to E)**. The development of macrocysts is a rarity nowadays. Bilateral involvement is common. The loss of periventricular white matter and coalescent cysts which may communicate with the ventricle results in a characteristic irregular outline of the ventricle. The recognition of cysts is important because their presence is associated with adverse clinical outcome.

Early Doppler studies may demonstrate increased mean velocities and lower RI of lenticulostriate vessels in preterm infants who develop PVL.[50,51]

Severe Hypotension in the Preterm Neonate

The thalami, brainstem, and cerebellum in the immature brain have high metabolic activity and hence are more susceptible to injury in severe hypotension. This manifests as hyperechogenicity of the injured brain at US imaging. Coexisting periventricular white matter injury and germinal matrix hemorrhage may be present[52] **(Figs. 23A to C)**.

Recent studies suggest that cerebellar infarction and hemorrhage in the preterm infant may not be as rare as once thought. Due to echogenicity of cerebellum, areas of infarction and hemorrhage can be easily missed on ultrasound. Transmastoid scanning may improve the sensitivity of sonographic identification.[36]

Certain normal variants must be kept in mind before interpreting the ultrasound scans as abnormal.

A periventricular echogenic halo or blush, parallels the posterior margin of the lateral ventricles in virtually all neonates, most prominently in premature neonates, and arises from the anisotropic effect of the vascular plexus and radial fibers coursing from the subependyma to the cortex. This is homogeneous, symmetric, and of lower echogenicity compared with the choroid plexus, lacks cysts, and is less conspicuous when viewed from the posterior fontanel. These features help distinguish the periventricular halo or blush from periventricular leukomalacia or hemorrhage. A striated pattern of the corona radiata and echogenic stripes external to the periventricular white matter paralleling the ventricles can be seen for the first few weeks of postnatal life in very preterm neonates, i.e. less than 28 weeks gestational age. These findings are likely due to the anisotropic effect of layers of migrating cells along radial glia fibers. Foci of increased echogenicity in the thalami are visible in one to two-thirds of neonates (more often in preterm neonates) on parasagittal images through the posterior fontanel and can mimic hemorrhagic or ischemic lesions. These are not as prominent on images through the anterior

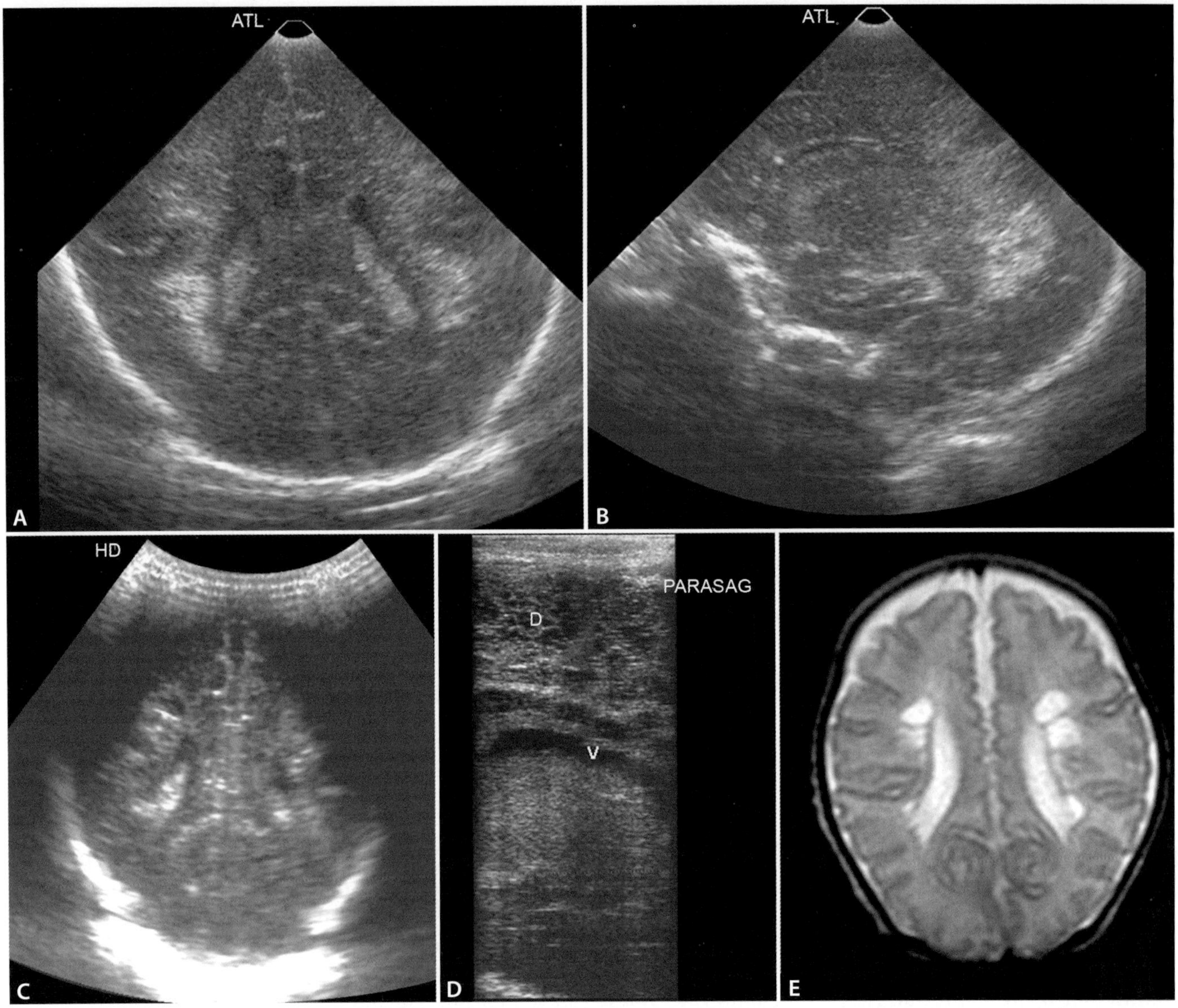

Figs. 22A to E: Serial cranial sonograms in a preterm neonate with birth asphyxia reveal periventricular areas of increased echogenicity most marked in the peritrigonal region on the initial coronal and sagittal scans (A and B); (C and D) Subsequent coronal and high resolution sagittal scans reveal partial resolution of the abnormal echogenicity with development of multiple small periventricular cysts. Axial T2W MR image (E) of the same child depicts the multiple periventricular cysts—consistent with cystic PVL.

fontanel, suggesting that these are due to the anisotropic effect of fibers from the posterior limb and genu of the internal capsule along the lateral margin of the thalamus or intrathalamic nuclear groups. However, diffuse hyperechogenicity of the basal ganglia and thalami may serve as a marker for brain injury.[40]

Sonography is less useful in evaluation of the term brain that has suffered anoxic-ischemic damage than premature brain because abnormalities are more often peripheral and not central and associated hemorrhage is less often present. Though the pattern of injury may vary with the severity of hypoxia, diffuse or focal lesions may occur anywhere in the brain parenchyma.[35,53]

Mild-to-moderate hypoxia: The primary locations of ischemic injury in the term neonatal brain are the intervascular watershed zones between the anterior and middle cerebral arteries and between the middle and posterior cerebral arteries or the border zone. The brain parenchyma appears echogenic in the distribution of the injury and there may be either accentuation or loss of gray-white matter interface, depending on the severity of injury. Subsequently, cystic changes develop **(Figs. 24A to C)**.

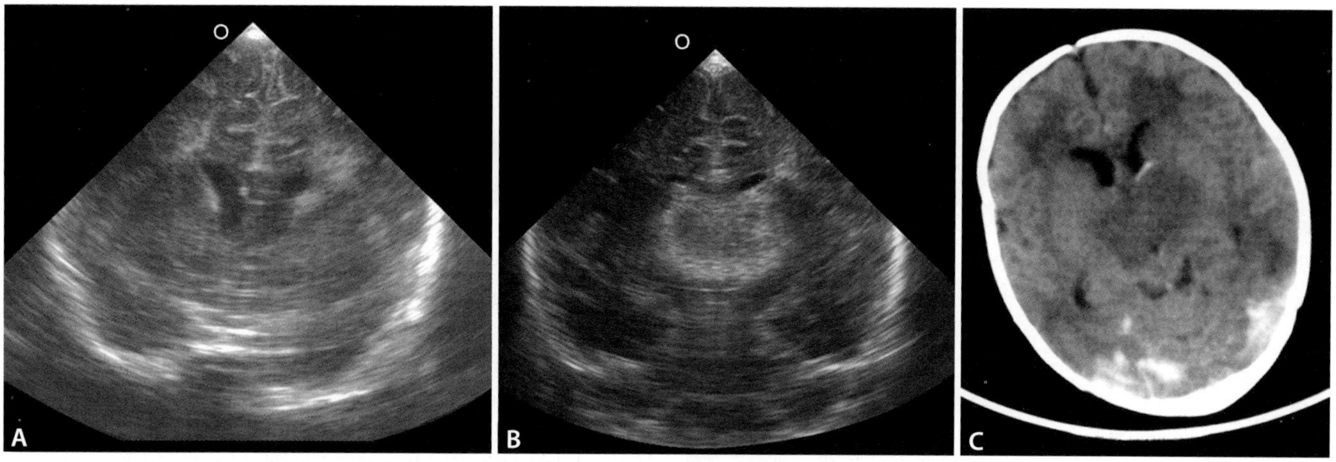

Figs. 23A to C: Coronal sonograms (A and B) showing abnormal bilateral periventricular echogenicity and markedly increased thalami echogenicity in a neonate with severe asphyxia; (C) The axial CT section of the same shows both the thalami to be hypodense due to hypoxic injury. Note the presence of postfossa hemorrhages as well (not seen US scan through anterior fontanel).

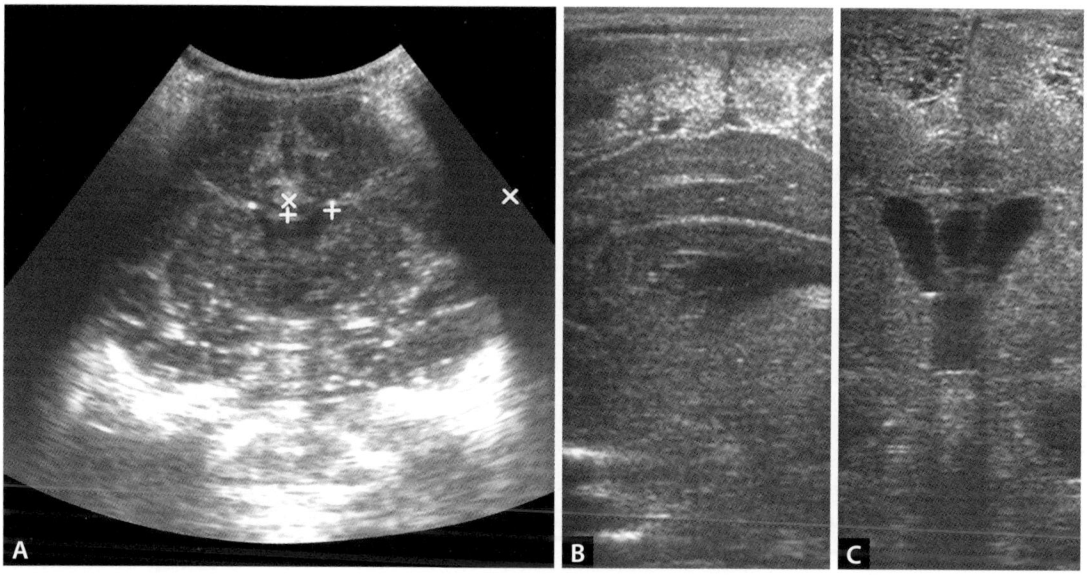

Figs. 24A to C: Routine coronal scan (A) of a term neonate with birth asphyxia appears unremarkable; however, subsequent high resolution sagittal scan (B) shows marked increase in cortical and subcortical echogenicity. A coronal high resolution scan at a later date demonstrates multiple subcortical cysts (C).

Severe hypoxia: The metabolically active tissues in the brain of the term neonate are most susceptible to injury in profound hypotension and include the lateral thalami, posterior putamina, hippocampi, brainstem, corticospinal tracts, and the sensorimotor cortex (perirolandic).[52] The thalami show diffuse increase in echogenicity **(Fig. 25)**. Subsequently, cystic changes may develop.

Diffuse Cerebral Edema

It is a common result of hypoxic ischemic events in full-term infants. Initially, the brain edema causes slit like ventricles with a diffusely echogenic brain. This echogenicity may cause silhouetting of the sulci, so that the sulci seem to disappear. The brain develops a diffusely reflective and featureless appearance due to a combination of edema and ischemic damage.

Doppler evaluation of severely asphyxiated infants has demonstrated earlier and at times, more focal abnormalities than on grayscale alone. Doppler studies may be helpful, showing low resistance indices (<0.6) in the anterior and middle cerebral artery complexes with increased diastolic flow in the first 48 hours of asphyxia

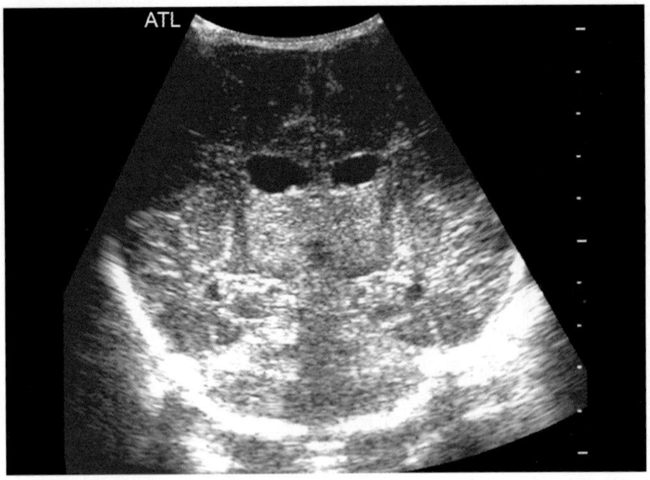

Fig. 25: Coronal sonogram showing increased echogenicity of bilateral thalami and basal ganglia in a term neonate with severe birth asphyxia.

insult. This correlates with adverse neurological outcome. As cerebral edema worsens, cerebrovascular resistance increases resulting in dampening of diastolic blood flow velocities. Several investigators have used Doppler, either to classify brain edema or to predict outcome. Some studies have shown that loss of diastolic flow, retrograde diastolic flow, and no detectable flow in the cerebral arteries did not all have a lethal outcome. Those with only loss or reversal of diastolic flow may survive with prompt and effective treatment.[35]

Extracorporeal Membrane Oxygenation

An extracorporeal membrane oxygenation (ECMO) is commonly used to treat term infants with respiratory insufficiency. The infants are continuously heparinized during the procedure and are at risk for intracranial hemorrhage. Baseline sonograms are performed prior to ECMO and patients with severe anoxeic-ischemic injury, large infarcts or intraventricular hemorrhage greater than grade 2 are not ECMO candidates. Daily ultrasounds are performed and any hemorrhage greater than grade 1 is cause for discontinuing ECMO. Since hemorrhages occurring while the patients are anticoagulated are less echogenic than hemorrhages in babies with normal clotting factors, a high index of suspicion should be maintained to notice any mass effect not seen on the previous day's neurosonogram.[16]

Post-traumatic Injury

Subdural and epidural hematomas can be a difficult diagnosis on sonography and they present as unilateral or bilateral hypoechoic fluid collections. Imaging through the post fontanel or foramen magnum may be needed for posterior fossa collection.[2,4]

Intracranial Infection

Both prenatal and postnatal infections are a significant cause of morbidity and mortality in infants. Diagnosis is almost always suspected on clinical grounds, the role of imaging being to support the clinical diagnosis and reveal complications of infection.

The most frequent congenital infections are caused by the **TORCH** complex. The resultant pathology, including parenchymal necrosis, vasculitis and gliosis are similar in all these, though the severity and extent of disease may vary.

Cytomegalovirus (CMV) infection is the most common congenital infection. Calcifications occur in a characteristic periventricular location, when these are surrounded by a hypoechoic ring like zone, the ultrasound finding is characteristic of CMV.[15] Calcifications may also occur in the basal ganglia, cortex or subcortical region. Mineralizing vasculopathy is visualized as branching calcification **(Fig. 26)**. Intracranial calcification is also seen in toxoplasmosis, which is the second most common congenital infection, with a predilection for basal ganglia, but more scattered calcification and periventricular calcification is also often seen **(Fig. 27)**.

Herpes simplex type 2 is common in the neonate, resulting in diffuse encephalitis with loss of grey white matter differentiation.

NEONATAL AND ACQUIRED INFECTIONS

Pyogenic Meningitis

Group B streptococci and *E. coli* are the most common bacterial organisms in the neonatal period and *H. influenzae* in infants (more than 3 months of age).

Sonography may be normal in uncomplicated cases. It demonstrates increased reflectivity of the cerebral sulci, secondary to leptomeningeal inflammation and pus.[54,55]

Cerebral vasculitis and thrombophlebitis may produce areas of **cerebritis** or **infarction** which are seen as echogenic areas in a segmental or gyral distribution.

Venous sinus thrombosis may also occur and can be detected using CDFI.[2] This may be associated with more complex patterns of brain injury, including venous ischemia and hemorrhage.

Extra-axial fluid collections are frequent findings in bacterial meningitis, especially *H. influenzae* infection.

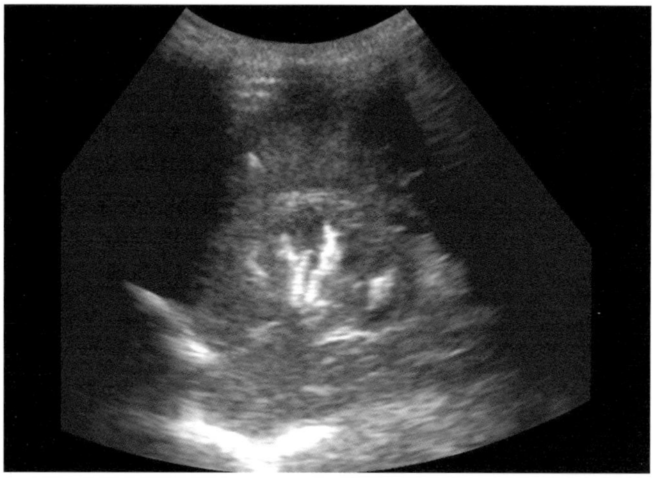

Fig. 26: Sagittal sonogram showing branching linear echogenicities in the basal ganglia consistent with mineralizing vasculopathy.

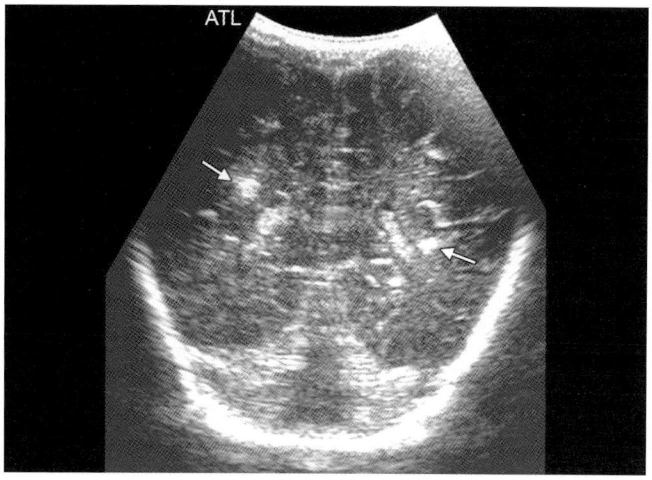

Fig. 27: Coronal sonogram showing bilateral periventricular echogenicities representing calcification in a case of CMV.

Subdural and subarachnoid collections may be echofree or may have low level echoes, the more reflective the collection, the more likely it is to represent empyema. CDFI may help separate subdural and subarachnoid collections. Vessels on the surface of the brain are compressed onto the surface of the brain in subdural fluid collection, whereas they traverse the fluid in subarachnoid collection, this is known as the 'cortical vein sign'.

Mild-to-moderate **ventriculomegaly** may occur as an early or late sonographic feature. In the acute stage, it probably represents a form of normal pressure hydrocephalus and is usually reversible. At a later date, it may occur due to obstruction to CSF flow at strategic points.

Involvement of the choroid plexus and spread to the ventricular system results in **ventriculitis** and hydrocephalus. The ventricular margins become more reflective, indicating generalized ependymitis. Particulate debris may be seen floating in the ventricles. Subsequently, septations and band adhesions appear resulting in complex multicompartmentalized hydrocephalus which is frequently resistant to effective shunting **(Fig. 28)**.

Abscess formation may occur in an area previously showing altered echogenicity due to cerebritis/infarction. This is seen as well marginated lesion with an echogenic rim and hypoechoic center. It may be associated with mass effect **(Fig. 29)**.

Tubercular Meningitis

Sonography in tubercular meningitis (TBM) may show echogenic sulci as in pyogenic meningitis. TBM can also result in basal or occasionally parenchymal calcification and communicating hydrocephalus.[56,57] Aqueductal block and infarcts have been more frequently observed in TBM than pyogenic meningitis. Granulomas may also be seen[58] **(Fig. 30)**.

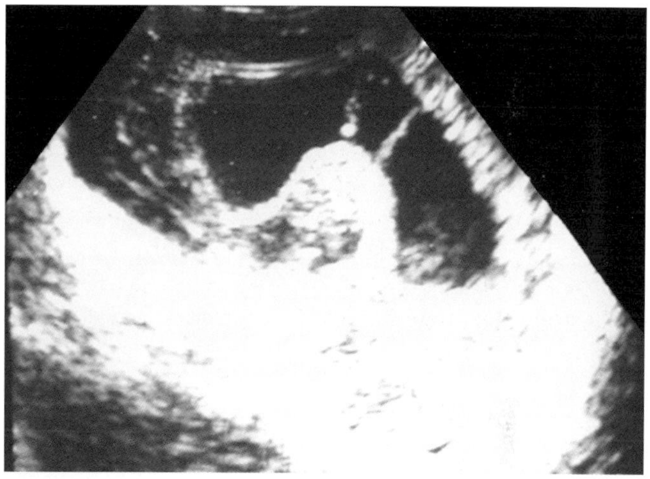

Fig. 28: Sagittal sonogram showing dilated lateral ventricle with multiple septations consistent with ventriculitis.

Neoplasms and Cysts

Neoplasms in the infant brain are rare and of all the tumors detected in the pediatric age group on CT, only about 4% present during the first year of life. The majority of the brain tumors under 1 year of age are supratentorial and therefore accessible by ultrasound **(Figs. 31A and B)**. The ultrasound appearance is variable and nonspecific and further evaluation is required to characterize these lesion. The major use of ultrasound is in intraoperative localization of tumors.

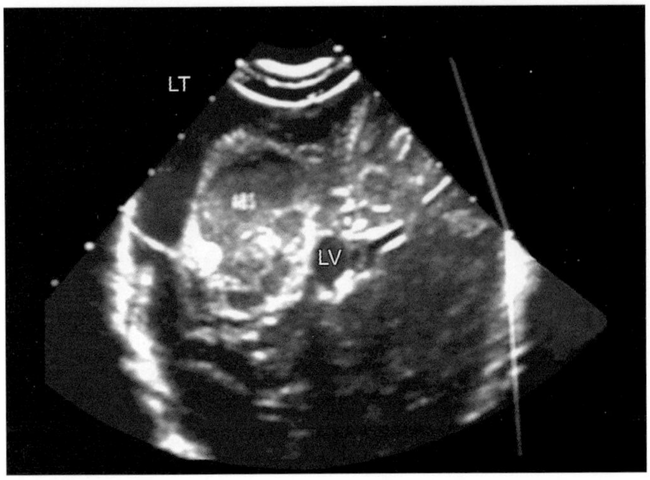

Fig. 29: Coronal sonogram showing a large round to oval lesion with hyperechoic walls and internal debris and mass effect s/o abscess in the left frontal lobe. A large subdural effusion is also present on the same side.

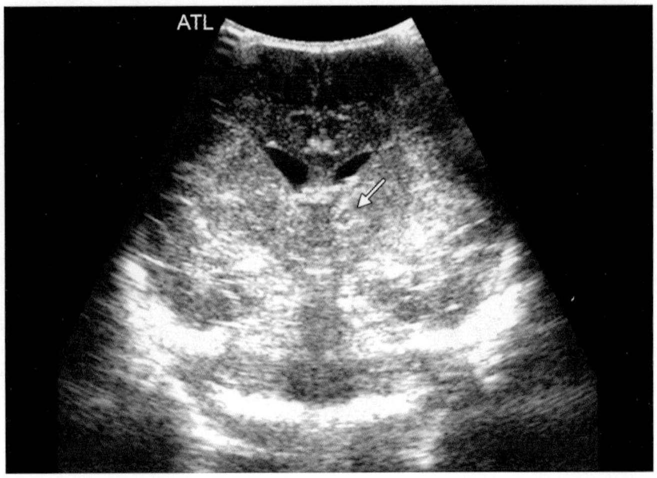

Fig. 30: Coronal sonogram in a patient with CSF findings s/o tubercular meningitis shows a small round hypoechoic granuloma with echogenic wall in the right thalamic region.

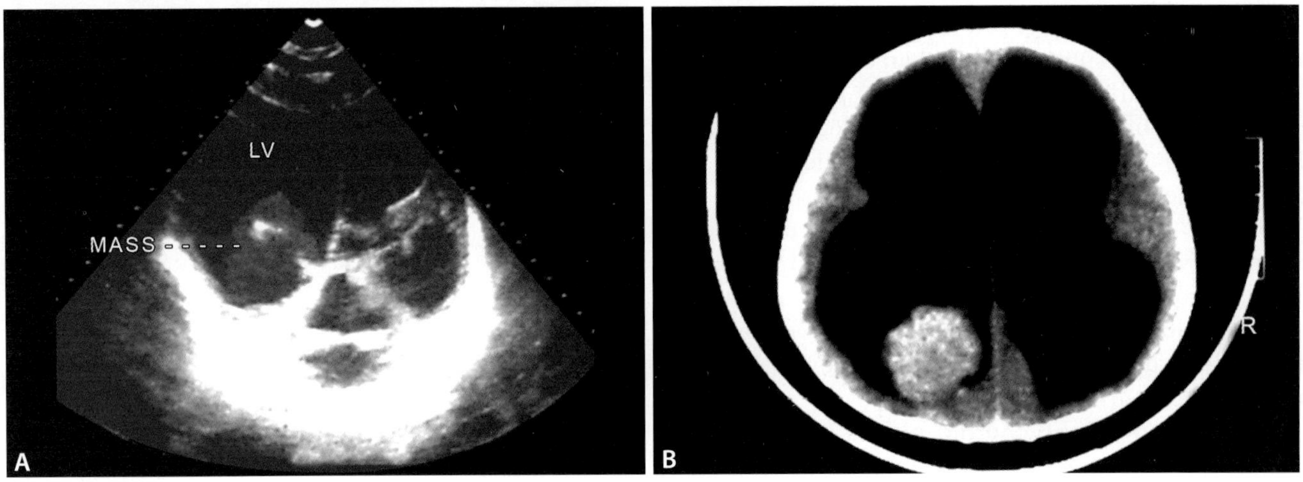

Figs. 31A and B: (A) Sonogram showing a mass in the left lateral ventricle with hydrocephalus; (B) CECT of the same patient showing an intensely enhancing intraventricular mass consistent with choroid plexus papilloma.

Cysts

Besides parencephalic cysts, the other commonly encountered cysts include arachnoid cysts, choroid plexus cysts and subependymal cysts.

Arachnoid cysts are the most common true cysts of the brain, but they account for only 1% of all space-occupying lesions in children. They are located in the anterior middle cranial fossa, suprasellar region, posterior fossa, quadrigeminal region, cerebral convexities and interhemispheric fissure in decreasing order of frequency. The cysts are seen as anechoic areas with discrete walls. Lesions abutting the ventricular system may cause obstructive hydrocephalus **(Fig. 32)**.

Choroid plexus cysts are common and usually incidental findings. They range in size from less than 4–7 mm and are usually unilateral and left greater than right.

Subependymal cysts are usually the sequelae of germinal matrix hemorrhage. They may also occur following infection, as a part of cerebrohepatorenal syndrome or as an isolated finding.

Although MR imaging is considered the gold standard for imaging the brain at all ages, some neonates may be too sick to be transported to the MR facility and hence have to rely on information obtained from neurosonography. Further, despite availability, one may not be able to get an MR examination done immediately or at the most

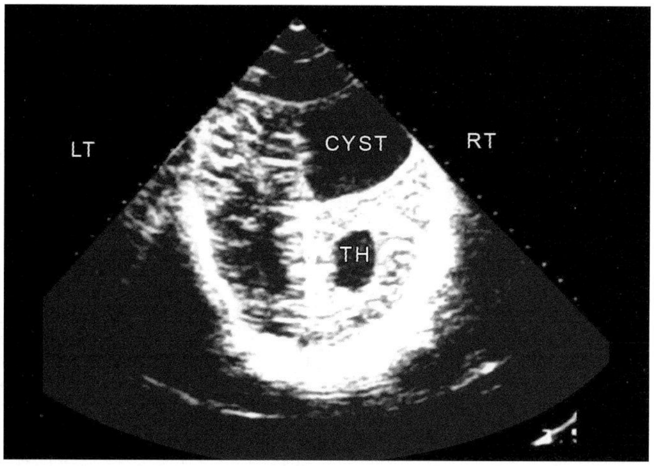

Fig. 32: Sonogram showing a large cyst in the right temporoparietal region with displacement of the cerebral hemisphere—Arachnoid cyst.

appropriate time. Hence, neurosonography continues to be the initial or sometimes the only examination in many neonates and infants. Thus, it is important to be aware of the normal anatomy and imaging appearances of various pathological conditions in order to be able to reach an appropriate diagnosis.

REFERENCES

1. DiPietro MA, Faix RG, Donn SM. Procedural hazards of neonatal ultrasonography. J Clin Ultrasound. 1984;14:361-6.
2. Kaske TI, Rumack CM, Harlow CL. Neonatal and Infant brain imaging in Diagnostic Ultrasound. In Rumack CM, Wilson SR, Charboneau JW (Eds): 2nd edn, Mosby 1998;1443-501.
3. Shuman WP, Rogers JV, Mack IA, et al. Real time sonographic sector scanning of the neonatal cranium: technique and normal anatomy. AJR. 1981;137:821-8.
4. Jaspan T. The neonatal brain, in Clinical Ultrasound a Comprehensive Test. In Meire H, Cosgrove D, Dewbury K, Farrant P (Eds): 2nd edn, 2001.pp.1055-6.
5. Veyrae C, Couture A, B and C. Pericerebral fluid collections and ultrasound diagnosis. Pediatr Radiol. 1990;20:236-40.
6. Dewbury KC, Bales RI. The value of transfontanellar ultrasound in infants. Br J Radiol. 1981;54:1044-52.
7. DI Salvo DN. A new view of the neonatal brain. Clinical utility of supplemental neurologic ultrasound windows. Radiographics. 2001;21:943-58.
8. Chadduck WM, Seibert JJ. Intracranial duplex Doppler: Practical uses in pediatric neurology and neurosurgery. J Child Neurol. 1989;4:577.
9. Allison JW, Faddis LA, Kinder DL, et al. Intracranial resistive index (RI) values in normal term infants during first day of life. Pediatr Radiol. 2000;30(9):618-20.
10. Taylor GA, Barnewolt CE, Duning PS. Excitotoxin induced cerebral hyperemia in newborn piglets: Regional cerebral blood flow mapping with contrast enhanced power Doppler US. Radiology. 1998;208:73.
11. Taylor GA, Sanders RC. Dandy-Walker syndrome. Recognition by Sonography. AJNR. 1983;1203-6.
12. Estroff JA, Pavad RB, Barnes PD, et al. Posterior fossa arachnoid cyst: An in utero mimicker of Dandy-Walker Malformation. J Ultrasound Med. 1995;14:787-90.
13. Kollias SS, Ball WAS Jr. Congenital malformations of the brain. In Bale Jr (Ed): Pediatric Neuroradiology Philadelphia: Lippincott-Raven 1997;110.
14. Yakovlev PI. Pathoarchitectonic studies of cerebral malformation III. Arrhinencephalies (holotelencephalies). J Neuropathol Exp Neurol. 1959;18:22.
15. Yakovlev PI, Wadsworth RC. Schizencephalies: A study of congenital clefts in the cerebral mantle I clefts with fused lips. J Neuropathol Exp Neurol. 1947;5:116.
16. Barr LL. Neonatal cranial ultrasound. Radiol Clin of North Am. 1999;37(6).
17. Tessler FN, Dion J, Vinuela F, et al. Cranial arteriovenous malformations in neonates color Doppler imaging with angiographic correlation. AJR. 1989;153:1027-30.
18. Pretorius DH, Russ PD, Rumack CM, et al. Diagnosis of brain neuropathology in utero. In Naidich, Quencer RM (Eds): Clinical Neurosonography Berlin: Springer-Verlag, 1987.
19. Dublin AB, French BN. Diagnostic image evaluation of hydrencephaly and pictorally similar entities with emphasis on computed tomography. Radiology. 1980;137:81-91.
20. Diebler C, Dulac D. Pediatric Neurology and Neuroradiology, Berlin: Springer-Verlag 1987.
21. Carey CM, Tullous MW, Walker ML. Hydrocephalus etiology, pathologic effects, diagnosis and natural history. In Cheek WR (Ed): Pediatric Neurosurgery, 3rd edn, Philadelphia: WB Saunders 1994;189-201.
22. Chowdhury V, Gulati P, Arora S, et al. Cranial Sonography in preterm infants. Indian Pediatrics 1992. p. 2.
23. Sauerberi EE, Digney M, Harrison PB, et al. Ultrasonic evaluation of neonatal intracranial hemorrhage and its complications. Radiology. 1981;139:677-85.
24. Levine MI. Measurement of growth of lateral ventricles in preterm infants with real time ultrasound. Arch Dis Childhood. 1981;56:900-4.
25. Davies MW, Swaminathan M, Churang SL, et al. Reference ranges for linear dimensions of the intra-cranial ventricles in preterm neonates. Arch Dis Child fetal Neonatal Ed 2000; 82:F218-23.
26. Perry RNW et al. Ventricular size in newborn infants. J Ultrasound Med. 1985;4:475-7.
27. Winkler P. Color encoded echographic flow imaging and spectral analysis of cerebrospinal fluid (CSF) in infants Part II CSF dynamics. Pediatr Radiol. 1992;22:31-42.
28. Seibert JJ, Mc Cowan TC, Chadduck WM, et al. Duplex pulsed Doppler US versus intracranial pressure in the neonate: Clinical and experimental studies. Radiology. 1989;171:155-9.
29. Bada HS, Miller JE, Menke JA, et al. Intracerebral pressure and cerebral arterial pulsatile flow measurements

in neonatal intraventricular hemorrhage. J Pediatr. 1982;100:291-6.
30. Taylor GA, Phillips MD, Ichord RN, et al. Intracranial compliance in infants evaluation with Dopper US. Radiology. 1994;191:787-91.
31. Taylor GA, Madsen JR. Neonatal hydrocephalus Hemodynamic response to fontanel compression-correlation with intracranial pressure and need for shunt placement. Radiology 1996;201:685-9.
32. Wolpert EM, Barnes PD. Clinical principles in pediatric neuroradiology. In MRI in Pediatric Neuroradiology. Philadelphia Mosby Year book 1992;41-80.
33. Very low birth weight outcomes of the National Institute of Child Health and human development neonatal network. Pediatrics. 1991;67:587-9.
34. Volpe JJ. Neurology of the Newborn. Philadelphia: WB Saunders 1987.
35. Rumack CM, Drose JA. Neonatal and Infant Brain Imaging in Diagnostic ultrasound 3rd Ed. Rumack Wilson Charboneau, Johnson (Eds) Mosby; 2005.pp.1623-702.
36. Hambleton G, Wigglesworth JS. Origin of intraventricular hemorrhage in the preterm infant. Arch Dis Child. 1976; 51:651-9.
37. Dykes F, Lazzara A, Ahmann I, et al. Intraventricular hemorrhage in newborn infant. Arch Dis Child. 1974;49:722-8.
38. Papile IA, Burstein J, Burstein R, et al. Incidence and evaluation of subependymal and intraventricular hemorrhage study of infants with birth weights less than 1500 gm. J Pediatr. 1978; 92:529-34.
39. Kirks DR, Bowic JD. Cranial ultrasonography of neonatal periventricular/intraventricular hemorrhage who, why, how and when? Pediatr Radiol. 1986;16:114-9.
40. Guillerman RP. Infant Craniospinal Ultrasonography: Beyond Hemorrhage and Hydrocephalus Semin Ultrasound CT MRI. 2010;31:71-85.
41. Babcock DS. Sonography of the brain in infants role in evaluating neurologic abnormalities. AJR. 1995;165:417-23.
42. Cooke RW. Early and late cranial ultrasonographic appearances and outcome in very low birth weight infants. Arch Dis Child. 1987;62:931-7.
43. Trounce JQ, Ratter N, Levene MI. Periventricular leucomalacia and intraventricular hemorrhage in preterm neonate. Arch Dis Child. 1986;61:1196-202.
44. Volpe JJ. Intracranial hemorrhage: Periventricular-intraventricular hemorrhage of the premature infant. In Volpe JJ (Ed): Neuro-Radiology of the Newborn 2nd edn, Philadelphia: WB Saunders 1987;311-61.
45. Volpe JJ. Current concepts of brain injury in the premature infant. AJR. 1989;153:243-51.
46. Taylor GA. Effect of germinal matrix hemorrhage on terminal vein position and patency. Pediatr Radiol. 1995;25:537-40.
47. Bergman I, Bauer RE, Barmada MA, et al. Intracerebral hemorrhage in the full term neonatal infant. Pediatrics. 1985; 75:486-96.
48. Chadha V, Mathur NB, Khaniju CM, et al. Periventricular hemorrhage in term germinal matrix. Indian Pediatrics. 1991; 28.
49. De Rinck J, Chatter AS, Richardson GPJ. Pathogenesis and evaluation of periventricular leucomalacia in infancy. Arch. Neurol. 1973;27:229-36.
50. Blankenberg F, Loh N, Norbash A, et al. Impaired cerebral autoregulation after hypoxic ischemic injury in extremely low risk weight neonates detection with power anal pulsed wave Doppler US. Radiology. 1997;205:563.
51. Bulas DI, Vezine GL. Preterm anoxic injury Radiologic evaluation. Radiol Clin N Am. 1999;27(6).
52. Chao CP, Zaleski CG, Patton AC. Neonatal Hypoxic Ischemic Encephalopathy. Multimodality Imaging Findings Radiographics. 2006;26;5159-72.
53. Daneman A, Epalman M, Blaser S, Jarrin JR. Imaging of the brain in full term neonates, does sonography still plays a role. Pediatric Radiol. 2006;36:636-46.
54. Han BK, Babcock DS, Mc Adams L. Bacterial meningitis in infants sonographic findings. Radiology. 1985;154:645-50.
55. Chowdhury V, Gulati P, Sachdev A, et al. Pyogenic meningitis sonographic evaluation. Indian Pediatrics 1991;26.
56. Das KM, Padmini P, Sachdeva S, et al. Sonographic evaluation of intracranial abnormalities in neonates and infants. IJR. 1(42):193-8.
57. Ganishan S, Dhawan SK, Mukherjee S, et al. Ultrasound in infectious meningitis. IJR. 1988;42(1):199-202.
58. Chowdhury V, Gulati P, Sachdev A, et al. Sonography in pyogenic and tubercular meningitis: A comparative study. Ind J Radiol Imagin. 1991;1:7-10.

CHAPTER 153

Inflammatory Diseases of the Brain

Vivek Gupta, Niranjan Khandelwal, Paramjeet Singh

INTRODUCTION

Role of imaging in CNS infections is supportive and helps to diagnose the involvement of the meninges, brain parenchyma and CSF spaces. The various imaging modalities available are computerized tomography (CT), conventional MRI pulse sequences and newer modalities like diffusion weighted imaging, MR spectroscopy, magnetization transfer imaging.

INVESTIGATIVE MODALITIES

CT is often the first modality of investigation in CNS infection because patient often presents with nonspecific signs and symptoms such as fever or seizures. CT can depict the late parenchymal changes in supratentorial lesions and complications such as hydrocephalus very well. The specific role of CT comes in evaluation for calcifications such as in congenital TORCH infections and calcifications in parenchymal granuloma. However, the CT findings in the early stage of infection are much nonspecific, evaluation of meningeal, cisternal and posterior fossa parenchymal lesions becomes difficult with contrast CT alone.

MRI plays a complementary role to the CT but is now the procedure of choice, because of lack of bony artifacts especially when visualizing the posterior fossa, has inherently excellent contrast resolution. MR is clearly superior to CT for demonstrating small lesions, white matter and meningeal pathologies. DWI is helpful in demonstrating complications of infections including early ischemia and infarction. Advances in MRI include proton spectroscopy which provides an in vivo assessment of the biochemical changes within inflammatory lesions and the surrounding brain.[1]

BACTERIAL INFECTIONS

The most common form of CNS infection is meningitis. Organisms can reach the meninges by five routes: (a) direct hematogenous spread, (b) passage through the choroid plexus, (c) rupture of superficial cortical abscesses, (d) penetrating trauma and contiguous spread from the infected sinuses and middle ear. Except for rare occasions, the diagnosis of meningitis is made from clinical signs and symptoms and the results of lumbar puncture. Imaging in meningitis is not performed routinely other than to ensure the absence of hydrocephalus or abscess formation before a lumbar puncture is performed. Neuroimaging is indicated if the clinical diagnosis is unclear, if the meningitis is associated with persistent seizures or focal neurological deficit.[1] On cross-sectional imaging thickened meninges showing continuous abnormal enhancement after contrast administration clinches the diagnosis of meningitis.[2] Contrast-enhanced MR is more sensitive imaging modality than contrast-enhanced CT in this regard **(Figs. 1A and B)**. Other imaging findings include inflammatory exudates in nonventricular CSF spaces, which are typically seen in granulomatous and fungal infections especially at the basal cisterns that can be hypo-, iso-, or hyperdense on CT and may show variable enhancement.

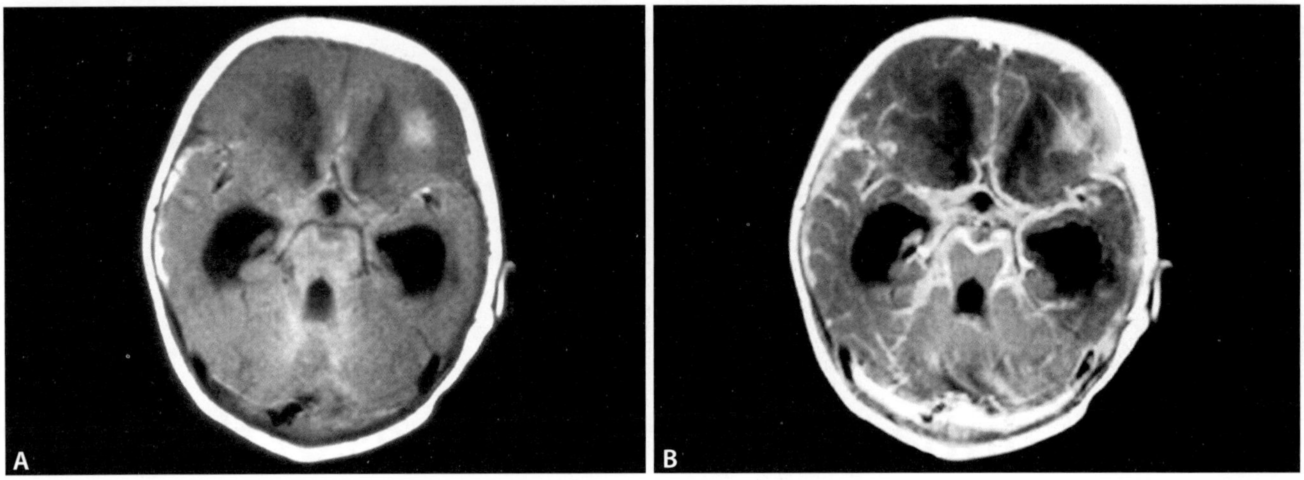

Figs. 1A and B: Meningitis: Noncontrast and contrast-enhanced short T1 MR sections showing intense leptomeningial enhancement in case of meningitis.

Once the meningeal infection is established, neurological sequelae can be caused by number of mechanisms. These include hydrocephalus, arteritis of penetrating cortical vessels, brain abscess formation, subdural effusion, subdural empyema, ventriculitis and venous thrombosis.

Hydrocephalus is demonstrated by all imaging modalities including ultrasound in the neonate. However, MR is most effective in localizing the level of obstruction.[3]

Subdural effusions are commonly encountered in meningitis due to *H. influenzae*. Unlike empyemas they are sterile fluid collections over the frontal and temporal lobes. They are usually not surgically treated as they regress along with the meningitis. On CT scan they appear isodense to CSF and may be slightly hyperintense to CSF on MR[4] **(Fig. 2A)**.

Subdural empyema **(Fig. 2B)** are associated with *Pneumococcus meningitis*. The reported incidence is 20% of all intracranial bacterial infections.[4] The cause of empyema is spread of infection from the paranasal sinuses, middle ear, calvarial osteomyelitis, infection following shunt placement or craniotomy or contamination of effusions. They are commonly located over the frontal lobes or close to the source of infection from the paranasal sinuses or middle ear.[5,6] On imaging studies empyemas are seen as widening of extracerebral spaces which appear as hypo-isodense crescentric or lentiform collection adjacent to the inner table **(Fig. 2B)**. On contrast administration (especially on CT) a thin curvilinear rim of enhancement is present demarcating the empyema. Mass effect may be evident with effacement of sulci, compression of ventricles and midline shift. In infants, transfontanelle sonography using 7–10 MHz transducer will show empyemas as hyperechoic collections often with fibrinous strands and a thick hyperechoic inner membrane. Sterile effusion on the contrary appear anechoic.[6] On MR, there are no signal characteristics which can distinguish empyema from nonpurulent collections, because they appear hyperintense to CSF on both T1- and T2-weighted images. It is important to remember that any extra-axial collection associated with sinusitis, otitis or orbital cellulitis indicates presence of empyema. Empyemas are generally unilateral, however reactive effusion due to *H. influenzae* are usually bilateral.[6]

Ventriculitis **(Figs. 3A and B)** is the term for inflammation of the ependymal lining of one or more ventricles. The cause of ventriculitis is due to possible retrograde spread of infections from the basal cisterns or due to a rupture of a periventricular abscess. Another possible source is via the choroid plexus. In neonates cranial sonography can demonstrate hyperechoic CSF or a proteinaceous debris in the dependent ventricle. On contrast-enhanced MR/CT, the ependymal lining of the ventricle shows intense enhancement which is pathognomonic of ventriculitis.[1,4]

Venous thrombosis can affect deep veins, cortical veins and dural venous sinuses as a complication of meningitis. Sinus thrombosis can be diagnosed on CECT as empty delta sign which is a triangle of decreased density in the posterior segment of the affected sinus.[4,7] On MR acute thrombus is seen as hyperintense structure on T1WI. Other than in the subacute phase thrombi, are difficult to image on MR.[1,4] MR venography by phase contrast technique is particularly useful in detecting venous thrombosis.[4] Arteritis occurs when the meningitis process spreads into perivascular space. Arteritis manifests as arterial infarcts

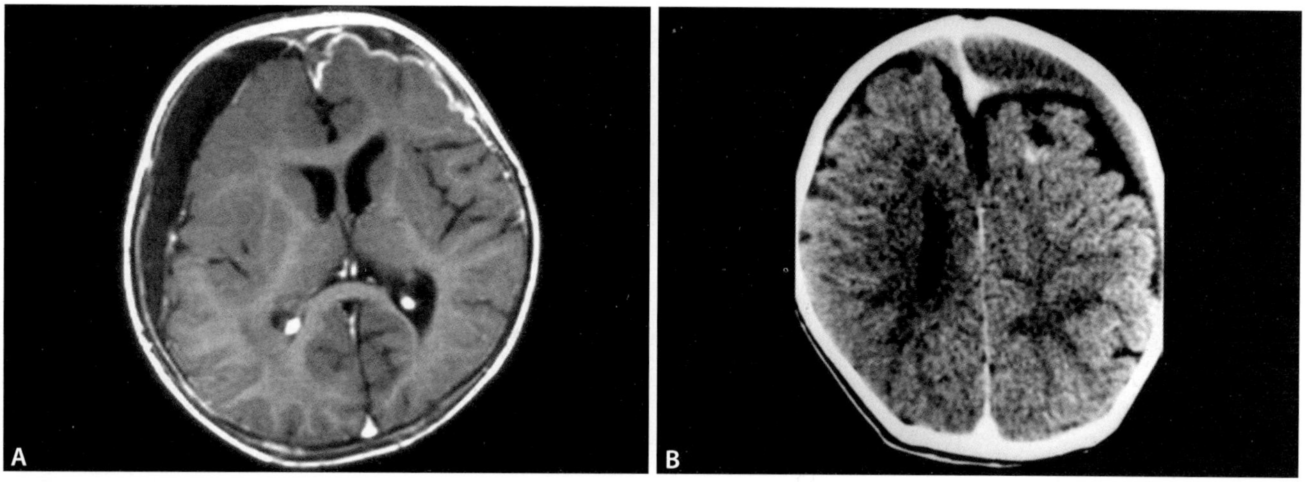

Figs. 2A and B: Sequelae of meningitis: (A) Subdural effusions in a patients of *Haemophilus influenzae* meningitis. Effusion appears as extracerebral collection over the frontal lobes which are isointense to CSF. Note leptomeningeal enhancement over the left frontal lobe; (B) Subdural empyema appears as a extracerebral collection which is of higher density than ventricular CSF in this CT scan section.

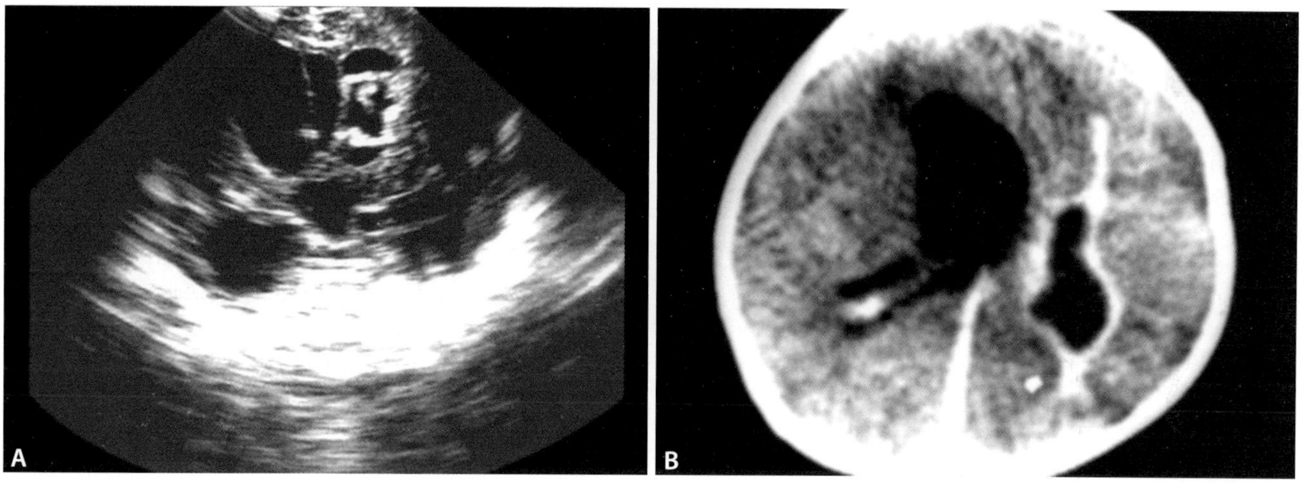

Figs. 3A and B: Ventriculitis on ultrasound (A) and CT scan (B): On ultrasound, there is increased echogenicity around the left lateral ventricle with internal septations. Ependymal enhancement on CT is the hallmark for diagnosis of ventriculitis.

which are seen as sharply demarcated areas corresponding to arterial territories on CT or MRI.[4]

Brain Abscess

It implies encapsulated pus within the brain parenchyma, usually secondary to acute pyogenic infection. Cerebral abscess is usually secondary to either trauma or paranasal sinus infection and an equal proportion is idiopathic. Other rare causes are post-surgical wound infection and septicemia. Most often brain abscess is solitary, but can be multiple in approximately 11–14% of cases and are usually secondary to cyanotic heart disease or middle ear infections. Infratentorial abscesses alone, or in association with supratentorial abscesses are invariably otogenic in origin **(Figs. 4A and B)**. Overall frontal and parietal lobes are the commonest sites for abscess formation. Cross-sectional imaging helps in the diagnosis, localization and in detecting complications of cerebral abscesses.

Abscesses Evolve in Four Stages

Stage I—early cerebritis stage: It consists of an inflammatory infiltrate of polymorphonuclear cells, lymphocytes plasma cells. Considerable edema is present around this infiltrate.

Stage II—late cerebritis stage: This is a stage when focal necrosis of the brain becomes better defined. Encapsulation begins as vessels proliferate around the necrotic area with increasing deposition of reticulin inflammatory cells and minimal amount of collagen.

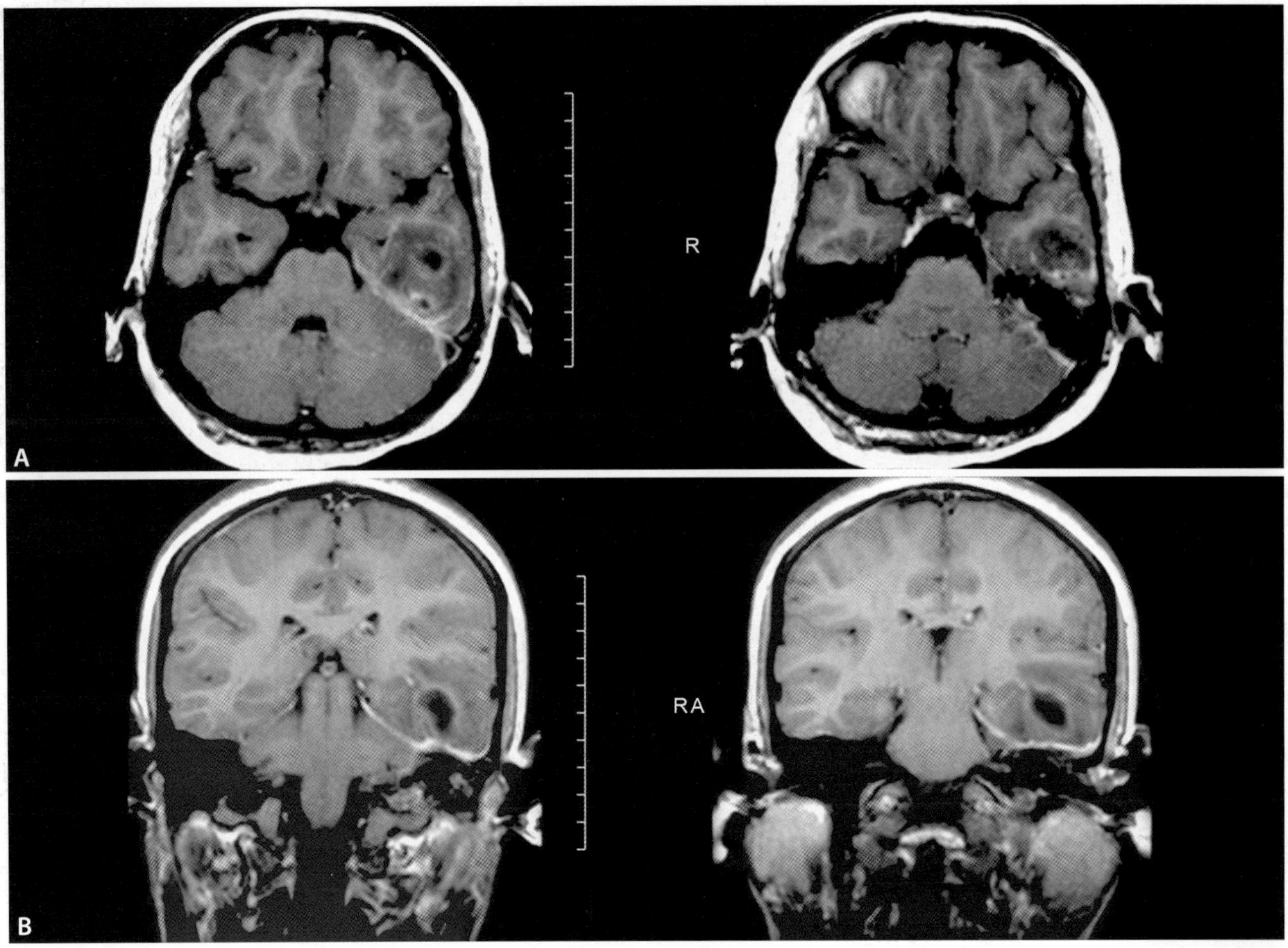

Figs. 4A and B: Otogenic brain abscess: Axial and coronal contrast-enhanced T1 WI showing enhancement within the middle ear cavity. There is enhancement of the leptomeninges over the petrous temporal bone. An ill-defined mixed intensity mass with peripheral rim-enhancing lesion is present in the overlying temporal lobe which is suggestive of an evolving brain abscess.

Stage III—early capsule formation: It is characterized by walling off the necrotic area by increasing deposition of collagen and reticulin. The capsule is better delineated than stage II. The surrounding edema tends to regress with partial resolution of the cerebritis.

Stage IV—late capsule formation: It is a stage when the encapsulation of the abscess by collagen deposition is complete. The abscess is well defined and smaller than stage III. The wall is better delineated and thicker towards the cortex than medially towards the ventricles, possibly due to the increased vascularity of the gray matter. These four stages evolve within 7–14 days.[1,7]

The imaging features mirror the evolutionary stages of abscess formation **(Figs. 5A to C)**.

On noncontrast CT scan abscess appear hypodense with a barely discernable hyperdense wall. On contrast administration the capsule or the wall of the abscess enhances and measures 5 mm or less in thickness. There is surrounding edema.[7]

On MR all four stages can be recognized.[1,8] Stage I is heterogeneous on T1 and T2WI with patchy enhancement after contrast injection. In stage II the abscess wall can be recognized as a hyperintense rim on T1WI. On T2WI the rim is hypointense. Contents of the abscess are heterogeneous on both sequences. Abscess wall is shown to be thicker in stage II than stages III and IV. The abscess wall enhances intensely in this stage. Contents of the abscess may also show enhancement. In stage III the abscess wall will be hyperintense on both T1- and T2-weighted sequences. Contents of the abscess are uniformly hypointense and hyperintense on T1- and T2-weight images, respectively. Abscess wall will enhance after contrast administration. Stage IV abscesses show isointense walls on T1WI which are hypointense on T2WI. Contents of the abscess are

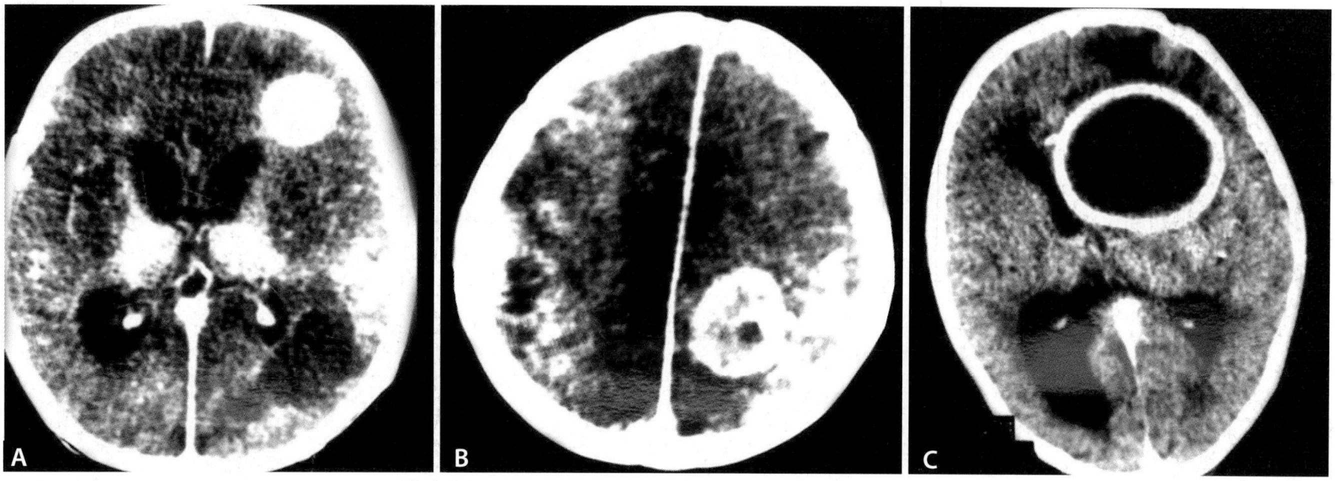

Figs. 5A to C: Stages of abscess formation: Axial CT sections from different patients show (A) An area of cerebritis in the left frontal lobe which appears as area of focal enhancement; (B) Stage of encapsulation and liquefaction. The lesion here shows a central hypodensity which is the area of liquefaction; (C) Formation of an abscess which appears as well-defined hypodense area with rim enhancement.

isohypointense on T1WI and hyperintense on T2WI; abscess walls enhance after contrast administration. Changes in the signal intensities in the wall of the abscess is believed to be reflecting the decreasing free water in the collageneous tissue.[8]

Role of protron MR spectroscopy lies in differentiation of abscesses from tumors.[9-12] Tumors show presence of choline, creatinine and NAA peaks whereas abscess show lipid peaks or amino acids together with a lactate peak. Attempts have been made recently to categorize MR spectral patterns with respect to underlying etiologic agents.[13] In this study, differentiation of anaerobic, aerobic or sterile brain abscess was attempted based on significant quantitative differences between lactate levels and ratios of lactate and amino acid peaks.

Complications of brain abscess include extension of the abscess into the ventricular system leading to ventriculitis; and subarachnoid spaces leading to purulent leptomeningitis. Daughter abscesses may develop when due to poorly developed capsule; abscess ruptures into the adjacent parenchyma.

CRANIAL TUBERCULOSIS

Central nervous system involvement occurs in 2–5% of all tuberculosis patients and in up to 15% of AIDS patients. Coexistent pulmonary tuberculosis is often seen in 25–83% of cases of CNS tuberculosis. Adult tuberculosis is most often a post primary infection whereas most cases in children are due to primary infection.[14] Intracranial tuberculosis manifests in three forms, viz. isolated meningeal involvement, isolated parenchymal form and compound parenchymal/meningeal lesions.

Tuberculous Meningitis

Tuberculous meningitis (TBM) is the most common form of presentation of CNS tuberculosis in children in India. The cause of (TBM) is thought to be rupture of a subependymal or subpial focus (rich focus) from an earlier hematogeneous dissemination into the CSF space.[14] Incidence of tuberculous meningitis is directly proportional to the prevalence of endemic tuberculosis. The diagnostic criteria of TBM on imaging are:[15]

1. Enhancing basal exudates,
2. Progressive hydrocephalus, and
3. Infarction in the striate cortex.

Basal Exudates

In tuberculous meningitis, there is a thick, gelatinous exudate around the brainstem, extending into the basal cisterns and into the sylvian fissures. Noncontrast CT scan or T1W MR images show these exudates as isodense (isointense) or hypodense (hypointense) areas in the basal cisterns.[1] Intense enhancement occurs after intravenous contrast administration **(*see* Figs. 1A and B)**. Exudates can be easily overlooked on T2W MR images because they will appear hyperintense similar to CSF and cannot be thus distinguished.[14] The degree of involvement of meninges over the convexities and in the depth of sulci are better appreciated on MR than on CT. Meningeal enhancement can extend over the cerebral hemispheres. Bhargava et al.[16] have graded the exudates as mild (+), moderate (++) and severe (+++). In mild grade, the cisterns are obliterated but do not enhance; in moderate grade, increased attenuations are seen outlining the obliterated cisterns and in severe grade, there are copious and dense exudates with increased attenuation filling and enlarging the cisterns. In their study this grading had a prognostic significance. Patients with severe degree of exudates had a longer duration of illness and carried a higher incidence of morbidity and mortality. Severe grade of exudates were seen to occur mostly in children.

Hydrocephalus

Communicating hydrocephalus is most commenly observed due to obstruction of flow of CSF by the exudates in the basal cisterns (e.g. suprasellar cisterns, cistern ambiens) and over the cerebral convexities. Uncommonly obstruction of the aqueduct by exudates results in non-communicatinghydrocephalus.Presenceofhydrocephalus may precede the obliteration of basal cisterns by several weeks and is frequently associated with poor prognosis especially in children. Presence of periventricular ooze suggests high pressure hydrocephalus. The progress of hydrocephalus can be followed up by sequential CT scans. The incidence of hydrocephalus increases with the duration of disease.[16-18]

Infarction

Inflammatory changes in arteries and veins result in formation of thrombi which in turn cause multiple infarcts. The middle cerebral artery territory is the most common area where infarcts due to meningeal tuberculosis occur. Involvement of the perforating vessels arising from circle of Willis is common and it results in infarcts of the basal ganglia. The area supplied by the medial striate and thalamoperforating arteries are specially affected in TBM and are termed as the medial TB zone as opposed to the area supplied by the lateral striate, anterior choroidal and thalamogeniculate arteries which is termed the lateral ischemic stroke zone.[18-20] Infarcts appear as low density regions on CT and as areas of prolonged T1 and T2 relaxation time on MR. Apart from the regions described above, infarcts can also occur in the cerebral cortex due to involvement of cortical vessels but these are less common.

Detection of ischemic infarcts by MR is significantly higher as compared with CT. MRI also helps in differentiating cerebritis from infarction because on diffusion weighted imaging (DWI) infarction will appear bright with matching area of decreased signal on apparent diffusion coefficient map. It is important to note that early cerebritis and infarction both appear as areas of increased signal intensity on conventional MR sequences, however, cerebritis will, in time, evolve into an abscess and arterial infarction will confirm to distinct topographical lesion corresponding to arterial territories.[2] In addition, a large number of these infarcts are hemorrhagic in nature on MR, finding which has not been well documented on CT scans. MR angiography may be a useful modality in follow-up of patients with vasculitis secondary to TBM. The findings are similar to those seen on autopsy or conventional angiogram and consist of a triad of narrowing of the arteries at the base of the brain, narrowed or occluded small or medium sized arteries associated with early draining veins and wide sweep of pericallosal arteries secondary to hydrocephalus.[18-20]

Parenchymal Tuberculous Granulomas

Tuberculous granuloma (tuberculoma) is the most common form of parenchymal lesion.[15] Granulomas of tuberculosis occur at all ages. These may be solitary or more commonly multiple **(Figs. 8 and 9)**. Infratentorial lesions are more common in children.[21,22] Parenchymal tuberculomas appear as multiple conglomerate punctate or ring enhancing lesions at the junction of gray and white matter.

On CT scan tuberculomas appear as low or high density ring lesions which are rounded or lobulated and enhance after contrast administration. The walls of these ring lesions are irregular and of varying thickness. There is moderate to marked perilesional edema frequently seen with parenchymal tuberculomas.[23,24]

MR features of individual tuberculomas are dependent on whether the lesion is noncaseating, caseating with a solid center or caseating with a liquid center **(Table 1)**.[24]

The noncaseating granuloma is hypointense on T1WI and hyperintense on T2WI. On contrast administration the lesion usually shows homogeneous nodular enhancement **(Figs. 6A to D)**. The caseating granuloma with a solid center **(Figs. 7A to D)** appears hypointense to isointense on T1 weighted images and isointense to hypointense on T2 weighted images. The wall of the caseating TB granuloma often has a striking hypointense rim on T2WI which enhances on administration of gadolinium. In vivo proton MR spectroscopy has shown presence of lipids in caseating granulomas which characterizes this lesion.

Caseating granulomas with central liquefaction of caseous material appears hypointense on T1WI and hyperintense on T2WI with a peripheral hypointense rim on T2WI **(Figs. 8A to C)**. Enhancement of the rim occurs after gadolinium administration as in the granulomas with a solid center and are indistinguishable from pyogenic abscess on the imaging characteristics.

Differential diagnosis of parenchymal tuberculoma includes cysticercosis, pyogenic and fungal lesions and foci of primary or metastatic neoplasia. Ring enhancing lesions on CT in patients presenting with epilepsy present

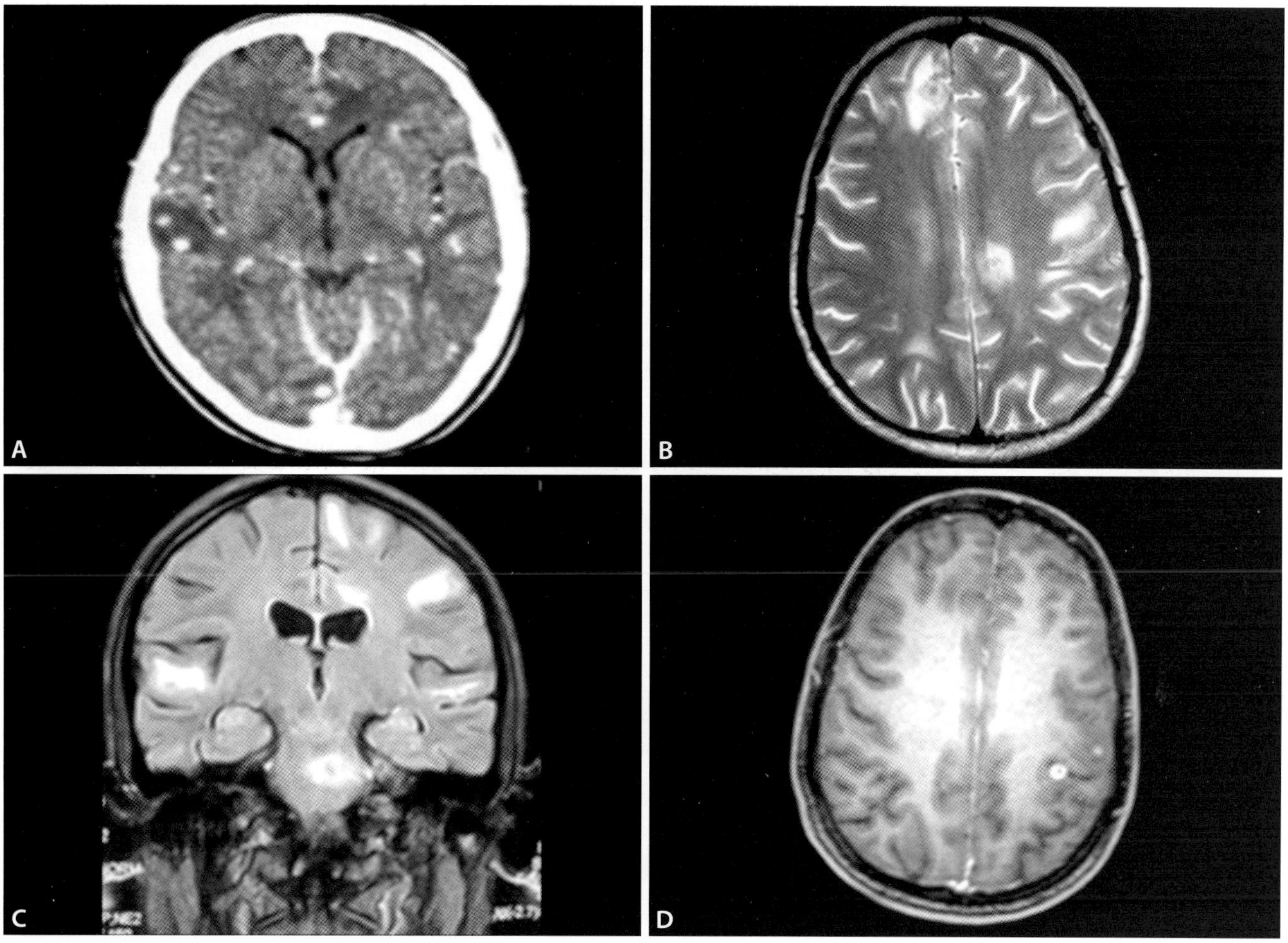

Figs. 6A to D: Tuberculous granuloma with no caseation (A) NCCT showing noncaseating granulomata in bilateral frontoparietal lobes showing nodular homogeneous enhancement. (B) T2W axial image (C) FLAIR coronal image and (D) T1 postcontrast image showing T2 hypointense lesions with perilesional edema showing nodular homogeneous postcontrast enhancement in left parietal lobe.

Table 1: MR features of intracranial tuberculoma.

Lesion	*T1WI*	*T2WI*	*Postcontrast T1WI*
Noncaseating granuloma	Hypointense	Hyperintense	Homogeneous nodular enhancement
Caseating granuloma with solid center	Hypo- to isointense core	Iso- to hypointense core with striking hypointense rim	Contrast enhancement of rim
Caseating granuloma with central liquefaction	Hypointense	Hyperintense with hypointense rims	Contrast enhancement of rim (resembling abscess)

a diagnostic dilemma since granulomas of cysticercus and tuberculosis both have similar morphological appearances.

Rajshekhar et al.[25] have reported that it is possible to distinguish between solitary cysticercus granuloma and tuberculous granuloma in patients presenting with seizures on the basis of clinical signs and radiological (CT) findings. In patients with tuberculoma there is evidence of raised intracranial tension with progressive neurological deficit. On CT scan the size of ring enhancing lesion is usually larger than 20 mm. Some of these may show irregular outlines, most of them cause midline shift. In contrast to this, neurocysticercus granuloma are less than 20 mm in size, rounded or oval in outline and appear as disks or rings. There is no significant mass effect. These findings based on the size and shape of lesions in their study had a specificity of 100% and 96% respectively. They have also stressed the role of repeat CT scans after 8–12 weeks of anticonvulsant therapy to rule out enlarging lesions which could be due to different etiologies. They advocated that all lesions larger than 20 mm should be biopsied to reach definitive diagnosis.

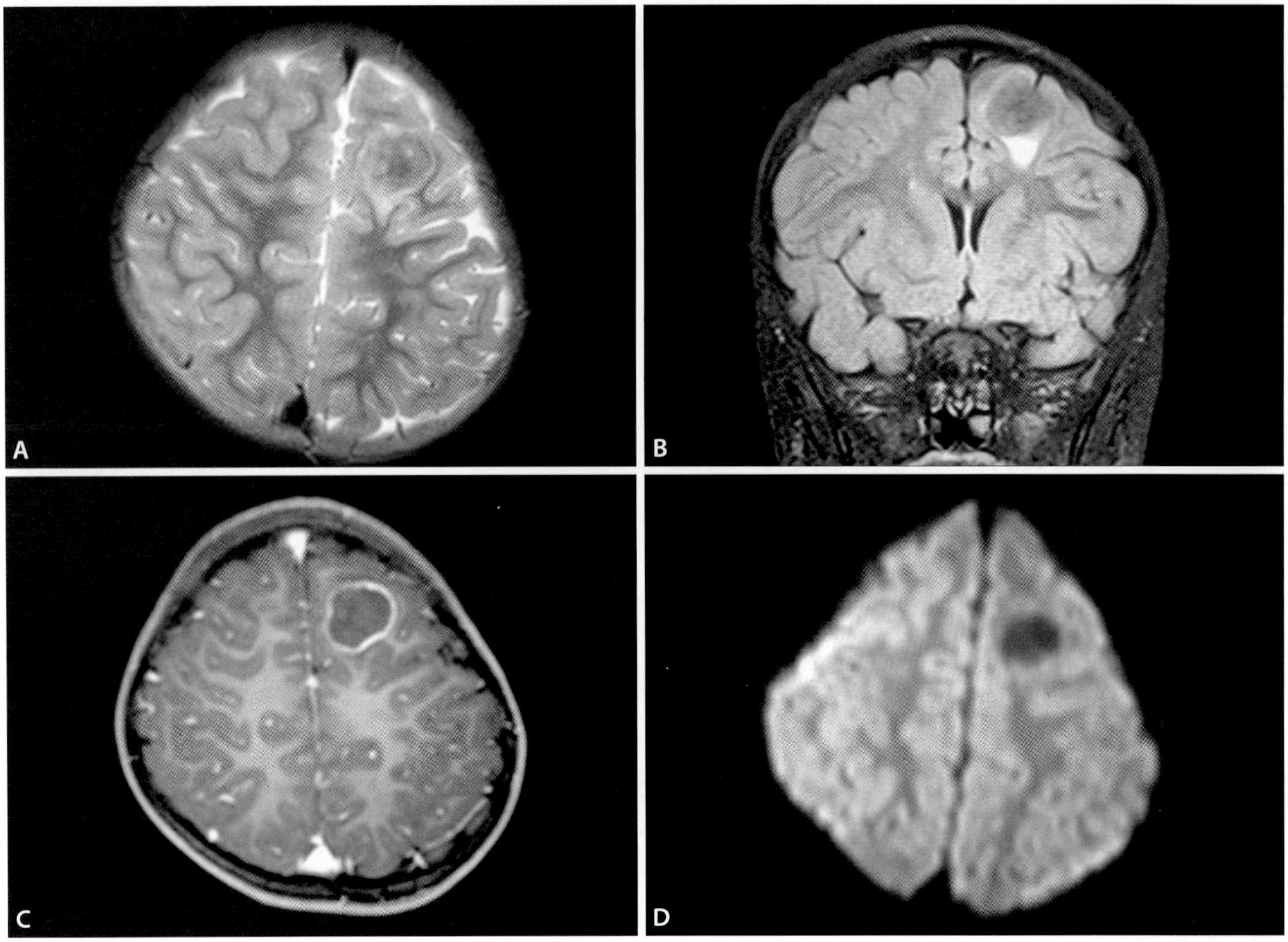

Figs. 7A to D: Tuberculous granuloma with solid caseation: (A to C) T2, FLAIR hypointense lesion in left high frontal lobe (A and B); (C) This lesion shows peripheral postcontrast enhancement; (D) The solid portion of the lesion shows no diffusion restriction on DW image.

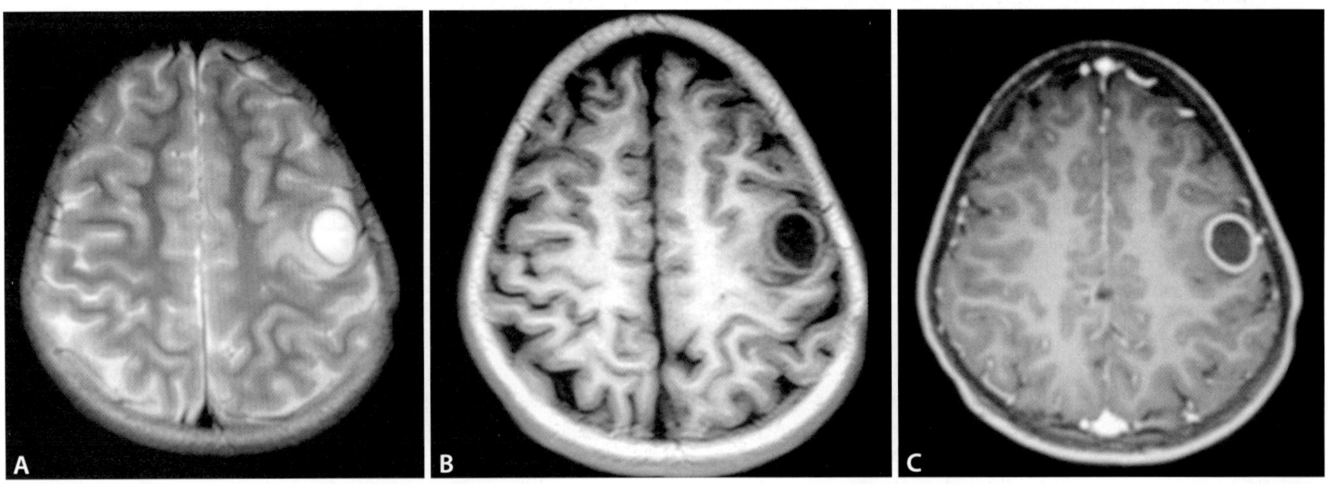

Figs. 8A to C: Tuberculous granuloma with liquid caseation: (A and B) T1 isointense and T2 hyperintense lesion in left high frontal lobe; (C) This lesion shows peripheral postcontrast enhancement.

In recent times, MR spectroscopy has been used with some success in distinguishing tuberculomas from pyogenic abscesses. Intracranial tuberculomas on protron MRS primarily show peaks from lipids at 0.9.1.3, 2.0 and 2.9 ppm **(Figs. 9A to F)**.[26] The major difference between spectra of tuberculomas and pyogenic abscess is that

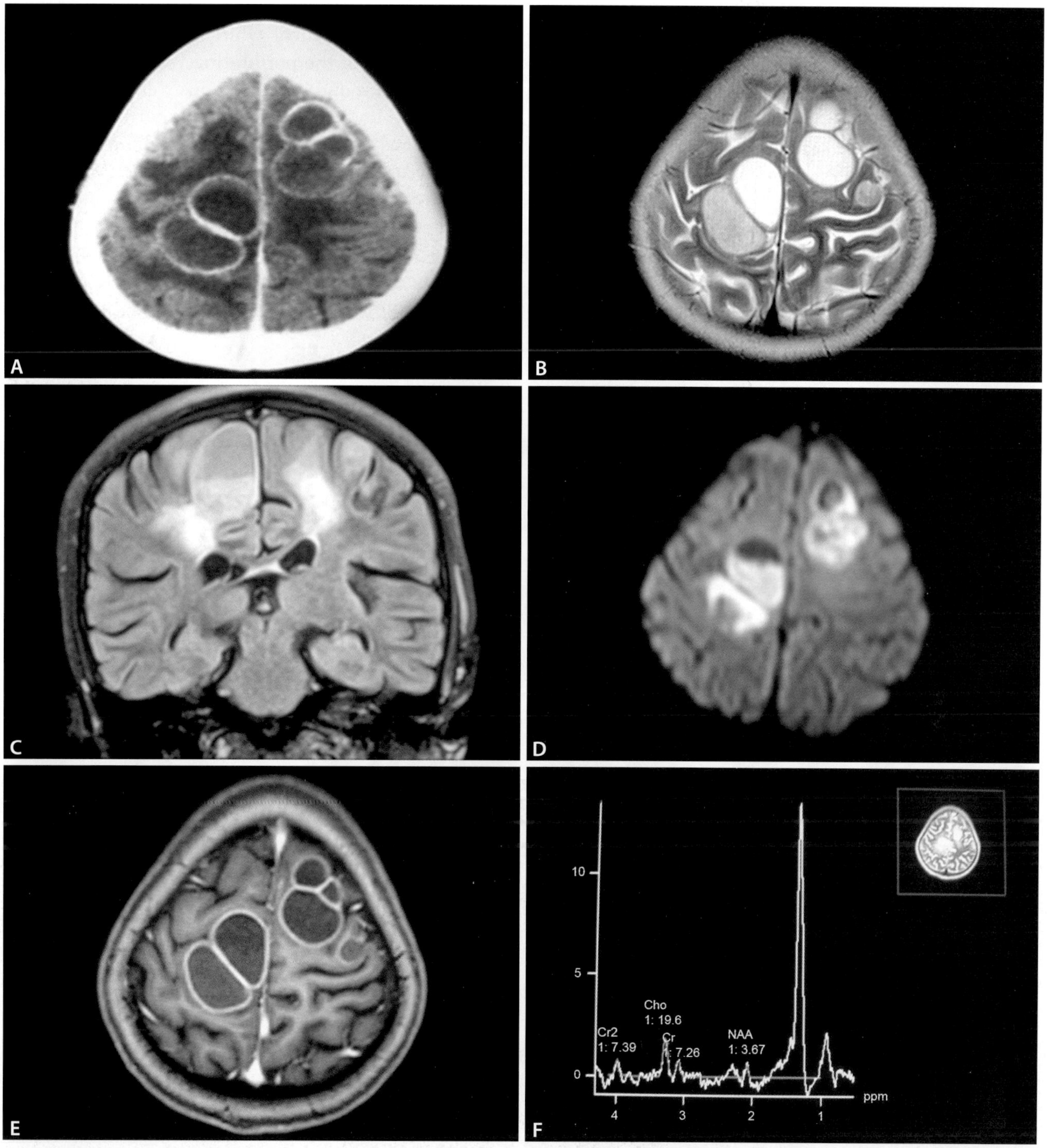

Figs. 9A to F: An 11-year-old child with multiple tubercular abscesses on antitubercular therapy: (A) CECT; (B) T2W1; (C) FLAIR; (D) DWI; (E) CEMR images showing multiple conglomerate ring-enhancing lesions in bilateral high frontoparietal lobes. Few of these lesions are showing restriction on DWI suggestive of partially treated lesions. Single voxel MR spectroscopy done at TE = 30 showing lipid peak at 1.3 ppm (F).

although lipid and lactate peaks are found in both conditions, an increased amino acid peak (choline peak) is found only in pyogenic abscesses **(Figs. 10A to C)**.[27]

Compound Parenchymal and Meningeal Tuberculosis

Meningeal and meningocerebral forms of tuberculous pathology of the brain can coexist and in one series they are the least common of all presentations.[23]

Rare presentation of intracranial tuberculosis includes tuberculous abscess and miliary tuberculosis. In general, true abscess formation is uncommon in CNS tuberculosis. Tuberculous abscess may be found more frequently in adults and immunocompromised patients.[21] Children are less commonly affected. Tuberculous abscess as opposed to tubercular granuloma is composed of pus teaming with tubercular bacilli which are few or absent in the latter. Tuberculous abscess is thin walled **(Figs. 9A to F)**. Walls are smooth and regular in thickness and indistinguishable from pyogenic abscesses on CT and MR although tuberculous abscesses are often multiloculated. Response to chemotherapy is variable as TB abscesses may not resolve and may have to be treated surgically.[28-30]

Miliary tuberculomas in the brain may be a feature of generalized miliary tuberculosis and the primary focus may be found in the lung or elsewhere. They are distributed in the cortical–white matter junction and in the distribution of the perforating vessels. They appear on CT as small round homogeneously enhancing lesions in the supra- and infratentorial compartments. On MR they appear as high intensity foci throughout the brain on T2WI. There is associated tuberculous meningitis. Their appearance may rarely precede the onset of meningitis. If treatment is successful the lesions may disappear. Paradoxical response to treatment may occur with the lesions increasing in size and new lesions appearing during the course of therapy.[31,32]

NEUROCYSTICERCOSIS

Pediatric neurocysticercosis should be considered an endemic disease in the third world countries. It assumes significance in the wake of its presentation in the form

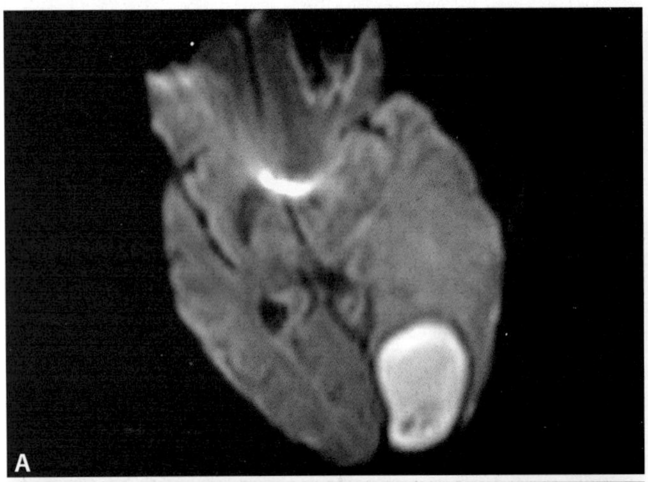

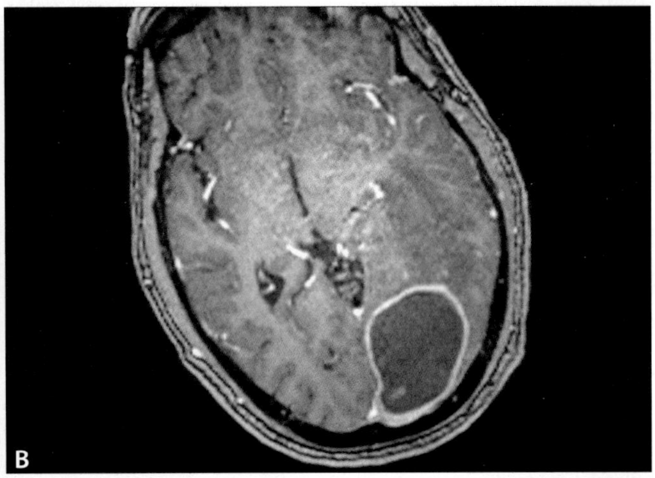

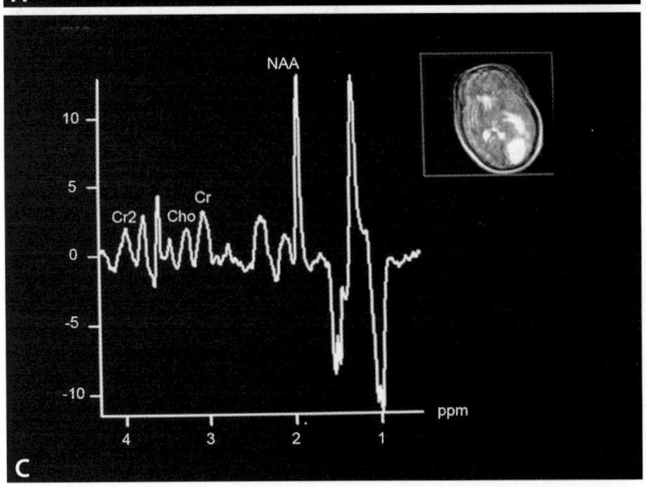

Figs. 10A to C: (A) The DW image shows restriction in the cavity of the lesion; (B) Pyogenic abscess in left occipital lobe; (C) Single voxel MR spectroscopy of pyogenic abscess at TE 30 shows lipid lactate peak at 1.3 ppm and presence of acetate (2.3 ppm) and succinate (2.5 ppm) peaks.

of one of the most common cause of focal epilepsy. The disease is transmitted by encysted form of *Taenia solium*. To become clinically manifested two hosts are needed to complete its life cycle. Humans are an intermediate host, acquiring the organism by accidental ingestion of tapeworm eggs from fecal contaminated substances. The eggs hatch in the small intestine, burrow into the mucosa and penetrate the venules. Mature larvae, or cysticerci, develop after 60–70 days.[33]

Clinical Features and Pathology

The expression of the disease is variable, although seizures have been reported in as high as 92% of patients. Headaches and focal neurological deficits are also common. Pathologically, four forms of cysticercosis have been described: (a) parenchymal cysticerci, (b) leptomeningitis, (c) intraventricular cysticerci, (d) racemose cysts.[1]

Parenchymal cysticerci are categorized according to Escobar's four pathological stages.[34]

Vesicular stage: The larva is seen as a small marginal nodule projecting into a small cyst containing clear fluid. The parasites are viable and elicit little or no inflammatory response in the surrounding tissue.On imaging a clearly marginated cyst with cyst fluid similar to the CSF signal intensity. A discrete, eccentrically placed scolex is seen. No contrast enhancement is seen in the cyst wall **(Figs. 11A and B)**.

Colloidal vesicular stage: As the larva begins to degenerate and the scolex shows signs of hyaline degeneration, the cyst shrinks in size, cyst fluid becomes turbid and cyst wall becomes thick with presence of surrounding inflammatory reaction. The cyst is slightly hyperintense on T1-weighted images and markedly hyperintense on T2-weighted images. There is associated contrast enhancement of cyst wall and perilesional edema.

Granular nodular stage: The cyst undergoes retraction and the scolex is transformed into a coarse mineralized granule and surrounding edema regresses gradually. The cyst may be seen as a nodular or a thick small ring-like enhancement. Occasionally, a target or bull eye appearance is seen with the calcified scolex in the center of the mass.

Nodular calcified stage: By this stage the granulomatous lesion has contracted to a fraction of its initial size. On NCCT scans, a small calcified nodule without mass effect or enhancement is typical **(Figs. 12A to C)**.

Leptomeningitic Form

It is seen on CT and MR scans as soft tissue filling the basal cisterns. After intravenous contrast administration, as with other granulomatous meningitides, there is marked enhancement of the subarachnoid space in the involved areas.The enhancement charecteristics of these granulomata are similar to those of parenchymal granulomata. Hydrcephalus and vasculitis are common with leptomeningitic form.[35]

Intraventricular Form

They are important to identify because affected patients can die from acute intraventricular obstruction. They are most commonly seen in the fourth ventricle followed by the lateral third ventricle and can migrate from one ventricle

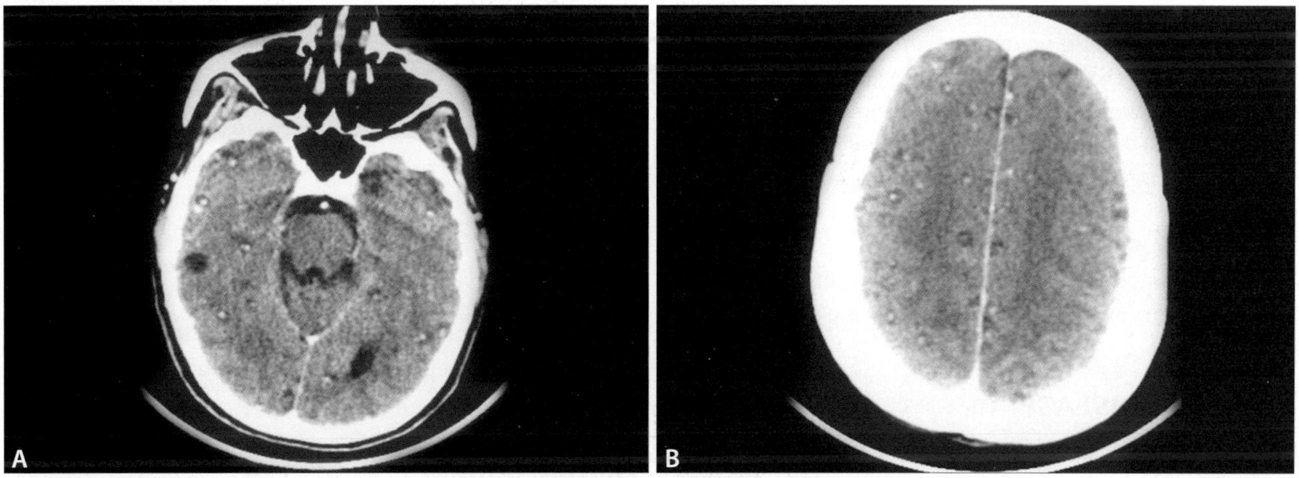

Figs. 11A and B: Diffuse intraparenchymal neurocysticercosis: (A and B) CECT axial sections showing multiple cystic attenuation lesions seen in bilateral cerebral hemispheres. These lesions are not associated either with perilesional edema or enhancement suggestive of vesicular stage of NCC. The scolices are seen as eccentric hyperdense foci within the cysts.

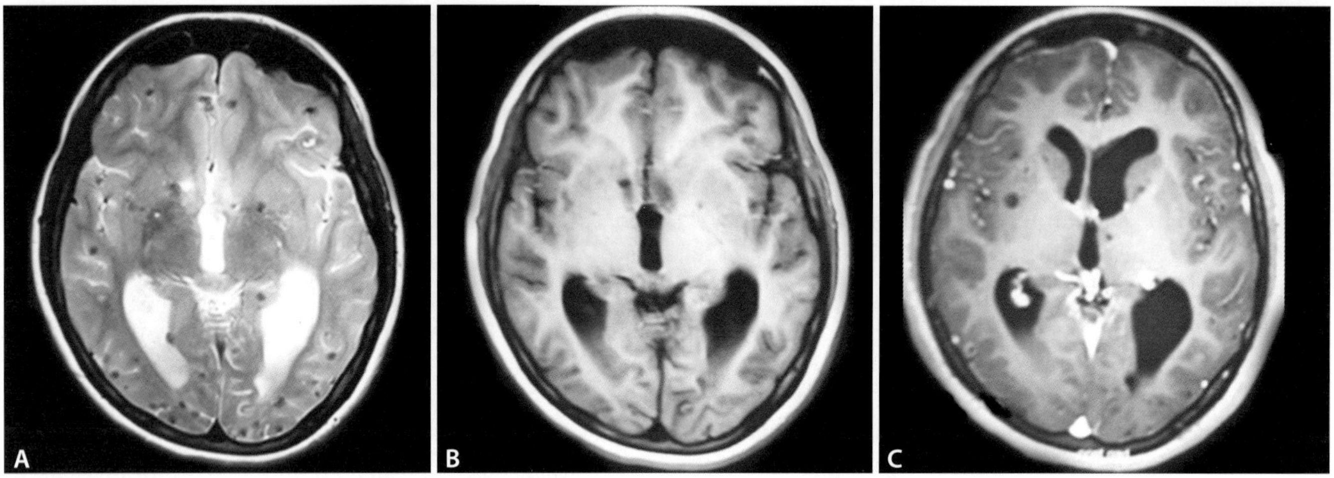

Figs. 12A to C: Calcified nodular stage of neurocysticercosis: (A to C) Multiple well-defined lesions that are hypointense on both T1 and T2W images with no definitive post-contrast enhancement.

to another ventricle and can be trapped in aqueduct of Sylvius to cause acute hydrocephalus. The MR imaging is superior to CT in imaging of these lesions. T1-weighted images 3 mm or less in thickness optimize detection of the scolex **(Figs. 13A and B)**. The use of steady state sequences such as constructive interference in steady state can also be useful in finding intraventricular or cisternal cystic lesions. Sagittal and coronal plane images allow better appreciation of fourth ventricular lesions.[34]

Racemose Cysts (Subarachnoid Form)

These are multilobular, nonviable (therefore lacking scolex) cysts located in the subarachnoid space. They are most commonly seen in the cerebellopontine angle, the suprasellar region, the sylvian fissures and the basilar cisterns. Although the lesions are sterile these lesions can grow by proliferation of cyst wall. On CT scans, large cystic lesions are seen which may enhance after contrast administration. On MRI, multiple cysts of varying size, clustered together like grapes are seen in the involved cisterns **(Figs. 14A to D)**. A combination of large cyst/cysts, multilobulation of a cyst, lack of mural nodule within the cyst, cisternal location and leptomeningeal enhancement on MRI strongly suggests that the lesion is caused by racemose cysticercus especially in endemic areas. A chronic leptomeningitis and arteritis may accompany these cysts.[1,34]

HYDATID DISEASE

Hydatid disease is caused by *Echinococcus granulosus* and less frequently by *Echinococcus multilocularis*. Human infection occurs by contact with definite host dog or by drinking or eating contaminated water or vegetables.

Ingested ova hatch in the gastrointestinal tract. Liberated embryos can then spread to virtually every organ or tissue via the portal and systemic circulation. They subsequently develop into cystic larva termed as hydatid cyst. CNS involvement occurs in 5% of cases as compared to liver (65–75%) and lung (15–20%). The cysts are usually unilocular, solitary and located in parietal lobes.[36]

CT shows presence of a thin-walled spherical CSF density cyst in the parietal area. Calcification of the wall is rare and enhancement is uncommon. The MR T2W sequence shows a typical thin low signal intensity rim surrounding a high signal intensity lesion **(Figs. 15A and B)**.

VIRAL ENCEPHALITIS

Encephalitis is defined as generalized and diffuse inflammatory disease of the brain with parenchymal infiltration of inflammatory cells either due to direct invasion (usually viral infections) or due to immune-mediated hypersensitivity process. Although a large number of viruses may effect the brain, all exhibit two common pathological processes—neuronal degeneration and inflammation. Imaging is required for early detection and accurate diagnosis because some patients may present with atypical clinical features and laboratory findings. MRI is widely accepted as a sensitive technique for the diagnosis of encephalitis and is very useful for detecting early changes.[37]

Herpes Simplex Encephalitis

Herpes simplex encephalitis (HSE) is the most common among sporadic encephalitis. HSV-1 causes 95% of all

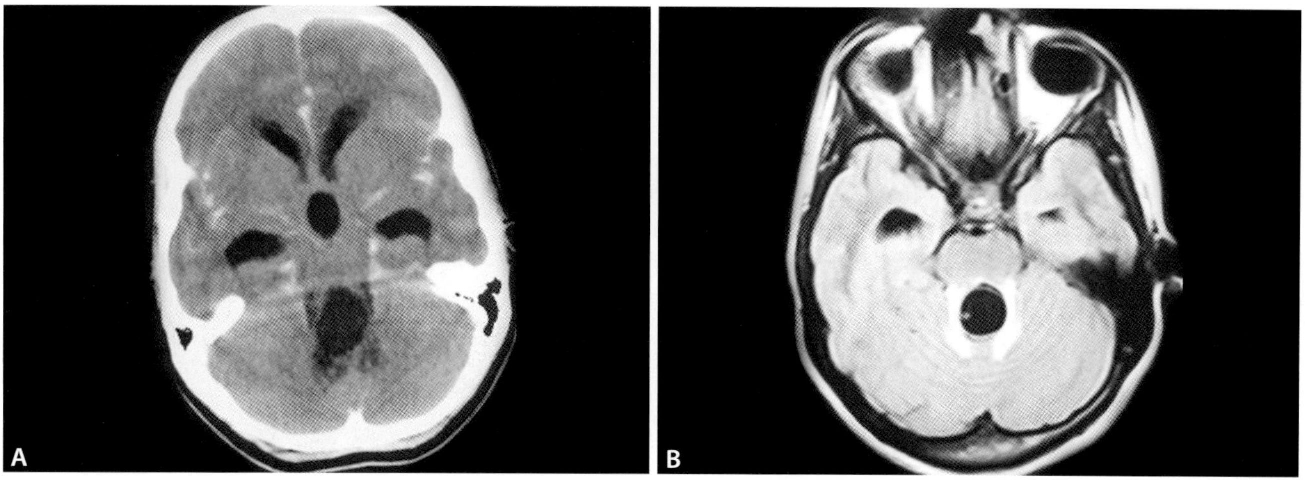

Figs. 13A and B: Intraventricular neurocysticercosis: (A) CECT image reveals presence of dilated supratentorial ventricular system and cystic lesion in fourth ventricle having enhancing eccentric nodular focus; (B) FLAIR image delineates the scolex in the cystic lesion.

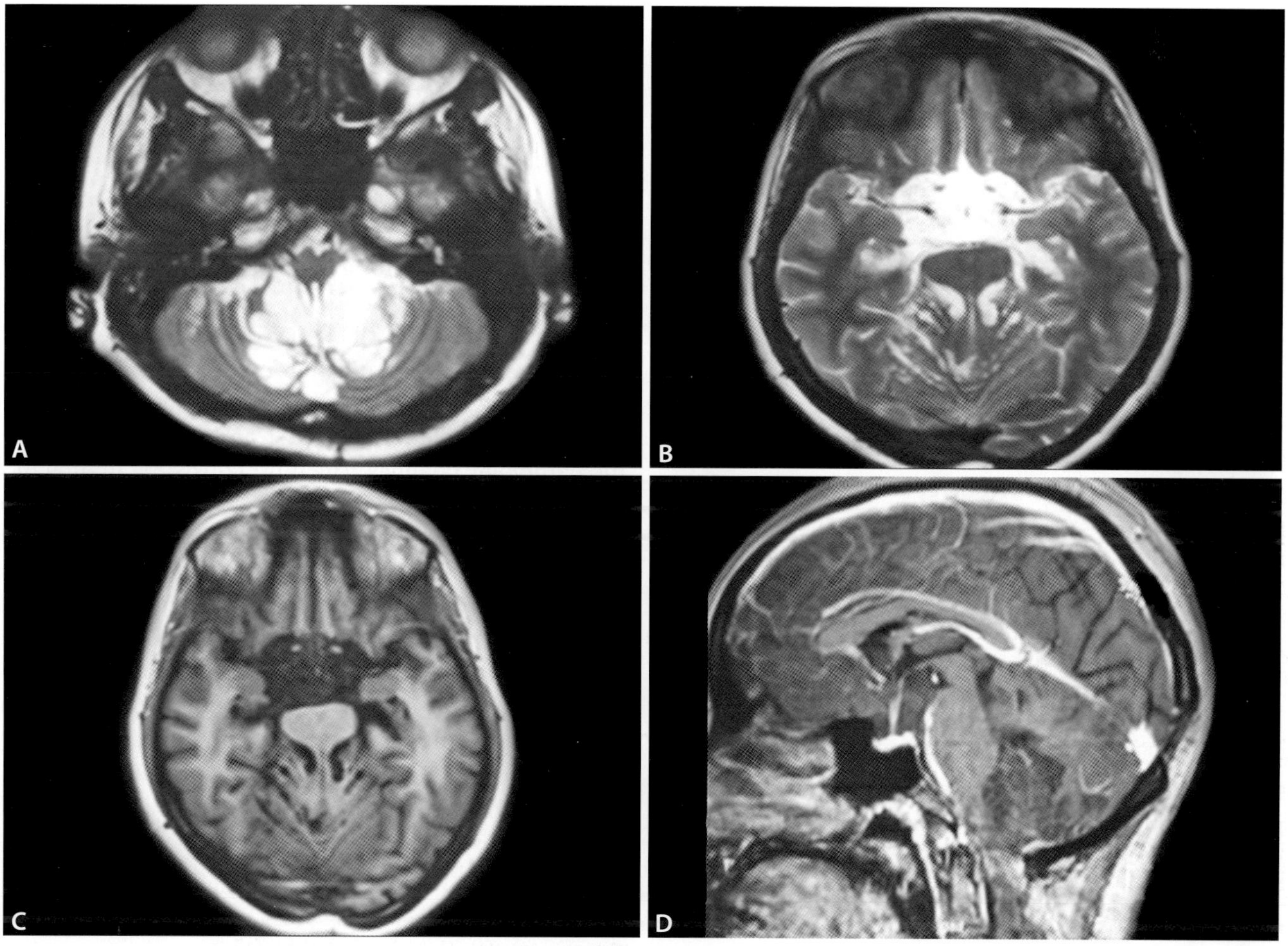

Figs. 14A to D: Racemose form of neurocysticercosis: (A to D) Multiple conglomerate cystic signal intensity lesions in bilateral sylvian fissures and basal cisterns.

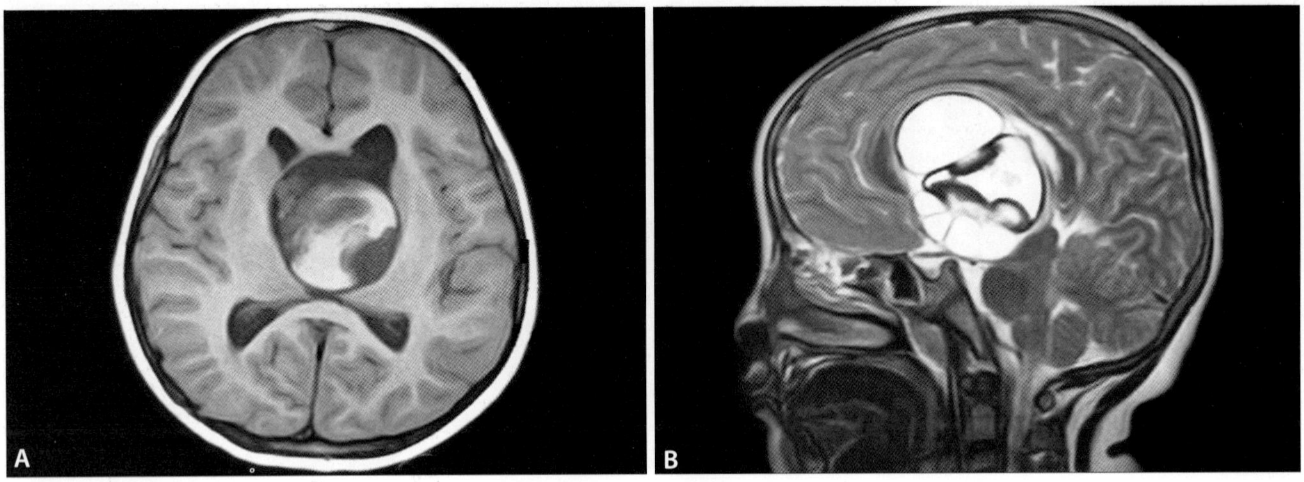

Figs. 15A and B: Suprasellar hydatid cyst: (A) T1 axial and (B) T2 sagittal images showing a large cystic lesion in suprasellar location surrounding T2 hypointense rim membranes within it.

herpetic encephalitis. Herpes simplex virus type 2 is the cause of neonatal herpes encephalitis. Initial HSV-1 infection occurs in oronasopharynx through contact via infected secretions. Later it invades along the cranial nerves (olfactory, trigeminal nerves). HSV-1 reactivation may occur spontaneously or be precipitated by various factors like local trauma, immunosuppression. The pathological hallmark of HSV encephalitis is hemorrhagic necrotizing encephalitis which results in severe edema and massive tissue necrosis. HSV-1 disease has a predilection for the limbic system and the lesions are localized to the temporal lobes, the insular cortex, subfrontal areas and the cingulate gyrus. HSV-1 encephalitis has a characteristic sequential bilaterality, i.e. initial lesions are unilateral but are followed by less severe contralateral disease. Changes appear earlier on MR than on CT. The findings include gyral edema in the involved regions which are better appreciated on T2WI and FLAIR sequences **(Figs. 16A and B)**. Contrast administration shows enhancement of the affected cortex and surrounding leptomeninges.

As the disease progresses T1 and T2 shortening develop secondary to hemorrhage and calcification.[38,39]

Herpes simplex virus-2 encephalitis is seen in neonates is acquired from infection in maternal genital tract. The virus destroys the brain leaving the pial glial membrane, ependyma and choroid plexus. Sonography of affected neonates show diffuse hyperechogenicity of the brain without ventricular compression. As the disease progresses, the ventricles dilate and the encephalomalacic brain shows increasing hyperechogenicity. On MR, the lesions are nonspecific with shortened T1 and T2 relaxation times in all sequences which persists for weeks or months. The changes are most marked in cortical gray matter.[38,39]

Japanese Encephalitis

Japanese B encephalitis (JE) is a major health problem in Southeast Asian countries. The JE virus belongs to the mosquito-borne flavivirus group and has an established endemicity, with frequent seasonal epidemics. The subclinical infections by JE virus outnumber the clinically overt disease. When clinically apparent, JE manifests as acute fulminant neurologic disease with fever, rapid development of focal neurologic signs, and unconsciousness, often resulting in death. Pathologic changes in the brains of acute JE patients are characterized by glial nodules and circumscribed necrolytic foci. These involve the thalami, sub-stantia nigra (SN), corpus striatum, cerebral cortex, brain stem, and cerebellum.

The imaging findings on CT and MR imaging reflect the pathologic changes. The most consistent finding in JE is bilateral thalamic lesions with or without hemorrhagic changes on MR imaging **(Figs. 17A and B)**. Hemorrhage in the thalami and basal ganglia is reported but is not a usual feature of JE. Although thalamic, SN and basal ganglia lesions are characteristic of JE. Temporal lobe involving hippocampus sparing rest of temporal lobe may also be seen. This and the concurrent involvement of the thalami, SN and basal ganglia allow differentiation from HSE.[40,41] Diagnosis of JE is confirmed by showing a fourfold rise in the antibody titer in a paired sample.

Post-varicella encephalitis occurs in <0.1% of children with a past history of chickenpox. Darling et al.[42] have shown that Varicella Zoster Virus (VZV) encephalitis takes two forms: (1) Bilateral, symmetric, hypodense, nonenhancing basal ganglia lesions on CT and nonenhancing low intensity lesion on T1WI and high signal intensity on T2WI

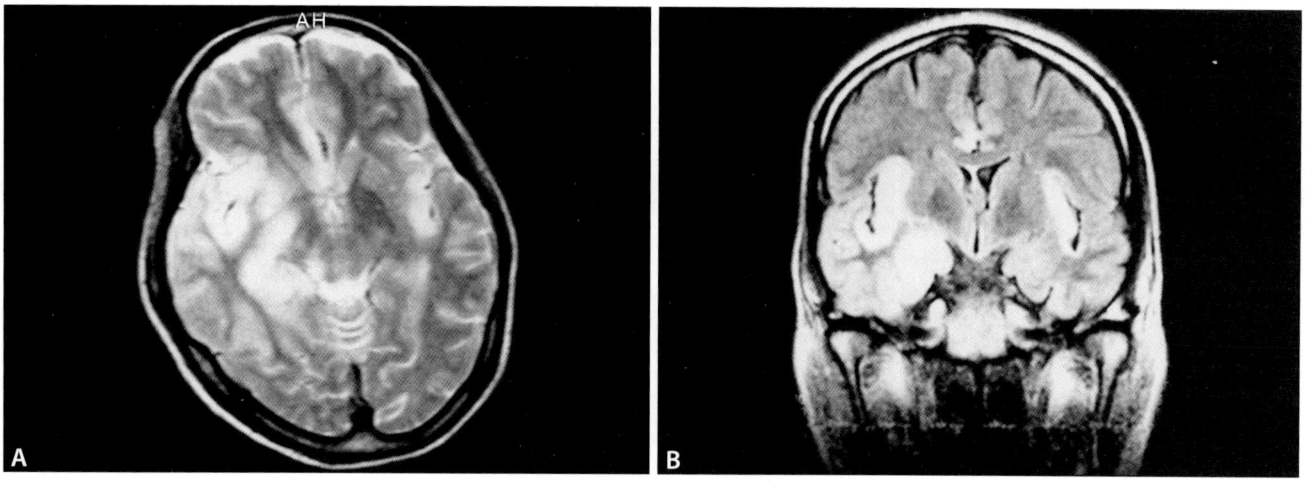

Figs. 16A and B: Herpes encephalitis: (A) T2W image and (B) FLAIR image showing hyperintensities involving bilateral medial temporal lobes, bilateral insular cortex and cingulate gyri.

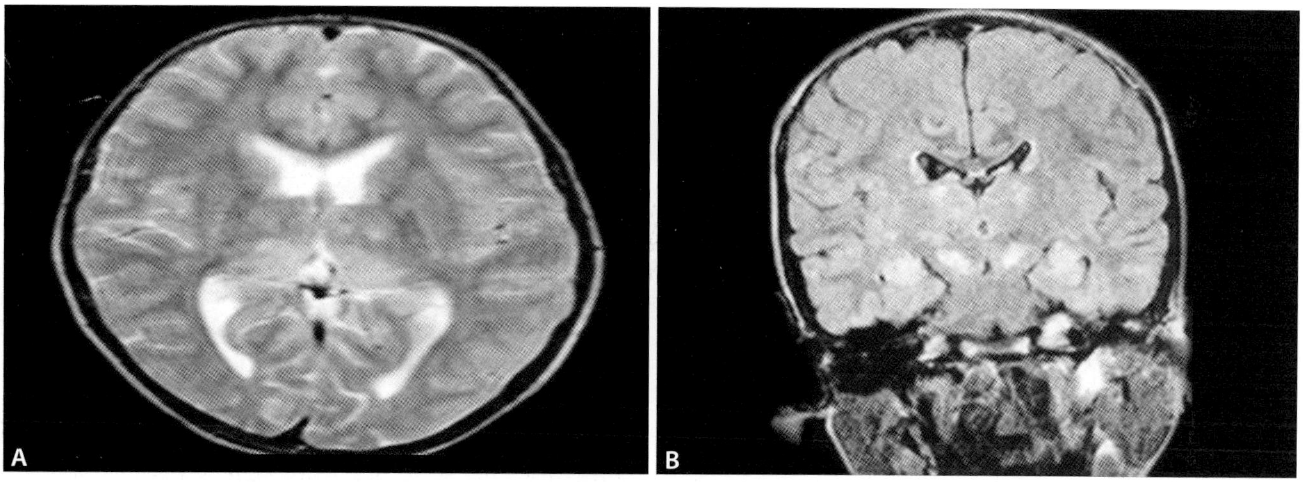

Figs. 17A and B: Japanese encephalitis: (A) T2W image and (B) FLAIR image showing hyperintensities involving bilateral thalami and substantia nigra.

on MRI, (2) Diffuse, multiple gray and white matter lesions of similar imaging characteristics.[42]

Subacute sclerosing panencephalitis (SSPE) is a slow progressive infection by measles virus (Morbilli virus genus). The condition manifests after a latent period of 3–9 years after measles infection. Boys are affected more than girls. MRI is more sensitive in detection of the lesion and in assessing the extent of the disease. In the early stages the lesion is usually located in the gray matter and subcortical white matter of the parietal and temporal lobes **(Figs. 18A to C)**. It is asymmetrical and bilateral. As the disease progresses, high signal intensity in the centrum semiovale and periventricular white matter is observed. In the final stages of the disease, diffuse cortical atrophy develops with T2 prolongation in the brainstem. Basal ganglia involvement is seen in 20–35% of affected patients.[43]

Acute disseminated encephalomyelitis (ADEM) is a delayed sequelae of viral encephalitis. It can occur following vaccination. It is a rare disease and has been reported as a sequelae with measles, varicella, smallpox, infectious mononucleosis, herpes zoster, mumps or influenza. Subcortical demyelination at gray-white matter junction is the hallmark of ADEM. It appears as areas of hyperintensity on T2WI in the periventricular white matter, centrum semiovale and corona radiata. The lesions are not surrounded by edema, are sharply demarcated and do not show mass effect. Contrast enhancement is variable. Involvement of spinal cord, cerebellum and brainstem may be present together with lesions in the deep cerebral nuclei mainly the thalamus, globus pallidii and putamina in about 50% of affected patients.[1]

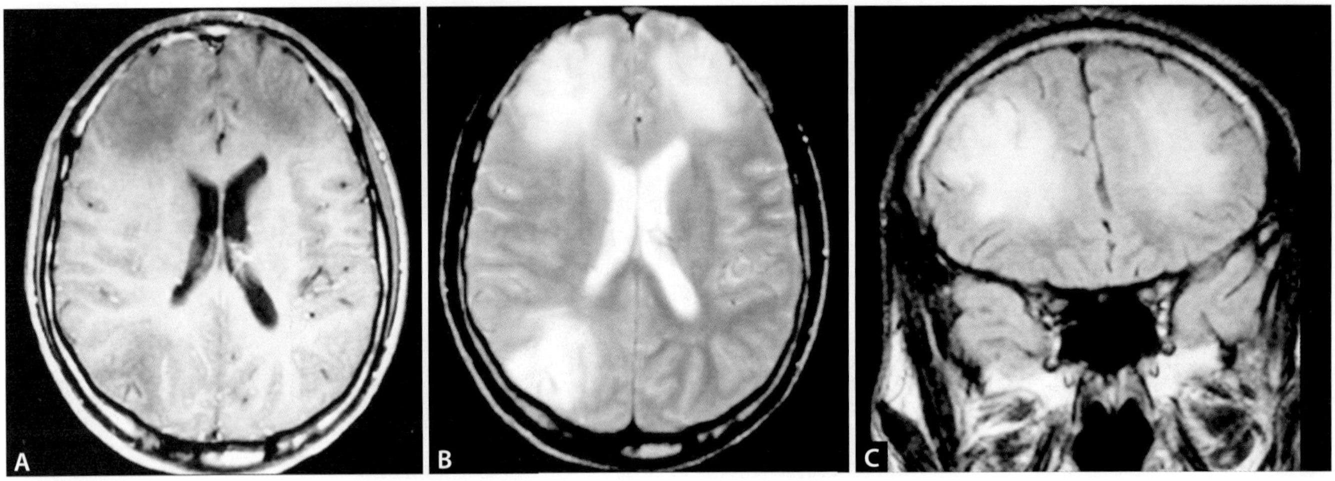

Figs. 18A to C: Subacute sclerosing panencephalitis: (A to C) T1 hypointense and T2 and FLAIR hyperintense lesions are seen in bilateral frontal and parieto-occipital lobe white matter.

DWI in Encephalitis

The MR appearance on DWI may be related to pathologic changes that occur following viral invasion. In the acute stage there are areas of congestion, perivascular cuffing and thrombus formation pathologically. These changes are responsible for the cytotoxic edema that leads to restricted diffusion and low ADC, changes that may not be picked up on conventional MR pulse sequences **(Figs. 19 and 20)**. In the late acute and early subacute stages, the components of vasculitis and perivascular cuffing diminish, so the proportion of diffusion restriction decreases and ADC starts to increase. At this stage due to vasogenic edema the number and extent of the lesion will be more marked in T2 and FLAIR images.[44]

CONGENITAL INFECTIONS

Infections of the fetal nervous system differ from those of older children and adults in that the age of the fetus at the time of insult is more important than the nature of insult. In general, infections during the first trimesters will result in congenital malformations whereas those that occur during the third trimester are manifested as destructive lesions.[1,45]

The transmission of infection is by two modes. Bacteria travel through the amniotic fluid whereas toxoplasmosis, syphilis and viruses usually pass through the placental circulation.

Cytomegalovirus

Congenital cytomegalovirus disease is the most common cause of CNS infection in neonates. It results from vertical transmission of the cytomegalovirus from the mother to the fetus transplacentally. It can cause hematologic, neurologic and developmental signs and symptoms.

Patients presumably infected during the first half of the second trimester, have lissencephaly with a thin cortex, hypoplastic cerebellum, delayed myelination, marked ventriculomegaly and significant periventricular calcification. Those infected in the middle of second trimester have more typical polymicrogyria, less ventricular dilatation. Patients infected near the end of gestation or in early post-natal period have normal gyral pattern and damaged periventricular or subcortical whitematter with scattered periventricular calcification **(Figs. 21A to E)**. When the findings of dystrophic calcifications, cortical malformations, myelination delay and cerebellar hypoplasia are present in a child with developmental delay or seizures, a diagnosis of congenital CMV is considered.[1]

Toxoplasmosis

It is the second most common cause of congenital CNS infections. The infection may be generalized or localized to the central nervous system. The CNS findings are choreoretinitis, hydrocephalus and seizure activity. The findings on cross-sectional imaging may be similar to those in CMV infection. Dystrophic calcifications located in basal ganglia, periventricular region and cerebral cortex are seen. Microcephaly, large ventricles and hydrocephalus can be seen. Absence of cortical and gyral malformations can be differentiating feature from CMV infection.

Neonatal Herpes Simplex Encephalitis

Herpes simplex virus-2 encephalitis seen in neonates is acquired from infection of maternal genital tract. The

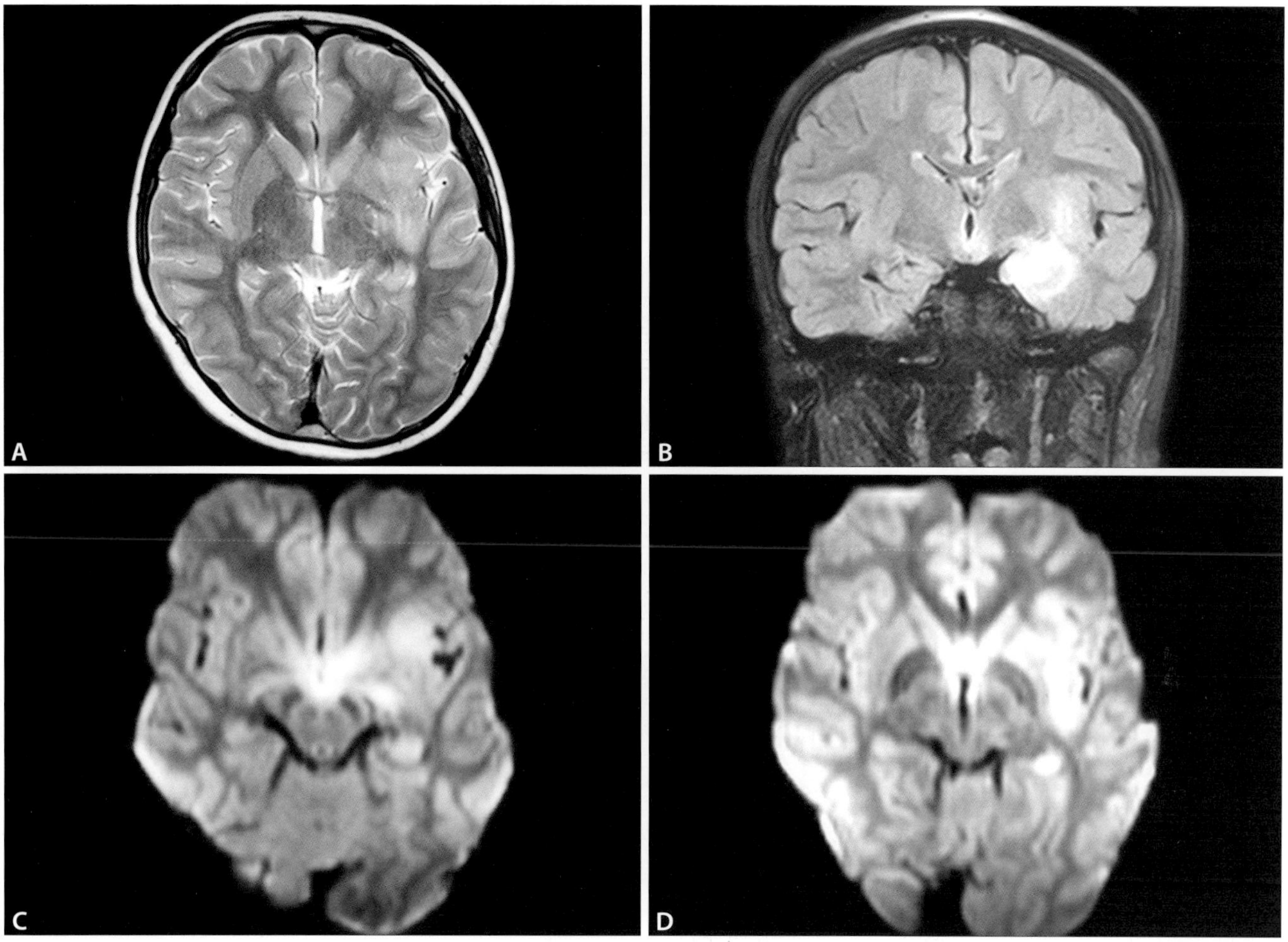

Figs. 19A to D: DWI in herpes encephalitis: Unilateral involvement in early stages on T2W and FLAIR images (A and B) of HSV encephalitis showing diffusion restriction (C and D) in the left medial temporal lobe and insular cortex.

virus destroys the brain leaving the pial glial membrane, ependyma and choroid plexus. Sonography of affected neonates show diffuse hyper-echogenicity of the brain without ventricular compression. On MR for the first two days, the lesions are patchy, widespread areas of prolonged T1 and T2 relaxation times in white matter, with restriction on DWI. Later the changes are seen in cortical gray matter. As the disease progresses, cortex shows thinning, the ventricles dilate and the encephalomalacia changes are seen in white matter and gyral or punctuate calcifications are seen.

Rubella

Congenital rubella is transplacentally transmitted infection. Risk of fetal damage is highest during the first trimester and decreases subsequently. Infection results in microcephalic brain with cortical and basal ganglia calcifications. CT show hypodensity through out the white matter together with calcification in periventricular region, basal ganglia and cortex. On MR multifocal bright lesions will be seen on T2WI with delay in myelination. Predilection of the virus for vascular endothelium may cause thrombosis or hemorrhagic infarction.

Congenital HIV Infection

HIV infection is a significant public health problem because of large number of HIV infected women who are having children. Nearly 80% of all childhood HIV infections are maternally transmitted, although only one third of HIV positive mothers pass on the infection. CNS manifestations are primarily of two types: Progressive encephalopathy and static encephalopathy. Neuro-imaging studies reveal meningoencephalitis, atrophy and calcific vasculopathy. HIV encephalitis results in diffuse cerebral atrophy (90% cases) and calcification of basal ganglia and subcortical white matter

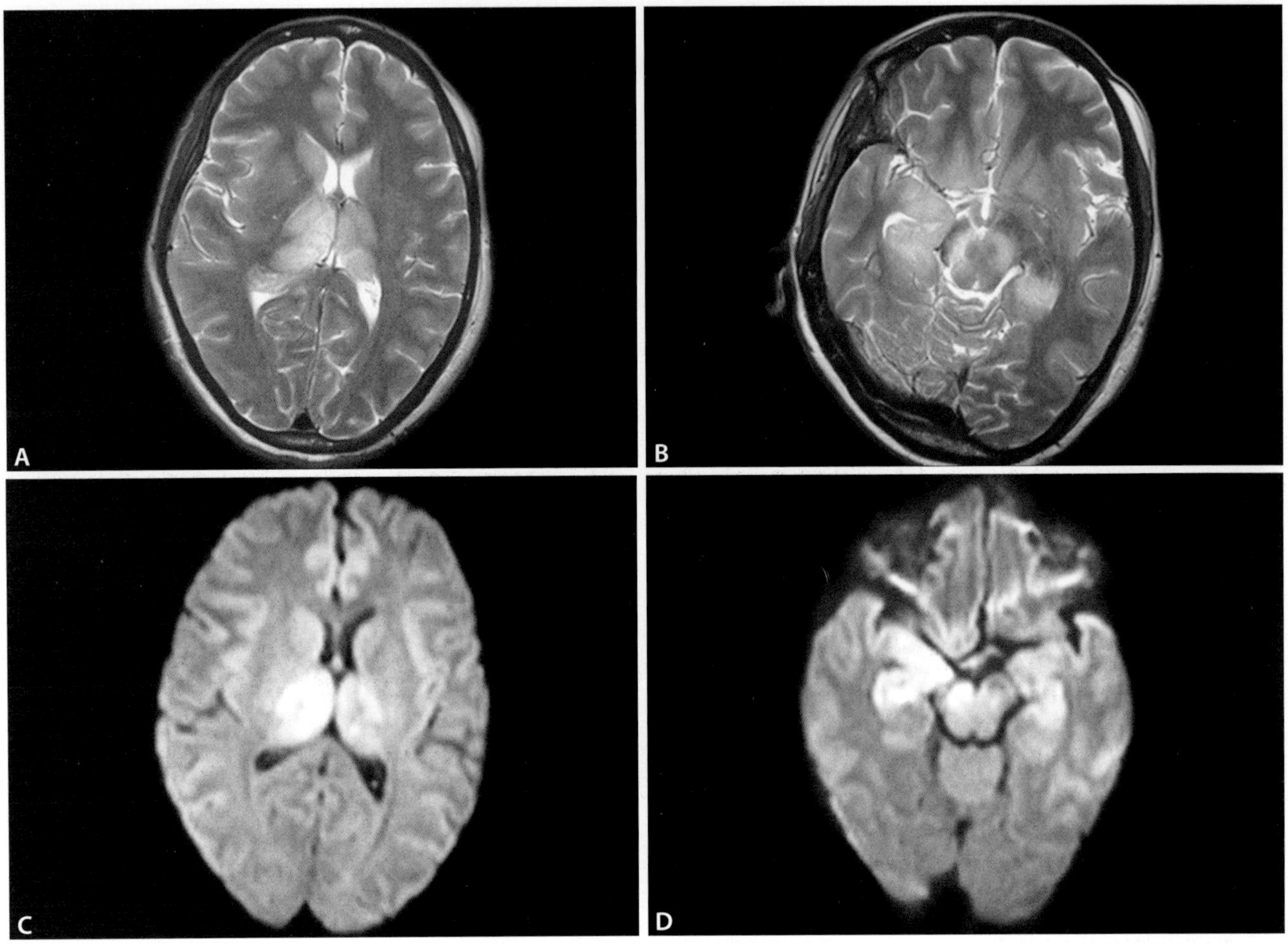

Figs. 20A to D: DWI on 3rd day of illness in Japanese encephalitis: (A and B) The T2W images showing involvement of bilateral hippocampi, substantia nigra and bilateral thalami; (C and D). The diffusion-weighted images showing restriction in the involved areas.

(33% cases). Calcification is seen in those infected in utero and hence usually never seen below 1 year of age. HIV vasculopathy can result in infarcts.[46-48]

In contrast to adults, opportunistic infections and tumors are relatively rare (15% of cases), the most common neoplasm being lymphoma reported with 5% incidence and CMV and PML are more common opportunistic infections. Proton MR spectroscopy has been used in pediatric patients. The NAA/Cr ratio is normal in static disease and significantly lower in progressive encephalopathy patients.[49,50]

FUNGAL INFECTIONS

Fungal infections are uncommon in children. Fungal infection can be classified in two broad categories: (i) those occurring in patients with lowered resistance as in diabetes, leukemia, lymphoma and in children on long-term cytotoxic, immunosuppressive or antibiotic therapy and (ii) those due to pathogenic fungi infecting immunocompetent children. The former infections are generally due to aspergillus, Candida and mucormycosis species and the latter are due to *Cryptococcus histoplasmosis* and blastomyces species.[1]

Fungal infections of the central nervous system (CNS) are being increasingly diagnosed both in immunocompromised and immunocompetent individuals. Sinocranial aspergillosis is more frequently described from countries with temperate climates, more often in otherwise immunocompetent individuals. Certain clinical syndromes are specific for certain fungal infections. The rhinocerebral form is the most common presenting syndrome with zygomycosis and skull-base syndromes are often the presenting clinical syndromes in patients with sinocranial aspergillosis. Subacute and chronic meningitis in patients with HIV infection is more likely to be due to cryptococcal infection.

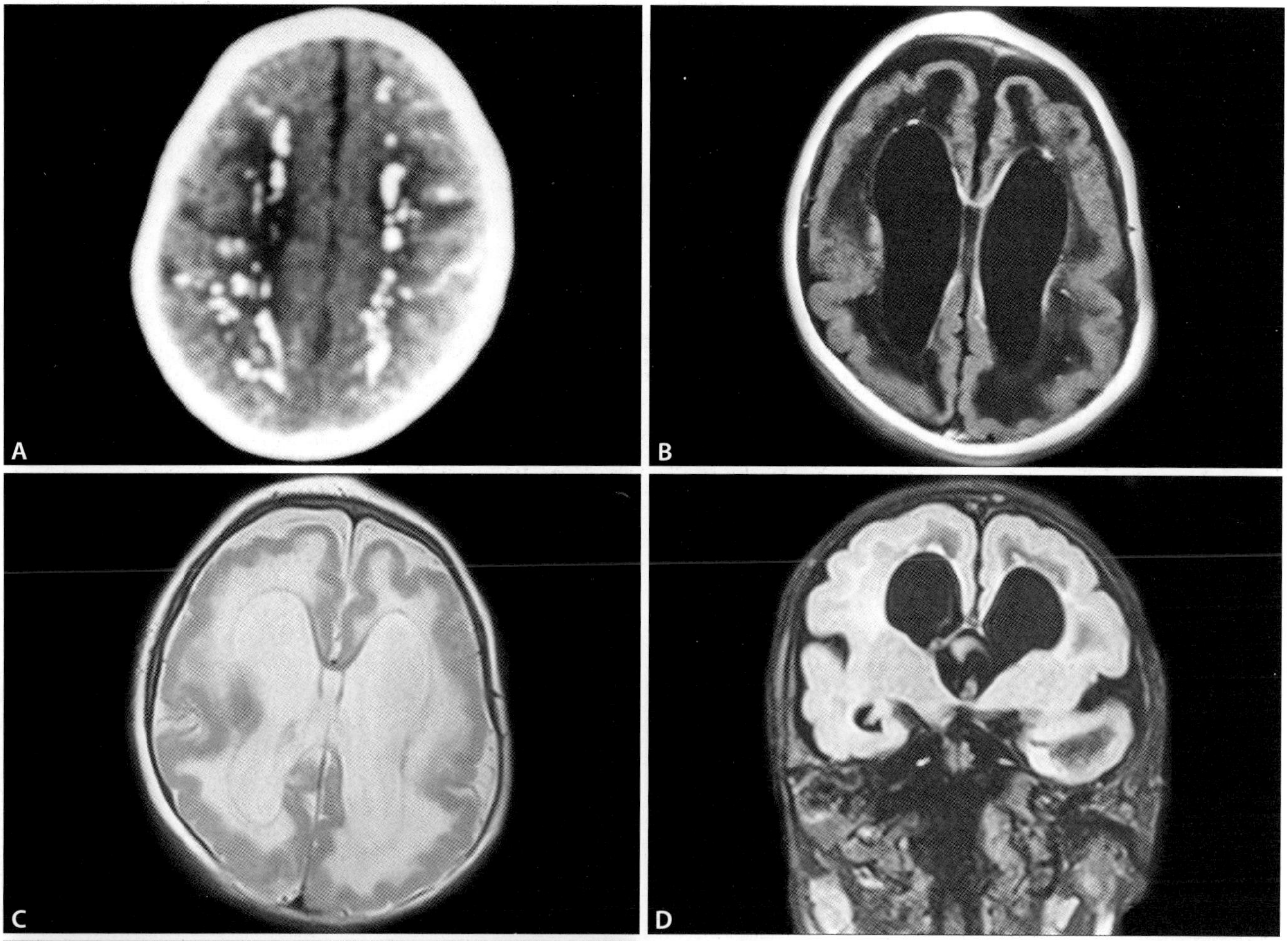

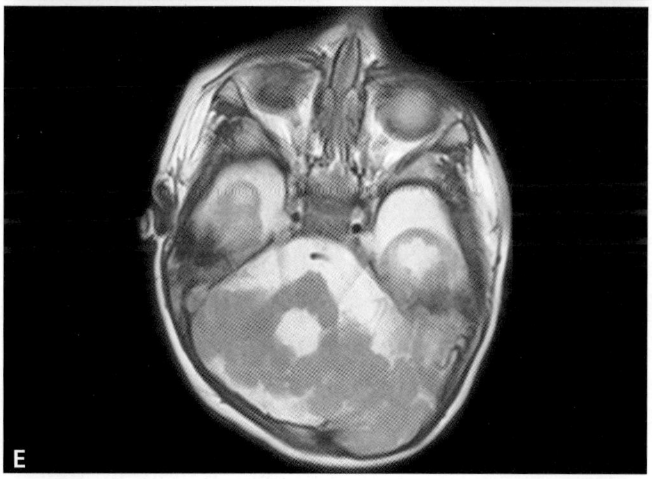

Figs. 21A to E: A 3-year-old with congenital cytomegalovirus infection: (A) NCCT image showing multiple periventricular calcifications; (B) T1 weighted image showing ventricular dilatation, periventricular hyperintensities and presence of thickened cortex with loss of sulcation in bilateral frontal regions; (C and D) T2W and FLAIR images showing hyperintensities in bilateral cerebral white matter; (E) T2W image showing cerebellar dysgenesis.

Aspergillosis

Aspergillus is saprophytic opportunistic ubiquitous fungi found in soil, plants. *Aspergillus fumigatus* is the most common human pathogen.[51]

CNS aspergillosis is a rare condition. The infection reaches the brain directly from the nasal sinuses or is hematogeneous from the lungs and gastrointestinal tract. Three pathological manifestations can occur with aspergillosis: infarction, abscess formation and meningitis.[52]

The most distinct imaging charecteristics on computed tomography or MR imaging are multiple lesions with infarction or hemorrhage in a random distribution due to the angioinvasive nature of the fungus. Aspergillus abscesses are usually hypointense on T1W images but areas of high signal intensity may be seen due to presence of iron, manganese, or methemoglobin. Hemorrhage occurs in approximately 25% of cases and contrast enhancement is usually minimal or absent. On T2W images peripheral low signal areas may be seen which correspond to areas of hemorrhages **(Figs. 22A to E)**. On diffusion-weighted images most lesions show peripheral areas of high signal intensity suggestive of restriction of diffusion that are interspersed with dark foci which can be due to susceptibility artifact due to hemorrhagic or iron products.[52,53]

Mucormycosis

Mucormycosis is a life-threatening opportunistic fungal infection caused by one of the members of the mucoraceae family. Rhizopus oryzae is the most common cause of infection.

When spores are converted into the hyphae, they become invasive, involve blood vessels and disseminate hematogenously or may spread through the paranasal sinuses into the brain and orbits. Diabetes comprise at least 70% of the reported cases. Infections can also be seen in patients of anemia, leukemia, uremia and severe burns and in those receiving steroid or chemotherapy. The rhinocerebral form is the most common infection. The organism may spread directly through the cribriform plate, via retrograde proliferation along vessels or through the superior orbital fissure or optic canal. Isolated CNS mucormycosis, a focal intracerebral infection, is rare and is most commonly seen in drug abusers.

Findings on CT and MR images include opacification of paranasal sinuses with absence of air fluid levels **(Figs. 23A to F)**. The finding of bony erosion of the

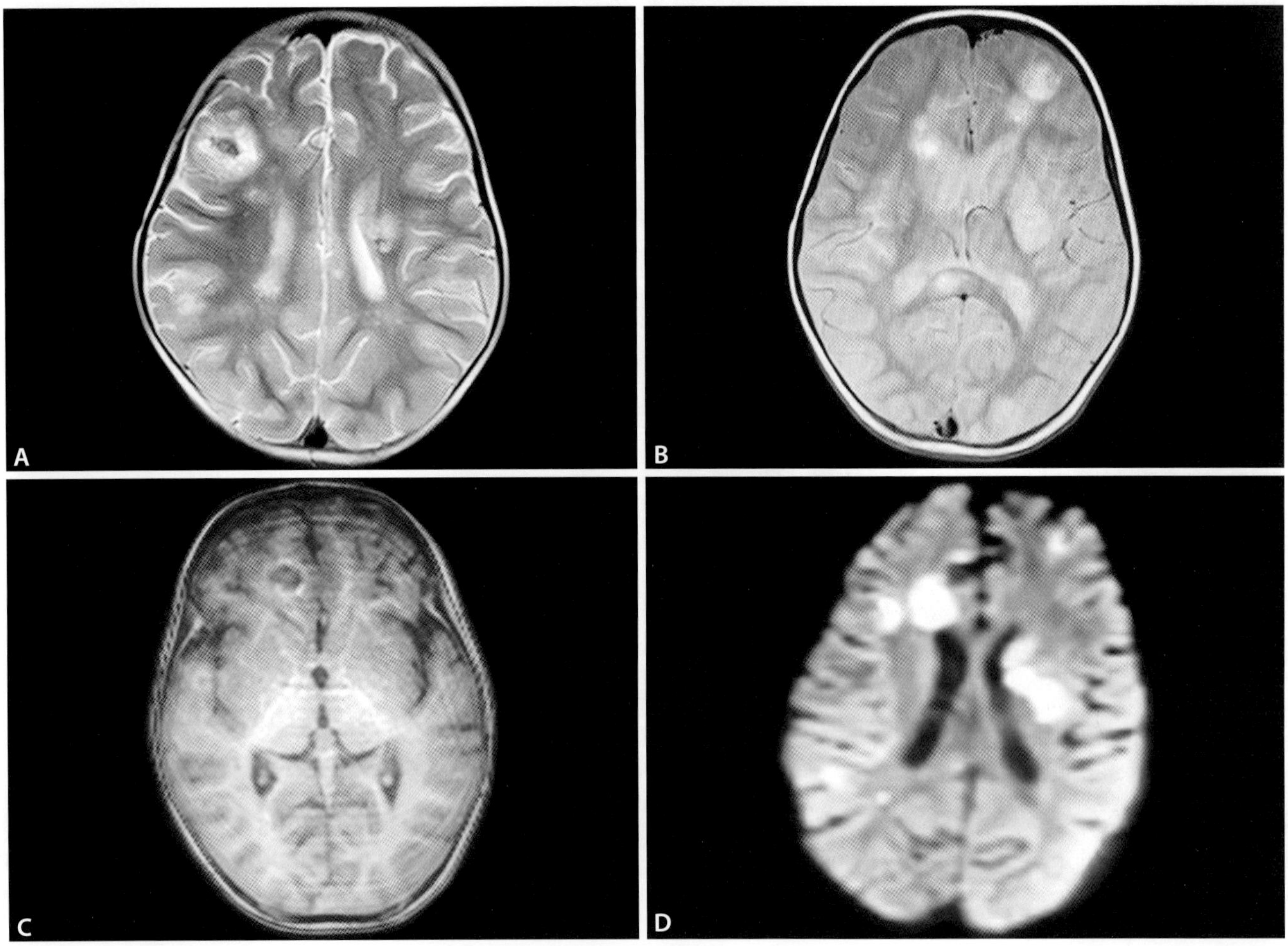

Figs. 22A to D

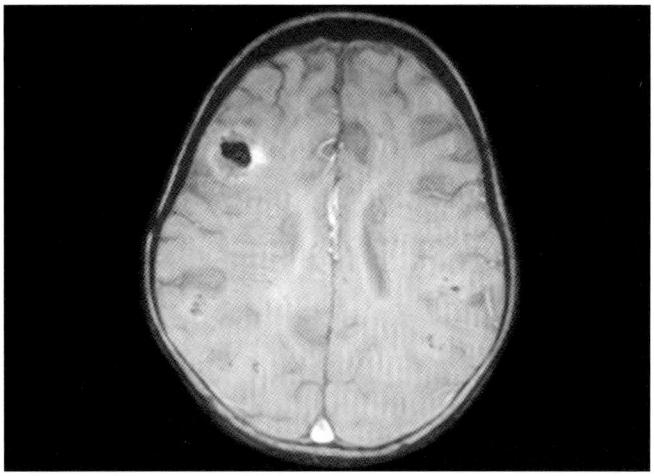

Fig. 22 E

Figs. 22A to E: A 5-month-old child with intracranial aspergillosis: (A to C) T2W and T1W images showing multiple well-defined lesions in the bilateral frontal lobes having T1 hyperintense and T2 hypointense wall; (D) DWI images show presence of diffusion restriction in the periphery of the lesions; (E) Susceptibility weighted imaging shows blooming of the wall of the lesions.

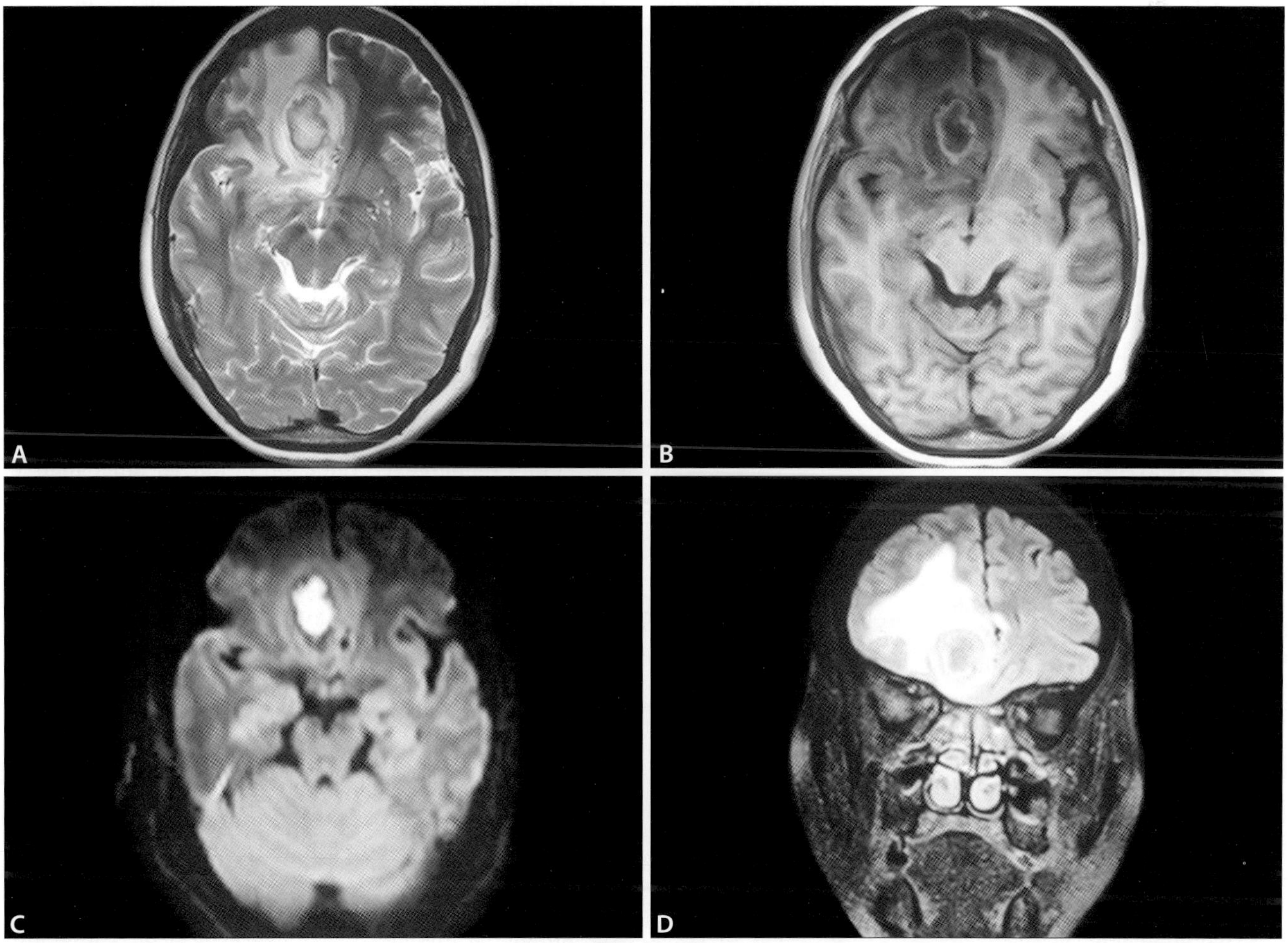

Figs. 23A to D

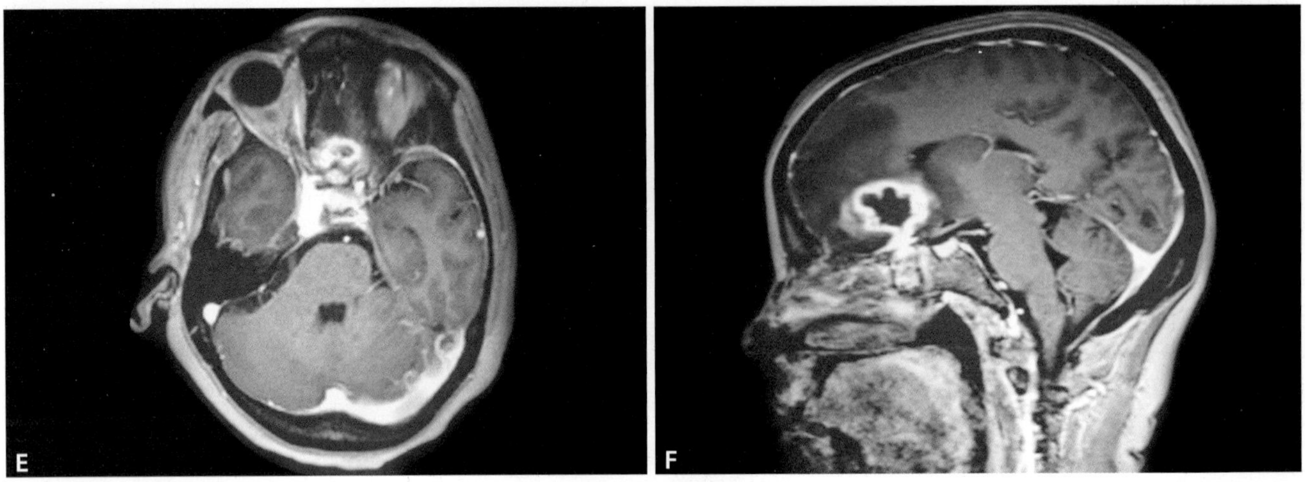

Figs. 23E and F

Figs. 23A to F: Fungal sinusitis with intracranial involvement: (A to C) Heterogeneous lesion with T2 hypointense rim and T1 isointense rim with central diffusion restriction; (D to F) The FLAIR image show hyperintense contents in the ethmoid sinuses with enhancement of the sinus contents, bilateral cavernous sinuses and wall of the frontal abscess.

sinuses is strongly suggestive of the diagnosis in the appropriate clinical setting. Sinus contents may have variable MR imaging charecteristics, from hypointensity to hyperintensity on T2WI. Intracranial findings include infarcts related to vascular thrombosis, mycotic emboli and fungal abscesses.[51,54]

CONCLUSION

Inflammatory diseases of the brain encompasses numerous causes. CT and MRI are the two main imaging modalities. Majority of lesions can be characterized for a specific disease based on imaging features along with clinical and biochemical information.

REFERENCES

1. Barkovich AJ. Infections of the nervous system. In: Benkovich AJ (Ed). Pediatric Neuroimaging, 4th edition. Lippincott Williams and Wilkins; 2005.pp.801-5.
2. Smirniotopoulos JG, Murphy FM, Rushing EJ, Rees JH, Schroeder JW. Patterns of contrast enhancement in the brain and meninges. Radiographics. 2007;27(2):525-51.
3. Friede RL. Developmental Neuropathology. 2nd edition. Berlin: Springer-Verlag; 1989.
4. Raybaud C, Girard N, Sevely A, et al. Neuroradiologic pediatrique (1). In Raybaud C, Girard N, Sevely A, et al (Eds): Radiodiagnostic-Neuroradiologic-Cppariel Locomotor Paris: Elsevier Science; 1996.p.26.
5. Moseley IF, Kendall BE. Radiology of intracranial empyema with special reference to computed tomography. Neuroradiol. 1984;26:333-45.
6. Courville CB. Subdural empyema secondary to purulent frontal sinusitis. Arch Otolaryngol. 1944;39:211-30.
7. Enzmann DR. Britt RH, Placone R. Staging of human brain abscess by computed tomography. Radiology. 1983;146:703-8.
8. Haimes AB, Zimmerman RD, Mrogello S, et al. MR imaging of brain abscesses. Am J Neuroradiol. 1989;10:279-91.
9. Kim SH, Chang KH, Song IC, et al. Brain abscess and brain tumor discrimination with in vivo H-1 MR spectroscopy. Radiology. 1997;204:239-44.
10. Marmer-Perez 1. Moreno A, Alonso J, et al. Diagnosis of brain abscess by magnetic resonance spectroscopy. J Neuro Surg. 1997;86:708-13.
11. Venkatesh SK, Gupta RK, Pal L, et al. Spectroscopic increase in choline signal is a non-specific marker for differentiation of infective/inflammatory from neoplastic lesions of the brain. J Magn Reson Imaging. 2001;14:8-15.
12. Luthra G, Parihar A, Nath K, Jaiswal S, Prasad KN, Husain N, et al. Comparative evaluation of fungal, tubercular, and pyogenic brain abscesses with conventional and diffusion MR imaging and proton MR spectroscopy. Am J Neuroradiol. 2007;28:1332-8.
13. Garg M, Gupta RK, Husain M, et al. Brain abscess, etiologic categorization with in vivo protron MR spectroscopy. Radiology. 2002;230:519-27.
14. Morgado C, Ruivo N. Imaging meningoencephalic tuberculosis. European J of Radiology. 2005;55:188-92.
15. Wallace RC. Brutons EM, Beret FF, et al. Intracranial tuberculosis in children CT appearance and clinical outcome. Pediatr Radiol. 1991;21:241-6.
16. Bhargava S, Gupta AK, Tandon PN. Tuberculous meningitis-A CT study. BJR. 1982;55:189-96.
17. Fischbein N, Dillon W, Barkovich A (Eds). Tuberculosis. In: Teaching Atlas of Brain Imaging. Thieme; 2000.pp.165-8.
18. Bonafe A, Manelfe C. Gomea MC, et al. Tuberculous meningitis, contribution of computerize tomography to its diagnosis and prognosis. J Neuroradiol. 1988;12:302.

19. Hsuh EY, Chi a LG, Shen We. Location of cerebral infarctions in tuberculous meningitis. Neuroradiol. 1992;34:197.
20. Reid H, Fallon RJ. Bacterial infections. In: Adams JH Duchen L (Eds). Greenfields Neuropathology, 5th edition. New York: Oxford University Press; 1992.pp.317-42.
21. Bhargava, Tandon PN. Intracranial tuberculomas: A CT study. Br J Radiol. 1980;53:935-45.
22. Welchman JM. CT of intracranial tuberculomata. Clin Radiol. 1979;30:567-79.
23. Jinkins JR. CT of intracranial tuberculosis. Neuroradiology. 1991;33:126-35.
24. Jinkins JR. Gupta R, Chang KH, et al. MR imaging of CNS tuberculosis. In: Goodman Pc. Jinkins JR (Eds): Imaging of Tuberculosis and Craniospinal Tuberculosis. Radiol Column N Am. 1995;33:771-89.
25. Rajshekhar V, Haran RPO, Prakash GS, et al. Differentiating solitary small cysticercus granulomas and tuberculomas in patients with epilepsy. J Neurosurg. 1993;78:402-7.
26. Gupta RK, Vatsal DK, Husain N, Chawla S, Prasad KN, Roy R, et al. Differentiation of tuberculous from pyogenic brain abscesses with in vivo proton MR spectroscopy and magnetization transfer MR imaging. Am J Neuroradiol. 2001;22:1503-9.
27. Tyson G, Newman P, Strachan WE. Tuberculous brain abscess. Surg Neurol. 1978;10,323-5.
28. Whitener DR. Tuberculous brain abscess. Report of a case and review of the literature. Arch Neurol. 1978;35:148-55.
29. Wouters EF, Hupperts RM, Vreeling FW, et al. Successful treatment of tuberculous brain abscess. J Neurol. 1985;232:118-28.
30. Yang PJ, Reger KM, Seeger JF, Carmody RF, Iacono RP. Brain abscess: An atypical CT appearance of CNS tuberculosis. AJNR. 1987;8:919-20.
31. Withman RR, Johnson RH, Roberts DL. Diagnosis of miliary tuberculosis by cerebral computed tomography. Arch Intern Med. 1979;139:479-80.
32. Gee GT, Bazan C III, Jinkins JR. Miliary tuberculosis involving the brain: MR findings. AJR. 1992;159:1075-6.
33. Osborn A (Ed). Infections of the brain and its things. In: Diagnostic Neuroradiology. New York: Mosby Year Book. 1994.pp.673-715.
34. Suss RA, Maravilla KR, Thompson J. MR imaging of intracranial cysticercosis: Comparison with CT and anatomopathologic features. AJNR. 1986;7:235-42.
35. Suh D, Chang K, Han M, et al. Unusual MR manifestations of neurocysticercosis. Neuroradiology. 1989;31:396-402.
36. Gupta S, Desai K, Goel A. Intracranial hydatid cyst: A report of five cases and review of literature. Neurol India. 1999;47:214-7.
37. Koelfen W, Freund M, Guckel F, et al. MRI of encephalitis in children: Comparison of CT and MRI in the acute stage with long-term follow-up. Neuroradiology. 1996;38:73-9.
38. Demaerel P, Wilms G, Robberecht W, et al. MRI of herpes simplex encephalitis. Neuroradiology. 1992;34:490-3.
39. Tien R, Felsberg G, Osumi A. Herpes virus infections of the CNS: MR findings. Am J Roentgenol. 1993;161:167-76.
40. Kumar S, Misra UK, Kalita J, et al. MRI in Japanese encephalitis. Neuroradiology. 1997;39:180-4.
41. Shoji H, Kida H, Hino H, et al. Magnetic resonance imaging findings in Japanese encephalitis. White matter lesions. J Neuroimaging. 1994;4:206-11.
42. Darling CR, Larsen MB, Byrd SE, et al. MR and CT imaging patterns in post varicella encephalitis. Pediat Radiol. 1995; 25:241-4.
43. Brismar J, Gascon GG, Yon Steyern KV, et al. Subacute sclerosing panencephalitis. Neurology. 1996;47:1278-83.
44. Kiroglu Y, Yunten N, Kitis O, et al. Diffusion-weighted MR imaging of viral encephalitis. Neuroradiology. 2006;48:875-80.
45. Barkovich AJ, Girard N. Fetal brain infections. Childs Nerv Syst. 2003;19:501-7.
46. Kauffman WM, Sivit CJ, Fitz CR, Rakusan TA, Herzog K, Chandra RS. CT and MR evaluation of intracranial involvement in pediatric HIV infection: A clinical-imaging correlation. Am J Neuroradiol. 1992;13:949-57.
47. Spreer J, Enenkel-Stoodt S, Funk M, Fiedler A, de Simone A, Hacker H. Neuroradiological findings in perinatally HIV-infected children. Rofo. 1994;161:106-12.
48. States LJ, Zimmerman RA, Rutstein RM. Imaging of pediatric central nervous system HIV infection. Neuroimaging Clin N Am. 1997;7:321-39.
49. Lu D, Parlakis SG, Frank Y, et al. Proton MR spectroscopy of the basal ganglia in healthy children and children with AIDS. Radiology. 1996;199:423-8.
50. Paralakis SG, Lu D, Frank Y, et al. Magnetic resonance spectroscopy in childhood AIDS encephalopathy. Pediatr Neurol. 1995;12:277-82.
51. Jain KK, Mittal SK, Kumar S, Gupta RK. Imaging features of central nervous system fungal infection. Neurology India. 2007; 55:241-50.
52. Tempkin AD, Sobonya RE, Seeger JF, et al. Cerebral aspergillosis: radiologic and pathologic findings. Radiographics. 2006; 26:1239-42.
53. Almutairi BM, Nguyen TB, Fansen GH, et al. Invasive aspergillosis of brain: radiologic–pathologic correlation. Radiographics. 2009;29:375-9.
54. Smith AB, Rushing JR. Central nervous system infections associated with Human Immunodeficiency Virus infection: Radiologic Pathologic Correlation. Radiographics. 2008;28: 2033-58.

CHAPTER 154

Pediatric Brain Tumors

Shailesh B Gaikwad, Ajay Garg

INTRODUCTION

Fifteen to twenty percent of all intracranial tumors occur in children under 15 years of age, with the peak occurrence between 4 years and 8 years of age. Only 1–2% of all brain tumors occur in children under 2 years of age.[1]

In neonates, brain tumors are uncommon and represent congenital tumors. They are most common in the supratentorial region than infratentorial region. Common primary brain tumors in the neonatal period are teratomas, embryonal tumors and congenital glioblastoma multiforme. In children between the ages of 2 years and 10 years, primary brain tumors are generally more benign and 70% of these are infratentorial in location.[2]

Most frequent supratentorial tumors in the cerebral hemispheres are astrocytic tumors (50%), embryonal tumors (15%) and ependymomas (15%). In the suprasellar region, 75% of tumors are craniopharyngiomas. Common tumors in the infratentorial region in the pediatric population are pilocytic astrocytoma, medulloblastoma, and ependymoma and brainstem glioma.

CLASSIFICATION OF CHILDHOOD TUMORS BASED ON TOPOGRAPHY[3]

The location of the tumor is a useful tool in the differential diagnosis and narrowing the list of possible tumors.

- *Cerebellum*:
  - Medulloblastoma
  - Pilocytic astrocytoma
  - Atypical teratoid/rhabdoid
  - Hemangioblastoma
- *Brainstem*:
  - Diffuse astrocytoma
  - Pilocytic astrocytoma
  - Anaplastic astrocytoma
  - Glioblastoma multiforme (GBM)
- *Fourth ventricle*:
  - Ependymoma
  - Medulloblastoma
  - Pilocytic astrocytoma
  - Choroid plexus papilloma
- *Cerebellopontine angle*:
  - Ependymoma
  - Choroid plexus papilloma
  - Astrocytoma
- *Cerebral hemispheres*:
  - Diffuse astrocytoma
  - Pilocytic astrocytoma
  - Anaplastic astrocytoma
  - Glioblastoma multiforme (GBM)
  - Pleomorphic xanthoastrocytoma
  - Primitive neuroectodermal tumor (PNET)
  - Ganglion cell tumors
  - Ependymoma
  - Oligodendroglial tumors
  - Atypical teratoid/rhabdoid
- *Lateral ventricle*:
  - Ependymoma
  - Choroid plexus papilloma (CPP)
  - Astrocytoma
  - Subependymal giant cell astrocytoma (SEGA)
  - Primitive neuroectodermal tumor (PNET)

- *Third ventricle*
  - Ependymoma
  - Astrocytoma
  - Choroid plexus papilloma
- *Pineal region*
  - Pineal cell tumor
  - Germ cell tumors
  - Glial tumors
- *Sellar region*
  - Craniopharyngioma
  - Germ cell tumors
  - Pilocytic astrocytoma
  - Hamartoma.

POSTERIOR FOSSA TUMORS

Medulloblastoma

Medulloblastoma (MB) is a malignant primitive neuroectodermal tumor and is the most common posterior fossa tumor in children, accounting for one-third of childhood pediatric tumors.[4] About three-fourths of MBs occurs in children 5–15 years old. Although much less common, the disease may also occur in adults, usually in the 3rd and 4th decades of life.

MBs are usually midline tumors and the most common site (80%) is in the region of the vermis and inferior medullary velum. A less frequent location, encountered in older patients, is the cerebellar hemisphere. Approximately 80% of patients with MB present with features of raised intracranial pressure and the most common symptoms include headache, nausea and vomiting. Cerebrospinal fluid seeding occurs in 10–30% of patients with MB.

Surgical resection, radiation therapy, and chemotherapy have substantially lowered the mortality associated with this tumor and a 5-year survival rate is now about 50–65%. However, dissemination at the time of diagnosis and recurrence remain major obstacles in achieving a cure.

Pathology

Medulloblastomas have long been classified into two chief histological variants, "classical" and "desmoplastic".[5] In classic MBs, densely packed cells in diffuse sheets have hyperchromatic, round or carrot shaped nuclei and scanty, ill-defined cytoplasm. In desmoplastic MBs, more often are found in adolescents or young adults, a nodular architecture is seen.

Imaging

MB is a well-circumscribed mass, centered near the midline and filling the fourth ventricle. Midline extension through the foramen of Magendie into the cisterna magna may occur, while lateral extension is uncommon. The tumor has characteristic hyperattenuation on unenhanced CT scans that reflects the hypercellularity and high nuclear-cytoplasmic ratio of the tumor cells.[4] MB show moderate to strong homogeneous enhancement on contrast administration. Cystic and necrotic degeneration is most commonly found in adult MBs. Calcification is seen in 20% of cases.

On MR imaging, these tumors are hypo- to isointense on T1WI and iso- to hypointense on T2WI **(Figs. 1A and B)**. Cysts, hemorrhage, necrosis and clump-like calcification are responsible for the signal heterogeneity on T2WI.[4] Enhancement after contrast administration is intermediate to strong **(Figs. 1C and D)**. Evidence of leptomeningeal metastatic spread is present in 33% of all cases at the time

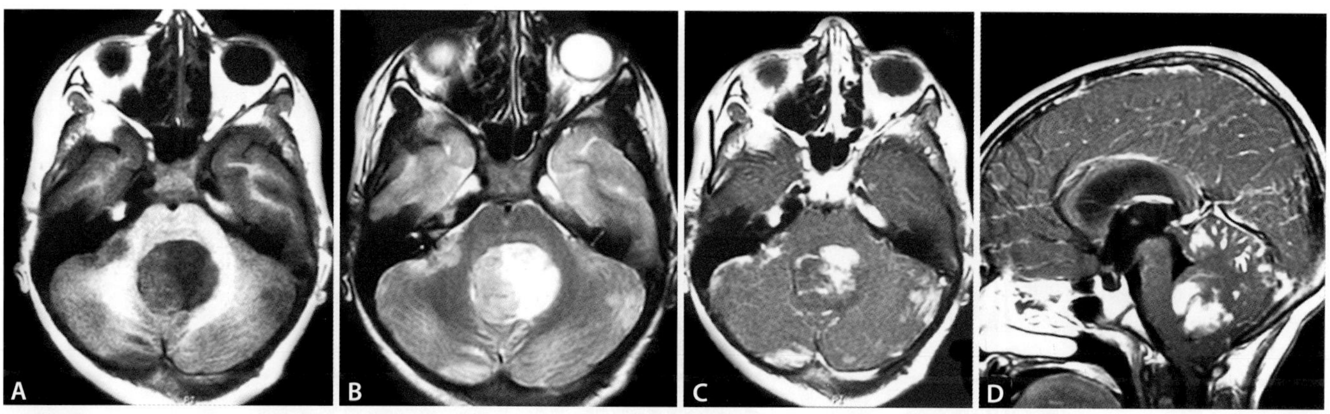

Figs. 1A to D: Medulloblastoma: Axial images show a vermian mass which is iso- to hyperintense on T1WI (A) and iso- to hypointense on T2WI (B). Post-gadolinium axial (C) and sagittal (D) T1WI show patchy enhancement within the mass and enhancement of the leptomeningeal deposits in right cerebellopontine angle cistern and cerebellar sulci.

of diagnosis and is well evaluated with contrast-enhanced MR imaging of the brain and the spine **(Figs. 1C and D)**.[4] Diffusion-weighted MRI in MB shows a marked increase in the signal intensity reflecting the dense nature of the tumor, which restricts the extracellular diffusion of water protons, and the high nuclear-to-cytoplasm ratio of these neoplastic cells, which limits intracellular motion.[6]

Combination of high density on NCCT and isointense-low signal on T1WI is believed to be highly suggestive of MB and this may help to differentiate it from other posterior fossa tumors.[7]

Pilocytic Astrocytoma

Pilocyticastrocytomas(PAs)arebenigntumorsofCNS(WHO grade I) and are of specific histologic type. They usually present in first two decades of life. They often arise from the cerebellum, hypothalamus, optic nerve, optic chiasm, brainstem and less commonly from cerebral hemispheres. Classically, cerebellar astrocytoma manifests with waxing and waning headache. Truncal ataxia, dysdiadochokinesia are other cerebellar signs. They have an excellent prognosis with 90% of patients having 25 years survival rate.

Pathology

Grossly, the pilocytic astrocytoma is usually sharply circumscribed, with a very narrow zone of microscopic infiltration. The tumor is partially cystic, often with a mural nodule supplied by capillaries that lack a complete blood-brain barrier (BBB). It has open tight junction in the endothelial cells with fenestration and therefore differs from low-grade astrocytomas. This fact and lack of BBB is the cause of both intense enhancement, as well as the source of production of the proteinaceous fluid that accumulates in the "cyst" of the tumor.

Imaging

Classically cerebellar PA present as a cystic mass with an enhancing mural nodule.[8] MR appearance is variable and nonspecific. Solid portion is hypointense on T1WI and hyperintense on T2WI. MR with contrast shows enhancement of the solid component **(Figs. 2A to D)**. Presence of fluid-fluid levels and waveforms from fluid pulsations are pathognomonic for cystic masses on MR. Other features of PA include the absence of accompanying edema.[8] Hemorrhage and intratumoral calcification is rare.

Ependymoma

Ependymomas are common tumors in children, comprising 10% of pediatric CNS neoplasms and 15% of posterior fossa tumors. The peak age at presentation is 1–5 years, with a smaller peak occurring in the fourth decade. Common presenting symptoms include nausea, vomiting, disequilibrium, and headaches, while common presenting signs include ataxia and nystagmus.

Pathology

Ependymomas are glial tumors arising from the cuboidal or columnar cells lining the ventricles and central canal. In the posterior fossa, they arise from the floor of the fourth ventricle with a tendency to fill it or track along its lateral recesses into the cerebellopontine angle. Subtypes of ependymoma include cellular, papillary, and myxopapillary forms. Typical gross pathology shows a lobulated mass, often with a cystic component. Histologic findings include perivascular pseudorosettes with ependymal cells organized around blood vessels. Less commonly, true rosettes are seen.

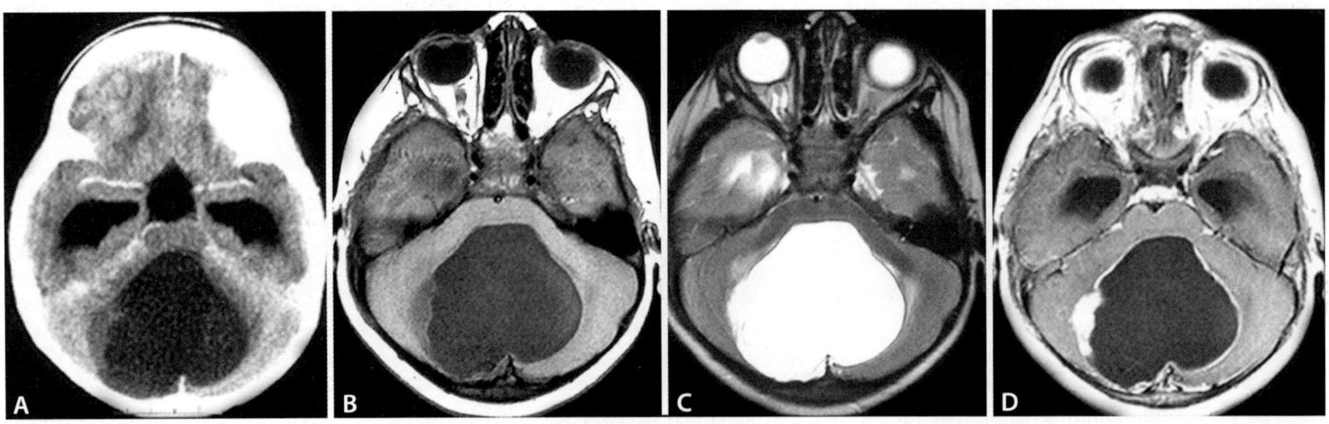

Figs. 2A to D: Pilocytic astrocytoma: NCCT (A) shows a cystic lesion in the vermis. A solid nodule of the tumor that is of lower attenuation than surrounding cerebellum is located within right lateral aspect of tumor. The cyst is hypointense on T1WI (B) and hyperintense on T2WI (C) and nodule show intense enhancement after gadolinium administration (D).

Imaging

On NCCT, ependymoma is iso- to hyperdense, with moderate enhancement after intravenous contrast.[9] Small intratumoral cyst and multifocal punctate calcification is common. Up to 45% of posterior fossa ependymomas contain calcifications. On MRI the typical appearance of posterior fossa ependymoma is a heterogeneous mass filling the fourth ventricle and causing obstructive hydrocephalus. MR signal characteristics of ependymoma are nonspecific and vary from hypointense lesion on T1WI, to hyperintense on T2WI (cysts, necrotic areas) with low intensity areas (calcification, hemorrhage) within the tumor mass **(Figs. 3A and B)**. Enhancement after administration of gadolinium is heterogeneous **(Figs. 3C and D)**. CSF seeding is found in small percentage of the cases. The distinguishing imaging feature for these tumors is their morphologic plasticity. These tumors have a tendency to conform to the ventricles that they are associated with and may indeed herniate through the ventricular foramina. An ependymoma may squeeze through foramen of Luschka into the cerebellopontine angle cistern.[9]

Brainstem Gliomas

Brainstem gliomas account for 10–20% of pediatric CNS tumors, and 75% of these occur before the age of 20 years. The majority (85%) are composed of high-grade fibrillary gliomas, which arise predominantly in the pons and less frequently in the medulla. There is no sex predilection, and children between 3 years and 10 years of age are commonly affected. Multiple cranial nerve palsies, pyramidal tract signs, ataxia and nystagmus are the usual presentation. Pontine gliomas have the worst prognosis.

Pathology

Brainstem gliomas can be divided into the diffusely infiltrative glioma and focal glioma.[10] On pathologic study, diffuse gliomas are infiltrative astrocytomas of varying grade, whereas the focal gliomas are frequently pilocytic astrocytomas. The former has a tendency for anaplasia, necrosis and hemorrhage. Except in tectal gliomas, hydrocephalus is uncommon in brainstem gliomas.

Imaging

Before the advent of MR imaging, radiographic diagnosis of diffuse glioma was based solely on indirect signs of subtle enlargement or morphologic distortion of brainstem on CT (i.e. flattening of ventral aspect of fourth ventricle or reduction of the diameter of prepontine cistern).[11] Contrast enhancement could be patchy, irregular, homogeneous or absent. CP angle cistern widening may be seen due to an exophytic component producing extra-axial effect.

MR imaging is useful for diagnosis and localization of the tumor. Diffuse glioma appears as poorly defined regions of low intensity on T1WI and high intensity on T2WI. Intratumoral heterogeneity is occasionally present, but cysts are not common. The signal changes may extend into the cerebellum and/or adjacent brainstem. The basilar artery is often engulfed by the anterior extension of the tumor. An undulating ventral border of the brainstem on sagittal image may be an indirect clue to the presence of the mass lesion. Contrast enhancement has been reported in approximately one-half of the cases and is often focal and nodular **(Figs. 4A to D)**.

Pilocytic brainstem gliomas are often well circumscribed and sometimes markedly exophytic. Exophytic component is readily identified on MR, due to its

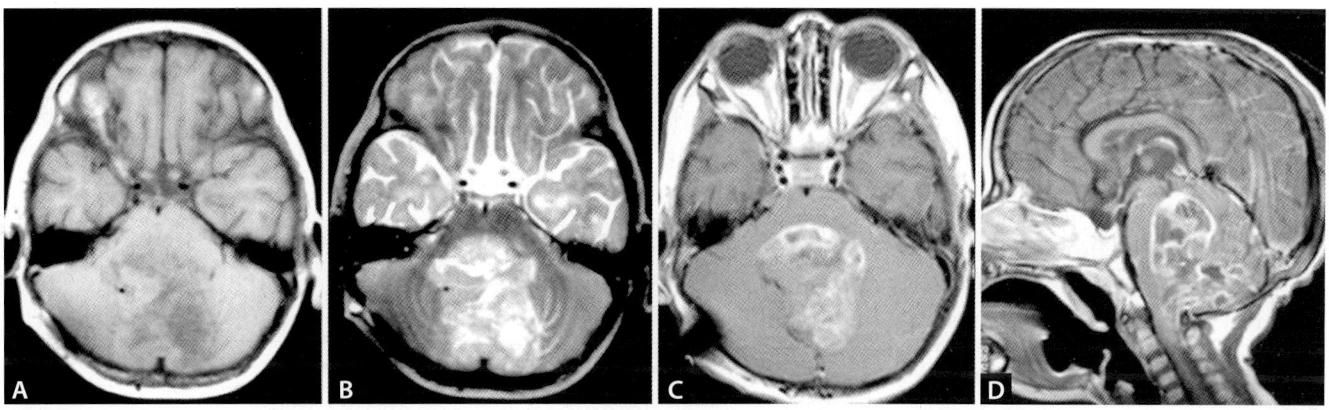

Figs. 3A to D: Ependymoma: Axial T1WI (A) and T2WI (B) show a heterogeneous mass filling the fourth ventricle. Post-gadolinium axial (C) and sagittal (D) T1WI demonstrate heterogeneous enhancement. The tumor is creeping through foramen of Magendie and reaching upper cervical canal.

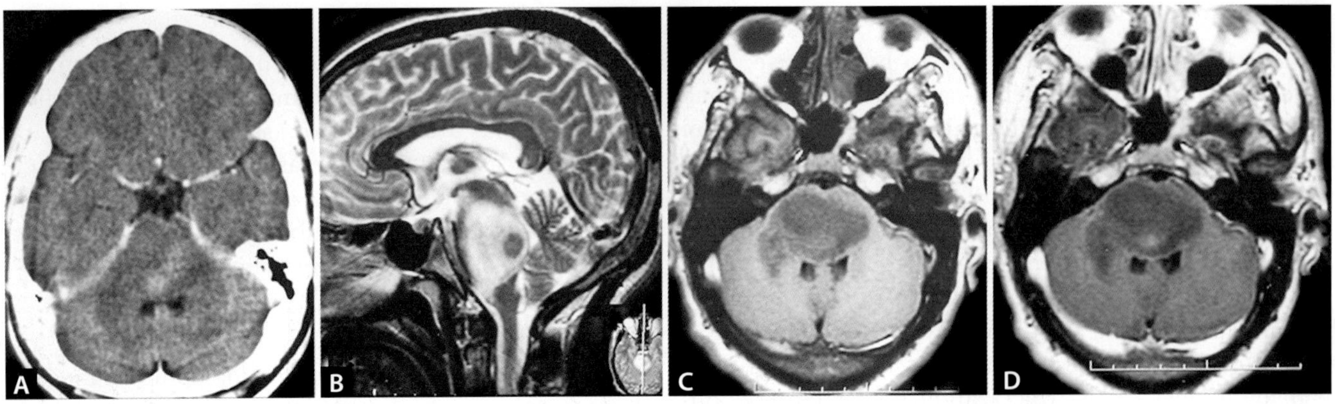

Figs. 4A to D: Diffuse pontine glioma: CECT (A), sagittal T2WI (B), axial T1WI (C) and post-gadolinium T1WI (D). The pons is expanded. Diffuse pontine glioma flattens fourth ventricle, envelops basilar artery, extends into right cerebellum and shows patchy enhancement.

multiplanar imaging capability. The dorsally exophytic lesions are grossly multicystic and often enhance intensely **(Figs. 5A and B)**. The presence of enhancement has not been correlated reliably with type or grade of malignancy.

Differential diagnosis includes encephalitis, tuberculoma, resolving hematoma, and vascular malformation.[11] MR can easily differentiate vascular malformation and resolving hematoma from brainstem tumor by demonstrating blood and blood breakdown products exquisitely.

Atypical Teratoid/Rhabdoid Tumor

Malignant rhabdoid tumor (MRT) is an extremely rare and highly malignant neoplasm of undetermined histogenesis. The term "rhabdoid" was used due to the similarity of these tumors to rhabdomyosarcoma under light microscopy. The tumor may arise at any site within the central nervous system, but 56% are located in the cerebellum and 17% are located in the cerebrum.[12] The hypothesis that the tumor is derived from the meningothelial cells may account for this predisposition to occur in the cerebellum where there are abundant meningothelial infoldings. The average age of presentation with primary MRT of the brain is 24.5 months (range 1 month to 12 years),[12] with a 3:1 male predominance. Clinical symptoms, although related to the location of the tumor, are often nonspecific and include lethargy, vomiting, failure to thrive, visual disturbances, and head-tilt. One-third of the patients have CNS dissemination of tumor at presentation. MRT has a strong tendency for subarachnoid dissemination.

Pathology

The tumor shows diffuse growth with areas of an alveolar or trabecular arrangement and an angiocentric pattern, with infiltration along the blood vessels.[13] All tumors, by definition, contain a population of rhabdoid cells and two-thirds contain fields that, taken in isolation, would be classical primitive neuroectodermal tumors (PNETs).

Imaging

The imaging features are nonspecific. Lesions are commonly large at presentation, with moderate-to-marked surrounding edema. On CT, these tumors are solid or mixed lesions.[14] The solid portion is hyperdense on NCCT. Areas of necrosis, cyst formation, hemorrhage and calcification may occur with various patterns of enhancement **(Fig. 6)**.[13] On MR, MRTs are hypointense on T1WI, isointense on PD and iso-hypo on T2WI with inhomogeneous enhancement. Meningeal enhancement and spinal tumor seeding are common, and hence, the spine should also be imaged.

Hemangioblastoma

Although hemangioblastoma occurs in young and middle aged adults, less than 20% occur in children. Approximately 25% are associated with von Hippel–Lindau disease (retinal detachment multiple cysts or tumors of kidney, lung, pancreas, liver and rhabdomyomas of the heart). The tumors are usually located in the cerebellum (83–86%). Other sites include spinal cord (3–13%), medulla (2–5%) and cerebrum (1.5%).[15]

Pathology

Classically, hemangioblastoma are well-circumscribed, cystic tumors with a mural nodule (60%), but may also be solid (40%).

Imaging

On NCCT, hemangioblastoma usually appears as a well-marginated, cystic lesion with a mural nodule.[9] The cystic

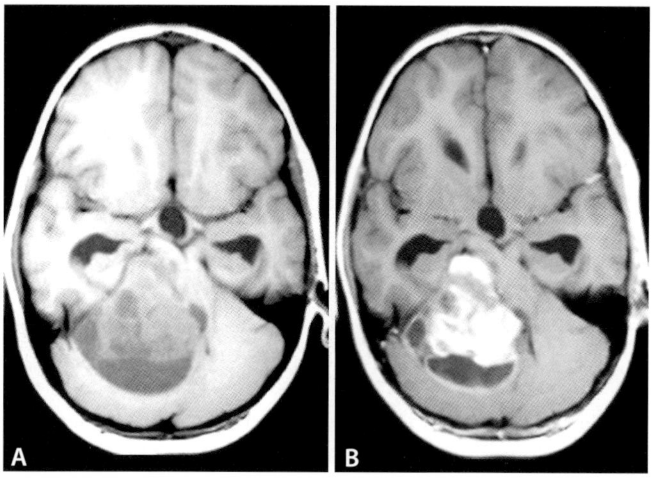

Figs. 5A and B: Dorsally exophytic brainstem glioma: Axial T1WI (A) shows a large tumor originating from posterolateral aspect of pons. The tumor is heterogeneous with cystic areas and shows heterogeneous enhancement (B).

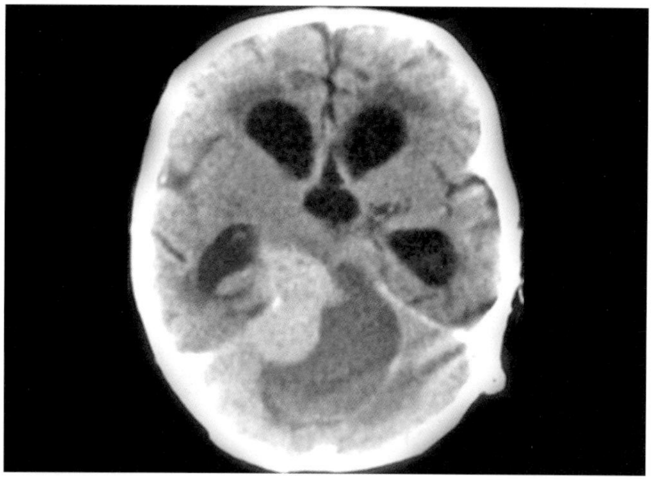

Fig. 6: Atypical rhabdoid tumor: CECT demonstrates a mixed density lesion in the vermis. The solid part of the tumor is densely enhancing.

lesion appears hypodense, while the mural nodule is isodense with the brain parenchyma. The mural nodule abuts the pial surface and show strong homogeneous contrast enhancement. Solid hemangioblastomas appear hyperdense on NCCT and show strong homogeneous enhancement **(Figs. 7A and B)**.

On MRI the cystic component of hemangioblastoma is either iso- or slightly hyperintense relative to CSF on T1-weighted image and hyperintense on T2-weighted image.[16] The nodule appears hypointense on T1WI and hyperintense on T2WI and enhances intensely after injection of gadolinium contrast material. Flow voids within and at the periphery of the tumor represent abnormal tumor vessels. The edema is usually slight or absent around this intra-axial tumor. On diffusion-weighted images, cystic portion of the tumor appears to be hypointense, reflecting increased diffusion properties of the cyst content. As on enhanced CT the solid portion of tumor shows marked enhancement.

The vascular component of the tumor shows homogeneous tumor blush at angiography. In patients with von Hippel–Lindau disease, the incidence of spinal hemangioblastoma is extremely high; therefore, it is mandatory to image the spine in these patients.

Epidermoid and Dermoid

Epidermoid and dermoid are generally considered congenital/developmental masses rather than neoplastic, arising from ectodermal heterotopia. Both cysts are lined with stratified squamous epithelium, with dermoids having additional mesodermal elements, such as hair, sebaceous and sweat glands.

Epidermoids are slightly more common than dermoids. They typically spread along the basal surfaces, with the cerebellopontine angles being the most common location, followed by parasellar sites. Epidermoids on CT appear as hypodense masses with irregular borders and have contrast enhancement rarely. Dense epidermoids have also been reported and calcification is occasionally seen. On MR, they have low signal on T1- and of increased signal on T2WI.[17] Occasionally, epidermoids are hyperintense on T1WI and then they need to be differentiated from the dermoid and lipoma. Chemical shift artifact is absent in epidermoids and also a fat saturation pulse sequence will suppress the high signal of dermoid and lipomas, but not of epidermoids. A lobulated mass with linear heterogeneities within the mass differentiates epidermoid from arachnoid cyst **(Figs. 8A and B)**. Diffusion-weighted imaging will show arachnoid cyst having diffusion characteristic of fluid, while epidermoids have diffusion characteristic of a solid lesion (similar to brain tissue).[18] Magnetization transfer techniques will show significant transfer of magnetization from solid matrix of the tumor to adjacent free water, but cysts show no magnetization transfer. Epidermoids are hyperintense on FLAIR while arachnoid cyst signal gets suppressed (iso-intense to CSF).

Dermoids are midline lesions, occurring in the parasellar, frontobasal region or posterior fossa (vermis or fourth ventricle). Dermoids on CT are essentially fat

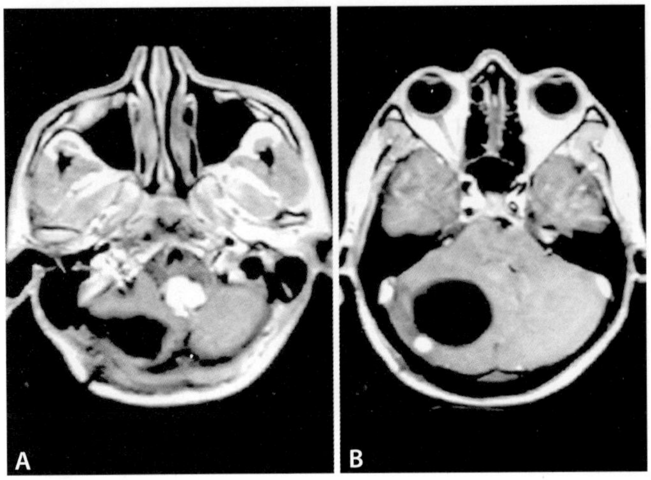

Figs. 7A and B: Hemangioblastoma: CECT at level of medulla (A) and pons (B) show a solid enhancing tumor in dorsal medulla and cyst with a mural nodule in the right cerebellar hemisphere.

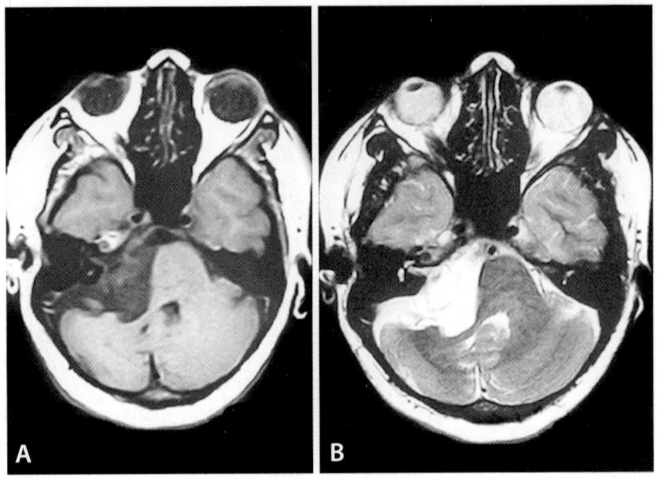

Figs. 8A and B: Epidermoid: Axial T1WI (A) and T2WI (B) show an extra-axial right cerebellopontine angle mass which is hypointense on T1WI and hyperintense on T2WI. The mass shows little internal heterogeneity.

density, extra-axial midline masses that do not enhance on contrast administration. They may be associated with bone defect in nasofrontal or occipital region that indicate the presence of a dermal sinus tract. CT is essential for detection of the calvarial defect, while MR delineates the tumor better. Tumor is hyperintense on both T1- and T2WI **(Figs. 9A and B)**. Chemical shift artifact is present similar to lipomas. However, dermoids are less lobulated than lipomas, and displace blood vessels and neural structures, in contrast to encasement of these structures by the lipomas.

SUPRATENTORIAL TUMORS

Tumors in supratentorial region are more common than infratentorial region in children below 2 years and those older than 10 years of age.

Cerebral Astrocytoma

Cerebral astrocytomas constitute approximately 30% of supratentorial tumors in children. Males and females are equally affected, with a slight peak at 8 years of age.

Pathology

In the supratentorial compartment, pilocytic astrocytomas often arise from hypothalamus, optic nerve, optic chiasm and less commonly in cerebral hemispheres.

Imaging

Imaging features are similar to the infratentorial astrocytoma. MR reveals deeply located hemispheric mass, which is hypointense and hyperintense on T1WI and T2W images respectively. Low-grade astrocytoma is homogeneous, well circumscribed with no associated hemorrhage or edema **(Figs. 10A and B)**. High-grade tumors are heterogeneous due to necrosis, intratumoral hemorrhage and vascularity.

Subependymal Giant Cell Astrocytoma

Subependymal giant cell astrocytoma (SEGA) occurs in 6–16% of patients with tuberous sclerosis and affects the region near the foramen of Monro eventually causing hydrocephalus.[19] This tumor is also known as "ventricular tumor of tuberous sclerosis". The peak age of occurrence is 8–18 years.

Imaging

CT shows hypo to isodense mass in the region of foramen of Monro. Hydrocephalus and focal calcification is common **(Fig. 11)**. Associated stigmata of tuberous sclerosis include presence of cortical tubers, calcified subependymal nodules and white matter lesions. On MRI, SEGAs show mixed signal intensities on T1- and T2WI. Most of them are isointense on T1- and hyperintense on T2WI.[19] Presence of subependymal nodules and also small multiple cortical hamartomas are easily identified on MR. Contrast enhancement is common with these tumors on both CT and MRI.

Ganglioglioma

Gangliogliomas are composed of neoplastic ganglion cells and glial cells in variable proportions. These tumors

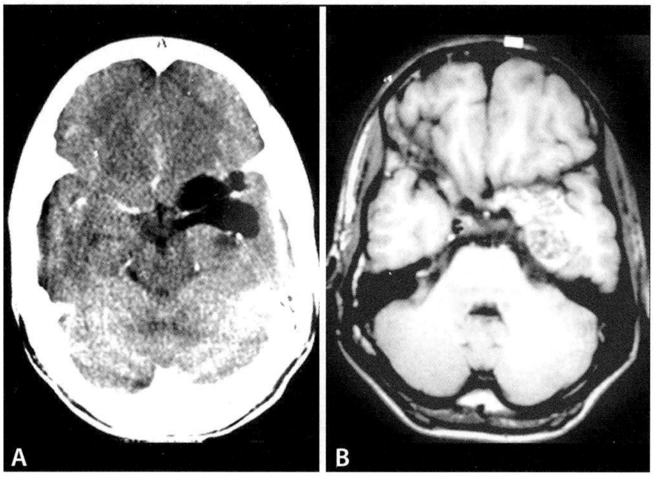

Figs. 9A and B: Parasellar dermoid: CT scans show a hypointense mass in left parasellar lesion (A) which is heterogeneously hyperintense on T1WI (B).

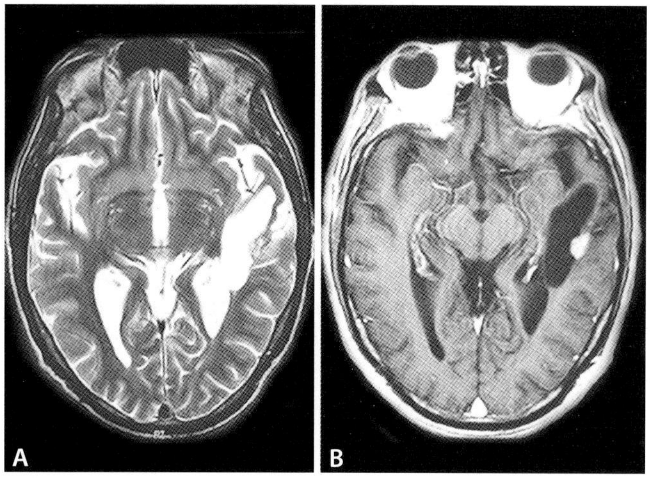

Figs. 10A and B: Supratentorial pilocytic astrocytoma: Axial T2WI (A) shows a well-defined cystic lesion in the left temporal lobe which is hyperintense with an isointense mural nodule on its lateral aspect. The mural nodule is showing dense enhancement on gadolinium administration (B).

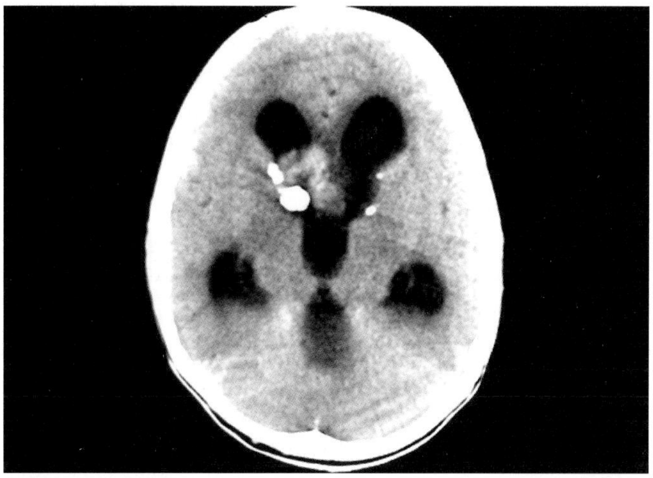

Fig. 11: Subependymal giant cell astrocytoma in patient with tuberous sclerosis. CECT shows heterogeneous intraventricular mass near foramen of Monro with calcified subependymal nodules.

account for 1–4% of all pediatric neoplasms of CNS. Most (80%) occur in patients younger than 30 years with a peak age of incidence between 10 years and 20 years. The temporal lobe (38%) is most commonly affected, followed by the parietal lobe (30%) and the frontal lobe (18%). Numerous other locations have been reported, including the brainstem, cerebellum, pineal region, spinal cord, optic nerve, optic chiasm, and ventricles. Gangliogliomas of the temporal lobe are commonly associated with the clinical presentation of medically refractory partial complex seizures. These tumors are the most common cause (40%) of chronic temporal lobe epilepsy.[20]

Imaging

NCCT reveals hypoattenuation mass (38%), mixed attenuation mass (32%), isoattenuating mass (15%) or hyperattenuating mass (15%). Calcification is seen in 30% of lesions.[21] Remo-deling of the skull may be seen if the neoplasm is located within the peripheral brain. Occasionally, the neoplasm may be com-pletely undetectable on CT. The enhancement is seen in 16–80% of gangliogliomas.[21]

The MR imaging appearance of gangliogliomas is also variable and nonspecific.[20,21] In general, the lesions are hypointense to isointense relative to gray matter on T1 and hyperintense relative to gray matter on T2 images. The solid-appearing components have an even more variable presentation at imaging. Some tumors may manifest as a hyperintense mass on T1WI. They commonly have at least some regions of high signal intensity on T2WI. Not all gangliogliomas are truly cystic despite a cyst like appearance, and the term *cystic* should be reserved for those that demonstrate a fluid-fluid level or pulsation artifact on MR images. Enhancement following intravenous administration of gadolinium contrast material is highly variable, ranging from nonenhancing to ring like to intense homogeneity.

Suggested imaging features for ganglioglioma include temporal lobe or posterior fossa location, involvement of both gray and white matter, combination of well-defined cystic and ill-defined solid components, calcification and enhancing nodule(s).

Supratentorial Ependymoma

Between 20% and 40% of childhood ependymomas are located in the supratentorial region. Male predominance is seen with a peak incidence between the ages of 1 year and 5 years.

Pathology

Histology is similar to infratentorial lesions. About 60% of the lesions are extraventricular and therefore subarachnoid seeding is uncommon. The incidence of cystic component in the supratentorial ependymomas is significantly greater than infratentorial ependymomas.

Imaging

The diagnosis of ependymoma should be considered in the presence of juxtaventricular hemispheric mass with focal calcification, cystic necrosis and heterogeneous enhancement **(Fig. 12)**. MR reveals heterogeneous mass due to presence of calcification, necrosis and intratumoral hemorrhage.[11] High-grade astrocytoma and PNET should be considered in the differential diagnosis.

Primitive Neuroectodermal Tumor

Primitive neuroectodermal tumors (PNETs) are malignant embroynal tumors occurring most commonly in the cerebellum of young individuals. The neoplasm is composed of primitive poorly differentiated neuroepithelial cells that appear as small blue cells, regardless of the location of the tumor or the type of focal cellular differentiation. The multipotential nature of the PNET cell is well-documented by morphologic evidence of ependymal, oligodendroglial, melanocytic, mesenchymal and photoreceptor differentiation. The most common location is the cerebellar vermis, where such tumors have long been known as medulloblastoma. PNETs constitute up to 25% of CNS tumors in children and have a high rate of proliferation and a tendency to metastasize throughout the leptomeninges. Medulloblastomas make up 85% of this group of tumors. Supratentorial PNETs are highly malignant tumors that have a much worse prognosis than medulloblastomas and include pineoblastomas, retinoblastoma, ependymoblastoma, cerebral neuroblastomas, ganglioneuroblastomas and medulloepithelioma. They are also recorded in the spinal cord and occasionally in brainstem. They account for less than 5% of supratentorial neoplasms in children. Children under 5 years of age are commonly affected.

Pathology

Supratentorial PNET most frequently occur in deep cerebral white matter and usually quite large at the time of presentation. Grossly, they have sharp margins with necrotic areas and foci of calcification. Subarachnoid seeding and distant metastases are frequent.

Imaging

The tumor is hyperdense to the normal brain on NCCT. Focal calcification, necrosis and hemorrhage have been reported in 10% of cases. Enhancement may be homogeneous, heterogeneous or ring like **(Fig. 13)**. Magnetic resonance imaging reveals a well-defined mass varying in signal intensity from homogeneous to heterogeneous.[22] Enhancement is variable. Presence of

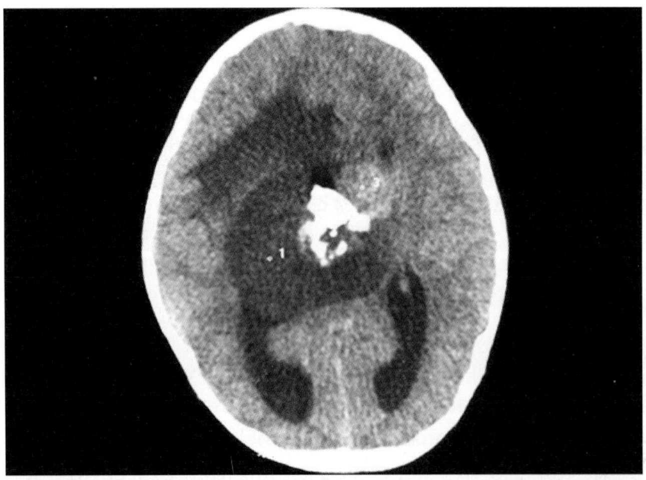

Fig. 12: Supratentorial ependymoma: CECT shows a juxtaventricular heterogeneous cystic and solid mass with areas of calcification and perilesional edema.

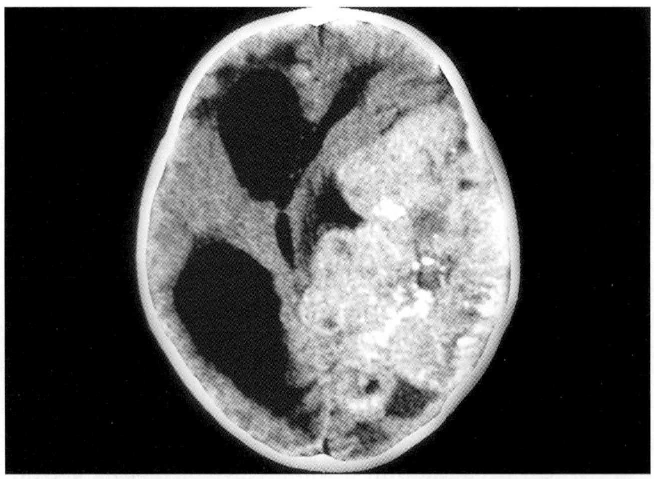

Fig. 13: Primitive neuroectodermal tumor: CECT shows a large hemispheric mass with foci of calcification.

a large mass with well-defined margins and markedly heterogeneous signal in a young child is highly suggestive of PNET.

Oligodendroglioma

Oligodendrogliomas are rare in children. They are typically slow growing hemispheric tumors with a propensity to involve the cortex. CT typically demonstrates a peripherally located hypodense tumor, however, intraventricular oligodendrogliomas have a tendency toward hyperdensity. Calcifications (40–90%), cysts (20%) and calvarial erosions (17%) have been identified on CT. MRI better delineates the tumor extent. The tumor usually is hypointense on T1WI and hyperintense or heterogeneous on T2WI. Distinguishing imaging features of oligodendrogliomas include gray and white matter involvement, the presence of calcification, and signal heterogeneity on MRI.[11]

Dysembryoplastic Neuroepithelial Tumors

Dysembryoplastic neuroepithelial tumors (DNETs) are benign lesions affecting young people and are clinically characterized by drug-resistant partial seizures and normal neurologic examination.[23] The temporal lobe is the most common site (62%), followed by the frontal lobe (31%) and parieto-occipital lobe (9%).[23] They may also arise within the caudate nucleus, cerebellum, or pons. Since cortical dysplasia is commonly seen with these tumors, perhaps they represent the tumoral form of cortical dysplasia or neoplastic transformation of a dysplastic area. These are stable and benign lesions.

Neuroimaging typically shows a predominantly cortical based well-demarcated lesion with gyral or nodular configuration. At CT, the tumor manifests as a hypodense mass that may occasionally have areas of calcification.[23] Remodeling of the adjacent inner table of the skull may also be seen.[23] They are hypointense on T1, hyperintense on T2WI and homogeneous in 57% of cases **(Figs. 14A to D)**. Edema and mass effect on midline structures are lacking, although they may be observed in cases of hemorrhagic complications. Some lesions may appear as an enlarged gyrus, producing a soap bubble appearance at the cortical margin. Sometimes DNETs show a multicystic appearance more commonly than do gangliogliomas. About one-third of DNETs enhance following intravenous administration of contrast material, which is typically focal and punctate.[23] Distinguishing features of DNET include a thick nodular or gyral configuration with little or no white matter extension is rarely seen in other glial tumors.[23]

Desmoplastic Infantile Ganglioglioma

Desmoplastic infantile ganglioglioma (DIG) is a voluminous, mixed ganglion and glial cell tumor (WHO grade I) with extensive desmoplasia and cyst formation.[24] Typically, the tumor is superficially located in frontal and parietal lobes. Growth into the subarachnoid space and adjacent meninges is uniformly present in these tumors. Barring isolated case reports, almost all cases have occurred in children less than 18 months of age.

The most striking imaging feature of DIG is its relatively large size. CT reveals a large tumor with formation of a large hypodense cyst and a hyperdense solid component, which enhances intensely. On MR, signal characteristics of the solid component have been variably reported as hypo-, iso- or hyperintense relative to gray matter. The cystic component has low T1 and high T2 signal. The solid component enhances markedly and typically is adjacent to the meninges.[25]

Differential diagnosis includes PNET, ependymoma and astrocytoma. DIG should be suggested in infants presenting as a large superficial cerebral mass with large

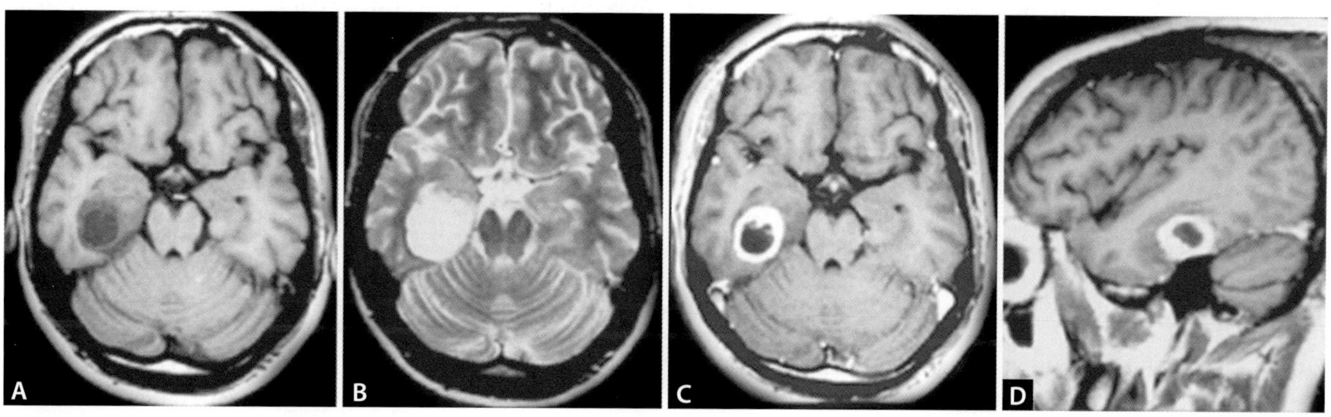

Figs. 14A to D: Dysembryoplastic neuroepithelial tumors: Axial T1W image (A) showing a predominantly cystic hypointense lesion in right medial temporal lobe. The lesion is heterogeneously hyperintense on T2WI (B) and shows thick ring enhancement (C and D).

cystic component and enhancing solid component adjacent to meninges. Its identification is important since it has a significantly better prognosis and different considerations relative to other infantile brain tumors.

SELLAR AND SUPRASELLAR TUMORS

Chiasmatic/Hypothalamic Gliomas

Gliomas of the hypothalamus and optic pathways represent 5% of pediatric brain tumors with 60% involving the optic chiasm and hypothalamus.[26] They represent 25–30% of pediatric neoplasm of suprasellar region. The vast majority are slow growing pilocytic astrocytomas, although malignant gliomas and in particular glioblastoma multiforme may occur, especially in adults. About 20–50% of these patients, have clinical evidence or family history of neurofibromatosis type 1 (NF1). It is almost impossible to determine the exact site of origin, since both hypothalamus and chiasm are involved regardless of origin. The mean age of presentation is 5 years. Patients usually present with visual symptoms, headaches and endocrine abnormalities.

Imaging

MR is examination of choice. The lesions tend to be solid with microcyst formation. They are usually iso- or hypointense on T1WI, hyperintense on T2WI and demonstrate enhancement with contrast. The sella is usually normal.

Craniopharyngioma

Craniopharyngiomas are complex epithelial tumors arising from remnants of Rathke's pouch. They most commonly arise in the suprasellar region (90%) and account for up to 10% of pediatric brain tumors. More than half of all craniopharyngiomas occur in children and young adults. A second, smaller peak occurs in middle-aged adults. Patients may present clinically with headaches, visual disturbances, and hypothalamic and pituitary dysfunction. On gross pathology, most craniopharyngiomas are cystic masses with cholesterol-rich fluid and calcifications. Clinicopathologically, two distinct subtypes are recognized: the adamantinous type, which tends to occur in children, and the squamous-papillary variant, which tends to occur in adults.[27]

Imaging

On CT, craniopharyngiomas can be cystic, mixed cystic and solid, or solid, and exhibit enhancement of more solid portions. Nodular or rim calcification is found in about 90% of cases **(Figs. 15A and B)**. Attenuation of the cystic

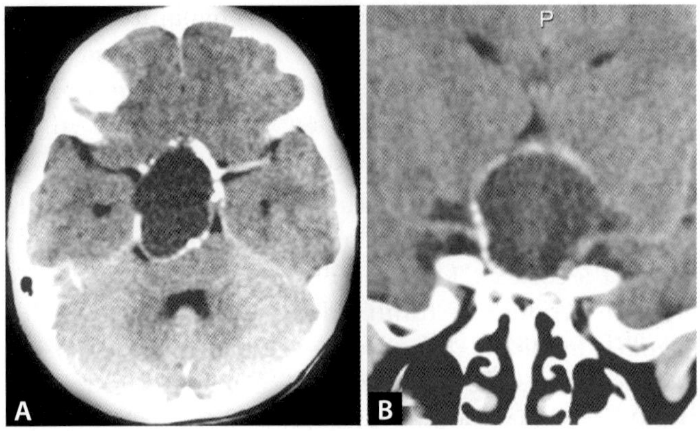

Figs. 15A and B: Craniopharyngioma: Axial (A) and coronal (B) contrast-enhanced CT through sella demonstrate a sellar and suprasellar cystic mass with calcifications at its margins and peripheral enhancement.

component is variable but is often slightly higher than CSF. The imaging characteristics of craniopharyngiomas on MRI are variable, reflecting wide range of components histologically composing these tumors. High-signal intensity on T1WI and T2WI is seen in cysts with high cholesterol content or/and subacute hemorrhage. Cysts containing large amount of keratin are hypointense on T1WI. Heterogeneous enhancement of the solid component has been noted on contrast-enhanced images. Encasement of vessels, a lobulated shape, presence of hyperintense cysts and recurrence favor adamantinous type of craniopharyngioma. A round shape, presence of hypointense cysts and predominantly solid appearance is seen with squamous-papillary tumors.

Despite benign histopathologic features, craniopharyngiomas are locally invasive, with projections of tumor extending into the adjacent brain. Hence, total resection of this tumor is often difficult and local recurrence at the primary site or in the contiguous brain may ensue, usually within 5 years.

Hypothalamic Hamartoma

The lesion consists of mature neuronal ganglionic tissue projecting from the hypothalamus down into the suprasellar cistern. It is usually attached to the mamillary bodies or tuber cinereum.[28] There is a definite male predilection. Presenting symptoms include precocious puberty, gelastic seizures, developmental delay and hyperactivity. It usually measures 1–2 cm in diameter.

Imaging

On CT, hamartoma is a round or ovoid isodense mass that projects into the suprasellar or interpeduncular cistern.

On MR, T1WI demonstrates a slightly hypointense mass in the suprasellar cistern, which abuts against the floor of the hypothalamus. The mass is generally isointense to adjacent gray matter and does not show enhancement after gadolinium administration **(Figs. 16A and B)**. T2WI demonstrates the mass to be isointense to adjacent gray matter and may contain patchy regions of slightly higher signal intensity.[28] The higher intensity areas may represent the gliotic areas seen histologically. These imaging findings are fairly characteristic and are helpful in differentiating the hypothalamic hamartoma from the more common suprasellar lesions such as craniopharyngioma and hypothalamic/opticochiasmatic glioma seen in children.

Pituitary Adenomas

Pituitary adenomas represent less than 3% of all pediatric intracranial tumors. In childhood, they are usually seen in adolescent males and are commonly macroadenomas, in particular prolactinomas, and they tend to be hemorrhagic.[29] Adenomas measuring 10 mm or less are referred to as microadenomas, and these tumors do not have suprasellar extension. Most microadenomas enhance less rapidly than surrounding normal pituitary tissue and therefore are seen as hypodense or hypointense areas on contrast-enhanced CT and MR studies, respectively. Macroadenomas are more common than microadenomas and enhance uniformly and intensely.

Arachnoid Cyst

Arachnoid cysts are congenital lesions of the arachnoid membrane lined by specialized cells that contain enzymes for secretory activity. Therefore, true arachnoid cysts expand by accumulation of CSF secreted by these cells. On the other hand, leptomeningeal cysts are caused by trauma or inflammation and represent merely loculation of cerebrospinal fluid surrounded by arachnoid scarring. Common locations are sylvian fissure, suprasellar, quadrigeminal, CP angle and posterior infratentorial midline cisterns, interhemispheric fissure, cerebral convexity and anterior infratentorial midline cisterns. Small arachnoid cysts are usually asymptomatic. Large midline lesions cause hydrocephalus. Sylvian fissure cysts are commonly associated with seizures and headache.

Imaging

Arachnoid cysts on CT and MR are well-defined homogeneous unilocular masses that are similar to CSF density on all imaging modalities and pulse sequences **(Fig. 17)**.[28] Large suprasellar cysts may cause hydrocephalus by obstructing the foramen of Monro. FLAIR is particularly useful in arachnoid cysts, because the signal should be completely suppressed if the contents represent CSF.[28] Pulsation artifacts may occasionally be seen within the large cysts and are revealed as focal streaks of hypointensity on T2WI.[28] Subdural and intracystic hemorrhages may complicate middle cranial fossa cysts, either following trauma or spontaneously.

PINEAL REGION MASSES

Germ cell tumors are the most common neoplasms of pineal gland that comprise about 3–8% of pediatric brain tumors.

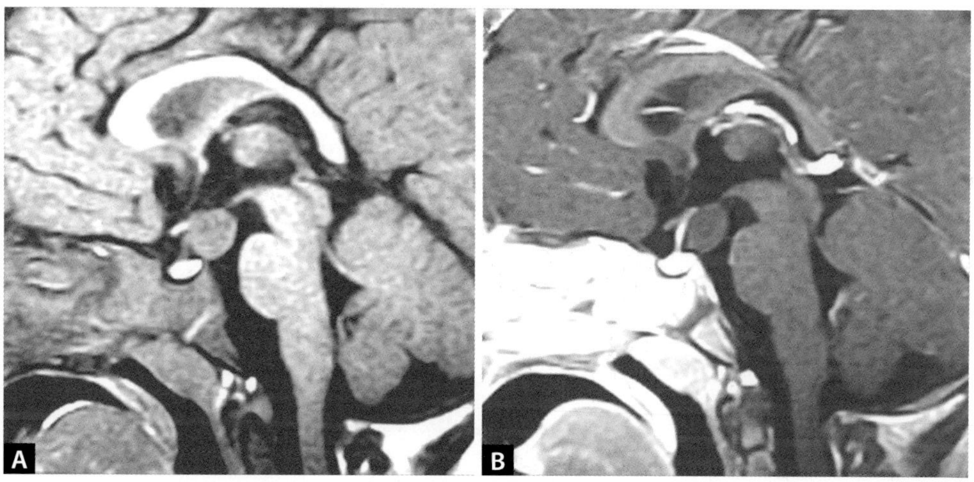

Figs. 16A and B: Hypothalamic hamartoma: T1WI sagittal images at the level of hypothalamus show a 1 cm mass in the suprasellar cistern abutting against floor of third ventricle. The mass is isointense to gray matter and do not show any enhancement after gadolinium administration (B).

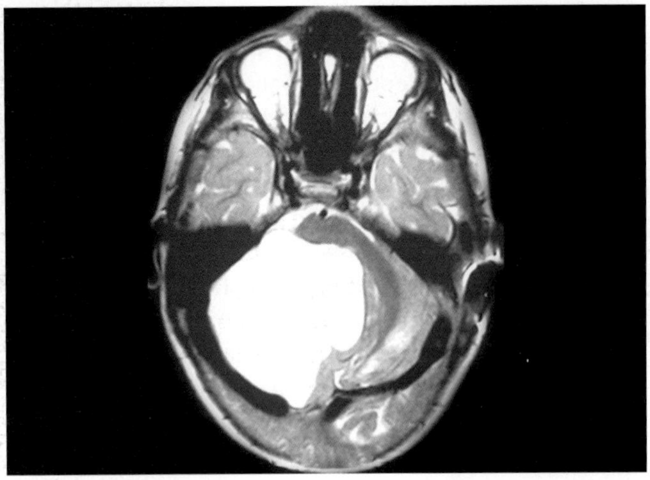

Fig. 17: Arachnoid cyst: Axial T2WI shows a well-defined extra-axial cyst in right cerebellopontine angle which is isointense to the CSF.

Germinomas

Germinomas are the most common germ cell tumors and also are the most common pineal mass. Pineal region accounts for more than 50% of germinomas. Suprasellar/hypothalamic region and basal ganglia are the other common sites for germinoma (35%). Synchronous pineal and suprasellar lesions occur in 6–12% of germinomas and are considered diagnostic.[30] Primary suprasellar germinomas have no sexual predilection, in contrast to pineal germinomas, which show a male predominance. Hydrocephalus and Parinaud syndrome are the common presentations of pineal germinoma. Subarachnoid seeding is frequent.

Imaging

Pineal germinomas are well-circumscribed relatively homogeneous lesions that are not separable from the pineal body itself. These are hyperdense on NCCT. Germinomas are typically low intensity (i.e. isointense to gray matter) on T2WI.[11] Intratumoral hemorrhage may be seen in these lesions. Germinomas and their metastases enhance markedly and homogeneously after IV contrast administration. Pineal germinomas do not calcify nor do they contain cysts, features that differ from those described for germinomas arising in basal ganglion.

Teratomas

The second most common pineal germ cell tumors are teratomas. They exclusively affect males and present in the first decade. Symptoms are similar to those of germinoma.

Pathology

Pineal teratomas are extremely heterogeneous masses with irregular and lobulated margins and are noninvasive in nature.

Imaging

On CT, these lesions are heterogeneous due to presence of fat, calcification, bone, hemorrhage, and cystic or necrotic areas. MR reveals a mass with variegated appearance. Both CT and MRI show heterogeneous or ring-like enhancement. Pineal teratomas may rupture either during surgery or spontaneously causing chemical meningitis. Malignant teratomas tend to invade surrounding structures, such as tectum, the brainstem and the splenium of corpus callosum.

Other Germ Cell Tumors

Choriocarcinoma, embryonal cell carcinoma, and endodermal sinus tumors are highly malignant tumors of pineal gland. Choriocarcinomas have a tendency to bleed, a feature which differentiates it from other pineal tumors on imaging. Serologic and CSF analysis for tumor markers can aid in specificity of preoperative diagnosis.

Pineal Parenchymal Tumors

Pineal parenchymal tumors account for less than 15% of all pineal region tumors. There are 2 types of tumors—pineocytomas and pineoblastomas. Both tumors arise from neuroepithelial cells of the gland itself.

Pineoblastomas appear predominantly in male infants and may be rarely associated with bilateral retinoblastomas. On MRI, the tumors show a heterogeneous pattern which is isointense to gray matter on T1WI and isohypointense to gray matter on T2WI due to cellularity of the tumor.[31] They exhibit intense enhancement.

Pineocytomas appear from 18 to 50 years of age and almost exclusively in females. On CT they appear as slightly hyperdense mass with a noticeable amount of calcification. On MRI the tumors appear homogeneous with high signal on T2WI and low to isointense signal on T1WI reflecting high amount of cytoplasm.[31] The tumors exhibit significant contrast enhancement, and for large tumors heterogeneity is observed.

Pineal Cysts

Cystic lesions of the pineal gland are found in 21–41% of autopsy series and 1.4–4.3% of cranial MR studies and are usually incidental. Pineal cyst development, small changes in cyst size, and cyst involution can all be seen on serial MR imaging without the development of specific symptoms. These lesions may, however, become clinically important for two reasons: first, pineal cysts may enlarge over time (because of either increased cyst fluid or intracystic hemorrhage) and become symptomatic. Second, benign-appearing cysts of the pineal gland may represent malignant or premalignant conditions. Rarely, pineocytomas may present as purely cystic tumors, or tumors may develop on the pineal cyst wall. The cysts are isointense to CSF on T1WI and slightly hyperintense with respect to CSF on T2WI.[32] Hemorrhage within the pineal cyst is rare and appears hyperintense on both T1WI and T2WI. On contrast study, a rim of normal pineal gland enhances around the cysts. Typical pineal cysts found incidentally on MR imaging may be followed clinically without further imaging.

EXTRAPARENCHYMAL TUMORS

Choroid Plexus Tumors

Choroid plexus papillomas (CPPs) and carcinomas originate from choroid plexus epithelium. They constitute 5% of supra-tentorial pediatric tumors and less than 1% of all primary intracranial neoplasms. CPPs are most frequent in the first year of life, and usually present with hydrocephalus. Choroids plexus carcinomas (CPCs) make up 30–40% of choroid plexus tumors and occur mostly during first 5 years of life. Focal neurologic deficit resulting from adjacent brain invasion is the frequent presentation of CPC. Male predominance is observed for both the tumors. Hydrocephalus frequently occurs with CPPs as a result of either the overproduction of CSF and/or occurrence of blockage in the subarachnoid cisterns or intraventricular pathways.

Pathology

In children, 80% of CPPs arise in the lateral ventricles; 16% in the fourth ventricle and 4% in the third ventricle. Fourth ventricle is the commonest site of adult CPP. Papillomas are very irregularly lobulated masses projecting into and enlarging the ventricular cavity. Foci of small hemorrhages and calcification may be found. Anaplastic papillomas frequently invade the brain and are difficult to differentiate from carcinomas. Metastasis through CSF pathways is common for both anaplastic papillomas and carcinomas.

Imaging

On NCCT, they are hyperdense or isodense relative to cortex, frequently contain prominent calcifications and display intense enhancement after IV contrast administration. On T1W MRI tumor usually have a lobulated margin and is iso- to slightly hypointense to gray matter. Areas of hypointensity within the tumor may represent calcifications or flow-voids. On T2WI the tumor may show a very heterogeneous hyperintensity due to presence of calcifications, flow-voids and iron from old hemorrhages.[33] Gadolinium administration will demonstrate enhancement throughout the tumor that may be heterogeneous in its pattern depending on degree of tumor calcification, vascularity and cystic changes **(Figs. 18A to D)**.

Anaplastic papillomas invade the ependyma and grow into the surrounding white matter, producing vasogenic oedema. They are more irregular in outline and closely resemble CPC.

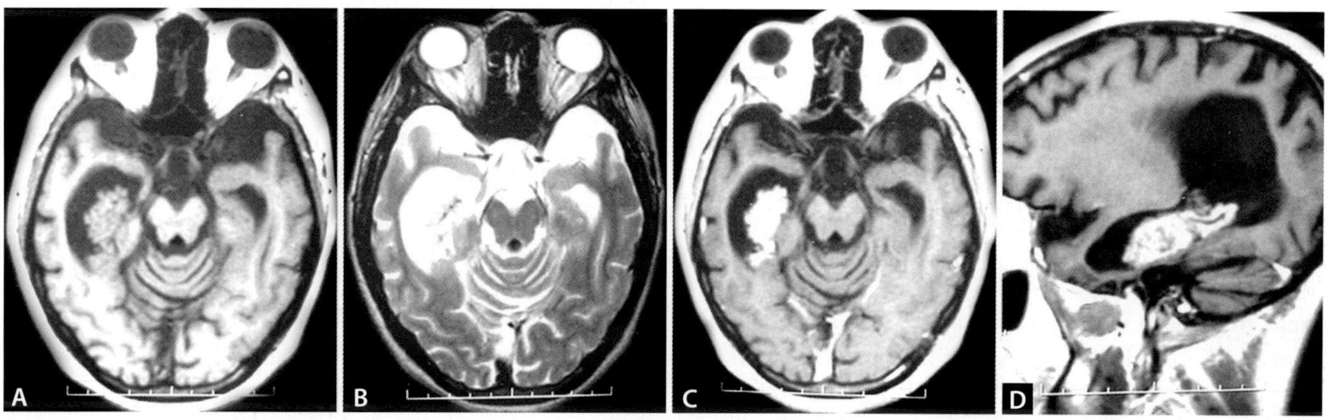

Figs. 18A to D: Choroid plexus papilloma: Axial T1WI (A) and T2WI (B) show a lobulated intraventricular mass in the temporal horn of right lateral ventricle. The mass is isointense to gray matter on T1WI (C) and hypointense on T2WI (D). The mass shows intense enhancement following gadolinium administration.

Compared to papillomas, CPCs are much more aggressive, irregular in contour, are of mixed density on noncontrast study and show variable enhancement. Cysts and hemorrhage are frequent. They almost always grow through the ventricular wall into the brain with associated oedema. Carcinomas are more heterogeneous on both T1WI and T2WI and may show evidence of intratumoral hemorrhage. Pathologically, carcinomas resemble PNET and ependymomas.

Meningiomas and Related Tumors

Childhood meningiomas represent 1–4.2% of central nervous system tumors and 1.5–1.8% of all intracranial meningiomas. Childhood meningiomas are associated with significant shorter survival due to limitation in surgical intervention, association with neurofibromatosis, increased incidence of sarcomatous change, large size of tumors and inability to use adjuvant radiotherapy and chemotherapy to treat the residual tumors.

Pathology

Pediatric meningeal tumors include meningioma, meningeal fibromas, meningeal sarcomas and meningeal melanomas. Sylvian fissure meningiomas are common, lack a dural attachment and originate from heterotopic meningeal rests within the brain. Significant percentage of pediatric meningiomas are intraventricular.

Imaging

The tumors are iso- to hyperdense on noncontrast CT and the solid portion shows diffuse enhancement on contrast injection. Heterogeneity is seen in about 50% of cases and is related to cystic changes and intratumoral calcification. A typical CT features should suggest a malignant tumor such as meningeal sarcoma or meningeal PNET. Intraventricular meningiomas originate from choroid plexus.[34]

On MR, meningiomas have well-defined margins, and are isointense on T1WI, and iso- to hyperintense on T2WI. Areas of cystic necrosis have prolonged T1 and T2 relaxation times. Solid portions show uniform enhancement on infusion of paramagnetic substance. Densely calcified areas may be of very low intensity on precontrast T1W images whereas less densely calcified areas may be iso- to hyperintense on T2WI. At angiography, meningiomas usually have dual blood supply, meningeal branches from both internal carotid and external carotid arteries may feed the tumor.

Leukemia and Lymphoma

Meningeal and parenchymal metastatic disease from leukemia and lymphoma are extremely uncommon. Meningeal enhancement after contrast administration is found in 5% of leukemic patients with CNS symptoms. Granulocytic sarcoma is a solid tumor found in association with systemic leukemia, usually the myelogenous type. It is postulated to arise from neoplastic cells that traverse the calvarial marrow to involve the dura, than pass through the perivenous adventitial tissue to invade the brain parenchyma. On CT granulocytic sarcomas appear iso- to hyperdense with uniform enhancement on contrast administration. The MR characteristics are variable, but in most cases the lesions are hypo- to-isointense on T1WI and iso- to slightly hyperintense on T2WI. The lesions enhance uniformly and intensely following contrast on both CT and MR.[28]

TUMORS OF THE ORBIT AND NECK

OCULAR TUMORS

Retinoblastoma

Retinoblastoma is the most common intraorbital malignancy of childhood. Autosomal dominant inheritance is found in 10% of cases that are frequently bilateral. About 2–5% of patients with bilateral retinoblastoma will eventually develop pineoblastoma, the term trilateral retinoblastomas is then applied. Bilateral lesions are seen in 31% and 33% are multifocal.

Majority (80%) of retinoblastomas occur in children below 2 years of age. Soft tissue sarcomas subsequently develop in 10–15% of affected patients. Leukocoria or 'cats eye reflex' is the usual clinical presentation in early childhood.

Imaging

A CT shows a retinal mass with ill-defined margins and commonly associated with calcification (95%). Intracranial extension occurs through scleral lymphatics along the optic nerves. CT is the imaging modality of choice to detect calcification and identification of the tumor. MR is useful for detection of intracranial extension.

Differential diagnosis includes Coats' disease, which is a degenerative proliferative disease of retina. Retinal detachment and subretinal hemorrhage is a common complication of Coats' disease. Larval granulomatosis is caused by *Toxocara canis* infection, and has CT appearance similar to Coats' disease. Both conditions lack calcification and therefore, could be differentiated from majority of retinoblastomas containing calcification. Persistent hyperplastic primary vitreous is also associated with leukocoria, retinal detachment and subretinal hemorrhage. Absence of calcification and hypoplastic affected globe are its major differentiating features from retinoblastoma.[35]

RETROBULBAR ORBITAL TUMORS

Vascular Tumors

Orbital hemangiomas and lymphangiomas are hamartomatous malformations. Capillary hemangiomas are the most common vascular masses, which typically present at birth and grow rapidly within first 6 months of life. They stop growing during the second year and subsequently involute over 5–6 years.

CT shows a diffuse, retrobulbar mass with ill-defined margins, present extraconally, intraconally or both. Contrast enhancement is diffuse. MR reveals a mass that is hyperintense to extraocular muscles and hypointense to fat on both T1WI and T2WI. Serpiginous flow void areas within the mass helps to differentiate it from malignant masses such as rhabdomyosarcomas. Orbital enlargement is seen frequently.

Lymphangiomas present between the ages of 1 and 15 years. Recurrent hemorrhages within the mass cause recurrent episodic proptosis. On CT lymphangiomas are heterogeneous, ill-defined masses with occasional phleboliths and heterogeneous enhancement. Recent hemorrhage appears hyperdense. On MR, lymphangioma appears as lobulated, multicystic mass, which is hypointense to muscle on T1WI and hyperintense to muscle on T2WI. Fluid-fluid levels, when present, are strongly suggestive of lymphangioma. Heterogeneous enhancement is seen on contrast administration. Cavernous hemangiomas are rare in children. They present as painless proptosis, which does not change with Valsalva maneuver, when compared with orbital varices. Cavernous hemangiomas are intraconal masses that spare the orbital apex and frequently have phleboliths within it. MR shows the mass as isointense on T1WI and hyperintense on T2WI compared to orbital muscles. Homogeneous contrast enhancement is noted on both CT and MR.[36]

Orbital Varices

Orbital varices are venous malformations located in the retrobulbar region. They present in older children or adulthood. Classical presentation is intermittent proptosis, which increases on Valsalva maneuver on lying prone or on bending forward. CT and MR show a mass with curvilinear configuration, phleboliths and dense enhancement after contrast administration. CT is a better modality since imaging can be performed during a Valsalva maneuver in short time.[36]

Neuroblastoma

Neuroblastoma is a common tumor of childhood, which involves the CNS either by direct extension, primarily in the spine, or blood-borne metastases. Neuroblastoma metastases commonly involve the orbit and calvarium and rarely the brain. Unenhanced CT scan may show multiple intracranial hyperdense masses, some of which mimic intraparenchymal lesions. Bony spicules are seen radiating centripetally from the calvarium. Splitting the coronal and sagittal sutures is another characteristic finding in neuroblastoma. Coronal images are useful to verify a dural extradural location of these lesions. Primary neuroblastoma originates in the sympathetic chain of upper cervical or skull base portion. On, MR, the tumor masses have intensity similar to soft tissues. Enhancement is marked and elevated periosteum also shows enhancement which helps to differentiate it from normal hemopoietic calvarium. Metastatic Ewing's sarcoma and leukemia cannot be differentiated from metastatic neuroblastoma to the skull base.[36]

Plexiform Neurofibroma

Plexiform neurofibroma is seen in the setting of NF1. They diffusely infiltrate the connective tissue and peripheral nerves of the orbit. Proptosis, visual loss, marked facial asymmetry, enlarged orbit and dysplastic adjacent greater sphenoid wing is commonly found. The mass may extend through the superior orbital fissure into the cavernous sinus. The masses are isodense to extraocular muscles on CT. MR is preferred to CT, since cavernous sinus involvement and other manifestation of NF1 can be assessed well even without contrast.[36]

Rhabdomyosarcoma

Rhabdomyosarcoma is a common childhood malignancy, only next to intracranial brain tumors and retinoblastoma. Orbit and nasopharynx are commonly involved, followed by paranasal sinuses and middle ear, constituting 40% of all rhabdomyosarcomas. Primary intracranial rhabdomyosarcomas are rare, although cranial involvement is common from extension of extracranial tumors. Rhabdomyosarcomas are classified into three major groups depending on the site of origin.

1. Parameningeal
2. Orbital
3. Other head and neck locations.

The parameningeal group consists of tumors originating in the middle nasopharynx, paranasal sinuses and nasal cavity. Prognosis is very poor since tumor in this location commonly invades the skull or spread through the foramina at the skull base.

Orbital rhabdomyosarcoma spread through orbital fissures in the cranium cavernous sinus and middle cranial fossa. The tumor is isodense on NCCT and enhances uniformly after IV contrast. Additionally, the involved foramina are expanded. MR findings consist of mass that is isointense on T1WI and hyperintense on T2WI as compared to muscle. Uniform enhancement is found following IV contrast. Fat suppression technique with contrast is preferred for better delineation of the tumor from fat and muscle.[36]

Juvenile Angiofibroma

These tumors are benign but locally invasive lesions that arise in the sphenopalatine foramen, nasopharynx or posterior nasal cavity. Adolescent boys are commonly affected. Local invasion is quite common.

Nasal obstruction and recurrent epistaxis are the frequent clinical presentation. Proptosis and cranial neuropathies are seen with intracranial extension of the tumor. CT shows a soft tissue mass in the nasopharynx/pterygopalatine fossa, with well-circumscribed margins and homogeneous enhancement following IV contrast. It produces anterior bowing of posterior maxillary wall sinus. Sphenoid sinus extension is quite common.

MR shows a mass that is iso- to hypointense on T1WI and iso- to hyperintense on T2WI as compared to muscles. Tumor vessels are seen as serpiginous flow void areas. Intense homogeneous enhancement of the tumor is a characteristic finding on IV contrast. Angiography reveals a very vascular tumor, mainly supplied by external carotid arteries. Endovascular embolisation may be carried out to reduce intraoperative blood loss.[37]

MAGNETIC RESONANCE SPECTROSCOPY IN BRAIN

Tumor Imaging

Magnetic resonance spectroscopy (MRS) is helpful in biochemical tissue characterization of tumors and differentiating radiation-induced necrosis from recurrent or residual tumor.

Positron-emission Tomography (PET) in Neuro-oncology

PET is relatively noninvasive modality to study regional cerebral physiology in patients with brain tumors. PET provides in vivo quantitative information about glucose, oxygen metabolism, blood flow, tissue drug uptake and receptor, and the effects of various therapeutic regimens.

Initial reports with 18-fluorodeoxyglucose (FDG) PET have suggested the possibility of grading cerebral tumors in vivo. High grade neoplasms show large increases in glucose metabolism and low grade neoplasms show hypometabolism.[20]

Thus, combination of PET with anatomic MR imaging or CT enhances the clinical usefulness of PET in neuro-oncology.

Diffusion-weighted Imaging

- Diffusion-weighted imaging derives image contrast from the movement of water molecules in tissues.
- Brownian motion—All molecules at temperatures greater than absolute zero experience random translation driven by their internal thermal energy.
- In the context of diffusion imaging, Brownian motion is also called self-diffusion or intravoxel incoherent motion.
- Thus, normal water motion results in decreased signal intensity, while reduced water motion that is, restricted water diffusion—Results in relatively increased signal.
- In routine clinical imaging, Diffusion weighting can be achieved with TSE, EPI, STE, SSFP and PSIF.
- Highly cellular tumors, such as lymphoma, PNET, cellular gliomas have a higher ADC than the normal brain parenchyma.
- Viable tumor shows normal-high SI on DWI (normal-decreased ADC).
- In areas of tumor necrosis, there is low SI on DWI and increased ADC.

Uses in Glioma Evaluation

- Grading of glioma.
- Stereotactic biopsy guidance.
- Distinguishing radiation necrosis from recurrent cancer.
- Determining prognosis and response to treatment.
- Gliomas—Higher grade-Increased angiogenesis-Increased rCBV.
- Mean rCBV ratio (obtained by division by contralateral WM value) is 4.82 in high grade gliomas and 1.83 in low grade gliomas. Proposed cutoff value for rCBV ratio is 2.93 and rCBF ratio is 3.57.

- High cerebral blood volume foci can be found in non-GD enhancing tumors.
- Helps to direct stereotactic biopsy to areas of increased rCBV, which are more aggressive and hence increased chances of malignant tissue retrieval.
- Radiation necrosis versus tumor recurrence are difficult to differentiates.

On conventional CT and MRI—as BBB breakdown, mass-effect and edema are common to both differentiate on Perfusion MRI-Irradiated areas reveal rCBV decrease in values, whereas rCBV increases in tumor recurrence.

NANOTECHNOLOGY

Imaging and Nanomedicine for Diagnosis and Therapy of CNS Tumors

Neuroimaging techniques have become increasingly important in assessing the biologic and physiological properties of brain tumors and neurologic lesions. Role of newer contrast media such as iron peroxide nanoparticle MR contrast or molecular agents based on therapeutic agents or tumor specific antibodies or agents is presently under evaluation. Superparamagnetic iron peroxide (SPIO) and utrasmall superparamagnetic iron peroxide (USPIO) nanoparticle MR contrast agents are being increasingly used in CNS for charactering particle delivery, monitoring trafficking of particles and cells and visualizing intracerebral tumors. Newer molecular imaging techniques should be integrated into brain tumor management to providing critical information that may significantly improve the survival and care of patients with brain tumors.[38]

Newly Codified Glial Neoplasms of the 2007 WHO Classification of Tumors of the Central Nervous System[39]

This new classification system proposed in 2007 has recognized three new entities:

1. *Angiocentric glioma (AG):* It is a slowly growing cerebral tumor that typically presents with seizures in children and young adults. It is characterized by monomorphous, bipolar tumor cells with typical perivascular growth pattern. The cell of origin of AG is not clear but the ultrastructural evidence points to an ependymal derivation. It is designated WHO grade I and can be completely cured by surgical resection.
2. *Polymyxoid Astrocytoma (PMA):* It is a solid, circumscribed tumor occurring mainly in the region of hypothalamus of young children. It is composed of monomorphous population of bipolar tumor cells within a rich background of myxoid with a conspicuous angiocentric arrangement. While PMA is considered a more aggressive variant of pilocytic astrocytoma, this relationship awaits further clarification. PMA has been designated WHO grade II.
3. *Pituicytoma:* The pituicytoma involves the posterior pituitary and or the stalk and affects young adults. It is solid in architecture and composed of spindle cells and presumably derived from pituicytes. Pituicytomas are indolent tumors and designated WHO grade I.

CONCLUSION

Central nervous system is the second most common site of pediatric neoplasm. Infratentorial tumors account for 52%, while 48% involve the supratentorial region. Aside from the initial recognition and characterization of these lesions, the mechanical effects and structural deformities resulting from intracranial neoplasms are also of great importance. Therefore, the neuroradiologists must be able to appreciate the consequences resulting from the combined effects of tumors and the associated oedema, many of which are potentially life-threatening, such as transtentorial herniation. For the optimal interpretation of MRI, it is essential for the neuroradiologists to be particularly familiar with neuropathology in addition to the requisite mastery of neuroanatomy since imaging abnormalities reflect pathologic findings in these lesions.

REFERENCES

1. Miltenburg D, Louw DF, Sutherland GR. Epidemiology of childhood brain tumors. Can J Neurol Sci. 1996;23(2):118-22.
2. McKinney PA, Parslow RC, Lane SA, et al. Epidemiology of childhood brain tumors in Yorkshire, UK, 1974-95: Geographical distribution and changing patterns of occurrence. Br J Cancer. 1998;8(7):974-9.
3. Karkavelas G, Tascos N. Epidemiology, histologic classification and clinical course of brain tumors. In: Drevelegas A (Ed): Imaging of Brain Tumors with Histological Correlation. New York: Springer; 2002.
4. Koeller KK, Rushing EJ. From the archives of the AFIP: Medulloblastoma: a comprehensive review with radiologic-pathologic correlation. Radiographics. 2003;23:1613-37.
5. Giangspero F, Bigner SH, Kleihues P, et al. Medulloblastoma. In: Kleihues P, Cavenee WK (Eds): Pathology and Genetics of Tumors of the Nervous System. Lyon: IARC Press 2000;129-37.
6. Kotsenas AL, Roth TC, Manness WK, et al. Abnormal diffusion-weighted MRI in medulloblastoma: Does it reflect small cell histology? Pediatr Radiol. 1999;29:524-6.
7. Tortori-Donati P, Fondelli MP, Rossi A, et al. Medulloblastoma in children: CT and MRI findings. Neuroradiology. 1996;38:352-9.

8. Lee YY, Van Tassel P, Bruner JM, et al. Juvenile pilocytic astrocytomas: CT and MR characteristics. Am J Roentgenol. 1989;152(6):1263-70.
9. Tortori-Donati P, Fondelli MP, Cama A, et al. Ependymomas of the posterior cranial fossa: CT and MRI findings. Neuroradiology. 1995;37(3):238-43.
10. Fisher PG, Breiter SN, Carson BS, et al. A clinicopathologic reappraisal of brainstem tumor classification. Identification of pilocytic astrocytoma and fibrillary astrocytoma as distinct entities. Cancer. 2000;89(7):1569-76.
11. Atlas SW, Lavi E, Fisher PG. Intra-axial brain tumors. In: Atlas SW (Ed): Magnetic Resonance Imaging of Brain and Spine, 3rd edition. Philadelphia: Lippincott. 2002;565-693.
12. Rorke LB, Packer R, Biegel J. Central nervous system atypical teratoid/rhabdoid tumors of infancy and childhood. Journal of Neuro-Oncology. 1995; 24:21-8.
13. Agranovich AL, Ang LC, Griebel RW. Malignant rhabdoid tumor of the central nervous system with subarachnoid dissemination. Surg Neurol. 1992;37(5):410-4.
14. Zuccoli G, Izzi G, Bachini E, et al. Central nervous system atypical teratoid/rhabdoid tumor of infancy: CT and MR findings. Clinical Imaging. 1999;23:356-60.
15. Ho VB, Smirniotopoulos JG, Murphy FM, et al. Radiologic-pathologic correlation: Hemangioblastoma. Am J Neuroradiol. 1992;13(5):1343-52.
16. Lee SR, Sanches J, Mark AS, et al. Posterior fossa hemangioblastomas: MR imaging. Radiology. 1989;171(2): 463-8.
17. Horowitz BL, Chari MV, James R, et al. MR of intracranial epidermoid tumors: Correlation of in vivo imaging with in vitro 13C spectroscopy. AJNR Am J Neuroradiol. 1990;11(2):299-302.
18. Bergui M, Zhong J, Bradac GB, et al. Diffusion-weighted images of intracranial cyst-like lesions. Neuroradiology. 2001;43(10):824-9.
19. Jelinek J, Smirniotopoulos JG, Parisi JE, et al. Lateral ventricular neoplasms of the brain: Differential diagnosis based on clinical, CT, and MR findings. Am J Neuroradiol. 1990;11(3):567-74.
20. Koeller KK, Henry JM. From the archives of the AFIP: Superficial gliomas: Radiologic-pathologic correlation. Armed Forces Institute of Pathology. Radiographics. 2001;21(6):1533-56.
21. Castillo M, Davis PC, Takei Y, et al. Intracranial ganglioglioma: MR, CT, and clinical findings in 18 patients. AJNR Am J Neuroradiol. 1990;11:109-14 (ganglioma).
22. Davis P, Wichman RD, Takei Y, et al. Primary cerebral neurocytoma: CT and MR findings in 12 cases. Am J Neuroradiol. 1990;11:115-20.
23. Daumas-Duport C, Scheithauer BW, Chodkiewicz JP, et al. Dysembryoplastic neuroepithelial tumor: A surgically curable tumor of young patients with intractable partial seizures. Report of thirty-nine cases. Neurosurgery. 1988;23(5):545-56.
24. VandenBerg SR, May EE, Rubenstein LJ, et al. Desmoplastic supratentorial neuroepithelial tumors of infancy with divergent differentiation potential ("desmoplastic infantile gangliogliomas"): Report on 11 cases of a distinctive embryonal tumor with favorable prognosis. J Neurosurg. 1987;66:58-71.
25. Fernandez C, Girard N, Paz Paredes A, et al. The usefulness of MR imaging in the diagnosis of dysembryoplastic neuroepithelial tumor in children: A study of 14 cases. Am J Neuroradiol. 2003;24:829-34.
26. Janss AJ, Grundy R, Cnaan A, et al. Optic pathway and hypothalamic/chiasmatic gliomas in children younger than age 5 years with a 6-year follow-up. Cancer. 1995;75(4): 1051-9.
27. Sartoretti-Schefer S, Wichmann W, Aguzzi A, et al. MR differentiation of adamantinous and squamous-papillary craniopharyngiomas. Am J Neuroradiol. 1997;18(1):77-87.
28. Atlas SW, Lavi E, Goldberg HI. Extraaxial brain tumors. In Atlas SW (Ed): Magnetic Resonance Imaging of Brain and Spine, 3rd edition. Philadelphia: Lippincott. 2002;695-772.
29. Poussaint TY, Barnes PD, Anthony DC, et al. Hemorrhagic pituitary adenomas of adolescence. Am J Neuroradiol. 1996;17(10):1907-12.
30. Sugiyama K, Uozumi T, Kiya K, et al. Intracranial germ-cell tumor with synchronous lesions in the pineal and suprasellar regions: Report of six cases and review of the literature. Surg Neurol. 1992;38(2):114-20.
31. Zee CS, Segal H, Apuzzo M, et al. MR imaging of pineal region neoplasms. J Comput Tomogr. 1993;15:56-63.
32. Lee DH, Norman D, Newton TH, et al. MR imaging of pineal cysts. J Comput Assist Tomogr. 1987;11(4):586-90.
33. Tomita T, Melone DG, Flannery AM. Choroid plexus papillomas of neonates, infants and children. Pediatr Neurosci. 1988;14:23-30.
34. Hope JKA, Armstrong DA, Babyn PS, et al. Primary meningeal tumors in children-correlation of clinical and CT findings with histologic type and prognosis. Am J Neuroradiol. 1992;13:1353-64.
35. Price HI, Batnitzky S, Danzinger A, et al. The neuroradiology of retinoblastoma. Radiographics. 1982;2(2):7-23.
36. Bilaniuk LT, Zimmerman RA, Newton TH. Magnetic resonance imaging - orbital pathology. In Newton TH, Bilaniuk LT (Eds): Radiology of the Eye and Orbit. Clavadel. 1990;531-84.
37. Lloyd GAS, Phelps PD. Juvenile angiofibroma imaging by MR, CT and conventional techniques. Clin Otolaryngeol. 1986;11:247-59.
38. LL Muldoon, PG Tratnyek, PM Jacobs, et al. Imaging and Nanomedicine for diagnosis and therapy in the central nervous system. Am J Neurorad. 2006;27:715-21.
39. Daniel J Brat, Bernd W Scheithauer, Gregory N Fuller, Tarik Tihan. Brain Pathology Vol 17, issue 3, July 2007; 319-24.

CHAPTER 155

Metabolic Disorders of the Brain

Sapna Singh, Veena Chowdhury

INTRODUCTION

Myelination begins during the fifth fetal month with the myelination of the cranial nerves and proceeds rapidly following the order of phylogenetic development—occurring first in the peripheral nerves then the spinal cord and lastly in the brain.[1] Myelin is composed of a bilayer of lipids (cholesterol and glycolipids) and large proteins. Although white matter diseases affect the myelin, there are now many studies which reveal that myelin is not the only brain tissue damaged in "demyelinating disease" as the oligodendrocyte is the cell responsible for wrapping the axon concentrically to form the myelin sheath.[2] With the addition of the magnetic resonance imaging (MRI) to the diagnostic armamentarium, it is possible to closely follow maturation and myelination of the neonatal and infant brain with a better understanding of the nature of diseases and a more precise histopathologic analysis. Cholesterol (fat) has a short T1 and protein also decreases the T1 value of water. The result is a shortening of T1 and an increased intensity (increased brightness) on a T1 weighted (T1W) MR image. Myelin lipids are hydrophobic; hence, when myelination occurs there is loss of brain water. This results in a decrease in T2 value in white matter and as a result a decreased intensity or darker appearance on T2 weighted (T2W) images. Thus, myelination will be seen as an area of increased intensity (brighter) on T1W images and decreased intensity (darker) on T2W images.[3]

Normal Myelination of the Brain

At birth, as seen on T1W images, myelination is present in the medulla, dorsal midbrain, cerebellar peduncles, posterior limb of internal capsule and ventrolateral thalamus[4] **(Figs. 1A to D)**. Maturation proceeds from the following:

- Central to peripheral
- Inferior to superior
- Posterior to anterior

The cerebellum is myelinated at 3 months of age with an adult appearance on T2W images.[5]

The pre- and postcentral gyri are myelinated at 1 month and maturation of motor tracts is complete by 3 months.

The pons matures from 3months to 6 months with maturation proceeding rostrally along the corticospinal tracts, cerebral peduncles through the posterior limb of internal capsule and central portion of the centrum semiovale.[6]

The optic nerves, tracts and radiations into the occipital white matter are myelinated by 3 months[7] and the anterior limb of internal capsule by 2–3 months. The subcortical white matter maturation starts at 3 months in the occipital region and proceeds rostrally to the frontal lobe.

Myelination in the corpus callosum can be a helpful landmark when estimating myelin development. Myelination begins in the splenium posteriorly at 4 months and is complete involving the genu anteriorly at 6 months.

MR Imaging at 1.5 T (Tables 1A and B)

Brain maturation occurs in an orderly manner commencing in the brainstem and progressing to the cerebellum and cerebrum. The changes appear at different times with T1 and T2W MR images possibly because of T1 shortening by the

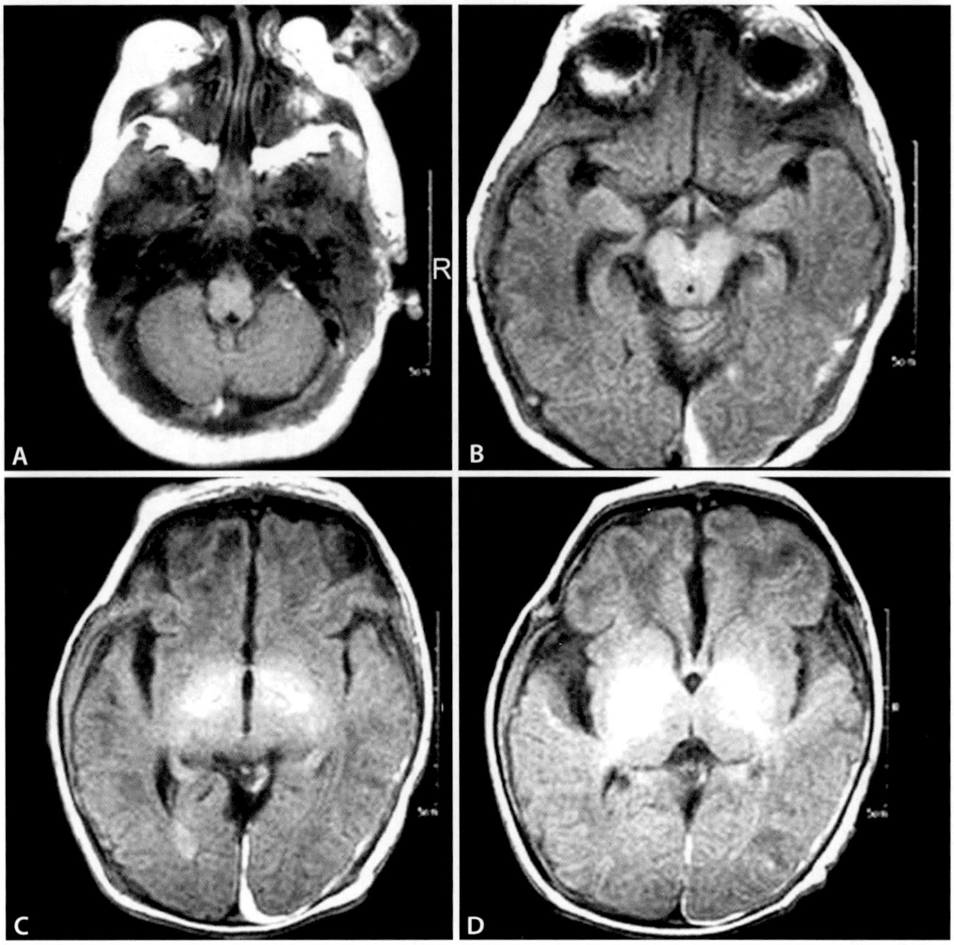

Figs. 1A to D: Axial T1W MR images in a newborn depicting normal myelination as an area of increased signal intensity (bright) in medulla (A), dorsal midbrain (B), ventrolateral thalamus (C) and in posterior limb of internal capsule (D).

Table 1A: Milestones: Normal myelination (1–6 months) (T1W images at 1.5 T).

Cerebellar white matter	3 months
Splenium	4 months
Genu	6 months
Adult	9 months

Table 1B: Milestones: Normal myelination (T2W images at 1.5 T).

Splenium	6 months
Genu	8 months
Anterior limb internal capsule	11 months
Frontal white matter	14 months
Adult pattern	18 months

components of the developing myelin sheaths. The difference in the maturation rate makes the T1W images more useful in the first 6–8 months and the T2W images thereafter.[8]

Thus, the early primary process of myelination from about 1–6 months is best evaluated using strongly T1W images (short TR/short TE). The T1W image will appear adult like at about 9 months. T2W images are better at depicting the associated changes of water loss that occur with myelination and may be helpful after 6 months of age.

On T1W images the sequential progression of myelination is seen and myelination is identified approximately 2 months earlier than on T2W images.[5,8]

Inversion recovery sequences also give excellent depiction of myelin deposition **(Figs. 2 and 3)** and may be extremely helpful in selected cases, the additional time needed to obtain them makes them less practical than SE sequences in the evaluation of young children.[5]

Graywhite Matter Differentiation

T2W spin echo pulse sequences can distinguish gray and white matter in infants and demonstrate early progression of myelination.

Although developmentally normal children show a spectrum of relative intensities of gray and white matter, their

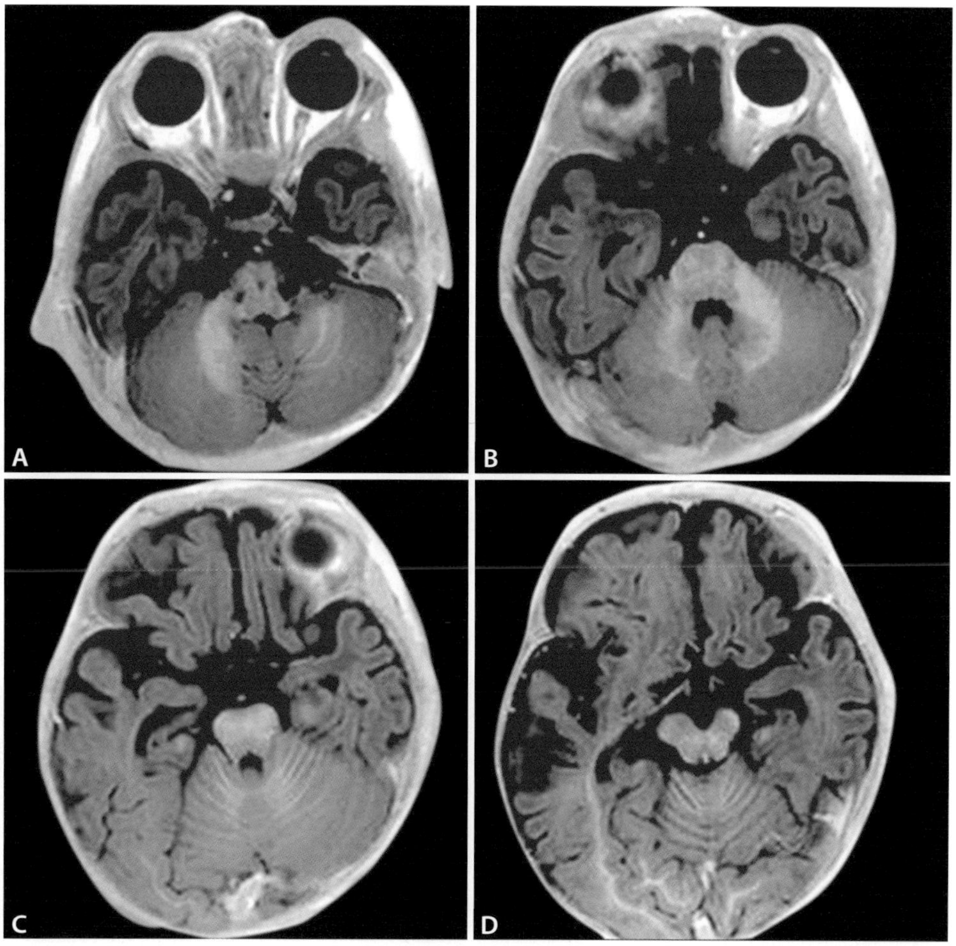

Figs. 2A to D: Inversion recovery images in a 9-month-old infant showing normal myelin deposition in medulla and inferior cerebellar peduncles (A), pons and middle cerebellar peduncles (B), cerebellum (C) and in midbrain (D).

graywhite matter patterns fall into three distinct groups: infantile, isointense and early adult.[7] At birth and first 6–8 months the "infantile" pattern shows reversal of the normal adult pattern seen on T2W images, i.e in neonates the white matter is hyperintense to gray matter. Children of the ages 8–12 months demonstrate the transient "isointense" phase with poor differentiation of gray and white matter. The early "adult" pattern where gray matter has higher intensity than white matter is seen in all children over 12 months and may be seen as early as 10 months of age.

METABOLIC DISORDERS

Metabolic disorders are classically divided into inborn errors of metabolism and acquired metabolic diseases. Acquired metabolic diseases usually occur in specific or suggestive clinical settings, such as kernicterus in neonatal hyperbilirubinemia, hypovitaminoses in malnutrition or neontatal hypoglycemia in premature infants. Toxic encephalopathies are special, exogenous forms of acquired metabolic diseases.

Inborn errors of metabolism represent a vast and complex group of pathologies. The cause is generally a mutation resulting in a biochemical alteration involving one or more metabolic pathways. The diagnosis of these disorders is often a challenge for all concerned with the care of the affected child. The presenting symptoms are usually nonspecific such as seizures, spasticity, ataxia, movement disorder or delay in achieving the developmental milestones. Biochemical tests and genetic analyses are often negative. As a result, at least 60% of children with the inborn errors of metabolism never receive a specific diagnosis despite extensive investigations.[8] Some methods of organizing the metabolic diseases from an imaging perspective are helpful to both the radiologist and the clinician as narrowing the differential diagnosis facilitates the clinical work-up. Many classifications exist, all of them with the aim of facilitating the systematic approach to these diseases.

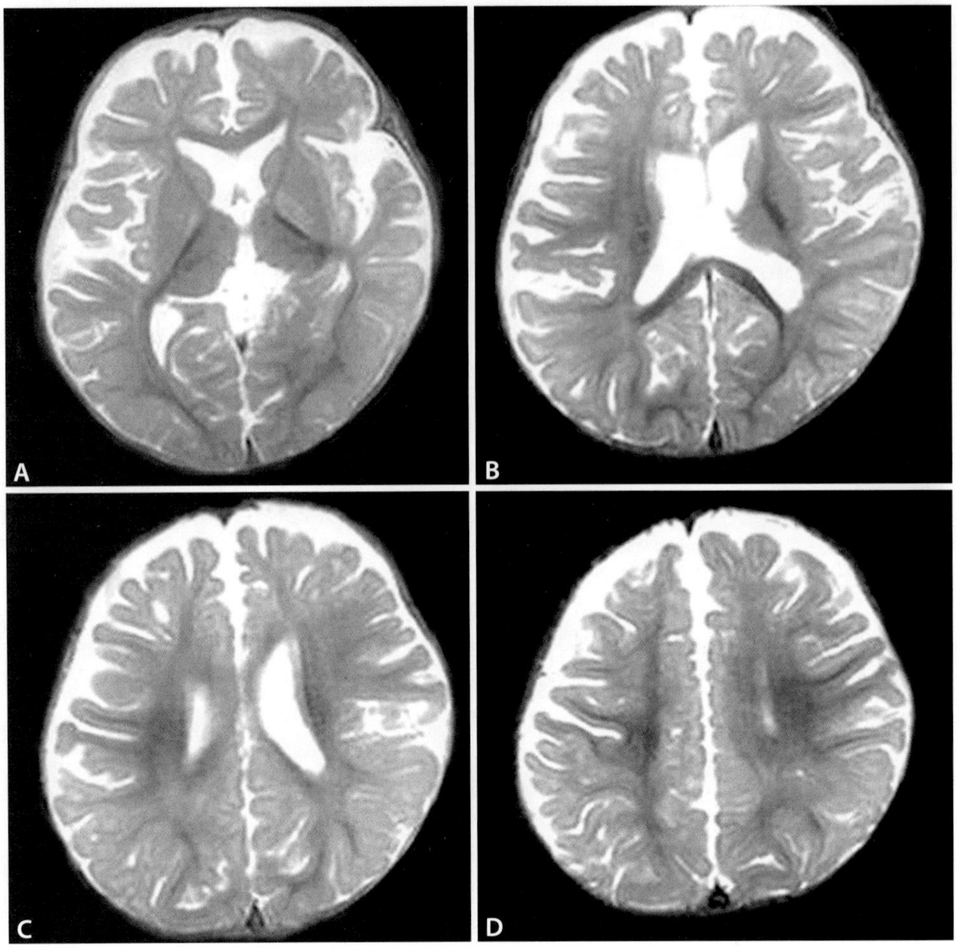

Figs. 3A to D: Inversion recovery images in a 9-month-old infant showing normal myelin deposition in posterior and anterior limbs of internal capsule, genu of corpus callosum and optic radiation (A), splenium of corpus (B) and peripheral white matter (occipital and parietal) (C and D).

Classification According to Cellular Organelle Dysfunction

The cellular organelles have distinctly different functions in the metabolism: the mitochondria are involved mainly in energy metabolism, lysosomes in the degradation of macromolecules (lipids, lipoproteins, mucopolysaccharides) and peroxisomes in both anabolic and catabolic functions.

Classification of Metabolic Disorders on the Basis of Organelle Disorder[9,10]

Lysosomal Storage Diseases with White Matter Involvement

- Metachromatic leukodystrophy
- Krabbe disease
- Niemann–Pick disease
- Fabry disease
- GM1 gangliosidosis
- GM2 gangliosidosis
- Mucopolysaccharidosis
- Fucosidosis
- Wolman disease and cholesterol ester storage disease Ceroid lipofuscinosis

Peroxisomal Disorders

- Zellweger syndrome
- X-linked adrenoleukodystrophy (ALD)
- Neonatal ALD
- Pseudoneonatal ALD
- Classic Refsum disease
- Hyperpipecolic acidemia
- Cerebrotendinous xanthomatosis
- Abetalipoproteinemia
- Rhizomatic chondrodysplasia calcificans punctata.

Mitochondrial Dysfunction with Leukoencephalopathy

- Leigh disease
- MELAS syndrome
- MERRF syndrome
- Kearns-Sayre syndrome

Disorders of Amino Acid and Organic Acid Metabolism

Canavan disease

White Matter Disorders with Unknown Metabolic Defect

- Pelizaeus-Merzbacher disease (PMD)
- Alexander disease
- Congenital muscular dystrophy (Fukuyama type).

Classification of Metabolic Disorders According to Brain Substance Involvement

The classification takes into account the dominance of substance involvement, i.e. gray matter, white matter or both within the brain. This is usually best shown by magnetic resonance imaging (MRI).

Leukodystrophies

Dysmyelinating diseases, or leukodystrophies, encompass a wide spectrum of inherited neurodegenerative disorders affecting the integrity of myelin in the brain and peripheral nerves. Diseases that present with white matter abnormalities are referred to as leukodystrophies. Leukodystrophies result from inherited enzyme deficiency that causes abnormal formation, destruction or turnover of myelin. Most of these disorders fall into one of three categories—lysosomal storage diseases, peroxisomal disorders and diseases caused by mitochondrial dysfunction. Each leukodystrophy has distinctive clinical biochemical, pathologic and radiological features **(Table 2)**.

Poliodystrophies

This group comprises diseases that present with predominantly gray matter abnormalities. Some degree of white matter involvement, however, is often present. Classical disease categories are respiratory chain disorders (so called 'mitochondrial diseases') and organic acidopathies.

Pandystrophies

The majority of the metabolic disorders fall into this category, since exclusive involvement of the gray or white matter structures is rare.

Following the classification according to the cellular organelle dysfunction, the metabolic disorders can be described as:

LYSOSOMAL STORAGE DISORDERS

Metachromatic Leukodystrophy

Metachromatic leukodystrophy (MLD) is the most common of all the familial leukodystrophies. It is an autosomal recessive disorder caused by a deficiency of the lysosomal enzyme arylsulfatase A.[11,12] This enzyme is necessary for the normal metabolism of sulfatides, which are important constituents of myelin sheath. Cerebroside sulfate (galactosyl sulfatide) abnormally accumulates within the white matter resulting in breakdown of the membrane of the myelin sheath, kidneys, gallbladder and other viscera. The accumulation of sulfatides within glial cells and neurons causes the characteristic metachromatic reaction. The name metachromatic is derived from the neuropathologic description of metachromatic staining

Table 2: Distinctive features of various leukodystrophies.

Disease	*Age of onset*	*Head size*	*White matter changes*	*Gray matter changes*	*Subcortical involvement*
Alexander disease	Less than a year	Large	Usually in frontal region	May show minimal changes	Early
Canavan disease	1–2 years	Large	Diffuse involvement	Cystic changes in gray matter	Early
Metachromatic leukodystrophy	1–2 years, 4–7 years (2nd peak)	Normal	Predominantly deep periventricular white matter	Often normal	Late
Adrenoleukodystrophy	5–10 years	Normal	Primarily occipital and splenium of corpus callosum	Normal	Late
PMD	Late infancy	Normal	Tigroid pattern	Normal	Early

which consists of a brownish or reddish color compared with the blue color of cell nuclei when stained with cresyl violet or toluidine blue.[13]

Metachromatic leukodystrophy is diagnosed biochemically on the basis of an abnormally low level of arylsulfatase A in urine, peripheral blood leukocytes or cultured fibroblasts. Diagnosis can also be made by sural nerve biopsy. Prenatal diagnosis can be achieved by assaying the activity of the enzyme in cultured amniotic fluid cells.

Clinical Features

According to the patient age three patterns of MLD are recognized—the late infantile, juvenile and adult forms.[14] The most common type is the late infantile variety, which usually manifests in children between 12 and 18 months of age and is characterized by motor signs of peripheral neuropathy followed by deterioration in intellect, speech and coordination. The disease progresses quickly and within 2 years of onset, gait disturbance, quadriplegia, blindness and decerebrate posturing may be seen. Disease progression is continuous and death occurs 6 months to 4 years after the onset of symptoms.[15] In the less common juvenile form, symptoms usually do not develop until 4 years of age. The clinical picture is similar to the late infantile form except that the child is old enough to manifest behavioral disturbances as well. There is impaired school performance and emotional lability. The neurological examination reveals cerebellar incoordination, pyramidal tract signs and decreased reflexes as in the lower extremities. In the uncommon adult form patients tend to present with dementia and progress to develop motor signs.

Pathologic Findings

At autopsy the surface of the brain appears atrophic, the white matter is shrunken and sclerotic and the ventricles are dilated. Changes in the peripheral nerve myelin explain the polyneuropathy noted in MLD. The hallmark of the disease is metachromatic granules (20–30 mm in diameter) presumably derivatives of cerebroside sulfate.[16]

Imaging Features

The typical CT appearance of MLD is a symmetrical lucency of the white matter, especially prominent in the centrum semiovale and in corpus callosum.[17] There is no evidence of inflammation or contrast enhancement and the cortical gray matter is spared **(Figs. 4A and B)**.

The characteristic MR features of MLD include symmetric confluent areas of high signal within the periventricular and cerebellar white matter on T2W images.[18,19] There is sparing of the subcortical U fibers until late in the disease **(Figs. 5A to C)**. *Thus, MLD is a progressive centrifugal white matter disease.* In the late onset (juvenile and adult forms) there is predominant involvement of the frontal white matter. In the late infantile form of MLD, the most common type, a posterior (occipital) predominance of signal abnormality has been reported with dorsofrontal progression of disease. Involvement of the corticospinal tracts may also be seen in the late infantile form of MLD. High signal intensity is seen on the long TR images along the path of corticospinal tracts in the posterior limbs of the internal capsules and brainstem. The corpus callosum is invariably affected and hypointensity may be seen within the thalami on T2W images. The so called tigroid pattern of demyelination with alternating areas of normal white

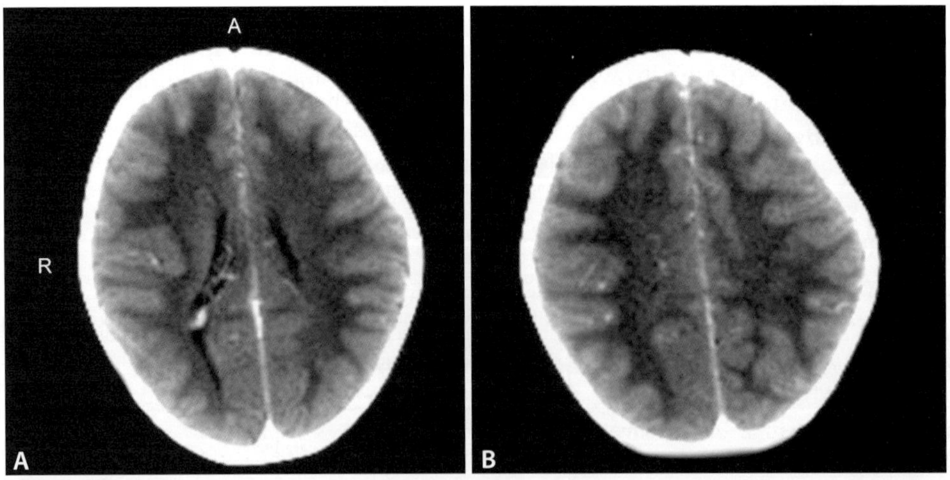

Figs. 4A and B: CT image in a 2-year-old child showing diffuse white matter hypodensity in periventricular location with relative sparing of the subcortical white matter—Metachromatic leukodystrophy.

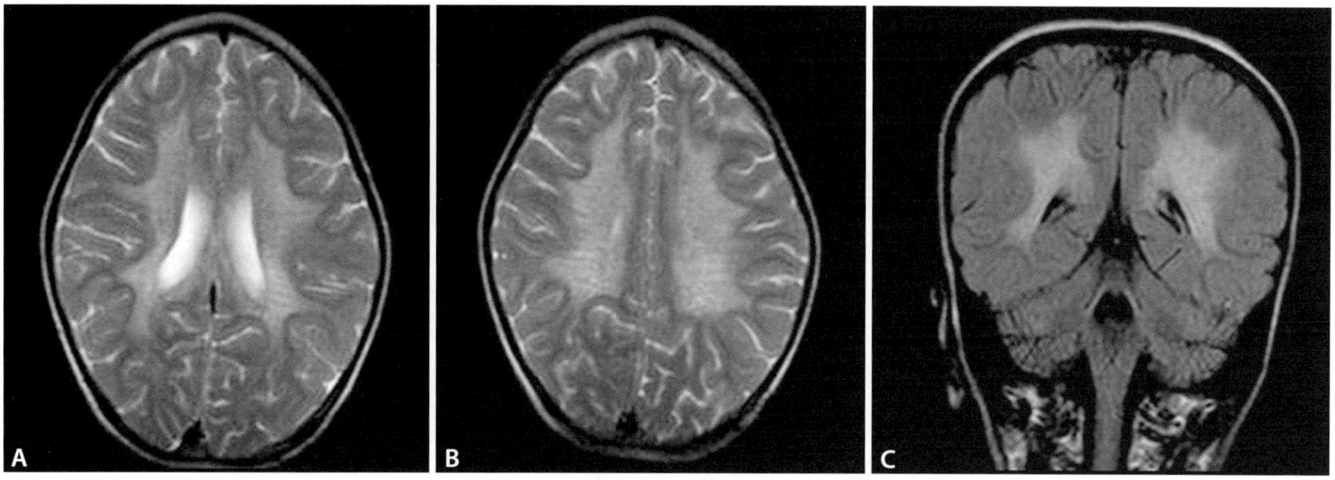

Figs. 5A to C: Axial T2W (A and B) and FLAIR coronal (C) MR images showing a symmetric pattern of high signal intensity in the deep periventricular white matter with relative sparing of the subcortical U fibers. The tigroid pattern of white matter involvement is well seen (B)—Metachromatic leukodystrophy.

matter within areas of demyelination may also be seen in the infantile form.[12,18] As the disease progresses the signal abnormality becomes more extensive and confluent with associated atrophy The corpus callosum (first the splenium then the anterior portions), the internal capsule and the deep hemispheric white matter are always involved **(Figs. 6A to D)**. In later stages, considerable atrophic dilatation of the lateral ventricles is seen. Atrophy may be the only finding in late adult onset cases **(Figs. 7A to C)**.

Diffusion-weighted images usually show signal abnormalities. Moderate hypersignal is seen in the presumed progression zone of the demyelinating process. In the late stages, diffuse hyposignal is seen. The tigroid pattern is also sometimes conspicuous on the diffusion weighted images.[20,21] Proton MR spectroscopy frequently demonstrates abnormality in the metabolic peaks before conventional MR imaging. The spectrum includes decrease NAA, abnormal elevation of choline, myoinositol and lactate peak **(Figs. 8A and B)**. The elevation of myoinositol is highly suggestive of MLD.[22]

Krabbe Disease/Globoid Cell Leukodystrophy (GLD)

Krabbe disease is an autosomal recessive disorder caused by a deficiency of lysosomal enzyme beta galactocerebrosidase, an enzyme that degrades cerebroside, a normal constituent of myelin. As soon as myelination commences and myelin turnover becomes necessary, cerebrosides accumulate in the lysosomes of macrophages within the white matter forming the globoid cells characteristic of the disease.[23] The abnormal accumulation of galactocerebroside and its derivative psychosine to toxic levels kills oligodendroglial cells. The genetic basis for the enzyme defect in Krabbe disease has been traced to a faulty gene on chromosome.[24] The diagnosis is made by demonstrating a deficiency of the enzyme in peripheral blood leukocytes.

Clinical Features

The clinical presentation of the disease varies with the age of onset.[25] In the early onset form, presentation is either before or at the age of 2 years while the late onset form presents after the age of 2 years. The early infantile form of the disease is the most common clinical form and has three phases. By 6 months of age the infant is irritable and hypertonic with spasticity and fever. Development fails to progress and the infant regresses neurologically. The second phase is characterized by rapid deterioration in motor function with chronic opisthotonos and myoclonic jerking accompanied by hyperpyrexia. In the third phase, the child appears decerebrate and has flaccid paralysis that culminates in death by 2 years of age.[26] The late onset forms have a variable clinical presentation with a slower progression of disease.[27,28]

In early onset GLD, CSF analysis always demonstrates an abnormally high protein level with a normal cell count. In the late onset form the protein level is not consistently high in CSF. Bone marrow transplantation has been shown to halt/reverse the neurologic manifestation of disease.[29]

Pathologic Findings

The brain is small and weighs only 600–800 g. The white matter is rubbery to firm but the cortex is relatively

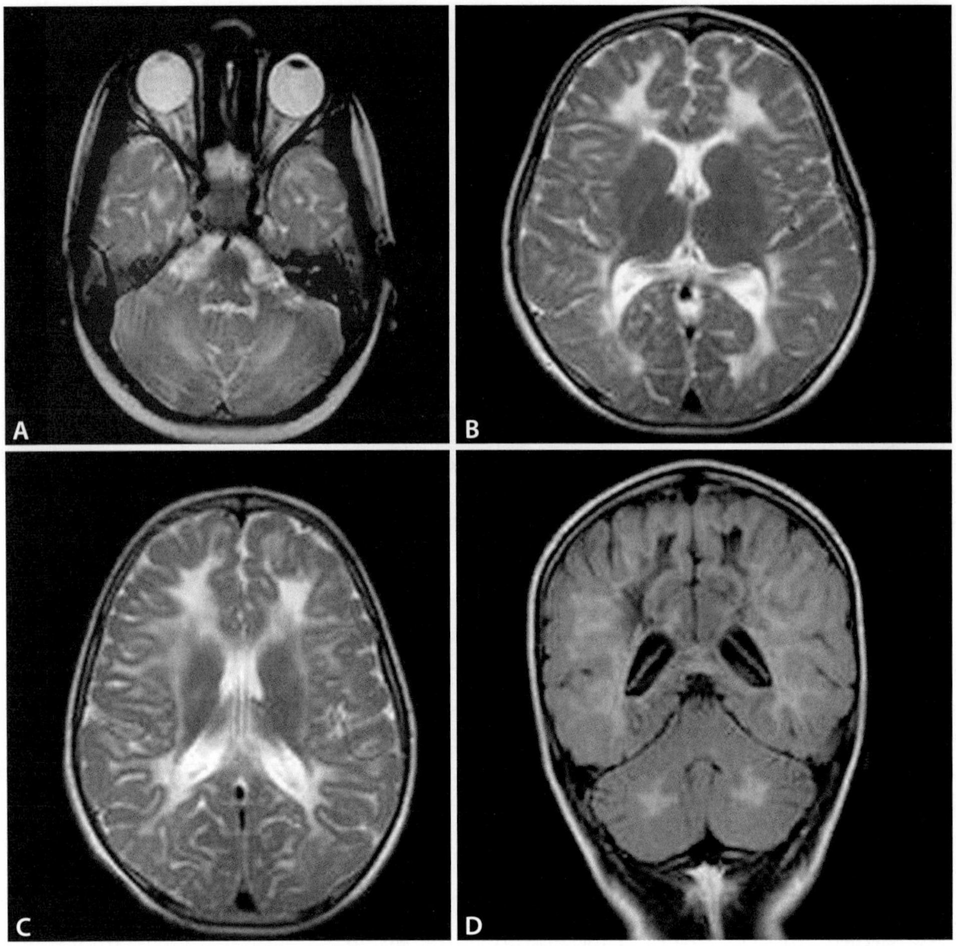

Figs. 6A to D: Axial T2W (A to C) and FLAIR coronal (D) MR images showing involvement of the deep periventricular white matter with relative sparing of the subcortical U fibers. There is involvement of the posterior limbs of internal capsule (B), the cerebellar white matter (A and D) and the splenium of the corpus callosum (D)—Metachromatic leukodystrophy.

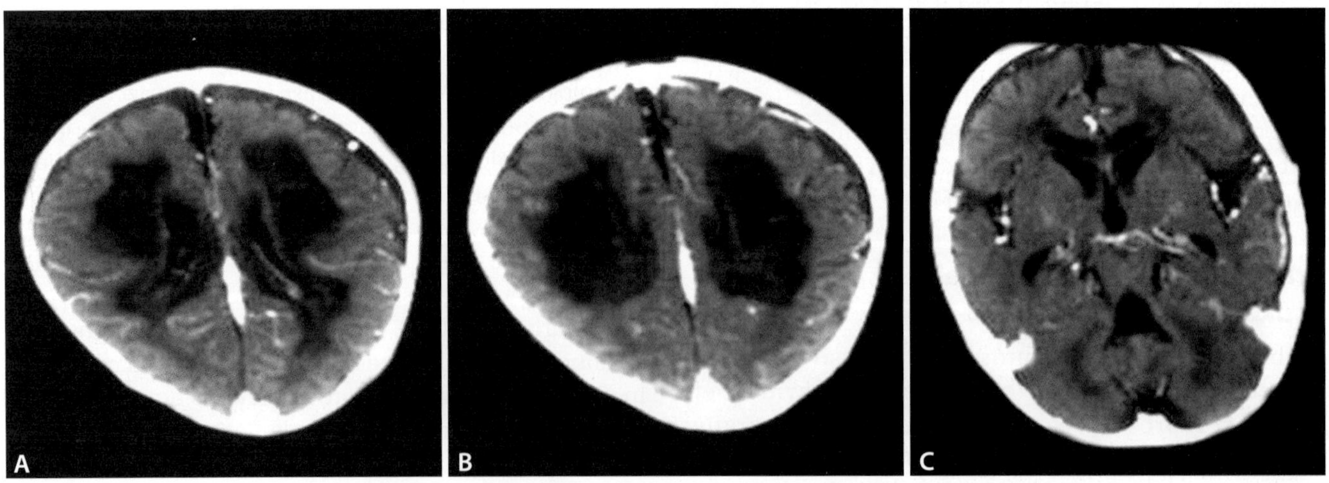

Figs. 7A to C: CT images in a 14-month-old-child showing symmetric lucency of the white matter especially prominent in the periventricular white matter, centrum semiovale with involvement of cerebellar white matter and corpus callosum. Cerebral atrophy and moderate enlargement of the ventricles is also seen—Metachromatic leukodystrophy.

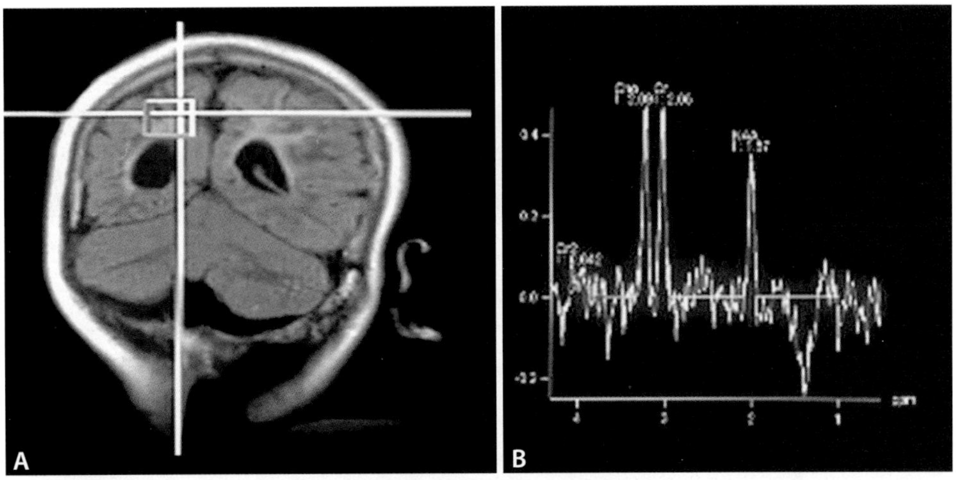

Figs. 8A and B: Coronal FLAIR images with voxel placement in the hyperintensity in frontal white matter show abnormal elevation of choline peak—An early finding in MLD.

unaffected. The pathologic hallmark of Krabbe disease is a massive accumulation of large multinucleated cells containing PAS positive material (globoid cells). There is complete myelin destruction with loss of oligodendroglia and marked astrogliosis.

Imaging Features

The CT findings in GLD range from white matter lucency to diffuse cerebral atrophy. The CT findings of hyperdense thalami, caudate nucleus and corona radiata are characteristic but not specific for the disease and have been shown to correspond to fine calcifications at autopsy. The most characteristic MR finding in both early and late onset forms of GLD is high signal intensity on T2W images found along the lengths of the corticospinal tracts. Additional findings in the early onset form include abnormal signal intensity within the cerebellar white matter[30,31] and deep gray nuclei (dentate, basal ganglia, thalamus) with progressive involvement of the parieto-occipital white matter and posterior portion of the corpus callosum[32] **(Figs. 9A to D)**.

The cerebellar white matter and deep gray nuclei are not involved in the late onset form. Classically, the subcortical U fibers are spared until late in the disease. Enhancement at the border between the white matter and arcuate fibers has been described but is not seen in most cases. The cranial nerves may be affected with evidence of thickened optic nerve seen on MR imaging and at autopsy.[33,34] Optic nerve atrophy has also been described in late onset form.[35] Late onset cases of GLD with primary involvement of the parietal periventricular white matter, splenium of the corpus callosum and corticospinal tracts may appear similar on imaging to adrenoleukodystrophy (ALD) However, auditory pathway involvement is characteristic of ALD and is not seen in GLD.[36] MR imaging of the spine shows diffuse hypersignal within the spinal cord parenchyma **(Fig. 9E)**. Nerve root enhancement may also be detected after intravenous contrast injection.[37]

Diffusion-weighted images, like MLD, may show prominent hypersignal along the presumed progression zone of the demyelinating process **(Figs. 10A to D)**. In the late stages, diffuse hyposignal is seen suggesting complete myelin loss.[38] Diffusion tensor derived anisotropy maps are useful as a quantitative evaluation of white matter abnormalities in these patients.[39] DTI scans are being studied as a potential tool for follow-up of patients before and after stem cell transplantation.[40] Perfusion MR techniques have also been used in the evaluation of white matter lesions in Krabbe disease. It shows a decreased intralesional CBV.

Sphingolipidosis

Sphingolipidoses involve abnormal metabolism and accumulation of sphingolipids. Deficiency of hexosaminidase alone results in GM2 gangliosidosis, the classic form of which is Tay-Sachs disease. Sandhoff's disease is caused by a deficiency in both hexosaminidase A and B. Clinical findings are identical to that of Tay-Sachs with additional findings of hepatosplenomegaly and bony deformities.[41]

Clinical Features

Onset of symptoms is between 3 and 6 months of age. The initial sign is an excessive startle reflex. A macular cherry red

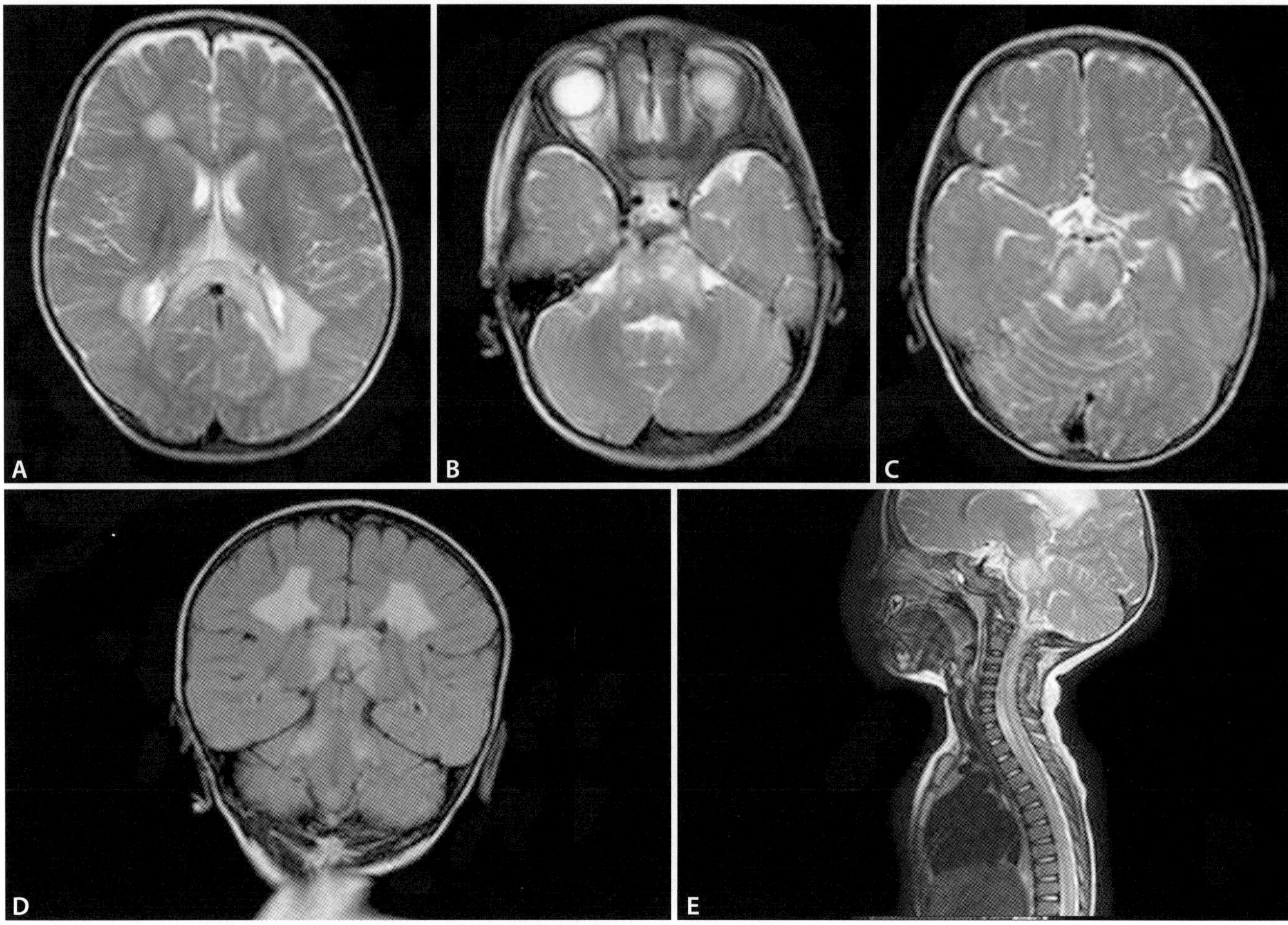

Figs. 9A to E: Axial T2W (A to C) and FLAIR coronal (D) MR images showing symmetric areas of white matter hyperintensity predominantly involving the parieto-occipital white matter with some involvement of the frontal white matter with relative sparing of the subcortical U fibers. Involvement of the splenium (A) and the corticospinal tracts (B and C) is seen. Sagittal T2W MR image of the cervicodorsal spine (E) reveals high-signal intensity within the spinal cord parenchyma—Late-onset Krabbe disease.

spot is almost always present at this stage and psychomotor regression then begins. Patients are macrocephalic and there is progressive psychomotor retardation, pyramidal and later extrapyramidal (choreoathetosis) signs and generalized tonic clonic seizures.

Imaging Features

The imaging findings in Tay-Sachs and Sandhoff disease are quite similar and the pattern is suggestive. CT examination of the brain shows hyperdensities within the basal ganglia and or thalami due to calcifications. MR imaging is sensitive in demonstrating the widespread white matter changes within the cerebral hemispheres. All the white matter structures are involved except for the corpus callosum, the anterior commissure and the posterior limbs of the internal capsules. The external and extreme capsules, the globi pallidi and the putamina are all abnormal. The involved basal ganglia structures (putamina, caudate nucleus) are somewhat swollen particularly initially during the disease course. The thalami are spared and show low signal on T2 weighted images **(Figs. 11A to C)**. The cerebellar white matter often shows signal abnormalities on the T2 weighted images, the hyperintensities are less prominent than supratentorially. Typically, no abnormalities are seen within the brainstem and spinal cord. The overall lesion pattern in a macrocephalic infant can be highly suggestive of the disease.

Diffusion-weighted images are usually quite unremarkable which suggest a slow demyelinating process. MR spectroscopy shows nonspecific alteration, the NAA peak is decreased and the choline peak is increased. No lactate is identified.

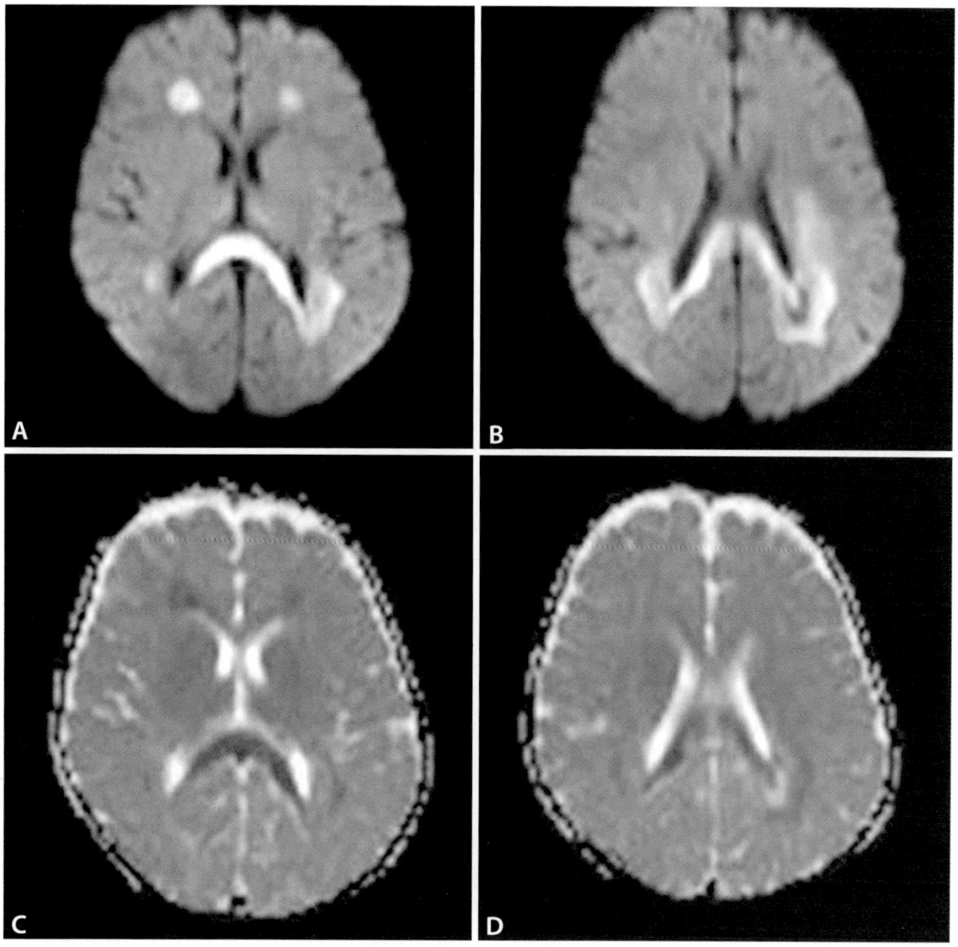

Figs. 10A to D: Diffusion-weighted MR (A and B) images in the same case showing a prominent hypersignal along the progression line of the demyelinating process reflecting the centrifugal gradient and the posteroanterior gradient of the disease process. ADC maps (C and D) reveal a hyposignal suggestive of a restricted pattern of diffusion—Krabbe disease.

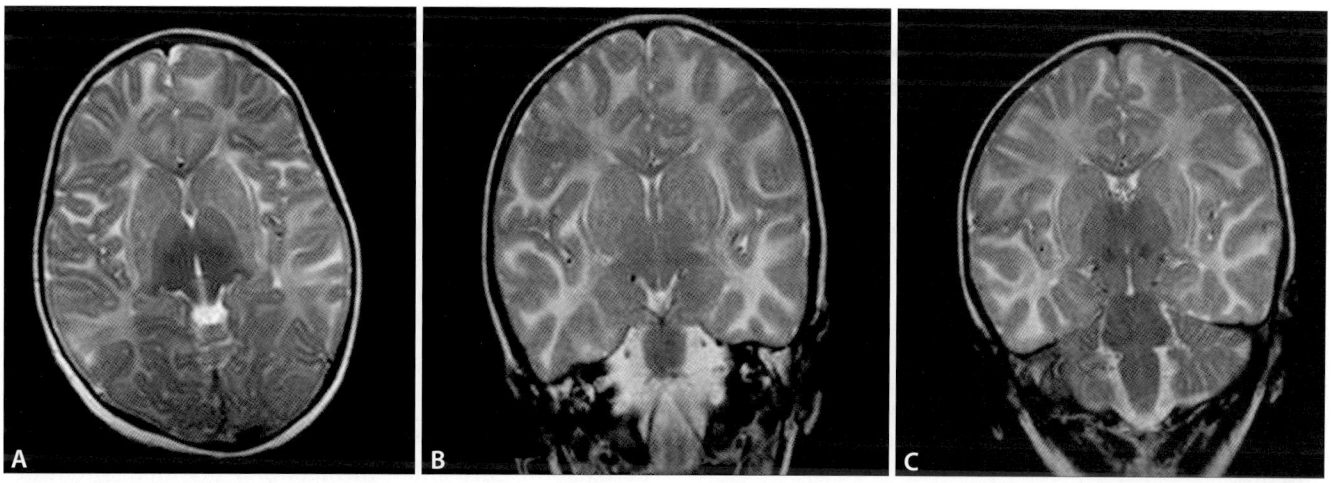

Figs. 11A to C: T2W axial (A) and FLAIR coronal (B and C) MR images showing extensive white matter changes in the supratentorial compartment with relative sparing of the infratentorial compartment. The basal ganglia (the putamina, caudate nucleus), the external and the extreme capsules are all abnormal showing a high signal (A and B). The claustra are well-delineated due to the involvement of the external and extreme capsules (A). The thalami are spared and show low signal on the T2W images—Tay-Sachs disease.

Fabry Disease

This is a X-linked recessive disorder due to deficiency of the lysosomal enzyme-galactosidase A, which results in accumulation of glycosphingolipids in the vascular endothelium, smooth muscles and neurons.

Clinical Features

It typically presents late in childhood but occasionally is not recognized until third or fourth decade of life.[16] Early manifestations include a punctate telangiectatic skin and mucous membrane lesion followed by fever, weight loss and pain in extremities and abdomen. Retinal, corneal and conjunctival abnormalities are present early in the disease. Cardiac disease develops with age and is typically worsened by a systemic hypertension secondary to vascular disease. Patients may eventually present with transient ischemic attacks or strokes secondary to small vessel ischemia and focal infarcts.

Pathologic Findings

Glycosphingolipids accumulate in the vascular endothelium particularly in the small vessels throughout the brain and spinal cord. Storage of lipids is seen within neurons of amygdala, hypothalamus and the brainstem. Focal infarcts are frequently found in the basal ganglia and central white matter.

Imaging Features

Early in the disease small areas of high signal intensity are seen on long TR sequences, most commonly in the basal ganglia and periventricular white matter.[42] The periventricular disease becomes more extensive and confluent with time and associated generalized loss of cerebral volume. Cerebral hemorrhage has also been reported.

Gaucher's Disease

Gaucher's disease includes several autosomal recessive *lipid storage diseases* in which there is a deficiency of the lysosomal enzyme glucocerebroside.

Clinical Features

Neurologic symptoms include seizures, developmental regression, spasticity, mental deficiency, incoordination and tics.

Imaging

CT and MR findings are similar to those of Fabry disease with atrophy, infarction and occasional hemorrhage.[43]

Mucopolysaccharidoses

In the mucopolysaccharidoses (MPS) impaired degradation of the various mucopolysaccharides (also known as glycosaminoglycans) cause variable combinations of coarse facies, short stature, bony defects, stiff joints, mental retardation, hepatosplenomegaly and corneal clouding. All forms of MPS are autosomal recessive except MPS type-II (Hunter syndrome) which is X-linked recessive. Imaging studies are usually performed when hydrocephalous or spinal cord compression is suspected. CT and MR usually reveals delayed myelination, atrophy, varying degrees of hydrocephalous and white matter changes.[44] In all types of MPS the white matter abnormalities are manifest as sharply defined foci in the corpus callosum and basal ganglia, isointense with CSF on all imaging sequences. These represent enlarged perivascular spaces filled with mucopolysaccharide or CSF. With progression of the disease, the lesions become larger and more diffuse and resemble a leukodystrophy, reflecting the development of infarcts and demyelination. The atrophy and white matter changes become more progressive with time. Affected patients are commonly macrocephalic from a combination of hydrocephalous and mucopolysaccharide deposition within the brain, meninges and skull.[45,46] A high incidence of intracranical arachnoid cysts has also been seen. The spines in MPS are usually imaged to determine the site and cause of cord compression which occurs frequently in MPS types IV and VI. The most common location for the cord compression is at the atlantoaxial joint. Atlantoaxial subluxation may occur in these patients as a result of laxity of the transverse ligament in conjunction with hypoplasia of the odontoid.

Magnetic resonance shows a shortened odontoid with a soft tissue mass of variable size with intermediate signal on T_1 and low signal on T2W images. The low signal on T2W images is a combination of unossified fibrocartilage and reactive changes. Another cause of cord compression at the C1–C2 level is dural thickening resulting from intradural deposition of collagen and mucopolysaccharides. This is seen as a thickening of the soft tissue proterior to the dens with consequent cord compression.

MR spectroscopy shows a decreased NAA/choline ratio and elevated glutamate glutamine and myoinositol.

PEROXISOMAL DISORDERS

Peroxisomes are small intracellular organelles that are involved in the oxidation of very long chain and mono-unsaturated fatty acids. Peroxisomal enzymes are also involved in gluconeogenesis, lysine metabolism and glutaric acid metabolism.

Neuropathologic lesions in the peroxisomal disorders can be divided into three major classes. The first group is characterized by defects in the formation and maintenance of white matter and X-linked adrenoleukodystrophy is the prototype. The second group is associated with migrational disorders and Zellweger syndrome is the classic example. The third group is associated with post developmental neuronal degenerations such as cerebellar atrophy seen in rhizomelic chondrodysplasia punctata.

X-linked Adrenoleukodystrophy

X-linked adrenoleukodystrophy (ALD) is a peroxisomal disorder that affects the white matter of the central nervous system, adrenal cortex and testes.[47] This is the best known and most frequent of the peroxisomal disorders. It is a true leukodystrophy with no involvement of the gray matter structures.

The genetic defect responsible for X-linked ALD is located in Xq28, the terminal segment of the long arm of the X chromosome. X-linked ALD is caused by a deficiency of a single enzyme, acyl CoA synthetase. The deficiency prevents the breakdown of very long chain fatty acids which then accumulate in tissue and plasma.[48] A rare form of ALD, neonatal ALD is an autosomal recessive disorder characterized by multiple enzyme deficiencies. Adrenomyeloneuropathy probably represents a phenotypic adult variant of adrenoleukodystrophy and is characterized by adrenal insufficiency.[49] Typically, the disease has slow progression, with survival into the eighth decade.

Clinical Features

The clinical features of X linked ALD include the onset of neurologic symptoms between the ages of 5 and 9 years with behavior problems, decreasing mental function, poor school performance, visual and hearing disorders progressing to motor signs and ataxia. The disease progresses to include seizures, spastic quadriplegia with death ensuing within the first few years of onset.[50]

Pathologic Findings

The histologic findings reflect the zones of activity seen on imaging studies. Three zones of demyelination are characteristically seen.[51] The central portion of the lesion reveals absent myelin sheaths and oligodendroglia with glial stranding and scattered astrocytes with no evidence of active disease. The next zone of involvement shows evidence of active inflammation with many macrophages filled with lipid. The outer zone is characterized by active myelin breakdown but no inflammatory changes.

Imaging Features

The CT and MR appearance of ALD is somewhat specific with symmetric areas of white matter abnormality in the peritrigonal regions and extending across the splenium of the corpus callosum[52,53] **(Figs. 12A and B)**. Demyelination then spreads outward and cephalad as a confluent lesion until most of the cerebral white matter is affected.[54] The subcortical white matter is relatively spared in the early stage but often becomes involved in the later stages. The progression pattern is thus centrifugal and posteroanterior **(Figs. 13A to C)**.

The central or inner zone which corresponds to irreversible gliosis and scarring is moderately hypointense on T1W MR imaging and markedly hyperintense at T2W imaging. The intermediate zone corresponding to active inflammation is isointense or slightly hypointense

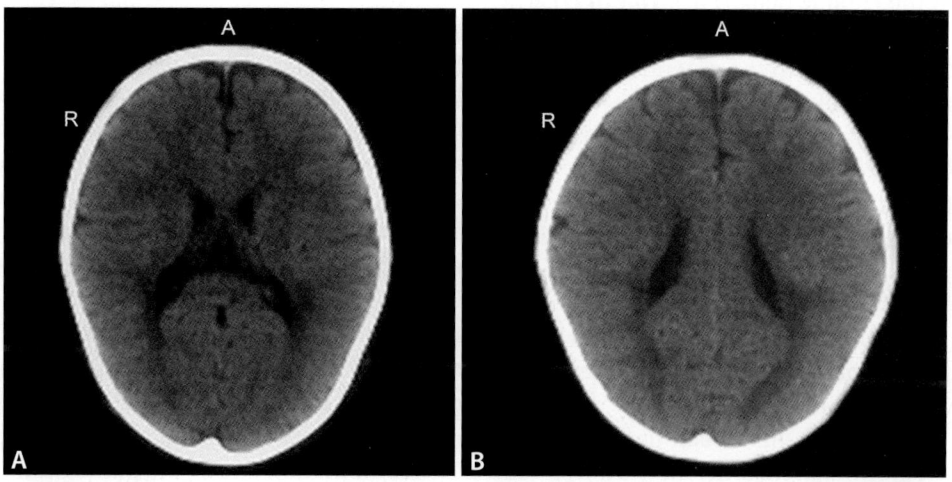

Figs. 12A and B: CT images in a child showing white matter hypodensity in the parieto-occipital and the peritrigonal areas—X-linked adrenoleukodystrophy.

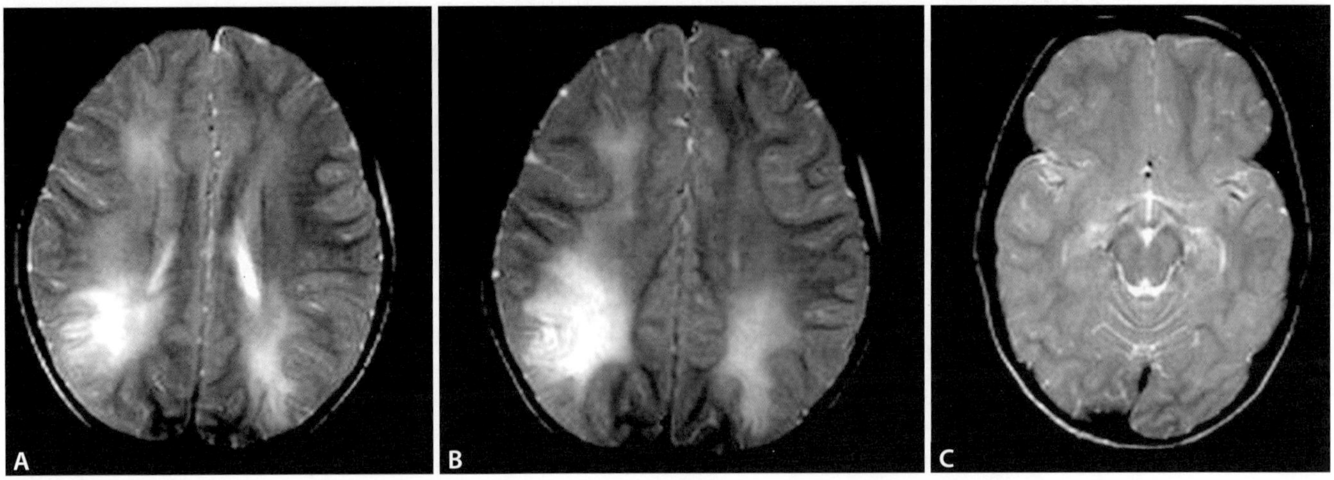

Figs. 13A to C: Axial T2W (A to C) MR images are showing extensive high signal abnormality in the peritrigonal regions in a bilateral symmetric pattern. Involvement of the corticospinal tracts is also seen (C)—X-linked adrenoleukodystrophy.

and rapidly enhances after administration of contrast **(Figs. 14A and B)**. The peripheral or outer zone representing the leading edge of active demyelination appears moderately hyperintense on T2W MR imaging and demonstrates no contrast enhancement.[55,56] Pontomedullary corticospinal tract involvement is a common finding in adrenoleukodystrophy and is uncommon in other leukodystrophies.[57] Atypical case of ALD with unilateral or predominantly frontal lobe involvement may occur.[58]

Diffusion-weighted MR images also reveal the three distinct zones in the cerebral hemispheric white matter lesions. The burned out zone is hypointense, the intermediate inflammatory zone is moderately hyperintense and the most peripheral demyelinating zone is very faintly hyperintense **(Figs. 15A to E)**. Proton MR spectroscopy typically shows a decrease in NAA peak and an increase in the choline peak **(Figs. 16A to D)**. The spectra may be abnormal before the conventional MR findings and studies have shown the potential of MRS for the prognostic assessment of ALD.[59-61]

Adrenomyeloneuropathy

Adrenomyeloneuropathy is not an independent disease entity, it is actually one of the clinical phenotypes of X-linked adrenoleukodystrophy. The age of onset is usually between 20 and 30 years but since both the clinical and the imaging findings are quite different from those in X-linked ALD, it is treated as a separate disease entity. Ataxia and paraparesis as well as peripheral neuropathy dominate the neurological presentation, mild cognitive disorder is often present as well. Adrenal insufficiency is a frequent associated clinical finding.

On MR imaging, the lesions are predominantly found within the cerebellum and the brainstem. Both structures are atrophic. The brainstem signal abnormalities are significant but the tegmental structures are relatively spared. The cerebellar white matter is diffusely abnormal. Involvement of the supratentorial white matter is limited mainly to the posterior limbs of the internal capsules and the splenium of the corpus callosum as well as the hemispheric white matter occasionally. Enhancement may also occur within the lesions after intravenous contrast injection. MR of the brain in adrenomyeloneuropathy may even be normal with neurologic involvement confined to the spinal cord and peripheral nerves.[62]

Zellweger Syndrome

Zellweger syndrome or cerebrohepatorenal syndrome, is an autosomal recessive disorder caused by multiple enzyme defects and characterized by liver dysfunction with jaundice, marked mental retardation, weakness, hypotonia and craniofacial dysmorphism.[63] It may lead to death in early childhood. The severity of the disease varies and is determined by the degree of peroxisomal activity.

MR imaging reveals diffuse demyelination with abnormal gyration that is most severe in the perisylvian and perirolandic regions. The pattern of gyral abnormality is similar to that seen in polymicrogyria or pachygyria.[64]

MR hallmarks of the disease are very markedly delayed myelination, brain atrophy, periventricular germinolytic cysts and bilateral symmetrical perisylvian cortical dysplasia (polymicrogyria) and gray matter heterotopias. The combination of these is pathognomonic of Zellweger syndrome.

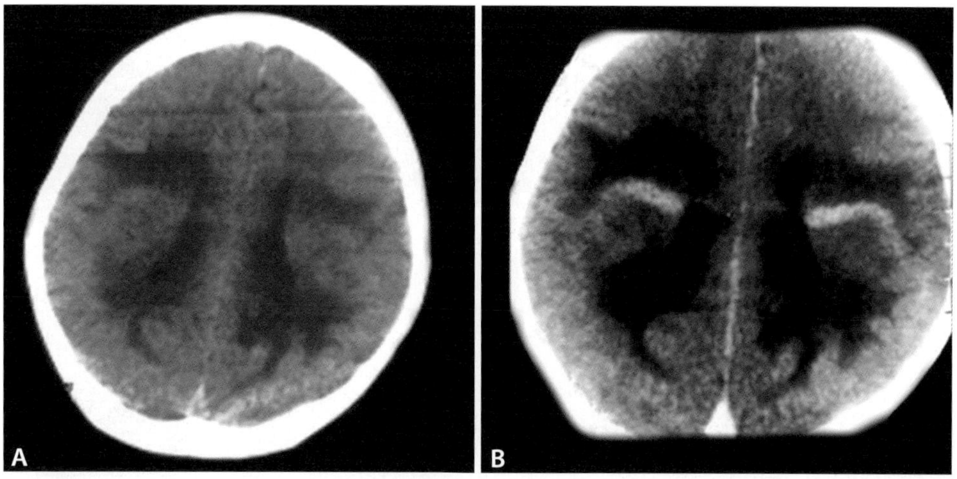

Figs. 14A and B: CT images showing symmetric areas of hypodensity in the peritrigonal regions extending across the splenium of the corpus callosum. These hypodensities are seen to extend outward and cephalad as a confluent lesion. Contrast enhancement is seen at the site of active inflammation—X-linked adrenoleukodystrophy.

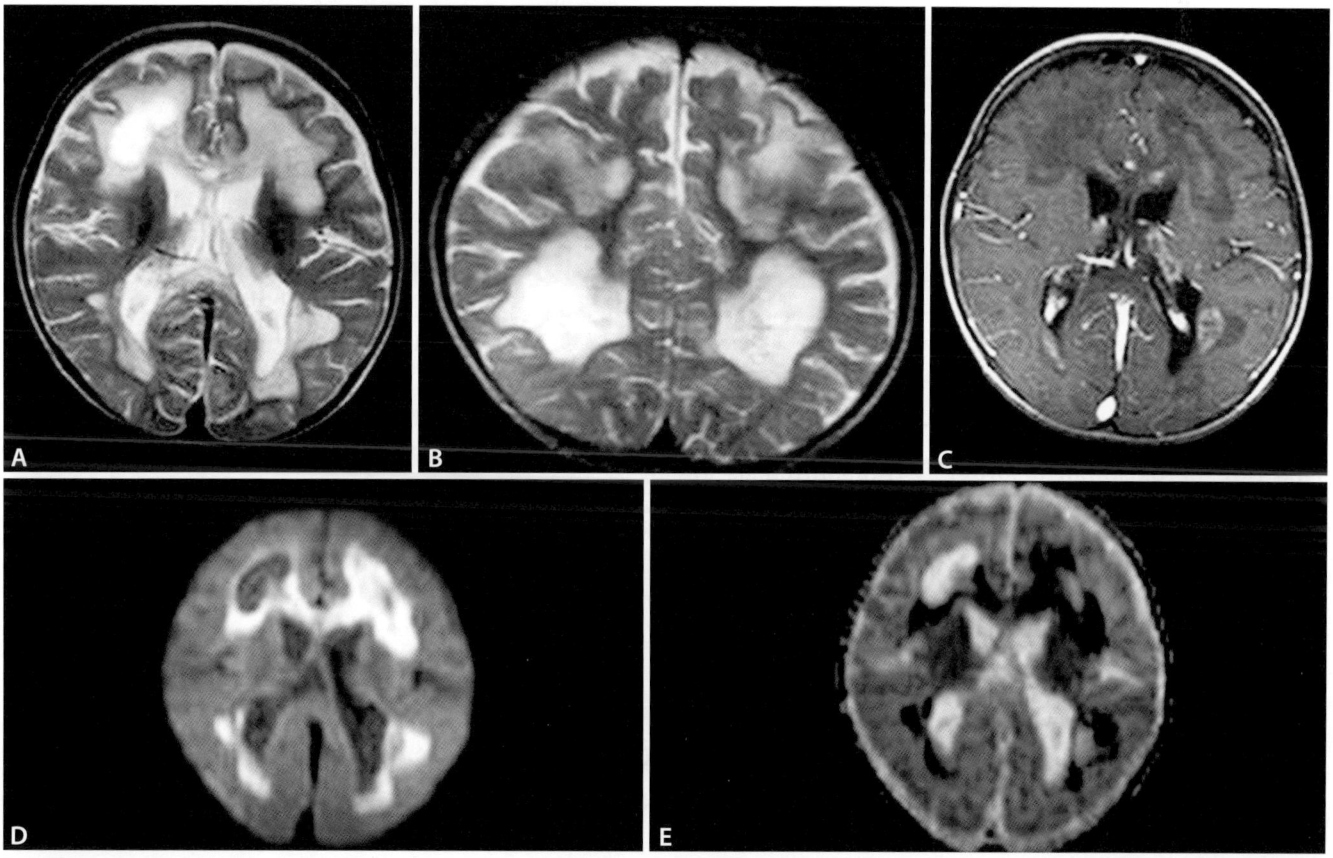

Figs. 15A to E: Axial T2W (A and B) MR images showing symmetrical parieto-occipital white matter lesions with sparing of subcortical U-fibers. The intermediate zone of inflammation shows enhancement on the postcontrast images (C). Diffusion-weighted images show isotropically restricted water diffusion within the intermediate zone (D) with faint hyposignal on the apparent diffusion coefficient image (E)—X-linked adrenoleukodystrophy.

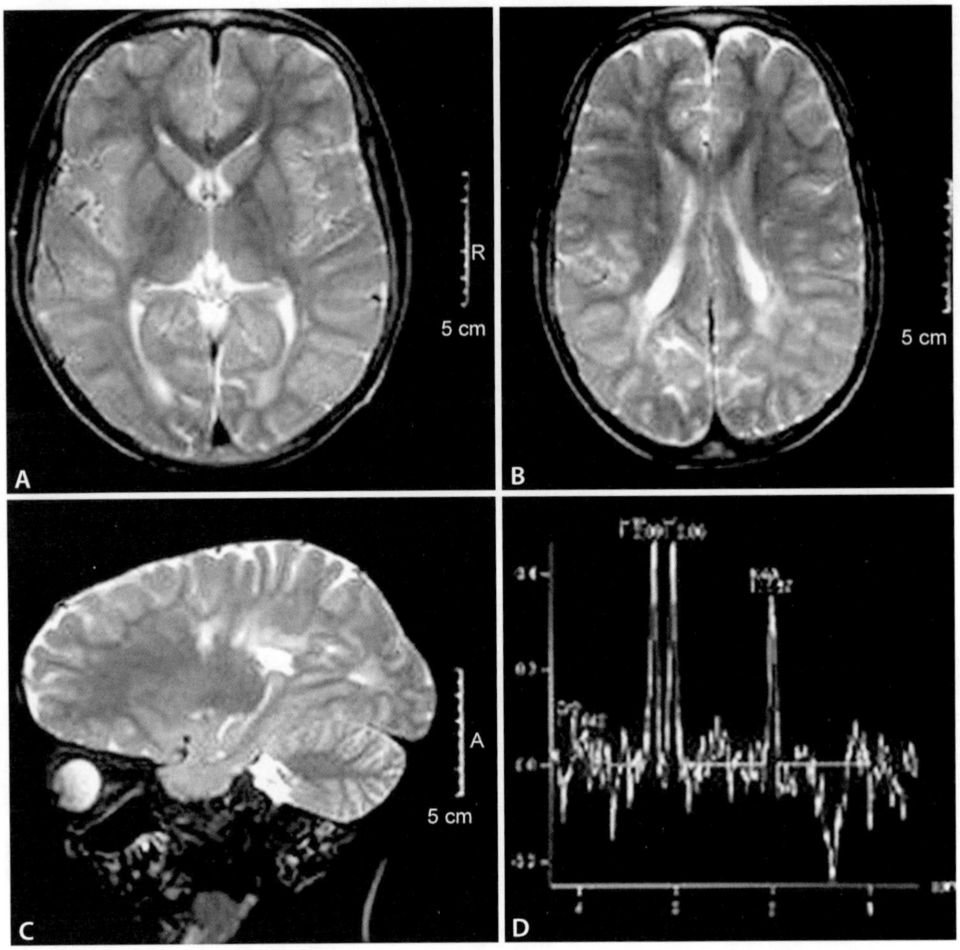

Figs.16A to D: MR spectroscopy with voxel placement in the demyelinating zone in the peritrigonal region reveals a decreased NAA and increased choline consistent with increased myelin breakdown—Adrenoleukodystrophy.

Refsum Disease

This rare peroxisomal disorder is transmitted as an autosomal recessive condition and is caused by a deficiency of phytanic acid 2 hydroxylase which causes phytanic acid to accumulate in the myelin.[16] The myelin thus affected has less viability. The infantile form is more severe. The affected children present with severe sensorineural deafness, retinitis pigmentosa, facial dysmorphism, hepatomegaly, growth retardation and mental retardation. MRI may show diffuse white matter hyperintensity in the brain and in the cerebellum on T2 weighted images. The involvement of the cerebellar white matter is more intense than in other conditions.

Cerebrotendinous Xanthomatosis

In this condition patients are deficient in a liver mitochondrial enzyme required for side chain oxidation of cholesterol to bile salts. The patients may show pyramidal and cerebellar signs and may have mental retardation and usually present xanthomas in the Achilles tendon, the knees and the elbows. CT may show decreased density in the cerebellum involving the region of dentate nuclei bilaterally. Hypointensity in the same areas is shown on MRI.[65]

Rhizomelic Chondrodysplasia Calcificans Punctata

This rare autosomal recessive disorder causes short limbs, dwarfism, abnormal facies, psychomotor retardation, congenital cataracts and joint contraction. These patients usually die within the first year of life. The radiographs show finely stippled epiphysis. T2 MRI may show periventricular white matter and subcortical changes, particularly in the occipital region.

UNCLASSIFIED LEUKODYSTROPHIES

Canavan Disease

Canavan disease (Canavan–van Bogaert–Bertrand disease) or spongy degeneration of the brain is an autosomal recessive disorder caused by deficient activity of the enzyme. N-acetylaspartylase, which results in accumulation of N-acetyl-aspartic acid in the urine, plasma and brain.[66,67] This is the only known disease with a defect in NAA metabolism.

Clinical Features

It usually manifests in early infancy as hypotonia followed by spasticity, cortical, blindness and macrocephaly.[68] Macrocephaly may not be apparent in the first few months of life but the head enlarges above the ninetieth percentile within 6 months to 1 year of age. Canavan disease is a rapidly progressive illness with a mean survival time of 3 years, although protracted cases do occur. Definite diagnosis usually requires biopsy or autopsy.

Pathologic Findings

Grossly the brain is heavy and soft with markedly increased water content. Canavan disease is characterized at pathologic analysis by extensive vacuolization that initially involves the subcortical white matter, then spreads to deep white matter. Normal myelin is absent and electron microscopy demonstrates increased water content within the glial tissue, described as having the texture of a wet sponge and dysmyelination.[69]

Imaging Features

The CT shows diffusely decreased attenuation of the cerebral and cerebellar white matter **(Figs. 17A and B)**. The disease has a centripetal progression. The MR imaging findings demonstrate diffusely decreased T1W signal and increased T2W signal within the white matter that corresponds to the CT abnormalities.[70] Typically, there is diffuse symmetric increased signal on T2W images throughout the white matter. Unlike metachromatic leukodystrophy or Krabbe disease the subcortical U fibers also are usually involved. The subcortical white matter appears swollen with broadening of the gyri. **Typically, there is diffuse, symmetric increased signal intensity on the T2-weighted images throughout the white matter with relative sparing of the internal and external capsules and corpus callosum.** The central white matter becomes involved with disease progression. High signal intensity is always seen within the globus pallidus, with frequent involvement of the thalamus and relative sparing of the putamen and caudate nucleus **(Figs. 18A to E)**. Cerebral and cerebellar atrophy is a late finding.

There is also evidence of restricted diffusion within the abnormal white matter structures (with increased signal on DWI and decreased signal on the ADC maps), likely related to myelin edema or a "gelatinous-like" state of the extracellular space.[71] **On MR spectroscopy there is a characteristic increase in NAA peak[72] (Fig. 19).**

Alexander Disease

Alexander disease or fibrinoid leukodystrophy is a rare disorder that occurs sporadically with no known pattern of inheritance.

Pathologic Findings

It is characterized at pathologic analysis by massive deposition of Rosenthal fibers seen as dense eosinophilic,

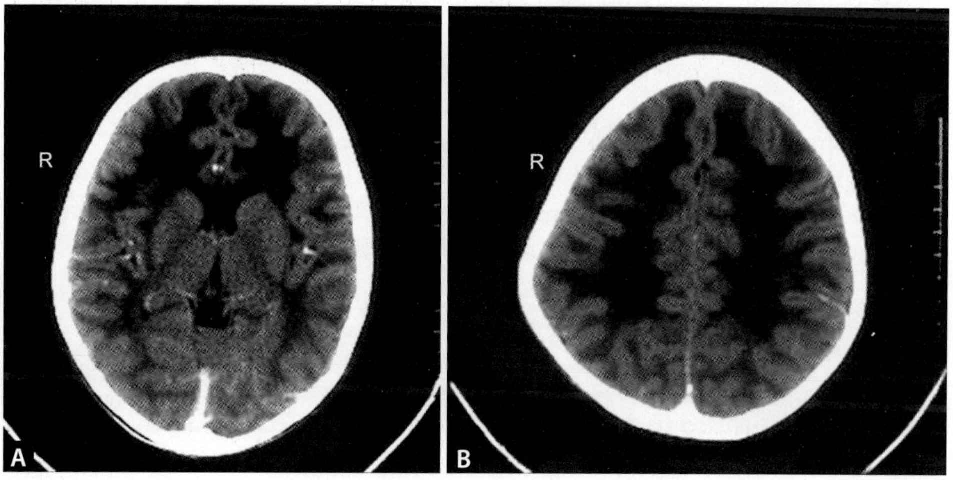

Figs. 17A and B: CT images in a child with macrocephaly showing diffuse white matter hypodensity with involvement of subcortical white matter—Canavan disease.

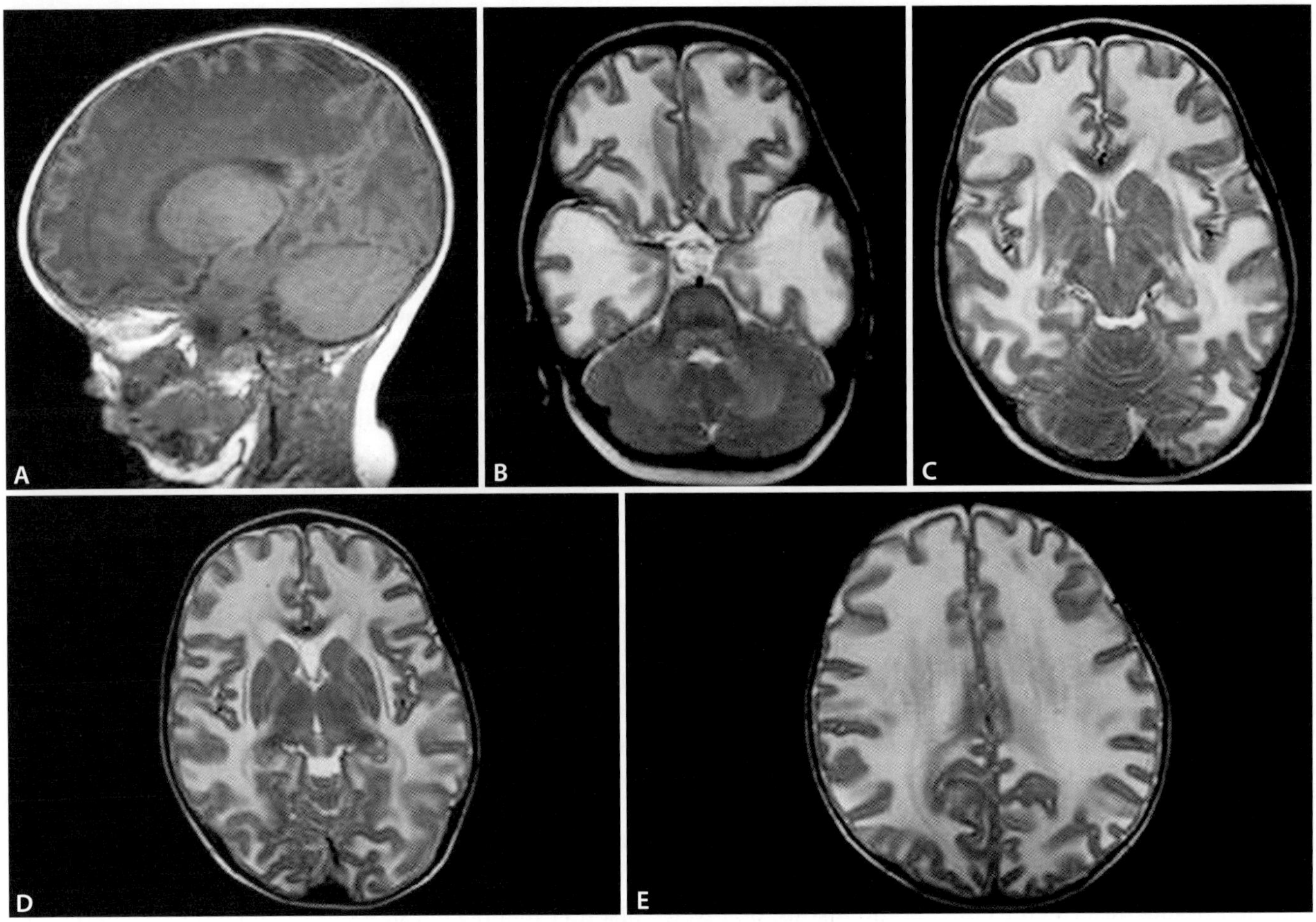

Figs. 18A to E: Sagittal T1W (A) MR image showing a widespread diffuse low signal throughout the cerebral white matter. Axial T2W (B and C) MR images reveal a high signal intensity in the white matter with extensive involvement of the subcortical U fibers.There is involvement of the cerebellar white matter and the brainstem (B and C). There is involvement of the globus pallidus with relative sparing of the corpus striatum (D).The subcortical white matter appears swollen with broadened gyri (E)—Canavan disease.

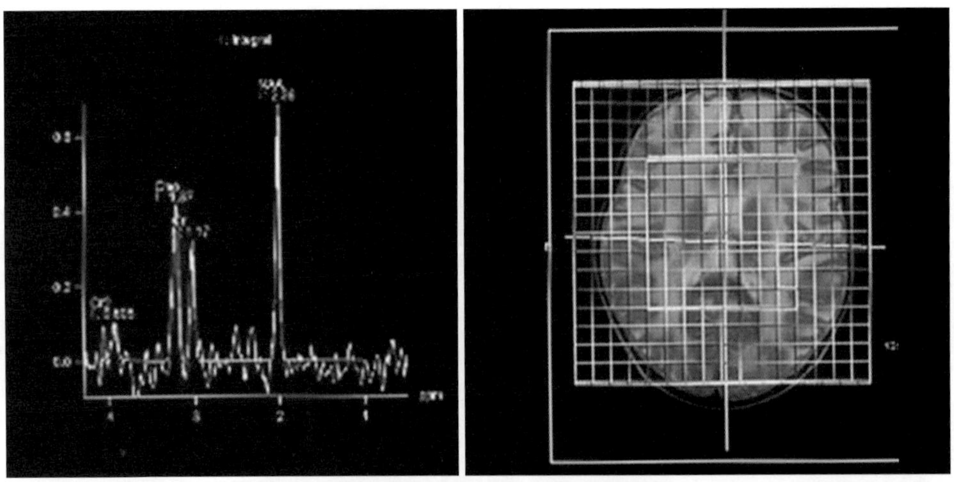

Fig. 19: MR image showing a characteristic increase in NAA peak—Canavan disease.

rod like cytoplasmic inclusions found in astrocytes in the subependymal, subpial and perivascular regions.[73]

Clinical Features

Three clinical subgroups are recognized. The infantile subgroup is characterized by early onset of macrocephaly, psychomotor retardation with seizures and death occurs within 2–3 years. The diagnosis is made on the basis of a combination of macrocephaly, early onset of clinical findings and imaging findings but definite diagnosis usually requires brain biopsy or autopsy.[74]

In the juvenile subgroup, onset of symptoms occurs between 7 and 14 years of age. Progressive bulbar symptoms with spasticity are common. In the adult subgroup, onset of symptoms occurs between the 2nd and 7th decade. The symptoms and disease course can be indistinguishable from those of classic multiple sclerosis in the adult subgroup.

Imaging Features

Alexander disease has a predilection for the frontal lobe white matter early in its course (Fig. 20). CT demonstrates low attenuation in the deep frontal lobe white matter. The characteristic frontal lobe areas of hyperintensity are seen on T2W MR imaging. The hyperintense areas progress posteriorly to the parietal white matter and internal and external capsules. The subcortical white matter is affected early in the disease course. Large cystic lesions are typically seen in the frontal and temporal regions. Enhancement is often seen near the tips of the frontal horns early in the disease course.[75] Contrast enhancement may also be seen along the ependymal linings of the lateral ventricles, within the basal ganglia or even the dentate nuclei **(Figs. 21A to E)**. Cystic dilation of the cavum septum pellucidum has been described. The occipital white matter and cerebellum are usually spared; however, involvement should not exclude the diagnosis. With disease progression, cavitation and atrophy of the white matter may be seen. Diffusion weighted MR images may reveal a restricted pattern of diffusion **(Figs. 22A to E)**. When there is diffuse white matter signal abnormality and swelling in a patient with macrocephaly, the differential diagnosis is mainly between Canavan and Alexander diseases. Brain biopsy is usually necessary to establish the diagnosis. MR spectroscopy may show a lactate peak, decreased NAA and elevated myoinositol.

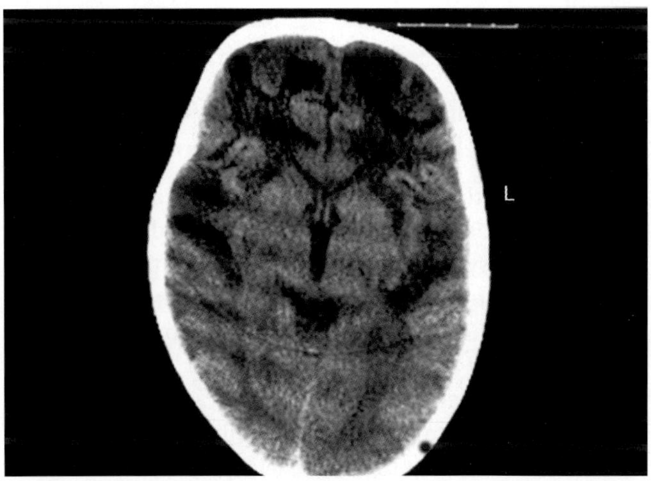

Fig. 20: CT scan showing bilateral symmetric low density areas within the frontal white matter and genu of the corpus callosum—Alexander disease.

Van der Knaap Disease/Megaloencephalic Leukodystrophy with Subcortical Cysts

This is one of the more recently identified leukodystrophies. It is also called infantile-onset spongiform leukoencephalopathy with a discrepantly mild clinical course or megaloencephalic leukodystrophy with subcortical cysts. The disease has an autosomal recessive inheritance. The onset of the disease is usually during the first year of life, but usually it is diagnosed several years later. Patients present with macrocephaly. The initial motor and mental development of the patients is either normal or slightly delayed. The disease is characterized by a slowly progressive course; in particular, ataxia, spasticity, gait disturbances and in the later stage of the disease, mental deterioration and seizures develop. No peripheral neuropathy is detected. Laboratory tests fail to demonstrate any specific metabolic abnormality. Histologically the findings are consistent with vacuolating myelinopathy.

The MR imaging findings are pathognomonic. The brain is diffusely swollen during the early stage of the disease. In the later stages, sulcal and ventricular enlargement may be present. **The white matter disease is always severe and it shows a clear centripetal progression pattern.** The peripheral white matter stuctures of the cerebral hemispheres are the most severely involved, including widespread disappearance of the subcortical U-fibers and the presence of large subcortical cyst formation in the frontoparietal and the temporal regions. *These subcortical cysts are best seen on the FLAIR images* **(Figs. 23A to C)**. These changes, as well as the initial slight sparing of the periventricular and subcortical white matter in the occipital regions suggest an additional anteroposterior

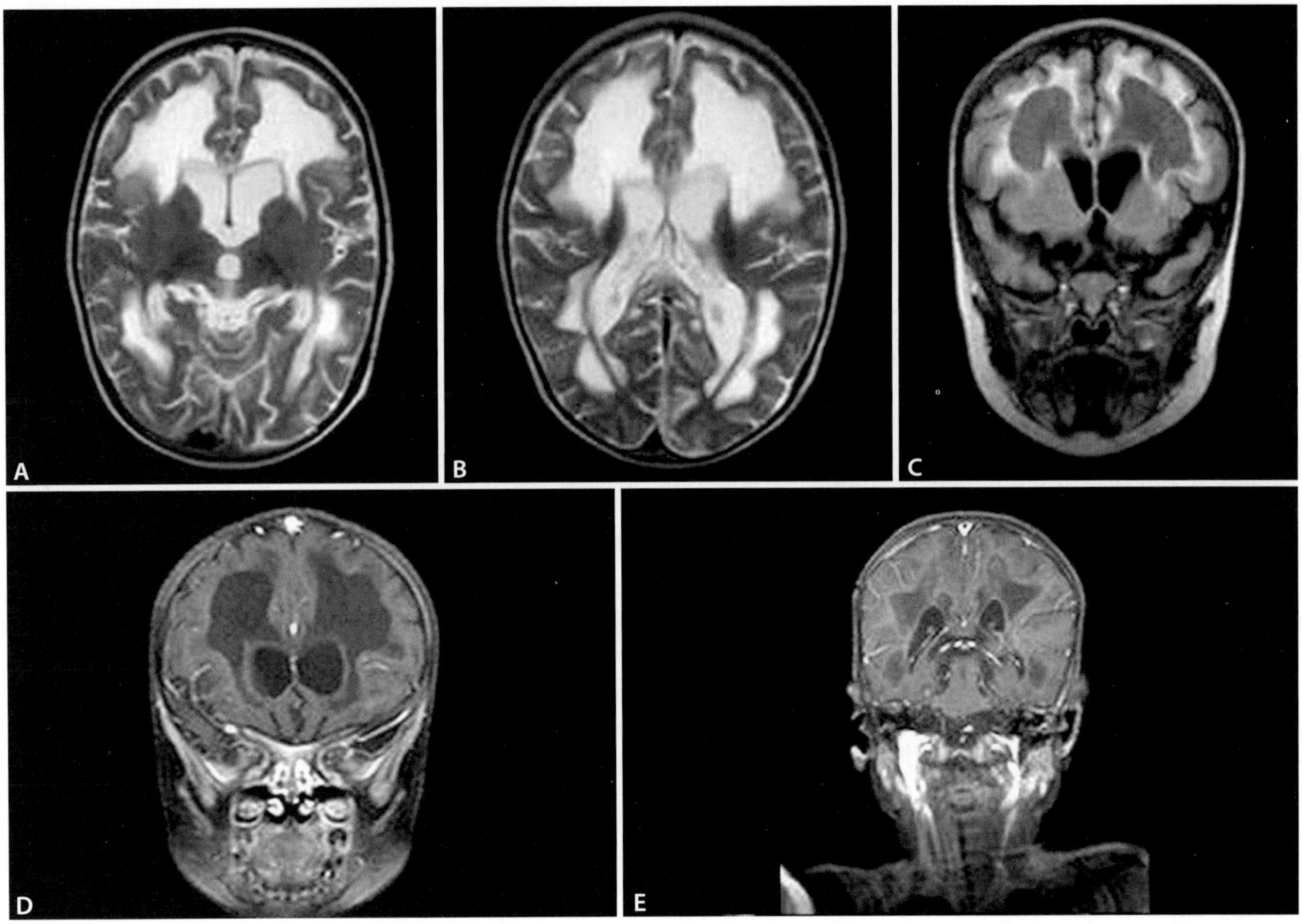

Figs. 21A to E: Axial T2-weighted (A and B) MR images revealing higher signal intensity in the frontal white matter than the parietal and occipital regions. FLAIR coronal (C) image showing involvement of the subcortical U-fibers. Postcontrast MR images reveal enhancement of the ependymal lining of the frontal horns and also of the bodies of lateral ventricles (D and E)—Alexander disease.

gradient. The deep white matter structures, the corpus callosum and the internal capsules are spared but the external and extreme capsules are involved **(Figs. 24A to E)**. The cerebellar white matter is involved but much less makedly than the supratentorial white matter structures. Subtle signal changes may be present within the brainstem along the pyramidal tracts. The cortical and deep gray matter structures are normal. No abnormal signal enhancement is seen within the brain parenchyma after intravenous contrast injection.

Diffusion-weighted imaging shows prominent hyposignal within the subcortical cysts and somewhat decreased signal within the affected white matter. No definite hypersignal is seen within the non-affected white matter structures or along the interface between the normal and abnormal areas.

The proton spectroscopic findings are nonspecific, the N-acetyl aspartate peak is decreased and the choline peak may be increased but no abnormal metabolites are demonstrated.

Vanishing White Matter Disease/Childhood Ataxia with CNS Hypomyelination

This is a recently described, distinct clinical radiological entity. The disease is typically of childhood onset. Initially, the psychomotor development of the patients is normal. Affected patients present with ataxia, spasticity, gait disturbance but only mildly impaired mental capacities. The clinical manifestation of the disease seems to be preceded by minor head trauma or infection, the same factors are also responsible for episodes of deterioration. During the later stages of the disease optic atrophy and mild epilepsy may develop. The disease is always progressive but the disease course varies. The severe forms lead to death at a relatively young age

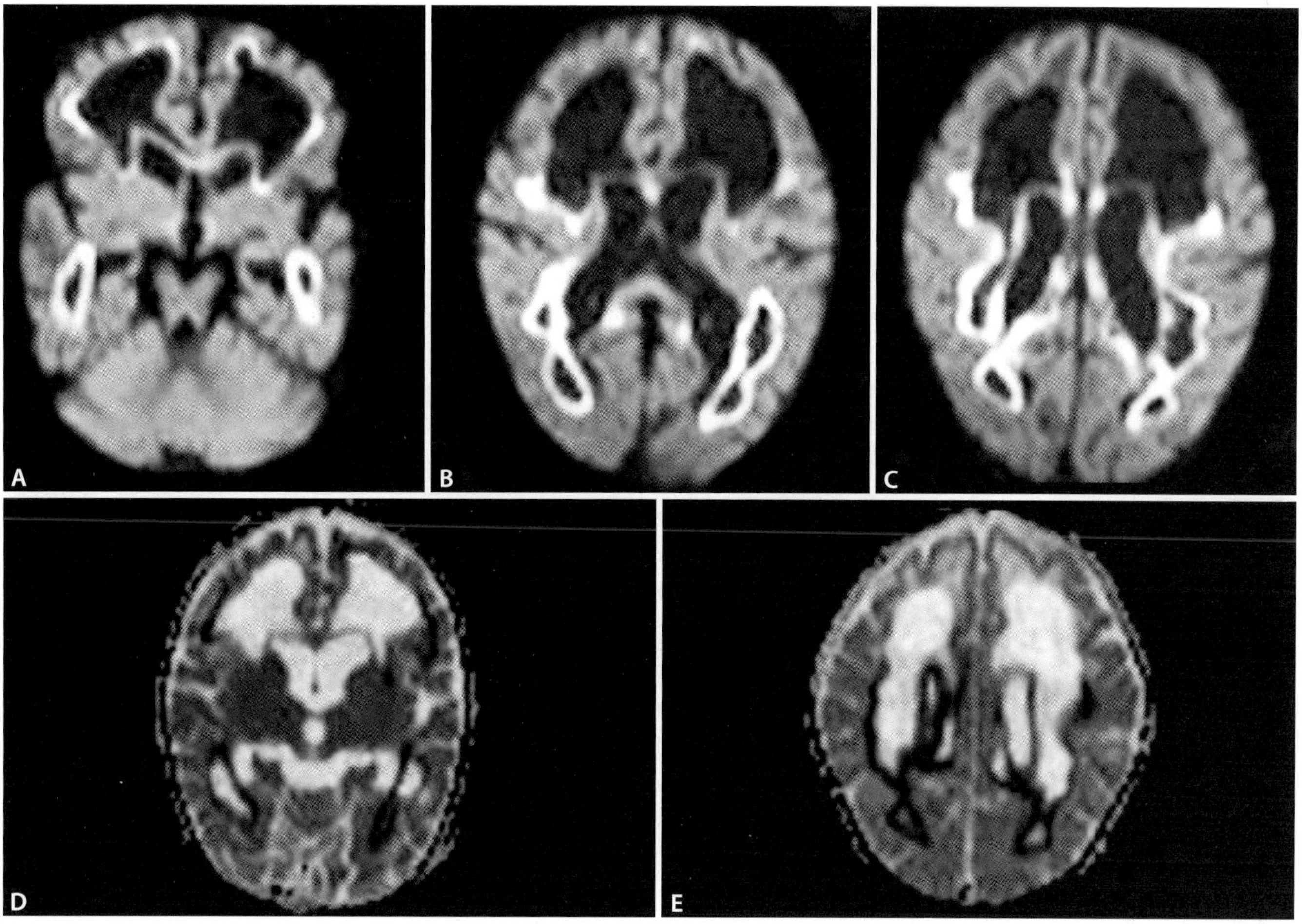

Figs. 22A to E: Diffusion-weighted MR (A to C) images revealing a restricted pattern of diffusion in the areas of signal abnormality with a hyposignal seen on the ADC maps (D and E)—Alexander disease.

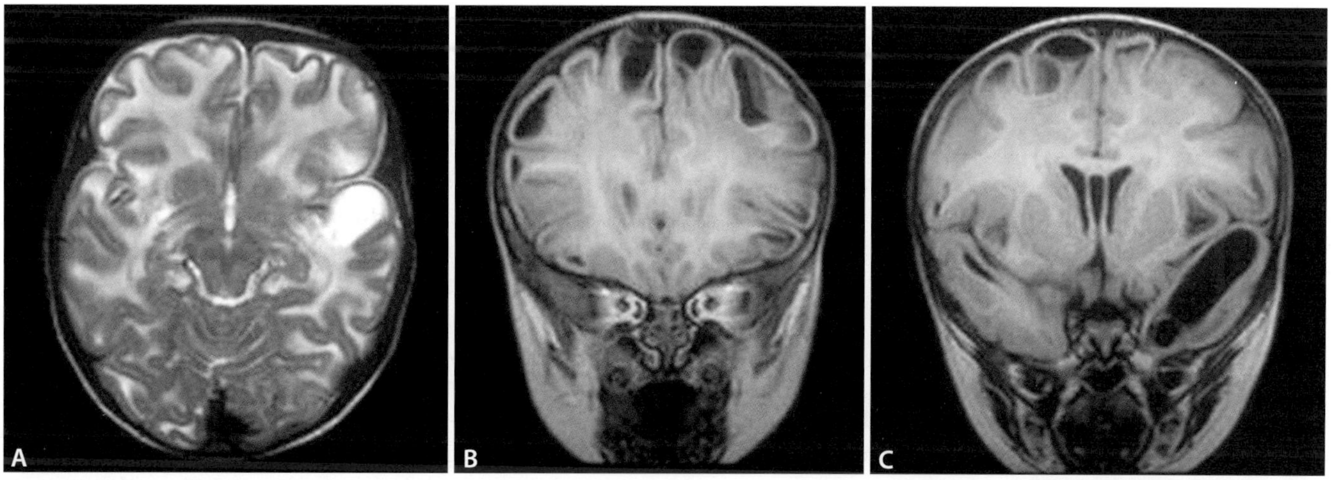

Figs. 23A to C: Axial T2W (A) and FLAIR coronal (B and C) MR images showing widespread involvement of the subcortical white matter. Subcortical cyst formation in the frontal and parietal regions is best seen on the FLAIR images (B and C)—van der Knaap disorder.

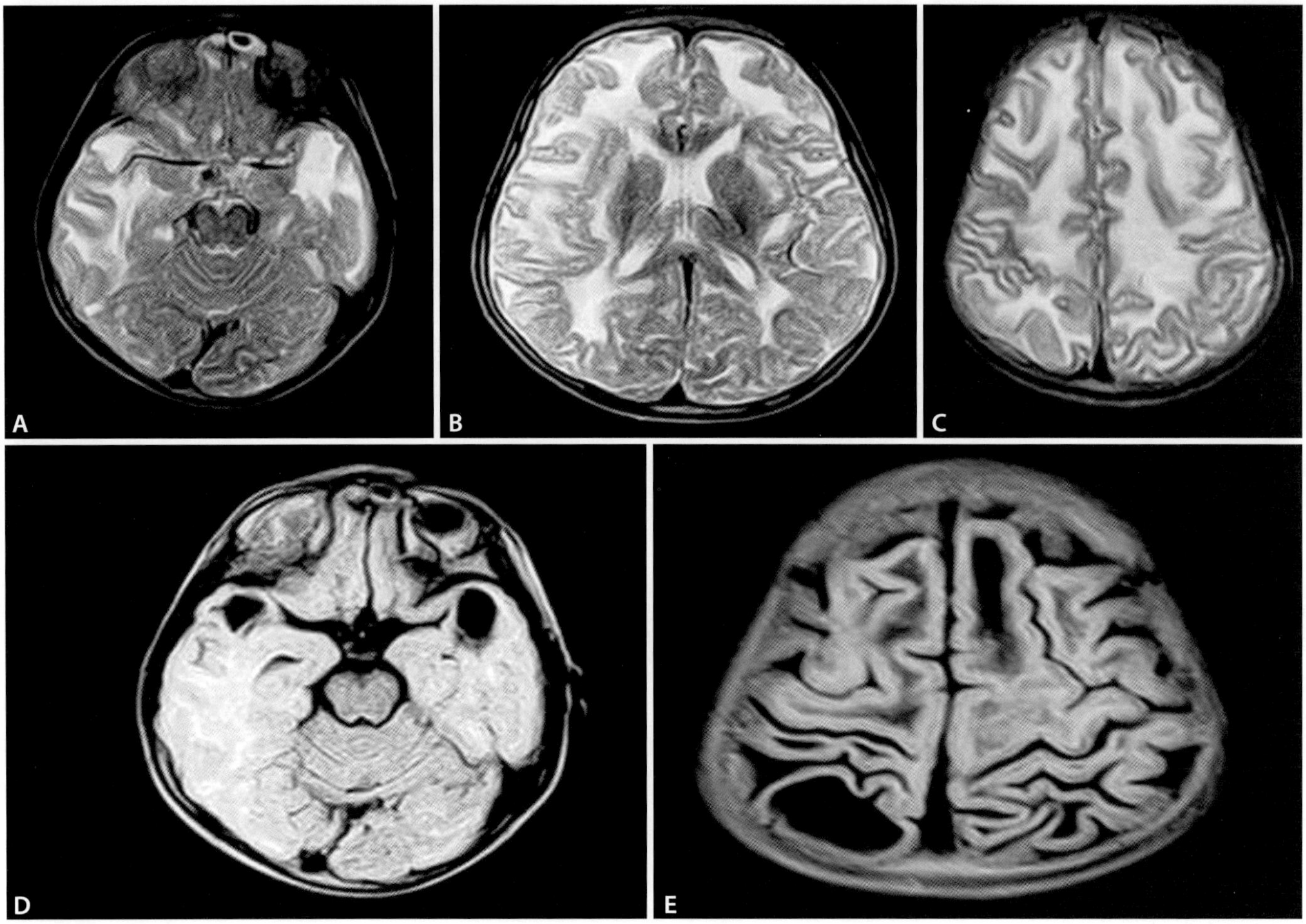

Figs. 24A to E: Axial T2W MR images (A to C) revealing extensive white matter changes with diffuse brain swelling with predominant involvement of the subcortical U-fibers (B and C). There is a relative sparing of the deep white matter structures, i.e. the corpus callosum and internal capsule (B). Signal changes are present in the brainstem along the pyramidal tracts (A) with relative sparing of the cerebellar white matter. Subcortical cyst formation is best seen on the FLAIR images (D and E)—van der Knaap disease.

(2–6 years) but patients with more moderate clinical phenotypes, live up to adulthood. A set of criterion were suggested by Van der Knaap et al. to identify children with vanishing white matter disease.[76]

- Normal or mildly delayed initial psychomotor development
- Neurologic deterioration with a chronic progressive and episodic course
- Presence of cerebellar ataxia and spasticity with relative preservation of mental function. Optic atrophy and epilepsy may occur
- Diffuse symmetric white matter involvement on MRI with all or part of white matter exhibiting a signal intensity similar to CSF.

The MR imaging findings are fairly characteristic. The brain appears to be slightly swollen but some of the gyri are somewhat broadened. The lateral ventricles show mild to moderate dilatation. *The white matter changes are very prominent; the signal properties of the affected myelin are practically identical to those of the CSF both on the T1 and T2 weighted images.* The posterior limbs of the internal capsules are often involved, whereas the anterior limbs are spared. The corpus callosum is also involved, with the exception of the outer rim. The cerebellum is usually slightly atrophic and the cerebellar white matter is mildly abnormal. In the brainstem, the posterior tegmental and the pyramidal tracts also show abnormal hypersignal. The gray matter structures including the basal ganglia are normal. MR spectroscopy of the affected gray matter shows decreased N-acetyl aspartate, normal or slightly increased choline, rather prominent lactate and glucose (at 3.43, 3.80 ppm) peaks.[77] The affected white matter shows decreased NAA, choline and creative peaks.

Aicardi–Goutieres Syndrome

This rare microcephalic disease is also called leukodystrophy with chronic CSF lymphocytosis and calcifications of the basal ganglia. The disease appears in the neonate or in early infancy. It is a relatively rapidly progressive, devastating disease, characterized by delayed development and spasticity leading to death in a few months or years.

Computed tomography is an essential diagnostic modality in this disease since it almost always demonstrates calcifications within the basal ganglia and the periventricular white matter. On MRI, the disease presents with an essentially superatentorial and very extensive white matter disease with possible cystic lesions in the temporal and parietal lobes. The internal capsules are some what less affected but are abnormal also. The brainstem and the cerebellar structures are spared.

Pelizaeus–Merzbacher Disease

Pelizaeus-Merzbacher disease, a sudanophilic leukodystrophy, is the best example of a hypomyelinating leukoencephalopathy. PMD has been linked to a severe deficiency of myelin specific lipids caused by a lack of proteolipid protein (PLP). This myelin specific proteolipid is responsible for oligodendrocyte differentiation and survival.

Pathologic Findings

The brain is usually atrophic particularly severe in the posterior fossa. Histologically, there is a profound lack of myelin. There is astrocytosis and lack of oligodendroglia. The residual myelin preferentially remains around blood vessels giving rise to characteristic "Tigroid" appearance. There is accumulation of sudanophilic droplets containing cholesterol and triglycerides in the white matter which is the histological hallmark of sudanophilic leukodystrophy.[78]

Clinical Features

PMD has traditionally been divided into classic and connatal forms[79] Classic PMD begins during late infancy with X-linked recessive inheritance. Connatal PMD is a rarer and more severe variant that begins at birth or in early infancy. This form has either X-linked or autosomal recessive inheritance. Patients with all forms of PMD present with clinical signs and symptoms including abnormal eye movements, nystagmus, extrapyramidal hyperkinesias, spasticity and slow psychomotor development.

Imaging Features

CT may demonstrate only atrophy. T2W MR findings reveal a nearly total lack of normal myelination with diffuse high signal intensity that extends peripherally to involve the subcortical U fibers, along with early involvement of the internal capsule **(Figs. 25A to C)**. Sometimes, the white matter demonstrates high signal intensity with small scattered foci of more normal signal intensity—a finding that may reflect the tigroid pattern of myelination seen on histology[80] **(Fig. 26)**.

Cockayne Syndrome

Cockayne syndrome is another sudanophilic leukodystrophy.[81] The affected children may be normal until late in infancy and may live long enough to develop dwarfism.

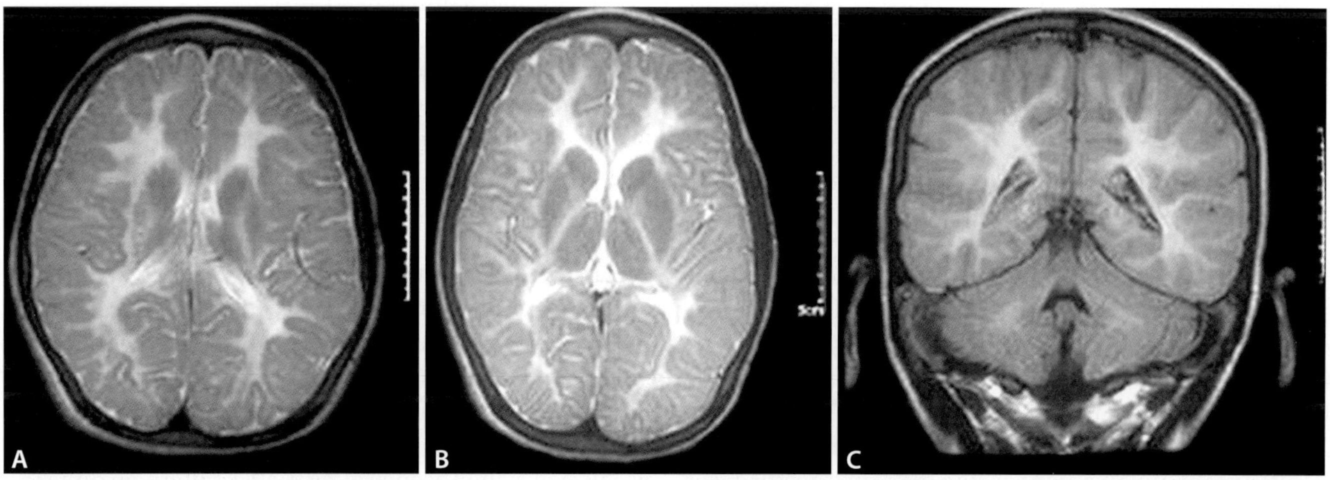

Figs. 25A to C: Axial T2W (A and B) and FLAIR coronal (C) MR images demonstrating diffuse high signal intensity within the white matter, including the posterior limbs of the internal capsules which should be myelinated at birth—Pelizaeus–Merzbacher disease.

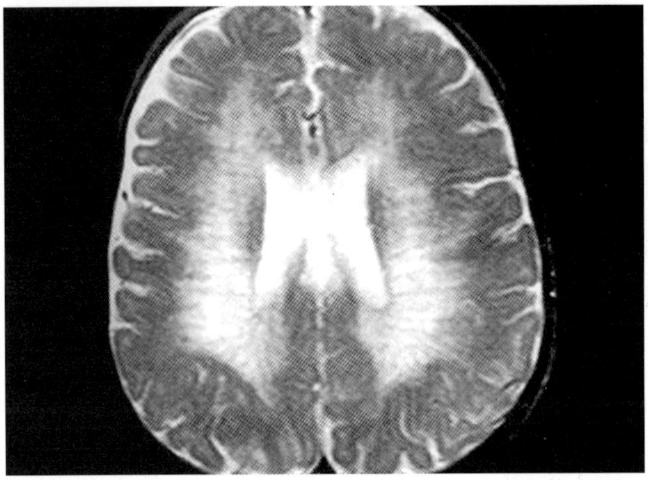

Fig. 26: Axial T2W MR image in an infant with slow psychomotor development with nystagmus and choreoathetoid movements revealing diffuse high signal intensity in the white matter with small scattered foci of more normal signal intensity within—Tigroid pattern of myelination seen in Pelizaeus-Merzbacher disease.

Transmitted as an autosomal recessive trait, this syndrome consists of growth retardation, mental retardation, microcephaly, retinopathy, cutaneous photosensitivity and ataxia. The pathologic changes are similar to other leukodystrophies. However a significant difference is that small vessels become involved by mural and extramural colloid deposits which frequently contain iron and exhibit striking calcification. The deposits occur chiefly in the basal ganglia, the cerebral white matter and the dentate nuclei of the cerebellum. There is extensive cortical calcification in both hemispheres.

MR Spectroscopy

Proton MR spectroscopy may reveal no abnormal peak consistent with the absence of sclerosis and well-preserved axons. Diffuse or focal reduction in NAA consistent with axonal damage may be seen in more severe cases.[82]

MITOCHONDRIAL DISORDERS/ DEFECTS OF THE RESPIRATORY CHAIN

Mitochondrial encephalopathy comprises a heterogeneous group of neuromuscular disorders caused by defect in the oxidative metabolic pathways of energy production, owing to a structural or functional mitochondrial defect. The so-called respiratory chain is a complex multiunit system within the inner membrane of the mitochondria. Multisystem involvement is the rule in the diseases related to defect of the respiratory chain. It is an important clinical diagnostic clue. In respiratory chain deficiencies, practically any organ or tissue in any combination may be involved. The most frequently affected organs are, however, the central nervous system and the muscles (both skeletal and visceral).

Mitochondrial Encephalomyopathy: Lactic Acidosis and Stroke-like Symptoms

Clinical Features

Patients with MELAS syndrome usually appear healthy at birth with normal development, then exhibit delayed growth, episodic vomiting, seizures and recurrent strokes and cortical blindness.[83] The age of onset is typically between 4 and 15 years but early infantile and adult forms have also been reported. No ophthalmoplegia or heart block is seen. These stroke like episodes are the result of a proliferation of dysfunctional mitochondria in the smooth muscle cells or small arteries giving rise to either permanent or reversible deficits. The disease course is progressive with periodic acute exacerbation. Systemic manifestations of the disease include cardiomyopathy and diabetes (both types 1 and 2)

Pathologic Findings

At electron microscopy, the affected tissue demonstrates an increased number of mitochondria which are enlarged and have lipoid inclusions. Serum and cerebrospinal fluid lactate levels are usually elevated.

Imaging Features

CT and MR findings of MELAS syndrome have been reported as multiple infarct like lesions, calcification of the basal ganglia and diffuse atrophy.[84,85] CT examination in MELAS frequently reveals basal ganglia calcifications. These infarct like lesions show low attenuation on CT and elongation of both T1 and T2 relaxation times on MR images, usually with a bilateral symmetric or asymmetric cortical and subcortical distribution. There is a posterior predilection for the lesions. The MELAS syndrome can be differentiated from cerebral infarct of vascular origin because the lesions are not restricted to a specific vascular territory and angiography reveals no vascular occlusion.[86] During the course of the disease lesions resolve with clinical improvement or residual atrophy while new lesions appear in other regions. This finding of migrating infarct like lesions in childhood is almost unique to MELAS.[87] Another useful sign is the absence of restricted pattern on diffusion weighted MR images which supports the hypothesis that the lesions are actually not of ischemic origin but rather secondary to metabolic crash or energy failure.

There may be generalized cerebral and cerebellar atrophy. The finding of multiple migrating infarct like lesions not limited to a specific vascular territory especially in the basal ganglia and the posterior part of the cerebral hemisphere in children suggest MELAS syndrome **(Figs. 27A to D)**. Muscle biopsy is important to confirm the diagnosis. MR spectroscopy may be a useful complementry test since a small amount of lactate is often detected even in apparently normal brain areas. Abnormally decreased FA values have been described in the abnormal brain areas and cervical spinal cord.[88]

Myoclonic Epilepsy with Ragged Red Fibers

Unlike MELAS syndrome, myoclonic epilepsy with ragged red fiber (MERRF) causes no strokes leading to cerebral infarcts.[89] The patients usually present with myoclonus, ataxia, weakness and generalized seizures.[90] The patients, have short stature and cardiac conductive defects.

Pathologic Findings

Muscle biopsy reveals ragged red fibers in skeletal muscles. This finding implies degeneration of granular fibers and a proliferation of mitochondria.

Imaging Features

The CT and MR show cerebral and cerebellar atrophy. MR findings may show hyperintense signal abnormalities in the white matter and deep gray matter **(Figs. 28A to C)**. CT may show calcification of the dentate nucleus and globus pallidus.

Kearns–Sayre Syndrome

First described by Kearns and Sayre, this mitochondrial disorder occurs more frequently in females and is inherited as an autosomal dominant tract.[91]

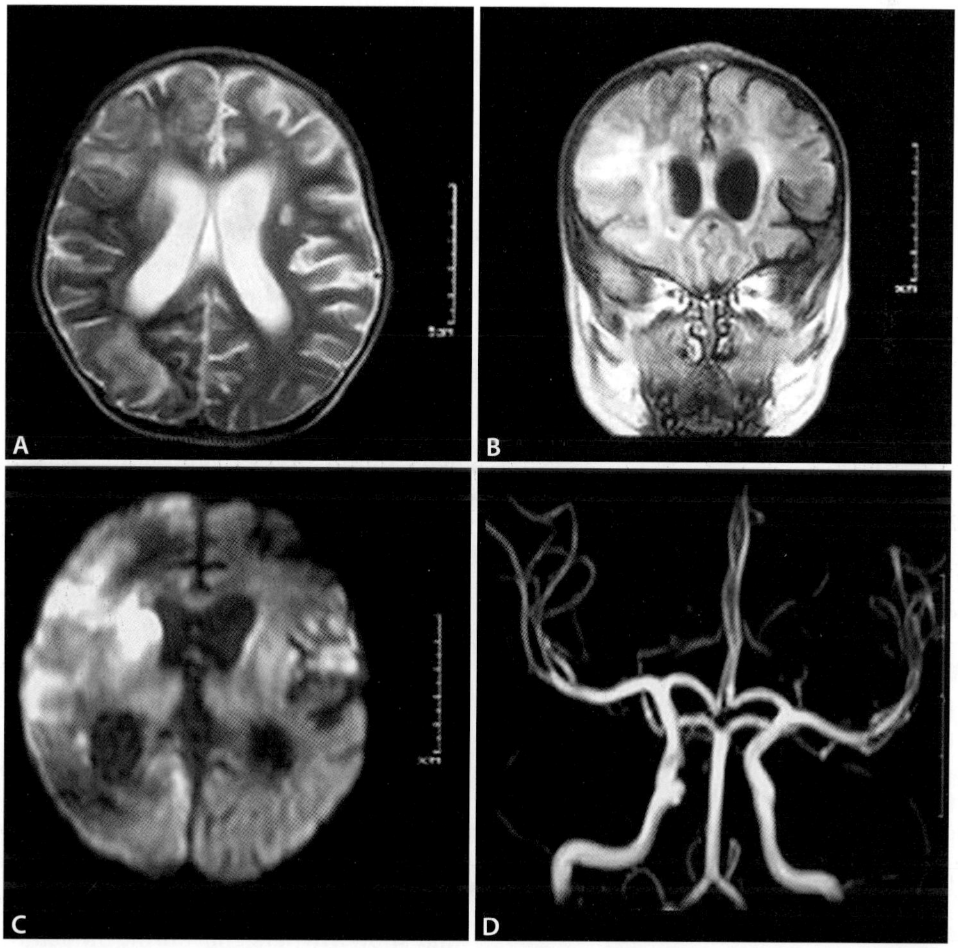

Figs. 27A to D: Axial T2W (A) and FLAIR coronal (B) MR images showing asymmetrical infarct-like lesions involving the subcortical white matter and basal ganglia. The lesions are not restricted to any specific vascular territory and show high signal on the ADC maps (C) MR angiography reveals no vascular occlusion (D)—Mitochondrial encephalopathy (MELAS).

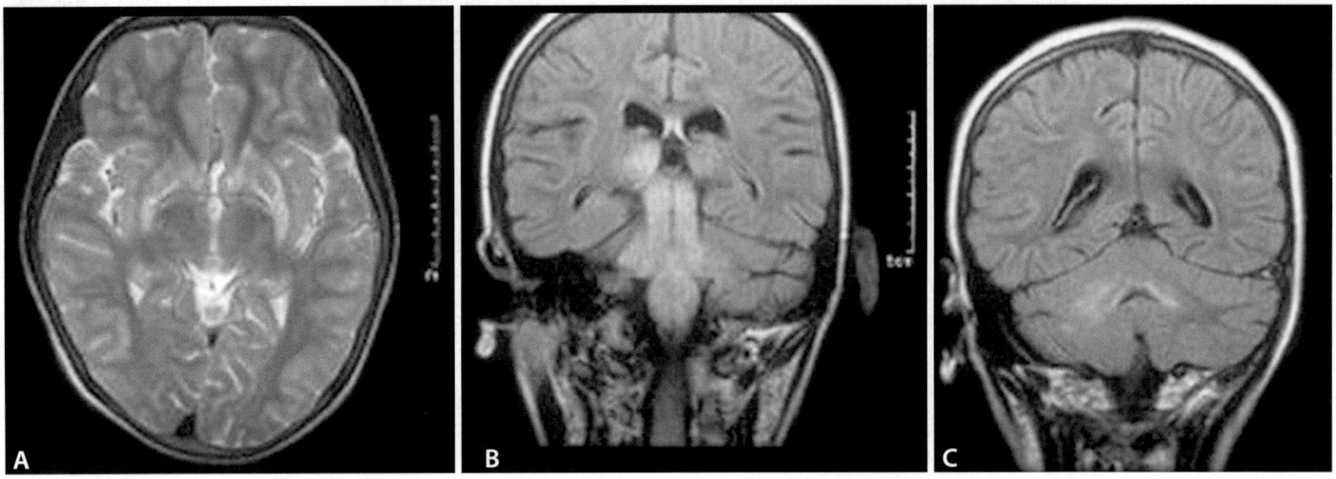

Figs. 28A to C: Axial T2W (A) and FLAIR coronal (B and C) MR images in a child showing symmetric areas of hyperintense signal abnormality involving the basal ganglia, brainstem and the cerebellar white matter—Mitochondrial encephalopathy.

Clinical Features

It presents as a triad of ophthalmoplegia, retinal pigmentary degeneration and complete heart block. There is short stature and frequently mental deterioration.

Imaging Features

MR findings in Kearns-Sayre syndrome reflect the pathology of spongiform degeneration and reveal high signal intensity on long TR images in the white matter with a predilection for involvement of peripheral U-fibers and sparing of the periventricular white matter.[92] Symmetric high signal on T2W images can be seen in basal ganglia. The cerebellar white matter and the dorsal brainstem may also demonstrate abnormal hyperintensity.[93] Diffuse atrophy is commonly seen involving the cerebrum and cerebellum.

Subacute Necrotizing Encephalomyopathy (Leigh Disease)

Leigh disease, or subacute necrotizing encephalomyopathy is an inherited, progressive, neurodegenerative disease of infancy or early childhood.[94] Affected infants and children typically present with hypotonia and psychomotor deterioration. Ataxia, ophthalmoplegia, ptosis, dystonia and swallowing difficulties inevitably ensue.[95] Acute respiratory failure may occur. Respiratory problems and ocular abnormalities (external ophthalmoplegia, nystagmus, strabismus) are suggestive clinical features.

Pathologic Features

Characteristic pathologic abnormalities include microcystic cavitation, vascular proliferation, neuronal loss and demyelination of the midbrain, basal ganglia and cerebellar dentate nuclei and occasionally of the cerebral white matter.[96]

Imaging Features

Typical MR finding in Leigh disease is the remarkably symmetrical involvement, most frequently in the putamen.[97] The lesions are also commonly found in the globus pallidus and the caudate nucleus but never in the absence of putaminal abnormalities.[98] Other areas of involvement include the paraventricular white matter, corpus callosum, substantia nigra, decussation of superior cerebellar peduncles, periaqueductal region, brainstem and the gray matter in the spinal cord[99] **(Figs. 29A to C)**. Loss of respiratory control in Leigh disease has been found to correlate with lower brainstem lesions (particularly situated in the periaqueductal gray matter and reticular formation of the medulla oblongata). Upper brainstem signal abnormalities are often transient and the associated respiratory difficulties resolve. The dentate nuclei frequently show abnormalities. White matter lesions in the cerebral hemispheres are usually patchy and predominantly subcortical. The important differential diagnosis is organic acidopathies but the presence of peculiar brainstem lesion in Leigh disease usually allows a confident differentiation.

Proton MR spectroscopy with voxel placement in the basal ganglia typically demonstrates an abnormal lactate peak with a decrease in NAA/Cr. Diffusion weighted images may show a hypersignal during the acute metabolic attacks within lesion areas in the brainstem, the basal ganglia and the dentate nuclei[100] **(Figs. 30A to D)**.

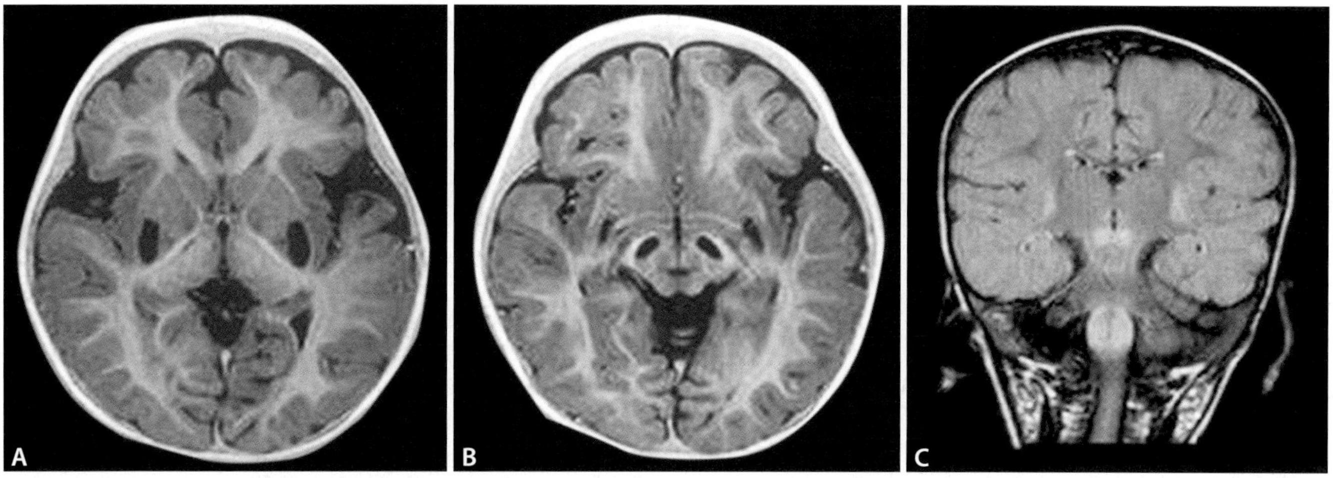

Figs. 29A to C: Inversion recovery (A and B) images showing bilateral symmetrical lesions involving the putamen (A), the substantia nigra and the periaqueductal region (B). FLAIR coronal MR image revealing lesions in the medulla in addition to putamen and midbrain. Lesions in the medulla correlate with the respiratory problems in these patients—Leigh disease.

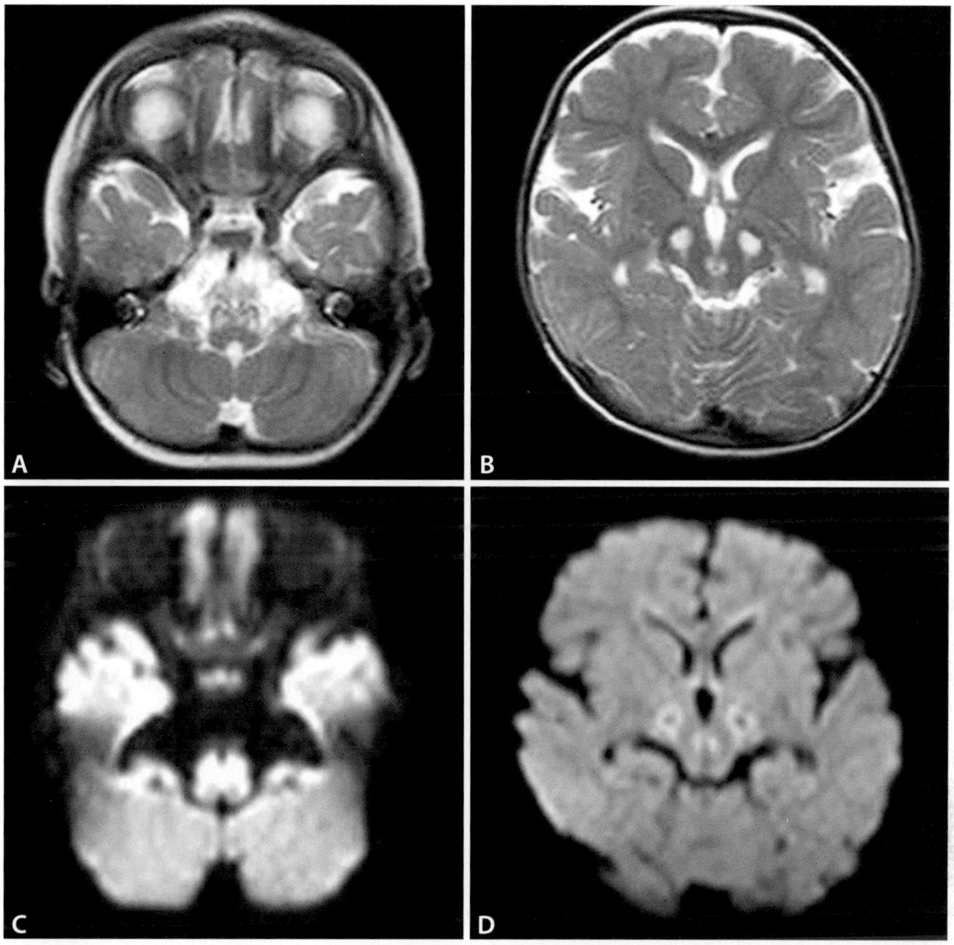

Figs. 30A to D: Axial T2W (A and B) images in a 20-month-old infant showing lesions in the medulla and symmetrical lesions in the substantia nigra and the periaqueductal region (B). These lesions reveal a restricted pattern of diffusion seen as hypersignal on the diffusion weighted images (C and D) during the acute metabolic crisis—Leigh disease.

LEBER'S HEREDITARY OPTIC NEUROPATHY

Leber's hereditary optic neuropathy (LHON) presents with rapidly progressive visual loss due to degeneration of the optic nerves. The disease typically occurs in young adults. No skeletal muscle involvement has been described in this disease. MR imaging usually shows signal abnormalities within the distal intraorbital optic nerves. Putaminal lesions and scattered white matter lesions within the centrum cerebral hemispheric white matter may also be present. ***See* Table 3** for mitochondrial disorders.

DISORDERS OF AMINO ACID METABOLISM/AMINOACIDOPATHIES

Urea Cycle Defects

The urea cycle is a complex metabolic process, the primary role of which is to convert the toxic ammonia in to non-toxic urea. Urea cycle defects are characterized by autosomal recessive inheritance except ornithine carbamoyl transferase deficiency, which is X-linked. The most common metabolic derangement in each disease entity is hyperammonemia and impairment of the metabolism of various amino acids (alanine, glutamine, citrulline and arginine). Some of the urea cycle defects present in neonates as a devastating metabolic disease of almost immediate postnatal onset. If the disease is of later onset (infantile, juvenile or adult), it may manifest with neurological signs and symptoms of acute or chronic encephalopathy. The urea cycle defects include carbamyl phosphate deficiency, ornithine transcarbamylase deficiency, citrullinemia and argininosuccinic aciduria.[101] Hyperammonemia induces brain swelling and Alzheimer type II changes in astrocytes and chronic elevation leads to neuronal degeneration.

Table 3: Mitochondrial disorders: Distinguishing clinical features and magnetic resonance findings.[16]

KSS	Ophthalmoplegia Retinal degeneration Heart block CSF protein >100 mg/dL	T2WI: High signal in U-fibers, thalami, dorsal brainstem, cerebellar WMT1 WI: high signal in basal ganglia
MERRF	Myoclonus, ataxia, weakness	T2 WI: High signal in deep GM and WM
MELAS	Episodic vomiting Cerebral blindness Hemiparesis, hemianopsia	T2 WI: High signal in subcortical WM, brainstem, basal ganglia, cerebellum infarcts (may not be in vascular territories)
Leigh	Respiratory failure Visual/auditory problems, ataxia, weakness	T2 WI: High signal in bilateral symmetric basal ganglia (particularly putamen), thalami, dorsal brainstem

MR imaging findings in neonates with urea cycle defects are dominated by the prominent brain swelling and white matter signal changes related to vasogenic edema. The myelinated white matter is less severely affected than the nonmyelinated areas **(Figs. 31A to H)**. Certain regions of the cerebral cortex and deep gray matter show prolongation of T1 and T2 relaxation times on MR, in particular the insular cortex (posterior more than anterior), perirolandic cortex and basal ganglia (particularly the globi pallidi) show early T2 prolongation and swelling. The differentiation from hypoxic ischemic injury can be made by the predominant globus pallidus and putaminal injury in urea cycle disorders in contrast to the predominant thalamic injury in hypoxic injury. MR spectroscopy reveals a characteristic elevated lactate (doublet centred at 1.33 ppm) and glutamate resonance at 2.2–2.6 ppm and at 3.75 ppm. The glutamate and glutamine resonances are best seen with short (20–30 ms) TEs.[102] As the case progresses, atrophy is often severe and may be multicystic.

Phenylketonuria

Classic phenylketonuria (PKU) is an autosomal recessive disorder caused by a deficiency in the enzyme phenylalanine hydroxylase which converts phenylalanine to tyrosine owing to which neurotoxic phenylketones accumulate. Two forms of phenylketonuria are known. The more frequent "classical" phenylketonuria is caused by the deficiency of the phenylalanine hydroxylase enzyme. The other more malignant and rare form is related to the deficiency of the tetrahydrobiopterin coenzyme which is also indispensable in the breakdown of phenylalanine into tyrosine.

The clinical and imaging manifestations of the two forms of phenylketonuria are different.

Clinical Features

Infants are normal at birth but in the first year of life manifest with progressive cognitive delay, microcephaly, spasticity, recurrent eczematous rash and a peculiar musty odour of the urine, skin and hair. Seizures occur in about 25% of untreated patients.

Imaging Findings

Imaging studies show primarily abnormal signal in the white matter that corresponds to the delayed and defective myelination. MR shows T2 prolongation that is predominantly found in the periventricular white matter in

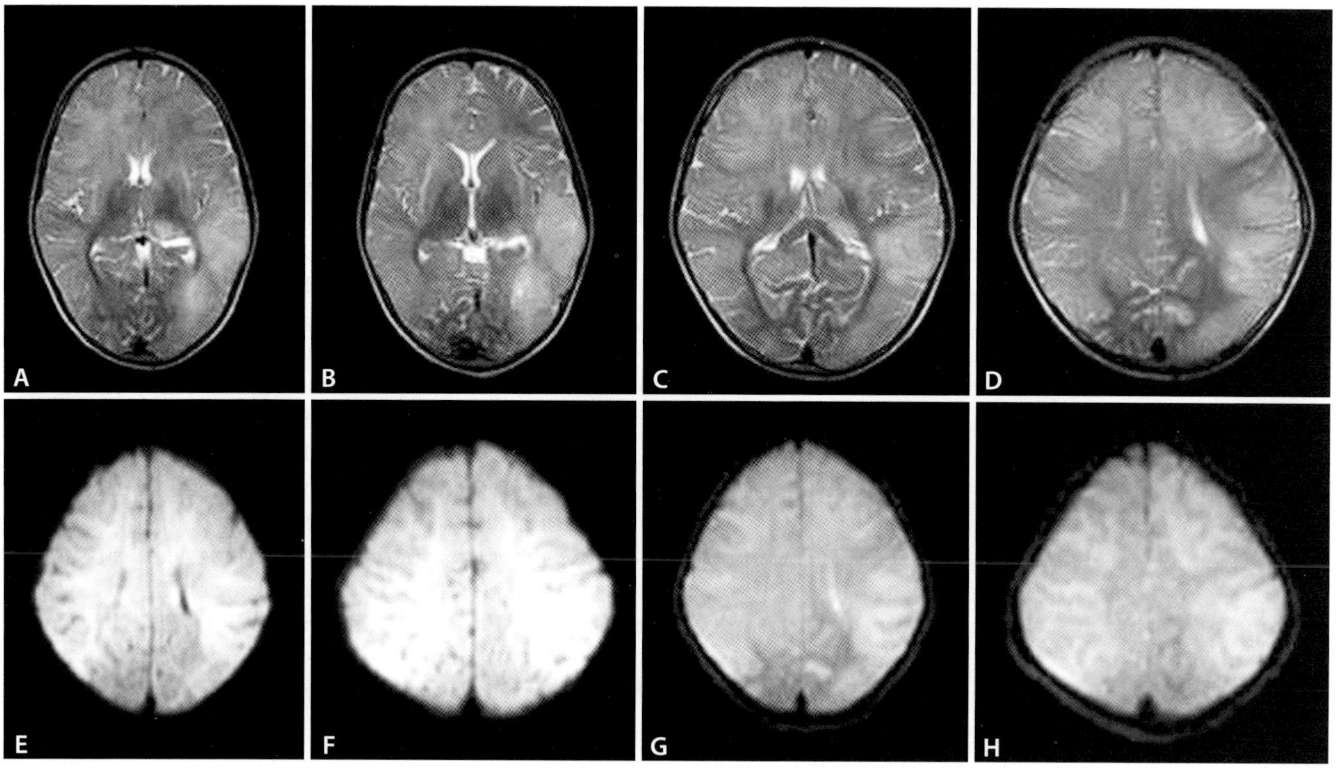

Figs. 31A to H: Axial T2W MR images (A to D) in a few-month-old infant showing a diffuse swelling of the brain. The unmyelinated white matter exhibits an abnormal increased signal intensity. There is a relative sparing of the myelinated optic radiation (B). Diffusion-weighted (E and F) images and ADC maps (G and H) do not reveal a restricted pattern consistent with vasogenic edema—Urea cycle disorder.

the initial stages.[103] The subcortical white matter is involved later. Diffusion-weighted MR images obtained in the acute phase will show a reduced diffusion in the affected white matter due to spongiotic changes of myelin.[104] Proton MR spectroscopy shows the presence of a peak from elevated phenylalanine at 7.37 ppm. The size of the peak is useful for monitoring response to treatment.[105]

Malignant Form of Phenylketonuria

In the malignant form, microcephaly and delayed development are also typical but the disease if not treated, often leads to death in early childhood. Neurologically, the patients present with prominent extrapyramidal signs (infantile parkinsonism, choreoathetosis) myoclonic and grand mal seizures. Progressive pyramidal and bulbar signs develop in conjunction with severe congnitive deterioration.

In the biopterin-dependent form of phenylketonuria, CT examination shows calcifications at the level of the putamina and/or the globi pallidi as well as along the cortical-subcortical junction area in the frontal regions somewhat similar to what may be seen in carbonic anhydrase II deficiency.

The MR imaging study shows signal changes within the calcified areas: hyperintense on the T1 and hypointense on the T2 weighted images. White matter lesions may be seen, sometimes, they are diffuse and in other cases focal with cystic degeneration in the parietal-occipital regions.

Maple Syrup Urine Disease

Maple syrup urine disease (MSUD) is a genetically heterogeneous disorder caused by abnormal oxidative decarboxylation of the branched chain amino acids leucine, isoleucine and valine. Four clinical phenotypes are distinguished: classical, intermediate, intermittent and thiamine responsive. The most severe form is the classical MSUD characterized by early postnatal onset and rapid progressive neurological deterioration leading to death, if untreated.

In the classic type, the infant is normal for about the first week. In the second week, the infant starts to eat poorly, fails to thrive, develops hypotonia, lethargy and vomiting. Urine, sweat and cerumen smell like maple syrup. The disease quickly progresses to coma, seizures and death, if untreated.[106] The severity of neurologic sequelae is strongly correlated with the duration of the acute toxic phase in the neonatal period. Conventional MR imaging shows diffuse swelling of the brain. This is mainly due to the vasogenic edema involving the nonmyelinated white matter structures. On the other hand, even more prominent signal changes are also present within the myelinated brain areas (posterior brainstem tracts, central cerebellar white matter, posterior limbs of the internal capsules) representing myelin edema secondary to vacuolating myelinopathy.

The **less severe** forms of the disease with higher residual enzymatic activity can present later in childhood with metabolic crisis resulting in lethargy, irritability, vomiting that may progress to stupor or coma. An intermittent form may present later in life as attacks of transient ataxia sometimes accompanied by cerebral edema. Tests during an attack show elevated leucine isoleucine and valine in blood as well as branched chain amino acids in urine. Chronic management relies on dietary restriction of branched chain amino acids.

Imaging Findings

The neonatal form typically presents on the seventh day after birth. The imaging findings may be normal in the first ten days of life. Because classic maple syrup urine disease presents in the neonatal period, it is one of the few metabolic diseases in which transfontanelle sonography may play a role in diagnosis. Cranial sonography may show a symmetric increase in the echogenicity of the periventricular white matter, basal ganglia and thalami.[107] The CT and MR findings are quite characteristic, revealing, profound localized edema seen as increased signal on T2 weighted images in the deep cerebellar white matter, dorsal brainstem, cerebral peduncles, inferior limb of the internal capsule, perirolandic white matter and the globi pallidi. The regions involved correspond to those that are myelinated or myelinating at the time of birth. Generalized edema of the cerebral hemispheres may be superimposed on the localized abnormailities particularly in the first weeks of life. Diffusion imaging is very useful in the acute stage as areas with MSUD edema (cerebellar white matter, dorsal brainstem, cerebral peduncles, costicospinal tracts, globi pallidi) show reduced diffusion with ADC values falling to 20–30% of their normal values. Myelin edema presents with isotropically restricted water diffusion; hence, there is high signal. The vasogenic edema is characterized by isotropically increased water diffusion which causes hyposignal on the diffusion-weighted images. **The sharp contrast between the diffusion-weighted imaging signal properties of these two edema types and the peculiar distribution of the pathological hypersignal (strictly limited to the myelinated white matter structures) results in a pathognomonic imaging pattern**. After the acute phase of the disease has resolved patients are left with a variable degree of brain damage dependent upon the time of initiation of the treatment. Proton MR spectroscopy in the acute phase of illness shows slight reduction of NAA and amino acid peak of leucine, isoleucine and valine at 0.9 ppm on short TE.[108]

The intermittent and intermediate forms of maple syrup urine disease have a more insidious clinical pattern. The first metabolic crisis may appear in late infancy or early childhood. The imaging findings also are less characteristic. Typically, brain atrophy, delayed myelination and pathological signal changes within the upper brainstem structures, the thalami, the globi pallidi and the centrum semiovale are observed. Diffusion-weighted imaging also shows signal abnormalities in these areas but they are often rather subtle **(Figs. 32A to E)**. From the imaging point of view, the intermittent form of maple syrup urine disease may, therefore, be somewhat similar to Canavan disease in the early stage but the clinical context and the laboratory findings allow easy differentiation.

In treated MSUD cases, the conventional MRI and the diffusion-weighted imaging findings rarely return to normal. Typically, variable but prominent residual abnormalities, including diffuse brain atrophy, delayed myelination and structural lesions are noted. The pattern of the structural lesions is very similar to those observed in the intermittent form of maple syrup urine disease. Changes are also present in the hypothalamic structures, the dentate nuclei and the cerebellar or the cerebral hemispheric white matter. Subtle residual diffusion weighted imaging abnormalities may also be noted. In successfully treated cases, MR spectroscopy shows improvement but total normalization of the branched chain amino acid peak complex is usually not achieved.

Classic Homocystinuria

Class homocystinuria is an autosomal recessive disorder caused by a defect in the enzyme crystathionine β synthetase resulting in elevations of homocystine and methionine. This results in intimal irregularities that cause arteriosclerosis, arterial thromboembolism and venous thrombosis in children and young adults.[109] The excess homocysteine generates superoxide and hydrogen peroxide, changes coagulation factor levels (encouraging clot formation), prevents small arteries from dilating, and causes proliferation of smooth muscle cells in arterial walls.

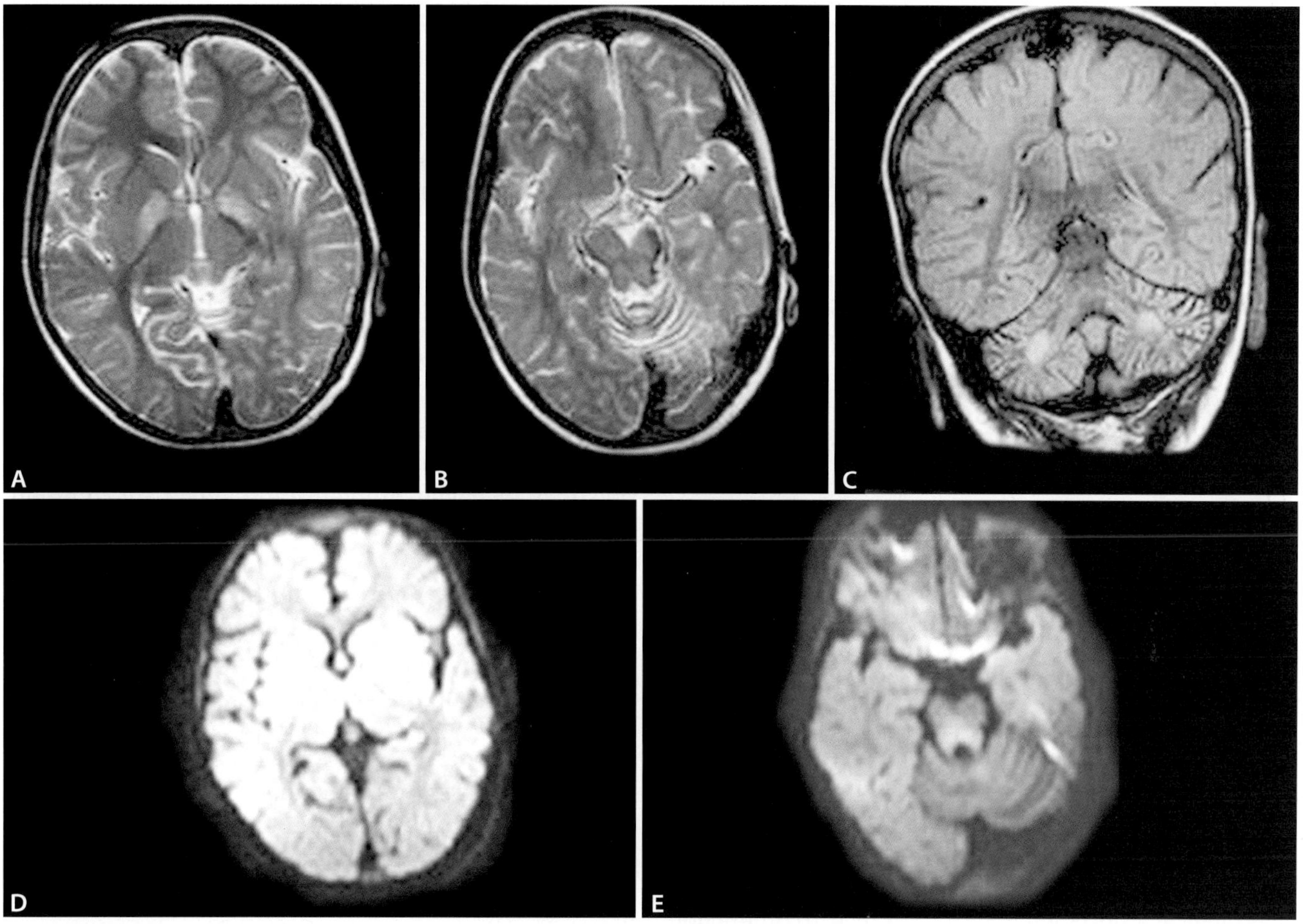

Figs. 32A to E: Axial T2W (A and B) and FLAIR coronal (C) MR images revealing symmetric areas of signal abnormality in the globus pallidi (A) dorsal brainstem (B) and the deep cerebellar white matter (C). Diffusion-weighted MR images (D and E) revealing restricted pattern of diffusion in the globi pallidi and dorsal brainstem—Intermittent form of maple syrup urine disease.

Clinical Features

The findings include dislocation of lens, osteoporosis, thinning and lengthening of long bones. Lens dislocation (ectopia lentis) is usually inferior which is the opposite of what is seen in Marfan syndrome. Untreated patients are at risk for seizures, psychiatric disorders, thromboembolic events including stroke myocardial infarction and pulmonary emboli.

Imaging

Imaging studies reveal multiple cortical-subcortical and lacunar infarctions both within the cerebral and the cerebellar hemispheres. The disease may also present with a less specific, diffuse white matter involvement and the pattern is suggestive of 'retrograde' demyelination.

Nonketotic Hyperglycinemia

This is caused by a defect in glycine cleavage with resultant accumulation of glycine in the plasma, urine and CSF. Two clinical phenotypes are known: the more common neonatal type, which is characterized by practically absent glycine cleavage system activity and the late onset (infantile and juvenile) form, in which some residual glycine cleavage system activity is present. The neonatal form presents as lethargy and poor feeding after starting the protein feeds. The patients are hypotonic (glycine is an inhibitor neurotransmitter at the level of the lower motor neurons) and have frequent myoclonic seizures. This quickly progresses to persistent seizures, encephalopathy and coma. Apnea is common and persistent hiccups have been described. The prognosis for the neonatal form is poor. The late onset form has a milder and rather nonspecific clinical presentation.

Imaging

The imaging hallmarks of nonketotic hyperglycinemia are callosal abnormalities and delayed myelination.[110]

The spectrum of morphological changes of the corpus callosum ranges from the rare true callosal dysgenesis to the more frequent callosal hypogenesis or hypoplasia but some degree of abnormality is always present. The delay in myelination is increasingly evident with the aging of the infant and is probably associated with global hypomyelination. Cortical gyral abnormalities have also been described. Acute hydrocephalus may contribute to the severe clinical picture. In the chronic stage of the disease, progressive atrophy of the brain develops.

MR spectroscopy is a useful adjunct to the MR work-up of patients with suspected nonketotic hyperglycinemia since the concentration of glycine is particularly elevated in the brain. Glycine resonates at the 3.55 ppm level. Proton MR spectroscopy reveals a glycine peak at 3.55 ppm. In order to separate the glycine peak from that of myoinositol which has a similar chemical shift, the spectrum should be obtained with a long echo time. The myoinositol peak disappears on the long echo time.

5, 10-Methylene-tetrahydrofolate Reductase Deficiency

5, 10-methylene-tetrahydrofolate reductase deficiency is the best known of the defects of folate metabolism. This form has an autosomal recessive inheritance.The onset of the disease is variable, it is more frequent in infants but later onset cases, including an adult form, are also known. Neurologically, developmental delay is seen in conjunction with signs of spinal cord (combined degeneration of the cord) and peripheral nerve involvement.

MR imaging in 5, 10-methylene tetrahydrofolate reductase deficiency may show rather prominent abnormalities in the brain. The cerebral white matter is diffusely abnormal, the lesions involve the corpus callosum, the external and extreme capsules, the laminae medullares and the anterior limbs of the internal capsules with sparing of the posterior limbs.[111] The corticospinal tracts within the centrum semiovale, the subcortical U-fibers in the occipital regions and the optic radiations are also spared. The basal ganglia and the thalami are normal but the globi pallidi show increased signal intensity on the T2-weighted images. Subtle signal changes may be present within the mesencephalon (hypersignal within the substantia nigra and the periaqueductal region) and the central tegmental tracts of the pons. The cerebellar white matter is not involved. Diffusion-weighted images show hypersignal within the white matter lesions, suggestive of vacuolating myelinopathy. The diffusion-weighted abnormalities (similar to the conventional MR imaging findings) may remain visible on follow-up studies even after a few years.

ORGANIC ACIDEMIAS

Many of the organic acidopathies fall into the group of devastating metabolic disease of the newborn, others have later and an often insidious onset. Typically, gray matter abnormalities dominate the imaging findings. White matter involvement may also be present which is usually less prominent. Occasionally, organic acidopathies present with a leukodystrophy like presentation but gray matter lesions are always conspicuous.[112]

Methylmalonic Acidemia

It is caused by a defect in methylmalonyl CoA mutase. Acidosis and hyperammonemia can be severe and a single attack can cause permanent cognitive disability. Seizures, spasticity, behavior problems and ataxia are common. Metabolic stroke with an acute decompensation can occur.

Imaging Findings During Metabolic Crisis

In methylmalonic aciduria, the most typical and often the sole abnormality is the symmetrical signal changes withintheglobipallidi,whichisassociatedwithswelling[112] **(Figs. 33A to C)**. The caudate nuclei, the putamina and the thalami are spared. The cortex is normal. During the acute metabolic crisis, diffusion-weighted images show hypersignal within the lesion areas. MR spectroscopy may show a small amount of lactate within the lesions. No disease specific metabolites are demonstrated.

Imaging Findings After Metabolic Crisis

The globus pallidus lesions undergo necrotic changes; they are markedly atrophic and continue to show hypersignal on the T2-weighted images. Sometimes, mild cerebellar atrophy may be present and subtle signal changes within the dentate nuclei suggest some damage too. In early onset cases, delayed myelination is frequently seen.

Differential diagnoses in bilateral globus pallidus disease without involvement of the other basal ganglia components include methylmalonic aciduria, kernicterus and carbon monoxide intoxication. In kernicterus, lesions of subthalamic nuclei are associated with the globus pallidus lesions. Carbon monoxide intoxication is usually encountered in suggestive clinical settings.

Management consists of vitamin $B_{1,2}$ supplementation and dietary protein restriction.

Propionic Acidemia

It is also a disorder of organic acid metabolism. It is a relatively common organic acidopathy. The deficiency enzyeme is propionyl coenzyme A carboxylase. Clinical

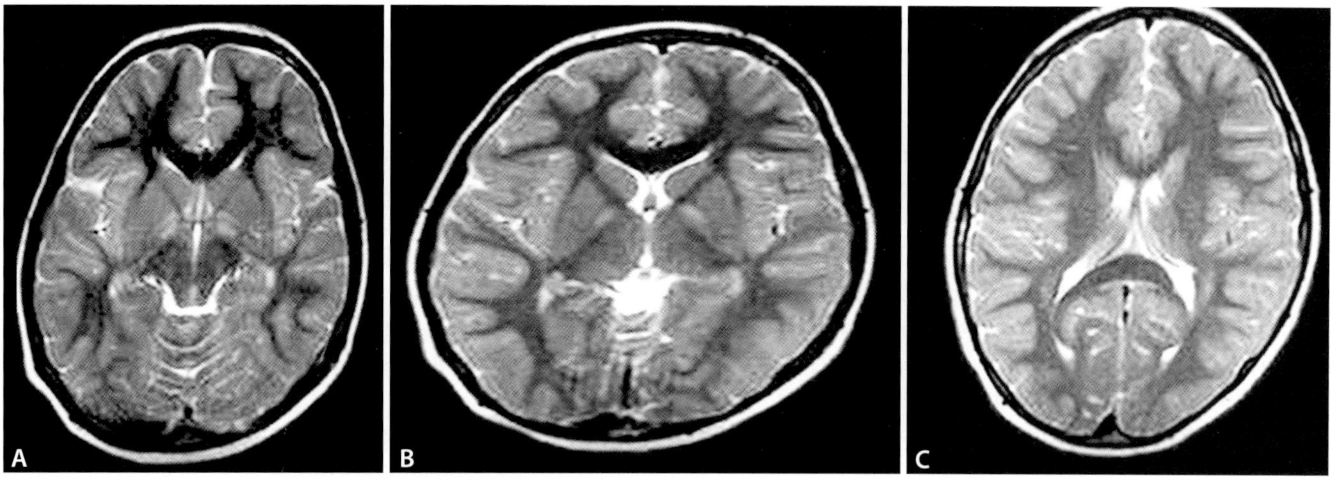

Figs. 33A to C: Axial T2W MR images showing symmetrical signal changes within the globi pallidi seen as a high signal (A and B); No other area of signal abnormality seen (C)—Methylmalonic acidemia.

features include cognitive disability, cardiomyopathy, pancreatitis, osteoporosis and movement disorders

Imaging Findings

During metabolic crisis diffuse brain swelling is seen. Signal abnormalities within the basal ganglia and the dentate nuclei are seen on the T2-weighted images. Subtle signal changes may be present within the pulvinar of the thalami. The cerebral and cerebellar cortices are also affected. The involved gray matter structures are swollen at this stage. White matter structures also show signal changes, mainly subcortically, including the subinsular areas (external and extreme capsules). The corpus callosum, the internal capsule and corticospinal tracts are spared. Diffusion-weighted images usually show moderate signal increase within the involved gray matter structures and the subcortical white matter.

MR spectroscopy demonstrates lactate within the lesion areas consistent with impairment of the energy metabolism resulting in anaerobic glycolysis. No disease-specific metabolites are identified.

Ethylmalonic Acidemia

Ethylmalonic aciduria typically presents with basal ganglia disease but patchy white matter lesions may also be present within the cerebral hemispheres. The signal changes within the heads of the caudate nuclei and the putamina are patchy and inhomogeneous. This may help to raise the possibility of the disease and differentiate it from other organic acidopathies. A distinct clinical feature of the disease is the widespread cutaneous petechiae and ecchymoses indicative of vasculopathy.[113]

Methylglutaconic Aciduria

The disease has at least four clinical phenotypic presentations. Type 2 has an X-linked inheritance, the others are autosomal recessive. The typical imaging presentation in types 1 and 4 of this metabolic disorder is, as in many other organic acidopathies, also the symmetrical bilateral basal ganglia disease.

Imaging Findings

During the acute stage of the disease, the basal ganglia are swollen and exhibit high signal on the diffusion-weighted images suggestive of cytotoxic edema. Sometimes, only the globi pallidi, the caudate nuclei and the anterior parts of the putamina are involved; posteriorly they are spared. With the progression of the disease, the putaminal abnormalities become complete. In some cases, ill defined, diffuse cerebral white matter signal changes are also present. During the metabolic crisis the cerebellar cortex and the dentate nuclei may also show signal abnormalities. Cerebellar atrophy is a very characteristic imaging finding. The vermis is usually more affected than the cerebellar hemispheres. **The association of cerebellar atrophy and basal ganglia disease is a suggestive imaging pattern of 3-methylglutaconic aciduria.**

On MR spectroscopy lactate is present within the lesion areas but no disease specific metabolite is identified.

3-Hydroxy-3-methylglutaryl (HMG)-Coenzyme a Lyase Deficiency

This is a relatively rare metabolic disorder of the L-leucine break down pathway. The disease may present with metabolic crises with hypoglycemia and ketoacidosis. MR imaging usually reveals nonspecific abnormalities.

Since the disease usually starts in the early postnatal period or in early infancy, initially the gray matter abnormalities are easier to depict, since the white matter is not myelinated. Later, as the brain myelination progresses, the white matter changes, which correspond to demyelination become more apparent. The gray matter abnormalities involve the basal ganglia and the dentate nuclei. They are fairly subtle in most cases and do not seem to lead to necrosis if the disease is appropriately treated. The white matter abnormalities within the cerebral hemispheres are sometimes patchy, but usually confluent. The subcortical U-fibers are often spared. Diffusion-weighted imaging shows faint hyper-signal within the involved white matter structures.

MR spectroscopy invariably demonstrates disease specific abnormalities with *two abnormal peaks at the 1.3 and 2.4 ppm levels.*

Glutaric Aciduria Type 1

Glutaric aciduria type 1 is usually an insidiously developing metabolic disease. The disorder may be diagnosed during a metabolic crisis, which is typically triggered by a febrile illness.

In the clinically mild phenotypes no parenchymal lesions may be seen. Patients with type 1 glutaric aciduria are usually macrocephalic. Another peculiar imaging finding is the bilateral enlargement of the sylvian fissures. They may correspond to arachnoidal cysts or disturbed and incomplete opercularization. They are usually bilateral but not necessarily symmetrical. Rarely, the abnormality is unilateral. These changes may be detected prenatally or in the early postnatal period by ultrasound. Macrocephaly and sylvian fissure abnormalities are present in both the clinically benign and malignant phenotypes.

Prominent brain atrophy may also develop. Chronic subdural hematomas are relatively frequently seen in type 1 glutaric aciduria without any evidence of significant head trauma in the clinical history.

The presence of bilateral sylvian fissure and temporal lobe CSF space enlargement and bilateral basal ganglia lesions in a macrocephalic child are almost pathognomonic of type 1 glutaric aciduria **(Figs. 34A to C)**. T2 prolongation is seen in the basal ganglia, most commonly the putamen, less commonly, the caudate and rarely the globus pallidus and periventricular white matter.[114]

MR spectroscopy may show lactate within the basal ganglia during the acute stage of the disease. Although the possible role of glutamine glutamate complexes in the pathogenesis of basal ganglia disease has been raised (glutamine 'excitotoxicity'or glutamine 'suicide') increased glutamine glutamate levels have not been demonstrated within the basal ganglia by *in vivo* MR spectroscopy. **Table 4** gives the differentiating features between various amino acid disorders.

METABOLIC DISORDERS PRIMARILY AFFECTING GRAY MATTER

Hallervorden–Spatz Disease

It is a rare metabolic disorder that is characterized clinically by progressive gait impairment, gradually increasing rigidity of all limbs, choreoathetoid movements,

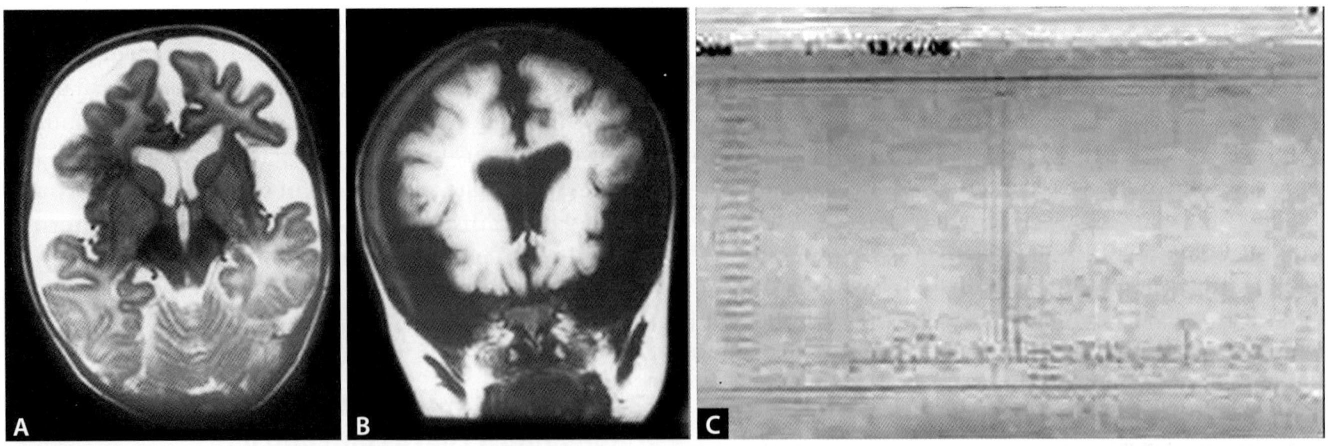

Figs. 34A to C: Axial T2W (A) and FLAIR coronal (B) MR images showing enlargement of bilateral sylvian fissures (A) with cysts in the temporal lobes (B) and signal abnormality in the bilateral putamen (A). Urine gas chromatography mass spectroscopy (C) revealing an abnormal glutaric acid peak—Glutaric aciduria type 1.

Table 4: Disorders of amino acid metabolism.[16]

Disease	*Imaging findings*	*Clinical findings*
Maple syrup urine disease	Swelling and increase signal T2WI: Brainstem, GP, cerebellum, posterior limb of internal capsule	• *Neonate*: Coma • Seizures • Respiratory failure
Glutaric aciduria type 1	Prominent extra-axial spaces, increase signal T2 WI: Bilateral caudate, putamen; delay in myelination	• Infancy/childhood • Encephalopathy • Macrocephaly
Phenylketonuria	Delay in myelination; increase signal T2WI; periatrial WM	• Normal at birth • Developmental delay • Varying severity
Nonketotic hyperglycinemia	Increase signal T2WI: Periventricular WM; delay in myelination	• Early infancy • Vomiting, seizures • Apnea
Urea cycle defects	Neonates: Brain swelling acute stages: Multifocal swollen areas cortex and subcortical WM chronic stages: diffuse atrophy, delay in myelination	• *Infancy*: Lethargy, coma • *Childhood*: Episodic lethargy, confusion, ataxia, dysarthria, coma

dysarthria and mental retardation. In the classic form onset of symptoms occurs before the age of 10 years while the atypical form has an older age of onset.

The striking pathologic finding in affected patients is rust brown pigmentation of the globus pallidus and zona reticulata of the substantia nigra. Iron is concentrated in these regions.

Imaging studies reflect the underlying pathology. Computed tomography scans show high or low density foci in the globi-pallidi. Magnetic resonance shows a pronounced hypointensity of both the globus pallidus and substantia nigra on T2W images resulting from iron deposition.

Imaging reveals a characteristic "eye of the tiger sign" with marked pallidal hypointensity peripherally and hyperintensity centrally. The hyperintense signal represents pallidal destruction and gliosis.

Neuronal Ceroid Lipofuscinosis (NCL)

These are among the most common progressive encephalopathies of childhood. Eight types have been described and are grouped together because of similar pathologic and clinical presentation. The first symptom is loss of vision followed by progressive dementia, seizures and progressive impairment of speech and motor function. Definitive diagnosis is made by chromosomal analysis or by electron microscopic analysis of lymphocytes from peripheral blood which show characteristic curvilinear deposits.

Imaging Findings

There is variable cerebral and cerebellar atrophy associated with high signal rims around ventricles and low signal intensity in the thalami and globi pallidi on T2 weighted images. The T2 changes appear to correlate with loss of myelin and gliosis of unknown origin. Thalamic atrophy develops later. MR spectroscopy shows a complete loss of NAA peak, marked reduction of creatine and choline and elevation of myoinositol and lactate in gray and white matter.[115] PET AND SPECT are useful in establishing the diagnosis in NCL. Severe reduction of metabolism in the cortical and subcortical structures have been shown in 18 fluorodeoxyglucose PET studies.

Rett Syndrome

Rett syndrome is a progressive neurodevelopmental disorder characterized by autistic like behavior, gait, ataxia, irregular respiration, seizures, dementia and microcephaly. On imaging, there is a global reduction in gray and white matter volumes with the largest reductions in the prefrontal, posterior frontal, anterior temporal cortices and the caudate nucleus. Proton MRS shows decreased NAA in older patients, more pronounced in gray matter than the white. The frontal and parietal lobes and insular cortex are the ones which are predominantly involved.

DISORDERS OF METAL METABOLISM

Wilson's Disease (Hepatolenticular Degeneration)

Wilson's disease results from an inborn error of copper meta-bolism and is transmitted in an autosomal recessive manner. It is characterized by a deficiency of ceruloplasmin, the serum transport protein for copper. As a result, copper is abnormally deposited in various tissues with resultant toxicity to these organs. Liver and brain are the most frequently involved with typical involvement of the lenticular nucleus.

Clinical Features

The peak age of presentation is between 8 and 16 years. Typical neurologic signs include tremor, rigidity, dystonia, gait difficulty incoordination and dysarthria. The Kayser-Fleischer ring, ring of green pigmentation in cornea, is virtually diagnostic of Wilson's disease.

Imaging

Typical sites of cerebral involvement are deep gray matter. Gray matter involvement is usually bilaterally symmetric in the putamen, caudate, thalamus, globus pallidus, dentate nucleus, pons and mesencephalon and the claustra. *Involvement of the claustra is a very characteristic finding and an important differential diagnostic clue in Wilson's disease.* The lesions are seen as hyperintensity on long TR images and reflect the pathologic changes of gliosis, edema and/or necrosis. *Mesencephalic involvement is characteristic, the so called "face of the giant panda sign"* **(Figs. 35A to C)**. This consists of high signal throughout the mesencephalon within the substantia nigra (mainly in the pars compacta) and the tegmentum of the mesencephalon in contrast with the normal or hypointense appearance of the red nuclei, the cerebral peduncles and the tectum. Some of these lesions appear to improve or reverse during treatment. In contrast to gray matter lesions, white matter lesions, if present are asymmetric, located in the subcortical regions and are commonest in the frontal lobes. The MR findings correlate well with neurologic findings. Lesion location is also useful. For example, dystonia correlates with putaminal lesions, dysarthria with both caudate and putaminal lesion and distractibility of gaze fixation with frontal lobe involvement. MR spectroscopy shows a decrease in all the metabolites.[116]

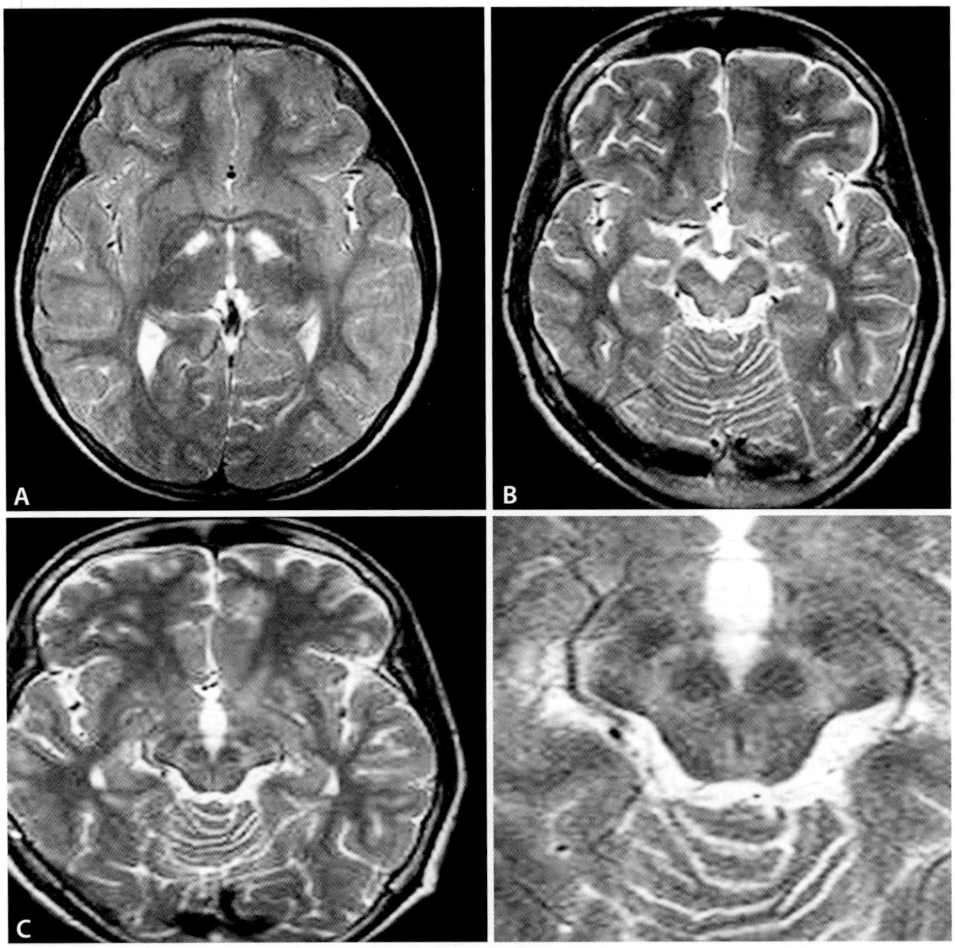

Figs. 35A to C: Axial T2W MR images showing symmetrical signal changes in the putamen seen as a high signal. High signal is also seen within the substantia nigra and tegmentum with sparing of the red nucleus and tectum (C) "face of giant panda sign"—Wilson's disease.

Menkes' Disease

Menkes' disease is related to a defect at the level of the membrane copper transport mechanism. One of the consequences of this is the impairment of the normal intestinal absorption of copper as a result of which a severe copper deficiency develops. On the other hand, transmembrane transport of copper is impaired, therefore, copper cannot be delivered to copper requiring enzymes, and hence copper is trapped and accumulated in connective tissues. Serum copper and ceruloplasmin levels are low. The most important manifestations of the disease are therefore connective tissue abnormalities and progressive degeneration of the central nervous system, the latter due to global failure of copper-requiring enzymes, in particular cytochrome C-oxidase.

The disease is of X-linked inheritance. The onset of the disease is neonatal but the patients are typically normal during the first 2 or 3 months of life. Then there is loss of milestones, convulsions, hypotonia followed by spasticity and eventually lethargy. Most affected children die during the first year of life. Menkes disease is often referred to as 'kinky hair' disease because of the peculiar appearance of the hair. Connective tissue abnormalities include bladder diverticula, inguinal hernia, loose skin, hyperflexible joints and vessel wall fragility.

At birth, the brain appears normal on MR imaging. During the course of the disease rapidly developing atrophy and prominent delay of the myelination become obvious. Shrinking of the brain can be so marked that spontaneous subdural fluid collections (hygroma, subdural hematoma) frequently develop. On the T1-weighted images the basal ganglia exhibit hypersignal, similar to what is seen in chronic hepatic encephalopathies, including Wilson disease. The cerebral vessels are usually tortuous and elongated; this can be seen on conventional images but is better appreciated on MR angiography.[117]

CONCLUSION

There are many different metabolic disorders, each of which has some distinctive features. MR imaging is highly sensitive in determining the presence and assessing the severity of underlying abnormalities in patients with metabolic disorders. Although the findings are often nonspecific, systematic analysis of the finer details of disease involvement may permit a narrower differential diagnosis, which the clinician can then further refine with knowledge of patient history, clinical testing and metabolic analysis. MR imaging has a role in monitoring the natural progression of various metabolic disorders and response to therapy.

REFERENCES

1. Holland BA, Haas DK, Norman D, et al. MRI of normal brain maturation. Am J Neuroradiol. 1986;7:201-8.
2. Hasegawa M, Houdou S, Mito T, et al. Development of myelination in the human fetal and infant cerebrum: a myelin basic protein immunohistochemical study. Brain Dev. 1992;14:1.
3. Barkovich AJ, Kjos BO, Jackson DE, et al. Normal maturation of the neonatal and infant brain: MR Imaging at 1.5T. Radiology. 1988;166:173-80.
4. Johnson MA, Pennock JM, Bydder GM, et al. Clinical NMR images of the brain in children: normal and neurologic disease. AJR. 1983;141:1005-18.
5. Dietrich RB. Maturation, myelination and dysmyelination. In Stark DD, Bradley WG (Eds): Magnetic Resonance Imaging, 3rd edition. Mosby; 1999.
6. Barkovich AJ, Jackson DE J. MRI assessment of normal and abnormal brain myelinization. MRI Decisions. 1989;19-25.
7. Dietrich RB, Bradley WG. Normal and abnormal white matter maturation. Seminars in Ultrasound, CT and MR. 1988;9:192-200.
8. Dietrich RB, Bradley WG, Zaragoza EJ, et al. MR evaluation of early myelination patterns in normal and developmentally delayed infants. Am J Neuroradiol. 1988;9:69-76.
9. Becker LE. Lysosomes peroxisomes and mitochondria: Function and disorder. Am J Neuroradiol. 1992;13:609-20.
10. Kendell BE. Disorders of lysosomes peroxisomes and mitochondria. Am J Neuroradiol. 1992;13:621-53.
11. Demaerel P, Faubert C, Wilms G, et al. MR findings in leukodystrophy. Neuroradiology. 1991;33:368-71.
12. Kim TS, Kim IO, Kim WS, et al. MR of childhood metachromatic leukodystrophy. Am J Neuroradiol. 1997;18:733-8.
13. Suzuki K, Armao D, Stone JA, Mukherji SK. Demyelinating diseases, leukodystrophies and other myelin disorders. Neuroimaging Clinics of North America. 2001;2:15-32.
14. Kolodny EH: Sulfatide lipidosis: Metachromatic leukodystrophy. In Scriver CR, Baedet AL, Syl W, et al (Eds): The Metabolic Basis of Inherited Diseases, 6th edition. New York NY: McGraw Hill, 1989.
15. Wolpert SM, Anderson ML, Kaye EM. Metabolic and degenerative disorders. In Wolpert SM, Barnes PD (Eds): MRI in Pediatric Neuroradiology. Mosby; 1992.
16. Nusbaum AO, Rapaleno, O Fung KM, Atlas SW. White matter diseases and inherited metabolic disorders. In Atlas SW (Ed): Magnetic Resonance Imaging of the Brain and Spine, 4th edition. Lippincott Williams and Wilkins; 2009.
17. Waltz G, Harik SI, Haufman B. Adult metachromatic leukodystrophy. Arch Neurol. 1987;44:225.
18. Faerber EN, Melvin JJ, Smergel DM. MRI appearances of metachromatic leukodystrophy. Paediatr Radiol. 1999;29: 669-72.
19. Nowell MA, Grossman RI, Hackney DB, et al. MR imaging of white matter disease in children. Am J Neuroradiol. 1988;9:503.
20. Sener RN. Metachromatic leukodystrophy. Diffusion MR imaging findings. Am J Neuroradiol. 2002;22(3):461-76.

21. Patay Z. Diffusion weighted MR imaging in leukodystrophies. Eur Radiol. 2005;15(11):2284-303.
22. Kruse B, Hanefeld F, Christen HJ, et al. Alterations of brain metabolites in metachromatic leukodystrophy as detected by localized proton magnetic resonance spectroscopy in vivo. J Neurol. 1993;241:68.
23. Suzuki Y, Suzuki K. Krabbe's globoid cell leukodystrophy: Deficiency of galactocerebrosidase in serum, leukocytes and fibroblast. Science. 1971;171:73-5.
24. Zlotogora J, Chakraborty S, Knowlton RG, et al. Krabbe disease locus mapped to chromosome 14 by genetic linkage. Am J Hum Genet. 1990;47:37-44.
25. Loes DJ, Peters C, Krivit W. Globoid cell leukodystrophy: Distinguishing early onset from late-onset disease using a brain MR imaging scoring method. Am J Neuroradiol. 1999;20: 316-23.
26. Demaerel P, Wilms G, Vendue P, et al. MR findings in globoid leukodystrophy. Neuroradiology. 1990;32:520.
27. Kolodny EH, Raghavan S, Krivit W. Late onset Krabbe disease (globoid cell leukodystrophy): Clinical and biochemical features of 15 cases. Dev Neurosci. 1991;13:232.
28. Lyon G, Hagberg B, Evard PH, et al. Symptomatology of late onset Krabbe's leukodystrophy: The European experience. Dev Neurosci. 1991;13:240.
29. Krivit W, Shapiro EG, Peters C, et al. Hematopoietic cell transplantation in globoid cell leukodystrophy. N Eng J Med. 1998;338:1119-26.
30. Barone R, Bruhl K, Stoeter P, et al. Clinical and neuroradiological findings in classic infantile and late onset globoid cell leukodystrophy (Krabbe's disease). Am J Med Genet. 1996;63:209-17.
31. Vanhanen SL, Raininko R, Santavilori P. Early differential diagnosis of infantile ceroid lipofuscinosis, Rett Syndrome and Krabbe's disease by CT and MR. Am J Neuroradiol. 1994;15:1443-53.
32. Choi S, Enzmann D. Infantile Krabbe disease: Complementary CT and MR findings. Am J Neuroradiol. 1993;14:1164-6.
33. Jones BV, Barron TF, Towfighi J. Optic nerve enlargement in Krabbe's disease. Am J Neuroradiol. 1999;20:1228-31.
34. Krabbe K. A new familial, infantile form of diffuse brain sclerosis. Brain. 1916;39:74-114.
35. Barker RH, Trautman JC, Younge BR, et al. Late juvenile onset Krabbe disease. Ophthalmology. 1990;97:1176-80.
36. Loes DJ, Hite S, Moser H, et al. Adrenoleukodystrophy: A scoring method for brain MR observations. Am J Neuroradiol. 1994;15:1761-5.
37. Vasconcellos E, Smith M. MRI nerve root enhancement in Krabbe disease. Pediatric Neurology. 1998;19:151-2.
38. Kim MJ, Provenzale JM, Law M. Magnetic resonance and diffusion tensor imaging in paediatric white matter diseases. Top Magn Reson Imaging. 2006;17(4):265-71.
39. Provenzale JM, Escolar M, Kurtzberg J. Quantitative analysis of diffusion tensor imaging data in serial assessment of Krabbe disease. Ann NY Acad Sci. 2005;1064:220-9.
40. Mc Graw P, et al. Krabbe disease treated with hematopoietic stem cell transplantation: serial assessment of anisotropy measurements—initial experience. Radiology. 2005;236: 221-30.
41. Okada S, McCrea M, O'Brien JS. Sandhoff's disease (GM2 gangliosidosis Type 2): Clinical, chemical and enzyme studies in five patients. Pediat Res. 1972;6:606.
42. Boothman BR, Bamford JM, Parsons MR. Magnetic resonance imaging in Fabry's disease. J Neurol Neurosurg Psychiatry. 1985;51:1240-1.
43. Mirowitz SA, Sartor K, Prensky AJ, et al. Neuro-degenerative diseases of childhood: MR and CT evaluation. J Comput Assist Tomogr. 1991;15:210-22.
44. Murata R, Nakajma S, Tanaka A, et al. MR imaging of the brain in patients with mucopolysaccharidosis. Am J Neuroradiol. 1989;10:1165-70.
45. Johnson MA, Desai S, Hugh Jones K, et al. Magnetic resonance imaging of the brain in Hurler syndrome. Am J Neuroradiol. 1984;5:816-9.
46. Walts RWE, Spellacy E, Kendell BE, et al. Computed tomography studies on patients with mucopolysaccharidosis. Neuroradiology. 1981;21:9-23.
47. Moser HW. Adrenoleukodystrophy: Phenotype, genetics, pathogenesis and therapy. Brain. 1997;120:1485-508.
48. Bezman L, Moser HW. The incidence of X-linked adrenoleukodystrophy and the relative frequency of its phenotypes. Am J Med Genet. 1998;76:415-9.
49. Griffin JW, Goren E, Schaumberg HH, et al. Adreno-myeloneuropathy: a probable variant of adrenoleukodystrophy. Neurology. 1977;27:1107-13.
50. Schaumburg HH, Powers JM, Raine CS, et al. Adrenoleukodystrophy: A clinical and pathological study of 17 cases. Arch Neurol. 1975;32:577-91.
51. Powers JM, Liu Y, Moser AB, et al. The inflammatory myelinopathy of adrenoleukodystrophy: cells, effector molecules and pathogenetic implications. J Neuropathol Exp Neurol. 1992;51:630-43.
52. Jensen ME. MR imaging appearance of adrenoleukodystrophy with auditory, visual and motor pathway involvement. Radiographics. 1990;10:53.
53. Kumar AJ, Rosenbaum AE, Naidu S, et al. Adrenoleukodystrophy: Correlating MR imaging with CT. Radiology. 1987;165:497.
54. Ono J, Kodaka R, Imai K, et al. Evaluation of myelination by means of T2 value on magnetic resonance imaging. Brain Dev. 1993;15:433.
55. Melhem ER, Breiter SN, Ulug AM, et al. Improved tissue characterization in adrenoleukodystrophy using magnetization transfer imaging. Am J Roentgenol. 1996;166:689-95.
56. Melhem ER, Loes DJ, Georgiades CS, et al. X-linked adrenoleukodystrophy: The role of contrast enhanced MR imaging in predicting disease progression. Am J Neuroradiol. 2000;21:839-44.
57. Barkovich AJ, Ferriero DM, Bass N, et al. Involvement of the pontomedullary corticospinal tracts: a useful finding in the diagnosis of X-linked adrenoleukodystrophy. Am J Neuroradiol. 1997;18:95-100.

58. Castellote A, Vera J, Vazquez E, et al. MR in adrenoleukodystrophy: atypical presentation as bilateral frontal demyelination. Am J Neuroradiol. 1995;16:814-5.
59. Tzika AA, Ball WAS, Vigneron DB, et al. Childhood adrenoleukodystrophy: assessment with proton MR spectroscopy. Radiology. 1993;189:467-80.
60. Warren DJ, et al. Magnetic resonance spectroscopy changes following hematopoietic stem cell transplantation in children with cerebral adrenoleukodystrophy. Dev Med Child Neurol. 2007;49(2):135-9.
61. Wilken B, et al. Quantitative proton magnetic resonance spectroscopy of children with adrenoleukodystrophy before and after hematopoietic stem cell transplantation. Neuropediatrics. 2003;34:237-46.
62. Fatemi A, et al. Magnetization transfer MRI demonstrates spinal cord abnormalities in adrenomyeloneurophathy. Neurology. 2005;64(10):1739-45.
63. Barkovich AJ, Peck WW. MR of Zellweger's syndrome. Am J Neuroradiol. 1997;16:1163-70.
64. Cheon JE, Kim IO, Hwang YS, et al. Leukodystrophy in children: a pictorial review of MR Imaging features. Radiographics. 2002;22:461-76.
65. Hokezu Y, Kuriyama M, Kubota R. Cerebrotendinous xanthomatosis: cranial CT and MRI studies in eight patients. Neuroradiology. 1992;34:308-12.
66. Matalon R, Michals K, Sebasta D, et al. Asparto-acyclase deficiency and N-acetylaspartic aciduria in patients with Canavan's disease. Am J Med Genet. 1988;29: 463-71.
67. Grodd W, et al. In vivo assessment of N-acetylaspartate in brain in spongy degeneration (Canavan's disease) by proton spectroscopy. Lancet. 1990;336(8712):437-8.
68. Patel PJ, Kolawole TM, Mahdi AH, et al. Sonographic and computed tomographic findings in Canavan's disease. Br J Radiol. 1986;59:1226-8.
69. Brismar J, Brismar G, Gascon G, et al. Canavan disease: CT and MR imaging of Canavan disease. Am J Neuroradiol. 1990;11:805-10.
70. McAdam HP, Gcycr CA, Done SL, et al: CT and MR Imaging of Canavan disease. Am J Neuroradiol. 1990;11:397-9.
71. Srikanth SG, et al. Restricted diffusion in Canavan disease. Child Nerv Syst. 2007;23(4):465-8.
72. Lyon G, Fattal-Valevski A, Kolodny EH. Leukodystrophies: Clinical and genetic aspect. Top Magn Reson Imaging. 2006;17(4):219-42.
73. Brrett D, Becker LE. Alexander's disease: a disease of astrocytes. Brain. 1985;108:367-85.
74. Shah M, Ross JS: Infantile Alexander disease: MR appearance of a biopsy proven case. Am J Neuroradiol. 1990;11:1105-6.
75. Trommer BL, Naidich JP, Dal Canto MC, et al. Noninvasive CT diagnosis of infantile Alexander's disease: Pathologic correlation. J Comput Assist Tomogr. 1983;7: 509-16.
76. Van der Knaap MS, Barth PG, Gabreels FJM, et al. A new leukoencephalopathy with Vanishing white matter. Neurology. 1997;48:845-55.
77. Sijens PE et al. ^{1}H chemical shift imaging, MRI and diffusion weighted imaging in vanishing white matter disease. Eur Radiol. 2005;15(11):2377-9.
78. Seitelberger F. Neuropathology and genetics of Pelizaeus-Merzbacher disease. Brain Pathol. 1995;5:267-73.
79. Silverstein AM, Hirsh DK, Trobe JD, et al. MR imaging of the brain in five members of a family with Pelizaeus-Merzbacher disease. Am J Neuroradiol. 1990;11:495-9.
80. Van der Knaap MS, Valk J: The reflection of histology in MR imaging of Pelizaeus-Merzbacher disease. Am J Neuroradiol. 1989;10:99-103.
81. Honkaniemi J, Kahari V, Latvala M, et al. Reversible posterior leukoencephalopathy after combination chemotherapy. Neuroradiology. 2000;42:895.
82. Kingsley PB, Shah JC, Woldenberg R. Identification of diffuse and focal brain lesions by clinical magnetic resonance spectroscopy. NMR Biomed. 2006;19(4):435-62.
83. Pavlakis SG, Philips PC, DiMauro S, et al. Mitochondrial myopathy, encephalopathy, lactic acidosis and stroke like episodes: a distinct clinical syndrome. Ann Neurol. 1984;16:481-8.
84. Barkovich AJ, Good WV, Koch TK, et al. Mitochondrial disorders: analysis of their clinical and imaging characteristics. Am J Neuroradiol. 1993;14:1119-37.
85. Allard JC, Tilak S, Carter AP. CT and MR of MELAS syndrome. Am J Neuroradiol. 1988;9:1234-8.
86. Kim IO, Kim JH, Kim SUS, et al. Mitochondrial Myopathy encephalopathylactic acidosis and stroke-like episodes (MELAS) syndrome: CT and MR findings in seven children. AJR. 1996;166:641-5.
87. Rosen L, Phillips S, Enzmann D. Magnetic resonance imaging in MELAS syndrome. Neuroradiology. 1990;32:168-71.
88. Ducreux D, et al. MR diffusion tensor imaging, fiber tracking and single voxel spectroscopy findings in an unusual MELAS case. Am J Neuroradiol. 2005;26(7):1840-4.
89. Wray S, Provenzale J, Johns O, et al. MR of brain in mitochondrial myopathy. Am J Neuroradiol. 1995;16:1167.
90. Fukuhara N, Tokiguchi S, Shirakawa K, et al. Myoclonus epilepsy associated with ragged red fibres (mitochondrial abnormalities): Disease entity or a syndrome? J Neurol Sci. 1980;47:117-33.
91. Kearns TP, Sayre GP. Retinitis pigmentosa, external ophthalmoplegia and complete heart block. Arch Ophthalmol. 1958;60:280-9.
92. Leutner C, Layer G, Zierz S, et al. Cerebral MR in ophthalmoplegia plus. Am J Neuroradiol. 1994;15:681-7.
93. Sandhu FS, Dillon WP. MR demonstration of leukoencephalopathy associated with mitochondrial encephalomyopathy: Case report. Am J Neuroradiol. 1991;12:375-9.
94. DiMauro S, Servidei S, Zeviam M, et al. Cytochrome C oxidase deficiency in Leigh syndrome. Ann Neurol. 1987;22:498-506.
95. Chi JG, Yoo HW, Chang KH, et al. Leigh subacute necrotizing encephalomyelopathy: Possible diagnosis by CT scan. Neuroradiology. 1981;22:141-4.

96. Berkovic SF, Karpati G, Carpenter S, et al. Progressive dystonia with bilateral putaminal hypodensities. Arch Neurol. 1987;44:1184-7.
97. KochTK, YeeMHC, HutchinsonHT, etal. Magneticresonance imaging in subacute necrotizing encephalomyelopathy (Leigh disease). Ann Neurol. 1986;19:605-7.
98. Medina L, Chi TL, DeVivo DC, et al. MR findings in patients with subacute necrotizing encephalomyelopathy (Leigh syndrome): Correlation with biochemical defect. Am J Neuroradiol. 1990;11:379-84.
99. Leigh D. Subacute necrotizing encephalomyelopathy in an infant. J Neurol Neurosurg Psychiatry. 1951;14:216-21.
100. Atalar MH, et al. Magnetic resonance spectroscopy and diffusion weighted imaging findings in a child with Leigh disease. Pediatr Int. 2005;47(5):601-3.
101. Chen YF, Huang YC, Liu HM, et al. MRI in a case of adult onset citrullinemia.Neuroradiology. 2001;43:845-7.
102. Connelly A, Cross JH, Gadian G, et al. Magnetic resonance spectroscopy shows increased brain glutamine in ornithine carbamoyl transferase deficiency. Pediatric Research. 1993;33:77-81.
103. Pearsen KD, Gean Marton AD, Levy HL, Davis KR. Phenylketonuria: MRI of the brain with clinical correlation. Radiology. 1990;177:437-40.
104. Phillips MD, Mc Graw P, Lowe MJ, Mathews VP, Hainline BE. Diffusion weighted imaging of white matter abnormalities in patients with phenylketonuria. Am J Neuroradiol. 2001; 22:1583-6.
105. Pietz J, Kreis R, Schmidt H, et al. Phenylketonuria findings at MR imaging and localized in vivo H- I MR spectroscopy of the brain in patients with early treatment. Raidology. 1996; 201:413-20.
106. Brismar J, Aqueel A, Brusmar G, et al. Maple syrup urine disease. Am J Neuroradiol. 1990;11:1219-28.
107. Fariello G, Dionisi-Vici C, Orazi C, et al. Cranial ultra-sonography in maple syrup urine disease. Am J Neuroradiol. 1996;17:311-5.
108. Jan W, Zimmerman R, Wang Z, et al. MR diffusion imaging and MR spectroscopy of maple syrup urine disease during acute metabolic decompensation. Neuroradiology. 2003; 45:393-9.
109. Rossi A, Cerone R, Biancheri R, et al. Early onset combined methylmalonic aciduria and homocystinuria. Neuroradiologic findings. Am J Neuroradiol. 2001;22:554-63.
110. Press GA, Barshop BA, Haas RH, et al. Abnormalities of the brain in non ketotic hyperglycinemia: MR Manifestations. Am J Neuroradiol. 1989;10:315-21.
111. AI Tawari A, Ramadan P, Neubauer D, et al. An early onset form of methylene terahydrofolate reductase deficiency: A report of a family from Kuwait. Brain Dev. 2002;24:304-9.
112. Brismar J, Ozand P. CT and MR of the brain in the diagnosis of organic acidemias. Experiences from 107 patients. Brain Dev. 1994;16(Suppl):104-24.
113. Ozand P, Rashed M, Millingtian D, et al. Ethylmalonic aciduria: an organic academia with CNS involvement and vasculopathy.Brain Dev. 1994;16(Suppl):12-22.
114. Brismar J, Ozand P. CT and MR of the brain in glutaric academia type 1: a review of 59 published cases and a report of 5 new patients. Am J Neuroradiol. 1995;16:675-83.
115. Brockmann K, et al. Localized proton magnetic resonance spectroscopy of cerebral metabolic disturbances in children with neuronal ceroid lipofuscinosis-Neuropediatrics. 1996;27:242-8.
116. Jayasunder R, Sahani A, Gaikwaid S, Singh S, Behari M. Proton MR spectroscopy of basal ganglia in Wilson disease: case report and review of literature. Mag Reson Imaging. 2002;20:131-5.
117. Jacobs DS, Smith AS, Finelli DA, et al. Menkes Kinky hair disease: characteristic MR angiographic findings. Am J Neuroradiol. 1993;14:1160-3.

AIIMS-MAMC-PGI's
Comprehensive Textbook of

Diagnostic Radiology

AIIMS-MAMC-PGI's Comprehensive Textbook of Diagnostic Radiology

SECOND EDITION

VOLUME 3

- **Chest and Cardiovascular Imaging**
- **Musculoskeletal and Breast Imaging**

Editors

Anju Garg MD
Director Professor and Head
Department of Radiodiagnosis
Maulana Azad Medical College
New Delhi, India

Arun Kumar Gupta MD FAMS
Professor and Head
Department of Radiodiagnosis
All India Institute of Medical Sciences
New Delhi, India

Manavjit Singh Sandhu MD FICR
Professor and Head
Department of Radiodiagnosis
Postgraduate Institute of Medical Education and Research, Chandigarh, India

JAYPEE

JAYPEE BROTHERS MEDICAL PUBLISHERS
The Health Sciences Publisher
New Delhi | London | Panama

Jaypee Brothers Medical Publishers (P) Ltd.

Headquarters
Jaypee Brothers Medical Publishers (P) Ltd.
4838/24, Ansari Road, Daryaganj
New Delhi 110 002, India
Phone: +91-11-43574357
Fax: +91-11-43574314
Email: jaypee@jaypeebrothers.com

Overseas Offices
JP Medical Ltd.
83, Victoria Street, London
SW1H 0HW (UK)
Phone: +44 20 3170 8910
Fax: +44 (0)20 3008 6180
E-mail: info@jpmedpub.com

Jaypee-Highlights Medical Publishers Inc.
City of Knowledge, Bld. 235, 2nd Floor, Clayton
Panama City, Panama
Phone: +1 507-301-0496
Fax: +1 507-301-0499
E-mail: cservice@jphmedical.com

Jaypee Brothers Medical Publishers (P) Ltd.
Bhotahity, Kathmandu, Nepal
Phone: +977-9741283608
E-mail: kathmandu@jaypeebrothers.com

Website: www.jaypeebrothers.com
Website: www.jaypeedigital.com

Inquiries for bulk sales may be solicited at: jaypee@jaypeebrothers.com

AIIMS-MAMC-PGI's Comprehensive Textbook of Diagnostic Radiology (Volumes 1 to 3)

First Edition: 2016
Second Edition: **2019**

ISBN: 978-93-5270-704-1

Printed at: Replika Press Pvt. Ltd.

Dedicated to

THE SUPREME BEING
Who so mercifully helps us to accomplish gigantic tasks
so smoothly, effortlessly and so beautifully

Associate Editors

VOLUME 1

SECTION 1: Neuroradiology including Head and Neck Imaging

Paramjeet Singh MD
Professor
Department of Radiodiagnosis
Postgraduate Institute of Medical Education and Research
Chandigarh, India

Vivek Gupta MD DM
Professor
Department of Radiodiagnosis
Postgraduate Institute of Medical Education and Research
Chandigarh, India

Shailesh B Gaikwad MD
Professor and Head
Department of Neuroimaging and Interventional Neuroradiology (CN Centre)
All India Institute of Medical Sciences
New Delhi, India

Ajay Garg MD
Professor
Department of Neuroimaging and Interventional Neuroradiology (CN Centre)
All India Institute of Medical Sciences
New Delhi, India

SECTION 2: Recent Advances and Applied Physics in Imaging

Sanjay Sharma MD DNB MNAMS FRCR FICR
Professor
Department of Radiodiagnosis
Dr Rajendra Prasad Centre for Ophthalmic Sciences
All India Institute of Medical Sciences
New Delhi, India

Ashu Seith Bhalla MD MAMS FICR
Professor
Department of Radiodiagnosis
All India Institute of Medical Sciences
New Delhi, India

Smriti Hari MD MAMS
Professor
Department of Radiodiagnosis
All India Institute of Medical Sciences
New Delhi, India

VOLUME 2

SECTION 3: Gastrointestinal and Hepatobiliary Imaging

Deep Narayan Srivastava MD MBA FAMS FICR
Professor
Department of Radiodiagnosis
All India Institute of Medical Sciences
New Delhi, India

Raju Sharma MD MAMS FICR
Professor
Department of Radiodiagnosis
All India Institute of Medical Sciences
New Delhi, India

SECTION 4: Genitourinary Imaging

Anupam Lal MD
Professor
Department of Radiodiagnosis
Postgraduate Institute of Medical Education and Research
Chandigarh, India

SECTION 5: Pediatric Imaging

Ashu Seith Bhalla MD MAMS FICR
Professor
Department of Radiodiagnosis
All India Institute of Medical Sciences
New Delhi, India

Sanjay Thulkar MD
Professor
Department of Radiodiagnosis
Dr BRA Institute—Rotary Cancer Hospital
All India Institute of Medical Sciences
New Delhi, India

VOLUME 3

SECTION 6: Chest and Cardiovascular Imaging

Sanjiv Sharma MD
Professor and Head
Department of Cardiac Radiology
Cardio-Thoracic Sciences Centre
All India Institute of Medical Sciences
New Delhi, India

Rashmi Dixit MD
Director Professor
Department of Radiodiagnosis
Maulana Azad Medical College
New Delhi, India

SECTION 7: Musculoskeletal and Breast Imaging

Anjali Prakash DMRD DNB MNAMS
Director Professor
Department of Radiodiagnosis
Maulana Azad Medical College
New Delhi, India

Contributors

Ajay Garg MD
Professor
Department of Neuroimaging and Interventional Neuroradiology (CN Centre)
All India Institute of Medical Sciences
New Delhi, India

Ajay Gulati MD MAMS
Additional Professor
Department of Radiodiagnosis
Postgraduate Institute of Medical Education and Research, Chandigarh, India

Ajay Kumar MD
Professor
Department of Radiodiagnosis and Imaging
Postgraduate Institute of Medical Education and Research, Chandigarh, India

Akshay Kumar Saxena MD Dip NBE
Professor
Department of Radiodiagnosis
Postgraduate Institute of Medical Education and Research, Chandigarh, India

Alpana Manchanda MD
Director Professor
Department of Radiodiagnosis
Maulana Azad Medical College
New Delhi, India

Amar Mukund MD
Associate Professor
Department of Radiodiagnosis
Institute of Liver and Biliary Sciences (ILBS)
New Delhi, India

Anil Chauhan
MBBS Board Certified in Radiology, USA
Fellow, Body Imaging
Department of Radiology
University of Texas MD Anderson Cancer Center, Houston, USA

Anil K Pandey PhD
Assistant Professor (Medical Physics)
Department of Nuclear Medicine
All India Institute of Medical Sciences
New Delhi, India

Anindita Sinha MD
Additional Professor
Department of Radiodiagnosis
Postgraduate Institute of Medical Education and Research, Chandigarh, India

Anish Bhattacharya DNB DRM MNAMS
Professor
Department of Nuclear Medicine
Postgraduate Institute of Medical Education and Research, Chandigarh, India

Anjali Prakash DMRD DNB MNAMS
Director Professor
Department of Radiodiagnosis
Maulana Azad Medical College
New Delhi, India

Anju Garg MD
Director Professor and Head
Department of Radiodiagnosis
Maulana Azad Medical College
New Delhi, India

Ankur Gadodia MD DNB FRCR
Consultant
Goyal MRI and Diagnostic Centre
New Delhi, India

Ankur Goyal MD DNB MNAMS
Assistant Professor
Department of Radiodiagnosis
All India Institute of Medical Sciences
New Delhi, India

Anmol Bhatia MD
Assistant Professor
Department of Radiodiagnosis and Imaging
Postgraduate Institute of Medical Education and Research, Chandigarh, India

Anuj Prabhakar DNB DM
Assistant Professor
Department of Neuroimaging and Interventional Neuroradiology (CN Centre)
All India Institute of Medical Sciences
New Delhi, India

Anupam Lal MD
Professor
Department of Radiodiagnosis
Postgraduate Institute of Medical Education and Research, Chandigarh, India

Arun Deep Arora MD
Former Senior Research Associate
Department of Radiodiagnosis
All India Institute of Medical Sciences
New Delhi, India

Arun Kumar Gupta MD FAMS
Professor and Head
Department of Radiodiagnosis
All India Institute of Medical Sciences
New Delhi, India

Arun Malhotra DRM PhD
Former Professor and Head
Department of Nuclear Medicine
All India Institute of Medical Sciences
New Delhi, India

Ashu Seith Bhalla MD MAMS FICR
Professor
Department of Radiodiagnosis
All India Institute of Medical Sciences
New Delhi, India

Atin Kumar MD DNB MNAMS
Professor
Department of Radiodiagnosis
Jai Prakash Narayan Apex Trauma Center
All India Institute of Medical Sciences
New Delhi, India

BR Mittal MD DRM DNB FICNM FAMS
Professor and Head
Department of Nuclear Medicine
Postgraduate Institute of Medical Education and Research, Chandigarh, India

Chandan Jyoti Das MD DNB MNAMS
Associate Professor
Department of Radiodiagnosis
All India Institute of Medical Sciences
New Delhi, India

Chandrashekhara SH MD DNB MNAMS
Associate Professor
Department of Radiodiagnosis
Dr BRA Institute—Rotary Cancer Hospital
All India Institute of Medical Sciences
New Delhi, India

Chirag Kamal Ahuja MD DM
Assistant Professor
Department of Radiodiagnosis and Imaging
Postgraduate Institute of Medical Education and Research, Chandigarh, India

Deep Narayan Srivastava MD MBA FAMS FICR
Professor
Department of Radiodiagnosis
All India Institute of Medical Sciences
New Delhi, India

Devasenathipathy Kandasamy MD DNB FRCR
Associate Professor
Department of Radiodiagnosis
All India Institute of Medical Sciences
New Delhi, India

Ekta Dhamija MD
Assistant Professor
Department of Radiodiagnosis
Dr BRA Institute—Rotary Cancer Hospital
All India Institute of Medical Sciences
New Delhi, India

Gaurav S Pradhan MBBS DMRD DNB
Director Professor
Department of Radiodiagnosis
Maulana Azad Medical College
New Delhi, India

Gurpreet Singh Gulati MD
Professor
Department of Cardiac Radiology
Cardio-Thoracic Sciences Centre
All India Institute of Medical Sciences
New Delhi, India

Hina Arif Mumtaz MD DNB
Former Senior Research Associate
Department of Radiodiagnosis
Postgraduate Institute of Medical Education and Research, Chandigarh, India

Jyoti Kumar MD DNB MNAMS
Professor
Department of Radiodiagnosis
Maulana Azad Medical College
New Delhi, India

Kartik Ganga MD
Fellow
Department of Cardiovascular Radiology and Endovascular Interventions
All India Institute of Medical Sciences
New Delhi, India

Kirti Gupta
MD Neuropathology Fellowship (St Jude, USA)
Professor
Department of Histopathology
Postgraduate Institute of Medical Education and Research, Chandigarh, India

Kumble S Madhusudhan MD FRCR MAMS
Associate Professor
Department of Radiodiagnosis
All India Institute of Medical Sciences
New Delhi, India

Kushaljit Singh Sodhi MD MNAMS FICR
Professor
Department of Radiodiagnosis
Postgraduate Institute of Medical Education and Research, Chandigarh, India

Kusum Joshi MD PhD
Professor and Former Head
Department of Histopathology
Postgraduate Institute of Medical Education and Research, Chandigarh, India

Mahesh Prakash MD MAMS FICR
Professor
Department of Radiodiagnosis
Postgraduate Institute of Medical Education and Research, Chandigarh, India

Manavjit Singh Sandhu MD FICR
Professor and Head
Department of Radiodiagnosis
Postgraduate Institute of Medical Education and Research, Chandigarh, India

Mandeep Garg MD FRCR
Professor
Department of Radiodiagnosis
Postgraduate Institute of Medical Education and Research, Chandigarh, India

Mandeep Kang MD DNB MAMS FICR
Professor
Department of Radiodiagnosis
Postgraduate Institute of Medical Education and Research, Chandigarh, India

Manisha Jana MD DNB FRCR
Associate Professor
Department of Radiodiagnosis
All India Institute of Medical Sciences
New Delhi, India

Manish Modi MD DM
Professor
Department of Neurology
Postgraduate Institute of Medical Education and Research, Chandigarh, India

Manphool Singhal MD DNB MNAMS
Additional Professor
Department of Radiodiagnosis
Postgraduate Institute of Medical Education and Research, Chandigarh, India

Mukesh Kumar Yadav MD
Assistant Professor
Department of Radiodiagnosis
Dr BRA Institute—Rotary Cancer Hospital
All India Institute of Medical Sciences
New Delhi, India

Naveen Kalra MD MAMS FICR
Professor
Department of Radiodiagnosis
Postgraduate Institute of Medical Education and Research, Chandigarh, India

Nidhi Prabhakar MD DNB
Assistant Professor
Department of Radiodiagnosis
Postgraduate Institute of Medical Education and Research, Chandigarh, India

Niranjan Khandelwal MD Dip NBE FICR FAMS
Former Head
Department of Radiodiagnosis
Postgraduate Institute of Medical Education and Research, Chandigarh, India

Pankaj Gupta MD DNB
Assistant Professor
Department of Radiodiagnosis and Imaging
Postgraduate Institute of Medical Education and Research, Chandigarh, India

Paramjeet Singh MD
Professor
Department of Radiodiagnosis
Postgraduate Institute of Medical Education and Research, Chandigarh, India

Pratik Kumar PhD Dip RP
Professor
Medical Physics Unit
Dr BRA Institute—Rotary Cancer Hospital
All India Institute of Medical Sciences
New Delhi, India

Priya Jagia MD DNB
Professor
Department of Cardiovascular Radiology
and Endovascular Interventions
All India Institute of Medical Sciences
New Delhi, India

Priyanka Naranje MD DNB MNAMS
Assistant Professor
Department of Radiodiagnosis
All India Institute of Medical Sciences
New Delhi, India

Punit Sharma MD
Former Senior Resident
Department of Nuclear Medicine
All India Institute of Medical Sciences
New Delhi, India

Radhika Batra MD DNB
Assistant Professor
Department of Radiodiagnosis
Maulana Azad Medical College
New Delhi, India

Radhika Srinivasan MD PhD
Professor
Department of Cytology and
Gynec-pathology
Postgraduate Institute of Medical Education
and Research, Chandigarh, India

Rajat Jain MD
Former Senior Resident
Department of Radiodiagnosis
Maulana Azad Medical College
New Delhi, India

Raju Sharma MD MAMS FICR
Professor
Department of Radiodiagnosis
All India Institute of Medical Sciences
New Delhi, India

Rakesh Kumar MD PhD
Professor
Department of Nuclear Medicine
All India Institute of Medical Sciences
New Delhi, India

Rakesh Kumar Vasishta MD FRCPath
Professor and Head
Department of Histopathology
Postgraduate Institute of Medical Education
and Research, Chandigarh, India

Rama Mohan Reddy MD (Nuclear Medicine)
Former Senior Resident
Department of Nuclear Medicine
All India Institute of Medical Sciences
New Delhi, India

Rashmi Dixit MD
Director Professor
Department of Radiodiagnosis
Maulana Azad Medical College
New Delhi, India

Sameer Vyas MD DM MAMS
Additional Professor
Department of Radiodiagnosis and Imaging
Postgraduate Institute of Medical Education
and Research, Chandigarh, India

Sanjay Sharma MD DNB MNAMS FRCR FICR
Professor
Department of Radiodiagnosis
Dr Rajendra Prasad Centre for
Ophthalmic Sciences
All India Institute of Medical Sciences
New Delhi, India

Sanjay Thulkar MD
Professor
Department of Radiodiagnosis
Dr BRA Institute—Rotary Cancer Hospital
All India Institute of Medical Sciences
New Delhi, India

Sanjeev Kumar MD
Assistant Professor
Department of Cardiovascular Radiology
and Endovascular Interventions
All India Institute of Medical Sciences
New Delhi, India

Sanjiv Sharma MD
Professor and Head
Department of Cardiac Radiology
Cardio-Thoracic Sciences Centre
All India Institute of Medical Sciences
New Delhi, India

Sapna Singh MD DNB MNAMS
Professor
Department of Radiodiagnosis
Maulana Azad Medical College
New Delhi, India

Satyam DNB MNAMS
Specialist
Department of Radiodiagnosis
Lok Nayak Hospital
New Delhi, India

SC Bansal MA MSc PhD
Former Lecturer
Department of Radiodiagnosis
Postgraduate Institute of Medical Education
and Research, Chandigarh, India

Shailesh B Gaikwad MD
Professor and Head
Department of Neuroimaging and
Interventional Neuroradiology (CN Centre)
All India Institute of Medical Sciences
New Delhi, India

Shamim Ahmed Shamim MD (Nuclear Medicine)
Assistant Professor
Department of Nuclear Medicine
All India Institute of Medical Sciences
New Delhi, India

Shashi Bala Paul PhD MAMS
Senior Scientist
Department of Radiodiagnosis
All India Institute of Medical Sciences
New Delhi, India

Shivanand Gamanagatti MD MAMS
Professor
Department of Radiodiagnosis
(Trauma Center Division)
All India Institute of Medical Sciences
New Delhi, India

Smita Manchanda MD DNB MNAMS
Assistant Professor
Department of Radiodiagnosis
All India Institute of Medical Sciences
New Delhi, India

Smriti Hari MD MAMS
Professor
Department of Radiodiagnosis
All India Institute of Medical Sciences
New Delhi, India

Subrat Kumar Acharya
DM FNASc FASc FNA JC Bose Fellow
Former Professor and Head
Department of Gastroenterology
All India Institute of Medical Sciences
New Delhi, India

Sudesh Prabhakar MD DM
Former Professor and Head
Department of Neurology
Postgraduate Institute of Medical Education
and Research, Chandigarh, India

Sudha Suri MD
Former Emeritus Professor
Department of Radiodiagnosis
Postgraduate Institute of Medical Education
and Research, Chandigarh, India

(Late) Sumedha Pawa MBBS MD
Director Professor
Department of Radiodiagnosis
Maulana Azad Medical College
New Delhi, India

Surabhi Vyas MD DNB MNAMS
Associate Professor
Department of Radiodiagnosis
All India Institute of Medical Sciences
New Delhi, India

Swati Gupta MD DNB FRCR
Assistant Professor
Department of Radiodiagnosis
Maulana Azad Medical College
New Delhi, India

Tulika Singh MD
Additional Professor
Department of Radiodiagnosis
Postgraduate Institute of Medical Education
and Research, Chandigarh, India

Ujjwal Gorsi MD
Assistant Professor
Department of Radiodiagnosis
Postgraduate Institute of Medical Education
and Research, Chandigarh, India

Uma Debi MD
Assistant Professor
Department of Radiodiagnosis
Postgraduate Institute of Medical Education
and Research, Chandigarh, India

Veena Chowdhury MBBS MD
Former Professor of Excellence
Department of Radiodiagnosis
Maulana Azad Medical College
New Delhi, India

Veenu Singla MD
Professor
Department of Radiodiagnosis
Postgraduate Institute of Medical Education
and Research, Chandigarh, India

Vikas Bhatia MD DM
Assistant Professor
Department of Radiodiagnosis
Postgraduate Institute of Medical Education
and Research, Chandigarh, India

Virendra Jain MD FRCR
Former Senior Resident
Department of Radiodiagnosis
Maulana Azad Medical College
New Delhi, India

Vivek Gupta MD DM
Professor
Department of Radiodiagnosis
Postgraduate Institute of Medical Education
and Research, Chandigarh, India

Preface

In 1996, a unique venture was jointly initiated by the faculty of Radiodiagnosis, All India Institute of Medical Sciences (AIIMS), New Delhi; Maulana Azad Medical College (MAMC), New Delhi; and Postgraduate Institute of Medical Education and Research (PGIMER), Chandigarh, India, to organize continuing medical education (CME) programs based on a series of imaging courses. An integral part of this endeavour was publishing books covering all organ systems. The aim was to provide state-of-the-art knowledge for postgraduate students as well as the practicing radiologists along with establishing a uniform pattern of teaching in radiology across the country.

The first series of seven imaging courses was successfully completed in the year 2000. A second series of these courses was then initiated in the year 2002 and was completed in 2004. This was also highly successful. The third series of seven extremely popular and successful courses covering all the organ systems and advances in physics was started in 2008 and was completed in 2013. Currently, the fourth series is underway.

Every course in each of the series has resulted in publication of a book. These books have been very popular amongst residents as well as among practicing radiologists.

Considering the popularity of these books, the editors, along with publishers, M/s Jaypee Brothers Medical Publishers (P) Ltd, New Delhi, India, decided to combine the individual books into three volumes—*AIIMS-MAMC-PGI's Comprehensive Textbook of Diagnostic Radiology*.

In keeping pace with newer developments in the field of diagnostic radiology and in order to cater to the contemporary needs of users, the second edition of *AIIMS-MAMC-PGI's Comprehensive Textbook of Diagnostic Radiology* is now being presented after a gap of three years since the previous edition of this book. It is anticipated that with such a complete coverage of all the subjects, the users will not have to refer to any other book during their routine learning of diagnostic radiology.

We are sure that residents and radiologists will find these comprehensive three volumes easy to handle and very useful in day-to-day practice.

We are once again grateful to all the contributors from the three apex academic institutions of India, i.e. AIIMS, New Delhi; MAMC, New Delhi; and PGIMER, Chandigarh, India.

We are thankful to M/s Jaypee Brothers Medical Publishers (P) Ltd, for helping us to make our dream come true.

Anju Garg
Arun Kumar Gupta
Manavjit Singh Sandhu

Acknowledgments

We would like to put on record our deep appreciation and gratitude:

To Professors Manorama Berry, Sudha Suri and Veena Chowdhury (Past Editors) the three pioneers who in 1996 took a bold initiative and started a unique teaching course now popularly known as AIIMS-MAMC-PGI's imaging course. Up to 2013, three series of these courses have been completed and the fourth series was started at the end of 2016. This course series has become extremely popular and every course is followed by the publication of a book which too is highly appreciated and popular.

To Professors Sima Mukhopadhyay, Sushma Vashisht and Niranjan Khandelwal who have been the Editors of past series and who contributed to organizing the earlier courses in their capacity as Heads of Departments.

To all the Associate Editors of the different course books who put in immense effort to bring the books out on time.

To all the Authors who contributed chapters without whom we could not have collected such an outstanding content of teaching and academic material.

To our respective hospitals for giving us the privilege and unique opportunity to work, which enabled us to amass data from patients and document images of diverse diseases that provide the reader with a wide spectrum of knowledge.

Our sincere and grateful thanks to Shri Jitendar P Vij (Group Chairman), Mr Ankit Vij (Managing Director), Mr MS Mani (Group President), Ms Chetna Malhotra Vohra (Associate Director–Content Strategy), Ms Pooja Bhandari (Production Head), Ms Kritika Dua (Senior Development Editor) and other members of M/s Jaypee Brothers Medical Publishers (P) Ltd, New Delhi, India, for their untiring coordination efforts in the production of this book.

We are very proud indeed at the culmination of two decades of these course series, to compile and present them together in the form of these three volumes of *AIIMS-MAMC-PGI's Comprehensive Textbook of Diagnostic Radiology*.

Contents

VOLUME 1

NEURORADIOLOGY INCLUDING HEAD AND NECK IMAGING, RECENT ADVANCES AND APPLIED PHYSICS IN IMAGING

SECTION 1: Neuroradiology including Head and Neck Imaging

SECTION 2: Recent Advances and Applied Physics in Imaging

VOLUME 2
GASTROINTESTINAL AND HEPATOBILIARY IMAGING, GENITOURINARY AND PEDIATRIC IMAGING

SECTION 3: Gastrointestinal and Hepatobiliary Imaging

SECTION 5: Pediatric Imaging

VOLUME 3
CHEST AND CARDIOVASCULAR IMAGING, MUSCULOSKELETAL AND BREAST IMAGING

SECTION 6: Chest and Cardiovascular Imaging

SECTION 7: Musculoskeletal and Breast Imaging

Section 6

Chest and Cardiovascular Imaging

CHAPTER 156

Chest Radiography and Sonography: Techniques and Anatomy

Mahesh Prakash, Manavjit Singh Sandhu

INTRODUCTION

Chest radiography is the most commonly performed radiological investigation around the world, and it forms an integral part of the routine study of individual case along with and as important as physical examination and laboratory investigations. The Chest radiograph nearly constitutes 50–60% of the total workload of the radiology department of any large or small general hospital. The cornerstone of the radiological diagnosis of the chest diseases is chest radiograph. All other radiological procedures including bronchography, computed tomography (CT) and magnetic resonance imaging (MRI) are strictly ancillary.[1]

Sonography of chest is relatively newer method to evaluate the diseases of thorax particularly useful for pleural and chest wall abnormalities and some pathologies of lungs The techniques and normal anatomy as demonstrated on plain chest radiographs and ultrasound have been discussed herewith.

CONVENTIONAL CHEST RADIOGRAPHY

Conventional film screen radiography using kV range of 50–85 depending on patient's build is the standard and most commonly used technique for chest evaluation. The benefits of this technique include low cost, high-spatial resolution, operation simplicity and dependability. The important factors that influence the contrast in the radiograph include kilovoltage, shape of sensitometric curve of film, exposure parameters and conditions of film processing. At low kV, the difference in attenuation by soft tissue and bone or air and bone is large, resulting in high contrast. Calcified lesions, pleural plaque, pulmonary nodules are well delineated in low kV radiograph. However, some of the limitations of conventional chest radiograph are given here:

- There is poor visibility of mediastinum, retrocardiac and subphrenic areas when lungs are well seen
- Lungs may be obscured by high contrast of bones
- Inadequate detail of airway and lung apices.

TECHNICAL ADVANCES

Following technical advances have been developed over the years to overcome limitation of the conventional chest radiograph:

- High kV technique
- New screen film combinations
- Beam equalization radiography
- Digital chest radiography.

High kV Technique

In this technique, we use more than 120 kV. The coefficient of X-ray absorption of bone and soft tissue approach each other at high kV and thus the lungs are not obscured by bones. It has better penetration of the mediastinum which provides more details of airway. Short exposure time with high kV allows less scatter radiation to reach intensifying screens and results in sharp details of structures within the lungs. However, high kV results in greater scatter radiation as compared to conventional radiography. Use of an air gap of 6 inches is required to reduce scatter radiation.[2]

New Screen Film Combinations

Fine details on radiograph is principally determined by screen film system. Generally, medium-speed system is preferred which provides better visualization of small vessels, fissures and depiction of abnormalities. The major advance in screen film system has been the introduction of faster rare earth phosphor screen and development of wide latitude film. The improved light emission from rare earth phosphor over traditional calcium tungstate crystal screen results in short exposure time and thus sharp image.

Another important development is the introduction of asymmetric screen film system, the asymmetric zero cross-over screen film system. It was introduced by Eastman Kodak in 1990 called insight thoracic imaging system.[3] This uses different emulsion on either side of film base and different front and back intensifying screens. In addition, layers of absorbing dye in the film base prevent crossover of light between two emulsions so that both screen film combinations operate independently. The front side has high resolution screen and high-contrast film emulsion. This combination optimizes visualization of fine details in lungs. The back side consists of high speed screen and film emulsion with low maximum density. This combination provides adequate visualization of high attenuating areas, e.g. mediastinum without overpenetration of lungs. Patient dose reduction up to 30% has been reported.[4]

Dupont in 1993 introduced an ultravision screen film system. In this system, screens use a high density rare earth phosphor (yttrium tantalate) which emits ultraviolet light that diffuses substantially less than the lower energy wave length visible light. The film emulsion used is symmetric.

These combinations of film screen system have provided increased information that can be recorded and displayed. The asymmetric system is slightly superior particularly for visualization of mediastinal and retro-diaphragmatic structures. The improved image sharpness achieved with these systems potentially can improve visualization of subtle parenchymal abnormalities.

Beam Equalization Radiography

Screen film system provides acceptable image-contrast of chest radiograph in most situations. However, the relatively narrow range of film sensitivity limits image contrast in poorly penetrated areas of chest. The technique of beam equalization radiography refers to varying the intensity of X-ray beam passing through various parts of chest so as to produce a chest radiograph with uniform density of areas with extremely variable attenuation differences on the same film. This can be achieved by two methods:

1. Interposing a customized filter unique to the patient that would attenuate the beam over the lungs and allow increased radiation exposure over the mediastinum.
2. Modulation of exposure for each part of the chest by electronic feedback system.

The first one lacks practicality, the latter one is the principle used in technique of beam equalization radiography that utilizes screen film receptors by increasing X-ray exposure in the thicker, denser part of chest while keeping the lung exposure unchanged, thereby reducing the dynamic range of intensities that ultimately reach the image recorder.[5,6]

Oldelft from Netherlands introduced in 1986 the Advanced Multiple Beam Equalization Radiography (AMBER) which is the only commercially available system for chest radiography. This system has horizontal X-ray fan beam which is divided into 20 adjacent beam segments, each of which is independently controlled by its own intensity modulator located in front of X-ray tube and corresponding exposure detector between patient and image recorder. As the fan beam scans the patient, the detector array measures local X-ray intensity passing through the patient and an electronic feedback mechanism dynamically adjusts each of beam modulators such that dense areas are imaged at higher exposure levels. This increases signal to noise ratio in the denser areas of chest and shifts the background film optical density in these areas onto higher contrast portion of H and D curve.

The advantages of this technique are as follows:

- Better delineation of mediastinum, retrocardiac and retrodiaphragmatic areas
- Improved visualization of lung apices in lateral view.

The reported disadvantage of AMBER are as follows:

- Decreased contrast between consolidation and normal lung
- Edge artefacts occur where there are abrupt changes in radiolucency, e.g. lung heart interface, lung diaphragm interface
- Dark halo around the heart may simulate pneumomediastinum
- Active imaging areas are limited to upright 14″ × 17″ orientation so it is not possible to acquire transverse image of chest
- Exposure parameter to be set manually
- Difficulty in comparing the radiograph of patient with previous one using conventional technique

- This system can not be used on bed side and for patient on stretcher
- Radiation dose is about 50% more than conventional chest radiograph.

The experience till date is not clearly indicative of the justification of additional expense even though images are more informative and this seems to have limited its popularity in clinical use.

Digital Chest Radiography

Advances in electronics and computer technology, over the past decades, have led to development of digital radiography or computed radiography system. This is different from conventional film-based analog system where the film is in direct contact with intensifying screen and there is no storage of information as digits in computer. In digital radiography, image detection can be completely separated from image display. The data of image is stored in the computer and can be retrieved, displayed, quantified, manipulated and hardcopied whenever required.[6]

Digital system using phosphor technique in which the entire receptor is exposed by conventional radiography equipment was introduced by Fuji in 1980 and is the most widely used technique for general digital radiography. This technique is based on reusable imaging plate coated with photostimulable phosphor material. When exposed to X-ray, a portion of X-rays is absorbed as to release stored energy as light and intensity of light measured and digitized. The resultant digital image is then preprocessed for contrast and spatial resolution before display. Imaging plate is ready for reuse after exposure to room light.

Introduction of selenium detector system is an important development in digital chest radiography. Unlike storage phosphor detector, which requires laser stimulation for image acquisition, selenium-based detectors capture image information as charge pattern and thus image can be read directly, eliminating image noise.[7,8] Also selenium is more efficient in detection of X-rays.

Flat panel detectors are relatively new development in the technology. Depending on the material, there are two types of flat panel detectors, indirect type uses a phosphor screen like cesium iodide to convert the X-ray to light photons. Direct flat panel detectors use instead a photoconductive layer, most commonly amorphous selenium, that converts X-ray energy directly to charge. By using flat panel detectors, patient dose can be reduced without degradation of image quality and multiple images can be acquired in a short time.[9,10]

Dual energy imaging is a new technique which utilizes a receptor with two layers, each of which records different energy components of X-ray beam and is possible for a computer to analyze and separate the components of dual energy in order to display both soft tissue and bone images of the same radiograph.[6] Dual energy imaging is one of the few areas in which digital radiography has proved of diagnostic advantage over conventional chest radiography.

Temporal subtraction imaging is used to improve the visual assessment of chest radiograph. This technique aims to selectively enhance areas of internal change by subtracting the patient's previous radiograph from the current one. Studies have shown that temporal subtraction improves the visual perception of subtle abnormalities such as pulmonary nodules, infiltrative opacities and diffuse lung disease.[11,12]

Digital tomosynthesis is a technique that has evolved from conventional tomography and solves many of the problems associated with conventional tomography. Digital tomosynthesis can produce an unlimited number of section images at arbitrary depths from single set of acquisition images. This technique is another method for improving detection of subtle lesions, such as pulmonary nodules.[13,14]

Digital Radiography and Chest

Major advantage of digital radiography lies in the control of display of optical density of radiographs in portable chest X-ray examination with dynamic range and control processing. It improves visibility of tubes and lines superimposed on the mediastinum. Although it may not offer any significant advantage over conventional film screen system, digital radiography improves visibility of normal lung structures, thus one has to be careful in distinguishing prominent blood vessels from interstitial disease. To avoid this misinterpretation, mild-to-moderate edge enhancement is required for better visualization of interstitial disease. Because of smaller size of digital radiograph, there is a definite learning curve to adjust to digital radiograph and one may have to interpret the film from a closer distance.

Numerous observe performance studies have shown that digital radiography can equal conventional film radiography in virtually any specific task. However, for this, post-processing of the digital image is required to match the digital radiograph to the task. A problem inherent in all forms of digital manipulation is that enhancement of the image for one purpose, degrades it for another.

There have been conflicting reports about whether digital chest radiography can be satisfactorily interpreted on high-resolution television monitors, as distinct from laser printed films. Recent studies suggest that 2K × 2K monitors may be adequate for making primary diagnosis on digital chest radiograph.

RADIOGRAPHIC PROJECTIONS

Posteroanterior View

The most satisfactory and standard radiographic view for evaluation of the chest is posteroanterior (PA) view with patient standing **(Fig. 1)**. Visualization of lungs is excellent because of inherent contrast of the tissues of the thorax.

The diagnostic accuracy of chest disease is partly related to the quality of radiographic images. It is incumbent on all radiologists to ensure that images on which their diagnostic impression is based are of the highest quality. Careful attention to several variables is necessary to ensure such quality.

Patient Positioning

Positioning must be such that the X-ray beam is properly centered, the patient's body is not rotated, and the scapulas are rotated sufficiently anteriorly so that they are projected away from the lungs. On properly centered radiographs, the medial ends of the clavicles are projected equidistant from the margins of the vertebral column.

Patient Respiration

Respiration must be fully suspended, preferably at total lung capacity (TLC). It has been shown that in erect chest radiographs, normal subjects routinely inhale to approximately 95% of TLC without coaxing;[15] thus, such radiographs can be of value in estimating lung volume, and by comparison with subsequent radiographs in appreciating an increase or decrease in volume as a result of disease.

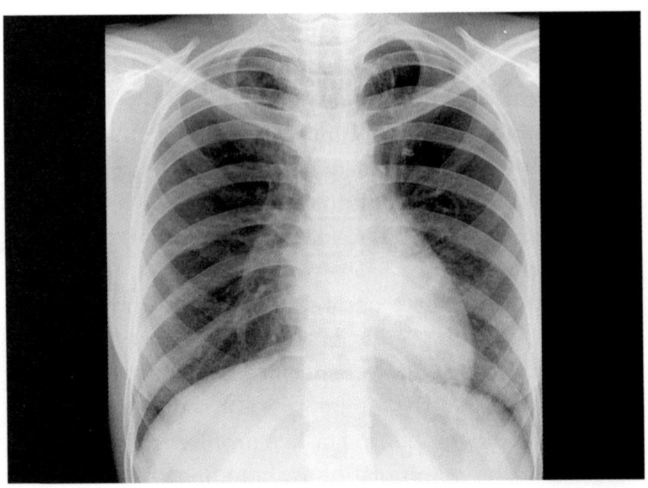

Fig. 1: Normal chest X-ray: Posteroanterior view in standing position.

Film Exposure

Exposure factors should be such that the resultant radiograph permits faint visualization of the thoracic spine and the intervertebral disks on the PA radiograph so that lung markings behind the heart are clearly visible. Exposure should be as short as possible, consistent with the production of adequate contrast. Unfortunately, all too frequently technical factors are such that optimal radiographic density is achieved over the lungs generally but without adequate exposure of the mediastinum or the left side of the heart, a tendency that seriously limits radiological interpretation, moderate overexposure can be easily compensated for by bright illumination; underexposure on the other hand cannot be compensated for by any viewing technique and since it prevents visualization of vital areas of the thorax, should not be tolerated in any circumstances. With perseverance, it is always possible to overcome problems of underexposure.

For a PA chest radiograph, the mean radiation dose at skin entrance should not exceed 0.3 mGy per exposure and the exposure time should not exceed 40 msec.[16] An optimally exposed radiograph presents the lung at a mid- gray level (average optical density, 1.6–1.9). (Optical density is a measurement of the ability of the film to stop light (film blackness), and it is equal to the logarithm of light incident on the film over light transmitted by the film ($D = \log I_O/I_t$).

The focal film distance should be at least 180 cm (72 inches) to minimize magnification (Focal film distance is the distance between the focal spot of the X-ray tube and the radiograph).[16]

Kilovoltage

A high kilovoltage technique appropriate to the film speed should be used;[10] for PA and lateral chest radiographs, the recommended kVp is 115–150 kVp. Since the coefficients of X-ray absorption of bone and soft tissue approximate each other in the higher kilovoltage ranges, radiographic visibility of the bony thorax is reduced with only slight change in the overall visibility of lung structures. Furthermore, the mediastinum is better penetrated, thereby permitting visibility of lung behind the heart and the many mediastinal lines and interfaces whose identification is so important to the overall assessment of both the mediastinum and lungs. This technique can produce chest radiographs superior in all respects to those obtained with other techniques in addition to better penetration of the mediastinum. High kilovoltage also results in lower radiation exposure than does lower kilovoltage. The only drawback of the high kilovoltage techniques is the diminished visibility of calcium that results from the lower coefficient of X-ray absorption; however this shortcoming has not proved troublesome in practice.

Grids and Filters

When using a grid, at least a 10:1 aluminum interspace grid with a minimum of 103 lines per inch recommended by the American College of Radiology.[16] An alternative option uses an air gap technique in which a space of 15 cm (6 inches) is interposed between the patient and the X-ray.[17] Since the air gap reduces radiation scatter by distance dispersion, no grid is required. When this technique is used, a constant focal film distance of 10 feet is recommended. In a comparative study of air gap and grid techniques, it was shown that the former can provide contrast equal to those obtained with grids[18] of the various combinations of distances possible. A focal distance of 10 feet with an air gap of 6 inches provides a good compromise. Patient exposure with an air gap technique was comparable to a no-grid, no-air gap technique and was less than that obtained with a grid.

Lateral View

The lateral view is the most important supplement to standard PA chest radiograph since much of the lung and mediastinum is hidden on the PA film. Right or left lateral view, depending on the area of interest closer to the film is obtained. The lateral view helps in localization of different lobes and segments and often this is the only view that will provide this information.[19] Important observations on lateral film of the chest include the clear spaces, vertebral translucency and outline of diaphragms. There are two spaces of increased translucency where both lungs lie closest. These are retrosternal and retrocardiac areas. Retrosternal space normally measures less than 3 cm at its widest point. Vertebral bodies normally are progressively more translucent caudally because of increase in the volume of aerated lung overlying the spine. Both diaphragms are visible throughout their length except the left anteriorly where it merges with the heart **(Fig. 2)**. The diaphragm of the side closer to the film is also more sharply defined. The ribs of the side away from the film appear wider.

Anteroposterior View

This is sometimes the only projection that is possible in very sick patients and usually it is obtained in wards and ICUs with portable X-ray machines. The quality is usually poor. In this view, the scapulae cannot be projected out of the lung fields. The ribs and clavicle are more horizontal and the heart is magnified as compared to the PA view **(Fig. 3)**. Anteroposterior (AP) view is, sometimes, very helpful in deciding whether a small questionable pulmonary opacity on the PA view is genuine, by altering its relationship to the overlying ribs and vascular shadows.[20] It is also useful in differentiating free and loculated pleural fluid.

Decubitus View

The cross-table lateral decubitus views are helpful in determining the confines of the cavity and demonstrating

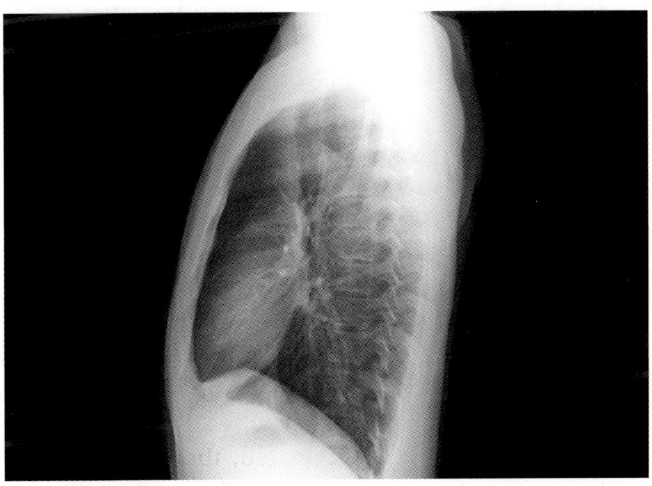

Fig. 2: Right lateral X-ray of normal chest.

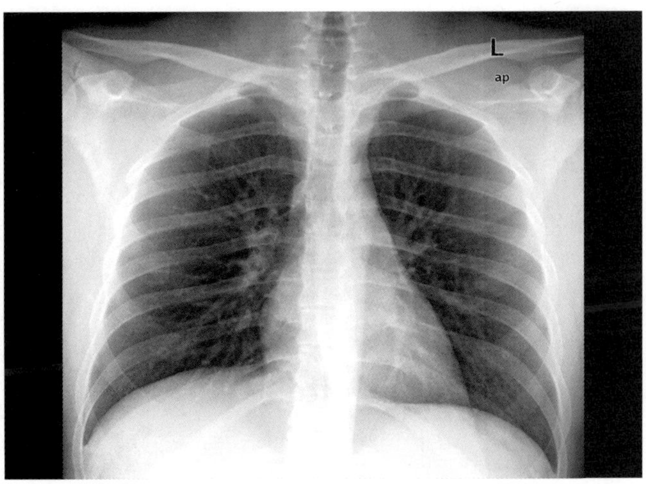

Fig. 3: Anteroposterior view of chest: The clavicle and ribs are more horizontal in position.

small pneumothorax or pleural effusions. The dependent hemidiaphragm normally rises considerably in this view.

Lordotic View

This view is obtained either with patient leaning backward in lordotic position or, more commonly, with cranial tilt of the X-ray tube. It is particularly useful for clear demonstration of lung apices. It is important in confirming middle lobe and lingular abnormalities. The clavicles are projected above the lung fields and anterior and posterior parts of the ribs usually overlap each other **(Fig. 4)**. The lower chest is highly distorted in this view.

Oblique View

Right or left posterior oblique views are obtained with degree of obliquity best determined with fluoroscopy. These are preferred to lateral views in case of bilateral disease, since the superimposition of two lungs is significantly obviated **(Fig. 5)**. The left posteroanterior oblique view is particularly useful for better demonstration of trachea and its divisions.

SPECIAL RADIOGRAPHIC TECHNIQUES

Inspiratory–Expiratory Radiography

Comparison of radiographs exposed in full inspiration and maximal expiration may supply useful information in two specific situations. The main indication is the investigation of air trapping, either general or local. The former is exemplified by asthma or emphysema. In both these abnormalities, diaphragmatic excursion is reduced symmetrically and lung density changes little between expiratory and inspiratory radiographs to demonstrate these features convincingly, expiration must be forced and preferably timed. When air trapping is local as in bronchial obstruction or lobar emphysema, the expiratory radiograph reveals decreased ipsilateral diaphragmatic elevation, a shift of the mediastinum toward the contralateral hemithorax and relative absence of density change involves bronchopulmonary segments.

The second indication for expiratory-inspiratory radiography is when pneumothorax is suspected and the visceral pleural line is not visible on the standard inspiratory radiograph or the findings are equivocal. In these situations, a film taken in full expiration may show the line more clearly.

Valsalva and Müller Maneuvers

The Valsalva and Müller maneuvers respectively consisting of forced expiration and inspiration against a closed glottis may aid in determining the vascular or solid nature of intrathoracic masses. A change in size indicates a vascular lesion. Lack of change in size, however, is not helpful, because it may occur with solid lesions or with insufficient effort. Although potentially helpful, these maneuvers are seldom used in clinical practice.

Bedside/Portable Radiography

The number of requests for radiographic examination of the chest with a mobile apparatus at a patient bedside has increased enormously since its introduction owing partly to the growth of intensive care units (ICUs) and partly to the introduction of complex cardiovascular surgical procedures that require close postoperative surveillance.

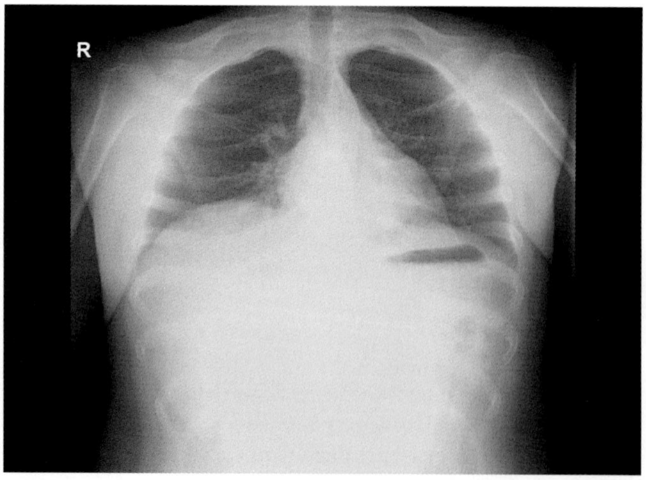

Fig. 4: Lordotic view of chest: The clavicles are projected superior to apex.

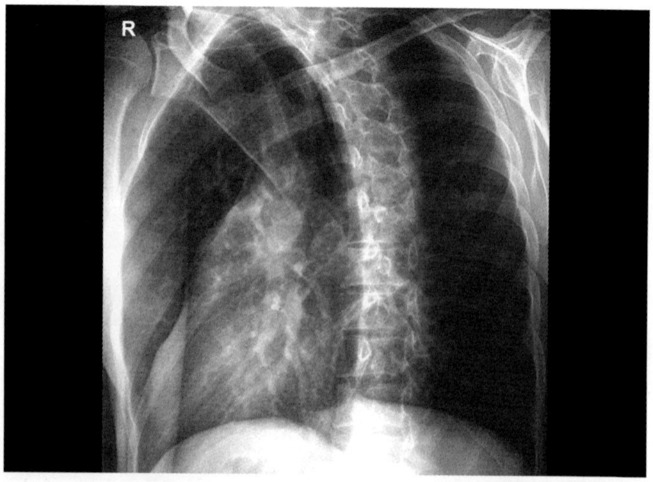

Fig. 5: Right oblique view of normal chest.

Such radiographs are almost invariably technically inferior to those obtained in the standard manner in the radiology department itself. This inferior quality derives from multiple factors, some of which are uncontrollable (e.g. the patient's supine position, a short focal film distance and the restricted ability of many such patients to suspend respiration or to achieve full inspiration). Other factors, however, including the technical ones used in the exposure, are subject to control.[21] Frequently, these radiographs are overexposed or underexposed, sometimes, to a degree that limits or even precludes recognition of the subtle changes that are so important in the radiologist either accepting an inferior product or arranging a repeat examination, with associated patient discomfort, increased radiation exposure and increased cost. Some of these problems can be minimized by using a wide latitude screen film combination. An alternative technique that is rapidly replacing the screen film combination for bedside radiographs is digital radiography, since it allows satisfactory images to be obtained over a wide range of X-ray exposures.

From the various studies in the literature, it seems reasonable to conclude that daily routine chest radiographs are indicated in ICU patients with acute cardiac or pulmonary problems, in patients receiving mechanical ventilation, patients admitted for cardiac monitoring, or ICU patients admitted because of extrathoracic disease. Chest radiographs are recommended after insertion of endotracheal tubes, central venous lines, chest tubes and intra-aortic balloons.[22-24]

NORMAL ANATOMY ON CHEST X-RAY

The normal Roentgen anatomy of the chest as seen on chest radiographs can be described in following headings:

Trachea

Trachea is a straight tube, midline in the upper part and deviates slightly to the right around the aortic knuckle. It shortens and deviates more to right on expiration. Its caliber is even with decreasing translucency as it is traced caudally. On plain chest radiograph, the upper limits of coronal diameters in adults are 21 mm (in females) and 25 mm (in males); sagittal diameters are 23 mm (in females) and 27 mm (in males).[25] The right tracheal margin (right paratracheal stripe) can be traced down to the right main bronchus. It is 4 mm or less in thickness and measured above the azygos vein.[26] The left paratracheal line is rarely visualized. After the age of 40 years, calcification of the cartilage rings of the trachea is a common finding.[27] The enlarged azygos vein, which lies in the angle between the right main bronchus and trachea, may be normally seen as a round opacity in the tracheobronchial angle in the supine chest film.

Tracheobronchial Divisions

The trachea divides into right and left main bronchus usually at D5 or D6 level in adults. The left main bronchus is longer and has more acute angle with trachea as compared to right main bronchus.

The right main bronchus divides into upper lobe bronchus and bronchus intermedius. The upper lobe bronchus divides into apical, posterior and anterior segmental bronchi. The bronchus intermedius divides into middle and lower lobe bronchi. Middle lobe bronchus has medial and lateral branches. The lower lobe bronchus has five branches: each for superior, anterior, lateral, posterior and medial basal segments of lower lobe. Absence of middle lobe on left side modifies the bronchial division on left side. The left main bronchus divides into upper and lower lobe bronchi. The upper lobe bronchus has two divisions: the upper division divides into apicoposterior and anterior branches to supply upper lobe, the lower division supplies the lingula with superior and inferior branches. The lower lobe bronchus on left side divides similar to the right side except the absence of separate medial basal branch. Major tracheobronchial divisions are illustrated in **Figures 6A and B**.

Lungs

The lungs are divided into three lobes on the right side and two lobes on the left side by the interlobar fissures. The major (oblique) fissures on both sides are similar. It runs obliquely forwards and downwards (upper portion facing forward and laterally and the lower portion facing backward and medially), passing through the hilum. On a lateral view, it starts at the level of fourth or fifth thoracic vertebra to reach the diaphragm 5 cm behind the costophrenic angle on the left and just behind the angle on the right side[28] **(Fig. 7)**.

The right lung has an additional fissure, the minor (horizontal) fissure. It can be drawn on chest PA film from right hilum to the sixth rib in axillary line **(Fig. 8)**. It separates the middle lobe from right upper lobe. There are some accessory fissures, which are occasionally seen. The azygos lobe fissure, so called because it contains the azygos vein on right and hemiazygos vein on left within its lower margin, is commonly seen on the right side with an incidence on 0.4%.[28] It appears as a hairline with slight

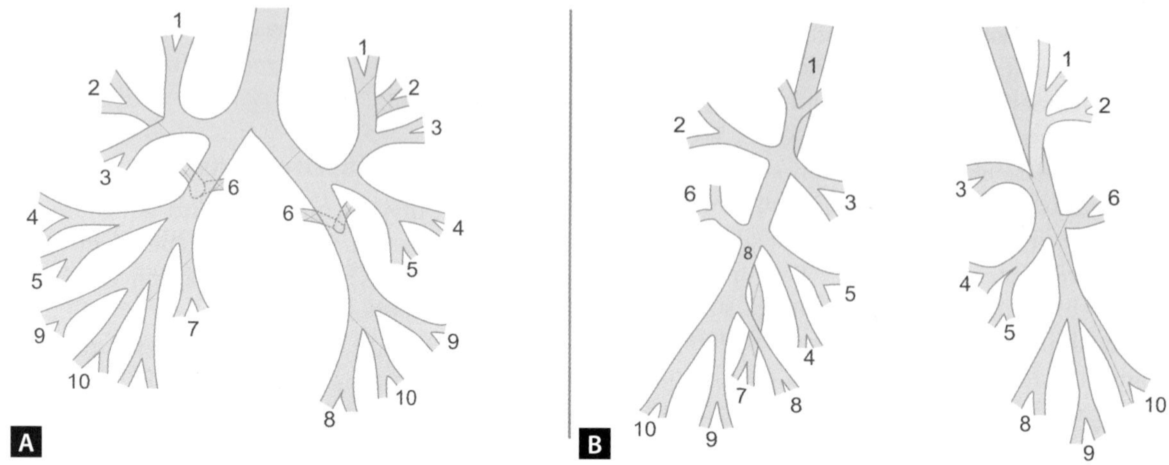

Figs. 6A and B: Diagrammatic representation of major tracheobronchial division as seen on frontal (A) and lateral (B) orientation. (1. Apical; 2. Posterior; 3. Anterior segments of upper lobe; 4. Lateral segment of middle lobe/superior lingula; 5. Medial segment of middle lobe/inferior lingula; 6. Superior; 7. Medial basal; 8. Anterior basal; 9. Lateral basal; and 10. Posterior basal segments of lower lobe)

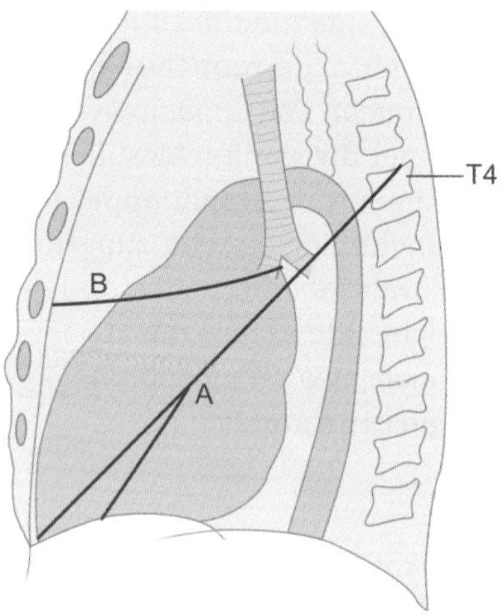

Fig. 7: Line diagram on lateral chest X-ray showing position of major (line A) and minor fissure (line B).

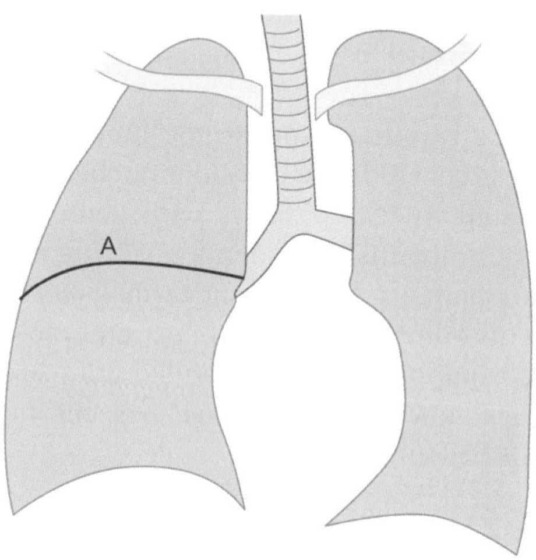

Fig. 8: Line diagram on chest X-ray (PA view) showing position of minor fissure (line A)

lateral convexity running across the right upper zone to end in a comma-like expansion (azygos vein) near the hilum. The azygos lobe is the area of the lung medial to the azygos fissure. The left-sided horizontal fissure, similar to the minor fissure on the right, separates the lingular from the other upper lobe segments. The superior accessory fissure separates the apical from the basal segments of the lower lobes. The inferior accessory fissure separates the medial basal from the other basal segments.

Bronchopulmonary Segments

Bronchopulmonary segments of individual lobes are based on the subdivisions of lobar bronchi. These segments represent the volume of the lung, which is supplied by an integral and relatively constant segmental bronchus and blood vessels. The boundaries between various segments are complex and with the rare exception of accessory fissure, the segments are not divided by septae. Although many pathological process may predominate in one segment or another, these usually never confirm precisely to whole of just one segment since collateral air drift occurs across segmental boundaries. However, information of segmental involvement in disease process is particularly important to surgeons since these segments can be removed separately. These bronchopulmonary segments are designated as per the divisions of segmental bronchi. There is a lot of overlap of bronchopulmonary segments on a PA view of chest but they project separately on a lateral view. Their approximate location, as seen on frontal and lateral radiographs, is illustrated **(Figs. 9A to D)**.

The radiographic density of the two lungs is symmetrical on a well-taken PA film. If the patient is rotated, the hemithorax closer to the film appears more radiodense. Both PA and lateral views are necessary to localise a lesion in one or more of the pulmonary segments. Since the normal bronchi are not visualised in the peripheral lung fields, it is difficult to make out the boundary of different pulmonary segments on plain radiographs of the chest.

Hilum and Pulmonary Vasculature

The structures contributing to the formation of the hilum are the pulmonary arteries and their main branches, upper lobe pulmonary veins, the major bronchi and lymph glands. Of all the structures in the hilum, only the pulmonary arteries and upper lobe veins significantly contribute to the hilar shadows on a plain radiograph. Normal lymph nodes are not seen. The left hilum is usually 0.5–2 cm higher than the right. Both hila are of equal density and size with a concave lateral border on PA film.

The diameter of the normal descending branch of right pulmonary artery is between 10–16 mm in males and 9–15 mm in females. The course of the pulmonary vessels can be described by dividing them into three zones depending upon their positions in the lungs, i.e. hilar, mid lung and peripheral. Mid-lung vessels extend from hilum up to 2 cm from the chest wall. Peripheral vessels are present in other 2 cm of the lung fields and these are rarely seen on a normal chest radiograph. The pulmonary veins have fewer branches and are straighter. The distinction between intrapulmonary arteries and veins is difficult and seldom useful so that they are collectively referred to as pulmonary

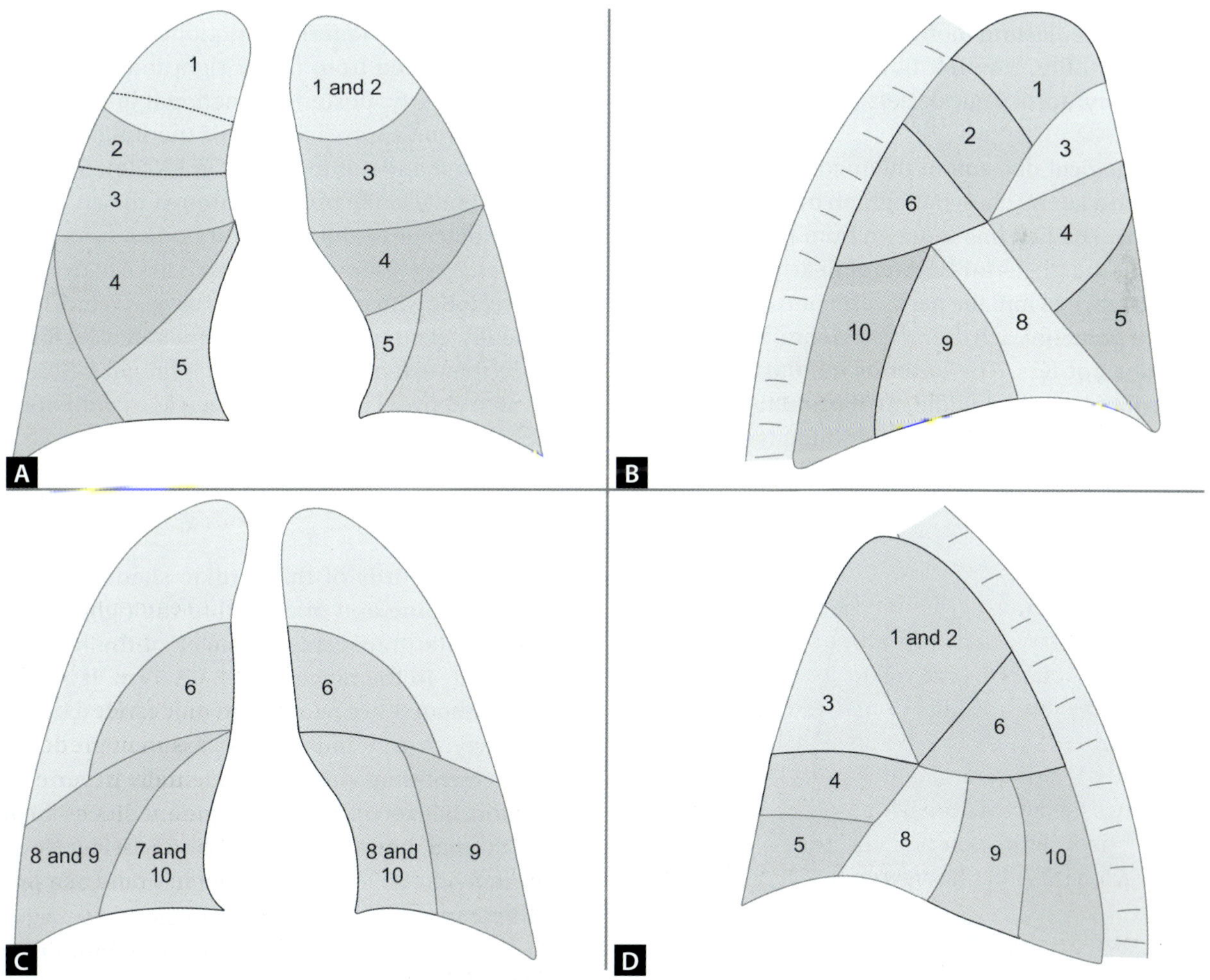

Figs. 9A to D: Line diagram showing approximate locations of various bronchopulmonary segments: (A) Upper and middle lobe/lingula on PA projection; (B) Lower lobe on PA projection; (C) Right lung on lateral projection; (D) Left lung on lateral projection (The segments numbers as per Figure in 6).

vasculature. The pulmonary vessels taper gradually as they proceed peripherally. On erect PA chest radiographs, the upper zone vessels are comparatively narrower than lower zone vessels because of the effect of gravity. The bronchial vessels are normally not seen on chest radiograph.

Pleura

Normal pleura is not visible on chest radiographs. The mediastinal surface of the pleura can occasionally be demonstrated near the midline in a well-penetrated chest radiograph.

Mediastinum

It is a space lying between two lungs. It is bounded by sternum anteriorly, dorsal spine posteriorly and pleural sacs on both sides. The borders of the heart and mediastinum are clearly defined except where the heart is in contact with the left hemidiaphragm. The bracheocephalic (innominate) vessels, superior vena cava and right atrium form the right mediastinal border. Rarely a dilated aorta may also contribute. The left border is formed by left subclavian artery, aortic knuckle, left atrial appendage and left ventricle.

The radiological division of the mediastinum can be ascertained on a lateral chest radiograph by two imaginary lines **(Fig. 10)**. The first line is drawn from the diaphragm upward along the posterior border of heart and anterior border of the trachea into the neck. A second line is drawn connecting a point on each thoracic vertebra, 1 cm behind their anterior borders. The anterior mediastinum is in front of the first line, the middle mediastinum is between the two lines and the posterior mediastinum is behind the second line.

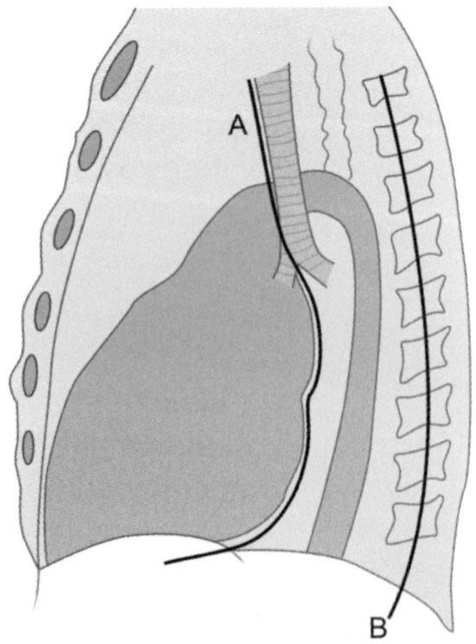

Fig. 10: Line diagram on lateral radiograph of chest showing division of mediastinum by A and B lines.

The anterior mediastinum contains thymus, heart with pericardium, great vessels and occasionally, aberrant thyroid. Middle mediastinum contains trachea and esophagus. Nerve roots and descending thoracic aorta are the main contents of posterior mediastinum. Normal lymph nodes and adipose tissue is seen in all divisions of mediastinum. Conventional PA and lateral views of the chest are the first radiological investigation in any suspected mediastinal abnormality. However, a lesion may not be detected if it is not large enough to cause contour abnormality in the lung-mediastinum interphase.

In neonates and young children, the normal thymus is seen as a triangular sail-shaped structure with well-defined borders, sometimes, wavy in outline. Its borders project from one or both sides of the mediastinum.

Mediastinal Lines and Interfaces

As the two lungs approximate anteriorly, four layers of pleura and anterior mediastinum separate them forming a septum called as anterior junctional line. On PA film this line is oriented from upper right to lower left of the sternum. Similarly, posterior junctional line is produced by the posterior approximation of the lungs behind the esophagus and anterior to spine. On PA film, the posterior junctional line usually projects through the air column of trachea. Adjacent to the vertebral bodies runs the para-spinal lines. Azygoesophageal recess is formed by contact of right lower lobe with esophagus and azygos vein. The recess is frequently identified on a well-penetrated PA film as an interface that extends from the diaphragm below to the azygos arch above. Typically, it is seen as a continuous arch concave to the right. It may be straight in young adults.[28] The paraspinal lines are usually 1–2 mm wide on PA film.

Heart

Normally two thirds of the cardiac shadow lies to the left of the midline and one-third to the right. In normal individuals, the transverse diameter of the heart on PA film is usually in the range of 11.5–15.5 cm. It is less than 11.5 cm in about 5% of people and only rarely exceeds 15.5 cm in heavy, stocky individuals. Assessment of cardiac size by determining cardiothoracic ratio is more useful. Cardiothoracic ratio of 50% is accepted widely as the upper limit of normal, however, it exceeds 50% in at least 10% of normal individuals.[29] The cardiothoracic ratio may be up to 60% in neonates.[30]

Diaphragm

In most individuals, it has a smooth dome shape. The peak or the highest point of the dome is medial. Flattening of the dome can be measured on PA view by dropping a perpendicular from midpoint of the dome to the line connecting costophrenic and cardiophrenic angles of the same side. The distance is normally greater than 1.5 cm.[31] In approximately 90% of normal individuals, the right hemidiaphragm is 1.5–2.5 cm higher than the left. In rest, either the domes are at the same level or the right diaphragm may be at the slightly higher level. The discrepancy in the levels of the diaphragms is related to the position of the cardiac apex and not to the position of the liver. A difference greater than 3 cm in the levels of two hemidiaphragms is significant.[32]

Sonography of Chest

Ultrasound of the chest is rapidly emerging valuable method in diagnosis of various thoracic diseases including pleural, chest wall and peripheral lung parenchymal pathologies.[33] The ultrasound examination of chest is very useful in critical care unit at bedside where standard radiography can be suboptimal due to various factors.[34] Other than diagnostic use, ultrasound can be used for guidance for FNAC/biopsy and placement of intercostal drainage tubes. The chances of successful thoracentesis increase when ultrasound used as guidance compared with physical examination.[35]

Ultrasound has several advantages, including its wide availability, better portability, absence of radiation, real time imaging and dynamic properties. The limitations of ultrasound are low resolution images and operator dependence.

The major indications of chest ultrasound are:

- Evaluation of pleural pathologies (effusion, hemothorax, empyema, pleural thickening, calcification, pleural mass, etc.)
- Diagnosis of pneumothorax
- Evaluation of opaque hemithorax
- Assesment of chest wall diseases (like neoplasms, hematoma, abscess, rib fracture)
- Assesment of diaphragmatic mobility
- To differentiate subpulmonic effusion with subphrenic collection
- Evaluation of peripheral lung parenchymal pathologies (consolidation, collapse, abscess and tumors)
- Evaluation of mediastinum (anterior mediastinal mass, lymphadenopathy, IVC thrombosis and pericardial effusion)
- Guidance for interventional procedures.

Ultrasound Technique

Appropriate ultrasound probe, proper patient positioning and placement of probe, are the important factors to get better result while doing chest ultrasound. Ultrasound of chest can be performed with any modern ultrasound machine equipped with curvilinear (3–5 MHZ) and high-resolution linear array probe (5–13 MHz). Curvilinear transducers convex shape has a wider field of view and provides visualization of deeper structures. Initially quick look of chest wall, pleura and lung can be done by curvilinear probe and once abnormality detected then detailed depiction of lesion should be done by high-resolution linear probe.[33,36] The lesion can be assessed by both grayscale and color Doppler imaging. Before doing chest ultrasound, it is important to review previous imaging including chest X-ray to localize the area of interest. It is useful to increase the rib space to facilitate the exam by asking the patient to elevate his/her arm above the head.[33]

USG gelly should be placed on the patient's skin to provide smooth slide to probe and airless interface. Scanning should be done in quite respiration to know the normal lung movement. The detailed assessment of lesion should be done in breath-hold particularly when using color Doppler. The various useful positions/methods are given below:

- *Sitting position:* Posterior chest is best imaged with patient sitting upright and putting probe in the intercostal space **(Fig. 11)**. It is useful to detect pleural effusion which gravitates to dependent position.
- *Lateral decubitus position:* The anterior and lateral chest may be assessed in the lateral decubitus position **(Fig. 12)**.
- *Suprasternal and parasternal position:* It is useful to evaluate superior and anterior mediastinum **(Fig. 13)**.
- *Supraclavicular access:* It allows the visualization of apex of lung and brachial plexus **(Fig. 14)**.
- *Subcostal position:* It is useful to examine diaphragm
- *Subxiphoid position:* Good to evaluate pericardial effusion and cardiac chambers **(Figs. 15A and B)**.

Changing to various positions may be difficult to critically ill patients who are usually in supine position with multiple leads/support devices.[37] In this situation, ultrasound should be done in supine position with ipsilateral hand put to chest towards opposite side.

Normal Anatomy

It is utmost important to know the normal sonographic appearance of the chest components for the diagnosis of any abnormality and interventional guidance.

Chest Wall and Pleura

The normal chest wall and pleura shows characteristic features on ultrasound.[38-39] There is, series of layers representing intercostal muscles which are hypoechoic

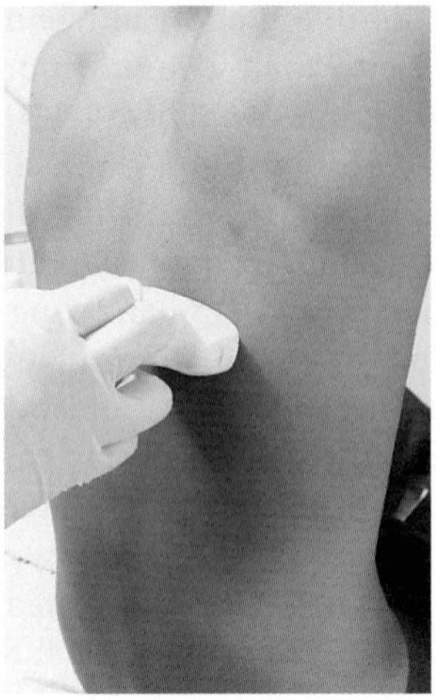

Fig. 11: Ultrasound probe and patient position for the examination of posterolateral chest wall.

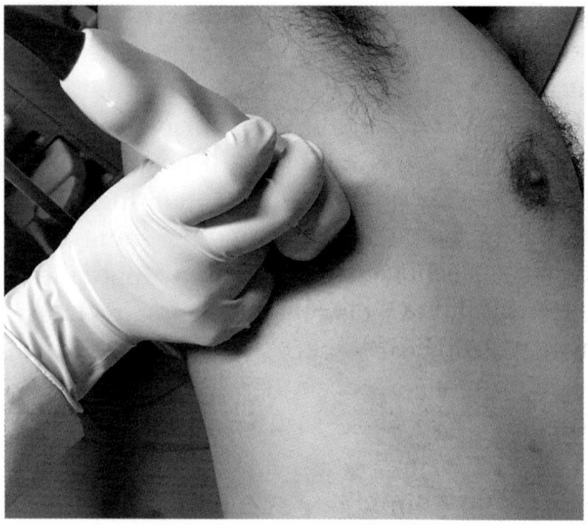

Fig. 12: Anterolateral chest ultrasound in decubitus position.

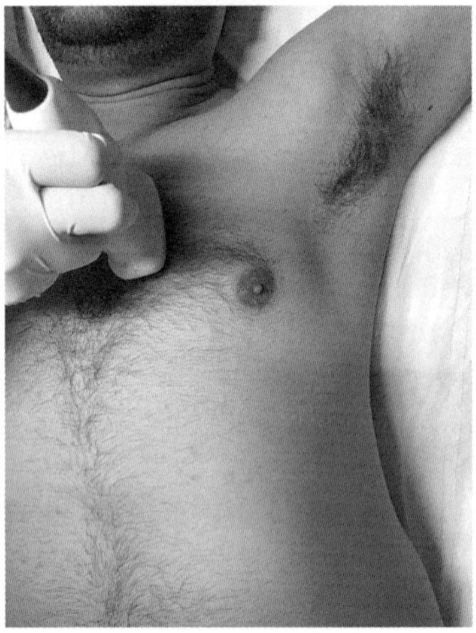

Fig. 13: Parasternal positioning of probe to evaluate anterior mediastinum, pleura and heart.

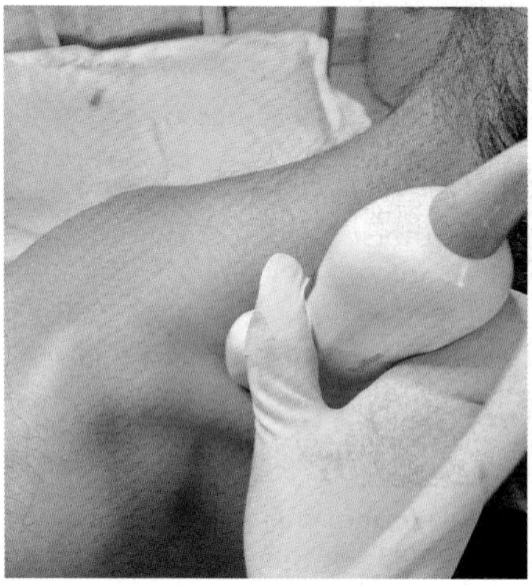

Fig. 14: Evaluation of lung apex by putting probe in supraclavicular location.

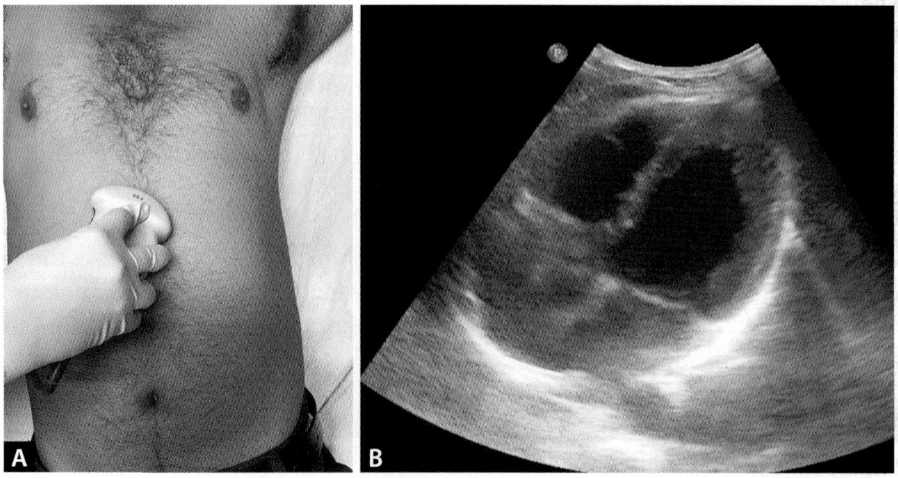

Figs. 15A and B: Subxiphoid position of ultrasound probe (A) and corresponding USG image (B).

and fascia seen as echogenic structure. Below the chest wall, the ribs appear curvilinear echogenic continuous structure with posterior acoustic shadowing **(Fig. 16)**. Posterior to rib, the pleura appears as thick approximately 2 mm echogenic line when imaged with 3–5 MHZ curvilinear probe. The high-resolution linear ultrasound probe is needed to differentiate parietal and visceral pleura which are seen echogenic lines deep to ribs **(Fig. 17)**. Both the layers of pleura can be seen sliding over each other during real time USG imaging.

Diaphragm

The diaphragm is seen as approximately 1-2 mm thick echogenic line which shows movement during respiration. Usually the diaphragm is located inferior to 9th rib when patient is in sitting position. Apart from the location of diaphragm subdiaphragmatic recesses should be evaluated **(Fig. 18)**.

Lung

The lung is air-filled and cannot be visualized deep to pleural lung interface. There are gross changes of acoustic impedance at this interface leading to horizontal artefacts which are seen as echogenic parallel lines. Additionally, comet tail artefacts which are vertically oriented can be seen in normal healthy individual **(Fig. 19)**. These artefacts are usually seen at the level of just above the diaphragm.

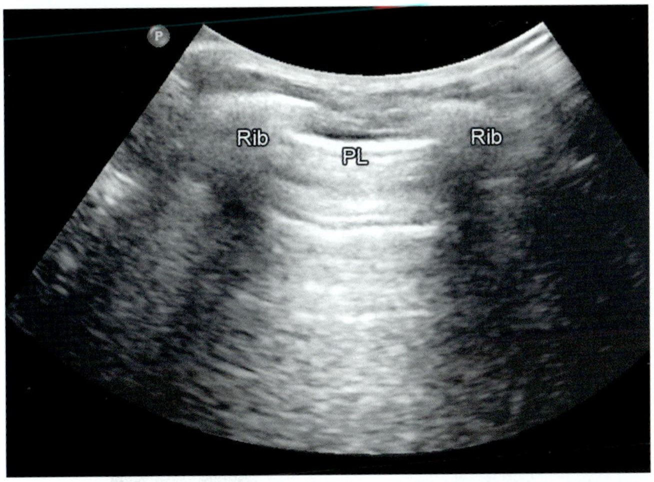

Fig. 16: Grayscale image of thoracic ultrasound by curvilinear convex probe showing wide view of components of thorax. Note made of acoustic shadowing of ribs and echogenic pleural line (PL).

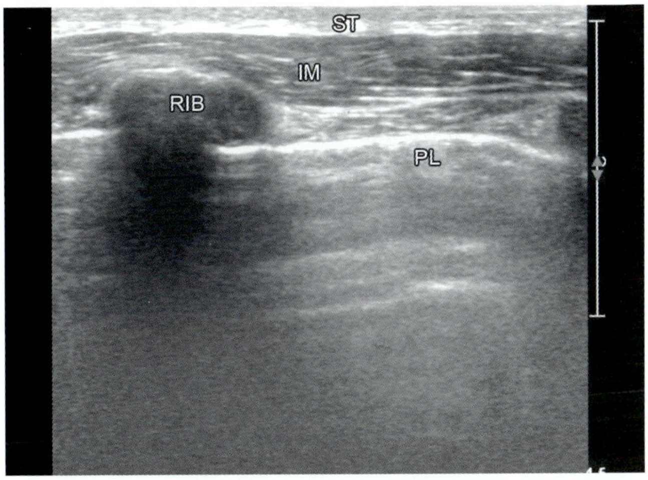

Fig. 17: Grayscale image by high-resolution linear ultrasound probe shows better visualization of structures of chest.
Abbreviations: ST: Subcutaneous tissue; IM: Intercostal muscles; PL: Pleural line.

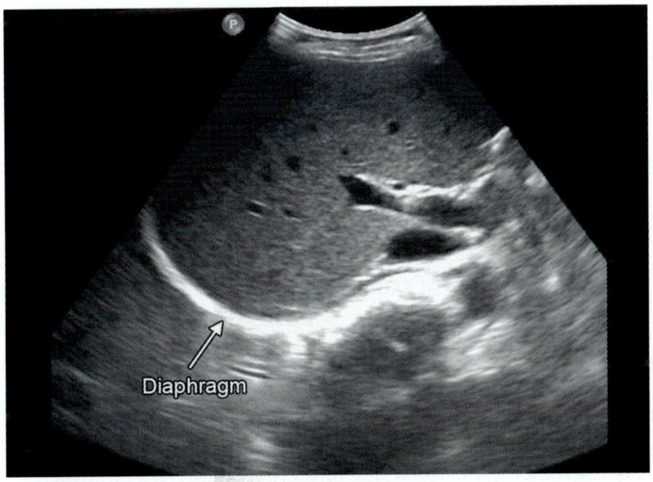

Fig. 18: Subcostal view ultrasound image shows echogenic (arrow) diaphragm.

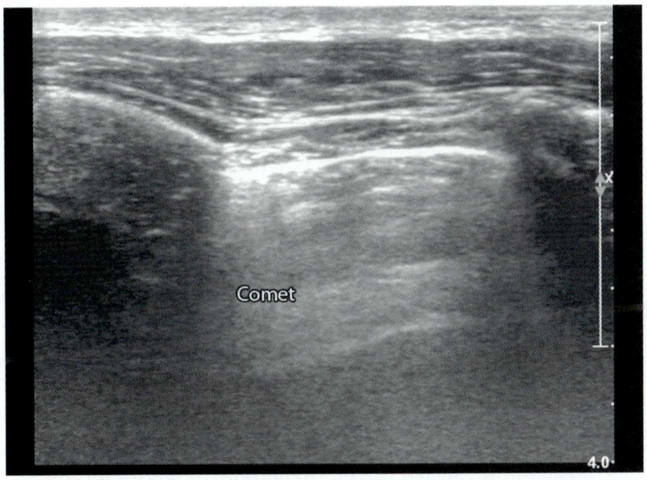

Fig. 19: Ultrasound image by linear probe shows comet-tail artefacts.

Heart

Identification of heart is important when planning for thoracentesis in left anterolateral aspect for safe puncture. The imaging features of heart on ultrasound depend upon axis and position of probe.

CONCLUSION

Chest radiography still remains the first investigation in the diagnosis of various chest diseases. Knowledge of normal anatomy has utmost importance in proper diagnosis of disease process on chest X-ray. Conventional radiograph may have technical limitation in some situations like critically ill patients in ICU; however, recent advances in electronics and computer technology have resulted in development of digital imaging which improves diagnostic quality of chest imaging.

Sonography of chest is emerging technique to evaluate the pathologies of chest which requires proper understanding of the techniques and anatomy of chest components.

ACKNOWLEDGMENT

We acknowledge the help of Dr Harish Bhujade for drawing line diagrams (***see* Figs. 7, 8 and 10**).

REFERENCES

1. Fraser RS, Muller NL, Colman N, et al. The normal lung. In: Fraser RS, Muller NL, Colman N, Pare PD (Eds). Diagnosis of Diseases of Chest (4th edition). Philadelphia: WB Saunders Co; 1999.
2. MacMohan H, Vyborny C. Technical advances in chest radiography. AJR. 1994;163:1049-59.
3. Bunch PC. Performance characteristic of asymmetric zero-crossover screen film system. SPIE Proc Med Imaging IV. 1992;1653:46-65.
4. Swension SJ, Grey JE, Brown LR, et al. A new asymmetric screen film combination for conventional chest radiology: evaluation of 50 patients. AJR. 1993;160:483-6.
5. Chotas HG, Floyd CE JR, Ravin CE. Film-based chest radiography: AMBER vs asymmetric screen film system. AJR. 1993;161:743-7.
6. Hansell DM. Technical consideration. In: Peter Armstrong, Alam G, Wilson, Paul Dee, David M Hansell (Eds). Imaging of diseases of chest (2nd edition). Mosby. 1995.pp.1-14.
7. Neitzei U, Maack I, Gunther-Kohfahl S. Image quality of digital chest radiography system based on selenium detector. Med Phys. 1994;21:509-16.
8. Chotas HG, Floyd CE JR, Ravin CE. Memory artifact related to selenium-based digital radiography system. Radiology. 1997;203:881-3.
9. Samei E, Flynn MJ. An experimental comparison of detector performance for direct and indirect digital radiography system. Med Phys. 2003;30:608-22.
10. Samei E. Performance of digital radiography detectors: factors affecting sharpness and noise. In: Samei E, Flynn MJ (Eds). Syllabus: categorical course in diagnostic radiology physics- advances in digital radiography. Oak Brook, III: Radiological Society of North America. 2003.pp.49-61.
11. Abe H, MacMahon H. Engelmann R, et al. Computer-aided diagnosis in chest radiography: results of large scale observer tests at the 1996–2001 RSNA scientific assemblies. Radiographics. 2003;23:255-65.
12. Okazaki H, Nakamura K, Watanabe H, et al. Improved detection of long cancer arising in diffuse lung diseases on chest radiographs using temporal subtraction. Acad Radiol. 2004;11:498-505.
13. Dobbins JT 3rd. Godfrey DJ. Digital X-ray tomosynthesis: current state of the art and clinical potential. Phys Med Biol. 2003;48:R65-106.
14. Godfrey DJ, McAdams HP, Dobbins JT 3rd. Optimization of the matrix inversion tomosynthesis (MITS) impulse response and modulation transfer function characteristics for chest imaging. Med Phys. 2006;33:655-67.
15. Crapo RA, Montague T, Armstrong J. Inspiratory lung volume achieved on routine chest films. Invest Radiol. 1979;14:137.
16. American College of Radiology: ACR standard for the performance of pediatric and adult chest radiography. American College of Radiology, Reston VA; 1997.p.27.
17. Jackson FI. The air gap and improvement, and an improvement by anteroposterior positioning for chest roentgenography. Am J Roentgenol. 1964;92:688.
18. Trout RD, Kelly JP, Larson VL. A comparison of air gap and grid in roentgenography of the chest. Am J Roentgenol. 1975;120:404.
19. Felson B. The Roentgen work-up. In: Felson B (Ed). Chest Roentgenology. Philadelphia: WB Saunders Co; 1988.
20. Flower CDR, Armstrong P. Techniques. In: Graingern RG, Allison D (Eds). Diagnostic Radiology, 3rd edition. New York: Churchill Livingstone. 1997.p.201.
21. Wandtke JC. Bedside chest radiography. Radiology. 1994;190:1.
22. Fong Y, Whalen G, Hariri RJ, et al. Utility of routine chest radiographs in the surgical intensive care unit. Arch Surg. 1995;130:764.
23. Gray P, Sullivan G, Ostryzniuk P, et al. Value of post-procedural chest radiographs in the adult intensive care unit. Crit Care Med. 1992;20:1513.
24. Hill JR, Horner PE, Primack SL. ICU Imaging. Clin Chest Med. 2008;29(1):59-76,vi.
25. Breatnach E, Abbott GC, Fraser RE. Dimensions of the normal human trachea. AJR. 1984;142:903-6.
26. Savoca CJ, Austin JHM, Goldberg HI. The right paratracheal stripe. Radiology. 1977;122:295.

27. Murfitt J. The normal chest: Methods of investigation and differential diagnosis. In: Sutton D (Ed). Textbook of Radiology and Medical Imaging, 4th edition. Churchill Livingstone. 1987;2:326-67.
28. Mukherjee S, Gupta R. Imaging in chest diseases. In: Pande JN (Ed). Respiratory Medicine in the Tropics, 1st edition. Delhi, Oxford University Press. 1998.p.90.
29. Muller NL. The normal chest. In: Muller NL, Fraser RS, Colman NC (Eds). Radiologic Diagnosis of Diseases of the Chest (1st edition) Philadelphia: WB Saunders Company; 2001.
30. Edwards DK, Higgins CB, Gilpin EA. The cardiothoracic ratio in newborn infants. AJR.1981;136:136.
31. Lennon FA: Simon 6. The height of the diaphragm in the chest radiographs of normal subjects. Br J Radiol. 1965;38:937.
32. Flower CDR, Verschakelan JA. The diaphragm. In: Grainger RG, Allison D (Eds). Diagnostic Radiology, 3rd edition. New York: Churchill Livingstone. 1997. p. 270.
33. Koh DM, Burke S, Davies N, Padley SP. Transthoracic US of the chest: clinical uses and applications. Radiographics. 2002;22(1):e1.
34. Yu CJ, Yang PC, Chang DB, Luh KT. Diagnostic and therapeutic use of chest sonography: value in critically ill patients. Am J Roentgenol. 1992;159:695-701
35. Weingardt JP, Guico RR, Nemcek AA Jr, et al. Ultrasound findings following failed, clinically directed thoracenteses. J Clin Ultrasound. 1994;22:419.
36. Havelock T, Teoh R, Laws D, et al. Pleural procedures and thoracic ultrasound: British Thoracic Society Pleural Disease Guideline 2010. Thorax 2010; 65 Suppl 2:ii61-76.
37. Feller-Kopman D. Ultrasound-guided thoracentesis. Chest. 2006;129:1709.
38. Diacon AH, Theron J, Bolliger CT. Transthoracic ultrasound for the pulmonologist. Curr Opin Pulm Med. 2005;11:307.
39. Tsai TH, Yang PC. Ultrasound in the diagnosis and management of pleural disease. Curr Opin Pulm Med. 2003;9:282.

CHAPTER 157

MDCT and MRI Thorax: Techniques and Normal Anatomy

Rashmi Dixit, Anjali Prakash, Alpana Manchanda

Imaging evaluation of thoracic disease invariably begins with a chest radiograph. Cross-sectional imaging is indicated not only for detailed evaluation of abnormalities seen on the radiograph but also to detect occult lesions not apparent on the radiograph especially when there is strong clinical suspicion of thoracic disease. Multidetector computed tomography (MDCT) remains the imaging method most widely used for the study of thoracic diseases due to its high spatial and temporal resolution, ease of performance and widespread availability. MR largely remains a problem-solving modality with emerging applications.

MDCT THORAX

CT TECHNOLOGY

Spiral CT systems introduced in the 1990s represented a significant advancement in CT technology allowing volumetric data acquisition as opposed to the discontinuous data acquisition in conventional CT.[1] In 1998, the first multidetector CT scanners ware introduced allowing simultaneous acquisition of four slices (or sections) with gantry rotation times which were as low as 0.55 s.[1] These scanners resulted in improvement in acquisition speed, Z-axis coverage, temporal and spatial resolution over the single slice spiral or helical CT scanners. Thus high-resolution, single-breath-hold imaging of the entire thorax became feasible.

Thereon MDCT technology has developed at a breath-taking pace, with increasing detector rows and decreasing tube rotation times. Currently, scanners with 128 and more active detector rows and gantry rotation times as low as 0.33–0.25 second per rotation are available. These scanners are able to scan the entire thorax in 2–3 seconds dramatically reducing motion artefacts.[1,2]

The best temporal resolution that is achievable in a single-source CT scan is half the rotation time of the scanner as this is the minimum data needed for image reconstruction close to the isocenter. With gantry rotation time of 0.3 s. The best possible temporal resolution is 125–150 ms. In recent years, further increase in spatial and temporal resolution has been made possible by the use of either wide area detectors or dual source CT systems.[2]

An area detector is a CT detector that is wide enough in the Z-axis to cover an entire organ such as the heart, kidney or brain without table movement. There are two CT systems providing a16 cm coverage at isocentre. One with a collimation of 256 × 0.625 mm and 0.28 s rotation time and the other with 320 × 0.5 mm collimation and 0.27s rotation time. These CT systems are useful for cardiac imaging as they cover the entire heart in a single axial scan without table movement avoiding the stair step or banding artefacts which may be seen with CT systems with lower detector coverage range. MDCT systems with lower detector range provide a Z coverage of up to 8 cm at isocentre so 2–4 image stacks, acquired in 2–4 consecutive heart beats are put together for volume coverage of the heart. These may be shifted or blurred with respect to each other due to insufficient temporal resolution or variation in cardiac motion from one cycle to next resulting in stair step or banding artefacts. However, on the flip side, all images acquired with an area detector may be affected by arrhythmias or ectopic beats during acquisition. Area detector systems have the ability to acquire dynamic volume data by scanning the same anatomic range repeatedly without table movement. This is useful for perfusion scanning of pulmonary nodules.[2]

Dual source CT (DSCT) systems use two X-ray tubes and detector systems positioned at 90° to each other which can simultaneously acquire data at the same Z-position. Dual source CT systems allow a significant improvement of temporal resolution to below 100 ms.[3] The third generation DSCT scanners acquire 2 × 192 slices with gantry rotation time of 0.25 s. Due to two X-ray tubes the best temporal resolution achievable in these CT systems is quarter of a gantry rotation as the two 90º segments acquired can be put together to give the required minimum 180º of scan data at the isocenter achieving temporal resolution of 0.66 s. Thus with dual source CT scanners, the entire thorax can be scanned within 0.3 s, almost eliminating respiratory and even cardiac motion artefacts.[1,4] They also allow a reduction in contrast dose.

DSCT systems with ECG triggering are useful for coronary imaging in one heart beat at very low dose. They are also excellent for comprehensive evaluation of acute chest pain or triple rule out studies and planning of trans aortic valve replacement (TAVR) procedures by providing adequate visualization of coronary arteries, aorta and iliac arteries.[5,6] The challenges with DSCT systems include cross- scattered radiation which, if not corrected, can produce artefacts and reduce contrast to noise ratio (CNR), and the limited scan field of view (SFOV) of the second detector. This was increased from 25 cm in the first generation to 35.5 cm in the third generation.[2] DSCT systems also provide dual energy applications which are discussed later.

CT ACQUISITION AND RECONSTRUCTION PROTOCOLS

Routinely, scans are acquired in the supine position in full inspiration to fully expand the lungs. This optimizes the contrast between the aerated lung and other normal high attenuation structures (e.g. vessels) and various abnormalities. Full inspiration also minimizes the occurrence of transient atelectasis which can be confounding at times. Scanning is generally done with thin collimation while images are reconstructed at a thickness slightly greater than the collimation to reduce noise in the reconstructed image. For example, in a 64 detector row scanner, the collimation is 64 × 0.625 or 64 × 0.5 (depending on vendor) while images can be reconstructed at 1, 3 and 5 mm thickness from the same data set.

The clinical indication dictates the choice of reconstruction. While 1 mm sections provide higher spatial resolution, a 3 mm thick slice has a better signal to noise ratio for the same acquisition dose. Thin section reconstructions are used for volumetric assessment and characterization of pulmonary nodules, pulmonary embolism and for evaluation of interstitial lung disease. Thin sections with 20–25% overlap are also used for 3D reconstructions. Thicker 3–5 mm sections are generally adequate for assessment of mediastinal masses, lung cancer staging, quick review and for archiving.[1,2,7]

Use of Iodinated Contrast Medium

Most thoracic CT examinations, except HRCT scans, are routinely performed with intravenous contrast. The aim of contrast administration is to opacify organs and delineate vessels within the area of interest. For most indications like lung cancer staging, evaluation of mediastinal masses or lymphadenopathy, a small-to-moderate amount of contrast medium, i.e. 60–120 mL of 300 mg I/mL at a slow injection rate of 1.5–3 mL/s with a long injection duration and scan delay of about 25 s produces adequate opacification of thoracic vessels. The contrast injection should ideally end about 5s before the MDCT acquisition and should be followed by a saline flush to reduce perivenous artefacts and improve the contrast bolus. A caudocranial direction of acquisition also minimizes perivenous artefacts.[7,8]

Window Settings and Reconstruction Algorithms[1,7]

Organs in the thorax have a wide range of densities or HU values ranging from –800 for the aerated lungs to +700 for the osseous structures like the ribs. A single window setting would be unable to represent these. A minimum of two-window settings are required, one to display the lung parenchyma and another to display the soft tissue structures of the mediastinum. Although the exact window settings may vary between institutions a window width of 300–500 HU and center of +40 HU is used for the mediastinum; while for the lungs, a wide window of 1200–1500. HU with a center of –600 HU is more appropriate. For evaluation of osseous structures, bone window settings at a window width of around 1500 and center of 450 are used in addition.

The choice of window settings is important as it can affect the approximate size of normal structures and pathology. The most accurate size measurement is done when the window level is half-way between the density of the structure to be measured and density of the surrounding tissue. Thus, the diameter of a pulmonary nodule will be underestimated if measured at soft tissue settings appropriate for the mediastinum. The smaller structures e.g. peripheral pulmonary vessels are more affected by inappropriate window settings than larger structures. Some authors recommend the use of specific window setting for certain conditions like use of wide window settings (600 HU - WW and 100–150 HU for window level) while interpreting routine CT scans of the chest to improve detection of unsuspected pulmonary embolism. Specific window settings have also been described for evaluation of airways and emphysema.

Each manufacturer provides several **reconstruction algorithms** to optimize visualization of various structures. The high frequency algorithm provides the best visualization of lung architecture while a standard smooth algorithm gives best soft tissue resolution and lowest noise for the mediastinum.

HIGH-RESOLUTION COMPUTED TOMOGRAPHY

High-resolution computed tomography (HRCT) is the use of thin section CT images (0.625–1.5 mm) with high spatial frequency reconstruction algorithm to detect and characterize diseases of pulmonary parenchyma and small airways.

Before the advent of multidetector CT routine CT chest and HRCT were strongly differentiated. The traditional HRCT protocol consisted of thin section CT obtained with 1 mm slice thickness at intervals of 10 or even 20 mm and reconstructed using high spatial frequency algorithms. The logic behind this protocol was that analysis of a diffuse parenchymal process did not require continuous coverage. The other reason being that the relatively higher doses required to achieve excellent signal to noise ratio and image quality did not result in an exponential increase in patient dose with discontinuous scanning. With the current MDCT scanners, each CT chest is an HRCT as the whole chest can be covered with narrow detector width of 0.5–1.25 mm and images reconstructed at 1–1.5 mm thickness with a high spatial frequency algorithm—the two essential factors that constitute an HRCT. Thus, in the past few years, discontinuous HRCT acquisition has been largely replaced by volumetric HRCT.[1,7,9] The factors responsible are:

- Volumetric HRCT can now be done at acceptable dose levels and doses have declined further with the use of reconstruction techniques such as iterative reconstruction. Discontinuous HRCT with 10 mm gap resulted in a dose of 0.7 mSv. Volumetric HRCT with 3D modulation and iterative noise reconstruction results in doses as low as 1.5–3 mSv as opposed to up to 7 mSv with volumetric HRCT in its early days. Hence increased dose is no longer a major concern.
- Volumetric scan allows easier and more precise delineation of disease distribution and comparison in follow-up studies.
- Subtle focal disease can also be detected which may be missed on the discontinuous scan. This may be especially useful when the diagnosis of ILD vs focal lung disease is not apparent clinically.

Modifications in Scanning Technique for HRCT[7,10,11]

Intravenous contrast is not required and, in fact, should be avoided as it may cause fallacious parenchymal opacification and interfere with interpretation.

Images are usually obtained in the **supine position in full inspiration** like routine scanning. In the normal lung effects of gravity on blood flow and gas volume, as well as some non-gravity, dependent effects can result in increase in attenuation and vessel size from anterior to posterior portion of the lung and may produce appearances similar to subpleural lines or atelectasis. In the **prone position**, these hydrostatic densities will disappear while true pathology will persist. The older publications with scans obtained on slower scanners with discontinuous technique reported the utility of prone scans in around 20% patients. This, however, is not the case with the current fast scanning technique. Prone scanning may be useful in a few selected patients with questionable subtle disease in dorsobasal area only, which would be critical in deciding the presence or absence of early disease, e.g. in a patient with asbestosis.

Addition of **expiratory scans** may be useful in the detection of focal or diffuse air trapping. In most cases with clinically significant small airway disease, mosaic attenuation may be visible on inspiratory scans, though much less conspicuous than expiratory scans. Diseases of the larger airways such as tracheobronchomalacia, however, will not be detected if only end inspiratory images are obtained.

High-quality HRCT examinations provide a spatial resolution of 0.5 mm and due to the high contrast within the lung parenchyma even structures as small as 0.2 mm can be seen well. Certain **modifications in reconstruction techniques** are important for achieving this:

- Use of **thin collimation** of 1 mm slice improves resolution and allows detection of important morphological features such as septal thickening, dilatation of airways, detection of small nodules, etc.

However, a slice thickness below 1 mm does not result in any significant improvement in spatial resolution while increasing image noise.

- Application of **high-spatial frequency reconstruction algorithm**: Standard reconstruction algorithms result in smoothening of the image by reducing visible image noise and increasing the contrast resolution. High-spatial frequency or 'sharp' high-resolution algorithms reduce image smoothening and increase spatial resolution. Tissue interfaces and anatomic margins, e.g. the pleura, fissures or septae appear sharper and small vessels and bronchi are better seen **(Figs. 1A and B)**.
- Use of a **suitably small FOV** decreases pixel size and thus increases spatial resolution. The field of view should be adjusted to the outer cortex of the ribs—this ensures that the field is restricted to the size of the lungs while no portion of the lung is cut-off. This results in a spatial resolution of 0.5–0.3 mm. Sometimes, targeted reconstruction of a particular lung or lobe may be done to further increase the spatial resolution for evaluation of minute abnormalities. However, here the resolution is limited by the intrinsic resolution of the detectors. Targeted reconstruction is generally a matter of personal preference and there is no definitive literature recommending its use.

ACQUISITION PROTOCOL AND CONTRAST OPACIFICATION FOR CT PULMONARY ANGIOGRAPHY[1,8,12]

The major factor to be considered for the technical success of a CT pulmonary angiography (CTPA) examination is excellent opacification of pulmonary vessels. The attenuation within the pulmonary arteries should be at least 250 HU to allow detection of filling defects and thrombi. A caudocranial acquisition is preferred as with this the basal portion will not show motion artefacts even in severely dyspneic patients. This is a common region for pulmonary emboli to lodge. Caudocranial acquisition also reduces perivenous streak artefacts. With the older generation of scanners which took about 20–25 s to scan the thorax 120–140 mL of 350–380 mg/mL iodine was required however with the latest MDCT scanners injected volume and iodine dose can be reduced markedly and 50 mL of contrast may be sufficient **(Figs. 2A and B)**. Scanners with capability of scanning at 70 kV are now available where the dose of iodine may be reduced to as low as 20 mL. In order to reduce radiation and optimize the contrast dose during CTPA the following should be done:

- Reduce KV from the routine 120 kV to 100 kV or even 80 kV if patient weighs less than 65 kg to take advantage of the K-edge absorption of iodine.
- Optimize flow rates to patient physiology, e.g. for old patients with possible altered left ventricular function, flow rate of 3 mL/s with high iodine concentration of 350–400 mg/mL is needed while in a young patient or a pregnant patient, a much higher flow rate of 5–6 mL/s will be required.[12]
- Calculate the correct contrast volume required: the acquisition time should be noted by setting the acquisition box in the scout. For a 128 slice scanner this is about 2s. Acquisition time is added to time for breath-hold instruction (generally 5s) and a reserve time of 5s which equals 12s (2+5+5) in this case. Using a flow rate of 4 cc/s total

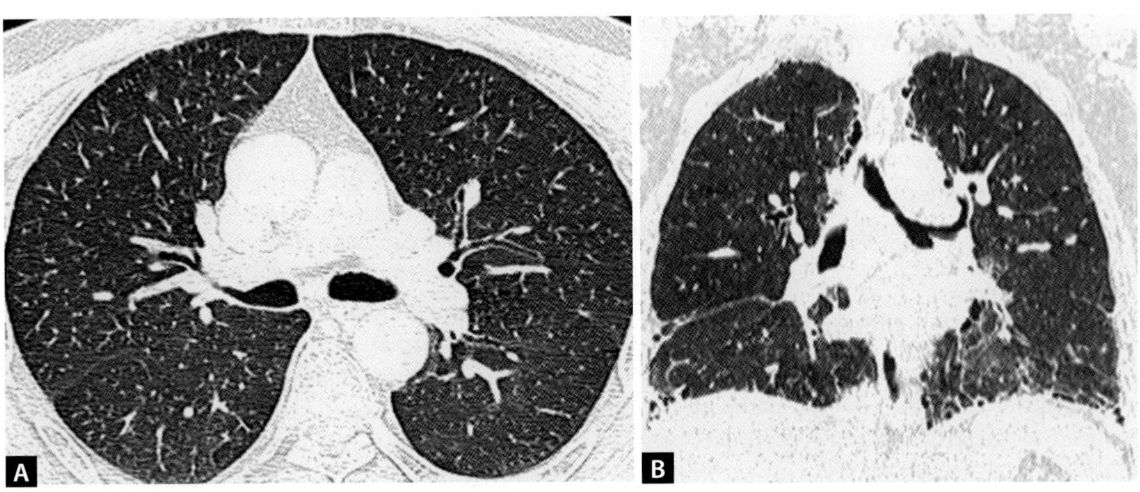

Figs. 1A and B: Normal HRCT: (A) 1 mm axial section from a volumetric spiral acquisition on a 128 slice MDCT scanner shows small vessels and bronchi in exquisite detail; (B) Coronal reconstruction in another patient shows the apicobasal gradient of interstitial lung disease.

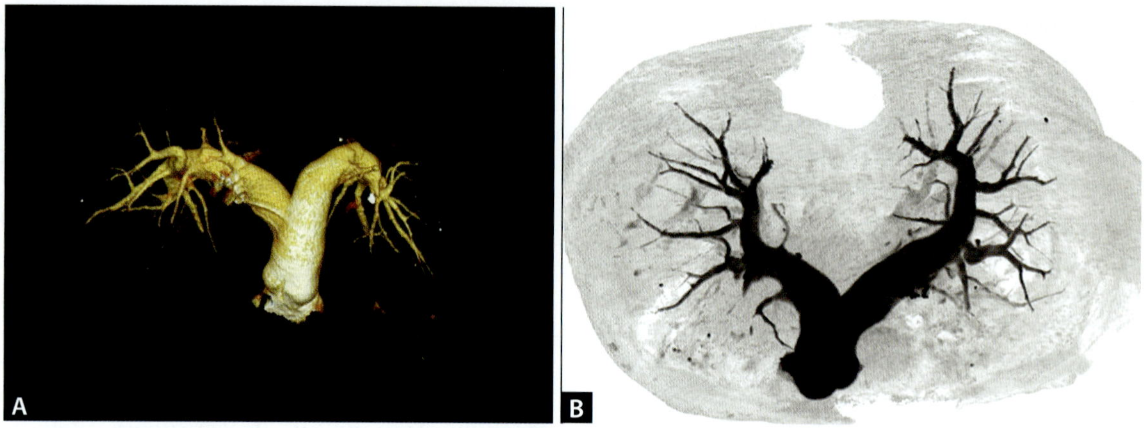

Figs. 2A and B: Normal CT pulmonary angiogram: Volume rendered (A) and MIP imaging displayed in the negative or angiographic mode (B) obtained with 30 mL of 350 mg I/mL contrast.

volume can be calculated as total time × flow rate (12 × 4 = 48 cc) for perfect vessel opacification. Scan should be triggered by bolus- tracking ROI in the main pulmonary artery with a trigger threshold of 80–120 HU.

- Holding of breath in deep inspiration or Valsalva maneuver is to be avoided to prevent **transient interruption of contrast medium**. This results in poor opacification of the pulmonary artery while the SVC and aorta are well opacified. Various mechanisms have been proposed for this, which include increased venous return of unopacified blood from IVC to right atrium resulting in poor opacification of pulmonary arteries. Opening of patent foramen ovale due to Valsalva maneuver is thought to be the other reason. Hence the patient should be asked simply to hold his breath and not to take a deep inspiration during acquisition.

EVALUATION OF THE AORTA AND CORONARY ARTERIES

Evaluation of the aorta and coronary arteries is discussed elsewhere in this book, however, ECG gating is mandatory for coronary artery evaluation and can also help to eliminate confusing artefacts at the aortic root in patients with suspected dissection.

EVALUATION OF PULMONARY VEINS

Evaluation of pulmonary veins may be indicated in suspected stenosis after radiofrequency catheter ablation treatment of chronic atrial fibrillation. A preprocedure CT is also indicated to map variant venous anatomy to enhance success rate of the procedure and to exclude atrial thrombi which are an absolute contra-indication for the procedure. This requires 70–85 mL of 300–370 mg I/mL contrast to be administrated at 4–5 mL/s, acquisition being triggered by bolus tracking ROI placed in the left atrium. ECG gating is not routinely required as the atria move much less compared with coronary arteries with cardiac motion and the pulmonary veins are much larger structures.[13]

EXTENDED CHEST PAIN PROTOCOL OR TRIPLE RULE OUT CT

In this case, the aim of contrast injection is to achieve opacification of the aorta, coronary arteries and pulmonary arteries simultaneously. 130–160 ml of 300–370 mg I/mL contrast medium is injected between 4–5 mL/s with bolus tracking in the ascending aorta. ECG gating is used to freeze cardiac motion of the coronaries and aortic root. The acquisition is done in the caudocranial direction to minimize streak artefacts from the SVC.[14]

POST-PROCESSING TECHNIQUES[1,11,15,16]

The goal of true isotropic imaging, i.e. each voxel with equal dimensions in all 3 axes was achieved with the introduction of modern MDCT scanners. This allows high-quality 2D and 3D reconstructions, converting CT from a 2D imaging modality to a volumetric or 3D imaging technique. Although, axial images remain critical to establish the diagnosis, these reconstructions are extremely useful for display of airways (including complex congenital abnormalities) vascular structures and distribution of pulmonary disease. Isotropic imaging has also helped the development of computer-aided detection and diagnosis programs. They increase diagnostic confidence, allow preprocedural planning for surgery or bronchoscopy and improve communication with clinicians and patients.

Multiplanar and Curved Multiplanar Reconstruction or Curved Planar Reconstruction (MPR and CMPR)

These are 2D post-processing techniques that can be used to obtain images in coronal, sagittal, oblique or even curved planes by reordering of voxels into a single voxel thick tomographic section, excluding the voxels outside the imaging plane **(Fig. 3)**. They allow viewing of a structure or abnormality in alternative planes, hence are useful when there are interpretative difficulties on axial sections. MPRs are useful for evaluation of large airways, vascular structures and to distinguish periarterialor peribronchial lesions from endoluminal ones. They are especially valuable for determining the craniocaudal length of airway stenosis which may be underestimated on axial images alone. They also allow accurate delineation of structures that run oblique to the axial imaging plane. Demonstration of centrilobular emphysema is facilitated as well. Coronal reformation helps to display of the distribution of parenchymal lung disease, e.g. the craniocaudal gradient in interstitial lung disease. Sagittal images can sharply delineate fissures and help to assess transfissural extension of disease.

Maximum Intensity Projection

Maximum intensity projection (MIPS) is a 3D reconstruction technique in which a ray is passed through the dataset and only pixels above a certain assigned value are used reducing the data to a single plane. (This lacks depth information). Slabs of 5–10 mm for thin MIPS or the entire dateset may be used for thick MIPS. In the thorax, it is used mainly for vascular imaging and for evaluation of small pulmonary nodules where it may help to distinguish small nodules from vessels and in precise delineation of nodule distribution **(Figs. 4A and B)**. In patients with mosaic attenuation, it can help in differentiation of ground-glass attenuation (normal vascular diameter) and mosaic perfusion (altered vascular diameter).

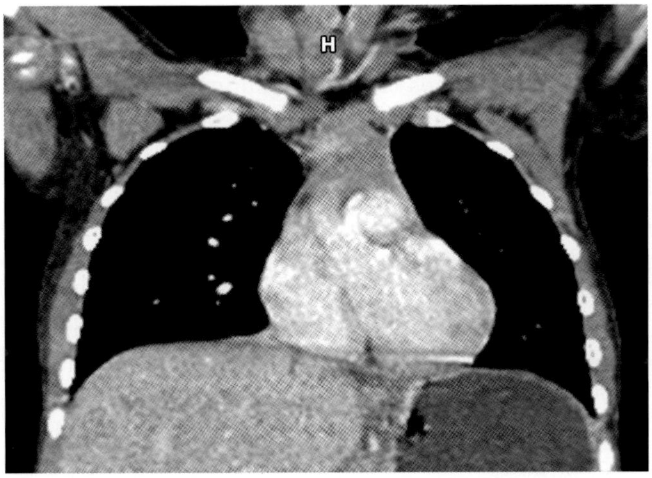

Fig. 3: Coronal multiplanar reconstruction at mediastinal window setting depicting the normal cardiac chambers.

Minimum Intensity Projection (MinIP)

This is similar to MIP hut only data below a certain value is displayed. It is useful to increase the conspicuity of low attenuation areas such as emphysema, air trapping or cystic changes **(Fig. 5)**. It is also useful for detection of ground-glass and linear attenuation patterns. Some authors have also found it useful to distinguish between bronchiectasis and honeycombing and for demonstrating bronchopleural fistula.

Shaded Surface Display

Shaded surface display (SSD) is a 3D surface-rendering technique that defines surface of tissue but does not provide any internal details. It is used in evaluation of airway abnormalities.

Volume-rendering

This is a unique 3D post-processing technique which displays depth information and 3D spatial relationships. A histogram representation of the entire dataset is done based on attenuation values. Voxels that are only partially filled with density of interest are also included. This is then manipulated to display internal and external perspective. The CT attenuation data can be mapped to brightness, color and opacity to display a particular structure of interest. Volume-rendered imagings can provide invaluable information because they preserve the 3D interrelationships of data. This is used extensively in the thoraxforangiographicexaminationsandairwayevaluation allowing evaluation of both central and peripheral airways and chest wall abnormalities **(Figs. 6A and B)**. Volume-rendering (VR) technique is extremely useful for evaluation of aneurysms and pseudoaneurysms, dissection, vascular slings and anomalous vessels. These images are valuable for preoperative planning. Imaging of the chest wall and thoracic cage benefits from VR because of the extremely complex anatomy of this region with a number of overlapping structures such as the shoulder girdle.

Virtual Bronchoscopy

Virtual endoscopic images of the airway are produced akin to bronchoscopy using surface and volume-rendering

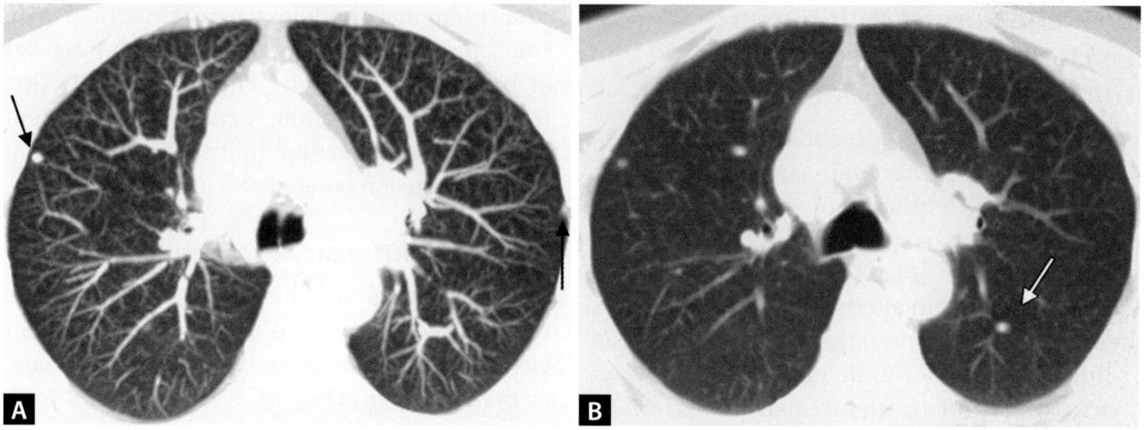

Figs. 4A and B: Axial MIP image at lung window settings (A) showing small nodules in the subpleural location on both sides (arrows) which are easily discerned from vessels. Note that one lesion that appears to be a small nodule in the apical segment of left lower lobe (arrow) on the 3 mm axial CT section (B) is actually a vessel on the MIP image.

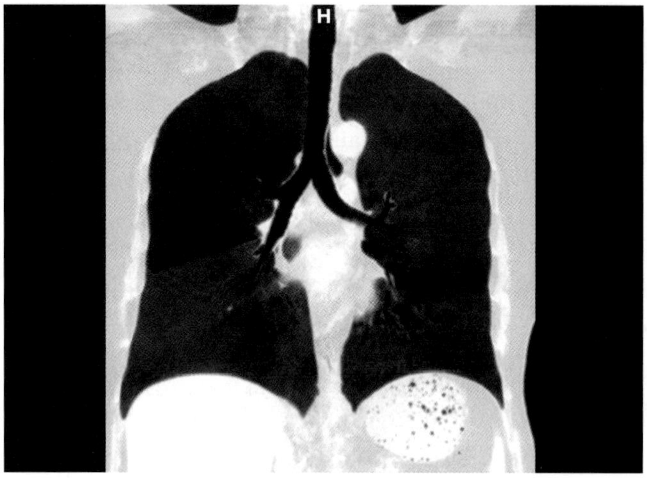

Fig. 5: Coronal MinIP image demonstrating not only the trachea, carina and central bronchi but also the smaller segmental bronchi.

techniques. The major advantage over conventional bronchoscopy is the ability to visualize the airway distal to an obstructing lesion **(Figs. 7A and B)**.

ADVANCED APPLICATIONS

Dual Energy CT: Thoracic Applications[1]

Dual energy (DE) CT allows differentiation of materials due to their different attenuation properties at different photon energies.[1] DECT requires simultaneous acquisition of data at two different kilo-Voltages, generally 100 kVp and 140 kVp. This can be achieved using a dual-source CT scanner with two X-ray tubes positioned at 90° to each other operating at two different kVs (Siemens) or a single-source CT with rapid KVs switching (GE) or a dual layer detector with different detectors absorbing different energies (Phillips). Recently, one vendor (Siemens) has introduced a single source twin beam dual energy CT which uses two filters one of tin (Sn) and the other gold (Au) to split a 120 Kv beam into a high-energy and low-energy beam respectively allowing DE acquisition.

Thoracic applications are based on the fact that the need for pre- and post-contrast images is eliminated and the computation of pseudomonoenergetic images. This avoids respiratory misregistration and reduces dose. For pulmonary nodule characterization, the generation of virtual noncontrast images thus allows exact enhancement to be measured. Iodine only maps of the lung parenchyma can also be generated to get a map of pulmonary blood volume and lung perfusion. This can help detect perfusion defects in acute and chronic thromboembolism providing a new functional aspect independent of thrombus visualization **(Figs. 8A and B)**.[17]

4D Scanning[18,19]

Dynamic 4D images to gain functional information on breathing mechanism can be obtained using physiologic respiratory triggers. Retrospective gating can be done using a cine mode where the table is still in one breathing cycle and then it is moved to cover a subsequent portion of lung. All the pieces of each respiratory phase are then put together to create a volume data set of the lung or tracheobronchial tree. The other technique is continuous acquisition of the whole chest in free shallow breathing. These can be acquired at low dose protocols with iterative reconstruction algorithms so that the radiation dose is not higher than an average low dose CT. Prospective gating similar to cardiac step and shoot is also becoming available.

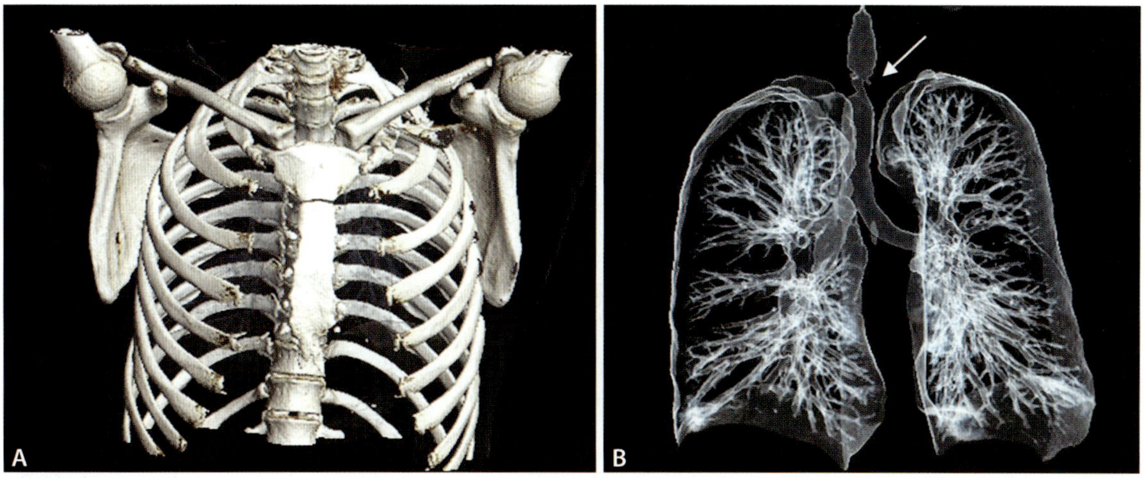

Figs. 6A and B: VRT images demonstrating the complex interrelationship between thoracic structures forming the thoracic cage (A) VRT image (transparency rendering) to show the central and peripheral airways. Note the area of narrowing in the trachea (arrow).

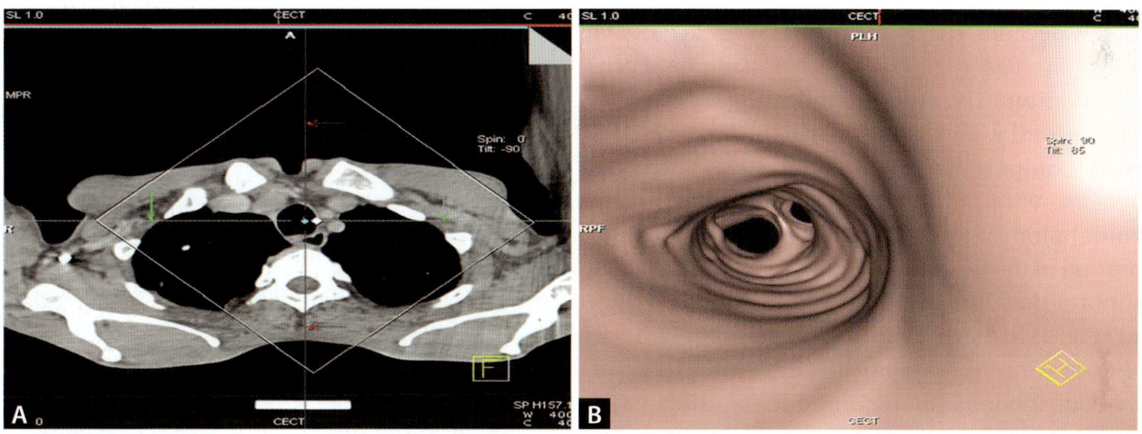

Figs. 7A and B: Virtual bronchoscopy image along with a source image showing the normal inner surface of trachea and the carina.

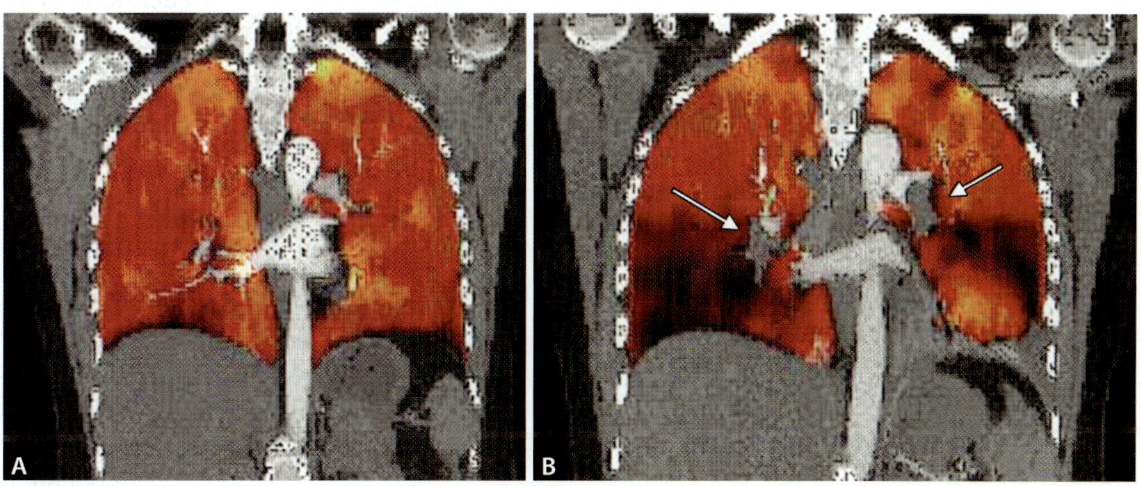

Figs. 8A and B: (A) Normal lung perfusion with DE acquisition displayed in a coronal format; (B) Large wedge-shaped perfusion detects due to pulmonary emboli in another patient (arrows).

Computer-aided Detection

This uses computer-based software for complex pattern recognition and employs a combination of image processing, segmentation and pattern classifiers to identify lesions like pulmonary nodules or emboli. Nodule volume quantification and quantification of pulmonary emboli can be done. Emphysema quantification has also been done by quantification of parenchymal lung density choosing a threshold value (usually below -950 HU) to identify emphysema. However, variation can occur due to differences in degree of inspiration, between contrast-enhanced and noncontrast scans and probably with the use of iterative reconstructions.[1,7,18,19]

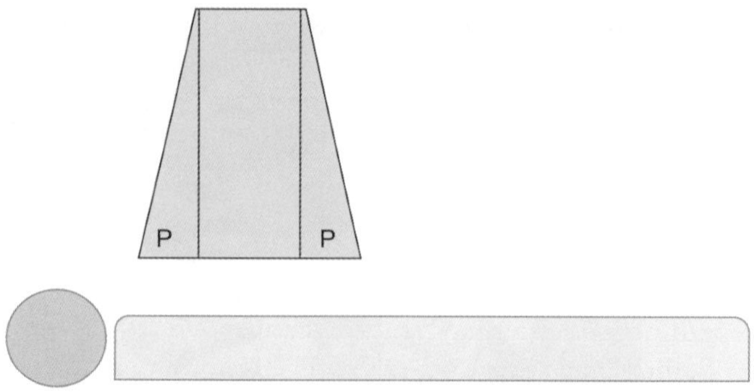

Fig. 9: Line diagram to show the trapezoidal dose profile along the Z-axis. The area outside the rectangle (P) on both sides represents the penumbra.

DOSE CONSIDERATIONS AND DOSE REDUCTION TECHNIQUES IN THORACIC CT[1,2,20]

In the past few decades, the utilization of CT for diagnostic purposes has increased exponentially raising concerns related to radiation exposure. Complicating this further is the fact that radiation exposure is higher with MDCT scanners as compared with a single slice scanners. This is because with multidetector CT the dose profile is trapezoidal along the Z-axis and only the central or umbral portion of the beam contributes to the image while the penumbral dose is wasted (also referred to as **over beaming) (Fig. 9)** In a single slice CT, on the other hand, in the entire dose contributes to image formation. However, the relative contribution of the penumbral region decreases as the number of simultaneously acquired slices increase thus a 128 slice CT results in less wasted radiation than a 4 slice CT. Gaps between detector elements in MDCT are another reason for decreased geometric efficiency and wasted dose as the photons falling in these regions do not contribute to image formation. Another problem with helical scanners is **over ranging**, i.e. irradiation beyond the imaged length is necessary in helical scanning for reconstruction of first and last images. This is larger with wider Z beam collimation (or larger number of detectors) offsetting improvement in dose efficiency of over beaming for shorter scan lengths. Modern CT systems now have **dynamic collimation diaphragms** such that the collimator opens asymmetrically at the beginning and end of an acquisition to eliminate radiation of tissues outside the range reducing this problem.

Dose Reduction Strategies

The first and foremost step in dose reduction is assessment of need. No CT should be performed without a valid indication and each study should be tailored to answer the specific clinical question at hand. Several technological advancements and modifications in technique can result in significant dose reduction. These are:

- *Tube current modulation using automatic exposure control or AEC*: Essentially, there are three methods available. Patient size-based modulation, Z-axis AEC and angular or X-Y-axis AEC. For patient size AEC, the appropriate current is selected by the system for the given patient size. Scanners assess the X-ray absorption profile over the patient's thorax during the topogram or scout acquisition and automatically choose the lowest tube potential for the patient and selected protocol. In the Z-axis or longitudinal modulation, the tube current is adjusted as the patient attenuation changes in the longitudinal direction or Z axis to ensure a constant image quality at each anatomical level. The angular tube current modulation adjusts the tube current as the tube rotates around the patient to compensate for attenuation changes as the view angle changes. The tube current is reduced at angles that are of less diagnostic importance. In most modern scanners automatic tube current modulation (A TCM) adapts the tube current in all 3 X-Y-Z-axes according to patient weight and can result in significant dose reduction while maintaining image quality.

  There are, however, two important considerations: determination of an acceptable level of image noise (this is generally preset by the manufacturer) and optimal patient position. The patient should be positioned centrally on the CT table ideally close to the isocenter prior to acquisition. This is because the use of automatic dose nodulation software in patients who are off the isocenter by as little as 3 mm may result in a 30% higher dose.

- *Tube current reduction in low dose examinations*: A 50% reduction in the tube current can reduce the effective radiation dose to half the original level. Several studies have demonstrated that the tube current time product or mAS may be reduced to levels as low as 40–70 mAS in chest CT without significantly affecting image quality since the lung is a high contrast organ. Most of these have been studies to detect pulmonary nodules in a screening setting. Some authors have demonstrated that common patterns of pulmonary diseases such as solid nodules, air space consolidation, airway and pleural diseases could be adequately demonstrated at 120 kV/40 mAS protocol using thin slices, high spatial frequency reconstruction kernel and standard filtered back projection (FBP) reconstruction. However ground-glass opacities and interstitial opacities require higher tube current or iterative noise reconstruction.
- *Tube potential reduction or low KV examinations*: The standard chest protocol is usually acquired at 120 kV, A low tube potential of 70–80 kV is useful in children and small adults due to the lower X-ray absorption profile. A tube potential of 80–100 kVp is also beneficial in adults when the area of interest is enhanced by iodinated contrast as for the thoracic aorta or pulmonary arteries. This is because the X-ray attenuation of iodine increases with the use of lower kV due to the K edge of iodine at 33 KeV. The X-ray attenuation of soft tissue depends only weakly on tube potential hence the contrast of vessels and tissue that take up iodinated contrast increases with respect to surrounding tissue increasing the contrast to noise ratio or CNR at the same dose. This effect can be utilized to either reduce radiation dose to patient or reduce the amount of iodinated contrast administered. A trade off while decreasing tube potential or voltage is that the mAs has to thus be significantly increased. Because of the lack of tube power reserves low kV scanning was limited to children and small patients. Recently new X-ray tubes with increased mA reserves and increased power at low kV have been introduced (VECTRON Siemens) which can extend this advantage to adults and obese patients. This may reduce radiation dose by as much as 52 %. Technologies that automatically adapt the tube voltage to the size and shape of the patient keeping in mind the power reserves of the tube are also available. This automatic tube voltage selection may reduce radiation dose in CT chest angiographies by as much at 38% compared to 120 KV protocol.
- *Use of a higher pitch*: Pitch is defined as table feed per rotation divided by the total width of the collimated beam. Using a higher table speed for a given collimation can significantly reduce patient dose if all other acquisition parameters are same. An important factor to take into account however is that in some modern scanners, e.g. Siemens and Phillips, an increase in table feed is automatically compensated by an increase in tube current to maintain the same effective tube current time product or **mAS effective** (defined as mAS/pitch). With these scanners an increase in pitch merely reduces examination time and not radiation dose. However, this may be very useful in sick, uncooperative patients in avoiding repeat examinations.
- *Use of filters*: These are of two types:
  - Beam shaping filters: Filters such as bowtie filters reduce ray intensity in the peripheral parts reducing radiation dose, especially skin radiation dose.
  - Spectral shaping: Spectral shaping by using a tin filter in the prepatient tube collimator box can significantly reduce patient dose in noncontrast lung examinations. The filter makes the beam 'harder' removing lower energy photons which would be absorbed in the patient without contributing to the image. This provision is available in the third generation dual source CT system. Low dose CT with spectral shaping and iterative reconstruction can reduce patient dose in quantitative lung CT and non-enhanced CT chest for pulmonary nodule detection to as low as 0.06 mSv when using 100 kv. This effect is however not valid for contrast-enhanced examinations as increased X-ray absorption of iodine at lower energies over compensates this. It also needs to be determined how well subtle features of lung parenchyma can be evaluated at such low doses.
- The length of coverage should be carefully planned so as not to extend the beyond the area of interest.
- Newer detector systems such as the solid state detectors have much higher detector efficiency than the conventional ionisation chamber-based detectors helping to reduce radiation dose.
- *Patient shielding*: Use of lead or lead free shields to protect areas outside the scan zone may help to reduce radiation exposure (e.g. thyroid and gonads). However, the use of bismuth breast shields to reduce radiation exposure to breast tissue during chest CT is not recommended as this increases image noise and artefacts. A similar breast dose reduction can be achieved by the methods already mentioned, such as tube current modulation.

- Newer reconstruction techniques: Newer reconstruction techniques that have become available can also help to reduce exposure indirectly as they help to reduce image noise making it possible to obtain diagnostic images with low dose examinations. CT images were traditionally reconstructed using the **filtered back projection (FBP)** technique. However, this requires a large amount of X-ray data to produce diagnostic quality images. The introduction of **iterative reconstruction (IR)** techniques into routine CT, made possible by the increased computational power of computers greatly enhances image resolution and reduces noise. In FBP increased spatial resolution is directly correlated with increased image noise while IR allows for decoupling of spatial resolution and image noise to a certain extent. (It maintains or enhances spatial resolution for high contrast objects while reducing noise in low-contrast areas). The first generations IR algorithms were image based IR, the second generation statistical weight based while the latest third-generation IR algorithms are model-based IR. It is reported that with the use of iterative reconstruction radiation dose could be reduced to less than 2 mSv for contrast-enhanced chest CT and to sub-mSv levels for noncontrast CT chest.
- Prospective ECG gating rather than retrospective gating for ECG gated examinations also reduces radiation exposure.

MAGNETIC RESONANCE IMAGING

The superior soft tissue contrast of MRI over CT ensures better tissue characterization in the evaluation of mediastinal masses, chest wall and diaphragm. In these areas, MRI already has an established role in diagnosis. However, most often it is performed subsequent to a CT examination not only due to the latter's faster image acquisition but also greater acceptance and familiarity among clinicians. The challenges to magnetic resonance imaging of the chest are due to its relatively longer acquisition times, motion artefacts related to respiratory motion and cardiac pulsations.

MR imaging of the lung especially is a very challenging field. This is because about 70% of the lung consists of air-filled spaces. Protons are localized within the tissues of the lung or blood vessels accounting for only 30% of the volume. The healthy lung thus has a tissue proton density which is about ten times lower than other tissues producing a signal that is 10 times weaker than other tissues even under perfect conditions.[21] The generation of MR signal from even these protons is hampered by two factors: the lung has countless air tissue interfaces which have very different magnetic properties leading to susceptibility artefacts with resultant loss of signal in structures such as alveolar septae and the pulsatile nature of blood flow. These problems are further compounded by artefacts due to respiratory and cardiac motion making lung one of the most difficult organs to image on MR. The susceptibility differences result in rapid dephasing of spins in gradient echo imaging hence pulse sequences with very short echo times (TE < 1–2 ms) are required. The magnetic field inhomogeneity increases with field strength hence even shorter TE's would be required for 3T systems offsetting the expected increase in SNR.[21]

Recently, there have been several advances in hardware and pulse design helping to overcome several of these limitations—such as multichannel MR systems, powerful gradients, parallel imaging, very short echo times, ultrafast turbo spin echo acquisitions, etc. These along with improved technology for k space sampling and development of contrast agents for perfusion and ventilation studies have put MR on the threshold of a radiation free alternative to CT in some clinical situations.[22-24]

TECHNICAL CONSIDERATIONS

Magnet Strength and Coils

For MRI of the thorax scanners with **a field strength** of 1.5 T and full parallel imaging capability are recommended. Chest MRI at 3T is more challenging because though theoretically, there should be an increase in SNR, this is offset by the faster signal decay due to susceptibility artefacts in the lungs. There are changes in relaxation times, increased magnetic field inhomogenity and increased SAR with 3T imaging hence modifications are required for imaging of the mediastinum, as well. The latest generation of MR scanners do provide some pretailored sequences for thoracic imaging allowing good quality images on 3T. Although field strength lower then 1.5 T has some potential advantages with respect to lung field homogeneity it requires signal averaging to improve SNR making imaging times unacceptably long.[21]

Along with the **spine coil** integrated in the table receive only **phased array body coils** are used over the chest. These increase SNR and allow parallel imaging reducing acquisition time. The coverage must be adequate in the craniocaudal and anteroposterior direction.[25]

Respiratory Motion

The availability of fast imaging sequences on modern scanners has ensured that most sequences can be acquired in less than 20 seconds. Thus, it is advisable to acquire images during a single breath hold or as a multibreath hold sequence. This minimizes blur associated with respiratory motion and is better than triggered or navigator sequences. The success of breath hold imaging can be significantly increased provided breath holding is rehearsed with the patient before lying down and the patient is informed about the frequency and duration of breath hold. If breath hold difficulty is anticipated, a MR compatible 2L nasal cannula oxygen can be provided to improve breath hold.[26] In patients who are unable to hold breath and for longer sequences synchronization of the image acquisition to the respiratory cycle is done. This can be done using respiratory or spirometric triggering or gating using external hardware such as pneumatic bellows or the signal of lung itself. Another method is to use navigator echoes to detect the motion of the diaphragm directly via MRI which can be used for retrospective gating of scans during free breathing.[21]

Cardiac Gating

Cardiac gating is useful to freeze cardiac motion for evaluation of cardiac and paracardiac lesions. ECG gating is preferred to peripheral gating because it freezes cardiac motion more reliably, eliminating pulsatility artefacts.[26]

PROTOCOL AND SEQUENCES

A basic protocol consists of noncontrast breath hold T1- and T2-weighted sequences without fat saturation. Gadolinium-based contrast agents are required for a number of indications such as evaluation of mediastinal and lung masses or pulmonary nodules, chest wall masses, pleural pathology, lung perfusion and evaluation of vasculature. A set of precontrast TIW images are acquired without fat saturation to facilitate detection of mediastinal nodes or masses surrounded by fat while postcontrast images are acquired with fat saturation. This may be done using the DIXON technique for a more homogeneous fat saturation near the neck. Identical parameters should be used for pre and post-contrast images when evaluating enhancement.[21,25] The postcontrast images can be acquired as a single post contrast T1W fat saturated sequence or as a dynamic contrast-enhanced examination (DCE) where multiple fast. 3D-T1W-GRE acquisitions are done after intravenous contrast.

Advantages of the dynamic technique include ability to show rate of enhancement over time, eliminating guess work about when maximal vascular or lesion enhancement will occur. The pattern of enhancement may help to increase specificity of diagnosis. In addition because exactly the same imaging parameters are used in the pre- and postcontrast acquisition, it is possible to measure relative ROI assessment of lesion hyperintensity and to subtract postcontrast images from precontrast which is very useful to assess enhancement in T1W hyperintense lesions.

The details of sequences used in MRI are summarized in **Table 1**. These sequences are obtained in the standard axial, coronal and sagittal planes. Additional planes may be used to optimize lesion characterization, e.g. to better characterize mediastinal or chest wall invasion acquisition can be planned to get images perpendicular or parallel to the site of invasion.

MR PULMONARY ANGIOGRAPHY

Heavily T1W 3D GRE FLASH/SPGR/FFE) sequences are used to obtain high resolution breath hold pulmonary angiograms. The shortest possible TR and TE is used with modest parallel imaging. Contrast is usually given via a pressure injector in a dose of 0.2 mL/kg body weight at 2–3 mL followed by a saline flush of 20 mL at 5 mL/sec. The acquisition is optimized to peak vascular enhancement using a test bolus or care bolus technique.

Alternatively a time resolved 3D sequence with echo sharing such as TRICKS/TREAT/TWIST can be used after intravenous injection of gadolinium, the so called "4D MRA" (3D over time). Acquisition times of 1.5 sec or less are possible so that multiple data sets in arterial and venous phases can be acquired **(Figs. 10A to D)**. The postcontrast images are subtracted from the precontrast images to enhance visualization of vasculature.[21,28]

MR PERFUSION IMAGING

MR perfusion of the lung or mediastinum is feasible using a time resolved low spatial resolution version of the time resolved pulmonary angiography sequence. With parallel imaging and view sharing spatial resolution can be enhanced. At a temporal resolution of <1s per 3D data set, this allows generation of passage kinetics curves and parametric maps of regional blood flow and blood volume. The contrast dose needed for a perfusion study is lower than that needed for a pulmonary angiography at 0.05 mL/kg followed by a 20 mL saline flush at 5 mL/sec. Generation of fully quantitative map of pulmonary blood volume PBV, pulmonary blood flow PBF and transit time (MTT) requires a deconvolution with arterial input function (AIF) measured in the larger arteries **(Figs. 11A and B)**. This may be challenging due to lack of linearity between local tissue contrast agent concentration and MR signal intensity. MR perfusion can provide information not just

Table 1: Sequences for lung and mediastinal MRI.[21,25,27,28]

Sl. No.		*Sequence*	*Vendor Acronym*	*Characteristics/Advantages*	*Uses*
1.	3D T1W GRE	GRE with parallel imaging/ slice interpolation	VIBE / THRIVE / LAVA	Covers entire thorax/lung in single breath hold at 5 mm slices	Pulmonary nodules masses
		With fat saturation (use Dixon for more homogeneous fat suppression)		Postcontrast imaging dynamic acquisition possible	• Airways • Dynamic for lung nodules • Dynamic lung volume • Tumor mobility for RT planning
		Heavily T1W 3D GRE	Flash 3D/FFE/SPGR	High spatial resolution for angiography (1.2 x 1 mm)	High resolution pulmonary angiography
		3D – GRE with echo sharing	TWIST/TRICKS/TRAK, etc.	Low spatial but high temporal resolution (<1–5 ms)	Lung perfusion and multiphase angiography
2.	Fast spin-echo T2W	Half fourier acquisition single shot TSE	HASTE/half scan FSE/½ NEXFSE	• Single/multibreath hold acquisition to cover entire chest • Low spatial, high temporal resolution • High SAR makes use at 3 T challenging	• Pulmonary infiltrates, bronchiectasis • Bronchial wall thickening
		• Rotating phase encoding • Central K space over sampling and inherent motion correction	BLADE/PROPELLOR/ Multivane	• Multibreath hold with moderate spatial resolution • Less motion artefacts from respiration and cardiac motion	• Pulmonary nodules and masses • Lymphadenopathy
		Conventional high resolution T2W/TSE	TSE/FSE	• Respiratory triggered acquisition during shallow breathing	Increased sharpness of lung pleural interphase
			Fat saturated FSE/BLADE, etc.		• Lymphadenopathy • Excellent for bone metastasis
3.	T2W GRE	Balanced steady state free precession (GRE)	True FISP/SSFE/FIESTA, etc.	*At short TR contrast is proportional to T2/T1*: • Single breath hold/free breathing Excellent anatomic information and soft tissue contrast Cine imaging possible *Disadvantages*: • High SAR • Susceptible to off resonance and field inhomogeneities resulting in banding artefacts especially at 3 T	• Effective for imaging blood and mucus (due to their long T2) • Differentiate masses/nodes vs vessels due to bright blood appearance • Respiratory mechanics diaphragmatic excursion • Relative tumor motion to assess mediastinal/chest wall invasion
			3D – bSSFP		Quick contrast free pulmonary angiogram Evaluation of pulmonary embolism without contrast
4.	STIR			Respiratory triggered sequence	Lymph node, bone metastases, lung nodule detection

Contd...

Contd...

Sl. No.		*Sequence*	*Vendor Acronym*	*Characteristics/Advantages*	*Uses*
5.	DWI (3 'b' values)	EPI		Respiratory triggered	Benign vs malignant pulmonary nodule/ masses, COPD
6.	Dual echo 2D GRE (T1 SPGR) In-opposed phase imaging (chemical shift)*		Turbo FLASH/FSPGR/TSE	Single breath hold imaging possible Detects microscopic fat	Useful for thymic hyperplasia vs neoplasm. Pulmonary hamartoma
7.	Double IR T2 cardiac gated		Double IR FSE 2/FSE 2/UFSE 2	Cardiac gated respiratory gated/breath hold	Exquisite anatomical information of mediastinal structures and cardiac chambers
8.	Double IR T1 cardiac gated		Double IR prep TSE T1/FSE 1/ SFSE T1	Fat saturation can be added	Exquisite anatomical information of mediastinal structures and cardiac chambers

*Some authors have reported that in and out of phase images from precontrast 3D–T1 SPGR with Dixon technique can provide similar information as a separate in—opposed phase sequence saving time.[21]

Abbreviations: bFFE: Balanced fast field echo (gradient echo sequence with steady state acquisition: (Philips); BLADE: Brand name/not an acronym (rotating phase encoding sequence; Siemens); FFE: Fast field echo (gradient echo sequence synonymous to FLASH; (Toshiba, Philips); FIESTA: Fast imaging employing steady-state acquisition (gradient echo sequence with steady state acquisition; GE); FLASH: Fast low-angle shot (GE; Siemens); FSE: Fast spin-echo (sequence; GE, Hitachi, Toshiba); GRE: Gradient echo (gradient echo sequence); Half scan: Half Fourier acquisition technique (Philips, Hitachi); HASTE: Half-Fourier short turbo spin echo (sequence; Siemens); LAVA: Liver acquisition with volume acceleration (a 3D gradient echo sequence with volume interpolation and RF fast saturation (GE); MRA: Magnetic resonance angiography; Multi Vane: Brand name/not an acronym (rotating phase encoding sequence; Philips); SPGR: Spoiled gradient echo recalled (sequence synonymous to FLASH; GE); SSFP: Steady state free precession (gradient echo sequence with steady state acquisition); STIR: Short tau inversion recovery sequence; THRIVE: T1 high-resolution isotropic volume excitation (a 3D gradient echo sequence with volume interpolation and RF fat saturation; Philips); TRAK: Time-resolved angiography using keyhole (a temporally resolved 3D gradient echo sequence with temporal resolution (3D+T) achieved by echo sharing; Philips); TRICKS: Time-resolved imaging of contrast Kinetics (a temporally resolved 3D gradient echo sequence with temporal resolution (3D+T) achieved by echo sharing; GE Philips; True FISP: True fast imaging with steady-state precession (gradient echo sequence with steady-state acquisition; Siemens); True SSFP: True steady state free precession (gradient echo sequence with steady state acquisition; Toshiba); TWIST: Time-resolved angiography with stochastic trajectories (temporally resolved 3D gradient echo sequence with temporal resolution (3D+t) achieved by echo sharing' Siemens); VIBE: Volumetric interpolated breath-hold examination (a 3D gradient echo sequence with volume interpolation and RF fat saturation; Siemens).

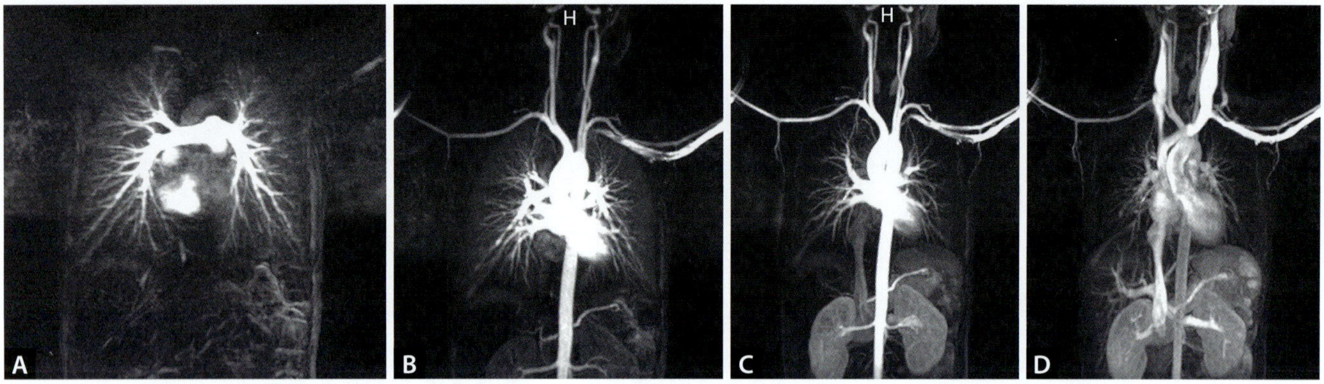

Figs. 10A to D: Multiphasic pulmonary angiogram using TWIST on a 3 T magnet. Note all the phases from the pulmonary opacification in the first image (A) to venous in the last image (D).

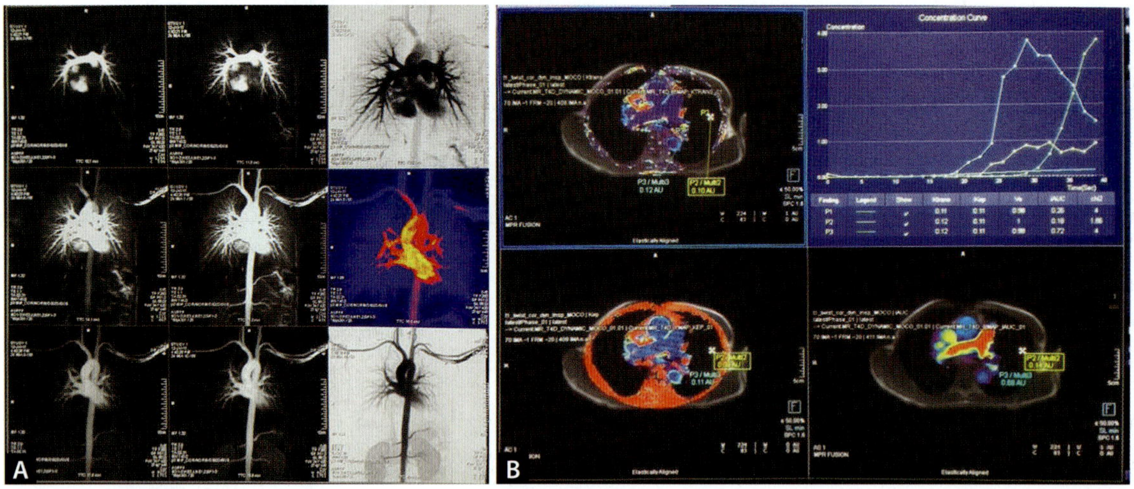

Figs. 11A and B: Multiphasic MR acquisition with generation of qualitative perfusion maps (A) and quantitative perfusion curves; (B) The yellow curve represents the pulmonary perfusion.

on presence or absence of perfusion but also on the time course of perfusion or capillary filling time. Delayed filling presumably via collaterals can be identified. Pulmonary hemodynamics and blood flow can also be analyzed using techniques developed for cardiac MRI.

Noncontrast methods proposed for assessing pulmonary perfusion include **arterial spin labeling techniques (ASL)**. Although several different variants of this have been proposed, they largely remain experimental.

OTHER ADVANCED/NEWER IMAGING TECHNIQUES

Ultrashort Echo Time Imaging

Ultrashort echo time (UTE) sequences that use radial K space sampling have recently become available. These shorten echo times to below 1 ms. At these very short TE (≤100 ms) the short T2 of the lung is less problematic and images with parenchymal sensitivity are possible. The resolution of these images is below the routine images, however they do make possible proton density contrast which allows visualization of parenchymal lung disease hitherto impossible with MRI.

Novel Contrast Methods and Ventilation MR

Ventilation is the second important aspect of gas exchange in the lung. 4D-MRI can visualize breathing motion and analyze lung volumes which have demonstrated excellent agreement with spirometric studies.

Direct visualization of lung ventilation can be done using hyperpolarized noble gases, sulfur hexafluoride or oxygen inhalation. Oxygen is paramagnetic, when the patient breathes in pure oxygen instead of air, it shortens the T1 of blood, plasma and tissue in the lungs resulting in an increase in signal. This can be used to generate parametric maps with ventilation and perfusion weighting.

Hyperpolarized noble gases like Xe-129 and He-3 can also be used to give high signal to noise images of lung ventilation. These techniques, however largely remain experimental.

CLINICAL APPLICATIONS OF MR THORAX

There are a number of emerging areas of thoracic imaging (besides cardiac applications) where MRI can play a significant role depending on the availability of expertise.

Mediastinum

MR can help to better characterize mediastinal abnormalities and masses. It is superior to CT in distinguishing solid from cystic masses, presence of hemorrhage and can help to detect both microscopic and macroscopic fat within the lesion. The detection of microscopic fat by chemical shift MR can help to distinguish between thymic hyperplasia (which has microscopic fat) from tumor (which lacks microscopic fat). Dynamic contrast enhancement patterns and low ADC values have been used to distinguish between benign and malignant lesions. Due to superior demonstration of fat planes and cine imaging capability MR can help to more accurately demonstrate lesion invasiveness, its relationship to critical vascular structures and discernment of mediastinal from paramediastinal lesions. Mediastinal and hilar nodes can be easily detected without the use of contrast however calcified nodes are difficult to detect.

Pulmonary Embolism and Pulmonary Hypertension

In a meta-analysis gadolinium enhanced MRA has a reported sensitivity varying from 77–100% and specificity of 95–98%.[30] The sensitivity is reported to be 100% for central and lobar arteries while it falls to 40% for subsegmental branches. MRA with MR perfusion has been shown to be highly accurate (98%) for detection of embolism with the perfusion sequence having a sensitivity of 100% and specificity 91%.[29,31] MR imaging using a combination of MRA and perfusion sequence allows differentiation between idiopathic pulmonary artery hypertension and secondary pulmonary artery hypertension due to thromboembolic disease. The latter shows features of segmental perfusion defects besides vascular change while the idiopathic variety shows a more diffuse and patchy perfusion pattern.[24,32] Even more importantly MR allows assessment of right ventricular dilatation, hypertrophy and estimation of cardiac strain and pulmonary artery pressures.[23]

Lung Cancer

In lung cancer imaging MR has a role in evaluation of Pancoast's tumors where it is reported to be more accurate than CT in demonstrating blood vessel and brachial plexus involvement. It is superior to CT for demonstrating pericardial, heart, mediastinal, vessel and chest wall involvement and may be indicated in specific situations as a problem-solving tool. MR may also be useful to distinguish between a central mass and postobstructive atelectasis, the latter showing higher signal intensity on T2W images, the central mass also shows lower ADC values than atelectasis **(Figs. 12A to D)**.[23,24]

Detection and Characterization of Pulmonary Nodule

MRI and CT have been reported to be equally accurate in distinguishing between benign and malignant pulmonary nodules in a recent meta-analysis.[32,33] For nodule detection noncontrast MR has significantly lower sensitivity (82.5%) as compared to MDCT (97%) but in detection of malignant nodules, there is no significant difference between the two techniques **(Figs. 13A and B)**. Nodules smaller than 5 mm are difficult to detect on MR. Malignant nodules have been reported to show lower ADC values than benign nodules. Enhancement characteristics can also be assessed using contrast-enhanced dynamic MR sequence. In and opposed phase imaging have been used to demonstrate microscopic fat in pulmonary hamartoma.[34]

Pneumonitis

In children with suspected pneumonitis MR can detect thoracic abnormalities such as consolidation, ill-defined nodules and effusions.[23,27] In a recent study, rapid lung MR has been reported to be comparable to MDCT in detecting thoracic abnormalities in pediatric patients with suspected pulmonary infection.[35] MR may be used in the follow up of pulmonary infections in order to reduce radiation exposure associated with CT.

Emphysema and Chronic Obstructive Pulmonary Disease

Researchers have attempted to use ventilation MR using He-3 to grade and characterise chronic obstructive pulmonary disease (COPD) with large wedge shaped or lobar defects being typical of advanced COPD. Alveolar filling time can be calculated using dynamic imaging of ventilation kinetics and alveolar size estimation may be done using ADC. MR perfusion can show perfusion defects correlating with severity due to hypoxic vasoconstriction.

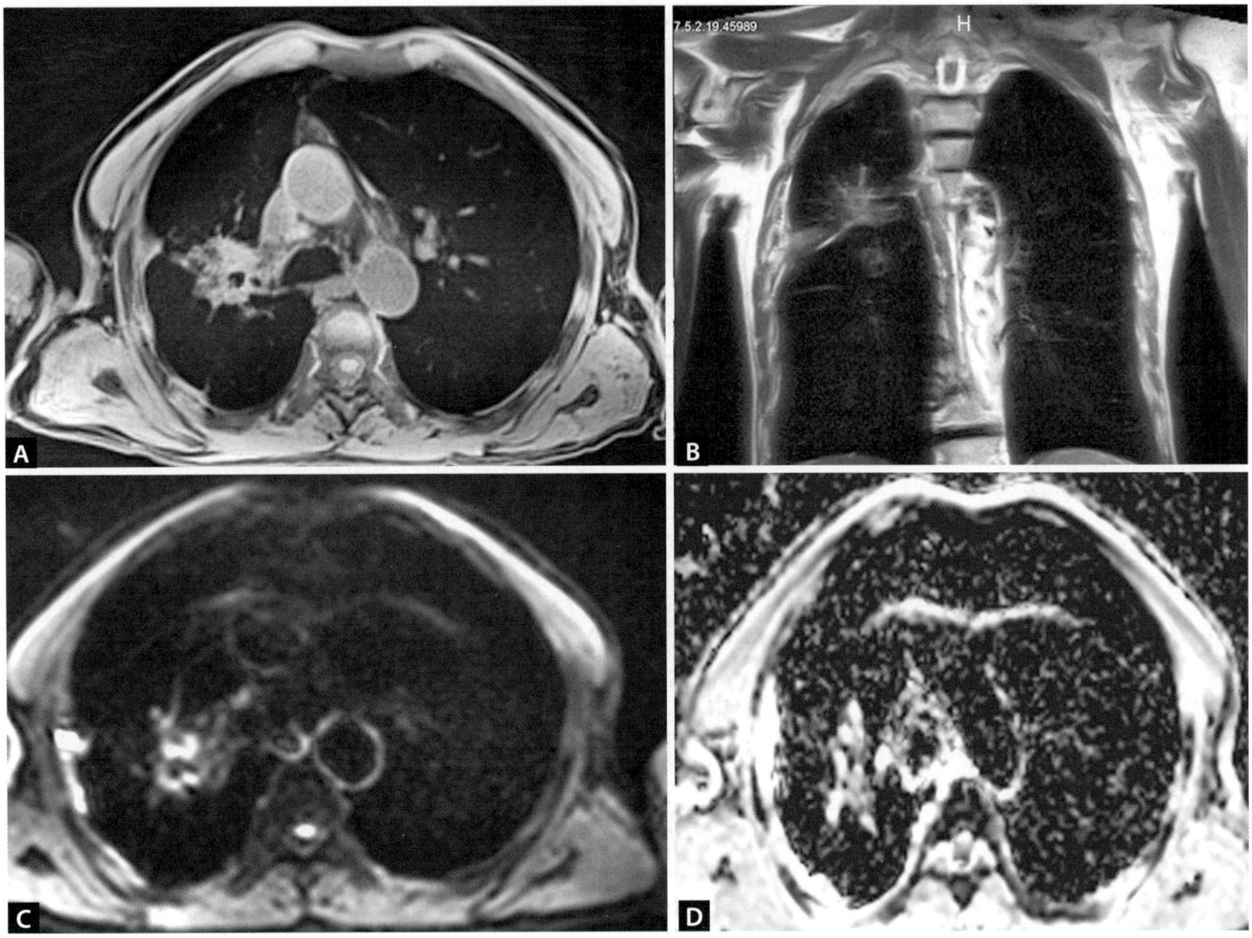

Figs. 12A to D: Axial T1(A) and coronal T2W (B) images in a case of lung cancer show a spiculated mass obstructing the right upper lobe bronchus with a pleural tail. DWI and ADC Map (C and D). Note the areas of diffusion restriction within the mass and in the pleura suggesting pleural spread.

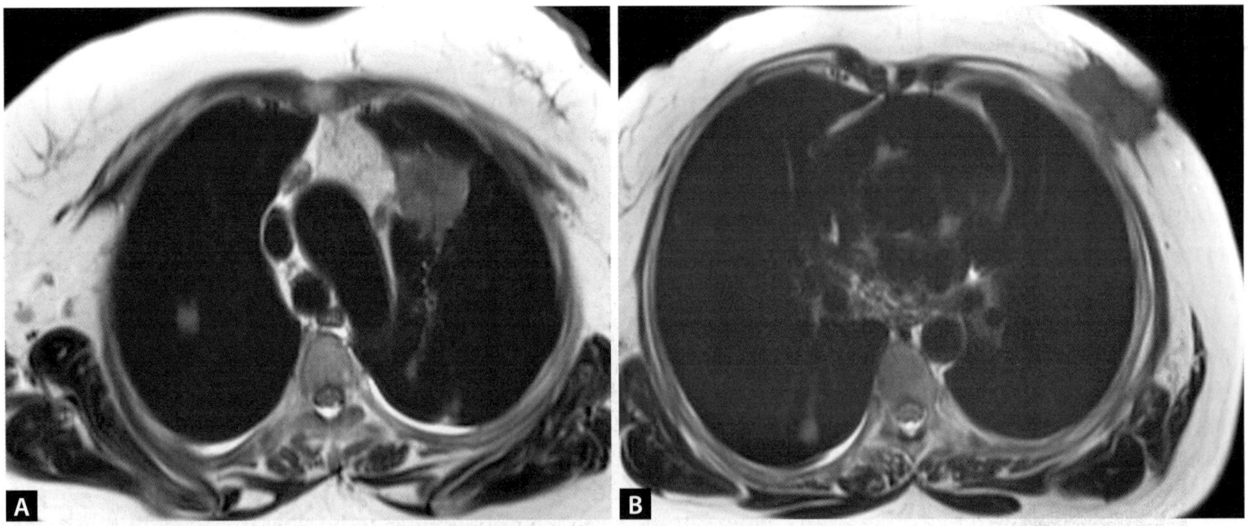

Figs. 13A and B: Axial T2W (HASTE) MR images show multiple lung metastases that appear hyperintense to skeletal muscle in a patient with carcinoma breast. Note the mass lesion in the right breast.

It can also evaluate diaphragmatic motion and dynamic lung volumes which are often altered in these patients.[23,27]

Cystic Fibrosis

Since patients with cystic fibrosis are young at presentation and require multiple examinations for follow-up MR-has been suggested as a tool for follow-up imaging. MR has been reported to be comparable to CT in detecting morphological lung changes while it is superior to CT in assessment of functional alterations. It is possible to visualize bronchiectasis, bronchial wall thickening, mucus plugging, air fluid levels and consolidation on MR. Functional assessment includes evaluation of respiratory mechanics, lung perfusion, blood flow and pulmonary ventilation using hyperpolarized gases for MRI.[22,24,27]

Interstitial Lung Disease

Three essential applications of MR have been suggested in literature—assessment of morphological changes and patterns, evaluation of inflammatory disease activity and effect of morphological changes on functional parameters. Consolidation, fibrotic changes, nodules, reticulation, etc. can be detected due to the increased T2W signal although subtle changes in subpleural region are difficult to detect. Post-contrast T1W images which increase the signal of the lung have been used to assess honeycombing. Dynamic MR and differences in T2W signal have been used to distinguish between active inflammation from fibrosis **(Figs. 14A and B)**.[27]

Pleura, Chest Wall and Diaphragm

MR can easily demonstrate pleural effusion, deposits and plaques of asbestosis. It is superior to CT in distinguishing pleural effusion from thickening and discernment of pleural invasion by tumours. Calcifications, a sign of benignity are however not well seen. MR is routinely used for evaluating chest wall masses to demonstrate the exact extent and invasion by the mass. MR can also be used to evaluate diaphragmatic pathologies like eventration, hernia and paralysis **(Figs. 15A to D)**.[25,27]

NORMAL ANATOMY

MEDIASTINUM

Normal mediastinal anatomy can be evaluated by analyzing CT or MR images at certain predefined anatomical levels due their characteristic appearance and landmarks.

Axial Sections (Cranial to Caudal)

Thoracic Inlet (Junction of Neck and Thorax)

Most mediastinal structures are vascular at this level. The internal jugular veins join the subclavian veins to from the brachiocephalic veins posterior to the clavicular heads. These veins are the most anterior and lateral vessels at this level. Medially lie the two common carotid arteries-while just posteriorly are the two subclavian arteries. The SCA cross over the first rib to exit the mediastinum and enter the axilla. The esophagus lies posterior or posterolateral to the trachea **(Fig. 16A)**.

Left Brachiocephalic Vein Level

The left brachiocephalic vein crosses the midline just beneath the manubrium to join the vertically oriented right brachiocephalic vein to form the superior vena cava. Between the brachiocephalic vein and the trachea are the three major branches of the arch of aorta—the innominate artery which is nearly midline, the left common carotid

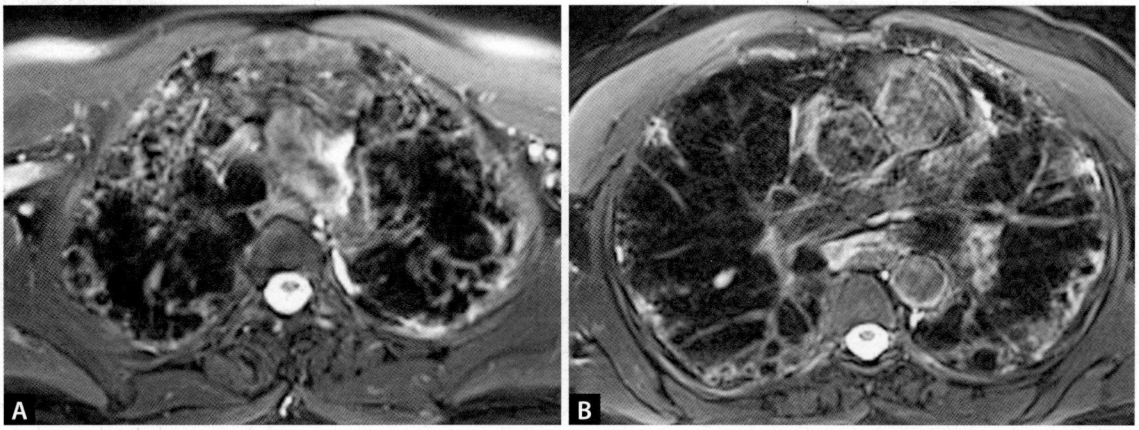

Figs. 14A and B: T2W images (FSE BLADE with fat saturation) show honeycombing in the subpleural regions of both lungs. Note some areas show higher signal, than the rest on the T2W images suggesting active inflammation according to some researchers.

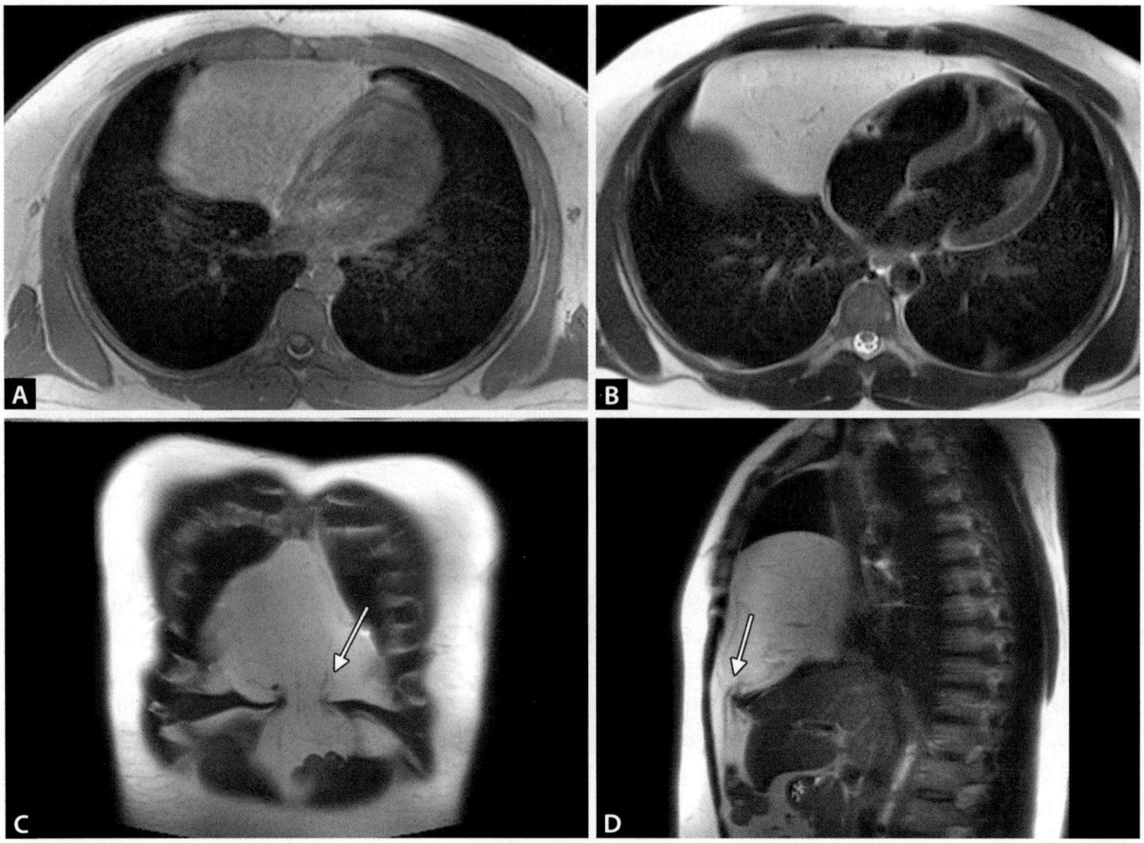

Figs. 15A to D: Axial T1W FLASH (A) and T2W HASTE (B) in a case of Morgagni's hernia show a paracardiac mass with signal identical to subcutaneous fat. The diaphragmatic discontinuity (arrows) through which the omentum is herniating into the thorax is well seen on the coronal and sagittal HASTE images (C and D).

artery which is slightly to the left and posterior and the left subclavian artery which is the most posterior and lateral vessel in close contact with the left upper lobe **(Fig. 16B)**.

Aortic Arch Level

The aortic arch traverses obliquely from right to left and anterior to posterior to left side anteriorly posteriorly just anterior to the trachea. The superior vena cava is seen in cross section adjacent to the anterior portion of the arch to the right side of trachea. The space posterior to the SVC, anterior to the trachea and lateral to the transverse aorta is the pretracheal space or anterior paratracheal space. Anterior to the great vessels and brachiocephalic veins is prevascular space. Both these spaces contain fat and small lymph nodes. Posterior or posterolateral to the trachea and anterior to the spine is esophagus **(Fig. 16C)**.

Azygos Arch-aortopulmonary Window Level

The azygos vein arches anteriorly from its location just anterior and slightly to the right of the spine to join the SVC. The entire arch may not be visible in a single section and occasionally this is poorly opacified leading to confusion with lymphadenopathy. The ascending aorta lies anterior to the trachea and descending aorta on the left posterolateral aspect of trachea. The ascending aorta in larger than the descending aorta measuring about 3.5 cm in mean diameter while the descending measures about 2.5 cm (this varies with age and sex). The aortopulmonary window is also seen at this level as a fat filled space. It is located between the inferior aspect of aortic arch superiorly and the superior aspect left pulmonary artery inferiorly. The contents of this important space include lymph nodes, left recurrent laryngeal nerve and the ligamentum arteriosum. The esophagus is seen anterior to the spine and posterior to trachea **(Fig. 16D)**.

Left Pulmonary Artery Level

The left pulmonary artery (LPA) is seen at a superior level compared to the main pulmonary artery and is located anterolateral to the left main bronchus at the level of

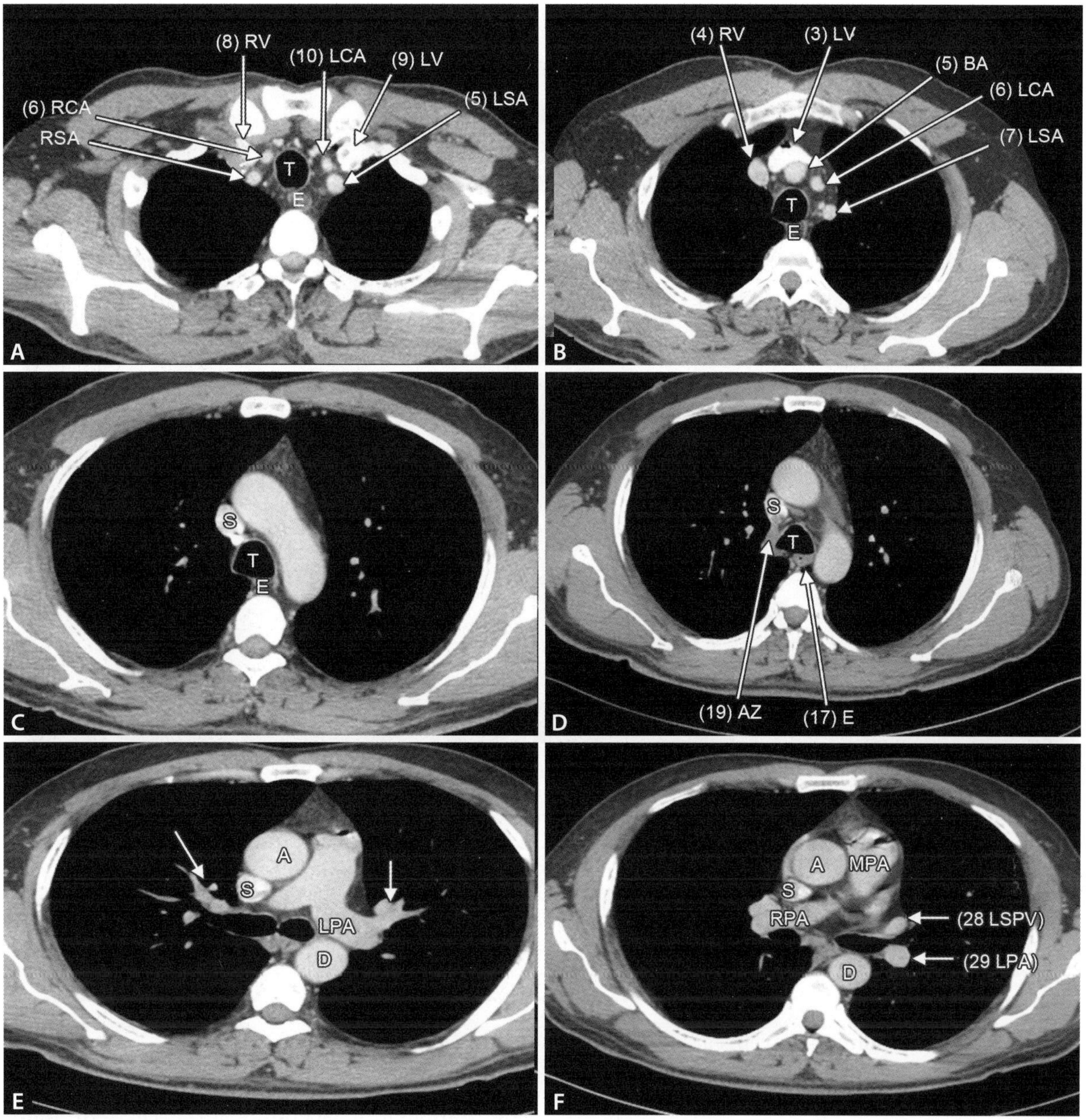

Figs. 16A to F: (A) Thoracic inlet level: The trachea (T) and esophagus (E) in midline. RV, Right brachiocephalic vein; RSA, right subclavian artery; RCA, right common carotid artery; LV, left brachiocephalic vein; LSA, left subclavian artery; LCA, left common carotid artery; **(B) Left brachiocephalic vein level:** Trachea (T), and esophagus (E); left subclavian artery (LSA); left common carotid artery (LCC); the right brachiocephalic vein (BRV) and left brachiocephalic veins (BLV) are anterior to the right brachiocephalic artery (BA); **(C) Aortic arch level:** The superior vena cava (S) and aortic arch lie anterior to the trachea (T) and esophagus (E). Anterior to the arch is the thymus, which has undergone fatty replacement; **(D) Azygos arch-aortopulmonary window level:** E, esophagus; T, trachea; the azygos vein (AZ) arches from a posterior position beside the esophagus to join the superior vena cava (S) crossing over the right upper lobe bronchus. The aortopulmonary window is between the ascending and descending aorta; **(E) Left pulmonary artery level:** To the left of the left pulmonary artery (LPA) lie the left superior pulmonary vein (zigzag arrow). The ascending (A) and descending (D) aorta and superior vena cava maintain their relative positions from the level above. The truncus anterior (TA), or right upper lobe pulmonary artery, is anterior to the right upper lobe bronchus. (arrow); **(F) Right pulmonary artery level:** S, superior vena cava; D, descending aorta; A, ascending aorta. The left superior pulmonary vein (LSPV) is anterior to the left main bronchus, and left pulmonary artery is posterior. The main pulmonary artery (MPA) divides into right pulmonary artery (RPA) and left pulmonary artery, which is more superior and not visible.

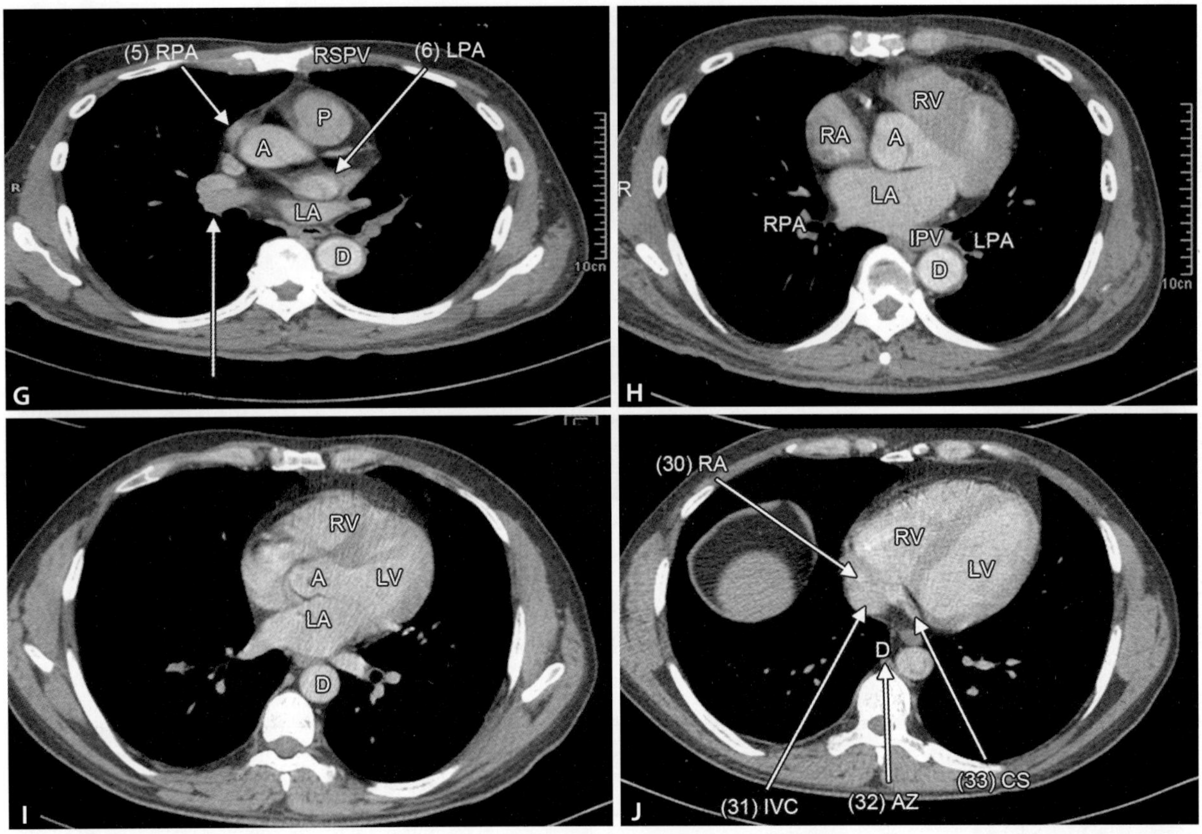

Figs. 16G to J: (G) Left atrial level: D, descending aorta; the right atrial appendage is anterior to the superior vena cava (S) and adjacent to the ascending aorta (A). The left atrial appendage is situated anterior and to the left of the left atrium, adjacent to the main pulmonary artery (P). The left atrium (LA) is the most superior and posterior chamber of the heart. Superior pulmonary veins enter the anterosuperior portion of the left atrium. **(H) Left atrial level** (at a caudal level). A, aortic root; D, descending aorta; IPV, left inferior pulmonary vein; LA, left atrium; LPA, left lower lobe pulmonary arteries; RA, right atrium; RPA, right lower lobe pulmonary artery; RV, right ventricle; **(I) Four chamber level.** A, aortic root; D, descending aorta; LA, left atrium; LV, lateral ventricle; RA, right atrium; RV, right ventricle; **(J) Three chamber level:** The left atrium is more cranial to this level and is not visible. The three visualized chambers are the right atrium (RA) with the IVC draining into it, right ventricle (RV), and left ventricle (LV). The coronary sinus (CS) is between the inferior vena cava (I) and the left ventricle. AZ, azygos vein; D, descending aorta.

carina. The left superior pulmonary veins are located just lateral to the posterior LPA. The right upper lobe bronchus can be seen arising from the right main bronchus at the level of carina. The right upper lobe pulmonary artery also called truncus anterior lies anterior to the right upper lobe bronchus. To the right of the esophagus lies the azygos vein. The hemi azygos vein lies to the left of the spine and parallels the course of the azygos vein. Along the posterior aspect of ascending aorta and anterior to the carina is a crescentic extension of the pericardium—the superior pericardial recess. It may contain a small amount of fluid or extend to more cephalad location and must not be confused with a lymph node or mass. Demonstrating continuity with the superior pericardial recess on contiguous sections can help to establish the true nature of a high riding pericardial recess **(Fig. 16E)**.

Right Pulmonary Artery Level

The main pulmonary artery (MPA) is situated anterior and to the left of ascending aorta. The right pulmonary artery courses posteriorly from the MPA between the SVC anteriorly and bronchus intermedius posteriorly. The right superior pulmonary vein lies to the right of the intra-pulmonary portion of RPA. Anterior to the left main and upper lobe bronchus lies the left superior pulmonary vein while posteriorly is the left lower lobe pulmonary artery **(Fig. 16F)**.

Left Atrial Level

In the upper sections, the right atrial appendage is situated anterior to the superior vena cava. It curves around the ascending aorta which is situated almost in the center of the mediastinum. The pulmonary artery out flow tract is located is located anterior and to the left of aorta. Posterior and to the left of the pulmonary artery outflow tract is the left atrial appendage (LAA)—roughly triangular in shape. The left main coronary artery courses in the fat between the LAA and aortic root. The right superior pulmonary veins drain into the left atrium just posterior to the superior vena cava **(Figs. 16G and H)**.

Four Chamber Level

All four cardiac chambers can be identified at this level. The left atrium is located posteriorly and is the most cranial of the chambers. On the posterolateral aspect inferior pulmonary veins can be seen entering the LA. The right atrium is situated anterior and to the right of the left atrium, which communicates with the right ventricle (RV) situated anteriorly and slightly to the left of RA. Just posterior and to the left of the RV lies the left ventricle. The right coronary artery may be seen in the right atrioventricular groove, the left circumflex in the left atrioventricular and left anterior descending coronary artery in the interventricular groove between the RV and LV **(Fig. 16I)**.

Three Chamber Level

At this level the left atrium, which has a more cephalad position is not visible. The right ventricle is seen just beneath the sternum, the left ventricle lying to the left posterolateral aspect. The right atrium is located posterior and to the right of right ventricle. The inferior vena cava opens into the inferior aspect of right atrium. Between the IVC and the left ventricle the coronary sinus can be seen opening into the right atrium **(Fig. 16J)**.

The normal axial anatomy on MRI can be seen in **Figures 17 and 18**.

Coronal and Sagittal Planes

These planes can be extremely useful for assessing the relationship between the mediastinal structures and their relationship with pathology. The anatomy is depicted in **Figures 19 and 20**.

Thymus

The thymus is situated anterior to the aorta and the pulmonary artery or right ventricular outflow tract in the prevascular space. It is usually best seen on a section through the aortic arch or great vessels. In children before puberty most of the mediastinum anterior to the great vessels is filled by the thymus. The size of the gland varies so much in this age group that it is not possible to decide if the gland is normal based on measurements alone, approximate symmetry is the norm. In addition, the normal gland appears to be moulded by the anterior chest wall and the great vessels **(Fig. 21)**. The size of the gland decreases with age. The average thickness of each lobe on CT decreases from 8–9 mm at 20 years to 5–6 mm at 50 years with the maximum thickness of each lobe being upto 15 mm.[1] The measurements are slightly greater on MRI probably because MR demonstrates thymic tissue replaced by fat as well. The craniocaudal measurements are 5–7 cm as measured on sagittal MR images. The density of the gland also changes from soft tissue attenuation prior to puberty to gradual fatty replacement so that above 40 years the attenuation is near, identified to fat making the gland indistinguishable from surrounding fat. Some streaky or modular densities may be seen representing residual thymic parenchyma. On T1W MR images the thymus has a signal similar to that of muscle and lower than that of mediastinal fat, with increasing age the signal of the gland increases approaching that of mediastinal fat. On T2W images the signal intensity differences are minimal and do not change with age **(Figs. 22A and B)**.

Lymph Nodes

Lymph nodes are distributed throughout the mediastinum. Normal lymph nodes are less that 10 mm in diameter in 95% cases. The remainder with a few exceptions being less than 15 mm. Retrocrural nodes (behind diaphragmatic crura) paraspinal nodes and those in the region of brachiocephalic veins are usually 6 mm or less. On the other hand, nodes in the aortopulmonary window, pretracheal, lower paratracheal and subcarinal compartment are often 6–10 mm in diameter. The nomenclature of mediastinal nodes should be in accordance with the international lymph node map in the TNM classification of lung cancer given by International Association for Study of Lung Cancer (IASLC).

Mediastinal Divisions on Cross-sectional Imaging[36,37]

Recently International Thymic Malignancy Interest Group (ITMIG) has introduced a new definition of mediastinal compartments to be adopted as a new standard with cross-sectional imaging. The three compartments as per this system are: (1) prevascular or anterior, (2) visceral or middle, (3) paravertebral or posterior **(Figs. 23A to D)**. The boundaries and contents of these are listed in **Table 2**.

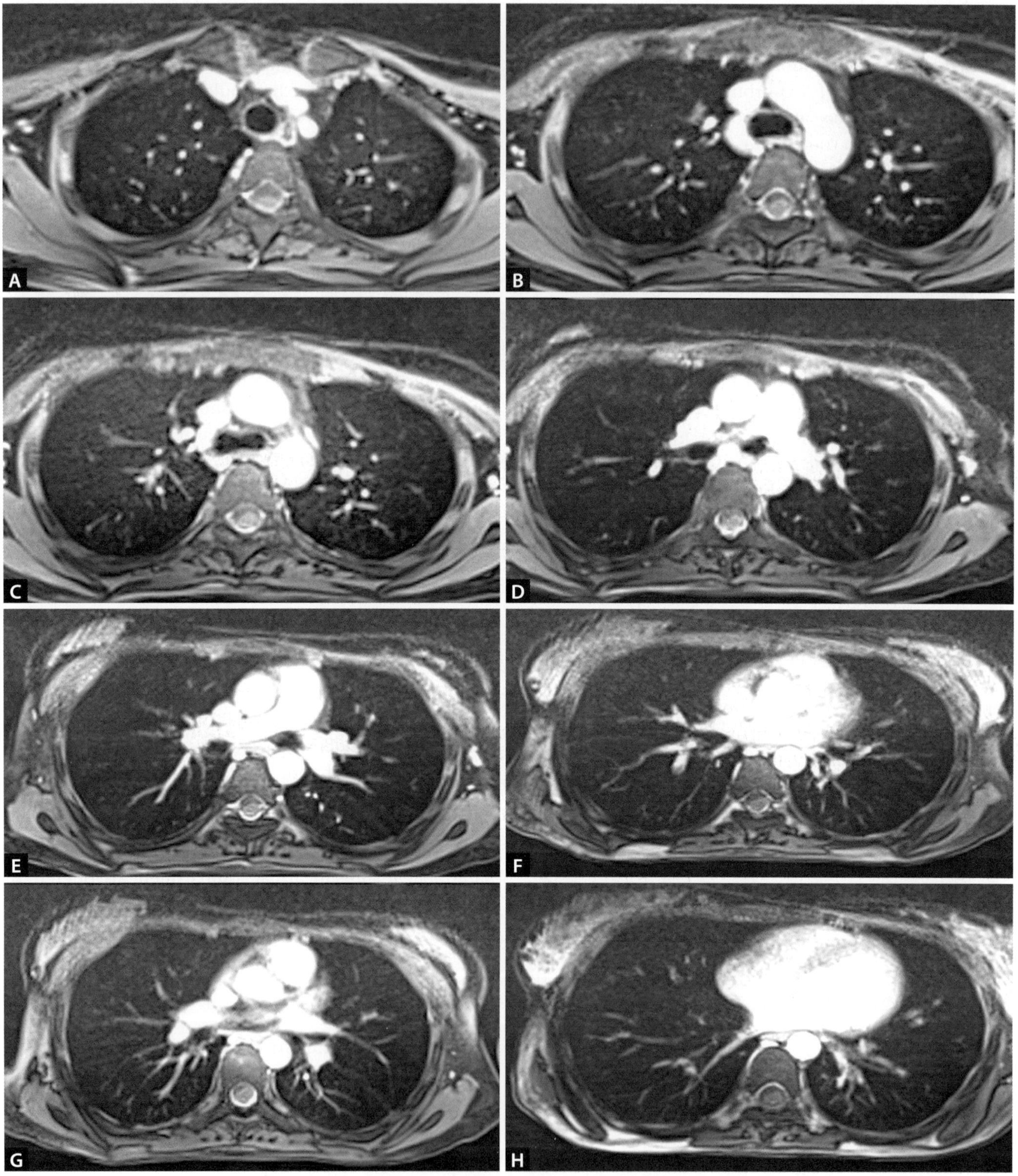

Figs. 17A to H: Postcontrast T1W (VIBE) images: Normal mediastinal anatomy on MR.

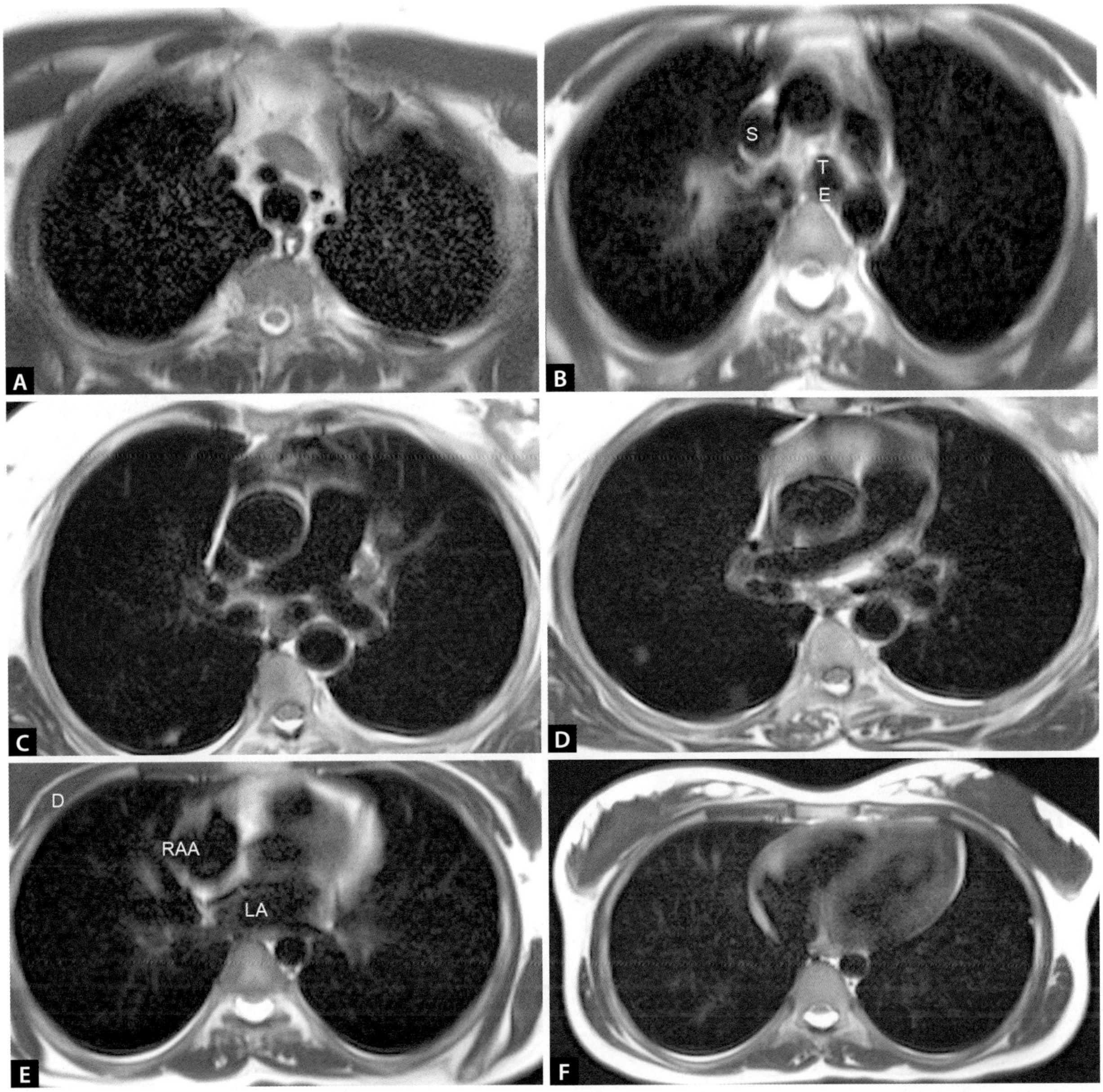

Figs. 18A to F: Representative HASTE axial images showing the normal mediastinal anatomy.

TRACHEOBRONCHIAL TREE [38,39]

The trachea is seen as a thin-walled air containing structure on axial CT scans lying anterior to the dorsal spine and esophagus. It is round or oval in shape with a slightly flattened posterior margin in about 25% patients. On expiratory scans, the posterior margin of the intrathoracic becomes more concave.

The normal dimensions of the trachea vary with the sex of the patient. In males, it ranges from 13 to 27 mm in transverse dimension and 13–27 mm in sagittal plane while in females the corresponding measurements are 10–21 mm and 10–23 mm. The tracheal index (coronal diameter in mm/sagittal diameter in mm) is approximately 1. Due to the angled course of the trachea a true perpendicular cross-section of its lumen is not obtained on axial CT images. The tracheal wall measures 3 mm in thickness. The posterior wall being thinner than the anterior wall. The cartilage within the anterior and lateral walls may appear slightly hyperdense as compared to surrounding soft tissue and fat. The cartilages may calcify in the elderly.

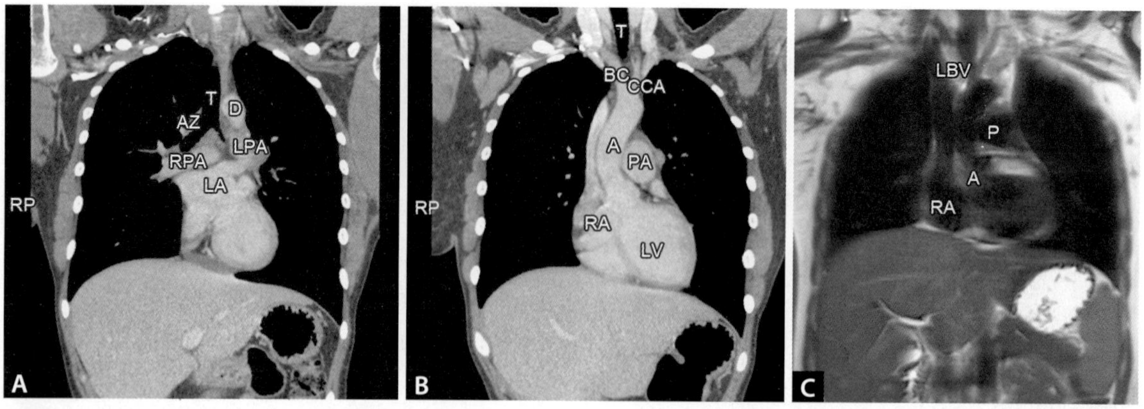

Figs. 19A to C: Coronal plane—CT at the level of carina (A) and at aortic outflow tract level (B) and corresponding MR (C): A, Aorta; LB, left brachiocephalic vein; LV, left ventricle; PA, pulmonary artery; RA, right atrium; LPA, left pulmonary artery; RPA, right pulmonary artery; D, descending aorta.

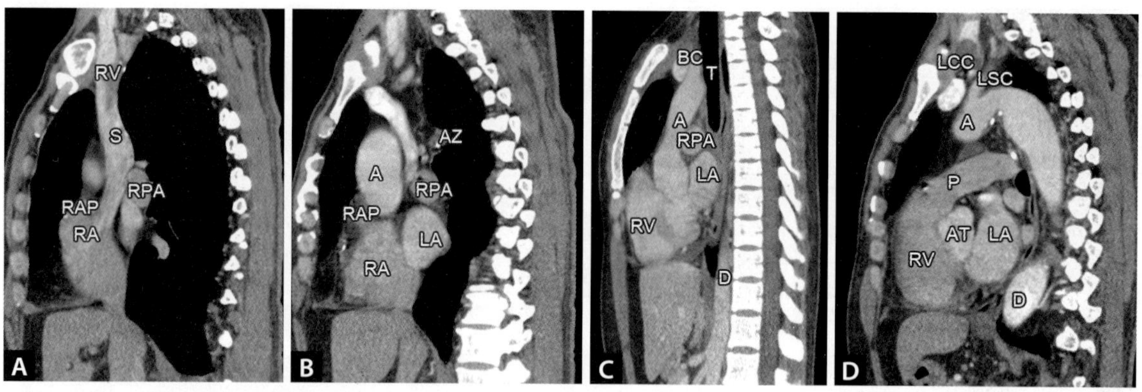

Figs. 20A to D: CT images: (A) Sagittal plane—superior vena cava level. RA, right atrium; RAP, right atrial appendage; RPA, right pulmonary artery; RV, right brachiocephalic vein; S, superior vena cava; (B) Sagittal plane—right atrial level. A, ascending aorta; AZ, azygos vein; LA, left atrium; RA, right atrium; RPA, right pulmonary artery; T, trachea; (C) Sagittal plane—aortic outflow tract level. A, ascending aorta; BC, brachiocephalic artery; D, Descending aorta; LA, left atrium; RPA, right pulmonary artery; RV, right ventricle; (D) Sagittal plane—pulmonary artery outflow tract level. A, ascending aorta; AT, aortic outflow tract; D, descending aorta; LA, left atrium; LCC, left common carotid artery; LSC, left subclavian artery; P, pulmonary artery (outflow tract); RV, right ventricle.

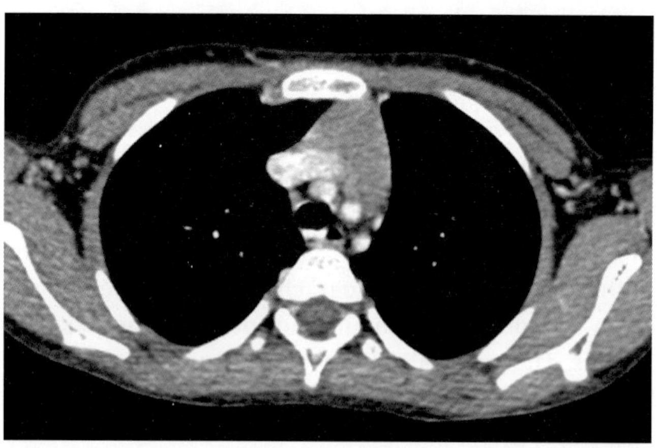

Fig. 21: Axial CT: Normal thymus in a 7-year-old boy seen as a triangular homogeneous soft tissue density anterior to the great vessels.

The trachea divides into the right and left main bronchi at carina. The right and left man bronchi course obliquely in the axial plane and are well seen on multiplanar reconstructions. On axial CT sections bronchi are seen as ring structures in cross-section while they appear as tubular structures when horizontally oriented.

The right upper lobe bronchus has a horizontal course and is seen just at or below the carina arising from the lateral aspect of right main bronchus. The anterior and posterior divisions of this, being horizontal in their proximal part are seen as tubular structures. The middle lobe bronchus arises from the anterior aspect of right main bronchus and is seen as a tubular structure due to its horizontal course. It divides into the medial and lateral segmental bronchi. At nearly the same level, the apical segmental bronchus

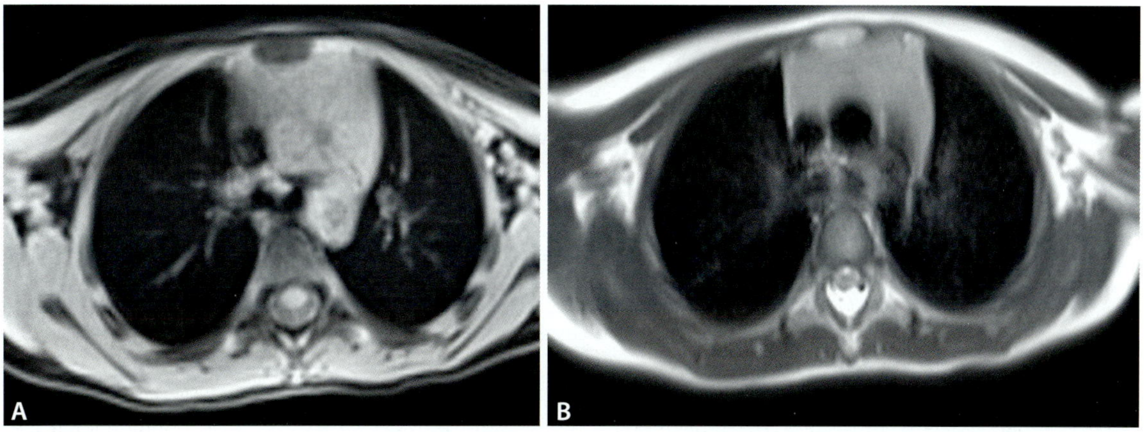

Figs. 22A and B: T1W FS (A) and T2W MR (B) images in a five-year-old demonstrate the thymus in the prevascular space appearing homogeneously isointense to skeletal muscle on T1 and hyperintense to skeletal muscle on T2.

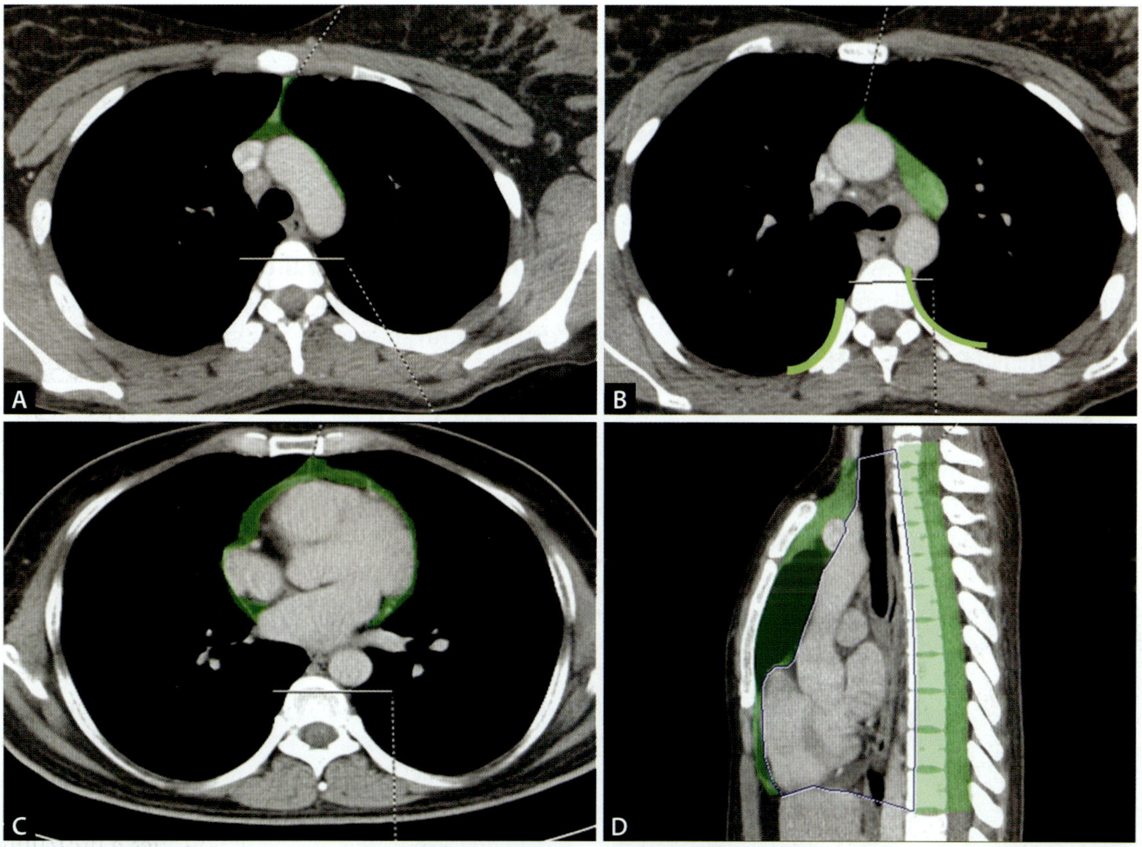

Figs. 23A to D: Axial and sagittal CT sections showing the mediastinal divisions according to the ITMIG classification. The prevascular space is depicted in green anteriorly. The horizontal line 1 cm behind the anterior vertebral imaging is the demarcation between the visceral and posterior mediastinal or paravertebral region which is again shaded in green.

of the lower lobe can be seen coursing posteriorly in the horizontal plane. The rest of the lower lobe bronchi are seen in cross-section below this level as they have a vertical course. The lung closely abuts the posterior aspect of the right main bronchus and the bronchus intermedius so that their posterior walls are clearly delineated as a thin stripe on axial CT images.

On the left side, the left upper lobe bronchus arises at a lower level than the right upper lobe bronchus with a horizontal course. The lingular bronchus courses

Table 2: International Thymic Malignancy Interest Group (ITMIG) classification of mediastinal compartments on cross-sectional imaging.

Compartment	*Boundaries*	*Major contents*
Prevascular	• *Anteriorly*: Sternum • *Posteriorly*: Anterior aspect of the pericardium as it wraps around the heart in a curvilinear manner • *Superiorly*: Thoracic inlet* • *Inferiorly*: Diaphragm • *Laterally*: Parietal mediastinal pleura	• Thymus • Lymph nodes • Left brachiocephalic vein • Fat
Visceral	• *Anteriorly*: Posterior boundary of the prevascular compartment • *Posteriorly*: Vertical line connecting a point on each thoracic vertebral body 1 cm posterior to its anterior margin** • *Superiorly*: Thoracic inlet • *Inferiorly*: Diaphragm	• Trachea, carina, esophagus, lymph nodes • Heart, ascending aorta, aortic arch, descending thoracic aorta, SVC intrapericardial pulmonary arteries, thoracic duct
Paravertebral	• *Anteriorly*: Posterior boundary of the visceral compartment • *Posteriorly*: Vertical line against the posterior margin of the chest wall at the lateral margin of the transverse process of the thoracic spine	• Thoracic spine • Paravertebral soft tissues

*The thoracic inlet is a thin plane demarcated by superior border of manubrium anteriorly, body of 1st thoracic vertebra posterosuperiorly and 1st ribs and their costal cartilages on each side.

** This line was chosen as the posterior boundary of the visceral compartment and the anterior boundary of the paravertebral compartment as most abnormalities in the posterior compartment are neurogenic masses that arise from the dorsal root ganglia/neurons adjacent to the intervertebral foramina.

anteriorly in the horizontal plane after arising from the upper lobe bronchus. The lower lobe bronchi have a roughly similar course as on **Figures 24A to F**.

LUNG SEGMENTS, FISSURES AND PLEURA[1,38,39]

Fissures are poorly seen on routine axial CT sections as avascular areas or broad bands as they represent subpleural regions with relative paucity of vessels. On HRCT sections, they are well seen as thin white lines and may be better appreciated on multiplanar reconstructions. **(Figs. 25A and B)**. The individual lung lobes and segments can be identified by their position within the hemithorax and their relationship to the segmental bronchi and fissures Segmental anatomy on CT is shown in **Figs. 26A to D**. The normal pleura and extrapleural spaces are not visible.

CONCLUSION

The increasing, almost universal use of CT for thoracic imaging and emerging applications of MR imaging makes it imperative that one is aware of the advancements, strengths and limitations of these techniques so that they can be tailored to answer the clinical question at hand while minimizing radiation exposure.

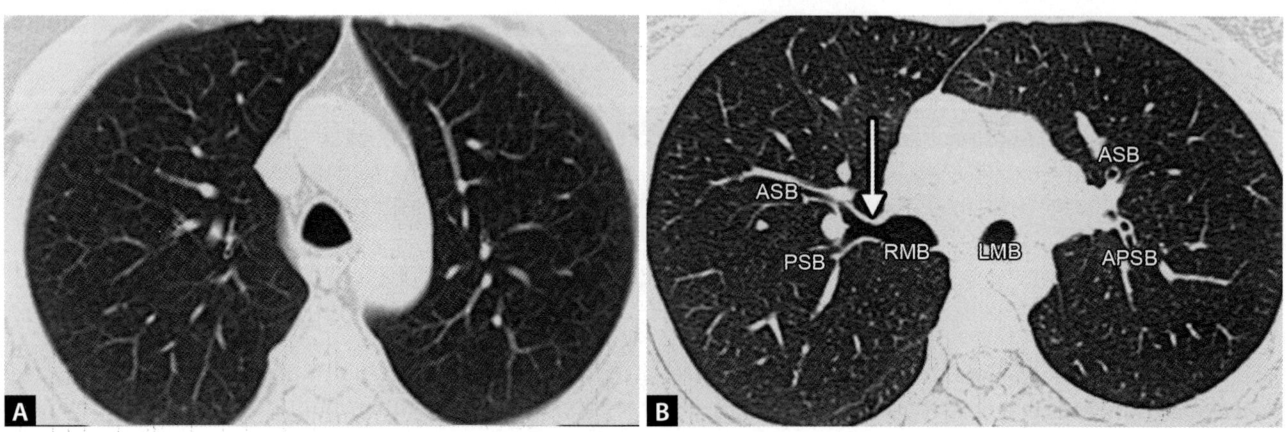

Figs. 24A and B

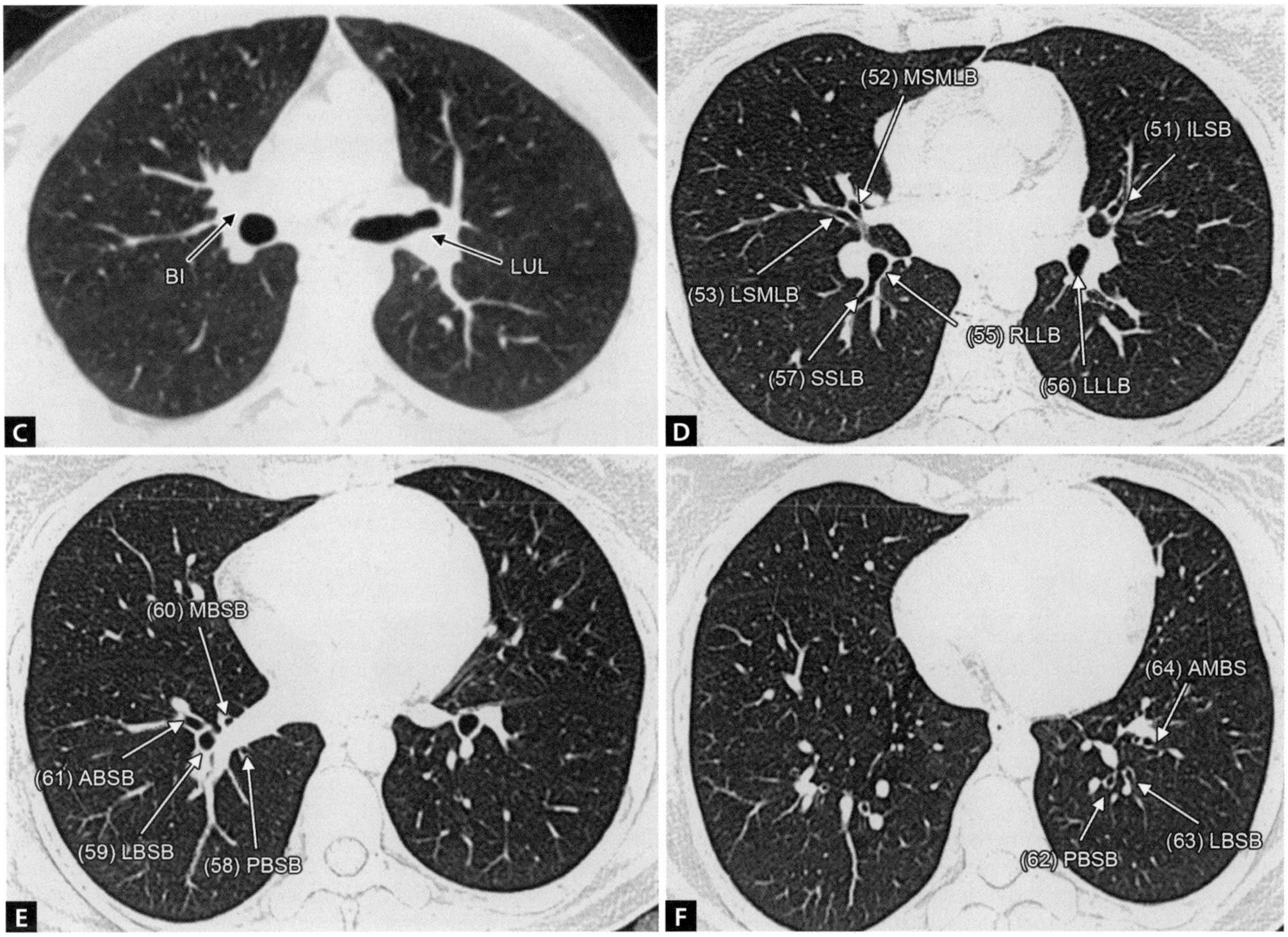

Figs. 24C to F

Figs. 24A to F: (A) Bronchial anatomy as seen on CT section just above the carina shows apical and apicoposterior segmental bronchi in cross-sections on right and left side respectively; (B) Section at the level of carina shows right and left main bronchi, right upper lobe bronchus I (arrow) and its division into anterior and posterior segmental bronchi; (C) Section just below carina shows bronchus intermedius on right side and left upper lobe bronchus arising from left main bronchus; (D) On the left side, lingular branch of upper lobe bronchus is seen. On right side, middle lobe bronchus and its divisions into medial and lateral segmental bronchi. The superior segmental bronchi of both lower lobes are also seen coursing posteriorly (E and F) Section at further caudal level shows major lower lobe segmental bronchi on both sides.

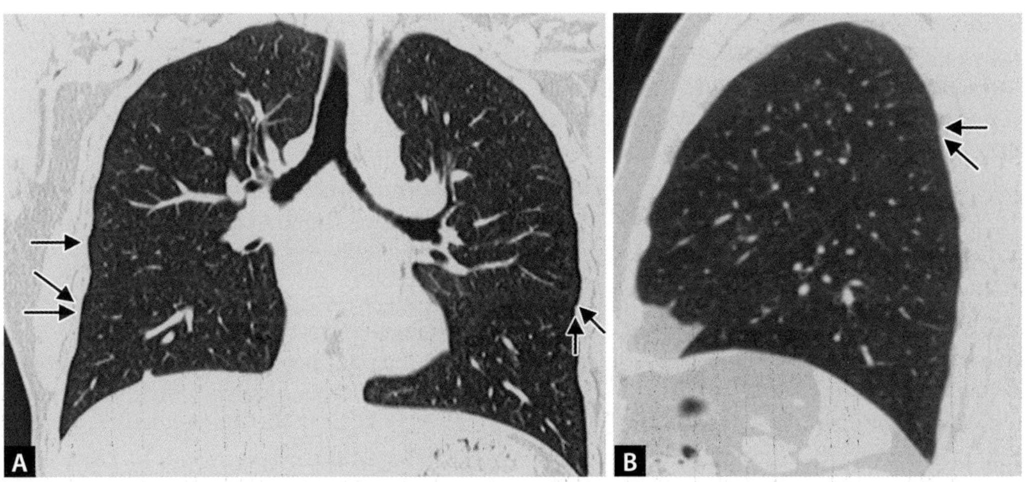

Figs. 25A and B: Coronal and sagittal CT sections in lung window showing the oblique fissures on both sides and the horizontal fissure on the right side (double and single arrows respectively)

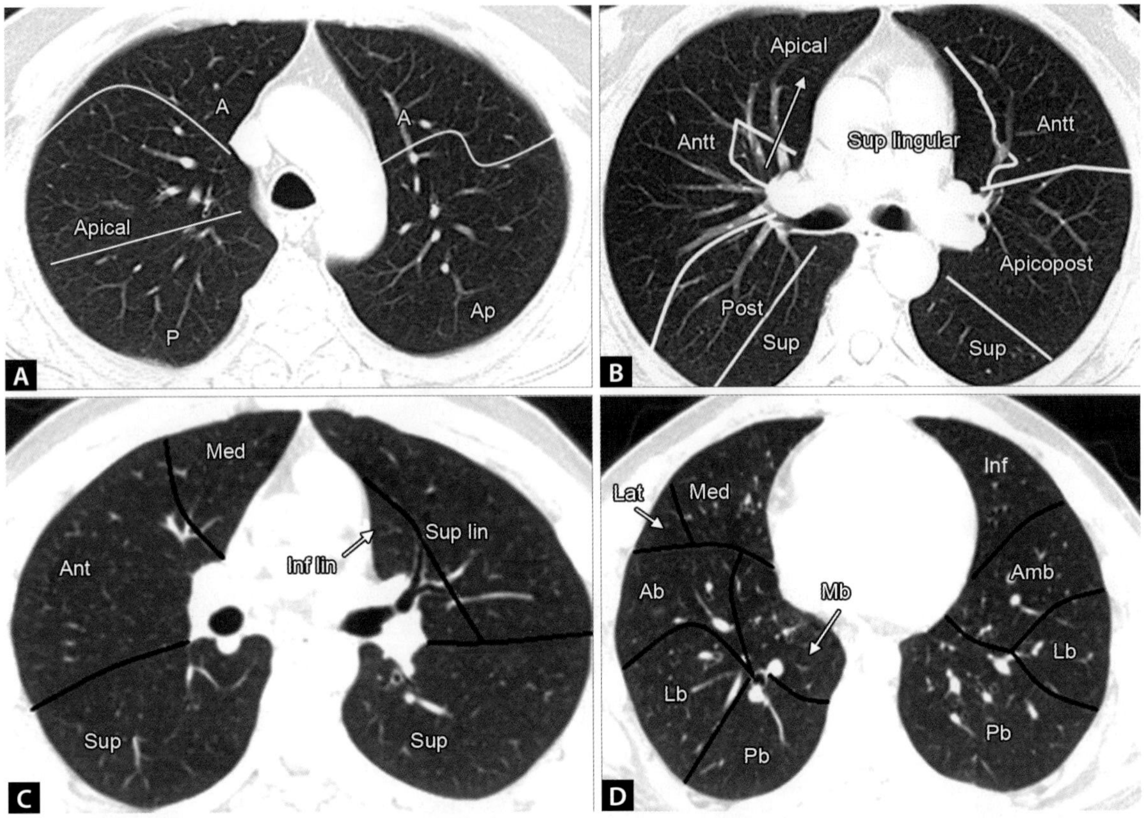

Figs. 26A to D: Normal segmental lung anatomy: (A) Section at the level of aortic arch; (B) Left pulmonary artery level; (C) Right pulmonary artery level; (D) Cardiac ventricular level. Apical: Apical segment of right upper lobe (S_1); P: Posterior segment of right upper lobe (S_2); Apicopost: Apicoposterior segment of left upper lobe (S_1+S_2); A: Anterior segment of right upper lobe (S_3); Lat: Lateral segment of right middle lobe (S_4); superior lingular segment (S_4); Med: medial segment of right middle lobe (S_5); Inf: inferior lingular segment of left upper lobe (S_5); Sup: Superior segment of right or left lower lobe (S_6); Mb: Medial segment of right lower lobe (S_7); Ab: Anterior segment of right lower lobe (S_8). Amb: Anteromedial segment of left lower lobe (S_7+S_8); Lb: Lateral segment of right or left lower lobe (S_9); Pb: Posterior segment of right or left lower lobe (S_{10}).

REFERENCES

1. Nair A, Aziz ZA and Hansell DM. Techniques in Thoracic Imaging. In: Adam A, Dixon AK, Gillard JH, Prokol S (Eds). Grangier and Alison's Diagnostic Radiology. 6th edition. 2015;149-83.
2. Thomas FG, Bernhard. CT technology for Imaging the Thorax: State of the Art. In: Schoepf UJ, Meinel FG (Eds). Multidetector-Row CT of the Thorax, Medical Radiology, 2nd edition, Springer, 2016;3-28. DOI 10.1007/978-3-319-30355-0_1
3. Hutt A, Tacelli N, Faivre JB, Flohr T, Duhamel A, Remy J, et al. Is bronchial wall imaging affected by temporal resolution? comparative evaluation at 140 and 75 ms in 90 patients. Eur Radiol. 2016;26(2):469–77.
4. Schulz B, Jacobi V, Beeres M, Bodelle B, Gruber T, Lee C, Bauer R, et al. Quantitative analysis of motion artifacts in high-pitch dual-source computed tomography of the thorax. J Thorac Imaging. 2012;27(6):382–6.
5. Morsbach F, Gordic S, Desbiolles L, Husarik D, Frauenfelder T, Schmidt B, et al. Performance of turbo high-pitch dual-source CT for coronary CT angiography: first ex vivo and patient experience. Eur Radiol. 2014;24(8):1889–95.
6. Wuest W, Anders K, Schuhbaeck A, May MS, Gauss S, Marwan M, et al. Dual source multidetector CT-angiography before Transcatheter Aortic Valve Implantation (TAVI) using a high-pitch spiral acquisition mode. Eur Radiol. 2012;22(1):51–8.
7. Tack D, Appiah V. Acquisition Protocol for Thoracic CT. In: Schoepf UJ, Meinel FG (Eds). In Multidetector-Row CT of the Thorax. Medical Radiology. 2nd edition. 2016;59-68. DOI 10.1007/978-3-319-30355-0_4.
8. Dominik F, Richard HL. Contrast Medium Injection Technique. In: Schoepf UJ, Meinel FG (Eds). In Multidetector-Row CT of the Thorax, Medical Radiology, 2nd edition. 2016;37-57. DOI 10.1007/978-3-319-30355-0_3
9. Mayo JR, Webb WR, Gould R, Stein MG, Bass I, Gamsu G, et al. High-resolution CT of the lungs: an optimal approach. Radiology. 1987;163(2):507–10.
10. Murata K, Khan A, Herman PG. Pulmonary parenchymal disease: evaluation with high-resolution CT. In: Nishino M, Boiselle PM, Copeland JF, et al. (Eds). Radiology. 2004;170:629–35.
11. Beigelman-Aubry C, Hill C, Guibal A, Savatovsky J, Grenier PA. Multi-detector row CT and postprocessing techniques

in the assessment of diffuse lung disease. Radiographics. 2005;25(6):1639–52. 25/6/1639 [pii].
12. Litmanovich DE, Tack D, Lee KS, Shahrzad M, Bankier AA. Cardiothoracic imaging in the pregnant patient. J Thorac Imaging. 2014;29:38-49.
13. Harald B, Heuschmid M, Andreas F. Kopp-Tubingen .Vascular: Pulmonary Veins. In: Medizin S, Heidelberg V (Eds). Dual source CT imaging. 2008;140-50.
14. Thorsten RCJ, Konstantin N, Christoph BR, Becker R. Munich-Grosshadern Vascular: Extended Chest Pain Protocol. In: Medizin S, Heidelberg V (Eds). Dual source CT imaging. 2008;130-9.
15. Eibel R, Türk T, Kulinna C, et al. Value of multiplanar reformations (MPR) in multi-slice spiral CT of the lung. Rofo. 2001;173(1):57–64.
16. Eibel R, Türk TR, Kulinna C, et al. Multidetector row CT of the lungs: multiplanar reconstructions and maximum intensity projections for the detection of pulmonary nodules. Rofo. 2001;173(9):815–21.
17. Kuettner A, Anders K, Lell M–Nuremberg E. Dual Energy: Virtual Non Contrast in Dual source CT imaging. Springer Medizin Veriag Heidelberg. 2008;242-51.
18. Dinkel J, Hintze C, Rochet N, Thieke C, Biederer J. Computed tomography of the lungs. A step into the fourth dimension. Radiologe. 2009;49(8):698–704.
19. Wielputz MO, Bardarova D, Weinheimer O, Kauczor HU, Eichinger M, Jobst BJ, et al. Variation of densitometry on computed tomography in COPD –influence of different software tools. PLoS One; 2014;9(11), e112898
20. Paul NS. Strategies for Dose Reduction and Improvement of image Quality in Chest CT. In: Schoepf UJ, Meinel FG (Eds). In Multidetector-Row CT of the Thorax, Medical Radiology, 2nd edition. 2016;29-36. DOI 10.1007/978-3-319-30355-0_2
21. Wild JM, Marshal H, Bock M, Schad LR, Jakob PM, Molinary MPF, et al. MRI of the lung (1/3): methods. Insights imaging. 2012;3:345-53. DOI 10.1007/s13244-012-0176x.
22. Kauczor HU, Zaporozhan JL, Ley S. Imaging of pulmonary pathologies. Focus on Magnetic Resonance Imaging. Proc Am Thorac Soc. 2009;6:458-63
23. Hochhegger B, de Souza VVS, Marchiori E, Irion KL, Souza Jr AS, Junor JE, et al. Chest magnetic resonance imaging: a protocol suggestion. Radiol Bras. 2015;48(6):373-80.
24. Henzler T, Bindert GS, Schoenberg SO, Fink C. Diffusion and perfusion MRI of the lung and mediastinum. Eur J Radiol. 2010;76:329-36.
25. Christine UL, White DB, Sykes AMG. Establishing a Chest MRI practice and its Clinical Application: Our Insight and Protocols. Published online 2014, doi: 10.4103/2156-7514.129288
26. Ackman JB. MR imaging of mediastinal masses, Magn Reson Imaging Clin Normal Am. 2015;23:141-64.
27. Mirasadraee JBS, Beer M, Molinary F, Hintze C, Bauman G, Both M, et al. MRI of the lung (3/3)-current application and future perspectives. Insights Imaging. 2012;3:373-86. DOI 10.1007/s13244-011-0142-z
28. Biderer J, Beer M, Hirsch W, Wild J, Fabel M, Puderbach M, Van Beek EJR. MRI of the lung (2/3). Why.... when...... how?. Insights Imaging. 2012;3:355-71. DOI 10.1007/s13244-011-0146-8.
29. Kluge A, Luboldt W, Bachmann G. Acute pulmonary embolism to the subsegmental level: diagnostic accuracy of three MRI techniques compared with 16-MDCT. Am J Roentgenol. 2006;187:W7-14.
30. Stein PD, Woodard PK, Hull Rd, et al. Gadolinium-enhanced magnetic resonance angiography for detection of acute pulmonary embolism: an in-depth review. Chest. 2003;124:2324-8
31. Kluge A, Loboldt W, Bachmann G. Acute pulmonary embolism to the subsegmental level: diagnostic accuracy of three MRI techniques compared with 16-MDCT. Am J Roentgenol. 2006;187(1):W7-14.
32. Nikolaou K, Schoenberg SO, Attenberger U, Scheidhler J, Dietrich O, Kuehn B, et al. Pulmonary arterial hypertension: diagnosis with fast perfusion MR imaging and high-spatial-resolution MR angiography-preliminary experience. Radiology. 2005;236:694-703.
33. Koyama H, Ohno Y, Kono A, et al. Quantitative and qualitative assessment of non-contrast-enhanced pulmonary MR imaging for management of pulmonary nodules in 161 subjects. Eur Radiol. 2008;18:2120-31.
34. Hochhegger B, Marchiori E, Dos Reis DQ, et al. Chemical-shift MRI of pulmonary hamartoma: initial experience using a modified technique to assess nodules fat. Am J Roentgenol. 2012;199:W331-4.
35. Sodhi KS, Khandelwal N, Saxena AK, Singh M, Aggarwal R, Bhatia A, et al. Rapid lung MRI in children with pulmonary infections: time to change our diagnostic algorithms J. Magn. Reson imaging. 2016;43:1196-206.
36. Carter BW, Benveniste MF, Madan R, Godoy MC, de Groot PM, Truong MT, et al. ITMIG Classification of Mediastinal Compartments and Multidisciplinary Approach to Mediastinal Masses. Radiographics. 2017;37(2):413-36.
37. Carter BW, Tomiyama N, Bhora FY, et al. A Modern definition of mediastinal compartments. J Thorac Oncol. 2014;9(9 suppl 2): S97-101.
38. Mukherjee S, Gupta R. Imaging in chest disease. In: Pande JN (Ed). Respiratory Medicine in the Tropics, 1st edition. Delhi, Oxford University Press, 90, 1988.
39. Amstrong P. The normal chest. In: Grainger RG, Allison D (Eds). Diagnostic Radiology, 3rd edition. New York: Churchill Livingstone, 207, 1997;1114-88.

CHAPTER 158

Basic Radiographic Pattern of Lung Diseases

Gaurav S Pradhan, Radhika Batra, Rashmi Dixit, Alpana Manchanda

Plain film radiography is the first and most frequently used radiological investigation in the diagnostic workup of chest ailments. Chest radiographs are one of the oldest noninvasive methods for identifying abnormalities in the chest.[1] Evaluation of a chest radiograph requires careful observation and a good understanding of chest anatomy. Many common clinical conditions can be evaluated with a chest radiograph for example pneumonia, pleural effusion, pneumothorax, rib fractures, pulmonary edema, etc. It is a quick, inexpensive and widely available investigation making it particularly useful in the emergency setting.

PATTERN RECOGNITION

Felson[2,3] popularized a pattern recognition approach to pulmonary disease, on the basis of classifying lung diseases as either alveolar or interstitial. An alternative approach to pattern recognition is the description of an abnormal radiograph and a differential diagnosis based on the radiographic features of the disease, rather than on its presumed histologic appearance. This system was endorsed by Felson[4] in 1989, who believed that it may be easier for radiologists to determine the correct diagnosis by describing the appearance of the radiograph, rather than by attempting to suggest the histology of the lesion. The basic radiographic signs as they indicate the fundamental nature of pulmonary disease are subdivided into three major sections:[5]

1. Increased radiographic density
2. Decreased radiographic density
3. Diseases of the pleura.

The basic difference in evaluating a chest radiograph as compared to high-resolution computed tomography (HRCT) chest is that on radiographs the diagnosis depends on the appearance of disease as opposed to HRCT images where diagnosis is virtually at histologic levels. A pulmonary opacity is defined as an area that preferentially attenuates the X-ray beam and therefore appears more opaque than the surrounding area.[6] There are various patterns of pulmonary opacities such as airspace opacities, atelectasis, nodules, ring shadows, linear and bandlike opacities and reticulonodular opacities.

Airspace Disease

Airspace Opacity

A small nodular opacity measuring about 4 to 10 mm in the alveoli may be the first radiological evidence of parenchymal pathology on chest radiograph **(Fig. 1)**. There can also be presence of remnant air in the alveoli and bronchioles seen as tiny radiolucencies within the nodule. The lucencies have been referred to as air alveolograms, although they do not correspond to alveoli **(Box 1)**.

Coalescence

Rapid dissemination of fluid through the collateral pathways of the lung into adjacent airspaces results in ill-defined margins of air space opacities. Asymmetric involvement of the lung results in an irregular area of consolidation with ill-defined margins **(Fig. 2)**.

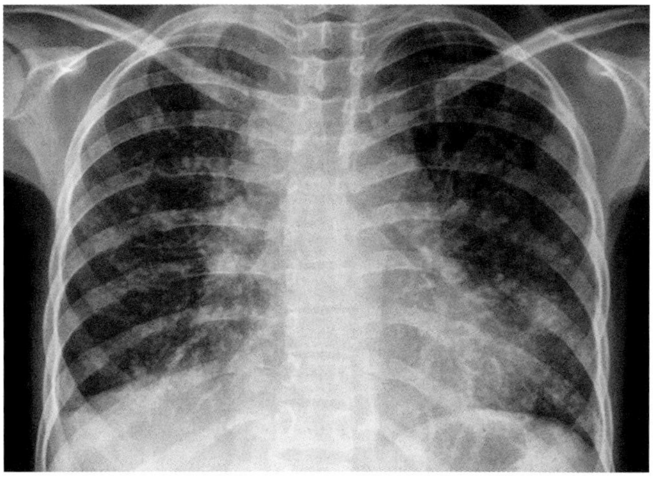

Fig. 1: Multiple nodular airspace opacities in bilateral lungs with areas of coalescence in left lower zone.

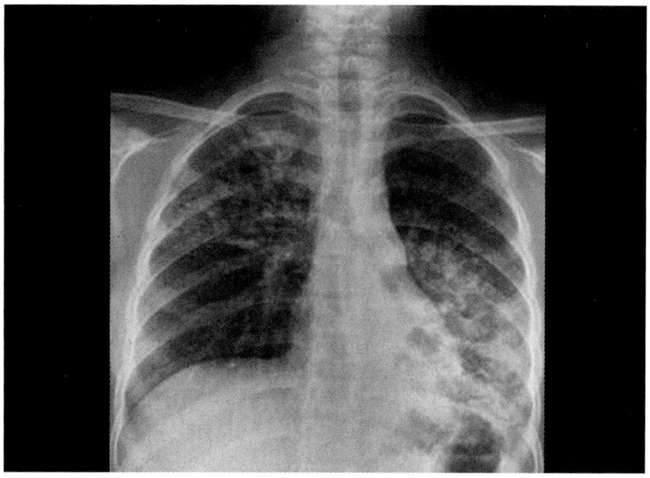

Fig. 2: Confluent airspace opacities in right upper, bilateral mid and left lower zones with areas of breakdown in left retrocardiac region.

Box 1: Causes of multifocal airspace opacification on chest radiograph.

- Infective pneumonia
- Eosinophilic pneumonia
- Organizing pneumonia
- Pulmonary edema
- Infarction due to pulmonary emboli
- Connective tissue disorders
- Alveolar proteinosis
- Pulmonary hemorrhage
- *Neoplasms*: Bronchoalveolar carcinoma, lymphoma, lymphangitis carcinomatosa
- Sarcoidosis
- Silicosis, coal workers' pneumoconiosis

Distribution Characteristics

Rapid spread of fluid or infection results in early coalescence of airspace opacities leading to widespread consolidation which is characteristically non-segmental in distribution, seen typically in pyogenic infections. Lack of segmental distribution is also seen with acute pulmonary edema. This is in stark contrast to segmental distribution observed in diseases spread through tracheobronchial route like aspiration pneumonias or those through hematogenous route like infarcts. The area of lung involvement in aspiration pneumonias depends on the patient's position at the time of aspiration.

Only certain diseases and not others appear to respect acinar boundaries. This is likely due to the viscosity of the consolidating medium. The inflammatory edema caused by some organisms, e.g. *Streptococcus pneumoniae*, is of low viscosity and therefore spreads rapidly via interalveolar pores, whereas that of others, such as *Mycobacterium tuberculosis*, may be of sufficient viscosity to prevent such ready dissemination.

Margination

The edge characteristics of airspace processes show poor margination. An example of the phenomenon is the "butterfly" or "bat's wing" appearance of acute airspace edema or hemorrhage **(Fig. 3)**. However, in acute diplococcal or *Klebsiella pneumoniae*, as the infection is propogated by centrifugal spread, the advancing margin of consolidation is sometimes smooth and sharply defined **(Fig. 4)**. When consolidation extends up to a pleural surface it may appear lobar.

Air Bronchogram

Presence of remnant air within the bronchi and its branches within the parenchymal opacity gives the radiologically important "air-bronchogram" sign. These bronchi stand out in contrast to opacified lung due to fluid or tissue filled alveolar spaces. It is important to remember that for air-bronchogram to be present, the bronchi need to be patent. The parenchyma may be airless when its air has been replaced by liquid or tissue (consolidation) or when it has been absorbed and not replaced (atelectasis). This sign originally described by Fleischner in 1927, was named the air bronchogram sign by Felson. It is most frequently encountered in pneumonia and pulmonary edema. Bronchoalveolar carcinoma, lymphoma, alveolar hemorrhage, fibrosis due to radiation and sarcoidosis can also present with this sign. In some diseases like pulmonary infarction, air bronchogram may be only temporary because of early filling of airway by blood or exudate.

Time Factor

The airspace opacification persisting for prolonged periods of time usually indicates persistent pathologies

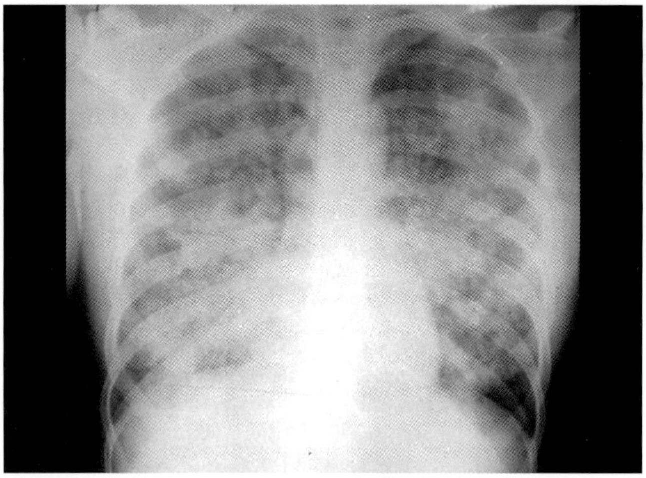

Fig. 3: Chest radiograph showing multiple patchy airspace opacities in bilateral lung fields giving rise to "Bat's wing" appearance in a case of pulmonary edema.

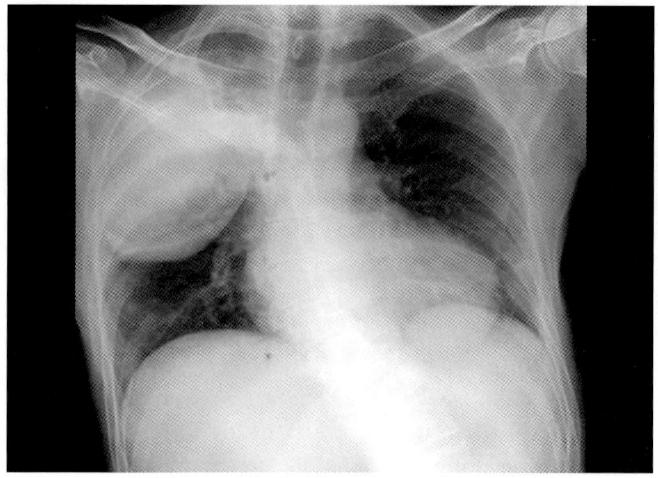

Fig. 4: Bulging fissure sign in *Klebsiella pneumoniae*.

like infection and neoplasm (bronchoalveolar carcinoma and lymphoma) as opposed to rapidly clearing or evolving opacities as seen in pulmonary edema, which clear with treatment of underlying heart failure.

Atelectasis

Air space opacity with resorption of air with no significant air replacement results in loss of lung volume. This is referred to as atelectasis or collapse. The natural tendency of the lung to collapse is opposed by the recoil of the chest wall outwards caused by the contraction of inspiratory muscles and diaphragm. Atelectasis can result due to mechanisms that interfere directly or indirectly with lung expansion. It can be divided into six types: resorptive, adhesive, compressive, passive, cicatrization and gravity dependent.[7]

When the lung is compressed by any space occupying lesion in the thorax such as pneumothorax, pleural effusion or a mass lesion in the pleural cavity, compressive atelectasis results. The distinction between compressive and passive atelectasis is not well defined, any space occupying lesion in the thorax may compress the lung or lead to passive retraction of the lung.

The most common form of atelectasis is caused by the resorption of gas from the alveoli.[5] When there is partial or total obstruction to flow of air from tracheobronchial tree to the alveoli, with inadequate air filling by collateral pathways, resorption atelectasis results. The lung becomes devoid of air within 24 hours of bronchial obstruction. Resorption atelectasis occurs rapidly when the patient is breathing pure oxygen as it is quickly absorbed from the alveoli. Mucous impaction in subsegmental bronchus and bronchiolitis obliterans due to repeated infections in early life can result in resorption atelectasis. It is also seen commonly after surgery and general anesthesia.[8]

When the compliance of the lung decreases because of it being diseased due to fibrosis, cicatrization atelectasis can develop. It is often associated with bronchiectasis. Cicatrization atelectasis can be seen with many conditions like idiopathic pulmonary fibrosis, sarcoidosis, chronic tubercular and fungal infections and collagen vascular diseases.

When there is deficiency of alveolar surfactant along with other coexistent factors, then even in the presence of a patent airway, atelectasis can occur. This is referred to as "non-obstructive" atelectasis or adhesive atelectasis. It is characteristically seen in respiratory distress syndrome of the newborn. It may also be seen in acute respiratory distress syndrome (ARDS), acute radiation pneumonitis and in postoperative patients.[8]

Gravity dependent atelectasis can occur in bedridden patients with shallow breathing. Gravity dependent alterations in alveolar volume may aggravate atelectasis in dependent parts of the lung.

'Plate like atelectasis' are the common linear opacities seen on a chest radiograph. These are usually 1 to 3 mm in thickness, 4 to 10 cm in length and are seen in the mid and lower lung zones. These shadows may be horizontal or oblique, single or multiple, unilateral or bilateral. These linear opacities are associated with diseases that limit diaphragmatic excursion, a frequent contributing factor being intra-abdominal disease (such as inflammatory conditions, ascites, etc.).

Direct and Indirect Signs of Collapse

The signs of lobar atelectasis are seen due to the opacity of a given lobe and the volume loss that results.[9-11] There can be direct and indirect signs. Direct evidence of presence of collapse can be inferred by displacement of lobar fissures which is the most reliable sign. Crowding of vessels and bronchi in a lobe can help in diagnosis if displacement of fissures is not apparent. Increased density of an atelectatic part of the lung usually becomes apparent when the collapse is almost complete.

Other indirect signs that may help us to suspect underlying collapse include elevation of part of diaphragm or hemidiaphragm usually seen in lower lobe collapse, whereas upper lobe collapse may be inferred by tracheal or upper mediastinal displacement. Lower lobe collapse may also be associated with cardiac displacement **(Fig. 5)**. Hilar displacement may also point to underlying collapse of lung. This is usually more evident with upper lobe collapse than with lower lobe collapse **(Fig. 6)**. Reduction of intercostal spaces with resultant rib crowding may occasionally be seen with chronic processes and old collapse. A change in the site of a parenchymal lesion, as seen after comparison with previous images, may result from atelectasis and is referred to as the **"shifting granuloma sign"**.

Compensatory hyperinflation of adjoining lung can also be seen with collapsed lung. The hyperinflation may occur over a prolonged period of time and may involve adjacent lobe or entire lung. There is resultant mediastinal displacement with paucity and spread out vascular markings when compared to contralateral lung. When a large portion of a lung becomes atelectatic, the tendency is greater for overinflation to involve the contralateral lung; this may progress to the stage in which the opposite lung displaces the mediastinum either generally or locally **(Fig. 7)**.

Local displacements occur in the three areas of the mediastinum, where the two lungs are separated only by loose connective tissue: (1) the anterior mediastinal compartment, at the level of the first three or four costal cartilages, limited anteriorly by the sternum and posteriorly by the great vessels; (2) the posterosuperior mediastinum, at the level of the third to fifth thoracic vertebrae, limited anteriorly by the esophagus and trachea and posteriorly by the vertebral column; and (3) the posteroinferior mediastinum, limited anteriorly by the heart and posteriorly by the vertebral column and aorta.

Lobar Atelectasis

Right upper lobe collapse—As the right upper lobe collapses, the lateral end of the horizontal fissure moves upwards and medially towards the superior mediastinum and the anterior end moves upwards towards the apex. The upper half of the oblique fissure moves anteriorly **(Figs. 8A and B)**.[12] Other radiographic findings associated with right upper lobe collapse include increased density in the upper thorax, silhouetting of the upper mediastinum, mediastinal widening, ipsilateral tracheal shift, elevated hilum, outward rotation of hilum or bronchus and juxtaphrenic peak **(Fig. 9)**. The "**Golden's S sign"** is seen with right upper lobe collapse due to a centrally located mass **(Fig. 10)**. The superiorly displaced, lateral and concave aspect of the "S" is formed by the minor fissure, while the inferiorly and medially located convex part is formed by the margin of the mass.[13]

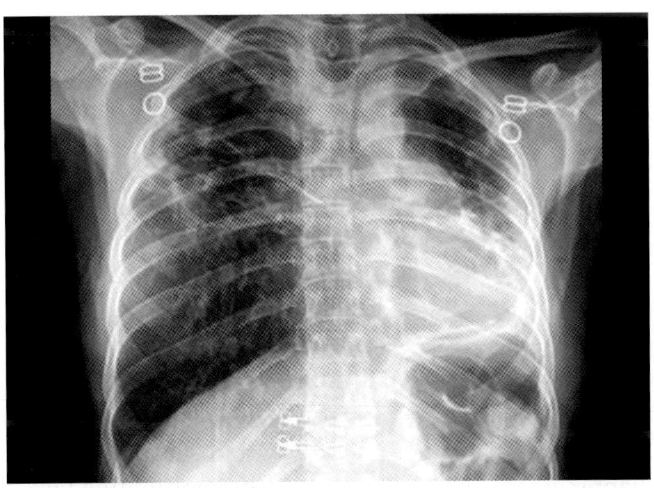

Fig. 5: Left lower lobe collapse with elevated left hemidiaphragm and ipsilateral mediastinal shift alongwith nodular and few fibrotic opacities in right lung field.

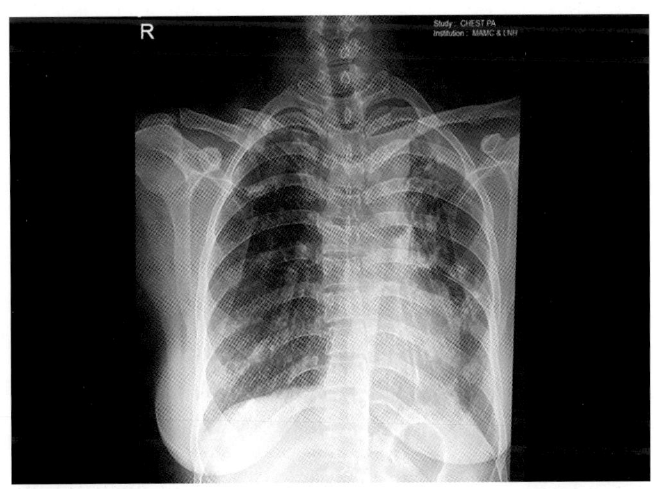

Fig. 6: Left upper lobe collapse with mild ipsilateral tracheal shift, pulled up left hilum and juxtaphrenic peak of left hemidiaphragm.

Right middle lobe collapse: It is seen as an increased density of the lung silhouetting the right heart border and the minor fissure is invisible. In this condition, the horizontal fissure and lower half of the oblique fissure move towards each other **(Figs. 11A and B)**.

Left upper lobe collapse: Left upper lobe collapse is seen as a hazy opacity in upper, mid and sometimes lower zones. Pulmonary vessels in the hyperinflated lower lobe are seen through the haze. On the lateral radiograph, it is seen as an elongated opacity extending from the paex and reaching the diaphragm. In left upper lobe collapse, there is vertical positioning and anterior and medial displacement of the major fissure **(Figs. 12A and B)**. Migration of the superior segment of the left lower lobe superiorly and anteriorly between the arch of the aorta and the collapsed lobe causes a crescent-shaped radiolucency around the aortic arch which is known as the "**Luftsichel sign" (Fig. 13)**.[14]

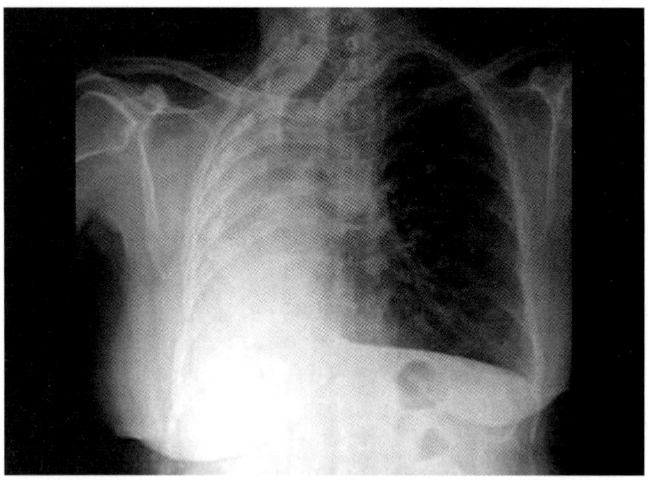

Fig. 7: Opaque right hemithorax with ipsilateral tracheo-mediastinal shift and compensatory hyperinflation of left lung—Complete right lung collapse.

Lower lobe collapse: In lower lobe collapse, there is posterior and medial displacement of the oblique fissure. It is seen as a triangular density in the retrocardiac location on a frontal radiograph, downward displacement of the hilum is seen **(Figs. 14 and 15)**.[15] The lower lobe pulmonary artery is also obscured on the frontal radiographs. The diaphragmatic contour is obscured and shift of the heart or mediastinum becomes apparent **(Fig. 16)**. The **"flat waist sign"**[16] can be seen with left lower lobe collapse where there is straightening of the left heart margin, aorta and pulmonary artery. With severe left lower lobe collapse the outline of the superior aortic knuckle may not be seen. On the lateral radiograph, lower lobe collapse may cause partial obscuration of the hemidiaphragm in its posterior aspect and the vertebral column appears to be progressively dense inferiorly.

Interstitial Pattern

Pulmonary interstitium encompasses support tissues within the lung and includes alveolar epithelium, pulmonary capillary endothelium, perivascular and perilymphatic tissues. It can be divided into the axial, parenchymal and peripheral interstitial spaces. The axial interstitial space is constituted by sheath of loose connective tissue around the bronchovascular bundles, the blood vessels, nerves and lymphatics lie in this space. Parenchymal interstitial space is a small space in the walls of the alveoli. Peripheral interstitial space is adjacent to the pleura. The interstitial involvement can

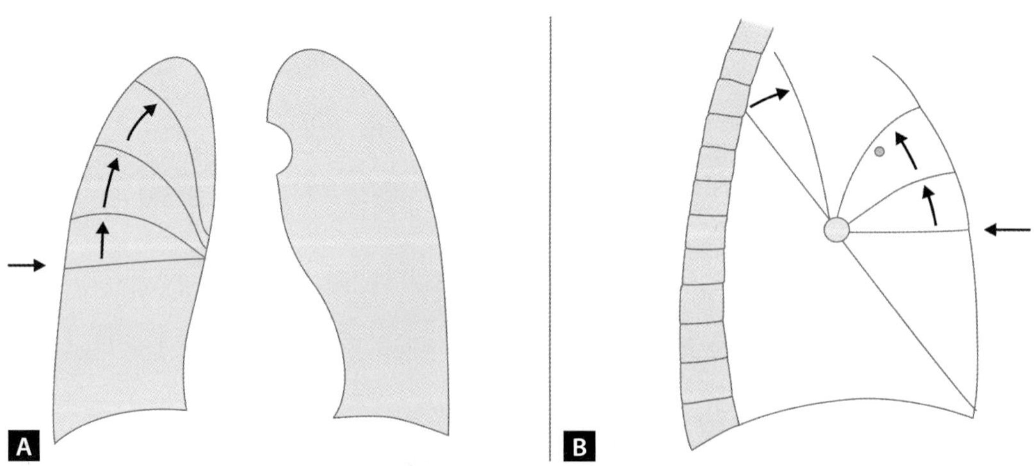

Figs. 8A and B: Right upper lobe collapse PA (A) and lateral (B) views: Horizontal fissure is drawn upward and curves towards the apex and mediastinum on PA view. On the lateral view there is upward displacement of the horizontal fissure with forward displacement of the oblique fissure above the hilum.

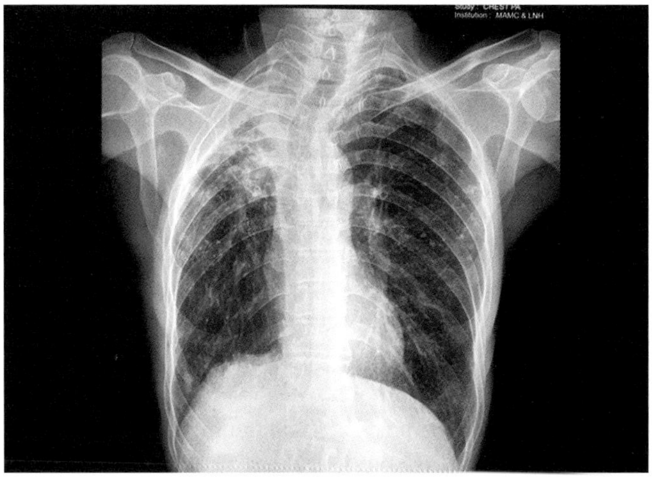

Fig. 9: Right upper lobe collapse with ipsilateral tracheal shift and pulled up right hilum. Multiple nodular calcific opacities are seen in bilateral lungs.

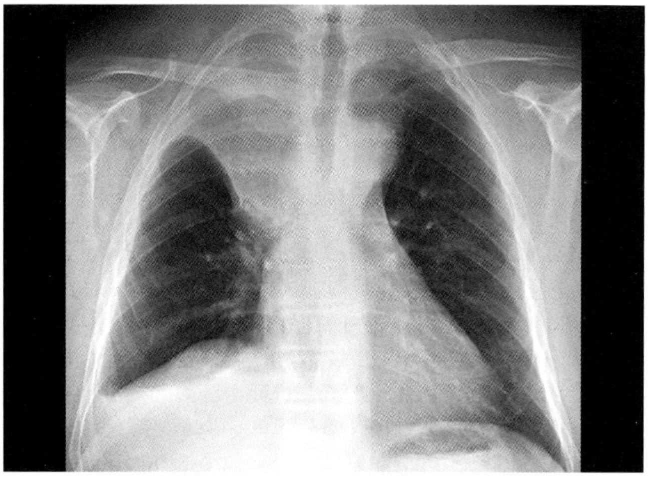

Fig. 10: Golden S-sign—centrally located mass causing right upper lobe collapse.

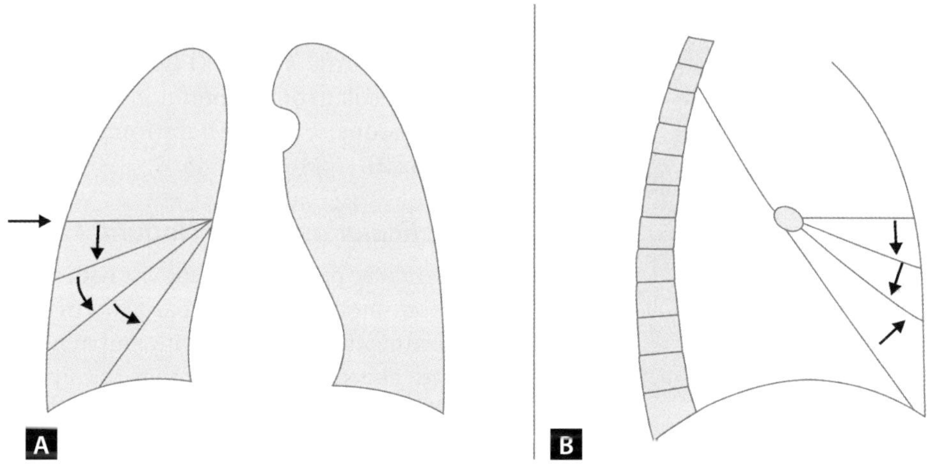

Figs. 11A and B: Right middle lobe collapse PA (A) and lateral (B) views: The horizontal fissure is displaced downwards on both views, on the lateral view there is forward displacement of the lower part of the oblique fissure.

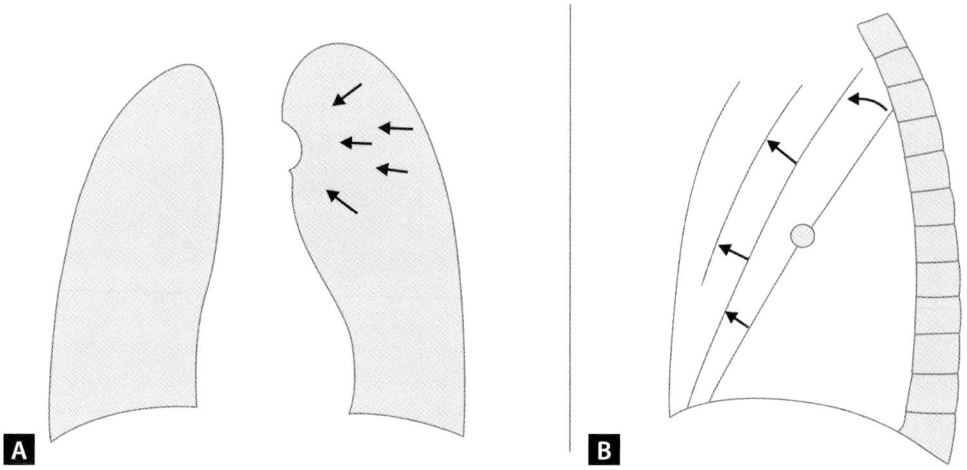

Figs. 12A and B: Left upper lobe collapse on PA (A) and lateral (B) views: Increased density is seen with increasing severity of collapse on PA view. The fissure moves forward on lateral view.

be in the form of reticular, nodular, reticulonodular and linear opacities. Inhomogeneous radiographic density can result because of primarily interstitial involvement. It is important to remember that alveolar air may be less but is not significantly compromised in interstitial disease and volume loss is not a feature of interstitial involvement as opposed to diseases with alveolar involvement.

Reticular Pattern

Reticular involvement is characterized by the development of thickening of interstitium around air containing cystic spaces. It can be further subdivided as fine, medium or coarse depending on the size. Fine reticulation implies a slender delicate mesh giving rise to ground-glass type of opacity. Medium reticular opacities enclose around 3 to 10 mm size of air spaces, whilst coarse reticulation encompass large cystic spaces of 1 cm or more. Honeycombing can result as a result of both medium and coarse reticulation and is seen in many conditions afflicting lung interstitium like fibrosing alveolitis, systemic sclerosis, rheumatoid lung, sarcoidosis, etc. **(Figs. 17 and 18)**. There is upper lobe predilection in sarcoidosis and eosinophilic granuloma while most of other disease entities displaying honeycombing have lower lobe preponderance.

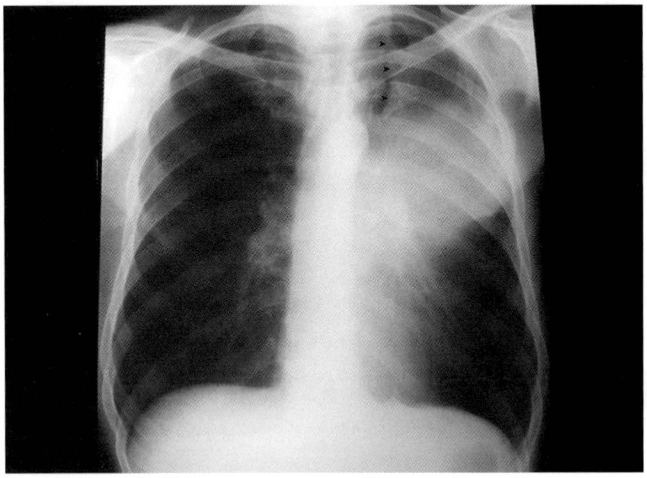

Fig. 13: *Luftsichel sign*: Crescent of hyperlucency seen in para-aortic location in left upper lobe collapse.

Nodular Pattern

Formation of various sized nodules in the interstitium can also occur. These nodules can be of varying sizes but are rounded and usually homogeneous in density. The sizes may vary from micronodular (less than 1 mm), small (1–3 mm), medium (3–5 mm) to large (more than 5 mm). Miliary tuberculosis is a classic example of widespread nodular interstitial involvement occurring as a result of blood-borne spread **(Fig. 19)**. Similar appearance can also result in other conditions like miliary carcinomatosis, sarcoidosis and inhalational diseases like silicosis **(Box 2)**.

Reticular as well as Nodular Pattern

Reticular pattern may coexist with nodular pattern due to disease etiology as well as progression. The disease may be interstitial to begin with and may have both nodular as well as reticular components as can be seen in sarcoidosis **(Box 3)**.

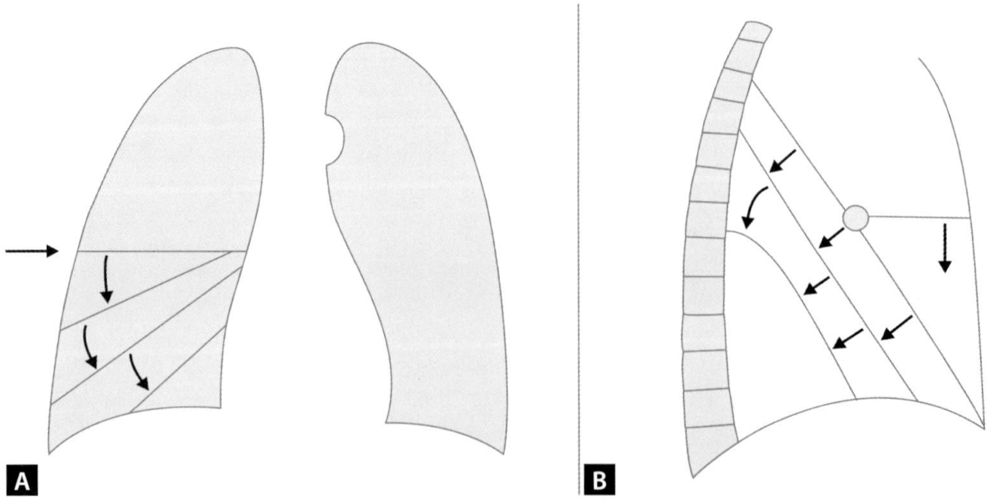

Figs. 14A and B: Right lower lobe collapse on PA (A) and lateral (B) views: Downward displacement of horizontal fissure is noted on PA view. The oblique fissure is displaced backwards on lateral view.

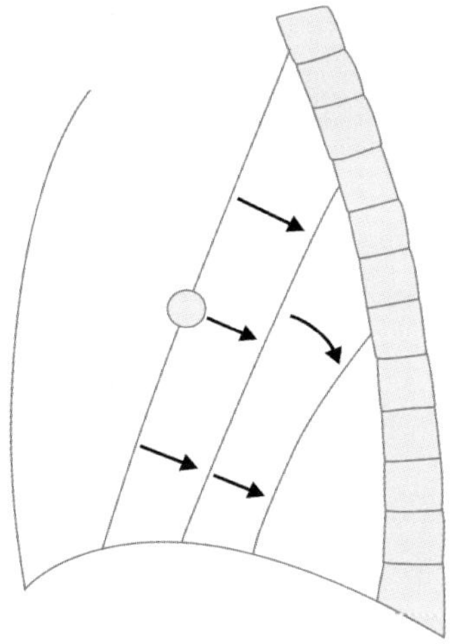

Fig. 15: Left lower lobe collapse on lateral view: No fissure is seen on the PA projection. Lateral view shows the oblique fissure to be displaced posteriorly.

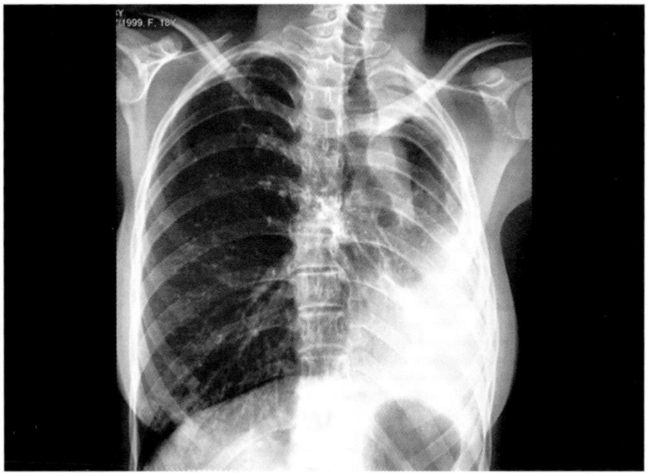

Fig. 16: Near complete collapse of the left lung with ipsilateral tracheomediastinal shift, obscured cardiac margins and left hemidiaphragm. Compensatory hyperinflation of right lung is seen which appears hyperlucent, few calcified granulomas are also seen in right lung.

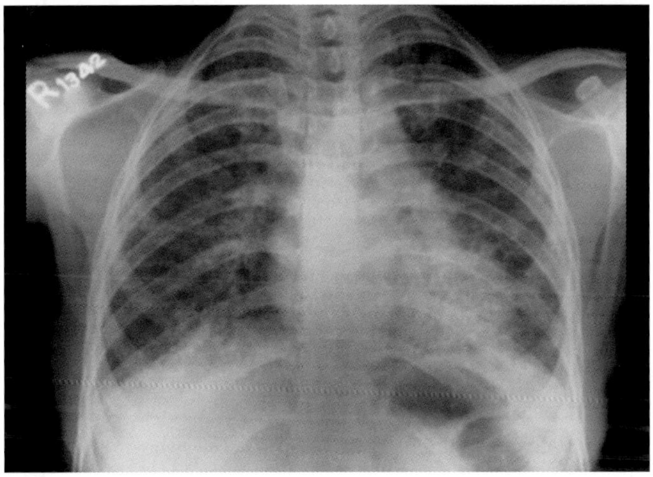

Fig. 17: Chest radiograph showing coarse reticular pattern in a patient with Idiopathic pulmonary fibrosis.

Combination of Airspace Opacities and Interstitial Pattern

Combined involvement of alveolar and interstitial compartments is commonly seen histologically. A similar pattern may be evident radiographically.[17] The disease affecting one compartment may spread to adjoining area with progression of disease. The disease may be interstitial to start with as seen with pulmonary edema, but with further rise of pulmonary venous pressures there is outpouring of fluid in alveolar spaces giving fluffy appearances. Similarly, in infective processes like staphylococcal pneumonias the disease initially involves the bronchial walls with resultant inflammation referred to as bronchiolitis. This leads to narrowing of smaller airways with consequent collapse and consolidation involving alveolar spaces.

This combination is also characteristic of certain infectious diseases of the lung—*Pneumocystis jirovecii* and cytomegalovirus. These two infections are characterized by diffuse interstitial pneumonitis, the disease then spreads into parenchymal airspaces, producing widespread alveolar consolidation **(Fig. 20)**. So, the diseases frequently coexist in interstitial as well as alveolar compartment.

Ring Shadows

Ring shadows can be seen in many conditions on chest radiography such as congenital causes including sequestered segment, bronchogenic cysts; infectious causes like bacterial abscesses, tuberculosis and *Pneumocystis jirovecii* pneumonia; connective tissue diseases like rheumatoid nodules, Wegener granulomatosis; neoplasms and bronchiectasis **(Fig. 21)**. The lesions may be single or multiple and of varying sizes.

Line and Band Shadows

Linear opacities with a diameter of more than 5 mm are referred to as band shadows whereas those with a diameter of less than 5 mm are called line shadows.[6]

Parenchymal Scarring

Linear shadows can be seen in a segment of lung that was the site of infectious disease and has healed through fibrosis. This may be seen in cases of healed upper lobe

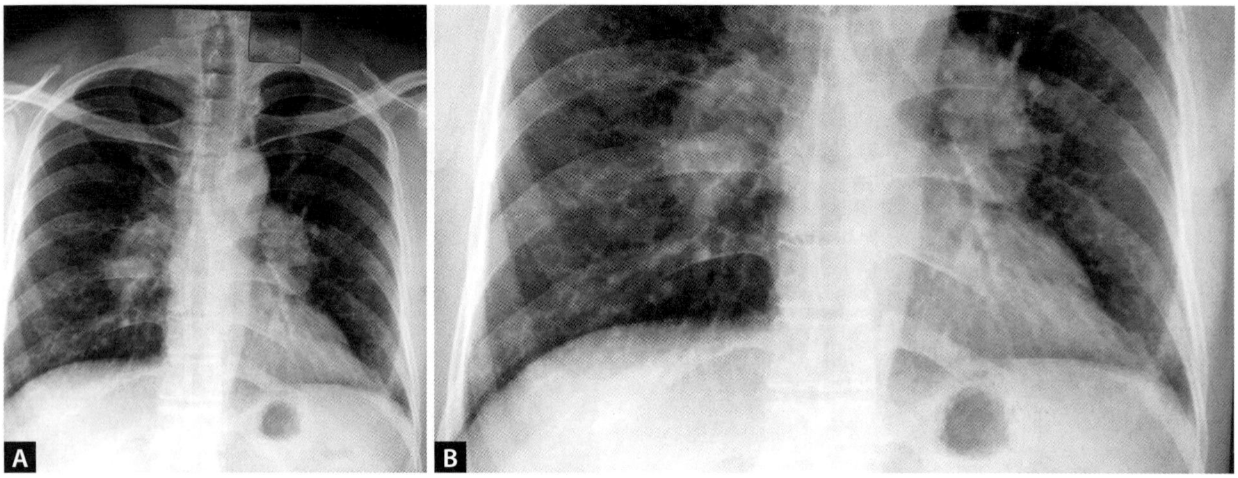

Figs. 18A and B: Bilateral hilar lymphadenopathy and reticular opacitites in bilateral lower zones in a case of sarcoidosis.

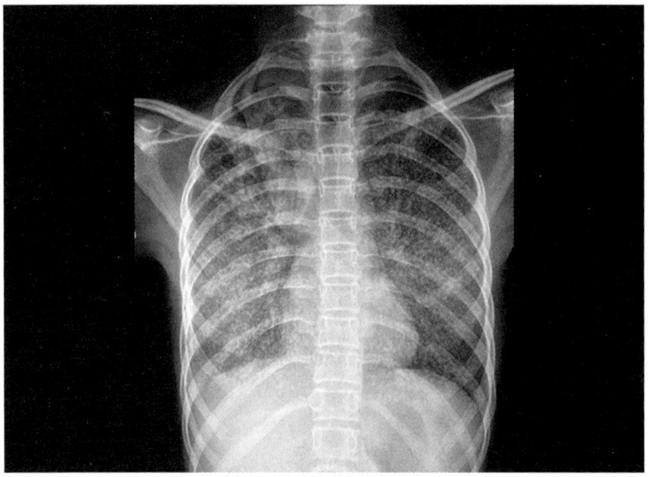

Fig. 19: Multiple small nodules seen scattered in bilateral lungs suggestive of miliary tuberculosis, subsegmental collapse of right upper lobe is noted.

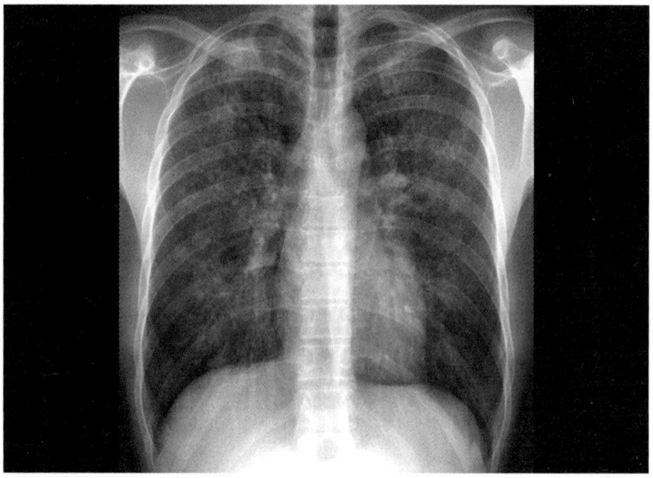

Fig. 20: *Pneumocystis jirovecii* pneumonia (PJP) showing reticular interstitial pulmonary pattern with few areas of airspace opacification, changes are more marked in perihilar location.

Box 2: Causes of miliary pattern on chest radiographs.

- Miliary tuberculosis
- Histoplasmosis
- Coccidioidomycosis
- Cryptococcosis
- Nocardiosis
- Viral infections
- Sarcoidosis
- Silicosis
- Siderosis
- Berylliosis
- Metastases
- Amyloidosis
- Alveolar microlithiasis

Box 3: Causes of reticulonodular opacities in bilateral lungs on chest radiography.

- Idiopathic pulmonary fibrosis
- Rheumatic lung disease
- Scleroderma, systemic lupus erythematosus
- Hypersensitivity pneumonitis
- Pneumoconiosis (Coal workers' pneumoconiosis, silicosis, asbestosis)
- Sarcoidosis
- Amyloidosis
- Mycoplasma, viral pneumonia
- Pulmonary edema
- Lymphangitic spread of carcinoma
- Hemosiderosis
- Lymphoid interstitial pneumonitis

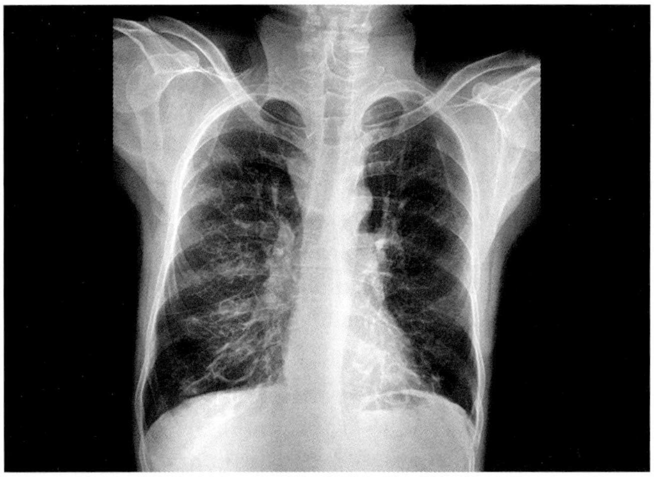

Fig. 21: Chest radiograph showing multiple ring shadows in bilateral lungs (right > left), with some showing thickened walls in a case of cystic bronchiectasis.

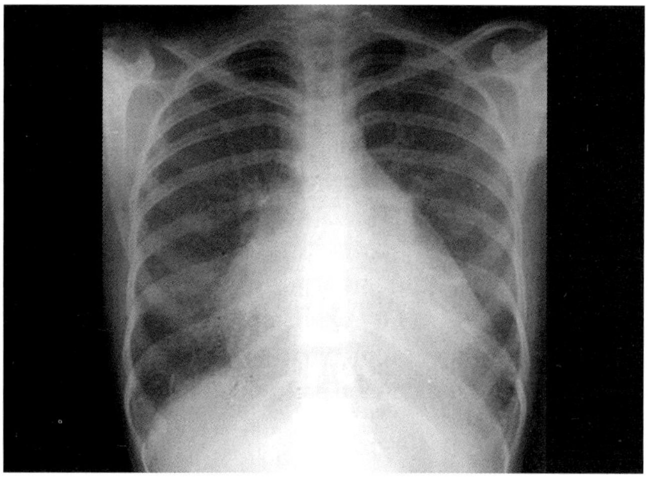

Fig. 22: Septal (Kerley B) lines seen in a case of mitral valve disease.

postprimary tuberculosis. It can also be seen in healed pulmonary infarction resulting in fibrous scarring secondary to lung necrosis . These linear shadows always extend to a pleural surface and this may be caused in part by an indrawing of the pleura by the scar.

Mucoid Impaction

Branching bandlike opacities pointing towards the hilum can be seen due to mucoid impaction and give rise to the "gloved finger" shadow. These are characteristically seen in allergic bronchopulmonary aspergillosis but can also be seen in many obstructive conditions like bronchial carcinoid, carcinoma lung, metastases, bronchial atresia, foreign body aspiration and benign strictures.

Septal Lines

Interstitial thickening involving the interlobular septae and bronchovascular bundle can lead to the development of primarily linear opacities.

Kerley first described septal lines on chest radiographs in cases of pulmonary edema.[18] They were named A, B and C lines as their anatomical basis was uncertain. Septal lines is a more appropriate term as increased fluid or tissue in the interstitium can result in linear opacities called Kerley B lines or rarely Kerley A or C lines **(Box 4)**.[19]

Kerley B lines are horizontal, peripheral nonbranching fine lines less than 2 cm long, seen typically at lung bases. These linear opacities are less than 1 mm thick, and lie roughly perpendicular to the pleural surface. They are commonly seen as a result of interstitial edema secondary to increase of pulmonary venous pressures, as in rheumatic heart disease and left ventricular failure **(Fig. 22)**.

Box 4: Causes of septal lines on chest radiograph

- Pulmonary edema
- Lymphangitis carcinomatosa
- Malignant lymphoma
- Sarcoidosis
- Pneumoconiosis
- Lymphoid interstitial pneumonitis
- Idiopathic pulmonary hemorrhage (late stages)

Kerley A and C lines are rare. Overlapping of Kerley B lines especially near pleural surfaces give rise to interlacing network of fine linear opacities referred to as Kerley C lines. Kerley A lines on the other hand, are slightly thicker than Kerley B lines and about 6 cm long, coursing from pleural interfaces to the lung hilum.

The Kerley B lines may be reversible in early stage of interstitial edema, with treatment of underlying cardiac pathology. However, these lines would persist if interstitial tissue pathology is irreversible, like in lymphangitic carcinomatosis, pneumoconiosis.

Tubular Shadows (Bronchial Wall Shadows)

The air column of the trachea, main bronchi, right intermediate bronchus, and left lower lobe bronchus is normally visible on well-exposed radiographs. Where these structures are in contact with aircontaining parenchyma their walls are also visible, their thickness being sufficient to cast a radiographic shadow. When tubular shadows are identified outside the hilar limits they constitute a definite sign of disease. Tubular shadows are doubleline shadows that may be parallel or slightly tapered as they proceed distally, and always follow the bronchovascular distribution.

Bronchiectasis is the most common cause of tubular shadows. The width of the air column separating them depends upon the severity of the bronchial dilatation. Since chronic bronchiectasis is often associated with atelectasis, multiple tubular shadows may be crowded together.

Tubular shadows may also be seen in the lungs of children with bronchial asthma. The tubular shadows seen in chronic bronchitis have been attributed to the accompanying bronchiectasis. Bronchial wall thickening may also be seen in pulmonary edema and in cases with neoplastic infiltration of the peribronchial tissues.

Line Shadows of Pleural Origin

In addition to the normal interlobar fissure lines, some line shadows that originate in the pleura indicate direct or indirect signs of disease. For example, with loss of lower lobe volume, the upper portion of the major fissure sweeps downward and medially and becomes visible on frontal radiograph as an obliquely-oriented shadow extending inferiorly and laterally from the lateral aspect of mediastinum above the hilum. Thickening of an interlobar fissure is caused more often by pleural edema than by pleural effusion. Since the pleural connective tissue layer is continuous with the interlobular septa, edema fluid also collects in the subpleural space. It not only thickens the interlobar fissures but also widens the pleural layer along the lung's convex surface.

The visceral pleural line is seen in pneumothorax **(Fig. 23)**. The double pleural line seen along either side of the mediastinum in cases of mediastinal emphysema is created by the combined thickness of parietal and visceral pleura displaced laterally by mediastinal gas.

Several other signs may aid in determining the nature of a pathologic process within the lungs.[5] To assess and interpret the ongoing process caused as a result of underlying disease, it is important to take into account ancillary findings that might prove contributory in the better understanding of the disease. These include position of fissures and hila on the chest radiograph and the characteristics of the lesion itself.

Position of Fissures and Hila

Frequently, displacement of the interlobar fissures and hila towards an area of increased density point to the presence of disease nearby like lung collapse **(Fig. 24)**. Displacement away from a lesion may be rarely seen because of volume expansion as in Friedlander's pneumonia (*Klebsiella*) where bulging fissure can be seen. This is due to the abundant exudates produced by the organism. It may also be seen with *Streptococcus pneumoniae, Mycobacterium tuberculosis* and plague pneumonia. Expansion of a lobe may also be seen with acute lung abscess, when air trapping by a check valve mechanism in the communicating airway distends the abscess cavity.

The interlobar fissures are an efficient barrier to the interlobar spread of parenchymal disease. A few diseases have a propensity for crossing pleural boundaries which is commonly seen with mycotic or actinomycotic infection of the lungs. In the latter, the organisms pass across visceral and parietal pleural layers and they may form abscesses leading to osteomyelitis in the chest wall.

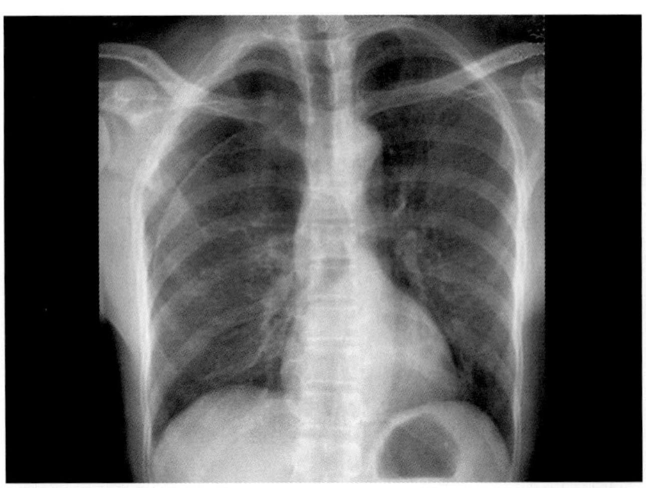

Fig. 23: Right-sided pneumothorax with passive atelectasis of right lung. Visceral pleural line is seen. Fractures of third to sixth ribs on right side.

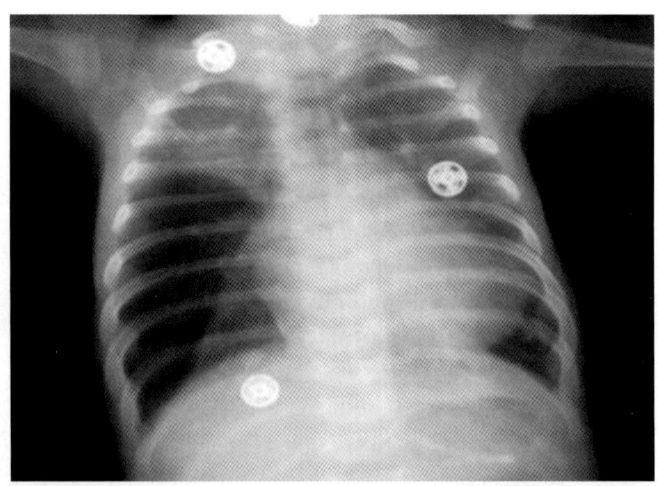

Fig. 24: Right upper lobe atelectasis showing increased density with upper displacement of transverse fissure. Atelectasis of posterior basal segment of right lower lobe.

Characteristics of the Lesion Itself

Single or Multiple

Primary malignant tumor of lung is characteristically solitary while metastatic disease frequently presents with multiple lesions. Pyemic abscesses are also multiple because of hematogenous spread.

Border

The smoothness of contour suggests benign disease and nodularity or lobulation indicates malignancy. A sharply defined contour is seen with acute airspace pneumonia that has extended to an interlobar pleural surface **(Figs. 25A and B)**, its margin is less distinct if it is formed by a spreading zone of confluent acinar lesions. A mass originating from the pleural space or extrapleurally, displaces the pleura and underlying lung inward such that the angle formed by the margins of the mass and the chest wall is obtuse. An intrapulmonary mass tends to be more sharply defined and forms an acute angle with the surrounding lung parenchyma.

Cavitation

A cavity is a gas-filled space, seen as a lucency or low-attenuation area, within pulmonary consolidation, a mass, or a nodule.[20] It sometimes contains a fluid level. Pulmonary cavities are mostly caused by tissue necrosis and expulsion of necrotic material into the bronchial tree **(Fig. 26)**. Rupture of a bronchogenic cyst or an *Echinococcus* cyst are exceptions where contents were originally fluid; as is infection of an existing cystic space, such as a bulla.

Wall thickness of the cavity, especially at its thickest part, can point to underlying disease process as being benign or malignant. Malignant lesions show a thick, nodular wall whereas benign lesions tend to have a thin, smooth wall. Nearly 85% of cavities with a wall measuring more than 15 mm in its thickest portion are malignant. If the thickest part of the wall is less than 5 mm, 95% are benign.[8] Presence of internal contents like aspergilloma, blood clot or floating membranes as seen with ruptured echinococcal disease giving rise to the **"water lily sign"** help in narrowing down the differential diagnosis.

Calcification

Presence of parenchymal lung calcification is a helpful indicator, usually pointing towards a benign process. Deposition of calcium in dead or non-vital tissue is referred to as dystrophic calcification, as is commonly seen in India in tubercular afflictions of the lung. Rarely calcification or ossification may occur in healthy lung as in metastasis from osteosarcoma. This is referred to as metastatic calcification.

Dystrophic calcification is fairly common in Ghon's focus as well as healed or old pulmonary tuberculosis and it may be solitary **(Fig. 27)**, localized or widespread **(Fig. 28)**. Popcorn or speckled calcification can also be seen in benign hamartomas. Calcification may be seen in other infective processes like histoplasmosis, post-chickenpox sequelae and miscellaneous conditions like arteriovenous malformations (phleboliths). Multiple ossific densities due to repeated hemorrhage can often be seen in patients

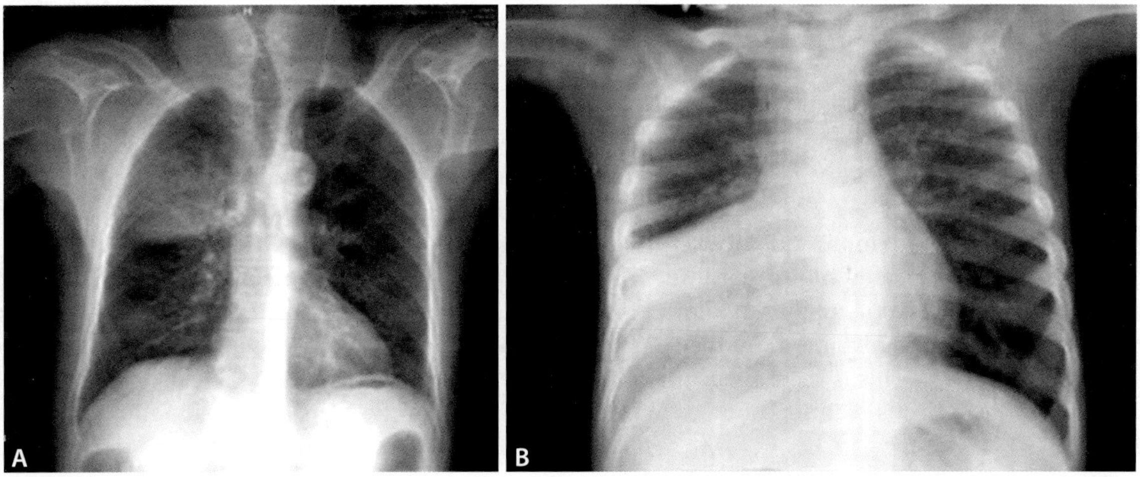

Figs. 25A and B: (A) Consolidation involving right upper lobe with poorly defined upper border; (B) Consolidation of right middle and lower lobes with smooth and sharply marginated upper border by the horizontal fissure. The right cardiac border and dome of diaphragm are silhouetted.

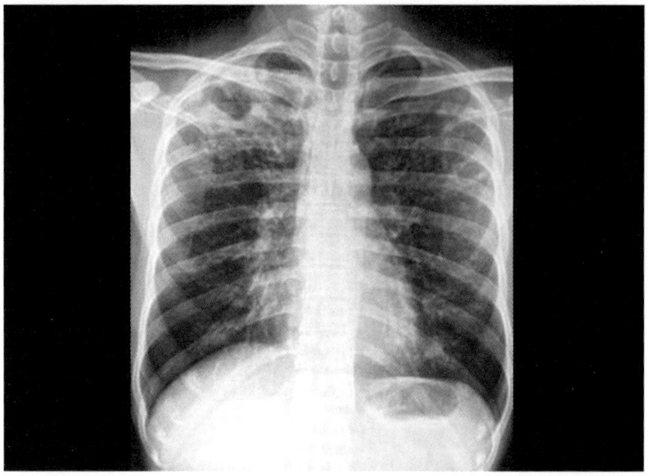
Fig. 26: Cavity in right upper lobe with surrounding consolidation. Multiple nodular opacities seen in bilateral upper and left mid zones.

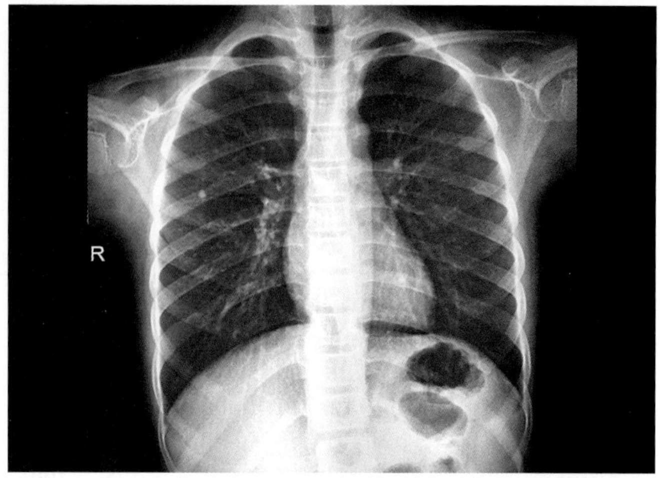

Fig. 27: Calcified granuloma in right mid zone.

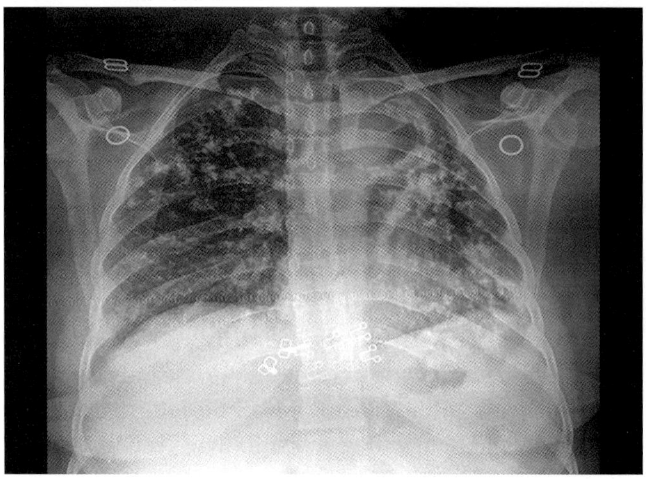
Fig. 28: Multiple calcified nodular opacities in bilateral lung fields with volume loss of left lung and an area of cavitation in left upper zone.

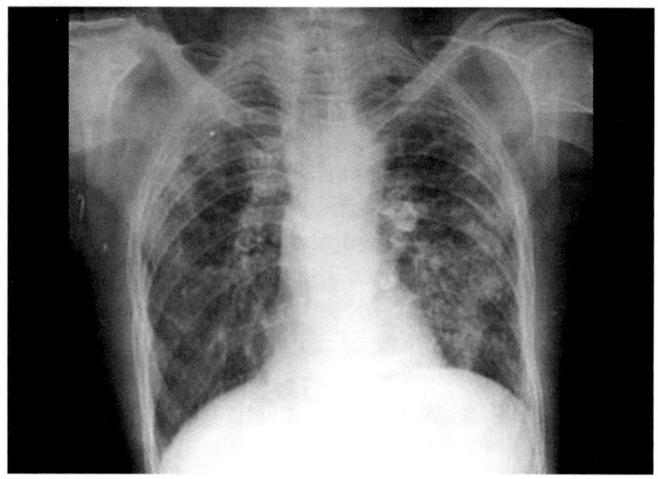
Fig. 29: In a case of sarcoidosis, chest radiograph shows multiple reticulonodular opacities and egg-shell calcifications in the hilar lymph nodes.

of mitral stenosis. In patients with alveolar microlithiasis and hyperparathyroidism cloudlike punctate calcification of the lung is seen.[21,22]

Irregular calcification in lymph nodes is frequently encountered in healing or healed tubercular infections. Rarely calcification results not in the substance but around the margins resulting in what is described as 'Egg shell' calcification **(Fig. 29)**. This is seen in occupational lung diseases like silicosis and coal workers pneumoconiosis.

Calcification of the pleura may occur and may be seen as a focal plaque of calcification or a long and broad sheet of calcification involving the visceral pleura. This can follow blood, purulent collections in the pleural cavity or tuberculous effusion. Rarely, parietal pleural calcification may be seen, typically involving diaphragmatic pleura as in asbestosis.

Physiological calcification of the tracheobronchial tree may occur in old age, seen more commonly in women. In younger patients however, it may point to an underlying hypercalcemic state. Costal cartilage calcification is also commonly seen on chest radiographs. Vascular calcifications may be evident along the aorta and coronary arteries. Main pulmonary arterial wall may occasionally show calcification in chronic pulmonary arterial hypertension.

Anatomical Basis of Disease

The site of involvement by a particular disease process in the lungs is influenced by certain physiological factors. The ventilation: perfusion ratio is different throughout the lung, primarily because of the influence of gravity. Gravity largely establishes the distribution of disease in aspiration pneumonia. The upper lobes are involved if aspiration occurs when the patient is supine, their posterior portions more frequently than the anterior. If the patient is erect, involvement of the lower lobes predominates. Aspiration occurs more readily into the right than left lung because the right main bronchus is more in line with the trachea. Blood-borne diseases predominate at the lung bases due to the greater perfusion of the lung bases in the upright patient. The hemodynamics of blood flow within the lungs causes embolic phenomena to also produce a peripheral distribution of disease. Pulmonary infarction occurs much more frequently in lower lobes than in upper lobes. Metastatic lesions occur more frequently in lower lobes. In bedridden patients, metastatic deposits do not show the usual anatomic bias and may predominate in upper zones. Pulmonary sequestration occurs almost exclusively in the lower lobes, most commonly in the posterior basal segment and on the left side than the right. The ground-glass opacity and reticulation of asbestosis shows basal distribution. Chronic idiopathic interstitial fibrosis and interstitial fibrosis of progressive systemic sclerosis are also predominantly basal in distribution.

Primary pulmonary carcinoma has an unexplained predilection for upper lung zones. The decrease in perfusion of the well-ventilated lung apices causes the apices to have a higher partial pressure of oxygen (pO_2) than the remainder of the lungs. The predilection of tuberculosis for the lung apices has been attributed to this difference in oxygen pressures. Upper lobe predilection is shown by silicosis, sarcoidosis, eosinophilic granuloma, and the conglomerate shadows of complicated silicosis and coal workers' pneumoconiosis.

The Silhouette Sign

This sign was described by Felson and helps in the localization and at times recognition of pulmonary disease. "An intrathoracic lesion touching a border of the heart, aorta or diaphragm will obliterate that border on the roentgenogram. An intrathoracic lesion not anatomically contiguous with a border of one of these structures will not obliterate that border". The sign is produced when the juxtaposed borders are of similar density. On a frontal radiograph, obscuration of specific contours indicate abnormalities in specific lobes, for instance if right superior mediastinum (superior vena cava) is obscured, the pathology is in the right upper lobe. Right heart border is obscured in right middle lobe involvement **(Fig. 30)** and right hemidiaphragm is obscured in right lower lobe involvement. The left superior mediastinum (aortic arch) is obscured in left upper lobe pathology, the left heart border in lingular involvement and the left hemidiaphragm or descending aorta in left lower lobe disease.[8]

The **"hilum overlay sign"** was described by Felson and helps in determining whether an opacity is within the hilum or anterior or posterior to it **(Fig. 31)**. If the opacity is situated within the hilum it will be obscured by the opacity from the proximal pulmonary artery and will appear inseparable from hilar structures. If hilar vessels

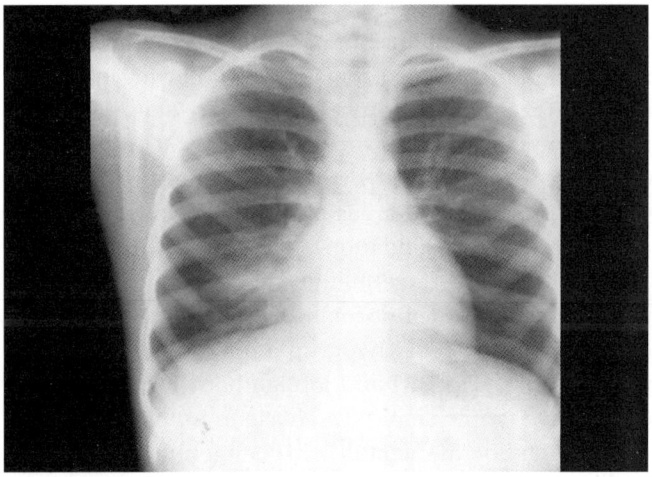

Fig. 30: "Silhouette sign"—right middle lobe consolidation obscuring the right cardiac border.

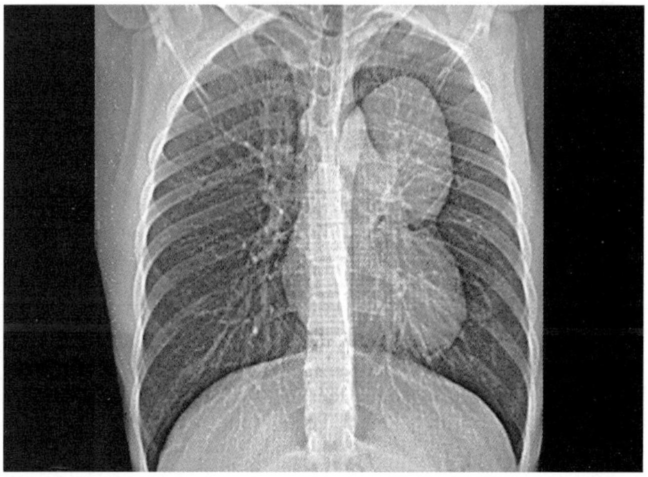

Fig. 31: Hilum overlay sign in anterior mediastinal mass, the hilar vessels are seen through the lesion.

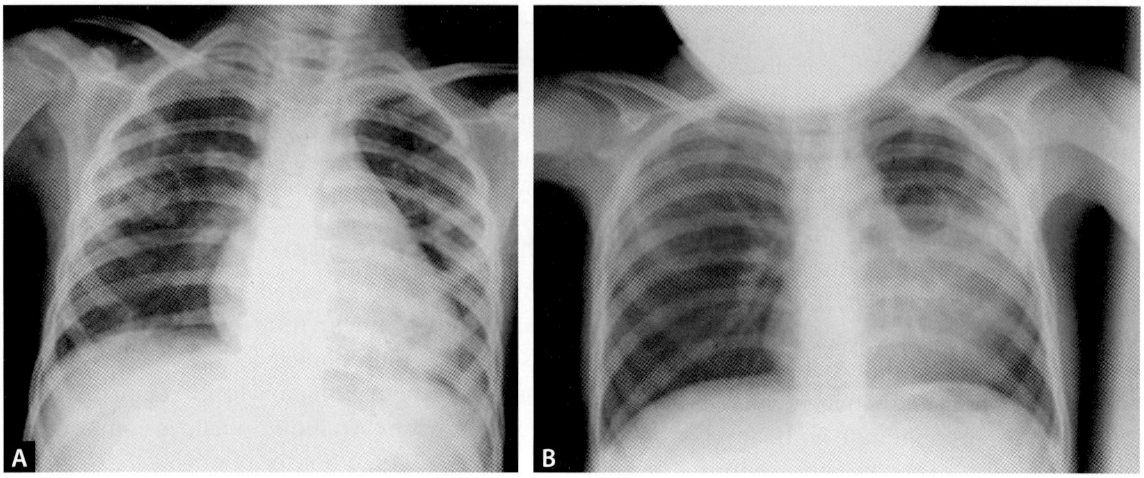

Figs. 32A and B: (A) Pneumatoceles in right lung field; (B) resolving staphylococcal pneumonia in left lung with pneumatocele.

are clearly seen through an opacity then it can be situated anterior or posterior to the hilum.[23]

Increased hilar size and density is seen with pulmonary artery enlargement. When pulmonary vessels are seen to converge on the lateral aspect of the hilum, it is referred to as the **"hilum convergence sign"** and is suggestive of vascular dilatation as the cause of hilar enlargement. The hilar angle shows its normal concave appearance.[8]

The **"cervicothoracic sign"** is used to differentiate between an anterior and posterior mass in the superior mediastinum. A posterior mediastinal mass is surrounded by lung tissue from all sides as the posterior part of the lung extends superior to the clavicle at the level of the thoracic inlet. Anterior mediastinal masses show ill-defined superior margins due to their anatomical contact with the soft tissues of the neck, either at or below the clavicle.[24]

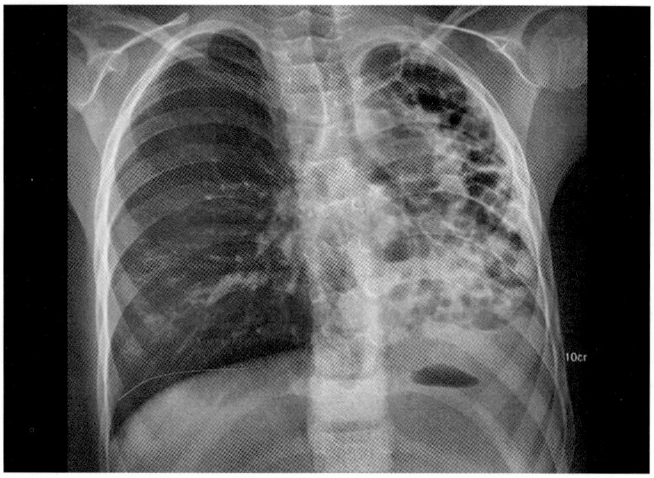

Fig. 33: Multiple cystic bronchiectatic opacities in left lung field with volume loss on left side and compensatory hyperinflation of right lung which appears hyperlucent

DECREASED DENSITY ON CHEST RADIOGRAPH

Diffuse increase in transradiancy of both lungs is seen in airway disease, constrictive bronchiolitis, asthma, emphysema, right to lung cardiac shunts like tetralogy of Fallot, Eisenmenger physiology or severe peripheral pulmonary arterial stenoses.

A focal increase in transradiancy can be seen in emphysema and bullous diseases, cysts, pneumatoceles and cavities. A bulla appears as a rounded focal lucency, 1 cm or more in diameter and is bounded by a thin wall. Multiple bullae may often be seen and are associated with other signs of pulmonary emphysema.[20] A cyst appears as a round parenchymal lucency with a well-defined interface with normal lung. Cysts have variable wall thickness but are usually thin-walled (2 mm) and occur without associated pulmonary emphysema. Cysts in the lung usually contain air but occasionally contain fluid or solid material.[20] Air cysts that develop following infections are known as "pneumatoceles" and are seen following *Pneumocystis jirovecii* or staphylococcal pneumonia **(Figs. 32A and B)** and hydrocarbon fluid aspiration.[6] Cavities are gas-filled areas of the lung within a nodule, mass or area of consolidation.

Unilateral hyperlucent lung can be seen with thoracic wall and soft tissue abnormalities, diminished perfusion of lung, compensatory hyperinflation of lung associated with collapse **(Fig. 33)** and foreign body impaction with obstructive emphysema.[6] Decrease in pulmonary blood volume may be associated with congenital defects like agenesis or hypoplasia of pulmonary arteries or acquired reasons such as thromboembolism.[25]

CONCLUSION

Chest radiography is an integral part of the diagnostic work-up of patients with respiratory disease. The natural contrast of the air containing pulmonary tissue provides a window which allows radiographic evaluation of diseases involving the lungs, tracheobronchial tree, and pleura. Computed tomography serves as an important adjunct to the plain film for the purposes of diagnosis and characterization of parenchymal lung disease.[26]

REFERENCES

1. Chest X-ray interpretation: Not just black and white. Pezzotti, William MSN, RN, ACNP-BC, CEN. Nursing. 2014;44:(1) p. 40-7.
2. Felson B. The roentgen diagnosis of disseminated pulmonary alveolar diseases. Semin Roentgenol. 1967;2:321.
3. Felson B. Chest Roentgenology. Philadelphia: WB Saunders, 1973.
4. Felson B. A new look at pattern recognition of diffuse pulmonary diseases. Am J Roentgenol. 1979;133:183-9.
5. Fraser RG, Pare JAP, Pare PD, et al. Diagnosis of Diseases of the Chest (3rd edn). Vol I: WB Saunders, 1988.
6. Hansell DM. Imaging of Diseases of the chest. 5th edition. St. Louis: Mosby Elsevier, 2009.
7. Collins J. Chest Radiology: The Essentials. 3rd edition. Philadelphia: Wolters Kluwer, 2015.
8. Webb WR. Thoracic Imaging: Pulmonary and Cardiovascular Radiology. 2nd edition. Philadelphia: Wolters Kluwer, 2010.
9. Woodring JH, Reed JC. Types and mechanisms of pulmonary atelectasis. J Thorac Imaging. 1996;11:92-108.
10. Proto AV, Tocino I. Radiographic manifestations of lobar collapse. Semin Roentgenol. 1980;15:117-73.
11. Woodring JH, Reed JC. Radiographic manifestations of lobar atelectasis. J Thorac Imaging. 1996;11:109-44.
12. Sutton D. Textbook of Radiology & Imaging. 7th edition. Edinburgh: Churchill Livingstone, 2009.
13. Golden R. The effect of bronchostenosis upon the roentgen-ray shadows in carcinoma of the bronchus. Am J Roentgenol. 1925;13:21-30.
14. Oktay Algın, Gökhan Gökalp, Uğur Topa. Signs in chest imaging. Diagn Interv Radiol. 2011;17:18-29.
15. Adam Grainger & Allison's Diagnostic Radiology, 6th edition. Philadelphia: Elsevier, 2014.
16. Kattan KR, Wlot JF. Cardiac rotation in left lower lobe collapse. 'The flat waist sign.' Radiology. 1976;118:275-9.
17. Felson B. A new look at pattern recognition of diffuse pulmonary disease. Am J Roentgenol. 1979;133:83.
18. Kerley P. Radiology in heart disease. BMJ. 1933;2:594-7.
19. Trapnell DH. The differential diagnosis of linear shadows in chest radiographs. Radiol Clin North Am. 1973;11:77-92.
20. Hansell DM, Bankier AA, MacMohan H, McLoud TC, Muller NL, Remy J. Fleischner Society: Glossary of Terms for Thoracic Imaging. Radiology. 2008; 246:697-722.
21. Brown K, Mund DF, Aberle DR, et al. Intrathoracic calcifications: radiographic features and differential diagnoses. Radio. Graphics 1994;14:1247-61.
22. Chai JL, Patz EF Jr. CT of the lung: patterns of calcification and other high-attenuation abnormalities. Am J Roentgenol. 1994;162:1063-6.
23. Felson B, Felson H. Localization of intrathoracic lesions by means of the posteroanterior roentgenogram; The silhouette sign. Radiology. 1950;55:363-74.
24. Kumaresh A, Kumar M, Dev B , Gorantla R, Venkata Sai PM, Thanasekaraan V. Back to Basics—'Must Know' Classical Signs in Thoracic Radiology. J Clin Imaging Sci. 2015;5:43.
25. Altinsoy B, Altintas N. Diagnostic approach to unilateral hyperlucent lung. JRSM Short Rep. 2011;2:95.
26. Kuhlman JE. Nonneoplastic Parenchymal Lung Disease. In: Haaga, Lanzieri, Sartoris, Zerhouni (Eds). Computed Tomography and Magnetic Resonance Imaging of the Whole Body, 3rd edition. Mosby, Vol I; 1998.

CHAPTER 159

Basic Patterns of Lung Disease on CT

Alpana Manchanda, Satyam, Gaurav S Pradhan, Jyoti Kumar

Computed tomography (CT) of the chest, especially high resolution computed tomography (HRCT) is the radiological imaging technique which best depicts changes in lung structure and is widely used for evaluating a variety of focal and diffuse lung disease. HRCT is superior to plain chest radiography in the detection and characterization of abnormalities due to the inability of plain radiographs to resolve small differences in lung density.

A CT "pattern" refers to a nonspecific finding or collection of findings suggesting one or more specific disease processes.[1] Various HRCT findings when taken together can represent typical patterns. The patterns, in conjunction with the anatomical distribution of findings along with clinical findings can narrow the differential diagnosis of diffuse lung disease, and in many cases indicate the correct diagnosis.[2]

HIGH RESOLUTION CT PATTERNS OF LUNG DISEASE

In order to successfully interpret the high resolution CT scan findings, it is important to follow a systematic approach with understanding of pathologic presentations of disease on HRCT.[3]

HRCT scan findings can broadly be classified into two groups:

1. Those manifesting as increased lung opacity
2. Those manifesting as decreased lung opacity

HRCT disease patterns, manifesting both as increased as well as decreased lung opacity can be further subclassified to simplify and thereby aid in differential diagnosis. At times, findings of increased and decreased lung opacity may be present on the same imaging study, suggestive of presence of two or more diseases or in certain cases be due to a pathologic process that manifests with both an infiltrative or obstructive process.

HIGH RESOLUTION CT SCAN FINDINGS MANIFESTING AS INCREASED LUNG OPACITY

HRCT scan findings manifesting as increased lung opacity can be further subclassified into the following abnormalities or patterns:

- Nodular pattern
- Linear and reticular pattern
- Ground-glass opacity
- Consolidation

Nodular Pattern: Nodules and Nodular Opacities

A number of diseases of the lung are characterized by multiple nodules as the primary abnormality. The term 'nodule' is used to describe a pulmonary opacity which is nearly circular, discrete, sharply defined or ill-defined ranging in size from 2 mm to 30 mm.[3] Nodules are usually further characterized according to their size, (uniform or variable) margin (sharply or poorly defined) density (solid or soft tissue vs sub-solid or ground-glass density), number and location. A small nodule is one which measures less than 1 cm, while a nodule 1 cm or larger in diameter is considered as a large nodule.[4]

The term 'micronodule' has been used by some authors to describe a very small, discrete, round, focal opacity. A variety of diameters have been used in the past to define a micronodule that is those with a diameter less than 7 mm, 5 mm, or 3 mm.[4]

The Nomenclature Committee of the Fleischner Society has recommended that the term micronodule be reserved for nodules less than 3 mm in diameter.[5] However, in patients of multinodular lung disease, the nodules are often of various sizes and except for miliary disease one does not usually come across cases characterized only by micronodules.

A nodular pattern is characterized on chest radiographs by innumerable, small, rounded opacities that are discrete and range from to 2 mm to 10 mm.[5] These are widespread but not necessarily uniformly distributed. On CT, the nodular pattern may be classified according to the three anatomic distribution of nodules, i.e. centrilobular, lymphatic or random, which will be discussed later.

The detection of pulmonary nodules on CT depends on their size, profusion, density and CT technique. Scan acquisition with narrow collimation is superior to thick section acquisition for detecting very small nodules as there is less partial volume effect which can average out the attenuation of tiny nodules.[6] The depiction of minute nodules on CT can be improved by the use of maximum intensity projection reconstructions of contiguous thin sections acquired by volumetric CT **(Figs. 1A and B)**.[7]

The HRCT evaluation of a patient with nodular lung disease is based on several findings and patterns.[8] These are:

- The craniocaudal distribution of nodules
- The appearance and attenuation of nodules
- The specific distribution of the nodules relative to lung structures.

The craniocaudal distribution of nodules helps in the differential diagnosis of nodular lung disease as certain diseases such as sarcoidosis and other granulomatous diseases are seen predominantly in the upper lobes while others such as hematogenous metastases tend to be lower lobe predominant **(Figs. 2A and B)**.

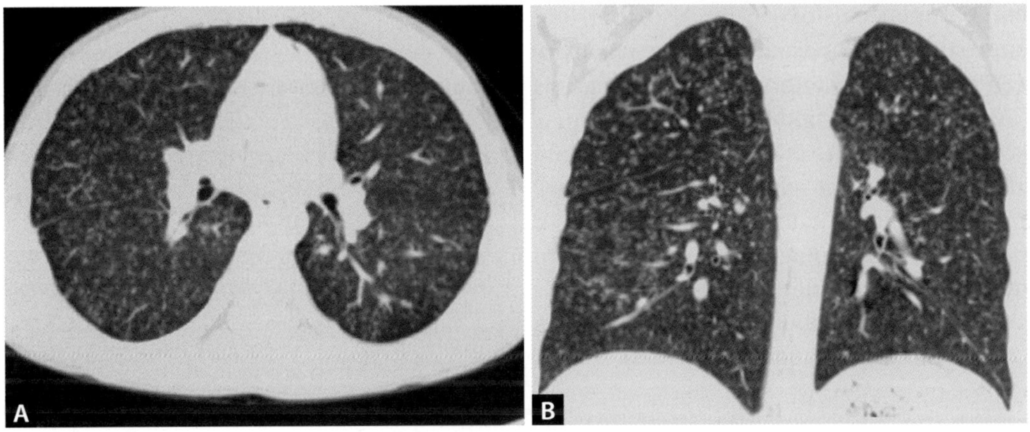

Figs. 1A and B: (A) Axial CT shows multiple, small, sharply defined nodules uniformly distributed in bilateral lung parenchyma; (B) Coronal reformatted CT MIP reconstruction delineates the miliary nodules better in bilateral lung fields.

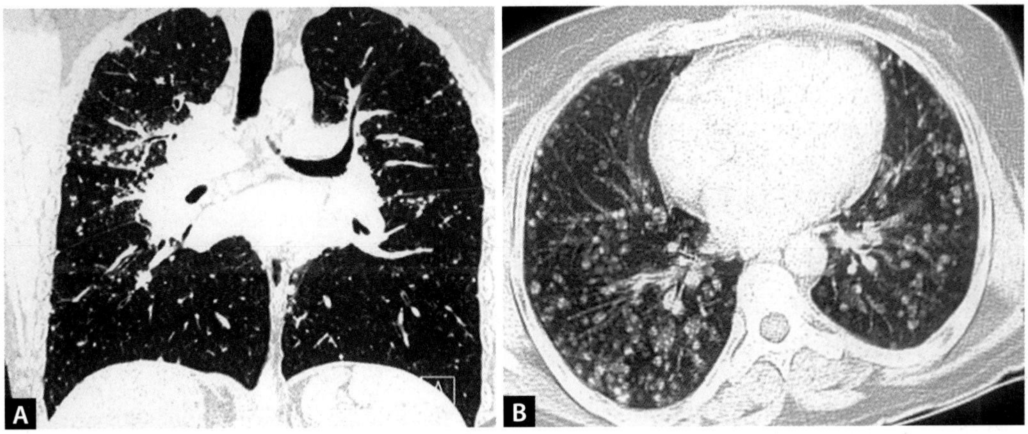

Figs. 2A and B: (A) Coronal MPR shows typical micronodules of sarcoidosis predominantly in bilateral upper lobes in perilymphatic distribution; (B) Axial CT shows multiple sharply defined random nodular opacities due to hematogenous metastasis.

However, the craniocaudal distribution of nodules should not be considered in isolation and should be used in combination with other findings. Some diseases may show overlap between the distributions (upper or lower lobe) and there may be variability among patients with the same disease.

The appearance of nodules may help to ascertain whether they are of interstitial or air space (alveolar) origin. Interstitial nodules are usually well-defined, of soft tissue (solid) attenuation and obscure the edge of vessels or other structures they are in contact with. Airspace nodules are typically ill-defined, and can be of homogeneous soft tissue attenuation (solid) or hazy and less dense than the vessels called ground-glass opacity (GGO). The following tables enumerate the differential diagnosis of multinodular lung disease based on sharpness of nodule margin **(Table 1)** and nodule attenuation **(Table 2)**.

Differentiating lung nodules into interstitial and airspace nodules on HRCT scan is not always accurate as many diffuse lung diseases involve both the interstitial and airspace compartments histologically. Also, there are many exceptions to the rule. For example, hypersensitivity pneumonitis (HP) which is an interstitial lung disease is characterized by very indistinct nodules **(Fig. 3)**.

In the assessment of diffuse nodular disease, *the anatomic distribution of nodules* relative to the secondary pulmonary lobule is diagnostic value on HRCT scans as it provides a focused differential diagnosis and is reflective of the pathophysiology of the underlying disease.

There are three specific distributions of small nodules in the secondary pulmonary lobule which can be distinguished on HRCT:

(A) Perilymphatic or lymphatic distribution, (B) Random, (C) Centrilobular distribution **(Figs. 4A to D)** are the representative schematic diagrams showing normal anatomy of the secondary pulmonary lobule and the various distribution patterns of nodules at the level of secondary pulmonary lobule. Recognizing one of these three distributions is fundamental to the HRCT interpretation of nodular lung disease and HRCT is found to be 90–95% accurate in determining the pattern present and formulating the correct differential diagnosis.[6]

Perilymphatic or Lymphatic Nodules

Diseases with perilymphatic distribution of nodules are characterized by involvement or spread through the pulmonary lymphatics.

Pulmonary lymphatics are normally found within the visceral pleura, the interlobular septa and along the veins and bronchovascular bundles. Hence, diseases which

Table 1: Differential diagnosis of nodular lung disease based on the sharpness of nodule margin.

Usually well-defined margins	*Usually ill-defined margins*	*Either well or ill-defined margins*
• Sarcoidosis • Metastases • Miliary infection (tubercular, fungal/viral)	• Hypersensitivity pneumonitis • Respiratory bronchiolitis • Follicular bronchiolitis	• Langerhans cell histiocytosis • Lymphoid interstitial pneumonia • Pneumoconioses
Amyloidosis	Infection (bacterial, fungal or viral)	
	Organizing pneumonia	
	Invasive mucinous adenocarcinoma (previously bronchioloalveolar carcinoma)	
	Aspiration	
	Pulmonary edema	
	Pulmonary hemorrhage	
	Metastatic calcification	

Table 2: Differential diagnosis of lung nodules based on nodule attenuation

Usually solid	*Usually GGO*	*Either solid or GGO*
Sarcoidosis	Hypersensitivity pneumonitis	Lymphoid interstitial pneumonia
Metastases	Respiratory bronchiolitis	Pneumoconioses
Miliary infections	Follicular bronchiolitis	Bronchopneumonia
Amyloidosis	Pulmonary edema	Invasive mucinous adenocarcinoma
Langerhans cell histiocytosis	Pulmonary hemorrhage	Organizing pneumonia
	Metastatic calcification	Aspiration

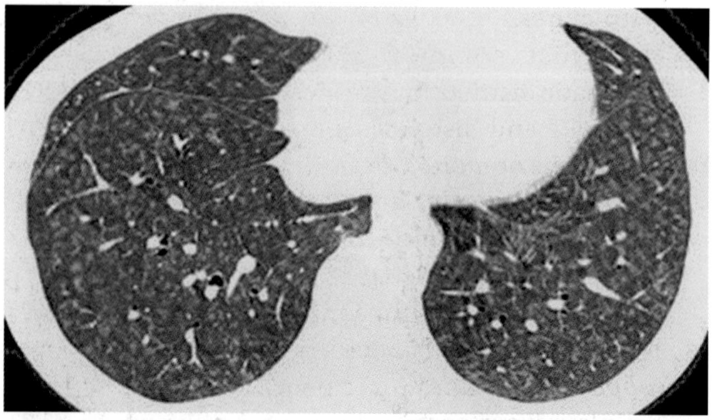

Fig. 3: Axial HRCT shows poorly defined ground-glass nodular opacities scattered in bilateral lower lobes in hypersensitivity pneumonitis.

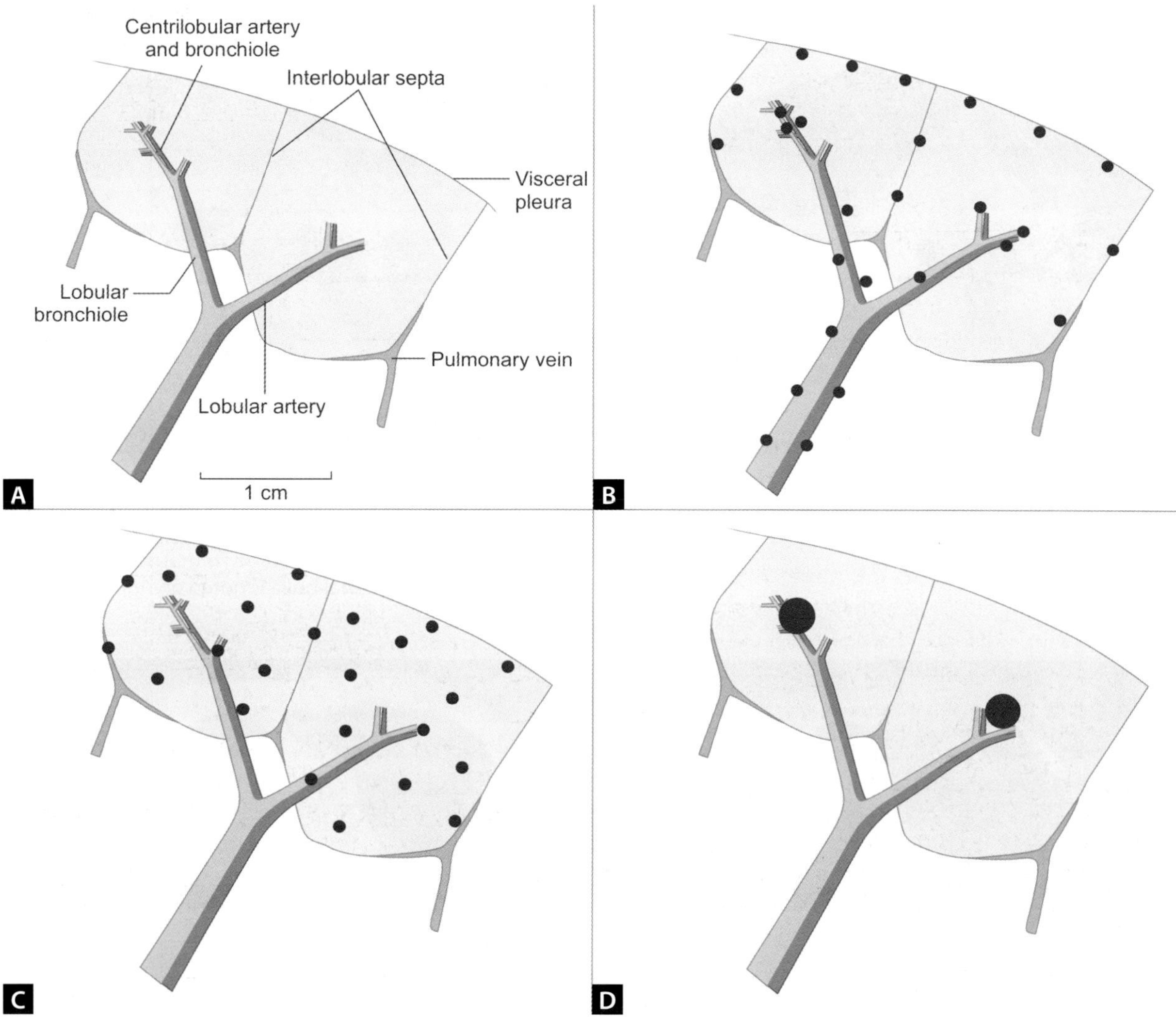

Figs. 4A to D: Schematic representations of distribution of nodules at the level of the secondary pulmonary lobule. (A) Normal anatomy of the secondary pulmonary lobule; (B) Perilymphatic distribution of nodules; (C) Random distribution of nodules; (D) Centrilobular distribution of nodules.

involve the lymphatics may produce nodules in relation to these structures.

The most common diseases which show a perilymphatic distribution are given in **Table 3**.

On HRCT and histologically, perilymphatic nodules are seen in one or more of the four locations:

i. *Peribronchovascular nodules* are seen individually or in clusters adjacent to large bronchi and vessels in the central lung regions, giving a nodular appearance to the walls of bronchi and arteries. There are most typically seen in sarcoidosis **(Fig. 5)**.

ii. *Subpleural nodules* are easily recognized beneath the pleural surfaces and adjacent to the interlobular fissures. Confluent subpleural nodules can result in the appearance of pseudoplaques. Subpleural nodules have been seen in around 80% of patients with silicosis or CWP and at least 50% of patients with sarcoidosis and also common with lymphangitic spread of carcinoma **(Fig. 6)**.[4]

iii. *Interlobular septal nodules* give the appearance of 'beaded' septa or nodular septal thickening. These are most frequent in patients of lymphangitic spread of carcinoma **(Figs. 7A and B)**.

Table 3: Differential diagnosis of perilymphatic nodules.[8]

• Sarcoidosis (common)
• Lymphangitic carcinomatosis
• Pneumoconioses—silicosis, coal-workers pneumoconiosis (CWP), berylliosis, talc, rare earth
• Lymphoid interstitial pneumonia (rare)
• Amyloidosis (rare)

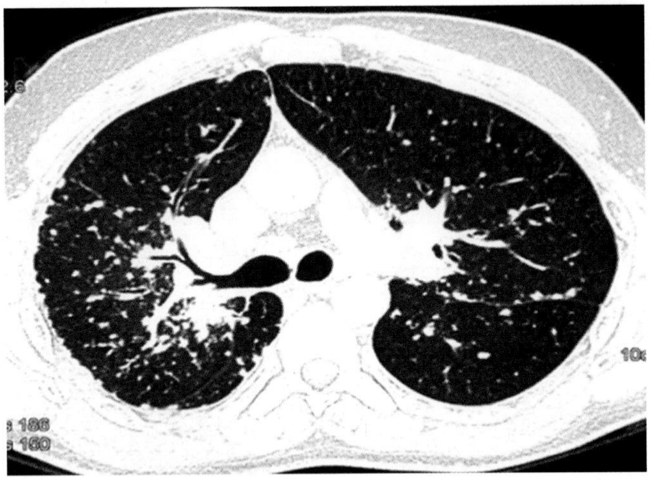

Fig. 5: *Nodular interlobular septal thickening*: Multiple granulomas in sarcoidosis in peribronchovascular, subpleural and centrilobular interstitium more marked in right upper lobe.

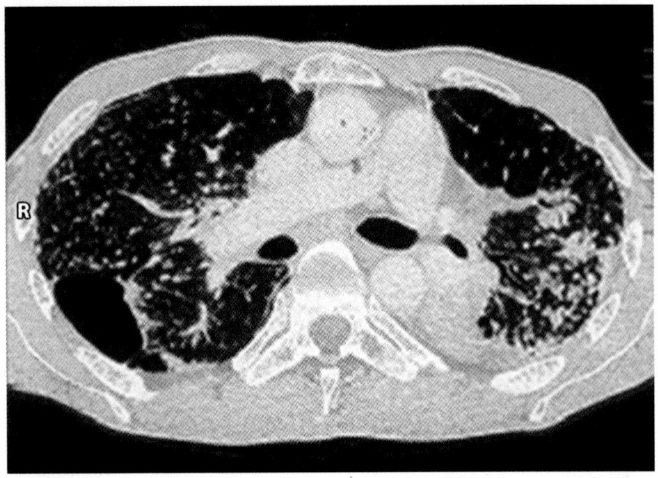

Fig. 6: *Perilymphatic distribution of nodules in silicosis*: Axial HRCT shows multiple small discrete and confluent micronodules in centrilobular and subpleural regions without tree in bud morphology. These are bilateral, symmetrical with upper lobe predominance. Subpleural bulla is noted on right side.

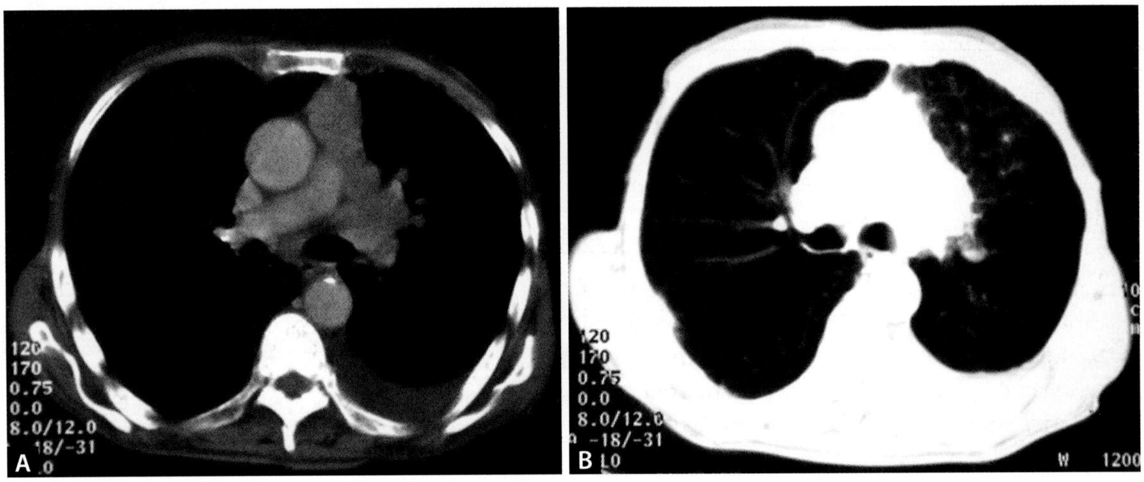

Figs. 7A and B: *Lymphangitis carcinomatosis*: Axial CT: (A) Mediastinal window shows a left suprahilar mass involving the left main bronchus, encasing the left main pulmonary artery with left pleural effusion; (B) Lung window depicts nodular interlobular septal thickening in the adjacent lung parenchyma.

iv. *Centrilobular peribronchovascular nodules* are also seen in relation to small airway and vessels in centrilobular location (center of pulmonary lobules), giving a beaded appearance to the centrilobular artery.

A combination of two of the above four possible sites has been described to be usually sufficient of perilymphatic nodules for diagnosis.[4] As perilymphatic nodules occur only in relation to these specific locations, the distribution of the nodules is patchy, with both normal and abnormal areas of lung regions seen on HRCT **(Table 4)**.[8]

Random nodules

Random nodules show a diffuse and homogeneous distribution with no particular distribution relative to the secondary pulmonary lobule. The nodules are seen in contact with interlobular septa, visceral pleural surfaces and in the center of the pulmonary lobule. In contrast to perilymphatic nodules which show a patchy distribution, random nodules are usually distributed uniformly throughout the lung parenchyma in a bilateral symmetric manner.[3] **Table 5** lists the differential diagnosis of random nodules.

Table 4: Typical pattern of involvement of the perilymphatic interstitium of some common diseases showing perilymphatic nodules.

	Sarcoidosis	***Silicosis***	***Lymphangitic Spread of carcinoma***
Site	• Upper lobe predominance • Diffuse distribution/lower lobe involvement also seen	May be diffuse but in mild disease may be seen in upper lobes	Upper or lower lobes or diffuse
Perilymphatic interstitium most commonly involved by nodules on HRCT	• Along central bronchi and vessels • In relation to major fissures	Centrilobular and subpleural in location	• Within thickened peribronchovascular interstitium, interlobular septa • Subpleural nodules less profuse
Size of nodules	Few mm to 1 cm	2–5 mm	Seen as beaded appearance of septum
Appearance of nodules	Usually well-defined	Well-defined	Septal thickening smooth/ nodular
Lung involvement	Patchy and asymmetric distribution of nodules	• More evenly distributed • Typical bilateral and symmetrical nodules	Variable-unilateral, patchy, bilateral or symmetric

Table 5: Differential diagnosis of random nodules.

- Hematogenous metastases
- Miliary tuberculosis
- Miliary fungal infections (coccidiomycosis, histoplasmosis)
- Disseminated viral infection
- Silicosis or coal-workers pneumoconioses (may occasionally appear random)
- Langerhans cell histiocytosis

Random nodules are smooth, sharply marginated and usually of soft tissue attenuation. A random pattern is most common in those diseases which show a hematogenous spread such as metastatic nodules. Metastatic nodules may show a basilar predominance due to a preferential blood flow to the lung base. Individual nodules may show a 'feeding vessel sign' consistent with their hematogenous origin **(Fig. 8)**. Metastatic nodules may be surrounded by a 'halo' of ground-glass attenuation which is typically seen in hemorrhagic metastasis such as due to choriocarcinoma.[9] In some patients with metastases, features of lymphangitic spread may be seen on HRCT along with metastatic nodules.

The size of the nodules may be useful in determining the most likely diagnosis. Metastatic nodules tend to be larger (range from a few millimeters to greater than 1 cm in size) and are frequently similar in size. While tiny well-defined nodules of a few millimeter are commonly due to miliary tuberculosis. Miliary tuberculosis may show an upper lobe predominance as the organism grows best where there is high oxygen tension which is present in the upper lobes. However, considerable overlap may be seen in the size of nodules that each disease produces. Miliary tuberculosis can result in nodules larger than 5 mm size.[8]

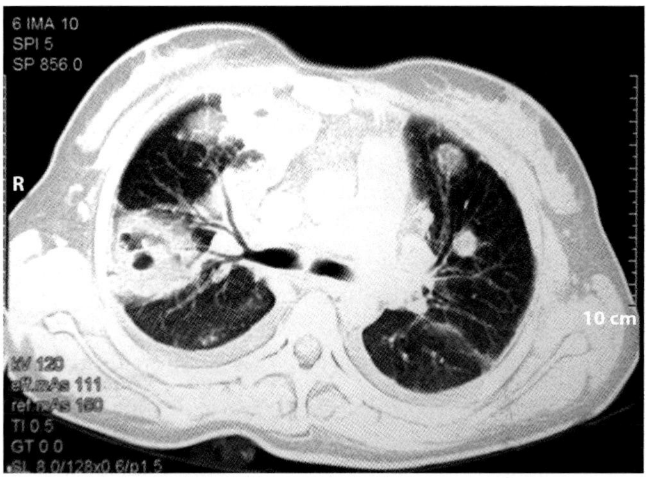

Fig. 8: *Feeding vessel sign*: Axial CT shows multiple variable sized nodules in angiocentric distribution scattered in bilateral lungs fields. Some of nodules show cavitation within.

A number of malignancies can result in a miliary pattern which can render the differential diagnosis to be difficult. This includes tumors such a renal cell carcinoma, head and neck cancer and testicular tumors which have their primary venous drainage in the lungs. In contrast, larger, less profuse metastatic nodules tend to be adenocarcinomas, typically originating from the lung, breast or the gastrointestinal tract. Less commonly, multiple cavitary nodules may be identified in patients with septic emboli, metastasis usually of squamous cell histology, Wegener's granulomatosis, rheumatoid lung disease, invasive fungal infections and pulmonary vasculitides **(Fig. 9)**.[1,9] Multiple irregular nodules in a bronchovascular distribution are characteristic of lymphoproliferative disorders, lymphoma, leukemia

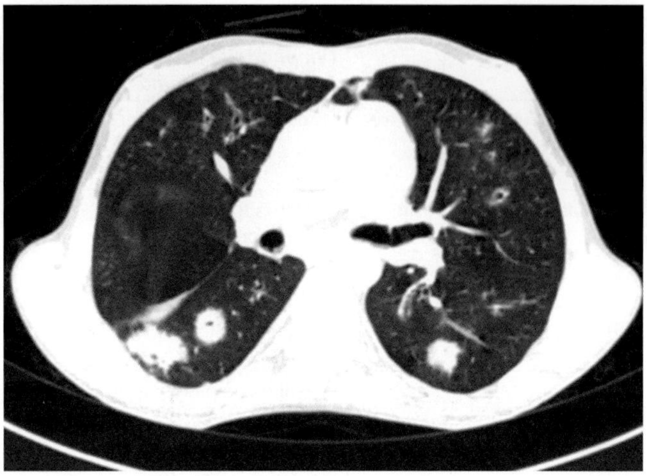

Fig. 9: *Cavitating nodules*: Axial CT in a patient of rheumatic heart disease reveals multiple nodules in bilateral lower lobes with central hypodensity consistent with septic emboli.

and Kaposi's sarcoma. When associated with thin walled cysts, randomly distributed nodules are suggestive of Langerhans cell histiocytosis.

When numerous, nodules in patients with sarcoidosis, Langerhans cell histiocytosis or silicosis may appear to be randomly and diffusely distributed and may be difficult to distinguish from the nodules of miliary infection or metastasis.[4]

Correlation with clinical history is important in the differential diagnosis of the nodular pattern. If patient has a known malignancy, the nodular pattern is diagnostic of hematogenous spread. If signs of infection such as fever or elevated counts are present, miliary tuberculosis or fungal infection is likely. However, it should be remembered that in the elderly or debilitated patients, miliary tuberculosis may be associated with very few symptoms.[8]

Centrilobular Nodules

Centrilobular nodules are distributed in the center of the secondary pulmonary lobule which contain the branches of the terminal bronchioles, their accompanying pulmonary arteries and supporting connective tissue with lymph vessels. Hence, centrilobular opacities can result from bronchiolar and peribronchiolar disease as well as from vascular and perivascular diseases.[2] They may be due to either interstitial or airspace abnormalities and may be dense (solid) or of ground-glass density and may range from a few mm to about a cm in size. They may be ill-defined or well-defined depending on the underlying disease process.

On HRCT, centrilobular nodular opacities show characteristic distributions which distinguishes them from other patterns. These are:

- The most peripheral centrilobular nodules show sparing of the visceral pleural surface. This is because the most peripheral pulmonary lobules are 5 to 10 mm from the pleural surfaces.
- The nodules appear evenly spaced from one another which is due to the similar size of the pulmonary lobules.[4,8]

Differential Diagnosis of Centrilobular Nodules

The differential diagnosis of centrilobular nodules depends on many findings:

- *Attenuation of centrilobular nodules:* (i) Ground-glass opacity (GGO), or (ii) Homogeneous soft tissue attenuation.
- *The overall distribution of nodules:* (Whether diffuse/symmetrical/patchy).
- Association with tree-in-bud (TIB) pattern.

Ground-glass opacity centrilobular nodules

Centrilobular nodules of ground-glass opacity may be seen as a result of airway disease or vascular disease, with ground-glass opacity centrilobular nodules due to airway disease being more common of the two. They typically reflect processes which produce peribronchiolar inflammation, infiltration or fibrosis without dense consolidation or obliteration of alveoli. **Flowchart 1** depicts the differential diagnosis of GGO centrilobular nodules.

Soft tissue attenuation centrilobular nodules

Centrilobular nodules of homogeneous soft tissue attenuation are characterized by inflammation or infiltration with consolidation of peribronchiolar alveoli or dense peribronchiolar fibrosis. There may be bronchiolar filling or impaction **(Fig. 11)** and the entire lobule may be involved with disease progression.[8] The differential diagnosis includes disease processes such as bronchopneumonia **(Fig. 12)**, aspiration **(Fig. 13)** and tumor, invasive adenocarcinoma (previously known as bronchioalveolar carcinoma). **Table 6** enumerates the differential diagnosis of soft tissue attenuation centrilobular nodules with their salient features.

Distribution of centrilobular nodules in differential diagnosis

When formulating a differential diagnosis of centrilobular nodules, the overall distribution of centrilobular nodules,

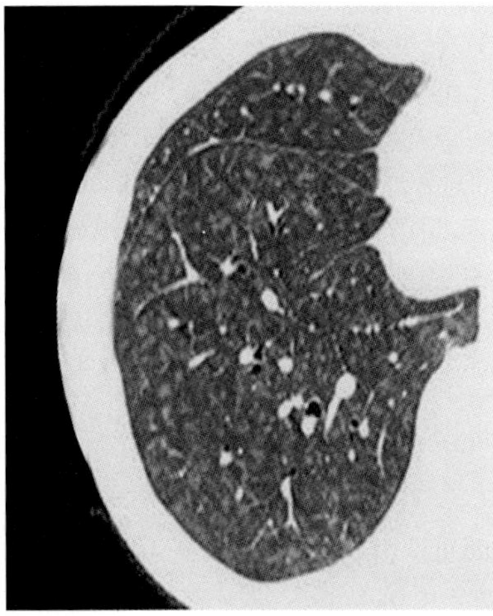

Fig. 10: Magnified axial HRCT image of right lung depicting diffuse ill-defined GGO nodules in subacute hypersensitivity pneumonitis.

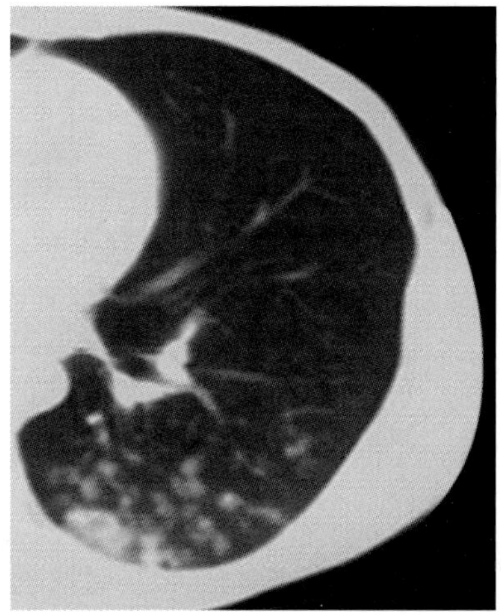

Fig. 11: *Soft tissue centrilobular nodules*: Axial CT image of left lung shows peripheral branching nodular opacities consistent with bronchiolar impaction.

Flowchart 1: Differential diagnosis of ground-glass opacity centrilobular nodules.[8]

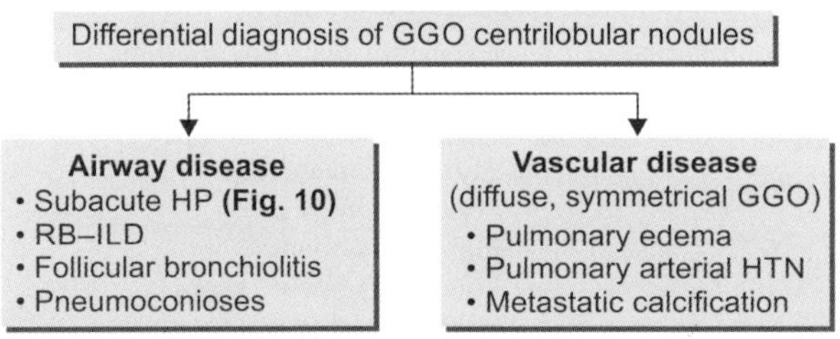

Abbreviations: HP: Hypersensitivity pneumonitis; RB-ILD: Respiratory bronchiolitis interstitial lung disease; GGO: Ground-glass opacity; HTN: Hypertension.

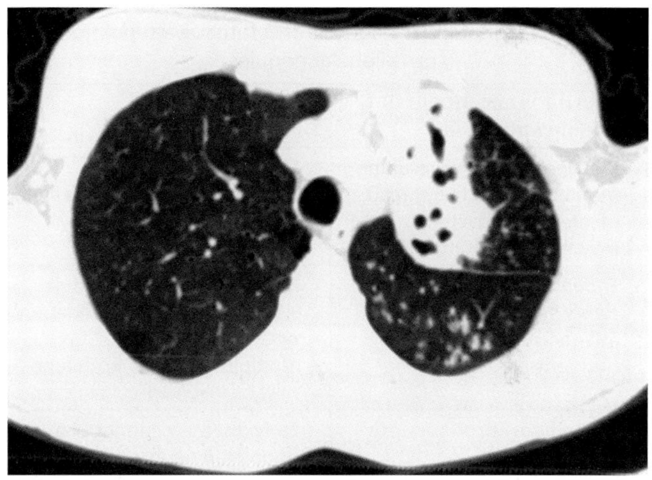

Fig. 12: *Airspace nodules in bronchopneumonia*: Axial CT reveals ill-defined soft tissue nodules in left lower lobe with collapse—consolidation of left upper lobe.

whether diffuse, symmetrical or patchy should be taken in conjunction with nodule attenuation (ground-glass or soft tissue attenuation). **Table 7** enumerates the differential diagnoses of centrilobular nodules based on overall distribution.[8]

"Tree-in-Bud" Pattern

Once nodules are characterized as being primarily centrilobular in distribution,further assessment is required to determine whether they have a "tree in bud" configuration or not.

"Tree-in-bud" (TIB) opacities are nearly always the result of inspissated secretions lodged within centrilobular bronchioles, which accounts for a branching configuration when coursing parallel to the CT scan plane. Normal bronchioles have a diameter of < 1 mm and a wall thickness < 0.1 mm which are below the limit of the spatial resolution of HRCT scan. The presence of inspissated secretions results in bronchiolar distension and increased density, allowing their direct visualization.[9]

The common radiological manifestation of the TIB pattern consists of centrilobular nodules of soft tissue attenuation connected to multiple branching linear structures of similar caliber, originating from a single stalk, which resembles the branches of a budding tree. **Figure 14** depicts the 'tree-in-bud' pattern.

On HRCT, the TIB pattern is well recognized by the presence multiple V or Y shaped branching linear opacities 1–2 mm in thickness and 1–2 cm in length, often associated with small nodules at the tips of their

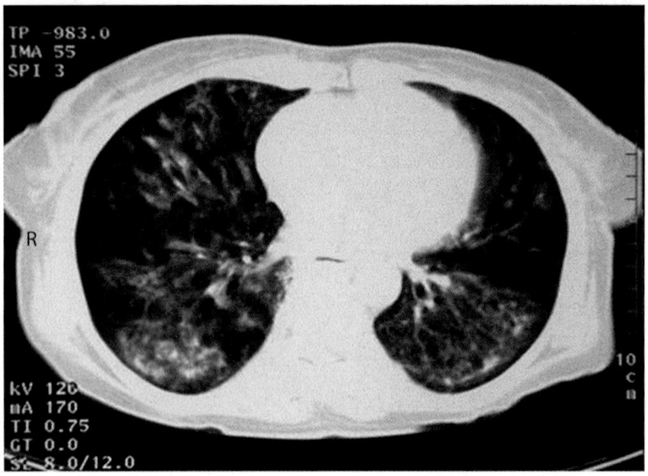

Fig. 13: Axial CT shows multiple discrete and confluent centrilobular nodules predominantly in bilateral lower lobes in aspiration pneumonitis.

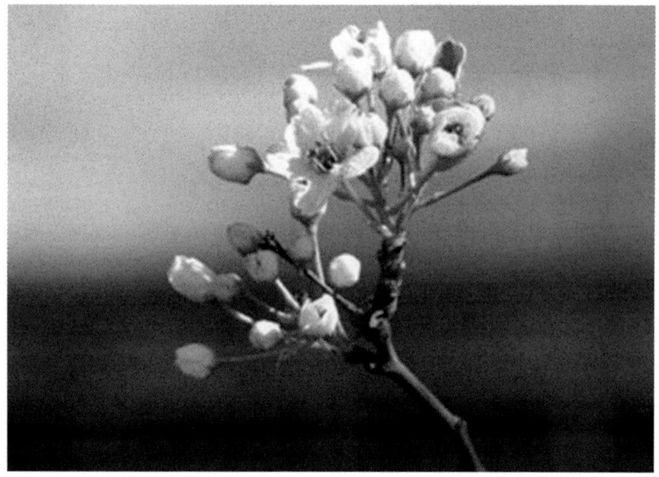

Fig. 14: Photographic representation of "tree-in-bud" pattern.

Table 6: Differential diagnosis of soft tissue attenuation centrilobular nodules.

Soft tissue attenuation centrilobular nodules	***Salient features***
• *Bronchopneumonia* resulting from endobronchial spread of infection—bacterial, mycobacterial, fungal, viral	• Most common cause • *Acute symptoms:* Nodules are focal, multifocal or patchy
• *Endobronchial spread of tumor* invasive mucinous adenocarcinoma (formerly BAC)	• Multifocal or patchy nodules ± larger areas of consolidation or GGO • Multiple lobes and both lungs may be involved
• *Langerhans cell histiocytosis*	• Early disease, centrilobular nodules in peribronchovascular distribution
• *Vascular diseases* (pulmonary edema, pulmonary hemorrhage)	• ± GGO or soft tissue attenuation nodules

Table 7: Differential diagnosis of centrilobular nodules based on distribution.

Distribution of centrilobular nodules	***Differential diagnosis***
Diffuse distribution	• Hypersensitivity pneumonitis (HP) • Respiratory bronchiolitis (RB or RB–ILD) • Follicular bronchiolitis • Atypical/viral infection • Pneumoconiosis • Pulmonary edema • Pulmonary hemorrhage • Pulmoary arterial hypertension
Upper or mid lung predominance	• HP • RB or RB–ILD • Langerhans histiocytosis • Pneumoconiosis
Lower lobe distribution	• Aspiration • Endobronchial spread
Patchy distribution	• Endobronchial infection (bacterial mycobacterial, fungal) • Invasive mucinous adenocarcinoma • Aspiration

branches. The HRCT finding of TIB is due to dilatation and impaction of centrilobular bronchioles by pus or mucus (branches) associated with small region of peribronchiolar inflammation (buds) and has a characteristic appearance **(Figs. 15A and B)**.[8]

The TIB pattern originally described in cases of endobronchial spread of *Mycobacterium tuberculosis* is highly suggestive of active tuberculosis. However, this pattern is now recognized as a CT manifestation of many diverse entities. **Table 8** enumerates the differential diagnosis of "tree-in-bud" pattern.[10]

The "tree-in-bud" pattern is most common due to infection with involvement of the small peripheral airways. It is not specific with regard to the type of infection, though bacterial and mycobacterial infections are seen most frequently. Bronchiectasis or bronchial wall thickening may be present depending on the cause or duration of the infection. In contrast, the non-infections causes of "tree in bud" pattern are relatively less common and include follicular bronchiolitis (usually in patients of connective tissue disease), mucoid impaction in asthma and allergic bronchopulmonary aspergillosis **(Fig. 16)**.[8]

Diagnostic Approach to Nodular Lung Disease

Differentiation of the three patterns of nodules (perilymphatic, random and centrilobular) on HRCT is essential to be able to formulate an appropriate differential diagnosis.

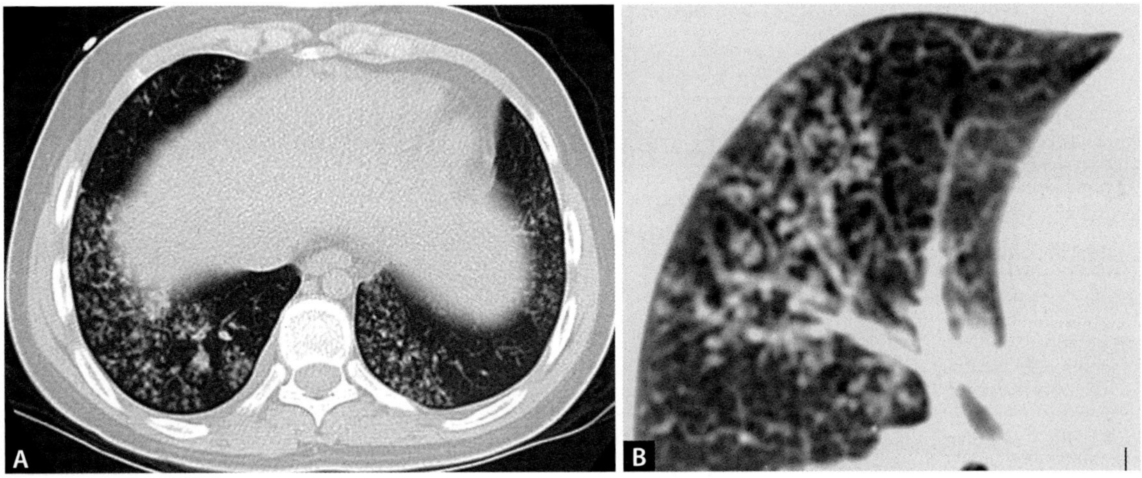

Figs. 15A and B: Tree-in-bud (TIB) pattern (A) Axial CT showing peripheral poorly defined small (2–4 mm) centrilobular nodules and branching linear opacities of similar caliber originating from a single stalk (TIB) pattern in bilateral lower lobes; (B) Magnified image depicting TIB pattern.

It is important to keep the following points in mind when identifying the pattern of nodules:

- Subpleural nodules are present in both perilymphatic and random patterns, but should not be present in patients with centrilobular nodules. If the distribution is not clear, then one should pay attenuation to the fissures and peripheral subpleural interstitium to determine if the nodules are present there.
- A diffuse distribution is typical of a random pattern, while a patchy distribution is typical of perilymphatic nodules. Centrilobular nodules may be either diffuse or patchy in distribution, depending on the underlying cause. For example, hypersensitivity pneumonitis (HP) is often diffuse while endobronchial spread of infection is typically patchy.
- When centrilobular nodules are present, one must ascertain the presence of "tree in bud" pattern. Infection is very likely when a "tree in bud" pattern is present, and when not present, the differential diagnosis depends on the attenuation and distribution of nodules.

Flowchart 2 depicts the algorithmic approach for distribution of small nodules on HRCT and their differential diagnosis.[8]

Linear and Reticular Pattern Opacities

Thickening of interstitial fiber network of lung by fluid, infiltration, fibrous tissue leads to increase in linear or reticular opacities on HRCT.

The reticular pattern consists of linear opacities that intersect one another at right angles, producing a mesh or netlike pattern.[3] On HRCT a reticular pattern almost

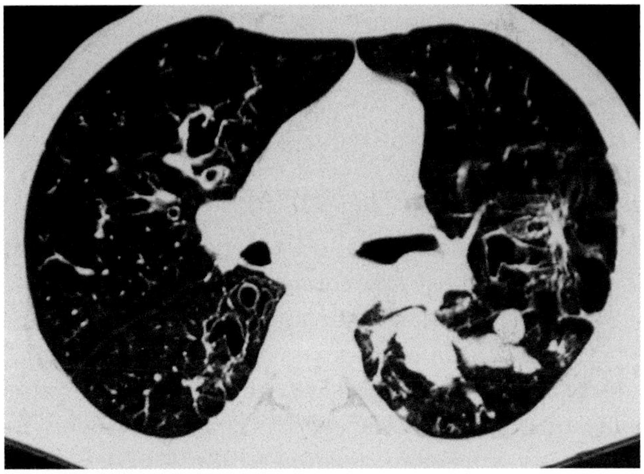

Fig. 16: Axial CT shows central bronchiectasis in bilateral lung fields with mucus filled bronchi in left lower lobe with centrilobular nodules in adjacent lung: Allergic bronchopulmonary aspergillosis.

Table 8: Differential diagnosis of "tree-in-bud" pattern

Infections
• Bacterial infections (*Staph. aureus, H. influenzae*)
• Mycobacterial infection (*M. tuberculosis*, MAIC)
• Fungal infections (airway invasive Aspergillosis)
• Viral infection (CMV, RSV)
Infectious variants (congenital/immunological/ idiopathic)
• Cystic fibrosis
• Kartagener's syndrome
• Allergic bronchopulmonary aspergillosis (ABPA)
• Obliterative bronchiolitis
• Panbronchiolitis
Aspiration
Inhalation

Abbreviations: MAIC: *Mycobacterium avium intracellulare*; CMV: cytomegalovirus; RSV: Respiratory syncytial virus.

Flowchart 2: Algorithm of distribution and differentials of multiple small nodules on HRCT.

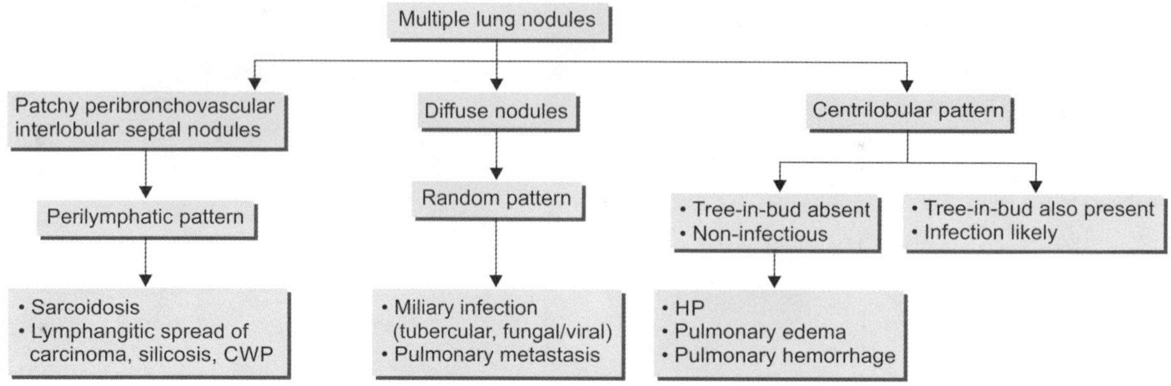

Abbreviations: HRCT: High-resolution computed tomography; HP: Hypersensitivity pneumonitis; CWP: Coal workers' pneumoconiosis.

invariably represents interstitial disease. It is a purely descriptive term (reticular - network) ranging from thickening of the interlobular septa to honeycomb lung destruction.[5] These reticular abnormalities are characterized into the following recognizable pattern on HRCT scan:[11]

- Interlobular septal thickening
- Honeycombing
- Intralobular interstitial thickening.

Interlobular Septal Thickening

Interlobular septa form the borders of the secondary pulmonary lobule. They comprise of connective tissue and contain pulmonary veins and lymphatics. These septa are around 0.1 mm in thickness and 1–2 cm in length. It is normal to find interlobular septae anteriorly or along mediastinal pleural surfaces.[3] The septae are seen when abnormally thickened, leading to the visualization of numerous septae. In the peripheral lung, the thickened septa of 1–2 cm in length are seen perpendicular to the pleural surface and may outline part or all of the secondary pulmonary lobule. On HRCT, the thickened interlobular septae are the counter part of Kerley B lines seen on chest radiographs.[12] The thickened interlobular septae outlining the pulmonary lobules appear polygonal in shape, are identified by the presence of a dot like branching centrilobular artery in the center. This characteristic relationship is valuable in identifying these structures on HRCT.

The terms septal lines or septal thickening may be used to describe interlobular septal thickening. Apart from interstitial lung disease, thickened interlobular septa may be seen in normal elderly patients and smokers.[11]

It should be kept in mind that the differential diagnosis of septal thickening is limited when it is seen as an isolated or predominant abnormality. Septal thickening can be characterized as smooth, nodular or irregular in morphology in different pathologic processes and recognizing this morphologic pattern is useful in differential diagnosis.[8,11]

Smooth septal thickening is present when the septae are thicker than normal and otherwise appears normal and are well-visualized on HRCT. It is usually a manifestation of pulmonary edema or lymphangitic spread of tumor with fluid or tumor infiltrating the lymphatics located within the septa. Irrespective of the cause, smooth interlobular septal thickening is often associated with smooth peribronchovascular and subpleural interstitial thickening which is most easily seen as thickening of fissures.[11]

In *pulmonary edema*, the smooth interlobular septal thickening may be diffuse and bilaterally symmetrical with basal predominance. Often the thickened septa are more defined in the apical and upper lobes as the interlobular septae are best developed in this region **(Fig. 17)**.[11]

Septal thickening in *lymphangitic spread of tumor* may be either smooth or nodular, with smooth thickening being more common. The abnormality may be unilateral or bilateral, asymmetric, patchy, having upper or lower lobe involvement. Both pulmonary and extra-pulmonary tumors (from breast, stomach, pancreas and prostate) can result in lymphangitic spread of tumor.[2,8]

Nodular septal thickening is most commonly seen in patients with sarcoidosis or lymphangitic spread of tumor **(Fig. 18)**. It reflects the lymphatic involvement within the septa, with the nodules representing clusters of granulomas or tumor nodules. In both conditions the nodules are seen in perilymphatic distribution.[13]

Sarcoidosis is often associated with architectural distortion which reflects the underlying pulmonary fibrosis. While lymphangitic spread of carcinoma is a non- fibrosing process which does not produce any architectural distortion.

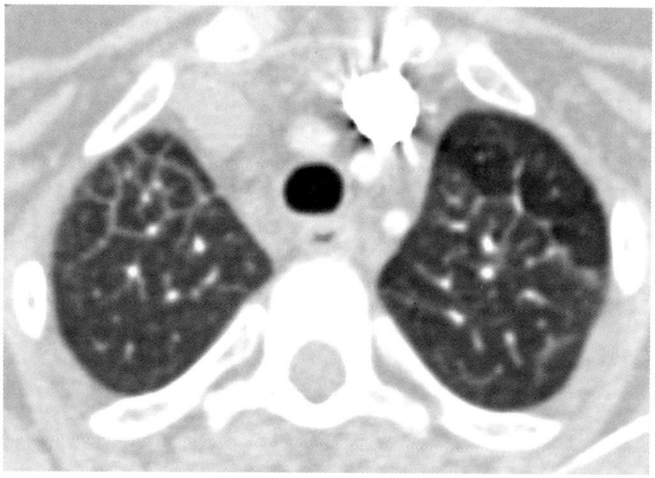

Fig. 17: *Smooth interlobular septal thickening*: Axial CT shows diffuse smooth interlobular septal thickening outlining pulmonary lobules with ground-glass opacity in bilateral upper lobes in a patient with pulmonary edema.

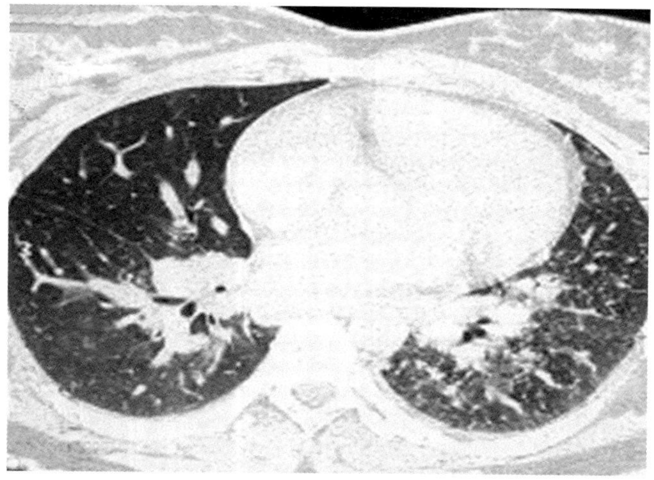

Fig. 18: *Perilymphatic distribution of nodules in sarcoidosis*: Axial HRCT shows multiple small nodules scattered in centrilobular, peribronchovascular and perilymphatic distribution. Micronodular beading is seen along major fissures.

Irregular interlobular septal thickening is usually seen in fibrotic lung disease with architectural distortion associated with fibrosis resulting in the septa to become jagged in appearance. On HRCT, other findings such as honeycombing, traction bronchiectasis are of importance in reaching a differential diagnosis **(Fig. 19)**.[13]

Flowchart 3 illustrates the algorithmic approach to the differential diagnosis of interlobular septal thickening when it is a predominant abnormality.[3,11]

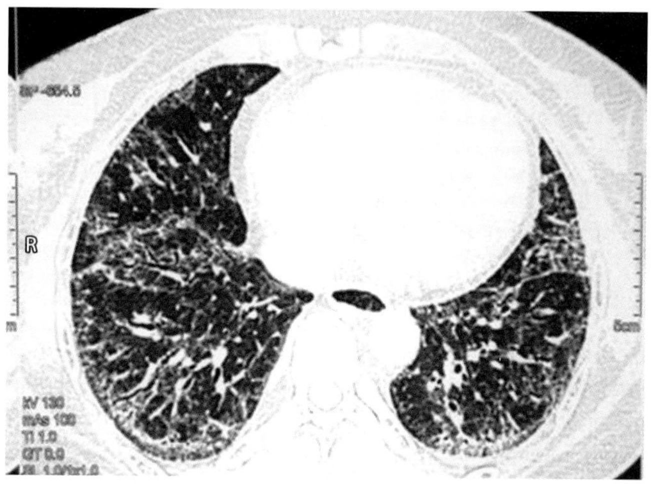

Fig. 19: *Irregular interlobular septal thickening*: Axial HRCT showing intralobular, interlobular and subpleural interstitial thickening involving bilateral lower lobes with traction bronchiectasis.

Honeycombing

Presence of honeycombing is the most specific HRCT sign of fibrosis, appearing as air-filled cystic spaces. This will be discussed later under the HRCT findings manifesting as decreased lung opacity.

Intralobular Interstitial Thickening

The intralobular interstitium refers to the interstitial network that supports the structures of the pulmonary lobules and does not include the interlobular septa. It is normally not visible on HRCT. It comprises mainly of the fine network of very thin connective tissue fibers within the alveolar walls or the parenchymal interstitium.[1]

Intralobular interstitial thickening is an early sign of fibrosis. It is a non-specific finding and may be associated with interstitial infiltration or inflammation in the absence of fibrosis. The term 'intralobular lines' is used to describe the presence of intralobular interstitial thickening. These lines are less than 5 mm long and form a fine lace like network and usually do not conform to the lobular anatomy. They are seen in all types of fibrotic lung disease, especially idiopathic pulmonary fibrosis usual interstitial pneumonia (UIP), nonspecific interstitial pneumonia (NSIP), pulmonary disease associated with collagen vascular diseases.

Intralobular interstitial thickening are usually associated with other features of lung fibrosis such as architectural distortion or tractional bronchiectasis. The term tractional bronchiectasis refers to the bronchial dilatation occurring as a result of interstitial fibrosis, whereby the bronchi appear irregular, but are not associated with any radiological evidence of bronchial inflammation, i.e. bronchial wall thickening or mucus impactions.

Flowchart 3: Algorithmic approach to differential diagnosis of interlobular septal thickening.

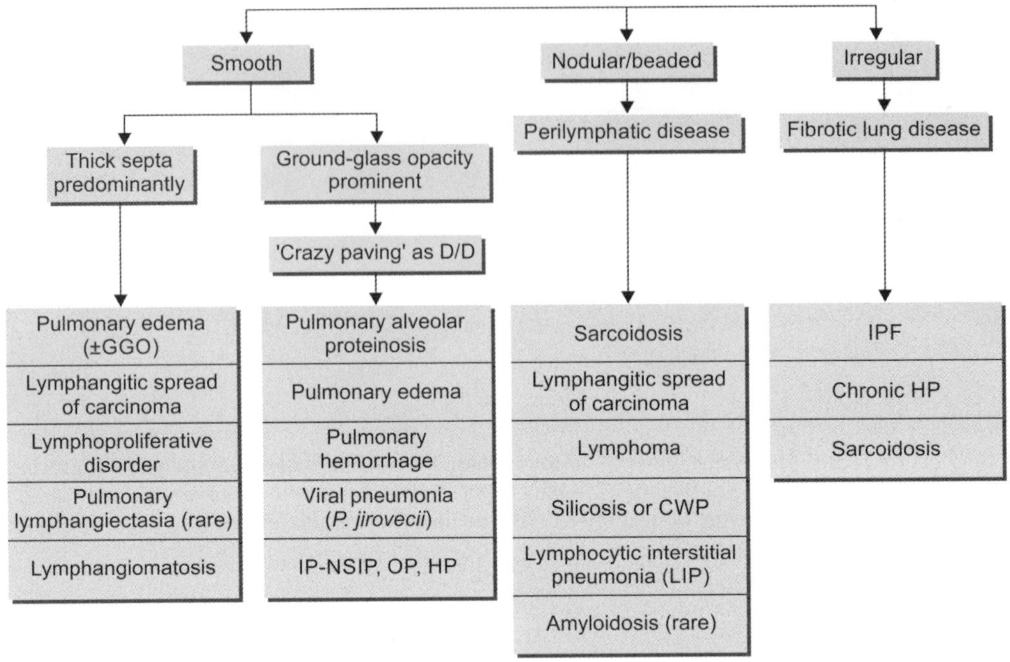

Abbreviations: D/D: Differential diagnosis; GGO: Ground-glass opacity; NSIP: Nonspecific interstitial pneumonia; OP: Organizing pneumonia; HP: Hypersensitivity pneumonitis; CWP: Coal workers' pneumoconiosis; IPF: Idiopathic pulmonary fibrosis.

Intralobular interstitial thickening may also be seen in other idiopathic interstitial pneumonias, pulmonary infections (viral pneumonias), pulmonary edema, pulmonary hemorrhage and lymphangitic carcinomatosis.

Irregular reticulation: Irregular reticulation is a non-specific finding and is said to be present when normal reticular opacities do not represent any of the other two patterns, i.e. interlobular septal thickening and honeycombing. They are known by various names like parenchymal bands and subpleural lesions. The presence of irregular reticulation is moderately specific for fibrosis.

Ground-glass Opacity

Ground-glass opacity (CGO) refers to the hazy increase in lung attenuation that does not obscure the underlying vessels or bronchial margins. It is a common but non-specific finding on HRCT. Ground-glass opacity results from volume averaging of morphological abnormalities that are too small to be clearly resolved by HRCT. It may reflect the presence of air space disease, interstitial disease, or a combination of both. It may be a manifestation of lung infiltration, active inflammation, or fibrosis and may also result from atelectasis.

Ground-glass opacity is a subjective finding on HRCT and may be difficult to recognize if it is minimal or involves the entire lung diffusely. However, it is mostly patchy or geographic in distribution, effecting some areas of lung and sparing other regions, thereby making it easier to recognize **(Figs. 20A and B)**. In cases where the presence of GGO is equivocal, comparing the attenuation of the lung parenchyma with air in the bronchi may be helpful. In normal individuals the density difference is marginal, while with GGO the airways appear "too black" within an area of lung (the 'black bronchus' sign).

Ground-glass opacity is a significant finding on HRCT and its presence indicates an ongoing active and potentially treatable/reversible disease. Its significance depends on the patient symptomatology (acute versus chronic), the distribution of GGO on HRCT, and the presence or absence of other findings on HRCT **(Fig. 21)**.

Differential diagnosis of ground-glass opacity: A large number of diseases can show GGO on HRCT. Knowing the duration of patients' symptoms (acute, subacute or chronic) is fundamental to the differential diagnosis with this HRCT appearance. **Tables 9** and **10** depict the differential diagnosis of GGO according to the clinical presentation and distribution.[14]

Pitfalls in Diagnosis of Ground-glass Opacity

There are several potential pitfalls in the recognition and diagnosis of GGO which a radiologist must be aware so as

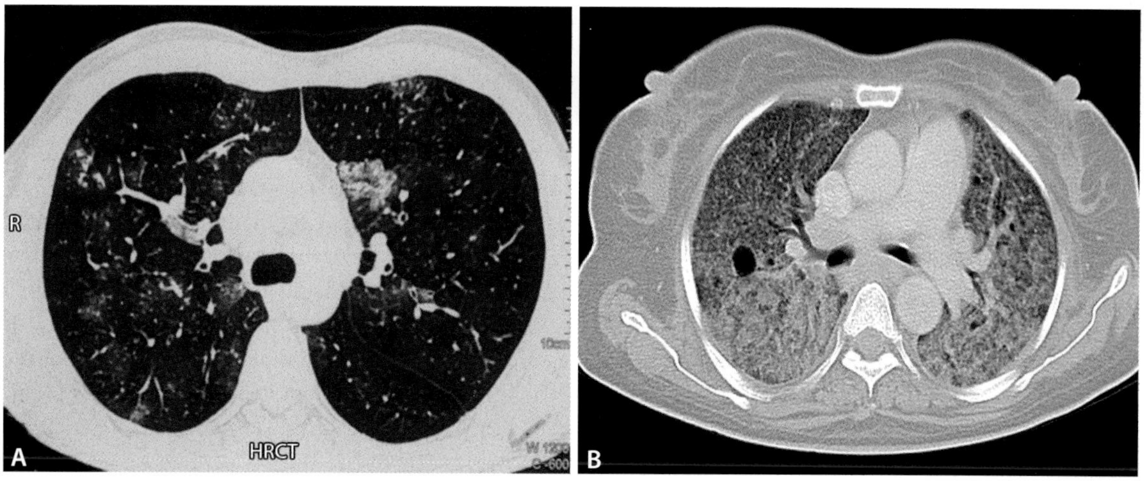

Figs. 20A and B: (A) Axial HRCT chest in a 40-year-old male with recurrent episode of cough, wheeze and blood eosinophilia reveal multiple patchy areas of transient GGO in bilateral lung fields which resolved following antihelminthic therapy—Loeffier syndrome; (B) Axial HRCT of *Pneumocystis jirovecii* infection in an HIV patient in the form of symmetric diffuse ground-glass opacity associated with cyst in right lung.

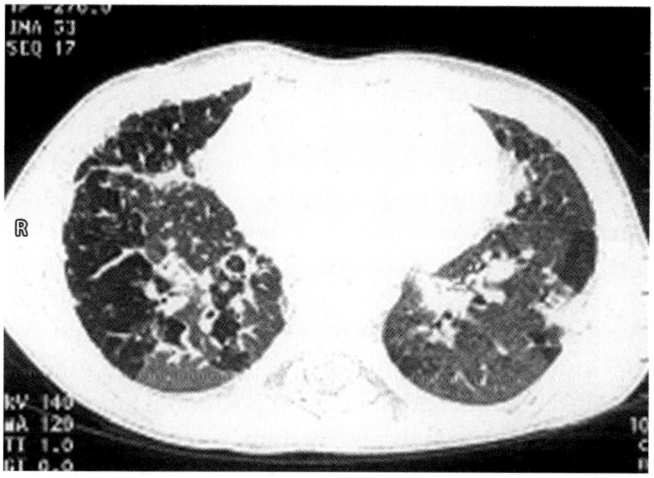

Fig. 21: *Acute hypersensitivity pneumonitis*: Axial HRCT shows extensive areas of ground-glass attenuation in bilateral lung fields.

to avoid misdiagnosis of the same. GGO may be spuriously diagnosed on HRCT in the following circumstances:

- In pediatric patients
- HRCT performed with thick collimation
- 'Dependent density' in the posterior lung in supine scanning which clears on prone scan
- Expiratory scans may mimic the appearance of GGO due to reduced amount of air in the alveoli on expiration.
- In scans showing patchy emphysema or other causes of hyperlucency such as airways obstruction and air trapping, normal lung regions can mimic the appearance of ground-glass opacity by appearing relatively dense which can be distinguished on expiratory scan.

Table 9: Differential diagnosis of GGO on the basis of clinical presentation.

Acute presentation
• Pulmonary edema • Pulmonary hemorrhage • All types of pneumonias (especially atypical pneumonia) – *Pneumocystis jirovecii* – Viral—cytomegalovirus (CMV) – Mycoplasma – Acute interstitial pneumonitis – Acute eosinophilic pneumonia • Hypersensitivity pneumonitis • Aspiration
Subacute or chronic presentation
• Nonspecific interstitial pneumonia (NSIP) • Pneumonia associated with collagen vascular disease • Desquamative interstitial pneumonia (DIP) • Respiratory bronchiolitis interstitial lung disease (RB–ILD) • Hypersensitivity pneumonitis (HP) • Organizing pneumonia (OP) • Chronic eosinophilic pneumonia • Chronic/recurrent aspiration • Adenocarcinoma *in situ* (formerly BAC) • Pulmonary alveolar proteinosis (PAP)

Table 10: Differential diagnosis of GGO on the basis of distribution.

Distribution of GGO	***Causes***
• Peripheral and subpleural	NSIP, DIP, OP
• Patchy and geographic	HP, OP, eosinophilic pneumonia
• Peribronchovascular	Sarcoid, OP, eosinophilic pneumonia
• Diffuse and extensive	HP

Abbreviations: GGO: Ground-glass opacity; NSIP: Nonspecific interstitial pneumonia; DIP: Desquamative interstitial pneumonia; OP: Organizing pneumonia; HP: Hypersensitivity pneumonitis.

Consolidation

Consolidation is characterized by abnormal dense opacification of the lung parenchyma with obscuration of the underlying vessels. It may be alveolar or interstitial in origin, though most commonly the alveolar air is replaced by fluid, cells, tissue or pus. Consolidation is detected both on plain radiography and CT, and may be visualized earlier on CT than plain radiographs.[6] HRCT provides useful diagnostic information regarding the distribution and characteristics of consolidated lung. But, the rate of change of consolidation should always be sought from serial chest radiographs. For example, rapid radiographic resolution in hours rather than days of diffuse lung opacification of acute onset is highly suggestive of pulmonary edema or hemorrhage.

The CT appearances of air space consolidation differ depending on the degree of involvement. The earliest findings consists of poorly marginated small nodules called acinar nodules approximately 7 mm in diameter which occur when single acini are replaced by fluid or tissue **(Figs. 22A and B)**. These are not true nodules and represent clusters of single acini filled with fluid, inflammatory cells or blood, depending on the disease process. With involvement of adjacent acini, the acinar nodules coalesce and may progress to lobular, subsegmental, segmental, lobar or multilobar areas of consolidation **(Figs. 23A and B)**. Unlike ground-glass opacity, on HRCT, consolidation results in an increase in lung opacity with underlying vessels being obscured. Air bronchogram are usually seen if the bronchi are patent.[15]

Differential Diagnosis

The differential diagnosis of consolidation overlaps considerably with ground-glass opacity. **Table 11** enumerates the differential diagnosis of consolidation with their salient features.[14]

The differential diagnosis of consolidation depends mainly on:

a. Duration of symptoms
b. Distribution of consolidation

Consolidation presenting in an acute condition is mostly seen in pneumonias and aspiration. The various causative organisms of pneumonia result in different patterns of parenchymal opacification on HRCT. Aspiration may be focal or patchy and typically involves the lower lobes and posterior upper lobes.

Perihilar "bat-wing" consolidation with sparing of the periphery of the lung is typical of pulmonary edema **(Fig. 23C)**. This pattern may also be seen with pulmonary hemorrhage, pneumonia such as *Pneumocystis jirovecii* pneumonia and inhalational lung injury. In patients of pulmonary edema, a perihilar distribution is most often seen when a rapid accumulation of fluid has occurred. Relative sparing of the lung periphery has been attributed to better lymphatic clearance of fluid in this region.[16]

Differential diagnosis of consolidation of chronic symptomatology include organizing pneumonia **(Fig. 24)**, chronic eosinophilic pneumonia, invasive adenocarcinoma, sarcoidosis, lymphoma, lipoid pneumonia, hypersensitivity pneumonitis, pulmonary infarction.[14,17]

Presence of focal consolidation within single or cluster of acini or a tree-in-bud pattern may help in reducing the differential diagnosis. But the differentiation of adenocarcinoma and organizing pneumonia may rarely be made with certainly on HRCT appearance alone and a tissue diagnosis is usually required.

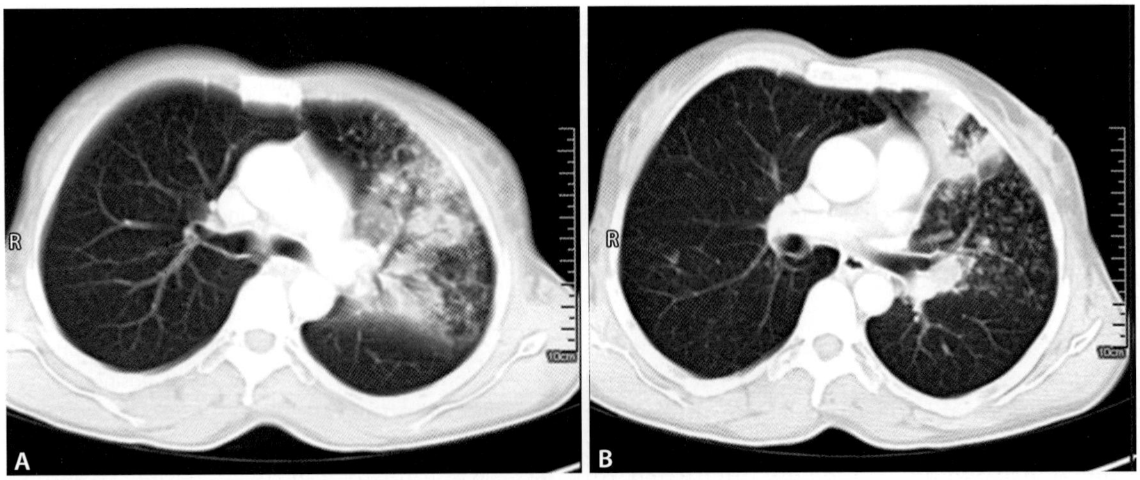

Figs. 22A and B: Axial CT shows consolidation with air bronchogram and adjacent airspace nodules in left upper lobe.

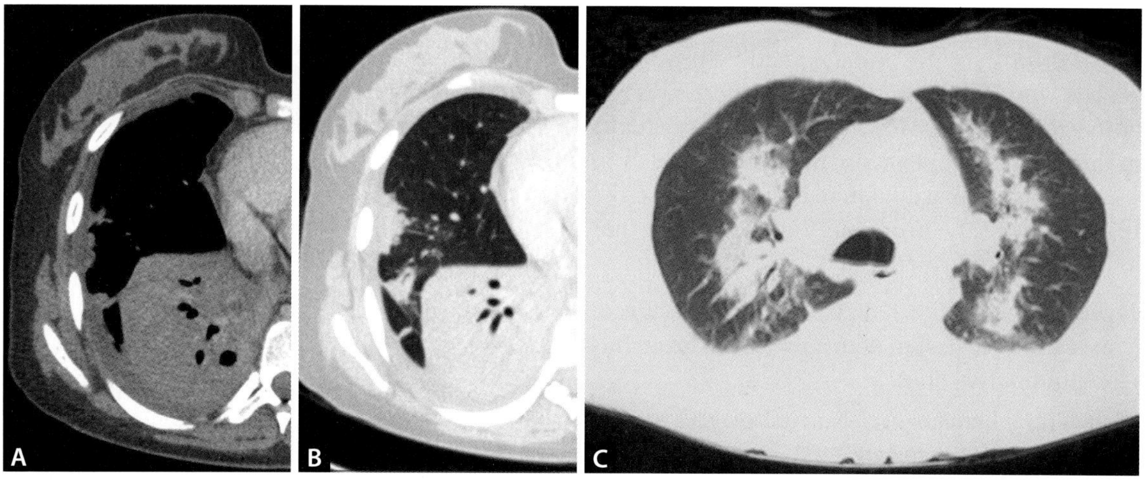

Figs. 23A to C: (A and B) Axial CT shows consolidation with air bronchogram in right lower lobe with subpleural smaller areas of consolidation and mild pleural effusion; (C) CT shows perihilar 'batwing' consolidation in pulmonary edema, with peripheral sparing.

Table 11: Differential diagnosis of consolidation.

Differential diagnosis	***Salient features***
Acute Consolidation	
Pneumonia (bacterial, mycobacterial, fungal, viral)	Patchy, nodular, lobular or diffuse, depending on the organism
AIP, ARDS	Patchy or diffuse
Pulmonary edema	Diffuse, GGO more common
Pulmonary hemorrhage	Patchy or diffuse, GGO more common
Acute eosinophilic pneumonia	Diffuse GGO more common
Radiation pneumonitis	Extent usually corresponds to radiation port
Subacute/Chronic Consolidation	
Organizing pneumonia (OP)	Mostly peripheral, may be mass like or reversed halo in some
Chronic eosinophilic pneumonia	Patchy or nodular, peripheral, resembles OP
Invasive mucinous adenocarcinoma	Diffuse, patchy or nodular
Nonspecific interstitial pneumonia (NSIP)	Patchy, subpleural GGO more common
Hypersensitivity pneumonitis (HP)	Patchy, GGO more common
Lipoid pneumonia	Patchy or lobular, low attenuation consolidation
Lymphoma	Focal, patchy or mass like in peribronchovascular distribution
Sarcoidosis	Patchy or mass like confluence of very small granulomas
Alveolar proteinosis	GGO more common, patchy or diffuse
Pulmonary infarction	Wedge-shaped, pleural-based

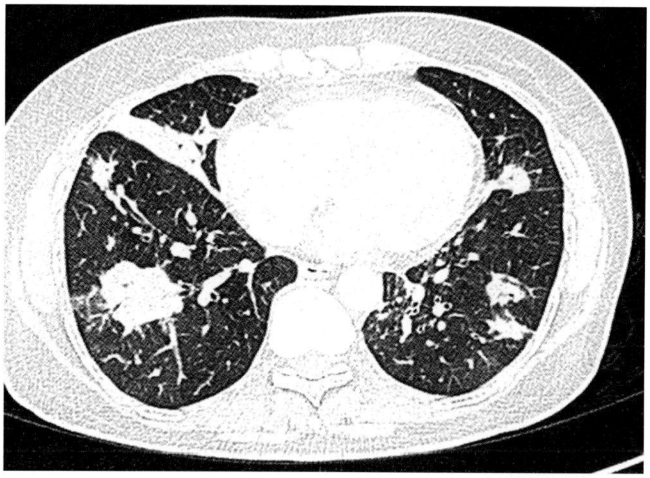

Fig. 24: *Organizing pneumonia*: Axial HRCT shows multiple focal consolidations with air bronchogram in peribronchial regions with surrounding GGO.

HIGH RESOLUTION CT SCAN FINDINGS MANIFESTING AS DECREASED LUNG OPACITY

Area of Decreased Attenuation with Walls

Various abnormalities associated with reduced attenuation in this sub-group include bronchiectasis, honeycombing, lung cysts, cystic lung disease and pneumatocele.

Bronchiectasis

Bronchiectasis is a chronic condition characterised by irreversible dilatation of the bronchi, usually associated with inflammation which occur secondary to bronchial obstruction, bronchial wall damage or parenchymal fibrosis.[18]

High Resolution CT Findings of Bronchiectasis

Bronchial dilatation is the most specific finding of bronchiectasis and is considered when the broncho-arterial ratio exceeds one . However, this may normally be seen in the elderly, people living in high attitude or in asthmatics. When bronchial dilatation is marked, the cross section appearance of the bronchus and artery together appears as a ring and is termed as the "signet ring" sign.

Lack of bronchial tapering: This is the earliest sign of bronchiectasis and is easiest to detect when the bronchus is seen in longitudinal section.

Visualization of peripheral airway: Normal airways are not visualized within 1 cm of the costal pleura. If visualized, then are considered abnormal and indicative of bronchiectasis. Airways may be seen within 1 cm of mediastinal pleura, but should not abut the mediastinal pleura.[3]

Mucoid impaction: Dilated bronchi when filled with fluid or mucous are easily appreciated on HRCT. They appear as gloved finger, V or Y shaped branching densities.

When oriented perpendicular to the scan slice, fluid or mucus filled dilated bronchi are visualized as nodular opacities. CT also demonstrates any atelectasis or hyperinflation distal to the impacted bronchi.

Types of Bronchiectasis

On the basis of morphological appearance on HRCT or pathology, bronchiectasis is classified into three types in increasing order of severity.

a. *Cylindrical or tubular bronchiectasis* is the mildest form which consist of uniformly dilated bronchi with smooth wall thickening **(Fig. 25A)**. They are often associated with chronic airway infections.[19,20]
b. *Varicose bronchiectasis:* In varicose bronchiectasis the bronchial lumen is characterized by alternating area of luminal dilatation and narrowing giving a beaded appearance with irregular or nodular wall thickening **(Fig. 25B)**. This is commonly seen in cystic fibrosis and allergic bronchopulmonary aspergillosis.[19,20]
c. *Cystic bronchiectasis:* Cystic or saccular bronchiectasis is the most severe form of bronchiectasis where the dilated bronchi terminate as a cluster of thin walled air-filled cysts **(Fig. 25C)**.[19] Air fluid levels may be present in the dependent portion of the dilated cystic bronchi. Cystic bronchiectasis often reflects an early childhood infection, is often patchy in distribution, and may be lobar.

More than one type of bronchiectasis may be seen in the same patient.

The radiologist has an important role in the detection and characterization, bronchiectasis and should be able to differentiate bronchiectasis from motion artifact (most commonly from cardiac pulsation in the middle and lingular lobes) and bronchial dilatation in acute lung disease.[19] CT has limited ability to determine the cause of bronchiectasis, but the distribution and pattern of disease can help suggest the most likely cause as given in **Table 12.**[15,21]

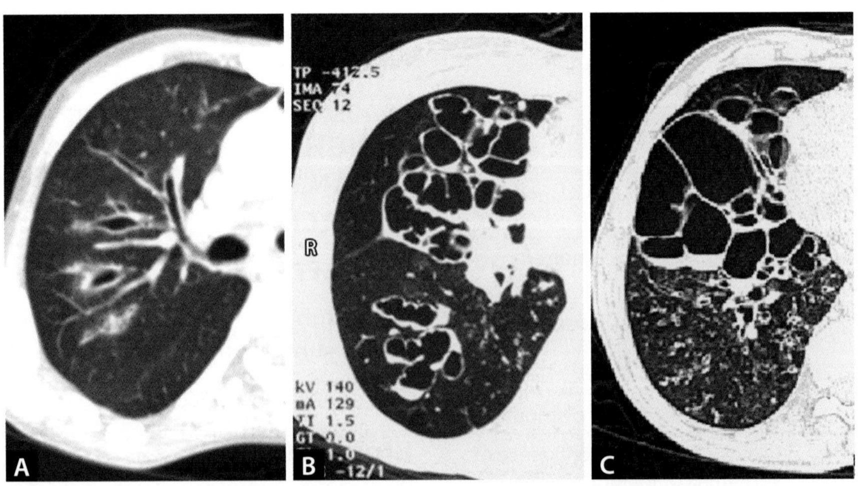

Figs. 25A to C: (A) Axial CT shows cylindrical bronchiectasis with bronchial wall thickening in right upper lobe with mucoid impaction in terminal bronchioles; (B) Varicose bronchiectasis with air-fluid levels in right lung; (C) Cystic bronchiectasis with air fluid levels and mucoid impaction in right lung.

Table 12: Distribution and pattern of bronchiectasis.

Distribution and pattern of bronchiectasis	*Likely etiology*
Bilateral upper lobe bronchiectasis Cystic fibrosis Allergic broncho-pulmonary aspergillosis	Bilateral symmetrical, central, upper lobe predominance Bilateral asymmetrical, central bronchiectasis, cylindrical or varicose type with mucoid impaction
Unilateral upper lobe distrbution	Most common with tuberculosis
Lower lobe distribution	Most common secondary to childhood viral infection
Right middle lobe and lingular distribution	Bronchiectatic form of atypical mycobacterial infection, immotile cilia syndrome, hypogammaglobinemia

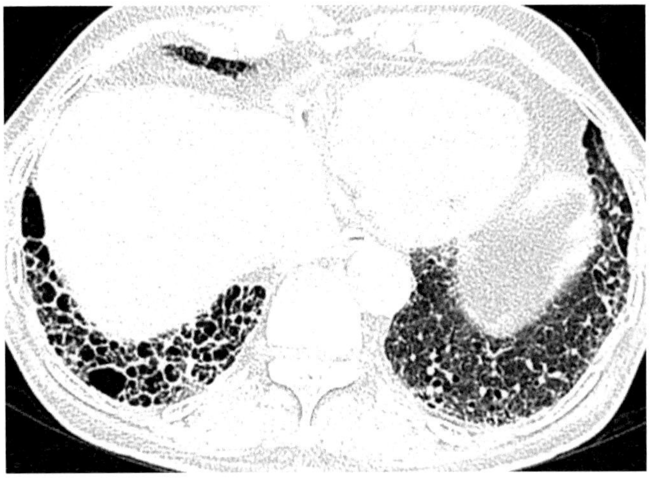

Fig. 26: HRCT image shows honeycomb cysts with predominance in right basal and subpleural region. The cysts are variable sized shows well-defined thick walls and occur in several layers.

Honeycomb Cysts

Honeycomb cysts are characterized by air containing space having thick walls that are lined by bronchiolar epithelium and fibrous walls. Pathologically honeycombing represents interstitial fibrosis with lung destruction and dilatation of peripheral air spaces and is the most specific HRCT sign of fibrosis. In patients with extensive disease (fibrosis), the stacked appearance of cysts resembles a 'honeycomb', hence the term honeycomb cysts.

Honeycombing produces a characteristic appearance on HRCT. Several HRCT findings must be present to make a confident diagnosis of honeycomb cysts, which are:

- Peripheral subpleural location of the cysts
- A layer or cluster of cysts which share walls
- Cysts are of air attenuation and appear lucent as compared to the normal lung parenchyma
- They range in size from few mm to 1 cm
- The cysts have clearly definable fibrous walls of 1–3 mm in thickness. This finding helps in distinguishing honeycombing from paraseptal emphysema or areas of subpleural air trapping **(Fig. 26)**
- The cysts appear as empty black holes with no vessels, bronchi or septations within the cysts
- The cysts of honeycombing do not branch. Branching cystic structures are likely to represent traction bronchiectasis
- Honeycomb cysts are associated with other signs of lung fibrosis such as architectural distortion, traction bronchiectasis, irregular reticulation and volume loss in the same lung region.

Significance of Honeycombing

Honeycombing on HRCT usually represents usual interstitial pneumonia (UIP) with the most common cause being idiopathic pulmonary fibrosis (IPF). The presence of lower lobe, subpleural honeycombing in such patients strongly suggests usual interstitial pneumonia—idiopathic pulmonary fibrosis (IPF) and obviates the need for surgical lung biopsy **(Figs. 27A to C)**.[3] However, number of other diseases show honeycombing on HRCT. **Table 13** gives the differential diagnosis of honeycombing on HRCT.

The honeycombing in these conditions may be indistinguishable on HRCT and require correlation with clinical, exposure or drug history to suggest the appropriate diagnosis.

Pitfalls in Diagnosis of Honeycombing

Paraseptal emphysema by virtue of its subpleural location may resemble honeycombing. But, there are several differentiating features between the two which are tabulated in **Table 14**.

Cystic Lung Disease

Lung disease may be characterized by cystic air spaces or lung cysts. Lung cysts are used to describe clearly defined air containing spaces that is 1 cm or more with a definable epithelial or fibrous usually less than 3 mm thick wall. Although the precise mechanism of cystic change is not understood, a check valve mechanism has been advocated in the pathologies of some cysts.[15] On chest radiography,

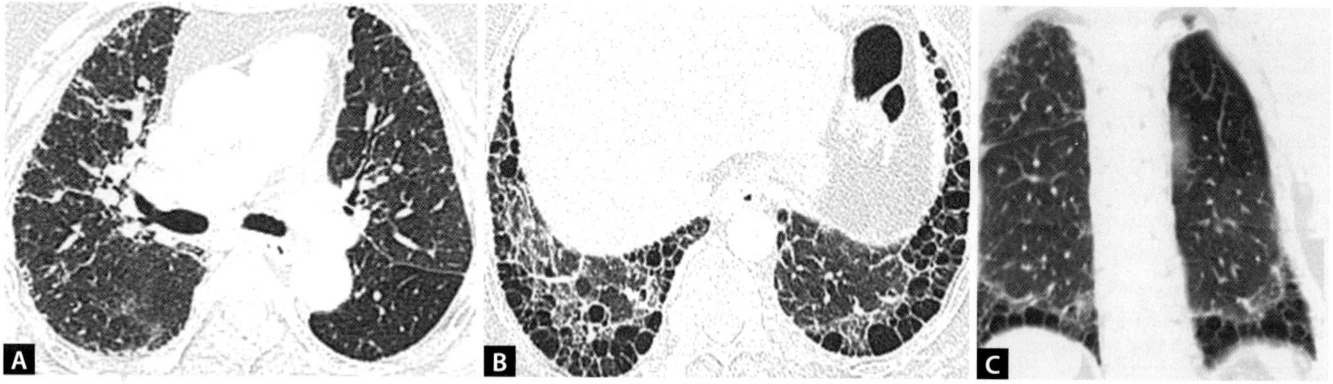

Figs. 27A to C: (A) Axial HRCT at the level of upper lobe bronchus shows mild septal thickening in bilateral lung parenchyma; (B) Axial HRCT through lung bases reveals extensive reticulation and honeycombing with lower lobe and posterior, peripheral predominance; (C) Coronal MPR image reveals an apicobasal gradient of abnormalities typical of UIP pattern.

Table 13: Differential diagnosis of honeycombing.

- Idiopathic pulmonary fibrosis
- Connective tissue disease (rheumatoid arthritis most common)
- Drug-related fibrosis
- Cyclophosphamide (common), nitrofurantoin
- Asbestosis

Table 14: Differentiating features of honeycombing and paraseptal emphysema.

Features	*Honeycombing*	*Paraseptal emphysema*
Layers	Cysts of one or more layer	Single layer only
Wall thickness	Thick walled	Very thin wall
Size	Small (few mm to 1 cm)	Large (up to several cm)
Distribution	Lower lobes	Upper lobes
Associated features	Traction bronchiectasis, irregular reticulation	± centrilobular emphysema
Overall lung volume	Volume loss	Increased

multiple cysts may not be identifiable and result in delicate reticular pattern due to the superimposition of their walls. **Table 15** gives the differential diagnosis of conditions characterized by lung cysts.[6] HRCT is often helpful in suggesting a diagnosis on the basis of their size, wall characteristics and distribution of the cysts.

Langerhans Cell Histiocytosis

It is a multiorgan disease with pulmonary involvement seen mostly in ages between 20 to 40 years in cigarette smokers. The predominant HRCT findings consists of cysts and nodules. The cysts are of irregular or bizarre shape, thin or thick walled may be of unequal sizes and show a predominant upper lung zone distribution with relative sparing of costophrenic sulci **(Fig. 28)**. Serial CT scan shows the natural history of the disease with nodules which cavitate, become cystic air spaces and finally coalesce.[22]

Table 15: Differential diagnosis of lung cysts.

- Langerhans cell histiocytosis (LCH)
- Lymphangioleiomyomatosis (LAM)
- Lymphoid interstitial pneumonia (LIP)
- *P. jirovecii* pneumonia
- Cavitating form of bronchoalveolar carcinoma
- Tracheobronchial papillomatosis
- Birt-Hogg-Dube syndrome
- Sarcoidosis
- Hypersensitivity pneumonitis (subacute)
- Elderly healthy individuals (>75 years)

Lymphangioleiomyomatosis (LAM)

It is a rare multi-organ disease that is almost exclusive to women of child bearing age and characterized by infiltration of airways and lymphatics by immature smooth muscle cells. Patients may present with dyspnea or recurrent pneumothorax. The typical HRCT pattern is of multiple, round, thin walled cysts which are diffusely distributed throughout the lungs, with involvement of the costophrenic sulci, the intervening lung parenchyma appears normal **(Fig. 29)**. Lymphangioleiomyomatosis (LAM) is not associated with nodules but pleural effusions are common.[22]

Lymphoid Interstitial Pneumonia

Lymphoid interstitial pneumonia (LIP) is a part of spectrum of pulmonary lymphoproliferative disorders characterized

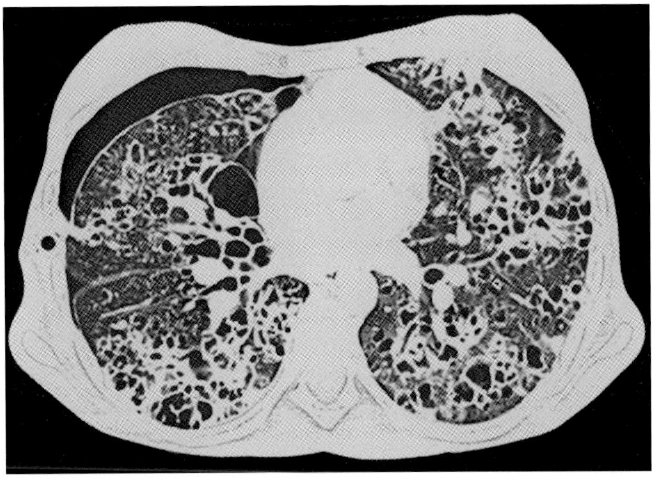

Fig. 28: Axial HRCT shows multiple thick wall cysts of varying sizes in bilateral lung parenchyma. A large thin wall cyst suggestive of bulla is seen along the right mediastinal pleura with associated pneumothorax: Langerhans cells histiocytosis.

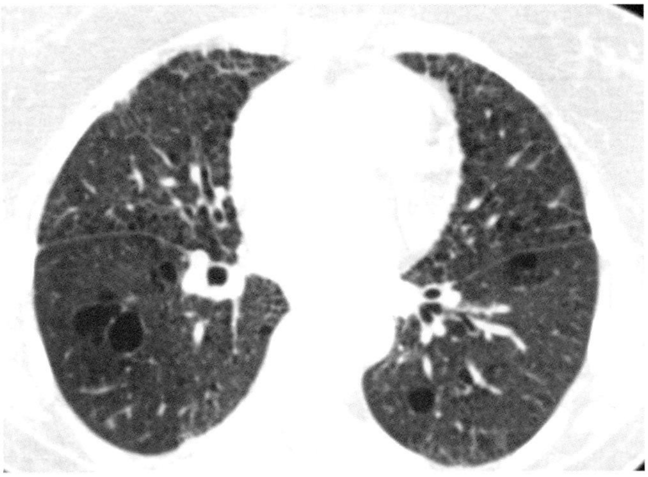

Fig. 29: Axial HRCT in early lymphangioleiomyomatosis shows subtle thin-walled cysts interspersed with normal lung parenchyma predominantly in lower lobes.

on HRCT by diffuse ground-glass opacities and ill-defined centrilobular nodules. Multiple thin walled cysts may be seen in the patients with LIP **(Fig. 30)**. They are usually associated with a history of connective tissue disease, especially Sjögren syndrome and immunosuppression. The cysts are less numerous in number than the cysts occurring in patients with histiocytosis or LAM. In patients with LIP, the cysts are seen mainly in the lower lobes with vessels often associated with wall of cysts.[20]

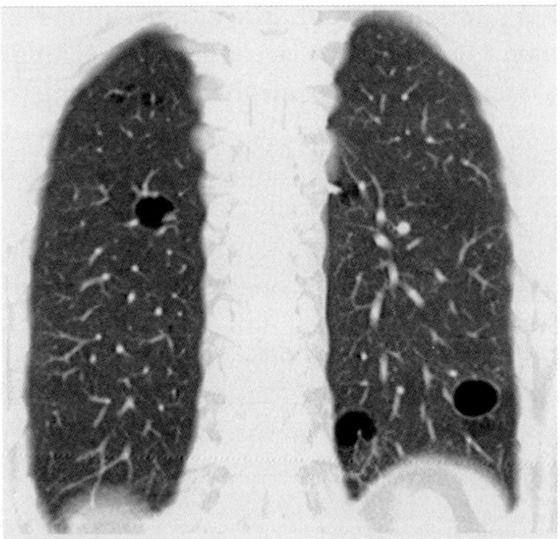

Fig. 30: Coronal MPR showing multiple bilateral thin-walled cysts (LIP) in a 40-year-old female of Sjögren syndrome having dyspnea on exertion.

Incidental Lung Cysts

Randomly scattered thin wall cysts have been seen as a normal finding in 25% of elderly patients older than 75 years on HRCT. The cysts ranging from 5 mm to 22 mm have been seen in all lobes in asymptomatic non-smoking individuals, likely to represent part of the aging process.[22]

DECREASED LUNG OPACITY WITHOUT DISCERNIBLE WALL

Emphysema

Emphysema is the permanent, abnormal enlargement of air spaces distal to the terminal bronchiole and is accompanied by destruction of the walls of the involved air spaces. It is the end result of several different processes such as cigarette smoking, enzyme deficiency and drug abuse. Emphysema result in focal areas of very low attenuation without well-defined walls which can be accurately diagnosed on HRCT.[23]

Emphysema is categorized according to the part of the secondary pulmonary lobule involved into the following types:

- Centrilobular emphysema
- Panlobular emphysema
- Paraseptal emphysema

Table 16 depicts the differences between the three types of emphysema.

Centrilobular emphysema (CLE) seen most commonly in the upper lobes manifests as multiple small areas of low attenuation without a perceptible wall, producing a punched out appearance. A centrilobular artery is often visible within the center of these lucencies **(Fig. 31)**. This appearance is diagnostic of CLE and biopsy is not required for diagnosis if the patient has a smoking history. HRCT is often more sensitive than pulmonary function

Table 16: Comparison of different types of emphysema.

Type of emphysema	***Causes***	***Distribution***	***HRCT appearance***
Centrilobular	Cigarette smoking	Upper lobes, central	Focal lucencies without visible walls
Panlobular	Alpha-1 antitrypsin deficiency, cigarette smoking	Lower lobes, diffuse	Generalized increase in lung lucency
Paraseptal	Cigarette smoking or idiopathic	Subpleural	Focal round, well-defined lucencies in a single layer with thin walls

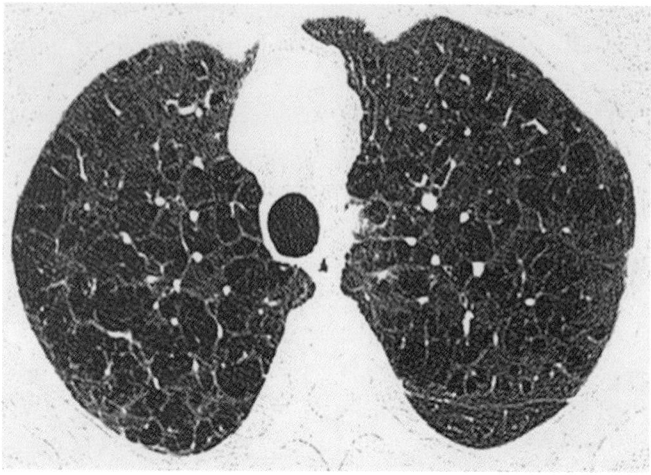

Fig. 31: Axial HRCT shows numerous small low-attenuation areas with ill-defined borders evenly distributed in bilateral upper lobes in centrilobular emphysema.

tests and is able to detect very early stage of centrilobular emphysema.[24]

Panlobular emphysema (PLE) is histopathologically characterized by complete destruction of the secondary pulmonary lobule and shows either diffuse or lobar distribution. On HRCT, it is seen as generalized lung lucency with attenuated small vessels with increased lung volume.[22]

Paraseptal emphysema (PSE) preferentially destroys the distal portion of the pulmonary acinus, hence, findings on HRCT are characteristically peripheral in distribution. On HRCT, paraseptal emphysema typically appears as air attenuation cysts seen in a single layer in the subpleural lung adjacent to the mediastinum and fissure **(Fig. 32)**. The cysts of PSE are outlined by a thin, discrete wall which may correspond to interlobular septa. As they are associated with smoking, they are often seen with centrilobular emphysema.

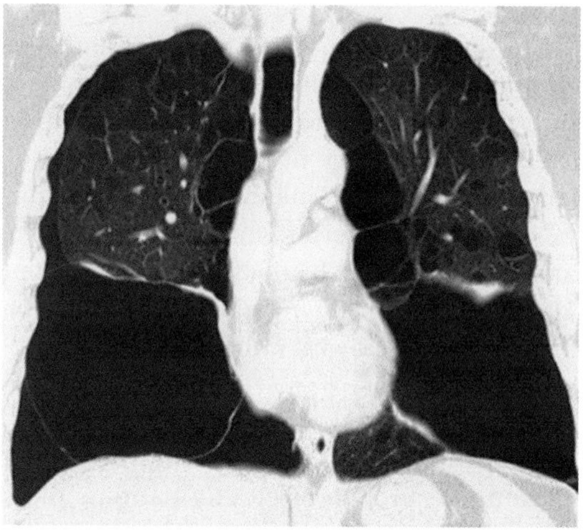

Fig. 32: Coronal MPR CT chest shows single layer of subpleural areas of low attenuation marginated by interlobular septa in bilateral upper zones along mediastinal pleural surface consistent with paraseptal emphysema. Large subpleural bullae in bilateral lower zones and small centriacinar emphysematous spaces are seen in bilateral upper and mid zones. A small pneumothorax is seen along the right lateral chest wall.

Bullous Emphysema

The term is used to refer to emphysema that is associated with large bullae. They occur most commonly in patients of paraseptal and centrilobular emphysema. A bulla is defined as a sharply defined area of emphysema that measures more than 1 cm in diameter. Walls of bulla appear as thin, hair-like on HRCT. **Flowchart 4** gives the algorithmic approach to cystic airspaces.

HRCT Findings Manifesting as Inhomogeneous Lung Opacity

Mosaic Attenuation Pattern

Inhomogeneous lung attenuation or mosaic attenuation pattern is a common finding on HRCT due to a wide range of causes that can involve the airways, pulmonary vasculature, alveoli and interstitium alone or in combination.[25] It is defined as heterogeneous areas of differing lung attenuation with well-defined borders. It is a CT pattern defined by the Fleischner society glossary as a "patchwork of regions of differing attenuation seen on CT of the lung" **(Fig. 33)**.[5] This pattern is a challenge for the radiologist to decide which are abnormal regions of lung, those of low attenuation or those of high attenuation or both. Non-uniform distribution of disease gives a mosaic pattern on imaging. Mosaic pattern of lung attenuation is the preferred terminology than the original terms of mosaic oligemia and perfusion and is caused by three categories of disease:[26]

Flowchart 4: Algorithmic approach to the diagnosis of cystic airspaces.

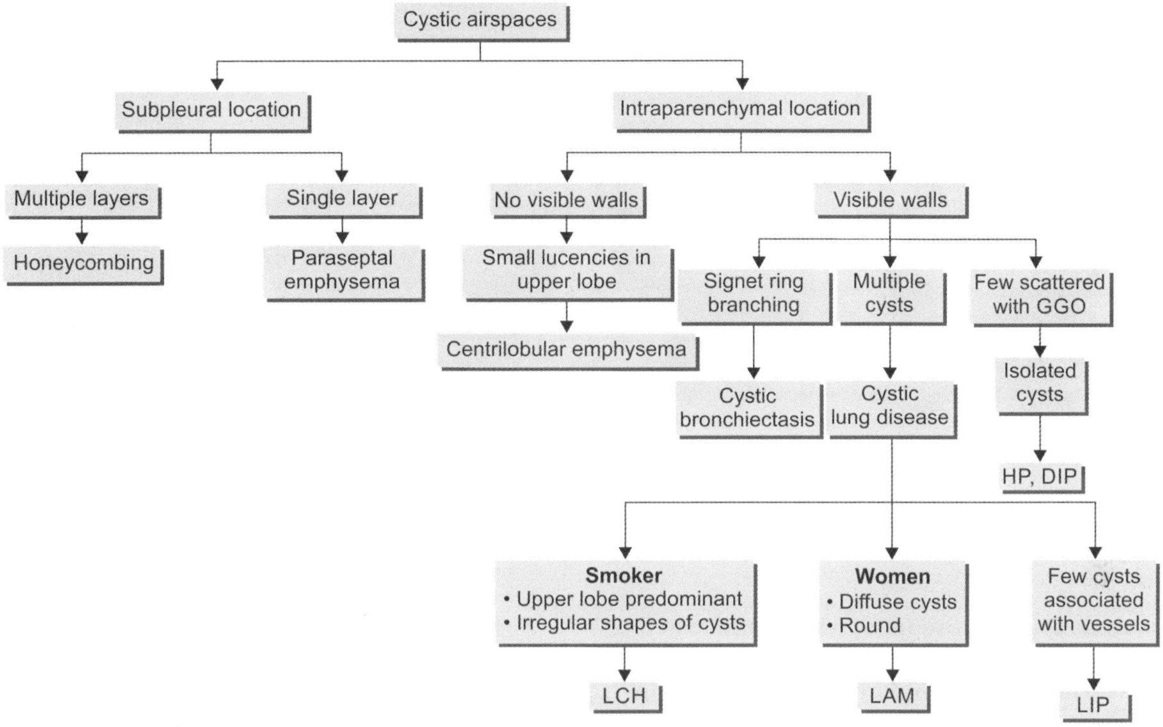

Abbreviations: GGO: Ground-glass opacity; LCH: Langerhans cell histiocytosis; LAM: Lymphangioleiomyomatosis; LIP: Lymphoid interstitial pneumonia.

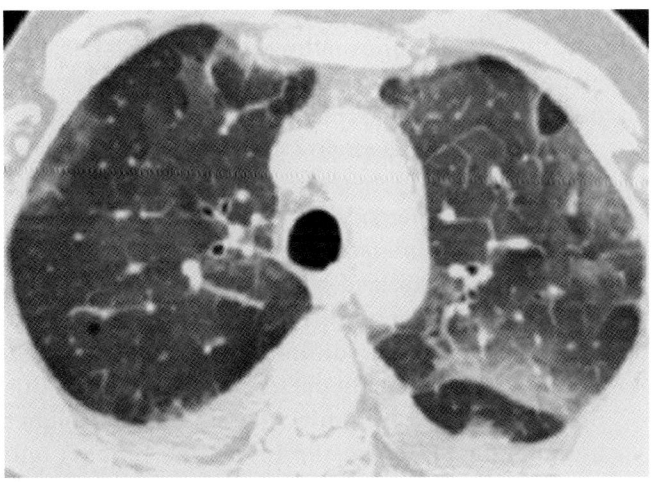

Fig. 33: Axial HRCT chest shows multiple geographic areas of GGO with low-attenuation areas showing reduced caliber of vessels within: Mosaic attenuation pattern.

1. Small airways disease
2. Pulmonary vascular disease
3. Infiltrative lung disease (parenchymal disease).

Small airways disease

Small airways are non-cartilaginous airways less than 2 mm in diameter, located from the eighth generation of airways down to the terminal and respiratory bronchioles. In the normal population, the small airways are not visible, but may be visible due to underlying disease.

Small airways disease can be classified as:

a. Primary bronchiolar disorders which includes:
   - Constrictive bronchiolitis
   - Cellular bronchiolitis
   - Diffuse panbronchiolitis
   - Respiratory bronchiolitis
   - Follicular bronchiolitis.
b. Bronchiolar involvement in diffuse interstitial lung disease, such as hypersensitivity pneumonitis.
c. Bronchiolar involvement in large airway disease, such as bronchiectasis or asthma.

Obstruction of small airways due to small airways inflammation is a common pathologic process and is usually reversible. In contrast; in constrictive bronchiolitis, the submucosal and peribronchiolar fibrosis leads to irreversible obstruction of the small airways **(Figs. 34A and B)**.

Pathophysiology of mosaic attenuation in small airways disease

Airway obstruction in small airways disease leads to hypoxia of underventilated lung resulting in reflux

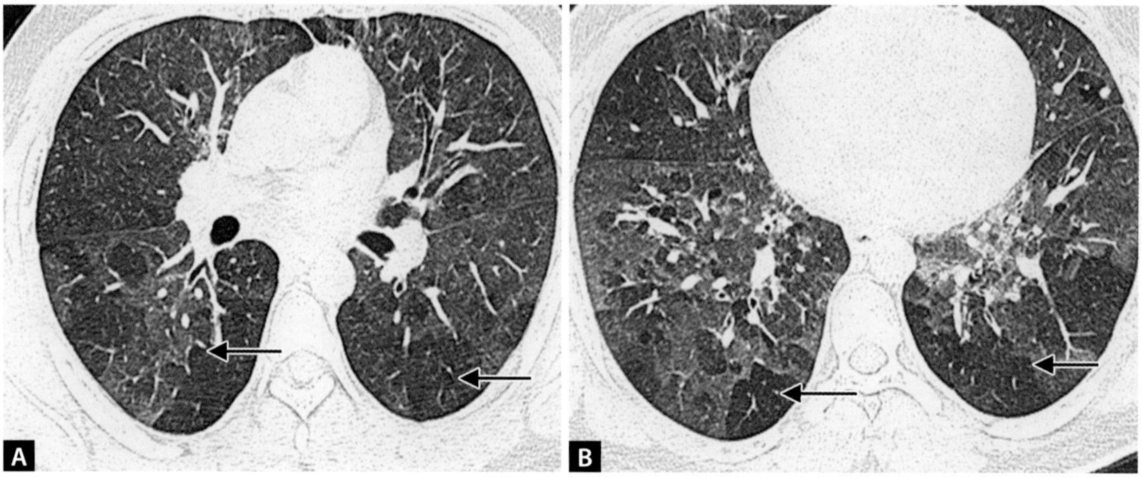

Figs. 34A and B: *Mosaic attenuation*: (A) Axial HRCT inspiratory scan showing patchy areas of mosaic attenuation seen as focal areas of reduced lung density with decreased vessel size within (arrows) along with normal appearing denser lung regions. Corresponding expiratory scan (B) Shows persistent lucency in same areas (arrows in B) confirming air trapping: Constrictive bronchiolitis in a patient of rheumatoid arthritis.

vasoconstriction and air-trapping which is reflected on HRCT as areas of decreased lung attenuation with reduced caliber of vessels as compared to normal lung. There is redistribution of blood flow to the uninvolved areas, which results in increase in attenuation and decrease in volume of the normally ventilated lung.

On CT scan, there are certain direct signs and indirect signs of small airways disease:

- Direct signs—thickened peripheral airways, dilatation of peripheral airways
- Indirect signs—air trapping, subsegmental atelectasis, mosaic lung attenuation, centrilobular nodules and tree in bud opacities.

The radiologist needs to look at the following structures on CT chest to ascertain the underlying cause of mosaic attenuation pattern:

i. *Peripheral vessels:* If these are smaller in the areas of decreased lung attenuation, then, it is either a vascular cause or small airways disease and not parenchymal disease (appearing on HRCT as GGO, reticular or reticulonodular opacities).

ii. *Heart and pulmonary vasculature:* Amongst the pulmonary vascular causes, mosaic attenuation is most commonly seen in pulmonary hypertension and pulmonary thromboembolism. In pulmonary hypertension, enlargement of the pulmonary trunk is suggestive of vascular cause of mosaic attenuation and right ventricular enlargement and hypertrophy seen on CT. In patients with left ventricular and/or left atrial dilatation, pulmonary edema may be the cause of mosaic appearance especially if interlobular septal thickening is present.

In pulmonary hypertension, the mosaic attenuation often manifests as scattered areas of low attenuation confined to the secondary pulmonary lobules **(Figs. 35A and B)**. While in pulmonary thromboembolism, the mosaicism is confined to segmental or subsegmantal distribution in the vascular distribution of thrombi.

iii. *Small airways:* Abnormally dilated or thick-walled airways in the lucent areas confirms small airways disease. In addition, presence of centilobular nodules along with mosaicism on CT is the clue to injury to small airways.

iv. *Parenchymal changes:* Mosaic attenuation pattern can be produced by interstitial lung disease (parenchymal disease) characterized by GGO, interlobular septal thickening. It may be seen in conditions, such as *P. jirovecii* pneumonia, diffuse alveolar hemorrhage, pulmonary edema, hypersensitivity pneumonitis or organizing pneumonia wherein areas of higher attenuation represent the interstitial process and areas of lower attenuation represent the normal lung.

v. *Air trapping:* Air trapping on expiratory HRCT is the best clue to the diagnosis of small airways disease. It refers to the regions of lung which do not show increase in attenuation or show little change in cross sectional area on expiration.

Pitfalls in classification[27]

- Areas of air trapping can be seen in normal patients and some degree of heterogeneity in lung parenchyma is seen on expiratory scan. One should inspect the posterior wall of trachea on CT scan. In case of

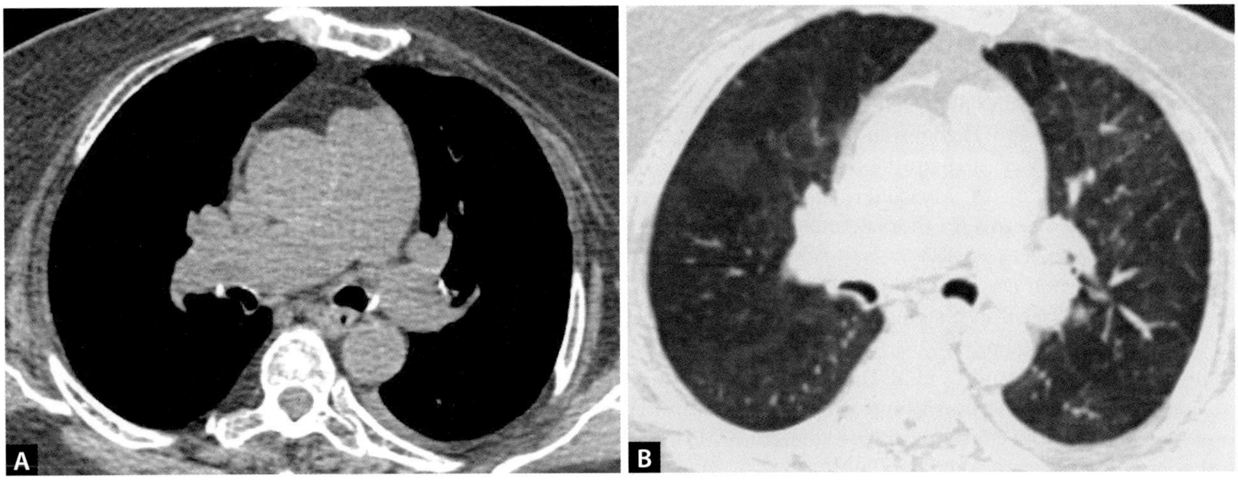

Figs. 35A and B: *CT chest mediastinal window*: (A) reveals dilated main pulmonary artery in patient of pulmonary artery hypertension; (B) lung window image reveals areas of mosaic attenuation in bilateral lung fields.

Flowchart 5: Algorithmic approach to inhomogeneous lung opacity mosaic attenuation pattern.

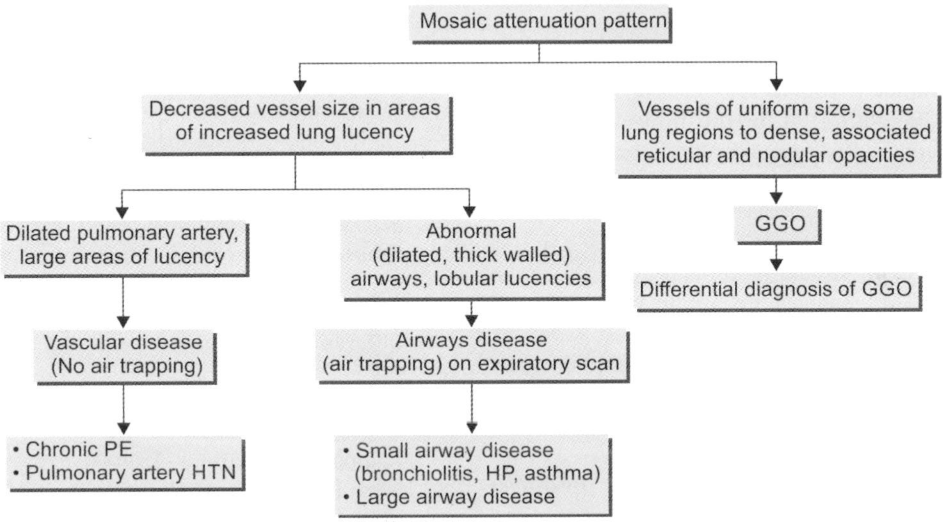

Abbreviations: GGO: Ground-glass opacity; PE: Pulmonary embolism; HTN: Hypertension; HP: Hypersensitivity pneumonitis.

acquisition during expiratory scan, the posterior wall of trachea shows bowing.

- Presence of air trapping excludes primary parenchymal disease unless there is suspicion of HP which has mixed features of both parenchymal and small airway disease.
- Rarely air trapping can occur in pulmonary vascular disease.

Flowchart 5 gives the algorithmic approach to mosaic attenuation pattern.

CONCLUSION

Lung disease can produce recognizable alteration in parenchymal anatomy on CT resulting in various patterns and distributions of abnormalities. However, the various patterns described are not always isolated findings on CT. They commonly occur in combination with other patterns and findings. Use of an organized algorithmic approach in conjunction with clinical data is essential in the evaluation of CT patterns of lung disease so as to formulate a differential diagnosis or reach a specific diagnosis.

REFERENCES

1. Collins J. CT signs and pattern of lung disease. RCNA. 2001;39(6):1115-35.
2. Elicker B, Pereira C, Webb R, et al. High resolution computed tomographic pattern of diffuse interstitial lung disease with clinical and pathological correlation. J Bras Pneumol. 2008;34(9):715-44.

3. Gotway MB, Reddy GP, Webb WR, et al. High-resolution CT of the lung: pattern of disease and differential diagnosis. Radiol Clin N Am. 2005.pp.513-42.
4. Webb RW, Muller NL, Naidich DP. HRCT findings: Nodules and nodular opacities in High resolution CT of the lung, 5th edition, Wolter Kluwer; 2015.pp.106-39.
5. Hansell DM, Bankier AA, McMohan H, et al. Fleischner society-glossary of terms for thoracic imaging. Radiology. 2008;246:697-722.
6. Hansell DM, Lynch DA, McAdams HP, et al. Basic HRCT pattern of lung disease in imaging of diseases of the chest. Mosby Elsevier; 2010.pp.153-204.
7. Remy JH, Remy J, Artaud D, et al. Diffuse infiltrative lung disease: clinical value of sliding. thin slab maximum intensity projection CT scans in the detection of mild micronodular pattern. Radiology. 1996;200:333-9.
8. Elicker BM, Webb RW. Nodular lung disease in fundamentals of high-resolution lung CT: Common findings, common patterns, common diseases, and differential diagnosis, 1st edition, Wolter Kluwer; 2013.pp.37-54.
9. Raoof S, Amchentsev A, Vlahos I, et al. Pictoral Essay: Multinodular disease: a high resolution CT scan diagnostic Algorithm. Chest. 2006;129(3):805-15.
10. Rossi SE, Franquet T, Volpacchio M, et al. Tree-in-bud pattern at thin-section CT of the lungs: radiologic-Pathologic Overview. Radiographics. 2005;25:789-801.
11. Webb RW, Muller NL, Naidich DP. HRCT findings: linear and reticular opacities in high resolution CT of the lung, 5th edition Wolters Kluwer; 2015.pp.74-105.
12. Collins J, Stern EJ. Signs and patterns of lung disease in chest radiology. The Essentials, 3rd Edition, Wolters Kluwer, 2015.pp.17-37.
13. Elicker BM, Webb RW. Reticular opacities in fundamentals of high-resolution lung CT: Common findings, common patterns, common diseases, and differential diagnosis, 1st edition, Wolters Kluwer; 2013. pp.17-36.
14. Webb RW, Muller NL, Naidich DP. HRCT findings: Parenchymal opacification in high resolution CT of the lung, 5th edition Wolter Kluwer. 2015. pp. 140-65.
15. Frauquet T. Non-neoplastic parenchymal lung disease in CT and MRI of the whole body. In: Hagga JR, Dogra VS, Forsting M, Gilkeson RC, Ha HK, Sundaram M (Eds). Volume 1, 5th edition, Mosby, Elsevier; 2009. pp. 863-926.
16. Pawa S. Basic patterns of lung disease in diagnostic radiology with chest and cardiovascular imaging. In: Chowdhury V, Gupta AK, Khandelwal N (Eds). Jaypee Brothers Medical Publishers, 3rd edition; 2010. pp. 28-59.
17. Elicker BM, Webb RW. Increased lung attenuation: Ground-glass opacity and consolidation in fundamentals of high-resolution lung CT: Common findings, common patterns, common diseases and differential diagnosis. 1st edition, Wolters Kluwer; 2013. pp. 59-70.
18. Grenier PA, Aubry CB. Airway disease and chronic airway obstruction in Grainger and Allson's Diagnostic Radiology: A Textbook of Medical Imaging, 6th edition, Churchill Livingstone, Elsevier; 2015. pp. 267-97.
19. Javidan NC, Bhalla S. Bronchiectasis. Radiol Clin N Am. 2009;47:289-306.
20. Webb RW, Muller NL, Naidich DP. HRCT findings: Air filled cystic lesions in high resolution CT of the lung, 5th edition, Wolters Kluwer. 2015.pp.165-86.
21. Cartier Y, Kavanagh PV, Johkoh T, et al. Bronchiectasis: Accuracy of high resolution CT in the differentiation of specific diseases. AJR. 1999;173:47-52.
22. Beddy P, Babar J, Devraj A. A practical approach to cystic lung disease on HRCT insights Imaging. 2011;2(1):1-7.
23. Webb RW, Muller NL, Naidich DP. HRCT findings: Decreased lung attenuation in high resolution CT of the lung. 5th edition, Wolters Kluwer; 2015. pp. 187-205.
24. Elicker BM, Webb RW. Decreased lung attenuation: Emphysema, mosaic perfusion and cystic lung disease in fundamentals of high-resolution lung CT: Common findings, common patterns, common diseases and differential diagnosis, 1st edition, Wolter Kluwer; 2013. pp. 71-82.
25. Kligerman SJ, Henry T, Lin CT, et al. Mosaic attenuation: etiology, methods of differentiation, and pitfalls. Radiographics. 2015;35:1360-80.
26. Stern EJ, Swensen SJ, Hartman TE, et al. CT mosaic pattern of lung attenuation: distinguishing different causes. AJR. 1995;165:813-6.
27. Ridge CA, Bankier AA, Eisenberg RL. Mosaic attenuation. AJR. 2011;197:W970-7.

CHAPTER 160

Imaging of Pulmonary Tuberculosis

Mandeep Garg, Anmol Bhatia, Naveen Kalra

INTRODUCTION

Tuberculosis (TB) is caused by *Mycobacterium tuberculosis*, and is responsible for significant morbidity and mortality, particularly in the countries of developing world.[1] As per the World Health Organization (WHO) data, in 2012 national programs on TB notified around 6.1 million cases of TB, 5.4 million of these being new cases. Of these, 2.5 million were sputum positive, 1.9 million were sputum negative, and 0.8 million were of extrapulmonary TB (EPTB); case type was not known in rest of the cases. India alone accounted for 26% of total cases of TB worldwide in 2012. TB causes significant mortality in Indian population, and kills two people every 3 min, and nearly a thousand persons every day.[2]

The disease course and clinical-radiological presentation is dependent upon and altered by nature of interaction between the mycobacteria and response by the body of the host. Due to variation of immune response of the body in some of the patient population, like immunocompromised and aging population, it is common to see various atypical clinical-radiological presentations. Also, the changing panorama where there tuberculosis can be encountered, as well as the resurgence of the disease around the world, and the changing clinical-radiological spectrum of the disease, justify the persistence of the concern in the radiology community to assess the imaging findings in pulmonary tuberculosis.

TB can affect any organ system, although the lungs are the commonest and often the initial organs to be involved. In the chest, after the lungs TB commonly affects the lymph nodes followed by pleura. The lymph nodes and pleural involvement are included under EPTB.[2]

CHANGING CONCEPTS OF RADIOLOGIC MANIFESTATIONS OF PULMONARY TB

The notion that the "clinical, pathologic, and radiologic findings of reactivation form of TB are quite different from those seen in primary form" has been challenged based on research related to DNA fingerprinting.[3] It has been found that samples from patients who are infected with epidemiologically different strains of TB have different restriction fragment length polymorphism (RFLP) patterns, while patients infected with epidemiologically similar strains have similar RFLP patterns. Therefore, the cases in which the samples have similar or related genotypes have usually been recently transmitted. Vis-à-vis, cases in which the isolates have different genotypes represent reactivation form of TB.[4]

A preliminary study on DNA fingerprinting showed that the radiologic findings are usually similar in patients having a primary or postprimary TB.[5] Therefore, period from contracting the infection to clinically obvious disease will not reliably predict the radiologic findings. The immune response of the patient is the sole forecaster of radiologic findings; with severely immunocompromized patients showing features of primary form, whereas immunocompetent patients showing propensity for the reactivation form of TB.[5]

ROLE OF IMAGING IN PULMONARY TUBERCULOSIS

- Making a diagnosis.
- Evaluating the treatment response and residual disease activity.
- Detecting the complications and sequelae.

RADIOLOGICAL PATTERNS OF PULMONARY TB

Radiological patterns may be considered under the following groups:

- Typical radiological patterns of primary TB.
- Postprimary TB or phtysis.
- Patterns encountered both in primary and/or post primary forms.
- Complications and sequelae of TB.
- Atypical patterns.

Typical Radiological Patterns of Primary TB

Four entities are known to occur in primary pulmonary TB: gangliopulmonary pattern; miliary pattern; tuberculous pleuritis; and involvement of tracheobronchial airway. The gangliopulmonary TB is seen only in primary TB while others are seen in both primary and postprimary TB. Gangliopulmonary form is characterized by the presence of enlarged lymph nodes in mediastinum and/or hila, with relatively less involvement of parenchyma (Ghon focus). This form preferentially occurs in children, and hence is known as "childhood-type TB". In areas where there is a low incidence of the disease, except for nonindigenous pediatric population, it has a high incidence of occurence in adults and older age groups.[6] Right paratracheal and hilar lymph nodes are the most commonly enlarged nodes seen in primary TB, although involvement of various other nodal stations in different combinations can be seen. The prevalence of lymph nodal enlargement decreases with increasing age.[7] On CECT, tuberculous nodes that are greater than 2 cm show central areas of low attenuation suggestive of caseous necrosis and peripheral rim enhancement **(Figs. 1A and B)**. In approximately two-thirds cases of primary TB in pediatric population, parenchymal lesions are encountered on the ipsilateral side of enlarged lymph nodes.[7] Lesions in parenchyma are typically located in the peripheral lung fields involving the subpleural locations.

The gangliopulmonary form of TB is usually self-limiting, with immunocompetent individuals usually remaining asymptomatic. Sometimes, the lone radiological finding is Ranke complex which includes both the parenchymal lesion (Ghon focus) and affected lymph nodes **(Fig. 2)**. The course in Gangliopulmonary form may be complicated in form of lymph node perforating in the bronchus, retro-obstructive pneumonia, and/or atelectasis (known as epituberculosis). Retro-obstructive pneumonia may evolve into a fibrotic lesion which may or may not be calcified. Destruction of the parenchyma of the lung result in fibrosis associated with traction bronchiectasis. In adults, the primary infection mostly causes parenchymal consolidation without lymphadenopathy **(Fig. 3)**. Cavitatory form is rarely encountered in children.

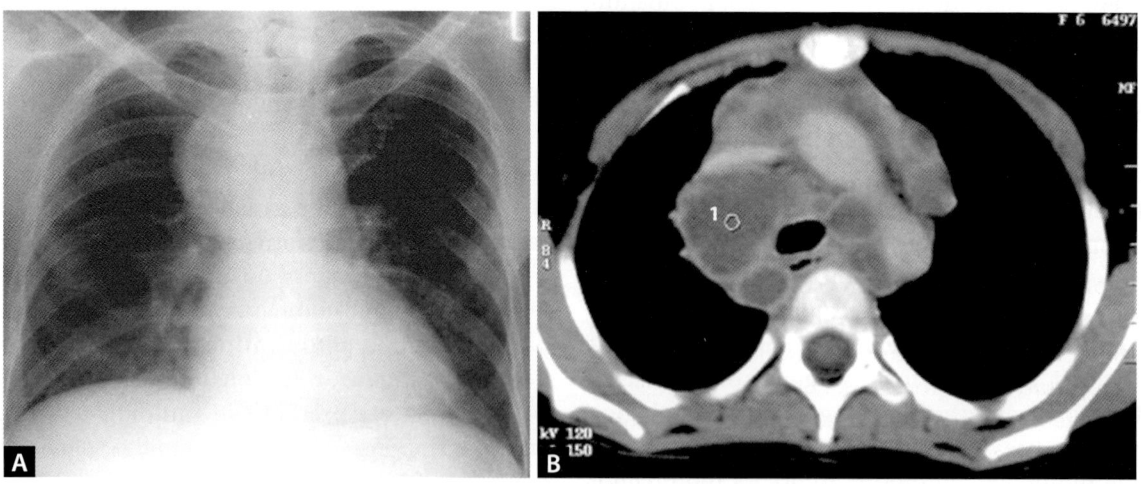

Figs. 1A and B: *Tuberculous mediastinal lymphadenopathy*: (A) Chest radiograph shows right paratracheal lymphadenopathy; (B) CECT reveals low density center with peripheral rim enhancement of the node. Similar but smaller nodes are also seen in the posterior mediastinum.

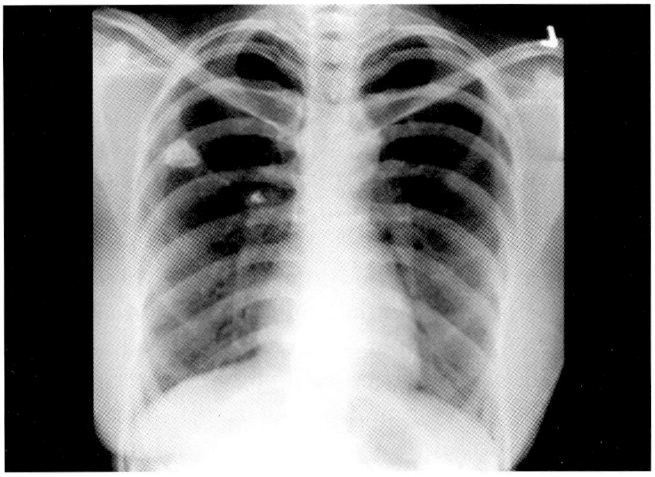

Fig. 2: *Ranke complex*: Chest radiograph shows a calcified lesion in the right upper zone along with calcification of the right hilar node and of the intervening lymphatic channel.

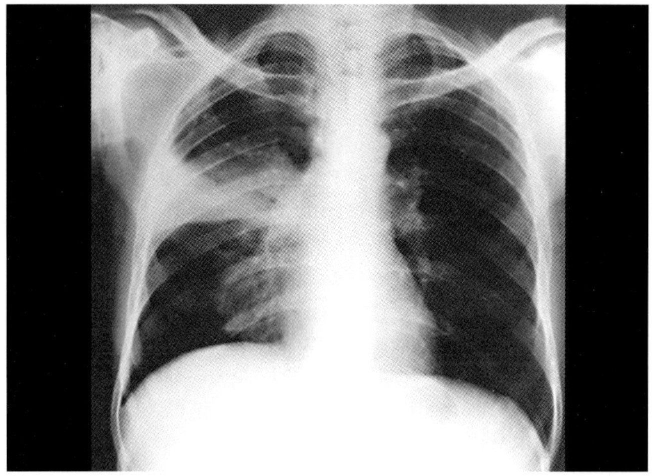

Fig. 3: Primary tuberculosis in a 40-year-old male. Chest radiograph shows multilobar consolidation of the right lung affecting the upper and lower lobes without lymphadenopathy.

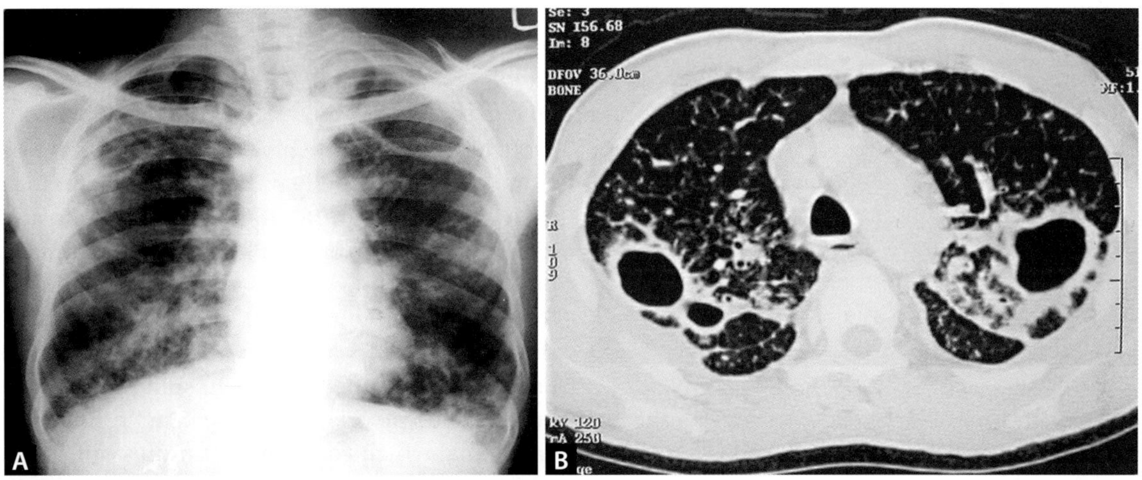

Figs. 4A and B: *Post primary tuberculosis*: (A) Chest radiograph shows cavitatory lesions in both the upper lobes and multiple ill-defined nodular opacities in both the lung fields; (B) HRCT section in the region of the upper lobes shows bilateral thick-walled cavities with surrounding consolidation.

Postprimary TB or Phtysis

This form evolves and progresses depending upon the status of acquired immunity, due to reactivation of residual dormant infective focus. It is mostly, but not always, a disease affecting adult population.[8] In pediatric population, it mostly occurs in adolescent children, particularly in girls at menarche.[7] This form of TB is characterized by caseous necrosis undergoing liquefaction, progressive lung destruction associated with fibrosis and formation of cavities. The lesions are typically located in the upper lobes (apicoposterior segments) and with a relative less degree of involvement of the lower lobes (superior segments). The areas of caseous necrosis undergoing liquefaction later on communicate with the adjacent airways resulting in formation of cavities **(Figs. 4A and B)**. The findings include parenchymal infiltrates in apicoposterior locations, cavities, pleural effusion, fibrotic areas causing lung parenchyma destruction, pulling up of hila/fissures, traction bronchiectasis, and pleural adhesions.[9] Cavitation may be seen in 40% cases in postprimary form radiographically. There may be thin and smooth walls as well as thick and nodular walls of the cavities. Air-fluid levels can be seen in 10% of cases with cavities,[10] which may because of superimposed infection by bacteria or fungus. Bronchogenic spread is characterized by multiple, ill-defined nodules, having a lobar/ segmental distribution, typically involving lower lung zones.[11] HRCT typically shows 2- to 4-mm sized nodules which are centrilobular in distribution presenting as sharply marginated branching structures within and around terminal and respiratory bronchioles giving "tree-in-bud" appearance **(Fig. 5)**.[12] Cicatrization atelectasis is a common finding following postprimary TB which presents as atelectatic changes in the upper lobe, retracted hilum, lower lobe compensatory hyperinflation, and ipsilateral tracheomediastinal shift. This may also be associated with pleural thickening in the apices along with fibrosis, proliferation of extrapleural soft tissues and subpleural atelectatic changes on CT.[13]

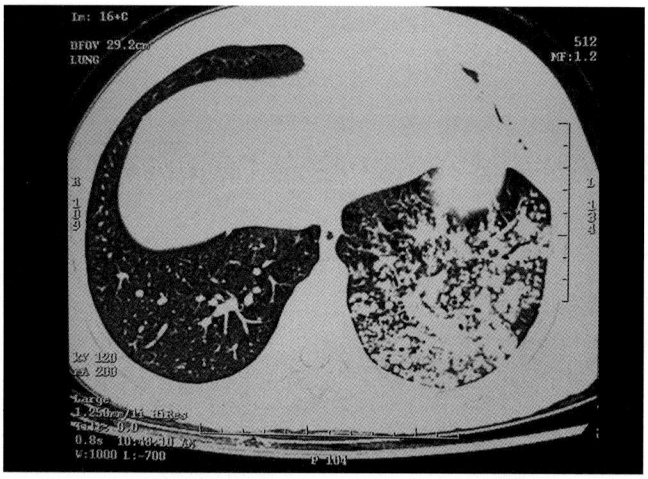

Fig. 5: Endobronchial spread depicted on HRCT. There is presence of extensive bronchiolar and alveolar ductal lesions with a typical 'tree-in-bud appearance' (arrow) in the right lower lobe.

Radiological Patterns Seen in Both Primary and/or Postprimary TB

Miliary TB

Miliary TB results from the hematogenous spread of the infection in lungs and other organs, resulting in innumerable tiny granulomas. Initially, skiagrams may be normal in up to 25–40% of patients.[14] CT helps in demonstration of the miliary nodules before they become perceptible on radiographs **(Figs. 6A and B)**. It shows a combination of both sharply as well as poorly defined, diffusely distributed 1- to 4-mm nodules in a random fashion commonly associated with thickening of the interstitium (both interlobular and intralobular septae).[15] A typical "snowstorm" appearance on Chest X-ray suggesting an evolution to adult respiratory distress syndrome has also been reported.[16] The second most common finding on HRCT in cases of miliary tuberculosis includes ground-glass opacities which represent small granulomas below the resolution of HRCT superimposed on exudative changes of the lung.[17]

Exudative Pleuritis

Pleural cavity may be involved from a caseating granuloma in parenchyma adjacent to pleural, or through hematogenous route. It is usually seen along with parenchymal and/or lymphadenopathy. It may however be seen sometimes in as the only radiologic finding 5% of adult patients suggesting primary TB.[18] CECT in shows smooth thickening with enhancement of parietal and visceral pleura resulting in split-pleura sign **(Fig. 7)**. Tuberculous pleurisy when localized results tuberculous empyema, which sometimes ruptures outside forming a

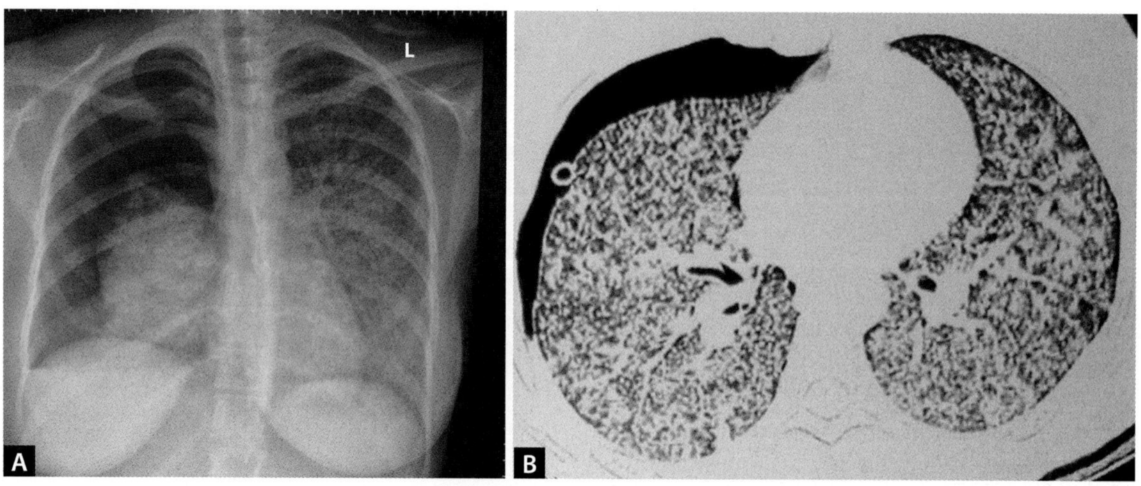

Figs. 6A and B: *Miliary tuberculosis*: (A) Chest radiograph shows diffuse fine micronodular opacities in both lungs. (B) HRCT demonstrates peribronchiolar and perivascular nodules with airspace consolidation in the superior segment of left lower lobe.

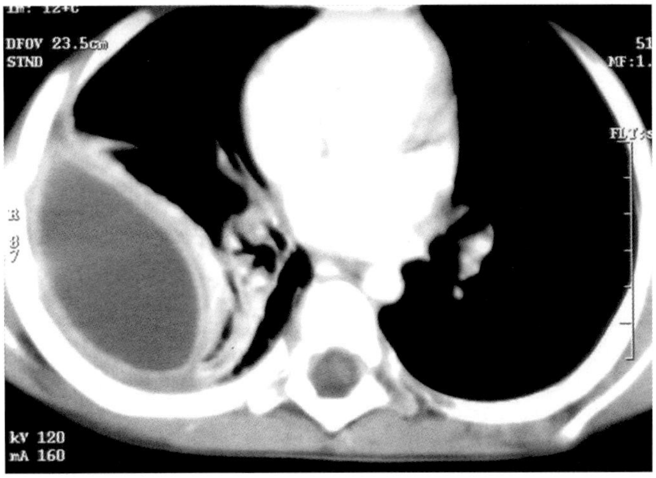

Fig. 7: *Empyema*: CECT chest depicting right pleural effusion with enhancing visceral and parietal pleura giving split-pleura sign.

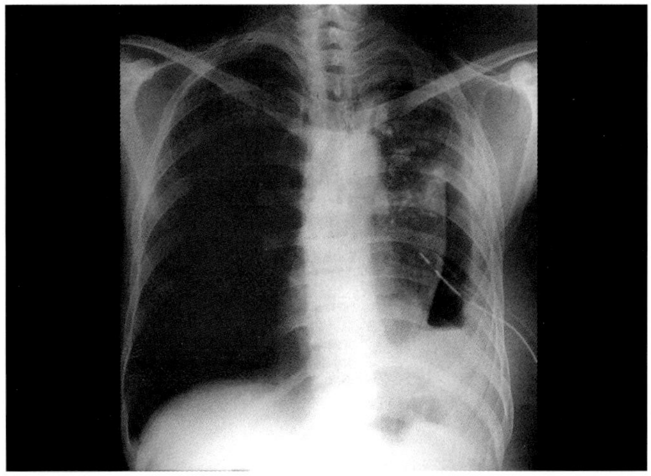

Fig. 8: Bronchopleural fistula in a patient with non-resolving hydropneumothorax on intercostals tube drainage. Chest radiograph shows left pleural effusion with an air-fluid level and partial atlectasis of the left lung.

subcutaneous abscess, called as empyema necessitans. Diffuse pleural thickening without any effusion suggests fibrothorax, and indicates disease inactivity. Pleural collection when communicates with the bronchial tree results in development of bronchopleural fistula and an air fluid level within **(Fig. 8)**. Diagnosis of bronchopleural fistula is suggested clinically by copious amount of sputum production by the patient, and radiologically by appearance of hydro-pneumothorax with changing air-fluid level as well as involvement of contralateral side. CT may demonstrate the communication between the collection in pleural cavity and bronchi or lung parenchyma.[19]

Tracheobronchial TB

Tracheobronchial TB is known to occur in 2–4% of patients of pulmonary TB.[20] It usually results from a perforation of enlarged lymph nodes into a bronchus,[21,22] although it may also result from lymphatic and hematogenous dissemination. The ulcerogranulomatous lesions in the involved submucosa; and granulomatous polypoidal growths are seen which result in fibrotic stenoses after healing, and later on postobstructive bronchiectasis **(Fig. 9)**. The acute form of tracheobronchial TB manifests as smooth or irregular thickening of the walls resulting in circumferential bronchial narrowing.[23] Encasement by the enlarged enhancing mediastinal nodes is also commonly seen in the active stage. Cicatricial bronchostenosis may occur lately following the healing of the focal infection involving the walls of bronchi. Chronic fibrotic stage shows circumferential symmetric thickening of the wall resulting in concentric narrowing of the bronchus.[24]

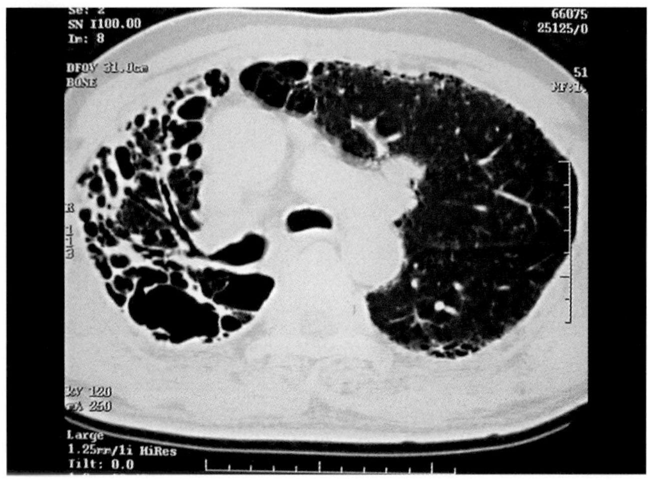

Fig. 9: *Bronchiectasis*: HRCT shows traction bronchiectasis in the right upper lobe.

Tuberculoma

Tuberculomas are usually the sequelae of healed form of primary TB, but can be seen in 3–6% of patients of postprimary tuberculosis as the only or the main finding.[25] These can be multiple or solitary, varying in size from 0.4 to 5 cm **(Figs. 10A and B)**. The possible pathogenesis resulting in tuberculoma formation include roundening of a contracted healing tubercular lesion, or a healed filled-in cavity.[25] Most of the tuberculomas remain static in size. Calcification is seen to occur in 20–30% cases in a diffuse or a nodular fashion.[26]

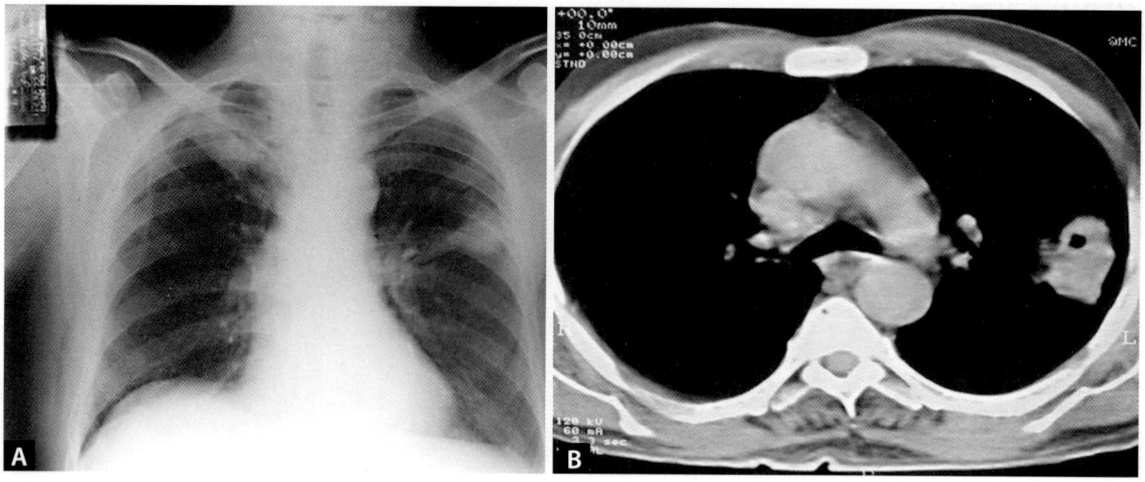

Figs. 10A and B: *Tuberculoma*: (A) Chest radiograph shows a pulmonary nodule in the left middle zone; (B) CECT of the chest shows eccentric cavitation of the nodule. CT-guided aspiration revealed caseous material positive for *Mycobacterium tuberculosis*.

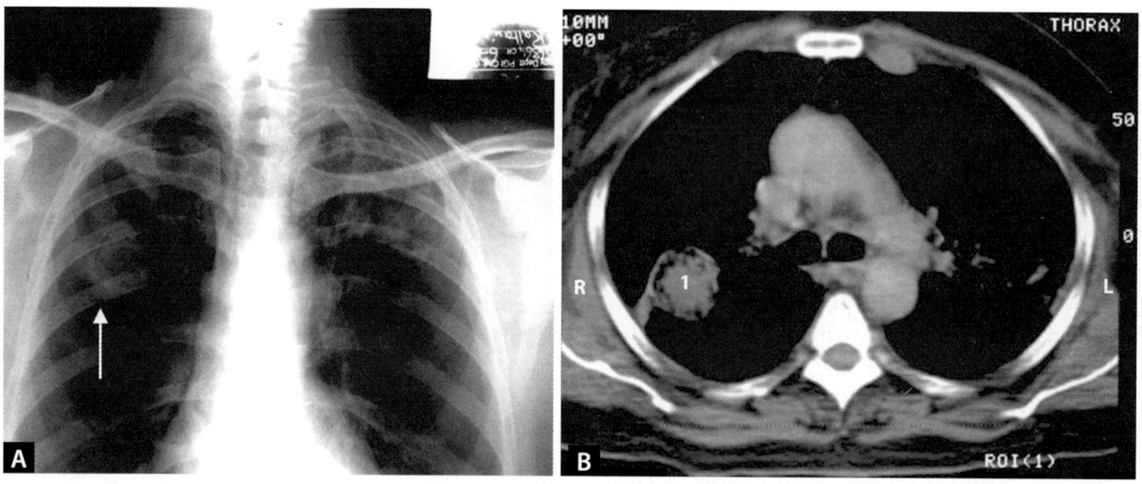

Figs. 11A and B: *Mycetoma in a cavity*: (A) Chest radiograph shows a cavity in the right upper lobe with a nodular lesion inside (arrow); (B) CECT of chest showing soft tissue filling the cavity with an air crescent anteriorly.

Complications and Sequelae of Pulmonary TB

A tuberculous cavity can be invaded by *Aspergillus* species resulting in an "aspergilloma" which consists of a bunch of entangled hyphae knotted together with cellular fragments and mucus. Thickening of the walls of the cavity or of the adjacent pleural lining are early radiographic findings seen suggesting the invasion of tubercular cavity. Radiographs show a nodular radioopacity or a mass which is separated from the adjacent wall by a crescent-shaped area of radiolucency or air **(Figs. 11A and B)**.[27]

Tuberculosis may predispose to the malignancy by local mechanism which is known as scar cancer, or there may be co-existence of TB and carcinoma. Malignancy may also cause tubercular reactivation, both by compromising the patient's immunity, and by erosion into an encapsulated focus. Hence, any predominant or an enlarging nodule on follow up imaging should raise a suspicion for coexisting carcinoma in tuberculosis patients.[28]

In the areas of active foci, pulmonary arteries and veins may demonstrate findings of vasculitis and/or thrombosis. There may be increased tortuousity of the bronchial arteries which commonly are hypertrophied in patients having bronchiectasis associated with TB or may be in parenchymal TB only **(Figs. 12A and B)**. Rasmussen aneurysm results when a tubercular cavity erodes the branch of pulmonary artery in the surrounding parenchyma **(Figs. 13)**.[29]

Broncholithiasis is an uncommon complication, and is a result of erosion of a calcified node in peribronchial location into the adjacent bronchus. CT shows a lymph node

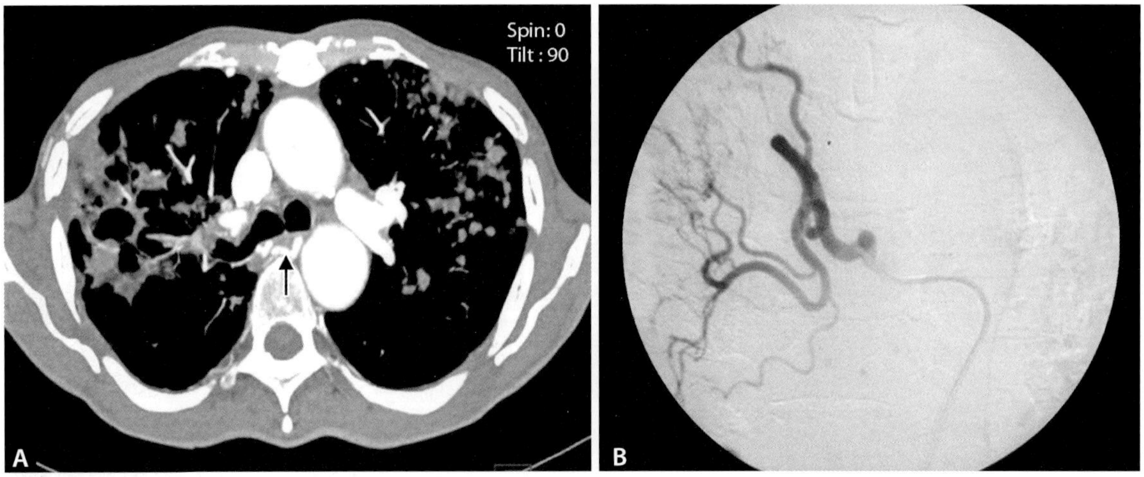

Figs. 12A and B: A 62-year-old man with pulmonary TB having massive hemoptysis. (A) Axial CECT image shows ostium of the enlarged right bronchial artery (arrow). Bilateral consolidation and multiple nodules are seen in both lungs. (B) Selective right bronchial angiogram shows enlarged and tortuous right bronchial artery.

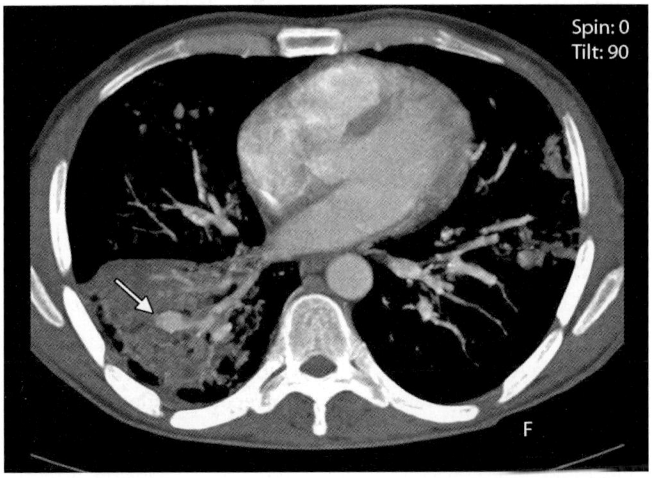

Fig. 13: *Rasmussen aneurysm*: Axial 10 mm MIP image in a patient with massive hemoptysis showing pseudoaneurysm arising from the branch of right pulmonary artery (arrow).

in endobronchial or peribronchial location which causes bronchial obstruction resulting in focal hyperinflation, atelectasis, obstructive pneumonitis, bronchiectasis, and branching opacities (obstructive bronchoceles).[30]

Esophageal involvement by TB from adjacent lymph nodes result in formation of strictures, fistulae between esophagus and mediastinum or airway, and traction diverticulae.[31]

Tuberculous pericarditis is seen to occur in 1% of cases of TB. It may result from the direct invasion of enlarged lymph nodes into the pericardium or by miliary spread of the infection. Pericardial thickening (with or without effusion) along with enlarged lymph nodes is seen on CT. Constrictive pericarditis characterized by fibrous or calcified pericardial thickening measuring >3 mm is seen as a delayed complication 10% of patients of tuberculous pericarditis **(Figs. 14A and B)**.[25]

Pneumothorax is seen in around 5% of cases of postprimary form, usually in severe cavitatory form of disease. It indicates severe and widespread lung involvement, and the inception of empyema and bronchopleural fistula.

Fibrosing mediastinitis in TB is an unusual complication which progresses slowly without obvious clinical symptoms. The findings on CT in fibrosing mediastinitis include a hilar or a mediastinal mass showing coarse calcification, narrowing of tracheobronchial tree, encasement of pulmonary and other mediastinal vasculature, sometimes presenting as a superior vena cava syndrome.[32]

Atypical Patterns

These are usually encountered in elderly and immunocompromised patients. Various factors which may alter the pathogenesis of the atypical patterns include:

- Deficient cellular immunity resulting in reactivation of TB (typical pattern)
- Reinfection or second primary infection can happen[33]
- Elderly subjects getting contracted by the disease for the first time.

A shift from the usual trail (reactivation) to an unusual trail is seen in cases where there is an exogenic reinfection or a second primary infection, thereby the presentation similar to what occurs in pediatric population.[34,35] These atypical radiographic findings like anterioinfiltrates, lymphadenopathy and exudative pleuritis can result in wrong initial diagnosis and thus delayed treatment.

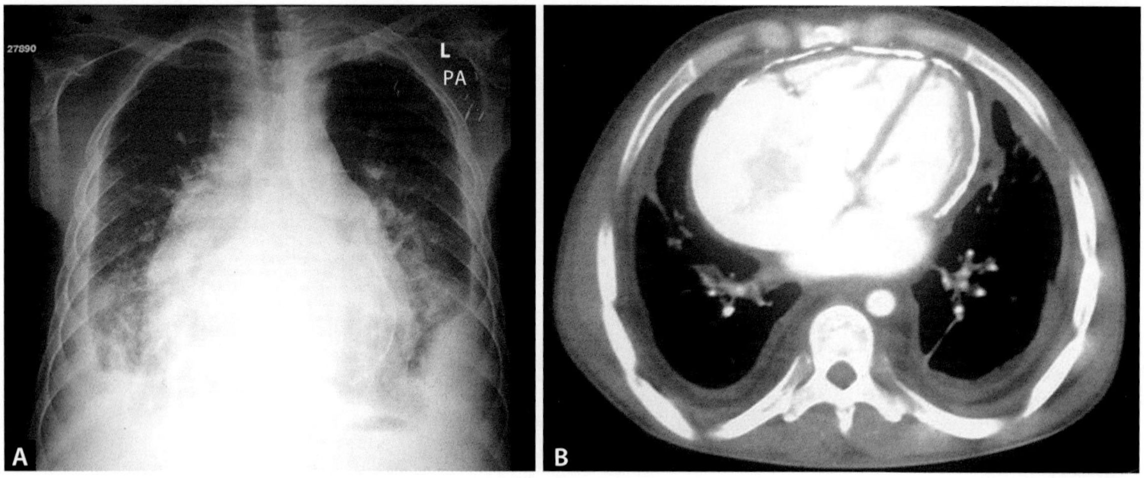

Figs. 14A and B: *Tuberculous pericarditis*: (A) Chest radiograph depicting curvilinear pericardial calcification over left heart border. (B) Axial CECT section showing thickened and calcified pericardium. Also noted is bilateral pleural effusion.

MRI in Pulmonary Tuberculosis

Several recent technical advances have helped MRI to overcome its main limitations (low proton density and low SNR) for characterization of pulmonary pathologies. MRI as a radiation free modality can be used for follow-up of the already known lesions in young patients to reduce radiation exposure.[36-38] MRI has been shown equivalent to CT for detection of lymph nodes, lung cavitation and pleural effusion having a sensitivity and specificity of 100%. Sensitivity and specificity of MRI has been shown to be up to 88.2% and 95.7% respectively for the detection of nodules in pulmonary tuberculosis, while a specificity of 92.9% and sensitivity of 100% for detection of consolidation.[39] However, high cost and limited availability are its main limitations.

PET/CT in Tuberculosis

PET/CT has a high sensitivity in detecting malignancies, infections and various inflammatory lesions. Hence, it has a potential role to play in the diagnostic algorithm and managing the patients of PUO.[40,41] However, due to high incidence of TB in Indian population, large number of false positive cases are commonly seen in patients on PET/CT during oncologic work-up. Hence, although PET/CT may not be very specific in tuberculosis, it can have a crucial role in assessment of suspected or known cases of TB. One approach which can increase the diagnostic accuracy for detection of TB involves use of combine F-18 FDG and C-11 acetate in combination. Amongst these two, C-11 acetate is taken up by malignant lesions but not by infective/inflammatory lesions.[42] FDG PET/CT can help in determining the activity in the lesions, thereby guiding for sampling from foci showing activity, detect occult foci at other places, as well as evaluate the response to treatment. Furthermore, new, radiotracers with more specificity, like antituberculous drug molecules labeled with positron-emitters may help in differentiating TB from malignancies and other infective/ inflammatory processes.

REFERENCES

1. Harkirat S, Anand SS, Indrajit IK, et al. Pictorial essay: PET/CT in tuberculosis. Indian J Radiol Imaging. 2009:18;141-7.
2. Bhalla AS, Goyal A, Guleria R, Gupta AK. Chest tuberculosis: Radiological review and imaging recommendations. Indian J Radiol Imaging. 2015;25:213-25.
3. Jeong YJ, Lee KS. Pulmonary tuberculosis: Up-to-date imaging and management. AJR. 2008;191:834-44.
4. Alland D, Kalkut GE, Moss AR, et al. Transmission of tuberculosis in New York City: An analysis by DNA fingerprinting and conventional epidemiologic methods. N Engl J Med. 1994; 330:1710-6.
5. Geng E, Kreiswirth B, Burzynski J, et al. Clinical and radiographic correlates of primary and reactivation tuberculosis: a molecular epide miology study. JAMA. 2005;293:2740-5.
6. Gyselen A, Uydebroeck M, Weyler J Epidemiologie. In: Demedts M, Gyselen A, Van den Brande P (Eds). Tuberculosis. Een blijvende uitdaging. Garant, Leuven-Apeldoorn. 1992; pp 17–30.
7. Leung AN, Muller NL, Pineda PR, et al. Primary tuberculosis in childhood: radiographic manifestations. Radiology. 1992;182:87-91.
8. Lamont AC, Cremin BJ, Pelteret RM. Radiologic patterns of pulmonary tuberculosis in the paediatric age group. Paediatr Radiol. 1986;16:2-7.

9. Palmer PE. Pulmonary tuberculosis: usual and unusual radiographic presentations. Semin Roentgenol. 1979;14:204-42.
10. Woodring JH, Vandiviere HM, Fried AM, et al. Update: radiographic features of pulmonary tuberculosis. Am J Roentgenol. 1986;146:497-506.
11. Hadlock FP, Park SK, Awe RJ, et al. Unusual radiographic findings in adult pulmonary tuberculosis. Am J Roentgenol. 1980:134:1015-8.
12. Im JG, Itoh H, Shim YS, et al. Pulmonary tuberculosis: CT findings—early active disease and sequential change with antituberculous therapy. Radiology. 1993;186:653-60.
13. Im JG, Webb WR, Han MC, et al:. Apical opacity associated with pulmonary tuberculosis: high-resolution CT findings. Radiology. 1991;178:727-31.
14. Kwong JS, Carignan S, Kang EY, et al. Miliary tuberculosis: diagnostic accuracy of chest radiography. Chest. 1996;110: 339-42.
15. Leung AN. Pulmonary tuberculosis: the essentials. Radiology. 1999;210:307-22.
16. Piqueras AR, Marruecos L, Artigas A, et al. Miliary tuberculosis and adult respiratory distress syndrome. Intensive Care Med. 1987;13:175-82.
17. Hong SH, Im JG, Lee JS, et al. High resolution CT findings of miliary tuberculosis. J Comput Assist Tomogr. 1998;22:220-4.
18. Choyke PL, Sostman HD, Curtis AM, et al. Adult-onset pulmonary tuberculosis. Radiology. 1983;148:357-62.
19. Westcott JL, Volpe JP. Peripheral bronchopleural fistula: CT evaluation in 20 patients with pneumonia, empyema or postoperative air leak. Radiology. 196:175-81.
20. Lee KS, Kim YH, Kim WS, et al. Endobronchial tuberculosis: CT features. J Comput Assist Tomogr. 1991;15:424-8.
21. Auerbach O. Tuberculosis of the trachea and the major bronchi. Am Rev Tuberc. 1949;60:604-20.
22. Smith L, Schillaci R, Sarlin R. Endobronchial tuberculosis. Serial fiberoptic bronchoscopy and natural history. Chest. 1987;91:644-7.
23. Moon WK, Im JG, Yeon KM, et al. Tuberculosis of central airways: CT findings of active and fibrotic disease. Am J Roentgenol. 1997;169:649-53.
24. Kim Y, Song KS, Goo JM, et al. Thoracic sequelae and complications of tuberculosis. Radiographics. 2001;21:839-58.
25. Sochocky S. Tuberculoma of the lung. Am Rev Tuberc. 1958;78:403-10. -
26. Lee KS, Song KS, Lim TH, et al. Adult-onset pulmonary tuberculosis: findings on chest radiographs and CT scans. Am J Roentgenol. 1993;160:753-8.
27. Fraser RS. Pulmonary aspergillosis: pathologic and pathogenetic features. Pathol Annu. 1993;28:231-77.
28. Snider GL, Placi B. The relationship between pulmonary tuberculosis and bronchogenic carcinoma: a topographic study. Am Rev Respir Dis. 1969;99: 229-36.
29. Santelli ED, Katz DS, Goldschmidt AM, et al. Embolization of multiple Rasmussen aneurysms as a treatment of hemoptysis. Radiology. 1994;193: 396-8.
30. Adler O, Peleg H. Computed tomography in diagnosis of broncholithiasis. Eur J Radiol. 1987;7:211-2.
31. Fraser RS, Muller NL, Colman N, et al. Diagnosis of diseases of the chest. Saunders, Philadelphia. 1999; pp 798-873.
32. Lee JY, Kim Y, Lee KS, et al. Tuberculous fibrosing mediastinitis: radiological findings. Am J Roentgenol. 1996;167:1598-9.
33. Stead WW, Lofgren JP, Warren E, et al. Tuberculosis as an endemic and nosocomial infection among the elderly in nursing homes. N Engl J Med. 1985; 312:1483-7.
34. Korzeniewska-Kosela M, Krysl J, Muller N, et al. Tuberculosis in young adults and the elderly: a prospective comparison study. Chest. 1994;106:28-32.
35. Umeki S. Comparison of younger and elderly patients with pulmonary tuberculosis. Respiration. 1989; 55:75-83.
36. Sodhi KS, Khandelwal N, Saxena AK, et al. Rapid lung MRI: Paradigm shift in evaluation of febrile neutropenia in children with leukemia: a pilot study. Leuk Lymphoma. 2016;57:70-5.
37. Sodhi KS, Khandelwal N, Saxena AK, et al. Rapid lung MRI in children with pulmonary infections: Time to change our diagnostic algorithms. J Magn Reson Imaging. 2016;43:1196-206.
38. Sodhi KS, Bhatia A, Khandelwal N. Rapid lung magnetic resonance imaging in children with pulmonary infection. Pediatr Radiol. 2017 May;47(6):764-5.
39. Sodhi KS, Sharma M, Saxena AK, et al. MRI in Thoracic Tuberculosis of Children. Indian J Pediatr. 2017 Jun; 10. doi: 10.1007/s12098-017-2392-3. [Epub ahead of print]
40. Meller J, Altenvoerde G, Lehmann K, et al. Fever of unknown origin—prospective comparison of 18FDG-imaging with a double head coincidence camera (DHCC) and Ga-67 citrate SPECT. Eur J Nuc Med. 2001; 28:OS387.
41. Meller J, Sahlmann CO, Scheel AK. 18F-PET and PET/CT in fever of unknown origin. J Nuc Med. 2007;48:35-45.
42. Liu RS, Shei HR, Feng CF. Combined 18F-FDG and 11C acetate PET imaging in diagnosis of pulmonary tuberculosis. J Nuc Med. 2002;43:127.

CHAPTER 161

Nontubercular Pulmonary Infections

Anju Garg, Swati Gupta, Jyoti Kumar

INTRODUCTION

Pulmonary infections or pneumonia are an important cause of morbidity and mortality especially in our country. Inflammatory disease of the lung may be referred to as either pneumonia or pneumonitis. Although these terms are used interchangeably, pneumonia usually implies an infection by pathogenic organisms whereas pneumonitis refers to a non-infective inflammatory process involving the alveolar wall.[1]

Community-acquired pneumonia (CAP) is an infection of the alveoli, distal airways and interstitium of the lungs that occurs outside of hospitals. ***Hospital-acquired pneumonia (HAP)*** is defined as a pneumonia not incubating at the time of hospital admission and occurring 48 hours or more after admission. ***Ventilator-acquired pneumonia (VAP)*** is defined as a pneumonia occurring more than 48 hours after endotracheal intubation. The term ***health care-associated pneumonia (HCAP)*** was introduced to include an already ill population of nursing-home residents, patients in long-term care, patients undergoing same-day procedures, patients receiving home or hospital based intravenous therapy, and patients undergoing dialysis. However, it has recently been removed by the 2016 Clinical Practice Guidelines of the Infectious Diseases Society of America and the American Thoracic Society.[2]

Patients with pneumonia commonly present with cough (with or without sputum), fever—often with chills, dyspnea and pleuritic chest pain. On physical examination, there may be tachypnea, with bronchial breath sounds and crepts on auscultation. In addition to these clinical features, an infiltrate on the chest radiograph or other imaging technique, with or without supporting microbiological data, is required for the diagnosis of pneumonia. The specific organism causing the infection can be established with certainty only in approximately 50% of patients, despite intensive laboratory investigation.

Although the specific diagnosis requires a microbiological workup, the radiologist plays a very important role in the workup of a suspected case of pulmonary infection. The radiologist can establish the presence of disease, localise and define the extent of disease, suggest an etiological diagnosis, recognize any underlying pathology, assess the response to treatment and establish the presence of complications.

IMAGING MODALITIES

Chest radiography and computed tomography (CT) are the most useful imaging modalities available for evaluation of a patient with known or suspected pulmonary infection.

A **chest radiograph** (posteroanterior view) is the basic and most useful imaging tool to establish the presence of pneumonia, determine its location and extent, and monitor its response to therapy. Further, the chest radiograph can suggest an etiological agent, prognosis, associated conditions, complications (cavitation, abscess formation, pneumothorax, pleural effusion), alternative diagnoses and sometimes guide invasive diagnostic procedures. Patients who are hospitalized for suspected pulmonary infection, but have negative chest radiography findings, should be presumptively treated with antibiotics and imaging repeated in 24–48 hours, as chest radiographs can be negative early in the course of the disease.

Computed tomography (CT) is not recommended for the initial evaluation of patients with pneumonia, but is recommended when there is a strong clinical suspicion of pneumonia that is accompanied by normal, ambiguous or non-specific radiography. It is a useful adjunct to conventional radiography in complicated cases or in patients in whom the response to treatment is unexpectedly slow. In these cases, the role of CT is to further characterize the complex pneumonias, look for complications and detect underlying disease within the lung or mediastinum. It also plays an important role in differentiating lung abscess from empyema.

Ultrasonography (US): In recent years, ultrasound has been used as an additional modality both, in the diagnosis, and follow up of patients with pneumonia.[3] Multiple studies have compared the findings in pneumonia on lung ultrasound (LUS) with chest radiography, and have shown that LUS is at least equivalent, if not superior to chest radiography.[4] Its use is specially recommended in the emergency setting, bedridden patients and in pregnant women and children because of its lack of ionizing radiation, portability (it can be done at the bedside) and repeatability.[5] It can also give quantitative and qualitative information about pleural fluid collections and serve as a guide for aspiration in cases of pulmonary infections.

Magnetic resonance imaging (MRI): With the recent advances in MRI, resulting in faster and shorter protocols, it has become possible to use MRI to diagnose pulmonary infection and its complications. MRI has been found to have a sensitivity and specificity equal to that of CT in the detection of pneumonia, with a better accuracy than chest radiographs. The major advantage of MRI is the lack of ionising radiation and therefore, it can be used as a non radiation alternative in children and pregnant patients. Challenges that remain are the need for sedation/anaesthesia in paediatric patients, cost and motion artefacts.[6,7]

RADIOGRAPHIC PATTERN

Pneumonias can be categorized according to their radiographic appearances. Although widely used, this categorization may have limited value because the same organism may produce several patterns and because patterns often overlap in an individual patient.

In **lobar/airspace pneumonia** the infective organism reaches the acini leading to a rapid production of abundant edema fluid with minimal cellular reaction. There is an initial peripheral localization but as the fluid increases in amount, it flows from alveolus to alveolus limited only by pleural boundaries, leading to a confluent involvement of the lung parenchyma.[8] Airspace disease is typically due to bacterial infection; however, some viruses can also cause this pattern.

On chest radiographs the classical appearance is a homogeneous non-segmental consolidation Eventually, the pneumonia may involve the whole lobe, but usually symptoms develop before the entire lobe is consolidated and antibiotic therapy, if started, halts the process. The consolidation is usually confined to one lobe, although multilobar involvement is not uncommon. Because the airways are not primarily affected, there is little or no volume loss and visible air bronchograms are common **(Fig. 1A)**.

On ultrasound, consolidated lung appears similar in echogenicity to liver or spleen—"hepatization" of the lung. Multiple bright dot-like structures and branching linear structures can be seen within the consolidated lung which represent scattered residual air in alveoli and bronchi—the "sonographic air bronchogram" **(Fig. 1B)**. These air bronchograms may show centrifugal movement with breathing.[9] Consolidation can be differentiated from atelectasis on the basis of this movement—the "dynamic air bronchogram". According to a recent study, dynamic air bronchograms have a 97% positive predictive value for pneumonia.[10]

On CT, airspace consolidation localizes in the middle and outer zones of the lungs and is seen as dense opacification with air bronchograms or air bronchiolograms. Areas of ground-glass attenuation may be seen around this denser airspace consolidation **(Figs. 1C and D)**.[11]

Lobar pneumonia must be distinguished from atelectasis and pleural involvement. Secondary causes of pneumonia like pulmonary edema, hemorrhage, or obstructed bronchi should be looked for. In lower lobes involvement aspiration pneumonia should be considered in appropriate clinical context. Non-infective causes of lobar pattern include acute interstitial pneumonia, radiation pneumonia, pulmonary alveolar proteinosis, organizing pneumonia, adenocarcinoma in situ (formerly bronchoalveolar carcinoma), and lymphoma.[12]

In **bronchopneumonia**, it is the mucosal surfaces of the bronchi and bronchioles that are affected, rather than the terminal airspace. There is development of a peribronchiolar focus of infection, which subsequently spreads along the intralobular airway to the alveolus, and then from one alveolus to another, until the pulmonary

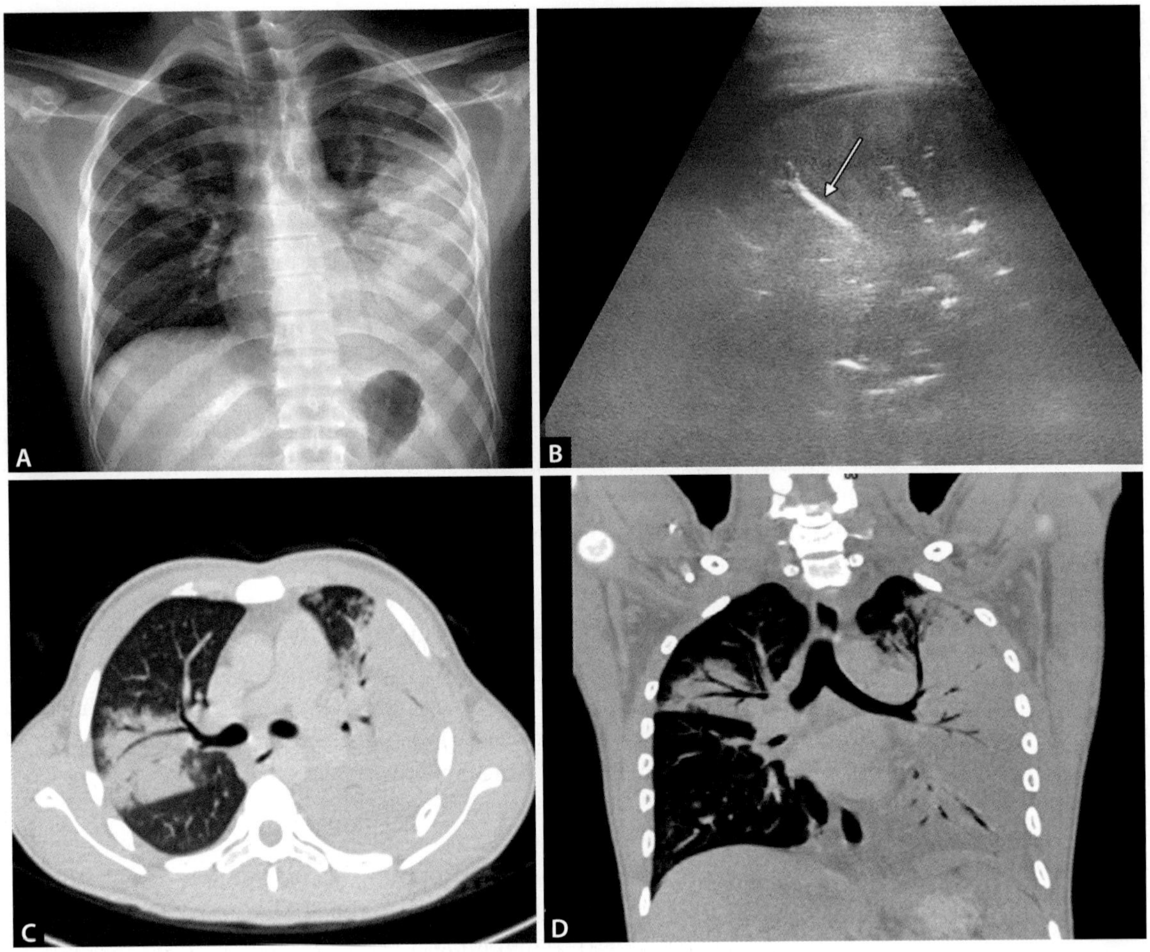

Figs. 1A to D: Airspace pneumonia: Chest radiograph (A) shows a homogeneous opacity in right mid zone, left mid and lower zone with air bronchogram within. Ultrasound image (B) showing lung parenchyma resembling liver (hepatization) with linear echogenic structure within representing air in bronchi—the sonographic air bronchogram (arrow). CT scan at lung window settings axial (C) and coronal reformat (D) shows airspace consolidation in the left lower lobe and right upper lobe with air bronchogram. Consolidation in right upper lobe is limited by major fissure.

lobule is partially or totally involved. A bronchopneumonia pattern is most commonly due to infection by staphylococcal or gram-negative organisms; anaerobic organisms may also cause this pattern of involvement.[13]

On chest radiographs, mild bronchopneumonia results in peribronchial thickening and poorly defined airspace opacities. More severe disease results in inhomogeneous, patchy, poorly defined opacities with absence of air bronchograms. The process is diffuse, as several foci of disease are often seeded at the same time, and frequently both lungs are involved **(Fig. 2)**. It is often difficult to make a radiographic distinction between lobar pneumonia and confluent bronchopneumonia.[13] On CT, consolidation which involves the terminal and respiratory bronchioles and adjacent alveoli results in poorly defined centrilobular nodular opacities measuring between 4 to 10 mm in diameter. When the infection extends to involve the

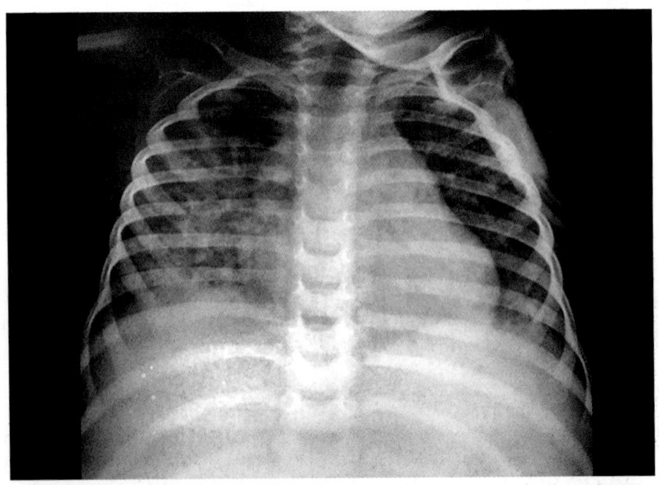

Fig. 2: Bronchopneumonia: Chest radiograph shows patchy opacities in right mid zone and bilateral lower zones.

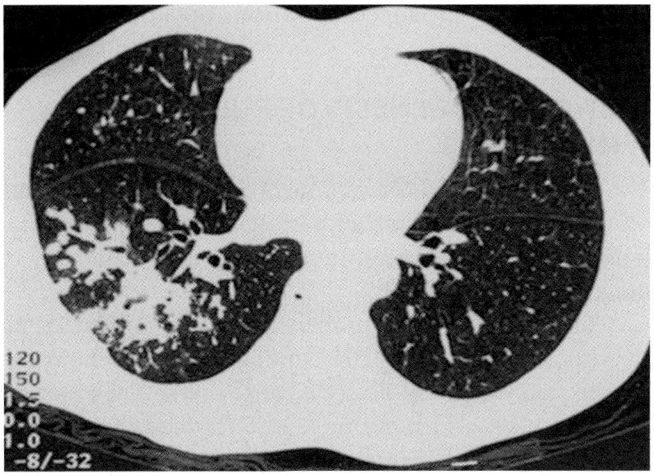

Fig. 3: Bronchopneumonia. CT scan shows acinar and centrilobular nodules along with lobular consolidation in right lower lobe.

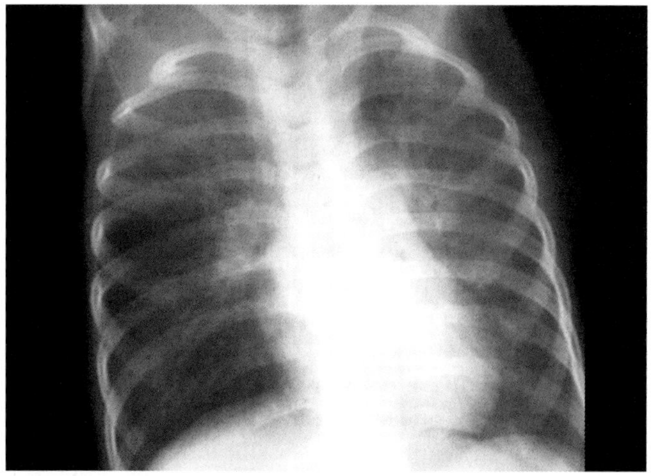

Fig. 4: Interstitial viral pneumonia: Chest radiograph showing bilateral poorly defined linear and nodular shadowing radiating from the hila with hyperinflated lung fields.

entire secondary lobule, lobular distribution of airspace consolidation is seen **(Fig. 3)**.[11] This pattern can also be seen in adenocarcinoma *in situ* (formerly bronchoalveolar carcinoma), hyperesoniphilic syndrome and lymphoma which can present as multifocal alveolar consolidation. In chronic cases, differential diagnoses include lipoid pneumonia, pulmonary alveolar proteinosis or radiation pneumonitis.[12]

In **interstitial pneumonia,** the infection results in diffuse edema of the airway walls along with inflammatory cellular infiltration which extends from the peri-bronchial tissues into the interlobular septa. The usual causes of acute interstitial pneumonia are viral or *Mycoplasma pneumoniae* infection.

The chest radiographs show generalized hyperaeration, widespread peribronchial thickening, increased reticular markings or small ill-defined nodules **(Fig. 4)**. On CT, the lesions are seen to be distributed in the central zone of the lung as well as middle and outer zones. There is thickening of bronchial walls, centrilobular shadows, acinar and lobular shadows **(Fig. 5)**. A predominantly ground-glass pattern may be seen.[11]

A **spherical or round pneumonia** is a well-circumscribed rounded consolidation, often pneumococcal in origin, which mimics a mass lesion.[14] It is seen more commonly in children and in the posterior segment of the lower lobes. It is thought to represent an early manifestation of the infectious focus that has spread centrifugally. An alternative theory is that round pneumonia occurs in children, because of underdeveloped pores of Kohn and the absence of canals of Lambert, which limits spread of the organism and results in a focal, round mass seen on

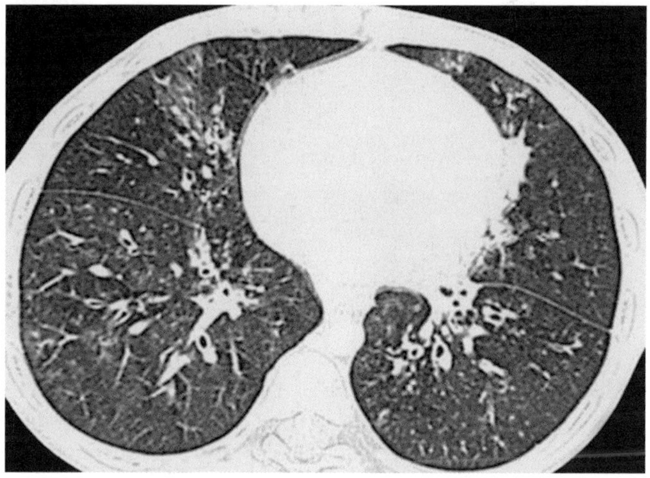

Fig. 5: Interstitial pattern of pneumonia: CT scan in a case of viral pneumonia shows focal areas of ground-glass attenuation with peribronchial thickening and centrilobular nodules.

radiographs and CT scans. As adults have fully developed canals of Lambert, this theory can also explain why round pneumonia is seen less often in adults.[15]

On chest radiographs, the appearance of a round pneumonia can vary from a small dense mass, to a large ill-defined rounded opacity **(Fig. 6)**. Margins may be smooth, irregular, lobulated, or even occasionally spiculated.[16] Air bronchograms can be seen in some cases but they are not specific for an infective process.

On CT scans, round pneumonia is seen as a heterogeneous mass of soft tissue attenuation that can have spicules, air bronchograms, pleural thickening and satellite lesions. The last two findings are found to be the most useful for diagnosis, while the presence or absence of air bronchograms does not help in distinguishing between malignancy and round pneumonia. Comparison with prior recent radiographs and short-term (3-7 days) interval follow-up are very useful in establishing the correct diagnosis.[14,16]

A **nodular pattern** may sometimes be seen as presence of random nodules in the lung parenchyma, which can occur due to hematogenous spread of disease **(Figs. 7A and B)** or granulomatous infection. Miliary TB, septic emboli, varicella zoster and some fungal infections can show a nodular pattern of lung infection.

In practice, these patterns may be of limited use as the radiological appearance may be indeterminate, the pathological and radiological classification can be varied and the pattern produced by various organisms is often inconstant.[17]

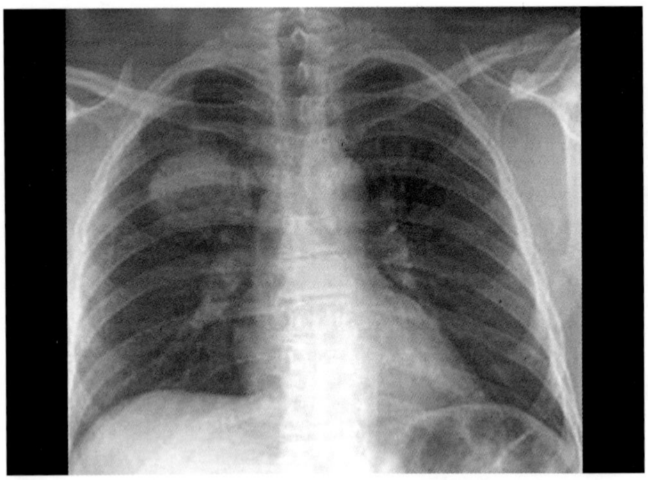

Fig. 6: Round pneumonia: Chest radiograph shows a rounded opacity in the right upper lobe containing an air bronchogram.

ETIOPATHOGENESIS OF PULMONARY INFECTIONS

The radiological manifestations of pneumonia are based on the etiopathological factors.[18] The type of pneumonic pattern and the consequent radiographic pattern is dependent on **(Table 1)**:

- The specific inherent properties of the organism, i.e. its virulence, its site of action and its mode of action, e.g. the staphylococcal bacteria cause marked destruction and abscess formation; *Klebsiella* leads to a more productive type of inflammation; a fungal or tubercular infection evokes a granulomatous response, etc.
- The route of entry of the organism has a significant influence on the radiographic appearance of the resulting pneumonia.
  - *Via the tracheobronchial tree:* By inhalation or aspiration. Inhalation, the most common route of entry of microorganisms, is in the form of droplet nuclei. The organisms reach the lower respiratory tract where they form a focus of infection and depending on the virulence, amount of inoculum and the state of the local and systemic defences of the host they can cause inflammation. The pneumonia caused by this route can be airspace, lobular or interstitial pneumonia.
  - *Via the blood vessels:* This kind of spread normally occurs in conjunction with an extrapulmonary source of infection which causes septicemia which in turn localizes in the lung. Radiographically,

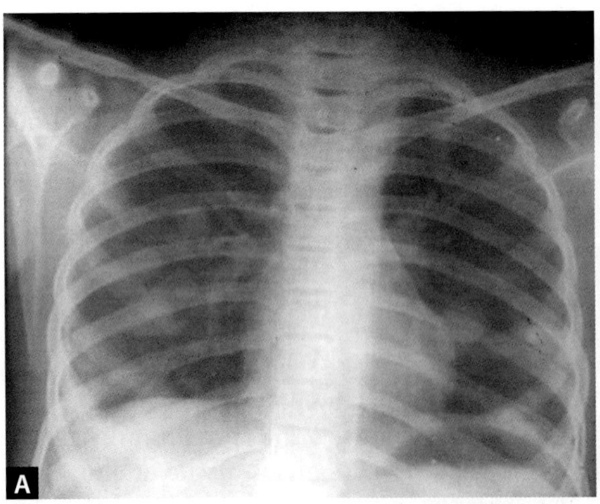
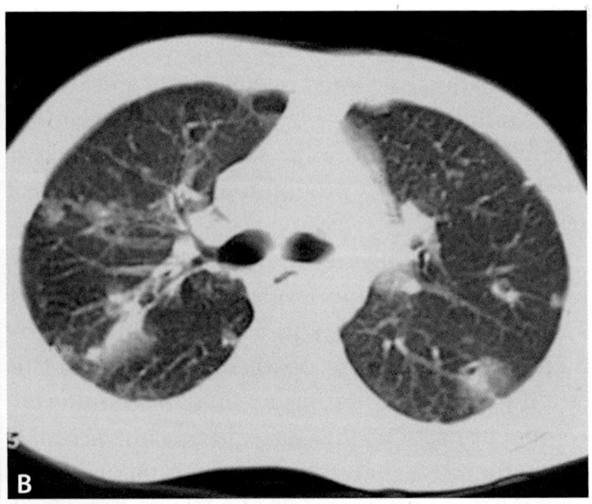

Figs. 7A and B: (A) Septic emboli seen as multiple nodular opacities scattered in both lung fields on a chest radiograph. (B) CT scan shows multiple nodular densities scattered in both lung fields, showing the "feeding vessel" sign. Few of the nodules show evidence of cavitation.

this is a random, patchy distribution with increased involvement of the basal segments due to preferential gravity related blood flow.
 - *Via direct spread* from infective lesions in the chest wall, across the diaphragm and from the mediastinum. The disease is usually localized to an area contiguous to the source and generally leads to formation of an abscess.
- Certain host factors also alter the classical appearance of a given pneumonia due to specific organism and should be evaluated to help narrow the radiographic differential diagnosis.
 - *Age:* In newborns, infection can be congenital or acquired.[19] Congenital infection is generally viral if due to transplacental spread. The acquired type is more often bacterial. Children are prone to respiratory infections with bronchiolitis and pneumonia as the common manifestations and are usually caused by viruses. In young adults, most pneumonias are viral or mycoplasmal in origin while pneumococcal is the most common bacterial infection. In middle age and beyond, streptococcal pneumonias become the leading cause and the incidence of non-bacterial pneumonia drops.[19]
 - *Immune status:* Immunosuppressed patients are unusually susceptible to infection with common pathogens and several microorganisms which are normally not pathogenic, e.g. *Pneumocystis jiroveci*, cytomegalovirus, etc. Differentiation between pneumonia, drug reaction, and parenchymal changes of pulmonary disease is difficult and often needs other investigations.
 - *Underlying lung disease:* A decrease in local resistance or a local obstruction leads to increased incidence of infection, e.g. bronchiectasis, sequestrated lung or chronic obstructive diseases. In emphysematous lungs, the pulmonary infection can often assume bizarre radiographic patterns due to the distorted emphysematous pulmonary parenchyma.[20]

The consolidation appears to have multiple cavities due to the underlying low attenuation emphysematous areas giving rise to a "swiss cheese appearance" **(Figs. 8A to C)**. These pseudocavities and pseudohoneycombing should be differentiated from true cavities and honeycombing. Resolution is often delayed in pneumonias associated with pulmonary emphysema.[21]

Table 1: Factors affecting pathogenesis of pneumonia.

Inherent properties of the organism	• Virulence • Site of action • Mode of action
Route of entry	• Via tracheobronchial route • Via the blood vessels • Via direct spread
Host factors	• Age • Immune status • Underlying lung disease • Systemic conditions • Aspiration pneumonia
Environmental factors	• Community acquired pneumonia • Nosocomial pneumonia • Infections in returned travellers

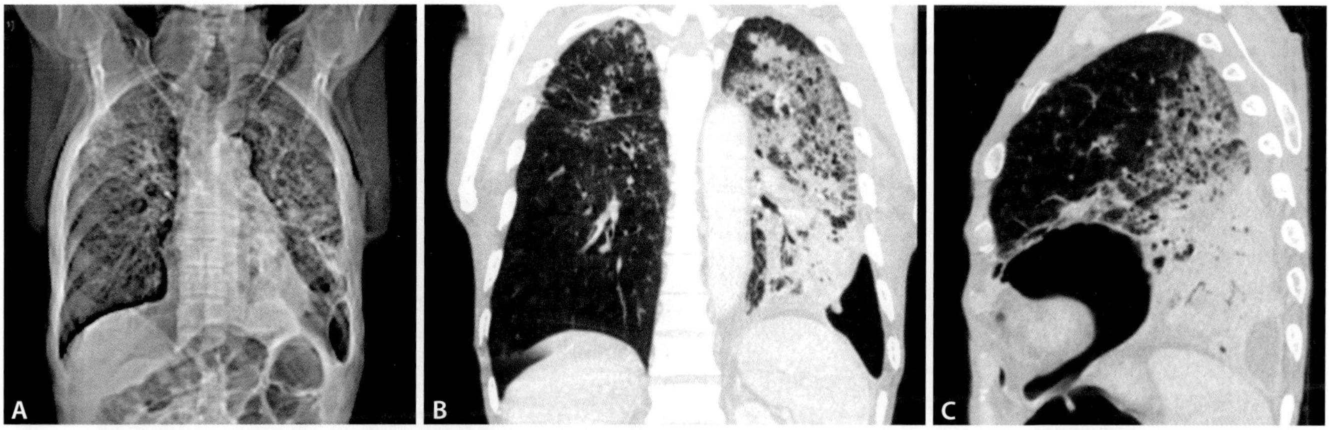

Figs. 8A to C: Chest radiograph (A) shows bilateral patchy opacities with a loculated left pneumothorax in a 60-year-old patient with emphysematous lungs. Coronal (B) and sagittal (C) CECT images show dense consolidation with air bronchogram in the left lower lobe, segmental consolidation in left upper lobe showing multiple small cysts within (Swiss cheese appearance), due to underlying centriacinar emphysematous changes with an associated small left pneumothorax. Few ground-glass opacities and apical nodular opacities seen in right lung.

- *Systemic conditions:* Diseases associated with increased lung infections are poor nutrition, diabetes, alcoholism, connective tissue disorders, malignancy and AIDS.
- *Aspiration pneumonia:* Occurs in patients with impaired consciousness, chronic debilitating diseases, structural abnormalities of the pharynx and esophagus, neuromuscular disorders, impaired swallowing mechanisms, indwelling tracheal or esophageal/gastric tubes and in postoperative patients, due to inhalation of bacteria, food, gastric contents, etc. leading to parenchymal inflammation or edema. It has several different pathophysiological aspects—bacterial pneumonia caused by the oral flora, chemical pneumonitis by gastric acid or exogenous lipids such as paraffin liquid and granulomatous reaction to foreign bodies. It occurs in the gravity dependent portions of the lung, so in recumbent patient it involves the posterior segment of the upper lobes and the superior segment of the lower lobes whereas in an erect patient, aspiration is more likely to involve bilateral basal segments, middle lobe, and lingular lobe. On imaging, it is often seen as a bronchopneumonia or bronchiolitis pattern **(Figs. 9A and B)**. Aspirated material may sometimes be seen in the bronchial lumen. A lung abscess may also be seen in bacterial aspiration.[22]

- *Environmental factors*:
  - *Community acquired infections (CAP):* Refers to pneumonia that develops in people in the community rather than in a hospital, nursing home, or assisted-living facility. The etiological causes of community acquired pneumonia are listed in **Table 2**.[23]
  - *Nosocomial infections (HAP and VAP):* It is paradoxical but true that pneumonia is more likely to occur in patients who are admitted to a hospital. This is because of the ease with which hospital strains of staphylococci and gram-negative bacilli can be acquired from other patients, hospital staff or inhalation therapy machines. Also, the frequent use of antibiotics in hospitalized patients suppresses the growth of normal respiratory flora, greatly increasing the susceptibility of treated patients to infection.[19] Causal organisms depend on onset of disease and host conditions **(Table 3)**.[24] A variety of radiographic patterns are seen, including airspace, interstitial and mixed compounding the problem. It is often difficult to distinguish atelectasis from hospital-acquired pneumonia, and the two may co-exist, although

Table 2: Common causative organisms of community acquired pneumonia.[23]

Bacteria	• *Streptococcus pneumoniae* • *Staphylococcus aureus* • *Chlamydia pneumoniae* • *Mycoplasma pneumoniae* • *Haemophilus influenzae* • *Klebsiella pneumoniae* • *Streptococcus pyogenes* • *Legionella pneumophilia*
Viruses	• Influenza virus • Respiratory syncytial virus • Adenovirus

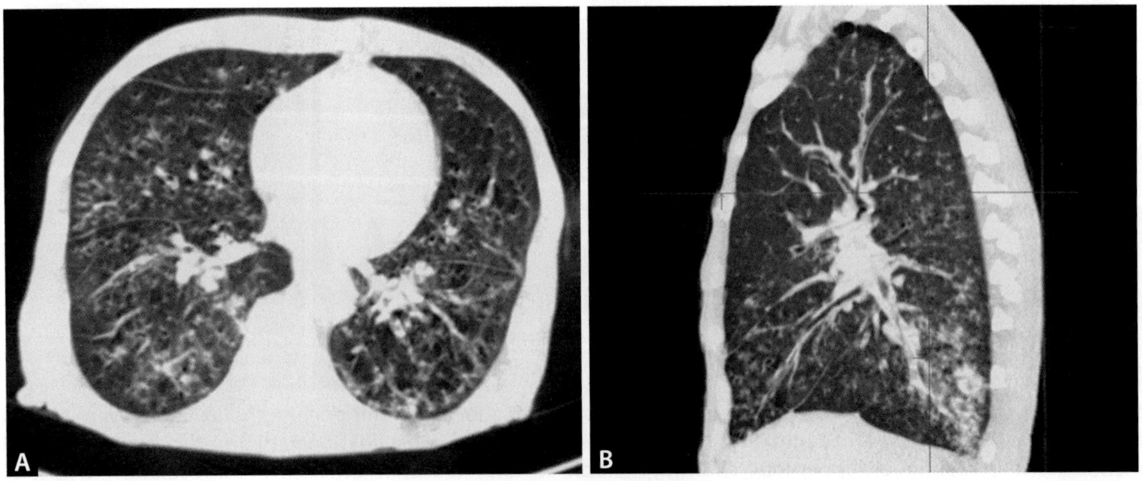

Figs. 9A and B: Axial (A) and sagittal (B) aspiration pneumonia: In a patient with carcinoma tongue, multiple confluent centriacinar opacities seen in posterior aspect of bilateral lower lobes and posterior segment of upper lobes, consequent to aspiration.

Table 3: Causative organisms of nosocomial pneumonia[24]

	Early onset (within 48–72 hours)	***Late onset (>72 hours)***
Hospital-acquired pneumonia	• *Haemophilus influenzae* • *Streptococcus pneumoniae* • Methicillin-sensitive *Staphylococcus aureus* (MSSA) • Enterobacteraciae (*Klebsiella, Escherichia coli, Serratia*) • Anaerobes • *Legionella*	• Organisms same as in early onset hospital-acquired pneumonia • *Pseudomonas aeruginosa* • Methicillin-resistant *Staphylococcus aureus* (MRSA)
Ventilator-acquired pneumonia	• *Streptococcus pneumoniae* • *Haemophilus influenzae* • MSSA • Enterobacteriaceae	• *Enterobacteraciae* • *Pseudomonas aeruginosa* • MRSA • *Acinetobacter* species

atelectasis often develops rapidly and may resolve rapidly.[25] The incidence of pneumonia in ventilated patients (VAP) can be as high as 20% with a high mortality rate.

Diagnosing pneumonia in ventilated or post-operative patients can be difficult. Portable chest radiography may not show basal consolidation in approximately one-fourth of patients following abdominal surgery.[26]

Pneumonia, edema, acute respiratory distress syndrome (ARDS), drug toxicity, atelectasis, infarction and hemorrhage have overlapping signs, so a confident diagnosis based on radiographic features alone is often impossible.[25,27] In patients with ARDS, CT may reveal areas of cavitation or empyema, not seen on chest radiographs and are suggestive of coexisting infection.[28] The use of ultrasound in correlation with clinical findings makes it an ideal tool for rapid diagnosis, especially in situations with unstable patients.

c. *Infections in returned international traveller:* Some pathogens are related to specific regions and locations. Travel to these regions may result in contracting travel related pulmonary diseases. Risk depends upon travel destination, activities undertaken and length of stay. High degree of clinical suspicion is of paramount importance in early diagnosis.[29]

SPECIFIC PNEUMONIAS

Bacterial Infections

Pneumococcal Pneumonia

Pneumococcal pneumonia is caused by *Streptococcus pneumoniae*. It is the commonest community acquired pneumonia and can occur at any age. The clinical presentation is in form of abrupt onset of fever, chills, cough and chest pain, often associated with bloody or rusty sputum. The organism tends to affect the terminal airways first and then disseminates to the surrounding segments giving rise to the classical unilateral airspace pneumonia **(Figs. 1 and 10)**. An air bronchogram is commonly present and this is a characteristic feature **(Fig. 11)**. The volume of the lobe usually remains unchanged. Classically, it causes a lobar pattern of consolidation but may sometimes even have a bronchopneumonic or interstitial pattern.[30] Occasionally, early during the disease, a spherical or round pneumonia may be seen, particularly in children. One study that investigated the radiographic appearance in 81 inpatients with culture documented pneumococcal pneumonia, demonstrated a lobar pattern of consolidation in 81% of patients. Lobar consolidation was focal in 48% and multifocal in 33%. A bronchopneumonic pattern was seen in 19% cases.[31]

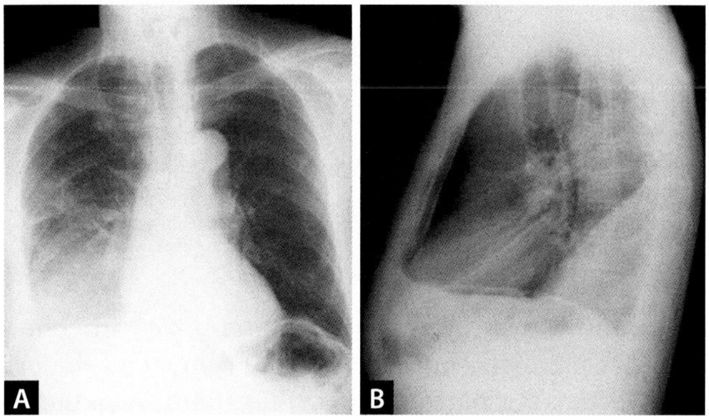

Figs. 10A and B: Chest radiographs PA view (A) and lateral view (B) Pneumococcal pneumonia involving the entire right lower lobe

Associated small pleural effusions may sometimes be seen, but empyema and cavitation are distinctly unusual. A very rare complication is pulmonary gangrene. Uncomplicated infection usually shows complete radiographic clearance within 10–14 days of appropriate

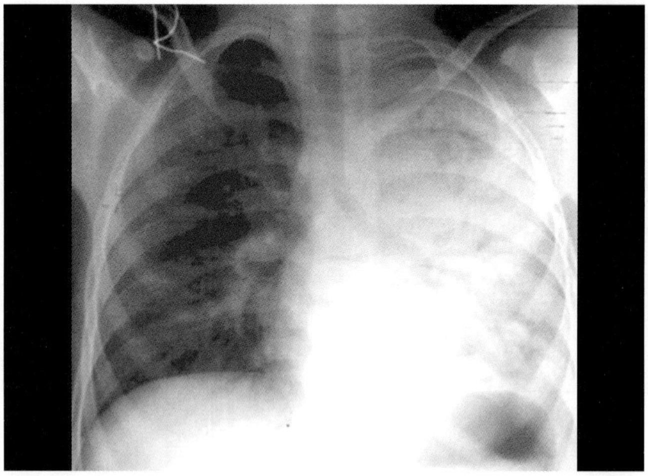

Fig. 11: Pneumococcal pneumonia involving almost the entire left lung with air bronchogram seen within

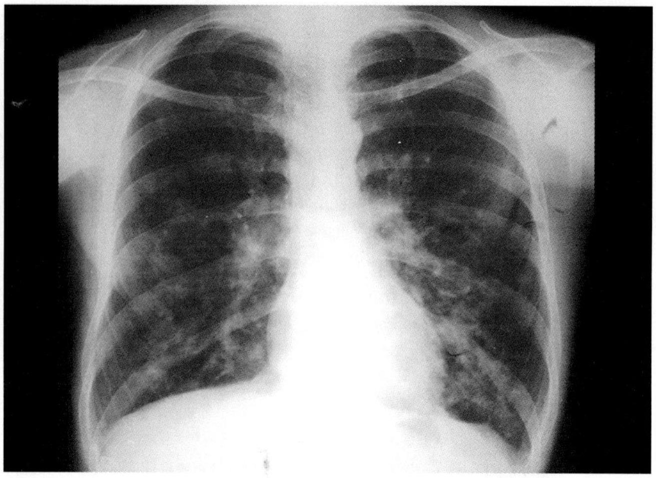

Fig. 12: Staphylococcal pneumonia showing patchy opacities in bilateral lung fields on background of emphysema.

treatment. The presence of multilobar disease is associated with increased morbidity and mortality.

Staphylococcal Pneumonia

It is caused by *Staphylococcus aureus*. The infection follows aspiration of organisms from the upper respiratory tract, occurring particularly in hospitalized patients. Staphylococcal pneumonia may be community acquired, particularly in infants and elderly individuals, often complicating influenza. Infection can also occur because of staphylococcal bacteremia.

The chest radiograph typically shows a bronchopneumonic pattern, initially involving the lower zones **(Figs. 2 and 12)**. The consolidation can spread rapidly and become confluent, resembling lobar pneumonia. Volume loss, early and large effusions, empyema and abscess formation are common **(Figs. 13A to D)**. Resolution is generally slower than pneumococcal infections and residual fibrosis can occur. Pneumatoceles **(Figs. 14A to C)** are more common in childhood than in adulthood, and may lead to pneumothorax.[32]

Septicemic staphylococcal infection occurs by hematogenous spread from endocarditis, thrombophlebitis or staphylococcal infection of indwelling catheters. It is also seen in drug addicts and immunocompromised patients. The usual radiographic and CT appearance is that of multiple pulmonary opacities **(Figs. 7 and 15)**. CT often shows more lesions than plain radiographs. The opacities may be of varying sizes, generally round (sometimes wedge-shaped or irregular), often show cavitation and have a lower zone predominance.[33] The "feeding vessel" sign i.e. a direct vessel leading up to the opacity can be seen on CT **(Figs. 15B and C)**. Accompanying pleural effusion and empyema are common features.

Gram-negative Pneumonias

These are caused by a great variety of organisms, the most important being the Enterobacteriaceae (notably *Klebsiella, Enterobacter, Escherichia coli* and *Proteus mirabilis*), *Pseudomonas aeruginosa, Acinetobacter* and *Haemophilus influenzae.* They are the most important cause of nosocomial infections and a major cause of morbidity and mortality in the hospital set-up. Very often, the affected patients have a known predisposing factor such as chronic obstructive pulmonary disease, a major medical condition like diabetes or history of recent surgery.

The organisms most commonly enter the lungs by aspiration, but pneumonia following inhalation of bacteria or spread by bloodstream is also occasionally seen. Aspiration is particularly important because the carriage of gram-negative organisms in the upper respiratory tract is greatly increased in debilitated patients in hospital.[17] The radiographic pattern is entirely nonspecific and ranges from small ill-defined nodules to patchy consolidation which may become confluent and resemble lobar pneumonia. Lower lobes tend to be predominantly affected; upper and middle lobe involvement may be seen in 50% of cases. Cavitation, pleural effusions and empyema are quite commonly associated **(Figs. 16 and 17)**.

The pneumonia caused by *Klebsiella pneumoniae* (also known as Friedlander's pneumonia) differs from other gram-negative pneumonias in that it is not uncommonly acquired outside the hospital and usually affects people

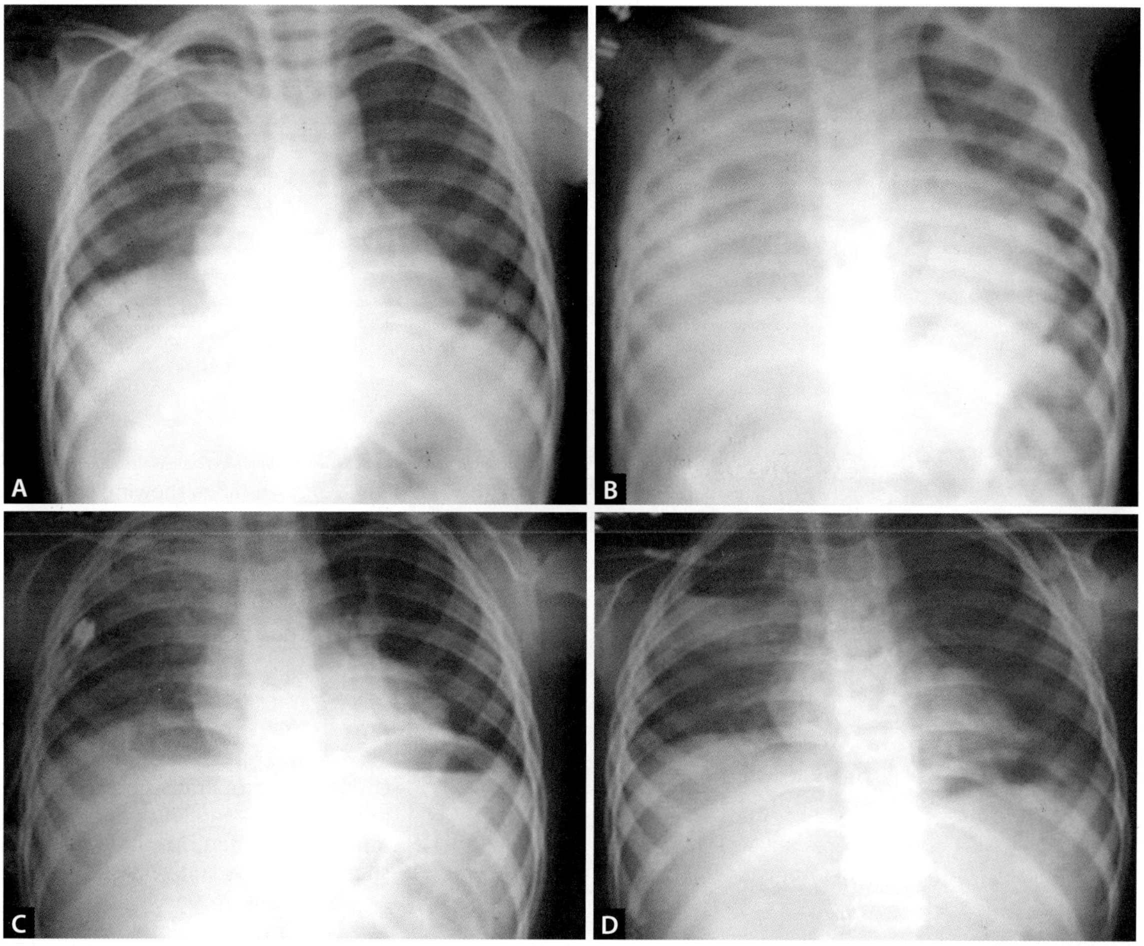

Figs. 13A to D: Serial chest radiographs of a 5-year-old child with a complicated staphylococcal pneumonia. (A) Areas of patchy consolidation in the right lung with evidence of volume loss. (B) 3 days later—complete opacification of right hemithorax was seen. A chest tube was inserted which drained pus. (C) Chest radiograph taken 2 days after chest tube insertion shows almost complete clearing of the empyema, however, there is an increase in the underlying patchy consolidation in right upper zone. (D) An abscess has developed in the right upper lobe.

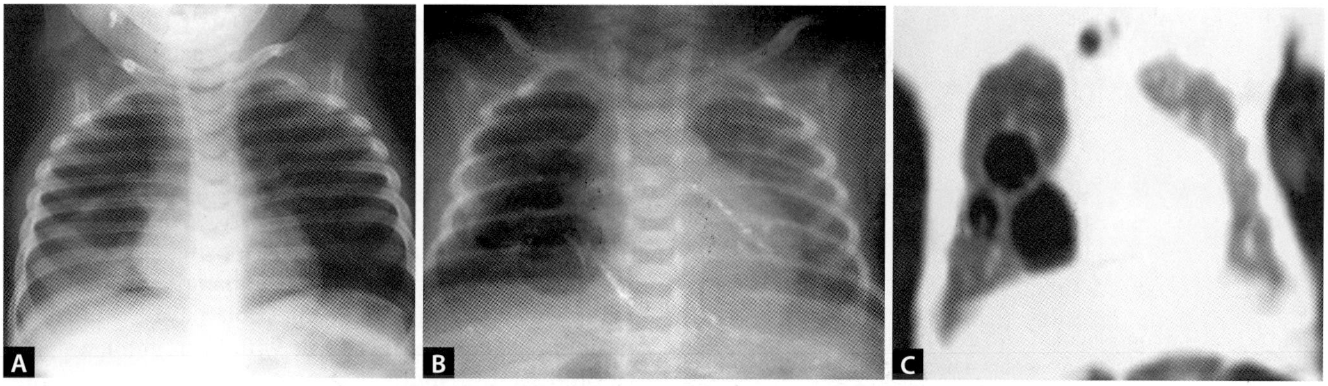

Figs. 14A to C: Chest radiograph (A) shows pneumatocele formation in a right lower lobe consolidation due to staphylococcal pneumonia. Chest radiograph (B) and CT scan—coronal reconstruction (C) in another infant showing multiple residual pneumatoceles following an episode of staphylococcal pneumonia

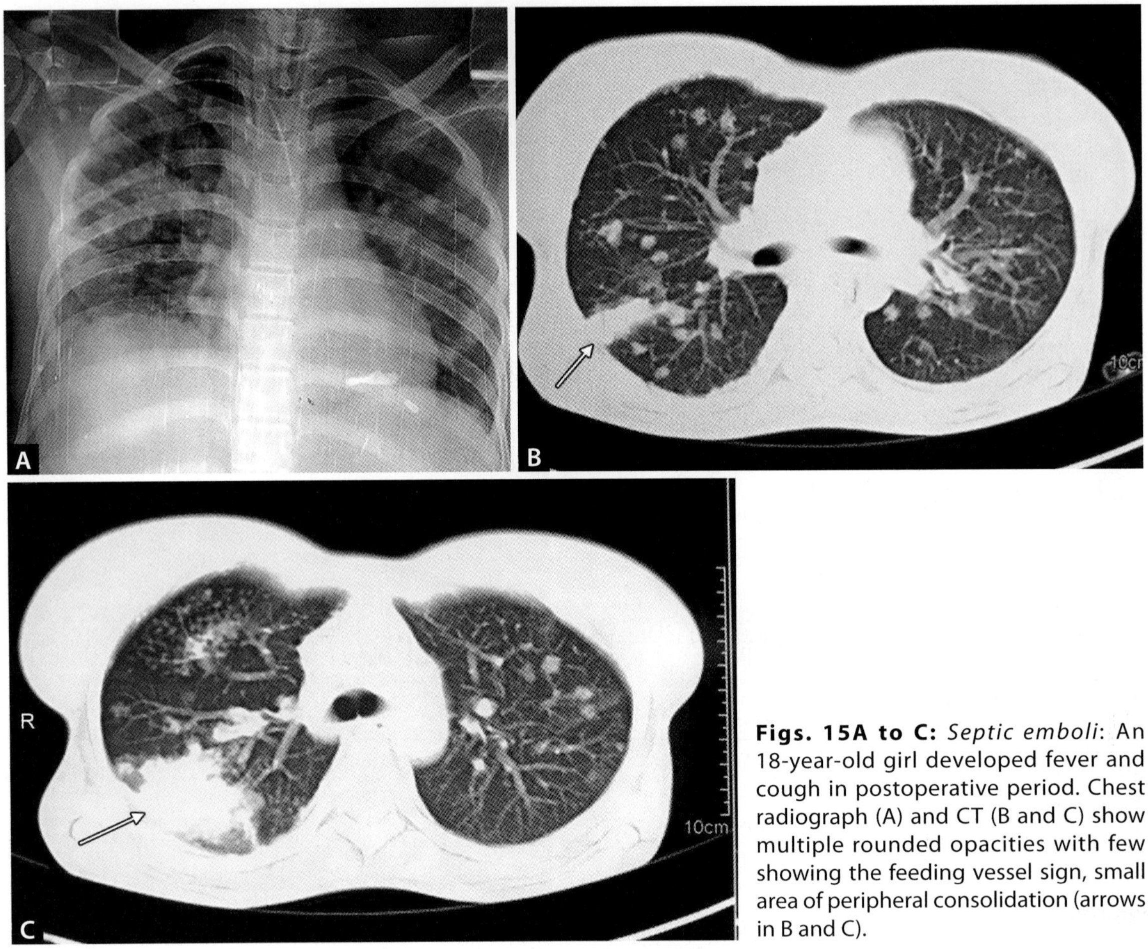

Figs. 15A to C: *Septic emboli*: An 18-year-old girl developed fever and cough in postoperative period. Chest radiograph (A) and CT (B and C) show multiple rounded opacities with few showing the feeding vessel sign, small area of peripheral consolidation (arrows in B and C).

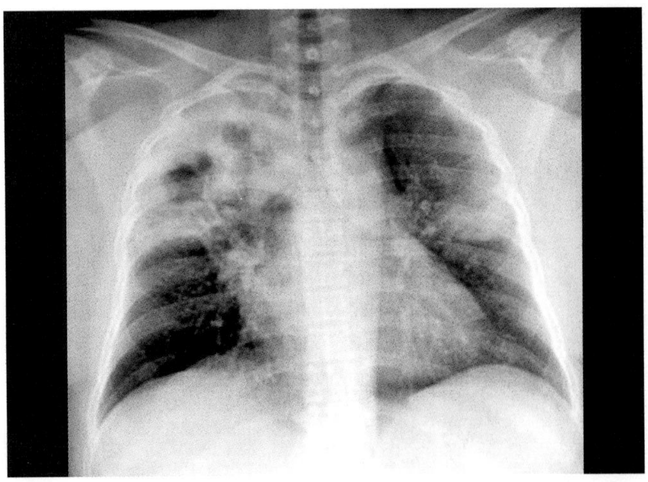

Fig. 16: Bilateral consolidation with extensive cavitation in the right upper lobe caused by gram-negative bacteria in a hospital setting.

with chronic debilitating illnesses or alcoholism. The symptoms include high fever, toxemia and resemble those of severe pneumococcal pneumonia. On chest radiography, the consolidations are also like those seen with *S. pneumoniae* pneumonia, i.e. a lobar pneumonia pattern. *Klebsiella pneumonia* has a tendency for the formation of voluminous inflammatory exudates leading to lobar expansion with resulting bulging of interlobar fissures **(Fig. 18)**, a greater tendency for abscess and cavity formation which are frequently multiple and large, and also a greater frequency of pleural effusion and empyema.[34]

Anaerobic Pneumonias

Most anaerobic lung infections result from aspiration of infected oral contents and obvious periodontal disease may be present in most patients.[20] Predisposing factors such as a recent episode of altered consciousness, dysphagia or alcoholism are frequent. The infection may be acute but is commonly subacute or chronic with prominent systemic symptoms and an indolent course. Anaerobic pneumonias are caused by a variety of organisms that are normally found in the oropharynx but which are abnormally aspirated into the lung including species of *Bacteroides*, *Clostridium*, *Fusobacterium*, *Peptococcus*, etc.[35]

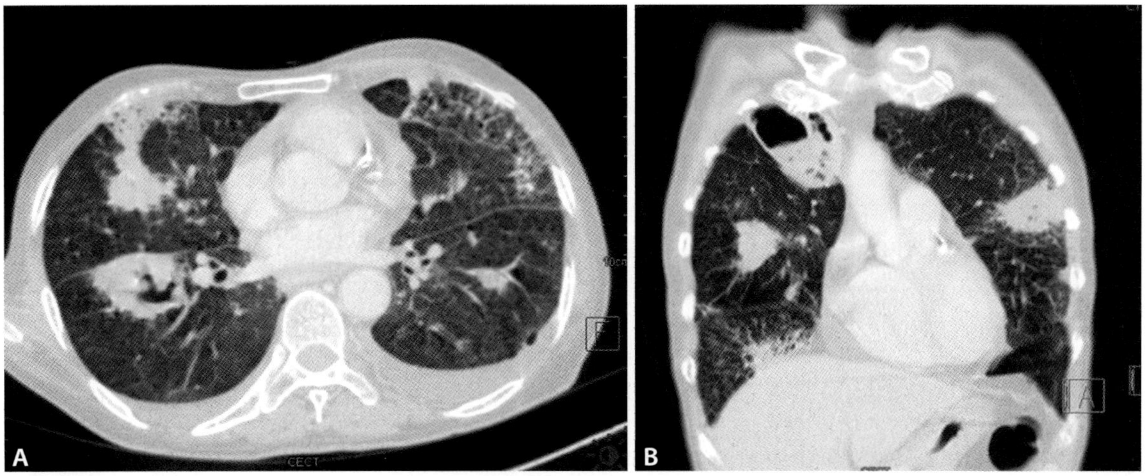

Figs. 17A and B: Axial (A) and coronal (B) CT showing multifocal areas of consolidation, bilateral ground-glass opacities and bilateral pleural effusions in a 65-year-old patient with *Pseudomonas* pneumonia in a hospital setting. Cavitation is seen in some of the consolidated areas.

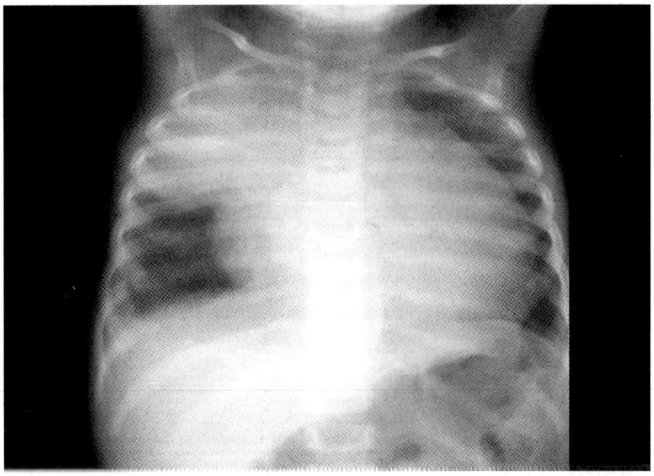

Fig. 18: Bulging fissure seen as downward convexity of the horizontal fissure in a case of consolidation of the right upper lobe with associated pleural effusion.

Following aspiration, the chest radiograph is frequently normal initially. The appearance of abnormality is delayed for 24 to 72 hours. Three types of radiographic appearances may be seen—pulmonary parenchymal infection, pneumonia with cavitation or a discrete lung abscess, each of which may be associated with empyema. These pneumonias commonly involve the superior and posterobasal segments of the lower lobe and/or posterior segment of upper lobe due to drainage of infected material from the mouth into these segments as the patient lies on his back (gravitational pneumonia). Involvement may be unilateral or bilateral. Heterogeneous opacities may be seen in the involved lobes. Multiple cavities may be seen within the area of consolidation due to severe lung necrosis or formation of lung abscess.

The other manifestation of an anaerobic lung infection is a focal cavitary mass with very little surrounding consolidation—the so called 'primary lung abscess'. The abscess may vary in size from 2 to 12 cm and characteristically has a thick, irregular wall **(Figs. 19 and 20)**. Hilar or mediastinal lymphadenopathy may accompany the lung abscess and such cases may closely resemble lung carcinoma.[36] Empyema is a common complication; may be large and may occur with or without radiographic evidence of pneumonia.[37]

Atypical Pneumonias

Atypical pneumonia or "walking pneumonia" is caused by atypical bacteria like *Mycoplasma pneumoniae*, *Chlamydophila pneumoniae* and *Legionella pneumophilia*. Some viral and fungal pathogens may also give rise to atypical pneumonia. Atypical community-acquired pneumonia (CAP) is characterized by prodromal upper airway symptoms, low grade fever, myalgias, dry cough and headache. There may also be associated extrapulmonary manifestations like diarrhea, abdominal pain, arthritis, facial rash etc. As the symptoms differ from those of typical pneumonia and are generally milder, they have been termed as atypical pneumonias. The importance of the atypical pneumonias is not related to their frequency (approximately 15% of CAPs), but to difficulties in their diagnosis, and their non-response to beta-lactam therapy.

Mycoplasma pneumonia is caused by *Mycoplasma pneumoniae* which is the smallest free-living organism,

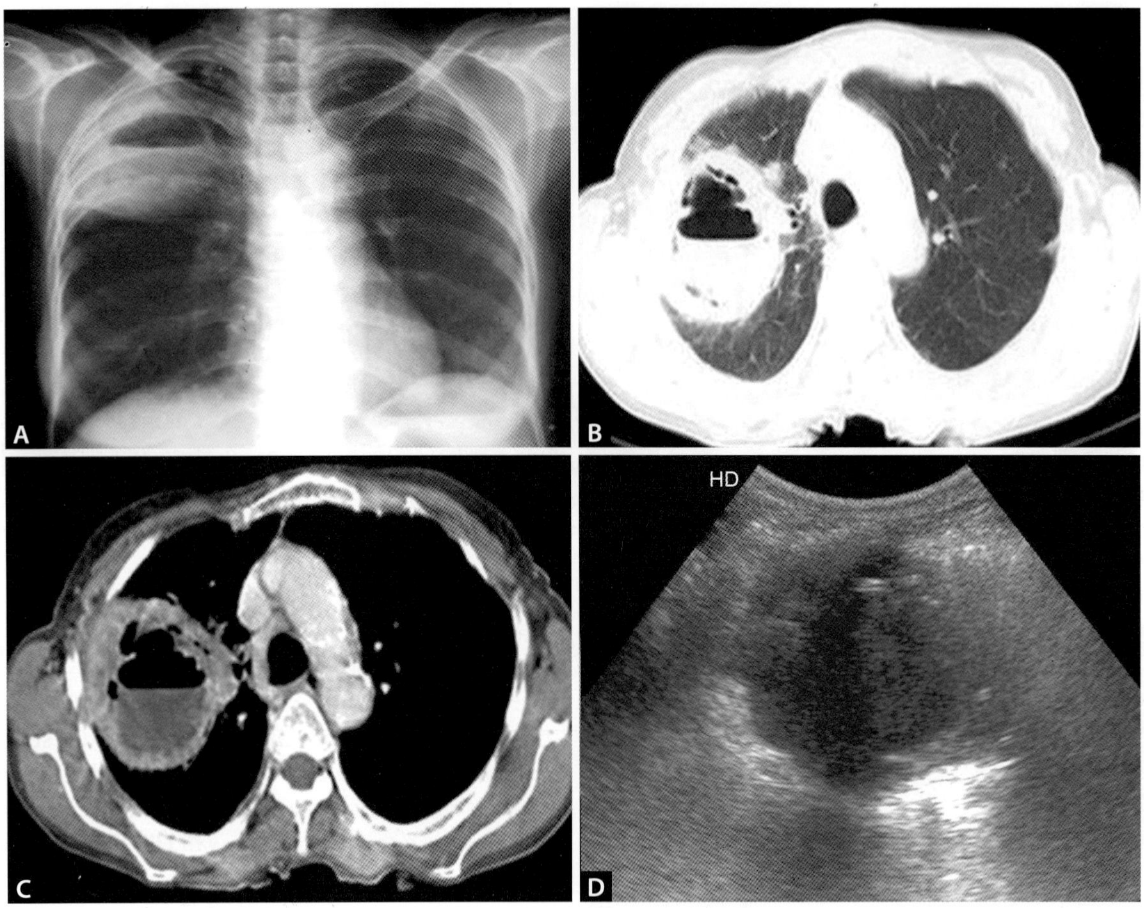

Figs. 19A to D: Anaerobic lung abscess in an alcoholic patient with poor orodental hygiene—Chest radiograph (A) CT scan at lung window settings (B) and mediastinal window settings (C). Lung abscess is seen in posterior segment of the right upper lobe with thick irregular walls. Ultrasound image (D) shows the abscess as an irregularly walled lesion with anechoic contents. This abscess was aspirated under US guidance.

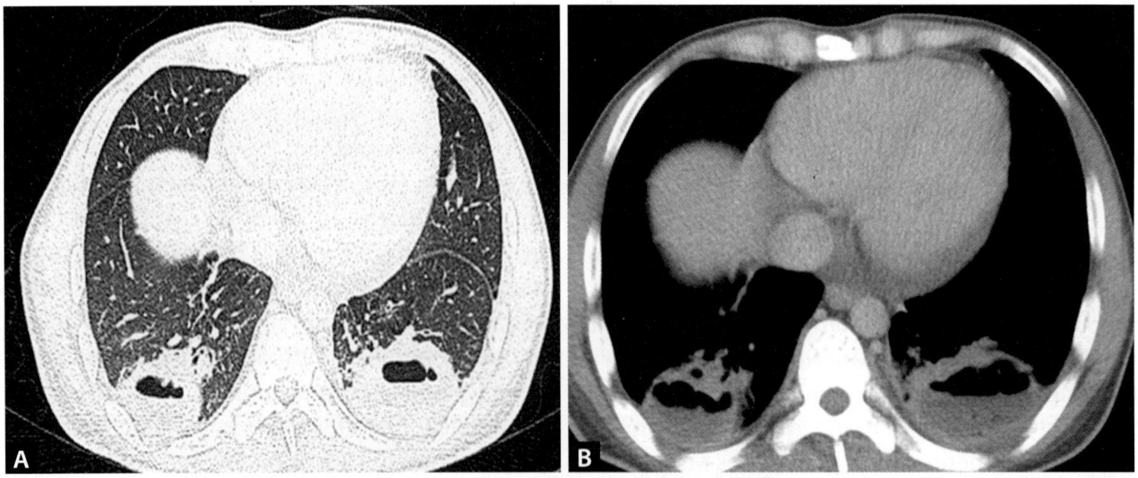

Figs. 20A and B: In a patient on ventilator, CT scan with lung window (A) and mediastinal window (B) settings, shows bilateral thick-walled abscesses seen in the posterior aspects of both lower lobes.

sharing some similarities with bacteria. It is a major non-bacterial cause of community-acquired pneumonias in the 20–40 year age group. Spread is via droplets, and the symptoms resemble a viral rather than a bacterial infection. The definitive diagnosis is serological and therefore, delayed and often retrospective. The radiological findings are very variable; the most common pattern is unilateral lower lobe involvement, beginning as a patchy/nodular, peribronchial consolidation that progresses to become sublobar or lobar and homogeneous **(Figs. 21A to C)**.[18] Sometimes the initial features are those of an interstitial process with small, irregular nodules and linear shadows.[38] Slow progression of this pattern to that of a typical consolidation is very suggestive of a mycoplasmal infection. Pleural effusion generally does not occur, and cavitation is rare. Nodal enlargement is common in children and is an unusual, but recognized, finding in adults. The CT findings consist of centrilobular nodules and branching linear opacities in a patchy distribution, thickening of the bronchovascular bundles and areas of lobular or segmental consolidation.[39]

Chlamydia pneumonia is caused by *Chlamydophila pneumoniae* and is a common cause of community-acquired pneumonia. It often affects children and young adults. The radiographic findings are non-specific with overlap of features with pneumonias from other organisms. The most common radiographic finding is airspace consolidation with interstitial infiltrates, combined interstitial and airspace infiltrates and pleural effusion.[40]

Legionella pneumonia is also known as Legionnaires' disease. It is caused by infection with any *Legionella* species, most commonly by *Legionella pneumophila*. It is seen more often in middle-aged and older adults, smokers, and those with chronic illnesses or a weak immune system. Infection occurs due to inhalation of airborne microscopic sources of contaminated water. It can be more severe than the other atypical pneumonias. The radiographic appearances may often lag behind the clinical picture and deterioration can be seen on imaging despite clinical improvement. The early radiographic and CT manifestations are nonspecific and similar to those found in community-acquired pneumonia from other bacterial origin. The chest radiograph shows asymmetric air space consolidation, more in middle and lower zones. Pleural effusion and mediastinal lymphadenopathy may be seen in a few cases. On CT, there is lobar or multilobar consolidation with adjacent ground-glass haze.[41,42]

Actinomycosis

Although previously grouped with the mycosis, *Actinomyces Israeli is* now regarded as a branching bacteria. It causes infection of the lung by aspiration or direct extension from abdomen or cervicofascial disease. The organism produces proteolytic enzymes that allow the infection to cross fascial planes. Therefore, the pneumonia readily spreads to pleura, producing empyema, and may spread extrapleurally to give rise to abscesses and sinus tracks in the chest wall, bones of the thorax, pericardium and mediastinum.[43] The chest radiograph usually shows an area of non- segmental airspace consolidation, commonly in the periphery of the lung and with a predilection for the lower lobes. If therapy is not instituted, an abscess may develop and infection may extend into the pleura. Pleural involvement manifests as pleural effusion, pleural thickening, or empyema formation but is seldom associated with large accumulations of fluid. Rib involvement causes lytic destruction with periostitis. Actinomycosis may

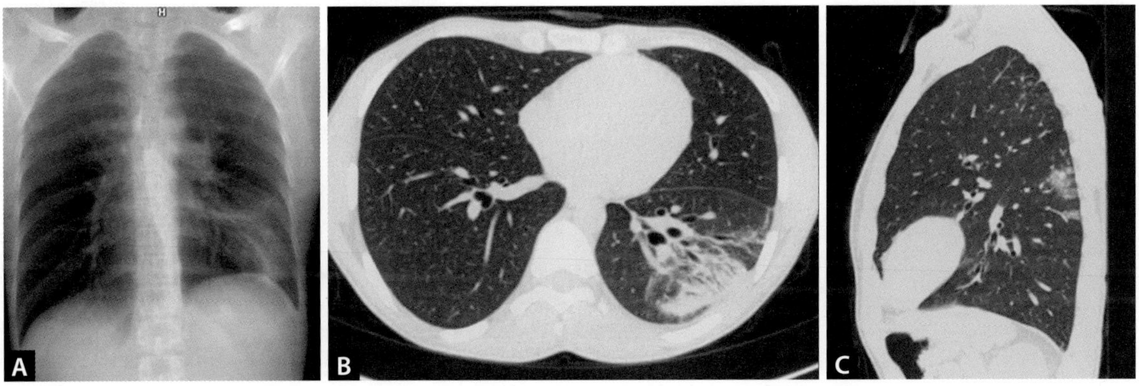

Figs. 21A to C: *Mycoplasma pneumoniae:* Chest radiograph (A) shows a homogeneous opacity in left lower zone. CT scan at lung window settings axial (B) and sagittal reformat (C) shows a peripherally based airspace consolidation in the left lower lobe with air bronchogram.

also present as a mass which may cavitate.[44] On CT, the typical findings are those of chronic low attenuation areas (representing actinomycotic or sulfur granules) with peripheral enhancement (representing granulation tissue in wall of abscess) and adjacent pleural thickening. CT can demonstrate chest wall, pleural, mediastinal and spinal invasion to advantage.[45] Associated mediastinal lymphadenopathy may be present.

Viral Infections

Viruses are a major cause of respiratory tract infection in the community, particularly in children. The usual mode of spread is by transmission by droplets. In infants and young children who are immunocompetent, respiratory syncytial virus, parainfluenza virus, adenovirus and influenza virus are the most common cause offenders, whereas in adults, influenza type A and B and adenovirus are more common.[46] Immunocompromised patients are susceptible to CMV and other herpes viruses.[47]

Viruses result in several forms of lower respiratory infections, which include tracheobronchitis, bronchiolitis, and pneumonia. The pneumonia usually begins in the distal bronchi and bronchioles and giving rise to the interstitial pattern of involvement. Parenchymal involvement initially involves the lung adjacent to the terminal and respiratory bronchioles, but spread throughout the lobule can occur. In elderly patients, rapidly progressive pneumonia may occur, with diffuse alveolar damage leading to a hemorrhagic pulmonary edema.

The imaging findings of viral pneumonias do not usually allow the diagnosis of a specific viral infection. Clinical features such as patient age, immune status, time of year, illness in other family members, community outbreaks; onset, severity and duration of symptoms, and the presence of a rash remain important aids in diagnosing viral pneumonia.

Chest radiograph shows reticular opacities that are often bilateral and diffuse in distribution. The associated bronchiolitis leads to hyperinflation of the lung fields **(Figs. 4 and 22)**. Presence of hilar lymphadenopathy is variable; it is common in measles pneumonia and infectious mononucleosis but rare with other viral pneumonias. Pleural effusions are not a prominent feature, although small ones do not negate the diagnosis. CT scan may show poorly defined airspace nodules (4–10 mm diameter), patchy areas of peribronchial ground-glass opacity and consolidation along with hyperinflation **(Figs. 5 and 22C)**. The combination of CT findings varies somewhat between the individual viral pneumonias and has been summarized in **Table 4**.

The progressive form of the pneumonia shows large areas of homogeneous or patchy, unilateral or bilateral airspace consolidation or poorly defined centrilobular nodules.[48]

Influenza and Parainfluenza Virus

Infections with influenza virus occur in epidemics, pandemics or sporadically. Influenza subtypes A and B are most commonly responsible for the severe outbreaks associated with pneumonia.

Swine Flu is caused by a strain of human influenza A (H1N1) virus which originated in Mexico in 2009 and spread to more than 190 countries, including India. In June 2009, the World Health Organisation had declared it a level 6 (highest level) pandemic. The virus causes a wide spectrum of respiratory illnesses, which range

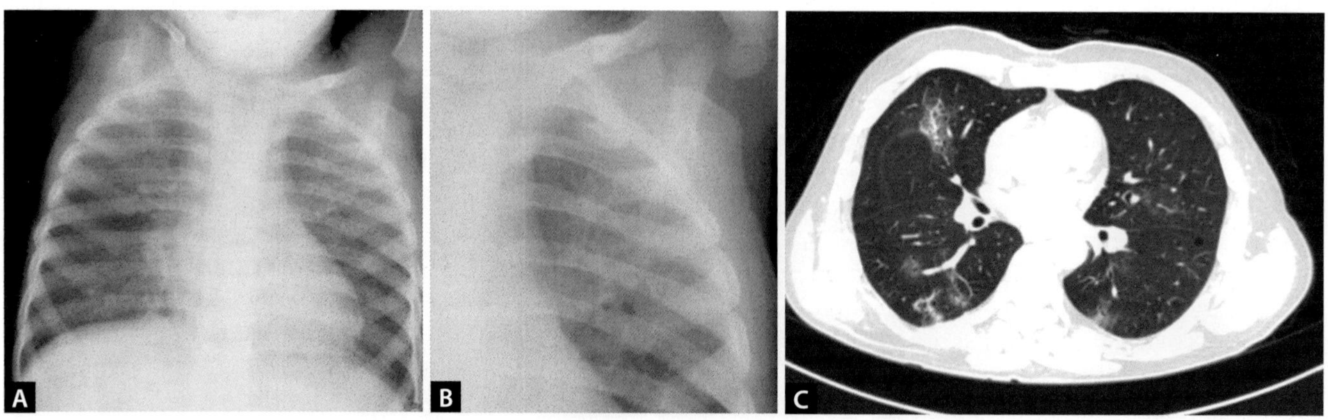

Figs. 22A to C: *Viral pneumonia*: Chest radiograph (A) with magnified view of left upper zone (B) shows hyperinflated lung fields with linear streaky opacities representing peribronchial thickening, nodular opacities. (C) Axial CT shows bilateral multifocal peripheral regions of ground-glass opacities in a case of non-specific viral pneumonia.

Table 4: Summary of CT findings in viral pneumonias.[46]

Cause of pneumonia	*Centrilobular nodules*	*Ground-glass attenuation with lobular distribution*	*Segmental consoliation*	*Thickened interloular septa*	*Diffuse ground-glass attenuation*
Influenza virus	+++	+++	+	---	+
Measles virus	++	+	+	---	+
Hantavirus	---	---	++	+	+++
Adenovirus	++	+	+++	---	---
Herpes simplex virus	+	+++	+++	---	+
Varicella-zoster virus	+++	+	---	---	---
Cytomegalovirus	++	++	+	+	++
Epstein-Barr virus	+	+	+	---	+

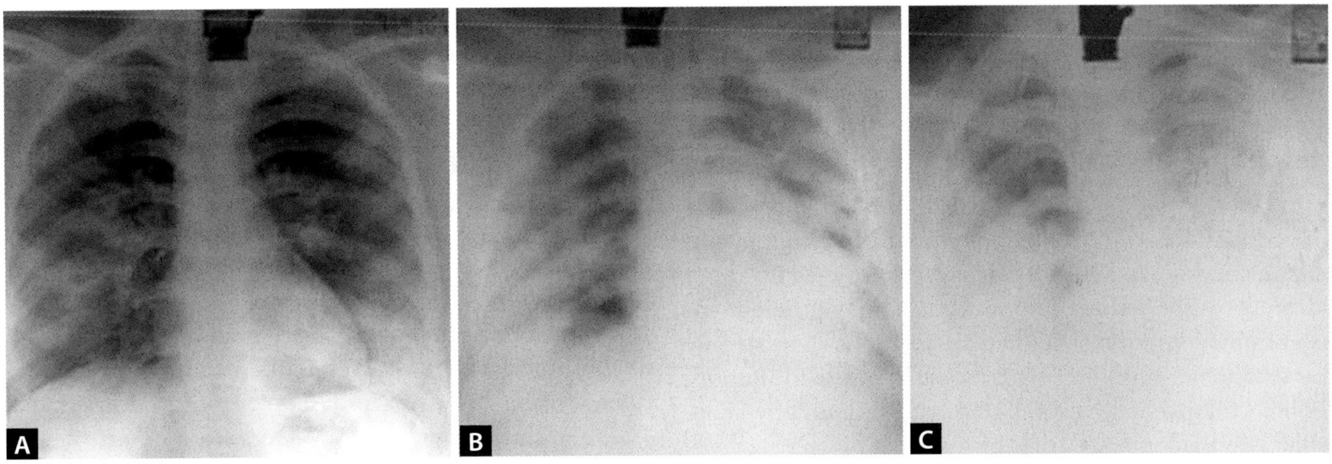

Figs. 23A to C: Serial radiographs of a 22-year-old female with swine flu. (A) At presentation areas of ill-defined consolidation seen in the lower zones. (B) Three days later, there is an increase in the consolidation. (C) A further 3 days later, there is extensive bilateral airspace consolidation like that seen in ARDS.

from mild febrile illness to severe respiratory distress.[49] Symptoms include fever, dry cough, myalgia and headache. The predominant radiological pattern in H1N1 pneumonia is bilateral ground-glass opacities and alveolar consolidation. The opacities are usually in the mid zone and bases in the chest radiograph, while on the CT they are mainly peripheral and peribronchovascular in distribution, with diffuse zonal involvement.[50] Pneumonia is more common in the very young, those over 65 years of age, in late pregnancy and in those with underlying disease. Pleural effusion is rare.[48]

An acute form of pneumonia with rapid progression, shows fast confluence of the consolidation caused by the diffuse alveolar damage, which may be homogeneous or irregular, unilateral or bilateral, giving rise to an ARDS type of picture **(Figs. 23 and 24)**.

Avian influenza or "bird flu" is caused by the H5N1 subtype of the influenza A virus. Human infection occurs as a result of close contact with infected birds, usually poultry or their products. Chest radiograph commonly shows multifocal consolidations. On CT, the most common findings consist of focal, multifocal, diffuse ground-glass opacities or areas of consolidation. Centrilobular nodules can be seen. There may be associated pseudocavitation, pneumatocele formation and lymphadenopathy.[51]

Severe Acute Respiratory Syndrome

Severe acute respiratory syndrome (SARS) is caused by a coronavirus, the SARS-associated coronavirus (SARS-CoV). It was recognized as a global threat in March 2003, after first appearing in Southern China in November 2002. It leads to a systemic infection clinically manifesting as a progressive pneumonia. Chest radiograph and CT show focal unilateral or bilateral areas of ground-glass opacities and/or consolidation. The areas of ground-glass opacity may be associated with thickening of the intralobular and interlobular septae.[17]

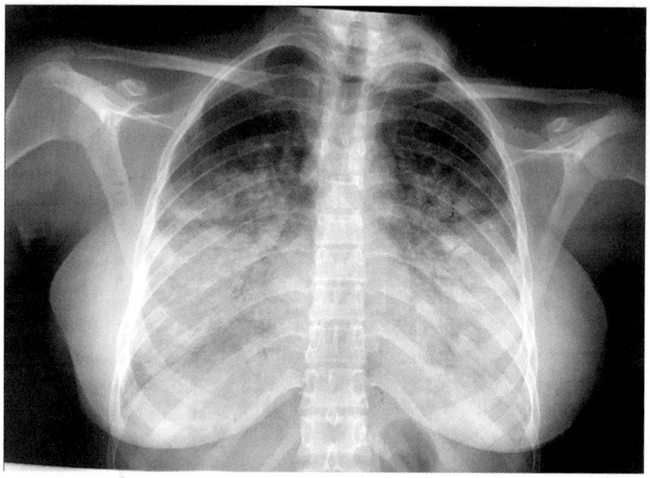

Fig. 24: *Swine Flu*: Confluent fluffy opacities due to alveolar consolidation in bilateral mid and lower zones in a young girl with swine flu.

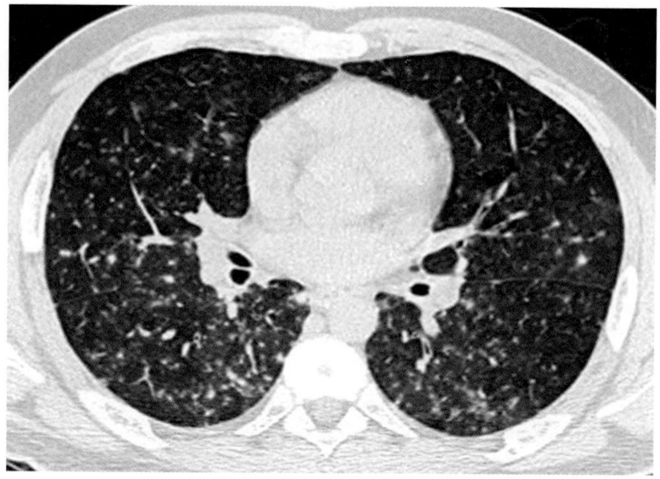

Fig. 25: *Varicella pneumonia*: Axial CT scan showing multiple nodular opacities scattered in bilateral lung parenchyma.

Respiratory Syncytial Virus

The respiratory syncytial virus (RSV) is a major cause of bronchiolitis and bronchopneumonia in infants and young children. In adults it can cause prolonged fever but it rarely causes serious complications, unless the patient is immunocompromised. Chest radiographs show streaky peribronchial infiltrates with associated hyperinflation. Lobar collapse or consolidation are occasionally seen. Hilar lymphadenopathy may be seen.

Varicella

Varicella pneumonia occurs more commonly in adults than in children. It has a specific radiographic appearance of multiple small, discrete acinar nodules scattered throughout both lung fields **(Fig. 25)**. Hilar lymph node enlargement may be present. HRCT findings mirror the radiographic abnormalities, but smaller nodules (1–10 mm) can be identified, few of them have a halo of ground-glass opacification representing hemorrhage. The nodules usually resolve in a week but may persist for months and in 2% of patients they may calcify.[17]

Adenovirus

The common cold virus—may sometimes cause pneumonia in epidemics. Radiographically, widespread scattered patchy/confluent opacities occur which are peribronchial in distribution. Hilar lymphadenopathy may occur. The infection can be highly damaging particularly if acute infection occurs before 2 years of age, causing bronchiectasis, obliterative bronchiolitis and in some cases Swyer-James/McLeod's syndrome.[52]

Fungal Infections

Fungi can be divided into two major groups according to the pathogenesis of infection: (1) Opportunistic invaders; (2) Primary pathogens.

1. Opportunistic invaders: These fungi invade debilitated or immunocompromised individuals and those with a pre-existing, diseased and scarred lung parenchyma. These include species like *Aspergillus, Candida,* and *Cryptococcus.*[13] In contrast to the primary pathogens, these organisms can be found throughout the world and usually are ubiquitous in the environment. In addition to saprophytic and invasive infection, some fungi (particularly *Aspergillus* species) can cause disease by inducing an exaggerated hypersensitivity reaction without invading tissue.

Aspergillosis

Aspergillus infections of the lung are caused by *Aspergillus fumigatus* which are ubiquitous fungi found throughout nature and may result in disease in susceptible hosts when inhaled. The pathogenesis of *Aspergillus* infection varies with quality and virulence of the inhaled organism and the status of the host defence mechanisms. Four varieties of pulmonary aspergillosis have traditionally been described.[53]

a. Aspergilloma—a saprophytic non-invasive infection of a pre-existing cavity.
b. Allergic aspergillosis—including allergic broncho-pulmonary aspergillosis (ABPA) and hypersensitivity pneumonitis caused by hypersensitivity to fungus.

c. Semi-invasive aspergillosis or chronic necrotizing aspergillosis a form of infection seen in patients with mild immunological suppression.
d. Invasive aspergillosis—an infection in immunocompromised hosts, which is invariably fatal without treatment.

Aspergilloma: Aspergilloma, also known as mycetoma is a ball of coalescent mycelial hyphae that typically colonize pre-existing chronic cavities. The pre-disposing causes can range from tuberculosis, sarcoidosis, cavities in rheumatoid lung or ankylosing spondylitis, etc. In most of the cases reported from India, there was a history of tuberculosis in the past or during detection.[54] Common clinical manifestations include cough and expectoration. Hemoptysis is frequent and has been reported in at least half of the cases. The mechanism of the bleeding is unknown; it has been attributed to friction between the fungus ball and the hypervascular wall, to endotoxins liberated from the fungus, and to a type 3 reaction in the cavity wall.[55]

On chest radiographs, an aspergilloma is seen as a round to oval mass of soft tissue density lying within a pre-existing cavity. As most of the pre-existing cavities colonised by the fungus are due to tuberculosis, mycetomas are most often found in the upper lobes or in the superior segment of the lower lobes. Typically, there is an airspace separating the fungus ball from the wall of the cavity resulting in a distinctive "air crescent sign" **(Fig. 26A)**. The air crescent sign is not specific to mycetoma formation, as it can also be seen in patients with blood clot within a pre-existing cavity, necrotic carcinoma, ruptured hydatid cyst and lung abscess with necrosis. If the mycetoma completely fills the cavity, it may obliterate the air crescent. The fungus ball is usually mobile within the cavity and this mobility can be demonstrated on a decubitus chest radiograph **(Fig. 26B)**. Thickening of a cavity wall may be an early sign of *Aspergillus* infection.

CT demonstrates to advantage the finding of a mobile intracavitary mass characteristic of aspergilloma. The fungus ball is a sponge like mass that contains irregular airspaces. The air crescent sign and the wall of the pre-existing cavity are well seen and fungal strands bridging the fungus ball and cavity wall may be seen **(Fig. 27)**. Mobility can be readily demonstrated by turning the patient although it is rarely necessary as the diagnosis is obvious in most cases. Occasionally, flecks of calcification may be seen within the mycetoma.[56]

Allergic aspergillosis is a result of hypersensitivity reaction that produces allergic bronchopulmonary aspergillosis (ABPA) or less commonly an extrinsic allergic pneumonitis, a Loeffler-like syndrome. The common symptoms of ABPA are cough, wheezing and associated allergic symptoms and radiographic findings include central bronchiectasis and mucoid impaction seen typically as branching opacities, usually central and in an upper lobe distribution—the "gloved finger sign". These opacities are commonly transient and recurrent but may occasionally remain unchanged or even grow overtime. CT shows the bronchiectasis and mucoid impaction very well **(Figs. 28 and 29)**.[57] The central distribution of bronchiectasis suggests the diagnosis of ABPA, even though it is not specific for the diagnosis. The findings of

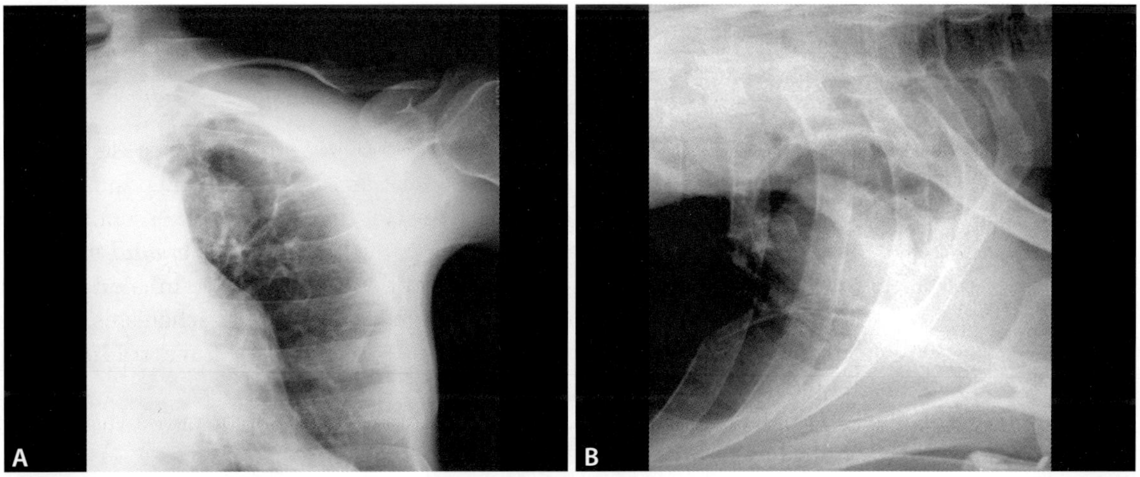

Figs. 26A and B: Frontal chest radiograph (A) shows a cavity containing an intracavitary fungus ball with a crescent of air above the mycetoma. Lateral decubitus view (B) shows the fungus ball lying in the dependant part of cavity suggesting movement of the mycetoma within the cavity.

ABPA overlap with other entities such as cystic fibrosis or post infectious bronchiectasis.

Hypersensitivity pneumonitis can occur with *Aspergillus* inhalation. It is seen on chest radiographs as a ground-glass opacity and/or diffuse small nodules. Sometimes recurrent transient opacities superimposed on a fine micronodular pattern may be seen.[58] Diffuse, small centrilobular nodules of ground-glass attenuation are seen on CT, which are characteristic of subacute hypersensitivity pneumonitis. Chronic hypersensitivity pneumonitis demonstrates traction bronchiectasis and interstitial thickening often associated with areas of ground-glass opacity and mosaic perfusion. The major differential diagnosis is idiopathic pulmonary fibrosis.[58]

Semi-invasive and *invasive aspergillosis* will be dealt in detail in a later chapter.

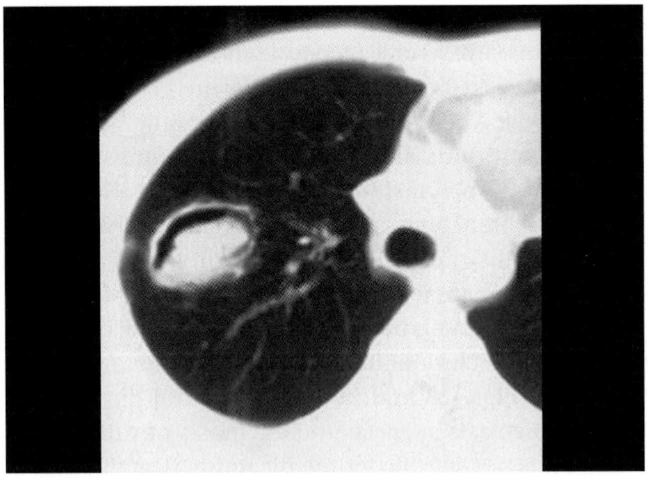

Fig. 27: *Aspergilloma*: CT shows the fungus ball lying in dependent portion of the cavity with a characteristic air-crescent sign.

Cryptococcosis

Cryptococcosis is caused by the fungus *Cryptococcus neoformans*. Although it can occur as pulmonary or disseminated disease in otherwise normal individuals, cryptococcosis is more frequently seen to affect immunocompromised patients. In the immunocompetent individuals, the radiographic findings can be single or multiple pulmonary nodules or areas of segmental or lobar consolidation. Cavitation and pleural effusion are rare. Hilar and mediastinal lymphadenopathy may be seen. Rarely a disseminated pattern of bronchopneumonia may be seen. Many patients with cryptococcal pneumonia have no symptoms and the pulmonary lesions seen radiographically heal spontaneously.[34]

2. Primary pathogens: Fungi that frequently infect healthy individuals constitute the primary pathogens. These include species like *Histoplasma*, *Coccidioides*, *Blastomyces*, and *Paracoccidioides*. They are natural inhabitants of North and South America and are not commonly found in the Indian subcontinent.[54,59]

Histoplasmosis

It is caused by the fungus *Histoplasma capsulatum* which is found in moist soil and in bird excreta in many parts of the world, but human infection is only seen with more frequency in parts of North America.[17] The radiographic picture closely resembles tuberculosis. In both, there is necrosis of pulmonary tissue followed by fibrosis and contraction. Parenchymal and/ or nodal calcification is commonly seen. Other manifestations can be pulmonary granulomas or small nodules scattered in both lung fields resembling military tuberculosis. An uncommon late

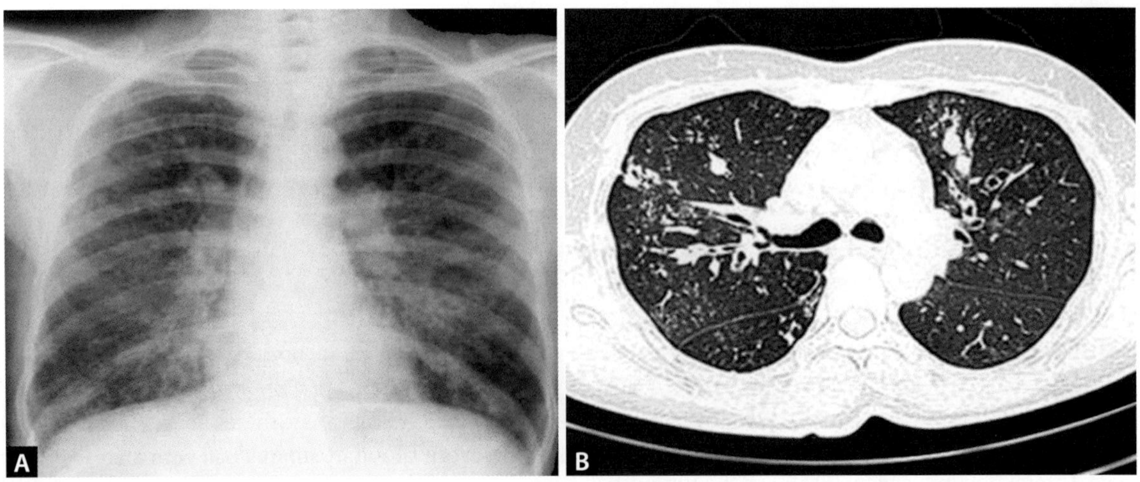

Figs. 28A and B: *Allergic bronchopulmonary aspergillosis (ABPA)*: Chest radiograph (A) and HRCT scan (B) showing bronchial thickening, central bronchiectasis and mucoid impaction within dilated bronchi and bronchioles in bilateral lung fields.

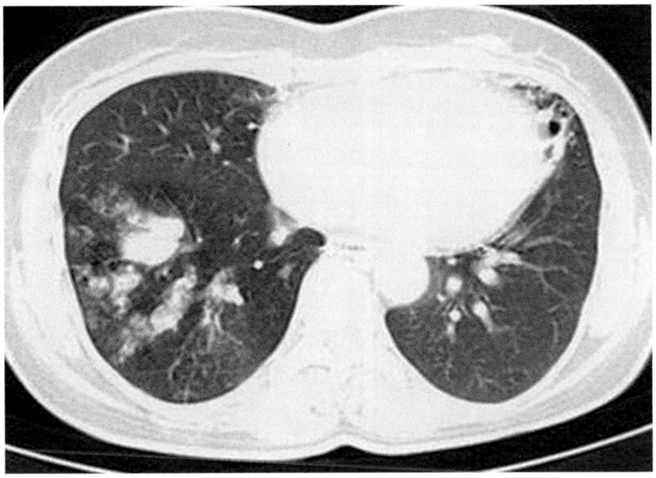

Fig. 29: CT scan in ABPA showing the characteristic "gloved finger" sign of mucoid-filled dilated bronchi in right lower lobe.

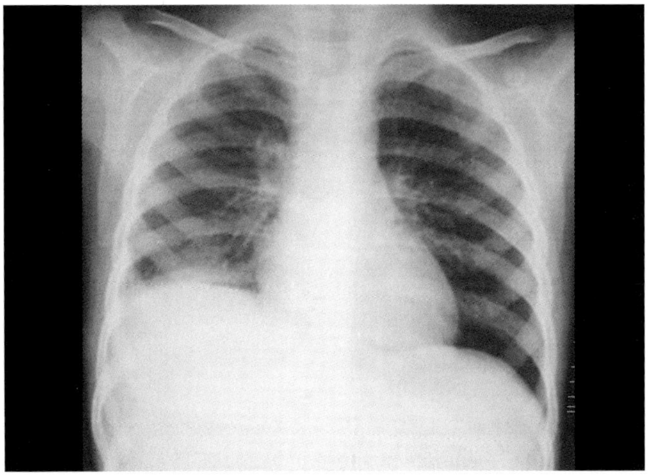

Fig. 30: Chest radiograph shows elevation of right dome of diaphragm with associated pleural effusion and basal consolidation. Ultrasound showed a subdiaphragmatic liver abscess.

manifestation of histoplasmosis is a fibrosing mediastinitis which can be well evaluated by CT.[17]

Coccidioidomycosis

It is caused by the fungus *Coccidioides immitis* and found principally in endemic areas in southwestern United States and northern Mexico. The most common radiological manifestation of primary coccidioidomycosis is a single or multiple foci of airspace consolidation. Thin walled cavities, pleural effusion and mediastinal lymphadenopathy may rarely be seen. Most patients of primary coccidioidomycosis recover within 3 weeks. Patients with persisting radiographic abnormalities after 6–8 weeks are considered to have chronic pulmonary coccidioidomycosis. The radiologic manifestations include lung nodules, cavities and rarely bronchiectasis and scarring. Apical fibrocavitary disease with lobar contraction, bronchiectasis and rarely calcification may resemble reactivation tuberculosis.[34]

Parasitic Infections

Protozoal Infections

Pleuropulmonary amebiasis is usually secondary to liver involvement.[60,61] Pleural effusion and lower lobe consolidation may be present contiguous to an amebic abscess in the liver or sub-diaphragmatic space, just as they may accompany any other suppurative process in these sites. Changes can occur at the base of either lung, because of the relationship of the liver to the diaphragm, but are much more frequent on the right. An amebic liver abscess may extend through the diaphragm into the pleural cavity, giving rise to an empyema. If it extends into the lung, it can cause pneumonia or a lung abscess.[62]

Chest radiographs may show an elevated hemidiaphragm, pleural effusion and/or thickening and basal atelectasis **(Fig. 30)**. If the abscess ruptures through the diaphragm, basal consolidation with cavitation may be seen. Fistulas may develop to airways, pericardium or rarely skin. The diagnosis can be established by ultrasound, CT or MRI and serological tests **(Figs. 31A to C)**.

Metazoal Infestations

Roundworm, hookworm and strongyloides infections: Many parasitic worms including Ascaris, Taenia, Ankylostoma, and Strongyloides pass through the lungs as part of their life cycle. In most instances, no pulmonary complications occur with any of these worms, but in a few patients, an allergic reaction takes place in the lung parenchyma, which manifests itself radiographically as dense migratory pulmonary consolidations without recognizable segmental distribution **(Fig. 32)**.[34,63] Blood and sputum eosinophilia are often present and the entity is therefore included as one of the causes of Loeffler's syndrome.[64]

Filariasis

The most common filarial worm to cause pulmonary manifestations is *Wuchereria bancrofti* which is responsible for elephantiasis. *W. bancrofti* can cause tropical eosinophilia, which is a syndrome consisting of cough, wheezing and severe blood eosinophilia. It is believed to occur due to an immunologic response to microfilariae rather than to a direct infection. The chest radiograph either be normal

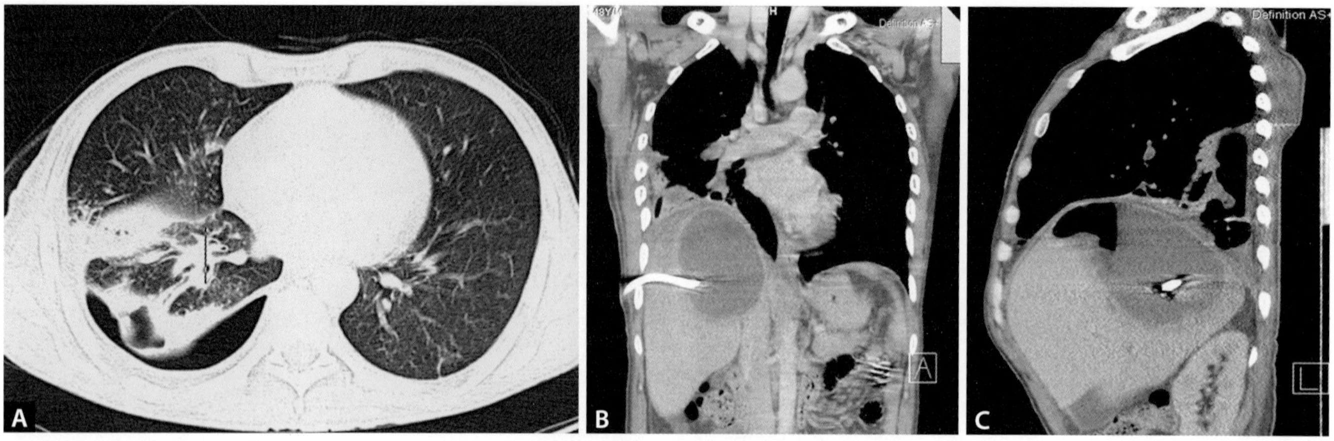

Figs. 31A to C: *Pleuropulmonary amebiasis*: CECT axial-lung window (A), coronal (B) and sagittal (C). *Mediastinal window*: A large abscess in the liver with a drain *in situ*, with a loculated pyopneumothorax and focal basal consolidation suggestive of an amebic liver abscess which has ruptured through the diaphragm.

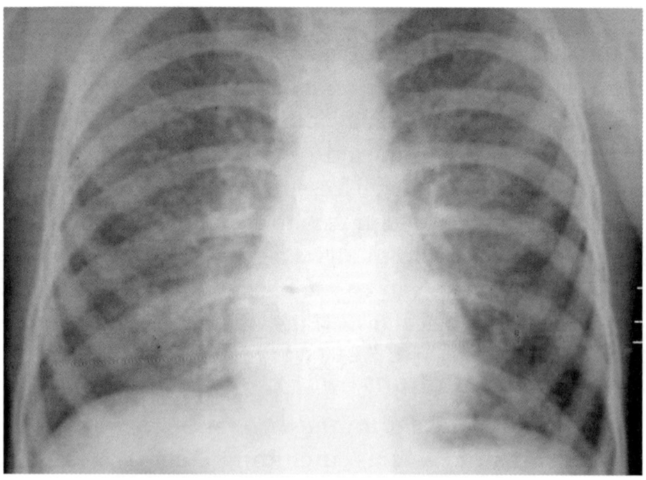

Fig. 32: *Tropical eosinophilia*: Chest radiograph shows diffuse nodular opacities in a child presenting with cough with a TLC of 40,000 cells/cc with 75% eosinophils.

or may show widespread fine nodular or reticulonodular shadowing, closely resembling military tuberculosis. Occasionally, localized consolidation may be seen.[65]

Echinococcus Infection/Hydatid Disease

Echinococcus infection is caused by a tapeworm *Echinococcus granulosus*. Humans are actually accidental hosts and acquire the infection by ingesting ova from fomites or contaminated water and by direct contact with dogs. Larvae develop in the host's duodenum, enter the bloodstream and travel to the end organs. Liver is the most common organ involved, followed by the lung. Cysts develop around this parasite in the end organs. The cyst wall consists of 3 layers: an outermost layer or the "pericyst" is a fibrotic capsule formed by the compression of the adjacent lung tissue. The cyst itself has a thin wall composed of 2 adherent layers, an outer ectocyst and an inner delicate lining—the endocyst. Multiple cysts are seen in approximately one third of patients and are bilateral in 20%.[66]

Unruptured pulmonary cysts are generally asymptomatic and may be discovered incidentally on a routine chest film. They are homogeneous, roughly spherical or oval, sharply demarcated mass lesions, ranging in size from 1–10 cm and occur more commonly in mid and lower zones **(Fig. 33A)**. CT scan shows the masses to be cystic in nature with a well-defined enhancing wall **(Fig. 33B)**. The internal contents are of water density and daughter cysts when present, are curved septations within the main cyst. The cysts are relatively pliant and mould to adjacent structures, resulting in indentation, lobulation and flattening. Calcification, which is a common feature of hydatid cysts in the liver, is very rare in lung cysts. Approximately, two-thirds of the cysts rupture. Cyst rupture may occur into the surrounding lung, airways or pleural space. If the pericyst ruptures, with the two inner layers remaining intact, air dissects between the pericyst and ectocyst giving rise to a crescent or meniscus sign. If there is disruption of the inner layers, a complex cavitatory lesion results which may show any of the following features like air fluid level, a floating membrane—water-lily sign **(Figs. 34A to C)**, a double wall, an essentially dry cyst with crumpled membranes lying at its bottom **(Fig. 35)**, or an empty cyst.[67] All these signs are particularly well seen on CT.[68] CT may also show air bubbles or blebs in the wall of a hydatid cyst which are specific for detection of rupture.[69] Secondary infection of

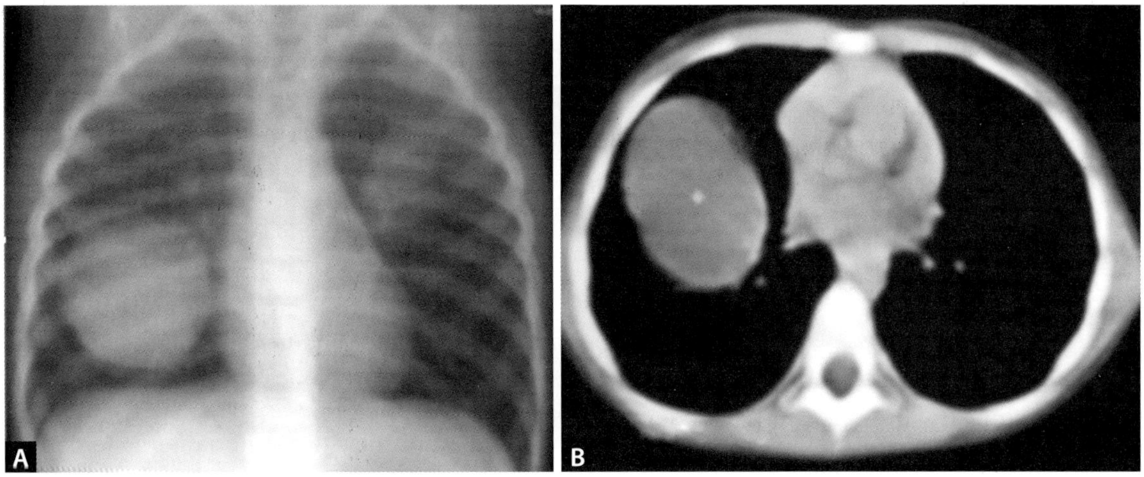

Figs. 33A and B: *Hydatid cyst*: Chest radiograph (A) shows a well-defined slightly lobulated mass in right lower zone and another oval shaped mass in left upper zone. CT scan (B) through the lower mass shows a homogeneous fluid density cyst.

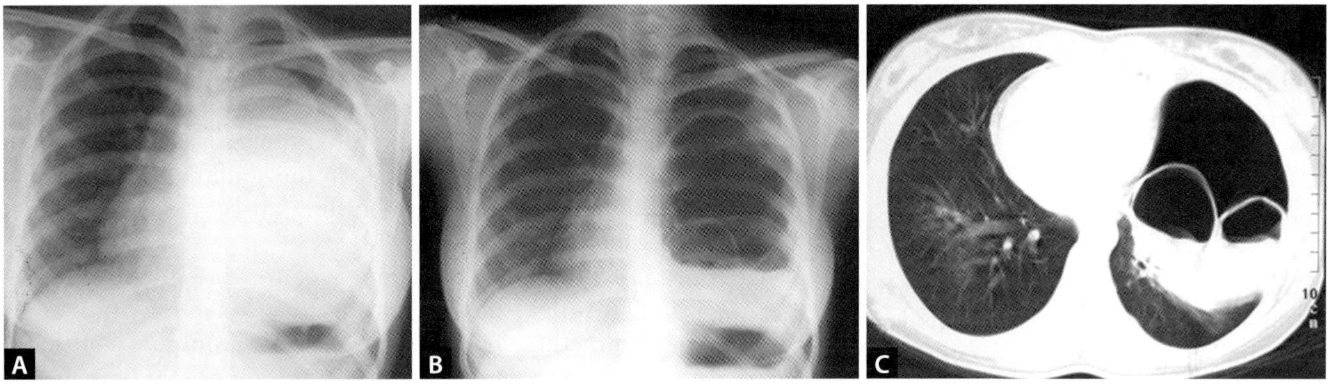

Figs. 34A to C: Chest radiograph (A) shows an unusually large unruptured hydatid cyst in left lung field, displacing the mediastinum to the right. After rupture, chest radiograph (B) and CT scan (C) show air-fluid level within the cyst with floating membranes—Water-lily sign.

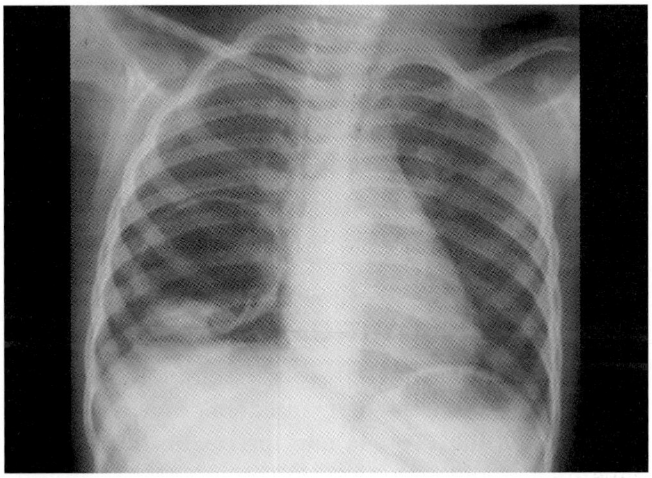

Fig. 35: Chest radiograph shows ruptured hydatid cyst with crumpled membranes lying at the bottom of the cyst.

a hydatid cyst may produce a lung abscess with or without surrounding consolidation. Rupture into the pleural space causes an effusion or if there is an additional airway communication, a hydropneumothorax.

MRI can display complex cysts contents well and the cyst membrane, whether collapsed or not, is clearly seen as a low intensity curvilinear structure on both T1W and T2W sequences. MRI and MDCT reconstructions may be particularly helpful in revealing the exact location of a hydatid cyst in relation to the diaphragm.[70,71]

COMPLICATIONS OF PNEUMONIA

Pleural Effusion and Empyema

Parapneumonic effusions complicate the course of 20–60% of patients hospitalized with bacterial pneumonia.[72] Effusions are quite common in staphylococcal and gram-negative pneumonias, much less common in pneumococcal pneumonias and distinctly unusual in viral and mycoplasmal infections.

Parapneumonic effusion progresses to empyema formation in 5–10% of patients, resolution occurs in the rest with antibiotic therapy. Progression to empyema in debilitated and elderly patients increases morbidity and likelihood of mortality.

The choice of modality for evaluation of effusion depends on the clinical context. Blunting of costo phrenic angle occurs in a chest radiograph with pleural fluid up to 200–500 mL.[73] Ultrasound is useful for detecting small amount of fluid (as little as 5 mL), loculations and viscosity.[74] On the other hand, CT allows detailed evaluation of complex fluid collections **(Fig. 36)**.

Hydropneumothorax

The appearance of gas in the pleural space together with fluid is usually iatrogenic in origin. It may be associated with a bronchopleural fistula casued by rupture of a pneumatocele or abscess, and is seen particularly with *S.aureus*, gram-negative and anaerobic infections.

Pneumatoceles

Pneumatoceles commonly follow staphylococcal infections in children (not so common in adults). They are thin- walled cavities of variable sizes **(Fig. 14)**. They are formed due to check valve obstruction between the lumen of a small bronchus and adjacent interstitium. They can resolve completely or persist for months in which case they are of no clinical significance unless they cause pressure on adjacent structures.

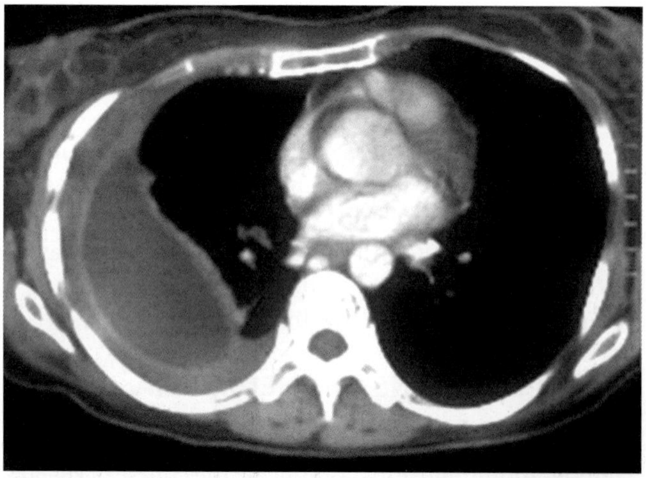

Fig. 36: CT scan in a case of empyema showing a homogeneous lenticular-shaped fluid collection based on the chest wall enclosed within thick enhancing pleura—split pleura sign.

Bronchiectasis

Bronchiectasis commonly occurs during the acute phase of pneumonia but resolves as the inflammation subsides.[75] Occasionally this can persist and act as source of hemoptysis or recurrent infections.

Pulmonary Abscess, Necrotizing Pneumonia and Pulmonary Gangrene

These conditions present a continuum caused by microbial infections, predominantly anaerobic microbes.[76] *Abscess* occurs due to cavitation secondary to necrosis in a variety of bacterial pneumonias, particularly those caused by *S. aureus*, gram-negative bacteria and anaerobes. Cavitation is also seen in amebic, fungal and metazoal infections, but it is rare with viral and mycoplasmal pneumonias. Abscesses that fail to establish airway communication do not cavitate and are undetected on chest radiographs, being isodense with surrounding consolidated lung. However, they can be seen on CT because of the low attenuation centre within the abscess **(Figs. 37A and B)**.

Necrotizing pneumonia is characterized by consolidation combined with peripheral necrosis and formation of multiple small cavities. In the continuum, necrotising pneumonia lies between lung abscess and pulmonary gangrene **(Figs. 38A to C)**.[77,78]

Pulmonary gangrene occurs due to progressive devitalization of pulmonary parenchyma. It is characterized by sloughing of a pulmonary segment or lobe as a consequence of thrombosis in branches of pulmonary and bronchial arteries supplying the necrotic area.[79] CECT shows obliteration of the pulmonary artery supply to the segment or lobe which has large cavities and necrotic parenchyma.[77]

Differential diagnosis of necrotizing pulmonary infections includes infected bullae, pleural empyemas and lung tumors.[76]

Miscellaneous Complications

Miscellaneous complications such as osteomyelitis, obliterative bronchiolitis and acute respiratory distress syndrome can occur.

DELAYED RESOLUTION OF PNEUMONIA

Non-resolving or slowly resolving pneumonia (NRP) refers to persistence of radiographic abnormalities beyond the expected time course and affects 10–20% patients hospitalized with community acquired pneumonia (CAP).[80]

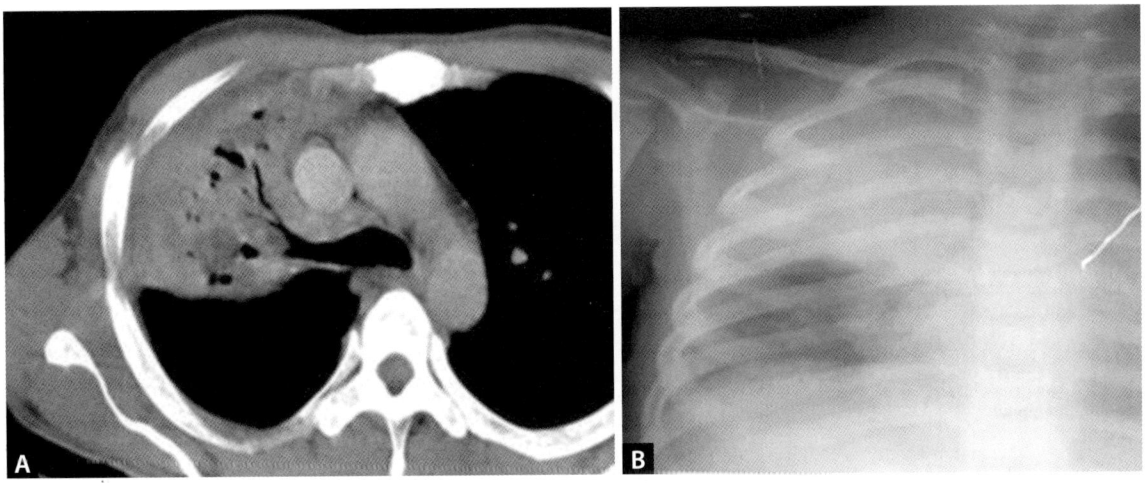

Figs. 37A and B: CT scan (A) demonstrates dense consolidation in the right upper lobe containing a focal region of low attenuation and gas consistent with necrosis and abscess formation not appreciated on chest radiograph (B)

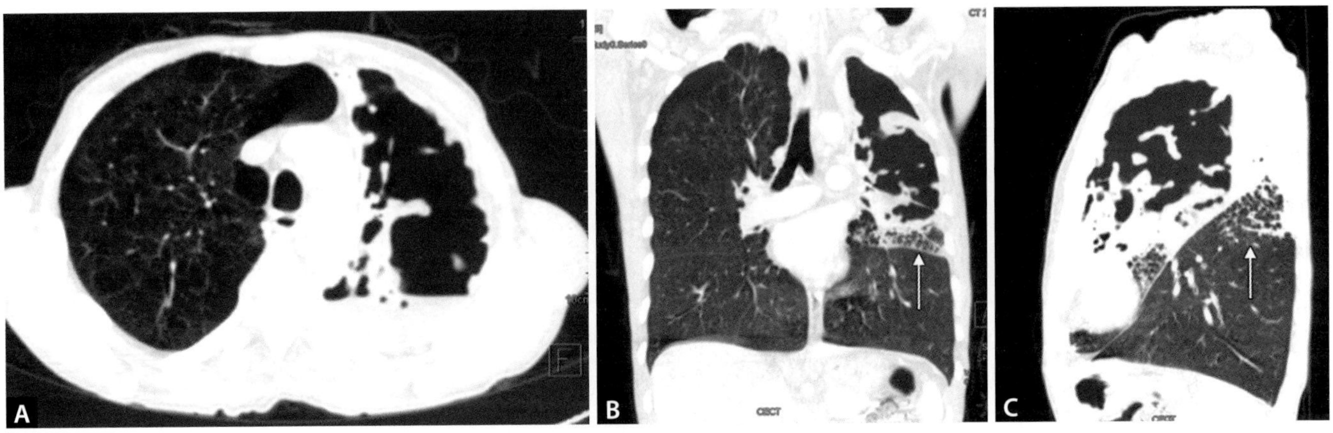

Figs. 38A to C: *Necrotizing pneumonia*: Axial (A), Coronal (B) and Sagittal (C) CECT in a 65 year old patient with emphysema shows consolidation of left upper lobe with marked destruction of the lung parenchyma with an air-fluid level. Adjacent areas of consolidation show small cysts within due to centriacinar emphysema (arrows in B and C)

It has been defined as either less than 50% clearing at 2 weeks or less than complete clearing after 4 weeks inspite of antibiotic therapy for a minimum period of 10 days.[81]

The various causes that can lead to non-resolving pneumonia are listed in **Table 5**.[82] Causes may be pathogen related or host related. The presence of complications is another cause of delayed resolution of pneumonia. Non-infectious diseases or "pneumonia mimics" as enumerated in the table can be misdiagnosed as pneumonia and thus be another reason for delayed resolution. In our country, tuberculosis is one of the most common cause for a non-resolving pneumonia **(Figs. 39A to D)**.[83]

Further evaluation in the form of CT chest, microbiological tests for etiological agent, bronchoscopy, biopsy and other tests specific to the suspected organisms/disease are required for these patients.

Diagnostic Algorithm in Patients Suspected with Pneumonia

An imaging algorithm for diagnosis of pneumonia has been suggested in **Flowchart 1**. In patients with mild disease, empirical treatment usually suffices, whereas in patients with severe disease, an aggressive approach is sometimes needed for identification of specific causative organism. Demonstration of the pathogen can be done by examination of stained smears of sputum, pleural fluid, by culture of respiratory secretions, blood or other biological material. Interventional procedures like transthoracic needle biopsy done, ultrasound or CT guidance are a reliable and cost-effective means to obtain material for culture.[84]

In cases with underlying co-morbidities or immuno-suppressed state of the host, specific treatment may be

Table 5: Causes of non-resolving pneumonia.

Factors	*Causes*
Pathogen-related	• Atypical organism • Resistant organism • Uncommon organism • Nosocomial infection
Host-related	• Severity of initial illness • Presence of comorbidities • Immunosuppressed state • Metastatic infection
Presence of complications	• Para-pneumonic effusion/empyema • Abscess • Gangrene
Non-infectious disease	• Neoplastic disorders (adenocarcinoma *in situ*, lymphoma, lymphangitis carcinomatosis, etc.) • Pulmonary embolism • Systemic vasculitis (Wegner's granulomatosis) • Connective tissue disorders • Drug-induced disorders (amodiarone, nitrofurantoin, methotrexate, etc.) • Cryptogenic organizing pneumonia • Eosinophilic pneumonia • Congestive cardiac failure

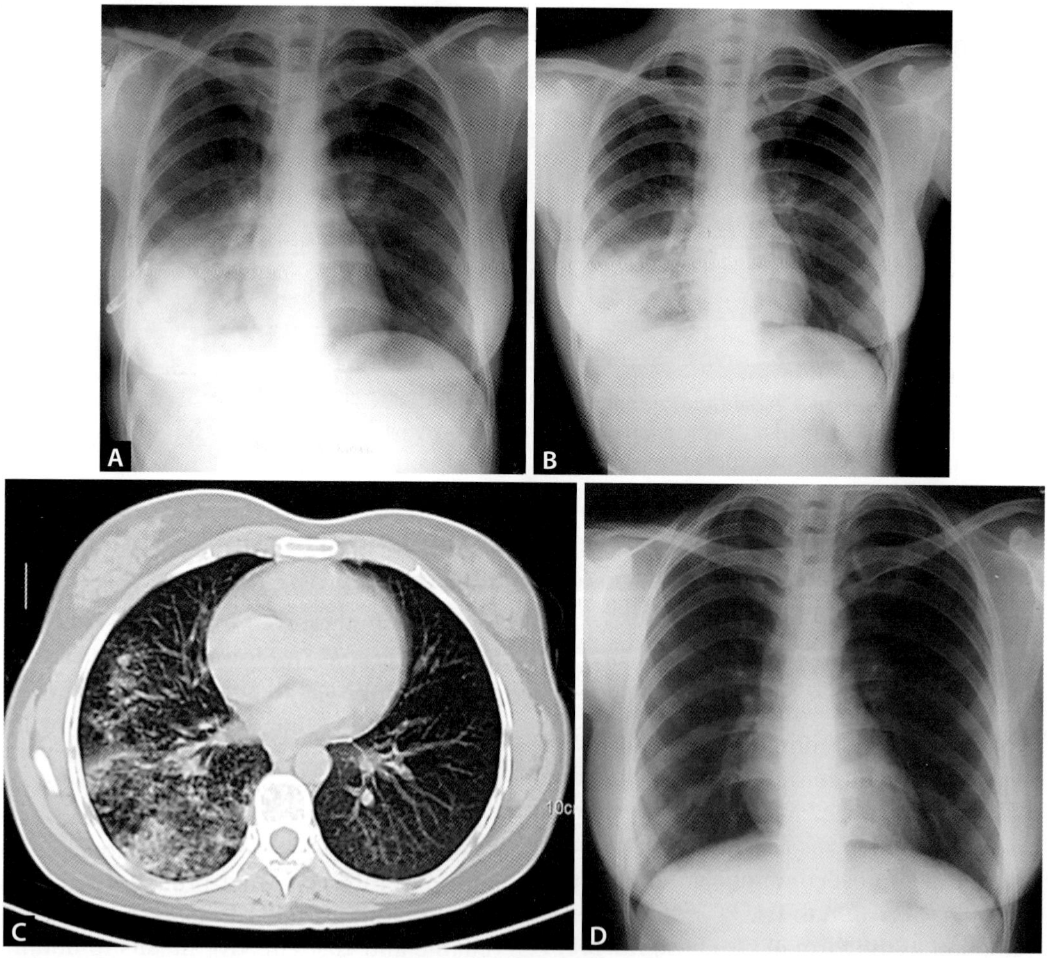

Figs. 39A to D: *Non-resolving pneumonia*: Chest radiograph (A) in a young 25-year-old girl with high-grade fever and cough, shows a right lower zone consolidation, which shows only partial clearance even after a prolonged course of antibiotics on chest radiograph (B) after 5 weeks. CT (C) showed multiple focal lobular alveolar and tree-in–bud opacities. ATT was started. Chest radiograph (D) after 4 weeks of ATT shows complete resolution.

Flowchart 1: Clinicoradiological algorithm for diagnosis of pneumonia.

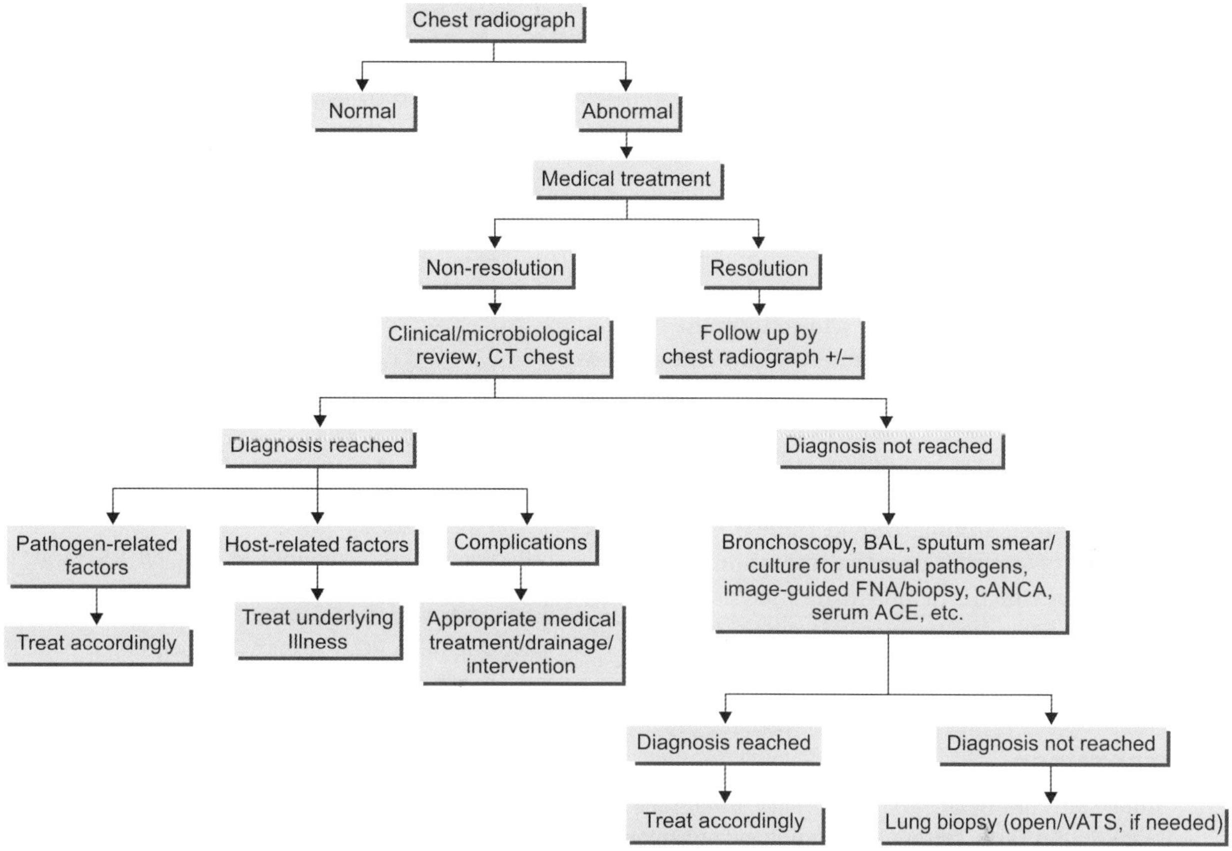

Abbreviations: BAL: Bronchoalveolar lavage; cANCA: Cytoplasmic antineutrophil cytoplasmic antibodies; ACE: Angiotensin-converting enzyme; VATS: Video-assisted thoracoscopic surgery.

Table 6: Summary of clinical and radiographic clues to the etiological diagnosis of pneumonia.[84]

Radiographic findings	***Clinical circumstance***	***Organism***
Segmental consolidation	Community-acquired	*S. pneumoniae, M. pneumoniae*
Lobar consolidation	Community-acquired diabetes	*S. pneumoniae* (2/3 of community-acquired pneumonias), *K. pneumoniae* Gram-negative bacilli
Round pneumonia	Community-acquired	S. pneumoniae
Bronchopneumonia	Hospital-acquired	*P. aeruginosa, S. aureus*, streptococci, gram- negative bacilli, anaerobes, *M. pneumoniae*, aspiration
Interstitial pneumonia	Community-acquired	Virus, *M. pneumoniae*
Cavitation/necrosis	Aspiration COPD	*S. aureus*, Gram-negative bacilli, anaerobes, *Actinomycosis*, *M. tuberculosis*, *Aspergillus*
Multiple cavitatory nodules	Drug addict, septicemia	*S. aureus*
Pneumatoceles	Postinfluenza	*S. aureus*
Empyema	Complication of pneumonia	*S. pneumoniae, S. aureus,* Gram-negative bacilli, *M. tuberculosis*
Chest wall invasion	Alcoholic	Actinomycosis, *M. tuberculosis,* Fungi
Lymphadenopathy		*M. pneumoniae, M. tuberculosis*

initiated accordingly. In cases of complicated pneumonia CT can assist in identify in the complication and hence aid management. If the disease is suspected to be a "pneumonia minic", specific and ancillary test may be needed to reach a conclusive diagnosis.

CONCLUSION

Chest radiography is the imaging technique of choice in evaluating patients with suspected pneumonia because of its low radiation dose, low cost, and wide accessibility. In daily practice, radiographs are used to confirm the clinical diagnosis of pneumonia, characterize the extent and severity of disease, search for complications, monitor the response to therapy, and examine for possible alternative or additional diagnoses. The radiographic pattern needs to be correlated with the clinical background to suggest an etiological diagnosis summarized in **Table 6**. CT scan has the advantage of superior contrast resolution and cross-sectional display which is helpful in the analysis of complex or slowly resolving cases, particularly when radiographic evidence of associated conditions and complications is equivocal.

REFERENCES

1. Padley SPG, Rubens MB. Pulmonary infections. In: David Sutton (Ed). Textbook of Radiology and Imaging. Edinburgh: Churchill Livingstone. 2003;1:131-60.
2. Kalil AC, Metersky ML, Klompas M, et al. Management of adults with hospital-acquired and ventilator-associated pneumonia: 2016 Clinical Practice Guidelines by the Infectious Diseases Society of America and the American Thoracic Society. Clin Infect Dis. 2016;63(5):e61-e111.
3. Alkhayat KF, Hasan M, Alam-Eldeen. Value of chest ultrasound in diagnosis of community acquired pneumonia. Egyptian Journal of Chest Diseases and Tuberculosis. 2014;63(4):1047-51.
4. Schenck EJ, Rajwani K. Ultrasound in the diagnosis and management of pneumonia. Current Opinion in Infectious Diseases. 2016;29(2):223-8.
5. Pereda MA, Chavez MA, Hooper-Miele CA, et al. Lung ultrasound for the diagnosis of pneumonia in children: A meta-analysis. Pediatrics. 2015;135(4):715-22.
6. Sodhi KS, Khandelwal N, Saxena AK, et al. Rapid lung MRI in children with pulmonary infections: Time to change our diagnostic algorithms. J Magn Reson Imaging. 2016;43: 1196-1206.
7. Liszewski M, Görkem S, Sodhi K, Lee E. Lung magnetic resonance imaging for pneumonia in children. Pediatric Radiology. 2017;47(11):1420-30.
8. Spencer H. The bacterial pneumonias. Pathology of the lung, 4th edn. Oxford: Pergamon Press. 1985. pp. 167-212.
9. Blaivas M. Lung Ultrasound in Evaluation of Pneumonia. Journal of Ultrasound Medicine. 2012;31:823.
10. Liechtenstein D, Meziere G, Seitz J. The dynamic air bronchogram: A lung ultrasound sign of alveolar consolidation ruling out atelectasis. Chest. 2009;135(6):1421-5.
11. Tanaka N, Matsumoto T, Kuramitsu T. High Resolution CT finding in Community-acquired Pneumonia. J Comput Assist Tomogr. 1996; 20(4):600-08.
12. Beigelman-Aubry C, Godet C, Caumes E. Lung infections: The radiologist's perspective. Diagn Intervent Imaging. 2012;93:431-40.
13. ER Heitzman. The radiological diagnosis of pneumonia in the adult: A commentary. Semin in Roentgenology. 1989;XXIV(4):212-17.
14. Rose RW, Ward BH. Spherical pneumonias in children simulating pulmonary and mediastinal masses. Radiology. 1973;106:179-82.
15. Wang N. Anatomy. In: Dial DH, Hammar SP (Eds). Pulmonary Pathology. New York: Springer Verlag. 1988;17-40.
16. Wagner AL, Szabunio M, Hazlett KS, et al. Radiologic manifestations of round pneumonia in adults. AJR. 1998;170:723-26.
17. Goodman PC, Wilson AG, Armstrong P, et al. Pulmonary Infections in Adults. In: Grainger RG, Allison D, et al (Eds). Diagnostic Radiology, Edinburgh: Churchill Livingstone. 2001;377-417.
18. Scanlon GT, Unger JD. The Radiology of Bacterial and Viral Pneumonias. RCNA. 1973;11(2):317-38.
19. Smith CB, Overall JC. Clinical and epidemiologic clues to the diagnosis of respiratory infections. RCNA. 1973;11(2):261-78.
20. Fein AM, Feinsilver SH, Niederman MS. Atypical manifestations of pneumonia in the elderly. Clin Chest Med. 1991;12:319.
21. Nambu A, Ozawa K, Kobayashi N, et al. Imaging of community-acquired pneumonia: Roles of imaging examinations, imaging diagnosis of specific pathogens and discrimination from noninfectious diseases. World J Radiol. 2014;6(10):779-93.
22. Franquet T, Giménez A, Rosón N, Torrubia S, Sabaté JM, Pérez C. Aspiration diseases: findings, pitfalls, and differential diagnosis. Radiographics. 2000;20:673-85.
23. Gupta D, Agarwal R, Aggarwal AN, Singh N, Mishra N, Khilnani GC, et al. Pneumonia Guidelines Working Group. Guidelines for diagnosis and management of community- and hospital-acquired pneumonia in adults: Joint ICS/NCCP (I) recommendations. Lung India: Official Organ of Indian Chest Society. 2012;29(Suppl 2):S27.
24. Kieninger AN, Lipsett PA. Hospital-acquired pneumonia: pathophysiology, diagnosis, and treatment. Surg Clin North Am. 2009,89(2):439–61. ix 10.1016/j.suc.2008.11.001.
25. Rubin SA, Winer-Muram HT, Ellis JV. Diagnostic imaging of pneumonia and its complications in the critically ill patients. Clin Chest Med. 1995;16;45.
26. Beydon L, Saada M, Liu N, et al. Can portable chest X-ray examination accurately diagnose basal consolidation after

abdominal surgery? A comparison with CT scan. Chest. 1994;106:221-35.
27. Winer-Muram HT, Rubin SA, Ellis JV, et al. Pneumonia and ARDS patients receiving mechanical ventilation: Diagnostic accuracy of chest radiography. Radiology. 1993;188:479.
28. Winer-Muram HT, Steiner RM, Gurney JW: Ventilator-associated pneumonia in patients with adult respiratory distress syndrome: CT evaluation. Radiology. 1998;208:193.
29. A Trimble, V Moffat, AM Collins. Pulmonary infections in the returned traveller. Pneumonia. 2017;9:1
30. Kantor HG. The many radiologic faces of pneumococcal pneumonia. AJR. 1981;137:1213.
31. Shah RM, Gupta S, Angeid-Backman E, et al. Pneumococcal pneumonia in patients requiring hospitalization: Effects of bacteremia and HIV seropositivity on radiographic appearance. AJR. 2000;175(6):1533-36.
32. Macfarlane J, Rose D. Radiographic features of staphylococcal pneumonia in adults and children. Thorax. 1996;51:539-40.
33. Naraqi S, McDonnel G. Haematogenous staphylococcal pneumonia secondary to soft tissue infection. Chest. 1981;79:173-75.
34. Armstrong P. Bacterial pneumonia. In: Hansell DM, Armstrong P, Lynch DA, et al (Eds). Imaging of Diseases of Chest. Philadelphia: Mosby. 2005. pp. 183-276.
35. Bartlett JG, Finegold SM. Anaerobic infections of the lung and pleural space. Am Rev Respir Dis. 1974;110:56-77.
36. Groskin SA, Panicek DM, Ewing DK, et al. Bacterial lung abscess: A review of the radiographic and clinical features of 50 cases. J Thoracic Imaging. 1991;6:62-67.
37. Landay MJ, Christensen EE, Bynum LJ, et al. Anaerobic pleural and pulmonary infections. AJR. 1980;134;233.
38. Putnam CE, Curtis AM, Aimeone JF, et al. *Mycoplasma pneumonia*: Clinical and roentgenographic patterns. Radiology. 1975;124:417.
39. Reittner P, Muller NL, Heyneman L, et al. *Mycoplasma pneumoniae* pneumonia: Radiographic and high resolution CT features in 28 patients. AJR. 2000;174:37-41.
40. Traver RD, Shawn DT, Heitkamp DE, et al. Radiology of community-acquired pneumonia. RCNA. 2005;43: 497-512.
41. Poirier R, Rodrigue J, Villeneuve J, et al. Early radiographic and tomographic manifestations of Legionnaire's disease. Can Assoc Radiol J. Published online May 4, 2017.
42. Kim KW, Goo JM, Lee HJ, et al. Chest computed tomographic findings and clinical features of legionella pneumonia. J Comput Assist Tomogr. 2007;31 (6): 950-5.
43. Mabeza GF, Macfarlane J. Pulmonary actinomycosis. Eur Respir J. 2003;21:545-51.
44. Frank P, Strickland B. Pulmonary actinomycosis. Br J Radiol. 1974;47:373-78.
45. Cheon JE, Im JG, Kim MH, et al. Thoracic actionomycosis: CT findings. Radiology. 1998;209:229-33.
46. Greenberg SB. Viral pneumonia. Infect Dis Clin North Am. 1991;5:603-21.
47. Waite S, Jeudy J, White CS. Acute lung infections in normal and immunocompromised hosts. RCNA. 2006;44:295-315.
48. Kim EA, Lee KS, Primack SL, et al. Viral pneumonias in adults: radiologic and pathologic findings. Radiographics. 2002;22:S137-49.
49. Chowell G, Bertozzi SM, Colchero MA, et al. Severe respiratory disease concurrent with the circulation of H1N1 influenza. N Engl J Med. 2009;361(7):674–9.
50. Abdelsalam M, Diab HS, Ragab Y. Radiologoical findings in patients with H1N1 influenza pneumonia. Egyptian Journal of Chest diseases and Tuberculosis. 2016;65(1):135-42.
51. Qureshi NR, Hien TT, Farrar J, et al. The radiologic manifestations of H5N1 avian influenza. J Thorac Imaging. 2006;21(4):259-64.
52. Teper AM, Kofman CD, Maffey AF, et al. Lung function in infants with chronic pulmonary disease after severe adenoviral illness. J Pediatr. 1999;134:730-33.
53. Gotway MB, Dawn SK, Caoili EM, et al. The radiologic spectrum of pulmonary Aspergillus infections. JCAT. 2002;26(2):159-73.
54. Panda BN. Fungal infections of lungs: The emerging scenario. Indian J Tuberculosis. 2004;51:63-69.
55. Johnson J. Pulmonary aspergillosis. Semin Respir Med. 1987;9:87-199.
56. Roberts CM, Citron KM, Strickland B. Intrathoracic aspergilloma. Role of CT in diagnosis and treatment. Radiology 1987;165:123-28.
57. Neeld DA, Goodman LR, Gurney JW, et al. Computerized tomography in the evaluation of allergic bronchopulmonary aspergillosis. Am Rev Respir Dis. 1990;142:1200-05.
58. Patel RA, Sellami D, Gotway MB, et al. Hypersensitivity pneumonitis: Spectrum of imaging findings. JCAT. 2000; 24:965-70.
59. Fraser RS, Pare JAP, Eraser RG, Pare PD. Infectious Diseases of Lungs in Synopsis of Diseases of Chest (2nd edn). WB Saunders and Co; Philadelphia. 1994;332-54.
60. Wilson ES. Pleuropulmonary amebiasis. AJR. 1971;111:518- 24.
61. Kinura K, Stoopen M, Reeder MM, et al. Amebiasis: Modern diagnostic imaging with pathological and clinical correlation. Semin Roentgenol. 1997;32:250-75.
62. Shamsuzzaman SM, Haschiguchi Y. Thoracic amebiasis. Clin Chest Med. 2002;23:479-92.
63. Bean W. Recognition of ascariasis by routine chest or abdomen roentgenograms. AJR. 1965;94:379-84.
64. Gelpi AP, Mustafa A. Ascaiasis pneumonia. Am J Med. 1968;44:377-89.
65. Udwadia E. Tropical eosinophilia. Prog Respir Res. 1975;7:35-155.
66. Beggs I. The radiology of hydatid disease. AJR. 1985;145:639- 48.
67. Von Sinner WN. Radiographic, CT and MRI spectrum of hydatid disease of chest: A pictorial essay. Eur Radiol. 1993;3:62-70.
68. Kervancioglu R, Bayram M, Elbeyli L. CT and MRI spectrum of hydatid disease. Acta Radiol. 1999;40:510-14.
69. Kokturk O, Ozturk C, Diren B, et al. Air bubble: A new diagnostic CT sign of perforated pulmonary hydatid cyst. Eur Radiol. 1999;9:1321-23.

70. Von Sinner WN. New diagnostic signs in hydatid disease; radiography, ultrasound, CT and MRI correlated to pathology. Em J Radiol. 1991;12:150-59.
71. Prieto A, Diaz A, Calvo J, et al. MR imaging of pulmonary hydatid disease. Eur J radiol. 1996;23:85-87.
72. Heffner JE. Infection of the pleural space. Clinics in Chest Medicine. 1999;20(3):607-20.
73. Blackmore CC Black WC, Dallas RV, et al. Pleural fluid volume estimation: A chest radiograph prediction rule. Acta Radiol. 1996;3:103.
74. Hirsh JH, Rogers JV, Mack LA. Real-time sonography of pleural opacities. AJR. 1981;136:297.
75. Nelson SW, Christoforidis AJ. Reversible bronchiectasis. Radiology. 1958;71:375.
76. Poole PS, Stark HE, Stark P. Necrotizing pneumonia, pulmonary abscess, and lung gangrene: multiple pathways to lung parenchymal destruction. Contemporary Diagnostic Radiology. 2011;34(13):1-6.
77. Reimel BA, Krishnadasen B, Cuschieri J, Klein MB, Gross J, Karmy-Jones R. Surgical management of acute necrotizing lung infections. Can Respir J. 2006;13:369–73. [PMC free article] [PubMed]
78. Penner C, Maycher B, Long R. Pulmonary gangrene: A complication of bacterial pneumonia. Chest. 1994;105:567-73. [PubMed]
79. Curry CA, Fish aEK, Buckley JA. Pulmonary gangrene: Radiological and pathologic correlation. South Med J. 1998;91:957–60. [PubMed]
80. Finich S, Chalmers JD. Brief clinical review: Non-responding pneumonia. EMJ Respir. 2014;2:104-11.
81. Kirtland SH, Winterbauer RH. Slowly resolving chronic and recurrent pneumonia. Clin Chest Med. 1991;12:303-18.
82. Kuru T, Lynch JP. Nonresolving or slowly resolving pneumonia. Clin Chest Med. 1999;20:623-51.
83. Jayaprakash B, Varkey V, Anithakumari K. Etiology and clinical outcome of non-resolving pneumonia in a tertiary care centre. J Assoc Physicians India. 2012;60:98-101.
84. Franquet T. Imaging of Pneumonia: Trends and algorithms. Eur Respir J. 2001;18:196-208.

CHAPTER 162

Pulmonary Manifestations in Immunocompromised Host

Mandeep Kang, Pankaj Gupta

INTRODUCTION

Immunocompromised hosts constitute a special group of patients who are predisposed to infections by both opportunistic and non-opportunistic organisms.[1] The number of individuals who are immunocompromised is growing steadily, not only because of the continuing human immunodeficiency virus/acquired immunodeficiency syndrome (HIV/AIDS) epidemic, but also due to the growing incidence of various kinds of malignancies and the increasing number of patients undergoing solid organ or bone marrow transplants. Pulmonary infections are a major cause of mortality and morbidity in this group of patients.[2-4] Diagnostic possibilities include infections (opportunistic or routine), hemorrhage, spread of underlying malignancy, chemotherapy or radiotherapy induced lung changes and conditions not directly related to the underlying disease process such as congestive heart failure or pulmonary embolism, therefore the development of a pulmonary infiltrate on the chest radiograph is an ominous sign which poses a considerable diagnostic challenge.[5]

This chapter will separately address two groups of patients which are: HIV/AIDS patients and non-HIV immunocompromised patients who have hematological malignancy or have recieved solid organ or hematopoietic stem cell transplantation.

HIV/AIDS

The epidemic of HIV and AIDS has affected the entire world. According to the World Health Organization (WHO) and Joint United Nations program on HIV/AIDS, it was estimated in 2007 that there are around 33 million people living with HIV infection throughout the world. Around twenty-five million deaths have occurred due to AIDS with opportunistic pulmonary infections accounting for a majority of these.[6] Pulmonary infections will occur in nearly all patients with HIV infection during the course of their illness at some time. HIV infection is associated with an increased risk for lung complications due to alterations in the host defenses in the lung, such as muco-ciliary functional abnormalities and impairment in the immune response to pathogens.[7] In the past several years, there have been various trends noted in the demographics as well as treatment of HIV patients, which have had an important impact on the incidence of various pulmonary complications.[3,8] A change in the epidemiology with higher rates of infection in women and children and lower rates of infection in intravenous drug abusers (IVDA) and homosexual or bisexual men has been reported. IVDA are far more likely to suffer recurrent *Staphylococcus aureus* infections, aspiration pneumonia, lung abscess, septic emboli and tuberculosis (TB). In IVDAs, the rates of bacterial pneumonia are more than twice of any other risk group, regardless of the CD4+ lymphocyte count. Tuberculosis is much more common in Africa and South-East Asia, and globally, is the major cause of mortality (13% according to estimates by the World Health Organization).[9] Kaposi's sarcoma (KS) is seen almost exclusively in homosexual males. In the subset of the patient population who have acquired the HIV infection through sexual contact, *Cytomegalovirus* (CMV) infection is seen more commonly.

With the introduction in 1989 of trimethoprim sulfamethoxazole (TMP-SMX) prophylaxis, there has been a marked reduction in the frequency of *Pneumocystis jeroveci pneumonia* (PCP), however opportunistic infections by atypical mycobacteria and CMV have increased in incidence.[8]

The introduction of combination antiretroviral therapy (ART) which effectively suppresses viral replication, has resulted in decreased viral loads and increased CD4+ lymphocyte counts thereby dramatically reducing the HIV-associated morbidity and mortality. Conversely, immune restoration which occurs with initiation of HAART has been associated with new clinical syndromes known variously as reversal syndrome, immune reconstitution syndrome or paradoxical response.[9]

Systematic Approach to Imaging Diagnosis

A systematic approach should be employed for the radiological evaluation of HIV/AIDS patients. The chest radiograph should be carefully analyzed for the pattern of abnormality.[10] This should then be integrated with the available demographic, clinical and laboratory information for interpretation. The clinical presentation of the patient is of vital importance as diseases which present acutely or in a more insidious fashion may demonstrate an identical pattern on the chest radiograph. Awareness of the CD4+ lymphocyte count is of critical importance as it predicts the vulnerability of the patient to specific opportunistic infections and malignancies.

CD4+ count less than 200 cells/mm^3 marks clinical AIDS in a HIV positive patient. If CD4+ counts are higher than 500 cells/mm^3, there is an increased risk of infection with virulent pathogens leading to recurrent community acquired bacterial pneumonias and reactivation TB. When the CD4+ counts are between 200 and 499 cells/mm^3, lymphoproliferative disorders and primary lung carcinoma are seen in addition to the above infections. PCP and disseminated TB occur with increasing frequency with a count less than 200/mm^3, however, the greatest risk of PCP is seen below a count of 100/mm^3. At profound levels of immune depression with CD4+ counts below 50 cells/mm^3, viral pneumonias (commonly CMV), atypical mycobacterial infection and disseminated fungal infections have a markedly increased frequency.[7,11]

Imaging Methods

After a thorough history and complete physical examination, the next steps in the evaluation of a symptomatic patient are a chest radiograph, sputum and various blood examinations. If the radiographic and clinical findings are nonspecific or unrevealing, computed tomography (CT) of the chest and fiberoptic bronchoscopy (FOB) with bronchoalveolar lavage (BAL) are the usual next steps. The indications for CT include: (i) evaluation of symptomatic patients with normal chest radiographs, (ii) characterization of abnormalities detected on the chest radiograph, (iii) assessment for complications of pneumonia such as development of empyema or lung abscess, (iv) staging AIDS related malignancies and (v) planning and guiding biopsy procedures. Computed tomography has been shown to be highly sensitive for the detection of disease and fairly specific in its characterization. Most importantly, a normal CT chest virtually rules out a pneumonia as the site of infection.[12,13] Bronchoalveolar lavage and transbronchial lung biopsy (TBLB) have been shown to have a high diagnostic yield for the diagnosis of both PCP and CMV infections.[14]

Radiological Pattern Approach to Diagnosis

A useful approach in the evaluation of a symptomatic patient is to identify the radiological pattern and correlate the differential diagnosis of the specific pattern with the clinical findings and CD4+ counts.

Normal Chest Radiograph

Chest radiographs may be normal in 10–39% of patients with proven PCP at initial presentation **(Figs. 1A and B)**.[3,4,8] About 6 to 17% of AIDS patients with pulmonary TB with positive sputum may also have normal radiographs.

Ground-glass Opacities

Ground-glass opacity (GGO) on high-resolution CT (HRCT) in a patient with HIV/AIDS is highly sensitive for the diagnosis of PCP and may be seen in 92% of patients **(Figs. 1A and B)**. Viral infections such as CMV or herpes may also present with GGO and tend to occur with severe degrees of immune depression. Lymphocytic interstitial pneumonia may also give rise to patchy GGO. In children, PCP presents at a much lower age (4–5 months) in comparison to lymphocytic interstitial pneumonitis (LIP). In comparison to children infected with PCP, children suffering from LIP generally tend to be older and less acutely ill.[16]

Consolidation

Focal segmental or lobar air space consolidation most likely represents a community acquired bacterial pneumonia.

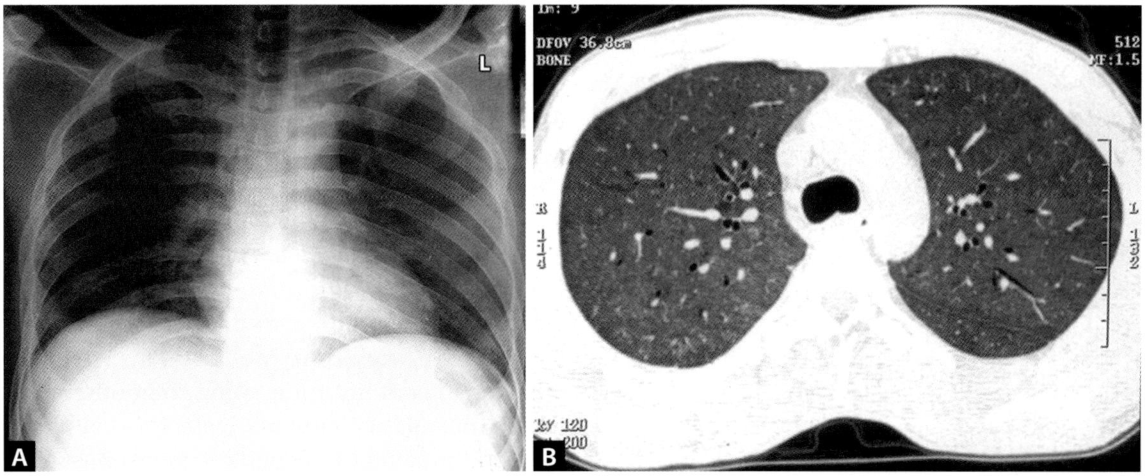

Figs. 1A and B: A 30-year-old HIV positive male with dry cough. (A) Chest radiograph is normal; (B) HRCT chest show disuse GGOs. Bronchoalveolar lavage demonstrated *Pneumocystis*.

Multiple areas of consolidation may be seen in TB or bacterial pneumonias with unusual organisms such as *Nocardia* or *Rhodococcus*.[3,8]

Multiple Pulmonary Nodules

A miliary pattern characterized by 1–3 mm nodules diffusely scattered in the lung parenchyma most commonly represents mycobacterial infection **(Fig. 2)**. In endemic areas, disseminated fungal infections such as *Histoplasma* and *Coccidioidomycosis* maybe the causative organisms. Larger nodules (<1 cm) associated with a reticular pattern are seen with CMV infections. *Cryptococcus* may also present with a reticulonodular pattern or as discrete nodules. Multiple subpleural nodules of 1–2 cm size with cavitation favor septic emboli. Larger nodules, associated with wedge-shaped, pleural based opacities are seen in invasive *aspergillosis*. These nodules may frequently show a 'halo' of surrounding GGO. Tuberculosis or atypical mycobacteria may also present with large nodules which are typically poorly marginated. Lymphoma may also present with large nodules as may metastases. The nodules in KS are typically clustered along the bronchovascular bundles.[3,7,8,11] A solitary pulmonary nodule with spiculated margins may represent a primary bronchogenic carcinoma.

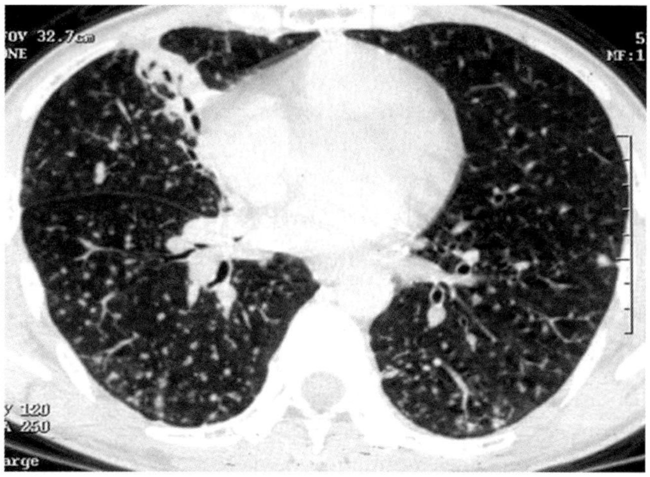

Fig. 2: A 23 year old HIV positive male with fever and cough. High resolution CT chest show multiple, 1–2 mm miliary nodules randomly scattered in the pulmonary parenchyma. Note the sub-segmental atelectasis in the RML with bronchiectasis. Sputum was positive for acid-fast bacilli.

Lymphadenopathy

The most common cause of hilar and/or mediastinal lymphadenopathy in a patient with AIDS are mycobacterial infections, either TB or atypical mycobacteria.[17] These lymph nodes classically show low density centers with rim enhancement post-contrast **(Fig. 3)**. Conversely, lymph nodes in KS and bacillary angiomatosis show intense enhancement reflecting their hypervascular nature. Mediastinal nodes with punctate calcifications are seen in disseminated *Pneumocystis* infection. Calcification may also be seen in the liver, kidneys and spleen in this situation. Unlike lymphoma in an immunocompetent host, lymphoma in an AIDS patient does not predominantly involve the lymph nodes, mediastinal or hilar lymphadenopathy is seen in only up to 25% of cases.

Pleural Effusion

The radiographic features of pleural effusion are generally unhelpful in narrowing the differential diagnosis. Large or

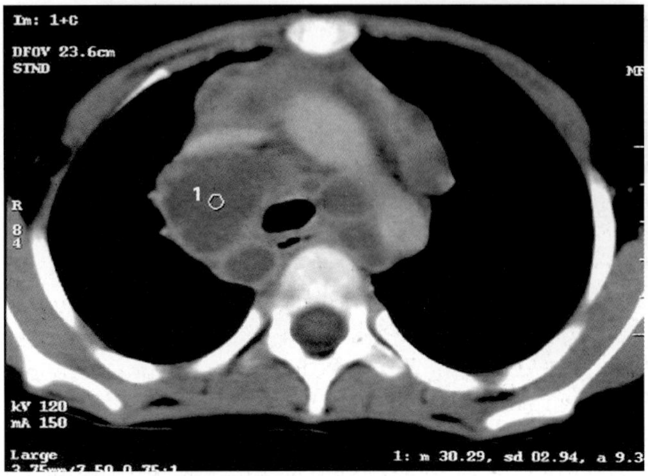

Fig. 3: A 40-year-old HIV positive female with fever and cough. Contrast-enhanced CT chest shows conglomerate, hypodense lymph nodes with rim enhancement in the pre- and paratracheal regions in a case of TB.

massive pleural effusions with predominantly lymphocytes on cytology are due to TB, while hemorrhagic fluid is suggestive of Kaposi's sarcoma (KS).

NON-HIV IMMUNOCOMPROMISED HOSTS

The number of non-HIV immunocompromised patients has significantly increased in the last two decades due to increase in the number of patients receiving solid organ or hematopoietic stem cell transplants, advances in cytotoxic therapy for various malignancies and immunosuppressive therapy.[18]

Organ transplantation is the most important treatment in end stage liver, kidney, heart and lung diseases. The immunosuppression caused by the anti-rejection medications render the solid organ transplant recipient vulnerable to a wide variety of infections causing significant mortality and morbidity. This group of patients is at further risk of pneumonia for several reasons which are as follows: (i) prolonged hospitalization, (ii) endotracheal tube injury to the trachea, and (iii) impaired clearance of respiratory secretions due to anesthesia and diminished cough. Lung transplant recipients are also at increased risk due to denervation of the lung and surgically impaired mucociliary transport.[4]

Cytotoxic chemotherapy causes neutropenia. As the granulocyte count declines, the risk of infections increases and the patient becomes susceptible to infections by pyogenic bacteria and fungi. The common organisms in the setting of neutropenia are bacteria including *Escherichia coli, Klebsiella, Pseudomonas aeruginosa, Staphylococcus aureus, Streptococcus pneumoniae* and *Streptococcus viridians* as well as fungi including *Aspergillus, Candida* and *Mucor*. Patients are most susceptible to bacterial infections in the early neutropenic phase. As neutropenia persists, fungal infections become more common.[3,18] Chemotherapy also causes defects in the humoral immunity which are associated with infections with encapsulated bacteria such as *Streptococcus pneumoniae* and Gram negative organisms such as *Haemophilus influenzae, Neisseria meningitidis* and *Pseudomonas aeruginosa*.[2]

Cellular immunity mediated by T-lymphocytes is affected in patients undergoing chemotherapy and solid organ transplant recipients. Defects in cellular immunity renders the patient susceptible to more unusual pathogens, including viruses (CMV, *varicella, herpes zoster*), protozoa, fungi (*Pneumocystis jirovecii, Aspergillus, Cryptococcus, Histoplasma*) and bacteria (*Legionella, Nocardia asteroides*).

Following solid organ transplant, in the first 4 weeks, infections are usually caused by nosocomial bacteria, or fungi in patients with prolonged neutropenia. At one to three months post-transplant, opportunistic pathogens such as PCP or CMV increase in frequency. One-half to all of the seronegative patients who receive a graft from a seropositive donor suffer from primary CMV infection. In the late post-transplant phase (>3 months), PCP remains a concern but mycobacteria and nocardia should also be considered.[13,18,19] After 6 months, the degree of immunosuppression required to prevent graft rejection dictates the frequency of infections.

In immunocompromised patients with hematological malignancies, the pulmonary involvement occurs in many ways, viz. (i) infection (ii) recurrence of the underlying hematological disease, (iii) adverse reaction to drugs, (iv) unrelated processes such as pulmonary emboli and (v) combination of the above mentioned processes. One-third of patients with hematological malignancies suffer a combination of at least two processes such as pneumonia caused by two different pathogens or a drug related pulmonary complication occurring along with infection. A reasonable differential diagnosis may be considered if one is aware of the host defenses that get compromised. Suppression in the number of granulocytes, B-lymphocytes, or T-lymphocytes is the most common pattern of impairment, though multiple types of cells may be frequently affected. A critical reduction in the number of each of these cell types predisposes to infection by a particular group of organisms. In these patients, most pulmonary complications, including drug-induced pulmonary disease and pulmonary emboli, are associated with fever that mimics infection. Noninfectious causes comprise one-fourth of the pulmonary complications.[20] With improved survival the late effects of treatment like second malignancy are becoming more common. Lately, due to better regimens, the incidence of radiation related complications have decreased.

Hematopoietic stem cell transplantation (HSCT) is now the treatment of choice for malignant diseases such as leukemias, aplastic anemia and congenital immunodeficiency syndromes. Pulmonary complications in these patients can be divided into two broad categories, i.e. HSCT nonspecific and HSCT specific complications. Hematopoietic stem cell transplantation specific pulmonary complications may develop in approximately half of transplant recipients.[21] Stem cells for HSCT may be obtained from patients own blood (autologous), related or unrelated donors (allogeneic), or may be obtained from peripheral blood, bone marrow or cord blood.[22] Complications related to the allogeneic HSCT are due to the toxicity of the conditioning regimen that includes chemotherapy with or without radiation.[23]

Imaging Approach

Chest radiographs remain the basic imaging investigation for the diagnosis of suspected pulmonary infection. However, early in the course of disease, chest radiographs maybe normal. Computed tomography has a higher sensitivity and allows diagnosis in the setting of a normal chest radiograph in patients with a high clinical suspicion for pneumonia. In a study by Heussel et al. 60% of pulmonary infections in febrile neutropenia were diagnosed by CT scans 5 days before radiographic abnormalities became evident.[24]

BACTERIAL INFECTIONS

Bacterial infections are responsible for most infections in HIV positive patients, having surpassed PCP. *S. pneumoniae* and *H. influenzae* account for most episodes of community acquired pneumonia in the general population. Recent hospitalization, antibiotic or steroid therapy are the predisposing factors for *Pseudomonas* infection. Unusual organisms such as *Rhodococcus* or *Bartonella* can also infect patients with AIDS. The radiological pattern of bacterial pneumonia does not differ from an immune intact host and consists of single or multiple sites of consolidation in a segmental or lobar distribution **(Figs. 4A and B)**. However, bilateral patchy opacities may be seen with certain organisms such as *Pseudomonas*. In contrast to immune intact individuals, there is a higher propensity for bilateral and multilobar disease in immunocompromised patients with a tendency for rapid progression as well as development of local and systemic complications, including cavitation, abscess formation and bacteremia. Pleural effusions may also occur.

In IVDAs, *Staphylococcus aureus* and Gram negative bacteria are common causes of generalized sepsis with secondary pneumonia. Septic embolic appear as multiple, bilateral, 1–2 cm nodules which frequently cavitate and are more numerous in the lower lobes.

Nocardia infection may be seen in solid organ transplant recipients in the late post-transplant phase (more than 1 year post heart-lung transplant).[4,25] It is also seen in diabetics and patients receiving steroid therapy. It most commonly appears as a solitary nodule or nodular infiltrate with cavitation. Pleural effusion occurs in up to 50% of cases.

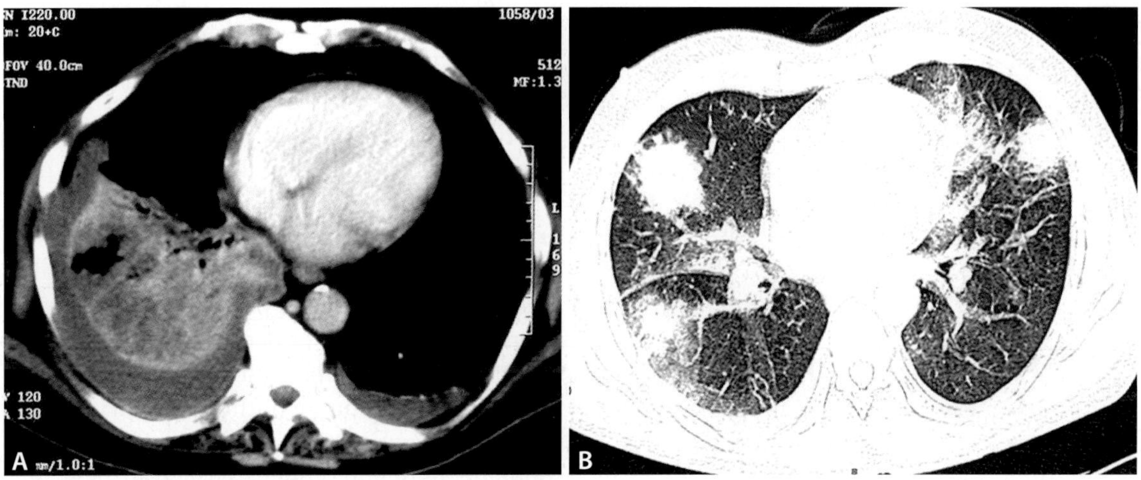

Figs. 4A and B: Bacterial pneumonia. (A) Airspace consolidation with air bronchograms and eccentric cavitation with associated pleural effusion; (B) Multifocal, bilateral, patchy airspace consolidation. Sputum culture revealed *Pseudomonas aeruginosa.*

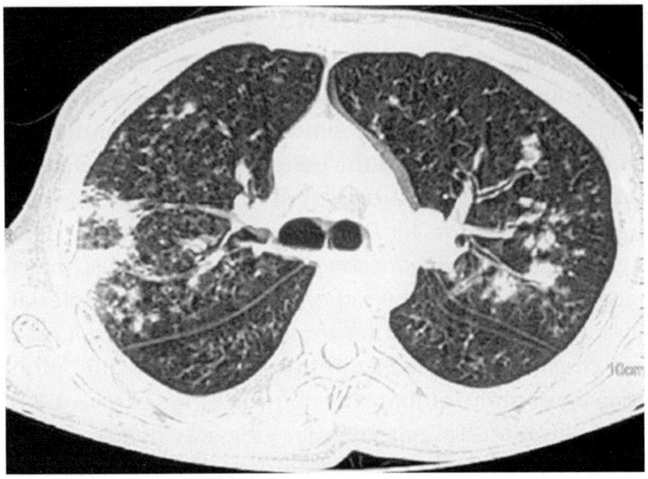

Fig. 5: A 50-year-old male post-chemotherapy presented with fever and dyspnea. High-resolution CT chest shows multifocal, patchy consolidation with centrilobular nodules and tree-in-bud appearance. Sputum was positive for *Streptococcus viridans*.

Pyogenic airways diseases viz. infectious bronchitis, bronchiolitis and bronchiectasis has increased in frequency in HIV positive patients. Chest radiographic findings in extensive bronchiolitis present an interstitial pattern with reticulonodular opacities distributed in a symmetrical fashion which mimics PCP. On CT, small nodular and branching Y-and V- shaped centrilobular opacities (tree-in-bud appearance) are seen which represent bronchioles impacted with inflammatory secretions **(Fig. 5)**. Similar imaging findings may be noted in viral and mycobacterial infections.

Bronchiectasis is commonly seen in association with HIV infection. It is thought to be a complication of prior lung infections. However, it has also been described in patients without history of previous infections and may represent an accelerated form of lung injury.[7]

Bacterial pneumonia affect 20–50% of HSCT recipients in the neutropenic phase.[26] Gram-negative organisms from the oral mucosa or gastrointestinal tract have been typically associated. However, more recently, Gram-positive organisms such as *Staphylococcus aureus* and coagulase negative *Staphylococcus* represent 60–70% of infections. The radiographic appearances include consolidation, ground-glass opacity, centrilobular, acinar and lobular opacities.

PNEUMOCYSTIS JIROVECII PNEUMONIA

Pneumocystis jirovecii is classified as a fungus and is an opportunistic eukaryote.[27] The incidence of *pneumocystis jirovecii* pneumonia (PCP) has decreased secondary to improved prophylaxis regimens and combined ART, however it still remains one of the most common AIDS defining illnesses as well as the most common cause of serious pulmonary infections in HIV positive patients.[3,27] In fact, at least one episode of infection with PCP will occur in most (more than 70%) of the patients with HIV/AIDS during the course of their illness. PCP occurs twice as frequently in homosexual males versus IVDAs. Also it affects males at twice the frequency of females. Although it can occur at any level of immune depression, it typically occurs at CD4+ counts below 200 cells/mm^3.

PCP has been reported in 33% of heart-lung transplant recipients, 3–10% of heart transplant, 0–11% of liver transplant and 6–14% of kidney transplant recipients. However, prophylaxis with TMP-SMX has dramatically reduced the incidence of PCP. The infection can occur at any time following solid organ transplant but commonly occurs in the 4th–6th month post-transplant and carries a mortality rate of 47%.[4,15]

PCP also affects patients with hematological malignancies undergoing intensive chemotherapy or HSCT. Its incidence is reported to be less than 10% in patients receiving HSCT.[6]

Clinically, affected patients present with a low-grade fever, dry cough and dyspnea. The initial symptoms may be subtle in HIV infected patients and be present even up to several weeks before diagnosis. This is in contrast to PCP in non-HIV patients in whom the presentation is more acute.[28] *Pneumocystis jirovecii* pneumonia classically presents on a chest radiograph with a bilateral, peri-hilar or diffuse, symmetric, interstitial pattern which may be ground-glass, reticular or granular in appearance. These opacities may progress to air space consolidation. The typical appearance on HRCT is extensive GGOs which histopathologically correspond to the presence of intra-alveolar exudates comprising fluid, debris and organisms **(Fig. 6)**. The ground-glass attenuation shows a patchy or geographical distribution with sparing of the subpleural regions. There may be a mosaic pattern with involved secondary lobules seen adjacent to uninvolved lung **(Figs. 7A and B)**. The parenchymal opacities have a predilection for the upper lobes which was earlier thought to be due to prophylaxis with aerosolized pentamidines. However, this upper lobe predominance is still prevalent in the present era of TMP-SMX prophylaxis. Thickening of the interlobular septal lines occurs in the subacute phase of the disease. Thin-walled cystic lesions may develop at any time during the course of the illness with an incidence of 10–34%. Cystic PCP is associated with a 35% risk for spontaneous pneumothoraces which are often refractory to treatment and may require surgical intervention. Although the radiographic abnormalities may clear within two weeks

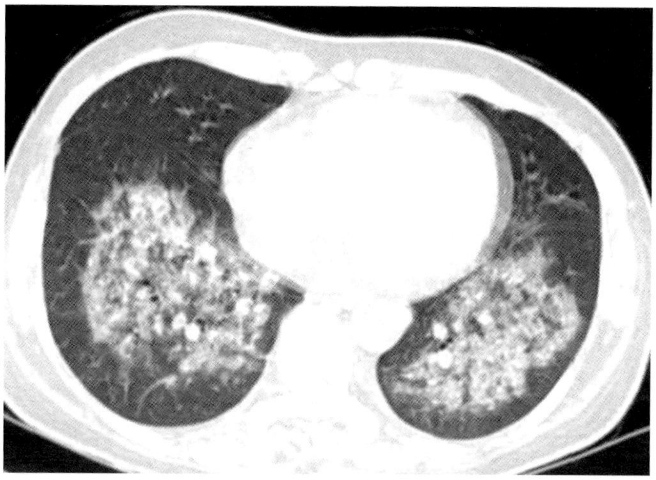

Fig. 6: A 45-year-old HIV positive lady presented with cough and dyspnea. High resolution CT chest shows typical, diffuse GGOs with subpleural sparing in both lower lobes in a case of *Pneumocystis* pneumonia.

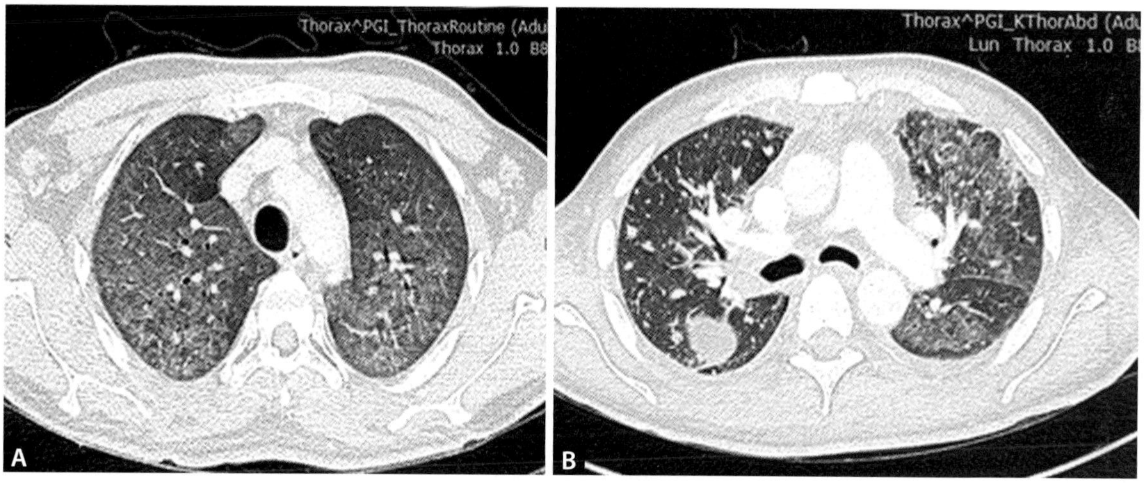

Figs. 7A and B: (A) A 30-year-old HIV positive male with dry cough of insidious onset. High resolution CT chest reveals diffuse GGOs with interstitial septal thickening giving a crazy paving appearance; (B) A 42-year-old HIV positive male with dry cough and low-grade fever. HRCT chest demonstrates involvement of the secondary lobules with sparing of adjacent lobules in the left lung. Note the nodules and focal consolidation in the right lung. Bronchoalveolar lavage demonstrated *Pneumocystis* in both the patients.

of therapy, it is not uncommon to see residual fibrosis or irregular cystic spaces.

Some patients may develop clinical symptoms and signs over months to years which is referred to as chronic PCP. This appears radiographically as thickened septal lines with honeycombing and traction bronchiectasis.[3,4,7,8] Rare presentations of PCP (5–10%) include focal lobar consolidation, nodules, mediastinal lymphadenopathy, bronchiectasis or pleural effusion.

MYCOBACTERIAL INFECTIONS

HIV/AIDS Patients

It has been estimated that there is a 50–200 fold increased risk of contracting TB by a HIV positive individual as compared to the general population in non-endemic areas. This risk increases for IVDAs and patients in endemic areas such as India and sub-Saharan Africa. Tuberculosis may accelerate the progression of AIDS. Prompt diagnosis and treatment are therefore critical. Tuberculosis may affect patients with HIV infection at any stage, however, the imaging findings are determined by the level of immune suppression. Early in the course of disease, when the CD4+ counts are >200 cells/mm^3, it usually manifests with the traditional pattern of reactivation TB with upper lobe opacities with cavitation and nodular bronchogenic spread **(Fig. 8)**. Pleural effusions are common. In severely immunocompromised individuals (CD4+ <200 cells/mm^3), the imaging appearance is reminiscent of primary TB with parenchymal consolidation and mediastinal

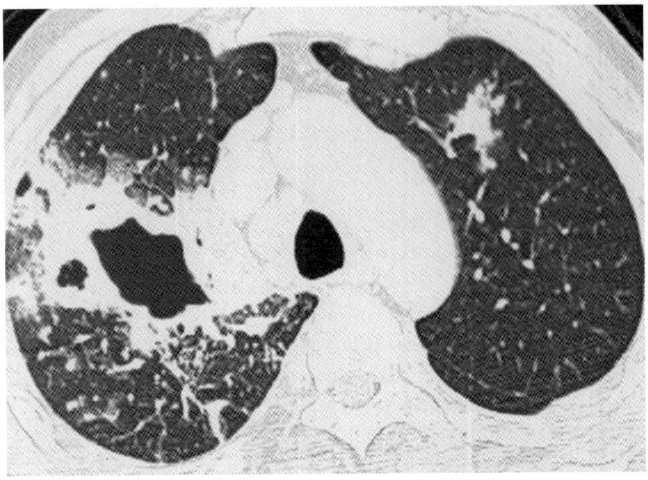

Fig. 8: A 32-year-old HIV positive lady presented with fever and productive cough. High resolution CT chest shows patchy, multifocal areas of consolidation with cavitation. Sputum was positive for acid-fast bacilli.

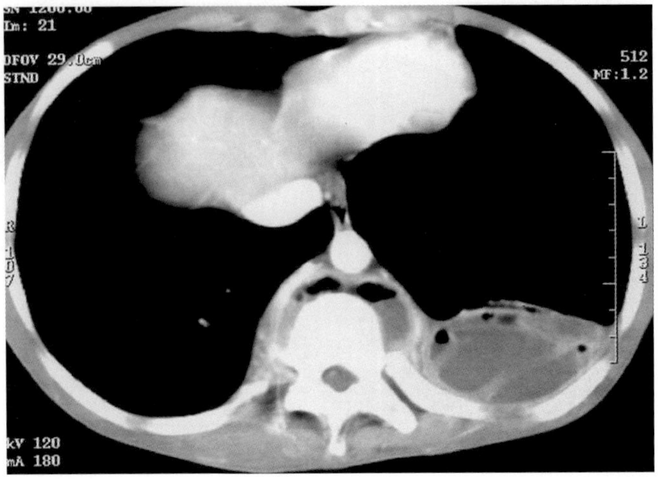

Fig. 9: A 23-year-old HIV positive male presented with fever, cough and back pain. Contrast-enhanced CT chest shows pre- and paraspinal fluid collections with multiple septae and enhancing walls due to spinal TB, miliary nodules were seen in the lungs.

lymphadenopathy which typically shows low attenuation centers with peripheral rim enhancement. A miliary pattern is also common. Atypical findings may be seen including diffuse infiltrates, multiple nodules, frequent middle and lower lobe involvement or even normal chest radiographs (14–20%). Compared to immunocompetent hosts, AIDS patients infected with TB are more likely to present with extra-pulmonary involvement (genitourinary system, bone marrow, central nervous system and lymph nodes) or systemic dissemination **(Fig. 9)**. These manifestations increase with increasing degrees of immune compromise: 70% of AIDS patients show extrathoracic disease when the CD4+ counts are <100 cells/ mm^3 as compared to 44% when CD4+ count is >300 cells/ mm^3. Almost half of the patients with extra-pulmonary involvement will show a miliary pattern in the lungs.[29] Tuberculosis can involve the central airways with stenosis and wall thickening. Involvement of the lower airways manifests as bronchiectasis or tree-in-bud appearance.

In patients who are put on ART, there may be worsening or appearance of new lymphadenopathy, lung parenchymal opacities or pleural effusion accompanied by fever. This is referred to as the immune reconstitution or the paradoxical syndrome. Patients who are severely symptomatic may benefit from steroid therapy.

Atypical mycobacterial infections are usually caused by *Mycobacterium avium intracellulare* (MAI) and less frequently by *Mycobacterium kansasii*. These usually occur when the CD4+ count is <50 cells/mm^3. *Mycobacterium avium intracellulare* infection commonly presents as disseminated disease with the gastrointestinal tract being the normal portal of entry. Imaging features are ill-defined nodules, multifocal consolidation, and cavities. Mediastinal lymphadenopathy may occur. The chest radiograph may be normal in roughly 20% of cases. *M. kansasii* commonly presents as focal alveolar consolidation.

The reversal syndrome has been recently described in HIV patients with MAI who are started on ART. This manifests as an acute febrile episode associated with new or enlarging lymphadenopathy.

HIV Negative Immunocompromised Patients

Solid organ transplant recipients are at increased risk of contracting TB with 50–100 times the incidence in the general population in the west. However, studies from India have reported a higher incidence, reflecting the endemic nature of the disease.[30] The infection may appear at any time after the surgery ranging from 1–96 months following transplant. Steroids and other anti-rejection medications affect cell-mediated immunity which is the primary means of controlling and eradicating mycobacterial infections. There is a high (40–64%) incidence of disseminated disease with pulmonary infection seen in approximately 40% of cases. The rate of progression is also faster than in the general population with higher morbidity and mortality.

The imaging appearance consists of cavitary upper lobe opacities in about one-third of patients. Another third demonstrate a miliary pattern **(Fig. 10)**. The rest may show a solitary lower lobe opacity, large nodule or pleural effusion. Lymphadenopathy is uncommon (3.5%).

Nontubercular mycobacterial infection is usually with MAI or *M. kansasii*. These account for a higher fraction of

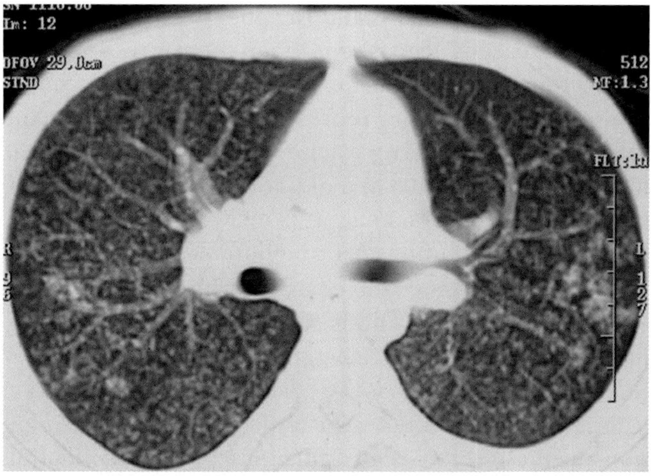

Fig. 10: A 35-year-old renal transplant recipient presented with fever three months after transplant surgery. High resolution CT chest shows multiple, 1–3 mm, randomly distributed nodules in both lungs with tree-in-bud appearance at places. Sputum was positive for acid-fast bacilli.

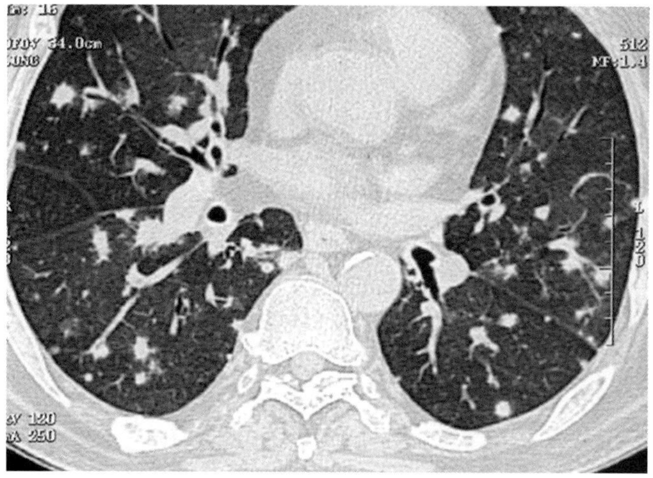

Fig. 11: A 42-year-old HIV positive male with fever. High resolution CT chest shows multiple, 5–8 mm nodules randomly distributed in both the lungs. Bronchoalveolar lavage showed CMV. Later autopsy confirmed cytoplasmic inclusion bodies.

mycobacterial infections in the transplant recipient: 25–43% of mycobacterial infections as compared to 5–10% in the general population. These usually present as multiple, moderate sized pulmonary nodules. Miliary nodules may be seen and are associated with a high mortality.

VIRAL INFECTIONS

Respiratory viral infections are commonly seen in HIV/AIDS patients with CD4+ counts <50 cells/mm^3. Cytomegalovirus is the most common viral pathogen with a reported incidence of up to 90% in advanced HIV disease.

The herpes group of viruses are the predominant viral pathogens in solid organ transplant recipients. Since these are most often reactivation infections of dormant organisms residing in the host or the transplant organ, they occur in the first few months post-transplant.

Although cytomegalovirus infection affects almost two-third of allogeneic HSCT recipients, CMV pneumonia develops in less than one-third of patients.[21] It typically occurs in the early phase and is associated with a high mortality rate of up to 85%. Infection with CMV is associated with increased susceptibility to bacterial, fungal and protozoal superinfections, increased risk of rejection and overall mortality.

The imaging appearance of CMV pneumonitis is classically that of diffuse ground-glass or patchy interstitial opacities resembling PCP. With severe infection, diffuse alveolar infiltrates may appear which mimic adult respiratory distress syndrome. Pulmonary nodules may be seen in about two-thirds of cases **(Fig. 11)**. Airway disease which manifests as bronchiectasis, bronchial wall thickening and bronchiolitis may be seen in a third of cases.

Herpes simplex (HSV-1, HSV-2) pneumonia is uncommon with a reported incidence of 0.8–10% in solid organ transplant recipients and 0.2% in AIDS patients.[3,4] The chest radiograph will demonstrate multifocal or diffuse consolidation. *Varicella zoster* is also a reactivation infection in the solid organ transplant recipient and usually manifests as disseminated disease. 5–15 mm, diffuse, ill-defined, nodular densities with fuzzy outlines are seen on chest radiographs.

Adenovirus and *respiratory syncitial virus* are common causes of viral community acquired pneumonia. Radiographs may show interstitial opacities, alveolar consolidation, nodules or pleural effusion.

FUNGAL INFECTIONS

Fungal pneumonias characteristically develop in patients who are neutropenic (from cytotoxic drugs and transplant recipients) or on corticosteroid therapy. The infecting organisms fall into two categories which are as follows: those that occur exclusively in immunocompromised hosts such as *Aspergillus*, *Candida* and *Mucor* species and endemic fungi with increased virulence in immunocompromised hosts such as *Histoplasma*, *Coccidioides*, *Cryptococcus* and *Blastomyces* species. Invasive aspergillosis and disseminated candidiasis are the most common agents, accounting for 80% of fungal infections in solid organ transplant recipients. Most will occur (80%) within two months post-transplant. The incidence varies from 5% in kidney transplant to 40% among liver transplant patients.

Fungal pneumonias are relatively uncommon in AIDS occurring in less than 5% of patients with the most common pathogen being *Cryptococcus*. The incidence of *Aspergillus* infection is increasing and almost exclusively occurs in AIDS patients who are neutropenic due to drugs such as zidovudine or ganciclovir or on steroids. Affected individuals are generally in an advanced stage of immune depression with CD4+ counts <50/mm^3. Although meningitis is the most common manifestation of *Cryptococcus* infections, active pulmonary infection is present in 40% of patients with cryptococcosis.

Fungal pneumonias are also common in patients undergoing chemotherapy for hematological malignancies during and following HSCT. Neutropenia is the most important risk factor.[28] Most common pathogen is *Aspergillus,* while *Mucor, Candida,* and *Cryptococcus* may also occur. *Aspergillus* infection has the greatest propensity to occur when the peripheral white cell count falls to less than 1,000/mm^3.

The radiographic abnormalities in angio-invasive aspergillosis consist of nodular or wedge-shaped opacities, frequently abutting the pleural surfaces. These often cavitate reflecting the angioinvasive nature of the fungus and may show central low density areas or the air crescent sign **(Fig. 12)**. The CT "halo" sign refers to GGOs surrounding a nodular opacity representing a rim of hemorrhage due to thrombosis within the adjacent vessels caused by the fungus and is an early sign of disease **(Fig. 13)**.[31] Although considered to be characteristic of angio-invasive aspergillus, the "halo" sign may also be seen with *Mucor, Candida,* CMV infections and Wegener's granulomatosis.[32] The "air-crescent" sign is seen when there is resorption of the necrotic tissue by returning neutrophils and is therefore is a relatively late sign, representing recovery from the infection.[33] Necrotizing tracheobronchial aspergillosis may be present in 10–30% of patients and may be seen on CT as nodular tracheal or bronchial wall thickening, or non-specific findings of bronchopneumonia.

Pulmonary mucormycosis may be seen in 0.2% of transplant recipients and is clinically and radiologically indistinguishable from *Aspergillus* infection. Pulmonary infection with *Candida* is rare, usually occurring as part of a disseminated infection. The radiologic appearances are nonspecific and consist of diffuse air-space consolidation or single or multiple, nodular infiltrates resembling *Aspergillus.*

Single or multiple, well-defined nodules with or without cavitation is the common radiological appearance of infection with *Cryptococcus.* Adenopathy and pleural effusion may be present. Atypical findings include diffuse pulmonary infiltrates, miliary nodules and areas of ground-glass haze.

Radiographic features in histoplasmosis include diffuse small nodules (usually <3 mm in size), miliary nodules or larger nodules around 1cm in size. Small pleural effusions and mediastinal lymphadenopathy may be seen. Chest radiographs may be normal in 35–50% of patients. In patients with coccidiomycosis, diffuse, small, nodular opacities are the most common radiographic manifestation. Thin-walled cavities which are characteristically seen in

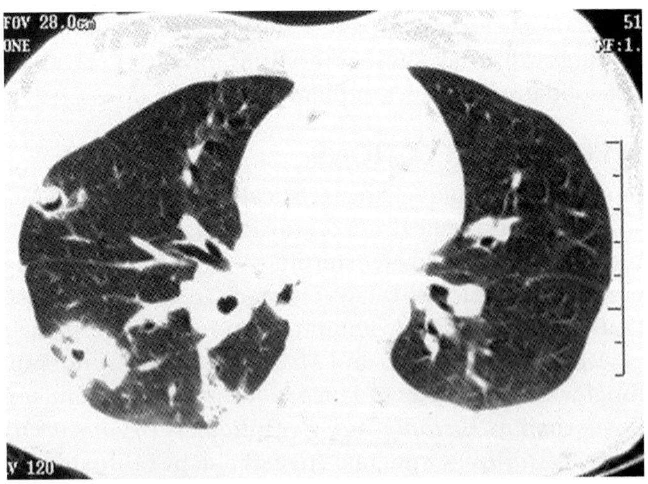

Fig. 12: A 28-year-old male presented with fever and chest pain following chemotherapy. High resolution CT chest shows multiple nodules with cavitations and air-crescent sign with wedge-shaped areas of consolidation. Computed tomography guided fine needle aspiration cytology revealed *Aspergillus.*

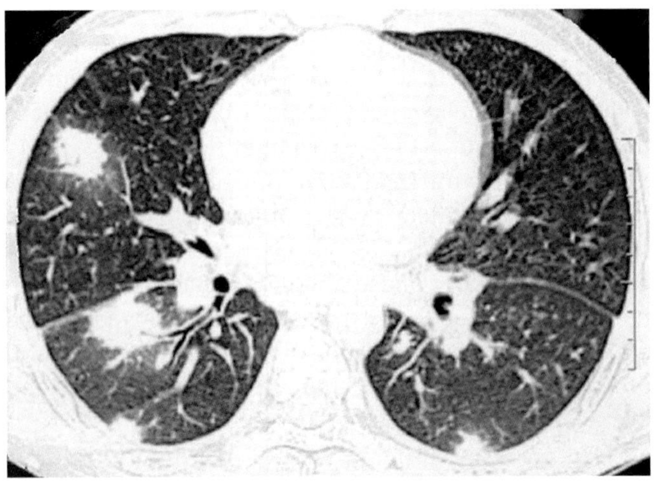

Fig. 13: A 40-year-old male (post-renal transplant) presented with fever and dyspnea. High resolution CT chest demonstrates multiple, bilateral, large nodules with surrounding ground-glass attenuation—the CT halo sign. Bronchoalveolar lavage revealed *Aspergillus.*

immunocompetent individuals are uncommon in the immune compromised host. Reports of infection with blastomycosis are rare. Pulmonary findings include focal alveolar infiltrates or bilateral patchy or nodular opacities.

NONINFECTIOUS MANIFESTATIONS OF AIDS

Kaposi's Sarcoma

Kaposi's sarcoma (KS) is a malignancy which almost exclusively occurs in bisexual and homosexual males with AIDS. It is also known to affect certain ethnic groups. Its incidence is decreasing in recent years due to greater awareness of safe sex habits and the introduction of ART.[33] The CD4+ counts in patients with KS are generally <100 cells/mm^3.

Kaposi's sarcoma is a multisystem disease that affects the skin, lymph nodes, lungs and the gastrointestinal tract. Characteristic findings of pulmonary KS are nodular thickening along the bronchovascular bundles, growing from the perihilar region to the periphery. The nodules may become coalescent, leading to dense air-space consolidation. Pleural effusion occurs in 30–89% of cases and may be unilateral or bilateral. Mediastinal lymphadenopathy is uncommon but when present, demonstrates characteristic enhancement following intravenous iodinated contrast.[34]

On MR, KS lesions demonstrate increased signal intensity on T1 weighted images, markedly reduced signal intensity on T2 weighted images with intense enhancement following gadolinium administration. On nuclear scanning, KS lesions are thallium avid, however, in contrast to infectious conditions they do not take up gallium, thereby allowing differentiation between the two conditions.

Lymphoma

Acquired immunodeficiency syndrome related lymphoma occurs in AIDS patients at an advanced stage of immune depression when CD4+ counts are <50 cells/mm^3. Most cases consist of non-Hodgkin's lymphoma, usually of high grade with an aggressive nature. Intrathoracic involvement is seen in 10% of cases and is typically extra-nodal. Pleural effusions are the most common radiographic abnormality. Diffuse, well-defined nodules, focal consolidation or mediastinal lymphadenopathy may also be seen.

Lymphocystic Interstitial Pneumonitis

Lymphocystic interstitial pneumonitis is a lymphoproliferative disorder characterized by infiltration of the pulmonary interstitium by lymphocytes, histiocytes and plasma cells. It is much more common in the pediatric population. The radiographic appearance consists of a diffuse, micronodular, interstitial pattern. On HRCT, the most common finding is of GGOs along with poorly defined centrilobular nodules. Cystic air spaces and interstial thickening may also be seen.

Post-transplant Lymphoproliferative Disorder

Post-transplant lymphoproliferative disorder is a spectrum of lymphoproliferative abnormalities ranging from a benign febrile illness with lymphadenopathy to a rapidly fatal malignant lymphoma. This may develop in 1–10% of transplant patients. The Epstein-Barr virus appears to be causally related to the development of PTLD. With current immunosuppressive regimes, the peak incidence of PTLD is in the third month following transplant.

Radiographically, PTLD manifests as one or multiple, uniform, non-enhancing masses in large organs including the lung, liver, kidney, bowel and brain. Lymphadenopathy may be seen in 15–37% of cases, either in isolation or in association with the organ masses. Endobronchial masses resulting in atelectasis have also been reported.[17]

NONINFECTIOUS MANIFESTATIONS IN HSCT

Noninfectious lung injury has emerged as a major cause of morbidity and mortality due to decline in infectious complications due to the widespread use of prophylactic broad spectrum antibiotics. The frequency of noninfectious complications is similar in allogeneic and autologous HSCT.[36] Definitive diagnosis of noninfectious complications is challenging as the clinical manifestations overlap with those of the infections and the difficulty in obtaining a histological diagnosis. Imaging studies particularly HRCT play a major role in the management of these patients. Noninfectious complications usually follow a time-line due to the underlying immunological status of the host. The neutropenic phase following HSCT lasts from 2 to 3 weeks. After allogeneic HSCT, the immunosuppressive phase continues for 1 year. This is divided into an early (up to 100 days) and a late phase which continues for one year or more.[37]

PRE-ENGRAFTMENT PERIOD

Noninfectious complications that occur during neutropenic (also known as pre-engraftment period) include idiopathic pulmonary syndrome (IPS), pulmonary edema, diffuse alveolar hemorrhage (DAH), and periengraftment respiratory distress syndrome (PERDS).[38]

Idiopathic Pulmonary Syndrome

It is defined as a diffuse lung injury without an infectious cause. Predisposing factors are pre-transplant chemotherapy and total body irradiation. It carries a high mortality. It progresses from an acute exudative to a subacute proliferative to a chronic fibrotic phase. HRCT findings are those of diffuse alveolar damage manifesting as focal or diffuse ground-glass opacity with density gradient towards the dependant regions. Consolidation is less common. Chronic phase is characterized by traction bronchiectasis and honeycombing. HRCT findings are thus nonspecific and IPS remains a diagnosis of exclusion.[39,40]

Pulmonary Edema

It is a common complication with a rapid onset, usually occurring in the 2nd or 3rd week after HSCT. Underlying mechanisms include GVHD, cardiac or renal dysfunction secondary to chemotherapy regimens, pulmonary vasculature hyperpermeability induced by total body irradiation, sepsis, cyclosporine A or fluid overload.[3,23.] CXR suggests a diagnosis when there are diffuse interstitial markings, peribronchial cuffing, perihilar haziness, ground-glass appearance and vascular prominence. HRCT features include perihilar ground-glass opacity or consolidation, thickening of interlobular septa, enlargement of pulmonary vessels and pleural effusions **(Fig. 14)**.

Diffuse Alveolar Hemorrhage

Diffuse alveolar hemorrhage (DAH) is the commonest noninfectious pulmonary complication in leukemia.[35] Around 20% of HSCT patients may develop DAH in the neutropenic phase.[21] The manifestations of DAH are secondary to pulmonary vessel damage by acute GVHD, pre-transplantation chemotherapy or total body irradiation. Clinical presentation is nonspecific, mild hemoptysis occurs in about two-third of the patients; frank hemoptysis is rare.[34] It carries a high mortality rate of about 80%. Early diagnosis and prompt steroid therapy improves survival. Bronchoalveolar lavage (BAL) may aid the diagnosis by demonstrating hemosiderin laden macrophages. Radiological findings are nonspecific. HRCT findings include widespread ground-glass opacity or consolidation with interlobular septal thickening (crazy-paving appearance) **(Fig. 15)**. The peripheral lungs are spared.

Peri-engraftment Respiratory Distress Syndrome

Peri-engraftment respiratory distress syndrome (PERDS) presents with diffuse capillary leak, cutaneous rash, and fever that occurs during the engraftment and neutrophil recovery phases. It is thought to result from proinflammatory cytokines released during engraftment. Autologous HSCT has a greater incidence of this complication. The HRCT findings of interlobular septal thickening with bilateral ground-glass opacities and perihilar or peribronchial consolidation and pleural effusions are indistinguishable from that of pulmonary edema and acute respiratory distress syndrome.[38]

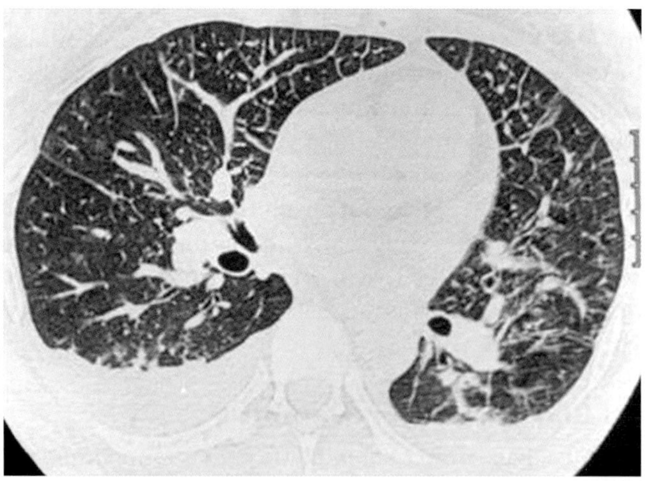

Fig. 14: A 38-year-old female following HSCT developed breathlessness. HRCT shows perihilar ground-glass opacity, thickening of interlobular septa, enlargement of pulmonary vessels and pleural effusion suggestive of pulmonary edema.

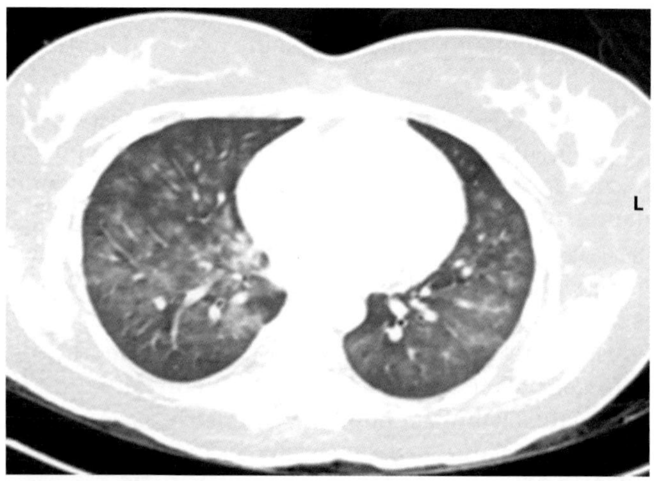

Fig. 15: A 28-year-old female with leukemia following HSCT complained of streaky hemoptysis. HRCT chest shows diffuse GGOs due to diffuse alveolar hemorrhage.

EARLY POST-TRANSPLANT PERIOD

During the early post-transplant period (30 to 100 days after HSCT), the neutrophil count has recovered. Impaired cellular and humoral immunity however persists. Reconstitution of the immune system leads to a reduction in the frequency of infectious complications as well. Noninfectious pulmonary complications during this period include acute GVHD, acute radiation injury and rarely, pulmonary cytolytic thrombi.

Drug-induced Lung Injury

Drug-induced lung injury occurs in around 10% patients with hematopoietic stem cell transplant. There are variable patterns of injury including nonspecific interstitial pneumonia, hypersensitivity pneumonitis, diffuse alveolar damage, and organizing pneumonia. The HRCT features are nonspecific and include diffuse ground-glass opacities, subpleural or peribronchial consolidation, centrilobular nodules and interlobular septal thickening.[38]

Acute GVHD

Graft versus host disease (GVHD) is a major cause of morbidity and mortality in patients following allogeneic HSCT and is secondary to immune reaction of the donor cells to the host tissues. Autologous transplant are not associated with acute GVHD. GVHD occurs in 20–75% of allogeneic HSCT recipients. Skin, liver, and gastrointestinal system are the primary targets. Lung involvement is uncommon and a broad spectrum of GVHD changes have been described histopathologically—ranging from acute injury to chronic irreversible damage.[41] HRCT demonstrates nonspecific changes including diffuse interstitial and alveolar opacities that mimic pulmonary edema.

Acute Radiation Pneumonitis

This complication occurs in patients who receive radiation therapy for intrathoracic lymphoma. Most patients are asymptomatic. More-over with modern techniques of radiation, the radiation related acute toxicity has reduced. The early stage changes (8-12 weeks after completion) are characterized by cellular infiltration composed predominantly of macrophages. On imaging, there is patchy consolidation in the radiation field that may coalesce to form a relatively sharp border conforming to the radiation portal. The late stage (6–24 months after completion) is characterized by fibrotic changes which appear on CT as parenchymal distortion and traction bronchiectases.[38]

Pulmonary Cytolytic Thrombi

Like GVHD, this is a rare pulmonary complication that occurs exclusively in allogeneic HSCT recipients. In fact, it may be a manifestation of GVHD. Children are primarily affected. A median onset of 72 days after HSCT has been reported.[38] Pathologically, there are intravascular thromboemboli composed of necrotic basophilic debris occluding the small and medium pulmonary vessels leading to surrounding alveolar hemorrhage or infarct. Multiple bilateral pulmonary nodules with surrounding ground-glass opacities are seen on HRCT.

LATE PULMONARY COMPLICATIONS

Late complications occur 3 months after HSCT. During this period, noninfectious causes are more common.[23] The most common complication during this period is chronic GVHD manifesting either as bronchiolitis obliterans, organizing pneumonia, or non-classifiable interstitial pneumonia. Air-leak syndrome (ALS), post-transplant lymphoproliferative disorder (PTLD), pulmonary veno-occlusive disease (PVOD), and pleuroparenchymal fibroelastosis are less frequently encountered complications.

Chronic GVHD

It occurs only in patients with allogeneic HSCT secondary to immune-mediated reaction of the donor T-lymphocytes against the host tissues.[41] Lung involvement is common unlike acute GVHD. It manifests either as organizing pneumonia (reversible with favorable prognosis) or bronchiolitis obliterans (irreversible).

Bronchiolitis Obliterans

It occurs most commonly in allogeneic HSCT for leukemia or aplastic anemia. About 10% of patients who develop chronic GVHD develop bronchiolitis obliterans. Factors that increase the risk include immunosuppression with methotrexate, chemotherapy or irradiation prior to HSCT and low serum immunoglobulins after HSCT. Pathologically, there is constrictive bronchiolitis with submucosal and peri-bronchiolar fibrosis. HRCT findings are best demonstrated on expiratory CT and include air trapping, mosaic perfusion and bronchial dilatation.[42]

Bronchiolitis Obliterans Organizing Pneumonia

The pathological hallmark is granulation tissue in the lumen of alveolar ducts and bronchioles followed by fibroblastic proliferation. HRCT findings include patchy, bilateral, multifocal areas of ground-glass opacity or consolidation in a peribronchial or subpleural distribution. Areas of consolidation tend to be multifocal, bilateral, peripheral and lower lobe predominant **(Fig. 16)**.[43]

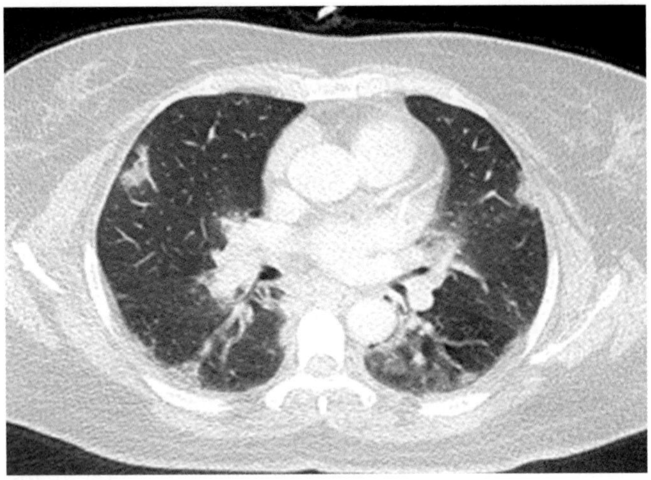

Fig. 16: A 47-year-old female with chronic myeloid leukemia. HRCT shows patchy, bilateral areas of ground-glass opacity and consolidation in a subpleural distribution. TBLB confirmed the diagnosis as BOOP.

Air-leak Syndrome

Air-leak Syndrome (ALS) is characterized by spontaneous pneumothorax, pneumomediastinum, pulmonary interstitial emphysema or subcutaneous emphysema in HSCT recipients. Typically, patients with ALS have chronic GVHD and bronchiolitis obliterans syndrome. On HRCT, the diagnosis of pneumothorax, pneumomediastinum and subcutaneous emphysema is straightforward; however, changes of interstitial emphysema are subtle and appear as linear lucencies along the bronchovascular bundles. Findings of bronchiolitis obliterans will also usually be evident.[44]

Pulmonary Veno-occlusive Disease

Pulmonary veno-occlusive disease (PVOD) is a rare complication that may be encountered following either autologous or allogeneic HSCT.[45] The diagnosis is based on a triad of pulmonary edema, pulmonary hypertension and normal pulmonary artery occlusion pressure. HRCT demonstrates main pulmonary artery dilatation, ground-glass opacities and smooth interlobular septal thickening.

Pleuroparenchymal Fibroelastosis

Pleuroparenchymal fibroelastosis is a rare complication with upper lobe involvement characterized by fibrotic thickening of the pleura and fibroelastosis of the subpleural parenchyma.[46]

CONCLUSION

Pulmonary infections are the most common complications in patients with HIV/AIDS patients and solid organ transplant/HSCT recipients and account for significant morbidity and mortality. It is important for the radiologist to demand and utilize all available clinical information such as signs and symptoms, degree of immunosuppression, risk factor for HIV infection and time period since solid organ or HSC transplant. In most cases, the clinical and chest radiograph findings are sufficient for confident diagnosis. However, chest radiographs may be normal or demonstrate subtle or nonspecific findings. Chest CT plays an important role in identifying the presence of disease and may specifically diagnose many conditions. Equally important, a negative HRCT chest virtually excludes active infectious disease.

REFERENCES

1. Afessa B, Green B. Bacterial pneumonia in hospitalized patients with HIV infection. Chest. 2000;117(4):1017-22.
2. Aronchick JM. Pulmonary infections in cancer and bone marrow transplant patients. Semin Roentgenol. 2000;35(2):140-51.
3. Daniel DM. Pulmonary infections in HIV/AIDS. Semin Roentgenol. 2000;35(2):124-39.
4. Miller WT. Pulmonary infections in patients who have received solid organ transplants. Semin Roentgenol. 2000;35(2):152-70.
5. Moore EH. Diffuse lung disease in the current spectrum of immunocompromised hosts (non-AIDS). Radiol Clin N Am. 1991;29(5):983-97.
6. World Health Organization/Joint United Nations programme on HIV/AIDS. Report on the global AIDS epidemic, 2008. *http:/ www.unaids.org*.
7. Beck JM. The immune-compromised host: HIV infection. Proc Am Thorac Soc. 2005;2:423-7.
8. Boiselle PM, Aviram G, Fishman JE. Update on lung disease in AIDS. Semin Roentgenol. 2002;37(1):54-71.
9. Grubb JR, Moorman AC, Baker RK, Masur H. The changing spectrum of pulmonary disease in patients with HIV infection on antiretroviral therapy. AIDS. 2006;20: 1095-107.
10. Huang L, Crothers K. HIV-associated opportunistic pneumonias. Respirology. 2009;14:474-85.
11. Castaner E, Gallardo X, Mata JM, Esteba L. Radiologic approach to the diagnosis of infectious pulmonary diseases in patients infected with the human immunodeficiency virus. Eur J Radiol. 2004;51:114-29.
12. Jasmer RM, Edinburgh KJ, Thompson A, Gotway MB, Creasman JM, et al. Chest. 2000;117:1023-30.
13. Kang E, Staples CA, McGuinness G, Primack SL, Muller NL. Detection and differential diagnosis of pulmonary infections and tumors in patients with AIDS: Value of chest radiography versus CT. Am J Roentgenol. 1996;166: 15-9.
14. Hartman TE, Primack SL, Muller NL, et al. Diagnosis of thoracic complications in AIDS: Accuracy of CT. Am J Roentgenol. 1994;162:547-53.
15. Shorr AF, Susla GM, O'Grady NP. Pulmonary infiltrates in the non-HIV infected immunocompromised patient: Etiologies, diagnostic strategies and outcomes. Chest. 2004;125:260-71.

16. Kuhlman JE. Pneumocystic infections: The radiologist's perspective. Radiology. 1996;198:623-35.
17. Greenberg SD, Frager D, Suster B, Walker S, Stavropoulos C, et al. Active pulmonary tuberculosis in patients with AIDS: Spectrum of radiographic findings. Radiology. 1994;193:115-9.
18. George R, Andronikou S, Theron S, du Plessis J, Hayes M, et al. Pulmonary infections in HIV-positive children. Pediatr Radiol. 2009;39:545-54.
19. Carignan S, Staples CA, Muller NL. Intrathoracic lymphoproliferative disorders in the immunocompromised host. J Thoracic Imaging. 1995;197:53-8.
20. Franquet T. High resolution computed tomography (HRCT) of lung infections in non-AIDS immunocompromised patients. Eur Radiol. 2006;16:707-18.
21. Mesurolle B, Tanaka N, Kosiuk J, Mignon F, Choquet S. The treated thorax in patients with hematological malignancies. In: Guermazi A (Ed). Radiogical imaging in hematological malignancies. Medical Radiology, Diagnostic Imaging. 1st edn. Berlin, Hiedelberg, Gemany. Springer-Verlag. 2004; pp. 443-72.
22. Rosenow EC, Wilson WR, Cockerill FR. Pulmonary disease in the immunocompromised host. I Mayo Clin Proc. 1985; 60(7):473-87.
23. Worthy SA, Flint JD, Muller NL. Pulmonary complications after bone marrow transplantation: High resolution CT and pathological findings. Radiographics. 1997;17:1359-71.
24. Hows JM. Status of umbilical cord blood transplantation in the year 2001. J Clin Pathol. 2001;54:428-34.
25. Mesurolle B, Tanaka N, Kosiuk J, Mignon F, Choquet S. The treated thorax in patients with hematological malignancies. In: Guermazi A (Ed). Radiogical Imaging in Hematological Malignancies. Medical Radiology, Diagnostic Imaging. 1st edition. Berlin, Hiedelberg, Gemany. Springer-Verlag; 2004. pp. 443-72.
26. Heussel CP, Kanczor HU, Heussel GU, et al. Pneumonia in febrile neutropenic patients and in bone marrow and blood stem cell transplant recipients: use of high resolution computed tomography. J Clin Oncol. 1999;17:796-805.
27. Huang L, Cattamanchi A, Davis L, den Boon S, Kovacs J, et al. HIV-associated *Pneumocystis* pneumonia. Proc Am Thorac Soc 2010;8:294-300.
28. Kramer MR, Marshall SE, Starnes VA, et al. Infectious complications in heart lung transplantation: Analysis of 200 episodes. Arch Intern Med. 1993;153:2010-6.
29. Spalgais S, Jaiswal A, Puri M, Sarin R, Agarwal U. Clinical profile and diagnosis of extra-pulmonary TB in HIV infected patients: routine abdominal ultrasonography increases detection of abdominal tuberculosis. Indian J Tuberc. 2013;60(3):147-53.
30. Soubani AO, Miller KB, Hassoun PN. Pulmonary complications of bone marrow transplantation. Chest. 1996;109:1066-77.
31. Gulati M, Kaur R, Jha V, et al. High resolution CT in renal transplant patients with suspected pulmonary infections. Acta Radiologica. 2000;41:1-6
32. Park YS, Seo JB, Lee YK, et al. Radiological and clinical findings of pulmonary aspergillosis following solid organ transplant. Clin Radiol. 2008;63:673-80.
33. La Ferla L, Pinzone MR, Nunnari G, Martellotta F, Lleshi A, Tirelli U, et al. Kaposi's sarcoma in HIV-positive patients: the state of art in the HAART-era. Eur Rev Med Pharmacol Sci. 2013;17(17):2354-65.
34. Davis SD, Henschke CI, Chamides BK, Westcott JL. Intrathoracic Kaposi sarcoma in AIDS patients: radiographic-pathologic correlation. Radiology. 1987;163(2):495-500.
35. Hildebrand FL Jr. Rosenow EC, Habermann TM, et al. Pulmonary complications of leukemia. Chest. 1990;98: 1233-9.
36. Brodoefel H, Faul C, Salih H, Vogel W, Fenchel M, Horger M. Therapy-related noninfectious complications in patients with hematologic malignancies: high-resolution computed tomography findings. J Thorac Imaging. 2013;28(1): W5-W1.
37. Tyndall A. Successes and failures of stem cell transplantation in autoimmune diseases. Hematology Am Soc Hematol Educ Program. 2011;(1):280-84.
38. Franquet T, Müller NL, Lee KS, Giménez A, Flint JD. High-resolution CT and pathologic findings of noninfectious pulmonary complications after hematopoietic stem cell transplantation. Am J Roentgenol. 2005;184(2):629-37.
39. Kantrow SP, Hackman RC, Boeckh M, Myerson D, Crawford SW. Idiopathic pneumonia syndrome: changing spectrum of lung injury after marrow transplantation. Transplantation. 1997;63 (8):1079-86.
40. Panoskaltsis-Mortari A, Griese M, Madtes DK, et al. An official American Thoracic Society research statement: noninfectious lung injury after hematopoietic stem cell transplantation—idiopathic pneumonia syndrome. Am J Respir Crit Care Med. 2011;183(9):1262-79.
41. Yousem SA. The histological spectrum of pulmonary graft-versus-host disease in bone marrow transplant recipients. Hum Pathol. 1995;26(6):668-75.
42. Ooi GC, Peh WC, Ip M. High-resolution computed tomography of bronchiolitis obliterans syndrome after bone marrow transplantation. Respiration. 1998;65(3): 187-91.
43. Yoshihara S, Yanik G, Cooke KR, Mineishi S. Bronchiolitis obliterans syndrome (BOS), bronchiolitis obliterans organizing pneumonia (BOOP), and other late-onset noninfectious pulmonary complications following allogeneic hematopoietic stem cell transplantation. Biol Blood Marrow Transplant. 2007;13(7):749-59.
44. Franquet T, Rodríguez S, Hernández JM, et al. Air-leak syndromes in hematopoietic stem cell transplant recipients with chronic GVHD: high-resolution CT findings. J Thorac Imaging. 2007;22 (4):335-40.
45. Mandel J, Mark EJ, Hales CA. Pulmonary veno-occlusive disease. Am J Respir Crit Care Med. 2000;162(5):1964-73.
46. Frankel SK, Cool CD, Lynch DA, Brown KK. Idiopathic pleuroparenchymal fibroelastosis: description of a novel clinicopathologic entity. Chest. 2004;126(6):2007-13.

CHAPTER 163

Pattern Approach to Interstitial Lung Disease and Imaging of Idiopathic Interstitial Pneumonias

Mandeep Garg, Uma Debi

Interstitial lung diseases (ILDs) are defined as a group of diffuse lung parenchymal diseases which result from damage to the lung parenchyma caused by different degrees of inflammation and fibrosis.[1] It refers to variable patterns/diseases characterized histologically by inflammatory infiltrate in the interstitium with variable degree of fibrosis. Correlation of clinical, radiological and pathologic features is often required to reach a correct diagnosis of ILD. According to the updated American Thoracic Society-European Respiratory Society classification, idiopathic interstitial pneumonias (IIPs) are ILDs of unknown etiology sharing common clinical features and can be categorized into (a) "chronic fibrosing IIPs" (idiopathic pulmonary fibrosis (IPF) and idiopathic nonspecific interstitial pneumonia (NSIP)), (b) "smoking-related IIPs" (respiratory bronchiolitis associated interstitial lung disease (RB-ILD) and desquamative interstitial pneumonia (DIP)), and (c) "acute or subacute IIPs" (cryptogenic organizing pneumonia (COP) and acute interstitial pneumonia (AIP)) and (d) "rare IIPs" (lymphoid interstitial pneumonia (LIP) and idiopathic pleura-parenchymal fibro-elastosis (IPPFE)) **(Table 1)**. In addition, another category "unclassifiable IIPs" has been proposed, which includes IIPs in which final diagnosis is not possible.[2]

IMAGING

Plain Radiography

It is an important part of initial imaging. During imaging interstitial pneumonias, the goals of chest radiograph interpretation are to determine the pattern of lung disease, recognize any change in lung volume and to determine any other accompanying abnormalities **(Fig. 1)**.

High Resolution Computed Tomography

High resolution computed tomography (HRCT) is required for evaluating the morphology and density of lung abnormalities and their location in relation to secondary pulmonary lobule. HRCT is much better than routine CT for this purpose. Previously sequential HRCT was performed in supine position with 1–2 cm spacing and 1 mm slice thickness. But this method is nearly obsolete now expect for follow-up imaging as it gives involves less radiation exposure to the patient. The development of multidetector CT scanners, capable of rapidly imaging the thorax using an isotropic technique has enabled another way in which HRCT scan may be obtained. HRCT scan can be obtained from thin-section (1–2 mm) reconstruction of volumetric data obtained by using multidetector CT, narrow detector width and with image reconstruction with a high spatial frequency algorithm. Expiratory scans should be performed in patients with obstructive disease at three or more levels. Prone scans may be needed to differentiate dependent densities from early changes of ILD.

ANATOMY OF THE SECONDARY PULMONARY LOBULE (MILLER'S)[3]

The secondary pulmonary lobule is the smallest unit of lung structure, which is demarcated by septae of connective

Table 1: Radiological features and differential diagnosis of the idiopathic interstitial pneumonias (IIPs).[2]

IIP Group and clinical radiologic pathologic diagnosis	***HRCT patterns***	***Typical HRCT distribution***	***Typical HRCT findings***	***HRCT differential diagnosis***
Chronic Fibrosing IIPs				
Idiopathic pulmonary fibrosis	Usual interstitial pneumonia	Peripheral, subpleural, basal	Reticular opacities, honeycombing, traction bronchiectasis, architectural distortion	Collagen vascular disease, hypersensitivity pneumonitis, asbestosis, sarcoidosis
Idiopathic nonspecific interstiial pneumonia	Nonspecific interstitial pneumonia	Peripheral, basal, symmetric	GGO, irregular lines, traction bronchiectasis, consolidation	Usual interstitial pneumonia, cryptogenic organizing pneumonia, desquamative interstitial pneumonia, hypersensitivity pneumonitis
Smoking IIPs				
Desquamative interstitial pneumonia	Desquamative interstitial pneumonia	Lower zone, peripheral predominance in most cases	GGO, reticular lines, cysts	Respiratory bronchiolitis—interstitial lung disease, nonspecific interstitial pneumonia, hypersensitivity pneumonitis
Respiratory bronchiolitis-associated interstitial lung disease	Respiratory bronchiolitis	Upper lung predominant	Centrilobular nodules, bronchial wall thickening, patchy GGO	Nonspecific interstitial pneumonia, desquamative interstitial pneumonia, hypersensitivity pneumonitis
Acute or Subacute IIPs				
Cryptogenic organizing pneumonia	organizing pneumonia	subpleural or peribronchial	Patchy consolidation or nodules, perilobular pattern reverse halo sign	Infection, aspiration pneumonia, eosinophilic pneumonia, nonspecific interstitial pneumonia, vasculitis, sarcoidosis, mucinous adenocarcinoma, lymphoma
Acute interstitial pneumonia	Diffuse alveolar damage	Bilateral or patchy	Consolidation, GGO, later traction bronchiectasis	Hydrostatic edema, pulmonary hemorrhage, acute eosinophilic pneumonia
Rare IIPs				
Lymphoid interstitial pneumonia	Lymphoid interstitial pneumonia	Lower lung predominant	GGO, centrilobular nodules, septal and bronchovascular thickening, thin-walled cysts	Nonspecific interstitial Pneumonia, sarcoidosis, Langerhans cell histiocytosis, lymphangioleiomyomatosis
Idiopathic pleura parenchymal fibro-elastosis	Idiopathic pleural parenchymal fibroelastosis	Peripheral, upper lung predominant	Pleural thickening, subpleural fibrotic changes or consolidation	Sarcoidosis, pneumoconiosis, postinfective pulmonary fibrosis, connective tissue disease, hypersensitivity pneumonitis

tissue. It is the smallest unit of the lung, which is visible on HRCT scan **(Fig. 2)**. The secondary pulmonary lobule is a polyhedron that depicts the smallest lung unit, which measures approximately 1–2 cm on one side and contains a few terminal bronchioles, which ultimately supply 5–15 pulmonary acini. Terminal bronchiole and centrilobular artery are present at the center of a secondary pulmonary lobule and pulmonary veins and lymphatics are present in the periphery. The interlobular septa in the periphery contain connective tissue, venules, and lymphatics. On HRCT, centrilobular artery and intralobular acinar arteries supplying a secondary pulmonary lobule can be discerned, while normal bronchioles supplying it cannot be. Centrilobular arteries measure approximately 1 mm in diameter. Intralobular acinar arteries measure approximately 0.5 mm in diameter. Normal bronchiole

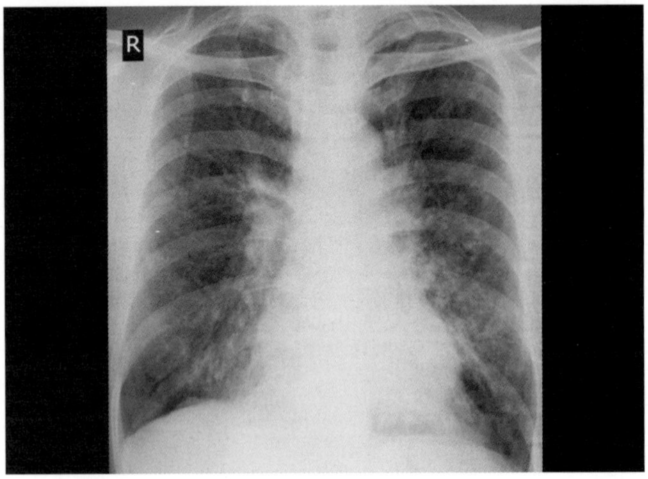

Fig. 1: Frontal chest radiograph posteroanterior view reveals reticulonodular opacities in bilateral lower lobes.

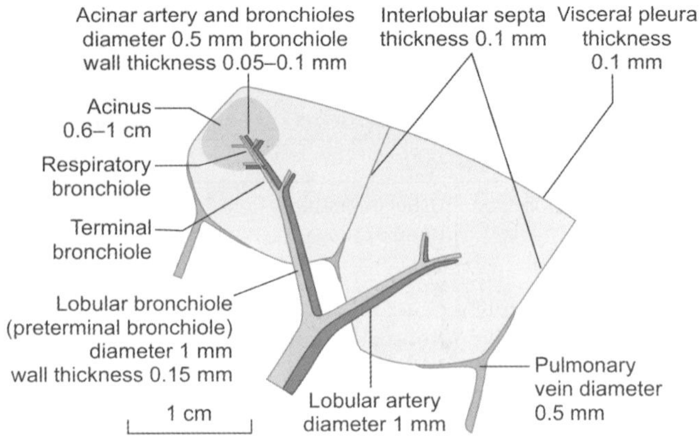

Fig. 2: Anatomy and dimensions of secondary lobule and pulmonary acinus. Two secondary pulmonary lobules in the lung periphery are illustrated along with the dimensions of their components.

supplying a secondary pulmonary lobule measure approximately 1 mm in diameter with wall thickness of approximately 0.15 mm, which is beyond the resolution of HRCT. However, abnormal thickening of the interlobular and intralobular septa, axial interstitium surrounding the bronchovascular bundles and subpleural peripheral interstitium should always be identified on HRCT.

The correct diagnosis of interstitial lung disease on HRCT depends on evaluating the morphology and density of the lung abnormalities and their distribution in relationship to the secondary pulmonary lobule. Lung abnormalities are first classified into four categories—increased lung attenuation, decreased lung attenuation, linear and reticular opacities, and nodules and nodular opacities.

Increased Lung Attenuation

It is classified into ground-glass opacity (GGO), consolidation, alveolar microlithiasis, metastatic calcification and granulomatous diseases (tuberculosis, silicosis, sarcoidosis). GGO is defined as mild increase in lung opacity, which does not cause obscuration of underlying vessel **(Fig. 3)**. It suggests an active or acute disease. Consolidation is defined as increased lung opacity, which causes obscuration of underlying vascular markings **(Fig. 4)**. Air bronchogram is characteristic finding seen in consolidation.

Decreased Lung Attenuation

It is categorized into mosaic perfusion, honeycombing, bronchiectasis, emphysema, pneumatoceles and lung cysts. Mosaic perfusion pattern is obtained due to differential attenuation of areas of lungs, caused due to differences in lung perfusion, either due to pulmonary vascular disease or airway disease. The pulmonary arteries are reduced in size in the lucent lung fields, which helps to distinguish mosaic perfusion from GGO **(Fig. 5)**. Honeycombing can be defined as clustered cystic airspaces, which have clearly definable walls and are most commonly seen in peripheral and subpleural lung **(Fig. 6)**. Bronchiectasis is localized, abnormal dilatation of bronchial tree usually segmental and subsegmental bronchi, which occurs as a result of airway inflammation, infections or impaired mucociliary clearance **(Fig. 3)**. Emphysema is known as irreversible abnormal enlargement and destruction of airspaces distal to terminal bronchiole **(Fig. 7)**. Lung cysts are well defined, thin walled (approximately 1–3 mm) air containing lesions. Multiple lung cysts are seen in diseases like lymphangioleiomyomatosis, Langerhans cell histiocytosis and lymphoid interstitial pneumonias.

Nodules and Nodular Opacities

HRCT classifies nodules into 3 categories depending on location, i.e. which portion of secondary pulmonary lobule is involved. Centrilobular nodules involve terminal/respiratory bronchioles **(Fig. 4)**. Perilymphatic nodules are seen in subpleural and peribronchovascular region. Random nodules have no particular anatomic distribution. Common causes of centrilobular nodules are infectious airway diseases, hypersensitivity pneumonitis and respiratory bronchiolitis. Perilymphatic nodules are seen in sarcoidosis, lymphangitic carcinomatosis, silicosis and coal worker pneumoconiosis. Random nodules are seen in tuberculosis, angioinvasive fungal infections and hematogenous metastasis.

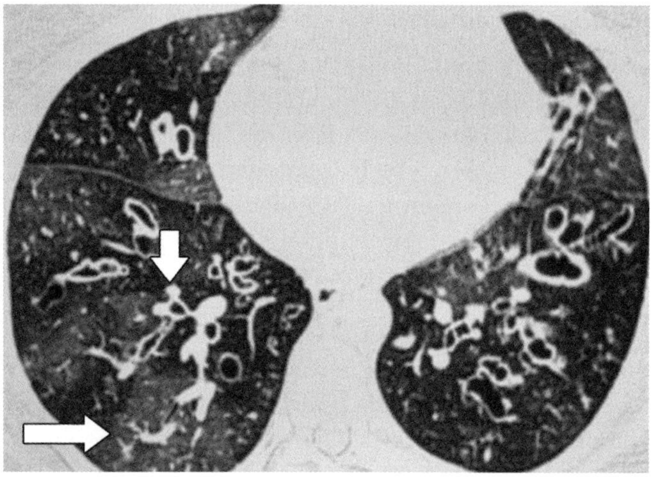

Fig. 3: Axial HRCT chest shows patchy areas of ground-glass opacity (long arrow) in bilateral lungs with varicose bronchiectasis, bronchial wall thickening and signet ring sign (short arrow).

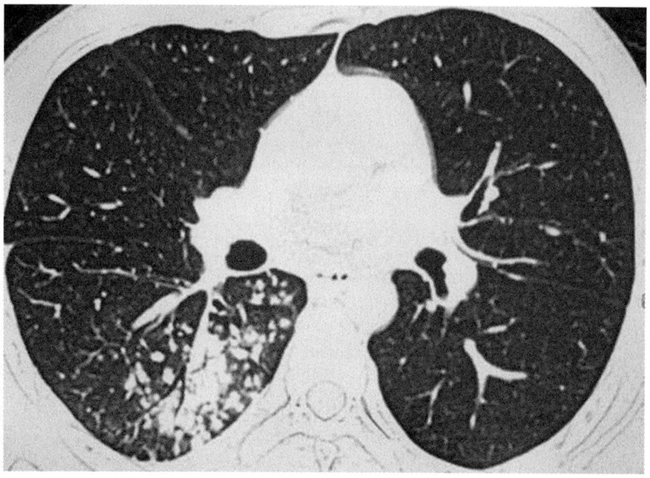

Fig. 4: Axial HRCT chest shows patchy areas of consolidation with air bronchogram in right lower lobe surrounded by multiple centrilobular nodules.

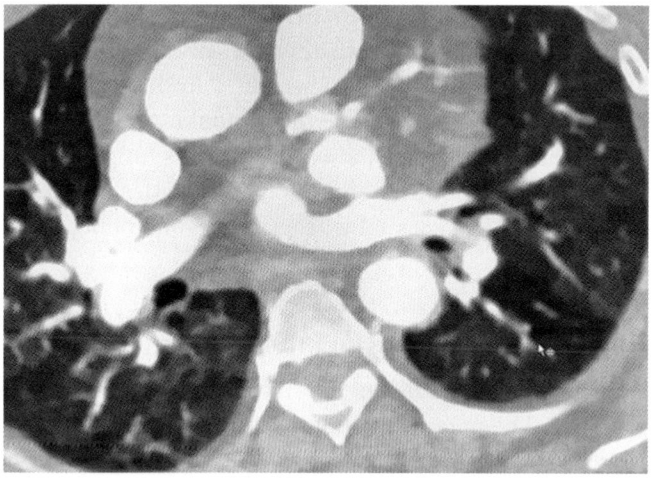

Fig. 5: Axial HRCT chest shows areas of mosaic perfusion in bilateral lungs.

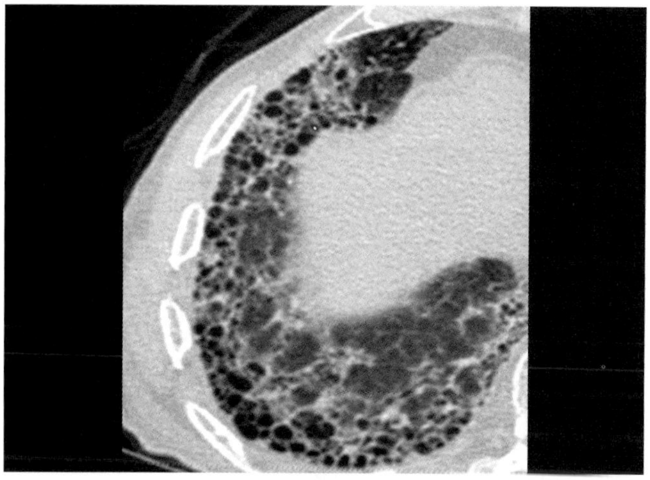

Fig. 6: Axial HRCT chest shows honeycombing consisting of multilayered thin-walled cyst.

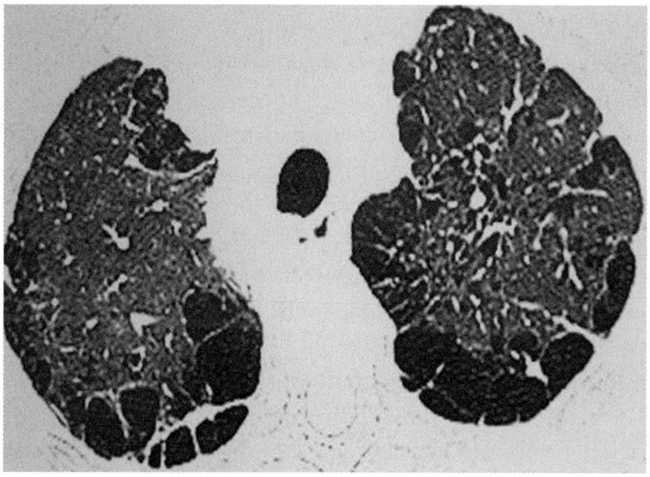

Fig. 7: Axial HRCT chest shows centriacinar and paraseptal emphysematous changes in bilateral upper lobes.

Linear and Reticular Opacities

These are categorized into intralobular septal thickening, interlobular septal thickening **(Fig. 8)**, parenchymal bands, peribronchovascular interstitial thickening and subpleural lines. Intralobular septal thickening is seen in IPF, chronic hypersensitivity pneumonitis, NSIP and asbestosis. Interlobular septal thickening is seen in lymphangitis carcinomatosis, LIP, IPF, sarcoidosis, pulmonary edema, silicosis, CWP, pneumocystis pneumonia. Parenchymal bands are linear opacities, which are several millimeters thick and approximately 2–5 cm in length. They are seen in patients with fibrosis. Crazy paving pattern is formed when there is concurrence of GGO with reticulations.

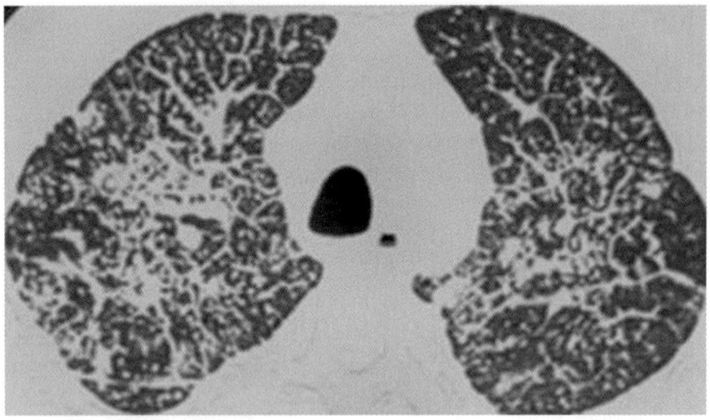

Fig. 8: Axial HRCT chest shows intralobular and interlobular septal thickening in bilateral upper lobes.

IDIOPATHIC INTERSTITIAL PNEUMONIAS

The final diagnosis of an IIP's should always be a consensus diagnosis made after evaluation by the chest physician, radiologist, and pathologist. The diagnosis may be altered as more details emerge from the patient's history, fine needle aspiration cytology, biopsy, bronchoalveolar lavage, or post-surgery lung histopathology. Lung damage similar to that seen in IIPs is also seen in diseases like connective tissue disorders, asbestosis, chronic hypersensitivity pneumonitis and drug reaction. The term idiopathic is used, when the cause of lung damage is not known and other known etiologies of lung damage have been excluded.

CHRONIC FIBROSING IDIOPATHIC INTERSTITIAL PNEUMONIAS

Idiopathic Pulmonary Fibrosis

Idiopathic pulmonary fibrosis (IPF) is a chronic fibrosing form of IIP, which is associated with the radiological or histopathological pattern of usual interstitial pneumonia (UIP). It occurs predominantly in older adult population and is associated with median survival of less than 5 years. The term IPF is used when other recognized causes of ILD have been excluded and there is UIP pattern seen on HRCT. IPF particularly excludes IIPs such as NSIP and DIP.[4] IPF is the most common ILD accounting for 25–50% of diffuse lung diseases. According to the current guidelines of American Thoracic Society and European Respiratory Society, an algorithm has been devised on the basis of which three levels of certainty can be assigned for UIP on the basis of HRCT findings (UIP, possible UIP, and inconsistent with UIP).[5]

Radiologic Features

Chest radiograph: Almost all patients of IPF who present with symptoms, have abnormal chest radiograph findings. The most common chest radiograph pattern is peripheral reticular opacities, which are predominant in the lower zones and are sometimes associated with honeycombing and volume loss of lower zones. Chest radiographs may sometimes also be normal.

HRCT: The diagnosis of UIP is usually made on the basis of clinical and imaging features, because of the high diagnostic accuracy of HRCT for cases of UIP.[4] Those cases without a confident HRCT diagnosis may require a biopsy. Characteristic HRCT features of UIP include reticular lines, traction bronchiectasis and bronchiolectasis, and honeycombing which are predominant in lower lobes and subpleural, peripheral lung. They may be associated with lower lobe volume loss **(Figs. 9A and B)**. GGO is much less common. Architectural distortion due to lung fibrosis is often seen. The HRCT findings of GGOs which occur in association with reticular opacities and traction bronchiectasis, always indicates lung fibrosis. Patients with preponderant reticular opacities or honeycombing on HRCT, usually progress despite being given treatment.[6]

Nonspecific Interstitial Pneumonia

Nonspecific interstitial pneumonia (NSIP) is less common than UIP. The mean age of patients at onset is about 40–50 years.[7] Onset of NSIP is gradual, but some patients may have subacute onset. Patients usually present with symptoms of breathlessness and cough. Histologic and radiologic findings of NSIP can be found in patients with drug-induced lung diseases, collagen vascular diseases and hypersensitivity pneumonitis. Hence, when HRCT pattern of NSIP is seen, these etiologies should be ruled out. In addition, HRCT features similar to those seen in NSIP may be seen in patients of organizing pneumonia, UIP and DIP and surgical biopsy may sometimes be required to differentiate them.

NSIP is further classified into two types: fibrotic or cellular subtypes. Fibrotic NSIP is more common than cellular subtype. On histology, interstitial thickening is mainly due to fibrosis with mild inflammation. In cellular NSIP, thickening of interstitium is due to infiltration by plasma cells and lymphocytes. Cellular NSIP has a better prognosis and usually shows response to corticosteroids.[8]

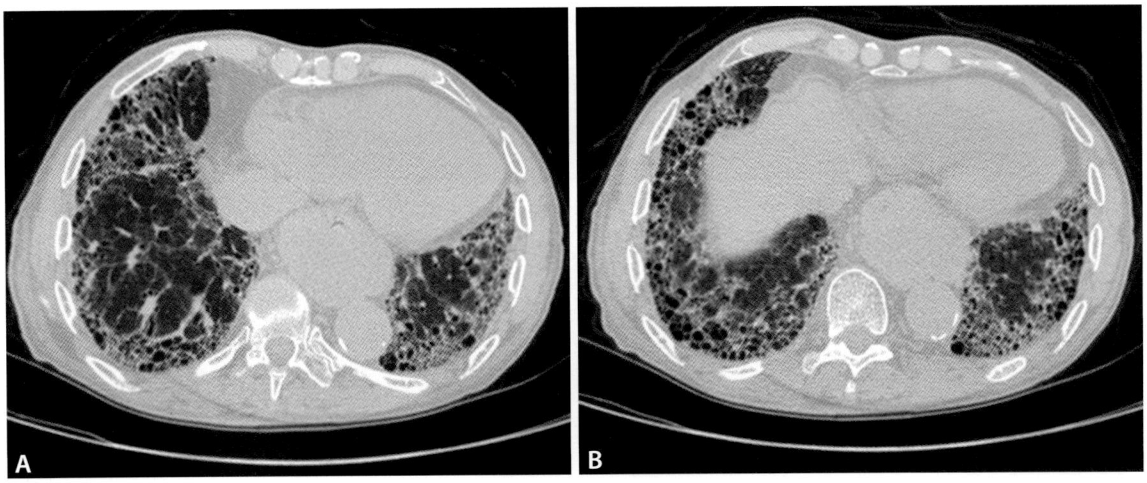

Figs. 9A and B: *Idiopathic pulmonary fibrosis (IPF)*: Axial HRCT chest shows intralobular and interlobular septal thickening with honeycombing and tractional bronchiectasis more pronounced in bilateral lower lobes.

It is sometimes difficult to differentiate fibrotic NSIP and UIP on histology. While fibrotic NSIP shows temporal homogeneity, UIP shows heterogeneity with collagen and fibroblastic foci, representing old and active disease together. This may aid in differentiating the two.[9]

Radiologic Features

Chest radiograph: NSIP shows infiltrates in bilateral lungs which are more common in lower zones.

HRCT features: The predominant HRCT finding of NSIP is GGO, which is usually bilateral, symmetric and preponderant in lower lobes and peripheral lung. Pathologically, GGO corresponds to homogeneous interstitial inflammation.[10] Irregular linear or reticular opacities are seen which may be associated with traction bronchiectasis or bronchiolectasis **(Figs. 10A and B)**. Honeycombing is rarely seen. Other occasional findings include nodules, pleural effusion, and hilar or meditational lymphadneopathy.

SMOKING-RELATED INTERSTITIAL PNEUMONIAS

RB, RB-ILD and DIP are currently thought of as a continuum of smoking-related lung diseases. There is similarity in their clinical, radiological and histological findings.[2] RB is asymptomatic and is detected at autopsy. RB-ILD is the term used when RB is associated with pulmonary symptoms or radiological findings. DIP represents the worst of this spectrum, in which imaging and histologic findings are more extensive.

Respiratory Bronchiolitis-associated Interstitial Lung Disease

Both RB and RB-ILD on histology show pigmented macrophages within first and second order respiratory bronchioles.[11] In RB-ILD, the degree of abnormality is generally more.[12] The course of this disease following smoking cessation generally improves.[13]

Radiologic Features

Chest radiograph: The most common abnormality in RB-ILD, on chest radiograph is thickening of the central or peripheral airway walls, which is seen in approximately 76% of patients. Ground-glass opacity is seen in 57% of patients.[14]

HRCT features: The common findings of RB-ILD include centrilobular nodules, patchy GGOs, and thickening of the central or peripheral airway walls **(Fig. 11)**. RB-ILD can be usually diagnosed in smokers with these HRCT findings, without the aid of lung biopsy.[5] The HRCT features of hypersensitivity pneumonitis may overlap with those of RB and RB-ILD. However, the centrilobular nodules, mosaic attenuation, air trapping and GGO found in hypersensitivity pneumonitis are usually more extensive. Additionally, almost all patients with hypersensitivity pneumonitis are nonsmokers.

Desquamative Interstitial Pneumonia

DIP is an uncommon interstitial pneumonia. It overlaps with RB-ILD in that the quality of the pigment-laden macrophages is identical, but their distribution and extent

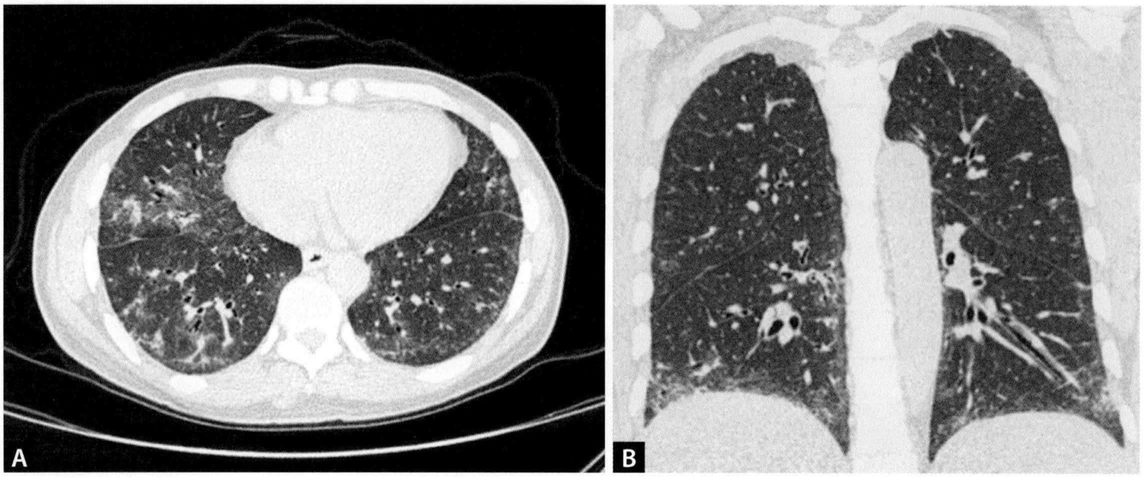

Figs. 10A and B: *Nonspecific interstitial pneumonia (NSIP)*: Axial and coronal HRCT chest shows bilateral patchy areas of ground-glass opacity and subpleural reticulations with mild-traction bronchiectasis in bilateral lower lobes. Fissural nodularity and fibronodular lesions seen are also seen in bilateral upper lobes and RML.

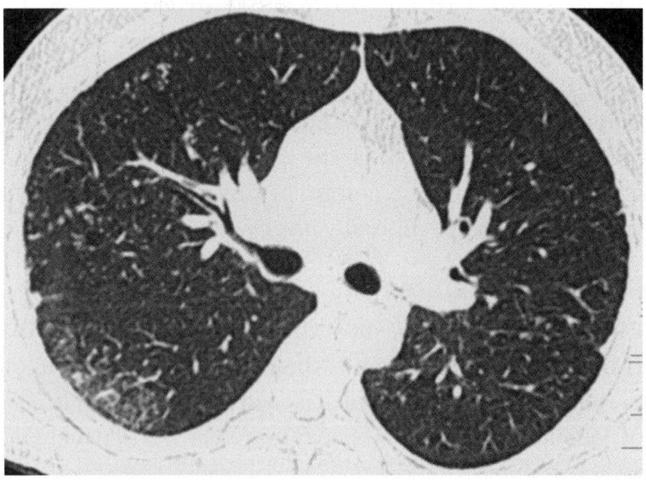

Fig. 11: *Respiratory bronchiolitis-interstitial lung disease (RB- ILD)*: Axial HRCT chest shows multiple ill-defined nodules in a chronic smoker with RB-ILD.

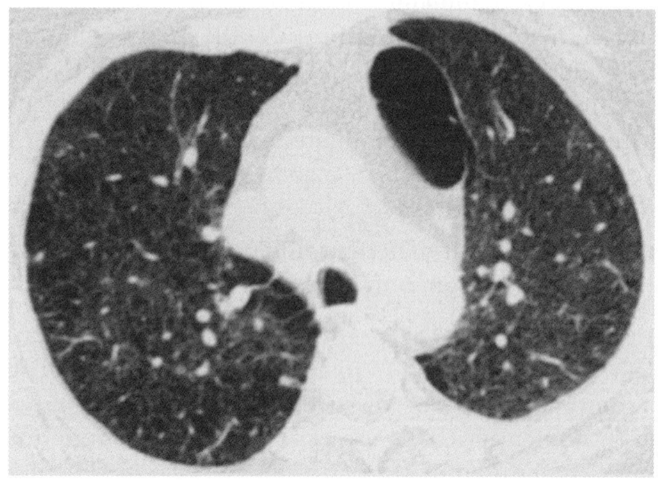

Fig. 12: *Desquamative interstitial pneumonia (DIP)*: Axial HRCT chest shows diffuse ill-defined bilateral symmetrical ground-glass opacification. Centrilobular emphysema with large left-sided bulla is also noted in this 45 years old heavy smoker.

differ, with pigment-laden macrophages being more diffuse and extensive in desquamative interstitial pneumonia.[2]

Radiologic Features

Chest radiograph: Chest radiograph may be normal in approximately 3–22% of cases of DIP. On chest radiograph, findings that can be seen are diffuse patchy GGOs, with predominance in lower zones and in periphery.[15]

HRCT: The most common and characteristic finding of DIP is GGOs, which are present on HRCT in all cases of DIP **(Fig. 12)**. This occurs due to the homogeneous accumulation of intra-alveolar macrophages and alveolar septal thickening. Mid and lower lobes predominance with peripheral distribution is seen in most of the cases. Reticular opacities are sometimes present. Well-defined and thin-walled cysts may be seen. The GGOs usually resolve with treatment. The main imaging difference between RB-ILD and DIP is the distribution of disease, which is predominantly centrilobular in RB-ILD and diffuse in DIP. Centrilobular nodules are uncommonly seen in patients of DIP. GGOs are usually patchier, less well defined, and less extensive in RB-ILD.

ACUTE AND SUBACUTE INTERSTITIAL PNEUMONIAS

Cryptogenic Organizing Pneumonia

Cryptogenic organizing pneumonia (COP) was previously referred to as bronchiolitis obliterans organizing pneumonia. However, cryptogenic organizing pneumonia is the preferred term because organizing pneumonia is the predominant feature and is responsible for the physiologic abnormalities and radiologic findings.

Radiologic Features

Chest radiograph: The most common chest radiograph findings in COP are unilateral or bilateral areas of consolidation.

HRCT: HRCT typically shows patchy, possibly migratory, unilateral or bilateral areas of consolidation or/and GGOs in a peribronchovascular or subpleural location **(Fig. 13)**. Air bronchograms with mild cylindrical bronchial dilatation may be frequently seen in areas of consolidation. Pleural effusions may uncommonly occur.[16] Nodules are seen in 30% of cases. They are usually small and present predominantly along the bronchovascular bundles. Reticular opacities may be sometimes present and signify histologic evidence of fibrosis.

Acute Interstitial Pneumonia

AIP is a type of interstitial pneumonia that progresses rapidly. On histology, there is presence of diffuse alveolar damage (DAD). The term acute interstitial pneumonia is used when there is DAD of unknown origin. Patients with AIP often have a clinical prodrome suggesting viral upper respiratory tract infection. Patients have hypoxemia which rapidly progresses to respiratory failure, with mortality rate of 50% or more. Treatment is generally supportive and mechanical ventilation is usually required.

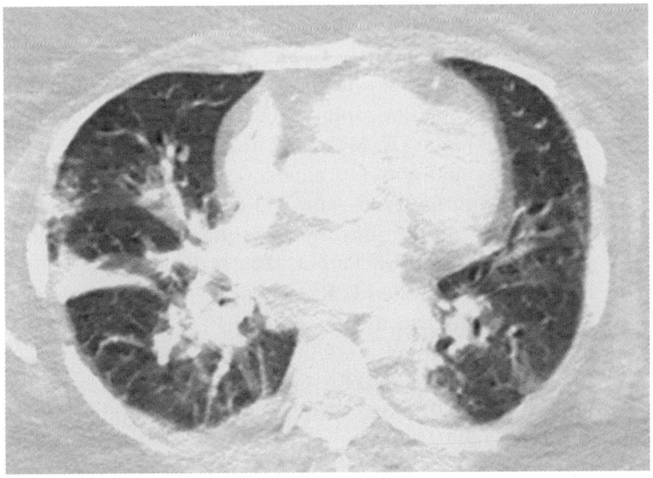

Fig. 13: *Cryptogenic organizing pneumonia (COP)*: Axial HRCT chest shows bilateral ill-defined ground-glass opacities with patchy areas of consolidation in bilateral upper lobes.

Radiologic Features

Chest radiograph: The chest radiograph shows patchy/diffuse areas of air space opacities bilaterally **(Fig. 14A)**.

HRCT: AIP is characterized by three stages, early exudative phase, subacute proliferative phase and chronic fibrotic phase. The first exudative phase of AIP, shows bilateral patchy GGOs with areas of focal sparing, often with consolidation in the dependent part of lungs **(Figs. 14B and C)**. While the later fibrotic stage of AIP shows distortion of bronchovascular bundles and traction bronchiectasis. AIP can progress to severe fibrosis with areas of honeycombing.[2] Few patients who survive this disease show progressive resolution of the areas of GGO and consolidation. On later HRCT scans, areas of hypoattenuation, reticular pattern, traction bronchiectasis and associated architectural distortion occurring predominantly in the nondependent part of lungs can be seen.

RARE INTERSTITIAL PNEUMONIAS

The recently created category of rare IIPs includes idiopathic LIP and IPPFE.[2]

Lymphoid Interstitial Pneumonia

LIP is a lymphoproliferative disorder, in which there is infiltration of lung interstitium predominantly by lymphocytes. The incidence of idiopathic LIP is low. LIP is most frequently associated with Sjogren's syndrome, autoimmune thyroid diseases, AIDS, and Castleman syndrome.

Radiologic Features

Chest radiograph: It is neither sensitive nor specific. Findings include bilateral basal reticular opacities and ill-defined nodules.[17]

HRCT: The predominant HRCT findings are usually GGO and perivascular cysts **(Fig. 15)**, sometimes leading to misdiagnosis of lymphangioleiomyomatosis. However, cysts related to LIP usually predominate in the lower lungs and around bronchi and vessels, in contrast to the diffuse distribution of cysts in lymphangioleiomyomatosis.

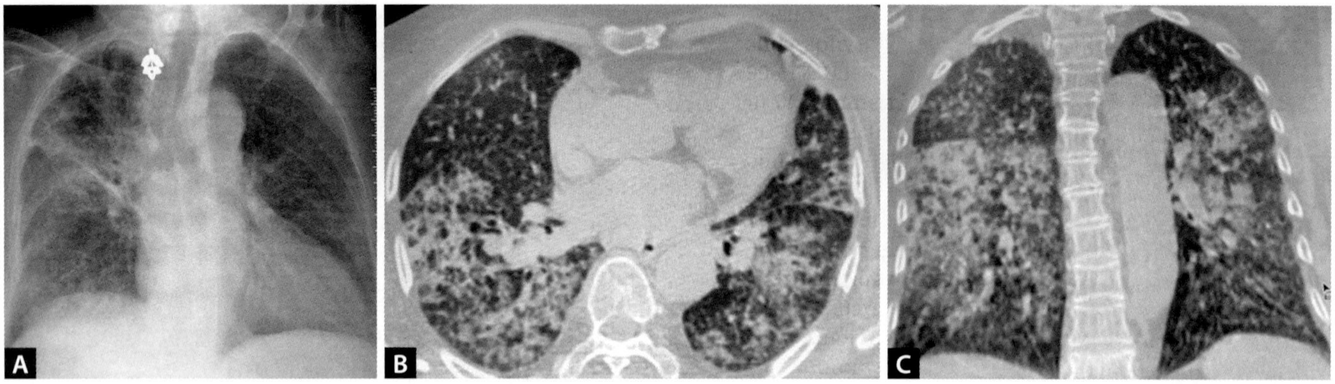

Figs. 14A to C: *Acute interstitial pneumonia (AIP)*: (A) Frontal chest radiograph posteroanterior view reveals bilateral airspace opacification with air bronchograms, with sparing of the costophrenic angles; (B and C) Axial and coronal HRCT shows bilateral diffuse ground-glass opacity and consolidation of the dependent lung.

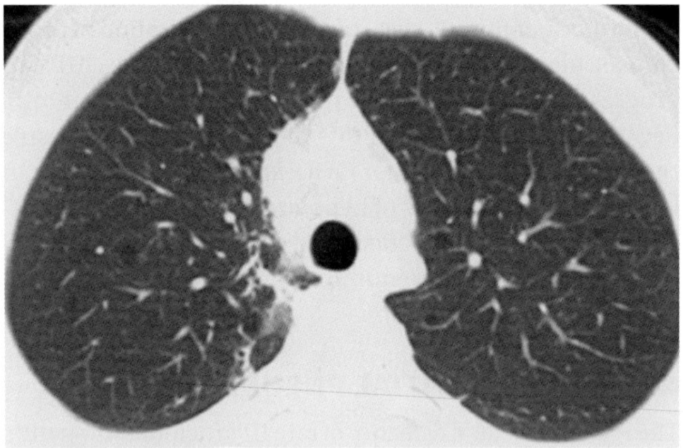

Fig. 15: Lymphoid interstitial pneumonia (LIP): Axial HRCT chest shows few thin wall perivascular cysts in bilateral lungs in a patient with AIDS and LIP.

Peribronchovascular and interlobular septae thickening are also seen frequently in cases of LIP. Centrilobular nodules may also be seen. Rarely, perivascular honeycombing can be seen.[18,19]

Idiopathic Pulmonary Fibroelastosis

This rare condition of IPPEE is diagnosed when there is upper-lobe predominant fibrosis involving the subpleural lung parenchyma and pleura. On histologic evaluation, intra-alveolar fibrosis is present and the fibrosis is elastotic.[20] Recurrent infections have been noted in half of patients. HRCT in patients with IPPFE is characterized by dense subpleural consolidation in the upper lobes. In addition, areas of traction bronchiectasis and architectural distortion may be seen.[21]

REFERENCES

1. American Thoracic Society/European Respiratory Society international multidisciplinary consensus classification of the idiopathic interstitial pneumonias. This joint statement of the American Thoracic Society (ATS), and the European Respiratory Society (ERS) was adopted by the ATS board of directors, June 2001 and by the ERS Executive Committee, June 2001. Am J Respir Crit Care Med. 2002;165(2):277-304.
2. Sverzellati N, Lynch DA, Hansell DM, et al. American Thoracic Society—European Respiratory Society Classification of the Idiopathic Interstitial Pneumonias: Advances in Knowledge since 2002. RadioGraphics. 2015;35:1849-72.
3. Hobbs S, Lynch D. The Idiopathic Interstitial Pneumonias: An Update and Review. Radiol Clin N Am. 2014;52:105-20.
4. American Thoracic Society. Idiopathic pulmonary fibrosis: Diagnosis and treatment—International Consensus Statement: American Thoracic Society (ATS), and the European Respiratory Society (ERS). Am J Respir Crit Care Med. 2000;161:646-64.
5. Mueller-Mang C, Grosse C, Schmid K, et al. What Every Radiologist Should Know about Idiopathic Interstitial Pneumonias? RadioGraphics. 2007;27:595-615.
6. Travis WD, Matsui K, Moss J, et al. Idiopathic nonspecific interstitial pneumonia: prognostic significance of cellular and fibrosing patterns—survival comparison with usual interstitial pneumonia and desquamative interstitial pneumonia. Am J Surg Pathol. 2000;24:19-33.
7. Flaherty KR, Thwaite EL, Kazerooni EA, et al. Radiological versus histological diagnosis in UIP and NSIP: survival implications. Thorax. 2003;58:143-8.
8. Ferguson EC, Berkowitz EA. Lung CT: Part 2, The Interstitial Pneumonias—Clinical, Histologic, and CT Manifestations AJR. 2012;199:W464-76.
9. Remy-Jardin M, Remy J, Gosselin B, et al. Lung parenchymal changes secondary to cigarette smoking: pathologic-CT correlations. Radiology. 1993;186(3):643-51.

10. Holt RM, Schmidt RA, Godwin JD, et al. High resolution CT in respiratory bronchiolitis-associated interstitial lung disease. J Comput Assist Tomogr. 1993;17(1):46-50.
11. Vassallo R, Ryu JH. Tobacco smoke-related diffuse lung diseases. Semin Respir Crit Care Med. 2008;29(6): 643-50.
12. Portnoy J, Veraldi KL, Schwarz MI, et al. Respiratory bronchiolitis-interstitial lung disease: longterm outcome. Chest. 2007;131(3):664-71.
13. An Official American Thoracic Society/European Respiratory Society Statement: Update of the International Multidisciplinary Classification of the Idiopathic Interstitial Pneumonias William D. Travis, Ulrich Costabel, David M. Hansell Am J Respir Crit Care Med. 2013;6(188):733-48.
14. Dalphin JC, Debieuvre D, Pernet D, et al. Prevalence and risk factors for chronic bronchitis and farmer's lung in French dairy farmers. Br J Ind Med. 1993;50(10):941-4.
15. Lynch DA, Travis WD, Müller NL, et al. Idiopathic interstitial pneumonias: CT features. Radiology. 2005;236:10-21.
16. Lee JS, Lynch DA, Sharma S, et al. Organizing pneumonia: prognostic implication of high-resolution computed tomography features. J Comput Assist Tomogr. 2003;27(2):260-5.
17. Johkoh T, Muller NL, Pickford HA, et al. Lymphocytic interstitial pneumonia: thin-section CT findings in 22 patients. Radiology. 1999;212(2):567-72.
18. Ichikawa Y, Kinoshita M, Koga T, et al. Lung cyst formation in lymphocytic interstitial pneumonia: CT features. J Comput Assist Tomogr. 1994;18(5):745-8.
19. Becker CD, Gil J, Padilla ML. Idiopathic pleura parenchymal fibro elastosis: an unrecognized or misdiagnosed entity? Mod Pathol. 2008;21(6):784-7.
20. Frankel SK, Cool CD, Lynch DA, et al. Idiopathic pleura parenchymal fibroelastosis: description of a novel clinicopathologic entity. Chest. 2004;126(6):2007-13.
21. Reddy TL, Tominaga M, Hansell DM, et al. Pleuroparenchymal fibroelastosis: a spectrum of histopathological and imaging phenotypes. Eur Respir J. 2012;40(2):377-85.

CHAPTER 164

Imaging of Interstitial Lung Disease of Known Etiology

Smriti Hari, Surabhi Vyas, Sanjay Sharma, Deep Narayan Srivastava

INTRODUCTION

Interstitial lung diseases (ILDs) are a group of disorders characterized by diffuse parenchymal lung abnormalities and clinically present with dyspnea, restrictive pulmonary function, and impaired gas exchange. The etiological cause is sometimes not known. The consensus statement on interstitial pneumonias classifies interstitial lung diseases into idiopathic interstitial pneumonias and those secondary to a known cause viz.[1]:

- Connective tissue diseases
- Granulomatous diseases (sarcoidosis)
- Infections
- Exposure related
- Miscellaneous.

The revised joint statement by American Thoracic Society/European Respiratory Society (2013) emphasised a multidisciplinary approach towards clinical, imaging and histopathological findings of ILDs and reclassified the Idiopathic interstitial pneumonias (IIP) in the following broad groups:[2]

1. Chronic fibrosing IIPs—idiopathic pulmonary fibrosis, idiopathic non-specific interstitial pneumonia
2. Smoking related IIPs—respiratory bronchiolitis, desquamative interstitial pneumonia
3. Acute or subacute IIPs—cryptogenic organising pneumonia and acute interstitial pneumonia
4. Rare IIPs—idiopathic pleuroparenchymal fibroelastosis, lymphoid interstitial pneumonia
5. Unclassifiable IIPs.

Although ILDs more commonly affect adults, some entities like Langerhans cell histiocytosis (LCH) hypersensitivity pneumonitis (HP), and idiopathic interstitial pneumonias (IIPs) are seen in children as well.[3] Diagnosis is based on history, clinical examination, pulmonary function tests, imaging in the form of chest radiographs and computed tomography and occasionally histopathology from lung biopsy.

In this chapter, we shall discuss the major imaging modalities, imaging nomenclature, followed by ILDs due to known cause and the idiopathic interstitial pneumonias.

PLAIN RADIOGRAPHY

The radiological diagnostic approach to ILDs classically begins with chest X-ray evaluation, which is done as a PA radiograph, though radiography is not sensitive in detecting changes associated with ILDs. In assessing diffuse lung disease, radiography may help in indicating:

1. Pattern of lung disease
2. Lung volume abnormalities
3. Additional findings like lymphadenopathy, pleural thickening/effusion, cardiomegaly, soft tissue or musculoskeletal involvement
4. Interval changes from previous imaging.

Common patterns seen on radiography include nodular pattern reticular pattern airspace disease, or a combination of these. Most commonly, a reticulonodular pattern is encountered.

- Nodular pattern is found in sarcoidosis, silicosis, coal worker's pneumoconiosis (CWP), miliary tuberculosis or fungal infection, berylliosis, and Langerhans cell histiocytosis (LCH).
- A reticular pattern is seen in idiopathic pulmonary fibrosis (IPF), asbestosis, collagen vascular disease, and chronic hypersensitivity pneumonitis.
- Airspace filling is the dominant pattern in cryptogenic organizing pneumonia (COP), eosinophilic pneumonia, alveolar proteinosis, vasculitis, and so called "alveolar sarcoidosis."

Volume loss:

- Involving the upper lobes—sarcoidosis, silicosis, chronic hypersensitivity pneumonitis, CWP, ankylosing spondylitis, radiation pneumonitis.
- Involving the lower lobes—asbestosis, IPF, and collagen vascular disease
- Lung volumes are preserved in LAM and LCH.

Mediastinal lymphadenopathy: It can occur with sarcoidosis or progressive systemic sclerosis (PSS). Pleural effusion points to rheumatoid disease, lupus erythematosus, or LAM.

Pleural plaques indicate asbestos exposure and the possibility that basal fibrosis could represent asbestosis.

Comparison with old radiographs can help to distinguish interstitial diseases—which typically run a subacute or chronic course—from acute diseases, such as infection or edema. It is also important in assessing progression and response to treatment.

However, chest radiography has substantial limitations viz.:

- Obscuration and overlap of various lung zones
- Limited contrast resolution, which impairs sensitivity to subtle alterations in lung density (e.g. ground-glass opacity or emphysema)
- Superimposition of the interstitial opacities within the lung which makes it difficult to characterize their shape and distribution.

Chest radiograph may be normal in 10–15% of proven infiltrative lung disease and may simulate changes of paraseptal emphysema and small-airway disease or may show non-specific findings.[4]

HIGH-RESOLUTION CT

High-resolution CT (HRCT) is routinely used in the assessment of ILD with the following common indications:

- Confirming presence, pattern, distribution, activity of disease
- Response assessment
- The selection site and type of biopsy
- Follow-up of on medical treatment
- Evaluation of associated conditions like emphysema, bronchiectasis, and bronchiolitis.

Details of the technique of HRCT have already been discussed in other chapters.

Anatomy of Secondary Pulmonary Lobule

- Secondary pulmonary lobule is the smallest anatomical unit of the lung visible on HRCT which on histology is the smallest area of lung parenchyma surrounded by connective tissue septa **(Fig. 1)**.[5] These septa, being 0.1 mm thick are only occasionally visible on HRCT.
- The secondary pulmonary lobule is shaped like a polyhedron measuring approximately 1 to 2.5 cm on a side containing few terminal bronchioles, which supply 3 to 12 acini. Pulmonary arterioles accompany the bronchioles.
- The interlobular septa contain connective tissue, venules, and lymphatics. Thickening of the interlobular and intralobular septae, peribronchovascular interstitium and subpleural interstitium is well identified on HRCT.
- Terminal bronchioles supplying a secondary lobule are not seen on HRCT.

CT interpretation in ILD takes in account the morphology, density and distribution of the lung abnormalities with respect to the secondary pulmonary lobule.

A glossary of terms that is used in HRCT interpretation is provided by the Fleischner Society and are summarized below:[6]

Air-trapping: Abnormal retention of gas within a lung or lung units following expiration.

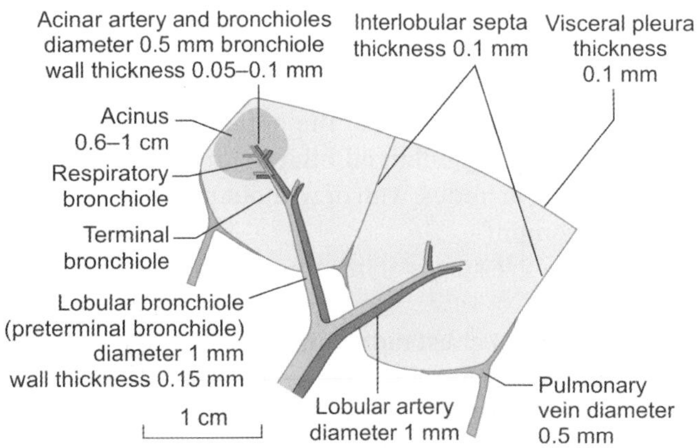

Fig. 1: Anatomy of secondary lobule and pulmonary acinus. Two adjacent secondary pulmonary lobules with their measurements and components.

Consolidation: An increase in lung opacity that results in obscuration of blood vessels.

Cyst: A clearly-marginated lucency with a wall that contains air, and no residual lung tissue. Emphysema is another cause of lucency in the lung, but an emphysematous space lacks clear margins and may contain some tissue strands, including blood vessels.

Ground-glass opacity: A hazy increase in lung opacity (compared with the density of normal lung) not associated with obscuration of underlying vessels.

Honeycombing: Cystic spaces ranging from several millimeters to several centimeters in diameter, characterized by thick, clearly definable fibrous walls, which typically are lined by bronchiolar epithelium.

Interlobular interstitial thickening: Abnormal thickening of the interlobular septae.

Intralobular interstitial thickening: Thickening of the intralobular interstitium, resulting in a fine reticular appearance to the lung parenchyma.

Nodule: A discrete, round, small opacity, ranging from 1 mm to 3 cm.

Reticulation: A network of linear strands of thickened interstitium.

Traction bronchiectasis: Bronchial dilation and irregularity occurring in patients who have pulmonary fibrosis, because of traction by fibrous tissue on the bronchial wall.

SARCOIDOSIS

Sarcoidosis is a chronic, multisystem disease of unknown etiology characterized pathologically by the presence of noncaseating granulomas.

- Commonly affects young and middle aged patients, females>males.
- Signs and symptoms—nonspecific, include fatigue, weight loss, and less commonly fever. About 50% of patients remain asymptomatic. Pulmonary manifestations[7] occur in 90% of the patients, in the form of symmetrically enlarged bilateral hilar and mediastinal lymph nodes, with or without lung parenchymal involvement.

There are five stages of intrathoracic abnormalities on radiography:[8]

Stage 0: Normal chest radiograph
Stage 1: Mediastinal and hilar lymphadenopathy
Stage 2: Lymphadenopathy with pulmonary parenchymal lesions
Stage 3: Pulmonary parenchymal lesions in the absence of hilar lymphadenopathy
Stage 4: Significant lung fibrosis with architectural distortion or bullae.

The main utility of this staging system is in predicting outcome.[9] However, interobserver concordance is the major limitation.

Imaging Features

Chest radiography—Hilar adenopathy is easily recognized on radiographs **(Fig. 2)**. Garland triad/1-2-3 sign/ Pawnbrokers sign, is the characteristic nodal involvement at the right paratracheal and bilateral hilar groups which may be identified on radiography.

CT–HRCT is the modality of choice:

- It is superior for demonstrating subtle mediastinal lymphadenopathy in the right paratracheal, aorto-pulmonary window and subcarinal region. In contrast to tubercular adenopathy, enlarged sarcoidosis lymph nodes tend to remain discrete, maintain their shape and do not have central necrosis. Sometimes, the nodes are calcified which may be amorphous, punctate, popcorn like, or eggshell-like peripheral.
- On HRCT, nodules are seen at initial evaluation in 90 to 100% of patients who have parenchymal abnormalities. They are small (5–10 mm), well-defined nodules **(Fig. 3)** occurring in a perilymphatic distribution in relation to the bronchovascular interstitium, pleural surfaces, interlobular septa, and interlobar fissures, predominantly in the upper and mid lungs. Miliary nodules may also occur. In about 15–25% of the patients, coalescing granulomas form large mass-like

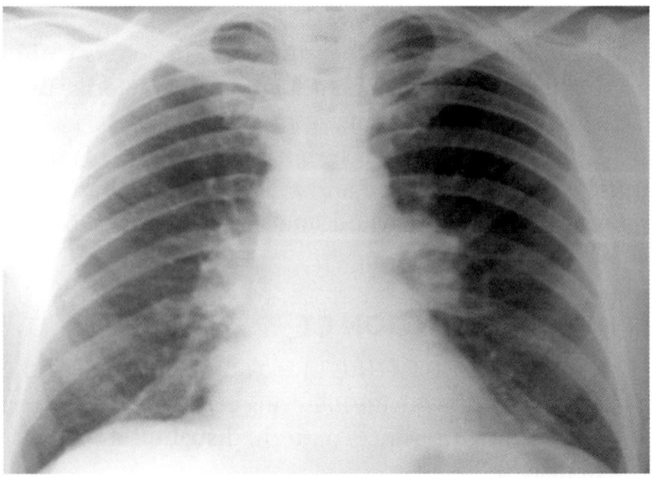

Fig. 2: Sarcoidosis: Frontal chest radiograph shows bulky, bilateral hilar lymphadenopathy.

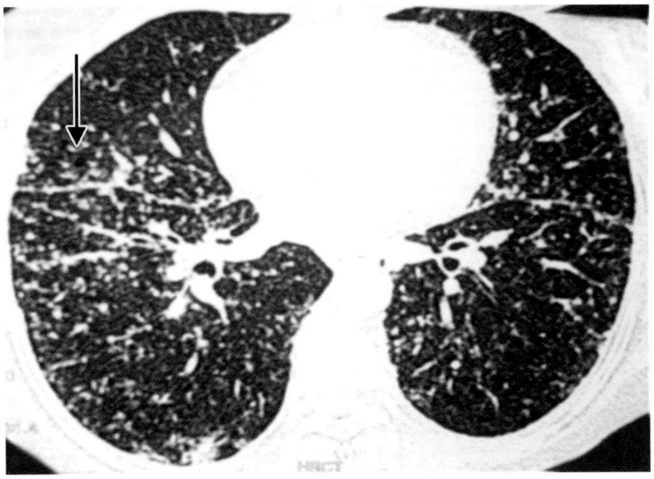

Fig. 3: Sarcoidosis: Axial HRCT shows numerous micronodules in subpleural, centrilobular and peribronchovascular distribution. Micronodular beading seen along the right major fissure (arrow).

nodules (1–4 cm in diameter), the so-called 'alveolar sarcoid pattern **(Figs. 4A and B)**.[10] When there are discrete nodules surrounding these confluent masses, it is termed as the "Galaxy sign". Unlike metastasis, these nodules are poorly defined and may contain air bronchogram within. Cavitating nodules are rare in sarcoidosis. The presence of cavitary disease should prompt exclusion of other conditions, such as vasculitis, tuberculosis, and necrotizing sarcoidosis.[11]

- Roughly 20% of the patients develop pulmonary fibrosis (Stage 4 disease): Conglomerated parahilar masses distorting bronchi and vessels **(Figs. 5A and B)**, traction bronchiectasis, septal thickening and honeycombing. The conglomerate masses near the hila with surrounding cicatricial emphysema resemble progressive massive fibrosis in complicated silicosis. Extensive calcification may be present within fibrotic granulomas.

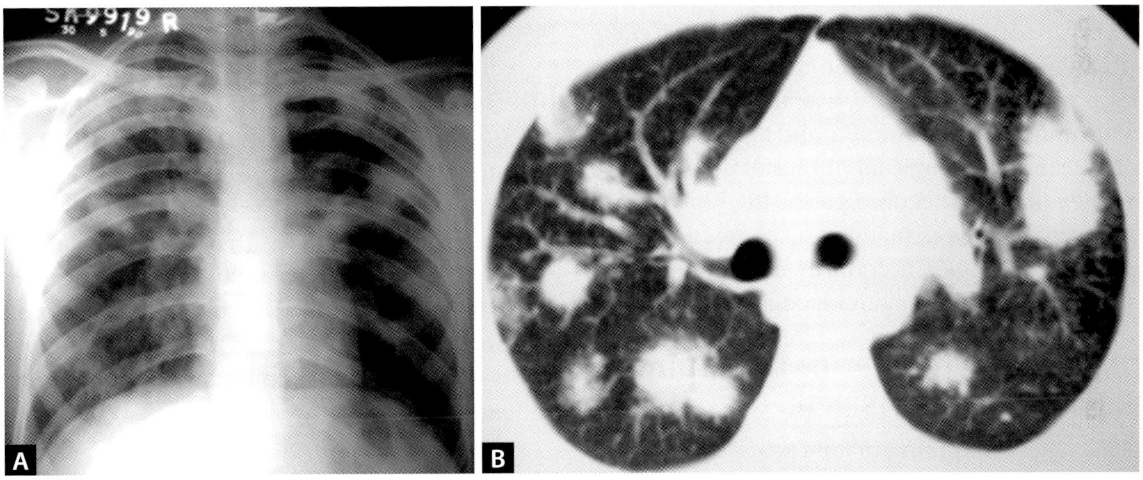

Figs. 4A and B: Alveolar sarcoidosis: (A) Frontal radiograph shows bulky hilar adenopathy and multiple lung nodules in bilateral upper and mid zones. (B) Axial CECT in the same patient shows well-defined, irregular parenchymal nodules indicating alveolar sarcoidosis.

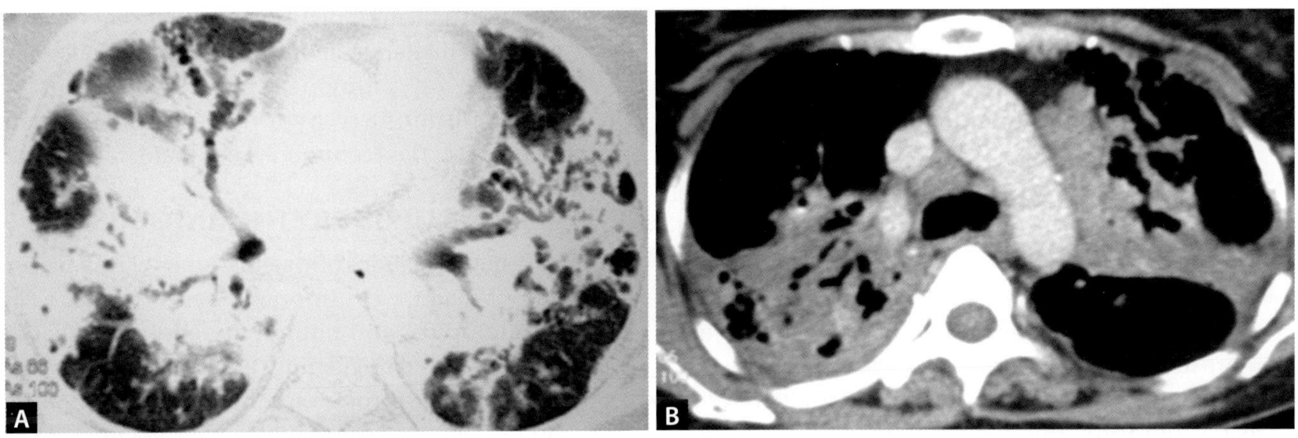

Figs. 5A and B : Sarcoidosis: (A) CECT chest (lung window) shows extensive, parahilar fibrotic masses with traction bronchiectasis, findings that indicate stage 4 disease; (B) CECT chest (mediastinal window) shows large fibrotic lesions, mediastinal adenopathy and irregularly thickened pleura.

- Airway involvement in the form of air trapping, mosaic attenuation and bronchial stenosis are non-specific findings, yet not uncommon.

Radionuclide scanning: Historically gallium scanning was performed for activity assessment, with limited specificity.[18] FDG-PET is used now-a-days for disease activity, location, and for prebiopsy planning.[12]

MRI has a role in evaluation of cardiac involvement of sarcoidosis.

CONNECTIVE TISSUE DISEASE (CTD) ASSOCIATED INTERSTITIAL LUNG DISEASE

Interstitial lung disease is re-frequently seen in patients with various collagen vascular diseases like systemic lupus erythematosus, rheumatoid arthritis, progressive systemic sclerosis, polymyositis and dermatomyositis, Sjögren syndrome and mixed connective tissue disease. At histopathologic examination, interstitial lung diseases associated with collagen vascular disease are diverse and include usual interstitial pneumonia, nonspecific interstitial pneumonia, COP, diffuse alveolar damage, lymphocytic interstitial pneumonia, and apical fibrosis.[13] The radiologic and pathological findings of CTD-ILD are identical to their idiopathic counterparts. HRCT has proved to be very sensitive in the detection and characterization of various histopathologically confirmed interstitial lung diseases in patients with collagen vascular diseases.

RHEUMATOID ARTHRITIS (RA) ASSOCIATED INTERSTITIAL LUNG DISEASE

About 5–40% of patients of rheumatoid arthritis (RA) have respiratory system involvement, including interstitial pneumonitis and fibrosis, rheumatoid (necrobiotic) nodules, COP, obliterative bronchiolitis, follicular bronchiolitis, and pleural effusion.[14] Interstitial pneumonitis and fibrosis are the most common pulmonary manifestations of rheumatoid arthritis with the later present in almost 5% of patients or radiography and 30–40% on HRCT.

Imaging Features

- UIP is the most common pattern of RA related ILD, with fine reticular pattern in early disease on radiography, with involvement of the lower lung zones. With disease progression, these reticulations become coarser and more diffuse in distribution. Honeycombing may also be seen in advanced disease. Similar to the findings at radiography, the predominant abnormality at HRCT consists of irregular linear opacities caused by a combination of thickening of interlobular and intralobular septa. Honeycombing is seen, most markedly near the diaphragm.
- NSIP is seen as the second most common pattern, with ground-glass opacities and microcyst formation.
- Acute interstitial pneumonia and organising pneumonia are less commonly seen patterns in RA- ILD.
- Drug-induced ILD may complicate the imaging appearance of RA-ILD with differentiation between the two possible on studying the temporal relationship only. Methotrexate is the most common causative agent.[15]

PROGRESSIVE SYSTEMIC SCLEROSIS (PSS)

Pulmonary involvement is commoner and more severe in systemic sclerosis than in other collagen vascular disease.[16] Interstitial fibrosis is the most common manifestation (in approximately 80% of patients). The histological features are those of NSIP or UIP, the former being more common and associated with worse prognosis.

Imaging Features

- Evidence of interstitial fibrosis has been reported at chest radiography in 20–65% of patients. Serial radiographs obtained over several years may show progressive loss of lung volume in addition to a worsening of the interstitial disease.
- HRCT frequently shows evidence of interstitial pneumonitis and fibrosis in patients who have normal or equivocal radiographic findings and may be used for monitoring the disease overtime. The abnormalities have a predominantly peripheral and posterior distribution **(Figs. 6A and B)**. The most common abnormalities that are seen on CT are peripheral and basal ground-glass opacities and fibrosis (often with subpleural sparing), pleural or pericardial effusion, esophageal dilatation, mediastinal lymphadenopathy, and sometimes pulmonary arterial dilatation that reflects pulmonary hypertension. Organizing pneumonia is a less commonly seen pattern in PSS-ILD.

SYSTEMIC LUPUS ERYTHEMATOSUS

Pulmonary manifestations of systemic lupus erythematosus (SLE) may be acute (pulmonary hemorrhage, acute lupus pneumonitis, and pulmonary edema), subacute (pleural effusion and thickening) and chronic (interstitial pneumonitis and fibrosis) manifestations. The most common radiologic abnormality is pleural effusion (25–35%). Pericardial effusion is seen in approximately 20% of patients and pulmonary parenchymal involvement in 20%.

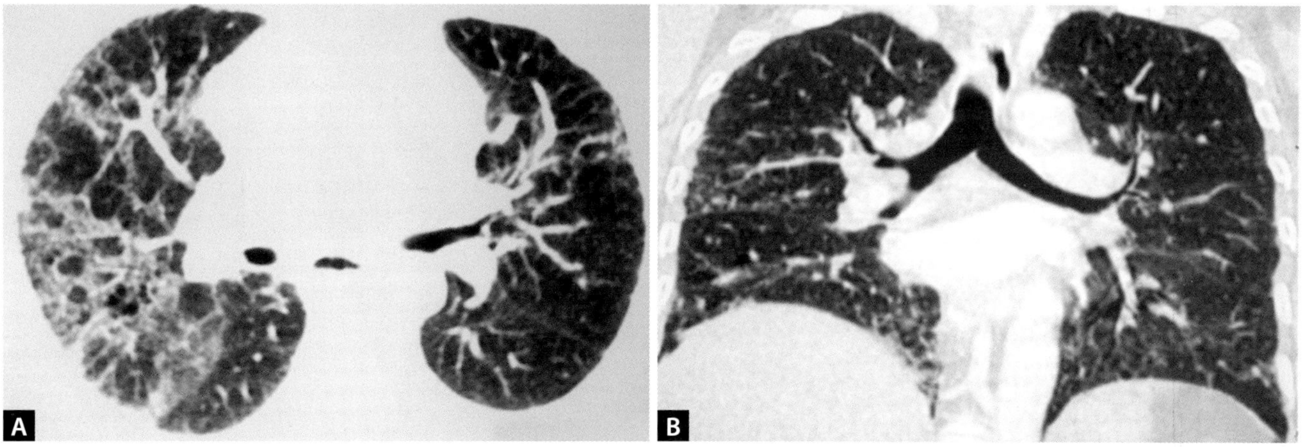

Figs. 6A and B: Progressive systemic sclerosis associated ILD: (A) Axial HRCT shows fine intralobular and interlobular septal thickening and ground-glass opacification in NSIP pattern. (B) Coronal multiplanar reconstruction shows the predominantly basal distribution of the patchy ground-glass opacities.

Imaging Features

- Ground-glass attenuation and consolidation on HRCT may be due to interstitial pneumonitis/fibrosis, acute lupus pneumonitis, hemorrhage, or, rarely, bronchiolitis obliterans organizing pneumonia (BOOP).
- Reticular pattern mainly involves the lower lung zones on radiography, and is seen in only about 3% of patients. On the other hand, HRCT may demonstrate the abnormalities in approximately 30% of patients. The interstitial abnormalities include interlobular septal thickening, irregular linear hyperattenuating areas and architectural distortion.
- Honeycombing is uncommon.
- Infections may occur secondarily, including community-acquired pneumonias, atypical pneumonia and tuberculosis.

POLYMYOSITIS AND DERMATOMYOSITIS

These are idiopathic inflammatory myopathies with pulmonary involvement in around 40% patients in the form of ILD, aspiration pneumonia, and infections.

The common pattern is that of NSIP followed by UIP and organizing pneumonia. Mostly a chronic, indolent course is seen in polymyositis, whereas acute and rapidly progressive course is more common in dermatomyositis.

HYPERSENSITIVITY PNEUMONITIS

Hypersensitivity pneumonitis (HP) is a diffuse granulomatous ILD caused by an abnormal immune response to various organic dusts. The clinical manifestations, radiologic and histological patterns are nonspecific and may be similar to other interstitial and small airway diseases.[17] A high index of suspicion, detailed exposure and occupational history is paramount in making the diagnosis. Still the causative antigen may remain unidentifiable in up to 40% of histologically proven cases of HP.[18]

Imaging Features

The radiologic findings vary with the stage of the disease. HP manifests in three phases: Acute, subacute, and chronic. Early in the course of the acute stage, the chest X-ray may be normal. Later, bilateral, patchy areas of consolidation appear, which may be diffuse or in the lower lung zones. Most characteristic findings during the subacute stage are multiple ground-glass opacities and poorly defined centrilobular nodules. These abnormalities frequently resolve if the antigenic exposure is stopped. If exposure is continued or repeated, the diffuse nodular or ground-glass pattern is replaced by a reticular pattern characteristic of interstitial fibrosis.

HRCT

- Acute and subacute stages—the predominant abnormalities on HRCT are patchy or diffuse bilateral ground-glass opacities **(Figs. 7A and B)** superimposed on poorly defined small centrilobular nodules in the middle and lower lung zones.
- The ground-glass opacities may be concentrated in the centers of the secondary pulmonary lobules with sparing of the periphery. Another frequent finding in patients with subacute disease is the presence of localized areas of decreased attenuation and vascularity. Such areas have a striking lobular distribution and show evidence of air trapping on expiratory images.

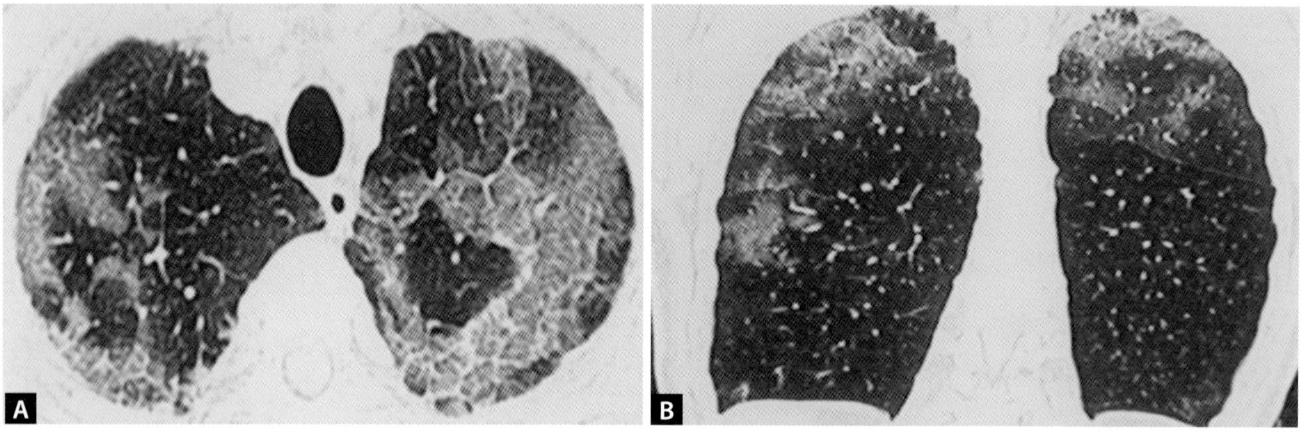

Figs. 7A and B: Acute hypersensitivity pneumonitis: (A) Axial HRCT shows extensive areas of patchy ground-glass attenuation; (B) Coronal multiplanar reconstruction shows the predominantly upper lobar distribution of the patchy ground-glass opacities.

- The HRCT differential diagnosis include DIP, alveolar proteinosis, lymphoid interstitial pneumonia (LIP) and respiratory bronchiolitis-associated interstitial diseases.
- Chronic HP shows reticulation, traction bronchiectasis and architectural distortion due to fibrosis with background changes of subacute HP. The reticulation may be random or subpleural and peribronchovascular in distribution. In a few cases, there is subpleural honeycombing resembling idiopathic pulmonary fibrosis, however the areas of air trapping and centrilobular nodules are rarely seen in idiopathic pulmonary fibrosis.[19]

SILICOSIS AND COAL WORKERS' PNEUMOCONIOSIS

Silicosis and coal worker's pneumoconiosis are ILDs related to exposure of dust-containing crystallized silicon dioxide and coal dust. A positive inhalational history with characteristic findings on imaging are often sufficient to make the diagnosis.

Imaging Features

HRCT—Small (2–5 mm), perihilar and dorsal lung zones centrilobular nodules with upper lobe predominance **(Fig. 8)**.[20] Miliary distribution can be rarely seen in these patients. Calcified lymphadenopathy (hilar and mediastinal) is common, sometimes with characteristic egg-shell calcifications.

- The nodules in silicosis patients tend to coalesce and initially form clusters, and later form large conglomerate masses, i.e. progressive massive fibrosis (PMF) **(Fig. 9)**. Conglomerate masses are seen more in apical and posterior segments of the upper lobes.

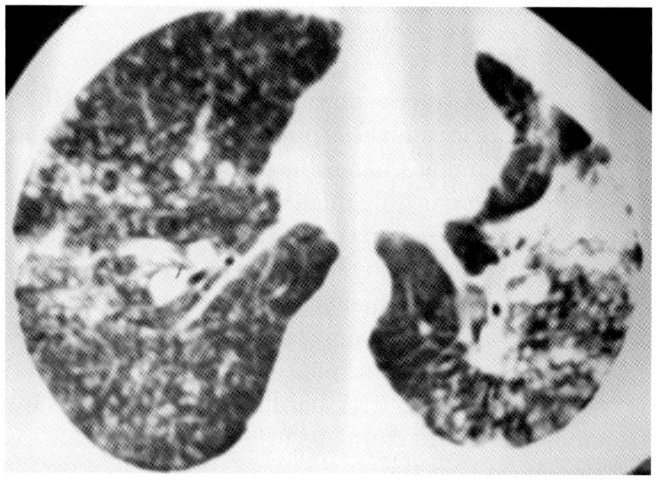

Fig. 8: Silicosis: Axial HRCT shows clusters of 5 mm of centrilobular and subpleural micronodules in a foundry worker with silicosis. Some of the nodules are seen aggregating into PMF masses.

- Associated peripheral parenchymal distortion with paracicatricial emphysema is common. PMF is typically bilateral and often symmetric. PMF lesions may uncommonly be calcified or show central cavitation which may result from ischemic necrosis or tuberculosis.
- On imaging, coal worker's pneumoconiosis and silicosis show overlapping features. The radiographic pattern of simple coal worker's pneumoconiosis include small 1–5 mm round ill-defined/granular nodules. Eggshell calcification is uncommon in the condition.[21]

ASBESTOSIS

Asbestos exposure is seen in miners, millers, persons employed in shipyards, and building trades. Asbestosis

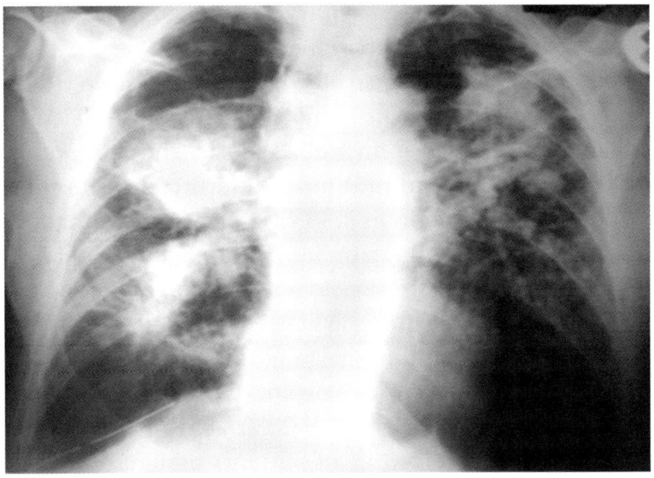

Fig. 9: *Advanced Silicosis with PMF*: Frontal chest radiograph shows large, parahilar fibrotic masses with surrounding cicatricial emphysema. As PMF progresses the number of nodules decreases because of their aggregation into fibrotic lesions.

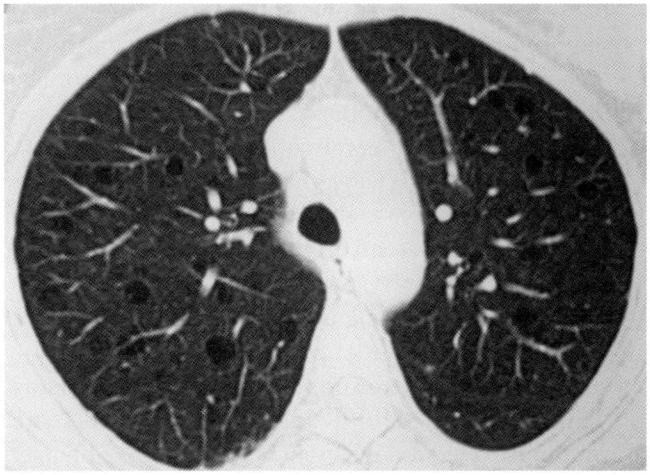

Fig. 10: Axial HRCT shows early LAM with subtle thin-walled cysts interspersed with normal lung parenchyma.

at plain chest radiography and HRCT is indistinguishable from other causes of lung fibrosis except when pleural plaques are visible, which then indicates asbestosis as the likely cause. In the absence of pleural plaques, the pattern of fibrosis alone in asbestosis is difficult to differentiate from UIP from other causes.

LYMPHANGIOLEIOMYOMATOSIS

Lymphangioleiomyomatosis (LAM) is characterized pathologically by interstitial proliferation of atypical smooth muscle and is a rare disease. Peribronchiolar proliferation causes distal air trapping and air-cyst formation.[22] It can occur in isolation or in association with tuberous sclerosis. It is restricted to women of childbearing age, and is not associated with smoking. Progressive dyspnea, spontaneous pneumothorax, chylothorax and hemoptysis are usual clinical presentations. Extrapulmonary manifestations include thoracic and abdominal lymphadenopathy, chylous ascites, pericardial effusion, renal angiomyolipomas, and lymphangiomatosis.

Imaging Features

Pleural and parenchymal abnormalities are clearly visualized on chest radiography in around 70% of the patients. A bilateral, symmetrical reticular pattern is seen involving all lung zones to a similar degree (80%) or the lower zones predominantly in the remaining 20% patients. Cysts can be identified in 50–60% of cases. Hyperinflation and expiratory air trapping are often found. Involvement of the lymphatics may cause obstruction and accumulation of chylous pleural effusions in 10–20%. Recurrent pneumothorax is a frequent complication (30–40%), due to spontaneous rupture of the thin-walled cysts.

- HRCT features of LAM are characteristic in the form of uniformly distributed multiple thin-walled cysts of 2 mm to 5 cm size, with intervening normal lung parenchyma **(Fig. 10)**. The wall thickness of the cysts is variable up to few millimeters.
- The main differential diagnosis on HRCT is LCH. However, the cysts in LCH typically involve the middle and upper lung zones, with sparing of the lung bases. In addition most patients with LCH also have nodules, a finding that is seen rarely in LAM. The presence of pleural effusion further helps to distinguish the cystic lung disease in LAM from LCH.

LANGERHANS CELL HISTIOCYTOSIS

Langerhans cell histiocytosis (LCH) refers to a group of diseases mostly affecting children with unknown etiology, in which Langerhans cell accumulate in one or more body systems like bone, lung, pituitary gland, mucous membranes, skin, lymph nodes, and liver. On the other hand, pulmonary Langerhans cell histiocytosis (PLCH) is a disease of adults affecting the lung, usually in isolation or less commonly in other organ systems.[23]

- Up to 100% of PLCH patients are current or former smokers and there is a slight male predominance. The peak is at 20–40 years of age.
- Extrapulmonary manifestations of PLCH (bone lesions, diabetes insipidus, and skin lesions) may occur in 5–15% of patients. About 20–25% patients are asymptomatic.

- Dry cough and dyspnea are common presenting complaints, followed by constitutional symptoms, such as weight loss, fever, night sweats, and anorexia. Spontaneous pneumothorax may occasionally be seen.
- A key histological feature of LCH is peribronchiolar nodules containing Langerhans cells and inflammatory cells in the early stages. With time, these nodules become fibrotic causing stellate peribronchiolar scars.
- Cessation of smoking is sufficient for stabilization of symptoms in most patients. Medical therapy includes corticosteroids which are the mainstay. Chemotherapeutic drugs such as vinblastine, methotrexate, and cyclophosphamide may be used in non-responders and in multi-organ involvement.

Imaging Features

Chest radiographs—show nodular or reticulonodular opacities predominantly in the upper lungs.[22]

- Costophrenic angles are spared.
- Lung volumes are preserved.
- With disease progression, cystic changes and bullae develop in the upper lungs and lung volumes increases.

HRCT—show characteristic findings of nodules and cysts predominating in the upper and mid lungs, with sparing of the bases. Early in the disease, peribronchiolar centrilobular nodules of 1 to 5 mm diameter predominate.

- With disease evolution, thick- or thin-walled cysts (usually less than 10 mm in diameter) are identified in 80% of the patients **(Figs. 11A and B)**. These cysts may be round, lobulated, irregular or bizarre in shape, often with normal intervening parenchyma. Rupture of cysts into the pleural space causes episodic pneumothorax. Longitudinal HRCT studies have shown progression of solid nodules to cavitary nodules to thick-walled cysts, and finally thin-walled cysts.[23]
- In patients showing isolated nodular disease on HRCT, the differential diagnosis includes sarcoidosis, silicosis, metastatic disease, and tuberculosis. The distribution in the upper and mid lungs and the centrilobular nature of the nodules in PLCH may in differentiation. Cystic changes may simulate the appearance of LAM; however, the cysts in LAM occur throughout the lung without sparing the lung bases and nodules are rarely seen. In both conditions, lung volumes are preserved and pneumothorax can occur.

The natural history of LCH is variable and unpredictable. Approximately, 50% of patients may have partial or complete clearing of radiologic abnormalities with symptom resolution. Follow-up CT scans may show regression of nodules, whereas any cysts that have formed are permanent. In 30–40% of patients, persisting symptoms are variable severity; scarring supervenes which results in reticulation, thickening of the cyst walls, and architectural distortion. In 10–20% patients, recurrent pneumothorax or progressive respiratory failure with cor- pulmonale occurs.

PULMONARY ALVEOLAR PROTEINOSIS

Pulmonary alveolar proteinosis (PAP) is a rare disease characterized by accumulation of abnormal proteinaceous material in the alveoli, causing hypoxemia, restrictive lung disease and a radiological appearance like pulmonary edema. Idiopathic PAP accounts for up to 90% of cases. Secondary PAP (5–10% of cases) is seen in patients with industrial inhalational exposure to silica particles, cement dust, aluminum dust, titanium dioxide, nitrogen dioxide, and fiberglass; underlying hematologic malignancy; or immunodeficiency disorders like cytotoxic

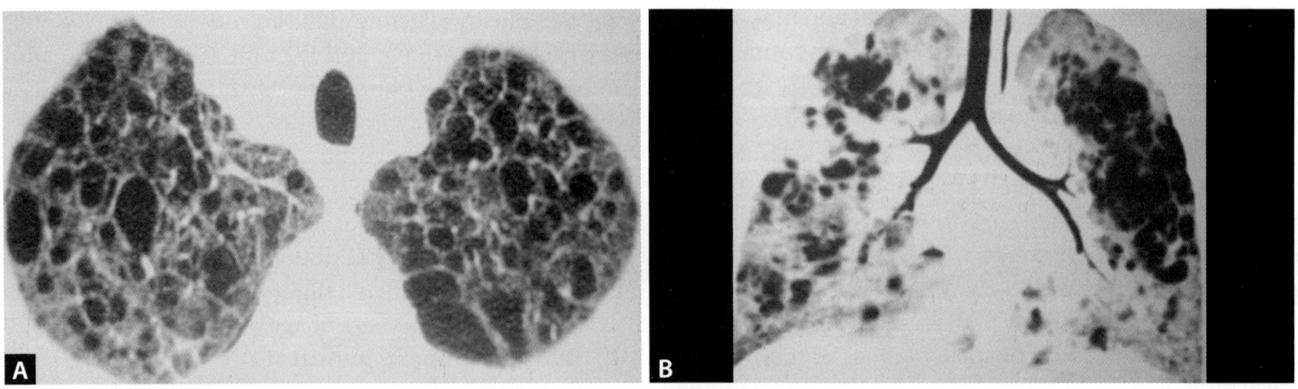

Figs. 11A and B: (A) Axial HRCT shows multiple, varying sized thick-walled cysts diffusely involving bilateral lungs; (B) Coronal multiplanar reconstruction shows the relative sparing of the bilateral lung bases.

or immunosuppressive therapy and human immunodeficiency virus infection.

Imaging Features

Chest radiography—Bilateral central and symmetric lung opacities, with relative sparing of the apices and costophrenic angles.

- Less commonly, radiographs show multifocal asymmetric opacities or extensive diffuse consolidation without any clear zonal predominance. Opacities may be ground-glass, reticular/reticulonodular, to consolidation with air bronchogram. Although the radiographic appearance of PAP may suggest pulmonary interstitial edema, pleural effusion and cardiomegaly are absent.
- There is often a discordance between marked radiographic abnormalities in the presence of more benign clinical symptoms (clinicoradiologic discrepancy).[24]

HRCT—bilateral, symmetric alveolar consolidation or ground-glass opacity, in a perihilar or hilar distribution. Geographic ground-glass attenuation, sharply demarcated from the surrounding normal parenchyma, with superimposed polygonal shape intra- and interlobular septal thickening **(Fig. 12)** creates the 'crazy paving' appearance.[25] The crazy paving appearance for alveolar proteinosis, although highly sensitive, is not specific.

- The radiological differential diagnosis includes diffuse alveolar damage superimposed on UIP, acute interstitial pneumonia, acute respiratory distress syndrome and bronchoalveolar carcinoma.

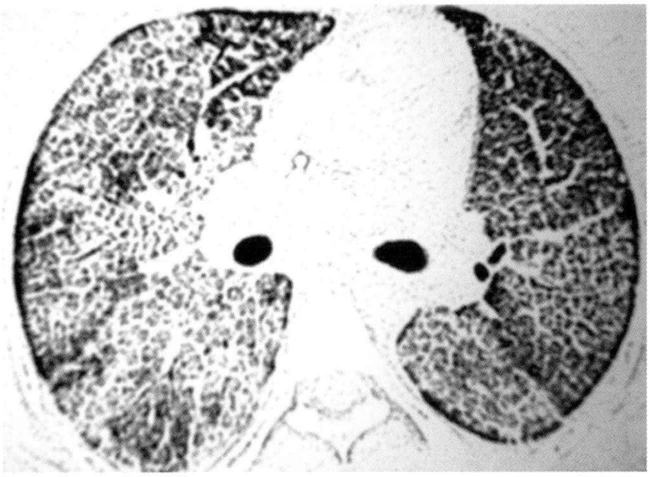

Fig. 12: *Pulmonary alveolar proteinosis (PAP)*: Axial HRCT shows classic findings of "crazy paving"; geographic ground-glass attenuation superimposed with thickening of interstitium producing polygonal opacities.

Sequential therapeutic whole-lung lavage is the main treatment in idiopathic PAP, which involves the use of saline solution and chest percussion to remove the lipoproteinaceous material from pulmonary alveoli. Post-therapeutic whole-lung lavage CT may reveal resolution of ground-glass opacity, however, the septal lines may still persist.

CONCLUSION

A whole gamut of conditions in the wide group of interstitial lung disease due to a known cause have similar clinical presentation. A meticulous history with regards to the offending allergens if any with thorough biochemical evaluation helps in narrowing down the diagnosis. A multidisciplinary approach with radiologist, pulmonary physician and pathologist is desired to achieve optimum care for such patients.

REFERENCES

1. American Thoracic Society/European Respiratory Society International Multidisciplinary Consensus Classification of the Idiopathic Interstitial Pneumonias. Am J Respir Crit Care Med. 2002;165:277-304.
2. Travis WD, Costabel U, Hansell DM, et al. An official American Thoracic Society/European Respiratory Society statement: Update of the international multidisciplinary classification of the idiopathic interstitial pneumonias. Am J Respir Crit Care Med. 2013;188(6):733-48.
3. Bokulic RE, Hilman BC. Interstitial lung disease in children. Pediatr Clin North Am. 1994; 41:543-67.
4. Epler GR, McLoud TC, Gaensler EA, et al. Normal chest roentgenograms in chronic diffuse. Infiltrative lung disease. N Engl J Med. 1978;298(17):934-9.
5. Webb WR. High-revolution CT of the lung parenchyma. Radiol Clin North Am. 1989;27:1085-97.
6. Hansell DM, Bankier AA, MacMahon H, et al. Remy J Fleischner Society: glossary of terms for thoracic imaging. Radiology. 2008;246(3):697-722.
7. Webb WR, Muller NL, Naidich DP. Standardized terms for high-resolution computed tomography of the lung: A proposed glossary. J Thorac Imaging. 1993;8:167-75.
8. Lynch JP, Kazerooni EA, Gay SE. Pulmonary sarcoidosis. Clin Chest Med. 1997;18:755-85.
9. James DG, Neville E, Siltzbach LE. A worldwide review of sarcoidosis. Ann NY Acad Sci. 1976;278:321-34.
10. Koyama T, Ueda H, Togashi K, et al. Radiologic manifestations of sarcoidosis in various organs. Radiographics. 2004;24(1):87-104.
11. Ichikawa Y, Fujimoto K, Shiraishi T, et al. Primary cavitary sarcoidosis: High-resolution CT findings. Am J Roentgenol. 1994;163 (3):745.
12. New Silva M, Nunes H, Valeyre D, Sverzellati N. Imaging of Sarcoidosis. Clin Rev Allergy Immunol. 2015; 49(1):45-53.

13. Kim EA, Lee KS, Johkoh T, et al. Interstitial lung diseases associated with collagen vascular diseases: radiologic and histopathologic findings. Radiographics. 2002;22 Spec No: S151-65.
14. Tanaka N, Kim JS, Newell JD, et al. Rheumatoid arthritis-related lung diseases: CT findings. Radiology. 2004;232 (1):81-91.
15. Vyas Surabhi. Connective tissue disorders and related interstitial lung disease: Imaging. In: Bhalla AS, Jana M (Eds). Imaging of interstitial lung diseases, Clinicoradiological series. 2017. The Health Sciences Publishers. P. 81-96.
16. Goldin JG, Lynch DA, Strollo DC, et al. Scleroderma Lung Study Research Group. High-resolution CT scan findings in patients with symptomatic scleroderma-related interstitial lung disease. Chest. 2008;134(2):358-67.
17. Glazer CS, Rose CS, Lynch DA. Clinical and radiologic manifestations of hypersensitivity pneumonitis. J Thorac Imaging. 2002;17:261-72.
18. Silva CI, Churg A, Müller NL. Hypersensitivity pneumonitis: spectrum of high-resolution CT and pathologic findings. Am J Roentgenol. 2007;188 (2):334-44.
19. CI, Müller NL, Lynch DA, Curran-Everett D, et al. Chronic hypersensitivity pneumonitis: Differentiation from idiopathic pulmonary fibrosis and nonspecific interstitial pneumonia by using thin-section CT. Radiology. 2008;246 (1):288-97.
20. Begin R, Ostiguy G, Fillion R, et al. Computed tomography scan in the early detection of silicosis. Am Rev Respir Dis. 1991;144:697-705.
21. Remy-Jardin M, Degreef JM, Beuscart R, et al. Coal worker's pneumoconiosis: CT assessment in exposed workers and correlation with radiographic findings. Radiology. 1990;177:363-71.
22. Abbott GF, Rosado-de-Christenson ML, Frazier AA, et al. From the archives of the AFIP: Lymphangioleiomyomatosis: Radiologic-pathologic correlation. Radiographics. 2005;25 (3):803-28.
23. Tazi A. Adult pulmonary Langerhans' cell histiocytosis. Eur Respir J. 2006;27 (6):1272-85.
24. Holbert JM, Costello P, Li W, et al. CT features of pulmonary alveolar proteinosis. Am J Roentgenol. 2001;176:1287-94.
25. Lee CH. The crazy-paving sign. Radiology 2007;243;905-6.

CHAPTER 165

Miscellaneous Interstitial Lung Diseases

Ashu Seith Bhalla, Manisha Jana

INTRODUCTION

This chapter includes a wide range of diffuse lung diseases (DLDs), not covered in the previous chapters. Some of them are interstitial lung diseases (ILDs), whereas some are diseases mimicking ILD. Since description of all of these is beyond the scope of this chapter, a pattern approach on High-resolution computed tomography (HRCT) will be followed. Uncommon DLDs presenting with ground-glass opacity (GGO), septal thickening and nodules is covered. This is followed by discussion of 'cystic lung diseases'.

DIFFUSE LUNG DISEASES PRESENTING WITH GROUND-GLASS OPACITY

Commoner DLDs presenting with a predominant GGO pattern have been discussed in detail in earlier capters. **Table 1** enlists less frequent etiologies.

Table 1: Uncommon DLDs presenting with GGO pattern.

Infections	• Interstitial pneumonia • Viral pneumonia • *Mycoplasma pneumoniae* • *Pneumocystis jirovecii*
Others	• Eosinophilic lung diseases • Lipoid pneumonia • Acute respiratory distress syndrome (ARDS) • Diffuse alveolar hemorrhage (DAH) • Pulmonary alveolar proteinosis (PAP)

INFECTIONS

Interstitial pneumonia[1,2] may appear as ill defined areas of GGOs. Severity can range from mild forms to those causing respiratory failure. A few more severe specific forms are described here.

Severe Acute Respiratory Syndrome

Severe acute respiratory syndrome (SARS) is an acute respiratory disorder caused by coronavirus. The pathology is alveolar damage and airspace edema.[3] Usual presenting symptoms are high-grade fever, dry cough and dyspnea usually within 10 days after SARS exposure. Chest radiograph reveals unifocal or multifocal consolidation. HRCT can show either GGO, consolidation or crazy paving appearance. The findings can either be unilateral or bilateral.

Swine Influenza (H1N1)

It is caused by Swine-origin influenza A (H1N1) virus. The pathology is a diffuse alveolar damage. Patients present with dry cough and dyspnea usually following a prodromal period of 2–7 days. Swine influenza is usually a mild disease but can be complicated by acute respiratory distress syndrome or secondary pneumonia. On HRCT, the predominant findings can be unilateral or bilateral GGO. Consolidations can be peribronchovascular or subpleural consolidations.

Mycoplasma Pneumoniae

It is a common cause of community-acquired pneumonia in children and young adults, caused by *Mycoplasma pneumoniae* (walking pneumonia). Usual presenting symptoms are fever and productive cough, nonspecific complaints, fatigue and myalgia. Chest radiograph can show diffuse reticulonodular opacities, peribronchial thickening or even frank consolidation. HRCT findings include centrilobular nodules, peribronchovascular and interlobular septal thickening, lobular or segmental consolidation **(Figs. 1A and B)**.

Pneumocystis jirovecii Pneumonia

This is the most common cause of opportunistic infection in HIV- infected patients. The causative organism is an atypical fungus *Pneumocystis jiroveci*. The clinical features depend on the immune status of the patient. While it presents as an acute illness with severe hypoxia and respiratory failure in an immunocompetent individual; the symptoms are more gradual in onset in HIV-infected patient. It is common in patients with a CD4 count <100.

Chest radiograph reveals a bilaterally symmetric perihilar reticulonodular pattern; which can progress to consolidation subsequently. HRCT reveals bilateral symmetric perihilar groundglass opacities **(Figs. 2A and B)**. In subacute stage of the disease, consolidation with septal thickening produces a 'crazy paving' pattern. Thin walled varying sized cysts can also develop in subacute stages; which can rupture and lead to spontaneous pneumothorax/pneumomediastinum.

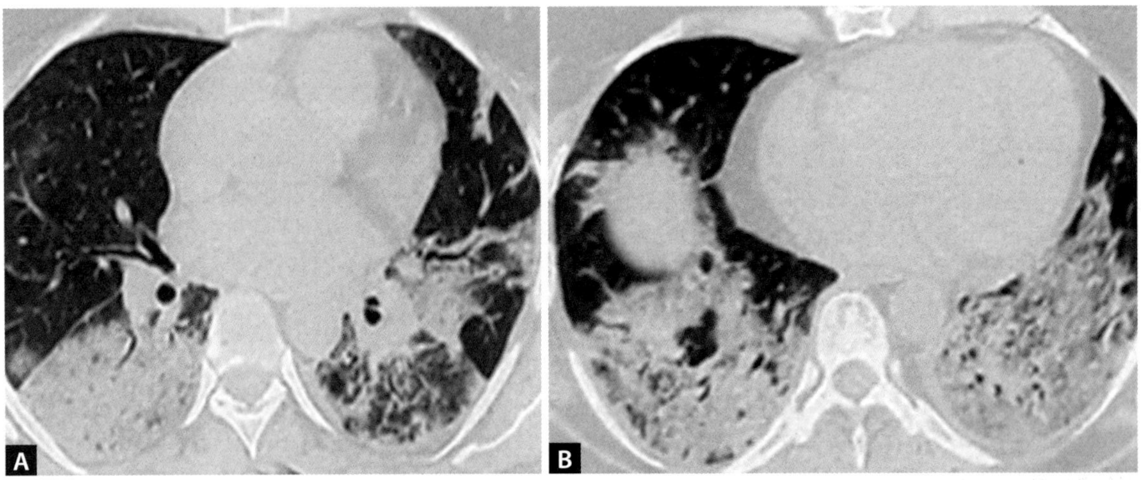

Figs. 1A and B: *Mycoplasma pneumoniae*: HRCT images reveal multifocal patchy consolidation in dependent locations.

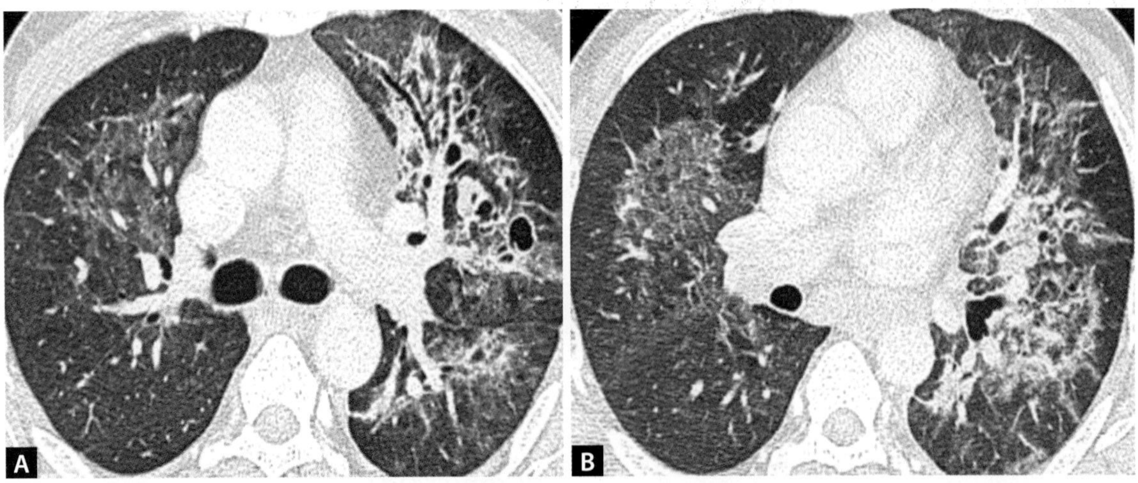

Figs. 2A and B: Subacute *Pneumocystis jirovecii* pneumonia: CT reveals central perihilar GGO with superimposed septal thickening and thin-walled cysts.

ACUTE RESPIRATORY DISTRESS SYNDROME

Acute respiratory distress syndrome (ARDS) is a diffuse alveolar damage resulting from variety of insults and requiring mechanical ventilation. The pathology is diffuse alveolar damage, increased capillary and alveolar permeability, leading to edema (interstitial and alveolar), followed by a phase of fibrosis. Three clinical phases are recognized-acute, subacute and chronic.[4,5]

Acute (Exudative) Phase

This is seen in the initial 7 days following insult. The chest radiograph can be normal in the first 24 hours. Over the next 2-3 days—extensive, bilateral air space opacification/ consolidation ("White lung") can develop. The consolidation can be patchy and multifocal. Radiographic criteria for diagnosis of ARDS include bilateral opacities (consistent with pulmonary edema), findings not explainable by pleural effusion, lung collapse or nodules. CT findings can appear by 12 hours. HRCT findings include GGO and consolidation having a diffuse or patchy distribution. Usually there is an apico-basal gradient, with more opacification of the lung bases.

Subacute (Proliferative) Phase

It is between one and two weeks, when there is conversion of alveolar exudates into cellular granulation tissue. Imaging in subacute phase shows an increasing consolidation in early phase, followed by appearance of interlobular septal thickening, "crazy paving pattern" and bronchiectasis and bronchiolectasis **(Figs. 3A and B)**.

Chronic (Fibrotic) Phase

It is seen two weeks or more following injury. Diffuse parenchymal fibrosis and architectural distortion ensue. HRCT reveals fibrosis, bronchiectasis, bronchiolectasis with distortion of airways and volume loss with bullae formation. Morphological changes may persist in survivors even when imaged months after the acute episode.

HYDROSTATIC PULMONARY EDEMA

Hydrostatic pulmonary edema is seen in cardiac failure or fluid overload due to accumulation of fluid in the extravascular compartment of the lung. There are two pathological phases—interstitial edema and alveolar filling.

Chest radiograph shows enlargement of upper lobe pulmonary veins (due to diversion of blood flow) in early phase. Later on airspace opacities with central/parahilar (batwing distribution) develop. CT reveals diffuse/patchy and parahilar GGO and smooth interlobular septal thickening **(Figs. 4A and B)**. Hydrostatic pulmonary edema has a preponderance towards involvement of the dependent areas; which differentiates it from increased permeability edema; which has more subpleural and peripheral distribution. Peribronchovascular interstitial thickening can appear as bronchial wall thickening or prominence of pulmonary vessels. In cardiogenic pulmonary edema, pulmonary arteries and veins appear dilated. Transudative pleural effusion is commonly seen.

DIFFUSE ALVEOLAR HEMORRHAGE

Diffuse alveolar hemorrhage (DAH) can be secondary to various causes, including coagulation disorders, collagen

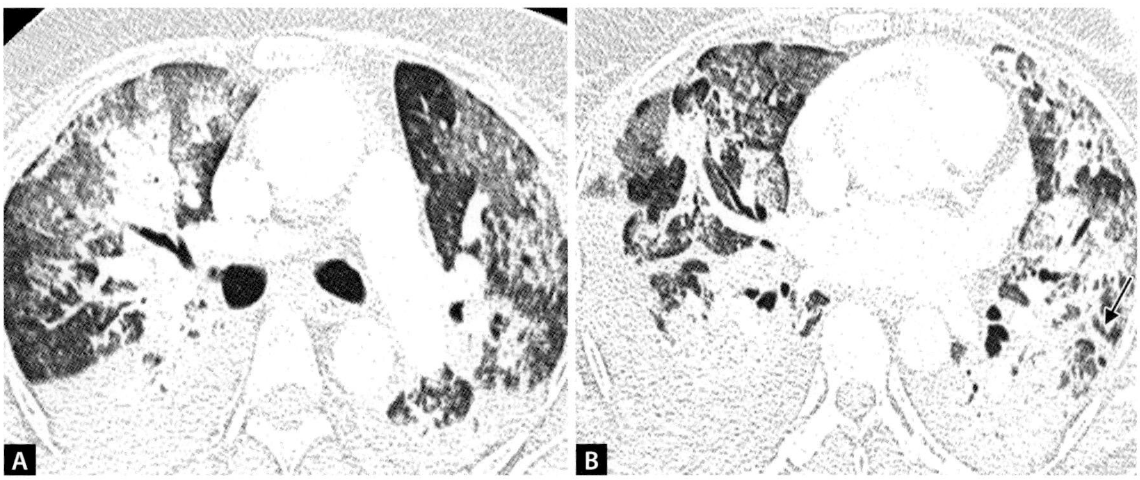

Figs. 3A and B: Acute respiratory distress syndrome in subacute phase. HRCT images reveal multifocal nonsegmental patchy consolidation and GGO with superimposed septal thickening (arrow). Bilateral pleural effusion is also present.

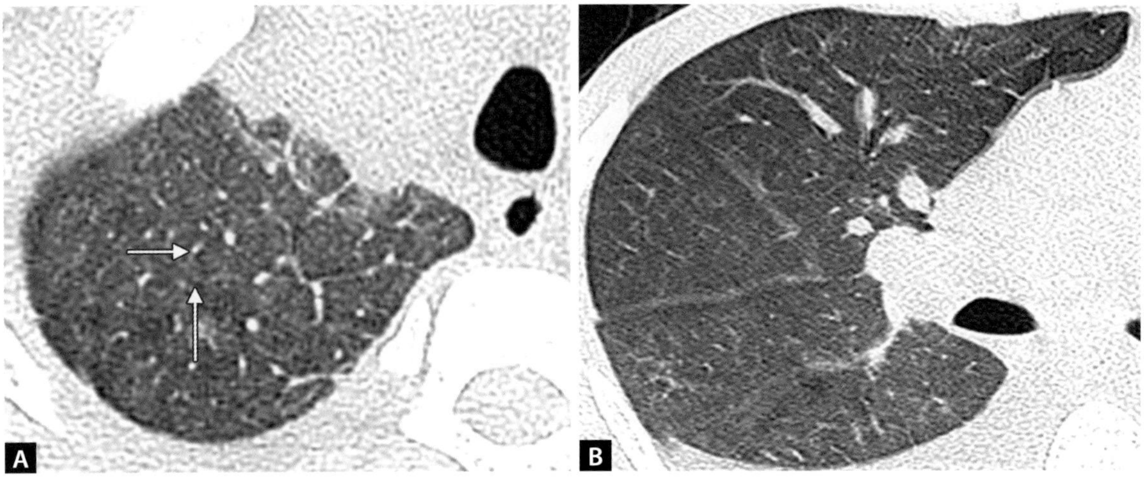

Figs. 4A and B: Hydrostatic pulmonary edema: HRCT images reveal smooth septal thickening (arrow), fissural thickening and right pleural effusion.

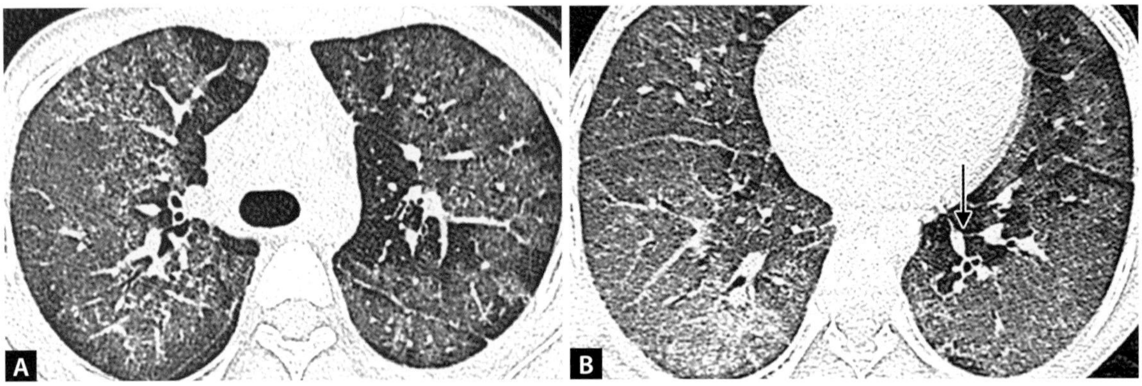

Figs. 5A and B: Diffuse alveolar hemorrhage in a 15-year-old male patient with anemia. HRCT images show diffuse GGO and septal thickening with sparing of lung bases and the periphery. Note the lobular sparing (arrow).

vascular disorders and vasculitis.[6] The isiopathic form is termed idiopathic pulmonary hemorrahge (IPH). The clinical presentation is variable; hemoptysis and anemia are some of the presenting symptoms. On pathology, three different patterns have been described—associated with pulmonary capillaritis, bland alveolar hemorrhage with no vasculitis and diffuse alveolar damage (DAD) related DAH. HRCT reveals bilateral GGO/consolidation having a lobular appearance and more involvement of dependent areas **(Figs. 5A and B)**. In most cause, the pulmonary changes are reversible, except in those with DAD.

EOSINOPHILIC LUNG DISEASE

Eosinophilic lung disease comprises of varied disease entities, which are characterized by pulmonary manifestations and eosinophilia (peripheral or tissue eosinophilia).[7] On the basis of etiolgy, they can be classified as—eosinophilic lung diseases of unknown cause, eosinophilic lung diseases of known cause and eosinophilic vasculitis. On the basis of clinical presentation, the folloing subtypes are describe.

Acute Eosinophilic Pneumonia (Figs. 6A and B)

It presents with fever and respiratory distress which shows immediate response to steroids. Usually there are >25% eosinophils in bronchoalveolar lavage (BAL) fluid. HRCT findings include bilateral patchy GGO and septal thickening. Ill-defined nodules and consolidation are other unusual findings.

Chronic Eosinophilic Pneumonia

It usually affects middle aged women, has an insidious onset and mild eosinophilia. HRCT shows GGO, peripheral nonsegmental consolidation with a upper lobe predominance.

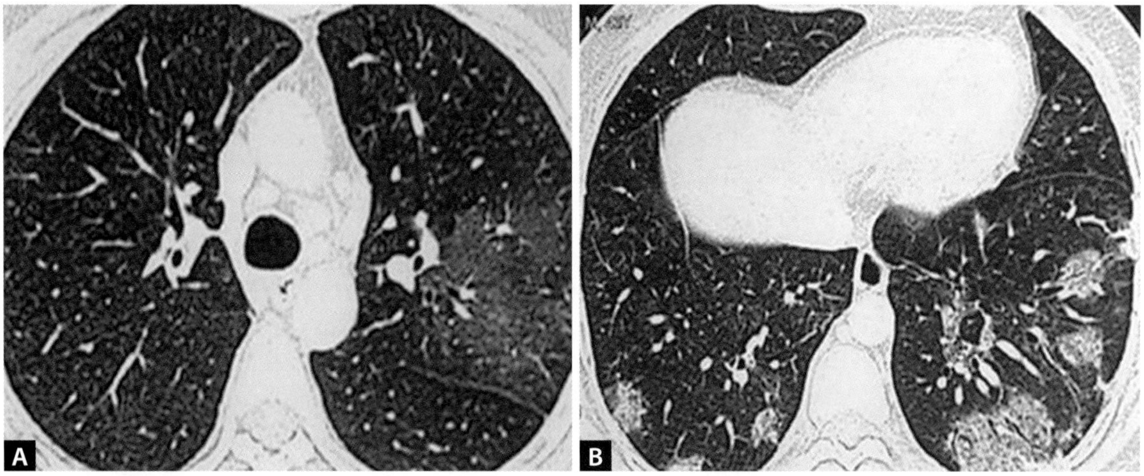

Figs. 6A and B: Acute eosinophilic pneumonia in a 30-year-old male with acute onset cough. HRCT images reveal bilateral peripheral ground-glass opacities.

Idiopathic Hypereosinophilic Syndrome

In contrast, usually affects males in their 30s and presents with multiorgan dysfunction. There is persistent eosinophilia without any demonstrable allergic or parasitic cause. HRCT shows a focal or diffuse nonlobar distribution of nodules, perinodular GGO and patchy GGO.

Other forms of eosinophilic lung disease include tropical pulmonary eosinophilia (TPE) which presents with ill-defined nodules, and eosinophilic bronchitis presenting with features of small airway disease.

LIPOID PNEUMONIA

Lipoid pneumonia is characterized by the alveolar accumulation of lipids.[8-10] It can be of three main types depending on the source and the presentation—exogenous acute, exogenous chronic and endogenous forms.

Acute Exogenous Lipoid Pneumonia

It is caused by inhalation/aspiration of large quantity of animal fats/mineral or vegetable oils. The radiological manifestations develop within 30 minutes to 24 hours. The findings include bilateral segmental or lobar GGO/consolidation; having a middle and lower lobe preponderance. Ill-defined nodules, pneumatoceles, pleural effusions are uncommon findings.

Chronic Exogenous Lipoid Pneumonia

It is cause by recurrent episodes of aspiration/inhalation. On imaging, segmental GGO/consolidation with a peribronchovascular distribution can be seen in the lower lobes. Other associated imaging findings are septal thickening or fibrosis. Sometimes the consolidation shows a mass like appearance with fat attenuation within **(Figs. 7A to D)**.

Endogenous Lipoid Pneumonia

It is caused by bronchial obstruction or chronic pulmonary infection causing accumulation of fat within intra-alveolar macrophages. In contrast to the exogenous form; endogenous "cholesterol pneumonia" usually does not show any fat attenuation on CT. It presents as a consolidation distal to a central obstructing lesion. The diagnosis is histopathologic.

PULMONARY ALVEOLAR PROTEINOSIS

Pulmonary alveolar proteinosis (PAP) is characterized by the alveolar accumulation of surfactant-like proteins.[11] It can be of three types—congenital, idiopathic (primary) and secondary: Secondary PAP is seen in patients of hematological malignancies, dust/metal exposure, chemotherapy or infection and responds well to treatment of the predisposing cause. Congenital form results from inherited disorders of surfactant proteins. Patients with PAP can have variable symptoms. They can either be asymptomatic, or can even present with an insidious onset of dyspnea, dry cough and easy fatigability.

Chest radiograph reveals bilateral symmetric or patchy airspace opacification. HRCT shows the 'crazy paving pattern', caused by GGO and septal thickening **(Figs. 8A and B)**.[11] The involvement of the lungs is usually patchy, with geographic/lobular sparing. Differential diagnoses include—pulmonary hemorrhage, pulmonary edema,

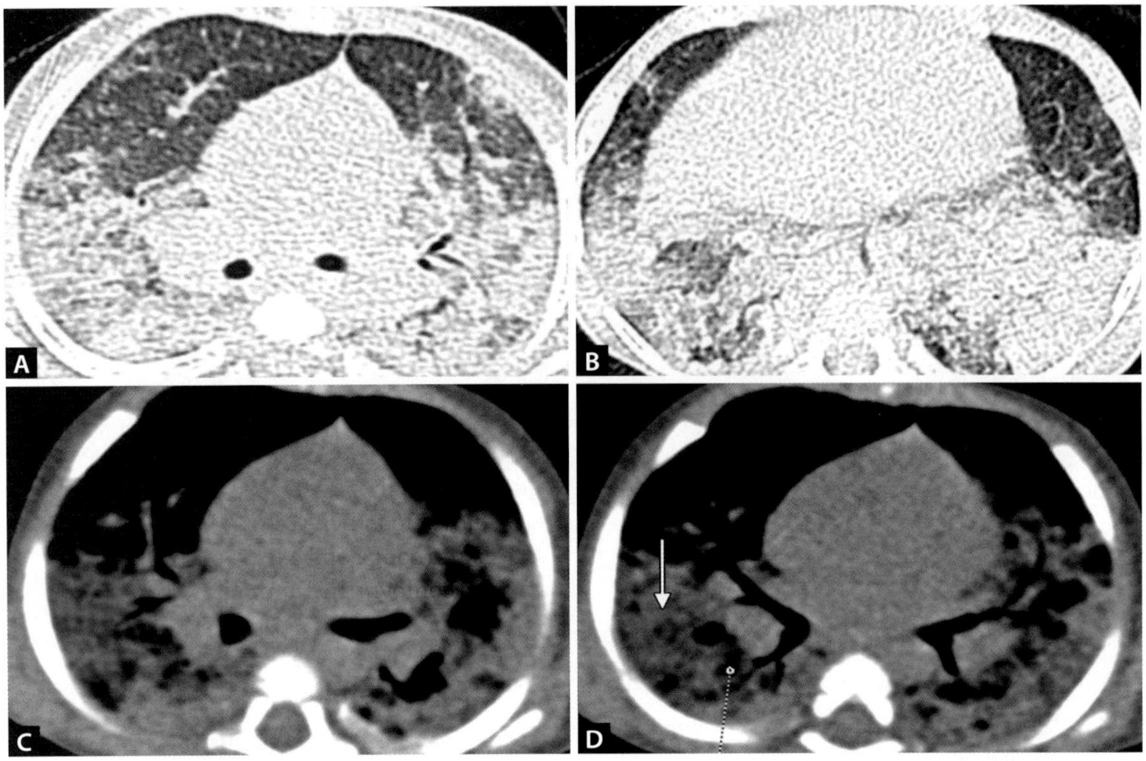

Figs. 7A to D: Exogenous lipoid pneumonia in a 7-year-old male child. HRCT images (A and B) reveal bilateral dense consolidation in dependent location. Soft tissue window images (C and D) reveal low attenuation areas within the areas of consolidation (arrow).

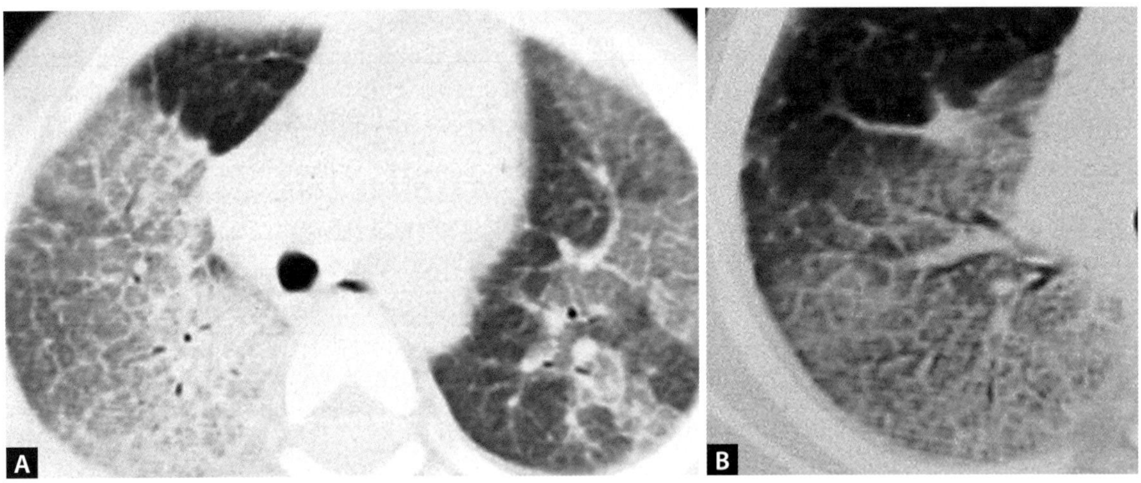

Figs. 8A and B: Pulmonary alveolar proteinosis pattern in storage disorder in a 6-year-old girl. CT images reveal diffuse 'crazy paving' pattern.

radiation exposure, drug induced, inhalation disorders, mucinous carcinoma, and storage disorders in children.

SEPTAL THICKENING PREDOMINANT DIFFUSE LUNG DISEASES

Uncommon DLDs presenting with septal thickening are listed in **Table 2**.

Lymphangitis carcinomatosa, Kaposi's sarcoma and lymphoma are covered elsewhere in this book.

PULMONARY LEUKOSTASIS

Pulmonary leukostasis is a complication observed in acute myeloid leukemia M4 (myelomonocytic type). When white blood cell count exceeds one lac/μL, leukemic cells start accumulating within the small vessels of lungs, heart, brain and testis; and clog these small vessels. The clinical and radiographic findings are often discordant.[12,13] Chest radiograph can either be normal even in the presence of severe dyspnea; or may show alveolar or interstitial opacities. CT may reveal thickened bronchovascular bundles and segmental ground-glass opacities **(Figs. 9A and B)**.

PULMONARY VENO-OCCLUSIVE DISEASE AND PULMONARY CAPILLARY HEMANGIOMATOSIS

Pulmonary veno-occlusive disease (PVOD) and pulmonary capillary hemangiomatosis (PCH) are rare disorders characterized by severe pulmonary arterial hypertension with normal pulmonary artery occlusion pressure and signs of pulmonary edema.[14-18] Although both are causes of pulmonary arterial hypertension the pathology in PVOD lies at the post-capillary level. There is fibrous occlusion of pulmonary venules. In PCH the problem lies at the capillary level [proliferation of alveolar capillaries (PCH)]. Definitive diagnosis is made on surgical lung biopsy.

The clinical features of both these entities include dyspnea on exertion, chronic cough, cyanosis, syncope and chest pain. In addition, hemoptysis is seen in PCH. The imaging findings **(Table 3)** are often quite characteristic **(Figs. 10A and B)**, in an appropriate clinical setting.

Diagnosing these entities on imaging in crucial; as administration of vasodilators on a presumptive clinical diagnosis of primary pulmonary hypertension can cause pulmonary edema in case of PVOD/PCH.

Table 2: Uncommon DLDs with predominant septal thickening.

Infections	• Atypical pneumonia—mycoplasma • *Pneumocystis jirovecii* pneumonia (PJP) • Severe acute respiratory syndrome (SARS)
Neoplastic	• Lymphangitis carcinomatosa • Lymphoma • Pulmonary leukostasis • Kaposi's sarcoma
Vascular	• Hydrostatic pulmonary edema • Acute respiratory distress syndrome (ARDS) • Pulmonary veno-occlusive disease (PVOD) • Pulmonary capillary hemangiomatosis (PCH)
Others	• Pulmonary alveolar proteinosis (PAP) • Diffuse alveolar septal amyloidosis • Diffuse alveolar hemorrhage (DAH)

PULMONARY AMYLOIDOSIS

Amyloidosis is characterized by the abnormal extracellular deposition of proteins. Thoracic involvement can be localized or a part of systemic disease. Three main patterns of pulmonary involvement are described—nodular parenchymal, diffuse alveolar septal and airway/tracheobronchial amyloidosis.[19]

Diffuse Alveolar Septal Amyloidosis

It is usually associated with systemic involvement; and presents with cough and dyspnea. The prognosis is poor; and progression to pulmonary hypertension and respiratory failure may ensue. Chest radiograph reveals well-defined small nodules and reticular opacities. HRCT findings **(Fig. 11)** include well-defined, small nodules, smooth septal thickening, bilateral basal consolidations,

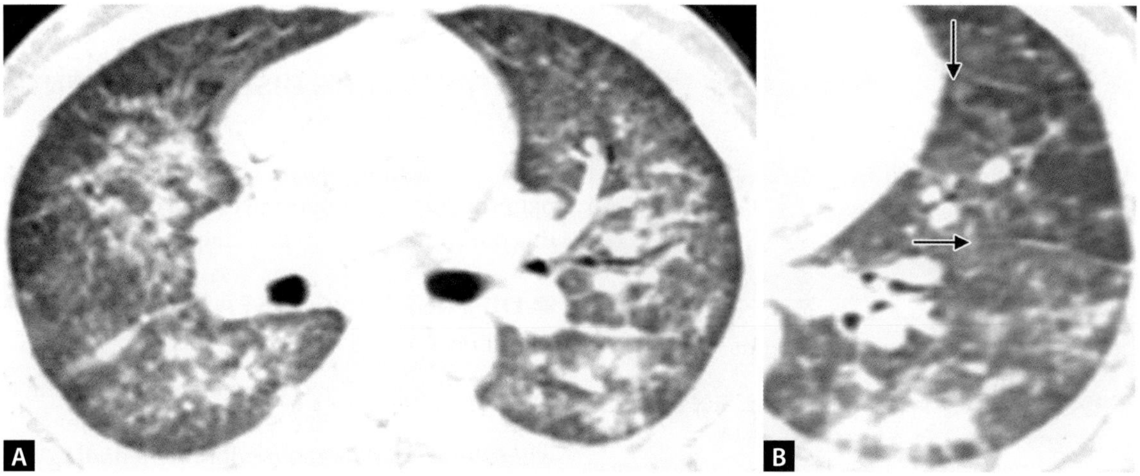

Figs. 9A and B: A 38-year-old male patient with AML having leukocytosis. CT reveals diffuse GGO, patchy consolidation and smooth septal thickening (arrow).

Table 3: Clinical and imaging findings of PVOD and PCH.

	PVOD	*PCH*
Gender predilection	M = F	F > M
Hemoptysis	Uncommon	Common symptom
HRCT	Dilated main pulmonary artery Smooth septal thickening Patchy ground-glass opacities Uncommon findings—multiple small nodules, consolidation in dependent lungs	Dilated main pulmonary artery Bilateral ill-defined ground-glass centrilobular nodules
Hemorrhagic pleural effusion	Uncommon	Common

Abbreviations: PVOD: Pulmonary veno-occlusive disease; PCH: Pulmonary capillary hemangiomatosis; HRCT: High resolution computed tomography.

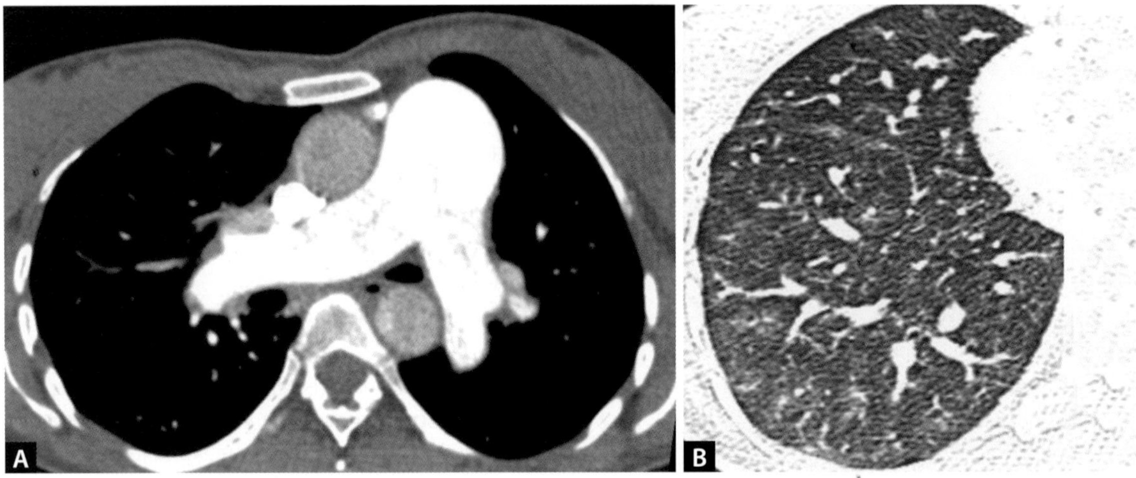

Figs. 10A and B: Pulmonary capillary hemangiomatosis in a 33-year-old lady with hemoptysis and PAH. CT reveals a dilated main pulmonary artery (A). HRCT image (B) reveals diffuse ground-glass nodules in the lungs.

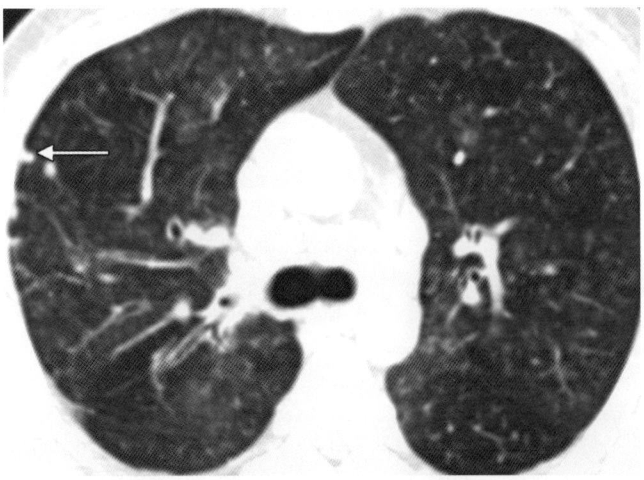

Fig. 11: *Pulmonary amyloidosis*: CT image reveals multiple small nodules, bronchovascular thickening, patchy GGO and peripheral bigger and well-defined subpleural nodules (arrow).

areas of punctate calcifications and occasional cysts and traction bronchiectasis.

DIFFUSE LUNG DISEASES PRESENTING WITH NODULES

Many diffuse lung diseases have a predominantly nodular pattern. These disorders have been discussed elsewhere in this book/previously in this chapter **(Table 4)**.

DIFFUSE LUNG DISEASES PRESENTING WITH CYSTS

Lung cysts are defined as small air containing lesions in lungs. Cystic lung diseases **(Table 5)** refer to a pattern where lung cysts are the predominant finding. These need to be differentiated from honeycombing, emphysema and cystic bronchiectasis.

Table 4: Uncommon ILDs presenting with nodules.

Centrilobular	*Random*	*Perilymphatic*
• Viral pneumonia, *Haemophilus, Chlamydia, Mycoplasma* • PCH	• Pulmonary nodular amyloidosis	• Lymphangitis carcinomatosa • LIP • Amyloidosis

Abbreviations: ILDs: Interstitial lung diseases; PCH: Pulmonary capillary hemangiomatosis; LIP: Lymphocytic interstitial pneumonia.

Table 5: DLDs presenting with cysts.

Cystic DLDs	*Mimics of lung cysts*
Pulmonary Langerhans' cell histiocytosis	Emphysema
Lymphangioleiomyomatosis (LAM)	Bronchiectasis
Tuberous sclerosis	Honeycombing
Birt-Hogg-Dubé (BHD) syndrome	
Cysts associated with other DLDs—LIP, DIP, PJP, any fibrosing ILD	

Abbreviations: DLDs: Diffuse lung diseases; LIP: Lymphocytic interstitial pneumonia; DIP: Desquamative interstitial pneumonia; PJP: *Pneumocystis jirovecii* pneumonia.

EMPHYSEMA

Emphysema is caused by permanent dilatation of the airspace distal to the terminal bronchioles with associated destruction of the alveolar wall. Three main types of emphysema are—centrilobular, panlobular and paraseptal.

Centrilobular Emphysema

It is the most common type, seen usually in smokers and affects lobules around the central respiratory bronchioles. HRCT reveals well-defined round lucencies in centrilobular portion of secondary pulmonary lobule. Borders of secondary pulmonary lobule are preserved.[20] Apices and lower lobe superior segments are usually more involved. CT is more superior to chest radiography to detect early disease.

Panlobular Emphysema

It is associated with α1-antitrypsin deficiency. Panlobular pattern can also be seen in advanced smoking-related emphysema and emphysema related to intravenous drug abuse. It affects the whole secondary lobule and on imaging seen as generalized diffuse decrease in CT attenuation, mainly in the lower lobe.

Paraseptal Emphysema

In paraseptal emphysema the destruction pattern is located in the periphery of the lung adjacent to the pleura or along the interlobular septa. Upper lung zones are more affected. On CT paraseptal emphysema is seen as small subpleural lucencies arranged as single tier of "cystic" spaces. Large emphysematous bullae may be seen and can cause pneumothorax.

COMBINED PULMONARY FIBROSIS AND EMPHYSEMA

Combined pulmonary fibrosis and emphysema (CPFE) is a relatively new entity, which is characterized by upper-lobe emphysema and lower-lobe fibrosis. On pulmonary function tests the typical findings include preserved lung volume and severely diminished capacity of gas exchange (DLco). Smoking, connective tissue disorders and mineral dust exposure are labelled as a few risk factors of this disease. It usually presents with symptoms of exertional dyspnea; and frequently complicated by pulmonary hypertension, acute lung injury and lung cancer. The prognosis is poor. This entity is defined radiographically by the presence of classic features of emphysema in the upper lobes and pulmonary fibrosis (mainly IPF/UIP) in the lower lobes. HRCT **(Figs. 12A to D)** shows upper-lobe centrilobular and/or paraseptal emphysema with multiple bullae and lower-lobe honeycombing with subpleural reticular opacities and traction bronchiectasis, and sometimes ground-glass opacities.[21,22]

PULMONARY LANGERHANS' CELL HISTIOCYTOSIS

Pulmonary Langerhans' cell histiocytosis[23-25] is preferred term for isolated pulmonary involvement; occurs most commonly in young adult smokers. The clinical features include dyspnea, nonproductive cough, fatigue, chest pain, weight loss or spontaneous pneumothorax. In children pulmonary LCH is usually seen as a part of multisystem involvement.

Imaging

Chest radiograph reveals bilateral diffuse symmetrical reticulonudolar opacities, which are predominantly distributed in upper zones. The lung volume is usually preserved. Small irregular-shaped nodules are seen in early disease; which later on cavitates and result in pneumothorax.

CT findings **(Figs. 13A to C)** depend on the stage of the disease. In early disease multiple small (1–10 mm in size), irregular-shaped nodules are seen. They have a distribution in centrilobular, peribronchial and peribronchiolar location. The nodules and cavitate. Cystic pattern dominates in later stage. These cysts are irregular, small (1–3 cm) and sometimes bizarre shaped. Nodules and cysts usually seen in upper/mid lung zone. The cysts

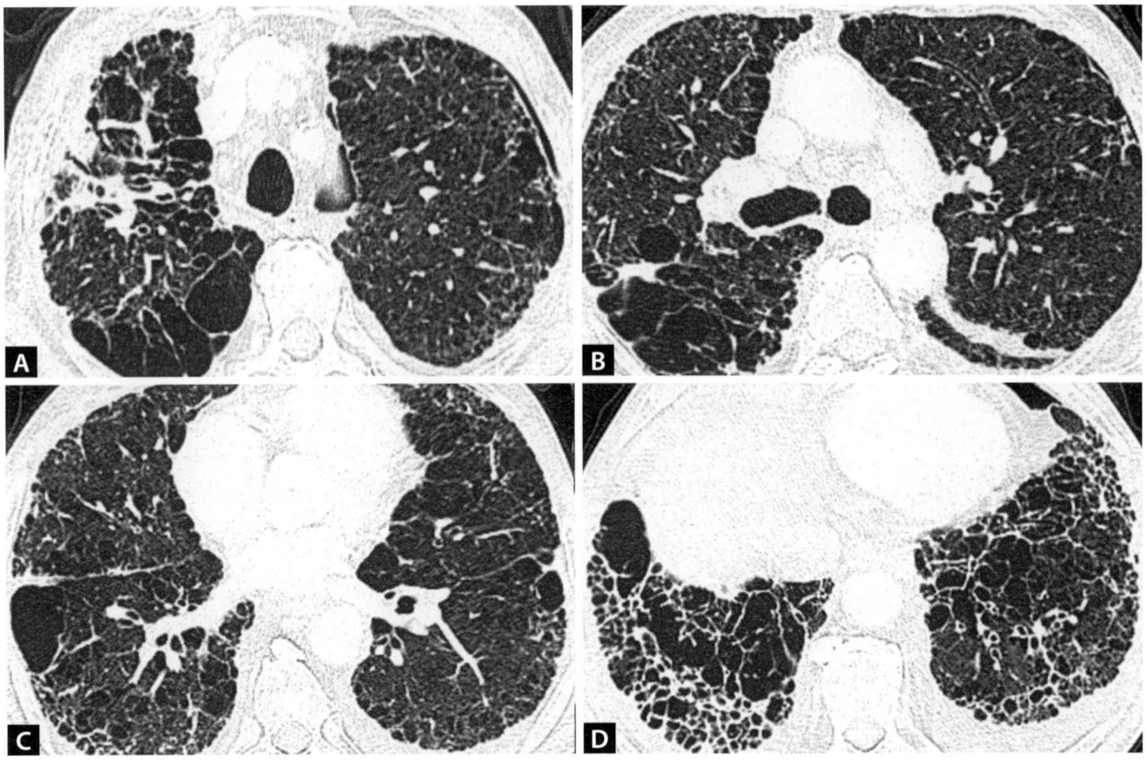

Figs. 12A to D: Combined pulmonary fibrosis and emphysema: HRCT images reveal upper-lobe centrilobular and/or paraseptal emphysema and lower-lobe honeycombing with subpleural reticular opacities.

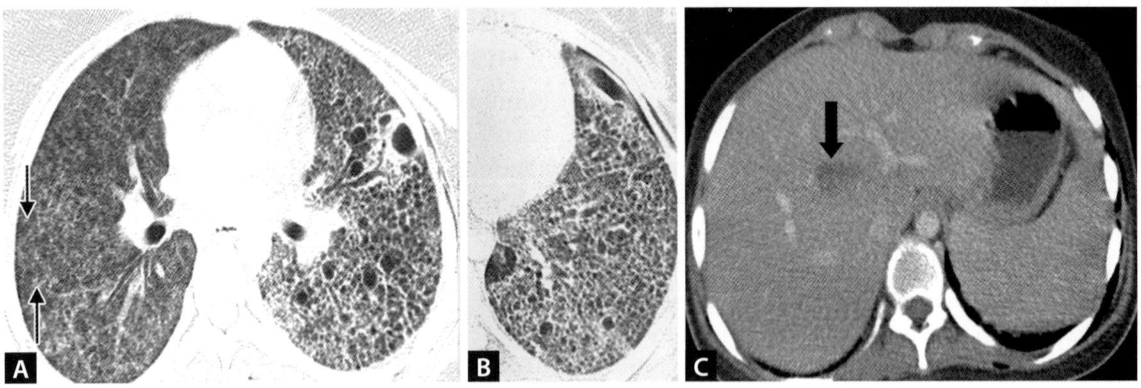

Figs. 13A to C: Langerhans' cell histiocytosis in a 16-year-old girl. HRCT images (A and B) reveal multiple irregular parenchymal nodules (arrow) in right lung and multiple cysts in left lung. Note left-sided pneumothorax. Soft tissue image (C) reveals focal a small hypodense liver lesion (block arrow).

can rupture and produce spontaneous pneumothorax (in 10-15%). When LCH is confined to the lungs, the prognosis is good.

LYMPHANGIOLEIOMYOMATOSIS

Lymphangioleiomyomatosis (LAM) is a disorder caused by abnormal smooth muscle and lymphatic proliferation. It can present either as sporadic form, or syndromic form (associated with tuberous sclerosis). In proven cases of tuberous sclerosis, about 30–40% patients can have LAM. Patients of tuberous sclerosis with LAM may not have the classical imaging triad of tuberous sclerosis (epilepsy, mental retardation and adenoma sebaceum). Sporadic form of LAM is commoner than syndromic form; and is seen almost exclusively in women of child-bearing age. Syndromic LAM can affect both males and females; although incidence is higher in females.

The pulmonary imaging findings of sporadic and syndromic LAM are similar. Chest radiograph may reveal bilateral reticular shadows with preserved lung volumes. HRCT **(Figs. 14A and B)** shows the presence of thin walled cysts uniformly distributed in lungs, and chylous pleural effusion. The parenchymal cysts are usually thin walled (less than 2 mm in size), uniform in size, randomly distributed without zonal predominance. The intervening lung parenchyma is usually normal. Rupture of cysts may cause pneumothorax; recurrence of pneumothorax is quite common. Hilar and mediastinal lymphadenopathy and pericardial effusion are other imaging findings.

Differential Diagnosis

LCH cysts are more irregular, bizzare shaped; intervening lung often abnormal, systemic manifestations commonly associated with pediatric LCH. LAM is a disease which is charecaterized by proliferation of peribronchovascular smooth muscle casuing air trapping and subsequent development of cysts.

TUBEROUS SCLEROSIS

Tuberous sclerosis is a genetic disorder having an autosomal-dominant inheritance. It affects multiple systems and the classic triad comprises of epilepsy, mental retardation and facial angiofibroma (adenoma sebaceum). While the disease equally affect men and women; pulmonary involvement is more commonly observed in females.

HRCT findings of tuberous sclerosis similar to those of those of LAM. Multiple uniformly distributed cysts and few small nodules (multifocal micronodular pneumocyte hyperplasia) may seen. Chylous pleural effusions usually not seen in tuberous sclerosis as compared to LAM.

BIRT-HOGG-DUBÉ SYNDROME

Birt-Hogg-Dubé (BHD) syndrome is a multisystem disease[26-28] caused by a deletion mutation on the FLCN gene (chromosome 17). The disease affects multiple organ systems, abnormalities include cutaneous angiofibromas, perifollicular fibromas, acrochordons, fibrofolliculomas; and renal masses. On imaging, multiple lung cysts are seen, along with multiple bilateral renal tumors (renal cell carcinoma, oncocytoma). Multiple lung cysts and secondary spontaneous pneumothoraces. CT reveals multiple small cysts **(Figs. 15A to D)** are located in lower zones, subpleural location. The cysts may be septated when they become large).

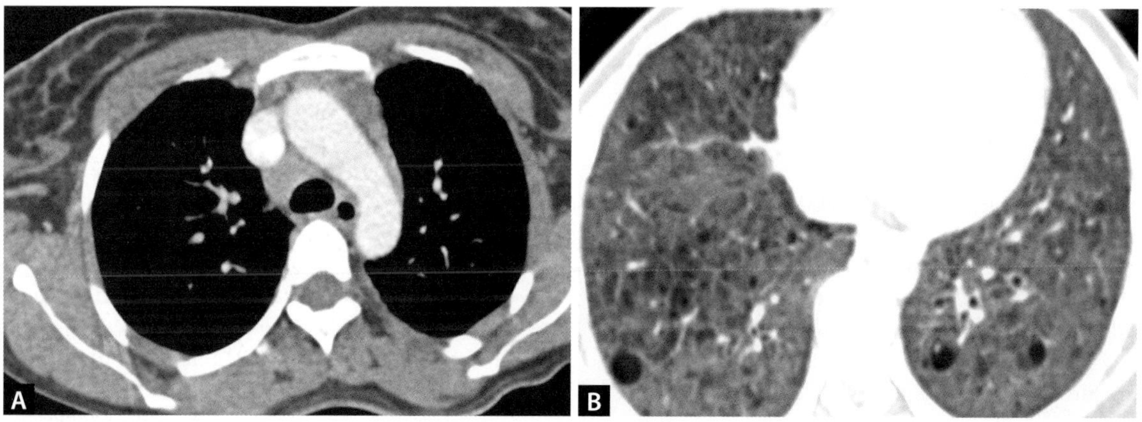

Figs. 14A and B: Lymphangioleiomyomatosis in a 30-year-old lady. Axial soft tissue window image (A) reveals mediastinal lymphadenopathy. HRCT image (B) reveals diffuse ground-glass opacities in both lungs; with scattered thin-walled cysts.

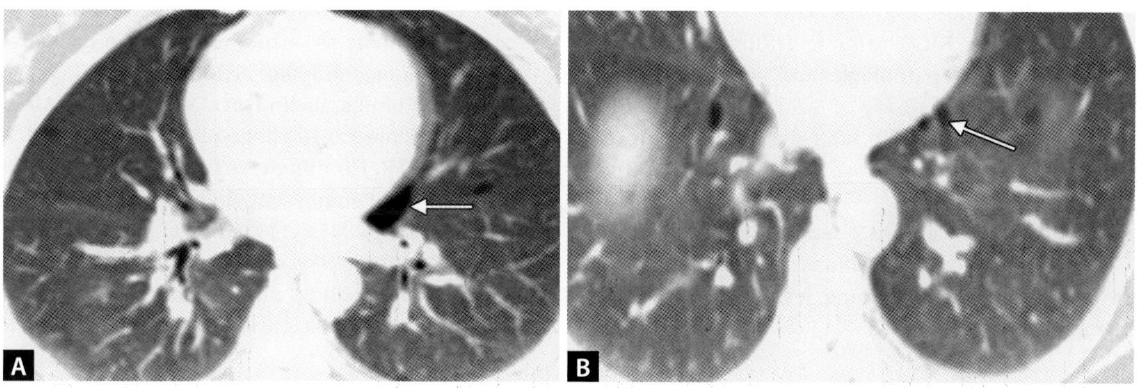

Figs. 15A and B

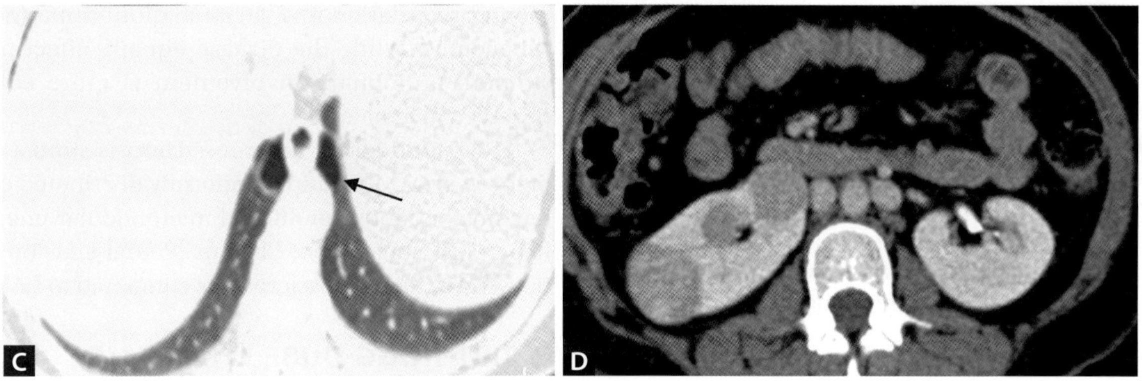

Figs. 15C and D

Figs. 15A to D: Birt-Hogg-Dubé syndrome in a 39-year-old lady. Note the thin-walled cysts in subpleural locations (arrows) and multiple solid enhancing right renal masses.

CONCLUSION

Diffuse lung disease is a complex disease with various etiologies; sometimes without any identifiable cause. While reaching a precise diagnosis requires a team effort and combination of clinical, laboratory and radiological findings; adoption of a pattern approach on HRCT can help the radiologist to narrow down the differential diagnoses.

REFERENCES

1. Franquet T. Imaging of pulmonary viral pneumonia. Radiology. 2011;260:1.
2. Kim EA, Lee KS, Primack SL, et al. Viral pneumonias in adults: radiologic and pathologic findings. Radiographics. 2002;22(Spec Issue):S137-49.
3. Cheung OY, Chan JW, Ng CK, et al. The spectrum of pathological changes in severe acute respiratory syndrome (SARS). Histopathology. 2004;45(2):119-24.
4. Chiumello D, Froio S, Bouhemad B, et al. Clinical review: Lung imaging in acute respiratory distress syndrome patients—an update. Crit Care. 2013;17(6):243.
5. Ashbaugh DG, Bigelow DB, Petty TL, et al. Acute respiratory distress in adults. Lancet. 1967;2:319-23.
6. Pnimack SL, Miller RR, Nestor L. Diffuse pulmonary hemorrhage: Clinical, pathologic, and imaging features. AJR. 1995;164:295-300.
7. Jeong YJ, et al. Eosinophilic lung diseases: A clinical, radiologic, and pathologic overview. Radiographics. 2007;27:617-39.
8. Betancourt SL, et al. Lipoid pneumonia: Spectrum of clinical and radiologic manifestations. AJR. 2010;194:103-9.
9. Gaerte SC, et al. Fat-containing lesions of the chest. Radiographics. 2002;22:S61-78.
10. Tamura A, Hebisawa A, Fukushima K. lipoid pneumonia in lung cancer: radiographic and pathologic features. J Clin Oncol. 1998;28:492-6.
11. Holbert MJ, Costello P, Li W, et al. CT features of pulmonary alveolar proteinosis. AJR. 2001;176:1287-94.
12. van Buchem MA, Wondergem JH, Kool LJ, et al. Pulmonary leukostasis: radiologic-pathologic study. Radiology. 1987;165(3):739-41.
13. Tanaka N, Matsumoto T, Miura G, et al. HRCT findings of chest complications in patients with leukemia. Eur Radiol. 2002;12(6):1512-22.
14. Frazier AA, Franks TJ, Mohammed TLH, et al. Pulmonary veno-occlusive disease and pulmonary capillary hemangiomatosis. Radiographics. 2007;27:867-82.
15. Mandel J, Mark EJ, Hales CA. Pulmonary veno-occlusive disease. Am J Respir Crit Care Med. 2000;162:1964-73.
16. Ito K, Ichiki T, Ohi K, et al. Pulmonary capillary hemangiomatosis with severe pulmonary hypertension. Circ J. 2003;67:793-5.
17. Masur Y, Remberger K, Hoefer M. Pulmonary capillary hemangiomatosis as a rare cause of pulmonary hypertension. Pathol Res Pract. 1996;192:290-5; discussion 296-9.
18. Dufour B, Maitre S, Humbert M, et al. High-resolution CT of the chest in four patients with pulmonary capillary hemangiomatosis or pulmonary veno-occlusive disease. Am J Roentgenol. 1998;171:1321-4.
19. Czeyda-Pommersheim F, et al. Amyloidosis: Modern cross-sectional imaging. Radiographics. 2015;35:1381-92.
20. Washko GR, Hunninghake GM, Fernandez IE, et al. Lung volumes and emphysema in smokers with interstitial lung abnormalities. N Engl J Med. 2011;364(10):897-906.
21. Lin H, Jiang S. Combined pulmonary fibrosis and emphysema (CPFE): an entity different from emphysema or pulmonary fibrosis alone. J Thorac Dis. 2015;7(4):767-79.

22. Cottin V, Nunes H, Brillet PY, et al. Combined pulmonary fibrosis and emphysema: a distinct underrecognised entity. Eur Respir J. 2005;26:586-93.
23. Abbott GF, Rosado-de-Christenson ML, Franks TJ, et al. Pulmonary Langerhans cell histiocytosis. Radiographics. 2004;24:821-41.
24. Sundar KM, Gosselin MV, Chung HL, et al. Pulmonary Langerhans cell histiocytosis: emerging concepts in pathobiology, radiology, and clinical evolution of disease. Chest. 2003;123:1673-83.
25. KoyamaM, Johkoh T, Honda O. Chronic cystic lung disease: diagnostic accuracy of high-resolution CT in 92 patients. Am J Roentgenol. 2003;180:827-35.
26. Birt AR, Hogg GR, Dube WJ. Hereditary multiple fibrofolliculomas with trichodiscomas and acrochordons. Arch Dermatol. 1977;113:1674-7.
27. Prachi P, et al. Thoracic CT findings in Birt-Higg-Dubé syndrome. Am J Roentgenol. 2011;196:349-52.
28. Souza CA, Finley R, Müller NL. Birt-Hogg-Dubé Syndrome: A rare cause of pulmonary cysts. AJR. 2005;185:1237-9.

CHAPTER 166

Mediastinum

Raju Sharma, Kumble S Madhusudhan, Arun Kumar Gupta

INTRODUCTION

Mediastinum is the space between the mediastinal pleura, extending from the thoracic inlet to the diaphragm, bounded anteriorly by the sternum and posteriorly by the paravertebral gutters and the ribs. There are no anatomical divisions or fascial planes that divide this space into compartments, and hence pathology from one compartment can spread to another and large masses are often multicompartmental. The division into radiographic compartments is done solely for the purpose of narrowing the differential diagnosis. This can be done by many methods, none of which are perfect.[1,2]

DIVISIONS OF THE MEDIASTINUM

Mediastinum is anatomically divided into superior and inferior compartments by a line extending from manubriosternal junction to lower margin of 4th dorsal vertebral body. The inferior compartment is further divided into anterior, middle and posterior mediastinum.[3] Felson modified this classification to include only three compartments, without any superior/inferior division.[4] This division into anterior, middle and posterior mediastinum is based on the lateral chest radiograph, by two lines drawn from thoracic inlet to diaphragm. The first line is drawn along the anterior margin of trachea and posterior margin of cardiac silhouette and the second line is drawn along the points 1 cm posterior to anterior margin of vertebral bodies. Many other classifications are also available in literature. However, these classifications are arbitrary and theoretical. Since most of the lesions of the mediastinum are detected on cross-sectional imaging, a CT or MRI based classification would be more appropriate. In 2014, Japanese Association for Research on Thymus (JART) defined CT based classification of mediastinum into four compartments.[5] This was later modified by the International Thymic Malignancy Interest Group (ITMIG), thus introducing new definitions and standards.[6,7] This divides the mediastinum into prevascular (anterior), visceral (middle) and paravertebral (posterior) compartments **(Table 1)**. All compartments extend superiorly from thoracic inlet to diaphragm inferiorly. This division has anatomical correlation, better distinguishes diseases and is less complicated.

IMAGING MODALITIES

The imaging modalities available to the radiologist to evaluate the mediastinum include chest radiograph, computed tomography (CT), sonography, magnetic resonance imaging (MRI), and positron emission tomography (PET). Occasionally barium swallow, digital subtraction angiography and scintigraphy are also used. The main role of imaging is in localization and characterization of the lesions. Further it also helps in staging of the tumors, assessing the surgical resectability and in guiding radiological interventions such as aspiration, biopsy and drainage.

Table 1: Classification of mediastinal compartments.

Classification of compartments	*Borders*	*Contents*	*Pathologies*
Prevascular	Posterior margin of sternum to anterior margin of pericardium	• Thymus • Fat • Lymph nodes • Left brachiocephalic vein	• Thymic—cysts, hyperplasia, carcinoma, thymoma, neuroendocrine tumor • Germ cell tumors • Lymph nodal—lymphoma, metastatic • Thyroid/parathyroid lesions
Visceral	Anterior aspect of pericardium to line along 1 cm posterior to anterior vertebral margins	• Nonvascular—trachea, carina, esophagus, lymph nodes • Vascular—heart, ascending thoracic aorta, aortic arch, descending thoracic aorta, superior vena cava, intrapericardial pulmonary arteries, thoracic duct	• Lymph nodal—lymphoma, metastatic • Tracheal lesions • Esophageal lesions • Duplication cysts • Vascular—cardiac, pericardial, great vessels
Para-vertebral	Posterior limit of visceral compartment to vertical line against the posterior margin of the chest wall at the lateral margin of the transverse process of the thoracic spine	• Thoracic spine • Paravertebral soft tissues	• Neurogenic tumors • Infection—discitis, osteomyelitis • Trauma—hematoma • Extramedullary hematopoiesis

Chest Radiograph

Chest radiograph is usually the initial modality used for evaluation of a mediastinal mass. Many mediastinal masses are discovered incidentally on chest radiographs done for other indications. Evaluation of a suspected mediastinal mass on a chest radiograph begins with the attempt to determine if the mass is mediastinal or pulmonary and then to place it in the appropriate mediastinal compartment.

A mediastinal mass on chest radiograph is usually sharply marginated with broad base towards the mediastinum. Its medial margin is not defined as it forms an obtuse angle with mediastinum. In contrast to this, intrapulmonary mass is often poorly defined, margins are spiculated, nodular or irregular, and it makes an acute angle with the mediastinum. Presence of air bronchogram within the mass lesion further points to intra-pulmonary location. Also bilaterality of the lesion and bone destruction of adjoining vertebra, rib or sternum favor mediastinal lesion.

Once the location in mediastinum is confirmed, the differential diagnosis of mediastinal mass starts with a classification scheme adopted by Felson. The mediastinum is conventionally divided into anterior, middle and posterior compartments on a lateral chest radiograph using two imaginary lines—the first line drawn along anterior border of trachea to back of the heart extending to the diaphragm and a second line joining a point 1.0 cm behind the anterior margin of the dorsal vertebrae **(Fig. 1)**. Space anterior to first line is anterior mediastinum, between first and second line is middle mediastinum and posterior to second line is posterior mediastinum.[1]

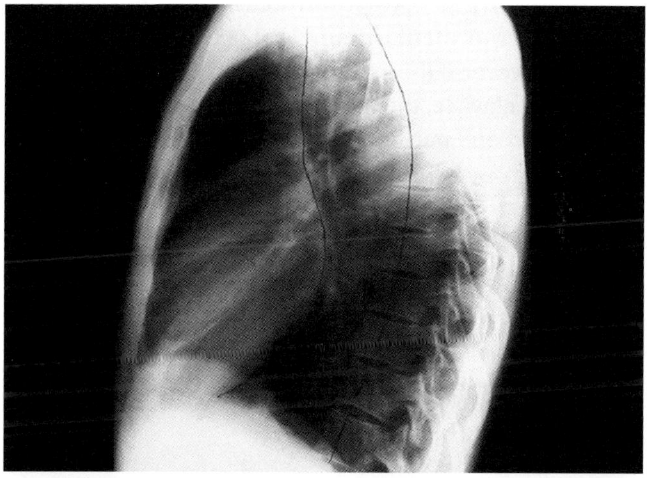

Fig. 1: Lateral radiograph showing the two lines that are drawn to divide the mediastinum into compartments. The first line is drawn along anterior border of trachea to back of the heart extending to the diaphragm and a second line joining a point 1.0 cm behind the anterior margin of the dorsal vertebrae. Space anterior to first line is anterior mediastinum, between first and second is middle and posterior to second line is posterior medisatinum.

Meticulous evaluation of frontal chest radiograph should be done for presence of silhouette sign, cervicothoracic or thoracoabdominal sign, effect of the mass on adjacent structures (e.g. trachea, paraspinal lines, ribs), the hilum overlay and convergence signs. These signs in combination are often more useful for localizing a mediastinal mass to different compartments rather than lateral chest radiograph.

The silhouette sign is useful for localizing a mediastinal mass to a particular compartment. It states that an intrathoracic opacity, if in anatomic contact with a border of the heart, the aorta, or the diaphragm will obliterate that border. This sign helps in locating the mediastinal mass lesion to appropriate compartment. An anterior mediastinal mass obliterates cardiac border **(Fig. 2)** and ascending aorta or overlaps aortic knuckle. A posterior mediastinal mass obliterates descending aorta and aortic knuckle but overlaps ascending aorta. A posterior mediastinal mass is often associated with adjacent rib or vertebral involvement. The hilum convergence sign states that when the vessels are seen converging to the opacity, it is an enlarged pulmonary artery but if the vessels are going through the opacity it is a mediastinal mass. The cervicothoracic sign says that when an opacity is seen extending above the clavicle with a clear margin, it is located in the posterior mediastinum and is entirely within the thorax. However, if the margins of this opacity disappear as it nears the clavicle, the mass is cervicothoracic, i.e. partly in the thorax and partly in the neck.

Computed Tomography (CT)

CT is the most often and widely used imaging modality for the evaluation of mediastinal masses. It is also the gold standard modality according to ITMIG. Although conventional radiographs can show recognizable abnormalities in many patients with mediastinal pathology, radiographs are limited in their sensitivity and ability to delineate the extent of mediastinal abnormalities and the relationship of masses to specific mediastinal structures. Multidetector CT provides excellent spatial resolution and helps identify normal mediastinal structures, opacified vessels, and vascular abnormalities and is often able to characterize masses based on their morphology (homogeneous or heterogeneous, cystic areas, calcification, fat components, enhancement pattern) and precisely localize them and assess their extent. The thin sections acquired allow multiplanar reconstructions which give an excellent depiction of anatomy.

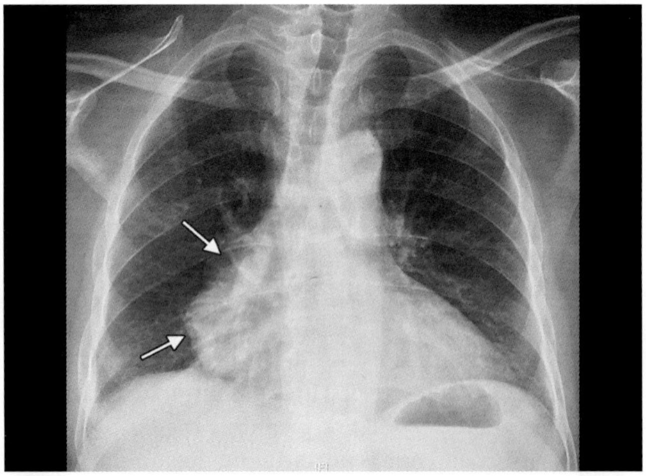

Fig. 2: Chest radiograph (PA view) showing a homogeneous mass in the right hemithorax (arrows) with broad base toward mediastinum and silhouetting the right cardiac margin suggesting anterior mediastinal mass. Hilum can be seen through the mass.

The indications for mediastinal CT can be divided into two broad categories: First, CT is commonly used to characterize a mediastinal abnormality suspected or diagnosed on plain chest radiographs. When a mediastinal contour abnormality is visible on plain films, CT should generally be the next imaging procedure performed. Secondly, CT is the most common imaging modality used to evaluate the mediastinum in patients who have normal chest radiographs yet there is a clinical reason to suspect mediastinal disease. For example, in the diagnostic workup of pyrexia of unknown origin to detect lymphadenopathy which could be due to tuberculosis, sarcoidosis or lymphoma. CT is done in patients with myasthenia gravis to detect thymic hyperplasia or thymoma, even when the chest radiograph is normal.[1,2]

Magnetic Resonance Imaging

The clinical indications for mediastinal MRI are increasing with the availability of better scanners and faster and new sequences. It is helpful in the differentiation of solid from cystic masses, for demonstration of septations in cystic masses and distinguishing benign cysts from cystic tumors. Primary uses of MRI include the evaluation of posterior mediastinal or paravertebral masses and neurogenic tumors, to detect neural foraminal and/or intraspinal extension and in differentiating thymic hyperplasia from thymoma.[8,9] It is also useful in the diagnosis of mediastinal abnormalities that are suspected to be vascular. In many other instances, however, MRI is best reserved as a secondary or problem-solving tool, in patients who have equivocal or confusing CT findings, or in whom specific anatomic information is required, which is less clearly demonstrated using CT. In such cases, a limited number of MR images can be helpful. MR provides multiple paradigms for lesion characterization, such as the T1 and T2 signal, presence or absence of diffusion restriction, etc. Recently the cine sequence has been reported to be useful in assessing invasion of surrounding mediastinal vessels and pericardium. In addition, it can be used as an alternative to CT in patients in whom iodinated contrast cannot be given or radiation risk has to be avoided. Another emerging role of MR is in the field of response assessment of tumors to chemoradiotherapy where it can be an alternative to PET-CT.

However, if MRI provides information that is merely equivalent to that given by CT, then CT is usually the more appropriate modality. It is more widely available, is less expensive, faster and is more suitable for imaging sick patients. However, CT and MRI are not competitive, but play a complementary role for many clinical problems.

DIFFERENTIAL DIAGNOSIS OF MEDIASTINAL MASSES

The most common lesions in anterior mediastinum include four Ts: Thymoma, Thyroid lesion, Teratoma and Terrible lymphoma. The key structures in middle mediastinum are lymph nodes, tracheobronchial tree and esophagus. Metastatic disease commonly affects lymph nodes in anterior and middle mediastinum. Posterior mediastinal masses are generally neurogenic tumors.[1,2,10]

The differential diagnosis of a mediastinal mass on CT is usually based on several findings, including its location and identification of the structure from which it is arising; whether it is single or multifocal (involving several different areas or lymph node groups), or diffuse; its size and shape and its attenuation (fatty, fluid, soft tissue, or a combination of these); the presence of calcification—its character and amount; and its enhancement following administration of contrast agents.

Rather than using the conventional compartment model, on CT, it is more appropriate to base the differential diagnosis of a mediastinal mass on directly observing the tissue or structure from which the mass is arising (e.g. lymph nodes, thymus, thyroid, parathyroid, trachea, esophagus, vertebral column). If this is not possible, then localizing the mass to specific regions of the mediastinum (e.g. prevascular space, pretracheal space, subcarinal space, anterior cardiophrenic angle, etc.) can be valuable in differential diagnosis. The differential diagnosis of masses arising in the prevascular area includes thymoma and other thymic tumors, cysts, lymphoma and other lymph node masses, germ-cell tumors, thyroid masses, parathyroid masses, fatty masses, and lymphangioma. The differential diagnosis of cardiophrenic angle mass includes pericardial cyst, fat pad, Morgagni hernia and occasionally thymoma and lymph node mass.[10] However, it is also important to remember that, although many pathologic processes have a typical location or locations, most can be seen in any part of the mediastinum.

The attenuation of mediastinal masses is also of primary importance in their differential diagnosis. Masses can be categorized as having fatty, low or high attenuation. Masses with fat attenuation value are composed primarily of or partially containing fat or lipid-rich tissues. These include lipomatosis and fat pads, thymolipoma, teratoma, lymphangioma and hemangioma, lipoma, liposarcoma, hernias, etc. Low-attenuation masses are usually cystic or fluid filled or contain some lipid. These include a variety of congenital or acquired cysts (bronchogenic, esophageal duplication, neurenteric, pericardial, and thymic); necrotic neoplasms, including lymphoma, cystic thymoma, germ-cell tumors, and lymph node metastases; lymphangioma and hemangioma; neurogenic tumors; thoracic meningocele and fluid collections, such as mediastinal abscess.[11-13]

High-attenuation masses generally contain calcium, have high iodine content, or are related to the presence of fresh blood. They include calcified lymph nodes secondary to granulomatous infection, sarcoidosis, silicosis, partially calcified primary neoplasms, including germ-cell tumors, thymoma, and neurogenic tumors, calcified goiter, calcified vascular lesions, goiter with high iodine content, and mediastinal hematoma.

The pattern of enhancement also aids in the differential diagnosis. Enhancing masses are highly vascular and include substernal thyroid and parathyroid glands, carcinoid tumors, hemangiomas, paraganglioma, Castleman disease, and a variety of partially necrotic, inflammatory, and neoplastic lesions in which some rim enhancement is visible.[2,14]

ANTERIOR MEDIASTINUM

Lesions of Thymus

Normal thymus is a bilobed triangular gland **(Fig. 3)** in the anterior mediastinum. Its size and morphology vary with age. In newborn, it is large and the size decreases with age. Normal thymus shows homogeneous attenuation on CT. Focal contour abnormality, heterogeneous attenuation on CT or signal intensity on MRI suggest thymic mass lesion.

CT remains the technique of choice following a standard chest radiograph when thymic lesion is suspected. Thymic enlargement is usually caused by tumor, most common being thymoma. Other lesions include thymolipoma, malignant lymphoma and carcinoid. Occasionally, thymic enlargement is caused by a thymic cyst and rarely by hyperplasia or infection.

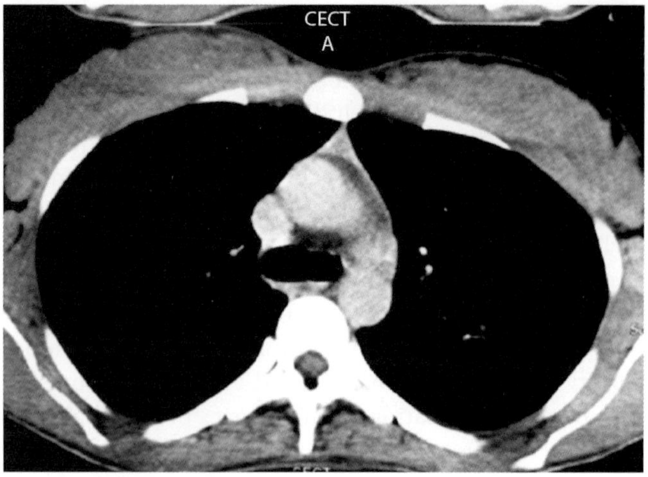

Fig. 3: Normal thymus: Axial CT scan showing the normal triangular configuration of the thymus gland in a young adult.

Thymic Rebound

Thymic rebound refers to thymic enlargement following atrophy from severe illness, steroid treatment or chemotherapy. This phenomenon is most marked in children, but it has also been seen in young adults. Following involution, the thymus grows back to its baseline volume within several months of the stressful episode. In about 12–25% patients it may exceed the baseline volume by 50%.[2] Because CT is more sensitive than plain chest radiographs for detecting thymic enlargement, thymic rebound is detected with greater frequency when patients are monitored with CT. CT or MRI show symmetrically enlarged but normal in shape and smooth outline of the gland with CT density and MR signal intensity being similar to normal thymic tissue.

In most patients with extrathoracic malignancies, thymic rebound is unlikely to cause concern or diagnostic confusion. Practically, thymic rebound is most problematic when it is seen in patients with malignant lymphoma who have been treated using chemotherapy. When an enlarged thymus is seen in such patients, it can be difficult to distinguish thymic rebound from recurrent lymphoma. However, when a patient with lymphoma shows thymic enlargement as an isolated finding after treatment with no adenopathy being visible, it is reasonable to follow the patient with the presumption that thymic rebound is responsible. However, in equivocal cases, chemical shift MRI and PET may be used to distinguish thymic hyperplasia from lymphoma. Thymic hyperplasia shows a signal drop on the opposed phase image whereas thymic tumors will not.[15] Diffusion weighted MRI can also be useful in distinguishing rebound hyperplasia from lymphoma because of the marked restriction of diffusion seen in the latter.

Thymic Hyperplasia

This is present in more than 50% of patients with myasthenia gravis. It is also seen in thyrotoxicosis, systemic lupus erythematosis, polyarteritis nodosa, Addison's disease, Hashimoto's thyroiditis. It is not recognized on chest radiograph; CT and MRI may show enlargement of both lobes but the normal shape of the gland is maintained and density and signal characteristics are same as normal thymus. In difficult cases, assessment may be done with chemical shift MRI due to the presence of interspersed fat within the thymic tissue.[15] Biopsy or surgery is rarely necessary. The normal thymus and thymic hyperplasia in the adult patient shows loss of signal on the opposed phase image due to the presence of microscopic fat **(Figs. 4A and B)**. A chemical shift ratio (thymus SI (OP)/ muscle SI (OP)/thymus SI (IP)/muscle SI (OP) has been found reliable. A CSR of 0.7 or less is suggestive of thymic hyperplasia whereas a CSI of 1 or more is suggestive of thymic tumor. This is not reliable in the pediatric patient as there may be insufficient amount of fat and the signal drop may not be seen. Normal thymic tissue and thymic hyperplasia can be avid on FDG PET-CT and this should not be mistaken as malignancy. Correlation with the CT and MR morphology can help in resolving this pitfall.

Thymoma

Thymoma is comprised of epithelial cells and lymphocytes, the proportion of each varies. It may be benign or malignant, but there is no distinction histologically, and therefore, the term invasive thymoma is used to describe a tumor which has spread beyond the capsule. Approximately 15–40% of thymomas are invasive.

Most are discovered between 40 years and 50 years of age, and there is no sex predilection. It is frequently associated with autoimmune disease, most commonly myasthenia gravis. About 35–40% of patients with thymoma have myasthenia gravis while 10–23% patients with myasthenia gravis have thymoma. Red blood cell aplasia is seen in 21–50% of patients and hypogammaglobulinemia in about 10% of patients.[16]

Most thymomas occur in anterior mediastinum, usually located anterior to ascending aorta, above the right ventricular outflow tract and main pulmonary artery, projects into hemithorax, less commonly extend on either side of the midline. Thymoma may project from

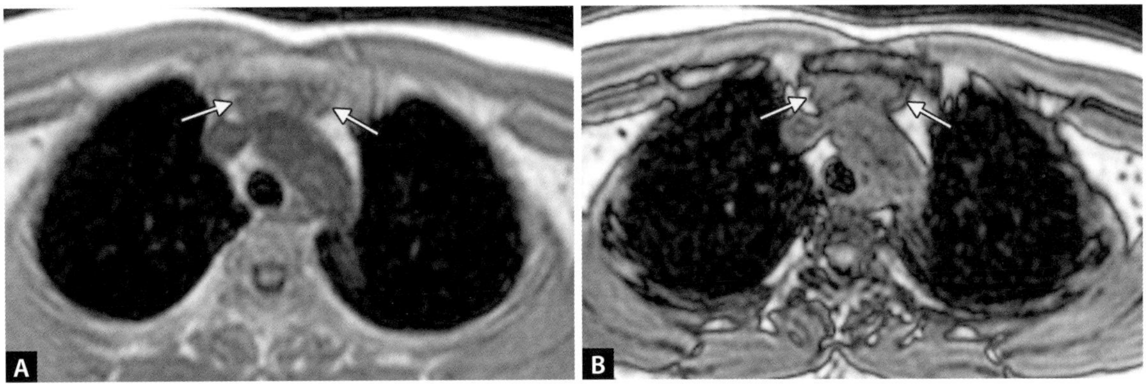

Figs. 4A and B: Thymic hyperplasia: Axial T1-weighted MR images with TE – 4.6 ms (in phase; A) and TE – 2.3 ms (in opposed phase; B) showing small lesion in the anterior mediastinum (arrows). The lesion showed a mean signal intensity of 448 in in-phase and 267 in opposed-phase, suggestive of thymic hyperplasia.

anterior mediastinum to adjacent middle and posterior mediastinum. Thymoma is seen as a spherical mass, characteristically arising from one lobe of the thymus, with smooth or lobulated outline, often silhouetting vascular or cardiac border. Thymomas are usually small and often obscured by surrounding mediastinal vessels and hence are difficult to see on chest radiograph.

CT is the most sensitive technique for detection of thymoma and lesions as small as 1 cm can be detected. The characteristic CT features include focal asymmetrical homogeneous soft tissue density mass, oval round or lobulated mass with sharply demarcated outline **(Figs. 5A and B)**, focal areas of calcification seen in nearly 25% and uniform contrast enhancement. Necrosis and hemorrhage may occur in one third of patients. It may appear cystic with discrete nodular components.

On MRI thymoma shows low to intermediate signal intensity on T1W and high signal intensity on T2W image. Heterogeneous signal intensity due to septation, cystic change or hemorrhage is common. MRI is indicated in patients with invasive thymoma to look for vascular invasion when there is contraindication to use intravenous contrast for CT examination.

The features that suggest invasive thymoma **(Figs. 6A to D)** on CT or MRI include poorly defined or infiltrative/lobulated margins, presence of cystic or necrotic areas, multiple calcific foci, definite vascular or chest wall invasion, irregular interface with adjacent lung or evidence of spread to ipsilateral pleura. Pleural spread may manifest either as discrete pleural nodules at a distance from the primary lesion **(Figs. 6A to D)** or as a sheet of neoplastic tissue extending from the primary lesion often mimicking pleural mesothelioma. Pleural effusion is uncommon despite frequent occurrence of pleural metastasis.[17-19]

The staging system proposed by Masaoka[18] is generally used to stage thymomas. The principal features of this staging system are as follows:
- Stage I: Tumor capsule is intact
- Stage II: Invasion of the tumor capsule or surrounding fat or mediastinal pleura
- Stage III: Invasion of surrounding organs (pericardium, great vessels, or lung)
- Stage IVa: Pleural or pericardial implants
- Stage IVb: Hematogenous or lymphogenous metastases

Thymic epithelial neoplasms were initially classified as (i) thymoma (benign tumor without invasion), (ii) invasive thymoma (benign tumor with invasion) and (iii) thymic carcinoma (malignant histology). Of all these, thymic carcinoma has the poorest prognosis with 5-year survival as low as 30%.[20] Differentiation of invasive thymoma from thymic carcinoma on imaging is difficult. World Health Organization (WHO) has classified thymomas based on histology to maintain uniformity.[21] This is shown in **Table 2**.

Thymolipoma

This is a rare benign tumor seen in any age group, which is composed of mixture of mature fat and normal looking or involuted thymic tissue.[22] It usually grows to a large size, and being pliable it moulds itself to adjacent mediastinum and diaphragm. It is often detected incidentally as a mediastinal mass or mimics cardiomegaly or lobar collapse on chest radiograph. It may change in shape or position on decubitus views.

CT shows presence of fat, thymic tissue and fibrous septae running through the lesion **(Figs. 7A and B)**. Calcification may be present. MRI shows imaging characteristics of fatty mass, i.e. increased signal intensity on both T1W and T2W images. Low signal intensity strands

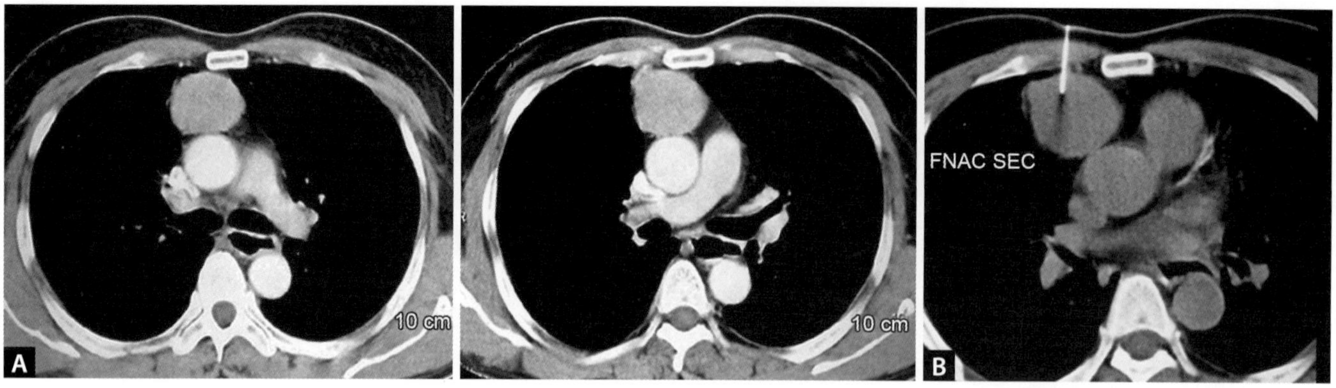

Figs. 5A and B: Thymoma: Contrast-enhanced (CE) CT (A) of a patient with myasthenia gravis showing a well-defined mass anterior to the ascending aorta suggestive of thymoma. CT-guided biopsy is seen in Figure B.

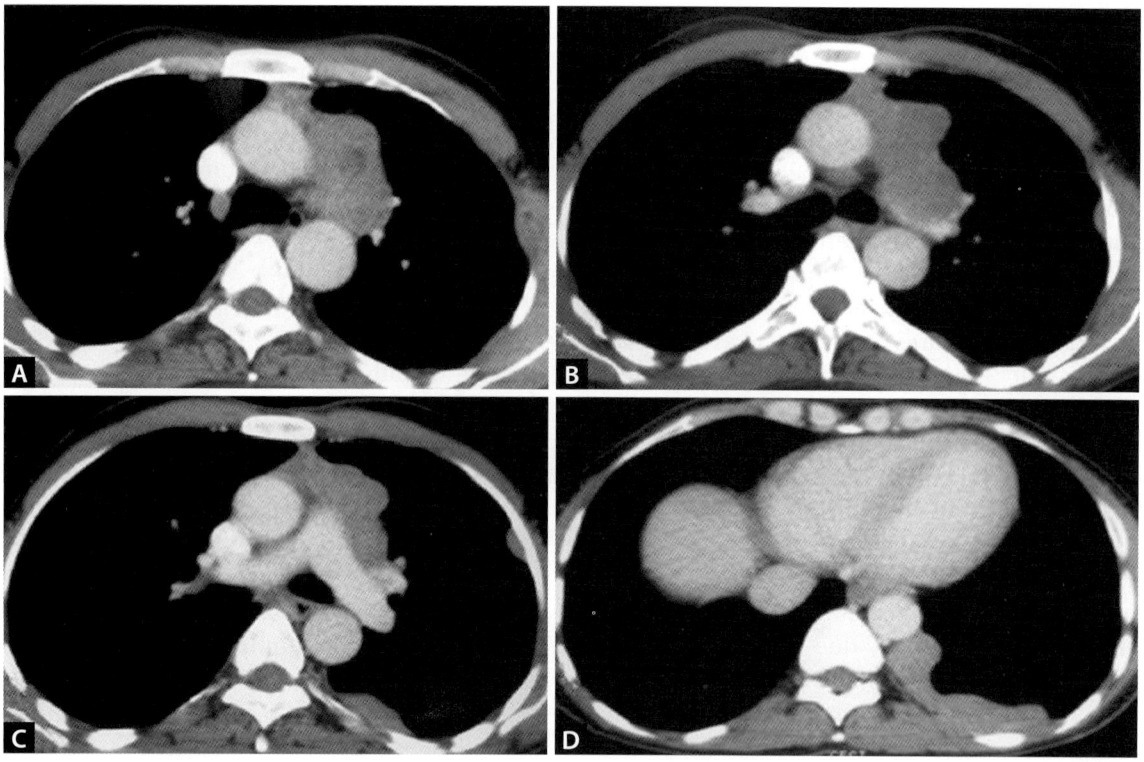

Figs. 6A to D: Invasive thymoma. CECT showing lobulated anterior mediastinal mass (A and B) with ill-defined fat plane with the ascending aorta and pulmonary artery. Nodular pleural metastases are also seen (C and D) suggestive of invasive thymoma.

may be seen coursing through the lesion, representing residual fibrous stroma or thymic tissue.

Thymic carcinoid

This is a rare tumor, thought to arise from thymic cells of neuroendocrine origin. Approximately 40% of patients have Cushing' syndrome as a result of tumor secretion of adrenocorticotropic hormone, and up to 20% have been associated with multiple endocrine neoplasia (MEN) syndromes I and II. They can be small, not detected on CT or MRI, or may be large **(Figs. 8A to C)** and aggressive with metastasis to distant site. This tumor is more aggressive than thymoma, often presenting in an advanced stage, and superior vena cava obstruction is more common with thymic carcinoid than with thymoma. Regional lymph node metastases and distant metastases may be seen, which may include blastic bone lesions. CT features are indistinguishable from invasive thymoma. The chest radiograph may be normal. Therefore, CT or MRI should

Table 2: WHO classification (4th edition) of thymoma.

Type	***Histological description***	***Frequency (%)***	***Association with myasthenia gravis (%)***	***Prognosis***
Type A	Spindle cell or medullary thymoma	4–7	17	Excellent 15-year survival in up to 100%
Type AB	Mixed thymoma	28–34	16	Good; 15-year survival 90%
Type B1	Predominantly cortical or lymphocyte rich thymoma	9–20	57	Good; 15-year survival 90%
Type B2	Cortical thymoma	20–36	71	Moderate; 20-year survival 60%
Type B3	Well-differentiated thymic carcinoma, epithelial thymoma or squamoid thymoma	10–14	46	Moderate; 20-year survival 40%
Type C	Heterogeneous thymic carcinoma	--	--	Poor; 10-year survival 28%

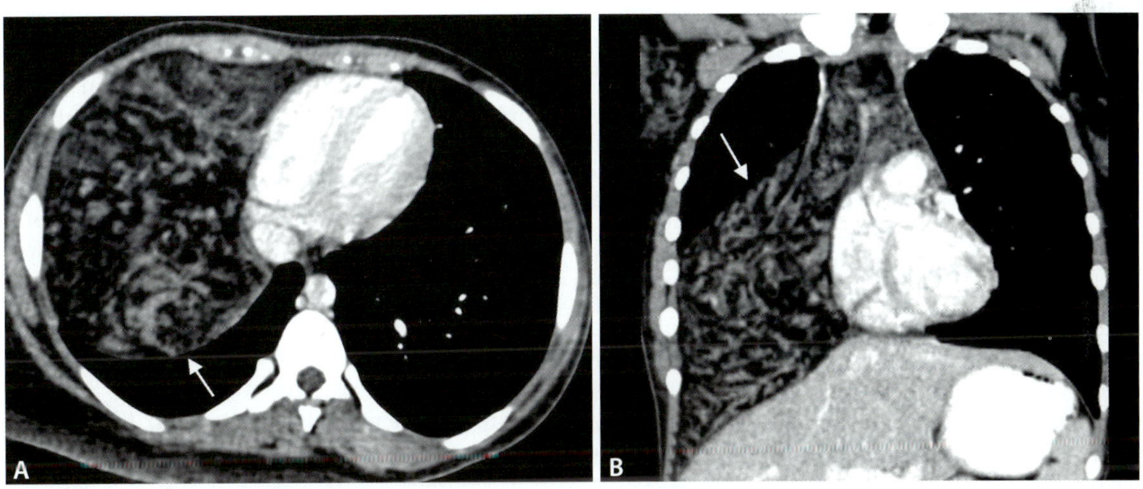

Figs. 7A and B: Thymolipoma: Axial (A) and coronal (B) contrast-enhanced CT images showing a large right-sided mediastinal mass (arrow) containing fat and soft tissue density, suggesting thymolipoma.

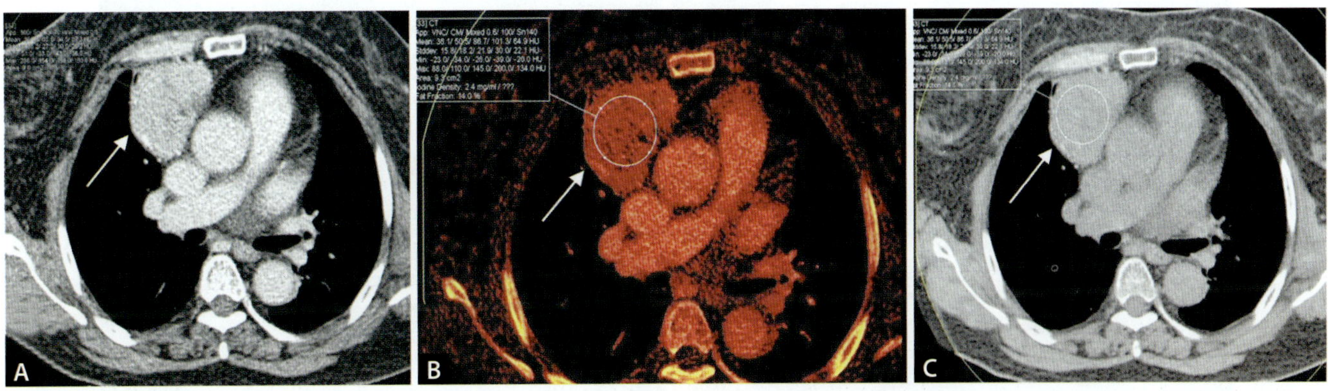

Figs. 8A to C: Thymic carcinoid: Monoenergetic (A), iodine (B) and virtual non-contrast (C) axial CT scans performed on dual energy scanner shows a homogeneously enhancing mass in the anterior mediastinum (arrow).

be done to look for a thymic mass in a patient with unexplained Cushing's syndrome. Octreotide radionuclide imaging or PET may be valuable in imaging these tumors.[2]

Thymic lymphoma

Hodgkin's disease has a predilection for involving the thymus gland in conjunction with lymph node involvement. It occurs in about one third of the patients either at the initial presentation or during relapse. This presents either as generalized thymic enlargement or as single or multiple focal masses along with mediastinal lymphadenopathy. Non-Hodgkin lymphoma (NHL) much less commonly involves the thymus. On CT and MRI the appearance of thymic mass mimics thymoma. The possibility of thymic lymphoma should be considered whenever a thymic mass is seen in combination with mediastinal lymphadenopathy. FDG PET-CT is more accurate than CT in the diagnosis of lymphomatous involvement in the mediastinum and thus is useful in staging of the disease.[7]

Thymic cyst

Thymic cysts can be either congenital or acquired. They account for 1% of anterior mediastinal masses. Acquired thymic cysts are generally associated with inflammation and have been reported following radiation therapy for lymphoma, in association with thymic tumors, and following thoracotomy. Congenital thymic cysts are usually unilocular, have a thin wall, and contain clear fluid. Acquired thymic cysts are often multilocular. Multilocular thymic cysts have been seen in children with HIV infection. The attenuation of thymic cysts is usually that of water but can be higher or lower depending on the presence of hemorrhage or lipid deposits. Calcification of the cyst wall can also be seen.

On chest radiograph, thymic cyst is seen as any other nonlobulated thymic mass with or without calcification of the wall. Ultrasonography demonstrates cystic nature of the mass. CT shows a thin walled, non-enhancing water density lesion. MRI shows typical characteristic of fluid i.e. low signal intensity on T1W and uniform high signal intensity T2W images with no restriction on the diffusion weighted image **(Figs. 9A and B)**. The cyst will show high signal intensity in both T1W and T2W images in the presence of hemorrhage. A thymic cyst with features of multiloculation, heterogeneous attenuation with thick wall and association of soft tissue component must be sampled or resected to exclude malignancy (cystic thymoma). Thymic cyst should be diagnosed with caution as cystic regions can be seen in a variety of thymic tumors, including thymoma and lymphoma.[1,2]

Germ-cell Tumors

These tumors are derived from the primitive embryonic germ cell layers, and account for 15–20% of mediastinal masses. They arise from cell rests within or in intimate contact with the thymus. They are classified as teratoma, seminoma, and nonseminomatous germ-cell tumor which include embryonal carcinoma, endodermal sinus tumor, choriocarcinoma and tumors with mixtures of these cell types. Mediastinum is the most common extragonadal primary site of these lesions. Malignant germ-cell tumors secrete beta human chorionic gondotropin and alpha-fetoprotein in 90% cases which can be used as markers to diagnose and monitor the tumor.[23-25] Serum lactate dehydrogenase may also be elevated, but it is less specific and may be elevated in other tumors like lymphoma.

Teratomas are the most common germ-cell tumors and are classified as mature, immature and malignant.

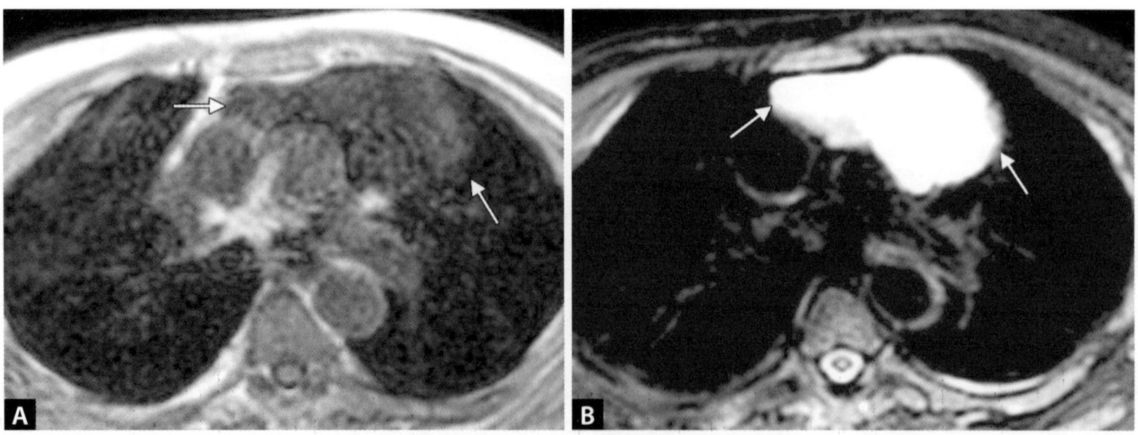

Figs. 9A and B: Thymic cyst. Axial T1-weighted (A) and T2-weighted (B) MR images showing a well-defined lesion in the anterior mediastinum (arrows) appearing hypointense on T1W and hyperintense on T2W, suggestive of a cyst.

Mature cystic teratomas are referred to as dermoid cyst which consists of predominantly ectodermal elements, such as skin, sebaceous material, hair and calcification. Benign teratoma contains elements of more than one of the three germinal layers. Mature teratomas and dermoid cysts account for majority of these lesions. They are seen at all ages, more common in adolescents and young adults, with females slightly outnumbering males. These are mostly asymptomatic and diagnosed incidentally. Occasionally, patient may present with symptoms due to local compression, rupture or infection.[2,23]

These lesions are usually seen as round or lobulated well defined mass, mainly to one side of the midline, located in anterior mediastinum, in front of the root of the aorta and main pulmonary artery. Calcification, ossification or even teeth and sometimes fat can be seen on chest radiograph.

On CT, these lesions are well encapsulated, may show curvilinear calcification of the wall and rim enhancement following intravenous contrast injection. The internal contents are inhomogeneous with variable density of water, fat and soft tissue **(Figs. 10 and 11)**. Presence of amorphous calcification, malformed teeth or bone, layering of fat and fluid within the mass confirms the diagnosis. Local invasion is the only criteria to suggest malignancy. The features of irregular outline of the mass with infiltration of the mediastinal fat, compression or invasion of the mediastinal vessels or airways on CT suggest malignant teratoma.[23-25] On MRI, fatty component shows hyperintense signal on T1 and T2 weighted images and shows chemical shift artefact. Cystic teratoma appears hyperintense on T2 weighted images with peripheral rim contrast enhancement. Occasionally, teratomas may rupture into the pleural space or in to the lung when the appearance becomes heterogeneous with poorly defined fat planes and spiculation mimicking malignant germ-cell tumors.[26] A fat fluid level in the pleural effusion has also been reported.

Malignant germ-cell tumors are usually seen in young adults, more common in men than in women, mostly in 3rd and 4th decades. They appear as irregular soft tissue mass, often with central areas of cystic degeneration or necrosis and even intratumoral calcification. They can invade the adjacent mediastinal fat, pleura or pericardium resembling CT or MR appearance of invasive thymoma or lymphoma. The only distinguishing feature is absence of transpleural droplet spread. Presence of lung metastases may help distinguish it from lymphoma.

Seminomas occur almost entirely in men with mean age at presentation of 29 years. They present as large smooth or lobulated, homogeneous soft tissue masses with obliteration of fat planes. They are sensitive to radiation and chemotherapy.

Nonseminomatous germ-cell tumors are seen as irregular, ill-defined heterogeneous masses on CT, with necrosis, hemorrhage and cystic areas. They have a poor prognosis and are associated with elevated levels of alfa fetoprotein.

Thyroid Mass

An intrathoracic thyroid mass is usually a multinodular colloid goiter or adenoma but occasionally may be a carcinoma. It is usually a downward extension of neck mass, the continuity between mediastinal mass and thyroid gland in the neck is an important diagnostic feature

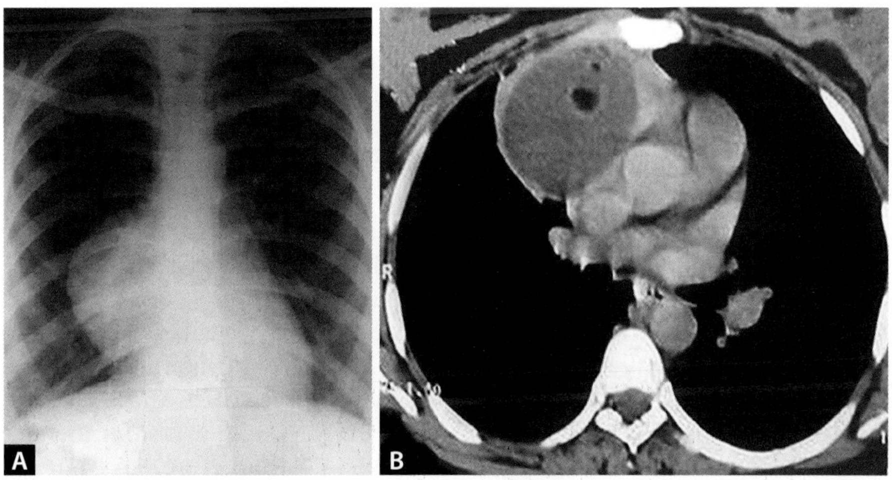

Figs. 10A and B: Teratoma: Chest radiograph (A) showing a large mediastinal mass in right paracardiac location obliterating the right heart border, suggesting its anterior location. Axial CT (B) shows a large well-encapsulated low-attenuating mass, with fat attenuation within it suggestive of teratoma.

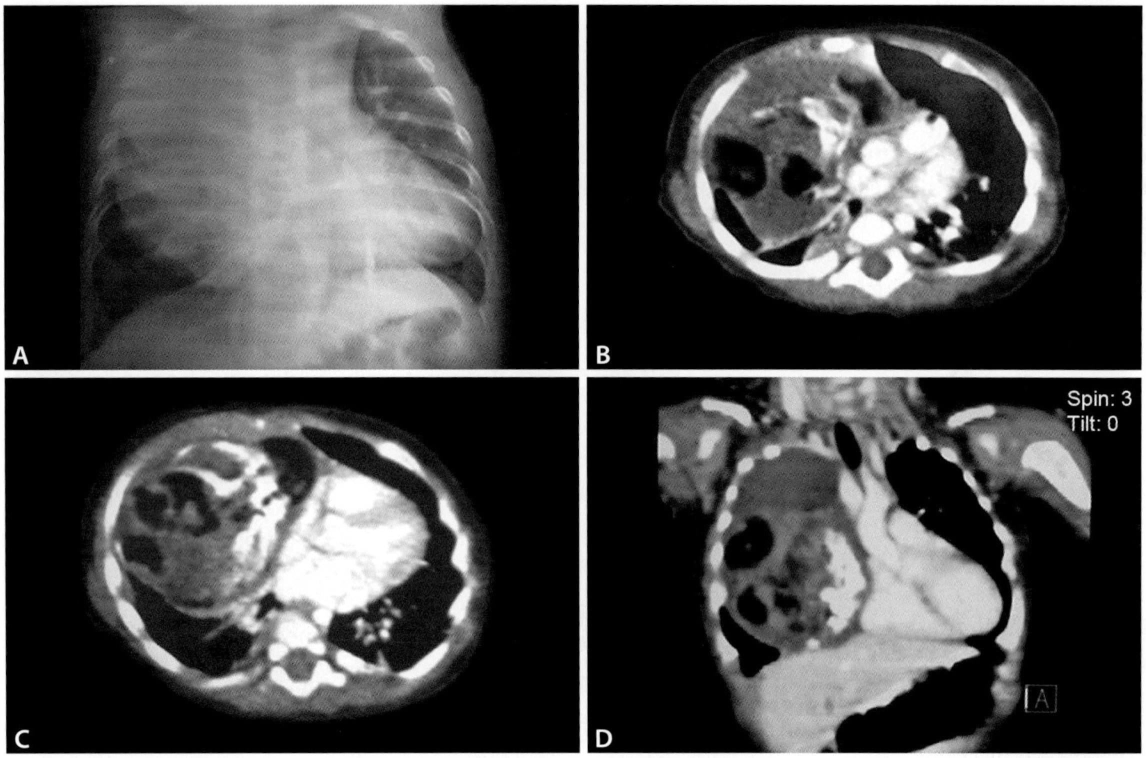

Figs. 11A to D: Teratoma: Chest radiograph (A) of a 3-month-old child showing a large mediastinal mass with foci of calcification, and contralateral mediastinal shift. Axial CT (B and C) and coronal reformatted image (D) show a large right-sided low-attenuating mass with calcification and fat within it. *Diagnosis*: Teratoma.

on chest radiograph and CT. An isolated thyroid mass in the mediastinum, arising from heterotropic thyroid tissue without any connection with thyroid in the neck is extremely rare. CT scan of the lower neck should always be done in the evaluation of mediastinal masses, especially those in the upper thorax.

On chest radiograph, this is seen as a well-defined spherical or lobular mass which may displace and compress trachea at the level of the thoracic inlet **(Figs. 12A to C)**. Dense amorphous calcification is seen on radiograph in 25% cases.

CT shows well-defined mass in the paratracheal region, continuous with thyroid gland in the neck with relatively high attenuation on non contrast CT which enhances homogeneously with intravenous contrast. Focal areas of calcification are seen in up to 75% cases, and low density areas may also be seen. The mass extends anterior to the trachea in 75% cases.[1,2] On MRI, signal intensity similar to muscle on T1W while heterogeneous increased signal intensity on T2W image is seen. However, it is not possible to distinguish adenoma from carcinoma from signal intensity. Radionuclide imaging is a sensitive and specific method of confirming thyroid nature of an intrathoracic mass, but is often unnecessary.

CT plays an important role in the preoperative assessment of substernal goiters. The surgical approach to these lesions depends on precise anatomic localization. Intrathoracic goiters should be removed for symptomatic relief as well as to reduce the risk consequent to acute hemorrhage or inflammation. Although anterior substernal goiters usually can be removed through a routine cervical incision, posterior mediastinal goitres may need a thoracotomy or a combined cervicothoracic incision depending on the size of the lesion.

Parathyroid Adenoma

Ten percent of parathyroid glands are ectopic in location. Two-thirds of these are present in the anterior mediastinum and are closely connected with thymus. Likelihood of an ectopic adenoma increases in postoperative patients who continue to have persistent hyperparathyroidism. Adenoma is usually homogeneous in density, often less than 2.0 cm in diameter and is difficult to distinguish from thymic remnant or lymph node on CT **(Figs. 13A and B)**. It may show cystic areas due to necrosis and hemorrhage. MRI shows intermediate signal intensity on T1W and marked hyperintensity on T2W image. Sestamibi radionuclide imaging is a sensitive

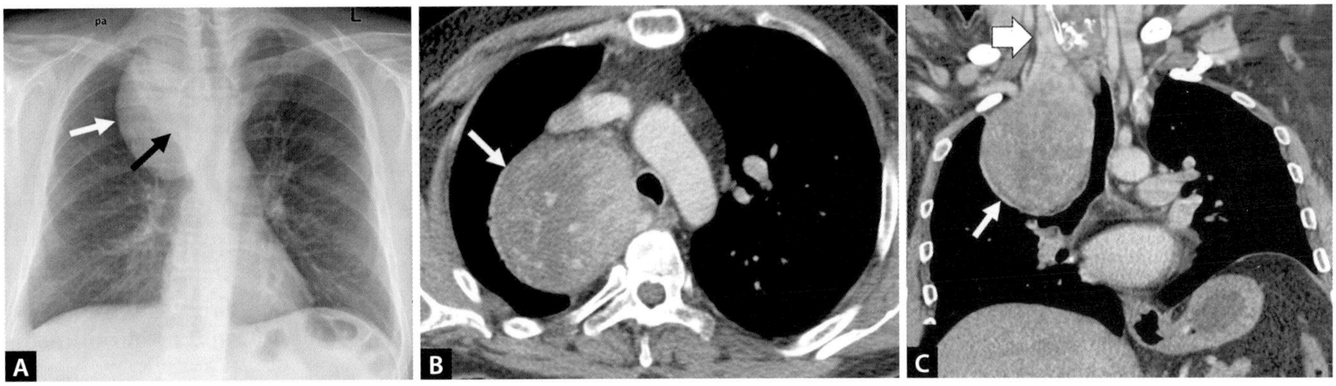

Figs. 12A to C: Thyroid mass: (A) Chest radiograph showing a right-sided mediastinal based mass (white arrow), indenting the trachea and not silhouetting the brachiocephalic vessel outline (black arrow) suggesting middle mediastinal location. Axial (B) and coronal (C) CT images showing heterogeneously enhancing mass in the middle mediastinum. Coronal image shows continuity with the right lobe of thyroid gland in the neck (block arrow) suggesting thyroid origin.

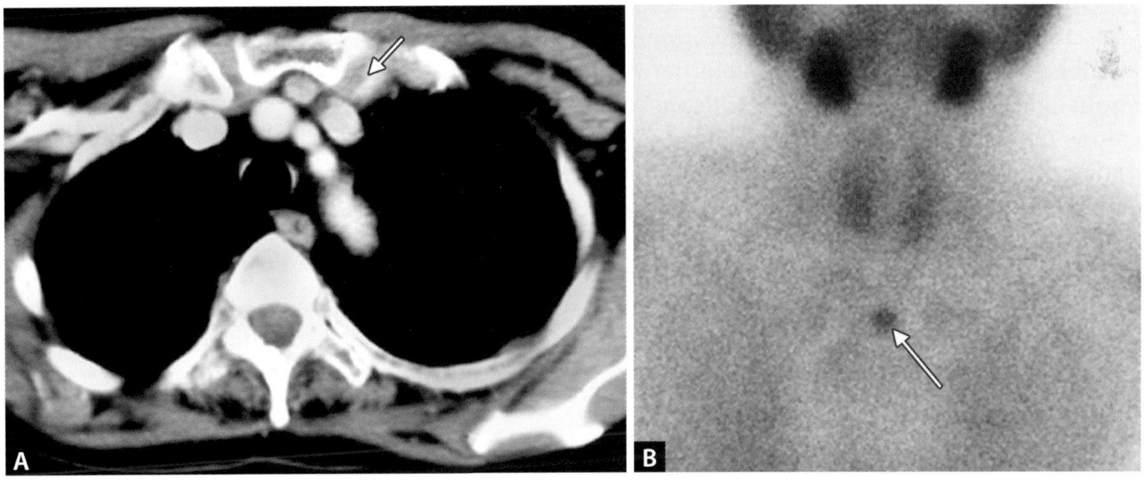

Figs. 13A and B: Parathyroid adenoma: Axial CECT (A) in a patient with hyperparathyroidism shows a small anterior mediastinal mass just behind the sternum. ^{99m}Tc Sestamibi scan (B) shows a small focus of increased uptake in the mediastinum confirming the diagnosis of an ectopic parathyroid adenoma.

technique to detect ectopic parathyroid adenomas **(Figs. 13A and B)**. Combined use of ^{99}mTcMIBI and MRI has been shown to be 89% sensitive and 95% specific for preoperative localization.[2,27] 4D multidetector CT is a recent advancement in the imaging of parathyroid lesions and is more sensitive than other imaging modalities.[28] The adenoma characteristically shows enhancement in the arterial phase with washout in the venous phase. A 'polar vessel' which may be a feeding artery or draining vein may also be seen in a hypervascular tumor.

Lymphangioma (Cystic Hygroma)

Lymphangioma is a rare benign lesion of lymphatic origin and represents 0.7–4.5% of mediastinal tumors; most are present at birth and are detected in the first 2 years of life. They are most common in the neck (75%) and axilla (20%). About 10% of cervical lymphangiomas extend into the mediastinum, but less than 5% of lymphangiomas are limited to the mediastinum itself.

They result from congenital malformation of the lymphatic system consisting of lymph channels and cystic lymph spaces lined by endothelium, containing clear or straw colored fluid. It grows slowly and commonly compresses surrounding tissues. It is a round, smooth mass with homogeneous attenuation value, sometimes lower than water. Septation is a common feature on CT, septae being thin or thick which enhance with intravenous contrast. MRI confirms the cystic nature of the lesion.

Patients may be asymptomatic because the mass is soft and yielding, but compression of mediastinal structures can result in chest pain, cough, or dyspnea. Because of a tendency for local growth, surgery is recommended. Lymphangioma can be seen in adults, with or without a history of incomplete resection as a child.

They are classified as capillary, cavernous, or cystic (hygroma), depending on the size of the lymph channels they contain. In adults, lymphangiomas are most common in the anterior (28–37%) or superior (16–36%) mediastinum but are also seen in the middle and posterior mediastinum. They can be quite large, ranging up to 30 cm in diameter.[2]

The imaging appearance of a lymphangioma is related to its type (i.e. cystic, cavernous, or capillary). On CT, cystic lymphangioma usually appears homogeneous and near to water in attenuation, but they can be of higher attenuation **(Figs. 14A to D)**. Lymphangioma may be variably composed of a combination of fluid, solid tissue, and fat; calcification is rare. Although they are usually well circumscribed and localized, they may appear to envelop mediastinal structures and insinuate between them. Lymphangioma may be associated with vascular malformations that are easily identifiable following the administration of intravenous contrast. Lymphangiomas composed of capillary-sized, thin-walled channels may appear as solid masses.

On MRI, heterogeneous signal is typical, with increased signal on T2-weighted images reflecting their fluid content. MR may also show an enhancing, multicystic, and multiseptated appearance; this suggests the presence of cavernous lymphangioma.

Other Vascular Tumors

Hemangiomas, hemangioendothelioma and hemangiopericytoma are other vascular tumors that occur in the mediastinum. Hemangiopericytoma is now considered identical to solitary fibrous tumor and the former term has been removed from the WHO classification.[29] Preoperative diagnosis of these entities is difficult. Mediastinal hemangiomas are most common in young patients, and about 75% present before the age of 35 years. Hemangiomas most commonly arise in the anterior and posterior mediastinum and may extend into the neck.

On CT, they are often heterogeneous in attenuation on unenhanced scans, and may occasionally show foci of fatty attenuation. Enhancement may be dense, multifocal or diffuse, and central or peripheral. Central enhancement is thought to be suggestive of this tumor. Phleboliths, thought to be pathognomonic, are visible in up to 10% of cases on plain radiographs. On CT, punctate calcifications are visible in 21% and phleboliths are visible in 7%. Hemangiopericytoma may appear on CT as a large, well-circumscribed, enhancing mass. It may have a predominance in the superior mediastinum.[1,2,14]

Pericardial Cyst

Pericardial or pleuropericardial cyst results from a defect in the embryogenesis of the celomic cavity. Their walls are composed of connective tissue and a single layer of mesothelial cells. Approximately 90% of pericardial cysts

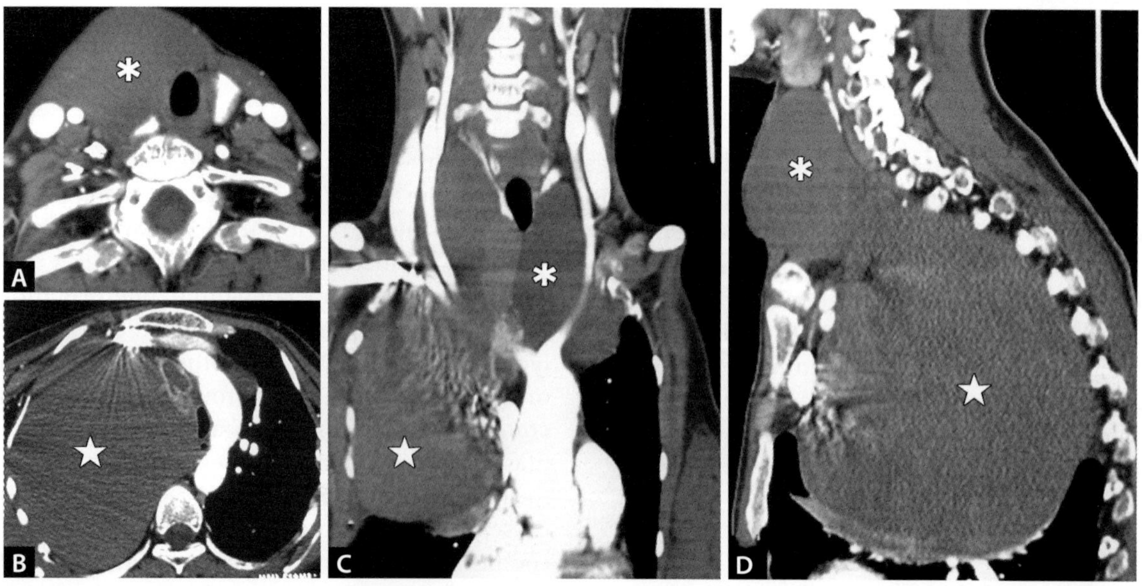

Figs. 14A to D: *Mediastinal lymphangioma*: Axial (A and B), coronal (C) and sagittal (D) contrast-enhanced CT scans showing a cystic lesion in the neck region (asterisk) with a large component in the mediastinum (star).

are in contact with the diaphragm, heart or chest wall. About 65% occur in the right cardiophrenic angle and 25% in the left cardiophrenic angle; 10 percent are seen at higher levels. They can be seen as high as the pericardial recesses at the level of the proximal aorta and pulmonary arteries. True cysts contains all layers of pericardium and do not communicate with pericardial space. They are usually asymptomatic and often an incidental finding on chest radiograph. CT is the diagnostic modality of choice and reveals their cystic nature **(Figs. 15A and B)**. They are sharply marginated, fluid attenuating lesions although pericardial cysts with high CT attenuation numbers have been reported.[2] Pericardial cysts are not always round and may assume different shapes when studied at different times. When small, they may sometimes be confused with enlarged cardiophrenic angle lymph nodes. Ultrasonography demonstrates cystic nature of the lesion. On MRI, they are hypontense on T1W and brightly hyperintense on T2W images. Hyperintense signal on T1W may be seen in case of proteinaceous contents. No contrast enhancement is usually seen. Peripheral calcification may be seen on CT due to repeated infection.[30]

MIDDLE MEDIASTINUM

Most developmental mediastinal cysts occur in the middle mediastinum and include bronchogenic, esophageal duplication and neuroenteric cysts. The distinction between these cysts may not be always clear and therefore, are classified as foregut cysts because these originate from embryologic foregut. A mediastinal cyst containing cartilage is bronchogenic, one with gastric epithelium is enteric while with seromucinous glands is probably respiratory in origin.[31]

Bronchogenic Cyst

It arises from abnormal budding of the ventral foregut and is histologically lined with ciliated respiratory epithelium, cartilage, smooth muscle, fibrous tissue and mucous glands. The common location is near carina or along right paratracheal wall. More than half of the patients present with symptoms like dyspnea, wheeze due to mass effect. The remaining are detected incidentally.

On chest radiograph, it is seen as well defined mass usually in close proximity to the major airways. CT shows well-defined mass with smooth or lobular outline, uniformly thin wall and fluid density **(Figs. 16A and B)**. Sometimes, it may show high density because of proteinaceous contents, mucin or hemorrhage. MRI features vary according to the cyst contents: uniform low signal intensity on T1W and high signal intensity on T2W similar to water, uniform high signal intensity on T1W and T2W images from proteinaceous contents and variable signal intensity in presence of hemorrhage. Post contrast, there is enhancement of cyst wall without internal enhancement.

Esophageal Duplication Cyst

It is a rare foregut malformation which may be indistinguishable from bronchogenic cyst, except for its location in close proximity to the esophagus. It is composed of a muscular coat and mucosa that resembles esophagus, stomach or small intestine. It occurs within the esophageal wall or may be adherent to the wall, but does not communicate with its lumen. It is spherical or tubular, usually located distally along the lateral aspect of the esophagus and has a thick wall.

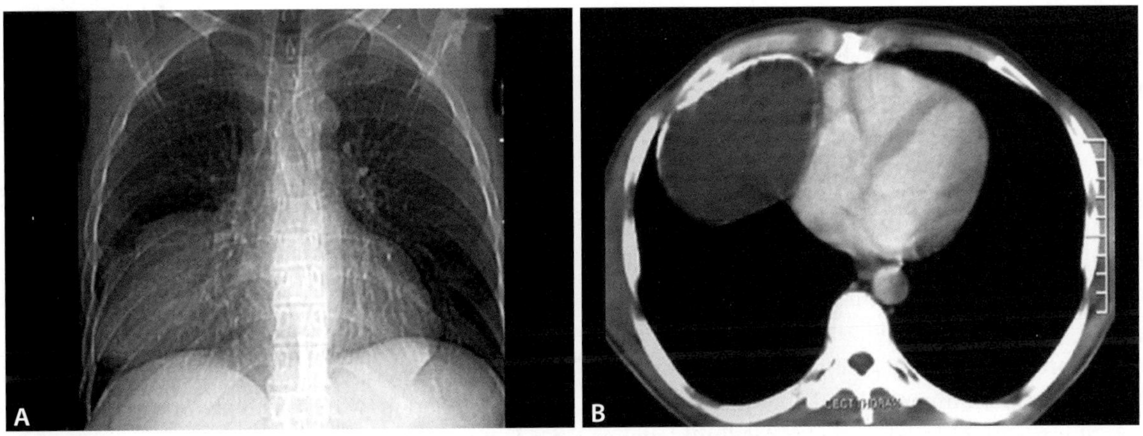

Figs. 15A and B: Pericardial cyst: Chest radiograph (A) showing a large right cardiophrenic angle mass; CECT (B) shows a fluid attenuating non-enhancing mass with peripheral rim calcification in right paracardiac location suggesting a diagnosis of pleuropericardial cyst.

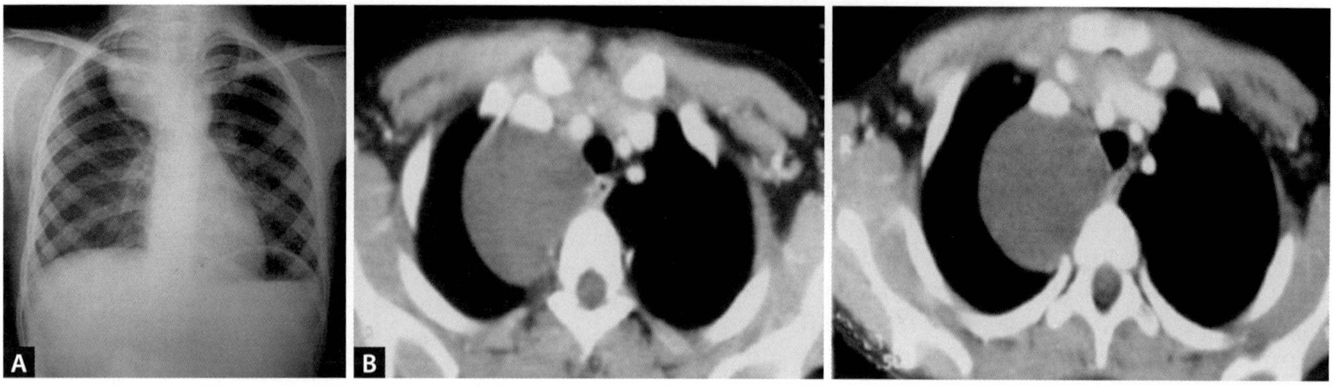

Figs. 16A and B: Bronchogenic cyst: Chest radiograph (A) showing a large right paratracheal mediastinal mass. Axial CT (B) shows a fluid-attenuating transcompartmental mass closely related to the trachea suggesting the diagnosis of a bronchogenic cyst.

Barium swallow examination may demonstrate extrinsic or intramural compression. CT shows spherical or tubular mass in close proximity to esophageal wall **(Figs. 17A to D)**, usually homogeneous with water density but may have soft tissue attenuation in presence of proteinaceous material or intracystic hemorrhage. MRI shows variable signal intensity on T1W image depending on intracystic contents and increased signal intensity on T2W image. The wall of the lesion is thick due to the presence of all the layers. Lesions accessible by ultrasonography (abutting chest wall) may show typical 'gut signature' of the wall (alternating hypoechoic and hyperechoic layers). This may be visualized on endoscopic ultrasound also. The cysts may contain ectopic gastric mucosa and ^{99m}Tc sodium pertechnetate may be useful in their diagnosis.

Neurenteric Cyst

It is a foregut cyst often associated with vertebral anomalies. It results from incomplete separation of the notochord (ectoderm) from foregut (endoderm) during early embryogenesis resulting in persistent communication between them. The cyst is lined by gastrointestinal mucosa and connected to the meninges through a midline defect in one or more vertebral bodies. Ectopic gastric mucosa may be seen in 60% cases.[30] The vertebral anomalies include hemivertebra, sagittal cleft of the vertebral body, butterfly vertebra and spina bifida. Neurenteric cysts occur in middle or posterior mediastinum, usually located above the level of carina. CT and MRI features are similar to those seen in other foregut cysts **(Figs. 18A to C)**. MRI is useful for optimally demonstrating extent of spinal abnormality and degree of intraspinal involvement.[13] Air-fluid level or air foci may be seen when there is communication with esophageal lumen.

Esophageal Lesions

A detailed discussion of esophageal pathology is beyond the scope of this chapter. Dilated esophagus as seen in achalasia, esophageal diverticuli, smooth muscle tumors (leiomyoma and leiomyosarcoma) of the esophagus and hiatus hernia may present as a mediastinal mass. Longitudinally oriented right sided mediastinal mass with air densities and food residue is suggestive of a dilated esophagus on a chest radiograph **(Figs. 19A and B)**. CT and barium swallow assist in making a specific diagnosis.

POSTERIOR MEDIASTINUM

The most common lesion in this location is neurogenic tumor, accounting for almost 90% of posterior mediastinal masses.[1,2]

Neurogenic Tumors

These tumors are classified in the following three groups:

- Tumors arising from nerve sheath include neurofibroma, schwannoma, malignant tumor of nerve sheath
- Tumors arising from sympathetic ganglia include ganglioneuroma, ganglioneuroblastoma and neuroblastoma
- Tumors originating from neuroectodermal cells located in relation to the autonomic nervous system include paraganglioma and pheochromocytoma.

Peripheral Nerve Tumors

These tumors are commonly seen in adults, and have no sex predilection. Most of these tumors are asymptomatic and often seen incidentally on chest radiograph. They usually arise from intercostal nerves close to the spine, near the junction of vertebral body with adjacent rib and

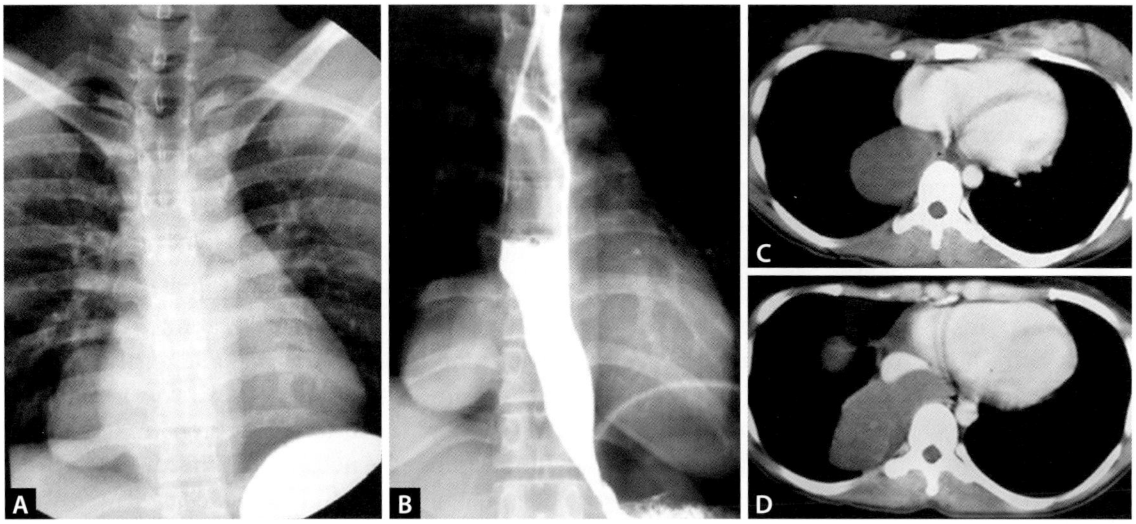

Figs. 17A to D: Esophageal duplication cyst: Coned down radiograph (A) showing a right paracardiac mass which is not silhouetting the cardiac border. Barium swallow (B) shows no communication of the esophagus with this mass. Axial CECT scans (C and D) show a fluid density mass intimately related to the esophagus, causing anterior displacement of the inferior vena cava. *Diagnosis*: Esophageal duplication cyst.

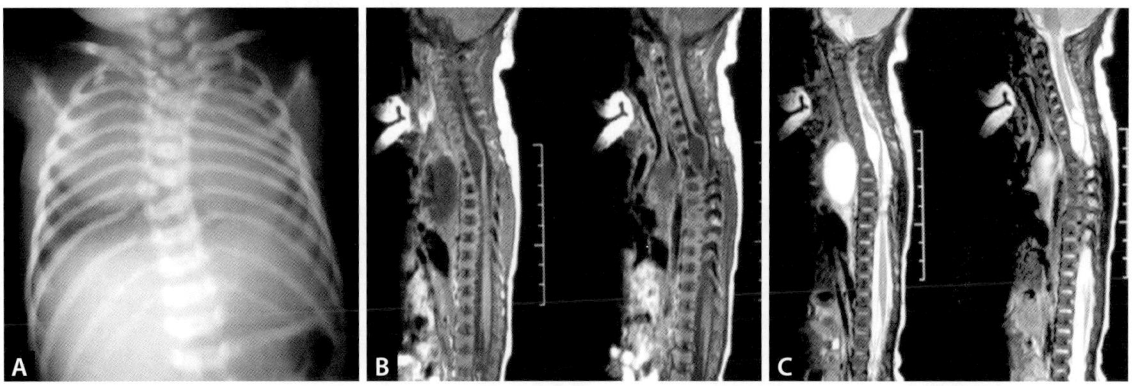

Figs. 18A to C: Neuroenteric cyst: Chest radiograph (A) shows a mediastinal mass, with congenital vertebral anomalies and scoliosis of dorsal spine. T1W (B) and T2W (C) sagittal images show a prevertebral mass with intraspinal extension which is hypointense on T1 and bright on the T2W image. *Diagnosis*: Neuroenteric cyst.

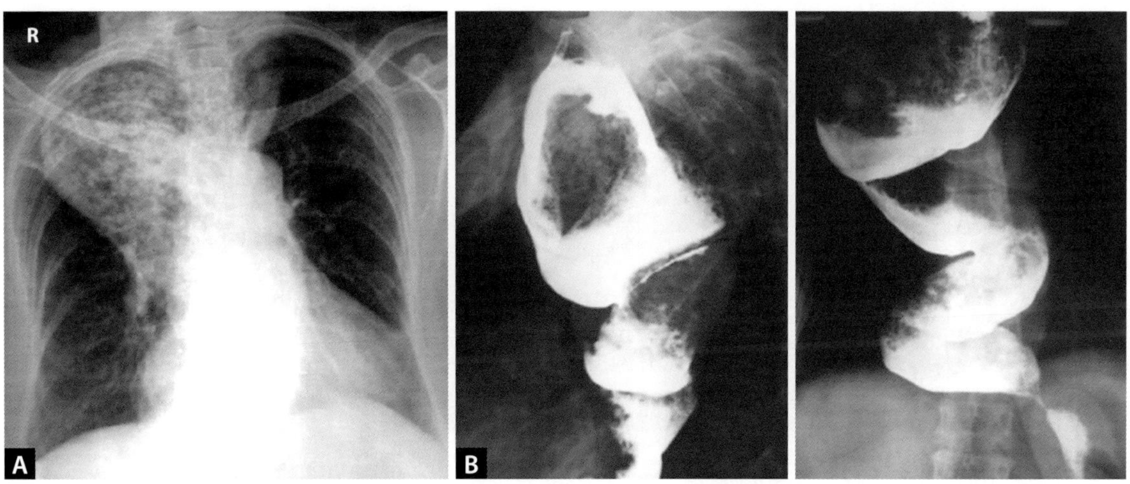

Figs. 19A and B: Achalasia cardia: Chest radiograph (A) shows a large right-sided mediastinal mass with air lucencies within it. Barium swallow (B) shows a grossly dilated sigmoid esophagus with a smooth narrowing at the lower end suggestive of achalasia cardia.

may extend through neural foramina into spinal canal (dumb-bell tumor).

Neurofibromas are unencapsulated tumors which result from proliferation of all nerve elements, including Schwann cells, nerve fibers and fibroblasts. They grow by diffusely expanding the parent nerve. More than 1/3rd of patients with neurofibromas may have neurofibromatosis type I (von Recklinghausen's disease). The plexiform neurofibroma infiltrates along the nerve trunk or plexuses. Schwannomas are encapsulated, arise from the nerve sheath, from Antoni A or B tissues. They grow eccentrically, along parent nerve and cause symptoms by compressing the nerve. They usually contain areas of cystic degeneration, hemorrhage and calcification.

Chest radiograph shows a well-defined posterior mediastinal mass **(Figs. 20A to E)** which may show pressure deformity of adjacent rib or vertebra, scalloped edge with preservation of cortex, thin and splayed apart ribs, widened intervertebral foramina or scoliosis of spine. They follow the axis of the involved nerve, commonly extending horizontally along the intercostal nerves.

CT shows a homogeneous density mass which enhances with intravenous contrast. Calcification is rare. Schwannoma on noncontrast CT shows low attenuation because of high amount of lipid content and cystic degeneration. Intraspinal involvement is better defined on MRI than on CT.

Neurofibroma shows variable signal intensity on T1W with characteristic target pattern consisting of higher signal intensity peripherally and low signal intensity centrally on T2W image. It enhances with gadolinium. Schwannoma shows inhomogeneous high signal intensity throughout the lesion on T2W corresponding to cystic degeneration and low to intermediate signal intensity on T1W image. The combination of coronal and axial imaging planes is a great advantage of MRI **(Figs. 20A to E)** and its ability to show spinal cord and its surrounding cerebrospinal fluid without the need of intrathecal contrast makes MRI, the imaging procedure of choice.[2,8,9] Two MRI signs have been described in the literature for neurogenic tumors. 'Fascicular sign', typically seen in schwannoma, indicates multiple fascicular bundles and is seen on T2W sequence as multiple ring-like lesions with central hypointensity. The 'target sign', seen more commonly in neurofibroma, appears as central hypointensity with peripheral hyperintensity within the tumor on T2W images.

Plexiform neurofibroma usually shows low attenuating infiltrative mass along the nerve on CT and low signal

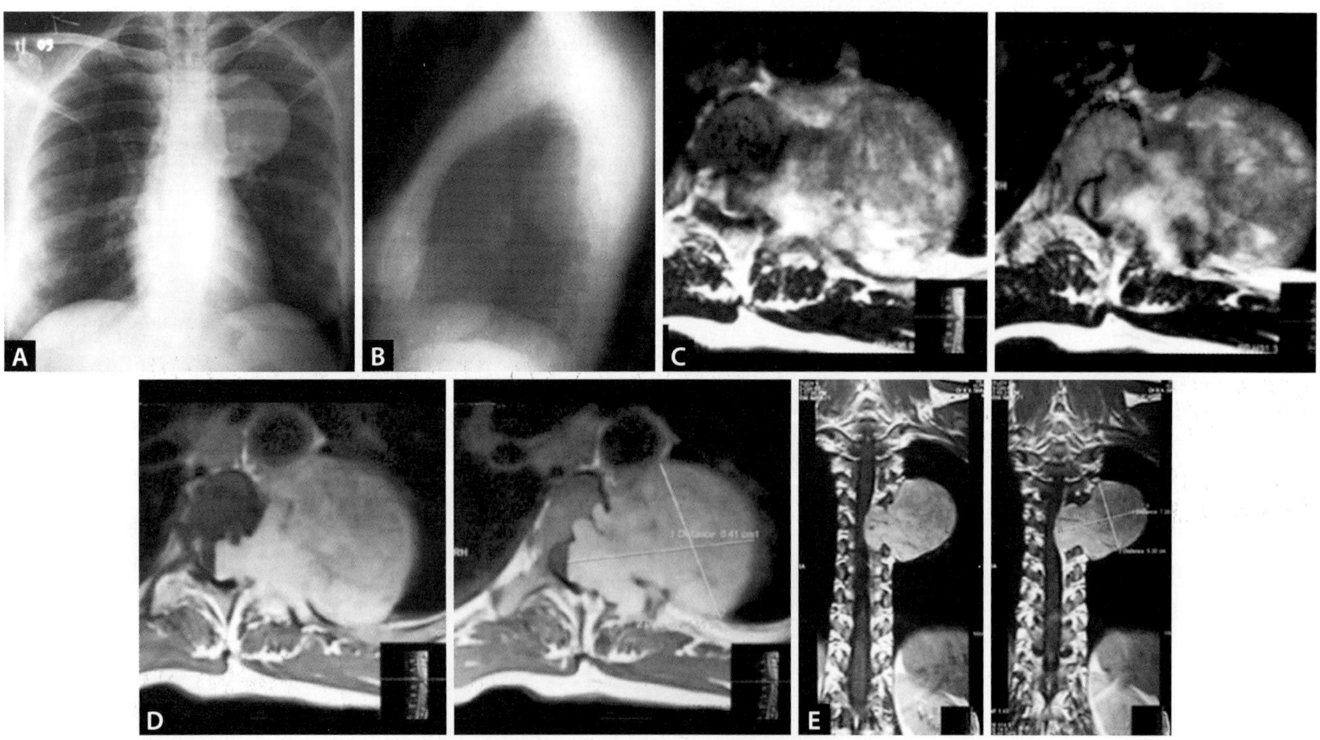

Figs. 20A to E: Neurogenic tumor: Chest radiograph frontal (A) and lateral (B) projection showing a posterior mediastinal mass. T2W (C) and post-gadolinium T1W axial (D) and coronal (E) images show an enhancing posterior mediastinal mass with intraspinal extension. The mass shows heterogeneous signal on T2W scan. *Diagnosis*: Nerve sheath tumor.

intensity on T1W and T2W images because of fibrous nature of the tumor. Malignant tumor tends to have poorly defined margins which may show bone destruction. Sudden increase in size of preexisting mass or development of heterogeneous signal intensity on MRI because of necrosis and hemorrhage, suggests malignancy. FDG PET-CT is useful in differentiating benign from malignant neurogenic tumors with SUV_{max} less than 2.5 suggesting benignity and more than 3.5 suggesting malignancy.[32]

Tumors from Sympathetic Ganglia

These include ganglioneuroma, ganglioneuroblastoma and neuroblastoma. Ganglioneuroma is a benign tumor, neuroblastoma is at the malignant end of the spectrum, while ganglioneuroblastoma is an intermediate form. These tumors are essentially tumors of childhood. The mediastinum is the second most common site for these tumors, the adrenal being the most common site.

These tumors are well-defined with smooth or lobulated outline located in the posterior mediastinum. Ganglineuroma and ganglioneuroblastoma usually extend vertically over three to five vertebrae lateral to the spine, may show broad base on the spine and cause pressure erosion of adjacent vertebra. CT shows homogeneous attenuation whereas MRI shows homogeneous and intermediate signal intensity on both T1W and T2W images.

Almost 10% of neuroblastoma may show stippled calcification that can be seen on chest radiograph. Evidence of widespread local invasion with tendency to cross midline, is characteristic of neuroblastoma. CT shows paraspinal mass with heterogeneous soft tissue attenuation because of hemorrhage, necrosis, cystic degeneration and calcification. MRI shows heterogeneous signal intensity on all pulse sequences and heterogeneous enhancement with gadolinium.[2,9]

Metaiodobenzylguanidine (MIBG) scintigraphy is useful for imaging neuroblastoma, especially to assess the extent of disease. However up to 30% neuroblastomas are not MIBG avid.

Paraganglioma

Paraganglioma (chemodectoma) is a rare tumor originating from neuroectodermal cells located in relation to the autonomic nervous system, especially in the region of the aortopulmonary window and the posterior mediastinum.

Paraganglioma appears as round, extremely vascular soft tissue mass that enhances markedly on contrast-enhanced CT. It is hypointense on T1W and hyperintense on T2W images, with flow voids within, indicating hypervascular nature.

Arteriography demonstrates large feeding vessels, pathologic vessels and intense tumor blush. MIBG scintigraphy shows increased activity and is a good technique to demonstrate paragangliomas.

MRI has largely replaced CT as an initial imaging modality in the evaluation of patients with suspected neurogenic tumors. Unfortunately, MRI is no more specific than CT in differentiating benign from malignant lesions.

Lateral Thoracic Meningocele

This is an anomalous herniation of spinal meninges through the intervertebral foramina. It usually (in 85%) occurs in association with neurofibromatosis type I. Patients present with back pain, neurological and/or respiratory symptoms. It is seen as well-defined paravertebral mass, scalloping and deforming adjacent ribs and vertebral body. Enlargement of intervertebral foramina is an important diagnostic feature. Kyphoscoliosis is often present. The features are indistinguishable from a dumb-bell nerve root tumor.

CT shows well circumscribed paraspinal mass of water attenuation, because bulk of it consists of cerebrospinal fluid. MRI shows low signal intensity on T1W and high signal intensity on T2W image, similar to CSF signal and it does not enhance with gadolinium.

Paraspinal Infection

Vertebral osteomyelitis can result in paraspinal abscess which may present as a mass lesion. The common causative organism in India is *Mycobacterium tuberculosis*, others being *Staphylococcus aureus* and anaerobic organisms. Plain radiograph of the dorsal spine may show narrowing of disk space with destruction of two or more contiguous vertebrae. CT shows heterogeneous attenuation of soft tissue density with rim enhancement with intravenous contrast. MRI shows low signal intensity on T1W and high signal intensity on T2W images. MRI with gadolinium defines the extent of inflammatory process better. MRI is preferred to CT because of its ability to see disc space, bone destruction, spinal canal and its contents.

Extramedullary Hemopoiesis

Extramedullary hemopoiesis is a compensatory mechanism for chronic anemias due to bone marrow dysfunction. Rarely, it causes paravertebral soft tissue masses typically bilaterally, along lower thoracic vertebrae, secondary to severe hemolytic anemia, particularly thalassemia and sickle cell disease. The best diagnostic clue is the presence of multiple lobulated posterior mediastinal masses with vertebral bodies which have prominent trabeculae. CT and MRI show fat density within the masses and there is no bony erosion. They show significant contrast enhancement. The masses are usually asymptomatic but neurological deficit may occur due to intraspinal extension. In difficult cases, marrow scanning may be done with ^{99m}Tc sulfur colloid and SPECT/CT to detect hemopoietic tissue and thus may avoid the need of biopsy.[7] The differential diagnosis includes nerve sheath tumors, varices, lymphoma and lateral thoracic meningocele.

Mediastinal Varices

Abnormal dilatation of veins in the mediastinum may occur in the setting of portal hypertension and obstruction of superior vena cava (downhill varices). They are seen as serpiginous enhancing vascular channels in or around the esophagus, in the portal venous phase. However, on a non-enhanced CT or arterial phase CT, they are unopacified and can mimic asymmetric thickening of esophageal wall, hiatus hernia or any mediastinal mass. On MRI they are seen as serpiginous flow voids on both T1W and T2W images.[2]

MULTICOMPARTMENT MEDIASTINAL MASSES/LESIONS

Mediastinal Lymphadenopathy

Mediastinal lymphadenopathy can occur in any mediastinal compartment **(Figs. 21 and 22)** but is more commonly seen in anterior or middle mediastinum. It can occur due to infection, neoplasm, sarcoidosis or reactive hyperplasia.[33,34]

It has been observed that most lymph nodes with a short axis diameter of more than 2.0 cm can be seen as mediastinal widening if they are present in the right paratracheal, aortopulmonary window and hilar region. Pretracheal, left paratracheal, subcarinal nodes may not be visible on chest radiograph even if they are larger than 2.0 cm. Right paratracheal lymphadenopathy is seen as uniform or lobular widening of right tracheal stripe, convexity of superior vena cava outline and increased density of superior vena cava almost equal to density of aortic arch. Left paratracheal nodes can cause recognizable mediastinal widening only when they enlarge to an extent as to project beyond the vascular pedicle. Nodes in the aortopulmonary area when enlarged significantly can cause a bulge in the angle between the aortic arch and main pulmonary artery. Subcarinal lymphadenopathy can be assessed by convex bulge of azygoesophageal line, increased opacity and lack of visibility of the medial wall of right main stem bronchus and bronchus intermedius, also may simulate appearance of left atrial enlargement. Posterior mediastinal lymph node enlargement causes localized displacement of the paraspinal and paraesophageal line. The features of hilar lymphadenopathy are overall hilar enlargement, lobular outline or round mass in the area of the hilum that does not contain major vessels.[2]

Lymph node enlargement on CT can be assessed by measurement of short axis diameter. Nodes less than 10 mm in short axis diameter are normal within 95th percentile. Nodes between 10 and 15 mm in short axis diameter may occur in subcarinal and tracheobronchial

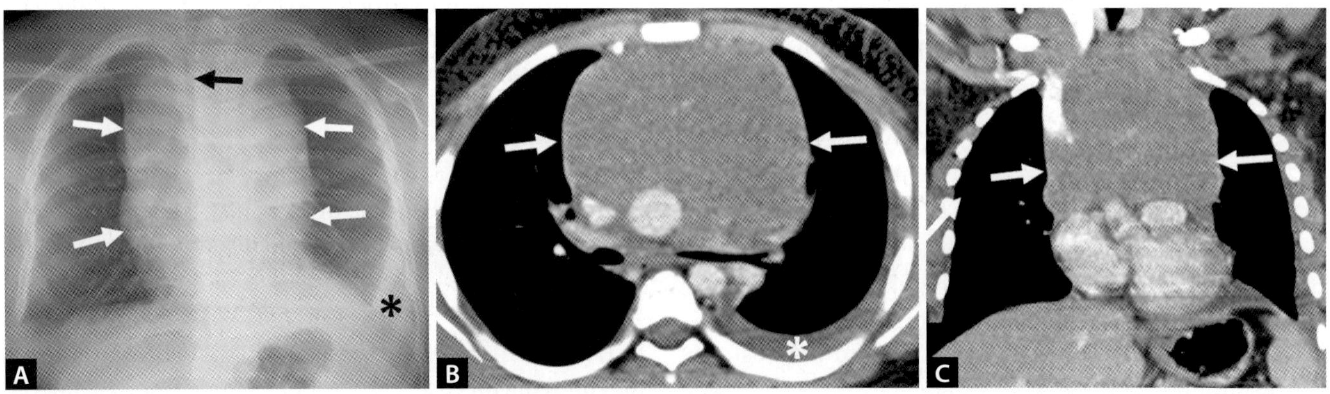

Figs. 21A to C: Mediastinal lymphoma: (A) Chest radiograph of a 20-year-old male presenting with respiratory distress showing mediastinal-based mass extending on either side of midline (white arrows), compressing and displacing the trachea (black arrow) and silhouetting cardiac margins suggesting anterior location. Left pleural effusion is noted (asterisk). Axial (B) and Coronal (C) CT images showing a homogeneous anterior mediastinal mass (arrows) and left pleural effusion (asterisk in B).

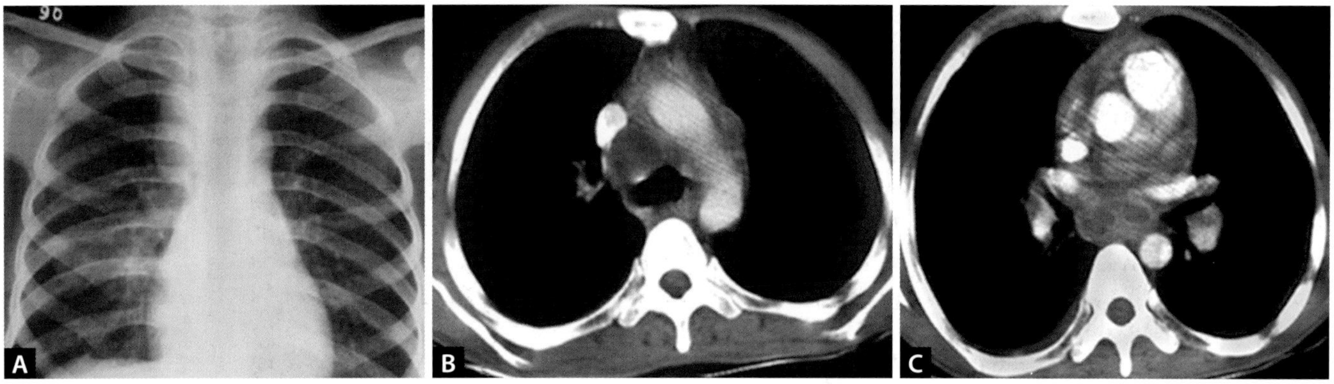

Figs. 22A to C: *Tuberculosis*: Chest radiograph (A) shows a right paratracheal mass with right middle lobe consolidation in a young boy presenting with pyrexia of unknown origin. Axial CECT scans (B and C) show necrotic lymph nodes with peripheral enhancement in right paratracheal and subcarinal location. *Biopsy*: Tuberculosis.

region in 5–7% of normal subjects. The CT features of lymph node enlargement are increase in size of individual nodes, focal bulge or lobulation of the interface between the mediastinum and lung, invasion of surrounding mediastinal fat, coalescence of nodes to form large mass or diffuse soft tissue density of the mediastinum obliterating fat planes. Hilar node enlargement on CT can be determined by presence of round soft tissue density which is too large to be blood vessel or nonenhancing mass larger than 5.0 mm in short axis diameter. Contrast-enhanced CT is necessary to distinguish between vascular structures and soft tissue mass. MRI is particularly useful when use of intravenous contrast is contraindicated to differentiate soft tissue signal intensity of lymph node enlargement against the signal void of air and of fast flowing blood on spin echo images.

Lymph node calcification is commonly seen in infective pathology like tuberculosis and fungal infection, may also be seen in other conditions namely sarcoidosis, pneumoconiosis, Castlemann's disease but rarely seen in neoplastic disease. Common patterns of calcification are coarse, irregularly distributed clumps within the node or homogeneous calcification of entire node. Peripheral ring like calcification of node, known as eggshell calcification is characteristic of sarcoidosis or in patients exposed to dust while working in coal or metal mines.

Low density areas within enlarged node due to necrosis are commonly seen in tuberculosis **(Figs. 22A to C)**. This may also be seen in fungal disease, infections in immunocompromised patients, and metastases particularly from testicular tumors.

Mild-to-moderate contrast enhancement is nonspecific, seen in tuberculosis, fungal disease, sarcoidosis or neoplasm. Low density area due to necrosis with peripheral rim enhancement is a characteristic feature of tubercular infection. Marked contrast enhancement is seen in metastatic disease, particularly from melanoma or primary in kidney or thyroid. Diffuse uniform enhancement is seen in Castleman's disease, a rare condition.[34]

CT and MRI provide comparable information; however, the distinct disadvantage of MRI is its inability to demonstrate calcification. Hilar node enlargement is easier to recognize on MRI, which is seen as distinct round or oval density with relatively high signal intensity against the background of signal void of air from bronchi and lungs.

Based on the morphology, site of involvement, presence of calcification, presence of associated lung or pleural pathology, it is possible to offer reasonable etiological diagnosis of lymphadenopathy.

Tuberculosis

Central low density with peripheral rim enhancement, loss of perinodal fat planes, obliteration of azygoesophageal recess suggest tuberculosis **(Figs. 22A to C)**. Associated area of pulmonary consolidation may or may not be present. On healing, the nodes usually become small with dense calcification.

Sarcoidosis

Discrete homogeneous enlargement, no necrosis, well-defined fat planes, classical site of involvement being bilateral hilar and right paratracheal in nearly two third of the patients are characteristic features.

Lymphoma

Anterior mediastinal and paratracheal nodes are more frequently involved **(Figs. 21A to C)**, lymphadenopathy is usually bilateral but asymmetrical. Isolated hilar node enlargement is rare and hilar adenopathy is usually seen along with mediastinal lymphadenopathy. Confluent mass of lymph nodes with irregular areas of necrosis, obliteration of fat planes encasement of vessels are specific features. Superior vena cava thrombosis, invasion of surrounding structures, pleural effusion, consolidation are commonly present.

Metastasis

There is no particular pattern or site of involvement of lymph nodes. However, invasion of pleura, pericardium or chest wall suggests metastasis.

Vascular Lesions

Various vascular abnormalities and anomalies can simulate mediastinal mass. These include right sided or double aortic arch, persistent left SVC or vertical vein, aberrant subclavian artery, dilatation of pulmonary artery, SVC, azygous and hemiazygous system, aortic aneurysm or dissection, SVC syndrome and mediastinal varix. Contrast-enhanced CT or MRI are essential for confirmation of diagnosis.

Aortic Aneurysm

Aortic aneurysms may present as mediastinal widening. This entity is discussed in detail in the chapter on aortic imaging. The most common site of thoracic aortic aneurysm is descending aorta, followed by aortic arch, ascending aorta being the least common. Aneurysm can be of two types: true aneurysm and pseudoaneurysm. True aneurysm occurs due to degeneration of elastic fibers of media. Due to loss of structural support, vessel dilates. True aneurysm contains all layers of the vessel wall. Pseudoaneurysm is the result of contained perforation of the vessel wall. Almost 70% of all thoracic aortic aneurysms are due to atherosclerosis, other causes include trauma, fungal infection and syphilis. The morphologic types are fusiform, saccular, dissecting or false. By definition a diameter more than 4.0 cm is taken as fusiform aneurysm.[2]

The common radiological features on chest radiograph are mediastinal widening/mass or enlarged segment of aorta with peripheral curvilinear calcification. Displacement and less frequently compression of esophagus, trachea and bronchi may be seen. Erosion of vertebrae or ribs may occur but is uncommon. Curvilinear or plaque like calcification is better seen on CT. Most of these aneurysms have lining thrombus with calcification. CT has excellent spatial resolution and both aortic wall and its associated complications are well seen. The availability of MDCT has improved diagnostic accuracy and reduced examination time. MRI is an excellent modality for assessing size and shape of aneurysm, demonstrating relationship of aneurysm to branch vessels and compression effects. MRI combines the strength of echocardiography, angiography and CT. Using spin echo and dynamic imaging techniques, combined with large FOV, MRI can fully characterize thoracic aneurysm and its complications.

Aortic Dissection

Spontaneous aortic dissection results from repeated trauma to the media, often in a patient with persistent hypertension, with development of intramural hematoma, localized to the media. As the hematoma evolves into a seroma, a rent can occur in the overlying intima, with subsequent establishment of a false lumen tracking down the media that communicates with true aortic lumen, also called dissecting aneurysm. The false lumen is usually between the inner one third and outer two-thirds of media. The dissection can extend in both antegrade and retrograde fashion. The dissecting channel usually spirals so that the false lumen lies anterior and to the right in ascending aorta, posterior and to the left in descending aorta. Cystic medial necrosis, Marfan's syndrome, hypertension are important predisposing factors.[1,2]

The chest radiograph is often abnormal but the findings are nonspecific. Superior mediastinal widening with distinctly undulating appearance of aorta, progressive change in aortic configuration on sequential radiographs, unexplained discrepancy between caliber of ascending and descending aorta suggest aortic dissection. The most specific sign is 1.0 cm or more displacement of aortic calcification inside the aortic contour on sequential chest radiographs. This sign is however, seen in a small percentage of patients.

CT and MRI are used to image aortic dissection. A detailed discussion of the imaging findings is given in the chapter on imaging the aorta. Transthoracic and transesophageal ultrasonography are proving increasingly useful in the diagnosis of aortic dissection.

Superior Vena Cava Obstruction

The most common cause of superior vena cava obstruction is compression and invasion by bronchogenic carcinoma either by primary tumor or lymphadenopathy. Other causes are metastatic disease, lymphoma, mediastinal fibrosis. The dilated collaterals, enlargement of azygous vein, and widened superior mediastinum can be seen on chest radiograph.

Contrast-enhanced CT is an excellent technique to show narrowing, filling defects in cava and collaterals besides providing information about the cause of obstruction. MRI also provides similar information with added advantage of multiplanar imaging and no need of contrast. The limitation of MRI is its inability to demonstrate calcification, an important feature in the diagnosis of granulomatous mediastinal fibrosis.

Abnormalities of the Mediastinal Fat

Mediastinal Lipomatosis

This is a benign condition in which exuberant deposition of unencapsulated fat occurs in the mediastinum. The etiology includes obesity, exogenous steroids, and Cushing's syndrome. The most common location is superior mediastinum, and it may be associated with enlarged epicardial and pericardial fat pad. The cardiophrenic fat pad may resemble a mass. Massive fat collection may be seen throughout the mediastinum in mediastinal lipomatosis. Chest radiograph may show smooth mediastinal widening without tracheal compression or displacement. The fat shows uniform low density on CT in the range of –70 to –130 HU, no soft tissue component or enhancement and it usually does not compress or invade adjacent structures.[2] MRI shows homogeneous hyperintense signal on T1W and T2W images with signal suppression on fat-saturated images.

Lipoma

This mediastinal tumor of fatty origin is uncommon, comprising less than 1% of all mediastinal masses. Benign as well as malignant fatty tumor appear as well-defined round or oval mass on chest radiograph. It is usually soft and moulds to the mediastinal contour, mimicking cardiomegaly. CT and MRI show uniform fat containing lesion with few strands of soft tissue within. Some liposarcomas may show inhomogeneous fat density with predominant soft tissue attenuation.

Herniation of Abdominal Fat

Herniation of omental fat through the esophageal hiatus, foramen of Morgagni or foramen of Bochdalek presents as focal fatty mass in the mediastinum. Bowel loops, liver, spleen and kidney may herniate into the thorax. Herniation through foramen of Morgagni almost always occurs on right side in the anterior mediastinum simulating cardiophrenic angle mass **(Figs. 23 and 24)**. Herniation through foramen of Bochdalek occurs often on the left side in posterior mediastinum presenting as diaphragmatic hump close to the spine. Diagnosis can be made on chest radiograph because of the characteristic location. Fat density with fine linear densities within, representing omental vessels on CT differentiates omental hernia from lipoma. Similarly on MRI **(Figs. 24 and 25)**, high signal intensity on T1W and moderately high signal intensity on T2W image (the characteristics of fat on MRI) with low intensity linear areas representing blood vessels, provide a specific diagnosis.

MISCELLANEOUS LESIONS OF THE MEDIASTINUM

Mediastinal Hemorrhage

Trauma to the aorta or one of its major arteries is a frequent cause of mediastinal hemorrhage. The other causes include dissecting aneurysm, rupture of the aneurysm, patient having bleeding diathesis or on anticoagulant therapy.

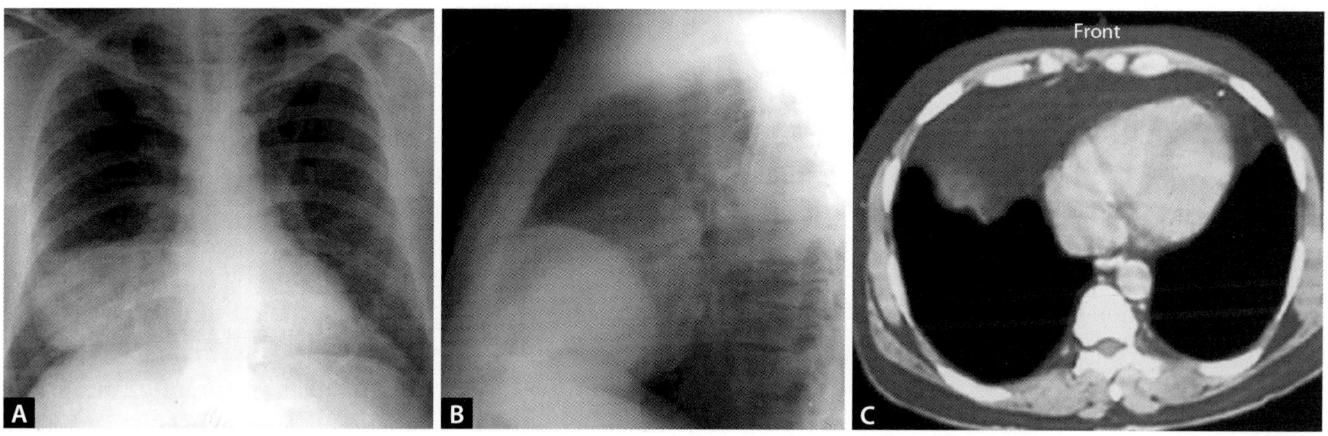

Figs. 23A to C: *Morgagni hernia*: Chest radiograph frontal (A) and lateral (B) projection showing an anteriorly located right cardiophrenic angle mass. Axial CECT (C) shows a fatty attenuating mass in this location, which shows vessels running through it. *Diagnosis*: Morgagni hernia containing omental fat.

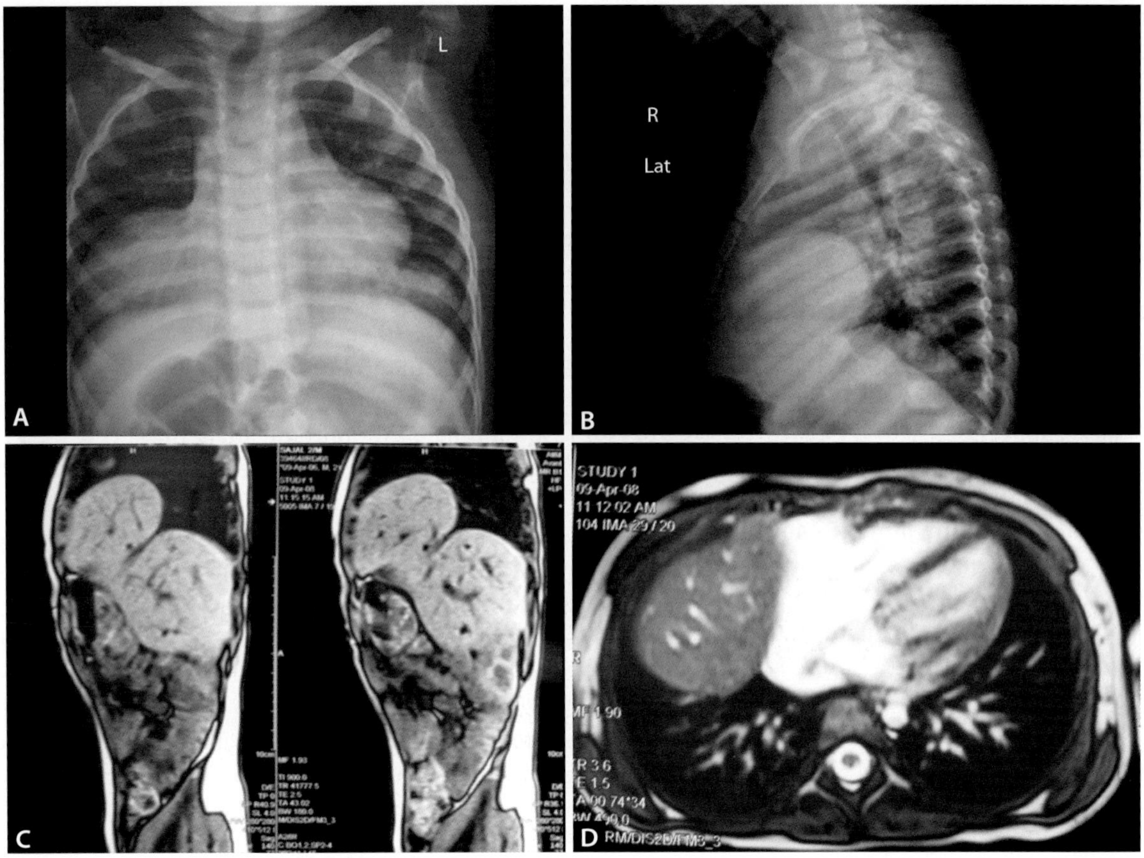

Figs. 24A to D: Morgagni hernia: Chest radiograph frontal (A) and lateral (B) projection showing an anteriorly located right cardiophrenic angle mass (C). T1W sagittal and T2W axial (D) MRI scans confirm the herniated liver in a Morgagni hernia.

Chest radiograph shows mediastinal widening. The blood may track along extrapleural space over the lung apices producing apical capping. It may rupture into pleural cavity or track into lung along perivascular, peribronchial sheath producing changes resembling pulmonary edema. Noncontrast CT shows streaky soft densities interspersed through mediastinal fat and high density associated with fresh hematoma **(Figs. 26A to C)**. The appearance of hemorrhage on MRI depends on the duration of bleed. In the acute phase, there is low signal intensity on T1W and high signal intensity on T2W images. As the days pass, signal intensity on T1W images increases and in subacute phase, both T1W and T2W images show high signal intensity. In chronic phase, signal intensity depends on the amount of water in the hemorrhage and degree of conversion from methemoglobin to ferritin and hemosiderin.[1,2]

Pneumomediastinum

Common causes include blunt chest trauma, asthma, mechanical ventilation, esophageal perforation, etc. Features of pneumomediastinum on chest radiograph are air outlining the left heart border, air dissecting under and medial to thymus outlining it distinctly, extrapleural tracking along upper surface of diaphragm, air between heart and diaphragm producing continuous diaphragm sign. Dissection of air along tissue planes overlying the mediastinal blood vessels, major airways or esophagus is better seen on lateral chest radiograph than in frontal view.

CT is more sensitive than chest radiograph, and shows streaky air densities in the mediastinal fat and around tubular structures like trachea and esophagus **(Figs. 27A and B)**. CT may also give a clue about the cause of pneumomediastinum. Differential diagnosis includes pneumothorax and pneumopericardium.[2]

Acute Mediastinitis

Acute mediastinal infections are uncommon and usually related to surgery, esophageal perforation, or spread of infection from adjacent regions. Infections may present as diffuse mediastinitis or mediastinal abscess, depending on their extent. Diffuse mediastinitis has a

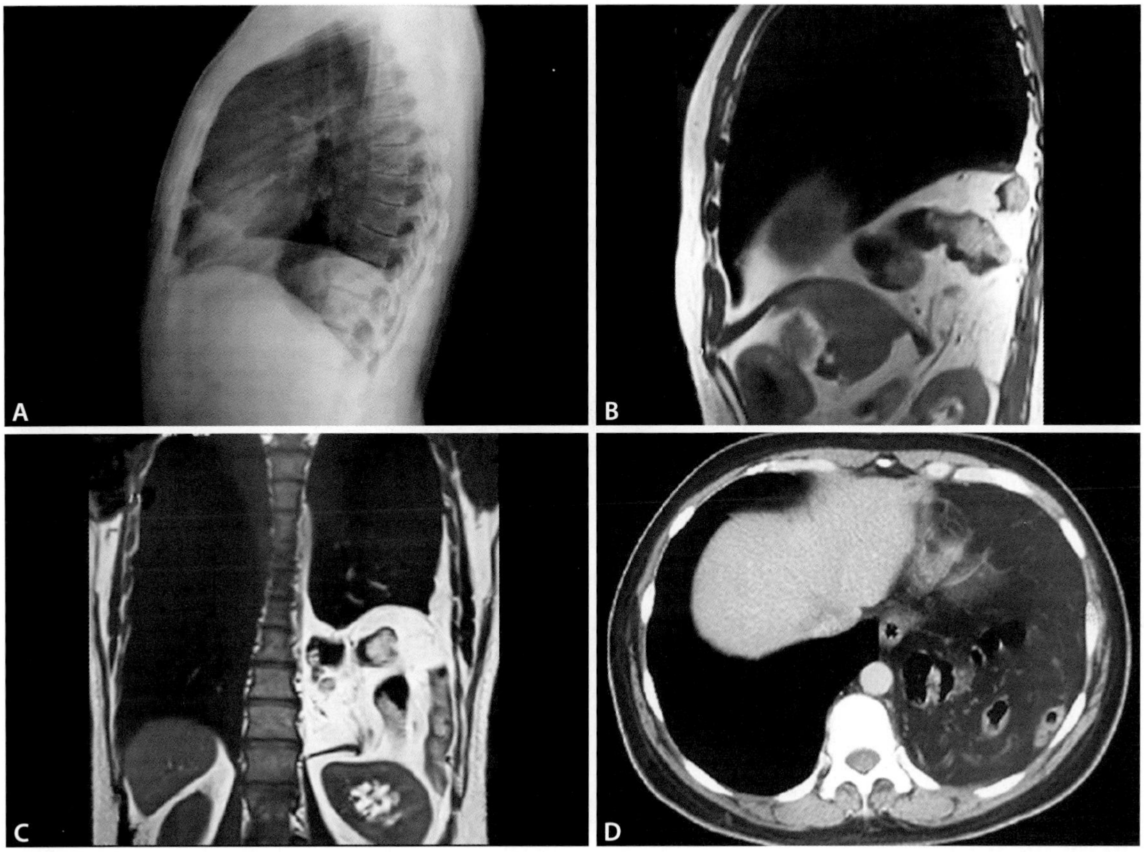

Figs. 25A to D: Bockdalek hernia: Chest radiograph (A) in lateral projection shows an apparent elevation of the left dome of diaphragm. Axial CT (B) shows fat and bowel loops in the left hemithorax. Coronal (C) and sagittal (D) T1W MR scans show herniation of mesenteric fat and bowel loops through a defect in the posterior part of the left dome suggestive of a Bockdalek hernia.

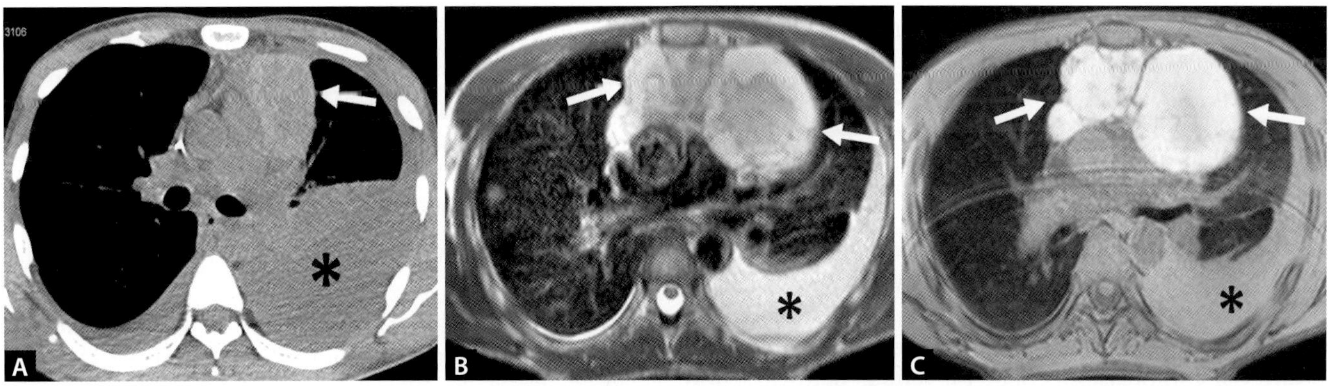

Figs. 26A to C: Mediastinal hematoma: (A) Axial noncontrast CT image showing hyperdense hematoma in the anterior mediastinum (arrow) with left pleural effusion (asterisk); (B and C) Axial T2-weighted (B) and T1-weighted fat saturated (C) MR images showing anterior mediastinal hematoma (arrows) appearing hyperintense on both sequences. Left pleural effusion is noted (asterisk).

relatively poor prognosis. Chest radiograph may show mediastinal widening, pneumomediastinum, pleural effusion, localized fluid collection and abscess formation. CT shows obliteration of fat planes and air bubbles in the mediastinum. The features seen on chest radiograph are better defined on CT.

CT is superior and the findings in mediastinitis include diffuse or streaky infiltration of mediastinal fat, localized fluid collections, pleural or pericardial effusion, lymph node enlargement, and compression of mediastinal structures.[1] Gas bubbles in the mediastinum, with or without associated fluid collections, are seen in up to

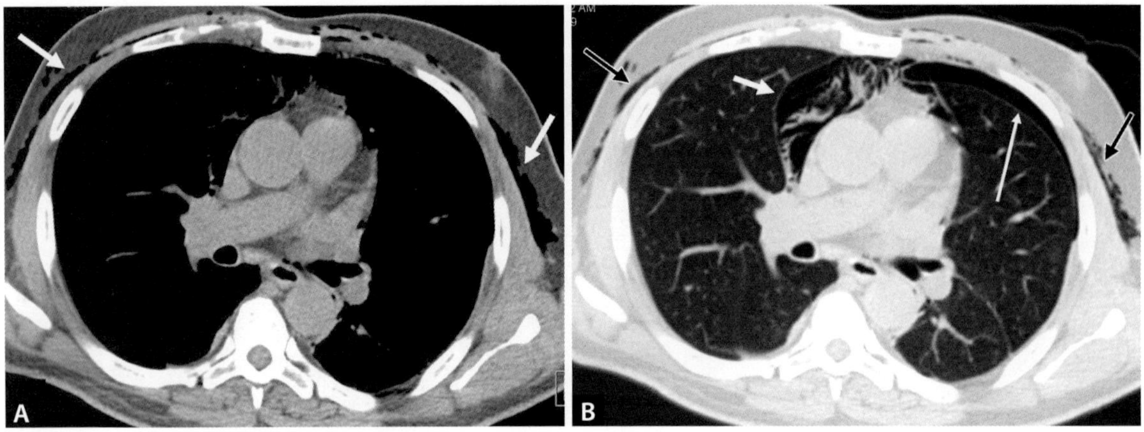

Figs. 27A and B: Pneumomediastinum: (A) Axial CT scan in mediastinal window shows air in chest wall (white arrows) suggesting surgical emphysema. Mediastinal air cannot be appreciated; (B) Lung window at the same level shows the pneumomediastinum clearly (white short arrow) along with left pneumothorax (long thin white arrow) and surgical emphysema (black arrows).

half of cases, and are an important finding. A localized fluid collection with an air-fluid level and an enhancing wall is suggestive of a mediastinal abscess. There may be a coexisting empyema or subphrenic abscess. Although most of the times diagnosis may be made on imaging, occasionally percutaneous image guided aspiration may be necessary.

Fibrosing Mediastinitis

Tuberculosis, histoplasmosis and radiation therapy are important causes of fibrosing mediastinitis. An idiopathic variety which is autoimmune in origin occurring in association with retroperitoneal fibrosis and orbital pseudotumor is also reported. Radiological features depend on the site and degree of lymphadenopathy and chest radiograph may show severity of obstructive phenomenon. Unilateral or bilateral hilar or mediastinal lymphadenopathy, often asymmetrical and mostly in superior mediastinum, narrowing of trachea and major bronchi, pulmonary oligemia due to narrowing of pulmonary artery are commonly present. Pulmonary consolidation resulting from bronchial, venous or lymphatic obstruction may be seen. CT features are lymphadenopathy with or without calcification, narrowing of airways, venous or arterial compression, collateral venous pathways, and obliteration of fat planes.

CT can diagnose and assess the severity of mediastinal fibrosis. Two distinct patterns of mediastinal involvement may be seen. A focal pattern present in 82% of cases is seen as a localized mass or masses of soft tissue attenuation, usually in the right paratracheal or subcarinal regions or hila, which frequently show calcification. A diffuse pattern of involvement is seen in 18% of cases and manifest as a diffusely infiltrating **(Figs. 28A and B)**, noncalcified mass, affecting multiple mediastinal compartments. In the presence of fibrosing mediastinitis, discrete enlarged lymph nodes cannot be identified.[2]

On T1-weighted MR images, fibrosing mediastinitis is typically seen as a heterogeneous, infiltrative mass of intermediate signal intensity. Its appearance on T2-weighted MR images is variable; regions of both increased and markedly decreased signal intensity are frequently seen in the same or in different parts of the mediastinum. Decreased signal intensity on T2-weighted images probably indicates the presence of calcification or fibrous tissue and hyperintense areas indicate more active inflammation. After the administration of Gd-DTPA, the mediastinal masses usually show heterogeneous enhancement. MRI is particularly valuable in assessing vascular patency without the need for intravenous contrast media. FDG-PET may show uptake in areas of active inflammation.

CONCLUSION

A wide spectrum of pathology can affect the mediastinum, and the radiologist plays a vital role in the clinical work up of mediastinal lesions. Many different classifications are available for mediastinal compartments primarily based on the radiograph with only the more recent one suggested by ITMIG being based on CT. Chest radiograph and CT are the primary imaging modalities and are invaluable for characterization and extent evaluation. MRI is used as a problem solving tool and can help differentiate atypical cysts from solid masses, distinguish thymic hyperplasia from thymoma and for the evaluation of posterior mediastinal lesions. The location of a lesion within the different mediastinal compartments and its imaging appearance help arrive at a precise diagnosis.

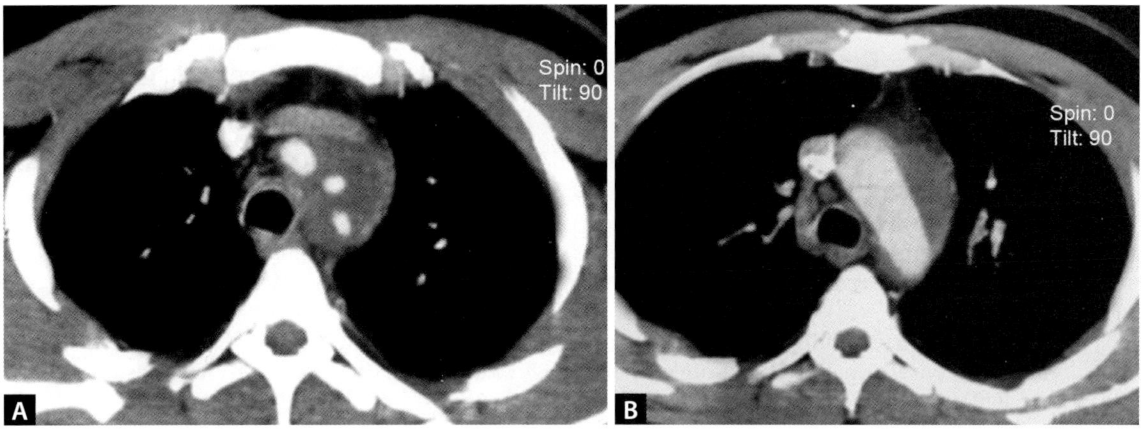

Figs. 28A and B: Mediastinal fibrosis. Axial CECT (A and B) showing a plaque-like soft tissue infiltrating the mediastinum and encasing the brachiocephalic trunk, left common carotid and the left subclavian artery. *Diagnosis*: Mediastinal fibrosis.

REFERENCES

1. Fraser R, et al. Fraser and Pare's Diagnosis of diseases of the chest, 4th edn. Philadelphia: WB Saunders.
2. Naidich, et al. Computed Tomography and Magnetic Resonance of the Thorax, 4th Edn. Lippincott Williams and Wilkins; 2007.
3. Gray's anatomy: Williams PL, Warwick R, Dyson M, Bannister LH. Splanchnology. In: Gray's anatomy. 37th edn. New York, NY: Churchill Livingstone; 1989.pp.1245-475.
4. Felson B. The mediastinum. Semin Roentgenol. 1969;4:41-58.
5. Fujimoto K, Hara M, Tomiyama N, Kusumoto M, Sakai F, Fujii Y. Proposal for a new mediastinal compartment classification of transverse plane images according to the Japanese Association for Research on the Thymus (JART) General Rules for the Study of Mediastinal Tumors. Oncol Rep. 2014;31(2):565-72.
6. Carter BW, Tomiyama N, Bhora FY, et al. A modern definition of mediastinal compartments. J Thorac Oncol. 2014;9(9 suppl 2):S97-S101.
7. Carter BW, Benveniste MF, Madan R, Godoy MC, de Groot PM, Truong MT, Rosado-de-Christenson ML, Marom EM. ITMIG Classification of Mediastinal Compartments and Multidisciplinary Approach to Mediastinal Masses. Radiographics. 2017;37(2):413-36.
8. Webb WR, Sostman HD. MR imaging of thoracic diseases: clinical uses. Radiology. 1992;182:621-30.
9. Erasmus JJ, McAdams HP, Donnelly LF, Spritzer CE. MR imaging of mediastinal masses. Magn Reson Imaging Clin North Am. 2000;8:59-89.
10. Laurent F, Latrabe V, Lecesne R, et al. Mediastinal masses: diagnostic approach. Eur Radiol. 1998;8:1148-59.
11. Jeung MY, Gasser B, Gangi A, et al. Imaging of cystic masses of the mediastinum. Radiographics. 2002;22(spec no):S79-93.
12. Kim JH, Goo JM, Lee HJ, et al. Cystic tumors in the anterior mediastinum. Radiologic-pathological correlation. J Comput Assist Tomogr. 2003;27:714-23.
13. Merten DF. Diagnostic imaging of mediastinal masses in children. Am J Roentgenol. 1992;158:825-32.
14. Macchiarini P, Ostertag H. Uncommon primary mediastinal tumors. Lancet Oncol. 2004;5:107-18.
15. Inaoka T, Takahashi K, Mineta M, et al. Thymic hyperplasia and thymus gland tumors: Differentiation with chemical shift MR imaging. Radiology. 2007;243(3):869-76.
16. Strollo DC, Rosado-de-Christenson ML. Tumors of the thymus. J Thorac Imaging. 1999;14:152-71.
17. Tomiyama N, Muller NL, Ellis SJ, et al. Invasive and noninvasive thymoma: distinctive CT features. J Comput Assist Tomogr. 2001;25:388-93.
18. Masaoka A, Monden Y, Nakahara K, Tanioka T. Follow-up study of thymomas with special reference to their clinical stages. Cancer. 1981;48:2485-92.
19. Jeong YJ, et al. Does CT of thymic epithelial tumors enable us to distinguish histologic subtypes and predict prognosis? Am J Roentgenol. 2004;183(2):283-9.
20. Azizad S, Sannananja B, Restrepo CS. Solid tumors of the mediastinum in adults. Semin ultrasound CT MRI. 2016; 37: 196-211.
21. Marx A, Ströbel P, Badve SS, et al. ITMIG consensus statement on the use of the WHO histological classification of thymoma and thymic carcinoma: refined definitions, histological criteria, and reporting. J Thorac Oncol. 2014; 9(5):596-611.
22. Nishino Mizuki, Simon K, et al: The thymus: A comprehensive review. Radiographics. 2006;26:335-48.
23. Moeller KH, Rosado-de-Christenson ML, Templeton PA. Mediastinal mature teratoma: imaging features. Am J Roentgenol. 1997;169:985-90.
24. Rosado-de-Christenson ML, Templeton PA, Moran CA. Mediastinal germ-cell tumors: radiologic and pathologic correlation. Radiographics. 1992;12:1013-30.
25. Drevelegas A, Palladas P, Scordalaki A. Mediastinal germ cell tumors: a radiologic-pathologic review. Eur Radiol. 2001;11:1925-32.
26. Madhusudhan KS, Sharma R, Gadodia A, Kumar A. Spontaneous rupture of benign mediastinal teratoma:

a report of two cases. Indian J Med Pediatr Oncol. 2012; 33(2):123-5.
27. Perez-Monte JE, Brown ML, Shah AN, et al. Parathyroid adenomas: accurate detection and localization with Tc-99m sestamibi SPECT. Radiology. 1996;201:85-91.
28. Kukar M, Platz TA, Schaffner TJ, et al. The use of modified four-dimensional computed tomography in patients with primary hyperparathyroidism: an argument for the abandonment of routine sestamibi single-positron emission computed tomography (SPECT). Ann Surg Oncol. 2015;22 (1):139-145.
29. Jo VY, Fletcher CD. WHO classification of soft tissue tumours: an update based on the 2013, 4th edition. Pathology. 2014;46(2):95-104.
30. Vargas D, Suby-Long T, Restrepo CS. Cystic lesions of the mediastinum. Semin Ultrasound CT MRI. 2016;37:212-22.
31. Kim Y, Lee KS, Yoo JH, et al. Middle mediastinal lesions: imaging findings and pathological correlation. Eur J Radiol. 2000;35:30-8.
32. Warbey VS, Ferner RE, Dunn JT, Calonje E, O'Doherty MJ. [18F] FDG PET/CT in the diagnosis of malignant peripheral nerve sheath tumours in neurofibromatosis type-1. Eur J Nucl Med Mol Imaging. 2009;36(5):751-7.
33. Kazama T, Faria SC, Varavithya V, et al. FDG PET in the evaluation of treatment for lymphoma: clinical usefulness and pitfalls. Radiographics. 2005;25:191-207.
34. Ko SF, et al. Imaging Spectrum of Castleman's Disease. Am J Roengenol. 2004;182(3):769-75.

CHAPTER 167

Imaging of Solitary Pulmonary Nodule

Sapna Singh, Anju Garg, Anjali Prakash

INTRODUCTION

A solitary pulmonary nodule (SPN) is defined as a well-defined round or oval lesion less than 3 cm in size surrounded at least partially by the lung parenchyma **(Figs. 1A and B)**. Lesions larger than 3 cm are called masses. There is no lymphadenopathy, atelectasis or pneumonia associated with SPN **(Figs. 2A and B)**.[1,2] However, practically, there is a lot of overlap between the two terms, SPN and mass, and many times are used interchangeably.

Differentiation between benign and malignant SPNs forms the goal of imaging. This differentiation is important because the overall mortality associated with lung cancer is about 85% and about 20 % of lung cancers are discovered in the form of SPN.[3] SPN is seen in about 0.2% of chest radiographs.[4]

SPURIOUS SPN

Pleural based and chest wall lesions, nipple shadow, skin nodules like neurofibroma, artifacts may be the causes of

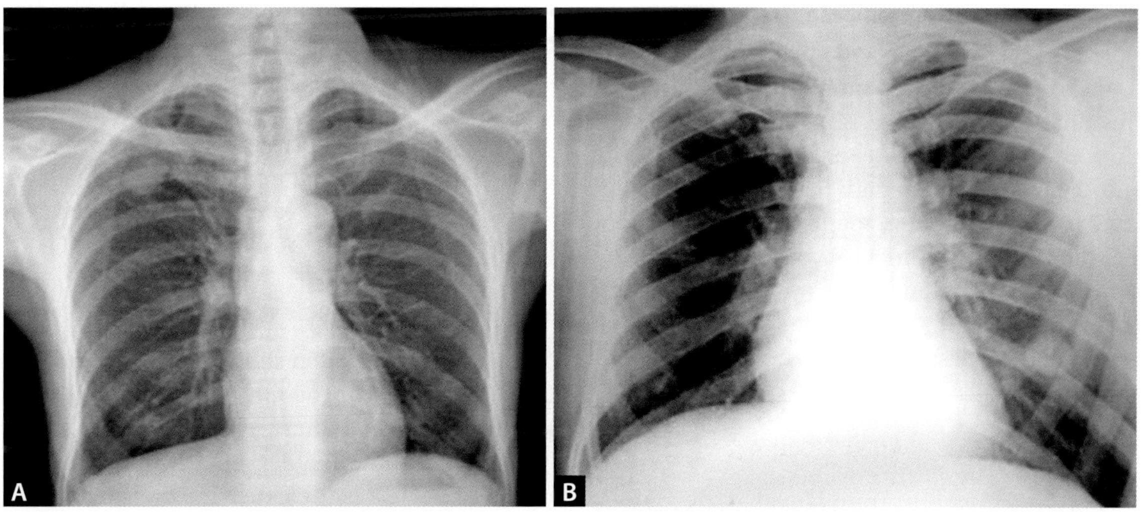

Figs. 1A and B: Chest radiographs in two patients showing a well-defined spherical lesion less than 3 cm in diameter surrounded by lung and not associated with lymphadenopathy, atelectasis or pneumonia. The lesions are seen in the right upper zone in one (A) and in the left lower zone in the other (B)—Solitary pulmonary nodules.

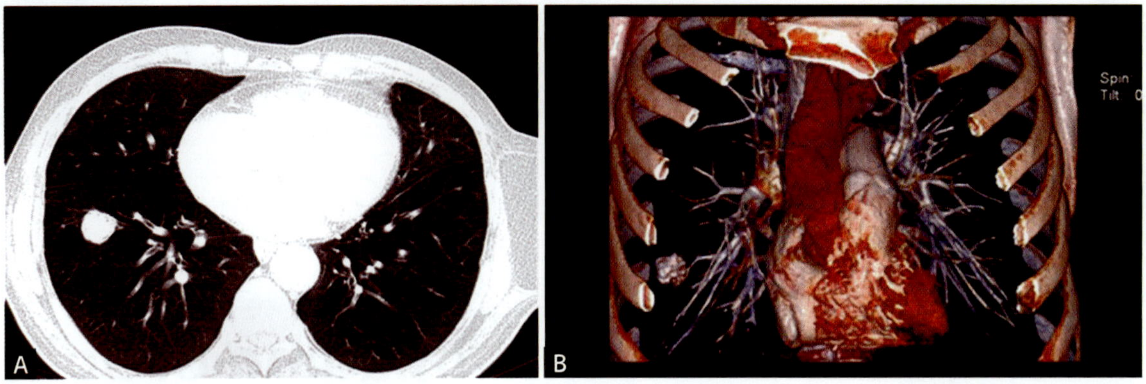

Figs. 2A and B: CT scan (A) in patient with suspected pulmonary embolism reveals an incidental SPN in the right lower lobe. VRT pulmonary angiogram image (B) showing the normal vasculature with the nodule in the lower lobe.

spurious SPNs, however oblique views, repeat radiographs or even CT at times may help to differentiate these from a true SPN **(Figs. 3A to C)**.

MORPHOLOGICAL CHARACTERISTICS OF SPN

Of the malignant lesions, adenocarcinoma is the most common carcinoma to give rise to a SPN though all the histological types may present as intrapulmonary nodules.[5,6] Of the benign nodules, granulomas and intrapulmonary lymph nodes account for 80% while hamartomas account for about 10% of the nodules.[6] Morphological characteristics of the nodule such as shape, size, margin, etc. have been used to differentiate between benign and malignant nodules.

Size

The larger the lesion, the more likely it is to be malignant **(Table 1)**. For a SPN to be detected on chest radiographs, it should be at least 9 mm in diameter while CT detects smaller lesions.[7] For a nodule ranging from 0.5-1 cm in diameter, the likelihood of cancer is about 35%, for nodules 1.0–2.0 cm in diameter it is 50%, and for a nodule more than 2.0 cm in diameter, the likelihood of it being malignant is 85% **(Figs. 4A and B)**.[8,9]

Though a very small lesion can turn out to be malignant, lesions larger than 3 cm in diameter are more likely to be malignant while those less than 1 cm are usually benign **(Figs. 5A and B)**.[8,9]

Shape

Benign lesions are usually round/oval with smooth margins, for example, hamartomas. Malignant lesions, on the other hand, tend to be irregular in shape, notched and lobulated **(Figs. 6A to C)**. Lobulation and notching are more indicative of a malignant lesion than a benign lesion.[10] A linear or angular shape may be seen in scars/atelectasis.

Table 1: Likelihood of malignancy related to nodule diameter.[9]

Diameter	*Malignancy Rate*
<1 cm	35%
1–2 cm	50%
2–3 cm	80%
>3 cm	97%

Location

About 70% of lung cancers are located in the right upper lobe, the right lung being a more common site for malignancy than the left lung.[11-13] While squamous cell carcinoma is more likely to be centrally located, adenocarcinoma is usually peripheral in location **(Figs. 7A to C)**.[14] Metastatic lesions usually involve the outer one third and bases of the lungs. *Location*, however, cannot be used as an independent predictor of malignancy because benign nodules are equally distributed throughout the upper and lower lobes.[15]

Edge Characteristics

Malignant lesions often show irregularity, spiculation and lobulation **(Fig. 8)**. The presence of spiculation is a strong predictor of malignancy. A radial extension of malignant cells, along the interlobular septa, lymphatics, small airways or blood vessels is the cause for the spiculation and has been likened to the spokes of a wheel or "corona radiata" or "corona maligna" or the "sunburst appearance" **(Fig. 9)**.[16-18]

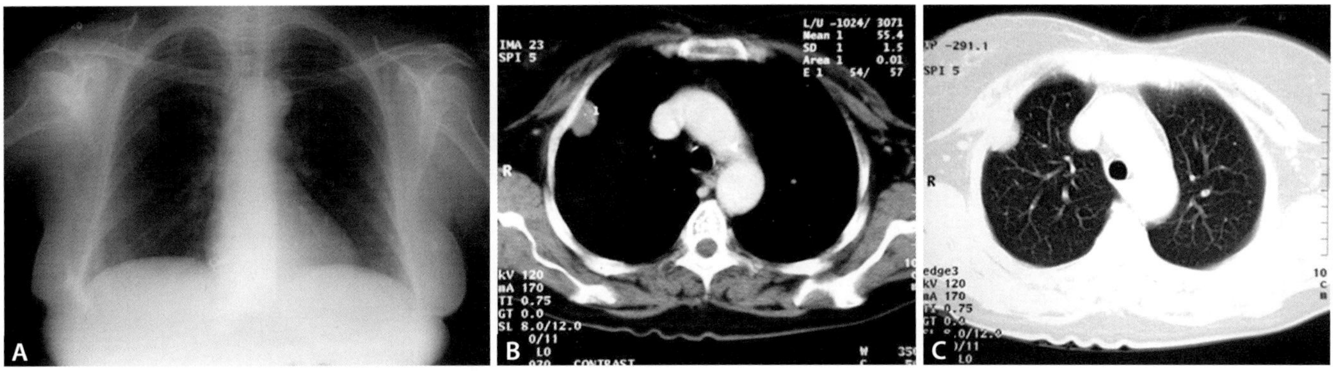

Figs. 3A to C: Chest radiograph (A) revealing a solitary nodule in the right lung. CT mediastinal window (B) and lung parenchymal window settings (C) reveal the lesion to be clearly pleural based—A case of pleural fibroma mimicking SPN.

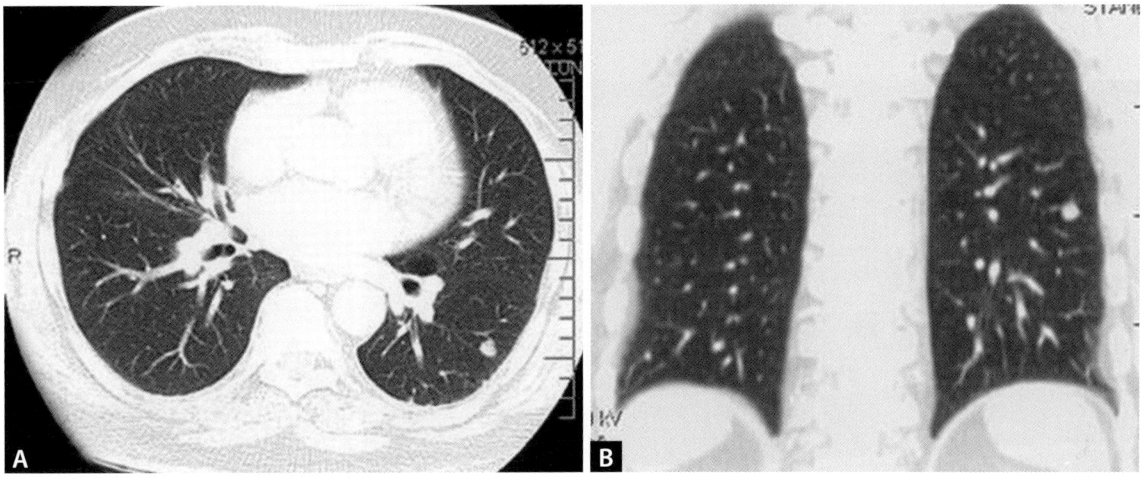

Fig. 4A and B: Chest CT scans showing a smooth, sharply marginated, rounded nodule in the left lower lobe with no evidence of calcification/cavitation. The small size of the lesion (<1 cm) makes malignancy less likely—Benign SPN/granuloma.

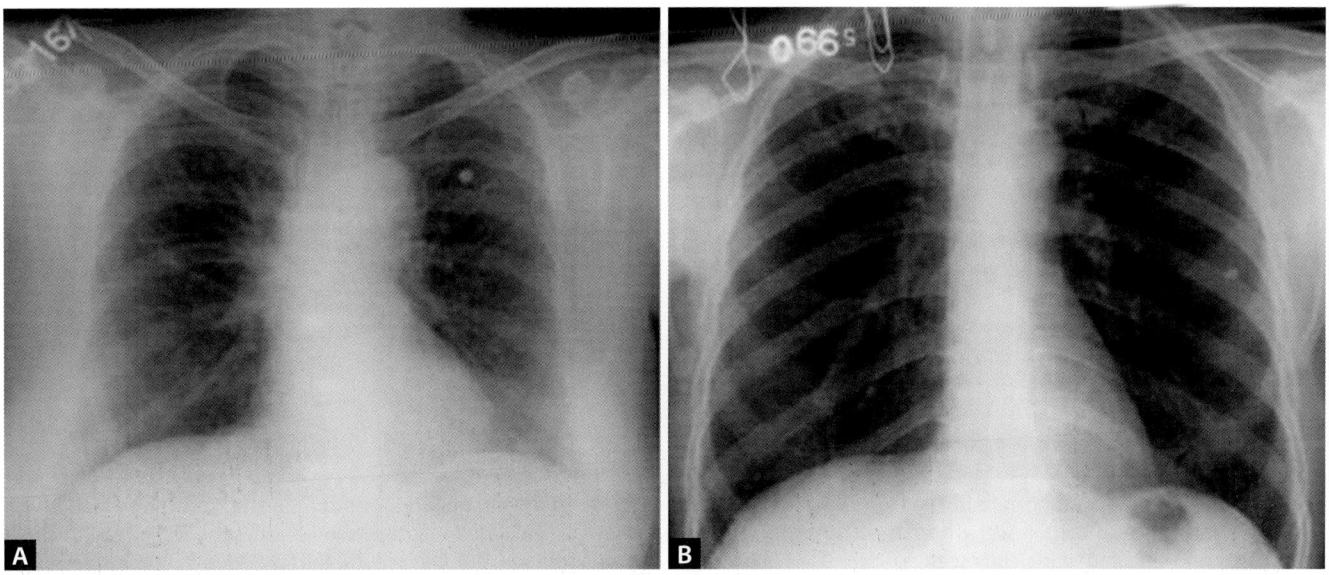

Fig. 5A and B: Chest radiographs in two cases showing well-defined nodules <1 cm clearly seen on plain radiographs due to being calcified—Benign SPNs/calcified granulomas.

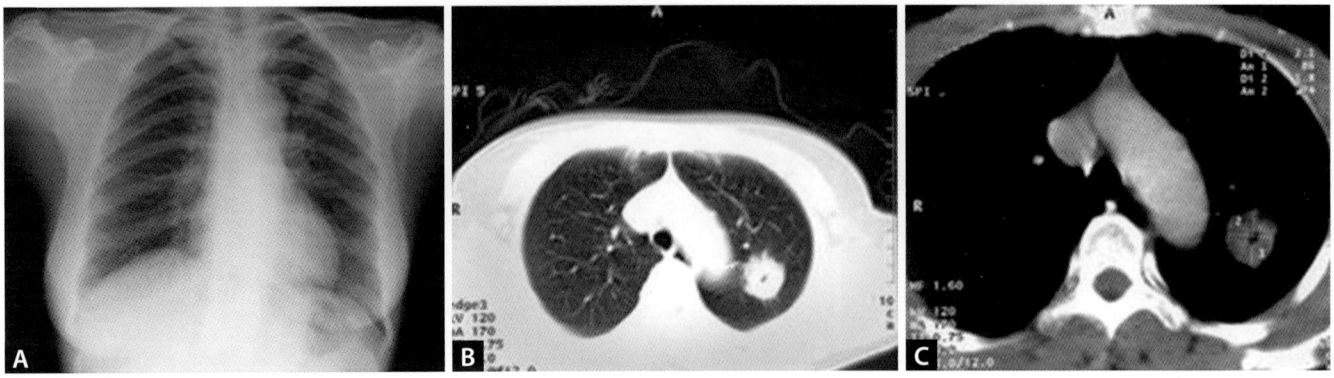

Figs. 6A to C: Chest radiograph (A) showing a nodule in the left upper lobe. The lesion is classified as a nodule because it is relatively well-defined, surrounded by lung, roughly spherical in shape and less than 3 cm in size. CT scan (B) showing the edge of the nodule to be ill-defined and lobulated with pleural tails extending to the pleural surface. The lesion measures 2.3 x 1.8 cm in size and shows evidence of central cavitation (C). The larger the nodule (>2 cm) the more likely it is malignant—Adenocarcinoma lung.

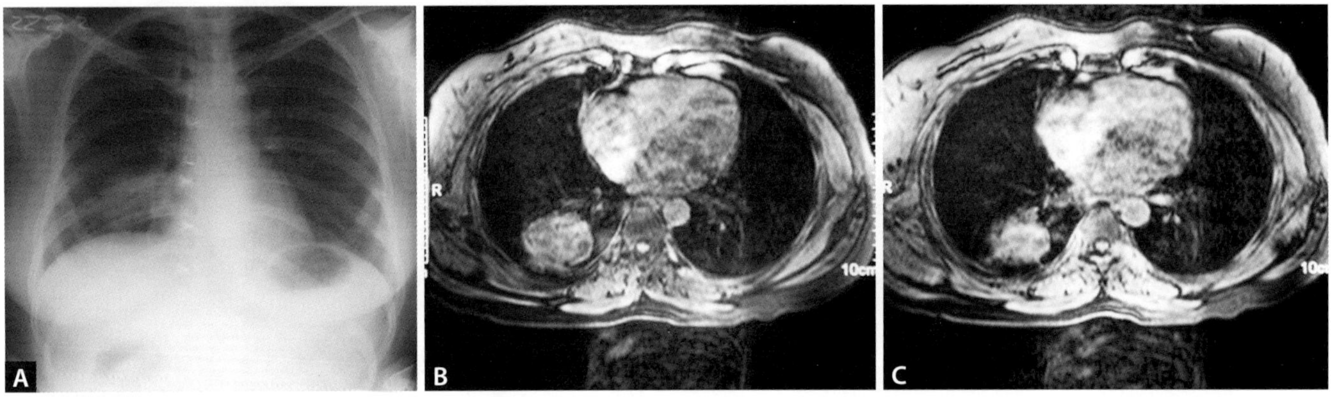

Figs. 7A to C: Chest radiograph (A) showing a solitary nodule in the right lower lobe. MR images in the same case (B and C) showing the large nodule in the right lung, it has irregular and spiculated margins—Adenocarcinoma manifesting as a peripheral SPN.

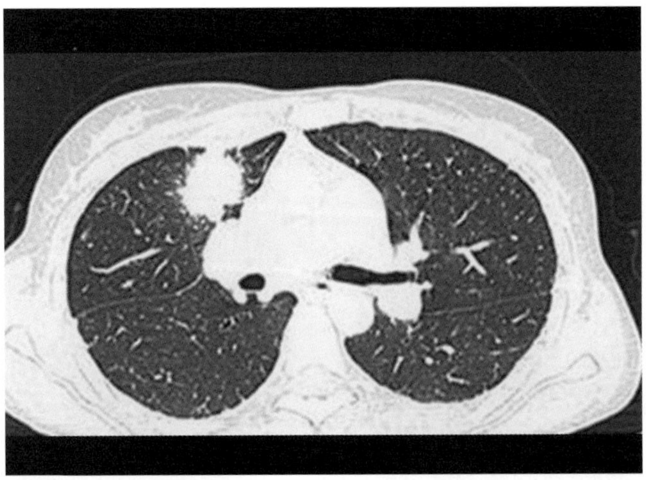

Fig. 8: CT scan showing a nodule in the right upper lobe. The nodule shows lobulations and evidence of notching. Edge irregularity and spiculation is clearly seen.

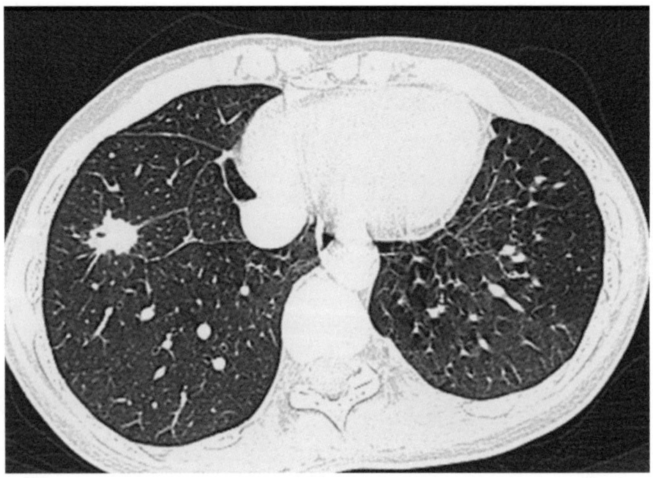

Fig. 9: CT chest showing a nodule in the right upper lobe with irregular, spiculated margins termed the "sunburst appearance" or corona radiata. Multiple pleural tails are seen extending from the mass to the pleural surface. A small eccentric cavitation is noted—Bronchogenic carcinoma.

In patients with adenocarcinoma and adenocarcinoma in situ (bronchioloalveolar carcinoma) it reflects the presence of fibrosis surrounding the tumor.[19] The fibrosis usually reflects a desmoplastic reaction and not a pre-existing lung fibrosis. Carcinoma can show the presence of a "pleural tail" or a "pleural tag" in which a thin linear opacity is seen extending from the edge of the lung nodule to the pleural surface. The presence of spiculation is more indicative of the lesion being malignant rather than pleural tail as pleural tail may also be seen with lesions which are benign such as granulomatous disease like tuberculosis.[20,21]

Presence of a Halo

Ground-glass opacity surrounding the nodule gives a "halo sign" to the nodule.[22] This peripheral non-solid component surrounding a nodule should not be confused with corona radiata.

Halo sign is seen in[23]:

- Invasive aspergillosis
- Adenocarcinoma
- Adenocarcinoma in situ (formerly Bronchioloalveolar carcinoma)
- Pulmonary hemorrhage

In lesions such as aspergillosis, the halo sign represents hemorrhage, while in malignancies it represents the lepidic spread of tumor.

INTERNAL CHARACTERISTICS

Calcification

Calcification is an important imaging feature that can be used to distinguish between benign and malignant SPNs.

Calcification in a Benign Nodule (Figs. 10A to D)

- Concentric rings of calcification (target calcification)
- Conglomerate foci of calcification involving a large part of the nodule (popcorn calcification)
- Homogeneous calcification/uniform calcification
- Dense central (bull's eye) calcification.

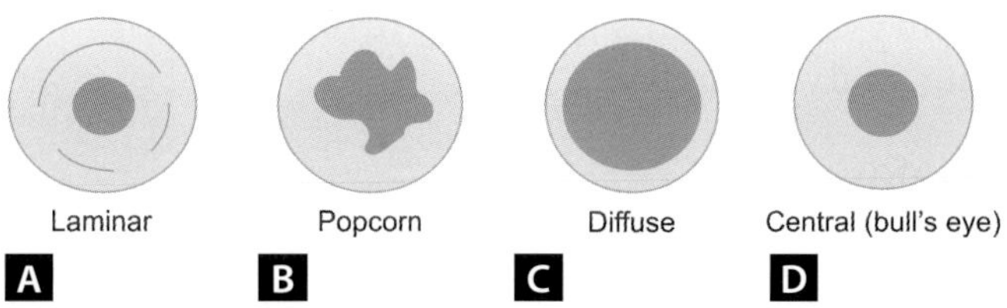

Figs. 10A to D: Calcification in benign module.

When any of these patterns is seen, the probability of the lesion being benign is almost 100%[24] **(Figs. 11A and B)**. Popcorn calcification is virtually diagnostic of cartilage containing tumors such as hamartomas **(Figs. 12A to C)**. Concentric (laminated) and uniform calcifications are suggestive of a calcified tuberculous or fungal granuloma.

Indeterminate Calcification

Eccentric calcification may be seen in a benign lesion which gets calcified in an eccentric fashion or when a benign calcified lesion is engulfed by a malignant lesion. Stippled/punctate calcification may be seen in both benign and malignant lesions and is thus classified as indeterminate.[25]

Calcification in a Malignant Nodule

A malignant nodule may show calcification which is diffuse and amorphous or psammomatous (in case of metastasis from mucin secreting tumors from the colon or ovary) or dystrophic (in areas of tumor necrosis).[25,26] Centrally located calcification in a spiculated SPN also suggests malignancy.[27]

Fat

The presence of fat (-40 to -120 HU) within a lesion is virtually diagnostic of a hamartoma **(Fig. 13)**. Other lesions that may show fat include lipoid pneumonia, lipoma and metastatic liposarcoma.[28]

Cavitation

Both benign and malignant SPNs can cavitate. A thick irregular cavity with wall thickness greater than 16 mm is likely to be malignant. About 95% of the nodules with wall thickness less than 5 mm are benign.[29] About 75% of the cavities with wall thickness 5–15 mm are benign. Cavitation usually occurs in squamous cell carcinoma, large cell carcinoma and adenocarcinoma while small cell cancers rarely show cavitation.

Air Bronchiolograms and Pseudocavitation

Air bronchiologram or bubble like lucencies or pseudo-cavitation may simulate cavities and are more commonly seen in malignant nodules (29%) than in benign nodules (6%).[30-32] Pseudocavitation results from sparing of alveoli and bronchi by tumor infiltration in malignant lesions.

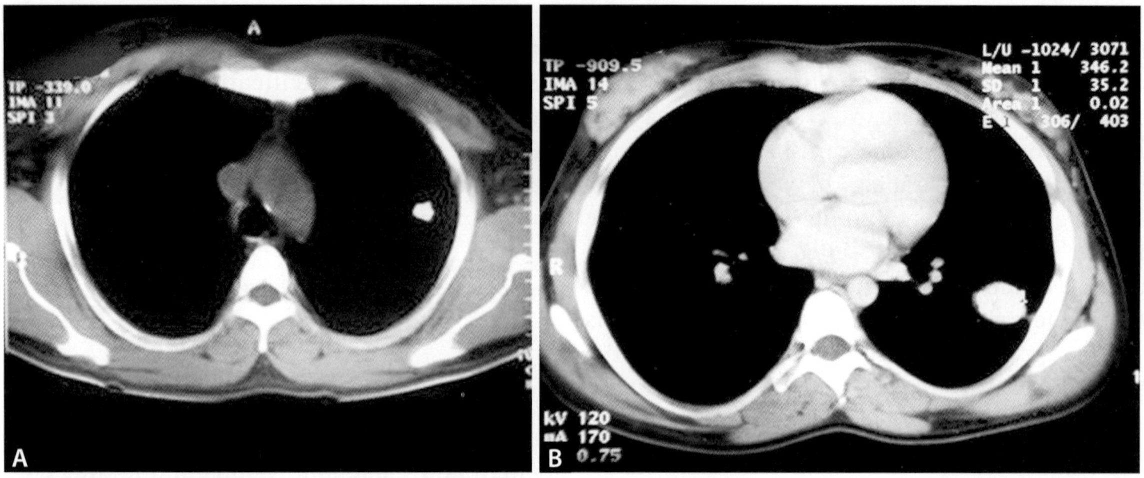

Figs. 11A and B: CT scans showing uniform homogeneous calcification in two cases of tuberculomas.

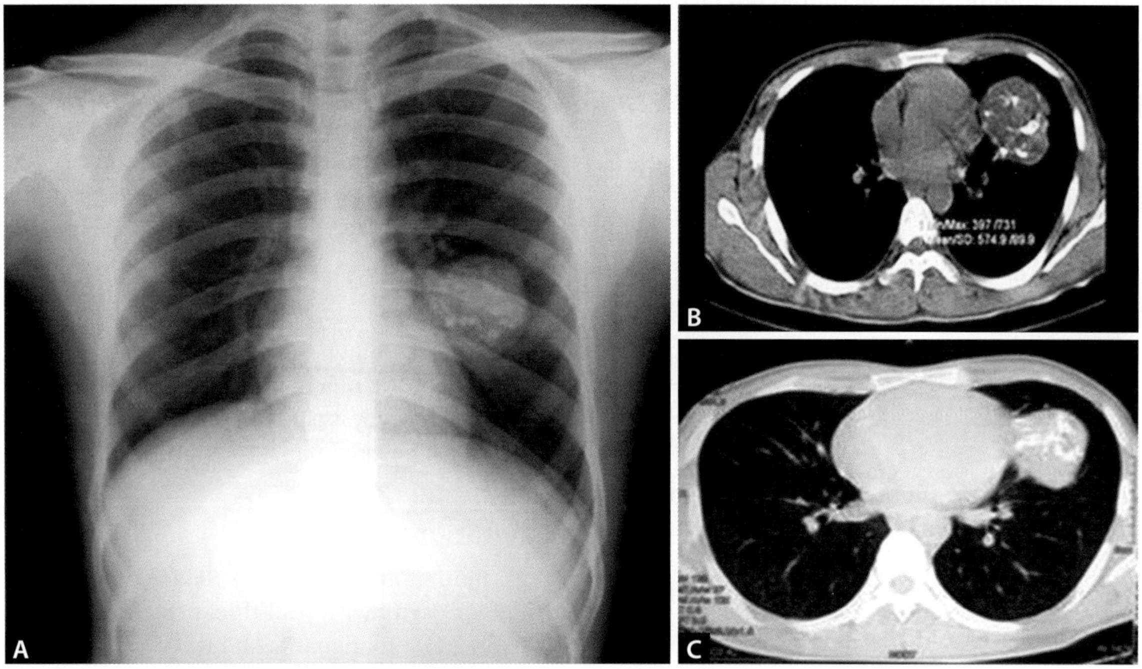

Figs. 12A to C: Chest radiograph (A) showing a large solitary nodule in the left lung with dense nodular foci of calcification within s/o characteristic popcorn calcification/central cartilage calcification. Noncontrast CT scan mediastinal window (B) showing a 3 x 3 cm nodule containing overlapping, randomly distributed small rings of calcification or the popcorn calcification and lung parenchymal window settings (C) reveal the nodule to be round in shape and sharply marginated—Pulmonary hamartoma.

Air Crescent Sign

An "air crescent" or "air meniscus" sign results from a peripheral halo of air between the intracavitatory mass and the cavity wall **(Figs. 14A and B)**. The commonest cause is a fungal ball, i.e. aspergilloma/mycetoma. Other causes include blood clot in a cavity, cavitatory carcinoma, complicated hydatid disease, Rasmussen's aneurysm, mucous plug in bronchiectasis and pulmonary gangrene.

Air-fluid Level

Presence of an air-fluid level within a lesion favours benignity such as a lung abscess or an infected cyst **(Figs. 15A to C)**. Intracavitatory hemorrhage or

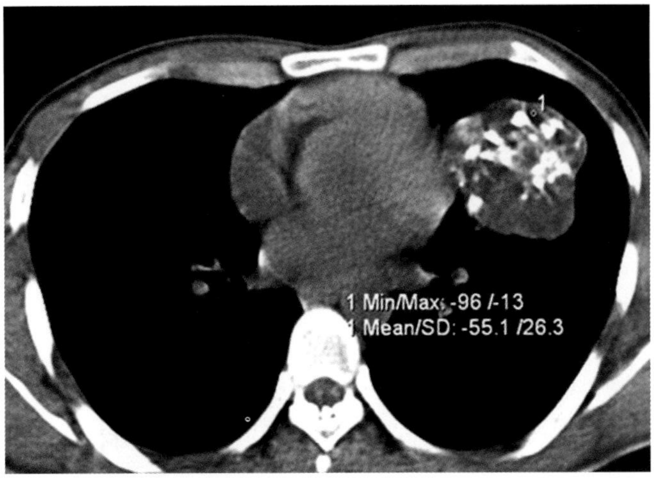

Fig. 13: Noncontrast CT scan showing foci of fat or negative attenuation (–50 to –100 HU) within the nodule in the left lung consistent with pulmonary hamartoma.

superinfection may rarely give rise to an air fluid level in cavitatory carcinoma.

OTHER CHARACTERISTICS OF SPN

Satellite Nodules

The presence of small nodules adjacent to a large nodule or mass favors a benign lesion such as tuberculosis and sarcoidosis. A cluster of small nodules seen within a segment or subsegment of the lung, 3–15 mm in diameter usually indicates a granulomatous process **(Figs. 16A and B)**. In sarcoidosis, the term "galaxy-sign" refers to the presence of multiple satellite nodules.

Feeding Vessel Sign

This refers to a small pulmonary artery directly leading to a nodule. A "feeding vessel sign" is seen in metastasis, septic emboli, arteriovenous fistula or infarct **(Fig. 17)**.[33,34]

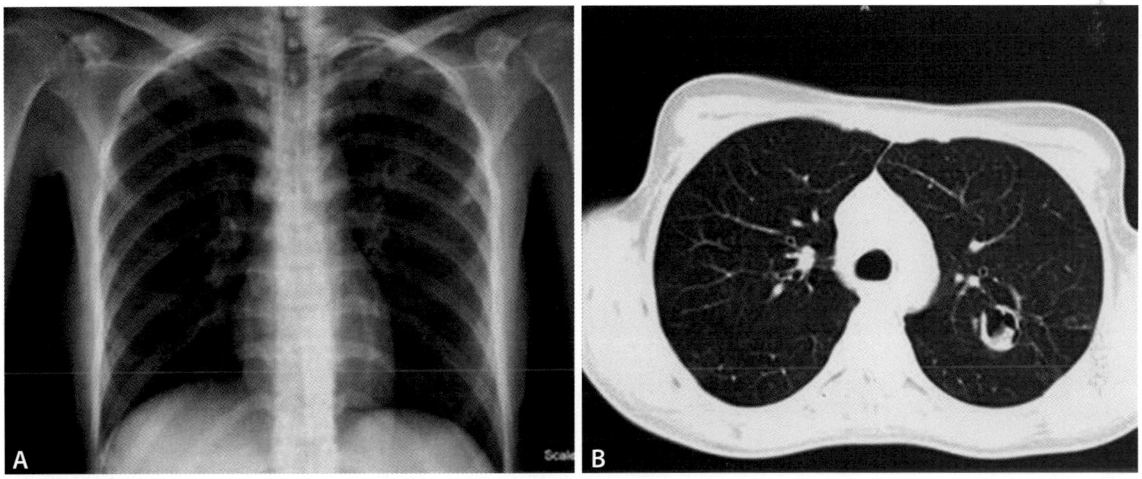

Figs. 14A and B: Chest radiograph (A) showing a small solitary lesion in the left upper lobe with a crescent of air between the intracavitatory mass and the cavity wall giving rise to the "air crescent" or air meniscus sign. CT scan (B) showing the same—Aspergilloma/mycetoma.

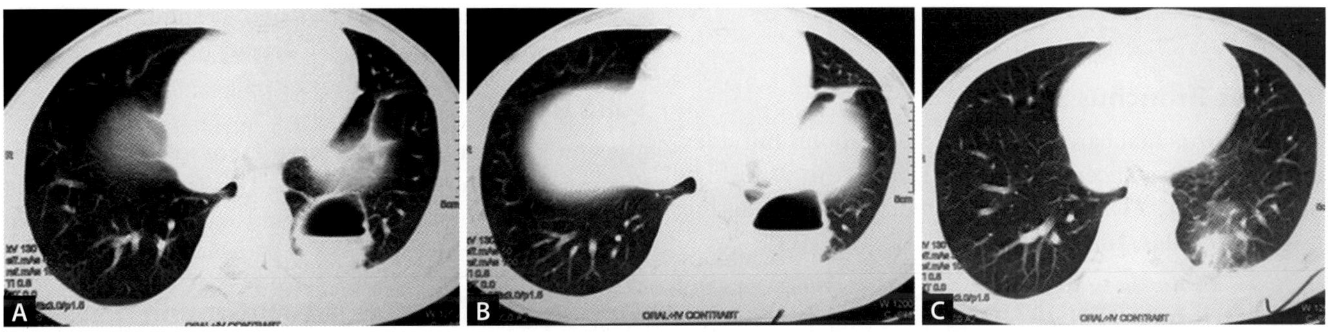

Figs. 15A to C: CT scans in a case showing a well-defined cavity with an air-fluid level with wall thickness <5 mm and surrounding consolidation—Lung abscess.

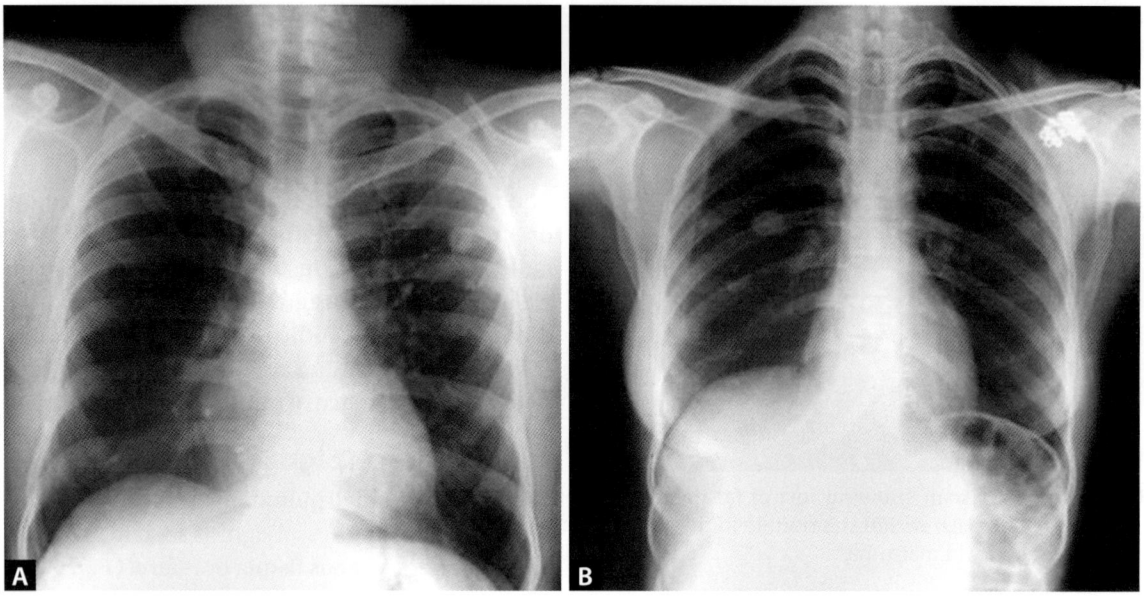

Figs. 16A and B: Chest radiograph in two cases showing a calcified tuberculoma with multiple small nodules adjacent to it in the left lung in one case (A) and the right lung in the other (B)—Satellite nodules predicting a benign disease.

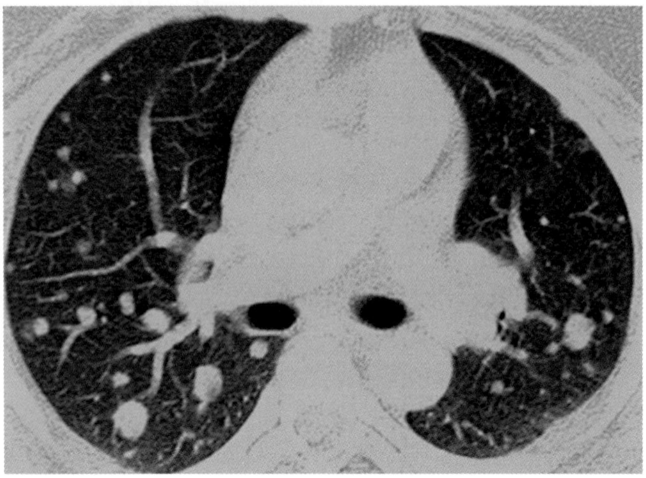

Figs. 17: CT scan in a case of hematogenous pulmonary metastases showing small pulmonary arteries directly feeding the nodules—"Feeding vessel sign".

Positive Bronchus Sign

When a bronchial carcinoma infiltrates around but does not occlude an adjacent bronchus it gives rise to a "positive bronchus sign".[35] This is seen as a patent bronchus entering the nodule **(Figs. 18A and B)**.

NODULE ATTENUATION

CT density of the nodule has been used to characterize nodules as benign or malignant based on the density measurement. Siegelman and co-workers suggested that a CT number above 164 HU represents benignity. Proto and Thomas gave a different cut off value of 200 HU above which the lesions could be diagnosed as benign.[36] The limitation of using cut-off value is that 6–7% of bronchial carcinomas may contain some type of calcification giving high value of CT density.[37] CT densitometry is not recommended for nodules greater than 3 cm, those with irregular or spiculated borders or those showing a growth rate compatible with bronchial carcinoma. To overcome these problems, Zerhouni used a reference phantom to provide a standard for density. The phantom simulated the shape, dimensions and density of the thorax at multiple levels to resemble the conditions under which SPN was measured.[38] If more than 10% of the voxels in the patient's nodule were higher in density than in the phantom nodule, the lesion was considered to be above the critical density level. Nodules have been classified as solid, partly solid and non-solid based on the CT density measurements.[39]

Solid Nodule

A lesion is said to be solid when it completely obscures the underlying lung parenchyma. This is the commonest type but less malignant as compared to the partly solid and non-solid nodules.[40,41]

Ground-glass Nodule (GGN)/Ground-glass Attenuation Nodule (GGAN)

Ground-glass nodule (GGN) is defined as a focal area of increased lung attenuation through which the pulmonary

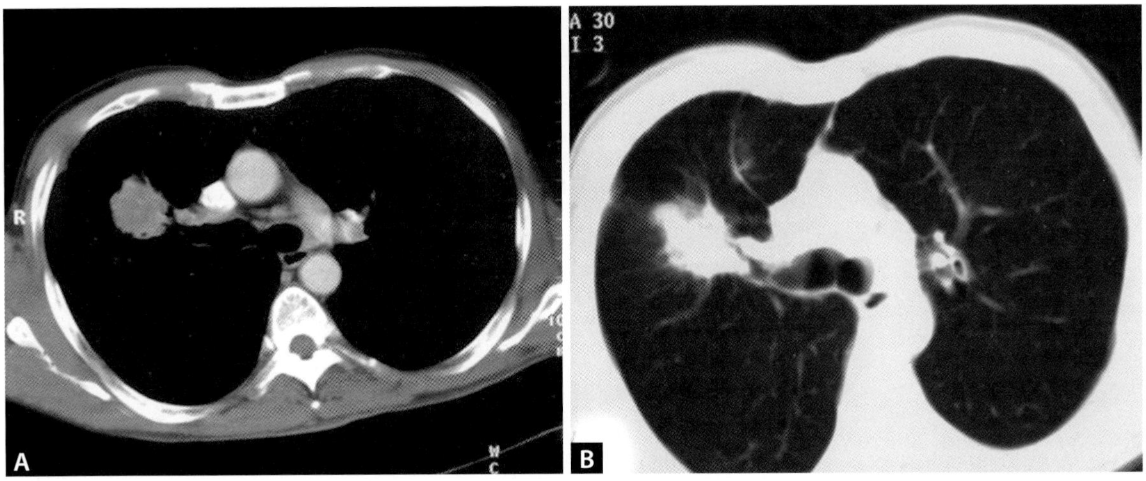

Figs. 18A and B: CT scans of the chest showing a pulmonary lesion abutting and narrowing the right upper lobe bronchus without completely occluding it. The positive bronchus sign in bronchogenic carcinoma.

vessels and bronchial structures, that is, the lung parenchyma structures can be observed.[42] Contiguous thin CT sections (1 mm) should be performed to establish lesions as true GGNs whenever possible to avoid the pitfall of interpreting them as solid or subsolid nodules.[43] Use of thick sections precludes accurate nodule characterization due to volume averaging.

Subsolid Nodules (SSNs)

This term includes both pure and part solid GGNs **(Figs. 19A and B)**. It is important to know the percentage of ground-glass versus solid components of subsolid lesions as greater the solid component, greater the chance of the lesion being an invasive adenocarcinoma with a poorer prognosis.

The incidence of malignancy in subsolid nodules has been estimated to be about 34% in comparison to the 7% seen in solid nodules.[44] Among the subsolid nodules, partly solid nodules have the highest rate of malignancy (63%) while pure ground-glass nodules have an incidence of 18%.[44]

Association of Nodule Attenuation with Adenocarcinoma

Adenocarcinoma which accounts for about 50% of all lung cancers presents more commonly as a solitary subsolid nodule (SSN) than the other histologic types of carcinoma. According to the IASLC (International Association for the Study of Lung Cancer), ATS (American Thoracic Society) and European Respiratory Society (ERS), adenocarcinomas can be classified as preinvasive and invasive.[45] Preinvasive lesions comprise atypical adenomatous hyperplasia (AAH) and adenocarcinoma in situ (AIS). These are lesions which typically exhibit growth along the alveolar surface called lepidic growth.[46] Atypical adenomatous hyperplasia (AAH) is a lesion which is purely ground-glass in attenuation and usually less than 1 cm in size.[47] Adenocarcinoma in situ (AIS) is a lesion with ground-glass attenuation and less than 3 cm in size. The invasive lesions include minimally invasive carcinoma (MIC) and invasive adenocarcinoma. Minimally invasive carcinoma (MIC) is defined as a lesion that shows a predominant lepidic growth with no necrosis, no lymphatic, vascular or pleural invasion, is less than 3 cm in size with an invasive component not more than 5 mm in any location.[45,46] MIA may be seen as ground-glass attenuation(GGAN) or partly solid nodule (PSN) on CT.[48] Classification of invasive adenocarcinoma as having a lepidic, acinar, papillary, micropapillary or solid pattern is based on the histological features. The MIA, AIS and lepidic forms may have both mucinous and non-mucinous forms **(Table 2)**. The term bronchioloalveolar carcinoma is now an obsolete term and should be called adenocarcinoma *in situ*.[49,50]

The solid component of a SSN is important as it predicts the prognosis of the patient, the solid component representing the invasive foci of adenocarcinoma. A direct correlation has been reported between presence of solid component, the size of the solid component and increasing attenuation with the invasiveness or aggressiveness of a subsolid nodule.[49,50] The higher the attenuation value of the subsolid nodule, the greater is the degree of invasion.

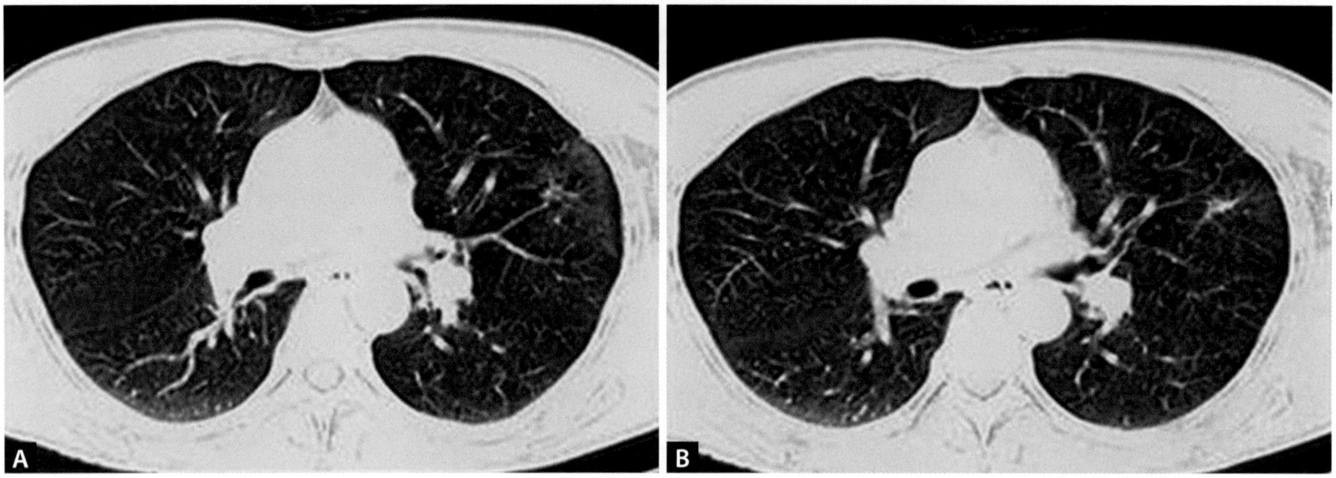

Figs. 19A and B: CT scans show an ill-defined central nodule along with ground-glass attenuation—Partly solid nodule.

Table 2: Correlation of the histological patterns with CT features of subsolid nodules[45,46].

2011 IASLC, ATS and ERS classification	*CT features*
• Atypical adenomatous hyperplasia (AAH) • Adenocarcinoma *in situ* (AIS)	• GGAN • GGAN with a possible solid component
• Minimally invasive adenocarcinoma (MIA) • Lepidic predominant adenocarcinoma • Invasive adenocarcinoma	• GGAN, partly solid nodule • Partly solid nodule, solid nodule • Partly solid nodule with a solid component, solid nodule

ASSESSMENT OF MALIGNANT POTENTIAL OF A SPN

Nodule Growth

An important criterion to differentiate between benign and malignant nodules is nodule growth. Previously, assessment of the size was done by measuring the maximum dimensions on posteroanterior and lateral radiography and also by matching circular standards printed on transparency with that of the nodule margin. However, such measurements are inaccurate. Nodule growth is also assessed by a volume doubling time (VDT) defined as the time in which the volume of a nodule becomes double. As the most common shape is spherical, the volume is calculated using the equation $4\pi r.^3$ A 26% increase in diameter is taken as a doubling in volume based on

$$VDT = [t \times \log 2]/\log (V_t/V_o)$$

Where V_o is the initial volume and V_t is the volume at time t.[51]

This formula is based on an exponential model of nodule growth, i.e. a 5 mm nodule will reach a diameter of 20.3 mm in 12 months if the doubling time (DT) is 60 days but will reach a diameter of only 7.1 mm in 12 months, if the doubling time is 240 days. Also the 26% increase in axial diameter taken as the volume doubling time is difficult to assess in case of nodules less than or equal to 5 mm in size because 5 mm nodule which doubles its volume increases in diameter by 1.25 mm only.[52] It has been seen that two-dimensional measurements obtained with electronic calipers are unreliable as compared to the three-dimensional measurements.

The volume doubling time (VDT) for malignant SPNs is rarely less than a month or more than a year (range 20–400 days).[53] Nodules with a doubling time less than 20 days and more than 400 days are considered benign. Also stability of nodule size over 2 years (730 days) has been considered to suggest benignity.[54] The radiologic pathologic correlation of partly solid and pure ground-glass attenuation nodule with the histologic spectrum of adenocarcinoma has been described.[55] It has been seen that small purely ground-glass opacity (nonsolid) nodules with malignant histologic features may have a mean volume DT of about 2 years while it is about 6 months for the solid cancers.[56] Subsolid nodules that have a higher likelihood of malignancy have a volume doubling time between the two extremes. Carcinoids and adenocarcinomas in situ may remain stable for more than two years. Therefore, the dictum that 2 year stability indicates a benign process should be used with caution.[57] Longer follow up is advisable for ground-glass nodules which have a longer doubling time.

Three-dimensional Volume Quantification

Three dimensional volume quantification utilizes the entire CT data to calculate nodule volume **(Figs. 20A and B)**.[58] Volume quantification method is able to detect smaller differences in nodule size than the two dimensional method. In order to separate/segment out the nodules from the lung parenchyma, threshold method is used, which takes into account the voxel attenuation above and below a particular threshold as nodule or parenchyma.[58,59] It is important to include the ground-glass component of a subsolid nodule in volume determination as ground-glass component has a high incidence of malignancy.[60] In the case of subsolid nodules, growth may occur in the form of an increase in size, an increase in attenuation, appearance of a solid component or increase in the size of the solid component. For optimal CT evaluation of subsolid pulmonary nodules, it is essential to obtain thin section CT.[61] Measurement of attenuation values on serial CT examinations is less variable than measurements of volume and diameter.[62] For these nodules, an increase in mass is calculated which is the product of mean volume and attenuation.

Computer-aided Diagnosis

The volume and morphology of nodules can be assessed by computer-aided diagnosis (CAD) that can act as a second reader. Identification of the nodule, size of the nodule, morphology and internal architecture of the nodule can all be studied with CAD. Differentiation of nodules with uniform attenuation from those with inhomogeneous attenuation called texture analysis can be undertaken with the help of computer-aided technique.[63] An association between nodule characteristics and rate of malignancy is also facilitated through this technique.

Image Registration

The follow up of the pulmonary nodules emphasizes the need for image registration techniques. Image registration entails superimposing image data or determining the spatial alignment between different images from the same modality at different points in times (intra-modality registration) or between different imaging modalities, such as CT, MR PET (intermodality registration). To correlate a nodule accurately on CT study with its matching counterpart on a subsequent CT, global registration of the thorax and the local registration of nodules and smaller structures need to be performed. An interactive system enables easy identification of corresponding structures on initial and subsequent CT studies, recording of nodules and their characteristics including volume and storage of image results for future analysis and documentation.[64]

Nodule Enhancement

Enhancement of the nodule can be assessed on CT to differentiate between benign and malignant solid SPNs.[65] Enhancement pattern can be studied by administration of iodinated contrast material intravenously (300 mg/mL at 2 mL/sec) with a pressure injector. The protocol consists of 3 mm images of the nodule at 1, 2, 3 and 4 minutes after contrast injection.[66,67] Enhancement value is obtained by subtraction of the precontrast value from

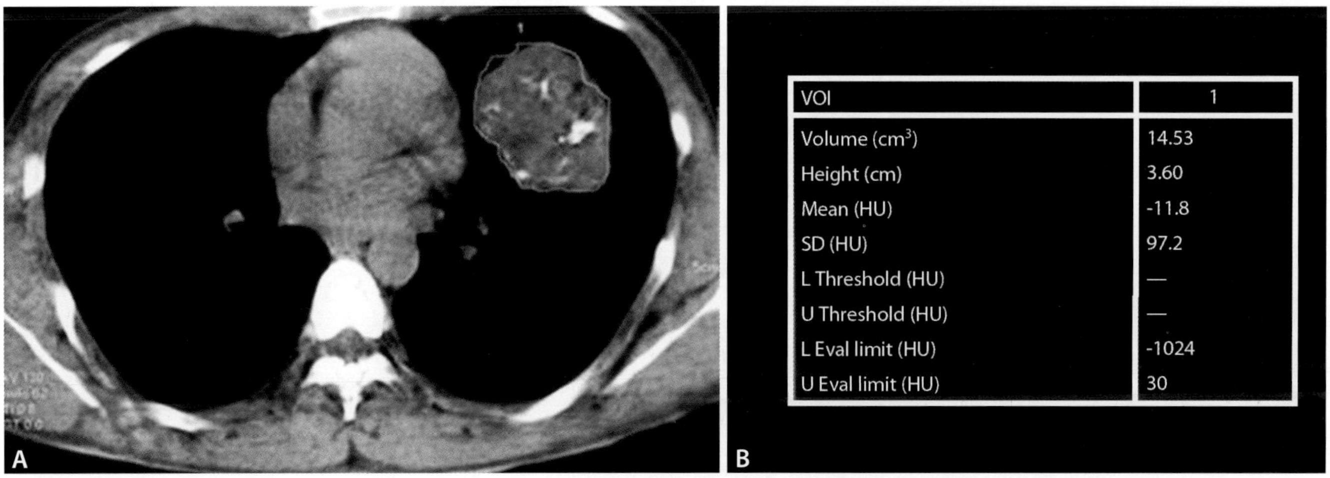

VOI	1
Volume (cm^3)	14.53
Height (cm)	3.60
Mean (HU)	-11.8
SD (HU)	97.2
L Threshold (HU)	—
U Threshold (HU)	—
L Eval limit (HU)	-1024
U Eval limit (HU)	30

Figs. 20A and B: Measurement of volume in a case of pulmonary hamartoma. The volume of the nodule is measured on each axial section and then summed to obtain the total nodule volume (B).

the peak enhancement. Measurements should be done on mediastinal window and the region of interest (ROI) should be so placed as to cover 70% of the diameter of the nodule **(Figs. 21A to C)**. A cut-off value of 15 HU for enhancement has been found to have a sensitivity of 98% and specificity of 58% for benignity with benign lesions showing enhancement <15 HU.[68] An enhancement of more than 20 HU is indicative of tumor neovascularity or malignancy **(Figs. 22A to C)**. The limitation of this technique includes its use in lesions smaller than 2 cm as larger lesions would have areas of necrosis and placement of cursor would be a problem. This technique is more applicable for lesions which are relatively spherical in shape and relatively homogeneous in attenuation with no large areas of necrosis, fat, calcification or cavitation **(Figs. 23A to C)**. Also, benign vascular tumors and granulomas show enhancement leading to a considerable overlap.[69] An analysis of combined wash-in and wash-out characteristics (studied at 15 minute delay) gives a more precise evaluation of the nodule enhancement.

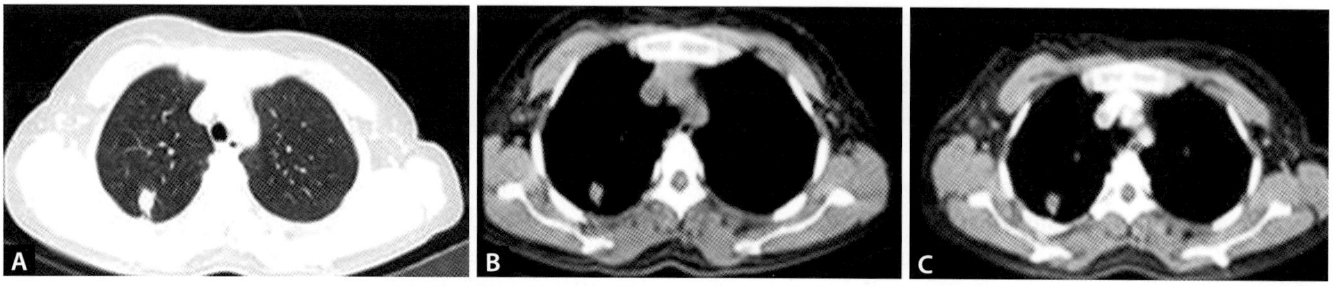

Figs. 21A to C: Lung parenchymal window settings on chest CT (A) showing a small (< 1 cm) smooth rounded lesion with a small pleural tail in the right upper lobe. Noncontrast and contrast-enhanced scans with mediastinal window settings (B and C) showing no enhancement of the lesion on the postcontrast scans—Benign lesion/tuberculoma.

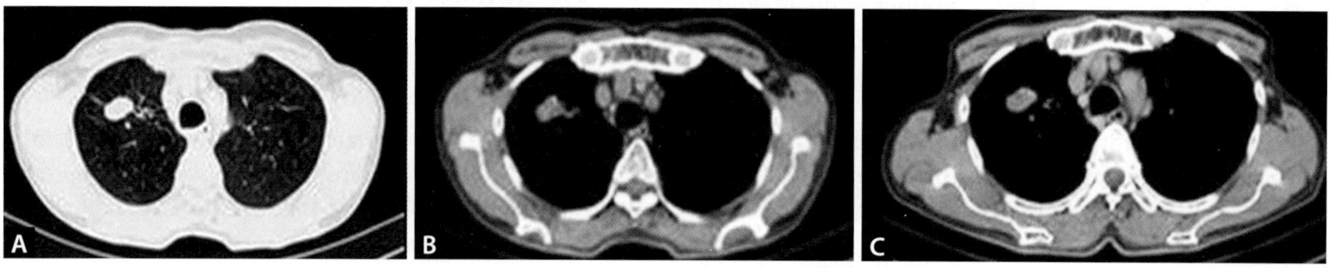

Figs. 22A to C: Lung parenchymal window settings (A) showing a small (1 cm) solitary lesion in the right upper lobe. The lesion is irregularly marginated with spiculated contour and multiple pleural tails. Noncontrast and contrast-enhanced scans with mediastinal window settings (B and C) reveal significant enhancement >15 HU on the postcontrast scans—Malignant lesion.

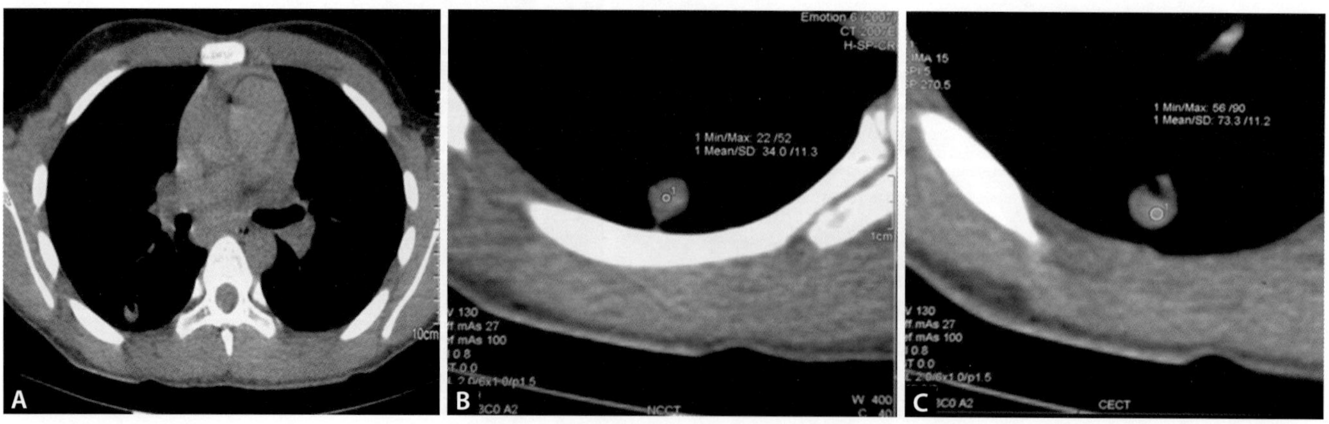

Figs. 23A to C: (A) CT scan image showing a lesion <1 cm in size in the right lower lobe with an eccentric cavitation. Pre- (B) and postcontrast (C) images reveal an enhancement of 34 HU (56-22 HU) suggestive of a malignant nodule.

For benign nodules:
- Wash in <25 HU
- Wash in ≥25 HU with a washout ≥31 HU
- Wash in ≥25 HU and a persistent enhancement without a washout.

For malignant nodules:[70]
- Wash in ≥25 HU
- Washout of 5–31 HU (not more than 31 HU).

The arterial supply of a nodule is via the bronchial arteries while the washout is via the bronchial veins. In the case of malignancy, a retarded flow in the intravascular and interstitial space accounts for contrast retention.[71] In the case of benign nodules, this washout takes place through relatively straight vessels and active lymphatic flow resulting in a significant washout. A persistent enhancement when seen in a benign nodule occurs due to the presence of fibrosis in the nodule, the fibrotic portion of the nodule retaining contrast for a long time without washout.

Table 3: LRs for selected radiologic features of nodules and patient characteristics.[76-78]

Feature or characteristic	*LR*
Spiculated margin	5.54
>3 cm	5.23
>70 years	4.16
Malignant growth rate	3.40
Smoker	2.27
Upper lobe location	1.22
<1 cm	0.52
Smooth margins	0.30
30–39 years	0.24
Never smoked	0.19
20–29 years	0.05
Benign calcification	0.01
Benign growth rate	0.01

Bayesian Analysis

The risk factor of the patients should be evaluated when a SPN is considered to be indeterminate in the initial examination. Age is an important factor in the evaluation with lung cancer being uncommon in patients younger than 40 years and being rare in those below 35 years of age (<1% of all cases).[72] The risk of developing cancer in male smokers is about 10 times than in non-smokers and the risk is related to the degree and duration of cigarette smoking.[73,74] A history of cancer in first degree relative, occupational exposure, exposure to asbestos, radon and uranium are other risk factors for the development of lung carcinoma.[75]

Bayesian analysis can be useful in the evaluation of these indeterminate solitary pulmonary nodules by allowing more precise determination of the probability of malignancy (pCa). Bayesian analysis uses likelihood ratio (LRs) for numerous radiological findings and clinical features associated with solitary pulmonary nodules to estimate pCa **(Table 3)**.

In a new Bayesian model that has been proposed, certain morphological features like edge have been added, criteria such as VDT, minimum HU and CT enhancement have been introduced as predictive features. The new model is an important update on Bayesian analysis and allows for a better differentiation between benign and malignant entities. [79]

Fluorodeoxyglucose Positron Emission Tomography

Nodule metabolism can be evaluated by functional imaging with fluorine 18 (^{18}F)- labelled fluorodeoxyglucose (FDG) positron emission tomography (PET). The technique is a measure of glucose metabolism and aids in the differentiation of benign and malignant nodules[80] **(Figs. 24A to D)**. A standardized uptake value (SUV) of more than 2.5 is usually seen in malignancy while a value less than 2.5 is seen in benign lesions. PET has a sensitivity and specificity of about 90% for detecting malignant nodules which are larger than 10 mm in diameter, but this high sensitivity and specificity is applicable to solid nodules. In the case of partly solid nodule (PSN) and ground-glass attenuation nodule (GGAN) FDG uptake cannot be used to reliably distinguish between benign and malignant lesions. PET has been found to have a sensitivity as low as 10% and specificity of about 20% for evaluating ground-glass opacities.[81] Also, FDG PET can give false negative results in the case of carcinoid tumors, mucinous adenocarcinomas and adenocarcinomas in situ and false positive results in the case of inflammation and infection.[82,83] There may be a respiratory mismatch between CT and PET images leading to an underestimation of the SUV with resultant false negative result. It has been suggested that a respiratory averaged CT, i.e. CT cine images obtained over different portions of the respiratory cycle rather than a mid-expiratory CT improves SUV quantification.

Transthoracic Needle Aspiration Biopsy (TNAB)

For a SPN with a high clinical suspicion of malignancy, surgical resection is the best option if the lesion is operable as needle biopsy does not alter management. If the biopsy result is positive, resection has to be done, a negative result

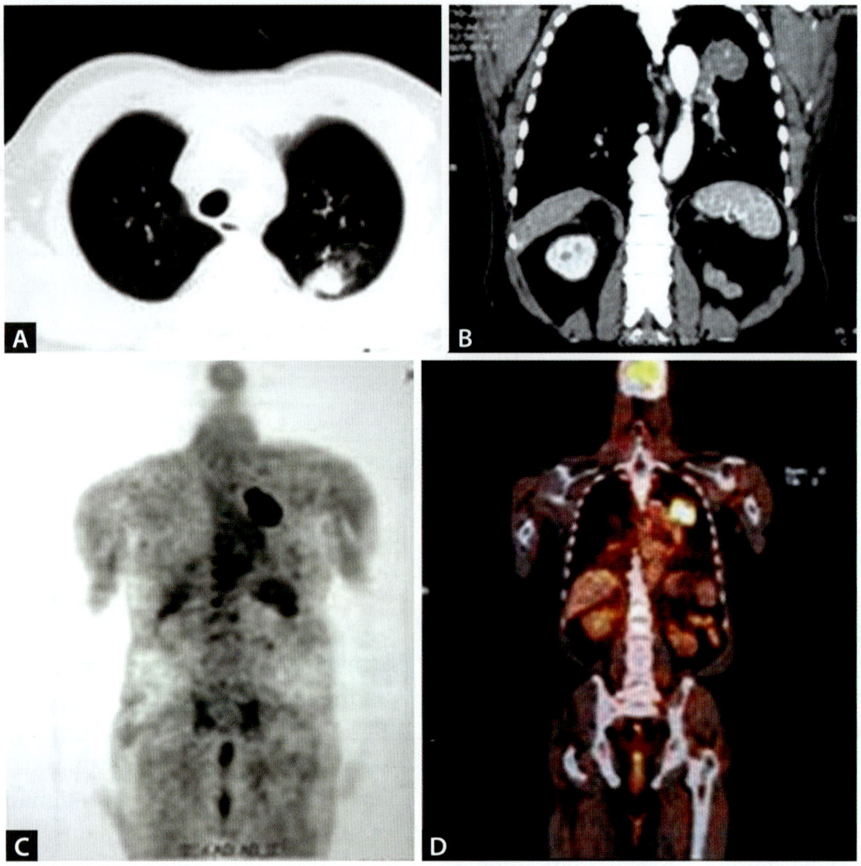

Figs. 24A to D: CT chest axial and MPR images (A and B) showing an irregularly marginated lesion with surrounding halo in the left upper lobe. FDG PET scans (C and D) in the patient showing an increased uptake and accumulation of FDG in the nodule—malignant lesion/ bronchogenic carcinoma.

does not exclude malignancy and has to be followed by resection if there is a high clinical suspicion of malignancy as the sensitivity of this technique is about 60% for lesions less than 2 cm in diameter **(Figs. 25A to D)**. The diagnostic yield further falls to 51% for GGO dominant lesions.[84] Thus, needle biopsy is usually indicated for inoperable SPN to confirm the histology. As compared to bronchoscopy, the complication rate of TNAB is high. Complications include pneumothorax and hemorrhage seen in about 5–30% of cases.[85]

Fiberoptic Bronchoscopy

Fiberoptic bronchoscopy (FOB) with transbronchial biopsy and washing has a limited role in evaluating SPN. Although transbronchial biopsy is accurate for assessing endobronchial lesions, the yield for peripheral nodules is less than 60 percent and is only 25 to 30 percent for a SPN smaller than 2 cm. The sensitivity of FOB is best when a bronchus leads directly to or is seen within the SPN (the positive bronchus sign).[35]

NEWER IMAGING TECHNIQUES FOR THE EVALUATION OF SPN

Dynamic MR Imaging

Blood patterns and tissue perfusion have been studied by dynamic MR imaging in liver, brain and breast. This technique can be used to characterize SPNs as well.[86] Signal intensity time curves are generated following intravenous injection of gadolinium and maximum relative enhancement ratio and shape of enhancement can be calculated from these. A ratio >0.15 indicates a malignant SPN, a ratio <0.80 indicates benign lesion and ratio between 0.8 and 0.15 usually indicates active infection. These MR indices are useful for differentiating between benign and malignant SPNs.[87,88]

Diffusion-weighted MRI Imaging

MRI has an inherent advantage in terms of tissue characterization. Tissue contrast attained using diffusion weighted imaging (DWI) is different from that obtained

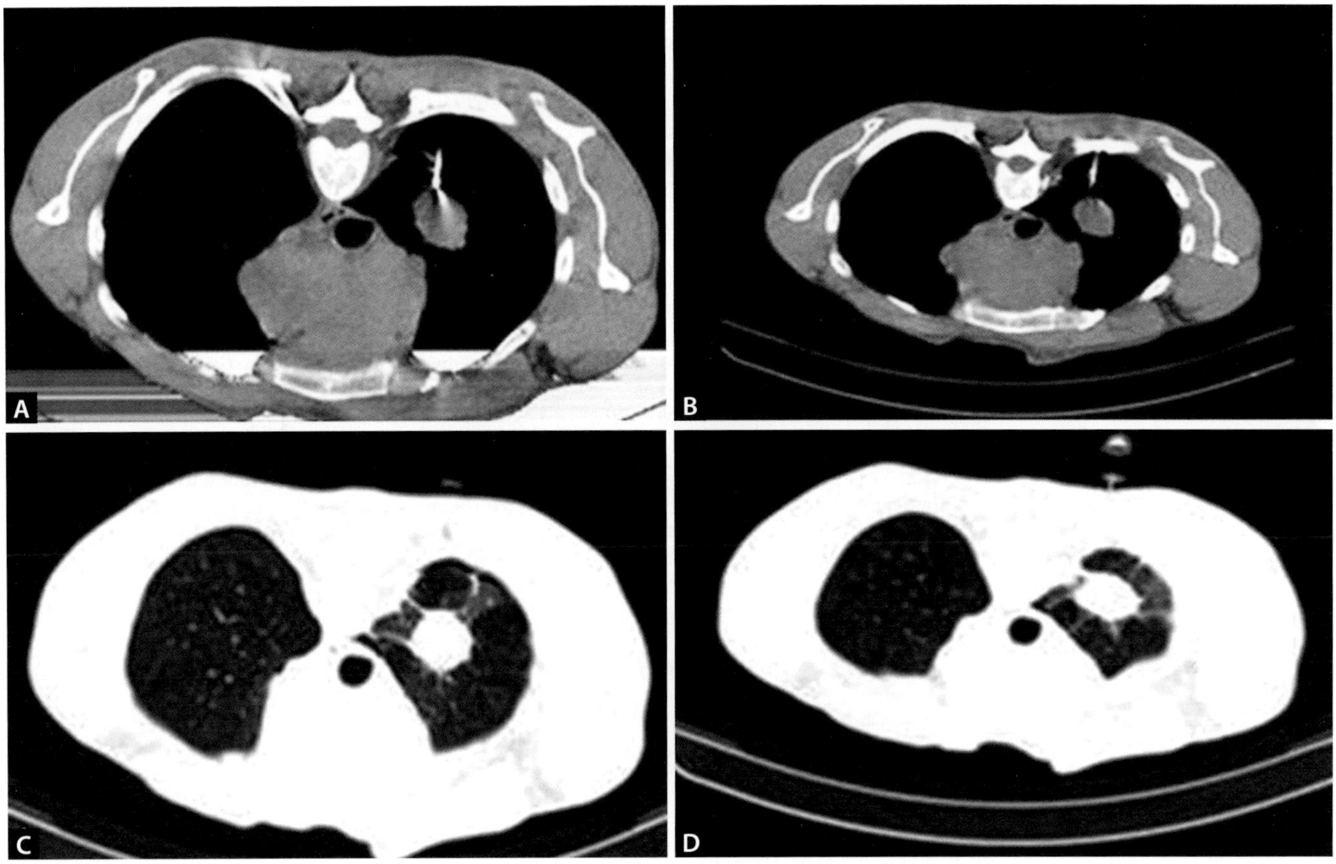

Figs. 25A to D: Transthoracic needle aspiration in a case of a nodule in the right lung with needle in situ (A and B) in prone position. The nodule is irregularly marginated with evidence of corona radiata and multiple pleural tails (C and D)—Bronchogenic carcinoma.

using conventional MR sequences. In a study by Satoh, et al difference between benign and malignant was based on a DWI scale graded from 1 to 5. These were: 1) nearly no signal intensity as seen in an almost normal lung; 2) signal intensity between 1 and 3; 3) Signal intensity almost equal to the spinal cord at thoracic spine; 4) higher signal than spinal cord; 5) much higher signal than that of the spinal cord. A score of 3 (a nodule with signal intensity equal to that of the spinal cord) was considered the threshold for differentiation between benign and malignant pulmonary nodules in their study.[89] Lower ADC values for malignant lesions has been reported helping in their characterization.

Dual Energy CT in the Evaluation of SPN

Angiogenesis of malignant nodules leads to a stronger enhancement of malignant tumors on CT. Iodine is the main ingredient of contrast medium and directly reflects blood flow. Iodine concentration maps can assess the vasculature and relative vascularity of pulmonary nodule. By single scanning after contrast injection, the degree of enhancement can be obtained without an additional non-enhanced scan. Iodine concentration in malignant nodules has been found to be significantly higher than benign nodules, thus allowing for the differentiation between benign and malignant nodules.[90] Owing to its material decomposition ability, DECT allows differentiation of calcification from enhanced tissue.

MANAGEMENT OF A SOLITARY PULMONARY NODULE

Following the Fleischner Society Guidelines of solid nodules in 2005[91] and the subsolid nodules in 2013[92-94] several modifications have taken place leading to the new guidelines of the Fleischner Society in 2017 **(Table 4)**.

The Fleischner Society guidelines are not for:

I. Patients with known primary cancer
II. Immunocompromised patients who are at risk of infection
III. Those at risk for metastasis
IV. Children and adults younger than 35 years

Table 4: Fleischner Society 2017 guidelines for management of incidentally detected pulmonary nodules in adults.*[95]

A: Solid nodules				
Nodule type	***Size***			***Comments***
	<6 mm (<100 mm³)	6–8 mm (100–250 mm³)	>8 mm (>250 mm³)	
Single: • Low risk	No routine follow-up	CT at 6–12 months, then consider CT at 18–24 months	Consider CT, PET/CT, or tissue sampling at 3 months	Nodules <6 mm do not require routine follow-up, but certain patients at high risk with suspicious nodule morphology, upper lobe location, or both may warrant 12-month follow-up
• High risk	Optional CT at 12 months	CT at 6–12 months, then CT at 18–24 months	Consider CT, PET/CT, or tissue sampling at 3 months	Nodules <6 mm do not require routine follow-up, but certain patients at high risk with suspicious nodule morphology, upper lobe location, or both may warrant 12-month follow-up
Multiple: • Low risk	No routine follow-up	CT at 3–6 months, then consider CT at 18–24 months	CT at 3–6 months, then consider CT at 18–24 months	Use most suspicious nodule as guide to management. Follow-up intervals may vary according to size and risk.
• High risk	Optional CT at 12 months	CT at 3–6 months, then at 18–24 months	CT at 3–6 months, then at 18–24 months	Use most suspicious nodule as guide to management. Follow-up intervals may vary according to size and risk

B: Subsolid nodules			
Nodule type	***Size***		***Comments***
	<6 mm (<100 mm³)	≥6 mm (>100 mm³)	
Single: • Ground-glass	No routine follow-up	CT at 6–12 months to confirm persistence, then CT every 2 years until 5 years	In certain suspicious nodules <6 mm, consider follow-up at 2 and 4 years. If solid component(s) or growth develops, consider resection.
• Part solid	No routine follow-up	CT at 3–6 months to confirm persistence. If unchanged and solid component remains 6 mm, annual CT should be performed for 5 years	In practice, part-solid nodules cannot be defined as such until ≥6 mm, and nodules <6 mm do not usually require follow-up. Persistent part-solid nodules with solid components ≥6 mm should be considered highly suspicious
Multiple:	CT at 3–6 months. If stable, consider CT at 2 and 4 years	CT at 3–6 months. Subsequent management based on the most suspicious nodule(s)	Multiple <6 mm pure ground-glass nodules are usually benign, but consider follow-up in selected patients at high risk at 2 and 4 years

*These are the new guidelines given by the Fleischner Society 2017 for incidentally detected pulmonary nodules in adult patients <35 years of age.[95]

Management in these groups should be based on the specific clinical situation and on a case-by-case basis.

Changes in the revised guidelines include:

1. The minimum threshold of the nodule for follow-up has been increased to 6 mm rather than 5 mm.
2. Follow-up intervals have been given a range rather than a precise time period.
3. The guidelines for solid and semisolid nodules are now included in one single table with specific recommendations for multiple nodules.

For multiple nodules, the subsequent management is based on suspicious nodule which may not be the largest nodule. Pure GGNs more than 10 mm, part solid GGN with solid component larger than 5 mm, bubbly appearance of reticulation, atypical subsolid nodules with spiculation should be interpreted with high degree of suspicion.

It has been recommended that thin CT sections of the thorax (≤1 mm) should be performed to enable accurate characterization of the small pulmonary nodules. Sagittal and coronal reconstruction should always be obtained. A low radiation dose technique is recommended for follow up CT scans with the use of dose modulation and iterative reconstruction techniques to reduce radiation. According to the ACR recommendations for screening CT, the CT dose index volume (CTDI vol) should not be more than 3 mGy.[96]

It is also recommended that the average of the long and short axis diameters rather than the maximum transverse diameter should be taken as it yields better results. All measurements should be rounded to the nearest mm rather than fractional millimeter measurements. It is stated that volumetric measurements can be performed instead of linear measurements with volume of 100 and 250 mm^3 corresponding to the 6 and 8 mm thresholds. Volumetric measurements should be performed with identical software versions.[95]

The differential diagnosis of a SPN is given in **Table 5**.

Table 5: Differential diagnosis of solitary pulmonary nodule.[97]

• **Malignant neoplasm:** – Carcinoma (squamous cell, small cell, adenocarcinoma, bronchioloalveolar carcinoma) – Lymphoma – Carcinoid – Pulmonary metastasis (colon, melanoma, renal cell, breast, osteosarcoma)
• **Benign neoplasm and neoplasm-like condition:** – Hamartoma – Chondroma – Fibroma
• **Infective causes:** – Round pneumonia – Abscess – Granuloma (fungal, mycobacterial)
• **Noninfectious inflammatory:** – Sarcoidosis – Rheumatoid arthritis – Amyloidosis – Wegener's granulomatosis
• **Airway and inhalational disease:** – Mucoid impaction (mucous plug) – Bronchial atresia – Cystic fibrosis – Conglomerate mass or progressive massive fibrosis (e.g. silicosis) – Lipoid pneumonia
• **Vascular lesions:** – Pulmonary artery aneurysm – Hematoma – Infarct – Arteriovenous malformation (AVM)
• **Congenital lesions:** – Sequestration – Bronchogenic cyst – Bronchial atresia
• **Idiopathic/Miscellaneous:** – Amyloidosis – Fluid filled bulla – Round atelectasis

MORPHOLOGICAL CHARACTERISTICS IN SPECIFIC LESIONS

Lung Malignancies

About 20% of lung cancers present as SPNs **(Figs. 26A and B)**. The most common type presenting as a nodule is adenocarcinoma. Bronchogenic carcinoma will show irregular, spiculated margins with absence of calcification. However, presence of calcification does not completely rule out malignancy as cancers may develop in a scar or granuloma which shows pre-existing calcification. The pre-existing calcification is usually of the stippled or eccentric type and occupies less than 10% of the nodule.

Metastasis

Though metastatic nodules are usually multiple, rarely these may present as solitary pulmonary nodule. Carcinoma of the colon, melanoma and carcinomas of the kidney and testicle may present with solitary metastasis **(Figs. 27A and B)**.

The metastatic nodules are usually sharply marginated though local invasion and surrounding hemorrhage may lead to the nodules being poorly defined. Metastatic lesions are predominantly seen in the lung bases because of greater blood flow. "Feeding vessel sign" may be seen in these nodules owing to a hematogenous origin because these nodules are usually seen at the tips of small arteries.[98]

Carcinoid Tumor

These account for 10–20% of SPNs. These are neuroendocrine tumors and two forms have been described: typical and atypical. Typical carcinoids account for 85–90% of these lesions and occur in the main, lobar or segmental bronchi in a central location. The atypical ones usually have a peripheral location with a worse prognosis than the typical variety.[99] Carcinoids can be intraluminal or extraluminal and are seen as well-defined, lobulated, round or notched with a smooth edge. Spiculation is rarely seen. Curvilinear or multiple nodular calcification may be seen. Rarely, dense ossification may be seen within the lesion.

A triad of:

- Well defined, lobulated round lesion
- Location adjacent to bronchial bifurcation
- Eccentric calcification

Is highly suggestive of bronchial carcinoid **(Figs. 28A to C)**.[100]

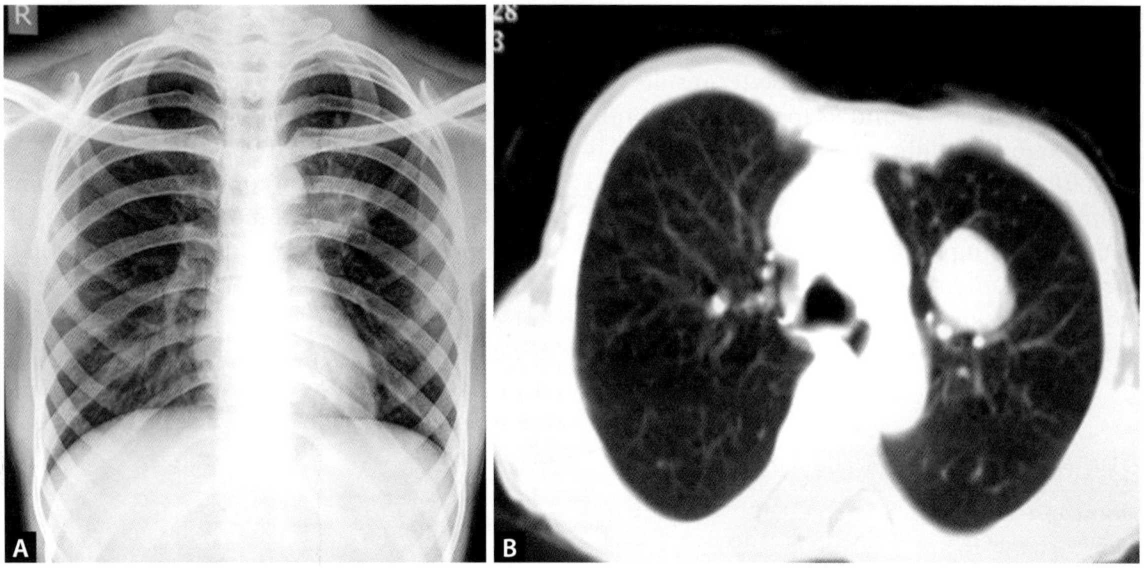

Figs. 26A and B: Chest radiograph shows a large nodule with irregular margins in the left upper lobe. Larger the lesion the more likely it is to be malignant—Bronchogenic carcinoma.

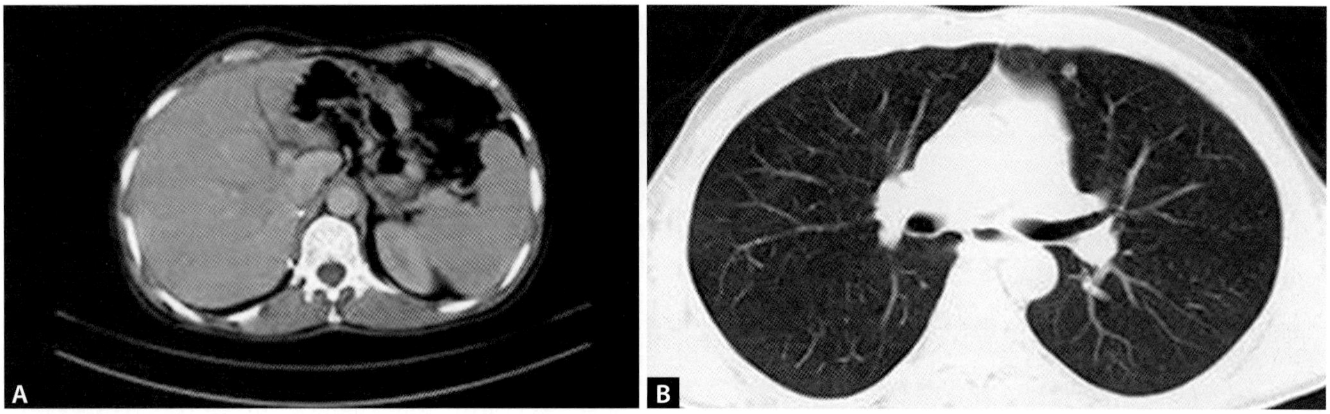

Figs. 27A and B: Follow-up CT scan (A) in a postoperative case of right renal cell carcinoma showing a small, smoothly marginated round solitary lesion in the left lung. The lesion is seen at the tip of a small artery (feeding vessel sign) (B)—Solitary metastasis in renal cell carcinoma.

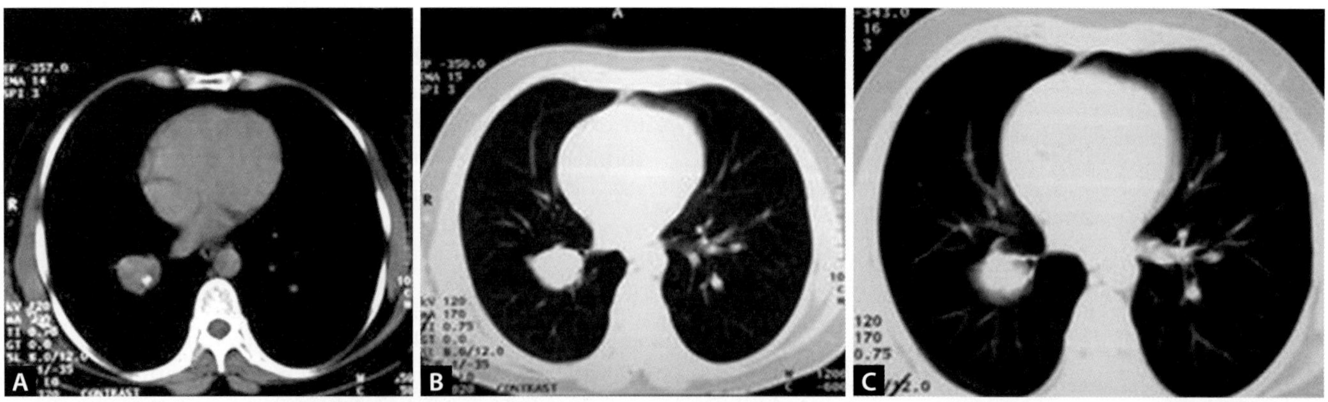

Figs. 28A to C: CT sections showing a well-defined rounded lesion in the right lung lying centrally in a perihilar location/vicinity of bronchial bifurcation with eccentric calcification noted within (A). Lung window shows the lesion to have a smooth edge with minimal lobulations (B). The right lower lobe bronchus shows the characteristic widening as it approaches the tumor (C)—Bronchial carcinoid.

Lymphoma

Both Hodgkin's and non-Hodgkin's lymphoma involves the lung in about 10–15% cases and is characterized by single/multiple nodules, masses or consolidation which may cavitate. Associated hilar and mediastinal adenopathy is usually present.[101]

Benign Neoplasms

Pulmonary Hamartoma

It is a benign pulmonary mass composed of cartilage, myxomatous connective tissue, fat, marrow, bone, smooth muscle in different amounts. 90% of the hamartomas have a peripheral location. These are seen as well-defined, round or lobulated nodules with a characteristic "popcorn calcification" owing to the cartilaginous and osseous component.[102] CT detects fat as areas with negative attenuation values. The presence of fat and calcification within a well-defined nodule is virtually diagnostic of a pulmonary hamartoma **(Figs. 29A to C)**.[103]

Other Benign Tumors

These may arise from epithelial or mesenchymal tissue. Carney's triad is a condition comprising of multiple pulmonary chondromas, extra-adrenal paragangliomas and gastric epitheloid leiomyosarcoma. This condition is seen in women less than 35 years of age, the presence of multiple cartilage tumors in the lung should warrant a search for the other tumors which are more lethal than chondromas.[104]

Infective Causes

Granuloma

The most common cause of granuloma is tubercular though other causes include histoplasmosis, cryptococcosis, coccidioidomycosis. These are seen as a solitary nodule 1–3 cm in diameter with a well-defined smooth regular margin and often showing calcification **(Figs. 30A to C)**. The patterns of calcification seen in a granuloma include amorphous, punctate, fleck-like or laminar, often subpleural in location, granulomas rarely show cavitation. Cavitation when seen should suggest reactivation.

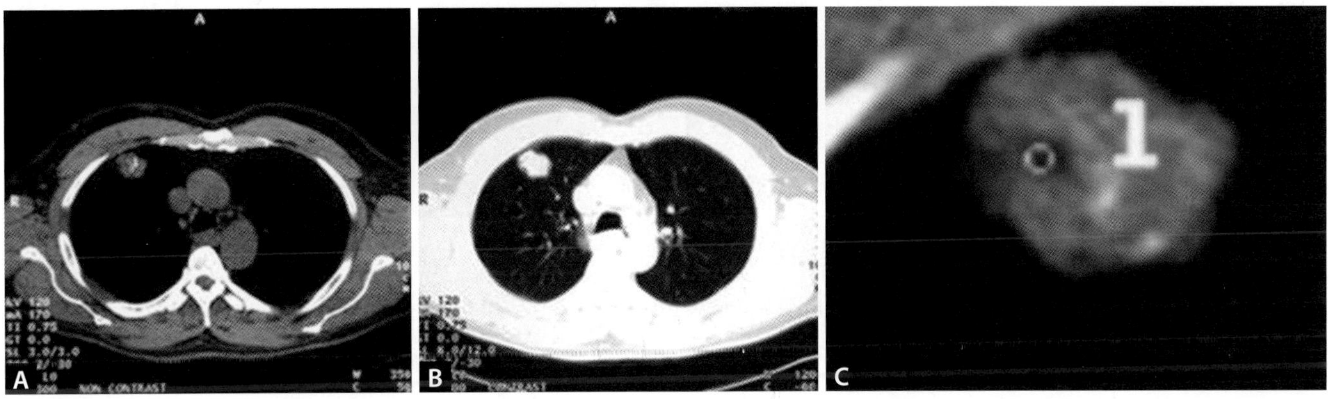

Figs. 29A to C: CT chest mediastinal (A) and lung parenchymal (B) window settings revealing a well-defined nodular lesion in the right upper lobe. The lesion shows fat attenuation (negative attenuation) values within. Magnified view of the lesion (C) showing the fat clearly and small specks of calcification in the lesion—Pulmonary hamartoma.

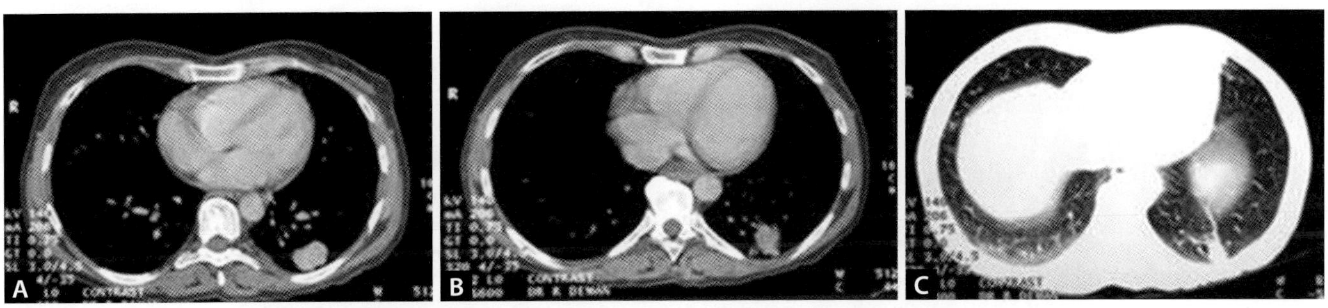

Figs. 30A to C: CT scans showing a single well-defined lesion 2 cm in size located subpleurally with no evidence of cavitation (A). The lesion shows evidence of multiple fibrotic strands around it (B and C)—Tuberculoma.

Hydatid Cyst

Caused by Echinococcus granulosus, the hydatid cyst is seen as a sharply demarcated, well-defined round or oval lesion with a homogeneous soft tissue density on radiographs **(Figs. 31A and B)**. The cysts occur more commonly in mid and lower lobes. An air-fluid level, water lily sign and rising sun sign are seen in cases of rupture of the hydatid cyst.

Mycetoma/Fungal Ball

A mycetoma results from saphrophytic invasion of a pre-existing cavity. The causes of the cavity in the majority of the cases is tubercular, but sarcoidosis, bronchiectasis, bulla, histoplasmosis, etc. may also result in a cavity in which the fungal mass develops. Matting of the aspergillus hyphae results in a fungal ball/mycetoma seen as a intracavitory mass in the upper lobe or superior segment of lower lobe usually. "Air-crescent sign" (air between the wall of the cavity and the fungal ball) is usually seen and is a diagnostic imaging finding **(Figs. 32A and B)**. CT shows a sponge like appearance of the mass with irregular air spaces.

Round Pneumonia

Round pneumonias are more commonly seen in children in cases of Streptococcus infection. Other causative organisms include K.pneumoniae, S.aureus, M.tuberculosis and fungi. On imaging round pneumonia appears as a focal round wedge shaped opacity in a peripheral location typically in the posterior lower lobe **(Figs. 33A and B)**. These have a predominant posterior

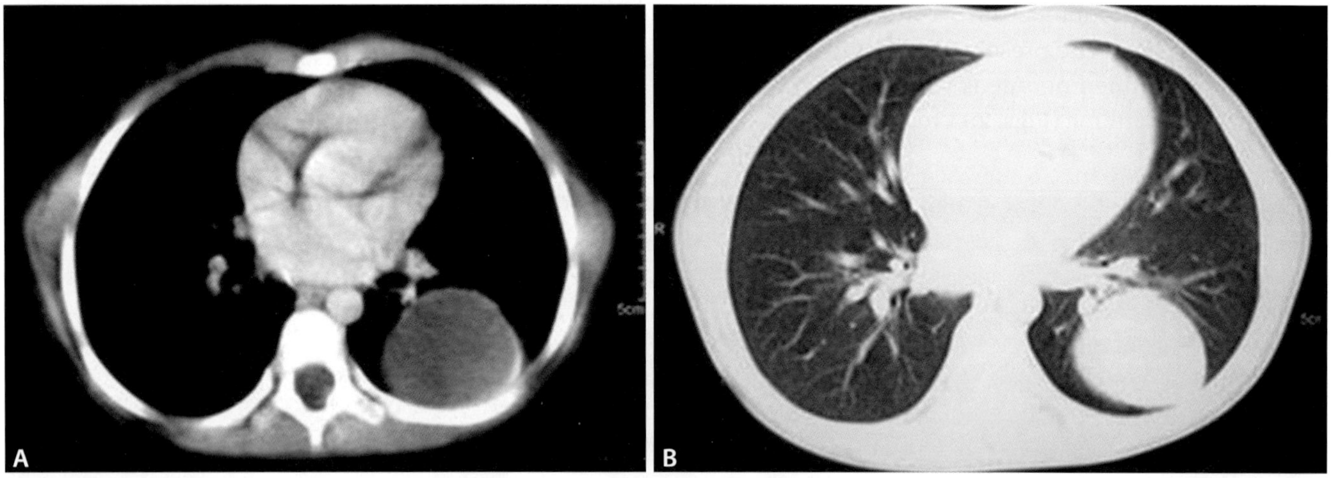

Figs. 31A and B: CT scan chest mediastinal (A) and lung windows (B) showing an oval, sharply marginated homogeneous fluid density cystic lesion in the left lower lobe—Hydatid cyst.

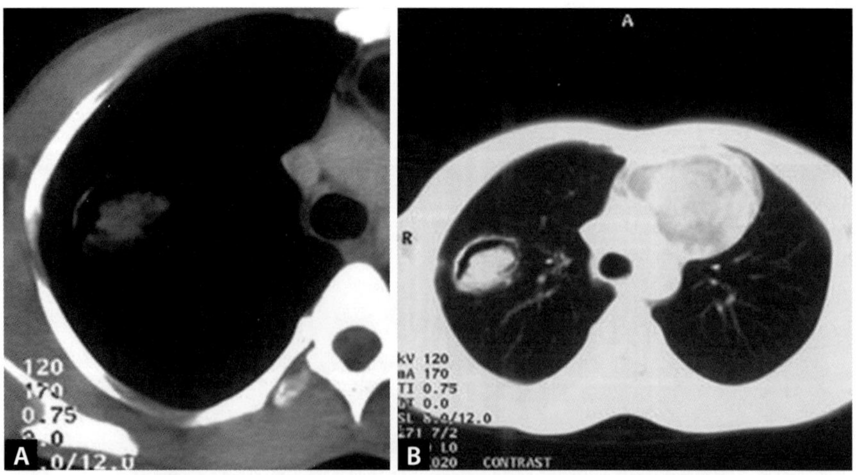

Figs. 32A and B: CT sections of the chest mediastinal and lung windows (A and B) showing the "air meniscus sign" seen as air crescent between the mass and the cavity in the right lung—Mycetoma.

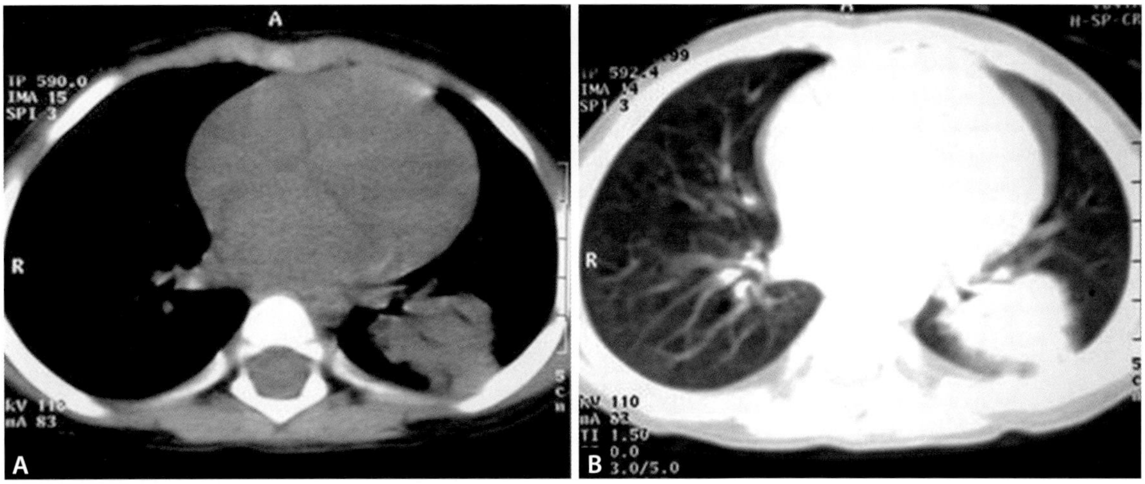

Figs. 33A and B: CT scan in a 2-year-old child showing a peripherally located wedge-shaped opacity with air bronchogram within the left lower lobe located posteriorly. The opacity is based against a focally thickened pleura—Round pneumonia.

distribution owing to the supine sleeping position of children while the gravity dependent passage of bacteria loaded fluid into the most dependent bronchus accounts for the lower lobe distribution. The underdeveloped pores of Kohn and the absence of canals of Lambert in children accounts for the sharp margins of the round pneumonia in contrast to the ill-defined margins of pneumonia seen in adults.[105] The centrifugal pattern of spread of the inflammation results in the lesion margin being sharply demarcated from the unaffected lung parenchyma **(Figs. 34A to C)**.

Lung Abscess

The etiology can be pyogenic, anaerobic bacteria or mycobacterial. Radiographs show an abscess as an ill-defined opacity with surrounding consolidation. An air-fluid level is seen in cases of communication with the bronchus. Contrast enhancement CT shows the abscess as a hypodense lesion with thick enhancing walls, shaggy margins and an air fluid level **(Figs. 35A to C)**.

Inflammatory Nodules

Rheumatoid Nodules

These are an uncommon manifestation of rheumatoid arthritis, may be seen as solitary or multiple nodules in the lung parenchyma.[106]

Airway or Inhalational Disease

Lipoid Pneumonia

Lipoid pneumonia is seen as an ill-defined nodule or mass in posterior lower lobe. Exogenous variety of lipoid pneumonia results from chronic aspiration of fat while the endogenous form occurs due to accumulation of lipid rich cellular debris distal to bronchial obstruction.

Vascular Lesions

Pulmonary Artery Aneurysm

Pulmonary artery aneurysm can present as a lung nodule.[107] Rasmussen aneurysm is seen in tuberculosis and is a mycotic aneurysm developing in the infectious cavity. Contrast-enhanced CT is diagnostic as the aneurysm is seen as a densely opacified nodular lesion in relation to lobar, segmental or smaller arteries **(Figs. 36A to C)**.

Pulmonary Vein Varix

A varix can result from a congenital defect of the wall, mitral valvular diseases or elevated pulmonary venous pressure. Radiologically, a pulmonary varix is seen as a round or oval density adjacent to the left atrium. Usually asymptomatic, a pulmonary varix can enlarge in response to high atrial pressure with resultant rupture and hemorrhage.

Arteriovenous Malformation

Arteriovenous malformation (AVM) is characterized by an enlarged artery feeding the nodule and a draining vein. Radiographs reveal the AVM as a well circumscribed nodule with a lobular outline, usually seen in the lower lobe, in a subpleural location. Contrast-enhanced CT reveals rapid enhancement and washout in the pulmonary AVM corresponding to the opacification and washout of the main pulmonary artery and right ventricle.[108]

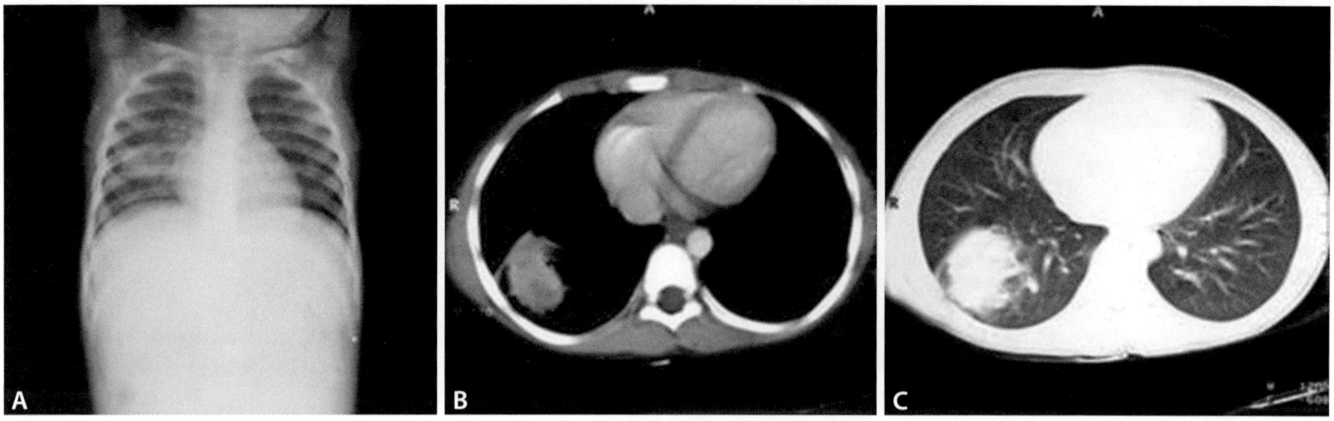

Figs. 34A to C: Chest radiograph (A) in a child showing a focal round nodule in the right lung. CT sections (B and C) showing an area of spherical consolidation in the right lower lobe with associated pleural thickening—Round pneumonia.

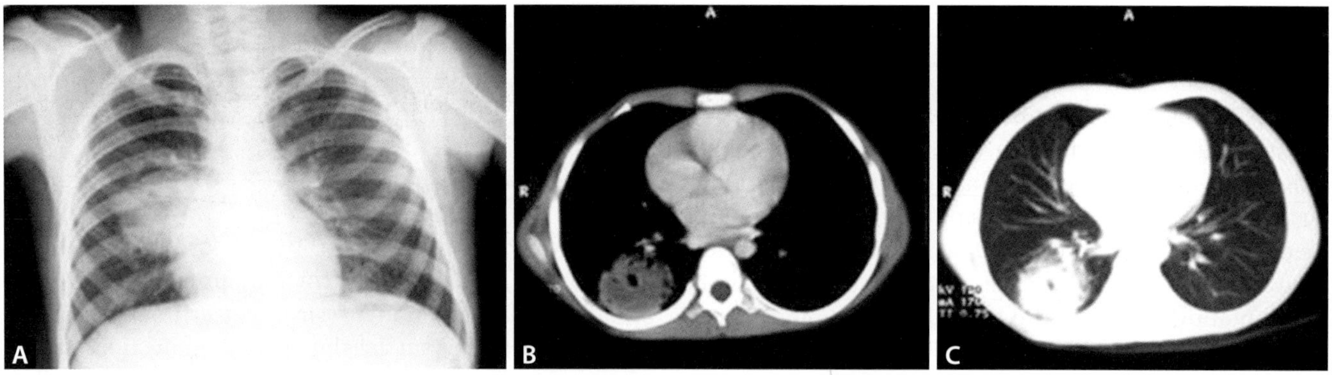

Figs. 35A to C: Chest radiograph (A) showing a focal round lesion in the right lung. A small air loculus is seen within. CT sections (B and C) showing a low attenuation lesion (i.e. fluid attenuation) lesion with enhancing wall. Multiple air loculi are seen in the center and in the periphery of the lesion (B). The margins are mildly irregular with surrounding consolidation (C)—Lung abscess.

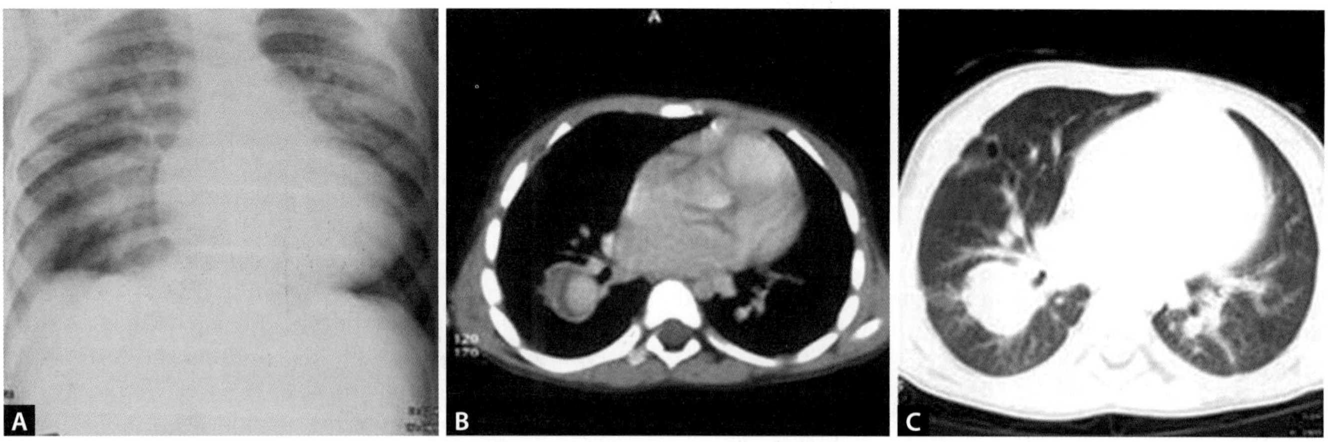

Figs. 36A to C: Chest radiograph (A) showing a sharply marginated solitary lesion located centrally in a perihilar location in the right lung (A). CT sections (B and C) showing an enhancing nodule in relation to a right interlobar pulmonary artery. A crescentic hypodensity is seen in the periphery of the lesion symptom of thrombus—Pulmonary artery aneurysm.

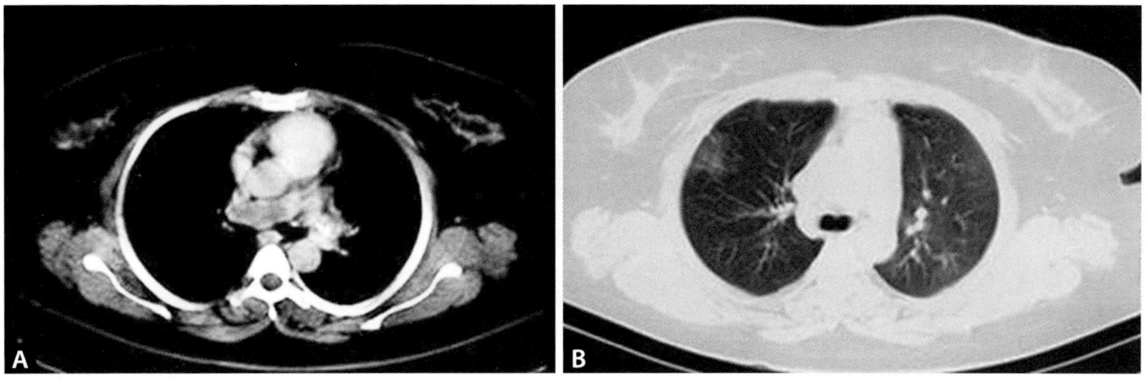

Figs. 37A and B: Contrast-enhanced CT (A) in a case of DVT showing a filling defect in the right pulmonary artery suggestive of thrombus. Lung parenchyma (B) shows a wedge-shaped pleural based opacity with surrounding halo symptoms of Hampton's hump in the right lung—Pulmonary infarction.

Pulmonary Infarction

A pulmonary infarct is seen as a wedge-shaped opacity in contact with the pleural surface known as Hampton's hump **(Figs. 37A and B)**. A halo sign due to adjacent hemorrhage or low attenuating areas due to necrosis may be seen. On contrast administration, feeding vessels may be seen and the periphery of the infarct may enhance owing to collateral flow. Cavitation of a pulmonary infarct occurs with infection of the bland infarct or with septic emboli. Pulmonary infarcts decrease in their size slowly over months what has been described as the "melting sign".[109]

Congenital Lesions

Pulmonary Bronchogenic Cyst

A bronchogenic cyst results from abnormal development of the lung bud. On the radiographs, it is seen as a well-circumscribed mass in a perihilar or subcarinal location. The fluid in the cyst can be serous, viscous and gelatinous or hemorrhagic. An air fluid level may be seen if the cyst is infected.

On CT, a variable density of the cyst ranging from water to soft tissue may be seen. The wall of the cyst is usually thin and smooth **(Fig. 38)**.

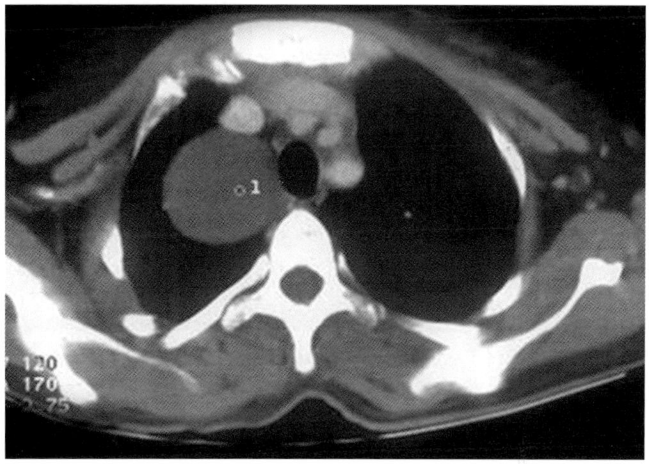

Fig. 38: CT scan showing a well-circumscribed cystic density lesion adjacent to the trachea on the right side. The cyst wall is thin and smooth—Bronchogenic cyst.

Sequestration

A disorganized area of pulmonary parenchyma without normal pulmonary arterial or bronchial communication is called sequestrated lung. It is of two types intralobar and extralobar. Intralobar, the more common form, occurs usually in the posterior basal segment of the left lower lobe adjacent to the diaphragm **(Figs. 39A to D)**.[110] The intralobar form has a normal pulmonary venous drainage and infections are common in this form. The extralobar variety is more commonly associated with other congenital anomalies, has its own pleural covering and is separate with a systemic venous drainage.

Miscellaneous

Round Atelectasis

Round atelectasis is a type of chronic atelectasis resembling a mass lesion. It is most often associated with asbestos related pleural disease but it may occur in association with other conditions like tuberculosis, other infections, Dressler syndrome and mesothelioma. According to one of the suggested mechanisms, the common event is pleural thickening and pleural exudates with the resultant effusion causing passive atelectasis of the adjacent lung. Fibrinous adhesions develop between the pleural surface of the atelectatic lung and the adjacent parietal pleura.

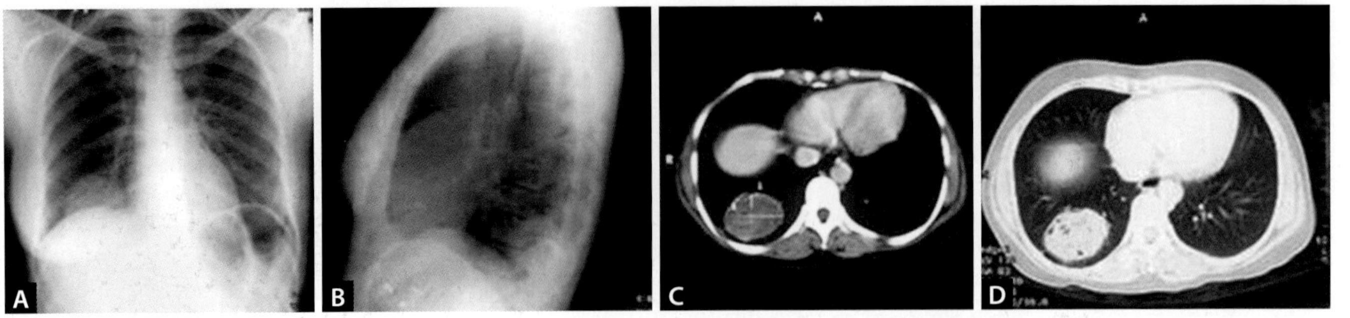

Figs. 39A to D: Chest radiograph frontal (A) and lateral projection (B) in a 35-year-female with recurrent chest infections showing a well-defined sharply marginated lesion in the posterior basal segment of the right lower lobe. CT sections (C and D) showing a hypodense well-circumscribed lesion with multiple air foci suggesting communication with adjacent bronchi due to infection—Pulmonary intralobar sequestration.

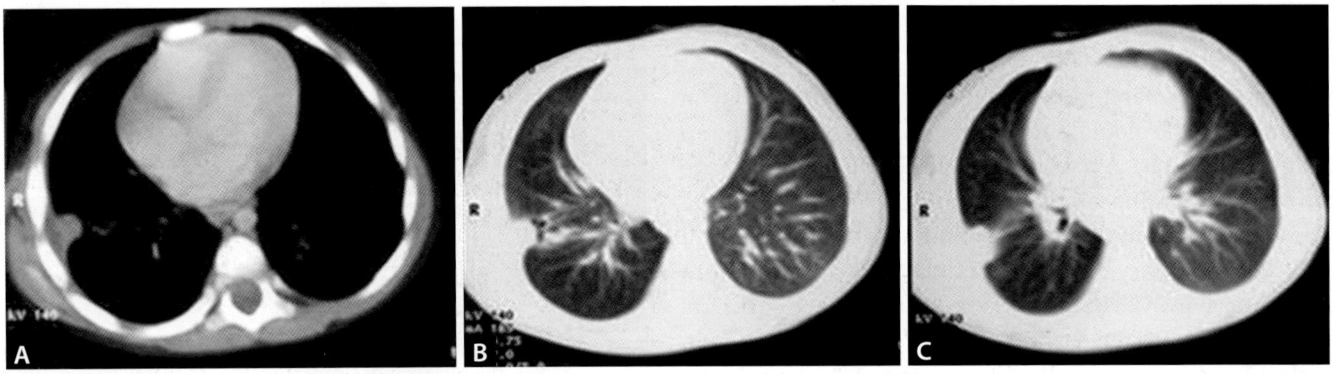

Figs. 40A to C: CT sections showing a peripherally located wedge-shaped opacity against thickened pleura (A). There is distortion and displacement of vessels adjacent to the opacity. The vessels are more numerous than normal in this portion (B) and have a characteristic curvilinear configuration (C)—Round atelectasis.

Another explanation is that as the pleural fibrosis matures, it retracts causing infolding and atelectasis of the lung parenchyma.[111]

On imaging, round atelectasis is seen as a peripheral opacity which is oval or wedge shaped. It is based against a thickened pleura with the edge pointing towards the hilum being ill-defined and irregular. Distortion, displacement of the blood vessels and bronchi which appear pulled towards the lesion forms a characteristic imaging appearance called the "comet tail" or "crow feet" appearance **(Figs. 40A to C)**. Air bronchograms and calcification may be seen.[112] Round atelectasis may show contrast enhancement. Though mostly static, it may shrink and rarely resolve spontaneously.

CONCLUSION

The workup and management of patients with SPNs relies on the imaging features and the clinical findings with the aim to differentiate benign lesions from small malignant tumors. One should strive not only to identify small malignant tumors where resection results in high survival rates, but also spare patients with benign disease from unnecessary surgery.

REFERENCES

1. Midthun DE, Swensen SJ, Jett JR. Approach to the solitary pulmonary nodule. Mayo Clin Proc. 1993;68:378-85.
2. Tuddenham WJ. Glossary of terms for thoracic radiology: recommendations of the Nomenclature Committee of the Fleischner Society. AJR. 1984;143:509-17.
3. Lillington GA, Caskey CI. Evaluation and management of solitary and multiple pulmonary nodules. Clin Chest Med. 1993;14:111-9.
4. Holin SM, Dwork RE, Glaser S, et al. Solitary pulmonary nodules found in a community wide chest roentgenographic survey. Am Rev Tuberc. 1959;79:427-39.
5. Austin JH, Garg K, Aberle D, et al. Radiologic implications of the 2011 classification of adenocarcinoma of the lung. Radiology. 2013;266:62-71.
6. Beigelman-Aubry C, Hill C, Grenier PA. Management of an incidentally discovered pulmonary nodule. Eur Radiol. 2007;17:449-66.

7. Kundel HL. Predictive value and threshold detectability of lung tumors. Radiology. 1981;139(1):25-9.
8. Zerhouni EA, Stitik FP, Siegelman SS, et al. CT of the pulmonary nodule: a cooperative study. Radiology. 1986; 160(2):319-27.
9. Webb WR. Radiologic evaluation of the solitary pulmonary nodule. AJR. 1990;154:701-8.
10. Volterrani L, Vegni V, Pieraccini MGC, et al. Small solitary pulmonary nodule and high resolution CT: a preliminary report. Eur Radiol. 1995;5:443-7.
11. Garland LH. Bronchial carcinomas: lobar distribution of lesions in 250 cases. Calif Med. 1961;94:7-8.
12. Swensen SJ, Viggiano RW, Midthun DE, et al. Lung nodule enhancement at CT: multicentre study. Radiology. 2000;214: 73-80.
13. Winer Muram HT, Jennings SG, Tarver RD, et al. Volumetric growth rate of stage I lung cancer prior to treatment: serial CT scanning. Radiology. 2002;223:798-805.
14. Quinn D, Gianlupi A, Broste S. The changing radiographic presentation of bronchogenic carcinoma with reference to cell types. Chest. 1996;110:1474-9.
15. Swensen SJ, Silverstein MD, Ilstrup DM. The probability of malignancy in solitary pulmonary nodules: application to small radiographically in determinate nodules. Arch Int Med. 1997;157:849-55.
16. Heitzman ER, Markarian B, Raasch BN, et al. Pathways of tumor spread through the lung: radiologic correlations with anatomy and pathology. Radiology 1982;144:3-14.
17. Zwirewich CV, Vedal S, Miller RR, et al. Solitary pulmonary nodule: High resolution CT and radiologic pathologic correlation. Radiology 1991;179:469-76.
18. Khan A, Herman PG, Vorwerk P, et al. Solitary pulmonary nodule: comparison of classification with standard, thin section and reference phantom CT. Radiology. 1991;179:477- 81.
19. Huston J III, Muhm JR. Solitary pulmonary opacities: plain tomography. Radiology. 1987;163:481-5.
20. Hill CA. "Tail" signs associated with pulmonary lesions: critical rappraisal. AJR. 1982;139:311-6.
21. Chen SW, Price J. Focal organizing pneumonia mimicking small peripheral adenocarcinoma on CT scans. Australas Radiol. 1998;42:360-3.
22. Gaeta M, Blandino A, Scribano E, et al. Computed tomography halo sign in pulmonary nodules: frequency and diagnostic value. J Thorac Imaging. 1999;14:109-13.
23. Primack SL, Hartman TE, Lee KS, et al. Pulmonary nodules and the CT halo sign. Radiology 1994;190:513-5.
24. Berger WG, Erly WK, Krupiniski EA, et al. The solitary pulmonary nodule on chest radiography: can we really tell if the nodule is calcified? AJR. 2001;176:201-4.
25. Grewal RG, Austin JH. CT demonstration of calcification in carcinoma of the lung. J Comput Assist Tomogr. 1994;18: 867-71.
26. Mahoney MC, Shipley RT, Corcoran HL, et al. CT demonstration of calcification in carcinoma of the lung. AJR. 1990;154:255-8.
27. Swensen SJ, Morin RL, et al. CT reconstruction algorithm selection in the evaluation of solitary pulmonary nodules. J Comput Assist Tomogr. 1995;19:932-5.
28. Ko JP, Naidich DP. Lung nodule detection and characterization with multislice CT. Radiol Clin North Am. 2003;41:575-97.
29. Woodring JH, Fried AM. Significance of wall thickness in solitary cavities of the lung: A follow up study. AJR. 1983;140: 473-4.
30. Lee Ks, Kim Y. Han J, et al. Bronchioloalveolar carcinoma: clinical, histopathologic and radiologic findings. Radiographics 1997;17:1345-57.
31. Kuriyama K, Tateishi R, Doi O, et al. Prevalence of air bronchograms in small peripheral carcinomas of the lung on thin section CT: Comparison with benign tumors. AJR. 1991;156: 921-4.
32. Kuii M, Templeton PA, White CS, et al. Evaluation of the air bronchogram sign on CT in solitary pulmonary lesions. J Comput Assist Tomogr. 1996;20(6):983-6
33. Milne EN, Zerhouni EA. Blood supply of pulmonary metastases. J Thorac Imaging. 1987;2:15-23.
34. Mori K, Saitou Y, Tominaga K, et al. Small nodular lesions in the lung periphery: new approach to diagnosis with CT. Radiology. 1990;177:843-9.
35. Singh SP. The positive bronchus sign. Radiology. 1998;209:251-2.
36. Proto AV, Thomas SR. Pulmonary nodules studied by computed tomography. Radiology. 1985;156:149-53.
37. Goldstein MS, Rush M, Johnson P, et al. A calcified adenocarcinoma of the lung with very high CT numbers. Radiology. 1984;150:785-6.
38. Zerhouni EA, Boukadoum M, Siddiky MA, et al. A standard phantom for quantitative CT analysis of pulmonary nodules. Radiology. 1983;149:767-73.
39. Heneschke CI, Yankelevitz DF, Mirtcheva R, et al. CT screening for lung cancer: frequency and significance of part solid and non-solid nodules. AJR. 2002;178:1053-7.
40. Li F, Sone S, Abe H, et al. Malignant versus benign nodules at CT screening for lung cancer: Comparison of thin section CT findings. Radiology. 2004;233:793-8.
41. Libby DM, Smith JP, Altorki NK, et al. Managing the small pulmonary nodule discovered by CT. Chest. 2004;125:1522-9.
42. Godoy MCB, Naidich DP. Overview and strategic management of subsolid pulmonary nodules. J Thorac Imaging. 2012;27:240-8.
43. Park CM, Goo JM, Lee HJ, et al. Nodular ground glass opacity at thin section CT: histologic correlation and evaluation of change at follow-up. Radiographics. 2007;27:391-408.
44. Kim H, Park CM, Koh JM, et al. Pulmonary subsolid nodules: what radiologists need to know about imaging features and management strategy. Diagn Interv Radiol. 2014;20:47-57.
45. Honda T, Kondo T, Murakami S et al. Radiologic implications of the 2011 classification of adenocarcinoma of the lung. Radiology. 2013;266(1):62-71.

46. Travis WD, Brambilla E, Noguchi M, et al. Diagnosis of lung adenocarcinoma in resected specimens, implication of the 2011 International Association for the study of Lung Cancer/ American Thoracic Society/European Respiratory Society classification. Arch Pathol Lab Med. 2013;137(5):685-705.
47. Park CM, Goo JM, Lee HJ, et al. CT findings of atypical adenomatous hyperplasia in the lung . Korean J Radiol. 2006;7(2):80-6.
48. Goo JM, Park CM, Lee HJ. Ground glass nodules on CT as imaging biomarkers in the management of lung adenocarcinoma. Am J Roentgenol. 2011;196:533-43.
49. Tsutani Y, Miyata Y, Nakayama H et al. Prognostic significance of using solid versus whole tumour size on high resolution computed tomography for predicting pathologic malignant grade of tumours in clinical stage IA of lung adenocarcinoma: a multicentric study. J Thorac Cardiovasc Surg. 2012;143(3):607-12.
50. Truong MJ, Ko JP, Rosi SE et al. Update in the evaluation of the solitary pulmonary nodule. Radiographics. 2014;34:1658-79.
51. Soubani AO. The evaluation and management of solitary pulmonary nodule. Postgrad Med J. 2008;84:459-66.
52. Wang YX, Gong JS, Suzuki K, et al. Evidence based imaging strategies for solitary pulmonary nodule. J Thorac Dis. 2014;6(7):872-87.
53. Collins VP, Loeffler RK, Twey H. Observations on growth rates in human tumors. AJR. 1956;76:988-1000.
54. Dunnick NR, Parker BR, Castellino RA. Differentiation of benign and malignant pulmonary nodules by growth rate. Radiology. 1962;79:221-32.
55. Godoy MC, Naidisch DP, Subsolid pulmonary nodules and the spectrum of peripheral adenocarcinomas of the lung: recommended interim guidelines for assessment and management. Radiology. 2009;253:606-22.
56. Aoki T, Nakata H, Watanabe H, et al. Evolution of peripheral lung adenocarcinomas: CT findings correlated with histology and tumour doubling time. Am J Roentgenol. 2000;174:763-8.
57. Yankelevitz DF, Heneschke CI. Does 2 year stability imply that pulmonary nodules are benign? AJR. 1997;168:325-8.
58. Revel MP, Lefort C, Bissery A, et al. Pulmonary nodules: preliminary experience with three dimensional evaluation. Radiology. 2004;231:459-66.
59. Kim H, Park CM, Woo S, et al. Pure and part solid pulmonary ground glass nodules: measurement variability of volume and mass in nodules with a solid portion less than or equal to 5 mm. Radiology. 2013;269:585-93.
60. Petrou M, Quint LE, Nan B, et al. Pulmonary nodule volumetric measurement variability as a function of CT slice thickness and nodule morphology. AJR. 2007;188:306-12.
61. Zhang L, Yankelevitz PF, Carter D, et al. Internal growth of non-solid lung nodules: radiologic-pathologic correlation. Radiology. 2012;255:199-206.
62. de Hoop B, Gietema H, Vande Vorst S, et al. Pulmonary ground glass nodules: increase in mass as an early indicator of growth. Radiology. 2010;255:199-206.
63. Girvin F, Ko JP. Pulmonary Nodules: Detection, Assessment and CAD. AJR. 2008;191:1057-69.
64. Wormanns D, Kohl G, Klotz E, et al. Volumetric measurements of pulmonary nodules at multi-row detector CT: in vivo reproducibility. Eur Radiol. 2004;14:86-92.
65. Littleton JT, Durizch ML, Moeller G, et al. Pulmonary masses: contrast enhancement. Radiol. 1990;177:861-71.
66. Zhang M, Kono M. Solitary pulmonary nodules: Evaluation of blood flow patterns with dynamic CT. Radiol. 1997;205:471-8.
67. Yamashita K, Matsunobe S, Tsuda T, et al. Solitary pulmonary nodule: Preliminary study of evaluation with incremental dynamic CT. Radiol. 1995;194:399-405.
68. Swensen SJ, Brown LR, Colby TV, et al. Lung nodule enhancement at CT: Prospective findings. Radiol. 1996;201:447-55.
69. Murayama S, Murakami J, Hashimoto S, et al. Noncalcified pulmonary tuberculomas: CT enhancement patterns with histological correlation. J Thorac Imaging. 1995;10: 91-5.
70. Jeong YJ, Lee KS, Jeong SY, et al. Solitary Pulmonary Nodule: Characterization with Combined wash in and washout features at Dynamic Multi detector Row CT. Radiol. 2005;237:675-83.
71. Yi CA, Lee KS, Kim EA, et al. Solitary pulmonary nodules: dynamic enhanced multi detector row CT study and comparison with vascular endothelial growth factor and microvessel density. Radiol. 2004;233:191-9.
72. Gadgeel SM, Ramalingam S, Cummmings G, et al. Lung cancer in patients <50 years of age: the experience of an academic multidisciplinary program. Chest. 1999;115:1232-6.
73. Guyatt GH, Newhouse MD. Are active and passive smoking harmful? Determination of causation. Chest. 1985;88:445-51.
74. Bach PB, Kaltan M, Thornquist MD, et al. Variations in lung cancer risk among smokers. J Natl Canc Inst. 2003;95:470-8.
75. Lee PN. Relation between exposure to asbestos and smoking jointly and the risk of lung cancer. Occup Environ Med. 2001;58:145-53.
76. Erasmus JJ, Mc Adams HP, Connolly JE. Solitary pulmonary nodules: Part-II. Evaluation of the indeterminate nodule. Radiographics. 2000;20:59-66.
77. Gurney JW, Lyddon DM, Mckay JA. Determining the likelihood of malignancy in solitary pulmonary nodules with Bayesian analysis Part II. Application. Radiology. 1993;186: 415-32.
78. Black WC, Armstrong P. Communicating the significance of radiologic test results: the likelihood ratio. AJR. 1986;147:1313-8.
79. Soardi GA, Perandini S, Molton M, et al. Assessing probability of malignancy in solid solitary pulmonary nodules with a new Bayesian calculator: improving diagnostic accuracy by means of expanded and updated features. Eur Radiol. DOI 10.1007/s00330-014-3396-2.

80. Sim YT, Poon FW. Imaging of solitary pulmonary nodule: a clinical review. Quant Imaging Med Surg. 2013;3:316-26.
81. Nomori H, Wattanbe K, Ohtsuka T, et al. Evaluation of F-18 fluorodeoxyglucose (FDG) PET scanning for pulmonary nodules less than 3 cm in diameter with special reference to CT images. Lung Cancer. 2004;45:19-27.
82. Lowe VJ, Fletcher JW, Gobar C, et al. Prospective investigation of PET in lung nodules (PIOPILN), J Clin Oncol. 1998;16:1075-84.
83. Huber KF, Buonocore E, Gould HR, et al. Differentiating benign from malignant lung lesions using quantitative parameters of FDG PET images. Clin Nucl Med. 1996;21:941-49.
84. Shimizu K, Ikeda N, Tuboi M, et al. Percutaneous Ct guided fine needle aspiration for lung cancer smaller than 2 cm and revealed by ground-glass opacity at CT. Lung Cancer. 2006;51(2):173-9.
85. Moore EH. Needle aspiration lung biopsy: A comprehensive approach to complication reduction. J Thorac Imaging. 1997;12:259-71.
86. Ohno Y, Hatabu H, Takenaka D, et al. Solitary pulmonary nodules: potential role of dynamic MR imaging in management: initial experiences. Radiol. 2002;224:503-11.
87. Kono M, Adachi S, Kusumoto M, et al. Clinical utility of Gd- DTPA-enhanced magnetic resonance imaging in lung cancer. J Thorac Imaging. 1993;8:18-26.
88. Guckel C, Schnabel K, Deimling M, et al. Solitary pulmonary nodules: MR evaluation of enhancement patterns with contrast enhanced dynamic snapshot gradient echo imaging. Radiol. 1996;200:681-6.
89. Satoh S, Kitazume Y, Ohdama S. Can malignant and benign pulmonary nodules be differentiated with diffusion weighted MRI? AJR. 2008;191:464-70.
90. Chae EJ, Song JW, Seo JB, et al. Clinical utility of Dual. Energy CT in the evaluation of solitary pulmonary nodules: Initial Experience. Radiology. 2008;249(2):671-81.
91. MacMohan MB, Austin JHM, Gamsu G, et al. Guidelines for management of small pulmonary nodules detected on CT scans: a statement from the Fleischner Society. Radiology. 2005;237:395-400.
92. Patel VK, Naik SK, Naidich DP, et al. A practical approach to the diagnosis and management of solitary pulmonary nodules: part 2-pretest probability and algorithm. Chest. 2013;143(3):840-6.
93. Naidich Dp, Bankier AA, McMohan H, et al. Recommendations for the management of subsolid pulmonary nodules detected at CT: a statement from the Fleischner Society. Radiol. 2013;266:304-17.
94. Vasquez M, Carter D, Brambilla E, et al. Solitary and multiple resected adenocarcinomas after CT screening for lung cancer: histopathologic features and their prognostic implications. Lung Cancer. 2009;64(2):148-54.
95. MacMahon H, Naidich DP, Goo JM et al, Guidelines for management of incidental pulmonary nodules detected on CT images: from the Fleischner Society 2017. Radiology. 2017 Jul;284(1):228-43. doi: 10.1148/radiol.2017161659. Epub 2017 Feb 23.
96. Kazerooni EA, Armstrong M, Amorosa JK, et al. ACR CT accreditation program and lung cancer screening program designation. J Am Coll Radiol. 2016;13(2 Suppl):R 30-34.
97. Armstrong P. Basic patterns in lung disease. In: Hansell DM, Armstrong P, Lynch DA, McAdams HP, (Eds). Imaging of Disease of the Chest. Philadelphia: Mosby. 2005;69-141.
98. Hirakata K, Nakata H, Haratake J. Appearance of pulmonary metastases on high resolution CT scans. Comparison with histopathologic findings from autopsy specimens. AJR. 1993;161:37-43.
99. Choplin RH, Kawanmoto EH, Dyer RB, et al. Atypical carcinoid of the lung: Radiographic features. AJR. 1986;146:665-8.
100. Muller NL, Miller RR. Neuroendocrine carcinomas of the lung. Seminar Roentgenol 1990;25:96-104.
101. Au V, Leung AN. Radiologic manifestations of lymphoma in the thorax. AJR. 1997;168:93-8.
102. Gjevre JA, Myers JL, Prakash UB. Pulmonary hamartomas. Mayo Clin Proc. 1996;71:14-20.
103. Siegelman SS, Khouri NF, Scott WW, et al. Pulmonary hamartoma: CT findings. Radiol. 1986;160:313-7.
104. Carney JA. The triad of gastric epitheloid leiomyosarcoma pulmonary chondroma and functioning extra adrenal paraganglioma: a five year review. Medicine (Baltimore). 1983;62:159-69.
105. Celebi S, Hacimustafaoglu M. Round pneumonia in children. Ind J Paed. 2008;75:523-5.
106. Cortet B, Flipo RM, Remy Jordin M, et al. Use of high resolution computed tomography of the lungs in patients with rheumatoid arthritis. Ann Rheum Dis. 1995;54:815-9.
107. Ferratti GR, Thony F, Link KM, et al. False aneurysm of the pulmonary artery induced by a Swan Ganz catheter: Clinical presentation and radiologic management. AJR. 1996;167: 941-5.
108. Spear BS, Sully L, Lewis CT. Pulmonary arteriovenous fistula presenting as spontaneous hemothorax. Thorax. 1975;30: 355-6.
109. Burkill GJ, Bell JR, Padley SP. Survey on the use of pulmonary scintigraphy, spiral CT and conventional pulmonary angiography for suspected pulmonary embolism in the British Isles. Clin Radiol. 1999;54:807-10.
110. Frazier AA, Rosado de Christenson ML, Stoker JT, et al. Intralobar sequestration: Radiologic pathologic correlation. Radiographics. 1997;17:725-45.
111. Carvalho PM, Carr DH. Computed tomography of folded lung. Clin Radiol. 1990;41:86-91.
112. O' Donovan PB, Schenk M, Lim K, et al. Evaluation of the reliability of computed tomographic criteria used in the diagnosis of round atelectasis. J Thoracic Imaging. 1997; 12:54-8.

CHAPTER 168

Imaging of Pulmonary Neoplasms

Priyanka Naranje, Mukesh Kumar Yadav, Chandan Jyoti Das, Arun Kumar Gupta

INTRODUCTION

Lung cancer is amongst the most common and most lethal cancers around the world. It represents about 13% of the new cancer cases and up to 28% of the cancer deaths.[1] It is the most common cancer in males in India with age averaged incidence ranging from 3.6 to 18.9 per 100,000 per year in different parts of the country.[2] Overall 5 years survival with this cancer is less than 15%. Most lung cancers are directly attributed to smoking. Reported highest incidence in smokers is 362 cases per 100,000 per year while the same in non-smokers is up to 21 cases only.[3] Passive smoking increases the risk of lung cancer by up to 30%. Exposure to nickel, cobalt, asbestos, radiation, pesticides also increases the risk of lung cancer. Lung is also the most common site of metastatic involvement from other extrathoracic malignancies; 20–54% of extrathoracic malignancies have pulmonary metastatic disease.[3] Synchronous and metachronous second lung malignancy occurs in about 2% of patients with lung cancer.[4]

A wide variety of imaging techniques are currently available for detection, diagnosis, and management of pulmonary neoplasms. Chest radiography is the primary imaging modality for detection of lung nodules and masses. Computed tomography (CT) and Positron emission tomography (PET) are most commonly used imaging modalities for further characterization, to define extent and along with non radiological modalities; for pre-treatment staging of the lung malignancies. Imaging is also required to assess the response to nonsurgical treatment and for follow up in treated patients. MRI has evolving role in evaluation of lung malignancies and is occasionally used as a problem solving modality and in assessment of treatment response.

WHO CLASSIFICATION[5]

Pulmonary neoplasms are classified pathologically according to 4th edition of WHO Classification 2015 which provides a standardized terminology for lung cancer **(Table 1)**. Previous classification of 2004 was based on resection specimens. In the present era, the therapeutic decisions are based on specific histologic and genetic characteristics of the tumor. Hence, in the 2015 classification system, whenever possible, *immunohistochemistry* is recommended for all cytology or biopsy or even resected specimens. For example, epidermal growth factor (EGFR) mutations, anaplastic lymphoma kinase (ALK) rearrangements and ROS1 are found in adenocarcinoma and these are effective targets for specific drugs such as EGFR tyrosine kinase inhibitors (Erlotinib, Gefitinib) or ALK inhibitors (crizotinib) in patients with advanced lung adenocarcinoma. Similarly, a pneumocyte marker such as thyroid transcription factor (TTF)-1 is desired to address primary versus metastatic adenocarcinoma.

CLINICAL FEATURES

Depending on the location, extent, size and histopathology of the tumor, various clinical manifestations are seen.

Table 1: 2015 WHO classification of lung tumors

Histologic Type and Subtypes
Epithelial tumors
• *Adenocarcinoma*: – Lepidic, acinar, papillary, micropapillary, solid, colloid, fetal, enteric – Invasive mucinous adenocarcinoma – Minimally invasive adenocarcinoma - Nonmucinous - Mucinous – *Preinvasive lesions*: - Atypical adenomatous hyperplasia - Adenocarcinoma *in situ* (formerly called BAC) • *Squamous cell carcinoma*: – Keratinizing, nonkeratinizing, basaloid – Preinvasive lesion - Squamous cell carcinoma *in situ* • *Neuroendocrine tumors*: – Small cell carcinoma – Large cell neuroendocrine carcinoma – *Carcinoid tumors*: - Typical carcinoid tumor - Atypical carcinoid tumor – *Preinvasive lesion*: - Diffuse idiopathic pulmonary neuroendocrine cell hyperplasia (DIPNECH) • Large cell carcinoma • Adenosquamous carcinoma • *Sarcomatoid carcinomas*: – Pleomorphic carcinoma – Spindle cell carcinoma – Giant cell carcinoma – Carcinosarcoma – Pulmonary blastoma • *Other and unclassified carcinomas*: – Lymphoepithelioma-like carcinoma – NUT carcinoma • *Salivary gland-type tumors*: – Mucoepidermoid carcinoma – Adenoid cystic carcinoma – Epithelial-myoepithelial carcinoma – Pleomorphic adenoma • *Papillomas*: – Squamous – Glandular – Mixed • *Adenomas*: – Sclerosing pneumocytoma – Alveolar adenoma – Papillary adenoma – Mucinous cystadenoma – Mucous gland adenoma
Mesenchymal tumors
• Pulmonary hamartoma • Chondroma • PEComatous tumors • Lymphangioleiomyomatosis • Congenital peribronchial myofibroblastic tumor • Diffuse pulmonary lymphangiomatosis • Inflammatory myofibroblastic tumor • Epithelioid hemangioendothelioma • Pleuropulmonary blastoma • Synovial sarcoma • Pulmonary artery intimal sarcoma
Lymphohistiocytic tumors
• Extranodal MALT lymphoma • Diffuse large cell lymphoma • Lymphomatoid granulomatosis • Pulmonary Langerhans cell histiocytosis • Erdheim–Chester disease
Tumors of ectopic origin
• Germ cell tumors (Teratoma) • Intrapulmonary thymoma • Melanoma • Meningioma NOS
Metastatic tumors

Contd...

Contd...

Source: This table is reproduced from the 2015 WHO Classification by Travis et al.[5]

Systemic symptoms of weight loss, anorexia and fever are common. Cough and hemoptysis are the most common clinical features of lung cancers. Hemoptysis may be streaky or massive at the presentation. Central tumors may present with wheeze and recurrent pneumonia due to bronchial obstruction. Advanced lung tumors with locoregional invasion of the pleura, chest wall or mediastinum may manifest with chest pain, brachial plexus neuropathy, Horner syndrome, phrenic or recurrent laryngeal nerve palsy, dysphagia or SVC obstruction. Besides, there are several paraneoplastic syndromes that may be associated with lung cancer such as Eaton-Lambart syndrome, subacute cerebellar degeneration, encephalomyelopathy, Cushing syndrome, hypertrophic pulmonary osteoarthropathy, etc. Some small peripheral lung cancers may be asymptomatic and only be detected incidentally or on screening. Signs and symptoms due to metastasis could be bone pain, neurologic symptoms or pathological fracture.

IMAGING MODALITIES

Conventional chest radiography and cross-sectional imaging techniques such as computed tomography (CT), magnetic resonance imaging (MRI) and PET-CT play a role in the detection, diagnosis, and management of pulmonary parenchymal neoplasms. Ultrasonography(US) including CEUS has specific utility in guided sampling of the peripheral based lung tumors.[6]

Chest radiography (PA view) is the primary modality for *detection* of the lung cancer **(Fig. 1A)**.[7] Any solitary pulmonary nodule (rounded opacity <3 cm) or mass (opacity > 3 cm with any shape/margins) in an adult may be a lung cancer unless it is proved otherwise.

CT is more accurate for detection of abnormality and it is a modality of choice for characterization of pulmonary neoplasms.[7] CT forms an integral imaging technique for staging the lung cancers. Advanced CT techniques such as dynamic perfusion CT,[8] dual energy CT[9] and dual-energy spectral CT imaging[10] as well as software based texture analysis[11] are new methods under evaluation for the characterization of lung tumors and help in distinguishing benign from malignant lesions. A routine CT protocol for the evaluation of suspected lung cancer should consist of a contrast-enhanced CT (CECT) of chest and upper abdomen including liver and adrenals.

PET provides functional information and hence it is generally more precise for overall evaluation of the disease extent. PET is not useful in T staging as its resolution is inferior and CECT is sufficient for this purpose. FDG uptake is also variable in tumors like invasive mucinous adenocarcinoma, carcinoid and small cell lung cancer and this may result in high false negative results on PET.[12,13] Conversely, false positive results may be seen in benign conditions like tuberculosis and sarcoidosis.[14]

PET is recommended as a single test for comprehensive preoperative evaluation of local and distant disease spread, with overall staging accuracy of more than 90%.[15] It is especially useful for mediastinal lymph node staging, differentiating benign from malignant pleural effusions[16] and detection of bone metastases.[17] In some patients, inflammatory lymph nodes may show PET uptake and cause false positive PET results. Similarly, because of the resolution issue, lymph nodes smaller than 5 mm cannot be reliably evaluated on PETCT.[18]

PET is also useful in monitoring of patients undergoing nonsurgical management. Modern conformal radiotherapy techniques require accurate delineation of the tumor volume for the treatment plans. PET-CT is now preferred for radiotherapy planning as it can differentiate the viable tumor from adjacent necrotic tissues or consolidations and hence, more accurate than CT based planning.[19] This characteristic of PETCT is also useful for planning image guided biopsies from viable area of the tumor.

For the assessment of response to chemotherapy, SUV monitoring is also more accurate and correlates better with patient survival than the RESIST size criteria used for conventional imaging techniques.[20] PET-CT is also useful to detect recurrences in treated patients, as it is more accurate in differentiating post-treatment changes from recurrences. However, radiation changes can sometimes show FDG uptake. To avoid false positive results, PET should be deferred until six months after the radiotherapy.

Magnetic Resonance Imaging[21]

Owing to the recent advances made in overcoming the challenges in MR acquisition of lung, current status of MRI is increasing in detection, characterization of pulmonary nodules, TNM staging and tumor response assessments. DWI as well as dynamic contrast-enhanced MRI have shown to be useful in distinguishing benign and malignant lung nodules. Using a cutoff ADC value of 1.1 $\times 10^{-3}$ mm^2/s, a sensitivity of 70% and specificity of 97% using a b value of 1000 s/mm^2 was seen in one study.[22] DWI can be used for early assessment of tumor response post chemotherapy **(Figs. 1B to E)**. Similarly, there are various dynamic MRI techniques for distinguishing malignant nodules from benign nodules, with reported sensitivities ranging from 94% to 100%, specificities from 70% to 96%, and accuracies >88%.[23,24] MRI useful for brachial plexus involvement in superior sulcus tumors and assessment of chest wall, diaphragmatic pleura, great vessel and cardiac involvement.

IMAGING FEATURES

Imaging features of the lung cancer are discussed under following headings: Peripheral tumors and central tumors.

Peripheral Tumors

Peripheral tumors are those arising beyond the segmental bronchi. Most commonly presents as nodule or mass with following characteristics.

Shape: Majority are spherical or oval in shape **(Fig. 2A)**. Superior sulcus tumors may resemble apical pleural thickening **(Fig. 2B)**.

Margins: May be well defined or ill defined. Uneven rate of growth in different parts of the tumor may produce lobulations **(Fig. 3A)**. One or more strands may be seen extending from the main mass into surrounding lung giving rise to spiculated appearance which is termed as 'corona radiata' **(Fig. 3A)**. Spiculations represent either tumor extension or desmoplastic reaction to the tumor. Spiculated margin is a useful sign to differentiate lung cancer from benign pulmonary nodules, although it may be rarely seen in granuloma and organizing pneumonia as well. A sharply defined spherical smooth edged nodule due to a carcinoma is rare. Sometimes, one or more linear strands may extend from a peripheral mass to the pleura known as 'pleural tail' **(Fig. 3B)**. It can be seen in both benign and malignant lesions and hence is not helpful in differentiating between the two.

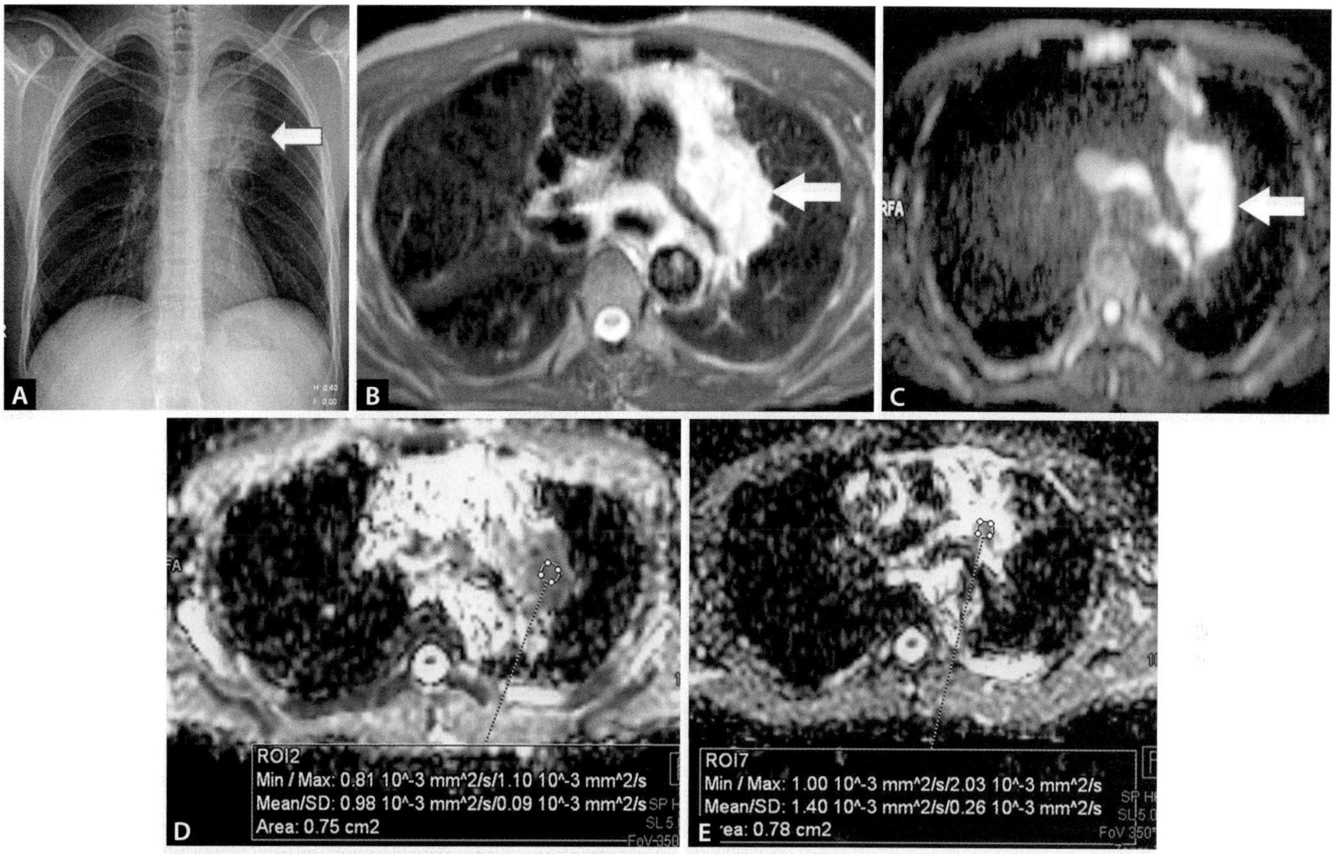

Figs. 1A to E: Diffusion weighted MRI in carcinoma lung: (A) Frontal chest radiograph showing mass in the left upper lobe extending in region of aortopulmonary window in a case of adenocarcinoma; (B) STIR axial image shows hyperintense mass in left upper lobe with mediastinal invasion; (C) Prechemotherapy DWI at b-1000 value, shows hyperintense signal in the region of mass with hypointense signal on corresponding ADC map; (D) ADC map shows a value of 0.98×10^{-3} mm^2/s suggestive of restricted diffusion; (E) Post-chemotherapy there is reduction in the size of the tumor with increase in the ADC value suggestive of good response to chemotherapy.

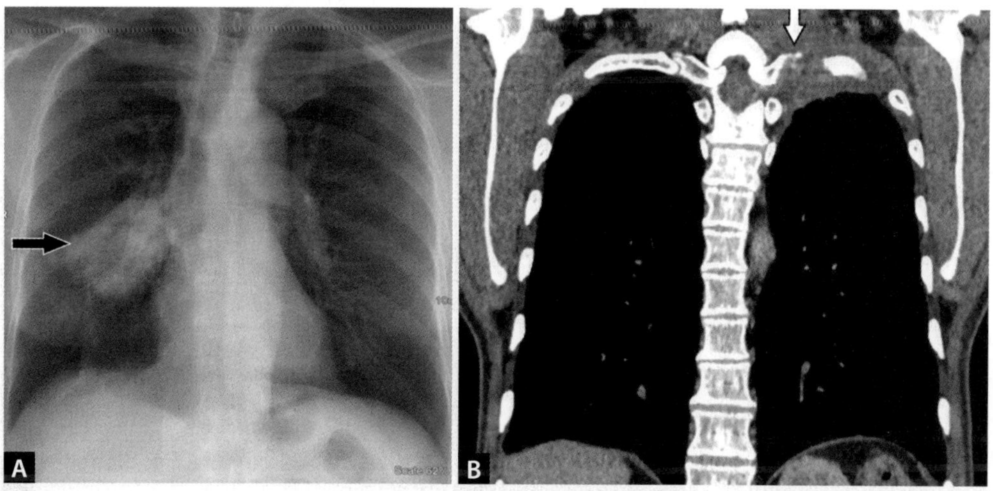

Figs. 2A and B: (A) Frontal chest radiograph showing an oval-shaped mass (black arrow) in right parahilar location in a case of squamous cell carcinoma; (B) Coronal CT image showing plaque-like thickening in the left apical region with adjacent rib erosion (white arrow) suggestive of superior sulcus tumor.

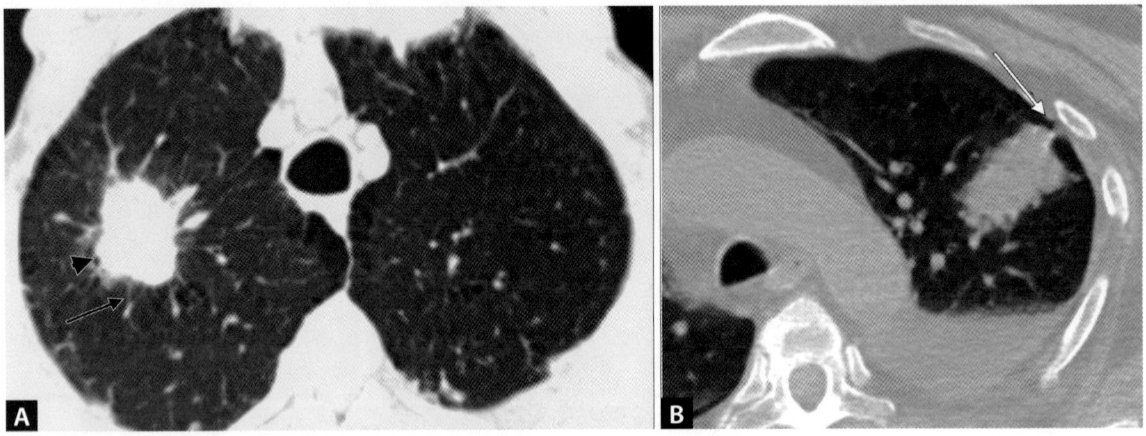

Figs. 3A and B: Corona radiata: (A) Axial CT image in a case of adenocarcinoma showing mass with multiple spiculations (arrow) as well as lobulations (arrowhead); (B) A small pleural tail is seen extending from the mass to pleura (arrow).

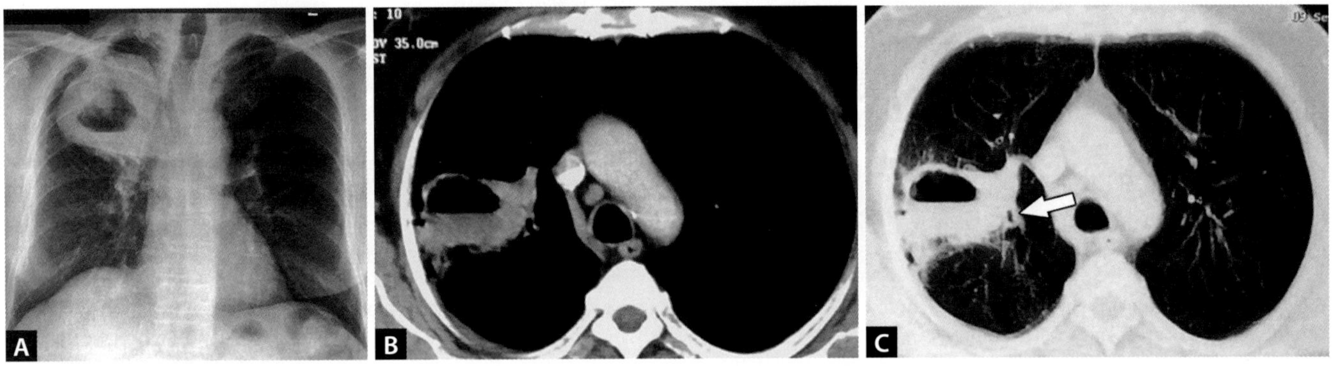

Figs. 4A to C: Squamous cell carcinoma: (A) Chest radiograph shows large cavitary lesion in right upper lobe with thick nodular walls and an air-fluid level; (B and C) CT scan of same patient shows right upper lobe cavity with irregular and nodular enhancing wall thickening with air fluid level. There is abrupt cutoff of bronchus at the tumor margin (arrow).

Cavitation: Best seen on CT. Most commonly seen in squamous cell carcinoma histology, however may be seen in any type of lung cancer. The wall of the cavity is usually >8 mm thick, may be smooth or more commonly is irregular and nodular **(Figs. 4A to C)**. Fluid levels may be seen within the cavity. It develops due to central necrosis, liquifection and emptying of the contents in the airways. Rarely, the cavity is seen as an air crescent, similar to the fungal ball. This appearance is caused by the air around an intracavitary tumor.

Calcification: Calcifications are rarely seen in lung cancers on chest radiographs; however, CT may demonstrate it in 6–10% patients.[25] These represent either preexisting granulomatous calcifications engulfed by the tumor or dystrophic calcifications developed in the areas of tumor necrosis. The dystrophic tumor calcification is usually amorphous **(Fig. 5)** or cloudy in appearance and located centrally while engulfed calcifications tend to be located at the periphery of the tumor. Tumor calcification may be seen in any type of bronchogenic carcinoma and there is no predilection for any specific histological subtype.[26]

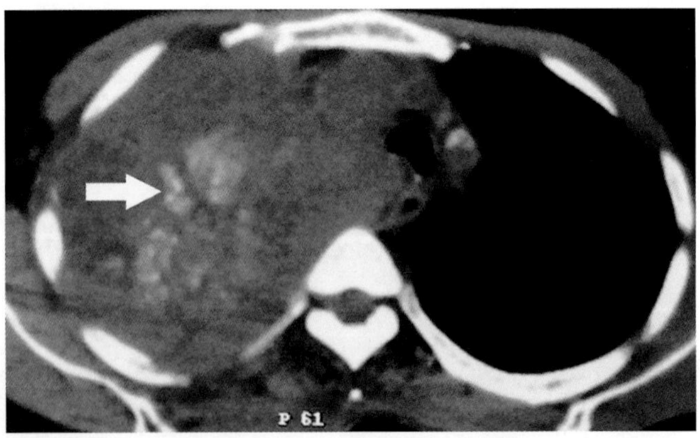

Fig. 5: Calcifications in lung cancer: NCCT shows large lung mass with fine, amorphous tumoral calcifications in a case of squamous cell carcinoma.

Consolidation pattern: Atypical presentation can be tumors with entirely ill-defined margins resembling consolidation/pneumonia on chest radiographs **(Figs. 6A and B)**, e.g. lepidic predominant adenocarcinoma [formally called bronchiolo-alveolar carcinoma (BAC)], invasive mucinous adenocarcinoma (formally called mucinous BAC). Persistent or recurrent consolidation at same site, air bronchograms, bubble-like lucencies or pseudocavitation, expansion of the consolidated lobe, Golden S sign, dilated fluid-filled bronchi are the features on CT/CXR suspicious of malignancy.

Ground-glass attenuation nodule: A feature of adenocarcinoma in situ, atypical adenomatous hyperplasia or minimally invasive adenocarcinoma which may present as pure ground-glass nodule **(Fig. 6C)** or part solid nodule and these tend to be slow growing tumors with better prognosis.[27] GGO surrounding a solid tumor may represent hemorrhage or inflammation or edema.

Other Findings

Bronchial carcinoma in segmental or distal bronchi may cause retention of mucoid secretions which is known as bronchocele or mucocele. On chest radiographs, these appear as tubular/oval densities with their stem pointing towards the hilum.

An abrupt cutoff of the bronchus at the tumor margin is highly suggestive of squamous cell carcinoma **(Fig. 4C)**.

Pancoast tumors may present as asymmetric apical pleural thickening with or without rib erosions which are better delineated on CT. Old tubercular fibrosis does not predispose to lung cancer. In so called scar carcinomas, the fibrous reaction follows, rather than precedes the carcinoma.

Growth rate: The round or oval shape of the opacity and slow growth on serial radiographs should raise the suspicion for malignancy. Growth rate of non-small cell lung cancer (NSCLC) is highly variable and related to histological subtype and smoking history, but not the presence of symptoms at diagnosis.[28] Lung cancers usually have doubling time between 1 and 18 months and a 26% increase in the diameter is equal to the doubling of tumor volume. Most lung cancers double in volume in 4 to 8 months, however, invasive mucinous adenocarcinomas tend to grow more slowly, and may even metastasize. Significant growth may be detected in as early as 2 months in smokers.

Central Tumors

Chest Radiograph Findings

Hilar enlargement: The cardinal imaging finding of a central tumor on chest radiograph is presence of hilar enlargement with or without distal collapse/consolidation of the lung. The hilar enlargement may be due to central tumor itself, enlarged lymph nodes, consolidation or combination of these **(Fig. 7)**.

Dense hilum sign: Sometimes, a small mass overlying the hilum may produce only an asymmetrically increased density of the hilum and this should raise a suspicion of tumor and a CECT is indicated.

Distal collapse: It is seen as homogeneous pulmonary opacity with volume loss, confined to one lobe. Air bronchogram however, is usually absent **(Figs. 8A to D)**. Displacement of the fissure towards the collapsed lung. 'Golden S sign' in right upper lobe collapse occurs due to central mass limiting the expected movement of the fissure and hence the medial aspect of fissure shows bulging contour. If there is retention of mucous in the collapsed lung bronchi, it may not lead to volume loss and rather an enlarged lobe 'drowned lung' may be visualized.

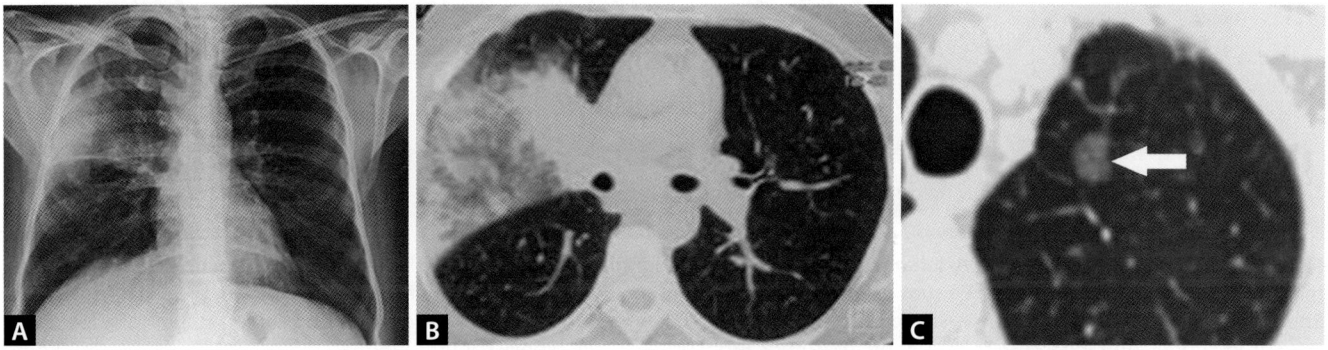

Figs. 6A to C: Lung cancer seen as non-resolving pneumonia: (A) Chest radiograph shows an airspace opacity in right upper lobe; (B) Corresponding CT shows consolidation and ground-glass opacity in right upper lobe. Endobronchial biopsy confirmed lepidic predominant adenocarcinoma; (C) Adenocarcinoma *in situ* presenting as focal ground-glass nodule in a different patient.

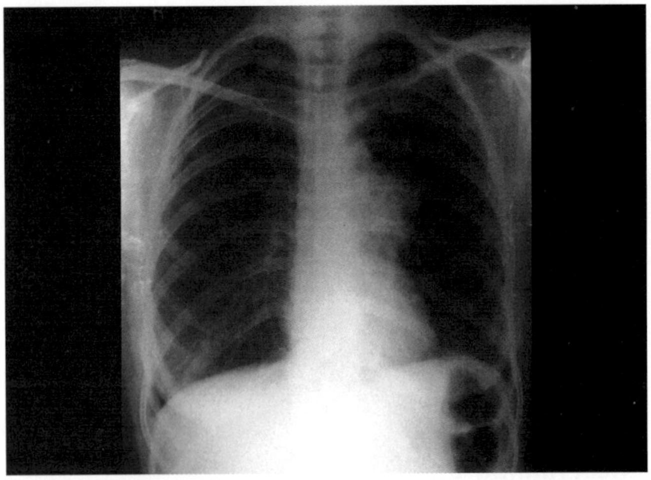

Fig. 7: Central lung cancer: Frontal chest radiograph shows increased density and enlargement of left hilum. Associated elevation of left hemidiaphragm is suggestive of mediastinal invasion and phrenic nerve palsy.

Consolidation: Inhomogeneous opacity persistent or recurrent in same lobe should raise a suspicion of central obstructing mass.

CECT Findings

Central lung cancers are seen as minimally enhancing soft tissue masses whereas distal collapse shows significant enhancement. Distended fluid filled bronchi may be seen as fluid bronchogram within the enhancing collapsed lung distal to the mass. Such an appearance should prompt a bronchoscopy, even when tumor is not visualized on CT. Delineation of the tumor separately from distal collapse consolidation cannot always be made on CT **(Figs. 8B and C)**. This may pose a difficulty in the confident initial diagnosis of lung cancer on CT. PETCT can demonstrate the central mass with FDG uptake separate from collapse. Accurate tumor delineation is an important requirement for radiotherapy planning. Dynamic perfusion CT can

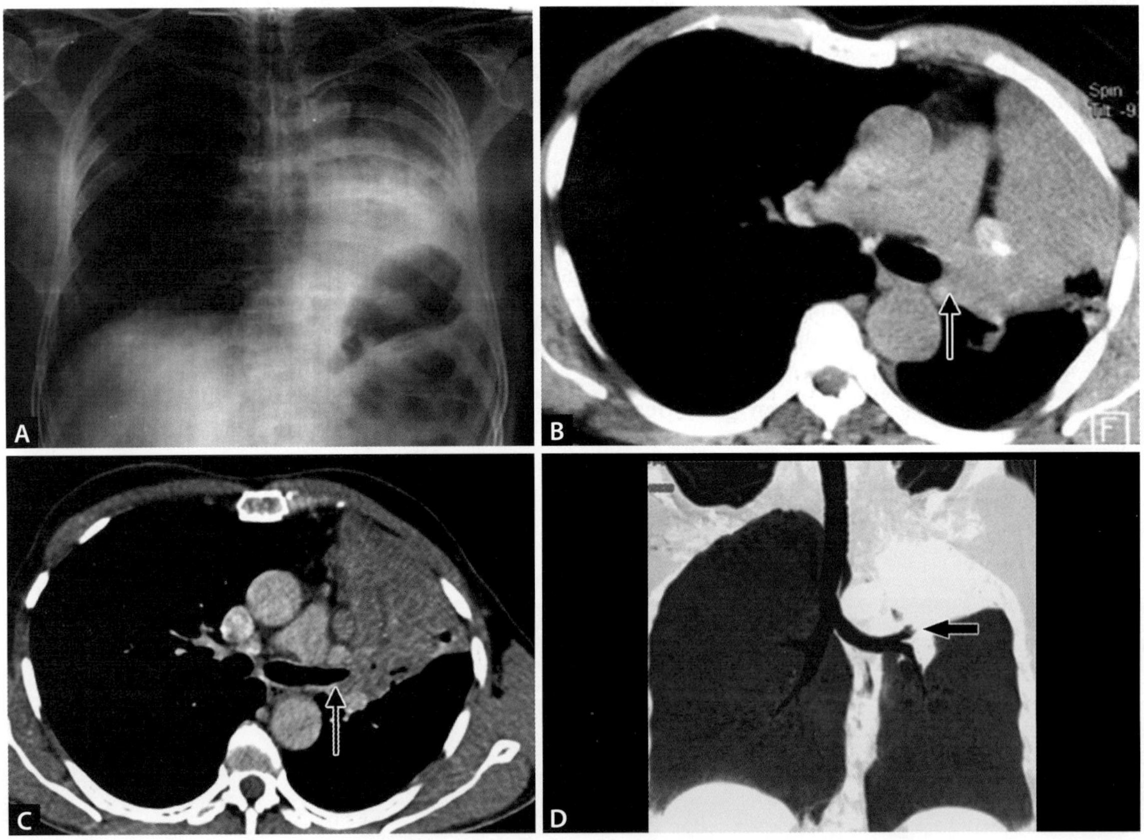

Figs. 8A to D: Central lung cancer with lobar collapse: (A) Chest radiograph shows signs of collapse of the left upper lobe with ipsilateral mediastinal shift; (B) Corresponding CT shows ill-defined mass occluding the left upper lobe bronchus (arrow) with distal collapsed lung. Endobronchial biopsy revealed squamous cell carcinoma; (C) CT scan of another patient showing cutoff of left upper lobe bronchus (arrow), left upper lobe collapse with no identifiable tumor. Bronchoscopy and biopsy confirmed squamous cell carcinoma; (D) Minimum intensity projection image in same patient, shows cutoff of the bronchus (arrow).

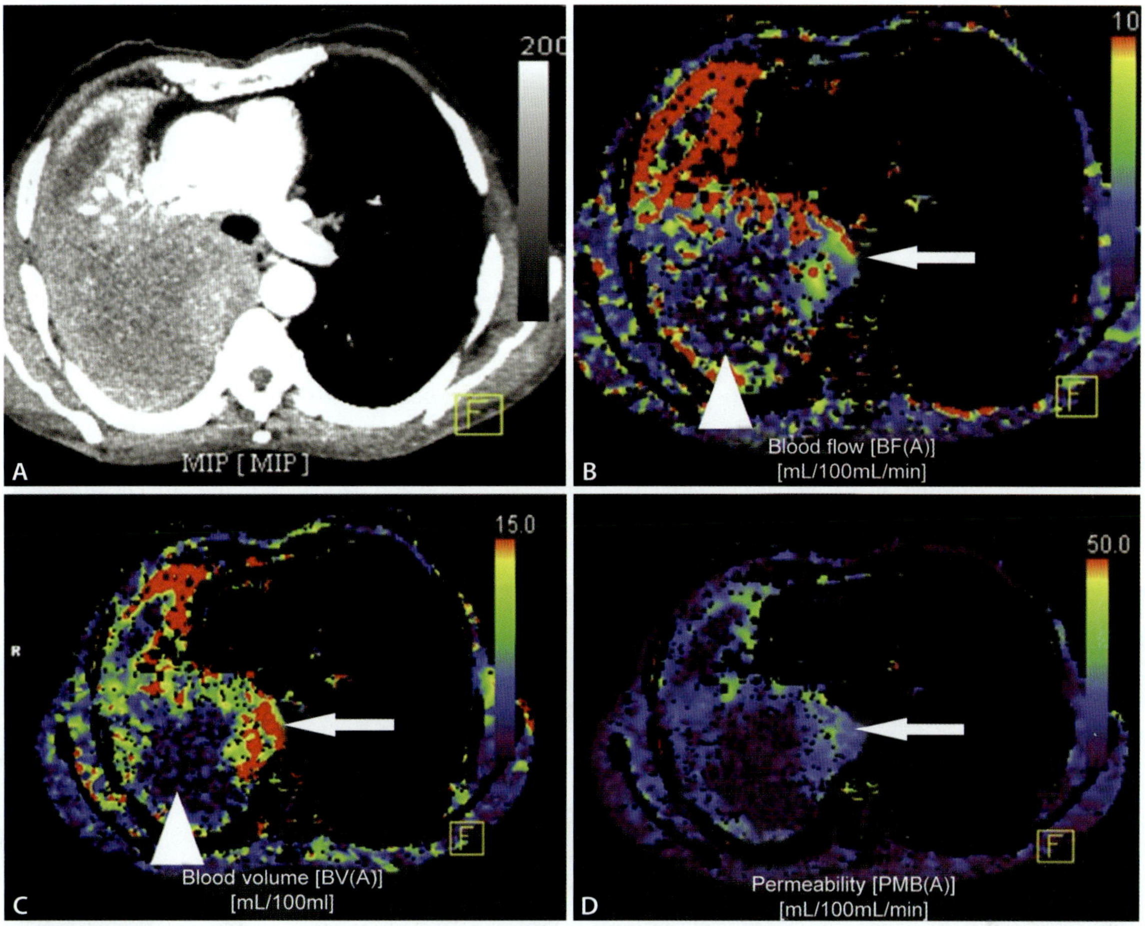

Figs. 9A to D: Dynamic perfusion CT lung: (A) MIP CT image shows heterogeneous mass in right lung and viable tumor tissue could not be confidently identified. CT perfusion blood flow color coded image (B) and blood volume image (C) shows increased blood flow and blood volume (areas depicted in red/yellow color) in the medial aspect of the mass suggestive of viable tumor tissue (white arrows). Minimal blood flow and volume in the central and lateral aspect of the mass suggesting necrosis (arrowhead); (D) Permeability image shows mildly increased permeability in medial aspect of the mass (arrow). CT-guided biopsy revealed adenocarcinoma.

help distinguishing between tumor mass and collapsed lung as well as demonstrate viable tumor tissue separate from necrotic non-viable area, thereby guiding proper CT guided needle placement for biopsy **(Figs. 9A to D)**.

RADIOLOGICAL CHARACTERISTICS BY CELL TYPE

Amongst the common subtypes of the lung cancers, adenocarcinoma accounts for 38.5% of the cases, squamous cell carcinoma 20%, small cell carcinoma 15% and large cell carcinoma 2.9% of cases.[29]

Adenocarcinoma

Adenocarcinomas are typically peripherally located tumor. These can either present as a localized ground-glass opacity or as solid nodule or mass. They are usually less than 4 cm in diameter and cavitation is rare (seen in only 4–6% lesions).[30] Adenocarcinomas are frequently associated with enlarged hilar and mediastinal lymph nodes, though not as massive as seen in small cell carcinomas. Pleural effusion is a feature of adenocarcinoma.

Invasive mucinous adenocarcinoma: Formally known as mucinous bronchioloalveolar carcinoma (BAC). It may present as a peripheral single pulmonary nodule/mass or multicentric or diffuse disease **(Figs. 10A and B)** or a localized parenchymal consolidation form in decreasing order of incidence. Characteristic bubble-like lucencies can be identified on CT within the mass.[30] Sometimes, air bronchograms and cavitation may also be seen. Hilar and mediastinal lymphadenopathy is uncommon.

Squamous Cell Carcinoma

These are more often centrally located within the lung and may attain greater size. Cavitation is seen in up to

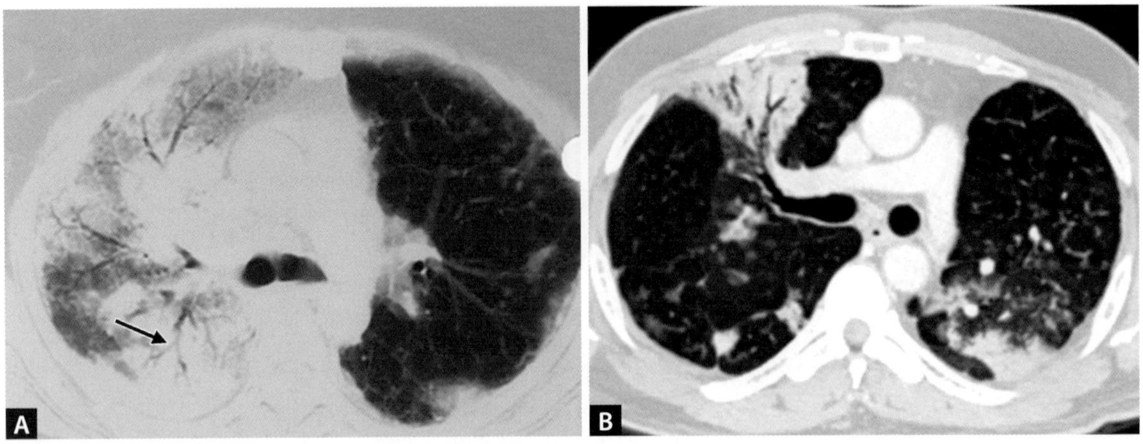

Figs. 10A and B: Invasive mucinous adenocarcinoma (formally known as invasive bronchoalveolar carcinoma): (A) CT shows pneumonic form of the cancer with extensive airspace opacities with characteristic stretching and narrowing of the bronchi (arrow) due to mass effect of the tumor; (B) Another patient showing multicentric pattern of disease.

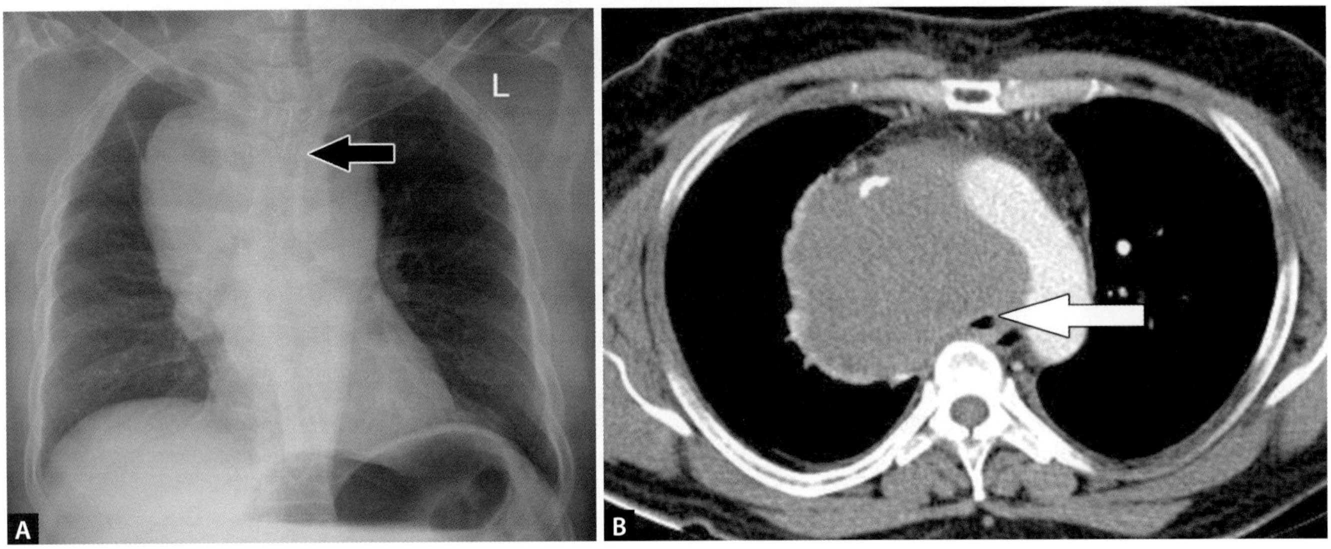

Figs. 11A and B: Small-cell carcinoma presenting as mediastinal mass: (A) Chest radiograph showing large mediastinal mass. A tracheal stent is seen as the mass was causing severe narrowing of the tracheal lumen; (B) Preprocedural CT shows large mediastinal lymphadenopathy with compression of SVC and trachea (arrow). No separate mass could be identified within the lungs.

82% cases.[30] Being central obstructive lesions, these tumors frequently produce segmental or lobar lung collapse **(Figs. 8B and C)**.

Small Cell Lung Cancer

This tumor is characterized by a high growth fraction and rapid doubling time. It represents the most malignant form of the neuroendocrine carcinomas of the lung. It is associated with poor prognosis as 60–70% of patients present with metastatic disease at the time of diagnosis.[31] These tumors most often present with massive enlarged mediastinal or hilar lymphadenopathy **(Figs. 11A and B)**. A large noncontiguous centrally located mass can be seen within the lung parenchyma and it rarely cavitates. Mediastinal invasion is common and seen in upto 68 % of cases[31] on CT. Sometimes only conglomerate mediastinal nodal mass may be present without detection of primary lung tumor.

Large Cell Carcinoma

It is a poorly differentiated non small cell carcinoma and is diagnosed in the absence of histopathologic features for adenocarcinoma or squamous cell carcinoma and presence of a large cell morphology. These are high grade tumors with rapid growth rate and tend to metastasize early to the mediastinum and brain.

SAMPLING FOR SUSPECTED LUNG CANCER

In a suspected lung cancer, if patient is producing sputum, the cytology assessment can often establish the diagnosis of malignancy. However, since the inception of 2015 WHO classification and new targeted treatment options, immunohistochemistry of the small biopsies or even cytology is indicated for further typing of the tumor. Bronchoscopy is used for evaluation and biopsy of most lung cancers. It is most useful for central tumors and diagnostic yield ranges from 81–90% for visible tumors.[32] Peripheral lesions can also be sampled using indirect bronchoscopic methods such as lavage, brushes, biopsy forceps or radial EBUS guided biopsy.[33]

CT-guided transthoracic FNAC or core biopsy **(Fig. 12A)** is accurate for the tumors not amenable to bronchoscopic visualization. However, non-diagnostic or nonspecific benign results are not reliable and repeat biopsy must be performed in these situations. Major complications include pneumothorax, hemotharax, hemoptysis, infection and air embolism. Peripheral lung tumors can be accessed under ultrasound guidance **(Fig. 12B)** and in case of necrotic tumors, a contrast enhance ultrasound may be used to differentiate between active areas and nonviable areas before sampling thereby increasing the accuracy of core needle biopsy.[6] CT or ultrasound guided biopsies are useful to obtain samples from metastatic sites of the lung cancer. In some patients with resectable disease on imaging, preoperative lymph node staging may be performed with mediastinoscopy and lymph node sampling and sometimes, with endoscopic or endobronchial ultrasound guided FNAC of mediastinal lymph nodes. Pleural effusions require thoracocentesis to determine if these are malignant. Video assisted thoracoscopic surgery (VATS) is frequently used for diagnosis, staging and occasionally, resection of the lung cancer.

STAGING OF LUNG CANCER

The TNM system remains the best prognosticator of lung cancer outcome and guides the treatment strategies. The 8th edition of Union for International Cancer Control and the American Joint Committee on Cancer (UICC/AJCC) TNM staging system of lung cancer[34] is recently published in January 2017 based on the recommendations of International Association for Study of Lung cancer (IASCL) **(Tables 2 and 3)**. This system is used to stage NSCLC, SCLC and bronchial carcinoids.

Imaging Modalities for the Staging of Lung Cancers

Chest radiographs and thin section CECT of the thorax and upper abdomen including liver and adrenals as well as supraclavicular areas are the basic imaging required for staging of the lung cancer. Multiplanar reconstructions are essential for the assessment of relationship of tumor with the fissure, adjacent cardiovascular structures and

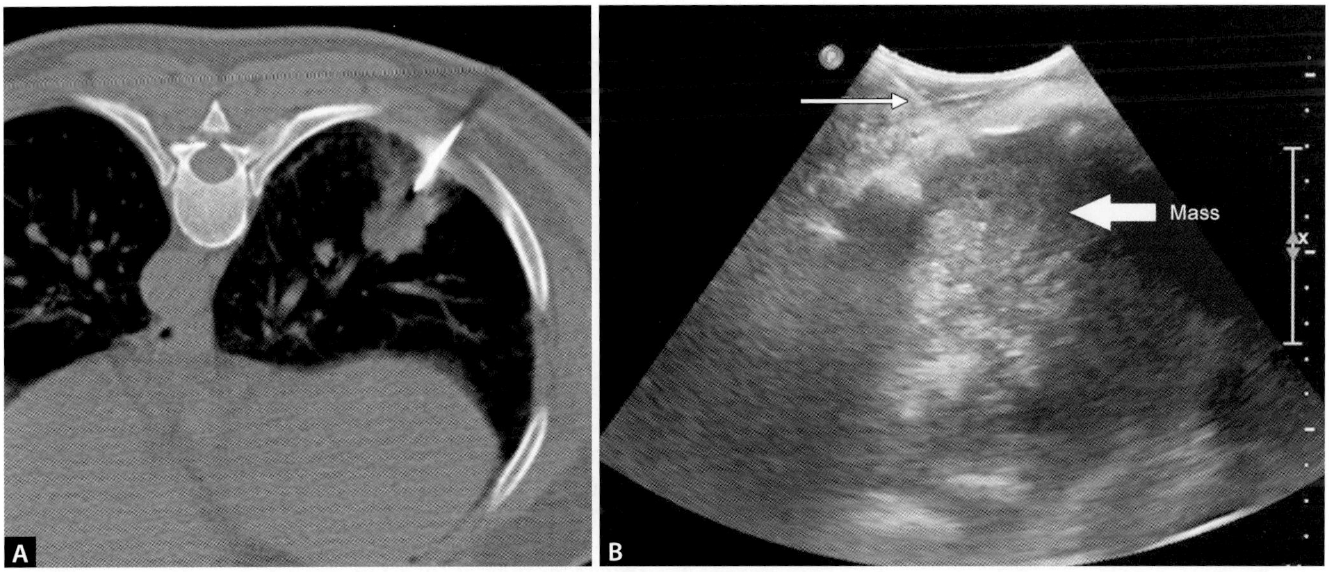

Figs. 12A and B: CT and USG guided biopsy of lung mass: (A) Prone CT image showing a coaxial needle in situ within a peripheral lung mass through which multiple biopsy cores were taken which revealed adenocarcinoma; (B) USG image of a large peripheral lung mass showing needle advanced through intercostal space (thin arrow) within the mass (thick arrow). Biopsy revealed squamous cell carcinoma.

Table 2: TNM descriptors.

T	*Primary tumor*
Tx	Cannot be assessed; Tumor in sputum/ bronchial washings not in imaging/ bronchoscopy
T0	No evidence
Tis	Carcinoma in situ
T1	≤3 cm surrounded by lung/visceral pleura, not involving main bronchus
T1a(mi)	Minimally invasive adenocarcinoma
T1a	≤1 cm
T1b	>1 to ≤2 cm
T1c	>2 to ≤3 cm
T2	>3 to ≤5 cm or Involves main bronchus without carina involvement or Visceral pleural invasion or Atelectasis/postobstructive pneumonitis extending to hilum
T2a	>3 to ≤4 cm
T2b	>4 to ≤5 cm
T3	>5 to ≤7 cm or Separate tumor in same lobe or Direct invasion of chest wall (includes parietal pleura and superior sulcus)/parietal pericardium/phrenic nerve
T4	>7 cm or Separate tumor in different lobe of ipsilateral lung or Invasion of heart/great vessels/diaphragm/ Mediastinum/trachea/carina/esophagus/ recurrent laryngeal nerve/vertebral body
N	***Regional lymph node***
Nx	Cannot be assessed
N0	No involvement
N1	Ipsilateral peribronchial and/or hilar nodes and intrapulmonary nodes
N2	Ipsilateral mediastinal and/or subcarinal nodes
N3	Contralateral mediastinal or hilar; ipsilateral/ contralateral scalene/supraclavicular
M	***Distant metastasis***
M0	No distant metastasis
M1	Distant metastasis is present
M1a	Tumor (s) in contralateral lung; pleural/ pericardial nodule/malignant effusion
M1b	Single extrathoracic metastasis
M1c	Multiple extrathoracic metastases, in one/ more organs

Table 3: Stage groups.

		N0	*N1*	*N2*	*N3*
T1M0	T1a	IA1	IIB	IIIA	IIIB
	T1b	IA2	IIB	IIIA	IIIB
	T1c	IA3	IIB	IIIA	IIIB
T2M0	T2a	IB	IIB	IIIA	IIIB
	T2b	IIA	IIB	IIIA	IIIB
T3M0		IIB	IIIA	IIIB	IIIC
T4M0		IIIA	IIIA	IIIB	IIIC
TxM1	M1a	IVA	IVA	IVA	IVA
	M1b	IVA	IVA	IVA	IVA
	M1c	IVB	IVB	IVB	IVB

exact localization prior to surgery. CT is the primary modality to assess the resectability of the tumor and for assessing the treatment options. However, the accuracy of the CT staging is poor when compared with surgico-pathological staging.[35] For tumor size measurement, the largest long-axis diameter must be measured using multiplanar reformation. Performance of CT alone for T staging is significantly lower than PET-CT, and precise T stages are provided in 68% and 86% respectively.[36] PET-CT is recommended gold standard for N staging of the lung cancer as CT, though highly sensitive for detection of lymph nodes, has low specificity for lymph node characterization into benign or malignant.[36] Also, CT data should be analyzed in conjunction with other modalities such as bone scan or PETCT for accurate M staging.

Salient Points

T Staging

- It includes measuring tumor size (largest long-axis diameter), invasion into adjacent structures and identification of satellite/separate nodule.
- It may be difficult to assess exact size of the tumor in presence of a postobstructive atelectasis/pneumonia and such lesion are considered T2.
- T1 and T2 tumors are most amenable for curative surgical resection. Parietal extension (T3) (rib bone lysis, extrapleural extension) is not a contraindication for surgery and some candidates may benefit from surgical intervention. Though conventionally T4 tumors are unresectable, some cases of T4 tumors may also be eligible for surgery (after a multidisciplinary discussion).[36]

Tracheobronchial Invasion

On CT, the bronchial invasion (T2) or tracheal invasion (T4) is seen as fixed smooth/nodular thickening of their wall. A bronchoscopic correlation is indicated whenever CT detects this finding.

Mediastinal Invasion

- Parietal pericardium/phrenic nerve involvement—T3
- Invasion of heart/great vessels/diaphragm/mediastinum/trachea/carina/esophagus/recurrent laryngeal nerve/vertebral body are categorized under T4.
- On CT/MRI, criteria for vascular invasion include complete circumferential encasement of a vessel **(Figs. 13A and B)** or presence of an intravascular enhancing focus of tumor. Loss of fat planes with the adjacent tissue may not represent actual invasion and such tumors may also be amenable for resection.
- If contact of the mass with the mediastinal vessel is more than 3 cm or more than 90 degree or there is parietal stiffness of the vessels, then it can be suggested as nonresectable; however, these findings needs surgical confirmation and hence a patient should not be deferred surgery on the basis of these imaging findings.
- Involvement of pulmonary veins or left atrium would be seen as hypodense filling defects within the intensely enhancing vessel/atrial chamber and it is categorized into T4 stage.

Pleural Invasion

- Crossing of the fissure by the mass classifies it into T2 **(Fig. 14A)**
- Involvement of parietal pleura makes it T3 lesion
- Distant or non-contiguous nodular pleural thickening—metastatic
- On CT, presence of definite pleural invasion is attributed when there is extension of tumor into the soft tissues beyond the pleura or associated rib bone lysis. Loss of extrapleural fat plane is also a sign of pleural invasion **(Fig. 14B)**. Mere presence of pleural effusion or contact with the pleura are not the signs for pleural invasion and diagnostic pleural fluid aspiration for malignant cytology or VATS guided pleural biopsy should be done to confirm the pleural involvement if it affects the therapy planning.

Chest Wall Invasion

Presence of extrapleural tumor tissue or extension into the ribs confirms the chest wall invasion and these are categorized as T3 lesions **(Figs. 15A and B)**.

MRI and PET-CT may be required for better delineation of chest wall invasion **(Fig. 15C)** as well as in cases of diaphragmatic involvement.

If a pancoast's tumor demonstrates involvement thoracic nerve roots, then it is a T3 stage. If it involves subcalvian vessels, vertebra, shows intraspinal extension **(Fig. 15D)** or involvement of lower cervical nerve roots (C8 and above) or cords of the brachial plexus, then T stage for such tumors would be classified as T4.

Satellite Nodules

Tumor with separate nodules in the same lobe is classified as T3.

Tumor with an ipsilateral nodule in another lobe—T4

Tumor with a nodule contralateral to the primary tumor—M1.

CT is highly sensitive to detect the nodules however lacks specificity. However, presence of separate nodule in same lobe as that of tumor is an indicator of poor prognosis and usually represents tumor nodule.

Lymphangitic Carcinomatosis

This finding *has not been addressed* in TNM staging criteria; however it is important to identify this because

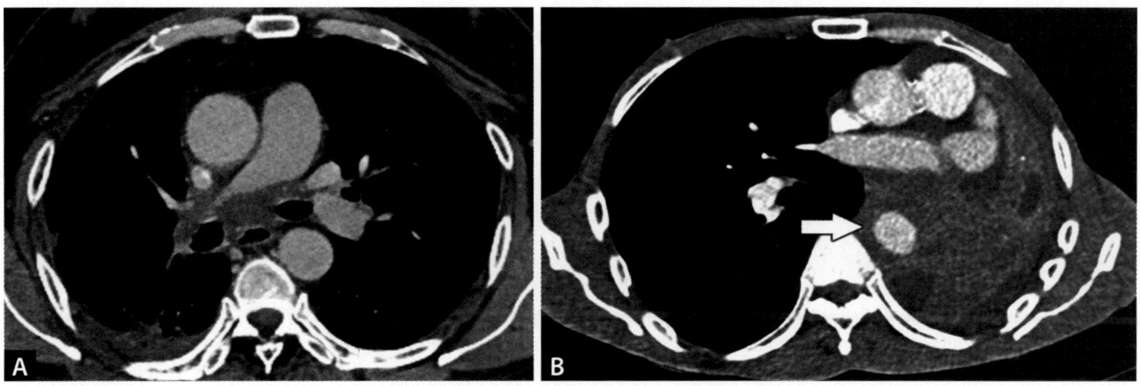

Figs. 13A and B: T4 tumors: (A) Central mass causing narrowing and circumferential involvement of right pulmonary artery suggestive of invasion; (B) Large left lung mass with circumferential invasion of aorta (arrow).

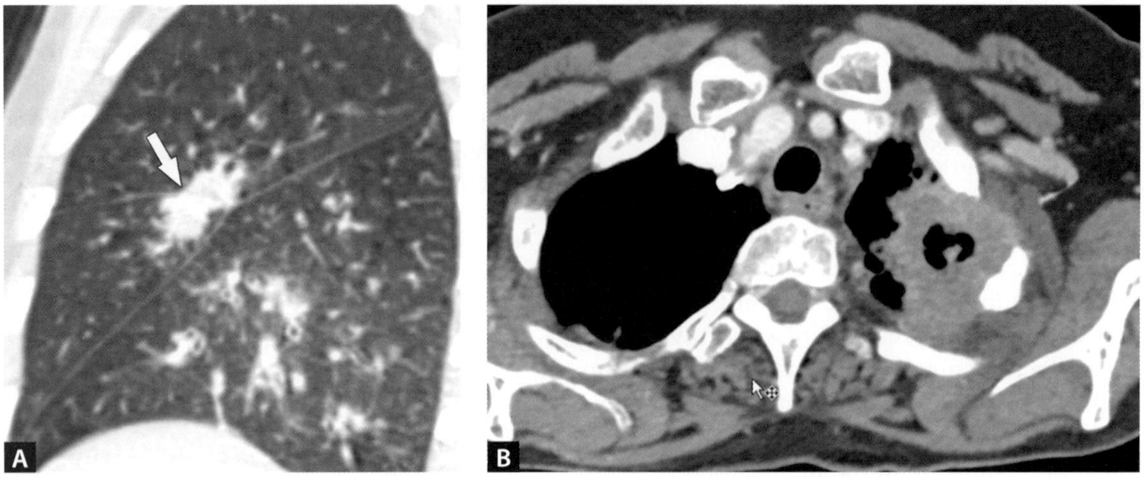

Figs. 14A and B: Invasion of fissure: (A) Sagittal CT image shows crossing of the horizontal fissure by a spiculated mass sign of invasion and T2 tumor; (B) Tumor is abutting the pleura with loss of extrapleural fat plane—A sign of chest wall invasion.

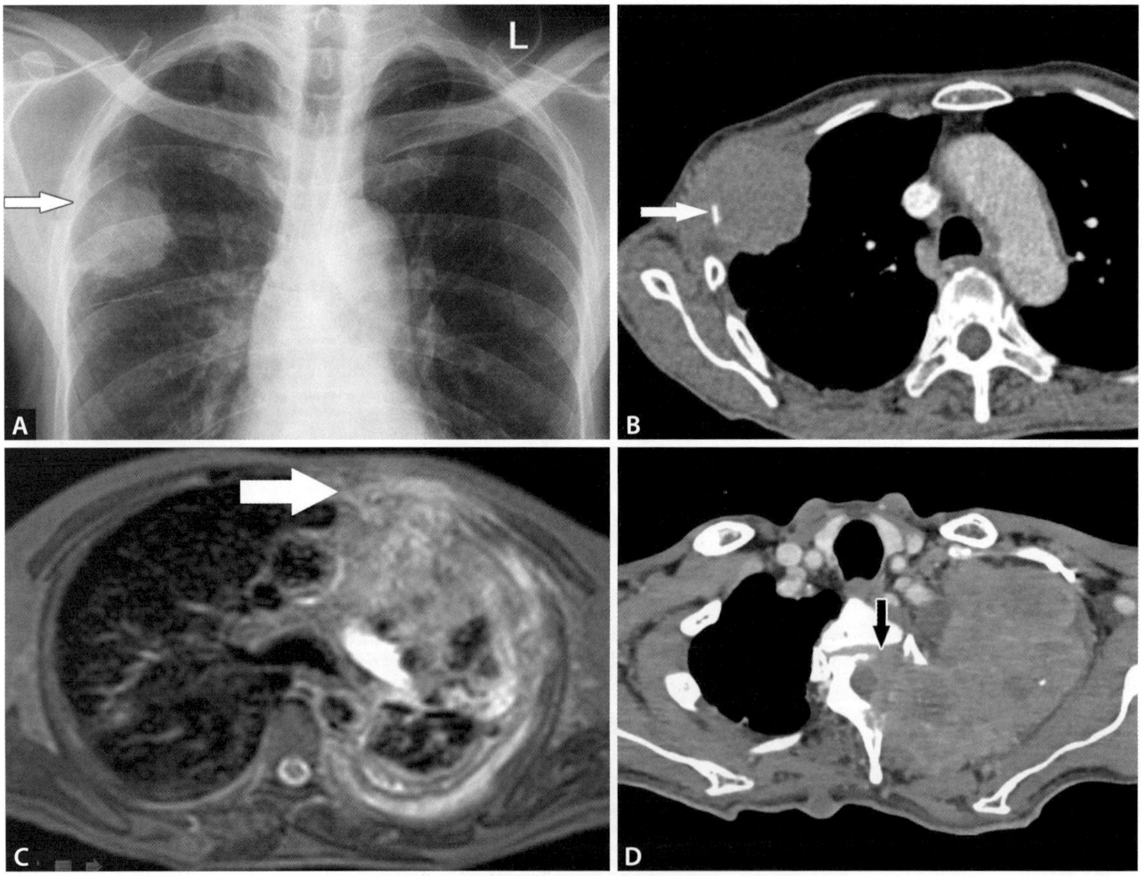

Figs. 15A to D: Chest wall invasion: (A) Frontal chest radiograph showing peripheral mass with nonvisualization of anterior end of second and third ribs; (B) CT shows a large right lung mass with contiguous invasion of the chest wall with rib destruction and extrathoracic soft tissue component (arrow); (C) Axial STIR MRI shows extension of the left upper lobe mass into the anterior chest wall muscles infiltrating the deep fibers of pectoralis muscle; (D) Intraspinal extension of left pancoast's tumor makes it T4 lesion.

presence of diffuse or more than one lobe involvement by lymphangitis carcinomatosis (LC) is a contraindication to surgery. Still, if same lobe as that of tumor is affected then it is not a contraindication.

On CT, it appears as nodular peribronchovascular and septal thickening which represents the perilymphatic extension of tumor nodules **(Fig. 16)**.

N Staging

On CECT, a hilar lymph node of more than 7 mm and mediastinal lymph node of more than 10 mm are considered involved. However, some studies have shown 40% normal sized lymph nodes up to 7 mm to be metastatic (such findings more commonly found in adenocarcinomas).

It should be reported according to 1 to 14 mediastinal lymph nodal stations described by IASLC.[37]

PET-CT is the gold standard for N staging with a high negative predictive value (>90%).[36]

M Staging

- *M1a:* Intrathoracic metastasis—pleural or pericardial nodules, contralateral lung nodule, malignant pleural/ pericardial effusion **(Fig. 17)**.
- *M1b:* Single metastatic lesion in an extrathoracic organ/ non-regional lymph node.
- *M1c:* Multiple metastasis.

Most common organs involved by metastasis include brain, bones, liver and adrenals **(Fig. 18)**. Liver is most commonly involved in small cell lung cancers and sometimes in cases of diffuse metastasis CT may not demonstrate any nodular lesions. Adrenal incidentalomas and metastasis may not be differentiated based on single phase CT alone and may require further imaging in the form of MRI/PETCT and at times even sampling. On CECT, peripheral irregular enhancement of the nodule with central necrotic area is highly suggestive of adrenal metastasis over an adenoma. CT and PET-CT are adequate in demonstration of the metastatic lesions, and histological confirmation should be done in most of the cases.

The CT report must always contain the TNM staging. If there is doubt about the correct T, N or M category then one should assign a lower category as well as stage.

TREATMENT OF LUNG CANCER

If detected in early stage, surgery remains mainstay of treatment for lung carcinoma in the form of either lobectomy, bilobectomy or pneumonectomy. Well defined lesions, away from fissures and no contiguous organ infiltration are the ideal lesions for surgery. However, tumors near carina, chest wall infiltration, or early mediastinal invasion can also be operated if there is no lymphadenopathy or metastatic lesions. Sleeve resection of tracheobronchial tree, chest wall reconstruction etc. are the adjunctive procedures in addition to primary surgery for such difficult lesions. A vast number of these patients will also be receiving chemo or radiotherapy or both. Involvement of trachea, pulmonary artery, aorta become contraindication for surgery. Hence involvement of these

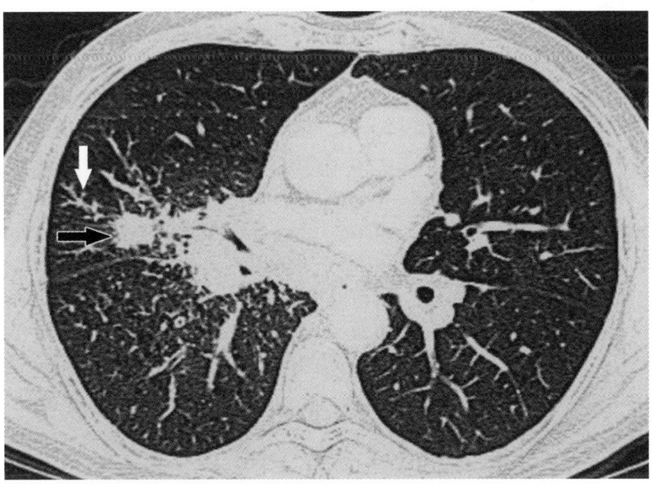

Fig. 16: Lymphangitis carcinomatosis: HRCT image showing a spiculated mass (black arrow) in right parahilar region adjacent peribronchovascular thickening and nodules (white arrow), also extending in right lower lobe.

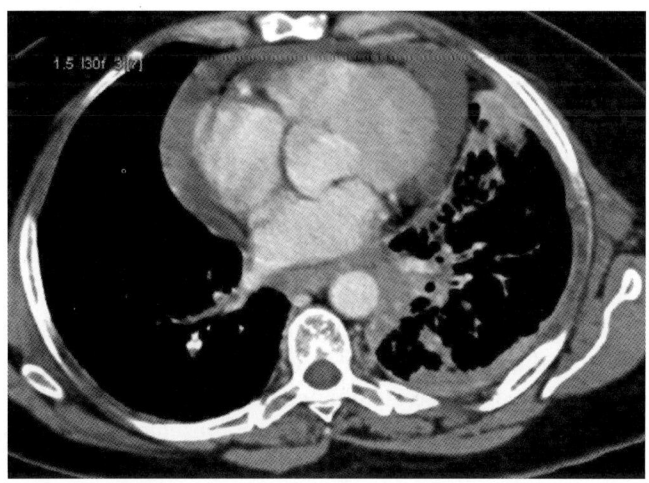

Fig. 17: Malignant pericardial and pleural effusion: CT axial image showing irregular left pleural thickening and mild pericardial effusion in a case of lung adenocarcinoma.

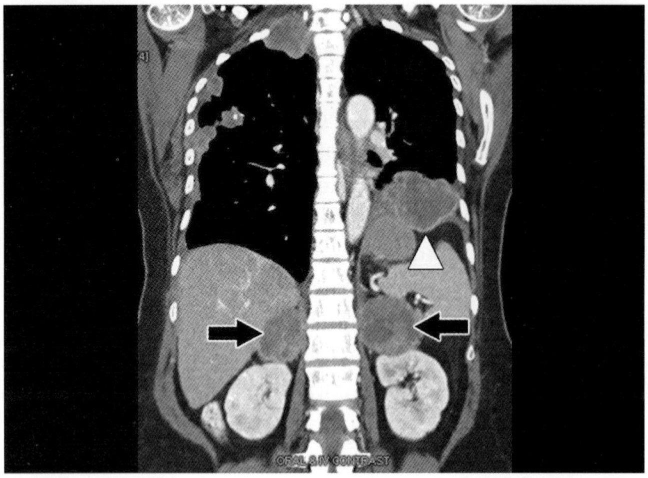

Fig. 18: Adrenal metastasis in disseminated adenocarcinoma lung (right apical tumor). Coronal CT image showing heterogeneous enhancing masses in bilateral suprarenal locations suggestive of adrenal metastasis (arrows). Note is also made of left invasive diaphragmatic metastatic deposit (arrowhead).

structures should be clearly documented in radiological reports.

Chemotherapy for carcinoma lung is different for different histological type of malignancy (squamous, adeno or small cell etc). The choice of chemotherapeutic agents also vary depending upon the presence or absence of many specific receptors, e.g. epidermal growth factor receptor (EGFR). Main therapeutic agents are cisplatin, etoposide, or gemcitabine, etc.[3] For some large (not disseminated) tumors chemotherapy may shrink the tumor to make it surgically resectable in follow-up period.

Conventionally for the cytotoxic drugs given for treatment of lung malignancies, Response Evaluation Criteria in Solid Tumors (RECIST) criteria are used for evaluating treatment response. It is suggested to read the recent RECIST criteria described by Eisenhauer EA et al.[38] and use this for assessing tumor response. However, for some newer (non-cytotoxic) chemotherapeutic agents the conventional RECIST criteria are not suitable as these drugs don't cause reduction in size. For these drugs newer evaluation criteria are being followed in randomized controlled trials (RCTs) which incorporate other imaging features like decrease in enhancement, increasing necrotic component etc. For such lesions even presence of few new lesions and initial increase in size of lesions are not strictly considered as progressive disease.

Patients with more advanced stage malignancies with invasion of major mediastinal structure or contralateral lymph nodes are usually offered supportive and palliative radiotherapy. There are many newer techniques to deliver radiotherapy in a more focused way to only the diseased area and avoiding adjacent normal lung thereby reducing radiation induced damage to the surrounding organs. These modalities are image guided radiotherapy (IGRT), intensity modulated radiation therapy (IMRT), conformational 3D radiotherapy and respiratory gated 4D CT techniques, etc.[39] Heart, esophagus and spinal cord are few of the more radiosensitive organs which need to be preserved more diligently and hence it is important on the part of the reporting radiologist to clearly define involvement of these structures by the neoplastic lesions so that during RT planning the treating radiotherapist is better equipped to avoid injury to these structures.

Radiofrequency ablation (RFA) is another option for those patients who have limited diseases but surgically unfit due to medical comorbidities.[40-43] Excellent results can be achieved for tumors less than 3–4 cm sizes. The complications of RFA can be pneumothorax, hemoptysis, pleural effusion, lung abscess etc. Another potential use of RFA is for treatment of isolated metastatic lesion in adrenal gland.[44]

SCREENING FOR LUNG CANCER

Screening for lung cancers was started based on the premise that if detected in early stage (stage 1 A) there is high survival rates for five years in these patients. In many previous randomized clinical trials (RCTs) which used chest X ray and/or sputum cytology for screening in chronic smokers, there was detection of many early stage cancers, however, there was no proven benefit regarding mortality rates.[45]

More recently many RCTs are going on in US and Europe (e.g. Mayo CT screening project, PLCO (Prostate, Lung, Colorectal and Ovary) and Early Lung Cancer Action Project (ELCAP) using low dose CT protocol (25–30 mAs). As CT is more efficient in detecting smaller nodules as compared to chest X-rays, the likelihood of detection of lung malignancies at earlier stages is more with CT as a screening tool. Few of these studies have evaluated the parameters and concluded that screening with CT for lung malignancies in high risk patient profile (age 55–80 and chronic smokers) provides significant decrease in mortality rates. Many of the societies have recommended that screening should be done in all elderly smokers (55/60 to 80 years) who smoke >30 pack cigarette per year. They have recommended strict criteria regarding definition of nodules, reporting format as well as guidelines for pathological evaluation and the treatment algorithms for such detected lesions in screening programs. The nodules detected during screening are typically smaller in size and represent less advance malignancies. Majority of these lesions will ultimately prove to be benign. High false positivity for these nodules to be cancers is a particular disadvantage. This problem is even more severe in areas with high prevalence of granulomatous diseases, e.g. in India. Careful evaluation of all the characteristics of these screening detected nodules is necessary to reduce the number of unnecessary biopsy or thoractomy. A nodule which is smaller than 10 mm is usually followed and subjected to biopsy when it shows suspicious growth pattern for malignancy. For larger lesions PET and CT guided biopsies are performed.

Till now there is no state sponsored lung screening program in India. This is partly attributed to high prevalence of granulomatous disease (TB) in our country in which imaging findings may mimic early cancers resulting in significant anxiety and resultant more invasive tests to prove the exact nature of these nodules; and partly due to lack of availability of sufficient imaging, pathology as well as surgical services which have got overburdened from various other diseases utilizing the already existing meager health care resources.

FOLLOW-UP IMAGING

Follow-up imaging for lung malignancies is done to detect treatment response. If patient has been treated with surgery and complete resection was feasible, then follow up imaging is done to detect recurrence and metastatic lesions. If patient has been treated with chemotherapeutic agents then follow up imaging is done to detect early response. This helps in deciding whether to continue with same treatment regime or should change it early to try other regimens. With few newer non-cytotoxic chemotherapeutic agents the clinical question of interest is to find whether there is progression or not. If no progression is there, then the same agent will be continued for further treatment otherwise a decision will be taken to change the agent quite early in course of treatment. Similarly imaging is also done to detect complications due to treatments. If patient is asymptomatic then chest X ray and clinical examination are sufficient. There is no standard protocol to follow these patients on CT, some centers do not prefer any follow up if patient is asymptomatic while other centers prefer every six monthly follow up.[46,47] Other expected changes are pleural thickening , crowding of ribs, ipsilateral mediastinal shift, etc.

Radiologists should be familiar with expected changes in imaging after some treatment. In the initial phase after lobectomy, there is presence of postoperative cavity with air fluid level **(Figs. 19A to C)**. The pneumothorax may be large in initial phase of postoperative time. In due course of time the cavity disappears with absorption of fluid and compensatory hyperinflation of the residual lobes.

Post-radiotherapy changes are seen as acute or chronic changes. In acute radiation pneumonitis there is appearance of ground-glass opacities within three months of completion in the radiation portal area. In chronic phase other changes are seen like consolidation, fibrosis, bronchiectasis or volume loss. The area of involvement shrinks with passage of time. The changes of radiation pneumonitis need to be differentiated from infective etiology. Infections usually conform to lobar or segmental anatomy; on the contrary the radiation changes conforms to the radiation field and may even cross fissures. However, for proper evaluation of these postradiation changes the radiologist should have complete information regarding the radiation field, type of radiation technique used e.g. IGRT, IMRT or conformal RT.[48,49] Small pericardial or

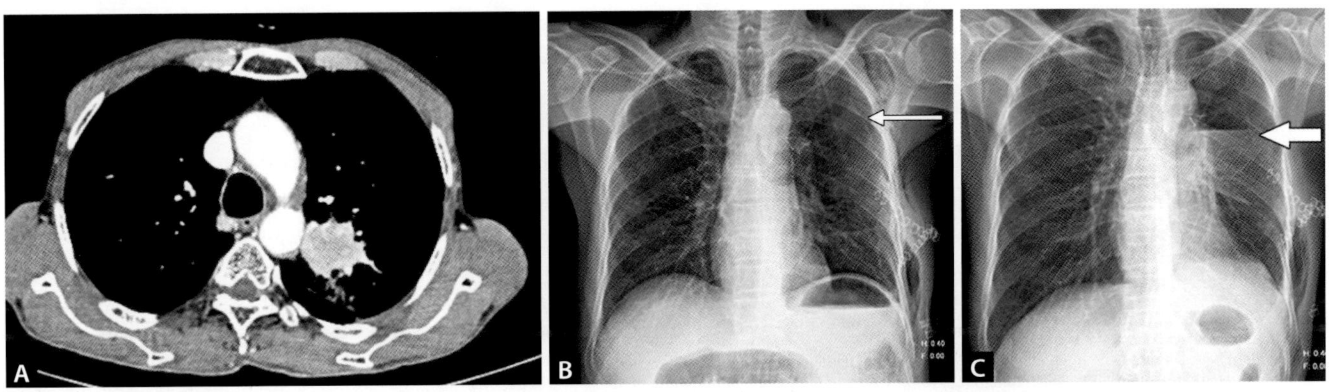

Figs. 19A to C: Normal postlobectomy appearance: (A) CT shows a stage IIA lobulated mass for which a left upper lobectomy was done; (B) Chest radiograph shows mild pneumothorax on postoperative day 4; (C) Postoperative day 14 radiograph shows air-fluid level in the pleural cavity in left upper zone which is normal finding after lobectomy.

pleural effusions are quite common after radiation therapy and they usually develop up to initial 9 months and resolve themselves by 12–16 months.

Other changes seen in post treatment period are drug toxicity and infections both of which may give similar radiological appearance. One of the commonly given drug, Geftinib, causes interstitial pulmonary fibrosis.[50] Almost all chemotherapeutic agents given in patients with NSCLC can cause lung fibrosis. The main imaging findings are ground-glass opacity, fibrosis and interstitial opacities.

RECURRENT LUNG CANCER

In lung cancer patients who have been treated, recurrences are more common at distant site as compared to the loco regional site.[47] The imaging findings in recurrence are usually similar to original tumors. The main imaging features of recurrent lesions are either developing mass or lymphadenopathy. Other features suspicious of recurrence are increasing hydropneumothorax in post-pneumonectomy patients, or appearance of a new air fluid level. Because of significant distortion of normal bronchial anatomy following lobectomy and post radiotherapy fibrotic changes, interpretation of CT examination in these patients become particularly challenging. Still there are few features which make one suspicious of recurrence are, emergence of new pulmonary nodule, or new bronchial stenosis, new or increasing soft tissue at hilum or enlarging mediastinal or hilar lymph nodes.[50] Similarly new appearance of pleural effusion after 6 months of radiotherapy also is a suspicious finding which needs aspiration to exclude recurrent lesion. In the areas of postradiation pneumonitis, new opacification of previously dilated and patent bronchi is also an important clue for recurrence of the disease.[51] When recurrence is suspected, PET is the most sensitive modality to diagnose the recurrence.

RARE LUNG MALIGNANCIES

Other uncommon lung malignancies are sarcomas and pulmonary blastomas. Few of these sarcomas are quite benign in course of disease, e.g. endobronchial fibrosarcoma and leiomyosarcoma. Other sarcomas which are quite aggressive in clinical behavior are rhabdomyosarcoma, osteosarcoma, chondrosarcoma, angiosarcoma and malignant fibrous histiocytoma, myxoid sarcoma, etc **(Figs. 20A and B)**. Sometimes there are sarcomatous component in non-small cell lung carcinoma (NSCLC) which are classified as carcinosarcoma, which have imaging appearance similar to non-small cell lung cancer (NSCLC). Out of these the angiosarcomas have a characteristic enhancement on CT as well as MRI.[52] Kaposi sarcoma are common in AIDS patients which show multiple nodular flame shaped opacities or linear peribronchial opacities . Other findings associated with Kaposi sarcoma are ground-glass opacities secondary to hemorrhage, lymphadenopathy or pleural effusion.[53] Pulmonary blastomas are usually found in children with solid masses having extensive cystic changes. Another separate entity pleuropulmonary blastoma show solid cystic masses which may mimic congenital lung lesion like cystic adenomatoid malformation or sequestration.[54]

Pulmonary blastoma arises from germ cell and classified under carcinosarcoma. These are usually found in children and young adults. On imaging, these are seen as single or multiple peripheral solid lung masses with cystic changes, cavitation and occasionally, calcifications.[55]

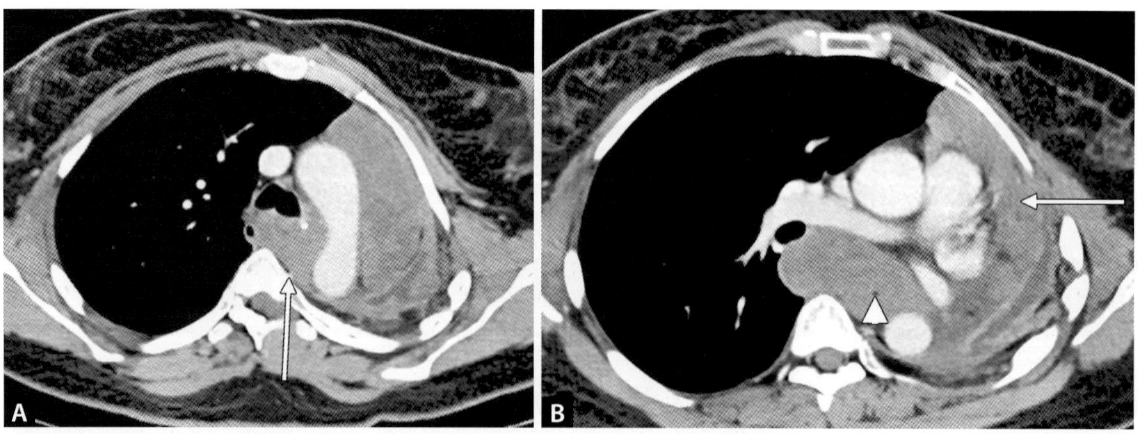

Figs. 20A and B: Myxoid sarcoma: Axial CT images of a 34-year-old female showing heterogeneous infiltrating mass involving the left main bronchus (arrowhead) with contiguous mediastinal extension (arrows) and complete collapse of left lung. Endobronchial biopsy was suggestive of myxoid sarcoma.

Pleuropulmonary blastoma is a separate entity seen in early childhood. These arise from primitive blastomatous tissues and develop in pre-existing congenital lung lesions like cystic adenomatoid malformation, sequestration or bronchogenic cysts. On imaging, these are seen as cystic-solid masses.[54]

PULMONARY LYMPHOMA

Primary Pulmonary Lymphoma

Most primary pulmonary lymphomas commonly arises from mucosa-associated lymphoid tissue commonly called MALT lymphoma, comprising up to 90% of cases although it is a fairly rare disease. Rest of the pulmonary lymphomas include diffuse large B-cell non-Hodgkin's lymphoma (NHL) followed by Hodgkin lymphoma (HL) usually from direct extension of mediastinal disease to involve parenchyma.[56,57]

There is lymphangitic spread at the periphery of these lesions leading to invasion of the adjacent pleura, vessels, and airways.[58] Main imaging findings on CT include nodules, masses, and/or nodular/mass like areas of ground-glass attenuation or consolidation (CT angiogram sign) with air bronchograms around bronchovascular distribution, hilar and mediastinal lymphadenopathy. Pleural effusion is uncommonly seen. They appear FDG avid in PET/CT scan in 50% cases. Patients tend to present around the 6th decade former or active smokers and has been associated with multiple autoimmune diseases such as Sjögren syndrome, rheumatoid arthritis, common variable immunodeficiency, concurrent lymphoid interstitial pneumonitis (LIP), chronic inflammation from smoking, and infections such as HIV and hepatitis C.[58,59]

The imaging picture on CT can be mimicked by sarcoidosis as it tends to show peribronchovascular distribution. Similarly polyangiitis (formerly Wegener granulomatosis), perilymphatic spread of metastatic disease and infection showing peribronchial consolidation can mimic MALT lymphoma. Clinical presentation and laboratory parameters can be helpful in narrowing the differential diagnosis.

Diagnosis is made usually by transbronchial, CT-guided percutaneous transthoracic biopsy or at times with a surgical biopsy. Immunohistochemical studies are required for definitive diagnosis to confirm a monoclonal B-cell population, which is positive for pan-B-cell antigens like CD19, CD20 and PAX-5.[5,60]

Treatment is usually with chemotherapy or immunotherapy (rituximab) with options of surgery and radiation therapy for localized disease. MALT lymphoma tends to recur in the lung in up to 50% cases within the first years after diagnosis. Although regional involvement of hilar lymph nodes does not affect prognosis, but presence pleural effusion or amyloid within the tumor signifies poorer prognosis.[57,60]

Secondary Pulmonary Lymphoma (SPL)

All the different forms of lymphoma may secondarily involve the lungs, but the mature B-cell neoplasms are the most frequent. Although a greater proportion of patients with HL rather than NHL have lung involvement, more NHL SPL is seen in clinical practice because NHL is more prevalent. Lymphomatous involvement of the lung itself is often asymptomatic and non-specific. However, B-symptoms of HL more often related to the presence of mediastinal lymphadenopathy.

Imaging findings are varied and nonspecific and include nodules <1 cm in diameter, solitary or multiple, mass/mass-like consolidation, bronchovascular thickening mimicking lymphangitis carcinomatosa, air bronchograms (NHL > HL) **(Figs. 21A and B)**. Mediastinal lymphadenopathy with nodules/masses with or without air bronchograms are the commonest HRCT features.[61,62] In HL, there is contiguous spread of the disease from the adenopathy to involve parenchyma whereas isolated lung disease without mediastinal involvement can occur in NHL.

Acquired Immune Deficiency Syndrome-Related Lymphoma (ARL)

Lymphoma is the second most common tumor occurring in patients with AIDS, after Kaposi's sarcoma. Most patients are symptomatic, presenting with cough and shortness of breath. This subset of patients usually develops aggressive B-cell lymphomas.[63]

Imaging findings include well-defined pulmonary nodules (0.5–5 cm) with or without cavitation or a large solitary pulmonary nodule/mass (2–5 cm), Pleural effusions is commonest thoracic manifestation followed by pericardial effusions, consolidation and/or ground-glass opacity. Combinations of nodules, effusions, adenopathy in a HIV positive patient is highly suggestive of ARL.[64]

Post-transplantation Lymphoproliferative Disorder

The post-transplantation lymphoproliferative disorder (PTLD) is a lymphoid/plasmacytic proliferation that occurs following solid organ or hematopoietic stem cell transplantation, manifesting as a spectrum of disorders ranging from polyclonal benign proliferations to monoclonal and monomorphic aggressive lymphomas.

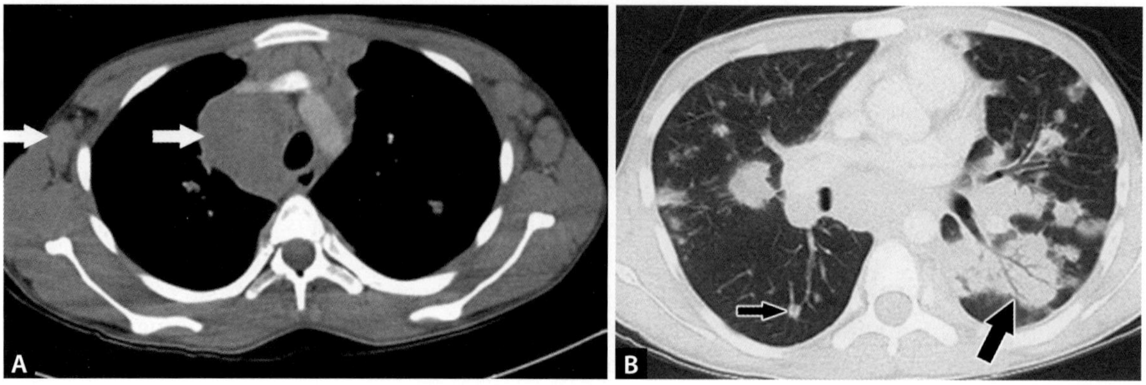

Figs. 21A and B: Secondary pulmonary involvement by lymphoma (nodular form): (A) Axial CT image mediastinal window shows homogeneous enlarged lymph nodes in mediastinum and bilateral axillae in a case of non-Hodgkin's lymphoma; (B) Multiple irregular lung nodules with air bronchograms (arrows) are seen in both lungs suggestive of lymphomatous involvement.

The etiology of PTLD is thought to be closely associated with EBV infection. PTLD is seen in less than 2% of all transplant cases and there is a clear association with the specific organ transplanted, with the highest incidence in lung transplantation (6–9%), followed by heart, liver and renal transplant. The majority of cases of PTLD occur within 2 years of transplantation, but it may be seen as early as 60 days post-transplant.[65]

The clinical presentation is variable and includes fever, lymphadenopathy, and abdominal pain with diarrhea, a mononucleosis-like syndrome and weight loss.

B-cell NHL is the most common type of lymphoma associated with PTLD. The most common imaging findings of PTLD are well defined usually multiple nodules (size range 0.3–5 cm), "halo sign" around nodules, patchy/focal consolidation or ground-glass opacity, more peribronchial/subpleural than diffuse distribution of nodules and lymphadenopathy.[66,67]

PULMONARY NEUROENDOCRINE NEOPLASMS

Pulmonary neuroendocrine neoplasms constitute approximately 20–25% of all invasive primary lung cancers. World Health Organization (WHO) in 2015 has grouped pulmonary neuroendocrine neoplasms into three histologic grades: Typical carcinoid as low-grade malignant neoplasm, atypical carcinoid as intermediate grade, and large cell neuroendocrine carcinoma (LCNEC) and small cell lung carcinoma (SCLC) as high-grade malignancies.[68,69]

Carcinoid Tumors

The respiratory tract is the second most common location after gastrointestinal tract, accounting for 20–30% of carcinoids.[70] They are indolent neoplasms with the potential to metastasize. Typical carcinoid is the least aggressive carcinoid type whereas atypical carcinoid is a more aggressive with 57% of affected patients present with lymph node metastases.[71]

Typical carcinoid is defined as a well-differentiated neoplasm with neuroendocrine histologic features, measuring 5 mm or more, exhibiting less than two mitoses per 10 high-power fields (HPF) or 2 mm^2, and no necrosis. The carcinoid is classified as atypical carcinoid when there are two to 10 mitoses per 10 HPF or necrosis, which is often punctate.[68] Most carcinoids are vascular lesions, and 30% of cases exhibit calcification.[72]

Most affected patients are adults although carcinoid is the most common malignant primary lung neoplasm till young adulthood.[71]

Most patients with centrally located neoplasms, present with symptoms like recurrent infections, cough, haemoptysis, and wheezing whereas peripheral tumors are asymptomatic and hence detected late.[69] Patients may present with Cushing syndrome and Carcinoid syndrome particularly patients with liver metastases. Carcinoid syndrome is characterized by skin flushing, bronchoconstriction, intractable diarrhoea, and right-sided heart disease.[73]

Imaging Findings

Carcinoids show a centrally located (hilar or perihilar), well-defined solitary 2–5 cm nodule more common in occur in the right lung (60%).[74] Atypical carcinoid tends to be larger and more peripheral than typical carcinoid.[75] Consider atypical carcinoid rather than typical carcinoid in older patients with well-defined peripheral nodule or central mass associated with lymph node or distant metastases. Multidetector CT demonstrates soft-tissue nodule located adjacent to airway[76] and may be completely endoluminal **(Figs. 22A and B)**, partially endoluminal, or may abut the

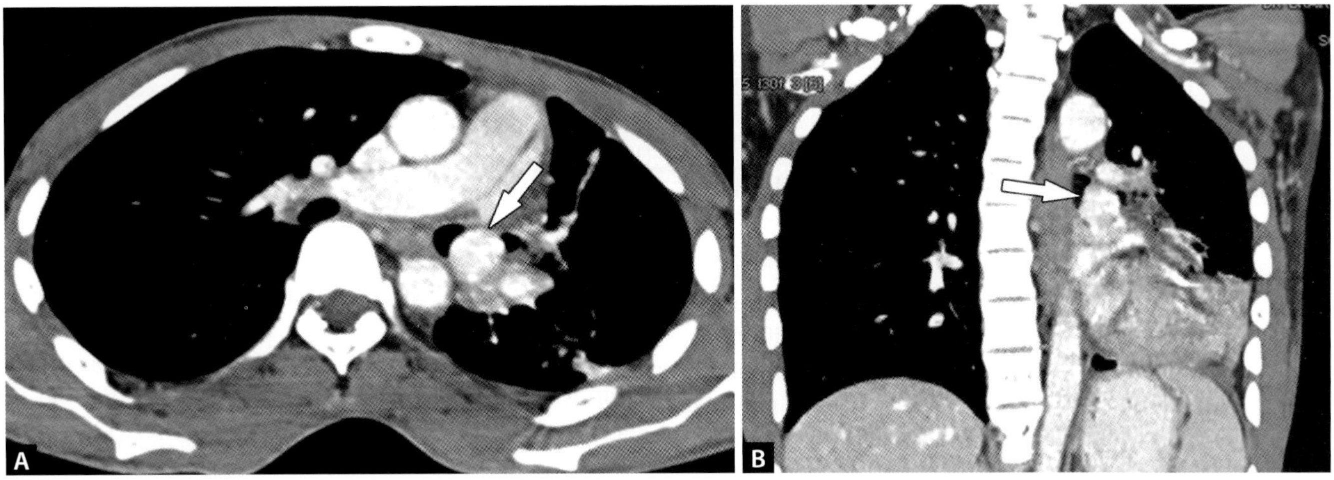

Figs. 22A and B: Typical carcinoid: (A and B) Intensely enhancing endoluminal nodule is seen in left main and lower lobe bronchus (arrows) with partial collapse of left lower lobe.

airway. Positive "bronchus sign" demonstrating bronchus leading directly to the tumor may suggest the diagnosis. CT may demonstrate variable degrees of tumor enhancement differentiating it from adjacent atelectasis **(Figs. 22A and B)** or consolidation.[74] Calcification may be seen. CT is also useful for detection of lymphadenopathy and metastases in the liver, bone, or adrenal glands.[77]

MR imaging usually shows lesions with high T2 and STIR (short inversion time inversion-recovery) signal intensity and intense enhancement during the systemic circulatory phase.[77] Indium 111 octreotide or lanreotide (short- and long-acting somatostatin analogs) scintigraphy can be useful for localization of occult tumors.[71] 68 Gallium DOTANOC scan is currently used to image the primary as well as lymph node metastasis (more sensitive investigation).[78]

The diagnosis of carcinoid tumor requires microscopic evaluation of tissue, which can be obtained with bronchoscopy or CT guided biopsy or thoracotomy.[76]

Large Cell Neuroendocrine Carcinoma

The LCNEC is defined as a high-grade non-SCLC with neuroendocrine histologic features, more than 10 mitoses per 10 HPF (median, 70 mitoses per 10 HPF), and necrosis. Most patients with LCNEC are heavy smoker male, with a mean age of 65 years (range, 44–82 years). Presenting symptoms are like other lung masses whereas paraneoplastic syndromes are rare.[69] The diagnosis of LCNEC is by surgical lung biopsy.

Imaging Findings

At imaging, LCNEC typically manifests as a large (13 to 92 mm), peripheral mass indistinguishable from other lung cancers and typically exhibits well-defined lobular margins.[79] Approximately one-fifth of LCNECs are centrally located and may be associated with pressure symptoms.[80] Necrosis, heterogeneous or peripheral enhancement, calcification, hilar and mediastinal lymphadenopathy.

Small Cell Lung Carcinoma

SCLC is the most common neuroendocrine lung neoplasm, representing 15–20% of invasive lung malignancies.[68]

SCLC is characterized by its small cell size, scant cytoplasm, finely granular nuclear chromatin, absent or faint nucleoli, extremely high mitotic rates (>10 mitoses per 10 HPF; median, 80 mitoses per 10 HPF), and extensive necrosis. The diagnosis is often established by image-guided or bronchoscopy biopsy. A panel of immunohistochemical stains including CD56, TTF-1, and Ki-67 is typically used to differentiate SCLC from other lung masses. The Ki-67 proliferation index is most helpful in separating SCLC from carcinoids.[69] SCLC occurs almost exclusively in smokers, and affected patients present with cough, hemoptysis, chest pain, and dyspnea. Constitutional symptoms, symptoms related to SVC invasion or extrapulmonary metastases. Patients with SCLC may also present with endocrine and nonendocrine paraneoplastic syndromes like SIADH and, Cushing syndrome, Eaton-Lambert syndrome, and encephalomyelitis.

Imaging Findings

On CT, SCLC typically manifests as a large central or mediastinal mass which are combination of the primary and associated lymphadenopathy. Bronchus cut-off sign, calcifications and pleural effusion may be present. The primary tumor may not be visible at times due to mediastinal lymphadenopathy.[81] Encasement or invasion of mediastinal structures, pleural effusion, pericardial thickening, pleural nodules, and metastases to the liver, adrenal glands, and bones may be seen.[81]

Diffuse Idiopathic Pulmonary Neuroendocrine Cell Hyperplasia (DIPNECH)

It is a preinvasive lesion of neuroendocrine group of tumors. On CT, it may present as mosaic attenuation secondary to expiratory air-trapping due to proliferation of neuroendocrine cells within bronchial/bronchiolar epithelium. Sometimes, it may manifest as multiple lung nodules or tumorlets (<5 mm).[82]

PULMONARY METASTASES

The lung metastasis is extremely common due to its high blood or lymphatics supply and through hematogenous and lymphatic routes. Lymphangitis carcinomatosis is a special form of lung metastasis where lymphatics in interlobular septa are clogged with tumor cells and appear nodular thickening of sepate on HRCT images. Most common cancers that metastasize to lungs include breast, colon, kidney, uterus, and head and neck are the most common primary sites with a pulmonary metastasis.[83] Cancers like choriocarcinoma, osteosarcoma, testicular tumor, melanoma, Ewing tumor, and thyroid carcinoma also frequently metastasize to the lung.[84] The early diagnosis of pulmonary metastases is crucial for treatment planning as well as for prognostication. MDCT is the most common imaging modality used for detection of possible pulmonary metastases. Typically, metastases appear well circumscribed soft tissue attenuation, rounded lesions, more often in the periphery of the lung of variable size, a feature which is of some use in distinguishing them from a granuloma.[85] A prominent pulmonary vessel (feeding vessel sign) can be seen heading into a metastasis **(Fig. 23A)**. The usual radiologic findings of a pulmonary metastasis include multiple peripherally located round variable-sized nodules (hematogenous metastasis) and diffuse thickening of the interstitium (lymphangitic carcinomatosis).[84] Among cases of multiple nodules detected with CT, 73% were reported to be pulmonary metastases.[86] The unusual radiologic features include cavitation **(Fig. 23B)** (squamous cell carcinoma, most often from the head and neck or from the lung), hemorrhage around the metastatic nodules (choriocarcinoma, angiosarcoma) **(Fig. 23C)**, pneumothorax (osteosarcoma), calcification (osteosarcoma **(Figs. 24A to C)**, chondrosarcoma, papillary thyroid carcinoma), air-space pattern, tumor embolism, endobronchial metastasis, solitary mass, dilated vessels within a mass, and sterilized metastasis. Innumerable small metastases (miliary pattern) may be seen in malignant melanoma, osteosarcoma, renal cell carcinoma, thyroid carcinoma and trophoblastic disease. Conversely, a pulmonary metastasis may be single in colorectal carcinoma, malignant melanoma, skeletal sarcoma and testicular carcinoma.[85] Adenocarcinoma metastases, rather than displace or destroy adjacent lung parenchyma, may grow in a lepidic fashion (spread along alveolar walls) resulting in pneumonia-like consolidation/air bronchograms.

PULMONARY HAMARTOMA

Hamartoma is the most common, slowly growing benign mesenchymal pulmonary neoplasm and represents about 6% of SPN detected on a CXR.[87] It consists of connective tissue elements such as fat, calcification, muscle, lymphatics. On CT, hamartomas typically manifest as well-circumscribed peripheral solitary pulmonary nodules or

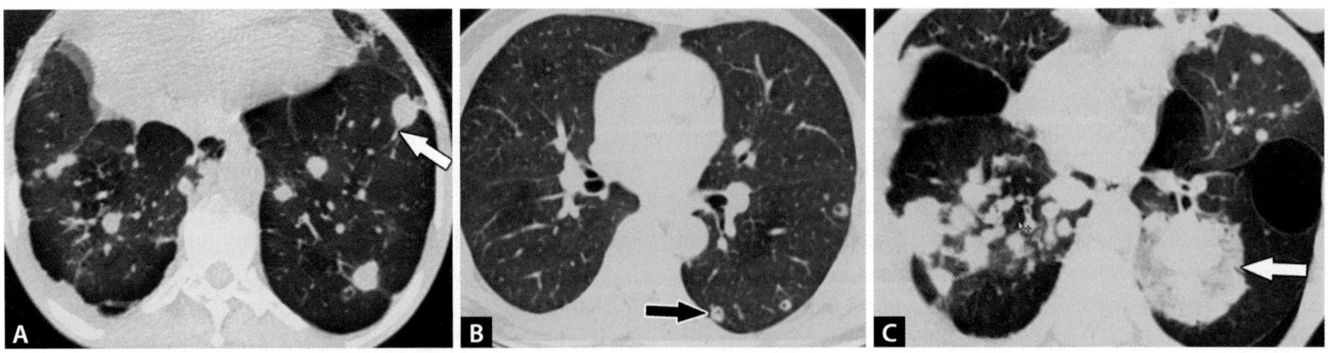

Figs. 23A to C: Pulmonary metastases: (A) CT lung window shows multiple well-defined nodules predominantly in peripheral lung with feeding vessel sign (arrow); (B) Cavitory metastases: CT of the patient with supraglottic squamous cell cancer shows multiple lung metastases in left lung showing cavitation (arrow); (C) Hemorrhagic metastases: CT of the patient with renal cell carcinoma shows multiple lung masses with ground-glass opacities around them (arrow), secondary to hemorrhages.

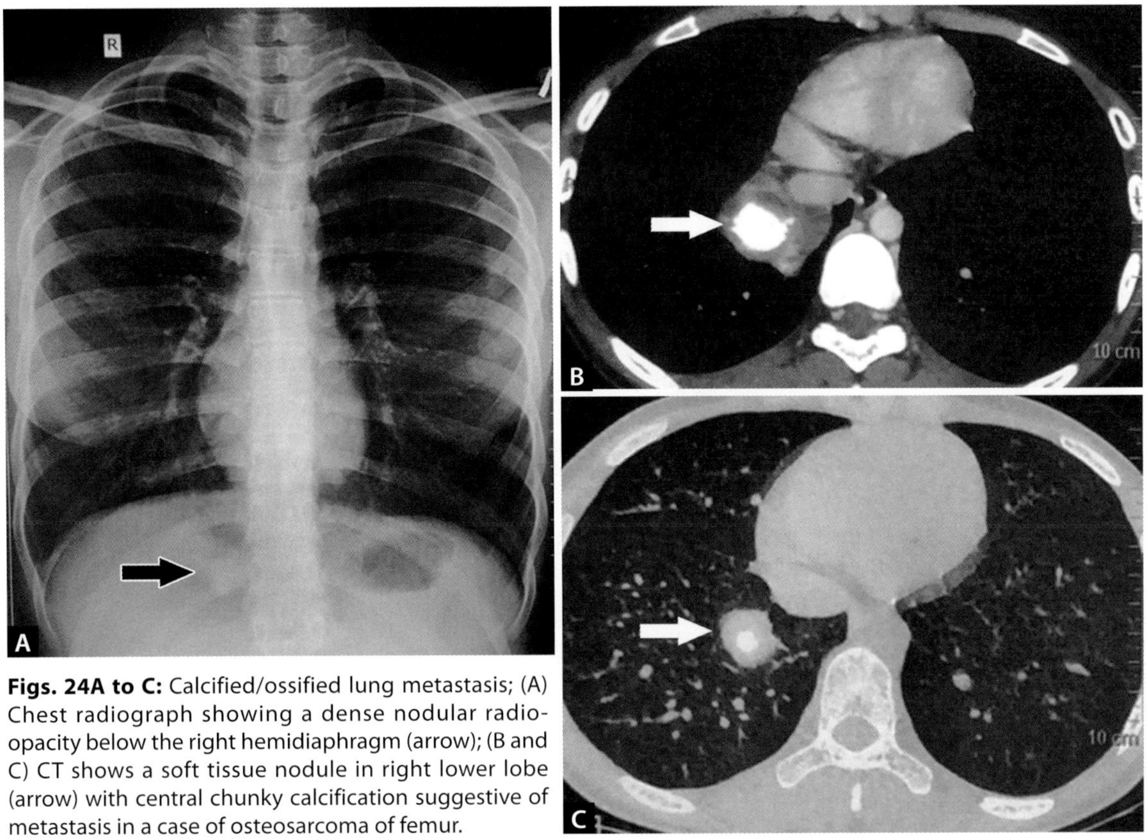

Figs. 24A to C: Calcified/ossified lung metastasis; (A) Chest radiograph showing a dense nodular radio-opacity below the right hemidiaphragm (arrow); (B and C) CT shows a soft tissue nodule in right lower lobe (arrow) with central chunky calcification suggestive of metastasis in a case of osteosarcoma of femur.

masses with smooth or lobular borders **(Fig. 25)**. 10% are central and endobronchial. Calcification is more common in larger lesions and is much better visualized on CT than on radiography. Although a characteristic popcorn pattern of calcification has been described, it is only present in 10–15% of cases. Internal fat, identified by Hounsfield units of -20 to -120 on CT, is present in 60% of cases. Identification of both internal fat and calcium is virtually diagnostic of a hamartoma. Following the administration of intravenous contrast, most lesions demonstrate heterogeneous enhancement.

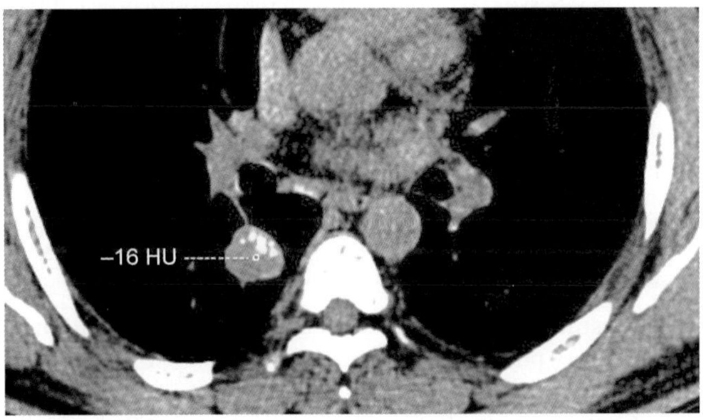

Fig. 25: Pulmonary hamartoma. A non-contrast CT axial image shows a well-defined nodule in peripheral aspect of right lower lobe with internal calcification and fat attenuation suggestive of a pulmonary hamartoma.

CONCLUSION

In conclusion, imaging is an integral part of management protocol for pulmonary neoplasms. A thorough knowledge of available imaging modalities and judicious utilization of these is necessary for optimal patient care. Chest radiography and CT are most commonly used modalities. MRI can be used as a problem solving tool. Survival in carcinoma lung depends on stage; an early detection and diagnosis can help in achieving surgical cure. Here, the cross sectional imaging play a key role in the assessment of malignancy. CT, being less expensive and more widely available than MRI, is more likely to remain as a principal modality for evaluation of this disease. PET-CT helps for further characterization and assessment of extent of disease. It is important that radiologists are familiar with the new 8th TNM staging system for accurate assessment of prognosis and treatment planning. FNAC, biopsy and image guided ablations (e.g. RFA) for lung tumors are major interventions performed, which need meticulous planning using various imaging modalities.

REFERENCES

1. Siegel RL, Miller KD, Jemal A. Cancer Statistics, 2017. CA Cancer J Clin. 2017;67(1):7-30.
2. Time trends in cancer incidence rates 1982-2010 [Internet]. 2013.
3. Schrump DS GG, Kelsey CR. Non Small Cell Lung Cancer. In: DeVita VT LT, Rosenberg SA (Eds), 8th edition. Philadelphia: Lippincott Williams & Wilkins; 2008. p. 896-946.
4. Xue X, Liu Y, Pan L, et al. Diagnosis of multiple primary lung cancer: a systematic review. J Int Med Res. 2013;41(6):1779-87.
5. Travis WD, Brambilla E, Nicholson AG, et al. The 2015 World Health Organization Classification of Lung Tumors: Impact of Genetic, Clinical and Radiologic Advances Since the 2004 Classification. J Thorac Oncol. 2015;10(9):1243-60.
6. Dong Y, Mao F, Wang WP, et al. Value of Contrast-Enhanced Ultrasound in Guidance of Percutaneous Biopsy in Peripheral Pulmonary Lesions. Biomed Res Int. 2015;2015:531507.
7. Batra P, Brown K, Aberle DR, et al. Imaging techniques in the evaluation of pulmonary parenchymal neoplasms. Chest. 1992;101(1):239-43.
8. Tacelli N, Santangelo T, Scherpereel A, et al. Perfusion CT allows prediction of therapy response in non-small cell lung cancer treated with conventional and anti-angiogenic chemotherapy. Eur Radiol. 2013;23(8):2127-36.
9. Zhang LJ, Yang GF, Wu SY, et al. Dual-energy CT imaging of thoracic malignancies. Cancer Imaging. 2013;13:81-91.
10. Hou WS, Wu HW, Yin Y, et al. Differentiation of lung cancers from inflammatory masses with dual-energy spectral CT imaging. Acad Radiol. 2015;22(3):337-44.
11. Dennie C, Thornhill R, Sethi-Virmani V, et al. Role of quantitative computed tomography texture analysis in the differentiation of primary lung cancer and granulomatous nodules. Quant Imaging Med Surg. 2016;6(1):6-15.
12. Heyneman LE, Patz EF. PET imaging in patients with bronchioloalveolar cell carcinoma. Lung Cancer. 2002;38(3):261-6.
13. Erasmus JJ, McAdams HP, Patz EF, et al. Evaluation of primary pulmonary carcinoid tumors using FDG PET. Am J Roentgenol. 1998;170(5):1369-73.
14. Chang JM, Lee HJ, Goo JM, et al. False positive and false negative FDG-PET scans in various thoracic diseases. Korean J Radiol. 2006;7(1):57-69.
15. Fischer B, Lassen U, Mortensen J, et al. Preoperative staging of lung cancer with combined PET-CT. N Engl J Med. 2009;361(1):32-9.
16. Gupta NC, Rogers JS, Graeber GM, et al. Clinical role of F-18 fluorodeoxyglucose positron emission tomography imaging in patients with lung cancer and suspected malignant pleural effusion. Chest. 2002;122(6):1918-24.
17. Song JW, Oh YM, Shim TS, et at. Efficacy comparison between (18)F-FDG PET/CT and bone scintigraphy in detecting bony metastases of non-small-cell lung cancer. Lung Cancer. 2009;65(3):333-8.
18. Lardinois D, Weder W, Hany TF, et al. Staging of non-small-cell lung cancer with integrated positron-emission tomography and computed tomography. N Engl J Med. 2003;348(25):2500-7.
19. Greco C, Rosenzweig K, Cascini GL, et al. Current status of PET/CT for tumour volume definition in radiotherapy treatment planning for non-small cell lung cancer (NSCLC). Lung Cancer. 2007;57(2):125-34.
20. Hicks RJ. Role of 18F-FDG PET in assessment of response in non-small cell lung cancer. J Nucl Med. 2009;50(Suppl 1): 31S-42S.
21. Koyama H, Ohno Y, Seki S, et al. Magnetic resonance imaging for lung cancer. J Thorac Imaging. 2013;28(3):138-50.
22. Mori T, Nomori H, Ikeda K, et al. Diffusion-weighted magnetic resonance imaging for diagnosing malignant pulmonary nodules/masses: comparison with positron emission tomography. J Thorac Oncol. 2008;3(4):358-64.
23. Schaefer JF, Schneider V, Vollmar J, et al. Solitary pulmonary nodules: association between signal characteristics in dynamic contrast enhanced MRI and tumor angiogenesis. Lung Cancer. 2006;53(1):39-49.
24. Kono R, Fujimoto K, Terasaki H, et al. Dynamic MRI of solitary pulmonary nodules: comparison of enhancement patterns of malignant and benign small peripheral lung lesions. Am J Roentgenol. 2007;188(1):26-36.
25. Grewal RG, Austin JH. CT demonstration of calcification in carcinoma of the lung. J Comput Assist Tomogr. 1994;18(6): 867-71.
26. Khan AN, Al-Jahdali HH, Allen CM, et al. The calcified lung nodule: What does it mean? Ann Thorac Med. 2010;5(2):67-79.
27. Aoki T, Tomoda Y, Watanabe H, et al. Peripheral lung adenocarcinoma: correlation of thin-section CT findings with histologic prognostic factors and survival. Radiology. 2001;220(3):803-9.
28. Mackintosh JA, Marshall HM, Yang IA, et al. A retrospective study of volume doubling time in surgically resected non-small cell lung cancer. Respirology. 2014;19(5):755-62.
29. Dela Cruz CS, Tanoue LT, Matthay RA. Lung cancer: epidemiology, etiology, and prevention. Clin Chest Med. 2011;32(4):605-44.
30. Hollings N, Shaw P. Diagnostic imaging of lung cancer. Eur Respir J. 2002;19(4):722-42.
31. Carter BW, Glisson BS, Truong MT, et al. Small cell lung carcinoma: staging, imaging, and treatment considerations. Radiographics. 2014;34(6):1707-21.
32. Acharya KV, Shenoy A, Holla R. Utility of Various Bronchoscopic Modalities in Lung Cancer Diagnosis. Asian Pac J Cancer Prev. 2017;18(7):1931-6.
33. Zhan P, Zhu QQ, Miu YY, et al. Comparison between endobronchial ultrasound-guided transbronchial biopsy and CT-guided transthoracic lung biopsy for the diagnosis of peripheral lung cancer: a systematic review and meta-analysis. Transl Lung Cancer Res. 2017;6(1):23-34.
34. Kay FU, Kandathil A, Batra K, et al. Revisions to the Tumor, Node, Metastasis Staging of lung Cancer: Rationale,

Radiologic Findings and Clinical Implications, 8th edn. World J Radiol. 2017;9(6):269-79.
35. Lewis JW, Pearlberg JL, Beute GH, et al. Can computed tomography of the chest stage lung cancer? Yes and no. Ann Thorac Surg. 1990;49(4):591-5; discussion 5-6.
36. Beigelman-Aubry C, Dunet V, Brun AL. CT imaging in pre-therapeutic assessment of lung cancer. Diagn Interv Imaging. 2016;97(10):973-89.
37. Detterbeck FC, Boffa DJ, Kim AW, et al. The Lung Cancer Stage Classification. Chest, 8th edition. 2017;151(1):193-203.
38. Eisenhauer EA, Therasse P, Bogaerts J, et al. New response evaluation criteria in solid tumours: revised RECIST guideline (version 1.1). Eur J Cancer. 2009;45(2): 228-47.
39. Ezhil M, Vedam S, Balter P, et al. Determination of patient-specific internal gross tumor volumes for lung cancer using four-dimensional computed tomography. Radiat Oncol. 2009;4:4.
40. Simon CJ, Dupuy DE, DiPetrillo TA, et al. Pulmonary radiofrequency ablation: long-term safety and efficacy in 153 patients. Radiology. 2007;243(1):268-75.
41. Sano Y, Kanazawa S, Gobara H, et al. Feasibility of percutaneous radiofrequency ablation for intrathoracic malignancies: a large single-center experience. Cancer. 2007;109(7):1397-405.
42. Lencioni R, Crocetti L, Cioni R, et al. Response to radiofrequency ablation of pulmonary tumours: a prospective, intention-to-treat, multicentre clinical trial (the RAPTURE study). Lancet Oncol. 2008;9(7):621-8.
43. Lanuti M, Sharma A, Digumarthy SR, et al. Radiofrequency ablation for treatment of medically inoperable stage I non-small cell lung cancer. J Thorac Cardiovasc Surg. 2009;137(1):160-6.
44. Mayo-Smith WW, Dupuy DE. Adrenal neoplasms: CT-guided radiofrequency ablation—preliminary results. Radiology. 2004;231(1):225-30.
45. Marcus PM, Bergstralh EJ, Fagerstrom RM, et al. Lung cancer mortality in the Mayo Lung Project: impact of extended follow-up. J Natl Cancer Inst. 2000;92(16):1308-16.
46. Younes RN, Gross JL, Deheinzelin D. Follow-up in lung cancer: how often and for what purpose? Chest. 1999;115(6):1494-9.
47. Bogot NR, Quint LE. Imaging of recurrent lung cancer. Cancer Imaging. 2004;4(2):61-7.
48. Koenig TR, Munden RF, Erasmus JJ, et al. Radiation injury of the lung after three-dimensional conformal radiation therapy. Am J Roentgenol. 2002;178(6):1383-8.
49. Aoki T, Nagata Y, Negoro Y, et al. Evaluation of lung injury after three-dimensional conformal stereotactic radiation therapy for solitary lung tumors: CT appearance. Radiology. 2004;230(1):101-8.
50. Munden RF, Swisher SS, Stevens CW, et al. Imaging of the patient with non-small cell lung cancer. Radiology. 2005;237(3):803-18.
51. Libshitz HI, Sheppard DG. Filling in of radiation therapy-induced bronchiectatic change: a reliable sign of locally recurrent lung cancer. Radiology. 1999;210(1):25-7.
52. Cox JE, Chiles C, Aquino SL, et al. Pulmonary artery sarcomas: a review of clinical and radiologic features. J Comput Assist Tomogr. 1997;21(5):750-5.
53. Bhatia K, Ellis S. Unusual lung tumours: an illustrated review of CT features suggestive of this diagnosis. Cancer Imaging. 2006;6:72-82.
54. Manivel JC, Priest JR, Watterson J, et al. Pleuropulmonary blastoma. The so-called pulmonary blastoma of childhood. Cancer. 1988;62(8):1516-26.
55. Weisbrod GL, Chamberlain DW, Tao LC. Pulmonary blastoma, report of three cases and a review of the literature. Can Assoc Radiol J. 1988;39(2):130-6.
56. Lee WK, Duddalwar VA, Rouse HC, et al. Extranodal lymphoma in the thorax: cross-sectional imaging findings. Clin Radiol. 2009;64(5):542-9.
57. Lee KS, Kim Y, Primack SL. Imaging of pulmonary lymphomas. Am J Roentgenol. 1997;168(2):339-45.
58. Kurtin PJ, Myers JL, Adlakha H, et al. Pathologic and clinical features of primary pulmonary extranodal marginal zone B-cell lymphoma of MALT type. Am J Surg Pathol. 2001;25(8):997-1008.
59. Huang H, Lu ZW, Jiang CG, et al. Clinical and prognostic characteristics of pulmonary mucosa-associated lymphoid tissue lymphoma: a retrospective analysis of 23 cases in a Chinese population. Chin Med J (Engl). 2011;124(7):1026-30.
60. Ahmed S, Kussick SJ, Siddiqui AK, et al. Bronchial-associated lymphoid tissue lymphoma: a clinical study of a rare disease. Eur J Cancer. 2004;40(9):1320-6.
61. Mentzer SJ, Reilly JJ, Skarin AT, et al. Patterns of lung involvement by malignant lymphoma. Surgery. 1993;113(5):507-14.
62. Lewis ER, Caskey CI, Fishman EK. Lymphoma of the lung: CT findings in 31 patients. Am J Roentgenol. 1991;156(4): 711-4.
63. Hamilton-Dutoit SJ, Pallesen G, Franzmann MB, et al. AIDS-related lymphoma. Histopathology, immunophenotype, and association with Epstein-Barr virus as demonstrated by in situ nucleic acid hybridization. Am J Pathol. 1991;138(1):149-63.
64. Blunt DM, Padley SP. Radiographic manifestations of AIDS related lymphoma in the thorax. Clin Radiol. 1995;50(9):607-12.
65. Bates WD, Gray DW, Dada MA, et al. Lymphoproliferative disorders in Oxford renal transplant recipients. J Clin Pathol. 2003;56(6):439-46.
66. Carignan S, Staples CA, Müller NL. Intrathoracic lymphoproliferative disorders in the immunocompromised patient: CT findings. Radiology. 1995;197(1):53-8.
67. Dodd GD, Ledesma-Medina J, Baron RL, et al. Posttransplant lymphoproliferative disorder: intrathoracic manifestations. Radiology. 1992;184(1):65-9.
68. Rekhtman N. Neuroendocrine tumors of the lung: an update. Arch Pathol Lab Med. 2010;134(11):1628-38.

69. Travis WD. Advances in neuroendocrine lung tumors. Ann Oncol. 2010;21 Suppl 7:vii65-71.
70. Pinchot SN, Holen K, Sippel RS, et al. Carcinoid tumors. Oncologist. 2008;13(12):1255-69.
71. Gustafsson BI, Kidd M, Chan A, et al. Bronchopulmonary neuroendocrine tumors. Cancer. 2008;113(1):5-21.
72. Jeung MY, Gasser B, Gangi A, et al. Bronchial carcinoid tumors of the thorax: spectrum of radiologic findings. Radiographics. 2002;22(2):351-65.
73. Fox DJ, Khattar RS. Carcinoid heart disease: presentation, diagnosis, and management. Heart. 2004;90(10):1224-8.
74. Chong S, Lee KS, Chung MJ, et al. Neuroendocrine tumors of the lung: clinical, pathologic, and imaging findings. Radiographics. 2006;26(1):41-57; discussion-8.
75. Soga J, Yakuwa Y. Bronchopulmonary carcinoids: An analysis of 1,875 reported cases with special reference to a comparison between typical carcinoids and atypical varieties. Ann Thorac Cardiovasc Surg. 1999;5(4):211-9.
76. Detterbeck FC. Management of carcinoid tumors. Ann Thorac Surg. 2010;89(3):998-1005.
77. Rosado de Christenson ML, Abbott GF, Kirejczyk WM, et al. Thoracic carcinoids: radiologic-pathologic correlation. Radiographics. 1999;19(3):707-36.
78. Caplin ME, Baudin E, Ferolla P, et al. Pulmonary neuroendocrine (carcinoid) tumors: European Neuroendocrine Tumor Society expert consensus and recommendations for best practice for typical and atypical pulmonary carcinoids. Ann Oncol. 2015;26(8):1604-20.
79. Jung KJ, Lee KS, Han J, et al. Large cell neuroendocrine carcinoma of the lung: clinical, CT, and pathologic findings in 11 patients. J Thorac Imaging. 2001;16(3):156-62.
80. Oshiro Y, Kusumoto M, Matsuno Y, et al. CT findings of surgically resected large cell neuroendocrine carcinoma of the lung in 38 patients. Am J Roentgenol. 2004;182(1):87-91.
81. Pearlberg JL, Sandler MA, Lewis JW, et al. Small-cell bronchogenic carcinoma: CT evaluation. Am J Roentgenol. 1988;150(2):265-8.
82. Benson RE, Rosado-de-Christenson ML, Martínez-Jiménez S, et al. Spectrum of pulmonary neuroendocrine proliferations and neoplasms. Radiographics. 2013;33(6):1631-49.
83. Coppage L, Shaw C, Curtis AM. Metastatic disease to the chest in patients with extrathoracic malignancy. J Thorac Imaging. 1987;2(4):24-37.
84. Libshitz HI, North LB. Pulmonary metastases. Radiol Clin North Am. 1982;20(3):437-51.
85. Collins J SE. Chest Radiology: The Essentials LWW Doody's all reviewed collection, illustrated ed: Lippincott Williams & Wilkins; 2008.
86. Padovani B, Mouroux J, Seksik L, et al. Chest wall invasion by bronchogenic carcinoma: evaluation with MR imaging. Radiology. 1993;187(1):33-8.
87. Gleeson T, Thiessen R, Hannigan A, et al. Pulmonary hamartomas: CT pixel analysis for fat attenuation using radiologic-pathologic correlation. J Med Imaging Radiat Oncol. 2013;57(5):534-43.

CHAPTER 169

Imaging of the Tracheobronchial Tree

Ashu Seith Bhalla, Smita Manchanda

INTRODUCTION

Airway is divided into the upper airway (above the thoracic inlet) and the lower airway (below the thoracic inlet). The lower airway is further divided into the large and small airways. This chapter focuses on the lower airways.

Large airways is a term used for airways which are >2 mm in diameter. This includes the:

- Central airway—trachea and main bronchi
- Peripheral airway—lobar, segmental, and proximal subsegmental bronchi.

Small airways refer to the distal airways, which are small in size (<2 mm in diameter) and lack cartilage and submucosal glands.

ROLE OF IMAGING (BOX 1)

Imaging plays a key role in diagnosis and planning management. The main role of imaging is to detect and localize the lesion (with respect to carina), delineate the exact length of the lesion (for stent placement as a therapeutic option), measure the degree of airway narrowing, and lastly to give a specific diagnosis, if possible. The current role of the various *imaging modalities* is detailed below.

Box 1: Role of imaging in evaluation of the tracheobronchial tree.

- Detection
- Localization—proximal and distal extent
- Etiology—extrinsic or intrinsic (mural or intraluminal)
- Length for abnormal segment
- Diffuse/focal
- Obstruction—fixed or dynamic
- Degree of narrowing
- Specific diagnosis, if possible

IMAGING MODALITIES

Chest Radiograph

Plain frontal and lateral chest radiographs are useful in acute obstructions such as foreign body and aspiration. These may occasionally demonstrate large masses involving the central airways. Areas of severe narrowing may also be appreciated. The effects of airway disease on the lung, i.e. consolidation, atelectasis or hyperinflation is well seen on plain films. Signs of bronchiectasis are also well described on plain radiographs **(Fig. 1)**. However, largely radiographs are unable to provide enough information for diagnosis or preoperative planning of patients.

Systemic Evaluation on Chest Radiograph

Refer **Box 2**.

Digital Tomosynthesis

Digital tomosynthesis (DTS) is a new technique using digital radiography and flat-panel detectors, which is based on the principle of geometric tomography.[1] DTS images represent sections through the anatomy that are generated and reconstructed from a set of projection radiographs. Because it removes overlapping clutter, there is improved visualization of thoracic abnormalities compared to radiography and better coronal plane resolution

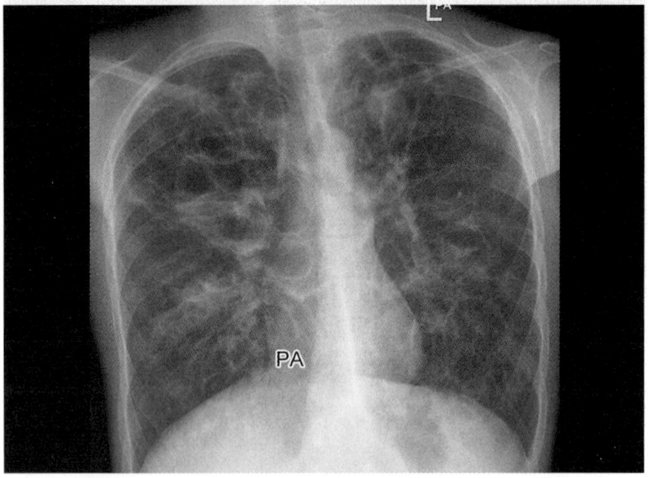

Fig. 1: Plain radiograph showing cystic lucencies and tram-track linear opacities in bilateral lung fields in a case of cystic fibrosis.

(Figs. 2A and B). The radiation dose to patients is less than that of chest CT.[2] The demonstration of the central airways is considered to be superior or equivalent compared with radiography.[1] In terms of airway evaluation this technique is useful in suspected cases of foreign body.

Multidetector Computed Tomography

Multidetector computed tomography (MDCT) is the investigation of choice for initial evaluation of suspected tracheobronchial tree pathology and for follow-up of these cases.[3] In the current generation of scanners, there is volumetric CT acquisition in a single breath hold and precise delineation of the entire tracheobronchial tree, including the distal airways can be done.[4]

Box 2: Systematic evaluation on chest radiograph.

- Tracheal caliber
- Mediastinal widening
- Asymmetric lung aeration
- Lung collapse/consolidation
- Length of tracheal narrowing
- Radiopaque foreign body
- Cardiac size
- Position of the aortic arch

Acquisition

Scans are routinely performed in deep inspiration in supine position. In a single breath hold of 6–8 seconds, the entire chest can be scanned without respiratory motion artifacts. Cardiac gating is not recommended and is not usually done.[3,5]

Although visualization of airways per se does not require contrast administration, IV contrast may prove helpful in some conditions; for example, differentiating a central mass from atelectatic lung.

CT acquisition technique has been summarized in **Box 3**. Until recently axial imaging by CT scan was the

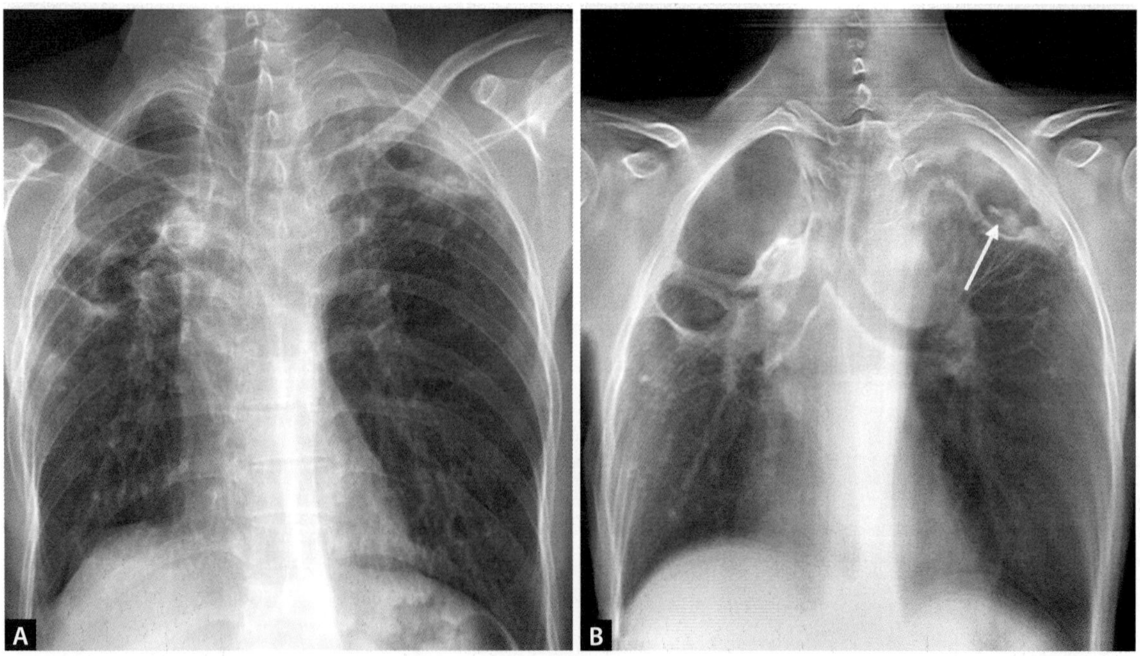

Figs. 2A and B: Digital tomosynthesis: Plain radiograph (A) reveals fibrocavitary lesions in bilateral upper lobes with suspicious fungal ball in left upper lobe cavity. DTS image (B) better depicts the central airways and fungal ball (arrow) as it removes overlapping clutter.

Box 3: CT acquisition technique.[6,7]

- Tube potential and tube current appropriate to patient size
- Use of tube current modulation
- *Scan area*: From the lung apices to the costophrenic sulci
- *Position*:
  - At isocenter to minimize radiation dose and optimize image quality
  - Supine
  - Prone (in specific cases)
- *Phase*:
  - Deep inspiration
  - *Expiratory (end expiration)*:
    - To demonstrate air trapping
    - Obtained throughout the lung fields or at selected 3 to 5 levels
    - Low dose (30–40 mAs)
  - *Dynamic (paired inspiratory and expiratory)*: In cases of tracheobronchomalacia
- Thin overlapping 0.5–1 mm sections acquired
- *Field of view*:
  - *Scan FOV*: Appropriate to patient size at time of image
  - *Reconstructed FOV*: Limited to the lungs with optimal spatial resolution for each patient (lung window)
- *Data sets*:
  - 5 mm width every 5 mm reconstruction interval at lung and mediastinal window settings
  - 1 mm width at 10 mm interval high resolution scans
  - Thin reconstruction at 1–1.5 mm slice thickness
- Retention of the radiation dose report in the radiological record

Abbreviation: FOV: Field of view.

accepted standard modality for diagnostic work-up for suspected airway pathology. However, MDCT has significantly enhanced the imaging of airways. The numerous reconstruction techniques have virtually revolutionized the way that CT images are viewed and interpreted.[4,6]

Of great concern is the potential of added risk resulting from increased radiation exposure especially when paired inspiratory-expiratory CT is performed. Cine imaging also has the potential for high radiation exposure.

The problem of additional radiation exposure can be reduced by routinely using reduced milliamperage whenever, feasible. This is especially true in young patients and those likely to require multiple follow-ups.

Diagnostic images of acceptable quality can be obtained with 80-100 mAs, and use as low as 40 mAs has been reported in thin patients. For the expiratory scans, a low-dose (30-40 mAs) technique should be used. Radiation exposure can be reduced further by using dose modulation techniques.

Acquisition in Special Situation (Tracheobronchomalacia)

There are various techniques described for the evaluation of tracheobronchomalacia; using either expiratory scans or coughing manuevers.[8] These include:

1. Paired end-inspiratory and end-expiratory MDCT: Scans at end inspiration and incremental scans at end expiration.
2. Paired end-inspiratory and dynamic expiratory MDCT: Scans at end inspiration and during expiration.
3. Cine MDCT combined with a coughing maneuver: Scans beginning at end inspiration which is followed by coughing movements.

Image Reconstruction

The various techniques available in MDCT scanners incude multiplanar reconstructions (MPRs), maximum intensity projections (MIPs), minimum intensity projections (minIPs) and internal rendering or virtual bronchoscopy (VB)[6,9-11] **(Figs. 3 and 4)**. The role of numerous reconstruction techniques is described in **Table 1**.

Quantitative CT Assessment of Airways

The lumen and area of airways can be measured quantitatively on CT images. With the use of MDCT scanners oblique reconstructions can be made in the axis and perpendicular to the axis of the airway.[12]

Box 4 summarizes the current role of MDCT in evaluation of airway pathology.

Endoscopic Ultrasound

Over the past decade, there has been a growing interest in the use of endoscopic ultrasound (EBUS) to diagnose to the central and peripheral lesions of tracheobronchial tree. EBUS has the unique capability to differentiate various layers of the bronchial wall.[13] Also pathologic changes both in and adjacent to airways can be assessed. Vessels can be readily identified and differentiated from lymph nodes. It has hence found a significant role in guided transbronchial needle aspiration (TBNA) of mediastinal nodes currently, the major limitation of EBUS guided TBNA is its high cost, and the need for special configuration of endoscopic probes to provide consistent positioning adjacent to bronchial walls.[3]

Magnetic Resonance Imaging

Magnetic resonance imaging (MRI) provides adequate visualization of the tracheobronchial tree up to lobar

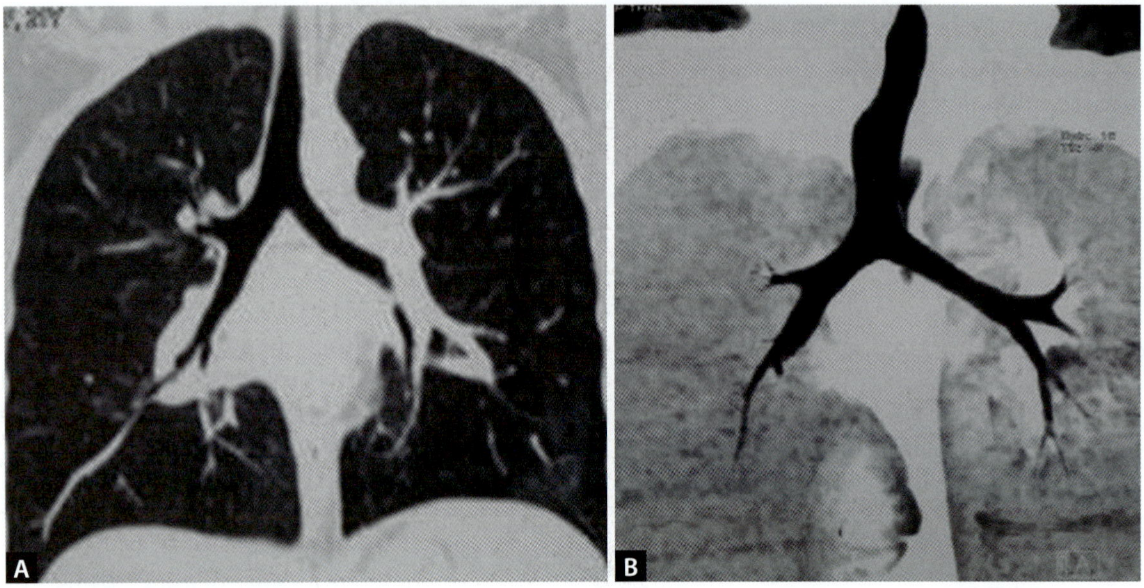

Figs. 3A and B: Coronal MPR (A) and coronal minIP (B) showing trachea, main bronchi and lobar bronchi.

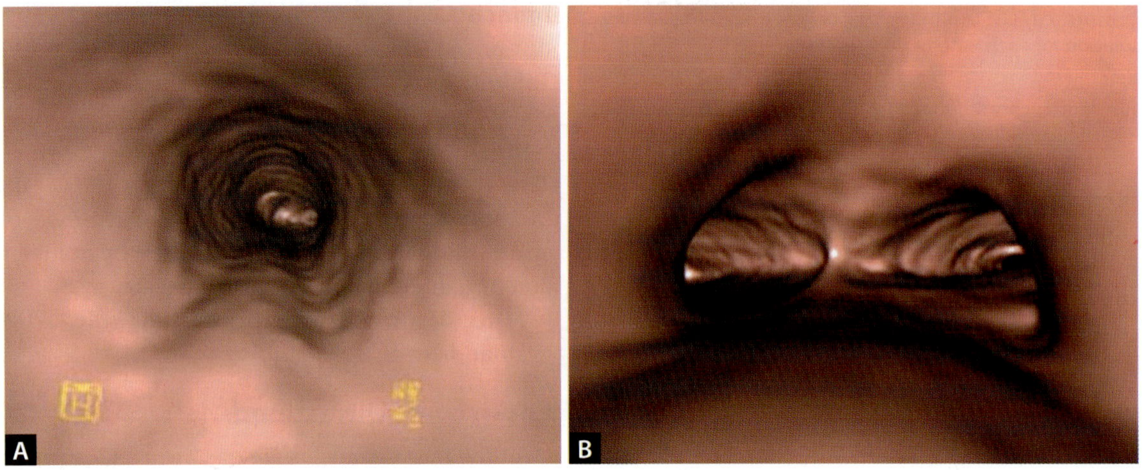

Figs. 4A and B: Virtual bronchoscopy images showing endoluminal view of normal trachea (A) and carina (B).

bronchi.[14] This is best seen on the coronal T1 TSE sequence **(Fig. 5)**. Mediastinal and hilar masses are also well evaluated on MRI with the superior depiction of vascular or cardiac invasion. MRI has also been used to demonstrate air trapping. There is an increasing use in those requiring repeated imaging such as cystic fibrosis and allergic bronchopulmonary aspergillosis (ABPA). The presence of mucus with high T1 SI and low T2 SI has been found to be highly specific for the diagnosis of ABPA in cystic fibrosis **(Box 5)**.[15]

NORMAL AIRWAY ANATOMY

The trachea is a cartilaginous and fibromuscular tube extending from the inferior aspect of cricoid cartilage to the carina, measuring 10–12 cm in length. It is divided into intrathoracic and extrathoracic parts. It contains 16–22 cartilaginous rings, which are incomplete posteriorly. The posterior portion of the tracheal wall, lying between the open ends of the tracheal cartilages, is a thin fibromuscular membrane termed posterior tracheal membrane.[16]

There is marked variability in the cross-sectional appearance of the trachea, which may appear rounded or oval (most common) or horseshoe-shaped trachea with flat posterior tracheal membrane (in about 25% of normal individuals).[16] Tracheal diameter can vary widely in anatomically normal persons. In men, tracheal diameter ranges from 13 to 25 mm (mean 19.5 mm) and in females it is slightly less, ranging from 10 to 21 m in the coronal

Table 1: CT reconstruction techniques (role in airway diseases).

Name	*Technique*	*Role*
MPR	• Multiplanar reconstruction • Evaluate in both mediastinal and lung window	• To visualize anatomical structures in reality • Airway stenosis • Resectability of bronchogenic carcinoma as well as hilar and mediastinal structures
minIP	• Minimum intensity projection • Thick slabs of 25–35 cm used to demonstrate entire TB tree	• Overall morphology of the tracheobronchial tree • Detecting airway stenosis (overestimates degree of narrowing) • Improved depiction of ground-glass pattern
MIP	Maximum intensity projection	• Improves detection of pulmonary nodules • Bronchiolar diseases, especially for patients with so-called tree-in-bud opacities • Size and location of vessels
VB	Virtual bronchoscopy	• Accurate reproduction of major endoluminal abnormalities • Assessment of airway stenoses • Unable to identify the causes of bronchial obstruction or detect mild stenosis, submucosal infiltration and superficial spreading tumors

plane (average 17.5 mm). In children variations in tracheal diameter at different levels can be as much as 20%. During forced expiration, there is invagination of the posterior tracheal membrane and the lumen becomes horseshoe shaped.

There is dichotomous branching with approximately 23 generations of branches from trachea to alveoli.

ANATOMIC VARIANTS

In adults, the most commonly encountered anomalies are either anomalous or supernumerary bronchi.[3] Other anomalies include agenesis, congenital bronchial atresia, bronchogenic cysts or even cogenital lobar obstruction. A clinically useful modified classification has been proposed by Wu et al. for these anomalies.[17]

1. *Anomalies arising from normal higher order bronchial divisions.* These include accessory superior segmental bronchi and axillary bronchi supplying lateral aspect of right upper lobe.
2. *Anomalies arising from sites typically lacking branches:* This group refers to tracheal bronchi, accessory cardiac bronchi and bridging bronchi.

The most common amongst these is *the 'tracheal or pig bronchus'*, seen in up to 1–2% of normal individuals.[18] Tracheal bronchus arises on the right side exclusively, and on endoscopy may be confused with tracheal diverticula or tracheoceles. CT readily identifies these **(Figs. 6A and B)**

The 'cardiac bronchus' usually arises from the bronchus intermedius, the origin being opposite and distal to origin of upper lobe bronchus **(Fig. 7)**. It is variable is size and in many cases is a blind ending stump; which does not aerate any lung parenchyma.

Box 4: Role of MDCT in evaluation of airway pathology.

- Workhorse of airway imaging
- Reconstructions definitely improve lesion evaluation compared to axial images alone
- MPR in both mediastinal and lung windows—length of stenosis
- VB does not have a distinct diagnostic utility, useful where fiberoptic bronchoscopy not available or not feasible
- minIP, volume rendered images useful in overall depiction of airway anatomy
- Excellent for congenital anomalies
- *Limitations of MDCT*:
  - Lesions smaller than 2–3 mm not detected
  - Difficult to differentiate between mucosal and submucosal lesions

Abbreviations: MPR: Multiplanar reconstruction; VB: Virtual bronchoscopy; minIP: Minimum intensity projection; MDCT: Multidetector computed tomography.

Box 5: Suggested MRI protocol for central airway evaluation.

1. *T1-weighted gradient sequence*:
   - *With fat supression (pre- and postcontrast)*: Axial
   - *Without fat supression*: Axial, Coronal
2. *T2-weighted fast spin echo sequence*:
   - *With fat supression*: Axial
   - *Without fat supression*: Axial
3. *T2-weighted sequence HASTE*: Coronal
4. *Diffusion-weighted sequence*: Axial (b0, 400, 800) (in cases of masses)

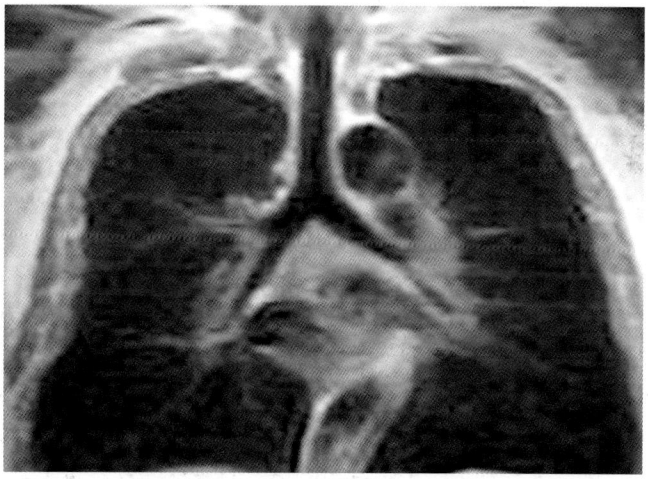

Fig. 5: MRI showing normal airway on T1W SE coronal image.

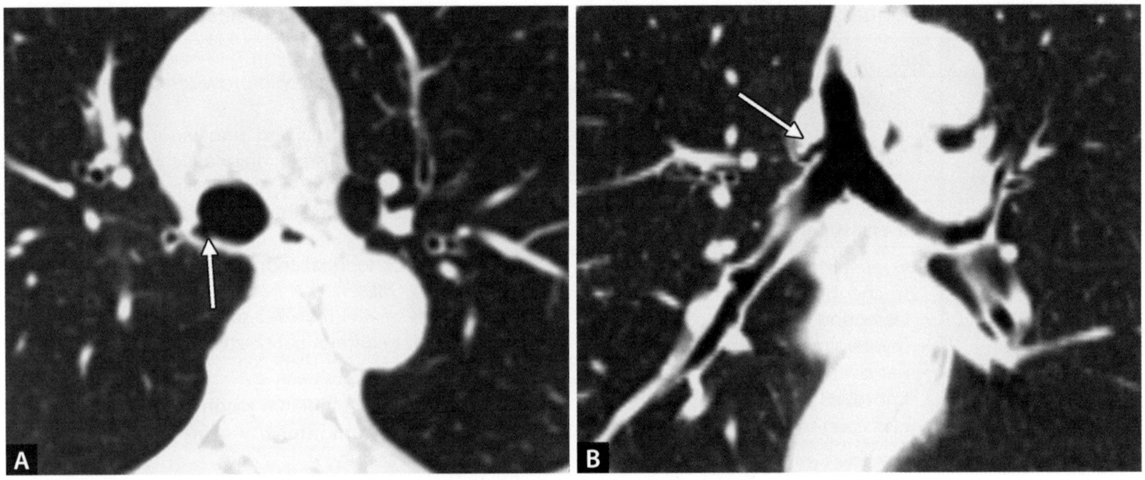

Figs. 6A and B: Tracheal bronchus: Axial (A) and coronal MPR (B) in lung window show the right upper lobe bronchus (arrow) arising directly from the trachea.

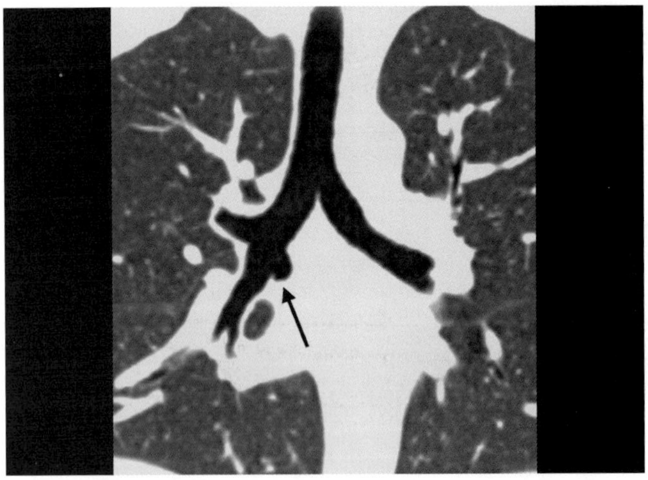

Fig. 7: *Cardiac bronchus*: Blind ending bronchial stump (arrow) arising medially from the bronchus intermedius.

3. *Anomalies associated with abnormalities of situs.* In this category, reversal of the right- and left-sided airways is the most commonly encountered form. Less frequent anomalies include bronchial isomerism, in which pattern of airway branching and pulmonary location is identical in both the lungs.

TRACHEOBRONCHIAL TREE PATHOLOGIES

Pathologies affecting the tracheobronchial tree can be broadly considered in three categories—those affecting the central airways, the peripheral airways and others involving the small airways. The levels of lower airway pathologies are described in **Figure 8**.

CENTRAL AIRWAYS

Central airway obstruction can occur because of extrinsic or intrinsic causes (which are further divided into mural and intraluminal causes). These are detailed in **Table 2**.

EXTRINSIC

A diverse variety of mediastinal masses or mass like lesions can cause extrinsic compression of the airways. These have been described in detail elsewhere.

INTRINSIC MURAL

Congenital

Tracheobronchomalacia

Tracheobronchomalacia (TBM) is characterized by weakness of the tracheobronchial walls and/or supporting cartilage. This results in a dynamic obstruction of the airway because of excessive collapse during expiration.[8,19] CT diagnosis **(Figs. 10A to C)** can only be made in paired scans (end inspiration and expiratory scan/during coughing) as described above in CT acquisition. It may be congenital or acquired due to prior intubation, trauma, prolonged extrinsic compression **(Figs. 11A and B)**, infection or chronic inflammation.[20]

Tracheal Stenosis

Congenital subglottic or tracheal stenosis occurs because of incomplete recanalization of the laryngotracheal tube. The various types of congenital tracheal stenosis include hypoplasia, funnel-shaped and segmental stenosis.[21]

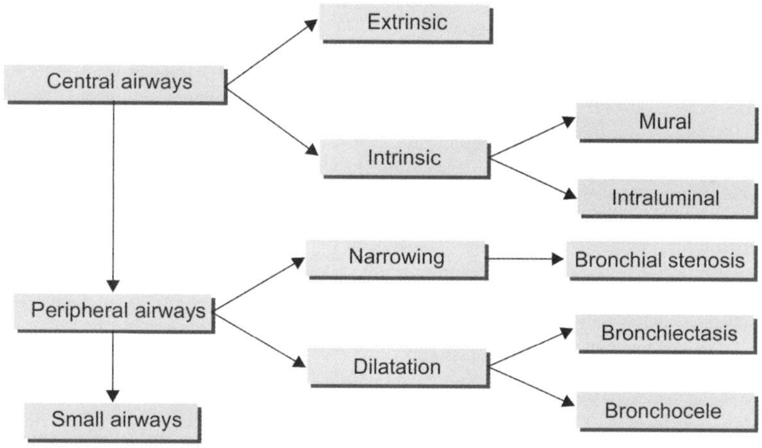

Fig. 8: Levels of lower airway pathologies.

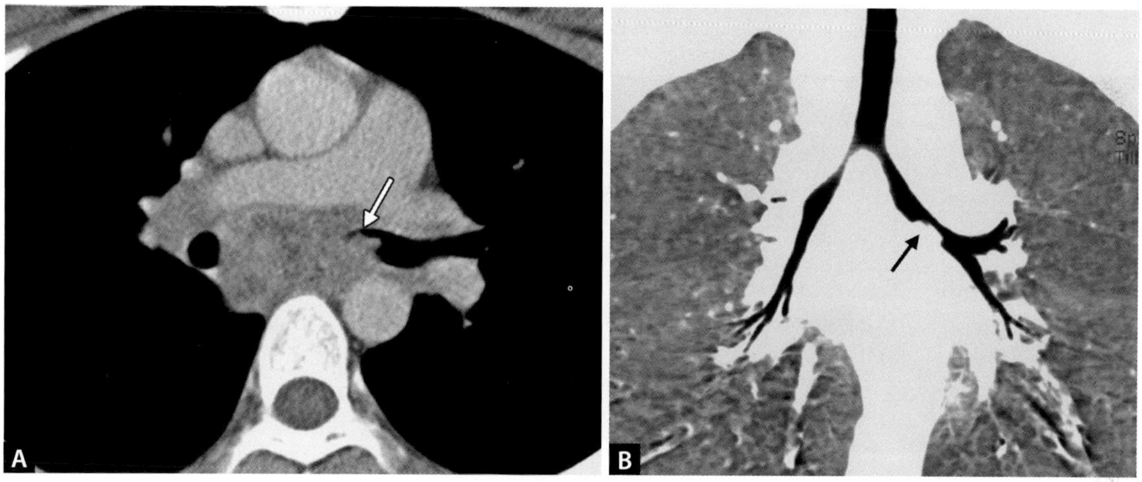

Figs. 9A and B: Extrinsic involvement by TB lymph nodes: Axial CT (A) and min IP (B) show necrotic subcarinal nodes extending into the left main bronchus (arrow).

Table 2: Etiology of central airway obstruction.

		Intrinsic	
Etiology	***Extrinsic***	***Mural***	***Intraluminal***
Congenital	• Vascular compression • Bronchopulmonary foregut malformations • Thoracic deformity • Vascular malformations	• Tracheobronchomalacia • Tracheal stenosis	
Inflammatory/ infective	• Lymph nodes **(Figs. 9A and B)** • Mediastinal abscess/cellulitis • Fibrosing mediastinitis	• Tuberculosis/fibrotic stricture • Vasculitis • Relapsing polychondritis • Post-intubation stricture • Sarcoidosis	• Granulation tissue • Broncholithiasis
Masses	• Lymphoma • Germ cell tumor • Vascular malformations		• Malignant tumors • Benign tumors
Miscellaneous		• Amyloidosis • Tracheopathia osteochondroplastica	• Mucus plugs • Foreign body • Clots

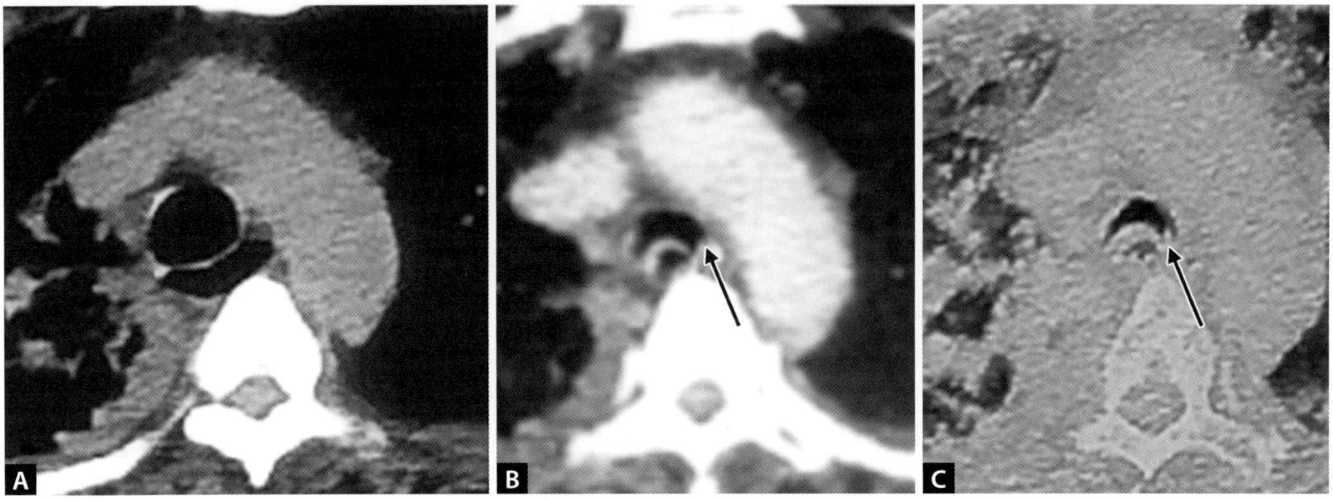

Figs. 10A to C: Tracheomalacia: Axial end-inspiration CT (A) shows normal appearance of trachea with collapse of the lumen during expiration (arrow in B and C).

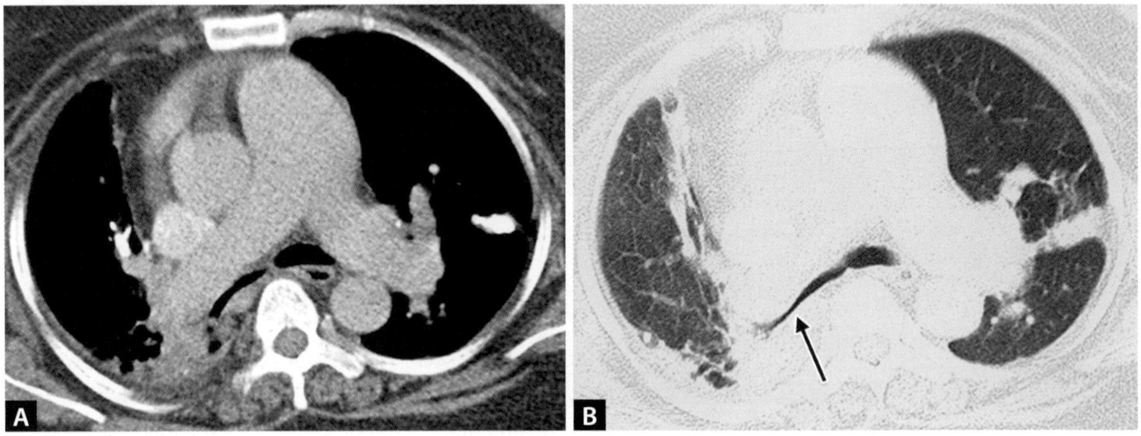

Figs. 11A and B: Bronchomalacia: Narrowing of the bronchus intermedius (arrow) because of chronic compression by enlarged pulmonary artery.

Inflammatory/Infective

Infections/Fibrotic Stricture

Inflammatory tracheal stenosis due to tuberculosis

Tubercular stenosis **(Figs. 12A to E)** is an endobronchial complication of pulmonary tuberculosis that can develop acutely at the time of infection or can become manifest years later. Endobronchial tuberculosis has been reported in 10–37% of patients with pulmonary parenchymal tuberculosis.[22] Tuberculosis typically involves the distal trachea and proximal mainstem bronchi **(Figs. 13A and B)**; isolated tracheal disease is rare.[23] Granulation tissue formation and subsequent fibrosis involving the airway causes luminal narrowing. Unlike active tuberculosis, which involves both mainstem bronchi equally, fibrotic TB usually involves the left main bronchus, perhaps because of its greater length. Evidence of associated mediastinal inflammation, in the form of enlarged mediastinal nodes or increased attenuation of mediastinal fat, may also be identified. CT findings are seldom specific. Findings that help differentiate tuberculosis from bronchogenic carcinoma include longer circumferential involvement and the absence of an intraluminal mass.[24] Focal infection may be responsible for tumor-like lesions when it produces granulation or endoluminal masses.

Fungal infections (Aspergillosis)

Airway disease caused by Aspergillus takes many forms, including saprophytic colonization, tracheobronchitis, ulcerative tracheobronchitis with or without pseudomembrane formation, and necrotizing (invasive) aspergillosis,[25] the latter being further divided into acute and chronic airway invasive forms. Multifocal or diffuse

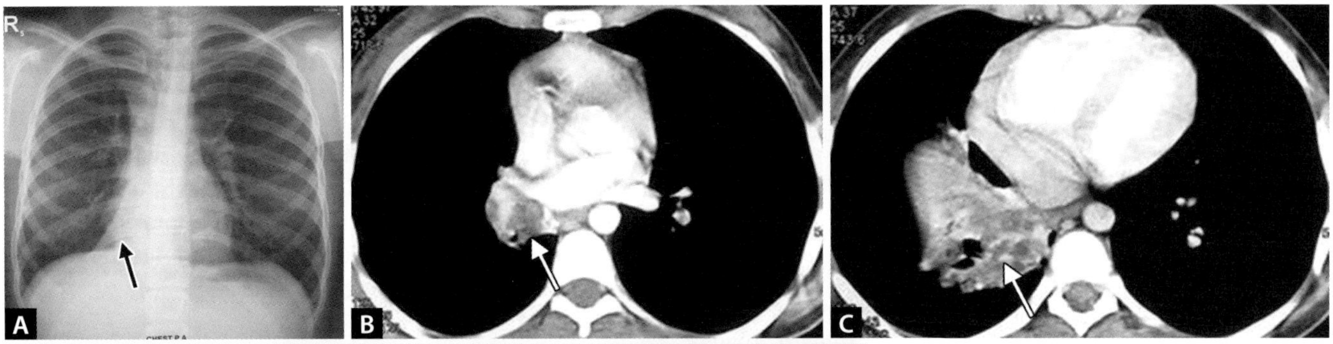

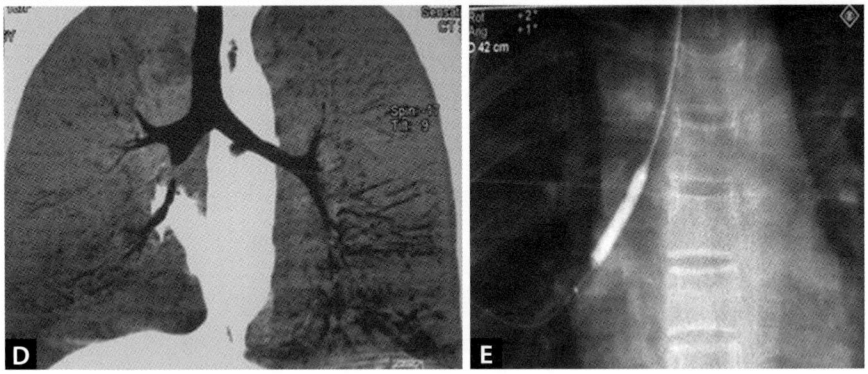

Figs. 12A to E: Tubercular stricture: Chest radiograph (A) of a 19 years old girl showing collapse of right lower lobe (black arrow). Axial CT (B and C) and coronal min-IP (D) demonstrates necrotic right hilar nodes (white arrows) narrowing the bronchus intermedius and lower lobe bronchus (black arrow). (E) balloon dilatation of the stricture was performed.

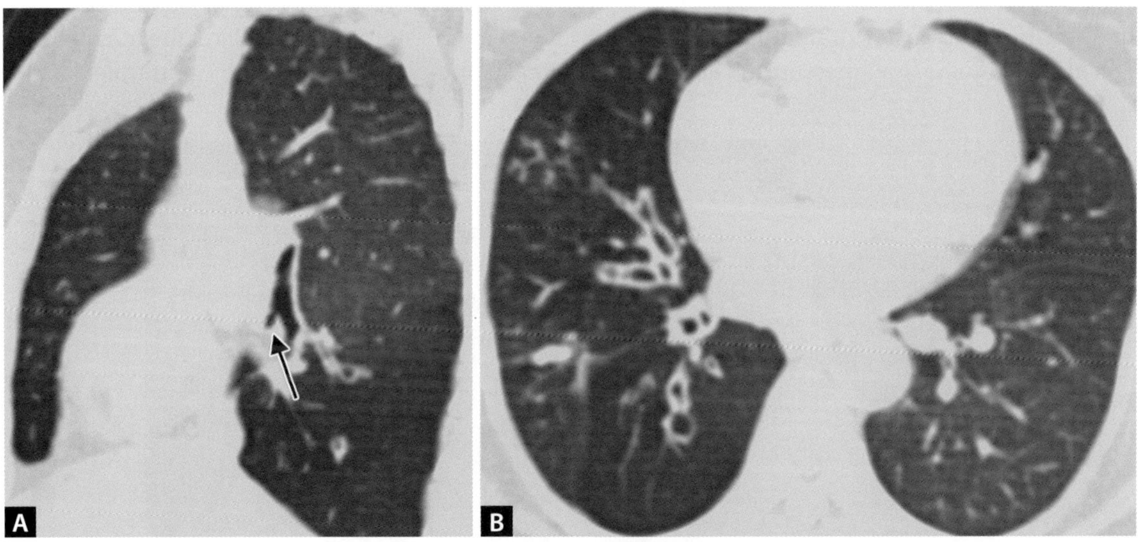

Figs. 13A and B: Post-tubercular bronchostenosis: Sagittal MPR (A) and axial CT (B) show narrowing of right middle lobe bronchus (arrow) with bronchiectatic changes in middle and lower lobes.

tracheobronchial wall thickening, causing luminal narrowing is seen on CT.

Rhinoscleroma

Rhinoscleroma is an insidious infectious granulomatous disease caused by Klebsiella rhinoscleromatis.[26] The involvement is characteristically of the upper respiratory tract; trachea and proximal bronchi may occasionally be involved. CT findings include diffuse nodular tracheobronchial wall thickening, causing luminal narrowing with mediastinal or hilar lymphadenopathy.[27]

Vasculitis

Granulomatous polyangitis (GPA)

Airway involvement in GPA includes bronchial stenosis, inflammation and pseudotumors.[28] Often, no correlation is seen between c-ANCA levels and the presence of tracheobronchial inflammation.

Relapsing Polychondritis

Relapsing polychondritis is a multisystem disease of unknown etiology characterized by recurrent inflammation of cartilage of nose, external ear, peripheral joints, larynx, trachea and bronchi.[29] It is ommonly seen in the third and sixth decades with initial involvement of larynx and subglottic trachea. Distal trachea and bronchi may be involved as the disease progresses. An acute inflammatory infiltrate in the cartilage and perichondrial tissue is seen on pathology. CT findings include increased airway wall attenuation in association with smooth tracheal or bronchial wall thickening. The increased attenuation may appear as frank calcification in later stages. There is characteristic sparing of the posterior membranous portion of the trachea.[30]

Post-intubation Stenosis

Among acquired strictures, the most common cause is injury resulting from intubation. Although investigators have estimated that complications occur in up to 10–15% of patients after intubation and up to 40% patients with tracheostomies, the incidence of serious complications after intubation has decreased dramatically since the introduction of high-volume/ low-pressure tubes.[31] The two principal sites for post-intubation stenoses are at the stoma or at the level of the endotracheal tube or tracheostomy tube balloon. Strictures result from pressure necrosis, which causes ischemia and subsequent scarring **(Figs. 14A to C)**. Other complications of intubation include tracheal rupture and tracheobrachiocephalic artery or tracheoesophageal fistulas. Stent placement remains one temporary option for treating such strictures, though optimal surgical technique is laryngotracheal resection and reconstruction.

Sarcoidosis

Tracheal involvement is rare and usually associated with laryngeal disease.[27] In sarcoidosis, airway involvement is usually in the form of bronchial involvement. It may be seen in up to 65% of patients with sarcoidosis on high resolution CT in the form of nodular or smooth wall thickening.[32]

Miscellaneous

Tracheopathia Osteoplastica

Tracheopathia osteoplastica is characterized by multiple small osteocartilaginous growths in the submucosa of the inner anterior and lateral walls of the trachea. Usually seen in asymptomatic elderly males. Multiple, small (1–5 mm

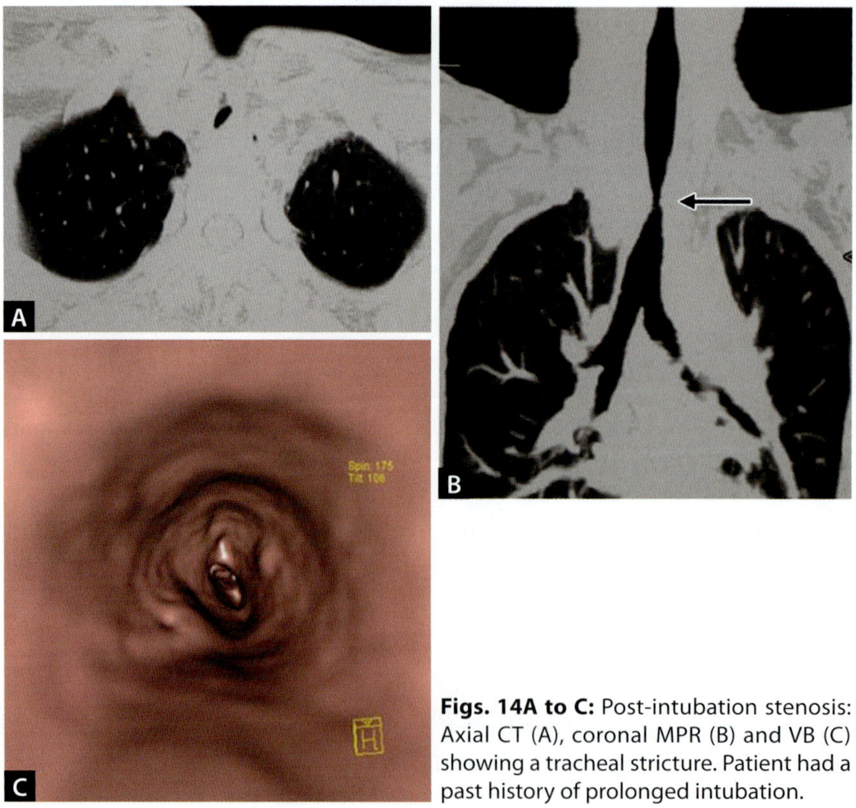

Figs. 14A to C: Post-intubation stenosis: Axial CT (A), coronal MPR (B) and VB (C) showing a tracheal stricture. Patient had a past history of prolonged intubation.

sized) irregular nodules (occasionally calcified are seen protruding into the tracheal lumen on CT **(Figs. 15A to C)**.

Amyloidosis

Amyloidosis entails a number of entities characterized by deposition of an autologous fibrillar protein and associated protein derivatives in extracellular tissue. Amyloidosis can be either primary (frequently associated with multiple myeloma or Waldenstrom macroglobulinemia) or secondary (in the setting of chronic inflammatory diseases including TB, cystic fibrosis, bronchiectasis, etc.).Within the lung, three types of localized amyloidosis have been identified—tracheobronchial, nodular and diffuse septal amyloidosis.[33] Tracheobronchial amyloidosis is the most common form of respiratory system involvement in patients with localized amyloidosis. Clinical presentation depends on the part of airway involved. Patients with proximal subglottic or laryngeal involvement typically present with hoarseness and stridor, distal trachea or mainstem bronchi involvement causes cough, wheezing, dyspnea.

CT images of tracheobronchial amyloidosis **(Figs. 16A to C)** appear as nodular thickening or focal mass partially or completely occluding airways; mimicking the appearance of benign or malignant tracheal neoplasms.[34] Mural calcifications are promiment features. In patients with recurrent infiltrates, bronchiectasis may develop.

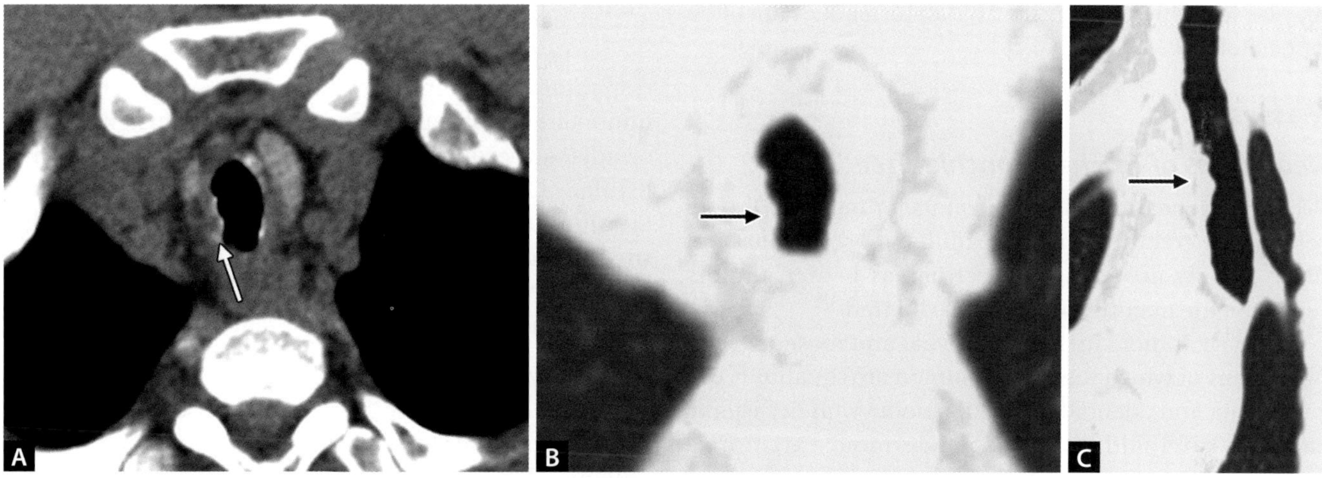

Figs. 15A to C: Tracheopathia osteoplastica: Axial CT (A and B) and sagittal MPR (C) showing multiple, small soft tissue nodules along the inner tracheal aspect with sparing of the posterior tracheal wall.

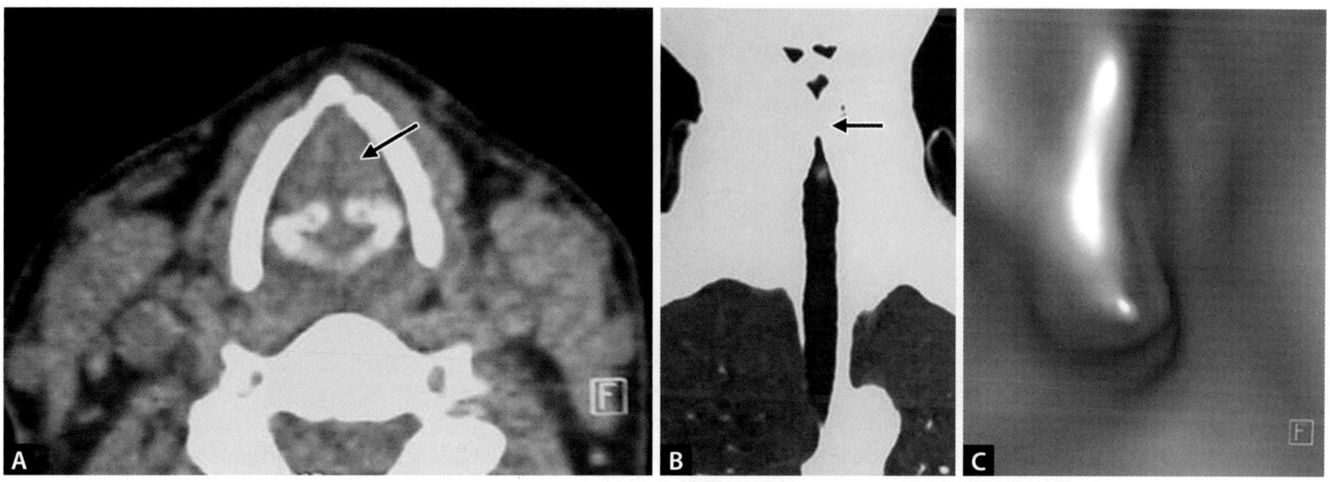

Figs. 16A to C: Amyloidosis: MDCT reveals diffuse wall thickening of the laryngeal wall and vocal cords with obliteration of the lumen (arrow).

INTRALUMINAL

Inflammatory/Infective

Granulation Tissue

Chronic inflammation of infective/noninfective nature can result in nonspecific granulation tissue forming bronchial obstructive lesions.

Broncholithiasis

In this condition, calcified lymph nodes erode into the tracheobronchial tree and it is a complication of granulomatous lymphadenitis. Patients may expectorate or aspirate the calcified material. On MDCT **(Figs. 17A and B)**, calcified focus is seen within the bronchial lumen without any mass. Peribronchial lymph node calcification may be seen and post-obstructive abnormalities are often associated.[3,35]

Masses

Neoplasms of Tracheobronchial Tree

Primary tracheal neoplasia accounts for only 1–2% of all respiratory tract tumors.[36] In adults, most (60–90%) of these tumors are malignant,[37] whereas benign tumors represent the majority of lesions in children.

Primary tumors include epithelial and mesenchymal neoplasms of which the most common are squamous cell carcinoma and adenoid cystic carcinoma with occasional cases of carcinoid and mucoepidermoid carcinoma. The most common benign lesions are hamartomas and bronchial papillomas. Secondary neoplasms are either metastases or, direct infiltration by adjacent mediastinal tumors (carcinomas lung, thyroid or esophagus).[36]

Clinical presentation is usually nonspecific with a significant overlap between the imaging appearances of benign and malignant lesions. The main role of imaging **(Figs. 18A to D)** is in delineation of tumor extent within the lumen, airway wall, and surrounding structures before treatment planning.

Malignant Tumors

Primary tracheal cancer is rare and seen commonly in middle aged/elderly males smokers. The prognosis of patients is poor, with the 5-year survival rate being 5–35%.[38]

Squamous cell carcinoma (SCC)

SCC is usually seen in smokers with up to one-third of the cases associated with other malignant lesions of the respiratory tract.[39] In approximately 10% of patients, these tumors are multifocal and extend into the mainstem bronchi or adjacent esophagus, resulting in esophagobronchial fistula.[39] CT **(Figs. 19A to C)** demonstrates a polypoid intraluminal mass of soft tissue density with irregular, smooth, or lobulated contours.[36] The relationships of the tumor with the tracheal wall vary from localized eccentric pedunculated lesions to circumferential invasion.

Adenoid cystic carcinoma

Adenoid cystic carcinoma (ACC) are low-grade malignancies that typically arise from the tracheobronchial mucous glands, most frequently on the posterolateral tracheal wall. These show a marked propensity for local,

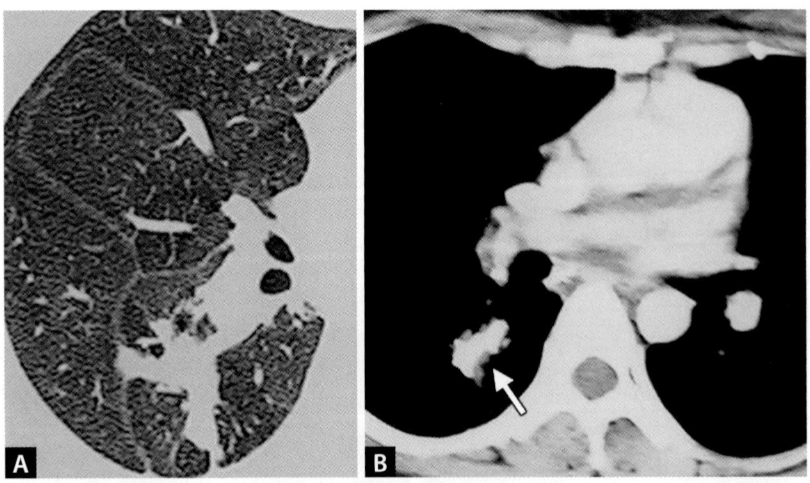

Figs. 17A and B: Broncholith: A branching tubular opacity is seen in the right lower lobe (A) of a 32-year-old woman with past history of tuberculosis. (B) On mediastinal window, the lesion is seen to be calcified (arrow).

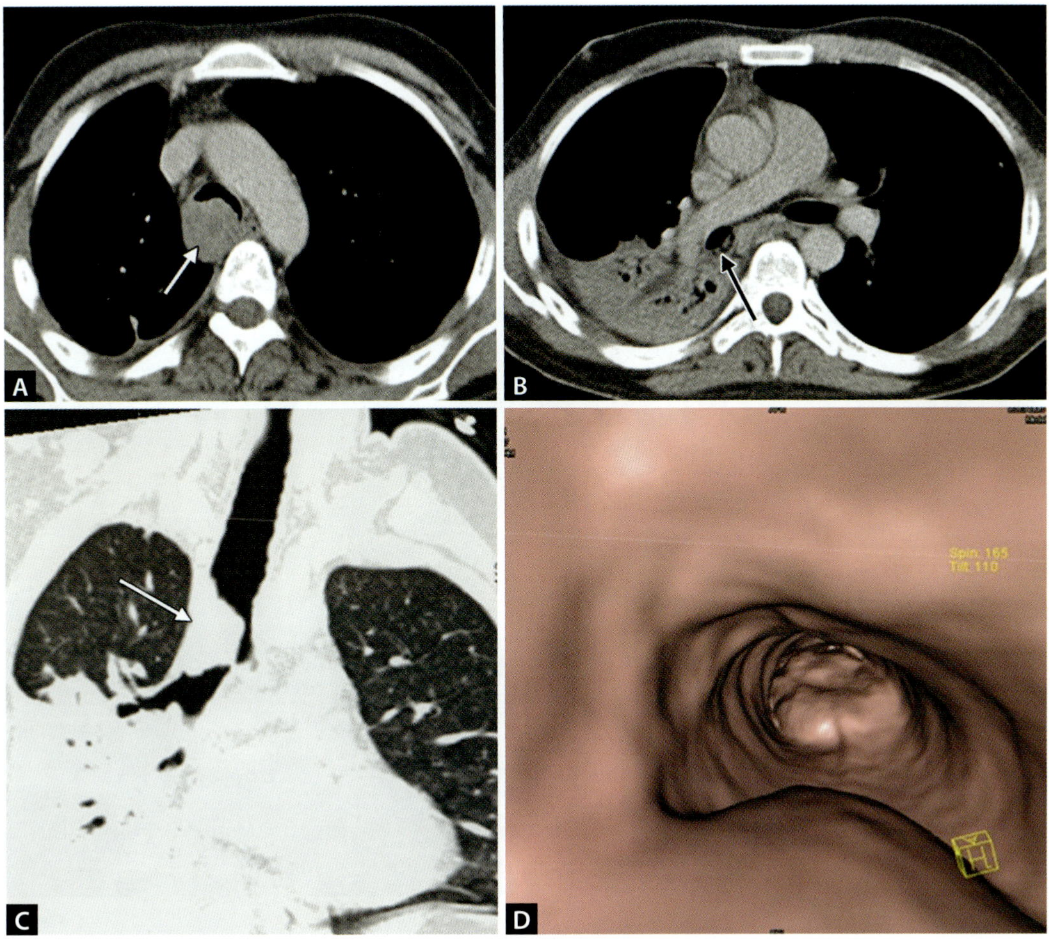

Figs. 18A to D: Tracheal mass: Axial CT (A and B), coronal MPR (C) and VB (D) showing a mass involving the trachea (white arrow). In addition, a low density lesion with air bubbles is seen in the right lower lobe with distal collapse suggestive of a mucous plug (black arrow in B).

submucosal and perineural invasion. Unlike squamous call carcinoma, no known association exists between smoking and development of ACC. CT appearances **(Figs. 20A and B)** include soft-tissue attenuating intraluminal mass which may infiltrate the mediastinal fat or localized stenosis because of circumferential wall thickening.[40]

Mucoepidermoid carcinoma

Mucoepidermoid carcinoma arises from the minor salivary glands lining the tracheobronchial tree.[41] Patients are less than 40 years old and usually present with obstructive airway symptoms. On CT, it is seen as a smooth, oval or lobulated, mildly enhancing endobronchial mass, often smoothly oval or lobulated.[42] Punctate calcifications are occasionally seen.

Malignancies of trachea or esophagus can also lead to the formation of acquired tracheoesophageal fistulas **(Figs. 21A and B)**.

Carcinoid tumors

Carcinoid tumors are neuroendocrine tumors, which arise from bronchial, or bronchiolar epithelium. They present a histologic spectrum of low-grade to high-grade neoplasms, with the highest grades merging with small cell carcinoma.[3] Most endobronchial carcinoids are central in location arising in the main, lobar, or segmental bronchi. On CT **(Figs. 22 and 23)**, they appear as a hilar mass or an endobronchial lesion. Classical findings have been described, of a well-defined round or lobulated tumor causing narrowing of the adjacent airway, associated with eccentric calcifications.[43] These often show intense enhancement.

Endobronchial metastases

Metastases to the bronchus can also present like an endobronchial mass. The metastases are usually from carcinoma breast, colon and kidney.

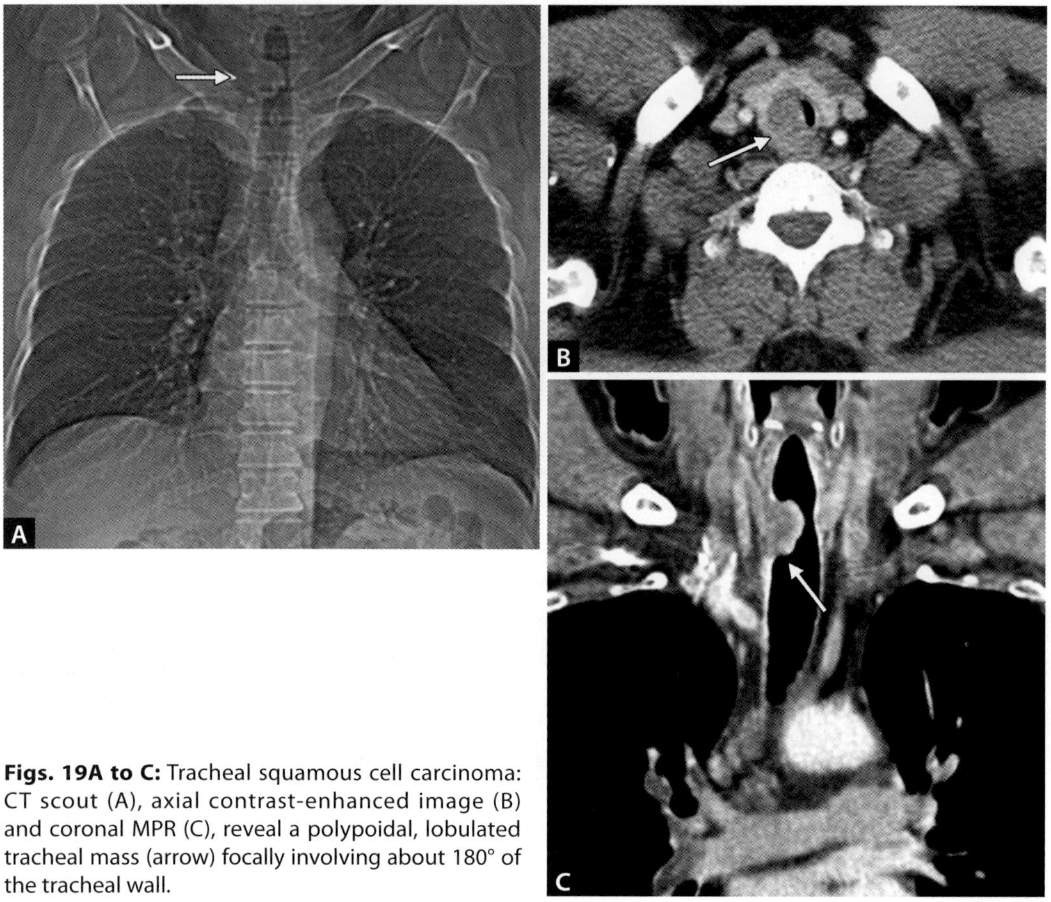

Figs. 19A to C: Tracheal squamous cell carcinoma: CT scout (A), axial contrast-enhanced image (B) and coronal MPR (C), reveal a polypoidal, lobulated tracheal mass (arrow) focally involving about 180° of the tracheal wall.

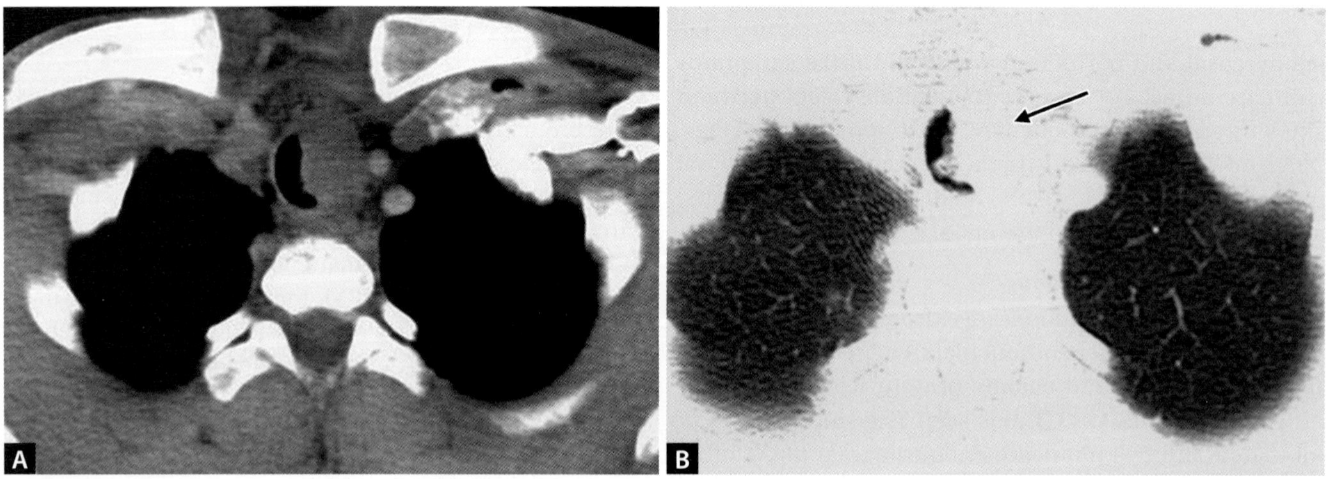

Figs. 20A and B: Tracheal adenoid cystic carcinoma: Axial contrast-enhanced CT in mediastinal window (A) and lung window (B) showing an irregular, soft tissue mass (arrow) with focal tracheal wall involvement. CT appearances of different tracheal tumors show significant overlap.

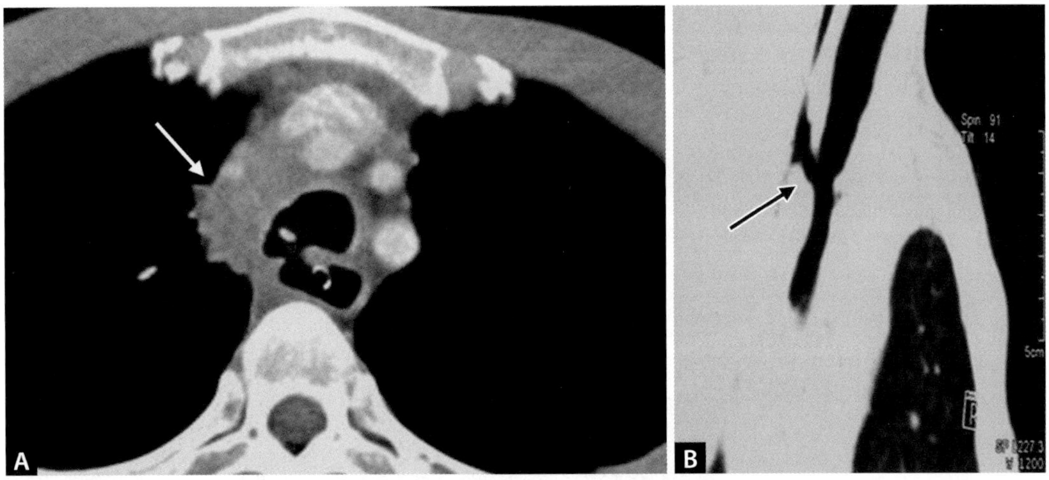

Figs. 21A and B: Tracheoesophageal fistula: Axial CECT (A) showing necrotic mediastinal nodes (white arrow) with a communication between trachea and esophagus. Sagittal MPR demonstrates the fistula (black arrow) well (B).

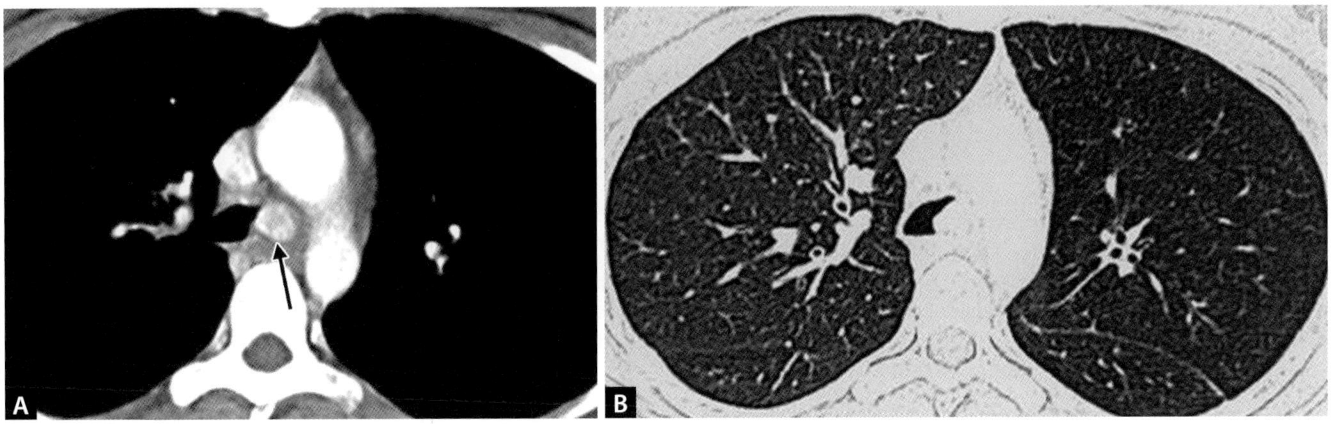

Figs. 22A and B: Carcinoid tumor: CT showing an intensely enhancing mass (arrow) involving the left main bronchus with hyperlucent left lung.

Benign Tumors

Benign tumors of the central airways are rare.[36] They can be of epithelial, mesenchymal, neural or composite origin. These tumors appear in clinical practice as the differential diagnosis of malignant lesions that are much more common.

Most common amongst these is the *squamous cell papilloma*. These most often occur in middle-aged male smokers, and typically involve the larynx or bronchi, tracheal involvement being uncommon. Involvement, when present, is limited to tracheal wall.[36] Papillomatosis is a condition associated with multiple papillomas. This condition typically affects children and young adults and is often limited to the larynx. It may involve the intrathoracic airways and also present with cavitating lung nodules and is referred to as *recurrent respiratory papillomatosis (RRP)* **(Figs. 24A and B)**. These lesions have a high propensity for recurrence and even malignant transformation.[44]

CT appearance may suggest the pathology of the neoplasm. Fat attenuation is seen in lipoma or hamartochondroma, while calcification may occur in hamartoma, chondroma or carcinoid. Presence of both fat and calcification suggests a hamartoma. High contrast-enhancement is seen in carcinoid, hemangioma, glomus tumor or fibroma.

MISCELLANEOUS

1. **Mucous plug/mucoid pseudotumor:** Mucus is the most common soft tissue mass within the airways. On CT scan **(Figs. 18 and 25)**, it is of low attenuation, nonenhancing, may contain small air bubbles and is not associated with cartilaginous ring disruption. Typically seen in the dependent portions of the airway it can move after coughing.
2. Other miscellaneous causes of focal airway narrowing include **foreign bodies (Figs. 26 and 27) and blood clot (Figs. 28A and B)**.

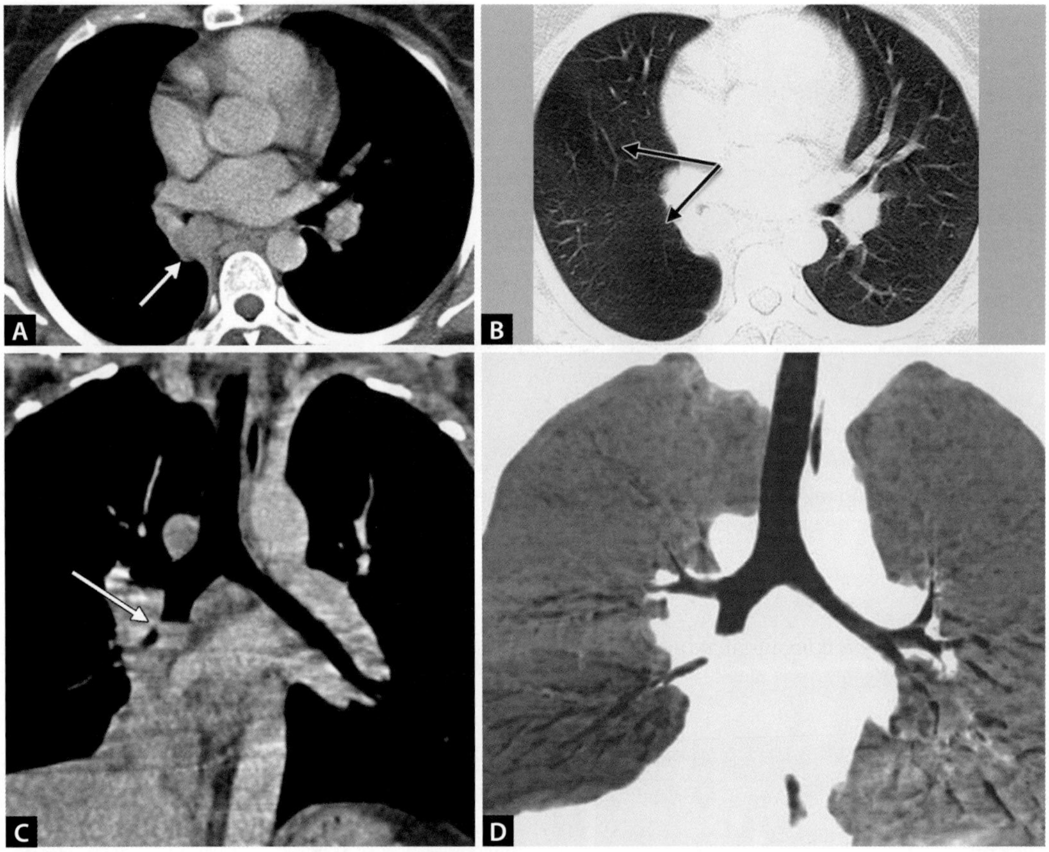

Figs. 23A to D: Carcinoid tumor. Axial CT (A and B), coronal MPR (C) and minIP (D) showing a lobulated mass (white arrow) involving the right bronchus intermedius with hyperlucent (black arrow) right middle and lower lobes. MinIP shows the craniocaudal extent of airway involvement the best.

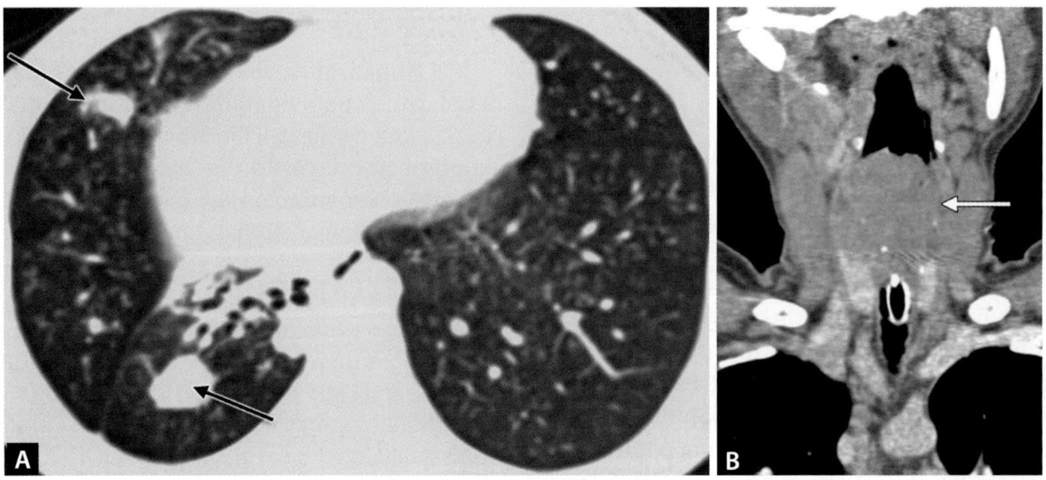

Figs. 24A and B: Recurrent respiratory papillomatosis: Multiple lung nodules (black arrow) and transglottic carcinoma (white arrow) in a young male with recurrent respiratory papillomatosis. The right lower lobe bronchiectasis is because of recurrent infections due to aspiration.

Prolonged increased intraluminal pressure can lead to the formation of acquired ***tracheal* (Figs. 29A and B) *and bronchial diverticula* (Fig. 30)**. Usually these are seen in COPD patients with chronic cough. Tracheal diverticulum is typically seen as an air filled outpouching from the right posterolateral tracheal wall.

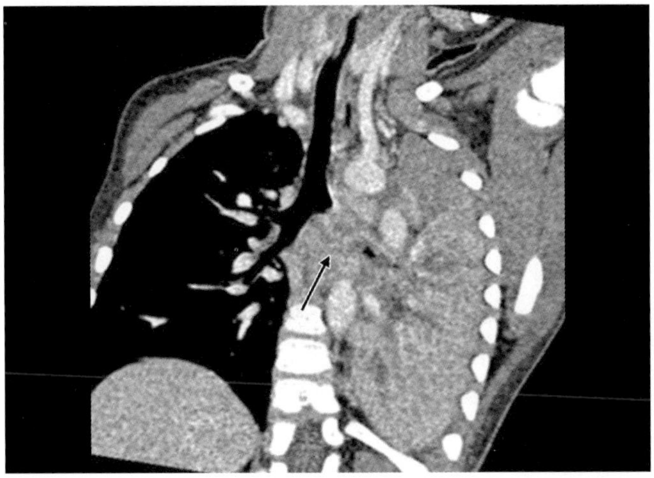

Fig. 25: Mucus plug: A fluid attenuating lesion is present in the left main bronchus (arrow) of an elderly male, with distal collapse of the left lung. These plugs can be successfully cleared bronchoscopically.

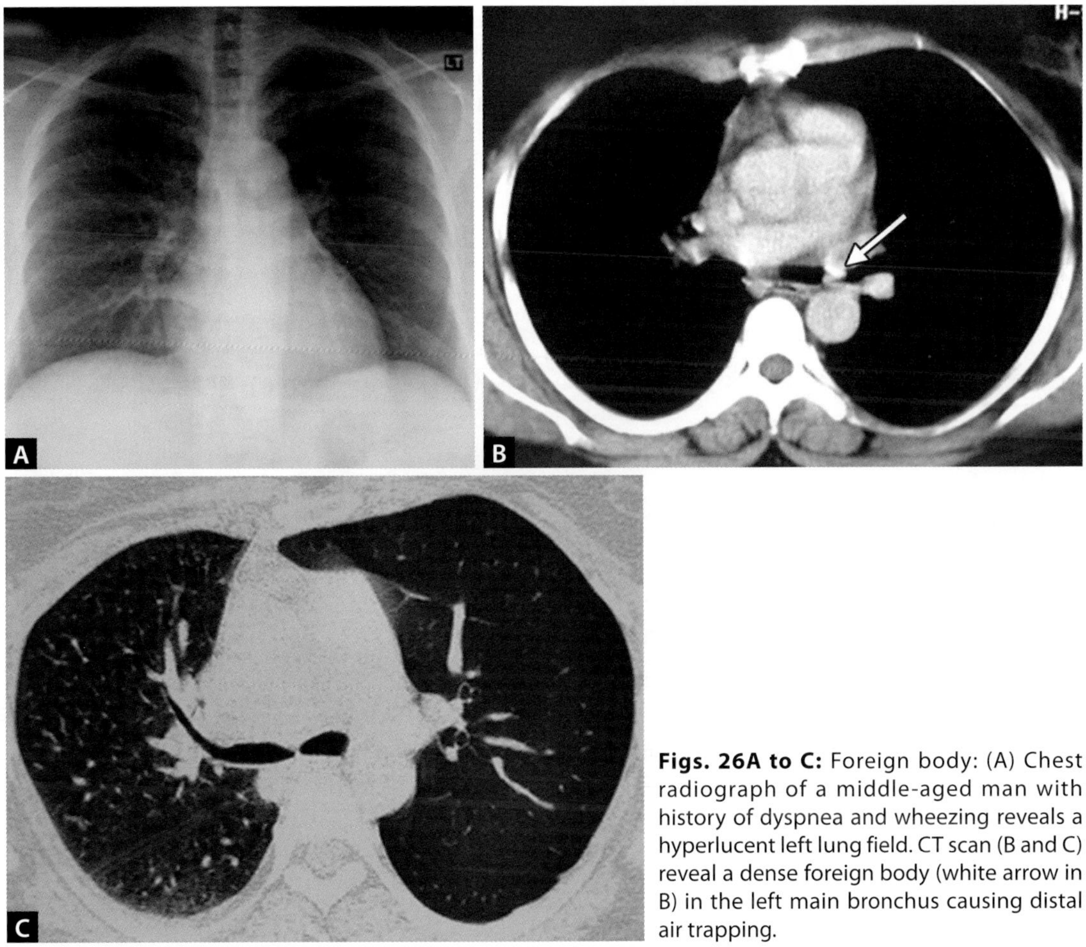

Figs. 26A to C: Foreign body: (A) Chest radiograph of a middle-aged man with history of dyspnea and wheezing reveals a hyperlucent left lung field. CT scan (B and C) reveal a dense foreign body (white arrow in B) in the left main bronchus causing distal air trapping.

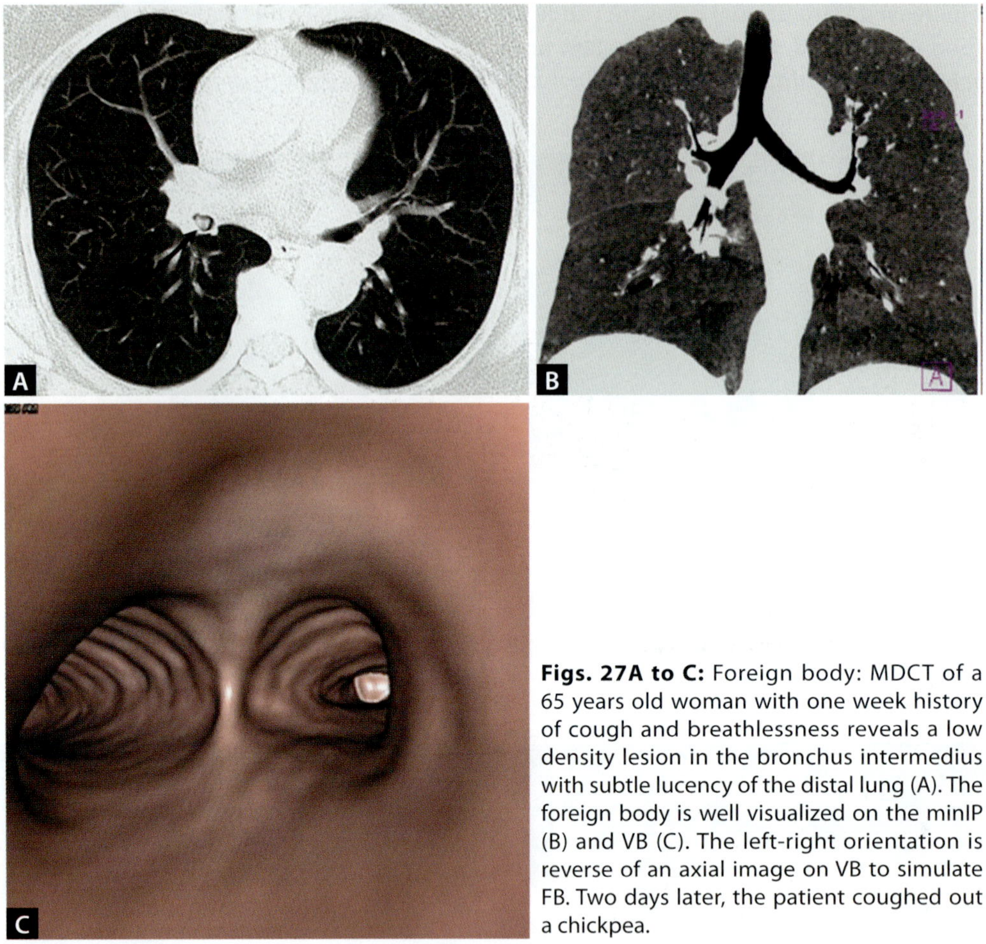

Figs. 27A to C: Foreign body: MDCT of a 65 years old woman with one week history of cough and breathlessness reveals a low density lesion in the bronchus intermedius with subtle lucency of the distal lung (A). The foreign body is well visualized on the minIP (B) and VB (C). The left-right orientation is reverse of an axial image on VB to simulate FB. Two days later, the patient coughed out a chickpea.

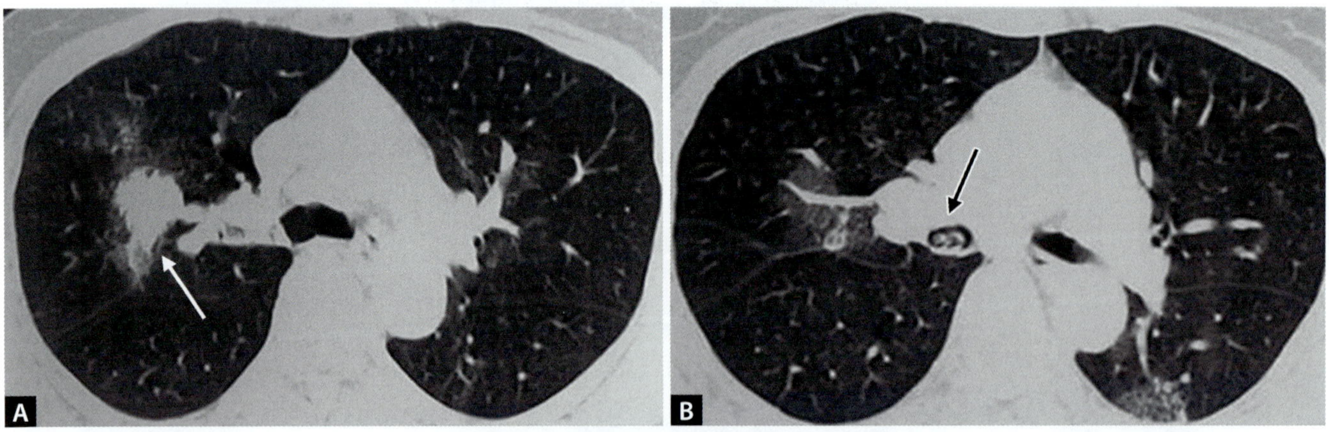

Figs. 28A and B: Blood clot: An elderly male presenting with hemoptysis. CT reveals a malignant mass in right upper lobe with surrounding hemorrhage (white arrow), and a blood clot (black arrow) in the right upper lobe bronchus. A blood clot resembles a mucous plug on imaging.

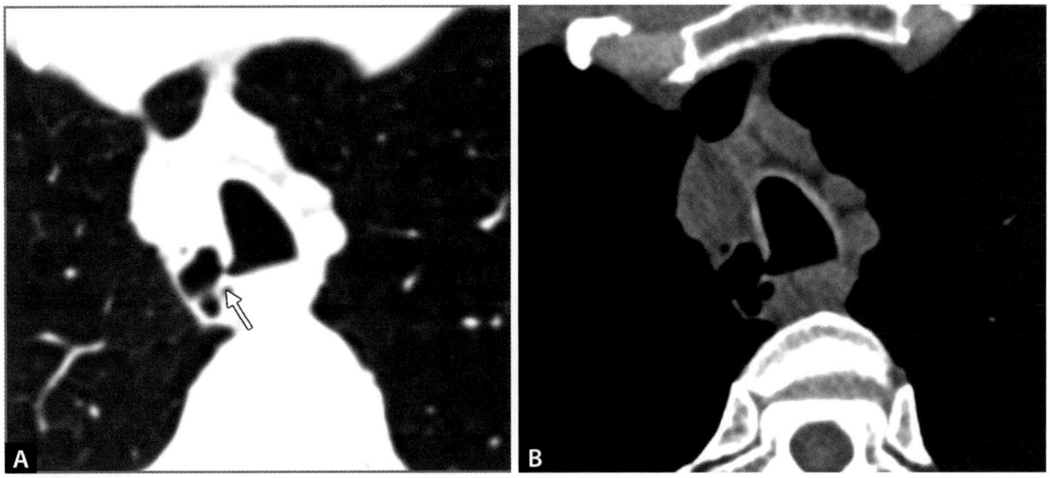

Figs. 29A and B: Tracheal diverticulum: Air-filled outpouching from the right posterolateral tracheal wall with small focal communication (arrow).

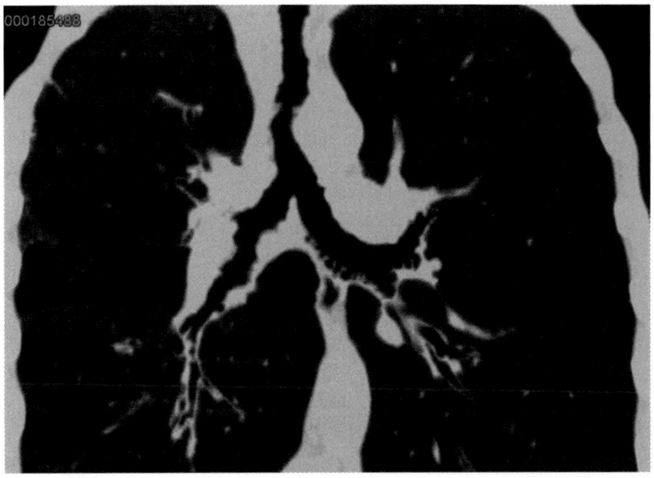

Fig. 30: Bronchial diverticulae. Multiple small diverticulae along the bilateral main and segmental bronchi with bronchial wall thickening and emphysematous changes in bilateral lung fields in a case of COPD.

PERIPHERAL AIRWAYS

BRONCHIECTASIS

Definition and Pathophysiology

Bronchiectasis is the localized, irreversible dilatation of the cartilage-containing airways or bronchi. It usually results from bronchial wall injury, bronchial lumen obstruction, and traction from adjacent fibrosis.[45] Obstruction and fibrosis are readily apparent on imaging. Bronchial wall injury and subsequent bronchiectasis can occur because of infection and, impaired host defense leading to recurrent infections, exaggerated immune response, congenital structural defects of the bronchial wall, and extrinsic insults damaging the airway wall.[46] Underlying mechanism of mucus plugging and superimposed bacterial colonization is common to these conditions.

Dilatation is classified by its gross appearance as tubular (cylindric), varicose, or cystic (saccular). These types are discussed in **Table 3** and shown in **Figures 31A to C**.

Clinical Features

Symptoms can be very nonspecific varying from mild cough or minimal dyspnea to chronic cough, abundant sputum production, progressive dyspnea, and repeated pulmonary infections. Chronic hypoxemia and hypercarbia can lead to digital clubbing, anemia, and weight loss. Other associated symptoms or manifestations include sinusitis, hemoptysis and pulmonary hypertension.[46]

Diagnosis is usually confirmed by spirometry and HRCT. The diagnostic workup may include a sweat electrolyte test, serum immunoglobulin levels, or serum *Aspergillus* antibody and precipitin, or even genetic testing according to the age of presentation and symptoms.

Imaging Findings (Figs. 1 and 32)

The imaging findings on *conventional radiography* are due to the bronchial wall thickening and are detailed in **Table 4**.

Table 3: Types of bronchiectasis.

Type of bronchiectasis	***Luminal dilatation***	***Wall thickening***
Cylindrical	Uniform	Smooth
Varicose	Alternating areas of dilatation and constriction (beaded appearance)	Irregular
Cystic	Uniform-dilated bronchus	Thick-walled bronchus terminates in a thick-walled cyst

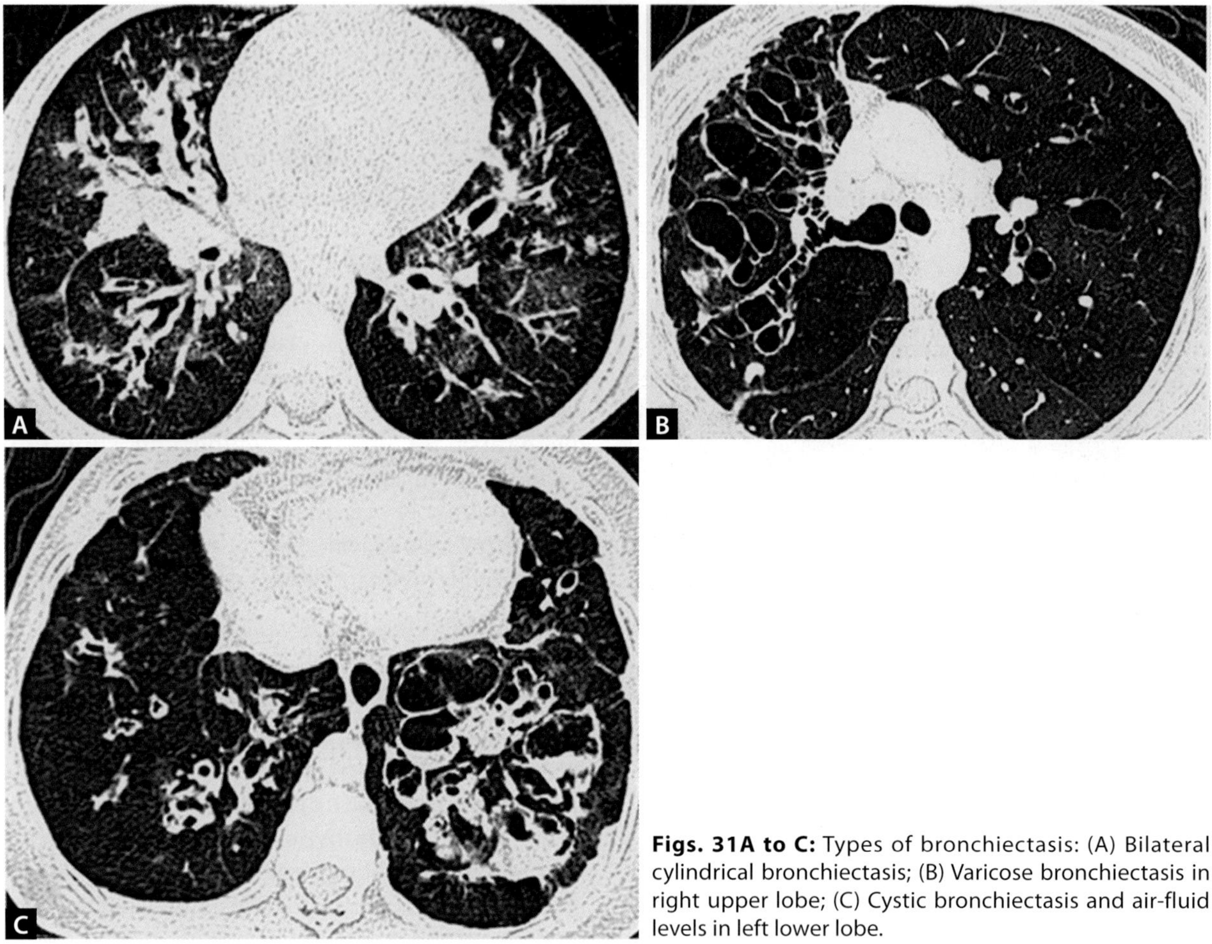

Figs. 31A to C: Types of bronchiectasis: (A) Bilateral cylindrical bronchiectasis; (B) Varicose bronchiectasis in right upper lobe; (C) Cystic bronchiectasis and air-fluid levels in left lower lobe.

HRCT is reliable to diagnose bronchiectasis. The key imaging features are due to bronchial dilatation and bronchial wall thickening and are detailed in **Table 5**. Bronchial wall thickening is seen in all cases of bronchiectasis, except those caused by congenital cartilage deficiency (William-Campbell syndrome, Mounier-Kuhn syndrome) or in allergic bronchopulmonary aspergillosis (ABPA).[46]

Etiology

The most common cause is postinfectious, followed by idiopathic bronchiectasis; bronchiectasis related to abnormal mucociliary clearance (cystic fibrosis and primary ciliary dyskinesia), and ABPA and systemic immunodeficiency.[47] Few of the common etiologies are discussed below.

Congenital Airway Wall Abnormality

There is abnormal physiologic clearing of mucoid excretions in congenital defects of cartilage, collagen, or other components of the bronchial wall. This predisposes to repeated infections and progressive bronchial dilatation.

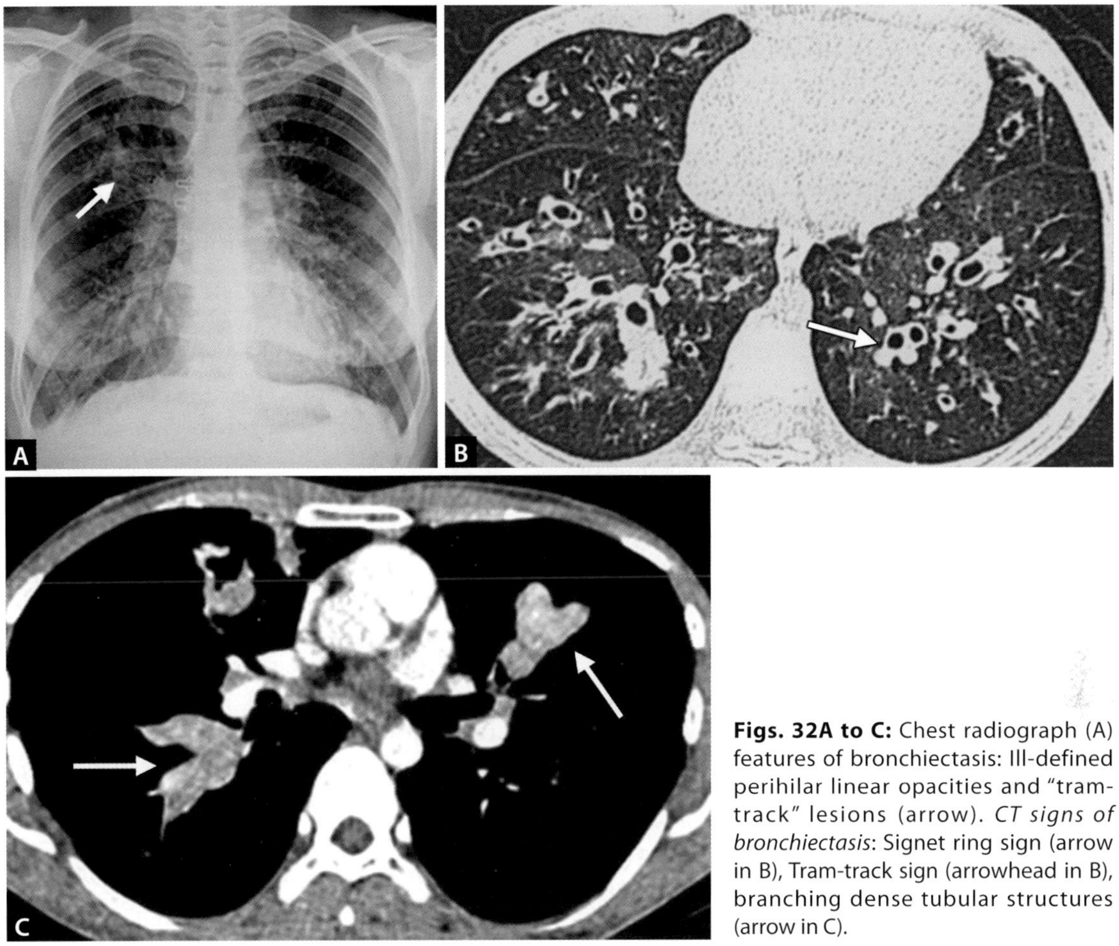

Figs. 32A to C: Chest radiograph (A) features of bronchiectasis: Ill-defined perihilar linear opacities and "tram-track" lesions (arrow). *CT signs of bronchiectasis*: Signet ring sign (arrow in B), Tram-track sign (arrowhead in B), branching dense tubular structures (arrow in C).

Table 4: Key radiographic features of bronchiectasis.

Imaging finding	***Etiology***
Ill-defined perihilar linear densities with indistinctness of the margins of the central pulmonary arteries	Bronchial wall thickening
Ill-defined ring shadows (bronchus seen end on)	Bronchial wall thickening
Tramlines or parallel lines along expected course of bronchi	Bronchial wall thickening in severe bronchiectasis
Elongated opacities ± calcified	Mucus plugging
Air-fluid levels in thick-walled cysts with surrounding consolidation	Superadded infection
Hyperinflation	Increased lung volume

Tracheobronchomegaly (Mounier-Kuhn Disease)

An uncommon disease presenting in males, in the fourth and fifth decades, it is believed to be congenital in origin. The common assocaitions include Ehlers-Danlos syndrome, Marfan syndrome, and generalized elastosis

Table 5: Key HRCT findings of bronchiectasis.

Imaging Finding	***Etiology***
Internal luminal diameter of one or more bronchi > diameter of adjacent artery	Bronchial dilatation
Lack of normal tapering of a bronchus	Bronchial dilatation
Visible bronchus abutting mediastinal pleura	Bronchial dilatation
Visible bronchus within 1 cm of pleura	Bronchial dilatation
Signet ring sign	Jewel: Artery abutting the Ring: Thick-walled dilated bronchus on axial view
Tram-track sign	Parallel, thickened walls of a dilated bronchus on a longitudinal section
Branching dense tubular structures	Mucus plugging of dilated bronchi and bronchioles
Centrilobular nodules, in a "tree-in-bud" pattern	Mucus-filled bronchiolectasis
Mosaic attenuation and air trapping	Coexisting constrictive bronchiolitis

(cutis laxa). Tracheobronchomegaly is characterized by pathological thinning of the muscle, cartilage, and elastic tissue of the airway walls. There is increased distensibility of the tracheal and bronchial walls with uniform dilatation of the tracheal and bronchial lumina predisposing to recurrent infections in the dependent lungs. Tracheal diameter more than 3 cm in both coronal and sagittal planes with central bronchiectasis but without airway wall thickening is seen on CT **(Figs. 33A and B)**.[46]

Williams-Campbell Syndrome

Williams-Campbell syndrome is a rare disease characterized by defect in the cartilage of the fourth-, fifth-, and sixth-generation bronchi. It maybe congenital or acquired (likely as a sequelae of prior adenovirus (measles and pertussis) infections). On CT imaging there is cystic bronchiectasis distal to the third-generation bronchi with ballooning on inspiratory CT and collapse on expiratory phase.[48]

Congenital Bronchial Atresia

There is congenital focal obliteration of the lumen of a segmental bronchus. This results in focal bronchiectasis and air trapping more distally. Usually identified as an incidental finding on a chest radiograph as an ovoid, tubular, or branching density. CT **(Figs. 34A to C)** shows the characteristic bronchial, branching nature, and distal air trapping. It should be differentiated from an acquired mucocele which is caused by focal scarring of a segmental bronchus (infective) or from an endobronchial lesion.[49] In case of an acquired mucocele an endobronchial neoplasm should be excluded.

Acquired Wall Abnormalities

Inflammation of the bronchial wall because of chronic infections, inhalational injury, and cellular infiltration in the setting of graft versus host disease can cause damage to the bronchial wall.

Mucociliary Clearance Abnormalities

In cystic fibrosis, the consistency of mucus is abnormal whereas primary ciliary dyskinesia and immotile ciliary syndrome are characterized by abnormalities of the structure and function of the cilia of the airway epithelium. This leads to ineffective mucus clearance and secondary colonization of the airway lumina by bacteria and repeated episodes of infections. There is upper lobe involvement in cystic fibrosis whereas in primary and acquired ciliary dyskinesia the bronchiectasis is worse in the lower lungs.[46] Primary ciliary dyskinesia (PCD) or immotile ciliary syndrome is caused by a defect in structure and function of the airway cilia and causes progressive bronchiectasis. Kartagener syndrome **(Figs. 35A and B)** or triad (situs inversus, bronchiectasis, and sinusitis) is seen in half of the PCD patients.[50,51] Bronchiectasis in PCD is primarily in the lingular, middle and lower lobes of the lung.

Hyperimmune Response

Hyperimmune response to internal or external antigens with inflammation of the airway wall and subsequent bronchiectasis can be seen in allergic bronchopulmonary aspergillosis, inflammatory bowel disease, rheumatoid arthritis, Sjögren disease and granulomatous polyangitis.

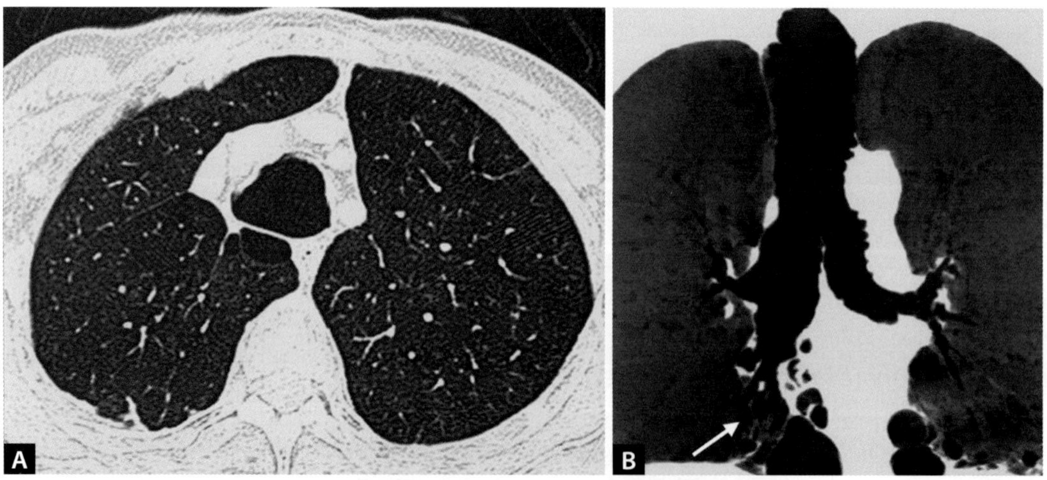

Figs. 33A and B: Mounier-Kuhn disease: CT reveals dilatation of the trachea and major bronchi. Bronchiectasis is seen in right lower lobe (arrow).

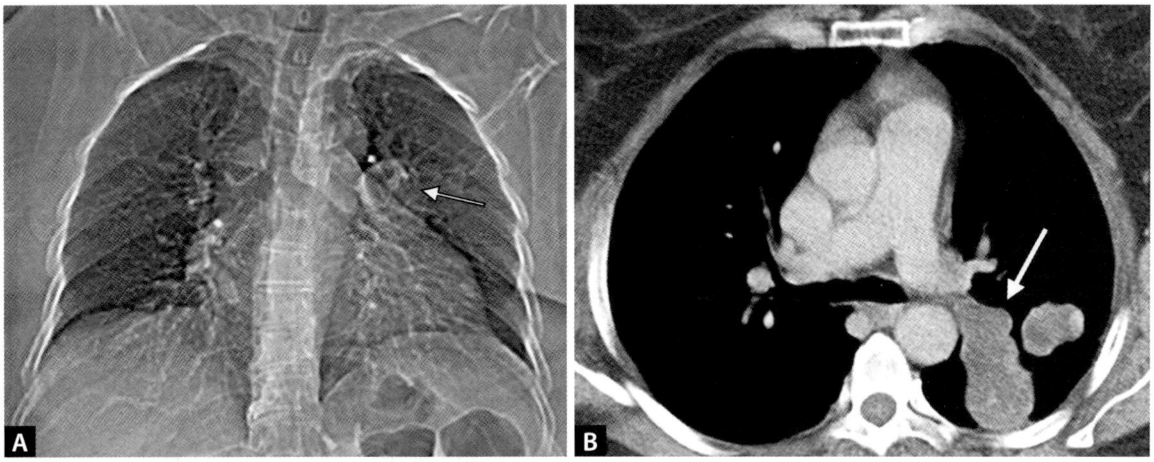

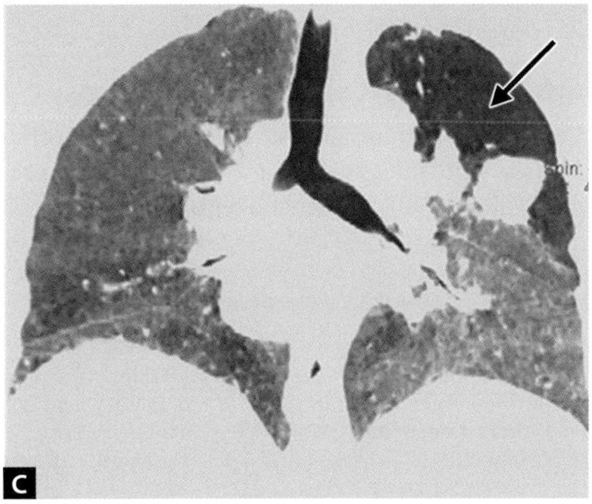

Figs. 34A to C: Congenital bronchial atresia: CT scout film (A) shows a well-defined left parahilar opacity (arrow). Mediastinal window (B) reveals a fluid-filled branching, tubular lesion (arrow) in the posterior segment of left upper lobe. MinIP (C) demonstrates the distal hyperinflation (arrow).

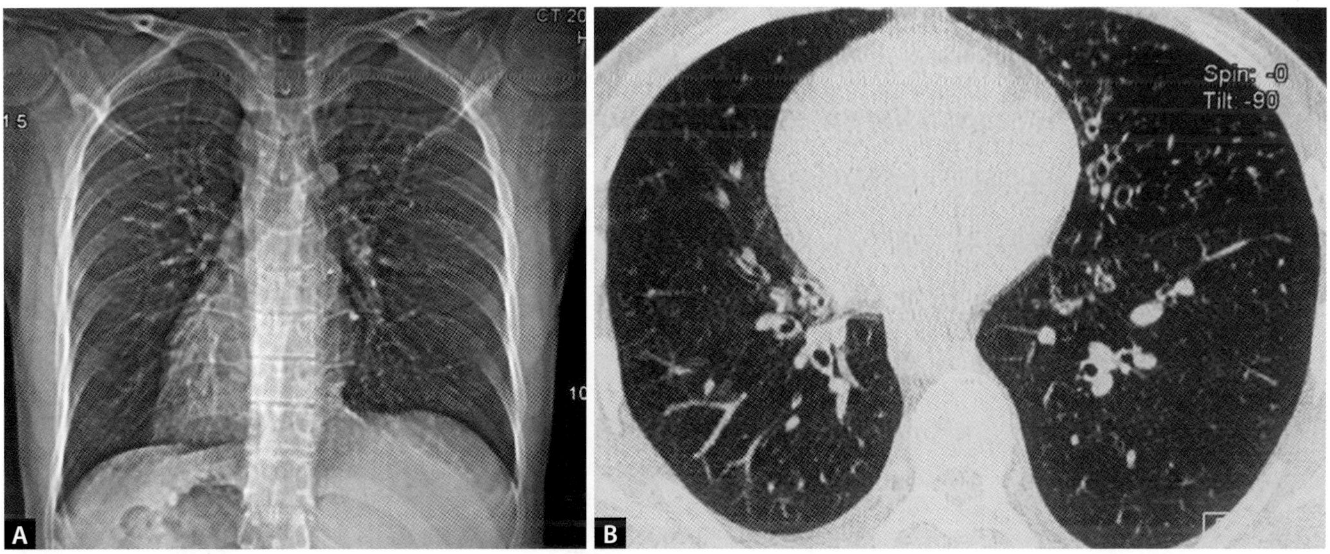

Figs. 35A and B: Kartagener syndrome: CT scout film (A) shows situs inversus. HRCT chest (B) reveals bilateral central bronchiectasis.

Allergic Bronchopulmonary Aspergillosis

Allergic bronchopulmonary aspergillosis (ABPA) is a hypersensitivity reaction to *Aspergillus fumigatus* antigens seen commonly in patients with atopic rhinitis, asthma, or CF. Patients present with fever, wheeze and expectoration of brown mucus plugs. Elevated serum IgE level, eosinophilia on peripheral blood smears, or positive skin reaction to *Aspergillus* antigen are seen on clinical evaluation. Mycelia can sometimes be identified in the expectorated mucus plugs. Imaging characteristically shows migratory consolidation early in the disease, usually involving the upper lobes. On HRCT **(Figs. 36A and B)**, there is central and upper lobe bronchiectasis, varicose or cystic subtypes. Inspissated mucus in the dilated central bronchi gives the classic finger in-glove appearance on the chest radiographs in more chronic cases.[46,50] There is atelectasis or hyperinflation of the lung distal to the impacted bronchi. In up to 20% of the patients, high-attenuation mucus may be seen.[52]

SMALL AIRWAYS

Small airway refers to the distal airways, which are small in size (<2 mm in diameter) and lack cartilage and submucosal glands. This includes the membranous (purely conducting) and respiratory bronchioles (conducting and gas exchange function). *Hence, the term bronchiolitis is used interchangeably with small airway disease (SAD).*

ROLE OF IMAGING IN EVALUATION OF SAD

CT is the mainstay of diagnosis as chest radiograph is often normal in early cases and also PFT derangements are evident only in advanced forms of the disease. The CT technique for evaluation of SAD has been described above **(Box 3)**.

CT SIGNS OF SMALL AIRWAY DISEASE

These include both direct and indirect signs and are detailed in **Table 6**.[53]

Table 6: CT signs of small airway disease.

Direct signs	*Indirect signs*
1. Centrilobular nodules with 'tree-in-bud' appearance (branching nodules; V or Y shaped) 2. Ground-glass opacities typically centrilobular or peribronchiolar in distribution 3. Bronchiolectasis (seen in chronic stages)	1. Air trapping (seen as areas of low attenuation, best on expiratory scans) 2. Atelectasis/collapse (less common)

CLASSIFICATION

Bronchiolitis is a term used to describe bronchiolar inflammation of diverse causes. The combined radiopathological approach is a commonly accepted classification system. According to this classification, there are two major types of small airway diseases.[54,55]

1. Inflammatory/cellular bronchiolitis
2. Constrictive/fibrotic bronchiolitis

Inflammatory/Cellular Bronchiolitis

Cellular bronchiolitis is characterized by inflammatory cellular infiltrates involving both the bronchiolar lumen and walls, usually associated with some degree of fibrosis.

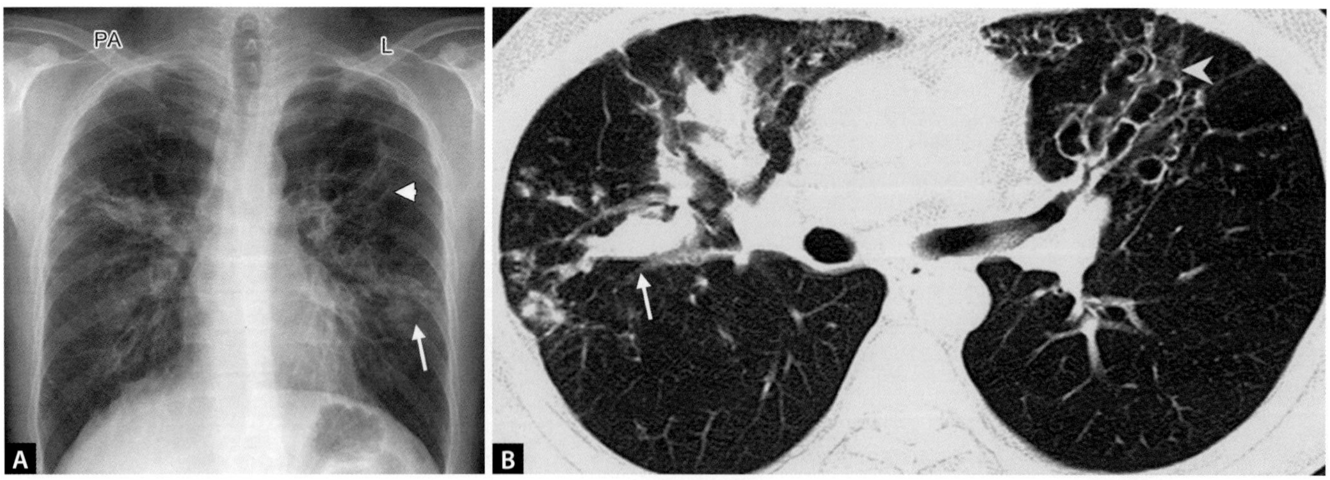

Figs. 36A and B: Allergic bronchopulmonary aspergillosis (ABPA): Chest radiograph (A) and CT scan (B) showing classical central, tubular bronchiectasis (arrowhead) with mucous plugging giving "finger-in-glove" appearance (arrow).

According to the clinical presentation, acute or chronic, and the predominant cell type, classification includes a number of specific etiologies, including—*infectious bronchiolitis, respiratory bronchiolitis (RB), follicular bronchiolitis, Asian panbronchiolitis, aspiration bronchiolitis; bronchiolitis associated with bronchiectasis and hypersensitivity pneumonitis.*

Smoking-related RB is the commonest of these forms followed by infectious diseases.[56] Follicular bronchiolitis is often of autoimmune etiology or associated with connective tissue disorders or immunodeficiency.

On imaging **(Box 6)** cellular bronchiolitis **(Fig. 37)** is characterized by the presence of centrilobular nodules, ground-glass nodules and bronchial wall thickening. RB **(Figs. 38A and B)** usually has fine nodules compared to infections where there is patchy distribution of larger and coarse nodules.

Constrictive/Obliterative Bronchiolitis

Obliterative bronchiolitis is characterized by irreversible circumferential submucosal fibrosis, which results in bronchiolar narrowing or obliteration in the absence of surrounding parenchymal inflammation or intraluminal granulation tissue. This narrowing of bronchiolar lumen may be due to collagen deposition, fibrosis or scarring of bronchiolar wall/peribronchiolar area.[57,58]

Conditions associated with constrictive bronchiolitis include—*post-infectious (Swyer-James or Macleod syndrome), inhalation of toxic fumes, autoimmune/connective tissue diseases, drug related, chronic allograft rejection associated with heart-lung or lung transplantation and graft-versus-host disease associated with bone marrow transplantation and idiopathic.*

Obliterative bronchiolitis is most frequently post-infectious (often viral) or connective tissue disease related (commonest being rheumatoid arthritis). Acute exposure to noxious fumes can also result in this form of lung injury.

Post-infectious *McLeod/Swyer James syndrome*, earlier thought to be unilateral is not uncommonly bilateral. On imaging, a unilateral (or bilateral) hyperlucent lung that demonstrates air trapping is seen.

Radiographically in obliterative bronchiolitis, hyperinflation is frequently apparent. The characteristic HRCT

Box 6: HRCT features of cellular/inflammatory bronchiolitis.

- Centrilobular nodules with or without "tree-in-bud"
- Ground-glass nodules
- Bronchial wall thickening

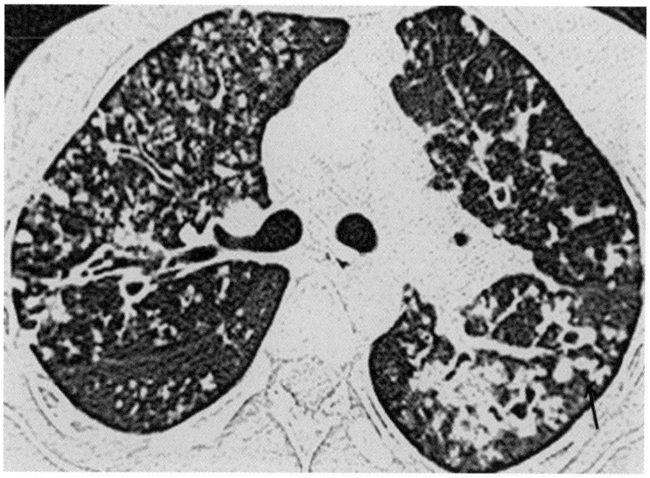

Fig. 37: Infectious bronchiolitis (tubercular): CT shows extensive "tree-in-bud" nodules (arrow) with bronchial wall thickening in bilateral lung fields.

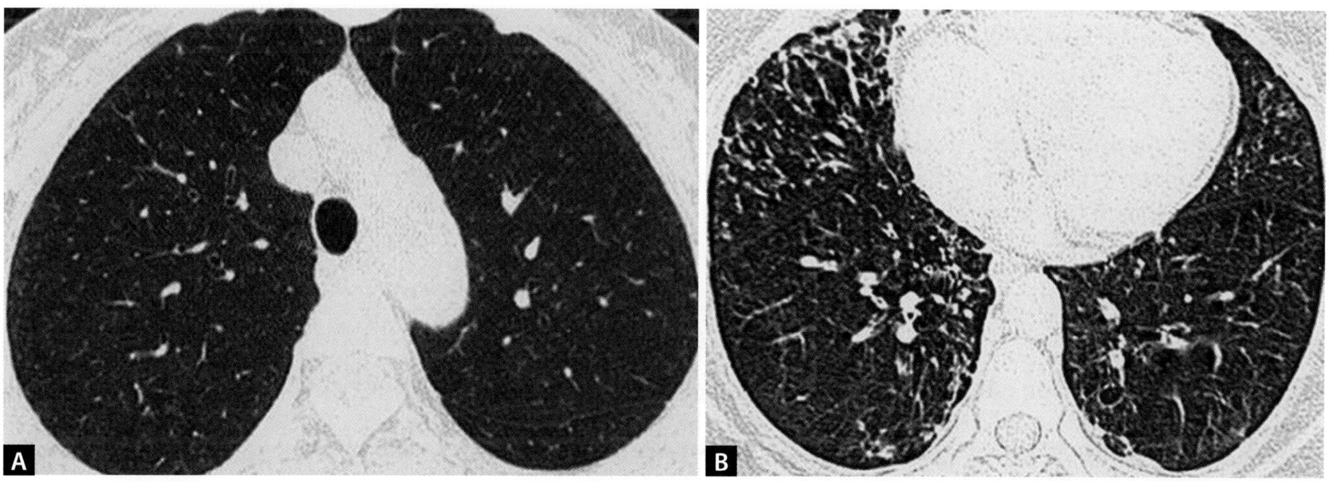

Figs. 38A and B: Respiratory bronchiolitis: CT scans of two different patients showing fine centrilobular nodules (A) with additional interstitial thickening in (B) (RB-ILD).

finding **(Box 7 and Fig. 39)** is air trapping and bronchiectasis/bronchiolectasis may also be occasionally seen. However, centrilobular nodules are rare.[58,59]

Box 7: HRCT features of constrictive/obliterative bronchiolitis.

- Air trapping
- Bronchiectasis/bronchiolectasis
- Centrilobular nodules are rare.

ASTHMA

Asthma is characterized by airway inflammation in response to a variety of stimuli resulting in bronchial hyper-responsiveness. Chronic inflammation results in smooth muscle thickening, neovascularity and fibrosis, leading to irreversible airway narrowing. Bronchiectasis may also result from chronic inflammation.

The clinical indications for CT in patients with asthma are limited and include identification of subtle radiographically occult airspace infection or treatable causes of airway inflammation, including ABPA and hypersensitivity pneumonitis and for documenting emphysema in smokers with asthma. CT may also be useful in excluding structural causes of localized wheezing, such as focal tracheal or mainstem bronchial lesions.

High-resolution CT findings in asthma include bronchial wall thickening, bronchial dilatation, and expiratory air trapping.[3,60]

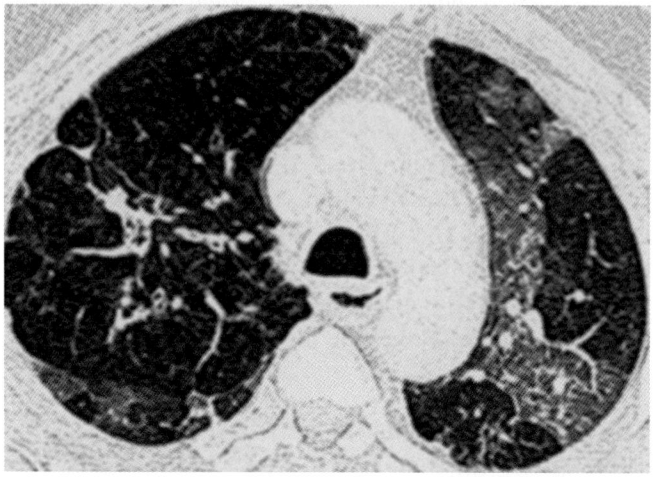

Fig. 39: Obliterative bronchiolitis: CT scan of 53-year-old patient with rheumatoid arthritis and dyspnea reveals bilateral areas of air trapping/mosaic attenuation.

CHRONIC OBSTRUCTIVE PULMONARY DISEASE

There is airflow limitation that is not fully reversible in chronic obstructive pulmonary disease (COPD) and is usually progressive. It results from variable mixture of airway obstruction (obstructive bronchiolitis) and parenchymal destruction (emphysema). Chronic bronchitis (clinical term) is characterized by presence of cough and sputum production for at least 3 months in each of two consecutive years. Pulmonary emphysema (pathologic term) is abnormal permanent enlargement of the air spaces distal to the terminal bronchiole, accompanied by the destruction of their walls. Expiratory scans well document the extent of central tracheobronchomalacia and peripheral small airway obstruction. There may be associated mild bronchiectasis. CT signs of small airways disease on CT are often present along with emphysematous changes **(Fig. 40)**.[61]

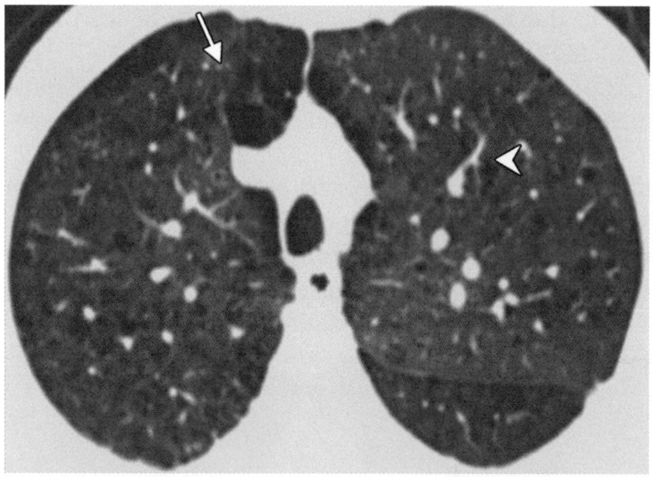

Fig. 40: Chronic obstructive pulmonary disease: CT scan of 35-year-old male smoker reveals paraseptal (arrow) and centrilobular (arrowhead) emphysema.

CONCLUSION

Tracheobronchial lesions include a wide range of abnormalities and MDCT is the modality of choice. Axial images should always be used with MPR and 3D reconstruction images for evaluating tracheobronchial disorders. MPR images are a useful adjunct and minIP gives good overview of airway. Virtual bronchoscopy can guide the bronchoscopist and may avoid bronchoscopy especially in children.

REFERENCES

1. Chou SSH, Kicska GA, Pipavath SN, et al. Digital Tomosynthesis of the chest: Current and Emerging Applications. Radiographics. 2014;34:359-72.

2. Dobbins JT 3rd, McAdams HP, Godfrey DJ, et al. Digital tomosynthesis of the chest. J Thorac Imaging. 2008;23(2):86-92.
3. Naidich DP, Webb WR, Muller NC, Vlahos L, Krinsky GA (Eds). "Airways" in Computed Tomography and Magnetic Resonance of the thorax, 4th edition. Lippincott Williams, and Wilkins, Philadephia, USA; 2007. pp. 453-556.
4. Sundarakumar DK, Bhalla AS, Sharma R, et al. Multidetector CT evaluation of central airways stenoses: Comparison of virtual bronchoscopy, minimal-intensity projection, and multiplanar reformatted images. Indian J Radiol Imaging. 2011;21(3):191-4.
5. Bankier AA, O'Donnell C, Boiselle PM. Respiratory instructions for CT examinations of the lungs: a hands on guideline. Radiographics. 2008;28:919-31.
6. Beigelman AC, Brillet PY, Grenier PA. MDCT of the Airways: Technique and Normal Results Radiol. Clin N Am. 2009;47(2):185-201.
7. American College of Radiology. ACR–STR practice parameter for the performance of high-resolution computed tomography (HRCT) of the lungs in adults. https://www.acr.org/~/media/ACR/Documents/PGTS/guidelines/HRCT_Lungs.pdf. Accessed on July 27, 2017.
8. Lee EY, Litmanovich D, Boiselle PM. Multidetector CT. Evaluation of Tracheobronchomalacia. Radiol Clin N Am. 2009;47(2):261-9.
9. Boiselle PM, Reynolds KF, Ernst A. Multiplanar and three-dimensional imaging of the central airways with multidetector CT. Am J Roentgenol. 2002;179:301-8.
10. Hooper KD, et al. Mucosal details at CT virtual reality: Surface versus volume rendering. Radiology. 2000;214:517-22.
11. Boiselle PM, Lynch DA. Anatomical airway imaging methods. In: Boiselle PM, Lynch DA (Eds). CT of the airways. Totowa (NJ): Humana Press; 2008. pp. 75-94.
12. Fetita CI, Preteux F, Beigelman-Aubry C, et al. Pulmonary airways: 3D reconstruction from multislice CT and clinical investigation. IEEE Trans Med Imaging. 2004;23: 1353-64.
13. Tanaka F, et al. Evaluation of tracheobronchial wall invasion using transbronchial ultrasonography (EBUS). Eur J Cardio Throac Surg. 2000;17:570-4.
14. Hochhegger B, et al. Chest magnetic resonance imaging: a protocol suggestion. Radiol Bras. 2015;48(6):373-80.
15. Dornes, et al. Allergic Bronchopulmonary aspergillosis in cystic fibrosis: MR Imaging of Airway Mucus Contrasts as a Tool for Diagnosis. Radiology. 2017. doi.org/10.1148/radiol.2017162350.
16. Gamsu G, Webb WR. Computed tomography of the trachea: Normal and abnormal. Am J Roentgenol. 1982;139:321-6.
17. Wu Ju, et al. Variant bronchial anatomy: CT appearance and classification. Am J Roentgenol. 1999;172:741-4.
18. Landing BH, Dixon LG. Congenital malformation and genetic disorders of the respiratory tract. Am Rev Respir Dis. 1979;120:151-85.
19. Fraser RS, Colman N, Müller NL, et al. Upper airway obstruction. In: Fraser RS, Colman N, Müller NL, Pare PD (Eds). Synopsis of diseases of the chest. 3rd edition. Philadelphia: BW Saunders; 2005. pp. 631-4.
20. Carden KA, Boiselle PM, Waltz DA, et al. Tracheomalacia and tracheobronchomalacia in children and adults: An in-depth review. Chest. 2005;127:984-1005.
21. Sundarakumar DK, Bhalla AS, Sharma R, et al. Multidetector computed tomography imaging of congenital anomalies of major airways: A pictorial essay. World J Radiol. 2011;3(12): 289-97.
22. Swensen SJ, Aughenbaugh GL, Douglas WW, et al. High-resolution CT of the lungs: Findings in various pulmonary diseases. Am J Roentgenol. 1992;159:971-2.
23. Arora A, Bhalla AS, Jana M, et al. Overview of airway involvement in tuberculosis. J Med Imaging Radiat Oncol. 2013;57:576-581.
24. Moon WK, et al. Tuberculosis of the central airways: CT findings of active and fibrotic disease. Am J Roentgenol. 1997;169:649-53.
25. Franquet T, et al. Necrotizing aspergillosis of large airways. CT findings in eight patients. J Comput Assist Tomogr. 2002;26:342-5.
26. Yigla M, Ben-Izhak O, Oren I, et al. Laryngotracheobronchial involvement in a patient with nonendemic rhinoscleroma. Chest. 2000;117(6):1795-98.
27. Grenier PA, Beigelman AC, Brillet PY. Nonneoplastic Tracheal and Bronchial Stenoses. Radiol Clin N Am. 2009;47(2):243-60.
28. Cordier JF, et al. Pulmonary Wegener's granulomatosis. A clinical and imaging study of 77 cases. Chest 1990;97: 906-12.
29. Trentham DE, Le CH. Relapsing polychondritis. Ann Intern Med. 1998;129(2):114-22.
30. Behar JV, Choi YW, Hartman TA, et al. Relapsing polychondritis affecting the lower respiratory tract. Am J Roentgenol. 2002;178(1):173-7.
31. Stark P. Imaging of tracheobronchial injuries. J Thoracic Imaging. 1995;10:206-19.
32. Lenique F, Brauner MW, Grenier P, et al. CT assessment of bronchi in sarcoidosis: endoscopic and pathologic correlations. Radiology. 1995;194(2):419-23.
33. O'Regan A, et al. Tracheobronchial amyloidosis. The Boston University experience from 1984 to 1999. Medicine. 2000;79: 69-79.
34. Kim HY, et al. Localized amyloidosis of the respiratory system: CT features. J Comput Assist Tomogr. 1999;23:627-31.
35. Conces DJ, Tarver RD, Vix VA. Broncholithiasis: CT features in 15 patients. Am J Roentgenol. 1991;157:249-53.
36. McCarthy MJ, Rosado-de-Christenson ML. Tumors of the trachea. J Thorac Imaging. 1995;10(3):180-98.
37. Macchiarini P. Primary tracheal tumors. Lancet Oncol. 2006;7:83-91.
38. Honings J, van Dijck JA, Verhagen AF, et al. Incidence and treatment of tracheal cancer: A nationwide study in the Netherlands. Ann Surg Oncol. 2007;14(2):968-76.
39. Grillo HC, Mathisen DJ, Wain JC. Management of tumors of the trachea. Oncology. 1992;6:61-7.

40. Kwak SH, Lee KS, Chung MJ, et al. Adenoid cystic carcinoma of the airways: Helical CT and histopathologic correlation. Am J Roentgenol. 2004;183(2):77-81.
41. Yousem SA, Hochholzer L. Mucoepidermoid tumors of the lung. Cancer. 1987;60(6):1346-52.
42. Kim TS, Lee KS, Han J, et al. Mucoepidermoid carcinoma of the tracheobronchial tree: Radiographic and CT findings in 12 patients. Radiology. 1999;212(3):643-8.
43. Naidich DP. CT/MR correlation in the evaluation of tracheobronchial neoplasia. Radiol Clin North Am. 1990;28:555-71.
44. Marchiori, et al. Laryngotracheobronchial papillomatosis: findings on computed tomography scans of the chest. J Bras Pneumol. 2008;34(12):1084-9.
45. Shoemark A, Ozerovitch L, Wilson R. Etiology in adult patients with bronchiectasis. Respir Med. 2007;191:1163-70.
46. Nejad CJ, Bhalla S. Bronchiectasis Radiol Clin N Am. 2009;47(2):88-306.
47. Muller NL, Fraser RS, Lee KS, et al. Diseases of the lung-radiologic and pathologic correlations. 1st edition (Chapter 15). Philadelphia: Lippincott Williams and Wilkins; 2003. pp. 280-1.
48. Hartman TE, Primack SL, Lee KS, et al. CT of bronchial and bronchiolar diseases. Radiographics. 1994;14:991-1003.
49. Kinsella D, Sissons G, Williams MP. The radiological imaging of bronchial atresia. Br J Radiol. 1992;65:681.
50. Martinez S, Heyneman LE, McAdams HP, et al. Mucoid impactions: Finger-in-glove sign and other CT and radiographic features. Radiographics. 2008;28:1369-82.
51. Brown DE, Pittman JE, Leigh MW, et al. Early lung disease in young children with primary ciliary dyskinesia. Pediatr Pulmonol. 2008;43:514-6.
52. Agarwal R, Khan A, Garg M, et al. Pictorial essay: Allergic bronchopulmonary aspergillosis. Indian J Radiol Imaging. 2011;21:242-52.
53. Jana M, Bhalla AS. Small Airway Disease: Imaging. In: Bhalla AS, Jana M. Imaging of interstitial lung diseases, 1st edition. Jaypee Brothers Medical Publishers (P) Ltd., 2017. pp. 331-41.
54. Pipavath SJ, Lynch DA, Cool C, et al. Radiologic and pathologic features of bronchiolitis. Am J Roentgenol. 2005;185(2):354-63 [review].
55. Pipavath SJ, Stern EJ. Imaging of Small Airway Disease (SAD) Radiol. Clin N Am. 2009;47(2):307-16.
56. Hansell DM, Nicholson AG. Smoking-related diffuse parenchymal lung disease: HRCT-pathologic correlation. Semin Respir Crit Care Med. 2003;24(4):377-92.
57. Myers JL, Colby TV. Pathologic manifestations of bronchiolitis, constrictive bronchiolitis, cryptogenic organizing pneumonia and diffuse panbronchiolitis. Clin Chest Med. 1993;14:611-22.
58. Edwards RM, Kisska G, Schmidt R, et al. Imaging of small airways and emphysema. Clin Chest Med. 2015;36: 335-47.
59. Burgel PR, et al. Small airway diseases, excluding asthma and COPD: an overview. Eur Respir Rev. 2013;22:128, 131-47.
60. Park CS, et al. Airway obstruction in asthmatic and healthy individuals: Inspiratory and expiratory thin-section CT findings. Radiology. 1997;203:361-7.
61. Zaporozhan JL, Kauczor HU. Imaging of Airways: Chronic Obstructive Pulmonary Disease. Radiol Clin N Am. 2009;47(2):331-42.

CHAPTER 170

Intensive Care Chest Radiology

Akshay Kumar Saxena, Kushaljit Singh Sodhi, Nidhi Prabhakar

INTRODUCTION

Imaging of chest in patients of intensive care unit (ICU) is a challenging job. Rapid and accurate interpretation of radiological investigations in these patients can make significant contribution in management of these critically sick patients. Since most of these patients are on life support devices, portable chest radiography is the most commonly performed radiological investigation. This is supplemented by portable ultrasonography and computed tomography (CT) in selected patients.

CHEST RADIOGRAPH

A chest radiograph is the most commonly requested radiology examination in the ICU. It is an essential supplement to physical examination, which is difficult to properly perform in an ICU setting, as most of these patients are uncooperative, unconscious and intubated.[1] Chest radiography is an economically viable investigation that can be performed rapidly with ease at the bedside of a critically ill patient. It can help in the diagnosis of a number of cardiopulmonary diseases. It is also used to evaluate monitoring and support devices.[2] Usually, upright posteroanterior and lateral views are performed for chest radiography. However, in the ICU, an antero-posterior (AP) radiograph is most commonly performed using a portable X-ray unit (portable radiography). The American College of Radiology has described a number of recommendations for the use of portable radiography in an ICU. The indications described by them include placement of enteric tubes, endotracheal tubes, central venous catheter, Swan-Ganz catheter, any other life support device or to evaluate any change in clinical status of the patient. Routine daily radiograph is not advised.[3]

Interpretation of chest radiographs for patients admitted in the ICU is a difficult task as the X-ray is not usually of optimum quality. The portable radiograph is taken with the patient usually in supine position and there is inconsistency in the technique from day to day. Patients are often critically ill and are monitored and supported by various medical devices which makes it still more difficult to obtain a good quality chest radiograph. Digital radiography in place of conventional portable chest radiography has gained acceptance in most centers because of consistent film quality and wide latitude of exposure possible with this technique which decreases the need for repeat examinations.

ULTRASOUND

While portable radiography is the mainstay of imaging for ICU patients, other modalities have started making an impact in management of these patients. Rapid strides in technology have now made available good quality portable color Doppler machines. Bedside sonography and color Doppler are now being increasingly used as imaging supplements for ICU patients. The indications may be broadly categorized as diagnostic thoracic, diagnostic non-thoracic, echocardiography and interventional procedures including vascular catheterization.[4-8] The diagnostic performance of sonography is seen to approach that of CT and exceed chest radiography especially for indications such as pneumothorax, qualitative reporting of pleural fluids and demonstration of consolidation. Quantitative reporting of pleural fluids as well as evaluation of the causes of septal edema is also possible with sonography, however these need more collaborative research for optimization.[9]

COMPUTED TOMOGRAPHY

While computed tomography (CT) scan is known to provide superior diagnostic information for chest diseases, its use for patients admitted in ICU has remained limited. This is because the patients admitted in ICU are dependent on life support devices and their transportation to CT scan room is hazardous. However, recent studies unequivocally reveal the potential of CT scan in providing superior diagnostic information and having impact on patient management. CT scan has been shown to change the therapeutic decision of patients in more than half of the cases. CT scan is also invaluable in rapid assessment of cerebral complications in the ICU patients.[10,11] Role of CT scan in imaging patients of pulmonary thromboembolism is discussed in details elsewhere in this book.

IMAGING OF CARDIOPULMONARY COMPLICATIONS IN ICU PATIENTS

Common cardiopulmonary complications, which can be visualized on imaging in patients of ICU, are atelectasis, aspiration, pneumonia, hydrostatic pulmonary edema, adult respiratory distress syndrome (ARDS) and barotrauma. By careful attention to the imaging pattern, the timing of the changes and the clinical setting, these entities may be correctly diagnosed.

Atelectasis

The most common cause of pulmonary opacities in the ICU is atelectasis. Atelectasis is frequently seen in postoperative and intubated patients. It often appears quickly and changes quickly. If unresolved in several days, secondary infection should be suspected. The most common locations of atelectasis are the left lower lobe, right lower lobe and right upper lobe. It is usually subsegmental. Atelectasis is classified as obstructive, cicatricial, compressive or adhesive. Obstructive atelectasis, which occurs due to impaired mucociliary clearance, retained secretions and altered consciousness, is the most commonly seen type of atelectasis in an ICU setting. If only the distal airways are blocked, peripheral areas of atelectasis are seen with crowding of bronchi and air bronchograms. However, if larger airways are obstructed, air bronchograms may not be visualized. A common cause of large airway obstruction leading to acute lung collapse is mucus impaction **(Figs. 1A and B)**. If acute lobar collapse is seen without an air bronchogram within the atelectatic area, mucoid impaction is usually the cause. This predicts a favorable response after bronchoscopy. Compressive atelectasis is caused due to mass effect on lungs, pleural fluid being the most common cause. Cicatricial atelectasis occurs secondary to lung fibrosis. Adhesive atelectasis is seen in premature neonates, due to inadequate production of surfactant. On CT, atelectasis is seen as areas of collapse with evidence of volume loss, like crowding of airways and vessels. Lung atelectasis shows higher attenuation on postcontrast CT, as compared to areas of consolidation due to pneumonia. This can help in differentiating the two entities.[2]

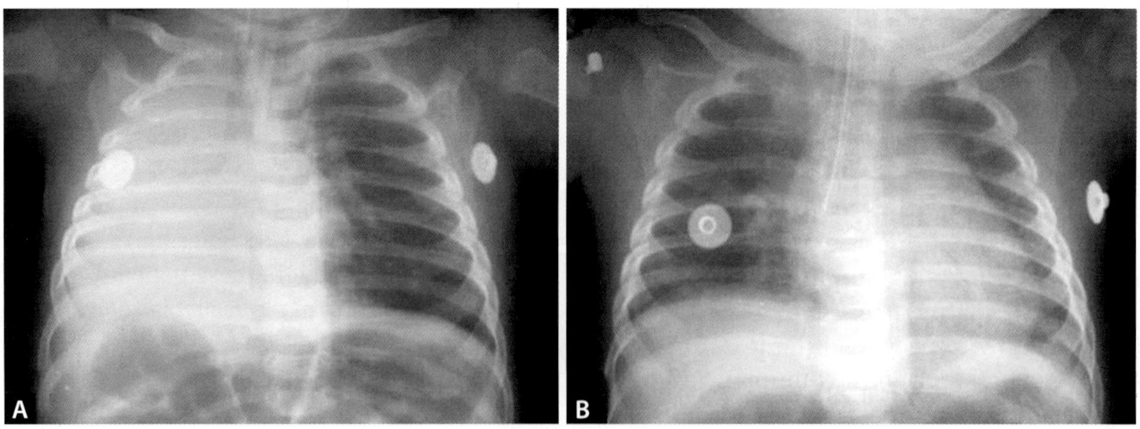

Figs. 1A and B: Atelectasis: (A) Chest radiograph of a child on mechanical ventilation reveals complete collapse of right lung; (B) Suction via the endotracheal tube followed by chest radiograph after few hours reveals re-expansion of the right lung.

Aspiration Pneumonitis

A depressed state of consciousness and a nasogastric tube, which disrupts the esophagogastric sphincter are the most frequent predisposing factors to aspiration pneumonia in an ICU patient. Aspiration can occur in spite of inflated cuff of endotracheal tube and has varying clinical presentation. Mild cases may not be clinically apparent while severe cases may cause respiratory distress. Aspirated contents may cause obstruction of airway, chemical pneumonitis or infective pneumonia.[12]

Chest radiography often shows patchy ground-glass or nodular opacities with areas of consolidation, in the dependent parts of the lungs (posterior segments of the upper lobes, and the superior, posterior basal segments of lower lobes).[2] These changes often occur within a few hours after aspiration and progress in the next 24–48 hours after which they regress. Persistence of opacities beyond this time is suggestive of aspiration pneumonia **(Fig. 2)**. On CT, patchy ground-glass opacities (GGOs), nodules and areas of consolidation in the dependent parts of lung are seen in cases of aspiration pneumonitis. *Tree-in-bud* pattern in dependent regions on CT scan is highly suggestive of aspiration.[12]

Pneumonia

Pulmonary infection is a major cause of morbidity and mortality in the ICU. Colonization of the upper airway is almost universal with prolonged hospitalization. The respirators and endotracheal tubes may act as a source and distributor of infected material. Aspiration is another risk factor for patients developing pneumonia.[12] This diagnosis is made when there is combination of fever, leukocytosis and sputum production, which is rich in white cell count and bacteria. Mixed anaerobic bacteria are the most common cause of pneumonia in the ICU. However, in the ventilated patients, aerobic gram-negative bacteria are also an important cause. Pneumonia is seen as areas of focal or multifocal consolidation on chest radiography and CT **(Figs. 3A and B)**. The infiltrates usually progress over several days, but their radiographic appearance is seldom as rapid as in atelectasis, aspiration or pulmonary edema.[2] Air bronchogram is usually seen. Lung infection

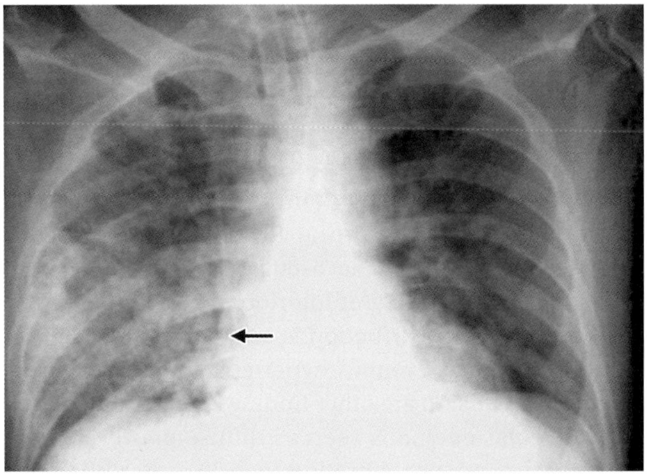

Fig. 2: Aspiration pneumonia: Chest radiograph showing patchy alveolar opacities predominantly involving the right lower zone (arrow).

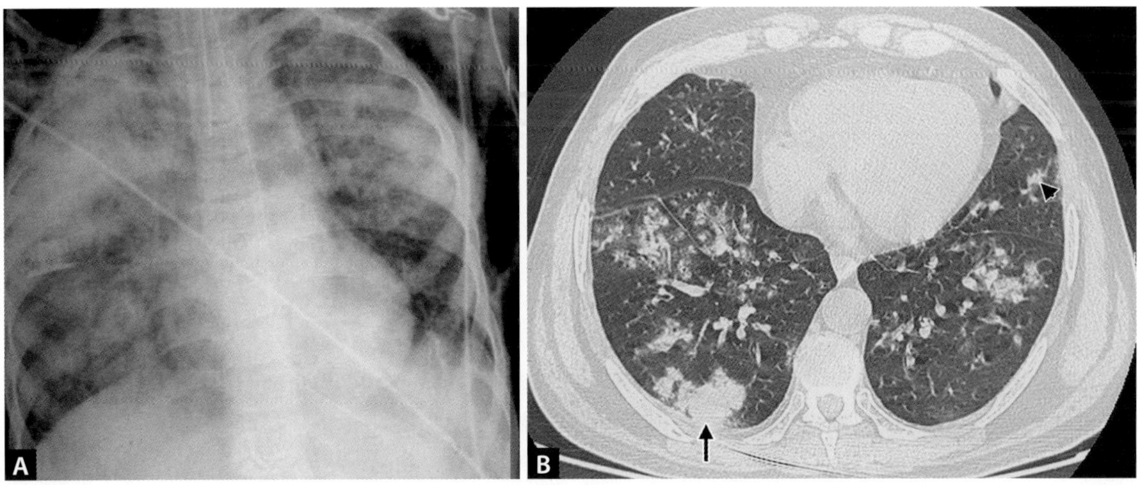

Figs. 3A and B: Pneumonia: (A) Chest radiograph in a 12-year-old male child shows patches of consolidation in both lungs suggestive of pneumonia. The patient was a diagnosed case of Bruton's disease; (B) CT chest in a 50-year old male patient shows multiple nodules (arrowhead) and areas of consolidation (arrow) in bilateral lungs suggestive of pneumonia.

secondary to septicemia may appear as nodules (which are peripheral and may be cavitatory) or wedge-shaped peripheral lesions on imaging.

Hydrostatic Pulmonary Edema

Hydrostatic pulmonary edema in an ICU patient may be due to various etiologies, which include renal failure, cardiac failure and overhydration.[12] The progression is often rapid and the response to therapy is equally rapid. The earliest change is congestion of vessels due to an increase in capillary hydrostatic pressure. As the pressure rises, lymphatics get congested and fluid gets accumulated in the interstitium around vessels and airways. This mechanism initially protects the lung against alveolar edema, which is caused due to leakage of fluid in alveoli. These sequences of changes can be appreciated on chest radiography. The first phase is 'redistribution' that is characterized by distension of upper lobar pulmonary veins. Subsequently, prominence of hila and loss of their definition is seen, followed by the appearance of septal lines (Kerley A and B) in lower lobes. Peribronchovascular thickening with hazy margins and thickening of interlobar fissures is seen in the later stage. Redistribution is only seen when there is chronic pulmonary venous hypertension. Cardiomegaly and pleural effusion are other findings seen on imaging.[13] Early alveolar edema is seen as diffuse poorly defined ground-glass opacities predominantly in perihilar and lower regions. This can progress to air space consolidation.

The diagnosis and management of hydrostatic pulmonary edema is commonly based on radiographic findings in appropriate clinical settings. However, recognizing the appearance of hydrostatic pulmonary edema on CT is also important, as edema may be seen on Chest CT done for other indications.[14] The HRCT findings include GGOs, smooth interlobular septal thickening, consolidation, increased vascular diameter, peribronchovascular thickening and pleural fluid **(Figs. 4A and B)**. The distribution of these findings is usually central and gravitational. In patients with an underlying disease such as emphysema, pulmonary edema can have atypical appearance and can mimic aspiration pneumonitis or pneumonia. Mitral regurgitation patients may have asymmetric pulmonary edema localized to right upper lobe.[2]

Noncardiogenic Pulmonary Edema

Noncardiogenic pulmonary edema is also called increased permeability edema. It is difficult to differentiate radiologically from the hydrostatic pulmonary edema and the two conditions may sometimes co-exist. The etiology of noncardiogenic pulmonary edema is diverse and includes thoracic (e.g. pneumonia, pulmonary contusion, aspiration, etc.) as well as extrathoracic pathologies (e.g. sepsis, shock, systemic inflammatory response syndrome, extra thoracic trauma, drug toxicity, etc.). Pathologically, there is diffuse alveolar damage secondary to the injury to alveolar capillaries and epithelium. The severe form of diffuse alveolar damage is ARDS. The 'Berlin definition' as created by ARDS definition task force, defined ARDS as respiratory failure (1) occurring within 1 week of a known clinical insult or new or worsening symptoms,

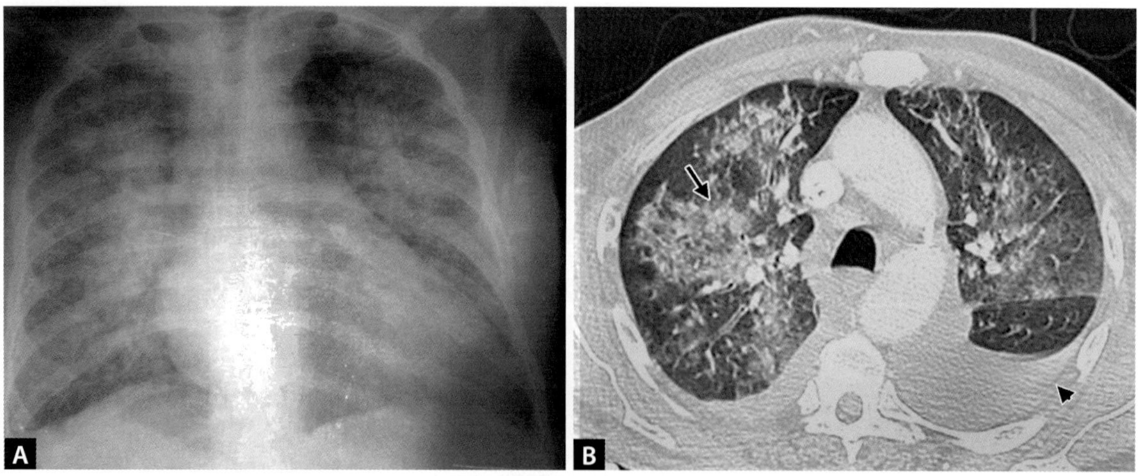

Figs. 4A and B: Hydrostatic pulmonary edema: (A) Chest radiograph of a postrenal transplant patient shows cardiomegaly and bilateral pulmonary consolidation with predominantly perihilar distribution; (B) CT chest in another chronic renal failure patient shows areas of ground-glass opacities and consolidation, predominantly in perihilar location (arrow) involving bilateral lungs suggestive of pulmonary edema. In addition, bilateral pleural effusion is seen (arrowhead).

(2) with opacities involving two or more quadrants on imaging (frontal radiograph or CT), (3) not attributable to cardiac failure or volume overload and (4) having arterial partial pressure of oxygen to fraction of inspired oxygen (Pa_2/ FiO_2) ratio of less than 300 mm Hg. These levels were further classified as mild ARDS (200–300 mm Hg), moderate ARDS (100–200 mm Hg) or severe ARDS (less than 100 mm Hg). The term 'acute lung injury' is now no longer used and has been replaced by 'mild ARDS'.[15,16]

The course of ARDS is a continuum of findings, which is frequently classified into proliferative, exudative and fibrotic phases. The radiographic findings frequently lag behind the onset of respiratory failure and chest radiograph may not be helpful in first few hours of illness. Pulmonary opacities coalesce to cause diffuse pulmonary opacification on radiograph or CT **(Figs. 5A and B)**. These opacities can last for a variable duration (days to months), which depends on the cause, severity, treatment and presence of associated complications such as aspiration and/or pneumonia. Chest radiograph findings may resemble hydrostatic pulmonary edema, however, patchy, peripheral distribution is more common in noncardiogenic than cardiogenic pulmonary edema. Radiographic changes are also slow in ARDS. The heart size is frequently normal in ARDS as compared to hydrostatic pulmonary edema. When ARDS is caused by extrathoracic causes, more symmetric pattern of GGOs is predominant and when ARDS is secondary to thoracic diseases, asymmetric GGOs and consolidation patches predominant. The prevalence of fibrotic changes early in the disease predict bad prognosis. The most common finding in survivors of ARDS is anterior fibrotic opacities.[17]

Pulmonary Embolism

In the critically-ill patient, there are numerous risk factors such as cardiac disease, obstructive airway disease, indwelling catheters, prolonged bed-rest, etc. which predispose the patient to pulmonary embolism. The diagnosis of pulmonary embolism can be very difficult when multiple factors can lead to respiratory distress. The most common chest radiographic findings are normal radiograph, pleural effusion, elevated hemidiaphragm, cardiac enlargement, pulmonary artery enlargement, peripheral consolidation and peripheral atelectasis **(Figs. 6A and B)**.[18] These radiographic signs are non-specific. In a patient with sudden onset respiratory distress, a normal radiograph is usually suggestive of pulmonary embolism. Ventilation perfusion scanning is of limited value in a critically ill patient as other accompanying conditions such as pneumonia, obstructive airways disease and pulmonary edema make definitive interpretation difficult in a majority of patients. Multidetector CT pulmonary angiography is emerging as imaging modality of choice for radiological evaluation of patients of pulmonary embolism. This topic is discussed in details elsewhere in this book.

Barotrauma

The term barotrauma refers to the deleterious effects of mechanical ventilation in the lungs. The most commonly recognized manifestation of barotrauma is the occurrence of extra-alveolar air collection due to airleak phenomenon. The overall incidence of barotrauma is approximately 3% in mechanically ventilated patients. Incidence varies depending on the presence of underlying lung diseases.[19]

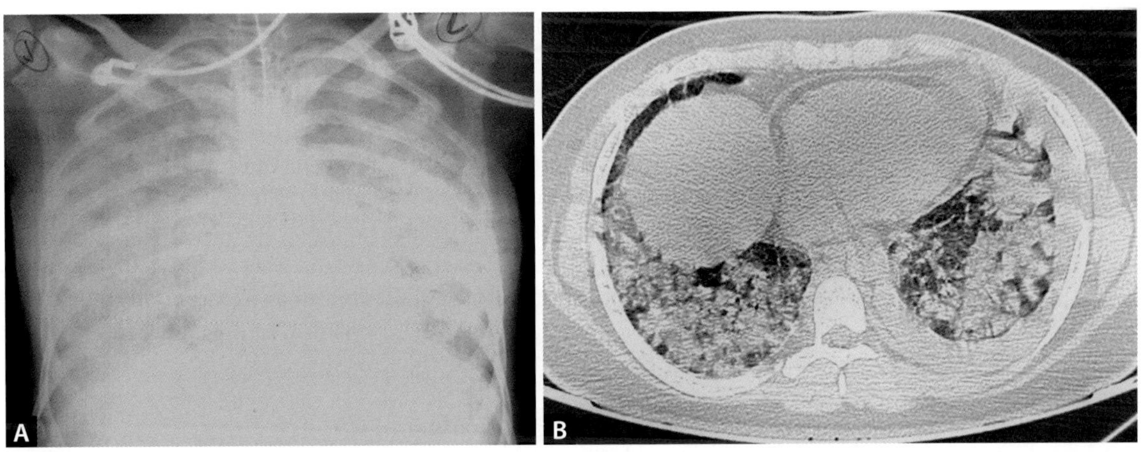

Figs. 5A and B: Acute respiratory distress syndrome: (A) Chest radiograph of a 7-year-old child shows bilateral diffuse airspace consolidation; (B) CT chest of a 25-year-old male, admitted in ICU and in sepsis, shows multiple areas of consolidation in bilateral lungs, predominant in the lower lobes due to ARDS. In addition, mild left empyema was noted.

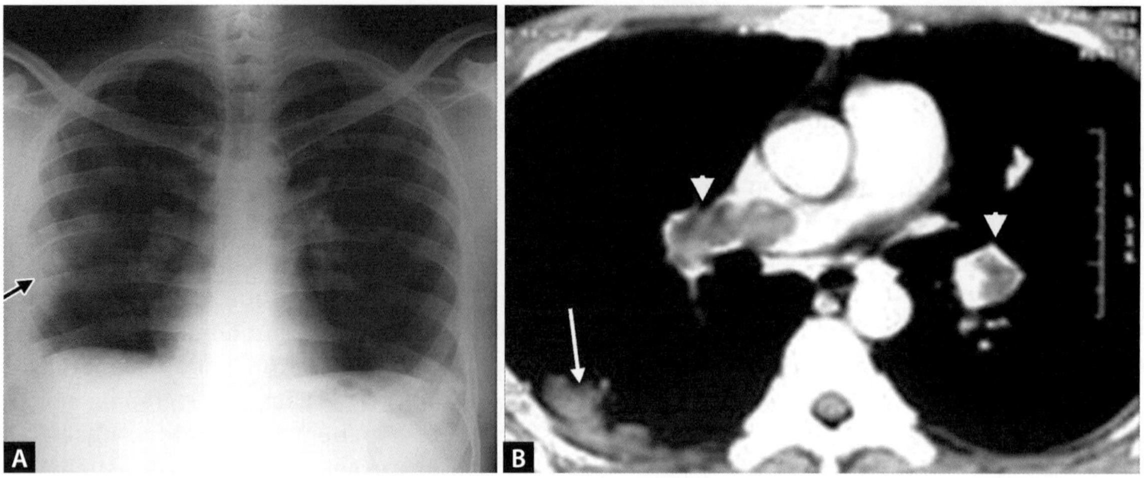

Figs. 6A and B: Pulmonary thromboembolism: (A) Chest radiograph of a 32-year-old male patient presenting with sudden onset shortness of breath. The right mid and lower zones show an ill-defined peripheral opacity (black arrow); (B) CT pulmonary angiography in the same patient shows thrombi in right and left main pulmonary arteries (white arrowheads). Infarction is seen in right lower lobe (arrow).

Pulmonary Interstitial Emphysema

Pulmonary interstitial emphysema (PIE) occurs due to increased alveolar pressure causing rupture of alveolar wall followed by dissection of air along the pulmonary interstitium upto the hilum (Macklin effect).[20] The air can subsequently reach mediastinum and pleural cavity to cause pneumomediastinum and pneumothorax. Radiographic findings of PIE include multiple lung cysts of variable size, lucent lines, which are directed toward the hilum, air around large vessels, subpleural air, intraseptal air and subpleural cysts. However, these findings may be subtle and may not be detected on radiography in the absence of opacified lung parenchyma. On CT, perivascular and peribronchial cysts or air within interlobular septa are seen. The 'line and dot' sign has been described on CT, which is due to air in the interstitium. The bronchovascular bundles are seen as 'lines or dots' (depending on their orientation with respect to plane of the CT) within the air lucencies **(Figs. 7A and B)**.[21]

Pneumomediastinum

Pneumomediastinum signifies presence of extraluminal air in the mediastinum. When occurring due to barotrauma, it may be accompanied by PIE. The radiographic findings in pneumomediastinum depend on the visualization of normal anatomic structures, outlined by the air in the mediastinum. These signs include the thymic sail sign, "ring around the artery" sign, double bronchial wall sign, continuous diaphragm sign, tubular artery sign and extrapleural sign. It is sometimes difficult to distinguish pneumomediastinum from pneumopericardium and medial pneumothorax. False positive diagnosis of pneumomediastinum may be made due to Mach band effect, which manifests as apparent radiolucency adjacent to convex border structures. In addition, normal anatomic structures (e.g. anterior junction line, major fissure) may occasionally mimic pneumomediastinum.[22,23]

Pneumothorax

Pneumothorax resulting from barotrauma is the most common life-threatening emergency in patients supported by mechanical ventilation. It may or may not always be preceded by pneumomediastinum. The diagnosis of pneumothorax, although of great clinical significance, is many times missed on the X-rays. This is because apicolateral accumulation of air is rather uncommon in the supine films.[24] Air preferentially accumulates in the anteromedial and subpulmonic recesses in the supine position.[24] The anteromedial air collection may cause sharp outline of contiguous mediastinal structures. Subpulmonic pneumothorax presents as a relatively lucent area in the left or right upper abdominal quadrant. Sometimes, the only radiographic sign of subpulmonic pneumothorax is deep lateral costophrenic angle (deep sulcus sign).[25] The air can also collect in apicolateral, posteromedial, inter lobar fissures and inferior pulmonary ligament.[24] The position of air collection is also modified by underlying lung diseases.

Tension Pneumothorax

Tension pneumothorax develops when one-way valve is formed between the lung and pleural cavity. This leads to an increase in intrathoracic pressure, due to accumulation

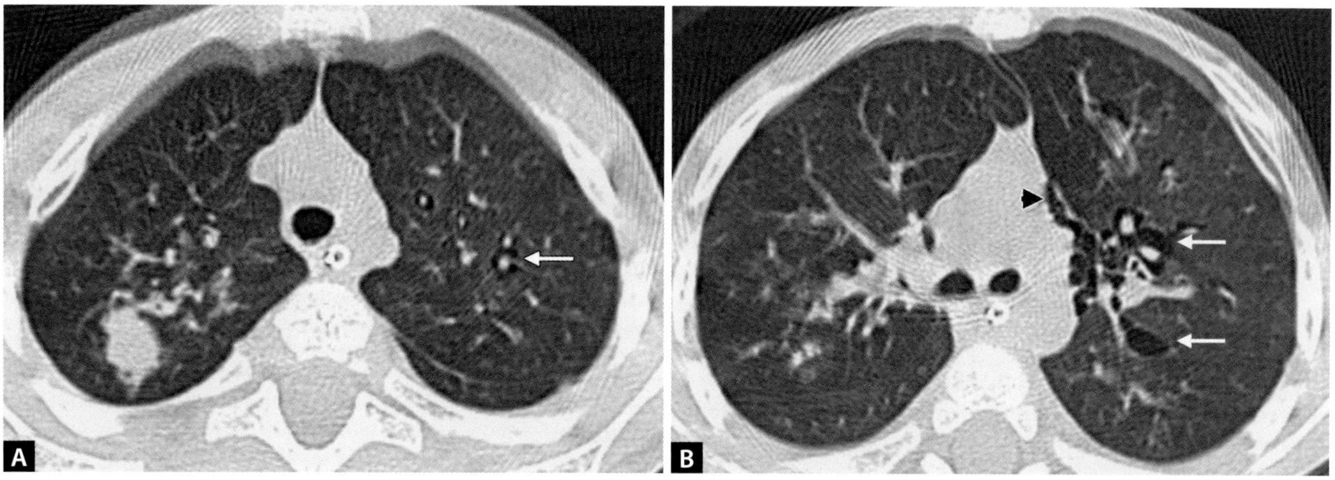

Figs. 7A and B: Pulmonary interstitial emphysema: (A and B) CT chest of a 7-month-old child showing air-filled cystic structures in pulmonary interstitium (arrows). The pulmonary vessels appear as line and dot-like structures within the interstitial air. These findings are suggestive of pulmonary interstitial emphysema. Pneumomediastinum (arrowhead) is also seen. In addition, few nodules and consolidation areas are seen in the right lung.

of air in the pleural cavity, during each respiratory cycle. Rapid progressive collapse of the ipsilateral lung and contralateral shift of mediastinum occurs. Venous return is obstructed, causing cardiac arrest.[26] Characteristic radiological features include flattening or inversion of dome of diaphragm and contralateral mediastinal shift **(Fig. 8)**.[12] Loculated tension pneumothorax is a complication of respiratory therapy in ARDS patients, in which there is accumulation of air, usually in an inferior subpulmonic or paracardiac location. This may occur even if there is a functioning ipsilateral chest tube. The only radiographic evidences of loculated tension pneumothorax may be subtle degree of mediastinal shift, slight flattening of the cardiac border and ipsilateral change of contour or depression of the diaphragm, which may be apparent only after comparison with previous radiographs. This loculated tension pneumothorax may lead to severe pulmonary and cardiovascular compromise even from a small volume of pleural air and rapid drainage is required. On few occasions, the diagnosis of tension pneumothorax in ARDS patient may only be apparent on CT scan.[27]

Subcutaneous Emphysema

From the mediastinum, air can travel along fascial planes into the subcutaneous tissues of the neck and chest wall and abdominal wall. The presence of air in the chest wall in patients receiving mechanical ventilation is often the first radiographic sign of barotrauma because the underlying pneumothorax may be impossible to detect in the supine portable radiograph.

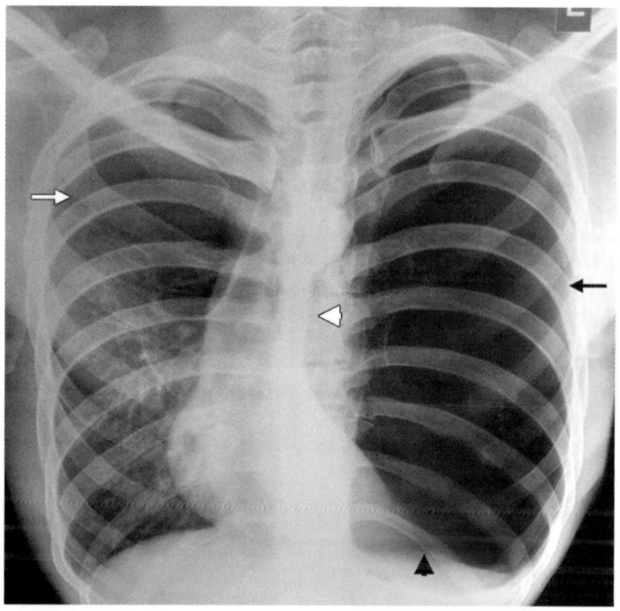

Fig. 8: Tension pneumothorax: Chest radiograph shows tension pneumothorax on the left side (black arrow) with complete collapse of left lung, flattening of the left diaphragm (black arrowhead) and contralateral mediastinal shift (white arrowhead). Large emphysematous bullae are seen on the right side in the upper zone (white arrow).

IMAGING OF SUPPORT AND MONITORING APPARATUS

A number of medical devices are used in the care of patients in the ICU. A good knowledge of their normal positions and complications is of vital importance to the radiologist and critical care physician.

Endotracheal and Tracheostomy Tube

Endotracheal intubation is done to provide short-term ventilatory support. Following endotracheal intubation, a radiograph should be obtained to ensure proper endotracheal tube placement. The ideal location for the tube tip is the mid trachea approximately 4 +/- 1 cm above the carina, in neutral head position **(Figs. 9A and B)**. Flexion or extension of the neck can alter the position by as much as 2 cm caudally or cranially respectively. Tubes placed too high may lead to inadvertent extubation or damage to the larynx. Tubes placed too deeply may irritate the carina or enter the main bronchus (usually right side).[12] Apart from localizing the endotracheal tube tip, the chest radiograph may also show contralateral atelectasis and ipsilateral hyperinflation and features of barotrauma. Following repositioning of the tube, re-expansion of the contralateral lung may take several hours to days. Endotracheal balloon cuff should not be inflated beyond the diameter of the trachea else it can lead to rupture or tracheal stenosis (as chronic complication). Esophageal intubation is usually clinically apparent, and leads to introduction of large amounts of air in gastrointestinal tract.[2]

Tracheostomy is done to provide long-term ventilation support. The tip of tracheostomy tube should be approximately at T3 level. The tube's position does not change with flexion or extension. The diameter of the tracheostomy tube should be approximately 2/3rd of tracheal diameter and the cuff should not dilate the tracheal wall. Pneumomediastinum may be noted sometimes even after uncomplicated tracheostomy tube placement.[2]

Chest Tube

Chest tubes may be malpositioned in approximately 10% of cases. Chest tube side holes are seen as interruptions of tube's radiopaque line on chest radiography. All these side holes must be located within the pleural space. If the tube is inserted into the lung parenchyma, a lung contusion may occur. This is seen as a new opacity adjacent to the chest tube on either radiography or CT. Sometimes, malpositioned chest tubes can injure the heart, major blood vessels, diaphragm or upper abdominal organs.[2] Hence, critical assessment of chest tube placement should be done to differentiate correct placement from aberrant position.

Venous Catheter

The tip of the central venous line should be within the superior vena cava, beyond the venous valves, to decrease the risk of thrombosis **(Figs. 10A and B)**. Presence of catheter tip in the lower SVC or at cavoatrial junction is associated with reduced thrombosis around the catheter.[28] However, the tip should not be within the atria to avoid arrhythmias and cardiac perforation.

Aberrant positioning of the venous catheters intra-arterially (usually subclavian artery or common carotid artery) is usually apparent because it leads to bright red oxygenated blood flowing from the catheter. However, in patients of sepsis and hypotension, this may not be so apparent. On an anteroposterior radiograph, if the venous catheter is noted above the level of clavicles, subclavian artery placement should be suspected.

Pneumothorax following subclavian vein catheterization is not uncommon because of the proximity of

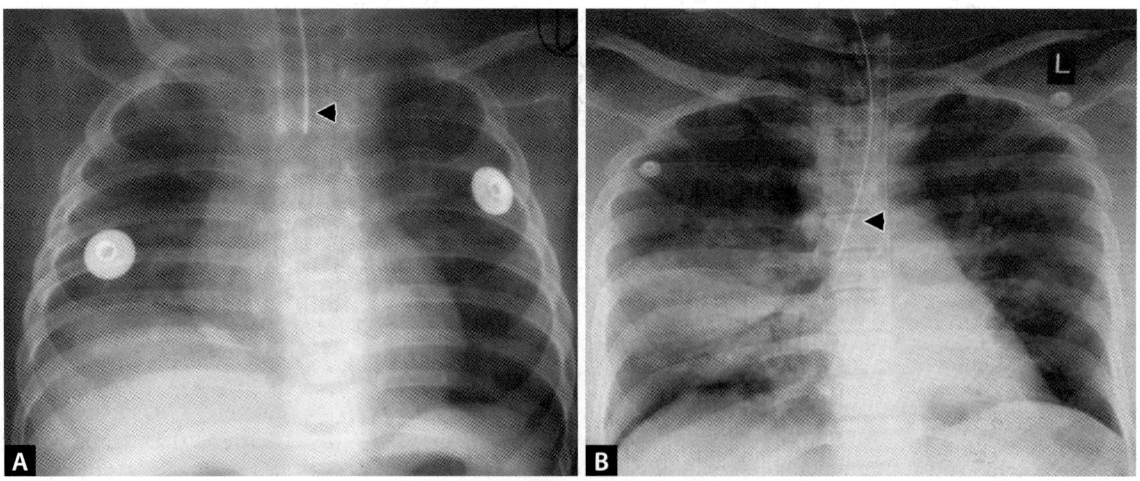

Figs. 9A and B: Endotracheal tube position: Chest radiographs showing (A) correct and (B) abnormal (right bronchial) positions of the endotracheal tube (arrowheads).

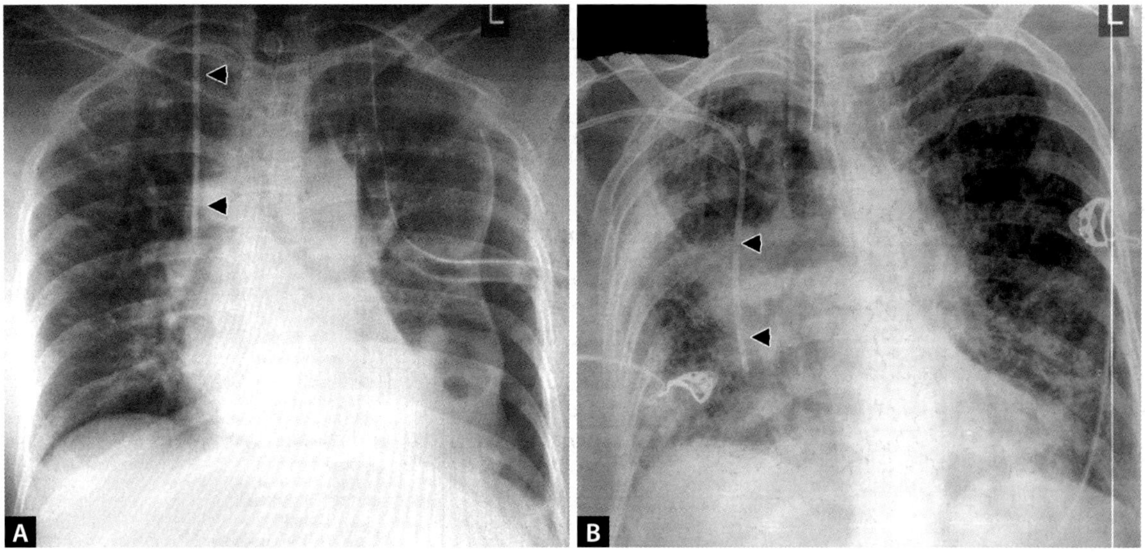

Figs. 10A and B: Central venous catheter position: Chest radiographs showing (A) correct and (B) deep positions of the venous catheters (arrowheads).

the apical pleura to the subclavian vein. Another complication is extravascular fluid collections. Widening of the mediastinum following catheterization usually indicates mediastinal fluid or blood accumulation due to venous laceration or extravenous insertion of the catheter. Rapidly developing pleural effusion may also occur due to faulty position.

Swan-Ganz Catheter

The flow directed balloon-tipped Swan-Ganz catheter measures the pulmonary capillary wedge pressure, pulmonary artery pressure and cardiac output. The Swan-Ganz catheter tip should be either within the right main pulmonary artery, left main pulmonary artery or proximal interlobar pulmonary arteries. On the radiograph, the catheter should be seen in the main pulmonary artery and not extending beyond the major hilar vessels. This is because the pulmonary arteries narrow in caliber as they extend from the hila. Thus, distal location of catheter may result in arterial occlusion and rupture. The chest X-ray should be scrutinized for any knots, which may complicate catheter removal.[12] Other complications similar to those seen in venous catheter placement such as dysrhythmias, cardiac perforation, pneumothorax or hemothorax may be also seen.

REFERENCES

1. Rubinowitz AN, Siegel MD, Tocino I. Thoracic imaging in the ICU. Crit Care Clin. 2007;23(3):539-73.
2. Bentz MR, Primack SL. Intensive care unit imaging. Clin Chest Med. 2015;36(2):219-34.
3. Suh RD, Genshaft SJ, Kirsch J, et al. ACR Appropriateness Criteria® Intensive Care Unit Patients. J Thorac Imaging. 2015;30(6):W63-5.
4. Beaulieu Y, Marik PE. Bedside ultrasonography in the ICU: part 1. Chest. 2005;128:881-95.
5. Beaulieu Y, Marik PE. Bedside ultrasonography in the ICU: part 2. Chest. 2005;128:1766-81.
6. Guillory RK, Gunter OL. Ultrasound in the surgical intensive care unit. Curr Opin Crit Care. 2008;14:415-22.
7. Lichtenstein DA. Ultrasound in the management of thoracic disease. Crit Care Med. 2007;35(Suppl):S250-61.
8. Nicolaou S, Talsky A, Khashoggi K, et al. Ultrasound-guided interventional radiology in critical care. Crit Care Med. 2007;35(Suppl):S186-97.
9. Ashton-Cleary DT. Is thoracic ultrasound a viable alternative to conventional imaging in the critical care setting? Br J Anaesth. 2013;111(2):152-60.
10. Aliaga M, Forel JM, De Bourmont S, et al. Diagnostic yield and safety of CT scans in ICU. Intensive Care Med. 2015;41(3):436-43.
11. Dorenbeck U, Bein T, Strotzer M, et al. Thoracic computed tomography in intensive care patients: evaluation of clinical usefulness. Anasthesiol Intensivmed-Not fallmed Schmerzther. 2002;37:273-9.
12. Hill JR, Horner PE, Primack SL. ICU imaging. Clin Chest Med. 2008;29:59-76.
13. Cardinale L, Priola AM, Moretti F, et al. Effectiveness of chest radiography, lung ultrasound and thoracic computed tomography in the diagnosis of congestive heart failure. World J Radiol. 2014;6(6):230-7.
14. Storto ML, Kee ST, Golden JA, et al. Hydrostatic pulmonary edema: high-resolution CT findings. Am J Roentgenol. 1995;165:817-20.

15. ARDS Definition Task Force. Acute respiratory distress syndrome: the Berlin definition. JAMA. 2012;307(23):2526-33.
16. Sweeney RM, McAuley DF. Acute respiratory distress syndrome. Lancet. 2016;388(10058):2416-30.
17. Desai SR, Wells AU, Rubens MB, et al. Acute respiratory distress syndrome: CT abnormalities at long-term follow-up. Radiology. 1999;210:29-35.
18. Elliott CG, Goldhaber SZ, Visani L, et al. Chest radiographs in acute pulmonary embolism. Results from the International Cooperative Pulmonary Embolism Registry. Chest. 2000;118(1):33-8.
19. Anzueto A, Frutos-Vivar F, Esteban A, et al. Incidence, risk factors and outcome of barotrauma in mechanically ventilated patients. Intensive Care Med. 2004;30(4):612-9.
20. Wintermark M, Schnyder P. The Macklin effect: a frequent etiology for pneumomediastinum in severe blunt chest trauma. Chest. 2001;120:543-7.
21. Donnelly LF, Lucaya J, Ozelame V, et al. CT findings and temporal course of persistent pulmonary interstitial emphysema in neonates: a multiinstitutional study. Am J Roentgenol. 2003;80(4):1129-33.
22. Zylak CM, Standen JR, Barnes GR, et al. Pneumomediastinum revisited. Radiographics. 2000;20:1043-57.
23. Bejvan SM, Godwin JD. Pneumomediastinum: old signs and new signs. Am J Roentgenol. 1996;166:1041-8.
24. Tocino IM, Miller MH, Fairfax WR. Distribution of pneumothorax in the supine and semirecumbent critically ill adult. Am J Roentgenol. 1985;144:901-5.
25. Gordon R. The deep sulcus sign. Radiology. 1980;136:25-7.
26. Watts BL, Howell MA. Tension pneumothorax: a difficult diagnosis. Emerg Med J. 2001;18(4):319-20.
27. Gobien RP, Reines HD, Schabel SI. Localized tension pneumothorax: unrecognized form of barotrauma in adult respiratory distress syndrome. Radiology. 1982;142:15-9.
28. Cadman A, Lawrance JA, Fitzsimmons L, et al. To clot or not to clot? That is the question in central venous catheters. Clin Radiol. 2004;59:349-55.

CHAPTER 171

Imaging in Thoracic Trauma

Atin Kumar, Shivanand Gamanagatti

INTRODUCTION

Thoracic injury is the third most common injury in the trauma patient after head and extremity injury. The mortality from thoracic injury with related complications ranges from 15–77% especially in the setting of multisystem trauma.[1] Thoracic injuries can potentially affect airway and breathing which are the two most important components responsible for early mortality in patients with torso trauma. The mode of injury can be blunt trauma or penetrating trauma. The chest wall remains intact in blunt trauma whereas its integrity is breached in penetrating trauma resulting in communication between the external environment and internal contents of the thorax, even if only transiently. Blunt trauma due to motor vehicle collision is the most common cause.

ROLE OF IMAGING

Imaging plays an important role in the diagnosis of the injuries due to thoracic trauma. After ensuring the hemodynamic stability of the patient, chest radiograph is obtained as the initial imaging evaluation during the primary survey.

The Chest Radiograph

It is usually obtained in the supine anteroposterior projection. It is a useful adjunct to rule out immediate life-threatening conditions like large pneumothorax, massive hemothorax, and hemomediastinum (mediastinal widening). Besides, it is also useful to detect lung injuries, osseous trauma and the position of various internal catheters, lines and tubes. However, it has multiple limitations including suboptimal patient positioning, magnification and distortion of mediastinum, overlap of soft tissue and lung parenchyma, inability to detect air-fluid level in the supine position besides being less sensitive in characterizing mediastinal and lung parenchymal injuries.

Ultrasound

Ultrasound of the chest is done as an extension of the Focussed Assessment with Sonography in Trauma (eFAST). This is also done alongwith the chest radiograph during the primary survey of the patient as part of initial evaluation and resuscitation. It is used to detect hemothorax, pneumothorax and hemopericardium. Pneumothorax is diagnosed on ultrasound by detecting loss of 'lung sliding sign'. When the chest is evaluated by ultrasound in a healthy patient, the parietal and visceral pleura are seen opposed to each other and appear as a bright echogenic line. This is the first air interface and acts as a barrier for the ultrasound beam. Beyond this line, the ultrasound beam is not able to penetrate and gets reflected back. Hence only reverberation artefacts and comet tail artefacts are seen deeper to this interface. With respiratory movements, the visceral pleura slides in a craniocaudal direction in relation to the parietal pleura. The ultrasound detects it as an inner bright echogenic line moving up and down. The reverberation artefacts and the comet tail artefacts also move with this line. This has been described as 'lung sliding sign'. When there is pneumothorax, the parietal and visceral pleura get separated by air. Now the ultrasound beam encounters air just after the parietal pleura and the first air interface is, therefore, the parietal pleura rather than visceral pleura. The beam is not able to penetrate beyond this and therefore the visceral pleura or the lung parenchyma which are deeper are not visualized. In this scenario, the echogenic bright line does not move with respiration as the air column in the pleural space is static. This leads to loss of 'lung sliding sign'. This is a marker of pneumothorax. It should be looked for in the most nondependent area like beneath the second intercostal space in parasternal location. The reverberation and the comet tail artefacts are also not well seen in pneumothorax.

Multidetector Computed Tomography

It is the modality of choice for detection of pulmonary, pleural, mediastinal and osseous abnormalities in the setting of thoracic trauma. However, it is done after the patient has been stablized hemodynamically. The current indications in patients of thoracic trauma include significant findings on a chest radiograph or eFAST, penetrating chest injury, suspicion of mediastinal vascular injury (aortic injury), significant osseous injuries on radiograph especially upper rib fractures or flail segments. It is also done in patients with dangerous mechanism of injury even when the chest radiograph and eFAST are normal. The CT is done as a part of torso imaging protocol combined with abdomen. At our center, we routinely do the CT chest in arterial phase to look for vascular injuries. A negative contrast CT examination virtually rules out any significant thoracic injury.

The following section describes the radiographic and CT findings of major lung parenchymal, pleural, mediastinal, diaphragmatic and chest wall injuries.

PULMONARY PARENCHYMAL INJURIES

Pulmonary Contusion

Pulmonary contusions are the most common cause of pulmonary opacifications in blunt chest trauma with a prevalence of 17–70%.[2] The causative force is direct injury to the lung parenchyma at the site of impact or in the opposite portion of the lung (contercoup injury). It represents a combination of parenchymal edema and hemorrhage secondary to alveolar membrane disruption. Patients may be asymptomatic (50%) or may have hemoptysis, fever, tachypnea, hypoxia and hypercarbia. The initial chest radiograph may be normal but the findings usually are evident within 6 hours. The contusions appears as unilateral or bilateral, ill-defined, focal or multifocal, patchy airspace opacity which is not confined by fissural boundaries (nonsegmental distribution). They are usually seen in the lung periphery adjacent to the site of lung trauma and frequently have associated bony injuries of ribs or spine except in pediatric patients where they often occur without overlying bony injuries. Lung bases are a preferred site due to increased basilar mobility. Air bronchograms are usually absent due to blood filling the airways. The maximal radiographic opacity is seen within 24–72 hours after which it gradually clears completely over the next 3–10 days.

CT is more sensitive than chest radiograph for detection of pulmonary contusions.[3] In CT also it appears as ill-defined areas of ground-glass opacity which readily cross pleural fissures **(Figs. 1A and B)**. The peripheral 1–2 mm of lung may show sparing especially in pediatric population.[4] Recently CT has been used to quantify the volume of contusion to predict the clinical course and outcome. Miller et al.[5] found contusion volume to be a direct predictor of subsequent development of acute respiratory distress syndrome (ARDS).

Pulmonary Laceration

Pulmonary laceration represents a tear of lung parenchyma secondary to penetrating injury, lung perforation from rib fractures or shearing forces caused by inertial deceleration. Clinically, it may manifest as hemoptysis. The lacerations are more common in children and young adults because of the greater flexibility of the chest wall causing higher likelihood of lung getting injured with blunt trauma.[6] They are not frequently identified on the initial chest radiograph because they get obscured by surrounding contusions. A chest CT is significantly more sensitive to detect and evaluate the extent of the pulmonary laceration than a conventional chest radiograph. Lacerations are usually ovoid. Radiologically, lacerations appear as ovoid lucent areas because of the elastic recoil of the lung with a thin rim of hyperdensity, representing a pseudomembrane. The laceration cavity may be filled with air (traumatic pneumatocele), blood (traumatic hematocele) or both with air and blood (traumatic hematopneumatocele). On CT, when air filled, they appear as localized air collections within areas of contusion **(Figs. 2A and B)**. After clearing of the adjacent lung contusion they are seen as thin-walled cysts filled with air or blood. The lacerations resolve slowly over a period of 3 weeks to a year. They may persist as a pulmonary nodule containing blood clots.

Potential complications include infection leading to pulmonary abscess, increased size of laceration or

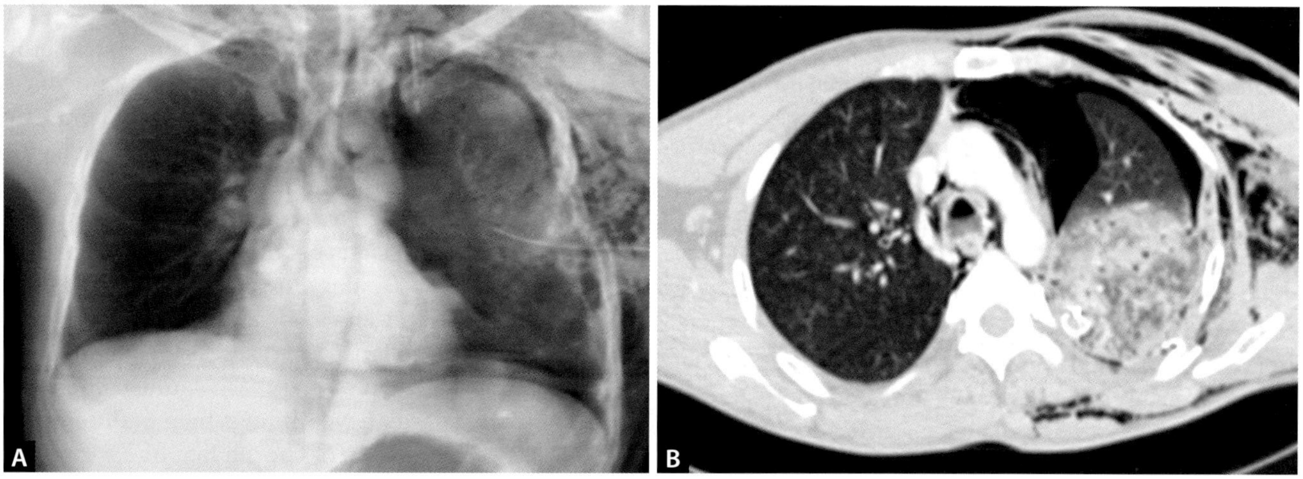

Figs. 1A and B: Pulmonary contusion: Thick coronal multiplanar reconstruction (A) and axial (B) CT images show homogeneous ground-glass density in left upper lobe of lung consistent with pulmonary contusion. Note presence of left pneumothorax and pneumomediastinum.

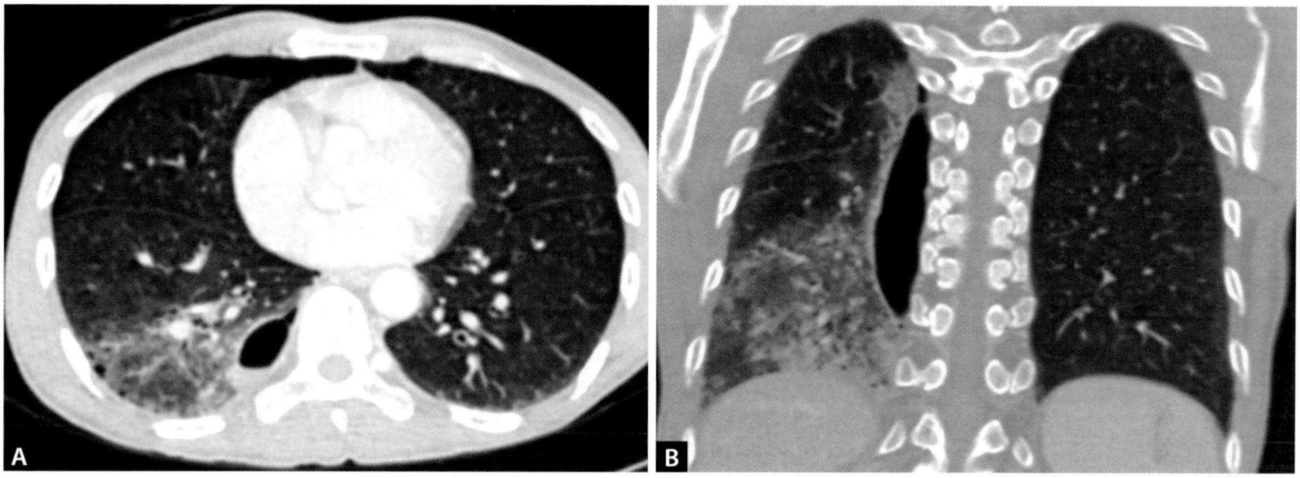

Figs. 2A and B: Pulmonary laceration: Axial (A) and coronal multiplanar reconstruction (B) CT images show an ovoid lesion with an air fluid level in paravertebral location of right lung representing laceration. Note the adjacent ground-glass density representing contusion and a small pneumothorax on right side.

development of bronchopleural fistula when the laceration communicates with a bronchus and pleural surface.[2,7] The abscess appears as thick-walled cavity with irregular inner margins and an air-fluid level. Broncholpleural fistula leads to persistent air leak which does not respond to chest tube placement. Abscess and bronchopleural fistula often require surgical or percutaneous drainage if the medical therapy fails.

Aspiration Pneumonitis

Aspiration pneumonitis is a frequent finding seen in post-traumatic patients especially those with head or maxillofacial injuries. It is important to differentiate aspiration pneumonitis from contusion because the management for the two entities is different. Aspiration produces "tree-in-bud" poorly defined centrilobular opacities usually in the dependent portions of the lung in contrast to contusions which appear as ill-defined areas of ground-glass opacity not respecting fissural boundaries with likely associated lacerations appearing as cysts **(Fig. 3)**. The CT "tree-in-bud" appearance of aspiration reflects aspirated material filling the distal small airways, whereas the confluent ground-glass opacity of contusion represents injury to the localized parenchymal area. The most frequently involved lung segments in aspiration include the superior and posterior basilar segments of the lower lobes and the posterior segments of the upper lobes. The classical "tree-in-bud" opacities are not easily visualized after few hours as they become confluent resulting in consolidative appearance except along the periphery where some isolated filled terminal bronchioles often persist.

Atelectasis

Lung collapse in the trauma patient can be separated broadly into the categories of obstructive, compressive, passive, and adhesive atelectasis. Obstructive atelectasis occurs due to obstruction of the airway by mucus plug, foreign body, blood or airway rupture. Compressive atelectasis occurs from mass effect of large contusions or traumatic lung cysts. Passive atelectasis occurs secondary to pneumothorax or hemothorax which disrupts the inherent elastic recoil properties of the lung **(Figs. 4A and B)**. It is the most common form seen in the setting of trauma. Adhesive atelectasis is caused by decreased surfactant production secondary to pulmonary contusion. Air bronchograms are often seen in all forms of atelectasis except from a central bronchial obstructive cause.

Radiologically atelectasis appears as a dense homogeneous opacity with signs of volume loss such as fissure deviation, bronchovascular crowding, ipsilateral hilar or mediastinal shift and elevated diaphragm. On contrast enhancement, the collapsed part shows greater enhancement due to crowded pulmonary vasculature compared to consolidation. These above findings help to differentiate atelectasis from contusion or consolidation.

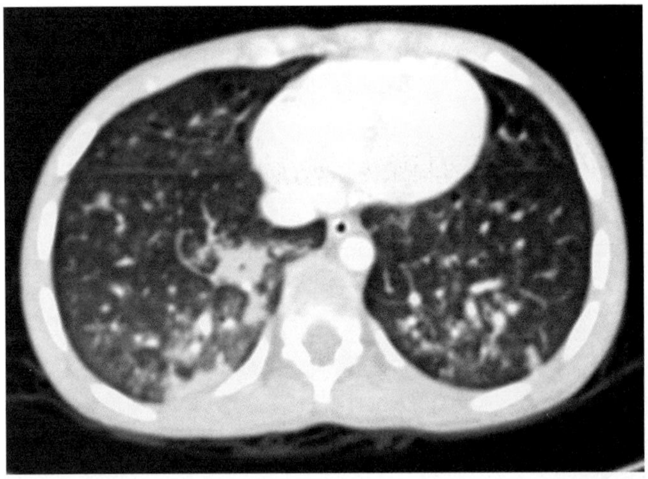

Fig. 3: Aspiration pneumonitis: Axial CT image shows poorly defined centrilobular nodules with some having 'tree-in-bud' configuration in the apical segment of right lower lobe.

Traumatic Lung Herniation

This uncommon entity occurs when a pleura covered part of lung herniates through a defect in the chest wall.[2,6] it is usually associated with a rib fracture. It is important to recognize this condition because if left untreated the herniation may increase secondary to positive pressure ventilation.

PLEURAL INJURIES

Pneumothorax

Pneumothorax is seen in 30–40% of all blunt chest trauma patients.[2] It is usually caused by alveolar rupture due to sudden increase in intrathoracic pressure associated with pleural tear. It may also be secondary to rib fracture with rib piercing the pleura and the lung. The diagnosis is first made on a chest radiograph. However, 30–50% pneumothoraces are missed on the radiographs which are usually taken in

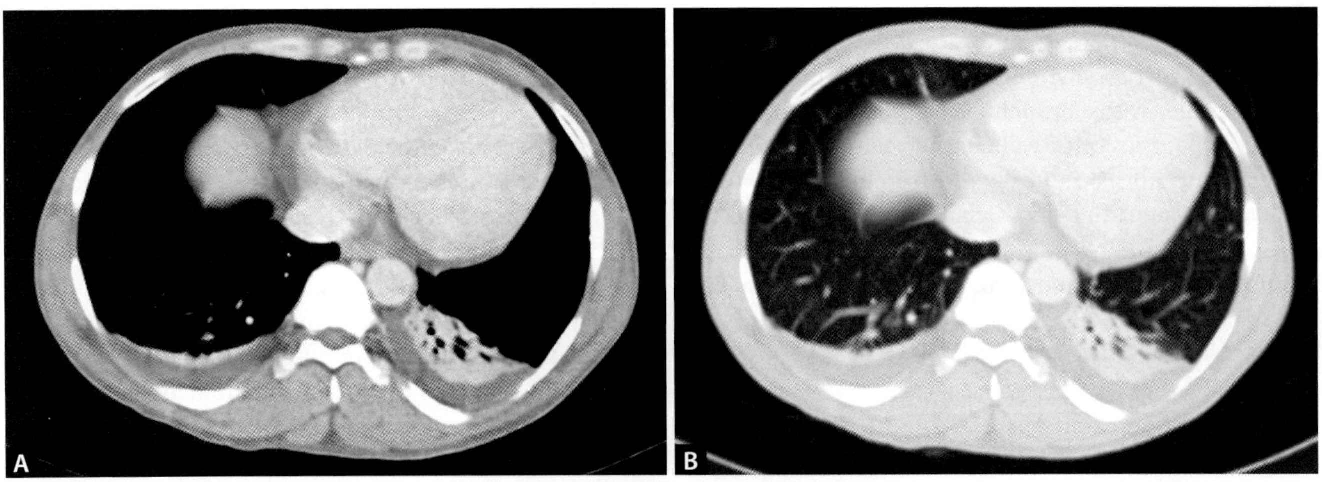

Figs. 4A and B: Atelectasis: Axial chest CT images in mediastinal (A) and lung (B) window shows passive atelectasis of left lower lobe segment with air bronchogram within secondary to pleural fluid. Also seen in right pleural fluid.

supine position in the setting of trauma.[6] These can be seen on CT and are called as 'occult pneumothoraces'. In the supine position air collects anteriorly and medially in the anterior costophrenic sulcus. The signs of pneumothorax on a supine chest radiograph are described in **Box 1**.

On an upright chest radiograph pneumothorax is seen as thin, sharply defined line that represents the visceral pleura. Lung markings are not seen beyond this line. False positive cases may be due to skin folds, large bullae, overlying tubes and catheters, bedding, scapular margin mimicking the pneumothorax. The correct diagnosis can be made by an upright expiratory chest radiograph or CT.

As described earlier in this chapter, eFAST has been increasingly used to detect pneumothorax and has shown very high sensitivity in experienced hands. Loss of 'lung sliding sign' confirms pneumothorax.

The clinical significance of a small pneumothorax which remains undetected on the chest radiograph or the eFAST is very low and does not warrant further radiographs in additional views except if the patient is on ventilation where even a small pneumothorax can quickly become life-threatening due to positive pressure ventilation.

CT is highly sensitive for detecting the pneumothoraces **(Fig. 6)**. Even evaluation of an abdominal CT often detects pneumothorax because of the tendency of the air to collect in the anterior costophrenic sulcus in the supine patient.

Chest tube placement is usually required in patients who are symptomatic, have >20% pneumothorax, in patients who are on ventilator or are likely to be put on ventilator or who have to undergo a lengthy operative procedure.

If the pneumothorax is persistent and does not completely respond to treatment including a chest tube placement, then malpositioned chest tube, tracheobronchial injury or a bronchopleural fistula needs to be ruled out on imaging.

Tension pneumothorax develops when the intrapleural pressure exceeds that of the atmosphere. This serious condition occurs when the pulmonary or bronchial injury acts as a one-way valve with air entering into pleural space without exit. This leads to pulmonary and cardiac compromise. It is a clinical diagnosis. However, there are signs to suggest tension pneumothorax on a radiograph **(Figs. 7A and B)**. These have been enumerated in **Box 2**.

If suspected, it warrants an immediate rapid decompression with a large bore needle followed by a chest tube placement.

Hemothorax

Hemothorax is seen in approximately 50% of patients of blunt thoracic trauma, especially those caused by penetrating trauma.[2] Source of bleeding is injury to pleura, lung parenchyma, mediastinum, diaphragm or with injuries to liver and spleen with associated diaphragmatic injury. Decubitus chest radiograph can detect as less

Box 1: Signs of pneumothorax on supine chest radiograph.

- Abnormally increased lucency in the lower chest or upper abdomen **(Fig. 5)**
- The 'deep sulcus' sign—abnormally wide and deep costophrenic sulcus
- The 'double diaphragm' sign—when air outlines the dome and anterior insertion of diaphragm
- Sharply outlined diaphragmatic or cardiac border
- Depression of hemidiaphragm

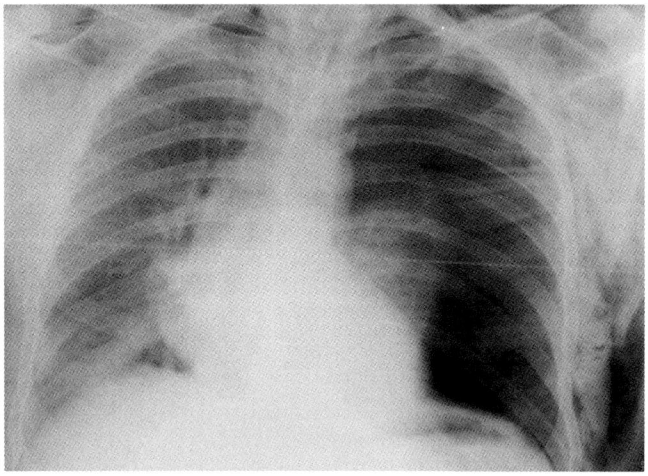

Fig. 5: Pneumothorax: Chest radiograph shows left-sided pneumothorax with clear visualization of lung border and deep sulcus sign. Also note subcutaneous emphysema along the pectoralis muscle.

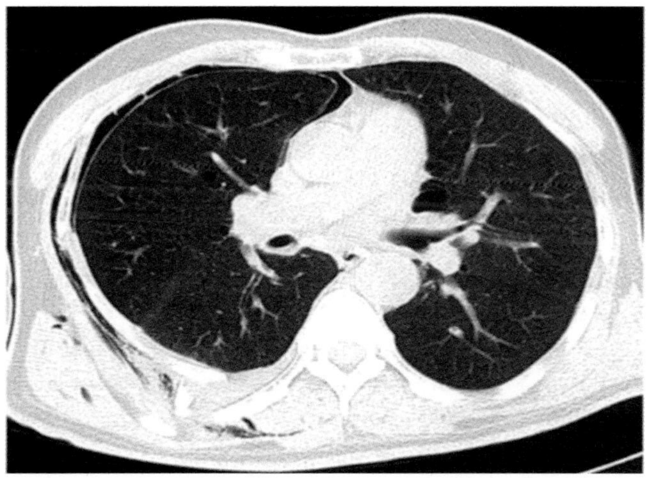

Fig. 6: Pneumothorax: Axial chest CT image shows minimal right sided pneumothorax. Rib fractures are seen posteriorly on right side.

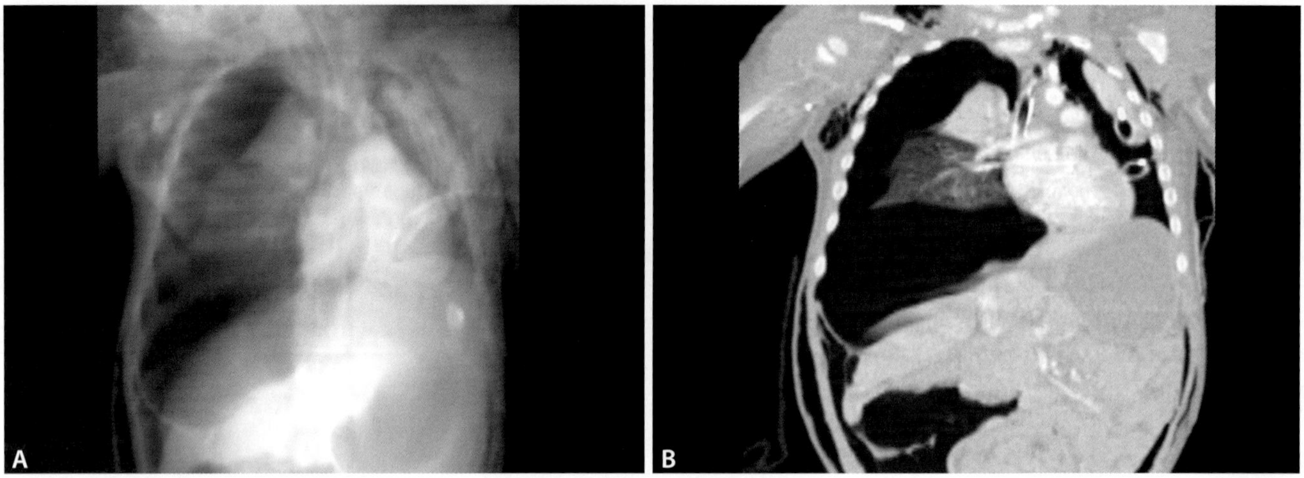

Figs. 7A and B: Tension pneumothorax: Coronal thick (A) and thin (B) multiplanar reconstruction CT images show right-sided tension pneumothorax with inversion of right diaphragm, collapsed left lung and mediastinal shift towards right.

Box 2: Signs of tension pneumothorax on chest radiograph in addition to presence of pneumothorax.

- Widening of lateral diameter of thorax
- Contralateral mediastinal shift
- Flattening or inversion of ipsilateral diaphragm
- Collapsed lung in the hilar region
- Deep sulcus sign
- Widening of intercostal spaces

as 5 mL of fluid in pleural space whereas blunting of costophrenic angle is seen on upright radiograph when approximately 200 mL of fluid accumulates in the pleural space. Progressive increase leads to the 'meniscus' sign, i.e. concave upward sloping of the fluid in the costophrenic angle **(Fig. 8)**. An air-fluid level indicates hemopneumothorax. However, in the setting of trauma since most often it is the supine radiograph which is acquired, the hemothorax is seen as increased opacity of the ipsilateral hemithorax with mediastinal shift to contralateral side **(Figs. 9A and B)**. eFAST is used to detect hemothorax with high sensitivity.

CT is highly sensitive for small amounts of pleural fluid and is also helpful in its characterization. A Hounsfield unit (HU) value of 35–70 represents hemothorax whereas HU less than 15 typically is seen in sympathetic pleural effusion which is seen in patients with hepatic, splenic or pancreatic injuries.

Other uncommon causes of pleural fluid in the setting of trauma include chylothorax which may occur secondary to injury to the thoracic duct, bilious effusion which is caused by biliopleural fistula secondary to hepatic and diaphragmatic injury and urinothorax which occurs secondary to renopleural fistula.

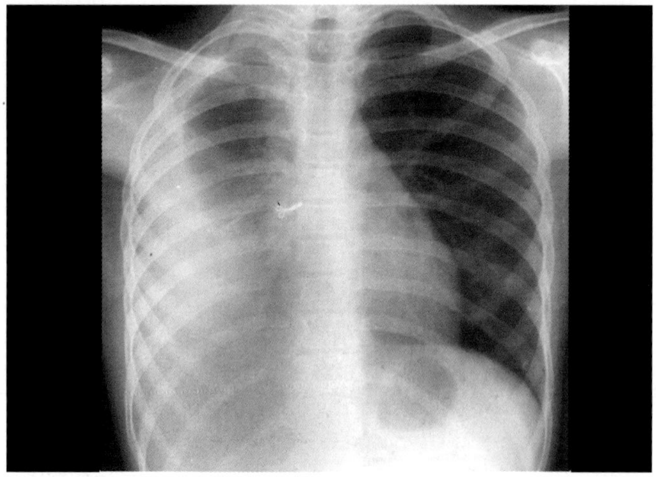

Fig. 8: Hemothorax: Chest radiograph in erect position shows right-sided pleural fluid with meniscus sign.

However, any fluid detected in the pleural cavity at presentation in a post-traumatic patient is considered as hemothorax unless proven otherwise and managed accordingly.

Source of bleeding can be venous which is usually self-limiting or arterial which usually progresses on follow-up imaging. Arterial bleed may also be seen on CT as active contrast extravasation usually from an intercostal artery.

It is also important to note the placement of the chest tube on CT. A malpositioned tube impinging into mediastinum, displaced into fissure or outside the pleura or in the lung parenchyma should be communicated to the clinician **(Fig. 10)**. A chest tube in the fissure may adequately drain a pneumothorax but is less effective for a hemothorax.

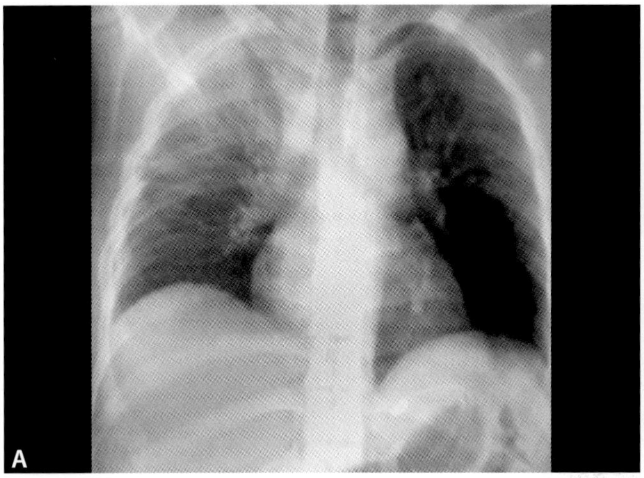

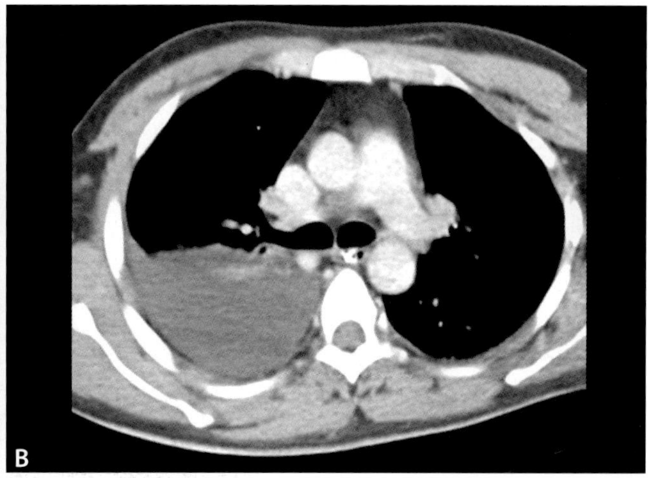

Figs. 9A and B: Hemothorax: CT thick coronal multiplanar reconstruction image (A) shows appearance of pleural fluid in supine patient appearing as diffuse haze of right hemithorax. CT axial image (B) shows moderate amount of right pleural fluid in dependent position. The fluid appears of high density signifying hemothorax.

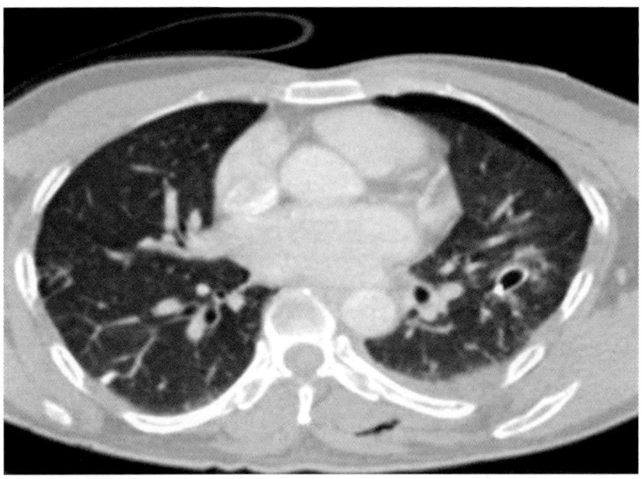

Fig. 10: Malpositioned chest tube: Axial CT image shows the tip of chest tube lying within lung parenchyma. Note small pneumothorax on left side.

INJURIES OF THE MEDIASTINUM

Tracheobronchial Injury

Tracheobronchial injuries are uncommon injuries occurring in 1–3% of blunt chest trauma and 2–9% of patients with penetrating chest trauma.[8] Penetrating injury accounts for 70% of tracheobronchial injuries and rest is from blunt trauma, iatrogenic from intubation or tracheostomy, foreign body aspiration, inhalation. Penetrating injuries most commonly involve the cervical part of trachea whereas blunt injury most commonly involves the intrathoracic part.[9] Right main stem bronchus is injured more commonly than the left side due to less protection from surrounding structures. The bronchial injuries usually occur within 2.5 cm of the carina whereas the tracheal injuries usually occur more than 2 cm above the carina.[10]

Box 3: Radiological signs of tracheobronchial injury.

- 'Double wall' sign—due to intramural air within the proximal airway[2]
- 'Fallen lung' sign—inferior falling of collapsed lung in the dependent portion due to complete disruption of the central airway
- 'Bayonet' sign—tapered air-filled bronchus[6]

Clinically, the diagnosis of tracheobronchial injury is often delayed in many patients because the airway column is maintained by the peribronchial tissue. Tracheal and proximal bronchial injuries result in pneumomediastinum whereas distal bronchial injuries result in pneumothorax.

On chest radiograph, presence of significant pneumomediastinum, persistent pneumothorax and atelectasis with increasing subcutaneous emphysema despite adequate chest tube placement should raise a doubt of airway injury. The classical radiological signs described for tracheobronchial injury are enumerated in **Box 3**.

CT with multiplanar reconstructions is superior to radiograph for detection of airway injury. The most direct sign on CT is demonstration of wall defect or deformity **(Figs. 11A and B)**. The tracheal lacerations are usually vertical and longitudinal and located at the junction of cartilaginous and membranous portion of the trachea whereas bronchial lacerations occur parallel to the cartilaginous rings. The indirect signs on imaging include an abnormal configuration of endotracheal balloon cuff, pneumomediastinum or pneumothorax and distal

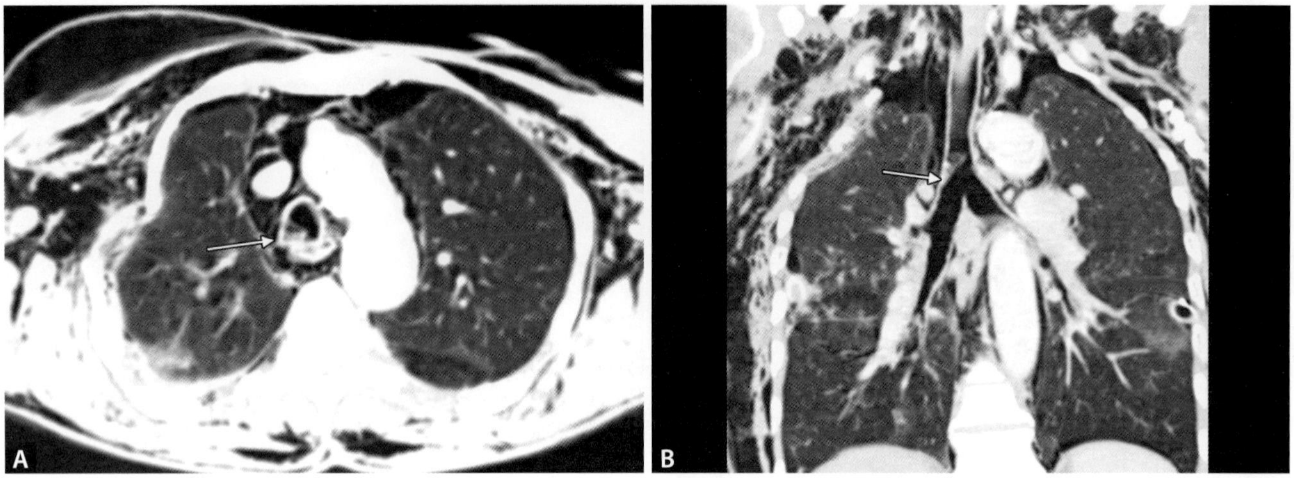

Figs. 11A and B: Tracheal injury: Axial (A) and coronal multiplanar reconstruction; (B) CT images show irregularity of right posterolateral wall of lower trachea (arrows) with formation of a luminal flap representing tracheal injury. Note the extensive pneumomediastinum and subcutaneous emphysema.

atelectasis. Multiplanar images with three-dimensional volumetric images as well as virtual bronchoscopy aid in the diagnosis of tracheobronchial injuries.

Esophageal Injury

Iatrogenic trauma due to endoscopic procedures is the most common cause for esophageal injury followed by penetrating trauma, toxic ingestions, emetic injury (Boerhaave's syndrome) and rarely blunt trauma. Early diagnosis and treatment is important as esophageal injury is associated with high morbidity and mortality. Radiological signs of esophageal perforation include cervical and mediastinal emphysema, pleural effusion, abnormal mediastinal contour due to leakage of fluid, hematoma or mediastinitis, leakage of oral contrast material into mediastinum or pleural space, and esophageal wall thickening. Mid to distal esophageal rupture causes right pleural effusion whereas lower esophageal or rupture of injury at gastroesophageal (GE) junction causes left pleural effusion. Contrast esophagography (radiographic or CT) followed by flexible esophagoscopy may be required to confirm and evaluate the site of injury **(Fig. 12)**.

Rarely, a traumatic tracheoesophageal, fistula may be formed. It is usually secondary to long-term use of an endotracheal or nasogastric tube.

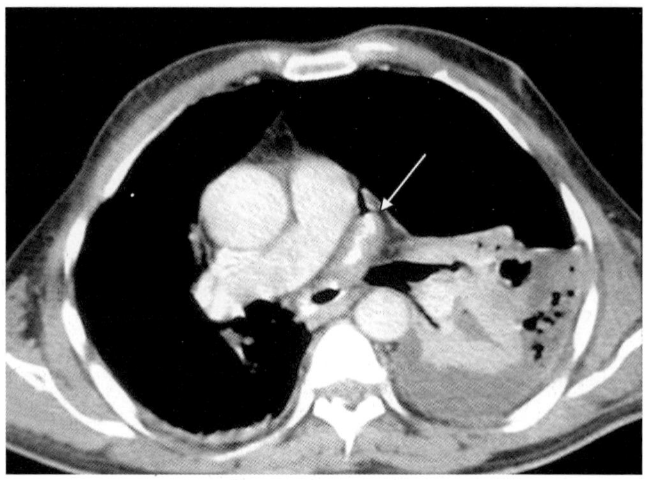

Fig. 12: Esophageal injury. Axial chest CT image shows leak of oral contrast (arrow) into mediastinum from a tear in the esophagus. Also seen is left pleural fluid with atelectasis of left lower lobe.

Pneumomediastinum

Pneumomediastinum can be due to intrathoracic and extrathoracic sources. Intrathoracic sources include injury to lung, tracheobronchial tree or esophagus whereas extrathoracic sources include head and neck and anterior retroperitoneum. The mediastinum and retroperitoneum communicate through the aortic and esophageal hiatus and at sternocostal attachments of diaphragm. Pneumomediastinum is not itself a dangerous condition but a sign of potentially more serious other injuries.

The most common cause of pneumomediastinum is air from rupture of alveoli due to increased alveolar pressure secondary to trauma. The leaked air dissects along the bronchovascular sheath and spreads into mediastinum. This phenomenon is known as 'Macklin effect'. The pneumomediastinum may increase in size with positive pressure ventilation. The CT appearance of Macklin effect is that of streaks of air along the bronchovascular bundles (similar to that seen in pulmonary interstitial emphysema) along with pneumomediastinum.[9,11]

Pneumomediastinum is visualized on anteroposterior chest radiograph as a lucency bordered by a thin white pleural line coursing along the pericardium and lateral mediastinum **(Fig. 13)**. It needs to be differentiated from pneumopericardium and pneumothorax. Pneumopericardium appears as more ovoid in shape than linear and does not extend above the level of aortic arch respecting the boundaries of the pericardium. Also the pericardium can be visualized in pneumopericardium. Medial pneumothorax may mimic pneumomediastinum but is usually associated with rib fractures and other evidences of pneumothorax. Also visualization of apparent septae favors a pneumomediastinum. Repeating the imaging in decubitus position confirms the diagnosis as the mediastinal air does not change in location whereas pneumothorax and pneumopericardium would show change in location of air. The pneumomediastinum may dissect into neck and soft tissues on increasing in size. The radiographic signs of pneumomediastinum are described in **Box 4**.

False-positive pneumomediastinum may be caused by 'Mach effect', where a thin linear lucency outlines the dense opaque cardiac silhouette. This is due to visual perception of edge enhancement and occurs at the level of the retina.

CT is most sensitive modality for detecting small amount of pneumomediastinum **(Figs. 14A and B)**.

Vascular Injury

Traumatic aortic injury is an important cause of morbidity and mortality in patients with blunt thoracic trauma. Early recognition and treatment is of utmost importance as early medical and definitive surgical treatment can improve survivability in these patients. The sites of aortic injury in descending order of frequency are—proximal

Box 4: Radiological signs of pneumomediastinum.

- 'Double bronchial wall' sign—visualization of both sides of bronchial wall due to air accumulating adjacent to bronchial wall
- 'Continuous diaphragm' sign—visualization of entire diaphragm from medial to lateral due to air trapped posterior to the pericardium at base
- 'Tubular artery' sign—air outlining the medial side of aorta with lung air outlining the lateral side
- 'Ring around the artery' sign—air outlining the pulmonary artery
- Elevation of the thymus especially in children

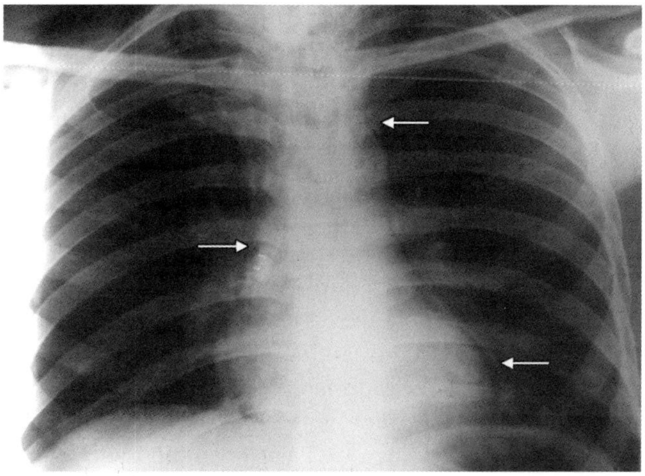

Fig. 13: Pneumomediastinum: Chest radiograph shows air outlining the mediastinum (arrows) on both sides. The air is seen above the level of aortic arch also (upper left arrow).

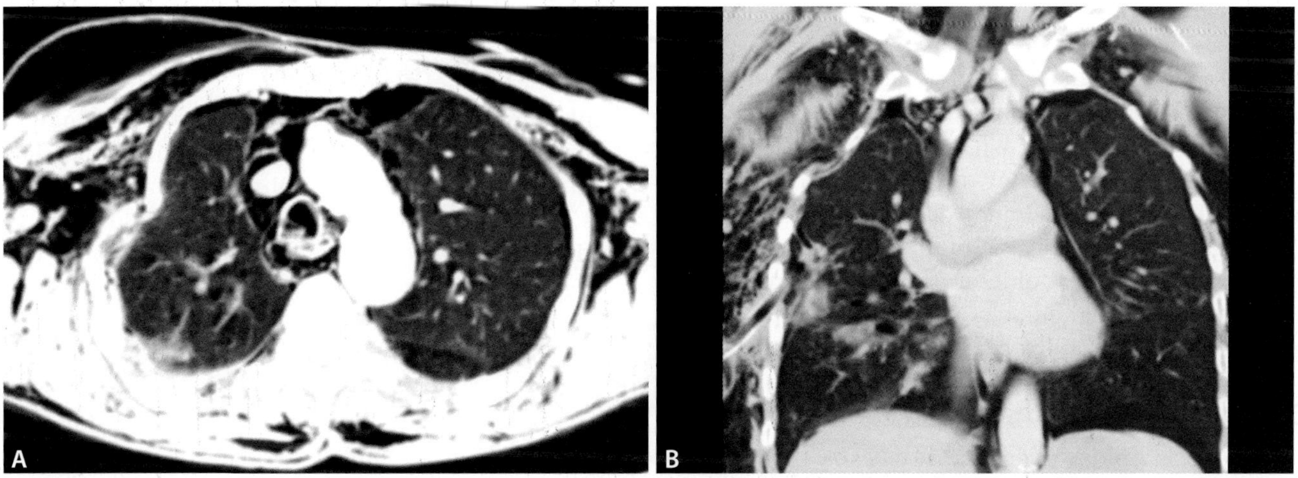

Figs. 14A and B: Pneumomediastinum: Axial (A) and coronal multiplanar reconstruction (B) CT images in a patient with tracheal injury (same patient as in Figure 11) shows extensive air in the mediastinum. The coronal image (B) shows the air to be present above the level of aortic arch and also tracking along the descending aorta inferiorly.

descending aorta at isthmus (90–95%), ascending aorta including aortic root, aortic arch and distal descending aorta.[10,12] It causes mediastinal hemorrhage especially in the periaortic region due to bleeding from small veins in the area or from vasa vasorum of the aorta.

Plain chest radiograph is the first investigation after initial resuscitative efforts. The findings on chest radiograph for possible traumatic aortic injury are shown in **Box 5**.

Mediastinal widening has a high sensitivity (90–100%) for mediastinal hematoma and associated aortic injury but the specificity is low (60%). False-positive diagnosis may be due to variety of causes including supine position, expiratory film, atelectasis, pleural effusions or lung injuries obscuring mediastinal margins, mediastinal tumors and mediastinal hemorrhage due to nonaortic causes like spinal fracture or spinal ligamentous injury. A negative plain chest radiograph has high negative predictive value of 90%. It should, however, be noted that rarely the radiograph may also be normal in aortic injury especially in intimal injuries.

Multislice CT with CT angiography is now the investigation for choice for detecting aortic injury. It has replaced catheter angiography for screening for aortic injury. Catheter angiography is reserved for doubtful cases and for interventional treatment. The American College of Radiology (ACR) appropriateness criteria recommends using CT angiography for evaluation of all suspected cases of traumatic aortic injury.[13] CT has been reported to have sensitivity of 100% and specificity of 96% for diagnosing aortic injury.[7] The signs of aortic injury on CT are enumerated in **Box 6**.

Multiplanar reconstructions (MPR) with volume rendering, and virtual angioscopy have been shown to aid in the detection of small rents. Thinner collimations used in CT have allowed detection of 'minimal aortic injuries' which include small intramural hematomas, intimal flaps and intimal thrombus.

Non-aortic vascular injury may also occur in thoracic trauma. These include injury to aortic arch branches, internal mammary artery, pulmonary artery and venous injuries. The spectrum of injuries include intimal tears, dissection, pseudoaneurysm, partial or total occlusion and arteriovenous fistula.

Box 5: Chest radiograph signs for possible aortic injury.

- Mediastinal widening
- Depression of the left mainstem bronchus
- Blurring of aortic contour
- Thickening of right or left paratracheal stripe
- Shift of trachea and nasogastric tube to the right
- Left hemothorax (effusion)
- Left apical pleural cap

Box 6: Signs of traumatic aortic injury on CT.

- *Direct signs*:
  - Active contrast extravasation
  - Pseudoaneurysm formation
  - Abrupt change in aortic diameter caliper
  - Aortic dissection
  - Intimal flaps or filling defects **(Figs. 15A and B)**
  - Aortic wall irregularity
- *Indirect signs*:
  - Indistinctness of mediastinal fat planes
  - Mediastinal hematoma
  - Periaortic hematoma

Cardiac and Pericardial Injury

The diagnosis of blunt cardiac injury relies on a high degree of clinical suspicion. Elevated cardiac enzymes with alterations in ECG findings in the setting of blunt thoracic trauma should raise a doubt of cardiac injury. Transthoracic echocardiography is the most appropriate modality for evaluation of the cardiac injury. If it is equivocal, then transesophageal echocardiography or cardiac MRI can be used as problem-solving tool. If contrast CT of the thorax has been done for evaluation of thoracic trauma, cardiac and pericardial injury manifestations include pericardial effusion/hemopericardium, pneumopericardium, contrast extravasation into pericardium or a decreased area of myocardial enhancement **(Figs. 16A and B)**.

Pericardial injury is most commonly on left side of pericardium parallel to phrenic nerve followed by diaphragmatic surface of pericardium. A large pericardial tear can cause cardiac herniation and death.

INJURY OF DIAPHRAGM

Diaphragmatic rupture and subsequent herniation of abdominal contents into thorax is nine times more common on left side than right due to the protective effect of the liver. On the right side most injuries to the diaphragm go unrecognized during the acute phase. In the interval phase, the abdominal viscus may not have herniated or the patient may have acclimatized to the presence of abdominal contents in the thorax. In the later phase, obstruction or strangulation presents with severe abdominal or chest pain. The injury may also be evident at a later stage in those patients who were earlier on positive pressure ventilation and have now been extubated. Chest radiograph may reveal nonspecific findings that include an indistinct or

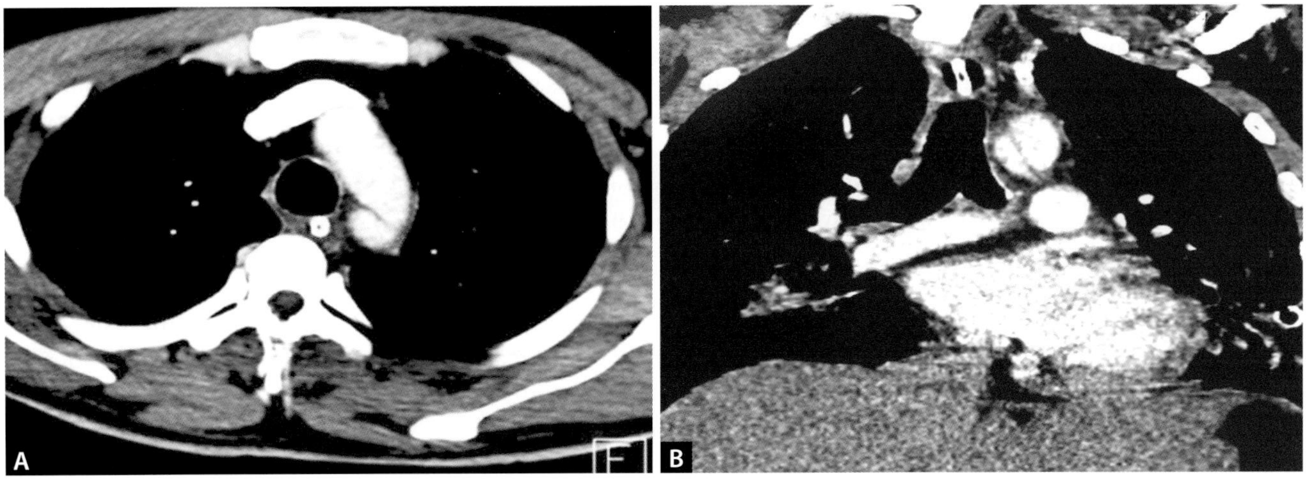

Figs. 15A and B: Aortic arch injury: Axial (A) and coronal MPR (B) CT images shows mild outpouching with an intimal flap in the aortic arch representing dissecting pseudoaneurysm.

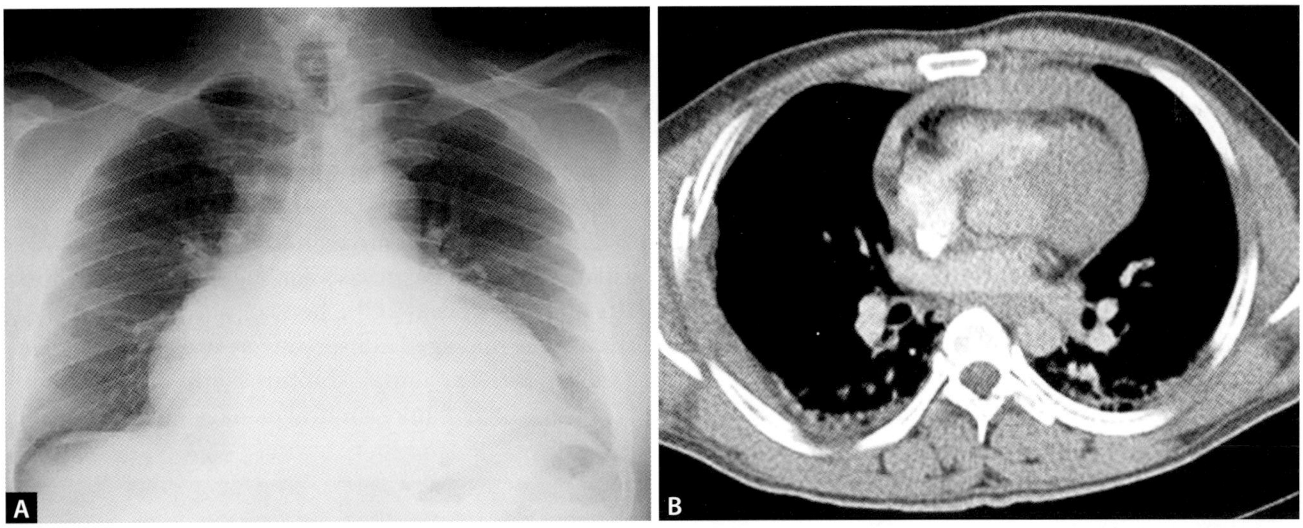

Figs. 16A and B: Hemopericardium: Chest radiograph (A) shows enlarged flask-shaped cardiac silhouette representing pericardial fluid. Axial CT image (B) in a different patient shows the hemopericardium. The patient was found to have ventricular wall injury peroperative.

elevated hemidiaphragm, pleural effusion, atelectasis with shift of the mediastinum to the contralateral side, hemothorax, pneumothorax or lower rib fractures. Specific findings are visualization of bowel loops or solid masses above the diaphragm and loss of the normal diaphragmatic contour. Detection of a nasogastric tube above the left hemidiaphragm is also a strong indicator. Contrast studies (barium meal or enema) can be used to clearly delineate the herniation.

The advent of MDCT with multiplanar reconstructions has significantly improved the sensitivity of CT in detecting diaphragmatic injuries. The various CT signs of diaphragmatic injury are given in **Box 7**.[14]

Box 7: Signs of diaphragmatic injury on CT.

- Focal diaphragmatic discontinuity or elevation
- Focal diaphragmatic thickening (retraction)
- Herniated abdominal contents into thorax
- 'Collar' sign
- 'Dependent viscera' sign

The 'collar' sign refers to the narrowed waist of a herniated intra-abdominal organ due to compression at the neck (diaphragm tear). In a healthy individual, the intra-abdominal organs such as spleen and stomach are seen to be separated by the costal margin by a layer of the diaphragm on cross-sectional imaging. However, if these organs have herniated through the diaphragm into the chest, then they appear to lie directly in contact with the posterior thoracic wall without the diaphragm intervening between them **(Figs. 17A and B)**. This has been described as the 'dependent viscera' sign. The 'dependent viscera' sign and the 'collar' signs are reported to be 100% specific.[15] MRI also has been reported to be highly sensitive in detecting diaphragmatic rupture.[16]

INJURY OF CHEST WALL

Rib fractures occur in approximately 50% of all blunt chest trauma and are the most common skeletal manifestation of injury. Isolated rib fractures are usually not clinically significant. However, multiple and bilateral rib fractures signify severe trauma and act as external manifestation of coexisting thoracic or abdominal injuries. Fractures of first three ribs occurs after severe trauma and is associated with injuries of brachial plexus or subclavian vessels. Fractures of lower three ribs is associated with intra-abdominal visceral organ injuries to kidney, spleen and liver. Further, due to the pain and immobility associated with rib fractures, the underlying lung is more prone to atelectasis and pneumonia. Rarely traumatic lung herniation, as described previously, can also occur. Chest radiography is much less sensitive than CT in detecting rib fractures. CT with three-dimensional volume rendering best depicts the rib fractures.

Flail chest occurs when there are atleast two sites of fractures on each of three or more consecutive ribs creating a flail segment which moves paradoxically with respiratory motion **(Fig. 18)**. It signifies significant chest trauma and is associated with atelectasis and pneumonia and often requires ventilator support or surgical intervention.

Sternal fractures are uncommon. The fracture typically involves the manubrium or body. CT is most sensitive for detection followed by lateral chest radiograph **(Figs. 19A and B)**. A retrosternal hematoma may be seen. A significantly displaced sternal fracture may be associated with underlying cardiac injury.

Fractures of the clavicle are classified according to their location. Group 1 fractures are most common (80%) and involve the mid-part of clavicle; group 2 fractures (15%) involve the lateral third of clavicle; and group 3 fractures (5%) involve the medial third of the clavicle **(Figs. 20A and B)**. Most fractures are managed conservatively although the surgical rate for distal third fractures is more as they have high rate of nonunion.

Sternoclavicular dislocations can be anterior or posterior. Anterior dislocation of clavicle is more common. It is usually not associated with significant injuries and is managed conservatively. Posterior dislocation of clavicle at sternoclavicular joint is more serious as the clavicle can cause injury of trachea, esophagus and mediastinal blood vessels.

Scapular fractures are seen with severe trauma and are usually associated with vascular and neurological injuries. Most fractures occur at the body or neck of scapula. They are usually managed conservatively except for displaced glenoid intra-articular fractures and juxta-articular fractures which require surgical management. Rarely there

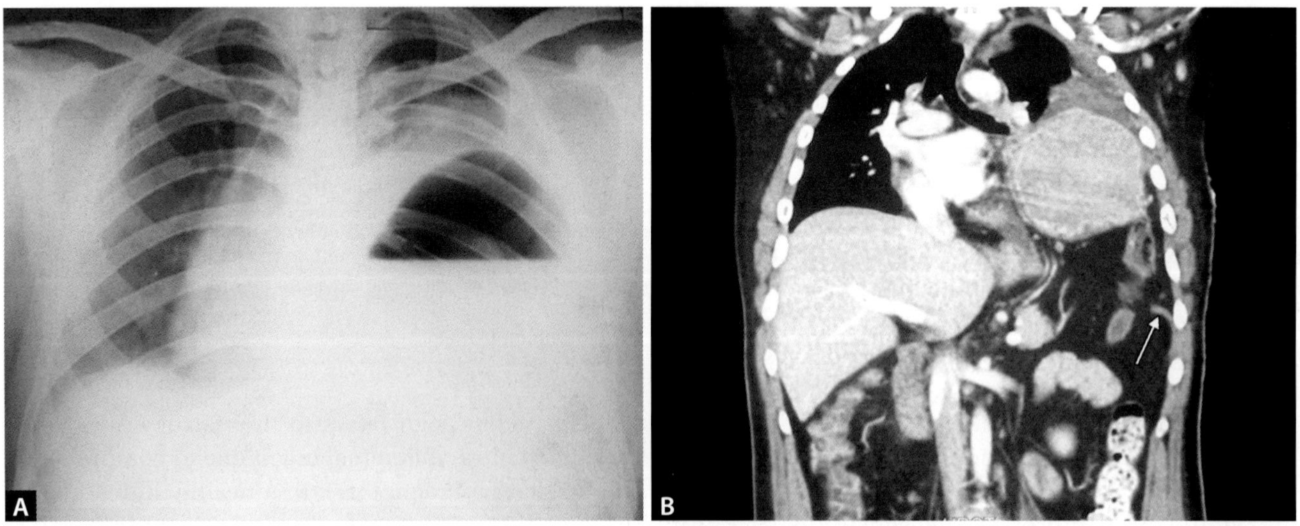

Figs. 17A and B: Diaphragmatic injury: Erect chest radiograph (A) shows indistinct left hemidiaphragm outline with large air-fluid level (of stomach) in left thoracic cavity with mediastinal shift towards right. Coronal MPR CT image (B) shows the left diaphragmatic hernia with thickened and retracted torn diaphragm (arrow).

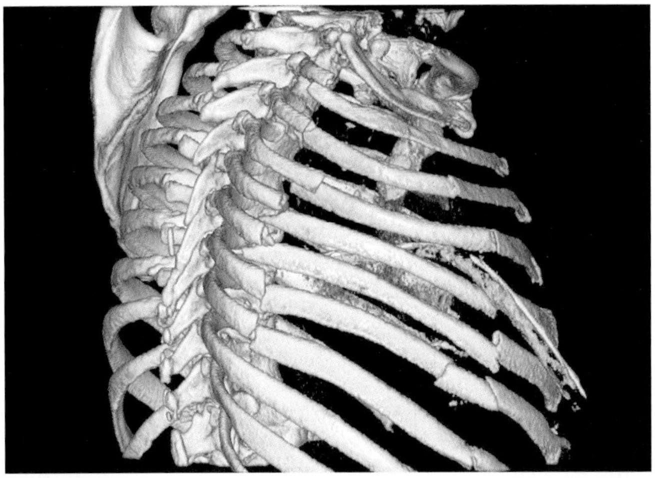

Fig. 18: Flail chest: Three-dimensional volume rendered CT image shows fractures of multiple ribs on right side with many ribs fractured at two places at lateral and posterior ends.

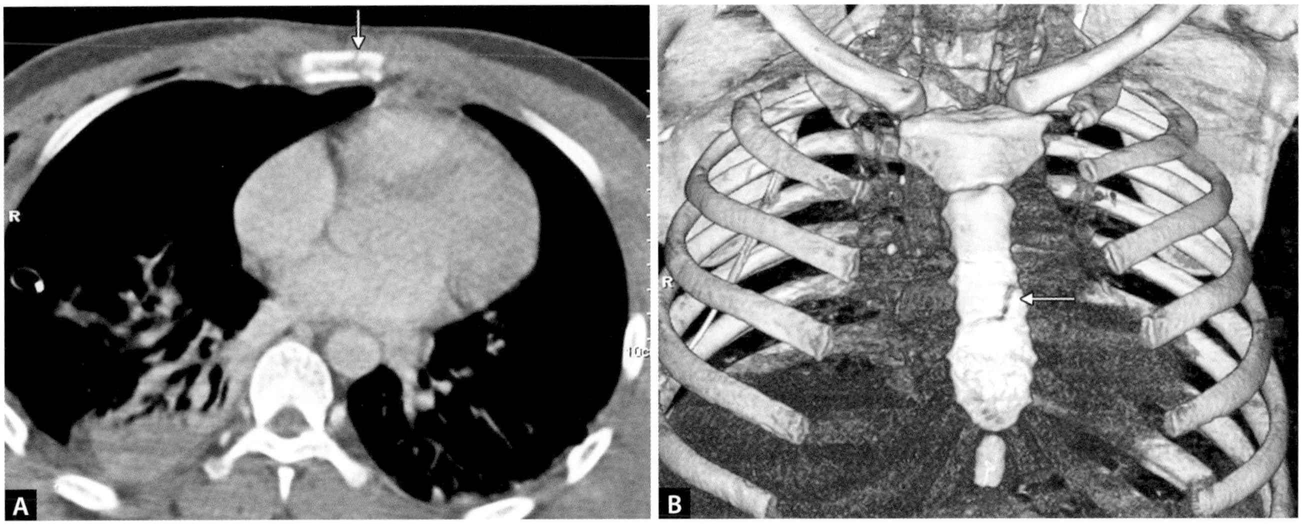

Figs. 19A and B: Sternal fracture: Axial (A) and volume rendered three-dimensional (B) CT images show fracture of mid body of sternum.

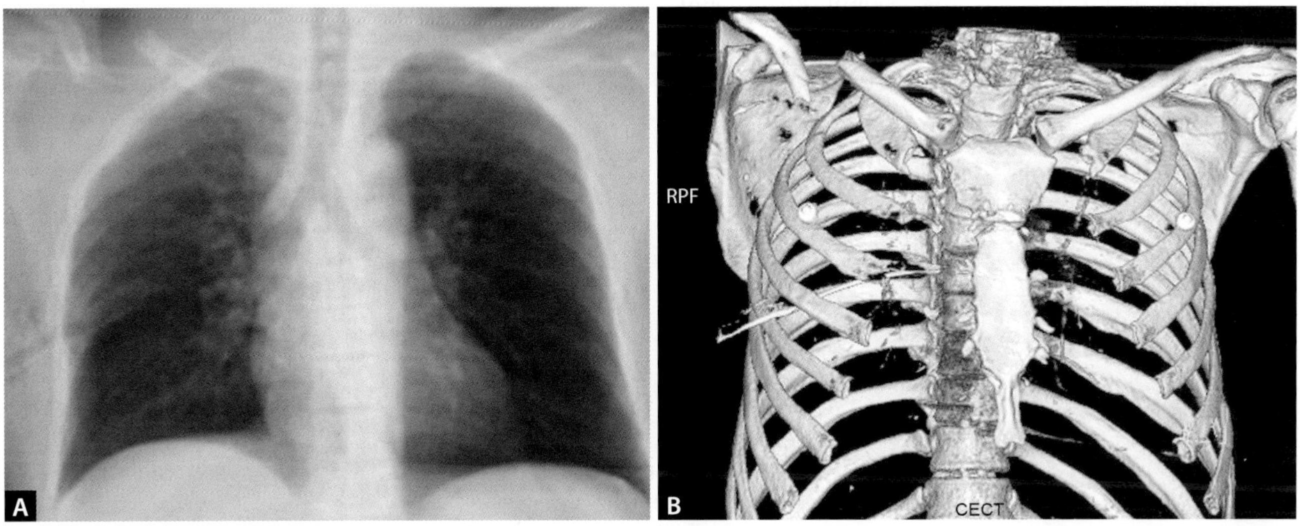

Figs. 20A and B: Clavicle fracture: Thick MPR (A) and volume-rendered three-dimensional (B) CT images show fracture of mid-part of right clavicle.

may be scapulothoracic dissociation in which scapula is displaced laterally. Multiplanar CT reconstructions are best to visualize the fracture fragments.

Spinal fractures may also be associated with thoracic trauma. The spinal fractures are easily seen on the multiplanar reconstructions of the CT done for chest. The fractures may be associated with significant neurological deficits in up to 60% of patients. MRI is indicated in patients with spinal trauma and associated neurological deficit for characterization of the spinal cord damage.

CONCLUSION

Diagnostic imaging quickly gives important information on extent and type of thoracic injuries from blunt and penetrating trauma. The chest radiograph is the 'first look' imaging modality and has a role in detecting some immediate life-threatening conditions like tension pneumothorax and massive hemothorax. Ultrasound is also used as a first line investigation for detecting hemothorax, pneumothorax and hemopericardium. Multislice CT has become the definitive modality which detects and characterizes the full extent of spectrum of thoracic trauma. MRI does not have any significant role in the setting of acute trauma except for evaluation of spinal cord in spinal injuries.

REFERENCES

1. Lomoschitz FM, Eisenhuber E, Linnau KF, et al. Imaging of chest trauma: radiological patterns of injury and diagnostic algorithms. European Journal of Radiology. 2003;48:61-70.
2. Miller LA. Chest wall, lung, and pleural space trauma. Radiol Clin North Am. 2006;44:213-24.
3. Costantino M, Gosselin MV, Primack SL. The ABC's of thoracic trauma imaging. Semin Roentgenol. 2006;41(3):209-25.
4. Donnelly LF, Klosterman LA. Subpleural sparing: a CT finding of lung contusion in children. Radiology. 1997;204:385-7.
5. Miller PR, Croce MA, Bec TK, et al. ARDS after pulmonary contusion: accurate measurement of contusion volume identifies high-risk patients. J Trauma. 2001;51:223-30.
6. Kaewlai R, Avery LL, Asrani AV, et al. Multidetector CT of blunt thoracic trauma. Radiographics. 2008;28(6): 1555-70.
7. Rivas LA, Fishman JE, Múnera F, et al. Multislice CT in thoracic trauma. Radiol Clin North Am. 2003;41(3):599-616.
8. Lee RB. Traumatic injury of the cervicothoracic trachea and major bronchi. Chest Surg Clin N Am. 1997;7:285-304.
9. Durso AM, Caban K, Munera F. Penetrating Thoracic Injury. Radiol Clin N Am. 2015;53:675-93.
10. Sangster GP, González-Beicos A, Carbo AI, et al. Blunt traumatic injuries of the lung parenchyma, pleura, thoracic wall, and intrathoracic airways: multidetector computer tomography imaging findings. Emerg Radiol. 2007;14:297-310.
11. Wintermark M, Wicky S, Schnyder P, et al. Blunt traumatic pneumomediastinum: using CT to reveal the Macklin effect. Am J Roentgenol. 1999;172:129-30.
12. Fishman JE. Imaging of blunt aortic and great vessel trauma. J Thorac Imaging. 2000;15:97-103.
13. Demehri S, Rybicki FJ, Desjardins B, et al. ACR Appropriateness Criteria: Blunt chest trauma—suspected aortic injury. Emerg Radiol. 2012;19:287-92.
14. Panda A, Kumar A, Gamanagatti S, et al. Traumatic diaphragmatic injury: a review of CT signs and the difference between blunt and penetrating injury. Diagn Interv Radiol. 2014;20(2):121-8.
15. Stanescu AL, Gross JA, Bittle M, et al. Imaging of blunt abdominal trauma. Semin Roentgen. 2006;41(3):196-204.
16. Barbiera F, Nicastro N, Finazzo M, et al. The role of MRI in traumatic rupture of the diaphragm. Our experience in three cases and review of the literature. Radiol Med. 2003;105(3):188-94.

CHAPTER 172

Imaging of Pleura

Anjali Prakash, Rashmi Dixit, Sapna Singh

INTRODUCTION

The pleura is a serous membrane of mesodermal origin that envelops the lungs, mediastinum, diaphragm and rib cage. It is composed of two layers—parietal and visceral. The lung is covered with visceral pleura, the parietal pleural covers the mediastinum, diaphragm and inner surface of thoracic cage. The layers are in continuity, both at the hilum and below, where they form the pulmonary ligament.

The parietal pleura is divided into costal pleura, diaphragmatic pleura, mediastinal and cervical pleura, based on its relationship to various regions of the thoracic cavity. The visceral and parietal pleural are separated by a potential space that normally contains only a few mL of fluid. As the thickness of the pleural space and its visceral and parietal pleura measures about 0.2–0.44 mm, it is only seen when parallel to the X-ray beam or outlined by air, extrapleural fat or fascia. This pleura is appreciated as:

1. The major, minor or accessory fissures, all of which (with the exception of azygous fissure) consists of two invaginated sheets of visceral pleura.
2. The junctional lines, which consists of four sheets of pleura (two parietal and two visceral), which are often more than a hairline thickness as both (particularly posterior) may contain fibrofatty tissue.

The vascular supply of the parietal pleural is from the systemic circulation, whereas the visceral pleural is supplied by branches of the pulmonary arteries and to a lesser extent by bronchial arteries. Lymphatic drainage of the visceral pleural is by a lymphatic plexus that covers the surface of the lung, just beneath the visceral pleural. This elaborate plexus connects to the bronchial lymphatics that drain centrally along the bronchovascular bundles to the pulmonary hilum. The parietal pleural is the primary drainage route for the pleural space and is lymphatically connected to the intercostal, internal mammary and mediastinal lymph node chains.

IMAGING MODALITIES

Chest radiograph is the initial screening radiological investigation when pleural disease or pulmonary disease is suspected. Chest frontal, lateral, decubitus views are helpful in detecting small amount of pleural effusion. Expiratory films may be required to visualize a small pneumothorax. The drawback is its limited ability to differentiate benign from malignant pleural disease. It is important to differentiate pleural from extrapleural disease and pulmonary disease.

Extrapleural masses usually displace the overlying parietal and visceral pleura resulting in an obtuse angle between the lesion and chest wall. Associated abnormalities include soft tissue mass or rib destruction. They are sharply marginated at the point they contact lung and displace pulmonary vessels away from them.

Pleural masses, arising from visceral or parietal pleura, usually remain confined to pleural space. The presence of an obtuse angle is common, unless the lesion is large. Large pleural lesions may have acute angle, where they meet the chest wall, although some pleural thickening is seen adjacent to them. Pleural lesions are also sharply marginated and displace pulmonary vessels away from them.

A peripherally placed pulmonary lesion will have acute angle with the pleural surface, unless there is pleural invasion, which could result is an obtuse angle. Pulmonary lesions are often ill defined along their inner aspect and may engulf, rather than displace vessels **(Table 1)**.

Ultrasonography is an efficient, 'point of care' imaging modality for evaluation of the chest wall and pleura because of the superficial location. It has low cost, bedside availability and involves no radiation. The indications and uses of chest ultrasound examination for pleural disease are:

- To clarify the nature of unknown pleural densities.
- To detect pleural effusion and to guide thoracocentesis and drainage, especially in minimal or loculated effusion.
- To differentiate subpulmonic effusion from subphrenic fluid accumulation.
- To detect pneumothorax in emergency setting.
- To localize pleural tumors/thickening and guide biopsy of the pleura.

Pleura is a superficial structure and hence seen with a high frequency linear tranducer applied directly over the chest—**the direct intercostal approach**. A sector probe (3.5 MHz) may be used for the lower aspect of pleura via the **abdominal approach**, with the liver and spleen providing an acoustic window. Normal pleura is identified just below the ribs and is seen on ultrasound as an echogenic line just beneath the chest wall **(Fig. 1)**. The air-filled lung covered by visceral pleura reflects the ultrasound beam producing the echogenic line that moves with respiration. This normal movement of lung surface is called '**gliding sign**'. This echogenic line represents the visceral pleura, with the parietal pleura appearing as a weakly echogenic, less distinct line, often obscured by artifacts. Using the abdominal approach, the diaphragm is seen as a bright curving echogenic line. An air-filled lung above it will cause specular reflection and mirror image reflection of liver or spleen on the left side **(Fig. 2)**. The presence of this mirror image implies presence of an air-filled lung and absence of pleural fluid above the diaphragm.

CT is the modality of choice in evaluating diseases of the pleura, especially pleural tumors. It is particularly helpful in determining chest wall, mediastinum and diaphragmatic involvement. CT allows differentiation of benign from malignant pleural disease except in very early disease. It can display anterior and paravertebral pleural plaques, areas not well seen on chest radiographs.

Table 1: Radiological differentiation of pleural, extrapleural and pulmonary lesion.

Features	*Pulmonary*	*Pleural*	*Extrapleural*
Incomplete border sign (radiograph)	Absent	Present	Present
Angle with chest wall	Acute	Obtuse	Obtuse
Epicenter	In lung	Along chest wall	Along chest wall
Pulmonary vasculature	Engulfs	Displace	Displace
Extrapleural fat displacement	-	Outwards	Inwards
Rib erosion	Unusual	Unusual	Usual

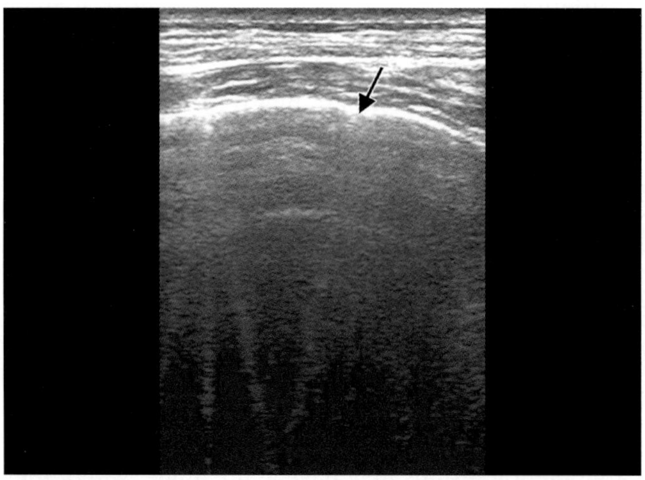

Fig. 1: Ultrasound chest direct intercostal approach: Echogenic line depicting the lung pleura interface.

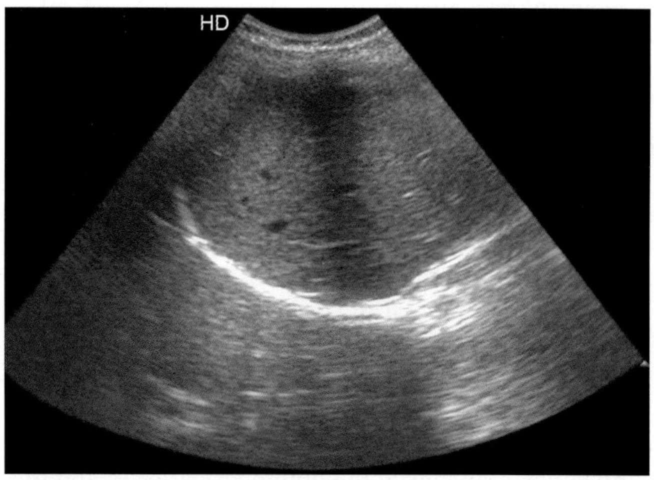

Fig. 2: Ultrasound chest-abdominal approach: Mirror image of liver seen above the diaphragm implying presence of air-filled lung.

For complete evaluation of the pleural surfaces the patient is scanned contiguously from the thoracic inlet to the L3 level. Pleural enhancement is best demonstrated with a delayed scan time of 45–60 seconds.

On HRCT the pleura may be identified when it forms the fissures. Depending on its obliquity to the imaging plane, a fissure appears as a thin, high density line or band. On conventional CT, the fissure is appreciated as an avascular band. Peripherally on CT and HRCT, there is a thin line–the intercostal stripe separating the lung margin and the fat lying inside the internal intercostal muscle **(Fig. 3)**. This line (the lung chest wall interface) connects the inner aspect of the ribs and is 1–2 mm thick. It comprises the two layers of pleura.

Subparietal pleural fat: Separates parietal pleura from endothoracic fascia. This is very thin in most locations, but can be markedly thickened over the lateral or posterolateral ribs, resulting in extrapleural fat pads.

Endothoracic fascia: This fibroelastic fascia covers the surface of the intercostal muscles and intervening ribs, blends with the perichondrium and periosteum of the costal cartilages. Posteriorly, it is continous with the prevertebral fascia that covers the vertebral bodies and intervertebral discs.

MRI suffers from the drawback of a poor signal to noise ratio in lung, cardiac and respiratory motion artefacts and susceptibility artifacts at air tissue boundaries. However, it is sometimes used as a problem solving tool.

Diffusion imaging (DWI) helps to non-invasively characterize various types of effusion. Diffusion weighted imaging can differentiate benign from pleural malignant disease with a cut-off ADC threshold being 1.52×10^{-3} mm^2/sec. This has a sensitivity of 71.4% and specificity of 100%. In cases where ADC is indeterminate, dynamic contrast-enhanced MRI improves the diagnostic confidence.[1]

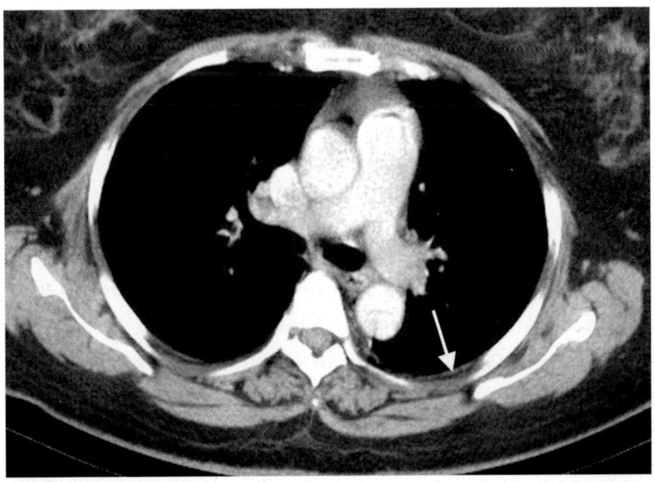

Fig. 3: CT: A thin white stripe (marked with arrow) between adjacent ribs represents the intercostal stripe, primarily representing the innermost intercostal muscle. This is anatomically absent in the paravertebral region.

MRI also plays an important role in the evaluation of extent of pleural neoplasm especially in areas like lung apices and diaphragm.

FDG-PET is complementary to CT in the evaluation of pleural tumors. It has an important role in staging pleural mesothelioma.

PLEURAL PATHOLOGY

Pleura may be affected by the following pathologies which may be linked to each other:

- Effusion
- Pneumothorax
- Pleural thickening
- Tumor
- Tumor-like conditions

PLEURAL EFFUSION

Fluid moves across the capillary membranes of the visceral pleura into the pleural space and is then reabsorbed by the lymphatic system. Changes in capillary permeability, hydrostatic and oncotic pressure or lymphatic function affects the balance between the formation and resorption of pleural fluid leading to accumulation of fluid in the pleural space.

The pleural fluid may be transudate, exudate, blood or chyle. All types of pleural effusion are radiographically identical, though clinical and biochemical features may help limit the differential diagnosis. Most pleural effusion are classified as exudates or transudates based on their chemical composition which is usually defined by thoracocentesis. The criteria most commonly used to separate transudative from exudative effusion are known as **Light's criteria.**[2] Pleural fluid is considered an exudate if one or more of the following criteria are met.

1. A ratio of pleural fluid protein to serum protein higher than 0.5.
2. A ratio of pleural fluid lactate dehydrogenase (LDH) to serum LDH leval that exceeds 0.6.
3. A pleural fluid LDH level more than two-thirds the upper limit of normal serum LDH.

Exudative effusion reflects the presence of a pleural abnormality associated with increased permeability of pleural capillaries. These effusions have high protein content. Common causes of exudative effusion include pneumonia with parapneumonic effusion, empyema, TB, pleuritis, neoplasm, pulmonary embolism, drug reaction, etc.

Transudative effusion is unassociated with pleural disease. It usually results from systemic abnormalities causing an imbalance in the hydrostatic and osmotic forces governing pleural fluid formation. These are low in protein and are usually bilateral. Common causes include CHF, pericardial disease, liver cirrhosis, renal disease, and hypoalbuminemia.

Bilateral effusions are usually transudates as they are secondary to generalized causes such as hypoproteinema. Some bilateral effusions may be exudates, e.g. those associated with metastatic disease, lymphoma, rheumatoid disease, systemic lupus erythematosus (SLE). Right-sided effusions are typically associated with ascitis, heart failure and liver abscess. Effusions associated with pancreatitis, pericarditis, esophageal rupture and aortic dissection tend to be left sided.

Massive effusions are most commonly due to malignant disease, especially metastatic (lung or breast), but may also occur in heart failure, cirrhosis, tuberculosis, empyema and trauma.

Specific Causes of Pleural Effusion

Congestive Heart Failure

Congestive heart failure (CHF) is the most common cause of transudative effusion, though exudative effusions may also occur. Pleural fluid accumulates in CHF because pulmonary interstitial fluid (due to edema) crosses into the pleural space. Bilateral effusions are seen is 70% of cases, if unilateral, it is usually right sided. A large unilateral pleural effusion should suggest an alternative diagnosis.

Renal Disease

Pleural effusion is seen with renal disease due to various causes.

- Renal failure with overhydration may result in transudative effusion, usually bilateral.
- Nephrotic syndrome may causel transudative effusions due to increased hydrostatic pressure and hypoalbuminemia resulting in decreased oncotic pressure.
- Uremia may result in fibrinious pleuritis and a bloody exudative effusion that is often unilateral and large. Pleural thickening may also be seen.
- Hydronephrosis due to retroperitoneal lesion may result in ipsilateral pleural effusion—which is rich in creatinine.
- Effusion may result from peritoneal dialysis, fluid enters the pleural space via diaphragmatic defects.

Radiation (Therapeutic)

Approximately 5% of patients having chest radiation develop a small exudative pleural effusion. This is usually in association with radiation pneumonitis the effusion being on the same side as that of radiation, develops within 6 months of radiation. It resolves slowly with time.

Dressler's Syndrome

Occurs in a few patients post myocardial infarction or cardiac surgery. It occurs 2–3 weeks after the event and is associated with chest pain, fever, dyspnea. Radiographs show pleural effusion (85%) lung consolidation and pericardial effusion. It is thought to be an immunologically mediated response. They are usually bilateral, when unilateral, it is usually left sided.

Pulmonary Embolism

Pleural effusion occurs in 30% of patients with pulmonary embolism. Usually associated with infarction, exudates (75%) are more common than transudates.

Pericardial Disease

Pleural effusion is common in patients with inflammatory pericardial disease. They are left sided in 70%. In patients with constrictive pericarditis, effusions or CHF may result from elevated left or right sided venous pressure.

Meig's Syndrome

Pleural effusion with ascitis and ovarian fibroma is the classical triad of Meig's syndrome. Other ovarian tumors may show similar presentation. It may be exudative or transudative. Resection of the tumor results in resolution of pleural effusion and ascitis.

Pancreatitis

Pleural effusion is associated with acute and chronic pancreatitis. The effusion shows high amylase levels. In acute pancreatitis, exudative effusion is seen, mostly on left side.In chronic pancreatitis, effusions are large and indolent. The pleural effusion is probably secondary to fistula formation following ductal rupture.

Chylothorax may result from rupture of thoracic duct or of a prominent lymphatic channel. Lymph may also accumulate as a result of oozing from pleural lymphatics or due to passage of chylous ascitis via diaphragm. Chylous effusion is associated with neoplastic etiology in majority[3] of cases, seen in patients with lymphoma, metastatic neoplasm. Chylothorax also develops following thoracic surgery chest trauma, inflammatory mediastinal lymph node disease, and in some developmental anomalies like lymphangioma, lymphangioleiomyomatosis. Traumatic chylothorax resolves over time as the thoracic duct heals. Reduction in lymph flow may be helpful. Ligation of duct is curative.

Chylous effusion contains intestinal lymph (i.e. chyle), which is high in protein and fatty acids and is low in cholesterol. It looks milky on naked eye examination. Chylothorax does not have a low CT number despite presence of fat as it is rich in proteins. A chylous effusion can show high signal intensity on T1WI. **Pseudochylous or chyleform effusion** contains cholesterol, but not chyle. It may be seen in patients with chronic inflammatory disease like to TB, rheumatoid arthritis. Chylous effusions may remain chronic for years.

Hemothorax

It refers to pleural fluid having a hematocrit of over 50% of blood hematocrit. On CT, hemothorax results in fluid with high attenuation (mostly higher than 50 HU) containing a dense clot or a fluid-fluid level, with the densest fluid posteriorly. Most of cases are traumatic in origin, others may be spontaneous, including rupture of aneurysm/dissection, pulmonary or pleural neoplasm, coagulopathy. Treatment includes drainage. Organization of hemothorax results in fibrosis and calcification. A resolving exudative effusion or hemothorax may deposit a clot of fibrin within the pleural space termed as fibrin body or pleural mouse. These appear 1–2 cm in diameter, mimicking a solitary nodule, localized to pleural space and are sometimes seen to move with change in patient position. They resolve or may remain stable for years.

IMAGING IN PLEURAL EFFUSION

Plain Radiographs

The radiological signs of a pleural effusion depend on the posture of the patient and distribution of fluid which may be free or loculated. The pleural space extends inferiorly below the visible lung, in relation to the diaphragm and ribs. Small amount of pleural fluid is not visible on erect radiograph as it collects under the lung. These small **subpulmonic** effusions are detected by ultrasound or CT.

In an upright subject at least 175 mL of fluid must be present to result in blunting of the lateral costophrenic angle on the frontal radiograph and rarely as much as 500 mL may be present without blunting **(Fig. 4)**. On a lateral decubitus film, as little as 10 mL fluid may be seen.

The classical signs of pleural effusion include—homogeneous opacification of lower chest with obliteration of costophrenic angle and the hemidiaphragm. The upper margin of the opacity is concave to the lung and is higher laterally than medially. The highest point of the "meniscus" reflects the true level of fluid **(Fig. 5)**. This is because the X-ray beam traverses a greater thickness of fluid at the periphery due to circumferential configuration of the pleural space around the air containing lung. Above and medial to the meniscus, there is a hazy increase in opacity owing to fluid behind and in front of the lungs.

Massive effusion can cause dense opacification of the hemithorax with contralateral mediastinal shift

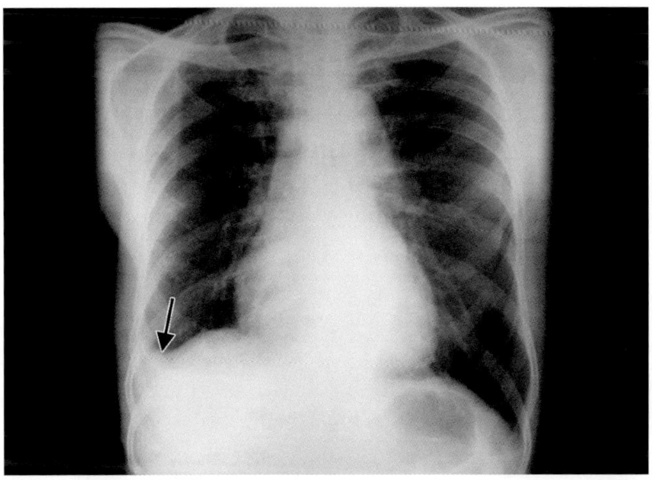

Fig. 4: X-ray chest PA view: Blunting of right costophrenic angle-pleural effusion.

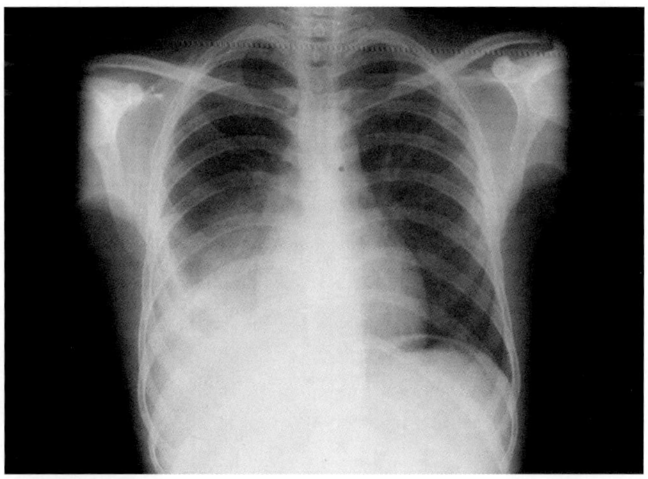

Fig. 5: X-ray chest PA view: Homogeneous opacification of right lower zone with obliteration of the right costophrenic angle and the hemidiaphragm. The upper margin of the opacity is concave and extends higher laterally "meniscus sign"—Pleural effusion.

(Figs. 6A to C) (Table 2). Shifted structures include the trachea, the heart, the azygoesophageal recess, producing a paravertebral retrocardiac density convex to the lung. Absence of mediastinal shift with a large effusion should raise the possibility of obstructive collapse of the ipsilateral lung or extensive pleural malignancy such as seen with mesothelioma or metastatic carcinoma.

Fluid entering into fissures may produce other opacities like middle lobe step or broad band with a curvilinear inner margin extending from midlung to chest wall, often becoming denser as it passes laterally.

On the frontal radiograph, fluid extending into the posterolateral major fissure typically results in an arcuate opacity, sharply defined medially and inferiorly. Fluid extending into the lateral aspect of the minor fissure and slightly separating the lobes, result in an opacity resembling a rose thorn (the thorn sign—**Fig. 7**).

As the lung is fixed medially, medial pleural fluid collections are usually smaller and more difficult to recognize. Medial fluid collection may be seen when effusions are large. More often, these accumulate in the posterior gutters, with thickening of the paravertebral stripe. The fluid collection may be triangular simulating lower lobe collapse.

Pleural fluid may accumulate in the subpulmonic space, allowing the lung base to float superiorly on a frontal radiograph. Subpulmonic effusion presents as a 'high hemi diaphragm' with an unusual contour that peaks more laterally **(Fig. 8)**. On the left side, 2 cm of separation of the lung base from the top of the stomach bubble is taken as an evidence of subpulmonic effusion, although distance may be variable. Most subpulmonic effusion are mobile with postural change. These are often transudates. On the lateral view, a subpulmonic effusion elevates the posterior lung, flattening its under surface, insinuates into the major fissure resulting in focal triangular thickening of the fissures, flattens the inferior contour of the lung anterior to the fissure which then angles sharply downward.

Fluid may accumulate between the lung and visceral pleura, a common finding in patients of heart failure. This is called 'lamellar effusion' and is not a true pleural effusion because it lies outside the pleural sac. It is a manifestation of waterlogged lung interstitium and is often accompanied by septal lines. Lamellar effusion is seen as vertical band of soft tissue density between the lung and chest wall above the costophrenic angle, this remains fixed with postural change **(Fig. 9)**.

Supine and semi-erect radiographs are less sensitive in showing pleural effusion. Signs of effusion on a supine radiograph are a hazy veil like opacity affecting the whole or lower part of hemithorax with preserved vascular opacities in the overlying lung **(Fig. 10)**. Additional signs include haziness of the diaphragmatic margins blunting of the costophrenic angle, a pleura apical cap which disappears in an upright film, thickening of the

Table 2: Causes of opaque hemithorax.

• Pleural effusion
• Consolidation
• Collapse
• Massive tumor
• Fibrothorax
• Pneumonectomy
• Lung agenesis

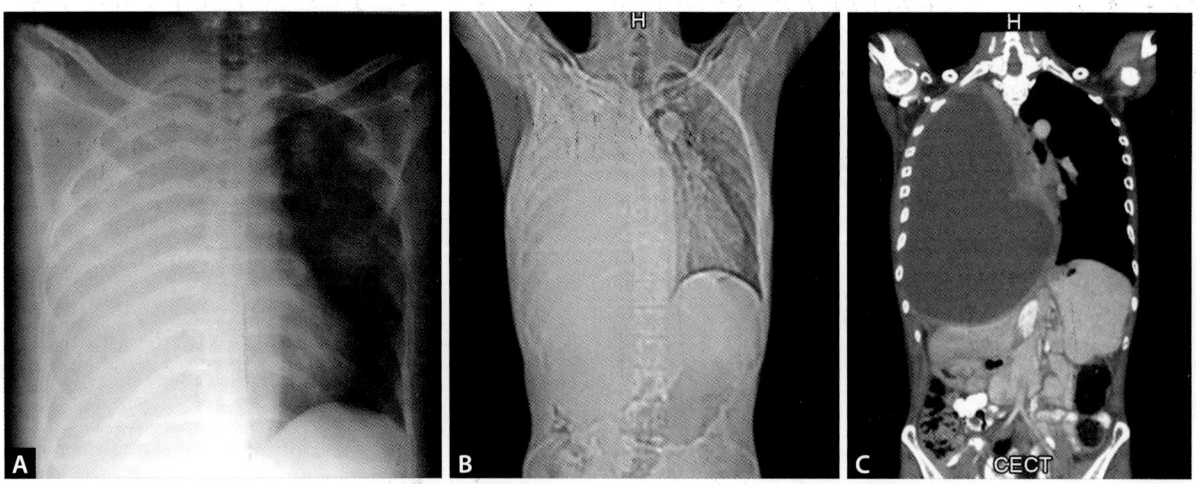

Figs. 6A to C: X-ray chest (A) Opaque hemithorax without shift of the mediastinum—scanogram (B) and coronal MPR (C) opaque hemithorax with shift of mediastinum and inversion of right hemidiaphragm in another patient.

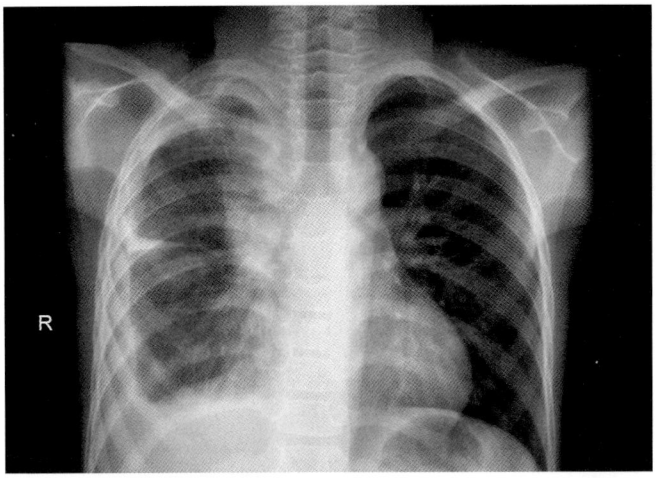

Fig. 7: Right pleural effusion is seen with associated mediastinal lymphadenopathy. Fluid is entering the minor fissure resembling a 'rose thorn'.

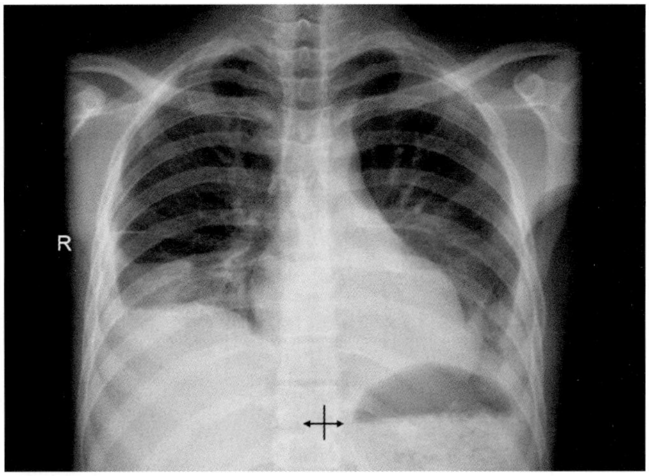

Fig. 8: Bilateral pleural effusion. Raised right hemidiaphragm with a lateralized apex suggestive of subpulmonic effusion.

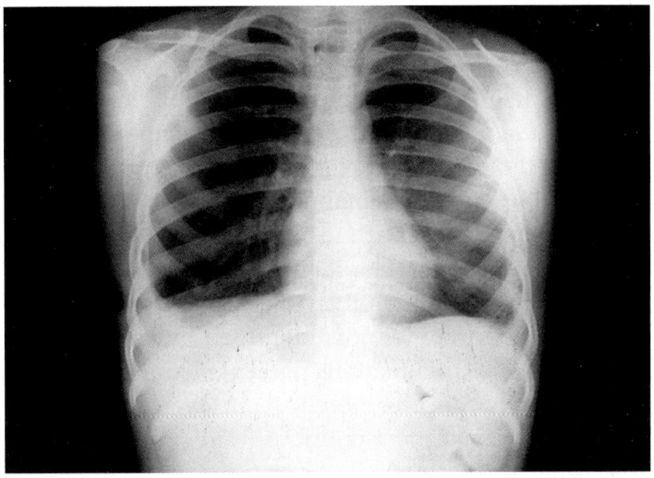

Fig. 9: Bilateral lamellar effusion with blunting of the costophrenic angles.

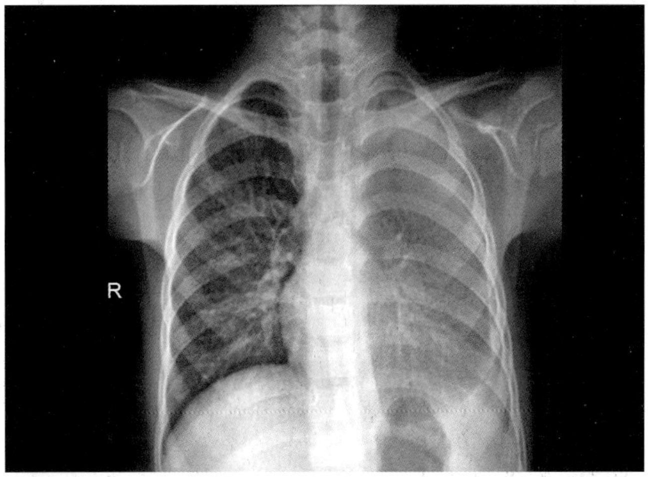

Fig. 10: X-ray chest: AP view (supine) shows a veil-like opacification of the left hemithorax with preserved vascular markings due to pleural effusion.

minor fissure and widening of the paraspinal interface. The lack of an air bronchogram and preserved vascular markings differentiate it from parenchymal disease such as pneumonia.

Loculated Pleural Fluid (Encysted/Encapsulated)

Fluid can loculate between visceral pleural layers in fissures or between visceral and parietal layers, usually against the chest wall. Loculated effusion usually occurs in association with exudative effusion, high in protein, such as those that occur in empyema, hemothorax or chylothorax.

The appearance of loculated pleural fluid on chest radiograph varies with its location and the radiographic projection used. It is sharply marginated when the surface is parallel to the X-ray beam and ill-defined when viewed en-face **(Figs. 11A and B)**. A collection loculated in the lateral pleural space will appear sharply marginated on the frontal radiograph and ill-defined on lateral film. For the effusion loculated anteriorly or posteriorly, the converse is true.

Fissural interlober loculation, seen particularly in heart failure produces the 'pseudotumor' or the 'phantom' tumor which can recur in the same place on repeated occasions. Pleural pseudotumors are transudates. Besides congestive

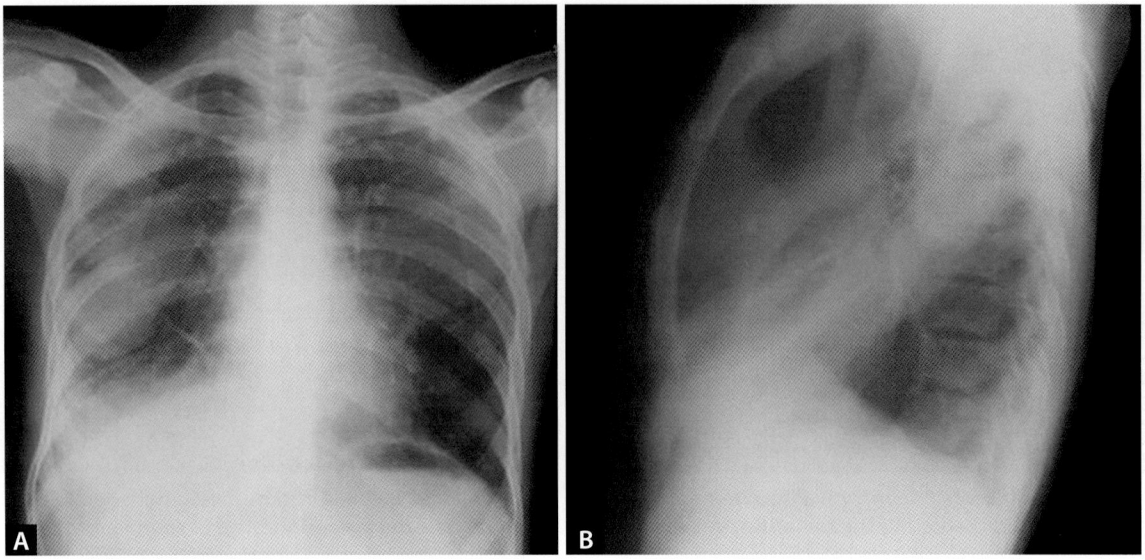

Figs. 11A and B: X-ray chest PA (A) and lateral (B)—opacities bilaterally with sharper medial margin and fading towards periphery-loculated fluid.

cardiac failure these are seen with renal failure and in cirrhotic patients. In the presence of pleural effusion, the elastic recoil of the lung causes each lobe to retract toward the hilum. This widens the fissure and can draw fluid into the fissure even in nondependent locations. The middle lobe, because it is the smallest lobe, has the greatest tendency to retract, and therefore the minor fissure is the most likely fissure to have a pseudotumor.[4]

Viewed in the lateral view, it is sharply marginated and biconvex, with a tail passing through the fissure. The en-face appearance depends on the thickness of the effusion. If it is relatively thin, it may produce a vague area of radio-opacity. If it has a certain thickness, it may appear clear edged and mass like. Sometimes encysted fluid in the right lower oblique fissure may be confused with middle lobe collapse. Features that favor a collapsed, consolidated middle lobe collapse include non-homogeneity, a straight or concave border in the lateral view, and a wedgelike outline with the base reaching the sternum. The presence of a dependent pleural effusion aids in recognizing a pleural pseudotumor. Fluid collections are rounded or lenticular and may show a tapering triangular opacity or 'beak' at the point they merge with the fissure. Fluid collections in the minor fissure appear sharply marginated and lenticular on both frontal and lateral views. Collection in the major fissure may be ill defined on the frontal view.

Ultrasound of Pleural Effusion

Ultrasonography is extremely sensitive to the presence of fluid, detecting even small amounts accurately. It is helpful in detecting subpulmonic and subphrenic effusion by noting the position and movement of diaphragm. USG is also useful in opaque hemithorax, to differentiate solid from fluid lesion and is mandatory before performing a thoracocentesis of an opaque hemithorax.

The US image of pleural effusion is characterized by echo free space between the visceral and parietal pleura **(Fig. 12)**. Visceral pleura is identified by movement of echogenic line with breathing,parietal pleura is identified by its position approximately 1 cm deep to ribs. The rough estimate of the amount of fluid can be made by measuring the maximum perpendicular distance between the lung surface and chest wall. The patient is supine and measurement is done in full inspiration. A 20 mm width has a mean volume of 380 mL ± 130 mL, 40 mm width would correspond to 1000 ± 330 mL.[5]

The sonographic characteristics of effusion may be helpful in differentiating transudates from exudates.[6] Pleural fluid, especially when it is a transudate is echo-free, though occasionally an exudates may also be anechoic. Exudative and hemorrhage effusions may be echogenic, complex and septated **(Fig. 13)**. The septae may be profuse giving rise to honeycomb appearance. These may not be well-appreciated on CT and may pose difficulty in tube drainage. Other sonographic features may be helpful in assessing the nature of pleural effusion such as associated consolidation favors empyema, while pleural nodules favor malignancy.

Ultrasound can be used to distinguish between pleural fluid, solid pleural or extrapleural lesions and

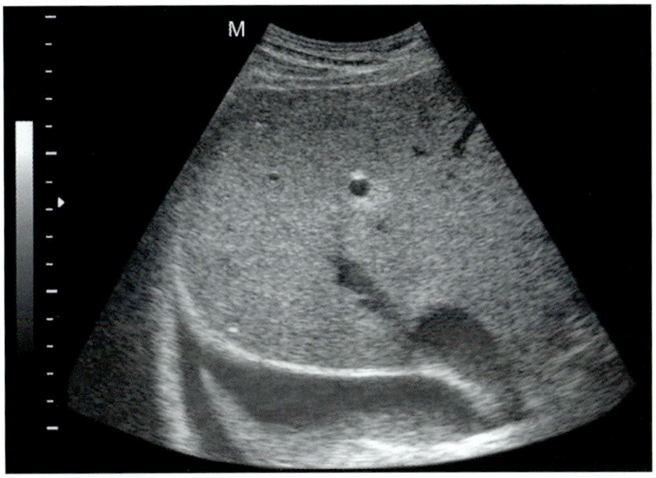

Fig. 12: Anechoic fluid in the right pleural space—seen on transabdominal ultrasound. Note absence of mirror image of liver.

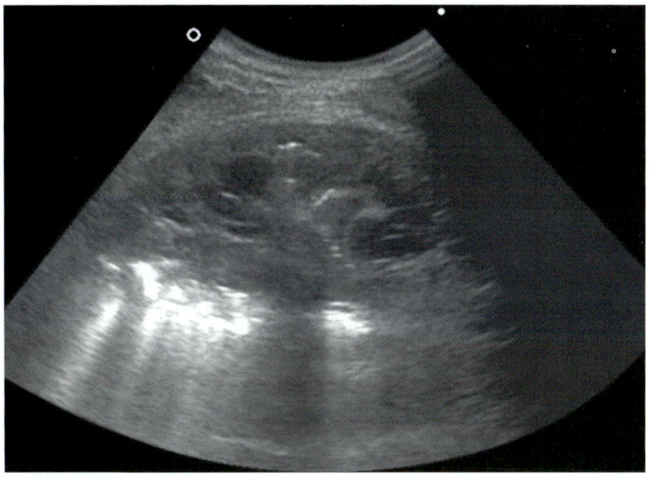

Fig. 13: USG chest shows multiseptated collection in the right pleural cavity.

peripheral lung lesions. Features that help distinguish a fluid from a solid echogenic lesion include changes in shape with breathing, presence of septa and fibrous strands and the movement of the components, induced by breathing. In peripheral lung lesions, the presence of fluid bronchograms and vessels on Doppler identify consolidation. Color Doppler signal in the fluid collection in the pleural space during respiratory or cardiac cycle is a pointer towards presence of fluid. Patients with pleural thickening do not show this sign **(Fig. 14)**.[7]

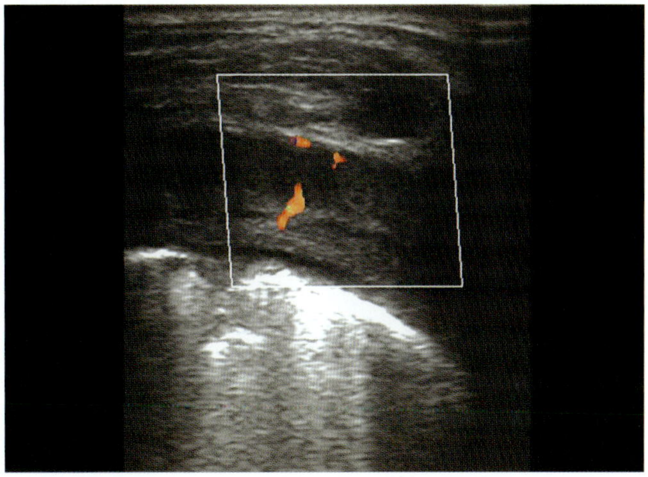

Fig. 14: Color Doppler depicting the "color fluid sign".

Computed Tomography of Pleural effusion

CT is sensitive in detecting pleural fluid and can distinguish between free and loculated fluid, identifying the extent and location of the loculation. It also allows differentiation of pleural from parenchymal pathology and the evaluation of underlying lung disease. Pleural morphology such as thickening or masses may also be studied by CT.

A pleural effusion appears as a dependent, sickle shaped opacity with a lower CT number than any adjacent pleura thickening or mass **(Fig. 15)** Most pleural effusions are near water attenuation on CT, ranging up to 20–30 HU regardless of cause.CT attenuation numbers alone do not allow a reliable distinction between an exudate and a transudate.[8] Distinguishing between the two is important for clinical management. The differentiation has to be made on the basis of thoracocentesis. The appearance of parietal pleura on CECT is of value in predicting the nature of pleural fluid collection. Visibility of enhancement of the parietal pleura indicates that it is thickened (enhancing pleura is thickened pleura) the presence of thickened parietal pleura is indicative that the fluid is an exudates. This is seen in up to 60% of exudative effusions and its accuracy in predicting the presence of exudates is nearly 100%. If pleural thickening is not present, an associated effusion may be a transudate or exudate.

CT findings of fluid loculation include a localized collection, an elliptical or lenticular shape/rather than crescentric, a non-dependent location (i.e. anterior, lateral or posterolateral) **(Figs. 16 and 17)**. If air is present within a loculated effusion, multiple septations may be seen, resulting in multiple localized air collections or air-fluid levels.

PLEURAL EFFUSION OR ASCITIS

Subpulmonic effusion and pleural fluid in the costophrenic angle can be seen below the lung bases on CT and mimic

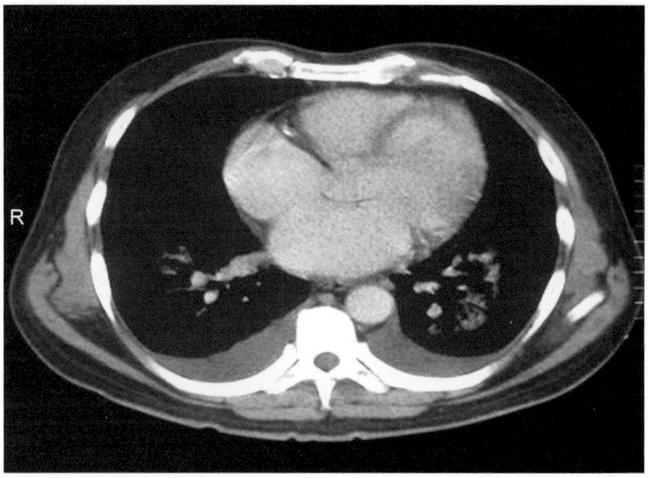

Fig. 15: CT-sickle-shaped opacity seen in dependent location—bilateral pleural effusion.

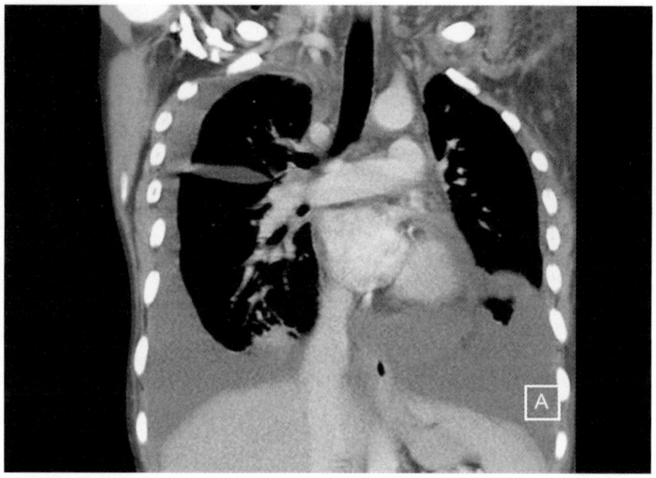

Fig. 16: Coronal MPR—bilateral pleural effusion, also tracking in the horizontal fissure.

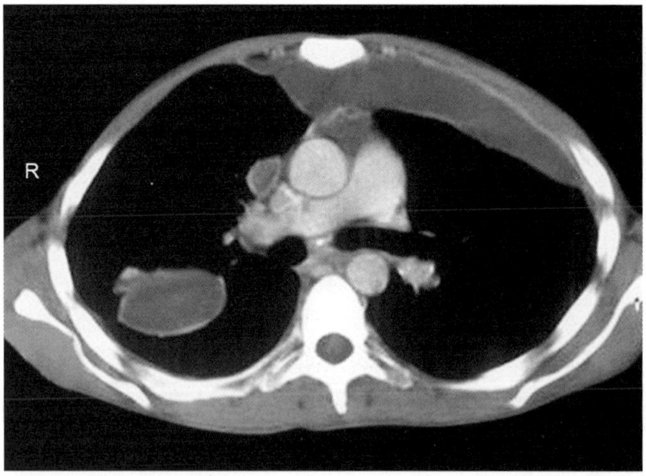

Fig. 17: CECT chest—loculated fluid along the chest wall anteriorly and horizontal fissure.

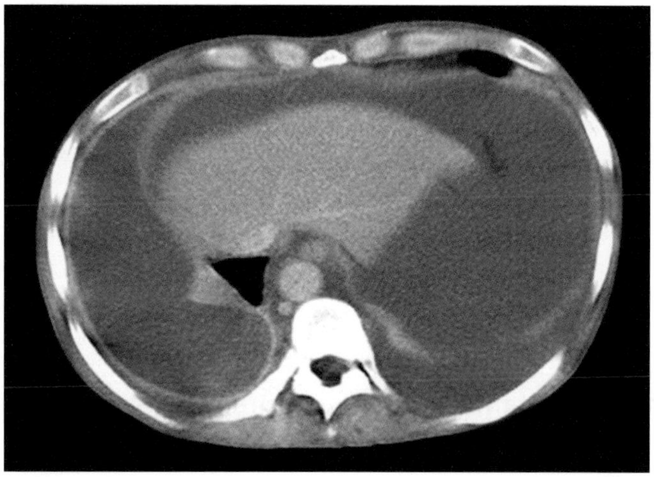

Fig. 18: Pleural effusion and ascitis in the same patient. Pleural fluid is seen medial and posterior and lateral to the crus of the diaphragm. Crus is displaced away from the vertebral body, better appreciated on the left side ascitis does the reverse. The displaced crus and diaphragm sign.

ascites. The parallel curvilinear configuration of the pleura and peritoneal cavities at the level of perihepatic and perisplenic recesses allows fluid in either cavity to appear as a crescentic collection displacing liver or spleen away from the adjacent chest wall. The two can be distinguished by certain signs.[9,10.]

1. **The 'displaced crus' sign**: Pleural fluid collections in the posterior costophrenic angle lie medial and posterior to the diaphragm and causes lateral displacement of the crus—away from adjacent vertebral body, ascitis does the reverse **(Fig. 18)**.
2. **The 'diaphragm sign'**: The most reliable sign to localize fluid is to identify its relationship to the diaphragm, if visible. The diaphragm is seen as uniform curvilinear structure of muscle density, fluid posterior or lateral to the diaphragm is pleural. A large pleural effusion will allow the lower lobe to float anteriorly and lose volume. On CT the posterior edge of the lower lobe, when surrounded by fluid, both anteriorly and posteriorly can appear to represent the diaphragm—pseudo- diaphragm **(Figs. 19A and B)**. On sequential scans at more cephalad levels, the density of atelectatic lower lobe becomes thicker, merges with the rest of lower lobe and often contains air-bronchograms.
3. **The 'bare area sign'**: Ascitic fluid is excluded from the bare area between coronary ligaments on the posterior aspect of the liver as the peritoneal space does not extend into this region.

Pleural fluid can be seen in the entire posterior costophrenic sulcus **(Figs. 20A and B)**.

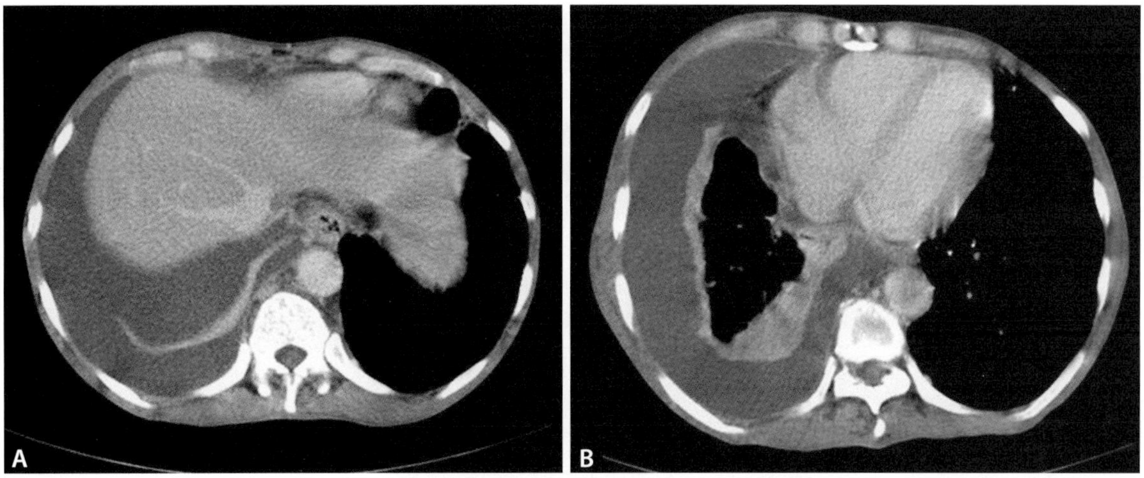

Figs. 19A and B: CT shows posterior edge of the right lower lobe as an arcuate density surrounded by fluid anteriorly and posteriorly resembling the diaphragm: (A) On sequential cephalad scan; (B) This is contiguous with the remainder of the lower lobe.

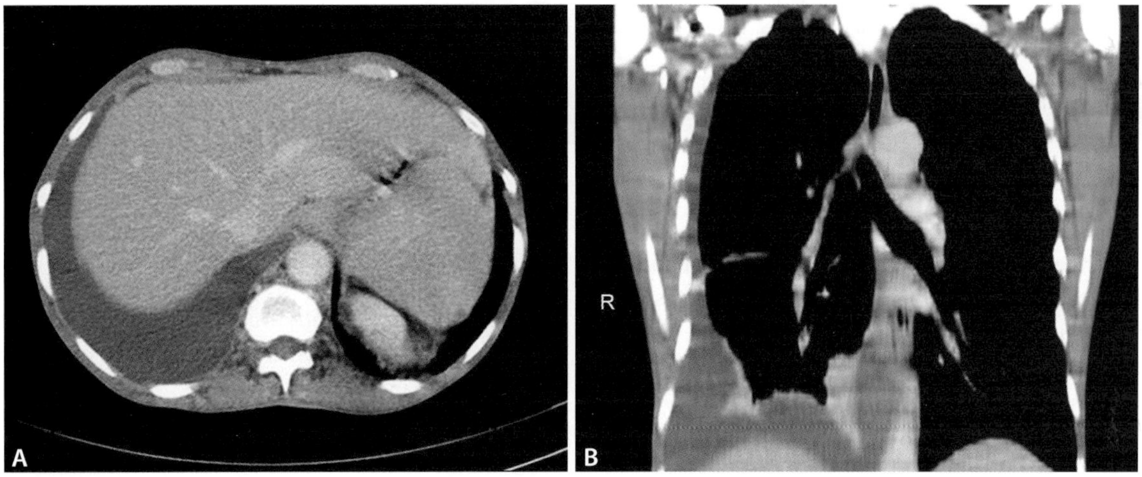

Figs. 20A and B: CT–axial (A), MPR (B), shows the pleural fluid occupying the entire posterior costophrenic sulcus, ascitis is excluded from this space due to lack of peritoneal reflection—bare area sign. Note that the interface with liver is hazy—interface sign.

4. **The 'interface sign'**: Pleural fluid can be distinguished from ascitis by the clarity of the interface of the fluid with diaphragm. With pleural fluid, the interface is hazy, whereas with ascitis it is sharp.

MRI of Pleural Effusion

Pleural fluid has a low signal on T1 and a high signal on T2 weighted images. Exudates give a higher signal than transudates on T2WI. A chylous effusion shows signal intensity similar to subcutaneous fat on T1W images. In the sub acute and chronic stage hematomas show a bright signal on T1WI, surrounded by a dark rim caused by hemosiderin.

MRI may be used to differentiate transudates from exudates. A gradual enhancement on delayed images of malignant pleural effusions after intravenous administration of GD-DTPA, in patients with lung cancer has been reported. Signal enhancement of the pleura indicates the presence of exudates while absence of the same suggests transudate. Non-invasive characterization of pleural effusion by means of DWI with single shot EPI technique may obviate the need for thoracocentesis with its associated patient morbidity. Most transudative effusions are isointense, while exudative effusions are hyperintense on DWI with b factor of 500 and 1000 s/min **(Figs. 21A to E)**. The ADC of exudative effusion is significantly lower than those of transudative effusions. The higher the protein content of pleural fluid, the less is the diffusion. The cellular content of exudates may also contribute to ADC values. At a cut off value of 3.6×10^{-3} mm^2/s, ADC has a sensitivity of 71% and a specificity of 63% for differentiating transudative from exudative effisions.[11,12]

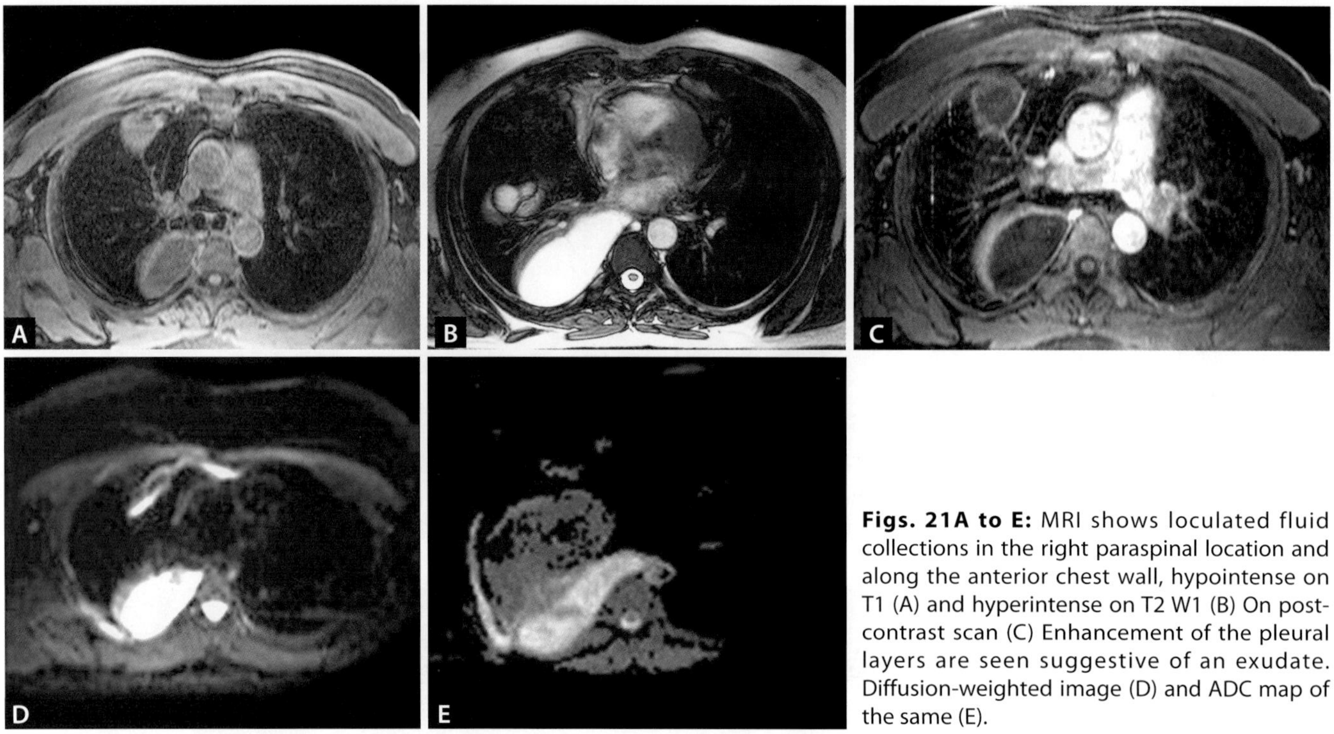

Figs. 21A to E: MRI shows loculated fluid collections in the right paraspinal location and along the anterior chest wall, hypointense on T1 (A) and hyperintense on T2 W1 (B) On post-contrast scan (C) Enhancement of the pleural layers are seen suggestive of an exudate. Diffusion-weighted image (D) and ADC map of the same (E).

Parapneumonic Effusion with Empyema

Pleural fluid accumulates in approximately 40% of patients with pneumonia. This is diagnosed by thoracocentesis and culture of the aspirated fluid. The term 'parapneumonic' effusion is used and it is classified into three stages of empyema. Progression from one stage to another does not necessarily take place.[13-18]

Simple Parapneumonic Effusion (Exudative Stage)

Simple parapneumonic effusion results from increased permeability of the visceral pleura occurring in association with pulmonary inflammation in patients with pneumonia. Effusions in this stage are usually sterile exudates and have a normal glucose level (> 40–60 mg/dL) and pH (>7. 2).They are usually dependent in location, do not show evidence of loculation, show a meniscus on plain radiographs and appear crescent shaped on CT. These usually resolve with antibiotic treatment of the pneumonia.

Empyema (Fibropurulent Stage)

The term empyema is used when a pleural effusion is infected, although the definition necessitates the presence of pus in the pleural space. Although most occur in association with pneumonia, approximately 10% are unassociated with obvious lung disease.

A large percentage of bacterial empyemas result from anaerobic infections. Common anerobic organisms include bacteroides, *Fusobacterium*. Common aerobic organisms are *Staphylococcus aureus*, *Streptococcus pneumoniae*, *Haemophilus influenzae*. Tuberculosis may also result in empyema.

Empyema is characterized by presence of infectious organisms in pleural fluid, increased white blood cells and polymorph nuclear cells, fibrin deposition along the pleural surfaces, a tendency for loculation, decreased glucose levels (<40 mg/dL) and (pH <7. 2) and increased LDH (>1000 IU/L).

In a patient who has pneumonia, presence of localized or loculated pleural effusion strongly suggests the presence of an empyema. On plain radiographs, empyemas often have a lenticular shape and tend to appear larger or better defined in one projection (e.g. frontal) than in other (e.g. lateral). On radiographs, an empyema containing air may be difficult to differentiate from a peripheral lung abscess abutting the chest wall. This distinction can be important to make because empyemas are often treated by tube thoracostomy in addition to systemic antibiotics, whereas most lung abscesses require antibiotics alone.

CT shows characteristic findings of empyema. It is seen in a non-dependent location with an elliptical or lenticular shape, with a sharp demarcation from the adjacent lung; the enhancing visceral and parietal pleural surfaces split apart by the fluid collection giving the-'**split pleura sign**' **(Fig. 22)**.

Empyemas show the thickened pleural layers as smooth and of uniform thickness when enhanced by contrast or outlined by air. Empyemas compress and displace adjacent lung and vessals. In patients with parapneumonic effusion or empyema, extrapleural fat is commonly thickened. The extrapleural fat adjacent to empyema may show increased attenuation with edema of chest wall muscles **(Figs. 23 and 24)**. In contrast to empyemas, lung abscesses are round and poorly defined owing to surrounding pneumonia, have shaggy walls or irregular thickness and tend to obliterate bronchi and vessals **(Figs. 25 and 26)**. The differences between a peripherally located lung abscess and empyema are enumerated in **Table 3**. Malignant neoplasms may arise in the walls of chronic long-standing empyemas, mostly in tubercular cavities. Non-Hodgkin's lymphoma, mesothelioma and rarely sarcoma may occur.

Organization Stage (Pleural Peel)

In patients with chronic empyema ingrowth of fibroblasts and organization can result in extensive pleural fibrosis and the development of an inelastic fibrotic pleural peel or fibrothorax. This can cause lung restriction and decreased lung volume—the trapped lung **(Fig. 27)**. Plain radiographs and CT show smooth pleural thickening. Extrapleural fat thickening is frequently visible on CT,separating the thickened parietal pleura from the intercostal muscle or rib. On CT a fibrothorax is defined as pleural thickening that extends >8 cm in craniocaudal direction, 5 cm laterally and with a thickness equal or more than 3 cm. Focal or extensive calcification is common with a tubercular etiology. Asbestos exposure related fibrothorax is usually bilateral and rarely calcified. An important finding in diagnosing pleural peel is reduction in the volume of the affected hemithorax **(Figs. 28A and B)**. A pleural peel may result from chronic pleural effusion and inflammation in the absence of infection, e. g. in cases of collagen vascular disease, uremia, etc.

Empyema Necessitans

Empyema can involve the chest wall directly and this is called empyema necessitatis or necessitans. Tuberculosis accounts for about 70% of these cases, other organisms like actinomycosis or nocardia have also been implicated. Extensive extrapleural fat thickening, edema and subcutaneous collections of pus can be seen on CT **(Figs. 29A and B)**.

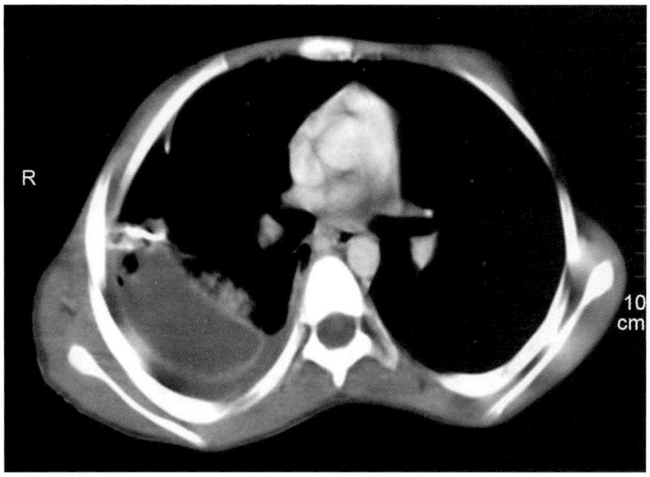

Fig. 22: Empyema CT show loculated collection in the hemithorax with enhancement of the visceral and parietal pleura—split pleura sign.

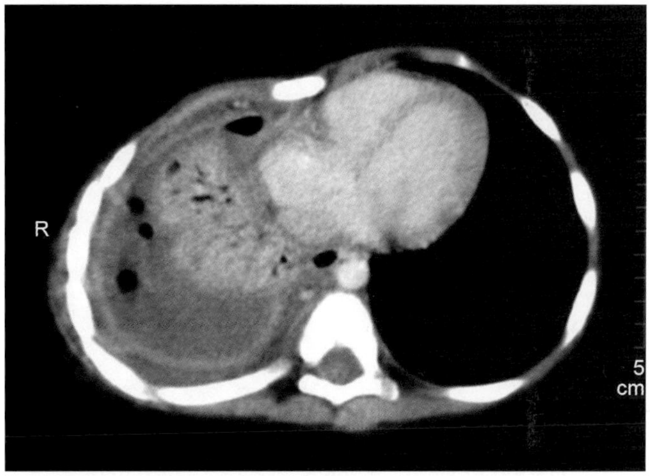

Fig. 23: Thickened enhancing pleura with proliferation of extrapleural fat on the right side. There are air loculi within the pleural cavity (post-intervention). Loss of volume with underlying consolidation is also noted.

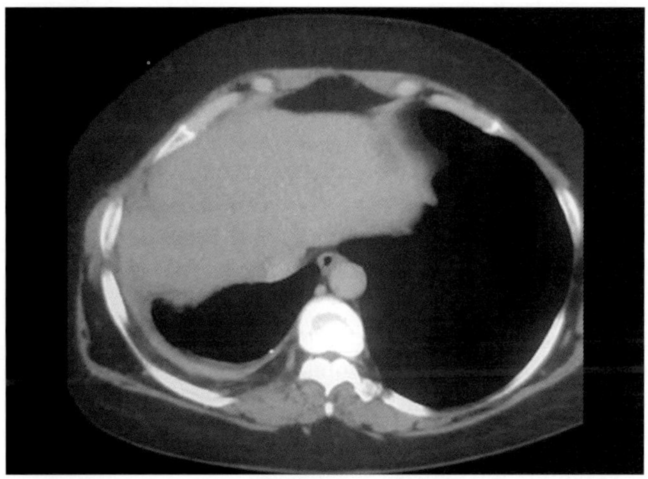

Fig. 24: CT—pleural thickening with proliferation of extrapleural fat.

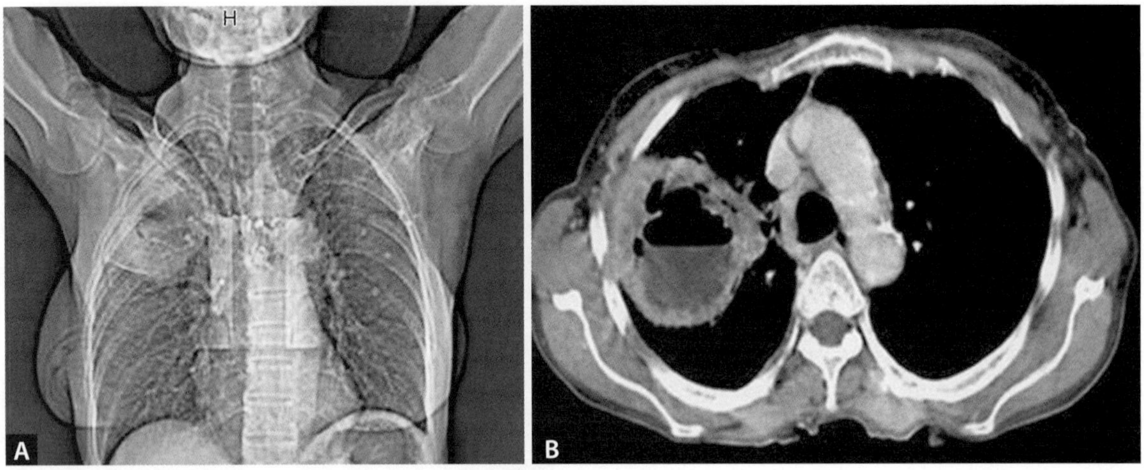

Figs. 25A and B: A large opacity with an air-fluid level with an acute angle with the chest wall with shaggy inner walls—lung abscess.

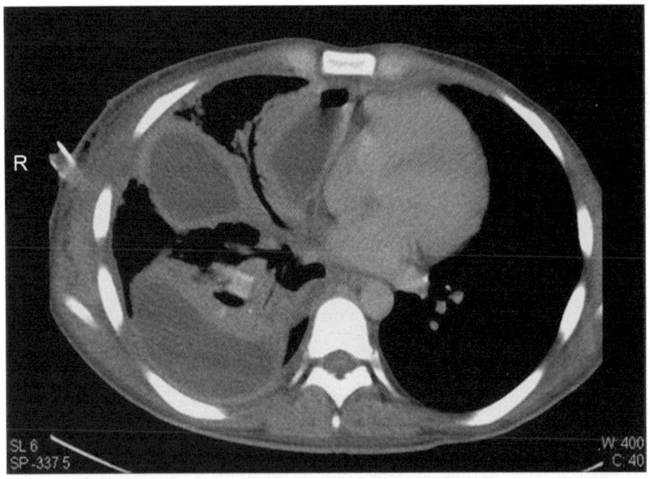

Fig. 26: CT chest—multiple loculated empyemas.

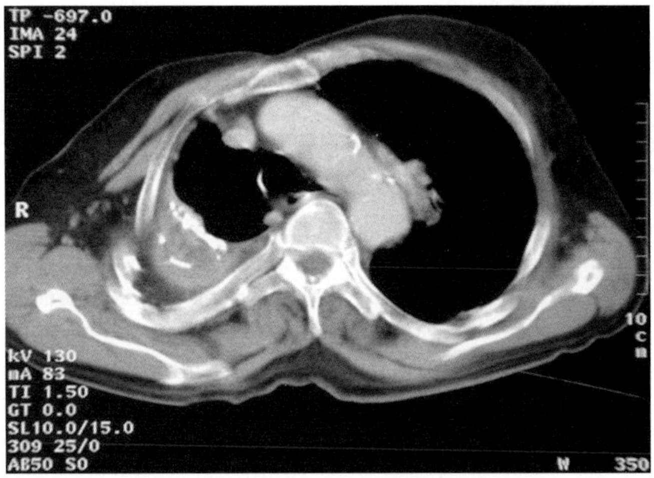

Fig. 27: CECT thorax: Calcified and thickened pleural layers on the right with a fluid collection between them and loss of volume indicative of fibrothorax—tubercular etiology.

Table 3: Differences between empyema and lung abscess.

Empyema	*Lung abscess*
Lenticular shape	Round shape
Uniform enhancing wall	Non-uniform thick wall
Compression of adjacent lung	Non-compression of surrounding lung
Obtuse angle with chest wall	Acute angles with chest wall
Separation of pleural layers	—

Tube Drainage of Empyema

Drainage of empyema is required if there is:

- Thick pus on thoracocentesis
- Positive gram stain
- Positive pleural fluid culture
- Pleural fluid glucose <60 mg/dL
- Pleural fluid pH <7.2
- LDH >1000 IU/L
- No response to antibiotics

Multiple septations within an infected or reactive fluid may be broken down by instillation of fibrinolytic agents such as urokinase. Indications for decortication include persistent sepsis despite appropriate antibiotic therapy and drainage, persistent thick pleural rind that appears to be trapping the underlying lung. CT can be used to determine the adequacy of chest tube drainage, the thickness of the pleural rind, the presence of loculi, and the extent to which the lung is trapped.

After thoracocentesis of a large pleural effusion, the re-expanded lung shows edema which persists for a few days. The lung sometimes fails to expand fully

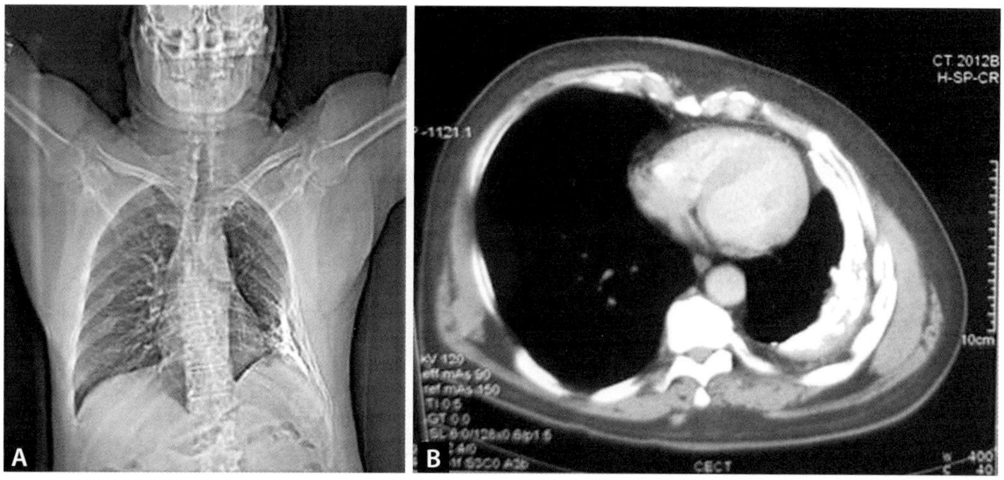

Figs. 28A and B: Chest X-ray (A), CT (B): Loss of volume on the left with extensive pleural thickening with calcification—fibrothorax.

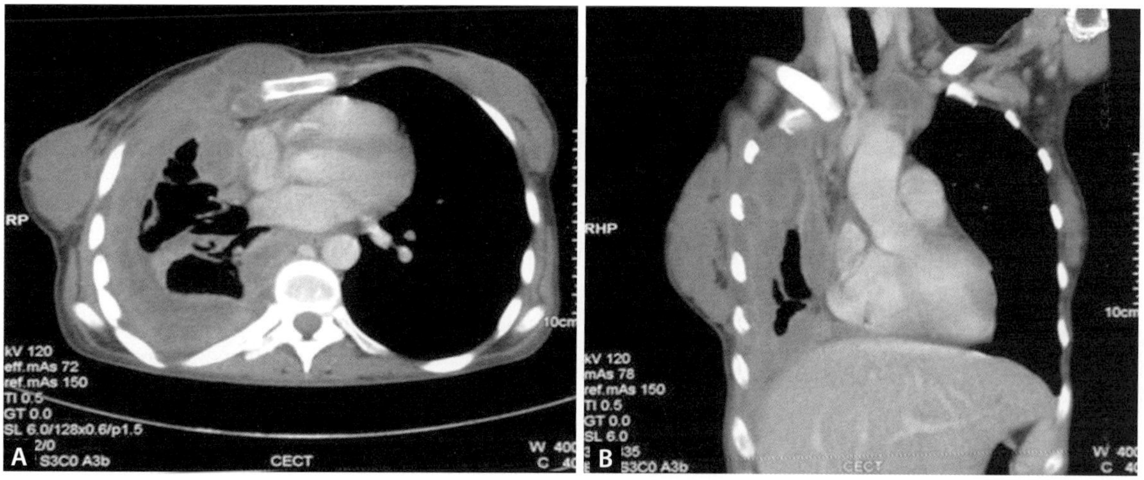

Figs. 29A and B: Empyema with direct extension into chest wall—empyema necessitans.

and a pneumothorax may persist. This usually occurs in patients with malignancy and is known as **"trapped lung"**. Metastatic implants on the visceral pleural surface prevents the lung from expanding. A trapped lung can also occur in cases of chronic empyema when a rind of thickened visceral pleura encases and contracts the underlying lung, preventing re-expansion of the lung despite adequate drainage of the empyema fluid. The other cause of persistent pneumothorax or hydropneumothorax is a bronchopleural fistula.

BRONCHOPLEURAL FISTULA

Bronchopleural fistula (BPF) is a communication between the pleural cavity and the bronchial tree. A parenchymal pleural fistula (PPF) refers to a fistula between pleura and parenchyma lung. In both these conditions there is a pneumothorax not attributable to trauma. Bronchopleural fistula results from rupture of the visceral pleura with a direct communication with the airway. It may occur following trauma or surgery or in association with necrotizing infections—empyema, TB, septic embolus and infected pulmonary infarct. Gas within a pleural fluid collection, in absence of a recent thoracocentesis is a presumptive evidence of empyema and BPF. It differs from pneumothorax in that the communication with the pleural space is via airways rather than the distal air spaces **(Figs. 30A and B)**. MDCT can detect bronchopleural fistula with the same or superior sensitivity as bronchoscopy **(Fig. 31)**.[19]

Postsurgical BPF

Following an uncomplicated pneumonectomy, the residual space contains air and fluid and there is ipsilateral mediastinal shift and elevation of the hemidiaphragm.

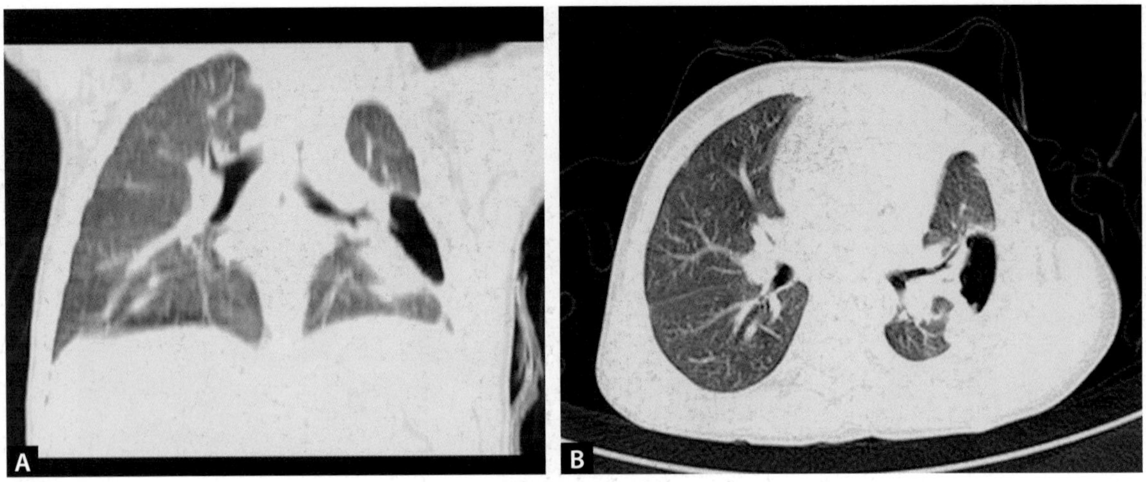

Figs. 30A and B: CT chest shows a loculated air containing space in the left pleural cavity that was not draining completely. A segmental bronchus is seen in close proximity to it—bronchopleural fistula.

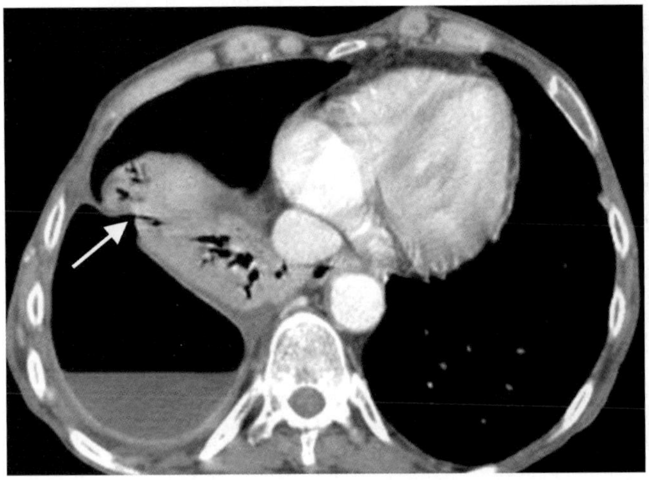

Fig. 31: CT chest-bronchus in communication with a hydropneumothorax—bronchopleural fistula.

Over 2–4 months, there is gradual resorption of air and increasing fluid accumulation, followed by organization and progressive movement of the mediastinum and hemidiaphragm, leading to obliteration of the space. BPF arises as an early complication, usually develops 7–10 days later with clinical deterioration, pneumonia, hemopytsis and the sudden expectoration of fluid and a persistent large air leak from the pleural drain. The diagnosis is made radiologically by the following signs:

- Return of the mediastinum to the midline.
- Presence of increasing air and decreasing fluid in the pneumonectomy space.
- Contralateral aspiration pneumonitis. If less than the whole lung has been removed, the main radiological sign is the sudden appearance of air-fluid level within the pleural space.

The delayed appearance of a fistula (>6 months after surgery) means tumor recurrence and is signaled by the appearance of air in the previously air free post-pneumonectomy space.

Infective BPF

This occurs in the setting of necrotizing pulmonary infection and is heralded by the appearance of an air-fluid level in the pleural cavity. The mimickers can be air introduced at thoracocentesis, pleuroesophageal fistula, herniated bowel and a subdiaphragmatic abscess.

PLEURAL THICKENING

Pleural thickening results as an end stage of infective or non-infective (e.g. asbestosis) processes. Generalized and gross pleural thickening is termed as **fibrothorax** and may cause significant ventilatory impairment.

On a chest radiograph pleural thickening appears as a fixed shadow of water density, most commonly located at the dependent parts of the pleural cavity **(Fig. 32)**. En profile it appears as a band of soft tissue density, with a sharp interface with the lung. Enface it is seen as an ill-defined veil like shadowing. Blunting of the costophrenic angle and tenting of the diaphragm are noted (On USG, benign pleural thickening is seen as homogeneous echogenic layer inside the chest wall **(Fig. 33)**. Pleural thickening, visible on radiographs and CT primarily affect the parietal pleura **(Table 4)**. On CT, it is seen as:

- A stripe of soft tissue density 1 mm more in thickness, internal to the ribs.
- A stripe of soft tissue density 1 mm or more in thickness, internal to the innermost intercostal muscle and separated from it by a thin layer of extrapleural fat.

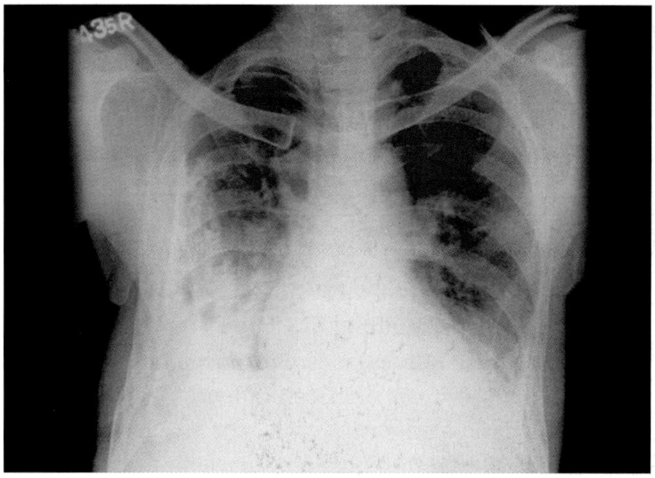

Fig. 32: Chest radiograph—diffuse pleural thickening bilaterally with calcification.

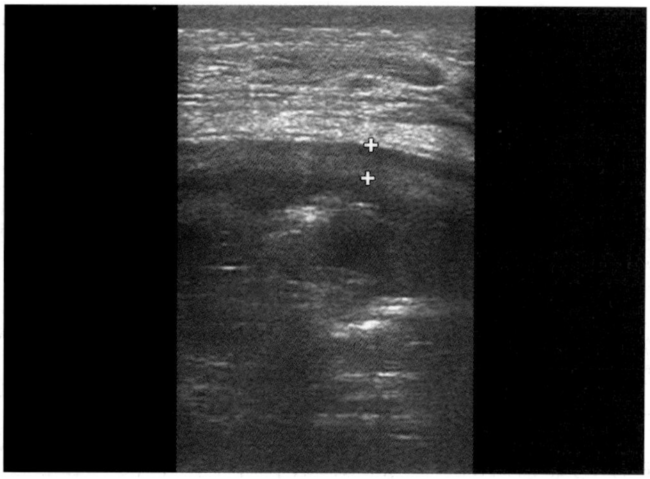

Fig. 33: Ultrasound chest—pleural thickening with minimal effusion.

Table 4: Pleural thickening—criteria.

• A stripe of soft tissue density 1 mm more in thickness, internal to the ribs or innermost intercostal muscle
• A distinct stripe in the paravertebral region >1 mm thickness
• Thickening of the normal extrapleural fat layer

- A distinct stripe in the paravertebral region 1 mm or more in thickness.
- Thickening of the normal extrapleural fat layer.

Diffuse pleural thickening may be seen unilaterally or bilaterally. The radiographic criteria used for diffuse pleural thickening are coverage of at least 25% of the total chest wall on a chest radiograph (50% if unilateral); and it must extend to a thickness of at least 5 mm in at least one site on the chest radiograph. [20]

CT criteria of diffuse pleural thickening includes, a continuous sheet of pleural thickening more than 5 cm wide, more than 8 cm in craniocaudal extent, and more than 3 mm thick.[21]

Visceral Pleural Thickening

This occurs almost always in association with parietal pleural thickening and effusion, empyema being the most common cause. Visceral pleural thickening alone is uncommon and may be seen in patients with lung disease, such as abscess or fibrosis. Visceral pleural thickening cannot be distinguished from parietal pleural thickening on chest radiographs, although it may appear as:

- Thickening of a fissure
- Separation of lung from adjacent ribs and chest wall, which may occur in association with contiguous lung disease. Both these signs may be seen in pleural effusions.

On CT, visceral pleural thickening may appear as either of the following:

- A distinct stripe of soft tissue at the lung surface in patients with pleural effusion and normal lung parenchyma.
- An enhancing stripe at the lung surface in patients with abnormal lung. Thickened visceral pleura enhances more than airless lung.

Pleural Apical Cap and Fibrous Thickening

Fibrous pleural thickening is common at the lung apex.[22] This may be secondary to tuberculosis or represent age related changes of unknown etiology. Apical caps may have a scalloped contour or be associated with tenting towards the lung **(Fig. 34)**. They can be unilateral or bilateral. Apical pleural caps need to be differentiated from companion shadows of upper ribs and from extrapleural fat.

Mimics of Pleural thickening

Normal structures may mimic the findings of pleural thickening or effusion.

Normal fat pads: Normal extrapleural fat is most abundant over the posterolateral 4th–8th ribs and can be several mm thick that extend into the intercostal space. In contrast to pleural thickening or effusion, normal fat thickening is typically symmetrical, smooth in contour, low in attenuation and unassociated with costophrenic angle blunting. On CT, extrapleural fat appears very low in density.

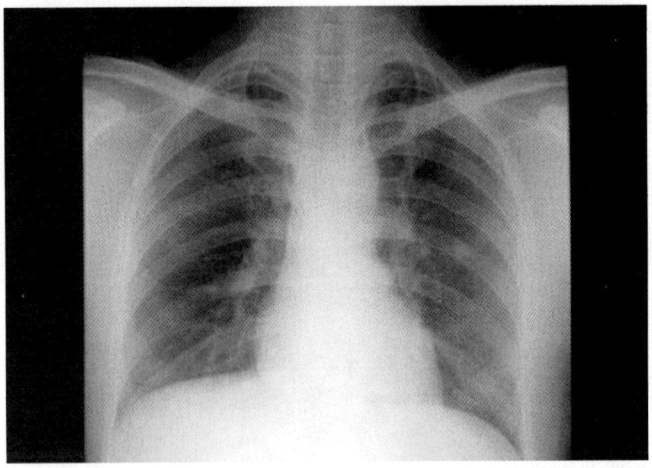

Fig. 34: Right pleural apical cap with soft opacities in left mid zone.

The subcostalis and transversus thoracis muscles: These are not seen on chest radiograph. On CT, a 1 to 2 mm thick line is seen internal to one or more ribs, along the posterior chest wall at the level of heart, representing the subcostalis muscle. Anteriorly, at the level of heart, adjacent to lower sternum or xiphoid process, the transversus thoracis muscle is nearly always visible on CT, internal to the anterior ends of ribs or costal cartilages. These muscles are smooth, uniform in thickness and bilateral.

Paravertebral intercostal veins: They may sometimes be seen in the paravertebral regions. Continuity of these opacities with azygous or hemiazygous veins may be visible these do not indent the lung surface, as pleural thickening would.

PLEURA AND ASBESTOSIS[23,24]

Asbestos-related neoplastic and nonneoplastic diseases of the lungs and pleura range from pleural effusion and pleural plaques to lung cancer and malignant mesothelioma. Pleural effusions are typically hemorrhagic exudates of mixed cellularity but do not typically contain asbestos bodies.

Pleural plaques are the most common manifestation of asbestos inhalation and occur 20–30 years after first exposure. Pleural plaques are seen in 3–14% of dockyard workers and in 58% of insulation workers. The pathogenesis of plaques is uncertain, but is postulated that fibers reach the pleura via lymphatic channels and cause an inflammatory response, which in turn leads to hyaline fibrosis along the parietal pleural surface. They usually arise from the parietal pleura but may arise from the visceral pleura. Plaques are seen over the diaphragmatic dome and the undersurface of the lower posterolateral ribs. Diagnosis is usually by chest-X-ray. The diameter of the plaques can vary from several millimeters to 10 cm. Any pleural or pericardial surface can be affected, but asbestos-related pleural plaques are usually in the lower 2/3 of the thorax and are bilateral. Calcification most often affects the parietal and diaphragmatic pleura (virtually pathognomonic) and spares the costophrenic sulci and apices **(Figs. 35A and B)**. The size and number are variable. Calcification may be the only evidence of exposure. Dense pleural fibrosis surrounding the entire lung and >1 cm in thickness can also follow asbestos exposure. It results from thickening and fibrosis of visceral pleura, which leads to fusion with parietal pleura.

Patients with pleural plaques are asymptomatic, there is no risk of malignant degeneration, but patients with pleural plaques may have an increased risk of developing mesothelioma and bronchogenic carcinoma compared with a control population matched for exposure but without pleural plaques. The plaques are most useful as a marker of asbestos exposure.

ASBESTOSIS PSEUDOTUMOR (ROUND ATELECTASIS)

The pathogenesis is thought to be due to an inflammatory reaction and fibrosis in the superficial layer of pleura. As the fibrous tissue matures, it contracts, causing pleura to fold into the lung, which in turn causes the atelectasis.

Chest radiograph shows a rounded peripheral "mass" with or without lung distortion. The CT features are of a round or oval mass that abuts the pleura, a "comet tail" of bronchovascular structures going into the mass, and thickening of the adjacent pleura. USG may show an echogenic line that extends into the mass from the pleura, representing the scarred invaginated visceral pleura **(Figs. 36A and B)**.

MRI shows a curved low signal intensity line caused by thickened indentation of visceral pleura. The main differential is malignancy of the lung. Stability or shrinkage of the mass with time suggests benignancy, but biopsy may be required.

PLEURAL CALCIFICATION

This is seen following asbestos exposure, empyema, tuberculosis, hemothorax. In the later two conditions calcification is irregular and resembles a plaque **(Figs. 37A and B)** or sheet and is contained within thickened pleura. It may occur anywhere but is most common in the lower posterior half of chest and is usually unilateral. Following tubercular empyema both parietal

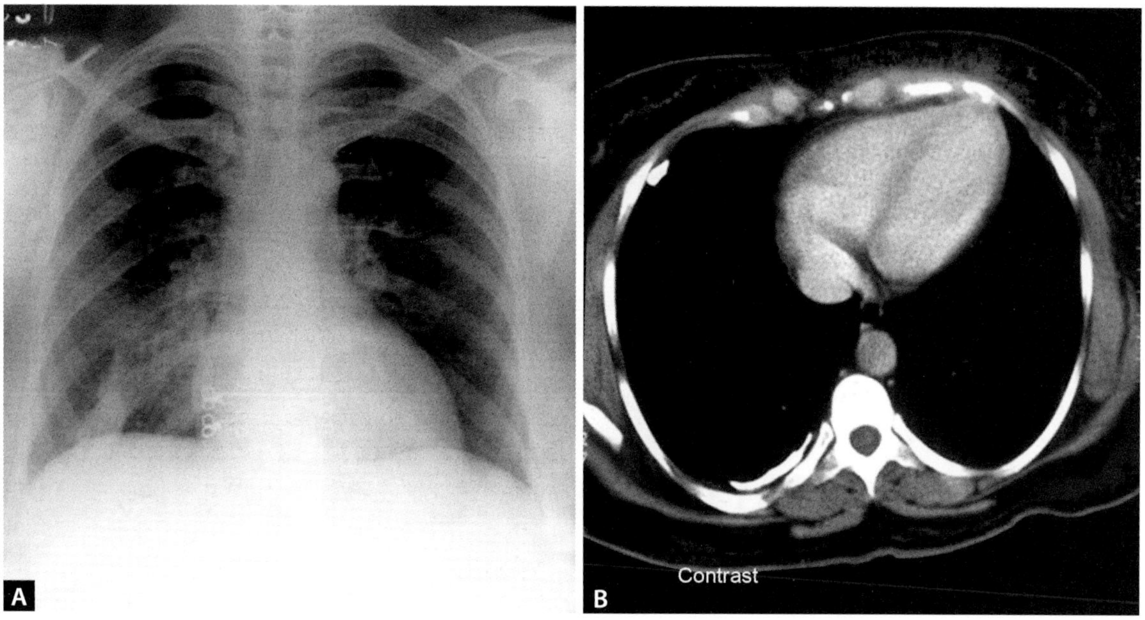

Figs. 35A and B: (A) X-ray chest—calcified pleural plaque on the right side; (B) CT chest—calcified pleural plaque seen in the right costal pleura and posteriorly along paraspinal gutter in a patient with history of asbestos exposure.

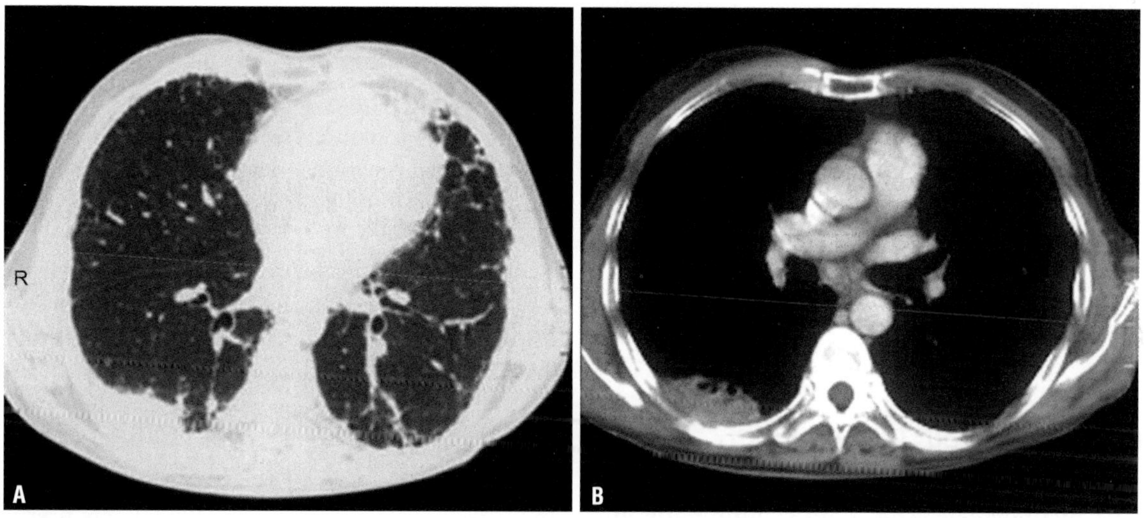

Figs. 36A and B: CT chest shows a peripherally based opacity on the right side with vessels curling up to it—round atelectasis.

and visceral pleura may be calcified. These layers are separated by a soft tissue opacity that may contain fluid for many years.

PNEUMOTHORAX

Air within the pleural cavities is referred to as pneumothorax. It is classified as spontaneous or traumatic. The causes of pneumthorax are summarized in **Table 5**.

Spontaneous Pneumothorax

These are classified as primary or secondary.

Primary Spontaneous Pneumothorax

It occurs without an antecedent cause in an otherwise healthy patient. It often occurs at rest, as a result of rupture of an apical subpleural bulla. The peak incidence is in young patients (20–40 years), men (80%), tall and thin patients and smokers (90%). Pain is common and a small pleural effusion is present in 10–20% manifested as an air-fluid level. It may be asymptomatic and detected incidentally. These patients are at increased risk of another pneumothorax.

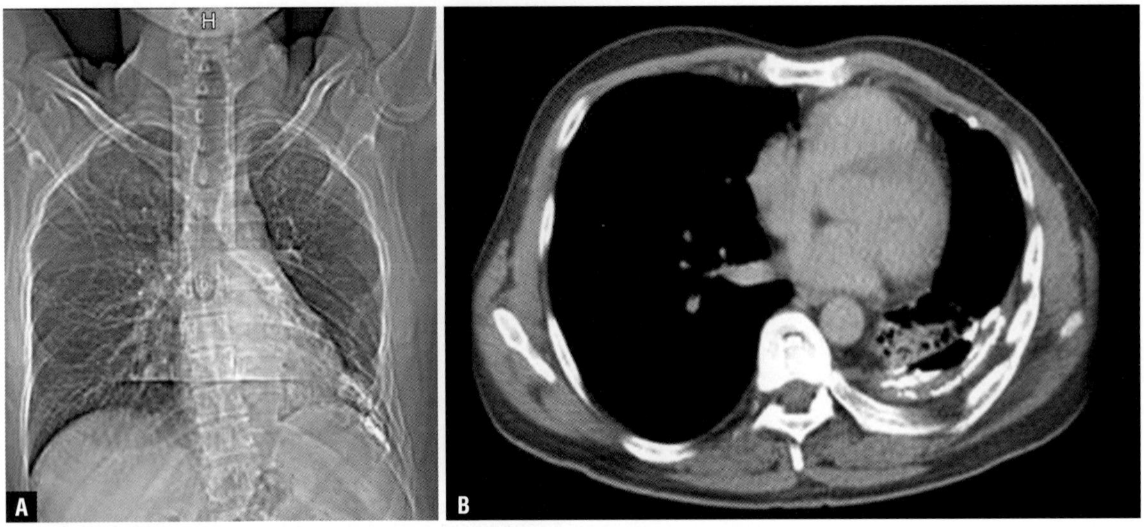

Figs. 37A and B: (A) Chest scanogram; (B) CT—pleural calcification with loss of volume—post-tubercular.

Table 5: Causes of pneumothorax in adult.

Spontaneous
• Primary spontaneous
• *Secondary spontaneous*: – Airflow obstruction—asthma, COPD, cystic fibrosis – Pulmonary infection—cavitary pneumonia, tuberculosis, fungal disease, AIDS, pneumatocele – Pulmonary infarction – Neoplasm—metastatic sarcoma – Diffuse lung disease—histiocytosis X lymphangioleiomyomatosis – Endometriosis (catamenial pneumothorax)
Traumatic
• Non-iatrogenic—ruptured esophagus/trachea, closed chest trauma (± rib fracture), penetrating chest trauma
• Iatrogenic—thoracotomy/thoracocentesis, percutaneous biopsy, tracheostomy, central venous catheterization

Secondary Spontaneous Pneumothorax

Occurs due to an underlying disease such as COPD, Langerhans histiocytosis. These are symptomatic and have a high recurrence rate.

Pneumothorax Ex-Vacuo

It is a rare cause of secondary spontaneous pneumothorax, occurring in patients with acute lobar collapse due to bronchial obstruction. Sudden collapse results in rapid decrease in intrapleural pressure adjacent to the collapsed lobe. This leads to gas, entering the pleural space. The resulting pneumothorax is seen adjacent to the collapsed lung.

Traumatic Pneumothorax

It can be caused by chest trauma (penetrating/non-penetrating, accidental or iatrogenic) or in patients on mechanical ventilation. Pneumothoraces with mechanical ventilation (due to high ventilator pressures) occurs due to alveolar rupture leading to interstitial emphysema, pneumomediastinum and rupture of pneumomediastinum into pleural subpleural location. Traumatic pneumothorax requires chest tube drainage.

Catamenial Pneumothorax

Pneumothorax, coincident with menstruation is rare. The symptoms start within 48 hours of onset of menses. Air may reach the peritoneum via vagina, uterus or the fallopian tubes. From there it may enter the pleural space via defect or diaphragm, common on the right. Endometrial implants may enter the pleural space by the same route. Endometrial implants involve visceral space and peripheral lung; the breakdown may result in pneumothorax.

IMAGING FINDINGS OF PNEUMOTHORAX

Radiograph

In an ***upright patient*** air usually collects first above the lung apex. The presence of a visible visceral pleural line is a key to diagnosis. This is visible as a very thin line at the pleural space with an avascular space above or lateral to it and one in the lung below and medial to it **(Figs. 38 and 39)**. Air may enter the fissure, outlining its pleural surface. In absence of underlying lung disease or adhesions; the partially collapsed lung maintains its normal shape. Lung markings are not seen peripheral to the pleural line. The visibility of pneumothorax is accentuated on expiration as there is increase in volume. Expiratory film or decubitus view with suspected side uppermost may demonstrate a small pneumothorax. Skin folds, hair, clothing, etc. may mimic the walls of bulla and visceral pleural line

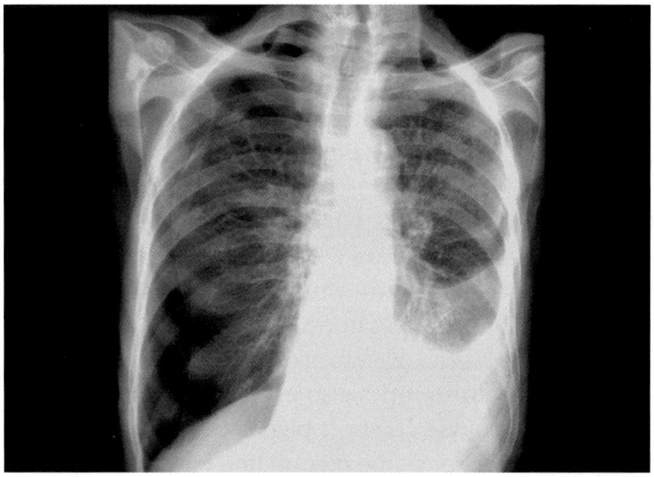

Fig. 38: Right-sided pneumothorax seen on chest skiagram as an avascular space, bounded by the visceral pleural line. Left pleural effusion is also seen.

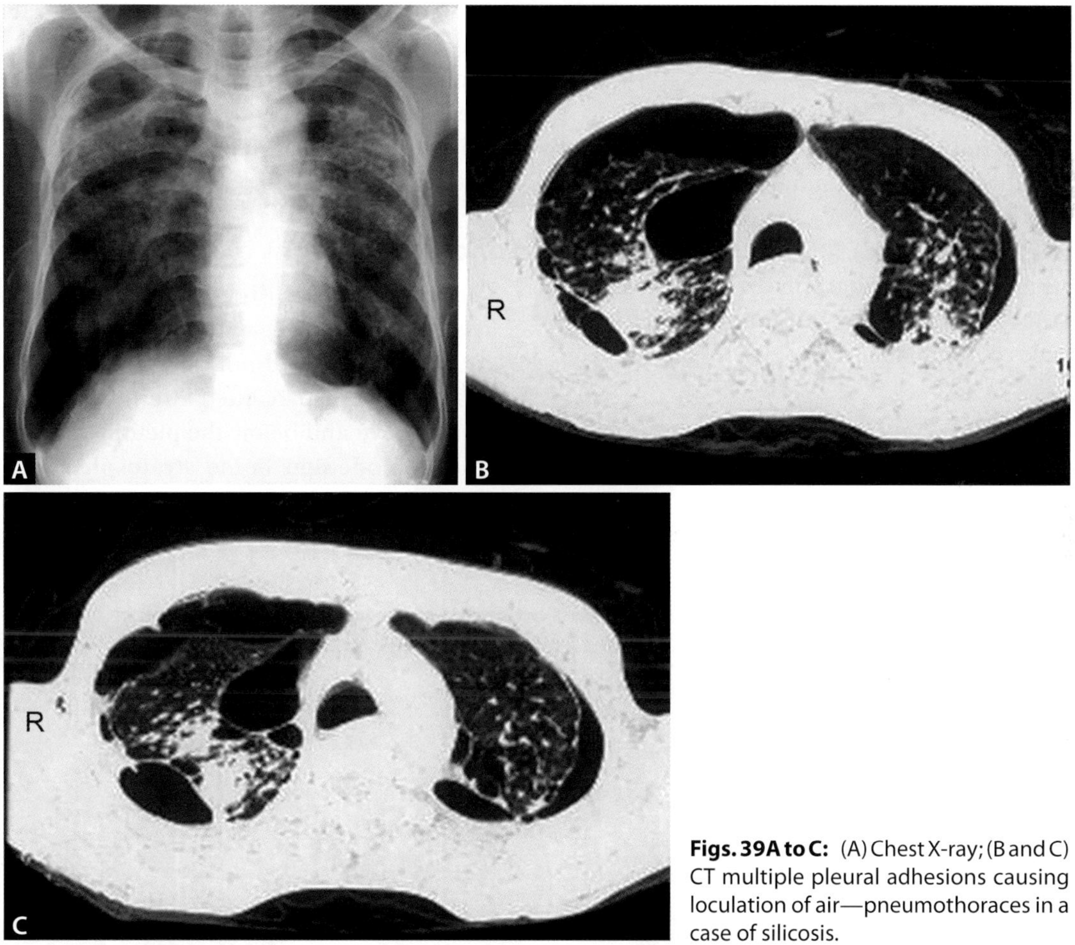

Figs. 39A to C: (A) Chest X-ray; (B and C) CT multiple pleural adhesions causing loculation of air—pneumothoraces in a case of silicosis.

of pneumothorax. Artefacts and skin folds can be distinguished from pneumothorax by extension of these beyond margin of chest cavity laterally located vessels. The margin of the skin fold is usually wider than the thin line of the visceral pleura. A repeat radiograph or an expiratory radiograph may be required in certain situation.

Distinction of a bulla from a pneumothorax is usually based on shape. Pneumothoraces are typically crescent shaped and taper towards the lung base. Bullae are rounded and have inner margin concave to the chest wall and do not conform to the costophrenic angle when they are at the lung base.

In ***supine patients***, free pneumothorax usually collects within the anterior pleural space. A visceral pleural line may be seen medially in some patients mimicking a pneumomediastinum. Pneumothorax in a supine patient may be inferred by the following:

- **Deep sulcus sign**: Costophrenic angle may appear abnormally deep and lucent because of air in the anterolateral pleural space **(Figs. 40 and 41)**.[25]
- **Increased lucency over the chest wall and abdomen**
- Visualization of the anterior costophrenic angle as an edge separate from the diaphragm, but parallel to it—**the double diaphragm sign.**
- **Increased sharpness of the hemi-diaphragm, cardiac border or mediastinum** (because it is outlined by air)
- A lumpy appearance at the cardiac apex, due to alteration in the shape of the epicardial fat pat.
- Air in the minor fissure.

Ultrasonography in Pneumothorax

Ultrasound is now routinely used to detect pneumothorax in emergency settings. Standard lung views are now part of **E-Fast ultrasound (Extended - focussed assessment with Sonography in trauma)**.[26] Ultrasound has higher sensitivity than chest radiograph in the diagnosis of pneumothorax, especially in identifying occult pneumothoraces of traumatic origin.

Technique of Ultrasound to Detect Pneumothorax[27,28]

A high frequency linear probe is used for analysing superficial structure such as pleura. Patients are scanned in supine positions, with the probe placed on the anterior chest wall in a sagittal plane at the 2nd intercostal space in the mid clavicular line. Two adjacent ribs are indentified by posterior shadowing behind them and bright hyperechoic pleural line in between them. This is termed the **'bat sign' (Fig. 42)**. In the supine position air rises to least dependent part of chest which is anteriorly. In a normal lung the visceral pleura will glide in a to and fro pattern over the parietal pleura with respiration. This is seen on dynamic ultrasound as horizontal sliding movement of pleural line, best seen over apex of lung.

M-mode is also used to detect this sliding movement. M-mode cursor is placed over the pleural line. The chest wall above the pleural line forms horizontal—the 'waves' and sliding pleural line forms a granular pattern—the 'Sand'. The resultant image of motionless chest wall and sliding pleura is **seashore sign (Fig. 43)**.

Reverberation artifacts are also seen as hyperechoic vertical lines that extend from pleura to edge of screen without fading. These are seen due to acoustic impendence differences.

Sonographic Signs of Pneumothorax

- **Absence of lung sliding in presence of pneumothorax**, visualized pleura will not be identified and movement of pleural line will not be present.[29,30] The M-mode tracing will display one pattern of parallel horizontal lines above and below the pleural line. This is termed the **'barcode sign'** or the **'stratosphere sign'**. **(Fig. 44)** This is an important sign as it has a negative predictive value of almost 100%. Presence of sliding sign rules

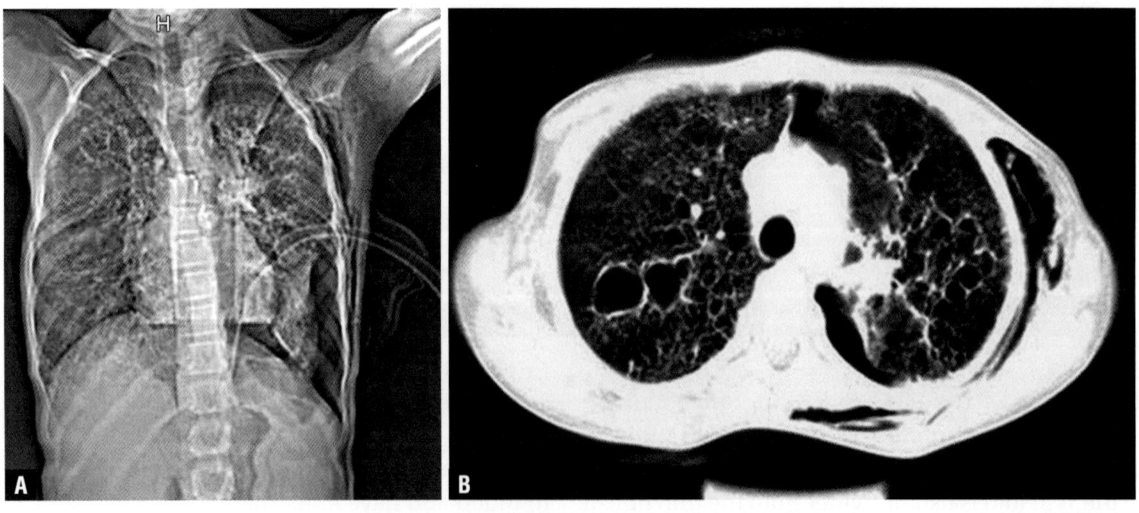

Figs. 40A and B: CT- topogram (A) demonstrates the deep costophrenic sulcus on the left and clarity of the left hemidiaphragm due to pneumothorax in a patient of lymhangioleiomyomatosis (B).

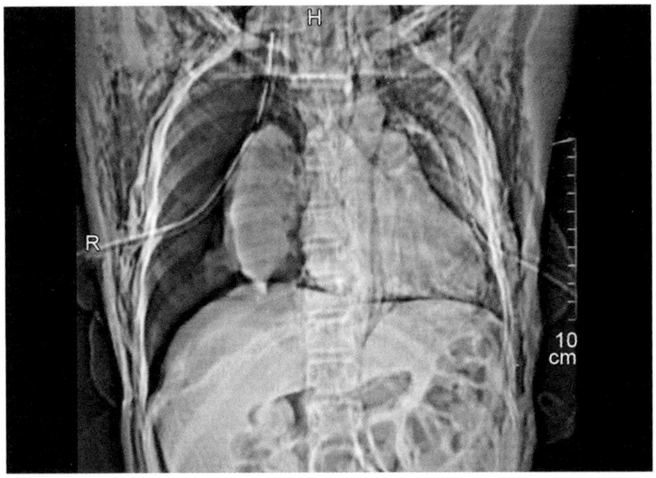

Fig. 41: Scanogram—traumatic pneumothorax. Note the clarity of the diaphragm and the deep costophrenic sulcus on the right side.

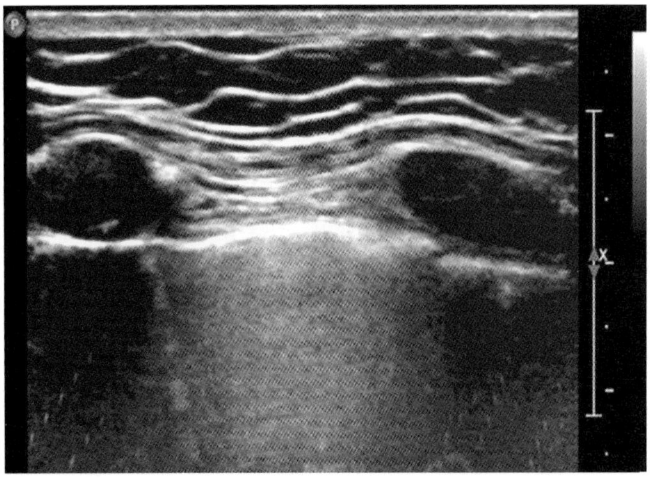

Fig. 42: Ultrasound chest transverse view intercostal approach—bright pleural line identified between two ribs-bat sign.

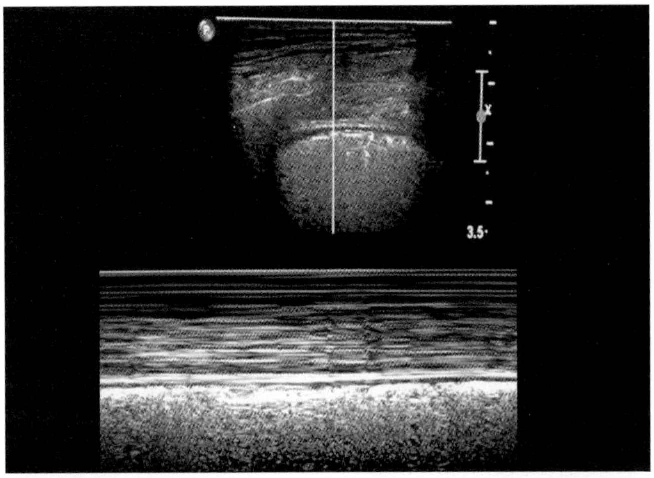

Fig. 43: M-mode—The chest wall above the pleural line forms horizontal —the'waves' and sliding pleural line forms a granular pattern—the 'Sand'-seashore sign.

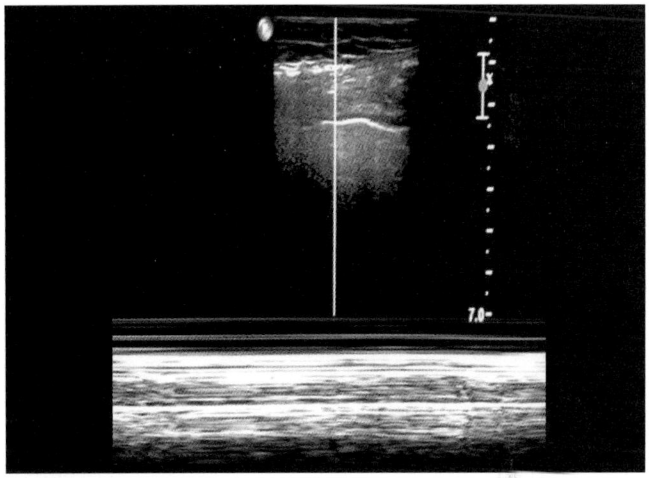

Fig. 44: M-mode tracing displays one pattern of parallel horizontal lines above and below the pleural line—'barcode sign' or the' stratosphere sign'.

out pneumothorax. Absence of lung sliding may be seen in other conditions like adult respiratoy distress syndrome, pulmonary fibrosis, etc.

Comet tail artifacts or B lines: These reverberation artifacts will be absent in pneumothorax. This is due to presence of air which does not allow sound to propagate. The negative predictive value of this sign is 98–100%.

- **Lung point sign:**[30] This indicates the border of pneumothorax and is useful to assess the size of pneumothorax which has therapeutic implications. At this point sliding and non-sliding lung will be seen together. On M-mode alternate seashore and barcode pattern will be seen. The probe is slowly moved from anterior part to lateral or posterior chest to locate the lung point. The more lateral this point is, the bigger is the pneumothorax.
- **Power slide sign:**[31,32] Power Doppler is sometimes used to detect sliding movement. This requires the probe to be steady and patient motionless to avoid artefacts. Absence of sliding indicates pneumothorax **(Fig. 45)**.

Computed Tomography

CT is extremely sensitive to the presence of air in pleural cavity. Lung Window settings should be used to detect pneumothorax. A pneumothorax is imaged as air in the pleural space outside the lung and visceral pleura **(Fig. 46)**. CT can be used to distinguish bullae from a

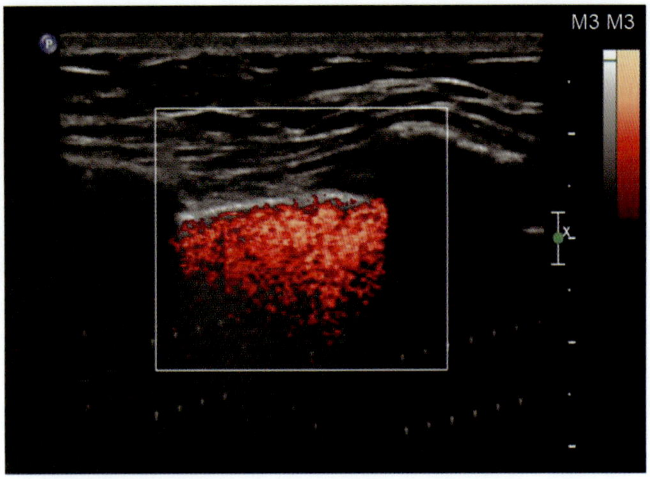

Fig. 45: Power Doppler—depicting normal sliding motion of lung. Absence of this sliding is seen in pneumothorax.

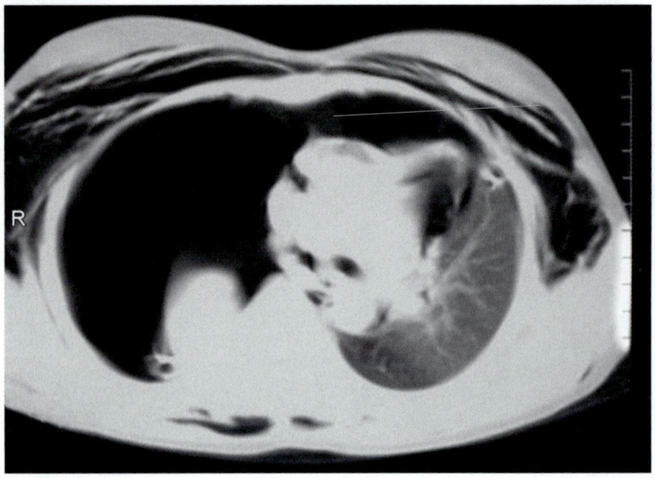

Fig. 46: Large right pneumothorax with passive collapse of the underlying lung, mediastinal shift to the opposite side. Extensive subcutaneous emphysema noted secondary to tube placement.

pneumothorax. Differentiating a medial pneumothorax from a pneumomediastinum may be difficult.

Tension Pneumothorax

This is a life-threatening emergency. It occurs when the pressure in pleural air exceeds atmospheric pressure for a significant part of the respiratory cycle. Tension has an adverse effect on gas exchange and cardiovascular performance causing a rapid deterioration in the patient's condition. It is most often seen in mechanically ventilated patients or in patients of chest trauma.

Tension pneumothorax is difficult to diagnose on chest radiographs **(Table 6)**. Shift of mediastinum away from side of pneumothorax may be seen in any large pneumothorax **(Fig. 47)**. Combination of this with clinical symptom of circulatory compromise is diagnostic. Downward displacement or inversion of hemidiaphragm, is a reliable sign of tension especially in a ventilated patient in whom mediastinal shift is absent. The condition must be urgently treated by immediate decompression of the pleural space.

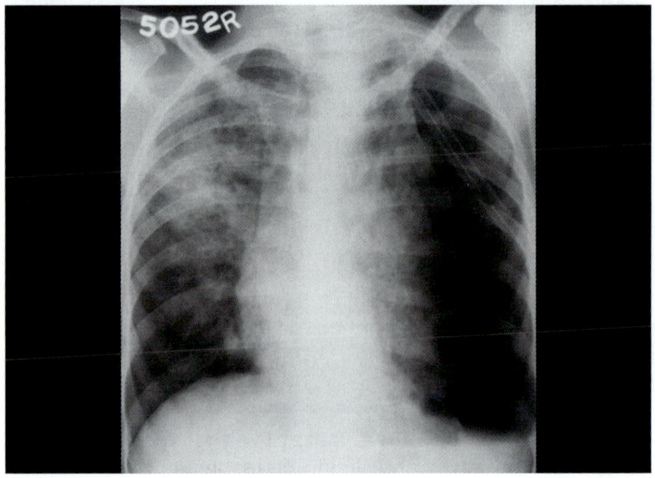

Fig. 47: X-ray chest—infiltrative opacities right uppper and mid zone, with left-sided pneumothorax—shift of the mediastinum to the right and flattening of left hemidiaphragm—tension pneumothorax.

Table 6: Tension pneumothorax.

Clinical diagnosis
Life threatening—immediate decompression required
Suggestive radiographic signs:
• Contralateral displacement of mediastinum
• Inferior displacement of the diaphragm
• Hyperlucent hemithorax
• Ipsilateral collapse

Size of Pneumothorax

A large pneumothorax may be differentiated from a small pneumothorax by the presence of a visible rim of more than 2 cm between lung margin and the chest wall at the level of the hilum. Pneumothorax may be calculated as percentage of the pleural space[33] as shown in **Figure 48**. A pneumothorax of >30% is generally considered to require treatment.

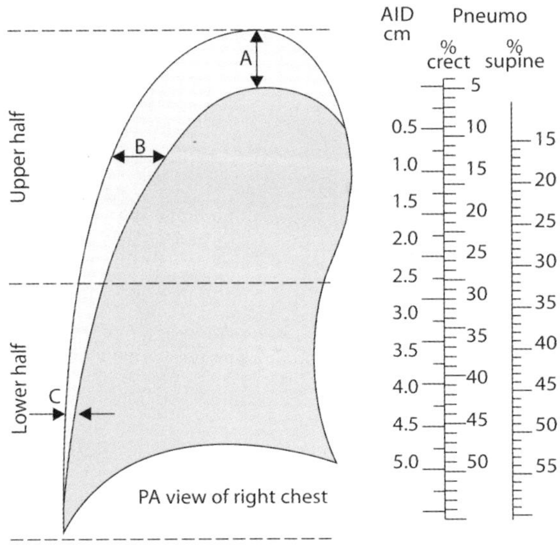

Fig. 48: Illustration depicting the calculation of size of pneumothorax. A = Maximum apical interpleural distance, B = interpleural distance at the midpoint of upper half of lung, C = interpleural distance at the midpoint of lower half of lung. Average interpleural distance AID = A+B+C/3 in cm.

PLEURAL NEOPLASM

The pleura may be involved by primary tumor or one of several metastatic neoplasms. **Metastatic disease is the most common pleural neoplasm.**[34]

Pleural neoplasm may present as pleural effusion or pleural thickening/mass.

Pleural Effusion

A malignant effusion is secondary to pleural involvement by tumor and contains malignant cells. Exudative effusion in patients with malignancy can reflect lymphatic or pulmonary venous obstructions by tumor or pneumonia. The most common causes are metastasis from lung cancer and breast cancer. Pleural fluid cytology is positive in 80–90% cases. Demonstration of tumor cells in pleural fluid is difficult but when present renders the primary disease as unresectable. Regardless of the cause, exudative effusions in a cancer patient requires treatment by drainage.

Pleural Thickening

Pleural thickening, in a patient of cancer with pleural effusion indicates the presence of exudates. Pleural thickening is seen in 30% of cancer patients. CT findings specific in diagnosing malignancy are:

1. Nodular pleural thickening.
2. Circumferential pleural thickening, surrounding the lung.
3. Mediastinal pleural thickening.

MESOTHELIOMA (MALIGNANT PLEURAL MESOTHELIOMA)[35-37]

Malignant pleural mesothelioma (MPM) is the most common primary neoplasm of the pleura. It is a highly malignant aggressive neoplasm of mesothelial cell origin. It occurs mainly in the pleura or peritoneum, but may arise in the pericardium or tunica vaginalis testis. There is a strong association between development of this neoplasm and asbestos exposure, particularly crocidolite. Approximately 5–7% of asbestos workers will develop it. A latency period of 20 to 40 years between exposure and development of tumor is seen. Symptoms include chest pain, dyspnea and weight loss with mean age at presentation of 60 years. Mesothelioma arises in relation to parietal pleura. It is classified pathologically as epithelial (50%), sarcomatous (25%) or mixed (25%). The epithelial type has a slightly better prognosis and is associated with pleural effusion.

Mesothelioma is characterized morphologically by gross and nodular pleural thickening, which can involve fissures. Hemorrhagic pleural effusion often occurs. It spreads by local infiltration of the pleura. The tumor can invade both visceral and parietal pleura and frequently extends to adjacent structures, such as chest wall, mediastinum and diaphragm, lymph node spread or metastasis to different organs such as liver, lung and kidneys can occur. The overall survival is related to the extent of the primary tumor.

Radiographic Findings of MPM

The most common plain radiographic findings are unilateral pleural effusion (30–95%) and concentric or lobulated pleural thickening **(Figs. 49 to 51)**.

Solid pleural lesions may vary from focal masses to diffuse thickening surrounding and encasing the entire lung surface. Extension into the interlobar fissure is common occurring in 40–86% patients. Distinct pleural masses without effusion are identified in less than 25% of patients. Benign calcified or noncalcified plaques may be present. Because of pleural thickening and mediastinal infiltration, the involved hemithorax may be normal in volume, despite presence of large effusion **(the frozen mediastinum sign).** The hemithorax may be reduced in volume because of restriction of lung expansion.

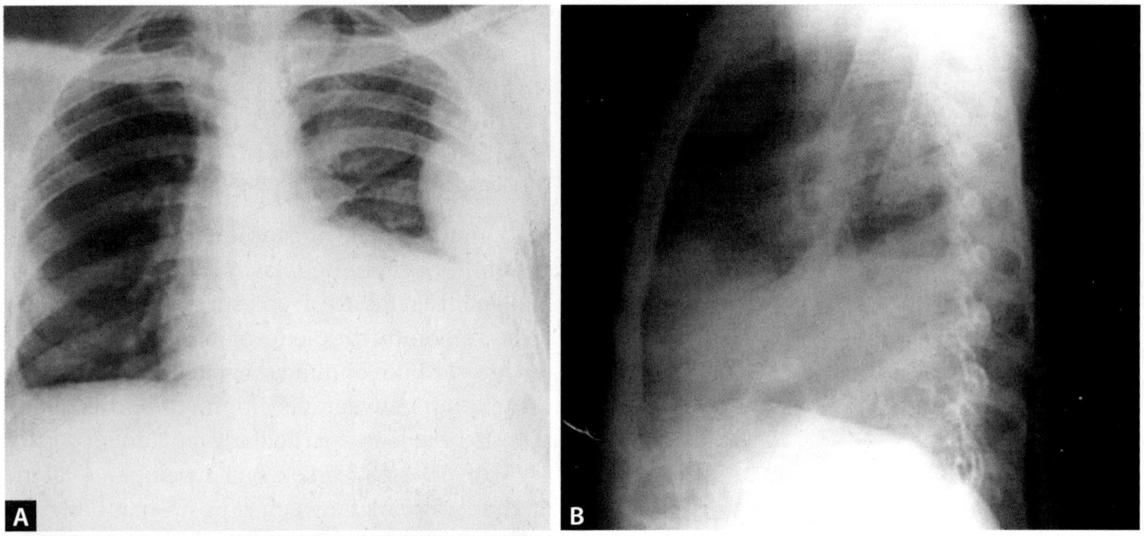

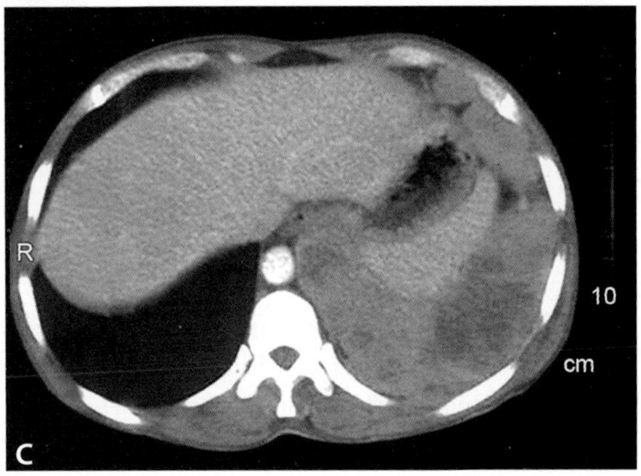

Figs. 49A to C: Chest X-ray (A and B) A nodular opacity noted along the left chest wall and lower zone. CT (C) shows, nodular pleural masses all along the pleural surface—malignant pleural mesothelioma.

Ultrasonography

Ultrasound will show pleural effusion and nodular soft tissue masses. The accuracy of US in detecting invasion of pleura and chest wall is high. US criteria of tumor invasion have been described. If the tumor is in contact with only visceral pleura it is UP1, if in contact with parietal pleura it is UP2 and with breech of pleura is UP3.

Computed Tomography

Computed tomography (CT) is the primary imaging modality for MPM. Major findings include nodular pleural thickening, unilateral pleural effusion,tumor invasion into the adjacent structures. Pleural thickening is circumferential/rind like with multiple nodules. Nodular concentric pleural thickening is highly suggestive of mesothelioma, rarely it may be thin and smooth. Calcified plaques are a sign of asbestos exposure; these are not a precursor to mesothelioma.

In early disease, pleural thickening may appear localized and discontinuous. As the disease progresses, pleural thickening becomes continuous, it increases in thickness and nodularity and the amount of fluid may decrease as pleural layers become fused.

In some cases, pleural effusion may be the only finding. The combination of an unexplained pleural effusion and pleural pain should raise the possibility of mesothelioma. Enhancement of the pleura after contrast administration can help differentiate tumor from adjacent fluid collections. Mesothelioma is visible most frequently along the lateral chest wall; mediastinal pleural thickening is seen with extensive disease. The abnormal hemithorax can appear contracted and fixed with little change in size during inspiration. Thickening of fissures, particularly the lower part of major fissures can reflect tumor infiltration or associated pleural effusion. Involvement of fissures is seen on CT in 85% of cases of mesothelioma.

The features that are helpful in distinguishing malignant from benign pleural disease are: Circumferential and nodular pleural thickening and mediastinal pleural thickening, parietal pleural thickening of >1 cm is not a helpful differentiating feature. Infiltration of adjacent

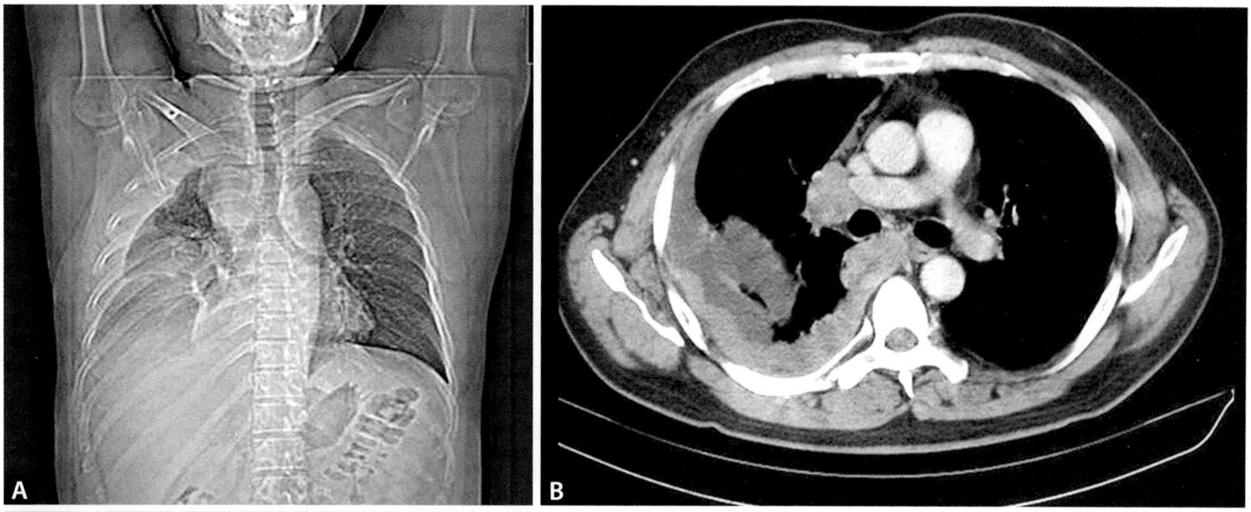

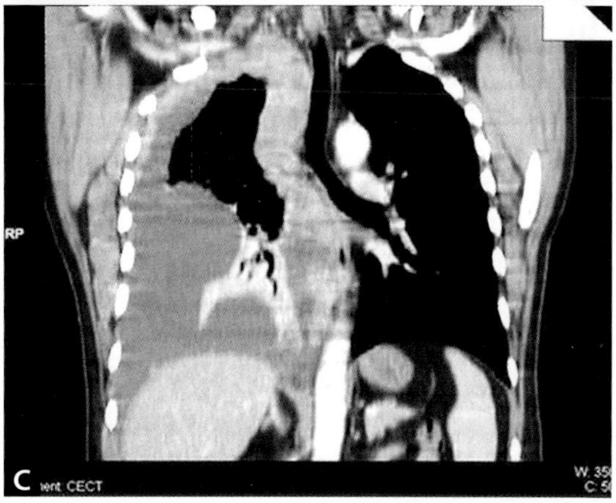

Figs. 50A to C: X-ray (A) CT chest (B and C)—circumferential and nodular enhancing pleural tumor with associated effusion. Extension into the mediastinal pleura and partial encasement of the right lung is suggestive of mesothelioma.

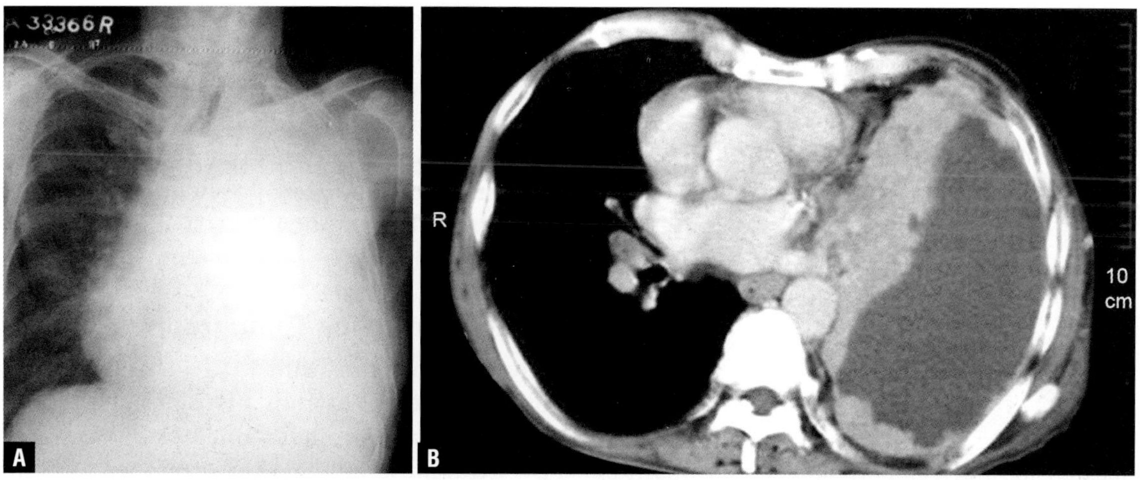

Figs. 51A and B: Chest X-ray (A)—opaque left hemithorax with shift of mediastinum to the right. CT scan (B) of the same patient shows nodular, thickened, enhancing pleura with associated effusion, malignant pleural mesothelioma.

structures like chest wall suggests malignancy. Some infectious process like tuberculosis can invade the chest wall, but do so at a single focus, rather than at multiple sites, as seen in malignant disease.

There is a TNM international staging system,proposed by the International Mesothelioma Interst Group for diffuse malignant pleural mesothelioma **(Table 7)**.[38] This new system emphasizes criteria that help in determining

Table 7: International Mesothelioma Interest Group TNM staging system.

TNM **T – Tumour** **TX:** primary tumour cannot be assessed **T0:** no evidence of primary tumour
T1a • Potentially resectable • Only parietal pleura • No mediastinal pleural involvement
T1b • Potentially resectable • Parietal pleura and • Scattered foci of mediastinal pleural involvement
T2 • Potentially resectable • Parietal and visceral pleural involvement, and /or • Pulmonary parenchymal involvement and/or • Diaphragmatic muscle involvement
T3 • Potentially resectable • Localized tumor extension into endothoracic fascia and/or • Localized non-transmural involvement of pericardium and/or • Localized extension into mediastinal fat
T4 • Unresectable • Multiple foci of extension into chest wall +/– rib destruction and/or • Extension through diaphragm into peritoneum and/or • Extension into contralateral pleura and/or • Extension into mediastinal organs and/or • Extension through pericardium +/– direct extension into heart
N – Nodes **NX:** nodes cannot be assessed **N0:** no evidence of nodal involvement **N1:** ipsilateral bronchopulmonary or hilar nodal involvement **N2:** subcarinal or ipsilateral mediastinal/internal mammary nodes **N3:** contralateral mediastinal/internal mammary nodes, or ipsilateral/contralateral supraclavicular nodes
M – Metastases **MX:** presence of metastases cannot be assessed **M0:** no evidence of metastases **M1:** distant metastases present
Stage groupings **Stage IA:** T1a, N0, M0 **Stage IB:** T1b, N0, M0 **Stage II:** T2, N0, M0 **Stage III:** T1 or 2, N1 or N2, M0 or T3, any N, M0 **Stage IV:** any T, any N, M1

local tumor extension and regional lymph node status in an attempt to identify patients with potentially curable early disease (T1 a and b); those who may benefit from surgery without necessarily being cured (T2 and T3); and patients with extensive local tumor spread (T4), extensive regional node involvement, or distant metastases for whom surgery would provide no benefit. The system therefore stratifies patients into prognostic groups.

CT criteria of resectability include:

- Preservation of extrapleural fat planes
- Absence of extrapleural soft tissue masses
- Normal CT attenuation values of adjacent structures
- Smooth inferior diaphragmatic surface.

CT criteria of unresectability include:

- Invasion of extrapleural soft tissue or fat
- Infiltration, separation, displacement of ribs by tumor
- Bone destruction
- Tumor encasing the diaphragm.

CT remains suboptimal because enlarged nodes do not imply nodal involvement. CT can also lead to underestimation of the extent of disease in early chest wall involvement.

Magnetic Resonance Imaging

Malignant mesothelioma has a slightly high signal intensity on T1WI, as compared to adjacent chest wall musculature, and moderately high signal intensity on T2WI. Mesotheliomas enhance on post gadolinium scans. Other findings include diffuse pleural thickening, pleural effusion and involvement of adjacent structures similar to CT.

MRI has been found to be superior to CT, in revealing invasion of the diaphragm, endothoracic fascia or solitary respectable focus of chest wall invasion. Diffusion MRI can also help to differentiate benign from malignant pleural disease. Presence of hyperintense pleural spots on high b value DW images called as "pleural pointillism" and has a sensitivity of 93% and a specificity of 79%.[39] The diagnostic accuracy of pleural pointillism is substantially better than that of mediastinal pleural thickness. Pleural pointillism can be used to provide guidance for biopsy or thoracoscopic evaluation. Perfusion MRI is a promising technique for assessment of perfusion, vascularity and permeability of tumors. Therapeutic effect of chemotherapy can be monitored with perfusion MRI.

Positron Emission Tomography

Functional imaging with FDG-PET has facilitated the non-invasive evaluation of tumor pathophysiology, metabolism and proliferation. Most mesotheliomas are FDG avid. Mesothelioma shows moderate to high FDG uptake involving areas of thickened pleura. Tumors at earlier stage tend to have focal or linear patterns of uptake, wheras the mixed and encasing patterns are indicative of more advanced disease. PET/CT increases the accuracy of overall staging and improves the selection of patients for extrapleural pneumonectomy as it detects more extensive disease and identifies occult distant metastasis.

The differential diagnosis of malignant mesothelioma includes benign causes of pleural thickening (such as post infection or diffuse pleural thickening) and metastatic adenocarcinoma. The lobulated outline, pleural effusion, or evidence of more advanced disease may help differentiate mesothelioma from diffuse pleural thickening.

Histologic or cytologic diagnosis is always required. Image guidance can be used to obtain the necessary tissue diagnosis, but spread along biopsy/drainage site is well documented, the differentiation between mesothelioma and metastatic adenocarcinoma is difficult even with biopsy. Immunohistochemistry and electron microscopy aid the diagnosis.

Pleural Metastasis

Metastatic disease accounts for the majority of pleural neoplasm. Approximately 40% of pleural metastases arise from lung carcinoma, 10% from lymphoma and remaining 30% from other primary sites. Several extrathoracic primary tumors like ovarian, uterine,gastrointestinal or pancreatic may metastasize to the pleura. In absence of a recognizable primary, metastatic adenocarcinoma is difficult to diagnose, because of histological similarity to malignant mesothelioma.

Invasive thymoma is an uncommon thoracic primary neoplasm with a propensity for pleural extension. This pleural implantation results in widespread pleural thickening and/or multiple discrete masses. It may be indistinguisble from mesothelioma, especially when anterior mediastinal component is small.

Malignant effusion is the most frequent manifestation of metastatic pleural disease and is often accompanied by solid tumor deposits of varying size **(Fig. 52)**. They may appear as solitary implant on the costal, diaphragmatic or mediastinal pleura or within the interlobar fissure.

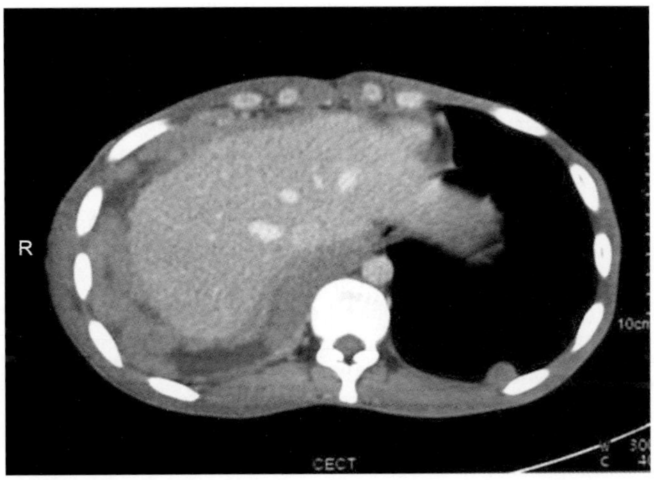

Fig. 52: CT multiple-enhancing pleural nodules—metastases.

Pleural Lymphoma

Involvement of pleura occurs in both Hodgkin and non-Hodgkin disease. Solid pleural lymphoma occurs as either a solitary nodule or as diffuse tumor infiltration. Associated exudative pleural effusion may be seen due to lymphatic obstruction and resolves with radiation. Marked thickening of extrapleural soft tissue may be seen with associated posterior mediastinal lymph node enlargement.

Localized Fibrous Tumor

Localized fibrous tumor (LFT) of the pleura was formerly known as benign mesothelioma, but it is not mesothelial in origin, and not always benign (30% are malignant).[40] About 50% of cases are encountered in patients in 6th–7th decade, with no gender predilection. It has no association with asbestos exposure. Patients are frequently asymptomatic, LFT is detected incidentally on chest radiographs. It can be associated with hypoglycemia (15%), chest pain or hypertrophic pulmonary osteoarthopathy (1/3rd of cases). These symptoms resolve with resection.

LFT arises from the visceral pleura in about 80%. They appear as solitary, well-circumscribed spherical ovoid, non-calcified lesions, contacting a pleural surface. The size ranges from less than 2 cm to 30 cm. They are often pedunculated and as a consequence may show change in position and shape during fluoroscopy.

LFT, when small has an obtuse angle at the pleural surface, when large angles can be acute. LFT can be seen within a fissure, mimicking appearance of loculated fluid. A "beak" or "thorn" sign is often seen on radiographs in patients with a LFT originating from or projecting into a fissure. Pleural effusion is not usually present. On CT, localized fibrous tumor appears as well-defined lobulated pleural mass **(Figs. 53A to C)**. Slight pleural thickening is usually visible adjacent to the mass. This is due to small amount of fluid accumulating at the pleural surface at the point of separation of visceral and parietal pleura by the mass. CT is useful in identifying masses arising from the interlobar fissure, which simulates a parenchymal lesion.On MR imaging, LFT may show low signal on both T1 and T2 weighted images or may have heterogeneous signal intensity reflecting the cellularity of these tumors. Surgical excision is the treatment with operative respectability being the most important predictor of clinical outcome.

TUMOR-LIKE CONDITIONS OF THE PLEURA

A tumor-like condition of the pleura is any non-neoplastic lesion of the pleura itself, or within the pleural space, that

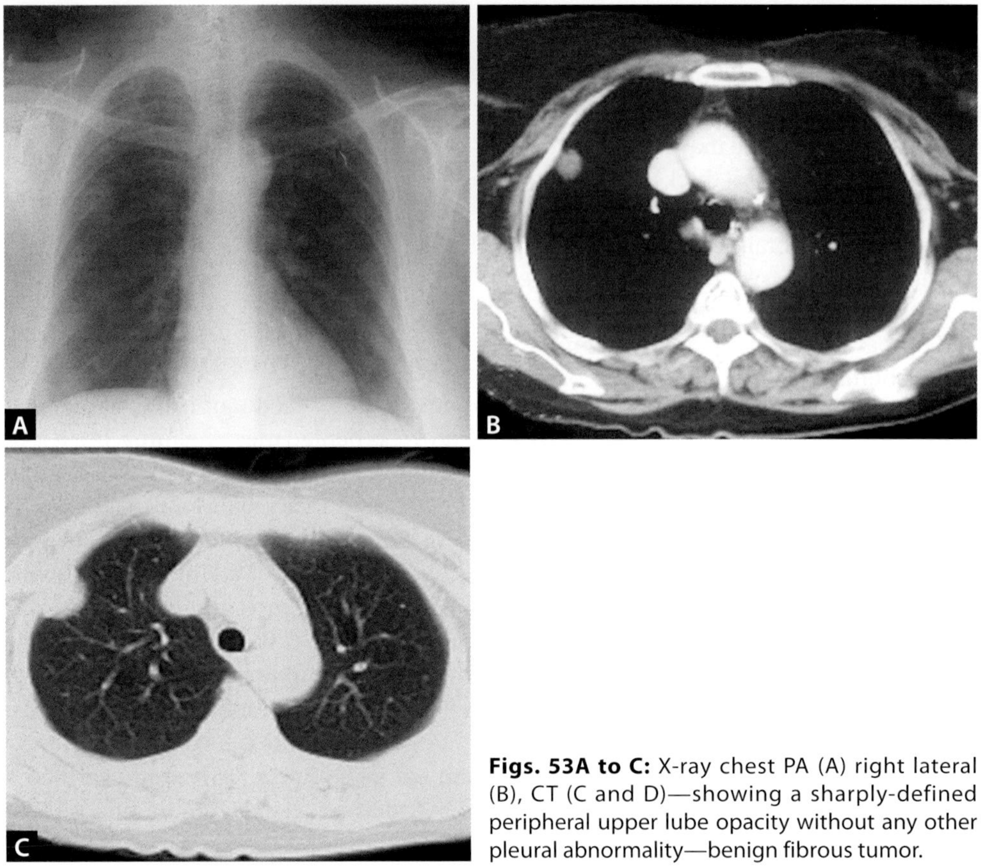

Figs. 53A to C: X-ray chest PA (A) right lateral (B), CT (C and D)—showing a sharply-defined peripheral upper lube opacity without any other pleural abnormality—benign fibrous tumor.

resembles a tumor.[3] These may be focal or diffuse. **Pleural plaque, thoracic splenosis, thoracic endometriosis** causing catamenial pneumothorax, and **pseudotumor** caused by pleural effusion are focal tumor-like conditions of the pleura. Diffuse tumor-like conditions of the pleura include diffuse pleural thickening and rare conditions such as **Erdheim-Chester disease** and **diffuse pulmonary lymphangiomatosis.** Erdheim-Chester disease is classified as non-Langerhans histiocytosis and is characterized by typical skeletal findings of femoral sclerosis, perirenal soft tissue halo. Diffuse pulmonary lymphangiomatosis is a rare condition, demonstrates diffuse pleural thickening, interlobular septal and peribronchovascular interstitial thickening, and mediastinal fat infiltration limited to the thorax.

REFERENCES

1. Coolen J, Keyzer FD, Nafteux P, et al. Malignant pleural disease: Diagnosis by using diffusion weight and dynamic contrast enhanced MR imaging initial experience. Radiology. 2012;263(3):884-92.
2. Parcel JM, Vives. Classic abbreviated and modified Light criteria; Chest. 1999;116:1833-6.
3. Sasson CS,Light RW.Chylothorax &pseudochylothorax. Clin Chest Med. 1985;6:163-71.
4. Walker CM, Takasugi JE, Chung JH, et al. Tumour like conditions of the pleura. Radiographics. 2012;32:971-85.
5. Eibenberger K, dock W, Ammann M, et al. Quantification of pleural effusions: Sonography versus radiography. Radiology. 1994;191:681-4.
6. Yang PC, Luh KT, Chang DB, et al. Value of sonography in determing the nature of pleural effusion: Analysis of 320 cases. Am J Roentgenol. 1992;159:29-33.
7. Wu RG, Yang PC, Kuo SH. "Fluid colour" sign-a useful indicator for discrimination between pleural thickening and pleural effusion. J Ultrasound Med. 1995;14(10):767-9.
8. Abramowitz Y, Simanovsky N, Goldstein MS, et al. Pleural effusion: Characterisation with CT attenuation values and CT appearance. AJR. 2009;192:618-23.
9. Halvorsen RA, Fedyshin PJ, Korobkin M, et al. Ascitis or pleural effusion? CT differentiation: four useful criteria. Radiographics. 1986;6:135-49.
10. Dwyer RA. The displaced crus: A sign for distinguishing between pleural fluid and ascitis on computed tomography. Comput Assist Tomog. 1978;2:598.
11. Baysal T, Bulut T, Gokirmak M. Diffusion weighted MR imaging of pleural fluid: Differentiation of transudative vs exudative pleural effusions. Eur Radiol. 2004;14:890-6.

12. Ivan N, Arsalan A, Akansel G, et al. Diffusion weighted MRI in the characterization of pleural effusions: Diag Interv Radiol. 2009;15(1):13-18.
13. Chen HJ, Yu YH, Tu CY, et al. Ultrasound in peripheral pulmonary air fluid lesions: Colour Doppler imaging as an aid in differentiating empyema and abscess. Chest. 2009;135(6):1426-32.
14. Kuhlman JE, Singha NK. Complex disease of the pleural space: Radiographic and CT evaluation. Radiographics. 1997;17:63-97.
15. Kuhlman JE. Complex disease of the pleural space: The 10 questions most frequently asked of the radiologist-new approaches to their answers with CT and MR imaging. Radiographics. 1997;17:1043-50.
16. Stark DD, Federle MP, Goodman PC, et al. Differentiating lung abscess and empyema: Radiography and computed tomography. Am J Roentgenol. 1983;141:163-67.
17. Leung AN, Muller NL, Miller RR. CT in differential diagnosis of diffuse pleural disease. Am J Roentgenol. 1990;154: 487-92.
18. Neff CC, vanSonnerberg E, Lawson DW, et al. CT follow-up of empyemas: Pleural peels resolve after percutaneous catheter drainage. Radiology. 1990;176:195-97.
19. Seo H, Kim TJ, Jin KN, et al. Multi-detector row computed tomographic evaluation of bronchopleural fistula: correlation with clinical, bronchoscopic and surgical findings. J Comput Assit Tomogr. 2010;34(1):13-8.
20. McLoud TC, Woods BO, Carrington CB, et al. Diffuse pleural thickening in the asbestos-exposed population. Am J Roentgenol. 1985;144:9-18.
21. Lynch DA, Gamsu G, Aberle DR. Conventional and high-resolution tomography in the diagnosis of asbestos-related diseases. Radiographics. 1989;9:523-51.
22. Renner RR, Pernice NJ. The apical cap: Semin Roentgenol. 1977;12:299-302.
23. Cugell DW, Kamp DW. Asbestos and the pleura—a review. Chest. 2004;125(3):1103-17.
24. Roach HD, Davies GJ, Attanoos R. Asbestos: when the dust settles an imaging review of asbestos-related disease. Radiographics. 2002;S167-84.
25. Gordon R. The deep sulcus sign. Radiology. 1980;136:25-7.
26. Kirkpatrick AW, Sirois M, Laupland KB, et al. Hand-held thoracic sonography for detecting post-traumatic pneumothoraces: The Extended Focussed Assessment with Sonography for Trauma (EFAST). J Trauma. 2004;57:288-95.
27. De Luca C, Valentino M, Rimondi M, et al. Use of chest sonography in acute care radiology. J Ultrasound. 2008;11:25-34.
28. Barillari A, Kiuru S. Detection of spontaneous pneumothorax with chest ultrasound in emergency department. Intern Emerg Med. 2010;1:253-5.
29. Lichtenstein DA, Menu Y. A Bedside ultrasound sign ruling out pneumothorax in the critically ill-lung sliding. Chest. 1995;108:1345-8.
30. Lichtenstein D, Meziere G, Biderman P. The lung point: An ultrasound sign specific to pneumothorax. Intensive care Med. 2000;26:1434-40.
31. Lichtenstein DA, Meziere G, Lascols N, et al. Ultrasound diagnosis of occult pneumothorax. Crit care Med. 2005;33:1231-8.
32. Cunnigham J, Kirkpatrick AW, Nicolaous, et al. Enhanced recognition of "lung sliding"with power colour Doppler imaging in the diagnosis of pneumothorax. J Trauma. 2002;52:769-71.
33. Choi BG, Park SH, Yun EH, et al. Pneumothorax size:correlation of supine anteroposterior with erect posteroanterior chest radiograph. Radiology. 1998;209: 567-9.
34. Dynes MC, White EM, Fry WA, et al. Imaging manifestations of pleural tumors. Radiographics. 1992;12:1191-201.
35. Wang ZJ, Reddy GB, Gotway MB, et al. Malignant pleural mesothelioma: Evaluation with CT, MR imaging and PET. Radiographics. 2004;24(1):105-19.
36. Yanamuro M, Gerbando VH, Gill RR, et al. Morphological and functional imaging of malignant pleural mesothelioma. Eur Radiol. 2007;64(3):355-66.
37. Nickell LT, Licchtenberger JP, Khorashadi L, et al. Multimodality imaging for characterisation, classification and staging of malignant pleural mesothelioma. Radiographics. 2014;34:1692-706.
38. Rusch VW. A proposed new international TNM staging system for malignant pleural mesothelioma: from the International Mesothelioma Interest Group. Chest. 1995; 108(4):1122-8.
39. Coolen J, Keyzer FD, Nafleux P, et al. Malignant pleural mesothelioma: Visceral assessment by using pleural pointillism at diffusion weighted MR imaging. Radiology. 2015;274:576-84
40. Rosado-de-christenson ML, Abbot GF, Mc Adams HP, et al. Localised fibrous tumours of the pleura. Radiographics. 2003;23(3):759-83.

CHAPTER 173

Imaging of the Diaphragm and Chest Wall

Ujjwal Gorsi, Sameer Vyas, Anupam Lal

EMBRYOLOGY AND ANATOMY

Diaphragm is a thin dome-shaped musculotendinous structure which serves two important functions: (1) it acts as a physical barrier between the thoracic and abdominal cavities, (2) It is the chief muscle of inspiration. Embryologically, it develops from septum transversum, pleuroperitoneal membranes, dorsal mesentery of the esophagus, and muscular body wall. Diaphragm develops during 4–12 weeks of embryogenesis.[1] The anteriorly placed septum transversum forms the central tendon of the diaphragm. Septum transversum fuses with pleura-peritoneal membranes and esophageal mesentery posteriorly and gets attached to the muscular body wall laterally to form diaphragm.

The peripheral muscular part of diaphragm arises from the margin of the thoracic outlet and is inserted into a trefoil-shaped central tendon. The muscular fibers arise from three sources and may be grouped into three parts, two slips from the back of the xiphoid (sternal part), muscle fibers arising circumferentially from inner surfaces of the cartilages and the adjacent parts of lower six ribs of each side interlocking with fibers of the transversus abdominis (costal part), and from the superior three lumbar vertebrae by the right and left crura (lumbar part) that unite anterior to the aortic hiatus to form the median arcuate ligament **(Fig. 1)**.[1,2] Lateral to the crura, the diaphragm arise from the arcuate ligaments (medial and lateral) which are the

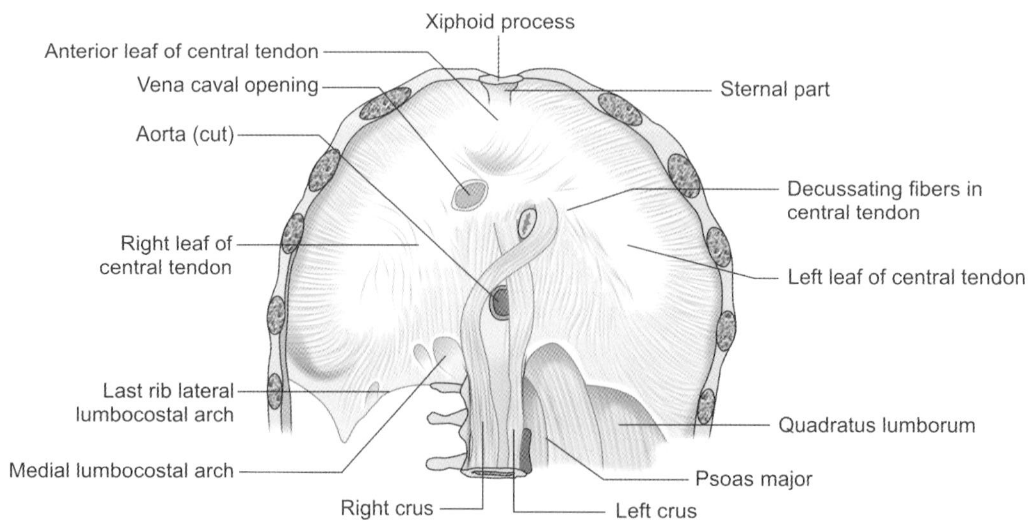

Fig. 1: Schematic diagram of diaphragm as viewed from abdominal aspect.

thickened fascia of the quadratus lumborum and psoas. The anterior muscle fibers are shorter than the posterior ones, which gives the diaphragm its characteristic dome-shaped configuration.

There are three openings in the normal diaphragm **(Fig. 2)**; aortic hiatus, esophageal hiatus and the hiatus for inferior vena cava (IVC). Aortic hiatus (osseoaponeurotic opening) is at level of 12th thoracic vertebra (T12). The aorta, thoracic duct, azygos and hemiazygos veins course through this hiatus. Decussation of the medial fibers of the right crus at level of T10 forms esophageal hiatus which gives passage to esophagus, vagus, sympathetic nerves and left gastric vessels. IVC hiatus is in the central tendon at level of T 8–9 and transmits IVC and branches of the right phrenic nerve. Nerve supply of the diaphragm is from left and right phrenic nerves, which arise from C3–C5 cervical nerves and have sensory as well as motor function.

FUNCTIONS

The main function of the diaphragm is to act as a muscle of respiration. It contracts along with sternocleidomastoid, scalene, and intercostal muscles which are the accessory muscles of respiration, during inspiration. This contraction causes expansion of thoracic cavity and reduces the intrathoracic pressure due to which air is drawn into the lungs. During expiration, along with elastic recoil of the lungs, diaphragm relaxes. The diaphragm, by increasing intra-abdominal pressure helps in urination, defecation and emesis. In addition diaphragm helps in preventing gastroesophageal reflux as it exerts external pressure at the esophageal opening.[1]

IMAGING MODALITIES

Imaging modalities for diaphragmatic disorders include plain radiography, fluoroscopy, ultrasonography, CT and MRI.

Plain Radiograph

Normal diaphragm is not separately identifiable on a chest X-ray. On a chest X-ray, usually the top of the abdominal cavity which normally represents the upper abdominal organs such as liver, stomach, spleen, or colon with the overlying diaphragm and is opaque on radiograph is spoken off as diaphragm. It is visualized as a distinct entity only if outlined by air on both the sides, i.e. on thoracic and abdominal sides **(Fig. 3)**. On inspiration, the domes of diaphragm are at the level of the sixth rib anteriorly and at or below the tenth rib posteriorly. The right hemidiaphragm is 1.5–2.5 cm higher than the left in most individuals. In about 9%, the two hemidiaphragm are at the same level, and the left hemidiaphragm is up to 1 cm higher than right in few normal individuals.[3] On lateral radiograph, both the domes project on each other. Right and left domes can be easily differentiated from each other by the fact that the anterior part of the left hemidiaphragm is mostly obscured by the

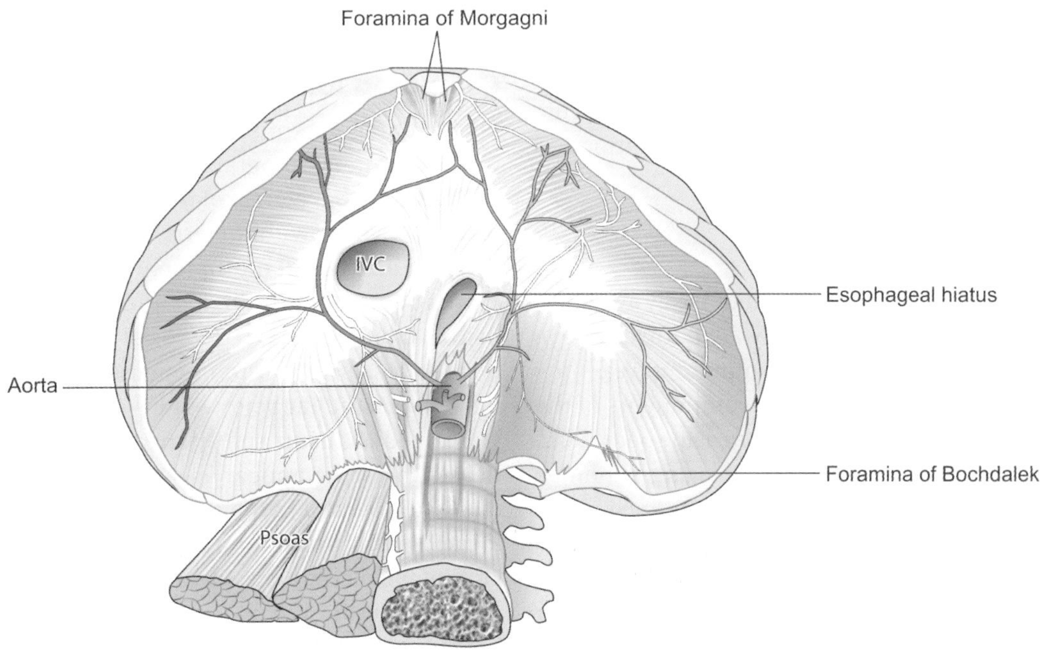

Fig. 2: Schematic diagram of diaphragm showing the hiatuses as viewed from its caudal aspect
Abbreviation: IVC: Inferior vena cava.

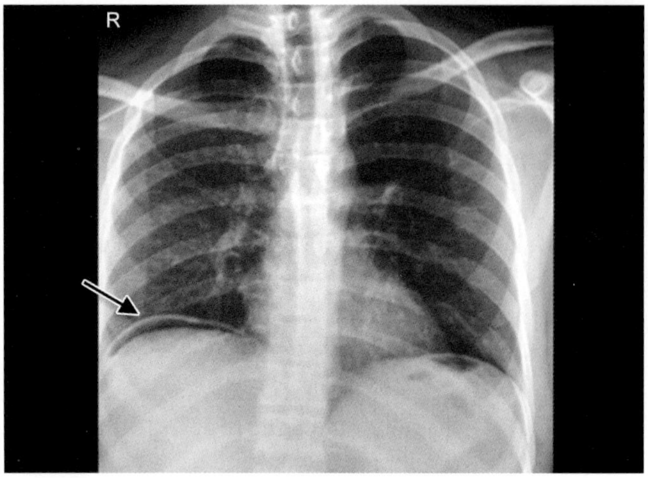

Fig. 3: Chest radiograph showing diaphragm (arrow) clearly identified because of pneumoperitoneum.

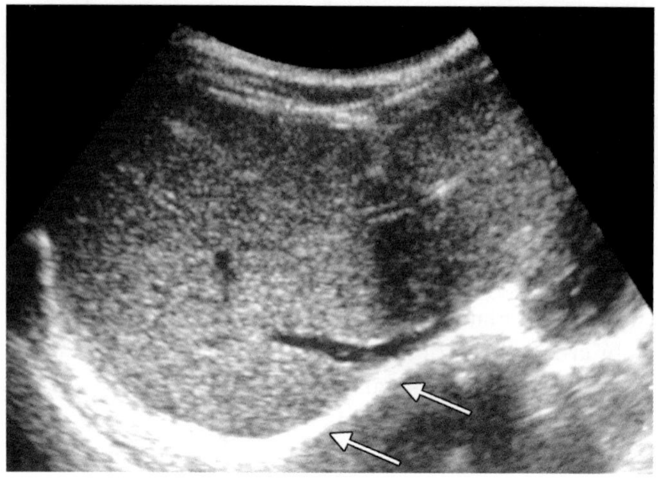

Fig. 4: The transverse ultrasound scan of right hemidiaphragm showing the diaphragm/lung interface as a thick curvilinear echogenic band (arrows). The triangular hypoechoic band between this and the liver is the peripheral muscular bundles of diaphragm.

heart, whereas the right dome can be seen in its entirety. On the left lateral view, the posterior part of the right dome projects under the left dome. The IVC stops at the right hemidiaphragm while stomach bubble or gas in splenic flexure is in close contact with the left hemidiaphragm. The distance between the dome of diaphragm and the top of the gastric air bubble of the left hemidiaphragm, is less than 1 cm in most of individuals (about 88%) and is best demonstrated in the lateral view.[2]

Fluoroscopy

The fluoroscopic sniff test is real time fluoroscopic assessment of motor function of diaphragm (excursion). It is commonly used in patients who have breathing difficulties following stroke or in patients who have suffered phrenic nerve palsy to look for absence of muscular contraction of the diaphragm during inspiration.[1]

Ultrasonography

Ultrasonography (USG) is cheap, portable, easily available, radiation risk free imaging modality. Structures above and below the diaphragm can be examined in real time using USG. Structural and functional components of the diaphragm can be assessed with USG even at the bedside. In children and young adults, it is preferred imaging technique for interrogating the diaphragm. Ultrasound visualizes the lateral and posterior parts of the diaphragm, instead of anteriorly located central tendon, which is examined by fluoroscopy. Transhepatic and trans-splenic sector scanning is the most appropriate technique to visualize the diaphragm **(Fig. 4)**. Pleural disease can also be used as an acoustic window to study the lateral parts of the dome. The diaphragm itself is seen as a thin hypoechoic line. The interface between diaphragm and liver (or spleen) appears as a thin echogenic line. The interface between diaphragm and lung appears as a stronger and thicker echogenic band. The diaphragm can be clearly visualized on USG when pleural effusion and ascites are present at the same time. B mode USG can assess both echogenicity and thickness of the diaphragm where as M mode ultrasound by assessing a specific site over time can evaluate excursion, velocity, and response to phrenic nerve stimulation.[4]

Computed Tomography

The diaphragmatic disorders are usually difficult to assess with computed tomography (CT) in axial plane, because of the tangential course of the diaphragm to the imaging plane. However, with the arrival of the multidetector CT (MDCT) and use of multiplanar reconstructions various diaphragmatic pathologies and injuries can be easily demonstrated **(Fig. 5)**.[5] The costal part of the diaphragm is frequently seen as a stripe of soft tissue between the aerated lung above and fat below. The sternal part is sometimes visualized as linear soft tissue densities anterior to the heart. The crura appear as smooth linear densities that decussate ventral to the aorta at the cranial level and are located lateral to the aorta at the more caudal level **(Fig. 6)**. Crus of the diaphragm extend up to third lumbar vertebra on the right side and up to second lumbar vertebra on the left side. As the right crus extend far below the left it can be mistaken for a lymph node.

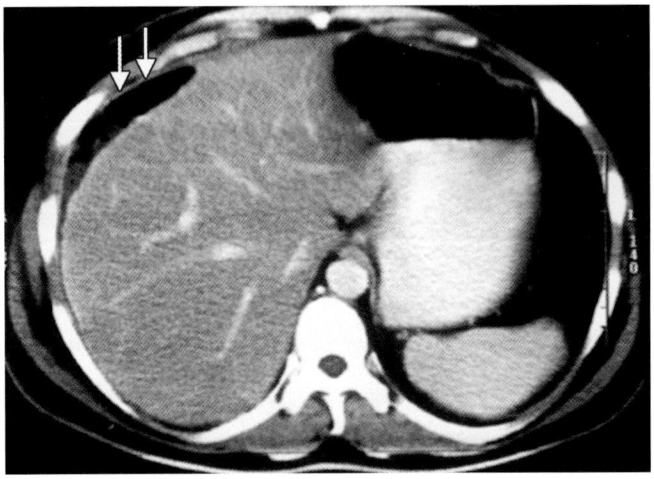

Fig. 5: Axial CT scan showing diaphragm (arrows) outlined by air present in the subphrenic abscess.

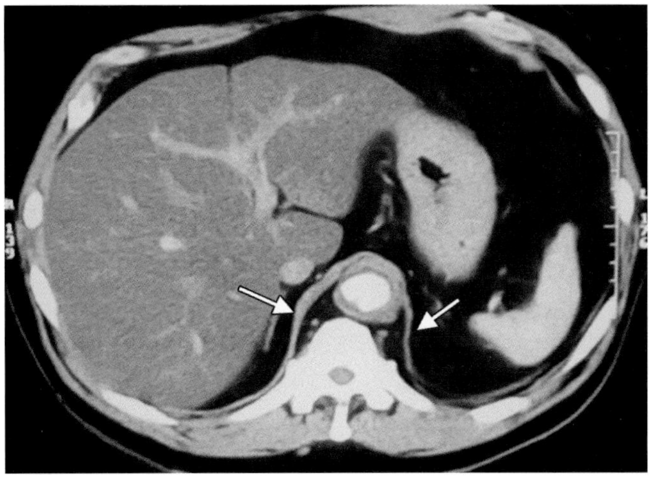

Fig. 6: Axial CT scan of abdomen showing diaphragmatic crura (arrows).

Magnetic Resonance Imaging

Coronal and sagittal MR images provide the best way to evaluate the relationship and involvement of the diaphragm to pathologic processes such as hernia, infection, and tumor.[6] MR can easily identify congenital, acquired and traumatic diaphragmatic hernias which commonly present as thoracic masses. In all MRI sequences, diaphragm has signal intensity which is lower than other skeletal muscles. It is excellent for demonstrating the extent and anatomic relationships of juxtadiaphragmatic tumors and can help to identify the location of peridiaphragmatic fluid collections. However, the respiratory motion may impair imaging of the normal diaphragm. In addition to morphologic abnormalities, MRI can be helpful in evaluating functional disorders of the diaphragm. With the advent of faster MR imaging, such as 'Gradient Recalled Echo' (GRE), it is possible to obtain sequential dynamic images of the diaphragm during real-time breathing, which can be viewed as cine loops.[6] This approach allows for the evaluation of diaphragmatic motion without the use of ionizing radiation. MRI allows quantitative evaluation, including the synchronicity, excursion, and velocity of motion of diaphragm.[7]

Radionuclide Scan

The role of radionuclide scans in assessing diaphragmatic pathology is limited. Most of the scans are performed for assessing diaphragmatic integrity in occult cases where the radiologic imaging is equivocal. Intraperitoneal injection of technetium sulfur colloid and subsequent scintigraphy has been shown to be a sensitive test for the diagnosis of diaphragmatic laceration. Radionuclide liver-spleen imaging with ^{99m}Tc sulfur colloid permits assessment of liver and splenic injuries and also their herniation into thorax in cases of traumatic diaphragmatic hernias.[8]

NORMAL VARIANTS

Scalloping

Appear as short curves of diaphragm which are convex upwards. It gives poly arcuate appearance and seen in approximately 5% individuals. They are commonly seen on the right side, and in patients with pulmonary emphysema or pneumothorax. Muscle slips: appear as small curved lines which are concave upwards and are common on the right side. They are commonly seen in tall, thin patients and in those with emphysema. Diaphragmatic humps and dromedary diaphragm: represents mild forms of eventration with incomplete muscularization of the hemidiaphragm but there is no muscle defect. They are commonly seen on right side and anteriorly.

Eventration

Eventration is a congenital anomaly with failure of muscular development of part or all of one or both hemidiaphragms. Total eventration of a hemidiaphragm is more common on the left side which is often associated with torsion or volvulus of the stomach **(Fig. 7)**. Partial eventration is more common on right side and frequently involves its anteromedial portion. On chest radiography, partial eventration is seen as a semioval or semicircular homogeneous opacity which has soft tissue density arising from the diaphragm.[2,3] On deep inspiration, eventration becomes more apparent as dorsal and lateral part of the diaphragm moves downward

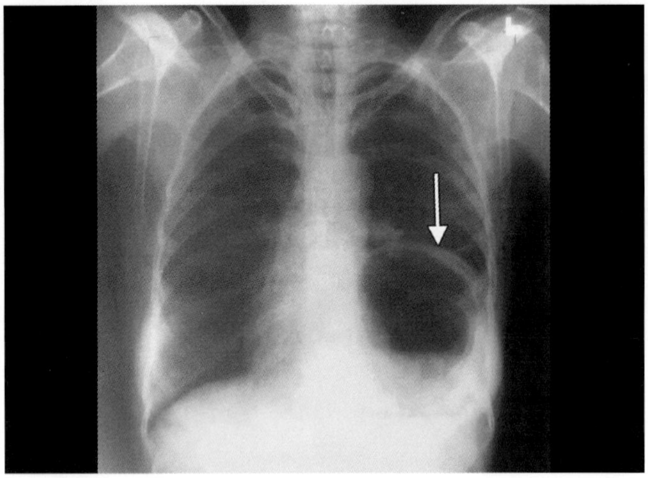

Fig. 7: Chest radiograph showing eventration of the left hemidiaphragm (arrow) with gastric volvulus.

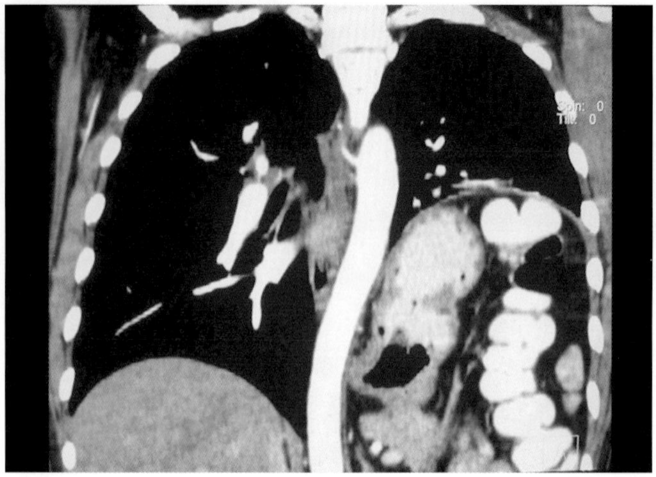

Fig. 8: Coronal reformats of multidetector CT showing eventration of the left hemidiaphragm with intrathoracic herniation of stomach and colon.

whereas convex segment may remain at the same level or shows upward movement. MDCT **(Fig. 8)**, USG and MRI may be required to differentiate eventration from mediastinal pericardial or pleural lesions. Differentiating an eventration involving a large part of a hemidiaphragm from a paralyzed hemidiaphragm and Morgagni hernia with herniation of liver or fat may not be easy at times. The paralyzed hemidiaphragm often has an adjacent area of atelectatic lung on chest X-ray whereas large eventration does not. This is due to the fact that an eventration still has some net inspiratory downward movement while a paralyzed hemidiaphragm has a paradoxical upward motion.

Accessory Diaphragm

It is partial duplication of a hemidiaphragm, almost always seen on the right side. It courses obliquely backward and upward and get attached along the third to seventh ribs. Part of the entire lower lobe is contained between the true and accessory hemidiaphragm. On the frontal view of the chest, the entire hemidiaphragm may be elevated and the heart and mediastinum are shifted to the affected right side. The adjacent right mediastinal margin is indistinct. On the lateral view, the accessory diaphragm appear as an oblique line rising posteriorly.[2]

Elevated Hemidiaphragm

Unilateral Elevation

Causes of a unilateral high hemidiaphragm are eventration, unilateral atelectasis, severe gastric distension, gross hepatomegaly, gross splenomegaly, obstructive emphysema of the contralateral lung, phrenic nerve palsy, subpulmonic effusion, subphrenic abscess, and ipsilateral pulmonary hypoplasia.[2,3]

Bilateral Elevation

Causes of a bilaterally high diaphragm are ascites, pregnancy, hepatosplenomegaly, large intra-abdominal tumors, poor inspiratory effort and causes of unilateral elevation present bilaterally.[2]

Low Lying Diaphragm

May be seen in cases of hyperinflated lungs, intrathoracic masses, and large pleural effusions.

Inversion of the Diaphragm

Represents reverse curvature of the diaphragm and can be partial or complete. It can occur with tension pneumothorax, large basal bulla, large pleural effusion or large tumors. The condition is usually seen on the left side as the right dome is somewhat protected by the underlying liver. An inverted diaphragm rises actively on inspiration and falls on expiration, resulting in paradoxical movement of the diaphragm and mediastinal shift toward the affected side during inspiration.

Peridiaphragmatic Collections

For localization of peridiaphragmatic collections, identification of the diaphragm is the key factor.[3] Accurate localization of a fluid collection in sub- or supradiaphragmatic location at times may be difficult on cross-sectional

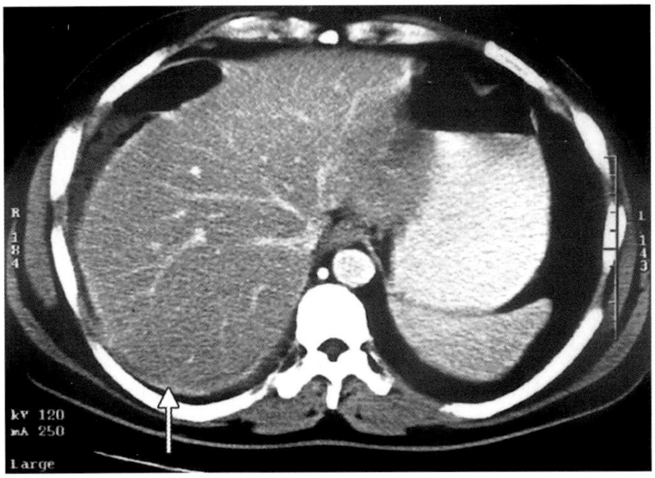

Fig. 9: Axial CT scan showing fluid collection anterior to the posterior aspect of the diaphragm (arrow) is subphrenic in location.

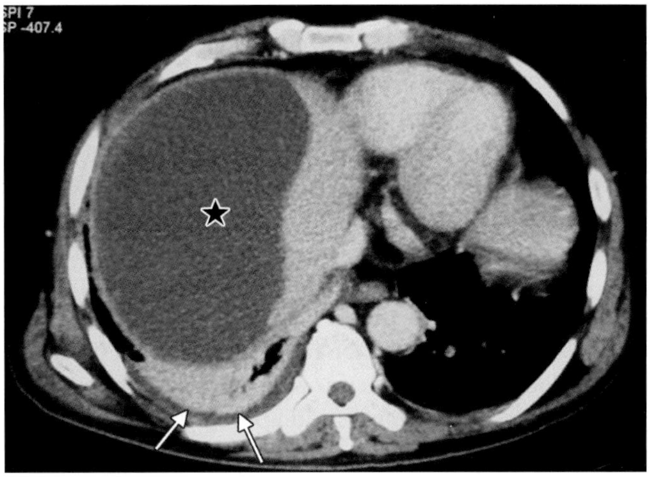

Fig. 10: Axial CT scan of the abdomen showing right pleural effusion (arrows) and subdiaphragmatic collection (star).

Table 1: Differences between ascites and pleural effusion on the basis of CT signs.

S. No.	*Feature*	*Ascites*	*Pleural effusion*
1.	Diaphragmatic circle	Center	Outside
2.	Displaced crus sign	Posteromedial	Anterolateral
3.	Bare area sign	Seen	Not seen
4.	Interface (abdominal viscera)	Sharp	Hazy
5.	Lung	Anterior	Surrounds
6.	Caudally	Increases	Decreases
7.	Cranially	Decreases	Increases

imaging. USG, CT and MRI are helpful in differentiating subdiaphragmatic (ascites) vs supradiaphragmatic (pleural) fluid **(Figs. 9 and 10)**.[9] On axial CT images, a number of CT signs are helpful in differentiating ascites from pleural effusion **(Table 1)**.

DIAPHRAGMATIC MOVEMENTS

Abnormal movement of the diaphragm during respiration is an important radiologic sign of diaphragmatic or juxtadiaphragmatic disease. Fluoroscopy, ultrasound and MRI may be employed for assessing diaphragmatic movements.[4,6] The normal amplitude of the motion ranges from 0.8 to 8 cm in normal, healthy, young adults. Most (77%) individuals may show asymmetry of diaphragmatic motion when observed on fluoroscopy, although the difference in excursion is usually less than 1 cm.[3] Minor asynchronous motion of the hemidiaphragm and even momentary minimal paradoxical movement may be seen. The dome also may move differently from the rest of the diaphragm. In the lateral decubitus position, the dependent hemidiaphragm rises higher than usual and its respiratory excursion is greatly exaggerated. Abnormal diaphragmatic movement can be classified into three types, paradoxical, complete or incomplete fixation. Paradoxical movement is the upward movement of the affected hemidiaphragm on inspiration instead of the normal descent; complete fixation is no movement of the affected hemidiaphragm during the respiratory cycle; and incomplete fixation is greatly decreased motion of the affected hemidiaphragm on respiration. These three types of abnormal movement can be seen in various conditions including paralysis, eventration, subphrenic abscess, traumatic diaphragmatic hernia, unilateral obstructive emphysema, and pneumothorax. Fluoroscopy and realtime ultrasonography are reliable in assessing diaphragmatic motion.

DIAPHRAGMATIC WEAKNESS AND PARALYSIS

Weakness or paralysis, of diaphragm may be due to central nervous causes or phrenic nerve involvement due to tumor invasion or thoracic surgery.[9] Paralysis of diaphragm is more often unilateral which is asymptomatic, and is found on imaging incidently. Bilateral diaphragmatic paralysis is mostly symptomatic, and may present with respiratory failure.

On chest radiograph, bilateral diaphragm paralysis is seen as the smooth elevation of the both hemidiaphragms and associated reduced volume of the lungs. The costovertebral and costophrenic sulci become narrow and deep. On lateral view, smooth elevation of diaphragmatic position may be better appreciated. At lung bases linear atelectasis may also be seen. In unilateral diaphragm paralysis, the left hemidiaphragm may lie at or above the right hemidiaphragm. If right hemidiaphragm is paralyzed, it lies more than the one interspace higher than the left side. A paralyzed hemidiaphragm is elevated entirely, including the posterior take off point, this feature helps in differentiating it from eventration. On fluoroscopic sniff test, if unilateral diaphragmatic weakness or paralysis is present, during quiet inspiration, deep inspiration, and sniffing weak side moves more slowly downwards (caudal) or paradoxically upwards (with paralysis).[9] The sniff test is not as useful in patients with bilateral paralysis. Ultrasonography and dynamic MRI are other modalities to assess weakness or paralysis of diaphragm.

DIAPHRAGMATIC HERNIAS

Abdominal viscera can herniate into the thoracic cavity through the diaphragmatic hiatus (sliding and paraesophageal hiatus hernia) or congenital defect (Bochdalek and Morgagni hernia).

Hiatal Hernia

It develops from a weakness or tear (rupture) of the phrenicoesophageal ligament. Sliding hiatus hernias are the most common type (99%) of diaphragmatic hernias. In sliding hernia, the gastroesophageal junction lies above the esophageal hiatus whereas in paraesophageal hernia, all or portion of the stomach herniates into the chest with gastroesophageal junction lying below the diaphragm. They can be diagnosed by barium examination but cross-sectional imaging (CT, MRI) may show the size, site and content of the hernia. Sliding hernia is diagnosed on barium study when pouch of stomach protrudes more than 2 cm above the hiatus, or three or more gastric folds passing across the hiatus and on CT when the hiatus is wide with diaphragmatic crura separated by more than 15 mm **(Fig. 11)**. In paraesophageal (rolling) hernia, the stomach herniates through widened esophageal hiatus or occasionally through separate diaphragmatic gap to lie alongside the lower esophagus.

Between the eighth and tenth weeks of fetal life, the diaphragm forms and the pleuroperitoneal canals close, dividing the celomic cavity into the abdominal and thoracic cavities. During the same period, the gastrointestinal tract elongates into the umbilical pouch and rotates on its return to the abdominal cavity. The left pleuroperitoneal canal closes slightly later than the right. The interrelationship of these two important developmental events results in the clinical spectrum of diaphragmatic hernias: Bochdalek hernia (posterolateral defect), Morgagni hernia (retrosternal defect), and Intrapericardial hernia (defect of central tendon).

Bochdalek Hernia

It is the most common congenital hernia and involves the posterior defects in the diaphragm caused by defective fusion or maldevelopment of the pleuroperitoneal membranes. Stomach, bowel and even spleen or kidney may herniate into the left hemithorax. On the right side, part of the liver may be found above the diaphragm. Bochdalek hernia occurs in one in 2000–5000 births with involvevment of left hemidiaphragm in 80% of the cases.[10,11] The chest radiograph may show aerated intrathoracic bowel loops and shift of mediastinum to opposite side **(Figs. 12 and 13)**. On CT, Bochdalek hernia often presents as fatty or soft

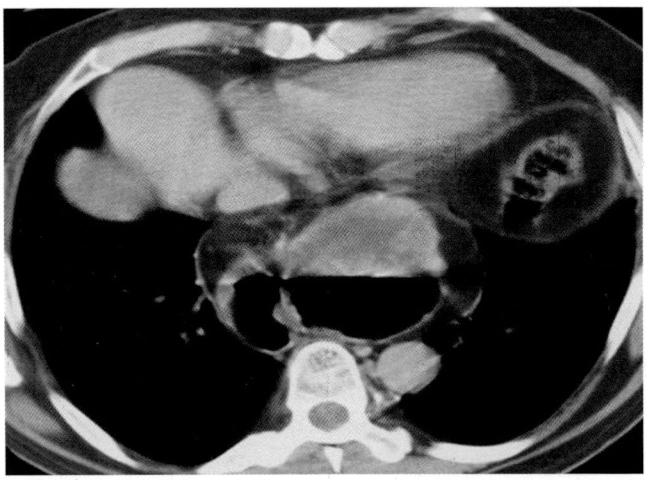

Fig. 11: Axial CT scan of upper abdomen showing large hiatus hernia.

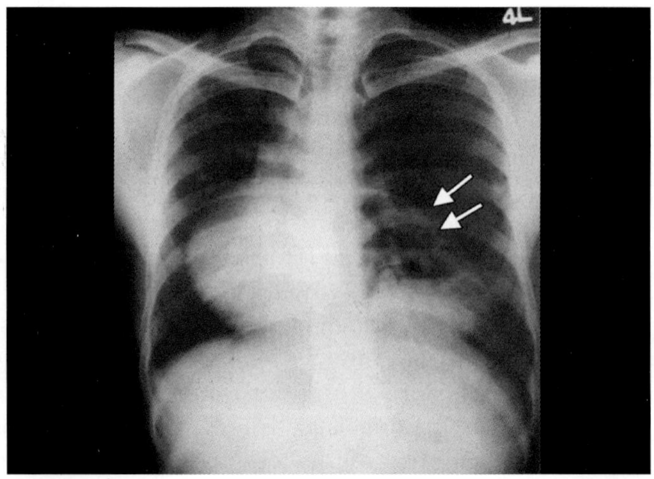

Fig. 12: Bochdalek hernia: Plain radiograph shows herniated bowel loops (arrows) into the thorax and right mediastinal shift.

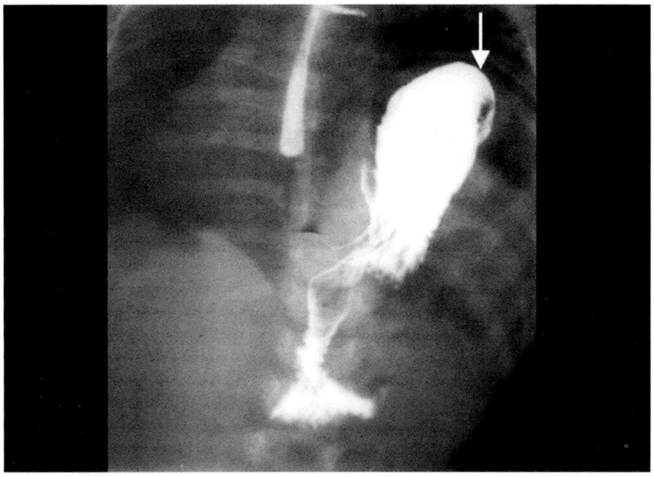

Fig. 13: Bochdalek hernia: Barium study showing herniation of stomach (arrow) into thorax.

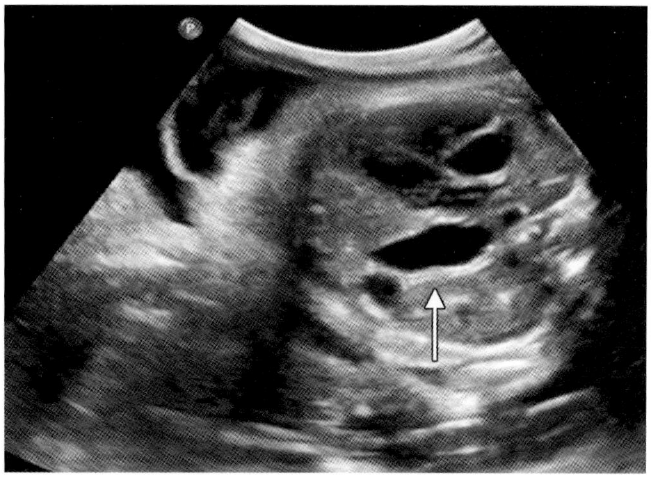

Fig. 14: Congenital diaphragmatic hernia: Antenatal ultrasound showing intrathoracic herniation of stomach (arrow).

tissue density mass which abuts the posteromedial aspect of either side of diaphragm. With the advent of CT, however, many small asymptomatic defects are being detected in adults. On the lateral chest radiograph,these hernias are seen as a smooth bulge with epicenter approximately 4–5 cm anterior to posterior costophrenic angle. Antenatal diagnosis of congenital diaphragmatic hernia on ultrasound is suspected when the fetal heart is displaced either by an intrathoracic solid mass (liver, kidney) or by a fluid filled structure (stomach, bowel) with decreased abdominal circumference **(Fig. 14)**.[10,11] MRI can also be extremely helpful modality to look for congenital diaphragmatic hernia **(Fig. 15)**. Pulmonary hypoplasia often results from compression of the fetal lung by the herniated viscera.

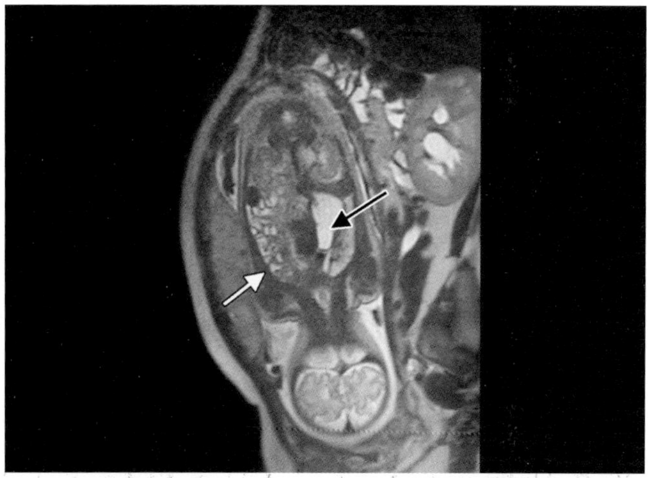

Fig. 15: Bilateral congenital diaphragmatic hernia: Antenatal T2-weighted MR image showing bilateral diaphragmatic hernia with intrathoracic herniation of stomach (black arrow) and bowel loops (white arrow).

Morgagni Hernia

It is commonly seen in adults and is mostly asymptomatic. It is due to the failure of fusion between the fibrotendinous elements of the sternal part and costal part of developing diaphragm. In Morgagni hernia, peritoneum or abdominal contents pass upwards through foramen of Morgagni in retro or para-sternal location into the thoracic cavity. In Morgagni hernia, weak area is congenital however the herniation of the abdominal contents is often acquired and conditions causing increase intra-abdominal pressure like severe effort, obesity and trauma. Morgagni hernia is mostly right sided because the the left sided defects are covered by heart and pericardium. On chest radiograph, a Morgagni hernia containing fat or liver presents as a rounded density occupying the right anterior cardiophrenic angle. Herniated organs and diaphragm defect are better evaluated by CT and MRI **(Fig. 16)**.

Intrapericardial Hernia

It results from herniation of abdominal viscera into the pericardial sac through a defect of the central tendon of the diaphragm but is extremely rare.

DIAPHRAGMATIC INJURY

Both blunt and penetrating injuries can injure diaphragm. Diaphragmatic injuries are usually caused blunt trauma or penetrating injuries. They occur in 0.8–8% after blunt trauma.[12] The confusing clinical and radiographic findings can delay the diagnosis. Tear is left sided in 70–90% and right sided in 10–30% in blunt trauma patients. This is attributed to the protection offered by the liver. The

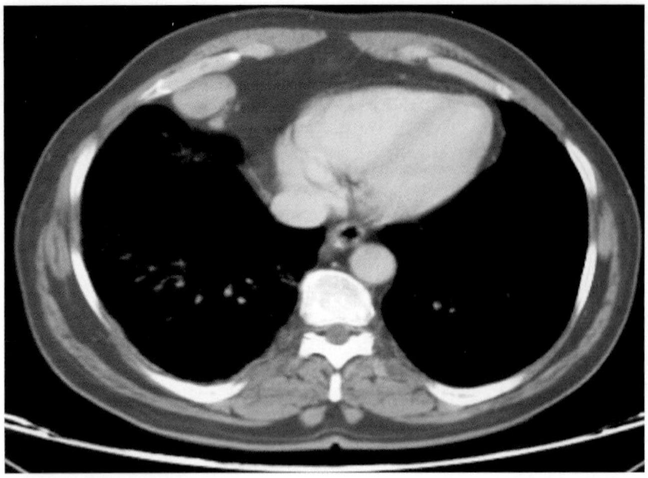

Fig. 16: Morgagni hernia: Axial CT scan of the abdomen showing fatty lesion with traversing vessels in right paracardiac region.

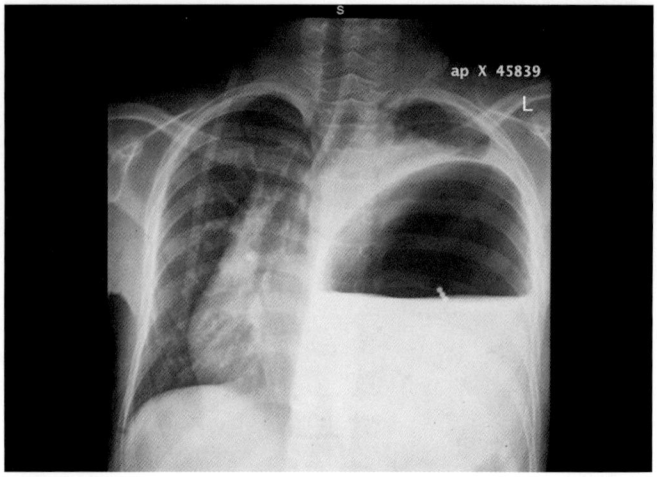

Fig. 17: Chest radiograph with left diaphragm tear showing intrathoracic herniation of the stomach with contralateral mediastinal shift.

stomach is the most commonly herniated organ, but bowel, spleen, liver and omentum can also herniate into the chest **(Fig. 17)**. The chest X-ray remains valuable in the acute phase for detection of diaphragmatic injuries, despite its technical limitations which include supine positioning, use of portable radiography and limited patient cooperation. Specific diagnostic findings of the injury include the following: asymmetry of a hemidiaphragm or changing hemidiaphragm levels, intrathoracic herniation of the hollow viscus which may be associated with focal constriction of the viscus at the site of the tear called collar sign. On left side, nasogastric tube may be seen above the hemidiaphragm.[6] Nonspecific X-ray finding are rib fractures, hemo- or pneumothorax, and atelectasis at the lung bases.

CT is usually the next imaging modality in trauma patients because of speed and global information provided. Multidetector CT (MDCT) with multiplanar reconstructions is very valuable diagnostic tool. MDCT features of the diaphragmatic trauma include direct visualization of injury, diaphragm thickening, segmental diaphragm non visualization, viscera herniation **(Figs. 18A and B)**, dependent viscera sign, the collar sign, and peridiaphragmatic active contrast extravasation.[12,13] Direct visualization of injury is often possible by depicting the free edge of the disrupted diaphragm. Isolated segmental nonvisualization of the diaphragm is highly sensitive but this sign must be used with caution when seen in isolation, especially in the elderly, in whom it can be a normal variant. Intrathoracic herniation of viscera has high specificity but have variable sensitivity. If an abdominal structure herniates through a diaphragm rent, the free edges of the diaphragm can constrict the herniated organ, and hence result in a "collar". The **collar sign (Fig. 19)** is an indication of intrathoracic herniation of abdominal contents even when its relative level does not clearly suggest so. When the diaphragm is torn, its constraints are released, and the viscera may lie "dependent" against the posterior chest wall as compared to the normal intact diaphragm which prevents the upper abdominal viscera from contacting the chest wall **(Fig. 20)**. The diaphragm is considered abnormally thickened by subjective comparison with the contra lateral side or diaphragmatic crus thickness more than 10 mm. In the presence of injury, intramuscular hematoma or edema or muscle retraction accounts for the abnormally thick diaphragm.

MRI is helpful in equivocal cases of diaphragmatic injury. Direct coronal and sagittal imaging with respiratory and cardiac gating may allow confirmation or exclusion of the diagnosis. Diaphragmatic signal may be interrupted due to the laceration hence confirm a traumatic diaphragmatic injury. [13] Barium studies allow confirmation of herniated intestine or stomach but are limited to evaluation of the hollow viscera. Fluoroscopic demonstration of severely decreased motion is highly suggestive but not diagnostic of injury. USG signs include herniation of viscera, diaphragm disruption, diaphragm non-visualization, and absent diaphragm excursion during the respiratory cycle.

TUMORS OF THE DIAPHRAGM

Tumors of the diaphragm are rare. The most common benign solid tumor is a lipoma **(Fig. 21)**. Benign tumors

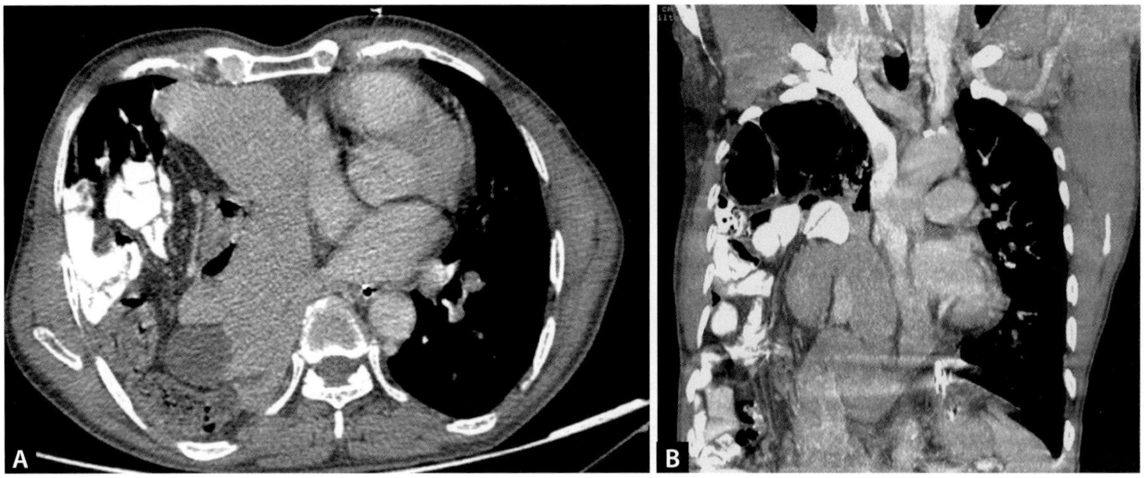

Figs. 18A and B: Traumatic right diaphragmatic hernia: (A) Axial and (B) coronal CECT sections show right diaphragmatic hernia with herniation of both hollow and solid viscera.

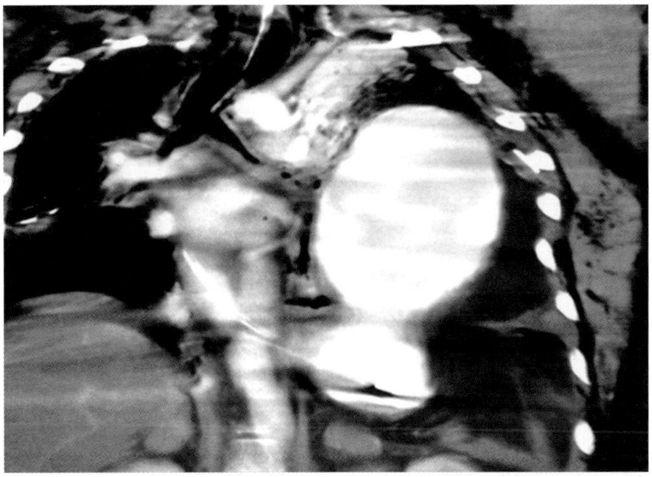

Fig. 19: Collar sign: MDCT with coronal reformation showing intrathoracic herniation of stomach through left diaphragmatic defect with constriction of stomach by the free edges of diaphragm at the site of herniation.

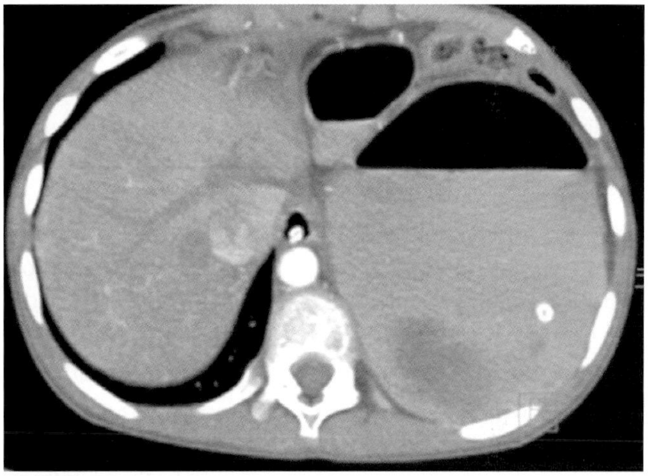

Fig. 20: Dependent viscera sign: CT axial sections showing intrathoracic herniation of the stomach through left diaphragmatic rupture and the stomach lying in a dependent position against the posterior ribs.

of the diaphragm may be removed surgically if there is a doubt about the diagnosis or they are symptomatic. Fibroma, angiofibroma, neurofibroma and neurilemmoma are the other benign tumors. The most common primary malignant tumor of diaphragm is rhabdomyosarcoma.[14] Metastatic neoplasms of the diaphragm may be due to direct invasion from tumors of adjacent organs. These include tumors of the lung, liver, stomach, colon pancreas, adrenal or liver. Cystic lesions of the diaphragm can be acquired or congenital. The most common benign cystic lesions of the diaphragm are bronchogenic or mesothelial cysts.[14] Acquired cysts include simple, fibrous lined and post-traumatic cysts. Hydatid disease and tuberculosis rarely cause inflammatory mass of the diaphragm. The majority of patients present with pleuritic chest pain. Radiographically, a mass which abuts the diaphragm is seen. Imaging modalities like CT and MRI are provide a specific diagnosis and look for extent of the tumor.

CHEST WALL

The chest wall structures are grouped into soft tissue and bony structures on the basis of the radiographic appearances. The soft tissue structures include muscles of the chest wall, breasts, fat, nerves, blood and lymphatic vessels. The bony structures include ribs, costal cartilages, sternum, clavicles and spine. Chest wall may be affected

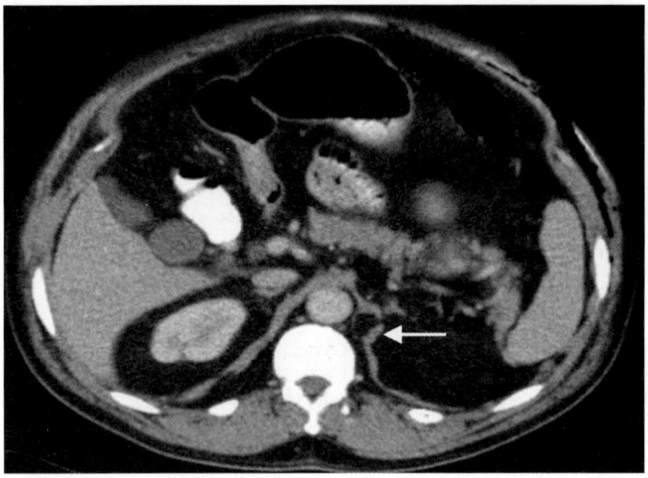

Fig. 21: Lipoma: CT axial sections showing well-marginated fat density lesion in the left crus of the diaphragm.

by a variety of disorders affecting these constituents. Chest radiography may be the first imaging study to suggest the presence of a chest wall mass given its widespread availability and utilization. However, it is difficult to detect, localize and characterize these disorders by means of conventional radiography alone most of the times and cross-sectional imaging such as MDCT and MRI, helps in the evaluation of these disorders and sometimes allow definitive diagnosis.[15] MDCT and MRI help in knowing the extent and character of the diseases. CT helps in better depiction of small calcifications and bone destruction whereas MRI in marrow involvement and soft tissue extension. Multiplanar imaging and three-dimensional (3D) reconstructions can be achieved with both modalities. Ultrasound generally provides less detailed information as compared to CT and MRI however it can be very helpful at times in localizing the lesion. It also helps in differentiating cystic and solid lesions and can characterize cystic lesions. It also provides imaging guidance for aspiration and biopsy when cytological/histopathological diagnosis is required. 2-[fluorine-18] fluoro-2-deoxyd- glucose (FDG) positron emission tomography (PET)/CT is not performed commonly to evaluate chest wall tumors, because many primary and secondary malignancies may demonstrate increased FDG uptake. PET/CT may be used, however, to determine the presence and extent of metastatic disease and assess response to therapy.[16]

Diseaes affecting chest wall can be grouped into congenital and developmental anomalies, inflammatory and infectious diseases and various primary and secondary tumors.[15]

CONGENITAL AND DEVELOPMENTAL ANOMALIES

Funnel Chest (Pectus Excavatum or Depressed Sternum)

It is the most common congenital anomaly affecting sternum. In this deformity, sternum is depressed and on each side ribs extent beyond the sternum anteriorly. Postero-anterior radiograph shows shift of the heart to the left, straightening of the left heart border with prominence of the main pulmonary artery segment, loss of the descending aortic interface, and an increase in the opacity in the right cardio-phrenic angle **(Figs. 22A and B)**.[15] The extent of sternal depression is evaluated easily at lateral radiograph and the severity can be best quantified with CT. MDCT is usually reserved for the individuals in whom surgery is planned. Severity may be graded using the Haller index. Haller index is ratio of the maximum internal transverse diameter of the chest divided by the minimum anteroposterior diameter. An index of >3.25 require correction surgically. Haller index ranges from 1.9 to 2.7 in normal children.[17]

Pigeon Chest (Pectus Carinatum)

It is less common than pectus excavatum. It may be congenital or acquired. In this condition, there is convex anterior protrusion of the sternum and costochondral joints and results due to disproportionate overgrowth of the costochondral cartilages. It is considered cosmetic deformity only and may be associated with family history, connective tissue disease and scoliosis.[18]

Poland Syndrome

In this syndrome, there is partial or total absence of pectoralis major muscles with ipsilateral hand and arm anomalies (particularly syndactyly). Radiograph shows an area of hyperlucency on the affected side and abnormal axillary fold. CT and MRI shows the absence of the muscles and associated anomalies.[15]

Cervical Rib

Cervical rib commonly originates from the seventh cervical vertebra. Usually, it is found in approximately 0.5% of the general population. In 90% of the cases its asymptomatic. It is seen as supernumerary rib that articulates with cervical-type transverse process which is horizontal as compared to upward-sloping thoracic transverse process of thoracic vertebra. MDCT helps in showing relationship between vascular compression and bony deformity.

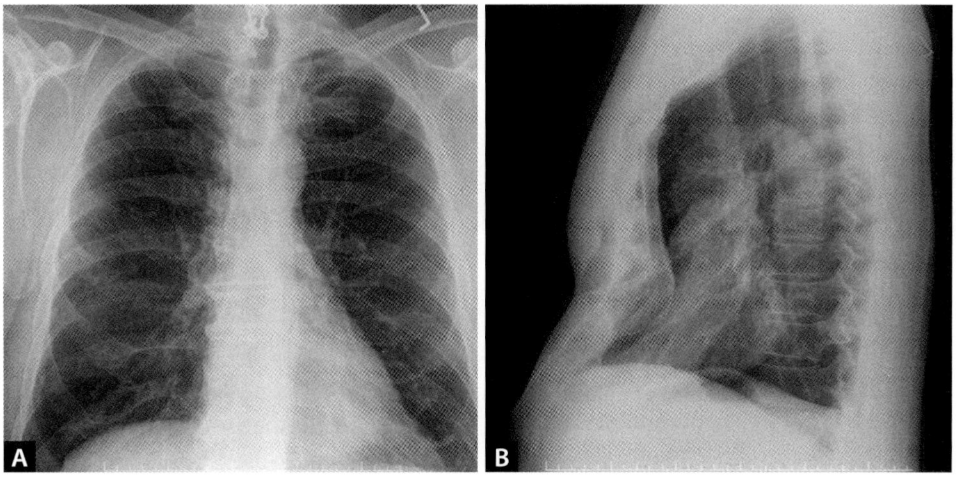

Figs. 22A and B: Pectus excavatum: (A) Posteroanterior and (B) lateral chest radiographs showing leftward displacement of the heart, straightening of the left heart border with severe depression of the sternum.

Clavicles

It may be hypoplastic in number of syndromes including cleidocranial dysplasia, Holt-Oram syndrome, pelvic-shoulder dysplasia, some trisomy disorders and progeria.

INFLAMMATORY AND INFECTIOUS DISEASES

Primary infections of the chest wall are rare, and are more common in setting of trauma, immunosuppression and diabetes mellitus. They occur more commonly secondary to infectious processes in the lungs or to pleural empyema (empyema necessitatis). Other causes are hematogeneous spread or iatrogenic (median sternotomy for cardiac surgery).

Cellulitis and Necrotizing Fasciitis

Infections of chest wall soft tissues range from cellulitis to infections of deeper soft tissues, including myositis, osteomyelitis, abscess, and necrotizing fasciitis. Cellulitis often appears more extensive on MR imaging than on other imaging modalities because of MR imaging's sensitivity for tissue edema. Cellulitis is characterized by high T2 signal in subcutaneous soft tissues.[19] Necrotizing fasciitis is a serious septic condition more common in immunocompromised, alcoholic, or diabetic patients. It affects subcutaneous fat and the superficial fascia and should not involve the underlying muscles. MRI shows the complete extent of the involvement and CT may show gas formation. In pyomyositis, predominant involvement is of muscles and MRI is the best imaging modality to assess intramuscular necrosis.

Pyogenic Osteomyelitis

Osteomyelitis of the chest wall is frequently associated with periosteal elevation, loss of planes of soft tissue and adjacent soft tissue masses. Common causative organisms are *Staphylococcus aureus* and *Pseudomonas aeruginosa*. CT and MRI can clearly depict the abnormality **(Figs. 23A and B)**. Median sternotomy is the main surgical approach to variety of cardiothoracic procedures. Poststernotomy complications can occur in less than 5% of the cases and include sternal dehiscence, mediastinitis, and osteomyelitis. They manifest usually 1–2 weeks after surgery. CT is useful modality for detecting and localizing retrosternal abscess. Acute mediastinitis at CT show inflammatory tissue replacing mediastinal fat.

Tuberculosis

Chest wall involvement in tuberculosis is commonly due to hematogenous route. However, it may occur as contiguous spread from underlying pleural or pulmonary involvement. It presents as destruction of bone and or cartilage with associated soft tissue mass **(Figs. 24A and B)** which may show rim enhancement and calcifications.

Fungal Infections

Actinomycosis and *Aspergillosis* may infect the chest wall. Actinomycosis may present as sinuses, massive thickening of the soft tissue, wavy periostitis, and underlying rib destruction. *Aspergilosis* involving the chest wall is associated with pulmonary involvement and cause permeative osteolytic destruction of underlying ribs.[15]

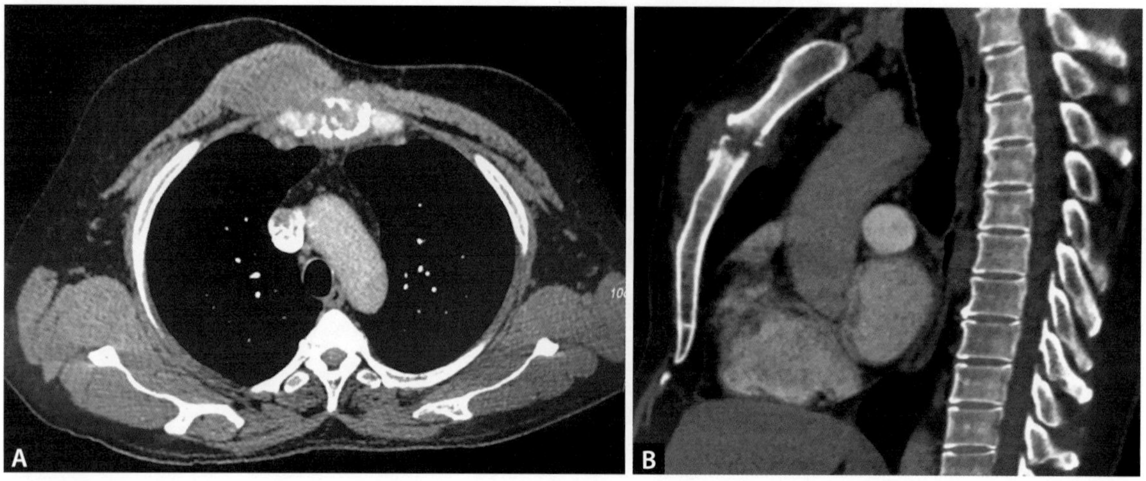

Figs. 23A and B: Sternal osteomyelitis: (A) Axial and (B) sagittal MDCT showing expansile lytic desctuction of sterum with associated soft tissue extending both anterior and posterior to sternum.

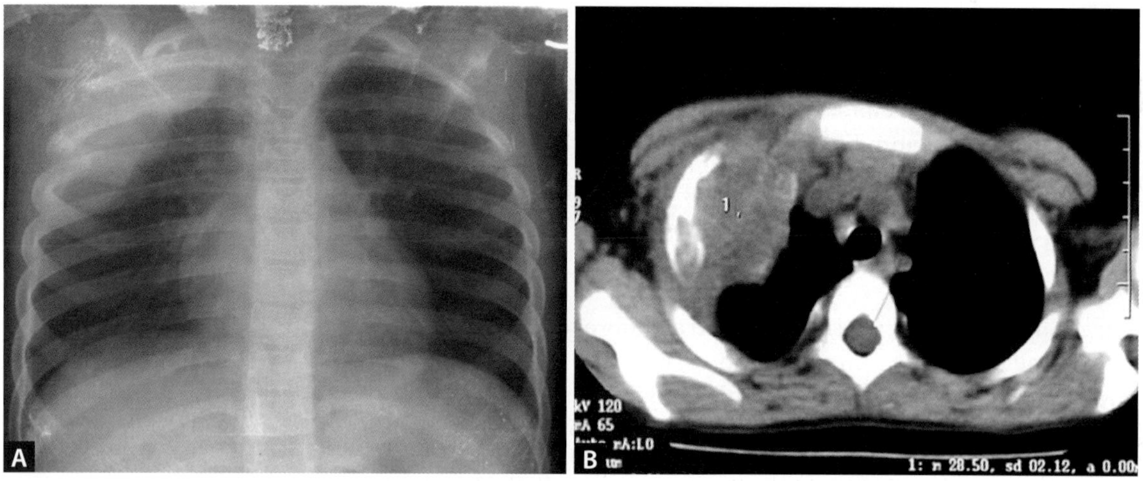

Figs. 24A and B: Chest wall tuberculosis: (A) Chest radiograph shows large right upper chest wall soft tissue with destruction of ribs; (B) CT shows expansion and destruction of rib with associated soft tissue. Aspiration from the soft tissue confirmed the lesion to be tubercular.

TUMORS OF THE CHEST WALL

Chest wall tumors represent approximately 5% of thoracic tumors.[21] These tumors are typically divided into categories based on the site of origin and tissue composition (osseous or soft tissue) as well as whether they are benign or malignant.[16,20] Greater than 50% of chest wall tumors are malignant, and most of these malignancies represent direct invasion by or metastasis from adjacent tumors of the lung, breast, pleura, and mediastinum. The most common primary malignancies of the chest wall are sarcomas, 45% of which arise from soft tissue and 55% of which arise from bone. Once a chest wall mass has been identified, the next step is to determine whether it is malignant or benign. A large soft-tissue mass with invasion into adjacent osseous and/or soft-tissue structures is nearly always malignant. Primary chondrosarcoma or osteosarcoma as well as their metastasis will show characteristic mineralization patter.[16] Benign osseous neoplasms do not result in extraosseous soft-tissue masses unlike their malignant counterpart and mostly exhibit nonaggressive radiological features.

Benign Osseous Tumors

Benign osseous tumors of the chest wall are less frequently encountered than malignant neoplasms. Most of these lesions are osseous or cartilaginous.

Fibrous Dysplasia

Present as fusiform enlargement with cortical thickening and increased trabeculation of involved bones. The ribs are commonly affected, followed by clavicle. This lesion appears lytic or mixed lesion with lytic regions and ground-glass matrix. Osseous erosion is generally not seen.

Osteochondroma

These tumors arise as aberrant growth of normal tissue. These tumors frequently involve costochondral junction of the ribs. Osteochondromas are pedunculated lesions arising from the surface of the bone **(Figs. 25A and B)**. Evaluation of the associated cartilaginous cap should be carefully evaluated, as caps measuring greater than 3 cm in children, greater than 2 cm in adults raises suspicion for malignant transformation.[22]

Aneurysmal Bone Cyst and Giant Cell Tumor

It may involve chest wall. In aneurysmal bone cyst (ABC), the most common sites of involvement is posterior elements of the spine whereas giant cell tumor involves sternum, clavicle and ribs.

Malignant Osseous Tumors

Malignant osseous tumors of the chest wall account for approximately 55% of all chest wall masses.[21] The most common primary malignancies include sarcomas, such as chondrosarcoma, osteosarcoma, the Ewing sarcoma family of tumors (ESFT) as well as multiple myeloma (MM) whereas metastatic disease and direct invasion from intrathoracic malignancies are the most frequent secondary causes.[20]

Chondrosarcomas

Chondrosarcoma is the most common malignant primary tumors of the chest wall. It frequently involves anterior chest wall originating from the costochondral arches or sternum **(Fig. 26)**.[23] Most of (90%) the tumors occur in the ribs, commonly along the upper five, adjacent to costal cartilage. These are primary lesions most of the times, however, approximately 10% arise from benign tumors which were preexistent. On chest radiograph bony destruction, irregular contours, and intratumoral mineralization are present. CT demonstrates well-defined, calcified soft-tissue masses with associated bony changes. MRI also shows characteristic features. On T1-weighted imaging, signal intensity of the lesion matches that of muscle signal intensity and on T2 weighted it is equal to or greater than that of fat and show heterogeneous enhancement post-contrast.

Osteosarcomas

Osteosarcomas account for 10–15% of malignant chest wall tumors. When osteosarcomas arise in a primary fashion from the chest wall, the most frequently affected structures include the ribs, clavicle, and scapula.[23] On T1-weighted images, the nonmineralized regions of osteosarcomas demonstrate variable signal intensity but are often hyperintense to muscle. On T2-weighted images, the nonmineralized regions demonstrate high signal intensity. Tumor mineralization is usually hypointense on both T1- and T2- weighted imaging. Heterogeneous enhancement after the administration of IV contrast is typical.[20]

Ewing Sarcoma

Ewing sarcoma of the chest wall presents either as a solitary mass or as multiple masses with an eccentric growth pattern. Ewing sarcoma can arise from rib, scapula, clavicle, or sternum but may originate from extra skeletal site.[23] These lesions commonly displace adjacent soft-tissue structures instead of encasement or invasion. They may arise in para-vertebral region and extend through the vertebral foramina. CT scans show a large ill-defined mass with an inhomogeneous enhancement caused by

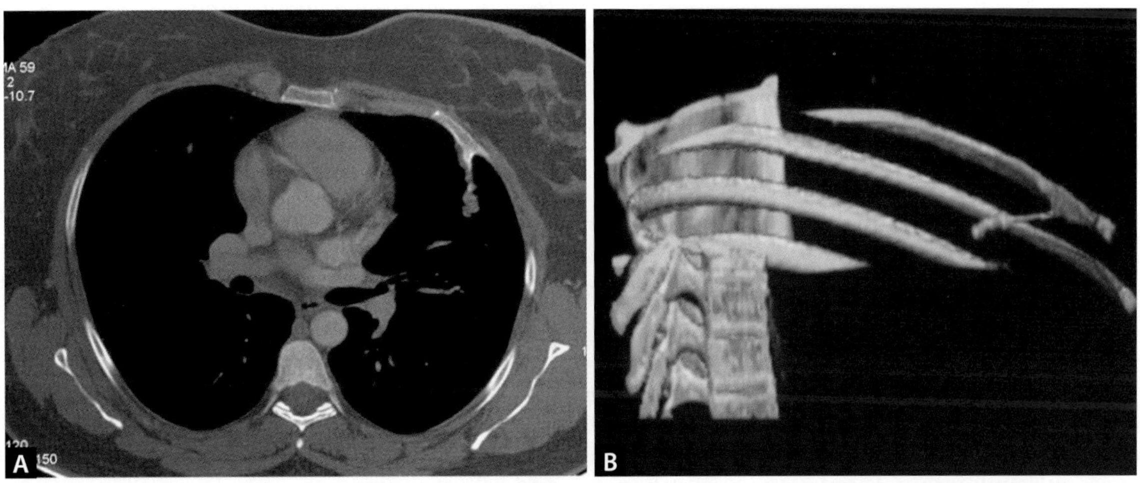

Figs. 25A and B: Osteochondroma: (A) Chest CT and (B) 3D bony reformat showing prick-like inward projecting intrathoracic osteochondroma with thickened overlying pleura.

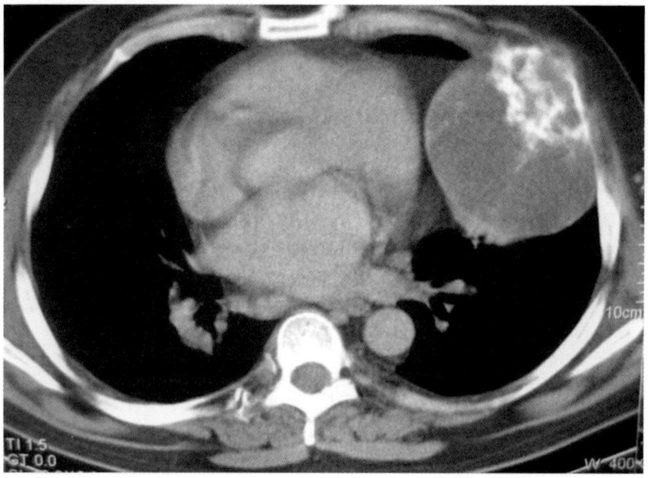

Fig. 26: Chondrosarcoma: Chest CT showing large expansile mass arising from the rib with matrix calcification and large associated soft tissue.

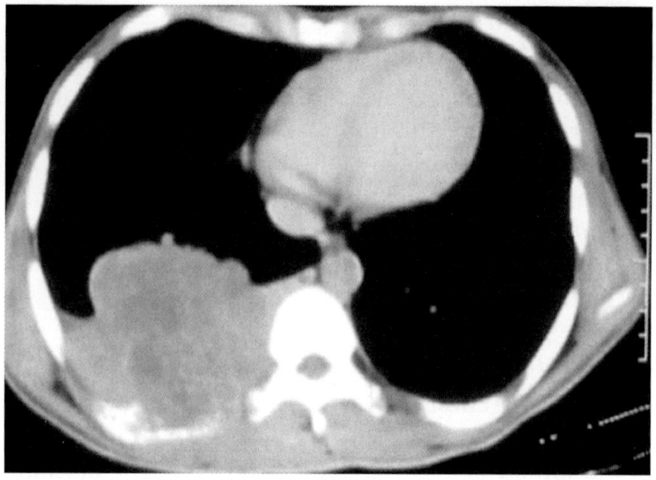

Fig. 27: Ewing sarcoma: Axial CT sections showing large heterogeneous chest wall lesion with erosion destruction of the posterior rib.

cystic degeneration. Mass lesion may be accompanied by calcification **(Fig. 27)**. These tumors generally have signal intensity equal to or greater than that of muscle on T1, in homogeneous high signal intensity on T2-weighted MR images and show marked enhancement. Small lesions are homogeneous where as large lesions have heterogeneous appearance with areas of necrosis and hemorrhage.

Multiple Myeloma

It may involve vertebral column, ribs, or clavicles and causes multiple osteolytic lesions with discrete margins. At MR imaging, lesions have low signal intensity on T1-weighted images on T2-weighted images have high signal intensity.

Soft Tissue Tumors

Malignant and benign soft tissue tumors of the chest wall are a heterogeneous group and can be divided into the following groups based on the tissue of origin: adipocytic, vascular, peripheral nerve sheath, fibroblastic-myofibroblastic, fibrohistiocytic, and cutaneous.[24]

Adipocytic

Lipoma

Lipomas are the most common soft tissue tumor and present as encapsulated masses composed of adipocytes that are similar to normal fatty tissue found within the chest wall. Lipoma has fat attenuation on MDCT, high signal intensity at T1-weighted imaging, and shows uniform signal loss at fat-suppressed MR imaging. Internal septations may be present and appear hypointense on T1-weighted images. After the administration of IV contrast, lipomas do not enhance, although internal septations may enhance when present.[24,25]

Liposarcoma

Liposarcomas are the second most common chest wall malignancy of soft tissue origin. These tumors constitute approximately 15% of all sarcomas, although only 10% of involve the chest wall.[23] Well-differentiated liposarcomas are typically composed of 50–75% adipose tissue, which results in high signal intensity on T1-weighted and low signal intensity on T2-weighted images. Depending on the volume of fat, it may be difficult to distinguish well-differentiated liposarcoma from lipoma. Features which suggest diagnosis of well differentiated liposarcoma are large tumors (size greater than 10 cm), thick internal septations, nodular regions of nonadipose tissue, and adipose tissue comprising less than 75% of the tumor.[26]

Vascular

Hemangioma and angiosarcoma

Hemangiomas have high signal intensity at T2-weighted imaging, demonstrates variable amounts of internal fat at multidetector CT and T1-weighted MR imaging, and frequently contains phleboliths **(Figs. 28A to C)**.[16] In contrast, angiosarcoma are heterogeneous, lack internal fat, are aggressive and invade adjacent structures. These tumors may be associated with chronic lymphedema and may exhibit findings related to their origin (such as fibrous thickening, soft-tissue nodules, and fluid collections) adjacent to the chest wall musculature.[23]

Peripheral Nerve Sheath Tumors

Benign nerve sheath neoplasms such as neurofibroma and schwannoma appear as low-attenuating soft-tissue masses which contain fat or cystic components. The "target"

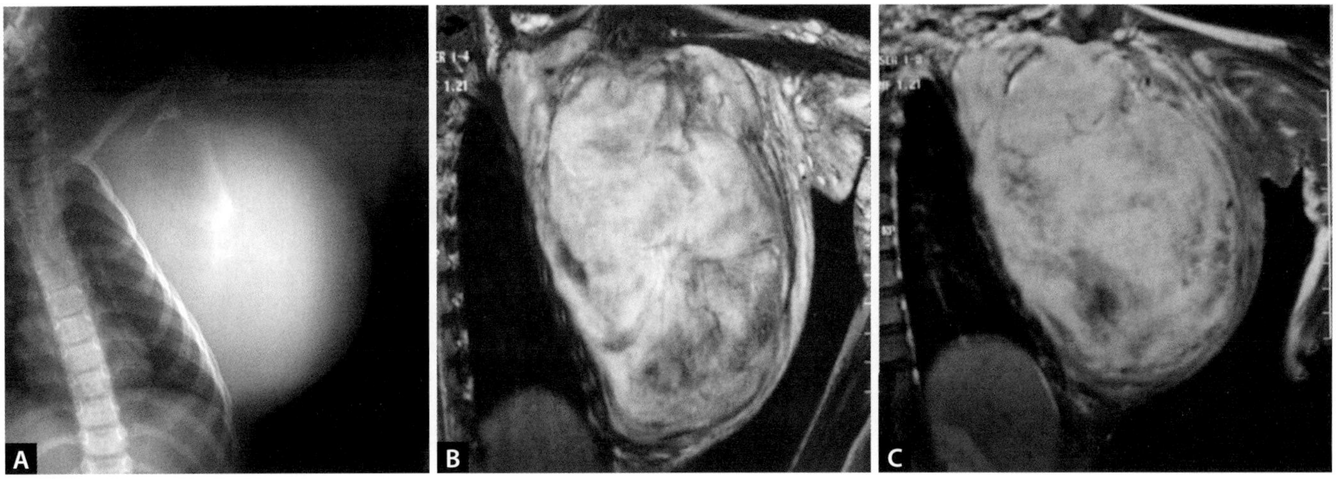

Figs. 28A to C: Child with large chest wall hemangioma: (A) Chest radiograph showing large well-circumscribed homogeneous soft tissue mass along lateral chest wall; (B) Coronal T2 and (C) postcontrast images showing heterogeneously enhancing chest wall lesion.

sign which is characterized by central low signal intensity and peripheral high signal intensity on T2-weighted MR images and central enhancement following the intravenous administration of gadolinium-based contrast material, and the fascicular sign, characterized by heterogeneous low signal intensity with a ring-like pattern on T2-weighted MR images, are frequently visualized.[16] The "split fat" sign, characterized by fat attenuation around the soft-tissue mass at multidetector CT, also may be seen. These radiologic signs are typically absent in malignant peripheral nerve sheath tumors which, when compared with benign nerve sheath neoplasms, demonstrate greater heterogeneity and aggressive behavior and invasion into surrounding structures.[23]

Fibroblastic–Myofibroblastic

Fibromatosis also known as desmoid tumor has been reported to primarily arise from the chest wall in 10–28% of cases.[23] Fibromatosis typically manifests as an ill-defined mass that grows in an infiltrative manner. On MR imaging, lesions has relatively homogeneous low to intermediate signal intensity on T1-weighted images whereas they appear more heterogeneous on T2-weighted images, low signal intensity bands have been reported in fibromatosis, and likely represent dense collagen bundles. Although fibromatosis may demonstrate moderate to marked heterogeneous enhancement, the collagen bundles do not enhance.[20]

Fibrohistiocytic

Undifferentiated pleomorphic sarcoma (UPS), also called malignant fibrous histiocytoma, is classified as a fibrohistiocytic malignancy and represents the most common malignant soft tissue neoplasm of the chest wall in adults.[26] At MDCT, UPS appears as a soft-tissue mass that involves the deep fascia or skeletal muscle and enhances heterogeneously after intravenous contrast material administration **(Figs. 29A and B)**. Involvement of adjacent osseous structures is common. Internal mineralization can often be identified in the peripheral aspect of the lesion after treatment. UPS demonstrates low signal intensity and is isointense to muscle on T1-weighted MR images. On T2-weighted images, UPS has intermediate to high signal intensity and is iso- to hyperintense to fat.

METASTATIC DISEASE

Osseous metastatic disease affecting the chestwall is typically encountered in the setting of extensive metastatic disease elsewhere in the body, but it may be seen early in association with aggressive primary malignancies. These lesions can manifest in many different ways, with some metastases demonstrating imaging characteristics specific to the primary malignancies from which they are derived. Soft-tissue metastatic disease typically is seen only in the setting of extensive metastatic disease elsewhere in the body, is considered an indicator of a poor prognosis.[16]

CHEST WALL INVASION BY THORACIC MALIGNANCY

The chest wall may be directly invaded by aggressive thoracic malignancies—typically lung cancer, breast cancer, pleural tumors, or mediastinal neoplasms. Although MR imaging and MDCT have been shown to have similar utility in the detecting chest wall invasion by lung cancer, MR imaging is considered to be superior due to better spatial resolution and soft tissue contrast.[16]

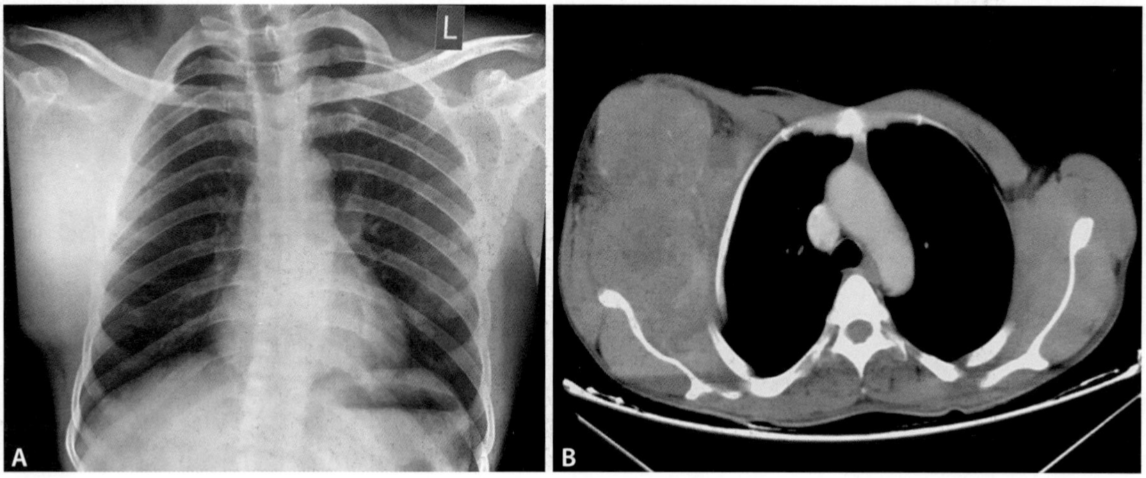

Figs. 29A and B: Undifferentiated pleomorphic sarcoma: (A) Chest radiograph showing large well-defined homogeneous mass along the right upper chest wall with no erosion or destruction of underlying bones; (B) CECT chest shows large heterogeneous soft tissue mass anterior to scapula with no bony involvement.

REFERENCES

1. Nason LK, Walker CM, McNeeley MF, et al. Imaging of the diaphragm: Anatomy and function. Radiographics. 2012; 32:E51-70.
2. Felson B: Chest Roentgenology. WB Saunders, Philadelphia. 1973.
3. Adam A, Dixon AK, Gillard JH, et al. Grainger and Allison's Diagnostic Radiology: A Textbook of Medical Imaging, 6th edition. Churchill Livingstone/Elsevier. 2014.
4. Sarwal A, Walker FO, Cartwright MS. Neuromuscular ultrasound for evaluation of the diaphragm. Muscle Nerve. 2013;47:319-29.
5. Shackleton KL, Stewart ET, Taylor AJ. Traumatic diaphragmatic injuries: spectrum of radiographic findings. Radiographics. 1998;18:49-59.
6. Gierada DS, Curtin JJ, Erickson SJ, et al. Diaphragmatic motion: fast gradient-recalled-echo MR imaging in healthy subjects. Radiology. 1995;194:879-4.
7. Kiryu S, Loring SH, Mori Y, et al. Quantitative analysis of the velocity and synchronicity of diaphragmatic motion: dynamic MRI in different postures. Magn Reson Imaging. 2006;24(10):1325-32.
8. May AK, Moore MM. Diagnosis of blunt rupture of the right hemidiaphragm by technetium scan. Am Surg. 1999;65:761-5.
9. Kharma N. Dysfunction of the diaphragm: Imaging as a diagnostic tool. Curr Opin Pulm Med. 2013;19(4):394-8.
10. Panicek D, Benson C, Gottlieb R, et al. The diaphragm: Anatomic, pathologic, and radiologic considerations. Radiographics. 1988;8(3):385-425.
11. Chavhan G, Babyn P, Cohen R, et al. Multimodality imaging of the pediatric diaphragm: Anatomy and pathologic conditions. Radiographics. 2010;30(7):1797-818.
12. Lochum S, Ludwig T, Walter F, et al. Imaging of the diaphtagmatic injury: a diagnostic challenge? Radiographics. 2002;22:S103-18.
13. Sliker CW. Imaging of diaphragmatic injuries. Radiol Clin N Am. 2006;44:199-211.
14. Kim MP, Hofstetter WL. Tumors of the diaphragm. Thorac Surg Clin. 2009;19:521-9
15. Jeung MY, Gangi A, Gasser B, et al. Imaging of chest wall disorders. Radiographics. 1999;19:617-37.
16. Carter BW, Benveniste MF, Betancourt SL, et al. Imaging evaluation of malignant chest wall neoplasms. Radiographics. 2016;36(5):1285-306.
17. Haller JA Jr, Kramer SS, Lietman SA. Use of CT scans in selection of patients for pectus excavatum surgery: a preliminary report. J Pediatr Surg. 1987;22:904-6.
18. Mak SM, Bhaludin BN, Naaseri S, et al. Imaging of congenital chest wall deformities. Br J Radiol. 2016;89(1061):20150595.
19. Lee TJ, Collins J. MR imaging evaluation of disorders of the chest wall. Magn Reson Imaging Clin N Am. 2008;16(2):355-79.
20. Carter BW, Gladish GW. MR imaging of chest wall tumors. Magn Reson Imaging Clin N Am. 2015;23(2):197-215.
21. Incarbone M, Pastorino U. Surgical treatment of chest wall tumors. World J Surg. 2001;25(2):218-30.
22. Zarqane H, Viala P, Dallaudière B, et al. Tumors of the rib. Diagn Interv Imaging. 2013;94(11):1095-108.
23. Tateishi U, Gladish GW, Kusumoto M, et al. Chest wall tumors: radiologic findings and pathologic correlation; Part 2. Malignant Tumors. Radiographics. 2003;23:1491-508.
24. Nam SJ, Kim S, Lim BJ, et al. Imaging of primary chest wall tumors with radiologic-pathologic correlation. Radiographics. 2011;31(3):749-70.
25. O'Sullivan P, O'Dwyer H, Flint J, et al. Soft tissue tumours and mass-like lesions of the chest wall: a pictorial review of CT and MR findings. Br J Radiol. 2007;80(955):574-80.
26. Kransdorf MJ, Bancroft LW, Peterson JJ, et al. Imaging of fatty tumors: distinction of lipoma and well differentiated liposarcoma. Radiology. 2002;224(1):99-104.

CHAPTER 174

Bronchial Artery Embolization

Ashu Seith Bhalla, Ankur Goyal

INTRODUCTION

Massive hemoptysis is an emergency; but even a small volume of hemoptysis can be life-threatening, especially in diseased lungs.[1,2] Lungs are supplied by two vascular systems; pulmonary arteries are involved in gas exchange and bronchial arteries provide oxygenated blood for nourishment.[3] Latter is a high-pressure circulation and is responsible for clinically significant hemoptysis in most of the cases.

Bronchial artery embolization (BAE) was first described by Remy et al. in 1974 as a measure to control hemoptysis.[4] Since then, the technique of BAE has evolved significantly and its clinical utility increased manifold. The procedure may be more aptly called *systemic artery embolization* because in addition to the bronchial arteries, the hypertrophied non-bronchial systemic collaterals are also embolized to control hemoptysis. A broader term of *endovascular embolization* would also include pulmonary arterial interventions to control hemoptysis. It is important to note that embolization is a palliative procedure and unless the causative disease is addressed, hemoptysis may recur.

PATIENT SELECTION

Hemoptysis is expectoration of blood, i.e. it originates from the respiratory tract. There is subjectivity in the literature regarding the grades of hemoptysis because the severity can be described in terms of volume of bleeding, duration of bleeding or its clinical impact. **Trivial hemoptysis** refers to blood-tinged sputum or few drops of blood. **Mild hemoptysis** means volume <100 mL/day or <50 mL/episode. **Moderate hemoptysis** refers to 100–300 mL/day or more than three bouts of at least 100 mL/day in a week. **Severe/Massive/Life-threatening hemoptysis** generally refers to either of the following:[2,5]

- Hemoptysis >300 mL/day.[1,2,6,7]
- Any volume hemoptysis leading to >1 g/dL drop in hemoglobin or >5% drop in hematocrit OR
- Any volume hemoptysis leading to respiratory failure ($SpaO_2$ <60%) OR
- Any volume hemoptysis leading to hypotension (systolic blood pressure <90 mm Hg).

Death from hemoptysis is rarely due to blood loss. Rather, it is the asphyxia caused from flooding of the airways and alveoli with blood, which is lethal.

MANAGEMENT APPROACH

For practical purposes, occasional blood-stained sputum can usually be managed conservatively but recurrent episodes of greater hemoptysis warrant intervention. Latter can be in the form of surgery or BAE. *BAE is the procedure of choice in patients with bilateral/extensive disease and in poor surgical risk patients.* In cases of episodic hemoptysis, BAE may be done electively in the quiescent phase to maximize the chances of technical success; rather than waiting for the patient to present in emergency. Massive hemoptysis is an emergency with high mortality and BAE is the management of choice in such a setting. Majority of the published literature on BAE includes patients with moderate-massive hemoptysis.

Surgery is the treatment of choice, if the pulmonary disease is localized and patients have adequate pulmonary reserve without comorbidities. Surgery is also indicated, if the hemoptysis is due to hydatid cyst, bronchial neoplasms or mediastinal vascular injuries.[1] *Even in surgical candidates, BAE has a role to reduce the intraoperative bleeding and especially if the patient presents in emergency department with massive hemoptysis.*

PATHOPHYSIOLOGY

In majority cases of non-cardiac hemoptysis, the source of bleeding is systemic circulation (bronchial arteries more commonly responsible than non-bronchial collaterals). This is because majority of the patients have chronic inflammatory lung disease. This leads to hypoxic vasoconstriction of the pulmonary arterioles in the areas of abnormality, which then incites hypertrophy of systemic arteries. These systemic arteries are recruited in order to participate in gas exchange through anastomoses with the pulmonary vascular system. The hypertrophic bronchial arteries are prone to rupture in the inflamed surroundings and since they are part of high pressure systemic circulation, this results in clinically significant hemoptysis.

In about 5% cases, the bleeding is from pulmonary vascular causes (pulmonary arterio-venous malformation, Rasmussen aneurysm, injury from Swan-Ganz catheter, etc.). Thus, most of the cases of significant hemoptysis result from systemic arterial source rather than pulmonary circulation.

INDICATIONS OF BAE

The common causes of hemoptysis requiring BAE are shown in **Table 1**.[2,8-10] and **Figures 1A to I** show examples of some of the common causes of hemoptysis.

It may be noted here that bronchial artery abnormalities are much less common in malignancies, whereas in infective/postinfective causes, these are usually hypertrophied. Thus, BAE is much more commonly done for non-neoplastic causes.[8,11] Majority of the published data on BAE is from Asia where TB (active disease/sequelae) is the most common cause of significant hemoptysis;[4,8-10,12-14] whereas sarcoidosis and cystic fibrosis are common indications in the west.[15,16] In addition, it is necessary to rule out cardiovascular (mitral stenosis, left heart failure, pulmonary embolism, aneurysm of aorta/pulmonary artery, iatrogenic injury by Swan-Ganz catheter) and systemic (bleeding diathesis, anticoagulation) causes of hemoptysis.

Table 1: Non-cardiac causes of significant hemoptysis.[7]

Post-tuberculosis (TB) sequelae: (fibrosis, bronchiectasis) ~30%	*Neoplasms:* Carcinoma, carcinoid, tracheobronchial lesions
Active TB: ~ 30%	*Vasculitis:* Granulomatosis with polyangiitis, Behçet's disease, SLE
Other inflammatory lung diseases: Bronchiectasis/bronchitis/ Aspergilloma/cystic fibrosis/ sarcoidosis/hydatid cyst	*Vascular causes:* Vascular malformations, post biopsy
Other lung infections: Non-tubercular infections, lung abscess	*Miscellaneous:* Pneumoconiosis, chronic obstructive pulmonary disease, and cryptogenic hemoptysis

PRE-PROCEDURE DIAGNOSTIC WORK-UP

The purpose of pre-procedure work-up is to identify the cause and site of hemoptysis. This would not only enable to exclude the cardiac and pulmonary vascular causes, but also to plan the embolization/surgical procedure. **Flowchart 1** depicts the diagnostic approach and management in a case with significant hemoptysis of pulmonary etiology.

Chest radiograph (CXR): Frequently performed as the first investigation and may be the only investigation feasible in emergency cases. Advantages include wide availability, low cost and can be done immediately. American College of Radiology (ACR) recommends a chest radiograph in the evaluation of all patients with hemoptysis, because it not only lateralizes the bleeding but may also identify the cause.[17] Radiographs are diagnostic in about 50% cases.[1]

Computed tomography (CT): Multidetector CT is the modality of choice for evaluation of hemoptysis. Contrast-enhanced CT (CECT) has the capability to detect airway, parenchymal as well as vascular causes of hemoptysis (**Figs. 1 and 2**). CT bronchial angiography (CTBA) provides a vascular roadmap by delineating the hypertrophied bronchial and systemic arteries **(Figs. 2A to H)** while CT pulmonary angiography (CTPA) acquisition can delineate the rarer pulmonary vascular causes of hemoptysis. As per ACR recommendations, CTBA is the next most appropriate investigation in patients with significant hemoptysis.[17] This technique has the potential to reduce the procedure time as well as improve the outcomes of BAE (by identifying the ectopic and uncommon arterial supply preprocedural). CTA has been found to reduce the rate of vascular catheterization failure in elderly patients.[18] A combined CTA for simultaneous evaluation of both systemic and

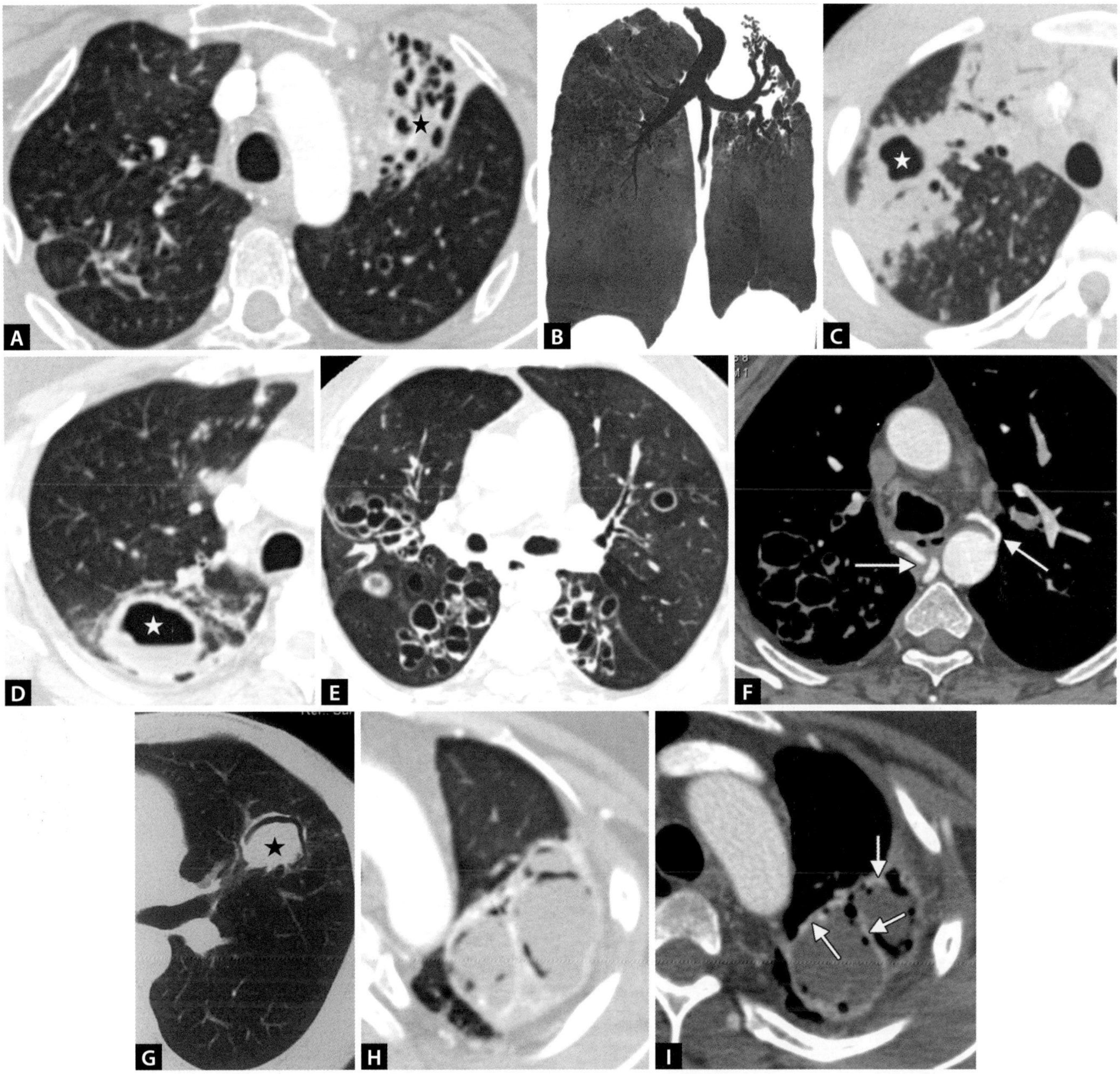

Figs. 1A to I: CT images showing common causes of hemoptysis: (A) TB sequelae (Fibrobronchiectasis and collapse left upper lobe (asterisk) and fibroparenchymal lesions right upper lobe); (B) Coronal MinIP image showing upper lobe predominant post TB fibrosis with bronchiectasis, volume loss and cavitation left upper lobe; (C) Active TB [thick-walled cavity right upper lobe (asterisk) with surrounding dense consolidation and centrilobular nodules]; (D) TB sequelae with superimposed pyogenic bacterial infection [Cavity (asterisk) with air-fluid level]; (E and F) Bilateral bronchiectasis with hypertrophied bronchial arteries (arrows); (G) Thin-walled cavity with aspergilloma (asterisk); (H and I) Chronic cavitary pulmonary aspergillosis with pleural thickening and vascularity in the walls of cavity (arrows).

pulmonary circulations in a single acquisition would be ideal and can be done by employing varying rates and concentration of contrast injection **(Figs. 2A to H)**.[19]

Fiberoptic bronchoscopy (FB): FB and CTA are complementary in the evaluation of hemoptysis and both should be done prior to BAE, in the elective setting.[20] CT is more useful to identify the cause while bronchoscopy is more accurate in localizing the site of active bleed. This is especially useful in case there is multifocal/bilateral lung disease. Bronchoscopy has the advantage that it can identify the bleeding endobronchial lesions, enable sampling as well as local ablation procedures. Such lesions may not

Flowchart 1: Approach to a patient with hemoptysis.

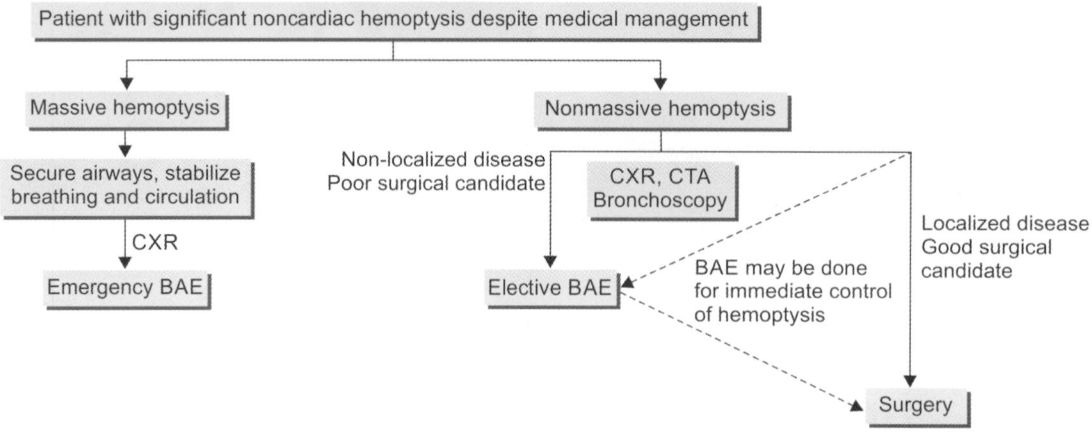

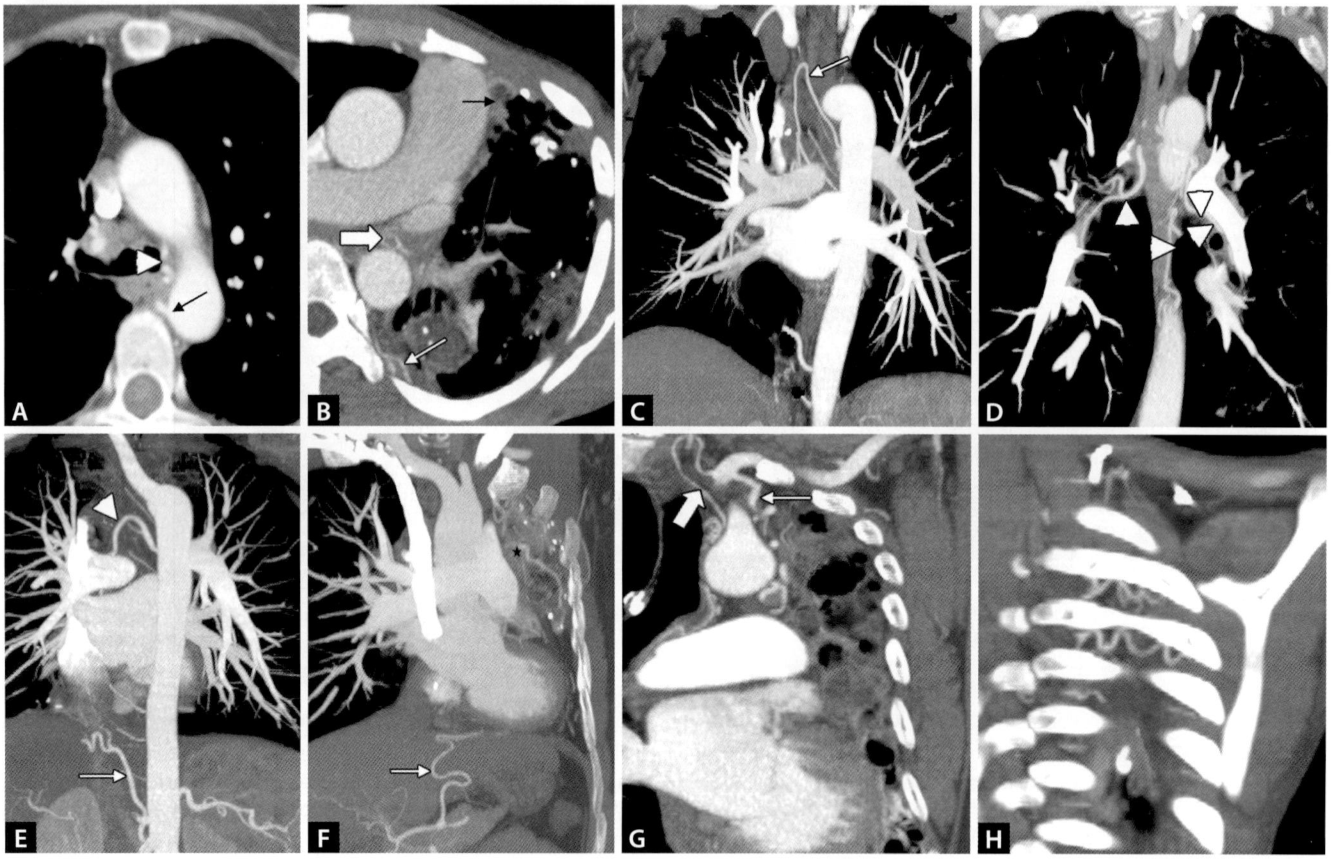

Figs. 2A to H: CT angiogram images showing hypertrophied bronchial arteries and NBSC: (A) RT-ICBT arises laterally from the descending aorta (black arrow). Left bronchial artery is seen around the left main bronchus (white arrowhead); (B) Left bronchial artery arises from anterior wall of aorta (solid white arrow). Also noted are NBSC from left internal mammary artery (black arrow) and tortuous left posterior intercostal artery (white thin arrow); (C) Combined CT angiogram coronal MIP image showing good opacification of both systemic and pulmonary arterial trees. The entire course of RT-ICBT is well seen (white arrow); (D) Multiple hypertrophied bronchial arteries (arrowheads); (E) Hypertrophied right bronchial (arrowhead) and inferior phrenic arteries (thin white arrow); (F) Hypertrophied left inferior phrenic artery (white arrow) and multiple chest wall collaterals (asterisk); (G) Coronal oblique MIP image depicts enlarged left costocervical trunk (solid white arrow) and internal mammary artery IMA (thin white arrow); (H) Tortuous hypertrophied left posterior intercostal arteries.

that well seen on CT and are usually not amenable to endovascular embolization. Furthermore, vasoconstrictive drugs can be administered locally to control bleeding. Intrabronchial antifungal agents can also be injected in cases of aspergilloma. The main problem in patients with massive hemoptysis is that blood/clots may fill up the bronchi and preclude further evaluation. Also, the feasibility of FB depends on the local availability as well as patient condition.

RELEVANT ARTERIAL ANATOMY

It is important to have a good understanding of the anatomy of the bronchial and commonly hypertrophied non-bronchial arteries so that the same may be communicated in the radiological report as well as guide management.

Bronchial Arteries

Bronchial arteries are systemic arteries which course along the branching of the major bronchi. This is a key finding which helps to distinguish (ectopic) bronchial arteries from non-bronchial systemic collaterals. The bronchial arteries supply the tracheobronchial tree (both intra- and extrapulmonary), regional lymph nodes, (visceral) pleura, esophagus, and vasa vasorum of aorta, pulmonary artery and vein.

Origin: Majority of the bronchial arteries are *orthotopic* i.e. arise from the descending thoracic aorta (DTA) between the superior border of T5 and inferior border of T6 vertebral levels **(Figs. 3A to H)**.[3] Angiographic landmark for the same is 1 cm above and below the crossing of left main bronchus over the DTA or just below the carina.[21] The frequency of orthotopic bronchial arteries varies depending on whether the study is based on CT, DSA or post-mortem; approximately 65% patients have orthotopic bronchial arteries.[3] If the origin is anywhere else from DTA or even from a branch of the aorta, but the course is parallel to the bronchial tree, then it is labeled as *ectopic* bronchial artery **(Figs. 4A to I)**. Practically, majority of the bronchial arteries arise from DTA between T4-T7 vertebral levels. Many variations can however occur, and ectopic bronchial arteries may arise from the inferior surface of aortic arch, internal mammary artery (IMA), thyrocervical and costocervical trunk, innominate artery, left subclavian artery and inferior thyroid artery, inferior phrenic artery or abdominal aorta.[22]

Cauldwell documented the variations in bronchial artery anatomy by describing nine patterns based on autopsy study of 150 cadavers.[23] Uflacker described 10 patterns of bronchial arterial anatomy based on angiography records of 72 patients.[24] However, what is more relevant is the information regarding number and origin of the hypertrophied bronchial arteries and pattern approach is not that helpful.

Right side: There are usually two bronchial arteries supplying the right lung. The first arises from DTA as a common intercostobronchial trunk (ICBT) with the third right posterior intercostal artery, and has a posterolaterally lying orifice **(Figs. 2A to H)**. **Right ICBT** is the most consistently seen artery at DSA. The initial course is oblique and upwards and can be seen on CT in the retro-esophageal region. Then the trunk divides, with the bronchial component hooking down and paralleling the branching of RT bronchus while the intercostal component ascends up and then traverses horizontally along the inferior border of the rib **(Figs. 3A to H)**. The second artery is the **common bronchial (CB)** that arises from the anterior surface and supplies both lungs by dividing into right and left bronchial arteries **(Figs. 3A to H)**. Depending upon the parenchymal abnormality, one or both the branches may be hypertrophied.

Left side: On the left side, a separate **left bronchial (LB)** artery is usually present, and arises from the anterior-left anterolateral surface of the aorta **(Figs. 2 and 3)**. Rarely the left bronchial artery may arise from the RT-ICB trunk but LB arising from left intercostal is not described.

On CT, bronchial arteries can be identified in the retroesophageal, retrotracheal, retrobronchial or aortopulmonary window locations **(Table 2) (Figs. 2A to H)**.

Table 2: Tips to identify abnormal bronchial and systemic arteries (NBSC).

• RT ICBT arises from right lateral wall of aorta and courses behind the right main bronchus
• RB or right branch of CB arise anterolaterally from aorta and course anterior to the RT main bronchus
• LB arises from anterior wall of aorta and may course anterior or posterior to left main bronchus
• Ectopic LB/RB arising from the arch course anterior to the corresponding bronchus
• Internal mammary arteries are hypertrophied in case disease is localized to anterior segments of upper lobes, RT middle lobe or lingual
• Right posterior intercostal arteries arise posterolaterally and left posterior intercostal arteries arise posteriorly from the aorta
• Posterior intercostal arteries are hypertrophied in case of posterior or posterolateral lung involvement.
• Inflammatory lung disease close to the lateral chest wall may recruit collaterals from lateral thoracic artery.
• Inferior phrenic arteries may hypertrophy in basal lung disease.

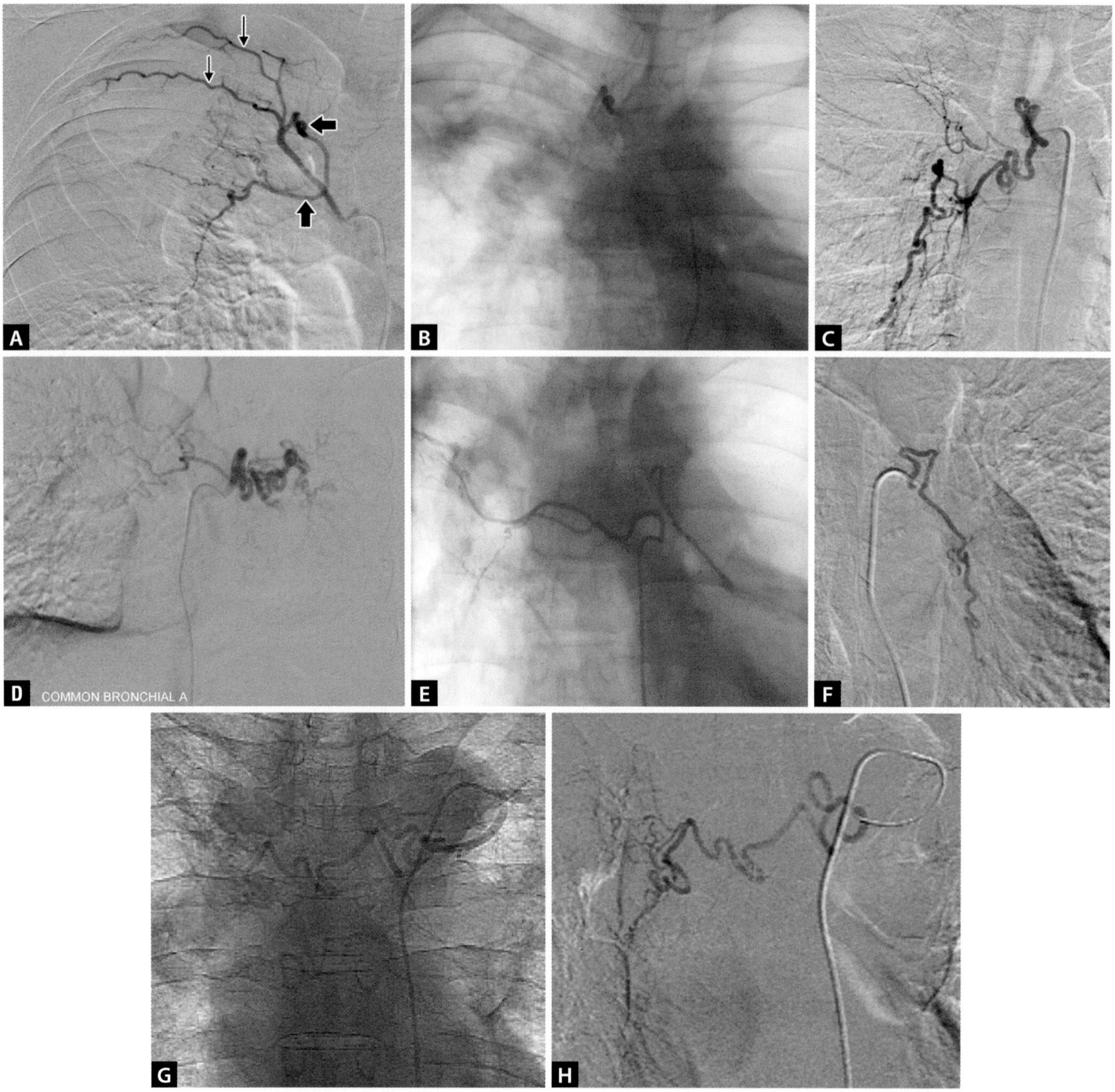

Figs. 3A to H: DSA images showing abnormal bronchial arteries: (A) Selective DSA run shows hypertrophied RT ICBT. The bronchial component is hypertrophied (solid black arrows) while the intercostal component is normal (thin black arrows), RB; (B) Stasis of contrast after superselective embolization; (C) Hypertrophied right bronchial artery; (D) Common bronchial artery with hypertrophied left component; (E) Common bronchial artery with right component more hypertrophied than left; (F) Hypertrophied left bronchial artery; (G) Ectopic right bronchial artery arising from the arch of aorta; (H) Superselective DSA run through microcatheter shows stable catheter position, just before embolization.

Bronchial arteries can have communications with other systemic arteries. Most important of such communication is that of RT ICBT with anterior medullary artery that contributes to vascular supply of the spinal cord through anterior spinal artery. The **anterior medullary arteries** have a characteristic 'hairpin' configuration, and follow a vertical course parallel to the spinal cord[25] **(Figs. 4A to I)**. These arteries, when they originate from D9 to D12, may communicate with the great anterior medullary artery (artery of Adamkiewicz). Other less commonly seen communications are with the subclavian artery and right coronary artery.[26,27]

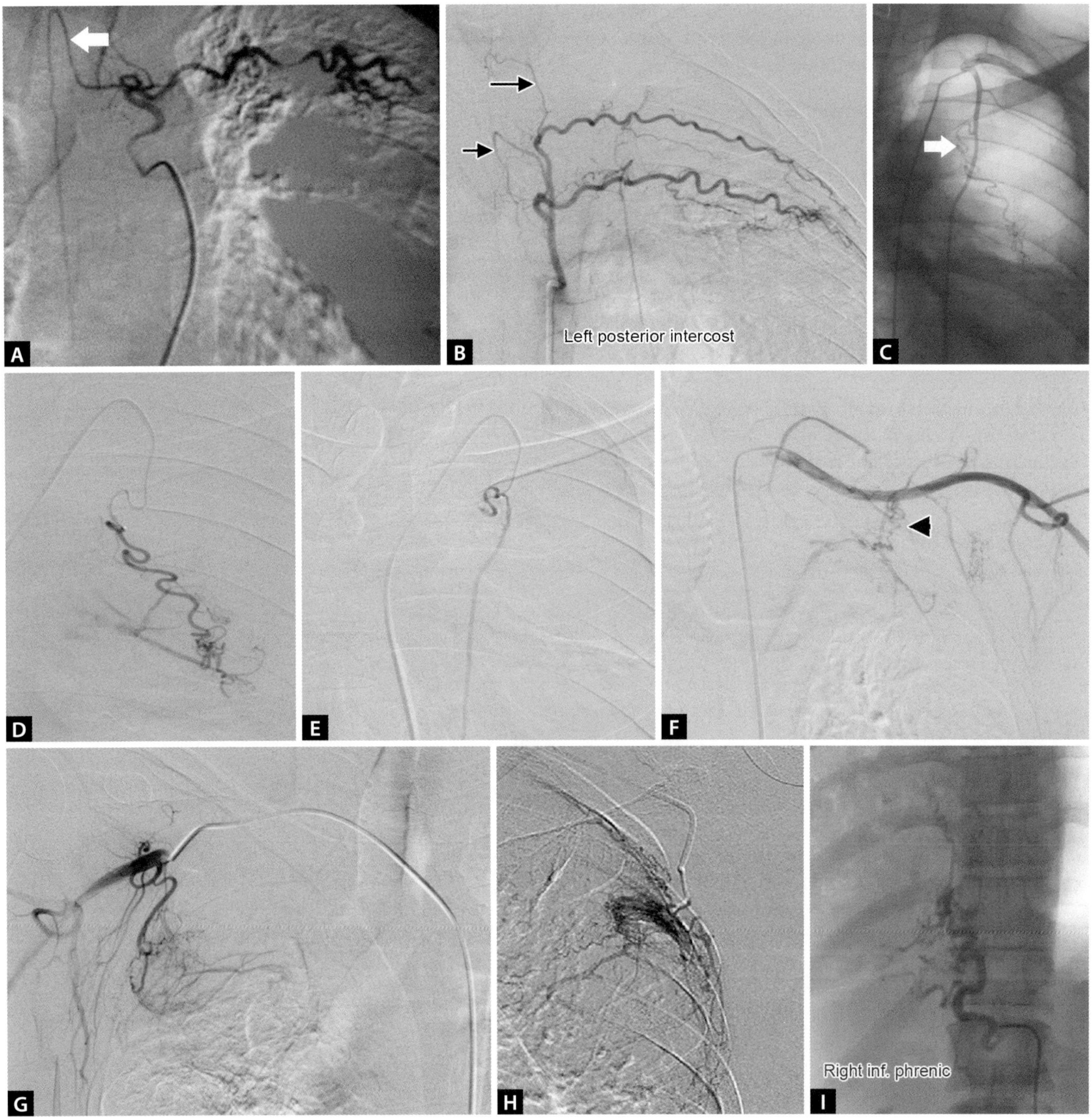

Figs. 4A to I: DSA images showing abnormal NBSC and communications with spinal artery: (A) Anterior medullary artery (solid white arrow) arising from left posterior intercostal artery; (B) Radicular arteries (thin black arrows) arising from left posterior intercostal artery; (C) Left subclavian artery (SCA) run shows abnormal branch arising from LT IMA; (D) Superselective catheterization of abnormal branch of LT IMA with stable catheter position and check run; (E) Postembolization run of the same; (F) Abnormal costocervical branch of second part of left SCA (arrowhead); (G) Abnormal pulmonary parenchymal blush from right superior thoracic artery (branch of first part of axillary artery); (H) Superselective catheterization of left superior thoracic artery; (I) Hypertrophied right inferior phrenic artery.

The other type of spinal arteries which may be seen are *radicular arteries*. These are small vessels which usually arise from the posterior intercostal arteries, do not have the 'hairpin' configuration, and supply the dorsal and ventral roots **(Figs. 4A to I)**. Radicular arteries are more commonly seen at DSA and are not considered to be a contradiction to embolization. Medullary arteries, on the other hand, are rarely seen but may give rise to cord ischemia, if inadvertently embolized.[1] Nevertheless, it is advisable to go superselectively beyond the origin of any spinal artery to prevent ominous complications.

Non-bronchial Systemic Collaterals

Non-bronchial systemic collaterals (NBSC) enter the lung parenchyma through adjacent pleura or the pulmonary ligament, and have a course that does not parallel the bronchial tree. The CT features that suggest the presence of NBSC include pleural thickening and presence of chronic inflammatory disease in the lung apex or base. NBSC may arise from the following:[13,28,29]

- Intercostal arteries in case of peripheral lung/pleural inflammation **(Figs. 2 and 4)**
- Branches of subclavian and axillary arteries (internal mammary, lateral thoracic, costocervical and cervicothoracic) in case of apical/anterior paramidline lung disease **(Figs. 2 and 4)**
- Phrenic arteries in case of basal lung disease **(Figs. 2 and 4)**
- Rarely left gastric artery.

Normal bronchial arteries have a diameter of <1.5 mm at their origin, and 0.5 mm at the level of the entrance into a bronchopulmonary segment. Indicators of abnormal bronchial arteries are[6,12,30] enumerated in **Table 3 (Figs. 5A to E)**. Systemic collaterals going into abnormal lung parenchyma are considered abnormal irrespective of diameter.

Table 3: Criteria to identify abnormal bronchial and systemic arteries (NBSC).

- *Hypertrophy:* Diameter at ostium >2 mm
- Increased tortuosity
- Bronchial artery traceable upto corresponding hilum on CT
- *DSA features:*
  - Neo- and hypervascularity in the form of abnormal vascular blush, dense soft tissue staining/parenchymal blush **(Figs. 5A to E)**
  - Shunting into the pulmonary vascular system (arterial or venous) **(Figs. 5A to E)**
  - Extravasation of contrast into the alveoli or bronchial tree
  - Pseudoaneurysm
- Any non-bronchial systemic collateral supplying diseased lung parenchyma is deemed abnormal

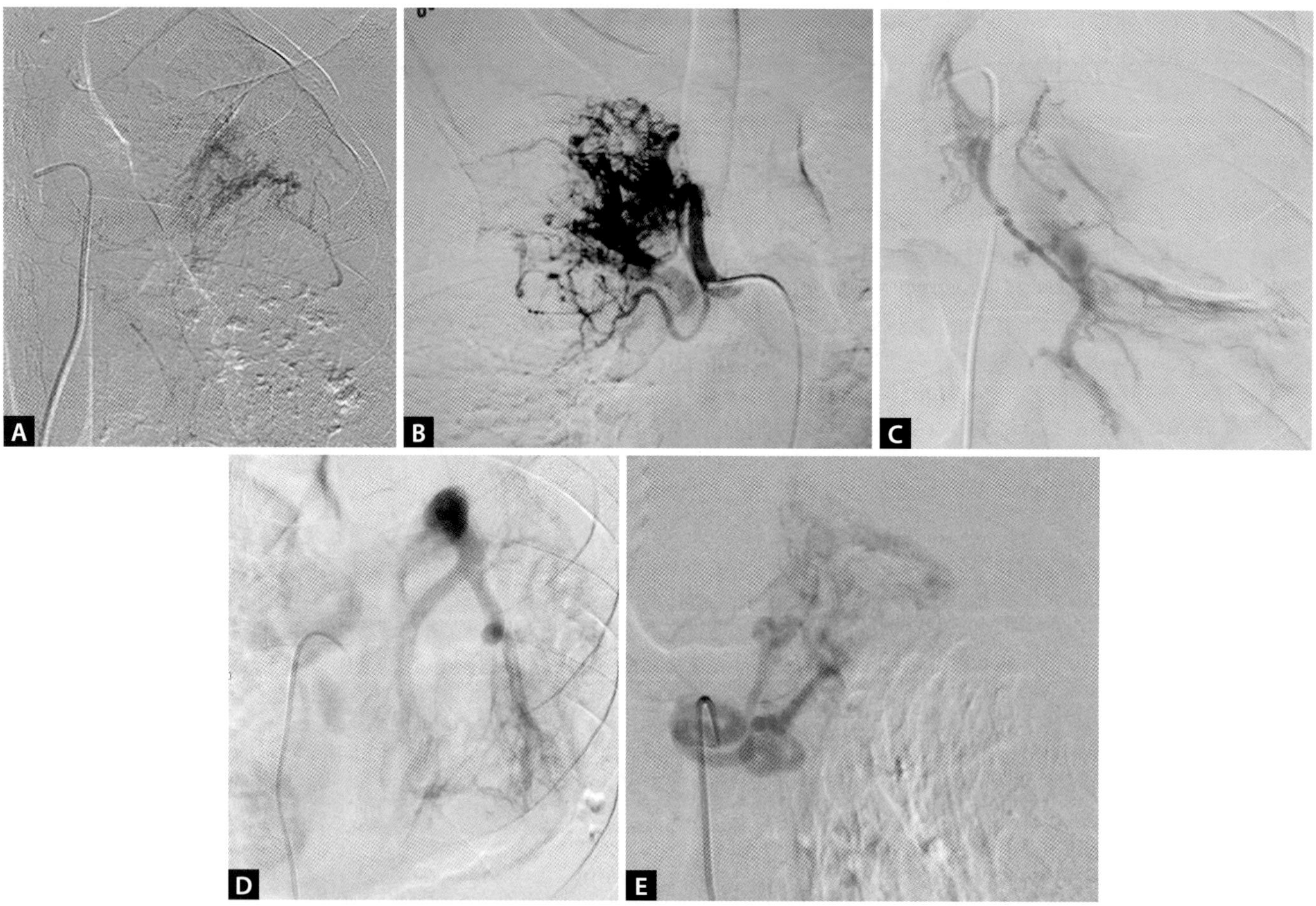

Figs. 5A to E: DSA features of abnormal bronchial arteries: (A) Abnormal parenchymal blush; (B) Hypertrophied right bronchial artery with dense vascular blush and shunting; (C) Vascular blush with shunting into pulmonary vein; (D) Delayed phase DSA run depicts shunting into pulmonary artery; (E) Hypertrophied tortuous left bronchial artery with pulmonary arterial shunting.

TECHNIQUE OF BAE

The first priority in patients with life-threatening hemoptysis is to maintain the airway, optimize oxygenation and stabilize the hemodynamic status. Blood tests for coagulopathy (Prothrombin time, platelet count) and renal dysfunction (blood urea, serum creatinine) need to be done before BAE. The technique of BAE is outlined in **Flowchart 2**.

Route: Transfemoral arterial access is routinely used to access the bronchial circulation. Transbrachial/ transaxillary access may be helpful in case of increased aortic tortuosity[8,9] and to selectively catheterize branches of subclavian artery. A long arterial sheath (carotid sheath) may also be used in case of tortuosity of the aortic arch. In case pulmonary angiography needs to be done, then common femoral vein access is used. 6F sheath is commonly used in adults while in young children, 5F access sheath is used.

Thoracic aortogram: After securing a vascular sheath in the femoral artery, the next step is usually to take flush aortogram using 5F angiographic pigtail catheter (having multiple side holes). The loop of the pigtail catheter is formed in the proximal DTA. About 25–30 mL of ~80% diluted contrast (concentration >= 300 mg iodine/mL) is injected at flow rate of 18 mL/s (~650 psi pressure) and patient is asked to hold breath. The contrast run is acquired in digital subtraction angiography (DSA) mode (3 frames per second), AP projection with wide field of view (FOV) after coupling the contrast inflow with fluoroscopic DSA acquisition. The aim is to identify all the abnormal bronchial and non-bronchial systemic collaterals from DTA so as to facilitate selective catheterization of the same **(Figs. 6A to E)**. The limitation of flush aortogram is that the opacification of subclavian arteries is suboptimal. So, either take separate subclavian artery runs or take the pigtail loop upto proximal arch. Problem with the latter technique is that contrast will unnecessarily go into the head and neck arteries. Due to several limitations of aortogram, this step may be omitted, if a good quality CT bronchial angiogram is available.

Superselective catheterization: The bronchial arteries are usually hooked using angiographic catheters having more than one curve such as RDC (renal double curve)/ cobra catheter **(Table 4)**. Reverse seeking catheter (like Simmons) may also be used, especially of there is sharp upward course from the origin. Once the artery is hooked, then check contrast run is taken. Using this roadmap, the main catheter is secured into the artery and then microcatheter (2.7Fr) is advanced through the main catheter (co-axial system). A multipurpose catheter or slip catheter may also be used to go selectively into the artery, by exchanging RDC/cobra over a long (~260 cm) guidewire.

In case of ICBT, attempt should be made to superselectively go into the bronchial component, unless the intercostal component is also abnormal **(Figs. 3A to H)**. Care must be taken to look for any contrast opacification of the anterior medullary artery **(Figs. 4A to I)**. Superselective catheterization by microcatheter enables delivery of embolizing agent specifically into the culprit branches with lesser risk of complications, and

Table 4: Commonly used catheters for selective cannulation.

Bronchial and intercostal arteries	RDC (double curve), Cobra (complex curve), Simmons (Reverse curve)
Subclavian artery and its branches	Picard, vertebral (Forward seeking simple curve angled-tip), headhunter (double curve)
Inferior phrenic artery	RDC, RC, Simmons

Abbreviations: RDC: Renal double curve; RC: Reverse curve.

Flowchart 2: Basic steps in the procedure of bronchial artery embolization.

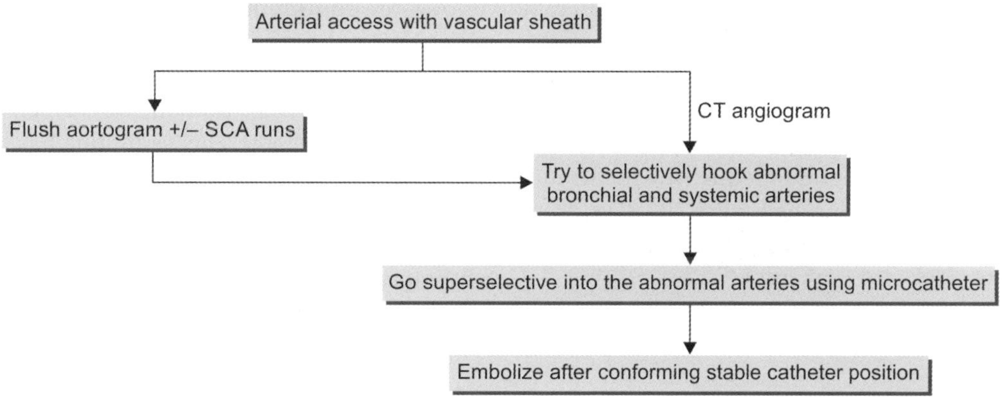

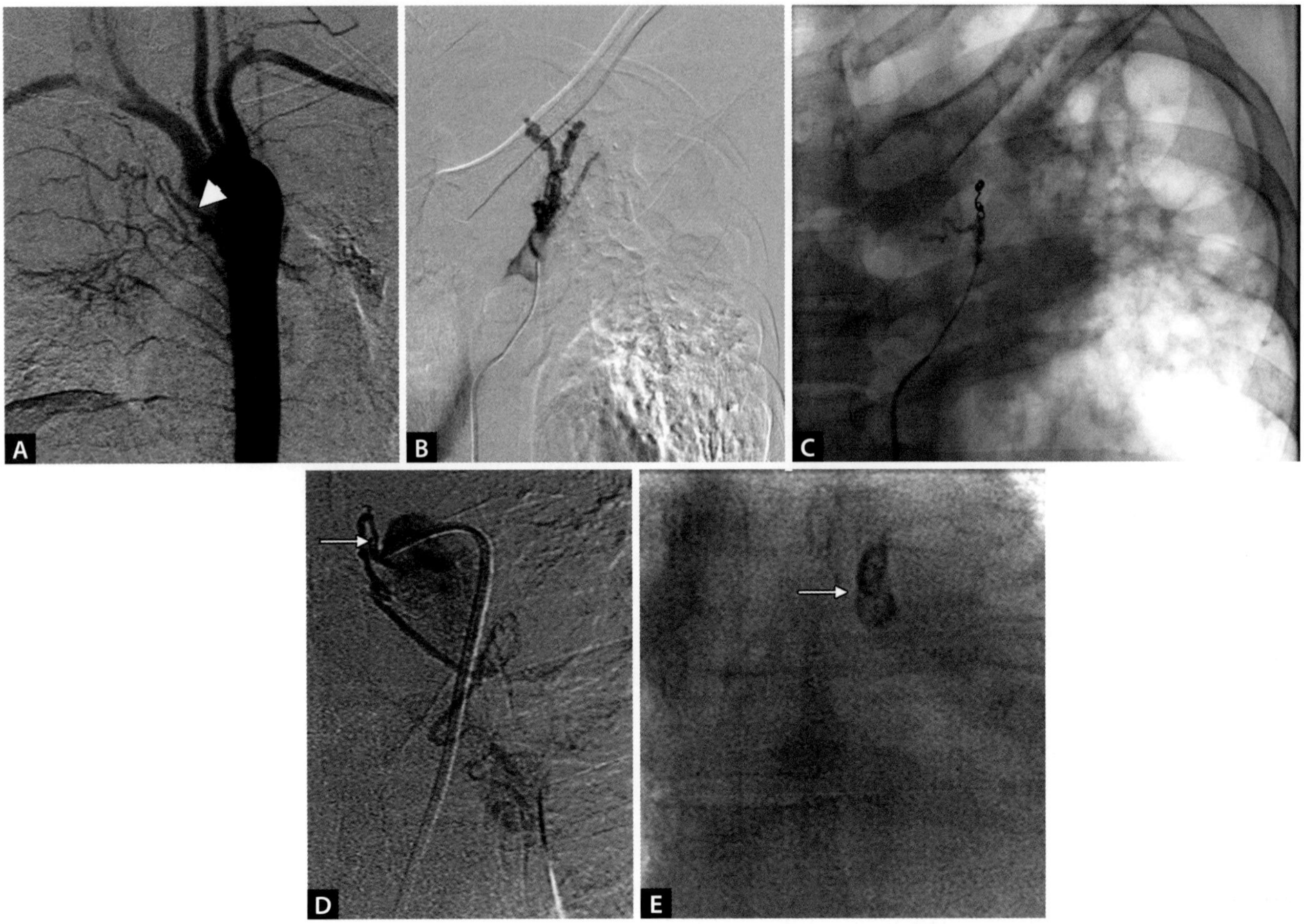

Figs. 6A to E: BAE technique and complications: (A) Flush aortogram shows hypertrophied RT-ICBT; (B) Superselective catheterization of left bronchial artery shows large shunt into the pulmonary vein; (C) Due to large size of the shunt and resultant potential of cerebral embolism, the shunt was blocked using microcoils; (D) DSA run shows shelf-like filling defect at the origin of ectopic left bronchial artery (suggesting dissection), caused by wire manipulation due to acute upward angulation; (E) Fluoroscopic spot image depicts contrast blob at the origin of this ectopic left bronchial artery (likely representing intramural hematoma in aortic wall).

thus providing better patient care.[8-10,31] Care should be taken not to create spasm or dissection while negotiating the smaller catheter.

Usually, the bronchial arteries are searched first, followed by any expected NBSC. Intercostal arteries can be searched by directing the RDC catheter posterolaterally for right-sided arteries and posteriorly for left posterior intercostal arteries. Subclavian artery branches are evaluated using Picard/vertebral catheter while phrenic may be hooked using RDC or RC catheter **(Table 4)**. The search for NBSC has been found to reduce the recurrence rates of hemoptysis.[7] A pre-procedural CTBA lays down the vascular roadmap for endovascular therapeutic interventions.

Again, attempt must be made to hook the hypertrophied branch of SCA using the main catheter and then go selectively into it using microcatheter **(Figs. 4A to I)**. If former is not feasible, then negotiation using microcatheter can be done after keeping the main catheter in subclavian artery itself, provided we use a large bore Tuohy-Borst sidearm adaptor (Y-connector). The latter allows for continuous flushing of the guiding catheter so as to avoid formation of thrombus in the dead space. Alternatively, a side hole can be created in a diagnostic catheter (at a distance from the tip), which can serve as an exit for microcatheter. This technique has been described to be helpful in the embolization of proximal subclavian arterial branches, when stable and selective position of the main catheter cannot be achieved.[32] In a similar fashion, catheters with pre-fabricated side holes can be used in difficult anatomical situations.[33] Before proceeding to the embolization of the target vessel, stability of the catheter tip and absence of backflow into the descending thoracic aorta should be confirmed by means of a test-injection using contrast medium.

Culprit arteries: The common culprit bronchial arteries in patients undergoing embolization are RB, RT-ICBT, CB, and LB (in descending order of frequency). Common NBSC are posterior intercostal and internal mammary arteries. Other branches of subclavian artery (like superior thoracic, lateral thoracic, costocervical and cervicothoracic), and inferior phrenic arteries may also be abnormal.

Embolizing agents: Particulate embolizing material are commonly used for BAE. Older literature describes use of gelatin sponge, but the current agent of choice is polyvinyl alcohol (PVA) particles. Gelatin sponge is readily available and inexpensive. Advantages of PVA over gelfoam include permanency of embolization (since gelatin sponge gets resorbed) and choice of different sizes **(Table 5)**. Gelfoam has the potential to cause more proximal embolization. Problems with PVA include tendency of the particles to clump in the microcatheter. Microspheres can overcome this problem because of hydrophilic nature and uniform size.[20] Commonly used size of PVA particles is 300–500 μ micron though use of all sizes from 150–1200 μ have been reported in literature. Particles smaller than 300 μ should ideally not be used because they can pass through the bronchopulmonary anastomoses and result in infarcts.[20] They may lead to occlusion of smaller branches resulting in bronchial or esophageal necrosis.[25]

Larger particles (500–700 μ) may be indicated in the presence of shunting. Shunting into pulmonary veins is potentially more dangerous than into the pulmonary arteries because of the risk of non-target systemic embolization. PVA/gelfoam is mixed with contrast and then injected under fluoroscopic guidance. It is important to monitor for slowing of flow and stasis so as to prevent any backflow/reflux of embolic material. 2 mL/1 mL syringes are routinely used for better precision. Intermittent contrast runs may be taken to look for any vascular anastomoses not previously visible. Always remember to empty the PVA column in the catheter before taking check runs.

PVA can also be used in conjunction with gelfoam. Former is used for distal embolization of the abnormal parenchymal bed and latter is typically used for proximal embolization. Recently, liquid embolic agents [glue, n-Butyl-2-cyanoacrylate (NBCA)] have been shown to result in better control of hemoptysis in case of bronchiectasis.[10] This has been attributed to lower rates of recanalization, compared with PVA. But use of glue calls for stable catheter position and need of greater expertise, owing to more chances of complications (distal necrosis, non-target complications due to reflux are more dangerous). Microcoils have been used uncommonly, and the chief indication is in case of pseudoaneurysms (provided microcatheter reaches upto the neck of the aneurysm) and large volume shunts **(Figs. 6A to E)**. Proximal coil embolization precludes repeat access in case of recurrence of hemoptysis due to distal collateralization.[34,35]

Table 5: Advantages and drawbacks of various embolizing agents.

Embolizing agent	***Advantages***	***Drawbacks***
PVA particles	• Relatively uniform size • Permanent • Different sizes available	• Tendency to clump • Costly
Microspheres	Better than PVA because do not clump	Costly
Gelfoam	Cheap, readily available	Heterogeneous particle size, temporary
Glue	• More permanent than PVA • Useful where significant shunting is there	Needs experienced hands and stable catheter position
Microcoils	• In case of pseudoaneurysms, markedly hypertrophied artery with large volume shunt • To protect parent vessel in case superselective catheterization not feasible	• Preclude future access • Expensive

Outcomes: The outcome of any interventional procedure is expressed in terms of technical as well as clinical success. The causes of technical and clinical failure of BAE have been listed in the **Table 6**. A pre-procedural CT angiogram enhances clinical success by depicting all the abnormal arteries. Few authors suggest a post-embolization flush aortogram to avoid missing a pathological vessel. The presence of NBSC is associated with higher rate of technical failures.[36]

Bronchial artery embolization is very effective in the treatment of acute hemoptysis. *Immediate clinical success* (significant reduction/cessation of hemoptysis within 24 hours of the procedure) is high (70-99%).[2] *Early recurrences*

Table 6: Causes of technical and clinical failure of BAE.

Causes of technical failure	*Causes of clinical failure*
• Patient not able to breath-hold/constantly coughing/expectorating. • Tortuous artery/acute angulation • Proximal/ostial narrowing • Aortic tortuosity may hamper stable catherization of subclavian artery branches • Failure to go beyond the origin of spinal cord branches	• Inability to embolize all culprit arteries • Presence of ectopic bronchial arteries • Pulmonary vascular causes

(within 1–3 months) suggest incomplete embolization, i.e. any abnormal vessel has been left untreated. This may be because of lack of complete search, ectopic origin or NBSC and too many hypertrophied arteries due to extensive collateralization. In latter scenario, it may be useful to split the embolization into two sessions, starting with the most abnormal arteries first, and bronchial arteries should be done prior to the NBSC.

Late recurrences occur due to recanalization of previously treated arteries or new recruitment of non-bronchial systemic collaterals.[8,31,36,37] This occurs, if the underlying disease is not simultaneously controlled, thus emphasizing the need to address the underlying disease medically or surgically. Superimposed infection on background TB sequelae, chronic cavitary pulmonary aspergillosis, and development of multidrug resistance TB (MDR-TB) can contribute to recurrence of hemoptysis in previously treated cases.[31,37,38]

Recurrences at long-term follow-up can be as high as 52% and the probability of recurrence increases with time. The chances of rebleed are more with aspergillomas and with cavitary lung disease.[4,24,31,38,39] Recurrences can again be effectively controlled with BAE, and thus repeat sessions provide for long-term control of hemoptysis.[13,36,37] It has been noted that patients who remain hemoptysis free for 3 years post-BAE have excellent prognosis, but those who rebleed, tend to bleed again and again.[13,16] It may be noted here that BAE is a palliative procedure to control hemoptysis and does not treat the underlying cause. Thus, wherever feasible and considered safe, surgery may be considered for definitive treatment.[12,16]

COMPLICATIONS

The most common complication after BAE is (transient) *chest/back pain*, being reported in up to 34.5% of cases.[2] This is likely related to ischemia of embolized systemic branches, and can be severe when intercostal arteries are embolized. Dissection of the bronchial artery or subintimal perforation and wire manipulation may lead to sudden chest pain **(Figs. 6A to E)**. There may be dissection of the aorta as well while negotiating a smaller catheter into its branch **(Figs. 6A to E)**. In such cases, intravenous fluid should be immediately started and blood pressure should be maintained. Usually, these dissections are non-progressive, but further catheter/wire manipulation in the vicinity of the injured segment should be avoided. The second most common complication is *dysphagia*, caused by embolization of esophageal branches, with a reported occurrence from 0.7 to 18.2%.[12] Spontaneous resolution of symptoms usually occurs.

The most devastating complication is *spinal cord ischemia* that has been reported to occur in 1.4-6.5 percent of patients.[6,12] This may lead to transient or permanent paraplegia, and thus any doubt of spinal artery anastomosis should become a red-flag. The occurrence of this complication can be reduced by using a superselective embolization technique and by performing regular check angiograms before and after administration of embolic agents. *Post-embolization syndrome* may occur and patient may develop fever, leukocytosis and chest pain. This is however a self-limiting complication seen in upto 30% cases.[7,10,14,24,36] *Rare complications* include aortic and bronchial necrosis, bronchial stenosis, unilateral diaphragmatic paralysis, pulmonary infarction (especially in patients who have suffered pulmonary artery embolism), left main bronchial-esophageal fistula, and non-target embolization (colon, coronary, foot and cerebral circulation)[40-43] In addition, contrast-induced nephropathy, hypersensitivity reactions, and groin hematomas may also occur.

CONCLUSION

Bronchial artery embolization is the treatment of choice in acute hemoptysis and can be performed in both emergency as well as elective settings. Knowledge of bronchial and non-bronchial systemic circulation is mandatory to reduce complications and to increase technical success. It is imperative to identify hypertrophied bronchial arteries and other systemic collaterals on CTA to enable successful embolization. BAE is a safe and effective procedure and can be done repeatedly for recurrent hemoptysis as well.

KEY MESSAGES

- The common diseases leading to significant hemoptysis include TB (sequelae and active disease), bronchiectasis and aspergillomas.

- BAE is the procedure of choice for patients presenting in the emergency setting with massive hemoptysis. Also, it is the treatment of choice for immediate control of any amount of hemoptysis in nonsurgical candidates.
- CT angiogram provides a vascular roadmap and bronchoscopy helps in localizing the site of active bleed in diffuse lung disease.
- Superselective catheterization aids in reducing the complications.
- Embolizing agent of choice in BAE is PVA particles (300–500 μ). Larger particles may be used in case of vascular shunts.
- Reactivation TB, MDR-TB and CCPA patients are more prone to develop recurrence of hemoptysis.

REFERENCES

1. Yoon W, Kim JK, Kim YH, et al. Bronchial and nonbronchial systemic artery embolization for life-threatening hemoptysis: a comprehensive review. Radiogr Rev Publ Radiol Soc N Am Inc. 2002;22(6):1395–409.
2. Panda A, Bhalla AS, Goyal A. Bronchial artery embolization in hemoptysis: a systematic review. Diagn Interv Radiol Ank Turk. 2017;23(4):307-17.
3. Walker CM, Rosado-de-Christenson ML, et al. Bronchial arteries: anatomy, function, hypertrophy, and anomalies. Radiogr Rev Publ Radiol Soc N Am Inc. 2015;35(1):32-49.
4. Remy J, Voisin C, Dupuis C. Traitement des hemoptysies par embolization de la circulation systemique. Ann Radiol. 1974;17:5-16.
5. Hayakawa K, Tanaka F, Torizuka T, et al. Bronchial artery embolization for hemoptysis: immediate and long-term results. Cardiovasc Intervent Radiol. 1992;15(3):154-8; discussion 158-9.
6. Wong ML, Szkup P, Hopley MJ. Percutaneous embolotherapy for life-threatening hemoptysis. Chest. 2002;121(1):95-102.
7. Anuradha C, Shyamkumar NK, Vinu M, et al. Outcomes of bronchial artery embolization for life-threatening hemoptysis due to tuberculosis and post-tuberculosis sequelae. Diagn Interv Radiol Ank Turk. 2012;18(1):96-101.
8. Bhalla A, Kandasamy D, Veedu P, et al. A retrospective analysis of 334 cases of hemoptysis treated by bronchial artery embolization. Oman Med J. 2015;30(2):119-28.
9. Agmy GM, Wafy SM, Mohamed SAA, et al. Bronchial and Nonbronchial Systemic Artery Embolization in Management of Hemoptysis: experience with 348 Patients. Int Sch Res Not. 2013;2013:e263259.
10. Woo S, Yoon CJ, Chung JW, et al. Bronchial artery embolization to control hemoptysis: comparison of N-butyl-2-cyanoacrylate and polyvinyl alcohol particles. Radiology. 2013;269(2):594-602.
11. Swanson KL, Johnson CM, Prakash UBS, et al. Bronchial artery embolization: experience with 54 patients. Chest. 2002;121(3):789–95.
12. Ramakantan R, Bandekar VG, Gandhi MS, et al. Massive hemoptysis due to pulmonary tuberculosis: control with bronchial artery embolization. Radiology. 1996;200(3):691-4.
13. Yu-Tang Goh P, Lin M, Teo N, En Shen Wong D. Embolization for hemoptysis: a six-year review. Cardiovasc Intervent Radiol. 2002;25(1):17-25.
14. Shao H, Wu J, Wu Q, SUn X, et al. Bronchial artery embolization for hemoptysis: a retrospective observational study of 344 patients. Chin Med J Engl. 2015;128(1):58-62.
15. Tom LM, Palevsky HI, Holsclaw DS, et al. Recurrent bleeding, survival, and longitudinal pulmonary function following bronchial artery embolization for hemoptysis in a US adult population. J Vasc Interv Radiol. 2015;26(12):1806–13.e1.
16. Fruchter O, Schneer S, Rusanov V, et al. Bronchial artery embolization for massive hemoptysis: long-term follow-up. Asian Cardiovasc Thorac Ann. 2015;23(1):55-60.
17. Ketai LH, Mohammed T-LH, Kirsch J, et al. ACR appropriateness criteria® hemoptysis. J Thorac Imaging. 2014;29(3):W19-22.
18. Khalil A, Fartoukh M, Parrot A, et al. Impact of MDCT angiography on the management of patients with hemoptysis. Am J Roentgenol. 2010;195(3):772-8.
19. Meena P, Bhalla AS, Goyal A, et al. Comparison of contrast injection protocols for simultaneous optimal opacification of systemic and pulmonary arteries in CT angiography of patients with hemoptysis. In Boston, USA; 2017.
20. Sopko DR, Smith TP. Bronchial Artery Embolization for Hemoptysis. Semin Interv Radiol. 2011;28(1):48-62.
21. Tanomkiat W, Tanisaro K. Radiographic relationship of the origin of the bronchial arteries to the left main bronchus. J Thorac Imaging. 2003;18(1):27-33.
22. Sancho C, Escalante E, Domínguez J, et al. Embolization of bronchial arteries of anomalous origin. Cardiovasc Intervent Radiol. 1998;21(4):300-4.
23. Cauldwell EW, Siekert RG. The bronchial arteries: an anatomic study of 150 human cadavers. Surg Gynecol Obstet. 1948;86(4):395-412.
24. Uflacker R, Kaemmerer A, Picon PD, et al. Bronchial artery embolization in the management of hemoptysis: technical aspects and long-term results. Radiology. 1985;157(3):637-44.
25. Marshall TJ, Jackson JE. Vascular intervention in the thorax: bronchial artery embolization for haemoptysis. Eur Radiol. 1997;7(8):1221-7.
26. Furnari ML, Salerno S, Rabiolo A, et al. Bronchial to subclavian shunt in a CF patient. A potential pitfall for embolization. J Cyst Fibros Off J Eur Cyst Fibros Soc. 2003;2(4):217-9.
27. Van den Berg JC, Overtoom TT, De Valois JC. Case report: bronchial to coronary artery anastomosis: a potential hazard in bronchial artery embolization. Br J Radiol. 1996;69(822):570-2.

28. Keller FS, Rosch J, Loflin TG, et al. Nonbronchial systemic collateral arteries: significance in percutaneous embolotherapy for hemoptysis. Radiology. 1987;164(3):687-92.
29. Sellars N, Belli AM. Non-bronchial collateral supply from the left gastric artery in massive haemoptysis. Eur Radiol. 2001;11(1):76-9.
30. Zhang JS, Cui ZP, Wang MQ, Yang L. Bronchial arteriography and transcatheter embolization in the management of hemoptysis. Cardiovasc Intervent Radiol. 1994;17(5):276-9.
31. Shin BS, Jeon GS, Lee SA, et al. Bronchial artery embolisation for the management of haemoptysis in patients with pulmonary tuberculosis. Int J Tuberc Lung Dis Off J Int Union Tuberc Lung Dis. 2011;15(8):1093-8.
32. Won JH, Park SI, Park KJ, et al. Microcatheter placement through a side hole created in a 5-F catheter into proximal subclavian arterial branches causing hemoptysis. J Vasc Interv Radiol. 2004;15(8):881-4.
33. Miyayama S, Matsui O, Akakura Y, et al. Use of a catheter with a large side hole for selective catheterization of the inferior phrenic artery. J Vasc Interv Radiol. 2001;12(4):497-9.
34. Barben J, Robertson D, Olinsky A, et al. Bronchial artery embolization for hemoptysis in young patients with cystic fibrosis. Radiology. 2002;224(1):124-30.
35. Saluja S, Henderson KJ, White RI. Embolotherapy in the bronchial and pulmonary circulations. Radiol Clin North Am. 2000;38(2):425-48, ix.
36. Chan VL, So LK, Lam JY, et al. Major haemoptysis in Hong Kong: aetiologies, angiographic findings and outcomes of bronchial artery embolisation. Int J Tuberc Lung Dis. 2009;13(9):1167-73.
37. Lee S, Chan JW, Chan SC, et al. Bronchial artery embolisation can be equally safe and effective in the management of chronic recurrent haemoptysis. Hong Kong Med J Xianggang Yi Xue Za Zhi. 2008;14(1):14-20.
38. Hwang H-G, Lee H-S, Choi J-S, et al. Risk factors influencing rebleeding after bronchial artery embolization on the management of hemoptysis associated with pulmonary tuberculosis. Tuberc Respir Dis. 2013;74(3):111-9.
39. Yoo DH, Yoon CJ, Kang S-G, et al. Bronchial and nonbronchial systemic artery embolization in patients with major hemoptysis: safety and efficacy of N-butyl cyanoacrylate. Am J Roentgenol. 2011;196(2):W199-204.
40. Ivanick MJ, Thorwarth W, Donohue J, et al. Infarction of the left mainstem bronchus: a complication of bronchial artery embolization. Am J Roentgenol. 1983;141(3):535-7.
41. Girard P, Baldeyrou P, Lemoine G, et al. Left main-stem bronchial stenosis complicating bronchial artery embolization. Chest. 1990;97(5):1246-8.
42. Chapman SA, Holmes MD, Taylor DJ. Unilateral diaphragmatic paralysis following bronchial artery embolization for hemoptysis. Chest. 2000;118(1):269-70.
43. Munk PL, Morris DC, Nelems B. Left main bronchial-esophageal fistula: a complication of bronchial artery embolization. Cardiovasc Intervent Radiol. 1990;13(2):95-7.

CHAPTER 175

Diagnostic and Therapeutic Interventions in Chest

Naveen Kalra, Mandeep Kang, Anupam Lal, Ujjwal Gorsi

INTRODUCTION

A wide range of procedures used in the diagnosis and treatment of diseases of the chest constitute image-guided thoracic interventions. Percutaneous interventional procedures in the chest were actually in use before the advent of imaging. Leyden did the first transthoracic needle lung biopsy in 1882 to confirm pulmonary infections.[1] Lung biopsy continued to be used during the first half of the 20th century for confirming the microbiological diagnosis of infectious lobar consolidation. In 1964, the first fluoroscopically-guided bronchial brush biopsy was described.[2] Around the same time, the technique of transthoracic fine needle sampling in the chest was established by Nordenstrom.[3] Percutaneous mediastinal procedures were adopted on a routine basis after the advent of CT. Percutaneous drainage of fluid collections in the chest was introduced in the late seventies. Better catheter designs and refinement of embolic agents established bronchial artery embolization as an accepted technique in the next decade. Good results with minimally invasive treatment of superior vena cava (SVC) obstruction were achieved with the development of specialized stents. The commonly performed thoracic interventional radiological techniques will be discussed in this chapter. Bronchial artery embolization will be discussed in another chapter.

IMAGE GUIDANCE MODALITIES

Modalities used for image guidance include fluoroscopy, cross-sectional imaging (ultrasound, CT and MRI) or a combination of both. Uni- or biplanar fluoroscopy was the first imaging technique which was used for the guidance of percutaneous transthoracic needle biopsy (TNB) and percutaneous drainage of fluid collections. The advantages of fluoroscopy include its wide availability, familiarity to most radiologists and real-time control of the procedure. Fluoroscopy may be used in combination with ultrasound for adjusting the tip of catheters introduced into fluid collections. Ultrasound is used for image-guided biopsies of the chest wall, pleural lesions, pulmonary lesions with parietal contact or lesions in the anterior or superior mediastinum. Using this technique, the peripheral pulmonary lesions can be successfully biopsied with very high success rates which are more than 90%.[4] The ultrasound probe should be oriented parallel to the intercostal space as this facilitates the biopsy of the peripheral pulmonary lesions. Other procedures which can be done under ultrasound guidance include percutaneous aspiration and catheter drainage. The advantages of ultrasound guidance are real-time monitoring, lack of ionizing radiation, easy availability, portability and the ability to target non-necrotic part of the lesion. CT guidance provides anatomical display of all the thoracic structures in detail and ensures accurate placement of the needle and drainage catheter. It helps to determine the optimal percutaneous entry point so as to avoid transgression of the pleural fissure or puncture of bullae, large vessels, bronchi and the esophagus. Helical CT has not been found superior to sequential scanning.[5] CT fluoroscopy combines the advantages of both cross-sectional imaging and real-time control and is now widely available. High rates of technical success have been reported with sensitivity ranging from 89–95% and specificity of 100%.[6] Studies have shown that using intermittent 'quick check' CT fluoroscopy between needle advancements instead of continuous fluoroscopy can reduce the radiation exposure. Recently PET-CT is being used to guide biopsies by providing information about the abnormal metabolic activity of primary neoplasm and metastases. There is scanty literature on usage of MR guidance for thoracic interventions due to limited availability of this modality and the requirement of especially designed needles compatible with MR scanners.

NONVASCULAR INTERVENTIONS

The various percutaneous nonvascular image-guided thoracic interventions are transthoracic needle biopsy, diagnostic thoracocentesis, drainage of fluid collections, pleurodesis, pneumathorax/bulla drainage, lung abscess drainage, pericardial effusion drainage, treatment of secondary pulmonary aspergilloma, endoluminal tracheobronchial stenting and thermal ablation of pulmonary malignancy.

Transthoracic Needle Biopsy of Pulmonary Lesions

Indications

Transthoracic needle biopsy (TNB) is most commonly done for the diagnosis of a solitary pulmonary nodule (SPN). TNB is also used for confirming metastatic lung disease, staging of lung cancer or extrathoracic malignancy, and sampling of suspected focal infections.[7,8]

Patient Evaluation

Before biopsy, every effort should be made to establish the identity of the lesion using non-invasive methods including review of old chest radiographs and thin section CT for nodule characterization. Some clinicians use 'pulmonary nodule calculators' based on clinical and radiological risk factors to estimate pretest probability of malignancy. Coagulation parameters should be checked for all patients to exclude bleeding diathesis.

Contraindications

There are no absolute contraindications to TNB. However, percutaneous biopsy should be strictly avoided in suspected vascular lesion (e.g. arteriovenous malformation, pulmonary varix) and hydatid cyst. Bleeding diathesis should be corrected prior to the procedure. Severe pulmonary hypertension is a relative contraindication because of the danger of persistent pulmonary hemorrhage. Emphysematous bullae in the planned biopsy route increase the risk of pneumothorax and should be avoided if possible. Severe pulmonary disease, (FEV less than liter), contralateral pneumonectomy, ventilator dependence and patient's inability to cooperate or hold breath are relative contraindications.

Image Guidance

The choice of image guidance modality is dependent on the availability of various techniques, the skill and preference of the interventional radiologist, and the site, size and other characteristics of the lesion to be targeted. Fluoroscopy is particularly useful for biopsies of nodules in the lower third of the lungs, where large respiratory excursions occur. Orthogonal views of lung nodule and the needle obtained either with a rotating C-arm or a biplane fluoroscopy help confirm proper positioning of the needle tip within the lesion. CT guidance is useful for lesions that are adjacent to hilum or mediastinum (to avoid injury to adjacent vascular structures, bronchi and esophagus), for small lesions and the lesions not clearly seen on fluoroscopy **(Figs. 1A and B)**. The use of US guidance is limited to masses that are apical, juxtadiaphragmatic or adjacent to the chest wall **(Figs. 2 and 3)**. PET-CT guidance may improve the success rate of image-guided biopsies if the functional information obtained from the PET study is used to position the tip of the biopsy needle into the area of highest metabolism **(Figs. 4A to D)**. Endobronchial ultrasound (EBUS) guided biopsy is a safer technique than the percutaneous methods. However, it is expensive, not widely available and is primarily the domain of the interventional pulmonologist.

Biopsy Technique

A wide range of needles can be used for percutaneous biopsy procedure. Needles can be classified by their calibre or gauge tip configuration and the mechanism of sample acquisition. Needle sizes can either be smaller gauge (20–25 gauge) or larger gauge (14–19 gauge). Smaller gauge needles result in lesser bleeding and reduce other complications as well. Larger gauge needles on the other hand are easier to direct and provide better samples for cytology and histology. Needles have different angles and bevel of the tip. The Chiba and spinal needles have bevel angle of 25 and 30° respectively. Greene and Franseen needles have 90° tips. Needle tips can also be aspiration (non-cutting) and cutting types. Aspiration needles such as the Chiba, spinal and Greene needles provides cellular material for cytologic evaluation of

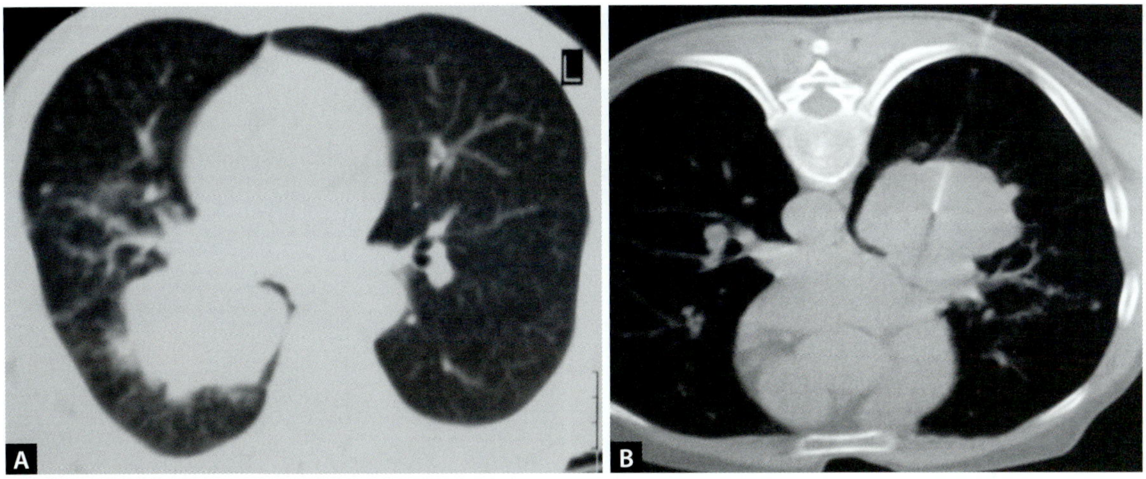

Figs. 1A and B: (A) Axial CT section of the chest at lung window settings shows a large mass with spiculated margins in the right hilar region; (B) Axial CT section of the chest in the prone position showing the needle *in situ* which has been placed in the mass after transgressing the lung parenchyma.

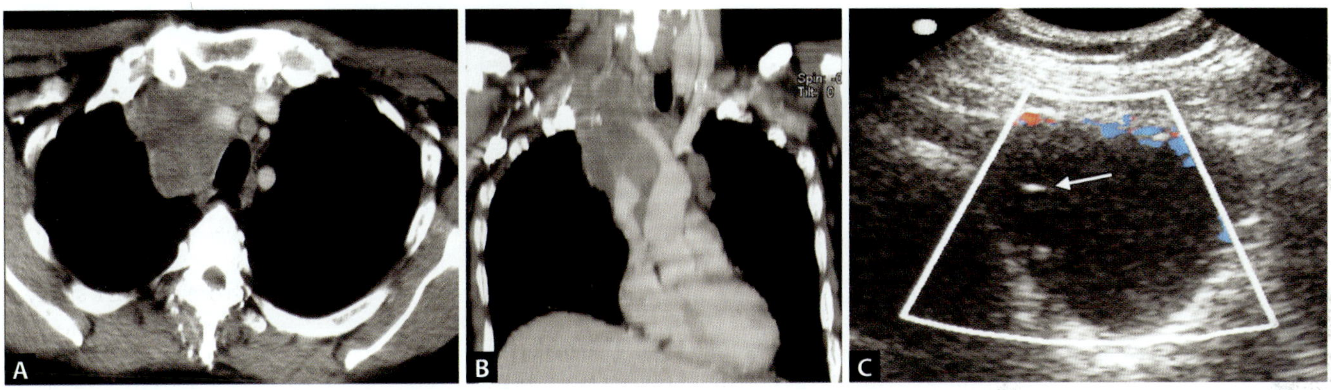

Figs. 2A to C: (A) Axial contrast-enhanced CT section shows an apical lung mass with loss of fat planes with the trachea and the brachiocephalic artery; (B) Coronal-reconstructed image showing the extent of the mass with lymph nodes in the neck region; (C) Color Doppler ultrasound showing the needle *in situ* (arrow). Doppler ultrasound ensures that there is no vessel in the course of the needle.

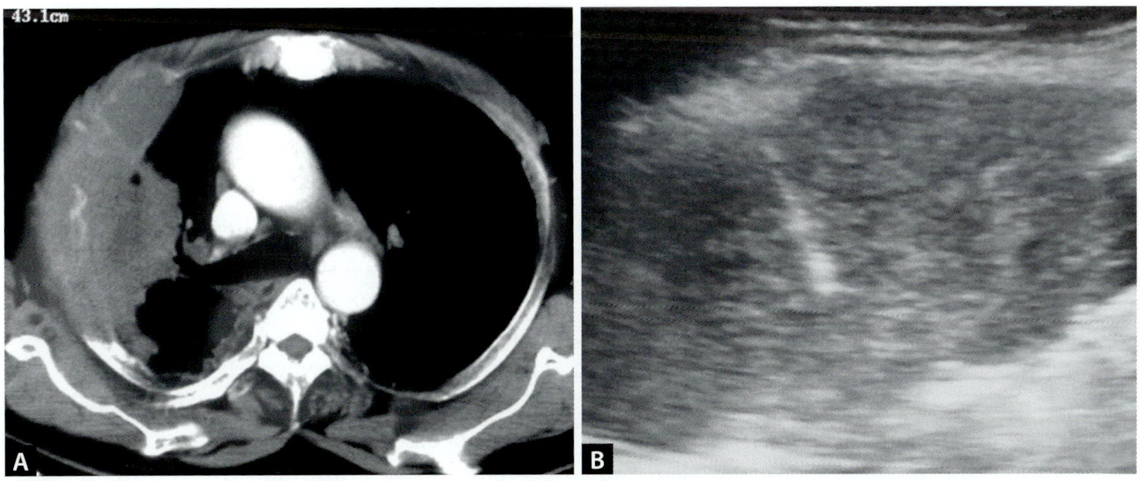

Figs. 3A and B: (A) Axial contrast-enhanced CT section shows a large peripheral mass with necrotic component in the right upper lobe with chest wall invasion and rib destruction; (B) Ultrasound image shows the entire extent of the needle which has been introduced percutaneously into the mass.

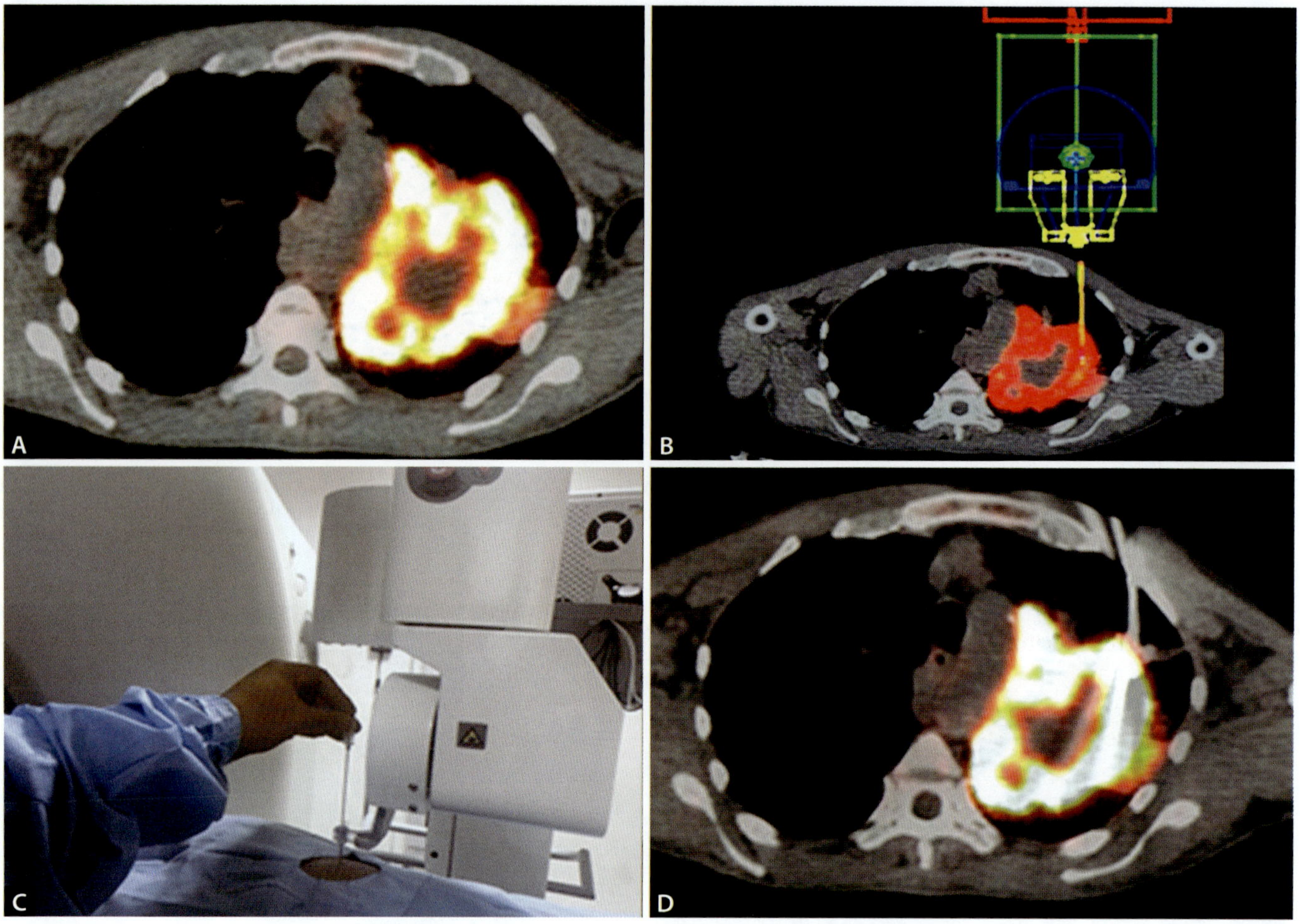

Figs. 4A to D: (A) Axial PET-CT functional image showing hypermetabolism in the periphery of the lesion in the left upper lobe of lung consistent with viable cells; (B) Planning of robotic arm-assisted trajectory for biopsy needle placement on robotic arm console; (C) Insertion of co-axial biopsy needle along the planned trajectory with the help of robotic arm needle navigation technique; (D) Check scan to confirm the tip of the semi-automated biopsy gun in the hypermetabolic region just before sampling.
Courtesy: Dr Rajender Kumar Basher and Dr BR Mittal, Department of Nuclear Medicine, PGIMER, Chandigarh.

malignancy. Cutting needle yield pieces of tissue for histologic analysis and can be used for the diagnosis of benign lesions, lymphoreticular malignancies, and in hospitals where experienced cytopathologists are not available. Needles can also be classified as manual, spring-loaded or automated.

The biopsy can be done with the single needle technique or the coaxial technique. As a rough guide, large easily accessible lesions lend themselves to the single needle technique whereas smaller lesions or lesions that require lengthy imaging procedures for correct needle placement are more easily accessible by the coaxial system. In the coaxial technique, an 18 or 19 gauge needle is initially advanced to the proximal edge of the lesion. A 22 gauge needle is then advanced through the guide needle to obtain a fine needle aspirate for cytology or else, a 20 gauge cutting needle is used for obtaining a core biopsy. Post procedural chest radiographs, one immediately after the procedure and another 4 hours later are obtained to rule out pneumothorax.

Complications

The most common complication of percutaneous lung biopsy is bleeding (hemoptysis, chest wall, parenchymal) **(Fig. 5)**. Hemoptysis occurs in about 5% of patients.[8] Usually, it is minimal manifesting as blood stained sputum. Rarely, however, it may be massive and may require bronchial artery embolization, balloon occlusion of the affected segmental bronchus or surgical resection.

The most complication requiring intervention is pneumothorax seen in 12–45% of the patients.[9] Having the patient lie with the puncture site dependent

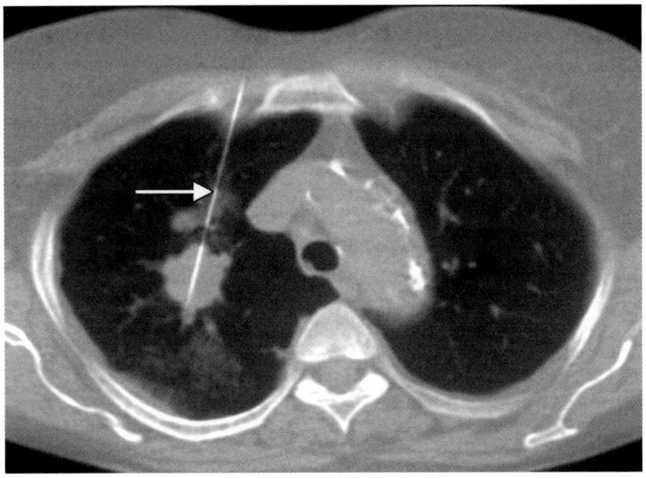

Fig. 5: Axial CT section shows a needle which has been placed in the lung nodule under CT guidance. There is presence of parenchymal hemorrhage along the needle tract (arrow).

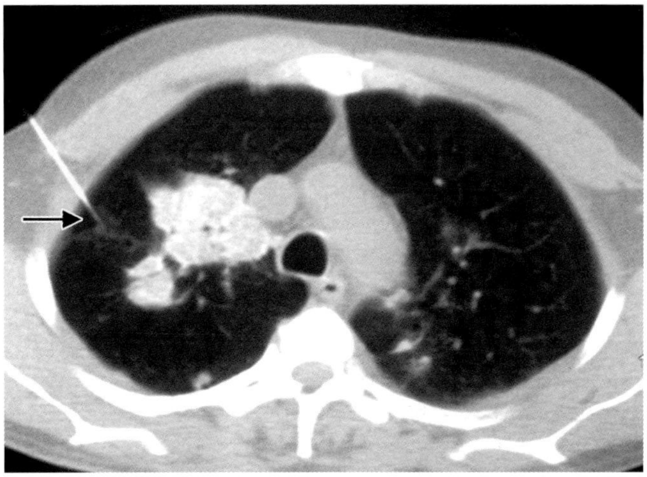

Fig. 6: Axial CT section shows presence of minimal pneumothorax at the site of needle entry. FNAC of the hilar mass was done under CT guidance in this patient (arrow). The pneumothorax was managed conservatively.

approximates the visceral puncture site with the parietal pleural and can decrease the rate of pneumothorax. 2–15% of pneumothoraces require treatment with chest tube placement **(Fig. 6)**. Large or symptomatic pneumothoraces can be treated with image-guided percutaneous placement of a small caliber catheter. The reported fatality rate of percutaneous lung biopsy is about 0.02%. The causes include tension pneumothorax, air embolism and pulmonary hemorrhage. Other uncommon complications include vasovagal reaction, lobar torsion and needle tract metastases. According to guidelines given by the Society of Interventional Radiology, a higher overall complication rate of 10% is acceptable for lung biopsies compared to 2% for all other organ systems.[10]

Results

Transthoracic needle biopsy of lung nodules is a relatively safe procedure with a high diagnostic yield. According to the guidelines for lung biopsy given by the Society of Interventional Radiology, an 85% success rate is acceptable.[10] TNB has an overall sensitivity of 70–100% in most series for the diagnosis of malignancy.[7,8] The yield for benign lesions, however is 50% or less since benign but non-specific results are not uncommon; this can be improved by performing both core biopsies and FNA of benign lesions.[11,12]

Transthoracic Needle Biopsy from Other Sites

Mediastinal masses may arise without any associated pulmonary mass and may represent metastatic disease. The best method of biopsy is determined by the location of the mass and its proximity to the vital structures. Biopsy of a mediastinal or hilar mass is usually performed under CT guidance as CT clearly shows the location of the mass and its relation to vital mediastinal structures, and allows selection of the optimal biopsy path. Ultrasound guidance can be used for large lesions which are in contact with the chest wall and where a safe acoustic window is available for lesion visualization and needle placement. Anterior mediastinal masses can be accessed by the parasternal **(Figs. 7A and B)**, suprasternal and trans-sternal **(Fig. 8)** approaches, while posterior mediastinal or subcarinal masses are accessed by the posterior paravertebral approach.[13-15] To avoid complications while using the parasternal approach, one should be aware of the anatomical location of internal mammary vessels. A direct mediastinal or extrapleural approach is preferred over a transpulmonary approach, as this reduces the risk of pneumothorax. Saline injection, 'salinoma,' can be used to widen the paravertebral or substernal extrapleural space for a direct mediastinal approach and is helpful in decreasing the incidence of post-biopsy pneumothorax.[16] A pleural space approach through an existing pleural effusion or an iatrogenically created pneumothorax has also been used for mediastinal biopsies.[17] According to the appropriateness criteria published by the American College of Radiology, nonradiologic mediastinal mass biopsy (bronchoscopically guided transbronchial FNA, transesophageal FNA, mediastinoscopy, thoracoscopy) may be safer and have higher yields compared to radiologic biopsy. However, the choices vary from institution to institution.

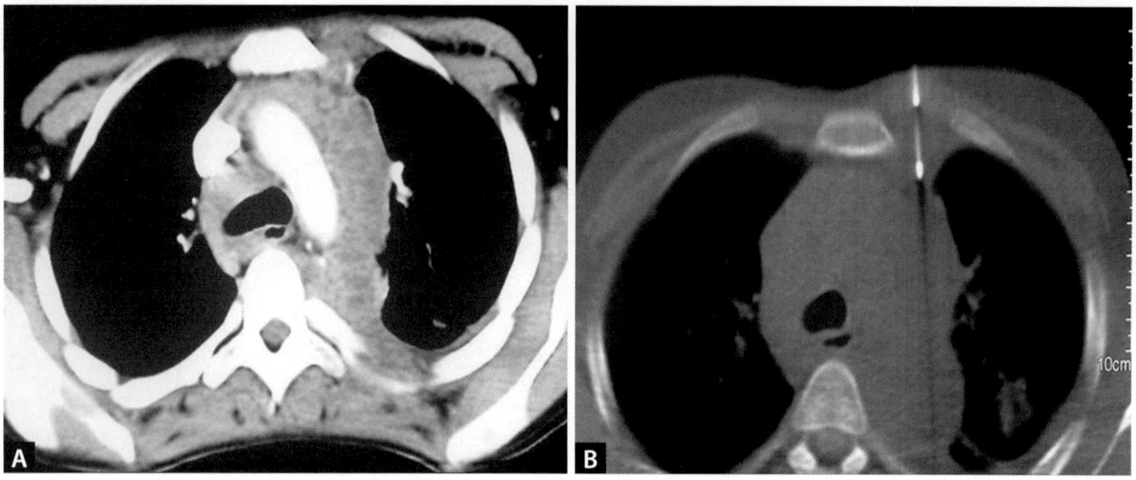

Figs. 7A and B: (A) Axial contrast-enhanced CT shows conglomerate lymph nodes in the prevascular and precarinal location; (B) CT-guided biopsy was done in this patient by the parasternal approach.

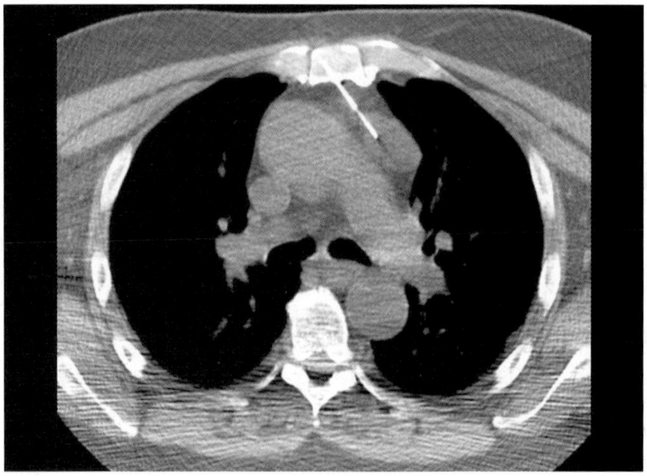

Fig. 8: CT-guided biopsy of the prevascular lymph node being done by the trans-sternal approach.
Courtesy: Dr Sanjay Gupta, MD Anderson Cancer Center, Houston, USA).

Percutaneous Needle Biopsy of the Pleura

Biopsies for diffuse disease are usually done without image guidance. Image-guided pleural biopsy is done for pleural masses or thickening with or without associated pleural fluid, small or loculated pleural effusions where thoracentesis has been nondiagnostic and where there are recurrent pleural effusions of unknown etiology. Most pleural biopsies are done using US guidance, although small pleural lesions require CT guidance for accurate needle placement. Solid masses or pleural thickening can be biopsied with the standard 16–20 gauge biopsy needle. Pleural effusions which are not associated with a discrete mass should be biopsied using a Cope needle system. Ultrasound guidance is able to localize even a small pleural effusion through which a core biopsy can be safely performed thus reducing the risk of pneumothorax. Complications such as pneumothorax, hemothorax, and laceration of diaphragm, liver or spleen have been reported in less than 1% of biopsies.[7]

Localization of a Nodule for Thoracoscopic Resection

Thoracoscopic resection has established itself as an effective method for diagnosing and treating a peripheral lung nodule that is near the visceral pleura. The radiologist can help by marking the lesion with a hook wire. The hook wire is inserted into the lesion through the guide needle of a coaxial system.[7]

Diagnostic Thoracocentesis

The most common indications for diagnostic thoracentesis are the evaluation of suspected infection or malignancy in the pleural space.[18,19] Sonographic guidance is used following a failed unguided thoracocentesis and when effusions are small or loculated. Using an aseptic technique an appropriate size needle (mostly 22 gauge; thicker up to 18 gauge for viscous collection) is inserted at a point where sonography shows the largest fluid dimension and the fluid is then aspirated. A post-procedure chest radiograph should be done to rule out a pneumothorax. Ultrasound guided diagnostic aspiration is successful in as many as 97% of cases.[20] The yield for cytological examination in documented malignant effusion has been reported to be approximately 50%. Pneumothorax rate is lower (0–3%) than that reported with blind aspiration (3–20%).[21]

Percutaneous Drainage of Pleural Space Fluid Collections

Image-guided percutaneous transthoracic catheter drainage of infected pleural collections is indicated in patients in whom diagnostic thoracocentesis shows frank pus, positive Gram stain on culture or a complicated parapneumonic effusion. Catheter drainage of pleural fluid is also performed for relief of symptoms (dyspnea, cough, pleuritic chest pain).

Empyema is an infected pleural collection caused by pneumonia, bronchiectasis, and/or trauma. Light[22] suggested three stages in the development of empyema. In the acute or exudative stage, although LDH and protein levels are raised, polymorphonuclear leukocytes, pH and glucose are normal. In this stage there is presence of a nonviscous, nonloculated effusion. Most of these collections resolve when appropriate antibiotic therapy is given. The subacute or fibrinopurulent stage is characterized by fall in pH ($\leq$7.00) and glucose ($\leq$40 mg/dL); at this stage, catheter drainage is usually required **(Figs. 9A to C)**. In the third or organizing stage, there is fibrin deposition and a pleural peel forms due to adhesion of visceral and parietal pleurae. In this stage, open thoracotomy and decortication is required for effective treatment.[19] Radiologic drainage is most effective in patients who have short duration of symptoms, free flowing or unilocular collections, absence of thick pleural peel and fluid that can be aspirated freely by needle insertion. Shankar et al.[23] found that radiologic drainage was more effective when on ultrasound the empyema was either anechoic or complex with diffusely distributed internal echoes and/or debris and no septations. On the other hand, empyemas which were complex and septated had a lower chance of successful percutaneous drainage. Postoperative empyemas, particularly those associated with bronchopleural fistula usually require open surgical procedure.

Most commonly, a combination of sonography and fluoroscopy is used for guidance. Fluoroscopy allows continuous monitoring of the course of needle, guidewire and catheter. Sonography is usually used for guidance of initial needle placement, and subsequent guidewire manipulations and catheter placement are performed under fluoroscopic guidance. For large collections, the entire procedure can be safely performed under sonographic control. CT is best used to drain loculated pleural collections, pleural fluid associated with underlying parenchymal fluid consolidation, and small less accessible collections.

Catheters ranging in size from 8–30 French are introduced by the Seldinger or trocar techniques. The catheter is placed in the most dependent part of the collection and is immediately attached to a water-seal pleural drainage system with or without suction. The water-seal system not only allows a unidirectional flow but also permits visual observation of an air-leak. The patient is assessed daily for therapeutic response, amount of drainage, and catheter patency. Periodic imaging is required to assess size of the residual collection and lung re-expansion. Chest radiographs usually suffice for non-loculated collections, but CT scanning may be needed for assessing loculated collections. The drainage catheter is removed when the drainage output is less than 10 mL per day, the patient's fever and leukocyte counts have decreased and resolution of the pleural collection is documented on imaging.

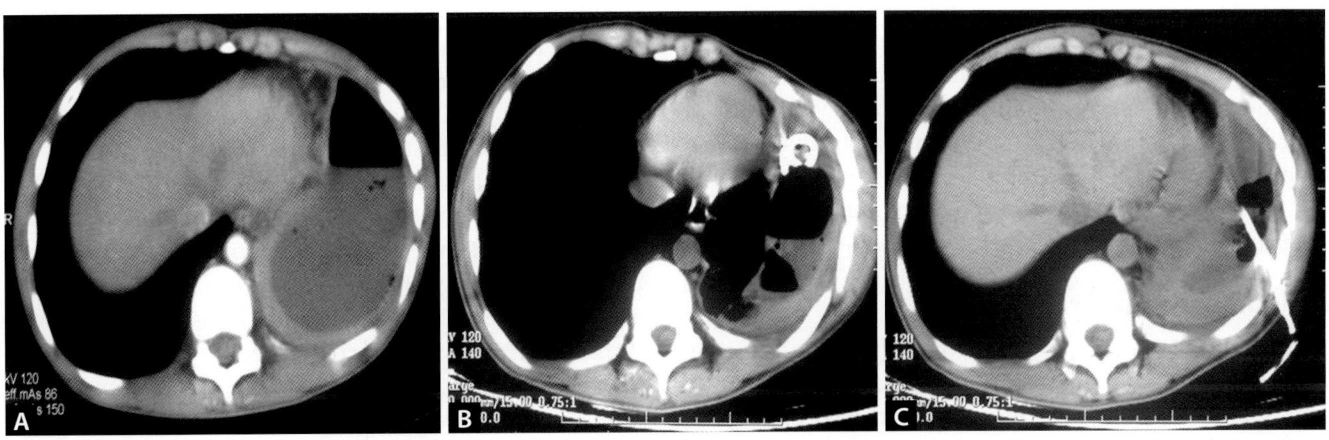

Figs. 9A to C: (A) Axial contrast-enhanced CT section showing a loculated collection with air-fluid level with enhancing pleura on the left side; (B and C) Axial CT sections done post-drainage show significant resolution of the collection after one week of drainage.

Poor drainage of pleural fluid and inadequate lung re-expansion may be secondary to improperly positioned or kinked catheter, complex fluid collection, multiple separate locules, a bronchopleural fistula, or airway obstruction. Undrained non-communicating loculi may require additional catheters. Occasionally, repositioning of catheter or conversion to a large bore catheter may help enhance drainage. A wire advanced through the catheter can be used to disrupt septae in multiseptate collections. Intrapleural administration of fibrinolytic medication (streptokinase, urokinase, or more recently tissue plasminogen activator) may aid in septated or loculated collections. Intrapleural fibrinolytic administration helps dissolve viscous fibrinous material and septations that interfere with drainage. In one protocol, 2–4 mg of t-PA in 10–20 mL saline is injected every 8 hours for several days with clamping of the tube after each instillation.[24] The reported clinical success rate is 62–100%.

Retrospective studies of radiologically guided pleural drainage procedures have shown success rates of 72–88%, which compare favourably with success rates of 66–83% reported in surgical literature.[19] Complications including bleeding due to intercostal vessel injury, pneumothorax, bronchopleural fistula, re-expansion pulmonary edema, and bacteremia are uncommon, seen in less than 2% of cases.[18,19]

Pleural Sclerotherapy or Pleurodesis

Recurrent malignant effusions can be managed by instillation of a sclerosing agent into the pleural space. This induces chemical pleurodesis. The procedure is performed by placing a catheter in the pleural space. When the catheter output drops below 100 mL/day and chest imaging shows drainage of fluid and re-expansion of the lung, sclerotherapy is performed. There should be adequate apposition of the visceral and parietal layers of the pleura for sclerosis to be effective. The agents used for this procedure include tetracycline, doxycycline, minocycline, bleomycin, diluted sodium hydroxide and talc.[18,19] A 20–50 mL of 1–2% lidocaine can be instilled into the pleural space before the sclerotic agent for analgesia. Reported success rates range from 62–90%, and no particular agent has been shown to be superior.[18,19]

Pneumothorax Drainage

The indications for pneumothorax drainage are large volume of the air pocket (>25% of the volume of one hemithorax), an enlarging pneumothorax indicating persistent air leak, tension pneumothorax, a diseased contralateral lung or any sized pneumothorax associated with shortness of breath or severe chest pain.[18,19] Most pneumothoraces drainages can be performed using fluoroscopic guidance. However, CT guidance may be used for small and loculated air collections. The pneumothorax may be approached in two ways, either through the first or second intercostal space in the midclavicular line or through the 4th or 5th intercostal space in the anterior axillary line in females and in males with bulky pectoralis muscles. The anterior approach has the advantage of allowing easier positioning of the catheter tip in the lung apex. The lateral approach allows real-time visualization of the pneumothorax and catheter insertion is then easily performed. Catheters ranging in size from 6 to 16 French are used and are connected to an underwater seal drainage with suction or to a one-way flutter (Heimlich) valve. There is need to confirm the correct catheter placement and reduction in the pneumothorax by doing a chest radiograph immediately after the drainage. The catheter is removed when the lung remains expanded on a follow-up chest radiograph obtained 2 hours after clamping the tube and there is no evidence of air leak. Success rates range from 87 to 93% with majority of pneumothoraces resolving within 24–72 hours.

Lung Abscess Drainage

Lung abscess represents an infected collection of the lung parenchyma. Primary abscesses are the result of aspiration and are caused by anaerobic bacteria. Secondary abscesses arise from adjacent infection or by hematogenous spread (e.g. pneumonia, lung cyst, septic emboli). Majority of lung abscesses respond to antibiotics, postural drainage and bronchoscopic lavage. Image-guided percutaneous catheter drainage is used for the treatment of lung abscesses that fail to resolve with medical therapy. A CT scan is done to assess the presence of pleural involvement and to plan a safe transthoracic route for catheter placement. Fluoroscopy, US or CT guidance can be used for performing the procedure. One should avoid traversing normal lung because of the risk of hemorrhage and bronchopleural fistula formation with empyema. The catheter should transverse the abnormal lung to avoid pneumothorax and collapse of normal lung. The patient should be positioned to keep the opposite hemothorax nondependent in order to avoid the aspiration of the abscess contents into the normal lung. As lung abscess drainage represents a controlled bronchocutaneous fistula, the size of the drainage catheter should not be more than 12–14 French to avoid large air leaks. The catheter is removed once clinical assessment and chest radiographs indicate resolution of abscess. 73–100% patients show resolution of the abscess after 10–15 days of drainage. However, complete collapse of the cavity may take longer up to 4–5 weeks as abscesses have thick walls.[3]

Mediastinal Abscess Drainage

Mediastinal abscess is a life-threatening infection which occurs subsequent to thoracic surgery or endoscopy. Mediastinal abscesses not considered for surgical drainage can be successfully drained percutaneously or by a transesophageal approach.[25] Drainage is usually done under CT guidance by a parasternal or paraspinous approach to avoid the lung. The few reported series indicate a success rate of 83–100% but 30 days mortality is high.[3]

Pericardial Effusion Drainage

Pericardial effusions require drainage when they impair the diastolic filling of the ventricles. Large pericardial effusions are caused by renal failure, metabolic or immunologic diseases, infection and malignancy. Pericardial catheter drainage is done under ultrasound guidance using a subcostal or subxiphoid approach with or without fluoroscopy. Drainage can also be done under CT guidance by the left anterolateral approach.[26]

Pneumatocele and Bulla Drainage

Percutaneous drainage of an infected or tension pneumatocele or bulla has been performed.[27,28] However, an air–fluid level within a bulla does not indicate infection and a percutaneous diagnostic aspiration should precede catheter insertion in doubtful cases **(Figs. 10A to C)**.

Secondary Pulmonary Aspergilloma

Intracavitatory aspergilloma may present with life-threatening hemoptysis and require a surgical resection. However, open thoracotomy may be contraindicated in patients with severe underlying pulmonary pathology. In such patients, transthoracic instillation of amphotericin B has been described. This technique has a reported success rate of 50% for resolution of aspergilloma and 75–100% for acute control of hemoptysis.[29]

Endoluminal Tracheobronchial Stenting

Tracheobronchial airway obstruction can occur due to a malignant or benign cause. Although surgery is the treatment of choice, balloon dilatation or stenting may be done as a palliative treatment in patients who have short life expectancy or extensive airway stenosis. Balloon dilatation results in rapid improvement of the respiratory function. However, relief of symptoms is often short lasting. Stents can be placed under image guidance or bronchoscopic control or by using a combination of both modalities. Tracheobronchial stenting has been successfully done for symptom palliation in patients with inoperable bronchogenic cancer, esophageal or tracheal tumors and metastatic tumors causing extensive compression or submucosal disease or tracheoesophageal fistula. It has also been done in benign conditions like post-intubation or post-anastomatic stricture, tracheobronchomalacia, fibrosing mediastinitis, relapsing polychondritis and amyloidosis. Helical CT is used for precise measurement of the diameter of the stenosis and for determining the location of the stenosis. Two types of stents are used: silicone stents (Dumon, Dynamic and others) and metallic stents (balloon expandable stents like Palmaz and Strecker or SEMS, self-expandable stents such as Gianturco, Wallstent, Ultraflex). As some of these stents have poor visualization on conventional fluoroscopy, CT fluoroscopy guidance may be used to ensure precise and real-time

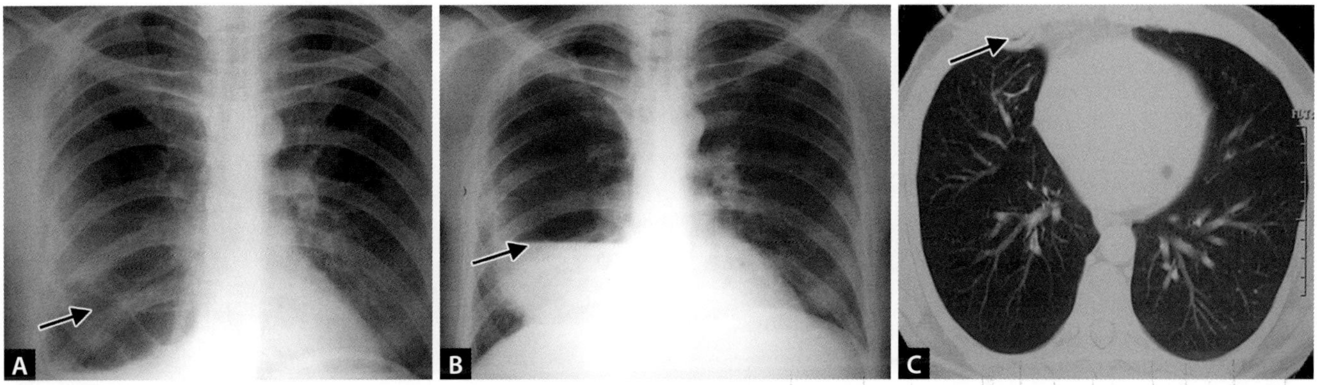

Figs. 10A to C: (A) Chest X-ray PA view shows multiple emphysematous bullae in the right mid and lower zones (arrow); (B) Chest X-ray PA view shows an air–fluid level in a large bulla in the right mid and lower zones (arrow) on follow-up; (C) Axial CT of the chest at lung window settings post-drainage shows the catheter *in situ* with resolution of the collection (arrow).

control on stent deployment. Placement of stents leads to immediate and significant decrease in symptoms and respiratory function improvement in majority (80–95%) of patients. Complications of stent placement are early or late stent migration, infection, tracheobronchial fistula, deformation or breakage of stent and stent obstruction by secretions, granulations or tumor overgrowth.

THERMAL ABLATION OF LUNG LESIONS

The three most commonly used ablative techniques in the lung are radiofrequency ablation (RFA), microwave ablation (MWA) and cryoablation. These ablative techniques are used in the management of inoperable nonsmall cell lung cancer (NSCLC) and in selected patients with pulmonary metastases. Surgical resection is the gold standard for the treatment of stage I NSCLC. Unfortunately, only about one-third of patients are suitable for surgical resection due to various comorbidities or poor cardiopulmonary reserve. Dupuy et al. reported the first clinical experience of percutaneous RFA of lung lesions in the year 2000.[30] RFA is a minimally invasive thermal energy delivery system. It delivers a high frequency alternating current supplied by a radiofrequency generator through a needle electrode placed in the tumor. The application of an alternating current results in ionic agitation and generation of frictional heat which ablates the tumor tissue. As air is a thermal insulator, the aerated lung has high electric impedance. Lung tumors are well suited for RFA as the surrounding normal lung parenchyma acts as an insulator for the heat energy delivered. Hence, less power input is required to achieve adequate ablation. By the same principle, pleural based lesions require more energy to treat and are associated with higher recurrence rates and complications. However, a longer approach traversing atleast 2 cm of aerated lung is recommended even for peripheral tumors to prevent air leak, chest pain and skin burns. When ablating lung tumors, tract cautery should be avoided to circumvent the risk of bronchopleural fistula formation.

The outcome of ablation is more promising in metastatic disease compared with primary malignancies and in lesions smaller than 3 cm in size. Most centers limit RFA to patients with five or fewer lesions and use 5 cm as the upper limit for size.[31] Contraindications for the procedure include lesions which are close to vessels (within 1 cm), poor lung function, presence of pacemaker and coagulopathy. The lesions are treated in a predetermined order, typically starting with the most dependent lesions as they may be obscured by blood from more anterior lesions as the treatment progresses **(Figs. 11A and B)**. CT done at this time shows the ablated lesion surrounded by ground-glass opacity (GGO). The treatment is considered technically complete when the entire tumor is surrounded by GGOs **(Figs. 12A and B)**. Complications of the procedure include pneumothorax, hemothorax, infective complications and tumor ablation syndrome. Symptoms of ablation syndrome include myalgia, fever and productive cough.

Follow-up imaging is done at 1 month and then at 3 months intervals for the first year. The criterion for complete resolution is reduction of the contrast enhancement compared with images taken before the procedure. A CT attenuation higher than 15 HU indicates disease persistence or relapse.[32] The postablation

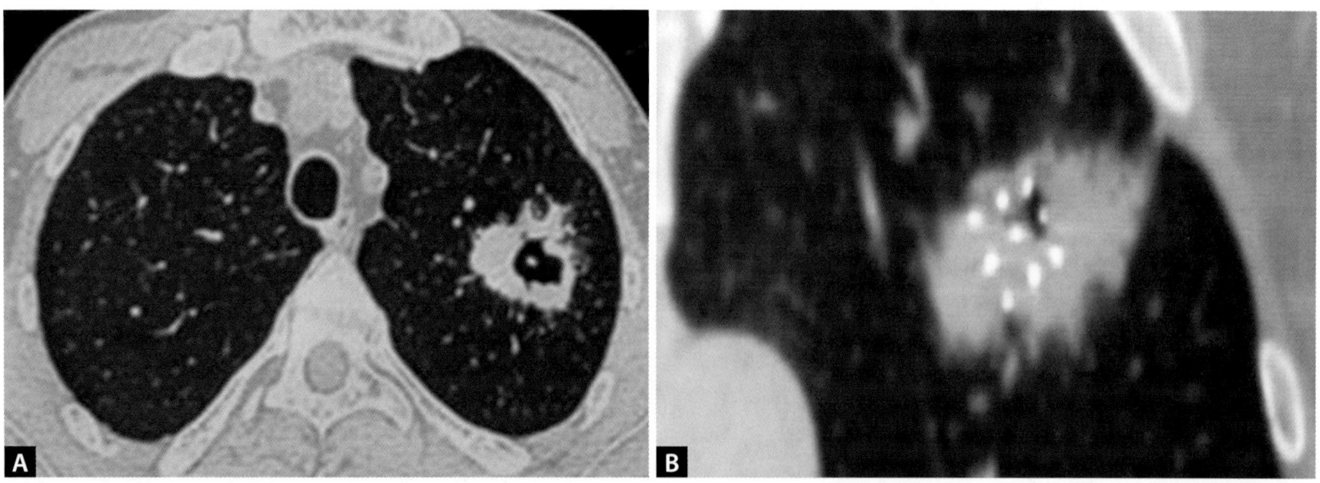

Figs. 11A and B: (A) Axial CT in the supine position at lung window settings shows a malignant cavitory nodule in the left upper lobe; (B) Coronal CT section during RF ablation shows the hyperattenuation with increase in the size of the nodule contributed by intraparenchymal hemorrhage.

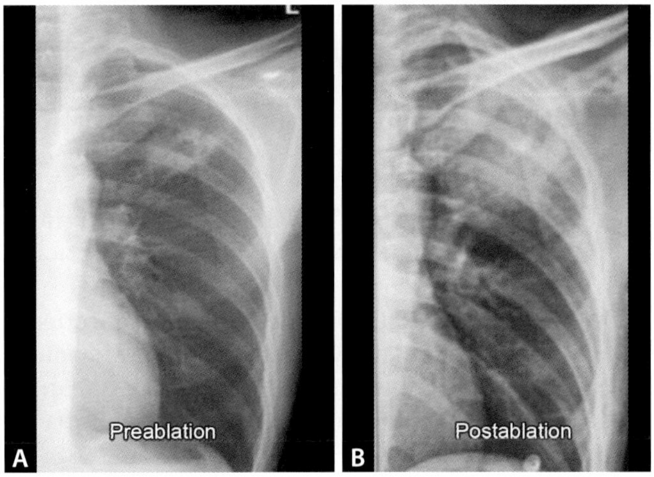

Figs. 12A and B: (A) Preablation chest X-ray showing cavitory lesion in left upper lobe; (B) Postablation chest X-ray showing a larger area of opacity due to the surrounding congestion and hemorrhage.

evolution of the lesion on imaging and histology is divided into three phases: early (<1 week), intermediate (1 week to 3 months) and late (>3 months) phases.[33] In the early phase, there are three layers of tissue seen on histology: an inner layer of thermal damage, a middle layer of alveolar congestion and an outer layer of congestion, hemorrhage and both damaged and viable cells. On CT the lesion is surrounded by an inner layer of GGO corresponding to the inner and middle layers on histology, and an outer thin, dense rim corresponding to the outer layer on histology. In the intermediate phase, there is granulation and fibrosis of the necrotic tissue. The size of the ablation zone may still exceed the size of the tumor in this phase. The benign periablational enhancement pattern still persists. In the late phase, the fibrous transformation is completed. The ablated area will be seen as fibrotic, nodular or cavitatory. CT done at this time should be taken as baseline examination in order to evaluate progression or recurrence. Even with PET-CT, an active lesion does not definitely represent tumor in the first three months.[34]

In the RAPTURE study (a prospective, intention-to-treat, multicenter trial), 106 patients (33 patients with primary disease, 73 patients with pulmonary metastases) with 183 lung tumors smaller than 3.5 cm were treated with RFA.[35] The study showed a 1-year overall complete response rate of 88% and a 2-year cancer-specific survival of 92% for primary disease. In another study of pulmonary metastases, RFA was found to be an effective treatment option for nodules less than 2 to 3 cm with a 4-year local efficacy of 89%.[36]

Microwave ablation is now becoming the favored technique for treating lung malignancies. It uses electromagnetic energy which is at a much higher frequency than RFA (300 MHz to 300 GHz). It delivers all the benefits of RFA and has several advantages.[37] The ablative zone is larger and is less susceptible to heat sink effect. The various benefits include consistently higher intratumoral temperatures, an improved convection profile, the capability of using multiple applicators, larger tumor ablation volumes and no need for grounding pads. Tumors smaller than 2 cm in maximal diameter are treated with a single applicator and tumors 2 cm or larger are treated with multiple antennae each powered by individual microwave generators. The reported cancer-specific 1-year survival is 83%, 2-year survival is 73% and 3-year survival is 61% for pulmonary tumors of mean size of 3.5 cm.[37]

Cryoablation works on the principle of freeze-thaw-freeze cycle. Pressurized argon gas is used to generate temperatures of less than –40°C and helium is used to increase the temperature to 20°C. There is cell rupture, protein denaturation and microvascular thrombosis-induced ischemia. One can accurately visualize the ablation zone as an 'ice ball' on CT scan. Presently, cryoablation is considered safer than RFA and MWA for lung tumors near the chest wall or mediastinum. The newer cryoablation devices have the cautery option unlike the older equipment which decreases the risk of bleeding complications like pulmonary hemorrhage, hemoptysis and hemothorax.[38] However, the potential risk of a severe systemic adverse effect, i.e. cryoshock still remains.

VASCULAR INTERVENTIONS

The various vascular interventions are bronchial artery embolization, pulmonary artery embolization, superior vena cava (SVC) stenting and percutaneous vascular foreign body retrieval. Bronchial artery embolization will be discussed in another chapter.

Pulmonary Artery Embolization

Pulmonary artery embolization is done for pulmonary artery aneurysms and pulmonary arteriovenous malformations (PAVMs). Aneurysms and pseudoaneurysms of the pulmonary arteries have several causes. The main pulmonary artery may be dilated by left-to-right shunts or pulmonary artery hypertension. Post-stenotic dilatation following pulmonary valve disease may mimic an aneurysm. Central pulmonary artery aneurysms are caused by congenital disorders or vasculitis. Multiple aneurysms may be seen with infection (e.g. Rasmussen's aneurysms in tuberculosis, following septic emboli, necrotizing pneumonia, syphilis). Large pulmonary artery aneurysms present with hemoptysis, chest pain or dyspnea or may be seen as an incidental finding on CT or chest X-ray.

Pseudoaneurysms are usually seen in the right middle or lower lobe arteries. Distal arterial rupture with pseudoaneurysm formation is a rare complication of Swan-Ganz catheter placement. The patients present with hemoptysis or a lung mass on imaging studies. Transcatheter embolization of the parent artery with coils or vascular plugs is the treatment of choice and is usually successful.

PAVMs occur sporadically or in patients with hereditary hemorrhagic telangiectasia (HHT), also known as Osler-Weber-Rendu syndrome. PAVMs may also occur secondary to trauma. HHT is an autosomal dominant disorder in which there are telangiectasias of the mouth and telangiectasias or AVMs of the brain, gastrointestinal treat (GIT), liver and lungs. Pulmonary AVMs are seen in 20–50% of patients with HHT and 60% have multiple lesions. Many patients present with epistaxis.

The majority (90%) of AVMs are simple and have single segmental arterial supply. The rest are complex and have multiple segmental arterial supply. They are usually found in the lower lobes. The PAVMs are direct communications between pulmonary artery branches and veins and thus cause a right-to-left shunt. This results in dyspnea, fatigue, hemoptysis, stroke or brain abscess. The primary indication for embolization of PAVMs is prevention of neurologic complications.

CT angiography is done to identify all feeding arteries. Pulmonary embolotherapy is the treatment of choice.[39] Many devices have been used for occlusion including coils and detachable balloons or vascular plugs **(Figs. 13A to D)**. Coils should be 1–2 mm larger than the artery being embolized and should be deployed near the nidus of the malformations. In small feeding arteries (<5 mm in diameter), detachable balloons may be preferred due to the precision of placement. Embolization is successful in more than 90% of patients. A post-embolization syndrome

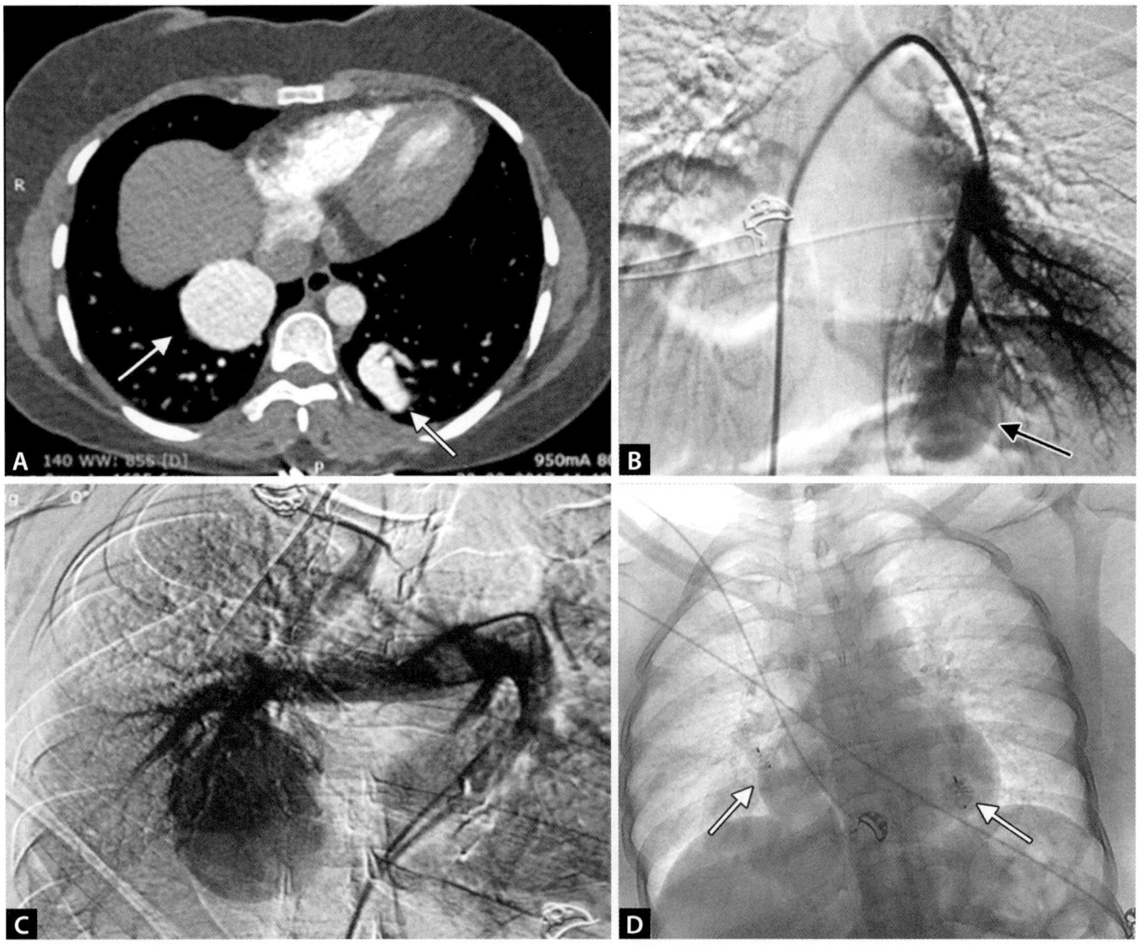

Figs. 13A to D: (A) Axial CECT showing pulmonary AVMs in lower lobes of both lungs (arrows); (B) Left pulmonary angiogram showing AVM in left lower lobe; (C) Right pulmonary angiogram showing large AVM in right lower lobe; (D) Post-embolization radiograph showing both vascular plugs (arrows).

with fever and chest pain is common. Complications occur in 10–20% of cases. Serious complications include paradoxical embolization of air or of the embolization device. All catheter and guide wire exchanges and coil introduction should be done 'under water' to avoid air embolism to the brain.

Endovascular Therapy of SVC Obstruction

The superior vena cava (SVC) may be obstructed as a result of luminal disease (thrombus or tumor), extrinsic compression (tumor or lymph node) or mural disease (intimal hyperplasia or tumor invasion). Fibrosing mediastinitis is a localized or diffuse infiltrative disease that may be idiopathic or may be caused by chronic infection. The SVC is involved in one-third of cases. Significant SVC or bilateral brachiocephalic vein stenosis or obstruction may lead to SVC syndrome. This is characterized by marked facial and neck swelling, bilateral arm swelling, cyanosis, shortness of breath, hoarseness and headache. Catheter directed therapy is considered only in patients with moderate to severe symptoms who fail to respond to less aggressive measures. SVC occlusion itself is rarely fatal and most patients die due to the underlying malignant disease. Therefore, the aim of treatment is only short-term palliation of symptoms. Long-term patency is required in patients with benign SVC obstruction. Intravascular stents are effective in both benign and malignant SVC obstruction. In patients with benign obstruction, PTA is done before stenting. It probes the degree of stenosis and localizes the level of maximum resistance within the stenosed segment. PTA is not done prior to stenting in malignant disease but should be done after stenting to establish optimal venous return. Relative contraindications to the procedure are preterminal patients with malignant disease, extensive chronic venous thrombosis, endoluminal tumor growth and upper limb paralysis. Complications include stent migration or misplacement, formation of *de novo* thrombosis and pulmonary embolism.

Percutaneous Vascular Foreign Body Retrieval

The percutaneous method of retrieval avoids thoracotomy and open heart surgery. The foreign bodies needing retrieval include lost central venous lines, Swan-Ganz catheters, ventriculoatrial shunts, port-a-caths, cardiac stimulator lines and pacemaker electrodes. Relative contraindications for retrieval are free-floating thrombus attached to the foreign body and chronic incorporation of the foreign body in a thrombus or vessel wall. The extraction is done by loop-snare technique, helical basket entrapment or the grasping forceps technique or a combination of the above. The reported success rate of closed percutaneous retrieval is >90%.[40]

CONCLUSION

There is a myriad of procedures that can be performed by the interventional radiologist in the chest. However there needs to be a close association between the radiologists, pulmonologists, oncologists, pathologists and thoracic surgeons to ensure the success of these procedures. The complication rate can also be kept low by following the prescribed guidelines for these interventions.

REFERENCES

1. Leyden OO. Uber infectiose pneumonie. Dtsch Med Wochenschr. 1883;9;52-5.
2. Hattori S, Matsuda M, Sugiyama T, et al. Cytologic diagnosis of early lung cancer: brushing method under X-ray television fluoroscopy. Dis Chest. 1964;45:129-42.
3. Ghaye B, Dondelinger RF. Imaging-guided thoracic interventions. Eur Respir J. 2001;17:507-28.
4. Middleton WD, Teefey SA, Dahiya N. Ultrasound-guided chest biopsies. Ultrasound Q. 2006;22:241-52.
5. Ghaye B, Dondelinger RF, Dewe W. Percutaneous CT-guided lung biopsy: sequential versus spiral scanning: A randomized prospective study. Eur Radiol. 1999;9:1317-20.
6. Gupta S. New techniques in image-guided percutaneous biopsy. Cardiovasc Intervent Radiol. 2004;27:91-104.
7. Tarver RD, Conces DJ Jr. Interventional chest radiology. Radiol Clin North Am. 1994;32:689-709.
8. Klein JS, Zarka MA. Transthoracic needle biopsy. Radiol Clin North Am. 2000;38:235-66.
9. Gupta S, Wallace MJ, Cardella JF, et al. Quality improvement guidelines for percutaneous needle biopsy. J Vasc Interv Radiol. 2010;21:969-75.
10. Cardella JF, Bakal CW, Bertino RE, et al. Quality improvement guidelines for image-guided percutaneous biopsy in adults. J Vasc Interv Radiol. 2003;14:S227-30.
11. Fraser RS. Transthoracic needle aspiration. The benign diagnosis. Arch Pathol Lab Med. 1991;115:751-61.
12. Greif J, Marmor S, Schwarz Y, et al. Percutaneous core needle biopsy vs. fine needle aspiration in diagnosing benign lung lesions. Acta Cytol. 1999;43:756-60.
13. Protopapas Z, Westcott JL. Transthoracic hilar and mediastinal biopsy. Radiol Clin North Am. 2000;38:281-91.
14. Gupta S, Gulati M, Rajwanshi A, et al. Sonographically guided fine-needle aspiration biopsy of superior mediastinal lesions by the suprasternal route. Am J Roentgenol. 1998;171:1303-06.
15. Gupta S, Wallace MJ, Morello FA Jr, et al. CT-guided percutaneous needle biopsy of intra-thoracic lesions by using the trans-sternal approach: Experience in 37 patients. Radiology. 2002;222:57-62.
16. Langen HJ, Klose KC, Keulers P, et al. Artificial widening of the mediastinum to gain access for extra pleural biopsy: Clinical results. Radiology. 1995;196:703-06.

17. Bressler EL, Kirkham JA. Mediastinal masses: alternative approaches to CT-guided needle biopsy. Radiology. 1994; 191:391-96.
18. Boland GW, Lee MJ, Silverman S, et al. Interventional radiology of the pleural space. Clin Radiol. 1995;50:205-14.
19. Klein JS, Schultz S, Heffner JE. Interventional radiology of the chest: Image-guided percutaneous drainage of pleural effusions, lung abscess, and pneumothorax. Am J Roentgenol. 1995;164:581-8.
20. Silverman SG, Saini S, Mueller PR. Pleural interventions. Indications, techniques, and clinical applications. Radiol Clin North Am. 1989;27:1257-66.
21. Collins TR, Sahn SA. Thoracocentesis: Clinical value, complications, technical problems, and patent experience. Chest. 1987;91:817-22.
22. Light RW. Parapneumonic effusions and empyema. Clin Chest Med. 1985;6:55-62.
23. Shankar S, Gulati M, Kang M, et al. Image-guided percutaneous drainage of thoracic empyema: Can sonography predict the outcome? Eur Radiol. 2000;10:495-99.
24. D' Agostino HB, Hurvitz D, Nall L, et al. Transcatheter fluid drainage. In: Valji K (Eds). Vascular and Interventional Radiology, Elsevier, 2006.pp.516-31.
25. Gobien RP, Stanley JH, Gobien BS, et al. Percutaneous catheter aspiration and drainage of suspected mediastinal abscesses. Radiology. 1984;151:69-71.
26. Szapiro D, Ghaye B, Dondelinger RF. Pericardial tamponade: CT-guided percutaneous drainage. J Interv Radiol. 1996;11:129-31.
27. Sewall LE. Franco AI, Wojtowycz MM, et al. Pneumatoceles causing respiratory compromise. Treatment by percutaneous decompression. Chest. 1993;103:1266-7.
28. Kalra N, Aiyappan SK, Jindal SL, et al. Image-guided percutaneous drainage of an emphysematous bulla with a fluid level. Indian J Radiol Imaging. 2010;20:34-6.
29. Giron J, Poey C, Fajadet P, et al. CT-guided percutaneous treatment of inoperable aspergillomas: A study of 40 cases. Eur J Radiol. 1998;28:235-42.
30. Dupuy DE, Zagoria RJ. Akerley W, et al. Percutaneous radiofrequency ablation of malignancies in the lung. Am J Roentgenol. 2000;174:57-59.
31. Roy AM, Bent C, Fotheringham T, et al. Radiofrequency ablation of lung lesions: Practical applications and tips. Curr Probl Diagn Radiol. 2009;38:44-52.
32. Akeboshi M, Yamakado K, Nakatsuka A, et al. Percutaneous radiofrequency ablation of lung neoplasms: Initial therapeutic response. J Vasc Interv Radiol. 2004;15:463-70.
33. Vogl TJ, Nour-Eldin NA, Albrecht MH, et al. Thermal ablation of lung tumors: Focus on microwave ablation. Rofo. 2017;189:828-43.
34. Bonichon F, Palussiere, Godbert Y, et al. Diagnostic accuracy of 18F-FDG PET/CT for assessing response to radiofrequency ablation treatment in lung metastases: A multicentric prospective study. Eur J Nucl Med Mol Imaging. 2013;40:1817-27.
35. Lencioni R, Crocetti L, Cioni R, et al. Response to radiofrequency ablation of pulmonary tumours: A prospective, intention-to-treat, multicentre clinical trial (the RAPTURE study). Lancet Oncol. 2008;9:621-28.
36. de Baere T, Auperin A, Deschamps F, et al. Radiofrequency ablation is a valid treatment option for lung metastases: experience in 566 patients with 1037 metastases. Ann Oncol. 2015;26:987-91.
37. Wolf FJ, Grand D, Machan JT, et al. Microwave ablation of lung malignancies: Effectiveness, CT findings, and safety in 50 patients. Radiology. 2008;247:871-9.
38. Lee KS, Erinjeri JP. Decision making in interventional oncology: Ablative options in the lung. Semin Intervent Radiol. 2017;34:176-81.
39. Mager JJ, Overtoom TT, Blauw H, et al. Embolotherapy of pulmonary arteriovenous malformation: Long-term results in 112 patients. J Vasc Interv Radiol. 2004;15:451-6.
40. Dondelinger RF, Lepoutre B, Kurdziel JC. Percutaneous vascular foreign body retrieval: experience of an 11 year period. Eur J Radiol. 1991;12:4-10.

CHAPTER 176

Chest X-ray Evaluation in Cardiac Disease

Sanjiv Sharma, Gurpreet Singh Gulati, Priya Jagia

INTRODUCTION

Chest radiography is an important imaging technique used for the assessment of heart disease.[1] A skilled interpretation of the chest radiograph may disclose important morphological changes and to some extent even indicate the functional status of the cardiovascular system. Despite the fact that it usually provides an indirect (inferential) information, and that other more specific imaging techniques for noninvasive cardiac imaging have now become available, the chest radiograph remains a widely available, economical and often the first examination performed in a patient with suspected cardiac disease. The size and shape of cardiac shadow can be determined and retained as a permanent record for future reference. A proper understanding of the normal anatomy is essential for correct interpretation of pathological states.

The evaluation of the chest radiograph must begin with the assessment of the situs. Normally, in the upper abdomen, the liver and the inferior vena cava (IVC) lie on the right side, and the gastric fundus and the spleen lie on the left side. The systemic venous atrium lies on the right side and opposite to the gastric fundus. This relationship is referred to as the "visceroatrial situs" meaning that the atrial situs almost always conforms to the situs of the upper abdomen, irrespective of the situs or position of the remainder of the heart. The right-sided bronchus is shorter, wider, and more vertically oriented than the left bronchus. The right lung is trilobed whereas the left lung is bilobed. This is referred to as the "bronchial situs". In addition, the ascending aorta is generally on the same side as the systemic venous atrium and opposite the side of the gastric fundus. The ipsilateral location of the ascending aorta and the gastric fundus is almost pathognomonic of corrected transposition of great vessels **(Fig. 1)**.

Situs solitus implies that the liver, IVC, right atrium, and right-sided bronchus are on the right side, and the gastric fundus, spleen, and left-sided bronchus are on the left side. The position of the cardiac apex is not directly related to the visceroatrial situs and may not correspond

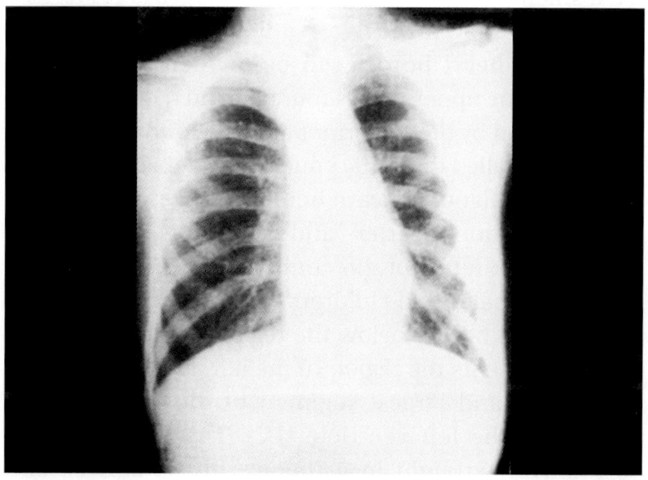

Fig. 1: Chest radiograph in a patient with corrected transposition of great vessels and pulmonary stenosis shows the absence of ascending aorta in the right upper cardiac border and a bulge along the left upper cardiac border obscuring the pulmonary conus. Peripheral pulmonary oligemia is also present.

with it. In addition, other issues to be considered include atrioventricular and ventriculoarterial connections, the loop of the aorta (dextroor levo), and the relation of cardiac chambers to each other.

CARDIAC SILHOUETTE

Cardiac Shape

Depending upon the build of the subjects, three types of shape are encountered in frontal projection. In hyposthenics, it is long and narrow, in hypersthenics, it is of transverse type, and in moderately built, it is oblique or globular in shape. In adults, 2/3rd of the heart lies on the left and 1/3rd on the right side of mid-line. In infants, the heart is of transverse or globular type, and the right heart is equal to the left. In infants and young children, there is enough thymic tissue to obscure the base of the heart and great vessels. By the age of 5–7 years, the globular infant heart attains the adult shape.

Cardiac Contour

Posteroanterior (PA) View

The right heart border consists of two segments. The upper segment is nearly vertical in normal young adults and is formed by the superior vena cava (SVC). The lower segment is usually convex and represents the lateral border of right atrium (RA) separated by a notch. In old age, the upper border may become convex due to the tendency of the aorta to dilate and elongate. The convexity represents the right lateral aspect of the ascending aorta. In hyposthenic subjects with a vertical heart, it is sometimes possible to see a small segment of the inferior vena cava (IVC) as a triangular shadow in the right cardiophrenic angle.

The left heart border can be divided into distinct segments. The uppermost is rounded and convex laterally and is formed by the posterior part of the transverse aortic arch, and is called the aortic knuckle or knob. Immediately below this, a flat or concave border is represented by the trunk of pulmonary artery and is called the pulmonary conus. Prominence of the conus is a normal variation in young females and children. A small concavity along the left heart border below the region of the pulmonary conus represents the region of the left atrial appendage. The lowest and largest segment of the left border is formed by the left ventricle (LV). This segment may be relatively straight in asthenics but is convex and rounded in hypersthenics. Diaphragmatic or inferior border is often not defined, but it may be seen in tall, asthenic-built subjects and is represented by the right ventricle (RV).

Right Anterior Oblique View

The anterior border from above downwards is formed by the transverse part of the arch of aorta, pulmonary trunk, RV and LV. The posterior border is formed by the left atrium (LA) above and RA below. The diaphragmatic surface is formed by the IVC, RA and RV.

Left Anterior Oblique View

The anterior border from above downwards consists of the innominate vein, SVC, ascending aorta, RA appendage and RV. The posterior border from above downwards includes a small part of LA and LV.

Lateral View

The anterior border is formed above by the RA appendage and below by the RV. The posterior border is formed above by LA and below by the LV.

Cardiac Size

The true size of the heart can only be assessed by orthodiagraphy with the help of an orthodiagraph. The method has now become obsolete. Conventional chest X-ray at a focus-film distance (FFD) of 6 feet provides some magnification and size of the heart is more than 1 cm greater in width than the orthodiagraphic measurements. If the FFD is doubled to about 12 feet, the measurements on the film are equal to those made on orthodiagraph. But this is not practical. Therefore, radiographic size at 6 feet is taken as a true representative size of the heart though there is some magnification.

Mathematical numerical cardiac measurement on chest radiograph has many variables, including age, sex, height, weight, race, occupation, phase of respiration, pulmonary and abdominal disease, which elevate or depress the diaphragm, and pose mathematical problems so that prediction tables are seldom used. The easiest method of measurement of cardiac size is to assess the transverse cardiothoracic ratio (CTR). This is the most adopted practical method though it is a rough estimate. This represents the ratio between the transverse cardiac diameter and the widest internal diameter of the thorax in PA view. The adult heart that measures more than half of the widest internal diameter of the chest is considered enlarged. In neonates, a ratio of up to 60%, and in infants, a ratio of up to 55% is taken as normal. The CTR may increase in the elderly probably due to infolding of the ribs which reduces the transverse thoracic diameter. Cardiomegaly has been graded as mild, moderate or severe by various authors based on the increase in the transverse diameter but these classifications are not widely used.

Cardiac Volume

Volume measurement is not done as a routine practice. It may be measured assuming the heart as an ellipsoid by the following formula:

$$V = l \times b \times d \times k \times m^3$$

V = Volume

l = Long or oblique diameter. This is drawn from the lowermost point of the heart on left side to the notch separating RA and right vascular shadow.

b = Broad diameter. It is obtained by joining the lower most point at the right cardiophrenic angle and uppermost point of the left vascular shadow.

d = AP diameter of the heart measured in lateral view. It is obtained by drawing a line from the point where the anterior border of the heart and sternum meet to the point of maximum convexity on the posterior surface of the heart.

m = Magnification factor

k = 0.63

Assessment of Chamber Enlargement

Right Atrium

When this is enlarged, the right heart border becomes more convex and also protrudes to the right away from the midline. The maximum convexity of right cardiac border >3 cm beyond right lateral vertebral border suggests RA enlargement. In early stages, only RA appendage fills the space between front of the heart and back of the sternum. The most reliable sign for the enlargement of the right atrium in the frontal chest radiograph is the increase in its height. In normal individuals, the distance between the top of the arch and the junction of the SVC and the right atrium is more than the distance between the latter and the right cardiophrenic angle. When the reverse happens, the right atrium is said to be enlarged **(Fig. 2)**.

Left Atrium

This chamber does not take part in the formation of any part of the cardiac border in frontal projection in normal subjects. It lies in the mid-line and in a posterior location. It usually enlarges posteriorly and to the right causing indentation and displacement of the esophagus posteriorly. With further increase in size, enlargement is in all directions except anteriorly. The LA may project beyond the LV producing localized convexity of the left border of cardiac silhouette just below the PAS. The earliest evidence of LA enlargement is seen as lifting up of the left main bronchus. But, this is difficult to appreciate on the chest radiograph. Subsequently, the carinal angle widens. The normal carinal angle ranges between 51° and 71°. With LA enlargement, it becomes right or obtuse angled. When enlargement reaches this stage, the chamber is often large enough to produce an oval shaped, localized density on the right side and projecting outside the lower right cardiac border. This can be seen in frontal projection as a double density within the cardiac shadow on the right side **(Fig. 3)**. With massive enlargement, LA forms the right cardiac contour almost throughout except superiorly in the upper part where SVC forms the right heart border

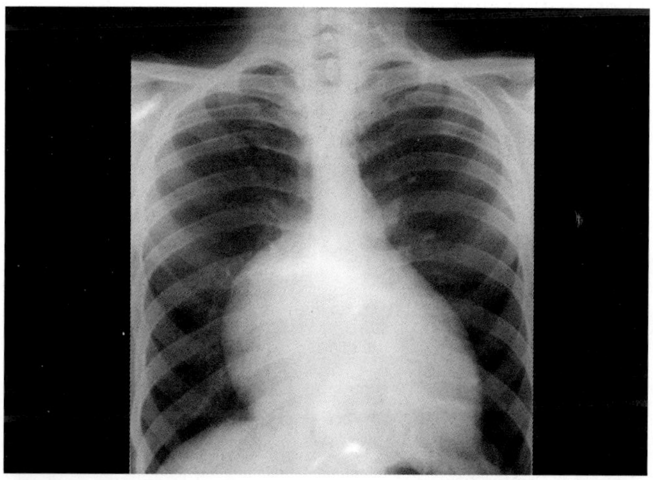

Fig. 2: Chest radiograph showing typical features of RA enlargement. Note that the height of the RA as seen by the distance between the junction of the SVC and RA, and the right cardiophrenic angle, is more than the distance between the top of the aortic arch and the junction of SVC and RA.

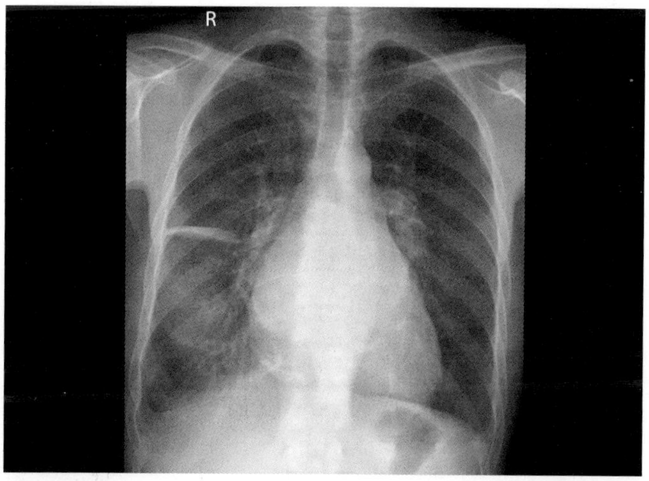

Fig. 3: Chest radiograph shows features of LA enlargement as seen by the double density in the mediastinum with widening of the carina. There is also evidence of bilateral hilar prominence with fluid in right fissure.

and inferiorly close to the diaphragm where the right atrium and, occasionally the IVC, form the right border. The enlarged LA can compress the left or occasionally the right bonchus and cause collapse, obstructive emphysema or rarely recurrent infection distal to the compressed lower lobe bronchus.

Left Ventricle

It enlarges to the left and posteriorly and only slightly to the right and anteriorly. Hypertrophy produces rounding of the cardiac apex whereas dilatation causes elongation either to the left or to the left and downwards, often combined with rounding of the apex **(Fig. 4)**. Rounding may also affect the left cardiac border when the LV gradually encroaches upon the pre-vertebral space. Left ventricular enlargement is best assessed in PA, LAO and lateral views.

Right Ventricle

It enlarges chiefly to the left and anteriorly . The outflow tract enlarges first and this is best seen in RAO and lateral views. When enlargement is significant, pulmonary conus becomes prominent in PA view. In some cases, the left border may be formed by this ventricle and may cause rotation of LV to the left with elevation of the apex **(Fig. 5)**. In lateral view, there is encroachment upon the retrosternal space in the upper part. This rotation tends to swing the aorta to the right, so that the aortic knucle becomes less prominent.

Aorta

The normal ascending aorta does not contribute to the cardiac silhouette in frontal projection. When dilated and elongated in old age, it bulges to the right beyond the SVC to form the right upper border. The most posterior part of arch of the aorta forms the left upper cardiac border and is called the aortic knob or knuckle. In infants and young children, the aortic knob is not well seen. However, its position can be indirectly inferred by the extrinsic impression of the knuckle on the lateral margin of the air-filled trachea. The aortic knuckle becomes more prominent, somewhat enlarged and may show curvilinear calcification in old age. The descending aorta can usually be seen as a straight line passing downwards and towards midline to the left of spine. The following should be looked for during the assessment of the aortic shadow:

- Is it a D-loop or L-loop?
- Is the aortic knuckle right or left sided?
- Is the aorta enlarged? If so, is there any disproportionate enlargement of the ascending or arch and descending aorta?
- Is there any calcification in the aorta? If so, its location (in the knuckle, descending thoracic or ascending aorta), pattern and extent.

Each of the above abnormalities has specific localizing value for the diagnosis.

PULMONARY VASCULATURE

Standard chest radiograph is a detailed record of the pulmonary vasculature. The pulmonary blood flow mirrors the pathophysiology of the heart since pulmonary blood vessels are clearly visualized on chest radiograph and the abnormal patterns of blood flow can be identified.[2]

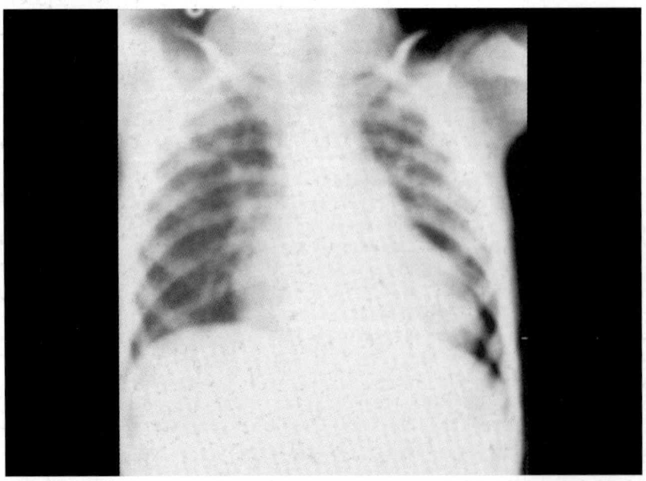

Fig. 4: Chest radiograph in a patient with a VSD shows LV enlargement, as evidenced by the concavity and elongation of the left cardiac border and rounding of the apex that is also shifted downwards and outwards.

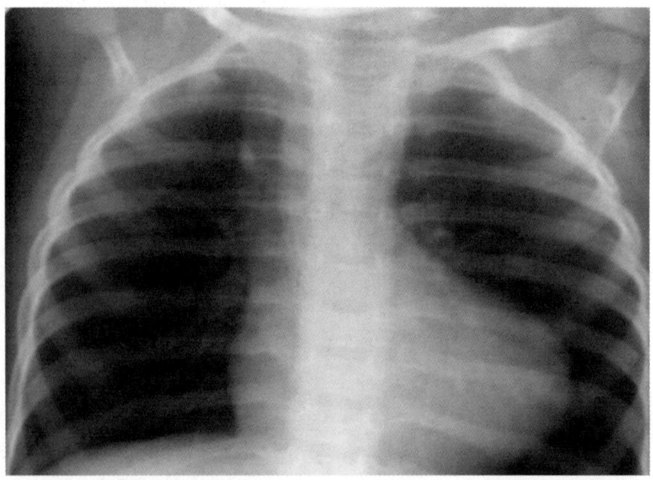

Fig. 5: Typical RV configuration is seen in this chest radiograph of a patient with TOF. There is elevation of the cardiac apex.

Normal Radiographic Anatomy

The analysis of pulmonary vascularity begins at the hilum. Pulmonary circulation begins at the pulmonary valve. The left border of main pulmonary artery (MPA) forms the floor of pulmonary segment. The normal pulmonary segment (PAS) is concave or straight. The enlargement of MPA causes a convexity of the PAS. MPA bifurcates within the mediastinum into the right (RPA) and left (LPA) pulmonary arteries. The intrapulmonary branches parallel the bronchi, divide in an orderly manner, and gradually taper towards the periphery. The arteries and bronchial branches are approximately the same diameter at any particular level with the ratio of 1:2:1. The LPA and left hilum are 1 cm above the RPA. The course of the pulmonary arteries is interlobular and intersegmental. The veins are wider, less well defined and branch less often than the companion arteries. These are located medial to the companion artery in the upper zones, overlap each other in the mid-zone and are lateral to the artery in the lower zone. The pulmonary veins converge in to the left atrium (LA) 2–3 cm below the hilum. The pulmonary arteries radiate from the hila above the pulmonary venous confluence. It is often difficult to differentiate the artery from the vein due to variable arterial supply and venous drainage. In normal individuals, the pulmonary arteries and veins in outer 1/3rd of lung are too small to be seen in chest radiograph.

The right hilum is formed by the confluence of the shadows of the right upper lobe pulmonary vein and the right descending pulmonary artery (RDPA). These form a right angle. The width of the pulmonary vessels depends on the flow. Normal RDPA has a straight outer border. A convexity suggests an enlargement and concavity suggests a diminished size. In children, the ratio of RDPA to trachea is <1.0.[2] In adults, the normal transverse diameter of RDPA just above the origin of right middle lobe branch or 1.25 cm distal to the origin of right upper lobe branch is 10–16 mm in males and 9–15 mm in females in deep inspiration.[3] In erect position, blood flow is greater to the lower lobe because of gravity and differential intra-alveolar pressure. The lower lobe vessels are 2–3 times larger than the upper lobe vessels. In the erect chest radiograph, vessels in first intercostal space are <3 mm in diameter and those just above the diaphragm are up to 6 mm in diameter.

Increased Pulmonary Blood Flow (Pulmonary Plethora)

This is defined as an enlargement of vessels due to increased flow. The width of the pulmonary vessels depends on flow as long as the vascular reserve is not exceeded. Beyond this, the size depends on flow and pressure or pressure alone. Increased pulmonary flow can be caused by high output states, left to right (L-R) shunts, and admixture lesions. The pulmonary veins also enlarge as pulmonary arterial blood flow increases. Blood vessels become visible in the outer one-third of the lungs. In larger shunts, there is recruitment of upper lobe vessels, so that the differential flow between the upper and lower lobe vessels is lost. There is a fair correlation between vessel enlargement and shunt size. Shunts with QP:QS >2:1 can be reliably detected. Very large volume shunts can also cause pulmonary venous hypertension (PVH).

Gooding compared the diameter of the RDPA and trachea in children up to 14 years of age. The ratio in normal children at any age was close to one. About 90% had diameters within 2 mm of each other, with one-third having diameters of the RDPA that was less than that of the trachea. When a L-R shunt was present, the diameter of the RDPA was never less than that of the trachea.[4,5]

Radiological Signs of Plethora (Fig. 6)

- The presence of shunt vessels, end-on vessels more than two times the diameter of the accompanying bronchus.
- Prominent upper and lower zone vessels.
- En-face vessels below the tenth posterior rib.
- Prominent vessels below the crest of the diaphragm.
- RDPA diameter more than that of the trachea.
- > 6 vessels in peripheral one-third of the lungs.
- RDPA > 16 mm in diameter.
- Prominent hilar vessels on lateral view.

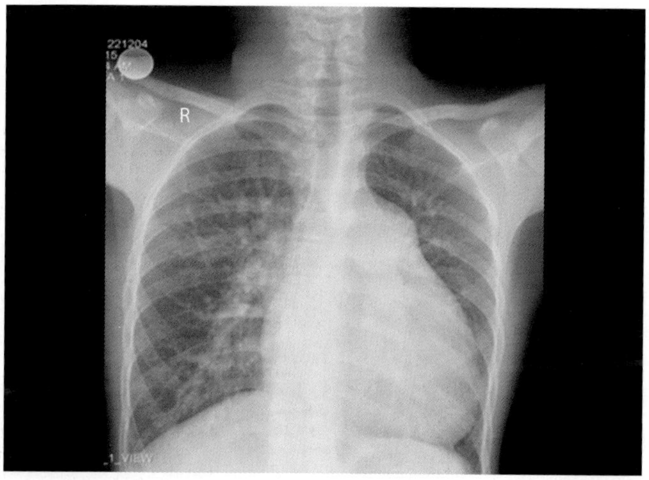

Fig. 6: Chest radiograph shows typical features of pulmonary plethora. Note the dilated pulmonary artery segment, increased caliber of the right descending pulmonary artery, and prominent end-on vessels in both lungs.

- In infants and children, generalised mottling may be seen. Plethora correlates with the size of L-R shunts better than the heart size.[6] With a normal or slightly increased heart size, QP:QS is >2:1 or 2:1 in 50%, with a larger heart, the shunt is >2:1 in at least 60% and with no plethora, the shunt is <2:1 in 100%. Assessment of plethora should not be based on measurements alone. However, measurements can be used in corroboration with a subjective impression.

Decreased Pulmonary Blood Flow (Pulmonary Oligemia)

It is difficult to diagnose pulmonary oligemia unless it is severe. Some normal persons may have small pulmonary vessels. Oligemia can be caused by pulmonary outflow tract obstruction and intracardiac right to left (R-L) shunts. The pulmonary arteries and veins are reduced in size, the central vessels become narrow, and peripheral arteries are not visible.

Radiological Signs (Fig. 7)

- Concave or absent MPA.
- Overall appearance of an over-penetrated film.
- <4 vessels in peripheral one-third of the lungs.
- Small hilar, lobar, segmental vessels.
- Decreased size and density of hilar vessels on lateral chest radiograph in the presence of cyanosis is suggestive of pulmonary oligemia.
- Enlarged bronchial and other systemic collateral arteries are seen in pulmonary atresia with ventricular septal defect (VSD) and in tetralogy of Fallot (TOF). These are seen as small, tortuous, non-tapering and disorganized vascular markings not radiating from the hilum and also not conforming to known branching patterns of the pulmonary vessels. The hila are not enlarged.

Pulmonary Arterial Hypertension (Fig. 8)

This may be primary or secondary to PVH, long-standing L-R shunts, pulmonary thromboembolic disease, respiratory disease, high altitude, drugs, and pulmonary arterial occlusion. It is said to be present, if the mean pulmonary artery (PA) pressure is >20 mm Hg. The PAH is graded as mild, moderate and severe with the PA mean pressure ranging from 20–29, 30–49, and >50 mm Hg respectively. The central vessels from the MPA to the second order branching vessels dilate and peripheral (lobar) vessels constrict. The transition between centrally dilated and peripherally constricted vessels is more lateral in L-R shunts. The pruning of the pulmonary arteries is defined as more than a 50% loss of the vessel diameter at any degree branching and is suggestive of PAH. Chronic PAH leads to calcification of the MPA and proximal branches. The presence of calcification is pathognomonic of PAH. The severity of central dilatation has a rough correlation with the severity of PAH. In the lower pressure ranges, the ratio of the size of the hemithoracic diameter to the size of the MPA shows an approximate correlation with PA pressure. Hyperkinetic → PAH → versus → Eisenmenger → PAH → In hyperkinetic PAH, peripheral vessels increase in size and number, and cardiac enlargement is proportional to the amount of L-R shunt. In Eisenmenger

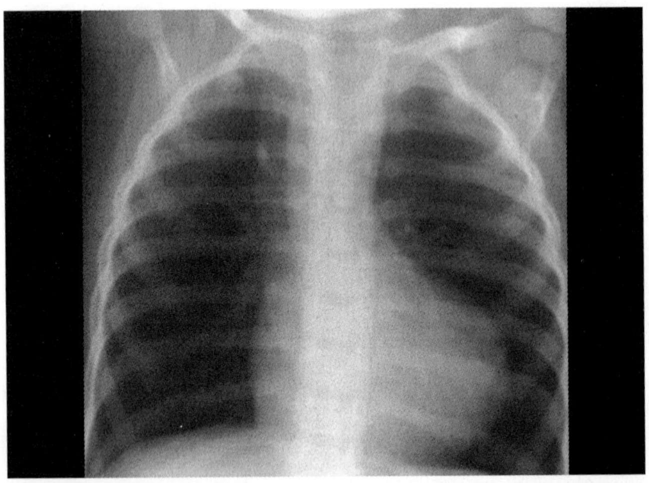

Fig. 7: Chest radiograph reveals typical oligemic lung fields. The hila are small in size, vascular markings are diminished in caliber, and the lungs appear hypertranslucent.

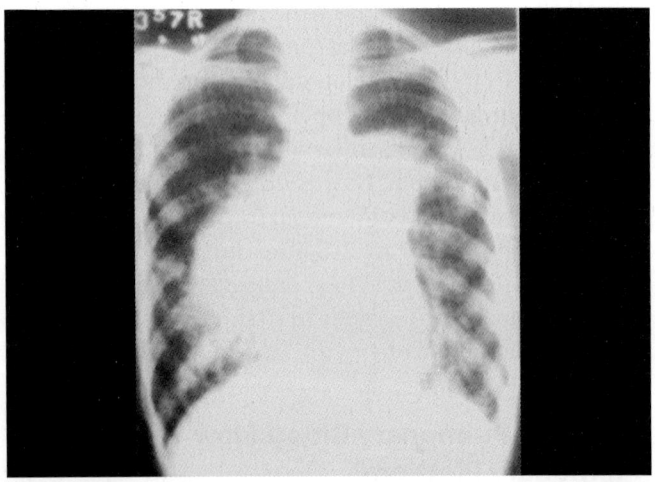

Fig. 8: A patient with primary PAH. The chest radiograph shows that the main pulmonary artery segment, and both pulmonary arteries are grossly dilated. There is a sharp transition between the centrally dilated hila and the vasculature of the peripheral lung fields.

PAH, peripheral vessels decrease, central vessels increase further in size, heart size decreases, and the right ventricle (RV) becomes more prominent.

Pulmonary Venous Hypertension

Pulmonary venous hypertension (PVH) is said to be present when the pulmonary capillary wedge pressure (PCWP) exceeds the normal range of 8–12 mm Hg. Progressive PVH produces changes reflecting the presence and severity of this disorder.

Stage 1: Redistribution/Cephalization of the Blood Flow (Fig. 9)

This may precede the clinical signs and symptoms. The venous pressure ranges from 13 to 19 mm Hg. The changes are characterized by constriction, blurring of lower zone vessels, effacement of hilar angle, and dilatation of upper lobe vessels. With increase in LA and PCW pressure, there is an increase in LA and PCW pressure. This results in an increase in the interstitial lung water and increased pulmonary lymphatic drainage, leading to "cuffing" of fluid around small bronchi. The increased interstitial water gravitates to dependent areas, causing increased interstitial pressure and vascular resistance at lung bases. Thus, blood is diverted to upper lobes leading to vascular redistribution. Exceptions to this pattern of redistribution are basal emphysema and pulmonary parenchymal diseases of the upper lobe.

Stage 2: Interstitial Edema (Fig. 10)

It is characterized by the presence of Kerley lines, peribronchial cuffing, background haze, septal and interstitial edema, and pleural effusion. The venous pressure ranges from 20 to 24 mm Hg.

Stage 3: Alveolar Edema (Fig. 11)

This occurs when the interstitial fluid accumulates at rates faster than it can be removed by the lymphatics. The venous pressure ranges from 25 mm Hg and above. Milking of edema fluid towards the hilum by the expanding lung imparts a "Bat's Wing appearance". However, a chronic lung disease and dependent posture may result in atypical patterns of edema. Pleural effusion occurs when pleural fluid formation by visceral pleura is faster than its absorption by the parietal pleura. This usually occurs when systemic venous pressure is also elevated, as in right heart failure. Several radiologic findings have been correlated with the level of PCWP in patients with acute and chronic heart failure.

Asymmetrical Pulmonary Blood Flow (Fig. 12)

This is due to the presence of vessels in one lung that are smaller than the other:

- ***Localized decrease:*** Pulmonary thromboembolism, chronic obstructive airway disease (COAD), arteritis, segmental stenosis.
- ***Unilateral decrease:*** Pulmonary artery branch atresia/ stenosis, hemi-truncus, TOF with unilateral pulmonary atresia.
- ***Unilateral increase:*** After shunt surgery (e.g. Blalock-Taussig shunt), Glenn shunt (on the side of shunt), PDA and anomalous origin of a pulmonary artery from the aorta.

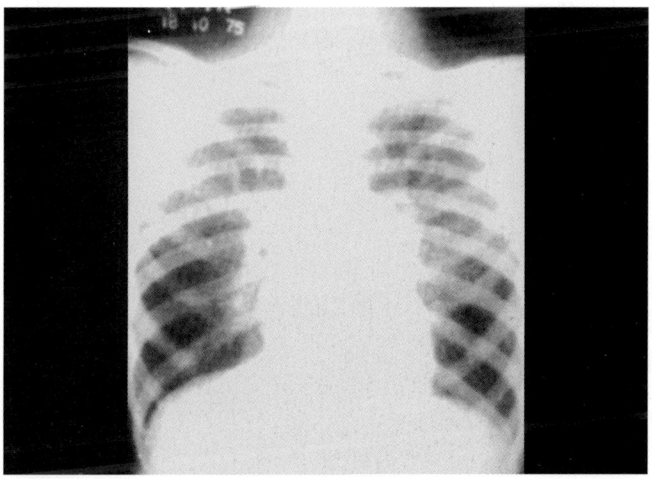

Fig. 9: Chest radiograph shows mild (grade I) PVH. There is cephalization of blood flow with increased caliber of the upper lobe vessels. Note that the patient has mitral stenosis, as evidenced by the enlargement of the LA and its appendage.

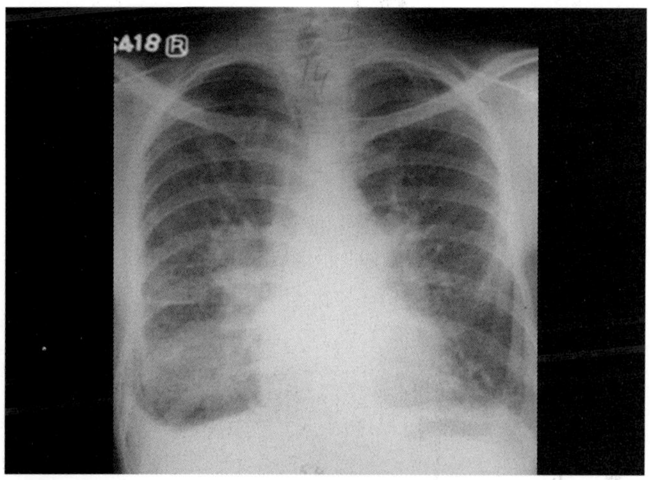

Fig. 10: Chest radiograph shows moderate (Grade II) PVH in a case of MS. Kerley's B lines are present in both costophrenic angles.

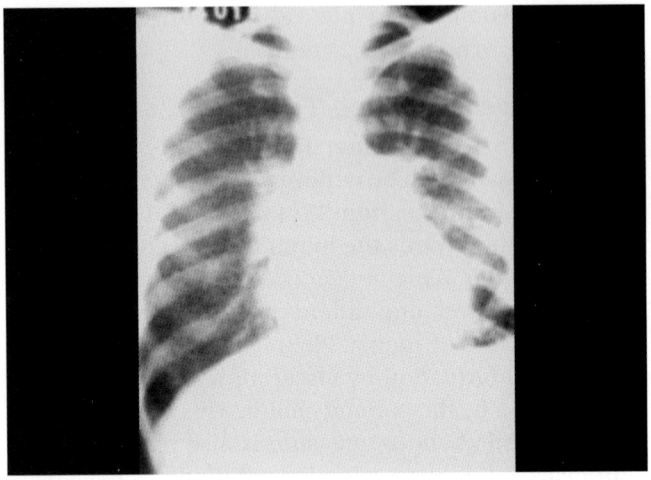

Fig. 11: Chest radiograph shows features of severe (grade III) PVH and PAH. In addition, there are miliary shadows in both lungs, due to the presence of secondary hemosiderosis.

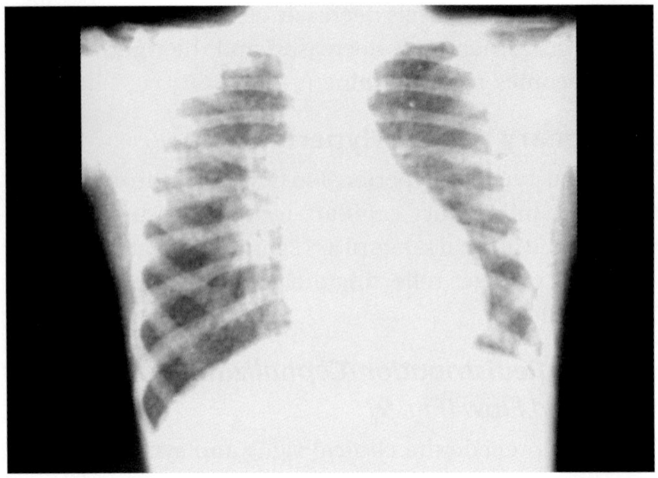

Fig. 12: This radiograph shows evidence of pleonemia, evidenced by the presence of increased vasculature on the right side and an inconspicuous left hilum with peripheral oligemia on this side.

Orientation of Pulmonary Outflow Tract

- *Towards left:* Valvular pulmonic stenosis
- *Towards right:* Transposition of great arteries

It is obvious from the above description that the chest radiograph is a mathematical record of the events produced by the cardiac disease. Its detailed, sequential interpretation provides important clues to the underlying heart disease and the functional impairment produced by it. The chest radiograph also serves as a useful method for follow-up after treatment in most cardiac conditions. Distinctive radiographic abnormalities in specific cardiac disorders will be dealt with in the following chapters.

REFERENCES

1. Radiology of the heart. In: Braunwald E (Ed). Heart Disease: A Textbook of Cardiovascular Medicine. WB Saunders, Philadelphia; 1992: pp. 204-324.
2. Coussement AM. Objective radiographic assessment of pulmonary vascularity in children. Radiology. 1973;109:649- 54.
3. Chang CH. The normal roentgenographic measurement of the right descending pulmonary artery in 1085 cases. AJR. 1962;87:929-35.
4. Roberts WC. Radiologic differentiation of common anomalies. In: Adult Congenital Heart Disease. 1988. pp. 191-219.
5. Moes CAF. Analysis of the chest in the neonate with congenital heart disease. RCNA. 1975;13:251-76.
6. Jefferson K, Rees R (Eds). Clinical Cardiac Radiology. Butterworth, London; 1980.

CHAPTER 177

Imaging Approach in Children with Congenital Heart Disease

Priya Jagia, Sanjiv Sharma, Gurpreet Singh Gulati, Sanjeev Kumar

INTRODUCTION

In children, severe congenital heart disease (CHD) is an important cause of mortality. Imaging is important to show the cardiac and vascular anatomy so that therapy can be planned. It is also useful in monitoring these children after surgery or endovascular interventions.

A correct diagnostic approach ensures that a functional diagnostic is made whereby correct decision in form of emergency surgery, endovascular intervention, medical therapy or just supportive measures can be arrived at. Approximately 75% cases of all CHD lesions either are not detected or do not have signs or symptoms warranting complete investigation in infants. Left-to-right shunts, even large, rarely present with serious respiratory or cardiac difficulty in first months of life, owing to high pulmonary vascular resistance.

There are nine congenital heart lesions, which account for most of the severe cyanotic heart disease in children. These can further be classified as follows, based upon pulmonary flow:

Group A: Lesions with decreased pulmonary blood flow:
1. Pulmonary atresia (PAt) or severe pulmonic stenosis (PS), with intact VSD.
2. Tricuspid atresia.
3. Pulmonary malformation of tricuspid valve.
4. Pulmonary atresia (or severe pulmonic stenosis) with VSD including tetralogy of Fallot (TOF).

Group B: Lesions with increased pulmonary blood flow:
1. Transposition of great arteries (TGA).
2. VSD with coarctation of aorta.

Group C: Lesions with severe pulmonary venous hypertension:
1. Total anomalous pulmonary venous return with obstruction (TAPVR).
2. Hypoplastic left heart (HLH).
3. Severe coarctation of aorta with intact ventricular septum.

PHYSICAL EXAMINATION

The conditions mentioned above might all cause cyanosis or respiratory distress or both in first few days of life itself. Patients with TGA, pulmonary atresia (or stenosis) and tricuspid atresia have marked cyanosis with minimal or no respiratory distress in neonatal period. On the other hand, respiratory distress is marked in TAPVR with obstruction and hypoplastic left heart syndrome with little cyanosis. In Ebstein's, child has cyanosis, tachypnea, pansystolic murmur and hepatomegaly which improves over first weeks of life.

RADIOLOGICAL APPROACH

Chest Radiograph

Chest radiograph is useful in the initial evaluation of a patient with a suspected CHD. It provides valuable information about the cardiac size, pulmonary vasculature, arterial and venous hypertension, the situs and the lungs. Echocardiography is a useful screening technique that allows real-time evaluation of each cardiac chamber in multiple orthogonal planes. It is noninvasive, easily available, provides a direct visualization of structural defects and also helps evaluate the attendant functional disturbances. The reports suggest that the results compare favorably with angiocardiography. Its major limitations include operator dependence and availability of a proper acoustic window. Recently, multi-slice computed tomography and magnetic resonance imaging are also being used in selected patients for optimal evaluation. Proper understanding of the imaging anatomy, image morphology in disease states, and the advantages and limitations of each technique is essential for its optimal utilization in a given patient or disease state.

A good quality chest radiograph still remains an important initial investigation for the evaluation of a patient with CHD. General principles in the interpretation of chest radiograph in CHD include a sequential evaluation of the cardiac size, chamber enlargement, aorta, status of pulmonary vasculature, assessment of the situs and other associated abnormalities. Chest radiographic abnormalities in various disease states are described below:

Left-to-Right (L-R) Shunt

Chest radiograph is useful in localizing the site of L-R shunts in CHD. If the aortic knuckle is enlarged, the shunt is extracardiac and if the aorta is normal, the shunt is intracardiac.

Large Aorta

If the aortic knuckle is enlarged disproportionate to the ascending aorta, the L-R shunt is caused by patent ductus arteriosus (PDA). The heart is usually normal or mildly enlarged with left ventricular (LV) configuration, aortic knuckle is obliterated or replaced by a bulge, pulmonary conus is enlarged, and lung vascularity is increased. In addition, pulmonary arterial hypertension (PAH) may be present. In a small group of patients, calcification may be present at the PDA site.

If the ascending aorta is enlarged disproportionate to the aortic knuckle, the L-R shunt is at the aortic root level. The causes include a ruptured aneurysm of the sinus of Valsalva, aortopulmonary window, and coronary arteriovenous fistula.

Ruptured aneurysm of the sinus of Valsalva (RSOV): The heart size is usually enlarged with a biventricular or LV configuration. An abnormal shadow of the aneurysm is usually present at the level of the aortic root. There may be curvilinear calcification in it. The aorta is enlarged with a disproportionate dilatation of the aortic root. The pulmonary conus is prominent and lung vascularity is increased. In addition, in symptomatic patients, some evidence of PVH is also present.

Usually, the right coronary sinus is involved and ruptures into the right ventricle. Simultaneous presence of pulmonary plethora and PVH is characteristic of an RSOV.

Aortopulmonary window: The heart size is usually enlarged with an LV configuration, there is disproportionate enlargement of the aortic root, pulmonary conus is prominent, lung vascularity is increased, and PAH is usually present.

Coronary arteriovenous fistula: The heart size is usually normal and there may be LV configuration. There is disproportionate enlargement of the aortic root, pulmonary conus is prominent and lung vascularity is normal or increased. Chest radiograph may be normal because the shunt is usually small.

Normal Aorta

Normal or apparently small aortic knuckle and inconspicuous ascending aortic shadow in a frontal chest radiograph in the presence of increased lung vascularity in a pink patient suggest an intracardiac L-R shunt. This shunt can be at pre- or post-tricuspid level.

Pre-tricuspid Shunt

The pre-tricuspid shunt is produced by an atrial septal defect or a partial anomalous pulmonary venous drainage.

Atrial septal defect (ASD): The heart size is usually normal. There may be mild cardiomegaly in approximately 25% of the patients. There is right atrial enlargement with right-sided configuration of the heart. Aortic shadow is normal in size with the ascending aortic shadow usually conspicuous by its absence in the upper right cardiac border. This sign is characteristic of an ASD. The heart appears to be shifted to the left and lung vascularity is increased. PAH may be present. The presence of associated anomalies may change this radiographic picture. Associated mitral valve disease should be suspected if LA/LA appendage is enlarged, PVH (especially if Kerley's lines) is present, or if the mitral valve is calcified. The association of ASD with mitral stenosis of rheumatic etiology is called "Lutembacher's syndrome". In patients over 40 years of age, a chest radiograph may show atypical features including the presence of LV configuration and distended upper lobe vessels due to left ventricular dysfunction which may be related to age, myocardial ischemia, or hypertensive heart disease.

Partial anomalous pulmonary venous drainage (PAPVD): This should be suspected if, in the presence of radiographic features of ASD, there is an abnormally enlarged shadow of superior vena cava (SVC) or an abnormally directed pulmonary vein is seen.

Post-tricuspid L-R Shunt

This results from the presence of a VSD. This is the most common form of acyanotic CHD. The findings on chest radiograph in VSD depend on the shunt size and the direction of predominant flow. In small <2:1 shunts, the chest radiograph may be normal. In presence of a large >2:1 shunt, the heart size is usually enlarged with a left or a biventricular configuration, and there is evidence of LA enlargement, a normal aorta, and increased lung vascularity. PAH may be present, In addition, there may be evidence of differential increase in lung vascularity in the right upper zone. In 3–5% of the patients, an associated right-sided aortic arch may be present.

Right-to-Left (R-L) Shunt

Although chest radiographic features of most of the following conditions can be characteristic, it is important to remember that typical features are not usually seen in most patients. As with L-R shunts, the size of the aortic shadow is important in the localization of R-L shunts.

Large Aorta with Decreased Lung Vascularity

Large aortic knuckle in the presence of cyanotic CHD and decreased vascularity is produced by tetralogy of Fallot (TOF), pulmonary atresia with VSD, tricuspid atresia, TGA with VSD and pulmonary stenosis (PS), double outlet right ventricle (DORV) with PS and allied conditions.

Tetralogy of Fallot: Etienne-Louis Fallot in 1888 described a tetralogy of defects, including pulmonary stenosis, a malaligned ventricular septal defect, overriding of the aorta and hypertrophy of the right ventricle. This is the most common form of cyanotic CHD in children. The pulmonic stenosis is usually infundibular in location. Additional valvular pulmonary stenosis and hypoplasia of the main pulmonary artery are also frequently present. The chest radiograph shows a characteristic picture produced by a normal heart size, RV configuration with an uplifted apex (coer-en sabot appearance), a large aortic knuckle, presence of pulmonary bay and pulmonary oligemia **(Fig. 1)**. A right-sided aortic arch is present in

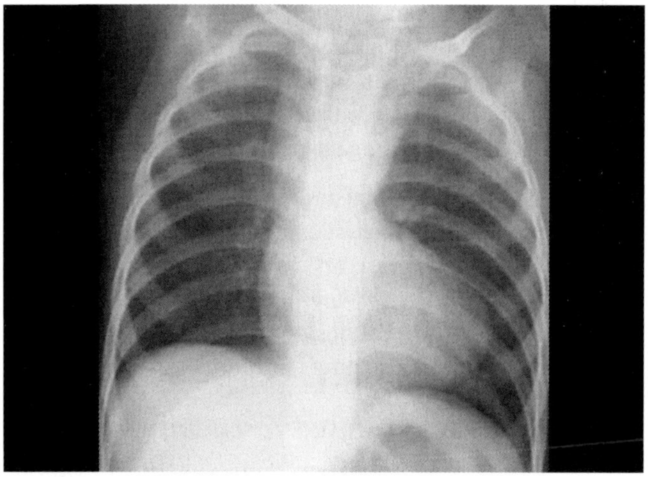

Fig. 1: Chest radiograph in tetralogy of Fallot. Cardiac size is normal with RV configuration. There is concave pulmonary bay and peripheral oligemia.

approximately 25% of the cases. In addition, characteristic criss-cross bronchial circulation may be present. Rarely, rib notching may be seen due to collateral flow. The heart size may be enlarged in the presence of tricuspid or pulmonary regurgitation, absent pulmonary valve, severe anemia, bacterial endocarditis, pulmonary atresia, or bacterial infections. Rarely, TOF may be associated with an absent pulmonary valve. This produces a pathognomonic appearance consisting of an enlarged heart, large central pulmonary arteries with peripheral oligemia in the setting of TOF. In addition, a host of lung abnormalities largely due to a defective bronchial cartilage and resultant tracheobronchomalacia may be associated. Occasionally, TOF may be associated with congenital absence of a pulmonary artery, left more commonly than right. When this happens, parenchymal lung abnormalities are frequently associated.

Pulmonary atresia with VSD: There is mild cardiomegaly RV configuration, a large aortic knuckle that frequently crosses the sternoclavicular joint into the neck, pulmonary bay, and peripheral oligemia. Aortic arch is right-sided in 30–40% patients. Bronchial collateral circulation is frequently present. Rib notching may be seen.

Tricuspid atresia: The chest radiographic picture depends on the relationship of great vessels, presence of PS, and the degree of RV hypoplasia. A typical picture is seen in only 15–20% of the cases and consists of a normal-sized or mildly enlarged heart, LV configuration, straight right heart border, some evidence of LA enlargement, enlarged aorta, pulmonary bay, and decreased vascularity, provided that there is PS and the great vessels are normally related **(Fig. 2)**. The aortic arch is right-sided in one-third of the cases. If the pulmonary arteries are not located in their normal position, an abnormal relationship of great vessels should be suspected. In the absence of PS, there is evidence of increased lung vascularity.

D-TGA, VSD and PS: A chest radiograph may superficially resemble TOF. The heart size is usually normal or may be mildly enlarged. The aortic knuckle is normal or the pedicle may appear narrow. Pulmonary artery segment is not present in the normal position and is located in a high and medial position. The lung fields are oligemic.

Small Aorta with Increased Vascularity

D-TGA: This is the second most common cause of cyanotic heart disease in infancy. It is caused by a ventriculoarterial abnormality in which the aorta originates from RV and PA from LV. The chest radiographic findings are characteristic, consisting of an enlarged heart, narrow pedicle, abnormally located pulmonary arteries, and increased lung vascularity.

The shape of the heart is typical and resembles an "egg-on-side" **(Fig. 3)**. There may be a differential increase in right lung vascularity, especially in the upper zone. This pathognomonic picture is seen in patients in whom there is no evidence of PS. The typical chest radiograph findings are seen in about half the patients.

Large Pedicle with Increased Vascularity

This combination is seen in truncus arteriosus, total anomalous pulmonary venous drainage (TAPVC), and tricuspid atresia without PS.

Truncus arteriosus: The heart is usually enlarged, there is LV configuration, the aorta is enlarged, pulmonary artery is not in its usual position, and lung vascularity is increased. The abnormal location of the PA may produce a characteristic picture described as "comma or water-fall" sign. This is more often seen on the left side. The aortic arch is right sided in about 50% of the cases.

TAPVC: This may be divided into four main groups according to the site or sites of connection, supracardiac, cardiac, infracardiac and mixed. The chest radiographic picture depends on the type of TAPVC. In supracardiac type, which is also the most common, the heart is enlarged, the pedicle is wide with a classical "figure of 8 or Snowman's" appearance, produced by the dilated left vertical and left innominate veins and the right SVC. The left atrium is small and there is increased flow, as evidenced by pulmonary plethora. In cardiac or mixed types, the picture may be nonspecific and consists of cardiomegaly, normal or enlarged aorta, and increased lung vascularity. Shadow of an enlarged abnormal pulmonary vein may be seen. The scimitar sign is seen in the infra-diaphragmatic type of TAPVC and is caused by the drainage of the right pulmonary vein into the IVC, hepatic or portal vein. This syndrome is often associated with hypoplasia or sequestration of the right lung.

Normal Aorta with Decreased Lung Vascularity

This combination can be seen in patients with Ebstein's anomaly, and valvular PS in failure.

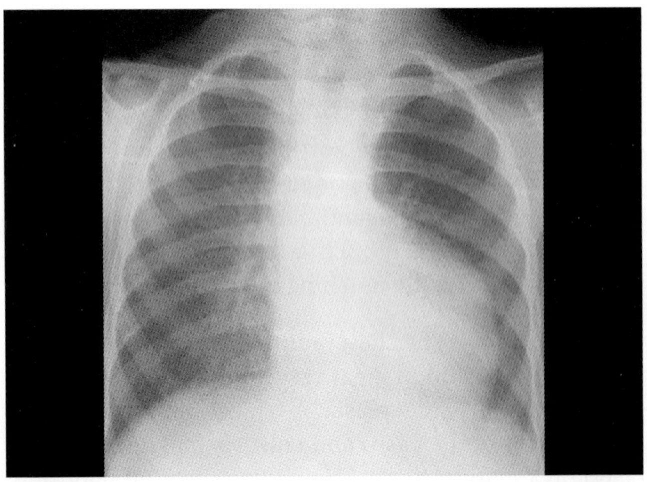

Fig. 2: Chest radiograph in tricuspid atresia. Note the straight heart border and right-sided aortic arch. Lung fields show peripheral oligemia.

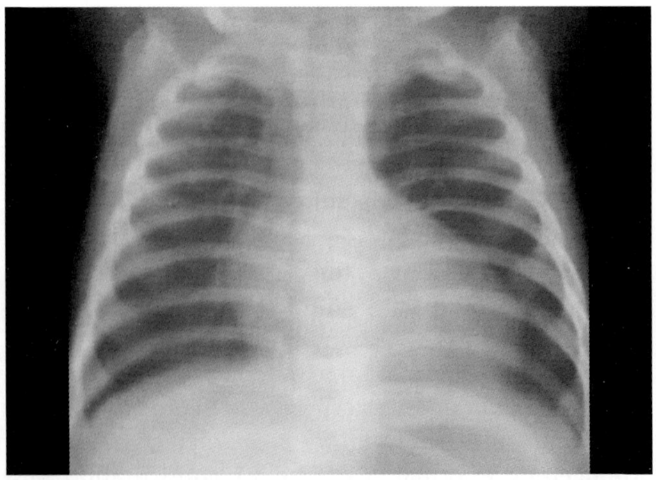

Fig. 3: Chest radiograph in transposition of great arteries. "Egg-shaped" heart is seen with narrow vascular pedicle.

Ebstein's anomaly: This produces a characteristic radiographic picture. There is cardiomegaly, evidence of RA enlargement, sharp, well-delineated cardiac margins, as if drawn by a pencil, normal aorta and pulmonary oligemia. It can superficially resemble pericardial effusion, valvular PS in failure, tricuspid regurgitation caused by chronic rheumatic heart disease (RHD), dilated cardiomyopathy (DCM), and Uhl's anomaly. The pulmonary vascularity is important in differentiating these conditions. In pericardial effusion, the lung vasculature is normal and no specific chamber enlargement is present. In RHD, there is PVH and tell-tale signs of the underlying valvular disease are always present. In DCM, there is evidence of PVH. LA and LV may be enlarged.

Valvular PS: A chest radiograph may be normal except for a prominent pulmonary conus till there is severe PS with congestive failure. In such cases, there is cardiomegaly, RA enlargement, a normal aorta, prominent pulmonary conus produced by post-stenotic dilatation of MPA and LPA, and peripheral pulmonary oligemia.

Other Conditions

Coarctation of aorta: This refers to a narrowing of the distal aortic arch and/or proximal descending aorta due to a discrete membrane or narrowing of the aortic isthmus. Findings on chest radiograph depend on the age of the patient, location of the coarct, ventricular function, competence of the aortic valve and associated abnormalities. In an uncomplicated isolated coarctation, the heart size is usually normal. There may be left ventricular configuration. The classical feature of bilateral notching of the posterior and inferior margins of the 4th-8th ribs is usually not seen in the first decade of life. The coarct segment is usually located in the juxtaductal region. Occasionally, it can be postductal and rarely preductal. Postductal or juxtaductal coarctation produces typical radiographic features in the cardiac configuration, ribs and aorta. Rib notching is caused by the hypertrophied intercostal arteries that run along the posterior and inferior margins of the ribs. In juxtaductal coarct, the fourth to eight ribs are usually involved. Coarctation proximal to the origin of the left subclavian artery results in unilateral right-sided rib notching. If the coarctation is proximal to an aberrant right subclavian artery, unilateral notching of the left ribs occurs. Abnormal appearance of the aorta is seen in most patients. The ascending aorta is slightly dilated. *Figure-of-3* appearance of the descending aorta is characteristic but not commonly seen. The upper convexity is formed by the dilated subclavian artery and the lower convexity by the post-stenotic dilatation of the descending aorta. Usually, a prominent or a flat knuckle is seen. If there is associated left ventricular decompensation, then PVH may be present.

Thus, it is obvious that the chest radiograph provides useful diagnostic information in the patient with CHD. These appearances are relatively easy to familiarize with. This, coupled with the universal availability of this imaging technique, makes it ideally suited as the first diagnostic investigation in the patient with suspected CHD. It has the unique ability to assess the pulmonary vasculature and the associated or coincidental lung or spinal abnormalities. These reasons also make it well suited for utilization as a follow-up technique after surgical or non-surgical intervention.

MULTISLICE CARDIAC CT

With advances in cross-sectional imaging in form of multislice CT and MRI, chest X-ray is no longer relied upon to make the diagnosis.

In all cases, where echocardiography has failed to provide sufficient information. Cardiac CT or MR needs to be performed to delineate the cardiac and vascular anatomy. This not only helps decide the treatment modality but also helps in planning surgery, if decided upon, and also to follow-up the postoperative cases. Both cardiac CT and MR are capable of providing anatomic and functional assessment of heart. But MRI is time consuming, and therefore may require lengthy period of sedation, which is not desirable in small children. But it has the advantage of being non-invasive and not involving any ionizing radiation. Hence, it can be repeated without risk of radiation, as necessitated in postoperative patients for follow-up.

Multislice cardiac CT has the advantage of widespread availability and needs very short time for image acquisition. It has a higher spatial resolution as compared to MRI and also is better for evaluation of lung parenchyma. ECG-gated cardiac CT allows delineation of otherwise mobile small structures in heart and also helps to rule out associated coronary artery anomalies. In children, however, the risks of ionizing radiation and those inherent to contrast media must be kept in mind before subjecting them to CT.

Short-term sedation for CT is often necessary especially in small children. At our institute, we have a policy of performing the pediatric CT in presence of an anesthetist and the child is admitted for a short period after CT for observation.

Nonionic contrast is used with a dose of 2–3 mL/kg body weight of child, and in infants is administered intravenously at rate of 1.5–2 mL/sec.

We routinely use dual source CT scanner (Siemens Medical Solutions, Germany) for cardiac CT. For children, a body weight based low dose protocol is used to limit the radiation exposure. Tube voltage of 80 KV has also been recommended for this purpose.

The entire thorax is scanned in 4–5 seconds, and hence the need for breath-hold is more or less obviated. ECG-gated CT scanning is advisable in cases with complex cardiac abnormality or when there is need to delineate an abnormal communication, so that motion artifacts are minimal. However, it is advisable to do ECG controlled tube current modulation whereby normal tube current is applied during motion-free diastole phase of cardiac cycle while much reduced current is applied during systole. An ECG gated study should only be performed when the advantages outweigh the risk of increased radiation in such study.

The scan delay is determined by bolus chase technique. In small children, the region of interest (ROI) is placed in right ventricle, if pulmonary arteries need to be evaluated and in LV, if aortic evaluation is required. Post-processing involves reconstruction of multiplanar reformation (MPR), maximum intensity projection (MIP) **(Fig. 4)** and volume-rendered (VRT) images **(Fig. 5)** on the dedicated workstation.

The greatest amount of anatomical delineation is obtained with MPR images.

CARDIAC MRI

As mentioned before, it gives excellent anatomical information without the use of ionizing radiation and contrast media **(Fig. 6)**. But it lacks the rapid acquisition of scans, and high spatial resolution offered by cardiac CT.

Small children need to anaesthetized prior to MRI. Use is made of small coil to cover chest of baby to provide highest signal to noise ratio.

For anatomic delineation, coronal, sagittal and axial nongated steady state free precession images covering the entire chest are taken. Vascular anatomy is best delineated by doing contrast-enhanced MR angiogram **(Fig. 7)**.

ECG-gated cine images in short axis from base of ventricle to apex help assess cardiac function and measure ventricular volume. Cine imaging across desired vascular planes can be done, e.g. along ventricular outflow tract, to rule out any stenosis or regurgitations **(Figs. 8 and 9)**.

Velocity encoded phase-contrast cine images assess blood flow velocity and volume. Systemic to pulmonary blood flow ratio (Q_p/Q_s) can be calculated by measuring flow in pulmonary trunk and ascending aorta.

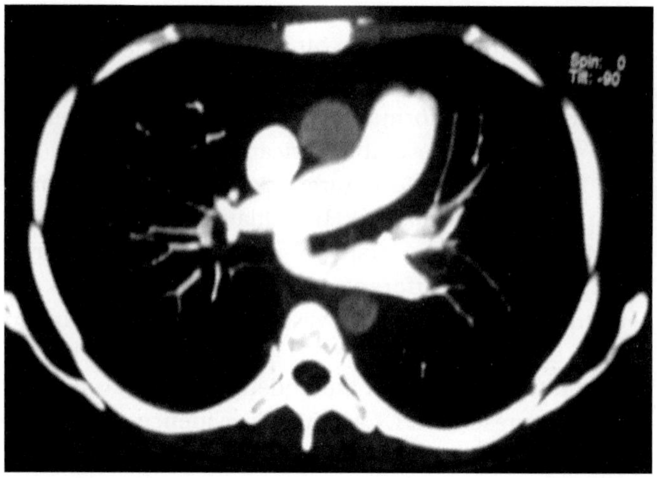

Fig. 4: LPA sling-axial CT image: MIP shows LPA arising from RPA and coursing behind trachea.

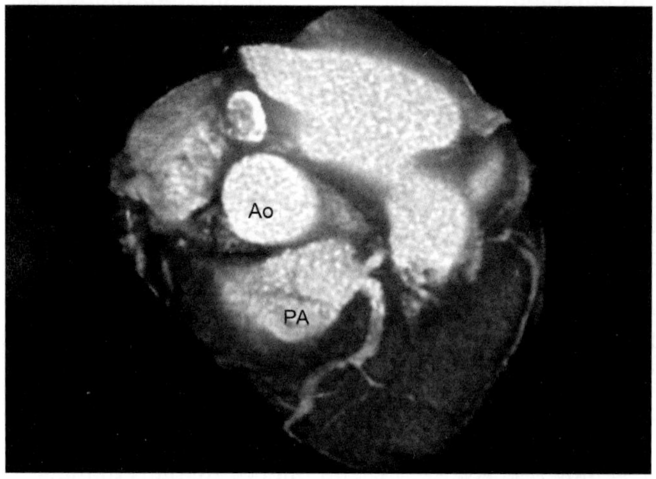

Fig. 5: Anomalous origin of left coronary artery from pulmonary artery (ALCAPA)—VRT image of coronary CT angiogram.

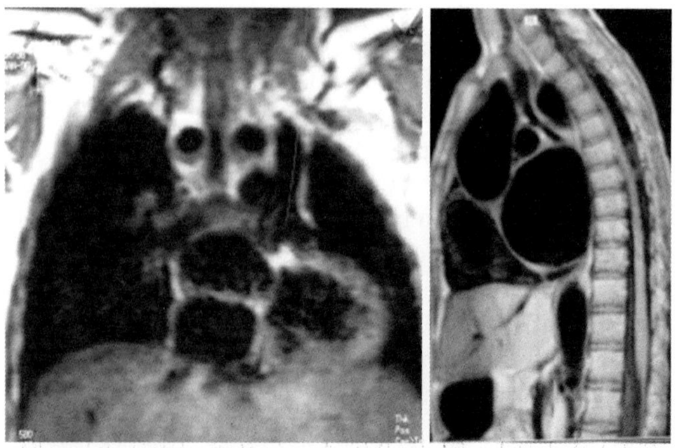

Fig. 6: Double aortic arch: Coronal and sagittal MRI-T1W image showing vascular structure on both sides of trachea.

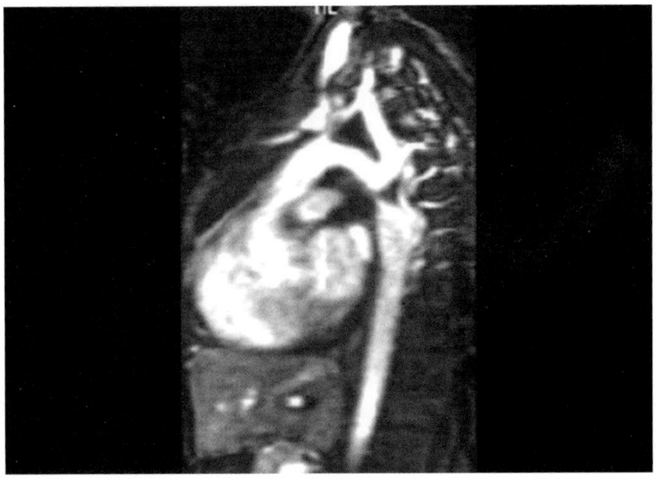

Fig. 7: Coarctation of aorta: Contrast-enhanced MR angiogram in oblique sagittal view shows coarctation just distal to left subclavian artery origin.

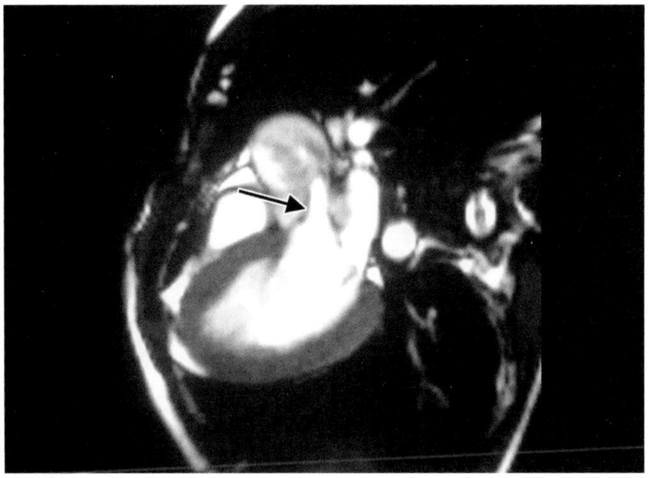

Fig. 8: Oblique sagittal cine MR image showing poststenotic jet in ascending aorta due to aortic stenosis.

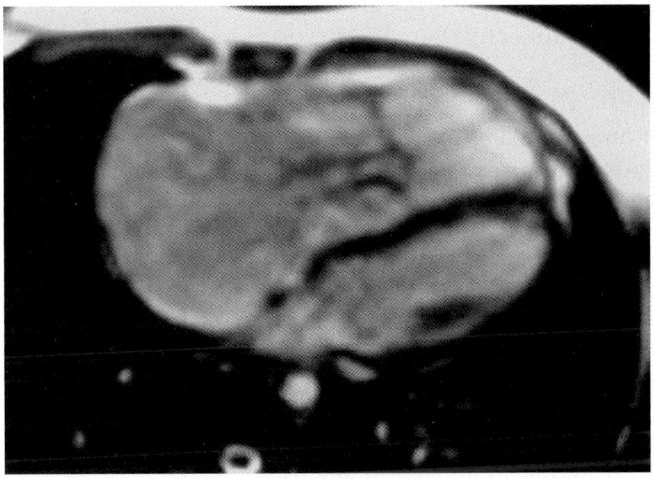

Fig. 9: Cine MR image in four-chamber view showing regurgitant jet in large RA in a case of Ebstein's anomaly, suggesting tricuspid regurgitation.

Pressure gradient (ΔP) across a stenosis can be calculated by measuring maximum poststenotic velocity (V_{max}) by using Bernoulli's equation:

$$\Delta P = 4\,(V_{max})^2$$

For cardiac tumors, ECG-gated spin echo T1W and T2W sequences are performed before and after administration of gadolinium contrast.

Common indications for cardiac CT and MRI in children with CHD are:

- Evaluation of vascular and cardiac anatomy
- Arterial blood supply to lungs (PA anatomy, AP collaterals) **(Figs. 10A and B)**
- Aortic arch abnormalities (Coarctation, interrupted aortic arch, vascular rings)
- Abnormal pulmonary venous drainage
- Abnormal coronary artery origin
- Quantification of ventricular volumes—in hypoplastic RV, hypoplastic LV
- Follow-up after surgery or intervention:
  - For shunt patency
  - Restenosis, aneurysm of aortic arch
  - For pulmonary artery stenosis
  - Valvular regurgitation, e.g. post-TOF repair
- Cardiac tumors.

Analyzing CT or MRI Images

The CT or MRI images need to be analyzed using a sequential segmental approach. This consists of following steps:

1. Determining cardiac sidedness (location of atrial chambers)
2. Identification of atria, ventricles and great arteries
3. Identification of venoatrial, atrioventricular and ventriculoarterial connections
4. Determination of cardiac position (in chest, apex orientation).

Anatomy

Cardiac sidedness is determined by position of morphological RA and this is independent of location of heart in chest, or position of ventricles and great vessels. In situs solitus, morphological RA lies to right of morphological LA.

Identifying atria is easy with the help of their respective appendages. Right atrial appendage is broad based and

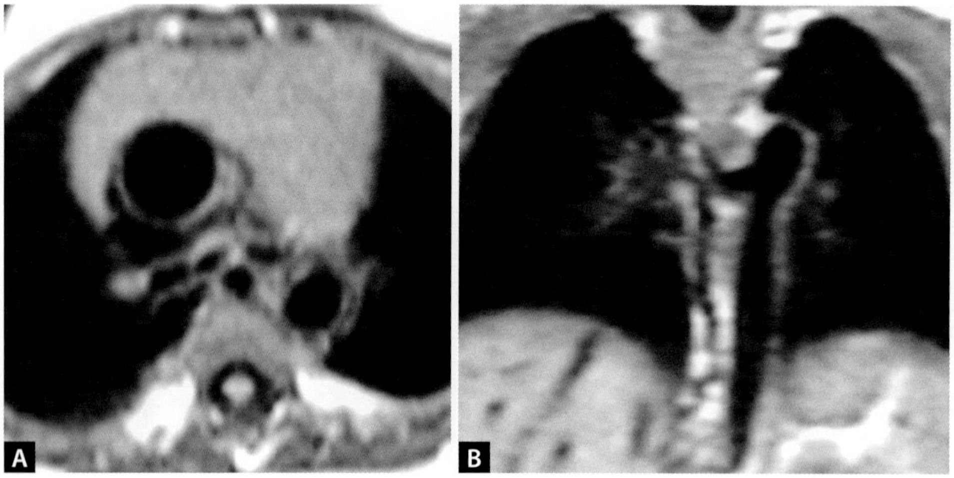

Figs. 10A and B: Spin-echo T1W axial MRI image showing small but confluent pulmonary arteries. Coronal image shows a large aortopulmonary collateral from descending thoracic aorta supplying right lung.

triangular while left atrial appendage has narrow base and is tongue shaped.

Ventricles have three parts—inlet, apex and outlet. Right ventricle shows atrioventricular discontinuity **(Fig. 11)** due to presence of supraventricular muscular crest. Right ventricle has tricuspid atrioventricular valve unlike bicuspid mitral valve of LV. Left ventricular trabeculae are fine while those is RV are few but coarse. Papillary muscles arising from septal surface, and moderator band crossing from septum to anterior papillary muscle are characteristic of RV.

Great arteries are identified by their branching pattern.

Bronchial branching pattern determines right or left sidedness. Right bronchus is superior to descending branch of RPA (epiarterial bronchus) while left bronchus traverses below the left upper pulmonary artery (hyparterial bronchus). The four pulmonary veins drain normally into left atrium.

The three systemic veins—superior and inferior vena cava and coronary sinus drain into right atrium.

Normal Connections

Venoatrial, atrioventricular and ventriculoarterial must be identified. Atrioventricular concordance and ventriculoarterial discordance is seen in complete transposition of great arteries. In corrected transposition of great arteries, there is both atrioventricular and ventriculoarterial discordance.

Extracardiac and intracardiac abnormalities must be identified. Extracardiac lesions include those associated with aorta (coarctation, PDA), Pulmonary arteries and veins (TAPVC, etc.).

Intracardiac lesions include atrial ventricular septal defects, conotruncal defects (truncus arteriosus, TOF), abnormal connections (single ventricles, d-TGA, C-TGA, double outlet RV).

Cardiac Tumors

Primary cardiac tumors are rare. MRI scores over CT in this entity because of its inherent tissue contrast. Gadolinium enhanced images help differentiate between tumor and thrombus. Cine imaging helps assess inflow or outflow obstruction and compression of adjacent vessels.

Follow-up after Surgery or after Endovascular Intervention

CT and MRI are useful to evaluate for:

- Patency of shunts/conduits and their caliber
- Complications such as aneurysms, restenosis, e.g. after aortic coarctation repair.

CARDIAC CATHETERIZATION

Cardiac catheterization and angiocardiography give physiologic and functional data besides revealing the morphology of the lesion **(Fig. 12)**. Though a detailed information of catheterization is beyond the scope of this chapter, there are certain things which must be kept in mind before taking up a child for this invasive procedure.

Firstly, the purpose of cath should clearly outweigh the risk of subjecting the ill child to this additional stress of contrast. The contrast must be limited to a maximum of 3 mL/kg body weight to ensure the safety of sick child.

With the advent of cardiac CT and MRI, cardiac catheterization is now limited to a few conditions where physiological information is required and pressure gradients need to be taken.

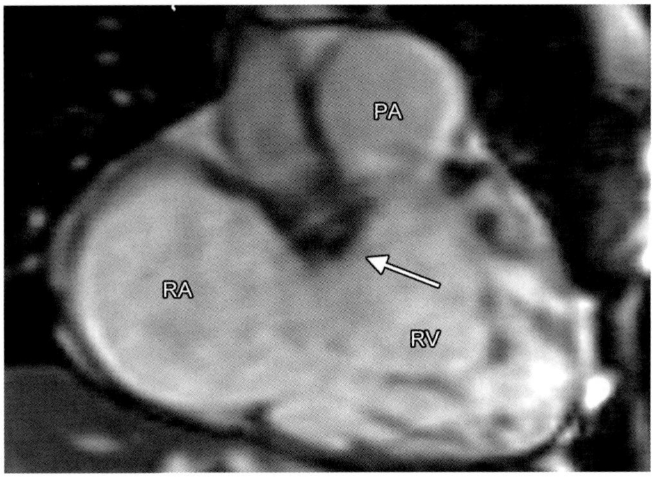

Fig. 11: MR image showing atrioventricular discontinuity in right ventricle due to supraventricular muscular crest (arrow), which is the distinguishing feature of RV.

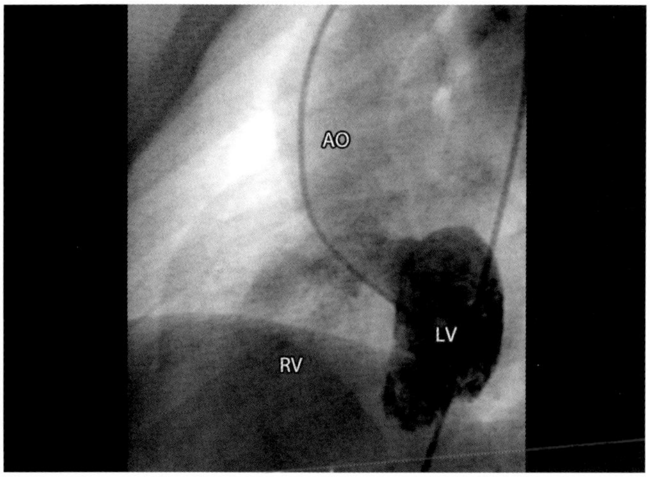

Fig. 12: Catheter angiogram image—injection through catheter in LV shows filling of RV by subaortic ventricular septal defect.

BIBLIOGRAPHY

1. Bıssoio RJ, Vincent WR. Diagnosis of congenital heart disease in first two weeks of life. California Med. 1969;110:200-6.
2. Chang CH. The normal roentgenographic measurement of the right descending pulmonary artery in 1085 cases. AJR. 1962;87:929-35.
3. Coussement AM. Objective radiographic assessment of pulmonary vascularity in children. Radiology. 1973;109:649- 54.
4. Elliot LP, Van Mierop LH, Gleason DC. Roentgenology of tricuspid atresia. Seminars in Roentgenol. 1968;3:399-409.
5. Elliott LP. Cardiac imaging in infants, children and adults, JB Lippincott Co., Philadelphia; 1991.
6. Flohr T, Stierstorfer K, Raupach R, et al. Performance evaluation of a 64-slice CT system with z-flying focal spot. Rofo. 2004;176:1803-10.
7. Goo HW, Park IS, Ko JK, et al. CT of congenital heart disease: normal anatomy and typical pathologic conditions. Radiographics. 2003;23:S147-65.
8. Gyepes MT, Vincent WR. Severe congenital heart disease in the neonatal period. AJR. 1972;490-500.
9. Jefferson K, Rees R. Clinical Cardiac Radiology, 2nd edn, Butterworth, London, 1980.
10. Kellenberger CJ, Yoo SJ, Buchel ER. Cardiovascular MR imaging in neonates and infants with congenital heart disease. Radiographics. 2007;27:5-18.
11. Leber AW, Knez A, von Ziegler F, et al. Quantification of obstructive and nonobstructive coronary lesions by 64-slice computed tomography: A comparative study with quantitative coronary angiography and intravascular ultrasound. J Am Coll Cardiol. 2005;46:147-54.
12. Leschka S, Alkadhi H, Plass A, et al. Accuracy of MSCT coronary angiography with 64-slice technology: first experience. Eur Heart J. 2005;26:1482-7.
13. Manghat NE, Morgan-Hughes GJ, Marshall AJ, et al. Multidetector row computed tomography: Imaging congenital coronary artery anomalies in adults. Heart. 2005;91:1515-22.
14. Moes CAF. Analysis of the chest in the neonate with congenital heart disease. RCNA. 1975;13:251-76.
15. Mollet NR, Cademartiri F, van Mieghem CA, et al. High-resolution spiral computed tomography coronary angiography in patients referred for diagnostic conventional coronary angiography. Circulation. 2005;112:2318-23.
16. Pugliese F, Mollet NR, Runza G, et al. Diagnostic angiography in patients with stable angina pectoris. Eur Radiol. 2006;16:575- 82.
17. Radiology of the heart. In: Braunwald E (Ed). Heart Disease: A Textbook of Cardiovascular Medicine. WB Saunders, Philadelphia; 204-34.
18. Raff GL, Gallagher MJ, O'Neill WW, et al. Diagnostic accuracy of noninvasive coronary angiography using 64-slice spiral computed tomography. J Am Coll Cardiol. 2005;46: 552-7.
19. Roberts WC. Radiologic differentiation of common anomalies. In: Adult Congenital Heart Disease; 1988. pp. 191-219.
20. Sharma S. Proceedings of symposium and workshops in Cardiovascular and Interventional Radiology. Springer-Verlag, Singapore; 1997.
21. Tsai-Goodman B, Geva T, Odegard KC, et al. Clinical role, accuracy and technical aspects of cardiovascular magnetic resonance imaging in infants. Am J Cardiol. 2004;94(1):69-74.

CHAPTER 178

Imaging in Ischemic Heart Disease

Gurpreet Singh Gulati, Sanjiv Sharma, Priya Jagia

INTRODUCTION

Ischemic heart disease (IHD) continues to be the leading cause of mortality in the developed countries. The prevalence in India has risen markedly in recent years, especially in urban areas.[1] Current estimates suggest that by 2020, India will have the largest burden of cardiovascular disease in the world, the bulk of which will be comprised of IHD. An accurate and early detection of the disease is crucial for the optimal management and prognostication of these patients.

The various components of IHD that need evaluation on imaging include: presence, extent and localization of ischemia, presence and size of myocardial infarction (MI), myocardium at risk, guidance for revascularization and follow-up, and quantification of myocardial function. Several noninvasive techniques, both traditional and advanced, are available for this purpose. Conventional modalities include echocardiography (ECHO), nuclear imaging and angiography. Over the last 15 years, ischemia imaging with cardiac magnetic resonance (CMR) and multi-detector CT (MDCT) technology has evolved extensively. This review focuses upon the utility of these newer modalities for evaluation of IHD.

PATHOPHYSIOLOGY OF ISCHEMIC HEART DISEASE

Myocardial Ischemia

Stenoses of an epicardial coronary artery leads to reduced perfusion and correspondingly diminished myocardial oxygen delivery. However, at rest, the equilibrium between perfusion, metabolism, and contractile function can be maintained even in moderate to severe stenosis. Therefore, these stenoses are asymptomatic at rest and cannot be detected using perfusion studies at rest. At stress (induced pharmacologically or by physical exercise), there is a three- to four-fold increase in contractile function, accompanied by a four-fold increase in oxygen demand and perfusion. Whereas, the flow in normal coronary arteries can be increased by vasodilation (induced by using either dipyridamole or more commonly, adenosine), moderate and severe stenoses become flow limiting, resulting in perfusion deficits, wall motion abnormalities, and symptomatic angina.

Different stress tests are clinically used to detect myocardial ischemia. In the progression of ischemia, successive myocardial events occur, known as the cascade of ischemia.[2] Initially, hypoperfusion is only detectable in the subendocardium. Further reduction of the blood flow due to more severe stenosis leads to transmural perfusion deficits. Progression of ischemia leads to diastolic, followed by systolic wall motion abnormalities. These can be detected by dobutamine stress ECHO/CMR. Finally, electrocardiographic changes can be detected and typical symptomatic angina may occur. As perfusion abnormalities are the first step in this cascade of ischemia, direct visualization of these perfusion deficits seems to be the diagnostic test of first choice in patients with suspected CAD. Both CMR and nuclear imaging techniques can measure myocardial perfusion.

Myocardial Viability and Myocardial Infarction

Viability is continued cell life. A myocyte is viable while alive and nonviable once irreversible cellular damage and cell death occurs. By this definition, histology is the ultimate method for inspection of individual cells. Myocytes may be viable in the setting of severely reduced or absent contractile function, resulting from either acute or chronic reduction in perfusion. Differences between the acute and chronic settings in terms of the potential for contractile recovery of myocardium are related to the underlying mechanisms of myocyte dysfunction. A number of indirect methods have been used to detect presence of living myocytes for the purpose of in vivo assessment of myocardial viability. As a result, in clinical practice and research settings, viability has been defined in accordance with the method used to indirectly demonstrate the presence of living myocytes, leading to a number of clinical definitions of viability. For example: (1) recovery of contractile function following revascularization; (2) response to inotropic stimulation (e.g. dobutamine ECHO or dobutamine MRI); (3) presence of glucose metabolism (e.g. fluoro-2-deoxygluclose (FDG) positron emission tomography (PET)); 4) presence of active cellular transport mechanisms (e.g. Tl-201 Single photon emission computed tomography (SPECT)); and presence of non-scarred (or more precisely, absence of scarred) myocardium (delayed enhanced MRI or DE-MRI).

Rationale for Ischemia and Viability Imaging

Although coronary artery luminal obstruction can be detected with catheter angiography or MDCT, assessment of myocardial perfusion helps to assess the functional relevance of the lesion. This is crucial to decide the need for revascularization, as coronary interventions should primarily be preformed where there is clinical evidence of myocardial ischemia associated with the coronary stenosis. Thus, even in patients with known intermediate stenosis of a coronary artery, there is frequently a need for stress testing to define whether the stenosis is hemodynamically significant. Also, there is a need to define the physiological significance of possible stenosis associated with highly calcified coronary arteries or in smaller stents that cannot be adequately resolved with current generation CT scanners.

Beyond establishment of a clinical diagnosis, an important value of stress perfusion imaging is in its ability to risk stratify patients. It is important to be able to separate low-risk group of patients from those at a high risk of sustaining subsequent cardiac events (cardiac death or MI), since it is towards the latter group that we direct our resources. This benefit of perfusion imaging has been well documented with nuclear cardiology techniques. A normal myocardial perfusion study is associated with a 0.3–1.0% annual risk of MI or cardiac-related death, in contradistinction to an abnormal study where the risk is five- to ten-fold.[3]

It is crucial to identify the myocardium that is viable and not infarcted. The presence of myocardial viability is especially important in patients with severe ventricular dysfunction, where the benefits of coronary revascularization may be questioned due to the increased risk of the procedure. Patients with viable areas clearly demonstrate survival benefit and improved quality of life after revascularization, as compared with those who do not.[4] The latter group may therefore be exposed to substantial operative risk without clear benefit.

IMAGING MODALITIES

Echocardiography

Echocardiography (ECHO) has emerged as the "workhorse" of cardiac imaging, since it is easily available, safe and quick and provides excellent information on morphology and function of nearly all cardiac structures. Stress ECHO has been shown to reliably demonstrate myocardial ischemia and helps to acquire prognostic data. There are two techniques for performing stress ECHO: (1) Detection of wall motion abnormalities induced with exercise/dobutamine; (2) Measurement of altered myocardial perfusion on contrast ECHO.[5] Myocardial contrast ECHO has been shown to be comparable to SPECT for the detection of CAD.[6] It is possible that the combination of stress perfusion and stress ECHO may improve accuracy of the technique.[7]

Limitations of ECHO include operator dependence with poor interobserver agreement. Also, an optimal acoustic window may not exist in every patient for detection of all wall motion abnormalities. The left ventricular apex, particularly in a large, hypocontractile left ventricle, may not be adequately assessed with this modality. In patients with MI, a mural thrombus may be difficult to distinguish from underlying myocardium on ECHO.

Nuclear Imaging

This is perhaps the most well established modality with a large body of literature available on its utility for detecting the presence of myocardial ischemia and infarction.

For detection of myocardial ischemia, the most common procedure is myocardial perfusion imaging (MPI) or single-photon emission computed tomography (SPECT). SPECT is a tomographic technique, providing 3-dimensional assessment of blood flow. Small amounts of radioactive material (including thallium-201, and the more recent available Tc-99m tetrofosmin and Tc-99m sestamibi) are injected intravenously and these tracers are taken up and retained in the heart tissue in proportion to regional blood supply. Usually, two scans are obtained after tracer injection, one at rest and one in which the agent is injected during exercise or medication-induced stress. Areas with reduced blood supply, either under resting conditions or following stress testing, indicate regions of scar or reversible perfusion alterations (ischemia), respectively. Additionally, an ECG-gated SPECT allows for assessment of LV function.

Positron-emission tomography (PET) has several technical advantages over SPECT, such as higher counting sensitivity, higher spatial resolution, and routine use of attenuation correction. PET (along with CMR) using metabolic tracers such as 18F-FDG (glucose analog), is currently regarded as the gold standard for tissue viability. Under normal conditions, fatty acids play a major role in the metabolism of the normoxic heart, while glucose becomes the major substrate for the myocardium under ischemic conditions. Therefore, PET imaging using metabolic tracers such as 18F-FDG enables detection of metabolic changes at the cellular level associated with ischemia. In clinical practice, 18F-FDG PET is often combined with flow tracers such as 13N-ammonia to assess myocardial perfusion. Although 18F-FDG PET imaging without flow tracer may work with reasonable sensitivity and specificity for detecting viable tissue, flow/metabolism combination would provide more comprehensive information on viability. The preserved or increased glucose utilization, and hence 18F-FDG uptake in hypoperfused and dysfunctional myocardium (flow metabolism mismatch) is regarded as a metabolic marker of cell survival and viability, whereas concordant reduction in both blood flow and 18F-FDG uptake is indicative of scar.

Limitations of nuclear imaging are discussed later, under "Evaluation of various components of IHD: Detection of myocardial ischemia".

Cardiovascular Magnetic Resonance Imaging (CMR)

During the past decade, significant advances have been made in the imaging speed, resolution, quality, and versatility of CMR. Reliable, reproducible CMR imaging can now be achieved as a result of advent of more rapid imaging acquisition along with breath-hold techniques, diaphragmatic navigator gating, and real-time imaging to counter the effects of respiratory motion. The availability of stress myocardial perfusion in mid 1990s, and steady state free precession (SSFP) imaging and DE-MRI at the start of the new millennium allows assessment of all aspects of ischemia, infarct and myocardial functional imaging in a single session of 45–50 min. There is growing evidence that CMR can be used at each step of the assessment of patients with IHD, from establishing the diagnosis to guiding the optimal therapeutic strategy through to risk stratification.

Other advantages of CMR are that it is operator independent and does not entail exposure to potentially nephrotoxic contrast or ionizing radiation. In the context of IHD, the high spatial resolution of CMR allows better detection of myocardial edema, subendocardial ischemia, subendocardial infarcts and microvascular obstruction.

IMAGING SEQUENCES

Stress CMR

There are two CMR techniques for assessment of myocardial ischemia: dobutamine stress MR (DSMR) and perfusion CMR. DSMR has not yet gained wide acceptance in the clinical arena because of concerns relating to patient safety and monitoring inside the MR scanner. Additionally, from a pathophysiologic point of view, perfusion CMR should be more sensitive than DSMR since decreased perfusion is the first step of the ischemic cascade.

For optimal first pass perfusion studies, a series of T1 weighted images need to be obtained every heart beat or every other heart beat while a bolus of contrast passes through the heart and myocardium. Gadolinium (dosage varies between 0.025 and 0.15 mmol/kg) is the most widely used contrast agent for perfusion CMR. After localizer images, the vasodilator stress agent is started IV (most commonly adenosine, in a dose of 140 mg/kg/min for 5 minutes before injection of gadolinium). By 3 minutes of the infusion, adequate vasodilator stress is usually achieved to allow performance of stress perfusion imaging. T1 weighted sequences are then used to visualise the passage of gadolinium. Areas of myocardial hypoperfusion will appear as areas of decreased signal intensity **(Fig. 1)**. Typical perfusion deficits tend to follow the perfusion territories of the coronary artery, affect the distal segments first (with few exceptions), are subendocardial (except most severe cases), last for several heartbeats beyond the initial rapid upslope of myocardial enhancement, and are not present at rest (except in MI). One needs to be aware of the various artefacts (including the most common susceptibility artefacts) that can interfere with the interpretation of true deficits. Perfusion CMR analysis is based on the time-intensity curves and can be performed in a quantitative, semi-quantitative, or qualitative fashion.

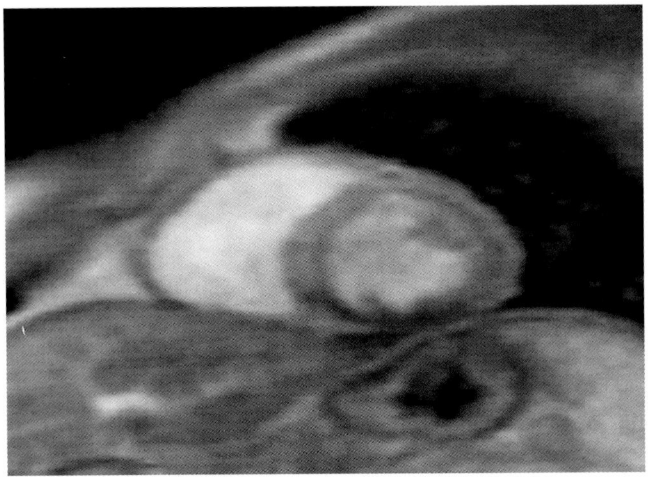

Fig. 1: Stress CMR perfusion—short axis image at the mid-ventricular level. There is a subendocardial perfusion defect (hypointensity) in the inferior wall, corresponding to right coronary artery (RCA) stenosis. The defect was not present at rest.

CMR for Viability

The standard CMR technique for detection of myocardial viability is DE-MRI. This was introduced in the late 1990's and is being increasingly regarded as the gold-standard for the detection of irreversibly damaged myocardium. The underlying concept is that infarcted tissue accumulates gadolinium and can be visualized as hyperenhanced or "bright" regions on T1-weighted images acquired at least 10 minutes after gadolinium injection **(Figs. 2A and B)**. Gadolinium is an inert extracellular contrast agent and the amount of contrast agent in a given tissue distribution volume determines the image signal intensity—the more contrast per distribution volume the higher the signal. In the normal myocardium, the tissue volume is predominantly intracellular. Because extracellular contrast media is excluded from this space by the intact sarcolemmal membrane, the volume of distribution of a contrast medium in normal myocardium is quite small (25% of water space), and one can consider viable myocytes as actively excluding contrast media. Therefore, the unifying mechanism for the hyperenhancement effect of nonviable myocardium may be regarded as being due to the absence of viable myocytes rather than any inherent properties that are specific for acutely necrotic tissue, collagenous scar, or other forms of nonviable tissue.

CMR for Myocardial Mass and Function

SSFP cine sequences provide high spatial resolution and a high contrast between the dark myocardium and the bright blood-pool and therefore are preferred for this purpose **(Figs. 3A and B)**: a stack of short-axis cine images (with a slice thickness of 8–12 mm) by which both ventricles can be covered without a gap in 1–2 breathholds. Either prospective or retrospective gating can be used with similar accuracy. The resulting section provides the typical volumetric and functional data for LV and RV including parameters such as EDV, ESV, SV, CO and filling rates. These calculations are done using the modified Simpson's rule. When both endo- and epicardial contours are drawn, ventricular mass and regional wall thickening can also be calculated.

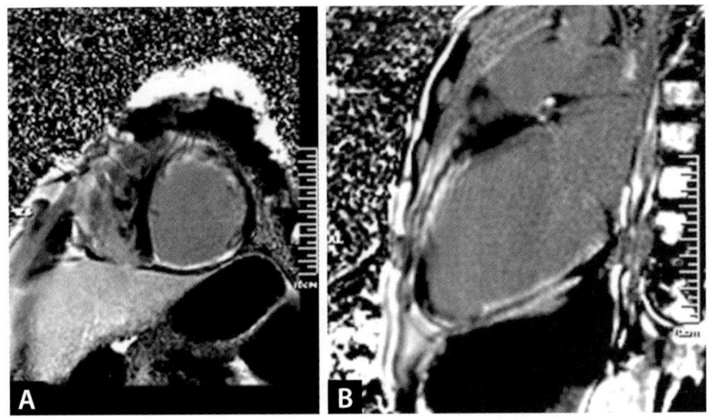

Figs. 2A and B: DE-MRI—short axis and vertical long axis views. There are transmural infarcts (hyperenhanced) in the anterior, anterolateral and anteroseptal segments (LAD territory), as well as in the inferior and inferolateral segments (RCA territory).

OTHER USEFUL SEQUENCES

T2-weighted turbo spin echo sequences are used to detect increased water tissue content as an indirect measure of tissue inflammation or edema and can be useful in the differentiation between acute and chronic MI between myocarditis and CAD.

Multidetector Computed Tomography (MDCT)

This modality has developed tremendously over the last decade to emerge as an excellent non-invasive tool for demonstration of coronary artery anatomy. Key technical requirements for coronary MDCT are high temporal resolution (which minimizes motion artifacts and is achieved through fast gantry rotation), high spatial resolution [which enables detailed depiction of the coronary anatomy (both the wall and lumen) and is achieved through thin collimation], fast continuous coverage (which enables imaging of the entire heart in one comfortable breath-hold), and synchronization to the heartbeat (which enables imaging during a consistent cardiac phase and is achieved through ECG gating).

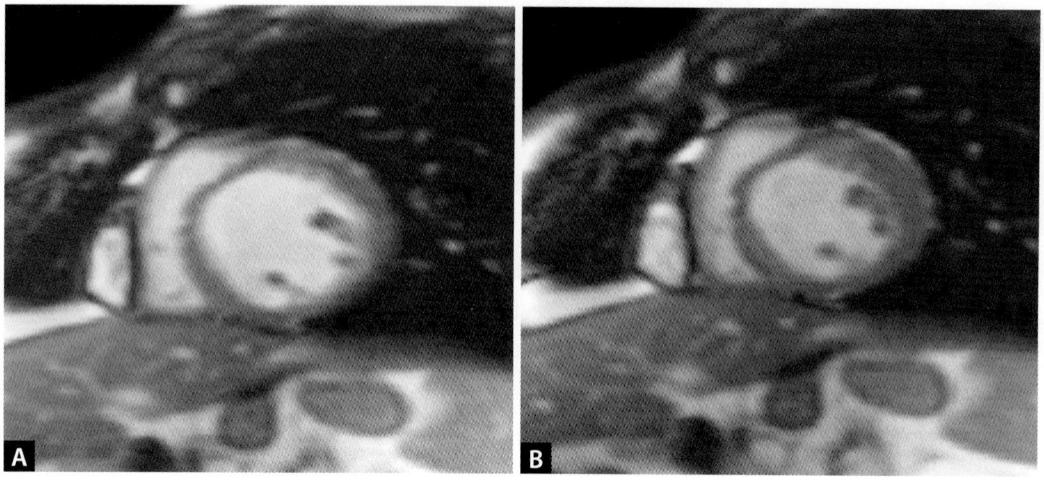

Figs. 3A and B: SSFP cine-CMR—short axis images in diastole (A) and systole (B). Thinning of myocardium is noted in the septal and anteroseptal segments (infarct in LAD territory). These segments do not thicken (akinesia) during systole. Also note reduced thickening (hypokinesia) in the inferolateral wall [left circumflex (LCx) artery territory].

There are two methods for ECG-gating on MDCT. A retrospective ECG-gated MDCT obtains different image sets at different times in the cardiac cycle in a spiral mode. While individual time windows of end-systolic and end-diastolic phases are usually used for adequate visualization of the coronary arteries at times where they present minimal velocity, one can also reconstruct the data for all phases of the cardiac cycle from the same original dataset. It is thereby possible to generate dynamic cine sequences of the whole heart and to select oblique reformatted planes along standard anatomic axis of the heart. These reconstructed data provide high quality images for the assessment of heart anatomy and ventricular function. A disadvantage of retrospective gated MDCT scanning is the higher radiation exposure. To circumvent this limitation, prospective ECG triggering (a step-and-shoot sequential scanning method) may be used. Image acquisition is timed to coincide with a predefined point in the cardiac cycle. The advantages of prospective ECG-triggering are speed and a reduction in radiation dose. One disadvantage is the need for a regular heart rate and rhythm.

In a patient with an irregular heart rate, image acquisition can be triggered at the wrong point in the cardiac cycle, resulting in misregistration artifact. In addition, sequential scanning yields single trans-axial slices rather than volumetric data, and z-axis resolution is suboptimal.

Cardiac MDCT scan is usually begun by obtaining a calcium score, scanning from the level of the tracheal bifurcation to the bottom of the heart. Exceptions are patients being scanned following revascularization [coronary artery bypass surgery (CABG) or stent placement]. The calcium score not only provides independent prognostic information, it also helps in determining whether a patient is a good candidate for coronary MDCT. There is no recommended absolute threshold coronary calcium score that precludes coronary MDCT. However, in a patient with very dense calcification along the length of the coronary vessels and at multiple branch points, it is extremely difficult to interpret MDCT images. For the contrast MDCT, scan range is the same as the calcium score. Scan range is increased to include the top of the chest in patients scanned after CABG. The heart is positioned at the isocenter, and images are reconstructed with a small field-of-view, to improve resolution. Contrast type, volume, rate, method of bolus (test or automatic bolus tracking) injection and scanner parameters vary depending on operator preference, particular vendor's equipment, scanner generation.

For 64 slice CT scanners, the patient's heart rate may need to be controlled. If the baseline heart rate exceeds 65 bpm, a beta-blocker—oral metoprolol 50 to 100 mg—45 minutes to 1 hour prior to the study is administered. If the rate still remains too high, IV metoprolol in 5-mg doses, up to a maximum of 20 mg may need to be given. It is important to use caution when administering beta-blockers to patients with asthma, severe aortic stenosis, atrio-ventricular block, or severe left ventricular dysfunction. With the higher temporal resolution available with dual source scanners, beta blockers are not usually indicated.

Up to the generation of scanners providing 16 slices per rotation, the ratio of non-conclusive studies was still in the range of 20 to 30% of the patients who had at least one coronary segment that could not be adequately evaluated despite the use of beta blockers. The advent of 64 slice scanners followed by new dual source and 256 (and 320) slice scanners have led to a quantum leap in temporal and spatial resolution with much higher performance allowing imaging patients with fast and irregular heart rates. Dual source scanners essentially double the speed of acquisition while maintaining the same spatial resolution of a 64-slice scanner.[8,9] With two X-ray beams and detectors rotating simultaneously on the same gantry, double the amount of data are acquired on each rotation. This increases the temporal resolution of the scan to 82 msec (1/4 gantry rotation time), which can be increased still further to 42 msec with multi-segment reconstruction. Furthermore, the ability of having each individual generator set to a different energy with different tissue penetration opens new perspectives in better tissue characterization that would potentially allow a better assessment of composition of vascular plaques. It is also possible using dual energy imaging to separate calcifications from contrast agent to generate images of the vascular lumens without interference from calcified plaques. Dual energy imaging has already been explored in peripheral vessels both for generating better calcium-free angiograms as well as assessing the tissue characteristics of vascular plaques. These techniques may also be applicable to coronary arteries in future.

Limitations of MDCT

- Need for a stable and well controlled heart rate
- Inadequate assessment of lesion severity
- Interference due to calcification in the vessel wall
- Need for iodinated contrast and radiation exposure.

The latter two aspects need to be weighed against the benefit of noninvasively depicting the coronary arteries. The risk of radiation exposure is more important in those cases in whom further functional nuclear assessment and, if necessary, invasive catheterization and interventions are required. With higher number of detectors (e.g. 64), images obtained with full spatial and temporal resolution over the complete heart cycle can easily deliver between 15 and 20 mSv. This is roughly double the radiation of conventional coronary angiogram that averages between 9 and 12 mSv.

There are various strategies to reduce radiation exposure. These include:

- Reducing dose to a level that is as low as reasonably achievable (the ALARA principle). The technologist can be instructed to only cover the area of the heart, instead of covering the whole chest. This can help reduce the exposure by half or more.
- Retrospective gating with pulsed radiation synchronous to the ECG that delivers lower radiation dose outside a selected window in diastolic phase. The radiation dose can be reduced significantly with ECG pulsing to approximately 10 mSv in men and 14 mSv in women.
- Lowering the tube voltage to 100 kV in patients with a normal body weight or body mass index.[10]
- Implementation of step-and-shoot cardiac CT is associated with an effective radiation dose of just 1–3 mSv.[11]
- A prospective gate window of 20% over diastole in patients with a heart rate around 60 bpm can reduce the total dose to the patient by 80%. At higher heart rates the reduction of dose may be less and still achieve 55–60% of dose reduction.

Recent publications have shown that by using prospective gating and proper imaging protocol, accurate images of the coronary arteries can be obtained at doses as low as 1 or 2 mSV.[12,13] With 256 detectors and higher, scanners can acquire full 3D images of the whole heart in a single rotation avoiding spiral averaging of multiple heart cycles. This can significantly reduce the dose down to 2.8 mSv with pulsed exposure over diastole and about 5 mSv for full dynamic assessment of LV function over the whole heart cycle.[14]

A more recent technical advance has been the introduction of a new dual source CT, generating 128 slices per detector system (instead of 64 slices per detector system in the earlier version). Besides having the fastest scanning speed for retrospective gating in spiral mode (43 cm/s) and highest temporal resolution (75 ms), the scanner operates at an extremely reduced radiation dose. For example, a spiral heart scan can be performed with less than 1 mSv, much lower than the annual radiation exposure from natural sources of 2–5 mSv.

EVALUATION OF VARIOUS COMPONENTS OF IHD

Coronary Artery Imaging

Conventional: X-ray angiography has the advantage of high spatial resolution (~ 0.3 mm) and temporal resolution (20 msec). However, it also has some important limitations: it is invasive, is a two-dimensional technique and does not provide any information about vessel wall structure or plaque morphology.

With CMR, despite the initial hype regarding its scope to image the coronary arteries, there are significant technical difficulties that preclude optimal coronary imaging: small vessel caliber, tortuous course, signal from surrounding epicardial fat and myocardium, near constant motion related to the cardiac and respiratory cycles and the fact that bulk of flow occurs in diastole (Which limits data acquisition time).

Coronary MDCT angiography produces high-quality images of the coronary arteries, in addition to defining their location and the extent of atherosclerotic involvement. Pooling of data from recent studies on accuracy of 64-slice CT and dual-source CT for the detection of coronary artery stenoses in patients with suspected CAD provided a sensitivity of 89% (95% CI 87–90), specificity of 96% (95% CI 96–97), and positive (PPV) and negative predictive values (NPV) of 78% (95% CI 76–80) and 98% (95% CI 98–99), respectively.[15-18] On average, 4.5% of segments (mainly distal segments or very small side branches) could not be evaluated. Importantly, the NPV was consistently high in all studies, indicating that the technique may be most suitable as a noninvasive tool to rule out significant CAD and avoid further imaging or invasive angiography **(Figs. 4A and B)**. Therefore, patients with low probability of CAD, with non-specific symptoms and/or non-conclusive functional tests such as exercise, stress ECHO or nuclear imaging are ideally suited for coronary MDCT.[19,20] Due to its ability to simultaneously assess the thoracic aorta, coronary arteries and the lungs, an ECG-gated MDCT of the chest may provide useful information in patients presenting with acute chest pain with intermediate probability for CAD and no enzyme or ECG changes **(Fig. 5)**. Hoffmann et al.[21] conducted a blinded, prospective study with 64-slice MDCT in this group of patients presenting to the emergency department. Among 103 consecutive patients, 14 patients were diagnosed clinically to have an acute coronary syndrome. Both the absence of significant coronary artery stenosis (73 of 103 patients) and non-stenotic coronary atherosclerotic plaque (41 of 103 patients) accurately predicted the absence of an acute coronary syndrome (NPV 100%). The PPV was rather low, indicating false-positive results in a considerable number of scans (47% for the detection of significant stenoses, 14/30 positive scans), and only a small percent age of patients with acute chest pain were actually included in the study (103 of 305 initially screened patients). Goldstein, et al.[22] randomized 197 patients with low-risk acute chest pain to an immediate 64-slice MDCT scan or 'standard of care' evaluation. CT was found to be safe, with no missed diagnosis of an acute coronary syndrome, faster (3.4 vs 15 hours until establishing the definitive diagnosis), and had lower cost ($1586 vs. 1872) compared with 'standard of care'.

MDCT is also suited for patients with intermediate probability for CAD where more traditional tests remain equivocal or in patients unable to exercise or undergo a stress test.

Coronary MDCT is also highly recommended for follow-up evaluation after CABG. Unlike invasive coronary angiograms, MDCT does not require accurate localization of ostia of venous grafts for selective contrast injections. Also, compared to native coronary arteries, grafts are larger in caliber, less mobile and away from heart. Pooled analysis of date from 180 patients showed the sensitivity, specificity, NPV and PPV of MDCT for graft stenosis/occlusion to be 97–100%, 95–100%, 92–99% and 99–100% respectively.[18] Only 0.7% of occluded and 6.4% of stenosed grafts were non-interpretable, proving MDCT to be an

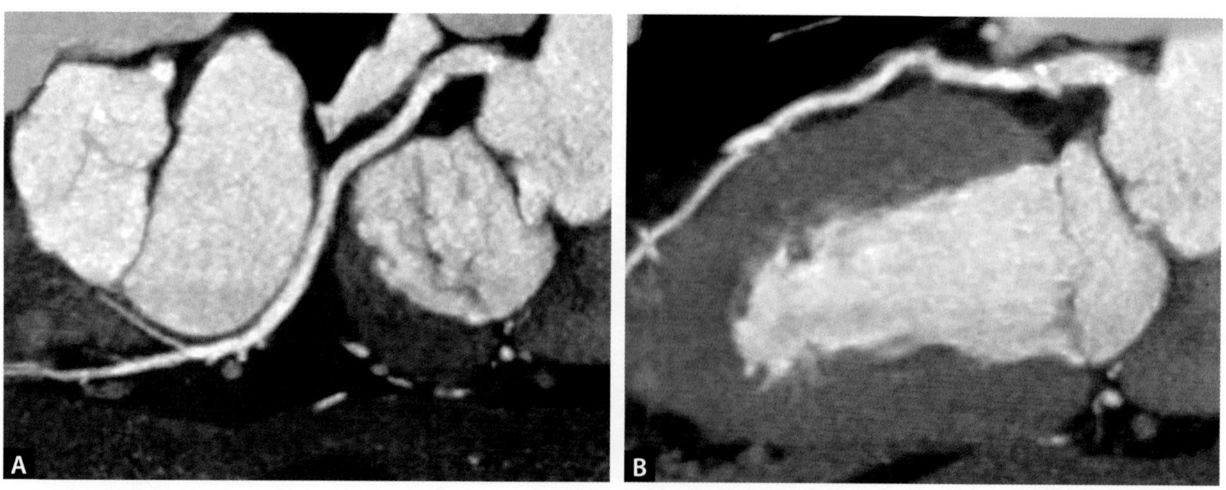

Figs. 4A and B: Coronary MDCT—curved multiplanar reconstructions along the RCA (A) and the LAD (B). There is no evidence of luminal obstruction (similar images were obtained for LCx), although calcified plaques are noted along the proximal and mid-LAD.

accurate and reliable test for detection of grafts stenosis as well as patency **(Figs. 6A and B)**. However, surgical metal clips may lead to artifacts that interfere with optimal visualization in some cases. Also, the native coronary artery visualization in CABG patients may not be adequate with MDCT due to extensive calcification.

Although in single, carefully selected cases (e.g. large diameter stents in a proximal vessel segment, low and stable heart rate, and absence of excessive image noise) coronary CT angiography may be a possibility to rule out in-stent restenosis, routine application of CT to assess patients with coronary stents is currently not recommended. Visualization of the stent lumen is often affected by artifacts, and especially the PPV is low.

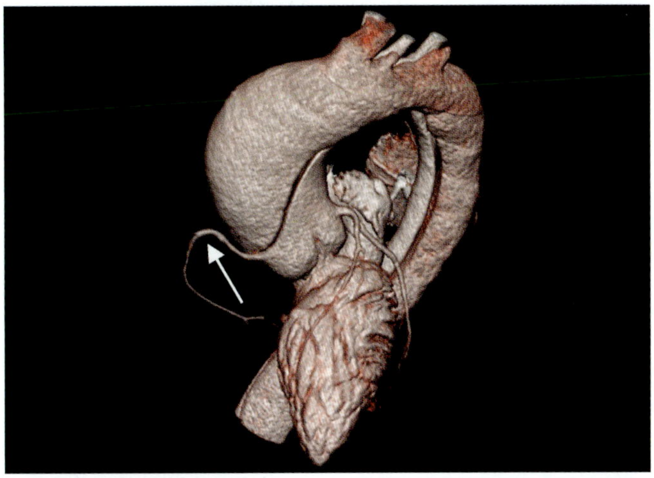

Fig. 5: ECG-gated thoracic MDCT in a patient presenting with acute chest pain, volume-rendered image. A type A aortic dissection, beginning in the aortic root and extending into the descending thoracic aorta, is seen. The RCA (arrow) is normal.

For evaluation of the origin and course of aberrant coronary arteries, invasive angiography may be limited. Because of the three-dimensional nature of the data set, MDCT is very well suited to detect and define the anatomic course of coronary artery anomalies and their relationship to other cardiac and non-cardiac structures **(Figs. 7A and B)**. Numerous case reports and several research papers have demonstrated that the MDCT analysis of coronary anatomy in these patients is straight forward and very reliable with an accuracy close to 100%.[23,24]

Plaque Imaging

Calcified Plaque

Coronary calcium is a surrogate marker for the presence and amount of coronary atherosclerotic plaque. Both EBCT and MDCT permit accurate detection and quantification of coronary artery calcium. The 'Agatston Score', which takes into account the area and the CT density of calcified lesions, is most frequently used to quantify the amount of coronary calcium in CT, and large population reference databases are available. With the exception of patients with renal failure, calcifications occur exclusively in the context of atherosclerotic lesions. The amount of coronary calcium correlates moderately closely to the overall atherosclerotic plaque burden.[25] On the other hand, not every atherosclerotic coronary plaque is calcified, and

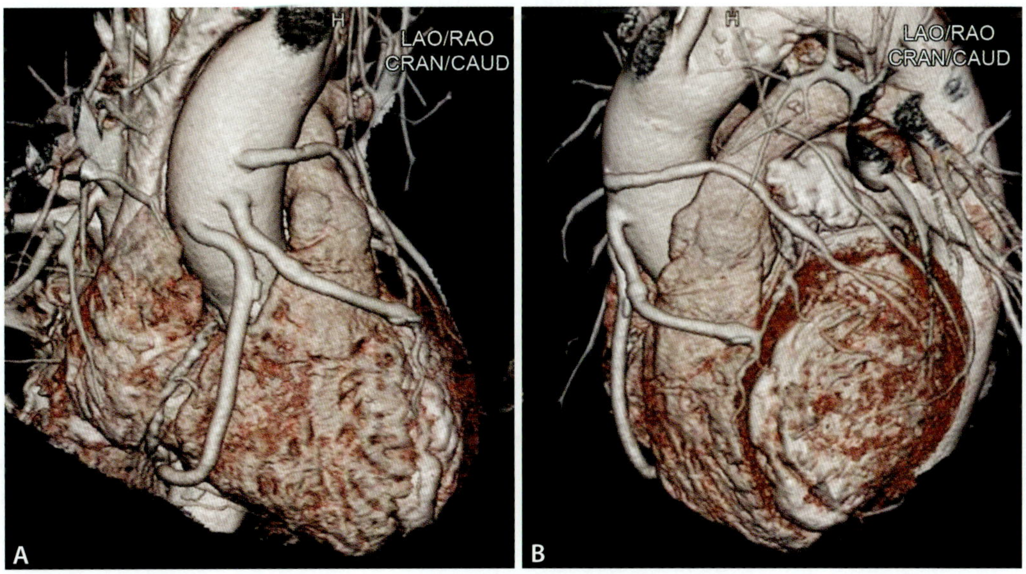

Figs. 6A and B: Coronary MDCT—postoperative CABG, volume-rendered images. There are three venous grafts, one each to the LAD, RCA and ramus intermedius. All grafts are patent.

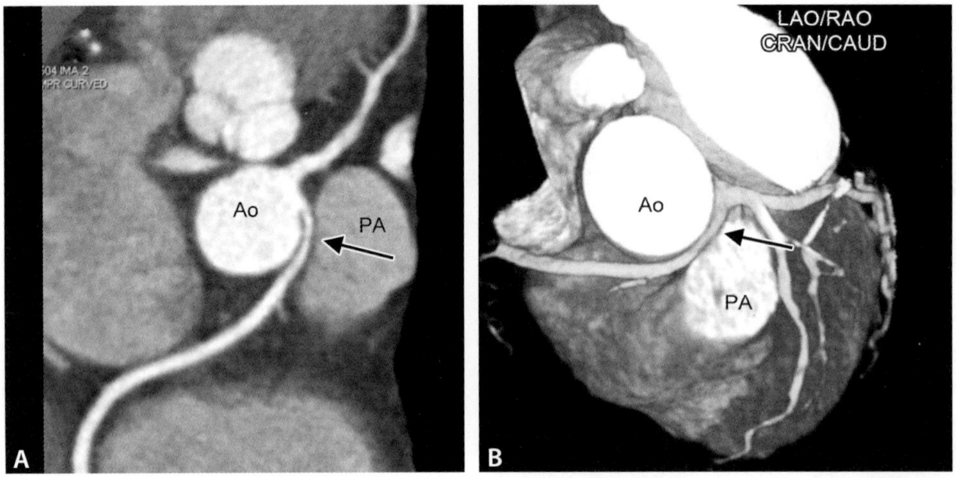

Figs. 7A and B: Coronary MDCT, curved multiplanar (A) and volume-rendered (B) images. The RCA (arrow) arises anomalously from the left coronary sinus, close to the origin of the left main coronary artery. It courses interarterially between the aorta (Ao) and pulmonary artery (PA).

calcification is a sign of neither stability nor instability of an individual plaque.[26]

In several trials, the absence of coronary calcium ruled out the presence of significant coronary artery stenoses with high predictive value.[25,27] However, even pronounced coronary calcification is not necessarily associated with hemodynamically relevant luminal narrowing. Therefore, even the detection of large amounts of calcium does not indicate the presence of significant stenoses and it should not prompt invasive coronary angiography in otherwise asymptomatic individuals.

Numerous prospective trials have demonstrated that the presence of coronary calcium in asymptomatic individuals is a prognostic parameter with strong predictive power for future hard cardiac events. A beneficial contribution of coronary calcium assessment to risk stratification can however, be most likely expected in individuals who seem to be at intermediate risk for coronary events (1.0–2.0% annual risk) on the basis of traditional risk factor analysis. The incremental value of calcium scoring may necessitate intensifying lipid lowering therapy in these patients. Unselected 'screening' or patient self-referral is not recommended, and the value of calcium scoring in individuals with very low (<1.0% annual risk) or very high risk (>2.0% annual risk) is discussed controversially.[25,27-29]

Although the coronary calcium score has been found to be progressive over time, only very preliminary studies are available that have linked progression of coronary calcium to cardiac event rates. Results concerning the influence of lipid-lowering therapy on the progression of coronary calcium have been inhomogeneous. Currently, there is no indication for repeated coronary calcium score measurements.

Non-calcified Plaque

There is growing interest concerning the ability of contrast-enhanced MDCT coronary angiography to detect, quantify and characterize non-calcified plaque **(Fig. 8)**. Data on the accuracy of CT angiography to detect non-calcified plaque are limited to a small number of studies that have compared CT angiography with intravascular ultrasound (IVUS). Sensitivities for the detection of coronary segments with plaque were found to be 80–90% (which, however, was mostly based on the detection of calcified plaque). Correlation of plaque area (r = 0.55) and plaque volume (r = 0.83) between CT angiography and IVUS was found to be moderate, and inter-observer variability is high.[30-32] It has been shown that the extent of remodeling of coronary atherosclerotic lesions can be assessed by CT. Some data are available concerning plaque characterization by CT. On average, the CT attenuation within 'fibrous' plaques is higher than within 'lipid-rich' plaques (mean attenuation values of 91–116 vs 47–71 HU).[30] There is however, large variability of these measurements, which currently prevents accurate classification of non-calcified 'plaque types' by CT.

Preliminary retrospective, small studies have used CT to investigate plaque characteristics in patients after acute coronary syndromes in comparison with patients with stable angina. They reported a higher fraction of non-calcified plaque and more positive remodeling in patients with acute coronary syndromes and in lesions responsible for cardiac events. One study found a significantly higher prevalence of plaque with a CT attenuation <30 HU in lesions associated with acute coronary syndromes when compared with stable lesions.[33] One analysis of 100 patients

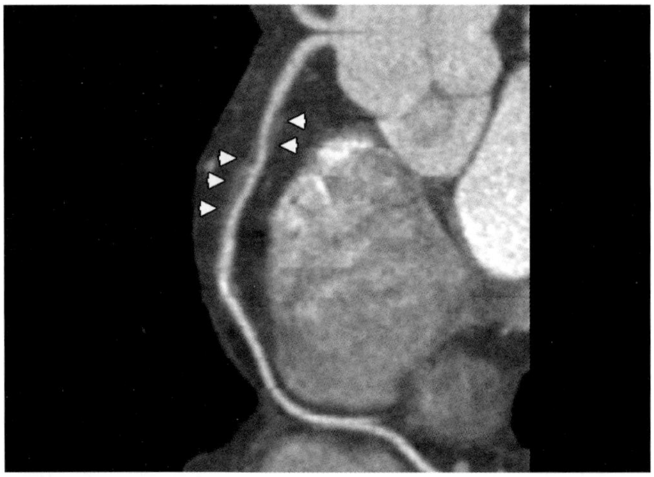

Fig. 8: Coronary MDCT—axial image. There is an non-calcified plaque (arrowheads) in the mid-RCA.

who were followed for 16 months after coronary MDCT angiography demonstrated a higher cardiovascular event rate in patients with nonobstructive plaque detected by MDCT compared with individuals without any plaque.[34] These initial observations suggest that there may be a potential value of plaque imaging by MDCT coronary angiography for risk prediction.

Detection of Myocardial Ischemia

Stress perfusion nuclear imaging has several significant limitations: the test is quite lengthy, since it usually requires a stress and a rest study to be performed in separate sessions. In addition, conventional cardiac nuclear imaging has poor spatial resolution and lacks the ability to perform quantitative measurement of perfusion. It also suffers from attenuation artifacts. More importantly, it exposes patients to significant doses of ionizing radiation. Finally, nuclear imaging lacks specificity for detection of CAD. Therefore, alternatives for conventional perfusion nuclear imaging would be clearly desirable.

Although PET perfusion imaging can overcome many of these limitations,[35] its complexity and cost, and the requirement to have either a cyclotron or a rubidium generator on-site, have prevented widespread use of the technique. CMR has proven to be a more practical alternative for stress perfusion imaging. Since the physiological half-life of gadolinium-based contrast agents is short, it is possible to repeat a rest perfusion scan several minutes after the stress study.

There are several important differences between the mechanism by which these two modalities assess myocardial perfusion. With Thallium-201 or TC-99m sestamibi SPECT, the signal intensity in the myocardium depends on the myocardial blood flow and the amount of viable cells extracting the tracer into the intracellular space. Therefore, areas with decreased myocardial perfusion as well as areas with a reduced number of viable cells result in reduced tracer uptake. In contrast, the myocardial signal intensity on CMR images during first-pass perfusion of a paramagnetic contrast agent depends on myocardial blood flow, vascular permeability, and the size of the extracellular space. The viability of myocardial cells does not affect signal characteristics. Thus, reperfused but infarcted myocardium appears dark on SPECT images, whereas it may be isointense to normal myocardium on first-pass CMR at rest.

Theoretical advantages of CMR perfusion imaging over nuclear SPECT are its significantly higher spatial resolution, allowing detection of subendocardial ischemia; the possibility to combine evaluation of myocardial ischemia with evaluation of contractile function and myocardial viability all within 30 minutes; and most importantly, the absence of radiation exposure. Several single-center studies and two smaller multicenter trials have been performed for the clinical evaluation of CMR perfusion imaging. The results of 12 of these single-center and the two multicenter trials were summarized in a meta-analysis.[36] In a total of 1183 patients (after exclusion of 50 patients secondary to unsuccessful CMR studies), this technique was found to have a sensitivity of 91% [95% confidence interval (CI) 88–94%] and a specificity of 81% (95% CI 77–85%) for detection of coronary artery disease. The major limitation of all these trials was their small size. Furthermore, there remains a lot of uncertainty and variation among doses of contrast agents, scanner hardware, and perfusion sequences. This limited the generalization of the findings.

The MR-IMPACT study by Schwitter et al.[37] is the largest published study on perfusion CMR in comparison with other modalities, across multiple CMR vendors and operators. This prospective double-blind randomized study of 241 patients compared the effect of five different contrast doses on image quality and diagnostic accuracy of perfusion CMR. It also compared the diagnostic accuracy of perfusion CMR at the best dose vs SPECT for detection of significant CAD using catheter angiography as reference standard. Perfusion-CMR at the optimal contrast dose (0.1 mmol/kg) had similar performance as SPECT, if only the SPECT studies of the 42 patients with this dose were considered ($P = 0.12$); however, diagnostic performance of perfusion-CMR was better vs. the entire SPECT population ($P = 0.013$).

Ingkanisorn et al. evaluated the prognostic role of adenosine perfusion CMR on 135 patients presenting to the emergency department with troponin-negative chest pain.[38] The perfusion abnormalities had 100% sensitivity and 93% specificity as the single most accurate component of the CMR examination. Compared to conventional risk factors, presence of perfusion abnormalities was a stronger predictor of future cardiac events. In ROC (receiver operator characteristic) analysis, adenosine CMR was a more accurate predictor than cardiac risk factors ($P < 0.002$). A negative perfusion CMR predicted an excellent prognosis at 1 year follow-up.

Despite these enthusiastic prospects, it is important to understand that perfusion CMR does have important limitations and contraindications, which will prevent unrestricted use in every patient. Patients with devices such as pacemakers and AICDs cannot undergo CMR. This modality will also not be tolerated well by claustrophobic patients. Image quality is significantly hampered by arrhythmias. The optimal performance of the technique is also associated with a steep learning curve. Finally, gadolinium-based contrast media have been associated with the development of nephrogenic systemic sclerosis in patients with renal failure.

Myocardial Viability

Human studies demonstrate that delayed enhancement magnetic resonance imaging (DE-MRI) is effective in identifying the presence, location, and extent of MI in both the acute and chronic settings. Additionally, DE-MRI provides scar size measurements that are closely correlated with PET, and provides results superior to SPECT in patients with subendocardial infarctions. This advantage of DE-MRI stems from its high spatial resolution. With a standard implementation, a voxel 6 mm in a typical DE-MRI image would represent an infarction of 0.16 grams. This level of resolution is more than 40 times greater than with SPECT. Hence, even micro infarcts, which cannot be visualized with any other technique, can be seen with CMR.

Another advantage of DE-MRI over nuclear imaging is that it provides direct visualization of both non-viable as well as the viable myocardium. Concurrently, in the setting of acute MI, DE-MRI can differentiate between acute infarcts with necrotic myocytes and acute infarcts with necrotic myocytes and damaged microvasculature (the latter being termed as "no-reflow" phenomenon). Microvascular obstruction appears as a dark rim of hypoenhancement within the hyperenhanced infarcted myocardium. A SPECT or PET scan would have simply identified this as being non-viable due to reduced tracer activity. The detection of myocardial segments with profound microvascular damage has an important bearing on outcomes of revascularization and prognosis of patients following acute MI.[39]

Presence of mural thrombus can be missed on ECHO, but is reliably picked up on DE-MRI as a hypointense mass overlying the intarcted ventricular wall **(Fig. 9)**. MRI is the only technique that can consistently demonstrate thrombus in patients following MI.

Kim et al. demonstrated the importance of CMR in the evaluation of myocardial viability.[40] They analyzed 50 patients with ventricular dysfunction who underwent DE-MRI before and after revascularization. About 80% had some regions of hyperenhancement on the pre-intervention CMR, while 38% had abnormal contractility. The likelihood of wall motion improvement was strongly correlated to the transmural extent of hyperenhancement. In patients without hyperenhancement, 78% of segments showed improved contractility after revascularization, compared to only 1 of 58 segments improving if there was more than 75% transmural hyperenhancement. In patients with myocardial hyperenhancement involving 51 to 75% of the wall, only 10% of revascularized segments showed improved contractility. This was an extremely important study with great impact on the therapeutic management of patient with LV dysfunction and hibernating myocardium, since it meant that it was possible to target revascularization to vessel supplying blood to a territory where functional recovery can be reliably predicted. The ability of CE-CMR to discriminate between viable and non-viable myocardium in the same region has important implications in the understanding of myocardial thinning,

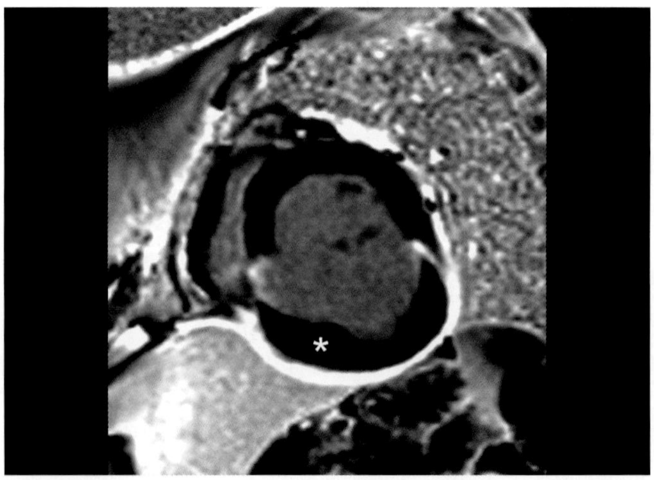

Fig. 9: DE-MRI—short axis view: There is a transmural infarct (hyperenhanced rim) in the inferior, inferoseptal and inferolateral segments (RCA territory). Overlying the infarct, there is a hypointense mural thrombus (*).

resulting in a paradigm shift. Conventional understanding is that very thin myocardium (<5 mm) represents essentially transmural infarction and hence is unlikely to recover function following revascularization.[41] With DE-MRI, studies have shown that even thinned myocardium can recover function, sometimes dramatically, if it does not show late enhancement.[42]

The ability of DE-MRI to detect and characterize myocardial scar has been compared to SPECT and PET. Kuhl et al. compared DE-MRI with combined PET/SPECT in their assessment of reversible myocardial dysfunction in patients with chronic IHD.[43] Sensitivity and specificity for the prediction of functional recovery at follow-up was 97 and 68% for DE-MRI and 87 and 76% for PET/SPECT. The positive predictive value was identical for both techniques (73%). However, DE-MRI achieved a higher negative predictive value (93 vs 77%, respectively), indicating that it may be superior to PET/SPECT for the identification of segments unlikely to recover function after revascularization. Both methods had a similar yield in the prediction of global functional improvement. Wagner et al. studied patients with suspected or known CAD who underwent both DE-MRI and SPECT and the results were validated with an animal model.[44] For transmural infarcts, both studies had similar rate of detection. However, of the 181 segments that had subendocardial infarcts on CMR, 47% were missed by SPECT. On comparison with PET in patients with ischemic heart failure, Klein and their colleagues showed that DE-CMR was superior for detection of subendocardial infarction.[45] The results of these studies are not surprising, since CMR has a higher spatial resolution, as described above. Accordingly, CMR is the current gold standard for myocardial viability assessment.

Myocardial Function

Cine-CMR is a robust noninvasive technique for assessment of regional and global systolic function of both ventricles. The development of segmented k-space techniques allows for breath-held cine-MRI, making possible a rapid acquisition of the entire ventricles in short axis. Since ventricular volume estimations are made without any geometrical assumption, this method is particularly well suited for remodeled ventricles in patients with IHD. Regional function can be equally well studied by cine-MRI both qualitatively and quantitatively, as it represents the best technique in defining endo- and epi-cardial borders.[46] Further, myocardial tagging is a novel technique for assessing complex mechanism of myocardial contraction and to quantify myocardial strain. Recently, the application of myocardial tagging has been shown to improve the accuracy of dobutamine CMR in both the evaluation of viability and the detection of significant coronary stenosis.[47,48] Finally, MRI is also able to assess diastolic function with phase velocity mapping.

CMR has been shown to have better inter-study reproducibility compared with ECHO in normal subjects and patients.[49] For these reasons, CMR is considered the gold standard for assessment of ventricular function.

RECENT ADVANCES ON CT FOR ASSESSMENT OF CORONARY ARTERY STENOSIS

Over the last 5 years. there has been rapid advancement in CT technology, with increasing number of detectors and gantry rotation time. These have led to application of functional MDCT techniques for better evaluatoin of coronary artery disease. Two of these techniques are myocardial stress CT perfusion and CT-derived fractional flow reserve (CT-FFR). They are currently under research evaluation for guiding clinical management in appropriately selected patients with suspected ischemic heart disease. Briefly, CT perfusion is a myocardial perfusion imaging technique that measures the amount of iodine contrast present within the myocardium, allowing one to create an attenuation map of the left ventricle analogous to a single-photon emission CT (SPECT) perfusion map.[50] FFRCT, in contrast, is a computational fluid dynamics modeling technique that can be applied to a CT coronary angiography (CTCA) dataset for estimating lesion-specific functional information of a coronary stenosis without requiring any protocol modifications.[51] Both CT perfusion and FFRCT are complementary to CTCA and offer greater specificity and positive predictive value for detecting hemodynamically significant coronary artery disease (CAD) compared with anatomic imaging alone. The two strategies are particularly valuable in guiding clinical management for patients with moderate stenosis (50–70%) detected on CTCA and in special circumstances when the accuracy of CTCA is compromised, such as in patients with coronary stents and heavily calcified arteries. Data from the FAME (Fractional Flow Reserve Versus Angiography for Multivessel Evaluation)[52] and FAME 2 (Fractional Flow Reserve (FFR) Guided Percutaneous Coronary Intervention (PCI) Plus Optimal Medical Treatment (OMT) verses OMT)[53] trials have demonstrated that invasive fractional flow reserve ischemic-guided revascularization reduce major adverse cardiac events (MACE), whereas angiographic strategies alone are ineffective for guiding revascularization. Functional CT imaging in combination with CTCA offers an opportunity for comprehensive noninvasive evaluation of coronary anatomy and function within a single imaging session, leveraging both the strong negative predictive value of CTCA in low-to-intermediate-risk patients and the higher specificity and positive predictive value of CT perfusion and FFRCT in intermediate- to high-risk patients.

In appropriately selected patients, CT perfusion and FFRCT are ready for clinical use in light of their demonstrated added value across four key domains: (1) improvement in accuracy for hemodynamically significant CAD, (2) safety and improvement in patient outcomes, (3) reduction in healthcare costs, and (4) streamlined diagnostic workflow.

FUTURE DIRECTIONS

Continuing technical developments should increase the clinical value of cardiac MDCT and CMR still further. Novel CMR techniques combining high temporal and spatial resolution may make it possible to produce accurate coronary artery assessments. For imaging of atherosclerotic coronary plaques, dual-source MDCT or spectral CT technology may replace the current CT methods for plaque characterization that rely on Hounsfield units. CMR contrast agents are also being developed to identify vulnerable plaques, by targeting mediators of neovascularization or macrophages in inflamed plaques.[54,55]

Although MDCT has emerged as a reliable tool for coronary imaging, an abnormal scan does not necessarily predict ischemia. In fact, since MDCT and perfusion imaging provide different and complementary information, their sequential use or hybrid imaging may provide useful incremental information. Combining noninvasive imaging modalities for assessments of cardiac perfusion, coronary morphology and myocardial function (e.g. hybrid MDCT-CMR or hybrid PET-MDCT) will give new insights into the mechanisms of cardiovascular disease. In one study, hybrid PET/CT was evaluated in patients with suspected CAD, which yielded a sensitivity and specificity of 90 and 98%, respectively, for the detection of hemodynamically relevant coronary artery stenoses.[56] This approach promises to have a significant impact on clinical decision making.

Appropriateness Criteria for Use of Cardiac MDCT and CMR in the Investigation of IHD

According to the appropriateness criteria established by the American College of Cardiology,[57] the use of MDCT is considered appropriate (with a score between 7 and 9 on a scale of 1 to 9) for IHD in the following situations:

1. Detection of CAD in patient with chest pain with:
   - Intermediate pre-test probability of CAD
   - ECG uninterpretable or unable to exercise
2. Evaluation of suspected coronary anomalies
3. Evaluation of acute chest pain syndrome in patient with:
   - Intermediate pre-test probability of CAD
   - No ECG changes and serial enzyme negative
4. Detection of CAD in patients with chest pain syndrome with:
   - Uninterpretable or equivocal stress test (Exercise, perfusion or stress ECHO)

CMR is considered appropriate in the following conditions involving CAD patients:

1. DSMR and perfusion CMR for both the detection of CAD in symptomatic patients with intermediate pre-test probability of CAD and either uninterpretable ECG or unable to exercise, and for the risk assessment in patients with stenosis of unclear significance on coronary angiography
2. Coronary MR angiography for the evaluation of suspected coronary anomalies
3. LV function assessment in patients following myocardial infarction or heart failure with poor ECHO windows or in patients with discordant information from prior tests
4. Evaluation of myocarditis or MI with normal coronary arteries
5. DE-MRI to evaluate myocardial necrosis, including no-reflow regions, in post-acute MI; to establish the likelihood of recovery of function with revacularization or medical therapy and to evaluate viability when SPECT or dobutamine stress ECHO has provided equivocal or indeterminate results.

CONCLUSION

Noninvasive cardiac imaging is now central to the diagnosis and management of patients with known or suspected IHD. However, neither MDCT or CMR will ever replace any of the existing modalities. ECHO can be performed as a bedside examination, which is a considerable advantage for acutely ill patients. Cardiac catheterization offers the option of simultaneously performing coronary interventions. Among the newer modalities, the pretest likelihood of disease becomes the most important determinant of the initial test. If the likelihood is very low, no testing is needed. However, if the likelihood is low, recent data suggest that assessment of early atherosclerosis is likely to be the most useful and cost-effective test. In patients who have an intermediate likelihood of CAD, stress perfusion with nuclear imaging becomes highly valuable; however, MDCT may emerge as the initial test of choice. MPS would then be used if the MDCT is inconclusive or if there is a need to assess the functional significance of a stenosis defined by MDCT. MDCT however, is not yet widely available and is limited in patients with dense coronary calcification. In older patients with a high likelihood of CAD, MPS may be the initial test of choice, since a high proportion of these patients have too much coronary calcium to allow accurate assessment of the presence of coronary stenoses. PET/CT or SPECT/CT could emerge as important modalities combining the advantages of each modality. While CMR currently lags behind CTA for noninvasive coronary angiography, it has already emerged as a highly effective method for assessing ventricular function, myocardial mass, and myocardial viability, and there is increasing use of this approach for clinical rest and stress perfusion measurements.

REFERENCES

1. Ahmad N, Bhopal R. Is coronary heart disease rising in India? A systematic review based on ECG defined coronary heart disease. Heart. 2005;91:719-25.
2. Nesto RW, Kowalchuk GJ. The ischemic cascade: Temporal sequence of hemodynamic, electrocardiographic and symptomatic expressions of ischemia. Am J Cardiol. 1987;59:23C-30C.
3. Iskander S, Iskandrian AE. Risk assessment using single-photon emission computed tomographic technetium-99m sestamibi imaging. J Am Coll Cardiol. 1998;32:57.
4. Bonow RO. Identification of viable myocardium. Circulation. 1996;94:2674-80.
5. Smanio PE, Watson DD, Segalla DL, et al. Value of gating of technetium-99 m sestamibi single-photon emission computed tomographic imaging. J Am Coll Cardiol. 1997;30:1687-92.
6. Bax JJ, Van der Wall EE, De Roos A, et al. Clinical nuclear cardiology. In: Zaret Bl, Beller GA (Eds). State-of-the-art and future directions. Philadelphia, Mosby; 2005. pp. 535-55.
7. Kaul S, Senior R, Dittrich H, et al. Detection of coronary artery disease with myocardial contrast echocardiography: Comparison with 99mTc-sestamibi single-photon emission computed tomography. Circulation.1997;96:785-92.
8. Matt D, Scheffel H, Leschka S, et al. Dual-source CT coronary angiography: Image quality, mean heart rate, and heart rate variability. AJR Am J Roentgenol. 2007;189(3):567-73.
9. Flohr TG, Schoepf UJ, Ohnesorge BM. Chasing the heart: New developments for cardiac CT. J Thorac Imaging. 2007;22(1):14-6.
10. Jakobs TF, Becker CR, Ohnesorge B, et al. Multislice helical CT of the heart with retrospective ECG gating: reduction of radiation exposure by ECG-controlled tube current modulation. Eur Radiol. 2002;12(5):1081-6.
11. Francone M, Di Castro E, Napoli A, et al. Dose reduction and image quality assessment in 64-detector row computed tomography of the coronary arteries using an automatic exposure control system. J Comput Assist Tomogr. 2008; 32(5):668-78.
12. Husmann L, Valenta I, Gaemperli O, et al. Feasibility of low-dose coronary CT angiography: first experience with prospective ECG-gating. Eur Heart J. 2008;29(2):191-7.
13. Husmann L, Valenta I, Kaufmann PA. Coronary angiography with low-dose computed tomography at 1.4 mSv Herz. 2008;33(1):75.
14. Kido T, Kurata A, Higashino H, et al. Cardiac imaging using 256-detector row four-dimensional CT: preliminary clinical report. Radiat Med. 2007;25(25):38-44.
15. Leber AW, Johnson T, Becker A, et al. Diagnostic accuracy of dual-source multislice CT-coronary angiography in patients with an intermediate pretest likelihood for coronary artery disease. Eur Heart J. 2007;28:2354-60.
16. Nikolaou K, Knez A, Rist C, et al. Accuracy of 64-MDCT in the diagnosis of ischemic heart disease. Am J Roentgenol. 2006;187:111-7.
17. Weustink AC, Meijboom WB, Mollet NR, et al. Reliable high-speed coronary computed tomography in symptomatic patients. J Am Coll Cardiol. 2007;50:786-94.
18. Schroeder S, Achenbach S, Bengel F, et al. Cardiac computed tomography: Indications, applications, limitations, and training requirements. Eur Heart J. 2008;29(4):531-56.
19. Pugliese F, Mollet NR, Runza G, et al. Diagnostic accuracy of non-invasive 64-slice CT coronary angiography in patients with stable angina pectoris. Eur Radiol. 2006;16(3):575-82.
20. Ohnesorge BM, Hofmann LK, Flohr TG, et al. CT for imaging coronary artery disease: Defining the paradigm for its application. Int J Cardiovasc Imaging. 2005;21(1):85-104.
21. Hoffmann U, Nagurney JT, Moselewski F, et al. Coronary multidetector computed tomography in the assessment of patients with acute chest pain. Circulation. 2006;114:2251-60.
22. Goldstein JA, Gallagher MJ, O'Neill WW, et al. A randomized controlled trial of multislice coronary computed tomography for evaluation of acute chest pain. J Am Coll Cardiol. 2007;49:863-71.
23. Kim SY, Seo JB, Do KH, et al. Coronary artery anomalies: Classification and ECG-gated multidetector row CT findings with angiographic correlation. Radiographics. 2006;26:317-33.
24. Schmid M, Achenbach S, Ludwig J, et al. Visualization of coronary artery anomalies by contrast-enhanced multidetector row spiral computed tomography. Int J Cardiol. 2006;111:430-5.
25. Budoff MJ, Achenbach S, Blumenthal RS, et al. Assessment of coronary artery disease by cardiac computed tomography: A scientific statement from the American Heart Association Committee on Cardiovascular Imaging and Intervention, Council on Cardiovascular Radiology and Intervention, and Committee on Cardiac Imaging, Council on Clinical Cardiology. Circulation. 2006;114:1761-91.

26. Schmermund A, Erbel R. Unstable coronary plaque and its relation to coronary calcium. Circulation. 2001;104:1682-7.
27. Greenland P, Bonow RO, Brundage BH, et al. ACCF/AHA 2007 clinical expert consensus document on coronary artery calcium scoring by computed tomography in global cardiovascular risk assessment and in evaluation of patients with chest pain: A report of the American College of Cardiology Foundation Clinical Expert Consensus Task Force (ACCF/AHA Writing Committee to Update the 2000 Expert Consensus Document on Electron Beam Computed Tomography). Circulation. 2007;115:402-26.
28. De Backer G, Ambrosioni E, Borch-Johnsen K, et al. European guidelines on cardiovascular disease prevention in clinical practice. Third Joint Task Force of European and other Societies on Cardiovascular Disease Prevention in Clinical Practice (constituted by representatives of eight societies and by invited experts). Atherosclerosis. 2004;173:381-91.
29. Naghavi M, Falk E, Hecht HS, et al. From vulnerable plaque to vulnerable patient— part III: executive summary of the Screening for Heart Attack Prevention and Education (SHAPE) Task Force report. Am J Cardiol. 2006;98:2H-15H.
30. Leber AW, Becker A, Knez A, et al. Accuracy of 64-slice computed tomography to classify and quantify plaque volumes in the proximal coronary system: A comparative study using intravascular ultrasound. J Am Coll Cardiol. 2006;47:672-7.
31. Schoenhagen P, Tuzcu EM, Stillman AE, et al. Non-invasive assessment of plaque morphology and remodeling in mildly stenotic coronary segments: comparison of 16-slice computed tomography and intravascular ultrasound. Coron Artery Dis. 2003;14:459-62.
32. Moselewski F, Ropers D, Pohle K, et al. Comparison of measurement of cross-sectional coronary atherosclerotic plaque and vessel areas by 16-slice multidetector computed tomography versus intravascular ultrasound. Am J Cardiol. 2004;94:1294-7.
33. Motoyama S, Kondo T, Sarai M, et al. Multislice computed tomographic characteristics of coronary lesions in acute coronary syndromes. J Am Coll Cardiol. 2007;50:319-26.
34. Pundziute G, Schuijf JD, Jukema JW, et al. Prognostic value of multislice computed tomography coronary angiography in patients with known or suspected coronary artery disease. J Am Coll Cardiol. 2007;49:62-70.
35. Di Carli MF, Hachamovitch R. New technology for noninvasive evaluation of coronary artery disease. Circulation. 2007;115:1464-80.
36. Nandalur KR, Dwamena BA, Choudhri AF, et al. Diagnostic performance of stress cardiac magnetic resonance imaging in the detection of coronary artery disease: a meta-analysis. J Am Coll Cardiol. 2007;50:1343-53.
37. Schwitter J, Wacker CM, van Rossum AC, et al. MR-IMPACT: comparison of perfusion-cardiac magnetic resonance with single-photon emission computed tomography for the detection of coronary artery disease in a multicentre, multivendor, randomized trial. Eur Heart J. 2008;29:480-9.
38. Ingkanisorn WP, Kwong RY, Bohme NS, et al. Prognosis of negative adenosine stress magnetic resonance in patients presenting to an emergency department with chest pain. J Am Coll Cardiol. 2006;47:1427-32.
39. Wu KC, Zerhouni EA, Judd RM, et al. Prognostic significance of microvascular obstruction by magnetic resonance imaging in patients with acute myocardial infarction. Circulation. 1998;97:765-72.
40. Kim RJ, Wu E, Rafael A, et al. The use of contrast-enhanced magnetic resonance imaging to identify reversible myocardial dysfunction. N Engl J Med. 2000;343:1445-53.
41. Cwajg JM, Cwajg E, Nagueh SF, et al. End-diastolic wall thickness as a predictor of recovery of function in myocardial hibernation: Relation to rest-redistribution T1-201 tomography and dobutamine stress echocardiography. J Am Coll Cardiol. 2000;35:1152-61.
42. John AS, Dreyfus GD, Pennell DJ. Images in cardiovascular medicine. Reversible wall thinning in hibernation predicted by cardiovascular magnetic resonance. Circulation. 2005;111:e24-e25.
43. Kühl HP, Lipke CS, Krombach GA, et al. Assessment of reversible myocardial dysfunction in chronic ischaemic heart disease: comparison of contrast-enhanced cardiovascular magnetic resonance and a combined positron emission tomography-single photon emission computed tomography imaging protocol. Eur Heart J. 2006;27(7):846-53.
44. Wagner A, Mahrholdt H, A Holly TA, et al. Contrast-enhanced MRI and routine single photon emission computed tomography (SPECT) perfusion imaging for detection of subendocardial myocardial infarcts: an imaging study. Lancet. 2003;361:374-9.
45. Klein C, Nekolla SG, Bengel FM, et al. Assessment of myocardial viability with contrast-enhanced magnetic resonance imaging: Comparison with positron emission tomography. Circulation. 2002;105:162-7.
46. Bellenger NG, Davies LC, Francio JM, et al. Reduction in sample size for studies of remodelling in heart failure by the use of cardiovascular magnetic resonance. J Cardiovasc Magn Reson. 2000;2:271-8.
47. Kramer CM, Malkowski MJ, Mankad S, et al. Magnetic resonance tagging and echocardiographic response to dobutamine and functional improvement after reperfused myocardial infarction. Am Heart J. 2002;143:1046-51.
48. Kuijpers D, Ho KY, van Dijkman PR, et al. Dobutamine cardiovascular magnetic resonance for the detection of myocardial ischemia with the use of myocardial tagging. Circulation. 2003;107:1592-7.
49. Grothues F, Smith GC, Moon JCC, et al. Comparison of inter-study reproducibility of cardiovascular magnetic resonance with two-dimensional echocardiography in normal subjects and in-patients with heart failure or left ventricular hypertrophy. Am J Cardiol.2002;90:29-34.
50. Rochitte CE, George RT, Chen MY, et al. Computed tomography angiography and perfusion to assess coronary artery stenosis causing perfusion defects by single photon

emission computed tomography: the CORE320 study. Eur Heart J. 2014;35:1120-30.
51. Koo BK, Erglis A, Doh JH, et al. Diagnosis of ischemia-causing coronary stenoses by noninvasive fractional flow reserve computed from coronary computed tomographic angiograms. Results from the prospective multicenter DISCOVER-FLOW (Diagnosis of Ischemia-Causing Stenoses Obtained Via Noninvasive Fractional Flow Reserve) study. J Am Coll Cardiol. 2011;58:1989-97.
52. Tonino PA, De Bruyne B, Pijls NH, et al. Fractional flow reserve versus angiography for guiding percutaneous coronary intervention. N Engl J Med. 2009;360:213-24.
53. De Bruyne B, Fearon WF, Pijls NH, et al. Fractional flow reserve-guided PCI for stable coronary artery disease. N Engl J Med. 2014;371:1208-17.
54. Flohr TG, McCollough CH, Bruder H, et al. First performance evaluation of a dual-source CT (DSCT) system. Eur Radiol. 2006;16(2):256-68.
55. Johnson TR, Nikolaou K, Wintersperger BJ, et al. Dual-source CT cardiac imaging: Initial experience. Eur Radiol. 2006;16(7):1409-15.
56. Namdar M, Hany TF, Koepfli P, et al. Integrated PET/CT for the assessment of coronary artery disease: a feasibility study. J Nucl Med. 2005;46:930-5.
57. Hendel RC, Patel MR, Kramer CM, et al. ACCF/ACR/SCCT/SCMR/ASNC/NASCI/SCAI/SIR 2006 appropriateness criteria for cardiac computed tomography and cardiac magnetic resonance imaging: a report of the American College of Cardiology Foundation Quality Strategic Directions Committee Appropriateness Criteria Working Group, American College of Radiology, Society of Cardiovascular Computed Tomography, Society for Cardiovascular Magnetic Resonance, American Society of Nuclear Cardiology, North American Society for Cardiac Imaging, Society for Cardiovascular Angiography and Interventions, and Society of Interventional Radiology. J Am Coll Cardiol. 2006;48(7):1475-97.

CHAPTER 179

Imaging in Cardiomyopathies

Priya Jagia, Gurpreet Singh Gulati, Sanjiv Sharma

INTRODUCTION

Cardiomyopathies (CMPs) comprise a spectrum of chronic progressive myocardial disorders which have distinct pattern of morphological, functional and electro- physiological changes. The expert consensus panel (2006) of the American Heart Association has proposed the following definition: "Cardiomyopathies are a heterogeneous group of diseases of the myocardium associated with mechanical and/or electrical dysfunction that usually (but not invariably) exhibit inappropriate ventricular hypertrophy or dilatation and are due to a variety of causes that frequently are genetic. Cardiomyopathies are either confined to the heart or are part of generalized systemic disorders, often leading to cardiovascular death or progressive heart failure-related disability".

CLASSIFICATION

Cardiomyopathies (CMPs) are broadly classified into: (1) Primary CMPs (genetic, nongenetic, acquired) comprise those few conditions that are either solely or predominantly confined to heart muscle. (2) Secondary CMPs are those group of conditions where the myocardial involvement occurs as part of a large number and heterogeneous variety of systemic disorders, usually affecting multiple organ systems.

This chapter will focus on those CMPs that can be diagnosed based upon the currently available imaging modalities. These include dilated, hypertrophic, restrictive, arrhythmogenic right ventricular and certain miscellaneous group of CMPs.

DIAGNOSTIC TECHNIQUES

It is important to detect exact cause of CMP as this determines the treatment and the patient survival. Echocardiography (ECHO) and radionuclide imaging alone cannot determine the exact etiology due to inadequate myocardial assessment (inferior spatial and contrast resolution and limited tissue characterization). Catheter angiography assesses only chamber lumen, with poor demonstration of myocardial changes. Also, significant overlap of features between CMPs frequently exists. Endomyocardial biopsy, though is the gold standard technique but has limitations in the form of sampling errors and poor sensitivity.

Cardiac multislice computed tomography (MSCT) can demonstrate ventricular function and some myocardial features. But **cardiac MR (CMR) is now considered the 'in vivo' gold standard imaging modality for the diagnosis and treatment monitoring of CMPs**. It provides high-resolution images of the heart in any desired plane without any radiation. Spin echo (SE) T1- and T2-weighted imaging allows for tissue characterization. Cine CMR helps assess cardiac morphology and function. Passage of gadolinium through the LV myocardium can be imaged during its first pass at rest and this provides important information about contrast kinetics of the myocardium. Delayed enhanced CMR (DE-CMR) helps to differentiate ischemic from nonischemic CMP. Late enhancement occurs in conditions where the extracellular volume is enlarged due to myocardial fibrosis, inflammation or edema. Delayed enhancement in non-ischemic myocardial disease does not correspond to any coronary artery territory and is often midwall rather than in subendocardial or transmural location.

All the various CMPs as described in this chapter are appropriate indications for performing a CMR examination, according to the recently published appropriateness criteria for CMR/cardiac CT.

DILATED CARDIOMYOPATHY

The anatomical abnormalities of dilated cardiomyopathy (DCM) include biatrial enlargement and increased size of the left (LV) and right (RV) ventricles **(Fig. 1)**. There may be pleural or pericardial effusion, SVC/IVC dilatation or ventricular thrombus. The functional abnormalities are in the form of segmental wall motion abnormalities or global dysfunction. Tagging sequences can help detect even subtle wall motion abnormalities mitral or tricuspid regurgitation, if present, can be well demonstrated on both ECG-gated CT and cine MR.

The pattern of enhancement in the myocardium can help differentiate LV dysfunction related to ischemia or nonischemic cardiomyopathy on CMR. Majority of DCM patients do not show contrast uptake. But in some patients, the late enhancement is seen in midmyocardium in a noncoronary pattern, which is clearly distinguishable from coronary artery disease (CAD). CMR helps in quantifying the effects of therapy in these patients.

Hypertrophic Cardiomyopathy

Hypertrophic CMP is characterized by significant myocardial hypertrophy which may be symmetric or asymmetric, when it is regional in distribution.

Asymmetric hypertrophy at the LV apex may not be evaluated with echo. Cardiac CT and CMR define the site and extent of hypertrophy, especially at LV apex.

Cardiac function and flow dynamics of the outflow in cases of hypertrophic obstructive cardiomyopathy (HOCM), including systolic anterior motion of mitral valve, are well seen on cine-CMR and cardiac CT images. Precise planimetric measurements of the left ventricular outflow tract (LVOT) area during systole can also be determined on CMR. Myocardial tagging on CMR identifies regional myocardial strain and shear abnormalities. DE-CMR demonstrates a pattern of contrast uptake in the areas of hypertrophy **(Fig. 2)** or at the RV insertion points on the septum. Patients showing hyperenhancement are at increased risk of sudden cardiac death. Bello et al. showed that patients with late enhancement usually will not respond to heart failure drug therapy and will need an implantable defibrillator. The CMR can help monitor the functional and anatomical outcome of surgical and pharmacological septal ablation.

The CMR is useful to screen the relatives of probands also.

Restrictive Cardiomyopathy

The World Health Organization (WHO) defines restrictive cardiomyopathy (RCM) as a myocardial disease characterized by restrictive filling and reduced diastolic volume of either or both ventricles with normal or near-normal systolic function and wall thickness and it accounts for nearly 5% of all primary heart muscle disorders.

The RCM is identified on CT and MRI by normal LV size and normal or mildly impaired systolic function,

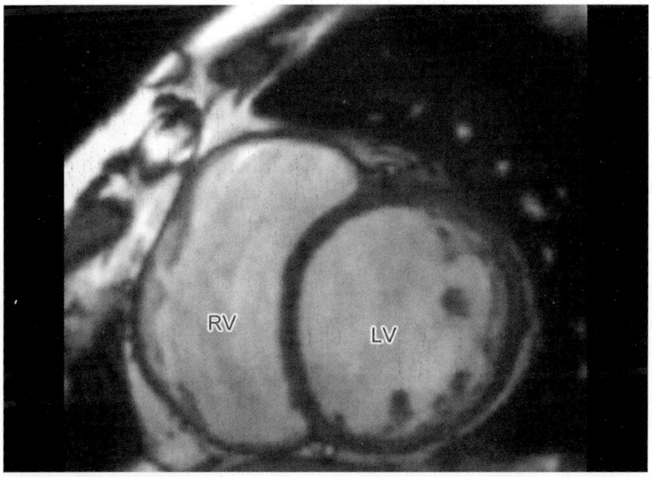

Fig. 1: Short axis image showing dilated right ventricle (RV) and left ventricle (LV) with thinned out walls in patient with dilated cardiomyopathy.

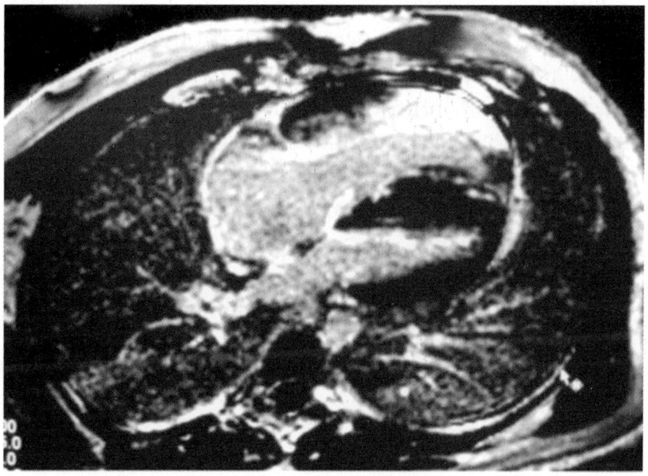

Fig. 2: Case of hypertrophic cardiomyopathy showing delayed dense enhancement in areas of hypertrophy in RV, interventricular septum and LV in this delayed enhanced four-chamber MR image.

abnormal severe diastolic ventricular function and biatrial enlargement **(Fig. 3)**. CMR can characterize tissue, identify anatomic .alterations and can quantify myocardial mass, ventricular volumes and ejection fraction, thus making it a useful modality for investigating infiltrative or restrictive CMPs.

Common infiltrative disorders of the heart include amyloidosis, sarcoidosis, hemochromatosis (or siderotic CMP), and endomyocardial fibrosis. Rarer causes include storage disorders such as Anderson-Fabry disease and Gaucher's disease.

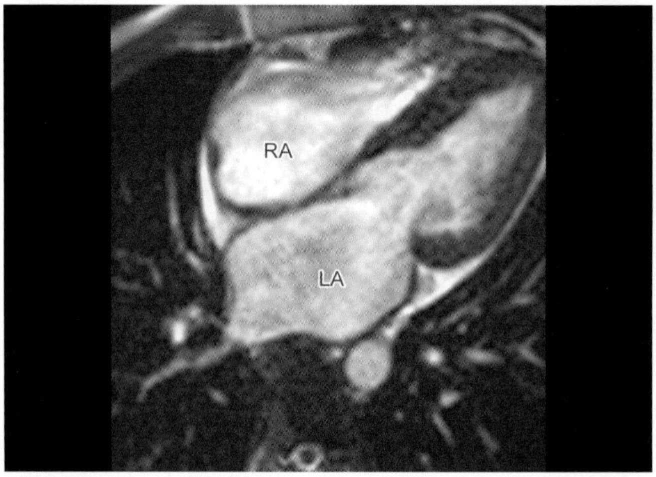

Fig. 3: Four-chamber spin-echo cardiac MRI showing typical biatrial enlargement with normal ventricular size in a patient with amyloidosis.

Amyloidosis

Cardiac amyloidosis is characterized by infiltration of interstitium with amyloid protein. Cardiac involvement is seen with most forms of amyloidosis, although it is most common and most often clinically significant with type AL amyloidosis (primary amyloidosis), often associated with multiple myeloma or other monoclonal gammopathies. It is the most common cause of RCM outside the tropics. In heart it leads to thickening of the left and right ventricular walls **(Fig. 4)**, sometimes associated with thickened atrial walls and the atrioventricular valves. On CT and CMR, the presence of these findings, in combination with pericardial and pleural effusions help to differentiate amyloidosis from hypertrophied myocardium. An increase in thickness of interatrial septum or posterior right atrial wall greater than 6 mm is quite specific for amyloid infiltration. There is a diffuse decrease in the myocardial signal intensity on both T1- and T2-weighted images. A ratio of myocardial to skeletal muscle signal intensity of < 1.0 at 20 ms TE is important feature of cardiac amyloidosis.

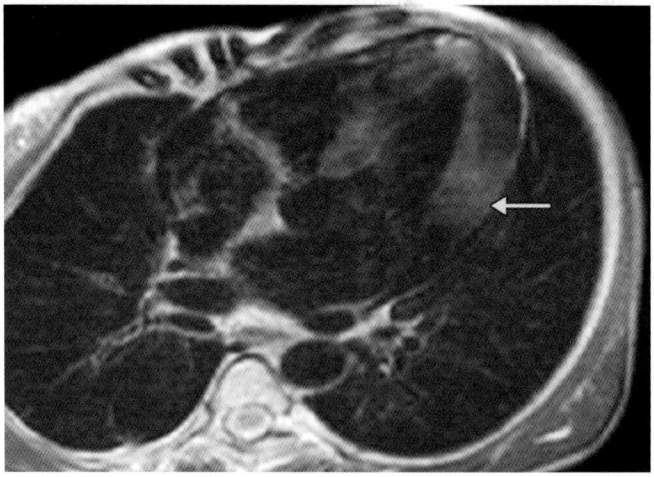

Fig. 4: Case of amyloidosis showing thickening of LV wall on T2 W image.

On DE-CMR, global contrast uptake **(Fig. 5)** is seen typically in the subendocardial location and does not match any specific coronary artery perfusion territory. Mahrholdt et al. reported that if more than 50% of LV myocardium nulls earlier than LV cavity and if this region is not in a coronary artery distribution territory, then the diagnosis of cardiac amyloidosis is highly likely. While performing the DE-CMR examination, the inversion time is shorter than normal and hence nulling occurs earlier. CMR can be used to follow-up the patients on drug therapy in amyloidosis.

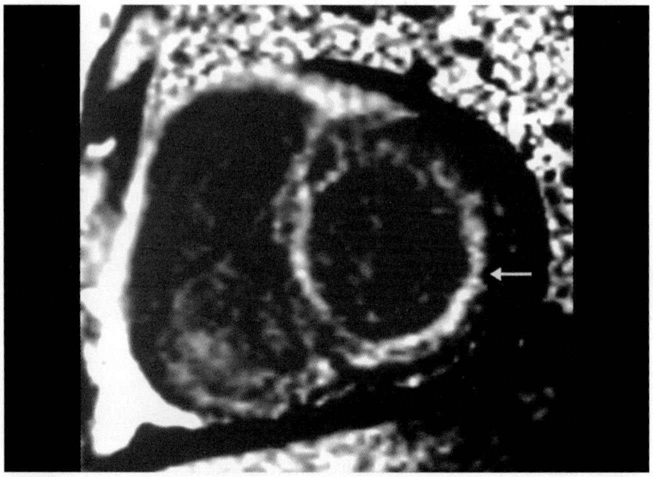

Fig. 5: Typical global subendocardial enhancement on DE-MRI image in short axis in amyloidosis.

Sarcoidosis

Heart is involved in about 25% of patients with sarcoidosis, but causes symptoms in only 5% of cases. An early diagnosis is important since early corticosteroid therapy can help prevent malignant arrhythmias, which can cause in sudden death. CMR is preferred since it shows characteristic abnormalities in cardiac sarcoidosis. In the acute phase, T2-weighted and early gadolinium enhanced images show focal areas of increased signal intensity. Confluent sarcoid granulomas show increased peripheral signal and low signal in the center on T2-weighted images **(Fig. 6)**. Focal myocardial thickening because of edema may be seen. Cine-CMR may show segmental wall motion abnormalities.

On DE-CMR, patchy or focal enhancement **(Fig. 7)** is seen which is often mid wall rather than subendocardial or transmural. The enhancement may be seen in the interventricular septum in basal region and sometimes in the LV wall. Sometimes, papillary muscle and RV wall may be involved. In later stages, features of DCM are seen.

Follow-up CMR can be done to see absent gadolinium uptake. CMR may also show associated features like pericardial effusion, mediastinal adenopathy, etc.

Siderotic (or Iron Overload) Cardiomyopathy

This is seen in patients with hemochromatosis or in those with inherited severe anemias like thalassemia where multiple and regular blood transfusions are required. CMR offers a noninvasive method for detecting heart iron deposition which can cause heart failure and arrhythmias.

CMR reveals an extensive myocardial signal loss on T1- and T2-weighted images, a finding which is more prominent on the T2* images. Focal signal loss is seen in dysfunctional myocardium, associated with a dark liver, which is enough to confirm the diagnosis of systemic hemochromatosis.

Measurement of myocardial T2* on CMR has been found to correlate with LV dysfunction, and has been chemically validated through various studies. CMR has been used for evaluation of different chelation regimes in these patients.

Endomyocardial Fibrosis

Endomyocardial fibrosis (EMF) is characterized by extensive subendocardial fibrosis, apical thrombus formation and progressive diastolic dysfunction. This disease entity is a common cause of RCM in the tropics. It involves the RV more commonly than the LV. The etiology is unknown, though eosinophilia and immunopathological processes are thought to play a role in its pathogenesis.

The CMR findings in EMF include high signal intensity along the endocardium of the apex on T2-weighted sequences, an overlying nonenhancing thrombus, and a distinct high signal intensity plane separating the thrombus from the underlying myocardium on gradient echo cine sequences. Cine-CMR show mitral and tricuspid regurgitation and obliterated apices of the ventricles **(Fig. 8)**.

The DE-CMR shows subendocardial hyperenhancement of the apex, related to endocardial fibrosis **(Fig. 9)**.

Anderson-Fabry Disease

It is an X-linked disorder of lysosomal metabolism, with accumulation of glycosphingolipid in various tissues. In cardiac variant of anderson-fabry disease (AFD), myocardial hypertrophy is the main feature. This hypertrophy appears to be similar to that seen in HCM, but on DE-CMR helps it differentiate from hypertrophic cardiomyopathy (HCM) since the pattern of enhancement is different, with basal inferolateral wall being the commonest segment showing enhancement. Also unlike

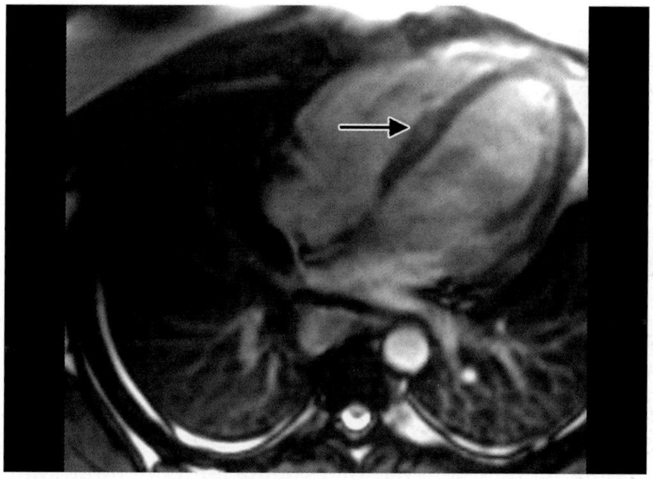

Fig. 6: T2W MR image showing a sarcoid granuloma in interventricular septum in four-chamber view.

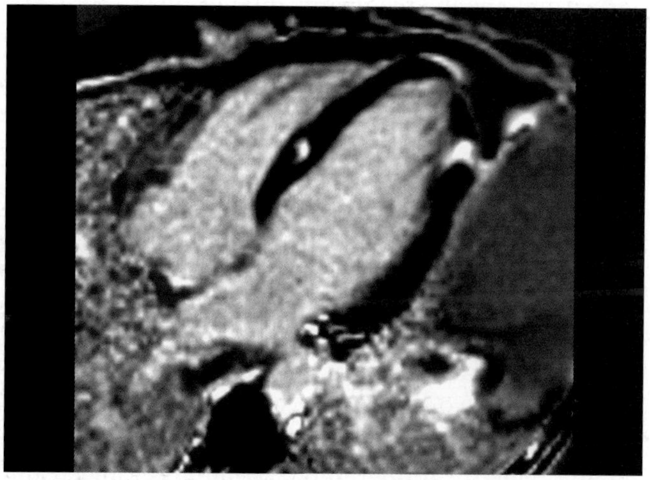

Fig. 7: Same case as in Figure 6—the granuloma shows enhancement on delayed contrast MRI.

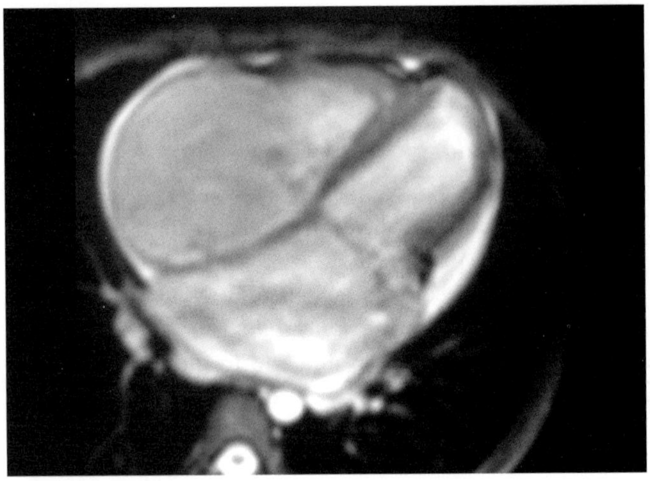

Fig. 8: Case of endomyocardial fibrosis showing obliteration of RV apex.

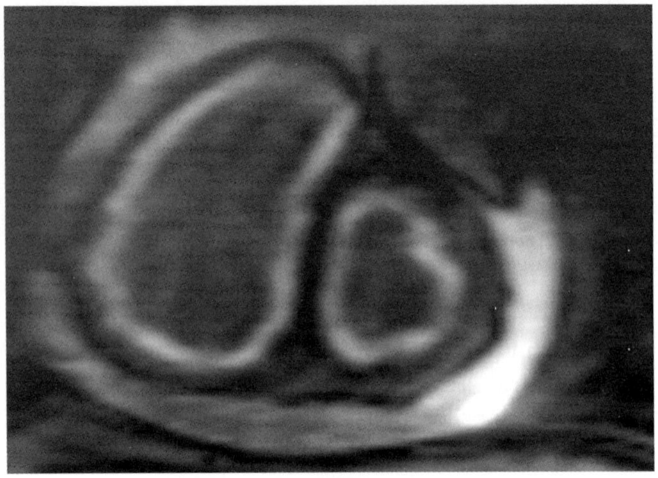

Fig. 9: Global subendocardial enhancement in this case of EMF suggesting gross fibrotic changes.

myocardial infarction, the subendocardium is commonly spared. Presence of myocardial scarring may imply that treatment with enzyme replacement therapy may be less effective at this stage, making a case for early initiation of this treatment before fibrosis has developed.

Tuberculosis

Myocardial tuberculosis is very rare, the reported autopsy incidence being 0.14–0.3%. Tuberculosis of the heart generally involves the pericardium and may result in constrictive pericarditis. Myocardial tuberculosis presenting as restrictive CMP is very unusual, with only 1 report till date. We have till now come across one case (not biopsy proven) of treated pulmonary tuberculosis presenting as restrictive CMP on ECHO. CMR showed diffuse myocardial thickening contiguous with the pericardial involvement and dilated atria. DE-CMR showed dense myocardial and pericardial enhancement.

Arrhythmogenic right ventricular dysplasia (ARVD): The ARVD has uncertain etiology and is marked by fibrosis and fatty replacement of the myocardium. It commonly involves the anterior wall of the right ventricle, in the so-called "triangle of dysplasia" (right ventricular subtricuspid area, the apex and the right ventricular infundibulum). It is more common in young males and has a familial occurrence. It leads to progressive right ventricular failure and dilatation, and is an important cause of sudden cardiac death due to ventricular arrhythmias. The diagnosis of ARVD is based on the presence of major and minor criteria encompassing genetic, electrocardiographic, pathophysiologic, and histopathologic factors. To fulfill the appropriate criteria for ARVD, patients must have either two major criteria, one major and two minor criteria, or four minor criteria.

The traditional imaging modalities used to evaluate right ventricular abnormalities include conventional angiography, echocardiography and radionuclide angiography. However, all of them have low sensitivity and specificity for diagnosing ARVD, primarily because of their inability to accurately characterize structural and functional abnormalities of the right ventricle. Also, all these imaging modalities are limited by a lack of spatial resolution in diagnosing the typical fatty and fibrofatty changes of the right ventricular myocardium. Endomyocardial biopsy suffers from sampling errors, since involvement generally occurs in a segmental fashion and also because it most commonly involves the anterior right ventricular wall, whereas biopsy specimen is usually obtained from the septum.

Due to its high resolution, large field of view and ability to quantify RV abnormalities, CMR has emerged as the imaging modality of choice in investigating ARVD. T1-weighted spin-echo images show fatty infiltration as bright signal **(Figs. 10A and B)** with thinning of the RV wall and dysplastic trabecular structures. Cine CMR shows decreased global function, regional wall motion abnormalities or aneurysms. Delayed enhancement CMR may show hyperenhancement in regions of fibrofatty replacement and thus may be useful to guide endomyocardial biopsy.

The CMR can help measure intramyocardial fat and thus help monitor evolution of the disease. However, it should be remembered that significant fatty infiltration occurs in more than 50% of normal hearts in elderly

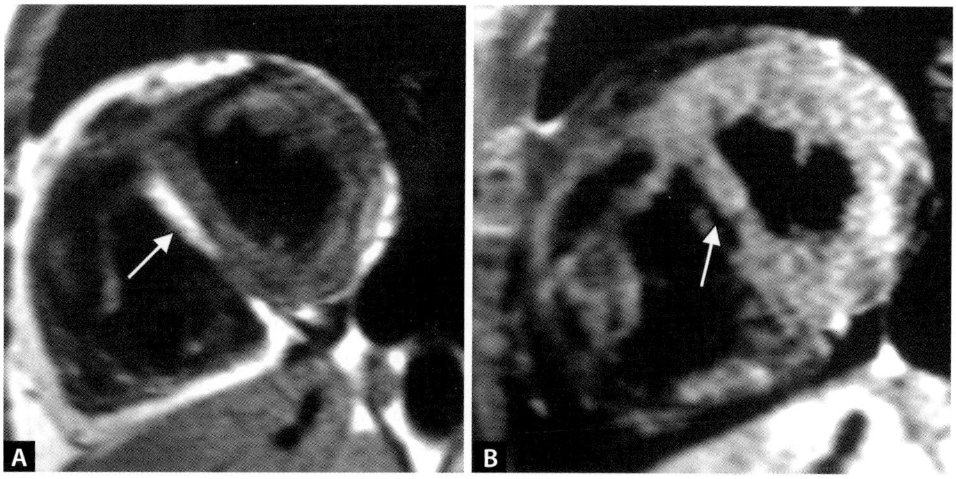

Figs. 10A and B: T1-weighted short axis image (A) showing bright signal along RV side in interventricular septum which nulls in fat-saturated images (B) confirming fatty infiltration.

people. Also in 15% of control subjects, some degree of intramyocardial fat is seen in anterior apex of right ventricle. So, focal wall motion abnormalities are considered to be a more reliable indicator of ARVD than presence of isolated intramyocardial fat.

Because first-degree relatives of individuals with ARVD have an increased chance of having the disease, with an increased risk of sudden death, CMR serves as an important tool for screening them for presence of preclinical disease.

Miscellaneous Myocardial Diseases

Left ventricular noncompaction: In this CMP, there is the persistence of deep intertrabecular recesses in communication with both the ventricular cavity and the coronary circulation. On imaging, the inner myocardial layer is spongy and less compacted compared to the outer compacted myocardium. Both CT and CMR image this differential compactness of the myocardium with superior spatial resolution, particularly in the ventricular apex where ECHO has inherent diagnostic limitations. The other common site of involvement is the lateral wall of the left ventricle. Lesser degrees of myocardial layering may also be seen in other CMPs. Peterson et al. reported that a noncompacted/compacted myocardium ratio of > 2.3 in diastole distinguished pathological noncompaction from other CMPs, with a specificity and negative predictive value of 99% each.

Takotsubo cardiomyopathy: The condition is likely thought to be due to stress related catecholamine upsurge causing cardiac dysfunction and is characterized by basal hypercontractile myocardium and a dyskinetic apex. Patients usually present with all clinical manifestations of an ST elevation myocardial infarction including chest pain, ECG changes and enzyme elevation. However, coronary angiography is normal. CMR is useful to show the reversible functional abnormalities as well as absence of any enhancement on DE-CMR, confirming noninfarcted myocardium.

Myocarditis: It is usually viral in origin and characterized by inflammation of the myocardium. Although spontaneous recovery is common, active myocarditis may occasionally lead to sudden death, and 5–10% of cases may progress to chronic dilated CMP.

Patchy involvement limits the use of myocardial biopsy for the diagnostic purposes. CT is not of much use in this entity. CMR may show focal areas of increased signal on T2-weighted images, representing active inflammation/edema. Both early and late gadolinium enhancement may be seen in areas of myocardial necrosis on histology. Cine CMR may show wall motion abnormalities. The late hyperenhancement is typically subepicardial and has 'nonischemic' pattern of distribution. It is known to occur predominantly in lateral free wall.

CONCLUSION

Cardiomyopathies are a heterogeneous group of myocardial disorders associated with distinct anatomical, functional and electrophysiological alterations of the heart. Traditional imaging techniques are limited in their assessment of the myocardium. **Cardiac MR has emerged as the investigation of choice for imaging in CMPs** and is likely to be even better utilized once improved techniques for myocardial characterization and assessment of contrast kinetics evolve further.

BIBLIOGRAPHY

1. Anderson LJ, Holden S, Davis B, et al. Cardiovascular T2-star (T2*) magnetic resonance for the early diagnosis of myocardial iron overload. Eur Heart J. 2001;22:2171-99.
2. Aso H, Takeda K, Ito T, et al. Assessment of myocardial fibrosis in cardiomyopathic hamsters with gadolinium-DTPA enhanced magnetic resonance imaging. Invest Radiol. 1998;33:22-32.
3. Bali HK, Wahi S, Sharma BK, et al. Myocardial tuberculosis presenting as restrictive cardiomyopathy. Am Heart J. 1990;120:703-6.
4. Blake LM, Scheinman MM, Higgins CB. MR features of arrhythmogenic right ventricular dysplasia. Am J Roentgenol. 1994;162:809-12.
5. Bogaert J, Taylor AM, Van Kerkhove F, et al. Use of inversion recovery contrast-enhanced CMR for cardiac imaging: Spectrum of applications. Am J Roentgenol. 2004;182:609-15.
6. Dariusch H, Fleuchter S, Suselbeck T, et al. Delayed hyperenhancement in a case of Takotsubo cardiomyopathy. J Cardiovasc Magn Reson. 2005;7:845-7.
7. Eichstaedt H, Danne O, Langer M, et al. Regression of left ventricular hypertrophy under ramipril treatment investigated by nuclear magnetic resonance imaging. J Cardiovasc Pharmacol. 1989;13:75-80.
8. Fattori R, Rocchi G, Celletti F, et al. Contribution of magnetic resonance imaging in the differential diagnosis of cardiac amyloidosis and symmetric hypertrophic cardiomyopathy. Am Heart J. 1998;136:824-30.
9. Felker GM, Thompson RE, Hare JM, et al. Underlying causes and long-term survival in patients with initially unexplained cardiomyopathy. N Engl J Med. 2000;342:1077-84.
10. Friedrich MG, Strohm O, Schulz-Menger J, et al. Contrast enhanced, magnetic resonance imaging visualizes myocardial changes in the course of viral myocarditis. Circulation. 1998;97:1802-9.
11. Friedrich MG. Magnetic resonance imaging in cardiomyopathies. J Cardiovasc Magn Reson. 2000;2:67-82.
12. Gardin JM, Dabestani A, Glasgow GA, et al. Echocardiographic and Doppler β observations in obstructed and non-obstructed hypertrophic cardiomyopathy. Am J Cardiol. 1985;56:614-21.
13. Hendel RC, Kramer CM, Patel MR, et al. ACCF/ACR/ SCCT/ SCMR/ASNC/NASCI/SCAI/SIR appropriateness criteria for cardiac computed tomography and cardiac magnetic resonance imaging. J Am Coll Cardiol. 2006;48:1-23.
14. Kimura F, Sakai F, Sakomura Y, et al. Helical CT features of arrhythmogenic right ventricular cardiomyopathy. Radiographics. 2002;22:1111-24.
15. Kubo N, Morimoto S, Hiramitsu S, et al. Feasibility of diagnosing chronic myocarditis by endomyocardial biopsy. Heart Vessels. 1997;12:167-70.
16. Maceira AM, Joshi J, Prasad SK, et al. Cardiovascular magnetic resonance in cardiac amyloidosis. Circulation. 2005;111:186-93.
17. Mahrholdt H, Wagner A, Judd RM, et al. Delayed enhancement cardiovascular magnetic resonance assessment of nonischemic cardiomyopathies. Eur Heart J. 2005;26:1461-74.
18. Maron BJ, Towbin JA, Thiene G, et al. Contemporary definitions and classification of the cardiomyopathies: An American Heart Association Scientific Statement from the Council on Clinical Cardiology, Heart Failure and Transplantation Committee; Quality of Care and Outcomes Research and Functional Genomics and Translational Biology Interdisciplinary Working Groups; and Council on Epidemiology and Prevention. Circulation. 2006;113:1807-16.
19. McKenna WJ, Thiene G, Nava A, et al. Diagnosis of arrhythmogenic right ventricular dysplasia/ cardiomyopathy. Task Force of the Working Group Myocardial and Pericardial Disease of the European Society of Cardiology and of the Scientific Council on Cardiomyopathies of the International Society and Federation of Cardiology. Br Heart J. 1994;71:215-8.
20. Ohneserge B, Flohr T, Becker C, et al. Cardiac imaging by means of ECG gated multisection spiral CT: Initial experience. Radiology. 2000;217:564-71.
21. Shimada T, Shimada K, Sakane T, et al. Diagnosis of cardiac sarcoidosis and evaluation of the effects of steroid therapy by gadolinium-DTPA-enhanced magnetic resonance imaging. Am J Med. 2001;110:520-7.
22. Varnava AM. Isolated left ventricular non-compaction: A distinct cardiomyopathy. Heart. 2001;86:599-600.
23. Vignaux O. Cardiac sarcoidosis: Spectrum of CMR features. Am J Roentgenol. 2005;184:249-54.
24. White RD, Obuchowski NA, Gunawardena S, et al. Left ventricular outflow tract obstruction in hypertrophic cardiomyopathy: Presurgical and postsurgical evaluation by computed tomography magnetic resonance imaging. Am J Card Imaging. 1996;10:1-13.

CHAPTER 180

Imaging Evaluation of Cardiac Masses

Gurpreet Singh Gulati, Priya Jagia, Sanjiv Sharma

INTRODUCTION

Cardiac masses comprise both the neoplastic and non-neoplastic lesions involving the heart. The latter group of lesions are more frequently encountered. Reaching an accurate diagnosis is important as management strategies vary depending upon the etiology. While non-neoplastic lesions usually respond well to conservative management, the neoplastic lesions often require surgical excision. Among the latter, defining the extra-cardiac extent of the lesion helps determine the treatment approach and prognosis. Additionally, it is necessary not to misinterpret normal cardiac structures and variants as cardiac masses. Hence, radiologists need to be familiar with the imaging appearances of various cardiac masses as well as normal structures and variants.

The advent and evolution of multidetector CT (MDCT) and MRI technology over the last 25 years has markedly improved our ability to evaluate and plan the optimal management of various pathological conditions of the heart. Prior to the availability of these modalities, the diagnosis of cardiac masses was difficult to make and often not possible antemortem. In this review, we discuss the clinical presentation, classification, modalities utilized for imaging along with the imaging features of various cardiac masses.

CLINICAL FEATURES

Cardiac masses are often detected incidentally on chest radiography or echocardiography (ECHO). Hence, a high degree of clinical suspicion is needed to make a reliable diagnosis. It should be noted, however, that symptoms related to cardiac masses are often non-specific and may not necessarily be cardiovascular in nature. At times, the presentation may even mimic a systemic illness. Often times, the symptoms are related to the anatomic location of the lesion rather than their histopathology. Therefore, a cardiac mass may be pathologically benign but may have a "malignant" clinical outcome. An example is a left atrial myxoma that may cause sudden cardiovascular collapse, if it obstructs the mitral valve, whereas an infiltrative malignant tumor may have a prolonged indolent course without producing any symptoms. Conduction disturbances (such as arrhythmia or heart block) and thromboembolic episodes may also be seen.

Imaging Techniques

An ideal imaging technique for cardiac masses should be able to provide holistic information regarding the nature, location, extent and hemodynamic abnormalities caused by the lesion. Importantly, it should be an accurate, operator-independent, reproducible, repeatable and a multi-planar technique with near isotropic resolution.

There is currently no single modality that possesses all the above characteristics. A multimodality approach is therefore, necessary in order to make an accurate and complete diagnosis.

Angiocardiography

Prior to the advent of non-invasive modalities, angiocardiography was the only modality available for detecting cardiac masses. Angiocardiography is however an indirect assessment based on the presence of a filling defect or a change in the luminal outline. It can often be misleading, and can easily miss small lesions and intramurally located masses. Further, it is invasive, and there is a real risk of embolization of dislodged tumor fragments during catheterization.

With the availability of non-invasive modalities that directly image the myocardium and can allow for tissue characterization, angiography is rarely indicated at present, and that too, in the following situations:

1. Suspicion of valvular or outflow tract obstruction by the mass, where catheterization may demonstrate a hemodynamically significant pressure gradient.
2. In vascular lesions, e.g. sinus of Valsalva (SOV) aneurysm or ventricular pseudoaneurysm.
3. Demonstration of coronary artery anatomy and tumor vascularity prior to surgery **(Fig. 1)**.
4. Performing endomyocardial biopsy for indeterminate lesions.

Both MRI and ECHO are capable of quantifying obstruction, MDCT can demonstrate coronary anatomy, while both MRI and MDCT can equally assess vascular lesions. Therefore, angiography can easily be avoided for these indications.

Echocardiography

Transthoracic (TTE) is universally acknowledged as the screening modality of choice in patients with suspected cardiac masses. It is non-invasive, cheap, quick and widely available. It is capable of providing most of the required

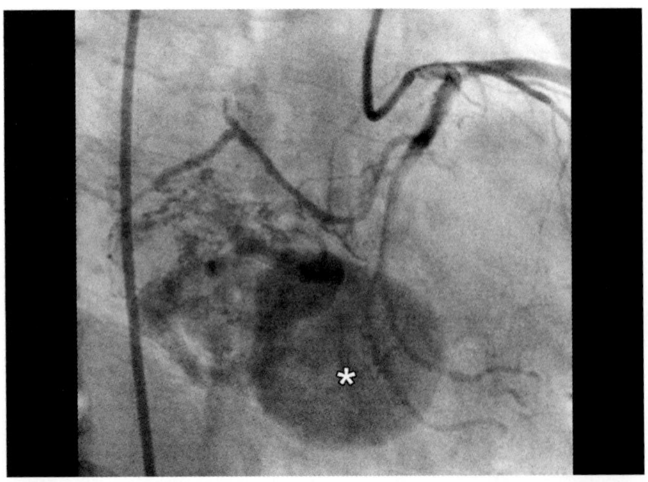

Fig. 1: Left coronary angiogram in a known case of right atrial myxoma. The atrial branches of the left circumflex artery are seen to supply a vascularized area within inter-atrial septum (representing the stalk) with an oval mobile mass (asterisk) that enhances immediately afterwards.

information regarding the lesion location, extent, mobility and hemodynamic consequences. It is especially useful for small, mobile lesions (e.g. valvular vegetation or tumor), since imaging is performed in real-time along multiple imaging planes. Image quality can also be substantially improved with use of tissue harmonic imaging. However, ECHO is operator-dependent, is suboptimal in patients with an inadequate acoustic window (obesity, emphysema or prior surgery), and may be limited in evaluation of lesions on right side of heart or those located away from chest wall. It is limited in assessing the extracardiac structures, which may be involved by intracardiac masses, or may themselves have a lesion that invades into the heart. Due to its limited ability for tissue characterization, ECHO is unreliable in suggesting the etiology, except in case of myxomas. Various authors have described an improved diagnostic yield of cardiac tumors with transesophageal echocardiography (TEE). This technique is superior to transthoracic echocardiography (TTE) for evaluation of small masses and lesions involving left atrium (LA), atrial appendage and inferior vena cava (IVC). TEE can detect the resolution or early recurrence of a tumor following medical or surgical therapy. However, this technique is invasive, complications may occur (related to the probe or drugs used) and some patients are not suited for the procedure (unstable angina, esophageal pathology or recent esophageal surgery).

Multidetector Computed Tomography

The development of multidetector computed tomography (MDCT) technology has dramatically improved the spatial and temporal resolution for cardiac imaging. Gating the cardiac images to the electrocardiogram (ECG) can be accomplished either by scanning or reconstructing raw data at the point of least cardiac motion. Due to its higher spatial resolution, MDCT is advantageous over MRI in that it generates three-dimensional images with nearly isotropic resolution. This allows for multiplanar reconstructions, which are useful for accurate demonstration of intra- and extra-cardiac masses, degree of myocardial or pericardial involvement, and associated lung abnormalities.[1,2] The volume rendered reconstructions provide a useful roadmap to the surgeon for tumor resection. Another distinct advantage of MDCT is its short image acquisition time. Current generation scanners also have large volume coverage with improved gantry rotation times, making these helpful in scanning unstable or pediatric patients. The latter often require deep sedation or even general anesthesia for doing MRI.

Compared to ECHO, MDCT has better soft tissue contrast and can definitively characterize fatty content and calcifications. While MDCT is as sensitive as MRI for detecting fatty content, it is superior to MRI for detecting calcification. The pattern of contrast enhancement on MDCT can also help to distinguish tumoral and non-tumoral masses to a certain extent. Overall however, MDCT is inferior to MRI for tissue characterization. A major advantage of MDCT over MRI and ECHO is its ability to assess coronary anatomy and rule out coronary artery disease, which make it a useful tool to evaluate older patients, who may require coronary artery bypass while undergoing surgical resection of cardiac tumors.

The major limitations to the routine use of MDCT include a relatively higher radiation dose, need for large volumes of intravenous contrast material and the high cost and limited availability of the technique. The former two limitations are however, being rapidly addressed by evolution in MDCT technology, leading to routine submillisevert scanning and low contrast requirements.

MRI

MRI has emerged as a useful tool for the detailed evaluation of cardiac masses, due to its ability to provide natural tissue contrast between flowing blood and surrounding structures, It is non-invasive, has a large field of view and allows for direct multiplanar imaging capability. It is better suited in suggesting the etiology, delineating the extent, relationship to adjacent structures, associated extracardiac lesions and presence of any hemodynamic effects. Tissue characterization ability is a distinct advantage of MRI over ECHO, allowing it to provide a tissue diagnosis in many cases. This is important since nearly half of all masses may be non-neoplastic and some of these may not even require surgical treatment. Also, many normal structures or variants that masquerade as mass lesions on ECHO can be resolved on MRI. MRI is particularly useful in detecting tumor recurrence, where ECHO may be of limited value due to a suboptimal acoustic window.

Compared to MDCT, MRI does not involve use of ionizing radiation or potentially nephrotoxic contrast (except for a small risk of causing nephrogenic systemic fibrosis with use of gadolinium in underlying severe renal insufficiency).

The major disadvantages of MRI include longer scanning period, susceptibility to motion artifacts, and requirement of a stable heart rate.

MR Imaging Sequences for Evaluation of Cardiac Masses

Conventional sequences may be limited in their diagnostic capability, due to presence of significant artifacts as a result of cardiac and respiratory motion, long examination times, and inadequate suppression of blood signal. Technical advances leading to newer imaging sequences have allowed for better spatial, contrast, and temporal resolution over the traditional imaging sequences. These have helped to enhance the capabilities of MRI in reliably diagnosing intracardiac masses.

Spin Echo (SE) Sequences

Compared to conventional SE imaging, segmented turbo (or fast) spin echo or single shot half-fourier spin echo (HASTE) sequences with double inversion recovery pulses lead to better suppression of blood signal, improving visualization of intracavitary masses.

Fat suppression techniques selectively saturate signal from fat and thus distinguish between high signal intensity (SI) lesions on the T1-weighted images (lipoma, exudative collection, thrombus).

Steady State Free Precession (SSFP) Sequences

Newer, faster, and short TE gradient echo sequences, with completely refocused gradients, (steady stage free precession or SSFP) provide excellent contrast-to-noise ratio. Due to their higher temporal resolution, mobile masses causing obstruction of a cardiac valve or the outflow tract of a ventricle, as well as the cardiac output and regurgitation volumes can be assessed using cine- SSFP MRI. The other advantages of SSFP techniques include better separation of myocardium from intracavitary blood, and reduction in examination time compared to SE acquisitions. The latter helps to optimize imaging in children and acute patients.

Contrast-enhanced Imaging

Myocardial perfusion and delayed enhanced imaging sequences are useful for evaluating the contrast enhancement characteristics of cardiac tumors.[3] Perfusion imaging can be useful to demonstrate increased tumor vascularity typical of malignant lesions such as angiosarcomas. Delayed enhanced imaging is useful to detect intramurally located lesions, distinguish tumors from thrombi, differentiate benign from malignant masses and identify areas of tissue necrosis. The usual dose of gadolinium used is 0.1 mmol per KBW.

Other Techniques

Myocardial tagging methods create a grid pattern on the myocardium and can thus help to differentiate contracting myocardial tissue from non-contractile tumor. This may help detect tumors of muscle consistency, such as rhabdomyomas. Phase-contrast imaging methods, being sensitive to slow flow, supplement SE techniques in distinguishing intra-cavitary mass lesions from a flow-related signal.

Classification (Table 1)

Cardiac tumors have a cumulative prevalence of 0.002–0.3% as determined in autopsy series.[4] Primary cardiac neoplasms include both benign and malignant histological types **(Table 1)**.[5] Importantly metastatic cardiac masses are nearly 20–40 times more prevalent than primary cardiac tumors. Secondary neoplasms can involve the heart by contiguous, hematogeneous, transvenous, or lymphatic spread. Non-tumorous masses include pathological conditions and various normal cardiac structures and variants that can present as a mass on imaging.

Table 1: Classification of cardiac masses.

1. Tumors A. *Primary*: a. *Benign*: i. Myxoma ii. Lipoma iii. Papillary fibroelastoma iv. Fibroma v. Rhabdomyoma vi. Hemangioma vii. *Others*: Pheochromocytoma, lymphangioma, teratoma b. *Malignant*: i. Sarcoma ii. Lymphoma iii. Mesothelioma B. *Secondary*: a. *Direct extension:* Lung cancer, breast cancer, mediastinal lymphoma b. *Hematogenous:* Malignant melanoma, lymphoma, leukemia c. *Transvenous*: Renal and hepatic tumors d. *Lymphatic:* Lymphoma, lung and breast carcinoma C. Paracardiac and extracardiac tumors
2. *Non-neoplastic lesions*: A. Thrombus B. Sinus of valsalva aneurysm C. Atrial septal aneurysm D. Pericardial cyst E. *Infective*: a. Valvular vegetation b. Hydatid cyst c. Tubercular
3. Normal structures and variants mimicking tumor

NEOPLASTIC LESIONS OF THE HEART

Primary

Benign Tumors

Myxoma: This is the most common benign tumor (50%) found in adults. These tumors usually present between the fourth and seventh decades of life. They arise from embryologic rests that get entrapped during the septation phase of cardiac embryogenesis. The classic triad of symptoms includes cardiac obstructive symptoms related to the obstruction of blood flow, embolic events, and constitutional symptoms such as fever, malaise and weight loss. Thromboembolic events occur in 35% of left-sided myxomas to the brain, kidney, spleen and extremities and 10% of right-sided myxomas to the lung. Friable and gelatinous myxomas are more likely to embolize than firm and fibrous lesions.[6] Pathologically, myxomas are gelatinous masses with calcification, necrosis and hemorrhage.

Approximately, 75% of myxomas are found in the LA, typically, in the interatrial septum in the region of the fossa ovalis; 20% of myxomas are located in the RA, and rare cases are found in the ventricles. Most lesions are sporadic. Carney's complex is an autosomal dominant disorder consisting of cardiac myxomas, hyperpigmented skin lesions and various extra-cardiac tumors.

The narrow stalk of myxomas may be difficult to appreciate on CT and MRI. The use of contrast-enhanced CT usually demonstrates the presence of a well-defined spherical or ovoid intracavitary mass, which typically has lobular contours and frequently calcified. Tumor attenuation is lower than that of the unopacified blood. The intravenous administration of contrast material helps better to define the lesion as a mass of low attenuation that is surrounded by enhancing intracardiac blood. Heterogeneity is a common feature of myxomas and is believed to reflect hemorrhage, necrosis, cyst formation, fibrosis or calcification.

Myxomas tend to show markedly increased signal intensity on the T2-weighted MR images. However, myxomas can show areas of decreased signal intensity due to presence of calcification or magnetic susceptibility artifacts caused by hemosiderin **(Fig. 2)**. Cine-MRI characteristically displays a mobile tumor which may prolapse through a cardiac valve. Contrast enhancement may be heterogeneous, and may be intense in highly vascular lesions.

Lipoma: They are the second most common benign cardiac tumors (10%), occur across a wide age range and

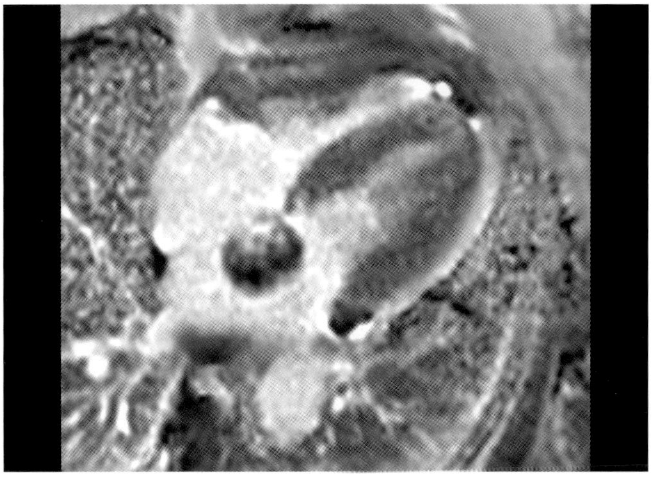

Fig. 2: Late gadolinium enhancement MRI in 4-chamber view in a case of LA myxoma. The lesion is attached to the interatrial septum, and shows heterogeneous enhancement.

are composed of mature adipose tissue.[7] Most lipomas are sporadic. Nearly 50% of lipomas arise subendocardially and the rest are epicardial or endomyocardial in location. The left ventricle (LV) and RA are the most frequently involved.

Both CT and MRI are highly specific and sensitive in the detection of lipomas. CT characteristically shows a homogeneous low density lesion of fatty attenuation. SE T1W MRI reveals a well circumscribed hyperintense lesion, whose SI is suppressed on fat-suppression technique. SI is slightly decreased on T2W images. As with soft-tissue lipomas, cardiac lipomas do not show enhancement with the administration of a contrast material.

Lipomatous hypertrophy of the interatrial septum (IAS), although not a true neoplasm, has been included in various reports of cardiac lipomas. This is defined as any fatty thickening of the IAS at the level of the fossa ovalis that exceed 2 cm in transverse dimension. It is seen in older, obese patients and is frequently associated with increased epicardial fat. It has a typical "dumb-bell" shape on imaging.

Papillary fibroelastoma: Papillary fibroelastomas are benign endocardial papillomas, composed of avascular fronds of connective tissue lined by endothelium. They comprise nearly 10% of all primary cardiac tumors. They usually affect the cardiac valves (more often the aortic and mitral valves) and account for approximately 75% of all cardiac valvular tumors.[8] Despite this predilection, these tumors are not known to cause valvular dysfunction. The tumor usually has a narrow stalk and is mobile.

Papillary fibroelastomas are usually not observed on CT or MR images as they are small (< 1.5 cm in diameter) and are attached to the moving valves.[8] MR imaging typically demonstrates the presence of a mass on a valve leaflet or on the endocardial surface. These tumors can create turbulence in the blood flow, which might be demonstrated with the use of cine MR imaging.

Fibroma: Fibromas are neoplasms that mainly affect infants and children, being the second most common tumors found in this age group after rhabdomyomas. These occur with increased frequency in patients with Gorlin syndrome. Grossly, the lesions are solid tumors, composed of fibroblasts with intervening collagen tissue. They arise within the myocardium (most commonly in the LV) and can grow to a size that obliterates the cavity. Usually these tumors are large in size, but may be nodular and discrete or infiltrative. Due to the potential risk of sudden death due to arrhythmias, surgery is the preferred treatment even in asymptomatic cases.

The use of CT shows fibromas as homogeneous masses with soft-tissue attenuation, which may be either sharply marginated or infiltrative. Calcification is often observed.[9] On MRI, these tumors are normally homogeneously isointense to hypointense relative to the myocardium as seen on T1- and T2-weighted images due to a dense, fibrous nature. For the same reason, these tumors often show delayed enhancement on gadolinium-enhanced MRI **(Figs. 3A and B)**.[10]

Rhabdomyoma: Rhabdomyomas are the most common cardiac tumors in infancy and childhood. About 75% of neonatal primary tumors are rhabdomyomas. These tumors are often associated with tuberous sclerosis in up to 50% of cases.[11] Most patients are asymptomatic, and rhabdomyomas generally regress spontaneously. As such, these lesions are not considered as true neoplasms but as hamartomas.These tumors originate within the myocardium, typically in the ventricles, and multiple lesions may be present in up to 90% of cases.

Rhabdomyomas appear isointense to marginally hyperintense as compared with the myocardium as seen on T1-weighted images and hyperintense as seen on T2-weighted images. Contrast enhancement is similar to that of myocardium.

In a child, the presence of a solitary, calcified, ventricular mass favors a fibroma whereas multiple tumors located in both atria and ventricles with other features of tuberous sclerosis favor rhabdomyomas.

Hemangioma: These are tumors of vascular origin composed of either capillaries (capillary hemangiomas) or cavernous spaces (cavernous hemangiomas). They comprise 10% of primary benign tumors of the heart. The

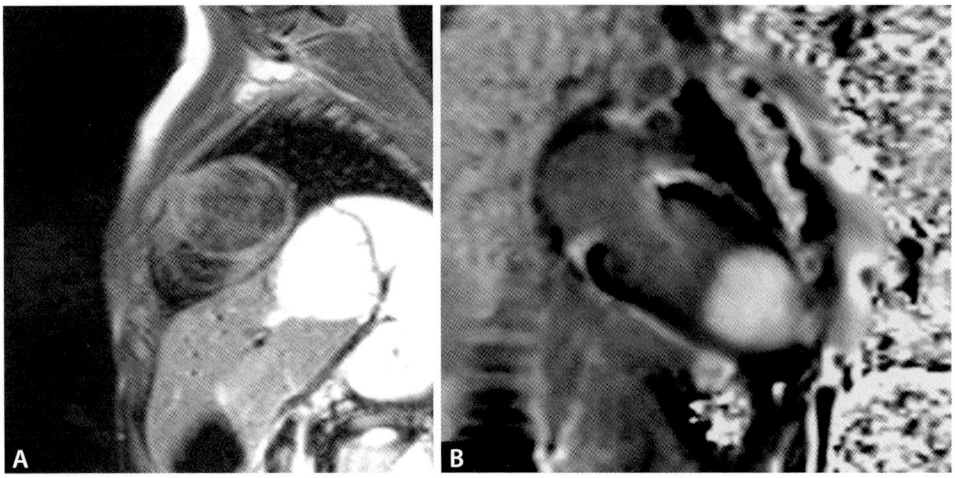

Figs. 3A and B: Short axis SE T2W fat-suppressed (A) and VLA delayed enhanced (B) MRI in a case of LV fibroma. The lesion is hypo-intense to myocardium on T2W, and enhances homogeneously following contrast injection.

tumors can be solitary, either in LV or RV or the IVS, or multiple masses. They may be intramural or intracavitary in location with roughly an equal frequency.

Cardiac hemangiomas are heterogeneous as depicted on pre-contrast CT images and are intensely enhanced as seen on contrast-enhanced CT images. On MRI, due to the presence of slow flow, they have a heterogeneous intermediate- to-increased SI on T1W images and high SI on T2W images. Like CT, the tumors usually enhance well after gadolinium administration.[12]

Pheochromocytoma: Cardiac location is extremely rare, usually in the distribution of the cardiac paraganglia. Most often, they are seen in the LA, either the posterior wall or the roof. They may arise from the IAS or along coronary arteries, the latter making surgical excision exceedingly difficult.

The initial screening for extra-adrenal paragangliomas is usually with MIBG scanning. CT usually shows a circumscribed, heterogeneous, low attenuation mass that enhances strongly with contrast. On MRI, the tumor is iso- to hypo-intense on T1W images. Increased SI on T1W images may be due to hemorrhage. It is markedly hyperintense on T2W images. Intense enhancement is usually noted with gadolinium. Non-enhancing areas may represent necrosis within the lesion.

Lymphangioma: These are benign lymph containing neoplasms. Most lesions occur in children. They may be associated with other lymphovascular masses of the neck or the mediastinum. The most common location is in the pericardial spaces. These tumors may present with cardiac tamponade. CT features have not been described. MRI demonstrates an increased SI mass on T1W and T2W images.

Primary cardiac teratomas are other rare pericardial neoplasms seen in children.

Malignant Tumors

These comprise 25% of primary tumors of the heart. Secondary cardiac involvement by extra-cardiac malignancies is more common. Primary tumors are often asymptomatic till they become large. Even then, the symptoms can be non-specific. The lesions include sarcoma, lymphoma and mesothelioma.

Sarcoma

Angiosarcoma: The most common cardiac sarcomas are angiosarcomas that comprise 37% of all cases.[7] These lesions are malignant mesenchymal tumors that arise from endothelial cells lining the lymphatics or blood vessels. They usually present with right-sided heart failure or tamponade as the tumors tend to occur in the RA and involve the pericardium. Presentation is late, and there is often the presence of metastases at the time of diagnosis, particularly to the lung. These tumors have been reported to occur over a wide age range. They have a poor prognosis, with a mean survival of 6 months following presentation. Metastasis most frequently occurs to the lungs. There are two morphological subtypes of the tumor: A well-circumscribed intracavitary mass, or a diffusely infiltrative lesion of the myocardium.

CT often shows the presence of a low-attenuation mass in the right atrium, which might be irregular or nodular. There may pericardial effusion or thickening. Cardiac sarcomas may have heterogeneous signal intensity as seen on MR images, with areas of high signal intensity as seen on T2-weighted images representing the blood-filled spaces within the neoplasm. A papillary or "cauliflower" appearance can be observed as a specific MR feature of angiosarcoma, with a nodular area of high signal intensity interspersed within areas of intermediate signal intensity as seen on T1- and T2-weighted images. In cases with diffuse pericardial infiltration, some investigators have described linear enhancement along the vascular spaces as a "sunray" appearance.[13] Perfusion MRI shows early and increased contrast uptake within the tumor **(Figs. 4A and B)**. Delayed contrast enhancement is heterogeneous on both CT and MRI.

Hemangiopericytomas are rare cardiac sarcomas that are indistinguishable from angiosarcomas on imaging.

Other cardiac sarcomas: Although angiosarcomas are the most common cardiac sarcomas, all types of sarcomas, including undifferentiated sarcomas, malignant fibrous histiocytomas (MFHs), leiomyosarcomas, osteosarcomas, lymphosarcomas, myxosarcomas, neurogenic sarcomas, synovial sarcomas, neurofibrosarcomas, and Kaposi's sarcomas can affect the heart. Although most angiosarcomas occur in the RA, the other sarcomas affect the LA more frequently, which is an important differentiating feature.[7]

Malignant fibrous histiocytomas consist of primitive mesenchymal, fibroblastic, and histiocytic cells arranged in a storiform pattern.[14] The most common location of MFHs is the LA where the tumors are usually attached to the posterior wall.[14] Distinguishing MFHs from a benign cardiac tumor might be difficult on a clinical and imaging basis, but MFH is far more aggressive and has a greater propensity for recurrence and infiltration. MR imaging demonstrates the presence of MFH as a mass with a nonspecific signal intensity as seen on T1- and T2-weighted images. A MFH arises from the posterior wall of the LA and can extend into the pulmonary veins. This finding would not normally be expected with a myxoma.

Leiomyosarcomas are malignant tumors of smooth muscle origin. Primary cardiac involvement is extremely uncommon. Most lesions (75%) arise in the superior vena cava (SVC) or the IVC and extend to the heart. Intracardiac lesions usually arise in the LA and may invade the pericardium.

Myxosarcoma is a rare form of primary malignant tumors that is very difficult to differentiate from a myxoma. The ratio between the incidence of myxomas and myxosarcomas is approximately 100:0.8 and the prognoses of the two tumor types are very different.[15] Myxosarcomas have local recurrences, involving the pulmonary artery, pericardium or pleura and distant metastases, with the brain being the site most affected.[15]

Lymphoma: Primary cardiac lymphoma refers to the one involving only the heart or pericardium.[16] These tumors are extremely rare, with a reported incidence of 0.15 to 1%. Although cardiac spread of extracardiac non-Hodgkin's lymphoma is more common, there is a recent increase in the occurrence of the primary form due to its association with AIDS.

Pathologically, most primary tumors are diffuse large B-cell lymphomas. It most commonly arises in the RA but may involve any chamber. Sometimes, large pericardial effusion or thickening may be the only finding. Cardiac mass may be a polypoidal or an infiltrative intramural lesion. The latter may be diffuse form of infiltration of lymphoma cells in the myocardium, mimicking classic hypertrophic cardiomyopathy.

CT images show cardiac lymphomas as hypo- or iso-attenuated infiltrative soft tissue masses as compared

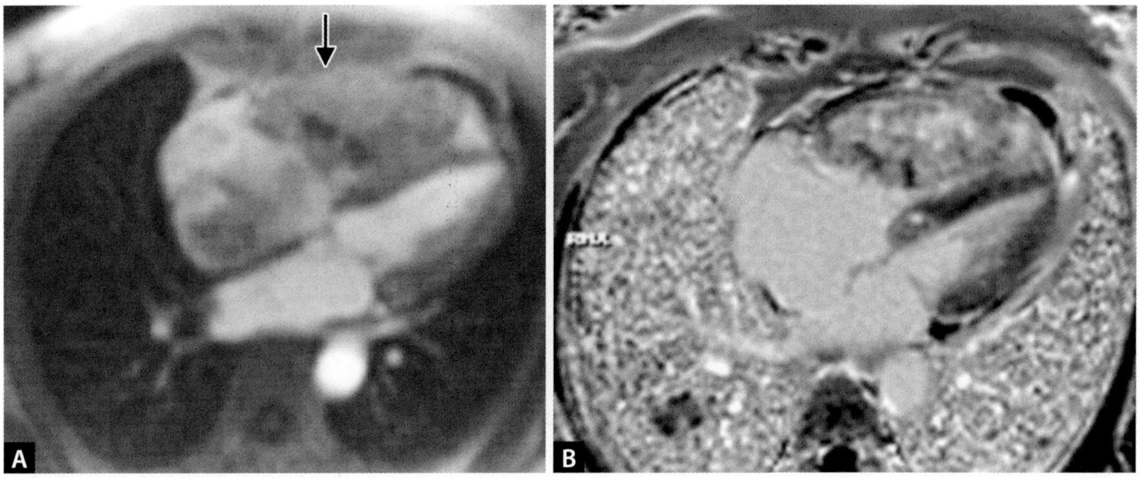

Figs. 4A and B: Rest-perfusion (A) and delayed enhanced (B) MRI in 4-chamber view, in a probable angiosarcoma of RV. There is early and increased contrast uptake in the lesion (arrow), that also shows heterogeneous enhancement on the delayed enhanced image.

with the myocardium, and the masses demonstrate heterogeneous enhancement after the administration of a contrast agent. On MRI, they usually appear as iso- to hypointense to cardiac muscle on both T1 and T2W images. They may be bright on T2W images. Contrast enhancement may be homogeneous, heterogeneous or minimal, with areas of low enhancement seen in the center of the lesion as compared with the periphery.

Pericardial mesothelioma: This most common primary pericardial neoplasm constitutes 15% of all malignant cardiac tumors. Unlike metastatic tumors to the pericardium, mesotheliomas are generally restricted to involvement of the pericardium without actually spreading to the cardiac chambers. There is no association with asbestos exposure.

Cross-sectional imaging helps to define the extent of the lesion and optimize the surgical approach. Contrast enhancement helps to differentiate the tumor from adjacent, normal myocardium. SI characteristics on MRI are nonspecific.

Secondary Neoplasms

Metastases to the heart are much more common than primary involvement, with an estimated ratio of 30:1.[17] In the presence of a malignant tumor, cardiac metastases are encountered in 11% of cases.[18] The tumors that most frequently metastasize to the heart are lung and breast cancers, melanomas and lymphomas.[18]

These lesions may involve the heart through direct extension or through hematogeneous, venous or lymphatic spread. Although imaging findings are not characteristic of any particular type of tumor, CT and particularly MRI is helpful in delineating the site and extent of cardiac and paracardiac involvement. The extent of involvement revealed by imaging may lead to a modification of the radiotherapy planning or the addition of chemotherapy.

The epicardium is the site most often affected by metastases.[17,18] Spread is mainly via a retrograde route through the mediastinal lymphatics, leading to implantation in the epicardial surface of the heart. Other tumors such as melanomas and sarcomas usually spread hematogeneously to the myocardium and epicardium through the coronary arteries, or less commonly, by the implantation of cancer cells through the vena cava.[18] Hematogeneous metastases in the heart and pericardium are normally accompanied by evidence of hematogeneous metastases in other organs. In particular, pulmonary metastases are usually present.[18]

Direct extension can occur with thymic, bronchial, breast and esophageal malignancies due to the proximity of the primary lesions to the heart. Invasion of the pericardium may be seen as interruption of the normal pericardial outline with nodular or diffuse pericardial thickening, hemorrhage, or effusion. Myocardial involvement is suspected when there is irregularity of the outline. Delayed enhanced MRI helps to demonstrate the extent of the cardiac invasion **(Figs. 5A and B)**. In addition, transvenous tumor spread relies on an extension of the tumor thrombus into the RA through the superior (lung cancers) or inferior vena cava (tumors from the kidney or liver) or an extension into the LA via the pulmonary veins. Both benign (uterine myoma, vessel wall leiomyoma) and malignant (hepatic, adrenal, renal and thyroid carcinoma)

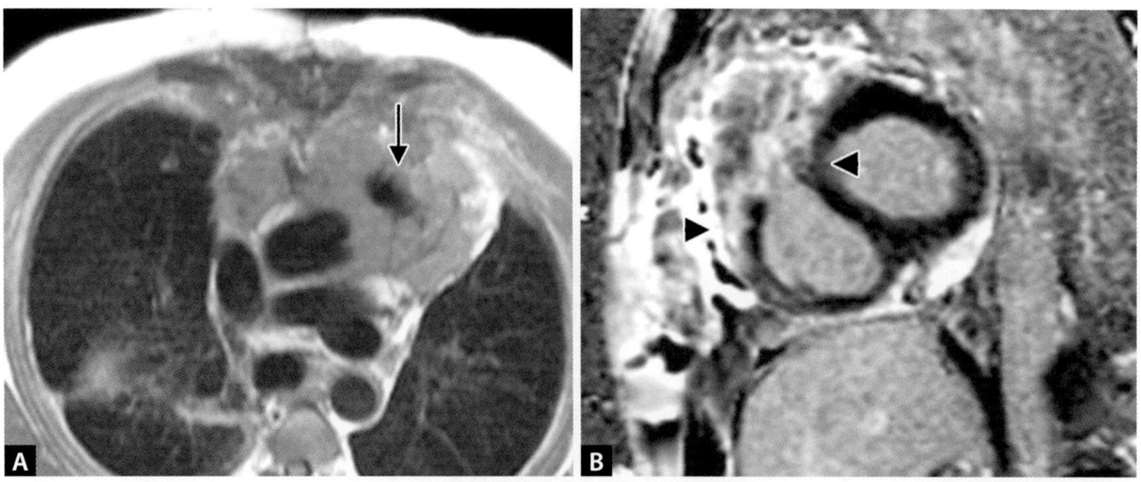

Figs. 5A and B: Axial SE T1W (A) and short axis delayed enhanced (B) MRI images in a patient with anterior mediastinal tumor. The mass is seen to encase and infiltrate the right ventricular outflow tract (irregular outline, arrow)) and extends up to the ascending aorta. Delayed enhanced image shows the heterogeneous mass also involves the RV myocardium and the upper IVS (arrowheads).

tumors can extend intracavally to the heart. This can cause caval or atrial occlusion. The tumor fragments may embolize distally with serious consequences. MRI is particularly suited to simultaneously demonstrate the primary site and its spread through the vena cava. This is helpful in planning the surgical treatment. Presence of intra-thrombus neovascularity on MRI may help to differentiate malignant from bland cavo-atrial thrombus.

Paracardiac and Extracardiac Tumors

These are mediastinal lesions that may extrinsically compress the cardiac structure or invade it. Anterior mediastinal masses include thymoma, thymolipoma, lymphoma, teratoma, terato-carcinoma and thyroid masses. Masses of neurogenic, airway (bronchogenic cyst or bronchial malignancy) or esophageal (carcinoma, duplication, leiomyoma) origin are the most common middle or posterior mediastinal lesions to about the heart. The direct orthogonal imaging capability of MRI makes it ideally suited to delineate the site of origin, extent and involvement of the heart by these tumors. CT and particularly MRI may localize the etiology by their ability to characterize tissue components. CT shows the presence of calcium and fat in germ cell tumors. On MRI, cystic lesions typically have a very high SI on the T2W images. High SI on T1W images may suggest high protein content, fat or hemorrhage within the lesion. Fat suppression techniques will distinguish fat, and GRE sequences will demonstrate hemosiderin deposits in chronic hemorrhage. Thymolipomas are anterior mediastinal lesions that usually conform to the shape of surrounding structures. CT and MRI characteristically display a mixture of fat and soft tissue within the lesion. Benign and invasive thymomas can, to some extent, be differentiated on MRI. The invasive thymomas tend to be more inhomogeneous, multinodular in appearance and less well-defined in outline.

NON-NEOPLASTIC LESIONS

Thrombus

Cardiac thrombi are more frequent than tumors and prompt recognition and appropriate treatment is important. Prior infarct (particularly in apical and interventricular septal location) and markedly depressed left ventricular systolic function predispose to thrombus formation in the left ventricular apical regions. These are most commonly and best diagnosed by transthoracic ECHO. Atrial fibrillation predisposes to thrombus formation in the LA appendage, whereas factors causing diastolic dysfunction (e.g. restrictive cardiomyopathy) or presence of mechanical valves, interatrial septal devices, and appendage occluder devices are other common factors leading to atrial thrombus formation that are best diagnosed by transesophageal ECHO. Thus presence of predisposing conditions along with a soft-tissue mass located in expected regions is the hallmark of echocardiographic diagnosis of intracardiac thrombi. Finding of a mass in the absence of predisposing conditions outlined above as well as of systemic hypercoagulable state make etiologic classification of a cardiac mass challenging by ECHO.

MRI, given its higher resolution, is able to better differentiate a cardiac mass based on its soft-tissue composition. Compared to ECHO, MRI has a higher sensitivity (90%) with a slightly higher specificity for detecting thrombus.[19,20] The signal intensity characteristics of a thrombus vary with MR imaging and are dependent on the age of the thrombus. An acute thrombus will appear bright as seen on both T1- and T2-weighted MR images, whereas a subacute thrombus will appear bright as seen on T1-weighted images with hypointense areas seen on T2-weighted images due to the paramagnetic effects of methemoglobin and shortening of the T2 relaxation times **(Figs. 6A and B)**. A chronic organized thrombus will exhibit hypointensity as seen on both T1- and T2- weighted images due to depleted water content.[20] Problems in differentiating thrombus and slowly flowing blood may frequently arise on SE MRI. GRE sequences are useful in this regard, since the thrombus always shows lower SI than blood. Also, on cine-GRE thrombus usually has a constant SI, whereas slowly moving blood continuously changes in SI. The other advantage of cine-GRE sequence is that it allows simultaneous assessment of the wall motion abnormalities. In cases where differentiation from tumor is difficult on MRI, imaging after administration of contrast with an inversion pulse to null normal myocardium may be useful (similar to the sequence for viability imaging, but imaging initiated at 3-5 minutes instead of waiting for at least 10 minutes). The thrombus should not show enhancement **(Figs. 6A and B)** whereas a tumor usually shows enhancement.[21] However, an organized thrombus may show some surface enhancement.

Aneurysm of Sinus of Valsalva

Sinus of valsalva (SOV) aneurysm is most commonly congenital in origin and caused by a deficiency of elastic tissue in the tunica media.[22] Rarely, it may be acquired secondary to aortic valve endocarditis or trauma. Most SOV aneurysms arise from the right and non-coronary sinuses. Unruptured SOV aneurysms are usually clinically

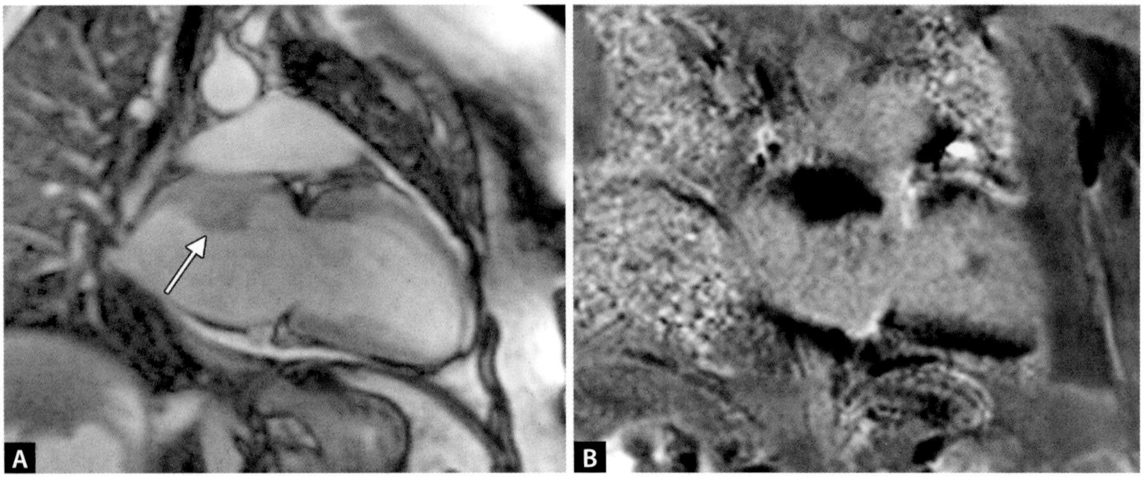

Figs. 6A and B: SSFP (A) and delayed enhanced (B) MRI in the vertical long axis view, in a patient with mitral stenosis. There is a mural thrombus in the posterosuperior wall of the left atrium. The lesion does not enhance in the 10 minutes following contrast administration (B).

silent and discovered serendipitously on ECHO as a vascular mass.[23,24] Rupture most often occurs into the RA or right ventricular outflow tract and may be a catastrophic event or present with rapid onset of heart failure caused by pronounced left to right shunting.

Although transesophageal ECHO is better for demonstration of site of communication of the aneurysm with a coronary sinus and its extension into a chamber wall (in case of unruptured aneurysms), it is an invasive technique and may be uncomfortable for the patient.

On CT, SOV aneurysm appears as a thin walled crescent shaped outpouching that is contiguous with the aortic root **(Figs. 7A and B)**. Occasionally, they are partially or completely thrombosed. MRI is very useful to confirm its vascular nature, by showing a signal void on SE sequences **(Figs. 8A and B)**. Both modalities are particularly useful for demonstrating extension into the adjacent cardiac chambers, valves and septum which can be difficult to fully evaluate with ECHO.

Atrial Septal Aneurysm

This is a localized protrusion of the primary component of the inter-atrial septum (IAS) through the fossa ovalis region, or a diffuse bulging of the entire septum into either of the atria. It may be associated with other congenital cardiac anomalies, or with acquired lesions that result in unequal pressures in the two atria. Due to thrombus formation in the concavity of the aneurysm, pulmonary or systemic embolic events may occur. Presence of an associated atrial septal defect may result in paradoxical embolism. Although, the diagnosis is usually made on ECHO, stagnant blood within aneurysm concavity may simulate a cystic tumor. Similar problems may result on SE MRI. Hence cine-SSFP MRI should be done and this shows blood flow within the aneurysm, as well as the mobility of the aneurysmal IAS.

Pleuropericardial Cyst

Though the most common pericardial mass lesion, these are very rare, the reported incidence being 1:100,000 of the general population. They are thought to be congenital in origin. The most common location is in the right cardiophrenic angle, although they may also be seen in left cardiophrenic angle and posterior mediastinum. Patients are usually asymptomatic, the lesion often being detected incidentally on imaging. Lesions are typically stable, and surgical excision is rarely required.

CT typically shows a well-marginated cyst of fluid attenuation **(Figs. 9A and B)**. There may or may not be a perceptible wall. MRI characteristically shows a well circumscribed, homogeneous paracardiac mass with iso- to hypointensity on T1W and hyperintensity on T2W images. Intracystic septae may be observed following paramagnetic contrast agent administration. The major role of MRI is in differentiating pericardial cysts from other mediastinal masses and thus avoiding an inadvertent surgery.

Infective Lesions

Valvular Vegetation

Due to their inferior temporal resolution compared to ECHO, valvular vegetations are not visible on MDCT and MRI unless they are large. These modalities are mainly indicated for detection of extent of peri-valvular invasion, including abscess and/or fistula formation. Vegetations

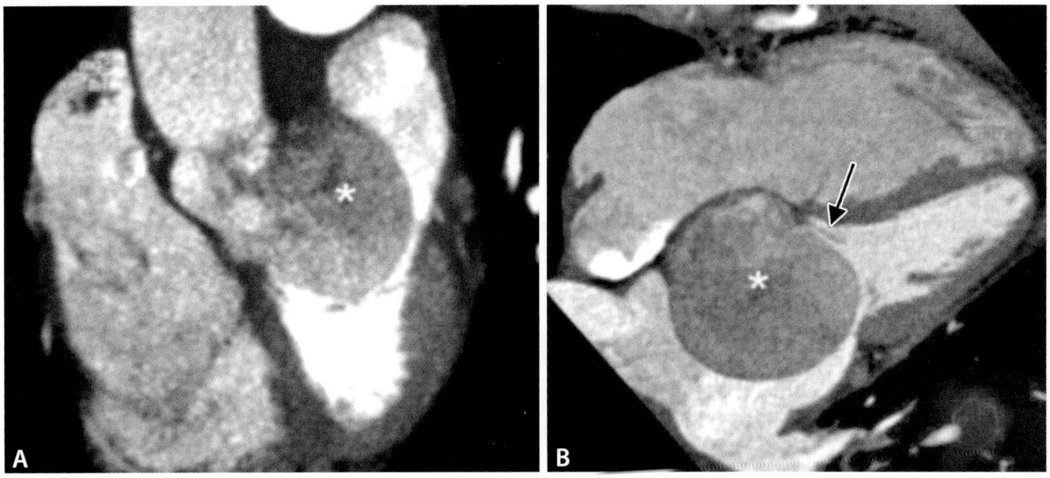

Figs. 7A and B: MDCT in a case of SOV aneurysm, sagittal (A) and 4-chamber (B) images. A round lesion (*) with heterogeneous enhancement in this early arterial phase (due to turbulent flow) arises from the aortic root and projects leftwards, posteriorly and inferiorly into LA. It also impinges on the mitral valve (arrow in Fig. B).

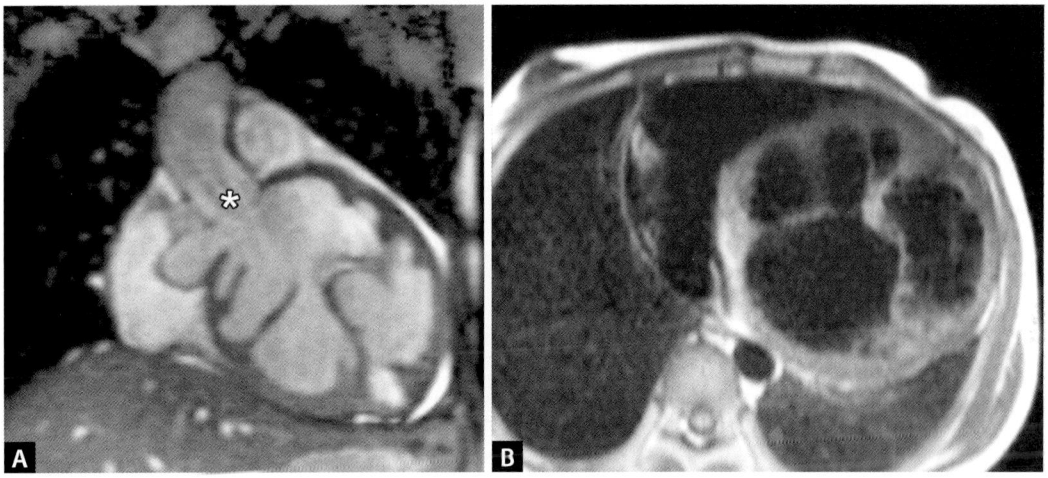

Figs. 8A and B: Coronal oblique SSFP (A) and axial SE T1W (B) MRI in a case of SOV aneurysm. The lesion arises from the aortic root (*), is multilobulated, and burrows into the interventricular septum. In (B), the lesion shows multiple large signal voids, consistent with its vascular nature.

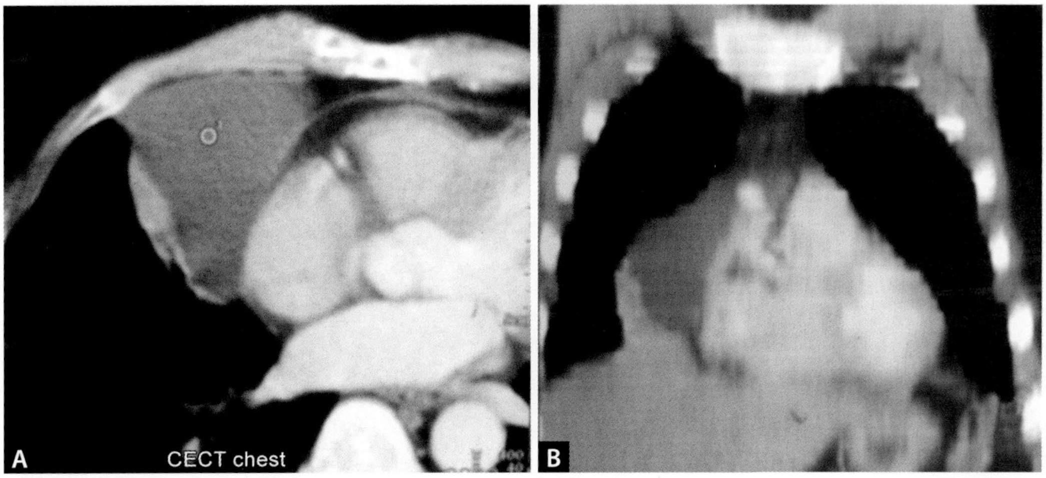

Figs. 9A and B: Axial (A) and coronal reformatted (B) contrast-enhanced CT images in pleuropericardial cyst. A well-marginated, fluid attenuation lesion with no rim enhancement is noted in its typical location (right cardiophrenic angle).

may be occasional findings when they appear as lesions intimately related to the valvular apparatus. Cine-SSFP MRI is useful to detect small lesions.

Hydatid Cyst

Cardiac hydatid cysts constitute 0.5–2% of all hydatid locations in the human body. The most common location is the LV (60%), followed by RV (10%), pericardium (7%), pulmonary artery (6%) and IVS (4%). Right sided lesions are seen to expand into the chamber cavity and subendocardially, while the left sided lesions more often grow subepicardially. The heart also can be secondarily affected by direct contact with hydatid cysts originating from the liver or the lung. These lesions are usually asymptomatic, and incidental detection is reported in 47% patients in one study. Symptomatic forms may compress the cardiac cavity or may rupture leading to anaphylaxis, tamponade or pericardial constriction.

Echocardiography, CT, and MRI can show the cystic nature of the mass and its relation to the cardiac chambers **(Figs. 10A and B)**. The cysts may be single or multiple, uniloculated or multiloculated, and thin or thick walled. More specific signs include calcification of the cyst wall, presence of daughter cysts and membrane detachment. CT best shows wall calcification. MRI depicts the exact anatomic location and nature of the internal and external structures and is the technique used for post-treatment follow-up. The appearance of a hydatid cyst on MRI is usually a characteristic oval lesion that is hypointense on T1-weighted images and hyperintense on T2-weighted images. MRI also demonstrates a thin low intensity peripheral rim on T2W images, reported to be a characteristic sign of a hydatid cyst **(Figs. 10A and B)**. This is thought to represent dense fibrous capsule from reactive host tissue.[24]

Tuberculoma

In tuberculosis, involvement of the heart apart from tuberculous pericarditis is extremely rare. The reported overall autopsy incidence of myocardial involvement ranges from 0.14 to 0.3%.[25,26] A tuberculoma, which is a mass like manifestation of the disease, is highly unusual and its description in the literature is confined to case reports.[26] The lesion most commonly involves the RA, close to SVC-RA junction or the RV. However, extensive infiltration of the myocardium, inseparable from pericardium and with the heart appearing literally "boxed in" has also been described. MRI usually demonstrates a homogeneous mass which is iso- to mildly hyperintense relative to the myocardium. The lesion is usually well defined with a sharp outline and without any flow voids. Delayed enhanced images may reveal homogeneous or heterogeneous enhancement. Lesions respond well to antitubercular therapy **(Figs. 11A and B)**.

VARIANT AND NORMAL ANATOMICAL STRUCTURES SIMULATING A CARDIAC MASS

Pericardium

The extension of the normal pericardial space into its various recesses and presence of small amounts of normally occurring pericardial fluid within them may lead to a false diagnosis of a pericardial or a vascular tumor. A

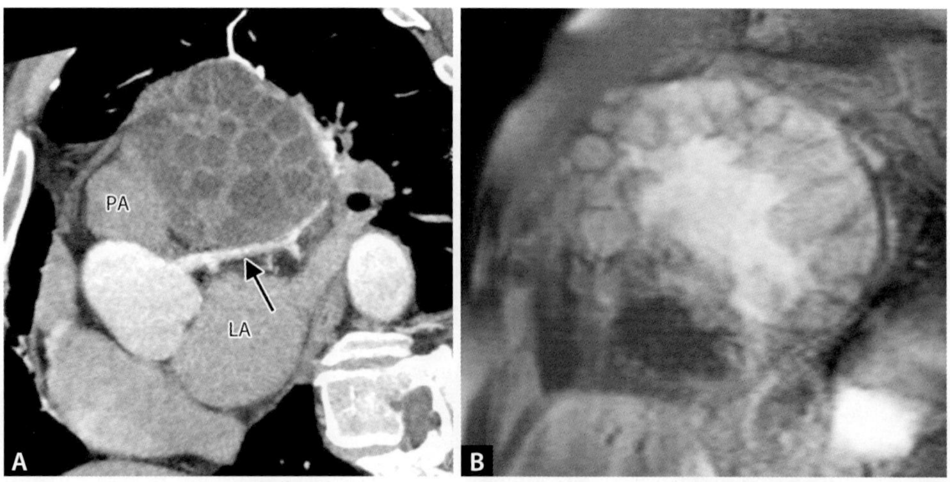

Figs. 10A and B: Short axis MDCT (A) and short axis SE T2W (fat-suppressed) MRI (B) images in a patient with hydatid cyst. The lesion shows multiple daughter cysts and abuts the PA, LA and the left circumflex artery (arrow). In (B) the typical hypointense rim to the lesion is seen.

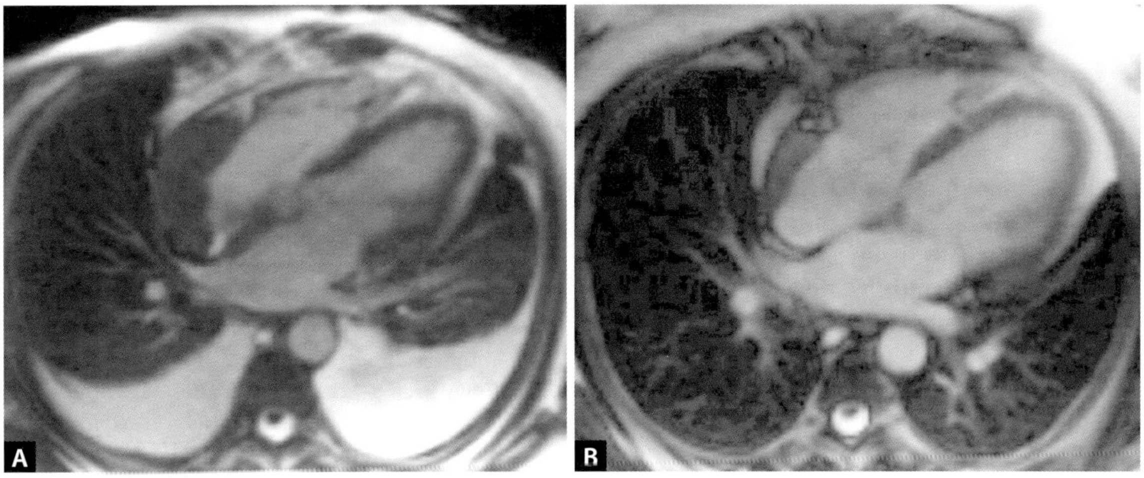

Figs. 11A and B: SSFP MRI in 4-chamber view in a case of RA tuberculoma, pre- (A) and 8 months post- (B) anti-tubercular therapy. There is a homogeneous, well-marginated right atrial mass that has significantly reduced in size following treatment. Pleural effusions have also disappeared.

typical example is a high extending superior pericardial recess that may simulate an enlarged lymph node, vascular tumor or an aortic dissection.

Left Atrium

The left atrial appendage is a tubular extension from the LA that is lined with thin, pectinate ridges, compared to the body of the LA that has a smooth endocardial outline. These ridges may be confused with thrombi. Also, other posterior mediastinal lesions such as cysts, esophageal tumors, and even a tortuous descending aorta may, at times, be misinterpreted as a LA mass. The multiplanar imaging capability of MDCT and MRI is useful in this regard to avoid a false-positive diagnosis.

Left Ventricle

False chordae and tendons are accessory structures that may appear as linear strands extending through the LV cavity, particularly on ECHO.

Right Atrium

The chiari network consists of fibrous strand-like structures arising from the region near the Eustachian valve and extending into the RA cavity. On MRI, these have a signal intensity (SI) similar to that of the mycocardium, and should not be misdiagnosed as a tumor or a thrombus. The crista terminalis is a prominent muscular ridge that runs along the posterior wall of the RA from the orifice of the SVC to that of the IVC. Embryologically, this represents the junction between the two parts of the RA that are derived from the sinus venosus and the embryologic atrium. It may present as a nodular mass on axial MDCT or MRI, but is resolved as a linear ridge on oblique coronal reconstructions.

Right Ventricle

The moderator band is a thin muscular band extending from the mid-portion of the IVS to the free wall of the RV across the cavity. It may enlarge and simulate a RV mass, particularly in patients with enlargement or hypertrophy. MDCT or MRI helps to delineate its points of attachment, with an attenuation/SI similar to that of the adjacent myocardium.

CONCLUSION

A high index of clinical suspicion supported by reliable non- invasive imaging is necessary to make a definite diagnosis of a cardiac mass lesion. It is imperative to differentiate between neoplastic, non-neoplastic and non-pathologic entities mimicking a mass, in order to avoid an inadvertent surgery. Although ECHO is universally accepted as the initial modality for evaluation of a suspected intracardiac mass, it has significant limitations. ECHO is the best modality, however, for valvular lesions.

MDCT is useful for vascular lesions, calcification and fat content, and for demonstration of coronary anatomy prior to surgery. It is also useful for staging malignant lesions. MDCT is distinctly superior to MRI in pediatric patients due to a significantly less scanning time. However, MDCT has significantly limited ability to characterize tissues compared to MRI.

Due to its superior contrast resolution and availability of multiple sequences (including perfusion and delayed enhancement), MRI is the ideal modality for complete evaluation of cardiac masses. It is capable of simultaneously assessing their nature, extent and hemodynamic consequences. MRI is particularly useful for differentiating thrombi from cardiac tumors. However, scanning time needs to be reduced by software modifications in order to improve image quality, obtain diagnostic images in small children and fast heart rates, and increase patient throughput. Adequate sedation remains a major requirement for a successful examination in a small child. This can be very difficult, at times. Despite these limitations, MRI is still the investigation of choice for providing a definitive diagnosis in a patient with a suspected cardiac mass. The higher signal-to-noise ratio of 3T MRI is expected to further improve the delineation of cardiac mass lesions with this modality.

REFERENCES

1. Kim EY, Choe YH, Sung K, et al. Multidetector CT and MR Imaging of Cardiac Tumors. Korean J Radiol. 2009;10(2):164-75.
2. Bogaert J. Cardiac masses. In: Bogaert J. Duerinckx AJ, Rademakers FE (Eds). Magnetic Resonance of the Heart and Great Vessels: Clinical applications. Chapter 10. Springer-Verlag, Berlin, Heidelberg, Germany. 2000:169-204.
3. Syed IS, Feng D, Harris SR, et al. MR imaging of cardiac masses. Magn Reson Imaging Clin N Am. 2008;16(2):137-64.
4. Sutsch G, Jenni R, von Segesser L, et al. Heart tumors: Incidence, distribution, diagnosis. Exemplified by 20,305 echocardiographies. Schweiz Med Wochenschr. 1991;121:621-9.
5. McAllister Jr HA, Fenoglio Jr JJ. Tumors of the cardiovascular system. Atlas of tumor pathology, 2nd series. Fascicle 15 Washington DC, Armed Forces Institute of Pathology. 1978;1-20:69-71.
6. Moriyama Y, Saigenji H, Shimokawa S, et al. The surgical treatment of 30 patients with cardiac myxomas: A comparison of clinical features according to morphological classification. Surg Today. 1994;24:596-8.
7. Burke A, Virmani R. Atlas of tumor pathology. Washington DC: Armed Forces Institute of Pathology. Tumors of the heart and great vessels. 1996;(3):79-90.
8. Edwards FH, Hale D, Cohen A, et al. Primary cardiac valve tumors. Ann Thorac Surg. 1991;52:1127-31.
9. Burke AP, Rosado-de-Christenson M, Templeton PA, et al. Cardiac fibroma: Clinicopathologic correlates and surgical treatment. J Thorac Cardiovasc Surg. 1994;108:862-70.
10. De Cobelli F, Esposito A, Mellone R, et al. Images in cardiovascular medicine. Late enhancement of a left ventricular cardiac fibroma assessed with gadolinium-enhanced cardiovascular magnetic resonance. Circulation. 2005;112:E242-3.
11. Webb DW, Thomas RD, Osborne JP. Cardiac rhabdomyomas and their association with tuberous sclerosis. Arch Dis Child. 1993;68:367-70.
12. Newell JD 2nd, Eckel C, Davis M, et al. MR appearance of an arteriovenous hemangioma of the interventricular septum. Cardiovasc Intervent Radiol. 1988;11:319-21.
13. Yahata S, Endo T, Honma H, et al. Sunray appearance on enhanced magnetic resonance image of cardiac angiosarcoma with pericardial obliteration. Am Heart J. 1994;127:468-71.
14. Okamoto K, Kato S, Katsuki S, et al. Malignant fibrous histiocytoma of the heart: Case report and review of 46 cases in the literature. Intern Med. 2001;40:1222-6.
15. Awamleh P, Alberca MT, Gamallo C, et al. Left atrium myxosarcoma: An exceptional cardiac malignant primary tumor. Clin Cardiol. 2007;30:306-8.
16. Cuotinsinger CR, Wilson J, Yoneda K. Primary cardiac lymphoma. Cancer. 1989;64:521-5.
17. Lam KY, Dickens P, Chan AC. Tumors of the heart. A 20 years' experience with a review of 12,485 consecutive autopsies. Arch Pathol Lab Med. 1993;117:1027-103.
18. Klatt EC, Heitz DR. Cardiac metastases. Cancer. 1990;65:1456-9.
19. Sechtem U, Theissen P, Heindel W, et al. Diagnosis of left ventricular thrombi by MRI and comparison with angiocardiography, computed tomography and echocardiography. Am J Cardiol. 1989;64:1195-9.
20. Sparrow PJ, Kurian JB, Jones TR, et al. MR imaging of cardiac tumors. Radiographics. 2005;25:1255-76.
21. Mollet NR, Dymarkowski S, Volders W, et al. Visualization of ventricular thrombi with contrast-enhanced magnetic resonance imaging in patients with ischemic heart disease. Circulation. 2002;106:2873-6.
22. Sasson L, Katz MG, Ezri T, et al. Ruptured sinus of Valsalva aneurysm complicated by myocardial ischemia: Pathogenetic mechanisms. Cardiovasc Pathol. 2006;15:291-3.
23. Pepper C, Munsch C, Sivananthan M, et al. Unruptured aneurysm of the left sinus of Valsalva extending into the left ventricular outflow tract: presentation and imaging. Heart. 1998;80:190-3.
24. Dursun M, Terzibasioglu E, Yilmaz, R, et al. Cardiad hydatid disease: CT and MRI findings. AJR. 2008;190:226-32.
25. Rose AG. Cardiac tuberculosis: A study of 19 patients. Arch Pathol Lab Med. 1987;11:422-6.
26. Gulati GS, Singh S, Arepalli CD, et al. Superior vena caval obstruction after complete resolution of cardiac tuberculoma. Clin Rad. 2008;63:605-9.

CHAPTER 181

Imaging Diagnosis of Valvular Heart Disease

Priya Jagia, Sanjiv Sharma, Gurpreet Singh Gulati

INTRODUCTION

Valvular heart disease is one of the most common group of cardiac disorders, largely due to the high prevalence of rheumatic fever in India. This disease most commonly involves the mitral valve, followed by the aortic, tricuspid and pulmonary valves in this order. The resultant lesions can result in stenosis, incompetence or both in the involved valve.

The objectives of imaging in valvular disease irrespective of its etiology include:

- Diagnosis of the valvular disease: Qualitative as well as quantitative assessment of all valves,
- Assessment of the hemodynamic effects of valvular disease on the pulmonary vasculature and ventricular function,
- Detection of associated pulmonary pathologies as a complication or coincidental to heart disease, and
- Follow-up after treatment.

The recent advances in imaging techniques for noninvasive evaluation of the cardiac diseases have helped better delineate the anatomic location of the disease, and study the impact of the resultant structural abnormalities on the hemodynamic and functional consequences on the cardiovascular system. These have also gone a long way in an improved understanding of the natural history of the disease processes. Accurate diagnosis is now possible with nonmethods. Chest radiograph is useful in the initial evaluation of the patient. It provides valuable information about the cardiac size, pulmonary vasculature, arterial and venous hypertension, and the secondary changes in the lungs. Echocardiography is a useful screening technique that allows real-time evaluation of each cardiac chamber in multiple orthogonal planes. It is noninvasive, easily available, provides a direct visualization of cardiac valves and also helps evaluate the attendant functional disturbances on the cardiac chambers. The stenosis and regurgitation, as well as the resultant derangement of ventricular function, including the size of the chamber, wall thickness, size of valvular orifice, trans stenotic pressure gradient or the regurgitant volume, can be reliably estimated by quantitative methods. The published reports suggest that the results compare favorably with the information obtained at cardiac catheterization and angiocardiography. Its major limitations include operator dependence and availability of a proper acoustic window. Now multislice computed tomography (MSCT) and cardiac magnetic resonance imaging (CMRI) are used in selected patients for optimal evaluation of the valvular heart disease and its hemodynamic consequences. Plain chest radiograph is useful in the initial evaluation of the patient. It helps aid the diagnosis and define the impact of the disease on the pulmonary vasculature. It is also useful in the assessment of the effect of treatment in a given patient. This technique is easily and widely available, and provides a reproducible and a permanent record of the patient. Therefore, it is widely used as the initial screening imaging technique in most patients. The chest radiographic abnormalities in various disease states are described here.

AORTIC VALVULAR DISEASE

The involvement of the aortic valve is characterized by LV hypertrophy in stenotic, and LV hypertrophy and dilatation in regurgitant lesions. The heart shows characteristic LV configuration in the form of rounding of cardiac apex, low apex and elongation of left border. Heart size is normal or minimally enlarged in stenotic lesions whereas it shows a moderate or severe enlargement in regurgitant lesions. Subtle cardiac enlargement in aortic stenosis is better detected on the lateral film and with volumetric measurements. Using the upper limit of normal (462 mL/m^2) for heart volume, LV enlargement confined to hypertrophy can only be detected with an accuracy of 79%. If one also takes into account other parameters of cardiac configuration, the false-negative rates are reduced to only 5%. The ascending aorta shows a typical post-stenotic dilatation in aortic stenosis (AS) whereas the dilatation is more diffuse and also involves the aortic knuckle in aortic regurgitation (AR). Aortic valve calcification is more frequently seen in AS with a bicuspid valve than in AS of rheumatic etiology. Calcification is best seen on fluoroscopy. The presence of calcification in the aortic valve is localized based on its characteristic location and movement. In presence of AR, the size of the heart roughly parallels the severity of regurgitation. Minimal LA enlargement and pulmonary venous hypertension (PVH) can be seen in aortic valve lesions. However, significant enlargement of LA indicates either an associated mitral valve involvement or left ventricular failure. A prominent LA appendage is virtually pathognomonic of rheumatic mitral valve disease. Frequently, AR and AS coexist **(Figs. 1 and 2)**.

MITRAL VALVULAR DISEASE

In mitral stenosis (MS), the heart size can be normal if assessed only by frontal projection. However, by volumetry, it is found to be enlarged in a majority of cases. Still a completely normal heart size can be seen in approximately 10% of the patients with critical MS **(Figs. 3 and 4)**. On the other hand, in mitral regurgitation (MR), the heart is generally enlarged with LV configuration and the size of the heart serves as a reliable indicator of the severity of MR. The radiographic picture can get modified in presence of TR **(Fig. 5)**, when there is a dominant enlargement of the right atrium with a less obvious PVH.

The hallmark of mitral valve disease is selective LA enlargement. Enlargement of the LA appendage (LAA) is pathognomonic of rheumatic etiology and can vary from a simple straightening of the left heart border to a large bulge in the typical site, immediately below the left main bronchus. Posteriorly, it can cause an indentation over the esophagus and may even deviate the middle descending aorta to the left (Bedford's sign). Rarely, LA or LAA may show calcification either in its wall or in the clot lining the wall. Valvular calcification, generally seen on fluoroscopy, strongly suggests a rheumatic etiology. In contrast, mitral annular calcification is often seen in age-related degenerative disease and in the postoperative patient after closed mitral valvotomy.

In MS, enlargement of LA may be mild or moderate but is rarely gross. In mitral regurgitation (MR), LA enlargement is usually gross or aneurysmal. In both MR as well as MS, the size of LA bears no correlation with the severity of the lesion as it is more dependent on the pliability of the

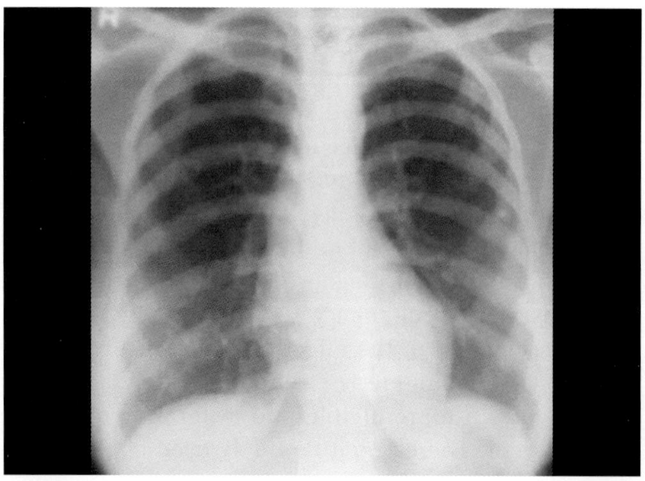

Fig. 1: Chest radiograph in a patient with valvular AS shows normal heart size, LV configuration, postdilatation of the ascending aorta and normal lung vasculature.

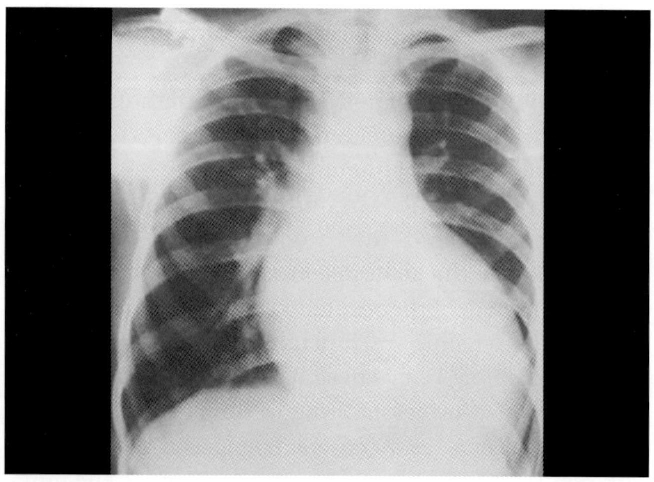

Fig. 2: Chest radiograph in a patient with AR shows a large heart, LV configuration, dilated aorta and mild PVH.

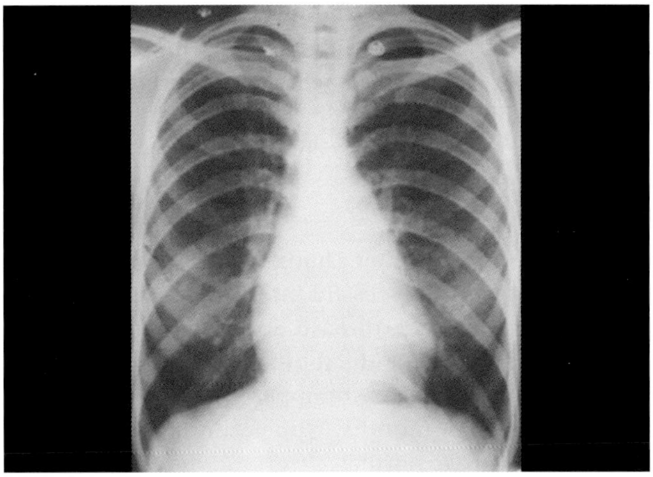

Fig. 3: Chest radiograph in a patient with MS shows normal heart size, LA enlargement and mild PVH.

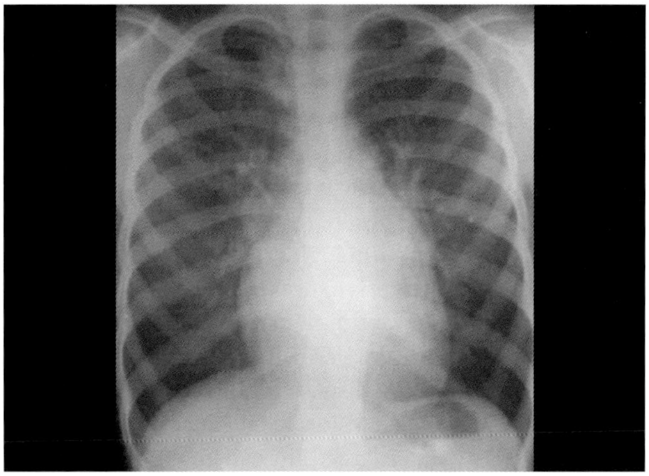

Fig. 4: Chest radiograph in a patient with MR shows a large heart, LV and LA enlargement, and mild PVH.

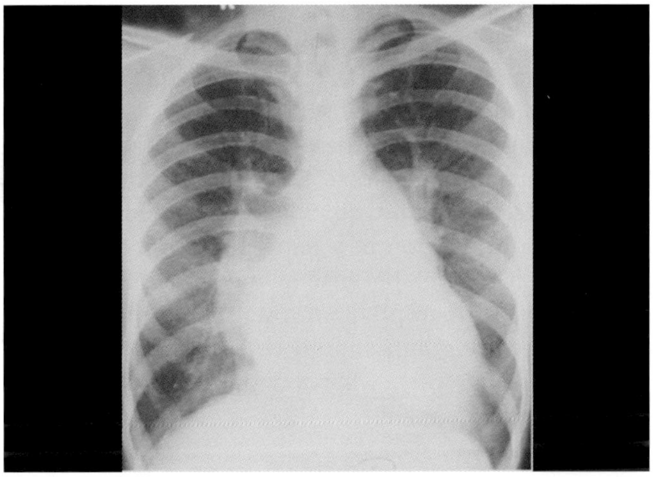

Fig. 5: Chest radiograph in a patient with MS and TR shows mild cardiomegaly, LA and RA enlargement and PVH.

atrial wall because of inflammation in rheumatic disease. The hemodynamic changes in the pulmonary circulation are sensitive indicators of the severity of disease in MS. Frequently, the mitral valve has a combined lesion. In such situations, it is usually not possible to assess the severity of each lesion by chest radiography alone. However, a dominant MS can be suggested by small heart and LA relative to the severity of PVH. A large heart and LA with relatively mild PVH changes suggests a dominant MR. Similarly, a concomitant involvement of aortic valve and tricuspid valve can be suggested if there is prominence of ascending aorta or right atrium (RA) respectively.

TRICUSPID VALVULAR DISEASE

The most common involvement of tricuspid valve is in the form of a functional regurgitation secondary to RV dilatation caused by the underlying mitral valve disease. Rarely, it is directly involved by the rheumatic process and results in regurgitation or, less commonly, stenosis. The characteristic radiological feature is a large RA. This chamber is most difficult to assess by plain chest radiography, especially when the other chambers are also enlarged. The increase in the height of the RA relative to that of the vascular pedicle provides the most specific index of its enlargement.

HEMODYNAMIC EFFECTS ON PULMONARY VASCULATURE

Mitral valvular disease and, to a lesser extent, the aortic valvular disease is characterized by a rise in the LA pressure which in turn leads to a rise in pulmonary capillary wedge pressure (PCWP). Depending on the severity of PVH, a series of changes may be seen on the chest radiograph. These changes have been discussed earlier and have been shown to bear a rough correlation with the pressure values obtained at cardiac catheterization. Sustained PVH causes obstructive changes in the small pulmonary arteries leading to an increase in pulmonary vascular resistance. This can result in reactive or organic pulmonary arterial hypertension (PAH).

Thus, a chest radiograph, in addition to indicating specific hemodynamic disturbances, can also help in predicting the severity of valvular lesion like in MS where these changes roughly parallel the severity of the disease. The relative accuracy of different roentgen signs in predicting severe MS (area of 1.0 cm^2 or less) is as follows:

- Kerley B lines—96%.
- Combined venous and arterial abnormalities in the pulmonary vascular pattern—97%.

- LA enlargement producing >12 cm^2 posterior deviation of the esophagus—83%.
- Either 1 or 2 plus 3—100%.

Associated Pulmonary Pathologies

A plain chest radiograph is useful in assessing most abnormalities of the lungs in a patient with valvular heart disease. Various lung pathologies, if present, can simulate or aggravate the symptoms in these patients. These can be vital in deciding the management strategy. These include pulmonary tuberculosis, chronic airway obstructive disease, interstitial lung disease, and pneumonia among others. Rarely, a cardiac lesion itself causes a pulmonary complication like an enlarged LA causing lobar collapse, consolidation, bronchiectasis, or obstructive emphysema.

Effects of Treatment during Follow-up

It is necessary to monitor the effect of treatment on the cardiac and pulmonary changes. Since valvular heart diseases generally run a protracted course and most patients lead a near normal life after surgical or other intervention, their follow-up requires close monitoring. Echocardiogram is best suited for this purpose because it can precisely quantify the hemodynamic effects of the valvular lesions. Chest radiographs are also useful for a ready comparison of the heart size and the status of the pulmonary vasculature.

Heart Size

In regurgitant lesions of aortic and mitral valves, the heart size generally serves as a good indicator for the severity of the disease. Once the diagnosis has been established, the patient can be followed-up by monitoring the heart size. Similarly, a postoperative reduction in heart size serves as a good indicator of successful outcome.

Left Atrial Size

Reduction in the size of LA indicates a favorable outcome in cases of mitral valve replacement or balloon dilatation. Therefore, a quantitative assessment of left atrial size in such patients can offer an easy way to assess the progress of such patients. Few methods adopted in the past include grading of the size of the left atrium according to the indentation on the esophagus; or by measuring the size of LA either on the lateral view by measuring the distance from the anterior border of the right pulmonary artery to the anterior wall of the esophagus, or on the frontal view by measuring the distance from the mid-point of the curvilinear margin of the double density to the midpoint of the inferior wall of the left bronchus. A measurement of more than 7 cm is seen in approximately 90% patients with LA enlargement. Left atrial size may not change if there is severe rheumatic involvement of left atrial wall and resultant fibrosis. Such cases should be assessed by echocardiography.

Other Changes

There are a host of other changes that can indicate an improvement after successful intervention, especially in presence of mitral valve disease. Some examples include:

- Interstitial edema disappears within days while diminution in the size of upper zone vessel may take weeks or even months. Upper zone vessels do not usually return to normal.
- In patients with PAH, the dilated pulmonary trunk may return to normal with successful treatment.
- Presence of a flat or concave left midcardiac border on chest radiograph may be seen after a closed mitral valvotomy or following a thrombus in the appendage. However, this sign has a poor predictive value of the presence of the latter. Echocardiographic examination can easily detect this complication during the course of the disease. Overall, chest radiographs are widely available, quick and cost-effective in the imaging evaluation of a patient with valvular heart disease. However, because of undisputed advantages of echocardiography, information available from a chest radiograph should be complemented with echocardiography, wherever possible, for optimal patient management.

ECHOCARDIOGRAPHY

This technique is useful in the evaluation of stenosis and regurgitation of all cardiac valves, prosthetic valve function, and in patients with infective endocarditis. It provides valuable information regarding the diagnosis, valvular morphology, etiology of the disease, identification and quantification of lesions, detection and evaluation of associated abnormalities, delineation of cardiac size and ventricular function. This technique detects structural abnormalities of the valve, including fibrosis, calcification, thrombus, or vegetation, and abnormalities of valvular motion, including immobile, flail or prolapsing leaflets, or prosthetic valve dehiscence. A full evaluation provides prognostic as well as diagnostic information, allows for risk stratification, establishes the baseline data for subsequent examinations, and helps guide and evaluate the therapeutic approach. Echocardiography may obviate the need for cardiac catheterization in selected patients.

Valvular Stenosis

Two-dimensional and Doppler echocardiography reliably identify and quantitate the severity of the stenotic lesions. MS is accurately assessed by planimetry of transthoracic or transesophageal 2D images, Doppler measurement of trans-stenotic gradient, and estimation of valve area. Prognostic information is obtained from assessment of the hemodynamic response to exercise and/or delineation of morphological characteristics, which may help guide the selection of therapeutic interventions. Although tricuspid stenosis is readily detected and assessed hemodynamically, the accuracy of Doppler measurements is less well validated but still preferred over other methods. AS is accurately quantified by Doppler measurements of gradients and estimation of valve area. Pulmonary valve gradients are similarly quantified. While still experimental, contrast injection may allow more accurate recording of stenotic jet velocities and, therefore, transvalvular gradients.

Valvular Regurgitation

This is, perhaps, the most sensitive technique for detection of native valve regurgitation. Precise assessment of the severity of regurgitant lesions is difficult using any invasive or noninvasive technique, and no perfect method is, yet, available to judge the relative accuracy of a given technique. By far, angiography is the most widely used gold standard for this estimation. The results of echocardiography correlate well with it. Doppler methods for detection of regurgitation are similar for the native and prosthetic valves. Methods include assessment of regurgitant jet characteristics (length, height, area, and width), effective regurgitant orifice area, and measurement of regurgitant flow volumes. Doppler echocardiography is also an excellent technique for the re-evaluation of regurgitant lesions after surgery and in determination of the timing and method of operative intervention. In the evaluation of patients with mitral valve prolapse, this technique is useful for diagnosis and risk stratification, by identifying leaflet thickening and LV dilatation.

Infective Endocarditis

Echocardiography is useful for the detection and characterization of the hemodynamic and pathological consequences of infection, including valvular vegetations, regurgitant lesions, ventricular function, and associated abnormalities such as abscess, shunt and ruptured chordae. Controversy remains on the role of echocardiographic characteristics of vegetations in predicting embolization, although vegetation size, mobility, identification of the involved valve(s), and detection of myocardial involvement are important for risk stratification and prognosis.

Prosthetic Valves

Valve replacement carries a subsequent risk of valve degeneration, thrombosis, pannus formation, development of regurgitant or stenotic lesions and endocarditis. Obtaining baseline postoperative studies can be useful for comparison with future evaluation of changes in ventricular function and hemodynamics in response to surgery. Assessment of prosthetic valve stenosis is best performed by a combined echocardiography and Doppler technique. Estimation of prosthetic valve regurgitation is often hampered by prosthetic shadowing, particularly in the mitral position. The transesophageal approach may be useful in such cases. Contrast injection may enhance the spectral recording of both right-sided regurgitant velocities as well as the extent of the regurgitant jet.

CARDIAC MAGNETIC RESONANCE IMAGING

Cardiac magnetic resonance imaging (CMRI) offers a unique advantage of providing an observer independent, noninvasive technique for demonstration of pathological anatomy, quantification of global and regional function of both ventricles, flow disturbances across the stenotic valve, estimation of regurgitant volume, measurement of blood flows, and for assessing myocardial perfusion. Optimal cardiac imaging requires some form of physiological gating. Acquisition of signals without gating gives poor images because of loss of signal from moving structures and due to variable position of the heart structures in relation to image pixels when the data is acquired indiscriminately. The accuracy of MRI can be improved by using small voxels, thin slices and very short echo delay time. Cine MRI can be used for evaluation and monitoring of ventricular function, mass and wall stress in patients with valvular heart disease.

The CMRI has certain attributes that make it useful for imaging this body system. Firstly, there exists a natural contrast between the blood pool and the cardiovascular structures due to lack of signal from the flowing blood during spin-echo MRI, and bright signal from flowing blood in gradient-echo sequences. The differential blood signal is strikingly different from that of the myocardium, and hence, there is a good edge delineation of the endocardium. As a result, no additional contrast material is required for demarcation of the blood pool. This ensures that MRI remains a noninvasive imaging technique.

Secondly, there is a wide range of soft tissue contrast on MRI images that provides characterization of the myocardial tissue. This tissue characterization is improved by the use of paramagnetic contrast material.

Thirdly, the imaging can be done in any plane.

Lastly, cardiac MRI is also useful in giving us the functional and hemodynamic information besides giving morphological details. It can demonstrate valvular stenosis and regurgitation on cine images with poststenotic and regurgitant jets seen as flow voids on bright blood images. Quantification of flow and gradient across the valve can be done using phase contrast techniques and ventricular analysis. Phase contrast method is principally based on the phase shifts of moving spins in the magnetic field gradient. The extent of phase shifts of moving spins is proportional to the velocity along the velocity-encoding direction. Velocity-encoding is performed by using bipolar gradient pulses. Its direction can be selected in any orthogonal or oblique axis of the body. Velocity-encoding of blood flow in each pixel provides 2D quantitative velocity mapping of the vascular system. Once velocity across a vessel is obtained, gradient can be derived using formula $\Delta = 4 (V_{max})^2$.

Valve Leaflet Morphology

This can be seen with both black blood and steady-state free procession (SSFP) images **(Fig. 6)**.

Aortic valve leaflets can be seen on 2 chamber and 4 chamber views **(Figs. 7A and B)** while tricuspid valve's anatomy can be well seen on long axis and short axis views. Aortic valve area can be calculated by direct planimetry. For pulmonic valve, a double oblique view of right ventricular outflow tract is used as a guide to planimetric visualization of pulmonary valve.

Valvular Stenosis

On cine images, leaflet movements appear to restricted and flow turbulence is seen in vessel/chamber in distal downstream **(Fig. 7C)**. For example, in valvular pulmonary stenosis, the turbulence and flow voids due to poststenotic jets are seen in main pulmonary artery.

Valvular Regurgitation

Signal void due to regurgitating blood is seen in the receiving chamber **(Fig. 8)**. Quantitative measurement

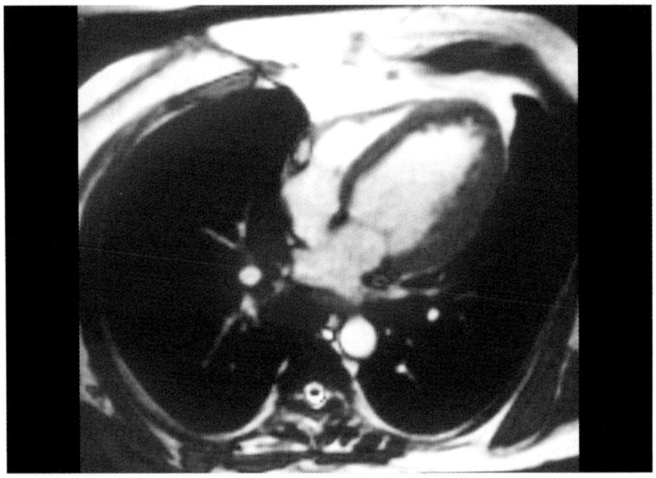

Fig. 6: Four-chamber SSFP MR image showing normal mitral valve in closed position.

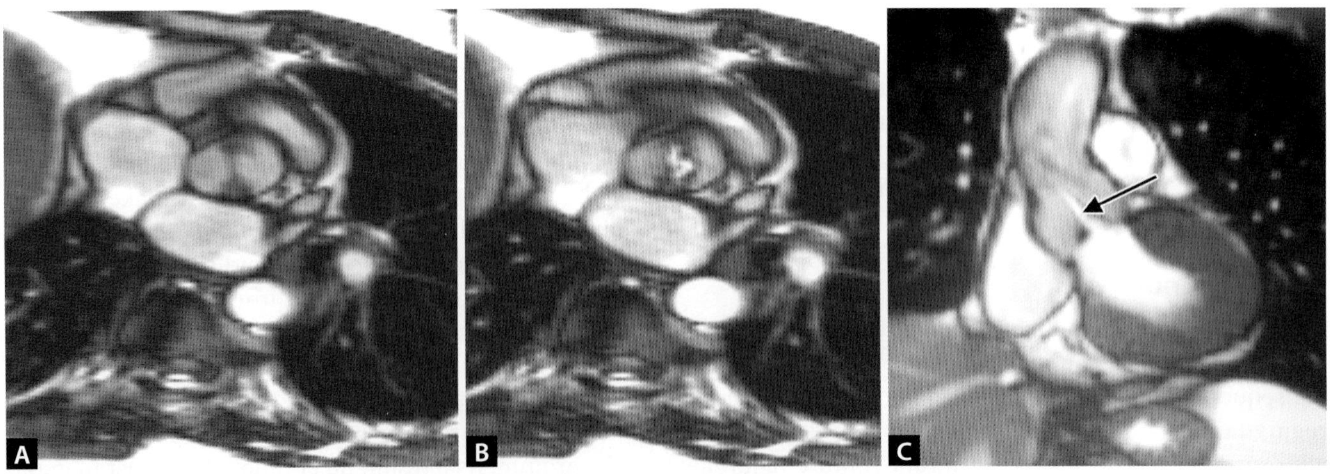

Figs. 7A to C: Bicuspid aortic valve seen in its short axis in diastole: (A) Aystole; (B) Planimetric measurement of aortic valve area can be done in the latter frame; (C) Oblique coronal view on cine bright blood MR image showing post-stenotic jet in ascending aorta in a patient with aortic valvular stenosis.

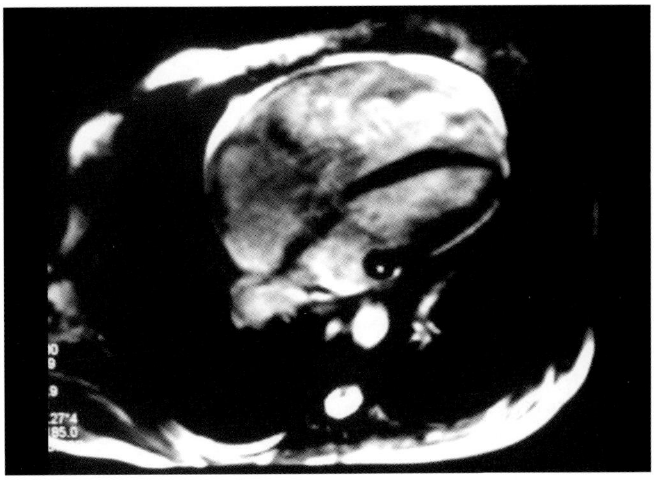

Fig. 8: Cine bright blood MR image in 4 chamber view showing jet due to tricuspid regurgitation, in right atrium.

of regurgitant volume can be done using volumetric or phase velocity methods or both. The difference between the end-diastolic and end-systolic volumes for a ventricle with a regurgitant valve includes both the forward stroke volume and the regurgitant volume. Because the forward or net stroke volume is equal to the volume ejected from the normal ventricle, the difference in stroke volumes between a regurgitant ventricle (e.g. LV with AR or MR) and normal ventricle (e.g. RV) is the regurgitant volume. The sum of the forward and regurgitant volume is called the total stroke volume of the regurgitant ventricle.

Phase-contrast techniques can be used to directly quantify the aortic and pulmonary regurgitation. For mitral and tricuspid regurgitation, a combined approach using phase contrast techniques and ventricular volume assessment is used. Velocity-encoded MRI is done to measure the systolic outflow from the LV at the level of the ascending aorta and diastolic inflow to LV at the level of the mitral annulus. The difference between the two is a measure of the volume of MR.

Valve Endocarditis and Tumors

Case reports have been published describing the use of MRI in evaluation of valve tumors. Cine images help identify the small valve vegetations and tumors. The regurgitation of valve, if present, can be also be quantified.

Prosthetic Valve

When prosthetic values are studied, they usually cause local signal loss and are not well seen. Early concerns regarding radio-frequency energy deposition and heating have, to date, been unfounded. Despite the increasing use of high gradient strengths for faster acquisition approaching close to physiological threshold for muscle and nerve stimulation limits set by FDA, there are no reports of MRI complications related to valve prosthesis. Valves that are strongly ferromagnetic (Starr-Edwards pre 6000 series valves), however, should not be scanned. Overall, MRI is well suited for the evaluation of a patient with valvular heart disease. A cooperative patient with a stable heart rate, that is not too fast or too slow and in normal sinus rhythm, is necessary for optimal image acquisition. Availability of the equipment, cost and familiarity of the operator and the treating physician will determine the optimal use of this modality.

COMPUTED TOMOGRAPHY

Multislice CT can, in single breath-hold, evaluate large volumes in orthogonal planes with a high signal-to-noise ratio. These features make imaging easier in children and in patients with any habitus.

The MSCT can identify cardiac calcification sensitively. It can be localized, characterized and quantified in the valves, chamber wall **(Fig. 9)**, pericardium and the coronary arteries. A negative MSCT used to assess coronary calcification has a strong negative predictive valve of 98% and excludes the need for coronary angiography in an elderly patient with valvular heart disease. Contrast enhancement is needed to evaluate the cardiac chambers and valves. CT can measure the cardiac chamber volume, wall thickness and myocardial mass. In addition, multi-slice CT can measure the cardiac output, ventricular mass and stroke volume. If only a single valve is regurgitating, the volume can be calculated by comparing RV and LV stroke volumes. ECG-gated CT images can help reconstruct cardiac motion throughout the cardiac cycle and the jets due to stenotic or regurgitant valves can be seen **(Fig. 10)**. With MSCT, it is possible to get stroke volumes and do ventricular analysis. CT is also useful in differentiating intracardiac thrombi from a tumor. Despite these advantages, the impact of CT techniques on valvular imaging is still evolving.

ANGIOCARDIOGRAPHY

In patients with valvular heart disease, cardiac catheterization provides data both confirmatory and complementary to noninvasive echocardiography and nuclear studies. Cardiac catheterization procedure includes pressure measurements in the cardiac chambers and the great vessels, oximetry in each chamber and resultant hemodynamic assessments, and angiography. Angiograms reveal typical diagnostic images in presence of stenotic **(Figs. 11 and 12)** and regurgitant **(Figs. 13 and 14)** lesions

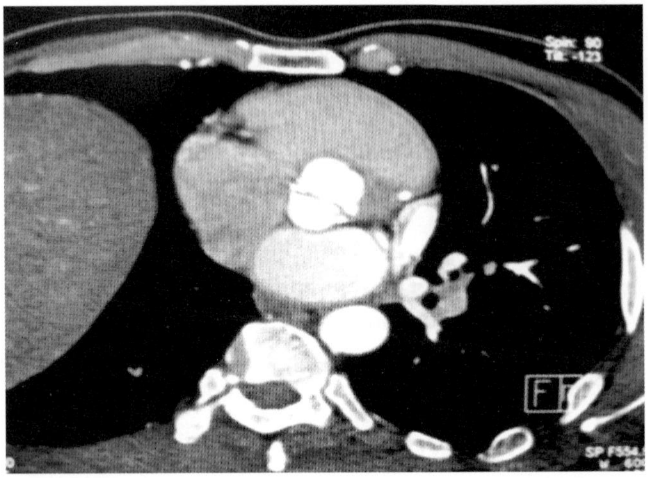

Fig. 9: Oblique axial CT image across the aortic valve showing bicuspid calcified valve.

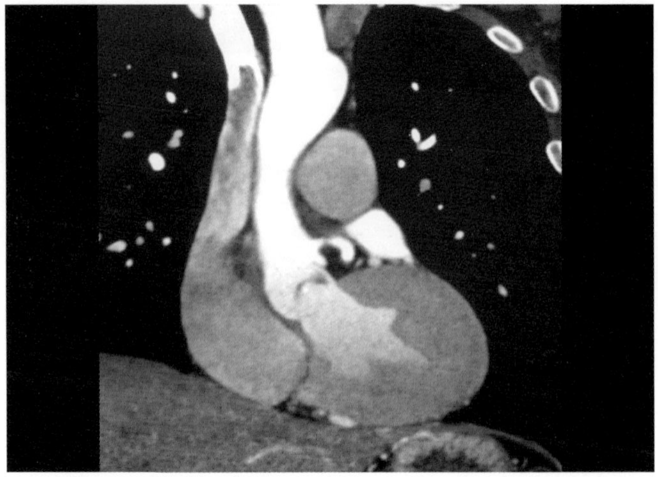

Fig. 10: Cine coronal image reconstructed from ECG-gated CT images shows doming of the bicuspid aortic valve in systole.

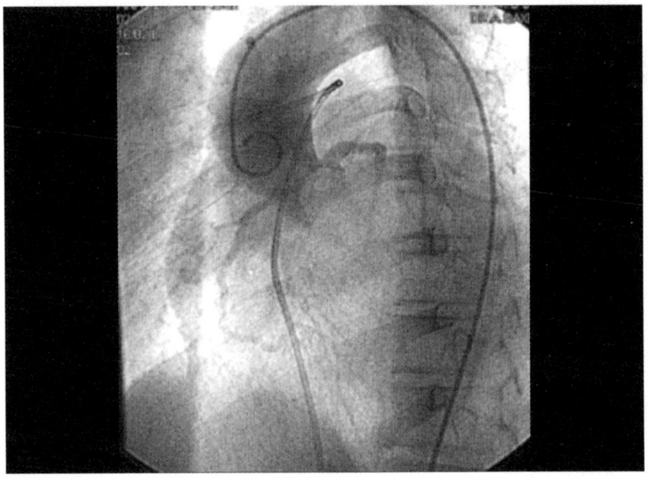

Fig. 11: Aortic root angiogram in the left anterior oblique (LAO) view in a patient with valvular AS shows doming of the aortic valve, restricted negative jet and poststenotic dilatation of the ascending aorta.

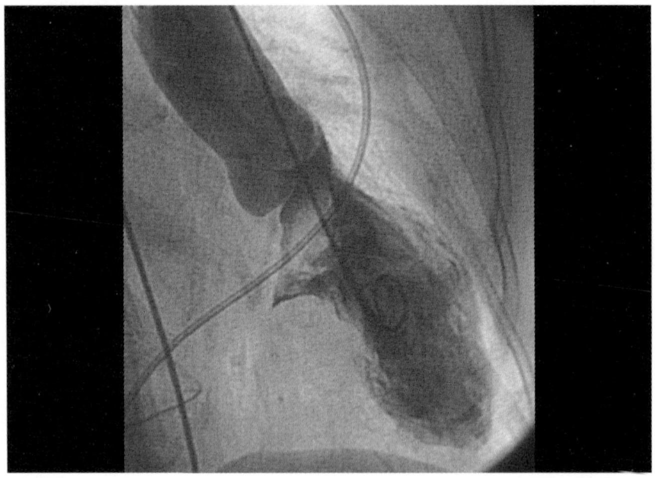

Fig. 12: LV angiogram in the right anterior oblique (RAO) view in a patient with MS shows doming of mitral valve, restricted negative bolus and no MR.

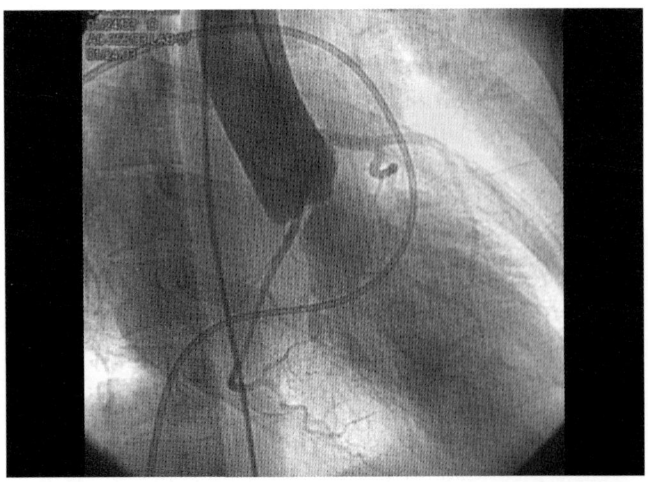

Fig. 13: Aortic root angiogram in the RAO view in a patient with severe AR shows opacification of the entire LV.

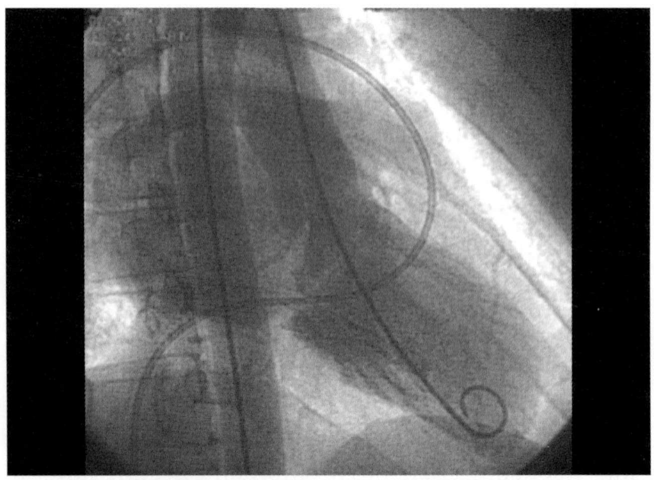

Fig. 14: LV angiogram in the RAO view in a patient with severe MR shows the opacification of the entire LV.

of all cardiac valves. The indications for angiocardiography are based on the assessment of risks versus benefits of the procedure. The availability and familiarity with noninvasive techniques, including echocardiography and MRI, has changed the indications of angiocardiography and all patients in whom surgical treatment is considered may not necessarily require angiography.

Whenever indicated, the overall benefits outweigh the risk of catheterization. At the present time, angiocardiography is not indicated in single valve pathologies in patients in whom coronary angiography is not required, and also in clear-cut double valve lesions in patients less than 40 years in age provided that the tricuspid valve is not involved. When performed, cardiac catheterization provides confirmation of the severity of valvular lesion, identifies associated coronary artery disease, quantifies the hemodynamic consequences of valvular lesions (such as pulmonary hypertension), and occasionally the acute hemodynamic response to pharmacological therapy. These may help select the optimal therapeutic strategy and define the risks of treatment. Valvular regurgitation may be assessed visually by determining the relative amount of the contrast medium that opacifies the chamber proximal to its injection. The estimation of regurgitation depends on the regurgitant volume as well as the size and contractility of the proximal chamber. In addition, cardiac catheterization is indicated whenever interventional catheter-directed treatment is planned.

CONCLUSION

A multimodality approach, using a combination of non-invasive techniques backed by a sound clinical assessment is usually adequate for the diagnosis and for defining the optimal management option in most patients. When choosing a given technique, it is important to keep in mind the availability, cost and familiarity of the operator and the other team members with its interpretation and pitfalls. Chest radiographs are useful for the initial evaluation and during follow-up after treatment in all patients. Echocardiography remains the mainstay for investigating these patients and planning their management strategy. Despite the fact that MRI and multislice CT are operator independent and are capable of providing excellent quality images along with information on the functional impairment caused by the valvular lesions in a noninvasive manner, their wider use in the diagnostic algorithm of these patients in most centers is still limited and investigational. Cardiac catheterization and angiography are indicated whenever coronary anatomy needs to be defined, in the evaluation of tricuspid involvement, in situations where a discrepancy between the clinical and imaging data exists and for interventional management of the lesions.

BIBLIOGRAPHY

1. Albers J, Nitsche T, Boese J, et al. Regurgitant jet evaluation using three-dimensional echocardiography and magnetic resonance. Ann Thorac Surg. 2004;78(1):96-102.
2. Cawley PJ, Maki JH, Otto CM. Cardiovascular magnetic resonance imaging for valvular heart disease: technique and validation. Circulation. 2009;119(3):468-78.
3. Chen JTT, Behar VS, Marris JJ, et al. Correlation of roentgen findings with hemodynamic data in pure mitral stenosis. AJR. 1968;102:280-92.
4. Chikos PM, Figley MM, Fisher L. Correlation between chest film and angiographic assessment of left ventricular size. AJR. 1977;128:367-73.
5. Higgins CB, Reinke RT, Jones NE, et al. Left atrial dimension on the frontal thoracic radiograph: a method for assessment left atrial enlargement. AJR. 1978;130:251-5.
6. Jefferson K, Rees S. Clinical Cardiac Radiology. Butterworths, London. 1973;230-9.
7. Kelley MR, Elliot LP, Schulman ST, et al. The significance of the dilated left atrial appendage in rheumatic heart disease. Circulation. 1976;54:146-53.
8. Murray JG, Brown AL, Anagnostov EA, et al. Widening of the tracheal bifurcation on chest radiographs: Value as a sign of left atrial enlargement. AJR. 1995;164:1089-92.
9. Newell JD, Higgins CB, Kelly MJ. Radiographic echocardiographic approach to acquired heart disease: Diagnosis and assessment of severity. Radiologic Clinics of North America. 1980;18:387-409.
10. Pouleur AC, le Polain de Waroux JB, Pasquet A, et al. Aortic valve area assessment: Multidetector CT compared with cine MR imaging and transthoracic and transesophageal echocardiography. Radiology. 2007;244:745-54.
11. Raphael MJ. Cardiac radiology: techniques and normal appearances In: Grainger RG, Allison DJ (Eds). Diagnotic Radiology, An Anglo American Textbook of Imaging. Churchill Livingstone, Edinburgh, 1992; pp. 431-45.
12. Sharma S, Kumar MB, Aggarwal S, Reddy VM, Kaul U, Rajani M, Venugopal P. Chest radiographs are unreliable in predicting thrombi in the left atrium or its appendage in rheumatic mitral stenosis. Clin Radio. 1991;43:337-40.
13. Vogel-Claussen J, Pannu H, Spevak PJ, Fishman EK, Bluemke DA. Cardiac valve assessment with MR imaging and 64-section Multi-detector row CT. Radio Graphics. 2006;26(6):1769-84.
14. Westcott JL, Ferguson D. The right pulmonary artery-left atrial axis line. A method for measuring left atrial size on lateral chest radiographs. Radiology. 1976;118:265-74.

CHAPTER 182

Imaging of the Pericardium

Jyoti Kumar, Sapna Singh, Anju Garg, Gaurav S Pradhan

INTRODUCTION

The initial approach to the evaluation of pericardial disease is usually performed with echocardiography and chest radiography. While echocardiography has its own advantages, namely high temporal and spatial resolution, easy availability, no involvement of ionizing radiation, it is usually limited by poor acoustic window, poor soft tissue characterization and operator variability. In addition, it can be very difficult to detect pericardial thickening or calcification.[1,2]

Computed tomography (CT) and magnetic resonance (MR) imaging techniques prove to be advantageous over echocardiography in the following respect: they provide excellent anatomic details, help in localizing pericardial pathology as well as depicting associated abnormalities of the lung and mediastinum. The advent of multidetector CT with its excellent temporal resolution helps us to image pericardium devoid of cardiac motion artifacts. Multiplanar reformats allow better visualization of pericardial pathology with easy communication to the referring physician.[3] A cinematic display of cardiac motion is now possible on CT with electrocardiography (ECG) gating and high resolution thin section images can be obtained. Increased sensitivity to detect calcification is another advantage of CT. MR imaging provides superior soft tissue characterization than CT and echocardiography. MR imaging can provide excellent display of cardiac motion in patients with regular heart rhythm.[3-6]

ANATOMY

The pericardium has an outer fibrous layer and an inner serous layer. The inner serosal layer is further composed of outer parietal and inner visceral layer. The outer parietal layer lines the inner surface of the fibrous pericardium and the inner visceral layer forms the epicardium.[7,8] Ligaments attach the outer pericardium to sternum and diaphragm. The serosal layer forms two complex sleeves as it reflects around major vessel. One of these sleeves enclose the aorta and pulmonary trunk and the other encloses the superior and inferior vena cava and the four pulmonary veins. These reflections form the sinuses and recesses **(Fig. 1)**. The transverse sinus is the channel in between these two sleeves around the arteries and veins and the oblique sinus is the channel behind the left atrium. The recesses are the blind ends of these sinuses **(Box 1)**. These

Box 1: Sinuses and recesses of pericardium.

- *Transverse sinus*:
  - *Superior aortic sinus*:
    - Anterior triangular extension
    - Posterior crescentic extension
    - Right lateral extension
  - Inferior aortic recess
  - Right and left pulmonic recesses
- *Oblique sinus*:
  - Posterior pericardial recess
- *Recesses of pericardial cavity proper*:
  - Right and left pulmonary venous recesses
  - Postcaval recess

sinuses and recesses can collect fluid within them in case of pericardial effusion. With the advent of MDCT, visualization of pericardial recesses without fluid accumulation is also possible with narrow collimation imaging.[8]

The normal pericardium can be seen as a thin line less than 2 mm in thickness.[7,9] On CT, it appears as a thin linear density surrounding the heart better visualized over the right ventricle **(Fig. 2A)**. It appears as a hypointense line on MR surrounded by epicardial fat on one side and mediastinal fat on the other side on T1-weighted, T2-weighted and gradient images **(Fig. 2B)**. Normally, up to 50 mL fluid may be present in the potential space created by two appossing serosal surfaces.[10]

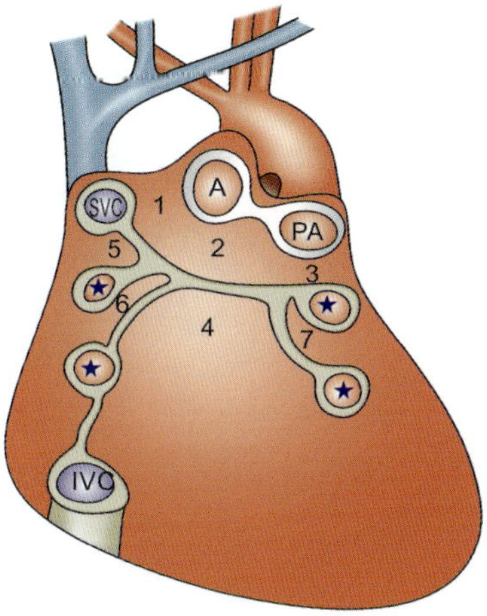

Fig. 1: Schematic representation of pericardium: Transverse sinus (2) with right and left pulmonic recesses (1 and 3). Oblique sinus (4) with its recesses—postcaval recess (5) and right and left pulmonary venous recesses (6 and 7).
Abbreviations: A: Aorta; PA: Pulmonary artery; SVC: Superior vena cava; IVC: Inferior vena cava; H: Pulmonary veins.

Transverse Sinus and Recesses

The transverse sinus lies behind the aorta and the main pulmonary artery and superior to the left atrium.

Superior Aortic Recess

The cranial most extent of this sinus is the superior aortic or superior pericardial recess. It can further be divided into posterior, right, and anterior portions depending on relationship with aorta. The posterior portion is seen as a crescentic fluid collection just posterior to the ascending aorta. It can be mistaken for a lymph node. The fluid in this posterior portion lies directly posterior to the aorta with no intervening fat. The crescent shape and fluid attenuation are other distinguishing features from lymph nodes. The anterior portion passes between the aorta and pulmonary artery, resulting in a triangular shape between them[8] **(Fig. 3A)**.

Inferior Aortic Recess

Inferiorly, the transverse sinus extends between the ascending aorta and the right atrium and forms the inferior aortic recess. This extends caudally till the level of the aortic valve annulus and lies anterior to the left atrium **(Figs. 4A and B)**.

Right and Left Pulmonic Recesses

Laterally, the transverse sinus ends in right and left pulmonic recesses **(Figs. 3B to D)**. The former lies inferior

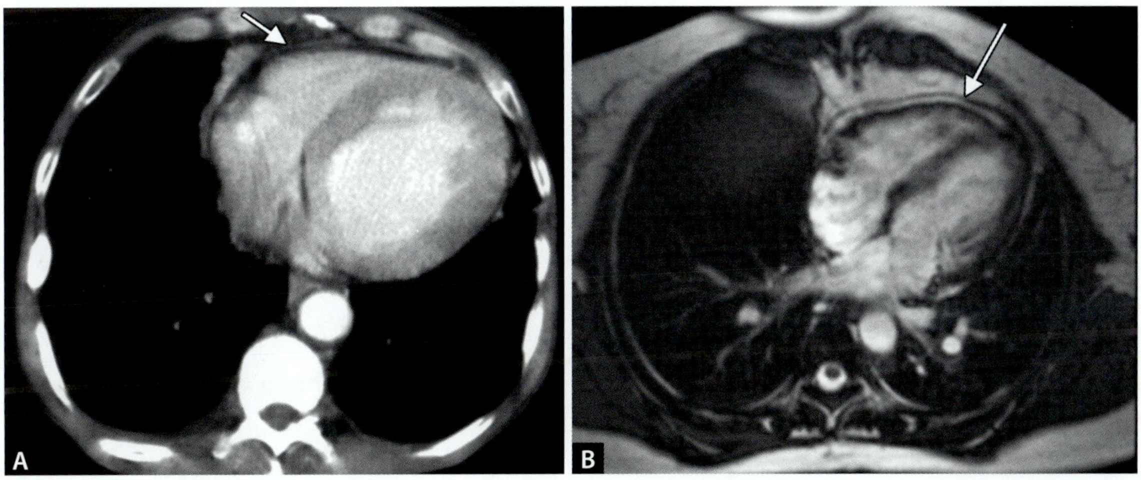

Figs. 2A and B: (A) Axial contrast-enhanced CT scan shows normal pericardium (arrow) outlined by epicardial fat and medastinal fat on either side. Note made of subsegmental atelectasis in right lung; (B) Short axis cine gradient echo MR image shows normal pericardium as a thin curved line (arrow) surrounded by bright epicardial and mediastinal fat on either side.

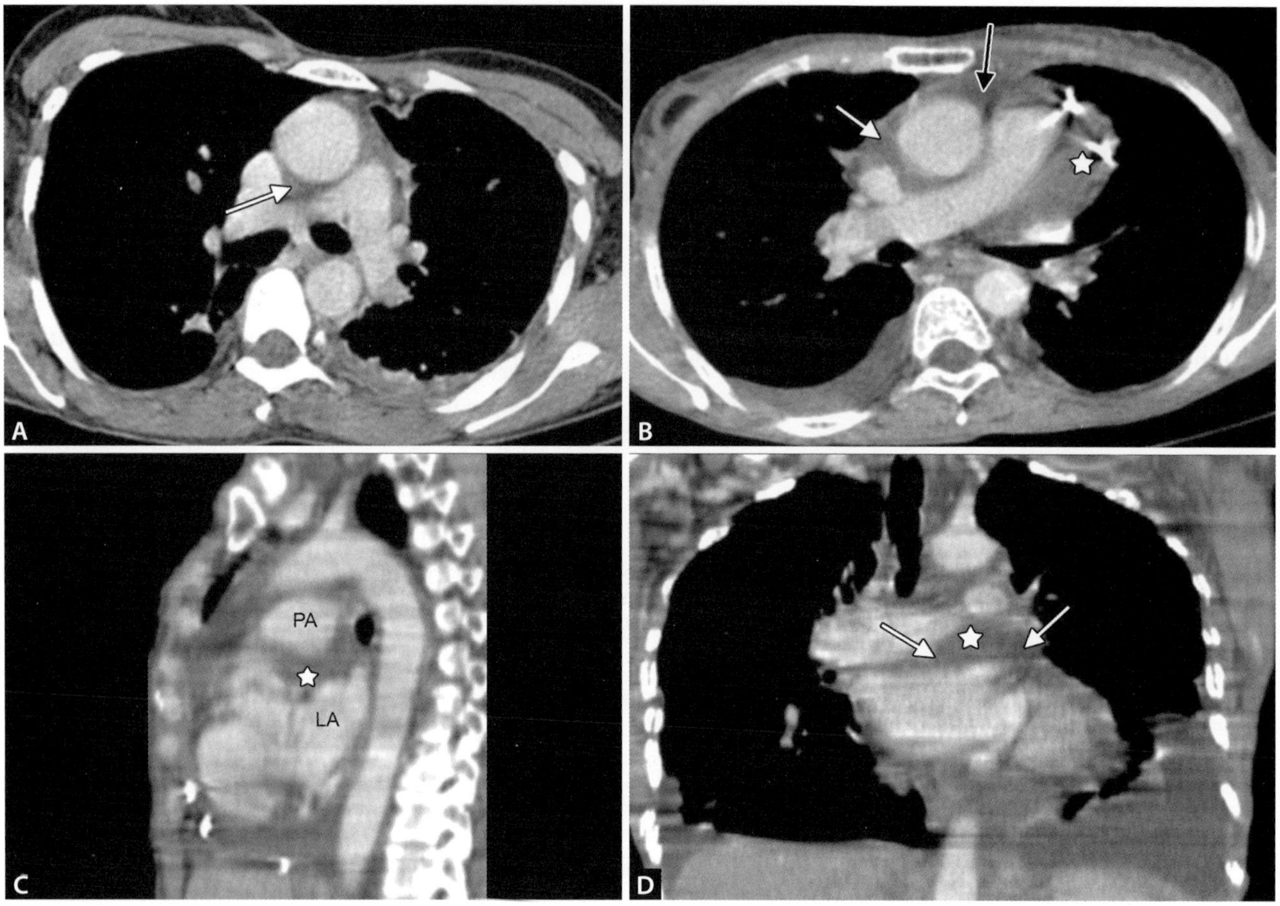

Figs. 3A to D: Axial CECT shows the posterior extension of the superior aortic recess posterior to the ascending aorta, as a crescentic fluid collection (arrow); (B) Axial CECT shows left pulmonic recess of the transverse sinus (star). Pericardial fluid is also seen in the anterior (black arrow) and right (white arrow) portions of the superior aortic recess. Note made of pericardial drainage catheter in situ; (C) Sagittal reformation shows the transverse sinus (star) between pulmonary artery (PA) and left atrium (LA). Note made of pericardial drainage catheter in situ; (D) Coronal reformation shows transverse sinus (star) along with right and left pulmonic recesses (arrows) at its right and left ends.

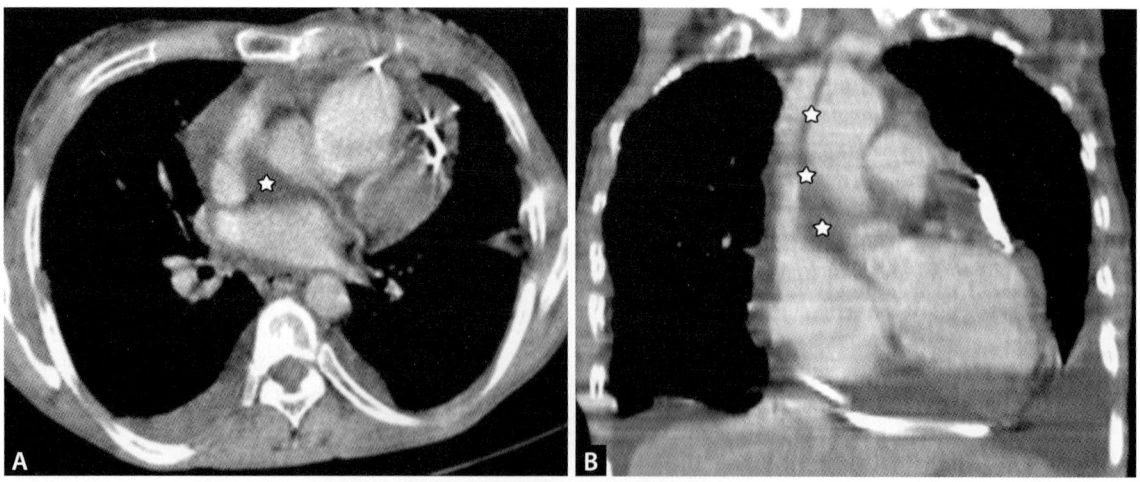

Figs. 4A and B: (A) Axial contrast-enhanced CT scan shows inferior aortic recess between the right atrium and aortic root (star). Note made of pericardial drainage catheter *in situ*; (B) Coronal reformation shows the vertical extent of the transverse sinus with its superior and inferior aortic recesses. (stars). Note made of pericardial drainage catheter *in situ*.

to the right pulmonary artery. The left pulmonic recess lies below the left pulmonary artery. Below this lies the superior pulmonary vein. Fluid within these recesses can sometimes simulate lymph nodes.[8,11]

Oblique Sinus and Recess

The oblique sinus lies superior and posterior to the left atrium and posteromedial to the superior pulmonary veins **(Figs. 5A and B)**. It is separated from the transverse sinus by a pericardial reflection between the right and left superior pulmonary veins. Since this lies just anterior to the esophagus, fluid here may be mistaken for esophageal lesions and sometimes even as bronchogenic cysts.

The cranial reflection is the posterior pericardial recess. This extends behind the right pulmonary artery and medial to the bronchus intermedius **(Fig. 5A)**. Fluid within this recess can mimic peribronchial or subcarinal lymph nodes.[6,10]

Recesses of the Pericardial Cavity Proper

Right and Left Pulmonary Venous Recesses

The right and left pulmonary venous recesses are recesses of the pericardial cavity proper, located between the superior and inferior pulmonary veins on either side.

Fluid in these pulmonary venous recesses can be mistaken for bronchopulmonary lymph nodes. These may be distinguished by the fact that fluid lies both anterior and posterior to the veins whereas lymph nodes lie only on one side and may narrow the vein.[11]

Postcaval Recess

The postcaval recess is another small recess from the pericardial cavity proper, lying posterior to the superior vena cava (SVC) and to its right.[11]

PHYSIOLOGY

The pericardium supports the heart and cardiac function in the following major ways:[12]

- It fixes the heart within the anterior mediastinum protecting it from surrounding organs
- Its elasticity limits excessive dilatation of cardiac chambers in response to increased preload
- It equalizes compliance between right and left ventricle. When stroke volume of left ventricle is altered due to elevated systemic vascular resistance, it helps in adaptation of stroke volume of the right ventricle accordingly (ventricular coupling)
- The respiratory changes in intrathoracic pressure are directly transmitted to the pericardial cavity and then to the cardiac chambers. The effect is greater on the right ventricle than on the left because of its thinner wall.

CONGENITAL PERICARDIAL ANOMALIES

Pericardial Cysts (Box 2)

These are rare lesions which result from pinching off of a portion of pericardium. They can be found throughout the mediastinum but the most common location is the right anterior cardiophrenic angle. A pericardial cyst elsewhere

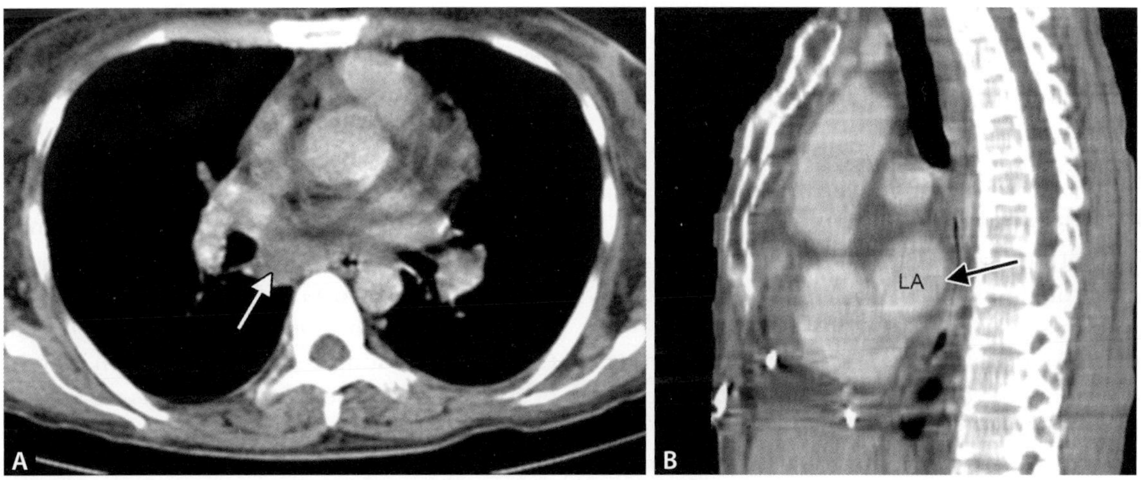

Figs. 5A and B: (A) Axial contrast-enhanced CT scan shows posterior pericardial recess of the oblique sinus (arrow) superior to the left atrium, medial to bronchus intermedius and posteromedial to the superior pulmonary veins; (B) Sagittal reformation shows the oblique sinus (arrow) between the left atrium anteriorly and the esophagus posteriorly.

Box 2: Pericardial cyst.

- Rare congenital lesion
- Most common location is right cardiophrenic angle
- Typical imaging features—well-defined cyst with thin wall, no internal septations, low signal on T1W MR and high signal on T2W MR images
- Mass effect and enhancement not seen unless infected

in the mediastinum may be difficult to differentiate from a bronchogenic or thymic cyst.[6] When these pericardial cysts have a residual communication with the pericardial space, these are called pericardial diverticulae.[7] This communication may however be difficult to delineate. Although usually asymptomatic, few patients may have chest pain, dyspnea, cough, pneumothorax, or fever.[10,13] Another rarer presentation may be due to bronchial compression.

The pericardial cyst is usually sharply demarcated round or ovoid mass in the region of right cardiophrenic angle silhouetting the cardiac border. The cyst may have a pointed upper border as it droops down into the cardiophrenic region from higher up. On cross- sectional imaging, it is a well-defined unilocular, thin walled homogeneous nonenhancing mass contiguous with the pericardium. Ultrasound can depict the cystic lesion adjacent to pericardium. On CT, it has fluid attenuation and on MR imaging, it matches the signal characteristics of water. Presence of proteinaceous contents within the cyst can result in occasional high signal on T1 weighted images. An important feature is that the cyst changes in size or shape with respiration or body position.[10] Additionally, a pericardial cyst should not normally cause mass effect on the heart. The cysts may get infected and then show peripheral enhancement or mass effect, which is otherwise not seen. Symptomatic and complicated cysts may need to be resected.[3]

CONGENITAL ABSENCE OF THE PERICARDIUM (BOX 3)

Compromise of the vascular supply to the pleuropericardial membrane results in congenital defects of the pericardium. Defect can be acquired after surgery or trauma also.[13]

Absence of the pericardium is rare. Absence of left pericardium is more common than complete absence.[3] Bilateral and isolated right sided defects are very rare. Pericardial defects are usually associated with defects in the parietal pleura through which lung can herniate. There may be other congenital anomalies along with pericardial defect which include cardiac anomalies (atrial septal defect, patent ductus arteriosus), and anomalies of the lung (bronchogenic cysts, pulmonary sequestration), chest wall (pectus excavatum) and diaphragm.[14] Patients are generally asymptomatic although vague chest pain can occur due to lack of fixation.[12-14] A focally deficient pericardium may allow a part of the heart to herniate through the hole. It most often involves the left atrial appendage. The left coronary artery may also be compressed by the herniation through this defect. This can rarely result in ischemia, especially during activity. In such situations, surgical closure or enlargement of the defect may be performed.[12]

Box 3: Congenital absence of pericardium.

- Rare anomaly
- Left-sided absence commoner than complete absence
- *Radiographic findings*:
  - Left ventricle and pulmonary artery displaced to left
  - Main pulmonary artery borders distinctly seen
  - Pulmonary artery/left atrial appendage may be prominent in partial absence
- *CT/MR findings*:
  - Leftward shift of cardiac axis
  - Prominent atrial appendage
  - Lung seen interposed between aorta and main pulmonary artery

In complete absence of left pericardium, left ventricle and pulmonary artery may be seen displaced to the left side on plain radiographs. The segments of the heart that make up the left heart border can be seen more distinctly. The medial and lateral borders of the main pulmonary artery are seen more clearly due to the absence of pericardium between the aorta and the pulmonary artery. In partial absence of the left pericardium, pulmonary artery or left atrial appendage may be prominent depending upon the location of pericardial defect.[13-15]

CT and MR may not depict the pericardium along its entirety. The pericardium may not be normally seen over the left atrial appendage and the left ventricle and should not be misinterpreted as pericardial defect.[7] The secondary signs, which include posterior and leftward shift of the cardiac axis, prominent atrial appendage and separation of the aorta and main pulmonary artery due to lung tissue interposition become more important features. Occasionally, lung tissue can be seen inferior to the heart, interposed between the heart and the diaphragm. The herniation may be intermittent; hence left lateral decubitus position of the patient can assist in diagnosing pericardial defects. Also, functional examination can pick up greater mobility of the cardiac apex which is otherwise essentially stationary in a normal cardiac cycle.[16]

PERICARDIAL EFFUSION

The various causes of pericardial effusion include heart failure, renal insufficiency, infection (bacterial, viral, tuberculous), neoplasm (carcinoma of the lung, breast, lymphoma, melanoma) and injury (trauma, myocardial infarction). Other causes may be hypothyroidism, connective tissue disorder, acquired immune deficiency syndrome (AIDS) or radiation pericarditis.[17]

The role of imaging is to confirm the presence and extent of fluid, to characterize the nature of fluid, to rule out pericardial inflammation, to determine its hemodynamic impact and to guide pericardiocentesis. Echocardiography is generally the first imaging modality to be used because of high sensitivity, specificity, easy availability and low cost **(Fig. 6A)**. Limited acoustic window may impair the utility of this modality in many cases. With exception of transesophageal echocardiography, it is not a reliable technique for estimating pericardial thickness and in assessment of loculated pericardial effusions. CT and MR provide a wider field of view and are superior in detecting the amount, nature and distribution of the fluid. Focal fluid accumulation may be seen posterolateral to the left ventricle and along the inferolateral wall of the right ventricle owing to their dependent locations. Superior pericardial recess is another common location of focal fluid accumulation.[12]

The size of a pericardial effusion may be semiquantitatively assessed by the thickness of fluid anterior to the right ventricle. Pericardial width of more than 4 mm may be regarded as abnormal. Using criteria established by echocardiography, a pericardial effusion may be quantified as small (<5 mm); moderate (5–10 mm); or large (>10 mm).[3,17,18] On a chest radiograph, pericardial effusion is suspected when there is diffuse cardiac silhouette enlargement without specific chamber enlargement. Filling of the retrosternal space, enlargement of normal cardiac borders, development of "flask" configuration and bilateral hilar overlay may be seen in larger effusions **(Fig. 6B)**. On the lateral projection, 'epicardial fat pad' sign is diagnostic of pericardial disease. This is positive when the anterior pericardial stripe, bordered by the epicardial fat and mediastinal fat on either side, is seen to be thicker than 2 mm. It may also be seen in the frontal view because of presence of abundant fat between the pericardium and pleura at the cardiac apex. This is seen as a radiolucent stripe internal to and parallel to the left lower cardiac border.[13] On a chest radiograph, pan chamber cardiac enlargement and large anterior mediastinal tumor may simulate pericardial effusion. On CT, the attenuation values of pericardial fluid are only of limited value. Serous effusions tend to have near-water attenuation values (<10 HU) **(Figs. 7A and B)**, while exudative effusions can range from 20 to 60 HU **(Figs. 7C and D)**. Chylopericardium can also present with low attenuation values but may be difficult to distinguish from transudative effusions. Acute hemopericardium can have attenuation values in the range of 60 to 80 HU, but if blood represents only a portion of the fluid, the attenuation values can then be similar to that of exudative effusions. Generally, 30 HU is a useful cut off between simple effusions and bloody or proteinaceous effusions.[7] It may sometimes be difficult to distinguish between pericardial effusion and thickening on CT which is better appreciated on echocardiography or MRI.

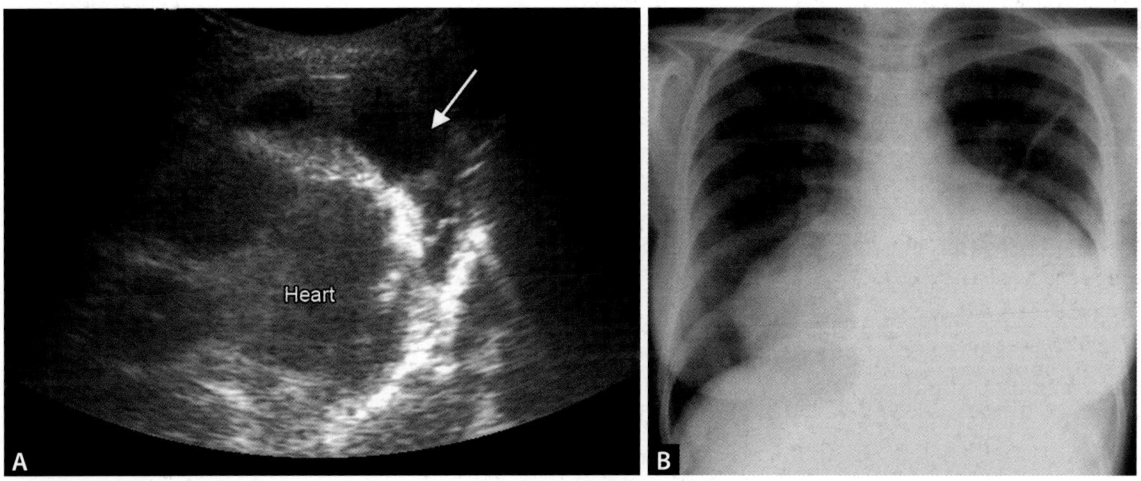

Figs. 6A and B: (A) Pericardial effusion: Ultrasound chest depicts fluid in the pericardial cavity (arrow); (B) Frontal chest radiograph shows enlarged 'flask'-shaped cardiac silhouette without specific chamber enlargement with bilateral hilum overlay sign. Both sides of the heart appear rounded and displaced laterally.

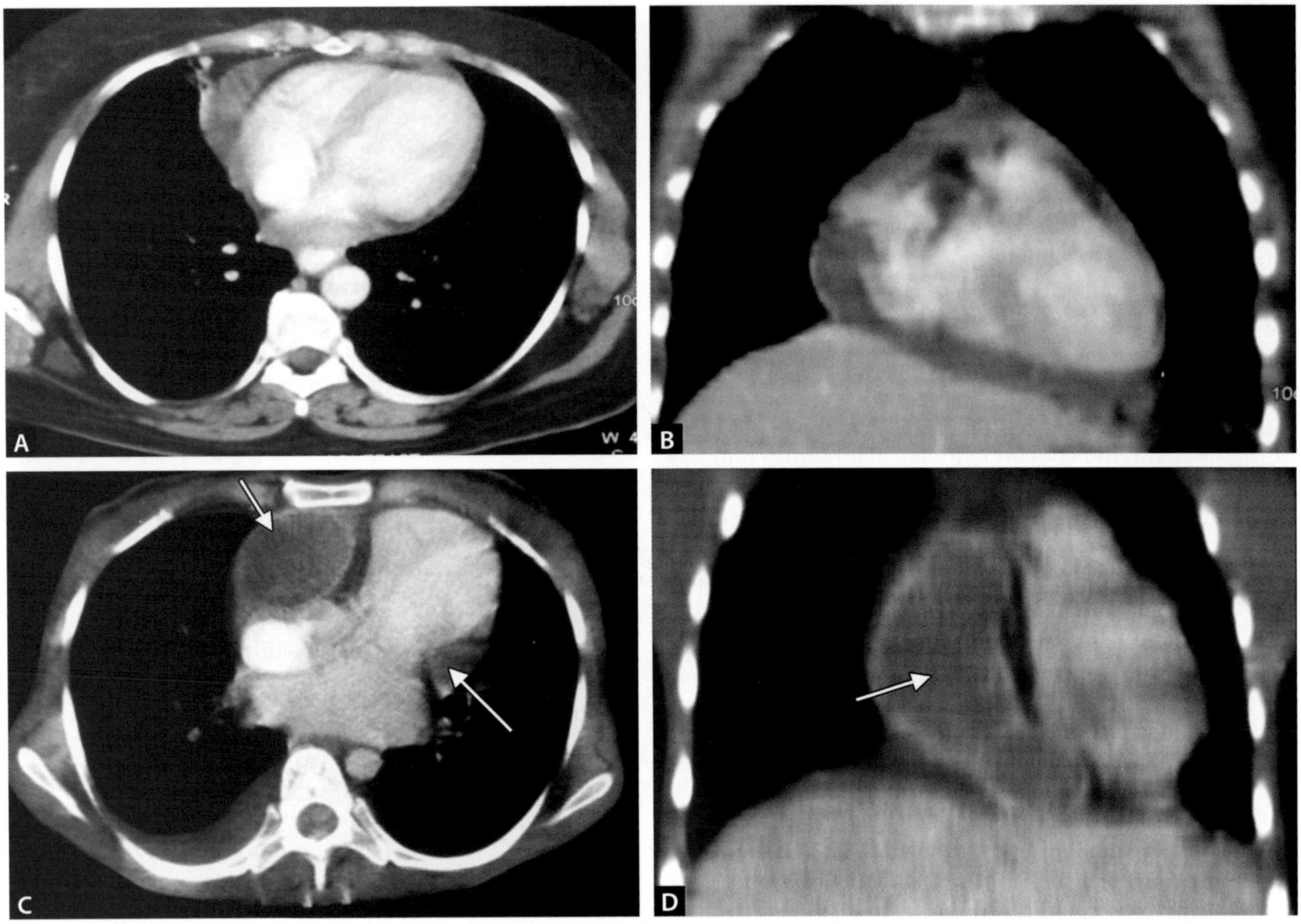

Figs. 7A to D: (A and B) Pericardial effusion: Axial CECT (A) and coronal reformation (B) show small simple pericardial effusion (HU = 10); (C and D) Exudative pericardial effusion: Axial CECT (C) and coronal reformation (D) shows high attenuation loculated effusion (HU = 45) (arrows) in atrioventricular groove in a case of tuberculous pericarditis.

MR imaging may be performed to further characterize pericardial effusions. Transudates have a low signal intensity on T1-weighted images and high signal intensity on T2- weighted images and GRE cine images **(Figs. 8A and B)**. Exudates have a higher signal intensity on T1-weighted images and low signal intensity on T2 weighted images due to high cellularity and protein content within **(Figs. 9A and B)**. Hemopericardium is characterized by high signal on T1-weighted images and may be low signal on T2-weighted images and GRE cine images. Hemorrhage or infection should be suspected on cine imaging when the effusion fluid is clearly complex and inhomogeneous, containing regions of different signal intensity.[19,20] The gradient images may better characterize a hemopericardium as they facilitate the visualization of fibrinous strands and presence of coagulated blood. The T1 and T2 signal intensity of a hemorrhagic pericardial effusion is dependent on the duration of the hematoma. However, certain artifacts like non-linear motion of pericardial fluid during cardiac motion may falsely cause high signal on T1-weighted spin-echo CMR even within a transudative effusion.[7,12] Effusion secondary to malignancy may have associated pericardial thickening and nodularity. MR is superior to CT in differentiating pericardial effusion from thickening. The high signal intensity on cine and T2-weighted images allows to clearly distinguishing between pericardial effusion and thickened pericardium which is low signal intensity on these sequences. In certain cases, double and triple IR sequences can aid in the differentiation between pericardial fluid and pericardial fat. Double IR images null the signal contribution of fluid, whereas triple IR images null the signal contribution of fat.[3] Delayed-enhancement imaging can demonstrate abnormal pericardial enhancement, indicative of inflammation or infection.[2]

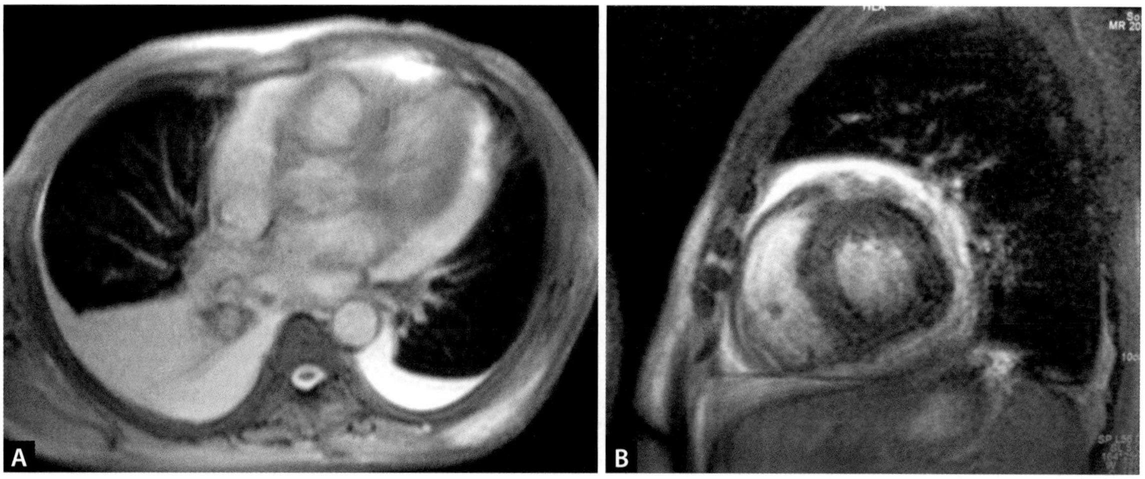

Figs. 8A and B: Pericardial effusion: Moderate simple effusion is seen on four-chamber (A) and short axis; (B) cine SSFP images. Bilateral pleural effusions are also seen.

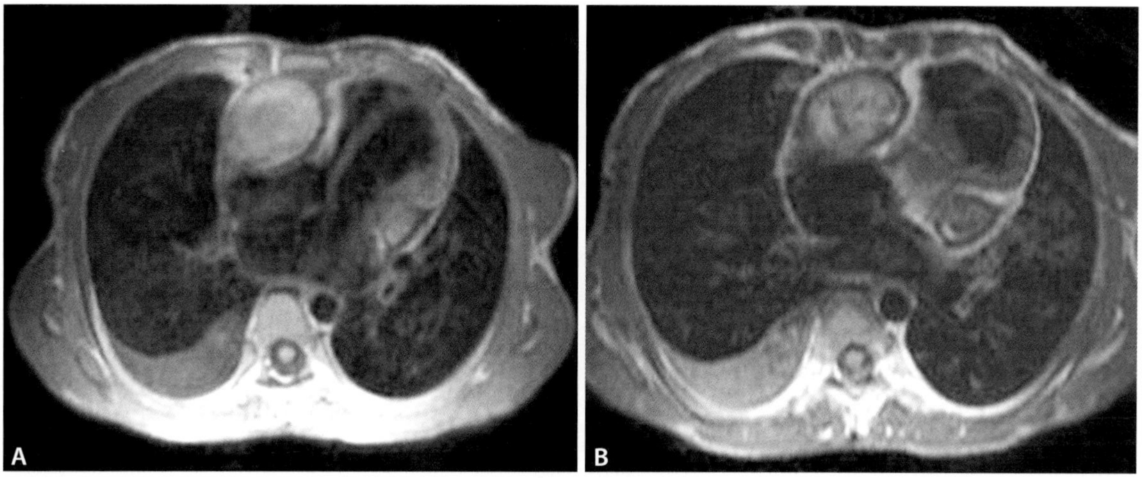

Figs. 9A and B: Exudative pericardial effusion (same case as in Fig. 8): Axial dark blood T1 and T2-weighted images show exudative effusion in the atrioventricular groove and associated pericardial thickening. It is seen as high signal intensity on T1-weighted images (A) with complex and inhomogeneous signal intensity on T2-weighted images (B). Note made of right pleural effusion.

CARDIAC TAMPONADE (BOX 4)

Slow accumulation of pericardial fluid may cause adaptive expansion of the pericardium with accumulation of up to 3 L of fluid without significant hemodynamic consequence.[21] However, in cases of rapid accumulation, as little as 100–200 mL of fluid may result in an effusion under tension or cardiac tamponade as pericardium has limited stretchability.[13] The resultant increased pericardial pressure is then transmitted to the cardiac chambers. Cardiac tamponade is a low cardiac output state due to excessive fluid in the pericardial space that compresses the heart. The diagnosis is generally made on clinical grounds and is confirmed by echocardiography where RV free wall can show collapse during diastolic phase, right atrium depicts collapse during late diastole/systole, greater respiratory variations and distended hepatic veins and inferior vena cava due to back flow.

Box 4: Cardiac tamponade.

- Life-threatening condition requiring urgent intervention
- Causes include trauma, cardiac surgery, inflammation, pericardial neoplasm, aortic dissection
- Speed of fluid accumulation key determinant of symptoms
- Clinical diagnosis confirmed on echocardiography
- Role of CT and MR limited to atypical/chronic cases

CT and MR have a limited role in the evaluation of acute cardiac tamponade; only long standing or less severe forms may sometimes be seen. CT and MRI may be helpful in non-emergent situations when echocardiographic findings are equivocal. The heart size, excluding the pericardial space is normal or decreased. This is contrary to restrictive cardiomyopathy and pericardial constriction in which the atria are typically enlarged.[2,3] The cavae and hepatic veins which are exterior to the pericardium dilate to accommodate back pooling of blood. Eventually, if pericardial pressure exceeds the ability of the circulation to fill the heart, the cardiac chambers especially right sided chambers collapse.[3]

Cine CT and MR imaging can show the dynamic features suggestive of tamponade. There is collapse of the right ventricular free wall in early diastole and collapse of the right atrial free wall in late diastole. This is because in early diastole less blood is present in the right ventricle than the right atrium, and so, the right ventricle has the least pressure to counteract the pressure of the pericardial effusion. In late diastole, the right atrium has less blood than the right ventricle, so the right atrium has less pressure. This collapse is especially evident during expiration which decreases right heart filling. Throughout the cardiac cycle there is enhanced intraventricular coupling from the taut pericardial space. This most often manifests as abnormal motion of the intraventricular septum. This is seen on cine images as septal rocking or sigmoid septum configuration. The diastolic dysfunction characteristic of tamponade is also well-evaluated on cine images.[3,7]

When cardiac tamponade is atypical, CT and MR may be better than echocardiography. In these unusual situations, the effusions tend to be loculated and exert mass effect on a part of the heart not well-visualized by transthoracic echocardiography, including the right atrium and left atrium.

Oftentimes, these effusions are malignant, postradiation, or postinfectious.[7]

PERICARDITIS

Nonconstrictive Pericarditis (Box 5)

Pericarditis is an inflammatory response of the pericardium which may be a result of various conditions, which include infections, uremia, rheumatic heart disease, systemic diseases like rheumatoid arthritis and sarcoidosis, postinfarction, malignancy and mediastinal irradiation. In about 30% of patients, it may be idiopathic.[12]

Box 5: Nonconstrictive pericarditis.

- Inflammatory response of pericardium involving pericardial thickening and effusion
- Enhancement of pericardium can be seen
- Findings may be localized to part of pericardium
- No features of constriction

In acute pericarditis, the pericardium may develop a small effusion and become slightly thickened. On contrast-enhanced CT and MRI, acute pericarditis shows enhancement of the pericardium, which can show smooth thickening **(Fig. 10)**. Acute (nonfibrotic) pericarditis enhances in the early arterial phase of contrast administration in contrast to chronic (fibrotic) pericarditis, which enhances late.[21] Associated small effusion may be seen. There are accompanying inflammatory changes in the pericardial fat which may be increased or stranded. On CT imaging, it may sometimes be difficult to differentiate a small effusion from pericardial thickening which may be resolved on echocardiography. Also, care needs to be taken for assessment of pericardium in its entirety as the findings may only be localized.

In chronic inflammatory pericarditis, the effusion may increase or pericardium can get more thickened. The thickened pericardium shows enhancement and may show an irregular contour. This may progress to fibrosing pericarditis which is non-enhancing and shows low-signal intensity on MRI. The latter may or may not be associated with constriction.[3,22]

Constrictive Pericarditis (Box 6)

Constrictive pericarditis is a condition in which cardiac function is impaired by a thickened, rigid and often calcified pericardium. This results in diastolic dysfunction of the heart and subsequent right heart failure. Clinical symptoms and radiological concordance are required to make this diagnosis. It can clinically mimic restrictive

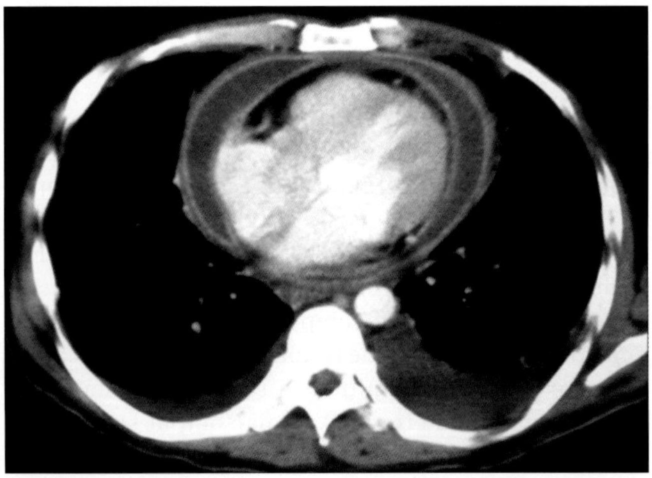

Fig. 10: Nonconstrictive pericarditis: Axial CECT shows enhancing thickened smooth pericardium with associated effusion in a known case of tuberculosis. Bilateral pleural effusions are also seen.

cardiomyopathy, hepatic disease, and congestive heart failure. The distinction between constrictive pericarditis and restrictive cardiomyopathy is very important, since the former would benefit from pericardial stripping and the latter would not. Constrictive pericarditis may be secondary to prior surgery, infection, trauma, radiation, uremia, connective tissue disorder, neoplasm or may be idiopathic.It is more often a sequelae to purulent and tuberculous pericarditis than viral amongst infectious causes.[23] Thickening may be localized involving only a portion of the pericardium, often overlying the right ventricle or may extend around the entire heart. The thickening is usually irregular. Calcified pericardium may be apparent on a chest radiograph **(Figs. 11A to D)**.

Box 6: Constrictive pericarditis.

- Reduced pericardial compliance leading to diastolic dysfunction
- Causes infection, radiation exposure, postoperative, etc.
- *Morphological findings*:
  - Pericardial thickening with calcification more over right ventricle
  - Unilateral/bilateral atrial enlargement
  - Dilated hepatic veins/IVC
  - Pleural effusion, ascites
  - Pericardial enhancement suggestive of residual inflammation
- *Findings on functional evaluation*:
  - Septal bounce on cine MR imaging
  - MR tagging technique—tag lines remain unbroken in case of pericardial lesions
- Dynamic MR imaging findings help distinguish constrictive pericarditis from restrictive cardiomyopathy

Both morphology and functional hemodynamic aspects are used to reach the diagnosis. CT and MR imaging findings center on the demonstration of global or focal thickened or calcified pericardium which is usually greater over the right ventricle, along with secondary morphologic signs of constriction. These include conical

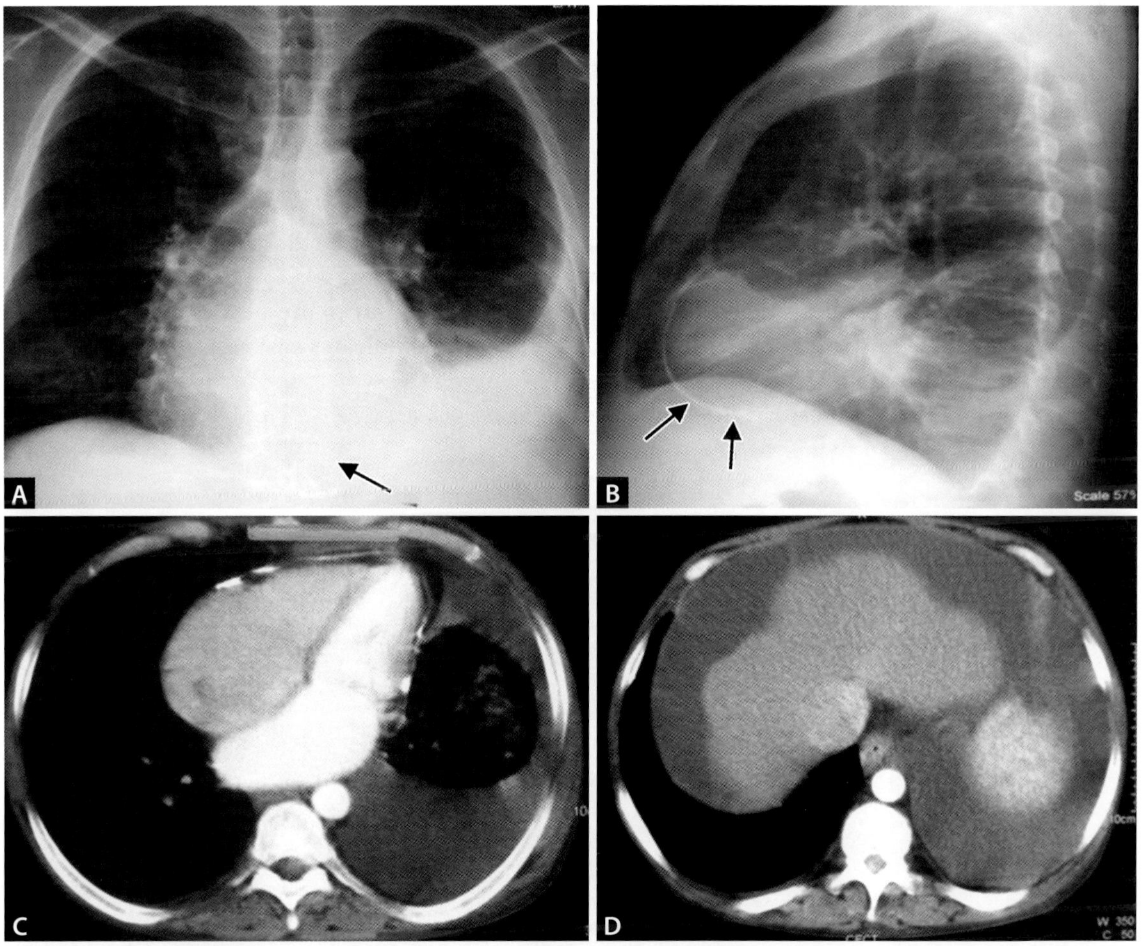

Figs. 11A to D: (A and B) Calcific constrictive pericarditis: In a patient with distant history of tuberculosis, posteroanterior (A) and lateral (B) chest radiographs demonstrate curvilinear calcification (arrows) along the lower left and diaphragmatic cardiac border; (C and D) Axial CECT shows global pericardial thickening with calcification. The ventricles are tubular shaped with dilated atria and IVC. Associated left pleural effusion and ascites noted. Liver appears congested with irregular outline suggestive of cardiac cirrhosis.

or tubular shape of either of the ventricles, sigmoid-shaped interventricular septum, enlargement of one or both atria, narrowing of one or both atrioventricular grooves and large inferior and superior vena cava in comparison with descending aorta[21,24,25] **(Fig. 12A)**. The diagnosis of pericardial constriction is absolutely certain if all these morphologic determinants are present. Any thickening of the pericardium more than a pencil-line is significant. Usually, pericardial thickness is greater than 4 mm although there is no direct relationship between the extent of thickness of the pericardium and its hemodynamic significance.[21,26] In the end stage fibrosing forms of constrictive pericarditis, the pericardium usually does not enhance after contrast administration. However, pericardial enhancement, which indicates residual inflammation, may be seen on delayed postcontrast imaging (>70 seconds postcontrast). A small amount of pericardial effusion may also be seen. Calcification of the pericardium is better visualized on CT and strongly suggests constriction of tubercular etiology.[13] However, presence of constriction and calcification are not always related. Atrial dilatation may or may not be seen depending on whether the entire pericardium is abnormal or just the anterior part. This is an insensitive finding as patients with restrictive cardiomyopathy may also demonstrate atrial dilatation. Pleural effusions, hepatic congestion, and ascites may also be seen. Other radiological stigmata of chest tuberculosis should also be looked for. Other causes of pericardial calcification include viral, uremic pericarditis, collagen vascular disease, postoperative setting, radiation exposure and asbestosis. It should be remembered that the diagnosis of pericardial constriction is made only in the appropriate clinical setting.[27]

Since the diagnosis of constriction is ultimately that of altered physiology, cine imaging is a more direct means of confirming the diagnosis. The most sensitive and specific finding is the septal bounce, best appreciated in inspiration. In a study by Francone, et al. septal bounce was seen in 85% of patients with constrictive pericarditis and in no patients without constriction.[28] It is most pronounced at the beginning of inspiration. During inspiration, the negative intrathoracic pressure results in more rapid right heart filling than the left. In early diastole the pressure in the right ventricle is transiently higher than the left, causing the septum to bow leftward due to enhanced ventricular coupling **(Fig. 12B)**. In mid diastole the left ventricular pressure once again becomes higher, pushing the septum rightward, and in late diastole the pressures equalize. The result is shivering of the ventricular septum or septal bounce.[3] Tagging cardiac MR techniques may be of use to depict fibrotic adhesions of pericardial layers **(Figs. 13A to C)**.

Underlying myocardium also needs to be evaluated in these cases as the presence of the myocardial factor (myocardial atrophy or fibrosis) is a contraindication to pericardiectomy, because of the risk of acute dilatation or rupture of one or both cardiac chambers following surgery.[21] Imaging also aids in planning surgery. The presence of a fat plane between the myocardium and pericardium indicates easier dissection.[29]

There are atypical forms of constrictive pericarditis. *Effusive constrictive pericarditis* represents a combination

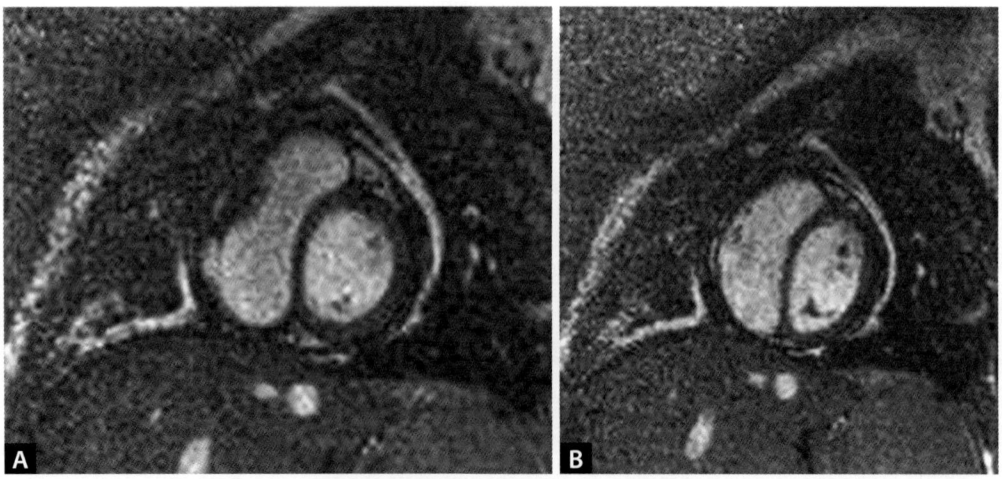

Figs. 12A and B: Short axis cine MR images in a patient with constrictive pericarditis in systole (A) and diastole (B) show straightening of the interventricular septum in diastole indicative of impaired right ventricular filling. Pericardium is focally thickened posterior to the left ventricle.

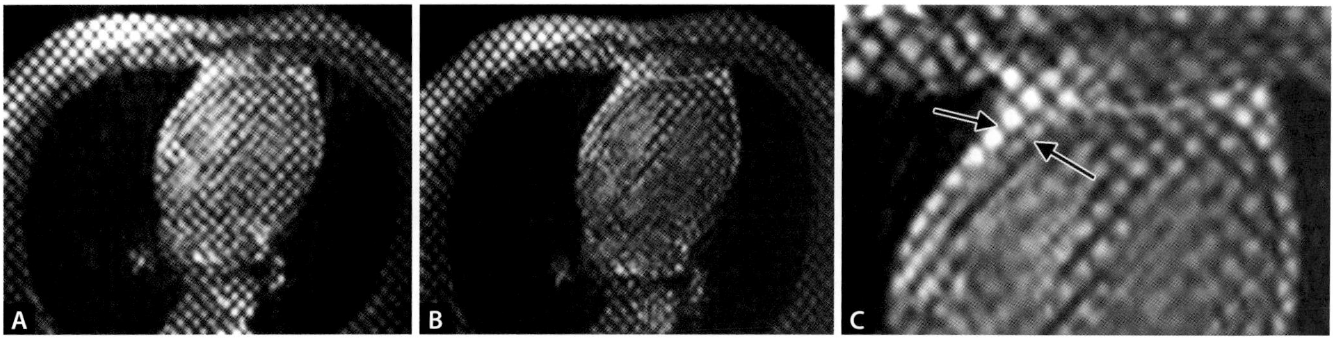

Figs. 13A to C: GRE tagging MR imaging in a healthy volunteer in axial plane. The continuity of the tags is lost during cardiac contraction because of shear motion between visceral and parietal layer of the pericardium [seen on the enlarged view (C)].

of pericardial tamponade and constrictive pericarditis. This is seen most often following radiation therapy. The typical clinical setting is that pericardial effusion is identified in a patient with symptoms of heart failure and despite drainage of the effusion, the patient continues to have abnormal pericardial dynamics. *Inflammatory constrictive pericarditis* results due to constriction during acute and chronic pericarditis which may be transient. There is accompanying enhancement of pericardium. *Focal pericarditis* may result in constriction if present in strategic location. *Occult constrictive pericarditis* refers to presence of constriction only when there is volume overload and not on routine examination.

PNEUMOPERICARDIUM

Pneumopericardium may result from blunt or penetrating trauma. Other rarer causes may be infectious pericarditis or from a gastrointestinal fistula, increased intrathoracic pressure as in asthma or barotrauma, with adjacent lung infection/cancer, esophageal rupture, cocaine abuse or liver abscess rupture. Pneumopericardium following pneumothorax or pneumomediastinum usually indicates a disruption of the pericardium. On erect chest radiographs, it is seen as a radiolucent band around the heart ('halo sign') limited superiorly by the pericardial reflection at the root of great vessels **(Fig. 14)**. Air may be seen in the transverse pericardial sinus giving the 'transverse band of air' sign. Lateral radiographs may show lucency of air behind the sternum and anterior to the base of heart and root of aorta ('triangle of air' sign).[30,31] In the setting of penetrating trauma, the presence of pneumopericardium should prompt investigation for potential cardiac laceration. Rarely, tension pneumopericardium may result in tamponade.[7] This may be seen as progressively decreasing cardiothoracic ratio. CT shows distension of SVC, IVC, hepatic veins, renal veins and periportal lymphedema.

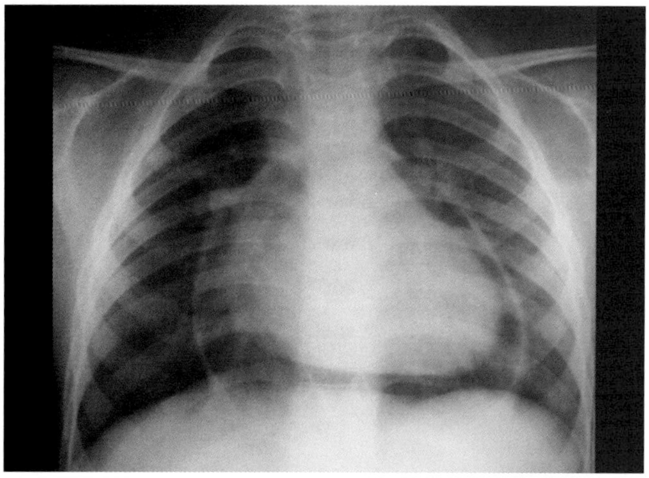

Fig. 14: Pneumopericardium. Posteroanterior chest radiograph shows radiolucent band of air surrounding the heart giving the 'halo sign'.

PERICARDIAL TUMORS

Metastases (Box 7)

Metastases to the pericardium are more common than involvement of pericadium by primary tumors.

Metastases to the heart and pericardium have been reported at autopsy in 10–12% of patients with known primary malignancies.[10] Pericardial metastases may result from contiguous spread from lung or mediastinum. Other modes may be lymphatic, hematogenous or transvenous route. The common sources of pericardial metastases are lung and breast cancer. Leukemias, lymphomas and melanomas are the other malignancies that can spread to the pericardium. Pericardial metastases when seen are a negative prognostic factor.

An effusion is the most common manifestation of metastatic pericardial disease. Pericardium can get irregularly thickened or a pericardial mass may be seen. To distinguish between inflammatory etiology and metastases (when effusion and thickening are the only findings), follow-up may be required. Pericardial invasion may be suggested when the pericardial line is not seen **(Figs. 15A and B)** and there is pericardial effusion. On MRI images, most deposits show low-signal on T1 and high-signal on T2- weighted images. Metastatic melanoma is an exception; high-signal intensity on T1-weighted images is virtually pathognomonic of this diagnosis.[2] The malignant tumor usually enhances significantly after the administration of contrast material.[6] Pericardium may remain intact adjacent to a primary mass. However, hemorrhagic effusion, seen as high-signal on spin echo MR images confirms the extension of the mass to the pericardium.[6,32] In a patient with a known primary tumor and pericardial effusion, other differential diagnoses are drug-induced and radiation-induced effusions.

Primary Pericardial Tumors

Primary pericardial tumors are rare. These include benign tumors (lipoma, benign teratoma, fibroma, and hemangioma) and malignant tumors (mesothelioma, lymphoma, sarcoma and liposarcoma, malignant teratoma). Although pericardial mesotheliomas are rare tumors accounting for less than 1% of all malignant mesotheliomas, they account for nearly half of primary pericardial tumors.[32]

Box 7: Pericardial metastases.

- Metastases are commoner than primary pericardial tumors
- *Mode of spread to pericardium*:
  - Direct spread
  - Lymphatic
  - Hematogenous
  - Transvenous
- *Imaging findings include*:
  - Pericardial effusion
  - Pericardial thickening
  - Pericardial mass
- Hemorrhagic pericardial effusion adjacent to a lung/mediastinal mass is suggestive of pericardial invasion.

Chest radiography in patients with pericardial mesothelioma typically demonstrates cardiac enlargement, evidence of pericardial effusion, an irregular cardiac contour or diffuse mediastinal enlargement. CT and MR may demonstrate hemorrhagic pericardial effusion accompanied by pericardial nodule or plaques. Lymphoma and sarcoma typically present with large masses accompanied by effusion.

Histopathology is usually necessary to achieve a definitive diagnosis of most pericardial tumors. The diagnosis of few tumors can be aided by specific signal and attenuation characteristics. Lipoma has low attenuation on CT images and high signal intensity on T1-weighted SE images. Presence of calcium or fat in a pericardial mass at CT suggests the diagnosis of a teratoma. Fibroma characteristically has low signal intensity on T2-weighted images with poor enhancement characteristics.[33,34]

Other entities that may simulate a pericardial mass are pericardial hematoma, coronary artery aneurysm and pericardial gossypiboma.[3,12] The signal characteristics of pericardial hematoma are age related. A coronary artery aneurysm should be suspected when a smooth enhancing mass is seen along the expected course of a coronary artery.[3] Pericardial gossypiboma should be considered in a patient with previous cardiac surgery.

CONCLUSION

Congenital disease, infection, injury, neoplasm may all affect the pericardium. Although echocardiography is often initially used to evaluate the pericardium, CT and MR are useful for further evaluation of the disease processes. With

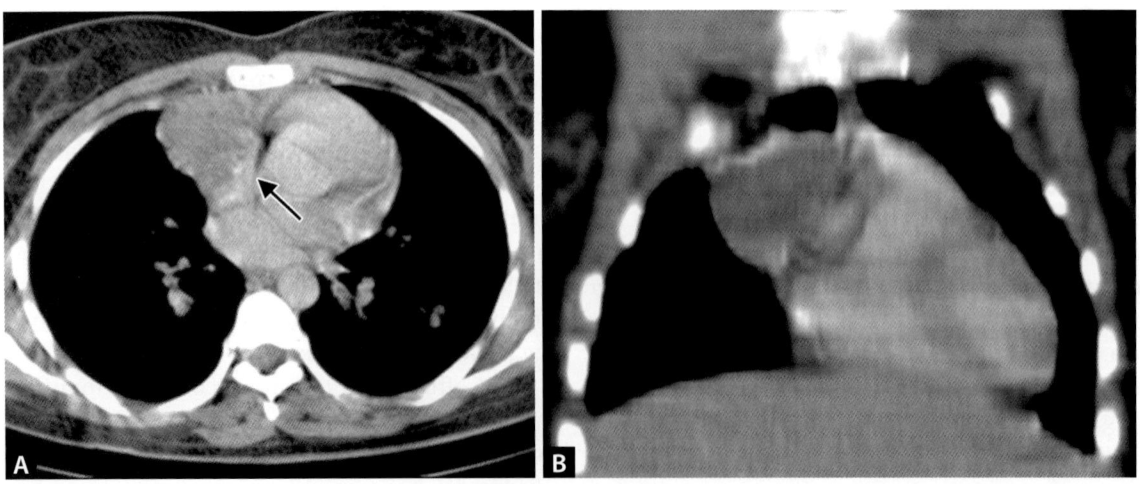

Figs. 15A and B: Axial CECT (A) and coronal reformation (arrow); (B) shows thymic carcinoma with direct invasion of the pericardium.

the advantages of a large field of view and high soft tissue contrast, these imaging modalities may help differentiate pericardial diseases, especially when echocardiography findings are equivocal.

REFERENCES

1. Gulati G, Sharma S, Kothari SS, et al. Comparison of echo and MRI in the imaging evaluation of intracardiac masses. Cardiovasc Intervent Radiol. 2004;27(5):459-69.
2. Grizzard JG, Ang GB. Magnetic resonance imaging of pericardial disease and cardiac masses. Magn Reson Imaging Clin N Am. 2007;15:579-607.
3. Misselt AJ, Harris SR, Glockner J, Feng D, Syed IS, Araoz PA: MR imaging of the pericardium. Magn Reson Imaging Clin N Am. 2008;16:185-99.
4. Budoff MJ, Achenbach S, Blumenthal RS, et al. Assessment of coronary artery disease by cardiac computed tomography: A scientific statement from the American Heart Association Committee on Cardiovascular Imaging and Intervention, Council on Cardiovascular Radiology and Intervention, and Committee on Cardiac Imaging, Council on Clinical Cardiology. Circulation. 2006;114(16):1761-91.
5. Coles DR, Smail MA, Negus IS, et al. Comparison of radiation doses from multislice computed tomography coronary angiography and conventional diagnostic angiography. J Am Coll Cardiol. 2006;47(9):1840-5.
6. Wang ZJ, Reddy GP, Gotway MB, Yeh BM, Hetts SW, Higgins CB. CT and MR imaging of pericardial disease. Radiographics. 2003;23:S167-80.
7. Lopez Costa I, Bhalla S. Computed tomography and magnetic resonance imaging of the pericardium. Semin Roentgenol. 2008;43(3):234-45.
8. Truong MT, Erasmus JJ, Gladish GW, Sabloff BS, Marom EM, et al. Anatomy of pericardial recesses on multidetector CT: Implications for oncologic imaging. Am J Roentgenol. 2003;181:1109-13.
9. Delille JP, Hernigou A, Sene V, et al. Maximal thickness of the normal human pericardium assessed by electron-beam computed tomography. Eur J Radiol. 1999;9:1183-89.
10. Oyama N, Oyama N, Komuro K, Nambu T, Manning W, Miyasaka K. Computed tomography and magnetic resonance imaging of the pericardium: anatomy and pathology. Magnetic Resonance in Medical Sciences. 2004;3(3):145-52.
11. Broderick LS, Brooks GN, Kuhlman JE. Anatomic pitfalls of the heart and pericardium. Radiographics. 2005;25:441-53.
12. Bogaert J, Francone M. Cardiovascular Magnetic resonance in pericardial diseases. J Cardiovasc Magn Reson. 2009;11(1);14.
13. O' Leary SM, Williams PL, Williams MP. et al. Imaging the pericardium: appearances on ECG-gated 64 detector row cardiac computed tomography. BJR. 2010;83:194-205.
14. Van Son JA, Danielson GK, Schaff HV, et al. Congenital partial and complete absence of the pericardium. Mayo Clin Proc. 1993;68(8):743-47.
15. Ellis K, Leeds NE, Himmelstein A. Congenital deficiencies in partial pericardium: Review with two new cases including successful diagnosis by plain roentgenography. Am J Roentgenol. 1959;82:125-37.
16. Psychidis-Papakyritsis P, de Roos A, Kroft LJM. Functional MRI of congenital absence of the pericardium. Am J Roentgenol. 2007;189:W312-W314.
17. Rajiah P. Cardiac MRI: Part 2, Pericardial disease. AJR. 2011; 197:W621-634.
18. Czum Jm, Silas AM, Althoen MC. Evaluation of the pericardium with CT and MR. ISRN cardiology 2014. http://dx.doi.org/10.1155/2014/174908.
19. Glockner JF. Imaging of pericardial disease. Magn Reson Imaging Clin N Am. 2003;11(1):149-62, vii.
20. Yared K, Baggish AL, Picard MH, Hoffmann U, Hang J. Multimodality imaging of pericardial disease. JACC Cardiovasc Imaging. 2010;3(6):650-60.
21. Rienmuller R, Groll R, Lipton MJ. CT and MR imaging of pericardial disease. Radiol Clin North Am. 2004;42(3): 587-601.
22. Kim JS, Kim HH, Yoon Y. Imaging of pericardial diseases. Clinical Radiol. 2007;62:626-31.
23. Imazio M, Brucato A, Maestroni S, et al. Risk of constrictive pericarditis after acute pericardiectomy. Circulation. 2011;124(11):1270-5.
24. Suh SY, Rha SW, Kim JW, et al. The usefulness of three-dimensional multidetector computed tomography to delineate pericardial calcification in constrictive pericarditis. Int J Cardiol. 2006;113:414-16.
25. Bogaert J, Francone M. Pericardial disease: Value of CT and MR imaging. Radiology. 2012;267(2):340-56.
26. Thavendiranathan P, Verhaert D, Wall MC, et al. Simultaneous right and left heart realtime, free-breathing CMR flow quantification indentifies constrictive physiology. JACC Cardiovasc Imaging. 2012;(1):15-24.
27. Verheart D, Gabriel RS, Johnston D, Lytle BW, Desai, MY Klein AL. The role of multimodality imaging in the management of pericardial disease. Circ Cardiovasc Imaging. 2010;3(3):333-43.
28. Francone M, Dymarkowski S, Kalantzi M, et al. Realtime cine MRI of ventricular septal motion: A novel approach to assess ventricular coupling. J Magn Reson Imaging. 2005;21(3):305-9.
29. Westwood MA, Moon JC. Cardiovascular magnetic resonance for pericardial disease. Indian J Radiol Imaging. 2007;17(2):133-36.
30. Ho ML, Gutierrez FR. Chest radiography in thoracic polytrauma. Am J Roentgenol. 2009;192:599-612.
31. Mirvis SE. Imaging of acute thoarcic injury: The advent of MDCT screening. Semin Ultrasound CT MRI. 2005;26: 305-31.
32. Grebenc ML, Christenson MLR, Burke AP, et al. Primary cardiac and pericardial neoplasms: radiologic-pathologic correlation. Radiographics. 2000;20:1073.
33. Fussen S, De Boeck BW, Zellweger MJ, et al. Cardiovascular magnetic resonance imaging for diagnosis and clinical management of suspected cardiac masses and tumours. Eur Heart J. 2011;32(12):1551-60.
34. Hoffmann U, Globits S, Frank H. Cardiac and paracardiac masses: Current opinion on diagnostic evaluation by magnetic resonance imaging. Eur Heart J. 1998;19:553-63.

CHAPTER 183

Imaging and Interventions of Aorta

Manphool Singhal, Kartik Ganga, Sanjeev Kumar, Vivek Gupta, Niranjan Khandelwal

INTRODUCTION

The word 'Aorta' is derived from *Latin* word*:* aorta, and *Greek*: aorte which means "a strap to hang (something by)". This term was first used by Aristotle while describing the aorta: how it seems to be 'suspended' above the heart.[1] The function of the aorta has been documented since the ancient times of Bible and Talmud, where it was noted as one of three major vessels entering or leaving the heart, and how it's perforation was linked to death.[2]

The aorta is the largest artery in the body which carries oxygenated blood from left ventricle to various organs of the body. It also functions both as a conduit and a reservoir. Its viscoelastic and compliance properties are responsible for the laminar blood flow during systole, and modulate continued forward flow during diastole.[3]

Aorta is an elastic artery and its wall consists of:

- *Intima:* A thin endothelial layer
- *Media:* The thickest layer consisting of smooth muscles, collagen and elastic fibers.
- *Adventitia:* The outermost layer of collagen and elastic fibers also containing vasa vasorum, nerves and lymphatics.

SEGMENTATION ANATOMY OF AORTA

Aorta is divided into the following parts **(Figs. 1A and B)**:

- **Root:** Comprises of 3 aortic sinuses and extending from aortic valve to sinotubular junction where it becomes the ascending aorta.
- **Ascending aorta:** Extends from sinotubular junction to the origin of brachiocephalic artery.
- **Arch of aorta:** Extends from origin of brachiocephalic artery to the origin of left subclavian artery.
- **Descending aorta:** Extends beyond the origin of left subclavian artery till aortic bifurcation at L4 level into common iliac arteries. It is further divided into thoracic and abdominal portions by the diaphragm, where the aorta passes through the aortic hiatus at D12 level.

A normal narrowing may be present just distal to left subclavian artery and proximal to ligamentum arteriosum called *isthmus*. Just beyond it, there may be a focal dilatation of the aorta, known as *aortic spindle*.

IMAGING OF AORTA: BASICS

Radiological evaluation of the anatomy and the pathology involving the aorta has undergone considerable refinement in recent years, which has been possible largely due to availability of multidetector CT (MDCT), dual source CT (DSCT) scanners and higher strength newer magnetic resonance imaging (MRI) and advanced software's. These modalities have largely replaced traditional contrast aortography.[4] Technological advances such as isotropic data acquisition with three-dimensional reconstruction capabilities, shorter acquisition times, improvement in processing and volume rendering have made it possible to visualize the aorta and its branches precisely. As a result, the role of catheter angiography is being restricted to special indications and to patients who may require catheter-based interventions.[5]

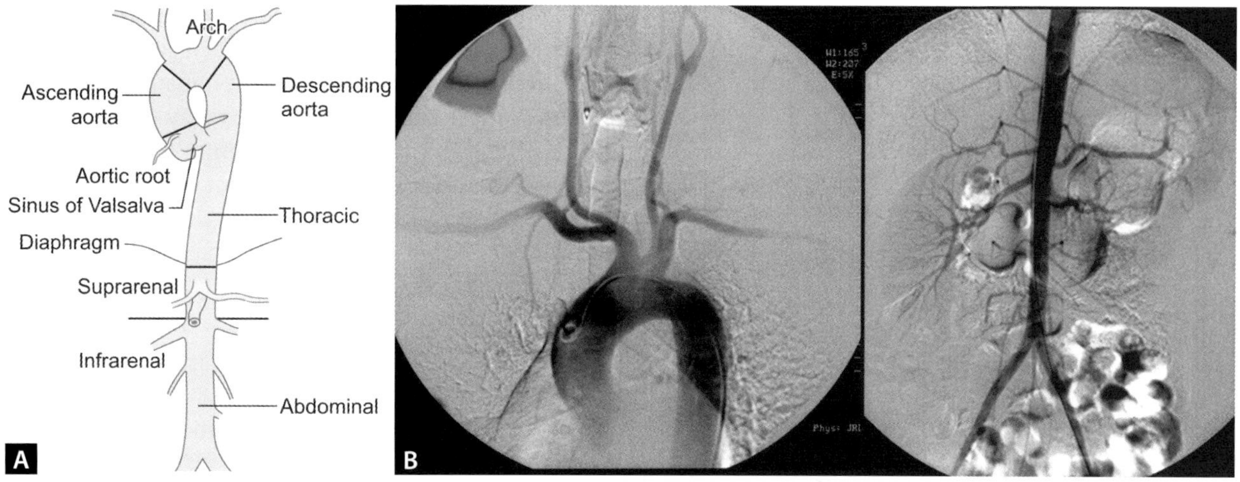

Figs. 1A and B: (A) Segmentation anatomy of aorta; (B) Normal angiographic anatomy: Arch and abdominal aortogram (DSA) shows normal branches.

Angiographic Anatomy

The aorta is broadly divided into thoracic and abdominal aorta **(Figs. 1A and B)**. The thoracic aorta begins at the aortic root just cranial to the aortic valve as the ascending aorta. It courses superiorly and to the left uptil the origin of the right brachiocephalic trunk where the aortic arch begins. The aortic arch continues cranially and posteriorly and gives rise to the left common carotid and left subclavian arteries. At this point, the aorta turns caudally and posterior to form the descending thoracic aorta. A normal narrowing called the *isthmus* may be present just distal to the left subclavian artery and proximal to the ligamentum arteriosum. The isthmus is commonly present in younger individuals and may be focal or extended over a long distance with a mild dilatation beyond it. It may form a small diverticulum called the *ductus diverticulum* **(Fig. 2)**. The descending thoracic aorta continues caudally in the posterior mediastinum slightly on the left side, anterolateral to the spine and posterolateral to the esophagus. It passes through the diaphragmatic hiatus at D12 level where it continues in the retroperitoneum on the left side as the abdominal aorta up to the iliac bifurcation. With age, the aorta shows enlargement of its diameter and tends to follow a more tortuous course.

The major branches which arise from the aorta are as follows:

- **Ascending aorta:** Right and left coronary arteries
- **Aortic arch:** Right brachiocephalic trunk (right subclavian and right common carotid artery), left common carotid artery and left subclavian artery

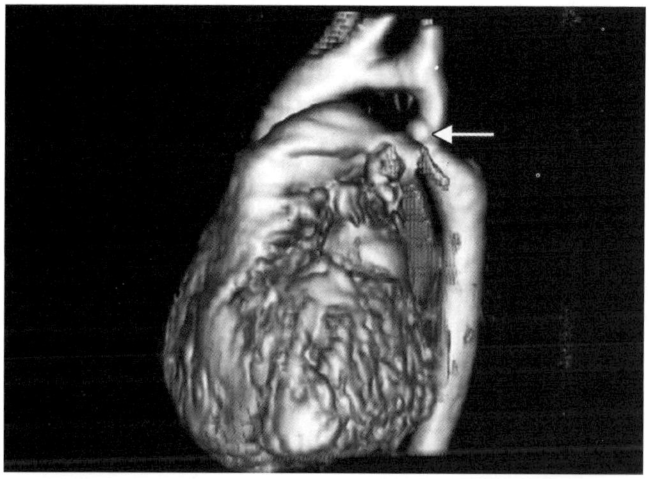

Fig. 2: Ductus diverticulum: CT angiogram (CTA) (Volume rendered-VR) shows isthmus and diverticulum (arrow).

- **Descending thoracic aorta:**
  - Visceral branches: Pericardial branches, bronchial arteries (one on the right and two on the left side), mediastinal branches and phrenic branches.
  - Parietal branches: Intercostal arteries and subcostal arteries
- **Abdominal aorta:**
  - Ventral: Unpaired: celiac axis, superior mesenteric artery and inferior mesenteric artery
  - Lateral: Paired—inferior phrenic artery, middle suprarenal artery, renal artery, testicular or ovarian arteries
  - Dorsal: Lumbar (5-Paired), median sacral (unpaired)
  - Terminal: Common iliac arteries (paired).

The Measurement (Diameter) of Aorta

The aortic diameter varies with body size, sex and ageing. The average mean diameter is as follows:[6]

Aortic root	:	3.6 cm
Aortic arch	:	3.5 cm
Proximal descending aorta	:	2.6 cm
Distal descending aorta	:	2.4 cm
Abdominal aorta	:	2.0 cm

The ratio of ascending and descending aorta is 2.2 (young) and 1.2 (elderly). In adults, the aortic diameter increases by approximately 0.1 cm per decade.

Normal Anatomic Variations

There are various normal anatomic variations involving the arch, brachiocephalic vessels and visceral branching patterns of the abdominal aorta. The most common variation is the common origin of brachiocephalic trunk and left common carotid artery which is seen in approximately 20% of the population **(Fig. 3)**. In about 5% of the population, the left vertebral artery arises directly from the aorta **(Fig. 3)**. In 1%, there is a common origin of both common carotid arteries and a paired brachiocephalic trunk. Aortic arch anomalies include aberrant origin of the right subclavian artery as the last branch of the thoracic aorta just distal to left subclavian artery (1%), right-sided aortic arch (1%), and aberrant origin of left subclavian artery (1%), etc.[7]

The most common variant of the abdominal aorta involves the origin of the hepatic artery. The left lobe of liver may be supplied completely or partially by the left hepatic artery originating from the left gastric artery (25%). The "replaced origin" of the right hepatic artery from the superior mesenteric artery (SMA) may be seen in 10% of the population. Rarely, the common hepatic artery may take origin directly from the SMA or the aorta or the celiac axis and SMA may have a common origin.[7]

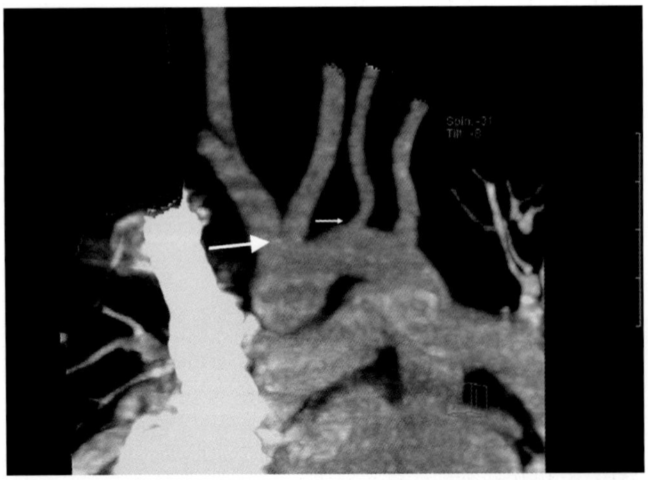

Fig. 3: MIP image of CTA showing common origin of right brachiocephalic and left common carotid arteries (thick arrow). Also seen is direct origin of the left vertebral artery from arch of aorta (thin arrow).

IMAGING MODALITIES

- *Noninvasive:*
  - Ultrasound (US): Transthoracic echocardiography (TTE), duplex scanning, color Doppler (CD), transesophageal echocardiography (TEE) and intravascular ultrasound (IVUS).
  - Computed tomography (CT): MDCT or DSCT
  - MRI: Three-dimensional contrast-enhanced MR angiography (3D CE-MRA), bright blood (steady state free precession-SSFP) imaging, various black blood inversion sequences, a short tau inverse recovery (STIR) and phase contrast (PC) sequences for flow quantifications
  - Nuclear fusion imaging: Nuclear fusion imaging (PET) with 18-flurorodeoxyglucose (18F-FDG) with either CT or MRI has increasing role now in the evaluation of systemic vasculitis, in the detection of vascular inflammation, delineating disease extent as well as treatment response evaluation
- *Invasive:* Catheter angiography—conventional or digital.

  In addition, plain radiographs of the chest and/or abdomen, barium swallow, etc. may suggest aortic disease and may provide some clues for further imaging.

Ultrasound

Ultrasound whether TTE or abdominal duplex scanning is the first noninvasive imaging modality for evaluation of aortic diseases and has sufficient accuracy for the purpose of diagnosis as well as surveillance. Technological improvement including combination of B-mode with pulsed wave Doppler and color flow mapping have increased the utility of US in the diagnosis as well as follow-up of aortic diseases. It is cost effective and portable with no hazards of ionizing radiation. However, the quality of the examination may be affected by patient factors such as bowel gas, obesity and it is highly operator dependent.

TEE and IVUS are two major advances in US that have modified preoperative aortic imaging.

Transesophageal Echocardiography

It has overcome many of the limitations of TTE and has a high degree of accuracy in skilled hands. One of the main advantages of TEE, especially in unstable patients, is that the examination can be performed safely and quickly at the bed side.

High resolution imaging of the thoracic aorta is possible with TEE. A 5 MHz one or two phased array transducer is mounted on the top of a gastroscope which is manipulated in the esophagus to get high resolution images of the thoracic aorta. The high image quality is possible because of close proximity to the heart and great vessels, absence of interposed air/bone and excellent acoustic coupling of the transducer face with the esophageal mucosa. In thoracic aorta imaging, TEE provides excellent information except for a 1–3 cm segment of the distal ascending aorta or proximal arch which cannot be imaged because of tracheal air; this is known as the "blind-spot".[8]

The limitations are that it requires a great deal of the physician's skill and it is not possible in patients suffering from esophageal stricture/tumors.

Intravascular Ultrasound

It is a relatively new imaging modality, used mainly during coronary and peripheral interventions. It provides 2D, cross-sectional images of the vessel lumen with good resolution. It allows evaluation of plaque morphology, vessel walls, and perivascular structures. It has not been used widely in aortic evaluation but it has the potential to provide useful information.[9]

Computed Tomography

The advances in CT technology have broadened its use for screening, diagnosis, endovascular treatment planning or preoperative evaluation and post-treatment follow-up of aortic diseases. It is more commonly used than MRI because of fast acquisition, high temporal and spatial resolution, and provision for ECG-gating especially for assessment of ascending aorta.[10-12]

CT Angiography Technique

With the advent of MDCT and DSCT scanners entire aorta and its branches can be imaged in a single breath hold with excellent image quality without venous contamination.[10]

Present scanners allow acquisition with radiation optimization with high temporal resolution (73 milliseconds-128DSCT).Newertechniqueslikeprospective triggering, ECG-based tube current modulation, body adaptive automatic dose calculation(exposure), excellent image quality with lower tube kilovoltage (kVp) setting by iterative images reconstruction algorithms have revolutionized the vascular imaging like never before.[10,13-15]

For ascending aorta evaluation ECG gating is usually desirable especially when imaging Standford type A dissection and aneurysm for simultaneous evaluation of coronary arteries, and for planning transcatheter aortic valve implantation (TAVI).

A typical protocol for image acquisition of entire aorta on a 64 MDCT/128 DSCT (which we routinely use at our institution) is given below, which can be customized according to the area of interest (thoracic or abdominal aorta).

Area coverage: The scan should cover area 3 cm above the aortic arch till the level of femoral heads, to include the entire aorta and the origins of its major branches. The imaging till proximal femoral arteries is essential for planning of endovascular treatment.

Contrast injection protocol: Since, the aorta is a large artery, dilution of contrast occurs rapidly thus a high rate of injection is required. If possible dual head pressure injector with saline chase is recommended to minimize/avoid artifacts caused by the high-density contrast in the superior vena cava. Flow rate should be 3–4 mL/second and volume should be calculated as follows:

$$\text{Flow rate} \times (\text{scan time} + \text{scan delay})$$

This should be followed by saline chase with the same flow rate for 5–6 seconds.

Acquisition of data: Since, imaging is to be done when the contrast density is maximum in the lumen, 'bolus chase' technique is preferred over fixed time delay, with threshold of contrast density kept between 100–200 HU (at level of ascending aorta) to trigger the acquisition with delay of 4–5 seconds to achieve maximum luminal enhancement **(Table 1)**.[16,17]

Data analysis: Data thus acquired can be reconstructed in axial or 3D images [maximum intensity projections (MIP), shaded surface display (SSD) or volume rendered technique (VRT)]. The 3D depiction of the entire aorta depicts the entire extent of the pathology in a single image and any number of desired projections can be made. This can be done with either VRT or MIP technique **(Figs. 4A to C)**. When detailed evaluation of pathology is required thin MIP up to 0.5 mm can be made and evaluated.

The major advantages of CTA over a digital subtraction angiography of the aorta are visualization of the wall and its surrounding changes. Pathologies like intramural

Table 1: Scan protocol for 128 DSCT angiography of the entire aorta.

Serial number	*CT coronary angiography scan parameters*	*Details of parameters*
1.	Scan area	3 cm above the aortic arch till the level of femoral heads
2.	Data acquisition technique	Bolus tracking technique (region of interest in the ascending aorta with preset of 100 HU)
3.	Scan delay	5 seconds after achievement of 100 HU
4.	Kilovoltage	100–120 KV according to body habitus, sex and age
5.	Tube current	Automatic exposure control system-based tube current modulation
6.	Detector collimation	2 × 64 × 0.6 mm
7.	Slice acquisition	2 × 128 × 0.6 mm by means of a z-flying focal spot
8.	Gantry rotation time	280 milliseconds
9.	Temporal resolution	75 milliseconds
10.	Reconstructed slice thickness	0.75 mm with a reconstruction increment of 0.5 mm
11.	Image window	Soft-tissue convolution kernel (B26f)
12.	ECG gating *(for ascending aorta only)*	Retrospective ECG gating with tube current modulation
13.	Image post-processing	Images construction in multiplanar, maximum intensity projection and volume rendering along with axial data set

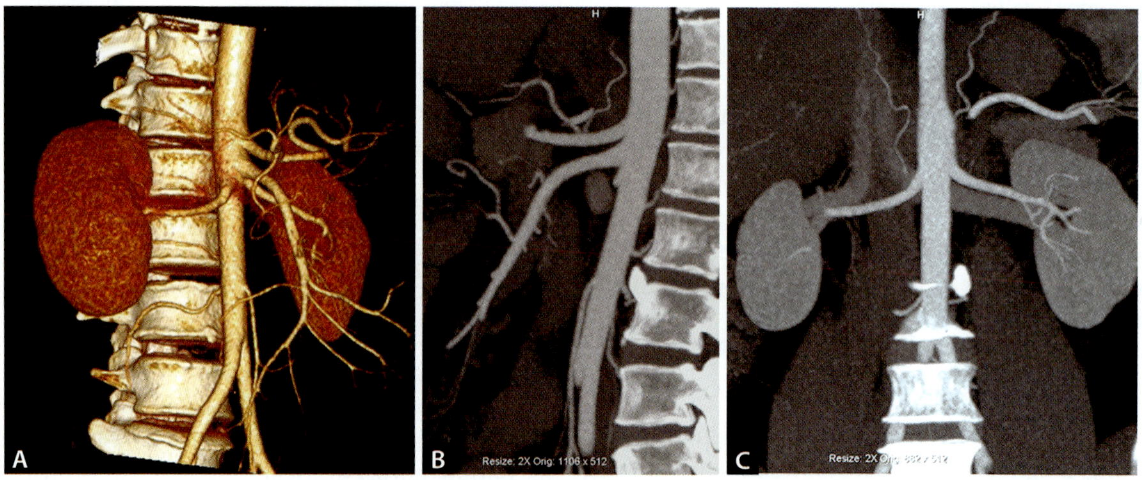

Figs. 4A to C: Normal abdominal CTA acquired on 128 DSCT: Volume rendering (A) and maximum intensity projection (B and C) projections showing major branches of aorta.

hematoma can be easily overlooked on digital substratction angiography (DSA). The other advantages being rapid imaging time, uniform arterial enhancement, lack of motion artifacts, identification of branch vessels, ease of use and it being less expensive. The major limitation includes lack of "flow quantification".

Magnetic Resonance Imaging and MR Angiography

Magnetic resonance angiography of the aorta offers certain advantages over CT angiography. Most important is that since it does not involve radiation, repeated examination can be done as required for follow-up, safely without any radiation concern.

One major advantage of MRI is that flow quantification and direction of flow can now be determined with advanced MR applications and MR angiography techniques.

Several techniques are available to image the aorta and can be broadly classified into:[11,12,18-22]

A. 3D contrast-enhanced MR angiography (3D CE-MRA)
B. White blood imaging—static and cine imaging
C. Black blood imaging—static imaging
D. Phase contrast (PC) sequences—for flow quantification.

3D Contrast-enhanced MR Angiography (3D CE-MRA)

3D CE-MRA is gadolinium-enhanced 3D gradient echo (3D-GRE) where thin contiguous image partitions are obtained in a single breath-hold. It uses heavily T1-weighted 3D-GRE technique and is the work horse for evaluation of vascular abnormalities of primarily thoracic aorta **(Fig. 5)**. It allows post-processing just like CT angiography and techniques like MIP reformation, volume rendering and multiplanar reformation of the images can be generated for analysis.[11,12,23]

It is done with injection of gadolinium-based contrast agents (0.1 mmol/kg body weight) with a flow rate of 2–5 mL per second, followed by a saline flush of 20 mL injected at the same flow rate immediately after contrast administration. Scan can be started after a fixed time interval as determined by doing a test scan using a small amount of contrast or by MR fluoroscopy method when contrast reaches left ventricle.

Bright Blood Imaging

Bright blood imaging provides images with blood having hyperintense signal that works on steady-state free-precession (SSFP) sequence (FIESTA, TrueFISP). It is a short TE and TR sequence, which provides very high and homogeneous intraluminal signal even in cases of turbulent flow because this sequence depends mainly on a function of the T2/T1 ratio **(Figs. 6A to D)**.

SSFP images can be acquired in both breath-hold and free-breathing manners, either with or without ECG-gating and navigator/respiratory trigger. SSFP can provide rapid bright-blood images with high-contrast resolution.

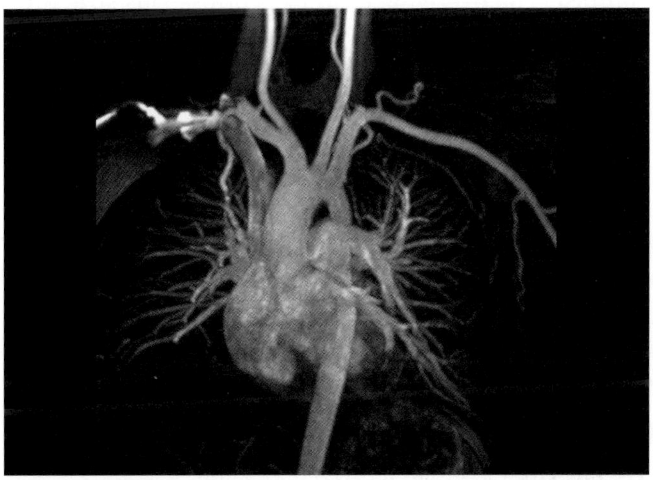

Fig. 5: 3D MIP image at 3T of contrast-enhanced MRA showing aortic arch, ascending and descending thoracic aorta and its major branches with high spatial resolution and without any artifacts.

SSFP sequences can also be acquired in a cine mode, and have become the foundation for cine imaging. Advantages are the higher signal-to-noise ratio (SNR), shorter imaging duration, and freedom from the reliance on inflow effects for signal generation. This sequence has benefited from the application of parallel imaging techniques, allowing high temporal resolution, large filed of view (FOV) imaging of the thoracic aorta, and left ventricular outflow during acceptable breath-holds as low as 5–6 seconds. The inherently high blood signal achieved using SSFP throughout a cine acquisition period has been shown to aid evaluation of aortic mural and valvular characteristics and allowing exclusion of aortic dissection. SSFP is the most promising of the "bright-blood" noncontrast-enhanced MR angiography techniques.[20-22]

Black Blood Imaging

Black blood employs the inherent contrast between the rapidly flowing blood (flow void) and aortic wall to generate images so that aortic wall is well depicted. It can be obtained either with spin echo (either conventional or echo-train spin-echo techniques) or double inversion recovery sequences. Short tau inversion recovery (STIR) sequence is restricted for demonstration of wall edema.[11,20,21] Usually image acquisition is with ECG-gating, exploiting the contrast between rapidly flowing blood and the aortic wall **(Figs. 6A to D)**.

Black blood imaging is recommended when analysis of aortic wall pathology is desirable such as mural hematoma and aortoarteritis. It may also be useful for the depiction of intraluminal abnormalities, such as dissection flaps and tumor thrombus.

Luminal signal void occurs because intravascular protons only produce signal if they are exposed to both a 90° excitation pulse and subsequent refocusing pulse while traveling through the image slice.[11,12] Therefore, low flow and entry/exit slice phenomena may produce high signal in the aortic lumen, artificially simulating wall disease, so before any conclusion is drawn all sequences and imaging planes need careful inspection and interpretation.

Phase Contrast (PC) Sequences

Quantification of aortic flow especially in aortic regurgitation, stenosis, congenital heart diseases and coarctation of aorta is required for management which is possible with PC sequences. It is based upon the principle that protons passing through a magnetic field gradient undergo a phase change in proportion to velocity, and this is utilized to measure the flow velocities within the aortic lumen during the entire cardiac cycle for measurement of forward flow, regurgitation and stenosis.[24-26]

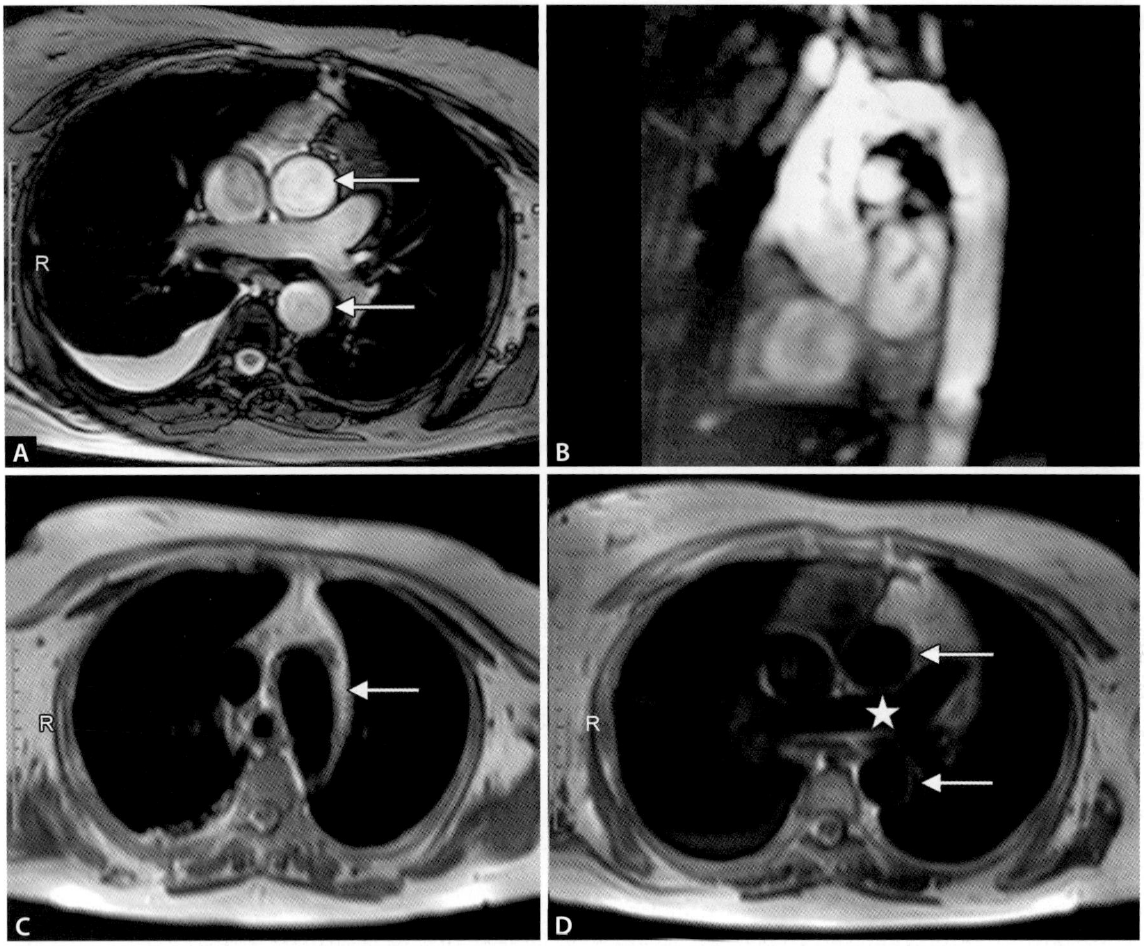

Figs. 6A to D: Axial (A) and "candy cane" view (B) SSFP images (bright blood images) at 3T through the thoracic aorta showing bright aortic lumen (arrows) due to sensitivity of the method to flowing blood; (C and D) Axial black blood double inversion recovery sequence images at 3T through the thoracic aorta showing dark aortic lumen with well-delineated arch (arrow in C), ascending and descending thoracic aorta (arrows in D) and pulmonary arteries (star in D).

18F-fluorodeoxyglucose (18F-FDG) with either CT or MRI

Fusion imaging of 18F-FDG PET with CT/MRI is now emerging as the modality of choice as it not only provides the anatomical imaging with high spatial resolution both also specific information about disease activity as 18F-FDG is a surrogate marker of increased activity of inflammatory cells. In specific it delineates extent of vascular inflammation and response to treatment in cases of aortitis. It also helps in selection of appropriate sites for biopsy—histopathologic confirmation of diagnosis.[27-29]

Catheter Angiography

It is the most definitive study in the evaluation of aortic disease. Both conventional angiography and DSA provide detailed anatomic information including aberrant origin of vessels. But DSA saves time, expenses on films and on contrast. The overlying bowel gas or osseous structures that obscure the area of interest is avoided. Contrast-related complications may be avoided by using CO_2 gas as contrast agent. Intravenous DSA, once the preferred noninvasive technique, has largely been discarded because of technical difficulties and poor contrast resolution. Nonetheless, it can be used in a limited way in acute settings like trauma. There has been progressive decrease in the size of catheter used from 6–7 French to 4–5 French, low flow rates and smaller arterial punctures with overall reduction in mortality and morbidity rate. All these factors have pushed the most invasive investigation to an outpatient procedure.[5]

Technique

A 5 or 6F arterial sheath is placed in the femoral or brachial artery by puncturing it with 18G puncture needle under strict aseptic precautions under local anesthesia: 2500 U of heparin is used normally for diagnostic studies. A 5F pigtail catheter is introduced over a 0.035"/0.032" guide wire in the ascending aorta (for arch study) 2.5 inches above the aortic valve or in the abdominal aorta (around T12) just above the origin of celiac axis. 25–30 cc of non-ionic contrast is injected at a flow rate of 12–14cc/sec through a power injector. A 45° LAO projection is taken for arch study and a straight AP and lateral views are taken for the abdominal aorta. Further studies like selective injection into branch vessels, lateral or oblique projection may be done depending upon the initial aortographic findings. After reviewing the entire study, the catheter and the arterial sheath are removed and pressure compression is applied at puncture site for 12–15 minutes till the bleeding stops.

Complications of Angiography

These are divided into three major categories: Reactions to contrast media, complications related to arterial puncture site and systemic complications related to arterial catheterization. A proper and carefully applied technique may reduce the complications rate to less than 0.1%.[30]

The contraindications of angiography include:

- Previous anaphylactic contrast reaction,
- Low cardiac output, and
- Anuria and bleeding diathesis.

INDICATIONS FOR IMAGING THE AORTA

Various diseases afflicting the aorta may warrant either noninvasive or invasive aortic imaging. The diseases can be classified as:

- *Congenital*:
  - Aortic arch anomalies
  - Coarctation
  - Aortic atresia
  - Aortic stenosis
- *Acquired*:
  - Aneurysms
  - Dissection
  - Aortitis
  - Trauma
  - Atherosclerosis.

CONGENITAL AORTIC ANOMALIES

Aortic Arch Anomalies

- Left aortic arch with aberrant origin of right subclavian artery **(Figs. 7A and B)**
- Right aortic arch
  - With mirror image branching
  - With aberrant origin of left subclavian artery
- Cervical arch
- Double aortic arch **(Figs. 8A and B)**

The detailed description and imaging findings are discussed in relevant chapters in this book.

Coarctation of Aorta

It is a congenital aortic narrowing in the region of the isthmus. It is more common in males (M:F = 4:1) and is rare in blacks. It is of two types:

1. Localized or adult or postductal or juxta-ductal type: It is the most common type where there is a short segment narrowing close to the ligamentum arteriosum. Coexistent cardiac anomalies are uncommon.
2. Tubular hypoplasia or infantile or preductal or diffuse type: There is hypoplasia of a long segment of the aortic arch after the origin of the brachiocephalic trunk. Coexistent cardiac anomalies are common.

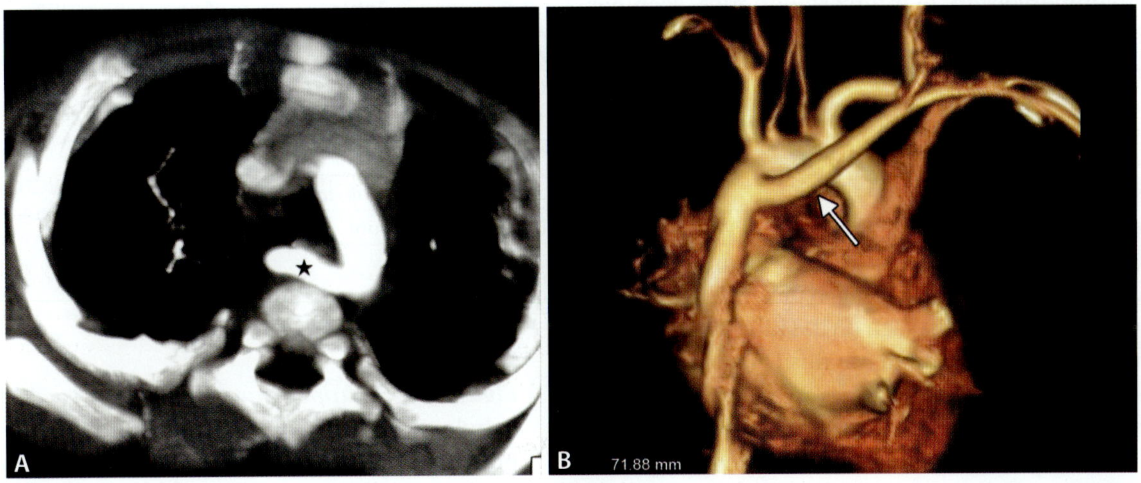

Figs. 7A and B: (A) MIP axial and (B) VR (posterior projection) shows aberrant origin of right subclavian artery (star and arrow) with retroesophageal course (star) from left-sided arch.

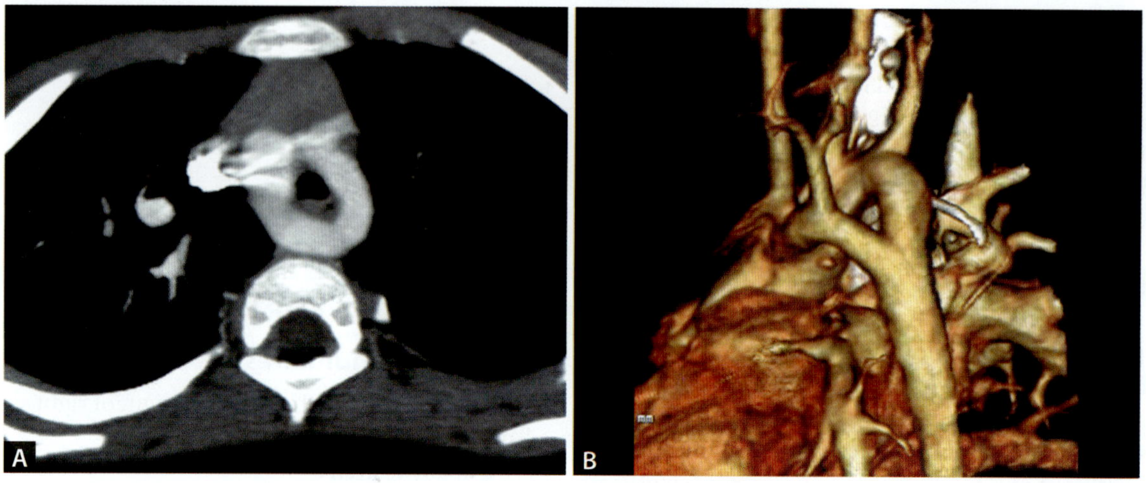

Figs. 8A and B: (A) MIP axial and (B) VR image (posterior projection) shows double aortic arch encircling trachea.

Associated Anomalies

- Bicuspid aortic valve (25–50%)
- *Cardiac shunts*:
  - Patent ductus arteriosus (PDA) (33%)
  - Ventricular septal defect (VSD) (15%)
- Turner's syndrome (13–15%)
- Cerebral berry aneurysms (5–7%)

A review of the natural history of coarctation revealed that of those patients who survived infancy, 20% were dead before the age of 20 years, 50% by 32 years and 90% by 58 years.[31] Most common causes of death are due to cardiac failure, aortic rupture, infective endocarditis, intracerebral hemorrhage, etc.

Hemodynamics in Adults

The collateral circulation distal to the coarctation is through the subclavian arteries and its branches like internal mammary artery to intercostal arteries, scapular artery to anterior spinal artery and transverse cervical artery to lateral thoracic artery.

Radiological Findings

Conventional X-ray Chest

- Rib notching **(Table 2)**: It usually takes several years to develop. It is due to pressure erosion by the enlarged and tortuous intercostal arteries. It is typically bilateral but asymmetrical and is best seen on the inferior aspects of the posterior thirds of 4th to 9th ribs **(Fig. 9)**. It will be seen only on the left side if there is an aberrant origin of the right subclavian artery below the coarctation and only on the right side if there is involvement of the left subclavian artery in the coarctation.
- Left ventricular hypertrophy.

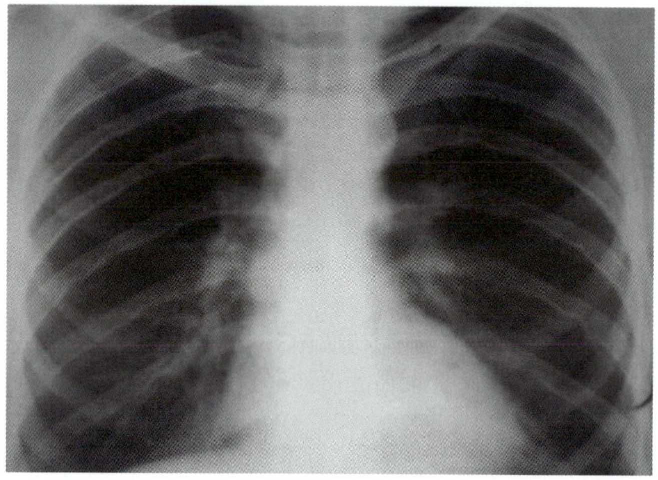

Fig. 9: Chest X-ray showing notching of posterior ribs bilaterally most prominent along inferior borders in a case of aortic coarctation.

Table 2: Causes of rib notching.

Aortic obstruction	***Pulmonary oligemia***
Coarctation	Fallot's tetralogy
Takayasu's arteritis	Pulmonary artery atresia
Thrombosis of abdominal aorta	*Miscellaneous:* • Chronic SVC or IVC obstruction • Intercostal AV fistula • Fallot's tetralogy • Pulmonary artery atresia
Subclavian artery obstruction	
Blalock-Taussig shunt	
Takayasu's arteritis	
Coarctation	

- *Figure of '3' appearance*: It is due to dilated left subclavian artery above the coarctation (CoA), a pinching at the site of CoA and the post-stenotic dilatation below.
- Small and flat aortic knuckle.

Angiography: It has been used for long to image CoA. A cardiac catheterization is also required to evaluate cardiac abnormalities and for the measurement of pressure gradient across the lesion. The CoA can usually be crossed from the femoral route but may require brachial artery catheterization in extreme stenosis. Multiple views are required in asymmetric lesions. The angiograms reveal the site, degree and size of the stenosis as well as the collateral circulation **(Figs. 10A to F)**.

Noninvasive Imaging

CTA, MRA and USG are often used in conjunction with angiography in the evaluation of coarctation. CT angiography can depict the morphology of the coarcted segment with good spatial resolution as well as status of aortic arch vessels and collaterals. However, it is not able to measure the gradient across the lesion, nor the direction of the flow. Still it is an important investigation for planning stent graft implantation and follow-up imaging after surgery **(Figs. 10A to F)**.

MRA now in addition to the anatomic details can give the information of the dynamics involved in the coarctation of aorta, noninvasively **(Fig. 11)**.

Phase-contrast velocity-encoded cine MR can give reliable information regarding flow velocity, flow volume and the pressure gradient across the stenosed segment. Also, it can give information regarding the collaterals and the direction of flow in them. Though this technique is promising, its use in routine clinical practise is limited because it also suffers from certain drawbacks like underestimation of flow volume and velocity and is also poor in small vessel assessment.

Management of Aortic Coarctation

Societal guidelines recommend that coarctation correction should be performed as early as possible (ideally as early as possible in childhood) to reduce the long-term morbidity and enhance survival.[32,33] The indications for corrective treatment are listed in **Box 1**. Percutaneous interventions and surgical correction are both acceptable

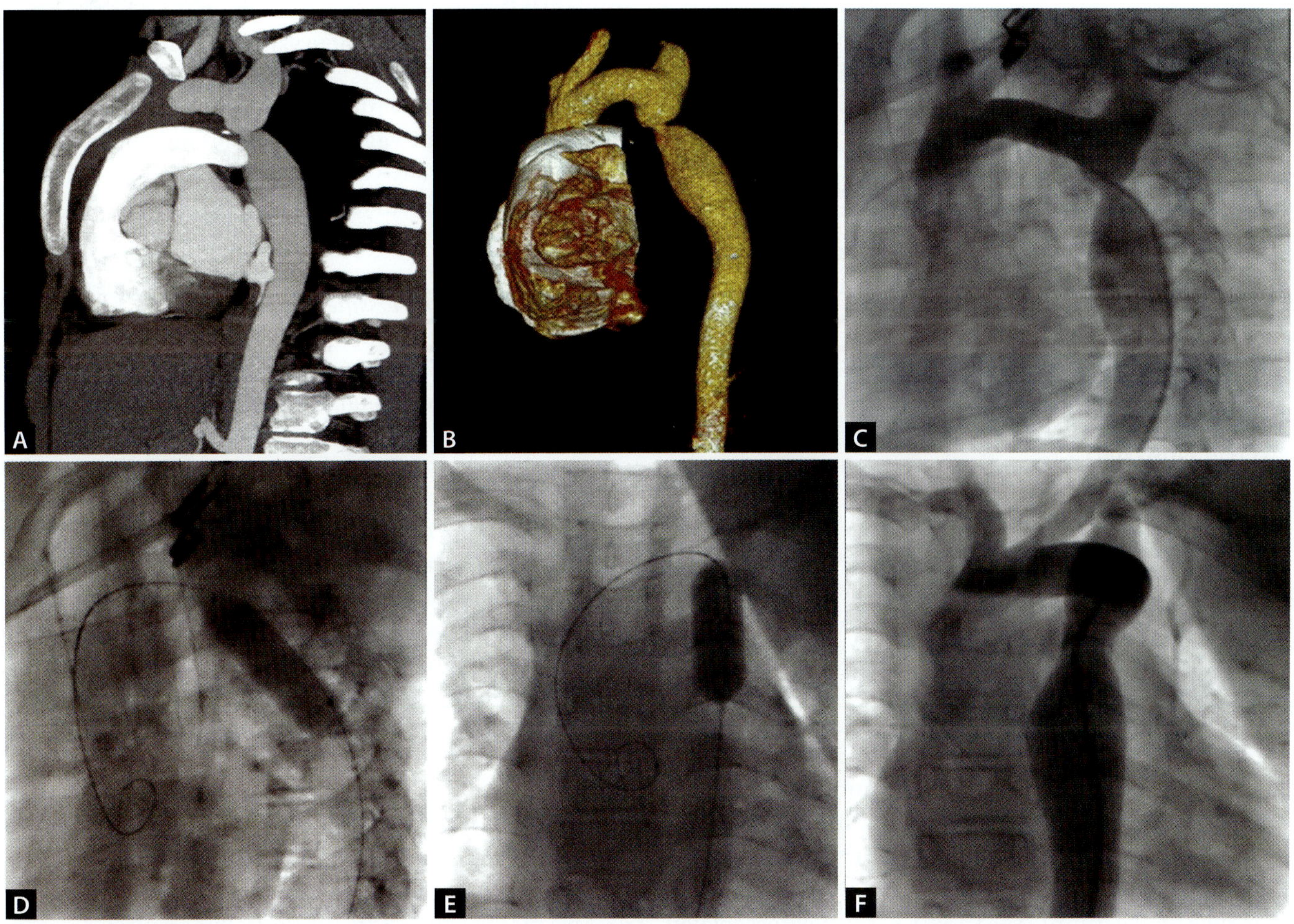

Figs. 10A to F: Balloon angioplasty of aortic coarctation: (A to C) Computed tomography and angiography showing coarctation of aorta; (D and E) Balloon angioplasty of the coarctation; (F) Postballoon angioplasty angiography showing significant reduction in severity of stenosis.

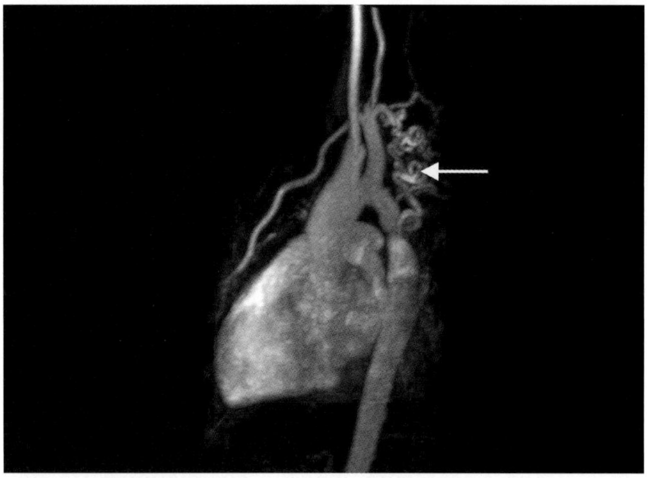

Fig. 11: MRA-MIP image lateral projection shows the coarctation, its length and the status of the aorta proximal and distal to it. Also note presence of collaterals seen on this MRA image (arrow).

Box 1: Indications for corrective treatment.

- Peak to peak (or maximum instantaneous) coarctation gradient ≥20 mm Hg
- Peak to peak coarctation gradient <20 mm Hg in the presence of significant coarctation with imaging evidence of significant collateral flow.

options for coarctation repair. A multidisciplinary team (i.e. cardiologist, interventionists, and surgeons) with experience in treating patients with congenital heart disease should be involved in deciding the management protocol and is dependent on the morphology, age, associated cardiac lesions as well as the availability of either an experienced interventionist or surgeon. A suggested algorithmic approach to manage coarctation is given in **Flowchart 1**.

Balloon angioplasty may also be performed as a palliative procedure in very sick patients as part of a staged protocol for initial stabilization of the patient.

Pseudocoarctation is a condition that results from an elongation of the distal aortic arch which, as it is fixed at the arterial ligament, bulges backwards above and below this point causing a 'double aortic' bulge. There is no hemodynamic obstruction. It may present as a mediastinal mass and the true nature can be demonstrated on CT or MRI. **Interrupted aortic arch** is a rare condition in which a localized atresia of the arch occurs distal to the left subclavian artery (Type A: 42%), **(Figs. 12A to C)** distal to the left common carotid artery (Type B: 53%) or distal to the brachiocephalic trunk (Type C: 5%). It is usually associated with various cardiac anomalies such as PDA and VSD.

ACQUIRED AORTIC DISEASES

In this section, imaging in particular reference to endovascular and surgical management of aortic aneurysms, pathologies causing acute aortic syndrome, surveillance of aortic aneurysms is discussed in detail.

Imaging of common inflammatory aortitis like Takayasu and IgG4 related aortitis are also described. Infective or mycotic inflammatory pathologies have been included in the aneurysm section.

AORTIC ANEURYSMS

An aneurysm is a localized or diffuse dilatation of an artery. Aneurysm is defined as a permanent focal dilatation of the artery having ≥ 50% increase in diameter compared with the expected normal diameter of the artery in question. Ectasia is arterial dilatation <150% of normal arterial diameter. Arteriomegaly is diffuse arterial dilatation involving several arterial segments, with an increase in diameter >50% in comparison with the expected normal arterial diameter.[34]

Incidence

The incidence of aortic aneurysm varies from 4% (60–70 years) to 11% (70 years and above) and is probably increasing. Patients with hypertension, coronary artery disease, peripheral vascular disease and those whose immediate family have aneurysms are at a higher risk of developing aortic aneurysms.

Classification

An aneurysm can be classified as:

- *True or false* **(Fig. 13)**: True aneurysms consist of all three layers of the arterial wall (intima, media, and adventitia) whereas false aneurysms are due to focal perforation of the aortic wall limited externally by the adventitia, perivascular connective tissue, or by hematoma.
- *Saccular or fusiform* **(Figs. 14A to D)**: Saccular aneurysms usually arise from a distinct portion of the aortic wall and have a mouth, while fusiform aneurysms involve the total circumference of an artery and have no distinctive mouth.
- *Congenital or acquired*: Acquired aneurysms are more frequent than congenital aneurysms.

Etiology

- Atherosclerosis (70–80%)
- Cystic medial necrosis (Marfan syndrome, Ehlers-Danlos syndrome.)
- *Mycotic/infective (2–2.5%)—usually saccular*:
  - Tuberculosis (typically affects thoracic aorta),

Flowchart 1: Approach to treatment of coarctation of aorta.

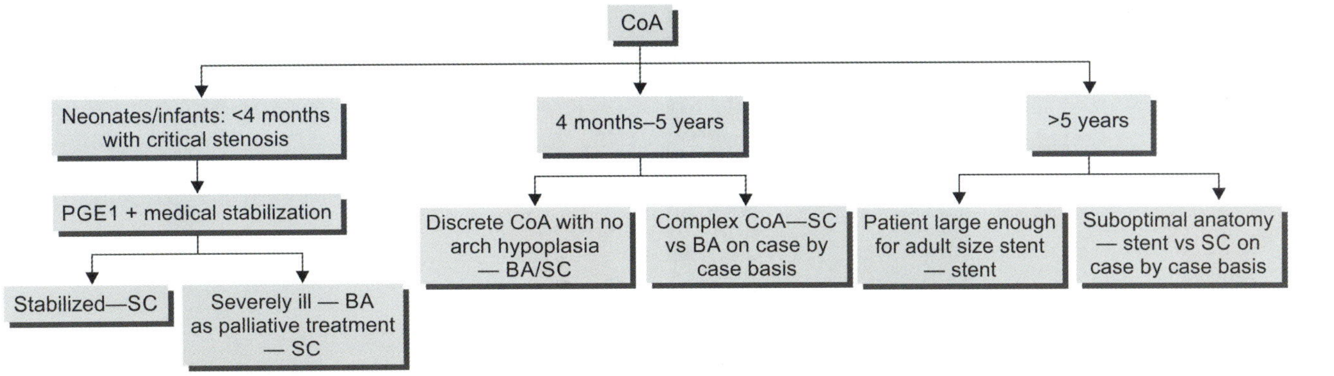

Abbreviations: CoA: Coarctation; PGE1: Prostaglandin E1; SC: Surgical correction; BA: Balloon angioplasty.

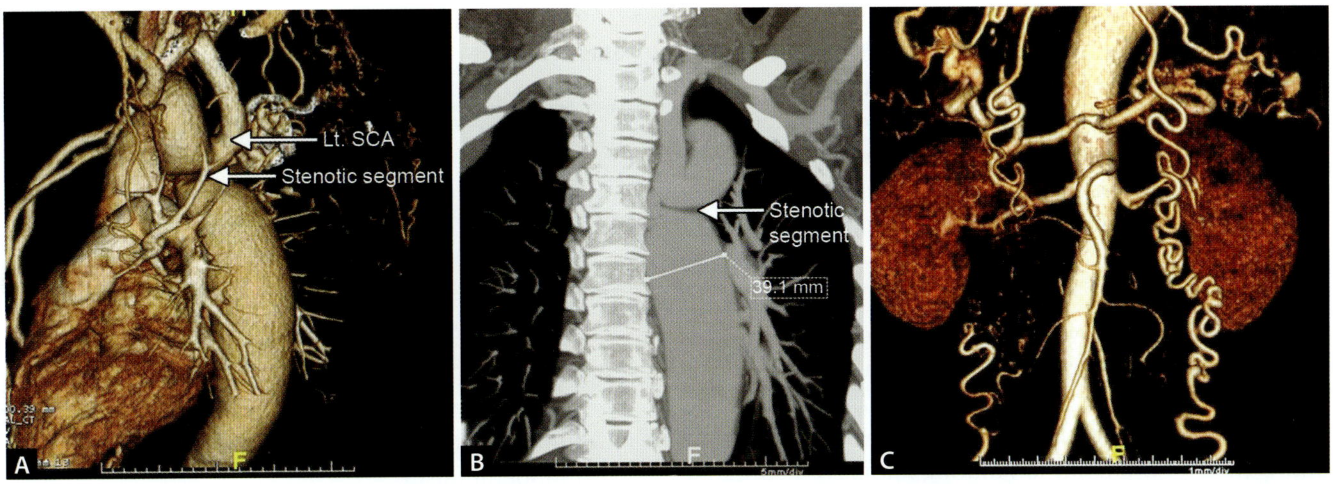

Figs. 12A to C: (A) CTA MIP image sagittal projection and (B) VR image show discontinuity of descending thoracic aorta just distal to origin of left subclavian artery; (C) Note extensive collaterals.

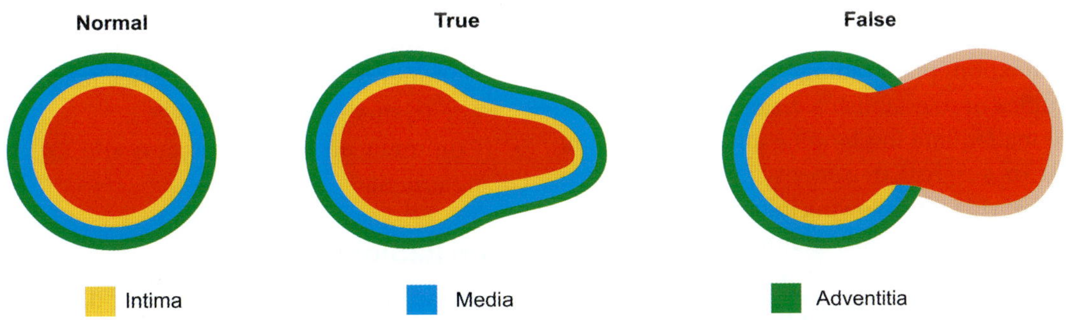

Fig. 13: Differentiation of true (covered by all layers) from false/pseudoaneurysm (arterialized periarterial hematoma).

  - Syphilis (90% affects ascending or arch of aorta)
  - Other infections (*Staphalococcus*, *Streptococcus*, salmonella infection)
- Vasculitis (Takayasu's and Giant cell arteritis)
- Spondyloarthropathies [Ankylosing spondylitis, rheumatiod arthritis (RA), psoriasis, Behcet's syndrome, Reiter's syndrome, Relapsing polychondritis]
- Post-traumatic (5–8%)—90% involving the isthmus and 8% in ascending aorta.

Growth Rates of Aneurysm

The mortality rate of untreated aortic aneurysms is unacceptably high and, once ruptured, it is almost 100%. Most aneurysms (80%) show progressive enlargement.

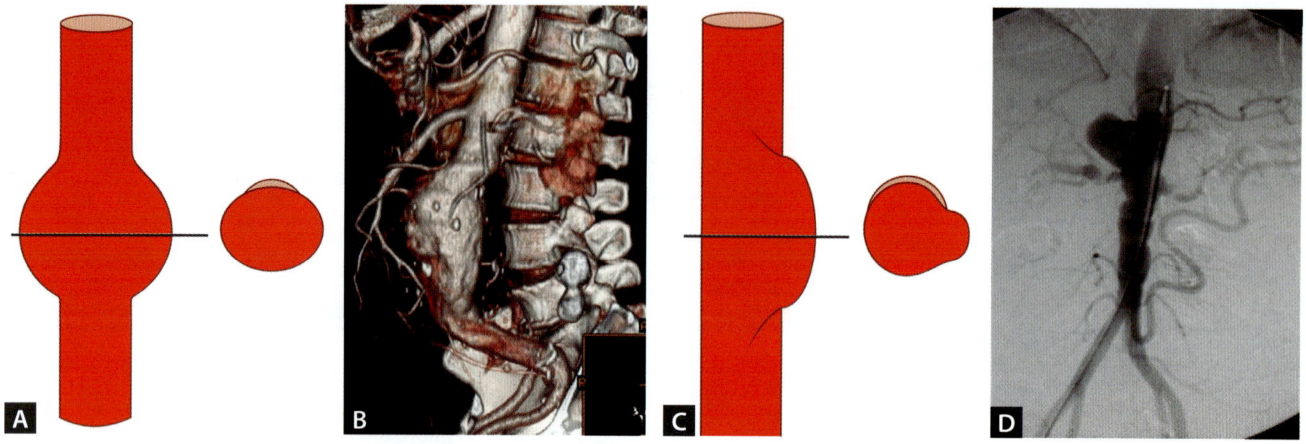

Figs. 14A to D: Images showing fusiform (A and B) saccular (C and D) aneurysms.

The rate of growth is significantly greater for aneurysms of the descending aorta, at 1.9 mm per year, than those of the ascending aorta, at 0.7 mm per year.[35] Larger the aneurysm, more rapid is the growth. As the size (radius) of aneurysm increases, the wall tension increases, which tend to further increase the size of aneurysm *(Laplace law)*.

Risk of Rupture

Diameter of the aneurysm is the best predictor of rupture risk. Other parameters associated with increased risk are type of aneurysm (Saccular > Fusiform), wall stress, rate of expansion, family history, hypertension, smoking and gender (more common among females). Estimated annular rupture risk of abdominal aortic aneurysm (AAA) is tabulated in **Table 3**.[35,36]

Diagnostic Imaging

Physical examination, plain radiography and ultrasound are usually sufficient to establish a diagnosis of aneurysm but these are inadequate in planning and implementing endovascular or surgical treatment. The preoperative imaging must provide the following information:[10,11,37]

- Location, size, angulations, craniocaudal extension and type of aneurysm.
- The maximum diameter of any dilatation, measured from the external wall of the aorta, perpendicular to the true axis of flow, and the length of the abnormally dilated aorta.
- Integrity of the wall, presence of intramural hematoma, penetrating ulcer and associated thrombus.
- Involvement of visceral arteries or adjacent structures.
- Associated anatomic variations.
- Unrecognized intra-abdominal/intra-thoracic conditions, e.g. cholelithiasis.

Table 3: Rupture risk per year of AAA in relation to diameter of aneurysm.

AAA diameter (cm)	*Rupture risk (%/year)*
<4	0
4–5	0.5–5
5–6	3–15
6–7	10–20
7–8	20–40
>8	30–50

- Complications of aneurysm, e.g. rupture, infection, thromboembolism.
- Measurements of aortic valve, sinuses of Valsalva, sinotubular junction, and ascending aorta in patients with presumed or documented genetic syndromes who are at risk for aortic root disease.
- Comments on coronary arteries for ascending aorta aneurysms.
- Comment on vascular access site for endovascular treatment.

Plain Radiography

Plain radiography may suggest a diagnosis of aortic aneurysm but information essential for preoperative planning cannot be obtained. Findings include:

- Widening of mediastinum; in a standard supine chest radiography, if the mediastinum measures >8 cm, it is highly suggestive of thoracic aortic aneurysm **(Fig. 15)**
- Localized dilatation of ascending aorta/knuckle/descending aorta with or without curvilinear calcification, **(Figs. 16A and B)**

- Depressed left main bronchus, tracheal displacement, obliteration of aorto-pulmonary window, cardiomegaly (thoracic aortic aneurysm) **(Figs. 17A to C)**
- Mural calcification, displacement of adjacent organs of gastrointestinal tract (GIT), vertebral erosion (abdominal aortic aneurysm) **(Figs. 18A and B)**.

Ultrasound

Ultrasound has sufficient accuracy to size aortic aneurysms for the purpose of diagnosis as well as surveillance to detect expansion **(Figs. 19A and B)**. It has the following advantages:

- It confirms the clinical diagnosis of an aneurysm.
- It serves as a screening modality for follow-up of patients with aortic aneurysms, especially abdominal aortic aneurysms.

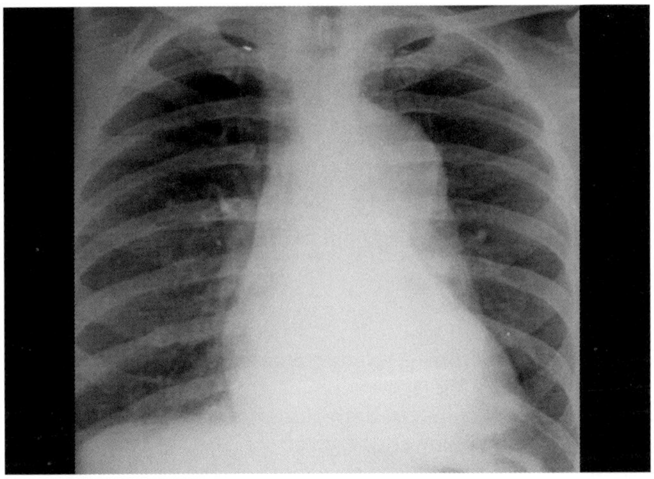

Fig. 15: Chest radiograph in a case of large thoracic aortic aneurysm showing mediastinal widening.

- It has a detection rate of 100% with size measurement within 4 mm of that obtained at surgery
- It is cost effective and portable.

The limitations of ultrasound are:

- It fails to provide reliable information regarding visceral artery involvement and craniocaudal extension.
- Obesity and intestinal gas hinder adequate evaluation, and
- Expertise and experience is required for providing other essential morphological information.

Transoesophageal echocardiography (TEE) and intravascular ultrasound (IVUS) have limited role in the diagnosis, however it may further modify the preoperative planning in aortic aneurysms. IVUS helps in accurate measurement of the aneurysm for selection of stent grafts during endovascular repair and helps in prevention of type I endoleaks.

CT and MRI

CT and MRI are the modalities of choice for imaging of aorta, however CT is preferred over MRI because of shorter scanning time and high temporal and spatial resolution. MR angiography is usually recommended for post-treatment evaluation. Computed tomography permits one to choose an imaging plane in any arbitrary space orientation, measure the tortuous aorta in true cross-section and obtain an accurate diameter. Breath-held dynamic contrast-enhanced MRI also allows rapid acquisition of images in any plane, independent of flow, however, disadvantages include non-visualization of calcifications and contraindications for MRI.[10-12,21,22,38]

In specific in cases of ascending arch aneurysm, ECG gated study should be considered for simultaneous evaluation of coronary arteries as significant CAD may be treated with by-pass grafts in one sitting.

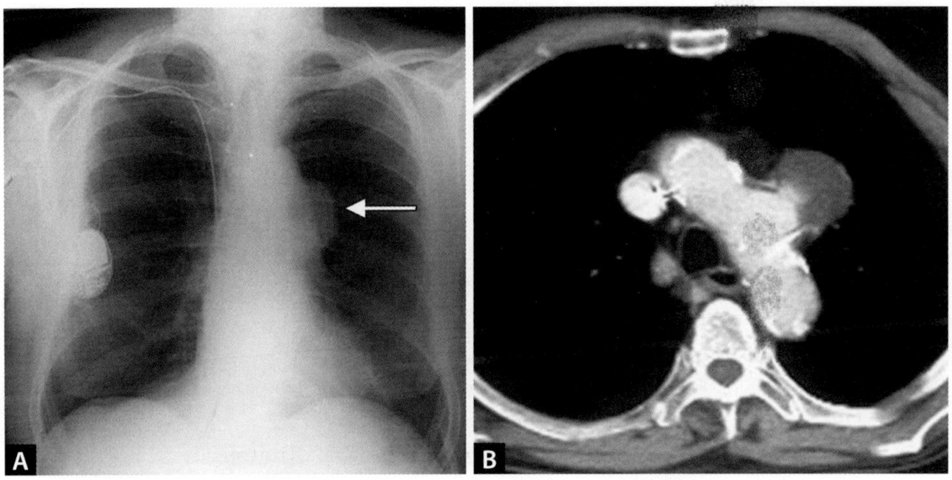

Figs. 16A and B: Chest radiograph in PA view shows prominent aortic kuncle (A), which on CTA (B) showed a peripherally thrombosed arch aneurysm with a penetrating ulcer.

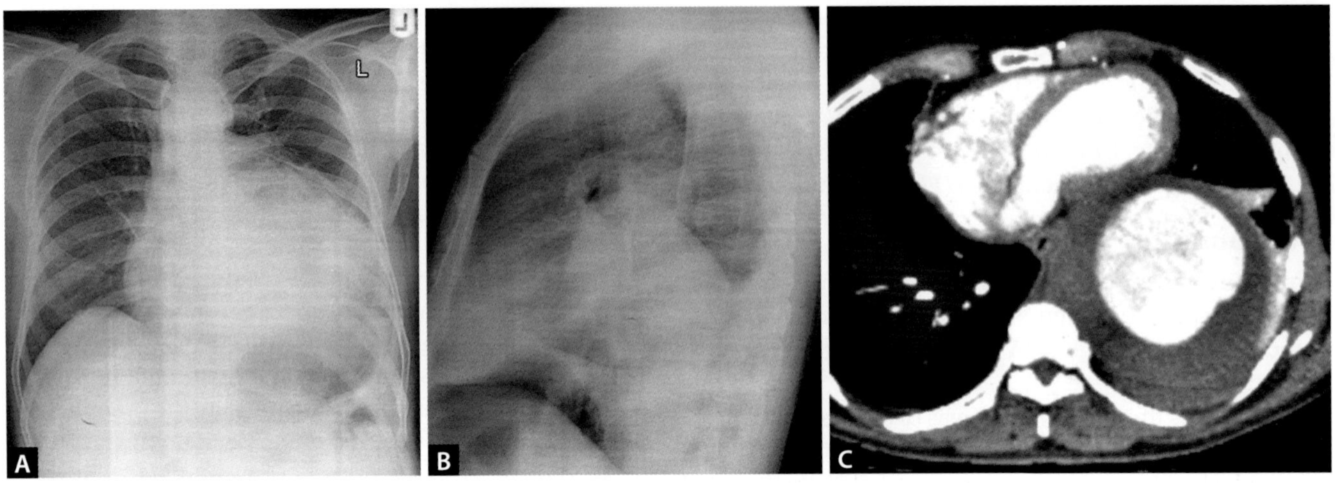

Figs. 17A to C: Chest radiograph in PA view shows cardiomegaly (A), which on lateral projection (B) shows a radio-opaque opacity overlying lower thoracic vertebra with loss of normal radiolucency. Subsequently on CTA (C) it was a large peripherally thrombosed DTA aneurysm.

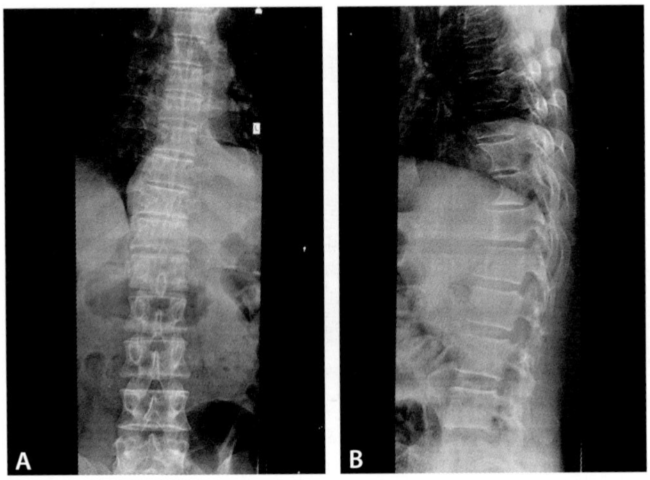

Figs. 18A and B: Front (A) and lateral thoracolumbar (B) spine radiograph shows a thoraco-abdominal mass-like lesion with well-defined lateral margins on both sides of spine. On lateral view anterior scalloping of lower dorsal vertebral bodies is prominently seen. On CTA it turned out to be a large mycotic aneurysm (Refer Fig. 23).

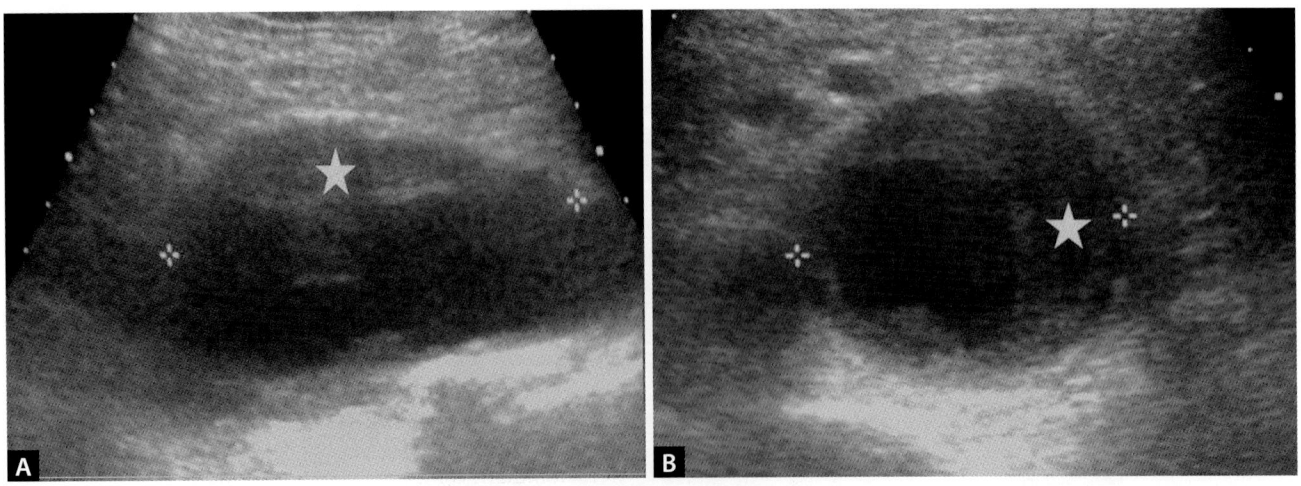

Figs. 19A and B: US abdomen longitudinal (A) and transverse (B) images show a peripherally thrombosed (along left lateral wall—stars) fusiform aneurysm of abdominal aorta.

Important Aneurysmal Features to be Assessed with CT or MRI[22,38,39]

- Proximal extent of the aneurysm whether it involves major vessels or aortic root. The surgical approach differs if there is involvement of major vessels **(Fig. 20)**.
- Distal extent of the aneurysm. Choice of the graft type depends on whether the aneurysm involves the common iliac vessels **(Figs. 21A to C)**.
- Congenital anomalies. The incidental anomalies like accessory renal artery or retroaortic/circumaortic left renal vein may warn an interventionist/surgeon to take due care during repair.

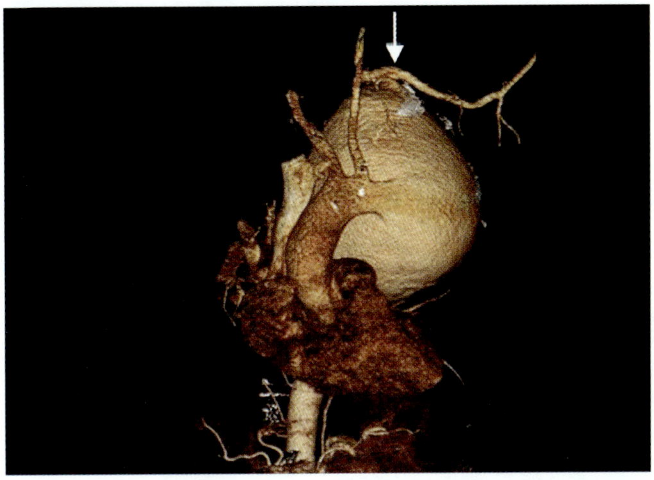

Fig. 20: Aortic Aneurysm: CTA-VR projection shows large saccular aneurysm arising from distal aortic arch and descending thoracic aorta. Note that this 64-slice VR projection clearly show origin of left subclavian artery from the aneurismal sac (arrow) and sparing of right brachiocephalic and left common carotid.

- *Etiology*: Based on imaging characteristics as whether it's inflammatory, mycotic or atherosclerotic (discussed in details later).

  Inflammatory aneurysm: It is variant of atherosclerotic aneurysm characterized by inflammatory and/or fibrotic changes in the periaortic regions **(Fig. 22)**. These changes are probably due to local autoallergic reaction to certain atherosclerotic plaque component. Aneurysmal repair is difficult in these patients because of fibrosis and involvement of important structures, e.g. ureter, GIT, vena cava, etc. CT or MRI demonstrates well-defined soft tissue mass with sharply defined margins surrounding the aneurysm in the anterolateral aspect with sparing of the posterior aspect. The contrast enhancement is variable. CT may rarely demonstrate infiltrative soft tissue mass with poorly defined margins or lobulated mass mimicking a pseudotumor. More details are enumerated in aortitis section.

  CT or MRI findings of mycotic aneurysm include **(Figs. 23A to C)**:
  - Saccular or irregular contour
  - Little or no mural calcification
  - Is adjacent to normal appearing aorta
  - Perianeurysmal fibrosis with or without air
- *Ruptured aneurysm*. CT or MRI demonstrates freshly hemorrhaged blood in the mediastinum/retroperitoneum and focal area of indistinctness in the aortic wall **(Figs. 24 to 26)**. The overall accuracy varies from 87–97%. Distinction between acute or chronic contained rupture is based on duration and severity of symptoms, the hematocrit and hemodynamic stability rather than on anatomic features demonstrated on CT/MRI.

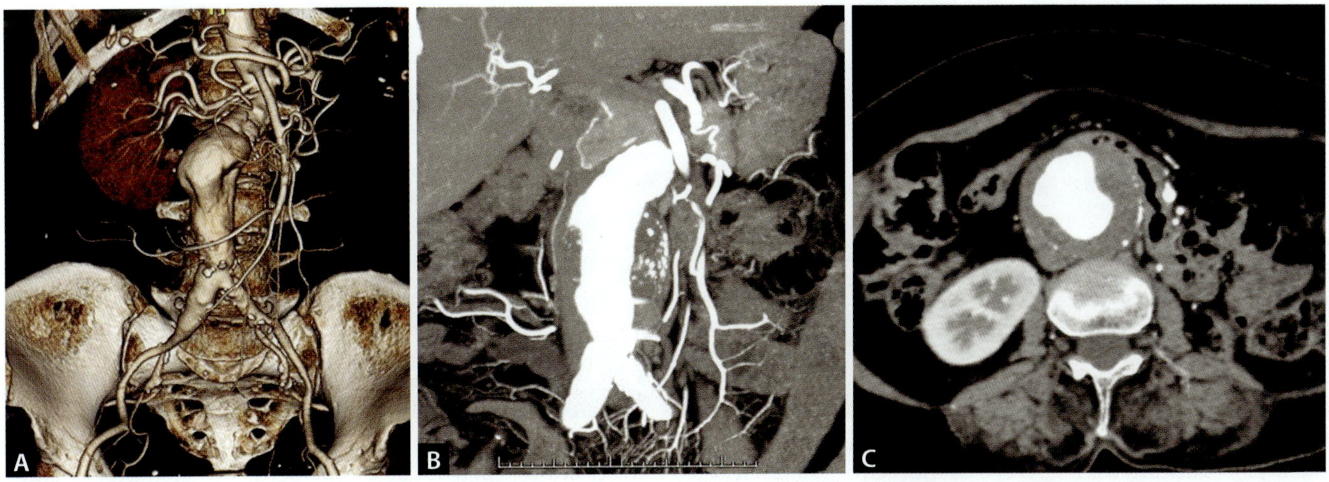

Figs. 21A to C: CTA-VR (A), MIP coronal (B) and axial (C) images demonstrate peripherally thrombosed fusiform infrarenal abdominal aortic aneurysm extending into both common iliac arteries.

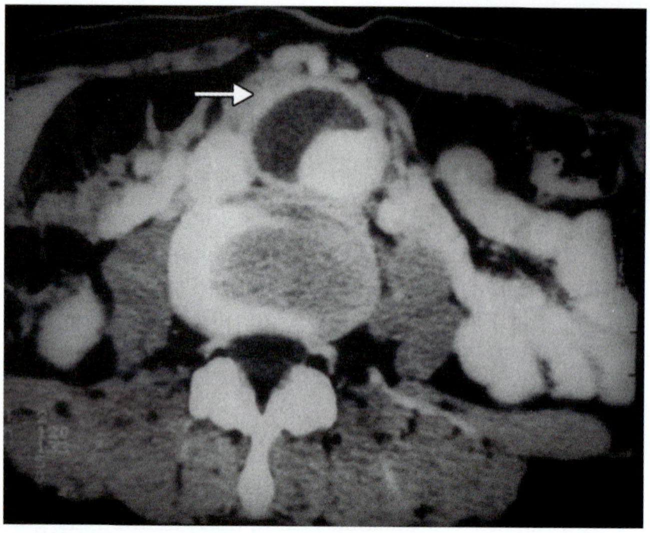

Fig. 22: Inflammatory aortic aneurysm: CECT shows a rind of soft tissue in right anterolateral aspect (arrow) of a partially thrombosed aneurysm (perianeurysmal fibrosis).

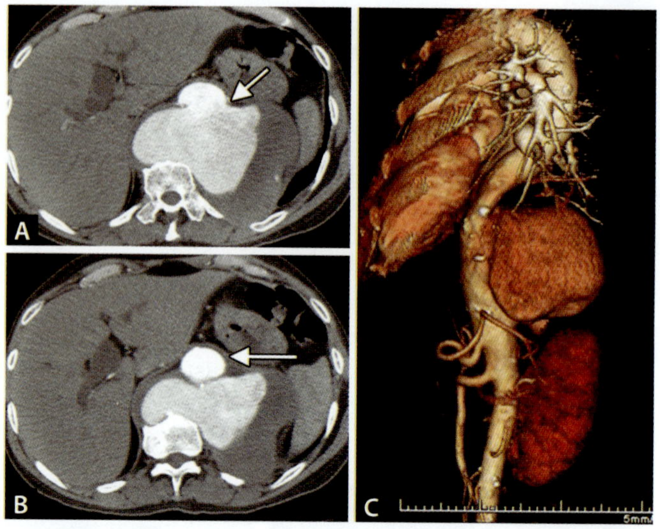

Figs. 23A to C: (A and B) CTA axial and (C) VR images show a large peripherally thrombosed juxta-diaphragmatic pseudoaneurysm (mycotic aneurysm) having lobulated outline with normal appearing anteriorly displaced aorta (thick arrow in B). Rent is posterior wall of aorta (thin arrow in A) is well seen. Note anterior scalloping of vertebral bodies (B). CTA pictures are of patient shown in Figure 18.

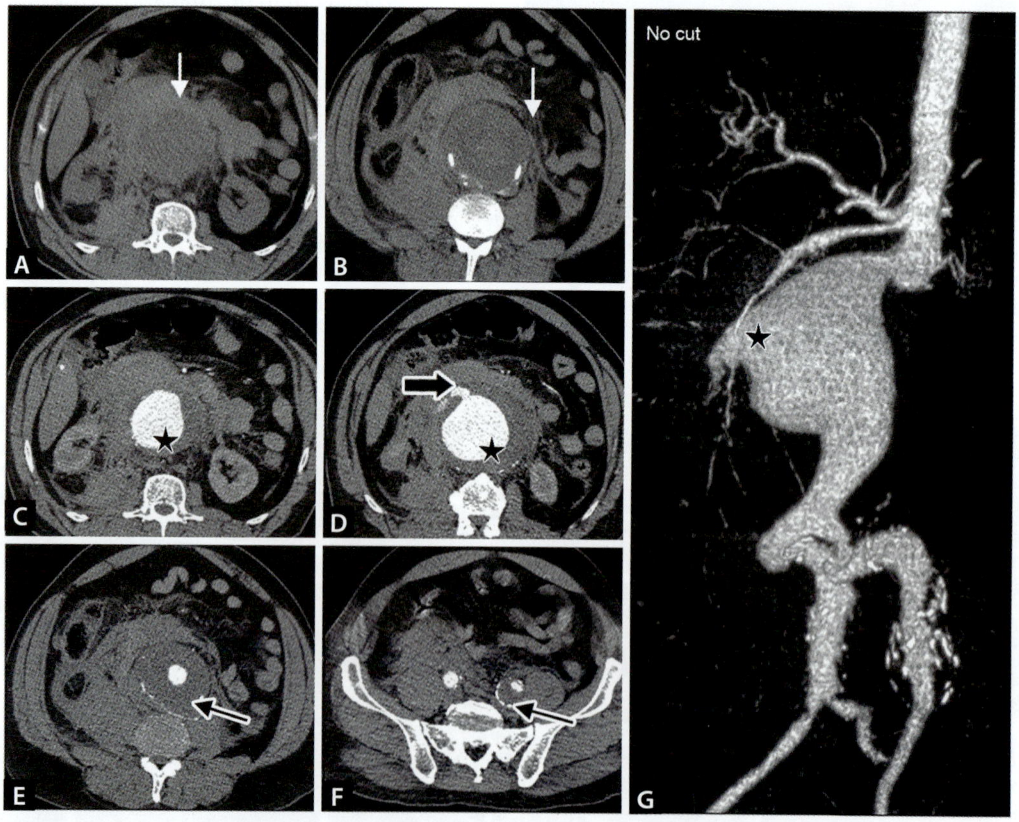

Figs. 24A to G: Noncontrast axial CT images (A and B), axial CTA (C to F) and VR (G) images shows fusiform infrarenal abdominal aortic aneurysm (black asterisk in C, D and G) with active contrast leak (block black arrow in D) associated hyperdense hematoma (black arrow in E and F) and associated significant periaortic stranding (white arrow in A and B). Patient expired on day 2 of admission and a diagnosis of IgG4 periaortitis was made on autopsy.

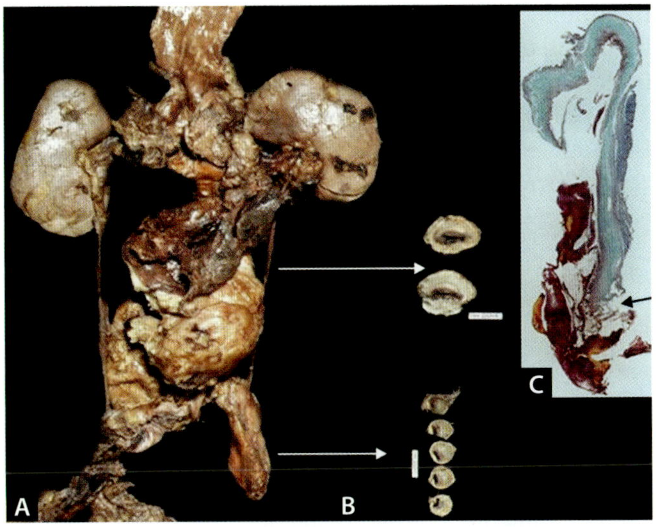

Figs. 25A to C: Autopsy specimen shows (A) gross specimen with evidence of blood collection in the area of aortic rupture confirmed (B and C) by cross-sections at the site of rupture and histopathology (arrow in C).
Courtesy: Professor Ritambra Nada, Department of Histopathology, PGIMER, Chandigarh, India.

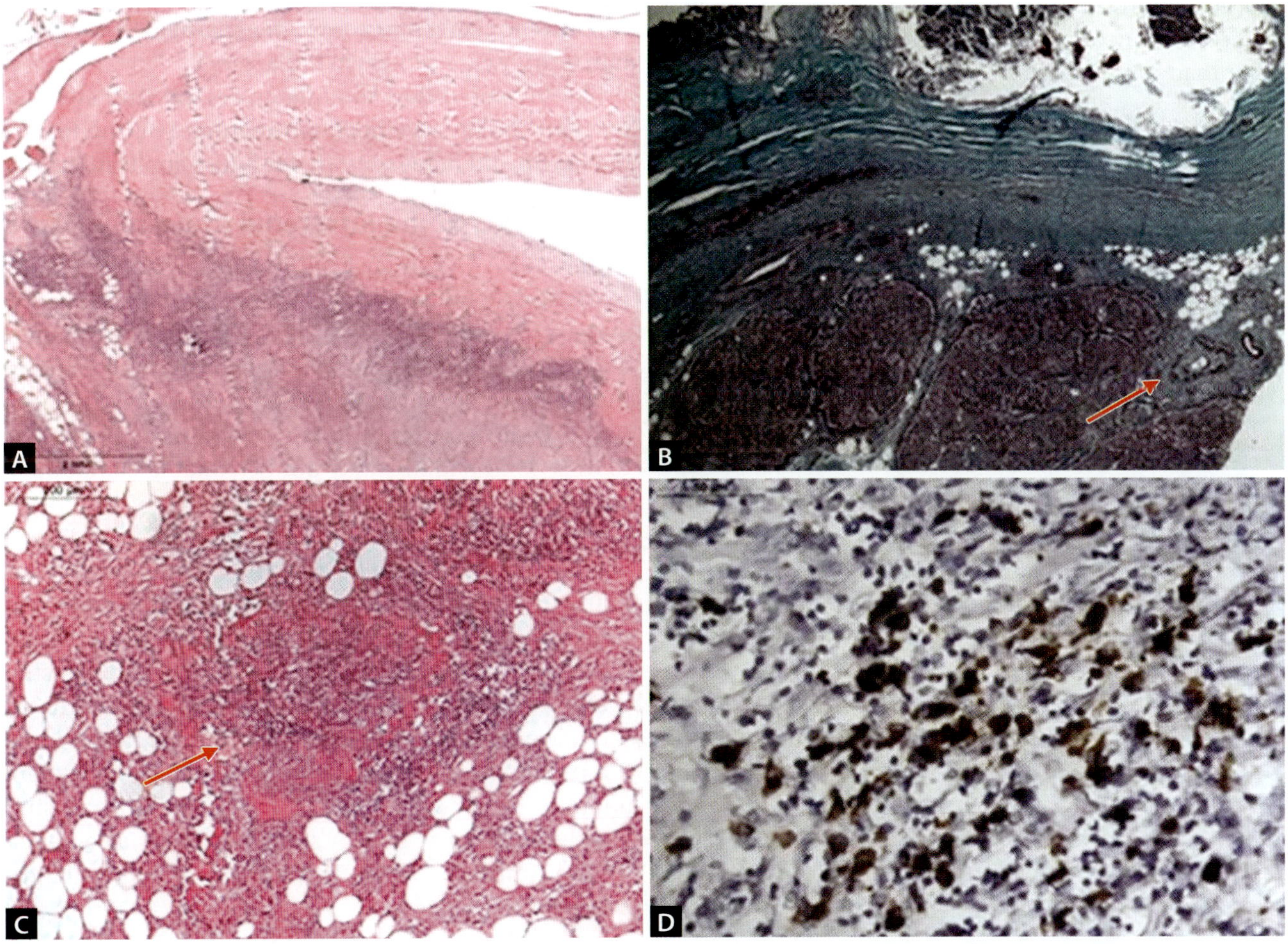

Figs. 26A to D: Photomicrograph shows (A) inflammatory periaortitis which had (B) evidence of fibrosis and venulitis (arrow). (C) shows obliterative venulitis (arrow) with immunohistochemistry (IHC) showing (D) IgG4 positive cells. Stains for CD3 CD 20 were negative (which are positive in aortoarteritis—not shown here).
Courtesy: Professor Ritambra Nada, Department of Histopathology, PGIMER, Chandigarh, India.

Catheter Angiography

Catheter angiography has limited role in diagnosis and follow-up aneurysms. However, with the advent of newer endovascular treatment methods, it has definitive role in preoperative evaluation and treatment planning of aortic aneurysms. It provides detailed arterial anatomy including aberrant origins, the location of the aneurysm relative to branch vessels and demonstrates occlusive lesions.

Surveillance of Small Abdominal Aortic Aneurysms

The risk of rupture of small (5 cm) AAA is low, and hence careful surveillance up to a diameter of 5.5 cm is safe, unless there is rapid expansion (1 cm/yea) or patient becomes symptomatic. Since benefits of early surgery over surveillance with later surgery are comparable, patient preference is important, especially for AAA 4.5–5.5 cm in diameter. The diameter of 5.5-cm appears to be an appropriate threshold for repair in an "average" patient based on the current evidences. For women, or AAA with greater than average rupture risk, elective repair at 4.5 cm to 5.0 cm is an appropriate threshold for repair.[40] Based on a recent individual-based meta-analysis of trials and observational studies with repeated AAA measurements over time, intervals of 3, 2, and 1 year(s) can be safely proposed for AAAs of 30–39, 40–44 and 45–54 mm diameter, respectively, with a rupture risk of1% in men. Women with 45 mm AAA had a risk of rupture equivalent to men with a 55 mm AAA, so a lower intervention threshold, rather than shorter intervals of follow-up, may be considered.[41]

Management of Aortic Aneurysms

Ascending Aortic and Arch Aneurysms

The treatment of ascending aortic and arch aneurysms remains surgical replacement. The extent of surgery depends on the status of the aortic valve, coronary arteries, and great vessels. Aortic valve replacement and complete arch replacement with re-implantation of the arch vessels may be required if the aortic valve is diseased or if the origins of the great vessels are involved. Hybrid debranching procedures as described in the section on dissection may be used in arch aneurysms where surgical grafts are placed to the great vessels from the ascending aorta followed by stent-graft placement across the arch from the ascending to the descending aorta.

Aneurysms of the Descending Thoracic Aorta

The relationship of the aneurysm to the arch vessels and the abdominal aortic visceral arteries determines the treatment. Involvement of these major aortic branches in the aneurysm increases the difficulty and morbidity of intervention. Complications of operative repair include a mortality rate of 5–10%, paraplegia due to spinal cord ischemia, renal failure, stroke and respiratory failure.[42]

An attractive alternative to open surgical repair is endovascular repair where the anatomy is suited for stent graft placement. Stent-grafts function by depressurizing the aneurysm sac. Anatomical prerequisites and the procedure itself are similar to those described in the section on aortic dissection.

Stent-graft repair of thoracoabdominal aneurysms requires either a hybrid procedure with surgical debranching of the abdominal aortic branches followed by stent-graft placement, or branched stent-grafts **(Figs. 27A to D)**. Debranching procedures are major surgical interventions, which increases the morbidity and mortality of the procedure. Branched stent-grafts are less invasive for the patient but are complex time-consuming procedures with the expertise for such procedures being available in only certain tertiary care centers in India.

Multilayered flow modulator devices and stents are currently being developed for treatment of true fusiform aneurysm and holds promise for future application.[43]

Aneurysms of the Infrarenal Abdominal Aorta

Infrarenal AAA which fulfil the criteria for treatment **(Box 2)** may be treated by placement of a stent-graft or surgery. The mortality rate is 3–6% for elective surgery and 25–50% for emergent repair of a ruptured aneurysm making endovascular treatment attractive. Careful preprocedural planning **(Table 4)** is paramount as up to 37% of all patients may not be suitable candidate for endovascular aortic repair (EVAR).[44]

Patients must meet several anatomic criteria to be eligible for a stent graft **(*see* Table 4)**. Three types of stent graft configurations can be used to treat infrarenal AAA depending on the anatomic suitability. Most patients treated with current devices receive bifurcated stent-grafts as shown in **Figures 28A to F**. Other alternatives include aortounilateral iliac graft with surgical femoral-femoral bypass.[45] This type is used when the patient's anatomy is not suitable for a bifurcated graft. A single stent graft (similar to DTA stent graft) may also be used in rare situations where the proximal and distal landing zones are adequate.

ACUTE AORTIC SYNDROME

Acute aortic syndromes (AAS) constitute a spectrum of conditions characterized by disruptions in the integrity of

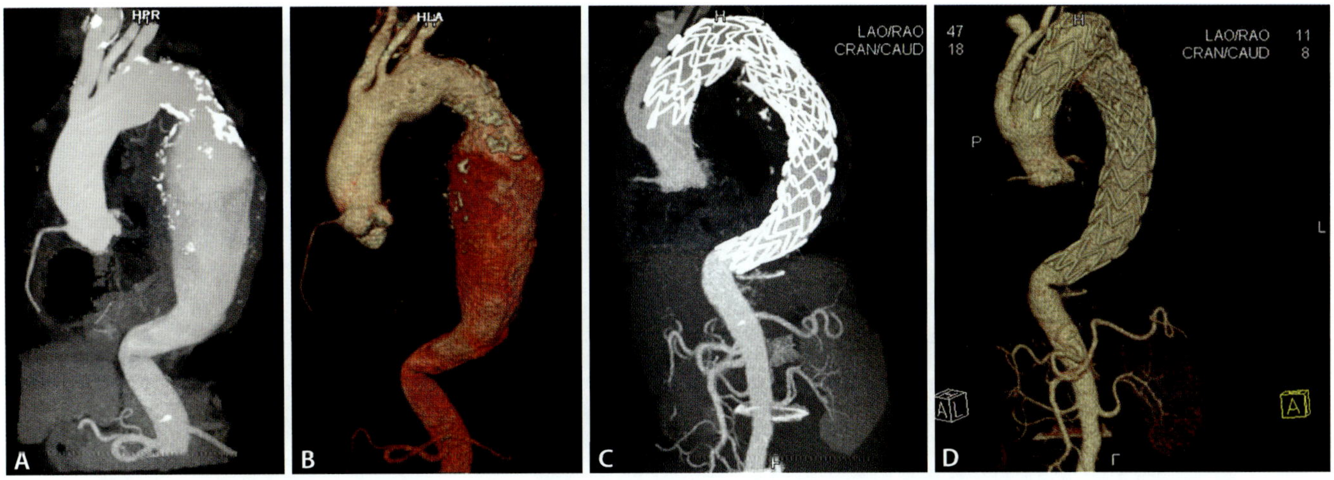

Figs. 27A to D: Descending thoracic aortic aneurysm treated with a stent graft after debranching to extend the proximal landing zone. (A and B) Oblique MIP and VRT computed tomography (CT) image showing the extent of the aneurysm; (C and D) CT of same patient 1 month after placement of a stent graft. The stent graft extends proximal and distal to the aneurysm with exclusion of the aneurysm sac. Transposed innominate artery to the ascending aorta is also noted.

Box 2: Indications for treatment of abdominal aortic aneurysms.

- AAA ≥5 cm diameter
- *Symptomatic aneurysms regardless of size*:
  - Contained-rupture AAA
  - Inflammatory AAA
- Rapidly expanding (>5 mm/yr) AAA
- High-risk for complication with open repair

the aortic wall presenting with acute pain as the leading symptom in most cases. They include classic aortic dissection, intramural hematoma, penetrating aortic ulcer, and aortic aneurysm rupture **(Fig. 29)**. Because of the life-threatening nature of these conditions, prompt and accurate diagnosis is paramount. Misdiagnosis of these conditions, usually because of confusion with myocardial ischemia, can lead to undue mortality. Benign conditions or findings that can mimic AAS on imaging studies are aortitis, atheromatous plaque, prior surgery of aorta, pericardial recess, remnant of a non-patent PDA, streak and motion artifacts on CT, and periaortic fat and hemiazygos sheath.[38]

Table 4: Eligibility criteria for interventional management of abdominal aortic aneurysm.

Criteria	*Favorable*	*Unfavorable*
Proximal aneurysm neck:		
• Diameter	<32 mm	>32 mm
• Length	>1.5 cm	<1.5 cm
• Angulation	<60°	>60°
• Morphological configuration	Cylindrical; Tapered	Reverse taper
• Calcification/thrombus	< 90% circumference involved	>90% circumference involved
Aneurysm sac:		
• Residual lumen	>18 mm	<18 mm
• Distal aortic diameter	>20 mm	<20 mm
• Extension	CIA not involved	CIA involved
Ileofemoral vessels:		
• CIA diameter	<25 mm	>25 mm
• Landing zone length	>10 mm	<10 mm
• EIA diameter	>6 mm	<6 mm
• Tortuosity	<90°	>90°
• Calcification/thrombus	<50% circumference involved	>50% circumference involved

AORTIC DISSECTION

Aortic dissection is the most common acute emergency affecting the aorta, occurring 2 to 3 times more frequently than acute rupture of an aortic aneurysm. The peak incidence is in the 6th and 7th decades of life, men are affected more than women. The clinical presentation is with acute onset of chest pain, congestive heart failure, abdominal pain, or stroke. Approximately 15–20% may be asymptomatic and incidentally diagnosed. The predisposing conditions are hypertension (70–90%), pre-existing aortic diseases (Marfan syndrome, coarctation) or aortic valve disease, aortitis, family history of aortic diseases, history of cardiac surgery, cigarette smoking, direct blunt chest trauma and use of intravenous drugs. Though the exact pathogenesis is somewhat controversial, the most accepted theory for long is that the initial event is a tear in the intima which allows blood to enter the aortic wall creating a true and false lumen. The demonstration

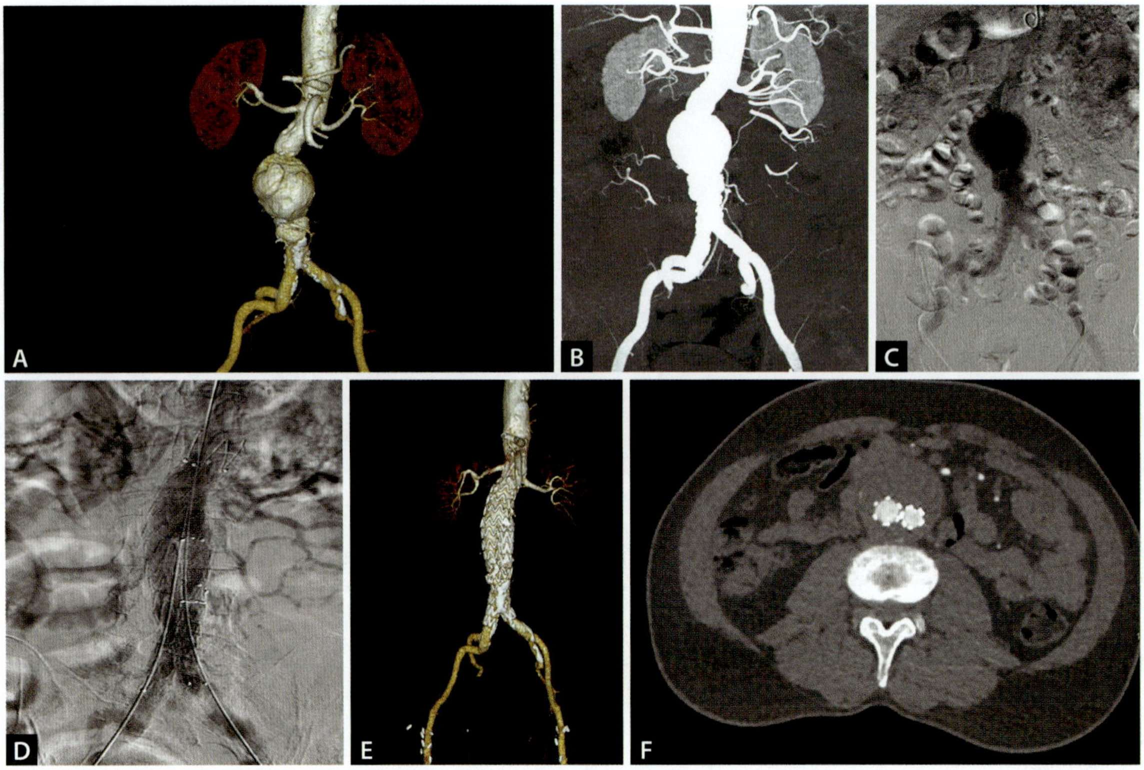

Figs. 28A to F: Infrarenal abdominal aortic aneurysm treated with a branched stent-graft: (A to C) VRT and MIP computed tomography images and aortogram showing a infrarenal abdominal aortic aneurysm; (D) Aortogram after deployment of stent graft shows exclusion of the aneurysm; (E) VRT computed tomography image of the same patient on 1 month follow-up; (F) Axial image showing good opacification of both limbs of the stent graft with aneurysm sac thrombosed.

of intimal flap is thus essential to make the diagnosis. It is now recognized that degeneration of the media leads to rupture of the vasa vasorum of the aortic wall which leads to dissecting hematoma between the media and adventitia which may or may not rupture through the intima into the aortic lumen. This explains the fact that no intimal tear is found at autopsy in a small number of cases of aortic dissection.[46]

Classification

The DeBakey classification categorized aortic dissections into:

- Type I (29–34%): Originates in the ascending aorta and extends to a variable distance beyond the aortic arch
- Type II (12–21%): Confined to ascending aorta
- Type III (50%): Originates distal to the left subclavian artery. It is subclassified into Type IIIA up to diaphragm and type IIIB: below diaphragm.

This classification has been replaced by 'Stanford classification' which takes into account of extent of dissection rather than location of entry site, and divided into type A (involving the ascending aorta) and type B (not involving the ascending aorta) **(Fig. 30)**. Approximately, 70% of dissections are type A and 30% are type B. Type A carries high mortality and morbidity and requires urgent intervention as compared to type B dissection, which is usually managed conservatively **(Table 5)**.[47]

IMAGING

The goal of imaging is not merely to detect presence and extent of AD but to define other important features:[38]

- Differentiation of true and false lumen
- Location of intimal tears
- Coronary artery ostia integrity (in type A)
- Aortic valve function
- +/– pleural or pericardial effusion.

There is no consensus as to which examination (s) should be used in the diagnosis of aortic dissections. The initial imaging should consist of a chest radiograph (CXR) and a transthoracic echocardiogram (TTE). Plain film findings include widening of the mediastinum and aortic contour, changes in aortic contour from prior examination(s), and displaced intimal calcification. However, a normal CXR does not exclude the diagnosis.

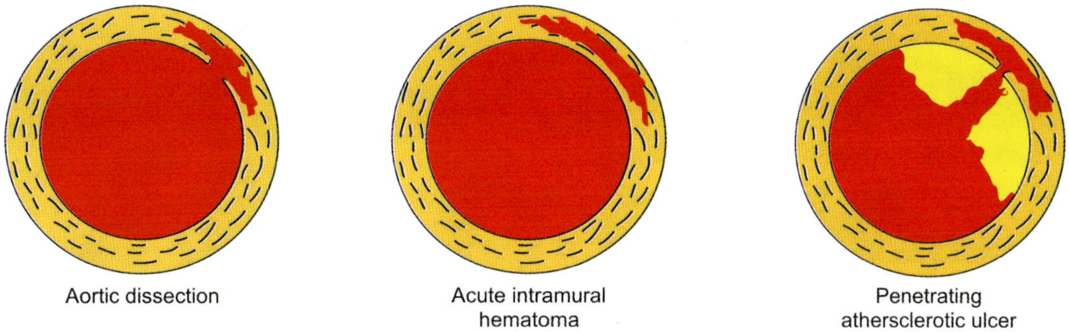

Fig. 29: Schematic diagrams demonstrating dissection, penetrating ulcer and intramural hematoma.

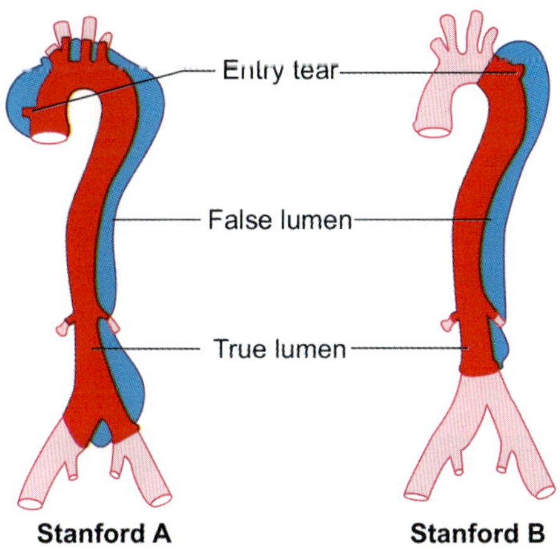

Fig. 30: Stanford types of dissections.

Table 5: Characteristics of Standford type A and type B aortic dissections.

Feature	***Type A***	***Type B***
Frequency (%)	65–70	30–35
Male:Female ratio	2:1	3:1
Average age (years)	50–55	60–70
Hypertension (%)	50	80
Atherosclerosis	+/–	+ +
Aortic insuffiency (%)	50	10
Intimal tear	Always present	Absent in 5–10%
Treatment	Urgent surgery	Usually conservative
Acute mortality (%)	90–95	35–50

TTE may show a pericardial effusion, adequately images the aortic valve and the aortic root but does not show the arch and descending aorta with confidence (blind spot). Transesophageal echocardiography (TEE) has overcome many of the limitations of TTE and has a high degree of accuracy in skilled hands. One of the main advantages of TEE, especially in unstable patients, is that the examination can be performed safely and quickly at the bed side, and can be used to monitor changes in-theater and in post-operative intensive care.

Computed Tomography

CT angiographic protocols typically begin with low-dose non-contrast CT to exclude the possibility of IMH, followed by contrast-enhanced ECG gated computed tomographic angiography. The coverage includes the entire thorax, abdomen, and pelvis to allow delineation of the extent of a flap and its extension into branch vessels and to evaluate for end-organ ischemia (e.g. bowel or kidneys), and possible extravasation **(Figs. 31 and 32)**.

The CT findings in aortic dissection include the following:

- *Precontrast images*:
  - Internal displacement of intimal calcification.
  - Visible intimal flap as a linear structure slightly higher in attenuation than surrounding blood.
  - High attenuation thrombosed false lumen, if acutely thrombosed.
  - Enlargement of long segment of the aorta
  - Pericardial, mediastinal and/or pleural hemorrhage, secondary to rupture.
- *Postcontrast images* **(Figs. 31 and 32):**
  - Contrast filled true and false lumen separated by intimal flap; false lumen typically seen in outer curvature of aorta.
  - Delayed enhancement of the false lumen because of slower flow.
  - Thrombosis of false lumen, with enhancement of only the true lumen.
  - Compression of true lumen by thrombosed false lumen.
  - Extension of dissection into branch vessels.
  - Ischemia/infarction of organs supplied by branch vessels from false lumen.

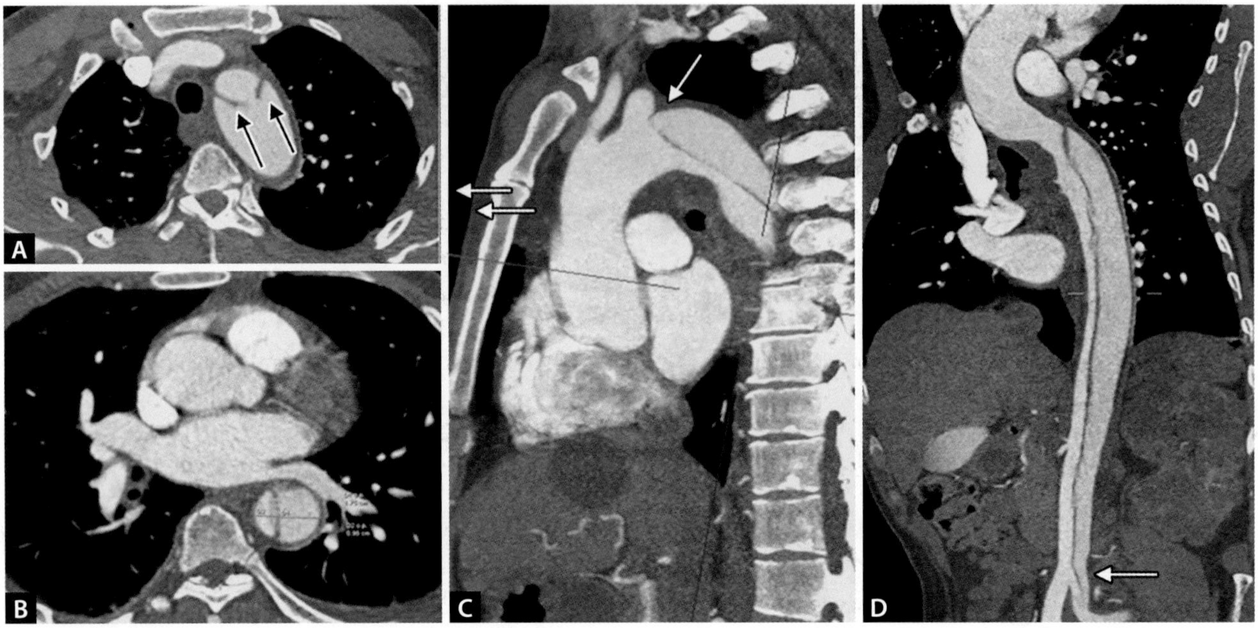

Figs. 31A to D: (A and B) CTA axial; (C) reconstructed sagittal and (D) stretched images shows type B dissection with entry point juxtaposed to the origin of left subclavian artery (arrows in A and C). Note "beak sign" with convex flap toward posterior false lumen (A). (D) Note extension of flap into the left common iliac artery.

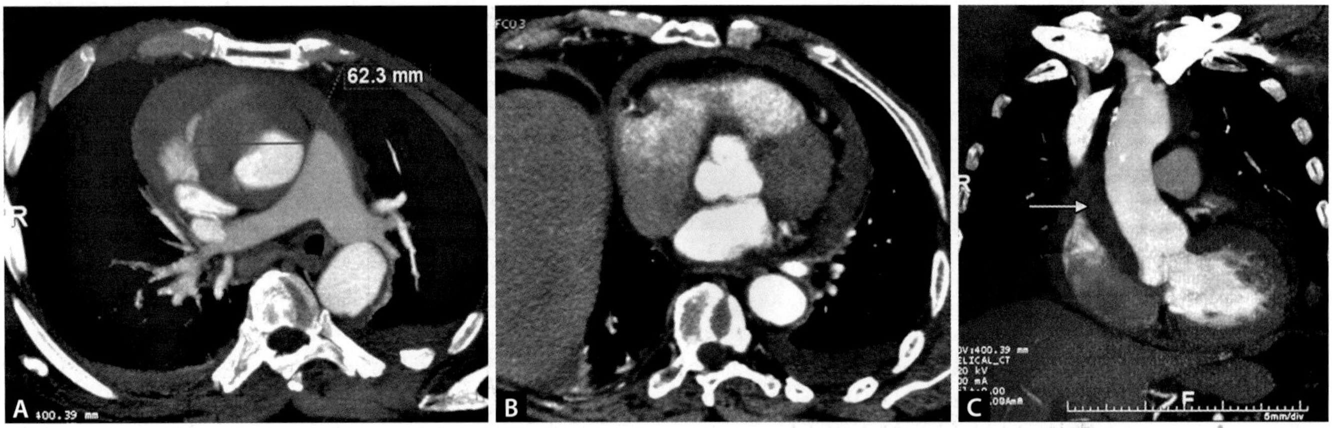

Fig. 32A to C: (A and B) CTA axial and oblique coronal images showing type A dissection with thrombosis of false lumen (A and C) with rupture into pericardial and right pleural cavities (A to C).

CT Signs of AD

Differentiation between true and false lumens of AD is important in planning of treatment with percutaneous endovascular grafts or surgical repair. It is critical to identify the lumen of origin of major branches such as coronary, carotid, renal and mesenteric arteries before treatment, as viscera supplied by false lumen are at risk when false lumen is spontaneously or surgically occluded **(Table 6)**.

The convex face of the intimal flap is usually towards the FL that surrounds the TL **(Figs. 31A to D)**. The FL usually has slower flow and a larger diameter and may contain thrombi. In Type A AD, the FL is usually located along the right anterolateral wall of the ascending aorta and extends distally, in a spiral fashion, along the left posterolateral wall of the descending aorta **(Figs. 32A to C)**. Slender linear areas of low attenuation may be observed in the FL, corresponding to incompletely dissected media, known as the 'Cobweb sign,' a specific finding for identifying the FL. Discrimination between the FL and TL is utmost important to identify collaterals perfused exclusively by the FL, as well as when endovascular therapy is considered.[48]

Table 6: CT features for differentiating true from false lumen.

S.No.	Features	True lumen	False lumen
1.	Continuity of lumen with lumen of uninvolved portion of aorta (Most reliable)	+	–
2.	Direction of free edges of the dissection flap at entrance tear	–	+
3.	Aortic Cobweb	–	+
4.	Outer wall calcification	+	–
5.	Beak sign	–	+
6.	Thrombosis	–/+	++
7.	Peak flow	Faster	Slower
8.	Size	Smaller and compressed	Larger and toward intimal concavity

If possible ECG-triggered CTA should be done for type A dissection for simultaneous evaluation of coronary arteries so that bypass grafts can be palced in one-sitting **(Figs. 33A and B)**.

Magnetic Resonance Imaging

It has been shown to be an effective alternative technique to CT for evaluation of aortic dissection with a reported sensitivity and specificity of 98%. MRI not only gives anatomical but also functional information required for treatment planning, however, because of ease of CT and its wider availability, CT is often the modality of investigation and MR is reserved for follow-up **(Figs. 34A and B)**.

Black blood imaging shows the intimal flap as thin linear structure in the aortic flow void. True lumen shows preservation of the flow void whereas the false lumen is seen as area of increased signal intensity because of turbulent flow.

Phase contrast images can be done to identify aortic insufficiency, intimal tear sites and to differentiate slow flow from thrombus in the false lumen. Combining black blood, bright blood with gadolinium-enhanced 3D MR angiography images can comprehensively give the required information.[19,24,38,49]

Aortography

It is highly accurate in the detection and evaluation of aortic dissection with diagnostic accuracy over 95%. The direct signs are identification of an intimal flap and a contrast filled true and false lumen. Indirect signs are aortic wall thickening, aortic regurgitation, compression of the true lumen, non-visualization of branch vessels and abnormal catheter position. False negative study may be seen when the false lumen is thrombosed, intimal flap not tangential to the X-ray beam, intimal tear proximal to the catheter and absence of intimal flap in some cases. Noninvasive imaging is more accurate in providing the diagnosis and therefore aortography is no longer used for the diagnosis of AD, except during coronary angiography or endovascular intervention.

Management of AD

Current classifications systems are not comprehensive at describing all the information pertinent to a surgeon/interventionist about the dissection. Information regarding chronicity of symptoms, location of primary entry tears, direction of flap extension (antegrade, retrograde, mixed), complications and patency of the false lumen are vital.

A mnemonic-based approach to the evaluation of aortic dissection was proposed by Dake et al.[50] The DISSECT classification system guides the radiologist through an assessment of six critical characteristics that facilitate a complete description of the most salient details that currently influence the selection of a treatment. The features of aortic dissection that are to be mentioned in the report are enumerated in **Table 7**.

Acute type A aortic dissection constitutes a surgical emergency since these patients are at high-risk for a life-threatening complication such as aortic regurgitation, cardiac tamponade, stroke, frank rupture and myocardial infarction. Medical management has a mortality of up to 50% as compared to the operative mortality of 7–36% in experienced centers.[51,52]

At certain advanced centers, a hybrid approach to the repair of type A aortic dissection, referred to as the "frozen elephant trunk repair," may be attempted. This involves combination of an open approach to surgically repair the ascending aorta, while deploying a stent-graft to manage the descending aorta.

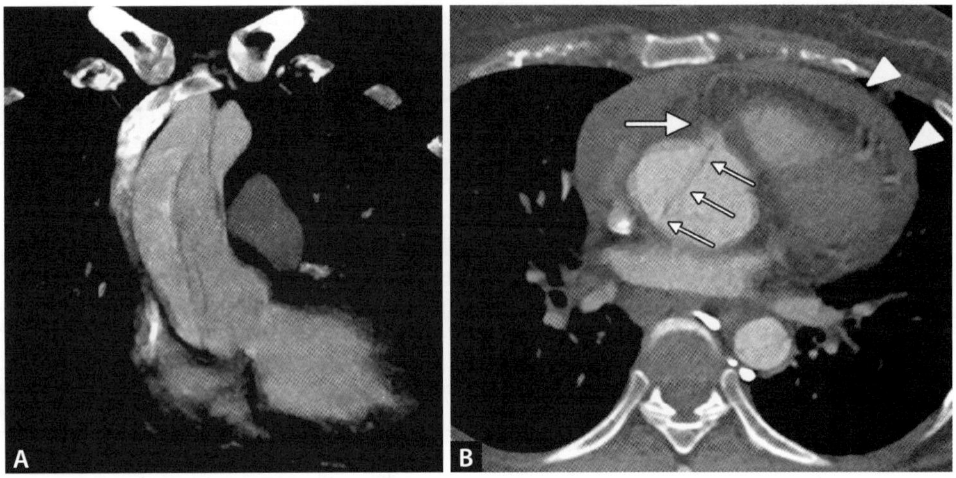

Figs. 33A and B: ECG –triggered CTA of ascending aorta oblique coronal and axial images show type A dissection (A and B) with intimal flap (thin arrows) extending into the ostia of right coronary artery (thick arrow). Note hemopericardium (arrowheads).

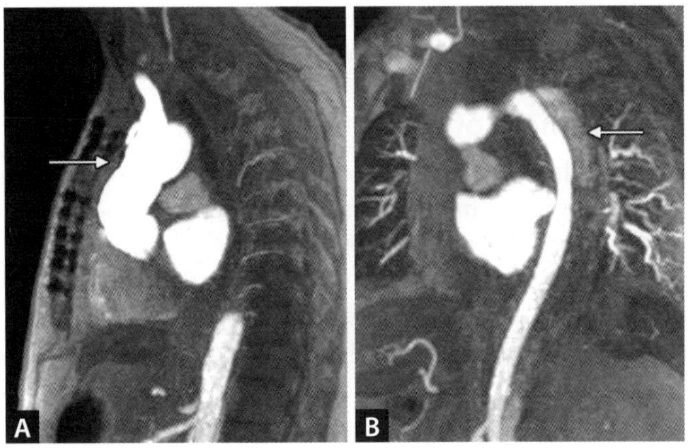

Figs. 34A and B: 3D CE-MRA oblique coronal views in a postoperative patient of type A dissection (post Bentall) show normally opacified ascending aorta (arrow in A) and faintly opacified false lumen (usually due to slow flow) in descending thoracic (arrow in B) and normally opacified true lumen.

Table 7: DISSECT classification.

D—Duration of symptoms	• *Acute*: <2 weeks from onset of symptoms • *Subacute*: 2 weeks to 3 months after symptom onset • *Chronic*: >3 months from initial symptoms
I—Intimal tear location	Ascending aorta, aortic arch, descending aorta, abdominal aorta, unknown
S—Sizes	Maximum aortic diameter at any level
SE—Segmental extent	Proximal entry and distal re-entry tear locations
C—Complications	• Cardiac tamponade • Rupture • Branch vessel malperfusion • Static and/or dynamic branch involvement with accompanying stroke, paraplegia, coronary, mesenteric, visceral, renal, and/or extremity symptoms • Progression of aortic involvement with proximal or distal extension of dissection • Involvement of aortic valve in case of type A dissection • *Other*: – Uncontrollable hypertension – Uncontrollable clinical symptoms – Rapid false lumen dilation – Overall trans-aortic enlargement of >10 mm within the first 2 weeks of initial diagnosis
T—Thrombosis of false lumen	Patent, completely or partially thrombosed

Type B dissection is generally managed initially with best medical therapy as given in **Box 3**.

Intervention (surgical or endovascular) for descending thoracic aortic dissection is reserved for patients who develop complications as described in **Table 7**.

Type B aortic dissection with such complications is associated with mortality rates that can exceed 60%. Interventional management consists of placing a stent graft over the proximal entry tear which has been shown to acutely depressurize the false lumen and restore normal flow in the true lumen **(Fig. 35A to F)**.

The endograft should be sized to the estimated diameter of the true lumen, not the overall diameter of the dissected aorta. Successful stent-graft exclusion in the thoracic aorta, or any other aortic segment, necessitates at least 15-mm proximal and distal "landing zones" of non-diseased aorta to achieve fixation and seal. However, in case the proximal landing zones are inadequate, there are strategies and techniques designed to "extend the landing

Box 3: Best medical management for aortic dissection.

Four main management goals for type B dissection patients either with or without surgical/interventional management:
1. Antihypertensive drugs to minimize the aortic wall shear stress caused by increased blood pressure.
2. Continued monitoring for high-risk clinical conditions/presence of complications which would require immediate treatment.
3. Serial imaging to detect signs of progression, re-dissection, or aneurysm formation.
4. Optimal pain management.

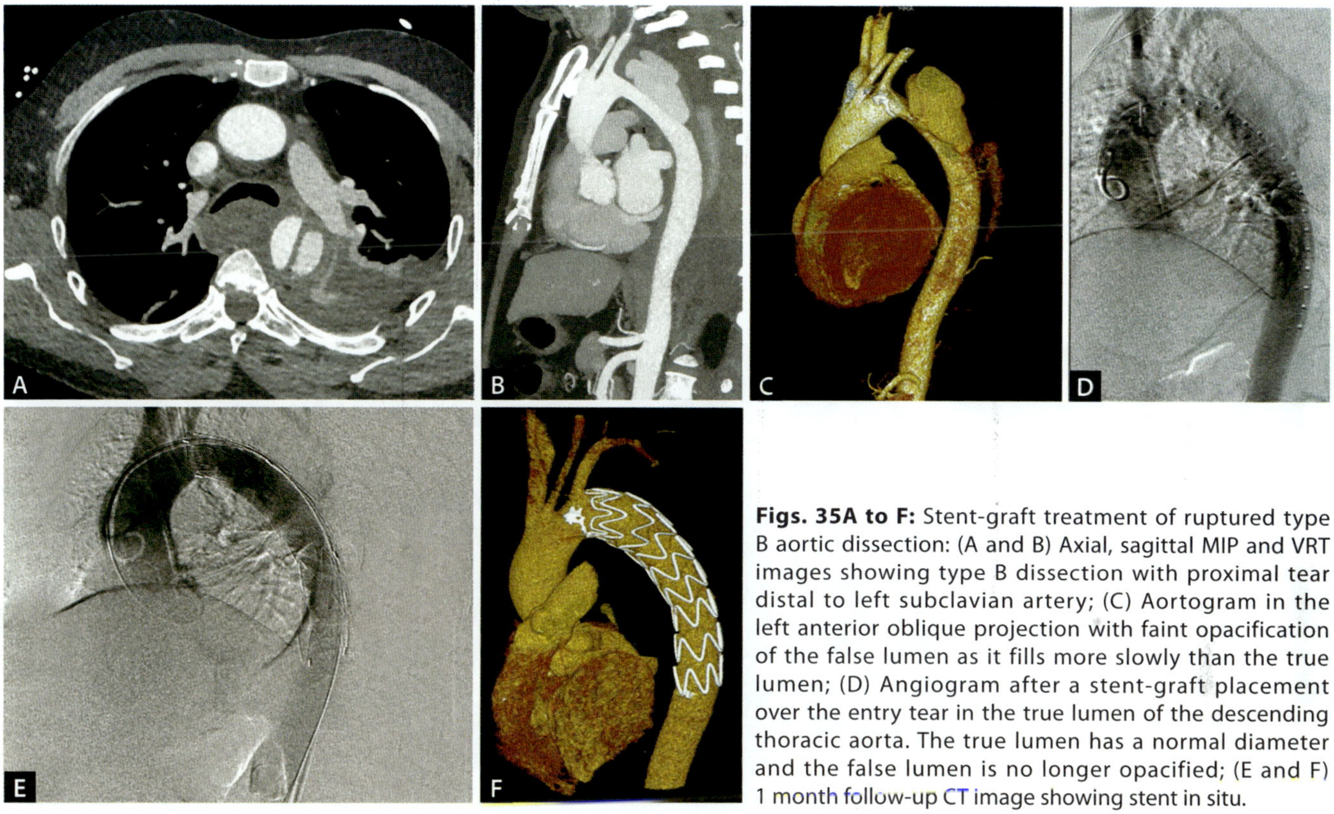

Figs. 35A to F: Stent-graft treatment of ruptured type B aortic dissection: (A and B) Axial, sagittal MIP and VRT images showing type B dissection with proximal tear distal to left subclavian artery; (C) Aortogram in the left anterior oblique projection with faint opacification of the false lumen as it fills more slowly than the true lumen; (D) Angiogram after a stent-graft placement over the entry tear in the true lumen of the descending thoracic aorta. The true lumen has a normal diameter and the false lumen is no longer opacified; (E and F) 1 month follow-up CT image showing stent in situ.

zone". These techniques may be endovascular (use of branched stent graft, chimney, or snorkel technique) or surgical debranching techniques to extend the landing zones. These techniques are known as debranching techniques. Using the classification proposed by Criado et al.[53] landing zones can be classified into 5 types **(Fig. 36)**. The complexity of procedures required to lengthen the landing zones increases as the landing zone of stent graft extends more proximally.

An endovascular procedure with proximal landing zones at Zone 3 and 4 is an optimal situation and requires no extra step for aortic interventions. A proximal landing zone involving zone 2 would require either coverage (and occlusion) or transposition of the left subclavian artery (LSA). If the left common carotid artery (CCA) origin (Zone 1) is involved, transposition to the right CCA via a carotid-carotid bypass can be performed. If the disease involves the full entire aortic arch, coverage of the innominate artery (IA) would be required along with transposition of the IA and left CCA to the ascending aorta **(Figs. 37A to E)**. Alternatively, branched stent graft or chimney techniques can be used in these cases in centers where expertise is available.

When critical organ ischemia is not relieved by occlusion of the proximal entry tear with a stent graft, bare stents can be placed from the true lumen of the aorta into the true lumen of the branch vessel to restore flow.[54] Another minimally invasive option is percutaneous fenestration of the aortic flap. This intentionally causes creation of a large distal exit tear, which decompresses the false lumen and relieves the dynamic obstruction of the true lumen. This is usually done as a lifesaving or as an adjunctive procedure as mortality with fenestration alone can be high. One of the ways to create a fenestration

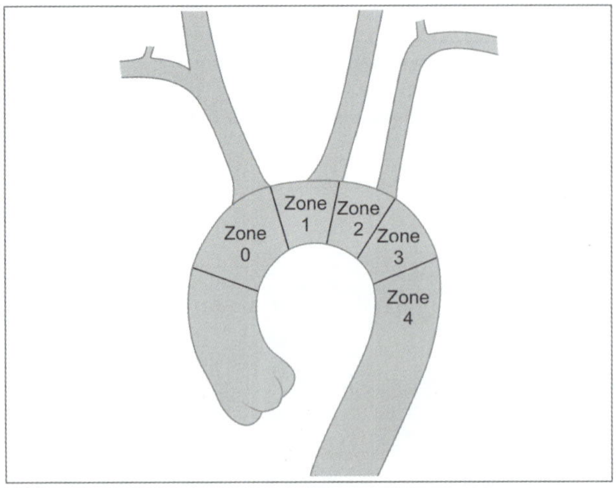

Fig. 36: Criado classification of aortic landing zones.

is to cross the intimal flap with an intravascular ultrasound to guide the puncture. This fenestration may then be enlarged using angioplasty balloons.

Delivery systems for thoracic stent-grafts tend to be large, so assessment of the femoral arteries, iliac arteries and abdominal aorta is necessary when evaluating a patient for one of these procedures. Surgical placement of a temporary graft to the common iliac artery or distal aorta (termed a *conduit*) may be required to deliver the endograft in patients with small or diseased pelvic arteries.

Although type B complicated aortic dissection can be handled by stent graft placement, with various adjunctive techniques, total surgical repair may be needed for those whose anatomy cannot support a stent-graft.

A summary of the prerequisites and challenges for interventional management is given in **Table 8**.

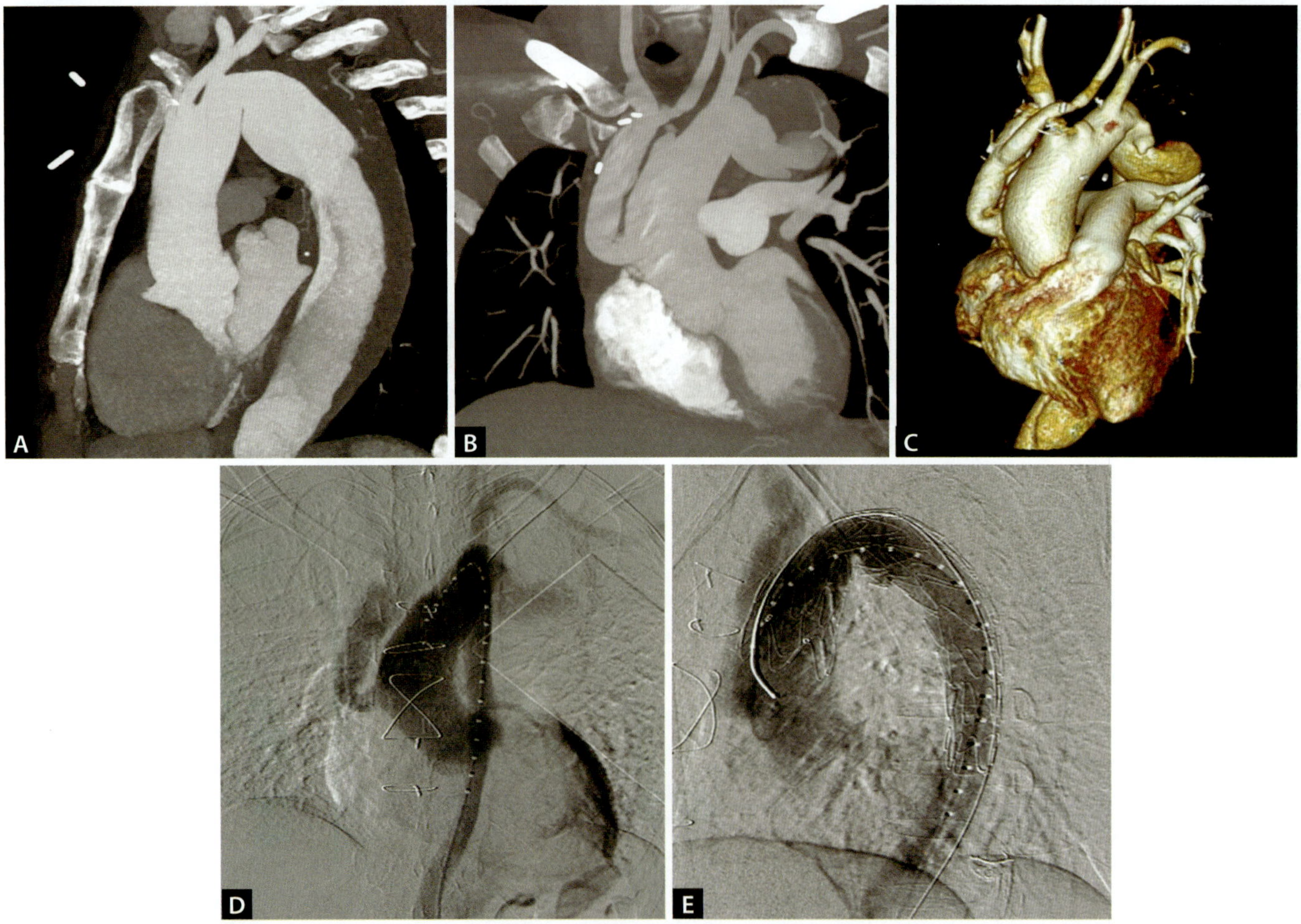

Figs. 37A to E: Stent-graft treatment with debranching technique of ruptured type B aortic dissection with unfavorable proximal landing zone anatomy. (A) Oblique sagittal image showing acute angulation of arch with proximal tear at the root of the left subclavian artery (not shown in image); (B to D) Oblique coronal, VRT images and aortogram showing innominate artery transposed to ascending aorta effectively "elongating the proximal landing zone". The left common carotid was transposed to the innominate artery; (E) Angiogram after a stent-graft placement over the entry tear in the true lumen of the descending thoracic aorta. The true lumen has a normal diameter and the false lumen is no longer opacified.

Table 8: Prerequisites for interventional management of dissection.

Proximal landing zone	• Atleast 1.5 cm normal aorta distal to left subclavian artery • If unavailable debranching procedures to extend the proximal landing zone
Distal landing zone	1.5–2 cm normal aorta above celiac artery
Landing zone diameters	Varies with device
Severe angulation of proximal or distal aorta	Longer landing zones needed which may necessitate debranching
Patency and caliber of pelvic arteries:	• Minimal external iliac/common femoral artery diameter required 7 mm • Smaller vessels may require direct access to common iliac artery or abdominal aorta via surgical conduit

Flowchart 2: Treatment strategy for dissection of aorta.

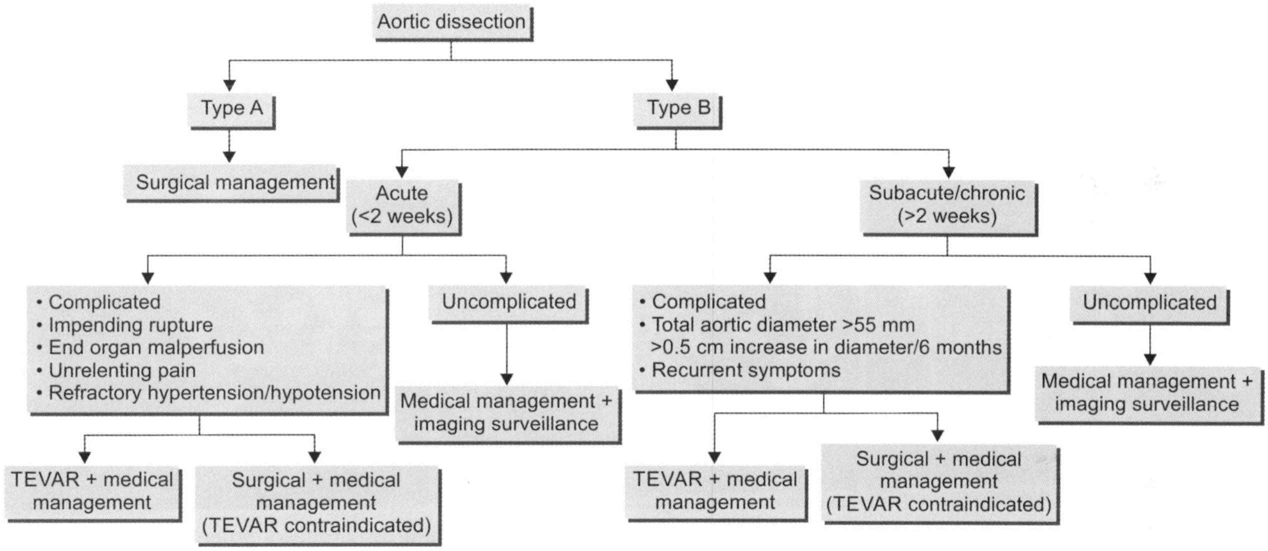

Abbreviations: TEVAR: Thoracic Endovascular Aortic Repair.

Endovascular intervention in patients with uncomplicated dissection may improve long-term outcomes by favorably influencing the dynamic relationship of the true and false lumen however, the results of multiple studies support a complication and patient-specific approach to type B dissection as the best treatment paradigm.

A suggested algorithmic approach to management of AD is given in **Flowchart 2**.

INTRAMURAL HEMATOMA

Intramural haematoma is diagnosed by the presence of a circular or crescent-shaped thickening of >5 mm of the aortic wall in the absence of detectable blood flow. It accounts for approximately 10 to 25% of AAS. IMH was first believed to be result of rupture of the vasa vasorum, allowing bleeding between the elastic lamina of the aortic media. However, recent findings suggest that at least some IMHs may be initiated by small intimal tears that are undetectable by current aortic imaging modalities and are often overlooked on gross inspection of the aorta at the time of surgery or autopsy.[55-58] IMH can be associated with several conditions, including spontaneous ("typical") aortic dissection, penetrating ulcer, aortic trauma, and iatrogenic dissection (cardiac catheterization, cardiac surgery).

Imaging features of IMH are ***(Figs. 38A and B)****:*

- Focal aortic wall thickening (crescentic > concentric)
- Preserved luminal shape with smooth luminal border
- Absence of dissection flap and false lumen
- Echolucent regions may be present in the aortic wall
- Central displacement of intimal calcium.

Predictors of complication and surveillance:

Maximum aortic diameter (>40–50 mm), wall thickness(>10–12 mm) and associated periaortic hemorrhage or pleural effusion has been described as a predictor of progression. IMH may weaken the aortic wall and either progress outward with aortic expansion and/or rupture **(Figs. 39A to C)** or inward with disruption of the intima-media,

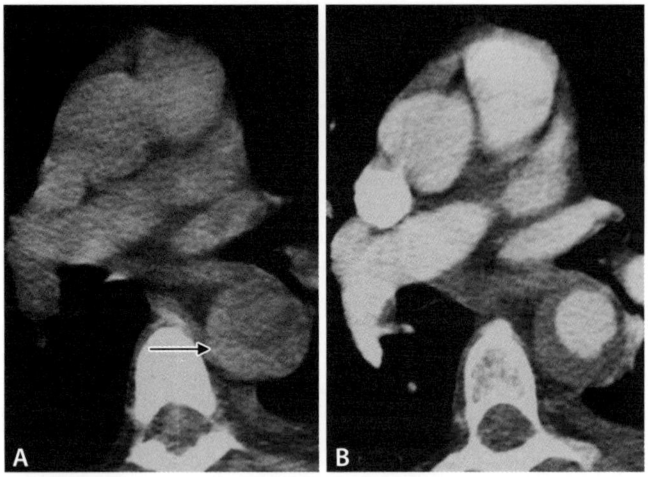

Figs. 38A and B: Noncontrast (a) axial and postcontrast CTA images show high density crescentic thickening along right posterolateral wall of distal descending thoracic aorta.

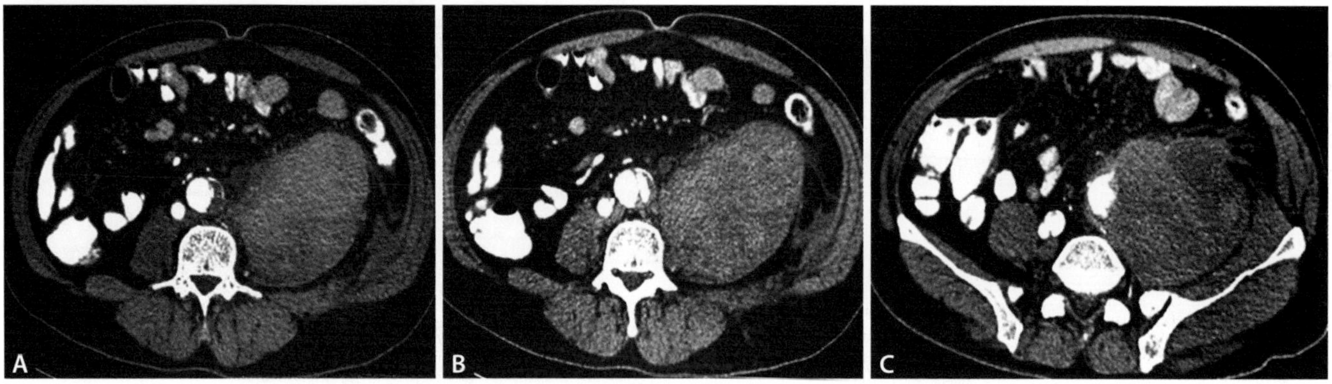

Figs. 39A to C: Serial CTA axial sections (craniocaudal) of distal abdominal aorta near bifurcation shows intramural hematoma along left lateral wall (A) penetrating ulcer (B) and rupture (C) leading to a large retroperitoneal hematoma (A to C).

resulting in typical aortic dissection. Therefore, serial imaging is necessary to rule out progression in patients who receive only medical treatment. Although there are no established guidelines for the optimal frequency and longitudinal duration for surveillance imaging of patients with IMH, Evangelista et al. on the basis of the significant dynamic evolution of IMH, recommended imaging at 1, 3, 6, 9, and 12 months from the time of diagnosis. Once stability has been documented, surveillance imaging may be annual.[59]

PENETRATING AORTIC ULCER

Penetrating aortic ulcer (PAU) is defined as ulceration of an aortic atherosclerotic plaque penetrating through the internal elastic lamina into the media.[60] These lesions represent 2 -7% of all AAS. Most common location of PAU is the middle and lower descending thoracic aorta, and less frequently noted in the aortic arch or abdominal aorta. Propagation of the ulcerative process may either lead to IMH, pseudoaneurysm, or even aortic rupture or an acute AD, and hence requires close follow-up.[61]

On noncontrast CT, PAU resembles an IMH. Contrast-enhanced CT is the technique of choice for diagnosis of PAU, which shows characteristic finding of localized ulceration, penetrating through the aortic intima into the aortic wall **(Figs. 39A to C)**. Focal thickening or high attenuation of the adjacent aortic wall suggests associated IMH. Limitation of MRI is that it is unable to detect displacement of intimal calcification, which frequently accompanies PAU.

Management of IMH and PAU

The management goals and treatment protocol for IMH and PAU are similar to type A and B AD. Surgery is advocated in patients with Type A IMH and ascending aortic ulcerations. Initial medical therapy is advocated in patients with type B IMH and descending thoracic aortic PAU. Some authors suggest that a symptomatic ulceration that is 20 mm in diameter or greater, or 10 mm in depth, should be managed aggressively.[62]

Complicated type B IMH with expansion of the hematoma, continued pain, development of hemorrhagic pleural effusion, or rupture requires more aggressive management with stent graft placement or surgery. The endovascular procedure is similar to that described for aortic dissection.

AORTITIS

Aortitis is an inflammatory condition of the aortic wall which can be infectious or noninfectious in origin. Imaging is required for assessment of aortitis and is crucial in establishing the diagnosis. CT, MRI and nuclear fusion imaging (PET CT/MRI) are the main imaging modalities for initial diagnosis and follow-up.[63,64]

Takayasu's Arteritis

Takayasu's arteritis (TA) is a necrotizing, obliterative and segmental primary large vessel panarteritis of unknown etiology that affects the aorta and its major branches including the pulmonary artery. It is most common in young Asian women and occurs about 10 times more commonly in women than in men. The etiologically factors implicated are previous tubercular infection, genetic factors and autoimmune mechanisms. The diagnosis of Takayasu's arteritis is often delayed because of a nonspecific clinical presentation. Ishikawa's criteria (sensitivity 60.4% and specificity 95%) and American College of Rheumatology criteria (sensitivity 77.4% and specificity 95%) have been widely used for diagnosis of this disease. Modified diagnostic criteria for Takayasu's arteritis by Sharma et al. have led to an early diagnosis of this condition thereby preventing high morbidity and mortality **(Table 9)**.[65,66]

The sensitivity and specificity using this modified diagnostic criteria is 92.5% and 95% respectively.

Incidence: 2.6 new cases/million/year
2.2% at autopsy

Pathology: TA is a T-cell-mediated panarterities which begins in adventitial vasa vasorum with inward progression. Destructive perivascular cuffing of vasa vasorum is

Table 9: Modified diagnostic criteria for Takayasu's arteritis, Sharma et al.[65]

Three major criteria	
1. Left mid subclavian artery lesion	The most severe stenosis or occlusion present in the mid portion from the point 1 cm proximal to the vertebral artery orifice up to 3 cm distal to the orifice determined by angiography
2. Right mid subclavian artery lesion	The most severe stenosis or occlusion present in the mid portion from the right vertebral artery orifice to the point 3 cm distal to orifice determined by angiography
3. Characteristic signs and symptoms of at least one month duration	These include limb claudication, pulselessness or pulse differences in limbs, an unobtainable or significant blood pressure difference (>10 mm Hg systolic blood pressure difference in limb), fever, neck, pain, transient amaurosis, blurred vision, syncope, dyspnea or palpitations
Ten minor criteria	
1. High ESR	Unexplained persistent high ESR >20 mm/h (Westergren) at diagnosis or presence of the evidence in patients history
2. Carotid artery tenderness	Unilateral or bilateral tenderness of common carotid on palpation. Neck muscle tenderness is unacceptable
3. Hypertension	Persistent blood pressure >140/90 mm Hg brachial or >160/90 mm Hg popliteal
4. Aortic regurgitation or annuloaortic ectasia	• By auscultation or Doppler echocardiology or angiography • By angiography or two dimensional echocardiography
5. Pulmonary artery lesion	Lobar or segmental arterial occlusion or equivalent determined by angiography or perfusion scintigraphy, or presence of stenosis, aneurysm, luminal irregularity or any combination in pulmonary trunk or in unilateral or bilateral pulmonary arteries determined by angiography
6. Left mid common carotid lesion	Presence of the most severe stenosis or occlusion in the mid portion of 5 cm in length from the point 2 cm distal to its orifice determined by angiography
7. Distal brachiocephalic trunk lesion	Presence of the most severe stenosis or occlusion in the distal third determined by angiography
8. Descending thoracic aorta lesion	Narrowing, dilatation or aneurysm, luminal irregularity or any combination determined by angiography: tortuosity alone is unacceptable
9. Abdominal aorta lesion	Narrowing, dilatation or aneurysm, luminal irregularity or aneurysm combination
10. Coronary artery lesion	Documented on angiography below the age of 30 years in the absence of risk factors like hyperlipidemia or diabetes mellitus

Presence of two major or one major and two minor criteria or four minor criteria suggests a high probability of Takayasu's arteritis.

followed by fibrosis and calcifications and leads to aneurysmal dilatations followed by stenosis of aorta and its branches. Arterial wall inflammation with adventitial mononuclear infiltration, multiple granulomas and perivascular cuffing of the vaso vasorum observed in early stages, followed by chronic fibrosis and wall calcification in later stages. Chronic necrotizing wall inflammation causes destruction of the media with resultant stenosis and/or aneurysm formations.[63,66-68]

Types[69] (Fig. 40)

- **Type I** involves only the branches of the aortic arch.
- **Type IIa** involves the aorta only at its ascending portion and/or at the aortic arch. The branches of the aortic arch may be involved as well. The rest of the aorta is not affected.
- **Type IIb** affects the descending thoracic aorta with or without involvement of the ascending aorta or the aortic arch with its branches. The abdominal aorta is not involved.
- **Type III** is concomitant involvement of the descending thoracic aorta, the abdominal aorta, and/or the renal arteries. The ascending aorta and the aortic arch and its branches are not involved.
- **Type IV** involves only the abdominal aorta and/or the renal arteries.
- **Type V** is a generalized type, with combined features of the other types.

Note: Involvement of the coronary and pulmonary arteries should be indicated as C(+) or P(+), respectively.

The commonly involved arteries are left subclavian artery (50%), left common carotid (20%), brachiocephalic, renal arteries, celiac trunk, SMA and pulmonary arteries (50%).

Imaging Findings

Almost all the available imaging modalities have some role in diagnosis and follow-up of TA, however, currently CT, MRI and/or PET CT/MRI are the main imaging modalities. Role of conventional angiography in diagnosis of TA is almost obsolete and restricted for interventional procedures.[70]

Early/acute stage: The arterial wall thickening **(Fig. 41)** can be detected on CT or MRI (Fat-suppressed T1-weighted postcontrast MR images) as soft tissue thickening encircling the aorta (swollen intima) with circumferential peripheral contrast enhancement (inflamed media and adventitia. On T2-weighted sequences mural edema is depicted as high signal. Nuclear fusion imaging (PET) with 18-flurorodeoxyglucose (18F-FDG) with either CT or MRI is now emerging as the initial diagnosis and assessment of disease activity with high sensitivity of 60-90% and specificity of 88–100% as 18F-FDG is a surrogate marker of increased activity of inflammatory cells.[70,71-73]

Chronic stage: The disease is characterized by development of aneurysm and linear stenosis of descending and abdominal aorta. There may be long diffuse or short segmental irregular stenosis with occlusion of the major branches of the aorta near its origin **(Fig. 42)**. There may be skip lesions, abundant collateralization, saccular or fusiform aortic aneurysm (10–15%) **(Fig. 43)**.[74,75] These findings can be seen on conventional angiography, CT angiography or MR angiography. Cross-sectional imaging, in addition, shows arterial wall thickening, mural calcium deposition and full thickness calcification which is very suggestive of chronic phase of disease.[76,77]

Management of TA

Active TA is treated with steroids or immunosuppressants before revascularization as revascularization during the

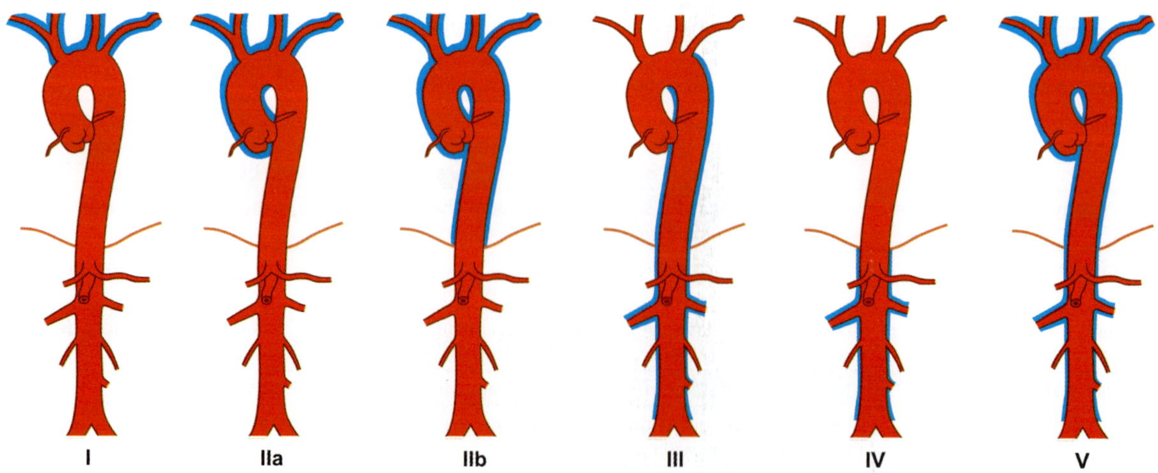

Fig. 40: Schematic diagrams show types of Takayasu's arteritis.

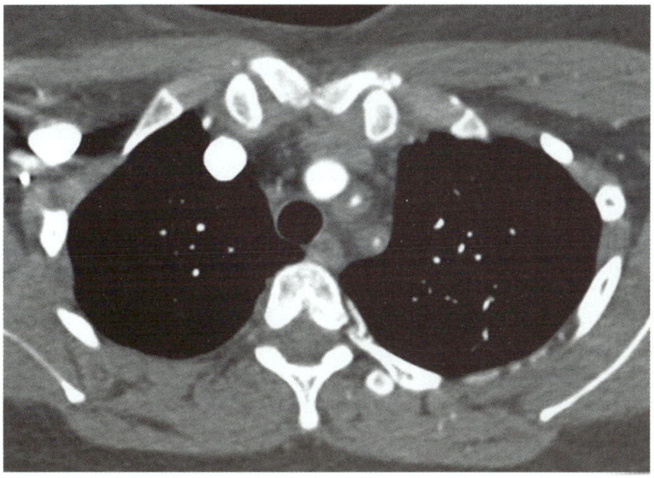

Fig. 41: Takayasu's arteritis: CTA source image showing circumferential mural thickening of the lateral common carotid and subclavian arteries.

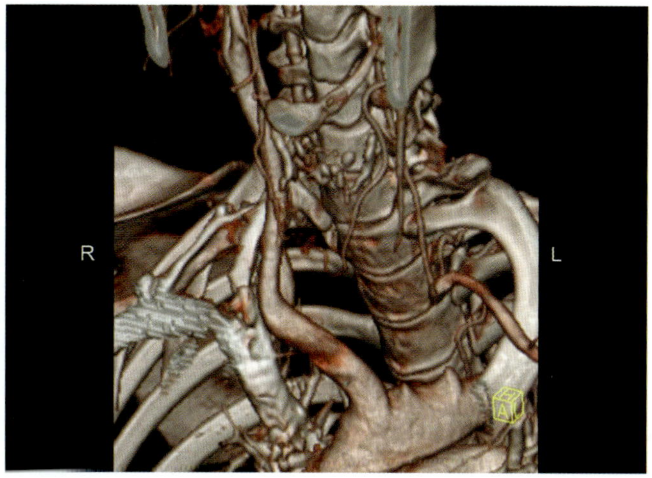

Fig. 42: Takayasu's arteritis: CTA VR image showing total occlusion of left common carotid and subclavian arteries just beyond their origins.

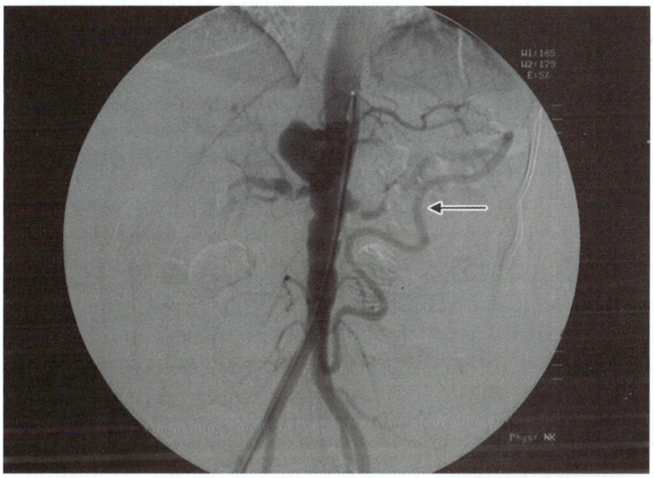

Fig. 43: Takayasu's arteritis: DSA shows aneurysmal dilatation of the abdominal aorta above renal arteries, irregular aortic contour, collaterals from IMA (arrow).

active phase can increase the risk of procedure-related complications, including restenosis and dissection.[78] Occlusion/restenosis rate of transluminal angioplasty with or without stent implantation in active disease is reported to be as high as 71.4% after a follow-up of 1.3 years.

Symptomatic TA is treated with revascularization of the affected vessels. In general, surgical bypass or endovascular intervention should be avoided during the active phase of TA, unless the presence of an acute life-threatening condition outweighs the risk any intervention including restenosis and dissection.[78,79]

Even in life-threatening situations (hypertensive encephalopathy, flash pulmonary edema and congestive heart failure), endovascular treatment is the treatment modality that carries the lowest risk of morbidity and mortality to the patient and should be considered before open surgical therapy. This is due to the fact that, surgical procedures are complicated by graft reocclusion, anastomotic site aneurysm and increased morbidity. The progressive inflammatory nature of TA has is also a widespread problem limiting use of reconstructive surgery.

In the chronic fibrotic stage, the principle of treatment is revascularization either by surgery or balloon angioplasty. Balloon angioplasty is a relatively simple and cost-effective method for relief of stenotic lesions in patients with TA **(Figs. 44A to D)**. It avoids the risks of anesthesia and shortens the hospital stay. Percutaneous angioplasty yielded excellent results with success rates ranging from 81% to 100% and low morbidity and mortality.[78]

The problem with balloon angioplasty is recurrence of the stenosis, which is however, easily tackled by a secondary reintervention. Studies also reported improved results with primary stenting; however, stenting is better reserved for flow limiting dissections or persisting stenoses after balloon angioplasty. Moreover, the presence of long segment juxta diaphragmatic stenosis involving the origin of visceral arteries, often in a young child precludes the use of a stent. The risk of stent occlusion is also higher due to protracted nature of the disease with waxing and waning of disease activity.

Immunoglobulin G4 (IgG4)-related Aortitis

IgG4 related diseases are of unknown etiology which can affect any organ from head to toe. It is characterized by diffuse or focal tumor like lesions with lymphoplasmacytic infiltrate enriched with IgG4 positive plasma cells and

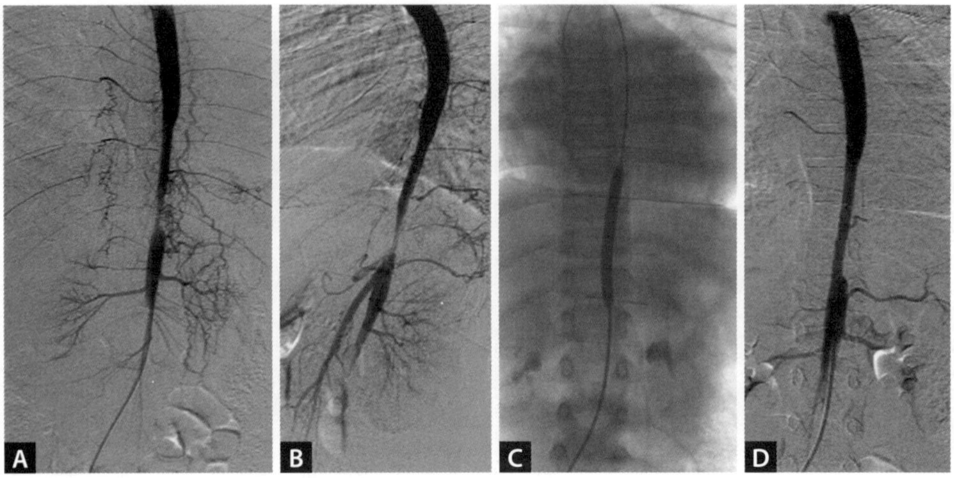

Figs. 44A to D: Balloon angioplasty in a patient of Takayasu's arteritis with heart failure: (A and B) Aortogram showing long segment tight stenosis of the juxta-diaphragmatic thoracic aorta; (C) Balloon angioplasty of the stenosed segment: (D) Postangioplasty aortogram showing significant reduction of degree of stenosis with reduction of the trans-stenotic gradient from 65 mm of Hg to 15 mm of Hg.

fibrosis. They are often associated with elevated serum IgG4 levels. It predominantly affects males in their 4–6 decades however exact incidence is unknown. It is a great mimicker with varying differential diagnosis on imaging, ranging from inflammatory lesions to malignancy.[81]

Recognition of imaging findings can suggest a diagnosis, which can be confirmed on serology, and histopathology. This is of paramount importance as the disease responds to immunosuppressive therapy. On pathology the lymphoplasmacytic cells are IgG4 positive with negative CD3 and CD20 staining which are markers for T-cell and B-cell related inflammation respectively and are positive in aortoarteritis.

On imaging a soft tissue like mass is seen encasing aorta and its branches, typically without any luminal compromise unlike aortoarteritis. The soft tissue is hypodense on CT **(Figs. 45A and B)** and demonstrates varying signal intensity on MR depending on degree and stage of fibrosis.[82] Contrast enhancement can be variable depending upon degree of fibrosis.

In long-standing cases aneurysmal dilatation of abdominal aorta and extensive wall thickening with or without periaortic inflammatory extension can be seen.[83] Rupture though uncommon with IgG4-related disease may be seen **(*Refer* Figs. 24 to 26)**.

18F-FDG PET-CT and CT are useful in detecting inflammatory activity in the aneurysmal wall **(Figs. 46A to D)** and assessing treatment response.[84]

AORTIC TRAUMA

Traumatic injuries to the aorta may result from either blunt (nonpenetrating, indirect) or sharp (penetrating, direct) trauma. Penetrating trauma is usually caused by stab or bullet wounds that puncture the aortic wall. Rare causes include misplacement of spinal fixation screws and lacerations from spinal fractures. Blunt aortic injuries (BAIs) are far more common and the aortic wall is damaged from the inside to the outside, from the intima to the adventitia.

Traumatic transaction of the aorta is a common cause of death in high-speed accidents. Sudden deceleration causes torsion and a shearing stress at the isthmus where the aorta is relatively fixed. "Osseous pinch" effect is due to pinching of the aorta between the manubrium and medial end of clavicle anteriorly and spine posteriorly. It is due to this pinch that there is posterior displacement of the heart which generates aortic torsion.[85] About 90% of traumatic tears occur around the isthmus. The other sites include: aortic arch with avulsion of brachiocephalic trunk (4.5%), ascending aorta (1%) and descending aorta (2.5%). These patients often have multiple injuries and pose a considerable challenge for early and rapid imaging.

Grading of Aortic Injuries[86]

- *Grade 0*: Normal mediastinum and normal aorta
- *Grade I*: Abnormal mediastinum and normal aorta. About 5–10% of blunt trauma of chest may have isolated mediastinal hematoma
- *Grade II*: Minimal aortic injury (differential diagnosis of ductus arteriosus remnant or atherosclerosis)
- *Grade III*: Confined aortic injury
- *Grade IV*: Aortic disruption.

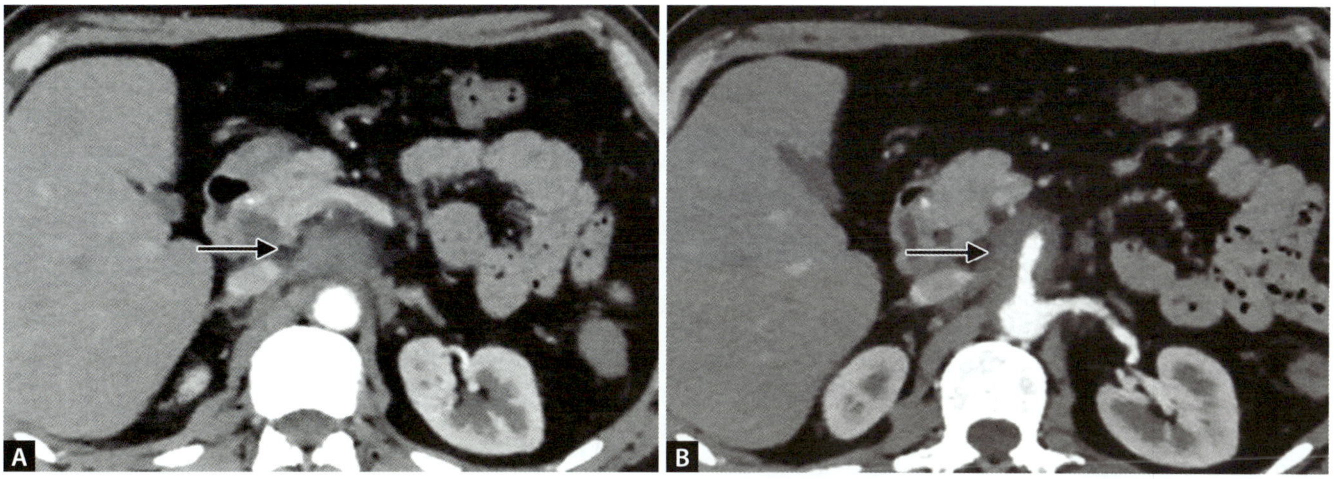

Figs. 45A and B: CTA axial images an ill-defined soft tissue is seen in preaortic location (arrow in A) which is encasing the celiac artery from its origin (arrow in B) without any luminal compromise.

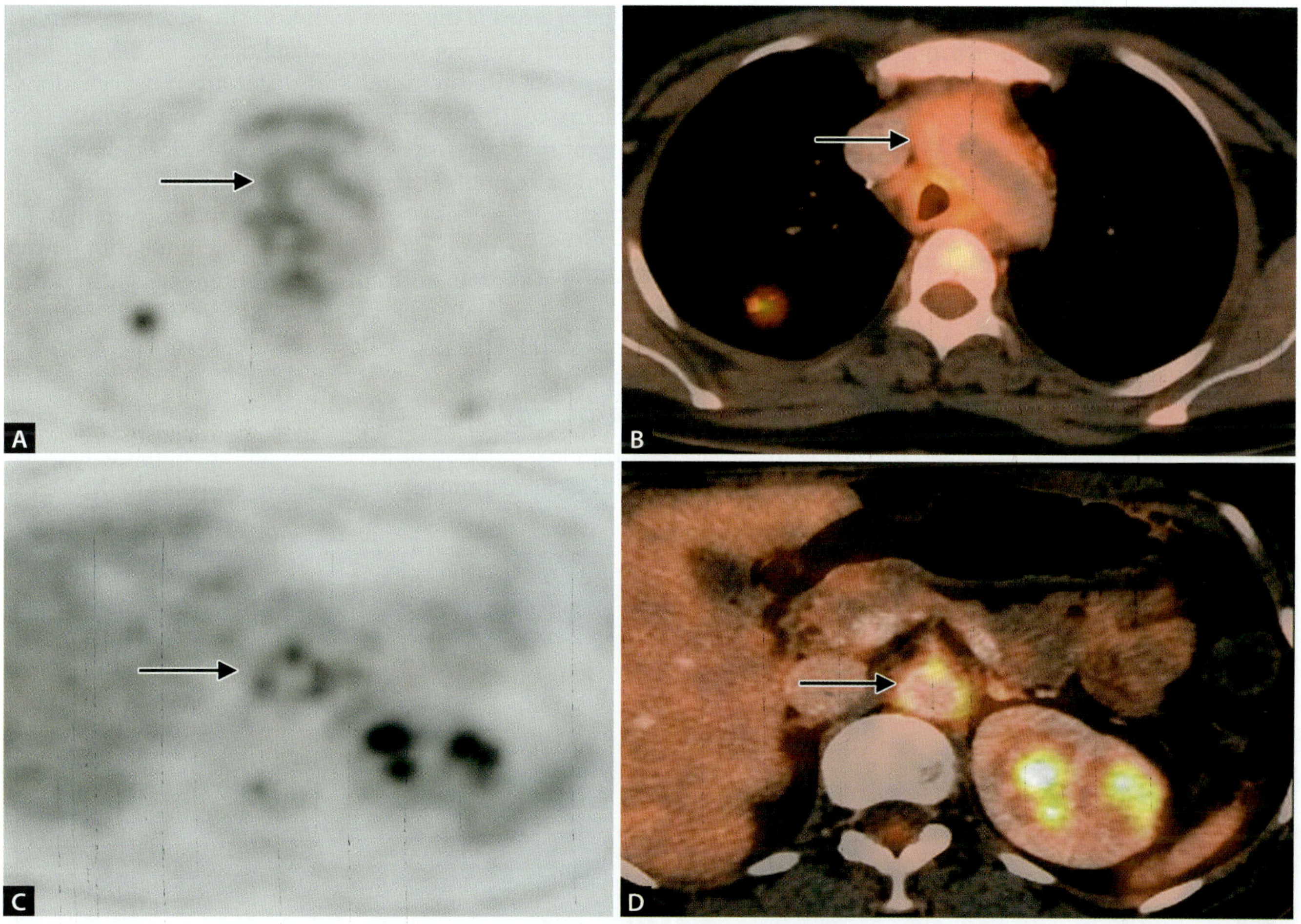

Figs. 46A to D: 18F-FDG PET and fused PET-CT images show increased activity in arch of aorta and abdominal aorta at the level of origin of celiac axis.
Courtesy: Dr Rajender Basher, Assistant Professor, Department of Nuclear Medicine, PGIMER, Chandigarh, India.

Imaging

The chest X-ray is a good screening tool for detection of mediastinal hemorrhage, but affords little as far as definitive diagnosis is concerned. An AP erect chest film with the patient leaning forward is ideal rather than a supine film with 90% sensitivity, 95% specificity and 95% negative predictive value.

The plain X-ray findings include widening of the superior mediastinum, an abnormal aortic contour, shift of the trachea to the right, inferior displacement of the left main bronchus, widening of left paravertebral stripe, etc.

Computed Tomography

Plain CT may demonstrate mediastinal hematoma. CECT may show an abrupt change in aortic contour, intimal flap, pseudoaneurysm, pseudocoarctation and extravasation of contrast. CTA shows 96.2% sensitivity, 99.8% specificity and 99.7% accuracy for the diagnosis of aortic injury.

Magnetic Resonance Imaging

In an acute setting of multiple injuries, MR is not recommended.

Aortography

It is the definitive mode of diagnosis but in view of the high sensitivity of CT, aortography is indicated only in selected cases of chronic aortic trauma.

Management of Thoracic Aortic Injury

The initial management of the patient with a contained aortic transection is stabilization of vitals. Patients with multiple injuries can be managed medically for several days or weeks until an intervention can be performed. The conventional therapy of aortic transection was surgery but stent-grafts are increasingly used to treat TAI and now the current procedure of choice **(Figs. 47A to D)**. All patients with external aortic contour deformity should be treated with endovascular stent graft as soon as possible and atleast before hospital discharge.

Its advantages include that it can be performed quickly and percutaneously in the patients who would be at high-risk for open surgical repair and cardiopulmonary bypass. The challenges faced in this population are similar to the challenges faced in treating type B AD and may be overcome using similar techniques.

ATHEROSCLEROSIS

Atherosclerosis is the most common disease involving the aorta. The changes of atherosclerosis are seen in almost all people beyond middle age although they often remain asymptomatic. The abdominal aorta below the renal arteries is the most common site of atherosclerosis and most patients with aortoiliac occlusive disease also have associated femoral and distal arterial occlusions. Reconstruction of the aorta and the iliac arteries by thromboendarterectomy, shunts, stents or angioplasties is an extremely satisfactory therapy for disabling arteriosclerosis obliterans of the aortoiliac system. CTA and DSA are the most effective imaging modalities for the demonstration of aorto iliac obstruction sites, distal run off vessels or collateral vessels and associated stenosis or occlusions of the major visceral arteries.

Pathology

Variable combination of changes of the intima of arteries with focal accumulation of lipids, complex carbohydrates,

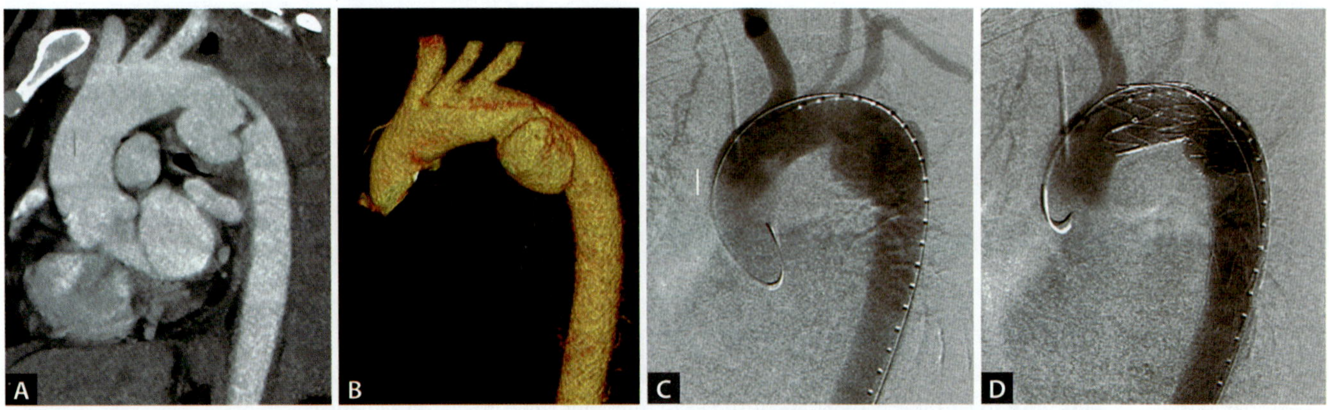

Figs. 47A to D: Stent-graft repair of traumatic aortic transection: (A and B) Computed tomography images showing transection with (A) pseudoaneurysm of the proximal descending thoracic aorta; (C) Angiogram prior to stent-graft placement shows in (A); (D) Angiogram following stent-graft placement. The pseudoaneurysm is excluded. Note that the left subclavian artery was sacrificed with its ostia covered by the stent graft.

blood and blood products, fibrous tissue and calcium are the hallmark of atherosclerosis. The disease is divided into:

- Early changes: Fatty streak and gelatinous elevation reflected on imaging as "smooth plaque".
- Fibroatheromatous plaque: It is seen on imaging as irregular plaque, plaque ulceration, etc. **(Fig. 48)**.
- The complicated lesion: Hemorrhage in the plaque, fibrogenesis leading to irregularity and tortousity, weakening of the wall leading to aneurysm formation and calcification **(Fig. 49)**. Stenosis and occlusion may be due to combinations of plaque, fibrosis and calcification.

Imaging

The gross morphological changes can be seen on all imaging modalities. These signs are:[07]

- Diffuse narrowing of the vessels
- Irregular vascular contours and diameters
- Nicks, filling defects and calcifications along the vessel wall
- Spotty or ragged density of the opaque contrast column
- Vessels that are generally large or tortuous or both.
- Saccular dilatations and aneurysm
- Stenosis and or frank occlusion of a vessel (obliterative arteriosclerosis)

Cross-sectional imaging may show a greater degree of luminal compromise, intimal atherosclerosis, mural thrombus and the surgeons may palpate a greater hardening of vessel wall than is seen on catheter angiograms.

Occlusion of the Aorto-iliac System

It may be the terminal event in slowly progressive arteriosclerotic stenosis and may be tolerated without medical attention. The blood flow through a vessel may be relatively adequate until the vessel diameter is reduced to about 70%. Acute occlusion may occur following emboli from heart, atherosclerotic plaques or aneurysms.

Complete Occlusion of Aorta

It rarely extends upwards to involve the renal arteries but at surgery, the renal and other visceral arteries are frequently found to be partially involved **(Figs. 50A to D)**. Syphilis, aortic dissection and atherosclerosis have been reported to cause complete aortic occlusion. 'Leriche syndrome' is due to complete occlusion of the terminal part of abdominal aorta and bilateral common iliac arteries.

Collateral Pathways

In stenotic or occlusive disease extensive collateral pathways open up.

- *Visceral collateral network:* The SMA and IMA form the major visceral collateral circulation.
  - Aortic occlusion above IMA: The SMA acts as the main affluent vessel through the left branch of middle colic artery into left colic branch of the IMA (effluent vessel). The "meandering mesenteric artery" or "central anastomotic artery" represents this communication **(Fig. 51)**.
  - Aortic occlusion below IMA: The IMA acts as a key source of collateral circulation via retiform anastomosis between superior hemorrhoidal branches and middle and inferior hemorrhoidal branches of the internal iliac arteries which may reconstitute the external iliac artery.
- *Parietal collateral network:* The parietal vessels that may be seen to bridge aortic occlusions are the

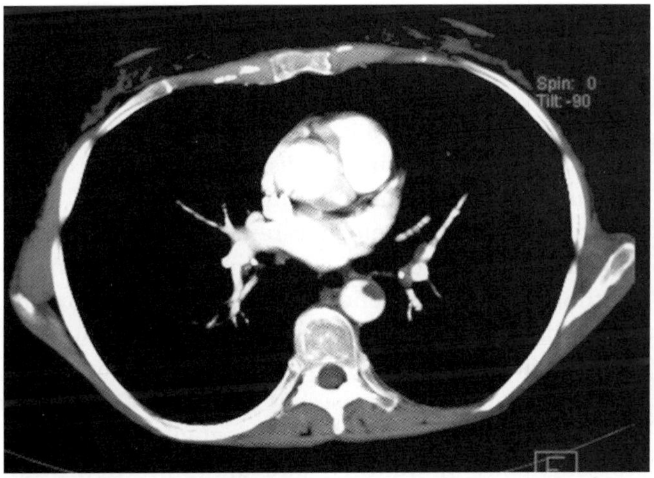

Fig. 48: Atheromatous aortic disease: CTA source image shows atheromatous plaque along anterolateral wall of aorta and projecting into the lumen.

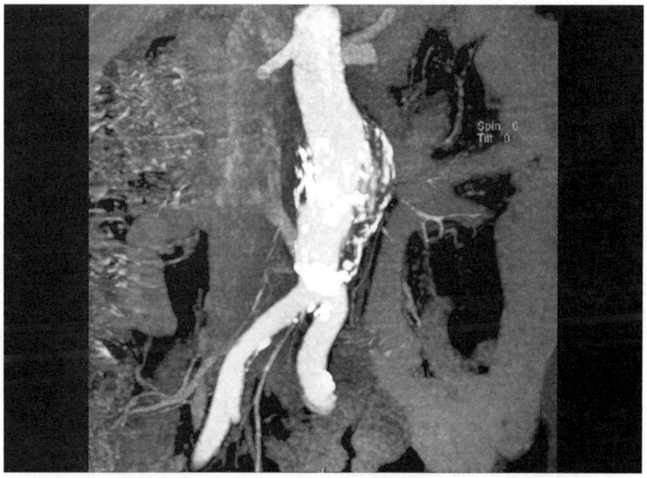

Fig. 49: Atheromatous aortic disease: Large plaque with circumferential calcifications, aortic dilatation and mural thickening.

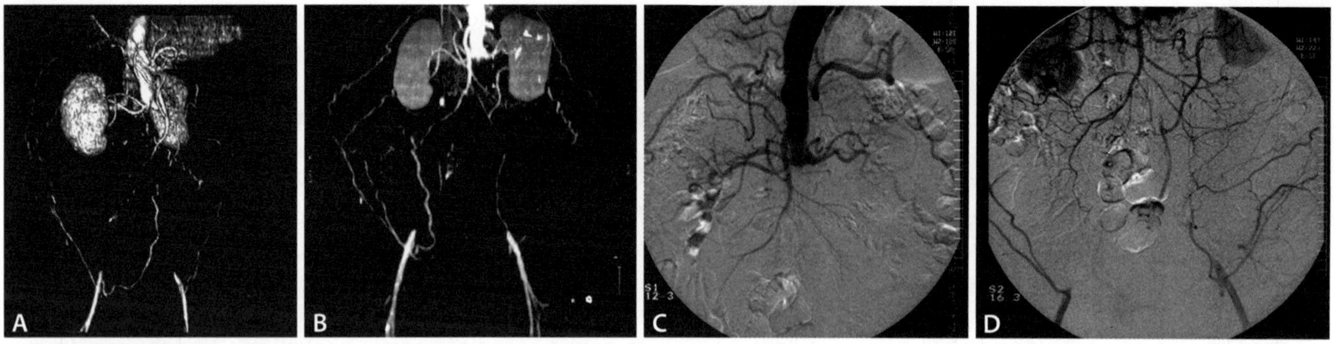

Figs. 50A to D: Atherosclerotic complete occlusion of aorta: CTA (A) and VR (B) MIP projections show complete block of abdominal aorta just distal to renal arteries with collaterals and run off to distal external iliac arteries. DSA (C and D) confirms the findings of CTA.

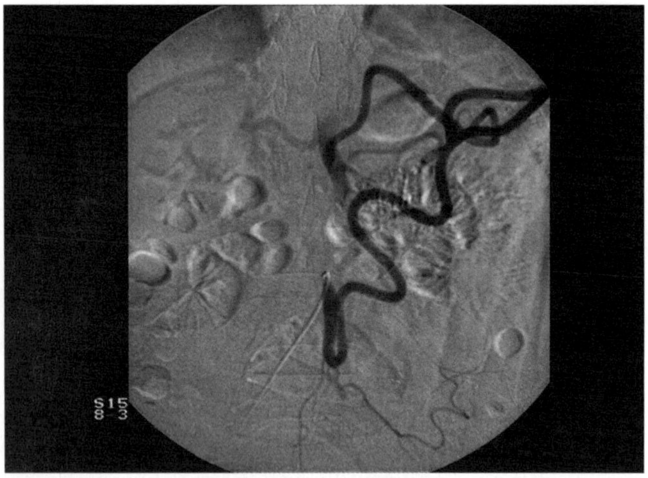

Fig. 51: Visceral collateral network: DSA shows IMA-SMA collateral network.

intercostals, subcostal, lumbar and median sacral branches of the aorta with iliolumbar, lateral sacral, superior gluteal and obturator branches of the internal iliac arteries, and deep iliac circumflex and medial and lateral circumflex branches of the external iliac and deep femoral arteries. Lumbar branches have anastomotic connections with iliolumbar and gluteal branches of the internal iliac artery. The epigastric arteries may form an important collateral circulation (Winslow's pathway), i.e. from the intercostals and internal mammary artery to the external iliac arteries through the epigastric arteries.

The indications for intervention in patients with occlusive disease of aorta are moderate to severe claudication, rest pain, acutely threatened limb and hemodynamically significant lesion proximal to a distal lesion for which revascularization is being attempted. Patients with mild claudication should undergo medical management with exercise therapy first. Surgical options including aortofemoral bypass, axillofemoral bypass, femoral-femoral bypass, and aortic endarterectomy are effective treatments but more morbid compared to endovascular approaches. Endovascular management includes balloon angioplasty with or without stenting. Stent placement is indicated for patients with obstructive dissection during balloon angioplasty, recanalization of total occlusions, or lesions that are likely to cause distal embolization. Stent-grafts may be used to exclude symptomatic ulcerated plaque, but otherwise currently have little role for aortic occlusive disease.

Postoperative Aorta

CTA or MRA is the preferred modality for evaluating postoperative aorta for demonstration of perigraft fluid collection and acute hemorrhage. It is also more informative in the diagnosis of graft infection, aortoenteric fistula, anastomotic pseudoaneurysm . These modalities are also very helpful in evaluating the efficacy of endovascular treatment in aortic diseases.[88]

CONCLUSION

Noninvasive imaging of the aorta has almost replaced invasive aortography. US is a good screening modality to confirm or exclude aneurysm, dissection, atherosclerosis etc. but additional anatomic information needs to be obtained prior to an elective repair or endovascular treatment. TEE provides additional information for the thoracic aorta except in the area of the proximal arch (blind spot). Contrast-enhanced CT should be used routinely both for preoperative and postoperative assessment of aortic diseases. At a reasonable cost and low-risk to patients, CT and CT angiography can provide the diagnosis, operability, and anatomic definition including concomitant intra-thoracic or intra-abdominal abnormalities. The recent advances in MR hardware, sequences and computational ability pose a real challenge to all imaging techniques. MR can now provide all the information needed for evaluating aortic diseases, anatomic as well as functional and gadolinium enhanced 3D MRA may replace catheter angiography for both preoperative and postoperative evaluation. Angiography is indicated to answer specific questions posed by the results of clinical examination and/or CT or MR imaging or as a prerequisite to endovascular intervention. Knowledge of indication of treatment (medical vs. interventional) of different aortic pathologies is of paramount importance. Surgery has been traditionally used in management of these patients however with increasing expertise and development of hardware, endovascular techniques have become the first line of management in many of these aortic pathologies.

ACKNOWLEDGMENTS

Dr Sreedhar BC, Fellow Interventional Radiology, PGIMER, Chandigarh for his active support in literature search and preparation of manuscript, Dr Chirag Jain, Fellow Neuro-Radiology, PGIMER, Chandigarh for his contribution to art work, Professor Ritambra Nada, Department of Histopathology, PGIMER, Chandigarh for pathology specimens and slides, and Dr Rajender Basher, Assistant Professor, Department of Nuclear Medicine, PGIMER, Chandigarh for providing PET-CT images.

REFERENCES

1. Douglas H. "Aorta". Online Etymology Dictionary. Retrieved 9 October; 2017.
2. Rosner F. Medicine in the Bible and the Talmud: selections from classical Jewish sources (Augm. ed.). Hoboken, NJ: KTAV Pub. House.1995.pp.87-96.
3. Goldstein SA, Evangelista A, Abbara S. Multimodality imaging of diseases of the thoracic aorta in adults: from the American Society of Echocardiography and the European Association of Cardiovascular Imaging: endorsed by the Society of Cardiovascular Computed Tomography and Society for Cardiovascular Magnetic Resonance. J Am Soc Echocardiogr. 2015;28:119-82.
4. Wolf YG, Zarins CK. Noninvasive aortic imaging. In: Bruce L Gewetz (Ed.) Philadelphia. W.B. Saunders. 2000;1:34-40.
5. Rosenblum JD, Leef JA. Aortography. In: Bruce L Gewetz (ed.) Philadelphia. W.B. Saunders. 2000;1:41-50.
6. Lucarotti ME, Shaw E, Heather BP. Distribution of aortic diameter in a screened population. Br J Surg. 1992;79:641-2.
7. Jaffee RB. Radiographic manifestations of congenital anomalies of the aortic arch. RCNA. 1991;29:319-34.
8. Shinley BR. Transesophageal echocardiography in the diagnosis of aortic disease. Seminars in US, CT and MRI. 1993;14:106-16.
9. Benenati JF. Intravasclar ultrasound: the role in diagnostic and therapeutic procedures. RCNA. 1995;33:31-50.
10. Kumamaru KK, Hoppe BE, Richard T, et al. CT angiography: Current technology and clinical use. Radiol Clin North Am. 2010;48:213-35.
11. Rajiah P. CT and MRI in the Evaluation of Thoracic Aortic Diseases. International Journal of Vascular Medicine. 2013. pp.16.
12. Litmanovich D, Bankier AA, Cantin L, et al. CT and MRI in diseases of the aorta. Am J Roentgenol. 2009;193:928-40.
13. Gutstein A, Wolak A, Lee C, et al. Predicting success of prospective and retrospective gating with dual-source coronary computed tomography angiography: development of selection criteria and initial experience. Journal of Cardiovascular Computed Tomography. 2008;2:81-90.
14. Gies M, Kalender W A, Wolf H, et al. Dose reduction in CT by anatomically adapted tube current modulation. I. Simulation studies. Medical Physics. 1999:26;2235-47.
15. Leschka S, Stolzmann P, Schmid F T, et al. Low kilovoltage cardiac dual-source CT: attenuation, noise, and radiation dose. European Radiology. 2008;18:1809-17.
16. Macari M, Israel GM, Berman P, et al. Infrarenal abdominal aortic aneurysms at multi-detector row CT angiography: intravascular enhancement without a timing acquisition. Radiology. 2001;220:519-23.
17. Cademaritiri F, Mollet N, van der Lugt A, et al. Noninvasive 16-row multislice coronary angiography: usefulness of saline chaser. Eur Radiol. 2004;14:178-83.
18. Czum JM, Corse WR, Ho VB. MR angiography of the thoracic aorta. Magn Reson Imaging Clin N Am. 2005;13:41-64.
19. Sakamoto I, Sueyoshi E, Uetani M. MR Imaging of the Aorta. Radiol Clin N Am. 2007;45:485-97.
20. Amano Y, Takahama K, Kumita S. Non-contrast-enhanced MR angiography of the thoracic aorta using cardiac and navigator-gated magnetization-prepared three-dimensional steady-state free precession. J Magn Reson Imaging. 2008;27:504-9.
21. Gebker R, Gomaa O, Schnackenburg B, et al. Comparison of different MRI techniques for the assessment of thoracic aortic pathology: 3D contrast enhanced MR angiography, turbo spin echo and balanced steady state free precession. Int J Cardiovasc Imaging. 2007;23:747-56.
22. Galizia MS, Bolen MA, Flamm SD. MRI of the thoracic aorta. Applied Radiology. 2015.pp.22-6 (www.appliedradiology.com)
23. Prince MR, Yucel EK, Kaufman JA, et al. Dynamic gadolinium-enhanced three-dimensional abdominal MR arteriography. J Magn Reson Imaging.1993;3:877-81.
24. Russo V, Renzulli M, Buttazzi K, et al. Acquired diseases of the thoracic aorta: role of MRI and MRA. Eur Radiol. 2006;16:852-65.
25. Russo V, Renzulli M, Palombara CL, et al. Congenital diseases of the thoracic aorta: role of MRI and MRA. Eur Radiol. 2006;16:676-84.

26. Hom JJ, Ordovas K, Reddy GP. Velocity-encoded cine MR imaging in aortic coarctation: functional assessment of hemodynamic events. Radiographics. 2008;28:407-16.
27. Lee YH, Choi SJ, Ji JD, et al. Diagnostic accuracy of 18F-FDG PET or PET/CT for large vessel vasculitis. Z Rheumatol. 2016;75:924-31.
28. Danve A, O Dell, J. The role of 18F-fluorodeoxyglucose positron emission tomography scanning in the diagnosis and management of systemic vasculitis. Int J Rheum Dis. 2015;18:714-24.
29. Glaudemans AW, de Vries EF, Galli F, et al. The Use of F-FDG-PET/CT for diagnosis and treatment monitoring of inflammatory and infectious diseases. Clin Dev Immunol. 2013;2013.623036.
30. Khandelwal N, Gupta S. Current concepts in imaging aortic aneurysms in Sanjiv Sharma (Ed). Recent advances in imaging and intervention in cardiovascular diseases. Singapore Springer. 1996;58-62.
31. Campbell M. Natural history of coarctation of aorta. Br Heart J. 1970;32:633-40.
32. Silversides CK, Marelli A, Beauchesne L, et al. Canadian Cardiovascular Society 2009 Consensus Conference on the management of adults with congenital heart disease: executive summary. Can J Cardiol. 2010;26:143-50.
33. Feltes TF, Bacha E, Beekman RH 3rd, et al. Indications for cardiac catheterization and intervention in pediatric cardiac disease: a scientific statement from the American Heart Association. Circulation. 2011;123:2607-52.
34. Hiratzka LF, Bakris GL, Beckman JA, et al. 2010 ACCF/AHA/AATS/ACR/ASA/SCA/SCAI/SIR/STS/SVM Guidelines for the diagnosis and management of patients with thoracic aortic disease. A report of the American College of Cardiology Foundation/American Heart Association Task Force on Practice Guidelines, American Association for Thoracic Surgery, American College of Radiology, American Stroke Association, Society of Cardiovascular Anesthesiologists, Society for Cardiovascular Angiography and Interventions, Society of Interventional Radiology, Society of Thoracic Surgeons, and Society for Vascular Medicine. J Am Coll Cardiol. 2010;55:e27-e129.
35. Davies RR, Goldstein LJ, Coady MA, et al. Yearly rupture or dissection rates for thoracic aortic aneurysms: simple prediction based on size. Ann Thorac Surg. 2002;73:17-27.
36. Brewster DC, Cronenwett JL, Hallett JW Jr, et al. Guidelines for the treatment of abdominal aortic aneurysms. Report of a subcommittee of the Joint Council of the American Association for Vascular Surgery and Society for Vascular Surgery. J Vasc Surg. 2003;37:1106.
37. LaRoy LL, Cormier PJ, Matalon TAS, et al. Imaging of abdominal aortic aneurysms. AJR. 1989;152:785-92.
38. Goldstein SA, Evangelista A, Abbara S, et al. Multimodality imaging of diseases of the thoracic aorta in adults: from the American Society of Echocardiography and the European Association of Cardiovascular Imaging: endorsed by the Society of Cardiovascular Computed Tomography and Society for Cardiovascular Magnetic Resonance. J Am Soc Echocardiogr. 2015;28:119-82.
39. Prince MR, Yucel EK, Kaufman JA, et al. Dynamic gadolinium-enhanced three-dimensional abdominal MR arteriography. J Magn Reson Imaging.1993;3:877-81.
40. Brewster DC, Cronenwett JL, Hallett JW Jr, et al. Guidelines for the treatment of abdominal aortic aneurysms. Report of a subcommittee of the Joint Council of the American Association for Vascular Surgery and Society for Vascular Surgery. J Vasc Surg. 2003;37:1106.
41. Bown MJ, Sweeting MJ, Brown LC, et al. Surveillance intervals for small abdominal aortic aneurysms: a meta-analysis. JAMA. 2013;309:806-13.
42. Walsh SR, Tang TY, Sadat U, et al. Endovascular stenting versus open surgery for thoracic aortic disease: systematic review and meta-analysis of perioperative results. J Vasc Surg. 2008;47:1094-8.
43. Zhang Y, Teng Z, Lu Q, et al. Management of complicated aortic aneurysms using multiple overlapping uncovered stents: mid-term outcome from a cohort study. Medicine (Baltimore). 2014;93:e209.
44. Sadat U, Boyle JR, Walsh SR, et al. Endovascular vs open repair of acute abdominal aortic aneurysms: a systematic review and meta-analysis. J Vasc Surg. 2008;48:227-36.
45. Kaufman JA, Geller SC, Brewster DC, et al. Endovascular repair of abdominal aortic aneurysms: current status and future directions. Am J Roentgenol. 2000;175:289-302.
46. William DM, Joshi A, Dake MD, et al. Aortic cobwebs: An anatomic marker identifying the false lumen in aortic dissection– imaging and pathologic correlation. Radiology. 1994;190:167-74.
47. Nienaber CA, vonKodolitsch Y, Nicholas V, et al. The diagnosis of thoracic aortic dissection by noninvasive imaging procedures. N Engl J Med. 1993;328:1-14.
48. LePage MA, Quint LE, Sonnad SS, et al. Aortic dissection: CT features that distinguish true lumen from false lumen. Am J Roentgenol. 2001;177:207-11.
49. Pereles FS, McCarthy RM, Baskaran V, et al. Thoracic aortic dissection and aneurysm: evaluation with nonenhanced true FISP MR angiography in less than 4 minutes. Radiology. 2002;223:270-4.
50. Dake MD, Thompson M, van Sambeek M, et al. DISSECT: a new mnemonic-based approach to the categorization of aortic dissection. Eur J Vasc Endovasc Surg. 2013;46:175-90.
51. Nienaber CA, Eagle KA. Aortic dissection: new frontiers in diagnosis and management: Part I: from etiology to diagnostic strategies. Circulation. 2003;108:628-35.
52. Hagan PG, Nienaber CA, Isselbacher EM, et al. The International Registry of Acute Aortic Dissection (IRAD): new insights into an old disease. JAMA. 2000;283:897-903.
53. Criado FJ, Barnatan MF, Rizk Y, et al. Technical strategies to expand stent-graft applicability in the aortic arch and proximal descending thoracic aorta. J Endovasc Ther. 2002;9(Suppl 2):II32-8.
54. Midulla M, Renaud A, Martinelli T, et al. Endovascular fenestration in aortic dissection with acute malperfusion syndrome: immediate and late follow-up. J Thorac Cardiovasc Surg. 2011;142:66-72.

55. Banning AP. Aortic intramural hematoma. N Engl J Med. 1997;337:1476-7.
56. Chao CP, Walker TG, Kalva SP. Natural history and CT appearances of aortic intramural hematoma. Radiographics. 2009;29:791-804.
57. O'Gara PT, DeSanctis RW. Acute aortic dissection and its variants.Toward a common diagnostic and therapeutic approach. Circulation. 1995;92:1376-8.
58. Park KH, Lim C, Choi JH, et al. Prevalence of aortic intimal defect in surgically treated acute type A intramural hematoma. Ann Thorac Surg. 2008;86:1494-500.
59. Evangelista A, Garcia-del-Castillo H, Gonzalez-Alujas T, et al. Diagnosis of ascending aortic dissection by transesophageal echocardiography: utility of Mmode in recognizing artifacts. J Am Coll Cardiol. 1996;27:102-7.
60. Bolger AF. Aortic intramural haematoma. Heart. 2008;94:1670-4.
61. Nathan DP, Boonn W, Lai E, et al. Presentation, complications, and natural history of penetrating atherosclerotic ulcer disease. J Vasc Surg. 2012;55:10-5.
62. Eggebrecht H, Plicht B, Kahlert P, et al. Intramural hematoma and penetrating ulcers: indications to endovascular treatment. Eur J Vasc Endovasc Surg. 2009;38:659-65.
63. Litmanovich DE, Yıldırım A, Bankier AA. Insights into imaging of aortitis. Insights Imaging. 2012;3:545-60.
64. Moyano JC, Magarolas MA, González EC, et al. Nonurgent aortic disease: clinical-radiological diagnosis of aortitis. Radiology. 2013;55:469-82.
65. Sharma BK, Siveski-Iliskovic N, Singal PK. Takayasu arteritis may be underdiagnosed in North America. Can J Cardiol. 1995;11:311-6.
66. Sharma BR, Jain S, Suri S, et al. Diagnostic criteria for Takayasu arteritis. International Journal of Cardiology. 1996;54(S):141-S147.
67. Restrepo CS, Ocazionez D, Suri R, et al. Aortitis: imaging spectrum of the infectious and inflammatory conditions of the aorta. Radiographics. 2011;31:435-51.
68. Kerr GS, Hallahan CW, Giordano J, et al. Takayasu arteritis. Ann Intern Med. 1994;120: 919-29.
69. Gotway MB, Araoz PA, Macedo TA, et al. Imaging findings in Takayasu's arteritis. Am J Roentgenol. 2005;184:1945-50.
70. Matsunaga N, Hayashi R, Sakamoto I, et al. Takayasu's arteritis. Protean radiologic manifestations and diagnosis. Radiographics. 1997;17:579-91.
71. Gornik HL, Creager MA. Aortitis. Circulation. 2008;117: 3039-305.
72. Kobayashi Y, Ishii K, Oda K, et al. Aortic wall inflammation due to Takayasu arteritis imaged with 18F-FDG PET coregistered with enhanced CT. J Nucl Med. 2005;46:917-22.
73. Meller J, Grabbe E, Becker W, et al. Value of F-18 FDG hybrid camera PET and MRI in early Takayasu aortitis. Eur Radiol. 2003;13:400-5.
74. Webb M, Chambers A, AL-N A, et al. The role of 18F-FDG PET in characterising disease activity in Takayasu arteritis. Eur J Nucl Med Mol Imaging. 2004;31:627-34.
75. Sharma S, Rajani M. Aortic occlusion in nonspecific aortoarteritis (Takayasu disease): incidence and spectrum of involvement. Australas Radiol. 1993;37:57-9.
76. Sharma S, Rajani M, Talwar KK. Angiographic morphology in nonspecific aortoarteritis (Takayasu's arteritis): a study of 126 patients from north India. Cardiovasc Intervent Radiol. 1992;15:160-5.
77. Sharma S, Sharma S, Taneja K, et al. Morphological mural changes in the aorta in non specific aortoarteritis (Takayasu's arteritis): assessment by intravascular ultrasound imaging. Clin Radiol. 1998;53:37-43.
78. Sharma S, Sharma S, Taneja K, et al. Morphologic mural changes in the aorta revealed by CT in patients with nonspecific aortoarteritis (Takayasu's arteritis). AJR. 1996;167:1321-5.
79. Keser G, Direskeneli H, Aksu K. Management of Takayasu arteritis: a systematic review. Rheumatology (Oxford). 2014;53:793-801.
80. Liang P, Tan-Ong M, Hoffman GS. Takayasu's arteritis: vascular interventions and outcomes. J Rheumatol. 2004;31:102-6
81. Hedgire SS, McDermott S, Borczuk D, et al. The spectrum of IgG4-related disease in the abdomen and pelvis. Am J Roentgenol. 2013;201:14-22.
82. Stone JH, Zen Y, Deshpande V. IgG4-related disease. N Engl J Med. 2012;366:539-51.
83. Kasashima S, Zen Y, Kawashima A, et al. Inflammatory abdominal aortic aneurysm: close relationship to IgG4-related periaortitis. Am J Surg Pathol. 2008;32:197-204.
84. Kasashima S, Zen Y. IgG4. IgG4-related inflammatory abdominal aortic aneurysm. Curr Opin Rheumatol. 2011;23:18-23.
85. Wintermark M, Wicky S, Schnyder P. Imaging of acute traumatic injuries of thoracic aorta. Eur Radiol. 2002;12:431-42.
86. Gavant ML. Helical CT grading of traumatic aortic injuries. RCNA. 1999;37:553-70.
87. Lipchick EO, Rogoff SM. The abnormal abdominal aorta: Arteriosclerosis and other diseases. In: Abrahams HL Little (Ed). Brown and Company, Boston. 1983;2:1057-78.
88. Sawhney R, Kerlan RR, Wall SD. Analysis of initial CT findings after endovascular repair of abdominal aortic aneurysms. Radiology. 2001;220:157-60.

CHAPTER 184

Imaging in Pulmonary Vascular Disease

Ujjwal Gorsi, Sanjeev Kumar, Kushaljit Singh Sodhi, Akshay Kumar Saxena

Pulmonary vascular diseases incorporate a large and distinctive group of pathologies which range from pulmonary thromboembolism to congenital malformations to vasculitides. The patient suffering from diseases of pulmonary vascular system can have a dramatic and acute onset of symptoms such as chest pain and dyspnea or an insidious onset and chronic course with symptoms ranging from fatigue, hypoxia dyspnea on exertion, and right heart failure.[1]

Imaging modalities available to evaluate diseases of the pulmonary vasculature include chest radiography (CXR), computed tomography (CT), magnetic resonance imaging (MRI), nuclear scintigraphy and transthoracic echocardiography (TIE).

ANATOMY

The pulmonary arteries carry deoxygenated blood from right ventricle to lungs and is primary circulation of the lungs other being bronchial circulation. Pulmonary arteries are low pressure system. The main pulmonary artery originates from the right ventricular (RV) outflow tract and divides into right and left branches before exiting the pericardium. Right and left pulmonary arteries give rise to lobar arteries and lobar arteries further divide into segmental and subsegmental arteries **(Figs. 1A and B)**.

The pulmonary veins are four in number: the right and left superior pulmonary veins and right and left inferior pulmonary veins in up to 70% individuals. Pulmonary veins bring oxygenated blood from lungs into

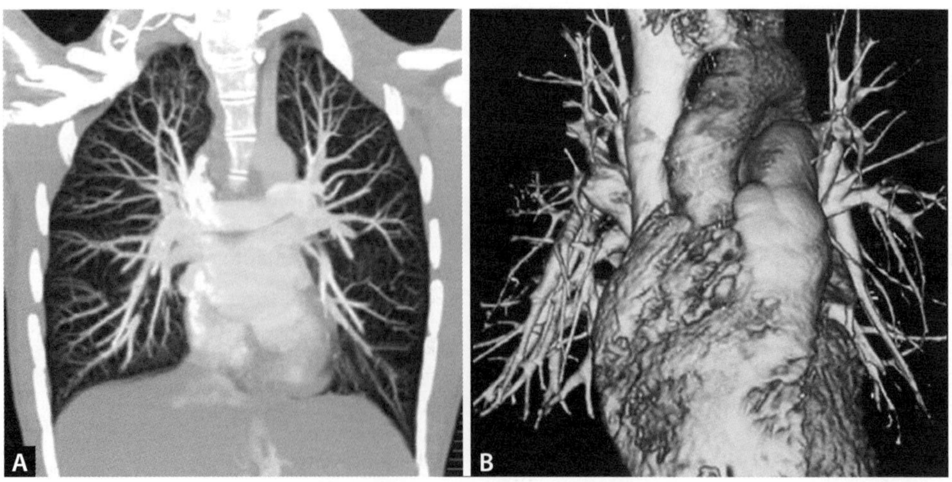

Figs. 1A and B: Normal pulmonary vasculature demonstrated on 64-row MDCT scanner. Coronal reconstruction using (A) maximum intensity projection and (B) volume-rendered technique demonstrate even the most peripheral pulmonary vessels with exquisite detail.

left atrium. Right upper and middle lobes are drained by right superior pulmonary vein whereas left upper lobe and lingula are drained by left superior pulmonary vein. The lower lobes are drained by inferior pulmonary veins. Anatomic variations are seen in approximately 38% of the population.[2] On left side, a common trunk may be present which is formed by the union of superior and inferior pulmonary veins. On right side, atypical anatomic pattern is less common. Single or multiple accessory veins may be present with independent drainage in to left atrium. The central portions of the pulmonary veins which open into the left atrium are intra pericardial.[2]

ACUTE PULMONARY EMBOLISM

Following coronary artery disease and stroke, pulmonary embolism (PE) is the third most common acute cardiovascular event disease.[3] PE commonly is the result of migration of deep vein thrombus from the lower limb veins. Diagnosis of acute pulmonary thromboembolism (PTE) has to be accurate and rapid as if left untreated outcome is dismal and needless treatment is associated with considerable morbidity. For both DVT and acute PE an annual incidence of 100–200 per 100,000 inhabitants has been reported.[4]

Clinical features of acute PE are nonspecific and often deceptive. It may remain asymptomatic or its first presentation can be sudden cardiac death. Hence imaging plays leading role in evaluation of patients suspected of having PE.

Massive PE is indicated by sustained systemic hypotension (systolic arterial pressure <90 mmHg for at least 15 minutes which is not due to cause other than PE) symptoms and signs of shock and chest pain.[5] Clinical scores such as Wells[6] and Geneva scores[7] are important scores which allows assessment of clinical pre-test probability of acute PE. Electrocardiography (ECG), D-dimer, chest radiograph and compression ultrasound of lower limbs are the initial investigations. D-dimer has a high sensitivity and very high negative predictive value and is raised in venous thromboembolism. It is considered the most important laboratory screening test for PTE. Ninety percent of PE originate from DVT in a lower limb.[8] For symptomatic DVT, compression ultrasound of veins of lower limb has a high sensitivity (>90%) and specificity (95%).[4]

If a diagnosis of PE is suspected based on clinical findings and evaluation of D-dimer, in patients with symptoms and signs of DVT, compression ultrasound is indicated specially in pregnant patient with suspected PE.[5] Patients suspected of PE, in whom compression USG shows thrombus in lower limb veins, can be started on anticoagulant treatment without further testing.[9]

Imaging Techniques

Chest Radiography

Chest radiography is useful to exclude other causes of acute chest pain when acute PE is suspected. It is important to exclude pneumonia, pneumothorax, pericardial effusion aortic dissection, and free intraperitoneal air as symptoms because of these entities may mimic those due to PE. In addition ventilation perfusion scan interpretation is dependent on whether the chest radiograph is normal or abnormal.[10]

Although chest radiograph is the first investigation performed in patients of suspected pulmonary embolism, unfortunately the radiographic features of acute pulmonary embolism are rather nonspecific. Findings which may be seen are Hampton hump (peripheral, wedge-shaped consolidation with a rounded medial margin representing infarct), Westermark sign (oligemia of lung beyond the occluded vessel), Fleischner sign (prominent central pulmonary artery) plate like atelectasis, small pleural effusion and elevated ipsilateral hemidiaphragm **(Fig. 2)**.[11] Not all patients with PTE have positive finding on chest X-ray. Normal chest skiagrams have been reported in the presence of PTE in 12–30% of patients.

Echocardiography

Echocardiography is important as it can exclude significant abnormalities like right ventricular dysfunction.

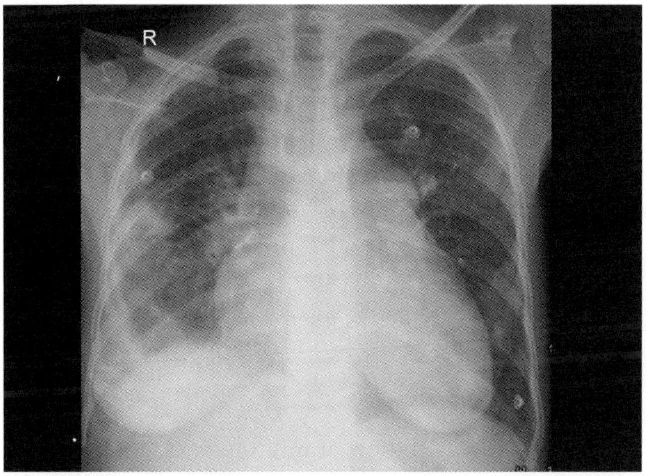

Fig. 2: Acute PE: Dilated central pulmonary artery with dilated right descending pulmonary artery proximally and acute cut-off. Dilated right-sided pleural effusion with peripheral wedge-shaped opacity in right middle zone symptoms of infarct.

Thrombolytic therapy is often recommended for the patients who are hemodynamically stable and who have right ventricular dysfunction on echocardiography. In addition associated right atrial and right ventricular thrombus may also be diagnosed with echocardiography. It also estimates pulmonary artery pressure thus guiding the management in these patients. Transesophageal echocardiography can demonstrate pulmonary arteries better than TTE. Though it is invasive. TEE can directly visualize thrombus in right pulmonary artery.

CT Angiography

CT pulmonary angiography is standard for diagnosis of PE as it is accurate, safe and can be performed rapidly. It has replaced catheter angiography for diagnosing PE.[10] It is considered the best imaging modality for those with intermediate or high clinical risk for acute PE and those with abnormal D-dimer values. PIOPED II (Prospective Investigation of Pulmonary Embolism Diagnosis) studied the accuracy of CTPA with V/Q and conventional pulmonary angiography. Sensitivity of 83% and specificity of 96% was shown in patients with a high pretest probability[12] of PE.[12] However scanners used in 4-, 8-, and 16-row scanners used in the PIOPED II study were 4-, 8-.or 16- row scanners, with rapid evolution of multidetector computed tomography (MDCT) even greater accuracy is achieved. Another advantage of CTPA is ability to detect alternative causes for clinical symptoms mimicking PE[1] unlike V/Q scan and catheter angiography.

For CTPA 80 to 100 mL of nonionic iodinated contrast is injected intravenously at a rate of 4 mL/s from an antecubital vein. To time optimal contrast delivery to the pulmonary vessels at the time of imaging, test bolus and automated bolus tracking techniques are very helpful. Test bolus technique is especially useful in patients who have delayed opacification of the pulmonary arteries due to poor cardiac function. Although, caudal to cranial scanning is often used to reduce effect of respiratory motion at the lung bases where more emboli are seen and more diaphragmatic motion occurs, the availability of ultrafast MDCT usually obviates this modification. Thin collimation allows is volumetric 1-mm slice reconstruction helping in multiplanar reconstructions and detailed analysis.[1]

Dual-Energy CT

With the implementation of multidetector CT scanners with two X-ray tubes (dual-source CT) and a single tube with two focal spots (dual-energy), both iodinated contrast material-enhanced and soft-tissue images from a single imaging examination can be obtained. This feature is useful in PE imaging as the area of perfused lung can be directly assessed and quantified in addition to the standard documentation of clot burden and presence of right heart strain.[13]

Dual-energy CT (DECT) permits functional data on lung perfusion (iodine distribution maps/lung perfusion blood volume [PBV] images). Which can quantitatively assess regional iodine density, a marker for pulmonary perfusion, and can be correlated to V/QSCAN or single photon-emission computed tomography (SPECT) V/QSCAN.[5,14] The diagnostic accuracy of iodine maps for occlusive acute PE is high but this is not the case for non-occlusive disease.[14] In addition dual-energy CT techniques has the potential to reduce contrast dose without compromising diagnostic capabilities.[15] Spectral CT can also be used to reduce both the iodine load and radiation dose to the patient. As shown by Szucs- Farkas et al. using a contrast injection of 75 mL (300 mg iodine per milliliter) and 80 kVp, images which were obtained were found to be equivalent to the standard dose of 100 mL (300 mg iodine per milliliter) and standard 100 kVp for diagnosing PE. The radiation dose was significantly less with this protocol (6.8 mSv for 100 kVp and 4.8 mSv for 80 kVp).[16]

Ventilation/Perfusion Scan

A ventilation/perfusion scan (V/Q scan) analyzes both the pulmonary blood flow and alveolar ventilation and is interpreted in correlation with a chest radiograph. It is an alternative test for patients who cannot undergo CTPA. The ability to detect PE on a V/Q scan can be improved by the addition of single-photon emission computed tomography imaging (SPECT imaging), which provides cross-sectional imaging of the lungs.[17] V/Q scans assess for perfusion defects without matched ventilation defects, the combination of which is suggestive of PE. V/Q scans are reported as normal, very low probability, low probability, intermediate probability, and high probability, on the basis of the number and sizes of unmatched defects as well as in correlation with the chest radiograph **(Figs. 3A and B)**. A normal V/Q scan indicates that chances of PE is <5% where as s high-probability V/Q scan indicates that chance of PE is >90%[18] where as the pretest probability of PE being present does not change with intermediate probability scan. In pregnant women, V/Q scan may be preferred rather than CTPA. The American Thoracic Society and the Society of Thoracic Radiology recommends that for pregnant women in whom PE is suspected but whose chest radiograph is normal, the V/Q scan should be performed. However, CTPA is to be carried out rather than a V/Q scan if abnormality is detected on chest radiograph.[19]

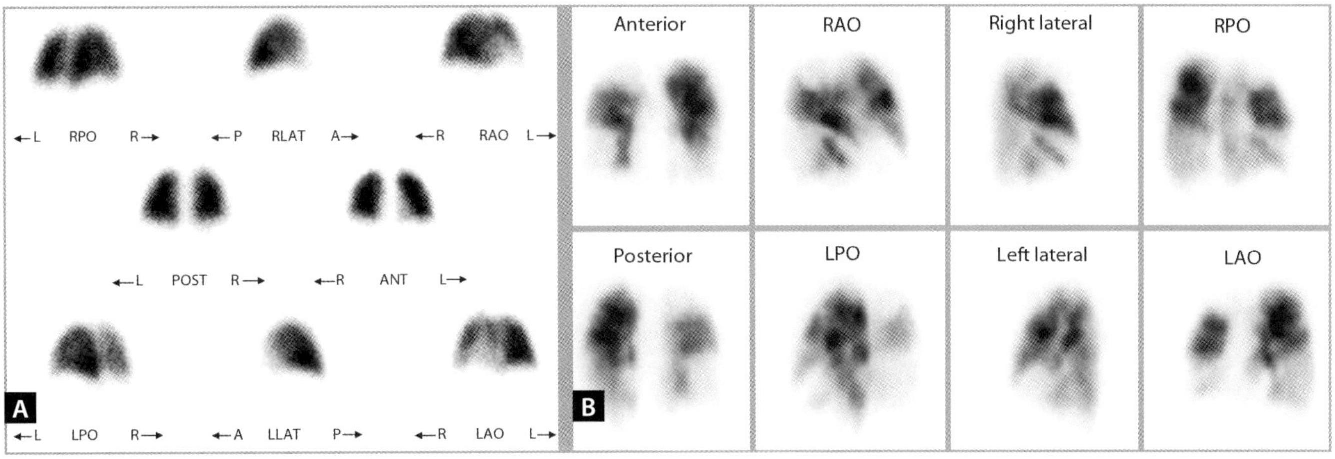

Figs. 3A and B: (A) Lung perfusion scan shows normal perfusion pattern; (B) Lung perfusion scan in another patient shows multiple large perfusion defects in both lungs, suggesting a high probability for pulmonary embolism.

Magnetic Resonance Imaging

MRI has undergone significant technical improvement with large coverage, faster sequences, and ability to perform high-resolution MR pulmonary angiography (MRPA), lung perfusion imaging and functional studies. MRPA consists of a three-dimensional (3D) heavily weighted-T1 gradient echo MRI sequences acquired during first-pass perfusion following intravenous injection of gadolinium via an injector pump to visualize the pulmonary arteries. Noncontrast-enhanced MRPA can be performed using SSFP free-breathing real-time imaging technique with additional navigator-gating, which is used to obtain the images in the same phase without the need for breath-hold[20] **(Figs. 4A to D)** In acute PE MRPA is not routinely used as CTPA is used routinely. PIOPED III study showed that a sensitivity of 78% and a specificity of 99% was achieved with MRPA when the studies were technically adequate a sensitivity of 92% and a specificity of 96% was shown when MRPA was performed along with MR venography. However, technically inadequate results were present in 52% of patients in this study. Conclusion from the study was that that MRPA should be considered only for patients for whom standard tests are contraindicated and only in those centers that routinely perform this study.[21]

Digital Subtraction Angiography

For the diagnosis of acute PE, CT angiography has largely replaced catheter angiography. Similar results are achiever with CTPA without the complications of catheter angiography noninvasively. Filling defect within main pulmonary arteries or their branches arteries or cut-off of a pulmonary artery branch is most accepted diagnostic sign of PTE[10] **(Fig. 5)**. Catheter angiography is now used only for therapeutic purposes including thrombolysis in setting of acute PE.

Imaging Features of Acute PE

CTPA is most common imaging modality used to image acute PE. Findings of acute PE on CTPA are described below though imaging features are similar on all angiographic studies.

Vascular Features

CTPA shows intravascular acute emboli with complete or partial vascular obstruction. In complete obstruction, the lumen is entirely occupied by thromboembolic material. Calibre of the vessel at the level of obstruction is either normal or enlarged as compared to chronic PTE **(Fig. 6)** In partial obstruction intraluminal central or eccentric filling defect are seen surrounded by contrast **(Figs. 7 and 8)**. The morphology of emboli varies according to whether the vessel is imaged in short axis ("rim" or "polo mint" sign) **(Fig. 9)** or long axis ("railway track" sign).[5] When analyzing small segmental branches for presence of emboli, in order to prevent obscuration of emboli by dense iodinated contrast, such window and level values should be chosen so that right heart structures such as trabeculations are visible.[1]

Parenchymal Features

Complete occlusion of the artery causes the complete loss of perfusion with distal infarct which manifest as triangular subpleural consolidation or ground-glass opacity with fine reticular areas **(Fig. 10)**. When obstruction is partial, there is reduced flow rate (oligemia) which causes nonuniform

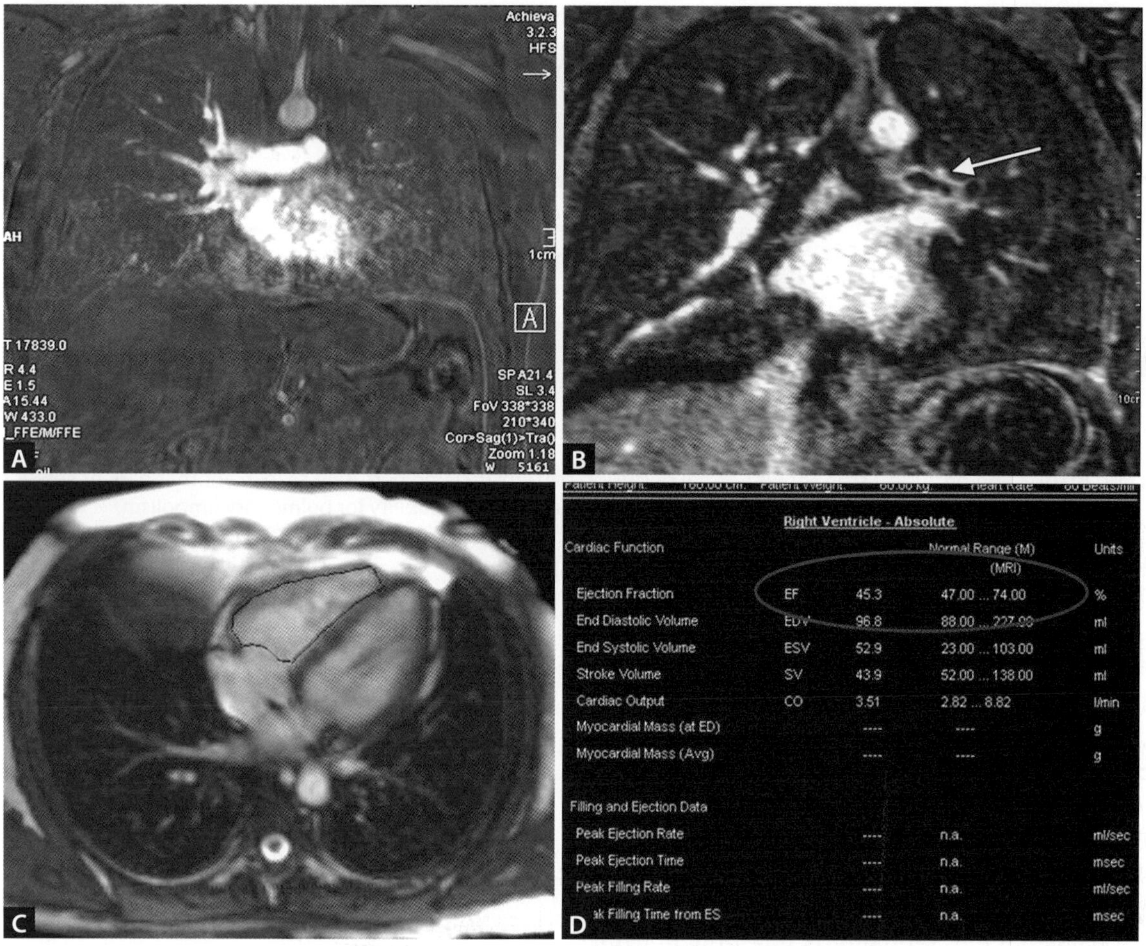

Figs. 4A to D: Acute pulmonary embolism: Coronal MRA images (A and B) showing acute thrombus in left pulmonary artery(arrow in B) with normal right pulmonary artery; (C) Cine steady-state free precession (SSFP) static image—calculation of RV function; (D) Argus values showing RV dysfunction with decreased EF (EF 43.55%) and mild strain.

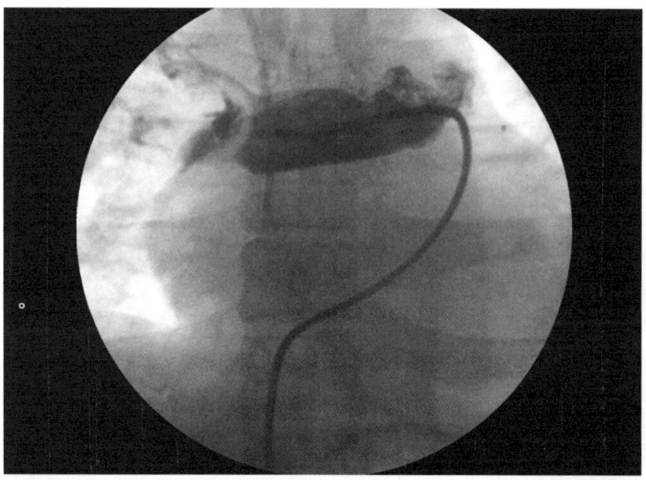

Fig. 5: Acute pulmonary embolism (PE): Catheter angiography of pulmonary artery confirming the filling defect in the right pulmonary artery typically forming concave margin suggestive of acute pulmonary embolism.

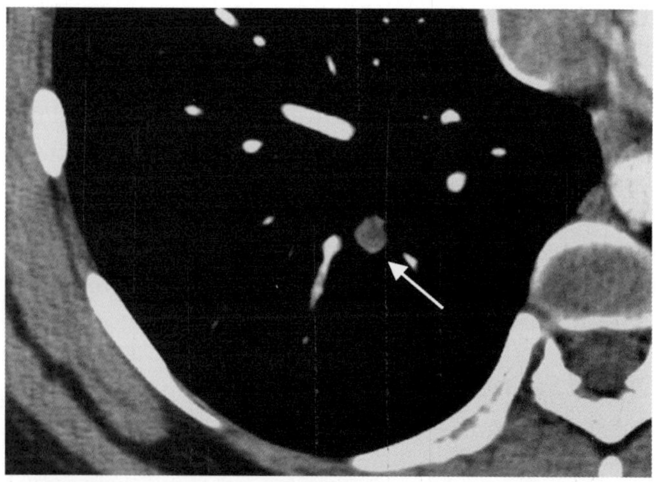

Fig. 6: Acute PE with complete obstruction. CTPA shows complete luminal occlusion with expanded vessel (arrow).

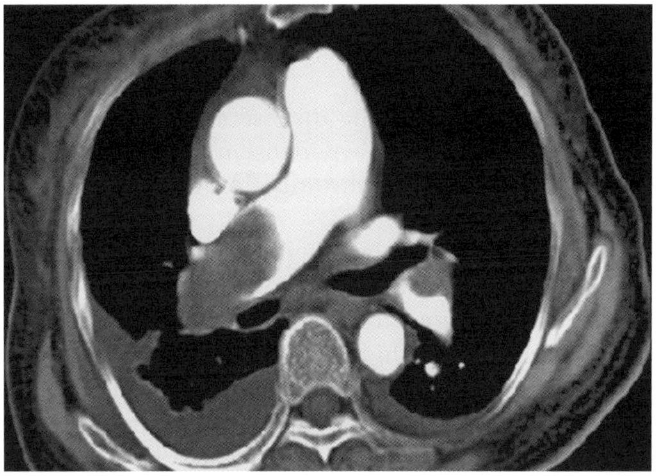

Fig. 7: Acute PE with partial obstruction: CTPA revealing filling defects in the right main pulmonary artery and left lower pulmonary artery branch with expansion of lumen symptoms of acute thrombus, as well as bilateral pleural effusion.

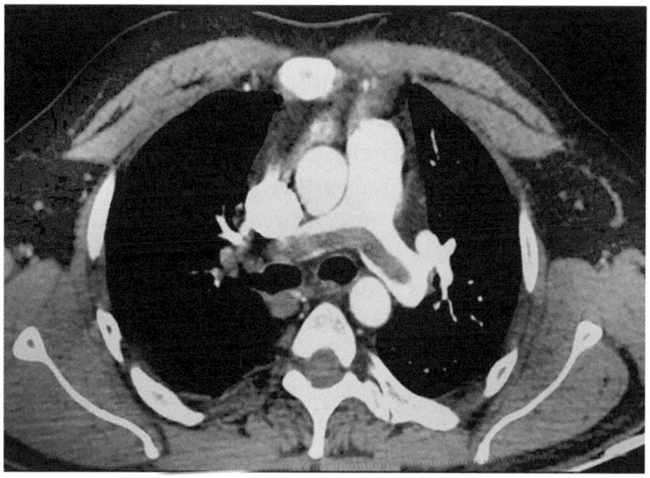

Fig. 8: Acute saddle pulmonary embolism: CTPA revealing a large pulmonary embolism that straddles the bifurcation of the pulmonary trunk extending into left and right pulmonary arteries.

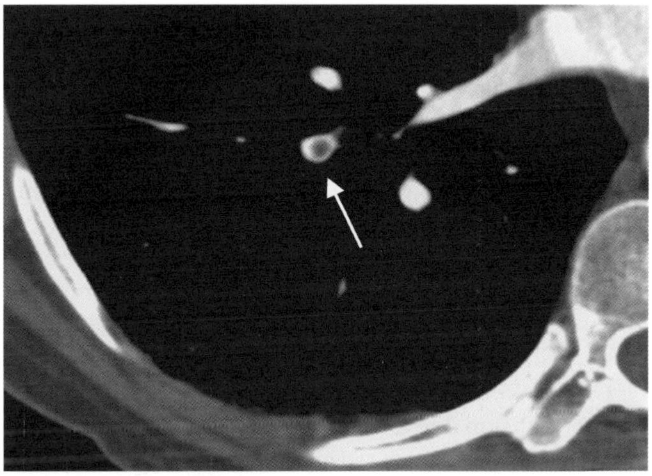

Fig. 9: Acute PE: Central filing defect in one of the branch of right lower lobar pulmonary artery (arrow) with contrast in periphery called as polo mint sign.

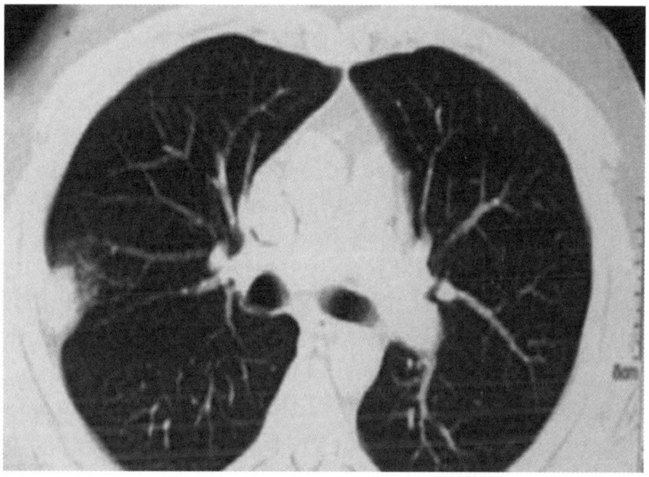

Fig. 10: Pulmonary infarct: CECT chest in a patient of acute PE shows characteristic peripheral wedge-shaped infarct.

arterial perfusion of the lung parenchyma with reduced vessel diameter patchy areas of low attenuation on CT or low signal on MRI (mosaic attenuation pattern). Atelectasis and pleural effusion may also be seen.

Cardiac Features

In acute PE, RV after load is rapidly increased as a result of obstruction to pulmonary arterial flow and the increase in PVR. Features of RV after load include dilatation of the right ventricle, bowing of the interventricular septum, dilatation of superior and inferior vena cava, dilatation of azygos vein, dilatation and reflux of contrast in the inferior vena cava and hepatic veins may also be present. Right ventricle dilatation is assessed commonly by RV/left ventricle (LV) ratio which can be calculated either on axial images or on a multiplanar reformatted four-chamber view. If the RV/LV ratio is >1.0 (on axial CT images) or >0.9 (on four-chamber view), RV dysfunction is suggetsted.[22] Artifacts that can limit assessment for acute PE on CTPA include flow artifacts which appear as transient interruption of the contrast column, image noise, motion and respiratory artifacts and partial volume averaging with surrounding structures.[1]

Non-thrombotic causes of PE are best evaluated with CT. These are rare as compared to venous thrombo-embolism. And include septic emboli, fat emboli, tumor emboli, venous air embolism, talc and cement embolism. Septic emboli contain microorganisms and appear as cavitatory nodules usually multiple and bilateral. Tumor emboli expand the involved pulmonary arteries if smaller they may appear as patchy ground-glass opacity, or as tree-in-bud appearance. Hepatocellular carcinoma, renal cancer, prostate cancer, breast cancer and gastric malignancy are known for producing tumor emboli.

Cement emboli is embolism of polymethyl methacrylate, which can enter the external venous plexuses during vertebroplasty. Branching tubular hyperattenuating opacities are seen on radiography and CT. Talc embolism can happen in patients who grind and inject oral medications, such as amphetamines into their veins.[17]

CHRONIC THROMBOEMBOLIC DISEASE

Chronic thromboembolic disease (CTED) results due to incomplete resolution and recanalization of acute emboli. There occurs organization and endothelialization of thromboembolic material which may appear as laminated thrombi, single bands parallel to the vessel (shelves) or complex web-like network as well as complete vascular occlusions. The pathophysiological basis explaining transition from acute to chronic thromboembolism is uncertain; however, failed thrombolysis, a localized inflammatory response and localized endothelial dysfunction are thought to be responsible.[23] CTED can occur without or with chronic thromboembolic pulmonary hypertension (CTEPH). CTEPH shares many of the imaging features with other etiologies of pulmonary hypertension along with few features specific to chronic PTE. Imaging features of chronic PTE will be discussed in the section of pulmonary hypertension.

PULMONARY HYPERTENSION

Pulmonary hypertension (PH) is defined as a mean pulmonary artery pressure (mPAP) of 25 mmHg or greater on right heart catheterization. A resting mean pulmonary arterial pressure of 20 mmHg or less is normal. Symptoms of PH vary greatly and are nonspecific. Dyspnea, syncope, and fatigue can be clinical manifestation of pulmonary hypertension. Right ventricular failure and subsequent death may be the consequence of untreated pulmonary hypertension.[24]

Classification

Pulmonary hypertension has been classified into following five groups by the World Health Organization (WHO) based upon etiology.[25]

- *Group 1:* Pulmonary arterial hypertension (PAH)
- *Group 2:* Pulmonary hypertension which is secondary to to left heart disease
- *Group 3:* Chronic lung disease and/or hypoxemia leading to pulmonary hypertension
- *Group 4:* Chronic thromboembolic pulmonary hypertension
- *Group 5:* Pulmonary hypertension secondary to multifactorial mechanisms or unknown etiology

Causes of pulmonary arterial hypertension in Group 1 to 5.

- *Group 1:* Idiopathic PAH, heritable PAH, drug-induced PAH, PAH associated with CTD, HIV, portal hypertension, CHD and schistosomiasis.
  Pulmonary veno-occlusive disease (PVOD) and pulmonary capillary hemangiomatosis (PCH) are included in 1′ and persistent pulmonary hypertension of the newborn (PPHN) is designated as 1″ because these entities have unique features which are different from other causes of PAH.
- *Group 2:* Valvular heart diseases, LV systolic and diastolic dysfunction and cardiomyopathies may lead to pulmonary hypertension and they are included in this group.
- *Group 3:* Lung diseases like COPD, ILD, chronic exposure to high altitude and few developmental lung diseases may lead to pulmonary hypertension. PH secondary to these diseases is included in this group.
- *Group 4:* Chronic thromboembolic disease may be associated with pulmonary hypertension (CTPEH). PH secondary to chronic PE is included in group 4.
- *Group 5:* This group comprises pulmonary hypertension due to varied etiologies. PH secondary to hematologic disorders (myeloproliferative disorders, splenectomy), systemic disorders (sarcoidosis, pulmonary Langerhans cell histiocytosis), metabolic disorders (glycogen storage disease, Gaucher disease, thyroid disorders), and other disorders (tumoral obstruction, fibrosing mediastinitis, chronic renal failure in patients undergoing dialysis) are included in this group.

Imaging Modalities

Imaging examinations that are useful in assessing of PH include chest radiography, transthoracic echocardiogram, CT/CTPA, MRI/MRA, ventilation perfusion scan and right heart catheterization. Many imaging features of PH are common irrespective of the etiologies on all imaging modalities which shall be discussed first. It will be followed by description of few features which are specific to a particular etiology.

Chest Radiography

As the symptoms and signs of PH are non-specific, chest radiography is usually the first imaging requested. In early course of the disease, chest radiography is usually normal but in advanced stage radiograph may show classic features of PH which include dilatation of central pulmonary arteries, dilated (15 mm in women and 16 mm in men) right interlobar artery, pruning of the peripheral arteries **(Fig. 11)**. On lateral radiograph, reduced retrosternal air space is easily appreciated which happens due to dilatation of right ventricle.[26] Radiograph may also show some of the causes of pulmonary hypertension, e.g. interstitial lung disease, emphysema and left-sided heart disease.

Transthoracic Echocardiogram

Transthoracic Doppler echocardiography is an investigation which is carried out routinely in patients suspected of having PH. Transthoracic Doppler echocardiogram can reveal the systolic pulmonary artery pressure. In patients with mild PH its accuracy and reliability is less.[17]

CT Pulmonary Angiography

The classic CTPA findings of pulmonary hypertension may be divided into three categories: Vascular, parenchymal and cardiac signs.

Vascular signs

Main pulmonary artery is assessed at the level of its bifurcation, orthogonal to its long axis on axial sections. Sensitivity of 87%, specificity of 89% and positive predictive value of 97%, is achieved for the presence of pulmonary hypertension with a pulmonary artery diameter of 29 mm or more.[27] A segmental artery-to-bronchus diameter ratio of 1:1 or more in three or four lobes has a specificity of 100% for the presence of pulmonary hypertension.[27] A main pulmonary arterial diameter greater than that of the ascending aorta is also signifies presence of PH. This sign has a positive predictive value of 96% and specificity of 92%, especially in young patients who are less than 50 years old **(Fig. 12)**.[28]

Parenchymal signs

Both lungs may show peripheral oligemia with areas of mosaic attenuation **(Fig. 13)**. Idiopathic pulmonary arterial hypertension[28] and pulmonary capillary hemangiomatosis may show centrilobular ground-glass nodules. Neovascularity is regarded as a manifestation of severe pulmonary hypertension.[29]

Cardiac signs

Findings of adaptation of right ventricle as well as its failure may be appreciated. These include right ventricular hypertrophy, (wall thickness of more than 4 mm), straightening or leftward bowing of the interventricular septum, right ventricular dilatation **(Fig. 14)**, decreased right ventricular ejection fraction; dilatation of the inferior vena cava and hepatic veins; and pericardial effusion.[24,30]

Ventilation/Perfusion Scanning

Ventilation/perfusion (V/Q) scanning is used as a screening in patients with pulmonary hypertension. Its

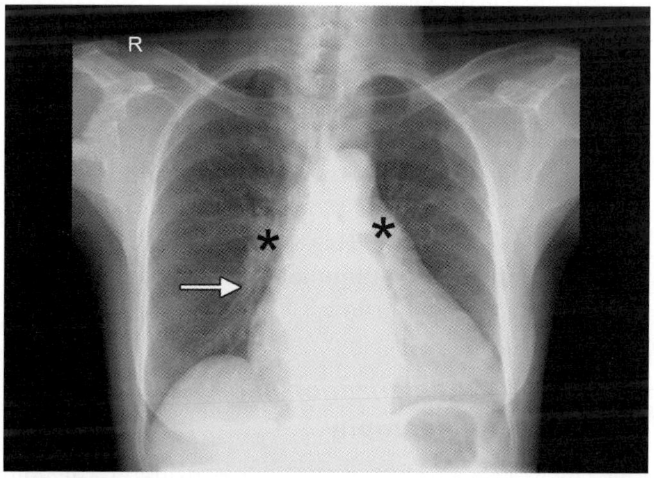

Fig. 11: Pulmonary hypertension: Posteroanterior chest radiograph showing dilated pulmonary arteries (stars), cardiomegaly, and rapid tapering (pruning) of right pulmonary artery (arrow). In addition, there is a decrease in the pulmonary vasculature in the periphery of the lung.

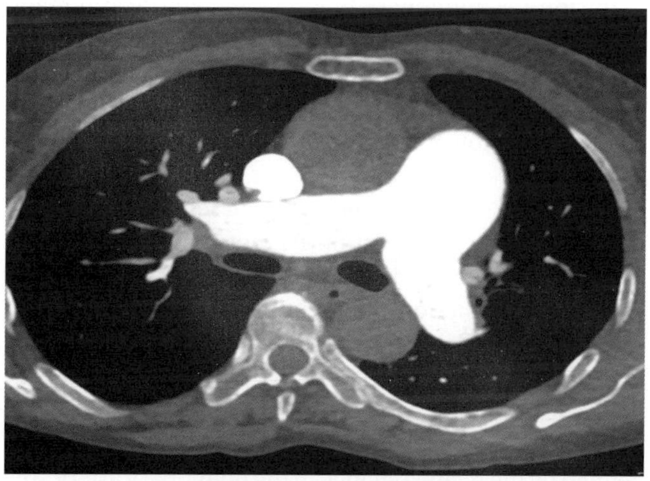

Fig. 12: Pulmonary hypertension: Pulmonary CT angiogram axial view shows dilated main, right and left pulmonary arteries consistent with the diagnosis of pulmonary hypertension.

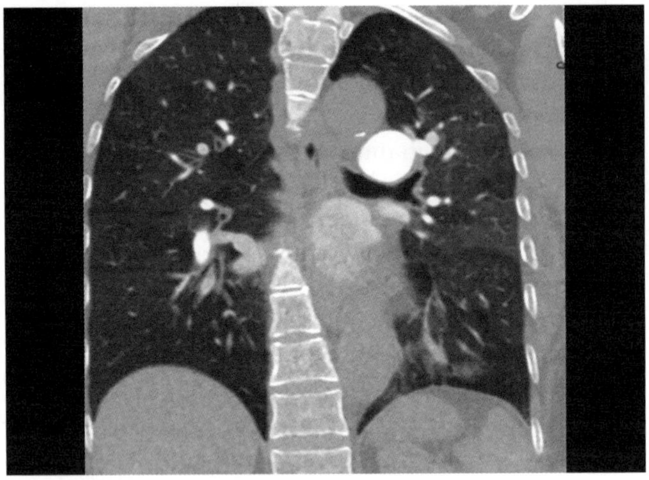

Fig. 13: Pulmonary hypertension: MDCT chest with coronal lung window showing multifocal areas of mosaic attenuation in bilateral lungs with peripheral oligemia.

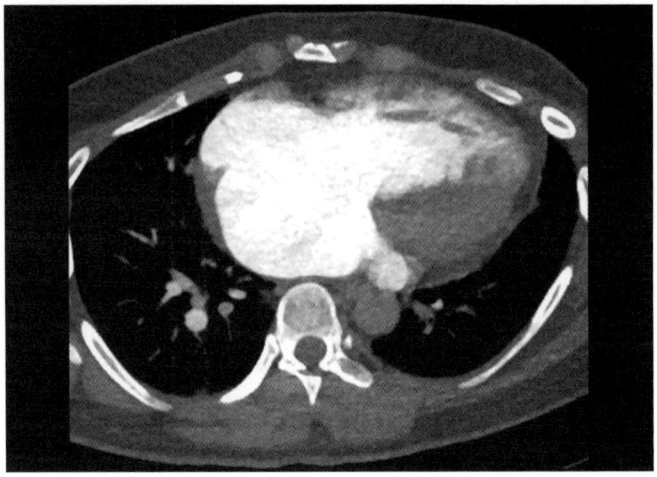

Fig. 14: Pulmonary hypertension: Contrast-enhanced computed tomography (CECT) chest shows cardiomegaly with dilatation of right atrium and right ventricle.

primary role is to identify patients with CTEPH. Sensitivity of >96% and specificity of >90% is noted when scan is interpreted according to modified PIOPED (Prospective Investigation of Pulmonary Embolism Diagnosis) criteria. If the V/Q scan is normal or of low probability CTEPH can be excluded with a sensitivity of 90–100% and specificity of 94–100%.[31]

Cardiac MRI and Pulmonary MRA

Advantage of MR imaging, relative to other imaging modalities is ability to assess both anatomy and function. This is accomplished by MR angiography (MRA) sequences for pulmonary artery anatomy, MR flow sequences and perfusion for pulmonary blood flow quantification, and cardiac MR imaging sequences for cardiac morphology and function. Morphologic findings of PH are demonstrated by pulmonary MRA and cardiac MRI. These features include dilatation of central pulmonary arteries, pruning of peripheral vessels, right ventricular hypertrophy, dilation of right ventricle and straightening or leftward bowing of the interventricular septum. Patients who have PH are followed with MRI and MRA so that early changes of right ventricle dysfunction may be picked before becoming clinical significant. MRA and MR perfusion may be used to diagnose CTEPH.[24,32,33] MRI can assess reduced pulmonary artery dispensability and heterogeneous flow in the main pulmonary artery. Pulmonary artery dispensability, as defined by the relative change in the pulmonary artery area throughout the cardiac cycle may be decreased in PH and is associated with poor outcome in patients who have PH.[34]

Right ventricular size, function and wall motion can be assessed with MR cine imaging which is considered the gold standard for the same. Ventricular mass of both ventricles can be determined with cine imaging. These values are then used to calculate a ventricular mass index (right ventricular mass/left ventricular mass). A ventricular mass index which is >0.6 is considered compatible with PH.[24,35] Functional abnormalities which may result in a patient of PH include right ventricular hypokinesis and dysfunction, paradoxical movement of the interventricular septum, reduced ejection fraction and stroke volume and increased end-diastolic volume. MR imaging can demonstrate all these functional abnormalities.[24,33,34] Enhancement at the insertion points of the right ventricle into the interventricular septum is depicted by delayed contrast MRI. Flow sensitive MRI can quantify the severity of cardiac shunt (intra and extra).[24,36] Hemodynamic alterations such as abnormal proximal PA flow patterns, decreased wall shear stress, and increased tricuspid regurgitation velocities which develop in patients of PH can be assessed with 4-dimensional multidirectional flow MRI. An abnormal blood flow pattern which is characteristic present in PH is a vortex blood flow pattern in the proximal main pulmonary associated with early-onset systolic retrograde flow.[37-40]

Right Heart Catheterization and Pulmonary Angiography

Right heart catheterization (RHC) is considered the gold standard for the diagnosis of PAH. It is performed to confirm the diagnosis of PH and also helps in assessing the severity of PH.[24] Catheter pulmonary angiography is now used only if therapeutic procedure is planned.

Etiologies of Pulmonary Hypertension

There are many etiologies for pulmonary hypertension[25] as enumerated earlier. Few of these have specific imaging findings in addition to the findings compatible with PH discussed above and will be discussed.

Idiopathic pulmonary arterial hypertension: Idiopathic pulmonary arterial hypertension is most common in women than men.[17] Both chest radiography and CT will show features of pulmonary hypertension already described. Centrilobular ground-glass attenuation which surrounds the enlarged and tortuous centrilobular arteries is a typical finding and may be appreciated on CT.[41] Rarely, small centrilobular nodules may also be noticed. Mosaic attenuation may be seen however its subtle as compared to the chronic PE.[41] CT may show pericardial effusion which is usually small.

Systemic-to-pulmonary (left-to-right) shunts: Left-to-right shunts such as atrial septal defect, ventricular septal defect and patent ductus arteriosus, increase the blood flow to pulmonary arteries. When pulmonary vascular resistance is similar or exceeds systemic vascular resistance Eisenmenger syndrome results with bidirectional or reversed flow in shunt. Eisenmenger syndrome may be associated with dilatation of the central pulmonary artery which may be massive, *in situ* thrombus formation with calcification may be noticed in Eisenmenger syndrome.[24,42]

Pulmonary capillary hemangiomatosis and veno-occlusive disease: In PCH diffuse proliferation of capillaries occurs in the pulmonary interstitium with the obstruction of venules. CT in addition to features of pulmonary hypertension shows centrilobular ground-glass nodules, and interlobular septal thickening.[43] PVOD is caused by intimal fibrosis and thrombosis of pulmonary vein which leads to pulmonary venous hypertension followed by PH. CT will show pleural effusion and interlobular septal thickening in addition to enlarged pulmonary arteries. In PVOD, the left atrium is normal in size unlike left heart mitral valve disease. Mediastinal lymph node may be enlarged. Biopsy is required for the diagnosis of PCH and PVOD. Vasodilators are contraindicated in both of these diseases because they can precipitate pulmonary edema which may be fatal.[17,43]

PH associated with left heart disease: Mitral valve pathology can lead to PH. Reduced blood flow through the mitral valve backs up into the left atrium, and then into pulmonary veins followed by pulmonary arteries which results in PH. CT will show an enlarged left atrium, interlobular septal and an enlarged main pulmonary artery.[24]

Chronic thromboembolic disease: Not all the patients with acute PTE go on to develop hypertension. Approximately 4% of patients with acute pulmonary embolism develop chronic thromboembolic pulmonary hypertension. Patients with chronic thromboembolic pulmonary hypertension become symptomatic only when at least 60% of the pulmonary arterial bed is obstructed.[24] It is important to diagnose that chronic thromboembolic disease is a cause of pulmonary hypertension as it may be treated with pulmonary thromboendarterectomy. The CTPA findings of chronic thromboembolic pulmonary hypertension include parenchymal and vascular signs, which are highly suggestive of the cause. Vascular findings in CTEPH include complete obstruction, indicated by a tapered occluded vessel, eccentric narrowing of pulmonary arteries with segments of post-stenotic dilatation **(Fig. 15)**, partial filling defects, indicated by obtuse mural margins with the vessel wall **(Fig. 16)** partial filling defect, indicated by the presence of webs or bands and collateral systemic supply **(Fig. 17)**. Parenchymal findings in CTEPH include scars from prior pulmonary infarction mosaic pattern of perfusion, **(Figs. 18A and B)**, cylindrical bronchial airway dilatation and systemic perfusion of the peripheral pulmonary arterial bed.[24]

CTPA is useful modality in assessing whether patients are candidates for surgery or not. If the main, lobar, or

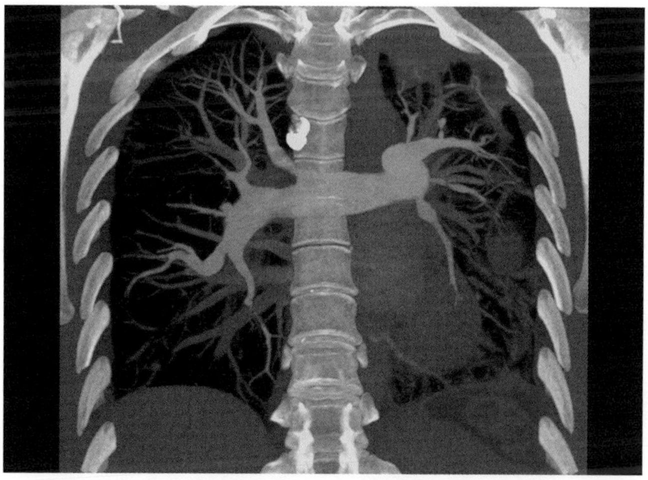

Fig. 15: Chronic thromboembolic pulmonary hypertension: CT pulmonary angiogram cornal reformatted image showing dilated central pulmonary arteries with eccentric narrowing of proximal right upper lobar pulmonary artery, posterior segmental branch of right lower, and left descending pulmonary artery with segment of post-stenotic dilatation (typical of chronic pulmonary thromboembolism), with relative oligemia in right middle and bilateral lower lobes.

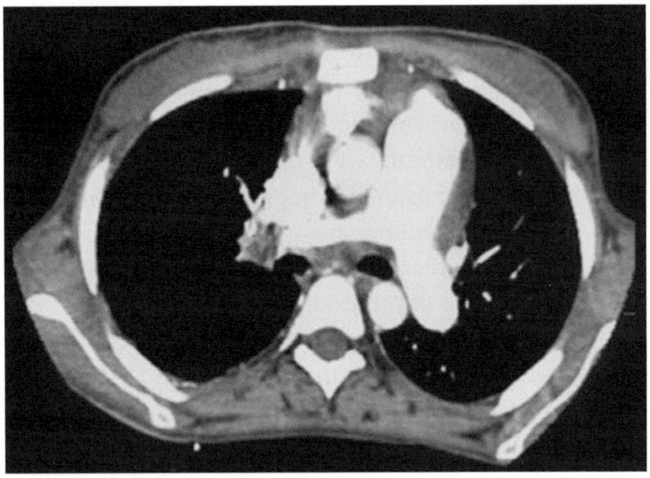

Fig. 16: Chronic pulmonary thromboembolism: Axial contrast-enhanced CT pulmonary angiography shows an attenuated right pulmonary artery with an eccentric thrombus, and irregular contours of intimal surface of main pulmonary artery and right pulmonary artery.

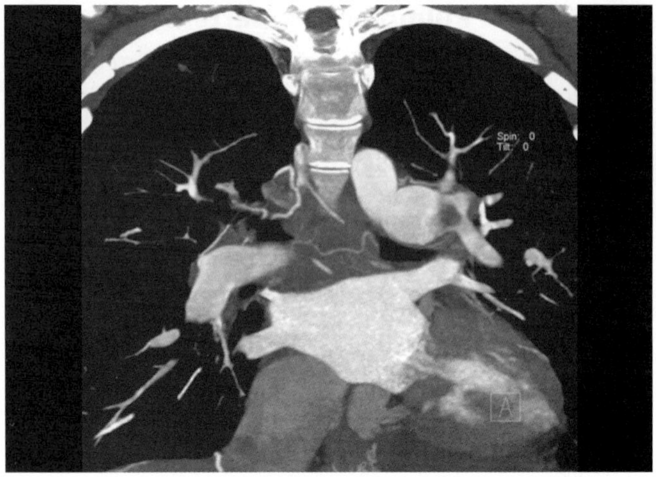

Fig. 17: Chronic pulmonary thrombolism: MDCT coronal reformation showing hypertrophied bronchial arteries.

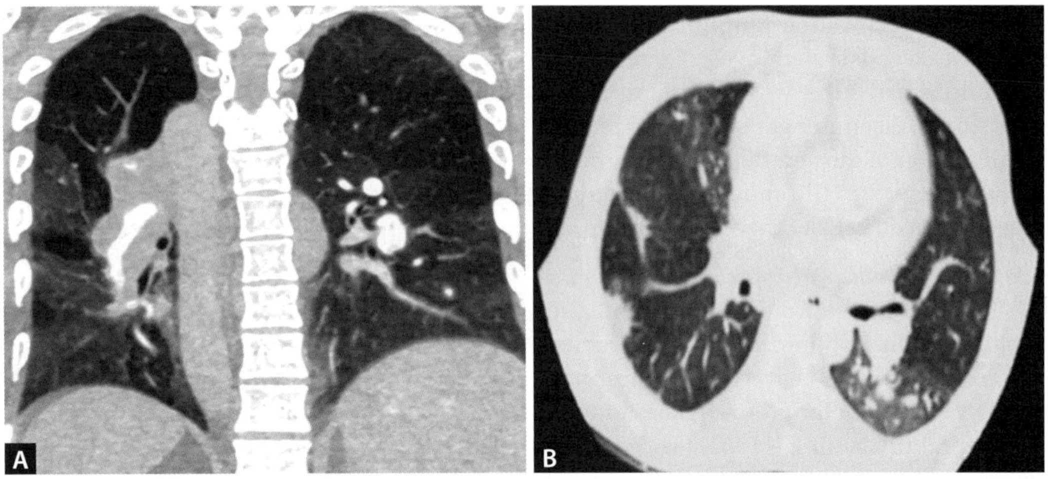

Figs. 18A and B: CT scan (lung window) in a case of chronic pulmonary thromboembolism shows (A) a mosaic perfusion pattern with wide regional variations in attenuation of the lung parenchyma and disparity in size of the segmental vessels. CT scan (B) in another patient shows mosaic attenuation with a peripheral parenchymal infarct and scar.

proximal segmental arteries are involved, patients are considered for resection whereas if distal segments are involved medical treatment is considered.

VASCULITIS

Vasculitides affecting the pulmonary arteries can be classified by the size of vessel that is involved. Takayasu arteritis and Behcet disease involve large-size vessels such as the aorta, arch branches, and central pulmonary arteries. Vasculitides that involve medium (visceral arteries) and small vessels (arterioles, capillaries, and venules) include granulomatosis with polyangiitis (GPA), antibasement membrane disease (Goodpasture disease, Churg-Strauss syndrome (CSS), and microscopic polyangiitis.[17]

Takayasu arteritis: Takayasu arteritis affect large elastic arteries. Young Asian women are most commonly affected. Disease usually involves aorta, arch branches. Involvement of pulmonary arteries may be seen in 50–80% of the patient population. In this disease, there is granulomatous inflammation of the arterial wall. Other histopathological features are proliferation of intima and fibrosis of the media and adventitia. These changes cause stenosis and occlusion of vessels, and may be associated with post-stenotic aneurysms. CT and MR show wall thickening of the aorta, aortic branches, and central pulmonary arteries early in the disease course **(Figs. 19A and B)** and stenosis, occlusion, and aneurysm formation later in the disease. Mural calcification can be seen on CT where as mural edema may be seen on MRI which is seen as high signal intensity on T2-weighted sequences on MR.[24,44]

Behçet disease: Behcet disease is a multisystemic vasculitis which presents with uveitis, oral and genital ulcerations, and involvement of multiple organ systems. In the lungs, it involves large, medium, and small vessels. The aorta is the most commonly involved vessel, followed by pulmonary vessels. CT and MRI may show wall thickening of the involved vessels. In addition, there is pulmonary aneurysm formation, which are usually multiple and bilateral. These aneurysms occur almost exclusively in men. Areas of focal vasculitis and infarction may be seen which appear as wedge-shaped or rounded peripheral areas of consolidation.[44,45]

PULMONARY ARTERY ANEURYSMS AND PSEUDOANEURYSMS

Pulmonary artery aneurysms and pseudoaneurysms are uncommon but can have catastrophic consequences.

True aneurysms: True aneurysms may be associated with connective tissue diseases such as Marfan's disease, Ehlers-Danlos syndrome, tuberous sclerosis, Behcet's disease and the Hughes-Stovin syndrome, in which both pulmonary artery aneurysms and pseudoaneurysms are seen that are typically central and at high-risk of spontaneous rupture. Some of the aneurysm can be idiopathic. Long-standing chronic thromboembolic pulmonary arterial hypertension, L-R shunts and pulmonary valve stenosis can cause dilatation of central pulmonary arteries which can be aneurysmal at times.[46,47]

Pseudoaneurysms: Pulmonary artery pseudoaneurysms are more common than true aneurysms. They may rupture spontaneously and require urgent management. They may be secondary to infections such as necrotizing pneumonia and tuberculosis (Rasmussen's aneurysms). Other etiologies include pulmonary arterial catheter trauma, e.g. Swan-Ganz catheters, septic pulmonary emboli, lung cancers and autoimmune vasculitides and penetrating trauma. Imaging findings of the underlying disease are usually apparent on radiograph and CT.[46,47] On plain chest radiography aneurysms and pseudoaneurysms may manifest as soft tissue nodule though they usually can not be diagnosed on radiography. On CECT, aneurysms and pseudoaneurysms show enhancement which matches the enhancement of adjacent pulmonary arterial branches **(Figs. 20A to C)**.[46,47]

PULMONARY ARTERIOVENOUS MALFORMATIONS

Pulmonary arteriovenous malformations (PAVMs) are arteriovenous (right-to-left) shunts between pulmonary artery and pulmonary vein with absence of intervening capillary bed. The site of shunt between the PA and PV is usually dilated and AVMs are more common in lower lung lobes. These can be congenital [e.g. in hereditary hemorrhagic telengectasia (HHT) syndrome] or acquired (e.g. traumatic, hepatopulmonary syndrome).[46,48] They can be solitary or multiple. Multiple bilateral AVMs are

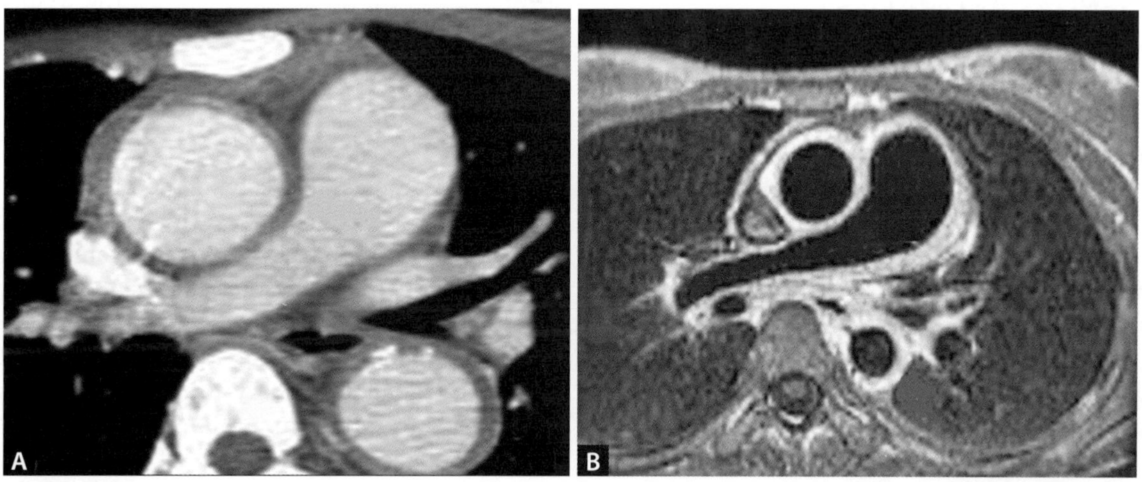

Figs. 19A and B: Takayasu arteritis—Involvement of aorta and pulmonary arteries: CT (A) shows thickening and enhancement of walls of aorta and pulmonary arteries. T2W MRI (B) shows thickening and edema of wall of aorta and pulmonary arteries.

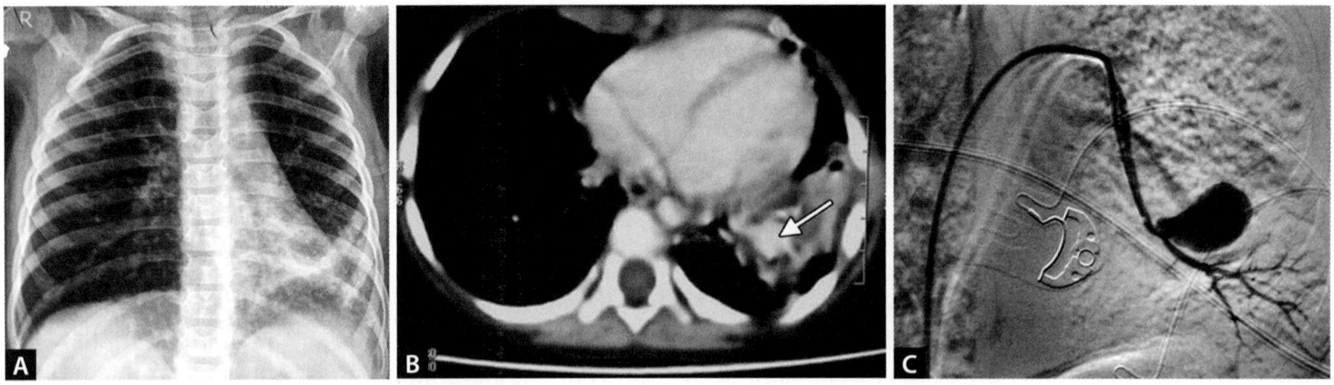

Figs. 20A to C: A four-year-child presented with fever and repeated episodes of hemoptysis. Radiograph (A) shows consolidation in left lower lobe . CECT chest (B) shows well-defined enhancing lesion (arrow) with in the necrotizing pneumonia consistent with the diagnosis of pseudoaneurysm. Catheter angiography of left lower lobar pulmonary artery (C) shows the pseudoaneurysm which was subsequently embolized using microcoils.

common in HHT syndrome. AVM can be simple when only a single feeder is present where as in complex AVMs, multiple feeding arteries are seen. Simple type of AVMs are commoner constituting 80–90% of pulmonary AVMs. Patients may be asymptomatic or may present with systemic oxygen desaturation, heart failure, ischemic or infectious emboli and hemorrhage (hemoptysis, hemothorax) due to rupture of the sac.[46,48]

On chest X-ray, AVM present as sharply defined lung nodules with one or more feeding artery and one or more draining vein.[46] CECT can demonstrate the number, size and site of these AVMs which is required before treatment by embolization **(Figs. 21A to E)**. Multiple bilateral AVMs are routinely found in HHT **(Figs. 22A and B)**. Catheter angiography is performed only for therapeutic purpose usually at the time of embolization.[46]

CONGENITAL ANOMALIES

A number of congenital anomalies can affect the pulmonary vasculature including proximal interruption of the pulmonary artery, pulmonary sling and partial anomalous pulmonary venous connection (PAPVC) syndrome. In proximal interruption of the pulmonary artery (right or left) is not present or terminates abruptly at the hilum. Collateral bronchial arteries supply the lung parenchyma. Cardiac defects are associated with interruption of the left pulmonary artery. Lateral chest radiograph will show the absence of the pulmonary artery and an ipsilateral small hemithorax. MRI/MRA or CT/CTPA will show these findings in details.[17,49] Pulmonary sling is formed when right pulmonary artery gives origin to left pulmonary artery which then courses between the trachea and the esophagus and supply the left lung. On chest radiography, the left pulmonary artery will appear as a nodular opacity posterior to the trachea. Both CT and MR will show the abnormal origin and the course of the left pulmonary artery.[17,49]

In PAPVC, an anomalous pulmonary vein drains into a systemic vein. On the left side, the left vertical vein will drain into either the left brachiocephalic vein or the coronary sinus. On the right side, an anomalous pulmonary vein may drain into coronary sinus, the azygos vein, superior vena cava or inferior vena cava. Scimitar syndrome refers to PAPVC to a systemic vein below the diaphragm, most commonly the inferior vena cava, which is associated with right pulmonary artery hypoplasia and a small right lung. Bronchial abnormalities, a horseshoe lung, sequestration, AVMs, and anomalous pulmonary systemic circulation may also be associated with scimitar syndrome. Radiography shows a tubular opacity adjacent to the right atrium coursing toward the diaphragm in scimitar syndrome, which is better depicted on CT and MRI **(Figs. 23A to C)**.[2]

MALIGNANT TUMORS

Malignant neoplasms involving the pulmonary include pulmonary artery sarcoma (PAS), metastases, and direct invasion of pulmonary arteries and veins by adjacent malignancy such as lung cancer. Metastatic disease is most commonly seen. PAS is rare and can be undifferentiated sarcoma or leiomyosarcoma. It usually involves the main and the proximal pulmonary arteries. PAS mimics PE and appears as an intraluminal filling defect on CTPA and MRA that spans the entire lumen of the pulmonary artery and often causes its expansion **(Figs. 24A and B)**. Lesions may enhance with contrast, but this may be difficult to

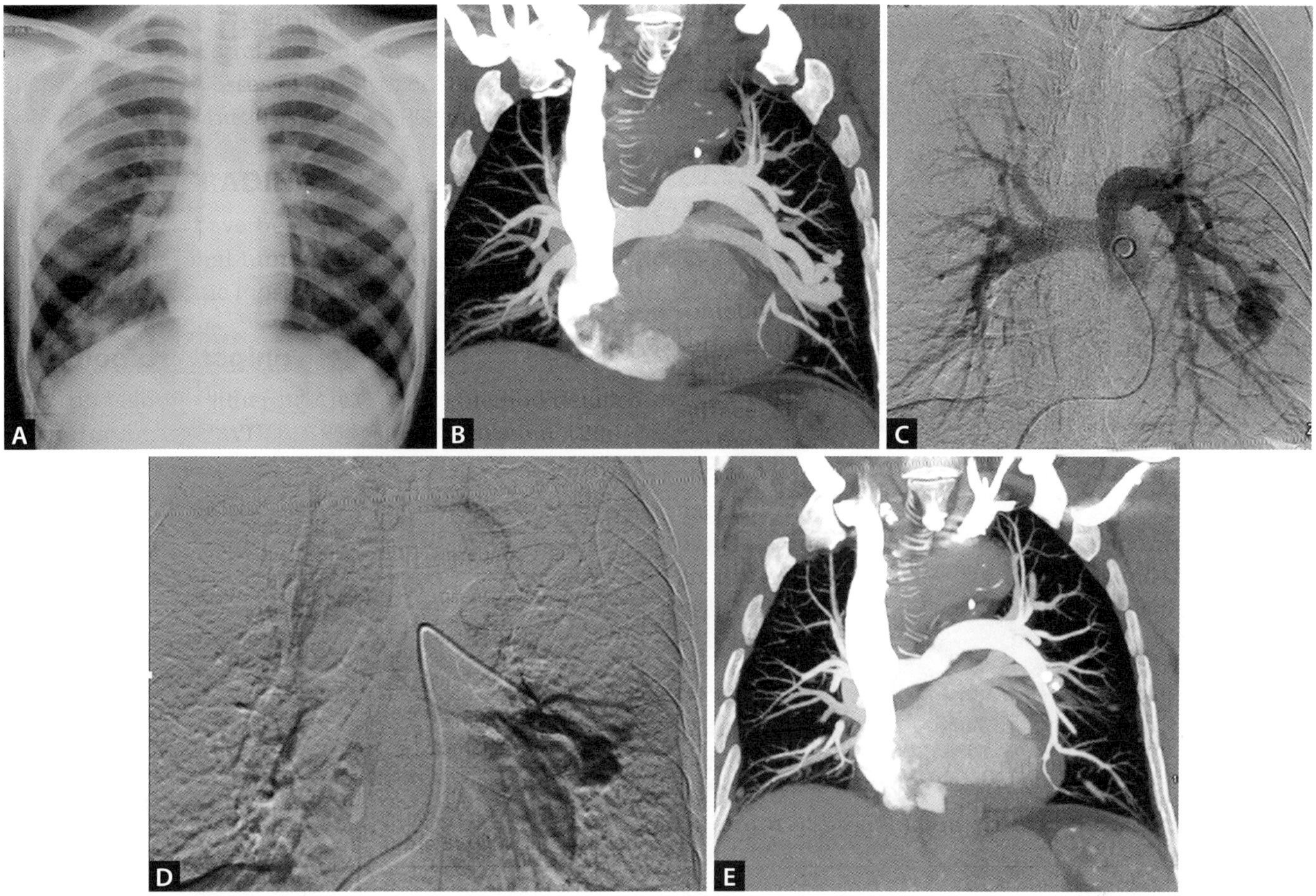

Figs. 21A to E: Solitary pulmonary arteriovenous malformation (AVM): Chest radiograph (A) shows solitary pulmonary AVM in right lower lobe with feeder vessel sign. Coronal CT pulmonary angiogram (B) in another patient showing solitary pulmonary AVM in left lateral basal segment with enlarged feeding artery and draining vein. Catheter pulmonary angiogram in main pulmonary artery (C) and on selective injection into feeding artery (D) showing similar findings as seen in DSA. Coronal CT pulmonary angiogram (E) postdeployment of vascular plug show no filling of pulmonary AVM.

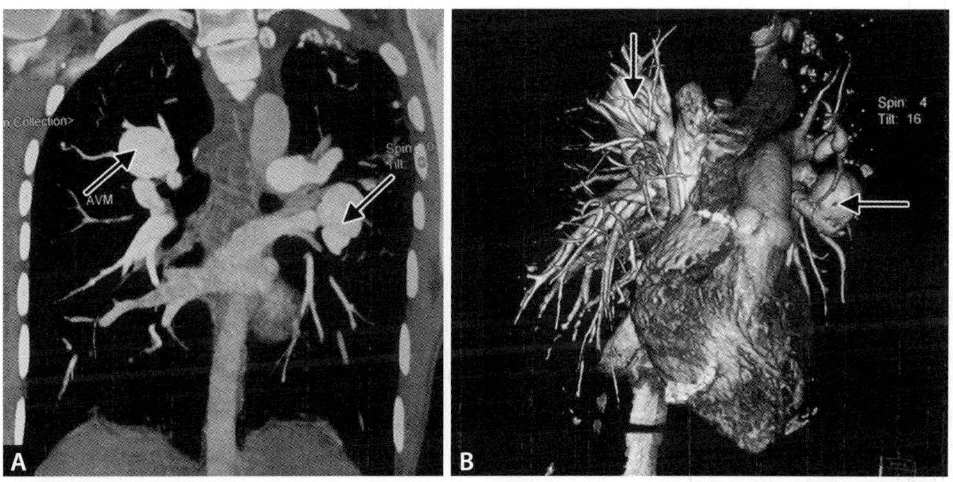

Figs. 22A and B: CT pulmonary angiogram—maximum intensity projection (A) and volume-rendered VR (B) images showing bilateral AVMs (arrows in A and B) in a patient of hereditary hemorrhagic telangiectasia.

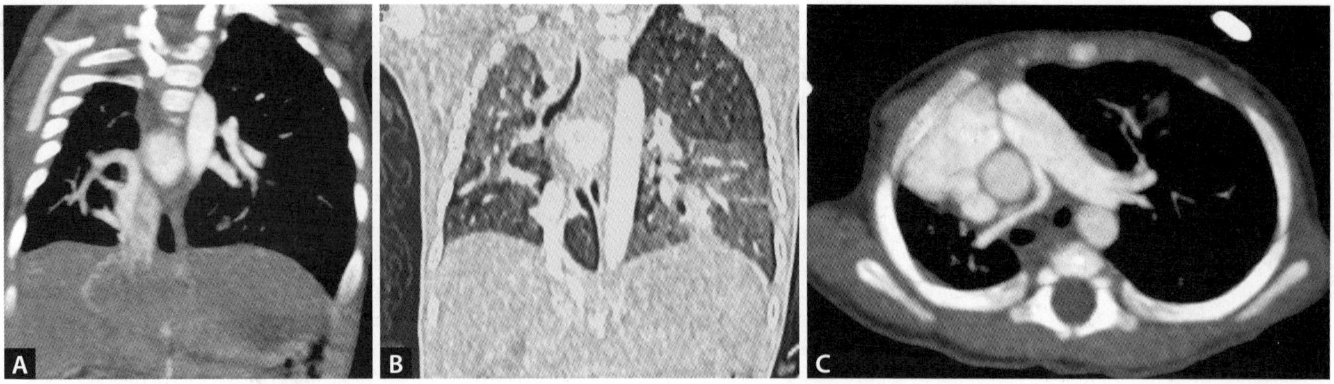

Figs. 23A to C: Scimitar syndrome: CT chest showing (A) abnormal drainage of right pulmonary veins into IVC; (B) Hypoplastic right lung with mosaic attenuation in bilateral lungs; (C) Hypoplastic right pulmonary artery.

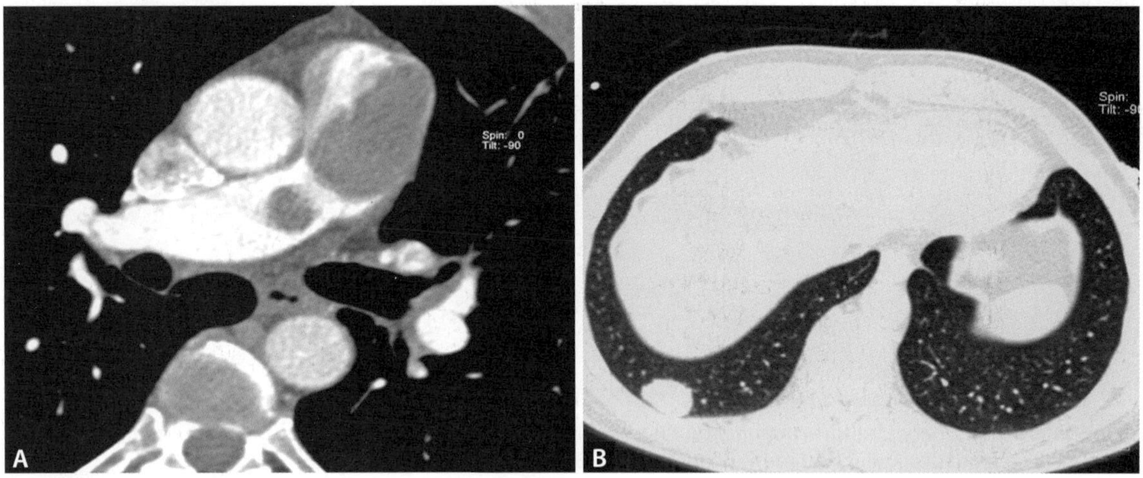

Figs. 24A and B: Pulmonary artery sarcoma: CT pulmonary angiogram (A) shows minimally enhancing main pulmonary artery mass with smaller similar lesion in right pulmonary artery. Lung section at a lower level (B) shows solitary metastasis in right lower lobe.

appreciate on CTPA. It can invade the adjacent lungs and the mediastinum. It may be hypermetabolic on PET-CT. Bland tumor thrombus may also be hypermetabolic on PET-CT; however, a maximum standard uptake value (SUV max) >2.25 is highly suggestive of tumor.[24,49,50]

REFERENCES

1. Cummings KW, Bhalla S. Pulmonary vascular diseases. Clin Chest Med. 2015;36:235-48.
2. Porres DV, Morenza OP, Pallisa E, et al. Learning from the pulmonary veins. Radiographics. 2013;33:999-1022.
3. Goldhaber SZ, Bounameaux H. Pulmonary embolism and deep vein thrombosis. Lancet. 2012;379 (9828):1835-46.
4. Konstantinides SV. ESC guidelines on the diagnosis and management of acute pulmonary embolism. Eur Heart J. 2014;35(45):3145-6.
5. Ruggiero A, Screaton NJ. Imaging of acute and chronic thromboembolic disease: state of the art. Clin Radiol. 2017;72(5):375-88.
6. Wells PS, Anderson DR, Rodger M, et al. Derivation of a simple clinical model to categorize patients probability of pulmonary embolism: increasing the models utility with the SimpliRED D-dimer. Thromb Haemost. 2000;83(3):416-20.
7. Wicki J, Perneger TV, Junod AF, et al. Assessing clinical probability of pulmonary embolism in the emergency ward: a simple score. Arch Intern Med. 2001;161(1):92-7.
8. Sevitt S, Gallagher N. Venous thrombosis and pulmonary embolism: A clinico-pathological study in injured and burned patients. Br J Surg. 1961;48:475-89.
9. Le Gal G, Righini M, Sanchez O, et al. A positive compression ultrasonography of the lower limb veins is highly predictive of pulmonary embolism on computed tomography in suspected patients. Thromb Haemost. 2006;95(6):963-6.
10. Sista AK, Kuo WT, Schiebler M, Madoff DC. Stratification, imaging, and management of acute massive and submassive pulmonary embolism. Radiology. 2017;284(1):5-24.
11. Abdelaziz MM, Wali SO, Hamad MMA, et al. Pulmonary embolism: A diagnostic approach. Annals of Thorac Medicine. 2006;(1):31-40.

12. Stein PD, Fowler SE, Goodman LR, et al. Multidetector computed tomography for acute pulmonary embolism. N Engl J Med. 2006;354(22):2317–27.
13. Fink C, Johnson TR, Michaely HJ, et al. Dual-energy CT angiography of the lung in patients with suspected pulmonary embolism: Initial results. Rofo. 2008;180(10):879-83.
14. Thieme SF, Becker CR, Hacker M, et al. Dual energy CT for the assessment of lung perfusion-correlation to scintigraphy. Eur J Radiol. 2008;68(3):369-74.
15. Delesalle MA, Pontana F, Duhamel A, et al. Spectral optimization of chest CT angiography with reduced iodine load: experience in 80 patients evaluated with dual-source, dual-energy CT. Radiology. 2013;267(1):256-66.
16. Szucs-Farkas Z, Christe A, Megyeri B, et al. Diagnostic accuracy of computed tomography pulmonary angiography with reduced radiation and contrast material dose: a prospective randomized clinical trial. Invest Radiol. 2014;49(4):201-8.
17. Sirajuddin A, François CJ, Kanne JP. Imaging studies for pulmonary vascular disease. Clinical Pulmonary Medicine. 2015;22(6): 307-21.
18. Bajc M, Albrechtsson U, Olsson CG, et al. Comparison of ventilation/perfusion scintigraphy and helical CT for diagnosis of pulmonary embolism; Strategy using clinical data and ancillary findings. Clin Physiol Funct Imaging. 2002;22:392-7.
19. Leung AN, Bull TM, Jaeschke R, et al. American Thoracic Society documents: an official American Thoracic Society/Society of Thoracic Radiology Clinical Practice Guideline—evaluation of suspected pulmonary embolism in pregnancy. Radiology. 2012;262:63546.
20. Kluge A, Luboldt W, Bachmann G. Acute pulmonary embolism to the subsegmental level: Diagnostic accuracy of three MRI techniques compared with 16-MDCT. Am J Roentgenol. 2006;187(1):W7-14.
21. Stein PD, Chenevert TL, Fowler SE, et al. Gadolinium-enhanced magnetic resonance angiography for pulmonary embolism: A multicentre prospective study (PIOPED III). Ann Intern Med. 2010;152(7):434-43. W142e433.
22. Furlan A, Aghayev A, Chang CC, et al. Short-term mortality in acute pulmonary embolism: Clot burden and signs of right heart dysfunction at CT pulmonary angiography. Radiology. 2012;265(1):283-93.
23. Lang IM, Pesavento R, Bonderman D, et al. Risk factors and basic mechanisms of chronic thromboembolic pulmonary hypertension: A current understanding. Eur Respir J. 2013;41(2):462-8.
24. Pena E, Dennie C, Veinot J, et al. Pulmonary hypertension: how the radioglogist can help. Radiographics. 2012;32:9-32.
25. Simonneau G, Gatzoulis MA, Adatia I, et al. Updated clinical classification of pulmonary hypertension. J Am Coll Cardiol. 2013;62:D34–41.
26. Fleischner FG. Pulmonary embolism. Clin Radiol. 1962;13: 169-82.
27. Tan RT, Kuzo R, Goodman LR, et al. Utility of CT scan evaluation for predicting pulmonary hypertension in patients with parenchymal lung disease. Medical College of Wisconsin Lung Transplant Group. Chest. 1998;113(5):1250-6.
28. Ng CS, Wells AU, Padley SPA. A CT sign of chronic pulmonary arterial hypertension: The ratio of main pulmonary artery to aortic diameter. J Thorac Imaging. 1999;14(4):270-8.
29. Sheehan R, Perloff JK, Fishbein MC, et al. Pulmonary neovascularity: A distinctive radiographic finding in Eisenmenger syndrome. Circulation. 2005;112(18):2778-85.
30. Van der Meer RW, Pattynama PM, van Strijen MJ, et al. Right ventricular dysfunction and pulmonary obstruction index at helical CT: Prediction of clinical outcome during 3-month follow-up in patients with acute pulmonary embolism. Radiology. 2005;235(3):798-803.
31. He J, Fang W, LV B, et al. Diagnosis of chronic thromboembolic pulmonary hypertension: Comparison of ventilation/perfusion scanning and multidetector computed tomography pulmonary angiography with pulmonary angiography. Nucl Med Commun. 2012;33:459-63.
32. Alassas K, Mergo P, Ibrahim el-S, et al. Cardiac MRI as a diagnostic tool in pulmonary hypertension. Future Cardiol. 2014;10:17-30.
33. Schiebler ML, Bhalla S, Runo J, et al. Magnetic resonance and computed tomography imaging of the structural and functional changes of pulmonary arterial hypertension. J Thorac Imaging. 2013;28:178-93.
34. Swift AJ, Rajaram S, Condliffe R, et al. Pulmonary artery relative area change detects mild elevations in pulmonary vascular resistance and predicts adverse outcome in pulmonary hypertension. Invest Radiol. 2012;47:571-7.
35. Iwasawa T. Diagnosis and management of pulmonary arterial hypertension using MR imaging. Magn Reson Med Sci. 2013;12:1-9.
36. Kondo C, Caputo GR, Masui T, et al. Pulmonary hypertension: pulmonary flow quantification and flow profile analysis with velocity-encoded cine MR imaging. Radiology. 1992;183:751-8
37. Reiter G, Reiter U, Kovacs G, et al. Magnetic resonance-derived 3-dimensional blood flow patterns in the main pulmonary artery as a marker of pulmonary hypertension and a measure of elevated mean pulmonary arterial pressure. Circ Cardiovasc Imaging. 2008;1:23-30.
38. Barker AJ, Rolda´n-Alzate A, Entezari P, et al. Four-dimensional flow assessment of pulmonary artery flow and wall shear stress in adult pulmonary arterial hypertension: Results from two institutions. Magn Reson Med. 2015;73:1904-13.
39. Rolda´n-Alzate A, Frydrychowicz A, Johnson KM, et al. Noninvasive assessment of cardiac function and pulmonary vascular resistance in a canine model of acute thromboembolic pulmonary hypertension using 4D flow cardiovascular magnetic resonance. J Cardiovasc Magn Reson. 2014;13:16-23.

40. Odagiri K, Inui N, Miyakawa S, et al. Abnormal hemodynamics in the pulmonary artery seen on time-resolved 3-dimensional phase-contrast magnetic resonance imaging (4D-flow) in a young patient with idiopathic pulmonary artery hypertension. Circ J. 2014;78:1770-2.
41. Rich S, Pietra GG, Kieras K, et al. Primary pulmonary hypertension: radiographic and scintigraphic patterns of histologic subtypes. Ann Intern Med. 1986;105:499-502.
42. Perloff JK, Hart EM, Greaves SM, et al. Proximal pulmonary arterial and intrapulmonary radiologic features of Eisenmenger syndrome and primary pulmonary hypertension. Am J Cardiol. 2003;92(2):182-7.
43. Frazier AA, Franks TJ, Mohammed TL, et al. From the Archives of the AFIP: Pulmonary veno-occlusive disease and pulmonary capillary hemangiomatosis. Radiographics. 2007;27:867-82.
44. Castaner E, Alguersuari A, Gallardo X, et al. When to suspect pulmonary vasculitis: radiologic and clinical clues. Radiographics. 2010;30:33-53.
45. Hiller N, Liberman S, Chajek-Shaul T, et al. Thoracic manifestations of Behçet disease at CT. Radiographics. 2004;24:801-8.
46. Gill SS, Roddie ME, Shovlin CL, et al. Pulmonary arteriovenous malformations and their mimics. Clin Radiol. 2015;70:96-110.
47. Nguyen ET, Silva CI, Seely JM, et al. Pulmonary artery aneurysms and pseudoaneurysms in adults: Findings at CT and radiography. Am J Roentgenol. 2007;188:W126-34.
48. Shovlin CL, Jackson JE. Pulmonary arteriovenous malformations and other vascular abnormalities. In: Mason RJ, Broaddus VC, Martin T, et al (Eds). Murray and Nadel's Textbook of Respiratory Medicine, 5th edn. Philadelphia: Elsevier-Saunders. 2010.pp.1261-82.
49. Castaner E, Gallardo X, Rimola J, et al. Congenital and acquired pulmonary artery anomalies in the adult: radiologic overview. Radiographics. 2006;26:349-71.
50. Lee EY, Khong PL. The value of 18 F-FDG PET/contrast enhanced CT in detection of tumor thrombus. Nuc Med. 2013;38:e60-5.

CHAPTER 185

Peripheral Vascular Diseases: Imaging and Interventions

Devasenathipathy Kandasamy, Shivanand Gamanagatti

INTRODUCTION

Peripheral vascular diseases (PVD) includes a wide spectrum of disease affecting the vessels of upper and lower extremity. The estimated prevalence of PVD increases with age which rises from 2.5% in the age group of 50–59 years to 14.5% in over 70 years of age.[1] Among the causes, atherosclerosis is by far the most common cause of PVD and commonly affects the lower limb. Atherosclerosis is the disease of the elderly, commonly affecting individuals more than 50 years of age. The common risk factors for developing atherosclerosis are smoking, diabetes mellitus, hyperlipidemia and hypertension. Other common nonatherosclerotic causes of PVD are Takayasu arteritis and Burgers disease, the former commonly affects the aortoiliac segment and the latter commonly affects the femoropopliteal and tibioperoneal circulation. PVD is less common in younger patients and common causes include trauma, thromboembolism and arteritis. Imaging plays an important role in the management of PVD because it is essential to know the arterial anatomy, extent and severity of pathology to choose the next appropriate step in management. Decades back, digital subtraction angiography (DSA) was the modality of choice for the diagnostic evaluation of PVD. However, in the current scenario, because of its invasiveness the role of DSA is usually limited to the endovascular interventional procedures. With the technological developments in Ultrasonography (USG), computed tomography (CT) and Magnetic resonance imaging (MRI) in the last few decades, the diagnostic evaluation of PVD has been taken over by these modalities.

Whenever PVD is suspected clinically, initial diagnostic evaluation is done using ankle-brachial index (ABI).[2] ABI is an effective method to detect significant stenosis and it is performed by measuring the systolic blood pressures at the level of ankle and arm in supine position. ABI less than 0.9 is suggestive of significant PAD in the lower extremity with the sensitivity and specificity of 79% and 96% respectively.[3] ABI between 0.9 and 1 is considered borderline. If there is extensive calcification of the arterial wall or reduced compliance of the vessel wall, ABI can be falsely elevated. Also ABI cannot assess the location and severity of the stenosis. Hence, ABI can be an effective screening method and further imaging is necessary for the detailed evaluation.

IMAGING MODALITIES

Digital Subtraction Angiography

Digital subtraction angiography used to be the diagnostic modality of choice decades ago which can show the arterial anatomy in great detail because of its superior spatial resolution compared to other modalities. It is a robust modality to show the flow dynamics across the lesion, distal run-off and it also provides an opportunity to perform interventional procedures in the same sitting. However, DSA has several limitations which eventually paved way to the newer modalities. It provides a 2D view of the vessels and hence the tortuosity and overlap can underestimate or overestimate the stenosis.[4] Other limitations of DSA are the need for invasive arterial access and associated complications, ionizing radiation and usage of iodinated contrast media.

Ultrasonography

Ultrasonography with color Doppler is another modality which can be of use in the evaluation of PVD. Apart from the grayscale (B mode), Doppler principle can be used to overlay color and generate graphical spectrum of the flow dynamics. It is safe, inexpensive, and widely available and can give functional information in the region of interest. Recent advances in the USG technology namely ultrafast Doppler made it possible to get spectral information in a large area rather than only from the sampling window. This technique allows the operator to get multiple spectral tracings over an area from a single data acquisition. Normal extremity artery shows a triphasic high resistance flow pattern with a preserved spectral window **(Figs. 1A to D)**. Whenever there is stenosis, B-mode USG shows vessel narrowing, the systolic flow rate across the stenosis increases and the flow changes from streamlined to turbulent **(Figs. 2A to C)**. This leads to increase in peak systolic velocity (PSV) which is the most sensitive parameter and spectral broadening causing obliteration of spectral window. To eliminate the variations in the PSV between vessel segments and patients, a ratio of PSV at the site of abnormality and at the normal proximal vessel is taken. The commonly used criteria to diagnose >50% stenosis is PSV ratio >2, PSV >200 cm/sec, color aliasing and spectral broadening.[5]

However, there are several shortcomings of color Doppler which made this modality less popular for the evaluation of PVD. The quality of the study depends on the operator, leading to moderate inter-observer agreement for the evaluation of aortoiliac and femoropopliteal segments.[6] The evaluation of aortoiliac segment is limited due to bowel gas and abdominal fat. The evaluation of infrapopliteal segments is usually challenging and time consuming. Because of the above reasons the complete

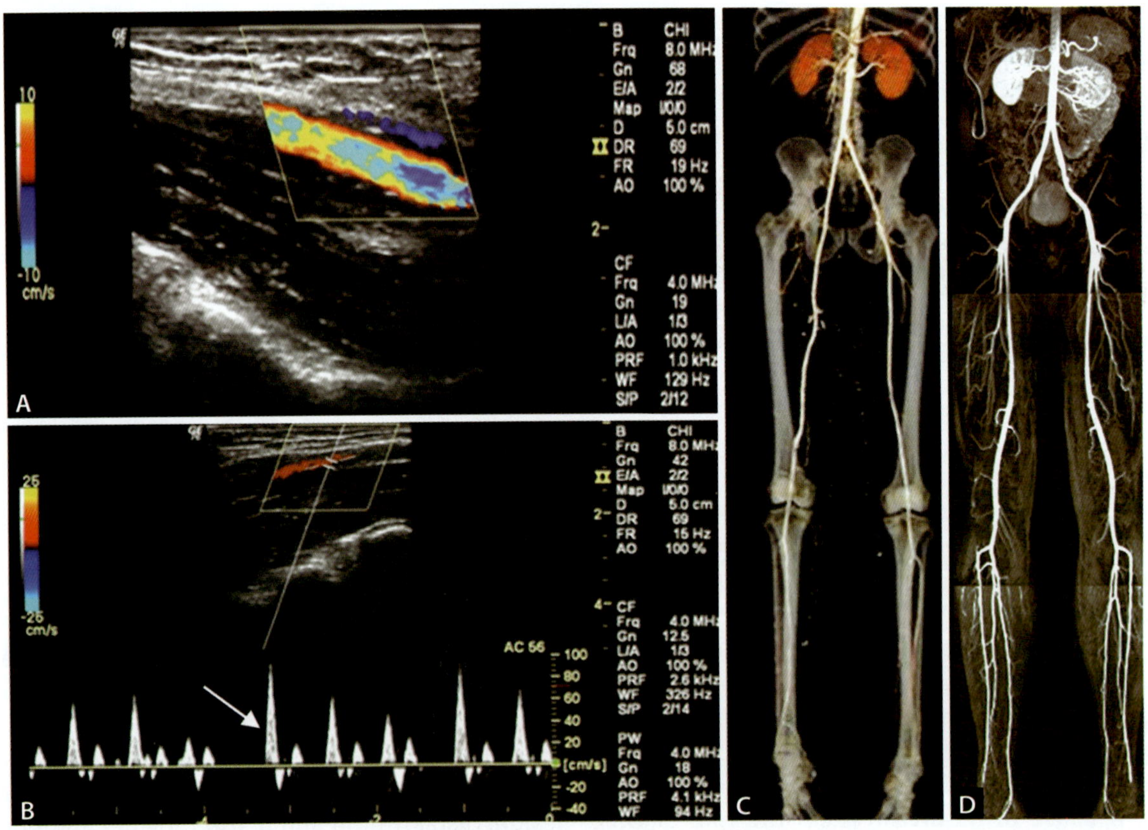

Figs. 1A to D: Normal lower extremity arteries on imaging. Color Doppler (A) with spectral tracing (B) of superficial femoral artery showing an uniform caliber artery which is showing typical triphasic flow pattern (arrow). Volume-rendered technique (VRT) image (C) showing normal appearance of abdominal aorta and bilateral lower limb arteries. The course, caliber and relationship of vessels with the bones are shown on the VRT image. Maximum intensity projection (MIP) image (D) acquired in three stations showing normal abdominal and lower extremity arteries.

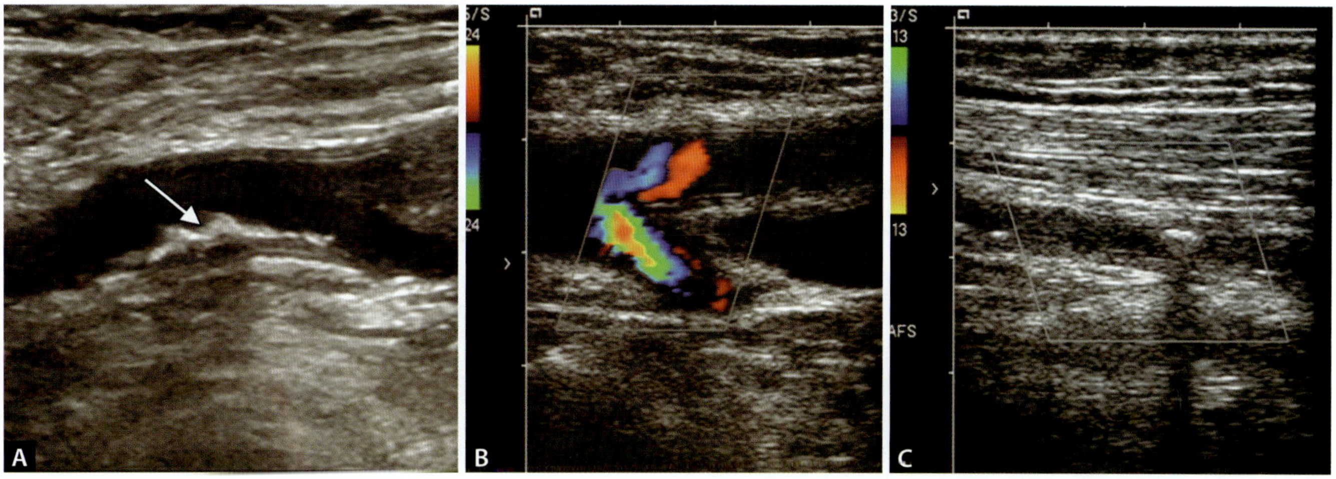

Figs. 2A to C: Arterial narrowing on color Doppler. B mode USG image (A) at the level of bifurcation of common femoral artery showing calcified plaques (arrow). Color Doppler image at the same level (B) and at the level of superficial femoral artery (C) showing no flow due to narrowing of the vessel.

evaluation of the entire arterial tree is not possible in many situations. Heavily calcified vessels cannot be evaluated using USG because of poor window. Another important limitation is that the sensitivity to detect the distal lesion in sequential stenosis is poor because of the change in arterial flow dynamics due to the proximal stenotic segment.

Computed Tomography

Computed tomography is currently one of the preferred modality to evaluate extremity arteries. The advent of multidetector CT has revolutionized CT angiography (CTA) leading to faster and high quality acquisition of images. Higher resolution compared to MRI and capability of 3D image generation are additional highlights. In the era of single slice CT scanners, optimal scanning of the entire extremity arterial tree in a single contrast injection was not possible. In the last decade due to the increase in the number of detector rows, more coverage per rotation of tube, faster rotation has made the evaluation of entire arterial tree from mid aorta till feet possible in the first pass of contrast (***see* Figs. 1A to D**). Faster scanning led to decrease in the contrast volume over years. With the current available scanning speed and lower dwelling time it is really critical to capture the peak enhancement of the arterial tree to obtain good quality images. The timing, rate of injection, contrast volume and the scanning speed of the scanner should be adjusted meticulously to avoid poor opacification of arteries. This is especially true in patients with stenosis or aneurysm where the blood flow is slow. The acquisition can be much faster than the leading edge of the contrast movement eventually resulting in scanning of unopacified arteries. Thus in the current generation scanners, there is a need to optimize the above said injector and scanner parameters to get the desired result. The typical scanning parameters are provided in **Table 1**.

Another factor which needs to be considered is the kVp of the scanning. Decrease in kVp increases the visualization of contrast and reduces radiation dose and thus 100–120 kVp scanning is recommended. Newer generation scanners have the capability of dual energy acquisition which opens up a wide range of applications such as accurate bone removal to generate high quality 3D images, automatic plaque characterization and removal which can give accurate stenosis measurements, reduction of streak artifacts and generation of optimum quality image sets with high contrast to noise ratio which has the potential to reduce radiation and contrast dose.

The 3D data of CT scan can be post processed to generate intuitive and clinically useful images. Maximum intensity projection (MIP) is a type of rendering in which the voxel with maximum value will be displayed from any point of view **(Figs. 3 and 4)**. The wall calcification and vessel contour are well-delineated on MIP and give an overview of the entire arterial tree. It can be used in two modes full-volume (thick) mode and sub-volume (thin) mode. Thin MIP is useful in depicting the inflow circulation (aortoiliac) so that the overlying abdominal visceral arteries are not visualized. Thick MIP is useful in showing the outflow circulation (femoropopliteal and tibioperoneal).

Curved planar reconstruction (CPR) is a specialized form of multiplanar reformat (MPR) in which the image can be reformatted in any curved plane. CPR is useful to visualize the entire length of artery in one image. It can also

Table 1: Typical injection protocol for CTA of lower extremity (for a 70 kg individual).

Contrast volume and rate	25 mL at 5 mL/s for 5 seconds followed by 120 mL at 4 mL/s for 30 seconds
Injection duration	35 seconds
Scanning time	40 seconds
Scanning delay after the arrival of contrast	3 seconds

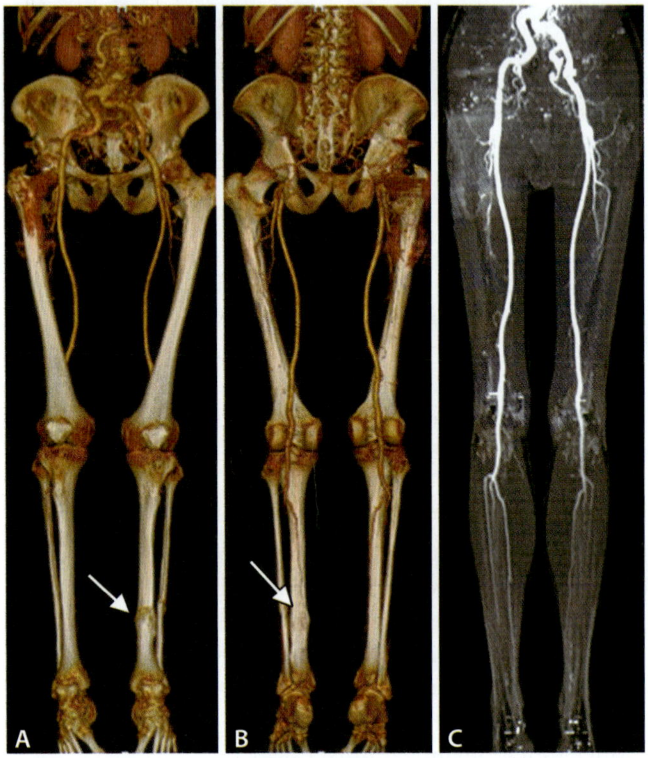

Figs. 3A to C: CTA—one stop shop technique in skeletal trauma. VRT images of CTA in front (A) and back (B) views showing fracture of both bones in the left leg (arrow). MIP image with bone removal of the same patient showing attenuated arteries in the left leg. CTA in this situation can provide information about the skeletal and soft tissue injuries apart from showing the detailed anatomy of the lower limb arterial tree.

be used to create orthogonal axial images perpendicular to the axis of the artery so that the stenosis measurements can be done accurately even in the presence of calcified plaques.

Volume-rendering technique (VRT) is a post-processing technique which can give 3D perspective of the entire volume. It is useful to provide spatial relationships with the adjacent structures such as collaterals and bone which is immensely helpful for interventional radiologists and surgeons **(Fig. 3)**. However, the distinction between

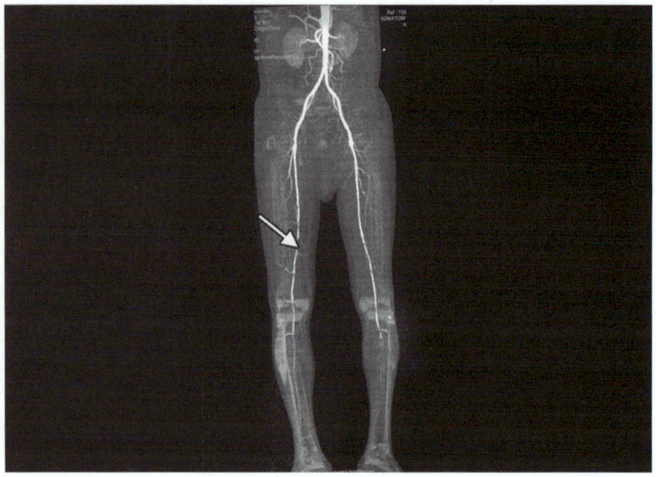

Fig. 4: Arterial narrowing on CTA: MIP image with bone removal of CTA data set showing short segment narrowing at the level of distal superficial femoral artery and good distal run-off. MIP image can provide an overview of the entire arterial tree on a single image based on the CTA data set which is otherwise huge.

the calcified plaque and vessel wall contour is not that well-visualized on VRT.

With the above post-processing methods especially the CPR along with axial images, stenosis can be easily categorized into mild (0–50%), moderate (50–70%) and severe (>70%).[7,8]

Magnetic Resonance Imaging

Magnetic resonance imaging has undergone several technological improvements over decades and with the current scanners it is possible to scan the entire arterial tree in a single injection of contrast. Advantage of MR angiography (MRA) as compared to CTA is that it can generate images without overlapping bones and calcified plaques without exposing the patient to ionizing radiation **(Figs. 1A to D, 5 and 6)**. Unique capability of MRI is that it can generate angiographic images without contrast media which comes handy in patients with chronic renal disease and patients with contraindication to contrast media. Because of superior background tissue suppression on 3 Tesla compared to 1.5 Tesla scanners, it is preferred for both contrast-enhanced MRA (CE-MRA) and non-contrast MRA studies.

CE-MRA is the most commonly performed, fast and robust MRA technique which depends on the T1 shortening effect of gadolinium-based contrast agents. Spatial resolution of CE-MRA is better than non-contrast MRA and artifacts are also less seen. CE-MRA sequence is a fast sequence with preferential filling of central k space which determines the contrast resolution of the image.

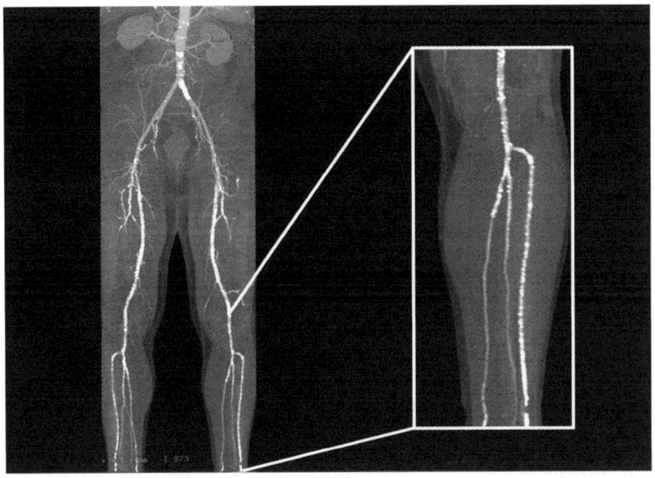

Fig. 5: Vessel wall calcification on CTA: MIP image of a CTA data set showing extensive vessel wall calcification involving the entire arterial tree. This is considered as a limitation of CTA in which the evaluation of vessel wall narrowing is known to be hampered by extensive calcifications.

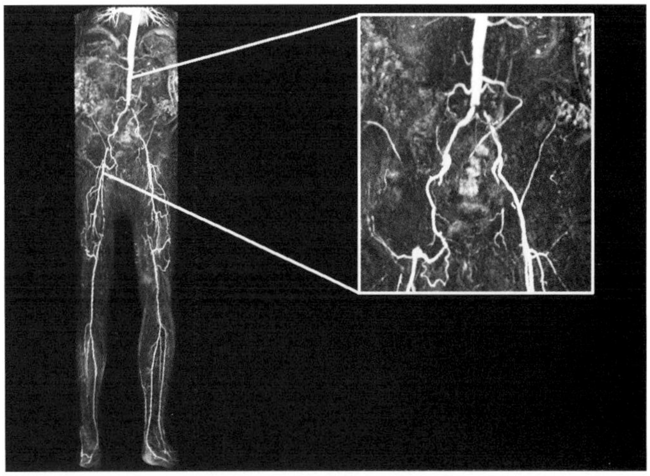

Fig. 6: Arterial narrowing on MRA: MIP image of MRA data set showing extensive atherosclerotic involvement of aorta and lower limb arteries. There is complete occlusion of bilateral common iliac arteries till superficial femoral arteries with good distal run-off. Extensive vessel wall calcifications do not hamper the vessel assessment on MRA which is an advantage over CTA.

Acquiring the entire lower extremity arteries without venous contamination is challenging. It is usually done in three stations namely aortoiliac, thigh and calf region and between the acquisitions the table has to move quickly to next station. This technique is called three station, moving table technique in which the contrast bolus is followed from aortoiliac to calf in the same order. Usually precontrast as well as post contrast volume sets are acquired and subtracted to obtain the MRA image. This DSA like subtraction using precontrast mask provides good background tissue suppression and showing only the vessels. The aortoiliac station is usually done with breath holding to minimize motion blurring. However, this method can sometimes lead to venous contamination in the third station resulting in nondiagnostic studies **(Fig. 7)**. There are different approaches described to overcome the venous contamination including thigh compression cuffs and pillow under the knee to slow down the venous return, non-contrast MRA for the calf station and acquiring calf station in a separate contrast injection.[9] Another technique which can be used to overcome venous contamination in calf is by performing time resolved MRA which generates images in every 1–2 seconds to differentiate arteries from veins. If the data is acquired during the inflow of contrast, ringing artifacts will degrade the image quality. Thus, the image acquisition should be performed during the plateau phase of the arterial enhancement. Hence the timing of contrast injection and start of scanning are of paramount importance. Typically 0.2 mmoL/kg body weight is the contrast dose used for lower limb MRA and it is injected at a rate of 2–2.5 mL/second followed by saline chase. One needs to be cautious in using contrast in patients with impaired renal function because they stand the risk of developing nephrogenic systemic fibrosis (NSF). The start of image acquisition can be either after an empirical delay or by performing a test bolus to know the arrival time of contrast or by MR fluoroscopic technique in which rapid real time images are taken and once the contrast arrival is ascertained, the MRA sequence is triggered manually.

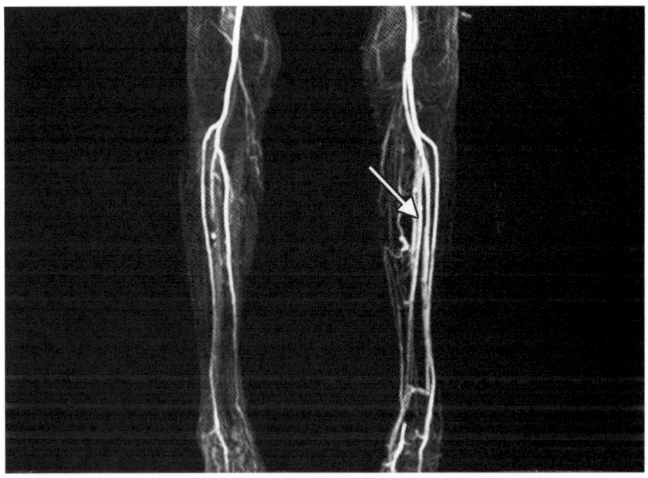

Fig. 7: Venous contamination in MRA: MIP image of MRA data set of bilateral legs showing venous contamination (arrow) in the left side. Venous contamination which usually occurs in the last station of data acquisition due to time delay can degrade the diagnostic quality of MRA.

There are various methods used to obtain non-contrast MRA in various parts of the body. Among those, time of flight (TOF), quiescent-interval single-shot (QISS) and fast spine echo (FSE) based gated subtraction MRA are commonly used for imaging extremity arteries especially if contrast injection is contraindicated. FSE-based subtraction technique suffers from motion which can degrade the image quality. However, it can be highly accurate if motion can be minimized. QISS MRA is another promising and robust method to evaluate extremity arteries which has been shown to have high sensitivity (85–97%) and specificity (95–98%) for the detection of significant stenosis compared to CE-MRA.[10–12]

IMAGING FEATURES CLINICAL ENTITIES

Atherosclerosis

Atherosclerosis is the most common cause of PVD affecting inflow or outflow circulation. Patients with significant aortoiliac disease present with buttock or thigh claudication and patients with femoropopliteal disease present with calf claudication. Isolated tibioperoneal circulation is a feature of diabetes in which patients usually present with calf and foot involvement. The role of imaging is to evaluate the location, arterial segment involved, length and severity of stenosis which is critical to decide on endovascular interventional therapy versus surgical therapy. Transatlantic Inter-society Consensus (TASC) Document on management of peripheral arterial disease (PAD) has categorized various stenotic lesions based on their length, severity and bilaterality into A, B, C and D and recommends the appropriate mode of treatment. The recommendations are shown in **Table 2**.

In patients with diabetes where there is extensive arterial wall calcifications especially in the tibioperoneal region, accurate evaluation of stenosis/occlusion may not be possible. MRA is a preferred imaging modality in these patients **(*see* Fig. 5)**.[13] With the emergence of dual energy CT, there is a potential to allow accurate distinction between arterial lumen and calcified plaque.

Table 2: TASC recommendations.

Type A lesions	Short length lesions—endovascular therapy is recommended
Type B lesions	Endovascular therapy is preferred unless other lesions in the same area necessitates surgical approach
Type C lesions	Generally longer lesions—surgical revascularization is recommended. Endovascular therapy, if the patient is a high-risk candidate for surgery
Type D lesions	Surgical revascularization is recommended in all

Atheroembolism and Thromboembolism

Atheroembolism is usually secondary to an ulcerative plaque in aortoiliac region leading to acute unilateral symptoms. The embolus usually occludes the smaller arteries of the leg. CTA can adequately evaluate the site of obstruction and also the probable source of embolus.

Thromboembolic events are generally from cardiac source, however paradoxical embolus from the systemic venous source is also a possibility. They are usually larger than atheroemboli and hence they occlude more proximal arteries in the femoropopliteal region. These patients need gated CTA of heart and thoracic aorta in addition to CTA of the extremity arteries to guide appropriate management.

Peripheral Arterial Aneurysm

Peripheral arterial aneurysms can co-exist with aortic aneurysm and they can be bilateral in almost 50% of patients.[14,15] Hence it is prudent to image the entire arterial tree from aorta till the toes. The size criteria for femoral artery aneurysm is >10 mm and popliteal artery is >7 mm.[16,17] Femoral artery aneurysms are usually secondary to trauma, arterial puncture or post bypass graft surgery. The initial evaluation is done using USG—color Doppler which can reliably diagnose the aneurysm and rule out other cystic lesions. The role of CTA is to provide more detailed visualization and detection of additional lesions.

Arteritis

Buergers disease and Takayasu arteritis are the most common arteritis affecting the extremity arteries. Other less common causes are giant cell arteritis, polyarteritis nodosa, Behcet's disease and Kawasaki disease. Buergers disease has strong association with smoking and usual age of presentation is around 40 years and they predominantly affect the small and medium-sized arteries (distal femoropopliteal and tibioperoneal circulation). Imaging studies show high-grade narrowing or complete occlusion of involved arteries with well-developed cork-screw collaterals because of slow progression of the disease.

Takayasu arteritis usually involves the large arteries such as arch vessels, aorta and iliac arteries with sparing of outflow circulation in the extremity. Young and middle aged females are usually affected. The role of imaging is to delineate the narrowing and assess the severity to direct appropriate management.

Popliteal Artery Entrapment Syndrome

It has 4 described types which is based on the extent of displacement of popliteal artery by the medial head of gastrocnemius muscle. The diagnosis can be made on USG in which narrowing can be demonstrated at the typical location and real time dynamic compression during dorsiflexion of foot can also be demonstrated. Similar findings can also be demonstrated on DSA.

Cystic Adventitial Disease

Cystic adventitial disease commonly affects the popliteal artery and seen in young patients. It leads to concentric or eccentric smooth narrowing of the involved segment. The underlying pathology is the mucin production in the adventitia of the arterial wall leading to narrowing. Although findings may be seen on USG, MRA is the modality of choice because of the ability to characterize mucin in the wall on T2-weighted images.

Imaging Strategy

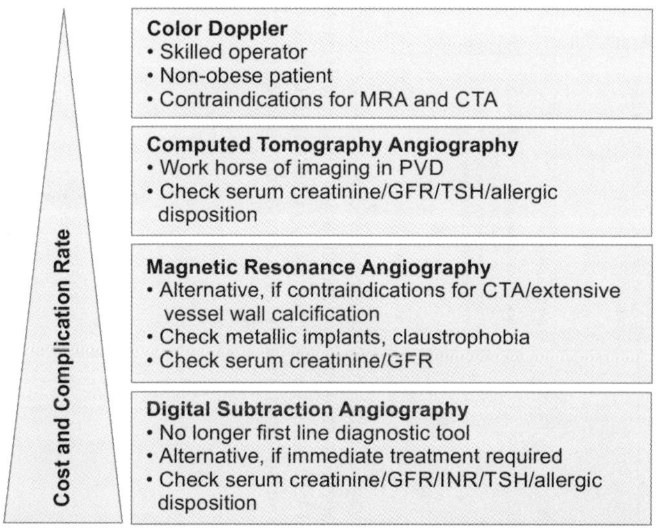

Abbreviations: PVD: Peripheral vascular disease; GFR: Glomerular filtration rate; TSH: Thyroid stimulating hormone; MRA: Magnetic resonance angiography; CTA: Computed tomography angiography; INR: International Normalized Ratio.

Interventions

Endovascular treatment provides a lower risk substitute to conventional surgery in many patients with multiple co-morbidities. Whenever possible, interventional treatments have become the first line of management in the treatment of PVD. Advances in interventional technology during the past few years have widened the choices for handling PVD percutaneously. The Inter-Society Consensus for the Management of Peripheral Arterial Disease (TASC) guidelines aimed to provide guidance on treatment decisions relating to the optimal revascularization strategy (endovascular versus surgical) based on the anatomic and clinical status of the patient **(Fig. 8)**.[18]

Noninvasive tests (ankle-brachial index) and arterial mapping (CT/MR angiography) done, prior to an endovascular treatment, help in localization of the disease and planning the procedure **(Figs. 9A and B)**.

Treatment Decision

The scheduling and necessity for revascularization depends upon the clinical settings. Three different clinical situations include:

1. Intermittent claudication
2. Critical limb ischemia
3. Acute limb ischemia

Most of the patients with intermittent claudication are managed by exercise and medical therapy. Interventional procedures are ascribed in circumstances, when these methods fail to improve quality of life and limb function.

In contrast, critical limb ischemia and acute limb ischemia impend the limb and warrants more imperative revascularization.

Types of Procedures

Balloon angioplasty and stenting are the key revascularization techniques. Latest advances in interventional treatments include, drug-eluting balloons, drug-eluting stents, plaque debulking devices (atherectomy) and devices for crossing tight chronic total occlusions.[19]

Results

In general, interventional therapies have better long-term durability for aortoiliac disease than femoral popliteal disease. Infrapopliteal revascularization has poor long-term results and is generally reserved for critical and acute limb ischemia.

Follow-up and Surveillance

Patients receiving any form of interventional revascularization measures need a planned surveillance strategy for follow-up care.

- Rigorous treatment of cardiovascular risk factors to avert myocardial infarction and stroke.
- Limb observation targets to identify restenosis and fresh disease elsewhere in the treated segments.

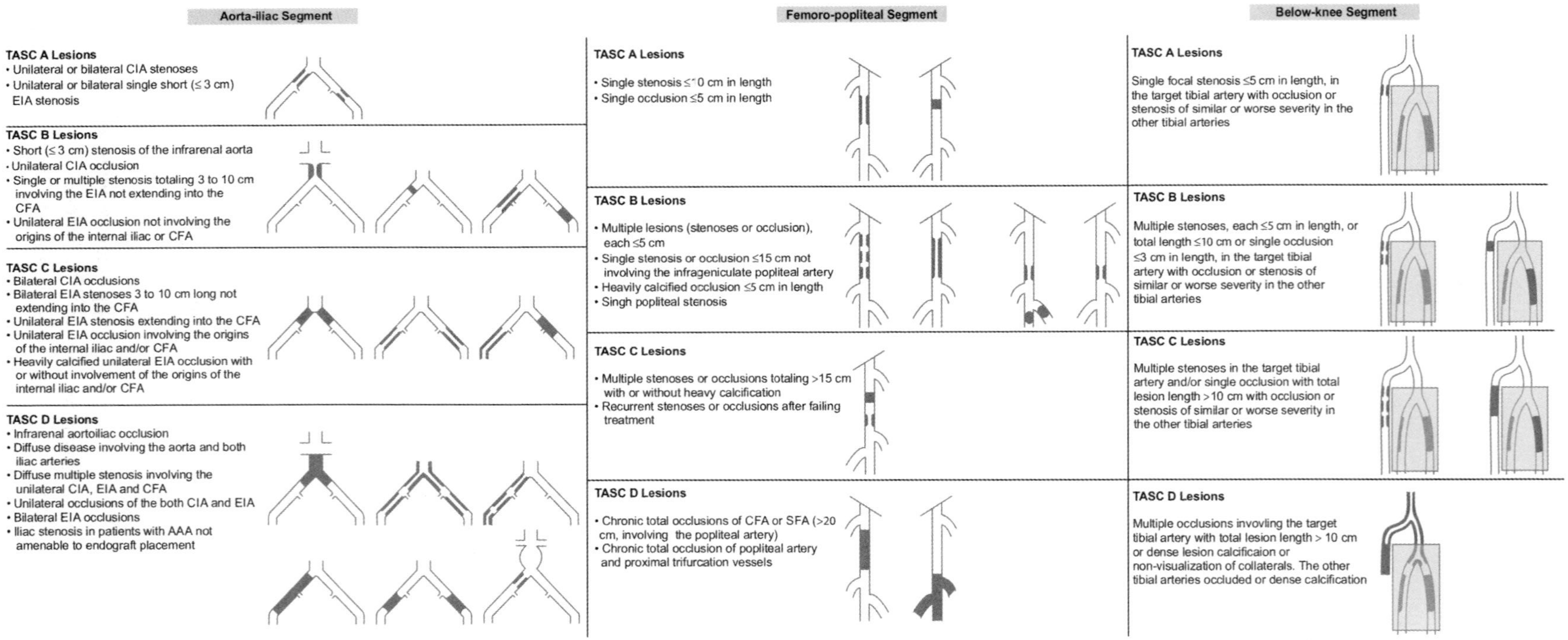

Fig. 8: TASC anatomic classification showing various patterns of disease based on extent of the disease at different segments of arterial tree. Used for treatment guidance regarding the optimal revascularization strategy (endovascular versus surgical) based on the complexity and location of the anatomic disease.
Abbreviations: TASC: Transatlantic Inter-Society Consensus; CIA: Common iliac artery; EIA: External iliac artery; CFA: Common femoral artery; AAA: Abdominal aortic aneurysm; SFA: Superficial femoral artery.

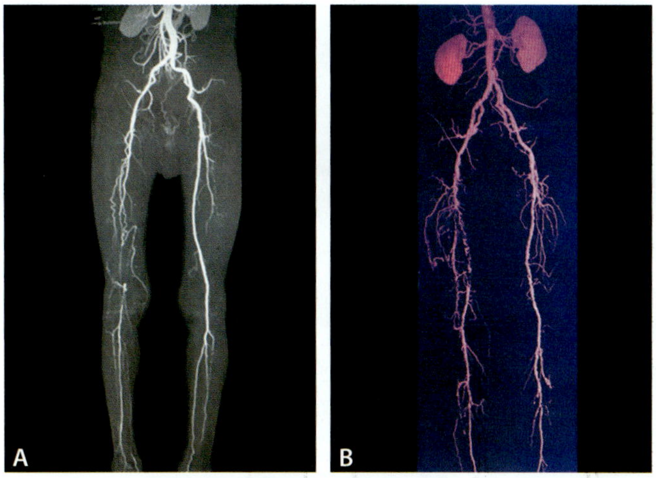

Figs. 9A and B: CT angiography (MIP and VRT) images of vascular mapping of bilateral lower limbs showing location of lesion and extent of the disease, important for planning the endovascular treatment.

Technique of Angioplasty

Definition: Percutaneous transluminal angioplasty (PTA) refers to deliberate opening (dilatation) of a vascular stenosis or occlusion using a balloon catheter.

Mode of action of PTA: Angioplasty causes rupture of the atherosclerotic plaque and a limited split or dissection of the vessel wall.

The split might spread in the vessel wall either in circumferential or longitudinal direction. Also, it may spread deep into the internal elastic lamina or into the media, keeping adventitial layer intact. Concentric arterial narrowing have good response to PTA, since the plaque and the vascular wall layers are split in an even fashion, whereas eccentric vascular lesions respond poor to balloon dilatation due to recoil of the normal elastic wall.[20]

A cutting balloon has got non-compliant balloon with fine fins fixed longitudinally on the outer surface of the balloon. These fins are devised to cut a lesion during balloon inflation, permitting a simpler angioplasty at lower inflation pressures. Cutting balloons are recommended for stenoses resistant to standard angioplasty.[21]

Stenting

Vascular stents are designed to provide an internal support for the vascular lumen. Stents has got following advantages:

- Quick, consistent, and constant expansion of the luminal diameter.
- Trapping of the weak plaque material that may possibly embolize after angioplasty.
- Removal of elastic recoil after angioplasty.

Preprocedure Work-up

- A comprehensive clinical and medical history must be taken. History regarding claudication symptoms, pertinent past history of cardiac and renal disease, risk factors for vascular disease such as diabetes, smoking and hypercholesterolemia. Also, history of contrast allergy must be obtained.
- Take history about present-day medication. Some of the medications may need to be stopped or modified prior to the procedure, such as, oral anticoagulants, antiplatelets and insulin.
- Evaluate all the fresh imaging findings to choose the proper site and direction of vascular access, i.e. ipsilateral versus contralateral approach, antegrade versus retrograde puncture.
- Review the appearance of the lesion on imaging that will help to plan the appropriate management, i.e. angioplasty versus stenting. In general, short segment narrowing/occlusions are likely to benefit satisfactorily to angioplasty.
- If there is renal dysfunction, IV hydration must be commenced a day prior to the procedure. Usage of iso-osmolar contrast agents is recommended.
- It is appropriate to discuss with the patient about treatment options (angioplasty versus surgery), results and the possible complications. Informed consent should be taken prior to the procedure.

Day of Procedure

- The patient reports to the vascular lab after fasting for 4–6 hours, however, clear fluids are allowed. The site of vascular access is cleaned and draped in a sterile manner.
- Close monitoring of the vital statistics (Pulse, BP, SPO_2) is done prior to the start of procedure and is continued till the procedure is completed.
- Patients are advised to start antiplatelet medicines (clopidogrel 75 mg/day, and aspirin 160 mg/day) 2 days prior to the procedure, which will help to diminish thrombotic events during the procedure.

Vascular Access

The site of vascular access is determined by the site of vascular lesion to be treated as determined by analysis of imaging studies prior to the start of procedure.

- For the lesions in iliac arteries (cranial to the inguinal ligament), an ipsilateral retrograde common femoral approach is preferred **(Fig. 10A)**.
- For the lesions caudal to the inguinal ligament:
  - Common femoral artery (CFA) and superficial femoral artery (SFA) till adductor canal level, cross

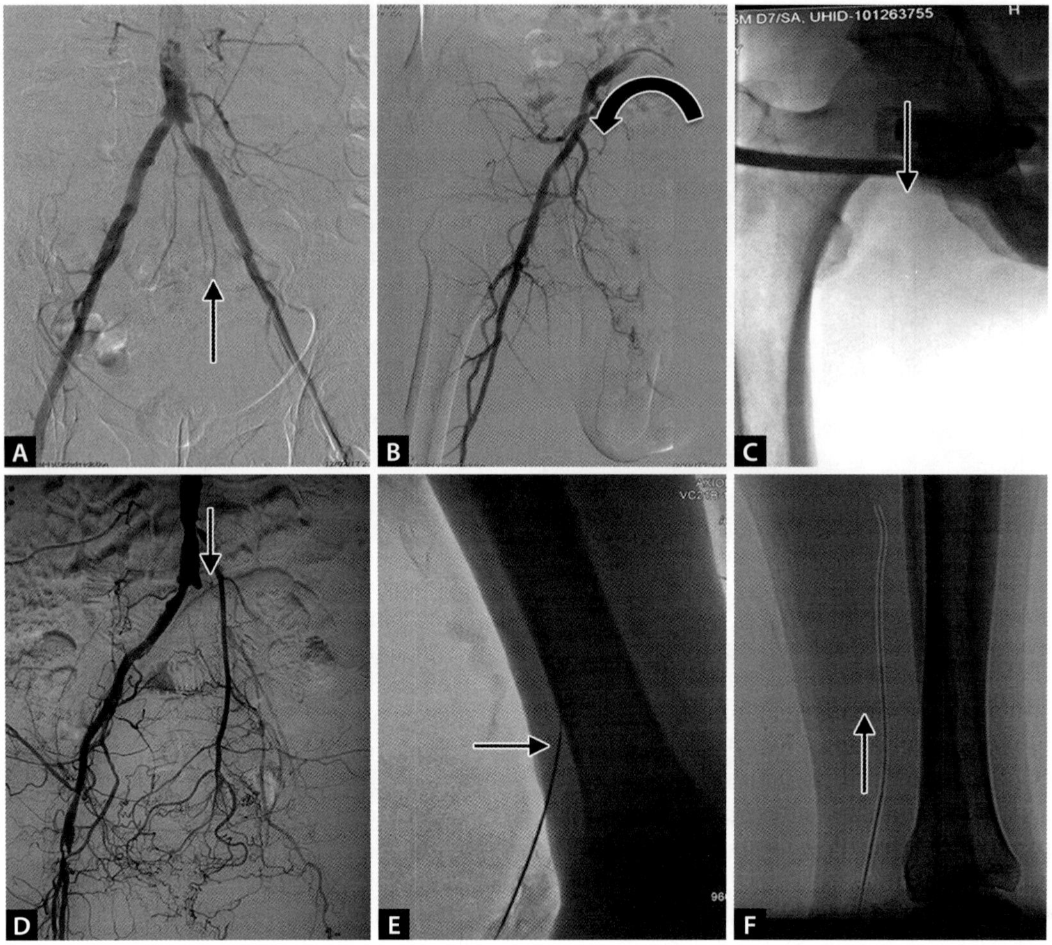

Figs. 10A to F: DSA spot images showing various types of vascular access: (A) Retrograde transfemoral approach; (B) Contralateral transfemoral access; (C) Antegrade transfemoral approach; (D) Brachial approach; (E) Anterior tibial approach; (F) Posterior tibial approach.

over techniques from contralateral femoral artery **(Fig. 10B)**.
- For distal SFA and beyond, the antegrade common femoral puncture is the preferred access route **(Fig. 10C)**.

- Other arterial access sites such as brachial artery **(Fig. 10D)**, the radial artery, the popliteal artery and the tibial arteries **(Figs. 10E and F)** may also be used to obtain vascular access.

Crossing of the Lesion[19]

- Appropriate size vascular sheath (preferably, 6F in common femoral access) is introduced into the access artery. If the contralateral approach is used, then crossover vascular sheath should be placed. The lesion is usually crossed using a combination of selective catheter and an atraumatic hydrophilic guidewire.
- Low molecular weight Heparin (3000–7000 IU) should be administered either in divided doses or as a single loading dose as per the institute practice.
- After crossing the lesion with guidewire, the catheter is pushed over the guidewire and the guidewire is withdrawn. If the catheter tip is in true lumen, one should start seeing the free flow of blood coming from the catheter hub. It is always good idea to aspirate blood and/or inject contrast medium to check the catheter position within the lumen.
- It is always important to ensure that the guidewire is long enough (use exchange guidewire of 260 cm) for exchanging the selective catheter, the balloon catheter or stent delivery system.
- It is important to take care that the guidewire is of appropriate diameter, which is recommended for the lumen of the balloon catheter or stent delivery systems.

For example, it is not feasible to introduce a stent delivery system devised for a 0.018-inch guidewire over a 0.035-inch guidewire.

- A choice of whether to treat the lesion by angioplasty alone or primary stenting could be made either prior to the start of procedure or after the initial angiographic images of the lesion location and appearance.
- Occasionally, choice of stenting is made, when angioplasty fails or makes the lesion worse.

Balloon Angioplasty (Figs. 11A to C and Table 3)

- A balloon catheter of suitable diameter and length must be chosen.
- Regarding balloon catheter size, there is a controversy whether to use oversized balloon or not in relation to the normal artery diameter. Most of the interventionists choose balloon catheters 10–20% larger than the native artery diameter.
- In case of uncertainty, it is a good idea to use a balloon catheter of lesser diameter than the artery as appreciated on a road map. This is to avoid selecting a balloon that is too big, which may cause vessel rupture.

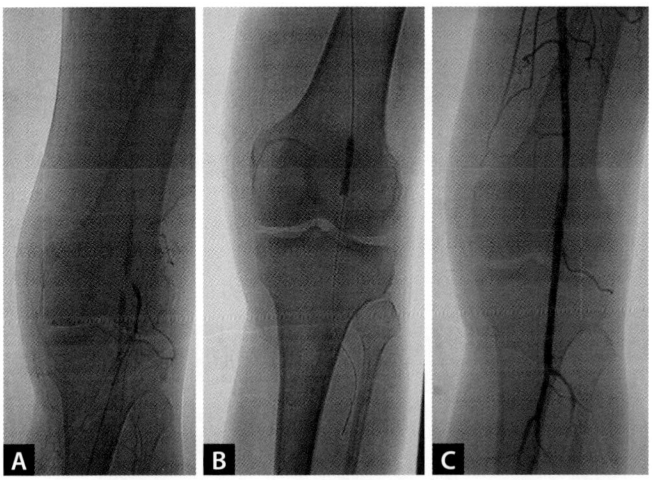

Figs. 11A to C: Image showing various steps of balloon angioplasty. Short segment occlusion of popliteal artery (A), crossed by the floppy end of hydrophilic guidewire followed by dilatation of the segment using balloon catheter (B). Final angiogram showing the opening of the occluded segment of popliteal artery (C).

Table 3: Recommended balloon catheter sizes.

Iliac segments	7–8 mm
Femoral segments	6 mm
Popliteal segment	4–5 mm
Below knee	2–3 mm

- Many interventionists choose the balloon catheter diameter using the "Eyeball technique" based on their clinical experience of the estimated diameter of the vessel to be treated.
- Regarding the length of the balloon catheter, length must be sufficient to include the entire length of the lesion. If an undersized balloon is chosen for a considerably longer lesion, several dilatations may be needed to cover the full length of the lesion, which could be time consuming.
- Proximal and distal radiopaque markers indicate the location of the balloon on the catheter.
- The balloon catheter is introduced over the guidewire under image guidance, steadily in smooth manner.
- Once the balloon is placed accurately across the lesion using the radiopaque markers as guidance, balloon catheter is slowly inflated using diluted iodinated contrast media.
- The inflation may be accomplished either by a 5 mL Luer-lock syringe or by mechanical inflation device having pressure measurement display.
- During balloon inflation, expansion starts from periphery of the balloon and extends gradually towards the middle as the lumen gets dilated. Frequently, the lesion creates a central waist on the balloon at the site of maximum resistance resulting in an hourglass configuration. The removal of the waist suggests effective dilatation of the stenosis.[22]
- There is no agreement about the ideal duration of balloon inflation. Balloon Inflation duration might range from a few seconds to a minute or more. However, the duration of balloon inflation does not matter in majority of cases.
- Usually, balloon dilatation is done from distal to proximal segments. At each station, after the balloon angioplasty, balloon should be fully deflated, so that it can be pulled easily to the next segment of narrowing.
- Pain is an important factor during balloon inflation and it should be closely observed. Generally, the balloon inflation produces some degree of pain due to stretching of the adventitia and this pain reduces following balloon deflation. However, when patient complains of continued pain following balloon deflation, one should suspect vessel rupture.
- Once, the entire length of stenotic/occluded segment is dilated, the balloon catheter should be withdrawn carefully, while keeping the guidewire across the site of angioplasty. It is very important to remember because by mistake if the guidewire is pulled out and the lesion entails additional management due to

unsatisfactory outcome or a complication (such as rupture/dissection), it may not be possible to go across the freshly treated lesion that may end in technical failure or a limb-threatening complication.

- Once the balloon catheter is removed over the guidewire, the vascular sheath should be aspirated for removal of the clots (if any) present inside the sheath and sheath is flushed with heparinized saline. Post-angioplasty angiogram must be obtained to assess the technical outcome and to look for complications (such as dissection/rupture/distal migration of ruptured plaque).
- Post-angioplasty angiogram should include the distal run of vessels (e.g. trifurcation and tibial vessels) along with angioplasty site to look for distal vessel occlusion due to distal migration of plaque material from angioplasty site.
- Once the angiogram looks acceptable, the guidewire and vascular sheath are removed. Manual compression is applied at the puncture site to achieve hemostasis.
- Sometimes, occlusion involves the origin of an artery (e.g. common iliac artery origin at the bifurcation), there is a hypothetical risk of creating an ostial stenosis of the contralateral vessel either by dissection or by dislodgment of plaque across the bifurcation. Hence, few interventionists ensure safety of the contralateral vessel by the placement of another balloon and is known as "kissing balloon technique" **(Figs. 12A and B)**. This is debatable and several interventionists do not advocate the use of this technique for treating ostial lesions at bifurcations.
- Similarly, if stenting has to be done for the lesion at bifurcation due to unsatisfactory angioplasty result, some operators choose to place a stent in the contralateral artery based on similar justification and is called as kissing stent technique **(Figs. 13A to C)**.[19,22]

How to Decide the Endpoint?

The angioplasty site must be cautiously assessed on the check angiogram to guarantee that the vessel is effectively opened with residual stenosis <30% as measured by pressure measurement using manometers. Another simple way of deciding the endpoint without pressure measurement is looking at the angiogram for disappearance of collaterals across the angioplasty site.

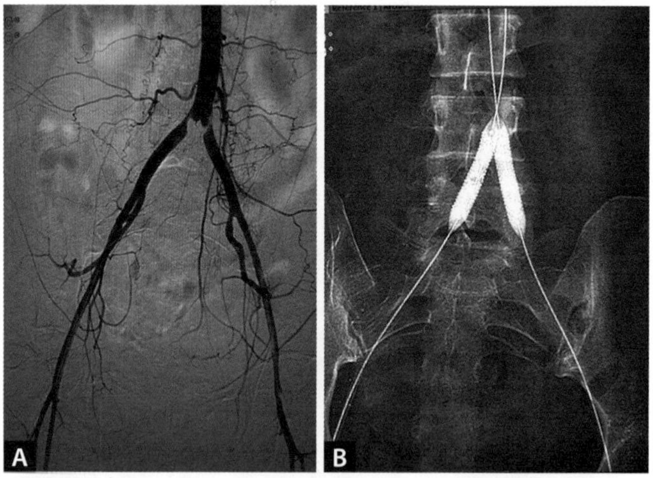

Figs. 12A and B: Kissing balloon technique: Digital subtraction angiography spot images showing (A) Ostial stenosis of bilateral iliac artery; (B) Managed by kissing balloon technique.

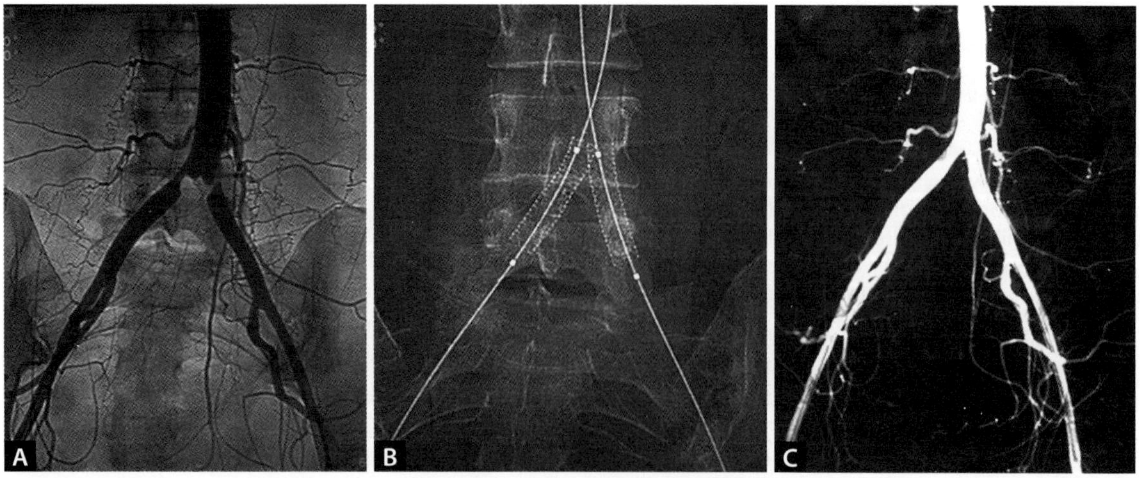

Figs. 13A to C: Digital subtraction angiography images showing kissing stent technique in the management of bilateral iliac ostial stenosis.

Subintimal Angioplasty (Figs. 14A to D)[23]

- In case of true lumen angioplasty, narrowing is negotiated by passing a guidewire through the true lumen of the vessel.
- Whereas in case of chronic tight occlusions, guidewire is intentionally negotiated through the wall of vessel (usually the subintimal space) rather than true lumen, and is known as subintimal angioplasty or also known as percutaneous intentional extraluminal recanalization (PIER).
- *Benefit of subintimal angioplasty:* Since we are doing angioplasty of the subintimal space, it provides a lumen that is free of atherosclerotic plaques as compared to true lumen angioplasty.
- In this procedure, combination of angled catheter (such as Picard catheter) and J-tip hydrophilic catheter is used for intentional passage of the guidewire into subintimal space. Just proximal to the site of occlusion, this catheter and guidewire combination is brought and forcibly pushed against the site of occlusion. During this forcible attempt to cross the occlusion, a loop of guidewire is created. This loop has to be advanced further, so that this loop dissects the intima and enter the subintimal space. Once, the loop enters the subintimal space, catheter and guidewire are progressively advanced distally till the entire segment of occlusion is traversed.
- When the loop has crossed past the distal limit of the occlusion, pull the guidewire to shorten the length of the loop. Now push the guidewire forward by rapid backward and forwards movements, so that guidewire re-enters the true lumen.
- Re-entry into the true lumen is complemented by sudden loss of resistance to passage of the guidewire
- If the catheter tip is in true lumen, one should start seeing the free flow of blood coming from the catheter hub. It is always good idea to aspirate blood and/or inject contrast medium to check the catheter position within the lumen.
- Once the guidewire position within true lumen is confirmed after re-entry, the dissection plane is dilated with an angioplasty balloon of a suitable size.[23,24]

Stents[19,22,25]

- There are two types of stenting technique and the prevailing indications for stenting differ depending upon the site of lesion.
- Types of stenting: Primary and secondary stenting.
- In primary stenting, stenting is done without preceding angioplasty. It is encouraged/suggested in few locations, such as stenosis involving ostium (renal artery stenosis, iliac artery stenosis) and malignant venous obstruction.
- In secondary stenting, stenting is done after the angioplasty especially when angioplasty results are poor due to elastic recoiling of wall or due to flow limiting dissection at angioplasty site.
- Stents may comprise of only metal known as bare metal stent or may comprise of a metallic stent covered with graft material, which is known as a stent-graft.

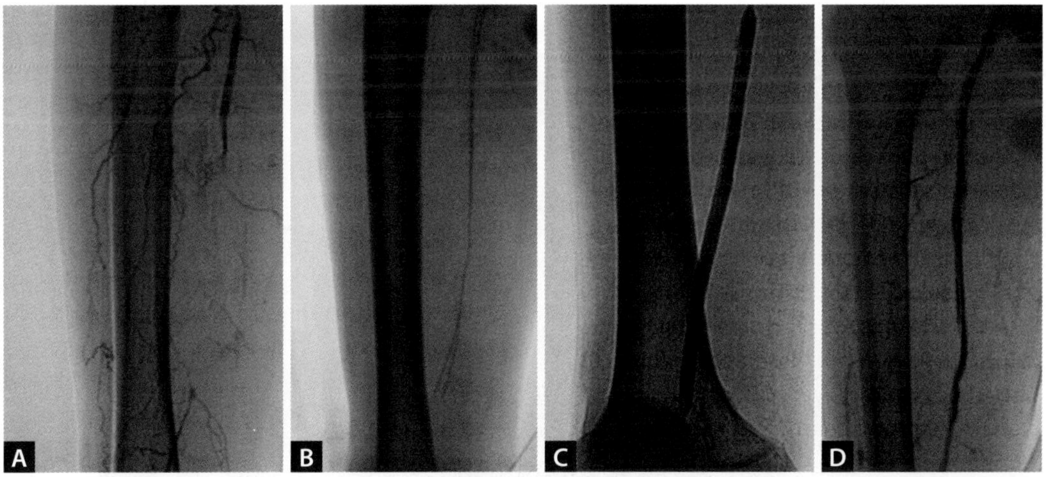

Figs. 14A to D: Digital subtraction angiography spots images showing technique of subintimal angioplasty (A). Long segment occlusion of superficial femoral artery, which was crossed by a loop of floppy end of hydrophilic guidewire into the subintimal space (B) and subsequently dilated by balloon catheter (C). Final angiogram showing the opening of the occluded segment of superficial femoral artery (D).

- Another method of classifying stents as balloon expandable and self-expandable, is based on their method of deployment.
- Balloon-expandable stents are valuable at sites where stent has to be deployed with highest accuracy (i.e. ostial lesions) **(Figs. 15A to D)**.
- As compared to balloon expandable stents, self-expanding stents have smaller profiles, are more flexible and are available in longer lengths. Hence, these are used for treating long segment tortuous occlusions like SFA occlusions **(Figs. 16A to C)**.
- Occasionally, self-expanding stents may require additional dilatation using balloon catheter of the equal diameter after deployment to assist their expansion to their full diameter. This is not required in case of balloon expandable stent, since they are deployed by balloon dilatation.

Complications[19,22]

Procedure-related complications (peri-procedural or post-procedural) are not uncommon and are commonly seen in elderly patients with diffuse disease and other comorbidities.[25]

The most common complications are puncture site complications such as hematoma and pseudoaneurysm formation which are easily managed by manual

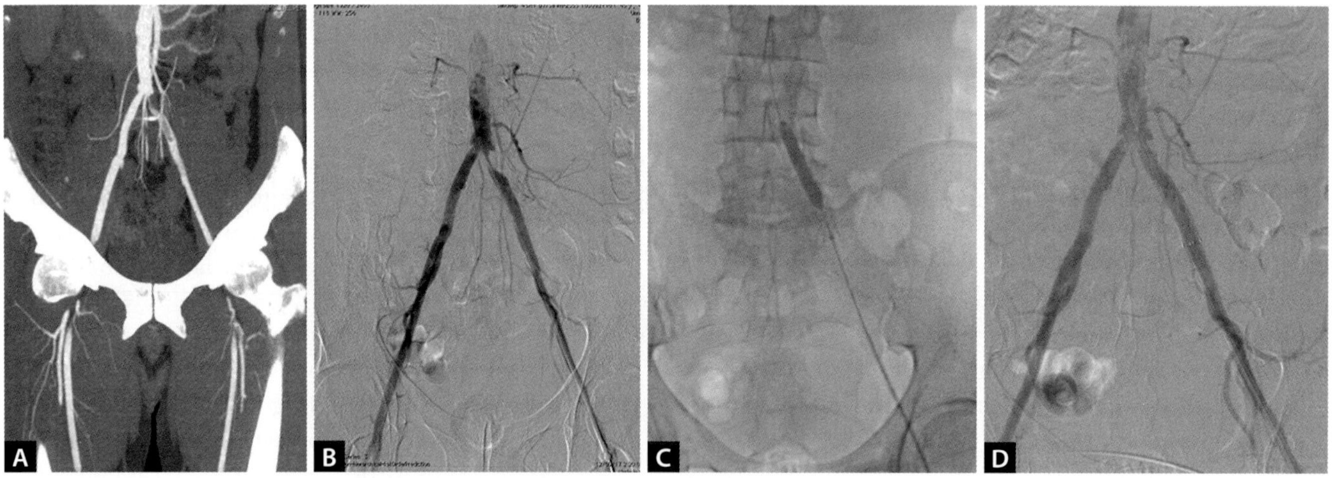

Figs. 15A to D: Images showing technique common iliac stenting using balloon mounted stent. Short segment occlusion of left common iliac artery involving the ostium (A and B), was initially crossed with floppy end of hydrophilic guidewire and subsequently managed by balloon mounted stent (C). Final angiogram showing the opening of the occluded segment of common iliac artery (D).

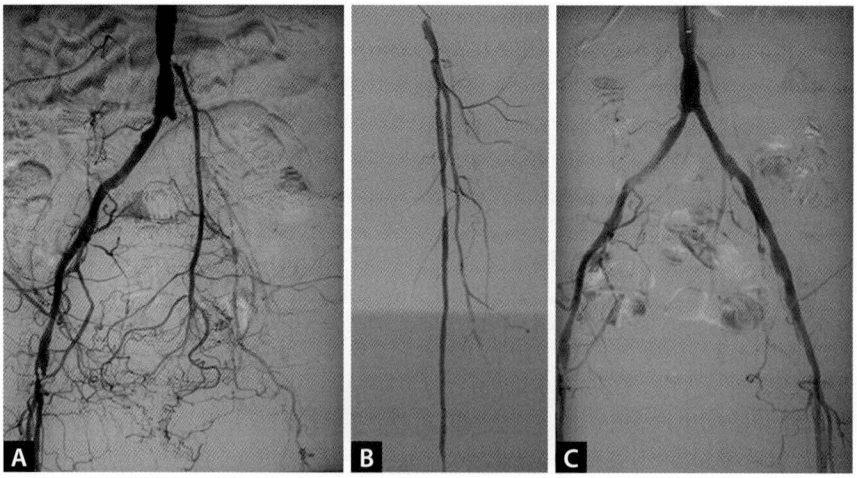

Figs. 16A to C: TASC type D lesion of left iliac segment managed by self-expandable stent. Long segment occlusion involving the left common iliac and external iliac arteries (A), with reformation of left common femoral and superficial femoral artery by collaterals (B), was subsequently managed by placing overlapping self-expandable stents across the occluded segment. Final angiogram showing the opening of the occluded entire segment of iliac artery (C).

compression. Occasionally, pseudoaneurysm needs to be managed by thrombin injection **(Figs. 17A to F)**.

The most serious complications include arterial rupture and distal plaque embolization.

Arterial Rupture

- It is the most serious complications and is seen <1% cases. If the rupture occurs in the periphery (infrainguinal), it is usually self-limiting and bleeding is controlled by local tamponade effect of the surrounding soft tissues. However, if the arterial rupture occurs above the inguinal ligament, it may be fatal because there is no tamponade effect by the surrounding area. If the patient complaints of severe pain, which continues even after balloon deflation and is accompanied by hypotension and tachycardia, one should suspect vascular rupture.
- Vascular ruptures below the inguinal ligament are usually self-limiting and require no specific treatment except for manual compression. Whereas arterial rupture above inguinal ligament needs immediate attention. Instant balloon re-inflation at the site of rupture to stop bleeding, followed by either placement of stent-graft across the rupture or shift the patient to operation theater for surgical repair **(Figs. 18A to C)**.

Distal Plaque Embolization

- Distal plaque embolization is another serious complication, which may lead to acute limb ischemia, tissue necrosis and amputation of limb. Certain amount of distal embolization occurs in most of the angioplasty procedures, however the volume of plaque embolization is high in iliac angioplasty.
- There is no specific treatment for this complication. Proper technique and careful patient selection are critical to circumvent this complication.

Stent-related Complications

- Stent migration during placement
- Stent fracture

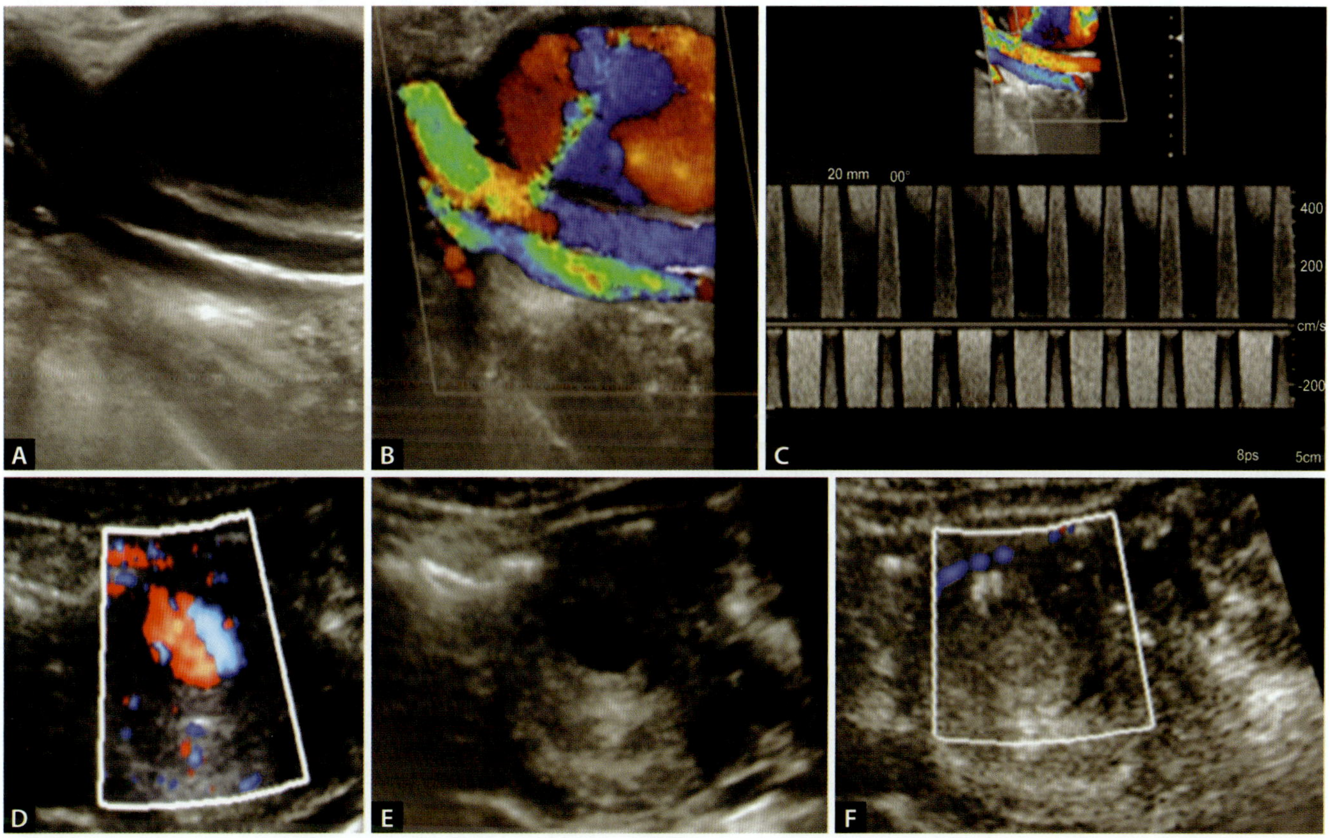

Figs. 17A to F: Post-angioplasty pseudoaneurysm complication management: Sonography with color Doppler images showing narrow neck pseudoaneurysm arising from the common femoral artery at the puncture site (A and B), with Yin-Yang spectral wave form at the neck of pseudoaneurysm (C), which was subsequently managed by percutaneous thrombin injection into the pseudoaneurysm and achieving complete thrombosis of the pseudoaneurysm (D to F).

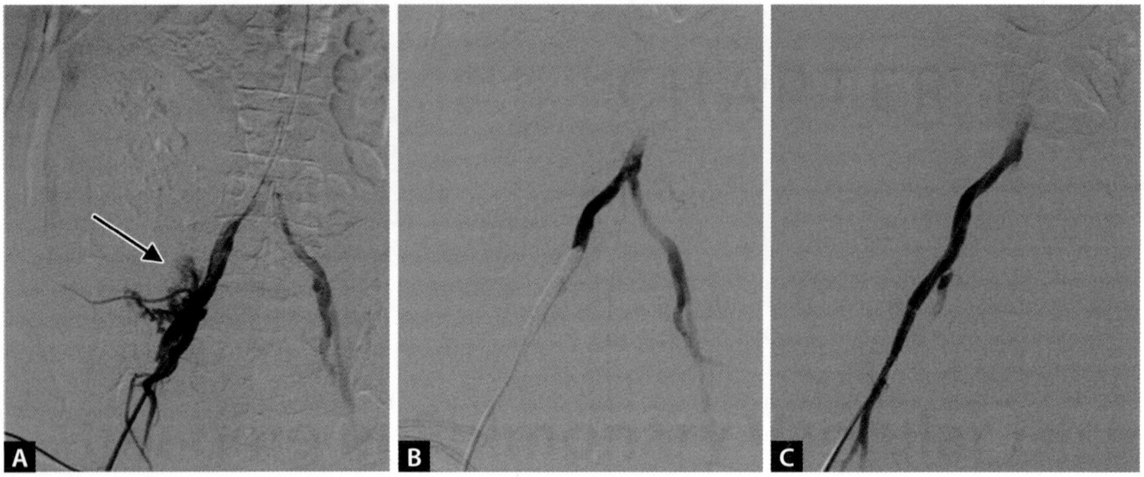

Figs. 18A to C: Post angioplasty complication of arterial rupture: DSA spot images showing rupture of the external iliac artery (arrow) following balloon angioplasty (A), which was subsequently managed balloon re-inflation for 10 minutes across the rupture site (B). Final angiogram showing the sealing of the ruptures site, maintaining the patency of external iliac artery (C).

Restenosis

Restenosis may occur following angioplasty alone or may occur within stents (in-stent restenosis). This restenosis may be due to disease progression or due to neo intimal hyperplasia. This restenosis is managed either by repeat angioplasty or repeat stenting.

Teaching Points

- Doppler sonography is used as screening modality in suspected peripheral vascular disease.
- CT angiography or MR angiography is needed to define disease extent and planning the treatment.
- Endovascular treatments offer low-risk alternative to surgery in majority of the patients.
- Angioplasty and stenting are the two most widely used treatment options.
- Antegrade access is generally preferable to contralateral access for infrainguinal lesions. Never withdraw the guidewire back across the lesion before the procedure is finished.
- Always check the run-off vessels at the end of the procedure for distal embolization.
- Stents are usually indicated if angioplasty results are unsatisfactory.
- Primary placement of stent is indicated in selected cases such as iliac artery occlusions and ostial renal artery stenoses.
- Proper patient selection and technique are two most important factors, which can prevent most of the complications.

REFERENCES

1. Selvin E, Erlinger TP. Prevalence of and risk factors for peripheral arterial disease in the United States: results from the National Health and Nutrition Examination Survey, 1999-2000. Circulation. 2004;110(6):738-43.
2. Pollak AW, Norton PT, Kramer CM. Multimodality imaging of lower extremity peripheral arterial disease: Current role and future directions. Circ Cardiovasc Imaging. 2012;5(6): 797-807.
3. Lijmer JG, Hunink MG, van den Dungen JJ, et al. ROC analysis of noninvasive tests for peripheral arterial disease. Ultrasound Med Biol. 1996;22(4):391-8.
4. Ota H, Takase K, Rikimaru H, et al. Quantitative vascular measurements in arterial occlusive disease. Radiographics. 2005;25(5):1141-58.
5. 2011 ACCF/AHA Focused Update of the Guideline for the Management of Patients With Peripheral Artery Disease (Updating the 2005 Guideline). J Am Coll Cardiol. 2011;58(19):2020-45.
6. Ubbink DT, Fidler M, Legemate DA. Interobserver variability in aortoiliac and femoropopliteal duplex scanning. J Vasc Surg. 2001;33(3):540-5.
7. Catalano C, Fraioli F, Laghi A, et al. Infrarenal aortic and lower-extremity arterial disease: Diagnostic performance of multi-detector row CT angiography. Radiology. 2004;231(2):555-63.
8. Schernthaner R, Stadler A, Lomoschitz F, et al. Multidetector CT angiography in the assessment of peripheral arterial occlusive disease: accuracy in detecting the severity, number, and length of stenoses. Eur Radiol. 2008;18(4):665-71.
9. Roditi G, Kusumawidjaja D. Magnetic resonance angiography and computed tomography angiography for peripheral arterial disease. Imaging. 2009;21(2):85-108.

10. Ward EV, Galizia MS, Usman A, et al. Comparison of quiescent inflow single-shot and native space for nonenhanced peripheral MR angiography. J Magn Reson Imaging. 2013;38(6):1531-8.
11. Hodnett PA, Koktzoglou I, Davarpanah AH, et al. Evaluation of peripheral arterial disease with nonenhanced quiescent-interval single-shot MR angiography. Radiology. 2011;260(1):282-93.
12. Amin P, Collins JD, Koktzoglou I, et al. Evaluating peripheral arterial disease with unenhanced quiescent-interval single-shot MR angiography at 3 T. Am J Roentgenol. 2014;202(4):886-93.
13. Foley WD, Stonely T. CT angiography of the lower extremities. Radiol Clin North Am. 2010;48(2):367-96, ix.
14. Crawford ES, DeBakey ME. Popliteal artery arteriosclerotic aneurysm. Circulation. 1965;32(4):515-6.
15. Friesen G, Ivins JC, Janes JM. Popliteal aneurysms. Surgery. 1962;51:90-8.
16. Wright LB, Matchett WJ, Cruz CP, et al. Popliteal Artery Disease: diagnosis and treatment. Radiographics. 2004;24(2):467-79.
17. Diwan A, Sarkar R, Stanley JC, et al. Incidence of femoral and popliteal artery aneurysms in patients with abdominal aortic aneurysms. J Vasc Surg. 2000;31(5):863-9.
18. Jaff MR, White CJ, Hiatt WR, et al. An update on methods for revascularization and expansion of the TASC lesion classification to include below-the-knee arteries: A supplement to the inter-society consensus for the management of peripheral arterial disease (TASC II): The TASC Steering Committee. Catheter Cardiovasc Interv Off J Soc Card Angiogr Interv. 2015;86(4):611-25.
19. Rholl KS, Durham JD, Sacks D, et al. Peripheral vascular interventions. In: Darcy MD, Vedantham S, Kaufman JA (Eds). Society of Cardiovascular and Interventional Radiology. 2nd edition. SCVIR. 2001.p.391.
20. Block PC, Myler RK, Stertzer S, et al. Morphology after transluminal angioplasty in human beings. N Engl J Med. 1981;305(7):382-5.
21. Bhat R, McBride K, Chakraverty S, et al. Primary cutting balloon angioplasty for treatment of venous stenoses in native hemodialysis fistulas: Long-term results from three centers. Cardiovasc Intervent Radiol. 2007;30(6):1166-1170-1172.
22. Vascular and Interventional Radiology: The Requisites. Mosby; 2004.p.744.
23. Bolia A. Percutaneous intentional extraluminal (subintimal) recanalization of crural arteries. Eur J Radiol. 1998;28(3): 199-204.
24. Reekers JA, Bolia A. Percutaneous intentional extraluminal (subintimal) recanalization: How to do it yourself. Eur J Radiol. 1998;28(3):192-8.
25. Pentecost MJ, Criqui MH, Dorros G, et al. Guidelines for peripheral percutaneous transluminal angioplasty of the abdominal aorta and lower extremity vessels. A statement for health professionals from a special writing group of the Councils on Cardiovascular Radiology, Arteriosclerosis, Cardiothoracic and Vascular Surgery, Clinical Cardiology, and Epidemiology and Prevention, the American Heart Association. Circulation. 1994;89(1):511-31.

Section 7

Musculoskeletal and Breast Imaging

CHAPTER 186

Diagnostic Approach to Focal Bone Lesions: Conventional Radiography, Computed Tomography and Magnetic Resonance Imaging

Shivanand Gamanagatti, Raju Sharma

INTRODUCTION

Focal bone lesions are broadly divided into three categories: benign, malignant (primary and secondary) and non-neoplastic. Plain radiographs are initial and most important imaging modality for the diagnosis and should be evaluated in systematic manner regardless of the pathology. Computed tomography (CT) and magnetic resonance imaging (MRI) provide complementary information that is extremely useful in the work-up of focal bone lesion. CT scan is particularly useful in evaluating the cortex and matrix. MRI is useful in determining the intramedullary extent, soft tissue extent of focal bone lesion and also play vital role in detecting skip lesions.[1]

General principles of focal bone lesion evaluation are as follows:

- Prior to the analysis of the radiographic features of focal bone lesion, certain clinical information is essential to narrow down the differential diagnosis, such as the age of the patient, the lesion's location and is it solitary or multiple?
- Within long bones, plane of the lesion must be determined with reference to longitudinal (epiphysis, metaphysis, diaphysis) and transverse (intramedullary, intracortical, surface) planes. Surface (juxtacortical) lesions may be parosteal or periosteal.
- Radiograph is essential for lesion detection and characterization. Radiograph should be systematically assessed for the following:
  - Pattern of bone destruction
  - Edge of lesion/zone of transition
  - Cortical response
  - Matrix mineralization.
- Nonaggressive versus aggressive pattern on radiograph is not always equivalent to benign versus malignant, e.g. osteomyelitis can have an aggressive pattern on radiograph.
- Do not "overdiagnose" a benign bone tumor and do not "underdiagnose" a malignant bone tumor.
- Do not misdirect the biopsy approach to the lesion so as to convert more conservative operation (compartment resection or limb salvage procedure) into more radical operation (amputation).
- Any skeletal lesion detected on well-penetrated radiograph rule out infection, eosinophilic granuloma, subchondral degenerative cyst, lesion related to metabolic bone disease, such as brown tumor, post-traumatic changes, such as stress fracture or is it normal variant.
- If the lesion is unchanged from old films (at least 2 years old), then consider for a clinical/radiographic follow-up of the patient.
- If there are multiple lesions rule out metastases especially in adults or other causes of multiple skeletal lesions, such as multiple enchondromas, multiple osteochondromas, fibrous dysplasia, fibrous cortical defects/nonossifying fibromas, sarcoidosis, etc.
- If there is solitary lesion, characterize the lesion further based on age, location, pattern of destruction, margins, cortical response, matrix, periosteal reaction.

AGE OF THE PATIENT

Most bone tumors have a tendency of occurring in a specific age group; so, the age of the patient is an important clinical information for the assessment of a bone tumor. The typical peak ages of different kinds of lesions are listed in **Table 1**. For example, simple bone cysts and chondroblastomas occur in people who are skeletally immature, while skeletally mature people are prone to giant cell tumors. Ewing sarcoma typically occurs in the second decade of the life of patients, while conventional osteosarcoma has two age peaks, one, arising de novo, in teenagers and the second, arising in pagetic or previously irradiated bone, in adults older than 50 years. A malignant bone lesion in an adult over 40 years old is more probable of being metastatic carcinoma, myeloma or metastatic non-Hodgkin's lymphoma rather than a primary bone sarcoma.[2]

Table 1: Bone tumors predilection for specific age groups.

• Metastatic neuroblastoma • Simple bone cyst • Fibrous cortical defect • Aneurysmal bone cyst • Ewing's sarcoma • Osteosarcoma • Giant cell tumor • Chondrosarcoma • Multiple myeloma • Metastasis	<2 years

LOCATION OF LESION (FIG. 1)

Most bone tumors, regardless of being benign or malignant in nature, occur most often in a characteristic location in the skeleton (i.e. axial vs appendicular skeleton or long vs flat bone). Thus, some tumors (e.g. osteosarcoma) have a predilection for sites of rapid bone growth, usually the metaphyseal region, while other tumors (e.g. Ewing's sarcoma) have a tendency of following the distribution of red marrow. Furthermore, a lesion in a long bone usually

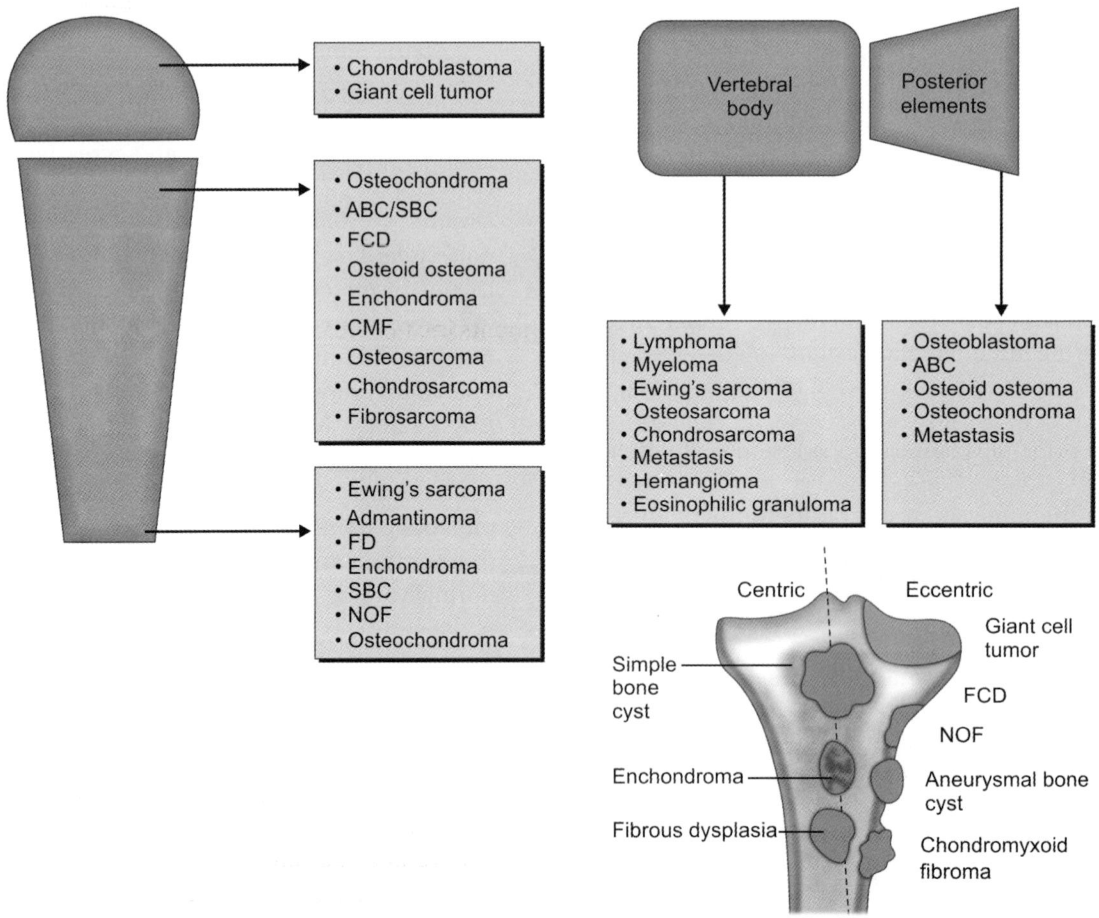

Fig. 1: Diagrammatic representation of the locations of various focal bone lesions.
Abbreviations: ABC/SBC: Aneurysmal bone cyst/simple bone cyst; FCD: Focal cortical dysplasia; CMF: Chondromyxoid fibroma; FD: Fibrous dysplasia; NOF: Nonossifying fibroma.

has a central location within the medullary cavity, while an aneurysmal bone cyst is located eccentrically in the medullary cavity **(Fig. 1)**. However, in short or thin tubular bones, such as the metacarpals, metatarsals, phalanges, and fibula, there can be involvement of the entire diameter of the bone, which sometimes makes it difficult to identify the part of the bone where the lesion started. An apophysis (a growth center that does not contribute to the length of a bone) is the equivalent of an epiphysis (a growth center at the end of a bone that does contribute to length); thus, one should use the "end-of-bone" differential list for a lesion in such sites as the greater trochanter of the femur and the tibial tubercle **(Fig. 1)**. Similarly, other growth centers, such as the patella, the small bones of the wrist, hindfoot, and midfoot, and the subarticular portions of flat bones, such as those around the sacroiliac joints and acetabuli in the pelvis and the glenoid of the scapula, are also end-of-bone equivalents.

The differential diagnosis can be narrowed down further if the patient's age is known. For instance, a lytic lesion in the epiphysis of a long bone of an adolescent is likely to be a chondroblastoma, whereas a lytic lesion at the end of a long bone in a young adult is likely to be a giant cell tumor. Ewing sarcoma and Langerhans cell histiocytosis have a predilection for the diaphysis of long bones in people younger than 20 years and a predilection for flat bones, such as the pelvis and skull in people older than 20 years, thus reflecting the normal change in the distribution of red marrow with the increase in the age of a person.

Some processes have a predilection for a particular bone and location, such as an adamantinoma and osteofibrous dysplasia for the anterior cortex of the tibia, periosteal desmoids for the posterior distal aspect of the femur, and hemangioma for vertebral bodies.[2]

PATTERN OF BONE DESTRUCTION

Three patterns of bone destruction have been described as follows **(Figs. 2A to C)**:[3]

1. Type I — Geographic bone destruction
2. Type II — Moth-eaten bone destruction
3. Type III — Permeative bone destruction

Geographic Bone Destruction

This type of bone destruction is the least aggressive form and suggests a slow growing lesion. It is seen as a well-circumscribed lytic lesion with a narrow zone of transition. The slow growth rate results in sharp demarcation between the destructive lesion and adjacent normal bone. The margin of the lesion represents the true histological margin of destruction, however, malignant lesions like metastasis or myeloma may also demonstrate a similar pattern.

This pattern is further divided into three subtypes:

1. Type IA — Geographic lesion with sclerotic margin
2. Type IB — Geographic lesion with no marginal sclerosis
3. Type IC — Geographic lesion with ill-defined margins.

Geographic Lesion with Sclerotic Margin

The slow growth of the lesion permits development of a reactive bone around the lesion so as to accommodate transmission of forces. The sclerotic margin may vary in thickness and is especially thick in lesions occurring in weight bearing bones like femur and tibia. This type of lesion is commonly seen in simple bone cyst **(Fig. 3A)**, enchondroma, chondromyxoid fibroma, Brodie's abscess, and fibroxanthoma. Fibrous dysplasia often displays a peripheral thick sclerotic rim resembling a "rind" of orange **(Fig. 3B)**. In some lesions like Brodie's abscess **(Fig. 3C)** and eosinophilic granuloma, the sclerotic rim is rather

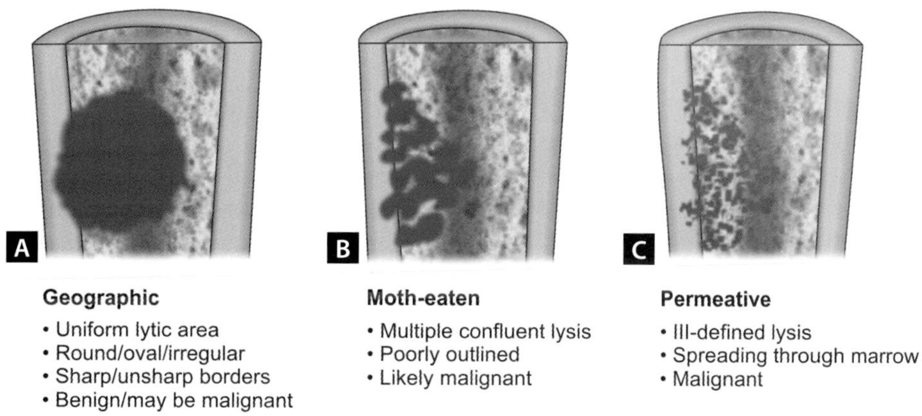

Figs. 2A to C: Pattern of bone destruction.

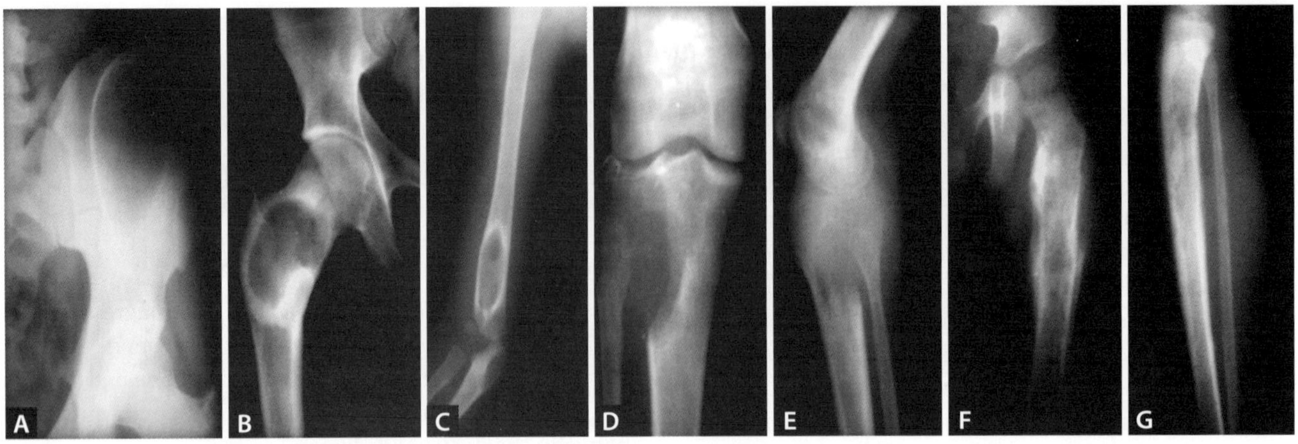

Figs. 3A to G: Patterns of bone destruction: (A) Type IA—geographic destruction with sclerotic margins in a simple bone cyst seen in the left iliac bone; (B) Type IA—geographic destruction with thick sclerotic margins, "rind sign", seen in fibrous dysplasia involving neck of right femur; (C) Type IA—geographic destruction with sclerotic margin which is fuzzy and facing peripherally, in Brodie's abscess involving lower end of humerus; (D) Type IB—geographic destruction with punched-out lesion seen in giant cell tumor involving upper tibia—note its typical eccentric subarticular position; (E) Type IC—geographic destruction with ill-defined margins seen in another patient of giant cell tumor involving upper tibia; (F) Type II—moth-eaten destruction seen in osteomyelitis involving left upper femur in a child—also note associated ingle lamellar periosteal reaction; (G) Type III—permeative bone destruction involving upper tibia with osteomyelitis—note the tunneling in the anterior cortex.

fuzzy and appears to be fading gradually into adjacent cancellous bone. The sclerotic rim is a mechanical adaptation designed to accommodate forces transmitted around the space-occupying mass.

Geographic Lesion with No Marginal Sclerosis

This type of lesion shows sharp margins with narrow zone of transition, referred to as a punched-out lesion with no sclerosis **(Fig. 3D)**. The margins seen on radiograph, reflects the true histological edge of the lesion. Giant cell tumor typically displays this pattern. Many lesions associated with type IA pattern may also show this pattern, e.g. bone cyst, enchondroma and chondroblastoma.

Geographic Lesion with Ill-defined Margins

This type indicates locally infiltrative process. The margins are poorly defined suggesting more aggressive pattern than type IB lesions **(Fig. 3E)**. The destructive process extends in the marrow between the trabeculae beyond the radiographic destructive edge. This type of lesion is seen characteristically in giant cell tumor, osteosarcoma, chondrosarcoma, fibrosarcoma, aneurysmal bone cyst, eosinophilic granuloma and osteomyelitis.

Moth-eaten Bone Destruction

This type of lesion is relatively more aggressive, suggesting more rapidly growing lesion. It is characterized by multiple small varying sized lytic lesions that coalesce and involve both cancellous and cortical bone **(Fig. 3F)**. In cancellous bone, normal trabeculae may be seen in between the lytic lesions while in cortical bone, the lytic lesion starts from endosteal surface and extends outwards. This may progress to complete cortical destruction with extension into adjacent soft tissues. The lesion has less well-defined margins with wide zone of transition and is more extensive on histopathology, than suggested on a radiograph. This pattern is usually seen in malignant neoplasms like reticulum cell sarcoma, osteosarcoma, chondrosarcoma, fibrosarcoma, round cell tumor (including Ewing's sarcoma) and also osteomyelitis.

Permeative Bone Destruction

This pattern represents the most aggressive form and suggests a rapidly destructive bone lesion. This type is characterized by multiple, tiny oval lucent lesions or lucent streaks mostly involving cortical bone **(Fig. 3G)**. Progressive cortical destruction occurs with exuberant cortical tunneling by osteoclasts, and the lesions are ill-defined. The highly aggressive nature does not allow bone to react and stop its further progress. These lesions are much more widespread than they appear on a radiograph. This type of lesion is seen in Ewing's sarcoma, reticulum cell sarcoma, high-grade chondrosarcoma, fibrosarcoma, angiosarcoma, leukemia and metastasis.

Combination and Changing Pattern

This is characterized by combination of type I A to C, type II or type III patterns in a single lytic lesion and suggests more aggressive local growth. This pattern is usually seen in some benign lesions, when they become active, undergo malignant change or fracture. Pressure from tumor growth or active hyperemia are some of the factors that contribute to this pattern. A changing pattern is discernible when a change in the nature of margin is observed radiographically over time.

MARGIN OF THE LESION AND RATE OF GROWTH

The margin of the lesion relates to the radiographic appearance of the interface between the lesion and adjacent normal bone. This is determined by reaction of the host bone to the lesion and rate of growth of the lesion. Well-marginated lesions have a narrow zone of transition **(Fig. 3A)** while poorly defined lesions have a wide zone of transition **(Fig. 3G)**. The aggressiveness and rate of growth of the lesion can be assessed from its margin. Sharply defined margin or a sclerotic margin suggests slow growth rate, while ill-defined margins indicate aggressive lesion and rapid growth rate. Some benign lesions may, however, show a rapid growth rate, and some malignant lesions may be slow growing and have well-defined margins. Therefore, assessment of radiographic margin does not always indicate benign or malignant nature of a lesion.[5,6] Aneurysmal bone cyst, eosinophilic granuloma, majority of giant cell tumors and chondromyxoid fibroma may display aggressive appearance on radiographs and yet be benign. On the other hand, malignant lesions like plasmacytoma and juxtacortical osteosarcoma are slow growing and may appear nonaggressive on plain radiograph. Treatment can also alter the appearance of malignant bone tumors; following radiation or chemotherapy they may exhibit significant sclerosis as well as a narrow zone of transition.[3]

Inflammatory lesions usually produce marked reactive bone formation compared with neoplasms. Typically, these lesions show a sclerotic margin with sharp inner border and hazy outer border. However, osteoid osteoma also shows extensive osteosclerosis around the margin of similar nature. Benign tumors or tumor-like conditions and slow growing malignant tumors usually show sclerotic rim with sharp outer and inner margins **(Fig. 3B)**. While inflammatory lesions show a sclerotic margin with sharp inner border and a hazy outer border **(Fig. 3C)**.

Sometimes, a lesion may demonstrate a scalloped margin. This occurs in lesions of cartilage, fibrous tissue, fat and vascular tissue, where the cells grow in clumps or lobules at different growth rate. The scalloped margin is seen typically in nonossifying fibroma. The assessment of growth rate on radiographs correlates well with virulence of organisms, host response, degree of spread of infection in inflammatory lesion and with aggressiveness of the tumors. However, the radiographic rate of growth is not synonymous with actual biological behavior and growth rate of the lesion as seen in acute osteomyelitis and Ewing's sarcoma. Both these lesions may show similar radiographic appearance of aggressive pattern of bone destruction. However, such an appearance develops in a relatively short period of time in acute osteomyelitis in contrast to Ewing's sarcoma which may take a longer period. Nonetheless, assessment of growth rate may help in narrowing the differential diagnosis.

CORTICAL RESPONSE

An intact cortex indicates slow growth. It may respond in various ways to the presence of a focal lesion. Cortical trabeculation implies a slow-growing, usually benign lesion, and is common in simple bone cyst (SBC) and giant cell tumor (GCT) **(Fig. 4A)**. Endosteal scalloping reects the lobular growth pattern of the underlying tumor, and is usually suggestive of a chondral **(Fig. 4B)** or brous lesion, but cannot differentiate between benign and malignant. Cortical expansion is a misnomer but implies that endosteal bone removal due to tumor occurs at a speed similar to the production of periosteal bone, which again indicates slow growth. In lesions which are more aggressive, the outer cortical layer may be too thin to be visible on plain films but is clearly evident on CT **(Figs. 4C and D)**.

Destruction of the cortex is suggestive of fast growth. The most aggressive malignant lesions usually penetrate the cortex even before the destruction is made evident on the radiograph. Apparent preservation of the cortex does not preclude extension of disease from the medulla. In saucerization, an extraosseous mass of tumor causes pressure erosion on the outer surface of the bone. It usually occurs with an apparently intact cortex **(Fig. 4E)**. Although the soft tissue mass may not be visible, its presence is implied by the the scalloping of the outer cortex. These last two entities, including the penetration of an apparently intact cortex and cortical saucerization, are most frequently found with malignant round cell tumors, particularly the Ewing's sarcoma.

MATRIX MINERALIZATION

Matrix refers to the acellular intercellular substance produced by the mesenchymal cells namely osteoblasts, cartilage cells, fibroblasts and this includes osteoid,

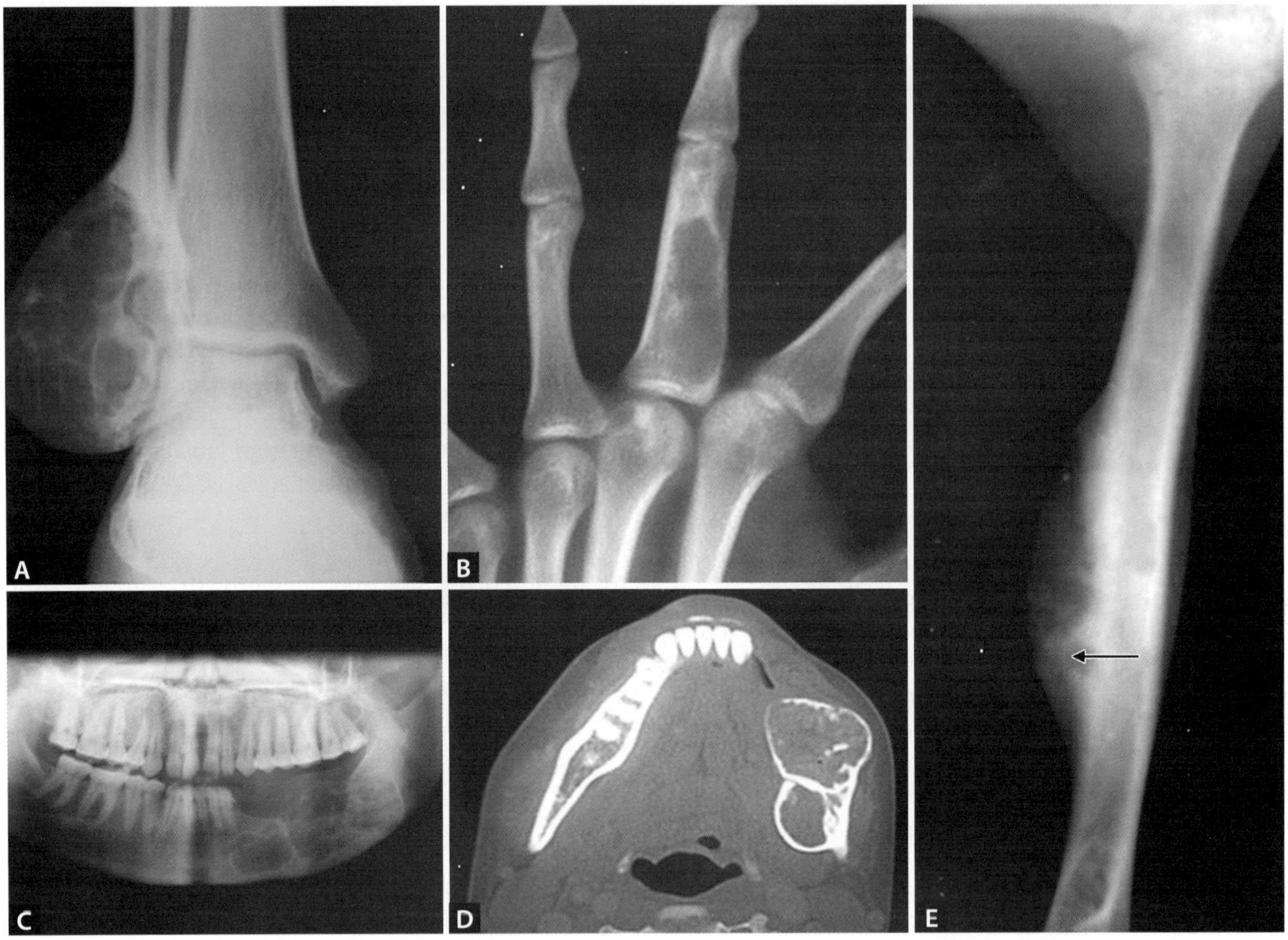

Figs. 4A to E: Cortical response: (A) Giant cell tumor showing expansile lytic lesion with intact cortex in lower end of fibula reaching up to subarticular location suggestive of cortical trabeculation indicating slow growth; (B) Enchondroma showing mildly expansile intramedullary lytic lesion in proximal phalanx causing endosteal scalloping indicating lobular growth; (C and D) Aneurysmal bone cyst showing expansile lytic lesion in body of mandible, cortical integrity is not well seen on plain radiograph. CT section of same patient showing the intact cortex around the expansile lytic lesion; (E) "Saucerization" (arrow) of the medial humeral diaphysis in Ewing's sarcoma caused by the pressure erosion of the soft mass.

chondroid, myxoid and collagen tissue. Matrix becomes visible on the radiograph only when it is mineralized sufficiently with calcium salts.[4]

Evaluation of matrix is valuable for two reasons:

1. Identification of particular configuration of matrix helps in suggesting specific diagnosis.
2. It is an indirect indicator of biological activity, e.g. transition from mineralized to nonmineralized matrix on follow-up radiographs indicates increased biologic activity and suggests this as an optimal site for biopsy.

The plain radiographs remain the best modality for assessing pattern of matrix mineralization; however, presence of subtle matrix mineralization can be seen only on computed tomography (CT).

Osseous Matrix

Osseous matrix is produced either by normal or tumor osteoblasts. The presence of bony trabeculae, appearing as thin interlacing radiodense struts within a lesion, is pathognomonic of a bone matrix. This occurs in myositis ossificans produced by normal osteoblasts, and in low-grade parosteal osteosarcoma produced by tumor osteoblasts. The osseous matrix may appear fluffy, amorphous, hazy **(Fig. 5A)** cloud-like or ivory pattern **(Fig. 5B)** on radiograph, when ossified sufficiently and is seen in high-grade osteosarcoma, parosteal osteosarcoma, and osteoblastoma.

Osseous matrix is also produced by modulation of fibroblasts into osteoblasts and occurs in fibrous dysplasia

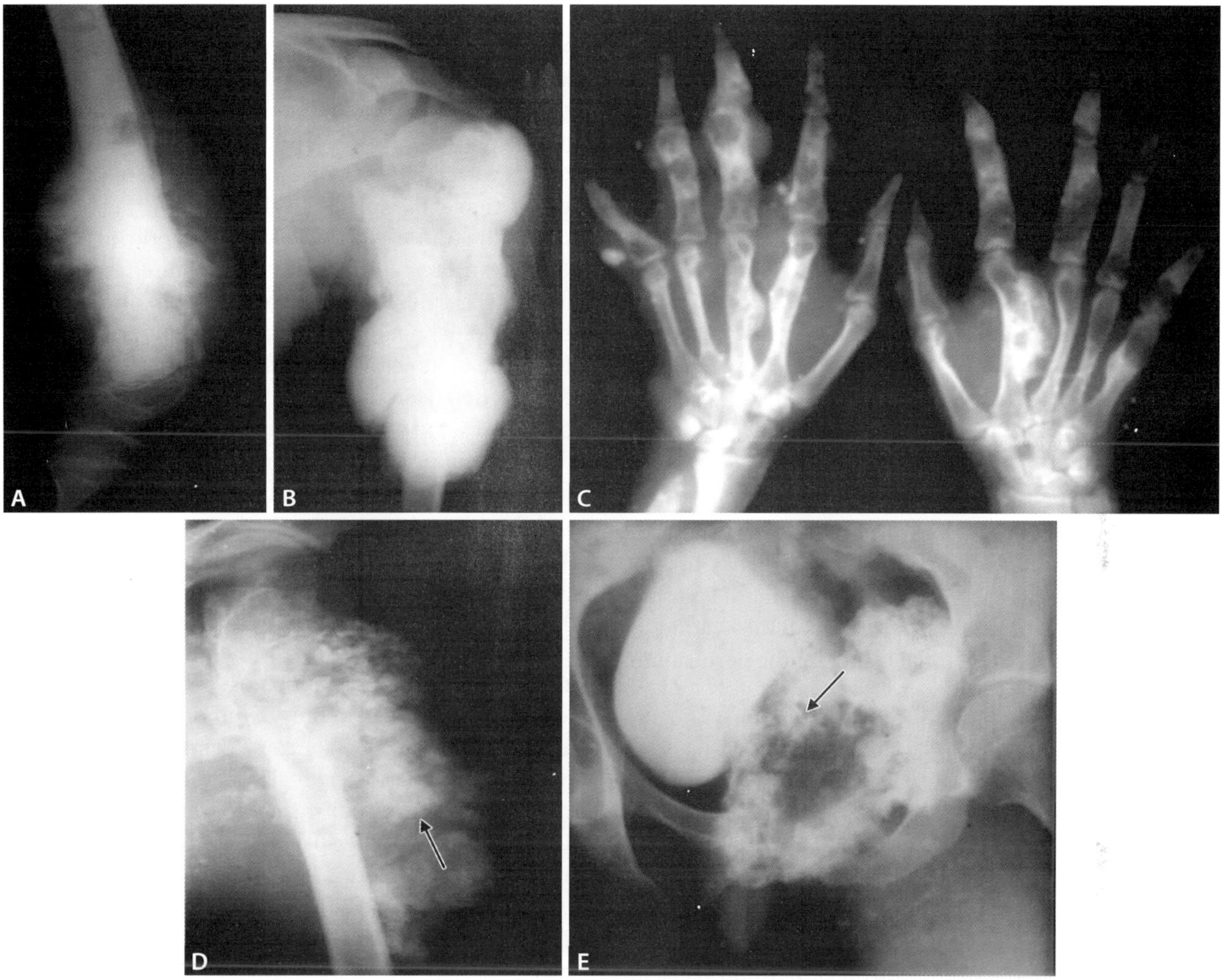

Figs. 5A to E: Patterns of matrix mineralization: (A) Cloud-like pattern of osteoid matrix in mid-diaphysis and ivory-like pattern in metaphyseal region of femur in osteosarcoma—note the single lamellar periosteal reaction along the anterior cortex; (B) Ivory-like pattern of osteoid matrix in a case of parosteal osteosarcoma involving proximal humerus—note that underlying humeral shaft can be seen through the tumor new bone in the lower part; (C) Punctate pattern of chondroid matrix in enchondromas involving multiple bones of hands in Maffucci's syndrome—note multiple phleboliths with soft tissue swellings suggestive of cavernous hemangiomas; (D) Flocculent and arc-like (arrow) pattern of chondroid matrix involving upper third of femur with sarcomatous change in diaphyseal aclasis; (E) Extensive flocculent and ring-like (arrow) chondroid matrix in chondrosarcoma involving left pubic bone, showing mass effect on urinary bladder.

and appears diffuse, hazy or poorly defined but not as radiodense as seen in tumor new bone. Necrosis of fat tissue may result in development of bone matrix which appears as clumps of radiodensity.

Cartilage Matrix

The cartilage matrix, when sufficiently calcified, is seen as flecks, punctate **(Fig. 5C)** or flocculated **(Fig. 5E)** in appearance (enchondroma, osteochondroma). When the cartilage matrix is sufficiently ossified, it shows appearance of arcs or rings **(Fig. 5D)** hazy, cloud-like or ivory-pattern. The punctate calcification of cartilage occurs in disrupted zone of provisional calcification while ring or arc appearance originates from disrupted enchondral bone formation. Both these patterns may exist alone or in combination. The ossified rings in cartilage tumor, suggests low-grade nature of the tumor.

PERIOSTEAL REACTION

Periosteum is like an envelope that separates the bone from surrounding soft tissues. This consists of two layers, the outer fibrous and inner cellular. It is firmly adherent to the underlying bone in adults but less so in children. Normally, periosteum is not visible and even when it is elevated, it cannot be appreciated on radiograph till mineralization occurs. The periosteal reaction can be stimulated by hyperemia, inflammation or spread of tumor. Its presence is an indicator of biologic activity and reflects the duration and intensity of underlying process.[5]

The type of periosteal reaction can be considered under three subgroups **(Fig. 6A)**:

1. Continuous
2. Discontinuous or interrupted
3. Complex.

Continuous Periosteal Reaction

Continuous periosteal reaction may occur either with intact or destroyed underlying cortex. It may be solid, single lamellar, multilamellar or parallel spiculated. An underlying inflammatory or neoplastic process incites hyperemia that activates fibroblasts to osteoblasts that produce osteoid and mineralized layers of new bone. It takes 10–21 days, from the initial insult, for the periosteum to be visible radiographically.

Single lamellar periosteal reaction **(Fig. 6B)** is seen as a thin 1–2 mm faint radiopaque line from the cortical surface and usually occurs in osteomyelitis, histiocytosis, some benign tumors, and healing fractures.

In multilamellated periosteal reaction **(Fig. 6H)**, there are multiple layers of concentric periosteal reaction resembling an onion skin. Repeated insults from underlying disease process with alternating periods of rapid and slow growth first result in ossified layer of periosteum to be elevated, and later subsequent layers of periosteum are formed as the lesion waxes and wanes during its progression. This type of periosteal reaction occurs in osteomyelitis, histiocytosis, aneurysmal bone cyst, Ewing's sarcoma and osteosarcoma. Interruptions in the lamellated periosteal reaction, indicates more aggressive behavior of the lesion.

Solid periosteal reaction **(Fig. 6C)** indicates a slow process and is almost always associated with benign pathology. This occurs as a result of ossified matrix filling the spaces between lamellations and cortex. This is seen as marked thickening of the periosteal surface of the cortex on plain radiographs. It may be smooth or irregular. Lesions that show solid periosteal reaction include osteoid osteoma and eosinophilic granuloma.

Undulating periosteal reaction **(Fig. 6D)** is a variant of solid periosteal reaction, seen in low-grade osteomyelitis, long-standing varicosities, pulmonary osteoarthropathy, and chronic osteitis but rarely in neoplasms.

Parallel spiculated continuous periosteal reaction represents an underlying malignant pathology. Bony spicules may appear perpendicular to the cortex—hair on end **(Figs. 6E and F)**, fan out in focal divergent manner—sunburst pattern **(Fig. 6G)**, appear to slope in a focal manner (velvet pattern), or show an unorganized pattern. The direction of the spicules is determined by the direction in which the tumor grows. This type of periosteal reaction suggests a more rapid process than lamellated or solid reaction. The spicules may show uniform, fine velvet-like pattern to long linear shadows with a gradual reduction in height in each direction along the shaft from the mid-zone of the reaction. Hair on end periosteal reaction commonly occurs in Ewing's sarcoma, osteosarcoma, metastasis and thalassemia. These spicules are composed of normal reactive bone. Loose areolar tissue between the spicules may be replaced by tumor tissue in Ewing's sarcoma, osteosarcoma and metastasis while these may be replaced by hyperplastic red marrow in thalassemia **(Fig. 6F)** and sickle cell anemia. Sunburst appearance is more often seen in osteosarcoma, osteoblastic metastasis and hemangioma **(Fig. 6G)**. In osteosarcoma, the divergent spicules are composed mainly of tumor bone but may also be composed of reactive bone or a combination of both. In velvet pattern of periosteal reaction, the spicules are short and sloped. This is seen rarely in chondrosarcoma. In unorganized form of periosteal reaction, the spicules are seen in various directions and indicate marked aggressive nature of the lesion, seen in Ewing's sarcoma as it extends into soft tissues.

Interrupted Periosteal Reaction

In this type, continuous mineralization of the periosteal reaction does not occur, resulting in the formation of Codman angles, buttresses or truncated lamellae.

Codman Angles

The periosteal reaction forms an angular configuration with underlying cortex, resembling two sides of an angle **(Fig. 6G)** and indicates an aggressive pathology. This is formed by elevation of the periosteum by tumor, blood, edema or pus. The angle of the triangle may or may not contain tumor. This is nonspecific, seen in both benign and malignant lesions.

Buttresses

In this type, solid reactive bone is formed at the lateral extraosseous margins of slowly growing bone lesions, the cortex beneath the buttress is frequently intact **(Figs. 6H and 7)**.

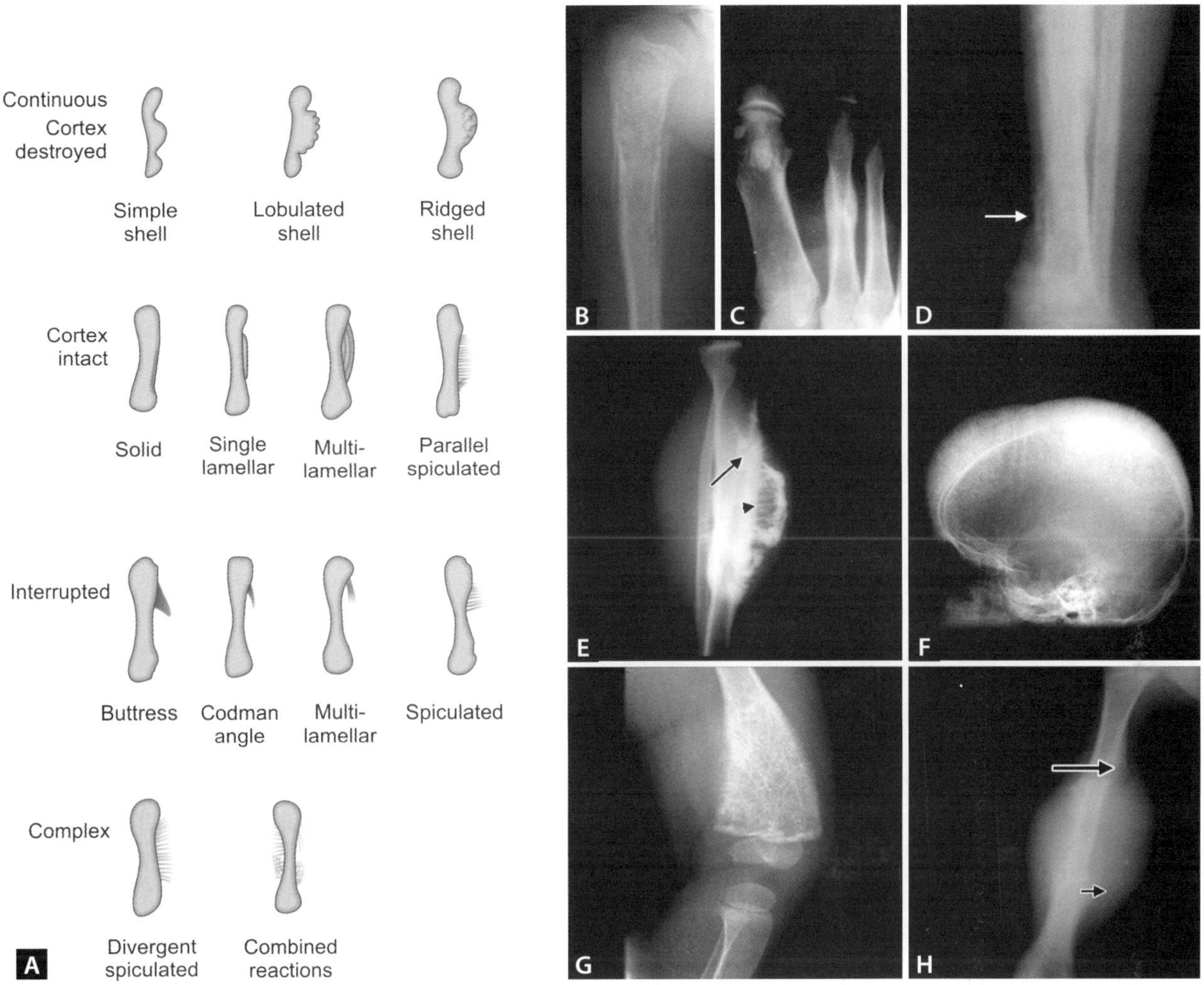

Figs. 6A to H: Various types of periosteal reaction: (A) Schematic diagram showing various types of periosteal reactions; (B) Single lamellar periosteal reaction in osteomyelitis involving upper-half of tibia—note type III—permeative bone destruction; (C) Solid periosteal reaction in stress fracture involving second metatarsal; (D) Undulating periosteal reaction (white arrow) in chronic osteomyelitis of tibia; (E) Parallel (hair-on-end) (arrow) and divergent (sunburst) (arrowhead) spiculated periosteal reaction in diaphyseal osteosarcoma of tibia—note ivory pattern of osteoid tumor matrix; (F) Hair-on-end periosteal reaction involving the skull vault in thalassemia with marked thickening of outer table in frontoparietal region; (G) Sunburst periosteal reaction with coarse and striated trabecular pattern seen in hemangioma involving distal femoral metaphysis in a child; (H) Complex periosteal reaction in Ewing's sarcoma of humeral diaphysis—note interrupted multilamellar (onion skin) reaction, buttress formation (long arrow) in the upper part and Codman angles (short arrow) in the lower part of the tumor both on medial and lateral aspects of bone.

Truncated Lamellae

In aggressive neoplasms and virulent infections, the lamellations are sometimes interrupted or truncated **(Fig. 6H)**, because they are resorbed faster than they can be formed.

Complex Periosteal Reaction

Complex periosteal reaction includes combinations of lamellated, divergent spiculated periosteal reaction, buttresses and Codman angles **(Fig. 6H)**. More extensive and complex the periosteal reaction, greater is the biologic activity of the underlying pathology.

SOFT TISSUE EXTENSION

Normally, the soft tissue shadow of muscle bundles when visualized on a radiograph is sharp with no displacement. It appears obscured when there is infiltration of intermuscular fat planes by inflammation, hemorrhage or tumor. It may show displacement by organized hemorrhage or abscess. Presence of fat density in a soft tissue mass suggests a lipoma **(Fig. 8A)**. Presence of phleboliths indicates hemangioma or angiomatous lesion (***see* Fig. 5C**). In myositis ossificans, focal rounded or streak-like areas of amorphous radiodensity are seen with areas of bone formation in the peripheral part as the lesion matures. Parosteal osteosarcoma also appears as an amorphous mass of increased density, but it matures earliest centrally in contrast to myositis ossificans. Both these lesions may or may not demonstrate a cleavage plane between the mass and underlying bone. Synovial sarcoma shows punctate clumps of calcific density and is usually present around a joint or along a tendon sheath **(Fig. 8B)**.[6]

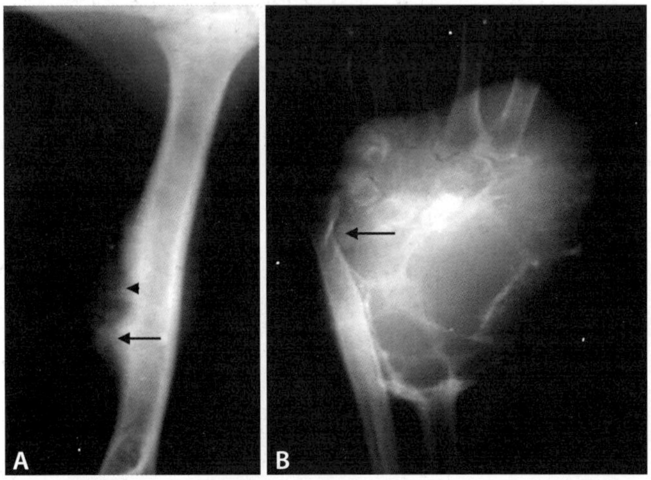

Figs. 7A and B: Saucerization: (A) Saucerization (arrowhead) of the medial humeral diaphysis in Ewing's sarcoma—note the buttress type (arrow) of periosteal reaction in the distal part; (B) Expansile, lytic, multiseptate lesion in a patient with giant cell tumor of lower end of radius—note saucerization (arrow) of lateral ulnar cortex due to soft tissue component of tumor and ridged shell periosteal reaction.

Soft tissue mass is often associated with primary bone tumor but less commonly with a secondary deposit. It may displace adjacent intermuscular fat planes **(Fig. 8C)** and may or may not erode the contiguous bony cortex.

MULTIPLICITY

Multiplicity of malignant lesions usually indicates metastatic disease **(Fig. 9A)**, multiple myeloma, or lymphoma. Very rarely, primary malignant bone lesions, such as Ewing's sarcoma or osteosarcoma, present as multifocal disease. Benign lesions, which tend to involve multiple sites, are polyostotic fibrous dysplasia, multiple osteochondromas, enchondromatosis **(Fig. 9B)**, Langerhans' cell histiocytosis **(Fig. 9C)**, hemangiomatosis, hemophilia pseudotumors **(Fig. 9D)** and fibromatosis.[7]

MISCELLANEOUS

Septations (Table 2)

Lytic expansile lesions often show septations which represent residual normal bone that has not been resorbed or destroyed. These include aneurysmal bone cyst, giant cell tumor, nonossifying fibroma, etc. These septations are left behind by the lobules of growing lesion that advance asymmetrically at a more rapid rate. The septae are thin in giant cell tumor **(Fig. 10A)** while they are thick in nonossifying fibroma and chondromyxoid fibroma **(Fig. 10B)**.[8]

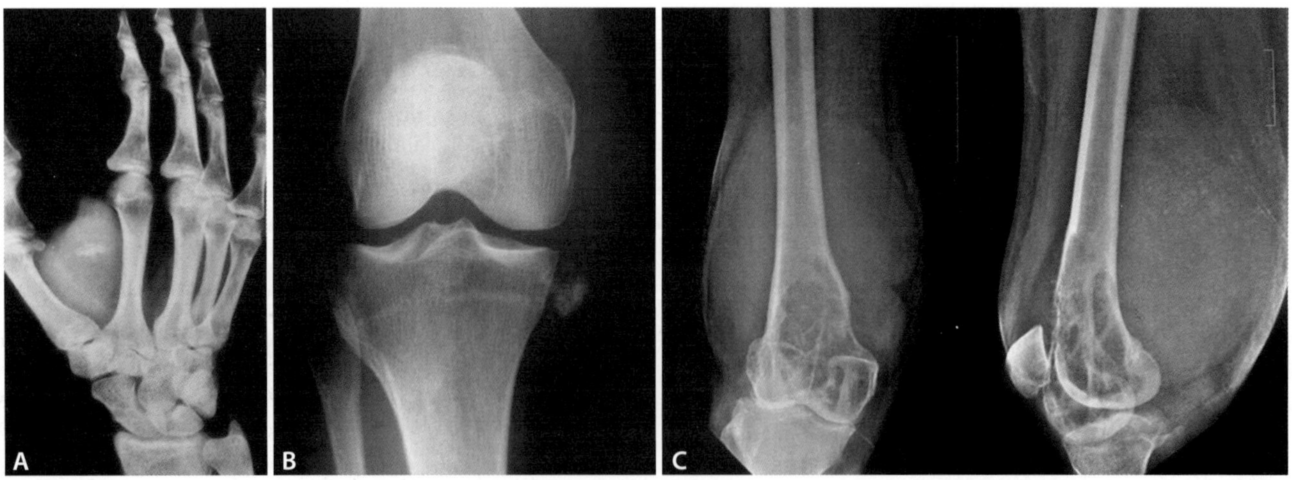

Figs. 8A to C: Soft tissue components: (A) Radiograph of hand showing low density lesion in 1st webspace (due to presence of fat density) suggests a lipoma; (B) Radiograph of knee joint showing punctate clumps of calcific density around the joint due to synovial sarcoma; (C) Radiograph of thigh including knee joint showing lytic destructive lesion in lower end of femur associated with large soft tissue component displacing the adjacent intermuscular fat planes.

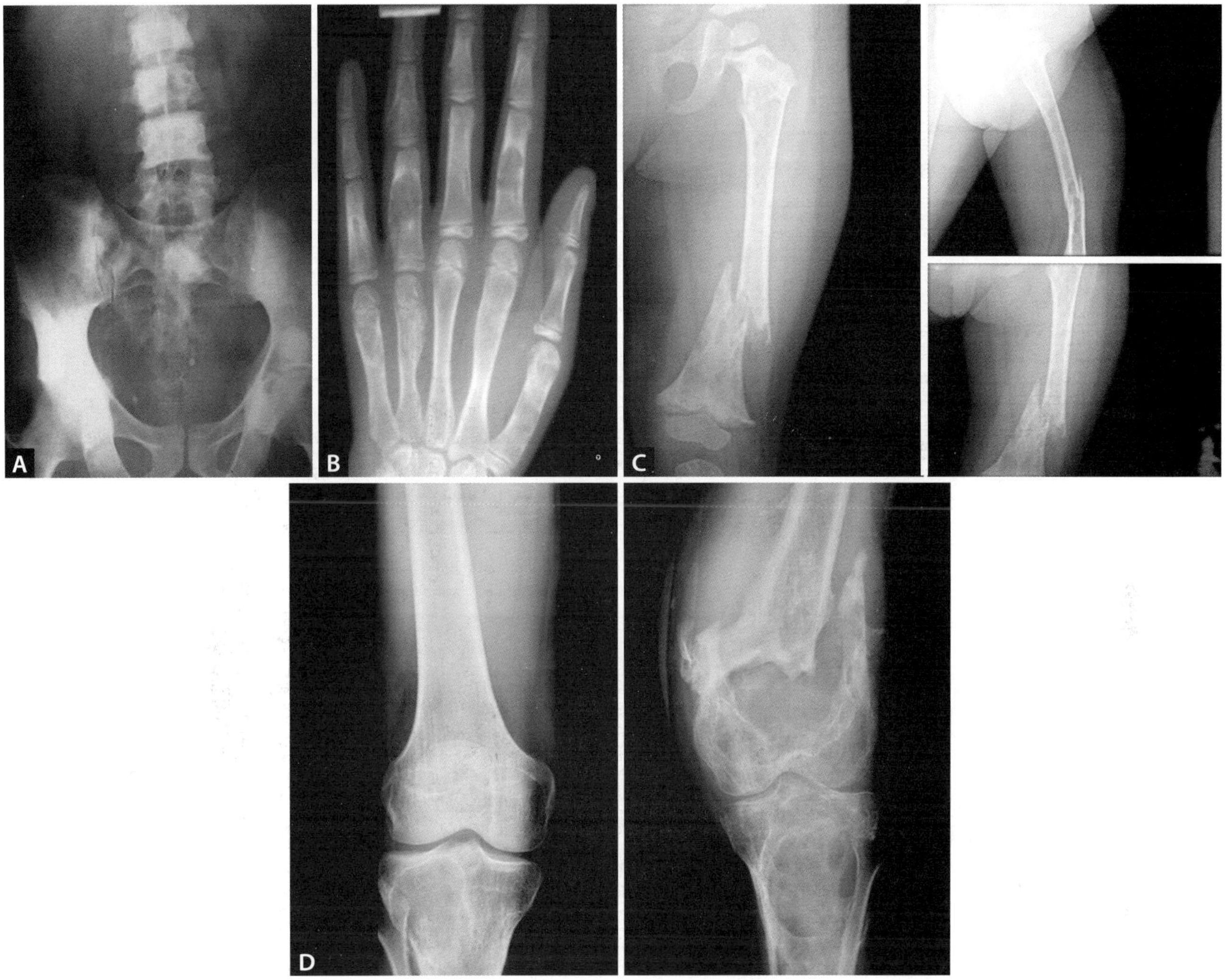

Figs. 9A to D: Multiplicity of lesions: (A) Multiple sclerotic lesions involving pelvis and lumbar spine in elderly patient suggestive of metastases; (B) Multiple intramedullary lytic lesions with chondroid type of calcification in short bones of hand suggestive of multiple enchondromatosis; (C) Multiple lytic lesions involving long bone both metaphysis and diaphysis with pathological fracture in a child suggestive of Langerhan's cell histiocytosis; (D) Multiple lytic lesions involving tibia and femur in patient with history of bleeding diathesis suggestive of hemophilic pseudotumors.

Table 2: Examples of septated lesions

Septations	*Lesions*
Coarse, thick	Chondromyxoid fibroma
Delicate, thin	Giant cell tumor
Delicate, horizontally oriented	Aneurysmal bone cysts
Lobulated	Nonossifying fibroma
Striated, radiating	Hemangioma

Saucerization

Some tumors invade the cortex of a tubular bone in such a way that the area of bone destruction resembles a saucer when the long bone radiograph is viewed in profile. Ewing's sarcoma and metastasis may show typical saucerization configuration. In Ewing's sarcoma, the tumor breaks through the cortex, extends subperiosteally and erodes from its paracortical location to produce saucerization **(*see* Fig. 7A)**. Metastasis also invade subperiosteal region in the same way as Ewing's sarcoma or may invade cortex directly. Large soft tissue masses may erode bone in a similar manner **(*see* Fig. 7B)**.[8]

Floating Fragment Sign

The fractured fragment may be seen within a radiolucent lesion. This fragment changes its location with change in extremity position, a characteristic feature seen in unicameral bone cyst. This sign is also known as "fallen fragment sign" **(Fig. 11)**. When the fractured fragment

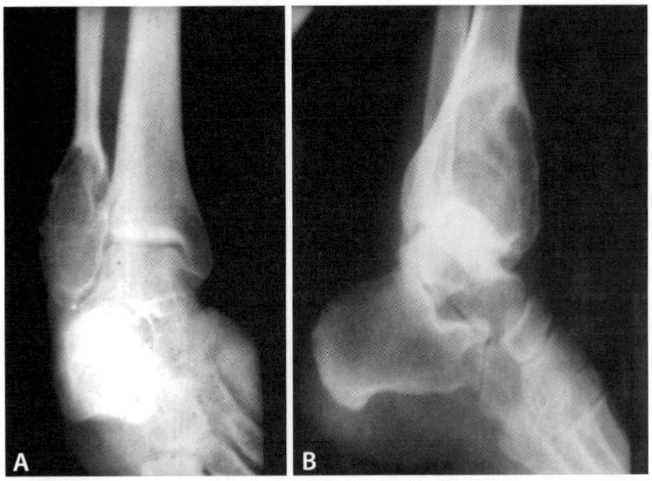

Figs. 10A and B: Septations: (A) Expansile, lytic, multiseptate lesion in a patient with giant cell tumor of lower end of radius—note saucerization of lateral ulnar cortex due to soft tissue component of tumor and ridged shell periosteal reaction; (B) Eccentric expansile lytic lesion showing thick septa and ridged shell reaction in chondromyxoid fibroma involving lower end of tibia.

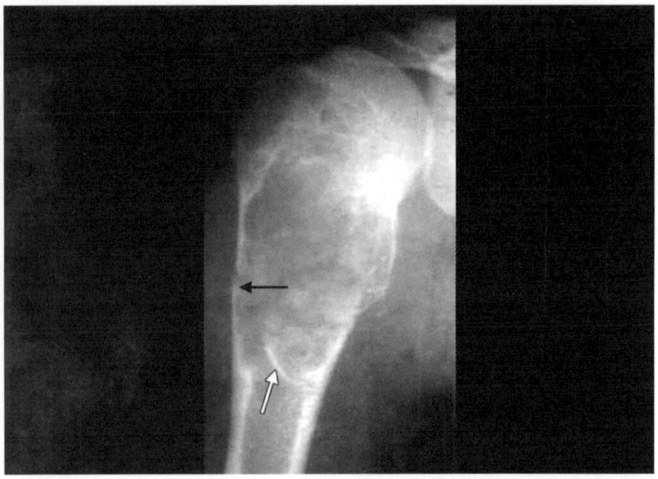

Fig. 11: Simple bone cyst involving humerus showing "fallen fragment" (black arrow) and "trap-door" (white arrow) signs.

remains attached at the fracture site, it is seen in the form of a trapped door due to hydrostatic pressure of the fluid contained within the cyst. This is called "trap door sign". Both these signs are typical of unicameral bone cyst.

BENIGN VERSUS MALIGNANT

Although it is sometimes very difficult to distinguish benign from malignant bone lesions on the basis of plain radiographys alone, however certain key characteristic features may favor one over the other. Benign tumors usually present with well-defined, sclerotic borders, a geographic type of bone destruction, an uninterrupted solid periosteal reaction and no soft tissue extension. Malignant lesions, on the other hand tend to demonstrate poorly defined borders with a wide zone of transition, a moth-eaten or permeative pattern of bone destruction, an interrupted periosteal reaction of the sunburst or onion-skin type, and an adjacent soft-tissue mass. As noted earlier, it should be kept in mind that some benign tumors can also exhibit aggressive features **(Table 3)**.[9]

Table 3: Benign lesions with aggressive features.

Lesion	*Radiographic presentation*
Osteoblastoma	Bone destruction and soft (aggressive) tissue extension similar to osteosarcoma
Desmoplastic fibroma	Expansive destructive lesion, frequently trabeculated
Periosteal desmoid	Irregular cortical outline, mimics osteosarcoma or Ewing's sarcoma
Giant cell tumor	Occasionally aggressive features—osteolytic bone destruction, cortical penetration, and soft tissue extension
Aneurysmal bone cyst	Soft tissue extension, occasionally mimicking malignant tumor
Osteomyelitis	Bone destruction, aggressive periosteal reaction. Occasionally, features resembling Ewing's sarcoma
Pseudotumor of hemophilia	Bone destruction, periosteal reaction occasionally mimics malignant tumor
Myositis ossificans	Features of parosteal or periosteal osteosarcoma
Brown tumor of hyperparathyroidism	Lytic bone lesion, resembling malignant tumor

When all the clinical and radiographic information concerning a patient with a bone lesion has been analyzed, the most important diagnostic decision is whether the lesion is definitely benign and not to be biopsied, but rather merely monitored or completely ignored (a "do not touch lesion") **(Table 4)**, or whether it has an ambiguous and an aggressive appearance and should be further investigated via percutaneous or open biopsy. The results of the histopathologic examination would then determine whether further management in a given case would be surgical, chemotherapeutic, radiotherapeutic or a combination of these.

COMPUTED TOMOGRAPHY ANALYSIS OF BONE LESIONS

Computed tomography (CT) provides greater morphological detail about the bone surrounding a lesion and

Table 4: Lesions that should not be biopsied.

Tumors and tumor-like lesions	Non-neoplastic conditions
Fibrous cortical defect	Avulsion fracture (healing phase)
Nonossifying fibroma	Bone infarct
Periosteal (cortical) desmoid	Bone island (enostosis)
Small, solitary focus of fibrous dysplasia	Pseudotumor of hemophilia
Myositis ossificans	Degenerative and post-traumatic cysts
Intraosseous ganglion	Brown tumor of hyperparathyroidism
Enchondroma in a short, tubular bone	Discogenic vertebral sclerosis

the application of this analysis is the same as the classic radiographic margin analysis. A well-defined lesion within the cortex is a sign of indolent growth while indication of cortical destruction or permeation is suggestive of aggressiveness. Like radiographic analysis, CT also has a grading system. Lesions contained in bone or by periosteal new bone are grade I and represent indolent processes. Lesions that partially or destroy cortex are called grade II. Penetration of the cortex or periosteal new bone exhibits aggressiveness. Grade III lesions completely penetrate through the cortex but display no localized bone destruction. These are highly aggressive, permeative lesions. CT margin is specifically useful when the tumor margin is not clearly visible on plain radiographs. This particularly applies to the lesions in vertebrae and flat bones such ilium, sacrum, and scapula **(Fig. 12)**.[6]

In the diagnosis of solitary bone lesions, CT is used primarily in order to obtain "radiographic" information, where conventional radiographs are unsuccessful due to limited contrast resolution, complex skeletal anatomy (e.g. spine, pelvis) **(Figs. 13A and B)**, or superposition of skeletal elements (e.g. scapula). Conventional tomography has been widely replaced by computed tomography, and with the recent advent of multislice techniques, it has developed into a "true" multiplanar modality. Computed tomography is superior to radiography in determination of the epicentre of a bone lesion (medullary, cortical, periosteal, parosteal). The site of origin characterises a special entity (e.g. nonossifying fibroma, periosteal chondroma), and influences the growth pattern of the lesion and therefore, it can determine whether the appearance of the lesion is more or less aggressive. The biologic activity of a lytic bone lesion is reflected in its pattern of bone destruction. Independent of the anatomic site of the lesion, CT can define the margins of an osseous defect in 360° survey, it can determine the exact width of the zone of transition between normal and abnormal bone, and it can detect delicate sclerotic reactions.

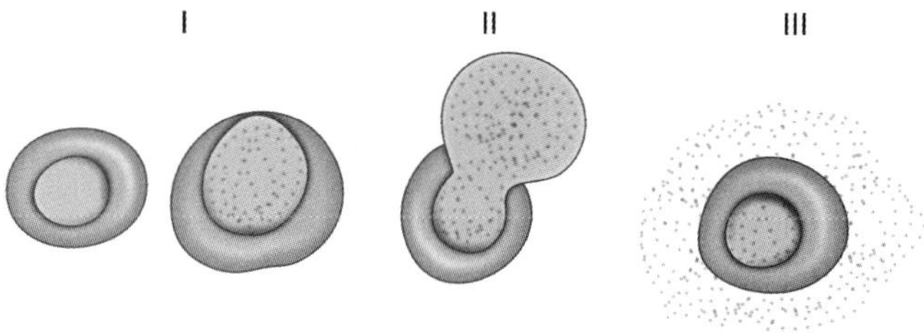

Fig. 12: Computed tomography grading system of bone lesions.

A major advantage that CT has over radiography probably is its superior delineation of cortical alterations, of which cortical expansion and remodeling, endosteal scalloping, and focal penetration represent the most common forms in benign bone lesions. Periosteal reactions represent another barometer of the biologic activity of bone tumors and tumor-like lesions. Computed tomography has the ability to depict periosteal reactions that might not be visible on radiographs because of superposition or limited contrast resolution. Furthermore, CT represents the most valuable imaging modality in detection of subtle matrix calcifications and can therefore help confirm the diagnosis of a bone- or cartilage-forming tumor.[10]

MAGNETIC RESONANCE IMAGING OF BONE LESIONS[11,12]

Magnetic resonance imaging is extremely sensitive to lesions that replace marrow and destroy bone. It shows the full extent of lesions and extension into soft tissues. Magnetic resonance imaging is of minor value in the estimation of the malignant potential of an osseous lesion. Although many bone tumors and tumor-like lesions present similar morphology at MRI, some entities can be diagnosed with good reliability. These include chondrogenic tumors **(Fig. 14A)**, solitary **(Fig. 14B)**, and aneurysmal bone cysts **(Fig. 14C)**, giant cell tumors, lesions containing fatty tissue and, to a certain extent, osteoid-osteomas and osteoblastomas.

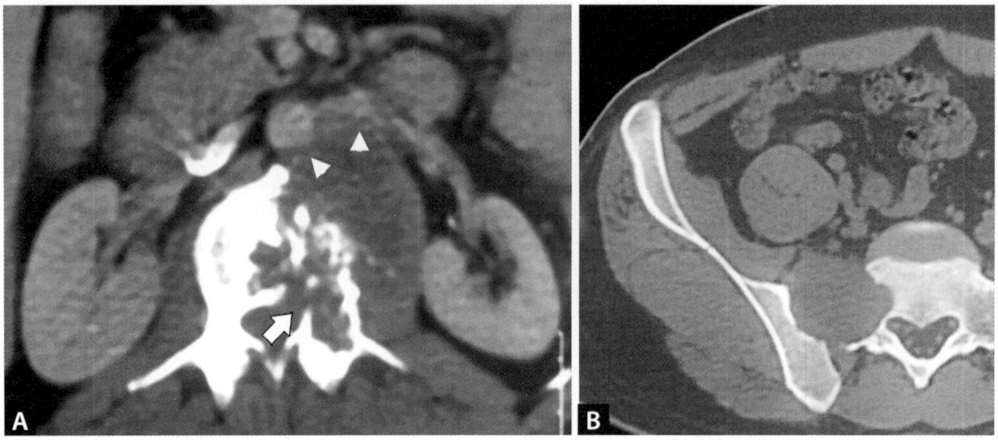

Figs. 13A and B: Role of CT scan in assessment of focal bone lesion: (A) Axial CT of the lumbar vertebra at the level of the renal hilum shows marked tumoral destruction of the left half of the vertebral body and the left pedicle, by a proven chondrosarcoma. Matrix mineralization and residual trabeculae are seen inside. The tumor is extending into the left psoas muscle and is lifting the aorta and the left renal vein anteriorly (arrowheads). The fat plane with the aorta is obliterated. Posteromedially the mass is extending into the spinal canal and causing an impression on the theca (arrow); (B) Axial CT section of sacrum showing expansile lytic lesion in right sacral ala, a case of giant cell tumor.

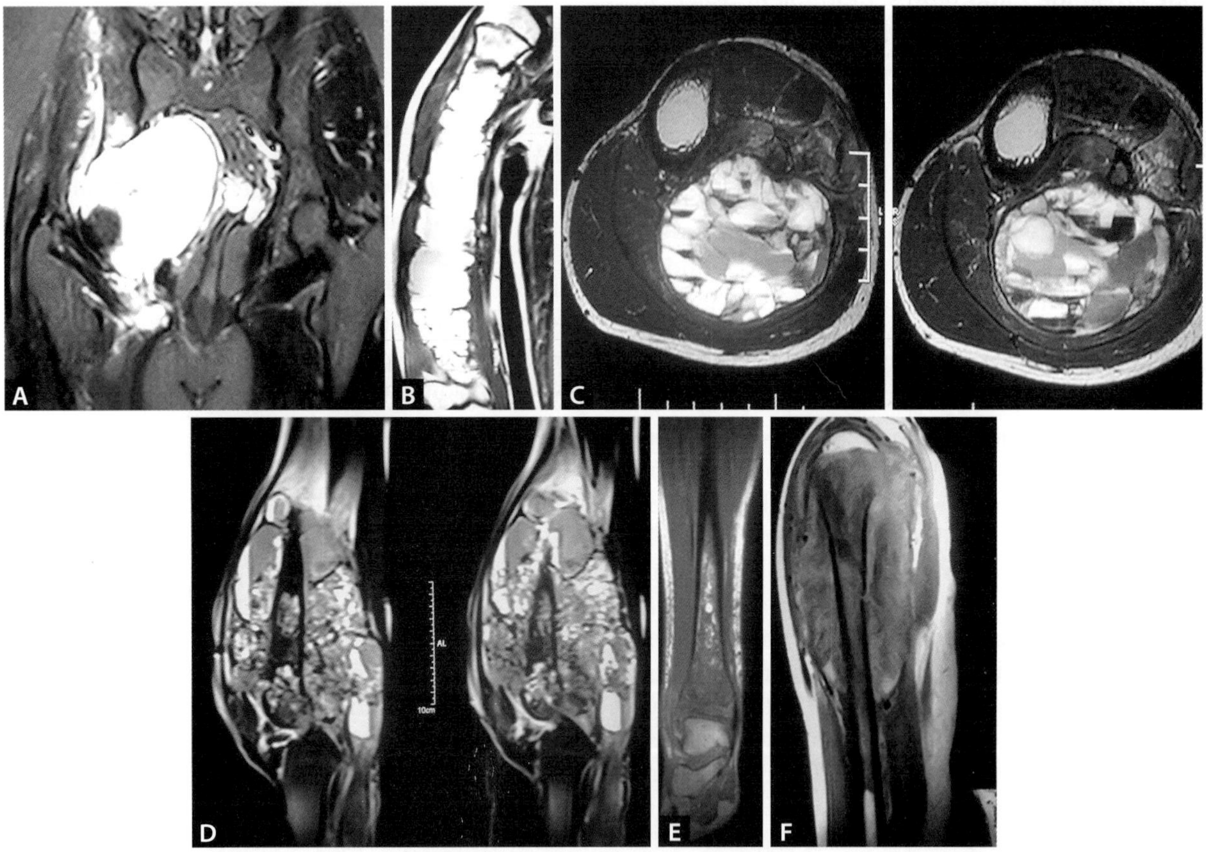

Figs. 14A to F: Role of MRI in assessment of focal bone lesion: (A) Coronal T2W MR image showing brightly hyperintense lobulated mass lesion arising from the right acetabulum in elderly patient suggestive of chondrosarcoma; (B) Coronal STIR MR image showing elongated hyperintense lesion involving the shaft of humerus in a child suggestive of simple bone cyst; (C) Axial T2W MR image showing expansile lesion with multiple blood fluid levels suggestive of aneurysmal bone cyst; (D) Sagittal T2W MR image of a patient with biopsy proven case osteosarcoma showing altered signal intensity involving the metaepiphysis of lower end of femur associated with large soft tissue component which is extending into knee joint; (E) Coronal T1W image of child with osteomyelitis showing heterogeneous signal intensity involving the diaphysis, metaphysis and epiphysis of lower end of tibia suggestive of aggressive lesion; (F) Sagittal T1W MR image of arm in patient with known case of osteosarcoma showing altered signal intensity involving upper end of humerus associated with large surrounding soft tissue component without obvious cortical destruction suggestive of transcortical infiltration.

The differential diagnosis for benign bone lesions surrounded by extensive marrow edema includes osteoid osteoma/osteoblastoma, chondroblastoma, Langerhans cell histiocytosis, and osteomyelitis. As a general (but not absolute) parameter, the greater the extent of surrounding marrow edema, the more likely is the bone lesion to be benign. Marrow edema may be present around malignant bone tumors, as well, in which case it constitutes the reactive zone of the tumor.

However, its main role on for preoperative staging of tumor extent and involvement of critical structures, such as joints and neurovascular bundles **(Fig. 14D)**.

Magnetic resonance is particularly useful in the evaluation of aggressive lesions, such as malignant tumors and infective lesions **(Fig. 14E)**. It displays transcortical infiltration a sign of highly aggressive lesions **(Fig. 14F)**. Magnetic resonance also depicts intratrabecular infiltration sign of infiltrative growth in case of malignant bone tumor. It also shows active tumor growth in periosteal and endosteal extension at tumor margins.

CONCLUSION

- The guidelines mentioned in chapter usually allow us to make accurate diagnosis or offer close differentials **(Flowchart 1)**.
- The pattern of bone destruction, margins, cortical response, location and site of lesion on radiographs helps in differential diagnosis of bone tumor and tumor like lesions.
- Because of high specificity in detection of lesion features, radiography is integrated with clinical findings that allows the differential diagnosis between neoplastic and non-neoplastic lesions including trauma (healing or stress fractures, myositis ossificans), infection (acute osteomyelitis Brodie's abscess), eosinophilic granuloma and such as brown tumors of hyperthyroidism.
- Radiography is insufficient in studying the lesions in complex anatomical sites such as spine, pelvis, and scapula nor does it define the intra- and extraosseous extent of the tumor. In such cases cross-sectional

Flowchart 1: Assessing focal bone lesion.

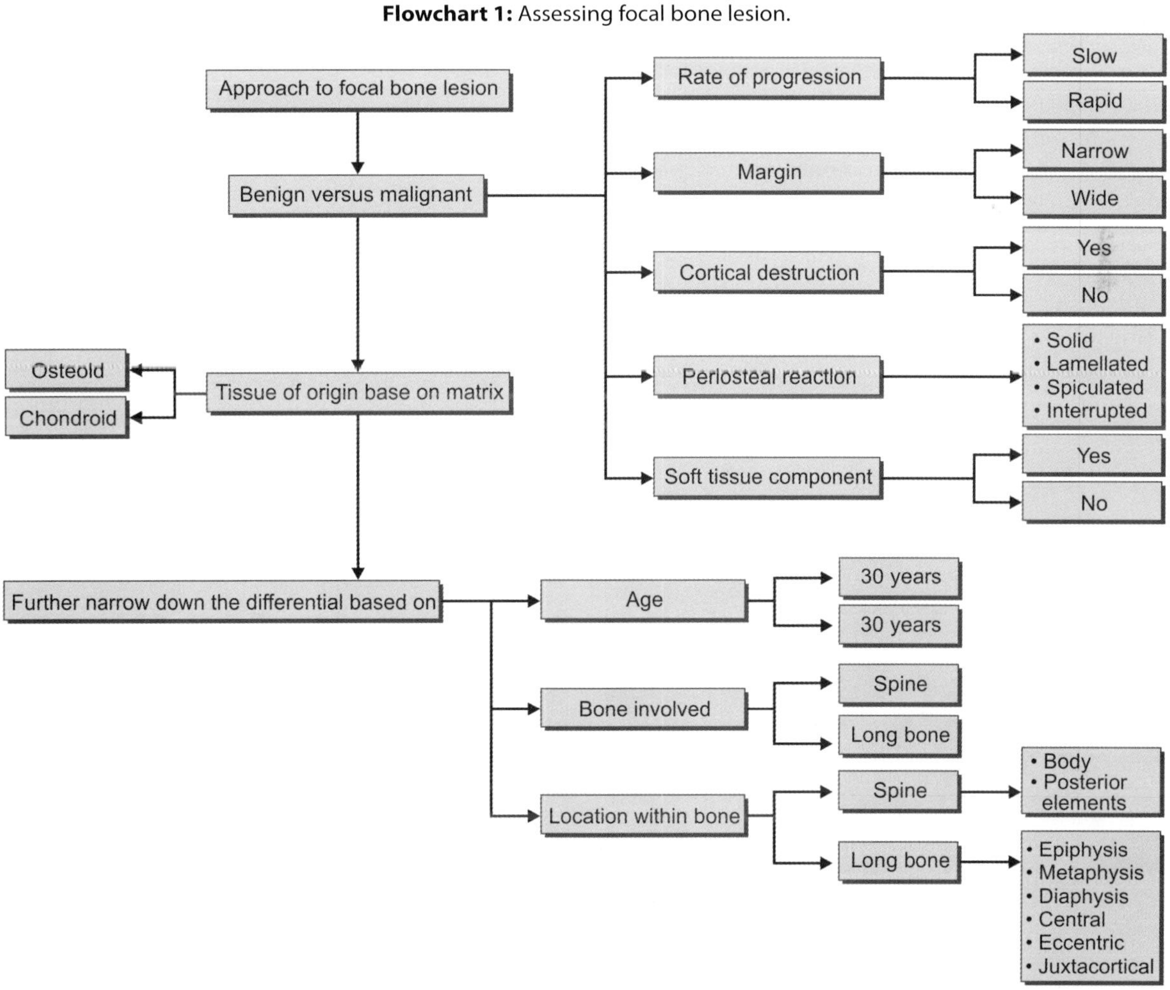

imaging such as CT and MRI helps defining the extent of lesions.

- The radiologist should never ever interpret the CT or MRI of a suspected bone tumor without first reviewing the plain radiographs. The orthopedic surgeon, radiologist and pathologist must collaborate to increase the accuracy of the diagnosis, thus improving the patient care.

REFERENCES

1. O'Donnel P. Evaluation of focal bone lesions: Basic principles and clinical scenarios. Imaging. 2003;15:298-323.
2. Miller TT. Bone tumors and tumor-like conditions: analysis with conventional radiography. Radiology. 2008;246(3):662-74. Epub 2008.
3. Madewell JE, Ragsdale BD, Sweet DE. Radiologic and pathologic analysis of solitary bone lesions. I. Internal margins. Radiol Clin North Am. 1981;19:715-48.
4. Sweet DE, Madewell JE, Ragsdale BD. Radiologic and pathologic analysis of solitary bone lesions. III. Matrix patterns. Radiol Clin North Am. 1981;19:785-814.
5. Ragsdale BD, Madewell JE, Sweet DE. Radiologic and pathologic analysis of solitary bone lesions. II. Periosteal reactions. Radiol Clin North Am. 1981;19:749-83.
6. Brown KT, Kattapuram SV, Rosenthal DI. Computed tomography analysis of bone tumors: Patterns of cortical destruction and soft tissue extension. Skeletal Radiol. 1986;15:448-51.
7. Priolo F, Cerase A. The current role of radiography in the assessment of skeletal tumors and tumor-like lesions. Eur J Radiol. 1998; 27(suppl 1):S77-S85.
8. Moser RP, Madewell JE. An approach to primary bone tumors. Radiol Clin North Am. 1987;25:1049-93.
9. Ma LD, Frassica FJ, Scott WW, Fishman EK, Zerhouni EA. Differentiation of benign and malignant musculoskeletal tumors: potential pitfalls with MR imaging. Radiographics. 1995;15:349-66.
10. Woertler K. Benign bone tumors and tumor-like lesions value of cross-sectional imaging. Eur Radiol. 2003;13:1820-35.
11. Pettersson H, Gillespy T 3rd, Hamlin DJ, et al. Primary musculo-skeletal tumors: Examination with MR imaging compared with conventional modalities. Radiology. 1987;164:237-41.
12. Zimmer WD, Berquist TH, McLeod RA, et al. Bone tumors: magnetic resonance imaging versus computed tomography. Radiology. 1985;155:709-18.

CHAPTER 187

Basic Principles and Current Concepts of Musculoskeletal Magnetic Resonance Imaging

Raju Sharma, Shivanand Gamanagatti

INTRODUCTION

Magnetic resonance imaging of the musculoskeletal system has made immense progress in the last two decades. The pace of innovation has been rapid and MR has become a versatile and virtually indispensable imaging modality for many musculoskeletal applications. Developments, such as high performance MR systems and optimized coil technology have led to improvements in spatial resolution and signal-to-noise and better cost-effectiveness of MR studies.[1] This in-turn has led to improved diagnosis in shorter period of time and better understanding of complex orthopedic disorders. This chapter aims to briefly outline the basic principles of musculoskeletal MRI and highlights the recent advances in this exciting and ever-changing specialty.

HARDWARE ISSUES

The basic prerequisites for optimized MR imaging of the musculoskeletal system are high spatial and contrast resolution and high sensitivity for the visualization of free water. Although high-field systems clearly have an advantage with regard to resolution, musculoskeletal imaging, for most indications, can be done on mid and low-field systems also. The ultra high-field systems (3 tesla) are now widely available and provide very high quality images of the musculoskeletal system. Faster gradients, improvements in surface coil design, and development of new and faster sequences have all contributed to the fact that MRI has become the modality of choice for evaluation of the musculoskeletal system.[1,2] The use of parallel imaging and motion reduction techniques like PROPELLAR and BLADE have further enhanced the image quality of MR images.[2] Scanners are now available which allow imaging in the weight bearing, upright position and also in flexion and extension (kinematic MRI). This allows evaluation of dynamic postural and functional changes in degenerated disks,[3] as well as dynamic evaluation of joints. Upright and kinematic MRI may detect minor neural foraminal compromise related to posture. However, these scanners are open configuration with low magnetic field strength which may compromise resolution and are therefore suitable for few niche indications.

Choosing the appropriate coil is important to obtain high quality images. The smallest coil possible, that allows the required anatomical coverage, should be used to get the maximum signal. Surface coils that can be placed on or close to the region of interest should be used. Most new coils are made with a phased array design. These are made of several smaller coils placed in a series and provide the combined advantage of high resolution images and a wide field of view. Eight channel coils are now available for musculoskeletal applications.

3 T IMAGING

3 T imaging has many advantages in the musculoskeletal system. Imaging at higher field strengths gives better signal to noise ratio (SNR), resulting in higher resolution images and shorter scan times. The SNR at 3 T is about twice that at 1.5 T and 3 T scanners are already being widely used for musculoskeletal imaging **(Fig. 1)**. Research studies

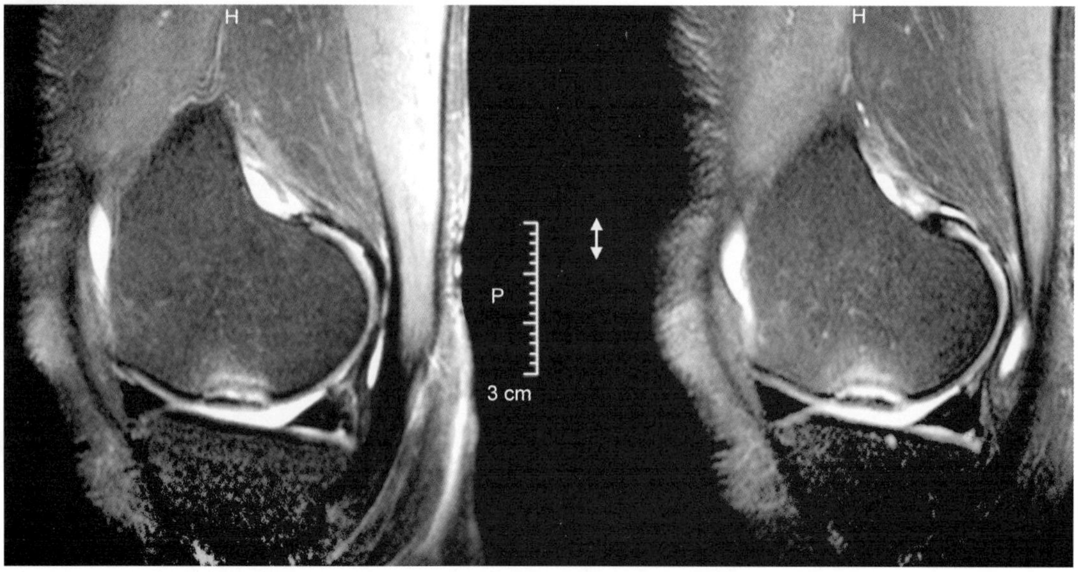

Fig. 1: Sagittal fat-suppressed T2W image acquired on a 3 tesla scanner shows a small detached ossific fragment in the articular surface of medial femoral condyle with fluid signal intensity between the fragment and the underlying bone, suggesting osteochondritis dissecans. The image has a high signal to noise ratio with excellent delineation of anatomy.

are being conducted at 7 T systems also. Not only SNR but also spatial resolution and the contrast to noise ratio can be enhanced on 3 T scanners. The collective benefit gives rise to better delineation of the small intrinsic structures of joints. Many studies have documented higher accuracy and greater degree of confidence using 3 T imaging, in the diagnosis of meniscal tears, defects in articular cartilage, triangular fibrocartilage pathology, etc. However, 3 T imaging is unlikely to replace the need for MR arthrography in lesions like labral tears.[2,4]

The sequences and protocols need to be modified for optimum imaging at 3 T. Improved sequence design and widespread use of parallel imaging are likely to improve the image quality at 3 T even further.

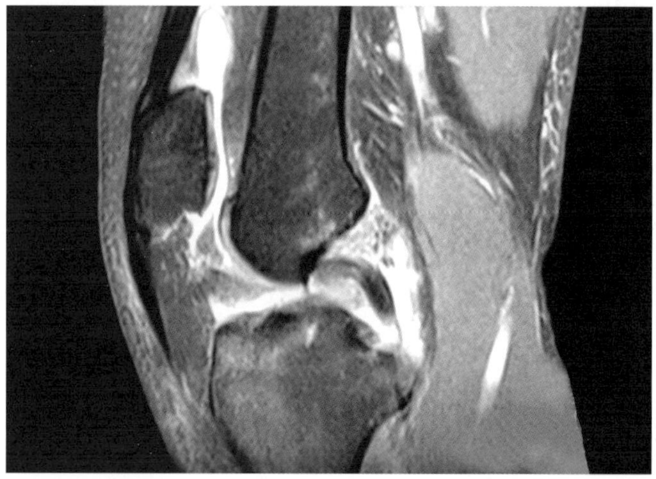

Fig. 2: Sagittal fat-suppressed (FS) proton density (PD) image shows good delineation of hyaline articular cartilage (gray signal intensity along posterior aspect of patella) and cruciate ligaments in the knee. Anterior cruciate ligament is disrupted with no normal fibers identified and there is buckling of PCL, suggesting complete ACL tear.

SEQUENCES

Many different options are available to image the musculoskeletal system. The aim is to get all the diagnostic information necessary in as short a time as possible. This can only be done by adopting a judicious protocol for which it is important to know the merits and demerits of the different types of sequences. It is a good practice to have a standard protocol tailored to a specific clinical indication for a given MR scanner. T1W sequence is good for delineation of anatomy and marrow pathology, proton density sequence for meniscal tears, articular cartilage **(Fig. 2)** and ligament pathology and T2W sequence for detecting soft tissue component of tumors **(Figs. 3A and B)**, edema, etc. For most musculoskeletal applications proton density and T2W sequences are coupled with fat suppression.

Fast Spin-echo Sequences

This group of sequences allows for much more rapid acquisition of images than the conventional spin-echo (SE) method. This is done by acquiring several samples in the time in which one sample is obtained in the conventional spin-echo technique. The time saved is directly proportional to the number of samples also known as the echo train length.[1] This decreases overall imaging time thereby decreasing the motion artifacts and

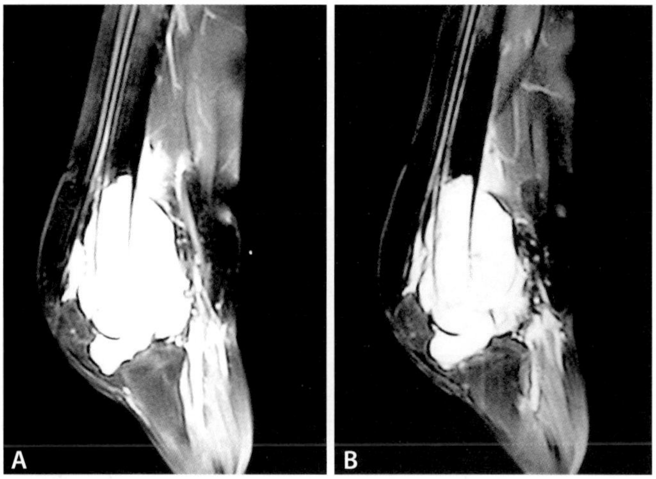

Figs. 3A and B: Sagittal FS T2W image of the knee gives excellent depiction of the extraosseous and intraosseous extent of the tumor in a case of osteosarcoma of the distal femoral end. Also note the intra-articular extension of the tumor.

increasing the throughput. Alternatively the time saved can be used for obtaining additional signal averages and increasing the matrix size to improve the signal and resolution, respectively.

However, the fast spin-echo sequences (FSE) technique has some disadvantages. Firstly the signal intensity of fat remains quite bright on these T2W images. As a result pathology in subcutaneous fat or marrow may be obscured, due to the similarity in the signal intensity of fat and fluid. This problem can be resolved by combining this technique with fat saturation **(Figs. 3A and B)**, which is now routinely employed.[1,2] Secondly the FSE technique can result in blurring along tissue margins when long echo train lengths are used. This may result in missing subtle pathology such as meniscal tears in the knee.

Gradient-recalled Echo Sequences

These sequences were originally developed to produce T2W images in less time than was possible with conventional SE techniques. They can be performed either with a 2D or 3D volume technique. In 3D imaging the signal from an entire volume of tissue is obtained at one time and this data can be partitioned into extremely thin slices such that the voxel dimensions are nearly isotropic.[2] This allows for high-resolution imaging and is especially useful when evaluating extremely small structures such as ligaments in the wrist. These 3D sequences also provide the ability to create reformatted images in virtually any plane. Ligaments and articular cartilage are particularly well demonstrated with these sequences. Dual echo steady state (DESS) is a 3D steady state GRE sequence with a good signal to noise ratio and strong T2 contrast. It is useful for the differentiation of synovial fluid and cartilaginous structures. Multiecho data image combination (MEDIC) is a multiecho GRE sequence that provides good T2-weighted images and has been found useful in joint imaging **(Fig. 4)**.

Gradient-recalled echo sequences (GRE) sequences are extremely sensitive to susceptibility effects. This is advantageous when searching for subtle areas of hemorrhage, detecting loose bodies and soft tissue gas. Conversely drawbacks of this effect include overestimating the size of osteophytes in spine imaging and gross artifacts when imaging patients with metallic hardware.

Fat-suppressed Sequences

Detection of a pathological process is often hindered by the presence of strong signal from neighboring adipose tissue. In such cases, suppression of the fat signal offers improved conspicuity and sensitivity.[1] Fat suppression is commonly employed with fast spin-echo T2W sequences on which fat is very bright. It is also frequently coupled with gadolinium enhanced images where the hyperintense signal from enhancing abnormalities may be masked by hyperintense fat. Fat-saturated T1W images are also used with gadolinium arthrography.

Two main techniques used to accomplish fat suppression are frequency selective (chemical fat saturation) and short tau inversion recovery (STIR) imaging. A problem with the frequency selective fat saturation is the potential for inhomogeneous suppression of fat signal. It relies on adequate separation of fat and water peaks, which occurs only at high-field strength (greater than 1 tesla) and hence it is not available on mid and low-field scanners.[1] The STIR technique relies on the relaxation properties of fat protons rather than their resonant frequency. It produces more homogeneous fat suppression, because it is not as sensitive to field inhomogeneity as the frequency selective technique **(Fig. 5)**. However, STIR sequence should not be used with intravenous or intra-articular gadolinium because the contrast agent has similar relaxation properties to fat protons and therefore its signal intensity may be saturated along with fat on the STIR images.

A third method of fat suppression is the DIXON technique or fat water separation technique. This is also based on the difference in the precessional frequency of protons in fat and water. However, unlike chemical fat sat it uses a spectrally nonselective radiofrequency pulse, with TEs that capture the phase difference between fat and water protons. When fat and water are in phase the signal is maximal and when they are out of phase

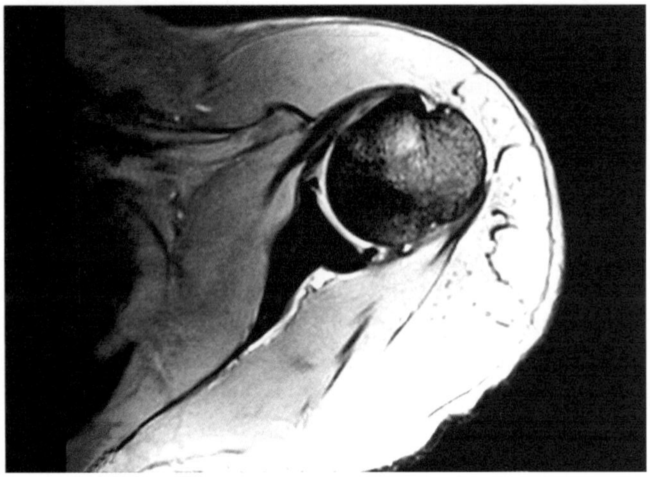

Fig. 4: Axial FS gradient-echo image (MEDIC) of the shoulder. Anterior and posterior glenoid labrum are well-seen.

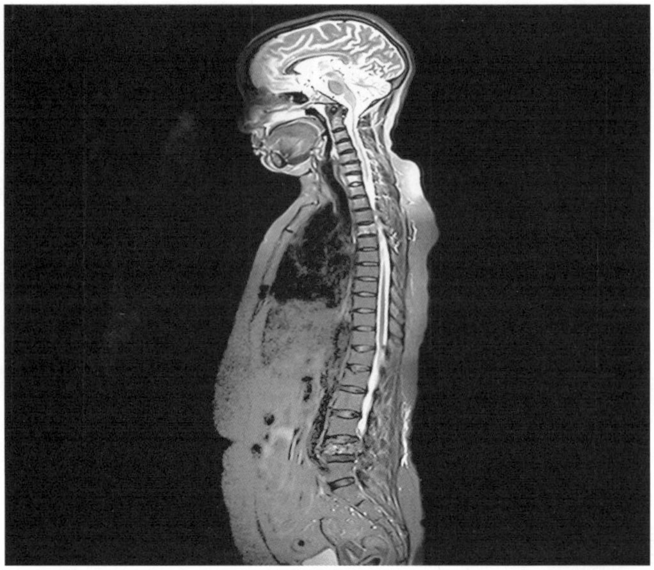

Fig. 5: Sagittal STIR image of the whole spine shows hyperintensity and decreased vertebral height involving multiple vertebrae, suggesting multiple metastases in a known case of malignancy. There is homogeneous suppression of fat.

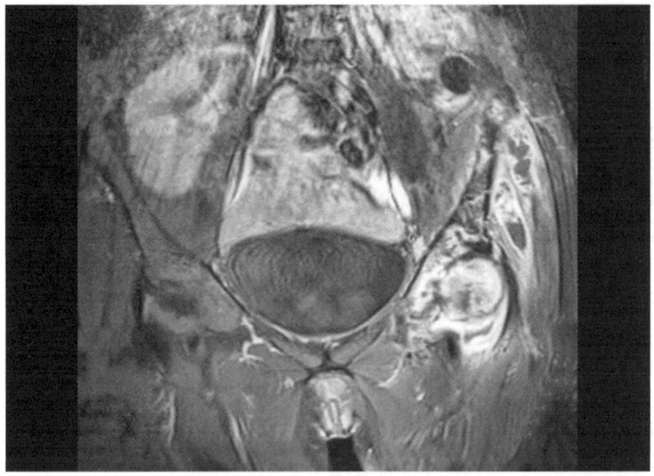

Fig. 6: Utility of contrast administration: Coronal FS postgadolinium T1W image shows abnormal synovial enhancement in a case of TB left hip with multiple rim-enhancing abscesses within the joint cavity and in the surrounding soft tissues.

there is destructive interference between fat and water magnetization vectors. At 1.5 T the TE for the in phase image is 4.6 msec or a multiple of 4.6 and the TE for the opposed phase image is 2.3 msec or a multiple of 2.3. The fat and water in phase and out phase images can be added or subtracted to produce water only or fat only images. This two point Dixon technique is sensitive to magnetic field inhomogeneity and to overcome this, a three point Dixon method has been developed where one in phase and two opposed phase images (one at. 2.3 msec shorter and another sequence with TE. 2.3 longer than the nominal TE) are acquired. The three images are analyzed and a phase map is generated from which fat only, water only and combined images can be created. This technique is called iterative decomposition of fat and water with echo asymmetric and least square estimation (IDEAL). The Dixon technique can be applied to regions of complex anatomy and can be used with spin-echo, fast spin-echo as well as GRE sequences. Its disadvantages include sensitivity to magnetic field inhomogeneity and potential blurring with fast spin-echo sequences.[2]

Role of Contrast

Gadolinium-DTPA is a paramagnetic compound and is a T1 contrast agent. For musculoskeletal applications it can be administered by the intravenous and intra-articular route. Its major application in musculoskeletal MRI is in the setting of infections **(Fig. 6)**, where it can help to distinguish cellulitis from abscess. It is used in evaluating bone tumors to differentiate cystic from solid lesions, for perfusion studies and for directing biopsy to the enhancing viable tumor rather than nonenhancing necrotic component.[1] Gadolinium is also useful in imaging postoperative spine to differentiate scar tissue from nonenhancing disk material.[2] MR arthrography is useful for the diagnosis of subtle pathology like labral tears.

Reduction of Metallic Artifact from Orthopedic Hardware

Patients with metallic implants and orthopedic hardware frequently need to be imaged. Although they are mostly MR compatible, they can give rise to significant artifact and image distortion. Radiologists should be aware of the steps that can be taken to reduce these artifacts. If there is any doubt of the MR compatibility of the prosthesis an alternative imaging modality should be used.

The degree of metal artifact is related to field strength and imaging at lower field magnets will decrease the metallic artifact. The long axis of the prosthesis should be positioned parallel to the external magnetic field (B0) to minimize artifacts. Other steps that can be taken to reduce metal artifact are aligning the frequency encoding direction along the long axis of the implant, increasing the receiver bandwidth and reducing the FOV. Fast spin-echo sequences with long echo train length are least susceptible to metal artifacts and should be preferred over gradient-echo sequences.[2]

NORMAL APPEARANCE OF MUSCULOSKELETAL TISSUES

It is useful to know the normal appearance of various tissues on different MR sequences and the optimal sequence for each, as this can be applied to any anatomical region. Cortical bone is dark on all sequences whereas the medullary cavity shows a variable signal depending on whether the marrow is hematopoietic or fatty. The distribution of red and yellow marrow changes with age. STIR, fat-suppressed FSE T2- and T1W sequences are ideal for imaging marrow pathology, whereas GRE sequences are not useful for bony evaluation. MRI is very sensitive to evaluation of occult osseous trauma when radiographs are normal and for early diagnosis of marrow infiltrative disorders and for this purpose STIR sequence is the most sensitive.[7]

Articular cartilage is dark gray on STIR and FSE T2W sequences and is bright on GRE sequences. Fibrocartilage like the menisci and glenoid labrum are dark on all sequences. Meniscal tears are best demonstrated on short TE sequences like T1 and proton density images.

Tendons are generally dark on all pulse sequences. Useful sequences are GRE T2*, T1 and FSE T2. Tendons are usually best imaged in the axial plane. Tears and tendonitis are seen as hyperintense areas but it is important to know some pitfalls for this finding. Tendons may show slightly increased signal intensity close to the site of osseous insertion. This is due to nontendinous fatty material getting interposed between tendon fibers. Another important cause is the magic angle phenomenon which can give rise to a hyperintense signal in the tendons that are oriented at 55° to the main magnetic field B°. However, this bright signal is seen only on the short TE images (T1W and proton density) and not on T2W images.[1] Common sites where this artifactual hyperintensity may be seen are the posterior tibial tendon in the ankle, rotator cuff in the shoulder and posterior cruciate ligament in the knee. Changing the position for instance imaging the ankle in 20° plantar flexion can help to overcome this artifact by changing the angle of the tendon with respect to the main magnetic field vector. In addition to hyperintense signal within the tendon, attention should also be paid to any thickening or fluid around the tendon as is seen in tenosynovitis.

Normal synovium is not usually visualized unless it is pathologically thickened. Postgadolinium T1W fat-saturated images are useful for delineation of thickened synovium. It may not be possible to distinguish hypertrophied synovium from synovial fluid on T2W and STIR images. Hypertrophied synovium is seen in tubercular and rheumatoid arthritis.

Muscle is of intermediate signal intensity on all sequences. T1W sequences are good to show the anatomy and detect subacute hemorrhage and fatty atrophy. T2W or STIR sequences are sensitive for the diagnosis of muscle strain, myositis and intramuscular tumors. These sequences are sensitive but unfortunately nonspecific for muscle pathology.

IMAGING OF ARTICULAR CARTILAGE

Articular cartilage imaging has become increasingly important in the setting of aging population where osteoarthritis is a leading cause of chronic disability. Accurate assessment of abnormalities has become essential with advanced surgical and pharmacological treatments proving to be useful in the management of cartilage pathology.

There are two types of cartilage assessment sequences based on their usefulness for morphological or compositional evaluation. To assess the morphology, standard spin-echo and gradient echo sequences, fast spin-echo and 3D spin-echo and gradient sequences are available.[5,6] These sequences allow the detection of morphological defects in cartilage and are also used for semiquantitative analysis. To assess the collagen and proteoglycan content of cartilage matrix, compositional assessment techniques like T2 mapping, d-GEMRIC, T1ρ mapping, sodium imaging and diffusion weighted techniques are available, but are mostly used at the research level.[2,7]

MORPHOLOGICAL ASSESSMENT OF CARTILAGE

On spin-echo T1W, proton density (***see* Fig. 2**) and T2W sequences articular cartilage is of intermediate signal intensity.[8] With both conventional and advanced MR techniques several investigators have reported a bilaminar and occasionally, a trilaminar appearance of articular cartilage on MRI. However, the laminar signals may not correspond to the histologic zones. Many MR artifacts like truncation, partial volume, chemical shift and magic angle can contribute to or obscure the laminated appearance. Routine MR evaluation of a joint includes conventional SE, FSE and GRE technique.[9] Fat suppression methods improve the contrast between the cartilage and fatty marrow. The cartilage appears bright due to an increase in the dynamic range. This technique is easily combined with the routine sequences to provide high contrast images of the cartilage. The use of 3D imaging methods in conjunction with FSE and GRE sequences allows for less than 1 mm slice thickness and greatly improved spatial resolution. Three-dimensional spoiled gradient in the steady state (3D SPGR) or 3D fast low-angle shot (FLASH) has been suggested to be one of the most useful techniques for assessment of cartilage lesions. Due to the availability of high-speed gradient MR imaging systems, interest has recently been renewed in steady-state free precession (SSFP), a rapid GRE imaging technique. SSFP has superior signal-to-noise ratio (SNR) compared with other GRE techniques and has excellent contrast behavior with varying dependence on T1 and T2. Synovial fluid appears bright due to its long T2. The limitation of this sequence is image degradation due to local magnetic field inhomogeneities at a long TR. 3D dual echo in the steady-state (DESS) images have been generated by combining images from first and second echoes in a steady state. These images show a high contrast between cartilage and joint fluid.[6,10]

Chondromalacia, osteoarthritic degeneration, osteochondral defects or inflammatory erosions are the common cartilage abnormalities seen on MR imaging.[8] Cartilage degeneration may be superficial or basal. The MR grading is mainly based on the depth of the abnormality (partial or full-thickness) which is seen as a focal signal alteration. Conventional MR techniques show 52–95% accuracy for lesion detection, which is higher for severe lesions. However, use of FSE 3D SPGR and delayed MR arthrography techniques have increased the sensitivity to early and surface lesions.[10]

Direct (joint injection) or indirect (intravenous injection with delayed imaging) MR arthrography is another cartilage imaging method and is especially useful for detecting superficial lesions. Indirect arthrography with intravenous administration of diluted gadolinium may be performed when direct arthrography is inconvenient or not logistically feasible. It is based on the concept that intravenous contrast over time will diffuse into the joint space, so that semi-arthrographic T1W images can be obtained. MR contrast agents do not produce signal themselves but affect the relaxivity of the surrounding structures; consequently a very low concentration can affect numerous surrounding molecules. The advantages are it does not involve a joint injection or fluoroscopic guidance. In addition vascularized or inflamed tissue will enhance with this method. It works best in joints like the wrist, ankle and shoulder but not in large joints like the knee.[2]

COMPOSITIONAL ANALYSIS OF CARTILAGE

The macromolecular network of articular cartilage consists of collagen and proteoglycans. The collagen provides the framework for the tissue and is the main source for tensile and shear strength, whereas glycosaminoglycans provide compressive strength.

T2 Mapping

T2 of hyaline cartilage is highly sensitive to alterations of cartilage matrix. A multiecho sequence is used to measure T2 values and a quantitative color coded map can be generated representing variations in T2 relaxation time within articular cartilage. Areas of early degeneration are seen as areas of higher T2 as compared to normal cartilage. T2 maps can be used to monitor the effectiveness of cartilage repair.[7,11]

d-GEMRIC

In this technique the joint is exercised for 10 minutes after the injection of Gd-DTPA and T1 mapping is done 90 minutes after the injection of Gd. The delay is required to allow gadolinium to penetrate the full thickness of the articular cartilage. It is based on the fact that ions in the interstitial fluid of cartilage are distributed on the basis of the concentration of negatively charged glycosaminoglycan molecules. When anionic molecules like Gd-DTPA enter cartilage they are distributed in areas where the concentration of glycosaminoglycans is low. The concentration of Gd-DTPA can be estimated by measuring T1, T1 mapping of cartilage after administration of Gd-DTPA allows quantitative assessment of glycosamine content. This technique may become the noninvasive method of assessing glycosaminoglycan content in cartilage after various methods of repair.[2,7,11]

T1ρ Mapping

This technique assesses both collagen and glycosaminoglycan content and can detect early degenerative changes.

However, an additional RF pulse has to be applied after the magnetization has been tipped in the transverse plane. It is a more time consuming technique and no large trials have been done using this method.[7,11]

MUSCULOSKELETAL TUMORS

MRI has a vital role in the detection, confirmation and preoperative evaluation of malignant and aggressive benign musculoskeletal tumors. Though plain radiographs are the initial modality for the diagnosis of bone tumors, MRI is indispensable for elucidation of the intra- and extraosseous extent of the tumor, its categorization as intra- or extra-compartmental, assessment of the neurovascular structures and the adjacent joint **(Figs. 7 to 10)**.[1] MRI is also the best technique to detect skip lesions, which are often missed by other imaging means. The plain radiograph is the modality most likely to yield a specific diagnosis **(Fig. 7A)**, whereas MRI is crucial for accurate local staging of a malignant tumor.

In general, musculoskeletal tumors have a nonspecific appearance on MRI and this modality is not reliable in determining the histology of bone tumors in most cases. Occasionally, it may enable a specific diagnosis on account of pathognomonic signal characteristics, for example vertebral hemangioma, soft tissue lipoma **(Figs. 8A and B)**, etc. Therefore one should be wary of interpreting the MR scan in a suspected tumor without reviewing the plain radiographs.

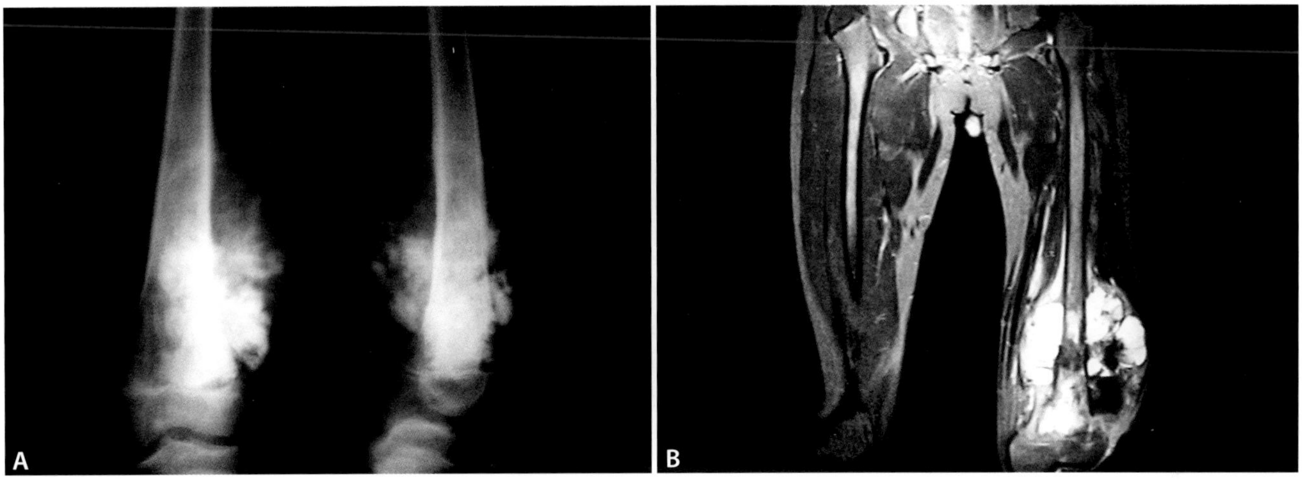

Figs. 7A and B: Frontal and lateral radiographs of the knee: (A) Osteosarcoma of the distal femoral metaphysis with permeative involvement and osteoid pattern of matrix mineralization extending into the soft tissues; (B) Coronal STIR image using body coil shows the complete extent of the tumor, which facilitates optimal surgical management.

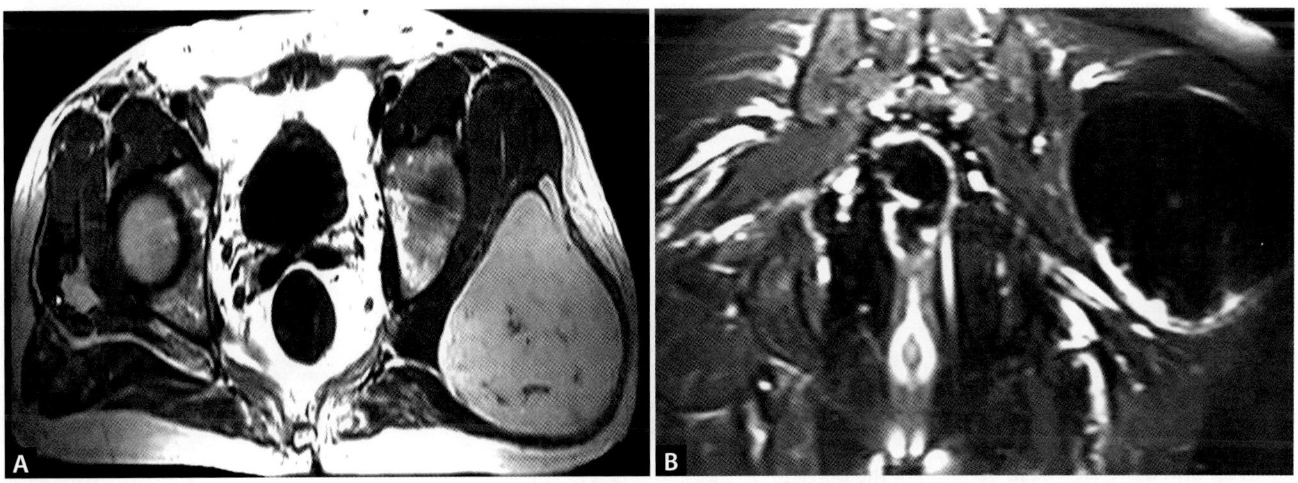

Figs. 8A and B: Axial T1W images: (A) A well-defined hyperintense mass lesion in the left gluteal region which completely looses signal on coronal fat-suppressed image; (B) Indicative of fat within, suggesting the diagnosis of soft tissue lipoma. Also note that the signal intensity of the lesion parallels that of subcutaneous fat.

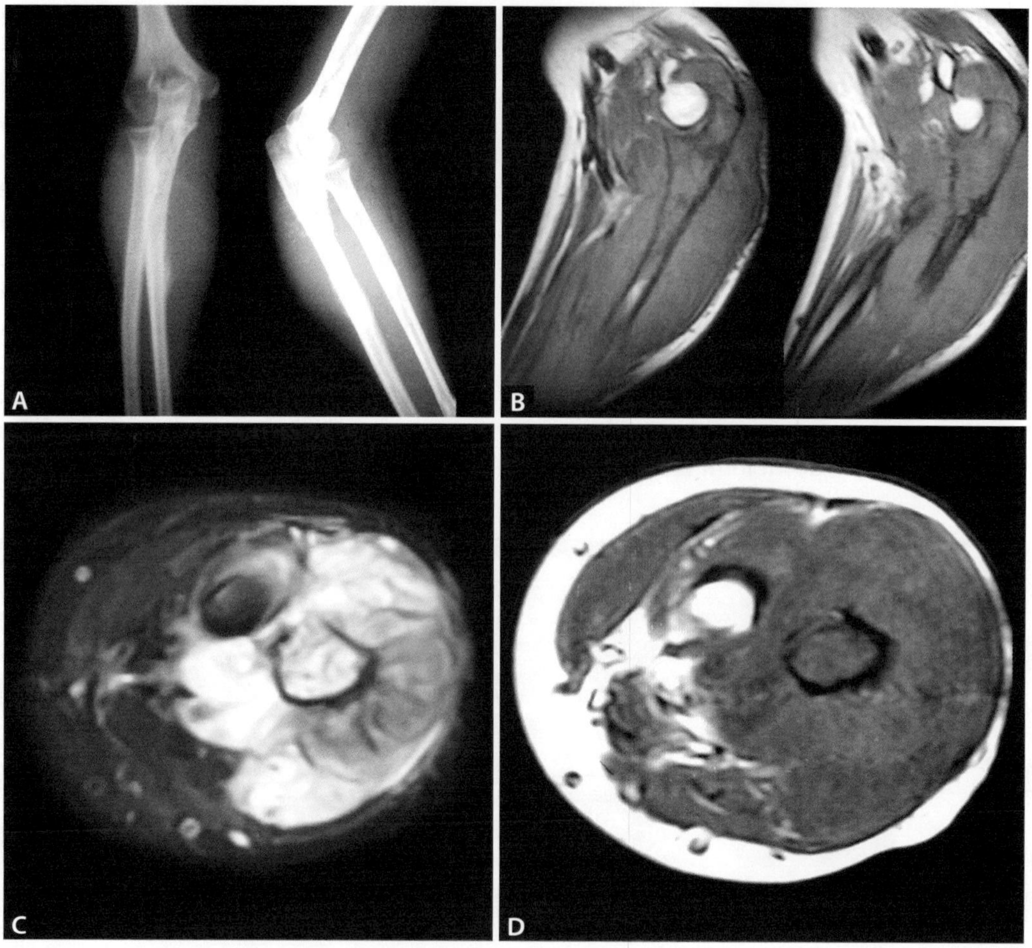

Figs. 9A to D: Frontal and lateral radiographs of the elbow (A) show permeative lytic bone destruction with ill-defined margins involving proximal ulna with Codman's triangle, cortical breech, soft tissue extension and osseous mineralization, suggesting osteosarcoma. Sagittal T1W image (B) clearly demonstrates the intraosseous extent and extension into surrounding soft tissues. Axial T2W (C) and T1W (D) images depict the extent of tumor, cortical disruption and soft tissue extension with sparing of the neurovascular bundle.

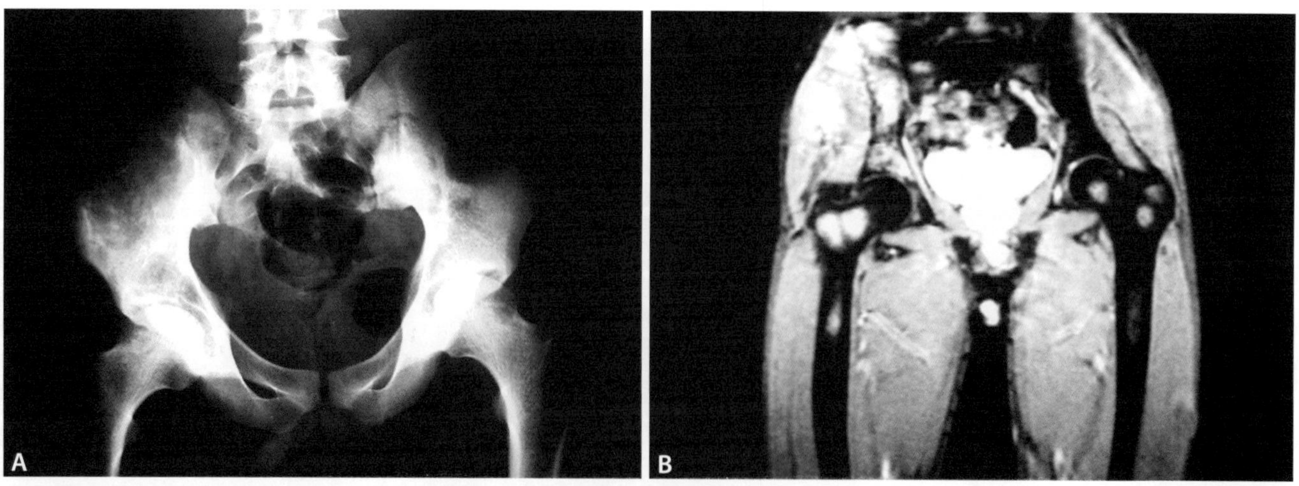

Figs. 10A and B: (A) Frontal radiograph of the pelvis shows an ill-defined permeative lytic lesion in the right iliac wing; (B) STIR coronal image clearly shows that there are multiple well-defined hyperintense lesions in bilateral femoral necks also, indicative of bony metastases. These lesions were not apparent on radiographs. The primary tumor was proven to be Ewing's sarcoma.

Magnetic resonance imaging may detect bone tumors, which are easy to overlook or are not visible on plain radiographs **(Figs. 10A and B)**. This is particularly true in the pelvis and sacrum and in patients with hematological malignancies. In patients with bone pain and a negative plain radiograph, MRI is more sensitive and specific than nuclear scan.[1]

All preoperative imaging of musculoskeletal tumors should be done before a biopsy is performed as it may aid in biopsy planning. Hemorrhage and edema resulting from a biopsy may alter the MR appearance and create difficulty in evaluating the lesion. The tumor should be imaged in at least two planes usually parallel and perpendicular to the long axis of the involved bone. The imaging protocol includes an initial large field of view T1W or STIR study using the body coil **(Fig. 7B)**. This is useful in detection of skip lesions and for planning subsequent sequences. Surface coil images are then obtained in the coronal or sagittal planes to display the extent of the lesion in all three dimensions. The accurate assessment of the craniocaudal extent and exact distance of the proximal and distal margins from a nearby landmark, such as a joint line is crucial for planning a limb-salvage procedure and selection of a suitable prosthesis.[1] Axial images best demonstrate the relationship of the tumor to the neurovascular bundle **(Figs. 9A to D)**. The elucidation of the intraosseous tumor extent as well as the skip lesions need inclusion of a T1W or STIR sequence. However, overestimation of the tumor extent may occur on STIR images due to peritumoral edema. The extraosseous extent is exquisitely demonstrated on a T2W sequence (***see* Figs. 3A and B**) due to the contrast provided by the low-signal muscles. Adjacent bright fat is best suppressed by a fat saturation technique to further increase the contrast on T2W images. MRI has a high negative predictive value for neurovascular or joint involvement by the tumor, though joint involvement tends to get over-diagnosed based on MRI. A GRE sequence is helpful in clear identification of the neurovascular bundle.[12]

USE OF ADVANCED MR TECHNIQUES IN TUMOR EVALUATION

Conventional MR is unable to provide a specific histologic diagnosis and is unreliable for differentiating benign from malignant neoplasms. Neoadjuvant chemotherapy is used in many bone tumors like osteosarcoma and Ewing's sarcoma. The evaluation of response to chemotherapy on routine MR is based on size reduction which is unreliable and may take time. These problems can be addressed by using techniques like dynamic contrast enhanced perfusion imaging, proton spectroscopy, diffusion imaging and in phase/opposed phase MR imaging.[13,14]

Dynamic Perfusion Imaging

T1W gradient echo sequence is repeated rapidly a number of times after an injection of gadolinium bolus (0.1 mmol/kg) followed by a saline chase. Timesignal intensity curves are generated in much the same way as is done in breast imaging. In general malignant tumors show greater enhancement at a faster rate **(Figs. 11A to D)** and a rapid wash out as compared to benign tumors.[13] This technique coupled with conventional MR, spectroscopy and DWI may help in narrowing the list of differential diagnosis, better assess the extent of disease, distinguish responders to chemotherapy from nonresponders and differentiate residual/recurrent tumor from radiation necrosis. The former enhance early and more rapidly whereas post-therapy changes enhance later and more slowly.[14]

Proton Spectroscopy

It can be performed using a single voxel technique with a point resolved spectroscopy sequence (PRESS) and echo time of 135 msec. The choline peak and choline/creatine ratio has been shown to distinguish benign from malignant bone and soft tissue tumors **(Figs. 11A to D)**. The voxel should be placed on areas showing early and intense enhancement. The caveat is that some metabolically active tumors like giant cell tumor may also show choline peak.[13]

Diffusion-weighted Imaging

Diffusion can be assessed both qualitatively and quantitatively and is a measure of tumor cellularity and cell membrane integrity. It can be used for detection and characterization of bone tumors as well as assess the response to chemotherapy. Diffusion-weighted imaging (DWI) sequences are done at different b values ranging from 0 to 1000. Typically benign lesions lose their signal intensity as b value increases whereas cellular tumors retain their signal intensity. Apparent diffusion coefficient (ADC) can be used for quantitative assessment. Low ADC values are seen in cellular tumors because of restricted diffusion.

DWI can also be used to assess response to chemoradiotherapy. Tumor necrosis caused by these modalities increases the ADC value which can be used as a surrogate marker for response.[14]

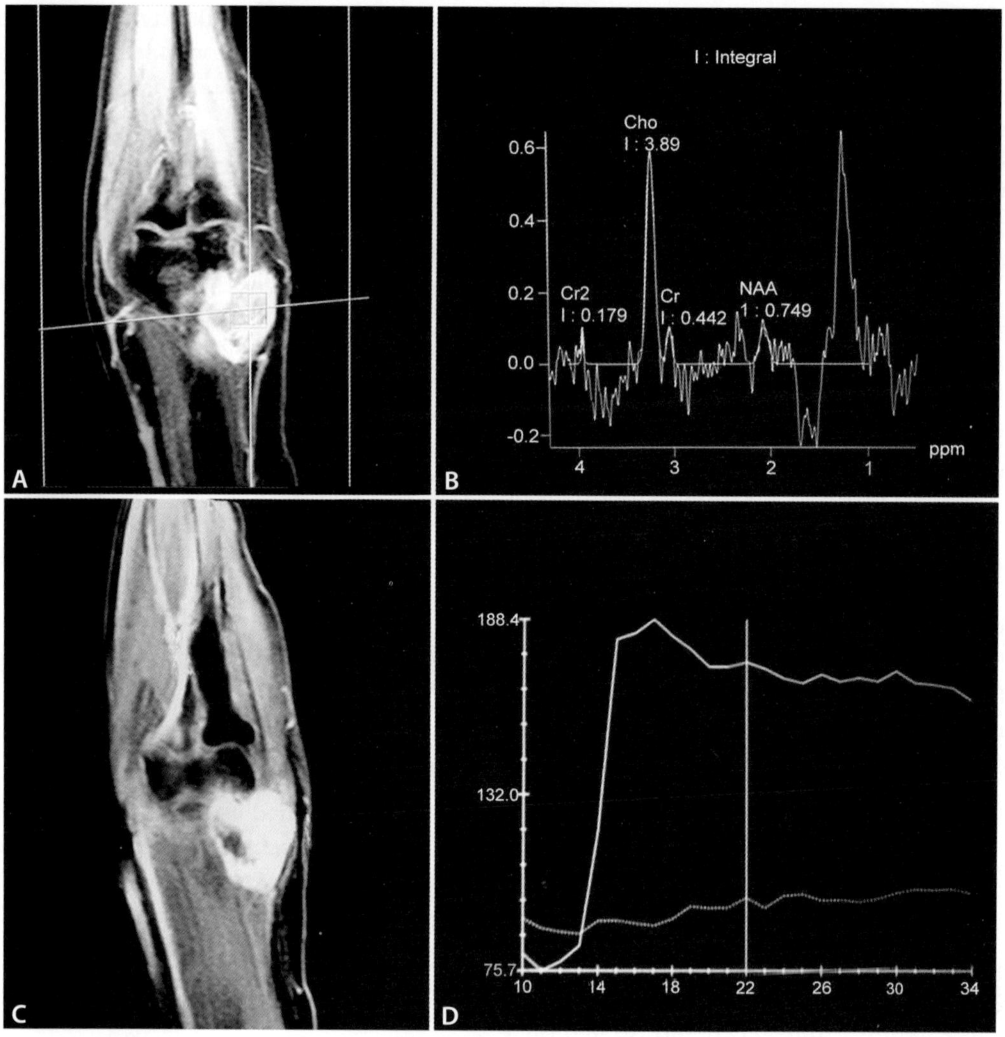

Figs. 11A to D: Coronal FS postgadolinium image (A) of the elbow showing the placement of voxel for single voxel MR spectroscopy in enhancing lesion seen in distal humeral metaphysis. There is elevated choline peak (B), suggesting malignant bone tumor. Coronal postgadolinium FS T1W image (C) of the elbow showing the placement of region of interest (ROI) for generation of perfusion map of the lesion to show contrast kinetics. Time signal intensity curve (D) of the same lesion shows rapid uptake and washout of the contrast, indicating malignant neoplasm.

MARROW IMAGING

Conventional radiographic techniques are very insensitive to marrow infiltration and tumors. CT may detect gross metastatic disease of the spine but is of limited use in imaging primary and metastatic neoplasms in the rest of the skeleton. Radionuclide bone scanning is insensitive to certain marrow neoplasms such as lymphoma and multiple myeloma. MRI has the major advantage of imaging the bone marrow directly and its excellent contrast resolution allows the differentiation of normal from infiltrated marrow.[1,2]

When diffuse marrow disease is suspected a survey of the entire spine, pelvis and proximal femora is performed, because this is where the bulk of the hematopoietic marrow exists. For a marrow survey the patient is positioned supine. The phased array coils are used for spine imaging and the body coil is used for the proximal femora and the pelvis. Sagittal images of the spine and coronal images of the pelvis and femora are most useful. Whole body MRI can now be routinely performed for metastatic survey and in marrow infiltrative diseases. There is a technique called DWIBS (Diffusion-weighted imaging with background suppression of fat signal) which is ideal for picking up foci of metastatic disease, lymphoma, etc. and may become a competitive modality for PET-CT. T1W and STIR images are most sensitive to marrow pathology.[1]

MRI can distinguish between hematopoietic or red marrow from yellow marrow. The normal distribution of red and yellow marrow and the conversion of red to yellow marrow occurs in a predictable manner based on age.[2] There is a vast array of marrow disorders that can be detected on MR imaging although the appearance may be nonspecific and only a differential diagnosis may be offered. However, MRI is excellent for establishing the presence of disease and also for directing biopsy to an appropriate site.

Important categories of marrow pathology include marrow proliferative disorders such as leukemia and myeloma and marrow replacement disorders such as metastases and lymphoma.[1] The usual appearance of marrow pathology is low signal intensity (equal to or less than muscle) on T1W scans **(Fig. 12A)** and variable but usually high signal intensity on T2W scans.

MRI is exquisitely sensitive for detection of metastatic disease and surpasses all other imaging techniques in this regard. A common clinical problem is the distinction between a metastatic deposits from an acute osteoporotic collapse, especially in a patient with a known primary tumor. Both may show a fractured vertebral body with replacement of normal marrow by low signal intensity on T1W scans. Features that suggest tumor are abnormal signal intensity extending into the pedicles and other posterior elements, involvement of the entire vertebral body by the abnormal signal intensity, associated soft tissue mass and multiple bone lesions. In osteoporotic fractures the abnormal signal intensity does not involve the entire vertebral body, but has a horizontal line or band separating the abnormal signal intensity from the normal fatty marrow signal.[1] It has been reported that GRE opposed phase sequence may be helpful based on the fact that some fat is still present in benign lesions such as osteoporotic fractures. Hence osteoporotic fractures are supposed to show lower signal intensity than the metastatic lesions. Diffusion weighted images (DWI) have also been successfully used for the purpose of this differentiation.[1] The vertebral lesions due to marrow infiltration by tumor become hyperintense on DWI **(Figs. 12B and C)** whereas osteoporotic collapsed vertebra remains hypointense. In and opposed phase images have also been used in this context. Collapse due to osteoporosis will retain some normal fatty marrow which will show loss of signal on the opposed phase image. On the other hand, metastatic and marrow infiltrative disease replaces the fatty marrow completely and hence does not show this signal loss **(Figs. 12D and E)**.

MR can also be used to monitor the response of marrow pathology such as leukemia and metastases to treatment. Serial MRI has been shown to be useful in confirming remission and detecting relapse in patients with leukemia.

MUSCULOSKELETAL INFECTIONS

Conventional radiographs remain the initial imaging modality of choice for suspected osteomyelitis. However, it is insensitive to the detection of early osteomyelitis. MR imaging scores over radiography, CT and scintigraphy in detection of early osteomyelitis. However, the MR appearance is nonspecific and similar to infiltrating neoplasms and stress fractures and the clinical context is important in reaching the correct diagnosis.[15] MR is also superior to other modalities in delineating the soft tissue involvement. The elucidation of the full extent facilitates preoperative planning of the maximal degree of debridement or the level of the amputation. Fat suppression techniques combined with gadolinium administration further increase the sensitivity for detection of involved areas. Contrast administration is also helpful in distinguishing abscess **(*see* Fig. 6)** from surrounding cellulitis, increasing the conspicuity of the sinus tracts by causing their walls to enhance and clearly demonstrating the nonenhancing sequestra within enhancing granulation tissue.[16]

In infants and children, involvement of the unossified physis and epiphysis is best shown by MR imaging.

INFLAMMATORY ARTHRITIS

Radiography has been the imaging modality of choice in rheumatoid arthritis (RA), primarily because of its reproducibility and feasibility. Currently MRI is being used widely for recruiting patients into clinical trials as well as monitoring disease progression over time, because of its advantage of simultaneous imaging of key structures other than bone (synovium and surrounding soft tissues) that are important in inflammatory arthritis. MRI is also a useful tool in evaluating patients with early rheumatoid arthritis. It can detect pre-erosive synovitis and can also identify early bone damage before it becomes apparent on radiography. In early rheumatoid arthritis, wrist and hand involvement is usually bilateral. Some authors perform bilateral MR imaging of the wrists or hands. However, it is preferred to study the dominant or more painful wrist in order to reduce the study time. The technical recommendations of the OMERACT (Outcome Measures in Rheumatoid Arthritis Clinical Trials) group for MR

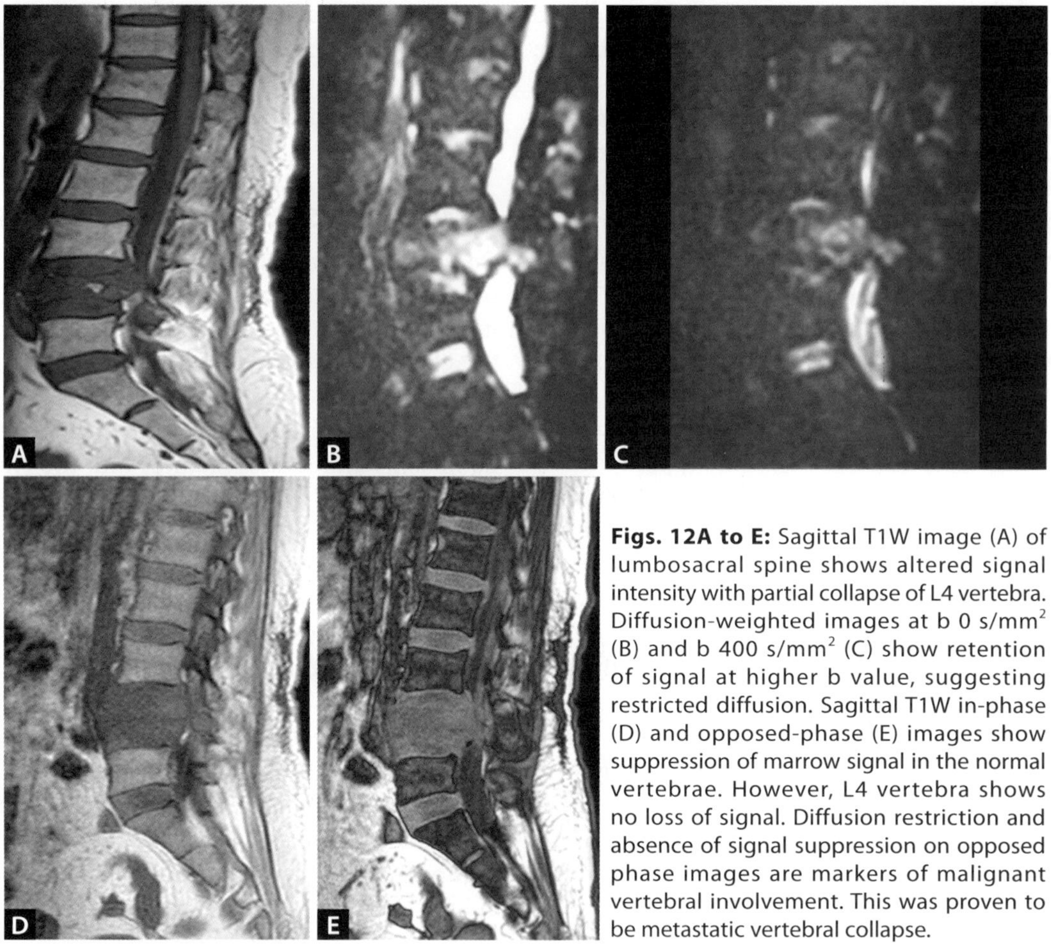

Figs. 12A to E: Sagittal T1W image (A) of lumbosacral spine shows altered signal intensity with partial collapse of L4 vertebra. Diffusion-weighted images at b 0 s/mm^2 (B) and b 400 s/mm^2 (C) show retention of signal at higher b value, suggesting restricted diffusion. Sagittal T1W in-phase (D) and opposed-phase (E) images show suppression of marrow signal in the normal vertebrae. However, L4 vertebra shows no loss of signal. Diffusion restriction and absence of signal suppression on opposed phase images are markers of malignant vertebral involvement. This was proven to be metastatic vertebral collapse.

imaging studies of RA patients should include at least the following sequences: (a) imaging in two planes (coronal and axial), (b) T1-weighted imaging before and after the administration of gadolinium, fat-saturated imaging is preferable after administration, and (c) a fat-saturated T2-weighted sequence or a STIR sequence.[17]

INTERVENTIONAL MR IMAGING

Due to restricted patient access on conventional high and midfield MR machines and unacceptable speed on the older low-field systems, MR imaging was not considered as a guidance tool for interventional procedures earlier. Since the introduction of open magnet designs offering a nearly free patient access, interest has now focused on interventional MR. In addition, short bore highfield systems presently allow satisfactory patient access combined with high performance imaging capabilities. A simultaneous creation of an adequate array of MR compatible instruments has made MR interventions viable.[18] Percutaneous biopsies and drainage procedures are currently the easiest procedures to be performed under MR control. These do not require dedicated hard or software modifications and are thus attractive and clinically useful.

Three types of magnets are clinically used for percutaneous biopsies: open low-field magnets [0.2–0.35 Tesla (T)], open midfield system (0.5 T) and closed short bore magnets (1–1.5 T). Improved patient access with open magnet allows interventions in any desired plane and patient position. To begin with, horizontally open magnets were used. Recently, experience with vertically open units has also been reported. Vertically open units permit unrestricted vertical and side access to the patient at the most homogeneous portion of the magnetic field. The other advantage is a horizontally directed main magnetic field along the long axis of the bore, which ensures that the needle trajectory is never parallel to the field.[19] In closed systems, instrument manipulation can only be performed with the patient outside the magnet. However, due to higher field strength, image quality as well as the imaging speed is better.

For instrument visualization the susceptibility artifact provided by the nonferromagnetic alloys of MR compatible needles is used. The size of the artifact is inversely proportional to the size of the instrument and directly proportional to the field strength and to the angle the instrument makes with the main magnetic field. Typically, biopsy needles are displayed as dark areas surrounded by a brighter rim.[20] Several vendors on the market offer MR compatible needles at present. Fine needles of 20–24G with different tip configurations and cutting needles of 14–18G are commercially available. The overall performance of a MR compatible needle is inferior to a stainless steel needle due to relatively blunt surfaces and softer alloys. For drainage procedures MR compatible sets consisting of MR compatible guidewires, dilators and drainage catheters are available.

Imaging protocol consists of fast localizers in three planes followed by a fast multislice T2W SE sequence. A postcontrast GRE sequence may be used to select the appropriate biopsy site. In the closed magnet, needle tracking is done by following a procedure similar to that used in CT guided interventions. After defining the target region, a T1W or T2W compatible grid is fixed to the skin of the patient to aid in selecting needle entry site. The angle and distance from skin to the lesion can be obtained by using standard scanner software. The needle track can be controlled step-by-step during advancement of the needle. In the open magnet, a palpating finger may be used instead of a grid for entry site. The instrument can be tracked by continuous repetition of a fast imaging sequence.[18]

Primary and secondary bone and soft tissue lesions can be accessed by MR guided interventional procedures. Due to its multiplanar capability, MR allows visualization of the entire planned biopsy pathway including orthogonal and oblique scans. Lack of ionizing radiation is an obvious advantage.[20] The unique advantage of MR interventions is in transcutaneous biopsy of bone marrow lesions of unknown origin, as their display and localization is possible exclusively on MR. However, the available armamentarium to perform MR guided transcortical bone biopsy is limited, though a MR compatible coaxial bone biopsy system has recently been developed.[18] Although lesion access by MR is good for appendicular skeleton, CT is preferred for biopsy of the axial skeleton due to superior spatial resolution.

CONCLUSION

The scope of musculoskeletal radiology has widened over the last few years and to a large extent this has been possible because of the exquisite detail provided by the versatile technique of MRI. Highfield MRI, diffusion weighted imaging, dynamic contrast enhanced imaging, MR spectroscopy and other advances have further enhanced the utility of this modality. However, elegant display of pathology alone does not suffice, as diagnosis based on images alone, especially MR images, is nonspecific. For the optimal use of this technology the radiologist must couple these images with an in depth knowledge of pathophysiology and clinical perspective so that he can guide the referring clinician appropriately. 'Seeing better' should be coupled with 'Knowing more' to make the optimum use of the high tech modality of MRI.[21]

REFERENCES

1. Helms CA, Anderson MW, Major NM, Kaplan P, Dussault R. Musculoskeletal MRI, 2nd edn. Philadelphia: WB Saunders Co; 2009.
2. Stoller DW. Magnetic resonance imaging in orthopaedics and sports medicine, 3rd edn. Lippincott Williams and Wilkins; 2007.
3. Zou J, Yang H, Miyazaki M, et al. Dynamic bulging of intervertebral discs in the degenerative lumbar spine. Spine. 2009;34(23):2545.
4. Ramnath RR. 3T MR imaging of the musculoskeletal system (Part II): clinical applications. Magn Reson Imaging Clin N Am. 2006;14(1):41.
5. Koff MF, Potter HG. Noncontrast MR techniques and imaging of cartilage. Radiol Clin N Am. 2009;47(3):495-504.
6. Strickland CD, Kijowski R. Morphologic imaging of articular cartilage. Magn Reson Imaging Clin N Am. 2011;19(2):229-48.
7. Choi JA, Gold GE. MR imaging of articular cartilage physiology. Magn Reson Imaging Clin N Am. 2011;19(2):249-82.
8. Suh JS, Lee SH, Jeong EK, Kim DJ. Magnetic resonance imaging of articular cartilage. Eur Radiol. 2001;11(10):2015-25.
9. Sonin AH, Pensy RA, Mulligan ME, Hatem S. Grading articular cartilage of the knee using fast spinecho proton density-weighted MR imaging without fat suppression. Am J Roentgenol. 2002;179(5):1159-66.
10. Reeder SB, Pelc NJ, Alley MT, Gold GE. Rapid MR imaging of articular cartilage with steady-state free precession and multipoint fat-water separation. Am J Roentgenol. 2003;180(2):357-62.
11. Crema MD, Roemer FW, Marra MD, et al. Articular cartilage in the knee: current MR imaging techniques and applications in clinical practice and research. Radiographics. 2011;31(1):37-61.
12. Peabody TD, Gibbs CP, Simon MA. Current concepts review—evaluation and staging of musculoskeletal neoplasms. J Bone Joint Surg Am. 1998;80(8):1204-18.

13. Costa FM, Canella C, Gasparetto E. Advanced magnetic resonance imaging techniques in the evaluation of musculoskeletal tumors. Radiol Clin North Am. 2011;49(6):1325-58.
14. Garner HW, Kransdorf MJ, Peterson JJ. Posttherapy imaging of musculoskeletal neoplasms. Radiol Clin North Am. 2011;49(6):1307-23.
15. Boutin RD, Brossmann J, Sartoris DJ, Reilly D, Resnick D. Update on imaging of orthopedic infections. Orthop Clin North Am. 1998;29(1):41-66.
16. D Towers J. The use of intravenous contrast in MRI of extremity infection. Semin Ultrasound CT MR. 1997;(18):269-75.
17. Narváez JA, Narváez J, De Lama E, De Albert M. MR imaging of early rheumatoid arthritis. Radiographics. 2010;30(1):143-63; discussion 163-5.
18. Adam G, Bücker A, Nolte-Ernsting C, Tacke J, Günther R. Interventional MR imaging: percutaneous abdominal and skeletal biopsies and drainages of the abdomen. Eur Radiol. 1999;9(8):1471-8.
19. Genant JW, Vandevenne JE, Bergman AG, et al. Interventional musculoskeletal procedures performed by using mr imaging guidance with a vertically open MR unit: Assessment of techniques and applicability. Radiology. 2002;223(1):127-36.
20. Ghelman B. Biopsies of the musculoskeletal system. Radiol Clin North Am. 1998;36(3):567-80.
21. Feldman F. Musculoskeletal Radiology: Then and Now. Radiology. 2000;216(2):309.

CHAPTER 188

Nuclear Medicine Imaging for Musculoskeletal Disorders

Rakesh Kumar, Punit Sharma, Arun Malhotra

INTRODUCTION

Musculoskeletal system is a dynamic organ system, which responds to systemic as well as to localized stress and hence apart from anatomical visualization, it requires physiological evaluation. Nuclear medicine techniques provide the physician with the physiologically detailed images that can give insight which cannot always be accomplished from plain radiograph or even with computed tomography (CT) and magnetic resonance imaging (MRI). The major advantage of nuclear medicine imaging stems from the fact that functional changes appear much before anatomical changes. Hence, nuclear medicine imaging allows early detection of diseases affecting musculoskeletal system. The present chapter summarizes the nuclear medicine techniques used for musculoskeletal imaging and their utility in various benign and malignant pathologies involving the musculoskeletal system.

BONE SCINTIGRAPHY

In spite of newer development in field of nuclear medicine, bone scintigraphy remains the most commonly employed method for musculoskeletal imaging. It is done with injection of bone seeking radiopharmaceuticals. These compounds are usually phosphonates labeled with ^{99m}Technetium (^{99m}Tc). The most widely used is ^{99m}Tc-Methylene diphosphonate (MDP). Others are ^{99m}Tc-Ethylene hydroxy diphosphonate (EHDP) and ^{99m}Tc-hydroxy methylene diphosphonate (HDP). The presences of p-c-p bonds make these compounds resistant to hydrolysis by bone phosphatases, thereby increasing the biological half life. Three to four hours after intravenous injection about 25–35% of radiotracer is retained in the normal adult skeleton, the rest is excreted in the urine via the kidney. These phosphorus containing complexes avidly attach themselves to the hydroxyapatite crystal surface by the process of chemisorptions.[1] Thus, they localizes at the site of direct and indirect osteoblastic activation. Autoradiographic studies revealed that the ^{99m}Tc-labeled phosphonates are mainly taken up in the mineral phase of skeletal bone at the site of reactive bone formation. This osteoblastic activation can be seen because of wide array of pathologies, thereby decreasing the specificity. The routine bone scintigraphy employs whole body anterior and posterior sweep images. In addition dynamic flow and pool images are acquired in selected cases.

SPECT AND SPECT-CT

Given the lack of anatomical information provided by planar bone scintigraphy, especially in regions of complex anatomy, additional methods are employed. Single photon emission tomography (SPECT) is being routinely used in such a scenario. It gives three-dimensional pictures and is beneficial in patients with normal planar images despite symptoms and in those with equivocal findings.[2] Single photon emission tomography imaging is most useful for evaluation of the thoracolumbar spine, skull and pelvis. These areas have extensive surrounding soft tissue and/ or complicated body contours, and thus superior image contrast provided by SPECT improves lesion detection. The decision to perform single field-of-view SPECT studies has been guided by suspicious findings on planar imaging or localized clinical symptoms. However, even with SPECT correlation with anatomical imaging is usually needed in many cases. SPECT-CT imaging with hybrid cameras has been introduced to overcome this shortcoming and to provide both anatomical and functional information in single setting.

PET AND PET-CT

In contrast to routine gamma camera imaging, positron emission tomography (PET) imaging is based on the detection of high energy (511 KeV) annihilation photons emitted by positron emitting radionuclides. The inherent physics of positron decay allows tomographic imaging without the need for collimators thereby improving the sensitivity and resolution. The lack of anatomical information on PET alone has been overcome with introduction of hybrid PET-CT. In fact, the availability of hybrid PET-CT systems has made PET alone redundant. Although, PET and PET-CT had greatest impact in the field of cancer imaging, its application for other areas including musculoskeletal disorders is being actively investigated. In clinical practice, most PET studies are performed with 2-[^{18}F] fluoro-2-deoxy- D-glucose (FDG), a glucose analogue. It is actively taken up by cells with increased glucose metabolic rate via specific glucose transporters (GLUT-1, GLUT-4) and is phosphorylated by hexokinases to FDG-6-phosphate, which is retained.[3] Nowadays, FDG is being increasingly used for imaging primary and secondary musculoskeletal tumors as well as infections. Another important tracer in context of skeletal imaging is ^{18}F-Flouride. It can also be used for quantitative studies of skeletal kinetics.[4] Although there are differences between ^{18}F-Fluoride and ^{99m}Tc-diphosphonate, it is probable that the mechanism of uptake in bone is the same, i.e. adsorption onto bony surfaces with predilection for sites of active bone formation.[5] The uptake of ^{18}F-Fluoride is approximately two-fold higher and its blood clearance is significantly faster compared with the ^{99m}Tc-diphosphonates, resulting in an increased bone-to-background ratio. In addition, PET offers high sensitivity and high resolution and therefore enables to perform highly accurate whole-body screening for metastases.[6]

MUSCULOSKELETAL TUMOR IMAGING

Metastasis

Skeletal metastasis is the most common malignant bone tumor. It affects approximately two-thirds of cancer patients, with breast cancer being the leading cause in women, prostate cancer in men, followed by lung cancer in both sexes. Accurate assessment of skeletal involvement is essential for optimal management of these patients.[7] Many patients with bone metastases are and may be identified during initial staging, routine follow-up, or investigation of rising tumor markers. For the past few decades, planar bone scintigraphy has been the most frequently performed imaging study in the evaluation of metastatic bone disease. Although scintigraphic findings alone are often nonspecific for skeletal pathologies, this technique reportedly has an exquisite sensitivity. Radiographs are found to be negative in 30–50% of patients with positive bone scan. Most common pattern of bone metastasis is multiple "hot" lesions distributed randomly throughout the skeleton.[8] A lytic metastasis usually presents as a photopenic area with increased activity at the edge of the lesion. False-negative results in bone scintigraphy are seen in avascular lesions, in the presence of rapidly growing pure osteolytic metastases with no reactive increased osteoblastic activity, or in lesions with low bone turnover (multiple myeloma, thyroid cancer). Specificity of BS is generally lower, due to a known increased blood flow and metabolic reaction of bone to a variety of disease processes, including osteoarthritis, trauma and inflammation. Therefore, further assessment with other imaging modalities, mainly CT and MRI and in some cases histologic confirmation may be required for precise diagnosis.[9]

Addition of SPECT has been reported to detect 20–50% more lesions in the spine compared with planar scintigraphy.[10] It increases both the sensitivity and specificity of bone scans (BS).[11] The use of SPECT for the assessment of suspicious vertebral lesions on planar BS had a negative predictive value of 98%. The sensitivity and specificity of bone SPECT for diagnosis of bone metastases are 87–92 and 91–93%, respectively.[12] The decision to perform single field-of-view SPECT studies has been guided by suspicious findings on planar imaging or localized clinical symptoms. Newly developed half-time wholebody SPECT protocols provide tomographic assessment of the entire skeleton within an acceptable image acquisition time, with subsequent improvement in sensitivity and an increased detection rate of asymptomatic small skeletal metastases.[13] However, even with SPECT correlation with high-quality anatomic images, CT, or MRI, may still be needed for diagnosis. Hybrid SPECT/CT devices equipped with multislice CT scanners further improves the sensitivity and specificity of BS. It has been shown to be superior to planar BS and SPECT for skeletal metastasis of breast and lung cancers.[14,15] Foci of increased tracer activity on BS suspicious as representing malignant bone lesions may not show any morphologic abnormality on CT as functional changes precede anatomical changes and therefore cannot be confirmed as such. The present consensus is to do SPECT-CT of suspicious planar BS lesions only if the lesion remains equivocal even after SPECT **(Figs. 1A to E)**.

Several studies have shown the superiority of the ^{18}F-Fluoride PET over BS for the diagnosis of skeletal metastases; the former demonstrated a higher number of the lesions and a higher contrast between normal and abnormal bone.[16] Although the superb resolution and high abnormal to normal bone ratio of ^{18}F-Fluoride PET can potentially lower the specificity, hybrid PET-CT imaging should help differentiate benign versus malignant lesions **(Figs. 2A to C)**.[17] ^{18}F-Fluoride has shown to be highly sensitive for detecting lytic and sclerotic bone metastasis in breast cancer,[18] prostate cancer[19] and lung cancer.[20] There has been the suggestion that ^{18}F-Fluoride could be more cost effective than the bone scan and that a case can be made for it replacing the bone scan.[21] Increased FDG activity at the sites of skeletal lesions represent active tumor itself, whereas increased ^{99m}Tc-MDP or ^{18}F-Fluoride activity represents a blastic activity/reparative process in response to tumor and destroyed bone. Compared with BS or ^{18}F-Fluoride, FDG-PET is reported to be more sensitive for lytic lesions and bone marrow disease but less sensitive for blastic lesions.[22] It has an additional advantage: the ability to assess extraskeletal metastatic disease, including muscle metastasis.[23] Recent data almost invariably have shown that BS is more sensitive than FDG-PET for detection of blastic/sclerotic lesion, whereas FDG-PET is more sensitive for lytic lesions and bone marrow involvement **(Figs. 3A to D)**.[24] The lower sensitivity of FDG-PET for detecting sclerotic lesions can be complemented by CT, which may obviate the need for BS.[25] At any rate, it seems generally agreed that the overall sensitivity of FDG-PET and BS for all lesions

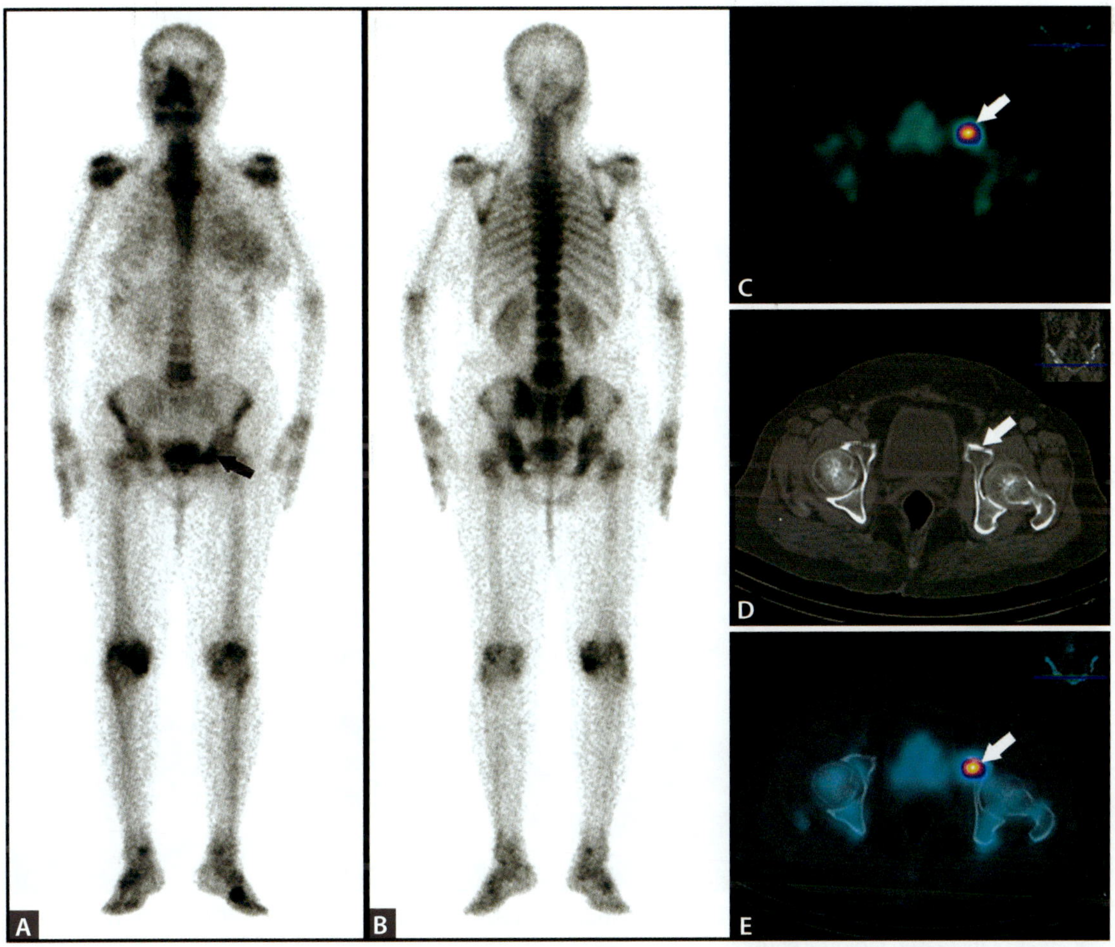

Figs. 1A to E: A 37-year-old carcinoma breast patient for staging. Planar bone scintigraphy (A and B) showed a suspicious focal uptake in left superior pubic rami (arrow). SPECT (C), CT (D) and SPECT-CT (E) images showed lytic lesion with increased tracer uptake (arrow) suggesting metastasis.

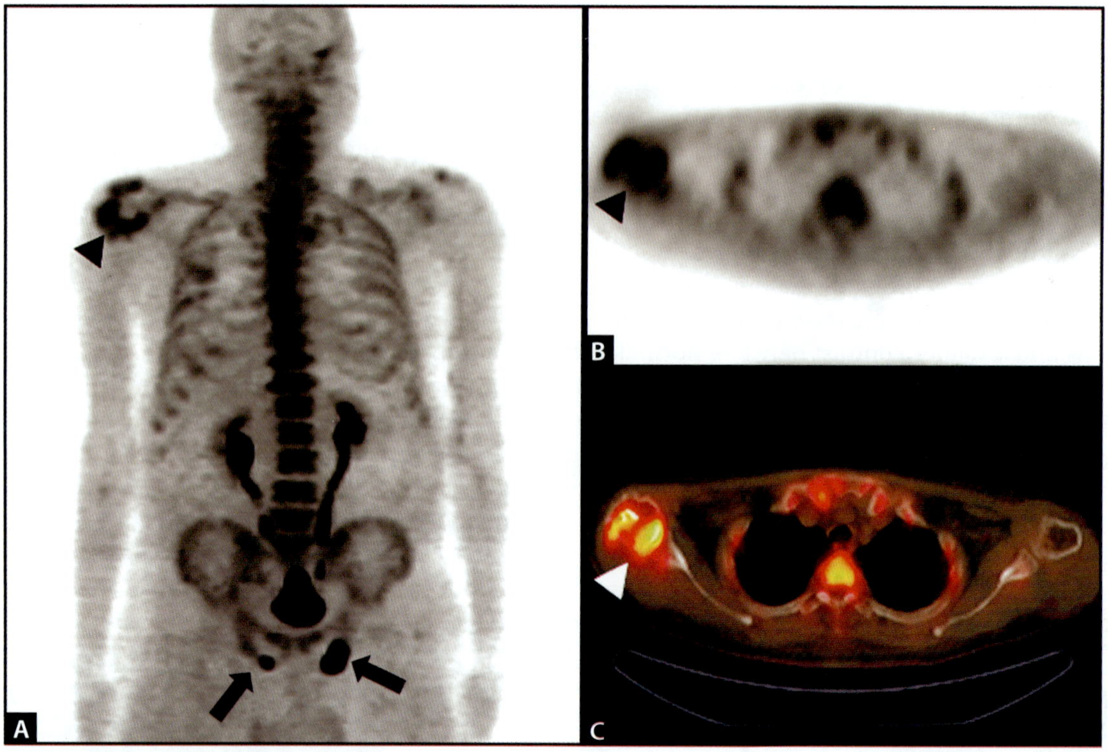

Figs. 2A to C: A 60-year-old male with carcinoma prostate and rising PSA. ^{18}F-Fluoride PET MIP images (A and B) shows focal tracer uptake in bilateral pubic ramii (arrows) suggestive of metastasis. Also noted was tracer uptake in right shoulder (arrowheads). On PET-CT images (C), this uptake was diagnosed to be degenerative change (arrowhead).

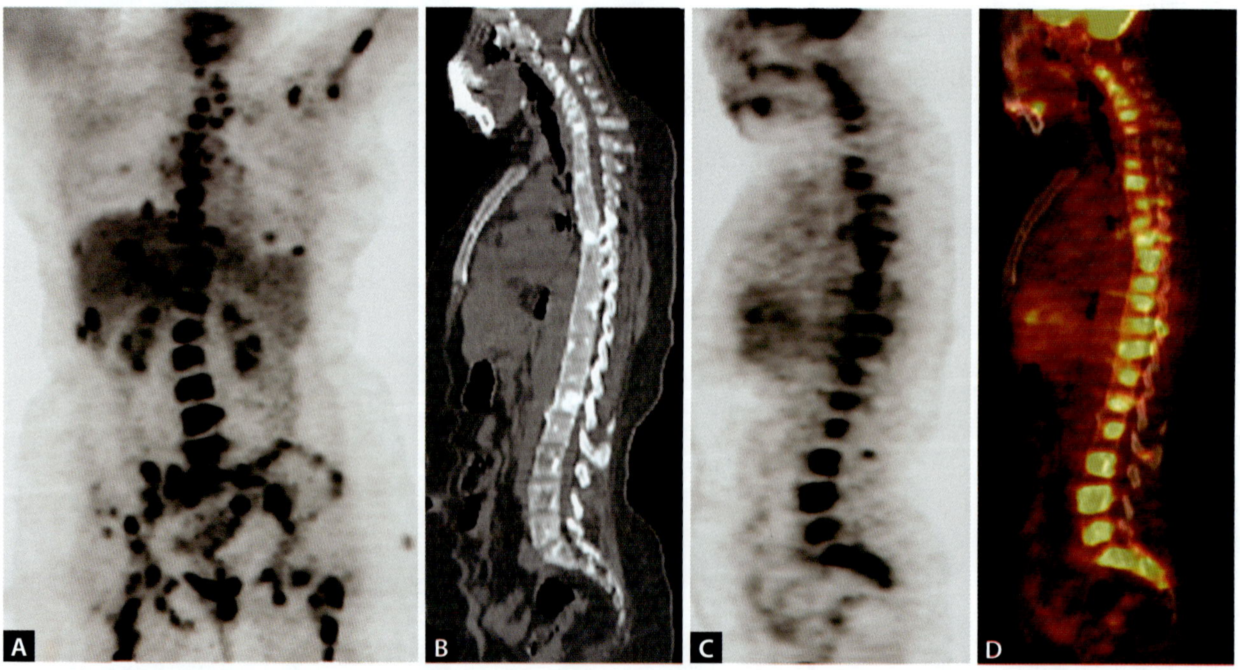

Figs. 3A to D: A 35-year-old female with known breast cancer underwent PET-CT scan for staging. ^{18}F-FDG whole-body projection image (A) shows focal areas of increased radiotracer uptake suggestive of metastases. Lytic sclerotic bone lesions and FDG uptake in multiple vertebrae in CT, PET and PET-CT sagittal sections (B to D). There are many lesions showing focal FDG uptake no sclerosis on CT suggestive of marrow metastases.

is comparable, but PET has a higher specificity, resulting in an overall higher accuracy. The utility of FDG PET-CT for bone metastasis has already been shown in breast cancer, lung cancer, lymphoma, multiple myeloma and neuroblastoma.[26-28] Another, very important advantage of FDG PET-CT is its ability to assess response to therapy in bone metastasis. Although BS has been used to assess the efficacy of treatment and to follow breast cancer patients, the early response to any treatment cannot be assessed by BS. Moreover, BS may show persistent increased activity even in treated lesions for several weeks to months. In most malignancies, FDG-PET has proved an effective modality for early assessment of therapeutic response by showing rapid reduction in FDG uptake by the tumors in responders following chemotherapy.[29] The changes in FDG standard uptake value (SUV) with therapy showed correlation with the overall clinical assessment of response as well as with the change in tumor marker value. Flare phenomenon which is considered to be a marker of response on BS has also been described on FDG-PET but only associated with antiestrogen therapy.[30]

Primary Malignant Tumors

The role of bone scintigraphy in primary malignant bone tumors is very limited. On three-phase BS, most primary malignant bone tumors are usually highly vascular with intense delayed radiotracer uptake that often extends beyond the margin of the bone with distorted and ill-defined outline. Although mild variations depending on the type of tumor exist, there is no single pattern specific for individual tumor. Basically, BS has no role in the initial diagnosis or assessment of the extent of primary malignant bone tumors for which MRI is considered the imaging modality of choice. Rather, whole body BS is generally reserved for evaluation of metastatic bone disease **(Figs. 4A and B)**. Although pulmonary metastases are occasionally identified on BS as focally increased soft tissue uptake, high-resolution CT is best suited for evaluation of pulmonary metastases.

Functional imaging with FDG-PET provides unique information with regard to the metabolic activity of bone and soft tissue tumors. This may help characterize indeterminate lesions and guide targeted biopsy of the most metabolically active area within larger tumors. This aspect is particularly important in many soft tissue and bone tumors which are of mixed grade and/or cell type. In one study with soft tissue tumors, there was a statistically significant difference in SUV between benign and malignant soft tissue lesions although there was considerable overlap between the two groups, with only

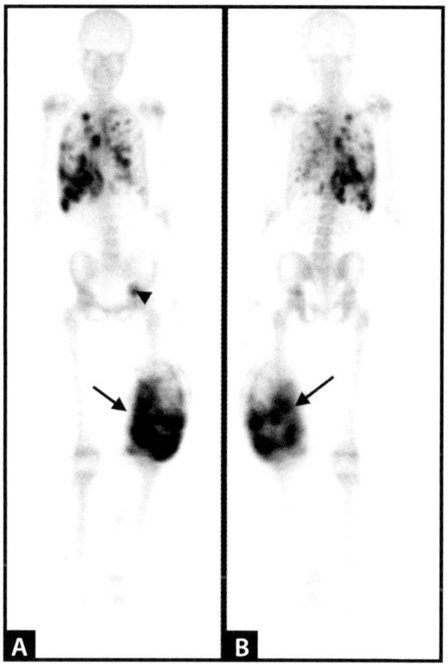

Figs. 4A and B: A 16-year-old male with osteosarcoma of left femur. Planar bone scintigraphy (A and B) shows mass in left femoral shaft with heterogeneous tracer uptake (arrows), consistent with primary tumor. In addition, it showed bone metastasis (arrowhead) and osteogenic pulmonary metastasis.

lipomas and hemangiomas consistently non-FDG avid.[31] Dual-time point PET imaging can be utilized to increase the accuracy of differentiating benign from malignant soft tissue lesions.[32] FDG-PET may also be used for more accurate staging of histologically confirmed tumors, in therapy response assessment to detect progression or regression of disease ahead of morphological change in the tumor and in the early detection of recurrent disease. The degree of FDG uptake by tumors pre- and post-therapy correlates well with histological response, often prior to demonstrable changes on anatomical imaging.[33] FDG-PET is also useful for the detection of tumor recurrence and has been found to be more sensitive than MR, especially when MR findings are equivocal.[34] SUV on FDG-PET is an important prognostic factor in most musculoskeletal tumors and has been shown to be a reliable independent prognostic indicator.[35,36]

Benign Tumors

Bone scan is a highly sensitive investigation for diagnosis of osteoid osteoma. A negative bone scan virtually rules out the diagnosis of osteoid osteoma. A three-phase bone scan shows increased blood flow and blood pool and a 'focal' area of intense uptake in delayed images.[37] Some surgeons have used intraoperative scintigraphic probes to localize osteoid osteoma. It addition bone scintigraphy has been used for detecting recurrence after radiofrequency ablation of osteoid osteoma. Other benign lesions, which can show increased uptake, are eosinophilic granuloma, aneurysmal bone cyst, chondroblastoma, enchondroma, etc. However, there is no specific pattern to make their diagnosis on BS alone. With the availability of hybrid SPECT-CT such diagnosis can be made with greater certainty employing the characteristic CT features of many such tumors.

INFECTION IMAGING

Acute and Chronic Osteomyelitis

Bone scintigraphy is used as a complementary imaging procedure in evaluation of infection. The classic findings are increased regional blood flow and blood pool with a corresponding increased uptake on delayed images. This is different from cellulitis where only increase in blood flow and blood pool in the soft tissue with no increased radiotracer uptake on delayed image is seen. ^{99m}Tc MDP has a high sensitivity (82–95%) and accuracy (90%) for detecting acute, uncomplicated osteomyelitis, becoming positive within 28–48 hours after the onset of symptoms. Compared with anatomic modalities, the radionuclide bone scan has the further advantage of detecting multiple foci of disease which can be seen especially in children. However, other conditions (e.g. fractures, neuropathic joints, arthritis) may mimic osteomyelitis on bone scanning alone, decreasing its specificity.[38] Although adding a fourth phase (24 hours image) is advocated to increase the specificity, with a high accuracy of 85%, the clinical results are not impressive.[39] In addition in pediatric population, BS can show reduced radiotracer uptake, which is attributed to increased pressure on blood vessels, stripping away of periosteum via the accumulation of pus and interruption of blood supply due to plugging and thrombosis. This can lead to a false negative study. About 30% of patients with acute osteomyelitis will progress to have subacute or chronic osteomyelitis **(Figs. 5A to E)**. Bone scan remains positive for months even after successful treatment of acute osteomyelitis. It is difficult to differentiate healing from chronic active disease.[40]

Other radiotracer, such as ^{67}Ga-Citrate and ^{111}In-oxine/^{99m}Tc-hexamethyl-propylene amine oxime (HMPAO) labeled leukocyte imaging has been extensively used in musculoskeletal infection, either alone or in combination with BS. ^{67}Ga-Citrate localize to the site of infection via several pathway including increased vascular permeability at site of infection, binding to lactoferrin and direct bacterial uptake.[41] Reported sensitivity for ^{67}Ga-Citrate scintigraphy ranges from 25–80%, with a specificity of 67%.[42] It has proven to be extremely useful in detecting infection in the immunocompromised population. It is usually done in combination with BS for musculoskeletal infection. However, ^{67}Ga-Citrate scintigraphy suffers from poor image quality, long scanning time and significantly higher patient radiation dose leading to decline in its use with advent of better tracers. Labeled leukocytes can overcome some of the disadvantages of BS. Its uptake is dependent on the chemotaxis of labeled leukocytes at the site of infection. ^{111}In-oxine/^{99m}Tc HMPAO labeled leukocyte imaging have shown increased specificity—up to 80–90%—compared to BS for detecting infection, particularly when complicating conditions are present. As the majority of leukocytes labeled are neutrophils, the procedure is most useful for identifying neutrophil mediated inflammatory processes, such as bacterial infections. It is less useful for those illnesses in which the predominant cellular response is other than neutrophilic, such as tuberculosis.[43] Additionally, in contrast to other locations in the skeleton, labeled leukocyte imaging is of limited value for detecting spinal osteomyelitis.[44] Also their performance requires the withdrawal of a large amount of blood (50 cc); it is also costly, labor intensive and has the inherent limitations related to personnel safety, including the risks of infection and cross contamination from handling blood products. All these factors limit their routine use. Additional use of SPECT-CT with BS, ^{67}Ga-Citrate and ^{111}In-oxine/^{99m}Tc HMPAO labeled leukocyte improves the specificity of these studies for detecting osteomyelitis.[45]

Diabetic Foot

Pedal ulcers with or without osteomyelitis is a very common complication in patients with long-standing diabetes. Foot osteomyelitis frequently presents without systemic illness and with no obvious clinical symptoms or signs, besides the ulcer and imaging studies are often needed to confirm the diagnosis. Although routinely performed, the accuracy of three phase BS for pedal osteomyelitis is modest with large prospective study demonstrating a sensitivity of 67% and specificity of 43%.[46] With the presence of associated Charcot arthropathy the diagnosis becomes more difficult. Addition of SPECT-CT in this scenario appears promising.[47] It can show focal bone destruction versus arthropathic changes, thereby clinching the diagnosis. Labeled leukocyte imaging may be more sensitive for detecting clinically unsuspected

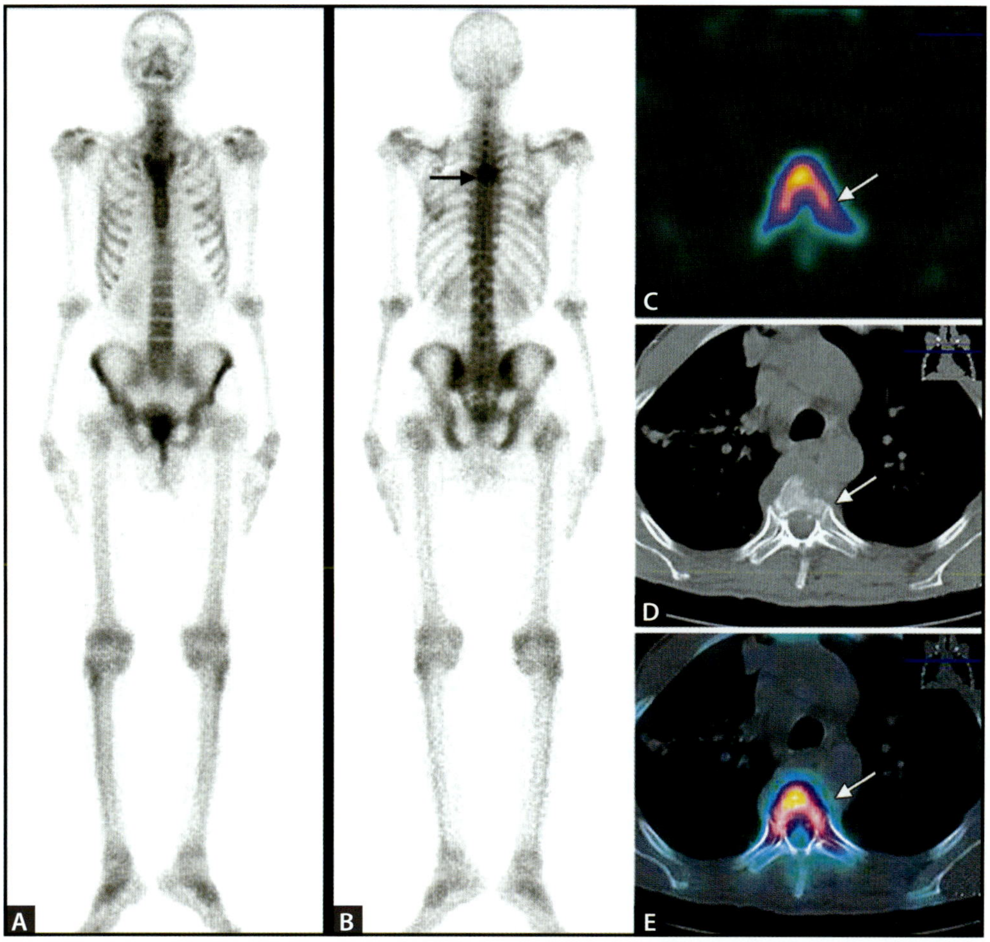

Figs. 5A to E: A 35-year-old male with backache. Planar bone scintigraphy (A and B) showed increased irregular tracer uptake in D6 vertebra (arrow). SPECT (C), CT (D) and SPECT-CT (E) images showed destructive changes in D6 vertebra with increased tracer uptake along with paravertebral fluid collection (arrow). The findings were highly suspicious for tuberculosis and confirmed at histopathology.

pedal osteomyelitis and is useful for monitoring response to medical therapy.[48] But a major drawback is the fact that even neuropathic joints may accumulate labeled leukocyte, hence not useful when both infection and Charcot joint coexists.[49]

Prosthetic Infection

With improving surgical techniques and availability of better prosthetics, the number of patients opting for the same is increasing. Although the clinical results of joint replacement surgery are usually excellent, these implants do fail. Aspetic loosening due to mechanical factors and inflammatory reaction to prosthetic components is the most common cause for implant failure followed by infection. Infection is perhaps the most serious complication of joint arthroplasty surgery, ranging in frequency from ~1 to 2% for primary implants to ~3 to 5% for revision implants.[50] Because their treatments are so different, the importance of distinguishing infection from aseptic loosening of a prosthesis cannot be overemphasized. Although BS is sensitive for detecting complications of prosthetic surgery, it cannot reliably distinguish among the causes for failure. Although routinely advocated, periprosthetic uptake patterns have not been found to be useful for differentiating infection from aseptic loosening.[51] Addition of ^{67}Ga-Citrate scintigraphy to BS only provides moderate improvement in accuracy.[52] Labeled leukocyte scintigraphy though theoretically presents the advantage of differentiating aseptic loosening from infection, the actual results has been variable.[53,54] Poor sensitivity is ascribed to the chronicity of the process, whereas poor specificity is ascribed to nonspecific inflammation. Addition of BS or marrow scintigraphy might improve the specificity of this test, though there is no general consensus.[55]

FDG PET-CT for Musculoskeletal Infection

Experimental studies have shown that mononuclear cells and neutrophilic granulocytes have increased FDG uptake when activated during the so-called respiratory burst, which they experience while fighting an infection.[56] This forms the basis for its use in musculoskeletal infections. It provides better resolution and shorter test duration compared to conventional radionuclide procedures, albeit with higher cost and radiation exposure. It should also be remembered that FDG is not specific for infection and increased FDG uptake also is observed in inflammatory arthritis, osteoarthritis, fractures, normally healing bone and degenerative changes.[57] For acute and subacute bone and soft tissue infections, sensitivities of 98% and specificities from 75 to 99% have been reported with FDG-PET.[58] It is especially useful in cases of chronic infections where BS has major limitations. It has been shown to be superior to labeled leukocyte imaging for chronic musculoskeletal infections.[59] Its specificity is higher, if recently (<4 months) traumatized or operated bone is excluded. Though initial results were excellent, FDG PET-CT appears to be less useful for diabetic foot infection.[60] It is inferior to labeled leukocyte imaging for this purpose. Moreover, altered glucose and insulin dynamic in these patients makes FDG technically challenging. Regarding FDG-PET in patients with the suspicion for total joint replacement infection initial studies showed promising results and reported sensitivities of 90% and specificities of 89% in the diagnosis of infected lower-limb prostheses.[61] Accuracy of FDG-PET was 96% for hip prostheses, 81% for knee prostheses and 100% for other orthopedic devices. However, when associated with loosening FDG-PET cannot differentiate between septic and aseptic loosening, as both conditions can cause increased FDG uptake.[62] The reason for the increased FDG uptake around the prosthesis in aseptic loosening is likely an inflammatory immune reaction to the prosthetic material. In a large series, the accuracy of FDG-PET for diagnosing infection of the failed prosthetic joint was low and varied between 47 and 71% depending on different criteria used to evaluate the images.[63] In fact, it was inferior to combined labeled leukocyte/marrow imaging in this series. It should be remembered that image interpretation in patients with prosthetic devices can be affected by attenuation-correction-induced artifacts. Therefore, it is necessary to examine the nonattenuated-corrected scans in these patients because they show less prominent reconstruction artifacts.[64]

MUSCULOSKELETAL TRAUMA

Stress Fractures

Stress fractures are two types: (i) fatigue fractures which are caused by repeated abnormal stress on normal bones, bone scan shows fusiform increased radiotracer uptake involving the posterior tibial cortex and (ii) insufficiency fractures resulting from normal stress on abnormal bone. The later are seen in patients with underlying bone disease such as osteoporosis, osteomalacia, Paget's disease, fibrous dysplasia, etc. Because clinical assessment usually is not definitive in these injuries, diagnostic imaging is often required. Plain-film radiography is usually the first examination performed when a stress fracture is suspected. Unfortunately, sensitivity of this method for stress fracture may be as low as 15%.[65] Bone scintigraphy, however, is extremely sensitive in detecting stress fractures because it assesses bone metabolism rather than bone anatomy. In fact for stress fracture at certain sites such as metatarsal bones, it is considered to be the reference method. Sacral insufficiency fractures have a classic appearance on BS , highly specific pattern of horizontal uptake in the body of the sacrum and vertical uptake in the alae, resulting in the "Honda," or "H," sign.[66] Addition of SPECT-CT is likely to improve the accuracy of BS, especially by improving the anatomical localization.

Shin Splints

The clinical entity shin splint is characterized by exercise induced pain and tenderness on palpation along the posteromedial border of tibia. It results generally from unaccustomed biomechanical stress on the tibiae. Shin splints are not fractures and can be distinguished from stress fractures by their linear activity rather than round or fusiform activity.[67] In addition, blood flow and blood pool images are almost always normal. Delayed images of bone scintigraphy demonstrate involvement of the posterior tibial cortex, longitudinally oriented uptake involving one-third of the length of the bone.

Fractures in Childhood

Very young children may present with failure to move a limb or joint. A history may not be available, especially in preschool children. Bone scans can identify unsuspected sites of fractures in such children. In addition, it can be useful to identify child abuse in children at risk. Radiological skeletal survey and wholebody scintigraphy does offer complementary information that is not available from either study alone.[68] More than 50% of such cases demonstrate diaphyseal injuries.[69] Rarely, fracture of the first rib may be the sole manifestation of abuse. Of course, knowledge of normal BS appearance for the age of child is essential for interpreting such a study.

Sport Injuries

The blood pool phase of bone scintigraphy is very important in detection of soft tissue injuries. Hyperemia is evident in the affected structure with delayed uptake apparent only if there is necrosis/calcification or close apposition of adjacent bony structures, as with tendonitis of the extensor and abductor pollicis tendons and the adjacent radius or tibialis posterior tendonitis and the medial malleolus. SPECT-CT adds by anatomically localizing the site of involvement. It can in addition guide the site of injection, when required.

METABOLIC BONE DISEASE IMAGING

Metabolic bone disorders represent a heterogeneous group of skeletal pathologies that can lead to global or focal changes in bone metabolism. The superior sensitivity of bone scintigraphy can be valuable for diagnosis, detection of complications and monitoring of treatment response **(Figs. 6A and B)**. The continuous improvement in gamma camera hardware and software with the addition of SPECT and more recently, hybrid SPECT-CT, has maintained a role for nuclear medicine methods in bone disease despite the improvements seen in morphologic imaging techniques.

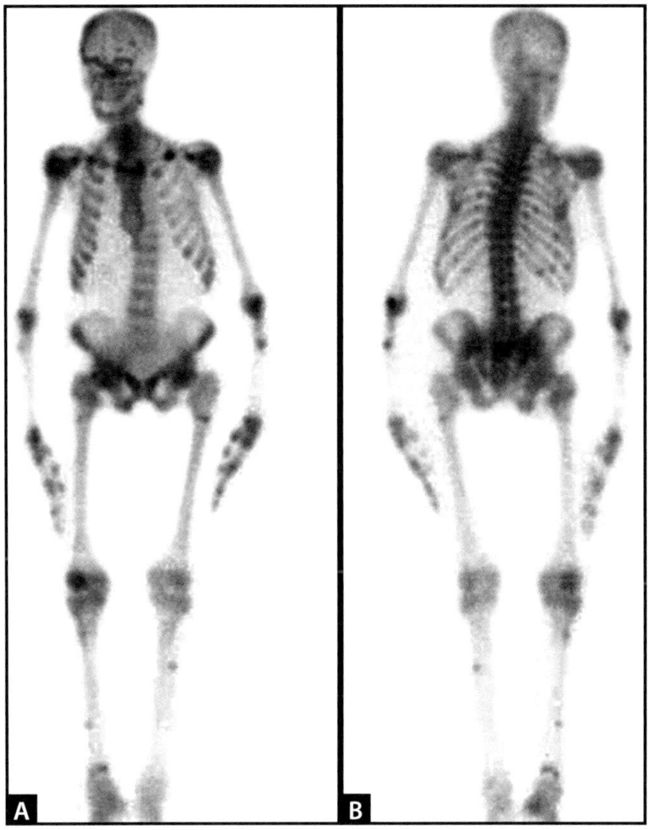

Figs. 6A and B: A 29-year-old female presented with multifocal body ache. Biochemical evaluation showed decreased serum calcium. Planar bone scintigraphy (A and B) images showed classical features of metabolic bone disease-increased bone to soft tissue activity, hot calvarium, tie sternum, nonvisualization of kidneys and multiple pseudofractures.

Paget's Disease

The initial step in Paget's disease is increased osteoclastic resorption, followed by compensatory osteoblastic activity and increased bone formation. Most patients with Paget's disease have polyostotic disease. Bone scans is a convenient way to evaluate the whole skeleton and has shown a greater sensitivity for detecting affected sites in symptomatic patients in comparison with radiographic skeletal surveys.[70] Characteristically, affected bones show intensely increased activity, extending from the end of a bone and spreading either proximally or distally, often showing a "V"-shaped leading edge. Many different patterns describing vertebral uptake have been reported as being specific for Pagetic involvement, including clover, heart and Mickey Mouse signs.[71] Apart from localizing the sites of multifocal involvement, another important use of BS is monitoring response to therapy (bisphosphonate). For this purpose, BS is better than measurement of serum alkaline phosphatase alone. The bone scan appearances can be unusual after successful bisphosphonate treatment, resultant heterogeneous uptake sometimes mimicking metastatic disease. As ^{18}F-Fluoride PET is better suited to assess bone mineral kinetics, it has also been used to monitor response to bisphosphonate therapy.[72]

Hyperparathyroidism

The diagnosis of hyperparathyroidism is biochemical and BS has no routine role in diagnosis. Bone scans are often used to help differentiate the causes of hypercalcemia, in particular, hyperparathyroidism vs malignancy, so that typical features of metabolic bone disorders may be recognized. The most common bone scan appearance is similar to a superscan from other metabolic bone disorders and uptake of diphosphonate in areas of ectopic calcification also may be seen. Multiple small focal areas of abnormal radiotracer uptake in bone scan are suggestive of pseudofractures in such patients.[73]

Renal Osteodystrophy

Renal osteodystrophy is due to a combination of bone disorders as a consequence of chronic renal dysfunction and often demonstrates the most severe cases of metabolic bone disease. It may comprise osteoporosis, osteomalacia, adynamic bone and secondary hyperparathyroidism in varying degrees. The most common bone scan appearance is similar to a superscan from other metabolic bone disorders. A clue in differentiating this type of scintigraphic pattern from others is that there may be a lack of bladder activity in view of renal failure. Quantitative measurements of bone metabolism in renal osteodystrophy using ^{18}F-Fluoride have been compared with bone histomorphometry and have shown a close relationship.[74]

Osteoporosis and Osteomalacia

Bone scans has no routine clinical role in the diagnosis of osteoporosis *per se* but is most often used in established osteoporosis to diagnose fractures, particularly at sites that are difficult to image with plain film radiography (e.g. sacrum, ribs) and may be particularly useful in the diagnosis of vertebral fractures. The characteristic appearance of this type of fracture is of intense, linearly increased tracer uptake at the affected vertebral level. In addition bone scan is extremely helpful in assessing the age of the fracture. Also other causes of bone pain can be reliably excluded in osteoporotic patients on BS. Osteomalacia on the other hand shows features similar to other metabolic bone disease. This is probably because of increased osteoid formation. The detection of pseudofractures with this technique is more sensitive than that with radiography.[75]

Bone Dysplasias

Fibrous dysplasia is characterized by a slow, progressive, replacement of the medullary cavity by fibrocollagenous tissue. There is usually intense hyperemia and intense uptake with well-delineated margins on BS. Failure of preservation of the bony outline differentiates fibrous dysplasia from Paget's disease. Identification of polyostotic involvement, which is often asymptomatic, is the main indication for BS.[76] In addition secondary complications in fibrous dysplasia can be demonstrated on BS. In several other uncommon congenital dysplasias, skeletal abnormalities are usually obvious radiologically. Bone scintigraphy can occasionally provide images that are of interest but, more importantly, reflect current physiological activity. The BS findings are variable depending on type and site of dysplasia. Additionally, BS might be used for monitoring therapy response.

Avascular Necrosis

Avascular necrosis (AVN) is a common condition affecting up to 30% of individuals with underlying medical conditions requiring steroids. Although the hip is most commonly involved AVN may affect many other bones, such as lunate (Kienbock's disease), navicular (Kohler's disease) scaphoid (post fracture) and jaw (post bisphosphonate therapy). Although MRI is the investigation of choice, a three phase BS provides useful information to diagnose AVN. A unique advantage of BS is its ability to identify AVN earlier than MRI (72 hours vs 6 day).[77] Up to 85% BS may be normal for first 48 hours, the femoral head then shows decreased activity ("cold") for a variable period followed by increased activity due to reparative process. BS is highly sensitive (98%) and specific (95%) for the diagnosis of AVN.[78] SPECT images improve sensitivity to detect AVN. SPECT-CT images are very useful especially when evaluating small bones.

Complex Regional Pain Syndrome (Reflex Sympathetic Dystrophy)

The complex regional pain syndrome (CRPS) comprises a spectrum of sensory, autonomic and motor features that predominantly affects the extremities. CPRS I occurs in absence of definable neurological abnormality. Radiological changes of bone resorption are late findings and hence three phase BS has been widely utilized in both the diagnosis and monitoring of treatment. The BS pattern of RSD varies significantly, depending upon the stage of the disease. In early stages, there is increased blood flow and blood pool with increased bone uptake on delayed images **(Figs. 7A to E)**. A characteristic feature is periarticular uptake of radiotracer. In later stages of RSD, bone scan shows normal or even decreased blood flow and blood pool but increased uptake on delayed images on the affected side.[79] In addition patients with BS abnormalities have higher response rate (90%) to systemic steroid therapy as compared to those without BS findings (36%).[80]

JOINT IMAGING

The role of bone scintigraphy is usually complementary to anatomical imaging for joint disease. The major role of bone scintigraphy is in the early detection of subclinical synovitis and monitoring its response to treatment.

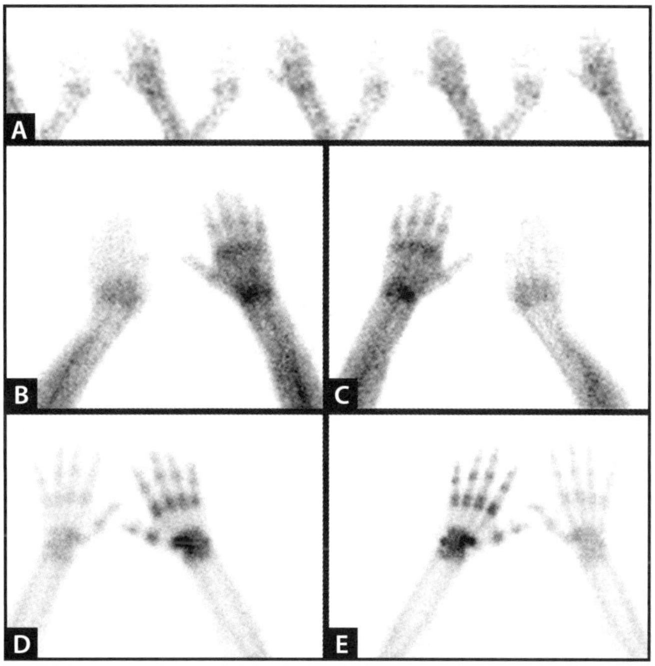

Figs. 7A to E: A 42-year-old male presented with swelling and pain in left hand 3 months after a minor surgery. Three phase bone scintigraphy showed increased blood flow (A) and pool (B and C) in left hand along with classical periarticular uptake in small joints (D and E) in delayed images, suggestive of complex regional pain syndrome (Reflex sympathetic dystrophy).

Scintigraphy is sensitive for the early detection of sacroiliitis, although MRI is used routinely. Three phase bone scans is as sensitive as MRI for identifying early rheumatoid arthritis. Bone scans is very sensitive for the diagnosis of septic arthritis and becomes abnormal much earlier than radiographs. Multiphase BS shows increased flow and blood pool in soft tissue and joint and diffuse increased uptake in bones around joints on delayed images. This is especially useful in pediatric population.

FUTURE DIRECTION

Further improvement in imaging technology and development of newer radiopharmaceuticals will keep on strengthening and redefining the role of nuclear medicine imaging. Routine use of SPECT-CT and PET-CT on one had will improve the accuracy and on the other hand will broaden the range of indications with respect to musculoskeletal imaging. Another exciting development is hybrid PET-MRI, which when clinically available might revolutionize musculoskeletal imaging providing high quality images (anatomical and functional) with less radiation burden. PET tracers such as ^{18}F-Fluoroestradiol, ^{18}F-Fluorothymidine, ^{18}F-Fluorocholine, etc. will improve the utilization of PET-CT for diagnosis, response monitoring and prognostication of musculoskeletal tumors. In addition, FDG as well as FDG labeled leukocyte PET-CT might gain more and more ground for infection imaging.

CONCLUSION

Despite challenges from morphological imaging, nuclear medicine imaging techniques continue to have a major role in a range of neoplastic, infective, inflammatory, metabolic and traumatic musculoskeletal diseases. In future, with widespread availability of hybrid modalities, its role in musculoskeletal imaging will continue to expand.

REFERENCES

1. Fogelman I. Skeletal uptake of diphosphonates: A review. Eur J Nucl Med. 1980;5:473-6.
2. Even-Sapir E. Imaging of malignant bone involvement by morphologic, scintigraphic and hybrid modalities. J Nucl Med. 2005;46:1356-67.
3. Kubota R, Yamada S, Kubota K, et al. Intratumoral distribution of uorine-18-uorodeoxyglucose in vivo: high accumulation in macrophages and granulation tissues studied by microautoradiography. J Nucl Med. 1992;33:1972-80.
4. Blake GM, Park-Holohan SJ, Cook GJ, et al. Quantitative studies of bone with the use of ^{18}Fluoride and ^{99m}Tc-methylene diphosphonate. Semin Nucl Med. 2001;31:28-49.
5. Schirrmeister H, Guhlmann A, Elsner K, et al. Sensitivity in detecting osseous lesions depends on anatomic localization: Planar bone scintigraphy versus ^{18}F PET. J Nucl Med. 1999;40:1623-9.
6. Schirrmeister H. Detection of bone metastases in breast cancer by positron emission tomography. Radiol Clin North Am. 2007;45:669-76.
7. Van der Wall H, Clarke S. The evaluation of malignancy: metastatic bone disease. In: Ell PJ, Gambhir SS (Eds). Nuclear Medicine in Clinical Diagnosis and Treatment. Edinburgh: Churchill Livingstone; 2004. pp. 641-55.
8. Krasnow AZ, Hellman RS, Timins ME, Collier BD, Anderson T, Isitman AT. Diagnostic bone scanning in oncology. Semin Nucl Med. 1997;27:107-41.
9. Tryciecky EW, Gottschalk A, Ludema K. Oncologic imaging: Interactions of nuclear medicine with CT and MRI using the one scan as the model. Semin Nucl Med. 1997;27:142-51.
10. Gates GF. SPECT bone scanning of the spine. Semin Nucl Med. 1998;28:78-94.
11. Savelli G, Mafoli L, Maccauro M, et al. Bone scintigraphy and the added value of SPECT (single photon emission tomography) in detecting skeletal lesions. Q J Nucl Med. 2001;45:27-37.
12. Kosuda S, Kaji T, Yokohama H, et al. Does bone SPECT actually have lower sensitivity for detecting vertebral metastasis than MRI? J Nucl Med. 1996;37:975-8.

13. Even-Sapir E, Flusser G, Lerman H, et al. SPECT/multislice low-dose CT: A clinically relevant constituent in the imaging algorithm of nononcologic patients referred for bone scintigraphy. J Nucl Med. 2007;48:319-24.
14. Sharma P, Singh H, Kumar R, et al. Bone scintigraphy in breast cancer: added value of hybrid SPECT-CT and its impact on patient management. Nucl Med Commun. 2012;33(2):139-47.
15. Sharma P, Kumar R, Singh H, et al. Indeterminate lesions on planar bone scintigraphy in lung cancer patients: SPECT, CT or SPECT-CT? Skeletal Radiol. 2011 Oct 16. [Epub ahead of print]
16. Petren-Mallmin M, Andreasson I, Ljunggren O, et al. Skeletal metastases from breast cancer: uptake of ^{18}F-fluoride measured with positron emission tomography in correlation with CT. Skeletal Radiol. 1998;27:72-6.
17. Even-Sapir E, Metser U, Mishani E, Lievshitz G, Lerman H, Leibovitch I. The detection of bone metastases in patients with high-risk prostate cancer: ^{99m}Tc-MDP planar bone scintigraphy, single- and multi-field-of-view SPECT, ^{18}F-Fluoride PET, and ^{18}F-Fluoride PET/CT. J Nucl Med. 2006;47:287-97.
18. Schirrmeister H, Guhlmann A, Kotzerke J, et al. Early detection and accurate description of extent of metastatic bone disease in breast cancer with fluoride ion and positron emission tomography. J Clin Oncol. 1999;17:2381-9.
19. Langsteger W, Heinisch M, Fogelman I. The role of uorodeoxyglucose, ^{18}F dihydroxyphenylalanine, ^{18}F-choline, and ^{18}F-Fluoride in bone imaging with emphasis on prostate and breast. Semin Nucl Med. 2006;36:73-92.
20. Schirrmeister H, Glatting G, Hetzel J, et al. Prospective evaluation of clinical value of planar bone scan, SPECT and ^{18}F-labeled NaF PET in newly diagnosed lung cancer. J Nucl Med. 2001;42:1800-4.
21. Hetzel M, Arslandemir C, Konig HH, et al. ^{18}F NaF PET for detection of bone metastases in lung cancer: Accuracy, cost-effectiveness, and impact on patient management. J Bone Miner Res. 2003;18:2206-14.
22. Cook GJ, Houston S, Rubens R, et al. Detection of bone metastases in breast cancer by ^{18}FDG PET: Differing metabolic activity in osteoblastic and osteolytic lesions. J Clin Oncol. 1998;16:3375-9.
23. Yilmaz M, Elboga U, Celen Z, et al. Multiple muscle metastases from lung cancer detected by FDG PET/CT. Clin Nucl Med. 2011;36(3):245-7.
24. Yang SN, Liang JA, Lin FJ, et al. Comparing wholebody (18)F-2-deoxyglucose positron emission tomography and technetium-99m methylene diphosphonate bone scan to detect bone metastases in patients with breast cancer. J Cancer Res Clin Oncol. 2002;128:325-8.
25. Even-Sapir E. Imaging of malignant bone involvement by morphologic, scintigraphic, and hybrid modalities. J Nucl Med. 2005;46:1356-67.
26. Cheran SK, Herndon JE, Patz EF. Comparison of wholebody FDG-PET to bone scan for detection of bone metastases in patients with a new diagnosis of lung cancer. Lung Cancer. 2004;44:317-25.
27. Antoch G, Vogt FM, Freudenberg LS, et al. Wholebody dual modality PET/CT and whole-body MRI for tumor staging in oncology. JAMA. 2003;290:3199-206.
28. Kushner BH. Neuroblastoma: a disease requiring a multitude of imaging studies. J Nucl Med. 2004;45:1172-88.
29. Stafford SE, Gralow JR, Schubert EK, et al. Use of serial FDG PET to measure the response of bone-dominant breast cancer to therapy. Acad Radiol. 2002;9:913-21.
30. Mortimer JE, Dehdashti F, Siegel BA, et al. Metabolic flare: indicator of hormone responsiveness in advanced breast cancer. J Clin Oncol. 2001;19:2797-803.
31. Aoki J, Watanabe H, Shinozaki T, et al. FDG-PET for pre-operative differential diagnosis between benign and malignant soft tissue masses. Skeletal Radiol. 2003;32:133-8.
32. Chen YM, Huang G, Sun XG, et al. Optimizing delayed scan time for FDG PET: comparison of the early and late delayed scan. Nucl Med Commun. 2008;29:425-30.
33. Evilevitch V, Weber WA, Tap WD, et al. Reduction of glucose metabolic activity is more accurate than change in size at predicting histopathologic response to neoadjuvant therapy in high-grade soft-tissue sarcomas. Clin Cancer Res. 2008;14:715-20.
34. Dimitrakopoulou-Strauss A, Strauss LG, Schwarzbach MH, et al. Dynamic PET ^{18}F-FDG studies in patients with primary and recurrent softtissue sarcomas: impact on diagnosis and correlation with grading. J Nucl Med. 2001;42:713-20.
35. Adler LP, Blair HF, Makley JT, et al. Noninvasive grading of musculoskeletal tumors using PET. J Nucl Med. 1991;32: 1508-12.
36. Ioannidis JP, Lau J. ^{18}F-FDG PET for the diagnosis and grading of soft tissue sarcoma: a meta-analysis. J Nucl Med. 2003;44:717-24.
37. Sartoris DJ. Skeletal system: The Requisites. St Louis: Mosby; 2001. pp. 110-44.
38. Palestro CJ, Torres MA. Radionuclide imaging in orthopedic infections. Semin Nucl Med. 1997;27:334-45.
39. Israel O, Gips S, Jerushalmi J, et al. Osteomyelitis and soft-tissue infection: differential diagnosis with 24 hour/4 hour ratio of ^{99m}Tc MDP uptake. Radiology. 1987;163:725-6.
40. Anderson SE, Heini P, Sauvain MJ, et al. Imaging of chronic recurrent multifocal osteomyelitis of childhood first presenting with isolated primary spinal involvement. Skeletal Radiol. 2003;32:328-36.
41. Palestro CJ. The current role of gallium imaging in infection. Semin Nucl Med. 1994;24:128-41.
42. Pineda C, Vargas A, Rodriguez AV. Imaging of osteomyelitis: current concepts. Infect Dis Clin N Am. 2006;20:789-825.
43. Fineman DS, Palestro CJ, Kim CK, et al. Detection of abnormalities in febrile AIDS patients with ^{111}In-labeled leukocyte and GA-67 scintigraphy. Radiology. 1989;170:677-80.
44. Whalen JL, Brown ML, McLeod R, Fitzgerald RH Jr. Limitations of indium leukocyte imaging for the diagnosis of spine infections. Spine. 1991;16:193-7.
45. Linke R, Kuwert T, Uder M, Forst R, Wuest W. Skeletal SPECT/CT of the peripheral extremities. Am J Roentgenol. 2010;194(4):W329-35.

46. Shults DW, Hunter GC, McIntyre KE, et al. Value of radiographs and bone scans in determining the need for therapy in diabetic patients with foot ulcers. Am J Surg. 1989;158:525-30.
47. Heiba SI, Kolker D, Mocherla B, Kapoor K, Jiang M, Son H, Rangaswamy B, Kostakoglu L, Savitch I, DaCosta M, Machac J. The optimized evaluation of diabetic foot infection by dual isotope SPECT/CT imaging protocol. J Foot Ankle Surg. 2010;49(6):529-36.
48. Newman LG, Waller J, Palestro CJ, et al. Leukocyte scanning with ^{111}In is superior to magnetic resonance imaging in the diagnosis of clinically unsuspected osteomyelitis in diabetic foot ulcers. Diabetes Care. 1992;15:1527-30.
49. Hayashida K, Ochi T, Fujimoto M, et al. Bone marrow changes in adjuvant-induced and collagen-induced arthritis. Interleukin-1 and interleukin-6 activity and abnormal myelopoiesis. Arthritis Rheum. 1992;35:241-5.
50. Hanssen AD, Rand JA. Evaluation and treatment of infection at the site of a total hip or knee arthroplasty. Instr Course Lect. 1999;48:111-22.
51. Aliabadi P, Tumeh SS, Weissman BN, McNeil BJ. Cemented total hip prosthesis: radiographic and scintigraphic evaluation. Radiology. 1989;173:203-6.
52. Love C, Tronco GG, Yu AK, et al. Diagnosing the infected prosthetic hip: an intraindividual comparison of three-phase bone, bone, gallium, bone/gallium, leukocyte, leukocyte/bone, and leukocyte/marrow imaging. Eur J Nucl Med Mol Imaging. 2007;34(suppl 2):(P)S384.
53. Pring DJ, Henderson RG, Rivett AG, Krausz T, Coombs RR, Lavender JP. Autologous granulocyte scanning of painful prosthetic joints. J Bone Joint Surg Br. 1986;68:647-52.
54. Wukich DK, Abreu SH, Callaghan JJ, et al. Diagnosis of infection by preoperative scintigraphy with indium labeled white blood cells. J Bone Joint Surg Am. 1987;69:1353-60.
55. Love C, Tronco GG, Yu AK, et al. Diagnosing lower extremity prosthetic joint infection: intraindividual comparison of leukocyte/marrow and leukocyte/bone imaging. J Nucl Med. 2007;48(suppl):62.
56. Mochizuki T, Tsukamoto E, Kuge Y, et al. FDG uptake and glucose transporter subtype expressions in experimental tumor and inflammation models. J Nucl Med. 2001;42:1551-5.
57. Beckers C, Jeukens X, Ribbens C, et al. ^{18}F-FDG PET imaging of rheumatoid knee synovitis correlates with dynamic magnetic resonance and sonographic assessments as well as with the serum level of metalloproteinase-3. Eur J Nucl Med Mol Imaging. 2006;33(3):275-80.
58. Stumpe KD, Dazzi H, Schaffner A, et al. Infection imaging using wholebody FDG-PET. Eur J Nucl Med. 2000;27:822-32.
59. de Winter F, van de Wiele C, Vogelaers D, de Smet K, Verdonk R, Dierckx RA. Fluorine-18 fluorodeoxyglucose positron emission tomography: a highly accurate imaging modality for the diagnosis of chronic musculoskeletal infections. J Bone Joint Surg Am. 2001;83-A:651-60.
60. Familiari D, Glaudemans AW, Vitale V, et al. Can sequential ^{18}F-FDG PET/CT replace WBC imaging in the diabetic foot? J Nucl Med. 2011;52(7):1012-9.
61. Zhuang H, Duarte PS, Pourdehnad M, et al. The promising role of ^{18}F-FDG PET in detecting infected lower limb prosthesis implants. J Nucl Med. 2001;42:44-8.
62. Reinartz P, Mumme T, Hermanns B, et al. Radionuclide imaging of the painful hip arthroplasty: positronemission tomography versus triple-phase bone scanning. J Bone Joint Surg Br. 2005;87:465-70.
63. Love C, Scott EM, Tomas MB, et al. Diagnosing infection in the failed joint replacement: a comparison of coincidence detection ^{18}F-FDG and ^{111}In-labeled leucocyte/^{99m}Tc-sulfur colloid marrow imaging. J Nucl Med. 2004;45:1864-71.
64. Goerres GW, Ziegler SI, Burger C, et al. Artifacts at PET and PET/CT caused by metallic hip prosthetic material. Radiology. 2003;226:577-84.
65. Donohoe KJ. Selected topics in orthopedic nuclear medicine. Orthop Clin North Am. 1998;29:85-101.
66. Sartoris DJ. Skeletal system: The Requisites. St Louis: Mosby; 2001.pp.110-44.
67. Barai S, Kumar R, Dhanpati H, et al. Bone scintigraphy in sports injuries. Ortho Today. 2003;5:29-32.
68. Mandelstam SA, Cook D, Fitzgerald M, et al. Complementary use of radiological skeletal survey and bone scintigraphy in detection of bony injuries in suspected child abuse. Arch Dis Child. 2003;88(5):387-90.
69. Kleinman PK. Shaken babies. Lancet. 1998;352(9130):815-6.
70. Fogelman I, Carr D. A comparison of bone scanning and radiology in the assessment of patients with symptomatic Paget's disease. Eur J Nucl Med. 1980;5:417-21.
71. Rotés-Sala D, Monfort J, Solano A, et al. The clover and heart signs in vertebral scintigraphic images are highly specific of Paget's disease of bone. Bone. 2004;34:605-8.
72. Installé J, Nzeusseu A, Bol A, et al. ^{18}F-Fluoride PET for monitoring therapeutic response in Paget's disease of bone. J Nucl Med. 2005;46:1650-8.
73. Sartoris DJ. Skeletal system: The Requisites. St Louis: Mosby; 2001. pp. 110-44.
74. Messa C, Goodman WG, Hoh CK, et al. Bone metabolic activity measured with positron emission tomography and ^{18}F-Fluoride ion in renal osteodystrophy: Correlation with bone histomorphometry. J Clin Endocrinol Metab. 1993;77:949-55.
75. Fogelman I, McKillop JH, Greig WR, et al. Pseudofractures of the ribs detected by bone scanning. J Nucl Med. 1977; 18:1236-7.
76. Fukumitsu N, Dohi M, Midda K, et al. Bone scintigraphy in polyostotic fibrous dysplasia. Clin Nucl Med. 1999;24(6):446-7.
77. Conway WF, Totty WG, McEnery KW. CT and MRI imaging of the hip. Radiology. 1996;198:297-307.
78. Collier BD, Carrera GF, Johnson RP. Detection of femoral head avascular necrosis in adult with SPECT. J Nucl Med. 1985;26:979-87.
79. Ruffin D. Natural history of reflex sympathetic dystrophy syndrome. J Nucl Med. 1984;25:423-9.
80. Kozin F, Genant HK, Bekerman C, et al. The reflex sympathetic dystrophy syndrome. II. Roentgenographic and scintigraphic evidence of bilaterality and of periarticular accentuation. Am J Med. 1976;60(3):332-8.

CHAPTER 189

Angiography and Interventions in Musculoskeletal Lesions

Deep Narayan Srivastava

INTRODUCTION

With increasing use of CT and MRI in the diagnosis of bone and soft tissue lesions, angiography is not being used as commonly as before; however, if the procedure is used properly in conjunction with other diagnostic studies, it can play a valuable role in the diagnosis and treatment of bone and soft tissue lesions. The role of angiointerventions and nonvascular musculoskeletal interventions is increasing and will be discussed.

TECHNIQUE

Diagnostic Angiography

The common femoral artery is the commonly used entry site for percutaneous approach, because of its accessibility, the ease of compression against the femoral head for hemostasis, and the low rate of complications when punctured. The left or right femoral artery is punctured by Seldinger technique and an arterial sheath is placed. Usually the contralateral femoral artery is used to approach the lesion in lower limb region. Through this arterial sheath angiographic catheter is advanced into the arteries supplying the lesion. A wide variety of preshaped 4/5 F angiographic catheters are available for selective and superselective catheterization. The catheter is placed selectively in the major vessel supplying the tumor and angiographic runs are taken with contrast medium injection. Various selective injections are taken depending upon the tumor supply.

Visualization of both the arterial and venous circulations is desirable in all cases. The radiographs/frames are obtained initially at two frames/second for three to four seconds followed by every 2 seconds for a total of 25–30 seconds. The amount of contrast injection depends on the size and location of the lesion.

Digital subtraction angiograms (DSAs) are superior to conventional angiograms since the superimposed bones, calcifications and also other limb supports in trauma patients can be subtracted resulting in better image quality because of which reliable evaluation of vascular supply of the lesion is possible.

Magnification angiograms are sometimes required for visualization of tiny vessels.

Angioembolization

The term embolization refers to the introduction of an embolic agent into a vessel through a selectively placed catheter to achieve therapeutic vascular occlusion. The advent of catheters with hydrophilic coating, microcatheters, torque control guide wires and various embolic materials has allowed precise and safe delivery of occluding agents to anywhere in the body using the blood vessels as a roadway. In certain situations, these embolizing materials are also injected into the lesion directly under image guidance without angiographic route.

The embolization is usually performed using the access used for diagnostic angiography. After the initial diagnostic angiography the angiographic catheter is advanced into the artery supplying the tumor before introduction of embolic material. The selective and superselective embolization is a safe interventional procedure for any vascular lesion. Sometimes small caliber catheters like microcatheters (2–3 F) are also used for this. It is also important to weigh the risks of the procedure against those of noninterventional and surgical therapies. The embolization should preferably be performed in angiography suite equipped with C-arm mounted image intensifier with digital subtraction angiography of high quality resolution. A portable ultrasound scanner is always useful in the assessment of nonpalpable arteries, veins and also for direct percutaneous puncture of lesion.

ANGIOGRAPHY IN BONE TUMORS

The role of angiography in bone tumors is limited because of the following reasons:

- If the definitive angiographic features of malignancy are present, it can be assumed that the lesion is malignant, but a normal arteriogram does not entirely rule out a malignancy.[1]
- It is often not possible to distinguish between various types of bone tumors from the angiographic features alone.

The angiographic features of malignancy include neovascularity, pooling or laking of contrast material, tumor stain or blush, encasement and occlusion of vessels, extension of the tumor vascularity outside the bone, displacement of vessels, arteriovenous shunts, abnormal draining veins, tumor invasion of veins, etc.

Neovascularity and pooling of contrast are important features of malignancy; however, these may also be present in some benign lesions like giant cell tumor, aneurysmal bone cyst, osteoblastoma, Paget's disease, benign nerve sheath tumor and certain hemangiomas **(Figs. 1 to 3)**. These lesions can easily be differentiated by their clinical and plain radiographic features.

The presence of a tumor blush does not indicate malignancy but may suggest the size and extent of the tumor. Angiography, however, does not always define the complete intraosseous extent of the tumor and skip metastases within the bone are not always seen.[2]

The angiographic information about the displacement or encasement of vessel is important if a radical local resection is planned in limb salvage surgeries.

Early arteriovenous shunting is not a reliable sign of malignancy, however, the identification of large abnormal draining veins is important to facilitate early ligation and prevent tumor embolization during surgery.[2]

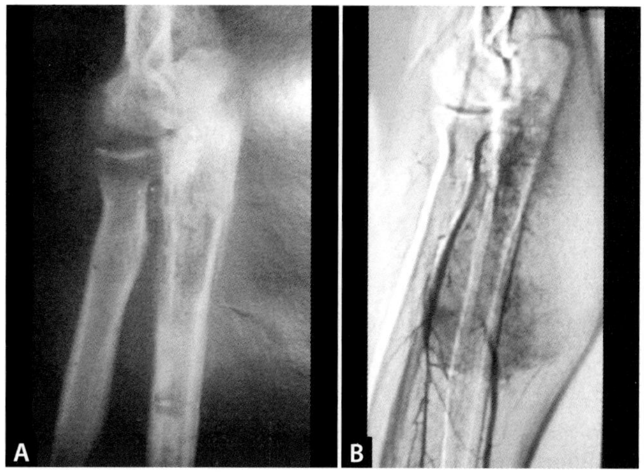

Figs. 1A and B: Ewing's tumor: (A) Lytic lesion with periosteal reaction and soft tissue mass of ulna; (B) Pooling of contrast material is seen on DSA.

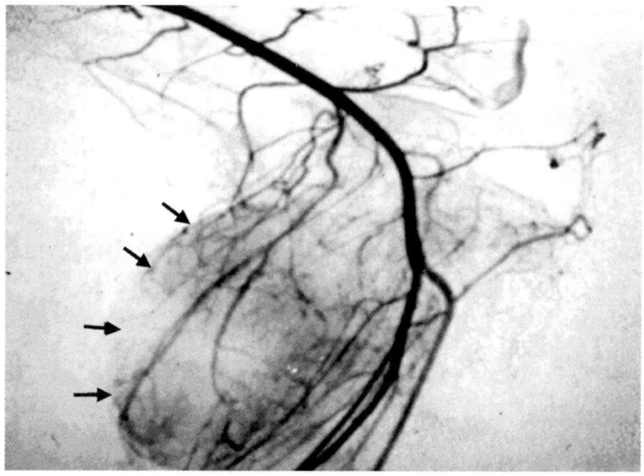

Fig. 2: Benign nerve sheath tumor: The DSA showing blush of contrast (arrows).

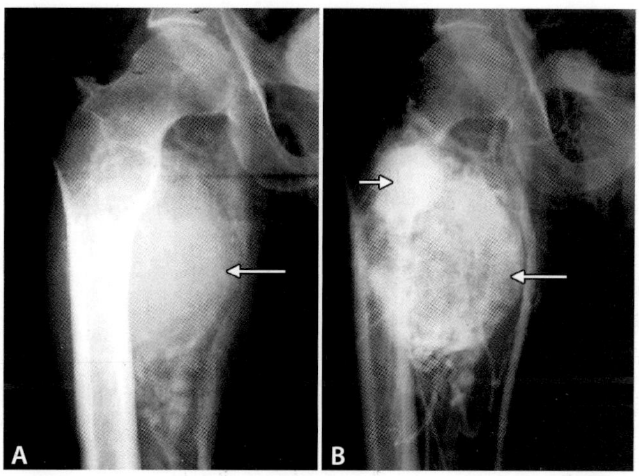

Figs. 3A and B: Angiography shows highly vascular mass with pooling of contrast in a case of hemangioma of femur (small arrow) with extraosseous component (large arrows).

Some bone tumors in which diagnostic angiography is sometimes indicated are discussed below.

Osteochondroma

These bone tumors because of their size and location may cause vascular complications in the form of thrombosis and pseudoaneurysms[3,4] as well as displacement of vessels. Angiography can show all these complications **(Figs. 4A and B)**. The tumor usually does not show hypervascularity or abnormal vessels.

Osteoid Osteoma

In the absence of classical roentgenographic findings, angiography can be helpful when the diagnosis is in doubt.[5] The angiographic feature is dense, circumscribed blush in the early arterial phase which persists in late venous phase. This feature differentiates it from osteomyelitis, Brodie's abscess and stress fractures that do not have the feature of dense vascular blush.

Osteosarcoma

Angiography can demonstrate that the tumor is malignant, and accurately define the degree of soft tissue extension, however, skip areas within the medullary canal are not always detected.[2] Magnetic resonance imaging (MRI) is useful in defining the intraosseous and extraosseous extent of the tumor and its anatomic relationship to nearby structures.

Giant Cell Tumor

Angiography can accurately define the intra as well as extraosseous extent of the tumor because the tumors are usually hypervascular and show neovascularity, intense blush and early venous filling. This is of particular importance in view of the high recurrence rate of the tumor and its ability to become malignant after treatment. The MRI is useful in the limb salvage surgeries in the assessment of extent of tumor and the anatomic relationship to nearby structures and joint.

Aneurysmal Bone Cyst

Angiography can differentiate aneurysmal bone cyst from giant cell tumor. On angiography, it is poorly vascularized tumor, devoid of arteriovenous fistulae and soft tissue invasion.[6] The clinical course and plain radiographic findings are very useful for the diagnosis of this lesion.

ANGIOGRAPHY IN BONE AND SOFT TISSUE LESIONS OF VASCULAR ORIGIN

Hemangioma

Hemangiomas can be grouped into four categories: capillary, cavernous, venous hemangiomas and arteriovenous malformations. Hemangiomas usually involve the soft tissues (most commonly skeletal muscles) but can also involve bones.[7] Arteriography can define the extent, degree of vascularity, source of vascular supply, local recurrence in follow-up case and differentiate from arteriovenous malformations.[8] Angiography may show mild to marked vascularity with coarse, irregular, enlarged arteries and pooling of contrast material **(Figs. 3 and 5)**. Arteriovenous shunting may be seen. The osseous hemangiomas may have dilated vascular spaces **(Figs. 3A and B)**. Venous hemangioma is rarely

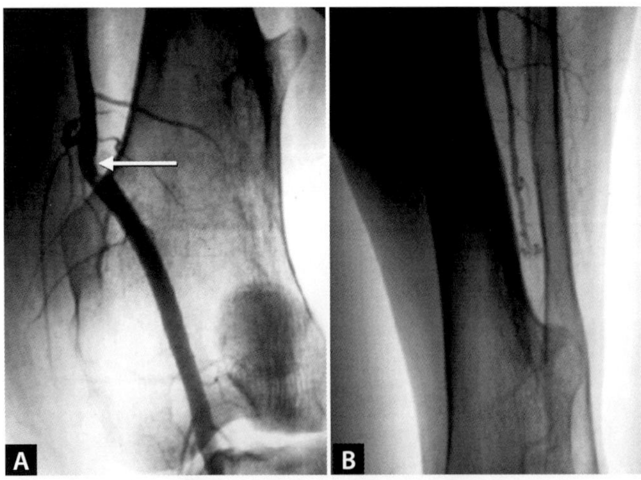

Figs. 4A and B: Multiple osteochondroma: (A) Displacement and narrowing (arrow) of femoral artery; (B) Thrombosis of leg vessels.

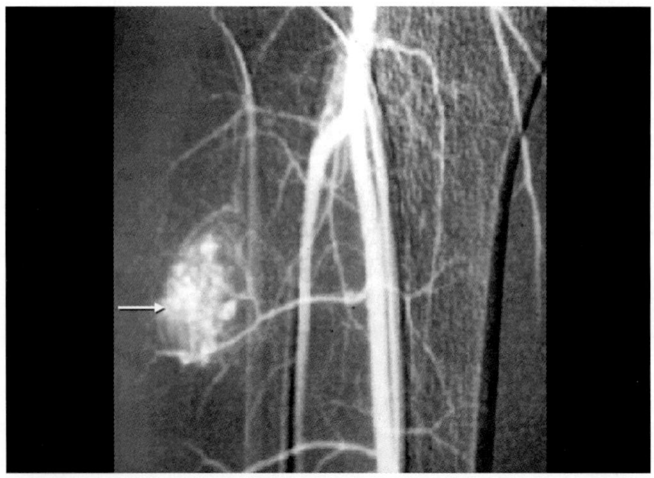

Fig. 5: Soft tissue hemangioma leg: Digital subtraction angiography shows fine vessels with some pooling of contrast (arrow). This painful lesion was successfully treated by percutaneous injection of sclerosing agent.

seen on arteriography but is usually seen on venography[9] **(Figs. 6A to D)**. Sometimes, it is difficult to ascertain the entire lesion on angiography.[9] The MRI is useful in depicting the full extent of the lesion and the relationship to surrounding structures **(Figs. 6A to D)**. Angiography sometimes cannot differentiate a benign hemangioma from a malignant vascular tumor.[8]

In cavernous hemangioma, arteriography demonstrates normal sized arteries that may show late venous staining on delayed films. They do not require treatment as they do not change with time and rarely bleed, but a common problem is local pain due to distention of the lesion or superimposed thrombosis. The embolization of regional arterial branches is not always useful, but injection of sclerosing agent by direct puncture technique has shown good results **(Fig. 5)**.

Klippel–Trenaunay syndrome (KTS) is a congenital vascular abnormality consisting of a cutaneous nevus, varicose veins and bone and soft tissue hypertrophy affecting one or more limbs. Venography is very useful in demonstrating the characteristic venous anomaly (KT vein), which is a large lateral superficial venous channel that often communicates with profunda femoris or iliac veins **(Figs. 7A to C)**. MRI with its multiplanar imaging abilities has the advantage of demonstrating the full extent of venous malformation and the status of muscle and soft tissues.[10]

Arteriovenous malformations (AVMs) tend to grow at the same rate as the individual, unlike the pattern of rapid growth and involution seen in hemangioma. The angiographic findings include enlarged, tortuous feeding arteries, a dense nidus of malformations and early opacification of draining veins. The AVMs are refractory to treatment. Mechanically disturbing a stable lesion (after surgical ligation or proximal embolization of feeding arteries) can result in significant worsening

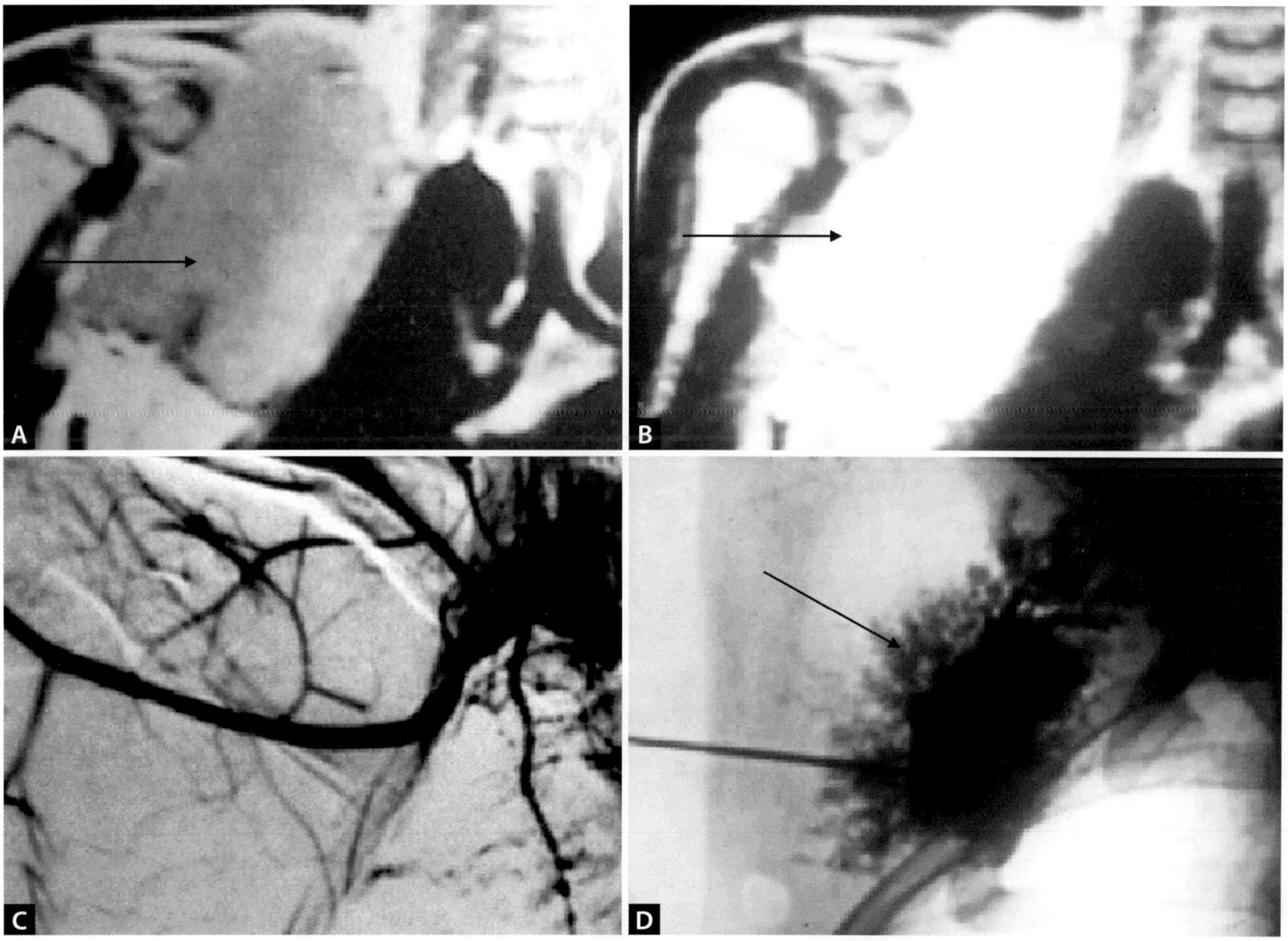

Figs. 6A to D: Venous hemangioma (arrow) of axilla with supraclavicular extension. The mass is mildly hyperintense to muscles on T1WI (A) Hyperintense on T2WI; (B) On DSA, the mass is not vascular with mass effect over axillary artery with splaying of its lateral thoracic and subscapular branches; (C) No early venous filling seen. Percutaneous aspiration and injection of contrast shows multiple dilated vascular spaces; (D) The pain disappeared and the size was reduced after injection of sclerosing agent through the same needle.

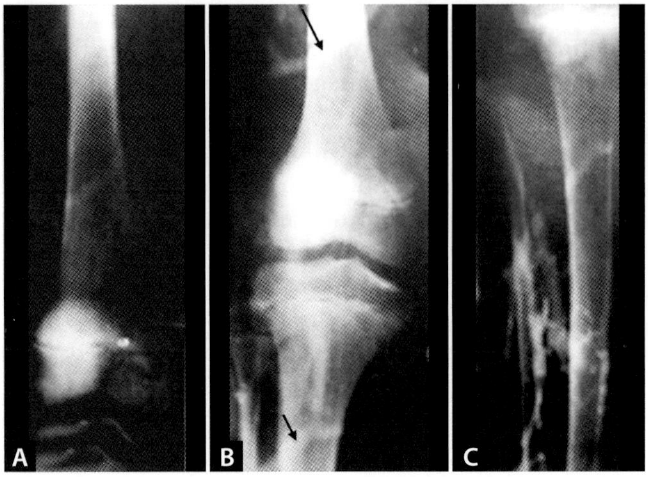

Figs. 7A to C: Ascending phlebogram showing two Klippel–Trenaunay veins, one communicating with the popliteal vein (small arrow), and the other with the superficial femoral vein (large arrow).

due to development of new collaterals. Transcatheter embolization close to nidus of the lesion has now attained a primary role in the management of AVMs, but proximal occlusion of feeding vessels by an endovascular embolic agent or surgical ligation will provide poor clinical result with recurrence **(Figs. 8A and B)**.[11,12] The angiography can tell about the size, number and location of these lesions **(Figs. 9A and B)**. In lesions of extremities, injection of sclerosing agent or alcohol by direct puncture technique is safe and useful.

Hemangiopericytoma

These are hypervascular tumors and are seen as a prolonged dense stain on angiogram.[13] There may be displacement of the major arteries **(Fig. 10)**.

Angiosarcoma

The angiographic features include highly irregular, tortuous arteries with pooling of contrast,[14] arteriovenous shunts and encasement of vessels.

ANGIOGRAPHY IN METASTATIC TUMORS IN BONE AND SOFT TISSUES

Most metastatic lesions have the same vascular characteristics that are exhibited by their primary tumors.[15] Angiography cannot distinguish between different types of metastases. It also cannot distinguish a primary osseous or soft tissue tumor from a secondary growth.

ANGIOGRAPHY IN PERIPHERAL TRAUMA

Angiography has an important role in the management of patients with suspected vascular injury both for diagnosis and treatment. Angiography is both sensitive and specific for the diagnosis of vascular injury (active bleeding, pseudoaneurysms and arteriovenous fistula) **(Figs. 11 and 12)**. Transcatheter embolization is effective, safe and can be a definitive therapy for suitable arterial injuries.

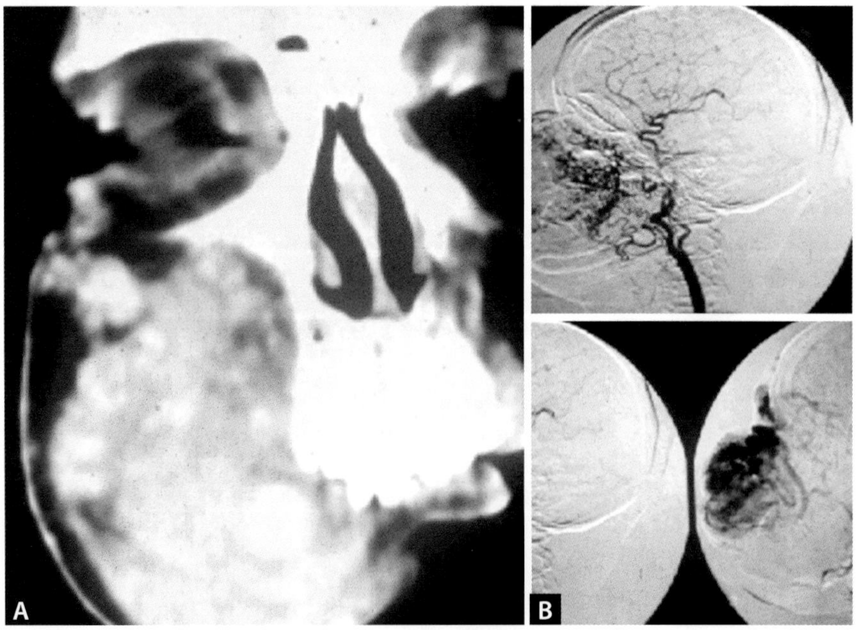

Figs. 8A and B: Arteriovenous malformations of cheek: (A) CT shows soft tissue vascular mass overlying maxilla, mandible, inferior orbital margin; (B) On DSA, the mass is supplied by branches of left external carotid artery with early venous filling.

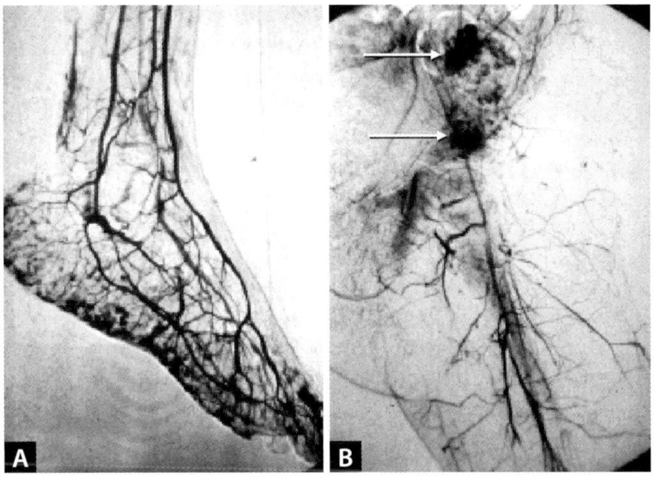

Figs. 9A and B: Multiple hemangiomas involving: (A) Left foot; (B) Gluteal muscles (arrows).

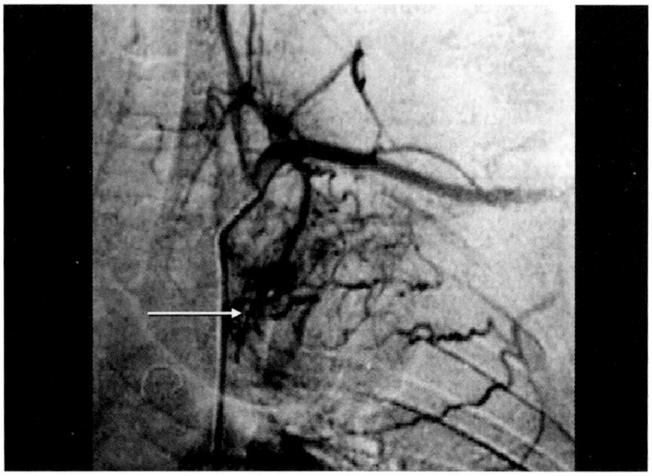

Fig. 10: Hemangiopericytoma: A well-demarcated hypervascular mass (arrow) with homogeneous blush seen on delayed images.

In arteriovenous fistula, early intervention is very useful. Early intervention in hemodynamically unstable patients with pelvic fractures is essential to reduce the morbidity of the injury.[16] In pelvic fractures, percutaneous embolization of uncontrolled pelvic hemorrhage is a lifesaving technique **(Figs. 12A and B)**. Small aneurysms can be treated by sonoguided manual compression or coil embolization **(Figs. 13 and 14)**. The intra-arterial thrombolytic therapy can also be used in arterial thrombosis **(Figs. 15A and B)**.

IMAGE-GUIDED INTERVENTIONS IN BONE AND SOFT TISSUE LESIONS

The commonly used image guided interventions are fine needle aspiration cytology and trucut biopsies, embolizations, intra-arterial chemotherapies, vertebroplasties, radiofrequency and laser ablation of benign bone lesions.

Aspiration Cytology and Biopsy

The role of aspiration cytology is limited since most lesions require biopsy. Percutaneous biopsy is less invasive, requires smaller dose of anesthetics and analgesics, causes minimal bleeding and biopsy tract contamination, and is a cost-effective method. However, it is less reliable in obtaining an adequate representative specimen for grading and further special studies. For heterogeneous tumors, very myxoid or cystic lesions and bone tumors without soft tissue component, a needle core may not give a high diagnostic yield. The hemangioma and arteriovenous malformations usually do not require histological confirmation because of characteristic imaging features. For biopsy various size trucut needles (11–18G) are used. For bone biopsy thick needles (11G) with diamond tip is preferred. Ultrasound guidance is always preferred though CT and fluoroscopy is required for vertebral and other bone lesions.

Embolization

Preprocedural Preparations

The patient must be informed about the procedure, benefits, alternative procedures and potential complications. The patient should be well hydrated and standby general anesthesia may be needed for uncooperative patients and children. Severe coagulopathy should be corrected and sometimes antibiotics are also given. The sedation is given during the procedure depending upon the type and duration of the procedure.

Indications

The indications of embolization in bone and soft tissue tumors are as follows :

- *To control hemorrhage*: If there is internal or external bleeding from the tumor, angioembolization is sometimes done as an emergency procedure.
- *To reduce peroperative bleeding*: It has been used in various soft tissue and bone tumors and hemangiomas to decrease intraoperative blood loss, which improves surgical vision and allows safer and faster surgery.[16,17] Voigt et al. reported the use of Gelfoam embolization in patients with deforming vascular malformations in the craniofacial area. The procedure allows reconstructive surgery to be carried out with decreased blood loss with good cosmetic results **(Figs. 16A and B)**.

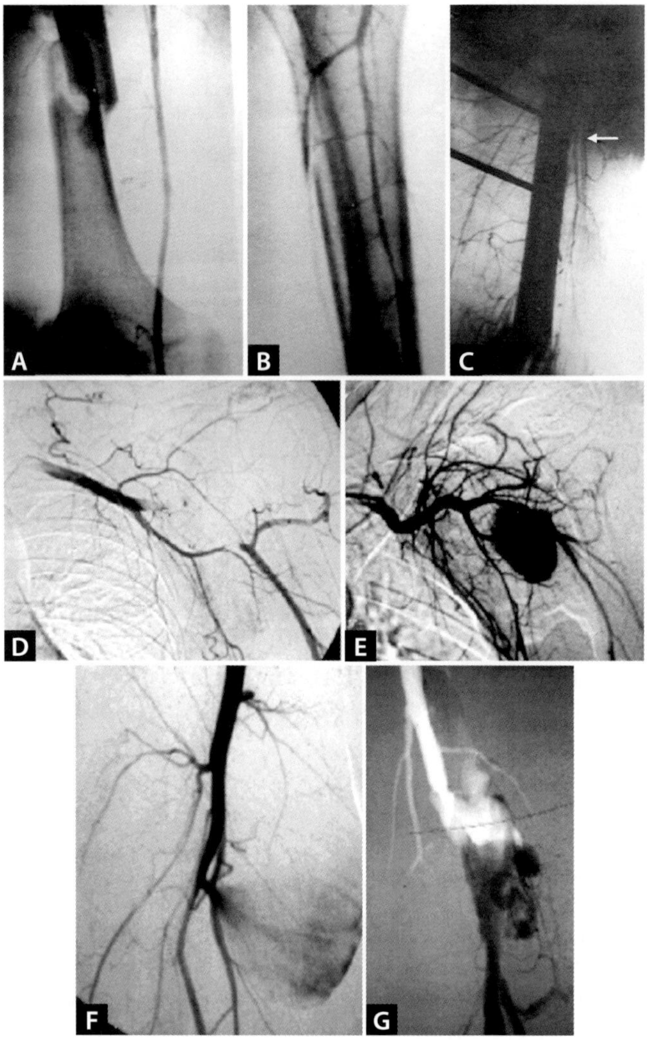

Figs. 11A to G: The DSA in different patients of trauma: (A and B) Fracture femur and fibula with patent arteries; (C) Fracture femur with thrombosed superficial femoral artery (arrow) with collaterals; (D) Soft tissue injury left shoulder with thrombosed axillary artery–brachial artery is filling from collaterals; (E) Large pseudoaneurysm from axillary artery; (F) Large pseudoaneurysm from right superficial femoral artery; (G) Arteriovenous fistula between popliteal artery and vein.

- *As palliative treatment*: In previously treated (surgery and/or embolization) cases of recurrent or residual arteriovenous malformations if intravascular access is difficult, direct puncture of the symptomatic lesion can be performed[18] by Chiba needle and alcohol or sclerosing agent can be injected directly in tumor bed (nidus) until flow is occluded. The embolization of the soft tissue tumors may result in severe, prolonged muscle pain if acute muscle ischemia takes place. Therefore, for palliation of pain in patients with inoperable tumors, embolization should be cautiously used.
- *To relieve from chronic pain due to tumors*: It has been reported that therapeutic arterial occlusion in pelvic tumors[19] and in metastatic deposits[16] gives symptomatic relief of pain. The major vessels of supply are embolized with Gelfoam followed by steel coils to occlude the vessels permanently **(Figs. 17A and B)**. Embolization with particles (transcatheter) or percutaneous instillation of sclerosing agent has been used to control pain associated with a peripheral hemangioma **(*see* Fig. 5)**.[20]
- *As a part of treatment*: In hemangiomas, angioembolization decreases the chance of recurrence **(Figs. 18A to C)**.[21] A study has shown that this not only decreases the size but also controls a persistent left-to-right shunt.[22]

Embolizing Materials

There are various types of embolizing materials available. The selection of the material depends upon the duration, extent and level of occlusion. The materials can be categorized as short, intermediate and long acting or as particulate or liquid agents depending upon the physical properties. The commonly used embolising materials have been listed in **Table 1**.

Complications

The common complications are postembolization syndrome in the form of nausea, vomiting, fever and pain due to tissue ischemia. The uncommon complications reported are inadvertent embolization, misplaced or migrated steel coils, abscess formation, spinal cord injury, aneurysm formation or vessel rupture.

Contraindications

The contraindications are patients with hemorrhagic diathesis and puncture site infection.

Intra-arterial Chemotherapy

Patients with sarcomas not amenable to cure by surgical resection alone can benefit from preoperative intra-arterial chemotherapy. Intra-arterial chemotherapy permits limb sparing resection with less morbidity **(Fig. 19)**.[23,24] In this chemotherapeutic drug is injected in tumor bed with the help of angiographic catheter placed in the artery supplying the tumor.

Percutaneous Vertebroplasty

Percutaneous vertebroplasty is a well-accepted interventional procedure for the treatment of painful

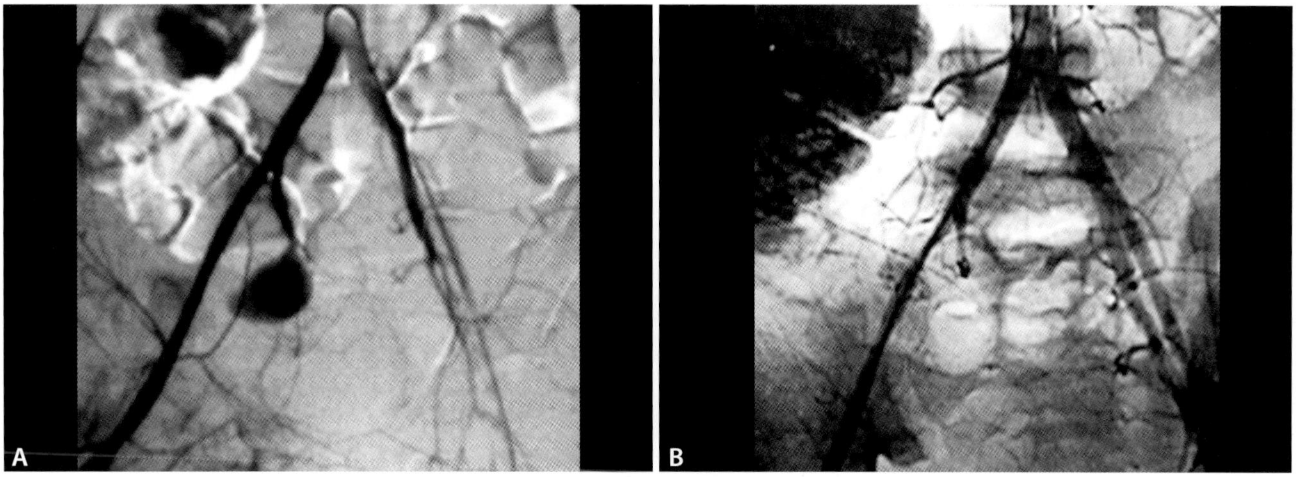

Figs. 12A and B: Post-traumatic pelvic bleeding: (A) DSA showing bleeding from right internal iliac artery trunk; (B) which stopped after steel coil embolization.

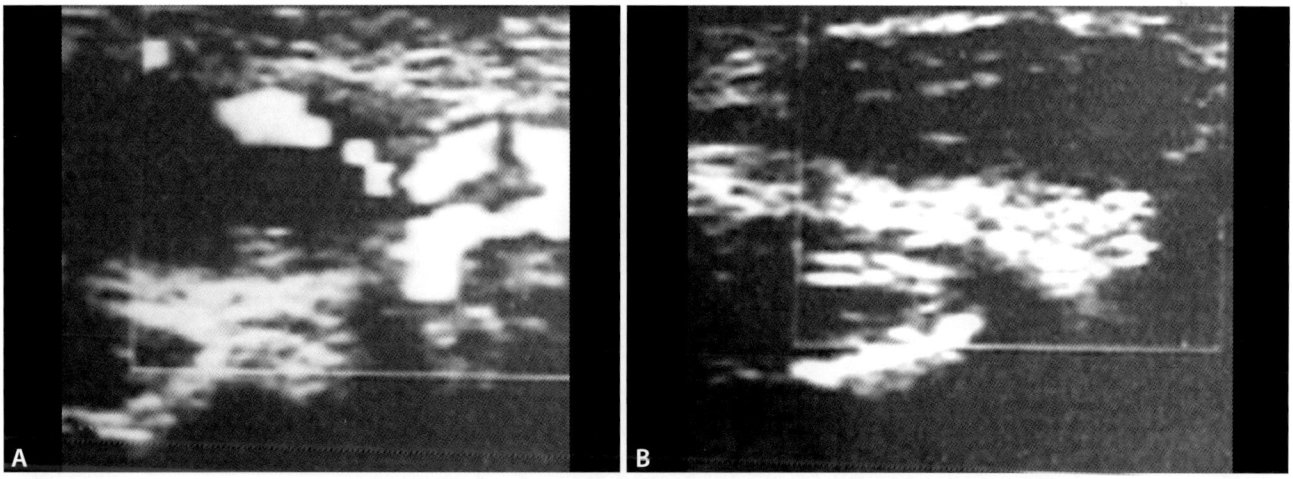

Figs. 13A and B: (A) Ultrasound showing pseudoaneurysm of femoral artery; (B) Developed after transfemoral arteriography, treated by manual compression.

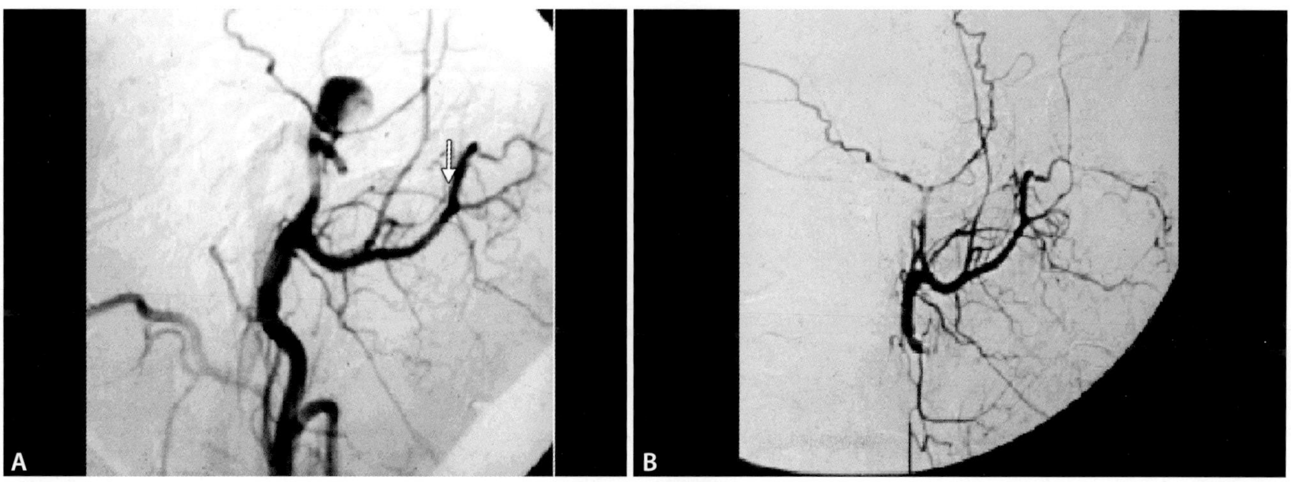

Figs. 14A and B: (A) Post-traumatic pseudoaneurysm from superficial temporal artery (arrow). This was treated by ultrasound-guided percutaneous coil embolization; (B) Post-treatment DSA is not showing aneurysm.

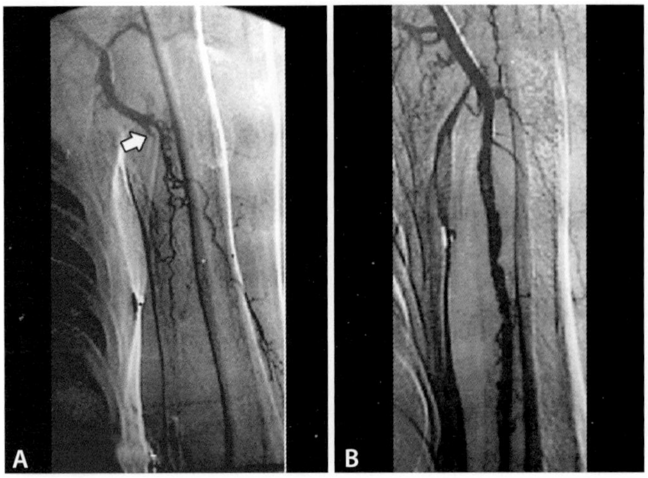

Figs. 15A and B: (A) Post-traumatic acute thrombosis (arrow) of brachial artery; (B) Recanalized after intra-arterial thrombolytic infusion.

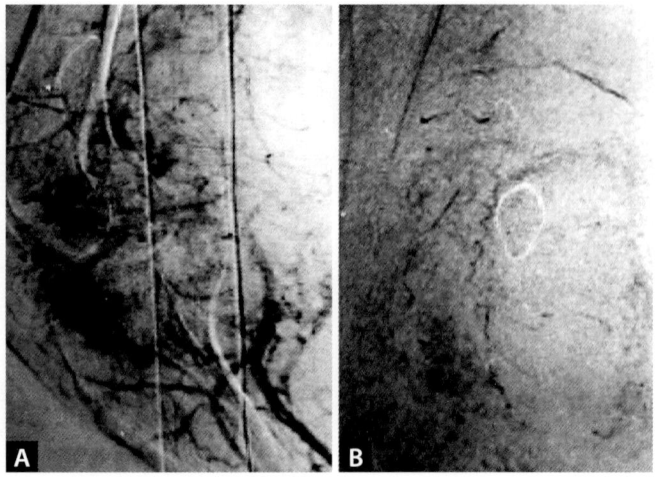

Figs. 16A and B: Preoperative embolization of a very large hemangioma around knee for reconstructive surgery. (A) Pre-embolization angiogram; (B) Post-embolization angiogram.

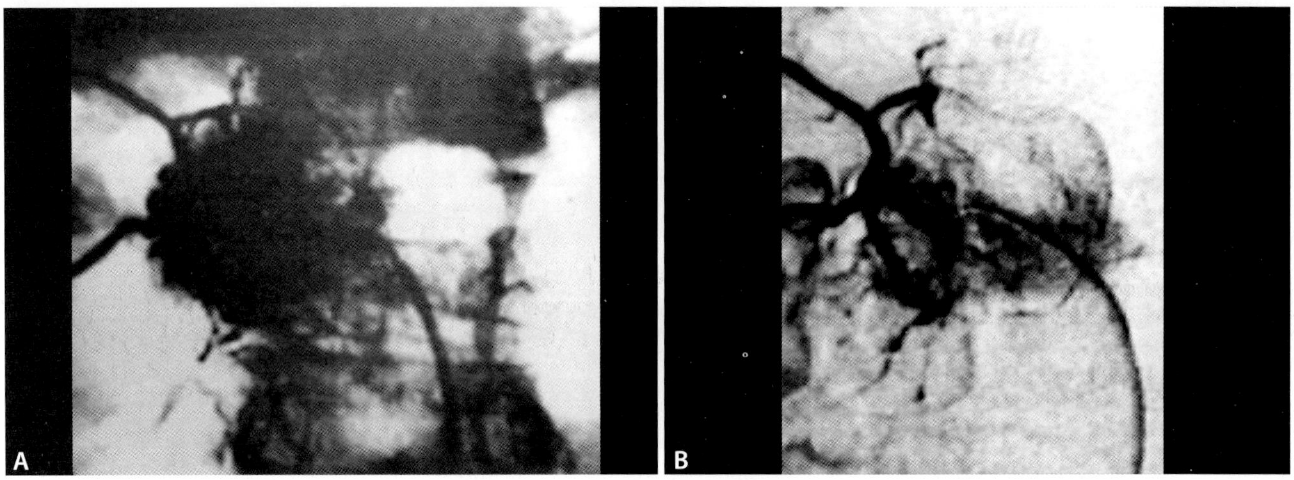

Figs. 17A and B: Painful metastatic deposit in the spine treated by therapeutic arterial occlusion. (A) Pre-embolization angiogram; (B) Post-embolization angiogram.

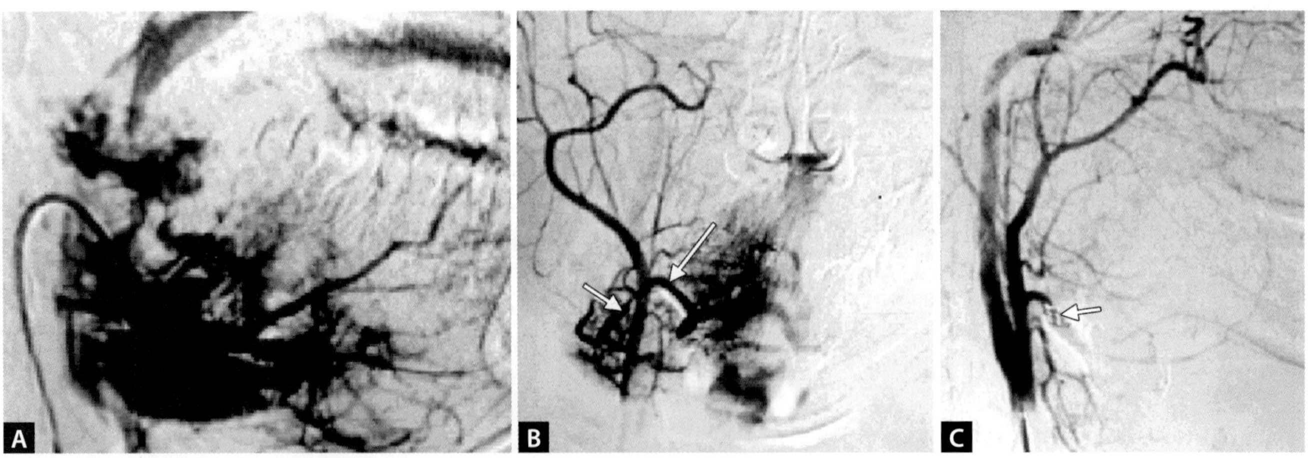

Figs. 18A to C: (A) Hemangioma submandibular region; (B) Supplied by right facial and lingual arteries (arrows); (C) The common origin of which embolized by steel coils (arrow).

Table 1: Commonly used embolizing materials.

Type of embolizing agent	*Examples and duration*
1. Particulate agents	• *Absorbable (temporary)*: – Autologous blood clot – Gelfoam • *Nonabsorbable (Permanent)*: – Polyvinyl alcohol particles – Microspheres
2. Mechanical agents	• *Nonabsorbable (Permanent)*: – Steel coils – Detachable balloons
3. Liquid agents	• *Nonabsorbable (Permanent)*: – Isobutyl 2-cyanoacrylate – Ethanol – Sodium tetradecyl sulfate

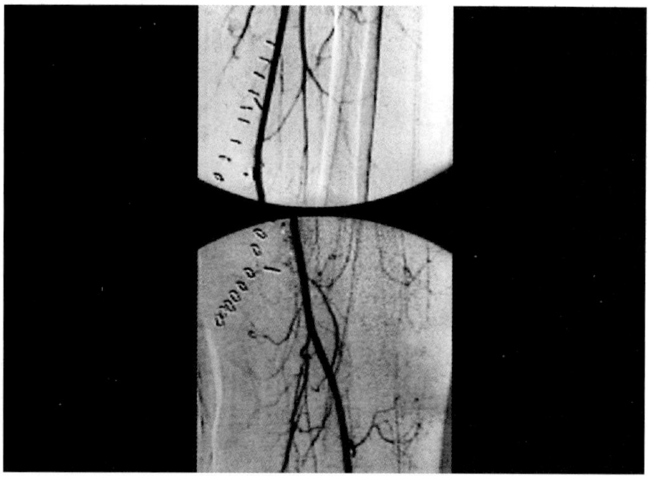

Fig. 19: Soft tissue sarcoma thigh. Postoperative angiogram was done to look for residual mass and intra-arterial chemotherapy.

vertebral lesions. The technique first introduced in 1984[25] for a vertebral hemangioma, has been subsequently used for the treatment of numerous lesions causing back pain associated with vertebral involvement like osteoporotic vertebral collapse, metastatic disease, multiple myeloma and symptomatic vertebral hemangiomas.

Technique

The procedure consists of instilling acrylic bone cement into the affected vertebra through a bone biopsy needle by a percutaneous approach. The cement consists of polymethylmethacrylate (obtained by mixing liquid monomer to the powdered polymer), which is mixed just before the injection. The cement is injected into the lesion after needle placement, under fluoroscopic control.[26] The cement polymerizes and subsequently sets, affording support to the vertebra **(Figs. 20A to C)**. The steps of the procedure are as follow:

I. Patient is placed in prone position on angiography/fluoroscopy table.
II. The procedure is performed under sterile conditions. The skin over the center of the pedicle is anesthetized with local anesthesia. A small skin incision is made and bone biopsy needle is positioned with its tip in the center of the mid point of the pedicle.
III. The needle is advanced under AP and lateral fluoroscopy till the junction of the anterior and middle third of the vertebral body. Approximately 6 mL of PMMA cement is injected.
IV. Patient is placed in supine position for three hours after the procedure and is discharged after 6 hours.

Results

Vertebroplasty results in relief of pain with decrease in analgesic use. It provides strength so prevents further collapse and pain relief by coagulating the tissue. The relief is obtained irrespective of the cause of pain, and is long lasting.[26]

Complications

The incidence of complications is less though various complications associated with the procedure are as follows:

- Cement leaks outside the vertebra are mostly inconsequential, but can cause local or radicular pain, neurological damage and pulmonary embolism.
- Inaccurate needle placement can injure nerve root or spinal cord.
- Pain exacerbation may occur due to substantial cement leaks.
- Rarely puncture site infection and bleeding may occur.

Future Directions

Although vertebroplasty can give considerable pain relief, it is not very useful in vertebral body height restoration. A new technique called kyphoplasty[27] involves the inflation of a bone tamp within the vertebral body to restore the height of the vertebra, and subsequently placing bone cement for augmentation of strength.

Vertebroplasty is becoming a well-established modality in the management of the aforementioned conditions, and is relatively safe.[28]

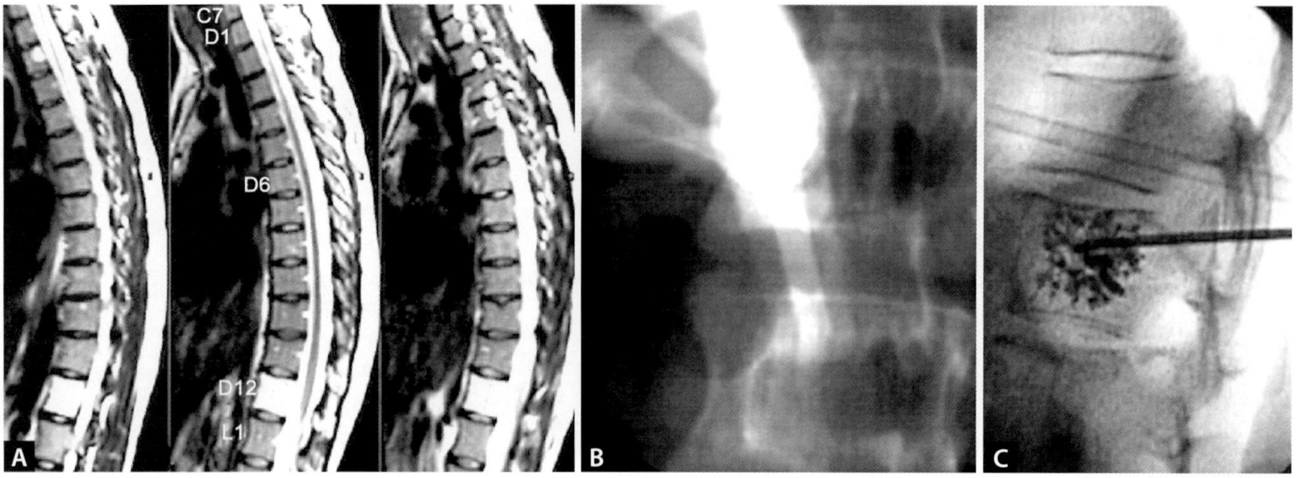

Figs. 20A to C: (A) A 30-year-old female with symptomatic D12 vertebral hemangioma, successfully treated with percutaneous vertebroplasty using polymethyl methacrylate bone cement. T2W pretreatment MR shows D12 vertebral body hemangioma; (B) The vertebroplasty needle is seen in position with (C) injected bone cement.

Percutaneous Treatment of Disk Herniation

Low backache is one of the major cause of chronic pain and morbidity. Treatment of herniated disk has evolved from open surgical techniques to minimally invasive or microtherapeutic procedures under local anesthesia. These include percutaneous laser disk decompression (PLDD), percutaneous ozone therapy, and percutaneous/endoscopic nucleotomy.

In PLDD, laser energy is delivered into nucleus pulposus by laser fiber, through a needle. The aim of PLDD is to vaporize a small portion of the nucleus pulposus. The ablation of this small volume results in reduction of intradiskal pressure, thus reducing the disk herniation[29] **(Figs. 21A to D)**.

In percutaneous ozone treatment, mixture of ozone-oxygen gas is administered into nucleus pulposus through the needle. This mixture has a direct effect on the proteoglycans of the nucleus pulposus, resulting in release of water molecules and subsequent degeneration of matrix and reduction of volume[30] **(Figs. 22 A to C)**.

Both PLDD and percutaneous ozone therapy are not used for uncontained herniations or sequestered disk. In both the procedures, patient is positioned prone and using either fluoroscopy or CT guidance a lumbar

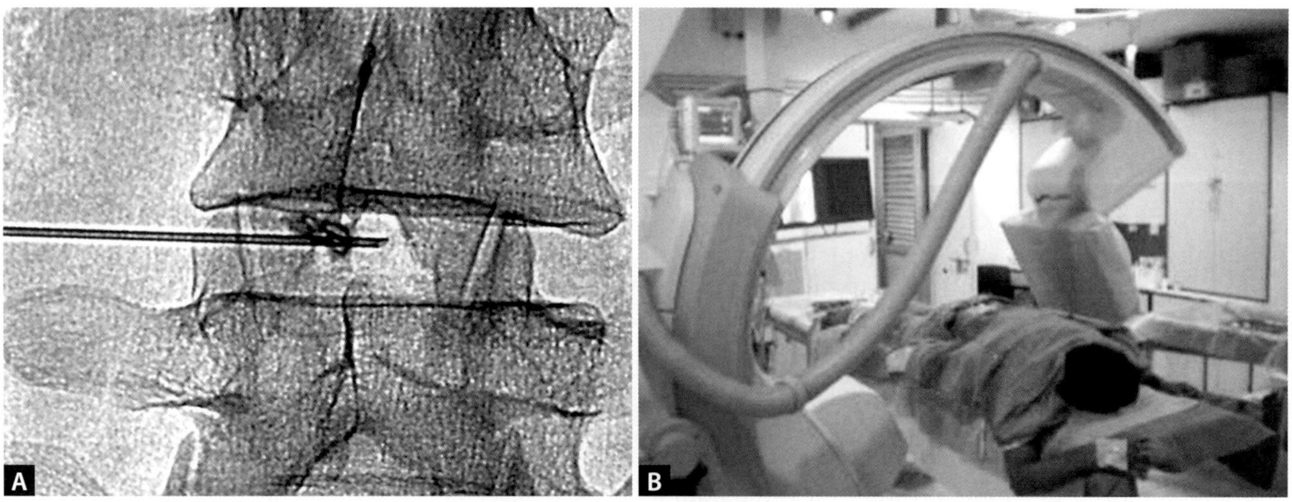

Figs. 21A and B

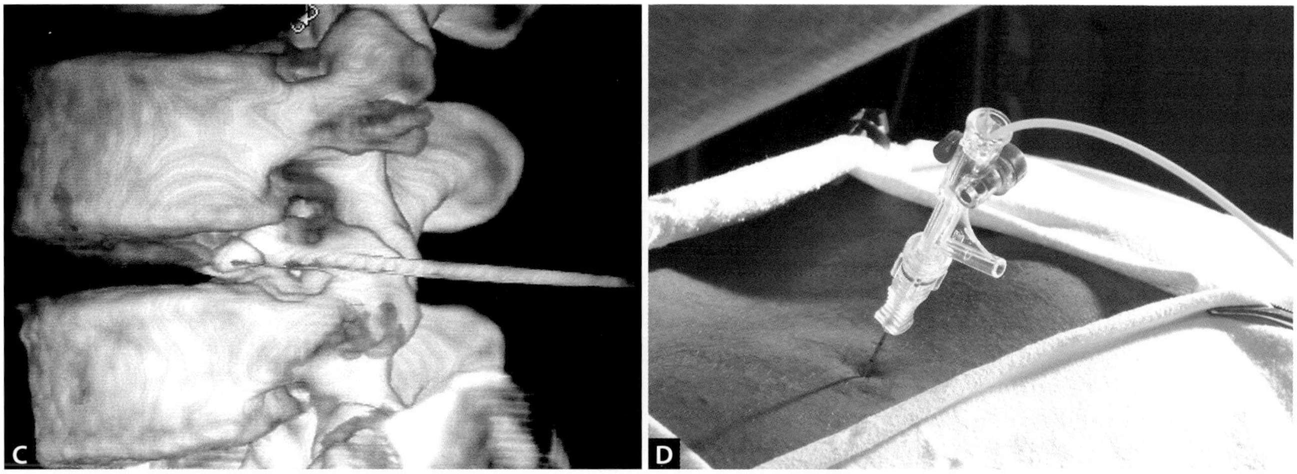

Figs. 21C and D

Figs. 21A to D: Percutaneous laser treatment of herniated disk: (A) A lumbar puncture needle is placed into the disk under fluoroscopy; (B and C) Needle position can be checked by doing rotation angiogram and 3D reconstruction image; (D) After proper position of needle, optical fiber is advanced through the needle and laser energy is deposited.

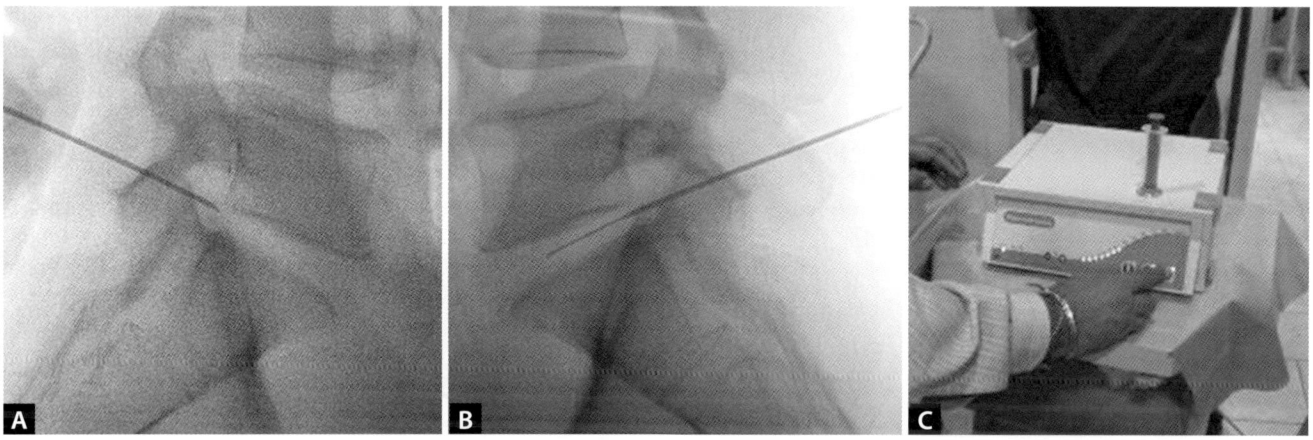

Figs. 22A to C: Percutaneous ozone treatment of herniated disk: (A and B) A lumbar puncture needle is placed into the disk under fluoroscopy; (C) Ozone gas is injected after preparing it from ozone generator machine.

puncture needle (18–21 G) is inserted into the center of the disk. After proper position of the needle, for PLDD, an optical fiber is advanced through the needle and proper laser energy is given. For ozone treatment, approximated 4 mL ozone-oxygen mixture is injected with an ozone concentration of 27 μg/mL.[31]

PERCUTANEOUS ABLATION OF BONE TUMORS

Percutaneous image guided tumor ablation with thermal energy source, such as radiofrequency, laser or microwave energy is used in the treatment of both benign (osteoid osteoma, osteoblastoma, enchondroma, etc.) and malignant (metastatic) lesions in place of surgery due to potential benefits, such as minimal invasiveness, reduced cost and morbidity.[32]

The procedure is performed with CT guidance either under general anesthesia or conscious sedation. A proper bone biopsy needle is placed into the lesion with the help of a hammer or a drill. Radiofrequency probe or laser fiber is introduced through the cannula and proper energy is delivered for ablation **(Figs. 23A to F)**.

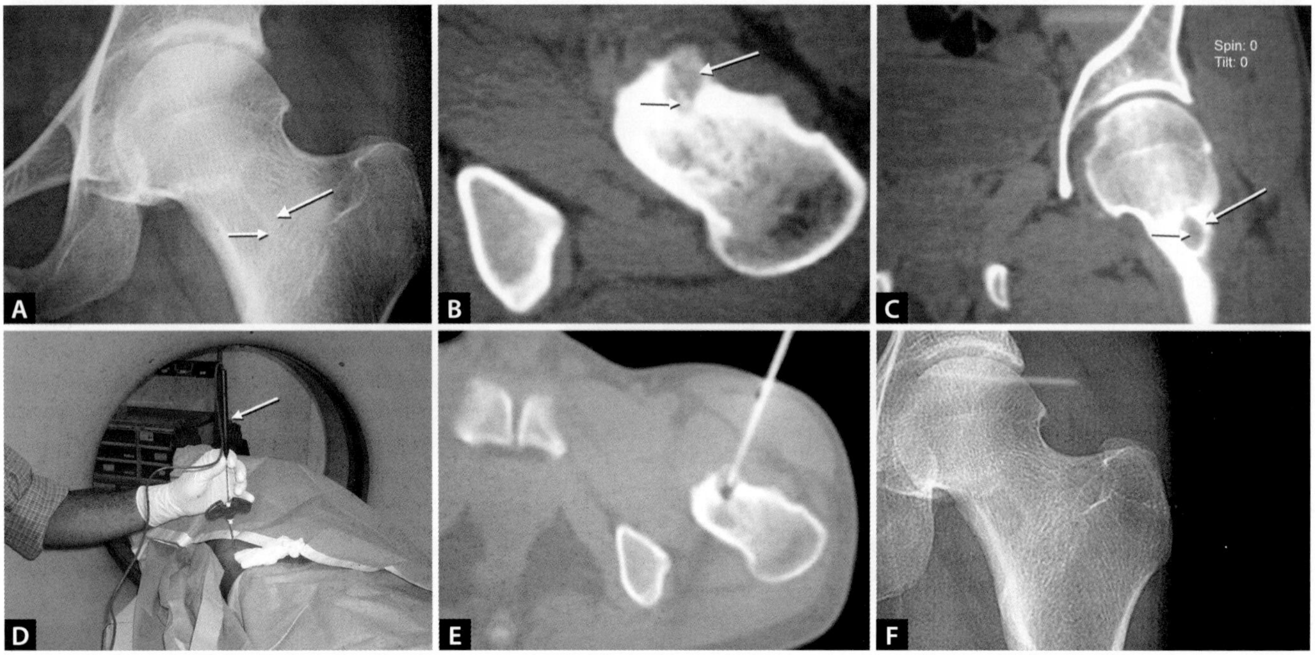

Figs. 23A to F: Percutaneous RF ablation of osteoid osteoma: Radiograph of left hip AP view (A), unenhanced axial (B) and coronal (C). CT images showing a small calcified nidus (small arrow) with surrounding sclerosis (long arrow). After placement of bone biopsy needle (small arrow) into the lesion under CT guidance the stylet was withdrawn and the RF probe (long arrow) was introduced (D). Axial CT image at the time of procedure (E) showing tip of the biopsy needle in the lesion. Post-treatment (1 week) AP radiograph (F) does not show nidus and patient is asymptomatic.

REFERENCES

1. Voegeli E, Uehlinger E. Arteriography in bone tumors. Skeletal Radiol. 1976;1:3.
2. Hudson TM, Haas G, Enneking WF, et al. Angiography in the management of musculoskeletal tumors. Surg Gynecol Obstet. 1975;141:11.
3. Han SK, Henein MHG, Novin N, et al. An unusual arterial complication seen with a solitary osteochondroma. Am Surg. 1977;43:471.
4. Gomez-Reino JH, Radin A, Gorevic PD. Pseudoaneurysm of the popliteal artery as a complication of an osteochondroma. Skeletal Radiol. 1979;4:26.
5. Lateur L, Baert AL. Localisation and diagnosis of osteoid osteoma of the carpal area by angiography. Skeletal Radiol. 1977;2:75.
6. de Santos LA, Murray JA. The value of arteriography in the management of aneurysmal bone cyst. Skeletal Radiol. 1978;2:137.
7. Bliznak J, Staple TW. Radiology of angiodysplasias of the limb. Radiology. 1974;10:35.
8. Levin DC, Grodon DH, McSweeney J. Arteriography of peripheral haemangiomas. Radiology. 1976;121:625.
9. Bartlely O, Wickbom I. Angiography in soft tissue haemangiomas. Acta Radiol. 1959;51:81.
10. Srivastava DN, Gulati M, Thulkar S, et al. Klippel-Trenaunay syndrome-unusual magnetic resonance features. Australasian Radiology. 1998;42:88.
11. Bjarnason H. Vascular embolotherapy. In: Ferral H, Bjarnason H, Qian Z (Eds). Synopsis of Castaneda's Interventional Radiology, 1st edn. Philadelphia: Lippincott Williams and Wilkins; 2001. pp. 27-45.
12. Rosen RJ, Riles TS. Arteriovenous malformations. In: Strandness D, van Breda A (Eds). Vascular Diseases: Surgical and Interventional Therapy. New York: Churchill-Livingstone; 1994. p. 1126.
13. Yaghmai I. Angiographic manifestations of soft tissue and osseous hemangiopericytomas. Radiology. 1978;126: 653.
14. Unni KK, Ivins JC, Beabout JW, et al. Haemangioma, haemangiopericytoma, and haemangio-endothelioma (angiosarcoma) of bone. Cancer. 1971;27:1403.
15. Yaghmai I. Angiography of bone and soft tissue lesions. New York: Springer; 1979.
16. Eric K, Hoffer, John J, Borsa, Robert D, Bloch, Arthur B. Fontaine. Endovascular Techniques in the Damage Control Setting. Radiographics. 1999;19:1340-8.
17. Feldman F, Cassarella WJ, Dick HM, et al. Selective intra-arterial embolisation of bone tumors–a useful adjunct in the management of selected lesions. AJR. 1975;123:130.
18. Voigt K, Schwenzer N, Stoeter P. Angiographic, operative, and histologic findings after embolisation of cranio-facial angiomas. Neuroradiology. 1978;16:424.
19. Doppman JL, Peusner P. Embolisation of arteriovenous malformations by direct percutaneous puncture. AJR. 1983;140:773.

20. Wallace S, Granmayeh M, de Santos LA, et al. Arterial occlusion of pelvic bone tumor. Cancer. 1979;43:322.
21. Hemmy DC, McGee DM, Armbrust FH, et al. Resection of a vertebral haemangioma after preoperative embolisation-a case report. J Neuro Surg. 1977;47:282.
22. Mitty HA, Kleiger B. Partial embolisation of large peripheral haemangioma for pain control. Radiology. 1978;127: 671.
23. Stanley RJ, Cubillo E. Nonsurgical treatment of arterio-venous malformations of the trunk and limb by trans-catheter arterial embolisation. Radiology. 1975;115:609.
24. Keus RB, Rutgers EJT, Ho GH, et al. Limb-sparing therapy of extremity sarcomas-treatment outcome and long-term functional results. Eur J Cancer. 1994;30A:1459-63.
25. Galibert P, Deramond H, et al. Preliminary note on the treatment of vertebral angioma by percutaneous acrylic vertebroplasty. Neurochirurgie. 1987;33:166-8.
26. Barr JD, Barr MS, Lemley TJ, et al. Percutaneous vertebroplasty for pain relief and spinal stabilisation. Spine. 2000;25:923-8.
27. Ledlie JT, Renfro M. Balloon kyphoplasty: one-year outcomes in vertebral body height restoration, chronic pain and activity levels. J Neurosurgery. 2003;98:36-42.
28. Afshin Gangi, Stephane Guth, Jean Pierre Imbert, et al. Percutaneous Vertebroplasty: Indications, Technique, and Results. Radiographics. 2003;23:e10.
29. Gupta AK, Narendra KB, Jayashree RS. Percutaneous laser disc decompression: Clinical experience at SCTIMST and long term follow-up. Neurology India. 2006;54:164-7.
30. Baabor MG, Vazques PF, Sanchez JA. Automated nucleotomy and nucleolysis with ozone. Acta Neurochir Suppl. 2011;108:97-101.
31. Cosma FA, Simonett L, Fabio de santis, et al. Minimally invasive oxygen-ozone therapy lumber disc herniation. AJNR. 2003;24:996-1000.
32. Ruiz Santiago F, Castellano Garcia Mdel M, Guzman Alvarez L, et al. Percutaneous treatment of bone tumors by radiofrequency thermal ablation. Eur J Radiol. 2011;77(1): 156-63.

CHAPTER 190

Tuberculosis of Bones and Joints

Gaurav S Pradhan, Veena Chowdhury

INTRODUCTION

Tuberculosis is widely prevalent in our country affecting all sections of the society, though it has been controlled to a great extent in the developed world.[1] Of all patients suffering from tuberculosis about three percent have skeletal system involvement.[2,3] Most of the skeletal tuberculosis is now caused by bacilli of human type as opposed to bovine bacilli in the past. Osteoarticular tuberculosis is second in frequency only to tubercular infection of spine.[4]

ETIOPATHOGENESIS

Osteoarticular tuberculosis begins in the synovium or in the metaphyseal spongiosa. Synovial infection can occur by contiguous spread or due to hematogenous spread. Hematogenous spread can occur from a lung primary or postprimary focus, or from any other visceral, lymph nodal source of infection. Simultaneous involvement of viscera, lymph nodes and parts of skeletal system suggest spread of infection through arterial blood supply. Lesion is usually destructive and accompanied by pus formation which may get calcified. The metaphyseal lesion may infect the joint through subperiosteal space, through capsule or through destruction of the epiphyseal plate. In contrast to pyogenic infections, sequestration and periostitis are not very common. Ischemic necrosis and endarteritis may result in very small sequestrum formation which is usually not radiologically visible. It may however become visible as a result of calcification. Marked exudative reaction is however a common feature. Granulation tissue spreads onto the free surface of cartilage eroding it in patches, insinuating between cartilage and subchondral bone, advancing from periphery to the center causing loosing and separation of cartilaginous tissue as it proceeds causing necrosis of cartilage with erosion of exposed bone. Marginal erosions are characteristic of tuberculosis in weightbearing joints, such as hip, knee and ankle. Wedge-shaped necrotic foci may become evident on either side of joint leading to the appearance of 'kissing sequestra'. Necrosed cartilage, fibrinous material form *rice bodies* in synovial joints, tendon sheaths and bursae.[5,6] Abscesses that form may track along fascial planes and result in sinus formation. Plaques of irregular bone, if present in walls of chronic abscess or sinus suggest diagnosis of long standing tubercular infection.

BCG osteitis that can occur following BCG vaccination runs a benign course with localization of the *Bacillus* in epiphysis and metaphysis with extension across growth plate. It resembles chronic osteomyelitis radiologically, but responds to ATT.

Synovial sheath infections are common with nontypical *Mycobacterium* [Other than *M. tuberculosis* and *M. bovis*], with history of trauma [puncture wounds], surgery, immune compromised status and exposure to contaminated marine life.

Tuberculosis has been seen as a late complication of implant surgery usually 6–12 months after operation. This has been attributed to extensive surgery, use of implants and favorable conditions for circulating mycobacteria like diabetes mellitus, corticosteroids and immune compromised status.[6,7]

Clinical Features

Clinical features include insidious onset, low-grade fever, anorexia, weight loss and night sweats. The patient may present with night pains, painful limitation of movement, muscle wasting, regional lymph node involvement and neurologic symptoms.

Weightbearing joints like hip, knee and ankle are commonly involved, though any part of the skeleton can get involved by the disease process.[8,9]

Radiological Features

Tubercular involvement of bone can be broadly divided into four stages:

1. Inflammatory edema and exudates (predestructive stage)
2. Necrosis and cavitation
3. Destruction and deformation
4. Healing and repair.

Tubercular infection in bones is said to develop two to three years after primary focus so the diagnosis is usually delayed, in contrast to pyogenic infections which are seen two to three weeks after clinical presentation. Further changes in bone on plain radiograph, are usually appreciable two to four months after onset of disease. The infection originates in the metaphysis and it can cross the growth plate. There is usually no sclerosis and small sequestra are absorbed. Diaphyseal lesions are rare and multiple cystic lucencies are rarer still.

Investigations include anteroposterior and lateral views of the involved region and radiograph of the chest.

Stage of synovitis: In early synovial disease there is soft tissue swelling and joint widening due to effusion and synovial hypertrophy. The first radiological sign may be juxta-articular osteoporosis. Patchy areas of trabecular or bony destruction may be evident. In the center of osteolytic lesion or cavity there may be sequestrum or calcification of the caseous tissue, giving appearance of an irregular soft, feathery, coke-like sequestrum [image en Grelot] **(Fig. 1)**. If there is secondary superadded infection, subperiosteal reaction may result. As a result of localized hyperemia growth plate may show overgrowth, especially in childhood.

Stage of arthritis: Later in the disease, the articular margin and bony cortices may be hazy (blurring and fuzzy) giving rise to "washed out appearance". With involvement of articular cartilage there is narrowing and reduction of joint space. Juxta-articular osteopenia, peripherally located osseous lesions and gradual narrowing of joint space are considered pathognomonic of tubercular osteoarthritis and are referred to as "Phemister triad" **(Fig. 2)**.

Early loss of articular joint space is more typically seen in rheumatoid arthritis and thus helps in differentiating from tuberculosis.

Stage of advanced arthritis: In advanced cases there is collapse of bone, subluxation or dislocation, migration of bone and resultant deformity of joint.[10,11]

With healing, there is remineralization and cortical and articular margins become distinct. Fibrous ankylosis may occur during healing phase. In contrast to pyogenic arthritis, the development of bone ankylosis is uncommon in tubercular arthritis.

Ultrasonography is helpful in the evaluation of large joints, like hip joint to demonstrate joint effusion, synovitis and capsular thickening. Synovial thickening can be seen

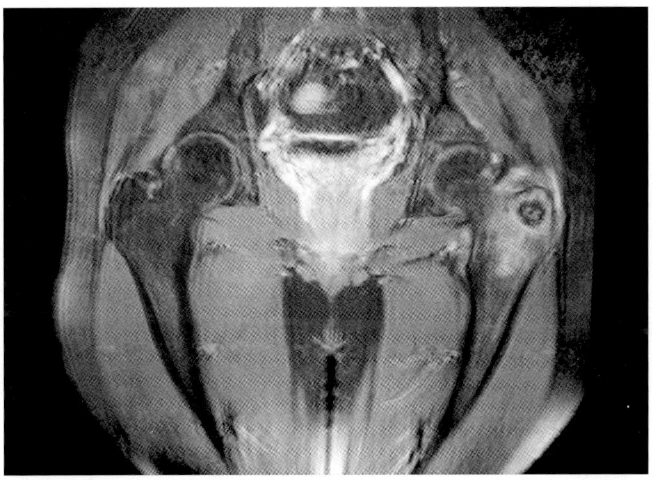

Fig. 1: In the center of osteolytic lesion in left femur, there is a small irregular sequestrum picked up on MRI [image en Grelot].

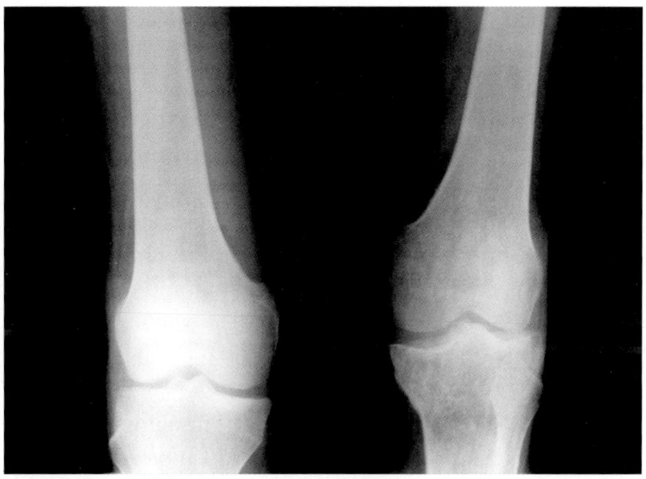

Fig. 2: Diffuse osteopenia with lytic lesion seen at the lateral articular margin of tibia with relative preservation of joint spaces in a case of tuberculosis of left knee.

as hypoechoic intra-articular soft tissue. Fluid in joint space and bursal fluid can be anechoic or hypoechoic (thick exudate). In tenosynovitis the synovial sheath along tendons is thick and heterogeneous with minimal fluid suggestive of chronic tenosynovitis. It can in addition indicate presence of associated soft tissue abscess like psoas abscess. It can also demonstrate cortical disruption, irregularity of articular margins and associated soft tissue swelling. Calcification in abscess, if any can also be seen. Further, evaluation of tendon sheaths and bursal spaces and smaller joints like wrist, hand, foot and ankle is also possible. Guided joint fluid aspiration or synovial biopsy is possible under ultrasound guidance.

Computed tomography scan is helpful in demonstrating lytic areas and marginal erosions much before plain radiographs.[12]

Swelling in soft tissues, granulation, exudations, abscess and early calcification can also be demonstrated much earlier. Joint space can also be better evaluated by CT scan.

The predestructive stage can be visualized by MRI and also probably by bone scans. The plain radiographs and CT scan are not likely to detect the stage of inflammatory edema and exudates.

Isotope bone scan or magnetic resonance imaging may reveal subclinical active lesion in forty percent of patients in addition to the presenting lesion. Out of technetium-99m, gallium-67 and indium-111 isotopes used in skeletal scintigraphy, technetium-99m is the most sensitive, though not specific. So a positive scan helps in localizing the suspicious region and is also helpful for follow-up.[18] Fluorine fluorodeoxyglucose-positron emission tomography (^{18}F-FDG-PET) has also been found useful in localizing tubercular disease and in differentiating soft tissue infection from osseous infection.[4,5,13]

Synovial hypertrophy is most commonly seen in osteoarticular tuberculosis, on magnetic resonance imaging. Hypointense areas on T2-weighted images suggesting hemosiderin deposition, rim of synovial lesions on pregadolinium T1-weighted images and fluid loculations with enhancing synovial rims and erosions on postgadolinium images may be helpful in characterizing the lesion as tubercular when the radiographs are normal **(Fig. 3)**.

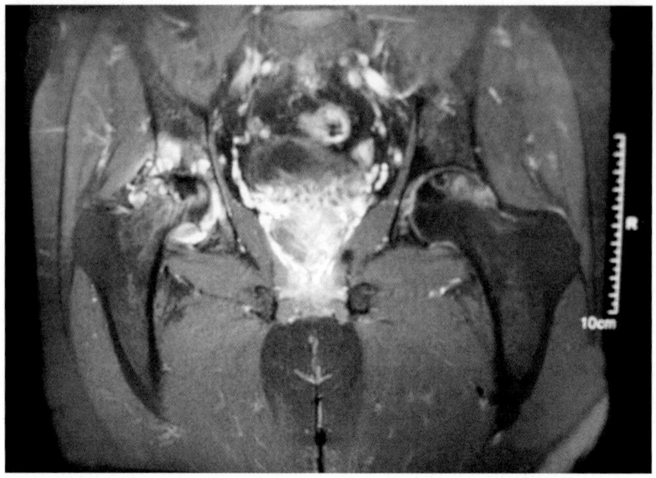

Fig. 3: Fluid loculations with enhancing synovial rims and erosions on postgadolinium images in a case of tuberculosis of right hip.

Certain characteristics that can be helpful on MRI are as follows:

- *Short tau inversion recovery* (STIR) imaging, inversion recovery (TR >2000 msec; TE >30 msec; TI = 120–150 msec): Fat-saturation technique that results in markedly decreased signal intensity from fat and strikingly increased signal from fluid and edema. Inversion recovery is an extremely sensitive tool for detecting tissue and marrow pathology. FSE-STIR sequence is used with most of our musculoskeletal protocols.
- The high signal of joint fluid on T2-weighted sequence makes it a sensitive method to detect joint effusion.
- Synovial proliferation due to tubercular arthritis may be hypointense on T2-weighted images and thickened synovium enhances vividly after gadolinium. Active pannus proliferating into the subarticular bone enhances on the postcontrast scans while chronic fibrosis does not enhance.
- Caseating granulomas with solid centers give a characteristic hypointense signal to the synovium on T2-weighted images.
- Chondral lesions and subchondral bone erosions may be visible at a stage when the joint space is still well preserved.
- *Penumbra sign* may be present. A thin intermediate signal intensity rim along the periphery of a bone or soft tissue abscess on unenhanced T1-weighted images may be seen, due to layer of granulation tissue along its wall. It is useful in identifying soft tissue abscesses.
- In the pelvis and extremities routine protocols include T1, STIR, and postgadolinium T1-weighted images. Section thickness used in the pelvis is 7 mm and in the extremities, 4 mm.
- Magnetic resonance imaging can be helpful in detecting bone marrow inflammation, intraosseous abscess, sequestrum, cortical destruction, cloaca and sinus tract formation **(Figs. 4A to C)**.

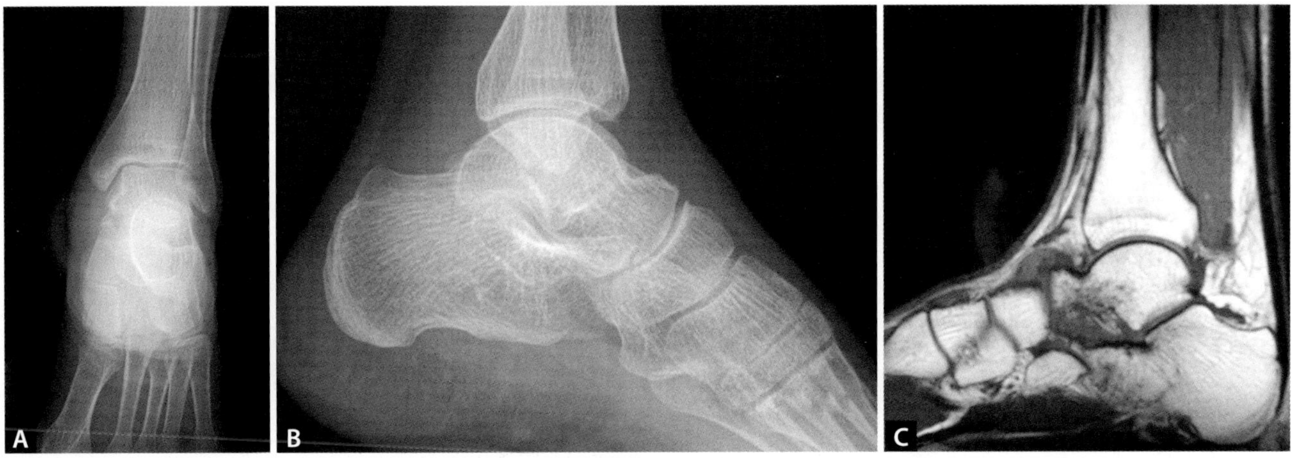

Figs. 4A to C: (A and B) Plain X-rays of ankle showing subtle osteolytic lesion in anterior aspect of talus on right side; (C) MRI showing markedly destructive lesion in anterior aspect of talus with associated soft tissue abnormality.

- Tenosynovitis may be seen in active (hygromatous) and chronic (serofibrinous) phase and bursitis may be seen as distended bursa or multiple small abscesses.[4,9,14]

Computed tomography guided aspirations and needle biopsy for difficult areas like sacroiliac joints may be helpful in obtaining tissues for diagnosis. Repeat imaging can be helpful in follow-up and if there is deterioration of clinical, laboratory or imaging features then a representative biopsy is mandatory from the area.

Skeletal TB involving parts of body other than spine can be classified according to region of involvement:

- *Tuberculosis* of joints—*Tubercular arthritis*
- *Tuberculosis* of long and flat bones—*Tubercular osteomyelitis*
- *Tubercular* of short tubular bones—*Tubercular dactylitis.*

TUBERCULOSIS OF JOINTS

Tubercular Arthritis

Hip

Lesions can arise in acetabulum, synovium, femoral epiphysis or metaphysis (Babcock's triangle) or spread to the hip from foci in the greater trochanter or ischium. If there is tubercular involvement of the upper end of femur (being entirely intracapsular), the joint is involved early in disease and there is destruction of articular margins of femoral head and acetabulum. Hip involvement is seen in about 15% of cases of osteoarticular tuberculosis.[15]

Tubercular lesion may also occur in the greater trochanter or the overlying bursa. The lesion may manifest as a surface erosion or lytic lesion in the greater trochanter. Tuberculosis of the greater trochanter may involve the overlying trochanteric bursa without involving the hip joint for a fairly long period of time.

Stage of synovitis: The patient may present with irritable hip with plain radiograph being normal **(Fig. 5)**. Displacement of fat planes and positive obturator sign occur due to flexion deformity (reduced obturator foramina size). This is followed by onset of soft tissue swelling and deossification. Radiologically significant osteoporosis appears 12–18 weeks after onset of symptoms.

Ultrasound, computed tomography and magnetic resonance imaging are more sensitive in this stage to detect increased joint space and accumulation of fluid. Investigations may be repeated, at three to six weeks interval, to help in establishing the diagnosis.

Differential diagnosis includes traumatic or non-specific transient synovitis, Perthes', slipped capital femoral epiphysis and low-grade pyogenic infections.

Stage of arthritis: There is deformity of the hip joint. In addition to osteoporosis localized erosions may be seen in periarticular region **(Fig. 6)**. The destruction of articular cartilage leads to erosion of acetabular margin and femoral head with reduction of joint space. Lesions can usually be picked up on computed tomography before they are apparent on plain radiographs.[7,9]

Stage of advanced arthritis: With progression of disease, there is destruction of articular cartilage, acetabulum, femoral head, capsule and ligaments. The capsule may also get thickened and contracted **(Figs. 7A to C)**. The upper end of femur may displace upwards and dorsally breaking the Shenton's line and leaving the lower part of acetabulum empty (wandering acetabulum) **(Fig. 8)**.

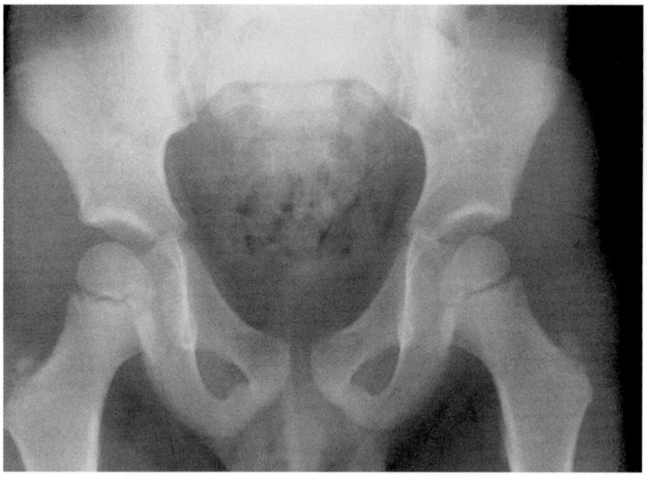

Fig. 5: Plain X-ray of pelvis showing relatively well-maintained hip joint on left side in an early case of tuberculosis of left hip with hip joint effusion on ultrasound.

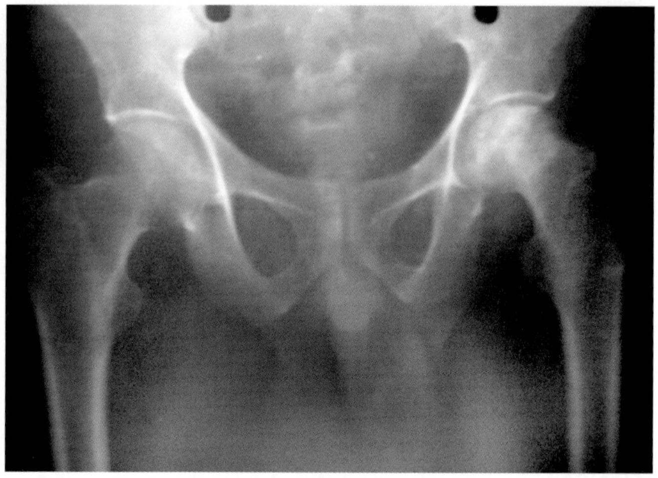

Fig 6: TB arthritis of left hip showing periarticular osteopenia, indistinct articular surfaces and erosions of femoral head and neck with relative preservation of joint space.

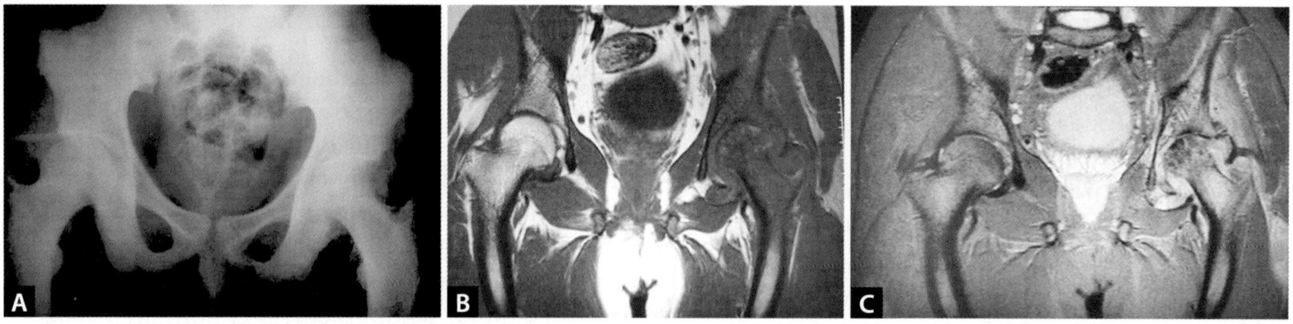

Figs. 7A to C: (A) Plain X-ray of pelvis showing erosion of the lateral aspect of femur head and neck with markedly reduced joint space on left side; (B and C) Altered marrow signal intensity in the left femoral head and neck appearing hypointense on T1 and hyperintense on STIR MR images.

Bone loss can lead to bird beak appearance with intra-pelvic protrusion. If femoral head, neck are grossly destroyed and collapsed in an enlarged acetabulum, this appearance is called "mortar and pestle" appearance **(Fig. 9)**.

Radiological classification for tuberculosis of hip (Shanmugasundaram) is useful in assessing relationship between various radiological types and functional outcome in which various radiological types have been described, such as normal (synovitis stage) wandering acetabulum, dislocated hip, Perthes' type, protrusio acetabuli, atrophic type and mortar and pestle type[16] **(Figs. 10A to C)**.

Knee

Tuberculosis of knee joint can occur in any age group. The most common symptoms are pain on movement of the knee joint, synovial effusion, palpable synovial thickening and restriction of mobility. Tenderness may be present in the medial or lateral joint line and patellofemoral segment of the joint. The knee joint has the largest intra-articular space and is involved in about 10% cases of osteoarticular tuberculosis. The initial focus may be in synovium or subchondral bone of distal femora, proximal tibia or patella.[17]

In synovial stage, there is osteoporosis, soft tissue swelling due to synovial effusion, thickened synovium and capsule. There may be distension of suprapatellar bursa on lateral radiograph of knee. Synovial infection in childhood can lead to effusion, osteoporosis, accelerated growth and maturation resulting in big bulbous squared epiphysis.[18] Synovitis can also cause widening of the intercondylar notch. Purulent material can accumulate in the joint space with destruction of articular cartilage secondary to the synovitis and metaphyseal and subarticular lesions can occur, both in femur and tibia.

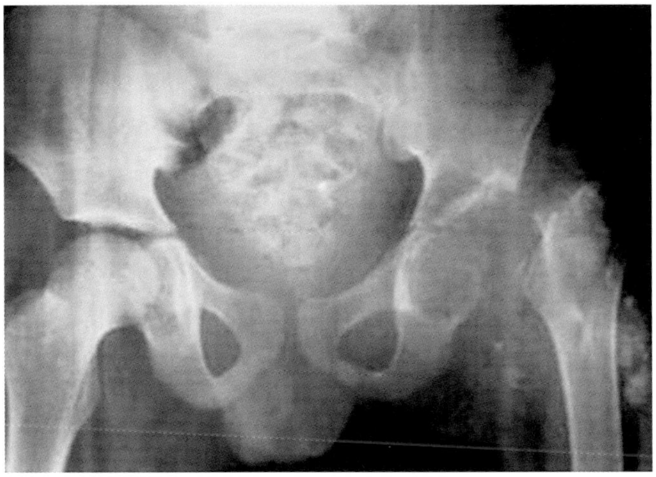

Fig. 8: Plain X-ray of pelvis showing destruction and subluxation of upper end of left femur, being displaced upwards and dorsally resulting in "wandering acetabulum".

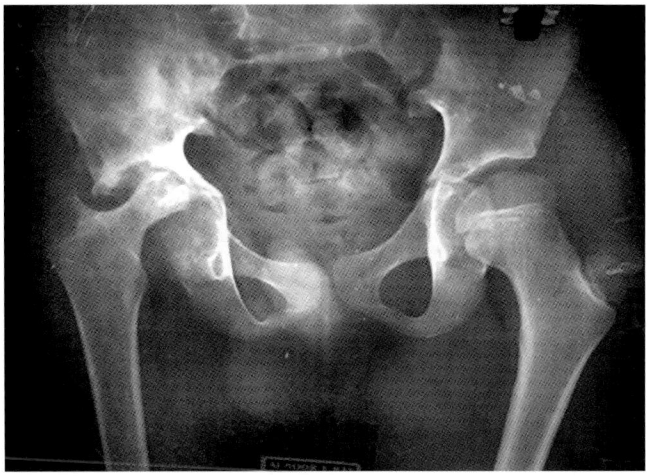

Fig. 9: Plain X-ray of pelvis showing gross destruction of right femoral head and neck with collapse contained within the enlarged acetabulum giving "mortar and pestle appearance".

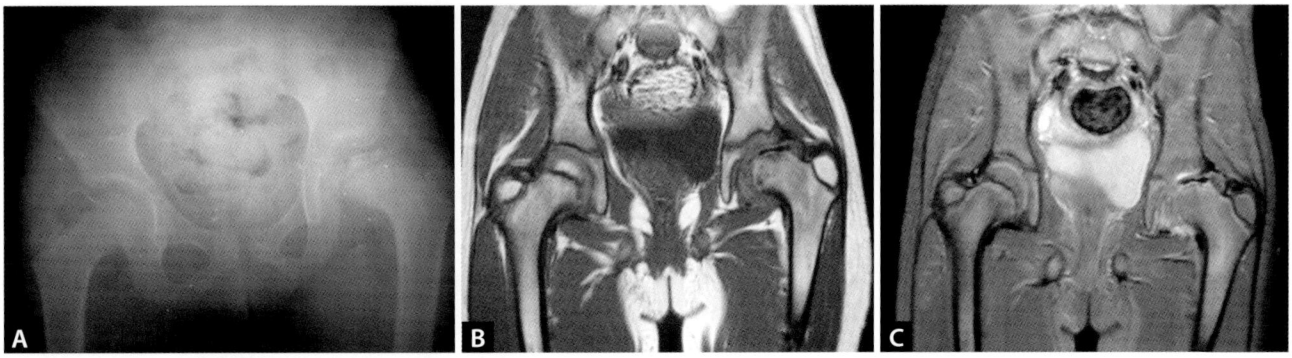

Figs. 10A to C: (A) There is evidence of irregularity, partial collapse and sclerosis of epiphysis of left femoral head suggestive of Perthes' type appearance in a case of tuberculosis of left hip joint; (B and C) Flattening of the left femur capital epiphysis in the same case, which appears diffusely hypointense on T1 and STIR suggestive of sclerosis with marrow signal alteration noted in the left femoral neck.

As arthritis sets in, there is loss of definition of articular surfaces, marginal erosions, decreased joint space and destruction of bones **(Fig. 11)**.

In advanced arthritis, there are osteolytic cavities with or without sequestra formation, marked reduction of joint space, destruction and deformity of joints. In advanced cases, there is triple deformity of the knee, that is lateral, posterior and superior displacement of tibia on femur.

The differential diagnosis includes juvenile rheumatoid arthritis, villonodular synovitis, osteochondritis dissecans and hemophilia.

Diagnosis is established by radiological examination which can show destructive lesions in the femoral or tibial condyles. Biopsy of the synovial membrane and aspiration of the joint fluid followed by smear, culture and guinea pig inoculation can confirm the diagnosis.

Ankle and Foot

Swelling, limp and pain may be the early presenting features in tuberculosis of ankle joint. The swelling is evident in front of the joint, around the malleoli and tendo-Achilles insertion. Marked osteoporosis with or without erosions and osteolytic lesions may be present in active stage of disease. There may be unsharpness of articular surfaces along with reduction of joint space **(Fig. 12)**.

In long-standing cases, gross destruction of bones and sinus formation can result. The ankle joint can show pathological anterior dislocation. Rarely, periosteal reaction may occur.

In tubercular affliction of foot, common involvement is seen of calcaneum, subtalar and midtarsal joints, anterior 2/3rds of calcaneum being commonly affected.

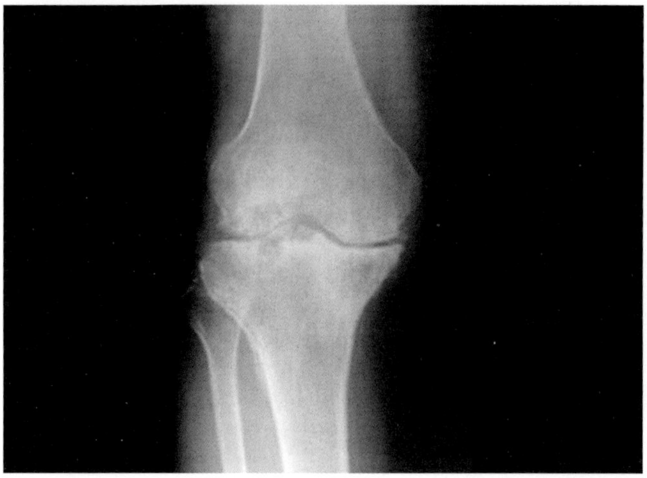

Fig. 11: Plain X-ray of knee joint showing juxta-articular osteopenia with fuzziness of articular margins numerous marginal erosions and loss of joint space.

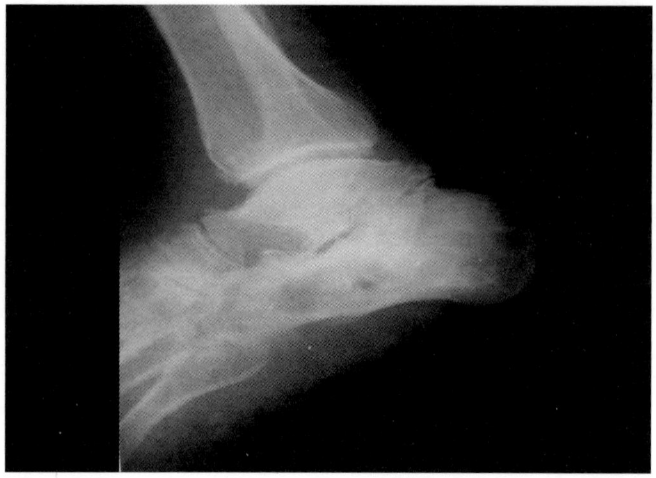

Fig. 12: Plain X-ray of ankle joint showing marginal erosions at subtalar joint with indistinct articular surfaces and loss of joint space.

Talus, metatarsal bones, navicular, cuneiform, cuboid can all get involved.[19] Radiograph can reveal presence of osteolyic lesion with or without coke-like sequestrum. Tubercular infection rapidly spreads across the inter-communicating synovial channels, so multiple bones are commonly involved **(Fig. 13)**.

Osteochondritis dissecans of talus can simulate a tuberculous lesion of the ankle.

The foot bones can have isolated tubercular lesions as in the os calcis or as diaphyseal foci in metatarsal bones (tubercular dactylitis). A subchondral lesion in the os calcis leading to talocalcaneal arthritis and peroneal spastic flat foot is a definite clinical entity. Talonavicular and naviculo-cuneiform lesions and calcaneocuboid joint involvement can also occur, particularly in diabetes mellitus. The tarsometatarsal articulation at Lisfranc's level and the metatarsophalangeal joint of the great toe can be other foci of involvement. Lesions very similar to tubercular lesions can occur in *Madurella* infection. Differential diagnosis should also include a neuropathic change in the foot, secondary to diabetes or leprosy.

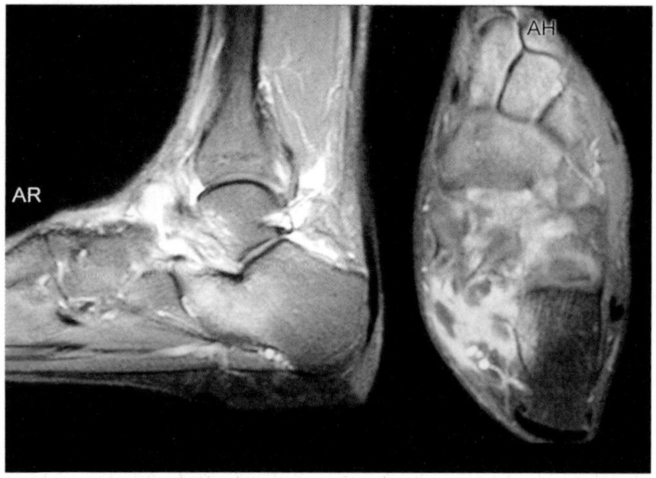

Fig. 13: MRI of ankle joint in a case of talocalcaneal tuberculosis showing bony destruction involving talus, multiple collections along with rim enhancement in the subtalar region with cloaca and sinus tract formation.

Shoulder

Tubercular disease involving the shoulder joint is rare. It is more frequent in adults and the incidence of concomitant pulmonary tuberculosis is high. The classical sites could be head of humerus, glenoid, spine of the scapula, acromio-clavicular joint, coracoid process and rarely synovial lesion. It can also be iatrogenic due to steroid injection given for a stiff shoulder with the mistaken diagnosis of frozen shoulder, particularly in diabetics. In the shoulder joint the initial tubercular destruction is typically widespread because of the small surface contact area of articular cartilage. The clinical presentation is with severe painful restriction of the shoulder movements, particularly abduction and external rotation, and gross wasting of shoulder muscles.[20]

Radiologically, there is osteoporosis with erosion of articular margins (fuzzy) with osteolytic lesion involving head of humerus, glenoid or both **(Fig. 14)**. The lesion may mimic giant cell tumor. The joint space involvement and capsular contracture are seen early in the disease. Sinus formation can also occur. In advanced cases, inferior subluxation of the humeral head and fibrous ankylosis may result **(Fig. 15)**. There is an atrophic type

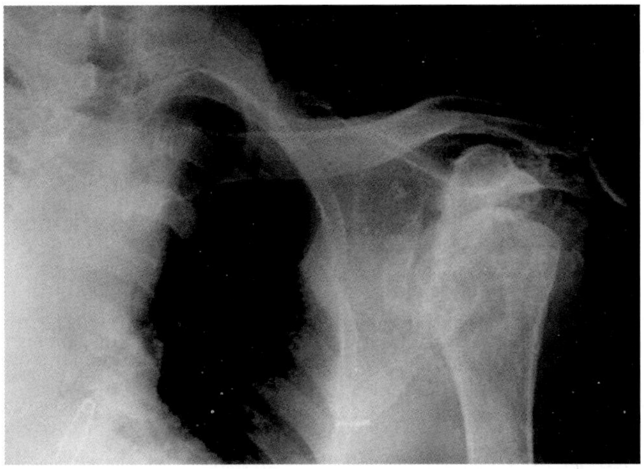

Fig. 14: Plain X-ray of left shoulder joint showing erosions and deformity of humeral head and acetabular margin with osteopenia and periarticular calcification.

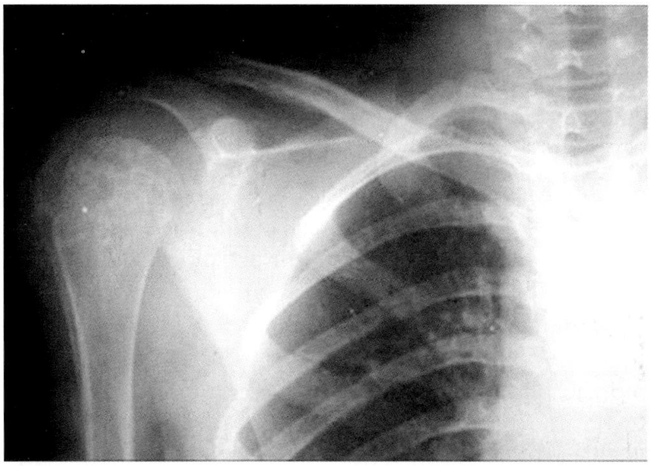

Fig. 15: Plain X-ray of right shoulder joint showing fuzzy articular margins and osteolytic lesions in proximal part of right humerus with pathological subluxation of head of humerus.

of tuberculosis of the shoulder in which the disease runs a benign course without pus formation called *caries sicca* and small pitted erosions on the humeral head may be seen. The classical dry type is more common in adults while the fulminating variety with cold abscess or sinus formation is more common in children.[21]

Since the joint space is small, multiple and large osseous destructive lesions are commonly seen. Magnetic resonance can show synovial lesions as well, besides the osseous lesions.

Differential diagnosis includes periarthritis of the shoulder, rheumatoid arthritis and post-traumatic shoulder stiffness. Aspiration of the shoulder and fine needle aspiration biopsy might be necessary to establish the diagnosis. The patient responds well to antitubercular drugs.

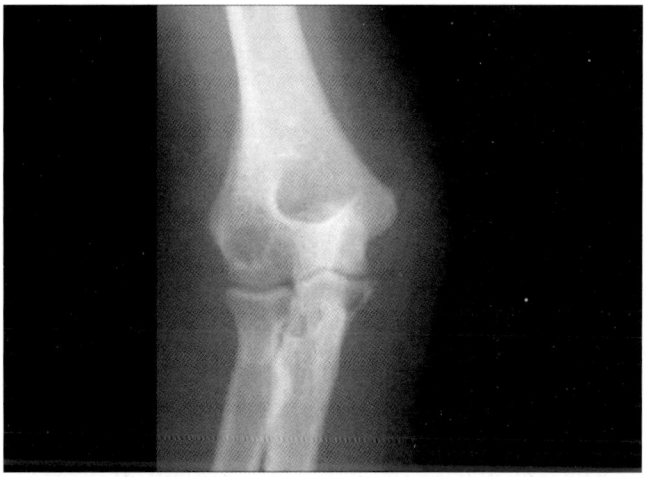

Fig. 16: Plain X-ray of right elbow joint showing multiple osteolytic lesions within the radius, ulna and capitulum.

Elbow

Tubercular involvement is seen in about 2 to 5% cases.

The most frequent sites of involvement are medial and lateral condyles of the humerus, articular surface of olecranon usually intra-articular but occasionally extra-articular and head of radius **(Fig. 16)**. Rarely the disease is synovial in origin.

Radiographic features in articular type include involvement of humerus and ulna, osteoporosis, blurring of articular cortex and early diminution of joint space while in the extra-articular type, ulna is involved most commonly with destructive lesions seen in olecranon or coronoid process.[9,21] Periostitis may also be seen.

Synovial thickening of the radiohumeral segment of the articulation can be present, particularly if the synovium is involved. X-ray examination is highly suggestive. Initially there is osteoporosis and blurring of articular cortex. Osteolytic lesions may be seen around the elbow joint. In advanced cases there is decreased joint space and subchondral bone destruction.[20,21] In infants and children, sequestra may be present. Periostitis is a common feature and most commonly affects the ulna. Pathological dislocation of elbow is very rare. The diagnosis can be confirmed by aspiration or biopsy of synovium from the lateral side.

Differential diagnosis includes osteochondritis dissecans of the humeral condyle and osteoid osteoma of the lateral condyle of the humerus which being intra-articular in location can be mistaken for tuberculosis of the elbow joint.

Wrist and Carpus

It is a rare site, usually affecting adults. The anatomical sites of the lesions may be in the radius or proximal row of carpal bones—scaphoid, lunate and capitate **(Fig. 17)**. Concomitant involvement of the sheaths of volar or dorsal tendons might also occur.

Radiographic features include intense osteoporosis, soft tissue swelling, erosions of articular margins and cartilage destructions, periosteal reaction and early appearance of ossification centers.

All carpal bones tend to get involved in adults while more localized lesions are seen in children. This is thought to be due to thicker articular cartilage in children.[22] With cartilage destruction, the carpal bones become crowded and adjacent bones tend to get involved. Intense demineralization is present in carpus, distal radius and ulna, metacarpals being usually spared. This serves as a differentiating feature from rheumatoid arthritis.

Biopsy of the wrist can be easily done from the dorsal route, when in doubt.

Sacroiliac Joints

These are affected more often in young adults than children and the involvement is usually unilateral. Sacroiliac (SI) joints infection is usually associated with tuberculosis of spine. Tenderness over the sacroiliac joint and compression and distraction tests are painful.

Radiographic features include irregularity and fuzziness of articular surfaces starting at the inferior surface. Sub-articular erosions may be present causing widening of joint space. Both the sclerosis and erosions predominate on the iliac side while punched out lesions may be seen in ilium or sacrum **(Figs. 18A to D)**.

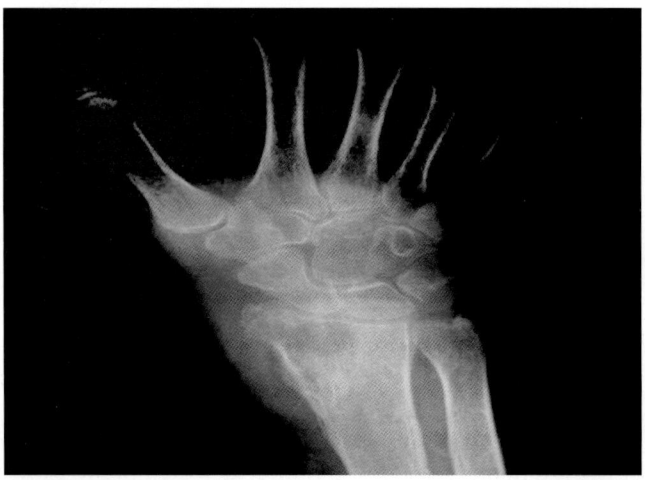

Fig. 17: Plain X-ray of right wrist joint showing irregular area of lytic destruction seen in distal metaphysis of radius with osteoporosis and soft tissue swelling.

Articular erosion cause widening of the joint space and infection is associated with abscess formation over the back of the joint which may later calcify. Tuberculosis at this uncommon site is frequently missed.[23] The cold abscess can be either intrapelvic or under the gluteus maximus muscle. Diagnosis is established by aspiration of pus or a fine needle aspiration biopsy. Antituberculosis therapy and protective bracing are the treatment of choice.

Magnetic resonance imaging is the ideal means of evaluating the complex anatomy of SI joints. Coronal imaging of the SI joints, parallel to the plane of the sacrum allows direct comparison of one SI joint to the other.[23,24]

Bone and joint tuberculosis occurs in 1–5% children who have untreated initial pulmonary tuberculosis. Spread to the skeletal system occurs during the initial infection via the lymphohematogenous route. The skeletal infection often becomes symptomatic within 1–3 years after the initial infection. Eighty-five percent of patients with tubercular dactylitis are younger than 6 years of age and its incidence among children with tubercular is reported to be 0.65–6.9%. Tubercular osteitis is one of the most common bacterial osteitis.

BCG is a vaccine of an attenuated bovine tubercular *Bacillus*. Although complications are unusual, generalized BCG infection and bone and joint infection can occur after BCG vaccination. Due to hematogenous spread of BCG infection to the skeleton, it is not usually associated with immunologic disorder and has a favorable prognosis.

Radiologically, BCG osteomyelitis affects children between 6 months and 6 years of age. It usually affects epiphysis and metaphysis of tubular bone especially around the knee, ribs, the sternum, the small bones of hand and feet. Lesions are more common on same side of the body as the vaccine was injected. Solitary lesions predominate and are seen as well-defined lytic foci.[1,8,23]

Diagnosis of osteitis after BCG vaccination is established according to criteria proposed by Foucard and Hjelmsted:

- BCG vaccination in the neonatal period
- A period of less than 4 years between vaccination and symptom onset
- No contact between the child and any adults with TB
- A consistent clinical profile
- Histopathology suggestive of TB.

TUBERCULOSIS OF LONG AND FLAT BONES

Tubercular Osteomyelitis

Tubercular osteomyelitis occurs in about 3% of patients with bone and joint tuberculosis. In 7% of them, the skeletal site of lesions are multiple. The most frequent

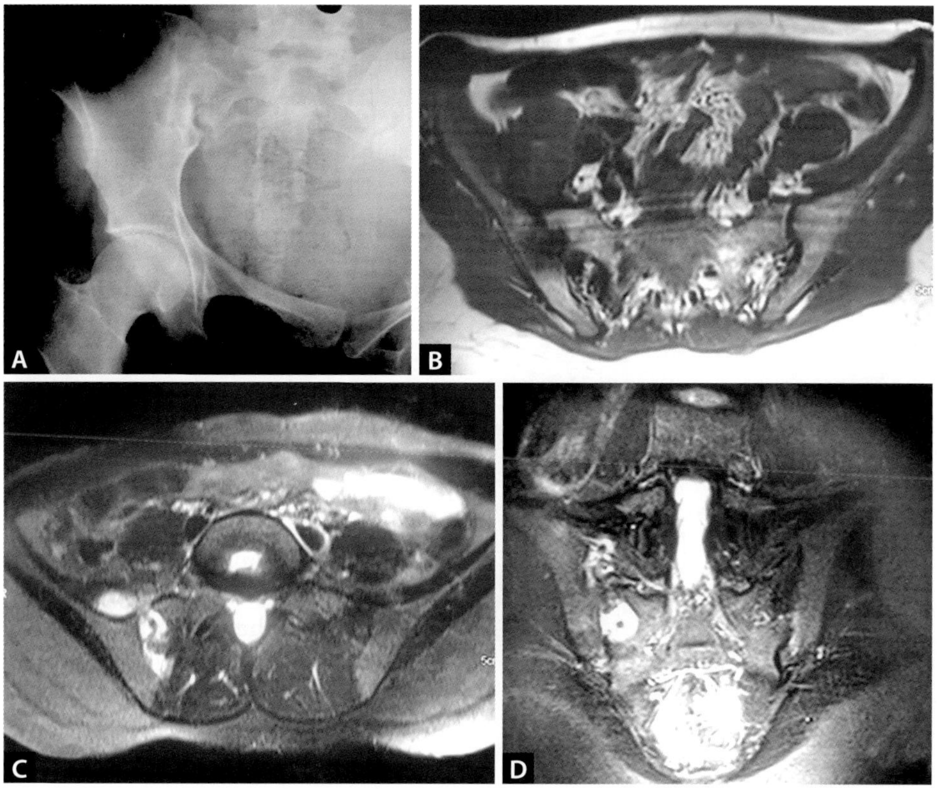

Figs. 18A to D: (A) Plain X-ray of pelvis showing large erosions with surrounding sclerosis at right sacroiliac joint; (B and C) Axial T1W and T2W images show hypointensity along iliac blade with hyperintense signal on T2 likely to be marrow edema with synovial proliferation with altered signal intensity in iliacus muscle; (D) STIR MR image showing hyperintense synovium in right sacroiliac joint.

sites are manubrium sterni, sternum and isolated spinous processes, spine of the scapula, ischium and fibula, but the diagnosis is frequently missed. The lesions tend to be simultaneous in onset and progression and generally affect persons with low immune resistance. Symmetric, well round, oval cystic lesions, with little or no periosteal reaction initially, may be present **(Fig. 19)**. In untreated cases, laminated periosteal reaction may be seen **(Figs. 20A to D)**. Sequestra formation is uncommon in adults, though in children large sequestra may be seen as the intraosseous vasculature is more prone to thrombosis. Joint involvement is rare as the lesions are diaphyseal or metaphyseal. Disseminated lesions may also present as bone cysts.[24,25] There is no sclerosis, abscess or sinus formation, so it is also called as closed cystic tuberculosis. A firm diagnosis can only be established by biopsy of the lesion. Antituberculosis regimens with curettage of the lesion are the treatment of choice.

Differential diagnosis includes polyostotic fibrous dysplasia, eosinophilic granuloma of the bone and enchondromatosis.

Isolated tubercular involvement of bone is rare (2–3% of all cases).

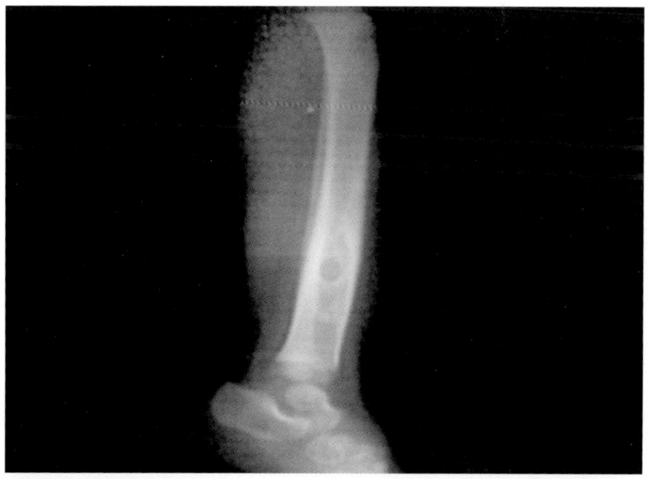

Fig. 19: Plain X-ray of right leg with ankle lateral view showing well-defined round osteolytic area seen in the shaft of tibia, in a case of diaphyseal tuberculosis.

Pathology

Bones are involved as a result of hematogenous spread from a primary focus, usually in the lung or the lymphatic system. Granulomatous lesion develops within the bone

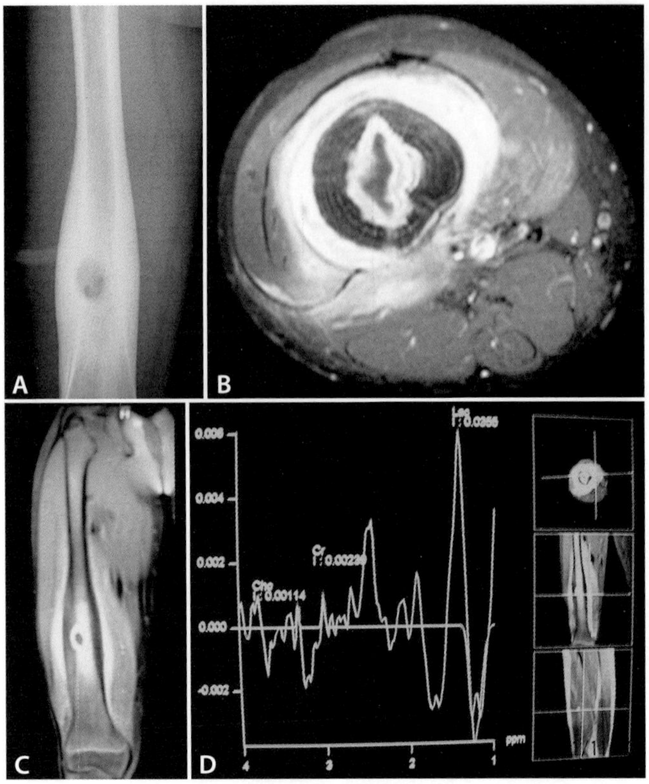

Figs. 20A to D: (A) Plain X-ray of right thigh showing well-defined round osteolytic area in the shaft of right femur, along with marked laminated periosteal reaction; (B and C) MR axial and coronal images showing intraosseous abscess in right femur, along with marked laminated periosteal reaction; (D) MR spectroscopic image showing prominent lactate peak in a case of diaphyseal tuberculosis.

at the site of deposition of the mycobacterium, usually metaphysis which is the site of infection. Earliest lesion appears as eccentric osteolytic lesion in the shaft near the epiphysis or metaphysis. Epiphyseal growth plate offers little resistance resulting in transphyseal spread of infections.

Two types of lesions have been described. Caseous exudative type in which there is destruction of bony trabeculae, softening and caseation necrosis followed by formation of tuberculous pus or cold abscess and granular type caries sicca where predominantly granulation tissue is formed with minimal caseation.

Tuberculosis of Long Bones

Two types of long bone TB occur:

1. Metaphyseal type in which oval or round focus in metaphysis ultimately crosses into the epiphysis and further to involve the joint, femur and tibia being the most commonly affected.
2. Cystic (diaphyseal type), it generally affects children and young adults. There is presence of well defined round or oval lytic areas involving and expanding the diaphysis. Large sequestra may be seen in diaphysis due to thrombosis of intraosseous vasculature in children. Tibia is the most common bone involved. Joint involvement is infrequent.

Solitary involvement is predominant although multifocal involvement can occur. Disseminated skeletal TB is rare, caused by widespread hematogenous dissemination.

Multiple cystic diaphyseal lesions can occur rarely. The condition is symmetrical in distribution with simultaneous onset, progression and regression. Multifocal tuberculous osteomyelitis also known as *osteitis cystica tuberculosa multiplex.*[25]

Multiple sites of involvement are seen in children, while in adults, involvement is more often confined to a single bone. The earliest lesion appears as an eccentric area of osteolysis in the metaphysis. Little or no surrounding reactive bone and local osteopenia are salient features.

The radiographic appearance may be somewhat different in children as compared to adults. In young patients, the lesions may be symmetrical and favor metaphyseal region. They are usually osteolytic and well defined, without sclerosis, and may show variable size while in adults, the lesions are smaller, located in the long axis of bone and may show well-defined sclerotic margins.

On MRI, early focus of altered marrow signal with irregular margins and cortical invasion with ill defined soft tissue may be seen. Eccentric lesion with cortical breach may show irregular breach or hyperintensity within the cortical black line while small communicating abscesses are better appreciated on postcontrast T1W images as enhancing rings of juxtacortical inflammatory tissue and are a strong predictor of tuberculosis.

Flat Bones

Ribs

Rib involvement is seen in about two percent cases of bone tuberculosis, adults being generally affected. Nearly one-third of patients will have pulmonary tuberculosis or tuberculosis at other sites. Patients may present with pain, tenderness and fluctuant chest wall swelling. There is bony rib expansion with punched out lesions and destruction which may be poorly marginated, posterior half of ribs being most commonly affected. Associated extrapleural soft tissue abscesses are commonly seen, e.g. cold abscesses tracking from spinal lesion **(Fig. 21)**. The abscess may present as chest wall discharging sinus.[5,7]

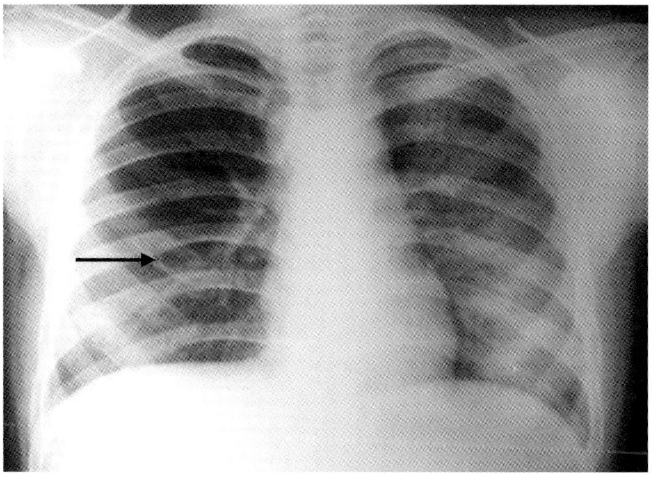

Fig. 21: Plain X-ray of chest showing lytic lesion involving anterior end of right 3rd rib in a case of rib tuberculosis.

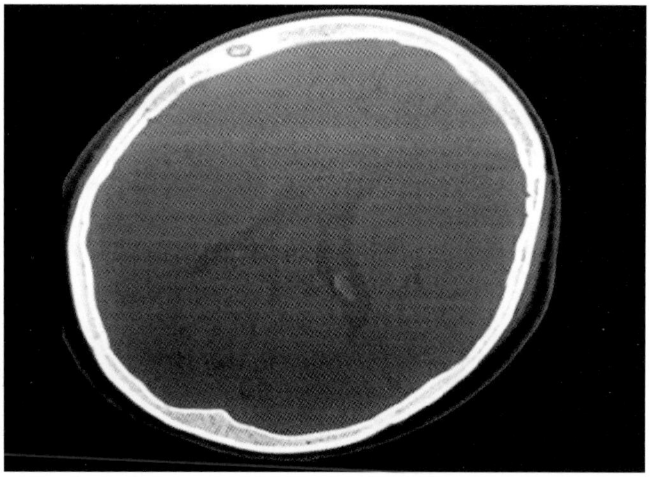

Fig. 22: Plain CT scan of cranium showing button sequestrum in the right parietal bone.

Scapula

Scapula is a rare site for tubercular infection. The infective focus may be present in acromion, spine, neck, superior or inferior angle of scapula. Patient presents with pain and swelling. CT and MRI are helpful in early detection of lesions.[23,24]

Sternum

Sternum is uncommonly involved, in about one and a half percent of cases. An irregular destructive lesion along with presence of retrosternal and presternal soft tissues mass may be seen. There is paucity of sclerosis or periostitis.[24]

Skull

Frontal bone is the most common site to be involved in bones of cranial vault. Ill-defined lytic lesion may be the only radiological feature seen with overlying cold abscess (Potts' Puffy tumor). Button sequestrum can also be sometimes seen **(Fig. 22)**. Facial bones and mandibular involvement is extremely rare.[8,9]

Pelvis

Isolated tubercular lesion may occur in iliac bone, ischial tuberosity and ischiopubic ramus. Ischial tuberosity involvement with the syndrome was earlier recognized as "weaver's bottom" in which the overlying bursa was inflamed with secondary involvement of bone. Concomitant involvement of sacroiliac joints is common. Radiologically, lytic lesions without surrounding sclerosis or periosteal reaction may be seen. Infection may extend to involve pubic symphysis **(Fig. 23)**.

Sternoclavicular Joint

Tuberculosis of the sternoclavicular joint is rare. It is usually seen in region of medial end and presents with a painful swelling. Cold abscess and sinus can result as a complication. MRI can be a useful modality to detect early erosions and associated soft tissue swelling. Biopsy may be necessary in doubtful cases. Differential diagnosis includes rheumatoid arthritis, multiple myeloma, metastasis and low-grade pyogenic infections.[11,14,24]

Acromioclavicular Joint

Tuberculosis of the acromioclavicular joint is also rare. It is usually seen in region of lateral end and presents with a painful swelling.[24]

Clavicle may rarely be involved without of adjoining joints. There may be diffuse thickening and honeycombing, multiple cystic cavities and sequestra formation like pyogenic infections. Biopsy may be necessary to confirm diagnosis.

TUBERCULOSIS OF SHORT BONES

Tuberculosis of short tubular bones is referred to as tubercular dactylitis. It is primarily a disease of childhood. The disease tends to affect short tubular bones distal to tarsus and wrist. The bones of the hands are more frequently affected than bones of the feet, proximal phalanx of the index and middle fingers and metacarpals of the middle and ring fingers being the most frequent locations.

Clinical features include soft tissue swelling, which may be followed by pain and numbness. They quite frequently

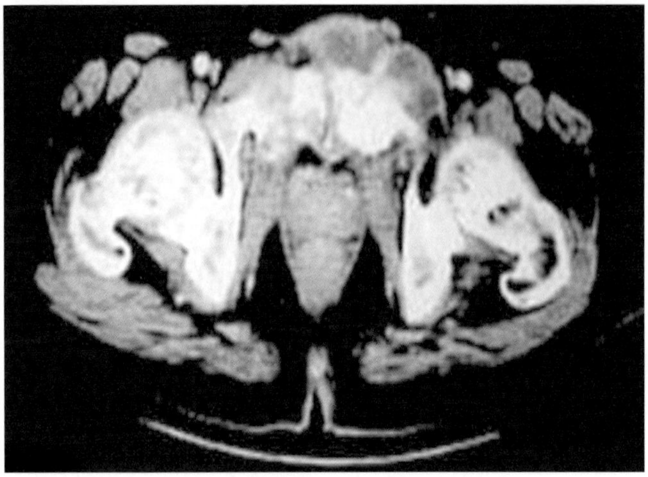

Fig. 23: Axial CT image showing bilateral pubic bone erosions with subcutaneous small cold abscess.

present as marked swelling on the dorsum of the hand and soft tissue abscess is normally a common feature.

Monostotic involvement is common, but multiple peripheral lesions may occur in 25% cases. It often follows a benign course without pyrexia and acute inflammatory signs, as opposed to acute osteomyelitis. Plain radiography is the modality of choice for evaluation and follow-up.

The radiographic features of cystic expansion of the short tubular bones have led to the name of "spina ventosa" being given to tubercular dactylitis of the short bones of the hand. This condition was first described by Boyer and Nelaton.[23] The term spina ventosa is derived from spina meaning short bone and ventosa meaning expanded with air.

Initial bony lesion is in the bone marrow. The disease is characterized by bone destruction and fusiform expansion of the bone large accompanied with raft fissure swelling. It is most marked in diaphysis of metacarpals and metatarsals in children. Periosteal reaction and sequestra are uncommon. Healing is gradual by sclerosis.[24]

Magnetic resonance imaging may demonstrate intraosseous involvement earlier than the other imaging modalities **(Figs. 24A and B)**.

This condition needs to be differentiated from syphilitic dactylitis in which there is bilateral and symmetric involvement, more periostitis, less soft tissue swelling and less sequestrations. Chronic pyogenic osteomyelitis and mycotic lesions in the foot bones have to be differentiated. The differential diagnosis also includes sarcoidosis, hemoglobinopathies and hyperparathyroidism.[24] Debridement and antitubercular regimen result in complete subsidence of the lesion.

Tuberculosis of Tendon Sheaths and Bursae

Any tendon sheath or bursa can be involved in tuberculosis. The most common sites are flexor tendon sheaths of hand, subacromial bursa, olecranon bursa and bursae under the medial head of gastrocnemius. In the volar aspect of the wrist, the classical presentation is a dumb-bell shaped swelling giving cross fluctuation and crepitus, due to melon seed bodies which are agglutinated protein nodules. The spread to these sites is normally from the neighboring bone or joint but it could be due to hematogenous spread. It can also occur from gravitational spread of the disease from the diseased area.[25]

Primary investigation to confirm the diagnosis of tenosynovitis and to reveal the degree and extent of tendon and tendon sheath involvement is ultrasonography. Sonograms can be quickly obtained along virtually any orientation and very high frequency transducers provide exquisite special and contrast resolution.

In chronic tenosynovitis, tendon and synovial thickening predominate, with relatively little synovial sheath effusion while in acute suppurative tenosynovitis, synovial sheath effusion is the predominant feature.[25]

Magnetic resonance imaging helps in delineating the precise extent of soft tissue involvement and any associated osseous or joint involvement. Three stages of tuberculous tenosynovitis have been described:

1. The hygromatous stage is characterized by the presence of fluid inside the tendon sheath without associated sheath thickening.
2. The serofibrinous stage is characterized by thickening of the flexor tendons and synovium, with multiple tiny hypointense nodules within the hyperintense synovial fluid on T2W images. These tiny nodules correspond to the rice bodies.
3. The fungoid stage is characterized by a soft tissue mass involving the tendon and tendon sheath.

Among bursal infections the most commonly affected locations are trochanteric, subacromial, subgluteal, and radioulnar wrist bursa.

Plain radiography may demonstrate local osteopenia due to hyperemia in long-standing bursitis or focal osteolytic bone destruction (e.g. greater trochanter or the humeral head) due to local pressure of the enlarged bursa. The wall of the distended bursa may contain calcifications, which may be visible on radiographs.[8,25]

On MRI, two patterns of involvement have been reported. A uniform distension of the bursa or multiple small abscesses in the bursa may be seen or low signal intensity material within the fluid-filled bursa on T2W

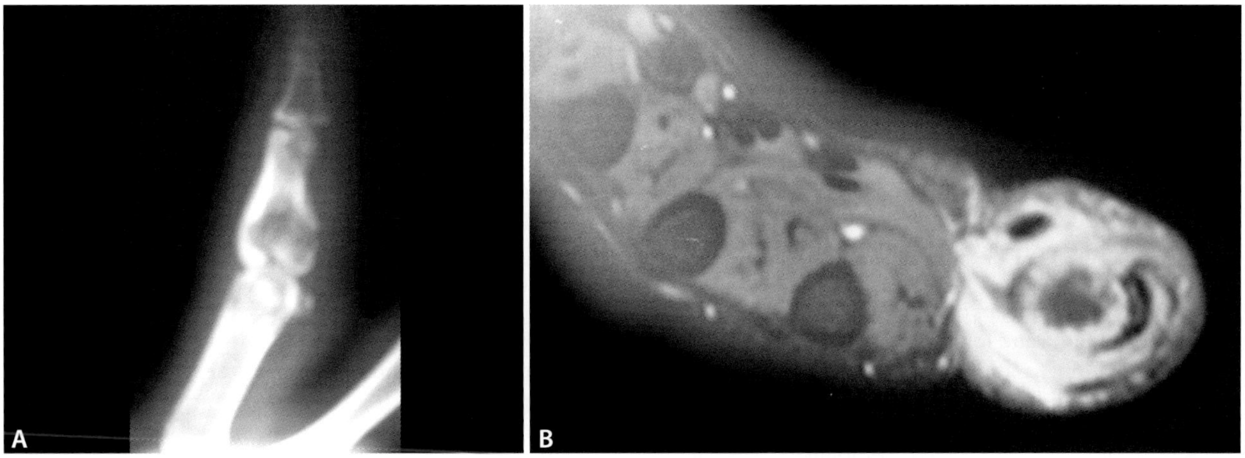

Figs. 24A and B: (A) Plain X-ray of right thumb showing cystic expansile lesion of the proximal shaft of proximal phalanx of right thumb with pathological fracture; (B) MRI of the same patient showing bone marrow inflammation along with marked enhancing synovium on postgadolinium images in a biopsy proven case of tuberculosis.

images may be seen due to the presence of caseous necrosis and fibrotic material.

Antituberculosis regimes coupled with excision of the synovial sheath and bursae are the treatment of choice.

Atypical Mycobacterial Infection

Infection due to atypical mycobacteria are also seen in specific clinical setting. Skin and pulmonary diseases are most frequent, however, skeletal changes may also be noted. The infection may be seen in immunocompromised patients, those with renal transplants or those receiving cortico steroids. Infection can lead to osteomyelitis, septic arthritis, tenosynovitis and bursitis.[20,23,25]

Radiologically, multiple lesions may be seen; metaphysis and diaphysis of long bones being usually affected. Discrete lesions may be present with sclerotic margins but osteoporosis is not marked. Abscesses and sinus tract can also be seen.

Tubercular Infection of Prosthetic Joint

Prosthetic joint infection may develop due to reactivation of tubercular arthritis for which the operation had been performed.[26] Arthrocentesis and specimens are required for establishing the diagnosis.

CONCLUSION

It is difficult to diagnose the disease in its earliest stage as the clinical and radiologic findings are nonspecific in initial stages. We should have a high level of clinical suspicion as the disease is endemic in our country. At this stage, cross-sectional imaging and histological examination can lead to correct diagnosis. In advanced cases, diagnosis is not much of a problem and imaging helps in supplementing and guiding therapeutic procedures.

REFERENCES

1. Yochum TR, Row LJ. Infection: non-suppurative osteomyelitis (tuberculosis). In: Essentials of Skeletal Radiology, 2nd edn. Williams and Wilkins; 1996.
2. Moore SL, Rafii M. Imaging of musculoskeletal and spinal tuberculosis. Radiol Clin N Am. 2001;39(2):329-42.
3. Bhan S, Nag HL. Skeletal tuberculosis. In: Surendra K Sharma: Tuberculosis, 2nd edn, Jaypee Brothers Medical Publishers (P) Ltd; 2009.pp.342-72.
4. Sawlani V, Chandra T, Mishra RN, et al. MRI features of Tuberculosis of peripheral joints. Clin Radiol. 2003;58:755-62.
5. Grainger and Allison's Vol 3, 4th edn: Churchill Livingstone Reprinted Edition; 2005.pp.2069-70.
6. Adam Greenspan. Orthopedic Imaging—A practical approach, 4th edn. Lippincott Williams and Wilkins; 2004. pp.798-9.
7. Tuli SM. Tuberculosis of the skeletal system. New Delhi: Jaypee Brothers Medical Publishers (P) Ltd; 1997.
8. David Sutton (Ed). Textbook of Radiology and Imaging Vol 2, 7th edn: Churchill Livingstone; 2003.pp.1166-71.
9. Donald Resnik, Mark J. Kransdorf: Bone and Joint Imaging, 3rd edn. Elsevier Saunders; 2005.pp.758-65.
10. Riddley N, Shaikh MI, Remedios, et al. Radiology of skeletal tuberculosis. Orthopedics. 1998;21(11):1213-20.
11. John Ebnezar. Textbook of Orthopedics, 3rd edn. Jaypee Brothers Medical Publishers (P) Ltd; 2006.pp.499-519.
12. Morris BS, Varma R, Garg A, et al. Multifocal musculo-skeletal tuberculosis in children: Appearances on computed tomography. Skeletal Radiology. 2002;31:1-8.

13. Yago Y, Yukihiro M, Kuroki H, Katsuragawa Y, Kubota K. Cold tubercular abscess identified by FDG PET. Ann Nucl Med. 2005;19:515-8.
14. Griffith JF, Kumta SM, Leung PC, et al. Imaging of musculoskeletal tuberculosis: A new look at old disease. Clinical Orthopedics and Related Research. 2002;398:32-9.
15. Babhulkar SS, Pande S. Tuberculosis of the hip. Clinical Orthopedics. 2002;398:93-9.
16. Shanmugasundaram TK. A clinicoradiological classification of tuberculosis of hip. In: Shanmugasundaram TK (Ed). Current concepts in bone joint tuberculosis. Madras: International Bone and Joint Club; 1983.
17. Hoffman EB, Allin J, Campbell JAB, et al. Tuberculosis of the knee. Clinical Orthopedics. 2002;398:100-6.
18. Lee AS, Campbell JAB, Hoffman EB. Tuberculosis of the knee in children. J Bone Joint Surg Br. 1995;77-B:313-8.
19. Dhillon MS, Nagi ON. Tuberculosis of foot and ankle. Clin Orthopedic. 2002;398:107-13.
20. Singh NV. Fundamental of Orthopedics, 1st edn, New Age International Publishers; 2011.pp.236-44.
21. Malaviya AN, Kotwal PP. Arthritis associated with tuberculosis. Best Practice Res Clin Rheumatol. 2003;17:319-43.
22. Gardam M, Lim S. Mycobacterial osteomyelitis and arthritis. Infect Dis Clin North Am. 2005;19:819-30.
23. Harisinghani GM, McLoud TC, Shepard JO, et al. Tuberculosis from head to toe. Radiographics. 2000;20(2):449-70.
24. Babhulkar SS, Pande S. Unusual manifestations of osteoarticular tuberculosis. Clinical Orthopedics. 2002;398:93-9.
25. Boutin RD, Brossmann J, Sartoris DJ, et al. Update on Imaging of Orthopedic Infections. Orthopedic Clinics of North America. 1998;29(1):41-65.
26. Kaya M, Nagoya S, Yamashita, Niiro N, Fujita M. Periprosthetic infection of the hip in a patient with no previous history of tuberculosis. J Bone Joint Surg Br. 2006;88:394-5.

CHAPTER 191

Nontubercular Bone and Joint Infections

Manphool Singhal, Niranjan Khandelwal

INTRODUCTION

Osteomyelitis refers to the infection of cortical bone and its marrow space. It is classified into three forms: acute, subacute and chronic. Subacute osteomyelitis is comparatively more insidious in presentation than the acute form. Chronic osteomyelitis is a continuous low-grade recurring infection. The pathogens responsible for osteomyelitis can be bacteria, viruses, mycobacteria or treponemes (syphilis). Most common among these is pyogenic osteomyelitis.[1,2] Plain radiographs, scintigraphy, ultrasonography (USG), computed tomography (CT) and magnetic resonance imaging (MRI), all are crucial in the diagnosis of osteomyelitis, but overall diagnostic accuracy does not exceed 80–90%.[3] Presence of previous or chronic osteomyelitis, adjoining soft tissue infection, fracture, surgery and prosthesis are some of the factors which create difficulty in the diagnosis.

IMAGING MODALITIES

Plain radiographs are the first imaging study required in the work-up of osteomyelitis. If cortical irregularity, periosteal reaction, deep soft tissue swelling and demineralization are detected, there might be no need for additional imaging to diagnose osteomyelitis.[3] However, merely 5% of radiographs are positive in the early course of disease. Less than one-third reveal abnormality by one week while 90% are positive only after 3–4 weeks.[4] This delay restricts the utility of plain radiographs in the early diagnosis of osteomyelitis.

Computed tomography has more advantages than conventional radiographs in terms of early detection of bony changes, better visualization of axial skeletal involvement (e.g. spine, pelvis, sternum) and better delineation of overlapping bony abnormalities like thick periosteal reaction or sequestra in chronic osteomyelitis.

Radionuclide scintigraphy is the most sensitive investigation available for the diagnosis of acute osteomyelitis though the specificity is not as good.[3] ^{99m}Tc labeled methylene diphosphonate (^{99m}Tc-MDP), hydroxymethylene diphosphonate (^{99m}Tc HMDP) and gallium 67 (^{67}Ga) citrate are the most commonly used radionuclide agents. The sensitivity and specificity for combined ^{99m}Tc ^{67}Ga scanning are 50% and 78%, respectively.[5] Indium 111 labeled leukocyte scanning (^{111}In WBC) has a higher sensitivity and specificity of 83% and 94%, respectively. Recently introduced Indium 111 labeled polyclonal immunoglobulin (IgG) has the highest sensitivity and specificity of 92% and 95–100%, respectively.[6,7]

Now with the advent of high resolution sonography equipment *ultrasonography* (USG) is being increasingly used for diagnosis of acute osteomyelitis. Positive findings can be detected much earlier than on plain radiographs. Deep soft tissue swelling is the earliest sign which can be detected within 2–3 days of onset. The other changes include periosteal elevation seen as a hyperechoic line and subperiosteal fluid collection **(Fig. 1)**. Cortical breech is seen as a focal defect in the cortex.[8] In a prospective study of 25 patients done to assess the role of ultrasound

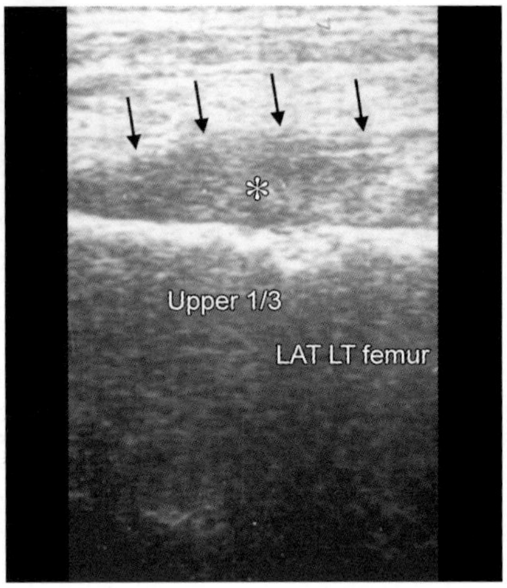

Fig. 1: Acute osteomyelitis: High resolution USG of femur shows periosteal elevation (hyperechoic line) with subperiosteal fluid collection (*).

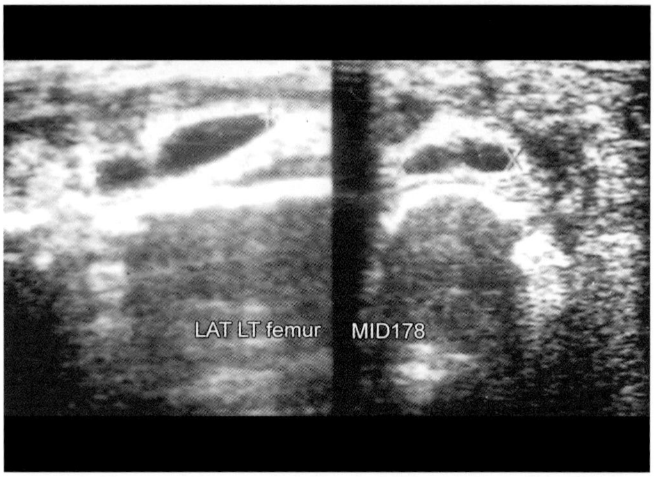

Fig. 2: High-resolution ultrasonography (USG) of femur (longitudinal and transverse) shows periosseous fluid collection in acute osteomyelitis.

in acute osteomyelitis, the authors found the presence of deep soft tissue swelling periosseous fluid **(Fig. 2)** and periosteal elevation has positive predictive value of 100% in first three days after the onset of symptoms.[9]

Ultrasonography is also an excellent method to detect presence of fluid in the joint which may be an indirect sign to suggest osteomyelitis especially of femur and humerus in an infant. In reactivation of chronic osteomyelitis, USG can demonstrate abscess or sinus tract formation in soft tissues which are characteristic of acute osteomyelitis. Ultrasonography guidance can also used for percutaneous aspiration of fluid from the joint or periosteal collection for diagnostic purposes **(Fig. 3)**.

Magnetic resonance imaging due to its multiplannar imaging capability, excellent tissue characterization and high resolution is now the imaging modality of choice for the early diagnosis of osteomyelitis and overlying soft tissue involvement.[10] It has a sensitivity and specificity of 92–100% and 89–100% respectively.[11] MRI is better than scintigraphy in evaluation of axial skeletal osteomyelitis because of better anatomical delineation.[12] In addition, MRI can distinguish soft tissue infection with periostitis from osteomyelitis.[13] More over the complications of osteomyelitis like soft-tissue and bone abscesses, physeal involvement, and septic arthritis can also be diagnosed which can help in further management, such as determining the need for percutaneous or surgical drainage in addition to antibiotic therapy.[14-16]

ACUTE OSTEOMYELITIS

Acute osteomyelitis is usually hematogenous in origin and generally follows skin infection. *Staphylococcus aureus* is the most common offending pathogen. Common age of presentation is 2–16 years with a male preponderance, the latter being attributed to greater exposure to trauma.

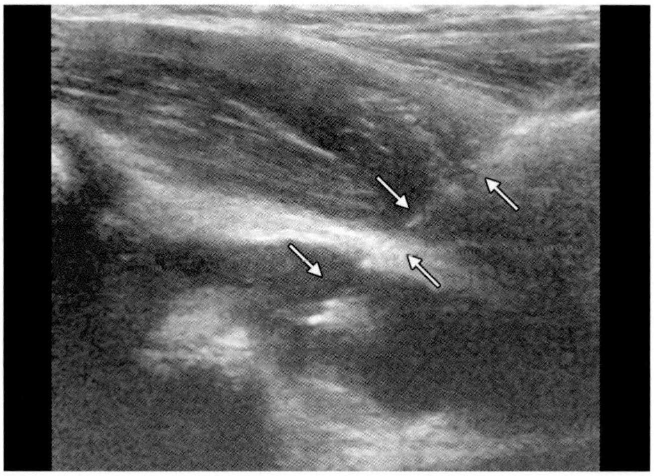

Fig. 3: USG-guided percutaneous aspiration of periosteal fluid. Note the needle *in situ* (arrows).

Clinical Features

The Clinical features differ in infants, children and adults, due to the structural and vascular differences of bone at these ages. The blood borne microbial emboli lodge in the metaphysis because of sluggish blood flow in this region. In children older than one year the epiphyseal plate hinders further extension of the infection **(Fig. 4)**, so the infection spreads laterally into the subperiosteal space or to the joint in which synovial reflections extend beyond the epiphysis to metaphysis, such as the shoulder and hip joints. In infants, small capillaries cross the epiphyseal

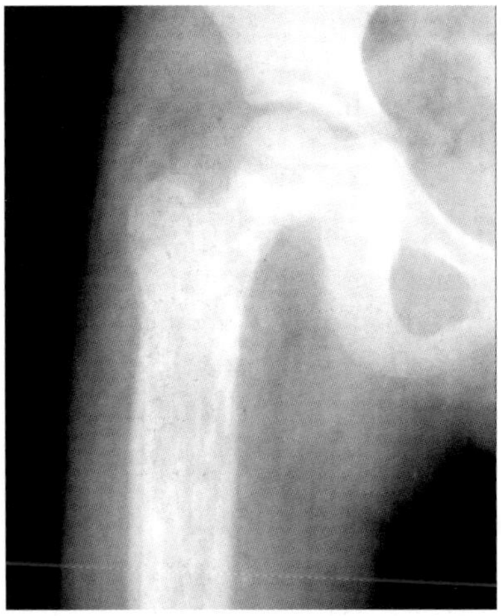

Fig. 4: Chronic osteomyelitis in a child: Radiograph of the right hip showing diffuse ill-defined lytic areas affecting the entire upper shaft of femur with cortical thickening. Note the sparing of epiphysis and the joint.

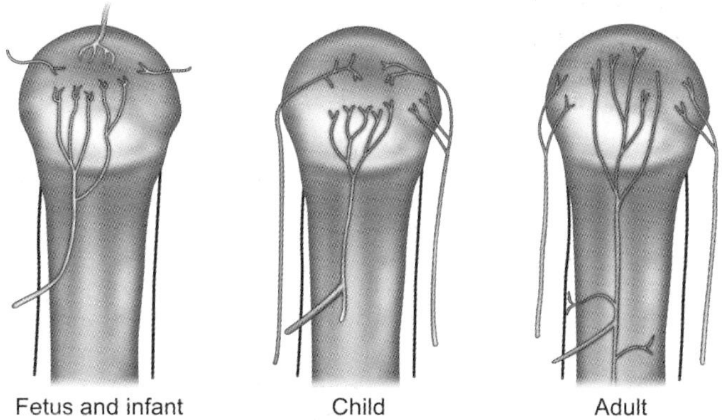

Fig. 5: Schematic diagram of vascular supply of the epimetaphyseal region in the infant, child and adult.

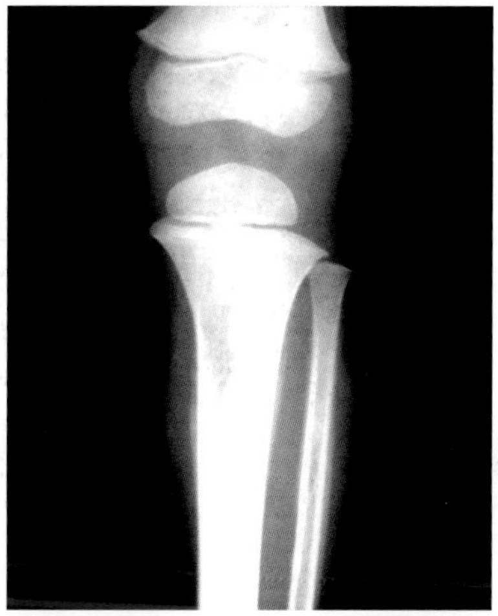

Fig. 6: Acute osteomyelitis of tibia: Radiograph of leg shows small lucencies in the metaphysis along with thin periosteal reaction.

growth plate, and thus, allow the infection to extend to the epiphysis and the joint. In adults, the epiphyseal plate is fused and thus, it fails to block the spread of infection from metaphysis to the adjacent joint. Thus, acute pyogenic arthritis is a frequent complication of osteomyelitis in infants and adults **(Fig. 5)**.

The infarcted bone is reabsorbed by formation of granulation tissue and the dead cortex usually forms sequestrum. Reparative new bone formation starts roughly 10 days after the onset of infection, and new bone is generally laid down along both periosteal and endosteal surfaces resulting in formation of involucrum. Cloacae appear at the site of dead periosteum.

Neonatal osteomyelitis offers few clinical signs despite multiple sites of its involvement, and hence, a complete skeletal survey is warranted in such cases.[17] Premature infants requiring umbilical catheterization are at higher risk for osteomyelitis.[18] Radionuclide bone scintigraphy is advocated in all patients with suspected neonatal osteomyelitis, following initial radiographs.[19]

A soft tissue component, subperiosteal abscess and dense involucrum are more striking in infants than in adults and children. This has been attributed to less rigid bone of infants and easy penetration of periosteum by the abscess.

Radiologic Features

The earliest radiographic changes are seen 7–10 days after onset of infection in the form of soft tissue swelling and small single or multiple osteolytic areas affecting the metaphysis **(Fig. 6)**. This is followed by elevation of the periosteum and layered new bone formation after 3–6 weeks. The periosteal reaction is typically lamellar and nodular.[2] The dead bone (sequestrum) also forms at 3–8 weeks. It appears dense since it does not participate in normal bone mineral metabolism because of loss of its vascular supply. Osteopenia in the surrounding bone due to hyperemia, enhances the density of the sequestrum. Once the acute phase has subsided, remodeling reverts the appearance of bone to normal in infants and children but sclerosis and cortical irregularity persists in adults.

Patients with sickle cell disease have an unusual propensity for *Salmonella* osteomyelitis. This infection is diaphyseal and difficult to differentiate from a bone infarct. Localized cortical fissuring or tunneling is a characteristic and early feature of this entity.[20]

The bone scintigraphy shows positive findings much earlier than plain radiographs, usually within 3 days and sometimes within 24 hours of onset of infection. Traditionally, "triple phase" bone scanning is done, using technetium ^{99m}Tc agents. The first phase shows the "blood flow", the second phase shows the "blood pool" of the inflamed region and the third phase, which is acquired after 2–4 hours, shows the uptake by bone. Osteomyelitis is "hot" on all phases. However, in patients presenting within 48 hours, the isotope bone scan may reveal a "cold" spot on account of vasospasm. A false-positive result can occur in degenerative disease, healing fracture and loose prosthesis. But these conditions do not show increased activity in early (I and II) phases, unlike osteomyelitis. Deep soft tissue infection with periostitis and diabetic osteopathy also cannot be differentiated from osteomyelitis on the basis of bone scanning alone.[3] MRI is considered superior to bone scan in distinguishing these two entities.

Magnetic resonance imaging is the modality of choice for early diagnosis of osteomyelitis. MRI features of osteomyelitis include low signal intensity on T1-weighted image and high-signal intensity on T2-weighted and fluid-sensitive images (fat-suppressed T2-weighted and STIR sequences) with postcontrast enhancement **(Figs. 7A to C)**. Intraosseous, subperiosteal, and soft-tissue abscesses, if present appear as well-circumscribed areas of focally decreased signal intensity on T1-weighted images with increased signal intensity equal to that of fluid on fluid sensitive sequences and rim enhancement on contrast T1-weighted images.[14,21,22]

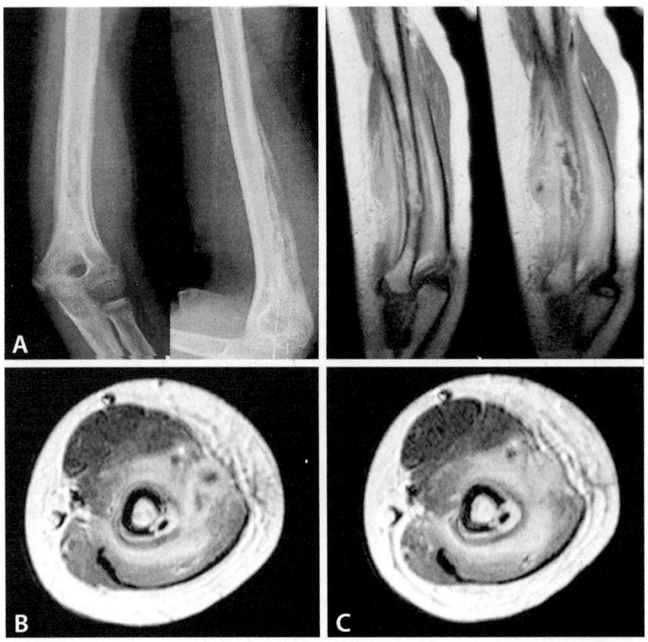

Figs. 7A to C: Acute osteomyelitis: Plain X-rays (A) show smooth periosteal reaction with cortical irregularity in the lower third of humerus. Postcontrast MR images sagittal (B) and axial (C) show cortical irregularity with break in the outline and periosseous fluid collection with increased signal in the adjacent soft tissues.

Magnetic resonance imaging has also been shown to be more sensitive and specific than isotope bone scanning in the detection, localization, and differentiation of osteomyelitis, cellulitis and abscess. Cellulitis and osteomyelitis may have similar soft tissue changes. However, in cellulitis, the bone is normal.[23]

LOCALIZED OSTEOMYELITIS (BRODIE'S ABSCESS)

Localized osteomyelitis or Brodie's abscess is a limited osteomyelitis caused either by organisms of low virulence or high resistance in the host. Most frequently, it occurs at one end of the bone, but it may also occur in the diaphysis. It is seen as a well-circumscribed osteolytic focus surrounded by a sclerotic margin **(Figs. 8A to C)**. Occasionally, a meta-physeal serpiginous channel with sclerotic border marks the tract of infection. This feature is considered characteristic of nontubercular etiology like *Staphylococcus, Streptococcus* or *Haemophilus*.[2] When the lesion is small, it may be difficult to identify on plain radiographs and CT/MRI may be required.

The close differential diagnosis of Brodie's abscess is an osteoid osteoma as on imaging both these condition closely simulate each other (T2 hyperintense nidus, sclerotic rim and bone edema), however, on T1-weighted MRI scans a 'penumbra sign' has been described as a discrete peripheral zone of marginally higher signal intensity than the abscess cavity and surrounding marrow edema/sclerosis, and of lower signal intensity than fatty bone marrow, which often enhances after contrast. This has been postulated to be due to the presence of active, vascular, inflammatory granulation tissue around the abscess.[24]

CHRONIC OSTEOMYELITIS

Chronic bone infections usually result from inadequately treated acute osteomyelitis or from infection following compound bone fractures. Pain, local swelling, discharge from wound, sinus formation and systemic signs and symptoms (fever, malaise, nausea and vomiting) may be present.

Conventional radiographs show cloacae, involucrum or sequestrum **(Figs. 9 and 10)**. There are sclerotic and lucent areas admixed with bony thickening and deformities. The radiographic impression regarding the

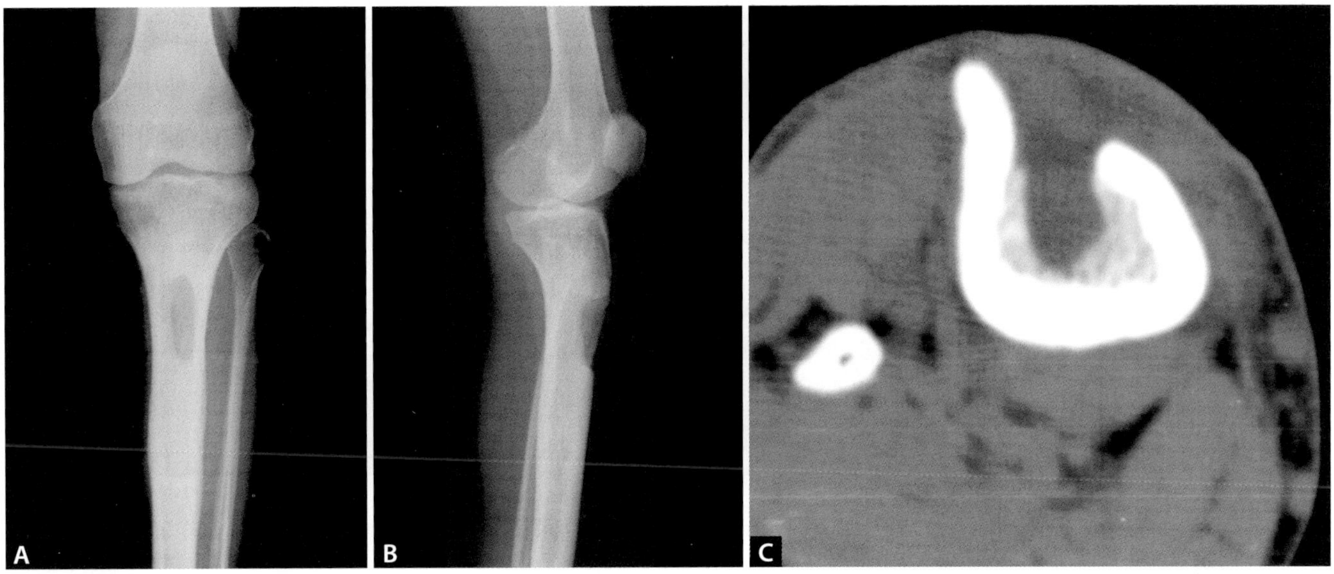

Figs. 8A to C: Plain X-ray (A and B) axial CT (C) showing Brodie's abscess in the upper end of tibia.

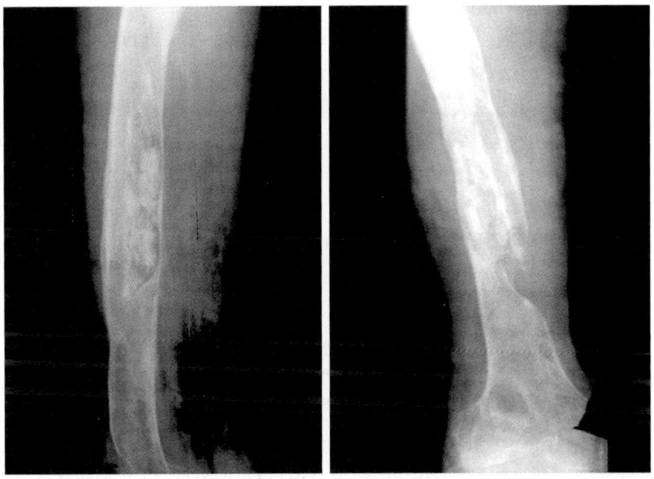

Fig. 9: Chronic osteomyelitis of the femoral bone: Diaphyseal lucent areas represent cloacae formation with sequestrum seen as radiodense opacities.

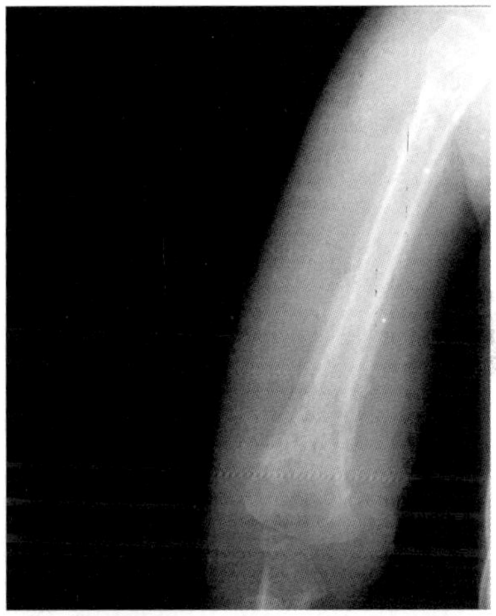

Fig. 10: Chronic osteomyelitis: Radiograph of right arm showing involucrum surrounding distal two-thirds of humerus.

activity of infectious process is often equivocal, and one relies heavily on clinical findings such as the presence of a sinus tract.[25] At times, it is imperative to review previous films as it may be difficult to differentiate inactive and active chronic osteomyelitis. In osteomyelitis of the skull, typically no sclerosis is seen **(Figs. 11A and B)**.

Scintigraphy is more useful in determining activity. Routine ^{99m}Tc-MDP scanning shows increased uptake, but is often non-diagnostic, since even after 1–2 years following successful treatment, a positive isotope bone scan is not uncommon.[3] ^{67}Ga has been recommended as the optimal agent. Following successful treatment ^{67}Ga uptake should decrease to a normal level.

MRI has been advocated as the imaging modality to distinguish regions of active infection from uninvolved marrow or fibrotic regions representing scars from previous infection or trauma.[25] Active foci of infection tend to have a low-to-intermediate signal intensity on T1W and high-signal intensity on T2W and fluid sensitive images which is in marked contrast to the low-signal of thickened, surrounding bone.[25,26]

Magnetic resonance imaging findings correspond to the pathologic features. On MR images the *involucrum*, manifests as a well-defined rim of low-signal intensity on all sequences surrounding the infected bone marrow.

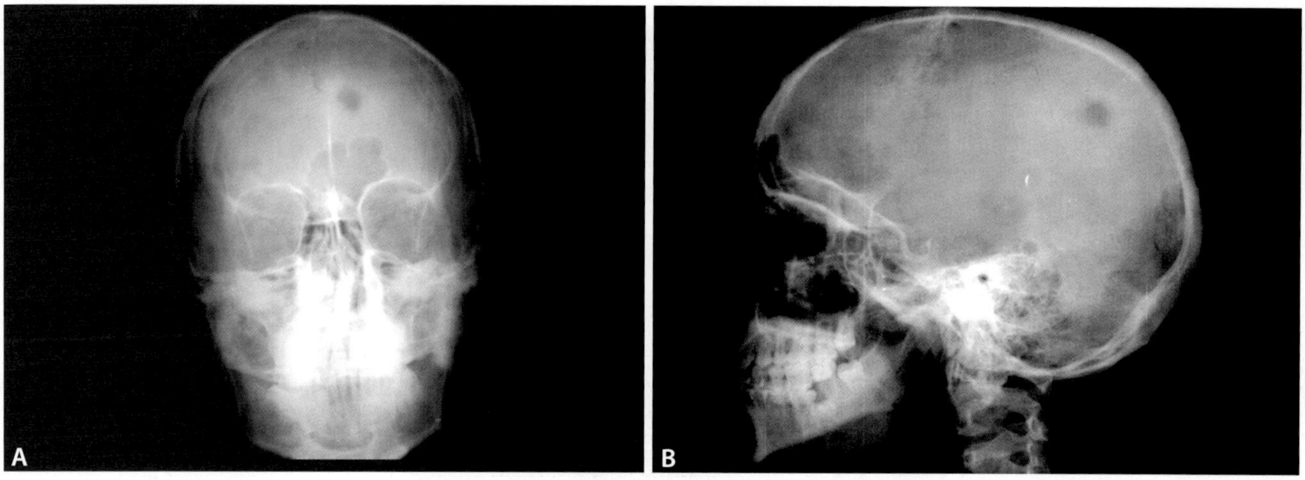

Figs. 11A and B: Chronic osteomyelitis of skull vault: (A) Anteroposterior and (B) lateral skull radiographs showing multiple lytic areas with no surrounding sclerosis.

Granulation tissue surrounding the infection appears as hypointense on T1W images, hyperintense on T2W and STIR images, and shows enhancement after Gd-DTPA.

Sequestrum is an isolated fragment of devitalized bone within an area of active infection shows signal intensity that of a sequestrum in all sequences.

Sinus tract is identified as a linear or curvilinear area of low-signal on T1W and high-signal on T2-weighted and STIR images extending in contiguity from the medullary cavity, with disruption of the cortex, to the skin.

Soft-tissue inflammation is visible as a bright signal on T2W and STIR images, which enhances after contrast. Sometimes soft-tissue abscess may also develop **(Figs. 12A to D)**.[25,26]

SCLEROSING OSTEOMYELITIS OF GARRE

Sclerosing osteomyelitis of Garre is a rare type of chronic osteomyelitis occurring in children and young adults, presenting with insidious onset of local pain. Symptoms recur at intervals for several years and then subside gradually. There is a predilection for involvement of mandible and shafts of long bones. Radiological appearance is of intense sclerosis resulting in thickened bone **(Fig. 13)**. Areas of frank bony destruction are rare. It is distinguished from Ewing's tumor by the absence of lamellations of periosteal reaction and permeative bone destruction.

SYPHILIS OF BONE

Syphilis is caused by *Treponema pallidum* and is of three types:

1. Congenital syphilis, present at birth or in early infancy
2. Late congenital syphilis
3. Acquired syphilis.

Congenital (Infantile) Syphilis

Congenital (infantile) syphilis is a systemic disease due to transplacental transmission of the spirochetes. Clinical features include, fever, failure to thrive, saddle nose, Hutchinson's teeth, etc. Serologic diagnostic tests include VDRL, FTA and ABS tests. Osseous abnormalities include luetic metaphysitis, diaphysitis and periostitis. Radiologically, the earliest change is in the metaphysis, with widening of the zone of provisional calcification. The epiphyseal plate appears wide and dense. The outstanding feature is symmetrical involvement of multiple bones especially at the upper end of tibia and lower end of femur. Symmetrical destruction of medial portion of the proximal tibial meta-physis (Wimberger's sign) is common and pathognomonic of syphilis **(Fig. 14)**.

The earliest diaphyseal change is focal cortical destruction. Later there may be extensive destruction of bone. Periosteal reaction can be solid or lamellated. In the skull, irregular, osteolytic lesions are seen.

Late Congenital Syphilis

In this condition, syphilitic bony lesions do not become evident until childhood or early adult life. The lesions are due to gumma or syphilitic endarteritis. There is minimal bone destruction which is overshadowed by extensive new bone proliferation. This results in diffuse thickening of cortical bone and lamellated periosteal reaction. This lesion causes typical thickening of the upper half of tibial cortex anteriorly and is called "Sabre tibia" **(Fig. 15)**.

Acquired Syphilis

Osseous changes in acquired syphilis manifest as dense osteosclerosis. Long bones and skull are most frequently

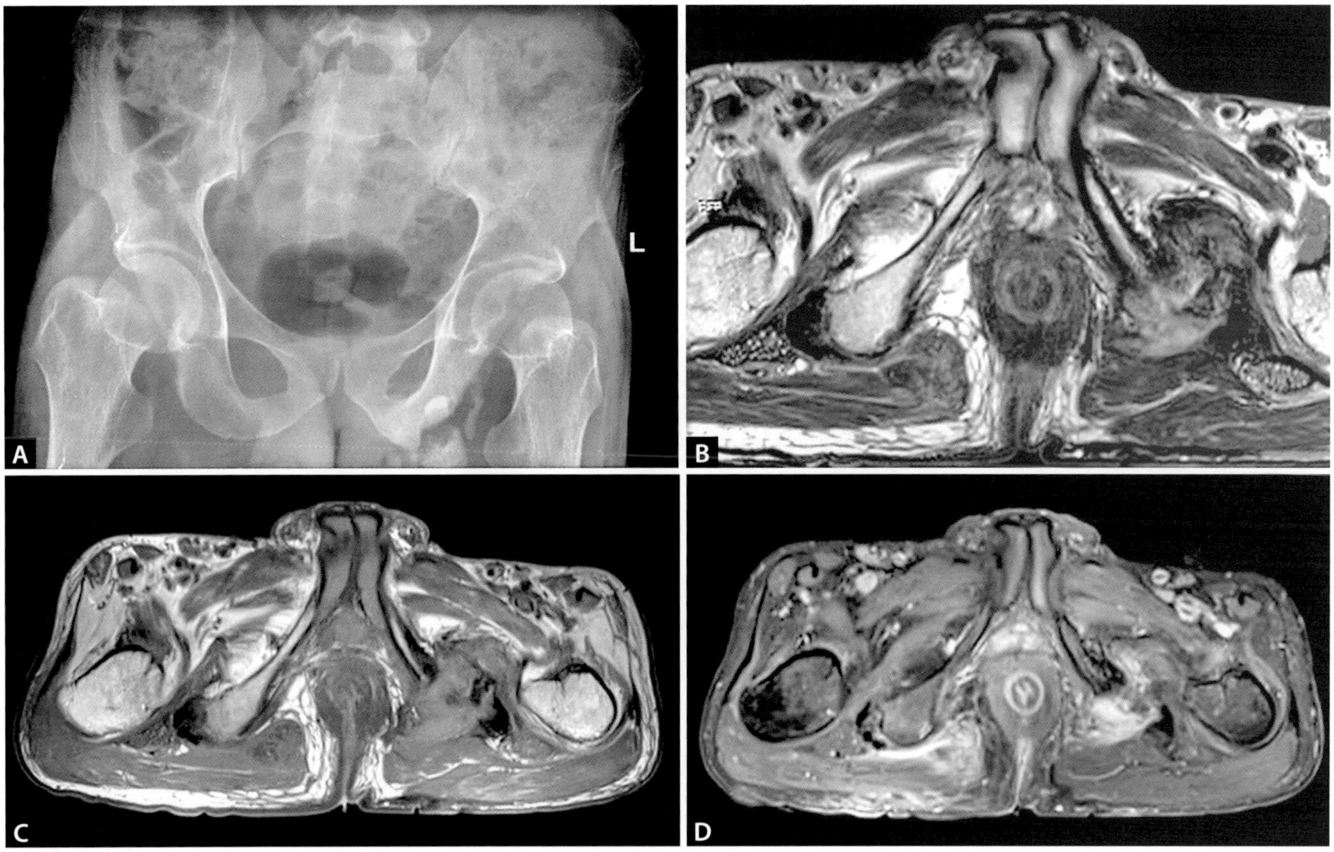

Figs. 12A to D: (A) Plain X-ray of hip joints reveal erosions along the inferior border of left ischium with sclerosis. Axial T2W (B), T1W (C) and postcontrast T1 fat-saturated (D) MRI images show a large area of lytic destruction involving the left ischium associated with a large inflammatory tissue which is of high signal on T2W and hypointense on T1W images involving the gluteal muscles. The marrow of the left ischium also show increased signal consistent with marrow edema. Few small peripherally enhancing collections are also seen representing abscesses. The gluteal muscles on the right side also show inflammatory changes.

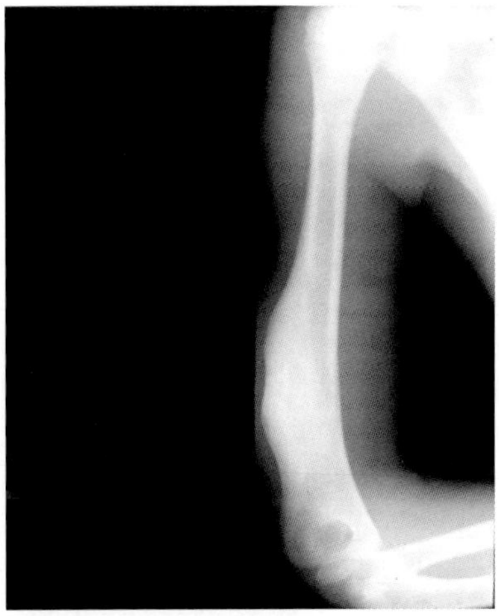

Fig. 13: Chronic sclerosing osteomyelitis of Garre: Long-standing osteomyelitis with endosteal thickening of cortex with obliteration of medullary cavity.

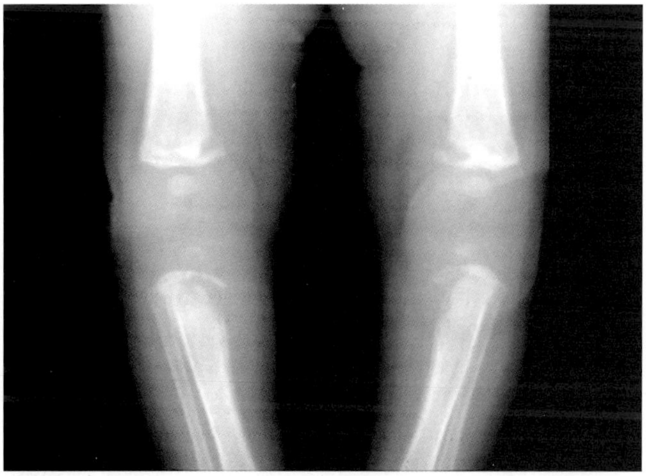

Fig. 14: Congenital syphilis: Radiograph of both knees of an infant showing symmetrical marginal destruction of medial aspect of tibia and femur in juxtaepiphyseal area and metaphyseal bands.

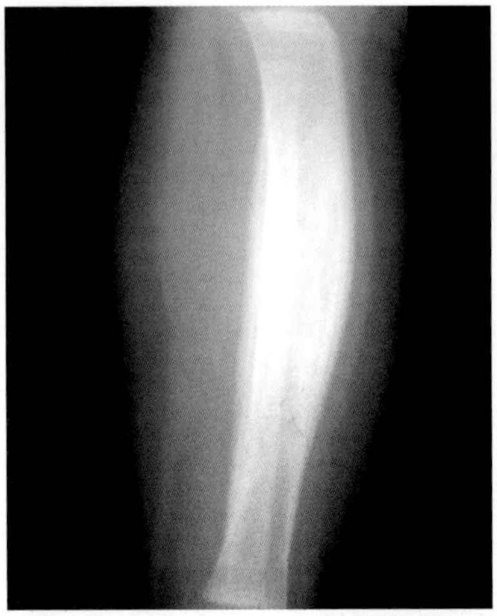

Fig. 15: Sabre tibia: Extensive cortical thickening affecting the shaft of tibia which is widened.

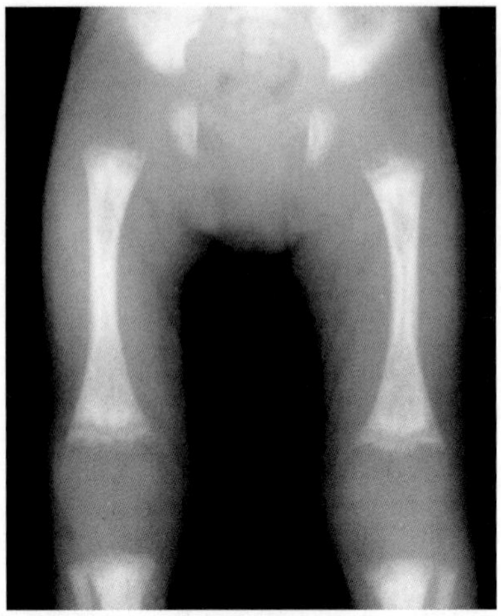

Fig. 16: Rubella: Radiographs of both lower limbs show the typical metaphyseal bands and trabecular irregularity in metaphysis extending longitudinally. Note absence of periosteal reaction.

involved. The earliest change is periosteal reaction. The affected bone shows thickened cortex with narrowing of medullary canal. Gummas cause osteolytic lesion of variable size and shape. The skull shows predominantly osteolytic lesions, and outer table is more often involved.

RUBELLA OSTEOMYELITIS

Congenital rubella infection occurs following maternal rubella in the early months of pregnancy. The characteristic radiological feature is metaphyseal lucent bands and trabecular irregularity, extending longitudinally from the epiphysis. It is seen in the upper and lower extremities, predominantly in the distal end of femur and proximal end of the tibia (Celery stalk appearance) **(Fig. 16)**. Bone changes can be confused with syphilis. Absence of periosteal reaction in congenital rubella helps in differentiating from congenital syphilis.

ACTINOMYCOSIS OF BONE

It is a chronic osteomyelitis caused by gram-positive organism, *Actinomyces israelii*, which grows in colonies and appear as yellow (sulfur) granules in pus. They are common saprophytes in the gastrointestinal tract and infection occurs after a dental procedure or trauma to mouth and jaw. The most common bones involved are vertebrae and mandible.

Radiologically, there is bone destruction without new bone formation. Vertebral osteomyelitis resembles tuberculosis, although disks are usually spared.[2] Ribs respond to actinomycosis by periosteal reaction and thickening, a feature which is most suggestive though, not diagnostic.

MADURAMYCOSIS

Maduramycosis is a form of chronic osteomyelitis due to granulomatous inflammation caused by a wide variety of pathogens, including fungi or actinomycosis. The infection occurs by entry of organism through minor trauma to skin, usually foot (Madura foot). The disease is painless and presents as swelling, sinus formation and marked deformity **(Figs. 17 and 18)**.

Radiologically, periosteal reaction is the most common lesion and is usually lamellated. The disease arises primarily in soft tissues and secondarily erodes the adjoining cortex and medulla. There is little, if any, osteopenia. The disease is painless, and characteristically, the sequestrum is absent.

LEPROSY OF BONE

Leprosy is a chronic granulomatous infection caused by *Mycobacterium leprae*. In lepromatous leprosy, the disease predominantly affects the skin, mucous membranes and the viscera. Bone involvement can rarely occur by direct lepromatous granulation tissue or by endarteritis causing bone infarcts. In tuberculoid (neural) type, there is predominant involvement of nerves which become thickened and nodular. The bone changes are secondary to neurotrophic disturbances causing recurrent trauma and infection which go unnoticed.

Radiographically, there is diffuse osteopenia and ill-defined small osteolytic areas with soft tissue swelling are seen. Periosteal reaction is rare. In later stages, erosions or resorption of phalangeal tufts are seen along with soft tissue atrophy **(Figs. 19A and B)**. Nonspecific changes,

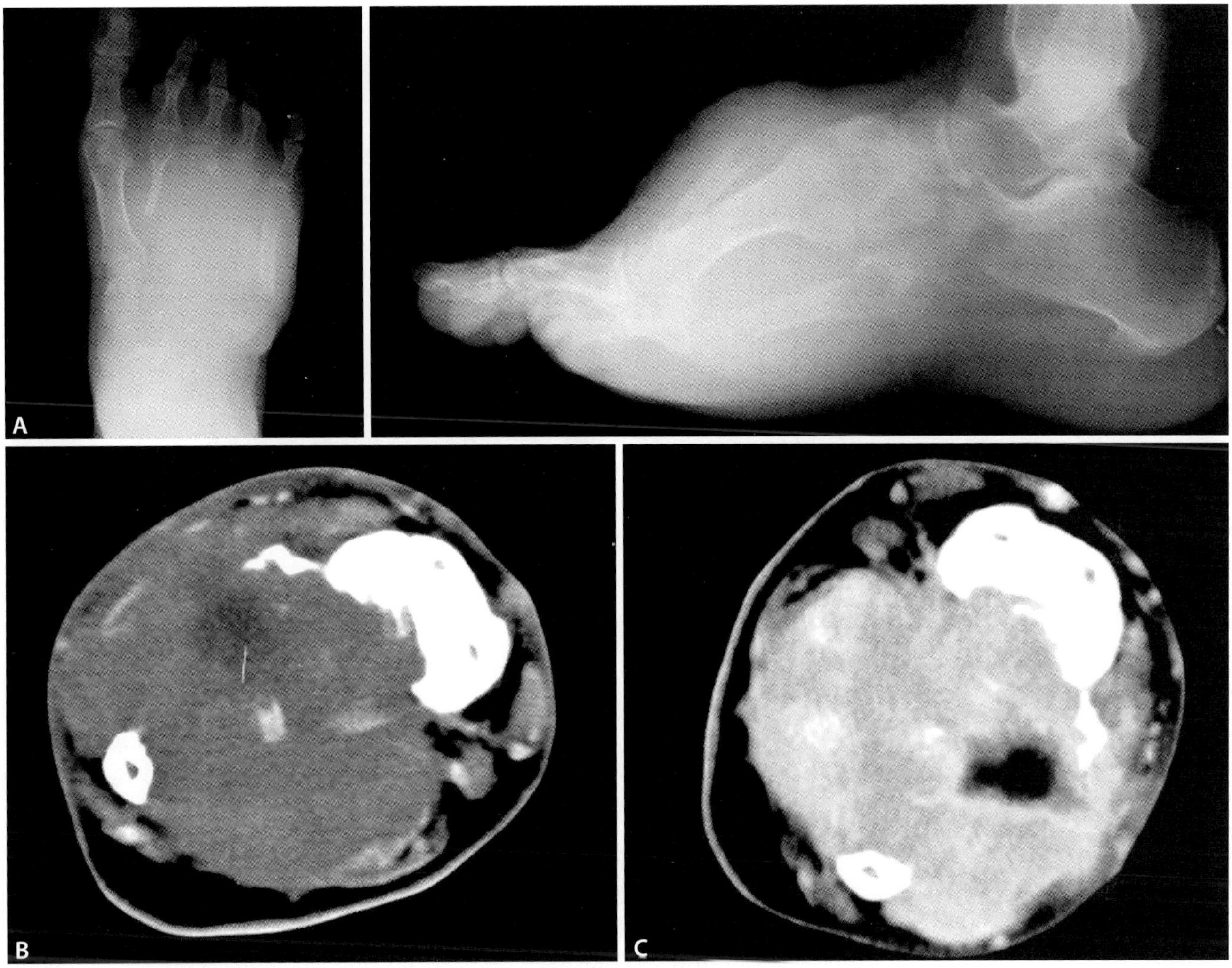

Figs. 17A to C: Maduramycosis: (A) Plain X-rays and (B and C) axial CT pre- and postcontrast images. There is a large soft tissue swelling in the foot with destruction of 2–4th metatarsals. On CT, an enhancing soft tissue lesion with secondary destruction of metatarsal shafts is seen.

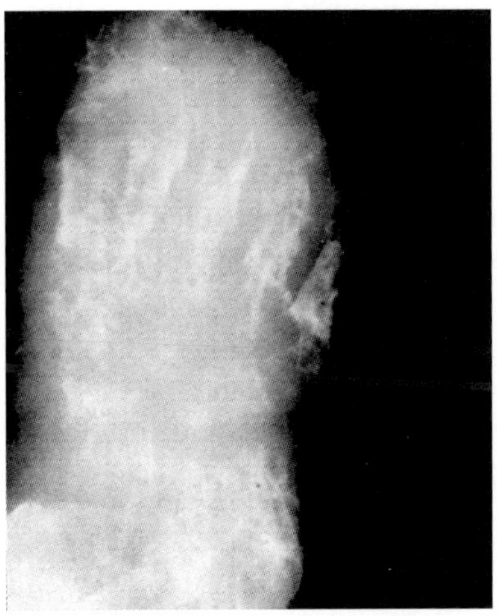

Fig. 18: Maduramycosis: Infiltrative destruction of the tarsal and metatarsal bones with large soft tissue component.

including soft tissue swelling and contractures are also seen. Calcification of nerves, if observed, is classical of leprosy. Nasal septal irregularity, thinning and perforation are not well appreciated on plain radiography, but these abnormalities are very well demonstrated on CT.

DIABETIC FOOT

Infection is the primary problem requiring hospitalization of diabetic patient with foot problems often necessitating amputation. Foot problems account for as much as one-fourth of hospital admissions among diabetic patients.[27] The pathological changes are often a combination of neuropathy, vasculopathy or infection.

Conventional radiographs show either osteomyelitic changes or neuropathic changes in the foot bones (sensitivity and specificity 75% each) **(Fig. 20)**.[28]

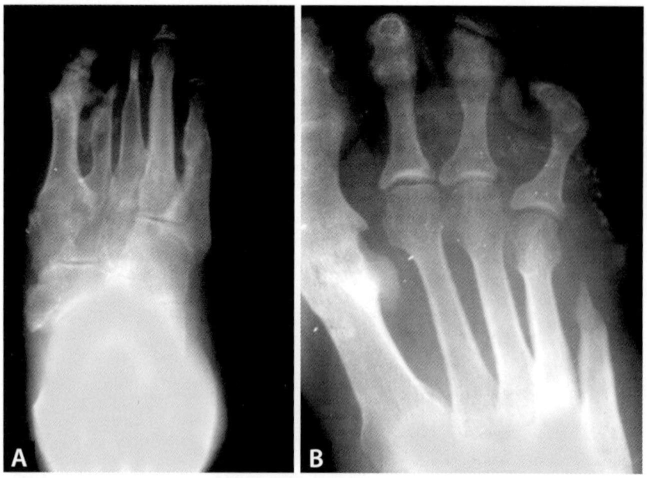

Figs. 19A and B: Leprosy: Osteopenia with 'licked candy appearance' of the metatarsals (A and B). Note the absence of the phalanges of the 5th toe (B) due to bony resorption.

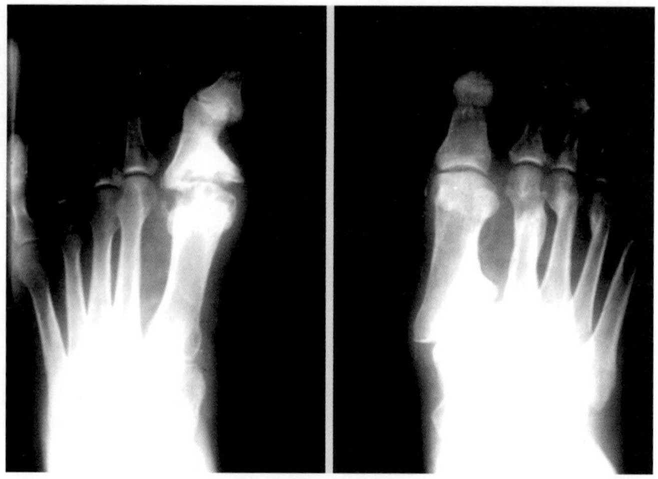

Fig. 20: Diabetic foot: There is narrowing of first metatarsophalangeal (right) and tarsometatarsal joint on left with articular erosion and marked sclerosis of adjacent bone. Lucencies in soft tissues are due to air.

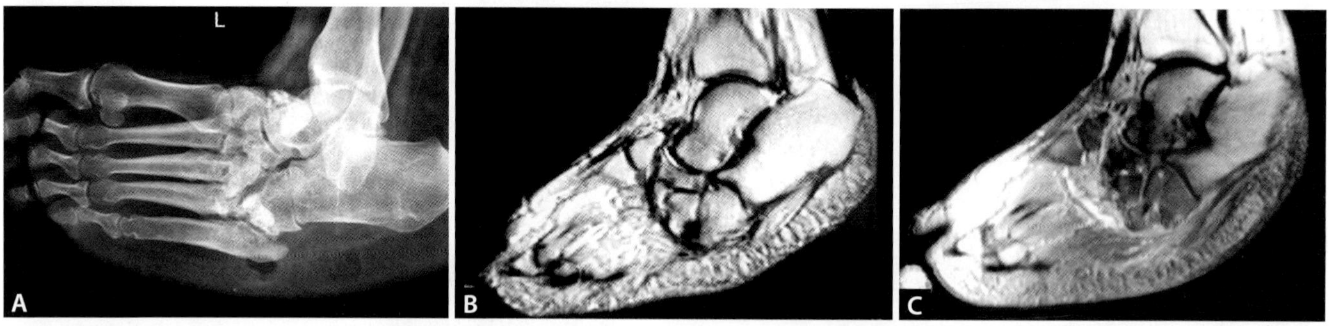

Figs. 21A to C: Diabetic foot: (A) Plain radiograph of foot shows dislocation of joints of midfoot and tarsometatarsal joints and with reduced joint spaces and erosions. The bones show mixed lytic and sclerotic areas; (B) T1W MRI image show dislocated-disorganized joints of foot with markedly hypointense areas of bony sclerosis; (C) Postcontrast T1W image shows thickened enhancing synovium at tarsometatarsal joints with enhancing muscles of plantar surface.

Scintigraphy can identify early osteopathy at a time when the conventional radiograph is normal, but its specificity is very low.[28] ^{111}In WBC scanning is more specific than ^{99m}Tc bone scan since it is not affected by increased bone turnover from neuropathy or fracture.[29]

Magnetic resonance imaging (MRI) can visualize marrow directly and is found to have the lowest false positive rate compared to both scintigraphy as well as plain radiography.[28] In neuroarthropathy, MRI typically shows a specific low signal from within the marrow space on T1W images and T2W images, although there are exceptions. This finding is consistently different from osteomyelitis where a high signal from the marrow space on T2W images is seen, however, concurrent infection in the adjacent soft tissues, synovium and muscles may reveal increased signal on T2W and STIR images which may enhance on post-gadolinium scans **(Figs. 21A to C)**. Since high signal on T2W images can also be caused by tumor, trauma or hemorrhage, MRI findings must be correlated with clinical findings and other imaging studies.

Soft tissue infection of foot occurs especially over pressure points, such as metatarsals where organisms enter via superficial ulceration. Gas may be noted in infective tissues, because of gas producing organisms, such as *E.Coli*, without implying the presence of gangrene.

HYDATID DISEASE

Bone involvement is rare accounting for 0.5–2% cases. The most commonly involved bones are the spine, pelvis, femur, tibia, ribs, skull, scapula, humerus and fibula.[30,31] The hydatid disease in the bone and joint begins in childhood and grows at a very slow rate and hence are seldomly diagnosed in childhood. The bone offers mechanical resistance; hence cyst cannot assume it is typical spherical shape and enlarges along the path of least resistance. Over the time, the trabeculae are absorbed and cortex is breached, resulting in fracture. This leads to the spread of the diseaseto surrounding structures and becomes symptomatic.

Hydatid disease should be suspected whenever cystic lesions are seen in the bone especially in the endemic areas.

The bone shows expanded medullary cavity with thinned out cortex with cortical breech or complete fracture. Typically, there is no periosteal reaction or new bone formation. On MRI, the infested bone reveals multiple cysts which exhibit medium-to-low signal on T1W images and high signal on T2W images **(Figs. 22A to D)**.[30,31]

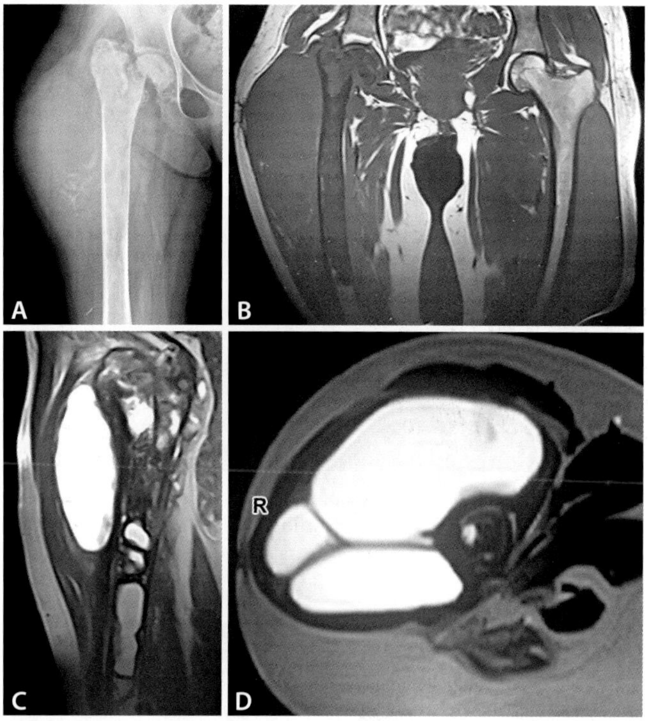

Figs. 22A to D: (A) Plain radiograph demonstrates expanded medullary cavity with endosteal scalloping in right femur and thinned out cortex. There is pathological fracture neck of femur with proximal migration of greater trochanter. A large soft tissue shadow is also seen along the lateral aspect with foci of calcifications; (B) Coronal T1W MR image showing altered marrow signal of medullary cavity (hypointense when compared to left femur) with a large hypointense lesion along lateral aspect of upper thigh. Note pathological fracture neck of right femur; (C) Sagittal T2W MR image showing multiple cysts in the medullary cavity of right femur with small cysts in adductor group of muscles and large cysts along lateral aspect of thigh; (D) Axial T2W MR image showing a multiseptated cystic lesion along lateral aspect of femur. Note a small cyst in the medullary cavity.

SEPTIC ARTHRITIS

Septic arthritis is usually hematogenous in origin but may follow local trauma, joint aspiration, soft tissue infection or periarticular osteomyelitis. Arthroscopic procedures are complicated by septic arthritis in 0.04–3.4% of patients.[7] *Staphylococcus aureus* is the most common invader followed by *N. gonorrhoea, Streptococcus, Haemophilus* and anaerobic organisms.[23]

Onset of bacterial arthritis is usually abrupt with high fever, chills and one or more severely tender swollen joints. Knee joint is most frequently affected (40–50%) followed by hip (20–25%), shoulder, wrist, elbow and ankle. Sternoclavicular, sacroiliac and manubriosternal joints are more often involved in intravenous drug abusers.

Bone scan is the investigation of choice for early diagnosis of septic arthritis. Although not specific, bone scanning is very sensitive and when negative can rule out the possibility of infected joint.[8] Computed tomography demonstrates bone changes much earlier than plain films and is superior in demonstrating the extent of infection. Magnetic resonance imaging is extremely sensitive in the depiction of joint fluid, cartilage damage, marrow changes and medullary bone destruction, but cannot differentiate infectious from noninfectious joint effusions.[32]

Radiological patterns are different in adults and infants. Plain radiographs are usually normal in early course of disease. Soft tissue swelling is the first radiographic sign of acute pyogenic arthritis. Hyperemia associated with pyogenic arthritis causes rapid, juxta-articular osteoporosis with disappearance of subchondral white line. Periarticular edema obliterates the adjacent fat planes. At this stage, effusion is identifiable. Earliest bone change occurs 8–10 days after the onset of infection.[33] There is loss of definition of the margins due to osteoporosis with small focal articular erosions followed by progressive destruction of cartilage leading to reduction in joint space. Untreated infection can lead to extensive bone destruction and loss of cortical outline. In later stages, subluxation or even dislocation can occur. With healing, sclerotic bone reaction occurs resulting in irregular articular surface. If the entire cartilage is destroyed, then bony ankylosis follows **(Figs. 23A and B)**.[34]

In infants and children, distention of joint capsule due to fluid can cause joint space widening and even subluxation, especially of the hip and shoulder. In neonates physiological ossification of femoral head is absent, thus plain radiographs are of limited value. Ultrasonography in such cases may reveal joint effusion with/without internal echoes **(Fig. 24)**. Thickened synovial membrane is seen

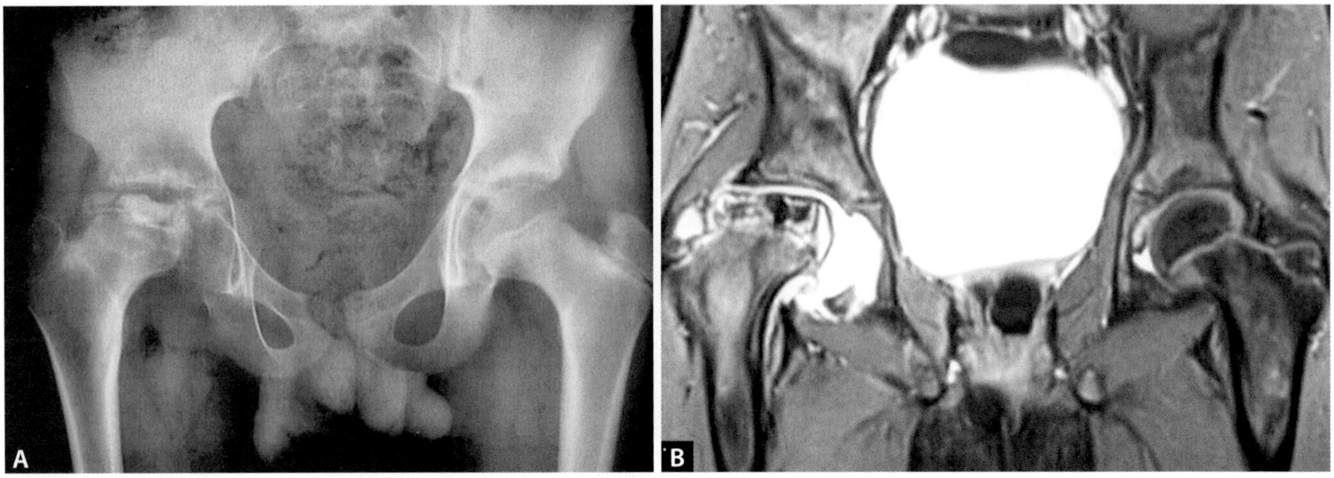

Figs. 23A and B: (A) Plain X-ray of hip joints reveal irregular articular margins of right femoral joint with sclerosis. The femoral epiphysis is massively destroyed with fuzzy outline; (B) Postcontrast T1W MRI image demonstrate thickened enhancing synovium with intraosseous abscesses in the femoral epiphysis and bone destruction. Also the marrow shows enhancement in the upper femur.

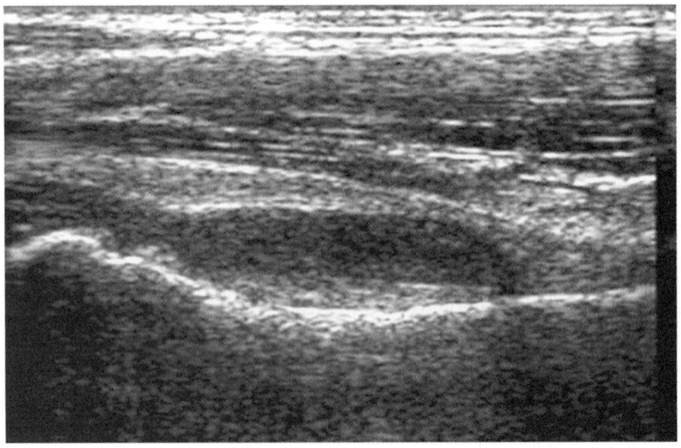

Fig. 24: USG image in an infant shows joint effusion in hip joint with dependent debris.

as irregular echogenic membrane surrounding the fluid. Joint effusion can also occur as sympathetic response to adjacent focus of osteomyelitis. Arthrocentesis with bacterial cultures is therefore essential in such cases to document joint infection.

In pediatric population distinguishing transient synovitis from septic arthritis is extremely important and in such cases the USG may not differentiate as both the conditions manifests as synovial thickening, joint effusions and alteration in surrounding soft tissues. MRI can differentiate these two conditions as in transient synovitis, there are minimal to almost nil marrow changes (high signal changes in T2W and STIR images which show postcontrast enhancement).[35]

Bone changes in gonococcal arthritis are indistinguishable from tuberculosis. Destruction is more rapid and serial films are helpful in distinguishing the two. Similarly, brucellar arthritic changes are also indistinguishable from tubercular joint; however, *Brucella* involves most commonly sacroiliac joints and usually unilaterally.[34] Fungal arthritis is most commonly due to *Candida*, coccidiosis and blastomycosis. Radiologically, there is soft tissue swelling, periarticular osteopenia, relative joint space preservation and bony erosions but differentiation from tuberculosis is difficult.

REFERENCES

1. Greenfield GB (Ed). Cardinal Roentgen Features Radiology of Bone Diseases, 5th edn. Philadelphia: JB Lippincott; 1990.
2. Edeiken J (Ed). Roentgen Diagnosis of Disease of Bone (4th edn). Baltimore: Williams and Wilkins. 1990.pp.973-1084.
3. Wegener WA, Alavi A. Diagnostic imaging of musculoskeletal infection. Roentgenography; gallium, indium-labeled white blood cell, gamma-globulin, bone scintigraphy. Orthop Clin North Am. 1991;22:401-18.
4. Wheat J. Diagnostic strategies in osteomyelitis. Am J Med. 1985;78:218-24.
5. Markel KD, Brown ML, Dewanjee MK, et al. Comparison of indium-labeled leukocyte imaging with sequential technetium-gallium scanning in the diagnosis of low-grade musculoskeletal sepsis: A prospective study. J Bone Joint Surg. 1985;67:465-76.
6. Rubin RH, Fischman AJ, Callahan RJ, et al. ^{111}In-labelled non-specific immunoglobulin scanning in the detection of focal infection. N Eng J Med. 1989;321:935-40.
7. D Angelo GL, Ogilive Harris DJ. Septic arthritis following arthroscopy with cost benefit analysis of antibiotic prophylaxis. Arthroscopy. 1988;4:10-4.
8. Esterhai JL Jr, Gelb I. Adult septic arthritis. Ortho Clin North Am. 1991;22:503-14.

9. Desai RV, Khandelwal N, Gupta S, Suri S, et al. Role of ultrasound in acute Osteomyelitis. Asian Oceanian Jr Radiology. 2001;6:159-65.
10. Modic MT, Pflanze W, Feiglin DHI, et al. Magnetic resonance imaging of musculoskeletal infections. Radiol Clin North Am. 1986;24:247-58.
11. Schanwecker DS, Braunstein EM, Wheat LJ. Diagnostic imaging of osteomyelitis. Infect Disease Clinics North America. 1990;4:441-63.
12. Modic MT, Feiglin DH, Piraino DW, et al. Vertebral osteomyelitis—Assessment using MR. Radiology. 1985;157:157-66.
13. Unger E, Moldfsky P, Gatenby R, et al. Diagnosis of osteomyelitis by MR imaging. Am J Roentgenol. 1988;150:605-10.
14. Morrison WB, Schweitzer ME, Batte WG, et al. Osteomyelitis of the foot: relative importance of primary and secondary MR imaging signs. Radiology. 1998;207:625-32.
15. Jaramillo D, Treves ST, Kasser JR, et al. Osteomyelitis and septic arthritis in children: appropriate use of imaging to guide treatment. Am J Roentgenol. 1995;165:399-403.
16. Beltran J, Noto AM, McGhee RB, et al. Infections of the musculoskeletal system: high-field-strength MR imaging. Radiology. 1987;164:449-54.
17. Brill PW, Winchester P, Krause AN, et al. Osteomyelitis in a neonatal intensive care unit. Radiology. 1979;13:83-8.
18. Mok M, Reilly RJ, Ash JM. Osteomyelitis in the neonate. Radiology. 1982;145:677-82.
19. Bressler EL, Conway JJ, Weiss SC. Neonatal osteomyelitis examined by bone scintigraphy. Radiology. 1984;152:685-8.
20. Rosen Ra, Morehouse HT, Karp JH, et al. Intracortical fissuring in osteomyelitis. Radiology. 1981;141:17-20
21. Connolly SA, Connolly LP, Drubach LA, et al. MRI for detection of abscess in acute osteomyelitis of the pelvis in children. AJR. 2007;189:867-72.
22. Karchevsky M, Schweitzer ME, Morrison WB, et al. MRI findings of septic arthritis and associated osteomyelitis in adults. Am J Roentgenol. 2004;182:119-22.
23. Cooper C, Cawley MI. Bacterial arthritis in an English Health district: A 10-year-review. Ann Rheum Dis. 1986;45:458-63.
24. Gulati Y, Maheshwari AV. Brodie's abscess of the femoral neck simulating osteoid osteoma. Acta Orthop Belg. 2007;73:648-52.
25. Quinn SF, Murray W, Clerk RA, et al. MR imaging of chronic osteomyelitis. J Compt Assist Tomogr. 1988;12:113-7.
26. Mason MD, Zlatkin MB, Esterhai JL, et al. Chronic complicated osteomyelitis of the lower extremity evaluation with MR imaging. Radiology. 1989;173:355-9.
27. Brodsky JW, Schneidler C. Diabetic foot infections. Orthop Clin North Am. 1991;22:473-89.
28. Yuh WT, Corson JD, Baraniewski HM, et al. Osteomyelitis of the foot in diabetic patients evaluation with plain film, ^{99m}Tc DMP bone scintigraphy and MR imaging. Am J Roentgenol. 1989;152:795-800.
29. Keenam AM, Tindel NL, Alavi A. Diagnosis of pedal osteomyelitis in diabetic patients using current scintigraphy techniques. Arch Intern Med. 1989;149:2262-6.
30. Pedrosa I, Saiz A, Arrazola J, et al. Hydatid Cyst: radiologic and pathologic features and complications. Radiographics. 2000;20:795-814.
31. Dhatt S, Singhal M, Tripathy SK, et al. Primary hydatidosis of femur: a case report and review of literature. Eur J Orthop Surg Traumatol. 2010;20:401-5.
32. Tang JSH, Gold RH, Besset LW, et al. Musculo-skeletal infection of the extremities: Evaluation with MR Imaging. Radiology. 1988;166:205-9.
33. Manaster BJ. Adult Chronic Hip Pain: Radiographic Evaluation. Radiographics. 2000;20:S3-25.
34. Ediken J (Ed). Roentgen diagnosis of diseases of bone, 4th edn. Baltimore: William's and Wilkins; 1990;(1):593-601.
35. Yang WJ, Im SA, Lim GY, et al. MR imaging of transient synovitis: differentiation from septic arthritis. Pediatr Radiol. 2006;36:1154-8.

CHAPTER 192

Tuberculosis of the Spine

Rashmi Dixit

INTRODUCTION

The spine is the most frequent site of osseous involvement by tuberculosis comprising in most series about 50% of cases.[1,2] The disease was first described by Sir Percival Pott in 1779, hence the name Pott's disease.[3] There has been a resurgence of the disease in the developed countries following the HIV pandemic.

Tubercular spondylitis is defined as an infection by *Mycobacterium tuberculosis* of one or more of the extradural components of the spine namely the vertebra, intervertebral disks, paraspinal soft tissues and epidural space.[4,5] It is associated with disproportionate amount of morbidity due to its tendency to produce significant deformity and neurologic complications therefore prompt diagnosis and treatment are of utmost importance.

PATHOPHYSIOLOGY

The spread of tuberculosis to the spine is usually by hematogenous route, whether by perivertebral arterial or venous plexi is still in debate, but the arterial route is generally considered more important.[2] Hematogenous seeding may arise from a primary focus in the lung or other extraosseous foci such as lymph nodes, GIT or any other viscera which may be active or quiescent.[6]

Lower thoracic and lumbar vertebrae are most often affected followed by middle thoracic and cervical vertebrae.[7] The C2–C7 region is reportedly involved in 3–5% of cases[8,9] and the atlantoaxial articulation in less than 1% of cases.[10-12] Usually two continuous vertebrae are involved but several vertebrae may be affected, skip lesions and solitary vertebral involvement may also be seen.[7] The so-called skip lesion or a second lesion not contiguous with the more obvious lesion is seen in 4–10% of cases.[4,13]

The infection begins in the cancellous area of the vertebral body commonly in the paradiscal location and less often in the centrum or anterior surface. The vertebral body becomes soft and gets easily compressed to produce either wedging or total collapse. Anterior wedging is commonly seen in the dorsal spine where the normal kyphotic curve accentuates the pressure on the anterior part of the vertebral body. This produces kyphus with a gibbus deformity.[6,7] Spread of infection can occur beneath the anterior longitudinal ligament, involving adjacent vertebral bodies.

As infection spreads to the adjacent disk, the disk space narrows. The intervertebral disk is avascular in adults and spread of infection to the disk can occur by extension through the subchondral bone via cartilaginous end plate or beneath the anterior or posterior longitudinal ligament to involve the peripheral disk. Disk space narrowing can also occur due to disk herniation into the weakened vertebral body with subsequent infection of the herniated disk.[6] The inter-vertebral disk, however, resists infection by *Mycobacterium tuberculosis* probably due to a lack of proteolytic enzymes in the *Mycobacterium* as compared with pyogenic infection.[14] The avascularity of the disk may prevent them from serving as an initial site of infection and it has been suggested that disk destruction begins only when two vertebral bodies are so involved that the disk loses its nutritional support.[2] Hence, disk space narrowing occurs later and is less marked in tubercular infection as opposed to pyogenic infection.[14-16] Although the vertebral body is involved more often than the posterior elements, these latter structures may be affected initially or predominantly in some persons.[17,18]

A marked exudative lesion due to hypersensitivity reaction to *Mycobacterium* results in formation of thick pus containing serum, leukocytes, caseous material, tubercle bacilli and bone fragments which tracks through the pre and paravertebral soft tissues forming pre and paravertebral abscesses. The exudate penetrates ligaments and follows the path of least resistance along fascial planes, blood vessels and nerves to distant sites from the original bony lesion as cold abscess. The abscesses may further extend into the spinal canal producing an epidural abscess and cord compression.[7]

CLINICAL FEATURES

Tuberculous spondylitis can occur in any age group but majority of the patients are under thirty years of age at the time of diagnosis. The disease is rare in the first year of life but when it occurs, it tends to be more severe with greater bone destruction and multiple vertebral involvement.[7,8] Symptoms and signs vary considerably.[4] Some patients may be afebrile and free of systemic symptoms until late stage of the disease, others may present with constitutional symptoms before symptoms related to the spine manifest. The usual presentation is with persistent spinal pain, local tenderness and limitation of spinal mobility.[4,7] The ESR is elevated in more than 80%[8] of cases and tuberculin skin test is usually positive.[19,20]

Paraparesis may be apparent in about 20–30% of all patients with spinal tuberculosis.[4,7] In the cervical region the incidence is much higher and over 40% cases may be associated with quadriparesis.[4,8] Paraplegia may be early onset, which develops during the active phase of the disease or late onset which may appear many years after the disease has become quiescent, even without any evidence of reactivation. Early onset paraplegia is usually due to cord compression by epidural abscess or granulation tissue, pathological subluxation or dislocation, sequestered bone or disk fragments. Nonmechanical causes include inflammatory cord edema due to vascular stasis and toxins or cord granulation tissue due to passage of tuberculous inflammation to the meninges and eventually the cord. Rarely paraplegia may be due to cord infarction due to endarteritis. Late onset paraplegia can occur due to dural fibrosis, severe kyphoscoliotic deformity, spinal canal stenosis, gliosis of cord or sequestra from vertebral body. Late onset paraplegia has a much less favorable prognosis than early onset paraplegia.[7]

LABORATORY INVESTIGATIONS[21-24]

Relative lymphocytosis, a low level of hemoglobin and a raised ESR are found in active tubercular disease. The mantoux test is nondiagnostic in an endemic region and may be negative in an immunodeficient individuals. The sensitivity of staining for acid-fast bacilli may vary from 25 to 75%. Culture of acid-fast bacilli requires a long incubation period of four to six weeks, although Bactec radiometric culture takes less than two weeks. The serological tests are non-diagnostic in lesions with a low level of bacilli. The immunoglobulin IgG and IgM titres show significant differences between the initiation of treatment and at three months later, but do not correlate with the stage, the recovery of the disease or the duration of antituberculous treatment. The polymerase chain reaction is an efficient and rapid method of diagnosis and can differentiate between typical and atypical mycobacteria. It analyses the expression of genes, even from the single cell. A positive result from a polymerase chain reaction is not a substitute for culture and not indicative of the activity of the disease, since it does not differentiate live from dead microorganisms and has been obtained from an 'ancient' sample of bone tissue.

IMAGING MODALITIES

Conventional Radiographs

Conventional radiographs are the usual initial investigation, but they are often negative in early disease **(Figs. 1A to D)**. More than 30–50% of mineral must be lost before a radiolucent lesion becomes conspicuous on the plain films and this takes about 2–5 months.[2,7] Plain films are also limited in the evaluation of areas such as craniovertebral junction, cervicodorsal junction, posterior neural arches and sacrum.

Nuclear Medicine Scintigraphy

Bone scintigraphy using technetium diphosphonate is an economical but nonspecific tool for early detection of tuberculous spondylitis.[25] Reported sensitivities vary from 87.5 to 95%.[25] Radiotracer uptake is usually increased in osseous tuberculous infection and may reveal multiple sites in disseminated disease—a nonspecific finding that may mimic metastases.[26,27] However, Lifeso and Weaver reported false-negative bone scan findings in 35% of plain film positive lesions.[28] The authors noted a high

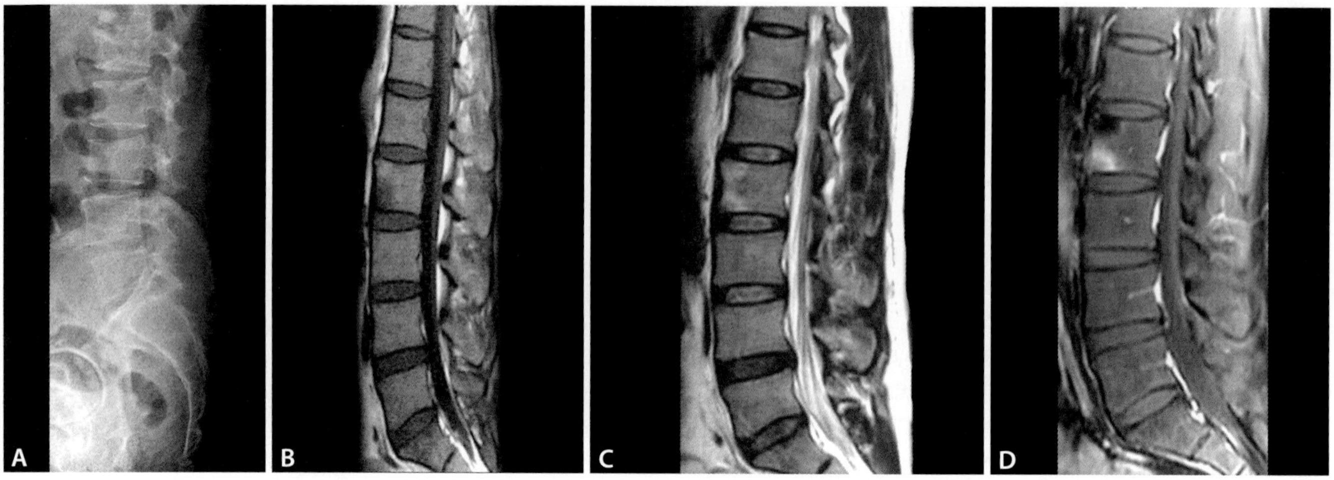

Figs. 1A to D: (A) Lateral radiograph L-S spine of a 25-year-old male presenting with low backache and fever reveals normal vertebrae and disk spaces; (B) T1W, (C) T2W, (D) Postcontrast T1W fat-suppressed sagittal images of the same patient show an area of signal alteration in the anteroinferior part of L2 vertebral body appearing hypointense on T1W, hyperintense on T2W images and showing patchy enhancement on the postcontrast images.

incidence of negative Gallium scans as well.[29] This may be explained by a purely lytic and avascular early phase of the disease. False-negative bone scans are seen with disseminated tuberculosis, cervical spine lesions and isolated neural arch lesions. Posterior neural arch lesions are more readily detectable when cross-sectional nuclear medicine imaging is performed.[2,26] The pitfalls of limited anatomic resolution, nonspecificity and false-negative examinations limit the use of scintigraphy in tuberculous spondylodiscitis. Also nuclear imaging techniques do not help distinguish between the different causes of sepsis, but they do help identify a focus of interest. Further imaging of the area in question, along with additional tissue sampling, can then be performed to aid in diagnosis.[30]

FDG-PET and PET-CT[31-35] have high sensitivity for detection of chronic osteomyelitis. Tubercular lesions are found to have increased FDG uptake in regions of active granulomatous inflammation with cold areas that represent necrosed tissue containing pus. PET/CT can also delineate the sinus tracks without the need for contrast instillation which is an added advantage of PET/CT. With the incorporation of contrast-enhanced computed tomography (CECT) in the PET/CT protocol, the complete extent of bone, bone marrow and soft tissue involvement can be delineated. Moreover, metabolically active disease can be distinguished from residual fibrotic tissue. As in oncological imaging, PET/CT plays a useful role in determining multiple occult foci of involvement in a single study. It can also serve as a valuable baseline for monitoring response to treatment and providing information on disease spread. It is also a useful tool to guide the site of biopsy or other interventional procedures.

Tuberculosis can be a common cancer mimick on PET/CT, producing uptake patterns that are indistinguishable from that of malignant processes. Though high standardized uptake values (SUVs) greater than 2.5 have been attributed to malignant lesions, high values (up to 21) have been seen in tuberculosis as well. Several groups have attempted to improve the specificity of an ^{18}F-FDG PET by imaging the abnormal sites at dual time points after its administration including additional delayed imaging at 90 to 120 minutes. At malignant sites, the FDG uptake continues to increase for several hours, which can be demonstrated by the increase in SUVs. On the other hand, in inflammatory lesions, uptake peaks at approximately 60 minutes after administration and the SUVs either stabilize or decline thereafter. Hence, Alavi et al.[35] concluded that imaging at 2 time points after FDG administration may help distinguish between malignant and inflammatory disorders. However, other authors have found equivocal results with dual point time imaging (45 and 120 minutes post FDG injection). They found that out of 15 patients a majority showed no reduction, a few showed mild reduction (up to 20%) and many showed an increase (from 10–40%) in SUV on the delayed images. Another approach to increase the diagnostic accuracy of PET is the combined use of ^{18}F-FDG and C-11 acetate as the latter accumulates in tumors and not in inflammatory lesions.

The exact role of FDG-PET and PET/CT in TB and other inflammatory diseases is evolving and is not as yet clearly defined. With the development of newer and more specific radiotracers like positron emitter labeled antituberculous drug molecules such as INH and rifampicin in the future, PET/CT may play a significant role in establishing an early diagnosis and effective monitoring of therapeutic response.

Computed Tomography

Technical innovations in last two decades such as multi row detector scanners have resulted in faster acquisition and processing times, thinner slice collimation, better resolution, isotropic voxels and allow high quality 3D-reformatted images to be produced. Computed tomography remains a versatile imaging modality for the evaluation of bone and soft tissue[4] and is extremely useful to assess the destruction of cancellous bone, cortical erosions, presence of bony fragments and soft tissue calcification.[36] The advantages of a CT examination in cases of tubercular spondylitis include—early detection of bone and soft tissue changes when plain films are normal, better anatomic localization and characterization of lesions, evaluation of areas difficult to evaluate on plain films such as cranio vertebral junction, cervicodorsal junction, sacrum and providing guidance for biopsy and surgical approach.[13,37] Computed tomography is also useful to demonstrate the exact extent of deformity in chronic cases.[36] In spinal disease, CT has a disadvantage that a routine examination may overlook lesions outside the chosen scan volume.[4] However, much larger volumes can now be covered with the use of multirow detector scanners though with an increased radiation burden **(Figs. 2A and B)**. For specific diagnosis of spondylitis CT is less useful than MR imaging as inflammatory marrow changes in the vertebral body, an early sign of infection are not well depicted on CT scanning.[38] In addition, soft tissue structures within the bony spinal canal are poorly delineated.[4,38] In the cervicothoracic region, epidural involvement may be missed even on CECT, without intrathecal contrast enhancement because of beam hardening artifacts. For this reason the effect of extradural disease on the thecal sac and its contained spinal cord and neural elements is difficult to evaluate properly.[38]

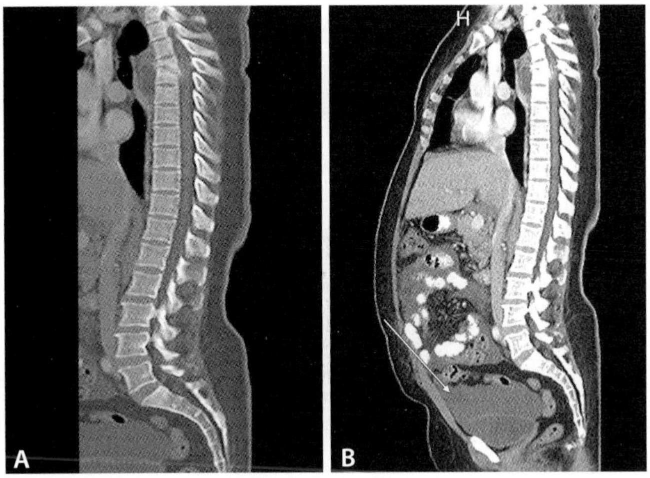

Figs. 2A and B: Sagittal reconstructions at bone (A) and soft tissue (B). Settings from a multislice CT acquisition for disseminated tuberculosis reveal reduction of disk space between D4 and D5, destruction of endplates and a peripherally enhancing prevertebral abscess due to tubercular involvement. Note the extended coverage and presence of free fluid in the abdomen (arrow).

Magnetic Resonance Imaging

The superiority of MR imaging in the detection and staging of inflammatory and infective disorders of the spine is generally accepted making MR the imaging modality of choice in these conditions.[38-40] Magnetic resonance imaging is extremely useful to detect disease in areas otherwise difficult to evaluate on plain films. The major advantages of MR imaging include multiplanar capability, the direct demonstration of early bone marrow involvement or edema and the unsurpassable assessment of spinal canal and neural involvement. Soft tissue and intraosseous abscesses are also well demonstrated on MR imaging.[38] Magnetic resonance imaging has higher sensitivity for early infiltrative disease including endplate changes and marrow infiltration than bone scan and plain films.[2] Because of its high sensitivity to detect marrow edema, MRI scores over CT in the detection of early disease as the earliest response to vertebral infection is the accumulation of water in extracellular bone marrow. This is best depicted on STIR and T1W images.[38] The changes at this stage, however, are nonspecific.

Skip lesions are more easily and more often detected by MR imaging as compared to CT because of its ability to screen the entire spine in a single examination. Incidence of multilevel noncontiguous vertebral tuberculosis is generally reported to be between 1.1% and 16%, but an incidence as high as 71.4% has been reported when using whole spine MR imaging **(Figs. 3A to D)**.[41] MR is also superior to CT for detection of epidural, meningial and cord involvement.[38,42] Planning the surgical approach can be facilitated by MR imaging because of the clear display of the extent of the active infection and its complications including involvement of neural arch.

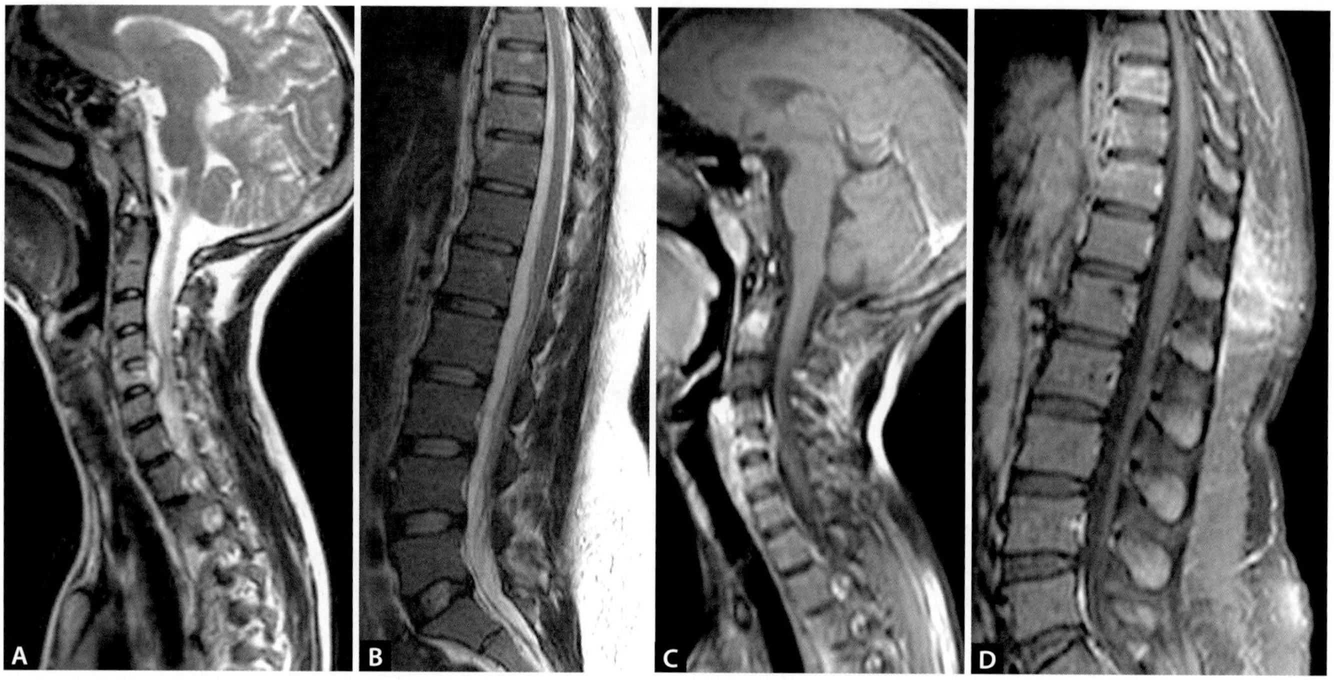

Figs. 3A to D: Sagittal T2-weighted images of the cervical (A) and lumbosacral spine (B) in a case of multifocal caries spine reveal hyperintense marrow signal in C5 and D8 to D11 vertebrae. A T2 hyperintense epidural soft tissue is noted at C5 and in the prevertebral region in the lower dorsal spine; (C and D) Postcontrast images reveal abnormal enhancement in the above vertebrae, and soft tissues. Additional foci of enhancement in C2 and postparaspinal soft tissues in the lumbar region are also seen. Note the relative preservation of the intervertebral disks.

While tuberculosis can be confidently diagnosed when the characteristic imaging features are present, at times it may be difficult to distinguish this from other causes of bone marrow edema in early stages and from other conditions such as metastases and myeloma in atypical cases. Diffusion weighted MR imaging has been applied in an attempt to distinguish between tubercular and neoplastic vertebral disease. In one study the authors concluded that DW-MRI and ADC values may help in the differentiation of spinal tuberculosis from other lesions of similar appearance. However, an overlap of ADC values was noted with metastatic disease, hence, these must be interpreted in association with clinical history and routine MR findings. Others found it to be of limited use.[43,44] MR imaging does have disadvantages. Calcification, the hallmark of tubercular infection and small bone fragments are not readily detectable by MRI. Gradient echo (T2*W) images demonstrate calcification better than spin-echo images. The low signal of calcification or bone fragments is more prominent on these images and closely matches calcification seen on CT. Demonstration of bone fragmentation on T2*W images is also considered characteristic of tuberculosis even in the absence of abscess formation.[45] Small bone fragments in an epidural abscess are important to detect when surgical management is being considered so that they can be accurately removed. The other disadvantage is that interventional procedures are difficult to perform with MR imaging.

IMAGING APPEARANCES

Imaging features in tubercular spondylitis consist of the vertebral, disk space and the soft tissue changes. Paravertebral abscesses are an important early feature of Pott's spine. Extension of tubercular spondylodiscitis to the adjacent soft tissues is common, incidence varying from 55 to 96%[1,4,46] and rarely may precede any visible vertebral lesion.[6] This extension usually occurs anterolaterally and is less often observed directly posteriorly in the peridural space.[6,46]

Associated changes in the spinal cord and rare variants of disease such as extraosseous extradural granuloma may be detected by modern imaging techniques.

CONVENTIONAL RADIOGRAPHS

The radiographic appearances vary depending on the initial focus of infection within the vertebra. There are mainly four sites of infection in the vertebra, i.e. paradiscal, anterior subperiosteal, central and appendiceal.

Paradiskal

This is the most common type of lesion, also called marginal, intervertebral, subarticular or metaphyseal lesion. The disease process most often begins in the anterior part of the vertebral body either superiorly or inferiorly adjacent to the endplate.[1,28] Two adjacent vertebral bodies are involved in about 50% of cases of tubercular osteomyelitis. There is demineralization and loss of definition of their dense margins or endplates. Little or no periosteal reaction or reactive sclerosis affect the remainder of the vertebra.[1,2,18]

As infection spreads, the adjacent intervertebral disk becomes involved with narrowing of the disk space **(Fig. 4)**. Disk space may also narrow due to lack of nutrition and prolapse of nucleus into the soft necrotic vertebral body. Rarely the disk space may remain intact for a long time. This makes the diagnosis difficult, since disk space narrowing constitutes an important diagnostic feature of infection and serves to differentiate tuberculosis from fracture, malignant disease, solitary myeloma and porotic collapse.[18]

With progressive destruction anterior wedging or collapse occur resulting in varying degrees of kyphosis. Scoliosis may occasionally be seen with asymmetric or unilateral destruction of vertebral bodies and disks and is virtually confined to the lower thoracic and lumbar vertebrae. This is not as frequent as kyphosis.[6]

Central

The central type of lesion starts in the center of the vertebral body. A lytic area with absence of normal trabeculae is seen in the central portion away from the disk margin **(Fig. 5)**. This gradually enlarges and the vertebral body may expand or balloon out like a tumor. In later stages concentric collapse occurs, almost resembling a vertebra plana. Paravertebral shadows may be absent or minimal. The disk space is either not affected or only minimally affected.[6,7,18]

Anterior Subperiosteal

This type of infection begins at the anterior vertebral margin underneath the periosteum and spreads beneath the anterior longitudinal ligament producing subtle anterior erosions of multiple vertebrae. The clinical symptoms are severe in relation to the minor radiographic abnormalities **(Figs. 6A and B)**. Disk destruction may be late and anterior erosions are difficult to detect on plain radiographs.

Appendiceal or Neural Arch Tuberculosis

The neural arch or vertebral arch includes the spinous process, the laminae, the transverse processes and the pedicle as well as the lateral masses of the atlas, as embryologically they are equivalent to the neural arch. Overall, the neural arch involvement is reported to range from 2–30% of cases usually in contiguity with vertebral body involvement.[4,13] Isolated involvement of the neural arch with complete sparing of vertebral bodies and intervertebral disks is rare, constituting less than 2% of all the cases of spinal tuberculosis in nonendemic areas and 5–10% in endemic areas.[4,47] Neural arch tuberculosis (NAT) is being increasingly recognized

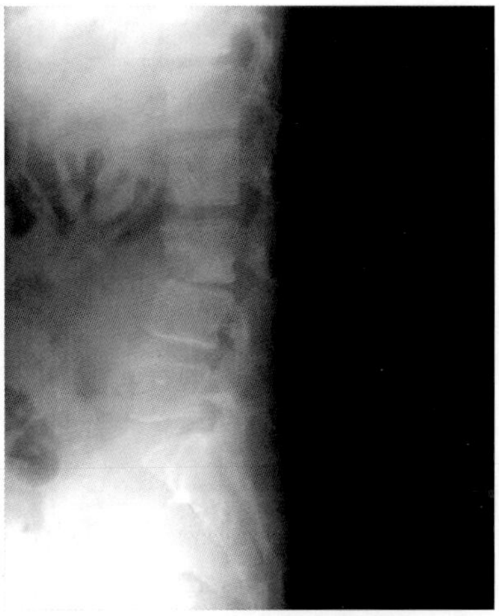

Fig. 4: Lateral radiograph L-S spine showing reduction of L3–L4 disk space with erosion of the anteroinferior aspect of L3 vertebral body—Marginal variety of caries.

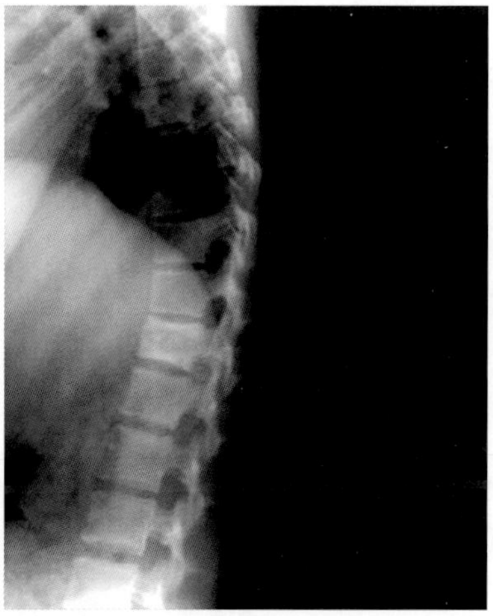

Fig. 5: Lateral radiograph D-L spine showing a lytic area with lack of normal trabeculae in the center of D12 vertebral body. There is mild reduction of vertebral height and minimal sclerosis, adjacent disk spaces are, however, normal—Central caries.

with the use of cross-sectional imaging as plain films are limited in the evaluation of the neural arch lesions. Both CT and MR are especially useful in the diagnosis of NAT **(Figs. 7A to C)**. Some authors have reported that NAT most commonly affects the cervical and upper dorsal spine unlike classical spinal tuberculosis which is most common at the lumbodorsal junction.[47] There is a tendency towards pedicular and laminar involvement in tubercular spondylitis whereas pyogenic spondylitis has a predilection for the facet joints.[48] The pedicle is usually the most common site of involvement, the

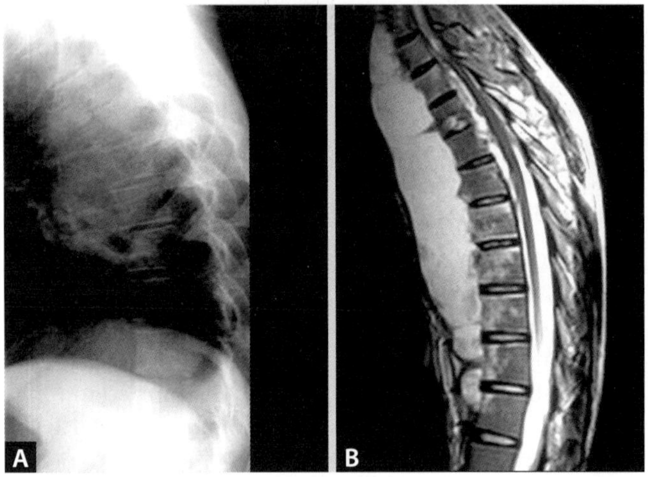

Figs. 6A and B: (A) X-ray dorsal spine lateral view in a patient with anterior subperiosteal caries show indistinct anterior cortices of multiple dorsal vertebrae; (B) Sagittal T2W MR of the same reveals the entire extent of pathology with patchy hyperintense signal in multiple dorsal vertebrae, erosions of the anterior cortices and a large prevertebral abscess. A small ventral epidural collection with dorsal displacement of the upper thoracic cord is also noted.

involvement usually being unilateral.[49,50] When there is bilateral involvement of the posterior elements associated with body involvement gross instability can lead to cord compression and paralysis. Radiographic findings in NAT include pedicular or laminar destruction, erosion of the adjacent ribs in the thoracic region or posterior cortex of the vertebral body with relative sparing of the intervertebral disks and a large paraspinal mass.[6]

Recognition of coexisting posterior and anterior involvement is essential for presurgical planning. Anterior stabilization relies on posterior stability, because decompression can lead to instability, anterior and posterior stabilization must be performed.[2] Cases of isolated NAT respond well to simple decompression and debridement followed by chemotherapy.[51] Paraplegia associated with NAT reportedly has a better prognosis than that with typical spinal tuberculosis.[47]

Associated bony changes in tubercular spondylitis seen on plain films include, unilateral large bridging osteophytes which may occur due to irritation of the bone by inflammatory process with periosteal new bone formation or due to ossification in ligaments. They are more common in the lumbar spine as it bears most of the body weight.

Abscess formation associated with tubercular spondylitis can produce soft tissue opacity on radiographs that appears out of proportion to the degree of osseous destruction. The opacity is commonly bilateral and uniform. It may be globular, which implies pus under tension or fusiform in morphology. Paravertebral abscess may be minimal in the central variety of tubercular lesion. An abscess in the cervical region presents as widening of

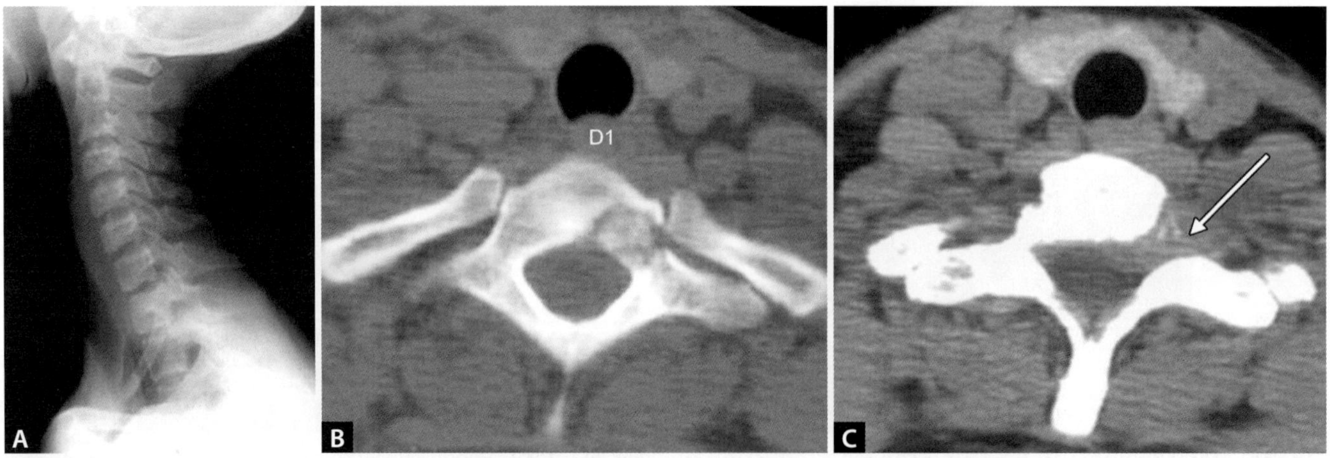

Figs. 7A to C: X-ray cervical spine lateral view with the shoulders pulled down reveals no abnormality (A); Axial CT sections bone (B); Soft tissue (C). Windows showing lytic lesions involving the left pedicle and posterior body of D1 vertebra. Associated soft tissue extending into the spinal canal is also seen (arrow)—Neural arch tuberculosis.

the prevertebral soft tissues **(Fig. 8)**. In the dorsal spine the posteromedial pleural line is displaced laterally by a paraspinal abscess and the abscess produces as typical fusiform shape called the "birds nest" appearance.[7] The aneurysmal effect may be found in Pott's disease associated with an anterior paravertebral or subligamentous abscess between D4 and D10 vertebrae, shallow erosions or gouge defects are found on the anterior and lateral surfaces of the vertebral bodies probably due to transmitted aortic pulsations. The intervertebral disks being resistant to pressure atrophy are spared.[6,7,18,52] An abscess at the dorsolumbar junction has an indistinct converging lower border and is referred to as a 'petering abscess' **(Fig. 9)**. In the lumbar region the abscess tends to track along the psoas producing bulging of the psoas outline.[6,7,52] Calcification in the paraspinal abscesses is considered pathognomonic of tuberculosis as nontubercular abscesses rarely calcify. Tuberculous abscesses of the psoas muscle calcify in two distinct patterns which are[6]—faint amorphous deposits and tear drop shaped calcification. With healing the calcification tends to become more dense and in rare instances may be seen to diminish or disappear on serial radiographs.[6]

The radiographic appearance of tuberculous spondylitis in **colored races**[1,52] may be different from the classical caries spine. In this setting there may be more frequent involvement of a single vertebral body with conspicuous preservation of adjacent disks, even when the vertebral body is totally destroyed. Cervical spine involvement and isolated involvement of the posterior spinal elements is also more commonly observed. Sclerotic changes and periosteal reaction mimicking nontubercular infection are also more frequently observed.[1] Cystic and multilocular patterns of involvement may be seen probably due to malnourishment and poor immunological status. However, in general, marked sclerosis, less destruction and collapse, small or no paravertebral abscess, more rapid clinical course should suggest a nontubercular etiology of an inflammatory spinal lesion on conventional radiographs.[53]

Computed Tomography

Four patterns of bone destruction have been described:[13] on CT, i.e. fragmentary—47% **(Fig. 10)**, osteolytic—33% **(Fig. 11)**, subperiosteal—10% **(Figs. 12A and B)** and well-defined lytic with sclerotic margins—10%. The fragmentary type is the most frequent and characteristic. This appearance consists of numerous residual small bone fragments embedded in a soft tissue mass. Similar appearance has also been described in involved areas of vertebral appendages.[47] The appearance is probably due to the fact that tuberculous inflammatory exudates lack proteolytic enzymes required to lyse bone.[13] Bone fragments may migrate into the surrounding structures including the spinal canal, paravertebral soft tissues and psoas muscles. These are easily detected by CT. Some authors describe that the vertebral bodies appear to have 'exploded' with peripheral bony fragments. This is in contrast to pyogenic spondylitis that shows multiple small erosions like a 'pepper pot' and no calcification. Disk space narrowing, multilevel involvement and kyphosis

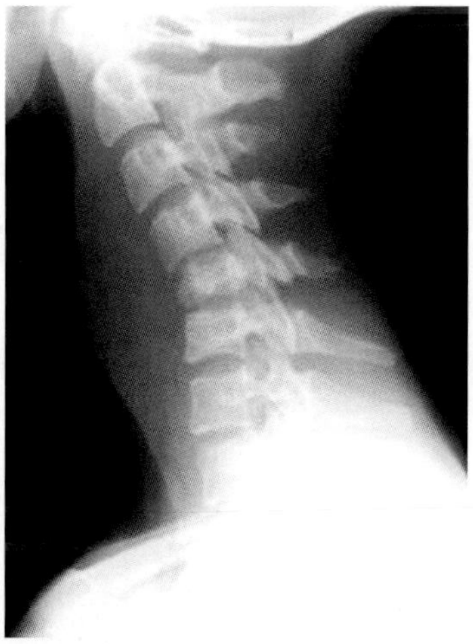

Fig. 8: Lateral radiograph cervical spine in a patient with caries C5 vertebra showing reversal of the cervical lordosis, widening of the prevertebral soft tissues and anterior displacement of the airway due to an associated abscess.

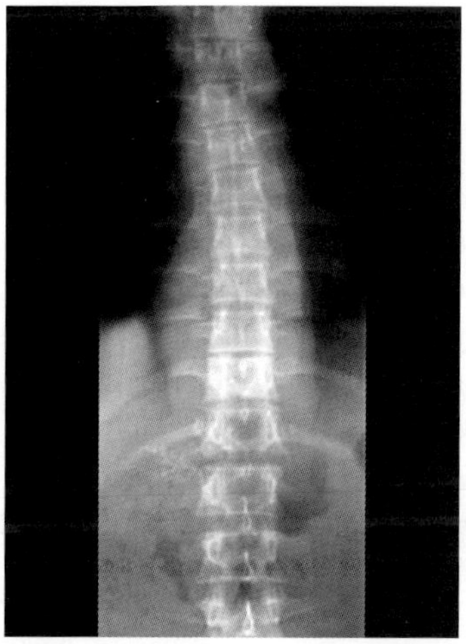

Fig. 9: X-ray D-L spine AP view of a patient with tuberculosis D10-D11 vertebrae showing a characteristic 'petering abscess' with indistinct inferior margins. Subtle amorphous calcification is seen on the right side.

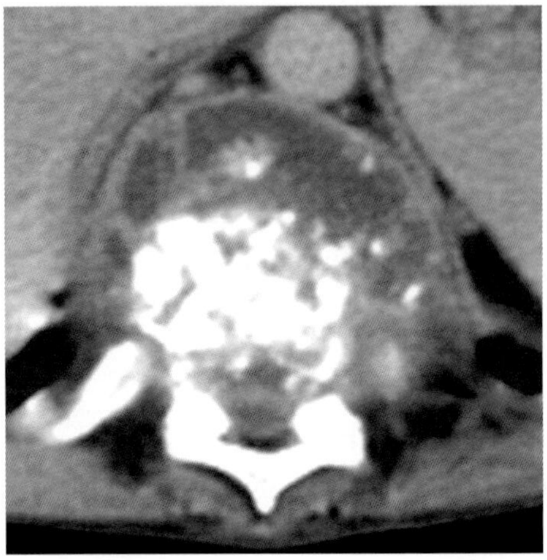

Fig. 10: Postcontrast axial CT scan showing characteristic fragmentary destruction of the vertebral body with an associated multiloculated pre- and paravertebral abscess.

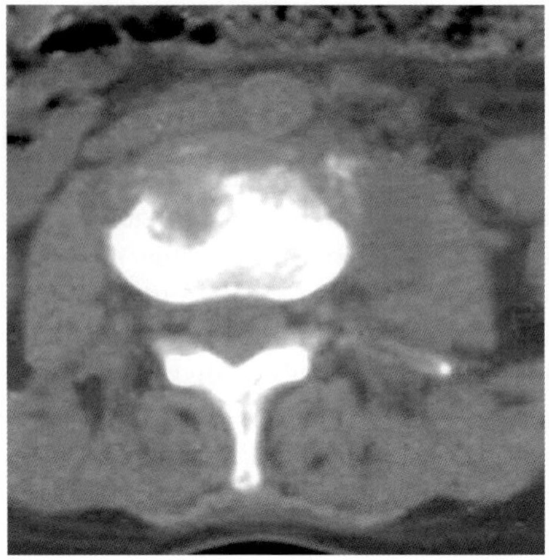

Fig. 11: Axial CT scan showing an osteolytic lesion in the anterior vertebral body in a case of caries spine.

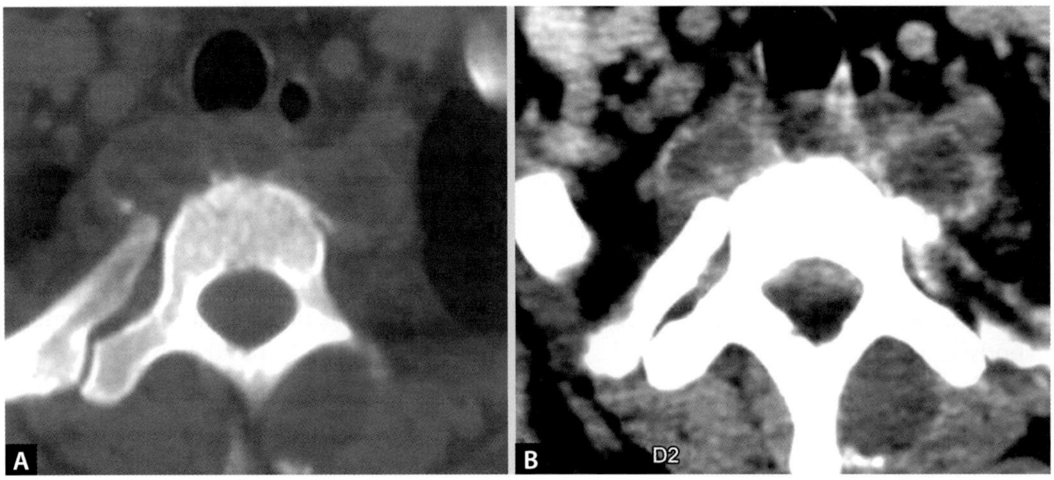

Figs. 12A and B: Axial CT scans—bone (A) and soft tissue (B). Window settings in a case of subperiosteal caries showing subtle erosions of the anterior cortex of the D2 vertebra. Associated collections are noted in the pre- and paravertebral soft tissues anteriorly. Note another collection in the left posterior paraspinal region.

are also demonstrated and are particularly well seen on multiplanar reconstructions.[4,36]

There is obliteration of the fat planes around the vertebral body early in the evolution of abscess formation.[4] Soft tissue abscesses are well-demonstrated on axial scans and multiplanar reconstructions.[4,13] These have been characterized by their CT attenuation values with high attenuation lesions being defined as granulation tissue and low density lesions defined as abscesses or caseous material. CT is ideally suited to demonstrate small amounts of calcification which are not visible on plain radiographs **(Fig. 13)**.[37]

The thick nodular rim of increased tissue attenuation of an abscess on a precontrast scan represents the

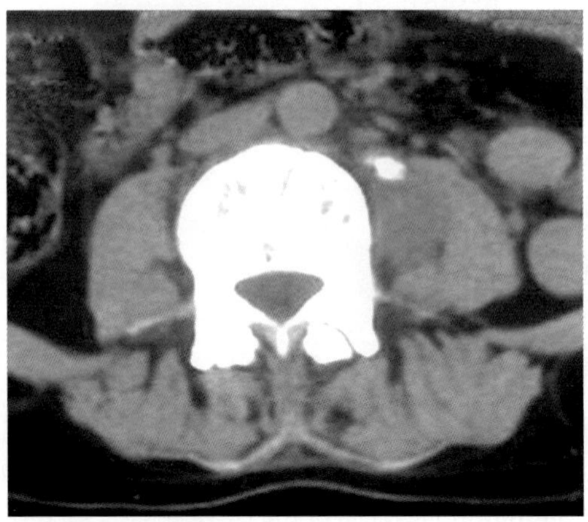

Fig. 13: Axial CT section showing a left psoas abscess with a small speck of calcification.

hyper-vascular, hypercellular fibrotic wall of the inflammatory cavity. Following intravenous contrast administration there is usually strong rim enhancement around low attenuation multiloculated collection. This is also called the '***rind sign***'.[6] Granulation tissue shows a more homogeneous enhancement **(Figs. 14A and B)**. CT can also demonstrate epidural extension of these soft tissue masses with cord compression. Small bone fragments which may be present some distance away from the actual site of vertebral destruction may be easily demonstrated by CT. It is especially important to localize such fragments prior to surgical removal.[13]

The combination of a multilocular and calcified paraspinal abscess with a thick, well-enhancing irregular rim in the presence of vertebral body bony fragmentation is a strong indication of tuberculous rather than pyogenic infection or neoplasm. CT findings though not always pathognomonic, facilitate guided biopsy procedures as well providing material for histo/cytopathology, AFB staining and culture in equivocal cases.[4,21,54-56]

Magnetic Resonance Imaging

T1-weighted images usually show a decreased signal within the affected vertebral marrow and loss of cortical definition of the affected vertebrae.[4,51] On T2-weighted images a relative increase in signal intensity is noted within involved vertebral bodies and disks. Disk involvement has been reported in 46–72% of cases and occurs relatively late compared to pyogenic spondylitis. The internuclear cleft within the disk is a normal finding in patients older than 30 years and its loss on imaging in combination with a high signal intensity are signs of inflammation **(Figs. 15A and B)**.[4] However, the intervertebral disk when uninvolved, will not show an increased signal on T2-weighted images.[46] Occasionally the disk space is preserved despite extensive bone destruction, the so-called ***floating disk sign***. In children the hydrated disks do not seem to form a good barrier to infection and are involved in most patients imaged.[36] Involvement posterior elements is also detected well by MR imaging and is more common in tuberculosis than pyogenic infections **(Fig. 16)**. Enhanced MR studies may demonstrate inhomogeneous enhancement in the region of marrow infiltration.

Paraspinal soft tissue masses are seen in approximately 71% of cases on MRI.[57] On T1W images loss of the uniform psoas muscle signal intensity and enlargement of the affected muscle indicate morphologic alteration of the paraspinal soft tissue. On T2W images there is an increase in signal intensity with paraspinal masses appearing hyperintense **(Fig. 17)**.[4,45,57] Postcontrast studies reveal thick rim enhancement around intraosseous and paraspinal soft tissue abscesses, which is more common in tuberculosis than in other spinal infections **(Fig. 18)**. More uniform enhancement is seen with granulation tissue or phlegmon. Neither an anterior paraspinal phlegmon nor an abscess encases the intercostal arteries in thoracic spinal tuberculosis as they barely penetrate the anterior longitudinal ligament.[58] MR is useful in delineating the communication between vertebral and paravertebral components of tuberculous spondylitis.[46] Epidural extension is detected by MRI in about 61% of involved vertebrae.[57] The soft tissue masses displace the thecal sac and the spinal cord is distorted. Postcontrast fat-suppressed T1W sequences are the best to demonstrate

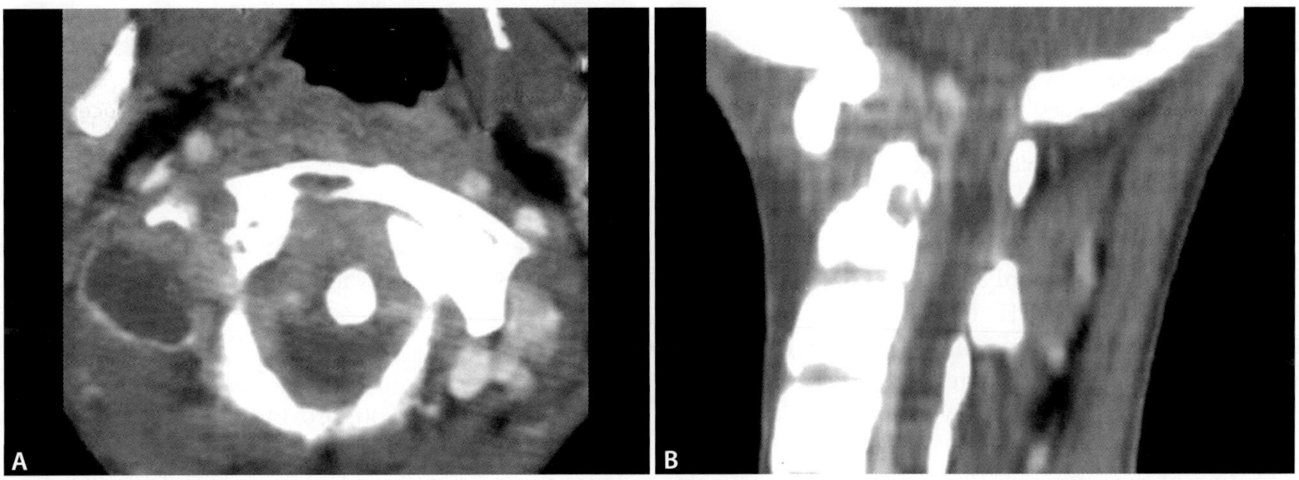

Figs. 14A and B: Axial postcontrast CT myelogram (A) with sagittal MPR; (B) in a patient with caries C1-C2 showing atlantoaxial dislocation with erosions of the right lateral mass of C1 and the dens. A peripherally enhancing abscess is noted on the right side while homogeneously enhancing granulation tissue is seen in the predental space.

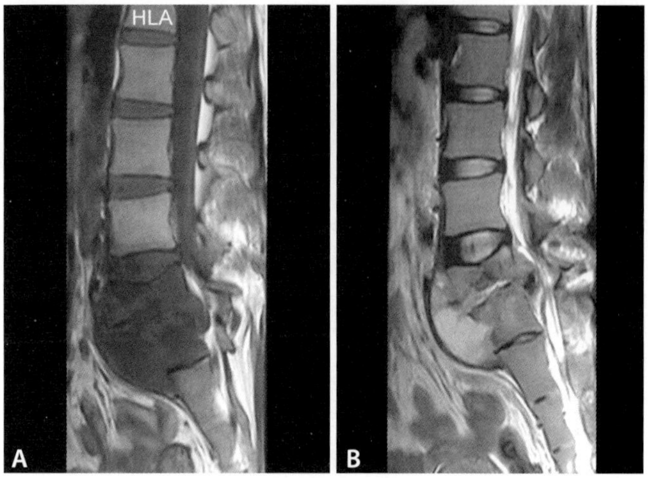

Figs. 15A and B: Sagittal T1W (A) and T2W (B). MR scans of a patient with tuberculosis L5-S1 show collapse of L5 vertebral body, hypointense marrow signal of L5-S1 and loss of cortical definition on the T1W image. The intervening disk space is reduced with hyperintense signal on the T2W image suggesting discitis. A prevertebral abscess lifting up the anterior longitudinal ligament and a small ventral epidural collection are also seen.

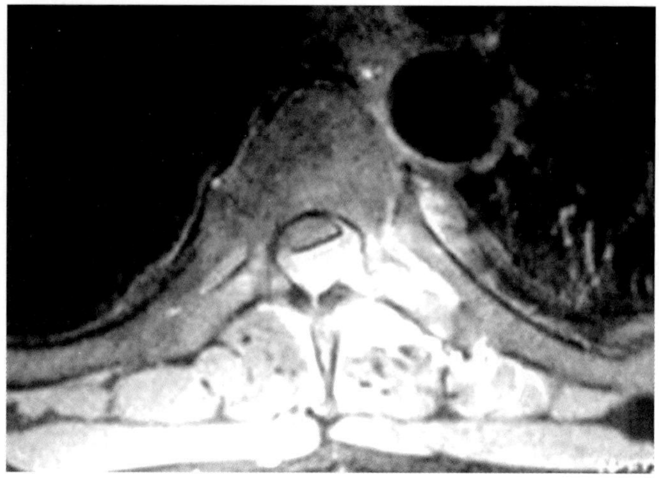

Fig. 16: Postcontrast T1W fat-suppressed axial MR section through a thoracic vertebra showing patchy enhancement in the left pedicle, lamina, transverse process and the adjacent rib. Homogeneously enhancing granulation tissue is noted in the left paraspinal region and dorsal epidural space displacing the cord anteriorly–NAT.

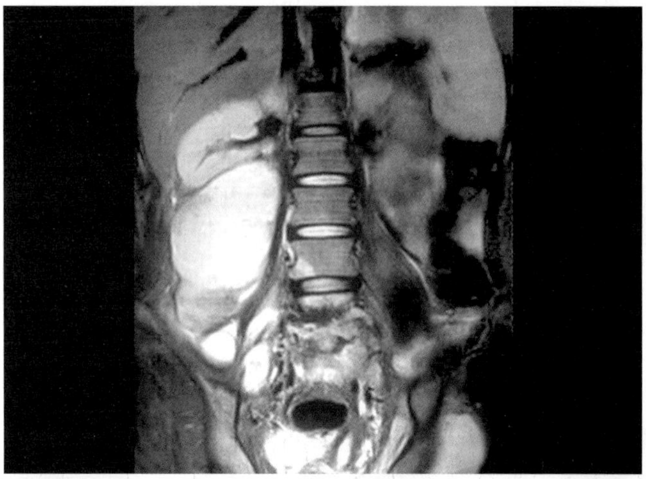

Fig. 17: STIR coronal scan in a patient with lumbosacral caries depicts partial collapse and hyperintense signal involving L4-L5 vertebrae. There is a disproportionately large psoas abscess on the right side lifting up the inferior pole of right kidney.

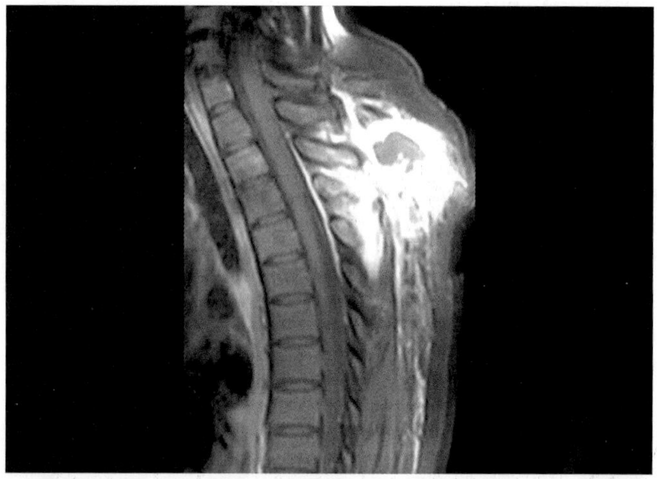

Fig. 18: Postcontrast T1W sagittal MR image of a patient with caries spine showing erosion of the spinous process of D3 vertebra with a large abscess showing thick peripheral rim enhancement.

meningeal and epidural inflammatory soft tissues, with improved definition of cord and nerve root compromise **(Figs. 19A and B)**.[29,39] Heavily T2W fast spin-echo sequences can also be used to provide a myelographic effect showing thecal sac compression.[57]

The MR imaging features, with high sensitivity and specificity for diagnosis of spinal tuberculosis[59] are disruption of the endplate, 100 and 81.4% respectively, paravertebral soft tissue shadow (96.8%, 85.3%) and a high signal intensity of the intervertebral disk on the T2-weighted image (80.6%, 82.4%). The overall sensitivity and specificity for diagnosis are 100 and 88.2%, respectively.

Cord Changes

Conventional radiographs provide little information if any, on the status of the cord and even CT cannot adequately assess the cord status. MR imaging on the other hand because of its superior soft tissue contrast provides invaluable information about the status of the cord.

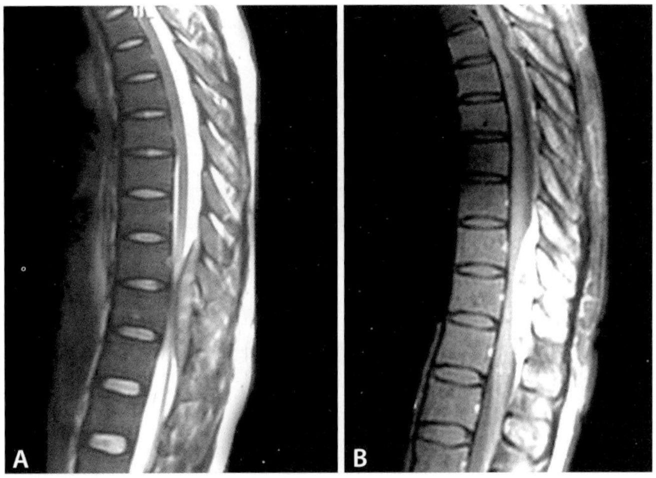

Figs. 19A and B: Sagittal T2W (A) and postcontrast fat-suppressed T1W (B) MR images in a patient with neural arch tuberculosis D-L spine show nearly homogeneously enhancing dorsal epidural granulation tissue with resultant cord compression. Note the abnormal enhancement in the adjacent spinous processes and interspinous region.

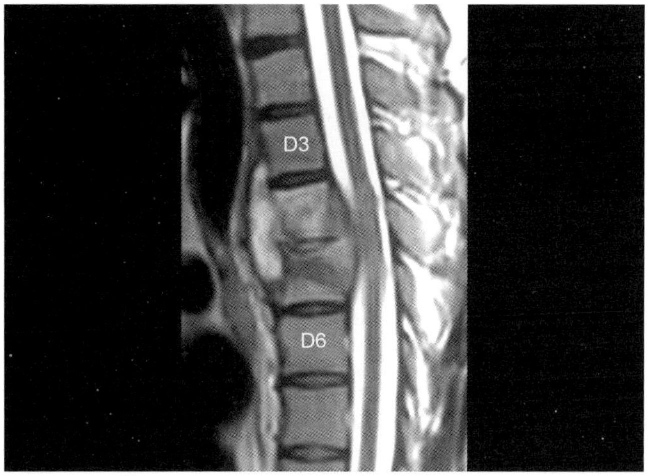

Fig. 20: Sagittal T2W MR scan of the cervicodorsal spine in a patient of caries D4-D5 shows reduction in disk space with altered marrow signal in the involved vertebrae and associated prevertebral and ventral epidural collections. The cord is mildly expanded at this level with T2 hyperintense signal due to cord edema.

Cord involvement often results in neurological deficit or paraplegia.

Paraplegia in patients with **active disease** may be caused by ***mechanical pressure*** on the cord by tubercular abscesses, granulation tissue, debris, internal gibbus or subluxation. The spinal cord seems to have some physiologic reserve to with stand pressure, particularly when pressure develops slowly as is the case with tuberculosis and 40–50% reduction in cord diameter is often compatible with good cord function. The midsagittal cord diameter and presence of CSF signal anterior to cord at the apex of the deformity at presentation have been shown to correlate with neurological deficit in a recent study. Ambulatory patients had greater cord dimensions and CSF signal persisting anterior to cord at the apex of the deformity in this study.[60] Unrelieved compression of the spinal cord results in loss of neurons, gliosis and demyelination of cord substance in the damaged segment.

Intrinsic changes in the spinal cord such as inflammatory edema or direct involvement of meninges and spinal cord by tuberculous infection may also lead to paraplegia .The changes in the spinal cord may be interpreted as edema of the cord, myelomalacia, atrophy of the cord and syringomyelia **(Fig. 20)**. Edema is seen as hyperintense signal on T2-weighted images but no signal alteration on T1 while myelomalacia shows a T1 hypointense signal (higher than that of CSF) as well and may be associated with thinning of the cord. A syrinx is a tubular, well-defined fluid filled region within the spinal cord. It is usually tapered to one, or both ends and can appear septated. The signal characteristics are typically those of CSF. Edema of the cord is compatible with good neurological recovery following treatment, while thinning of the cord with syrinx or myelomalacia leads to poor cord function. Mild atrophy of the cord is observed even when there is a successful neurological outcome.[36,61] Rarely a small tuberculoma of the cord may be responsible for neurological deficits presenting as spinal tumor syndrome **(Figs. 21A and B)**.[61]

According to some authors MR findings may also be a useful guide to treatment strategy. Patients ,with neurological deficit, in whom MR shows a relatively preserved cord with evidence of myelitis or edema and a predominantly fluid collection in the extradural space, respond well to conservative treatment, if mechanical compression is the only cause of the neurological deficit. Early surgical decompression is indicated when MRI shows that the extradural compression is due to granulation tissue or caseous tissue, with little fluid component compressing the spinal cord and with features of edema of the cord, myelitis or myelomalacia.[21] **Paraplegia** with **healed disease**[21] may occur when the initial lesion has healed with a residual severe deformity, even after a gap of 10–20 years. It is produced by stretching the spinal cord over an internal anterior bony projection, producing gliosis. MRI shows severe atrophy of the cord and/or syringo-hydromyelia, or constricting scarring of and around the dura **(Figs. 22A and B)**. Reactivation of the disease is found in 30–40% of

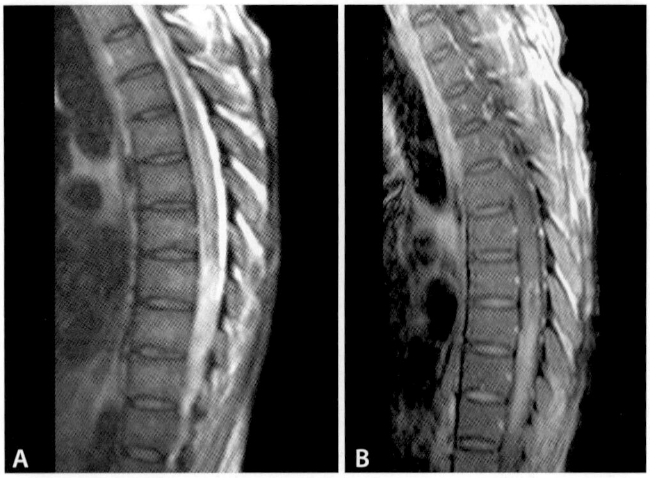

Figs. 21A and B: T2W (A) and postcontrast T1W (B): Sagittal images of a patient with tubercular myelitis reveal cord swelling and edema appearing hyperintense on the T2-weighted image with patchy enhancement on the postcontrast image.

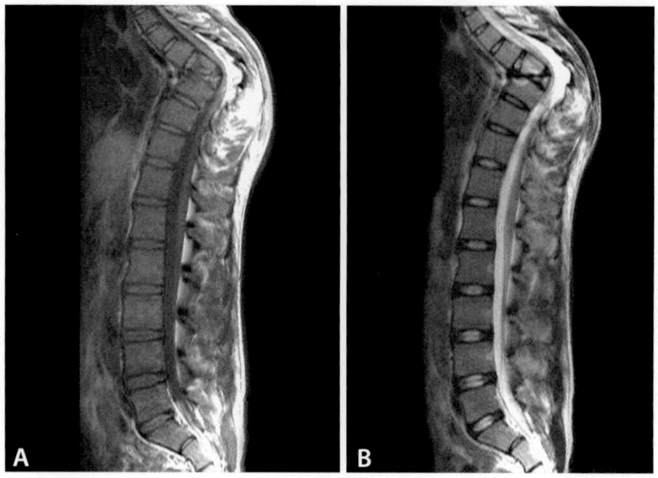

Figs. 22A and B: T1W (A) and T2W (B) images of the dorsolumbar spine in an old treated case of tuberculosis spine reveal near complete destruction of D8 vertebra and partial destruction of the adjacent D7 and D9 with fatty marrow signal and gross kyphotic deformity. There is resultant stretching and thinning of the cord but no signal change suggestive of cord atrophy. Note the fibrofatty proliferation along the dorsal epidural space appearing hyperintense on both T1 and T2W images.

cases on exploration. Symptomatic severe stenosis of the lumbar canal and ossification of the ligamentum flavum adjacent to severe kyphosis may produce an incomplete neurological deficit.

ATYPICAL SPINAL TUBERCULOSIS[21]

The typical paradiscal tubercular lesion is well-described, easily recognized and treated. Atypical spinal tuberculosis is defined as compressive myelopathy with no visible or palpable spinal deformity and without the radiological appearance of a typical vertebral lesion. Such lesions are relatively uncommon, and are difficult to diagnose and treat in the early stages with more chance of neurological complications. Atypical lesions may present as an intraspinal tubercular granuloma, involvement of the neural arch, compressive myelopathy in single vertebral disease, a concertina collapse of a vertebra or a sclerotic vertebra. Granulomatous lesions of the epidural, intradural, or intramedullary spaces present as a compressive myelopathy, the ***spinal tumor syndrome***, without obvious radiological signs. Tubercular granuloma should be considered in the differential diagnosis of spinal tumor syndrome in zones endemic for tuberculosis.

Extraosseous extradural granuloma is a rare variant that leads to a extradural granulomatous lesion in the absence of bone involvement. The route of infection is most likely hematogenous. This manifestation is more common in men than women, in the dorsal epidural space and in the thoracic segment. Clinically compressive radiculomyelopathy is evident. On pathologic examination a granulomatous membrane is found ensheathing and compressing the spinal cord or cauda equina.[6] This variety of disease may be easily diagnosed by MR imaging. Epidural tubercular lesions appear to be isointense to cord on T1W images and have mixed signal intensity on T2W images. Enhancement after gadolinium will be uniform if the inflammatory process is phlegmonous in nature or peripherally enhancing if abscess formation or caseation has occurred **(Figs. 23A to C)**.[5] Epidural tuberculous abscess may occur as primary lesions or may be seen in association with arachnoiditis, myelitis, intramedullary tuberculoma, etc.[62]

Post-treatment Follow-up

Conventional Radiographs

While on treatment, sequential radiographs can be repeated to assess the degree of healing. However, radiological evidence of healing is appreciated late on routine radio-graphs. It lags behind by about three months.[21] Evidence of bone destruction or loss of vertebral height may progress till 14 months after starting treatment and should not necessarily be considered an adverse feature.[63] Soft tissue paravertebral masses may also progress while on treatment reaching a maximum size within 1.5 months, although they may take up to 15 months to resolve. Although MRC trials (Multicenter randomized controlled trials of Medical Research Council,

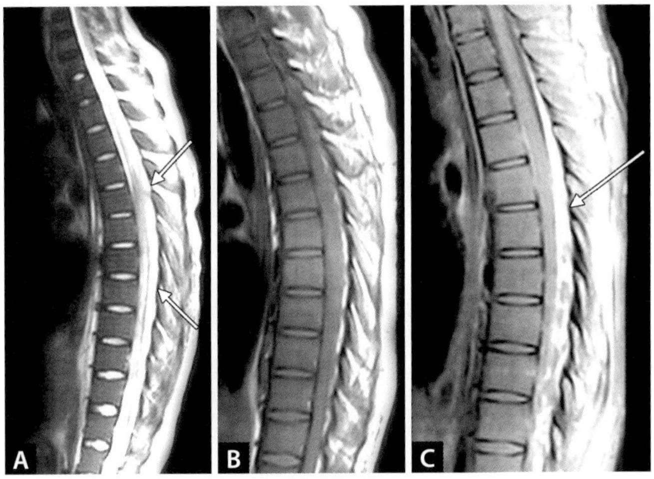

Figs. 23A to C: Extraosseous extradural granuloma: Sagittal T2W (A) T1W (B) and postcontrast (C). MR images show normal vertebral and intervertebral disk morphology and signal intensity pattern. A long segment, crescentic dorsal epidural abscess showing heterogeneous signal on T1W and T2W images with irregular peripheral contrast enhancement (arrows) causing anterior displacement of thecal sac is seen.

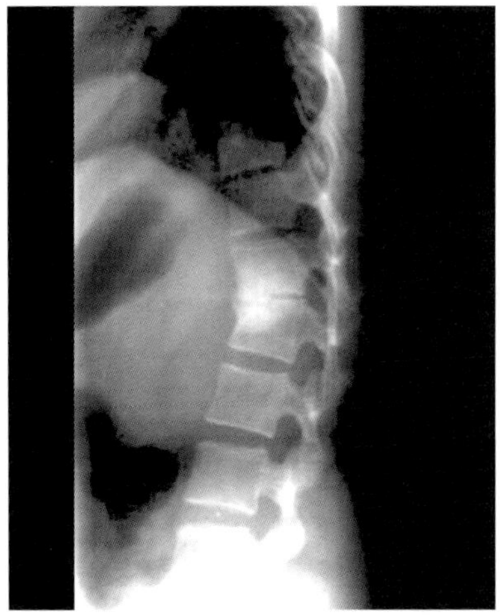

Fig. 24: Lateral radiograph D-L spine in a case of healing tuberculosis shows reduced disk space between D12 and L1 vertebrae with sclerosis adjacent to the vertebral end plates.

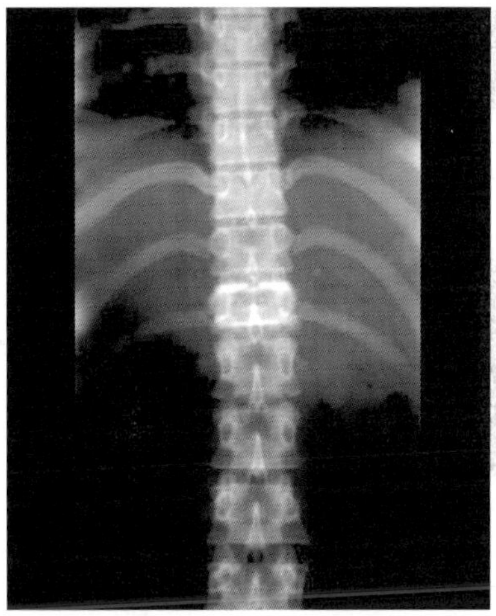

Fig. 25: X-ray D-L spine AP view showing sclerosis of D12 vertebra giving the appearance of ivory vertebra in a patient with healing caries.

UK) have shown persistent changes in plain radiological appearances of the vertebral column up to three years after completion of treatment, these changes were attributed to new bone formation and ankylosis.[64] Signs of healing include static lesion or regression of a lesion on serial radiographs, well-defined outlines of the lesion, evidence of sclerosis **(Fig. 24)** and fusion of adjacent vertebral bodies forming a large block of osseous mass. Increased density of the vertebral body in association with healing can lead to the appearance of an ivory vertebra. The phenomenon is usually evident in the lumbar region **(Fig. 25)**.[6] Calcific debris which progresses to fusion on serial films may be seen as early as 3 weeks, although it can take up to 27 months for any evidence of fusion to appear.[63] Fusion of contiguous vertebrae has long been regarded as the surest sign of healing of spinal tuberculosis although there is no actual proof of this **(Fig. 26)**.[63]

In the absence of reliable serological and immunological markers of healing, the 'healed status' is achieved if there is clinical and radiological evidence of healing with no recurrence after two years.[21] It is, however, well known that reactivation of disease may occur years later.

PET/CT[65]

A few recent studies suggest that ^{18}F-FDG-PET may be useful for discriminating residual and nonresidual spinal infection after treatment.

Computed Tomography

Features of resolution such as increase in vertebral bone density, with reduction in the size of paraspinal soft tissue masses as edema and inflammatory exudate subside are readily apparent on sequential CT examinations.[4] The inflammatory reaction in the bone marrow, however, is not well depicted **(Figs. 27A and B)**.[38]

Magnetic Resonance Imaging[40,48,57]

Post-therapy follow-up can also be done with MR. The earliest sign of healing is a reduction in the amount of inflammatory soft tissue. Increasing soft tissue mass,

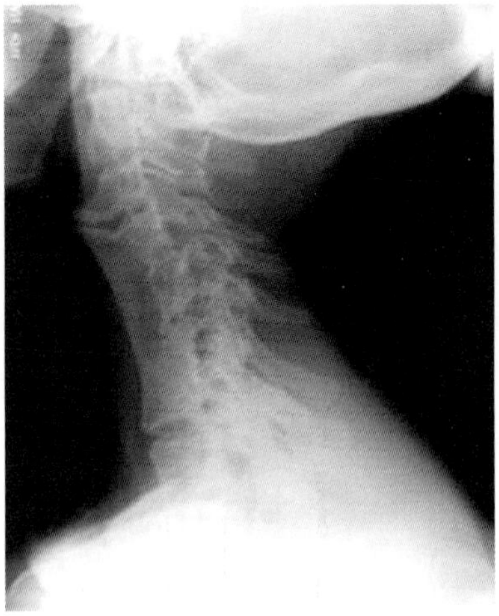

Fig. 26: Lateral radiograph of the cervical spine shows fusion of multiple cervical vertebral forming a large osseous block in a patient with healed tuberculosis of the cervical spine.

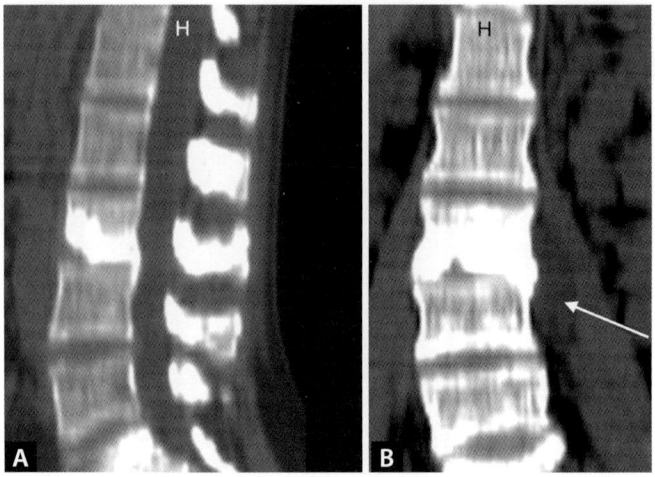

Figs. 27A and B: Sagittal and coronal CT reconstructions of the lumbar spine of a patient on ATT showing sclerosis of the inferior body and end plate of L1 vertebra with reduced L1-L2 disk space suggestive of healing disease (arrow).

bony destruction or an alteration in signal intensity do not indicate failed treatment. A high-signal intensity rim on the T1W sequences at the edge of the osseous lesion represents healing **(Fig. 28)**. A progressive sequential increase in signal intensity on T1W images has been found to correlate well with resolving symptoms and clinical signs **(Fig. 29)**. Reduction in gadolinium enhancement and eventual loss of enhancement are useful signs of healing. However, persistent or increasing enhancement are not necessarily indicative of either deterioration or treatment failure. MR imaging is also useful in the detection of reactivation of old tubercular spondylitis. The change of signal from low signal in healed tuberculosis to high signal on T2W images suggest active disease. Reactivation may present with an isolated psoas abscess without evidence of bony lesions.

The exact role of MR in the follow-up of spinal tuberculosis is not defined.

In a study[66] where follow-up MR spine examinations were performed between 6 and 12 months after starting ATT, a significant proportion of patients had radiological evidence of persistent disease activity in the form of infective discitis, vertebral body abscess, vertebra body edema or multifocal intraosseous abscess with persistent cord compression. Both the British and American Thoracic Societies, based on the evidence of the MRC trials, advocate short course chemotherapy (six months) for adult uncomplicated fully sensitive spinal TB. However, the authors felt that in a significant proportion of patients, longer durations of treatment (more than 6 months) may be required as their MR scans were abnormal even though there was apparent disease resolution clinically.

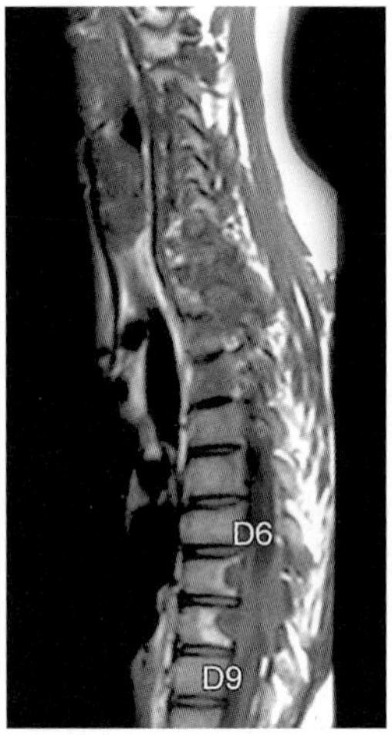

Fig. 28: Sagittal T1W MR image of the cervicodorsal spine of a patient after 3 months of ATT shows erosions of the posterior cortex of D7-D8 vertebrae. These lesions show marginal hyperintense signal signifying healing lesions.

In another study[67] where parallel follow-up of the clinical (weight, analgesic intake and neurological status), laboratory, and imaging outcome of nineteen patients treated for spinal tuberculosis was done it was suggested that the laboratory inflammatory syndrome, i.e. elevated CRP and ESR should disappear after 3 months of treatment and that patients should recover their previous clinical status after 6 months of treatment. On MRI, all epidural abscesses disappeared within 9 months, but importantly, many lesions remained visible on MRI at the end of treatment, i.e. 12 months (15% of initial paravertebral abscesses and 25% of vertebral edematous signals) despite

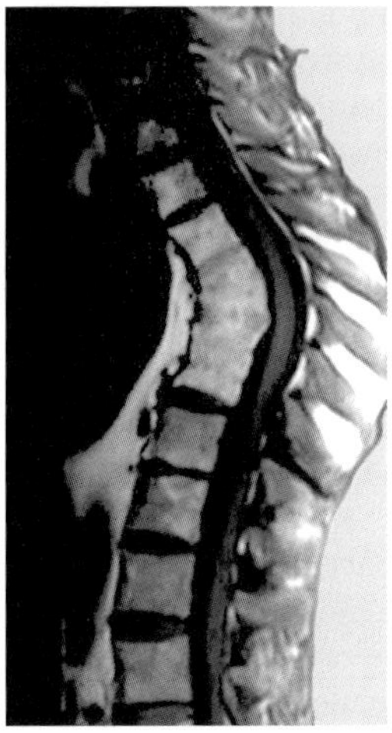

Fig. 29: Sagittal T1W MR of the dorsal spine in a patient with healed caries spine shows kyphosis with complete absence of disk space between multiple dorsal vertebrae which appear hyperintense on the T1W image due to fatty replacement.

the favorable clinical outcome with a mean follow-up of 25 months. The authors suggested that the persistence of MRI abnormalities after 12 months of treatment does not require further treatment in patients who have a favorable clinical and laboratory outcome. MRI alone cannot determine when treatment should be stopped. Repeat MRI is probably not necessary in patients who have a clinical and laboratory improvement during treatment.[67]

Although both these studies have evaluated only a limited number of patients they highlight the fact that there is currently no guidance on soft tissue or vertebral changes noted on MR spine examination, during the course of, or after antituberculous therapy. Furthermore, time course studies of the MR changes of spinal TB need to be performed to achieve consensus on the interpretation and use of this powerful modality in the follow-up of spinal TB patients.[66]

DIFFERENTIAL DIAGNOSIS

The differential diagnosis of tubercular spondylodiscitis includes pyogenic and fungal infections, degenerative disk disease, brucellosis, neoplasms, etc.

Clinical findings usually allow a differentiation of infection from *degenerative spondylosis*, but vertebral infection with radicular pain may be misdiagnosed as degenerative disease if the patient is afebrile. With degenerative disease, the disk space is usually not markedly narrowed and on MR imaging disk dessication is manifested as low signal intensity on T2W images. After intravenous contrast, infected disks enhance strongly whereas degenerated disks only occasionally enhance to a small degree.[17]

When infection is considered, a history of chronicity and insidious progression suggests tubercular rather than *pyogenic infection*. In tuberculosis, lack of sclerotic and reactive changes with prominent osteoporosis are seen on plain films. On MR imaging relative preservation of disk, with involvement of multiple contiguous vertebrae, involvement of entire body, loss of cortical definition, more frequent involvement of posterior elements, a well-defined paraspinal region with abnormal signal intensity, disproportionally large paraspinal masses, especially with calcification or a thick rim of enhancement, subligamentous spread to three or more vertebral levels and presence of skip lesions favor a tubercular etiology. However, differentiation from pyogenic infection can at times be difficult.[1,17]

Like tuberculosis the course of *brucellosis* is indolent. Characteristic features of brucellar spondylitis include gas within the disk, only minimal associated paraspinal soft tissue mass, absence of gibbus deformity and predilection for the lower lumbar spine. On MR images, vertebral body morphology and cortical margins are intact despite evidence of osteomyelitis.

Sarcoidosis can produce findings identical to those of tuberculosis including multifocal vertebral lesions with paraspinal masses.[1]

When a solitary vertebra is involved, differentiation from *metastatic disease* in adults and from *eosinophilic granuloma*, in children may be difficult. Spinal lesions such as *lymphoma* that affect consecutive vertebrae or neoplasms such as *multiple myeloma* and *chordoma* that involve contiguous vertebrae and disks can add to the diagnostic difficulty.[1,2,4]

Bizarre infections such as fungal disease and spinal echinococcosis cannot be easily distinguished from tuberculosis or neoplasms.

The morphologic and pathophysiologic changes encountered in spinal tuberculosis are the most severe among infective spondylitides and are also the most varied. Conventional radiographs are the usual initial imaging investigation. However, early in the disease and in atypical cases such as isolated NAT, plain films may be negative and if the clinical suspicion of tubercular infection is strong MR imaging which is the technique of choice should be considered. The wider availability of CT, high sensitivity and ability to assist in diagnosis by accurately targeting lesions for guided biopsy make it a useful alternative diagnostic tool for early diagnosis when MR is not available.

A delay in diagnosis may lead to irreversible neurologic sequelae and spinal deformity in a high percentage of cases. Hence, a multidisciplinary approach to tubercular spondylitis is essential to ensure prompt assessment of the location, extent and character of spinal pathology to positively affect the clinical management in a timely fashion.

REFERENCES

1. Yao DC, Sartoris ADJ. Musculoskeletal tuberculosis. Radiol Clin N Am. 1995;35(4):679-89.
2. Moore SL, Rafi M. Imaging of musculoskeletal and spinal tuberculosis. Radiol Clin N Am. 2001;39(2):329-42.
3. Pott P. Remarks on that kind of palsy of the lower limbs which is frequently found to accompany a curvature of the spine. London J Johnson; 1779.
4. Sharif HAS, Morgan JL, Mona S, et al. Role of CT and MR imaging in the management of tuberculous spondylitis. Radiol Clin N Am. 1995;33(4):787-804.
5. Gupta RK. Tuberculosis and other non-tuberculous bacterial granulomatous infections. In: Gupta RK, Lufkin RB (Eds). MR Imaging and Spectroscopy of Central Nervous System Infection. Kluwer Academic/Plenum Publishers; 2001.pp.95-146.
6. Resnick D. Osteomyelitis, septic arthritis and soft tissue infection: mechanism and situations. In: Resnick D (Ed). Diagnosis of Bone and Joint Disorder, 4th edition. Philadelphia: WB Saunders; 2002. pp. 2377-480.
7. Bhan S, Nag HL. Skeletal tuberculosis. In: Sharma SK, Mohan A (Eds). Tuberculosis. Jaypee Publishers; 2001. pp.237-60.
8. Hsu LC, Leong JC. Tuberculosis of the lower cervical spine C2-C7. J Bone Joint Surg Br. 1984;66(1):1-5.
9. Martin NS. Tuberculosis of the spin: A study of results of treatment during the east twenty-five years. J Bonc Joint Surg Br. 1970;53:613.
10. Fang D, Leong JCY, Fang HSV. Tuberculosis of the upper cervical spine. J Bone Joint Surg Br. 1983;65:47.
11. Lal AP, Rajshekar V, Chandy M. Management strategies in tuberculous atlantoaxial dislocation. Br J Neurosurg. 1992;6:529-35.
12. Tuli SM. Tuberculosis of the craniovertebral region. Clin Orthop Res. 1974;104:209.
13. Jain R, Sawhney S, Berry M. Computed tomography of vertebral tuberculosis: patterns of bone destruction. Clinical Radiology. 1993;47:196-9.
14. Chapman M, Murray RO, Stoker DT. Tuberculosis of the bones and joints. Semin Roentgenol. 1979;14:266-82.
15. Weaver P, Lifeso RM. The radiological diagnosis of tuberculosis sof the adult spine. Skell Radiol. 1984;12: 178-88.
16. Kahn DS, Pritzker KPH. Pathophysiology of bone infection. Clin Orthop. 1973;96:12-9.
17. Sharif HAS, Aideyan OA, Clark DC, et al. Brucellar and tuberculous spondylitis: Comparative imaging features. Radiology. 1989;155:419-25.
18. Golding FC. Tuberculosis of bone. In: Shanks CS Kerly P (Eds). A Textbook of X-ray Diagnosis by British Authors. 3rd edition. 1959.pp.274-89.
19. Jalleh RD, Kuppuswamy L, Mahayiddin AA, et al. Spinal tuberculosis—A five year review of cases at the National Tuberculosis Centre. Med J Malaya. 1991;46:269.
20. Fam AG, Rubenstein J. Another look at spinal tuberculosis. J Rheumatol. 1993;20:1731.
21. Jain AK. Afresh look at an old disease. J Bone Joint Surg [Br]. 2010;92-B:905-13.
22. Negi SS, Khan SF, Gupta S, et al. Comparison of the conventional diagnostic modalities, baltec culture and polymerase chain reaction test for diagnosis of tuberculosis. Indian J Med Microbiol. 2005;23:29-33.
23. Jain AK, Jena SK, Singh M, et al. Evaluation of clinico-radiological, bacteriological, serological, molecular and histological diagnosis of osteoarticular tuberculosis. Indian J Orthop. 2008;42:173-7.
24. Tuli SM. Tuberculosis of the spine: a historical review. Clin Orthop. 2007;460:29-38.
25. Pandit HG, Sonsale PD, Shikare SS, et al. Bone scintigraphy in tuberculous spondylodiscitis. Eur Spin J. 1999;8:205-9.
26. Desai S. Early diagnosis of spinal tuberculosis by MRI. J Bone Joint Surg Br. 1994;76:863.
27. Nocera RM, Sayle B, Rogers C, et al. Tc-99m MDP and indium-111 chloride scintigraphy in skeletal tuberculosis. Clin Nucl Med. 1983;8:418-20.
28. Weaver P, Lifeso RM. The radiological diagnosis of tuberculosis in the adult spine. Skeletal Radiol. 1984;12:178-86.
29. Lifeso RM, Weaver P, Harder E. Tuberculous spondylitis in adults. J Bone Joint Surg Am. 1985;67:1405-13.
30. Burrill J, Williams CJ, Bain G, Conder G, Hine AL, Rakesh R. Tuberculosis: A radiologic review. Radiographics. 2007;27: 1255-73.
31. Harkirat S, Anand SS, Indrajit IK, Dash AK. Pictorial essay: PET/CT in tuberculosis. Indian J Radiol Imaging. 2008;18(2):141.
32. D'Souza MM, Sharma R, Tripathi M, Mondal A. F-18 Fluorodeoxyglucose positron emission tomography/ computed tomography in tuberculosis of the hip: A case report and brief review of literature. Indian J Nucl Med. 2011;26(1):31-3.
33. Hustinx R, Smith RJ, Benard F, et al. Dual time point fluorine-18 fluorodeoxyglucose positron emission tomography: a potential method to differentiate malignancy from inflammation and normal tissue in the head and neck. Eur J Nucl Med. 1999;26(10):1345-8.
34. Zhuang H, Pourdehnad M, Lambright ES, et al. Dual time point ^{18}F-FDG PET imaging for differentiating malignant from inflammatory processes. J Nucl Med. 2001;42:1412-7.
35. Alavi A, Lakhani P, Mavi A, et al. PET: a revolution in medical imaging. Radiol Clin North Am. 2004;42:983-1001.
36. Andronikou S, Bindapersad M, Govender N, Waner JI, Segwe A, Palliam S, Shenxane O, Mngomezulu V. Musculoskeletal tuberculosis-imaging using low-end and advanced modalities for developing and developed countries. Acta Radiol. 2011;52(4):430-41.
37. Buxi TBS. Computed tomography in spinal tuberculosis. Ind J Radiol Imag. 1993;3:291-3.

38. Stabler A, Reiser MF. Imaging of spinal infection. Radiol Clin N Am. 2001;39(1):115-35.
39. Maiuri F, Iaconetta G, Gallicchio B, et al. Spondylodiscitis Clinical and Magnetic Resonance Diagnosis. Spine. 1997;22:1741-6.
40. Sharif HAS. Role of MR imaging in the management of spinal infections. Am J Roentgenol. 1992;158:1333-45.
41. Kaila R, Malhi AM, Mahmood B, Saifuddin A. The incidence of multiple level noncontiguous vertebral tuberculosis detected using whole spine MRI. J Spinal Disord Tech. 2007;20(1):78-81.
42. Sharif HAS, Clark DC, Aabed MY, et al. Granulomatous spinal infections MR imaging. Radiology. 1990;177:101-7.
43. Palle L, Reddy MB, Reddy KJ. Role of magnetic resonance diffusion imaging and apparent diffusion coefficient values in the evaluation of spinal tuberculosis in Indian patients. Indian J Radiol Imaging. 2010;20(4):279-83.
44. Pui MH, Mitha A, Rae WI, Corr P. Diffusion-weighted magnetic resonance imaging of spinal infection and malignancy. J Neuroimaging. 2005;15(2):164-7.
45. Gupta RK, Agarwal P, Rastogi H, et al. Problems in differentiating spinal tuberculosis from neoplasm on MRI. Neuroradiology. 1996;38:S97-104.
46. Mendonca RA. Spinal infection and inflammatory disorders. In: Atlas SW (Ed). Magnetic Resonance Imaging of the Brain and Spine, 3rd edition. Lippincot Williams and Wilkins. 2002.pp.1855-972.
47. Rahman NU, Jamjoom A, Jamjoom ZAB, et al. Neural arch tuberculosis: Radiological features and their correlation with surgical findings. Br J Neurosurg. 1997;11(1):32-8.
48. Loke TKL, Ma HT, Chan CS. Magnetic resonance imaging of tuberculous spinal infection. Australas Radiol. 1997;41:7-12.
49. Kumar K. Clinical study and classification of posterior spinal tuberculosis. Int Orthop. 1985;9:147-52.
50. Raglan R, Abdelwahan F, Braffman B, et al. Posterior spinal tuberculosis—a case report. AJNR. 1990;11:612.
51. Abdelwahan IF, Camins MB, et al. Vertebral arch or posterior spinal tuberculosis. Skeletal Radiol. 1997;26:737-40.
52. Jacobs P, Renton P. Periosteal reaction; bone and joint infections; sarcoid. In: Sutton D (Ed). Textbook of Radiology and Medical Imaging, 4th edition. Churchill Livingstone; 1987.pp.71-2.
53. Richards AS. Non-tuberculous pyogenic osteomyelitis of the spine. Can Assoc Radiol J. 1960;11:45-9.
54. Kang M, Gupta S, Khandelwal N, et al. CT-guided fine-needle aspiration biopsy of spinal lesions. Acta Radiol. 1999;40:474-8.
55. Mondal A, Misra DK. CT-guided needle aspiration cytology (FNAC) of 112 vertebral lesions. Indian J Pathol Microbiol. 1994;37:255-61.
56. Francis IM, Das DK, Luthra UK, et al. Value of radiologically guided fine needle aspiration cytology (FNAC) in the diagnosis of spinal tuberculosis: a study of 29 cases. Cytopathology. 1999;10:390-401.
57. Gouliamos AD, Kehasgias DT, Lahanis S, et al. MR imaging of tuberculous vertebral osteomyelitis: Pictoral review. Eur Radiol. 2001;11:575-9.
58. Hong SH, Ja-Young Choi, Lee JW, RaKim N, Jung-Ah Choi, Kang HS. MR imaging assessment of the spine: Infection or an imitation? Radiographics. 2009;29:599-612.
59. Danchaivijitr N, Temram S, Thepmongkhol K, Chiewvit P. Diagnostic accuracy of MR imaging in tuberculous spondylitis. J Med Assoc Thai. 2007;90:1581-9.
60. Dunn R, Zondagh I, Candy S. Spinal tuberculosis: magnetic resonance imaging and neurological impairment. Spine (Phila Pa 1976). 2011;36(6):469-73.
61. Kumar R. Spinal tuberculosis: with reference to the children of northern India. Childs Nerv Syst. 2005;21(1):19-26.
62. Trivedi R, Saksena S, Gupta RK. Magnetic resonance imaging in central nervous system tuberculosis. Indian J Radiol Imaging. 2009;19(4):256-65.
63. Boxer DI, Pratt C, Hine AL, et al. Radiological features during and following treatment of spinal tuberculosis. Br J Radiol. 1992;65:476-9.
64. Tenth report of the Medical Research Council Working Party on Tuberculosis of the Spine: A controlled trial of six-month and nine-month regimens of chemotherapy in patients undergoing radical surgery for tuberculosis of the spine in Hong Kong. Tubercle. 1986;67:243-59.
65. Kim SJ, Kim IJ, Suh KT, Kim YK, Lee JS. Prediction of residual disease of spine infection using F-18FDG PET/CT. Spine. 2009;22(34):2424-30.
66. Cormican L, Hammal R, Messenger J, Milburn HJ. Current difficulties in the diagnosis and management of spinal tuberculosis. Postgrad Med J. 2006;82(963):46-51.
67. Le Page L, Feydy A, Rillardon L, Dufour V, Le Hénanff A, Tubach F, et al. Spinal tuberculosis: a longitudinal study with clinical, laboratory, and imaging outcomes. Semin Arthritis Rheum. 2006;36(2):124-9.

CHAPTER 193

Noninfective Inflammatory Arthritis

Mandeep Kang, Mahesh Prakesh

INTRODUCTION

Noninfective inflammatory arthritides comprise a group of different, mostly systemic disorders that have one important feature in common; inflammatory granulation tissue eroding and destroying articular cartilage. The noninfective inflammatory arthritides include rheumatoid arthritis (seropositive) and the seronegative spondyloarthropathies namely, ankylosing spondylitis, psoriatic arthropathy, Reiter's syndrome and enteropathic arthritis. Although radiologic manifestations of the arthropathies reflect pathologic alterations, joints can react to disease only in limited ways and therefore, different pathologic conditions may exhibit similar radiologic features. Many of these are nonspecific, but certain combinations are more likely than others to occur in a particular disease; thus one may consider the "predictive value" of a radiologic feature relative to the clinical condition.[1] A systematic approach with evaluation of various radiological abnormalities helps in arriving at the correct diagnosis. Various features to be evaluated include:

a. Distribution of affected joints
b. Presence of soft tissue swelling
c. Bone density
d. Cartilage space narrowing
e. Reactive bone formation
f. Site and character of erosions
g. Subarticular cystic lesions
h. Presence of soft tissue calcification
i. Joint deformities.[2]

RHEUMATOID ARTHRITIS

Rheumatoid arthritis (RA) is the most common inflammatory arthritis affecting approximately 0.5–1% of the world's adult population. It is a progressive, chronic, systemic inflammatory disease affecting primarily the synovial joints which can lead to considerable disability and morbidity. Rheumatoid arthritis may develop at any age, but the peak age of onset is between the 4th and 6th decades. Women are three times more likely to be affected than men.[3] The etiology is unknown but appears to be multifactorial. There is a genetic predisposition with over 70% of patients expressing HLA-DR4. A role for factors like smoking and infectious agents has also been suggested in the etiology.[4] Although any synovial joint in the body may be affected, the classical presentation is of a symmetrical polyarthritis affecting the small joints of the hands and feet. However, it may be asymmetrical in 20–25% of cases.[1] Large joints which are commonly involved include the ankle, knee and shoulder. The axial skeleton is later and less often affected, with the exception of the cervical spine. Characteristically, joints which communicate with one another tend to be affected together, e.g. uniform tricompartmental involvement in the knee joint and simultaneous involvement of the distal radioulnar and radiocarpal joints.[2]

Over the past couple of decades, there has been a paradigm shift in the management of RA which has resulted in significantly improved prognosis. Presently, the management involves two main strategies, to start treatment as early as possible and to frequently assess disease activity to monitor response to therapy. New biologic therapies have also emerged, such as the antitumor necrosis factor drugs to supplement the conventional disease modifying antirheumatic agents.[5]

The spectrum of disease manifestations of RA is protean. The 1987 diagnostic criteria of the American College of Rheumatology are commonly used for the diagnosis of this disease **(Table 1)**.[6] However, these criteria are not readily applicable in patients with early disease, hence in recent years, the role of imaging like MR and ultrasound has gained in importance.[7,8]

Pathophysiology

The rheumatoid factors are anti-gamma-globulin antibodies which are elaborated by the synovium in response to unknown antigens. These antibodies are believed to be the initiating factor that triggers RA. Immune complex deposition in the synovium activates the complement system with invasion by neutrophils and macrophages. This leads to synovial proliferation, pannus formation and ultimate cartilage and subchondral bony destruction. In advanced cases, there may be fibrous ankylosis which may be followed by bony ankylosis.[9, 10]

Rheumatoid factors (RF) are found in the serum and synovial fluid in 70–80% of patients with a clinical diagnosis of RA. They may be found in the synovial fluid even when the serum is negative. However, they may also be found in the synovial fluid of patients with non-rheumatoid disorders, therefore, only high titres of RF in a joint effusion suggest RA. Early in the course of the disease, the rheumatoid factors may initially be negative and later become positive.[3]

Table 1: The traditional diagnostic criteria (1987) of the American College of Rheumatology for the diagnosis of RA.

• Morning stiffness in and around joints that lasts at least 1 hour before maximal improvement.
• Soft tissue swelling of at least three joints that is observed by a physician.
• Swelling (arthritis) of the metacarpophalangeal, proximal interphalangeal or wrist joints.
• Symmetrical swelling (arthritis).
• Subcutaneous rheumatoid nodules.
• A positive test for rheumatoid factor.
• *Radiographic signs:* Erosions or periarticular osteopenia in hand or wrist joints.

Imaging

The radiologic features of RA may be divided into "early" and "late" changes. The detection of early changes is important because new disease modifying therapies are more effective when used before severe disability has occurred. Since early changes are nonosseous in nature, sonography and MR imaging can detect disease earlier than conventional radiography and CT. Secondly, in the present scenario, RA is treated aggressively with disease modifying drugs, hence osseous changes are delayed.[4]

Radiographic Features

The earliest changes include joint space widening and soft tissue swelling.

Joint space widening: It is the earliest but a transient radiographic abnormality, sometimes, lasting for only a few weeks. This finding is due to edema and swelling of the synovium and joint effusion. Joint space widening is best detected at the metacarpophalangeal (MCP) joints, especially in the 5th digit.[11]

Soft tissue swelling: It represents a combination of joint effusion, synovial edema, and proliferation and tenosynovitis which invariably precedes cartilaginous and osseous changes. In the hand, periarticular fusiform swelling may be seen over the proximal interphalangeal (PIP) and 2nd and 5th MCP joints. Soft tissue swelling over the 3rd and 4th MCP joints may be appreciated as a local increased density. Soft tissue swelling over the ulnar styloid may be better detected on radiographs rather than clinical examination and is due to involvement of the extensor carpi ulnaris sheath. Soft tissue swelling over the radial styloid may be seen due to involvement of the radiocarpal joint.[12] In the feet, the soft tissue changes are less evident radiographically but may be seen over the 1st and 5th metatarsal heads. There may be blurring and obliteration of the pre-Achilles fat pad and blurring and thickening of the Achilles tendon.[2]

In the knee, there may be lateral bulging of the fat lines over the distal femur on AP radiographs. On lateral views, there is distension of the suprapatellar bursa with blurring of its surrounding fat lines. In the elbow, the anterior and posterior fat lines are displaced away from the joint on the lateral view.[12]

Osteopenia in RA: It is of two types: Local juxta-articular osteopenia is due to synovial inflammation and hyperemia and is seen early in the course of the disease. Generalized osteopenia is due to limitation of movement due to pain, muscle wasting or steroid therapy and is therefore seen late in the disease.[2] Osteopenia is seen more often as the disease progresses and 80% of patients demonstrate osteopenia by 2 years after onset of symptoms. It is a precursor of erosive disease and may mask early erosions. Assessment of osteopenia may be difficult and comparison between normal and abnormal joints in the same patient is helpful. However, it is subjective and there may be interobserver as well as intraobserver variability in the assessment. Generalized or solitary terminal phalangeal sclerosis may be seen in up to 35% of patients with RA and other arthropathies and may be seen before any other abnormality.[12]

Joint space narrowing: It is due to destruction of the articular cartilage and is virtually always uniform **(Fig. 1)**. It may be more apparent than real in the presence of flexion deformities, and an oblique view may be required to assess the space. Uniform narrowing with an intact subchondral cortex is however not specific for RA as it may also be seen in the seronegative spondyloarthropathies or connective tissue diseases. Presence of uniform narrowing on the other hand is an important feature of RA that helps differentiate it from osteoarthritis in which the joint space narrowing is characteristically nonuniform or segmental.[1]

Subperiosteal bone apposition: It is uncommon in adult RA and is almost always subtle. When present, it may be seen at the site of capsular or tendon attachments and probably reflects the effect of tenosynovitis. This relative lack of periosteal reaction, despite advanced and often dramatic joint destruction is a hallmark of the disease and is so

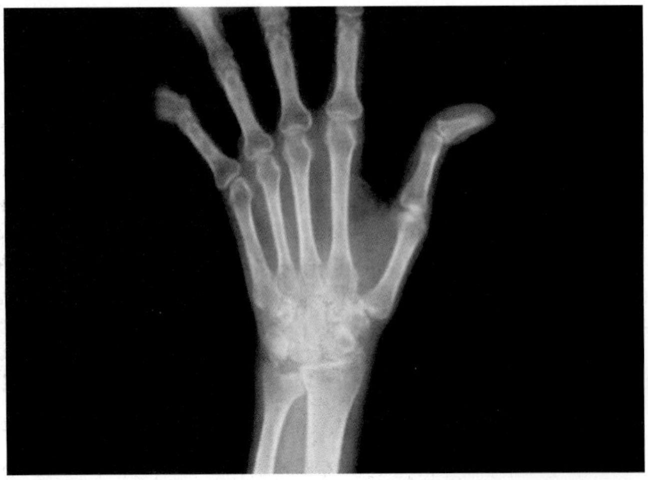

Fig. 1: X-ray hand reveals the early changes of rheumatoid arthritis with classical juxta-articular osteopenia and uniform narrowing of the distal radioulnar, radiocarpal and intercarpal joints. Subluxations at the 1st MCP and IP joints cause the classical "Hitch-hiker's" deformity.

characteristic that the presence of exuberant periosteal reaction should suggest an alternate diagnosis.[2]

Erosions: They are the most important diagnostic feature of RA but may not be seen when the patient presents initially. Their incidence rises from less than 40% at 3 months from symptom onset to 90–95% at 10 years of disease.[12] The detection of erosions indicates irreversible joint damage. The earliest sites of cortical surface erosions are at the bare areas of bone between the edge of the articular cartilage and the attachment of the joint capsule and therefore their distribution is related to the anatomy of the joint.[13]

In the hands, erosions usually involve the wrist, MCP and PIP joints. The DIP joints are usually spared. Erosions involve a larger area on the proximal side of the PIP joints due to the larger bare areas on this side of the joint. At the MCP joints, the erosions develop first and most extensively in the metacarpal heads and are most evident at the radiovolar aspect of the 2nd and 3rd MCP joints. The 5th metacarpal may demonstrate the earliest erosions on its lateral aspect. In the interphalangeal (IP) joint of the thumb, erosions generally develop at the ulnar side of the volar aspect of the base of the distal phalanx. The ulnar styloid is commonly eroded due to inflammation in the prestyloid recess. There may be large erosions of the radius at the distal radioulnar joint. Erosions occur throughout the carpus and may be followed by fusion. However, bony ankylosis is uncommon in other joints in adult rheumatoid arthritis.[3]

In the feet, erosions appear earlier and are most often seen at the 5th MTP joint. The metatarsal heads erode before the bases of the proximal phalanges, particularly on the medial plantar aspect, although the lateral aspect of the 5th metatarsal head may be eroded. A characteristic site for erosion in the tarsus is at the posterosuperior aspect of the calcaneum above the insertion of the Achilles tendon. However, tarsal erosions are less often seen in RA as compared to the seronegative spondyloarthropathies.[12] Bone erosions may also develop at extra-articular sites including the upper posterior ribs and ischial margins.[2]

Radiologically, early marginal erosions appear as cortical defects or an indistinctness of the subchondral cortex. This erasure or loss of the cortical white line is first seen on the radial aspect of the 4th and 5th metacarpal heads. If seen *en face*, erosions appear entirely within the bone giving a cystic appearance **(Fig. 2)**. Some may be deep or pocketed.

Erosive change is less common in the large joints. There may be a superficial surface irregularity in the presence of diffuse joint narrowing **(Fig. 3)**. In the hip, the medial joint space is characteristically involved with

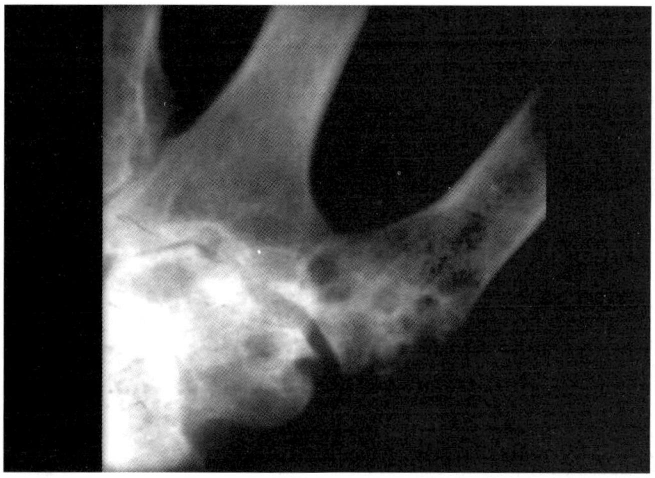

Fig. 2: Rheumatoid arthritis: Magnified view of the CMC joints demonstrates multiple erosions in the bases of the metacarpals and trapezium giving a cystic appearance.

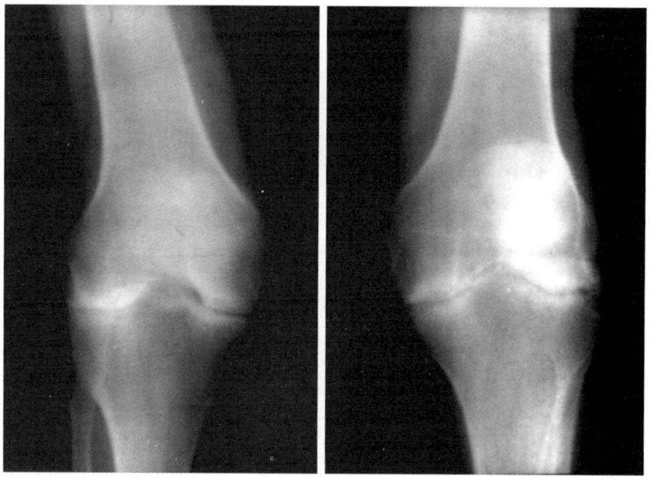

Fig. 3: X-ray both knee joints in a case of RA reveals diffuse osteopenia with uniform narrowing of the joint spaces. Note the lack of irregularity of the articular margins.

medial migration of the femoral head causing protrusio acetabuli. This is in contrast to OA which generally involves the superior compartment of the hip joint.[1]

Rarely, large intraosseous defects or pseudocysts may be seen in patients with massive synovial proliferation. It is hypothesized that these form due to the high intra-articular pressure which exceeds the intraosseous pressure resulting in migration of synovial fluid into the underlying subchondral bone. Invariably, there is destruction of the adjacent joint cartilage. Pseudocysts may attain sizes up to 2–3 cm, are usually oval to round, with regular outlines or slightly scalloped margins.[13]

Late Changes

Alignment deformities at joints may result from local synovitis weakening the capsule and tendonitis preventing normal musculotendinous actions causing subluxations and dislocations. Tendons may also rupture in the region of eroded bone. Thus, rotator cuff tears result in upward subluxation of the eroded humeral head. Subluxation at the MCP joints leads to ulnar deviation which is seen in 50% of patients with chronic disease. There is also increasing palmar flexion due to ulnar deviation of extensor tendons. Other classical deformities in the hands are the "boutonnière" deformity due to flexion at the PIP joint with extension at the DIP joint. The reverse is seen with the "swan-neck" deformity due to PIP joint extension and DIP joint flexion. Flexion at the 1st MCP joint with hyperextension at the interphalangeal joint results in the "Hitch-hiker's thumb". There may also be dislocation of the carpus causing a bayonet deformity at the wrist.[3]

In the feet, there may be lateral deviation of the toes, especially hallux valgus **(Fig. 4)**. The hallux sesamoids sublux between the 1st and 2nd metatarsal heads and the transverse arch flattens due to ligamentous laxity.[12]

Severe erosive change leads to marked *destruction and narrowing of the joint spaces* with extreme irregularity and destruction of the subchondral bone **(Fig. 5)**. In the hands, the bone ends are often reciprocally eroded and there may be telescoping of the fingers. There is resultant arthritis multilans which may also be seen in other conditions such as erosive OA and multicentric reticulohistiocytosis.[2]

Gross *loss of bone* at the femoral head results in a "bird's beak" appearance. There may be pointing of the adjacent bone ends at the acromioclavicular joints with resorption of the distal clavicles.

Stress fractures may occur due to normal stress on bone with decreased elastic resistance. *Giant synovial* cysts may develop, particularly originating from the knee joint and presenting in the calf. They may also occur around the shoulder, elbow and hip where they may protrude into the pelvis. Rheumatoid arthritis can attack any synovial joint and there may be involvement of the laryngeal joints, sternomanubrial or temporomandibular joints.[2]

Pulmonary involvement may lead to pleural effusions, pulmonary nodules (30%) or interstitial fibrosis (predominantly lower lobe). Pulmonary nodules are usually associated with subcutaneous nodules over the extensor surfaces of the elbows or other joints. Secondary osteoarthritis may complicate RA in weight-bearing joints. Reactive sclerosis and new bone formation is not marked in these joints.[12]

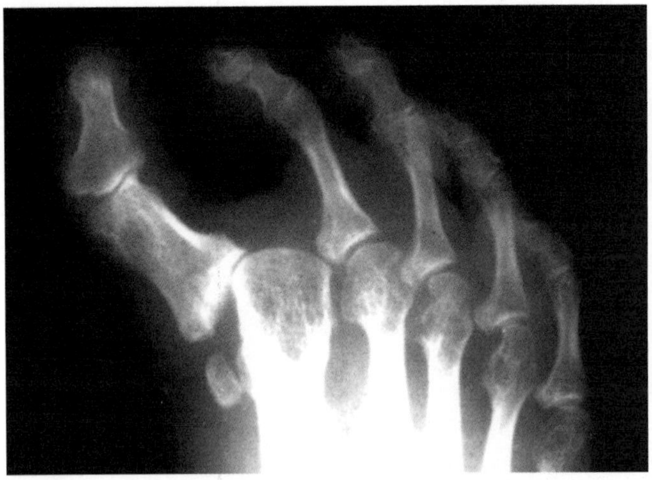

Fig. 4: X-ray of the forefoot shows more advanced changes of RA with gross erosions of the metatarsal heads with subluxations at the MTP and IP joints with hallux valgus.

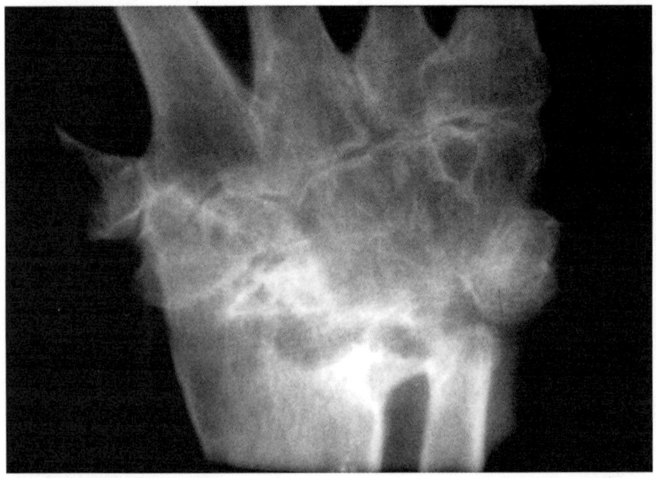

Fig. 5: Magnified view of the wrist joint demonstrating late changes of RA with severe osteopenia, gross destruction of the distal ends of the radius and ulna with ankylosis of the carpal bones.

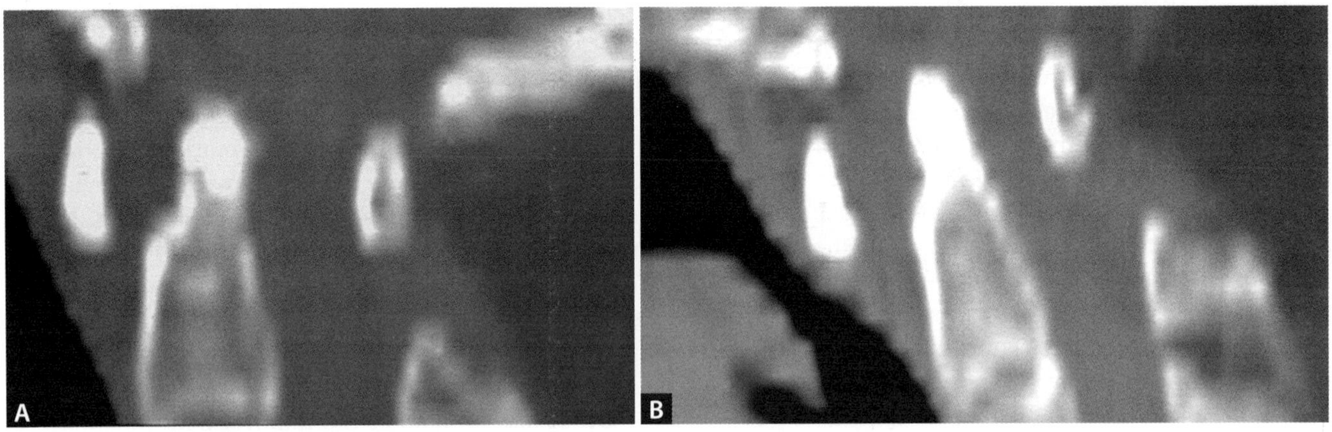

Figs. 6A and B: Sagittal reformatted 3D CT images of the craniovertebral junction in (A) extension and (B) flexion show increase in the atlantoaxial distance on flexion with erosion of the odontoid peg due to RA.

Axial Skeleton Involvement

The spondylitis of RA is distinctive in that it has a predilection for the cervical region. Thoracic or lumbar involvement is distinctly uncommon. Osteoporosis, disk narrowing and end plate irregularity are seen with only a little reactive new bone formation in the upper cervical vertebrae in contrast to osteoarthritis which involves the lower cervical vertebrae. Facet joint erosions may lead to subluxations at multiple levels in the upper cervical spine giving a step ladder appearance.[3]

Atlantoaxial (AA) subluxation is seen in up to 20–25% of patients with chronic RA and is primarily due to laxity of the transverse ligament (which is responsible for maintaining the integrity of the AA joint) with or without erosion of the odontoid. Separation between the anterior border of the odontoid and the posterior surface of the anterior arch of the atlas in flexion of more than 2.5 mm in adults or 4 mm in children is considered diagnostic of AAD **(Figs. 6A and B)**. Although it can be visualized on plain radiographs, 3D CT and MR give a better depiction of both the soft tissue and bony involvement **(Figs. 7A to D)**.[13] The eroded odontoid may at times fracture. Resorption of bone at nonarticular surfaces occurs at the spinous processes which become short, sharp and tapered.[2]

Occasionally, the sacroiliac joints exhibit minimal erosions with joint space narrowing, however reactive sclerosis as seen in ankylosing spondylitis, is typically absent. Rarely, there may be ankylosis of the SI joints.

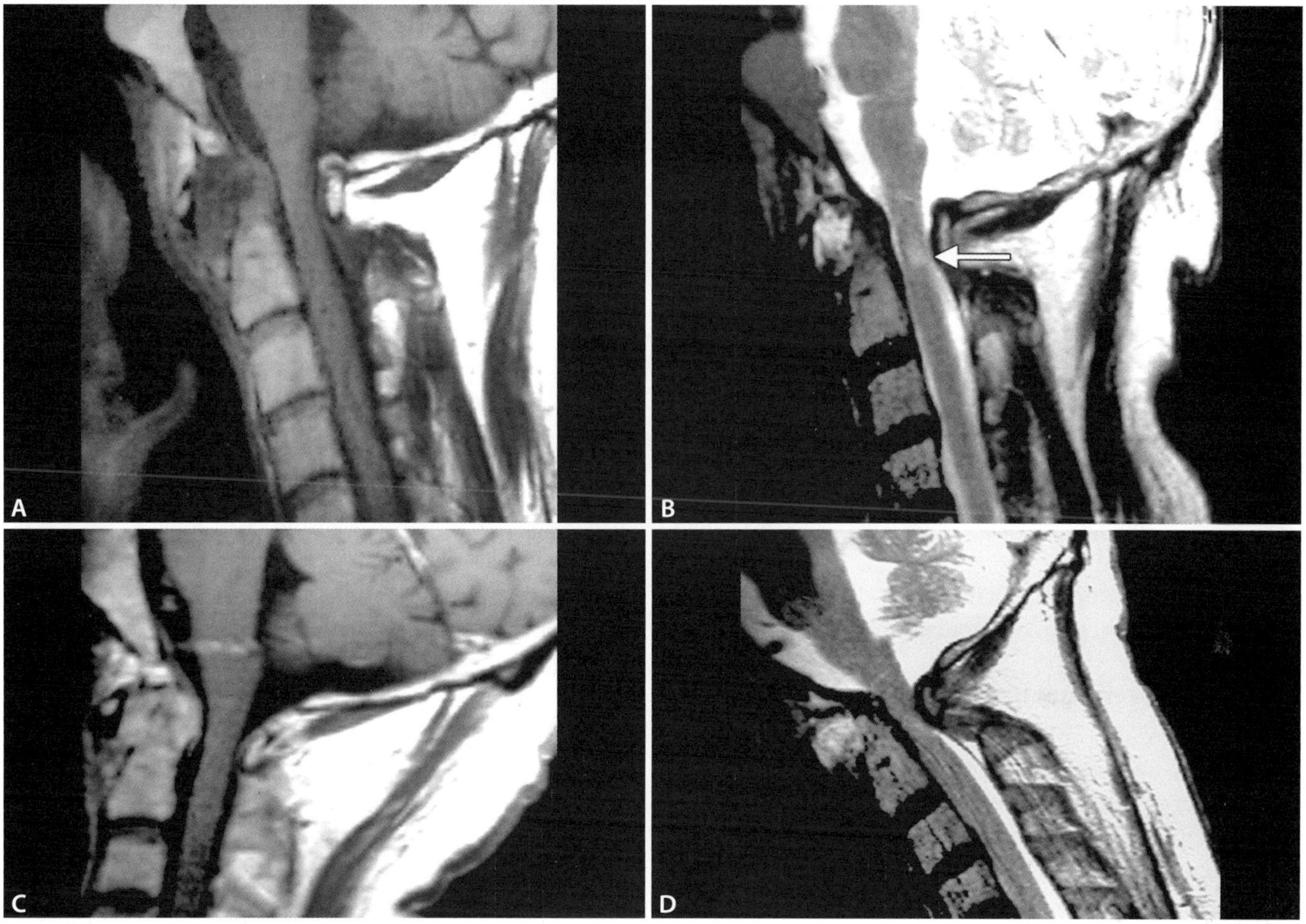

Figs. 7A to D: MR of the craniovertebral junction in a case of RA with AAD: (A) T1- and (B) T2-weighted images in neutral position reveal erosion of the odontoid with pannus which appears hypointense on T1 and hyperintense on T2-weighted sequences. Hyperintense signal is seen within the cord at this level due to ischemia/edema; (C) Postgadolinium, there is significant enhancement of the pannus; (D) T2-weighted image in flexion demonstrates compression of the cord due to posterior displacement of the odontoid peg.

OTHER IMAGING MODALITIES

Ultrasonography

With the advent of high resolution linear transducers, (7.5 MHz and higher), ultrasonography (USG) may be used for detection and monitoring of joint and soft tissue inflammation and bone damage. A number of studies have demonstrated the ability of USG to detect early synovial inflammation in the form of synovial thickening and joint effusion. Power Doppler has the capability to detect and measure changes in the vascularity of the synovium due to inflammation **(Figs. 8A and B)**. Ultrasonography contrast agents have the potential to increase the sensitivity of power Doppler by increasing the signal from the synovial vessels.

The joint margins can be assessed for the presence of erosions. It has been demonstrated that USG is more sensitive than conventional radiography for detection of erosion in the small joints of the hands and feet.[14] The internal structure of the tendons can be assessed and their integrity or rupture demonstrated by dynamic scanning. Leakage of synovial fluid may also be demonstrated, e.g. a ruptured Baker's cyst which needs to be differentiated from other causes of calf pain, such as deep vein thrombosis or muscle tear. USG can also be used to monitor response to therapy. Following treatment, USG can detect reduction in the synovial inflammation and vascular flow parameters.[15] Several studies have compared power doppler with MR imaging for the detection of early arthritis. A prospective study that followed 60 patients showed that USG was more sensitive than MR in detecting synovitis.[16] In another study, sonography was found to be a valuable tool, however, CEMR was superior in evaluating synovial proliferation and erosions.[17] Disadvantages of USG

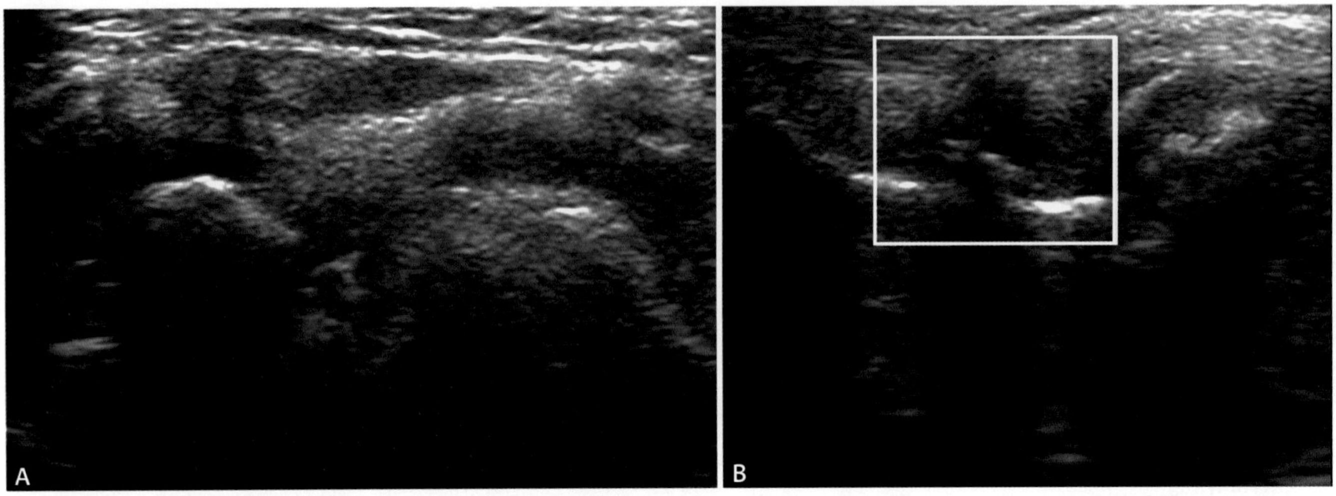

Figs. 8A and B: (A) Ultrasound image of the carpal bones shows diffuse synovial thickening in a case of RA; (B) Power Doppler in another case shows synovial thickening extending along the tendon sheaths with increased vascularity.

include the user dependent nature of the modality and the long time required to evaluate multiple joints.

Computed Tomography

Computed tomography (CT) is not frequently used routinely in RA as it is inferior to MR and USG for the detection of early disease along with the disadvantage of using ionizing radiation. It can demonstrate the presence of erosions, particularly in the carpal and tarsal bones. It can also show joint space narrowing or ankylosis. A recent study has reported comparable performance of CT with MR for the evaluation of synovitis and tenosynovitis using contrast enhanced CT with digital masking of the bone.[18] However, its main use lies in the diagnosis and management of upper cervical spine abnormalities, particularly for the evaluation of atlantoaxial subluxation.[13]

Radionuclide Scanning

Scanning with ^{99m}Tc-MDP is highly sensitive for detection of the inflammatory changes of arthritis but shows poor specificity. In RA, isotopes are at least 70% more sensitive than conventional films and may be used to monitor response to therapy.[9] Findings include increased flow in the synovium in the early or blood pool phase and increased uptake in the delayed 3 hours scans.

Magnetic Resonance Imaging

Over the last two decades, magnetic resonance imaging (MRI) has come to be considered to be the best imaging modality for RA, despite being expensive and time consuming. The Outcome Measures in Rheumatoid Arthritis Clinical Trials (OMERACT) MR imaging study group is an international, multidisciplinary group set-up for the purpose of standardizing techniques and definitions of joint pathologies in RA.[5] According to their recommendations, a MR scan for RA should include at least the following: (i) imaging in two planes (axial and coronal), (ii) T1-weighed sequences before and after gadolinium and (iii) A fat-saturated T2-weighted or a short inversion recovery (STIR) sequence. MR is also a useful imaging modality for the follow-up of RA to evaluate progression or remission. The typical progression in RA from the stage of synovitis followed by bone marrow edema and finally bony erosion are well demonstrated on MRI.[5]

Synovial Imaging

Magnetic resonance is considered to be the gold standard for synovial imaging. Inflammatory changes within the soft tissues of the joints which precede the development of erosions and which are not detectable on plain radiographs are well demonstrated on MR.[19] It has been reported that using the enhancement of MCP and PIP joints as a positive diagnostic criteria, RA could be diagnosed with a sensitivity of 96% and accuracy of 44%.[7] The OMERACT group defines synovitis as an area in the synovial compartment with increased contrast enhancement whose thickness exceeds the width of the normal synovium.[5] Magnetic resonance depicts irregular thickening of the synovium which is of intermediate signal intensity (SI) compared to darker fluid on T1 and high signal intensity on T2-weighted spin echo sequences. Fat-suppressed T2-weighted sequences more clearly delineate disease extent. Postgadolinium, there can be significant rapid enhancement of the inflamed synovium unlike joint effusion which does not enhance in the early phase. Images obtained more than 10 minutes after gadolinium show diffusion of gadolinium into the synovial joint fluid resulting in increased signal intensity.[5] Active synovitis is best visualized on postcontrast fat suppressed T1-weighted images and there is indirect evidence suggesting that the degree of postcontrast enhancement correlates with the degree of inflammation.[13] Fibrotic pannus and pannus with hemosiderin deposition shows low SI on T1- and T2-weighted images and do not enhance on postgadolinium images.

Quantification of synovial volume has been shown to play an important role in the diagnosis and follow-up of RA. The baseline synovial volume has been found to correlate significantly with the number of new bone erosions at 1 year follow-up.[5,19]

Bone Marrow Edema

Bone marrow edema has been reported to be a distinctive finding in RA, especially in the early phase. It manifests as ill defined, high SI on fat suppressed, T2-weighted and STIR images with enhancement following gadolinium **(Fig. 9)**. It has been found in 39–75% of patients with RA with disease duration of less than 1 year.[5] It is usually found in the subchondral bone and can be seen alone or surrounding bone erosions. It is currently considered as a forerunner of erosions. Some studies have shown the high association of bone marrow edema at baseline with erosions 1 year and 6 years later.[20]

Erosions

On MR, erosions are seen as a focal loss of normal SI from cortical or subchondral bone on T1 and focal regions of high SI on T2-weighted or STIR images **(Figs. 10A and B)**. Erosions replace marrow fat and contain inflamed synovium which enhances with gadolinium and are thus easily differentiated from other interosseous fluid filled cystic lesions.[21]

In early RA, MR can identify bone erosions in 45–72% of patients with disease of less than 6 months duration, compared with 8–40% on radiography.[5,8] This is important as MR can assist in making an early diagnosis of RA, allowing treatment to be instituted early in the course of disease. It is also important to identify those patients in whom progressive disease is not seen as these patients do not require aggressive treatment protocols. In one study, 82% of patients without erosions at baseline MR imaging had no radiographic erosions at 2-year follow-up.[5]

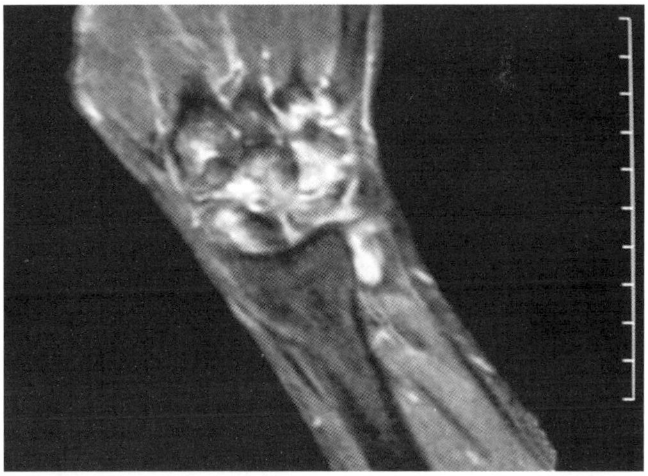

Fig. 9: Coronal STIR image shows ill-defined areas of high signal intensity in the carpal bones due to bone marrow edema.

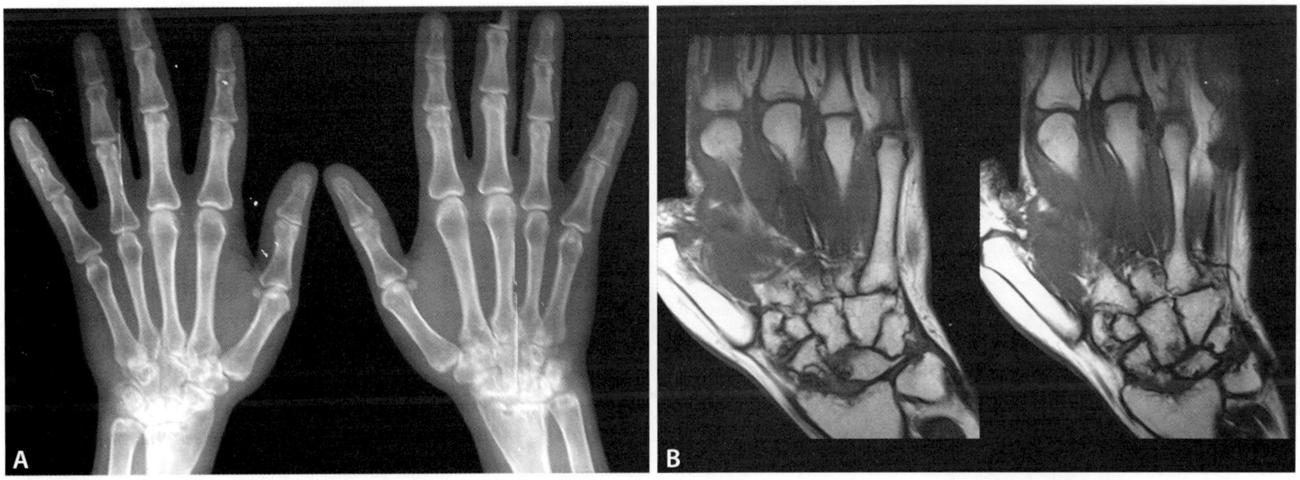

Figs. 10A and B: Patient with RA: (A) X-ray both hands PA view shows diffuse loss of the joint spaces at the radiocarpal, intercarpal and CPC joints; (B) T1-weighted coronal image demonstrates multiple erosions in the carpal bones, distal ulna and radius.

Tendons and Ligaments

Rheumatoid arthritis can involve the ligaments or tendons directly which results in predisposition to rupture. Increased signal on T2-weighted spin echo and STIR sequences indicates tendon involvement and may be due to erosion, invasion by pannus or partial tear. Thinning or thickening of the tendon is also abnormal.

Tenosynovitis can be diagnosed by the presence of fluid in the tendon sheath, tendon sheath thickening or enhancement. The extensor carpi ulnaris is the most frequently involved tendon.[21] Tenosynovitis of the flexor tendons of the wrist results in an increase in carpal tunnel volume, which leads to mechanical pressure and compression of the median nerve which can also be inflamed resulting in Carpal-Tunnel syndrome. Axial images are most useful for assessing the anatomic characteristics of the Carpal-Tunnel.

Intraosseous cysts show low SI on T1 and high SI on T2-weighted images and may not enhance in the immediate postcontrast phase.[4]

Intra-articular loose bodies are frequently seen due to the destructive inflammatory process and include cartilaginous and osseous fragments. A subset of loose bodies is called "rice bodies" as they resemble polished rice. They are now recognized as a characteristic feature of RA. They may contain collagen, fibrinogen, fibrin, fibronectin, mononuclear cells, blood cells and amorphous material.[4]

Large Joints

Though involvement of large joints usually occurs after established disease elsewhere, MRI is more sensitive in picking up early change. In the glenohumeral joint, rotator cuff tears, joint effusion, giant synovial cysts and early erosions are best evaluated on MR imaging. Similarly, involvement of the hip joint with detection of joint effusion, pannus, erosions and articular cartilage destruction is well depicted on MRI **(Figs. 11A and B)**.[19]

SCORING SYSTEMS FOR RHEUMATOID ARTHRITIS

Radiographic images demonstrate the structural damage in the patient at a given point in time. Radiographic abnormalities were initially used to develop an index of damage that was used to assign patients to four stages. However, by the early 1960s, it was realized that assigning a single score for all radiographic abnormalities lacked sensitivity for detecting disease progression and various scoring systems were developed which separately rated the severity of erosion and joint space narrowing. Larsen developed a global scoring method that incorporated erosions, osteoporosis and soft tissue swelling in a single score. Various modifications of the global or composite methods have been extensively used to describe the course of articular damage in RA and evaluate response to therapy.[22] However, the scoring methods are not precise measurements, they reflect individual readers and the error of individual scores is considerable. Also, the expected progression of structural damage in untreated RA is impossible to determine. None of the attempts to describe course so far have taken into account the effect of treatment. Development of an accurate, easily reproducible and easily carried out quantitative measurement of bony erosion and cartilage destruction is required.

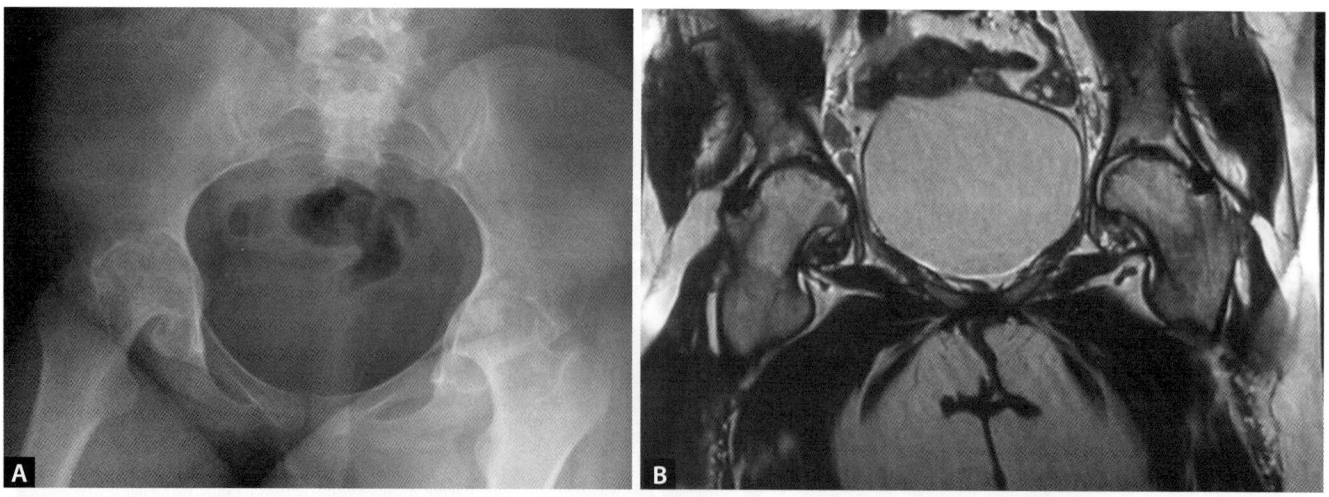

Figs. 11A and B: (A) X-ray pelvis of a patient with RA shows uniform loss of joint space with irregularity of the articular surface in bilateral hip joints. Note the medial migration of the femoral heads; (B) Coronal T2-weighted image better demonstrates the erosions. Note the bone marrow edema manifesting as ill-defined hyperintense signal.

On MRI at present, the most frequently used method is the OMERACT rheumatoid arthritis magnetic resonance imaging score (RAMRIS). In this, the synonitis is assessed in three wrist regions: distal radioulnar joint, radiocarpal joint and the intercarpal, carpometacarpal and MCP joints on a scale of 0–3. A score of 0 is normal, while score of 1 (mild), 2 (moderate) or 3 (severe) reflect the maximum volume of enhancing synovium. Similarly, bone marrow edema is scored from 0 to 3 based on the volume 0: no edema, volume 1: 1–33%, volume 2: 34–66% and volume 3: 67–100% of bone that is edematous. Erosions in the carpal bones, distal radius and ulna and the bases of the metacarpal bones are scored separately. The scores range from 0 to 10 on the basis of the volume of erosion in the assessed bone in increments of 10%. The maximum score in the wrist is 150.[23] However, using the RAMRIS score is difficult, requiring years of dedicated work, is subject to high interobserver variability and is not practical in clinical practice.

Scoring methods have been effective in establishing benefit from drug treatment and will continue to examine the benefit of new drugs in the years to come. Development of a simple, easy to use, accurate and reproducible method would be a powerful tool for both the physician and the clinical investigator.

JUVENILE IDIOPATHIC ARTHRITIDES

A number of separate disorders can lead to chronic arthritis in children; however, there is as yet no uniformly accepted classification for these diseases. The International League of Associations of Rheumatologists (ILAR) task force did attempt to establish classification criteria,[24] however, they are not in universal use.

Juvenile-onset Adult Type (Seropositive) Rheumatoid Arthritis

Seropositive juvenile rheumatoid arthritis (JRA) accounts for 5–15% of juvenile idiopathic arthritis (JIA). The onset is during adolescence and there is a strong female preponderance. It is a peripheral erosive polyarthritis which is nearly identical with adult RA. Large joints, such as the knee and hips may be affected.

Seronegative Chronic Arthritis

In this subgroup, systemic or articular symptoms and signs develop in the absence of positive serology for rheumatoid factor:

a. Classic systemic disease represents 20% of children with JIA. It occurs in children under the age of 5 years. Both sexes are equally affected. These children present with an acute febrile onset with anemia, hepatosplenomegaly, lymphadenopathy, anorexia, weight loss and chronic recurrent arthralgias. Erosive arthritis is uncommon.
b. *Pauciarticular* type is the most common type of JIA accounting for nearly half the cases. Four or less joints are involved, usually the large joints such as the knee, elbow and ankle. It typically affects young girls.
c. *Polyarticular* type represents approximately 20% of JIA. It may occur at any age and is more common in females. It is symmetric and involves the large and small joints as well as the cervical spine. Growth retardation is common due to premature fusion of the epiphyses and there may be associated mandibular hypoplasia with antegonial notching.

Generally, the prognosis in JIA is good with lesser than 20% children having progressive destructive disease. The pathophysiology is virtually identical to the adult form with synovial inflammation and increased production of joint fluid with effusion. Pannus is less extensive than adult RA but still produces significant cartilage and bony destruction.[3,10,25]

Radiologic Features

The knee is the most common joint to manifest radiographic abnormalities followed by the ankle, wrist, hand, elbow, hip, shoulder, cervical spine, sacroiliac (SI) joints and sternoclavicular joint.[25] Early changes include soft tissue swelling and osteopenia which may be juxta-articular or diffuse. In early stages, it is probably due to hyperemia, but later, disuse atrophy and steroids contribute to it. Band-like metaphyseal lucent zones (growth arrest lines) may be evident. Pathological fractures may occur.[10] Periostitis appears within weeks after the onset of symptoms and is usually seen along the shafts of the proximal phalanges, metacarpals and metatarsals.[3]

Later, there is uniform loss of joint space and articular erosions **(Figs. 12A to C)**. Progressive destruction can lead to bony ankylosis. Fusion at the carpometacarpal joint of the index and middle fingers is characteristic as are multiple fused cervical vertebrae.[3]

The most distinctive radiographic findings are seen as a result of altered growth patterns. There is accelerated bone maturation with early fusion of epiphyses and bone shortening secondary to hyperemia.[10] This results in large expansile (ballooned) epiphyses while the adjacent metaphysis and diaphysis appear gracile and constricted.[3] Muscle atrophy is generally a prominent feature **(Fig. 13)**.

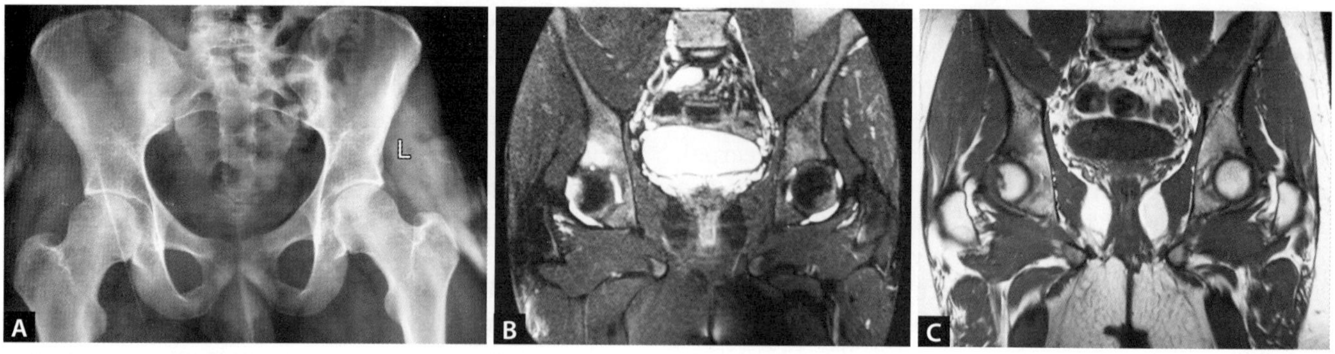

Figs. 12A to C: A 12-year-old boy with JIA: (A) X-ray of the pelvis shows mild narrowing of the joint spaces in bilateral hips; (B) Coronal T2-weighted image demonstrates the presence of joint effusion and ill-defined hyperintense signal in the acetabulum signifying bone marrow edema; (C) Coronal T1-weighted image shows bone erosions in bilateral hip joints.

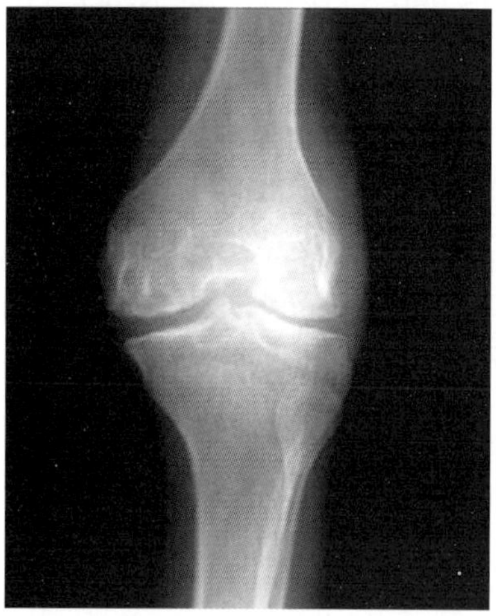

Fig. 13: Juvenile rheumatoid arthritis: X-ray knee joint AP view reveals diffuse osteopenia with large squared femoral condyles, widening with irregularity of the intercondylar notch and subchondral lucencies. Note the reduction in the soft tissue bulk.

In the carpus and tarsus, the bones show accelerated maturation, crowding with joint space narrowing and an abnormal angular shape (squashed carpi). The cervical spine is often affected with erosions at the apophyseal joints (usually at C2–3) leading to ankylosis. The associated vertebral bodies fail to develop. AAD is said to occur rarely in children with seronegative disease. The intervertebral disks are narrowed and fusion may occur. There may be ankylosis of the SI joints. Late in the course of the disease, secondary degenerative changes may occur.[12]

Radiographs are useful for diagnosis, staging and follow-up and for exclusion of other causes of pain, such as fractures, tumors or congenital disorders. However, they mostly depict late manifestations and indirect signs of synovial disease. Ultrasound is a quick, safe and radiation free modality which can directly image the synovium for evidence of proliferation or hypervascularity.[26] It can also depict joint effusion or provide guidance for aspiration to exclude septic arthritis. In a study on 30 patients, USG was found to be more sensitive than clinical assessment for the detection of synovial effusion and thickening in cases of JIA.[27] In another study, it was found that power doppler sonography was highly accurate in monitoring the therapeutic response in cases of JIA.[28]

Magnetic resonance remains the imaging modality of choice for evaluating the early changes of JIA because of its ability to allow direct visualization of nonossified portions of epiphyseal cartilage.[10] It clearly depicts joint effusion, cartilage changes, synovial proliferation, bony erosion or synovial cysts. With long standing JIA of the knee, synovial proliferation over the meniscal surfaces leads to meniscal attenuation with eventual meniscal hypoplasia or atrophy.[25,29]

Radiographic evidence of synovitis may be seen in trauma induced synovitis, septic arthritis or tubercular arthritis. These disorders are monoarticular in contrast to JIA and history of trauma or acute onset may serve to differentiate them from JIA. If tubercular arthritis involves multiple large joints, it may be indistinguishable from JIA. In hemophilic arthropathy, repetitive bleeding into the joint induces synovial inflammation and hypertrophy with a radiologic picture closely resembling JIA.

SERONEGATIVE SPONDYLOARTHROPATHIES

Seronegative spondyloarthropathies (SSA) are a group of seronegative arthritic diseases affecting multiple organ systems with clinical and radiological overlap and a significant genetic component. They are characterized by the absence of rheumatoid factor, peripheral arthropathy and sacroiliitis with or without spondylitis. A classification criteria for the entire group of SSA has been developed.

These criteria are inflammatory spinal pain or synovitis, together with at least one of the following: positive family history, urethritis, inflammatory bowel disease, psoriasis, acute diarrhea, alternating buttock pain, enthesopathy or radiographically evident sacroiliitis.[30]

ANKYLOSING SPONDYLITIS

Ankylosing spondylitis (AS) is a chronic, progressive inflammatory arthritis principally affecting the synovial joints of the spine and adjacent soft tissues as well as the SI joints, although peripheral joints, such as the hips, shoulders and knee may also be involved.[3] There is a strong association with HLA-B27 with more than 90% of patients with AS having this antigen. It has been shown that AS will develop in 0.6–1.3% of persons who are positive for HLA-B27. 65% of patients of psoriasis with spondylitis or inflammatory bowel disease with spondylitis also have HLA-B27 and it has been postulated that the antigen is essentially related to spinal changes.[12]

The disease is common in males (4:1) though recently it has been realized that women may be more commonly affected than thought earlier. Women are more likely to have clinical manifestations without radiographic evidence of disease. The onset of disease is generally between 15 and 35 years.[10]

The classical clinical description of AS is of an insidious onset with low back pain persisting for more than 3 months. Back stiffness is worse after periods of inactivity and there may be pain over the gluteal and sacroiliac regions. Radiographic evidence of sacroiliitis is required for the definitive diagnosis of AS, but may take several years to appear. Various extra-articular features may be present of which the most common is acute anterior uveitis. Others include aortitis, aortic regurgitation, pulmonary fibrosis, cardiac conduction defects, arachnoiditis and amyloidosis.[31] Pulmonary involvement can result in cavitation with fibrosis in bilateral lung apices mimicking tuberculosis.[10]

Pathophysiology

Histologically, the synovitis of AS is identical to that of RA. There is a predisposition to develop ankylosis via cartilage metaplasia, endochondral ossification, fibrosis and formation of woven bone. The enthesopathy consists of destruction of ligaments, tendons and local bone with inflammatory infiltrate. This heals by deposition of new bone at the tendon/ligament interface causing bone proliferation at nonarticular sites, syndesmophytes and capsular ossification.[12] It has been suggested that there is a genetic predisposition which allows an antigen or other triggering factor to reach the synovium and incite an inflammatory response. This response includes activated lymphocytes which liberate tumor necrosis factor alpha (TNFα) and other cytokines leading to destruction of tissue.[31]

Radiologic Features

Sacroiliac Joints

The classic sacroiliitis is bilateral and symmetrical. In about 10% of cases, the sacroiliitis may be unilateral or asymmetrical at presentation but eventually becomes bilaterally symmetrical. Changes occur in both the synovial and ligamentous (superior and posterior) parts of the SI joints. The earliest radiographic findings are a loss of or blurring of the subchondral cortex. This is followed by small (rat-bite) erosions which are worse along the iliac aspect of the joint. These cause widening of the joint space with hazy margins **(Figs. 14A and B)**. This is followed by larger erosions, subjacent sclerosis and joint space narrowing as irregular new bone bridges the joint space with eventual ankylosis and resolution of the sclerosis.[1,2,10,12]

The modified New York criteria for grading sacroiliitis established in 1994 are as follows:[32]

Grade 0 : Normal findings
Grade 1 : Suspicious changes
Grade 2 : Minimal abnormality (small localized erosions or sclerosis without alteration in joint width)
Grade 3 : Unequivocal abnormality
Grade 4 : Total ankylosis.

Joint changes are assessed using prone views with cephalad angulation or oblique views. However, CT is more sensitive than radiographs in depicting small and early erosions and joint space changes.[31] Recently, it has been suggested that dynamic CEMR may be even more sensitive than CT in detecting sacroiliitis.[33] Magnetic resonance findings include erosions, subchondral sclerosis, bone marrow edema, intra-articular hyperintensity on T2 and T2*-weighted images and enhancement within the joint cavity **(Figs. 15A and B)**. Radionuclide scanning shows nonspecific increased uptake in the presence of active sacroiliitis.

Spine

Spinal involvement classically starts at the dorsolumbar or lumbosacral junction with subsequent progressive involvement of the rest of the spine in an ascending manner. In females, the cervical region may be initially affected. Erosions initially occur at the vertebral margins

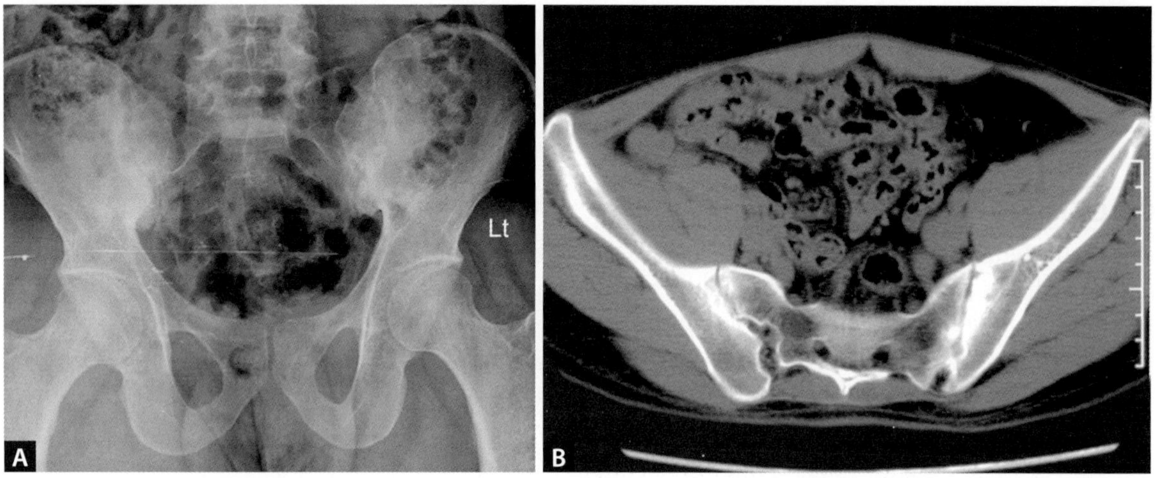

Figs. 14A and B: Sacroiliitis in ankylosing spondylitis: (A) X-ray pelvis AP view shows mild irregularity with subarticular sclerosis in both SI joints; (B) Axial CT section of the SI joints of the same patient shows irregularity of the articular surfaces with subarticular sclerosis which is more marked in the iliac blades.

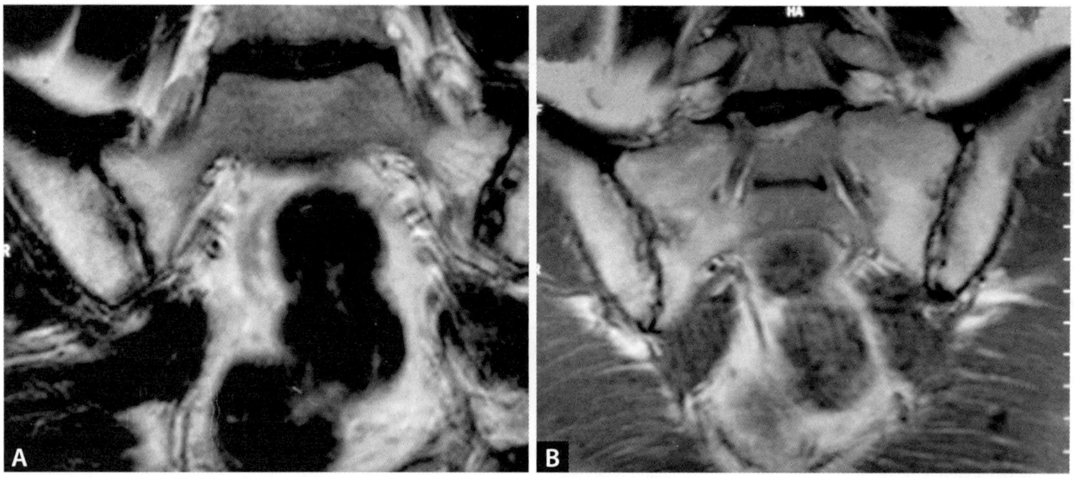

Figs. 15A and B: Ankylosing spondylitis: (A) T1- and (B) T2-weighted coronal images show irregularity of the cortex, discrete subchondral erosions, irregular thinning of the articular cartilage and reactive subarticular bone marrow edema and fatty change.

at the site of attachment of the outer fibers of the annulus fibrosus (Romanus lesions) with adjacent sclerosis (shiny corner sign). In adolescents, these erosions can be large mimicking an infectious process (erosive spondylitis). Healing of these erosions or laying down of bone beneath the anterior longitudinal ligament causes "squaring" of the vertebral bodies, best appreciated on lateral radiographs of the lumbar spine. Exuberant new bone formation may even cause anterior convexity of the vertebral body (barrel shaped vertebrae).[3,12,31]

As the disease progresses, there is syndesmophyte formation along the anterior and anterolateral aspects of the body due to ossification in the annulus. Syndesmophytes are paravertebral in location and vertically oriented in contrast to the osteophytes seen in degenerative disease, which are horizontally directed. The syndesmophytes seen in AS are classically marginal, symmetrical, fine and delicate. Ankylosis of multiple vertebrae by syndesmophytes gives the bamboo spine appearance. Similar ossifications may be seen in the interspinous ligaments and facet joints resulting in the dagger and tram-track signs respectively **(Figs. 16A and B)**. Facet joint ankylosis is the major factor causing loss of spinal mobility.[1-3,10]

Studies have shown than MR can detect active enthesitis in the spine before Romanus lesions are seen on radiographs. Magnetic resonance shows an abnormal area of low signal intensity on T1WI which is hyperintense on T2WI and enhances postcontrast.[31]

Spinal fractures are common in the spine through the porotic bone just beneath the endplates. Two categories have been described, the traumatic fractures and stress fractures. Traumatic fractures occur after spinal fusion even with trivial trauma and are of the unstable category with involvement of all three columns. Stress fractures typically occur near the cervicothoracic and thoracolumbar junctions, with development of sclerotic pseudoarthrosis with destruction of the disk and vertebral endplates (Andersson lesion) resembling an infective diskitis.[12,31]

Cauda equina syndrome can result from arachnoiditis with large posterior dural diverticula causing osseous defects in the laminae. CT and MR imaging may show peripheral clumping of nerve roots, prominent arachnoid diverticulae, laminar erosions and dural calcifications.[12,31]

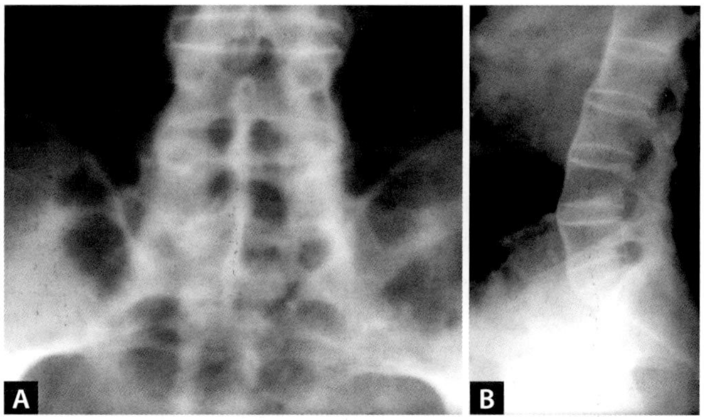

Figs. 16A and B: Ankylosing spondylitis—X-rays lumbosacral spine: (A) AP and (B) lateral views reveal the classical appearance of the bamboo spine on the lateral view and the dagger and tram-track signs on the AP view with bilateral ankylosis of the SI joints.

Atlantoaxial subluxation can occur but it is much less common than RA. There may be dramatic resorption of bone from the anterior aspects of the lower cervical vertebral bodies.[2]

Peripheral Joints

Ankylosing spondylitis is the only seronegative spondylo-arthropathy where large joint involvement is not so uncommon. In general, the arthropathy resembles RA with a few differences. Shaggy periostitis and ankylosis are more common, whereas osteoporosis, erosions and joint space narrowing are less prominent.[12]

The hip joints are involved in up to 50% of patients with AS. Radiographic changes include concentric joint space narrowing, axial migration, cuff like osteophytes on the femoral head and protrusio acetabuli with eventual joint fusion **(Figs. 17A to C)**. The shoulder is the next commonly involved joint and shows narrowing of the acromioclavicular and glenohumeral joint spaces and a hatchet deformity on the humeral head due to enthesitis of the rotator cuff tendon.[31] Small joint involvement is rare and is characterized by an asymmetric distribution, subtle erosions and proliferative bone changes at the involved joints.

Enthesopathies at tendinous and ligamentous insertions can cause erosions with marked sclerosis.[3] These can be commonly seen at the iliac crest, ischial tuberosity (ischial whiskering) and the calcaneum.

PSORIATIC ARTHROPATHY

Psoriasis is a chronic inflammatory disease of the skin which may be associated with a chronic inflammatory arthritis in 5–8% of cases. The incidence is highest between

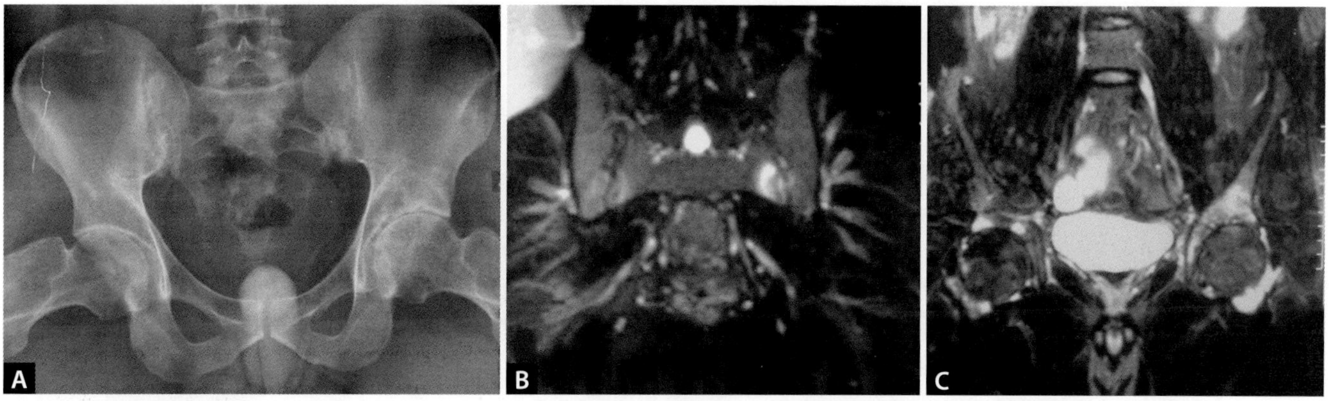

Figs. 17A to C: A 32-year-old male with ankylosing spondylitis: (A) X-ray pelvis shows bilateral sacroiliitis with rat-bite erosions and fuzzy, irregular margins. Note the narrowing of the joint space with erosions in the left hip joint; (B) Coronal STIR image shows bilateral sacroiliitis with bone marrow edema; (C) Coronal T2-weighted fat-saturated image demonstrates the narrowing of the left hip joint space, erosions and bone marrow edema.

20 and 39 years in males and 40–59 years in females with an equal male-to-female ratio. The etiology is unknown. Histologically, a chronic synovitis may cause joint destruction with inflammation of the tendon and ligamentous insertion sites (enthesitis).[31]

Skin lesions are usually seen on extensor surfaces, scalp and lumbosacral areas and are sharply demarcated, dry, erythematous plaques with a silvery scale. Clinically, patients with PA can be broadly classified into three groups:[3,12,31]

1. Mono or oligoarthritis with enteritis
2. Peripheral polyarthritis resembling RA and
3. Predominant axial disease resembling AS with or without peripheral joint disease. This is rare, occurring in only 5% of patients.

The skin lesions precede the arthritis in 70% of patients; however, arthritis may precede skin lesions in 15% of cases. In another 15%, the two appear concomitantly.[12] The joints commonly involved are the knee, DIP and PIP joints of the hands and feet, MTP and MCP joints and the ankles. Sacroiliitis may be seen in 35 to 50% and spondylitis in 30–40% of cases.[34]

Radiologic Features

The radiologic features are quite characteristic and the diagnosis can be strongly suggested based on the presence of bone erosions and prominent bone proliferation which is the most distinguishing feature in this condition.

The hands and feet are most commonly involved in proriatic arthropathy (PA). A fusiform soft tissue swelling is seen involving the entire digit (sausage digit). The involvement may be unilateral, if bilateral, it is asymmetric. All the joints of a single row may be affected. The bone density is preserved. Bone erosion typically begins at the margins of the joint and proceeds along the articular surface (surface erosion) or progresses along the joint capsule away from the joint along the metaphysis (enthesitic erosion).[31] This leads to a pencil like tapering of the ends of the small bones. The joint space may be widened due to fibrous tissue deposition and bone resorption due to severe surface erosions resulting in the "pencil-in-cup" appearance. The enthesitic erosions along with bone proliferation may give an irregular outline to the metaphyses or may widen the end of bone (mouse-ears sign) **(Figs. 18A and B)**.[3] Nail changes may be associated with resorption of the terminal tufts or the distal phalanges may become sclerotic. Calcaneal erosions with fluffy periosteal reaction may be seen at both the posterosuperior and posterior plantar aspects. Periosteal reaction along the diaphysis of the short tubular bones is common. In the advanced stages, there may be "arthritis mutilans" which is a term used to describe severe destruction of the joints of the hands and feet associated with extensive bone resorption.[12]

The sacroiliac joints may be involved in up to 50% of patients with PA and the involvement is usually bilateral. It may be symmetric or asymmetric and ankylosis is relatively uncommon. Involvement of the spine may occur in the absence of sacroiliitis and is more common in males than females. It is characterized by coarse, asymmetric paravertebral ossification (nonmarginal syndesmophytes) in the dorsolumbar region in contrast to the symmetric,

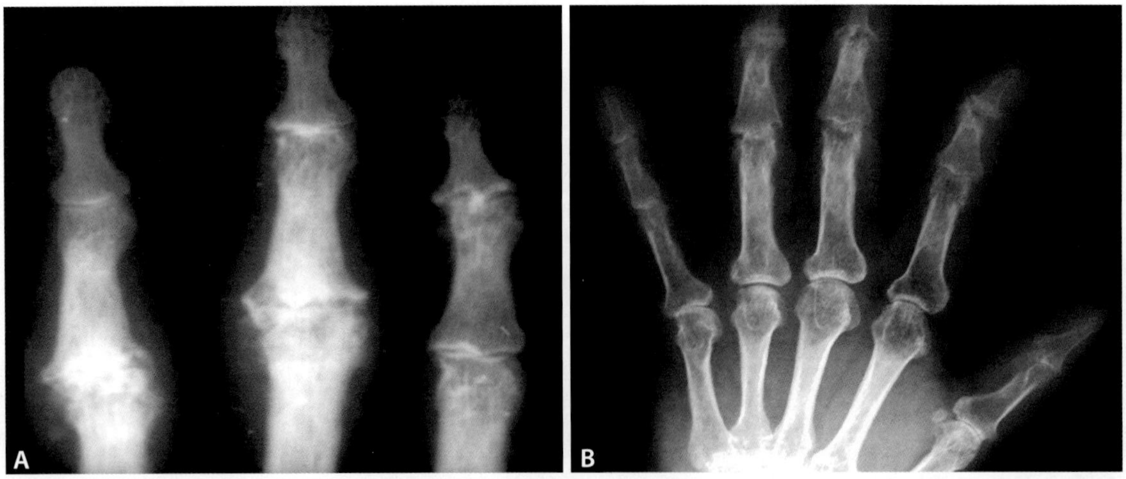

Figs. 18A and B: X-rays of the hands—magnified views reveal: (A) Fusiform soft tissue swelling with gross erosive changes at the DIP and PIP joints. Note the subperiosteal bone apposition causing widening of the bone ends; (B) Erosive changes at the PIP and DIP joints with a "pencil-in-cup" appearance. These features are characteristic of psoriasis.

fine marginal syndesmophytes seen in AS.[1,3] These may be unilateral with skip areas. The anterior surface of the vertebral bodies is spared and squaring of the bodies is distinctly uncommon. There may be diffuse, ill-defined, paravertebral ossification. Isolated cervical involvement may be seen with apophyseal fusion and AAD.[31]

Magnetic resonance frequently shows signal changes in the soft tissue and bone marrow related to the enthesitis reflecting inflammatory changes.[35]

REITER'S SYNDROME

Reiter's syndrome (RS) is a sexually transmitted disease commonly affecting young men which is characterized by arthritis, uveitis and conjunctivitis. In Europe, a similar syndrome occurs in association with bacillary dysentery.[3,12]

Skeletal involvement may eventually occur in up to 80% of cases. There is a peripheral asymmetric arthritis with a predilection for the joints of the lower limbs especially the feet where erosions occur at the heels, MTP joints and IP joint of the great toe. The DIP joints are rarely involved (in contrast to PA). Periostitis may be fine and lamellar in acute cases or fluffy and irregular in chronic cases. Reactive calcaneal spurs occur in 20% of patients.[2,12]

Sacroiliitis may develop in about 50% of cases and may be unilateral or asymmetrical in contrast to AS where it is classically bilaterally symmetrical **(Figs. 19A to C)**. Ankylosis is also less common. Coarse, asymmetric syndesmophytes similar to those seen in psoriatic arthropathy may occur, especially in the thoracolumbar region but occur less frequently.[1,3]

ENTEROPATHIC SPONDYLOARTHROPATHY

This group comprises arthritides associated with inflammatory intestinal diseases, such as ulcerative colitis, regional enteritis (Crohn's disease) and Whipple's disease. HLA-B27 is present in most patients with spinal involvement.[3] There are two distinct types of joint involvement:

1. A spondylitis and sacroiliitis which is indistinguishable from ankylosing spondylitis may be seen in 6% of patients with inflammatory bowel disease and may even precede the development of bowel disease. Syndesmophyte formation, squaring of vertebral bodies and apophyseal ankylosis is seen similar to AS. The sacroiliitis is bilateral and symmetric. These changes do not correlate with the activity of the gut disease and may continue to worsen even if the gut disease becomes quiescent.
2. A peripheral asymmetrical arthropathy with non-specific features of soft tissue swelling and local periostitis. The activity of the arthropathy approximates the activity of the bowel disease.[12]

CRYSTAL DEPOSITION ARTHROPATHY

Gout

Gout is a metabolic disorder characterized by recurrent episodes of arthritis which results from a disturbance of urate metabolism with the deposition of monosodium urate (MSU) crystals in the joints and soft tissues. Primary gout is caused by inborn defects of either purine metabolism or the renal tubular secretion of urate. Secondary gout is caused by acquired disorders that result in increased turnover of nucleic acids (e.g. myeloproliferative disorders), by acquired defects in renal excretion of urates or due to certain drugs like cyclosporine.[36]

Men in the age group of 40–50 years are commonly affected; however, gout also occurs in postmenopausal women. Four stages are seen clinically:[37]

1. Asymptomatic gout—presence of hyperuricemia.
2. Acute gouty arthritis—episodes of monoarticular peripheral acute arthritis, involving the 1st MTP joint

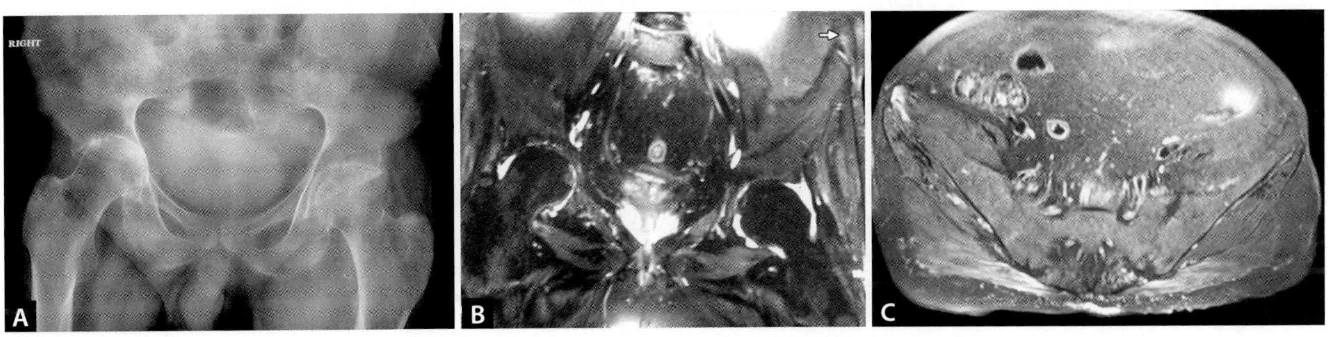

Figs. 19A to C: A 32-year-old male with Reiter's arthropathy: (A) X-ray pelvis shows bilateral sacroiliitis with narrowing and irregularity of the right hip joint; (B) Coronal T2-weighted fat-saturated image shows fluid in bilateral hip joints with erosions and narrowing of the left hip joint; (C) Axial T2-weighted fat-saturated image shows asymmetric ankylosis of the sacroiliac joints.

of the great toe in 75% of cases. Later, the arthritis may be polyarticular and chronic and a phase of chronic gouty arthritis results.

3. Intercritical gout—is the symptom free period between acute attacks.
4. Chronic tophaceous gout—is characterized by the deposition of monosodium urate crystals (tophi) in tendons, ligaments, cartilage, bone and other soft tissues including synovium or in the subcutaneous tissues in a para-articular location.

Definitive diagnosis involves the demonstration of MSU crystals in the synovial fluid which are needle shaped and show strong negative birefringence under polarized light microscopy.[3]

Imaging

Gout has several characteristic radiographic features, but these are seldom seen these days as it takes 4-6 years for gout to cause radiographically evident disease and most patients are correctly diagnosed and treated successfully before that.[1]

The classic findings are the presence of sharply marginated, round to oval erosions, which are oriented in the long axis of the bone, often with sclerotic borders or overhanging edges **(Fig. 20)**. These are initially periarticular in location, but may later extend into the joint. There is a predilection for the 1st MTP joint; however, other joints, such as the ankles, knee, elbow and wrist joint may also be affected. Spinal involvement is unusual but the sacroiliac joints may be involved in 5–13% of cases. The bone density is preserved till the late stages of the disease. Punctuate bone sclerosis owing to intraosseous deposition of tophi may be seen resembling enchondromas.[12] There is uneven articular space narrowing due to cartilage destruction. Para-articular tophi cause asymmetric "lumpy-bumpy" soft tissue swellings which frequently show fluffy calcification in the presence of renal disease **(Fig. 21)**. These tophi may saucerise the underlying bone. Chondrocalcinosis may be seen because up to 40% of patients with gout have concomitant CPPD deposition disease. Nephrolithiasis may be seen in 20% of cases.[1]

On MR, an inflamed joint will show joint effusion and para-articular edema with enhancement of the para-articular structures postcontrast. Tophaceous deposits have a low to intermediate SI on T1 and a low (if calcified) or high SI on T2-weighted images.[36]

CALCIUM PYROPHOSPHATE DIHYDRATE CRYSTAL DEPOSITION DISEASE

Calcium pyrophosphate dihydrate (CPPD) crystal deposition disease is characterized by acute, subacute or chronic joint inflammation with deposition of CPPD crystals in hyaline and fibrocartilage and other soft tissue structures. CPPD crystals are weakly birefringent on polarized light microscopy. The disease may cause intermittent acute attacks of arthritis when it is called pseudogout.[2]

The classic triad consists of pain, cartilage calcification and joint destruction. Chondrocalcinosis can occur in any joint but commonly involves the medial and lateral compartments of the knee, the triangular cartilage and lunotriquetral ligament in the wrist and the symphysis

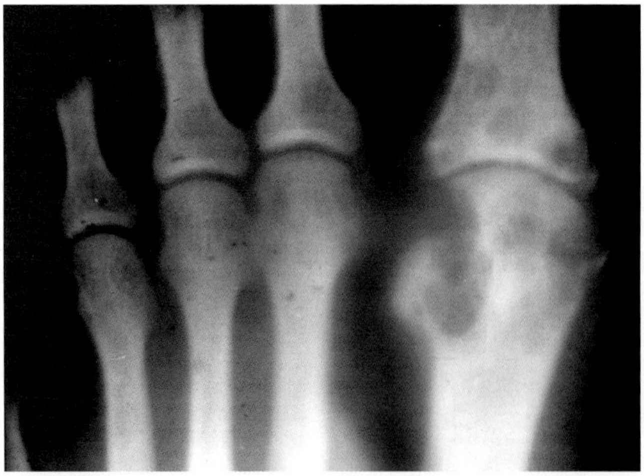

Fig. 20: X-ray of the first MTP joint shows well-defined periarticular erosions with overhanging edges classical of gout.

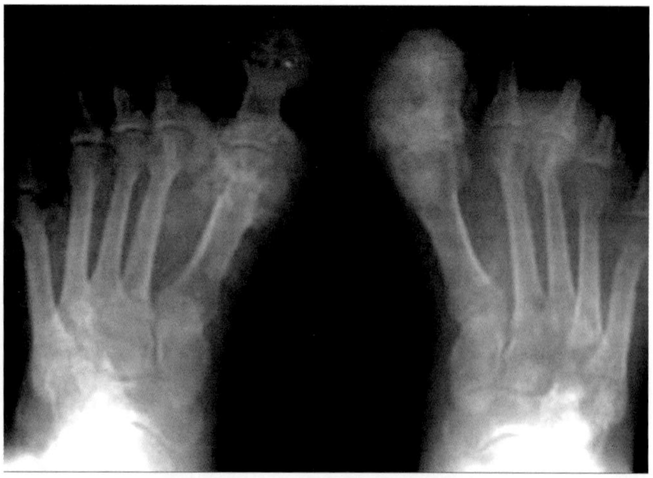

Fig. 21: X-ray both feet shows advanced changes of gout with multiple soft tissue tophi, some of which are calcified. Gross periarticular erosions are seen in both 1st MTP joints. Note the saucerization of the left 1st proximal phalanx due to overlying soft tissue tophi.

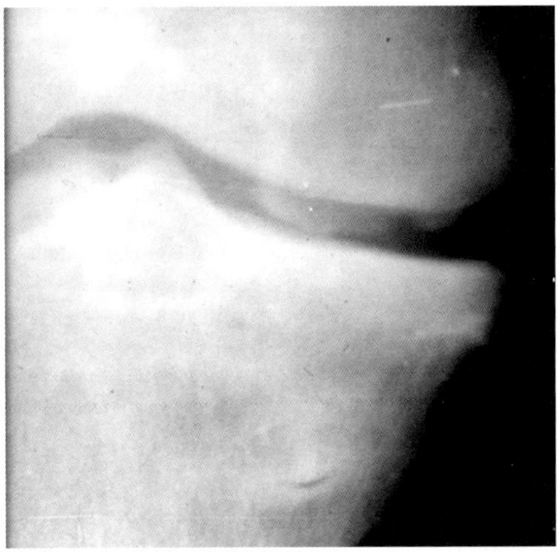

Fig. 22: Magnified view of the knee joint demonstrating chondrocalcinosis.

pubis **(Fig. 22)**. When CPPD crystals occur in the soft tissues, such as the rotator cuff, they cannot be differentiated from calcium hydroxyapatite crystals which occur in calcific tendonitis.[1]

The arthropathy of CPPD is a degenerative joint disease caused by the crystals eroding the cartilage. However, CPPD has a tendency to involve the shoulder, elbow, wrist and the patellofemoral compartment of the knee, sites which are not usually involved by degenerative joint disease. Occasionally, CPPD arthropathy may accelerate and severe destruction occurs to such an extent that it mimics a neuropathic joint.[2]

REFERENCES

1. Helms CA. Arthritis. In: Helms CA (Ed): Fundamentals of Skeletal Radiology. Philadelphia: WB Saunders; 1989.pp. 135-76.
2. Martel W. Diagnostic radiology in the rheumatic diseases. In: Kelley WN, Harris ED Jr, Ruddy S, Sledge CB (Eds): Textbook of Rheumatology. Philadelphia: WB Saunders; 1982.vol 1. pp.580-621.
3. Greenspan A. Inflammatory arthritides. In: Greenspan A (Ed). Orthopaedic Radiology: A Practical Approach, 3rd edition. Philadelphia: Lippincott Williams and Wilkins; 2000.pp. 453-78.
4. Sommer OJ, Kladosek A, Weiler V, Czembirek H, Boeck M, Stiskal M. Rheumatoid arthritis: A practical guide to state-of-the-art imaging, image interpretation and clinical implications. Radiographics. 2005;25:381-98.
5. Narváez JA, Narváez J, De Lama E, De Albert M. MR imaging of early rheumatoid arthritis. Radiographics. 2010;30:143-65.
6. Arnett FC, Edworthy SM, Block DA, et al. The American Rheumatism Association 1987 revised criteria for the classification of rheumatoid arthritis. Arthritis Rheum. 1988;31:315-24.
7. Sugimoto H, Takeda A, Hyodo K. Early stage rheumatoid arthritis: prospective study of the effectiveness of MR imaging for diagnosis. Radiology. 2000;216:569-75.
8. Østergaard M, Ejbjerg B, Szkudlarek M. Imaging in early rheumatoid arthritis: roles of magnetic resonance imaging, ultrasonography, conventional radiography and computed tomography. Best Pract Res Clin Rheumatol. 2005;19(1):91-116.
9. Imhof H, Nobauer-Huhmann IM, Gahleitner A, et al. Pathophysiology and imaging in inflammatory and blastomatous synovial diseases. Skeletal Radio. 2002;31(6): 313-33.
10. Resnick D. Rheumatoid arthritis and the seronegative spondyloarthropathies: Radiographic and pathologic concepts. In: Resnick B (Ed): Diagnosis of Bone and Joint Disorders. Philadelphia: WB Saunders; 2002.pp.837-90.
11. Renner WR, Weinstein AS. Early changes of rheumatoid arthritis in the hand and wrist. Radiol Clin North Am. 1988;26:1185-93.
12. Renton P. Diseases of joints. In: Sutton D (Ed): Textbook of Radiology and Imaging, 7th edition. Churchill Livingstone; 2002. vol. 2.pp.1201-45.
13. Resnick D. Rheumatoid arthritis. In: Resnick D (Ed): Diagnosis of Bone and Joint Disorders. Philadelphia: WB Saunders; 2002.pp.891-987.
14. Wakefield RJ, Gibbon WW, Conaghan PG, et al. The value of sonography in the detection of bone erosions in patients with rheumatoid arthritis: a comparison with conventional radiography. Arthritis Rheum. 2000;43:2762-70.
15. Brown AK, Wakefied RJ, Conaghan PG, Karini Z, O' Connor PJ, Emery P. New approaches to imaging early inflammatory arthritis. Clin Experiment Rheumatol. 2004; 22(Suppl 35):S18-25.
16. Backhaus M, Kamradt T, Sandrock D, et al. Arthritis of the finger joints: A comprehensive approach comparing conventional radiography, scintigraphy, ultrasound and contrast enhanced magnetic resonance imaging. Arthritis Rheum. 1999;42(6):1232-45.
17. El-Miedany YM, Housny IH, Mansour HM, et al. Ultrasound versus MRI in the evaluation of juvenile idiopathic arthritis of the knee. Joint Bone Spine. 2001;68(3):222-30.
18. Polster J, Winalski CS, Sundaram M, Lieber ML, Schils J, et al. Rheumatoid arthritis: Evaluation with contrast enhanced CT with digital bone masking. Radiology. 2009;252(1):225-31.
19. Tehranzadeh J, Ashikyan O, Dascalos J. Advanced imaging of early rheumatoid arthritis. Radiol Clin North Am. 2004;42:89-107.
20. McQueen FM, Benton N, Perry D, et al. Bone edema scored on magnetic resonance imaging scans of the dominant carpus at presentation predicts radiographic joint damage of the hands and feet six years later in patients with rheumatoid arthritis. Arthritis Rheum. 2003;48(7):1814-27.
21. McQueen F, Beckley V, Crabbe J, et al. Magnetic resonance imaging evidence of tendinopathy in early rheumatoid arthritis predicts tendon rupture at six years. Arthritis Rheum. 2005;52(3):744-51.

22. Larsen A. How to apply Larsen score in evaluating radiographs of rheumatoid arthritis in long-term studies. J Rheumatol. 1995;22:1974-5.
23. Østergaard M, Peterfy C, Conaghan P, et al. OMERACT Rheumatoid Arthritis Magnetic Resonance Imaging Studies: core set of MRI acquisitions, joint pathology definitions, and the OMERACT RA-MRI scoring system. J Rheumatol. 2003;30(6):1385-6.
24. Petty RE, Southwood TR, Baum J, et al. Revision of the proposed classification criteria for juvenile idiopathic arthritis: Durban, 1997. J Rheumatol. 1998;25:1991-4.
25. Buchmann RF, Jaramillo D. Imaging of articular disorders in children. Radiol Clin North Am. 2004;42:151-68.
26. Doria AS, Kiss MH, Lotito AP, et al. Juvenile rheumatoid arthritis of the knee: Evaluation with contrast-enhanced color Doppler ultrasound. Pediatr Radiol. 2001;31(7): 524-31.
27. Kakati P, Sodhi KS, Sandhu MS, Singh S, Katariya S, Khandelwal N. Clinical and ultrasound assessment of the knee in children with juvenile rheumatoid arthritis. Indian J Pediatr. 2007;74(9):831-6.
28. Shanmugavel C, Sodhi KS, Sandhu MS, Sidhu R, Singh S, Katariya S, Khandelwal N. Role of power doppler sonography in evaluation of therapeutic response of the knee in juvenile rheumatoid arthritis. Rheumatol Int. 2008;28(6):573-8.
29. Lamer S, Sebag GH. MRI and ultrasound in children with juvenile chronic arthritis. Eur J Radiol. 2000;33(2):85-93.
30. Dougados M, van der Linden S, Juhlin R, et al. The European spondyloarthropathy study group preliminary criteria for the classification of spondyloarthropathy. Arthritis Rheum. 1991;34:1218.
31. Bennett DL, Ohashi K, El- Khoury GY. Spondyloarthropathies: Ankylosing spondylitis and psoriatic arthritis. Radiol Clin North Am. 2004;42:121-32.
32. van der Linden S, Valkenburg HA, Cats A. Evaluation of diagnostic criteria for ankylosing spondylitis: A proposal for modification of the New York criteria. Arthritis Rheum. 1984;27(4):361-8.
33. Bollow M, Braun J, Hamm B, et al. Early sacroiliitis in patients with spondyloarthropathies: Evaluation with dynamic gadolinium-enhanced MR imaging. Radiology. 1995;194(2):529-36.
34. Boumpas DT, Illei GG, Tassiulas IO. Psoriatic arthritis. In: Klippel JH (Ed). Primer on the rheumatic diseases, 12th edition. Atlanta: Arthritis Foundation; 2001.pp.233-8.
35. Weishaupt D, Schweitzer ME, Alam F, et al. MR imaging of inflammatory joint diseases of the foot and ankle. Skeletal Radiol. 1999;28:663-9.
36. Monu JUV, Pope TL. Gout: A clinical and radiological review. Radiol Clin North Am. 2004;42:169-84.
37. Resnick D. Gouty arthritis. In: Resnick D (Ed). Diagnosis of Bone and Joint Disorders. Philadelphia: WB Saunders; 2002.pp.1519-59.

CHAPTER 194

Nontubercular Infections of the Spine

Sameer Vyas, Manavjit Singh Sandhu

INTRODUCTION

Spinal infections result from several infectious pathologic agents with wide and varied clinical presentations.[1-6] Several factors can make people more vulnerable to spinal infections, including immunodeficiency secondary to human immunodeficiency virus (HIV) infection or intravenous drug abuse, old age, chronically debilitated individuals, the widespread use of broad-spectrum antibiotics, the use of corticosteroids and immunosuppressive drugs and parenteral alimentation. The recent development of medical technologies has enhanced the ease of detection and the options for definitive management of spinal infections. Ironically, technologic advances have also promoted the occurrence of spinal infections by increasing the number of patients with iatrogenic immunosuppression, enhancing the life expectancy of patients with chronic medical illnesses, and increasing the complexity of spinal procedures and therefore the potential for infectious complications.[7,8]

PATHOGENESIS OF SPINAL INFECTIONS

The pathogens can reach the spine by four principal routes of spread: (a) the arterial hematogenous route from distant septic foci, (b) the venous hematogenous route, (c) contiguous spread from neighboring infected organs such as the oropharynx, pleural space of the lung, and thoracic or abdominal wall, and (d) direct inoculation (iatrogenic during surgery or interventional procedures).[1,3,6] Iatrogenic spinal infections constitute 2.5% of all spinal infections. The infection risk of open surgery is reported to be approximately 3–13%. Myelography, discography chemonucleolysis, vertebroplasty, and kyphoplasty are other known causes of spinal infection.

Vertebral bodies and intervertebral discs are most frequently affected with primary or secondary involvement of the epidural space, posterior elements, and paraspinal soft tissues. The pathogenesis of spinal infections can be explained on the basis of the vascular anatomy of the vertebral column. The vasculature of the vertebral bodies and intervertebral discs changes significantly with age. The most accepted hypothesis is that vertebral osteomyelitis results from hematogenous spread from an infected microembolus in the arterial system becoming lodged in one of the metaphyseal arteries resulting in infarction and subsequent infection. Osteomyelitis is most frequent at the endplates because of the greater number of arteries in this location. Anterior subchondral vertebral region is the usual site of infection within the vertebra corresponding to the area rich in arterial supply.[1] Also pre-existing foci of infection within the body and a high incidence of streptococcal and tubercular spinal infection favor the theory of hematogenous route of infection. The early infectious lesion occurs in the anterosuperior subchondral region of the vertebral body and subsequently extends through the endplate. Further dissemination may occur via subligamentous spread of infection with resulting anterior vertebral body scalloping or rupture of anterior longitudinal ligament **(Fig. 1)**.

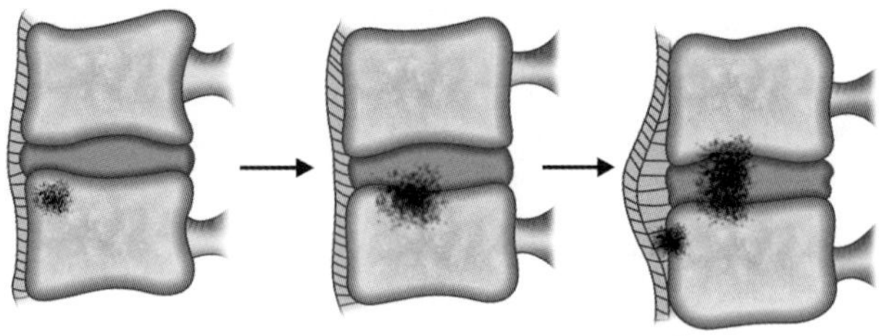

Fig. 1: Pathophysiology of vertebral osteomyelitis—the focus of infection usually begins in the anterosuperior subchondral region and subsequently extends to involve the adjacent disc and vertebral body. Anterior subligamentous spread may also occur.

The pathogenesis of disc space infection differs in the adults and in children. In children, the intervertebral discs receive nutrition by blood vessels that pass through the cartilaginous endplates of adjacent vertebral bodies. Hence, any infection involving the vertebral endplates easily extends to the adjacent disc space, whereas this is not so in the mature adult spine, where the nutrition of the nucleus pulposus occurs primarily by the process of diffusion.[1]

IMAGING OF SPINAL INFECTIONS

The various modalities available for evaluation of patients with suspected spinal infection are plain radiography, radioisotope scanning, computed tomography, myelography or CT myelography, and magnetic resonance imaging. A wise selection of the modalities is essential for timely patient management, as untreated spinal infections can lead to crippling and even life-threatening situations. Comparison of various imaging modalities in infections is illustrated in **Table 1**.

Plain Radiography

Plain radiographs are often done first in patients with suspected spinal pathology. Unfortunately the changes on plain radiographs appear quite late (2–8 weeks) after the onset of infection. It is possible to suggest a positive diagnosis, if changes are present on plain radiographs; however, there is a significant overlap of findings on radiographs between various infections. Atypical radiographic features at times make it difficult to differentiate infective spinal conditions from other noninfective causes, such as spondylodiscitis degenerative changes and metastases.[2,5] The plain radiographic features of spinal infection **(Figs. 2 to 4)** may include demineralization, loss of definition of endplate margins, narrowing of intervertebral disc space, associated soft tissue swelling (paraspinal or epidural soft tissue masses), and

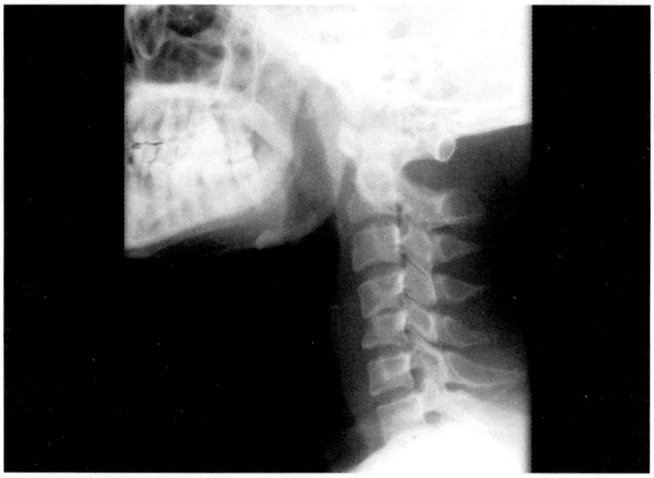

Fig. 2: Bacterial osteomyelitis involving the cervical vertebrae: Plain X-ray cervical spine lateral view showing anterior erosion of C5 vertebra, prevertebral soft tissue mass and early loss of disc space height between C4 and C5.

Table 1: Comparison of imaging modalities in infections.

	Advantages	*Disadvantages*
Plain radiograph	Readily available Inexpensive	30–50% loss of bone density before becomes abnormal Poor sensitivity
Computed tomography	Detects bony changes and surrounding extent	Lacks sensitivity of magnetic resonance imaging
Magnetic resonance imaging	Evaluation of the bone marrow, and neural structures	Hard to distinguish trauma/neoplasm from infection/new from old disease
Radionuclide scanning	Scans whole skeleton, sensitive earlier in disease than radiograph and computed tomograph	Expensive Long acquisition time, hard to distinguish overlying soft-tissue infections

eventually destructive changes of the vertebral end plate and the vertebral body (spinal deformity, frank vertebral destruction).[1,5,6] Paraspinal extension of the infective process may be appreciated as widened retropharyngeal or retrotracheal space in the cervical region, displacement of paraspinal lines in the dorsal region and evidence of unilateral or bilateral paravertebral psoas abscesses in the lumbar region.[9-12]

Healed or healing processes may be seen on plain radiographs as areas of sclerosis, reactive new bone formation, spur formation, bony bridging or vertebral fusion. Limitation of plain radiographs is most evident when it comes to differentiate between chronic vertebral

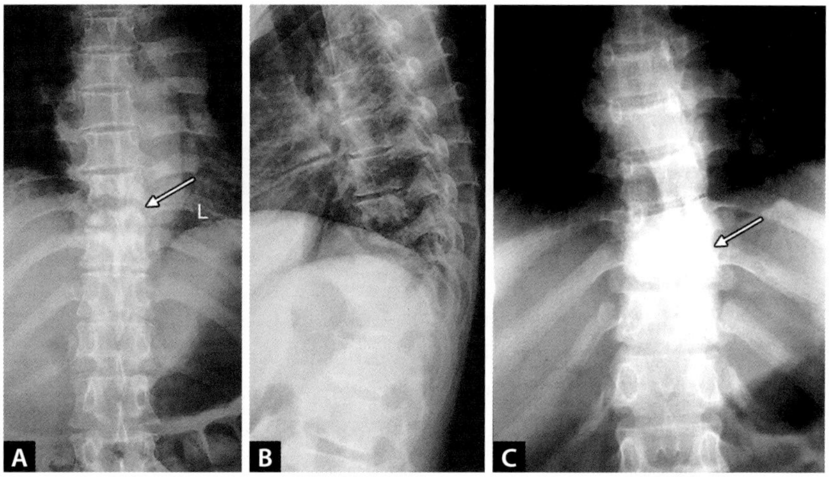

Figs. 3A to C: X-ray dorsal spine anteroposterior (A) and lateral view (B) showing contiguous endplate destruction at D8-9 intervertebral disc space and decrease in height of D9 vertebral body, features suggestive of pyogenic spondylodiscitis. The follow-up X-ray dorsal spine anteroposterior view (C) demonstrating healing as evidenced by ankylosis of two adjacent vertebrae.

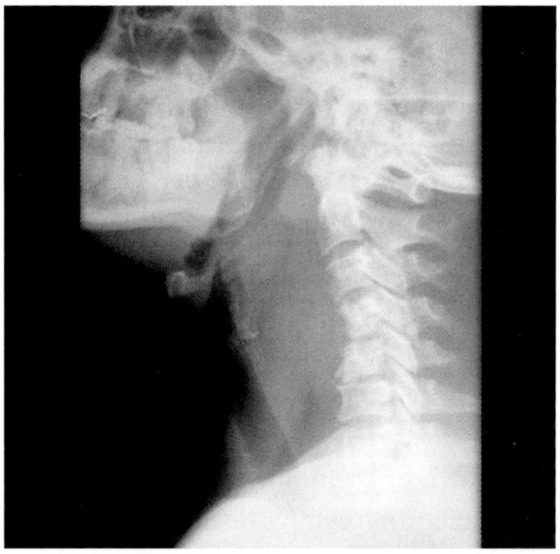

Fig. 4: Case of infective spondylodiscitis in middle aged female, X-ray cervical spine lateral view showing decreased disc space at C4–C5 level with destruction of anterior vertebral body of C4 vertebra and large prevertebral abscess.

osteomyelitis, discogenic degenerative end plate changes, and the presence of superimposed infection in the setting of chronic degenerative disc disease.[2,9]

Radioisotope Scanning

Radionuclide imaging frequently is part of the diagnostic work-up of musculoskeletal infection.[13-18] Isotope scanning is a very sensitive technique for early diagnosis of spinal lesions which is ubiquitously available and relatively inexpensive. Radionuclides most commonly used for detecting inflammatory changes of the spine are technetium-99m (^{99m}Tc) phosphate complexes, gallium 67 (^{67}Ga) citrate, and indium 111 (^{111}In)-labeled white blood cells. A three-phase Technetium-99m diphosphonate bone scan can be valuable in the diagnosis of vertebral osteomyelitis and is positive within hours to days after the onset of infection. It shows increased activity in all phases.

Radionuclide imaging is sensitive to infection, but this is a highly nonspecific tool and cannot differentiate infection from other causes of increased uptake like trauma (healing fractures), sterile inflammatory reactions, loosened prosthetic devices, arthritis or tumor. Combined, or sequential, bone (Technetium-99m) and gallium imaging is the dual tracer technique used for diagnosing complicating osteomyelitis and can differentiate infection from increased bone mineral turnover. Gallium-67 scans are specifically used to localize areas of inflammation.[14] ^{67}Ga binds to leukocytes which migrate to the area of inflammation. These leukocytes bind to various proteins at the site of the pathology. A gallium scan is usually obtained in conjunction with a technetium scan. If gallium scan is congruent or hotter than ^{99m}Tc scan, infection is implied and if ^{67}Ga scan is noncongruent or colder it implies that no infection is present. The overall accuracy of sequential bone/gallium imaging is about 65–80%. The gallium-67 combined with ^{99m}Tc MDP is useful in the diagnosis of vertebral osteomyelitis and has an accuracy similar to that of MRI.[13] The combined accuracy of technetium and gallium scan has been reported to be as high as 94%.[8] Labeled leukocyte imaging is not useful for detecting spinal osteomyelitis in contrast to other areas in the skeleton, because 50% or more of all cases of vertebral osteomyelitis present as nonspecific areas of decreased, or absent, activity. The radionuclide study takes time to perform (hours to days).

Single photon emission computed tomography (SPECT)/CT has been found to be very useful in musculoskeletal infection. The three dimensionality of a focal process can be further enhanced by the use of (SPECT).[13,15] SPECT may reveal abnormalities not seen on the planar images. SPECT/CT provided precise anatomic localization and delineation of the extent of the infection. The CT component of the test improved specificity by excluding active bone infection and by identifying bone abnormalities, other than infection, responsible for increased tracer uptake.

FDG-PET is a promising alternative to bone and gallium imaging for diagnosing spinal osteomyelitis. It may be especially useful and superior to MRI for distinguishing true infectious spondylodiscitis from severe granulation-type degenerative disc disease, and in patients who had previous surgery and suffered from high-grade infection in com-bination with a paravertebral abscess and in those patients with low-grade spondylitis or discitis. The specificity of the test, however, was adversely affected by the presence of spinal implants.[18]

Computed Tomography

Computed tomography (CT) entails a much better evaluation of the extent of bone destruction **(Figs. 5A and B)**. Involvement of vertebral body and the posterior elements is easily identified by cross-sectional imaging. Destruction of disc space and presence of disc space gas are additional features that CT can pick-up. Identification of pre- or paravertebral soft tissue mass and extent of spread into the epidural space with subsequent thecal sac deformity can be well appreciated on CT. Chronic stages of infection may reveal extensive osseous destruction, sequestrum and marked heterotropic bone formation. Paravertebral abscesses with psoas involvement are easily identified after contrast administration. Intravenous contrast-enhanced CT may show ring enhancement of an epidural abscess causing posterior displacement of the dural sac. The use of helical and multislice CT scans with reformatted images in the sagittal and coronal planes has proved to be extremely useful.[9] CT may also be used to guide various diagnostic and therapeutic procedures.

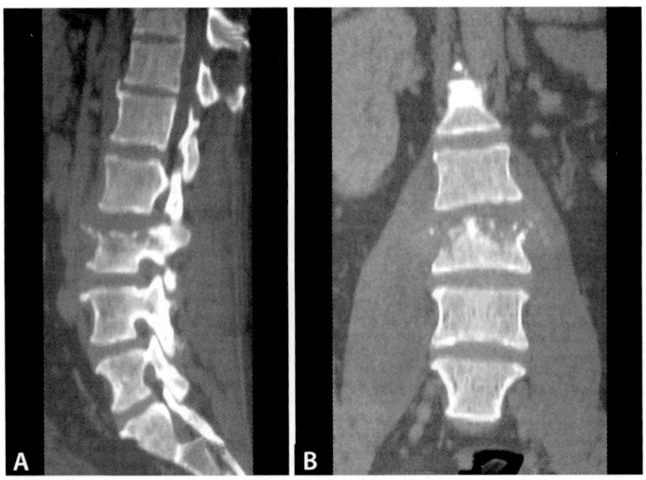

Figs. 5A and B: NCCT lumbar spine sagittal (A) and coronal (B) reformat images showing better depiction of bony changes. There is superior endplate destruction of the L3 vertebra with involvement of the L2–L3 intervertebral disc.

Myelography/CT Myelography

In these days, the use of myelography is limited and is used where MR is unavailable or contraindicated. Encroachment on the spinal canal due to any infectious process may lead to thecal sac abnormality which can be identified by these techniques. Myelography is an invasive investigation with its complications related to the puncture site, such as infection and CSF leakage with additional risk of exacerbating cord compression and contaminating additional spinal compartments. Thus, myelography alone or with CT is not the preferred imaging modality in patients with suspected spinal infection.

Magnetic Resonance Imaging

Magnetic resonance imaging (MRI) is the imaging modality of choice for infective lesions of the spine because changes on MRI precede any other radiographic changes, detects marrow inflammation and has superior spatial resolution in imaging the spinal cord and nerve roots.[19-28] MRI has high sensitivity in early stages and with its known multiplanar capabilities and better soft tissue contrast, MRI provides a much better definition of the paravertebral and epidural extension of the disease.[25] Several MR imaging patterns and SI alterations have been described to be indicative of spinal infection including decreased disc height, disc hypointensity on T1-weighted MR images, disc hyperintensity on T2-weighted MR images, disc enhancement, effacement of the nuclear cleft, and erosion of the vertebral endplates on T1-weighted MR images.[20,21]

Use of I/V gadolinium-DTPA allows better definition of the extent of spinal inflammatory lesions. Also paramagnetic contrast better defines the paravertebral and intraspinal extension of disease. MRI is also a valuable tool in evaluation of postoperative spinal infections.

MR imaging has a reported sensitivity of 96% and an accuracy of 94% in vertebral infections.[9] Although MRI is an excellent diagnostic tool, it may overlook vertebral osteomyelitis in the absence of a localized study site, in the early course of disease, and in the presence of sclerosis.[17]

In addition to the diagnostic capabilities of various modalities CT and fluoroscopy can be used to guide percutaneous aspiration or biopsy in patients of suspected spinal infections. US/CT-guided catheter drainage of large paraspinal/psoas abscesses can also be undertaken.

TYPES OF INFECTIONS

Vertebral bodies and intervertebral discs are most frequently affected with primary or secondary involvement of the epidural space, posterior elements, and paraspinal soft tissues. In Asia and Africa, tuberculosis has been and still is the leading cause of spinal infections, mostly affecting the younger population. A small percentage of cases can be attributed to nontubercular bacteria, fungal and parasitic causes.[8]

The various nontubercular infections of the spine can be grouped under the following subheadings:

1. Bacterial (pyogenic) and nonpyogenic (e.g. brucellosis, actinomycosis, nocardiosis).
2. Viral infections, e.g. human immunodeficiency virus (HIV), cytomegalovirus and herpes simplex.
3. Fungal, e.g. coccidioidomycosis, cryptococcosis, blasto-mycosis, aspergillosis, candidiasis.
4. Parasitic, e.g. hydatid disease, cysticercosis.

Pyogenic Bacterial Infections

Suppurative infections of the spine comprise only 2–5% of all osteomyelitis. A higher incidence is seen in the debilitated, diabetics and in elderly. *Staphylococcus aureus* accounts for more than half the cases of infection. Other organisms responsible for infection include *Streptococcus, Pneumococcus,* gram-negative organisms like *E. coli, Pseudomonas, Salmonella* (in sickle cell disease) and *Klebsiella*. Spine is a common site for infection in IV drug abusers (mainly by *Pseudomonas*) along with sacroiliac and sternoclavicular joints involvement.

Hematogenous spread is common. Blood-borne pathogens may reach the spine either by antegrade flow through the nutrient arterioles of the vertebral bodies or by retrograde flow through the paravertebral Batson venous plexus. There is usually a history of recent primary infection of the skin, urinary tract or the upper respiratory tract, recent surgery or instrumentation. Patients typically present with severe back pain which is constant and aggravated by movement. Other symptoms include fever, malaise and local tenderness. Development of neurological symptoms usually indicates the spread of infection to the epidural space. Lower lumbar spine involvement may lead to hip pain and contractures. Uncommonly, even radicular pattern of pain may be seen. Examination reveals local tenderness and restriction of movement. ESR is invariably raised. Diagnosis of spinal infection can be established with positive blood cultures (less than 25% of cases), percutaneous needle biopsy sampling of the infected vertebral body or disc performed under fluoroscopic or CT guidance (in 68% to 86% of cases) and an open surgical biopsy procedure can be performed in cases in which percutaneous biopsy sampling fails, is nondiagnostic, or cannot be performed. Spinal osteomyelitis is most common in lumbar region (48%), followed by the thoracic spine (35%) and is less common in the cervical spine (6.5%) and sacrum. Infection involves the vertebral body rather than the appendages.

Radiological findings on plain radiographs usually lag behind the symptoms by 2–8 weeks. Infection usually starts anteriorly in the subchondral area of the vertebral body; thus, the earliest finding is rarefaction of the endplates. Later frank erosions, scalloping and destruction of vertebral endplates is noted. Following this, there is loss of disc space height as the infection spreads to involve the adjacent vertebrae. In most patients, only two vertebrae are involved. Rarely, the infection is confined to one vertebral body. Vertebral destruction occurs and collapse may result with accompanying soft tissue swelling in pre- and paravertebral location. Reparative process can begin as early as 4–6 weeks after the onset of radiologic change and is heralded by increasing sclerosis, reactive new bone going on to spur formation, bony bridging or ankylosis of the adjacent vertebrae. Rarely, ivory vertebrae and soft tissue calcification may be found. Radionuclide scanning may be used to localize the exact site of infection and to search for multifocal lesions.[14]

Computed tomography (CT) plays a minor role in cases with bony or soft tissue components. CT findings of vertebral osteomyelitis include (i) detection of erosion or bone destruction and fragmentation and (ii) presence of adjacent soft tissue swelling with obliteration of fat planes around the vertebral body. CT diagnosis may be problematic if soft tissue lesions are seen in the absence of fragmentation or if fragmentation is seen without associated soft tissue swelling as in the case of previously treated or inactive discitis or hypertrophic degenerative disease. Diagnosis of vertebral osteomyelitis can also be difficult if pathognomonic features of other specific disease entities are present like acute vertebral fractures, metastatic or degenerative disease. Intradiscal or vertebral gas is an extremely uncommon finding in spinal infection and may be detected in clostridial or streptococcal infections. At about 10–12 weeks, an osteoblastic response may occur with sclerotic new bone formation. This is more a feature of pyogenic than tubercular osteomyelitis. Vertebral body ankylosis or fusion may be seen with the process of healing. However, if the therapy is inadequate, collapse with spinal deformity resulting in instability of the vertebral column may occur.

Magnetic resonance scanning is the imaging modality of choice for evaluation of patients with vertebral osteomyelitis.[22-27,29,30] The findings on MR are characteristic and occur early in the disease. A constellation of findings of MR **(Figs. 6 to 8)** indicates pyogenic infection and helps differentiate it from some of the other disease processes like TB.[30] These include the following:

1. The vertebra usually show homogeneous areas of altered signal intensity (low signal intensity on

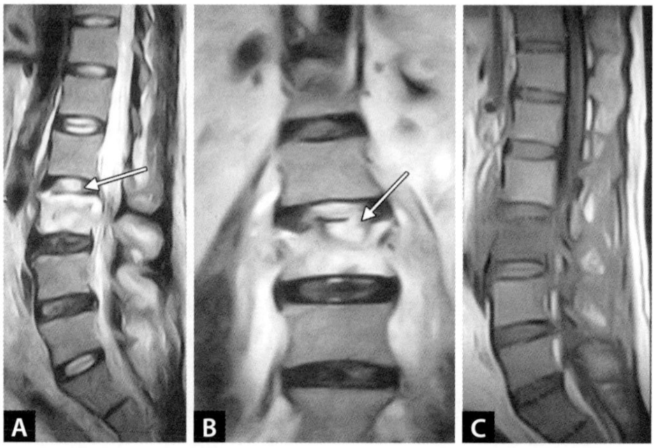

Figs. 6A to C: MRI lumbar spine sagittal coronal, T2W and T1 images show abnormal signal intensity (arrows) of L3 vertebra, contiguous L2–L3 intervertebral disc and surrounding soft tissue in a case of pyogenic spondylodiscitis. In addition, there is loss of intranuclear cleft.

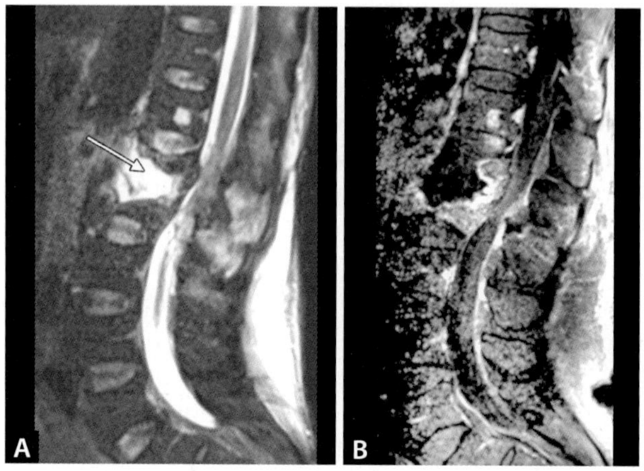

Figs. 7A and B: MRI lumbar spine sagittal T2W (A) and T1 fat-saturated postcontrast (B) images show destruction of L1–L2 intervertebral disc and contiguous vertebral bodies with T2 hyperintense soft tissue that is showing peripheral contrast enhancement and having intraspinal epidural extension in a case of pyogenic spondylodiscitis.

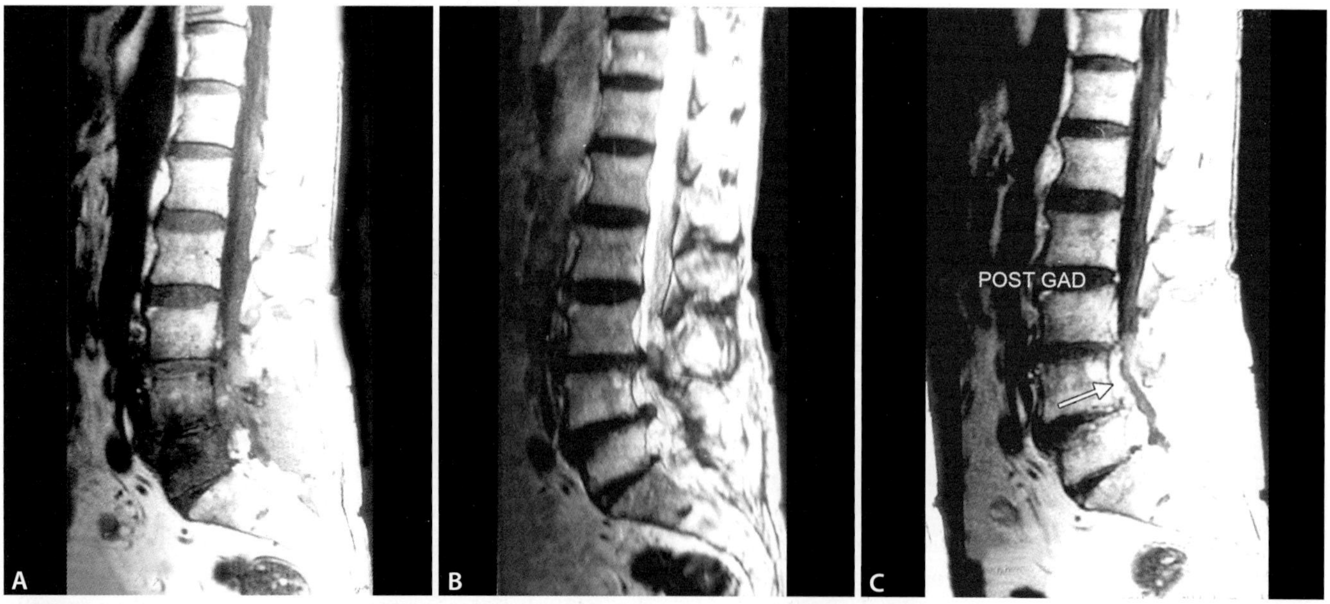

Figs. 8A to C: T1W sagittal image (A) of the lumbosacral spine shows a decreased signal from L4 and L5 vertebrae with reduced intervening disc space. T2W image (B) shows increased signal intensity involving more than half of the L5 vertebral body. Contrast-enhanced T1W sagittal image (C) showing enhancement of the osseous lesion as well as the inflammatory epidural mass (arrow).

T1-weighted images and high signal intensity on T2-weighted images), but usually at one of the vertebral body metaphyses. These signal alterations mainly represents edema and often precede the destructive changes.
2. The intervertebral disc usually show hyperintensity on T2-weighted imaging, with abnormal configuration (absence of the internuclear cleft). The height of the intervertebral disc may be reduced.
3. Loss of a margin between disc and vertebral bodies on T2-weighted images.
4. Diffuse and homogeneous enhancement is seen in the affected marrow and discs.
5. Variable extension of the process into the paraspinal region. The presence of epidural extension and associated meningeal inflammation can be better demonstrated with contrast.
6. Osseous and extra-axial abscesses showing restricted diffusion on diffusion-weighted imaging.

Magnetic resonance imaging may able to differentiate tuberculous spondylitis from pyogenic spondylitis.[22,23] A well-defined paraspinal abnormal signal, a thin and smooth abscess wall, subligamentous spread to three or more vertebral levels, and multiple vertebral or entire body involvement were more suggestive of tuberculous spondylitis than pyogenic spondylitis. Diffusion-weighted magnetic resonance imaging has limited usefulness for differentiating spinal infection and malignancy.[24] It is also possible to differentiate between pyogenic infection and other nonpyogenic granulomatous infections involving the spine, based on clinical and imaging features as described in **Table 2**.[22,23,31]

Pyogenic Disc Space Infections

In adults, since the disc is avascular, hematogenous infection is rare. Most infections occur by contiguous spread from vertebral osteomyelitis or by direct inoculation of bacteria into the disc at the time of surgery or percutaneous procedures like discography, percutaneous discectomy and chemonucleosis. *Staphylococcus aureus* is the most common organism implicated and presentation is usually with back pain. Erythrocyte sedimentation rate (ESR) is elevated, but this is not a very useful marker especially in postoperative cases where ESR remains elevated even up to 6 months.

Radiographic features include decreased disc space height and reactive sclerosis of adjacent endplates. Isotope scanning may show increased uptake but it may also be due to recent surgery or percutaneous manipulation. MRI has become the modality of choice for evaluating disc space infection. Septic discitis demonstrates disc space narrowing on MRI. The vertebral endplates are indistinct and show low SI on T1WI. On T2WI and proton density

Table 2: Differentiating features of infectious spondylitides.

Features	***Tubercular***	***Pyogenic***	***Brucella***
Associated with pulmonary site	Yes	No	–
Site of predilection	Dorsolumbar	Lower lumbar	Lower lumbar
Onset of symptoms	Insidious	Acute	Acute
Progression	Slow	Rapid	Rapid
Multifocal involvement	Yes	No	Infrequent
Vertebral body height	Destroyed	Destroyed	Preserved
Posterior elements	May be involved	Spared	Spared
Subligamentous spread	Common	May be seen	No
Disc destruction	Late	Early	Early
Intradiscal gas	Infrequent	May be seen	Frequently
Paraspinal and epidural extension	Common	Common	Uncommon
Paraspinal mass	Large	Small	Small
Enhancement of paraspinal mass	Peripheral	Patchy	Patchy
Calcification in paraspinal mass	Yes	No	No
Spinal deformity	Common	Uncommon	No
Bone sclerosis	No*	Yes*	Yes

*Caucasians show a greater tendency to new bone formation in pyogenic infection. This is not so in Asians and Blacks where such changes are seen in tuberculosis and vice versa

images, the vertebral endplates may be of increased signal intensity but the major finding in the disc space is an abnormal high signal.[32]

Paraspinal soft tissue thickening and edematous changes in the paraspinal musculature are also seen. In fact the earliest MR finding in pyogenic septic discitis is obliteration of fat planes between the paraspinal musculature and the outer margin of the disc. Diagnosis is usually confirmed by percutaneous disc aspirates which can be cultured for organisms.

Spinal Infections in Children

Infections of the spine in children consist of osteomyelitis and the so-called spondyloarthritis or discitis. The hallmark of radiographic diagnosis is disc space narrowing with destruction of the two adjacent vertebral body surfaces.[33]

Localization of infection to the osseous and articular structures of the vertebral column is not as common in children as adults. The most common route of contamination of the spine is by a hematogenous pathway, either by an arterial route or Batson's paravertebral venous system. The arterial pathway can be implicated by the localization of early infection in the subchondral region of the vertebral body, where numerous arterial loops are present. Infection may also be distributed along the course of the ascending and descending nutrient branches of the posterior spinal artery. The direction and extent of flow through the valveless venous plexus are significantly influenced by changes in intra-abdominal pressure, which may account for the contamination of the spine that may be observed in a child with urinary tract and other pelvic infections.[33]

Infection of spine may also occur secondary to spread from a contiguous contaminated source or from direct implantation. Subligamentous spread of infection with subsequent bony invasion is more characteristic of tuberculosis than pyogenic infection. Direct implantation of organisms can occur during punctures of the spinal canal. Postoperative infection may develop following laminectomy or other instrumentation, such as scoliosis repair. The cervical spine may be infected by direct extension from prevertebral abscesses, especially those associated with sharp foreign bodies in the pharynx.

Vertebral and disc infections account for approximately 2–4% of all cases of osteomyelitis with equal incidence in boys and girls. The symptoms include fever, malaise, weight loss, back pain, which may be intermittent or constant, or hip contracture, which occurs secondary to psoas muscle irritation. The erythrocyte sedimentation rate (ESR) is elevated, but serum leukocyte count may be normal and organisms may not be recovered from blood cultures.

Magnetic resonance imaging is the modality of choice for early diagnosis of vertebral osteomyelitis. MR imaging is more sensitive in the detection of vertebral osteomyelitis than either conventional radiography or CT scan and nuclear scintigraphic studies. Soft tissue extension from spinal osteomyelitis in the form of epidural abscess or paravertebral abscess is well demonstrated by MR imaging and enhanced CT scan. Following treatment, a radiodense "ivory" vertebra may be seen. The affected disc space may remain relatively intact, or complete bony ankylosis may occur.

Childhood Disc Infection or Discitis

Until about 7 years of age, profuse anastomoses exist between the intraosseous spinal arteries, preventing devascularization and infarction of large portions of the metaphysis when septic emboli occlude a metaphyseal artery. This tends to limit the extent of metaphyseal and osseous infection to the cartilaginous endplate at either end of the vertebra. Hence, hematogenous spread to the pediatric spine tends to be limited to the disc space. Additionally, the pediatric disc retains vascularity, unlike in adults, and occasionally blood-borne pathogens may lodge directly in the disc space in children, without any involvement of the metaphyseal endplates.[1] This is different from the adult form of infection and has a good prognosis. Natural course of the disease is slow and self-limiting following medical therapy. The posterior elements of the vertebrae are not involved and paravertebral soft tissue masses are absent.The mean age at presentation is 6–8 years. Diagnosis is often delayed due to nonspecific nature of complaints. Clinically there may be low-grade fever, malaise and irritability, and the child might refuse to walk, stand or sit. ESR is frequently elevated.

Radionuclide ^{99m}Tc or gallium scan is useful modality which shows an increased uptake in the affected area, and this is positive well before the plain radiographic changes appear. Plain films show decreased disc space height and at a later stage vertebral endplates might be eroded or irregular with or without sclerosis. Seventy-five percent of the discitis are seen in lumbar or dorsal region, rarely in the cervical spine. At times two levels may be involved. MRI detects the lesion early and shows abnormal signal from the disc spaces and discs (increased on T2WI) with reduction in disc height seen best on sagittal images.[34]

Differential Diagnosis of Spinal Infection

Spinal infections may be mimicked by degenerative and inflammatory spinal diseases.[1,2,25] Conditions, such as discogenic vertebral body degeneration in the inflammatory phase (Modic type 1 degeneration), acute cartilaginous node, ankylosing spondylitis, neuropathic spine, dialysis-related spondyloarthropathy, and neoplasm may lead to alterations in signal intensity that may be mistaken for infection. Lack of abnormally increased signal intensity of an associated disc on T2-weighted images and a lack of soft-tissue involvement are characteristic findings of Modic type 1 degeneration and conversely endplate destruction, increased disc signal intensity on T2-weighted images, or a paravertebral or epidural abscess are indicative of infectious spondylitis. Acute cartilaginous node may be distinguished by concentric ring of high signal intensity around the node on T2-weighted images, involvement of only one endplate and no diffuse signal intensity abnormality of the disc. Ankylosing spondylitis can be differentiated by presence of spinal ankylosis and fracture that extends into the posterior column (Andersson lesion). Neuropathic spine is characterized by vacuum phenomenon, facet involvement, lower signal intensity of disc and bone marrow on T2-weighted images whereas in dialysis-related spondyloarthropathy vertebral marrow shows hypointense signal on both T1- and T2WI.

Postoperative Spondylodiscitis

Postoperative spondylodiscitis is an infrequent complication of lumbar disc surgery.[1] The typical clinical presentation is recurrent pain after initial postoperative relief, muscle spasm and fever. The most probable cause is intraoperative contamination rather than hematogenous spread, although either may occur. The imaging findings appear several weeks after the initial symptoms. MR may be helpful earlier, but it is usually not possible to reliably diagnose infection until 3 weeks after surgery. The disc space infection can be diagnosed in the postoperative spine by triad of intervertebral disc space enhancement, annular enhancement, and vertebral body enhancement when found in conjunction with appropriate laboratory findings, such as an increased ESR.[1] Contrast enhancement and signal changes in the intervertebral disc or the vertebral end plates can be seen both in the setting of discitis and in normal postoperative asymptomatic patients. MR imaging may be useful for the exclusion rather than the confirmation of postoperative spondylodiscitis by showing absence of signal changes in the vertebral endplates, contrast enhancement of the disc, or enhancing paravertebral soft tissues.

Epidural Space Infections

The frequency of epidural abscess has been increasing. Epidural abscess usually manifests itself by intense pain, which could be localized over the infected level or be spread diffusely over the spine. The pain could be even more disabling than the concomitant neurologic deficit. The epidural space can become infected either by contiguous spread of an infective process from the surrounding bone, intervertebral disc or adjacent soft tissue abscesses or by direct inoculation of organisms into the epidural space following use of indwelling epidural catheters. At times hematogenous spread of microorganisms may occur. Unchecked epidural infections can be dangerous often leading to cord compression and paralysis. Hence, it is important to diagnose and treat this entity early.

Contrast-enhanced MRI provides the best evaluation of such patients. Besides its ability to distinguish the cord from the thecal sac, it offers easy identification of paraspinal soft tissues and extension and involvement of the bone marrow. T1W images can show a soft tissue mass displacing the thecal sac away from the bone. On T2W images, epidural abscesses are defined clearly on sagittal planes as hyperintense extradural lesions. The epidural abscess and the dural sac are usually separated by hypointense stria corresponding to the leptomeninges. Gadolinium enhancement in epidural abscesses is of two types, a peripheral enhancement with a central hypointense area corresponding with the true abscess with fluid contents **(Fig. 9)** and a second, homogeneous enhancement corresponding with the inflammatory

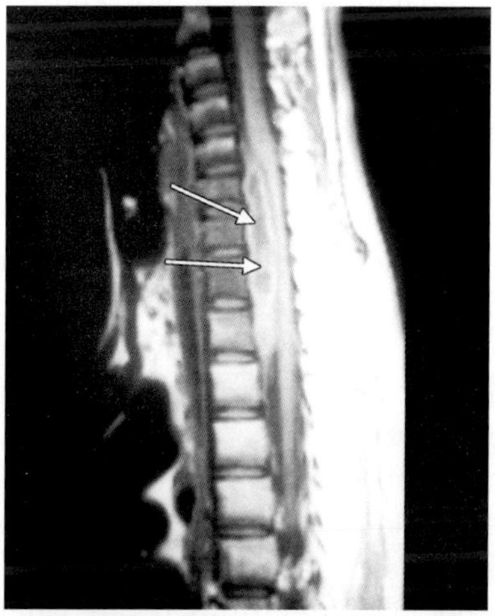

Fig. 9: Sagittal MRI scan in a patient with a large epidural abscess in the dorsal spine showing peripheral enhancement following gadolinium administration with hypointense central areas representing purulent contents.

tissue without purulent contents. Fat suppression techniques improve the sensitivity further by eliminating the possible confusion between high signal of fat and similar signal from gadolinium.

Nonpyogenic Bacterial Infections

Brucellosis

Brucellosis or undulant fever is a granulomatous nontubercular infection which is caused by gram-negative rods of *Brucella* species. Brucellosis is a zoonosis disease that affects animals as the primary host (e.g. camels, sheep, goats) and humans as the secondary host. The organisms are usually transmitted by the consumption of uncooked meat or unpasteurized dairy products.[35] Vertebral infection occurs in about 6–12% of cases of brucellosis. The presenting signs and symptoms of spinal brucellosis are nonspecific and similar to those associated with other forms of spinal osteomyelitis. The symptom onset of spinal brucellosis tends to be subacute, and the radiologic manifestations are nonspecific, with some similarity to cases of tuberculosis.[36] The main problem in the diagnosis is its differentiation from other infective processes particularly tuberculosis which is the most common cause of spinal infection in India. However, the proliferative changes associated with bony repair in brucellosis are not seen in tuberculous infection, and deformities of the spine, which are common in TB, are rarely seen with brucellosis. Radionuclide bone scans are highly sensitive in demonstrating areas of involvement in patients with *Brucella* infection who have musculoskeletal complaints. Spine is the most common site for skeletal brucellosis. Spinal infection with brucellosis can be focal or diffuse. In the focal form, the osteomyelitis is located in the anterior aspect of the vertebral endplate (classically superior endplate of L4 vertebra) at the discovertebral junction. In the diffuse form, the infective process involves initially the entire vertebral body and ultimately extends to involve the neighboring discs and vertebrae. The lower lumbar spine is most frequently affected.

Plain radiographs mainly show a focal lesion at the superior endplate with a maintained vertebral body architecture. Associated sclerosis is frequently seen. Disc space reduction with presence of gas in disc is a hallmark of brucellosis not seen in tuberculosis. Paravertebral soft tissue abscesses are less commonly associated and spinal deformity is rare when compared with tuberculosis.

Computed tomography confirms the presence of focal or diffuse disease in brucellosis. Findings of bone sclerosis, localized endplate destruction simulating Schmorl's nodes, loss of muscle/fat plane and disc space gas when seen point to a *Brucella* infection, whereas large paraspinal abscesses with enhancing rim, calcification, or bone fragments suggest tubercular nature of infection. On MR, the above findings are further corroborated with evidence of an intact vertebral morphology, normal posterior elements and a focal lesion which shows a decreased SI on T1W images and moderately increased SI or T2W images. Disc destruction is early. There is only a moderate extension into the paraspinal and epidural space by granulation tissue and/or edema and spinal deformity is infrequent.

Actinomycosis

Actinomyces species are gram-positive, filamentous bacteria that are most commonly associated with chronic draining infections. Spinal involvement is rare and generally the result of contiguous spread from adjacent sites of infection, especially the lungs and sinuses. Vertebral destruction with deformity is uncommon with *Actinomyces* infection.[37]

Actinomycotic infection of the spine is caused by anaerobic organisms and is usually seen in debilitated persons. Mandible and spine are most commonly affected. Osseous involvement results from extension of soft tissue infection. Radiological manifestations include lytic lesions with surrounding sclerosis involving several vertebrae and frequently sparing the discs. Posterior elements and ribs are frequently involved, with associated paravertebral abscesses which are not as large as seen in tuberculosis and do not show calcification. Presence of sinus tracts leading to the skin along with above findings suggests the diagnosis.[37]

Nocardiosis

Nocardia are filamentous, branching, gram-positive aerobic bacteria. They are normally found in the soil and are associated primarily with pulmonary infection in immunocompromised patients. Spinal involvement is rare with nonspecific radiological findings—there are only about a dozen cases reported in the literature—and occurs both by direct extension of intrathoracic infections and through hematogenous spread.

Viral Infections

Spinal Infections in AIDS

The most frequent causative agent of bacterial spinal infections in patients with HIV is *S. aureus*, as in immunocompetent patients. The manifestations may be isolated or a combination of osteomyelitis, discitis, epidural spinal phlegmon or abscess, paraspinal abscess, or myelitis. The presence of complete prevertebral soft tissue involvement, absence of posterior elements involvement, diffuse bone destruction, and absence of marginal sclerosis are signs of pyogenic spondylodiscitis, whereas nonpyogenic infection manifestations are the presence of focal lytic bone involvement, marginal sclerosis, and paraspinal soft tissue masses.[38]

Use of gadolinium-enhanced T1-weighted images is recommended in the investigation of spinal infections because it increases the conspicuity of epidural disease and is essential for the detection and delineation of intradural disease. In cases of spondylodiscitis, the involved disc and adjacent vertebral bodies typically show enhancement to various degrees. Homogeneous enhancement of epidural or paraspinal soft tissue masses is consistent with the presence of a phlegmon, whereas ring enhancement is seen with abscesses.

Fungal Infections

Fungal infections of the spine are infrequent and tend to occur in patients with predisposing conditions or, rarely, as a consequence of iatrogenic interventions. Examples of comorbid conditions usually seen in patients with fungal spinal infections include prolonged corticosteroid administration, immunosuppression after organ transplantation, severe systemic illness associated with malnutrition and multiple antibiotic use, HIV infection, diabetes, alcohol or intravenous drug abuse, and parenteral nutrition.

Fungal infections of the spine include aspergillosis, coccidioidomycosis, cryptococcosis, *Candida* and blastomycosis. Following inhalation of spores, these involve the spine by a hematogenous route. Radiologically, each fungal infection does not have any distinctive features of its own. Most of them resemble tubercular infection, but a few characteristic features have been described for some of the infections.

Aspergillosis

Aspergillus, a ubiquitous species of fungus, is usually pathogenic only in patients with impaired immune defences. *Aspergillus* typically invades the spine from a contiguous site of infection (usually pulmonary) but can also be spread hematogenously. Though rare, *Aspergillus* vertebral infections have been reported in immunocompetent hosts as well.[39] Differentiation must be made from tuberculosis, which can closely mimic aspergillosis of the spine, using serologic testing. The radiographic features, including osseous and disc space destruction and a paraspinal mass, resemble those of tuberculosis.[39]

Coccidioidomycosis

Coccidioidomycosis is caused by *Coccidioides immitis*, a filamentous fungus which infects the lung primarily and disseminates throughout the body in about 0.5% of patients. Osseous involvement is seen in 10–50% of which spine is the most common site.[40] Plain radiographs usually reveal multiple erosive defects involving vertebral bodies and appendages. Disc space is usually preserved and spinal deformity is uncommon. Paraspinal masses and adjacent rib involvement is common. Differentiation from tuberculosis can be made by the presence of skull lesions, which, although common in coccidioidomycosis, are rare in tuberculosis.[39]

Lumbar spine is commonly affected. MR appearances of the lesion are that of hypo- to hyperintense SI on T1WI and on T2WI the lesions are almost always hyperintense. Following gadolinium injection, the lesions which are hypo- to isointense on T1W sequence show enhancement.[40] Ring enhancement may be seen in intraosseous abscesses. Presence of paraspinal masses, epidural spread and subligamentous spread are similar to those seen in tuberculosis.

The absence of hyperintensity within the intervertebral discs on T2-weighted images and the preservation of the intranuclear cleft are findings associated with nonpyogenic or TB spondylitis.[41] These are, however, nonspecific findings that have been reported in cases of pyogenic disease as well. Other nonpyogenic infections caused by *Nocardia,* Actinomycosis, *Echinococcus* and Coccidioidomycosis may also spare the intervertebral disc. The pathogenesis of absence of hyperintensity within the intervertebral disc is unclear and may be multifactorial. The imaging findings may reflect an absence of fungal invasion, an altered inflammatory reaction within the infected disc, or an intrinsic characteristic of either the disc before infection (e.g. degenerated disc) or of the invading fungi (e.g. paramagnetic elements).[41]

Cryptococcosis (Torulosis)

Cryptococcosis is a serious disease of worldwide distribution caused by *Cryptococcus neoformans*, an organism that has an unusual predilection for the central nervous system. This fungus can be recovered from soil, pigeon droppings, fruit, and human intestinal tract and skin. The disease is generally acquired by the respiratory route through inhalation of aerosolized spores. The development of *Cryptococcus* infection in patients with compromised immune defences is well known. Patients undergoing renal transplantation are particularly susceptible.

Disseminated cryptococcal infection may result in osseous involvement in 5–10% of patients and spine is commonly involved. Radiologically, nonspecific well-defined osteolytic areas with sclerotic margins are seen involving the vertebral body and posterior elements **(Figs. 10A to C)**. Again, multifocal involvement and large paraspinal soft tissue abscesses may be present making the picture at times indistinguishable from tuberculosis.[39]

Blastomycosis

This infection caused by *Blastomyces dermatitidis* enters the body by a skin wound or the respiratory tract. Skeletal changes can occur because of hematogenous seeding, or by direct extension from an overlying cutaneous lesion. The commonly affected osseous sites are the vertebrae, the ribs, the tibia, the carpus, and the tarsus. The radiologic features are not specific.

All age groups can be affected, but the disease appears to have a predilection for those in the second through fifth decades of life. The infection may be self-limited or may progress to dissemination. Disseminated disease produces generalized symptoms of fever, malaise, anorexia, and night sweats. Secondary osseous involvement is common, with the spine being a prime target. Vertebral involvement produces a destructive lesion often associated with a large paraspinal mass. The lower thoracic and lumbar spine is most often the site of the infection. Blastomycosis of the spine must be distinguished from tuberculosis and coccidioidomycosis. In tuberculosis the posterior elements of the vertebral body are not infected, whereas in coccidioidomycosis and blastomycosis all bony elements of the spine may be involved.[39] Also blastomycosis frequently involves the adjacent ribs and unlike coccidioidomycosis or actinomycosis, the disc space is frequently involved in blastomycosis. Additionally, blastomycosis has a greater tendency to produce cutaneous fistulae.[30] The definitive diagnosis is typically made through positive cytology or histologic examination of biopsy specimens.

Candidiasis (Moniliasis)

Of the various *Candida* species, *Candida albicans* is most commonly associated with human disease. *Candida* infection of the musculoskeletal system occurs typically in intravenous drug addicts and when host resistance is depressed. Infants, children, and adults can be affected. Osteomyelitis can occur in one or more sites. Common patterns of distribution include involvement of a single long bone, the sternum, or two consecutive vertebral bodies. Usually, the lumbar spine is the region affected.

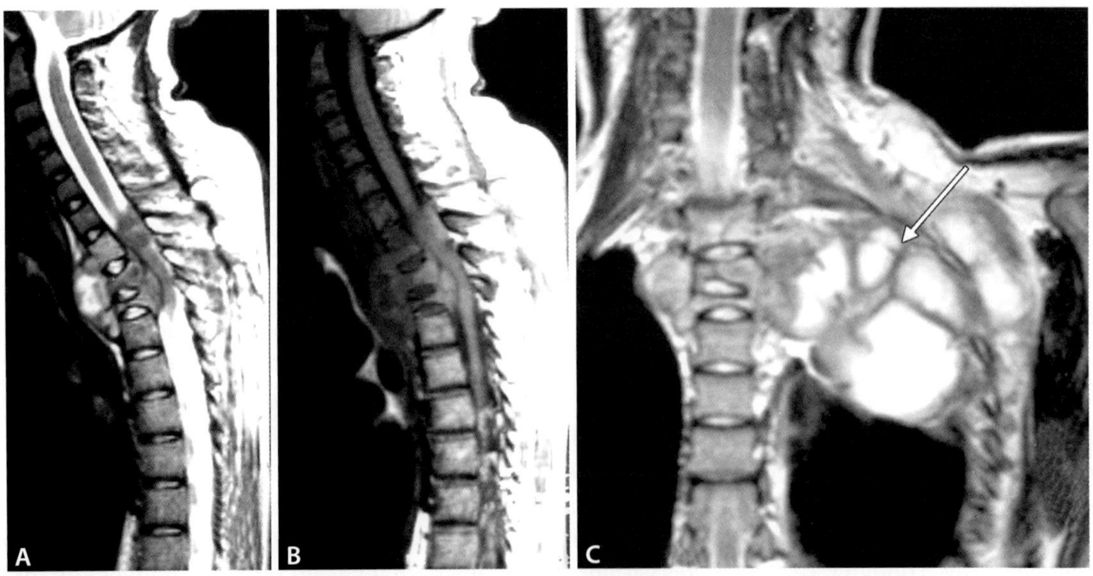

Figs. 10A to C: T2 (A), T1 (B) sagittal, and T2 (C) coronal MR imaging in a case of cryptococcosis of the dorsal spine showing multiple contiguous vertebral involvement of the upper dorsal spine with vertebral destruction and prevertebral, epidural and posterior paraspinal abscesses with compression of the adjacent cord and relatively preserved disc spaces.

Radiographic findings include soft tissue swelling, joint space narrowing, irregularity of subchondral bone, and more widespread changes of osteomyelitis.[30] Granulomas usually are not apparent at surgery. Aspiration of synovial fluid or biopsy of synovial membrane with isolation of *Candida* confirms the diagnosis.[39]

Parasitic Infections

Echinococcosis or Hydatid

Echinococcosis occurs throughout South America, the Arabian Peninsula, Australia, New Zealand, Indian subcontinent and East Africa. The principal host is the dog, whereas sheep and humans are the intermediate hosts. Ingestion of ova and absorption by the bowel is the major route of transmission. Echinococcosis or hydatid disease of the bones is rare, accounting for approximately 0.5–4% of all patients.[30] Spinal involvement by hydatid disease is seen in about half of these patients. In the spine, sacrum and lower dorsal vertebra are commonly involved. The primary infection from the medullary cavity in the vertebral body spreads to involve the pedicles and laminae.[42] Hydatid disease in the bones differs from disease elsewhere in the soft tissues in that the cysts are always multilocular. Growth occurs along the line of least resistance particularly along the intertrabecular spaces with the formation of diverticulated cysts that may form by exogenous vesiculation. Enlargement of the larvae results in dilatation of the bony spaces of spongiosa and resorption of cancellous bone. Expansion is relatively slow with a smooth well-defined sclerotic margin. Erosion through the periosteum into the adjacent soft tissues proceeds without subperiosteal new bone formation. Extension into extradural space or paraspinal tissues may occur. Contiguous involvement of the rib is a feature.

Spinal hydatid has been classified into: (i) primary cyst in the cord, (ii) intradural cyst, (iii) extradural cyst, (iv) hydatid disease of the vertebrae, and (v) paravertebral hydatid disease. Mid dorsal and lumbosacral levels are most commonly affected. Plain film findings include a uni- or multiloculated lytic expansile bone lesion with marginal sclerosis involving the vertebral body, posterior elements and even the adjacent ribs with paraspinal soft tissue mass. Disc space is preserved as the disease propagates beneath the periosteum and ligaments.[39] The findings are at times nonspecific and indistinguishable from other benign cystic bone lesions or metastatic disease.

CT signs are nonspecific and often reveal bone lysis extending into the posterior elements, adjacent vertebrae, disc space and epidural space, creating a picture of spondylitis. However, costal involvement and lack of enhancement following contrast administration suggest hydatid disease. CT is superior to MR in demonstrating calcified lesions.

On MR, cysts demonstrate inhomogeneous low signal intensity on T1W images and high signal on T2W images **(Figs. 11A to D)**. T2W images are not helpful in differentiating quiescent from active stage of the cysts. MRI may demonstrate intradural extension to better advantage than CT without the need for subarachnoid contrast.

Cysticercosis

Cysticercosis is caused by the pork tapeworm *T. solium*. Humans are an intermediate host for these worms and are infested by eating raw or poorly cooked infected pork or contaminated vegetables. Embryos penetrate the intestinal wall and travel to the subcutaneous tissues, muscles, viscera, and the central nervous system. Intramuscular cysts and calcifications can be clinically palpated. On conventional radiographs and CT, dead calcified cysticerci can be identified in the paravertebral muscles and soft tissues as small linear rice shaped calcifications measuring approximately 5–8 mm with long axis running parallel to the paravertebral muscle fibers. CT scan can also reveal innumerable, round, low attenuating cysts, 5–7 mm in diameter with no enhancement following contrast administration. Scolices can be demonstrated as small foci of high attenuation located eccentrically within the cysts.[39]

Amongst the different forms of spinal cysticercosis, leptomeningeal form seen as cysts in the subarachnoid space is the most common.[43] Cysts may also be seen in the epidural, subpial and intramedullary location. On MRI, intramedullary lesions are seen as focal cystic lesion showing peripheral enhancement and cord edema **(Figs. 12A to C)**.

CONCLUSION

Magnetic resonance imaging is the imaging modality of choice for the evaluation of spinal infection because of the capability of multiplanar imaging, direct evaluation of the bone marrow, and simultaneous visualization of the neural structures. However, inflammatory lesions of the spine are often indistinguishable on imaging and there is frequent overlap of radiological findings amongst different types of infections. So it is essential to recognize atypical MR imaging findings of spinal infection; and imaging features of other noninfectious inflammatory

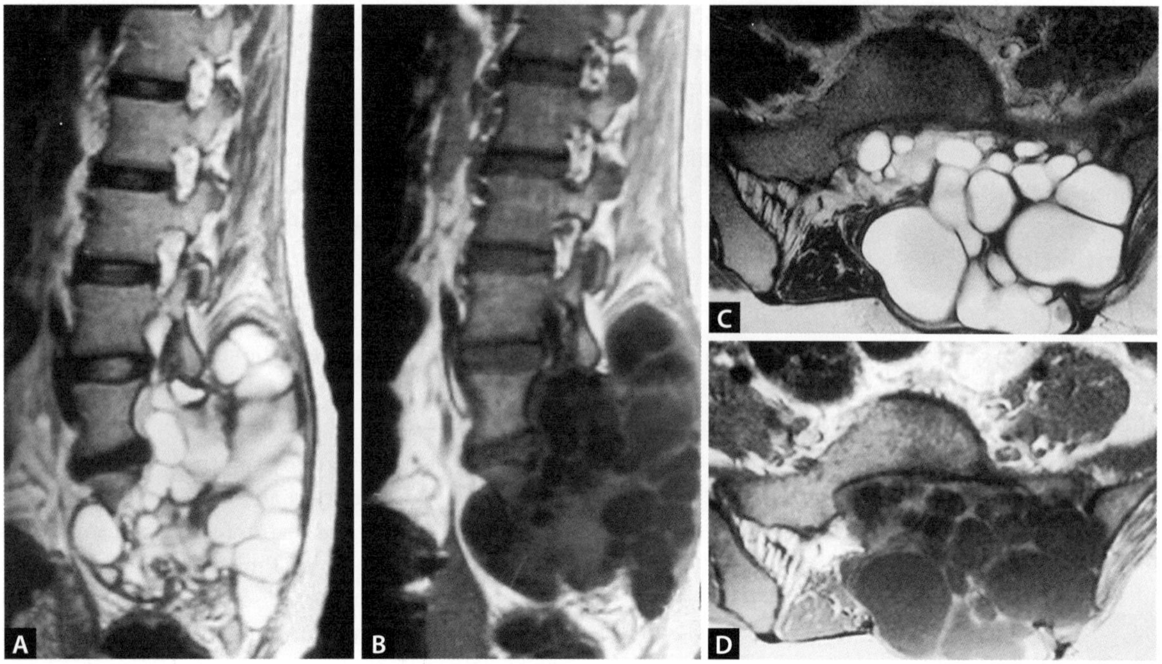

Figs. 11A to D: MRI lumbosacral spine parasagittal T2W (A), T1W (B), axial T2W (C) and T1W (D) images show large multiloculated, cystic, expansile lesion involving posterior arch elements of L5 and sacrum demonstrating a having both osseous and extraosseous components. The cysts show peripheral T2 hypointense wall and central fluid signal in a case of spinal hydatid.

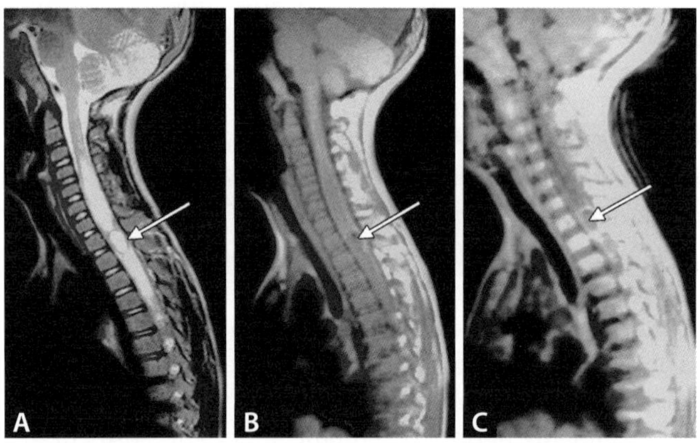

Figs. 12A to C: MRI sagittal T2W (A), T1W (B) and postcontrast T1W (C) images show intramedullary ring enhancing lesion with T2 hypointense rim and associated cord edema in a case of intramedullary neurocysticercosis.

diseases and degenerative disease that may mimic spinal infection to avoid misdiagnosis and inappropriate treatment.

REFERENCES

1. DeSanto J, Ross JS. Spine infection/inflammation. Radiol Clin North Am. 2011;49:105-27.
2. Hong SH, Choi JY, Lee JW, Kim NR, Choi JA, Kang HS. MR imaging assessment of the spine: infection or an imitation? Radiographics. 2009;29:599-612.
3. Tins BJ, Cassar-Pullicino VN. MR imaging of spinal infection. Semin Musculoskelet Radiol. 2004;8:215-29.
4. Balériaux DL, Neugroschl C. Spinal and spinal cord infection. Eur Radiol. 2004;14(Suppl 3):E72-83.
5. Jevtic V. Vertebral infection. Eur Radiol. 2004;14(Suppl 3):E43-52.
6. Tali ET. Spinal infections. Eur J Radiol. 2004;50:120-33.
7. Tandon N, Vollmer DG. Infections of the spine and spinal cord. In: Winn R (Ed). Youmans-Neurological Surgery, 5th edn. Saunders; 2004. pp. 4363-94.
8. Wisneski RJ. Infectious disease of the spine. Orthop Clin North Am. 1991;22:491-8.
9. Varma R, Lander P, Assaf A. Imaging of pyogenic infectious spondylodiscitis. Radiol Clin North Am. 2001;39:203-13.
10. Colmenero JD, Jiménez-Mejías ME, Sánchez-Lora FJ, Reguera JM, Palomino-Nicás J, Martos F, et al. Pyogenic, tuberculous, and brucellar vertebral osteomyelitis: a descriptive and comparative study of 219 cases. Annals of the Rheumatic Diseases. 1997;56:709-15.
11. Digby JM, Kersley JB. Pyogenic non-tuberculous spinal infection: an analysis of thirty cases. J Bone Joint Surg Br. 1979;61:47-55.
12. Butler JS, Shelly MJ, Timlin M, et al. Nontuberculous pyogenic spinal infections in adults. A 12 year experience from a tertiary referral center. Spine. 2003;31:2695-700.
13. Palestro CJ, Love C, Schneider R. The evolution of nuclear medicine and the musculoskeletal system. Radiol Clin North Am. 2009;47:505-32.
14. Love C, Patel M, Lonner BS, et al. Diagnosing spinal osteomyelitis: a comparison of bone and 67Ga scintigraphy

and magnetic resonance imaging. Clin Nucl Med. 2000;25:963-77.
15. Sarikaya I, Sarikaya A, Holder LE. The role of single photon emission computed tomography in bone imaging. Semin Nucl Med. 2001;31:3-16.
16. Turpin S, Lambert R. Role of scintigraphy in musculoskeletal and spinal infections. Radiol Clin North Am. 2001;39:169-89.
17. McEwan L, Wong JC. Nuclear medicine imaging in early vertebral osteomyelitis: still of clinical utility. Australas Radiol. 2000;44:454-7.
18. Stumpe KDM, Zanetti M, Weishaupt D, Hodler J, Boos N, von Schulthess GK. FDG positron emission tomography for differentiation of degenerative and infectious endplate abnormalities in the lumbar spine detected on MR imaging. Am J Roentgenol. 2002;179:1151-7.
19. Maiuri F, Laconetta G, Gallicchio B, et al. Spondy-lodiscitis–clinical and magnetic resonance diagnosis. Spine. 1997;22: 1741-6.
20. Ledermann HP, Schweitzer ME, Morrison WB, Carrino JA. MR imaging findings in spinal infections: Rules or myths? Radiology. 2003;228:506-14.
21. Thrush A, Enzmann D. MR imaging of infectious spondylitis. Am J Neuroradiol. 1989;11:1171-80.
22. Harada Y, Tokuda O, Matsunaga N. Magnetic resonance imaging characteristics of tuberculous spondylitis vs pyogenic spondylitis. Clin Imaging. 2008;32:303-9.
23. Chang MC, Wu HTW, Lee, Liu CL. Tuberculous spondylitis and pyogenic spondylitis. Comparative magnetic resonance imaging features. Spine. 2006;31:782-8.
24. Pui MH, Mitha A, Rae WI, Corr P. Diffusion-weighted magnetic resonance imaging of spinal infection and malignancy. J Neuroimaging. 2005;15:164-70.
25. Mellado JM, Pérez del Palomar L, Camins A, Salvadó E, Ramos A, Saurí A. MR imaging of spinal infection: atypical features, interpretive pitfalls and potential mimickers. Eur Radiol. 2004;14:1980-9.
26. Forrester DM. Infectious spondylitis. Semin Ultrasound CT MR. 2004;25:461-73.
27. Hetem SF, Schils JP. Imaging of infections and inflammatory conditions of the spine. Semin Musculoskelet Radiol. 2000;4:329-47.
28. Sharif HS. Role of MR imaging in the management of spinal infections. Am J Roentgenol. 1992;158:1333-45.
29. Sharif HS, Clark DC, Aabed MY, et al. Granulo-matous spinal infections: MR imaging. Radiology. 1990;177: 101-7.
30. Scott W Atlas (Ed). Magnetic Resonance Imaging of the Brain and Spine, 4th edn. Lippincott Williams and Wilkins. 2009;(2):1647-739.
31. Jung NY, Jee WH, Ha KY, Park CH, Byun JY. Discrimination of tuberculous spondylitis from pyogenic spondylitis on MRI. Am J Roentgenol. 2004;182:1405-10.
32. Smith AS, Weinstein MA, Mizushima A, et al. MR imaging characteristics of tuberculous spondylitis vs vertebral osteomyelitis. AJNR Am J Neuroradiol. 1989;10:619-25.
33. Mahboubi S, Morris MC. Imaging of spinal infections in children. Radiol Clin North Am. 2001;39:215-22.
34. Heller RM, Szalay EA, Green NE, Horev GD, Kirchner SD. Disc space infection in children: magnetic resonance imaging. Radiol Clin North Am. 1988;26:207-9.
35. Al-Sous MW, Bohlega S, Al-Kawi MZ, et al. Neurobrucellosis: Clinical and neuroimaging correlation. Am J Neuroradiol. 2004;25:395-401.
36. Sharif BS, Aideyan OA, Clark DC, et al. Brucellar and tubercular spondylitis: Comparative imaging features. Radiology. 1989;171:419-25.
37. Young WB. Actinomycosis with involvement of the vertebral column: case report and review of the literature. Clin Radiol. 1960;11:175-82.
38. Bureau NJ, Cardinal E. Imaging of musculoskeletal and spinal infections in AIDS. Radiol Clin North Am. 2001;39:343-55.
39. Chhem RK, Wang S-C, Jaovisidha S, et al. Imaging of fungal, viral, and parasitic musculoskeletal and spinal diseases. Radiol Clin North Am. 2001;39:357-78.
40. Erly WK, Carmody RF, Seeger JF, et al. Magnetic resonance imaging of coccidioidal spondylitis. Int J of Neuroradiology. 1997;3:385-92.
41. Williams RL, Fukui MB, Meltzer CC, et al. Fungal spinal osteomyelitis in the immunocompromised patient: MR findings in three cases. Am J Neuroradiol. 1999;20:381-5.
42. Patel SB. Hydatidosis of central nervous system. In: Rao KS (Ed), Diagnostic Radiology and Imaging; 2003. pp. 1113-9.
43. Leite CC, Jinkins JR, Escobar BE, et al. MR imaging of intramedullary and intradural-extramedulary spinal cysticercosis. Am J Roentgenol. 1997;169:1713-7.

CHAPTER 195

Degenerative Disease of the Spine and Joints

Jyoti Kumar, Sumedha Pawa

INTRODUCTION

Degenerative joint disease is the most common and widespread form of arthritis. Degenerative joint disease is a general term to describe degenerative alterations in any type of articulation, i.e. synovial, cartilaginous or fibrous. It is a disease of the whole joint in which all articular structures are affected. Osteoarthritis (OA) has a greater predilection for involving certain joints while sparing others. For example, it is highly prevalent in the spine and knees. Imaging evaluation of OA has become especially important because of the prevalence of the condition, the increased life span of the population, and the newer treatments that are being developed.

DEGENERATIVE DISORDERS OF THE SPINE

Degenerative diseases of the spine are a ubiquitous collection of conditions that represent some of the most common indications for advanced imaging studies. Degenerative changes may arise in the vertebrae, intervertebral discs, facet joints and ligaments. Degeneration at various sites is linked to each other since the main common pathogenetic factor is chronic overload. The intervertebral articulation consists of a three-joint complex consisting of the amphiarthrodial endplate-disc-endplate joint of the anterior column and the two diarthrodial facet joints of the posterior column supported by ligaments and muscle groups. In the cervical spine, uncovertebral joints (joints of Luschka) are the other lateral articulations between the vertebral bodies. The intervertebral disc space consists of the inner nucleus pulposus, outer annulus fibrosus, and hyaline cartilaginous endplates. The ligaments consist of the anterior and posterior longitudinal ligaments (ALL, PLL), ligamentum flavum (LF) and interspinous ligaments. Since involvement of one site predisposes the other sites to degenerative changes owing to altered biomechanical forces, patients often present with degenerative changes in multiple sites.[1,2]

Imaging Modalities

Magnetic resonance imaging (MRI) is often the modality of choice in evaluation of spine because of its superior soft tissue contrast. Computed tomography (CT) demonstrates superior spatial resolution and improved conspicuity of osseous and calcified structures.[3]

Complementary tests in evaluation of degenerative spine include radiography, discography, conventional myelography, CT myelography, and nuclear scintigraphy. Plain films are inexpensive, widely available and give a panoramic view of the entire spine. Bones can be directly visualized and functional information regarding alignment and stability can be obtained with upright dynamic films in flexion-extension and lateral bending. Myelography is reserved only for patients with contraindications to MRI or in whom subtle instability is suspected but not confirmed by other examinations. Discography is reserved for selected patients before intervention or when the diagnosis of discogenic pain must be confirmed.[2]

Weight-bearing CT or MRI may be done by axial loading performed in supine position. A hydraulic compressor is placed below a patient's feet and over the shoulders to apply a variable axial load. This simulates static mechanical forces acting on the spine in the upright position. Dedicated upright open MR scanners can determine axial load by gravity, patient's weight and spine morphology without artificial stimulation. Dynamic flexion extension is also possible in these units.[2] Dynamic plain films, weight-bearing CT or MRI have been used for the study of spinal stenosis. Previously occult abnormalities, including disc herniation, ligamentous infolding, subluxations may all be demonstrated using kinematic MRI. Functional information regarding vertebral stability may also be provided on dynamic examination.

Pathophysiology

Pathogenetic mechanisms are multiple and chronic overload is the most important factor. The other causes are sequelae of acute trauma, metabolic, toxic, genetic, vascular or infectious. The distribution of axial load determines the common sites of spine degeneration. In the cervical spine, it is C5–C6 and C6–7 levels as these are the sites of lordosis inversion. The dorsal spine is rarely involved as it is less mobile and less involved in dynamic load. In the lumbar spine, L4–5 and L5–S1 are the sites of highest dynamic and static overload and hence most predisposed to degenerative changes.[2]

In patients with degenerative changes of the spine, there are multiple mechanisms that act in combination to produce pain.[4] These are as follows:

- Biochemical mediators of inflammation resulting from disc degeneration and herniation.
- Mechanical compression of nerves by bone, ligament or disc material.
- Instability or abnormal motion with associated disc degeneration and facet arthropathy.
- Disruption of free nerve endings in the outer annular fibers.

Anatomy of Intervertebral Disc

The intervertebral disc has an inner nucleus pulposus and an outer annulus fibrosus and is bordered by cartilaginous endplates. The nucleus pulposus consists of hydrated proteoglycans supported by network of elastin and collagen type 2 fibers. Over time, the gelatinous proteoglycans is replaced by fibrocartilage. The nucleus is eccentrically located and more closely related to the posterior surface of the intervertebral disc. The annulus is composed of outer and inner layers. The outer layer consists of dense collagen type 1 fibers and is anchored to the vertebral endplates by perivertebral ligaments. The inner annulus is composed of fibrocartilage and collagen and attaches to the cartilaginous endplate. The collagen in the inner annulus is less plentiful than in the outer ring. The annular fibers become progressively more compact centrifugally. The outermost fibers are the densest, known as Sharpey's fibers. The nucleus pulposus converts much of the axial force into radial force and functions to spread the load evenly over the adjacent endplate. Cartilaginous endplates are composed of hyaline cartilage. These are usually not well discernible on imaging. Surrounding the cartilaginous endplate is a ring of dense bone, the ring apophysis that fuses to the vertebra in the second decade of life. Fetal and infantile disc is well vascularized but these branches soon atrophy and the adult disc becomes avascular. It obtains its nutrition by diffusion from vertebral endplates.[3]

The normal intervertebral discs are of slightly lower signal intensity than bone marrow on T1-weighted images and with higher T2 signal. The annulus is seen as a peripheral region of low signal intensity on T2W images and nucleus pulposus is hyperintense. A horizontal internuclear cleft of fibrous tissue containing collagenous, elastic and reticular fibers may normally be seen on T2WI in over 90% of patients over 30 years of age and is considered a paraphysiologic change.[1,2] On T1WI, the distinction between the nucleus and annular fibers is less discernible **(Figs. 1A to C)**, similar to CT.

Degenerative Disc Changes

The intervertebral disc undergoes marked changes with aging, which must be distinguished from degenerative changes in the disc. The incidence of degeneration increases with age, but most discs in normal aging individuals do not show changes in height and morphology that characterize degenerating discs. With aging, small concentric and transverse tears may develop in the annulus. The composition of the intervertebral disc may change with decrease in glycosaminoglycans and increase in collagen; and hence a decrease in affinity for water. Therefore, aging can reduce the signal intensity of the disc by a few percent. However, loss of high signal intensity on T2WI or loss of disc height cannot be entirely attributed to aging.[5]

Degenerating discs may undergo dehydration, fissures, bulging and herniations. On MR, the earliest appearance of degeneration of the nucleus is dessication, manifest as low signal intensity on T2-weighted images instead of high signal of normally hydrated discs **(Fig. 2)**. Although it is

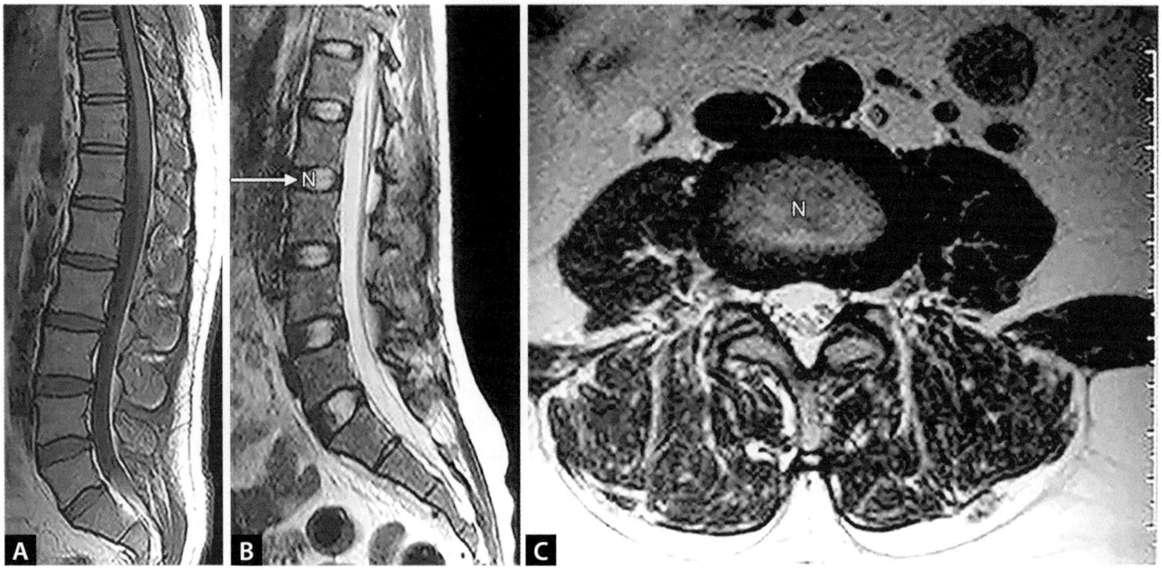

Figs. 1A to C: Sagittal T1-weighted (A); T2-weighted (B); and axial T2-weighted (C) MR images of lumbosacral spine show normal intervertebral disc that is slightly lower signal intensity than bone marrow on T1-weighted images and with higher T2 signal. The annulus is seen as a peripheral region of low signal intensity on T2W images (arrow) and nucleus pulposus (N) is hyperintense. A horizontal internuclear cleft is seen on T2W sagittal image.

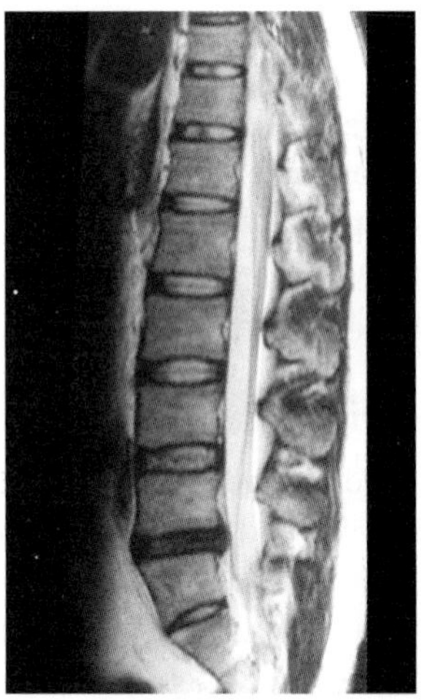

Fig. 2: Sagittal T2-weighted MR image of lumbosacral spine shows decreased T2 signal of L4/5 disc with loss of differentiation between nucleus and annulus fibrosus suggestive of disc desiccation. Note made of transitional vertebra.

usually asymptomatic, it suggests disc overload and is a precursor to further degenerative abnormalities.[1,2] There is progressive loss of disc height. The one morphological feature that characterizes disc degeneration is annular radial tears. Development of annular radial tears results in shrinkage of fibrocartilage in the nucleus pulposus and replacement by dense fibrous tissue and cystic spaces. The disc becomes more and more fibrous and disorganized with no clear distinction between nucleus and annulus.[4] Negative pressure produced by abnormal spaces pulls in gas, predominantly nitrogen resulting in vacuum disc phenomenon **(Figs. 3A and B)**. The disc may show linear or patchy low signal intensity either due to gas or sometimes, calcification. When occasionally fluid may be pulled instead of nitrogen, there may be paradoxical high signal appearance of the disc on T2WI instead of the low signal intensity of dessicated disc. Associated disc narrowing and endplate changes and osteophytes are pointers that this seemingly hydrated disc is a degenerated disc. With progress of degeneration, disc calcification may occur. This can appear as increased or decreased signal on T1WI. Paradoxical high signal on T1WI may be seen depending on the amount and state of calcium.[4,6]

Annular disruption is a critical factor in degeneration. Annular fiber degeneration may result in tears: (i) type 1 circumferential or concentric tears, (ii) type 2 radial tears, and (iii) type 3 transverse tears. Concentric tears are tears that run longitudinally along the plane of collagen fibers and precede annular bulging. These are seen as focal hyperintense areas in the external aspect of the annulus. Transverse tears are ruptures of Sharpey's fibers adjacent to the ring apophyses and can be seen in normally hydrated disc. Radial tears are linear rupture of the annulus fibers extending from the nucleus pulposus traversing the entire inner-to-outer dimension of the annulus and correlate with shrinkage and disorganization of the nucleus. This can progress to more severe disruption and disc herniation.

Megnetic resonance is less sensitive than cryomicrotomy or discography in detecting radial tears.[5] On MRI, radial tears appear as hyperintense transverse band into the annulus on MRI **(Figs. 4A and B)**.[1,2] These high intensity zones (HIZ) may enhance suggesting ingrowth of granulation tissue. However, presence of HIZ or even their enhancement is no more thought to be correlated with the acuity of the tear.

Disc Herniation

Herniation is the term used most commonly to describe the displacement of disc material. It can involve displacement of the nucleus pulposus, endplate cartilage, fragmented apophyseal bone or annular tissue beyond the normal confines of the disc space.

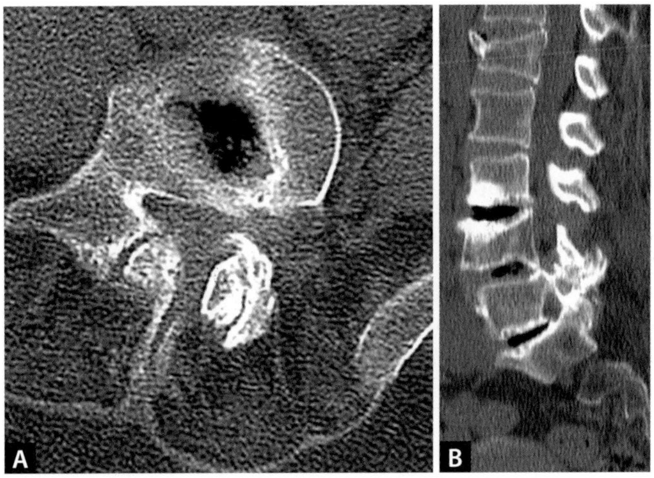

Figs. 3A and B: Axial CT (A) and sagittal multiplanar reformatted CT (B) images show vacuum phenomenon seen as air within multiple intervertebral discs. Note also made of marked hypertrophy of the left facet joint seen on the axial image and wedge compression fracture of L1 vertebra on the sagittal image.

To bring uniformity to reporting of disc degeneration, North American Spine Society, American Society of Spine Radiology, and American Society of Neuroradiology combined their committees, yielding a consensus paper on nomenclature of disc degeneration.[7]

Disc herniation is localized displacement of the disc material, involving less than 50% of the circumference of the disc. In contrast, disc bulge by definition is not herniation and is the term used when there is a smooth circumferential extension of the disc margin beyond the boundary of the adjacent vertebral endplates in greater than 50% of the disc circumference. This is usually less than 3 mm beyond the edges of the vertebral body. The annulus fibrosus is grossly intact, although weakened due to tears in the oblique collagen bridges between the concentric annular fibers. The concentric fibers are intact. On MR, there is uniform circumferential extension of the outer disc margin. There is usually loss of height of the involved disc space and desiccation of the nucleus pulposus **(Figs. 5A and B)**.[1,2,8] Apart from degeneration, disc bulge has several etiologies—normal variation, ligamentous laxity, vertebral body remodeling because of osteoporosis or even partial volume averaging.[6]

Disc herniation can be classified into disc protrusion and disc extrusion. When the greatest distance between the edges of the disc material beyond the disc space is less than the distance of the edges at the disc base in all planes, it is referred to as disc protrusion. The disc protrudes through a defect in the inner annulus but the outer annular fibers are intact. Protrusions may be classified as focal or broad, based on their degree of disc involvement. It is

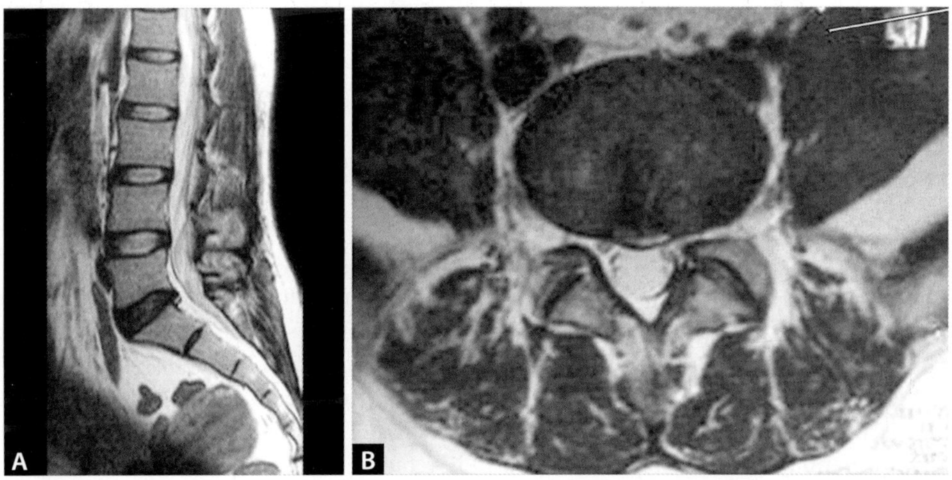

Figs. 4A and B: Sagittal (A) and axial (B) T2-weighted MR images of lumbosacral spine depict disc desiccation with annular tear seen as high intensity zone at L5/S1 level.

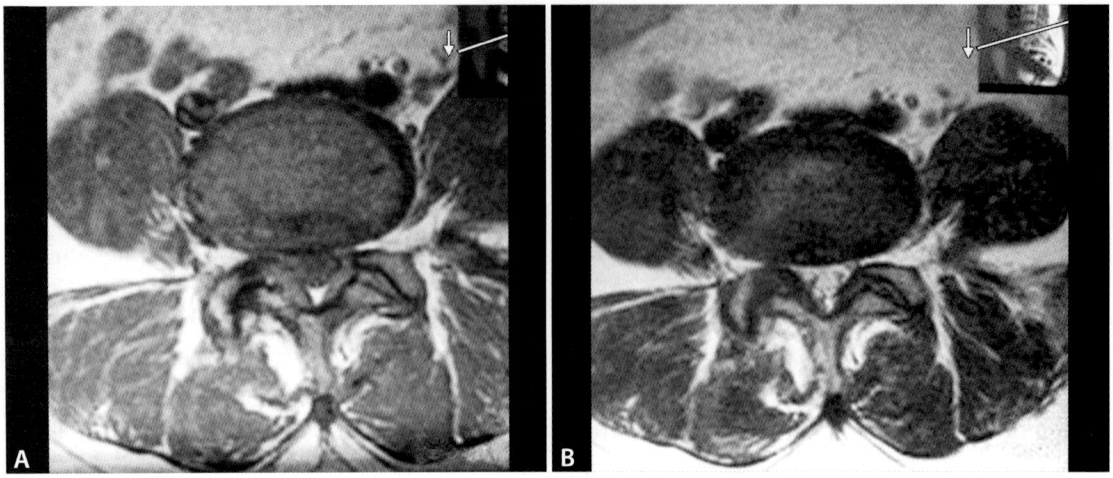

Figs. 5A and B: Axial T1- (A) and T2-weighted (B) images at L4-5 level show diffuse disc bulge with ligamentum flavum hypertrophy resulting in canal and lateral recess stenosis (arrow). Note that ligamentum flavum are better discernible on T1 rather than T2-weighted image (arrow).

termed a focal protrusion when it involves less than 25% of the disc circumference, whereas the term broad-based protrusion is used when it involves between 25 and 50% of the disc circumference **(Figs. 6A and B)**.[1,2,8]

When the distance between the edges of the disc material beyond the disc space is greater than the distance between the edges of the base in at least one plane, it is called disc extrusion **(Figs. 7A to C)**. The extruded disc suggests complete rupture of the annulus fibrosus. Disc extrusions may be further classified into migrated or sequestrated discs. The disc that displaces away from the site of extrusion but still maintains continuity with the parent disc is known as a migrated disc. Sequestrations are disc extrusions that get detached from the parent disc. This is clinically very relevant as a sequestered disc may be a contraindication to minimally invasive therapies, such as a microdiscectomies, percutaneous radiofrequency ablations, or the use of intradiscal steroids.[1,2,8]

Other descriptions of intervertebral disc herniations may also be described according to their relationship with the posterior longitudinal ligament. They may be categorized as subligamentous (disc herniation is ventral to the PLL), transligamentous (disc has extended through the PLL), or extraligamentous (disc has herniated in a region not bounded posteriorly by the PLL. This terminology is used when PLL can be seen as a distinct structure. Normally, it may be difficult to distinguish the PLL from the outer annulus and the dura. The relationship to PLL is related to the sagittal location of the abnormality. In the midline, PLL is firmly attached to the posterior vertebral body and no potential space exists between the two. In the paramidline location the PLL narrows and is not firmly attached to the vertebral body and a potential space exists between the two, known as the anterior epidural space. This is the space where disc fragments are frequently trapped.[8]

In the axial plane, it is classified into various zones as central, subarticular (lateral recess), foraminal and extraforaminal (far lateral). The medial edge of the facet articulations and the borders of the pedicles or the neural formina are used for anatomic landmarks, although they may be difficult to interpret on axial images as they are curved structures.[8]

The axial classification is useful, as it describes the herniation relative to the various exiting and traversing nerves. Lumbar disc herniations generally produce symptoms involving the nerve root inferior to the level of herniation as it compresses the transiting inferior root. However, an extraforaminal or foraminal disc herniation may compress the exiting root at the same level. In the cervical spine, disc herniations tend to involve the nerve root at the same level. This information is important to determine whether patient's symptoms are attributable to MR imaging findings, for preoperative planning and to avoid surgery at the incorrect spinal level.[1]

Magnetic resonance is the most frequently used technique for evaluation of disc herniation as it has high inherent soft tissue contrast. Contrast MRI is usually not required and is more used in postoperative examinations to differentiate residual and recurrent herniations from scar tissue. It may also be used sometimes in the preoperative setting to detect annular tears and inflammatory processes that may accompany acute disc dessication-like facet joint synovitis and radiculitis. It may also help differentiate herniation from neurinoma. Computed tomography is unable to detect early disc dessication.

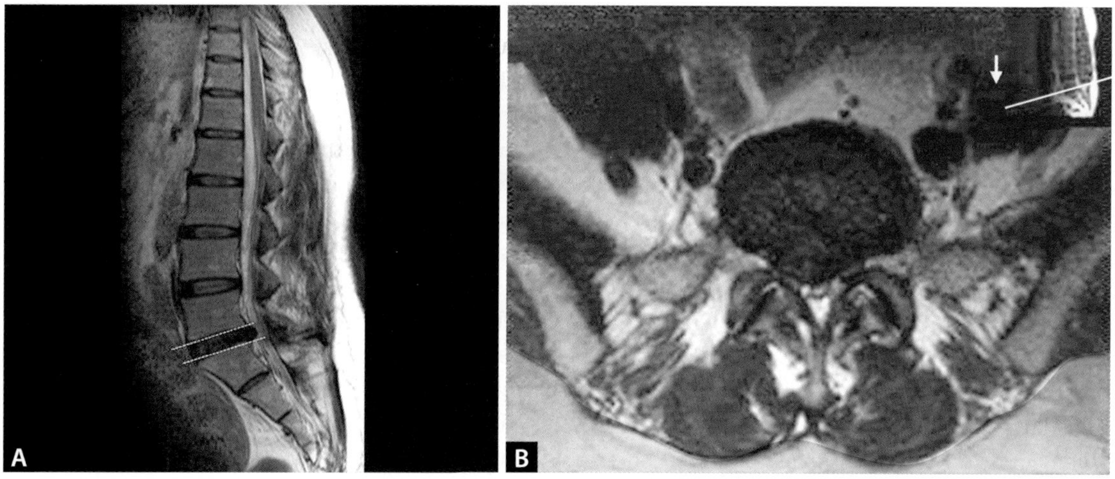

Figs. 6A and B: Sagittal (A) and axial T2-weighted (B) MR images depict broad based disc protrusion at L5/S1 level. On the sagittal image, the herniated disc is seen to lie within the confines of the disc margins (arrow).

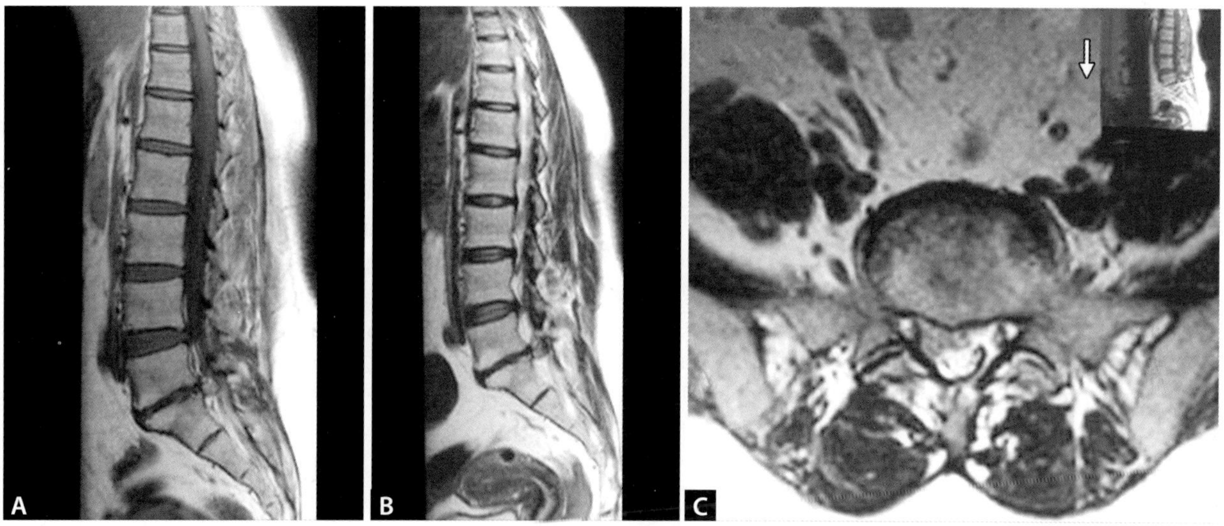

Figs. 7A to C: Sagittal T1 (A), sagittal T2 (B) and axial T2-weighted (C) MR images reveal markedly decreased disc space between L5/S1 with disc extrusion that is seen to extend beyond the confines of the disc space on the sagittal image. On the axial image, the extruded disc is seen to impinge on the traversing S1 nerve root on the right side. Note the type 2 endplate marrow changes seen as bright signal (arrow) on both T1- and T2-weighted sagittal images.

It can detect advanced changes like disc space narrowing and sclerotic endplate changes. Computed tomography is more sensitive than MR for detecting the presence of transdiscal gas, predominantly nitrogen. This is known as the vacuum phenomenon and is very specific for disc degeneration and is only rarely encountered in infective discitis.[1] Computed tomography is also more accurate in detection of discal calcification and posterior osteophytes which may have therapeutic implications. On MRI, bright T1 signal may be found with mild to moderate intradiscal calcium deposition.[1,2]

Imaging studies with 6–12 months follow-up have demonstrated that nearly 63% of disc herniations may show spontaneous reduction in size. This may be due to dehydration, fragmentation and phagocytosis of the disc material. This is greatest in extrusions and sequestrations.[2,9]

Radiology is also involved in interventional techniques for therapeutic purpose, e.g. automated discectomy, percutaneous laser disc decompression, intradiscal oxygen-ozone injection. Their success rates range from 70 to 80% with minimal potential complications.[2]

Endplate Changes

These are a reflection of abnormal stresses—loading or motion stresses. According to Michael Modic, endplate changes can be classified into three categories.[4]

Modic type 1 changes (vascular pattern) correspond to active inflammation, showing decreased signal on T1WI and high signal on T2WI. Type 2 changes (fatty pattern) reflect fatty infiltration and show bright signal on both T1- and T2-weighted images **(Figs. 7A and B)**. Type 3 changes (sclerotic pattern) are seen in advanced chronic stage, and correspond to bone sclerosis. This is seen as decreased signal on both T1 and T2-weighted images. These changes are also apparent on radiographs and CT **(*see* Fig. 3A)**.[1,2] Sometimes, more than one type of Modic change can be seen at the same level.

The relationship with degenerative disc disease is probably caused by multiple factors—common biomechanical factors, raised mechanical stresses on the endplates induced by disc dehydration and disc metabolism changes. Endplate alterations can also induce disc changes as disc is an avascular structure supplied by metabolite diffusion from endplate cartilage. The relative lack of blood supply and sparse cell population within the nucleus results in limited ability to recover from metabolic or mechanical injury.[2]

Type 1 may progress to type 2 changes or rarely may revert to normal. Type 1 and type 2 changes may occasionally progress to type 3 changes. Type 1 Modic changes have been positively correlated with back pain. According to Chung et al.[10] asymptomatic type 1 changes when present are generally focal, involve the anterosuperior endplate and involve midlumbar spine. In contrast, in symptomatic individuals, these are confluent changes superior and inferior to a degenerated disc, and usually seen in the lower lumbar spine.

Sometimes type 1 changes may be so extensive that the imaging appearance may simulate infective etiology. However, in infectious process, there is hyperintensity of the disc on T2WI with enhancement, paraspinal or epidural inflammation and erosion or destruction of endplate. Subchondral enhancement may be seen in both cases.[1,2] Sclerotic type 3 changes can be rounded and mimic blastic metastatic disease on radiographs and CT. However, the degenerative endplate changes are seen abutting the endplate and there are associated features of disc degeneration like disc narrowing and vacuum phenomenon.[6]

Focal herniations of discs through cartilaginous endplates may produce Schmorl's nodes. In most cases, these are remote occurrences of no clinical consequence. However, some of them may be traumatic in etiology and can be related to episodes of sudden pain when MR may show endplate edema representing endplate fracture.[1]

Most Schmorl's nodes occur after axial loading and result in extrusion of nucleus pulposus through the endplate rather than biomechanically stronger annulus fibrosus. Additional predisposing factors are intrinsic abnormalities of the endplate due to vascular channels or notochordal remnant defects. Patients with straight rather than concave endplates are also more predisposed due to less favorable axial loading.[3]

On CT, Schmorl's nodes are seen as focal indentations in the endplate in continuity with the intervertebral disc. There may be surrounding endplate sclerosis. On MR, we can see direct continuity of the disc material into the region of the endplate defect. In acute/subacute cases, there may be increased T2 signal, typically following the contour of the endplate which may also demonstrate enhancement.[3]

Disease of Facets, Uncovertebral Joints and Ligaments

The facet or zygoapophyseal joints are synovium lined joints. They are oriented nearly in the sagittal plane in the cervical spine and approximately 40 degrees in the sagittal plane in the lumbar spine. Like other synovial joints, these are predisposed to arthropathy with alterations of articular cartilage. Facetal joint changes may be primary or secondary to disc degeneration. The latter is believed to be the main inciting factor for facet osteoarthritis. Secondary to disc degeneration, increased loading on facets and increased mobility at a segment can contribute to facet arthropathy. Facet tropism (asymmetry) and more sagittal orientation of facets greater than 45 degrees are other hypothesized causes. It has been postulated that facetal joint degeneration is more likely associated with patient symptoms as this is less frequently found in asymptomatic individuals compared to disc degeneration. Patients usually present with axial pain. computed tomography is more sensitive in detecting early changes than MRI. The imaging findings include joint space narrowing, subchondral sclerosis and cyst formation, osteophyte formation, vacuum phenomenon and hypertrophy of the articular processes **(Figs. 8A and B)**. In addition, MR imaging can demonstrate edema in the adjacent posterior elements and soft tissues.[1]

In the lumbar spine, facetal degeneration is accompanied by ligamentum flavum hypertrophy contributing to secondary spinal canal stenosis. This is due to fibrosis and loss of elasticity of the ligament. These ligaments are best assessed on T1-weighted images as these are difficult to differentiate from cortical bone on T2WI **(Figs. 5 and 9)**. In the lumbar spine, posterior

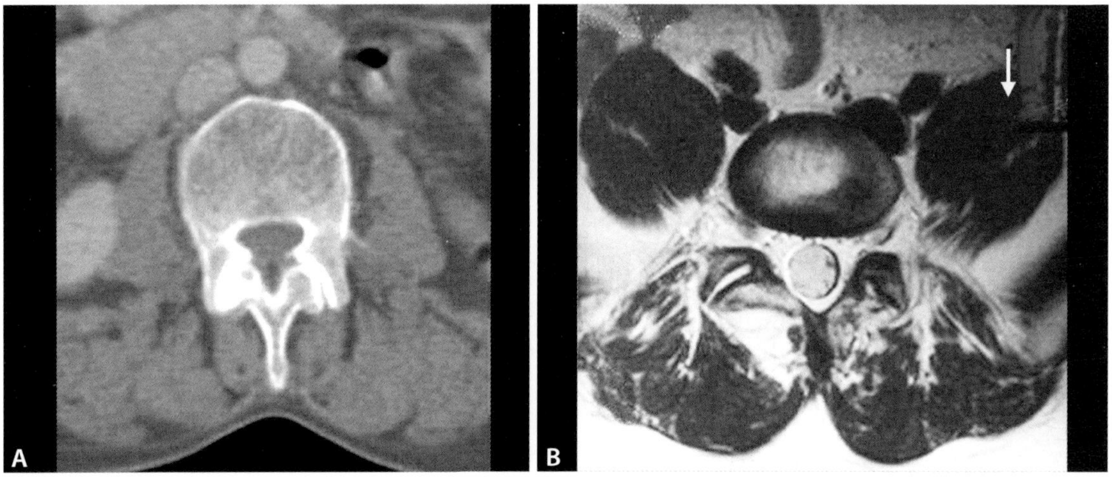

Figs. 8A and B: (A) Axial CT image depicts right facet arthrosis seen as erosions, sclerosis and decreased joint space; (B) T2-weighted axial image of another patient with facet arthritis shows increased fluid within the right facet joint with accompanying paraspinal muscle atrophy (arrow).

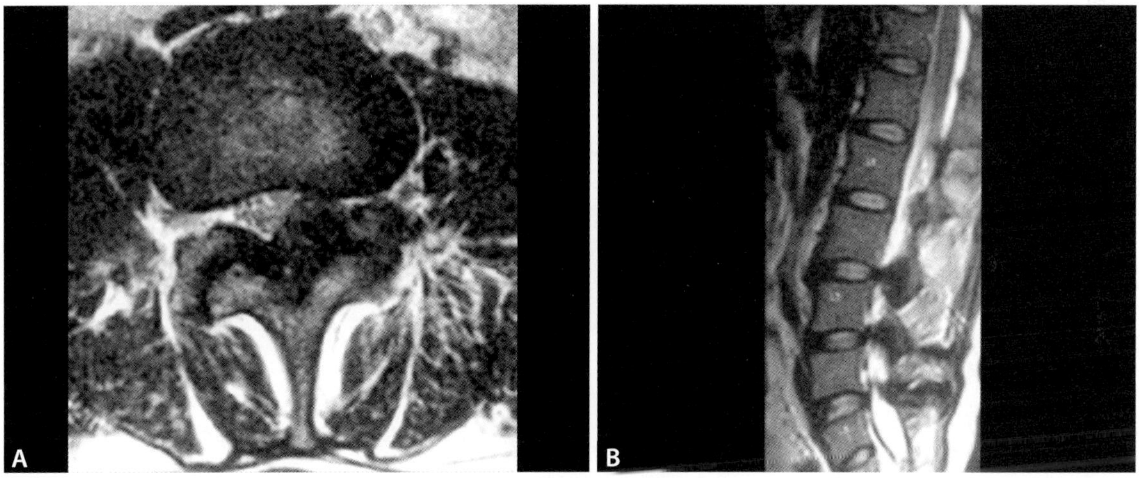

Figs. 9A and B: Axial (A) and sagittal T2W (B) MR images show facetal degenerative changes more marked on the left in the axial image with evidence of ligamentum flavum hypertrophy resulting in narrowing of the spinal canal at L3–L4 and L4–L5 levels.

paraspinal muscle atrophy also frequently accompanies facet joint degeneration **(Fig. 8B)**.[1,3]

Juxta-articular cysts may also be seen accompanying facet degeneration, most commonly at L4/5, frequently with degenerative spondylolisthesis. These may represent synovial cysts, ganglion cysts or cysts of the ligamentum flavum. It is often difficult to differentiate between these entities by radiologic, pathologic or surgical means. Anterior cysts are more likely to be associated with symptoms than posterior cysts as the former project into the spinal canal or neural foramina.[3]

On MRI, these cysts are generally high signal intensity on T2WI. Some portions may be low SI on T2WI due to calcification or gas. Adjoining facet joints may show increased amount of fluid within. These may be treated surgically or percutaneously, while spontaneous regression is also known.[1,3]

In the cervical spine, in addition, uncovertebral joints can undergo degeneration **(Figs. 10A to C)**. These develop between the uncinate processes of the lower vertebrae and the lateral margin of the superior vertebrae and are found from C2-3 level to C6-7 level. These are variable joints, not present at all levels and not seen in the infants. These joints are lined with cartilage, which is presumably continuous with the adjacent cartilaginous endplate. These are clinically important as degeneration of these joints plays an important role in foraminal stenosis and nerve root compromise in the cervical spine.[3]

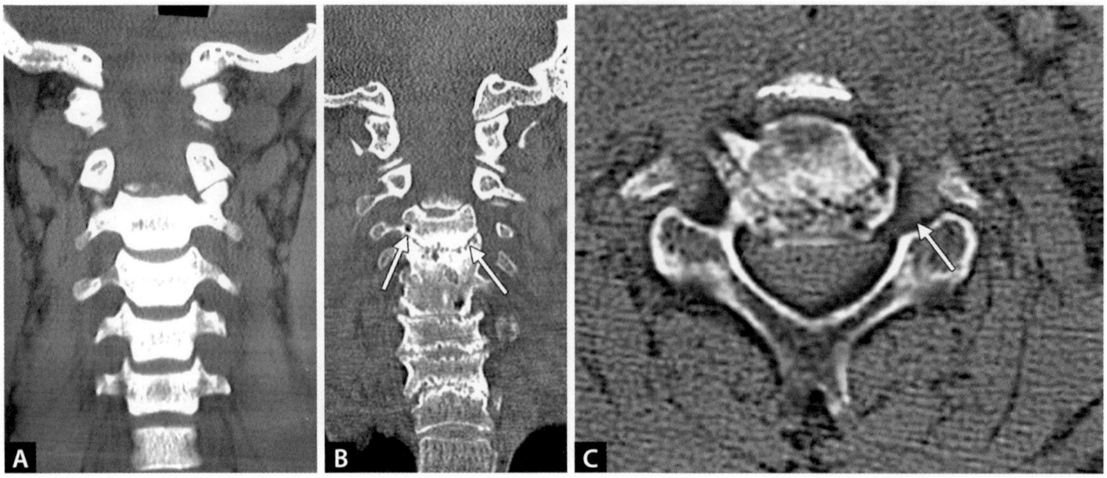

Figs. 10A to C: Coronal reformatted CT image (A) shows normal uncovertebral joints in cervical spine. Coronal reformatted CT image in another patient with extensive spinal degenerative changes (B) depicts marked arthrosis involving uncovertebral joints as well as endplate changes (arrows). Axial CT image (C) of the same patient depicts uncovertebral arthrosis with neural foraminal narrowing (arrow).

Narrowing of the intervertebral disc may lead to abnormal contact between spinous processes, leading to degeneration of the spinous processes and interspinous ligaments. This may result in interspinous pseudoarthrosis and cyst formation and has been termed Baastrup's phenomenon. There is localized tenderness that is exacerbated with extension and relieved with flexion, anesthetic injections or surgical excision. Redundant interspinous ligaments, interspinous bursae, or hypertrophic degeneration may extend anteriorly, contributing to spinal canal stenosis.[3]

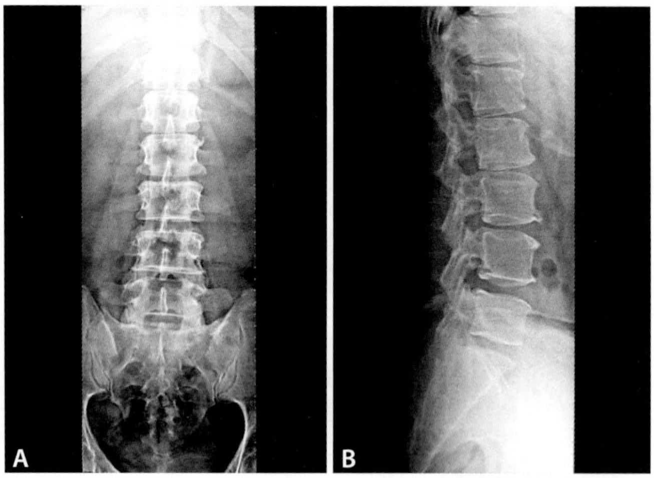

Figs. 11A and B: Lumbar spine AP and lateral radiographs depict marginal osteophytes at L2–L4 levels with relatively preserved disc spaces.

Spondylosis Deformans and Intervertebral Osteochondrosis

Degeneration of the disc affects both the nucleus and the annulus simultaneously. The imaging appearance depends on the predominant component.

Spondylosis deformans essentially affects the annulus fibrosus and adjacent apophyses. The classic sign of spondylosis deformans is osteophytosis. Osteophytes are bony spurs that originate on the anterolateral aspect of the vertebral bodies a few millimeters from the margins of the disc space **(Figs. 11A and B)**. Increased vertebral motility due to weakening and radial degeneration of annular fibers and resultant traction on Sharpey's fibers stimulates osteogenesis. Initially, osteophytes have a triangular horizontal extension (in contrast to syndesmophytes in seronegative arthropathies which are vertically oriented). In more advanced cases, osteophytes become hooked and grow more vertically. These may fuse together on either side of the disc space to form bridging osteophytes. The mucoid matrix of the disc becomes fibrous; however disc height is normal or only slightly decreased and the disc margins are regular. Posterior osteophytes, although less common, are clinically more relevant because of possible compression of neural structures. They have a triangular shape with marginal location. Large posterior osteophytes may result in spinal stenosis, with compressive myelopathy, especially in the cervical region.[1-3]

Spondylosis deformans is considered a paraphysiological change as it is found in 60% of women and 80% of men after the age of 50 years. They may be considered pathologic when severe or symptomatic.[2] Plain films are adequate for the diagnosis of spondylosis. Computed tomography and MRI, although can depict osteophytes are useful for other associated degenerative changes or to establish relationship between osteophytes and neural structures.

In contrast to spondylosis, vertebral osteochondrosis is a pathological process, although not always symptomatic. It involves primarily the nucleus pulposus and vertebral end plates. There is accompanying fissuring of the annulus fibrosus. Early disc changes seen on sagittal FSE T2WI include loss of normal T2 hypointensity within nucleus. Late changes include further decreasing signal within the nucleus pulposus, loss of distinction between nucleus pulposus and annulus fibrosus, disc space narrowing, disc bulges, vacuum phenomenon and endplate changes. Posterior osteophyte formation may also occur at this stage.[2] Computed tomography can detect later changes, including disc calcification, gas within disc space and also aid in differentiating oseophytes from degenerated disc.[3]

Complications of Degenerative Spinal Disease

Spinal and Foraminal Stenosis

Lumbar canal stenosis is the most common acquired disorder in elderly population, caused by degenerative changes and primarily manifesting after the 6th decade of life. Congenital stenosis presents earlier in life with multilevel involvement and fewer degenerative changes.[1]

Congenital stenosis is seen in patients with disorders such as achondroplasia and mucopolysaccharidosis or may be idiopathic. It is usually related to short pedicles, short laminae or sagittal orientation of facet joints. Any superimposed pathological process is much more likely to cause symptomatic compression. Acquired stenosis is most commonly due to degenerative changes and usually involves the cervical and lumbar spine. The central canal may be narrowed anteriorly by degenerated disc, posterior bulging of posterior longitudinal ligament or posterior osteophytes and posteriorly by facet joints and ligamentum flavum.[1,3] Other less common causes of acquired spinal canal stenosis include ossification of the PLL (OPLL) and /or LF (OLF) and epidural lipomatosis.

Although absolute measurements may not be clinically relevant in all cases, the diagnosis of spinal canal stenosis should be considered if the anteroposterior diameter of the cervical and lumbar canals is less than 12 mm and in the thoracic region if it is less than 10 mm. Stenosis may also be considered if the ratio between canal sagittal diameter and vertebral body sagittal diameter is <0.8. More than objective canal measurements, it is the subjective evaluation of canal morphology and relationship between containing and contained structures that correlates better with patient's symptoms. Epidural fat is reduced or disappears. Multiple anterior and posterior notches can be observed on the dural sac, with disappearance of the subarchnoid space and narrowing of the spinal cord. The stenosis is severe if CSF signal is completely effaced on axial T2WI or CT myelogram images.[1,2]

In severe lumbar canal stenosis, sometimes "redundant nerve roots" is seen as enlarged and swollen cauda equina. This may be due to radicular venous congestion, ischemia and edema.[2]

Myelopathy is the most serious complication of canal stenosis. It is thought that continuous pinching of the cord can result in chronic hypoperfusion and result in demyelination and neuronal death. Increased intramedullary signal on T2WI is seen **(Fig. 12)** that indicates the presence of edema, chronic ischemia, myelomalacia, or rarely syringomyelic cavitation. Enhancement on T1WI may confirm the abnormality. Low signal on noncontrast T1WI suggests a poor prognosis. However, it must be remembered that absence of abnormal signal does not rule out myelopathy, as clinical and electrophysiological criteria may be more sensitive. ADC maps and diffusion tensor imaging may improve the sensitivity in detecting subtle changes, but decrease the specificity.[3]

Facet hypertrophy, PLL thickening or disc herniation can lead to encroachment of lateral recesses. This is best evaluated on axial images and is found most commonly at L4–5 level. The normal sagittal diameter of the lateral recess is >5 mm; when this space is less than 4 mm, it is considered stenotic.[2,3]

Disc and facet degeneration can also project into the neural foramina, causing their narrowing. Remodeling of

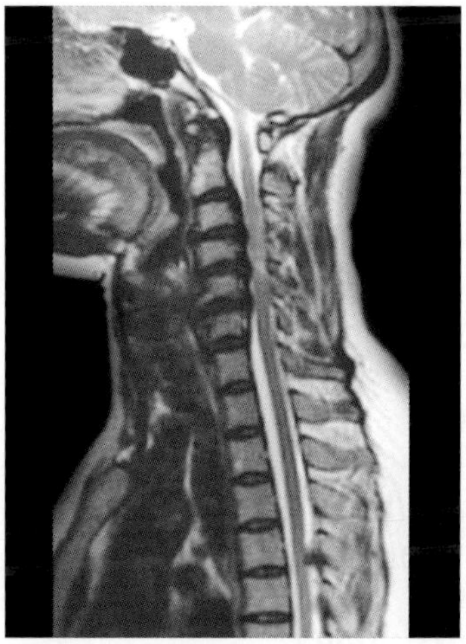

Fig. 12: Sagittal T2-weighted image of the cervical spine shows multiple disc bulges and posterior longitudinal ligament thickening resulting in thecal sac indentation with hyperintense signal within the cord suggesting myelopathy.

the endplates secondary to disc degeneration results in wider and shorter vertebral body and this may also cause narrowing of the spinal canal, lateral recesses and neural foramina. Loss of disc height may result in anterosuperior slippage of the facet joint and narrow the craniocaudal diameter of the foramen and hence, contributing to neural foraminal narrowing. In the cervical spine, neural foraminal narrowing is most commonly caused by uncovertebral osteophytes. Lumbar neural foramina are well seen on both axial and sagittal MR images whereas cervical neural foramina are best evaluated on axial MR images.[1,3] On sagittal MRI, foramen is seen as an ovoid structure, filled with cerebrospinal fluid and fat. Mild narrowing is seen as a "keyhole" appearance. Moderate narrowing effaces the inferior portion of the foramen at the level of the disc. Severe narrowing results in effacement of the fat in the foramen. There may be loss of fat around the exiting nerves and thecal sac. There may be effacement of contrast or CSF around nerve roots in the lumbar cistern. Inflammatory changes around the entrapped nerve may enhance on gadolinium administration. It must be remembered that correlation with symptoms of radiculopathy is essential to diagnose nerve root impingement.[3]

Computed tomography is the gold standard for evaluation of bony abnormalities, and is accurate for identifying posterior osteophytes and calcification of ligaments. Magnetic resonance imaging depicts the disc pathology and nervous structures clearly.[2]

Spinal cord or nerve root compression is a dynamic phenomenon that worsens in erect position or with certain movements. The stenosis can become more evident or sometimes, may only be evident during weight bearing or dynamic examination.[2,3]

Scoliosis and Kyphosis

Asymmetric degenerative disc changes can result in degenerative scoliosis **(Fig. 13)**. This tends to produce a positive feedback loop that tends to accelerate the degenerative changes on one side. Compared to idiopathic scoliosis, degenerative scoliosis is usually short segment and most often occurs in the lumbar spine. Also, loss of lumbar lordosis and spinal and foraminal stenosis are more common with degenerative scoliosis. Thoracic kyphosis in adults is frequently secondary to asymmetric degeneration in the anterior portions of the discs.[3]

Segmental Instability

Disc degeneration can lead to narrow disc space and buckling of ligamentum flavum which can further result in an unstable vertebral segment. Resultant malalignment may result in anterolisthesis, posterolisthesis, rotolisthesis (rotational spondylolisthesis) or lateral spondylolisthesis. Degenerative rotolisthesis occurs classically secondary to disc degeneration and results in canal and foraminal stenosis. It may also occur secondary to asymmetric facet degeneration. Anterolisthesis occurs mostly at L4–5 level, secondary to facet degeneration. In patients with degenerative scoliosis, lateral and rotolisthesis is often encountered.[3] Posterolisthesis, which is associated with facet and disc degeneration, is frequent at more mobile spine segments such as the cervical and upper lumbar spine.[2] The typical sites of degenerative spondylolisthesis are L3–4 and L4–5, because of more sagittal orientation of facet joints.

Spondylolisthesis may also result from pars interarticularis defects (spondylolysis) and the most common is the isthmic type of spondylolysis. This is most commonly seen at L5 and L4 vertebrae and is a defect in pars interarticularis which is considered a fatigue fracture. Other less common causes of spondylolisthesis are acute trauma, congenital dysplasias, tumors and iatrogenic causes. Spondylolisthesis due to pars defect may be distinguished from degenerative spondylolisthesis on imaging. The former depicts canal widening at the involved level **(Figs. 14A to C)** whereas the latter demonstrates canal narrowing at the affected level because of slippage of the posterior arch and facet hypertrophy.[1,2]

Secondary to segmental instability, hypertrophy of the ligaments, facet osteoarthritis, and osteophyte formation, may develop which have an additive effect on narrowing of the spinal canal and foramina. These osteophytes may aid in stabilizing the spinal segment, which may be shown on kinematic MR imaging.[3]

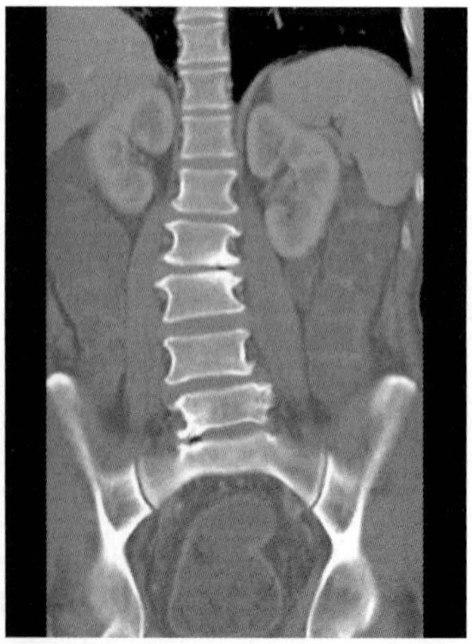

Fig. 13: Coronal reformatted CT image reveals laterally directed osteophytes on the concavity of scoliosis with vacuum phenomenon at multiple levels.

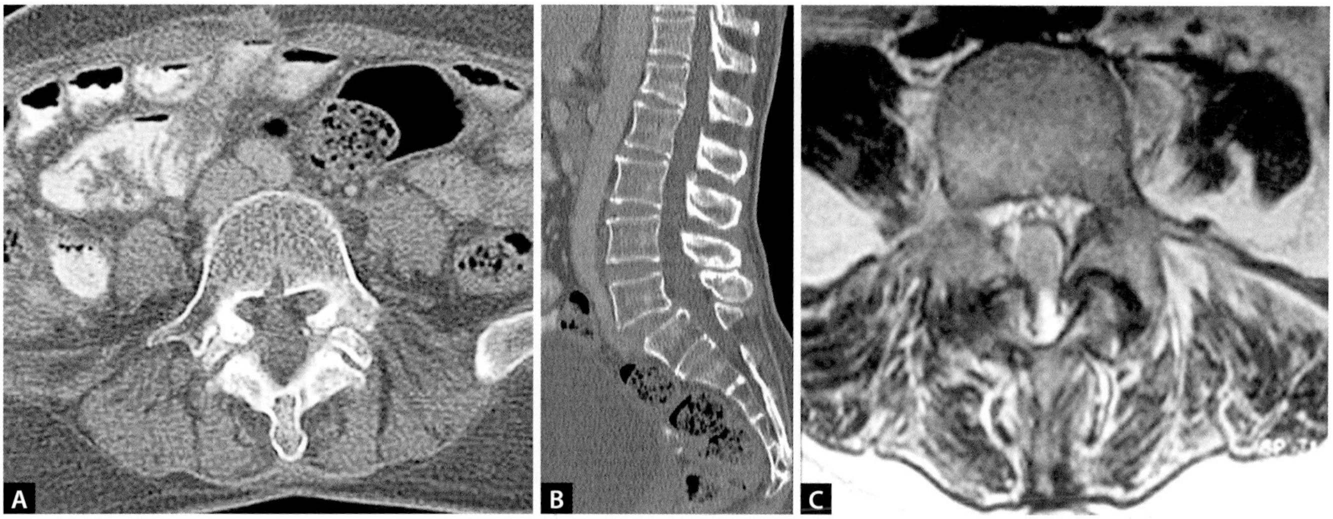

Figs. 14A to C: Axial (A) and sagittal reformatted CT (B) images reveal lysis of pars interarticularis of L4 with spondylolisthesis of L4 over L5 resulting in widening of the AP diameter of the spinal canal. T2-weighted axial MR image (C) of another patient shows break involving pars interarticularis of L4 with widening of spinal canal.

Vertebral body movement may be seen on flexion, extension and lateral bending radiographs where instability may be diagnosed as loss of alignment of one or more vertebral lines. Other radiographic signs are vertebral slippage, variations in pedicle length, narrowing of neural foramina, and loss of disc height. Conventional MRI has a limited role. It may show displacement and pseudobulging of disc at the involved level. Axial loaded CT or MRI or upright MRI can provide functional information regarding vertebral stability.[2]

Clinical Implications

Clinical features and imaging findings need to be always evaluated together to plan appropriate therapeutic strategy as symptoms and imaging findings do not always correlate well. Roudsari and Jarvik[11] concluded that imaging is not necessary with low backache in patients who have no signs or symptoms of systemic disease and who have no clinical suspicion for serious spine problems. However, if there is no clinical improvement after medical/noninvasive therapy at one month follow-up, imaging must be cosidered. Spinal stenosis and radiculopathy should also be evaluated by imaging if symptoms persist for more than one month.

DEGENERATIVE DISEASE OF JOINTS

Prevalence and Incidence of Osteoarthritis

Osteoarthritis has a predilection for certain joints while sparing others. For example, in the hands, the distal interphalangeal, proximal interphalangeal, and carpometacarpal joints are frequently affected, whereas the wrists are rarely affected. Other frequently affected joints include knee, hip and metatarsophalangeal joint. The ankles and elbows are usually spared.[12]

Approximately 32.5% of adults aged 30 years and older have radiographic evidence of osteoarthritis in the hand in at least one joint.[13] According to data from the Framingham study, radiographic knee osteoarthritis occurs in at least 33% of persons aged 60 years and older.[14]

Another feature of osteoarthritis is the higher prevalence and more often generalized distribution in women than in men. For most joints, before the age of 50 years, men have a higher prevalence of the disease than do women. After age of 50 years, women have a much higher prevalence of disease than do men. The reasons for this gender difference may be related to the hormone deficiency that develops in women around age of 50 years.[12]

Imaging Modalities

- *Conventional radiography:* It is the initial examination performed in routine evaluation of degenerative arthritis. It is a sensitive and cost-effective modality, therefore, appropriate for large scale studies and follow-up of patients. However, it does not directly demonstrate the articular cartilage and soft tissues of the joint.
- *Magnetic resonance imaging:* MR imaging provides excellent soft tissue contrast. With its ability to differentiate tissues according to their biochemical

properties and to obtain images in multiple planes, MRI is the optimal modality to assess pathologic conditions of joints. MR imaging allows direct visualization of the articular cartilage, inflamed synovium, other soft tissues like joint-capsule, menisci, and ligaments noninvasively. It is also valuable in treatment planning for chondral lesions and in following cartilage reconstructions longitudinally. It may reduce the need for more costly and invasive diagnostic arthroscopy. Whenever accurate evaluation of surface changes is needed, arthrographic techniques may be done. MR imaging and MR arthrography is being increasingly done to obtain detailed information about the status of the degenerated joints prior to prosthetic replacement. MR imaging reliably shows the whole spectrum of osteoarthritic changes accurately.

- *Computed tomography:* CT provides excellent contrast resolution and has the advantage of allowing excellent display of the bones of the affected joint. CT arthrography, an excellent tool for measuring cartilage thickness, may be done when MR arthrography is not possible (e.g. not available, claustrophobia, metallic implants). It has the inconvenience of radiation exposure and is limited to evaluation of surface lesions only. DECT is a promising technique with potential application in evaluation of tendons, ligaments and can aid in reduction of metal artifacts.[15]
- *Radionuclide scintigraphy:* ^{99m}Technetium scintigraphy is a very sensitive method that reveals increased indicator uptake in very early stages of OA and allows evaluation of compartment distribution. Because of the poor specificity of these changes, scintigraphy is used only as a screening method and for follow-up studies.

Pathogenesis

The joints are used over and over again. Whether this use constitutes a dynamic trophic and healthy effect on joints or an injurious effect depends on the activities involved and the vulnerability of the underlying joint. Most daily activities, even if performed repeatedly over many years, do not produce sufficient injury to a joint to cause osteoarthritis. Joints become susceptible to injury and subsequent osteoarthritis when local factors in the joint combine with systemic vulnerabilities.[12]

Hyaline articular cartilage loss is a signature event in osteoarthritis. Articular cartilage is a complex structure that consists of a gel extracellular matrix composed of 80% water and 20% solids that include collagens (mainly type II), proteoglycans, and noncollagenous proteins.[14] The unique biomechanical properties of articular cartilage in response to mechanical loading result from the flow of water through the intercellular matrix. Mature chondrocytes seldom divide but remain metabolically active, synthesizing and turning over matrix proteoglycans. A complex network of cytokines and growth factors secreted by synovial lining cells and by chondrocytes controls the level of matrix synthesis and degradation. Aggrecan is a macromolecule consisting of small highly negative charged glycosaminoglycan chains that are forced into close proximity and electrostatic repulsion by the collagen II chains interwoven through the matrix. The electrostatic repulsion of aggrecan gives cartilage its compressive stiffness. In early osteoarthritis, despite an increased production of aggrecan and matrix in general, the net concentration of aggrecan in cartilage falls as degradation outweighs synthesis. Eventually, superficial fibrillation and cracking of the matrix occur, which are followed by focal disintegration and ulcerations of cartilage.[16]

Deep to cartilage loss is an increased quantity of subchondral bone. Bone grows into the calcified cartilage. At the joint margins, chondral structures form at sites of tension, and endochondral ossification occurs in these structures, producing chondro-osteophytes, so called "osteophytes". Osteophytes form in areas of low stress, increasing the surface area of the articular cartilage, thereby, decreasing the stresses that are experienced by the joint and increase joint stability. They commonly form at the margins of the joint where increased vascularization of subchondral bone stimulates endochondral ossification.[12,16] Synovial hypertrophy and fibrosis are seen in most joints affected by osteoarthritis, and local synovitis affects 20–30% of diseased joints. Synovial involvement in osteoarthritis may contribute to disease by serving as the source of cytokines such as interleukin-1 that may turn off chondrocyte-mediated cartilage matrix synthesis and trigger synthesis of degradative enzymes, by secreting excess synovial fluid that makes the joint-lax and vulnerable to injury.[12]

A sound knowledge of the pathophysiology of degenerative arthritis is important for understanding disease progression and its timely management.

The causes of OA include systemic factors, such as genetics, estrogen use and bone density, and biomechanical factors that affect the joints, including muscle weakness, obesity, joint-laxity, and alignment.[17]

Systemic Risk Factors

Osteoarthritis is a disease of aging, but age alone does not cause osteoarthritis; rather, the vulnerabilities of the joint that occur as part of aging make the joint susceptible to disease.

There is a higher percentage of hand and hip osteoarthritis due to inheritance than knee osteoarthritis.[18] It is likely that multiple genes confer an increased risk for osteoarthritis. It is increasingly likely that the genetic predisposition to osteoarthritis will be based on a variety of physiologic vulnerabilities, including alterations in minor collagens within cartilage, changes in enzymes or their activators within cartilage, variations in cytokines, or growth factor profiles in cartilage and genes that dictate joint shape and structure.[12]

Osteoporosis and osteoarthritis are inversely associated—persons with high-bone density are at high-risk for osteoarthritis.[19] A part of, but not all, of this relationship between high-bone density and osteoarthritis is explained by obesity causing osteoarthritis and also being strongly associated with high-bone density. Attrition and perhaps even low-bone density are associated with the progression of osteoarthritis, and it seems likely that high-bone density contributes only to the initial occurrence of disease and not necessarily to its progression.[20]

Inconsistent data exist on the relationship of estrogen deficiency to osteoarthritis in women. Women have a high-risk for osteoarthritis after about age of 50 years, much higher than the risk for men. Studies have been inconsistent regarding whether estrogen replacement therapy eliminates that risk. Preliminary data suggest that nutritional deficiencies may increase the occurrence or progression of osteoarthritis, including low-level intakes of vitamin C, vitamin E, and vitamin D.[21]

Local Joint Vulnerabilities

Factors that affect joint shape are likely to have an important role in causing osteoarthritis, especially in the hip. Developmental abnormalities occurring during infancy or childhood that leave a hip-joint misshapen and that increase local stresses to cartilage in that hip-joint predispose to hip osteoarthritis in early adulthood. The three types of congenital and developmental abnormalities that are most commonly implicated are congenital dysplasia, Legg–Perthes disease, and a slipped capital femoral epiphysis. Although these abnormalities are rare in childhood, milder forms may be more common and may account for a large percentage of osteoarthritis of the hips in adults.[22]

A major injury to a joint can cause permanent damage to many of the structures within a joint and can serve as the incipient lesion of osteoarthritis.[12]

An important interplay occurs between systemic and local joint vulnerabilities. Injury to the knee in an adolescent is unlikely to cause osteoarthritis quickly, if at all. In contrast, older joint is more vulnerable to major injury than the younger joint.[23] Limb malalignment markedly increases the risk of progression of knee osteoarthritis.[16]

Extrinsic Factors Acting on the Joint

- *Obesity*: Persons who are overweight have a higher prevalence of knee osteoarthritis. Weight probably increases the risk for knee osteoarthritis by increasing the amount of mechanical load across a joint. Indeed, every pound of weight is multiplied threefold to sixfold in terms of its effect on knee loading. Although, obesity markedly increases the risk for knee osteoarthritis, its relationship to hip osteoarthritis is not as strong.[24] By distributing the weight-bearing load more broadly, hip-joints may be protected against the effects of being overweight.
- *Muscle weakness*: As a consequence of disease, persons with osteoarthritis have weakness in the muscles that bridge, the diseased joint. Affected persons become relatively inactive, leading to muscular atrophy. Also, direct neurologic messages transmitted by a swollen joint through afferent impulses inhibit the maximal contraction of muscles bridging joints, leading to apparent weakness. This weakness most likely accounts for much of the disability and may increase the risk of progression.

Joint Overuse from Occupations and Athletics

The normal joint is built to withstand the considerable dynamic loading that occurs with daily activities. It provides healthy trophic influences to cartilage and other joint structures.[25] When activity is excessive or when normal activity acts on a vulnerable joint, joint injury and eventually osteoarthritis occur. Two examples are athletic and occupational activities.

Prolonged continuous activity may injure the joint when it is past the point where joint protective mechanisms are effective.[24,26]

Particular types of activities that occur in a variety of jobs pose a high-risk of later development of osteoarthritis. Examples include jobs that require regular knee bending and lifting or carrying heavy loads, which predispose to knee osteoarthritis. In men, such jobs may account for as much osteoarthritis as obesity.[27]

Most studies of runners have suggested that they are not at especially high-risk for knee osteoarthritis. This may not be true for nationally competitive professional runners who are more likely to have hip osteoarthritis.[24]

Radiographic–Pathologic Correlation

Altman et al.[28] defined OA as "a heterogeneous group of conditions that lead to joint symptoms and signs which are associated with defective integrity of articular cartilage, in addition to related changes in the underlying bone and at the joint margins". The need to separate idiopathic (primary) OA from OA that is related to an underlying condition (secondary) was stressed. Articular degeneration occurs without a pre-existing insult in primary OA, or as a result of previous injury or underlying condition in secondary OA.[29]

The most typical pattern of OA is the presence of reparative changes in both the stressed and nonstressed aspects of the joint. In the stressed segment of the joint, cartilage damage is evidenced by thinning of the cartilage rim and development of erosions and ulceration. Such damage is followed by hypervascularity of the articular cartilage. The radiologic picture is characterized by joint space loss. Subchondral infraction, compression and necrosis of bone trabeculae lead to bone sclerosis on radiographs.[30,31] Other subchondral changes, such as formation of cystic lesions as a result of either synovial fluid intrusion or bone contusion, occur in the stressed segment.[31-33]

In the nonstressed segment, reparative changes lead to osteophytosis.[34] Osteophyte formation is the most characteristic feature in OA. They commonly form at the margins of the joint where increased vascularization of subchondral bone stimulates endochondral ossification.[15] Osteophytes can be classified as marginal, central, periosteal, and capsular or synovial depending on their origin. Marginal and central osteophytes develop through endochondral ossification after vascularization of subchondral bone marrow. Periosteal osteophytes form from a process resembling appositional bone growth due to stimulation of periosteal membrane; capsular osteophytes develop in reaction to capsular traction forces.

Subchondral sclerosis: It is believed to be caused by redistribution of stress that results from progressive cartilage loss. Subchondral sclerosis occurs at these sites as a result of deposition of new bone on pre-existing trabeculae and trabecular microfractures with callus formation.

Subchondral cysts: They appear between thickened subchondral trabecula. Cysts often are multiple, and, histologically, can contain myxoid and adipose tissue, occasional cartilage with surrounding fibrous components and are bordered by peripheral sclerotic bone.[35] Proposed theories of the pathogenesis of cyst formation include bony microcontusions that leads to extension of synovial fluid into the subchondral bone through tiny gaps in the articular surface,[36] or the proliferation of myxomatous tissue within the bone narrow.[35]

Radiologically, the marginal osteophytes represent lips of new bone around the joint edges **(Fig. 15)**. Osteophytes of the central type lead to new bone formation in the center of the joint and therefore may produce an irregular contour of the joint surface. Radiographs of periosteal osteophytes reveal an area of thickened cortex. This type is most common at the medial aspect of the femoral neck, where it is called buttressing. Capsular osteophytes extend along the direction of capsular pull.

Besides the articular surface itself, other articular structures, such as ligamentous and capsular tissue may undergo severe degenerative changes, including thickening, disruption and distortion, which lead radiographically to deformation, malalignment and subluxation of the joint. Degenerative lesions also occur in intra-articular fibrocartilaginous tissue, such as menisci in the knee or the labra in hip and shoulders.

Fragmentation of the cartilaginous or osseous surface, especially in advanced disease can lead to the formation of intra-articular bodies, which may be either embedded on the surface or loose in the joint cavity. Depending on their size and location, intra-articular bodies can cause joint inflammation with clinical symptoms and acceleration of osteoarthritis.

The radiographic appearance of OA in different joints varies, being dependant on anatomic relationships and the stress to which each joint is subjected. The two

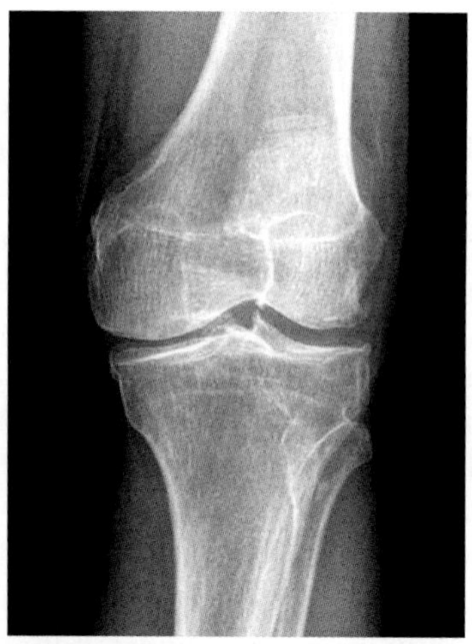

Fig. 15: AP radiograph of the knee shows marginal osteophytes, seen as lips of new bone near the lateral edge of knee-joint and tibial spiking in a case of degenerative arthritis.

weight-bearing joints that are affected most frequently by OA, are the hip and the knee.

HIP OSTEOARTHRITIS

Radiographic Views

Standard views performed include a supine anteroposterior (AP) view of the pelvis, an AP view of the hip, and a frog lateral view of the hip with the patient rolled towards the affected side.[37] In the anteroposterior view, the femur should be placed in 15–20 degrees of internal rotation to best visualize the femoral neck. In the frog-leg view the femur is in 45 degrees of abduction. The superior aspect of the joint space is visualized but with a different projection of the femoral head. Neither anteroposterior nor frog-leg views allow assessment of the anterior and posterior part of the joint space. Therefore, anterior and posterior oblique views (between 30° and 45°) are additionally recommended. All of these views except the frog-leg view can also be obtained under weight-bearing conditions, which provides more accurate measurement of the joint space.

The "false profile" view that was first described by Lequesne and Laredo[38] in 1961 has been proposed as a more sensitive view for diagnosing cartilage space narrowing than conventional AP views. The "false profile" view is an oblique lateral view of the hip obtained in the erect position. A recent series compared cartilage space narrowing that is seen on conventional AP radiographs and "false profile" radiographs. Of the cases with doubtful or no narrowing seen on the AP view, nearly 75% showed detectable narrowing on the "false profile" view. It is recommended in addition to conventional AP views, to help detect early cartilage space narrowing in patients who have a clinical suspicion of OA.[38]

Radiographic Appearance

In 1991, the American College of Rheumatology subcommittee on criteria for OA summarized the findings from a multicenter study and suggested clinical and radiographic criteria for reporting OA in symptomatic patients.[39] These included: (i) cartilage space narrowing; (ii) osteophytosis; (iii) subchondral cysts; (iv) subchondral sclerosis; (v) femoral neck buttressing; and (vi) femoral head remodeling. Of these, cartilage space narrowing was the most sensitive, but least specific. Medial femoral neck buttressing, when seen, was the most specific. Osteophytosis had the best overall balance of high sensitivity and specificity in detecting hip OA. When using radiographs to assess progression of hip OA, combining cartilage space narrowing with subchondral cysts or subchondral sclerosis produces the best sensitivity.[40]

Asymmetric joint space narrowing: It is the most reliable sign of OA in the hip-joint. Distinctive patterns of nonuniform loss of articular cartilage lead to the classic patterns of femoral head migration which can be categorized into three different patterns: (i) superior migration, (ii) medial migration, and (iii) axial migration.

Superior Migration Pattern

Superior migration is the most common pattern and is seen in 78% of patients who have OA.[41] This can be subdivided into superolateral and superomedial types. The superolateral type is characterized by unilateral and asymmetric changes, including narrowing of the superior joint space, which causes the femoral head to move superiorly. In more advanced disease, flattening of the superolateral aspect and lateral displacement of the femoral head lead to widening of the inferomedial joint space. In the pressure zone on the lateral and outer aspect of the femoral head and acetabulum, sclerosis, cyst formation and osteophytes also can be seen. In the femoral neck, medially thickening of the cortex (buttressing) accompanies these findings **(Fig. 16)**.

Superomedial migration in most cases occurs bilaterally and in contrast to the superolateral pattern, is more frequent in men than women. After superior movement of the femoral head with narrowing of the superior joint space and progressive head deformity,

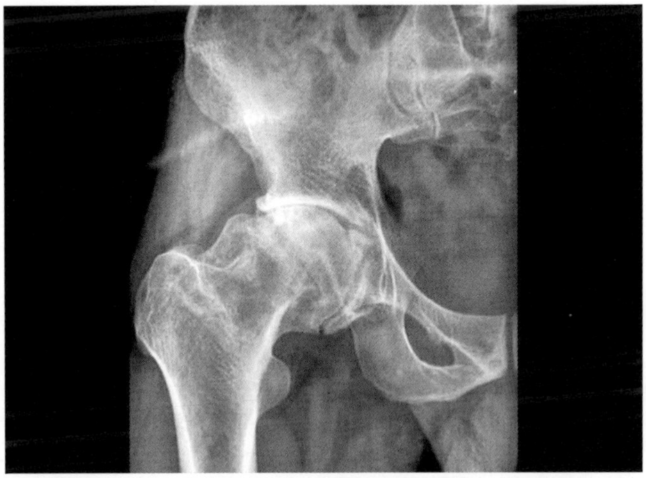

Fig. 16: AP radiograph of the right hip joint shows marked reduction in joint space on the right side, more along the superior joint space with osteophytes, subchondral sclerosis and cysts. Note made of cortical buttressing on medial femoral neck.

broad based osteophytes begin to fill in the apparently widened medial part of the joint space. The femoral head flattens progressively at the superior aspect. These changes produce apparent displacement of the femoral epiphysis. Other findings in this particular migration pattern are osteophytes and cystic lesions on the lateral and outer aspects of the femoral head and acetabulum in association with subchondral sclerosis. Buttressing can occur on the medial as well as lateral side of the femoral neck. The differential diagnosis of the superior migration patterns is quite limited and includes calcium pyrophosphate dihydrate (CPPD) crystal deposition disease and osteonecrosis, both associated with secondary degenerative changes.

Medial Migration Pattern

Medial migration of the femoral head can be observed in about 22% of all patients with osteoarthritis.[41] This pattern frequently shows bilateral and symmetric changes and is more common in women than in men. Radiographically, joint space loss in the medial aspect with consequent widening of the lateral aspect of the joint space is the most typical finding. Some cases also reveal acetabular protrusion. Osteophytes develop on the lateral and medial sides of femur and acetabulum, and cystic lesions are mostly small. Buttressing can occur on the medial side of the femoral neck. For the medial migration pattern, Paget's disease and osteomalacia with additional degenerative changes are included in the differential diagnosis.

Axial Migration Pattern

Concentric loss of joint space is the characteristic finding in the axial migration pattern but it is not specific **(Fig. 17)**. This pattern is infrequent and may cause problems in differential diagnosis, as diffuse and symmetric joint space loss is also present in various other abnormalities, such as rheumatoid arthritis and infection. The presence of osteophytes and sclerosis as well as the absence of erosions and osteoporosis adjacent to the joint may be helpful for differentiation. Even if osteophytes and sclerosis are combined with axial migration of the femoral head, other primary diseases, such as ankylosing spondylitis, CPPD crystal deposition disease, and secondary OA superimposed on rheumatoid arthritis, Paget's disease or osteonecrosis must be excluded.[36]

Uniform loss of cartilage indicates a primary disorder of cartilage rather than loss secondary to abnormal mechanical stress. This disorder could be either an inflammatory process or a deposition process. Inflammatory disease will usually cause erosive changes and aggressive destruction of cartilage. Some inflammatory arthropathies may lead to new bone proliferation in the form of ossification of ligamentous attachments or ankylosis. Deposition arthropathies usually cause slow degeneration of cartilage and secondary osteoarthritic changes.

Subchondral sclerosis: It occurs at these sites because of deposition of new bone on preexisting trabeculae and trabecular microfractures with callus formation. The areas of subchondral sclerosis that are visible on radiographs are smaller than areas of low signal that are identified on MR imaging.

Subchondral cysts: Cystic spaces appear between thickened subchondral trabecula. They vary from 2 to 15 mm and are often multiple. They can contain myxoid and adipose tissue, occasional cartilage with surrounding fibrous components, and are bordered by peripheral sclerotic bone.[35] Subchondral cysts in the acetabulum have been referred to as "Eggers" cysts.[15]

The term "intraosseous ganglion" is used to describe acetabular lesions that contain gelatinous fluid. The combination of a mass and erosion of the adjacent superolateral acetabulum is characteristic, although non-specific for paralabral cysts (ganglia). A more specific finding is gas within the soft tissue mass, apparently due to nitrogen tracking from the joint. MR imaging showed these juxta-acetabular soft tissue masses to have intermediate signal intensity on T1 and proton density images and high signal intensity on T2-weighted images. The signal intensity of the fluid within the ganglion may be greater on T1-weighted images than that of the joint fluid because of the cyst's greater protein content.[42]

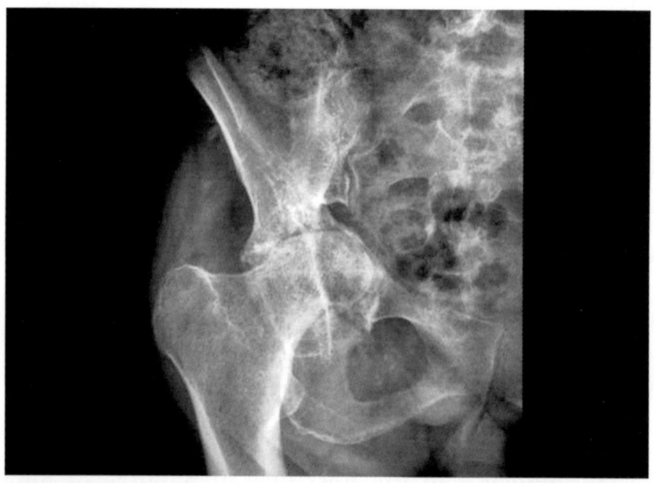

Fig. 17: AP radiograph of the right hip joint shows marked reduction in joint space on the right side, with axial migration of the femoral head and accompanying osteophytes.

Osteophytosis: Marginal osteophytes occur at the periphery of the femoral head or the margins of the fovea. Central or interior osteophytes extend from the subarticular surface. On radiographs they appear as flat or button-like osseous projections that cause contour deformities of the articular surface. They may be misdiagnosed as intra-articular bodies. Central osteophytes form at the acetabular fossa and partially or completely enclose it. Periosteal or synovial osteophytes form as osseous outgrowths from periosteum or synovial membranes. This is most apparent in the medial femoral neck where production of cortical thickening or a line of new bone formation occurs which is termed "buttressing".[43,44] Buttressing bone is believed to be due to altered stress loads on the femoral neck, possibly from increased neck shaft angle or decreased femoral neck diameter. It is most commonly seen with OA and less often with avascular necrosis. Identification of this finding makes the diagnosis of inflammatory arthritis unlikely, since it is rarely seen in patients who have RA or psoriasis.[39,43]

Osteophytes, sclerosis and cystic lesions are not specific finding for OA. These changes also can be seen in CPPD crystal deposition disease and neuropathic osteoarthropathy, most commonly combined with marked collapse of the femoral head, and in ankylosing spondylitis, which shows a characteristic femoral osteophyte extending across the femoral head-neck border.

There may be some difficulty in differentiating between medial osteophytes and loose articular bodies in the acetabular fossa. A linear radiodense shadow favors osteophytes, whereas a circular intra-articular shape makes a loose body much more likely than an osteophyte.

Rapid Destructive Osteoarthritis

Rapid destructive osteoarthritis (RDO) is an uncommon subset of hip OA that results in striking bone and cartilage loss, usually within a matter of weeks to months. Pain is severe and progressive. Rapid destructive osteoarthritis (RDO) most often affects elderly women and is usually unilateral. It is postulated that RDO is likely multifactorial and results from increased levels of bone resorptive enzymes or the use of anti-inflammatory drugs or intra-articular corticosteroids.[45,46] Watanabe et al. postulated that RDO is triggered by mechanical factors, such as insufficiency fractures caused by osteopenia, posterior pelvic tilt, and mild acetabular dysplasia, and progresses to end-stage disease by inflammation that is due to granulation tissue.[47]

Lequesne[48] noted rapid destructive osteoarthritis to be defined by cartilage space narrowing of at least 2 mm per year, whereas in the commonly seen form of OA, cartilage space narrowing of 0.8 mm is noted yearly. Rapid, marked bone loss from the femoral head and acetabulum occurs.[49] Osteophytes are small or absent and buttressing bone is absent; cyst like changes and sclerosis are typical features. Radiographic evidence of osteoporosis may be present. The radiographic features may mimic osteonecrosis with secondary OA, RA, seronegative arthropathies, infection, or neuropathic arthropathy.

Treatment of RDO is joint replacement. Exclusion of septic arthritis and neuropathic arthropathy is of critical importance preoperatively.[15]

KNEE OSTEOARTHRITIS

Radiographic Views

A large array of radiographic examinations are available for evaluating the three compartments of the knee. Generally, the goal is to provide a tangential view of the weight bearing joint so that the thickness of the cartilage space can be assessed. Standard radiographs for evaluation of knee OA include anteroposterior (AP) standing, posterior-anterior (PA), lateral, and tangential patellar views. The anteroposterior radiograph is obtained with the patient supine with the central ray directed 5 degrees in a cephalad direction. The lateral view may be obtained with the knee-flexed (20–35°) or as a cross table radiograph with the knee fully extended. All three joint space compartments can be assessed with these two views. The tunnel view (a frontal view with the knee flexed about 50°) provides additional information about the intercondylar tubercles and the posterior surface of the femoral condyles.[1] The nonweight-bearing tunnel view may demonstrate cartilage loss that is not visible on routine PA, oblique and lateral views or on standing views.[50]

For accurate assessment of joint space loss, weight-bearing radiographs may be helpful. These views reliably show the extent of joint space loss and the degree of angulation and subluxation (varus or valgus).[51] Complete evaluation of the femoropatellar joint, however, requires additional views: (i) The Merchant view is obtained with the patient in the supine position with the knee-flexed in a 45 degrees angle. The tube should be angled 30 degrees toward the floor, (ii) Sunrise view—the patient lies in the prone position with the knee-flexed 90 degrees or more and the X-ray beam strikes the articular surface tangentially and so provides information about the joint space. In this view the patella is deeply situated within the intercondylar fossa **(Figs. 18A to C)**.

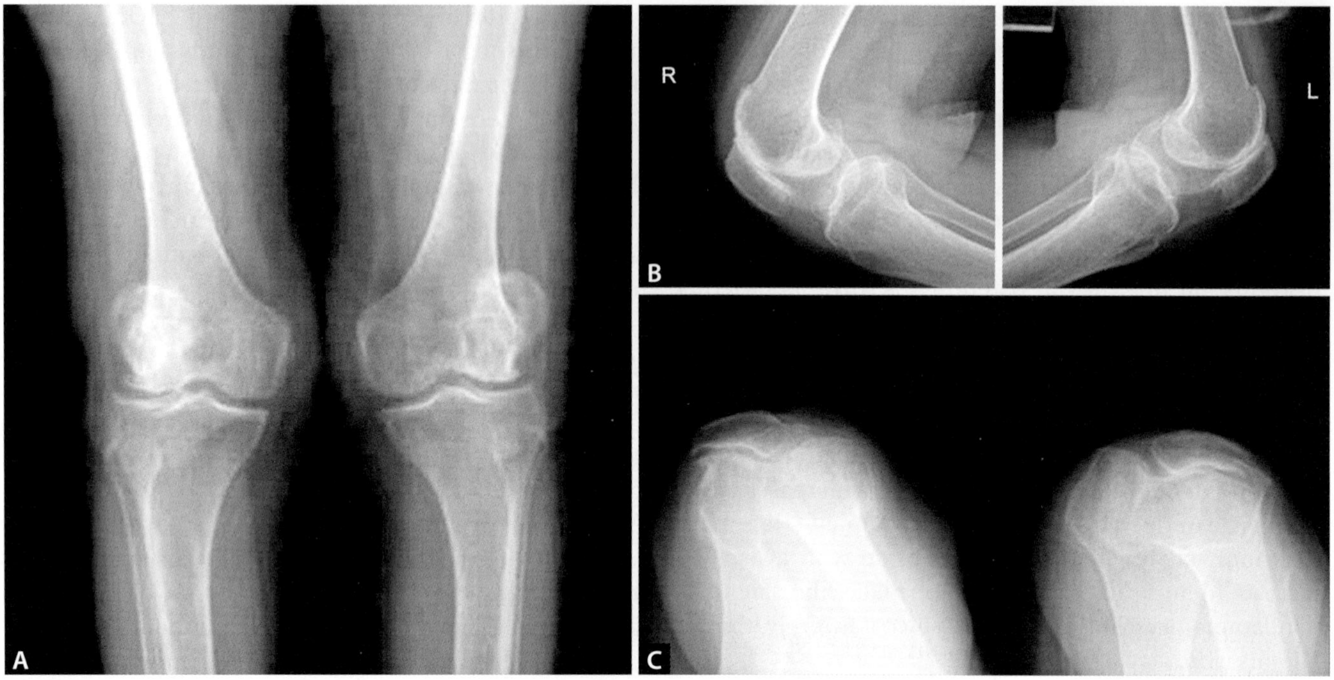

Figs. 18A to C: AP (A), lateral (B) and sunrise (C) views of both knees depict marginal osteophytes involving femorotibial articulation. Degenerative changes are more marked at patellofemoral compartment with osteophytes, subchondral sclerosis and asymmetric reduction in joint space.

The standing view of the legs is an important study for the evaluation of osteoarthritic deformity and is especially valuable for planning osteotomy correction. The view is obtained using a long cassette to include the hips to the ankles. The patient stands with weight equally distributed on both legs and the patellae directed forward. In a normal individual, the mechanical axis (a line drawn from the center of the femoral head to the center of the ankle) passes just medial to the center of the knee-joint. The distance from the mechanical axis to the center of the knee helps quantify the deformity in millimeters and is termed the 'mechanical axis deviation'.[15]

Radiographic Findings

The knee-joint can be divided into three compartments: the lateral femorotibial, medial femorotibial and patellofemoral compartments. In most cases only one or two of these compartments show evidence of osteoarthritic changes. Involvement of all three compartments is rare. Most commonly the medial femorotibial part is involved either alone or along with the patellofemoral compartment.

Cartilage Space

Asymmetric joint space loss of varying severity is the cardinal feature **(Fig. 19)**. The normal cartilage space on a standing view is 3 mm or more. Ahlback[52] defined cartilage space narrowing on standing views as a cartilage space of less than 3 mm, or less than half the width of the same area in the opposite normal knee, the other compartment of the same knee, or by the presence of cartilage space narrowing on weight bearing as compared with nonweight-bearing views. Buckland-Wright et al.[53] classified cartilage space narrowing (on macroradiographic studies), based on the cartilage space width, as mild (3 mm), moderate (between 3 mm and 1.5 mm), and marked (<1.5 mm).

Osteophytes

Four areas of knee osteophyte formation have been described, marginal, intercondylar, tibial spine, and internal. Marginal osteophytes are frequently seen at the femoral and tibial margins of the joint as well as in advanced cases at the intercondylar tubercles. The central type of osteophytes, most common at the femoral condyles, can be misinterpreted as intra-articular bodies.

Subchondral Sclerosis

Cartilage space narrowing is accompanied by subchondral cysts and sclerosis at femoral and tibial locations, most commonly at the tibial plateau.

Increased stress across a compartment may be associated with subchondral sclerosis. A technique called "fractal signature analysis" has been used to study the structure of the subchondral bone on 5 × microfocal radiographs.[54] The structure of the medial tibial subchondral bone was altered in patients who had OA; the abnormality correlated with the degree of cartilage space narrowing. Sclerosis in the subchondral bone of the tibia and femur suggest severe cartilage loss and should suggest the severity of the disorder, even when the cartilage space does not seem to be narrowed.

The patellofemoral compartment is affected frequently in OA, most commonly in combination with involvement of the medial femorotibial compartment **(Figs. 20A and B)**. Osteoarthritis related changes in the patellofemoral space rarely occur in isolation; if such changes are seen, other underlying processes should be excluded.

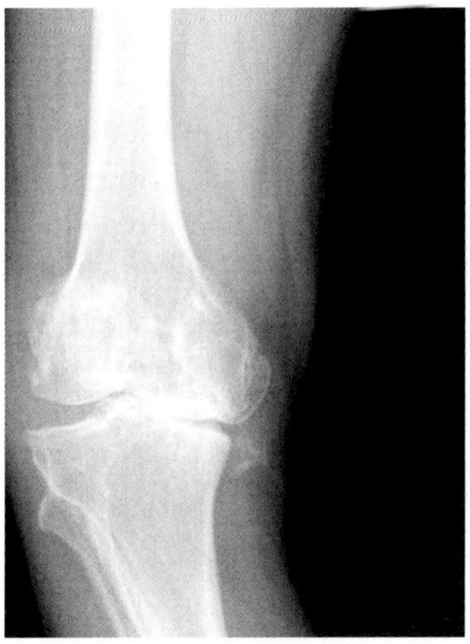

Fig. 19: AP radiograph of the knee shows marginal osteophytes with marked reduction in medial joint space with subchondral sclerosis and cysts.

The patellofemoral findings include joint space loss with deformity at the patellar articular surface in severe cases and osteophytes, which can involve an extensive area at the superior and inferior aspects of the posterior patellar surface **(Figs. 18A to C)**.

Other abnormalities are increased sclerosis at the dorsopatellar surface and subchondral cystic lesions. Two more changes which are nonspecific and found also in other diseases, frequently occur in osteoarthritis: (1) In severe patellofemoral compartment disease, a scalloped cortical defect of the anterior femoral surface as a result of mechanical attrition produced by the patella in a fully extended knee, (2) Bone proliferation at the site of osseous attachment of the quadriceps tendon. Radiographically known as the "tooth sign", this finding consists of hyperostotic changes at the anterior-superior surface of the patella.[55]

Malalignment

In advanced osteoarthritis, angulation and subluxation at the knee joint can occur. Varus and valgus deformities are diagnosed on weight-bearing films. If a line is drawn through the midpoints of the femoral head and the talotibial joint, it should bisect the knee-joint between the intercondylar tubercles. If the axis lies medial to the intercondylar tubercles, the more frequent varus deformity is present; if it lies lateral, a valgus deformity is present. Varus alignment is more often seen in patients who have

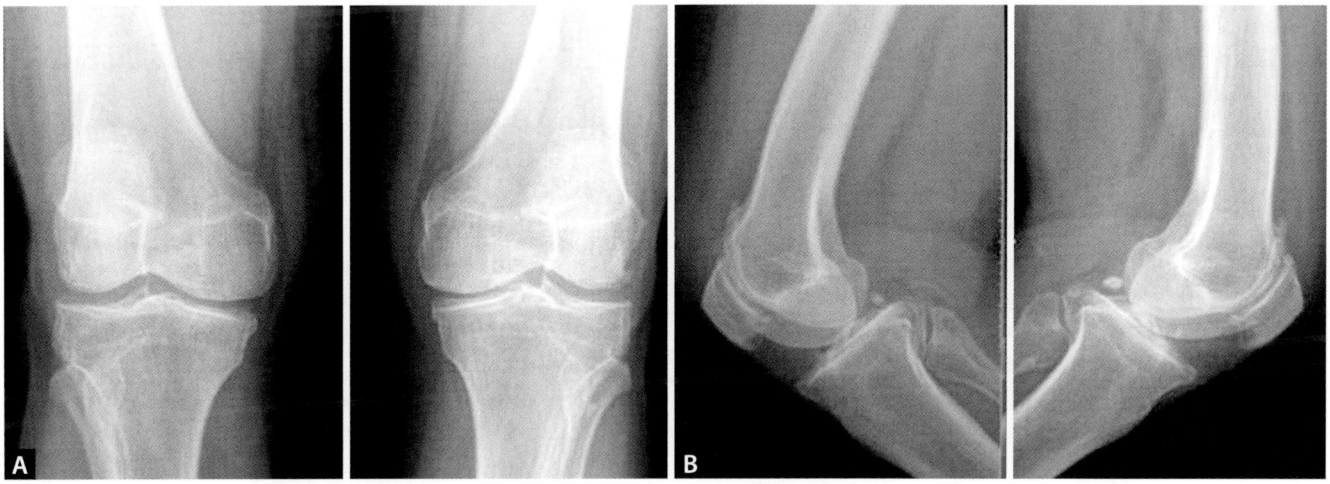

Figs. 20A and B: AP (A) and lateral (B) radiographs of both knees show degenerative arthritis involving medial femorotibial and patellofemoral compartments in the knee joint.

OA than in those who have RA. Varus alignment increased the risk of medial OA progression; valgus alignment increased the risk of lateral progression.[16]

Additional signs include small joint effusions, intra-articular bodies of different sizes and bone proliferation. Sclerosis and flattening of the fabella are signs of sesamoid involvement.

Differential Diagnosis

Distribution of abnormalities among the three joint compartments of the knee can be helpful in establishing the differential diagnosis. Unicompartmental or bicompartmental disease is more typical of OA than is tricom-partmental involvement. Pathologic changes in the medial femorotibial compartment usually indicate OA, whereas the lateral femorotibial space also can be affected in rheumatoid arthritis and CPPD crystal deposition disease.[34]

Symmetric involvement of both femorotibial spaces more frequently is observed in rheumatoid arthritis, ankylosing spondylitis and joint infection. Entities, such as hyperparathyroidism, CPPD crystal deposition disease and chondromalacia patellae may produce isolated femoropatellar disease.[56]

The differential diagnosis of sclerosis, cysts and osteophytes includes CPPD crystal deposition disease (large cystic lesions, fragmentation and deformity) and gout (erosions without joint space loss).[57]

Radiographic Grading of Osteoarthritis

Radiographic grading of OA typically includes assessment of osteophytes and cartilage space narrowing. Other features, such as sclerosis and cyst formation, have lower reproducibility.[58] Clinical and laboratory assessment also may be included.[38]

Of the features of OA, cartilage space width is the most sensitive radiographic measurement for detection of change over time. The reproducibility of cartilage thickness measurement is critical to the follow-up of subjects. Reproducibility in measuring cartilage space relates to several factors, including variations in patient positioning on follow-up visits and measurement technique. Ravaud et al.[59] evaluated the reproducibility of measuring the medial compartment cartilage space in healthy subjects and osteoarthritic patients. The reproducibility was greatest if patient positioning techniques were used with fluoroscopy. The assessment of cartilage space narrowing of the tibiofemoral articulation has higher intraobserver reproducibility than the assessment of sclerosis and cyst formation. Greatest interobserver reproducibility was found for evaluation of osteophytes.[59]

Amongst some specific grading systems, the Kellgren and Lawrence system was the first standardized method for assessing knee OA on radiographs.[60] This system uses a global score. Radiographic features that were believed to be indicative of OA included osteophytes from the joint margins or tibial spines, periarticular ossicles (usually at the proximal interphalangeal or distal interphalangeal joints), cartilage space narrowing with sclerosis of subchondral bone, subchondral "pseudocystic areas", and altered shape of bone ends. Critics of this method noted that greater emphasis was placed on osteophytes than on cartilage space narrowing.[58]

Nagaosa et al.[58] developed an atlas of line drawings of the knee to be used for grading OA in that joint. This atlas included osteophytes and cartilage space narrowing as separate criteria. The use of line drawings (rather than radiographs) allows only one of these abnormalities to be presented on each illustration so that analysis of osteophytes, for example, is not influenced by the presence of cartilage space narrowing. Cartilage space narrowing was assessed separately for men and women.

Altman et al.[61] developed an atlas of individual radiographic features in OA.

SHOULDER OSTEOARTHRITIS

Osteoarthritis of the shoulder may be primary or secondary to other disorders such as RA, chronic rotator cuff tear, trauma, CPPD arthropathy, avascular necrosis, or congenital malformations. Primary OA was believed to be rare so that an underlying cause should be sought in most cases. Phillips and Kattapuram, however, noted that primary OA may not be as rare as many observers have stated.[62]

Radiographic evaluation of the shoulder includes a 40 degrees posterior oblique, external rotation view, internal rotation AP, and scapular lateral ("Y") views. These may be supplemented by outlet views (Y view with 10° caudal angulation), AP angled views for impingement, and axillary views.

The normal alignment of the humeral head with relation to the glenoid on posterior oblique images places the medial epiphyseal-metaphyseal junction of the humerus at about the inferior aspect of the glenoid rim. Thus, an arc normally can be drawn from the medial aspect of the humerus to the lateral aspect of the scapular border. The degree of upward displacement of the humerus could be classified by degrees depending on the position of the humeral baseline to the glenoid.

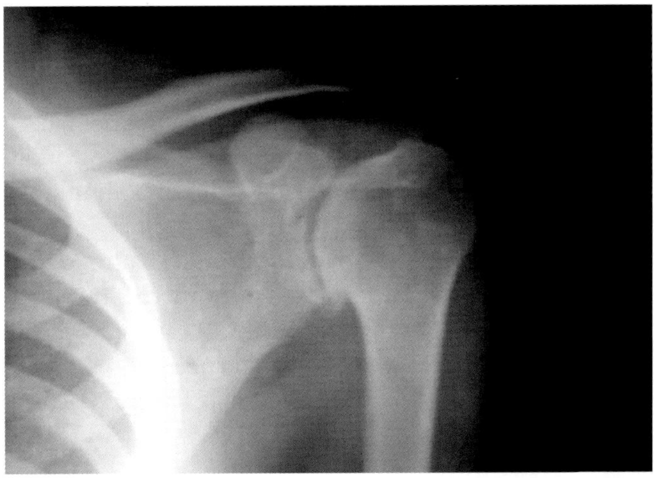

Fig. 21: AP radiograph of left shoulder shows osteophytes with subchondral sclerosis and cysts in patient with degenerative changes.

Normally, the acromiohumeral distance is at least 7 mm and the glenohumeral cartilage space measures about 4 mm.[63]

Radiographic findings of primary OA are similar to osteoarthritic findings in large joints elsewhere. Formation of osteophytes occur along the articular margin of the humeral head and the line of attachment of the labrum to the glenoid. The osteophytes predominate along the anterior and inferior aspects of the humeral articular margin and the lower two-thirds of the glenoid circumference **(Fig. 21)**. Marginal osteophytes develop around the anatomic neck and may be prominent medially. In addition, articular eburnation of the humeral head causes subchondral sclerosis, which can be associated with bony erosions. Eventually, the humeral head becomes flat and enlarged and subluxes posteriorly which results in secondary posterior glenoid erosion. Computed tomography may be useful in preoperative planning to assess glenoid bone stock and the degree of posterior bone loss.[64,65]

ROTATOR CUFF TEAR ARTHROPATHY

Neer et al.[66] postulated that the condition arose from a series of nutritional and mechanical factors that begin with rotator cuff tear. The condition is the end-stage of a series of degenerative changes in the glenohumeral joint. The degenerative changes in the rotator cuff lead to instability and wear and tear of the glenohumeral joint and arthritis. Basic calcium phosphate crystals are generated that induce synovial hyperplasia and secretion of enzymes with subsequent destruction of collagen-containing structures. The clinical syndrome is usually seen in elderly women and is bilateral in more than half of the cases.[67]

Characteristic features of cuff tear arthropathy include elevation of the humeral head with articulation between the humerus and acromian, rounding of the greater tuberosity, cartilage space narrowing and osteophytes formation at the glenohumeral articulation, soft tissue swelling, and calcification with a distended subacromial bursa sometimes visible.[63] Humeral subluxation may be associated with glenoid, acromial, or coracoid wear. CT may be useful to document the degree of bone erosion and subluxation. Magnetic resonance is the investigation of choice.

Medical treatment of cuff-tear arthropathy may be used in mild cases; the use of prostaglandins to inhibit the effects of basic calcium phosphate crystal is being explored. Surgical treatment usually consists of hemiarthroplasty.[68,69]

HAND AND WRIST OSTEOARTHRITIS

Osteoarthritis of the hand is most often seen in middle-aged, postmenopausal women. In descending order, the most common areas of involvement are the distal interphalangeal (DIP) joints, the base of the thumb, the proximal interphalangeal (PIP) joints, and the metacarpophalangeal (MCP) joints.[70] There is a relative symmetry of distribution in both hands.[71] Clinically apparent bony nodules about the DIP joint are called Heberden's nodes; similar features about the PIP joints are called Bouchard's nodes. Most investigators consider these nodes to be palpable osteophytes.[72] Hallmarks of OA of the hand are cartilage space narrowing, subchondral sclerosis, osteophytosis, and subluxation. Cyst formation is rare. Erosion and ankylosis are not typically present.

According to the American College of Rheumatology subcommittee, combining radiographic findings by rows of joints was more sensitive and specific for diagnosing OA of the hand than evaluating individual joints.[73]

Interphalangeal Joints

Multiple joint involvement of the DIP and PIP rows are characteristic features of OA; DIP joint involvement is significantly more common than PIP joint involvement.[70] The highest incidence of hand OA is in the second DIP joint. DIP joint involvement may occur in the absence of PIP involvement; however, it is rare to see solitary PIP changes.

Cartilage loss results in characteristic apposition of the subchondral bone with undulating osseous contours. The wavy contours of the base of the distal phalanx resemble the wings of a seagull—the gull wing sign **(Fig. 22)**.[74] The osteophytes are marginal with narrow, spike-like bony growths extending proximally from the distal phalanx in the DIP joint and extending proximally from the base of the middle phalanx in the PIP joint.[36] There is a predilection for dorsal and volar osteophyte formation, that are, therefore, more apparent with steep oblique and lateral views of the hand.

The osteophytes are continuous with the adjacent cortical and cancellous bone, and, therefore, should not be confused with the irregular new bone formation that is seen in psoriatic arthritis.[74] Subluxation of the joint line usually occurs in the radial and ulnar directions and produces a characteristic zigzag appearance. In contrast, in RA, dorsal or volar subluxation is seen.

Thumb Base

The base of the thumb consists of four trapezial articulations: trapeziometacarpal, trapezioscaphoid, trapezial-index metacarpal, and trapeziotrapezoid. Radiographic changes of OA of the wrist essentially involve only the trapeziometacarpal joint or, less often, the trapezioscaphoid joint **(Fig. 23)**. If degenerative changes are seen at trapezioscaphoid joint, 84% of these patients have coexisting involvement of the trapeziometacarpal joint.[75]

Degenerative changes that are seen in isolation at the trapezioscaphoid joint, however, suggest other causes, including CPPD and RA.

Base of thumb OA can be diagnosed with a high degree of accuracy with standard AP, lateral, and oblique views along with Eaton and Littler's basal joint stress view. This view provides clearer visualization of all trapezial facets. It is a PA 30 degrees oblique view of both thumbs under stress; the patient pushes the radial sides of both thumbs together.

It has been postulated that chronic loading leads to progressive instability and laxity of the trapezial ligaments, which leads to trapezial tilt away from the trapezoid. This tilt causes abnormal shear forces on the trapeziometacarpal joint, which possibly leads to OA.[76]

Metacarpophalangeal Joints

Osteoarthritic changes in the second through fifth MCP joints are classically associated with other arthropathies, such as RA, CPPD, and hemochromatosis or with certain occupations where there is repetitive stress on these joints. Although changes in the MCP joints are common, they are less prominent than changes that are seen in the interphalangeal joints. Cartilage space narrowing seen with OA in the MCP joints tends to be uniform. Marginal osteophytes are smaller than in the interphalangeal joints and subchondral cysts are generally small.

Erosive (Inflammatory) Osteoarthritis

Erosive OA is seen predominantly in the hands of postmenopausal women. Large joint involvement is

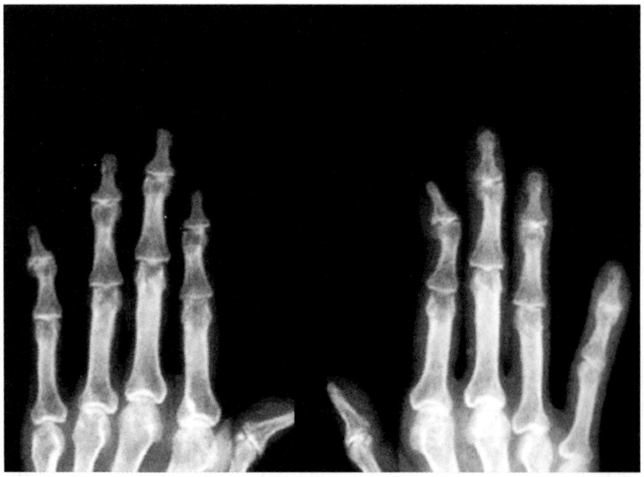

Fig. 22: PA radiograph of both hands depict degenerative changes involving multiple DIP joints. Note is made of Gullwing sign at DIP of right index finger along with radial subluxation. Ulnar subluxation is seen at left little finger DIP which produces a characteristic zig-zag appearance.

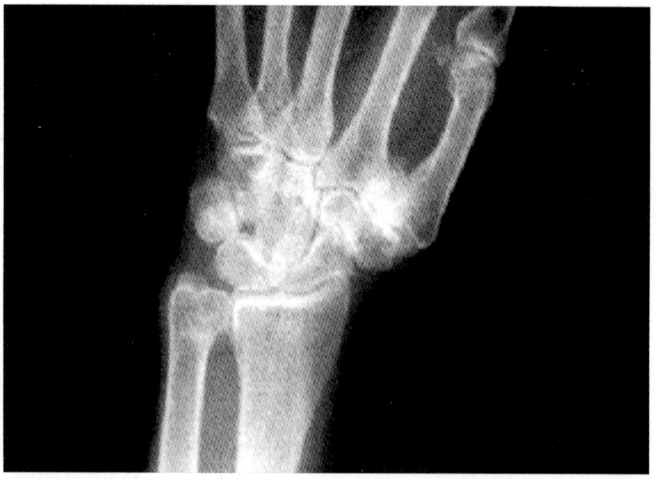

Fig. 23: Standard PA radiograph of the wrist shows joint space narrowing and osteophyte formation that involves the trapezium—1st metacarpal joint with less severe involvement of the trapezoidal-index metacarpal joint. Notice the radial subluxation of the first metacarpal.

rarely reported in the shoulder, hips, knees, spine and metatarsophalangeal joints.

The distribution of joint involvement is nearly identical to noninflammatory OA of the hand with bilateral involvement of the interphalangeal joints, and, to a lesser degree, the trapeziometacarpal, trapezioscaphoid, and MCP joints. The central erosions that are most commonly seen in the interphalangeal joints are characteristic of erosive OA. Eventually, there may be intra-articular bony ankylosis of one or more interphalangeal joints. Clinical evaluation should distinguish this from rheumatoid arthritis and psoriatic arthritis.[77,78]

FOOT AND ANKLE OSTEOARTHRITIS

Osteoarthritis of the ankle is usually secondary to previous fractures or ligamentous injury,[79] often with interruption of the ankle mortise. Chronic repetitive stresses, from occupational or sports activities, and tarsal coalition or surgical fusion of adjacent joints may lead to OA of the ankle. Radiographic findings include asymmetric cartilage space loss, subchondral sclerosis, and cystic changes and osteophytosis. Weight-bearing views have been suggested to better demonstrate cartilage space loss.[79] A bony excrescence form the dorsal aspect of the talus near the head-neck junction is believed to be due to capsular traction and can be seen in athletes; it is not an indicator of OA.

Osteoarthritis of the first metatarsophalangeal joint is termed "hallux rigidus". It occurs twice as often in women as in men, and may be bilateral. Progression of the disorder leads to painful restriction of dorsiflexion of the great toe and a characteristic dorsal osteophyte. There is also loss of joint space. Suggested causes include congenital factors, such as a long first metatarsal, an irregular ball and socket joint, osteochondritis dissecans, dorsiflexion of the toe, pronation of the foot, and trauma.[80]

SECONDARY OSTEOARTHRITIS

Secondary OA is a response to underlying cartilage damage from trauma, arthritis, infection, metabolic conditions or other causes. Several of these underlying conditions may be discovered by careful assessment of radiographs. In particular, OA in an atypical distribution for primary OA or osteoarthritis in young patients should suggest an underlying cause. Osteoarthritis of shoulders, MCPs or elbows should be suspect for secondary OA.[15]

CONCLUSION

Osteoarthritis is a disease affecting all joint structures, not just hyaline articular cartilage. It develops as a consequence of injurious activities acting on a vulnerable-joint. The correlation between structural changes of the joint and patient's symptoms is poor. Radiographically, there is considerable discordance between the presence of osteoarthritis and symptoms in the affected joint. One important reason is that radiographs do not image well the structures that are innervated by pain fibers. These structures include the synovium, the joint capsule, the periphery of the meniscus, ligament insertion sites, and periosteal bone.[81] The finding that these structures are uniquely affected in patients with pain, forms the basis of performing MR imaging prior to any major joint replacement, to see the involvement of various structures.

Natural history of back pain is also poorly understood and causes of low backache remain unknown in majority of cases. Nonspecific imaging findings may often be encountered in asymptomatic subjects and findings seen in symptomatic patients do not necessarily correlate with symptoms.[1] The diagnosis should always be based on combined information from clinical findings and imaging studies for determining appropriate patient management strategy.

REFERENCES

1. Rumboldt Z. Degenerative disorders of the spine. Sem Roentgenol. 2006;41(4):327-62.
2. Gallucci M, Limbucci N, Paonessa A, Splendiani A. Degenerative disease of the spine. Neuroimaging Clin N Am. 2007;17(1):87-103.
3. Malfair D, Beall DP. Imaging the degenerative diseases of the lumbar spine. Magn Reson Imaging Clin N Am. 2007;15(2):221-38.
4. Modic MT, Ross JS. Lumbar degenerative disk disease. Radiology. 2007;245(1):43-61.
5. Kaplan RT, Czervionke LF, Haughton VM. Degenerative Disease of the Spine. In: Scott W Atlas (Ed). Magnetic Resonance Imaging of the Brain and Spine Vol II, 4th edn. Philadelphia, Lippincott Williams and Wilkins; 2002.
6. Miller TT. Imaging of disk disease and degenerative spondylosis of the lumbar spine. Semin Ultrasound CT MR. 2004;25(6):506-22.
7. Fardon DF, Milette PC. Nomenclature and classification of lumbar disk pathology. Recommendations of the Combined task Forces of the North American Spine Society, American Society of Spine Radiology, and American Society of Neuroradiology. Spine (Phila Pa 1976). 2001;26(5):E93-E113.
8. Costello RF, Beall DP. Nomenclature and standard reporting terminology of intervertebral disk herniation. Magn Reson Imaging Clin N Am. 2007;15(2):167-74.
9. Bozzao A, Gallucci M, Masciocchi C, Aprile I, Barile A, Passariello R. Lumbar disk herniation: MR imaging assessment of natural history in patients treated without surgery. Radiology. 1992;185(1):135-41.

10. Chung CB, Vande Berg BC, Tavernier T, Cotten A, Laredo JD, Vallee C, Malghem J. End plate marrow changes in the asymptomatic lumbosacral spine: frequency, distribution and correlation with age and degenerative changes. Skeletal Radiol. 2004;33(7):399-404.
11. Roudsari B, Jarvik JG. Lumbar spine MRI for low back pain: indications and yield. Am J Roentgenol. 2010;195: 550-9.
12. Felson DT. An update on the pathogenesis and epidemiology of osteoarthritis. Radiol Clin North Am. 2004;42:1-9.
13. Lawrence RC, Helmick CG, Arnett FC, et al. Estimates of the prevalence of arthritis and selected musculoskeletal disorders in the United States. Arthritis Rheum. 1998;41:778-99.
14. Felson DT, Naimark A, Anderson J, et al. The prevalence of knee osteoarthritis in the elderly. Arthritis Rheum. 1987;30(8):914-8.
15. Karçaaltincaba M, Aktas A. Dual-energy CT revisited with multidetector CT: review of principles and clinical applications. Diagn Interv Radiol. 2011;17(3):181-94.
16. Gupta KB, Duryea J, Weissman BN. Radiographic evaluation of osteoarthritis. Radiol Clin North Am. 2004;42:11-41.
17. Felson DT, Lawerence RC, Dieppe PA, et al. Osteoarthritis: New insights. Part 1: The disease and its risk factors. Ann Intern Med. 2000;133(8):635-46.
18. Spector TD, Cicuttini F, Baker J, et al. Genetic influence on osteoarthritis in women: a twin study. BMJ. 1996;312:940-4.
19. Dequeker J, Boonen N, Aerssens J, et al. Inverse relationship osteoarthritis—osteoporosis: What is the evidence? What are the consequences? (editorial). Br J Rheumatol. 1996;35:813-20.
20. Zhang Y, Hannan MT, Chaisson CE, et al. Bone mineral density and risk of incident and progressive radiographic knee osteoarthritis in women: the Framingham study. J Rheumatol. 2000;27:1032-7.
21. McAlindon TE, Felson DT, Zhang Y, et al. Relation of dietary intake and serum levels of vitamin D to progression of osteoarthritis of the knee among participants in the Framingham study. Ann Intern Med. 1996;125:353-9.
22. Lane NE, Lin P, Christiansen L, et al. Association of mild acetabular dysplasia with an increased risk of incident hip osteoarthritis in elderly white women. Arthritis Rheum. 2000;43:400-4.
23. Ross HP, Adalberth T, Dahlberg L, et al. Osteoarthritis of the knee after injury to the anterior cruciate ligament or meniscus: The influence of time and age. Osteoarthritis Cartilage. 1995;3:261-7.
24. Felson DT, Zhang YQ. An update on the epidemiology of knee and hip osteoarthritis with a view to prevention. Arthritis Rheum. 1998;41:1343-55.
25. Grodzinsky AJ, Levenston ME, Jin M, et al. Cartilage tissue remodeling in response to mechanical forces. Ann Rev Biomed Engr. 2000;2:691-713.
26. Croft P, Coggon D, Cruddas M, et al. Osteoarthritis of the hip: An occupational disease in farmers. BMJ. 1992;304:1269-72.
27. Anderson J, Felson DT. Factors associated with osteoarthritis of the knee in the first National Health and Nutrition Examination Survey (NHANES). Am J Epidemiol. 1988;128:179-89.
28. Altman R, Asch E, Bloch D, et al. Development of criteria for the classification and reporting of osteoarthritis. Classification of osteoarthritis of the knee. Diagnostic and Therapeutic Criteria Committee of the American Rheumatism Association. Arthritis Rheum. 1986; 29(8):1039-49.
29. Bancroft LW, Peterson JJ, Kransdorf MJ. Cysts, geodes, and erosions. Radiol Clin North Am. 2004;42:73-87.
30. Cameron HU, Fornasier VL. Trabecular stress fractures. Clin Orthop Rel Res. 1975;11:266.
31. Havdrup T, Hulth A, Telhag H. The subchondral bone in osteoarthritis and rheumatoid arthritis of the knee: A histologic and microradiographical study. Acta Orthop Scan. 1976;47:345.
32. Freund E. The pathological significance of intra-articular pressure. Edinburgh Med J. 1940;47:192.
33. Jaffe HL. Metabolic, Degenerative and Inflammatory Diseases of Bones and Joints. Philadelphia, Lea and Febiger; 1972.735.
34. Resnick D, Niwayama G. Degenerative disease of extraspinal locations. In: Resnick D (Ed). Diagnosis of Bone and Joint Disorders, 3rd edn. Philadelphia, WB Saunders; 1995. p. 1263.
35. Milgram JW. Morphologic alterations of the subchondral bone in advanced degenerative arthritis. Clinical Orthop Rel Res. 1983;173:293-312.
36. Resnick D. Degenerative diseases of extraspinal locations. In: Diagnosis of bone and joint disorders. Vol. 3, 2nd edn. Philadelphia, WB Saunders; 1988. pp. 1365-479.
37. Yochum T, Rowe LJ. Essentials of skeletal radiology, Vol. 1, 2nd edn, Baltimore (MD). Williams and Wilkins; 1996.
38. Lequesne MG, Laredo JD. The faux profile (oblique view) of the hip in the standing position. Contribution to the evaluation of osteoarthritis of the adult hip. Ann Rheum Dis. 1998;57(11):676-81.
39. Altman R, Alarcon G, Appelrouth D, et al. The American College of Rheumatology criteria for the classification and reporting of osteoarthritis of the hip. Arthritis Rheum. 1991;34(5):505-14.
40. Altman RD, Fries JF, Bloch DA, et al. Radiographic assessment of progression in osteoarthritis. Arthritis Rheum. 1987;30(11):1214-25.
41. Resnick D. Patterns of migration of the femoral head in osteoarthritis of the hip. Roentgenographic-pathologic correlation and comparison with rheumatoid arthritis. Am J Roentgenol Radium Ther Nucl Med. 1975;124(1):67-74.
42. Haller J, Resnick D, Greenway G, et al. Juxta-acetabular ganglionic (or synovial) cysts: CT and MR features. J Comput Assist Tomogr. 1989;13(6):976-83.
43. Dixon T, Benjamin J, Lund P, et al. Femoral neck buttressing: A radiographic and histologic analysis. Skeletal Radiol. 2000;29(10):587-92.
44. Moore RJ, Fazzalari N, Manthey BA, et al. The relationship between head-neck-shaft angle, calcar width, articular cartilage thickness and bone volume in arthrosis of the hip. Br J Rheumatol. 1994;33(5):432-6.

45. Yamamoto T, Bullough PG. The role of subchondral insufficiency fracture in rapid destruction of the hip joint: A preliminary report. Arthritis Rheum. 2000;43(11): 2423-7.
46. Komiya S, Inoue A, Sasaguri Y, et al. Rapidly destructive arthropathy of the hip. Studies on bone resorptive factors in joint fluid with a theory of pathogenesis. Clin Orthop Rel Res. 1992;284:273-82.
47. Watanabe W, Itoi E, Yamada S. Early MRI findings of rapidly destructive coxarthrosis. Skeletal Radiol. 2002; 31(1):35-8.
48. Lequesne M. Rapidly progressing destructive diseases of the hip. Ann Radiol (Paris). 1993;36(1):62-4. [in French]
49. Rosenberg ZS, Shankman S, Steiner GC, et al. Rapid destructive osteoarthritis: Clinical, radiographic, and pathologic features. Radiology. 1992;182(1):213-6.
50. Resnick D, Vint V. The "tunnel" view in assessment of cartilage loss in osteoarthritis of the knee. Radiology. 1980;137(2):547-8.
51. Jonsson K, Buckwalter K, Helvie M, et al. Precision of Hyaline cartilage thickness measurements. Acta Radiol. 1992;33:234.
52. Ahlback S. Osteoarthritis of the knee. A radiographic investigation. Acta Radiol Diagn (Stockh). 1968;(Suppl 277):7-72.
53. Buckland-Wright JR, Macfarlane DG, Jasani MK, et al. Quantitative microfocal radiographic assessment of osteoarthritis of the knee from weight bearing tunnel and semiflexed standing views. J Rheumatol. 1994;21(9): 1734-41.
54. Buckland-Wright JC, Lynch JA, Macfarlane DG. Fractal signature analysis measures cancellous bone organisation in macroradiographs of patients with knee osteoarthritis. Ann Rheum Dis. 1996;55(10):749-55.
55. McAlindon TE, Snow S, Cooper C, et al. Radiographic patterns of osteoarthritis of the knee joint in the community: The importance of the patellofemoral joint. Ann Rheum Dis. 1992;51(7):844-9.
56. Resnick D. Letter to the editor. J Bone Joint Surg [Am]. 1982;64:633.
57. Ledingham JM, Preston BJ, Doherty M. Cystic changes in the head of the fibula in osteoarthritis. J Bone Joint Surg [Br]. 1993;75:429.
58. Nagaosa Y, Mateus M, Hassan B, et al. Development of a logically devised line drawing atlas for grading of knee osteoarthritis. Ann Rheum Dis. 2000;59(8):587-95.
59. Ravaud P, Giraudeau B, Auleley GR, et al. Variability in knee radiographing: Implication for definition of radiological progression in medial knee osteoarthritis. Ann Rheum Dis. 1998;57(10):624-9.
60. Kellgren J, Lawrence J. Radiological assessment of osteoarthrosis. Ann Rheum Dis. 1957;16:494-501.
61. Altman R, Hochberg M, Murphy WA, et al. Atlas of individual radiographic features in osteoarthritis. Osteoarthritis Cartilage. 1995;3:3-70.
62. Phillips Jr WC, Kattapuram SV. Osteoarthritis: with emphasis on primary osteoarthritis of the shoulder. Del Med J. 1991;63(10):609-13.
63. Pons-Estel BA, Gimenez C, Sacnun M, et al. Familial osteoarthritis and Milwaukee shoulder associated with calcium pyrophosphate and apatite crystal deposition. J Rheumatol. 2000;27(2):471-80.
64. Green A, Norris TR. Imaging techniques for glenohumeral arthritis and glenohumeral arthroplasty. Clin Orthop Rel Res. 1994;(307):7-17.
65. Walch G, Boulahia A, Boileau P, et al. Primary glenohumeral osteoarthritis: Clinical and radiographic classification. The Aequalis Group. Acta Orthop Belg. 1998;64(Suppl 2):46-52.
66. Neer II CS, Craig EV, Fukuda H. Cuff-tear arthropathy. J Bone Joint Surg Am. 1983;65(9):1232-44.
67. Jensen KL, Williams Jr GR, Russell IJ, et al. Rotator cuff tear arthropathy. J Bone Joint Surg Am. 1999;81(9):1312-24.
68. Zeman CA, Arcand MA, Cantrell JS, et al. The rotator cuff-deficient arthritic shoulder: Diagnosis and surgical management. AJ Am Acad Orthop Surg. 1998;6(6):337-48.
69. Weiss JJ, Good A, Schumacher HR. Four cases of "Milwankee shoulder" with a description of clinical presentation and long-term treatment. J Am Geriatr Soc. 1985;33(3):202-5.
70. Chaisson CE, Zhang Y, McAlindon TE, et al. Radiographic hand osteoarthritis: Incidence, patterns, and influence of pre-existing disease in a population based sample. J Rheumatol. 1997;24(7):1337-43.
71. Lane NE, Bloch DA, Jones HH. Osteoarthritis in the hand: A comparison of handedness and hand use. J Rheumatol. 1989;16(5):637-42.
72. Alexander CJ. Heberden's and Bouchard's nodes. Ann Rheum Dis. 1999;58(11):675-8.
73. Altman R, Alarcon G, Appelrouth D, et al. The American college of Rheumatology criteria for the classification and reporting of osteoarthritis of the hand. Arthritis Rheum. 1990;33(11):1601-10.
74. Martel W, Stuck KJ, Dworin AM, et al. Erosive osteoarthritis and psoriatic arthritis: A radiologic comparison in the hand, wrist, and foot. Am J Roentgenol 1980;134(1):125-35.
75. North ER, Eaton RG. Degenerative joint disease of the trapezium: A comparative radiographic and anatomic study. J Hand Surg Am. 1983;8(2):160-6.
76. Bettinger PC, Linscheid RL, Cooney III WP, et al. Trapezial tilt: A radiographic correlation with advanced trapeziometacarpal joint arthritis. J Hand Surg Am. 2001;26(4):692-7.
77. Belhorn LR, Hess EV. Erosive osteoarthritis. Semin Arthritis Rheum. 1993;22(5):298-306.
78. Smith D, Braunstein EM, Brandt KD, et al. A radiographic comparison of erosive osteoarthritis and idiopathic nodal osteoarthritis. J Rheumatol. 1992;19(6):896-904.
79. Harrington KD. Degenerative arthritis of the ankle secondary to long-standing lateral ligament instability. J Bone Joint Surg Am. 1979;61(3):354-61.
80. Shereff MJ, Baumhauer JF. Hallux rigidus and osteoarthrosis of the first metatarsophalangeal joint. J Bone Joint Surg Am. 1998;80(6):898-908.
81. Dye SF, Vaupel GL, Dye CC. Conscious neurosensory mapping of the internal structures of the human knee without intra-articular anaesthesia. Am J Sports Med. 1998;26:773-7.

CHAPTER 196

Skeletal Disorders of Metabolic and Endocrine Origin

Alpana Manchanda, Arun Kumar Gupta

Metabolic bone disease encompasses a diverse group of disorders associated with altered calcium and phosphorus homeostasis.[1,2] Although many of these disorders are quite common, they may be difficult to distinguish on the basis of history, physical examination and imaging studies.[1,2]

To the clinician, metabolic bone disease is often silent until the patient presents with fracture, the ultimate complication of many metabolic disorders. Other patients may however, present with a clinical history of back pain and a nonspecific radiologic finding of generalized osteopenia.[3] At this stage prior to fracture, accurate diagnosis is crucial. Understanding their diverse manifestations on imaging studies may allow early diagnosis.

The manifestations of endocrine derangements in the skeletal system depend on the age of the patient at the time of presentation. In general, skeletal manifestation in childhood and infancy consist of disturbances in growth and maturation and in adulthood, disturbances in maintenance and metabolism.

DISORDERS OF METABOLIC ORIGIN

The most common types of metabolic bone diseases are acquired disorders; nonetheless, rare forms frequently are genetically based and cause intrinsic alterations in the bone cell population.

The various metabolic bone disorders may be grouped according to their underlying defects:

- Defect in osteoid formation—Scurvy
- Defect in mineralization—Rickets/Osteomalacia
- Disorder with increased bone resorption—Hyperparathyroidism (HPT)
- Disorder with no defect in mineralization and osteoid formation but decreased bone mass—Osteoporosis
- Miscellaneous—Fluorosis, heavy metal poisoning, hypervitaminosis. **Table 1** lists the metabolic profile with reference values.

Table 1: Metabolic profile–reference values.

1.	Serum calcium	8.7–10.2 mg/dL
2.	Ionized calcium	4.5–5.3 mg/dL
3.	Serum phosphorus	2.4–4.1 mg/dL
4.	Alkaline phosphatase	223–635 U/L
5.	Vitamin D	>25 ng/mL
6.	Serum parathormone	8–51 pg/mL
7.	Serum ascorbic acid	<0.6 mg/100 mL

RICKETS AND OSTEOMALACIA

Rickets in children and osteomalacia in adults are a group of bone disorders in which there is incomplete mineralization of normal osteoid tissue. Both conditions usually result from an abnormality in vitamin D metabolism. The biochemical and histological abnormalities are identical in the two conditions while skeletal manifestations differ depending upon the age of the patient at the time of onset of disease.

Vitamin D is a steroid hormone which in normal individuals is produced by skin exposure to sunlight and obtained from the diet.[4] To attain its active form, vitamin D must undergo two hydroxylations, first in the liver and second in the kidneys **(Fig. 1)**. The primary function of vitamin D is to maintain calcium and phosphate homeostasis, thereby ensuring normal mineralization of the skeleton. The target areas for vitamin D action include bone, gastrointestinal tract, kidneys and parathyroid gland.[1,4,5]

Causes

Rickets and osteomalacia occur due to many causes **(Table 2)**, most common being due to dietary deficiency of vitamin D called vitamin D deficient rickets or nutritional rickets. Many abnormalities in vitamin D metabolism can potentially result in rickets and osteomalacia. These include malabsorption syndromes, hepatobiliary diseases, renal diseases, drugs and neoplasms.[1,4]

Clinical Features

Clinical findings of rickets and osteomalacia are highly variable and depend on the etiology and severity of the disorder, as well as the age of patient at the time of presentation.[1,4,5] In the first six months of life, rickets can present with tetany or convulsions. In most children with rickets, skeletal growth is stunted and they present with swollen, tender joints. With advanced disease, they may present with irritability, weakness and bony deformities. The most notable clinical finding is soft tissue swelling occurring around the growth plates due to hypertrophied cartilage. Clinically, enlargement of wrists and costal cartilage are most suggestive of the disease with a specificity of 81% and 64% respectively.[6]

In adults, findings of osteomalacia are more subtle. Initial symptoms include fatigue, malaise or bone pain. With advanced disease, proximal muscle weakness and abnormal gait may be present.[1,5] Typical manifestations of osteomalacia consist of bone pain especially in the hips and muscle weakness.

Biochemical Findings

On laboratory evaluation, the serum calcium and phosphorus may be normal or slightly reduced while serum alkaline phosphatase levels are increased.

Pathology of Rickets and Osteomalacia

There is remarkable similarity in the biochemical and histologic abnormalities in rickets and osteomalacia. The characteristic changes of rickets are identified in the growth plates prior to closure while abnormalities of osteomalacia are seen in the mature areas of trabecular and cortical bone.

In order to understand the changes of rickets, the general structure and organization of growth plate is discussed briefly. The growth plate is a complex structure which is located at the ends of long bones and situated between the epiphysis and metaphysis.[4] Although it is

Table 2: Causes of rickets and osteomalacia.

Abnormalities of Vitamin D Metabolism	
1.	*Deficiency conditions*: • Dietary deficiency of vitamin D • Lack of exposure to ultraviolet light
2.	*Absorption defects*: • Gastrointestinal malabsorption • Biliary atresia • Small bowel bypass surgery
3.	*Hepatic diseases*: • Cirrhosis • Hepatitis
4.	Anticonvulsant therapy
5.	*Renal insufficiency*: • Type I vitamin D-dependent rickets (VDDR) • Type II VDDR
Rickets and Osteomalacia Secondary to Phosphate Loss	
1.	X-linked hypophosphatemia, genetic (Vitamin D resistant rickets)
2.	Primary hypophosphatemic rickets, acquired
3.	*Renal tubular acidosis*: • Type I (distal) renal tubular acidosis (RTA) • Type II (proximal) RTA
4.	Tumor-associated phosphate deficiency
5.	Chemotherapeutic drug induced rickets
Miscellaneous	
1.	Metaphyseal chondrodysplasia (Schmid type)
2.	Hypophosphatasia
3.	Atypical axial osteomalacia

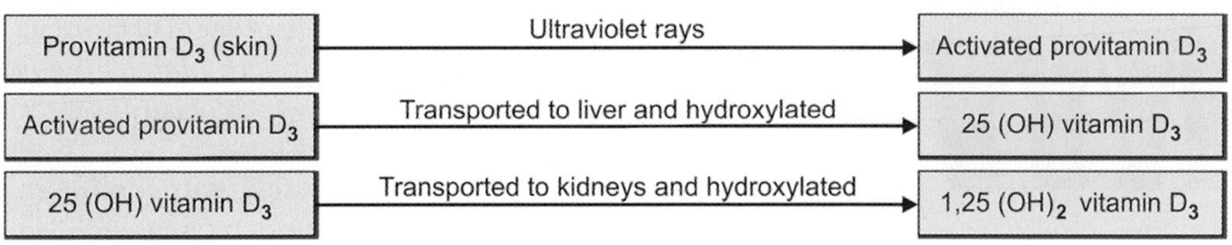

Fig. 1: Pathway for activation of vitamin D_3.

adjacent to the epiphysis, functionally it is part of the shaft. Histologically, the cellular arrangement of the normal growth plate is characterized by order, with progressive increase in the number and size of cartilaginous cells from the epiphysis to metaphysis. The normal epiphysis has four zones. From the epiphyseal ossification center towards the shaft the various zones are—the resting zone, proliferating zone, hypertrophic zone and zone of primary and secondary spongiosa. The hypertrophic zone is further subdivided into zones of maturation, degeneration and provisional calcification **(Fig. 2)**.

In rickets, there is disorganization of the growth plate and adjacent metaphysis. The resting and proliferative zones of the cartilaginous growth plate are not significantly altered from the normal pattern. However, the zone of maturation is grossly abnormal with a disorganized increase in the number of cells and a loss of normal columnar pattern. This cell mass results in an increase in length and width of the growth plate. Overall, there is diminished quantity of calcified osteoid and an increase in uncalcified osteoid which casts increased radiolucency on the radiographs.

Osteomalacia results from insufficient, delayed or defective mineralization of cortical and spongy bone. Histologically, it is characterized by abnormal quantities

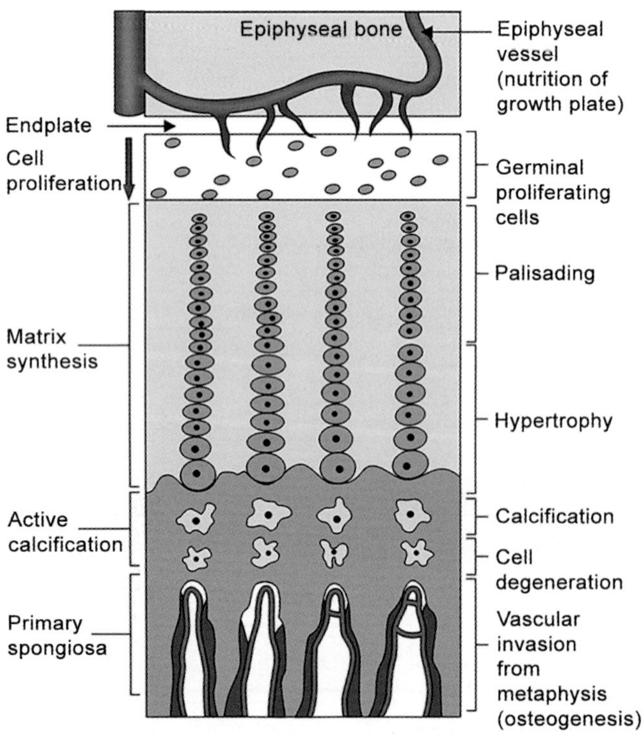

Fig. 2: Structure of the growth plate showing normal cellular organization.

of inadequately mineralized bone matrix called osteoid, coating the surfaces of trabeculae and lining the haversian canals in the cortex. These layers of osteoid are often referred to as osteoid seams. Osteoid seams are not pathognomic of osteomalacia and may be found in other active metabolic states associated with high bone turnover. However, there is an increase in both the number and width of the osteoid seams in osteomalacia.

Radiological Features

Although there is a significant overlap between rickets and osteomalacia, their radiologic findings are quite different and hence, they will be discussed separately.

RICKETS

In the earliest stage, rachitic changes are not detectable radiologically. Biochemical and histologic changes develop several weeks prior to the appearance of the conclusive changes in the radiographs.[7]

The most common and nonspecific radiologic finding in patients of rickets is osteopenia.[1,4,5] Characteristic changes occur at the open growth plate.[5] These changes are best seen in those areas showing most active growth. The distal ends of radius and ulna are the optimal site for the demonstration of the earliest lesion.[7] Significant changes are often seen in the ulna when the radius appears to be normal as the distal ulnar growth plate grows more rapidly than the distal radius. Therefore, the ulna is a more sensitive indicator of rickets at the wrist.

Radiographic abnormalities reflect the disordered proliferation of cartilaginous cells in the zone of hypertrophy along with the deficient mineralization in the zone of provisional calcification.[4,5] The zone of provisional calcification is a band of calcification which marks the end of the radiolucent growth plate and beginning of the radiographically calcified metaphysis.

As the rachitic changes are more advanced at the fastest growing growth plates, radiographs of the most active sites should be undertaken. In order of decreasing activity, the most active growth plates are costochondral junction of the middle ribs, the distal femur, the proximal humerus, both ends of tibia, and the distal ulna and radius.

The characteristic radiologic features of rickets seen at the end of long bones in order of occurrence are:

1. *Widening of the growth plate* is the *earliest specific radiologic change* which occurs as a result of increase in cartilaginous cell mass.[4]
2. *Irregular metaphyseal margins* (paint brush metaphyses) occurs due to fraying and disorganization of the spongy bone in the metaphyseal region.

3. Further progression of the disease leads to *widening and cupping* of the *metaphysis* **(Figs. 3A and B)**. This can be explained by the protrusion of the bulky mass of cartilaginous cells in the zone of hypertrophy into the poorly mineralized metaphysis. Cupping of the distal end of the ulna in younger infants is not necessarily abnormal as it has been observed in some nonrachitic infants during the first months of life.[7] Cupping is common in both ends of the fibula and the distal ends of the ulna and tibia. Metaphyseal cupping is however never found in the bones of the elbow.[8]
4. Similar process occurs on the epiphyseal side of the growth plate. The defective maturation and mineralization results in an *epiphysis* that is *osteopenic* and has irregular, indistinct borders and shows *delayed appearance of ossification centers.*
5. The shafts of long bones may appear normal when changes are first detected in the metaphysis. *Rarefaction* of the *shaft* becomes evident a few weeks later due to loss of mineral content. The cortex becomes thin with a coarse texture.
6. *Skeletal deformities* are the most common complication detected radiologically, appearance and location of which depend on age and the part in which disease develops.[4]
   i. *Skull*: It is particularly affected in the early months of life as it has to accommodate the rapidly growing brain. There is excess osteoid deposition in frontal and parietal regions and posterior flattening due t o supine posture of the infant. This results in squared configuration of the skull known as "craniotabes" **(Fig. 4A)**.
   ii. *Long bones*: In early childhood, more rapid growth occurs in the long bones and bowing deformities of arms and legs are common which can be related to the sitting position assumed by infants and children. Bowing also is a result of displacement of the growth centers owing to the asymmetrical musculotendinous pulls on the weakened growth plate[9] **(Fig. 4B)**. Bulbous enlargement of the costochondral junctions, particularly those of the middle ribs can be seen (rachitic rosary **Fig. 4C**), which can indent the pleural surface or even the thymic shadow.[6]
   iii. *Spine*: Scoliosis and vertebral end plate deformities may develop in older children as the effects of weight bearing become more important. Scoliosis coupled with bending deformities of long bones results in an overall decrease in height of the child.
   iv. *Pelvis*: The protrusion of the hip and spine into the soft pelvis produces a triradiate configuration of the pelvis. Such a pelvic deformity may cause considerable difficulty during parturition.
   v. *Fractures*: In long standing cases of rickets, trivial trauma may result in fracture of the weakened undermineralized bone **(Figs. 5A and B)**.

In severe malnutrition, rickets may be associated with scurvy and protein deficiency.

Signs of Healing Rickets

Radiological evidence of healing is seen within 2–3 weeks of adequate therapy and total recalcification is usually complete in two months.[10] The signs of healing rickets are:

- Reappearance of the dense zone of provisional calcification. This is the first evidence of healing and

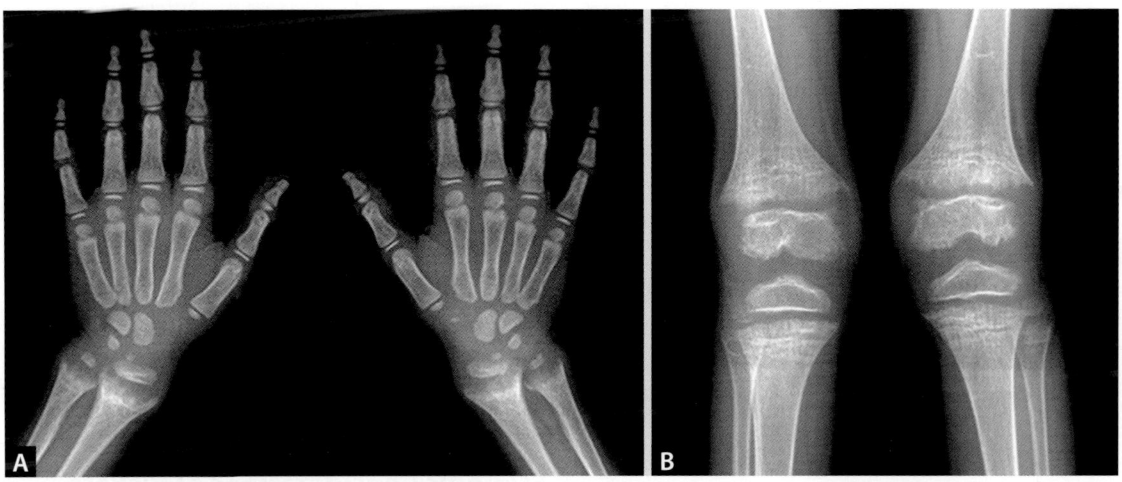

Figs. 3A and B: Rickets: X-ray bilateral wrists and knees AP view: Typical changes of active rickets consisting of fraying, irregularity of distal radius and ulnar metaphysis and distal femoral and proximal tibial metaphysis with widening of the growth plates at the wrists and knees. The adjacent epiphysis and diaphysis are osteopenic.

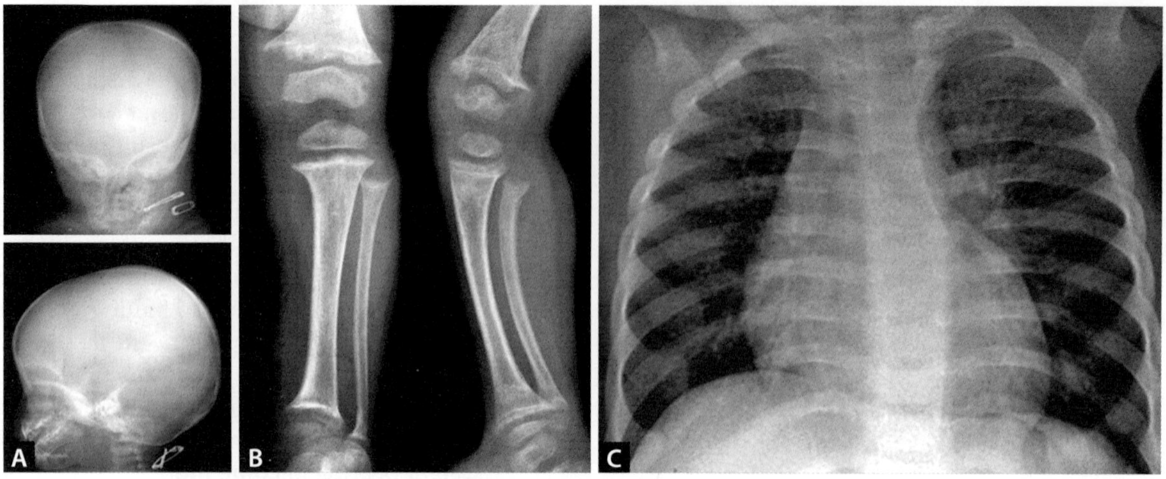

Figs. 4A to C: Skeletal deformities in rickets: (A) Squared configuration of the skull in the neonatal period: "Craniotabes"; (B) Marked anterior bowing of the tibia and fibula with rachitic changes. The visualized bones are osteopenic; (C) "Rachitic rosary": Widened anterior ends of ribs due to hypertrophy of costochondral junction.

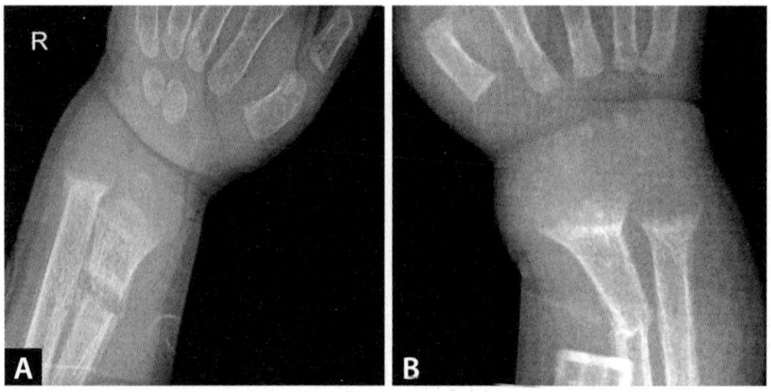

Figs. 5A and B: X-ray wrists of two infants with rickets. The bones are markedly osteopenic with fracture of distal ends of radius in both.

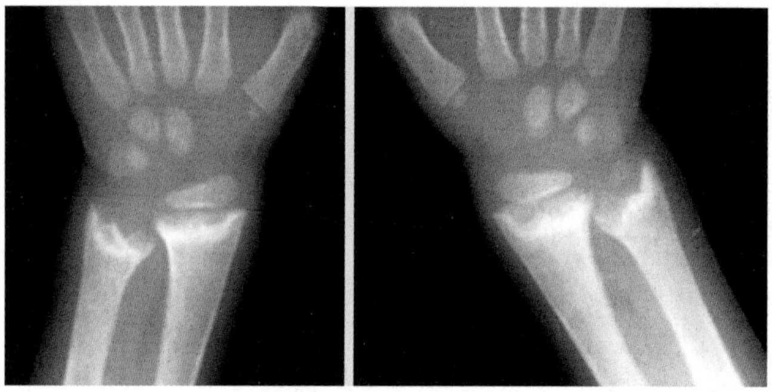

Fig. 6: Healing rickets: X-ray B/L wrists showing reappearance of the dense zone of provisional calcification at the metaphysis.

is seen radiologically as a transverse line of increased density which appears beyond the visible end of shaft with a metaphysis interposed between the two radiolucent areas **(Fig. 6)**. Further mineralization of the osteoid unites this with the metaphysis.

- Increase in cupping of the healing metaphysis is seen as compared to the cupping seen in the active stage of rickets.
- Recalcification of the subperiosteal osteoid may produce a thick envelope of cortex that surrounds the shaft. This thick, opaque envelope along the shaft may be of uniform density or lamellated.
- Epiphyseal ossification center which were ill-defined and osteopenic in the active stage of rickets become sharply defined in the healing stage. In severe cases, the ossification centers may become invisible during the active stage of rickets and reappear when they are recalcified during healing, erroneously suggesting a rapid advance in skeletal maturation.

When the patient is on intermittent or inadequate treatment, the process of calcification and repair is irregular. Radiologically, patchy sclerosis of the metaphysis is seen, sometimes with alternating sclerotic and lucent bands.

Sequelae

Complete healing and restoration of normal structures is the rule in rickets even when severe changes are present during the active stage.[7]

Central rarefaction of ossification centers and cortical thickening of tubular bones may remain for a long time. Bowing and angulation deformities are not uncommon due to weakened bones.

Etiologic Considerations of Rickets

Once the radiographic diagnosis of rickets is made, an attempt must be made to determine a possible etiology.

The causes can be:

I. Abnormalities of vitamin D metabolism
II. Secondary to renal tubular loss of phosphate
III. Conditions in which there is no known abnormality of vitamin D metabolism or calcium-phosphorus homeostasis.

ABNORMALITIES OF VITAMIN D METABOLISM

Renal Osteodystrophy

Renal osteodystrophy is a term which is used to describe the bony changes in patients with chronic renal insufficiency. In children, end stage renal disease is commonly due to loss of renal parenchyma because of structural abnormalities of the urinary tract. While, in adults, chronic glomerulonephritis is the main cause.

Due to chronic renal disease there is phosphate retention along with impaired ability to form 1,25 dihydroxy vitamin D_3. Low levels of vitamin D and an excess of phosphate stimulate an excess parathyroid hormone resulting in secondary hyperparathyroidism.

Radiographic changes in renal osteodystrophy, therefore, reflect a combination of different processes including rickets/osteomalacia, secondary hyperparathyroidism and osteosclerosis. Radiological changes in rickets have already been described. The characteristic radiological changes in secondary hyperparathyroidism consists of bone resorption which may be subperiosteal, intracortical, endosteal or subligamentous; presence of brown tumors; soft tissue and vascular calcification. Increased bone density or osteosclerosis is either focal or diffuse **(Fig. 7A)** and is commonly seen in the spine but also occurs in the pelvis ribs, skull and tubular bones. The characteristic appearance of the spine is called "rugger jersey spine" because of its resemblance to the striped jersey worn by rugby players and is caused by increased bone deposition in the vertebral endplates **(Fig. 7B)**.

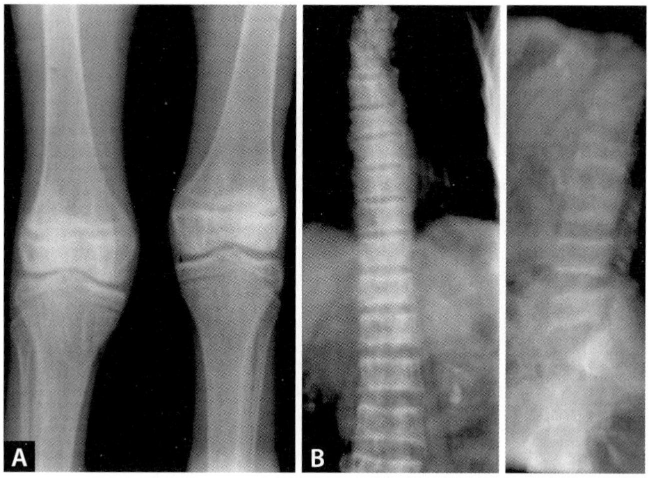

Figs. 7A and B: Renal osteodystrophy: (A) X-ray B/L knees showing knock knee deformity and patchy sclerosis at the distal femoral and proximal tibial metaphysis with slight widening of the growth plate; (B) Characteristic "rugger jersey spine" appearance in a patient of chronic renal failure with nephrolithiasis in the left kidney.

Hereditary Vitamin D-dependent Rickets

Vitamin D-dependent rickets (VDDR) should be considered when rickets presents in early infancy and other usual causes such as inadequate vitamin D intake, intestinal malabsorption, liver disease or kidney disorders have been excluded.

Two forms have been described which involve problems with the formation or function of $1,25(OH)_2D_3$.

Type I VDDR

Type I disorder results from a deficiency (genetic defect) of the renal enzyme 1-alpha-hydroxylase, which converts $25(OH)D_3$ to $1,25(OH)_2D_3$. Therefore, the blood levels of $25(OH)D_3$ are normal while those of $1,25(OH)_2D_3$ are decreased.

Clinical presentation is early, often by 3 months of age, with most patients being symptomatic by one year of age. The disease is differentiated from X-linked hypophosphatemic rickets by the presence of convulsions and muscular weakness. Rachitic bone changes may be severe, rapidly progressive and accompanied by pathologic fractures.[4] Healing occurs with physiologic doses of 1,25 dihydroxy vitamin D_3. This disorder is also known as *pseudovitamin D deficiency rickets* as patients with this condition respond to large doses of vitamin D or physiologic doses of 1,25 $(OH)_2D$ with resolution of the clinical, biochemical and radiographic abnormalities.

Type II VDDR

In this type of VDDR serum levels of $1,25(OH)_2D_3$ are elevated, thereby indicating an end organ resistance to $1,25(OH)_2D_3$. It is also known as *calcitrol resistant rickets* (CRR) and is a rare autosomal recessive disorder characterzed by severe rickets, growth retardation, severe dental changes and alopecia from early infancy. The diagnosis of type II VDDR should be suspected from the unusual association of severe rickets and alopecia.

RICKETS AND OSTEOMALACIA SECONDARY TO PHOSPHATE LOSS

A number of rachitic and osteomalacic syndromes have been identified of both congenital and acquired origin which share one or several renal tubular abnormalities. Rickets or osteomalacia results from hypophosphatemia secondary to impaired renal tubular resorption of phosphate resulting in phosphate loss. These disorders were described by Albright, Fanconi and associates who also reported that rickets was resistant to vitamin D therapy in these patients.[4]

X-linked Hypophosphatemia

X-linked hypophosphatemia *(or familial vitamin D—resistant/refractory rickets)* is the most common form of renal tubular rickets and osteomalacia. It is genetically transmitted in an X-linked dominant trait. The syndrome is characterised by lifelong hypophosphatemia. The basic defect lies in impaired reabsorption of phosphate from proximal tubules.[4] In addition, the conversion of $25(OH)D_3$ to $1,25(OH)_2D_3$ is also impaired. Serum calcium levels are in the normal range while the serum inorganic phosphate levels are persistently low. Rickets generally develops between 12 and 18 months of age.

Clinical Features

Clinical features include bowing of legs, limb deformities, short stature and premature fusion of cranial sutures leading to skull deformities. Dental abnormalities are also seen.

Biochemical Findings

It is characterized by low serum phosphorus, normal serum calcium, normal parathyroid hormone (PTH) and elevated levels of alkaline phosphatase.

Radiological Features

Radiographically, the rachitic changes may be mild to moderate with bowing of long bones seen, particularly in the lower limbs. Coarsening of trabecular pattern is seen with increasing age. In adults, generalized increase in bone density, especially of the axial skeleton is characteristic. The spine and pelvis may show changes in the form of calcification and ossification in the paravertebral ligaments, ligamentum flavum, iliolumbar and sacroiliac ligaments. The spinal changes may resemble those of ankylosing spondylitis or diffuse idiopathic skeletal hyperostosis (DISH). However, the sacroiliac joints in X-linked hypophosphatemia show no bone erosions in contrast to that seen in ankylosing spondylitis. The appendicular skeleton also shows multiple sites of new bone formation at various muscle and ligament attachments. Osteoarthritis is common, particularly in the ankle, knees, wrists and sacroiliac joints.

The above radiographic findings in the axial and appendicular skeleton are distinctive and the diagnosis may be suggested prior to the clinical recognition of the disorder.

Renal Tubular Acidosis

Renal tubular acidosis (RTA) comprises a group of tubular transport defects characterized by inability to appropriately acidify the urine with resultant metabolic acidosis. The underlying abnormalities consist of an impairment of bicarbonate resorption or excretion of hydrogen ions or a combination of both. Detailed biochemical tests are essential for reaching at a correct diagnosis in RTA.[11]

Type I (Distal) RTA

It is characterized by persistent severe metabolic acidosis with continuous bicarbonaturia and is an important cause of severe rachitic abnormalities.[11] In untreated cases nephrocalcinosis/renal calculi are formed.

Type II (Proximal) RTA

This type of RTA may occur in children in an isolated form or as part of global proximal tubular dysfunction called *Fanconi's syndrome.* In this condition, phosphaturia of tubular origin is associated with glycosuria, various aminoacidurias, in addition to bicarbonaturia. Unlike type I RTA, children with type II RTA do not progressively accumulate acid.[11] Rachitic deformities and nephrocalcinosis are uncommon in isolated proximal RTA but are common in Fanconi's syndrome.

Tumor-associated Rickets and Osteomalacia

Tumor-associated rickets and osteomalacia (also termed *oncogenic osteomalacia*) is a syndrome characterized by hyperphosphaturia, with resultant hypophosphatemia, decreased levels of $1,25(OH)_2D_3$ (refractory to vitamin D_3 administration) and various neoplasms.

The syndrome is more common in adults than children. The tumors are benign, of connective tissue origin, located either in soft tissues or bones. They are typically vascular and often show foci of new bone formation.

Patients with this syndrome frequently have generalized muscle weakness and proximal myopathy. Radiographic changes of rickets and osteomalacia may be advanced at the time of initial presentation.

The cause of rickets in association with these tumors has been attributed to the secretion of a humoral agent termed 'phosphatonin' which directly inhibits the absorption of phosphates in the proximal tubule.[12] The tumors are usually small, benign and of vascular origin (hemangiopericytoma), but there is now known to be a wide spectrum of tumors, some of which may be malignant.[13]

Biochemically, serum calcium is normal with marked decrease in serum phosphate. These patients are resistant or refractory to vitamin D. However, resection of the tumor results in the reversal of metabolic, clinical and osseous abnormalities.

Chemotherapeutic Drug-induced Rickets

High doses of a chemotherapeutic agent, '*Ifosfamide*' used in the treatment of solid tumors, especially in children have been known to result in Fanconi syndromes with hypophosphatemic rickets.[12] This complication is seen as a result of nephrotoxic metabolites of the drug and may be irreversible.[12] Renal toxicity is predominantly tubular, although glomerular abnormalities may also occur. Any part of the nephron may be damaged by ifosfamide. The major cause of rickets and osteomalacia is hyperphosphaturia with resultant hypophosphatemia.

SYNDROMES WITH THE RADIOGRAPHIC APPEARANCE OF RICKETS OR OSTEOMALACIA BUT WITHOUT ABNORMALITIES OF VITAMIN D METABOLISM OR RENAL TUBULAR DYSFUNCTION (PHOSPHATE LOSS)

Hypophosphatasia

Hypophosphatasia is a rare disorder that is genetically transmitted that may resemble rickets both clinically and radiologically. However, the serum calcium and phosphorus levels are normal. The characteristic diagnostic features are as follows:

- Defective skeletal mineralization, resembling rickets radiologically.
- Low serum alkaline phosphatase level (in contrast to rickets in which it is increased).
- Increased amounts of phosphoethanolamine, an amino acid, in the blood and urine.

A wide spectrum of clinical severity is noted with most patients being diagnosed in infancy and childhood. The most severely effected neonates usually die soon after birth. *Radiologically,* there is reduced mineralization. Fractures with deformity and shortening may suggest a dwarfing syndrome. Radiographic changes at the growth plate may be seen soon after birth, are similar to those of rickets but show characteristic multiple radiolucent extensions into the metaphysis that represent uncalcified bone matrix.[4] Coarse trabecular pattern, bowing deformities with or without healing fractures may be present. Wormian bones and craniosynostosis may be present.

Metaphyseal Chondrodysplasia (Schmid Type)

It is a disorder in which there is generalized symmetric disturbance of enchondral bone formation, primarily at the metaphysis.[4] It is manifested in childhood as short stature, bowing of the long bones and has a benign course. The radiographs show widening of the growth plate. Multiple, small, bony projections extend from the metaphysis into the growth plate. In contrast to the usual rickets, the metaphysis is well mineralized and may show increased density.[4] There is absence of Looser's zones. The serum calcium, phosphorus and alkaline phosphatase levels are normal. Spontaneous improvement occurs and patients do not respond to vitamin D therapy.

Atypical Axial Osteomalacia

It is a rare condition in which the radiographic abnormalities are confined to the axial skeleton, with sparing of appendicular sites. A dense, coarse trabecular pattern is most marked in the cervical region. The lumbar spine, pelvis and ribs are also involved. Looser's zones have not been identified in this condition.[12] The biochemical findings are normal with no response to vitamin D therapy.

OSTEOMALACIA

The term osteomalacia literally means *"soft bones".*

Radiological Changes

The radiological findings of osteomalacia are often nonspecific.[4] Correlation with appropriate laboratory and clinical data are often required for reaching at a correct diagnosis. The major skeletal changes observed are:

- *Osteopenia:* It is the most common radiologic sign due to decreased bone mineral content.[4] It is usually uniform involving all the bones.
- *Coarse indistinct trabecular pattern:* It is in combination with generalized osteopenia suggestive of osteomalacia.[4] An overall decrease in number of bony trabeculae within all the bones enhances the contrast of the remaining trabeculae giving a coarse, mottled appearance **(Figs. 8A and B)**.
- *Cortical involvement:* The cortices of long bones become thin, with indistinct definition, especially on the endosteal surface.
- *Pseudofractures or Looser's zones:* These are a more specific but less common manifestation of osteomalacia.[14] Looser's zones are linear areas of under mineralized osteoid that occur in a bilateral

and symmetric distribution[14,15] **(Figs. 9A and B)**. They are oriented at right angles to the cortex.[10] The characteristic sites include:

- Axillary margins of scapula
- Superior and inferior pubic rami
- Inner margins of the proximal femur
- Posterior margins of the proximal ulna
- Ribs.[4,15]

Looser's zones are considered to be either insufficiency type stress fracture or due to vascular pulsations acting on the softened bone.[6,12] However, in contrast to fatigue type stress fractures, pseudofractures do not necessarily involve weight bearing bones and may remain unaltered over long periods of time. True fractures may develop later at these sites because they represent areas of weakened bone[12] **(Fig. 10)**. In addition, Looser's zones show mild to moderate sclerosis with an absence of callus. Radiolucent areas similar to pseudofractures may be seen in bones affected by Paget's disease and fibrous dysplasia.[12,14]

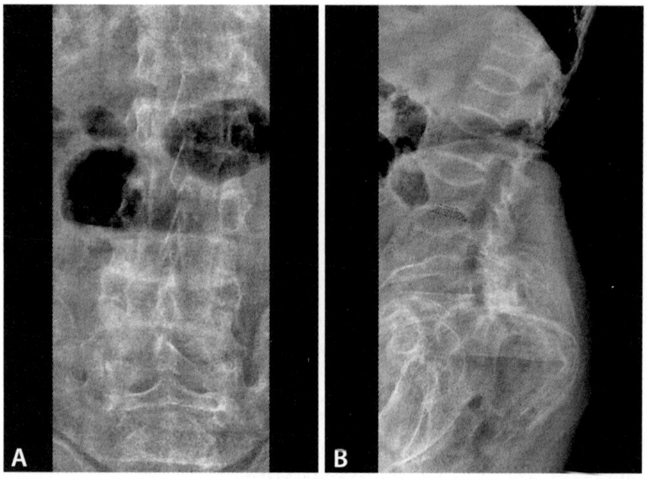

Figs. 8A and B: X-ray lumbosacral spine AP and lateral views reveal marked diffuse osteopenia with reduced vertebral height with biconcave appearance giving cod-fish appearance. The sacral spine is acutely kyphotic—Osteomalacia.

The terms *Milkman's fracture, increment fracture and Umbauzonen* have also been used to describe osteomalacic pseudofractures.[4,6] Pseudofractures occur at sites of increased stress and therefore, accelerated bone turnover. The osteoid which is laid down in the replacement process is inadequately mineralized, which accounts for its radiolucent appearance **(Fig. 11)**.[4,12]

Pseudofractures may be identified by radionuclide bone scan or MR imaging before being evident on radiographs.[12]

Bone scintigraphy has been found to be more sensitive than blood biochemistry and radiographic findings in the detection of osteomalacia. The typical features of osteomalacia seen on whole body scintigraphy are widening of mandible, rachitic rosary sign, the tie sign of the sternum, pseudofracture sign and prominent epiphysis of the knees.[16]

- *Bony deformities:* These occur mainly in weight bearing joints. In the pelvis, there is medial acetabular migration (protrusio acetabulae) and inferior displacement of sacrum thereby producing a triradiate shape of the pelvis[11] **(Figs. 12A and B)**. Both the femur and tibia show bowing deformity, vertebral bodies may

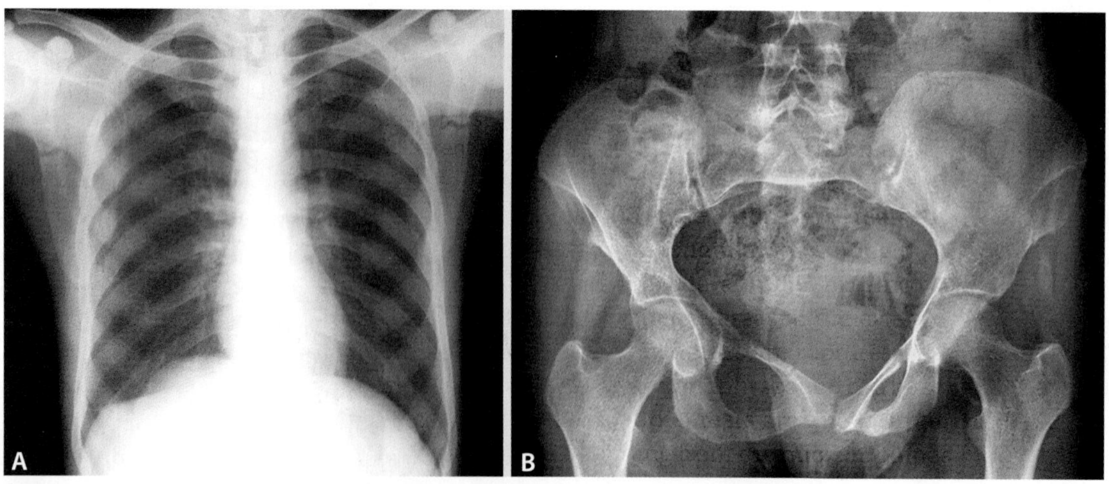

Figs. 9A and B: (A) Chest radiograph showing typical appearance of Looser's zone in bilateral lateral and medial borders of scapulae and ribs; (B) X-ray pelvis (AP) showing characteristic appearance of Looser's zones in bilateral superior pubic rami and mild right protusio acetabuli with resultant asymmetric shape of the pelvic cavity.

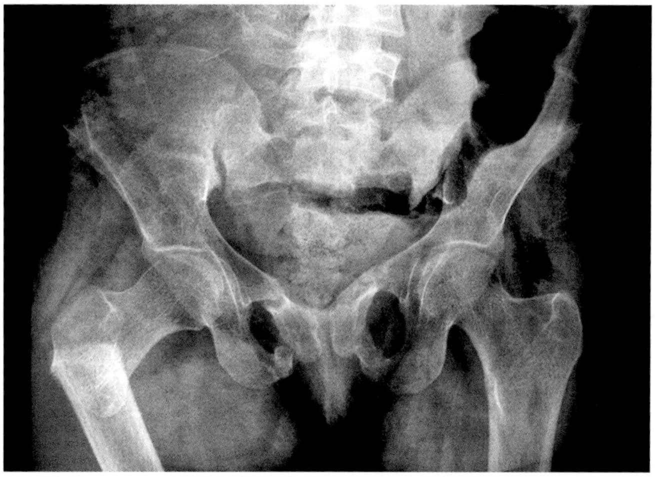

Fig. 10: X-ray pelvis (AP) in a 28-year-old female with sudden onset pain over right thigh following trivial trauma reveals fracture of upper end of the right femur. The visualized bones are osteopenic with coarse trabecular pattern. Looser's zones are seen in bilateral superior and inferior ramii—Osteomalacia.

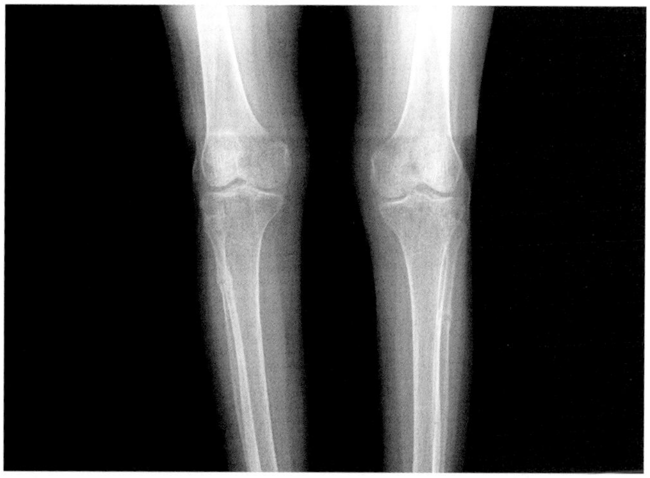

Fig. 11: Radiograph bilateral legs (AP) showing Looser's zone in upper 1/3rd bilateral fibula with surrounding sclerosis. There is osteoporosis with cortical thinning of the bones.

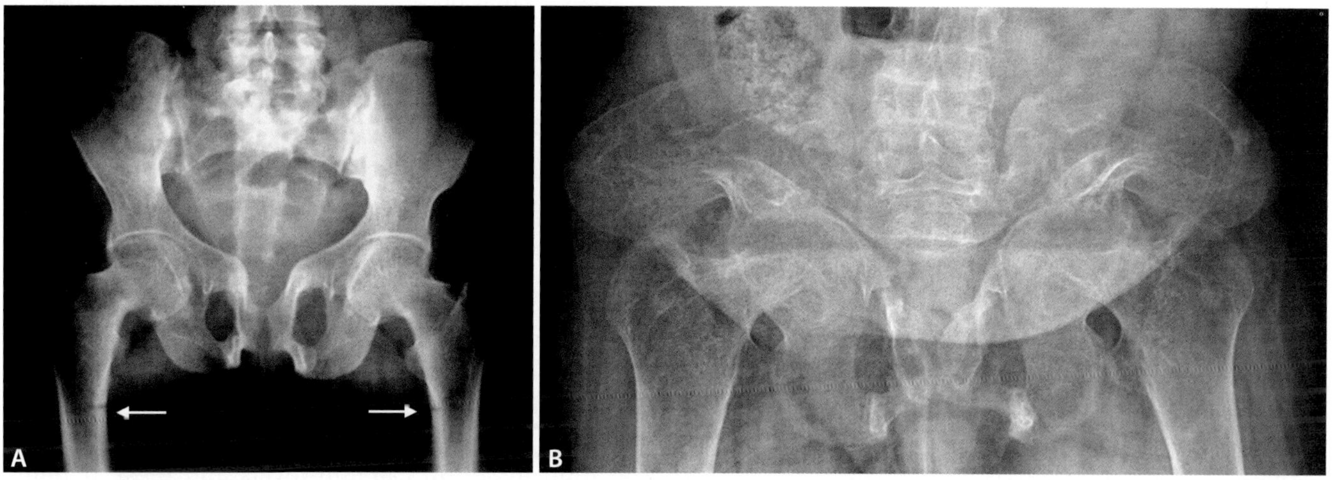

Figs. 12A and B: Pelvis AP in two different patients of osteomalacia: (A) Looser's zones in bilateral symmetric distribution in inner margins of proximal femora and superior and inferior pubic rami; (B) Severe osteomalacic changes with triradiate pelvis due to bilateral protrusio acetabuli and inferior displacement of sacrum. The visualized bones are markedly osteoporotic. Old healed Looser's zones are seen in bilateral superior and inferior pubic rami.

develop a biconcave shape and kyphoscoliosis is not an uncommon finding. Basilar invagination of the skull may occur.[11]

Radiographs of the spine in osteoporosis (characterized by decrease bone mass but there is no defect in mineralization) and osteomalacia may appear to be similar but they can be differentiated on the basis of coarse and indistinct trabeculae in osteomalacia while the trabeculae are thin and sharp in osteoporosis. Also, the spinal deformity in osteomalacia is uniform unlike osteoporosis wherein it is nonuniform.[4]

HYPERPARATHYROIDISM

Hyperparathyroidism is a pathological state characterized by excessive production of parathyroid hormone. In the normal state, parathyroid hormone promotes release of calcium into the blood from the bone. It also stimulates extensive bone remodeling. Alterations of parathyroid function cause a breakdown in calcium homeostasis leading to characteristic pathologic and radiologic abnormalities.[17]

Hyperparathyroidism is divided into primary, secondary and tertiary types.

Primary HPT

Primary HPT is characterized by increased parathyroid hormone secretion occurring as a result of abnormality in one or more of the parathyroid glands. The cause in most cases is a single parathyroid adenoma (90% of cases); less common causes include double adenomas (4%), hyperplasia of multiple glands (6%) and parathyroid carcinoma (<1%).[18] Hyperplasia of the parathyroid glands can occur as an isolated finding or as part of multiple endocrine neoplasia (MEN) syndromes.

Secondary HPT

Secondary HPT is associated with abnormalities in function of the parathyroid glands induced by a sustained hypocalcemic stimulus. The most common cause is chronic renal failure. Occasionally, malabsorption states and dietary abnormalities leading to hypocalcemia may be responsible.[19]

Tertiary HPT

Tertiary HPT occurs in patients with long standing secondary HPT who develop autonomous parathyroid function and hypercalcemia.

Pathophysiology

The clinical, pathological and radiological manifestation of HPT can be understood by understanding the interrelated roles of PTH and vitamin D in the regulation of calcium metabolism.

Parathyroid hormone influences many tissues in the human body and is essential for the proper transport of calcium and other ions in bone, intestine and kidney. The synthesis and secretion of PTH is regulated by the ionized serum calcium level. The normal serum calcium levels are maintained within a normal physiologic range by the intestines and kidneys which balance intake and excretion. Ninety-nine percent of the elemental calcium is bound to the skeleton and PTH works to increase the serum calcium by increasing the resorption with liberation of calcium and phosphorus.

In the kidneys, PTH inhibits resorption of phosphate in the proximal and distal tubules. This causes decrease in the plasma phosphate concentration which in turn helps to maintain the serum calcium level. PTH also increases the renal tubular reabsorption of calcium.

Parathyroid hormone has no documented direct effect upon intestinal calcium absorption. PTH along with a decreased serum calcium and phosphate stimulate synthesis of 1,25 dihydroxy vitamin D; the primary mediator of intestinal calcium and phosphorus absorption and also acts on bone to produce resorption. Thus, functioning renal tissue is critical to the metabolism of both PTH and vitamin D and is a major target organ for the action of these hormones **(Fig. 13)**.

Therefore, there exists a negative feedback loop between serum calcium and PTH. An abrupt fall in serum calcium will actively stimulate PTH secretion. Other factors affecting PTH secretion include Al, Mg and Li levels and the secretion of histamine, cortisol, calcitonin and cyclic AMP **(Fig. 14)**.

Clinical Features

The clinical features of primary HPT relates to hypercalcemia which results from:
- increased intestinal absorption of calcium
- increased bone turnover
- increased tubular resorption of calcium.

Patients may present with tiredness, lethargy, polyuria, anorexia or nausea, or to bone or renal complication.

The true incidence of primary HPT is not known but biochemical screening identifies the condition in unsuspected persons. It is found at all ages from birth to old age, with the highest incidence between 20 and 60 years, with women being affected two to four times more often than men.[10]

There appears to be a relationship between the severity of the disease and the type of symptoms that predominate. Patients with renal calculi are younger, have a chronic course and are associated with hyperplasia of the parathyroid gland. Those with bone changes have a subacute progressive course characterized by a marked elevation in serum calcium levels and these patients generally have adenomas.[19]

Nephrolithiasis is the most common clinical manifestation, followed by hypertension, peptic ulcers, pancreatitis, psychiatric disorders and bone pain.[20]

Biochemical Findings

In most cases the diagnosis of hyperparathyroidism can be made on the basis of clinical symptomatology and laboratory tests. Sustained elevation of serum calcium and serum parathormone levels are the most accepted means for the establishment of diagnosis of primary HPT.[17] Multiple measurements of serum calcium are often recommended due to the variations in the amount of circulating parathyroid hormone at any given time. Also, hypercalcemia is a feature of other disease states such

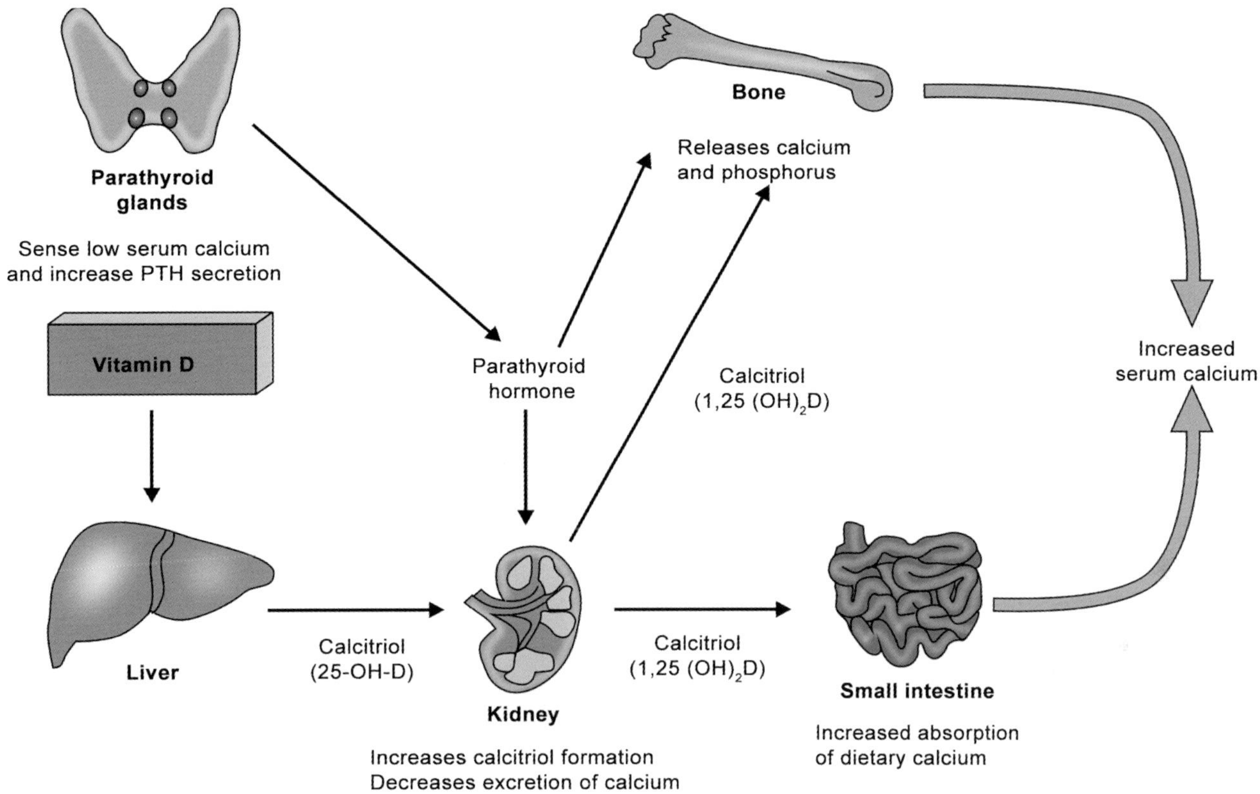

Fig. 13: Overview of vitamin D metabolism.

as malignancy, endocrinological disorders, secondary to drugs, granulomatous disorders, etc. **(Table 3)**. Ten to twenty percent of patients with malignancy have levated serum calcium levels (normal ref range = 9–11 mg%) with majority of these patients having direct involvement of the skeleton by a malignant lesion.[21]

The term pseudohyperparathyroidism is referred to the syndrome consisting of hypercalcemia of malignancy in the absence of demonstrable skeletal metastasis or primary hyperparathyroidisim.

Elevated urinary cyclic AMP and elevated alkaline phosphatase levels signify increase in bone turnover and skeletal involvement.

In secondary HPT, the plasma calcium levels are normal or low and the serum inorganic phosphate levels are high (chronic renal failure) or low (intestinal malabsorption).

Radiological Approach

The value of radiological studies in primary and secondary HPT lies not in the initial diagnosis, but in assessing the severity of the condition and in noninvasive localization of the parathyroid glands prior to surgery as well as in the follow-up of the patient.[19]

Radiological Findings

The skeletal changes in hyperparathyroidism are characteristic and reflect the histologic changes of increased resorption of cortical and cancellous bone with substitutive fibrosis. Conventional radiography can assess the extent of bone involvement and the presence of bone changes is an accepted indication for parathyroid surgery in primary HPT.[19] The bone changes of primary and secondary HPT are identical, except for the associated changes of renal osteodystrophy in secondary HPT.

BONE RESORPTION

The incidence of bone lesions varies from 30 to 40%.[19] The initial bone changes may not be seen on radiographic or gross pathologic examination, although, microscopic evaluation shows osteoclastic activity.[17] Bone resorption is a hallmark of HPT and is one of the effects of increased PTH production. The bone resorption is due to increased osteoclastic activity and can be detected on the subperiosteal, intracortical, endosteal, subchondral and trabecular surfaces. Overall cortical bone is affected more severely than cancellous bone. These changes are reflected

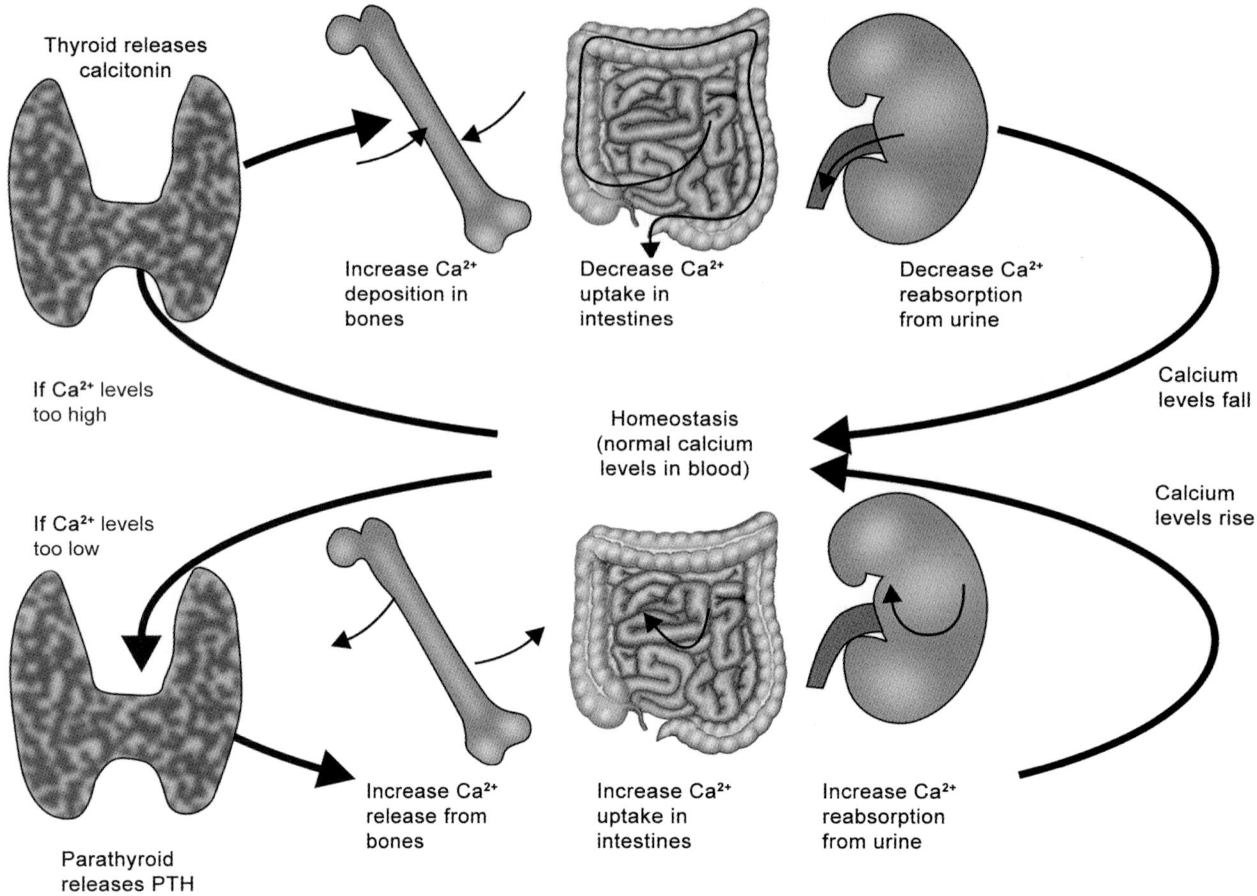

Fig. 14: Role of parathyroid hormone (PTH) and calcitonin in the regulation of calcium metabolism.

radiologically by poor definition of cortical surfaces, increased cortical striations ("tunneling"), cortical thinning and distortion and blurring of trabecular bone.[19]

Subperiosteal Resorption

Subperiosteal resorption of cortical bone is considered pathognomic of HPT.[17,19] Although it may be seen at various skeletal sites, the earliest and best recognized changes are seen in the hands.[22] The earliest site of subperiosteal resorption is the radial aspect of middle phalanges of middle and index fingers **(Figs. 15A and B)**. Some authors have cited the earliest radiographic evidence of superiosteal resorption to occur in the terminal tufts of the fingers.[19,22] Loss of fine cortical outline around the tufts results in a mesh like or woven appearance, with significant erosion of tufts being more obvious in advanced cases. A distinctive pattern of band-like appearance of acroosteolysis may be seen in the terminal phalanges of the hands (less commonly the feet), consisting of band-like radiolucent areas that may separate the tuft and the base of the phalanx separately.

Other sites of subperiosteal resorption include the medial aspect of the proximal end of tibia, humerus and femur; superior and inferior margins of the ribs and lamina dura surrounding the teeth[22] **(Fig. 16)**. Loss of lamina dura once considered pathognomic of HPT is now considered as nonspecific as it may accompany dental sepsis, fibrous dysplasia, Paget's disease, osteomalacia and other endocrine disorders.[17,22] Subperiosteal resorption may also occur in the marginal areas of joints, particularly in the hands and feet, and may mimic erosive changes of rheumatoid arthritis or other inflammatory arthropathies. A feature to differentiate the erosions in HPT from that of rheumatoid arthritis is that they are located slightly away from the joint margin and are almost always associated with typical subperiosteal resorption of the adjacent phalangeal tufts.

Intracortical Bone Resorption

Intracortical bone resorption or tunneling is one of the hallmarks of rapid bone resorption wherein groups of

Table 3: Differential diagnosis of hypercalcemia.

Malignancy
• Solid tumors (primarily breast cancer) • Hematologic disorders • Myeloma • Lymphoma • Leukemia
Enocrinological Disorders
• Primary hyperparathyroidism • Multiple endocrine neoplasias (types I and II) • Ectopic hyperparathyroidism (malignancy predominantly lung cancer) • Secondary hyperparathyroidism (renal failure) • Hyperthyroidism • Hypoadrenalism
Drugs
• Vitamin A intoxication • Vitamin D intoxication • Thiazides • Calcium • Milk alkali syndrome • Dialysis
Granulomatous Disorders
• Sarcoidosis • Tuberculosis • Histoplasmosis • Beryliosis • Rheumatoid arthritis
Pediatric Disorders
• Infantile hypercalcemia • Hypophosphatasia
Miscellaneous
• Immobilization • Paget's disease

osteoclasts tunnel through the Volkman's and haversian canals.[19] This finding is also not specific for HPT and may be seen in hyperthyroidism, acromegaly and disorders causing rapid osteoporosis. They are radiographically seen as tiny linear striations within the cortex parallel to the long axis of the bone, best seen in the tubular bones of the hand and feet, especially in the cortex of the second metacarpal. Intracortical resorption of bone is almost always associated with subperiosteal resorption **(Fig. 17)**.

Richardson et al. quantified the degree of intracortical tunneling in the metacarpal shafts and found it to be a sensitive indicator of the extent of bone disease in HPT.[19,22,23] This method known as the "cortical striation index" requires detailed magnification radiographs.[19,22] A grading system is used to determine the degree of cortical striation present in the first and second metacarpal of each hand.

Grade 0 — Solid cortex with up to one striation.
Grade 1 — Mild increase in striations.
Grade 2 — Increased striations, but with involvement of less than 50% of the cortex.
Grade 3 — Extensive striations throughout the cortex.

The second and third metacarpal of each hand are graded separately. In normal individuals the "mean cortical index" is one or less than one. Increased striations are seen in patients with primary HPT, renal osteodystrophy and osteomalacia. The importance of cortical striation measurement in patients with HPT is in monitoring the response to treatment.[19]

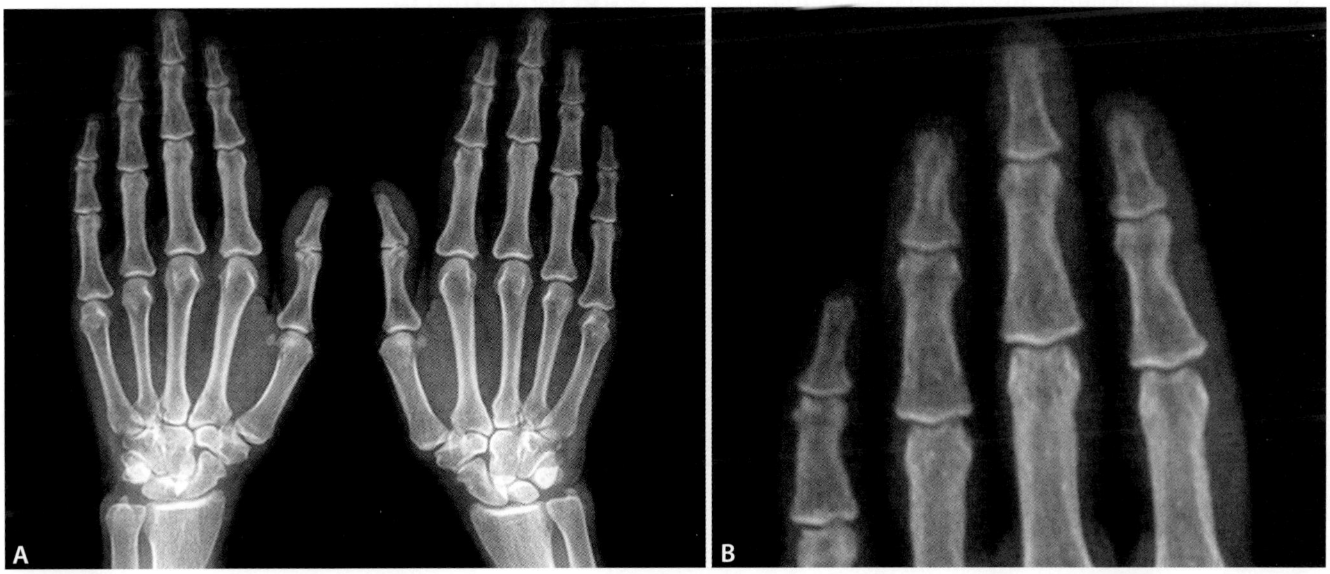

Figs. 15A and B: Hyperparathyroidism: (A) Hands showing resorption of the subperiosteal bone on the radial aspect of the middle phalanges of the index and middle fingers with magnified view; (B) Showing minimal resorption of the tufts of terminal phalanges as well.

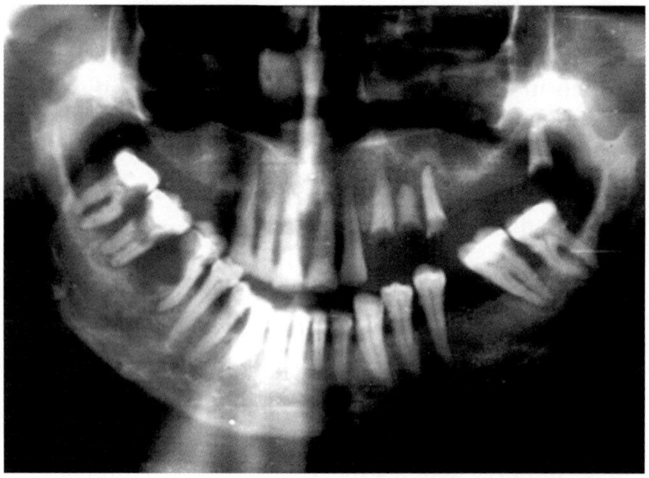

Fig. 16: Pantomogram showing extensive subperiosteal resorption with loss of lamina dura in a patient with parathyroid adenoma.

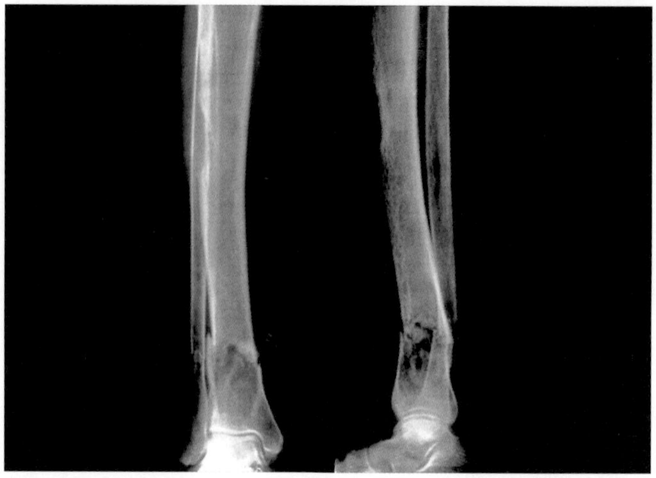

Fig. 17: Anteroposterior and lateral radiograph of leg shows resorption of anterior tibial cortex, intracortical striations and brown tumor with pathological fractures—HPT.

Endosteal Bone Resorption

It leads to cortical thinning, scalloping and irregularity of the endosteal surface, especially in the bones of the hand. Endosteal bone resorption may occur more commonly in conjunction with subperiosteal and intracortical resorption rather than an isolated finding.

Subchondral Bone Resorption

Subchondral bone resorption is a common manifestation of hyperparathyroidism, particularly in the joints of the axial skeleton, such as the sacroiliac, sternoclavicular, acromioclavicular joints, pubic symphysis and discovertebral junctions causing surface irregularity and increase in joint space.[19,22] The changes are most severe in the distal clavicles. The peripheral joints may also show subchondral bone resorption and these changes may mimic infective arthritis.

Subphyseal Bone Resorption

In children with primary or secondary HPT, irregular radiolucent areas may appear in the mataphysis adjacent to the growth plate. This finding is reminiscent of the abnormalities accompanying rickets.[21]

Subligamentous and Subtendinous Bone Resorption

Resorption of bone occurs at sites of tendon and ligament attachment to bone. The frequently involved sites are femoral trochanter, ischial and humeral tuberosities, elbow, inferior surface of calcaneus and inferior aspect of distal end of clavicle.

Trabecular Bone Resorption

Trabecular resorption occurs throughout the skeleton in HPT, especially in the advanced stages of the disease, though changes in the skull vault are characteristic.[17,19] Osteoclasts on the surface of bone dissect through the center of trabecula giving a stippled, mottled, granular appearance termed radiologically as *"salt and pepper skull"*[17,19] **(Fig. 18)**. The definition of outer and inner table is lost. Focal areas of osseous thickening in the cranial vault may be observed on radiographs as well-defined or poorly defined radiopaque areas.

BROWN TUMORS

They are also known as *osteitis fibrosa cystica or von Recklinghausen disease of the bone*. Brown tumors are cystic lesions within bone and are an end result of extensive bone resorption.[17] They have initially been described characteristic of primary hyperparathyroidism, but seen with increasing frequency in secondary hyperparathyroidism as well.[22] They represent hemorrhage and deposition of breakdown products of hemoglobin. Brown tumors may cause swelling, pathological fracture and bone pain in the skeletal system. Histologically, the cavities are filled with fibrous tissue and osteoclasts with necrosis and hemorrhagic liquefaction. *Radiographically* brown tumors are seen as lytic, expansile, cystic lesions which are often multiple. They appear as well defined lesions of the axial or appendicular skeleton and are frequently eccentric or cortical in location **(Figs. 19A and B)**. The common sites of involvement are the mandible, clavicle, ribs, pelvis and tubular bones.[17,19,23]

Other manifestation of HPT are generally present, although occasionally a brown tumor may be the only finding radiologically. With removal of the parathyroid adenoma, brown tumors may demonstrate healing with sclerosis.[19,23]

The presence of multiple osteolytic lesions in an elderly patient with complaints of bone pain is suggestive of a mitotic/metastatic etiology. However, other etiologies such as multiple myeloma or brown tumor should be considered and serum phosphate, calcium and PTH levels and serum protein electrophoresis should also be checked.

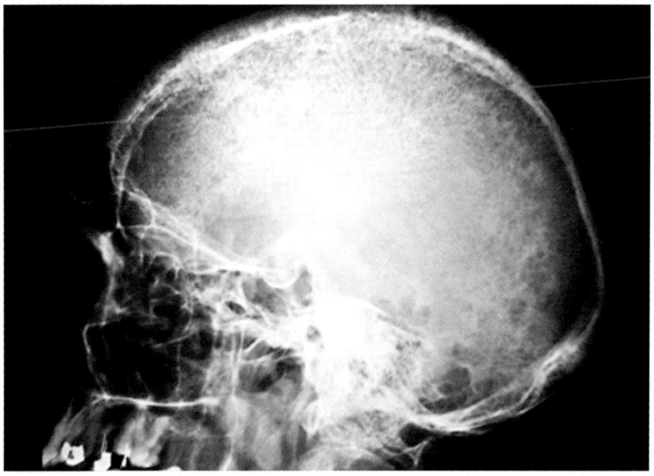

Fig. 18: Osteoporosis with loss of definition of inner and outer tables of the skull causing a classical mottled appearance of the skull vault—"Salt and pepper skull".

Brown tumors with hemorrhagic or cystic component in weight bearing bones are associated with a higher risk of pathological fracture. MR imaging can aid in determining hemorrhage and cystic component and indirectly in estimation of fracture risk.[24]

It has been seen that there is a risk of pathological fracture when the brown tumor involves more than two-thirds of the cortex of the long bone, especially in the weight-bearing area. Preventive internal fixation is indicated if the tumor involves more than two-thirds of the cortex of the weight-bearing long bone.[25]

In the past, advanced cases of hyperparathyroidism presenting with severe bone resorption was not an uncommon finding. However, use of more sophisticated diagnostic techniques along with an increased awareness of this condition, have led to an earlier diagnosis, when the degree of bone resorption is somewhat limited.[17] Fine detail and magnification skeletal radiography in primary HPT will not only detect mild disease but will also reveal intracortical, endosteal and trabecular resorption.[17]

The combined effect of all the patterns of bone resorption is generalized osteopenia in a majority of patients.[17,22] On radiographs, osteopenia is frequently a subjective finding that is difficult to interpret and is identifiable only after 30–50% of mineral content is lost. This difficulty can be overcome by using quantitative bone mineral analysis which will indicate not only the degree and rate of bone loss in the disease but also partial recovery of the loss that is seen after successful parathyroidectomy.[17]

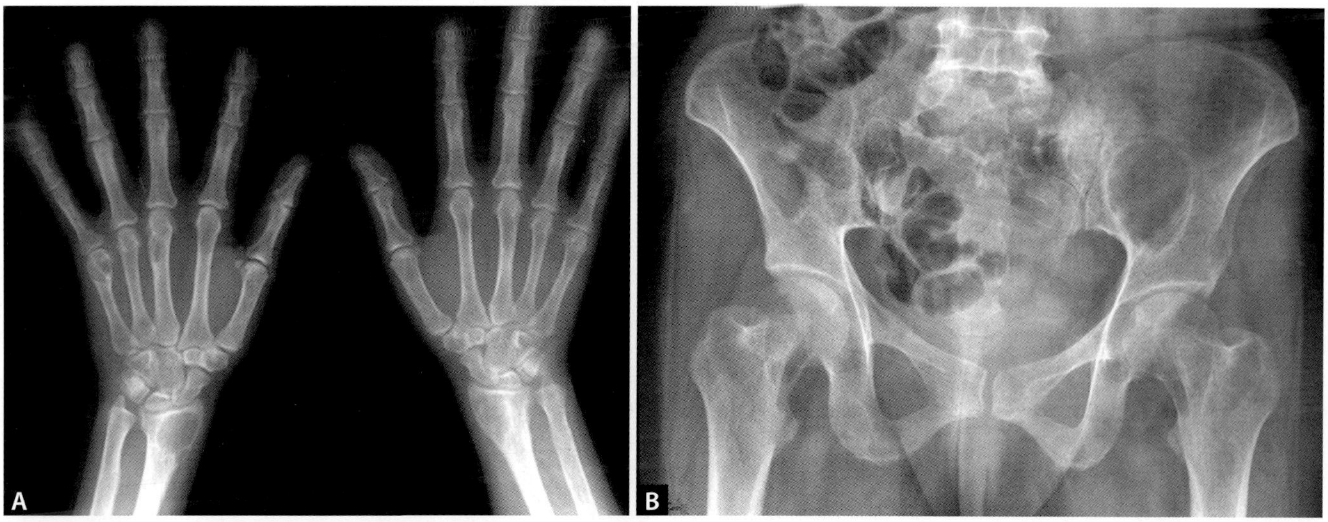

Figs. 19A and B: (A) X-ray bilateral hands in primary HPT showing multiple, well-defined, expansile lytic lesions in lower end of radius, head and distal ends of 3rd and 5th metacarpals of right hand; (B) A large well-defined, oval lytic lesion with sclerotic rim in left iliac bone with multiple smaller ill-defined lesions in bilateral ischium—Brown tumors.

JOINT DISORDERS

Erosive arthropathy of the hands, wrists and shoulders may occur in patients with HPT, simulating rheumatoid arthritis. These changes are almost always associated with typical subperiosteal resorption of the phalanges and occur on the ulnar aspect of metacarpal heads unlike rheumatoid arthritis.

Another feature that is more common in primary hyperparathyroidism is chondrocalcinosis or calcification in hyaline cartilage or fibrocartilage. This occurs due to calcium pyrophosphate dihydrate (CPPD) crystal deposition. It may also occur in chronic renal disease, although its frequency is much lower than in primary HPT. Radiologically, chondrocalcinosis is seen in 18–40% patients with primary HPT.[17,22] Chondrocalcinosis may be seen in hyaline cartilage and fibrocartilage of the knee, symphysis pubis and triangular cartilage of the wrist.[20] The deposition of crystals may lead to episodes of pseudogout. In contrast, soft tissue and vascular calcification is more common in secondary HPT than in primary HPT.

OSTEOSCLEROSIS

Increased bone density or osteosclerosis may be seen due to stimulation of osteoblastic activity by PTH in addition to its osteoclastic activity. The bone sclerosis can be either focal or diffuse.[22] In patients with secondary HPT a diffuse increase in bone density is seen while in patients of primary HPT bone sclerosis is localized or patchy. Focal bone sclerosis is apparent in the metaphyseal regions of the long bones, the skull or the vertebral endplates. In the evaluation of hyperparathyroidism, one must keep in mind that osteosclerotic changes may also occur as a manifestation of healing, either spontaneous or as a result of treatment.[26]

RENAL OSTEODYSTROPHY

Renal osteodystrophy is a term applied to the bone changes present in patients with chronic renal failure. In chronic renal failure, secondary HPT often co-exists with rickets, osteomalacia, osteosclerosis and osteoporosis as part of spectrum of findings called renal osteodystrophy. The skeletal changes of primary and secondary HPT are identical, except for associated changes of renal osteodystrophy seen in secondary HPT. **Table 4** highlights the features differentiating primary from secondary HPT.

The most common cause is chronic glomerulonephritis.[27] It can also result from bilateral chronic pyelonephritis, often associated with vesicoureteric reflux. In both conditions small contracted kidneys are an evidence of the end stage renal disease. The findings in renal osteodystrophy in children and adults are distinctive.

The most common finding in secondary HPT of renal osteodystrophy is subperiosteal resorption although other manifestations may be seen. The osseous resorption has shown to increase from 10% in the early stage of disease to 50–70% after 3–9 years of dialysis.[27] Conversely, following parathyroidectomy bone resorption has shown to regress. Calcification of arteries, articular cartilage and periarticular tissues also occurs in renal osteodystrophy.

Osteosclerosis may occasionally be the only manifestation of renal osteodystrophy. It has a predilection for the axial skeleton **(Fig. 20)**, with deposition of bone in the subchondral areas of the vertebral bodies. This results in the appearance of radiodense bands across the superior and inferior vertebral margins known as "rugger jersey" spine appearance. Other sites of osteosclerosis include

Table 4: Primary versus secondary hyperparathyroidism (HPT).

Primary HPT	*Secondary HPT*
Consists of skeletal features of HPT only	Skeletal features of HPT with features of renal osteodystrophy (rickets/osteomalacia and osteosclerosis)
Skeletal changes are less florid	More florid
Sclerosis rarely seen	Commonly seen
Brown tumors are more common	Less common
Chondrocalcinosis more common	Less common
Soft tissue and vascular calcification are less common	More common

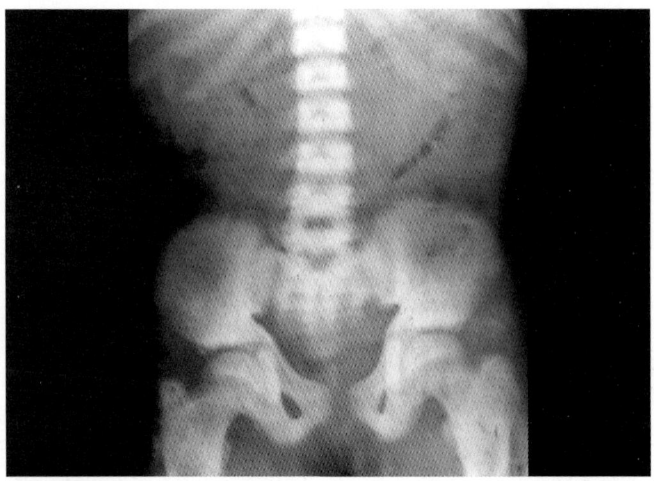

Fig. 20: Renal osteodystrophy: Diffuse increase in bone density of the pelvis and lumbar vertebrae with coarsened trabecular pattern.

the pelvis, ribs and clavicles **(Fig. 21)**. It also involves the metaphysis of long bones and the skull.

Osteopenia has been reported in up to 85% of patients in renal osteodystrophy and is the end result of effect of osteomalacia, bone resorption and a decrease in bone quantity (osteoporosis).[27]

In children, metaphyseal changes resembling rickets are seen. This together with cortical erosions can give rise to the "rotting fencepost" appearance, particularly in the femoral neck. Slipped capital epiphysis may also be seen as a complication, most commonly involving the proximal femur.

RENAL LESIONS

Renal tubular dysfunction results from the direct effect of parathyroid hormone on the kidney and is corrected by parathyroidectomy. Renal calculi have been reported in 50% patients. These calculi are often small and the patient often presents with a renal colic.

NEPHROCALCINOSIS

This is less common than renal calculi. Deposition of calcium is generally in the region of the renal pyramids **(Fig. 22)**, but forms no diagnostic pattern. Uremia is a major cause of death in untreated HPT.

PARATHYROID LOCALIZATION

The standard treatment for primary hyperparathyroidism is surgical removal of the abnormal parathyroid gland or glands.[19,28] This is because untreated HPT leads to bone loss, renal calculi and nephrocalcinosis. The presence of bone changes is an accepted indication of parathyroid surgery in primary HPT.[19]

Following parathyroidectomy the subperiosteal resorption resolves, bone turnover decreases and bone density improves. Patients with nephrolithiasis develop fewer newer stones and renal function improves. Patients with peptic ulcer disease improve and symptoms of depression, weakness and fatigue often disappear.[19]

Preoperative localization of abnormal parathyroid is not routinely advocated by all surgeons due to a high success rate of 90–95% in localizing the lesion in previously unoperated patients.[28] However, imaging can assist the surgeon in preoperatively identifying a persistent or ectopic parathyroid adenoma or parathyroid hyperplasia, thereby increasing surgical success from 60 to 90%.[28]

PREOPERATIVE LOCALIZATION TECHNIQUES

The noninvasive tests for parathyroid localization are:

- High resolution ultrasound
- High resolution computed tomography (HRCT)
- Magnetic resonance imaging (MRI)
- Dual isotope thallium-201 chloride - technetium-99m subtraction scanning
- Technetium-99m sestamibi scintigraphy
- Single photon emission computed tomography (SPECT)
- Parathyroid digital subtraction angiography
- Selective venous sampling.

The success of all these techniques, except venous sampling depends to a varying degree on the size of the abnormal gland.

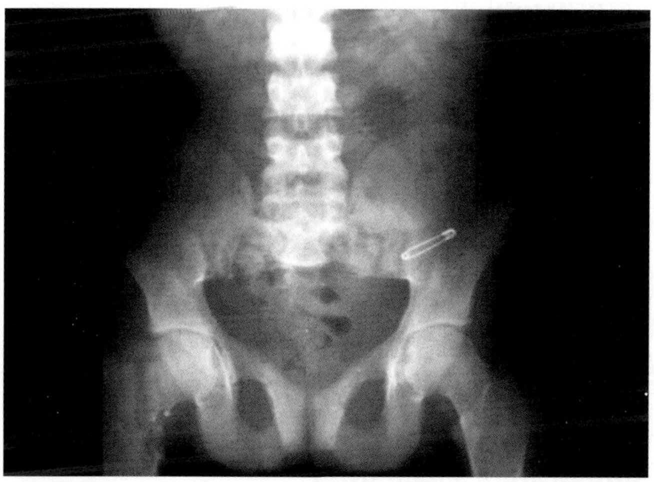

Fig. 21: Typical features of renal osteodystrophy in form of osteosclerosis of the axial skeleton with osteomalacic changes in the pelvis.

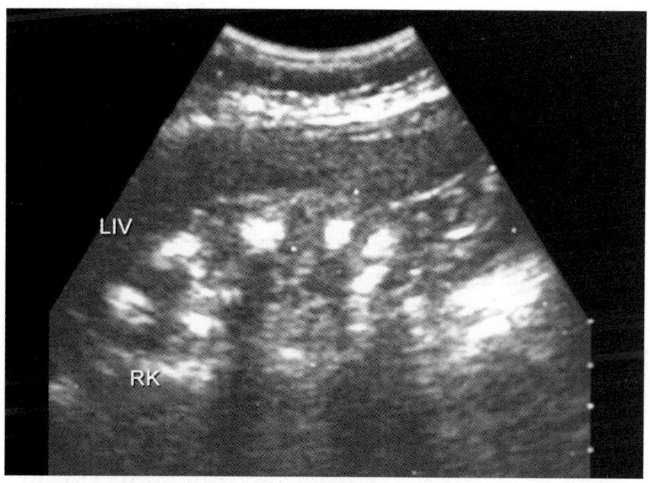

Fig. 22: Ultrasound of the right kidney shows medullary nephrocalcinosis in a patient of secondary HPT.

ANATOMICAL AND PATHOLOGICAL CONSIDERATION IMPORTANT FOR LOCALIZATION

Embryology and Anatomy

In the majority of population (84%), the parathyroid glands are four in number—two superior and two inferior. The glands are symmetrical, with the superior parathyroid glands usually lying posterior to the junction of upper and middle thirds of the thyroid and the inferior parathyroid glands just below the lower poles of the thyroid. Three to five percent population have 5 glands, and 1–3% have 3 glands. Supernumerary glands are seen approximately 3–5% of time.[29]

The superior parathyroid glands are derived from the fourth branchial pouch along with the lateral lobes of the thyroid. The inferior glands arise from the third branchial pouch along with thymus gland. These embryologic relationships help to explain the normal and variable anatomic location of the superior and inferior parathyroid glands. The superior parathyroid glands being closely related to the thyroid gland undergo minimal descent and their position are relatively constant.[18] More than 90% glands are located deep in relation to the mid portion of the superior pole of the thyroid near the cricothyroid junction.[29]

The incidence of ectopic parathyroid glands is 20%. Ectopic superior parathyroids may be found within the thyroid gland (1–2%), in retrotracheal or retroesophageal location (1% cases), within the carotid sheath (1% of cases) or may descend into the posterosuperior mediastinum (5% of cases). The inferior parathyroid glands along with the thymus decend a greater distance and therefore are more variable in location but most commonly are located inferior, posterior or lateral to the lower thyroid pole (69%). Ectopic inferior parathyroid glands are more common and can lie anywhere from the angle of the mandible to the pericardium, i.e. along the path of migration of the thymus.[30] They can be found more inferiorly in the neck, in the thymic tongue or in the cervical portion of the thymus gland (29%). Persistent hypercalcemia after parathyroid surgery can be due to mediastinal parathyroid glands in as many as one-third of cases.

Surgical Treatment

Definitive treatment of primary hyperparathyroidism involves the surgical excision of hyperfunctioning parathyroid glands. In the past, this was achieved with bilateral neck exploration and removal of the enlarged gland or glands. Improved presurgical imaging localization, intraoperative PTH assays and hand-held gamma detectors have made the selective excision of hyperfunctioning parathyroid glands possible.[18]

Over the past decade, the development of minimally invasive techniques to parathyroid surgery has made accurate preoperative localization of parathyroid disease absolutely critical for effective surgical treatment.

Currently practiced minimally invasive techniques include unilateral open parathyroidectomy, video-assisted parathyroidectomy and videoscopic parathyroidectomy. All of these techniques involve a more focused approach wherein the procedure is limited to the abnormal parathyroid gland, thereby reducing the operating time substantially.[29] The extent of minimally invasive parathyroidectomy is often guided by rapid intraoperative PTH testing. A greater than 50% drop in the serum PTH to normal or near-normal levels 10 minutes after parathyroid resection is suggestive of a single parathyroid adenoma as the cause of primary HPT.[18] Thus, the primary benefit of preoperative imaging studies is the accurate determination of uniglandular disease to help select patients most appropriate for unilateral and minimally invasive approaches.

A National Institute of Health consensus panel on primary hyperparathyroidism revised parathyroid surgery guidelines for asymptomatic patients in 2002. Surgery is indicated if one or more of the following factors are present like: a serum calcium level 1.0 mg/dL above the upper limit of the normal range, a 24-hour urinary calcium level of more than 400 mg, creatinine clearance reduced by 30%, a bone mineral density T-score of less than –2.5 SD measured at any site, age of less than 50 years and undesirability or impossibility of medical surveillance.[29]

Parathyroid Imaging

High resolution sonography and ^{99m}Tc-sestamibi scintigraphy are the main imaging techniques for preoperative location of parathyroid adenomas, with similar sensitivities and specificities for solitary adenoma detection by these techniques.

Localization accuracy improves when both sonography and scintigraphy are obtained preoperatively. Contrast-enhanced CT and MRI can also effectively locate parathyroid adenomas but are less commonly used for preoperative location and are more commonly used in the setting of failed parathyroidectomy, for the detection of suspected ectopic (mediastinal) glands.[29]

Sonographic Evaluation

Ultrasonography is the modality of choice for preoperative localization of the pathological gland in all patients of proven HPT. Transducers of 12–15 MHz are used for imaging giving a tissue resolution of 1–2 mm. Solid lesions can be differentiated from blood vessels. High resolution sonography is an established procedure with a sensitivity of 80% and specificity of 90% in detecting cervical parathyroid adenomas.[19]

Normal parathyroid glands are 2–7 mm in length, 2–4 mm in width, and 0.5–2 mm in thickness and weigh 35–55 mg.[30] They are normally not visible on ultrasound, CT or MRI.

Most cases of primary hyperparathyroidism are caused by a single parathyroid adenoma (90%). Hyperplasia of all four glands (6%), double adenomas (4%) and rarely parathyroid carcinoma are the other causes. Adenomas are considerably larger, having a mean mass of greater than 10 times the normal parathyroid gland and are thus often identified at cross-sectional imaging.[27]

At sonography, *parathyroid adenomas* are typically seen as homogeneously hypoechoic solid masses. This is due to the compact cellularity of the gland that is characteristic of adenomas at sectioning.[29] They may sometimes have a hyperechoic capsule. The echogenicity of vast majority of parathyroid adenomas is substantially less than that of thyroid tissue; normal thyroid parenchyma having a characteristic sonographic appearance of homogeneous medium to high level echoes. Around 90% of adenomas are found at the poles of the thyroid gland and are easily discernable sonographically **(Figs. 23A and B)**. Imaging of the lower poles can be enhanced by asking the patient to swallow, which momentarily raises the thyroid gland in the neck. They are usually oval or bean shaped, but larger adenomas can be multilobulated.

Parathyroid carcinomas are usually larger than adenomas, on an average measuring more than 2 cm as compared to 1 cm for adenomas. Carcinomas generally have a lobulated contour, heterogeneous echotexture and cystic components. However, they may be indistinguishable from parathyroid adenomas in all imaging studies except when local invasion of neighboring structures is present.[19]

When parathyroid gland enlargement is not found in the region of the thyroid, the entire neck from mandible to suprasternal notch should be examined sonographically, including the retrotracheal region via a lateral approach.[28] However, ectopic parathyroid glands in the neck may be missed on ultrasonographic evaluation. Ultrasonography cannot be used to identify mediastinal parathyroid adenomas. Rarely, parathyroid adenomas may be intrathyroid in location. These are completely surrounded by thyroid tissue and are oriented with their greatest dimension in the cephalocaudal direction. Sonographicaly, they are well visualized because they are hypoechoic in contrast to the echogenic thyroid parenchyma. However, percutaneous biopsy may often be required to reliably differentiate an intrathyroid adenoma from a thyroid nodule.

Grayscale imaging should be supplemented by color and power Doppler imaging to look for feeding vessels and vascularity of suspected adenomas seen at initial grayscale imaging. As per recent literature, color and power Doppler imaging commonly show a characteristic extrathyroidal feeding vessel (typically a branch off the

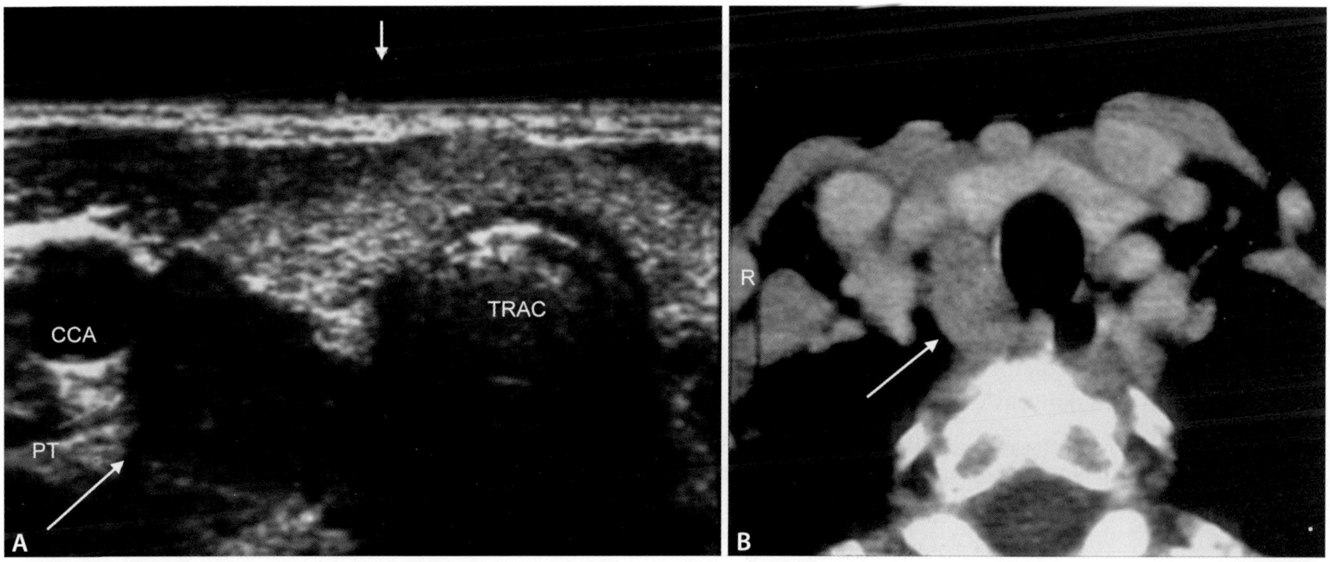

Figs. 23A and B: (A) Transverse ultrasound scan reveals a hypodense mass posteroinferior to the right lobe of thyroid in a patient with parathyroid adenoma; (B) Contrast-enhanced computed tomography (CECT) also shows a hypodense solid mass in the same location.

inferior thyroidal artery), which enters the parathyroid gland at one of the poles. Internal vascularity is also commonly seen in a peripheral distribution. The artery feeding the adenoma tends to branch around the periphery of the gland before penetrating deeper, resulting in a characteristic arc or rim of vascularity. In addition, color Doppler sonography of the overlying thyroid gland may show an area of asymmetric hypervascularity that may help to locate an underlying adenoma. When grayscale and Doppler imaging fail to show an abnormal parathyroid gland, graded compression of subcutaneous tissues and strap muscles may show a relatively incompressible gland which may help differentiate an adenoma from surrounding soft tissue. This technique is often helpful in detection of ectopic glands in the lower neck.[29]

Hyperplasia is also a more difficult diagnosis to make sonographically because the single gland size is generally much smaller than an adenoma. However, similar to adenomas, compact cellularity may render hyperplastic glands hypoechoic relative to the overlying thyroid.

Pitfalls in Interpretation

Normal cervical structures such as perithyroid veins, esophagus and longus colli muscles of the neck can simulate parathyroid adenomas, producing false positive results during neck sonography. Performing real time sonography in multiple planes, color Doppler flow imaging and use of certain maneuvers by the patient help to differentiate the above normal structures from a suspected parathyroid adenoma. Pathologic structures that are potential causes of false positive results include thyroid nodules and cervical lymph nodes.

Several features may help in distinguishing lymph nodes from adenomas. An echogenic fatty hilum usually indicates a benign lymph node. At color Doppler examination, lymph nodes are supplied by small hilar vessels, whereas a polar, peripheral distribution of color flow is commonly seen with parathyroid adenomas.

Concomitant thyroid disease also contributes to imaging pitfalls. Enlarged multinodular thyroid gland can limit the sonographic evaluation of parathyroid adenomas. Anatomy is distorted and posterior nodules may mimic parathyroid disease. Posterior thyroid nodules can have a similar sonographic appearance to intracapsular parathyroid glands, although the typical vascular pattern of a parathyroid adenoma is uncommonly seen in thyroid nodules.[29]

Thyroid nodules more often show a heterogeneous echotexture with calcification and or cystic changes;[28] while parathyroid adenomas are of a homogeneous, hypoechoic echogenicity. A hyperechoic capsule favors a parathyroid adenoma. However, these sonographic features are inconsistent and it may not be always possible to differentiate abnormal parathyroid glands from lymphadenopathy and thyroid masses.

Percutaneous Aspiration/Biopsy

Fine needle aspiration cytology of the parathyroid masses has increased the specificity of sonography by reliably differentiating parathyroid pathology from thyroid nodule and cervical lymph nodes. In addition to the cytologic or histologic analysis of the specimen, the aspiration can be diluted with 1 mL of saline and analyzed for PTH by radioimmunoassay.[19]

Although PTH aspiration is rarely necessary for routine cases, this procedure can be particularly helpful in cases in which prior thyroid or parathyroid surgery has distorted neck anatomy or when preoperative confirmation of unusual-appearing or ectopic glands is needed. A theoretic complication of the procedure is seeding of abnormal parathyroid tissue along the biopsy track, resulting in an entity known as parathyromatosis. This has been described in cases of recurrent hyperparathyroidism after parathyroidectomy in which the capsule of the parathyroid gland was disrupted during the procedure.

Although it is primarily used as a therapy to treat tertiary hyperparathyroidism (most often in the setting of renal failure), sonographically guided parathyroid ablation with ethanol is a potential treatment option for patients with primary hyperparathyroidism. The procedure involves placement of the needle in the parathyroid gland and slowly injecting a volume of ethanol equal to approximately 50% of the volume of the gland until the absence of blood flow to the gland is confirmed on color Doppler sonography.[29]

Contrast-enhanced Computed Tomography

Contrast-enhanced computed tomography (CECT) has a sensitivity of up to 87% in detecting parathyroid adenoma. It is superior to sonography in patients with failed parathyroidectomy, in cases of altered anatomy and in delineating ectopic mediastinal parathyroid masses, thereby aiding in operative planning. Computed tomography has the advantage of larger field of view and ability to image all areas of neck and mediastinum. The advent of spiral CT has enabled excellent visualization of neck vasculature and their separation from other neck structures[19] **(Figs. 24A and B)**.

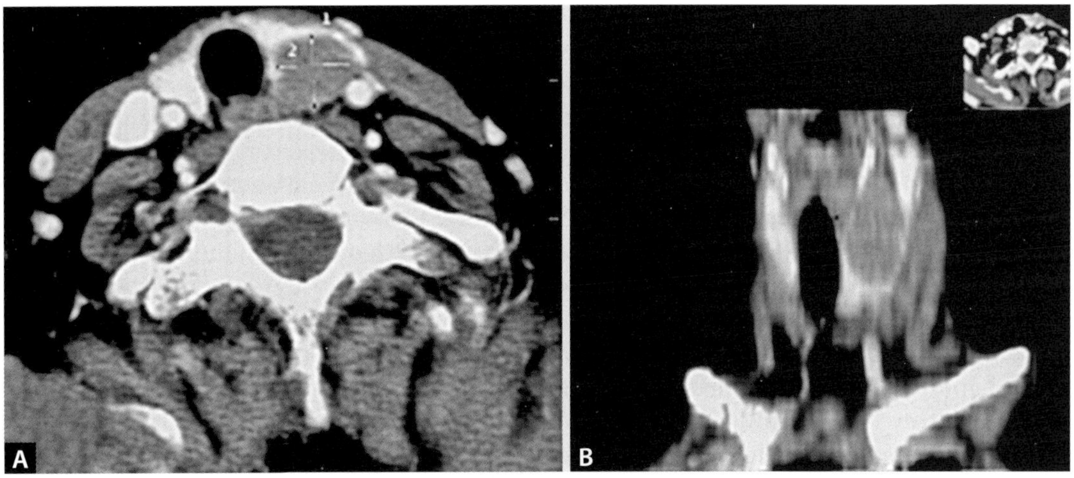

Figs. 24A and B: Axial CT section (A) and coronal reconstruction (B) shows a solid mass posterior to the left lobe of thyroid extending to the inferior part of neck in a patient of multiple parathyroid adenomas.

Magnetic Resonance Imaging

Magnetic resonance imaging (MRI) is less commonly used for preoperative localization than sonography and scintigraphy though it has similar sensitivity to other techniques in the detection of abnormal parathyroid tissue. MR imaging is the accepted modality for localizing parathyroid lesion in persistent or recurrent hyperparathyroidism, despite previous parathyroidectomies with a sensitivity of 88%.[30] Magnetic resonance imaging has an equally high sensitivity when the gland is in the mediastinum.[30]

On MR scans, parathyroid adenomas are soft tissue masses that are of low to medium signal intensity on T1-weighted images, are medium to high signal intencity on T2-weighted images and show moderate enhancement on gadolinium enhanced images. Approximately 10–35% of enlarged glands do not have high signal intensity on T2-weighted images. This may be due to fat content, hemorrhage or fibrosis. The size of the gland is the most important factor affecting detection on MRI.[30]

The typical signal intensities of abnormal parathyroid gland on T1-weighted and T2-weighted images may not be distinguishable from lymph nodes. This differentiation is more often based on topography and shape of the structures. A location medial to the carotid sheath is mostly due to parathyroid while nodes are located laterally.[19]

Parathyroid Scintigraphy

Nuclear medicine computer subtraction images of thallium and technetium can aid in the localization of the abnormal parathyroid gland. This technique relies on the differential uptake of the two isotopes by the thyroid and parathyroid glands. Thallium-201 chloride accumulates in tissues with high blood flow which includes both thyroid and parathyroid glands as well as in thyroid nodules and parathyroid adenomas. Technetium-99m accumulates only in the thyroid. Digital images are produced with each isotope. The technetium scan is then subtracted from the thallium leaving an image of only the parathyroid concentration of thallium.

The primary disadvantage of nuclear medicine techniques is limited spatial resolution. The maximum resolution of thallium-technetium scanning is 7–8 mm and it is very difficult to detect glands weighing less than 500 mg with this technique.[28]

The *radiopharmaceutical of choice* for imaging parathyroid enlargement is *^{99m}Tc sestamibi.* ^{99m}Tc sestamibi has replaced ^{201}Tl for parathyroid scintigraphy because of superior image quality, more favorable dosimetry, and improved detection sensitivity with its use. Three general techniques of radionuclide scintigraphy are commonly used for the detection and visualization of hyperfunctioning parathyroid glands that are as follows: single-phase dual isotope subtraction imaging, dual-phase single-isotope imaging and a combination of the two. In *dual isotope subtraction imaging technique,* one radiopharmaceutical (^{99m}Tc sestamibi) is used for visualization of the hyperfunctioning parathyroid gland and the thyroid gland and a second (^{123}I or ^{99m}Tc pertechnetate) is used for visualization of the thyroid gland only. The second set of images is then digitally subtracted from the first set. Evidence of residual radioactivity on the subtraction image represents a hyperfunctioning parathyroid gland. Disadvantages of this subtraction method include the necessity of two radionuclide injections and of a cooperative and immobile patient, identically positioned for the two studies. In addition, there is an increased likelihood of artifacts on images obtained with digital subtraction. Dual agent studies with ^{99m}Tc sestamibi and iodine 123 or ^{99m}Tc pertechnetate subtraction have produced a sensitivity of 95% for adenomas and 64–80% for hyperplastic glands.[28] The *single-isotope dual-phase imaging technique* was proposed on the basis of the frequently observed difference between the rate of ^{99m}Tc sestamibi washout from the thyroid gland and the rate of washout from hyperfunctioning parathyroid glands, which is typically slower. This technique requires a single injection of ^{99m}Tc sestamibi, followed by imaging at approximately 10–15 minutes and 1.5–3 hours after the injection. Increased mitochondrial content in parathyroid adenomas is believed to be responsible for the observed sestamibi concentration. Due to the high sensitivity of sestamibi scintigraphy (82–100%), it is generally considered the standard initial imaging modality to detect a parathyroid adenoma.

Single-photon Emission Computed Tomography

Single-photon emission computed tomography (SPECT) is a technique whereby images of diseased glands which have absorbed a radioactive marker can be obtained. It increases the sensitivity and specificity by 2–3% over routine sestamibi scanning. SPECT can be performed anytime within the first several hours after a patient is injected with sestamibi. SPECT is used with increasing frequency as it provides three dimensional information (lateral, superoinferior and anteroposterior). The major reason for the superiority of SPECT is the improved contrast resolution (target to background). The fusion of CT images with SPECT images, either by using software or by performing the studies sequentially on hybrid SPECT/CT imaging systems, has the advantage of combining the physiologic three-dimensional information from SPECT and anatomic information from CT. The most important use for SPECT scanning is when ordinary sestamibi scans are inconclusive or when a more detailed anatomic localization is required such as when patients are being reoperated.[19]

HYPOPARATHYROIDISM

The most common cause of hypoparathyroidism is excision or trauma to the parathyroid glands during thyroid surgery.[17] It can also occur as idiopathic hypoparathyroidism in which the parathyroid glands are absent or atrophied.

It usually occurs in childhood, with girls being affected more commonly than boys. The disorder may be characterized by the presence of circulating antibodies to the parathyroid, adrenal and thyroid glands, supporting the concept that idiopathic hypoparathyroidism may be part of a generalized autoimmune disease.

Rare forms of hypoparathyroidism are seen after radiation damage to the gland and as a response of an infant to HPT in the mother owing to transplacental transport of calcium with suppression of fetal parathyroid activity.

Clinical Presentation

Patients with hypoparathyroidism usually present with neuromuscular dysfunction precipitated by hypocalcemia.[14] Premature closure of the growth plate may lead to short stature. Dental abnormalities may occur in the form of delay or failure of tooth eruption.

Biochemical Findings

Laboratory findings in hypoparathyroidism consist of decreased serum levels of PTH and calcium with elevated phosphate levels.

RADIOLOGICAL FINDINGS

- The most common finding in hypoparathyroidism is bony sclerosis, which may be focal or generalized.[14,17] Localized osteoslerosis is more common, reported in 23% of patients while generalized osteosclerosis is seen in 9%.[21] Bones involved more commonly are pelvis, proximal femur, vertebral bodies.
- Other findings include calvarial thickening, hypoplastic dentition.
- Band-like areas of increased radiodensity in the metaphysis of long bones may also be seen in hypoparathyroidism.
- The abnormalities in the spine resemble those of diffuse idiopathic skeletal hyperostosis (DISH) including calcification and ossification of the anterior longitudinal ligament and spinal osteophytes. The sacroiliac joints are generally spared. This feature along with lack of erosive arthropathy differentiates it from ankylosing spondylitis.
- Subcutaneous calcification may be seen around the hip and shoulder joints.
- Calcium deposition in the basal ganglia a characteristic finding and occasionally also seen in the cerebrum

and cerebellum. It is also a feature of pseudohypoparathyroidism. It is also seen in infectious disorders such as toxoplasmosis and cytomegalic inclusion disease, in Fahr's syndrome (ferrocalcinosis), after radiation therapy and exposure to toxic substances such as carbon monoxide.[21]

PSEUDOHYPOPARATHYROIDISM

Pseudohypoparathyroidism (PHP) is an inherited disorder that manifests as end-organ resistance to parathyroid hormone rather than from deficient secretion of the hormone. This may be due to a defect in the adenylcyclase-cyclic AMP system in the renal tubules and bones. It is transmitted as an autosomal dominant trait and shares many features with hypoparathyroidism.

Clinical Findings

The patients are usually short, obese, mentally retarded and may have brachydactyly.[14,17]

Pseudohypoparathyroidism is more frequent in women than men and is usually diagnosed in the second decade of life.

Biochemical Findings

Hypocalcemia and hyperphosphatemia are seen similar to that in hypoparathyroidism. However, the levels of serum PTH are elevated.

Radiological Findings

- The best known sign of PHP is *shortening of the fourth metacarpal*: Although not specific for PHP as it is also seen in pseudopseudohypoparathyroidism (PPHP), this is a characteristic finding **(Fig. 25)**.

  The metacarpal sign has been used to determine whether this shortening is present. To use the sign a line is drawn tangential to the heads of the fourth and fifth metacarpals. Normally, the line does not intersect the third metacarpal bone or just contact its distal aspect. The sign is considered positive if the line intersects the third metacarpal, indicating disproportionate shortening of the fourth and fifth metacarpal bone. Other congenital conditions with positive metacarpal sign are basal cell nevus syndrome, multiple epiphyseal dysplasia, Beckwith-Wiedemann syndrome as well as acquired conditions such as juvenile chronic arthritis, sickle cell anemia with infarction, trauma and neonatal hyperthyroidism. This sign may be unreliable in diagnosing PHP and PPHP as the third metacarpal may also be short in these conditions.[21]

  Other radiological findings in PHP are similar to those of hypoparathyroidism and consist of bony sclerosis, soft tissue calcification, dense metaphyseal bands, calvarial thickening and basal ganglia calcification. Basal ganglia calcification is more common than in idiopathic hypoparathyroidism **(Fig. 26)**.[27]
- *Soft tissue calcification and ossification*: This occurs in approximately 55% of patients with PHP and is seen commonly in the hands and feet. The calcifications may be present at birth and are superficial in location and usually periarticular in distribution.
- Radiographic findings of secondary hyperparathyroidism may be seen in some patients with PHP.

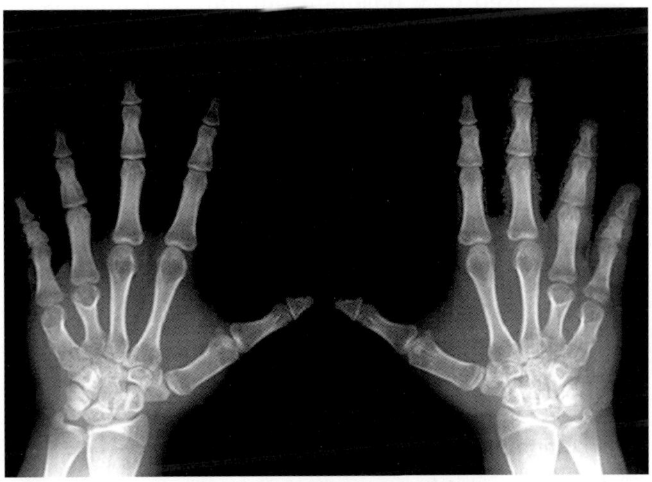

Fig. 25: Shortening of fourth and fifth metacarpal bones seen in both hands in a patient of pseudohypoparathyroidism (PHP) along with shortening of the middle phalanges of the fifth fingers.

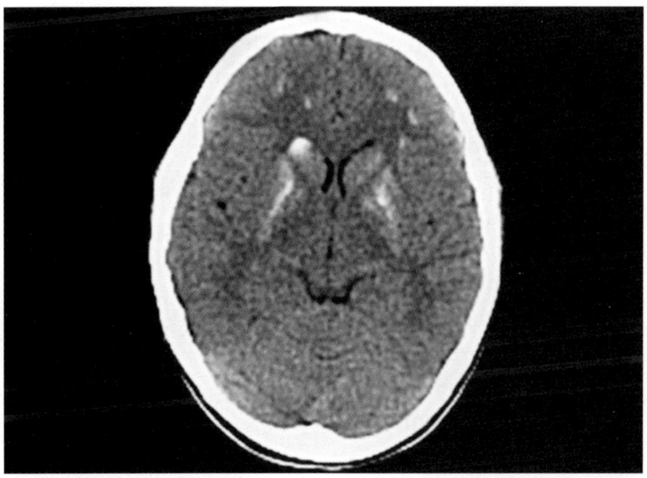

Fig. 26: PHP-Axial CT section of the cranium reveals calcification in bilateral basal ganglia and frontal lobes in a 13-year-old child.

- In addition to short metacarpals, metatarsals; phalanges may be short and exostoses and cone shaped epiphysis may be seen. The exostoses are frequently located centrally and project at right angles to the bone and differ from the appearance of multiple hereditary exostoses in which the outgrowths are usually directed away from joints.
- Growth deformities in the form of bowing of long bones may be seen.

PSEUDOPSEUDOHYPOPARATHYROIDISM

This is the result of incomplete genetic manifestation of PHP and like PHP is caused by an end organ resistance to PTH. Pseudohypoparathyroidism and PPHP share most of their clinical and radiological features. The main difference between the two is that patients with PPHP are normocalcemic.

Radiographic abnormalities of the hand in PHP and PPHP are almost identical except for a relatively higher rate of occurrence of short distal phalanges in PHP and relatively shorter metacarpals in PPHP.[17]

The differential diagnosis of short fourth metacarpal includes Turner's syndrome and physeal trauma. Other radiologic features of PHP may resemble fibrodysplasia ossificans progressiva or multiple hereditary exostosis syndrome.

DISORDERS OF ENDOCRINE ORIGIN

Normal skeletal maturation requires the presence of certain hormones in addition to vitamin D and other metabolites. The principal endocrine glands that influence this process are pituitary, thyroid, adrenals and gonads. Deficient production of hormones from any of these glands may disturb normal skeletal maturation and ossification. **Table 5** lists the normal reference values.

The various skeletal disorders of endocrine origin may be grouped as:

- *Disorders due to excessive corticosteroids*:
  - Hypercortisolism
- *Growth hormone disorders*:
  - Acromegaly
  - Gigantism
- *Thyroid disorders*:
  - Hypothyroidism
  - Hyperthyroidism
- *Gonadal disorders*:
  - Hypogonadism
  - Hypergonadism.

Table 5: Endocrine profile–reference values.

1.	Serum cortisol	Fasting (8 am–12 noon): 5–25 µg/dL 12 noon–8 pm: 5–15 µg/dL 8 pm–8 am: 0–10 µg/dL
2.	Serum ACTH	6–76 pg/mL
3.	Serum TSH	0.34–4.25 µIU/mL
4.	Free T3	2.4–4.2 pg/mL
5.	Total T4	5.4–11.7 µg/dL
6.	Serum growth hormone	0.5–17 ng/mL
7.	*Serum LH*: • Follicular phase • Ovulatory phase • Luteal phase	 2–15 IU/L 22–105 IU/L 0.6–19 IU/L
8.	*Serum FSH*: • Follicular phase • Ovulatory phase • Luteal phase	 3–20 IU/L 9–26 IU/L 1–12 IU/L
9.	*Serum free testosterone*: • Male • Female	 47–244 pg/mL 0.6–6.8 pg/mL
10.	Serum calcitonin (male/female)	3–26 pg/mL; 2–17 pg/mL

HYPERCORTISOLISM

Hypercortisolism or *Cushing's syndrome* is the clinical manifestation of exposure to excessive amounts of cortisol-like corticosteroids (glucocorticoid). It is caused by a tumor of the adernal glands (adenoma, carcinoma), ectopic ACTH production by a tumor (bronchial carcinoma) or iatrogenically by treatment with glucocorticoids. Cushing's disease caused by a basophil pituitary adenoma is an uncommon cause of hypercortisolism. Hypercortisolism is most frequently the result of excessive administration of exogenous corticosteroids.[31]

The effects of glucocorticoids on the skeleton are numerous and complex and consist of inhibition of bone formation, stimulation of bone resorption by osteoclast, decrease in intestinal absorption and increase in renal excretion of calcium and decrease in synthesis of collagen. The net result of hypercortisolism on the musculoskeletal system are osteoporosis, osteonecrosis and muscle wasting.[31]

Radiological Findings

- Generalized loss of bone density (osteoporosis) occurs which is more prominent in the spine, pelvis, ribs and cranial vault as trabecular bone is affected more severely than cortical bone.

- There is accentuation of primary trabeculae, with central endplate depressions in the vertebral bodies giving them a biconcave fish like appearance.
- Increased radiodensity of the superior and inferior margins of compressed or collapsed vertebral bodies is a characteristic feature due to exuberant callus formation, called marginal condensation, resulting from the combination of insufficient compressive microfractures and subsequent healing **(Figs. 27A and B)**. Exuberant callus may also be seen at fracture sites in long bones and ribs. Although the vertebral end plate sclerosis with osteoporosis is typical of hypercortisolism, in most cases it may be indistinguishable from generalized osteoporosis resulting from other causes such as hyperthyroidism, hyperparathyroidism, acromegaly, hypogonadism.

4. Local regions of osteonecrosis may be seen especially after treatment with exogenous corticosteroid. The typical sites of avascular necrosis are femoral and humeral heads which may be involved months or years after the corticosteroid treatment has begun or end.

Hypercortisolism during skeletal immaturity suppresses growth, resulting in a short child with osteoporosis, truncal obesity and delayed bone age. Osteonecrosis at growing epiphyses may lead to abnormal development at the ends of bone and eventually result in early development of degenerative osteoarthropathy.

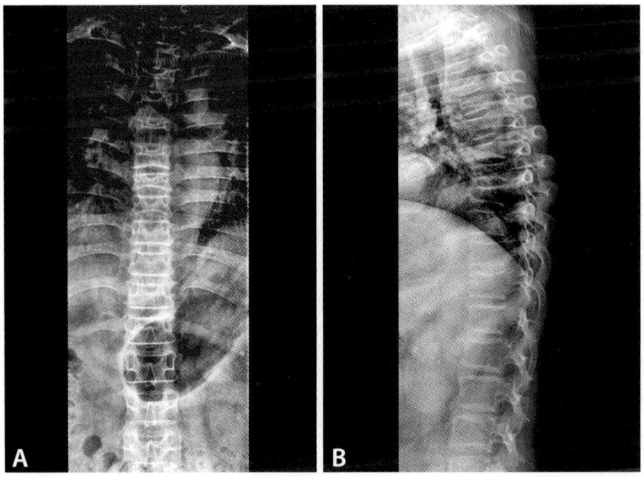

Figs. 27A and B: Cushing's syndrome due to increased ACTH production in a 16-year-old. X-ray dorsolumbar spine (AP) and (lateral) views reveal reduced height of vertebral bodies with endplate sclerosis and osteoporosis.

HYPOPITUITARISM

This is due to deficiency of anterior pituitary hormones, particularly growth hormone resulting from damage to the pituitary gland by neoplasms, infections, vascular insults or posttherapeutic ablations. If the deficiency in growth hormone occurs in combination with deficiencies in other pituitary hormones, it is called panhypopituitarism.[31]

Radiological Findings

- There is delay in skeletal maturation manifested radiologically by a delay in appearance and closure of epiphysis.
- Skeletal growth is retarded.
- There is overall loss of bone density due to decreased bone formation.

HYPOTHYROIDISM

Deficiency of thyroid hormones (T3 and T4) produces a spectrum of musculoskeletal abnormalities termed 'cretinism' in infants, 'juvenile myxoedema' in children and 'myxoedema' or 'hypothyroidism' in adults.[20] The deficiency may result from disorders that affect the thyroid gland (primary hypothyroidism) or from a deficiency of thyroid stimulating hormone (secondary hypothyroidism). Primary hypothyroidism occurs as a result of thyroiditis, neoplastic disorders, thyroid ablation or disturbances in iodine metabolism.

Clinical Findings

Clinical manifestations of hypothyroidism vary according to the age of the patient at the time of presentation.[14] In infants there is mental retardation and developmental abnormalities as thyroid hormone is essential for postnatal growth. In children; mental retardation, obesity, developmental delay, growth retardation, lethargy and constipation may be seen. The clinical presentation in adults includes fatigue, lethargy, paresthesias, dry coarse skin and hair, constipation and bradycardia.

Radiological Findings

The radiologic findings also depend on the patient's age at presentation.

Congenital hypothyroidism is characterized by delayed skeletal maturation with bone age lagging behind the chronological age. This is evident by short stature and the late appearance of epiphyseal ossification centres. Bone age can be assessed by getting a plain radiograph of the knee.[31] Normally, the distal femoral epiphysis is usually ossified at 36 weeks gestational age and the proximal tibial epiphysis at 38 weeks gestational age. Decreased size or absence of distal femoral or proximal tibial epiphyses is a marker for intrauterine hypothyroidism. When they appear, the ossification centres are deformed and irregularly shaped (*epiphyseal dysgenesis*). These changes are bilateral and symmetrical. Such changes in the hip must be differentiated from bilateral Perthes disease and multiple epiphyseal dysplasia.There is also delayed closure of the epiphyseal plates in hypothyroidism.

In the *skull,* the sutures may remain open and show the formation of intrasutural (Wormian) bones. The sella is either small and bowl shaped in young children or large, rounded in older children. The paranasal sinus are underdeveloped.

In the *spine,* anteriorly wedged bullet-shaped vertebral bodies are seen, especially at the thoracolumbar junction, where kyphosis may develop.

In the *pelvis,* the incidence of slipped capital femoral epiphysis is increased. The pelvis is often narrow with coxa vara deformities.

In adult hypothyroidism, skeletal manifestations are usually mild. Generalized osteoporosis is the most common finding.

HYPERTHYROIDISM

Hyperfunction of the thyroid gland usually occurs as a result of Graves' disease (toxic diffuse goitre) or toxic multinodular goitre.[20] Excessive production of thyroid hormones, both triiodothyronine (T3) and thyroxine (T4) by the overactive gland cause a hypermetabolic state. This results in increase in both formation and resorption, with bone resorption being dominant.[14] Catabolism of protein and loss of connective tissue manifests as muscle wasting.

Hyperthyroidism in children causes accelerated skeletal maturation and advanced bone age. In adults it causes generalized osteoporosis leading to vertebral fractures and kyphosis.

Clinical Findings

Patients may present with weakness, fatigue, nervousness, weight loss, tachycardia, palpitations, diarrhea or intolerance to heat.[14] Myopathy is a common clinical feature of hyperthyroidism whose symptoms may mimic that of arthritis. Muscle wasting is also known to occur especially in the proximal muscle groups.[31]

Biochemical Findings

Biochemical findings show elevated levels of calcium, phosphorus and alkaline phosphatase and elevated urinary calcium.

Radiological Findings

Skeletal finding in hyperthyroidism are more common in men and patients with radiologic abnormalities having had the disease for at least five years.

- *Osteoporosis* is the most common radiological finding particularly in the spine, pelvis, skull, hands and feet. Older patients show rapidly progressive generalized osteoporosis. It has been seen that the progression of thyrotoxic osteoporosis is much more rapid than post-menopausal osteoporosis,[31] even though the two are radiologically indistinguishable. An overall decrease in bone density is seen as a result of bone resorption. Changes in the spine are more common in the dorsal and lumbar vertebrae and consist of biconcave vertebral bodies, wedge deformities and resultant kyphosis. Fractures may also occur, especially in femoral neck.
- The predominant radiographic pattern of increased osteoblastic and osteoclastic activity consists of *cortical tunneling or striations*. This is more evident in the tubular bones of the hand and feet occurring in up to 50% of patients.[20]
- *Thyroid acropachy* is a rare complication that occurs in 0.5–1% of patients after treatment for hyperthyroidism by surgery or antithyroid medication.[14,31] It may appear years after the initial presentation of hyperthyroidism and the patients are often euthyroid but may be hypo or hyperthyroid. The cause is unknown with no apparent age or gender predilection. Patients may present with exophthalmos, soft tissue swelling of the fingers and toes, pretibial myxoedema or clubbing.[14,31]

The radiologic findings of thyroid acropachy are virtually diagnostic and consist of dense, solid, periosteal new bone formation with feathery margins. The periostitis is commonly seen in an asymmetric distribution and is most prominent along the radial margin of metacarpals and phalanges in the diaphyseal region. Uncommonly, long bones may be involved. The bony changes are not progressive.[31]

Thyroid acropachy must be distinguished from hypertrophic osteoarthropathy, a very painful condition wherein the long bones are considerably more likely to be involved than are hands and feet and the feathery contour is absent. Another differential of thyroid acropachy is pachydermo-periostitis where the periostitis effects the long bones more than the hands with extension of the periosteal new bone to the metaphysis and epiphysis. There is associated soft tissue prominence of the hands with bilateral symmetrical periosteal bone formation in tibia, fibula, radius and ulna.[32] The radiological appearance of venous stasis, leukemia, osteomyelitis may mimic thyroid acropachy but differentiation is usually possible on the basis of characteristic clinical presentation of these disorders.[14] Fluorosis is associated with more extensive abnormality of the axial skeleton and long bones, while leukemic acropachy is particularly prominent in the terminal phalanges.[32]

HYPERGONADISM

Hypergonadism may be caused by overproduction of sex hormones by the testes or ovaries or by the overproduction by the adrenal cortex. In congenital adrenal hyperplasia, a deficiency in the synthesis of cortisol leads to high levels of ACTH. A secondary effect of high ACTH leads to excessive levels of adrenal sex steroids. A central nervous system lesion may also lead to gonadotropin excess and hypergonadism.

The skeletal manifestation of hypergonadism in the child is precocious growth and maturation. The epiphyseal ossification centers appear early. The long bones grow rapidly and the growth plates close early. Although there is initial precocious growth spurt, the early closure of the growth plate results in short stature, with a tall child becoming a short adult.[31] The morphology of the skeleton is otherwise normal.

HYPOGONADISM

Hypogonadism may be secondary to low production of gonadotropins (luteinising hormone, follicle stimulating hormone) from the pituitary, or deficient production of hormones by the gonads themselves.[20] The latter is termed 'primary gonadal deficiency' and, when present in growing boys is referred to as *eunuchoidism. Turner's syndrome* is a female sex-linked disorder in which there is ovarian dysgenesis due to an XO genotype. In older women, primary gonadal deficiency occurs with menopause.

Radiological Findings

The radiographic features of hypogonadism in males consist of:

- Generalized decrease in bone density.
- Delay in skeletal maturation which manifests in the form of delayed closure of epiphysis. This results in long extremities with relatively short trunks.

Turner's Syndrome

- More than 50% of the patients do not have any radiographic abnormalities. In the remaining patients, skeletal maturation is usually normal until 15 years of age, following which delayed epiphyseal closure becomes evident, particularly in the apophysis of the iliac crests[20] and unusually long and slender tubular bones in the extremities.
- There may be depression or slanting of the medial tibial plateau with concomitant overgrowth of the medial condyle of the femur.
- The fourth and fifth metacarpals are often short producing a positive metacarpal sign. The heads of the third and fourth metacarpals may appear flattened and cubitus valgus may be seen. This is seen in 50% of patients.
- Other findings include narrow ribs, small sella turcica, hypertelorism and android pelvis.

GROWTH HORMONE DISORDERS

Growth hormone disorders occur as a result of excess or deficient production of growth hormone.

ACROMEGALY

Acromegaly results from excessive production of growth hormone (somatotropin) in a skeletally mature individual. It is usually caused by a pituitary adenoma that produces growth hormone autonomously. Elevated serum growth hormone reactivates endochondral bone formation, stimulates periosteal bone formation along with connective tissue proliferation leading to characteristic clinical and radiological features.

The overgrowth of bone in association with enlargement of soft tissue is particularly prominent in the acral parts (hands, feet, lower jaw) of the skeleton leading to the term acromegaly for this condition.[33]

Clinical Findings

Acromegaly is typically seen in the third or fourth decade of life with an equal incidence in men and women.

The clinical features are distinctive and include coarse facial features, thick skin, poor dental occlusion, thick calvarium, deepening of voice, lantern jaw, prominent tongue, broad hand and feet and organomegaly.[14] Rheumatologic complaints like backache and arthropathy are common.

Definitive Diagnosis

The definitive diagnosis of acromegaly is made by measurement of 24 hours serum growth hormone levels and demonstration that growth hormone secretion is not suppressed by an oral glucose challenge. Measurement of serum levels of insulin-like growth factor 1 (IGF-1 or somatomedin C) is a sensitive screening test.[31]

Radiological Findings

The radiographic findings of bony and soft tissue overgrowth are quite characteristic in patients of acromegaly.

- Collagen tissue demonstrates a marked response to excessive amounts of growth hormone which manifests in the form of thickening of the skin. *Soft tissue thickening* is classically seen in the heel pads and digits. The measurement is obtained by calculating the shortest distance between the calcaneus and plantar surface of the skin **(Fig. 28)**. According to Kho and associates, the thickness of the heel pad in acromegaly is related to the severity and chronicity of disease and is correlated with serum levels of growth hormone (GH).[33] Values greater than 23 mm in men and 21.5 mm in women are suggestive of acromegaly and values greater than 25 mm in men and 23 mm in women are diagnostic, if local causes of skin thickening are excluded.[33]
- In the *skull, changes* include:
  - Thickening of the cranial vault
  - Prominence of the supraorbital ridges and zygomatic arches
  - Prominence of the external occipital protuberance
  - Enlargement of the sella turcica with distinctive changes
  - Prominence and enlargement of the frontal and maxillary sinuses
  - Excessive pneumatization of the mastoid
  - Enlargement and elongation of the mandible with widening of the mandibular angle.
- *Abnormalities in the hands and wrists* include soft tissue thickening of fingers, thickening and squaring of the phalanges and metacarpals, tabulation or overconstriction of the shafts of the phalanges, abnormally wide articular spaces, bony excrescences at sites of tendon and ligament attachment to bone and prominence of the ungual tufts which may assume a spade-like appearance.[33] An increase in soft tissue **(Fig. 29)** and bony measurements at certain specific sites have been described. One such measurement in the *Sesamoid index* which is the greatest product of the medial first metacarpophalangeal sesamoid and its maximum perpendicular diameter. This index greater than 40 mm in men and 32 mm in women is suggestive of acromegaly. No single measurement is specific for acromegaly and the concomitant findings which are suggestive of acromegaly include:
  - Increased phalangeal soft tissue thickness ≥27 mm (men) (at proximal mid phalanges) ≥26 mm (women)
  - Widening of second metacarpophalangeal joint >2.5 mm in men and women
  - Bone excrescences and marginal spurs
  - Increased width of phalanges
  - Large sesamoid index >40 mm (men) >32 mm (women)
  - Increased interstyloid distance.
- The abnormalities in the *vertebral column* in acromegaly consist of:
  - Elongation and widening of vertebral bodies
  - Anterior and lateral osteophytes
  - Increased height of intervertebral disk
  - Scalloping of the posterior margins of vertebral bodies
  - Increased thoracic kyphosis
  - Exaggerated lumbar lordosis.

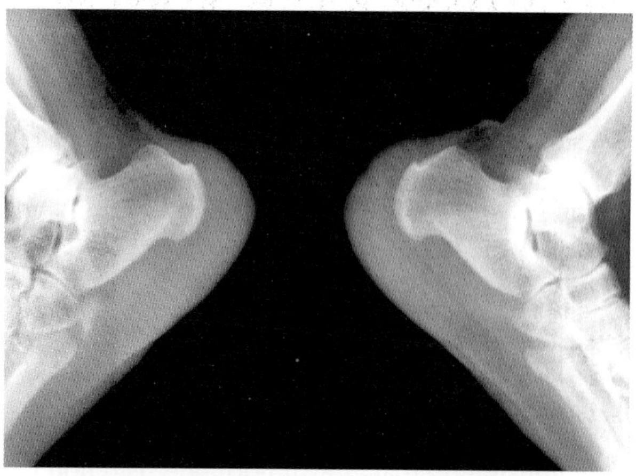

Fig. 28: Acromegaly with increase in soft tissue thickness of the heel pad.

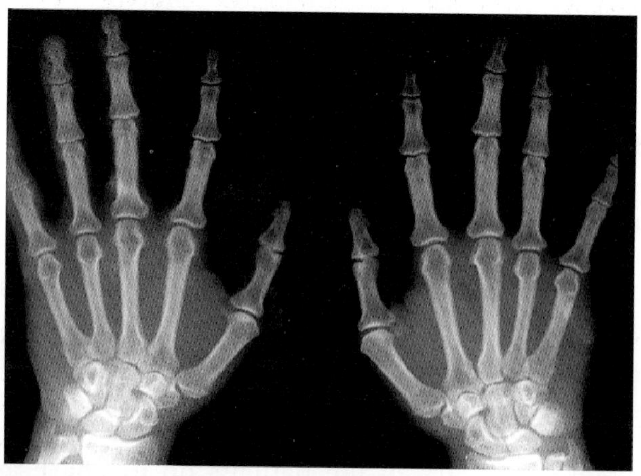

Fig. 29: Acromegaly: There is enlargement of the soft tissues with thickening of fingers and prominent joint spaces due to cartilage hypertrophy. The distal phalanges show the characteristic arrow head appearance, more marked in the first finger.

- *Thoracic cage abnormalities* consist of an enlarged thorax due to elongation of ribs and prominence of costochondral junction.
- In *pelvis*, in addition to articular alteration in sacroiliac joints and hip, enlargement and beaking of symphysis pubis is seen.
- In the *feet*, the radiographic changes resemble those in hands with:
  - Soft tissue enlargement
  - Prominence of tufts and base of terminal phalanges
  - Bone proliferation at sites of tendon and ligament attachment like undersurface of calcaneum.
- *Articular abnormalities* are most frequently seen in the knees, hip and glenohumeral joints. Proliferation of chondrocytes in the articular cartilage result in widening of articular space seen at metacarpophalangeal, metatarsophalangeal and interphalangeal joints.

In the later stages of the disease cartilaginous and osseous degeneration occurs leading to secondary degenerative changes. Superficially, the appearance of acromegalic arthropathy is similar to osteoarthritis, but the joint spaces tend to be widened rather than narrowed. The distribution of involvement usually includes the large joints and the lumbosacral spine which are normally spared by osteoarthritis.

GIGANTISM

Excess of growth hormone during skeletal development results in gigantism, which is a rare condition. The direct hormonal stimulation of activity at the growth plates and other sites of bone formation by growth hormone leads to progressive enlargement of length and width of the bones. The most striking feature of patients with gigantism is extreme height with normal body proportions.[31] An autonomously functioning pituitary adenoma is the most common cause of gigantism. Unless treated, the growth hormone excess continues after growth plate closure with patients of gigantism developing progressively more striking features of acromegaly.[31]

SCURVY

Scurvy is the result of long-term deficiency of vitamin C. Infantile scurvy is found in infants fed on pasteurized or boiled milk formula, since the pasteurization and boiling processes destroy the vitamin C content.[7,20] Scurvy is rare before six months of age as for scurvy to manifest itself the deficiency must be present for at least four to six months.[20] It is seen much less frequently than rickets.[34]

Clinical Findings

Scurvy usually occurs in 6 months to 2 years age group. Child presents with progressive irritability, with tender, edematous limbs. Subcutaneous and mucous membrane hemorrhages occur and a secondary anemia may develop. Scurvy is rare in adults, being seen in patients suffering from chronic severe malnutrition.

Biochemical Findings

Serum ascorbic acid <0.6 mg/100 mL.

Pathophysiology

The pathological changes seen in scurvy are the result of depression of normal cellular activity.[20] There is suppression of osteoblastic activity resulting in cessation of normal bone formation. However, bone resorption continues leading to the development of osteoporosis.

At the growth plate, although cartilage proliferation is decreased, mineralization is unimpaired, resulting in the zone of provisional calcification becoming wide and dense. Similar changes occur around epiphyseal ossification centres, resulting in a thin ring of *increased* density surrounding the *epiphysis*. Vascular invasion of the zone of provisional calcification is arrested and with suppressed osteoblastic activity there is decreased formation of bony matrix. Thus, the trabecular bone mass is decreased in the zone of primary and secondary spongiosa. This is seen radiographically as a *transverse band* of *radiolucency* adjacent to the zone of provisional calcification. This zone, called Trümmerfeld zone represents an area of weakened bone and shows a tendency to fracture. The zone of provisional calcification extends beyond the margins of the metaphysis, resulting in periosteal elevation and marginal spur formation. Large subperiosteal hemorrhages resulting in soft tissue edema occur in late stages of the disease.

The optimal sites for detection of scurvy in the skeleton are bones of the lower extremities. Diagnostic changes may be demonstrable at the knees when minimal changes are present at the wrists.[7]

Radiological Findings

Radiographically, characteristic signs are seen which reflect the pathological changes occurring as a result of lack of vitamin C.

- Osteoporosis
- *White line of Frankel* is the dense, white line in the zone of provisional calcification at the growing metaphysis.

- Beneath the Frankel's line is a radiolucent zone in the metaphysis called *Trummerfeld zone or Scorbutic zone*, due to lack of mineralization of osteoid **(Fig. 30)**.
- The epiphysis is small, sharply marginated by a sclerotic rim while the central portion is more radiolucent, called *Wimberger's sign*.
- Finally, as the metaphysis is weakened, it is prone to fractures, which manifest themselves at the cortical margin, giving rise to *Pelkan's spur*.
- In addition, due to capillary permeability, *subperiosteal hemorrhages* occur which may give rise to periosteal elevation and subsequent new bone formation, particularly following treatment. The hemorrhages are most often seen in the ends of long bones, such as femur, tibia, humerus. Upon healing, the subperiosteal hemorrhages calcify and cast shadows of increased density in the soft tissues surrounding the bone **(Fig. 31)**.

The above findings constitute the classic signs of infantile scurvy. These changes are less apparent as the patient ages. On healing, all changes are reversible on vitamin C therapy though a single growth arrest line may remain in the metaphysis as a residual of Frankel's line.

FLUOROSIS

Chronic ingestion of excessive amounts of fluoride results in fluorosis, with a fluoride concentration in excess of 8 parts per million (ppm) in drinking water.[34]

The alterations in bone metabolism in fluorosis are not clearly understood but seem to be multifactorial. A generalized increase in bone density is seen which is due to osteoclastic response to the fluorine rather than fluorine deposition *per se*.[10] The synthesis of normal collagen is also disturbed.

Clinical Findings

Clinically, there is marked variation in presentation. The most pronounced feature is mottled dental enamel. Bone changes produces few symptoms. However, exceptionally high levels of fluorine may be associated with crippling stiffness and pain.[10]

Radiographical Findings

Radiographically the changes are diffuse osteosclerosis, osteophytosis and calcification/ossification in ligaments.

- *Osteosclerosis* involves all bones but is most marked in the spine, pelvis and ribs **(Figs. 32A and B)**. Initially, there is a thickening of the bony trabecular pattern which then progresses to a dense, uniform, symmetrical sclerosis that obliterates the bony architectural landmarks. The skull and tubular bones of the appendicular skeleton are relatively spared in the sclerotic process. The only change in the calvarium may be a sclerosis of the base of the skull and posterior clinoids.[34]

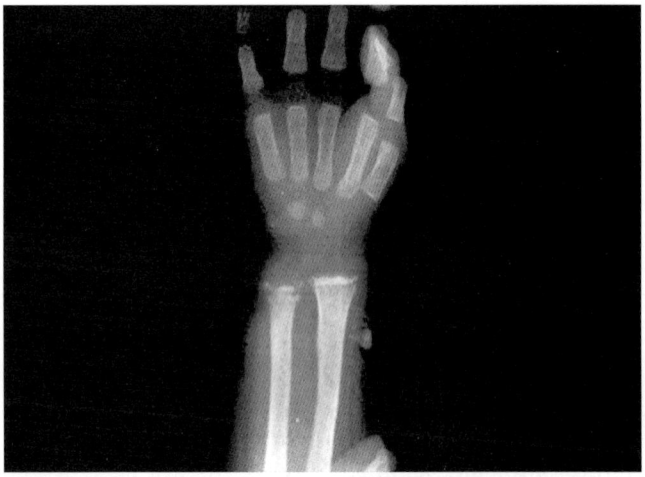

Fig. 30: Scurvy: X-ray wrist AP view reveals increased density of the zone of provisional calcification (Frankel's line) with a lucent zone beneath it (Trummerfeld zone) in the distal radial and ulnar metaphysis.

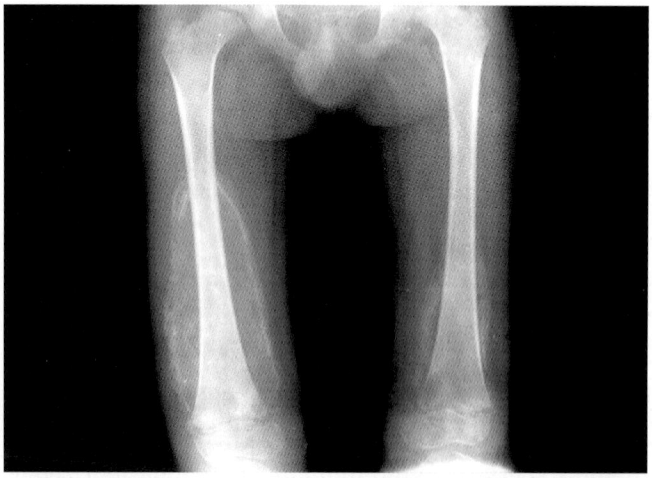

Fig. 31: Calcified subperiosteal hemorrhages seen along bilateral femoral shafts, more extensive on the right side—Healing scurvy.

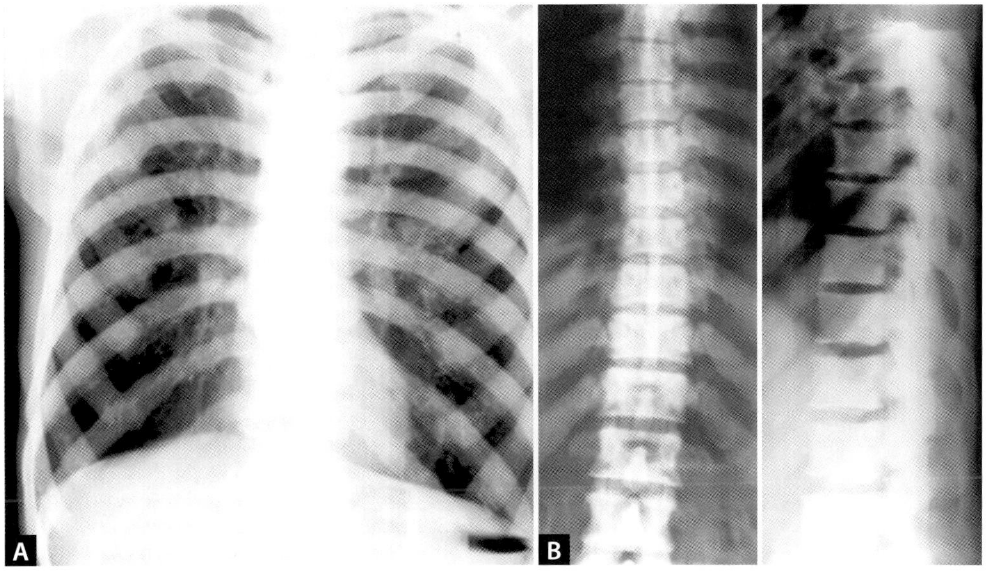

Figs. 32A and B: Fluorosis: (A) Frontal chest X-ray reveals diffuse osteosclerosis; (B) Osteosclerosis and osteophytosis of the dorsal vertebral bodies with posterior longitudinal ligament ossification.

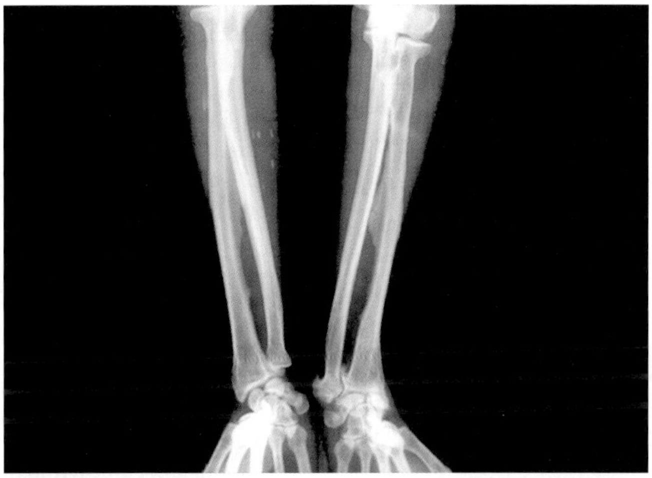

Fig. 33: Interosseous membrane ossification—Diagnostic of fluorosis.

- Thickening of the cortex of the affected bones occur at the expense of the medullary cavity.
- The inferior margins of the ribs may show characteristic irregularity/fringed appearance called "rose thorn appearance."
- *Ligamentous calcification* and *ossification*; particularly of sacrospinous and sacrotuberous ligaments is another characteristic radiographic feature.
- *Ossification* in the *interosseous membranes* of paired bones is *diagnostic* **(Fig. 33)**.
- *Osteophytosis* of the vertebrae can be severe and at times encroach on the spinal canal and intervertebral foramina. Paraspinal and intraspinal ligament ossification is known to occur and may cause compressive myelopathy **(Fig. 34)**.

To conclude, plain radiographs are the primary imaging tools for the evaluation of suspected skeletal disorders of metabolic and endocrine origin. By and large these disorders involve the skeleton as a whole. The radiographic changes are therefore predominantly diffuse or at least multifocal involving many areas of the skeleton. An understating of the diverse manifestations of these disorders including their findings on imaging help us reach an early diagnosis.

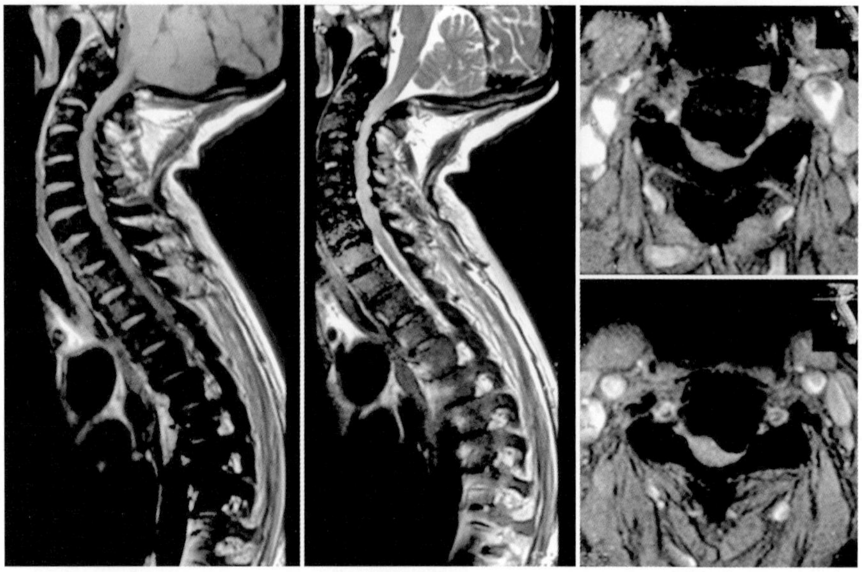

Fig. 34: Fluorosis: T1W and T2W sagittal MR scans of cervicodorsal spine reveals diffuse decrease in marrow signal intensity of vertebral bodies, appearing more hypointense than intervening intervertebral discs consistent with sclerosis. The vertebral bodies show osteophytic changes. Axial images depict ossification of posterior longitudinal ligament with resultant spinal canal stenosis.

REFERENCES

1. Mankin HJ. Metabolic bone disease. J Bone Joint Surg Am. 1994;76:760.
2. Reynolds WA, Karo JJ. Radiologic diagnosis of metabolic bone disease. Orthop Clin North Am. 1972;3:521.
3. Pitt M. Osteopenic bone disease. Orthop Clin North Am. 1983;14:65.
4. Pitt MJ. Rickets and osteomalacia are still around. Radiol Clin North Am. 1991;29(1):97.
5. Mankin HJ. Rickets, osteomalacia and renal osteodystrophy: Part I. J Bone Joint Surg Am. 1974;56:101.
6. Rowe LJ, Yochum TR. Nutritional Metabolic and Endocrine Disorders. In: Yochum, Rowes (Eds). Essentials of skeletal Radiology, 3rd edition. Lippincott Williams and Wilkins. 2005;2:1497-545.
7. Silverman FN. Dysostoses, miscellaneous syndromes and metabolic abnormalities. In: Silverman FN, Kuhn JP (Eds). Caffey's Pediatric X-ray Diagnosis, 9th edn. Mosby. 1993;2:1746-81.
8. Kottamasu SR. Metabolic Bone diseases. In: Silverman FN, Kuhn JP (Eds). Caffey's Pediatric X-ray Diagnosis, 10th edn, Mosby. 2003;2:2242-68.
9. Pitt MJ. Rickets and osteomalacia. In: Resmick D, Krausdorf MJ (Eds). Bone and Joint Imaging, 3rd edn. Elsevier Saunders. 2005;2:563-75.
10. Murray RO, Stoker DJ. Skeletal disorders of metabolic and endocrine origin. In: Sutton D (Ed). Textbook of Radiology and Imaging, 4th edition. Churchill Livingstone. 1987;1:229-63.
11. Gupta AK. Rickets and osteomalacia. In: Berry M, Chowdhury V, Suri S, Mukhopadhyay S (Eds). Diagnostic Radiology—Musculoskeletal and Breast Imaging, 1st edition. Jaypee Brothers Medical Publishers; 1998. pp. 162-75.
12. Pitt MJ. Rickets and osteomalacia. In: Resnick D (Ed). Diagnosis of Bone and Joint Disorders, 4th edition. WB Saunders Company. 2002;2:1901-45.
13. Adams Judith E. Metabolic and endocrine skeletal disease. In: Adams A, Dixon AK (Eds). Grainger and Allison's Diagnostic Radiology A Textbook of Medical Imaging, 5th edition. Churchill Livingstone Elsevier. 2008;2:1083-113.
14. Lenchik L, Sartoris DJ. Orthopaedic aspects of metabolic bone disease. Orthop Clin North Am. 1998;29(1):103-34.
15. Steinbach HL, Noetzli M. Roentgen appearance of the skeleton in osteomalacia and rickets. AJR. 1964;91: 955.
16. Chuang TL, Kuo JL, Chang XY, et al. Scintigraphic evidence of osteomalacia: Usefulness and typical signs. Ann Nucl Med Sci. 2007;20:115-20.
17. Resnick D. Parathyroid disorders and renal osteodystrophy. In: Resnick D (Ed). Diagnosis of Bone and Joint Disorders, 4th edn WB Saunders Company. 2002;2:2043-111.
18. Eslamy HK, Ziessman HA. Parathyroid scintigraphy in patients with primary hyperparathyroidism: ^{99m}Tc sestamibi SPECT and SPECT /CT. Radiographics. 2008;28:1461-76.
19. Chowdhury V. Hyperparathyroidism. In: Berry M, Chowdhury V, Suri S, Mukhopadhyay S (Eds). Diagnostic Radiology-Musculoskeletal and Breast Imaging, 1st edition. Jaypee Brothers Medical Publishers; 1998. pp. 186-200.
20. Volger JB, Kim JH. Metabolic and endocrine disease of the skeleton. In: Grainger RG, Allison DJ, Adam A, Dixon AK (Eds). Diagnostic Radiology. A Textbook of Medical Imaging, 4th edn. Churchill Livingstone. 2001;3:1925-66.
21. Resmick D. Parathyroid disorders and renal osteodystrophy. In: Resmick D, Krausdorf MJ (Eds). Bone and Joint Imaging, 3rd edition. Elsevier Saunders. 2005;2:603-22.
22. Hayes CW, Conway WF. Hyperparathyroidism Radiol Clin North Am. 1991;29(1):85-96.

23. Richardson ML, Pozz-Mucelli RS, Kanter AS. Bone mineral changes in primary hyperparathyroidism. Skeletal Radiol. 1986;15:85-95.
24. Sahan MH, Guner S, Guner SI. Radiological findings in the primary hyperparathyroid case with multiple brown tumors: a case report. East J Med. 2008;13:30-4.
25. Su AW, Chen CF, Huang CK, et al. Primary hyperparathyroidism with brown tumor mimicking metastatic bone malignancy. J Chin Med Assoc. 2010;73(3):177-80.
26. Greenspan A. Hyperparathyroidism. In: Greenspan A (Ed). Orthopaedic Imaging: A practical approach, 4th edition. Lippincott Williams and Wilkins; 2004. pp. 837-42.
27. Young WR. Metabolic and Endocrine disorders affecting bone. In: Sutton D (Ed). Textbook of Radiology and Imaging, 7th edition. Churchill Livingstone. 2003;1:1351-69.
28. Larson TC, Smith MM, Chong WK, Martin WH. Imaging of the thyroid and parathyroid glands. In: Hagga JR, Lanzieri CF, Gilkeson RC (Eds). CT and MR Imaging of the Whole Body, 4th edition. Mosby. 2003;1:663-90.
29. Johnson NA, Tublin ME, Ogilvie JB. Parathyroid imaging: Technique and role in the preoperative evaluation of primary hyperparathyroidism. AJR. 2007;188:1706-15.
30. Mc Dermott VG, Spritzer CE. Parathyroid and thyroid glands. In: Stark DD, Bradley WG Jr (Eds). Magnetic Resonance Imaging, 3rd edition, vol III. Mosby, Inc; 1999. pp. 1807-20.
31. Chew FS. Radiologic Manifestations in the musculoskeletal system of miscellaneous endocrine disorders. Radiol Clin North Am. 1991;29(1):135-47.
32. Resnick D. Pituitary Disorders. In: Resnick D (Ed). Diagnosis of Bone and Joint Disorders, 4th edn. WB Saunders Company. 2002;3:2003-25.
33. Resnick D. Pituitary Disorders. In: Resnick D (Ed). Diagnosis of Bone and Joint Disorders, 5th edn. WB Saunders Company. 2005;2:589-96.
34. Greenfield GB. Epiphyseal region. In: Greenfield (Ed). Radiology of Bone Diseases, 5th edition. JB Lippincott Company; 1990.p.235.

CHAPTER 197

Osteoporosis

Mukesh Kumar Yadav, Vivek Gupta, Niranjan Khandelwal

DEFINITION

Osteoporosis is the most common of all metabolic bone disorders and has been defined by the World Health Organization (WHO) as "a skeletal disease, characterized by low bone mass and microarchitectural deterioration of bone tissue, with a consequent increase in fragility of the bones and susceptibility to fracture".[1] Histologically, the disorder is characterized by a decrease in cortical thickness and in the number and size of the trabeculae of cancellous bone. Individual trabecular plates may be fractured or trabecular connectivity may be reduced. There is no abnormality in the structure of organic matrix (osteoid), nor is there any defect in mineralization. Thus, osteoporosis can be readily distinguished histologically from osteomalacia, in which mineralization of osteoid is impaired and the ratio of organic matrix to mineral is increased.[2]

PATHOGENESIS

Bone remodeling (its formation and resorption) is a continuous process. It is normally regulated by systemic and locally produced agents and metabolic, nutritional and mechanical factors. The normal balance between bone formation and resorption results in maintenance of skeletal mass. In osteoporosis, the bone mass is decreased, indicating that the rate of bone resorption must be more than that of bone formation.[2]

A decrease in bone mass is also a consequence of aging. Skeletal growth is complete by the end of adolescence, but even after closure of the endochondral growth plate, bone mass increases by radial growth until peak bone mass is achieved at about the age of 35 years. After a short interval of balanced bone metabolism, bone resorption begins to exceed bone formation and skeletal mass decreases. The rate of bone loss differs in different areas of skeleton. In both sexes, after the age of 40–50 years, there is a slow rate of loss of cortical bone of about 0.3–0.5% per year; because of its higher metabolic activity, it is higher for trabecular bone, about 1.5% per year. The rate of bone loss in women also may be accelerated around the time of menopause which is likely to be due to estrogen deficiency. The cumulative loss of bone mass ranges from 20% to 30% in men and 40% to 50% in women.[2]

CLASSIFICATION

Cause Unknown

- Primary osteoporosis (senile, postmenopausal)
- Juvenile osteoporosis.

Causes Known[3]

Endocrine Disorders:
- Acromegaly
- Adrenal atrophy in Addison's disease
- Cushing's syndrome
- Eating disorders
- Endometriosis
- Gonadal insufficiency (primary or secondary)

- Hyperparathyroidism
- Hyperprolactinemia
- Hyperthyroidism
- Hypogonadism
- Type 1 diabetes mellitus
- Nutritional disorders
- Tumor secretion of parathyroid hormone-related peptide.

Gastrointestinal Disease:
- Alcohol-related liver diseases
- Celiac disease
- Chronic active hepatitis
- Chronic cholestatic diseases
- Gastrectomy
- Inflammatory bowel disease
- Jejunoileal bypass
- Malabsorption syndromes
- Pancreatic insufficiency
- Parenteral nutrition
- Primary biliary cirrhosis
- Severe liver disease.

Marrow-related Disorders:
- Amyloidosis
- Hemochromatosis
- Hemophilia
- Leukemia
- Lymphoma
- Mastocytosis
- Multiple myeloma
- Pernicious anemia
- Sarcoidosis
- Sickle cell anemia
- Thalassemia.

Organ Transplantation:
- Bone marrow
- Heart
- Kidney
- Liver
- Lung.

Miscellaneous Causes:
- Ankylosing spondylitis
- Chronic obstructive pulmonary disease
- Congenital porphyria
- Epidermolysis bullosa
- Hemophilia
- Idiopathic hypercalciuria
- Idiopathic scoliosis
- Multiple sclerosis
- Rheumatoid arthritis
- Immobilization.

Genetic Disorders:
- Hypophosphatasia
- Osteogenesis imperfecta
- Homocystinuria
- Ehlers-Danlos syndrome
- Marfan's syndrome.

Drugs-associated with Bone Loss:
- Aluminium
- Anticoagulants
- Anticonvulsants
- Cigarette smoking
- Cytotoxic drugs
- Excessive alcohol
- Excessive vitamin A
- Glucocorticoids and adrenocorticotropin
- Gonadotropin-releasing hormone agonists
- Heparin
- Lithium
- Tamoxifen (in the premenopausal patient)
- Beta carotene
- Bile-acid binding resins.

PRIMARY OSTEOPOROSIS

Type I (postmenopausal) osteoporosis: It occurs in women between 51 and 75 years of age with accelerated and disproportionate loss of trabecular bone. Fractures of vertebral bodies and distal forearm are common. Biochemically both circulating parathormone and 1,25$(OH)_2$ vitamin D are reduced.

Type II (senile) osteoporosis: It occurs in both sexes over 70 years of age. There is proportionate loss of both cortical and trabecular bone and the fracture sites are also those which contain both types of bone, i.e. femoral neck, proximal humerus, proximal tibia and pelvis. Biochemically circulating parathormone is increased but 1,25$(OH)_2$ vitamin D is reduced.

JUVENILE OSTEOPOROSIS

Juvenile osteoporosis is a rare disease which occurs in children between 8 and 15 years. Clinical features include bone pain, fractures with minimal trauma (mostly metaphyseal fractures of distal tibia and vertebral crush fractures), reduced bone density at areas of new bone growth and loss of height. Spontaneous recovery occurs within 4–5 years, but deformities may persist. Biochemical investigations are normal and most forms of treatment are ineffective.

ENDOCRINE CAUSES

Glucocorticoid excess: Cushing's syndrome or glucocorticoid excess from exogenous or endogenous sources results in osteoporosis. There are a number of mechanisms responsible for this, and it has been shown by various studies that both dose and duration of steroid treatment correlate with bone loss. Glucocorticoid induced bone loss predominantly affects the trabecular bone. Once osteoporosis develops in adults with Cushing's syndrome, the abnormality may persist indefinitely even after the cause is removed.

Hypogonadism: Whether due to primary gonadal failure or secondary to gonadotropin deficiency, hypogonadism is associated with osteoporosis, particularly of trabecular bone. It is a well-known fact that estrogen is important in preventing bone loss in normal premenopausal women, and estrogen deficiency due to any cause can lead to osteoporosis.[4] Similarly testosterone deficiency appears to be the major factor responsible for reduced bone mass in men.[4]

Thyrotoxicosis: Significant bone loss is rare in thyrotoxicosis due to its early diagnosis and treatment. Both bone formation and resorption is increased in this disorder, but the formation is unable to match the resorption which leads to reduced bone mass.

Hyperprolactinemia: In women with hyperprolactinemia, reduced estrogen secretion is the key factor for osteoporosis. Even in men with hyperprolactinemia there is reduced bone density due to associated hypogonadism.

Diabetes mellitus: In insulin dependent (type 1) diabetes mellitus, there is reduction in the bone mass. The mechanism is not clear. Though the calcium levels are high, there is reduced tubular reabsorption of phosphate that may be a contributing factor for osteoporosis. A primary decrease in bone formation due to reduced insulin action has also been postulated.

Hyperparathyroidism: Generalized loss of bone density is a prominent feature in primary or secondary hyperparathyroidism which is followed by endosteal resorption. Osteoporosis may be seen in patients with primary hyperparathyroidism who may not have subperiosteal resorption or brown tumor or elevated serum alkaline phosphatase. Increased osteoclastic activity is responsible for osteoporosis.

Malignant Diseases

Several malignant tumors may cause diffuse osteopenia. Multiple myeloma is the most common. Others tumors include lymphoma, leukemia, systemic mastocytosis, etc. The neoplastic plasma cells secrete osteoclast activating factor which may be involved in mediating bone loss. Heparin or possibly other agents released by mast cells or lymphoma cells may be the effector molecule for osteoporosis.

Immobilization

Increased bone resorptions resulting from decreased weight bearing is the cause of bone loss.

Drugs

Long-term heparin administration potentiates PTH mediated bone resorption and activation of collagenase which leads to bone loss. Ethanol may also cause or contribute to bone loss. There is a long list of medications associated with bone loss.

Genetic Abnormalities in Bone Collagen Synthesis

Osteogenesis imperfecta (brittle bone syndrome) is described under four types. Type I osteogenesis imperfecta is an autosomal dominant form characterized by mild-to-moderate bone fragility, blue sclerae and premature deafness. Type II is a lethal perinatal disorder. Type III is characterized by severe bone fragility, progressive bone deformity and white sclerae. Type IV shows features of type I with white sclerae. Defective gene encoding leading to decreased collagen formation of type I leads to osteoporosis. It is postulated that what is now diagnosed as idiopathic or postmenopausal osteoporosis is due to defect in these genes (*COLI A1* and *COLI A2*) in absence of other features of osteogenesis imperfecta.

Osteoporosis also occurs in patients with homocystinuria due to cystathionine synthetase deficiency, an autosomal recessive trait associated with ectopia lentis, various deformities of the extremities, mental retardation, decreased pigmentation of hair and skin and thromboembolism. The osteoporosis may be due to the effect of homocystine or other metabolites in interfering with cross linking of collagen.

In Marfan's syndrome, an autosomal dominant disease, osteoporosis is due to defective collagen formation. It is characterized by arachnodactyly, posterior scalloping of vertebral bodies, high arched palate, lenticular subluxation and dissecting aneurysm.

GASTROINTESTINAL DISEASES

In diffuse liver diseases, malabsorption or defective metabolism of vitamin D can cause osteopenia. Primary biliary cirrhosis is a well-known example. In addition many other gastrointestinal diseases are associated with osteoporosis.[3]

ORGAN TRANSPLANTATION

Organ transplantation as the effective therapy for end-stage diseases of kidney, lung, liver and cardiac patients have improved, the number of transplant patients have increased to a great extent in the world. These patients require lifelong medications, such as steroids, immunosuppressant drugs and anticoagulation. Varying mechanisms are responsible for osteoporosis in these patients.[3]

CLINICAL FEATURES

Osteoporosis becomes clinically significant when bone mass is reduced to the extent that the skeleton is insufficient to perform its normal function. Generalized skeletal pain is uncommon, and between fractures most patients are free of symptoms. Pain usually results from collapse of vertebra especially in the dorsal and lumbar regions, typically acute and often radiates around the flank into the abdomen. These may occur even with trivial trauma. The collapse fractures usually cause anterior wedging of the vertebrae and result in loss of height with kyphosis (dowager's or widow's hump). Scoliosis is also common. Although recurrent episodes of vertebral collapse, increasing spine deformity and loss of height are common, the cause in any one subject is not predictable, and there may be intervals of several years between fractures.[2]

INVESTIGATIONS

Bone Mineral Analysis

With the advent of bone mass measurement, the fracture risk in osteoporosis can be quantified before the fracture occurs. This is the major advancement in the field of osteoporosis.

The advances in radiologic sciences have allowed the development of various noninvasive, accurate and sensitive techniques for determining the mineral content of bone.[6] These include as follows:

- Standard radiography
- Radiogrammetry
- Photodensitometry
- Compton scattering
- Neutron activation analysis
- Single and dual photon absorptiometry
- Dual energy X-ray absorptiometry
- Quantitative computed tomography
- Quantitative ultrasound
- Magnetic resonance imaging
- Multidetector computed tomography.

Standard Radiography

Qualitative assessment of bone mineral content from standard radiographs of skeleton is usually based on subjective criteria. The assessment is commonly done on metacarpal, calcaneum, talus, femoral neck, vertebral bodies, etc. The findings are as follows:

- Generalized osteopenia, most prominent in the axial skeleton, especially the vertebral column **(Fig. 1A)**.
- Thinning and accentuation of cortices.
- Accentuation of primary trabeculae with thinning of secondary trabeculae.
- Changes in vertebral body shape—wedge shape, biconcave and compression **(Fig. 1B)**.
- Insufficiency fractures due to normal stress on weakened bone. Sacrum, supra-acetabular regions, os pubis, etc. are common sites. The fracture may be occult radiographically and detected on CT or scintigraphy.
- Fractures at other sites (especially wrist and hip).

The major disadvantage is that it is subjective and gets affected by body habitus, radiographic exposure factors, the presence of overlying soft tissue and patient positioning. Approximately more than 30% bone loss must be there to be appreciated on plain radiographs.[2,6]

Magnification radiography by either optical or direct geometric means has a small but significant role in the assessment of osteoporosis. Subperiosteal and intracortical

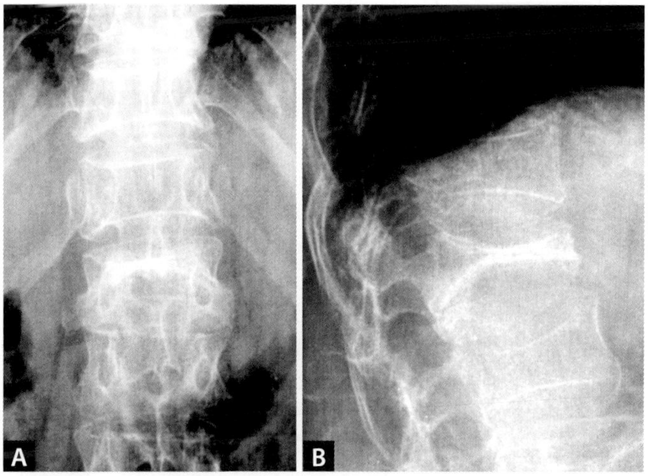

Figs. 1A and B: Radiograph of dorsolumbar spine AP view (A) and lateral view (B) demonstrate decreased bone density with thinning of vertebral endplates which appear as fine dense lines in contrast to the center of the vertebral body and the presence of multiple biconcave vertebrae.

bone absorption, even subtle, may be appreciated on magnification radiography.

Radiogrammetry

Radiogrammetry is one of the simplest methods of quantitative bone mineral assessment. Conventional AP radiograph of a tubular bone (like metacarpal) is taken. The cortical thickness on either side of medullary space is measured with a measuring device, and their sum is expressed as the combined cortical thickness (CCT). This technique is most commonly used at midshaft of second metacarpal. Cortical bone volume is calculated from the CCT. However, it does not reliably reflect absolute bone mineral content and does not measure intracortical bone porosis. This technique too, is imprecise and insensitive.

Photodensitometry

In this technique, images of bone of interest and of reference aluminum wedge of known density are exposed on the same film. The optical density of the bone is then compared with that of the wedge with photodensitometer. This provides information comparable to that of single photon absorptiometry but with slightly lower precision, sensitivity and accuracy.

Neutron Activation Analysis

In this method, neutrons from an accelerator or reactor bombard a small fraction of the total ^{48}Ca in the body, changing it to ^{49}Ca which is a radioactive isotope. By counting its activity, total calcium content of the body is estimated. The precision and accuracy are in the order of 2–5%. However, it does not clearly reflect the state of trabecular bone and does not correlate well with spinal mineral measurements. Another disadvantage is relatively large radiation dose (200–300 mrem).

Compton Scattering

This technique measures the absolute density of a volume of tissue based on its electron density and is the only method other than computed tomography that can measure purely trabecular bone. It is based on measurement of scattered radiation from a source of 100–700 keV gamma rays and is used for calcaneum, spine and radius. The precision of this method is about 3–5% and radiation dose varies from 200 to 2000 mrem. At present, it is largely a research tool.

Single Energy Photon Absorptiometry

Single energy photon absorptiomerty (SPA) technique requires a gamma ray source (^{125}I), a detector and intervening electronics that measure the beam attenuation through bone and express the result in bone mineral per sqcm scanned. Usually the radius is measured at two sites, the mid diaphysis which consists of nearly 100% cortical bone, and the distal radial metaphysis which contains about 75% cortical bone and 25% trabecular bone.

This technique is useful in population study. The precision of coefficient of variance (CV) of this technique is about 2% and the accuracy about 6% along with low radiation exposure (less than 10 mrem). However, because of dosimetric and statistical considerations, the low energy ^{125}I source cannot be used for body parts thicker than the forearm. A major clinical limitation of this technique, therefore, is that it reflects the status of peripheral long bone and measures primarily the cortex.

Dual Energy Photon Absorptiometry

Dual energy photon absorptiomerty (DPA) technique utilizes radioisotope that emits photons at two different energy levels. The chief advantage is that the gamma ray energy of the source is higher (^{153}Gd with photons of 42 and 100 keV), and it has a uniform path length. The lumbar spine from L1 to L4 is usually scanned. This technique yields integral of all mineral within the scan path including the vertebral bodies, endplates and posterior elements. The major disadvantage is that vertebral compression fractures with callus formation, kyphoscoliosis, articular facet hypertrophy, diskogenic sclerosis, marginal osteophytosis and extraosseous calcification (aorta) are also included in the integral measurement and may result in inaccurate and poorly reproducible vertebral measurements. In healthy subjects, the precision is in the order of 2–3% with accuracy of 4–10% of coefficient of variance. The usual radiation dose is about 15–20 mrem. It is also used to determine total body mineral content.

Dual Energy X-ray Absorptiometry

The WHO, In 1994, defined the threshold levels for the diagnosis of osteopenia and osteoporosis with dual energy X-ray absorpiometry (DXA). Consequently, DXA measurements are currently the standard of reference for the clinical diagnosis of osteoporosis with bone densitometry. DXA has the distinguishing feature of making use of an X-ray beam composed of two different photon energies. Practically, the intensities of high-energy and low-energy photons are analyzed separately after the protons have passed through bones and soft tissue. With use of a particular computing algorithm, the attenuation values of soft tissues are subtracted, leaving only the attenuation values of bone. Technical developments in

DXA in recent years include fan-beam X-ray sources and a bank of detectors. Fan-beam scanners use wider beams (as compared to previously used pencil width X-ray beam) that permit more rapid scanning (approximately 3–5 minutes per site; times are similar for wholebody scans), improved image quality, and a spatial resolution of 0.5–0.7 mm. The measurements provided by DXA are bone mineral content (in grams) and the projected area of the measured site (in square centimeter). Dividing bone mineral content by the area yields bone mineral density (BMD) (in grams per square centimeter).[7] As a consequence, the bone size has a significant effect on the measurement of areal BMD, which results in systematic overestimation of density in larger bones and underestimation of density in smaller bones. BMD is expressed in terms of standard deviation (SD) as a T-score and a Z-score. The T-score describes the difference between the BMD of the patient being examined and the mean BMD of a standard young adult population (20–30 years of age), and refers to the peak of bone mass. The Z-score shows the difference between the patient's BMD and the mean BMD of age- and gender-matched controls. The Z-score is particularly important in patients aged 75 years or older. The WHO classifies BMD on the basis of the T-score as normal (≥ –1.0), osteopenia (< –1.0 but > –2.5), osteoporosis (≤ –2.5), and severe osteoporosis (≤ –2.5 with a fragility fracture).[8] This definition is applied to DXA measurements made **(Table 1)** in the lumbar spine, proximal femur, and forearm, but not to measurements made with other techniques (e.g. quantitative CT) or to DXA measurements made at other anatomic sites (e.g. calcaneus).

Bone mineral density examinations have three principal roles, namely the diagnosis of osteoporosis, the assessment of patients' risk of fracture, and monitoring response to treatment. BMD is a strong predictor of fracture risk, accounting for 75–85% of bone strength. The risk of fracture increases approximately 1.5-fold for each SD decrease from age-adjusted BMD.[9] A helpful list of clinical indications for performing a bone density examination was published by the International Society for Clinical Densitometry (ISCD)[10] and is summarized in **Table 2**.

There are many advantages of central DXA as summarized in **Table 3**.[11]

Dual energy X-ray absorptiometry is the only procedure which can be used with fracture risk assessment tool or FRAX, which is particularly helpful in identifying patients who are at higher risk for fracture.[12] The fracture risk assessment tool or *FRAX* provides an estimate of fracture risk on the basis of the BMD of the femoral neck; the patient's age, sex, height, and weight; and seven clinical risk factors (previous fracture, having a parent who had a hip fracture, current smoking, glucocorticoid use, rheumatoid arthritis, secondary osteoporosis, and ingestion of three or more units of alcohol daily). If this information is entered along with the name of the manufacturer of the DXA scanner used and the algorithm estimates the 10-year probability of a major osteoporotic fracture (hip, spine, proximal humerus, or distal forearm).[12]

Recently, a study was published to establish age-specified bone mineral density (BMD) reference range for

Table 1: The World Health Organization (WHO) definitions of osteoporosis and osteopenia.[5]

Terminology	*T-score definition*
Normal	T ≥ –1.0
Osteopenia	–2.5 < T < –1.0
Osteoporosis	T ≤ –2.5
Severe osteoporosis	T ≤ –2.5 in the presence of one or more fragility fractures

Table 2: Indications for bone mineral density (BMD) testing.

- Women aged 65 and older
- Postmenopausal women under age 65 with risk factors
- Men aged 70 and older
- Adults with a fragility fracture
- Adults with a disease or condition associated with low bone mass or bone loss
- Adults taking medication associated with low bone mass or bone loss
- Anyone being considered for pharmacological therapy
- Anyone being treated, to monitor treatment effect
- Anyone not receiving therapy in whom evidence of bone loss would lead to treatment

Table 3: Clinical advantages of hip and spine DXA.

- Proven ability to predict fracture risk
- Consensus that BMD results can be interpreted using WHO T-scores
- Proven for effective targeting of antifracture treatments
- Effective for monitoring response to treatment
- Basis of new WHO algorithm for predicting fracture risk
- Short scan times
- Easy patient set-up
- Low radiation dose
- Good precision
- Acceptable accuracy
- Availability of reliable reference ranges
- Stable calibration
- Effective instrument quality control procedures

Indian females using dual-energy X-ray absorptiometry.[13] Peak BMD was observed between 30 and 35 years at the hip, lumbar spine and radius. Compared with age-matched US females, BMD of lumbar spine was significantly lower for our subjects in all age groups. Prevalence of osteoporosis among women aged older than 50 years was significantly higher based on Caucasian T-scores as opposed to using peak BMD/standard deviation values from the population under review at lumbar spine but not at femoral neck.

However, DXA, a two-dimensional technique, has some inherent limitations. It cannot distinguish between cortical and trabecular bone or discriminate between changes due to bone geometry (e.g. increases in the third dimension). Nor can it help those due entirely to increased bone density (within a fixed volume of bone).

Apart from axial skeleton (lumbar spine and proximal femur) DXA scan can also be done at peripheral sites like distal radius and calcaneus. The calcaneus is particular useful for monitoring changes in BMD secondary to treatment as it contains high percentage (95%) of metabolically active trabecular bone.

According to ISCD guidelines measurement by validated peripheral DXA (pDXA) devices can be used to assess vertebral and global fragility fracture risk in postmenopausal women, however its ability to predict vertebral fracture is weaker than central DXA and heel QUS. There is not sufficient evidence yet to support this position for men. Radius pDXA in conjunction with clinical risk factors can be used to identify a population at very low fracture probability in which no further diagnostic evaluation may be necessary. Central DXA measurements at the spine and femur are the preferred method for making therapeutic decisions and should be used if possible. However, if central DXA cannot be done, pharmacologic treatment can be initiated if the fracture probability, as assessed by radius pDXA (or DXA) using device specific thresholds and in conjunction with clinical risk factors, is sufficiently high. However, pDXA devices are not clinically useful in monitoring the skeletal effects of presently available medical treatments for osteoporosis.[10] ISCD has also issued guidelines for use of DXA in children and adolescents.[10] **Table 4** lists comparison of different bone densitometry techniques.[11]

Quantitative Computed Tomography

Quantitative computed tomography (QCT) is an addition to the field of bone mineral analysis. Quantitative CT differs from DXA as it provides separate estimates of trabecular and cortical bone BMD as a true volumetric mineral density in milligrams per cubic centimeter. This method uses a mineral calibration phantom that is placed in the CT scanner with the patient and provides corrections for machine drifts. A lateral computed radiograph (scout view) is first obtained for localization and then single axial scans are obtained through the midplane of two to four lumbar vertebral bodies **(Figs. 2 and 3)**. Quantitative readings are obtained from a region of interest over trabecular bone encompassing 3–4 cm^3 of each vertebral body and from four different reference solutions in the phantom. These readings are averaged and used to calculate the mineral density of trabecular bone in mineral equivalents of K_2HPO_4 (mg/cm^3).[14,15] In addition to estimating the bone mineral density, QCT now, can also determine the future risk of osteoporotic fractures.

The precision of this method is 1–3% for single energy (80 kVp) and 3–5% for dual energy (80 kVp/140 kVp) techniques with accuracy of 5–10%. The radiation dose is approximately 2 Sv.

The theoretic advantages of QCT over other modalities include: (i) transaxial display of data permitting

Table 4: Comparison of different bone densitometry techniques.

	Central DXA	*Peripheral DXA*	*QCT*	*QUS*
Compatible with WHO T-scores	√	X	X	X
Proven to predict fracture risk	√	√	√	√
Compatible with new WHO fracture risk algorithm	√	X	X	X
Proven for effective targeting of treatment	√	?	?	?
Suitable for patient follow-up	√	X	√	X
Stable calibration	√	√	√	X
Good precision	√	√	√	X
Reliable reference ranges available	√	?	?	?

Keys: (√) Indicates where an alternative technique is known to perform in a comparable manner to central DXA. (?) Indicates where our knowledge is limited by an absence of suitable studies. (X) Indicates that alternative types of measurement are definitely unsuitable in these roles.

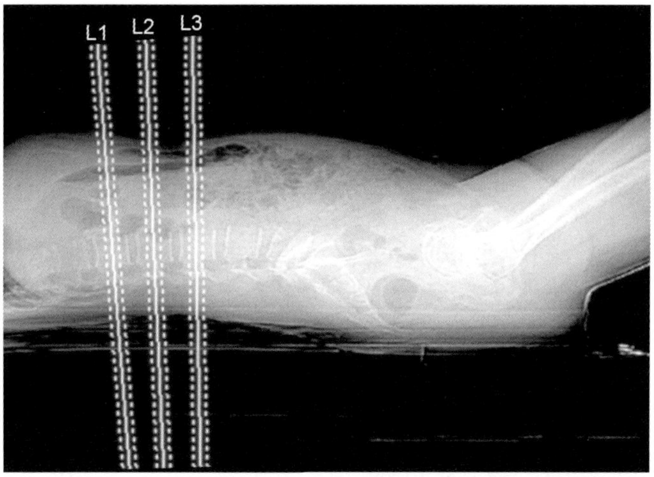

Fig. 2: Lateral topogram (scout view) shows automatic determination of midvertebral slices of L1–L3.

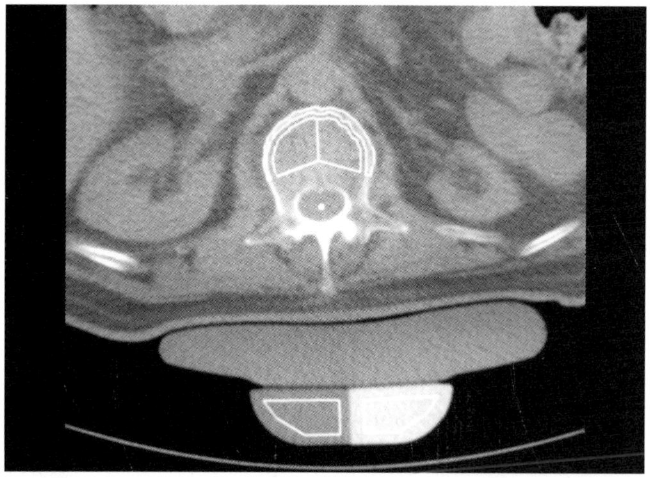

Fig. 3: Midvertebral slice on QCT shows automatic contour determination separating cortical (outer semicircle) and trabecular bone (inner semicircle). Note the phantom and calculation marker.

identification of the anatomy and separate measurement of cortical, cancellous, or integral bone mineral, (ii) capability of determining the linear absorption coefficient for a readily defined volume of bone and thereby, providing a measure of density, and (iii) in the dual energy mode, the ability to determine mineral content with high accuracy in the presence of variable fat and soft tissue content.[16]

Quantitative CT is excellent for predicting vertebral fractures in postmenopausal women and serially measuring bone loss, generally with better sensitivity than projectional methods (such as DXA) because it selectively assesses the metabolically active and structurally trabecular bone in the center of the vertebral body. This selective assessment of trabecular bone also makes quantitative CT sensitive in measuring changes over a short follow-up period. The main theoretic advantages of quantitative CT over DXA are (a) the exclusion from the measurement of structures that do not contribute to spine mechanical resistance, yet contribute to DXA BMD values and (b) the possibility of selectively measuring trabecular tissue, the most metabolic active tissue and the main determinant of compressive strength in the vertebrae.[17] Spine trabecular BMD by QCT can be used to monitor age-, disease- and treatment-related changes.[18]

There have been fewer fracture prediction studies using QCT than those where DXA is applied, thus this area requires more research. In postmenopausal females QCT of the spine has been found to perform as well as, if not better than, DXA in the prediction of vertebral fractures.[19] However, the use of spine QCT to predict hip fracture has not been substantiated yet.[18]

The ISCD position statements regarding QCT is that spinal trabecular BMD as measured by QCT has at least the same ability to predict vertebral fractures as AP spinal BMD measured by central DXA in postmenopausal women. There is lack of sufficient evidence to support this position for men. There is lack of sufficient evidence to recommend spine QCT for hip fracture prediction in either women or men.

Central DXA measurements at the spine and femur are the preferred method for making therapeutic decisions and should be used if possible. However, pharmacologic treatment can be initiated if the fracture probability, as assessed by QCT of the spine in conjunction with clinical risk factors, is sufficiently high.

Trabecular BMD of the lumbar spine measured by QCT can be used to monitor age, disease, and treatment related BMD changes.

The disadvantage of QCT is that accuracy of BMD decreases to 20–25% in elderly osteoporosis populations.[20]

The authors analyzed bone mineral content in 100 normal Indian females (unpublished data) with mean age of 38.27 ± 11.12 years using QCT in their institute by linear regression. Normal Indian female has BMD of 217.87 – (1.6 × age of the patient) and normal Indian male has BMD of 221.01 – (1.5 × age of the patient). BMD is bone mineral density in mg/cm^3. The mean annual rate of trabecular bone loss was 1.10% for normal Indian females and showed more than two fold increase in 50–60-years range (1st menopausal decade). The trabecular bone loss at age 70 reached 3.19% **(Figs. 4 and 5)**.

In a study of 55 patients of prostate cancer who underwent orchidectomy the author found that a

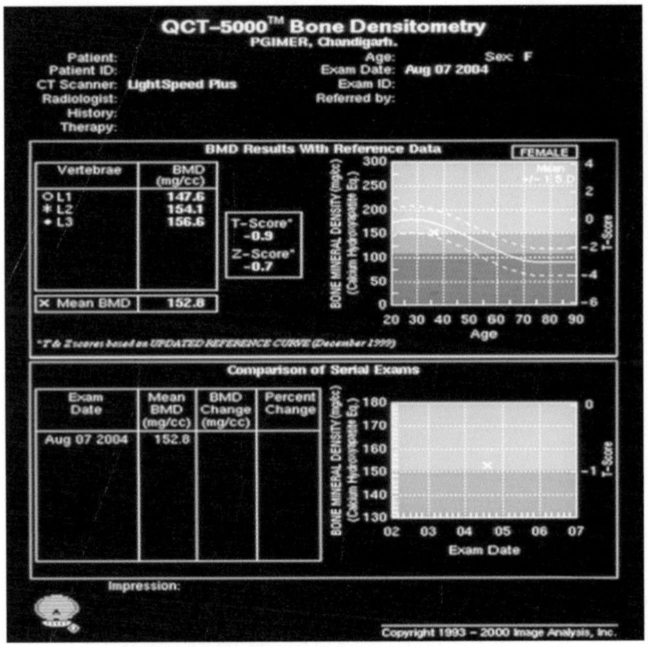

Fig. 4: QCT determination of BMD of a normal 36-year-old female with mean BMD of 152.8 mg/cc with T-score of –0.9 and Z-score of –0.7.

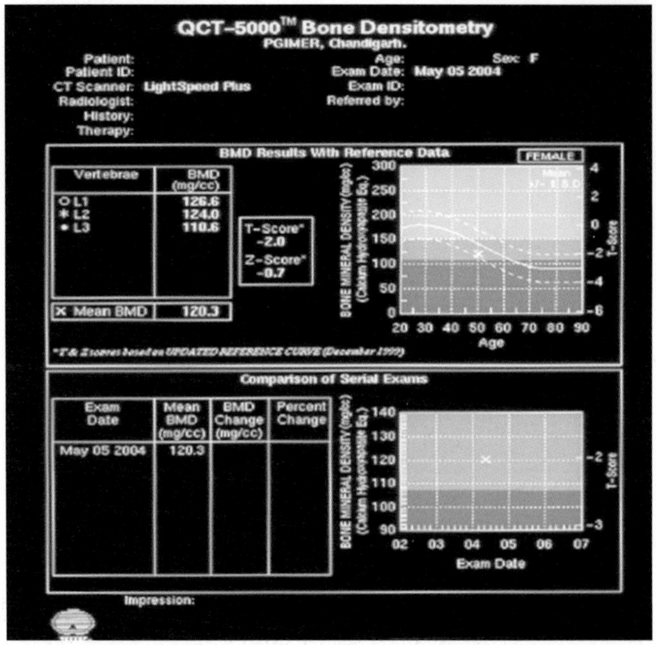

Fig. 5: QCT determination of BMD of a osteopenic 50-year-old female with mean BMD of 120.3 mg/cc with T-score of –2.0 and Z-score of –0.7.

statistical reduction in vertebral trabecular bone mineral density was observed in all patients within six months of orchidectomy.[21] Average BMD decreased by 16.5 ± 8.6 mg/cc (13.8%) **(Figs. 6 and 7)**.

In another group of female patients of progressive systemic sclerosis (n = 17), who were to undergo low dose steroid therapy, a pre- and post-therapy QCT was done to determine the effect of low dose steroids on bone mineral density. The author found a significant decrease in trabecular bone mineral density at all vertebral levels with an average decrease of 26.54% (unpublished data).

The authors also studied the correlation between biochemical bone markers and bone mineral density (BMD) by using both QCT and DXA scanners of the same subjects done on the same day and to compare their findings in diagnosing them as osteoporotic or normal. They found that in the total population there is strong correlation only between bone marker osteocalcin and DXA-lateral. In males only there was no correlation between the bone markers and BMD findings by QCT and DXA scanners. In females both pre- and postmenopausal, there is strong correlation only between osteocalcin and DXA-AP and lateral but not with QCT and crosslaps. Whereas, in only postmenopausal females there is strong correlation between osteocalcin and all the densitometric modalities, e.g. QCT, DXA-AP and DXA- lateral but no correlation with crosslaps.[22]

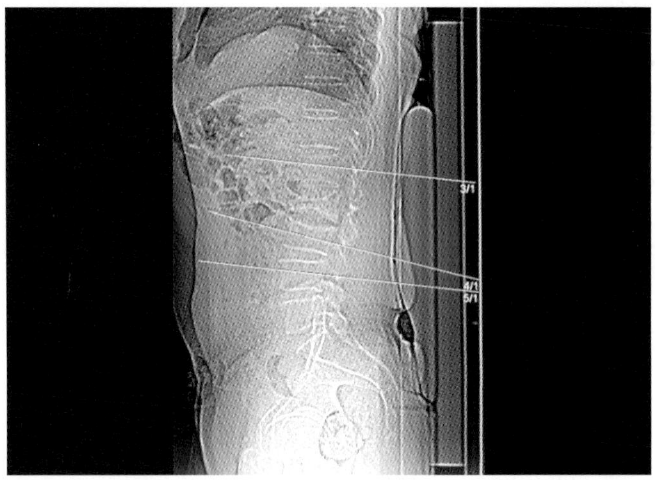

Fig. 6: Lateral topogram (scout view) shows midvertebral slices taken at L1–L3 vertebrae. Collapsed vertebra (L2 in this case) can be skipped manually.

Another study has been done by the authors regarding comparison between the QCT and the DXA scanners in the evaluation of BMD in the lumbar spine. In both the scanning modalities there is direct correlation between age and osteoporosis as with increasing age the incidence of osteoporosis increased in all the groups. But QCT has been found to be more efficacious than DXA scan in the diagnosis of osteoporosis, i.e. QCT helps discriminate

Osteo-Evaluation Result of L3

9216/04 — Male, 65 Years
603 IMA, 4, 19-July-2004, 10:29:06

Bone Mineral Density of L3 [mg Ca-HA/mL] (and Pixel Standard Deviation):

	Left	Right	Total
Trabecular	47.4 (39.8)	103.1 (36.3)	75.6 (47.2)
Cortical	205.9 (91.7)	220.2 (64.8)	212.3 (81.1)

A

OSTEO-Evaluation Summary

9216/04 — Male, 65 years
16-July-2004, 10:28:37

Bone Mineral Density [mg Ca-HA/mL] (and Pixel Standard Deviation):

Vertebra	Scan Number	Trabecular	Cortical
L4	5	14.7 (31.3)	137.4 (70.4)
L3	4	75.6 (47.2)	212.3 (81.1)
L1	3	36.5 (31.7)	104.3 (49.2)
Average		42.3	151.3
Standard Deviation		25.2	45.2

B

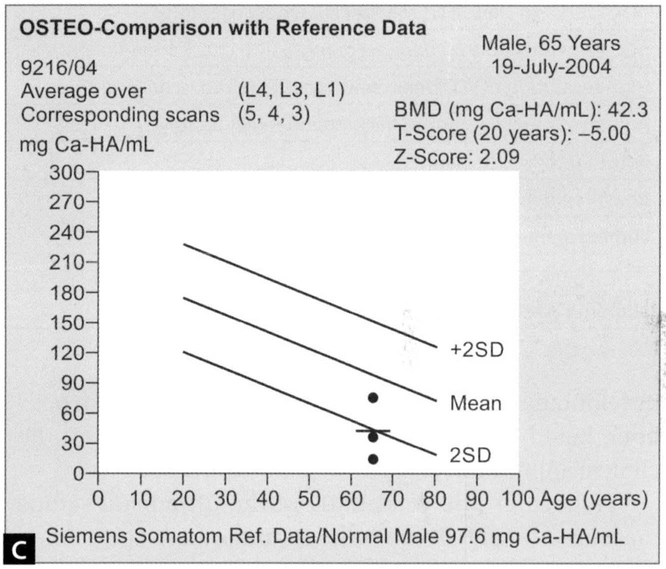

Figs. 7A to C: QCT determination of BMD of a 65-year-old postorchidectomy male patient at an individual vertebra (A) and average of 3 lumbar vertebrae (B and C).

between normal subjects and those with osteoporosis better than DEXA-Lateral and DEXA-AP.[23]

Although spinal quantitative CT has several advantages with respect to DXA technique, it also has several disadvantages, including a high radiation dose **(Table 5)**, poor precision that limits its applicability to longitudinal assessments, high costs for quantitative CT scanners, a high degree of operator dependence, the need for a considerable amount of space and limited scanner access. Moreover, axial quantitative CT is used only for the assessment of spine volumetric BMD because the complexity of the hip architecture has precluded the development of reliable methods of densitometric assessment in this clinically important region. The World Health Organization (WHO) has defined osteoporosis in terms of bone densitometry as a *T*-score "at or below" 2.5. This applies only to DXA of the lumbar spine, femoral neck, total hip and distal 33% radius. The definition does not apply to other anatomical sites (e.g. calcaneus) or to other densitometric techniques, such as quantitative ultrasound or QCT, in either a central or peripheral site. This is not surprising as DXA provides a composite measurement of integral trabecular and cortical bone, whereas QCT of the lumbar spine measures vertebral body trabecular BMD which will show a more rapid age-dependent decrement than that measured by DXA.[24] Therefore, the WHO criterion of a *T*-score of "at or below" 2.5 applied to spinal QCT would lead to earlier age of diagnosis of osteoporosis and over-classification of the number of people suffering from the disease.[25] Felsenberg and Gowin suggested that subjects with a BMD below 80 mg hydroxyapatite/cm^3 could be classified as osteoporotic and those with a BMD between 80 and 120 mg/cm^3 as osteopenic.[26]

Over the last decade technical developments in CT technique has resulted in development of dedicated peripheral CT scanners which are smaller, more mobile and less expensive than whole body CT scanners to assess peripheral skeletal sites.

Peripheral QCT is most commonly applied to the non-dominant forearm. Accurate and consistent positioning of the forearm and reference lines are essential in any longitudinal or multicenter studies for comparable results.

Peripheral QCT has been used more widely than central QCT in pediatric research to assess bone

Table 5: Radiation exposure of QCT protocols18 and other procedures involving ionizing radiation for comparison.

Technique	*Voltage (kV)*	*Time current product (mAs)*	*Approximate effective dose (mSv)*
Single slice QCT spine L1–L3 10 mm slice thickness	80	120	<0.2
	120	200	Approx 1.0
3D QCT spine L1 and L2 (10 cm scan length)	120	100	Approx 1.5
3D QCT proximal femur (15 cm scan length)	120	200	Approx 2.5–3
pQCT forearm clinical CT scanner (10 cm scan length)	120	100	<0.01
pQCT forearm/tibia on dedicated single slice pQCT scanners per slice	<70	<1	<0.003
High resolution pQCT forearm (XtremeCT) (15 cm scan length)	60	1	<0.005
Annual naturally occurring background radiation (UK)			2.7
Return transatlantic flight			0.08
Chest radiograph			0.02
Lumbar spine radiograph			0.7
CT imaging, e.g. abdomen/pelvis			2.5–4
Radionuclide bone scan			3

development in healthy children and in those at risk for poor bone health.[27,28] The ISCD has issued guidelines on the clinical application of pQCT in children in 2008.[27]

Trabecular and total BMD of the ultradistal radius measured by pQCT can be used to monitor age-related BMD changes.

Quantitative Ultrasound

Ultrasound has been successfully used for many years for nondestructive material testing. Both scattering characteristics and ultrasound velocity changes have been used to evaluate mechanical competence and detect the presence of damage in both materials and structures. Ultrasound variables are speed of sound (SUS) and broadband ultrasound attenuation (BUA). These quantitative ultrasound (QUS) parameters are associated with the material properties of trabecular bone, as well as with failure load of the proximal femur. QUS of bone is performed at substantially lower frequencies, i.e. between 200 kHz and 1.5 MHz and signals are acquired in transmission mode. In addition to assessing bone density these variables reflect parameters, such as elasticity and microarchitecture which are important in assessing fracture risk in osteoporotic subjects. US is currently being performed at peripheral sites like patella, fingers, tibia and calcaneum. The calcaneum is the most favored site as it is a weight bearing bone and composed almost entirely of trabecular bone. The ultrasound wave is produced in the form of a sinusoid impulse by special piezoelectric probes, and is detected once it has passed through the medium; there are two distinct probes, emitting and receiving, and the skeletal segment for evaluation is placed between them.

Quantitative US results can be expressed as absolute values or as T-scores and Z-scores, thanks to well-established and validated normative reference curves, allowing bone loss to be followed up over time.[29] It has been demonstrated that the WHO criteria simply cannot be used with quantitative US.

Many studies are available which highlight the fact that the ultrasound variables like SUS and BUA are independent predictors of fractures risk even after adjustment for bone density.[30,31] The false-negative report is up to 10% as the typical sites of bone density like lumbar spine or hip are not directly measured on QUS. It can be used as an initial screening modality for osteoporosis.[32]

The main advantage of ultrasound is lack of ionizing radiation.[33] It is less expensive than X-ray technology and is portable. Therefore, QUS has a potential for wider applicability, including preventive screening for osteoporosis. However, the major disadvantage is that there is no standardized method of calibration and expression of measurement results since QUS devices employ diverse technology and different methods of calibration.

Currently, US assessment is used as a screening tool, with confirmation of diagnosis by means of DXA evaluation. Several studies have confirmed the usefulness of quantitative US in predicting osteoporotic fractures of the calcaneus, particularly in elderly women aged 65–70 years or older.[34]

The current ISCD guideline about QUS are that validated heel QUS devices predict fragility fracture in postmenopausal women (hip, vertebral, and global fracture risk) and men over the age of 65 (hip and all nonvertebral fractures), independently of central DXA BMD. Heel QUS in conjunction with clinical risk factors can be used to identify a population at very low fracture probability in which no further diagnostic evaluation may be necessary. However, if central DXA cannot be done, pharmacologic treatment can be initiated if the fracture probability, as assessed by heel QUS, using device specific thresholds and in conjunction with clinical risk factors, is sufficiently high. However, QUS cannot be used to monitor the skeletal effects of treatments for osteoporosis.[10]

High-resolution Bone Imaging

The importance of assessing the microarchitectural make-up of addition to its mineral density in the context of osteoporosis has been emphasized in a number of publications. Currently, the best suited modalities meeting these requirements in vivo are high resolution peripheral quantitative imaging (HR-pQCT) and magnetic resonance imaging (MRI). Whereas HR-pQCT is limited to peripheral skeleton regions like the wrist and ankle, MRI can also image other sites like the proximal femur but usually with lower spatial resolution.

Magnetic Resonance Imaging

Magnetic resonance imaging (MRI) is an emerging technology for acquiring high-resolution images of cortical and trabecular bone in vivo. It is a noninvasive modality and does not require ionizing radiation. Therefore, it is suitable for the assessment of bone structure in a clinical setting. In MRI, the bones are usually depicted with a negative contrast relative to the high background signal from bone marrow. Information regarding structure, topology, and orientation of the trabecular bone network as well as cortical thickness and area can be extracted from the images by applying digital postprocessing techniques. Since the requirements for the analysis and measurement of trabecular versus cortical bone are different, these will be discussed separately.

Trabecular Bone Assessment Using

Signal to noise and spatial resolution: In MRI, spatial resolution and SNR are tradeoff parameters and it is not clear yet whether enhancing resolution at the expense of SNR increases or decreases detection sensitivity and what errors are incurred by imaging at anisotropic resolution. Li et al. investigated the effect of limited spatial resolution and noise on structural parameters.[35] The authors noted systematic changes in the derived structural parameters when the SNR decreased below a certain threshold. They also showed that these errors at smaller SNR levels can be corrected if simple linear transformations are used, thereby allowing the data to be normalized. Numerous efforts have been made to develop trabecular bone imaging of peripheral sites, such as the radius, tibia and calcaneus. Recently clinically useful images of femur (the deeper structure) are obtained by Krug et al.[36] In principle, two main types of pulse sequences can be used for bone imaging. Namely, spin-echo (SE) based pulse sequences and gradient-echo (GE) based pulse sequences. In order to choose a suitable pulse sequence for bone MRI, a few guidelines have to be considered. Firstly, a 3-dimensional (3D) excitation usually provides higher SNR than a 2D sequence. Secondly, the gradient-echo has to be acquired immediately after the excitation pulse in order to avoid signal loss due to T2 relaxation. Finally, the imaging time has to be in a clinically feasible range. The simplest sequence that fulfills the aforementioned requirements is a basic gradient-echo sequence. Further improvements of SNR efficiency can be made by fully balancing all magnetic gradients during one repetition. The so-called balanced steady state gradient-echo pulse sequence (bSSFP) maximizes SNR efficiency but is also very prone to magnetic field inhomogeneities. Krug et al. pointed out some advantages of this signal attenuation.[37] Smaller trabeculae that would normally disappear due to partial volume effects were enhanced and thus visible due to increased signal cancelation using bSSFP compared to a spin-echo approach.[38] Therefore, due to its very high SNR efficiency, SSFP has become the sequence of choice among gradient-echo based pulse sequences for trabecular bone imaging.[39,40] Furthermore, imaging time was considerably reduced by employing accelerated image acquisition techniques (parallel imaging).

Image analysis: Image analysis of trabecular bone images in MRI involves several postprocessing steps; mainly the outlining of the trabecular bone region of interest (ROI), the correction of the coil sensitivity, bone/marrow segmentation and structural calculations.

Image postprocessing: There are many different approaches for extracting structural information from 3D images of the trabecular bone. The most fundamental parameter in MRI is related to bone volume fraction (BVF) and is also denoted BV/TV (a bone volume to total volume fraction).

Trabecular bone analysis: Structural parameters are commonly divided into three classes, including scale, topology and orientation.[41,42] Scale is primarily described by the volume of bone in a ROI and the thickness of the trabeculae or the spacing between the trabeculae. Topology can be assessed by investigating the plate- or rode-like structure of the network. And finally orientation methods characterize the degree of anisotropy of the structure.

Carballido-Gamio et al. introduced a new technique to provide a complete assessment of scale, topology, and anisotropy using geodesic topological analysis (GTA). It was further demonstrated that GTA combined with BMD allowed for better discrimination than BMD alone (AUC = 0.95; $p < 0.001$).[43] For treatment monitoring, it is important to analyze the same trabecular sections at baseline and follow-up in order to detect small changes in the fine trabecular structure.

Cortical Bone Assessment Using MRI

Cortical bone thickness is an important determinant of the strength of bone as demonstrated by Hyun et al.[44] They have demonstrated significant differences in cortical thickness of postmenopausal osteopenic vs osteoporotic women which underscores the significance of geometric measurements of the cortical bone. Similarly, Techawiboonwong et al. showed that the bone water content was increased 65% in the postmenopausal group compared to the premenopausal group.[45] The differential water content may be due to presence or absence of marrow in the cortical pores. For efficiently imaging the intracortical microstructure, ultrashort echo times (UTE) have to be employed.

Pulse sequences: Hyun et al acquired MR images of the distal radius at 1.5 tesla using a 3D fast gradient recalled echo (FGRE) pulse sequence featuring an in-plane resolution of 0.16×0.16 mm^2 and 2 mm slice thickness.[44] Goldenstein et al. chose slightly different parameters on 3 T MR scanner in a prone position using a quadrature wrist coil with a balanced steady state free precession (bSSFP) pulse sequence (pulse sequence parameters were 512×384 matrix, 60° flip angle, 122 Hz/pixel BW, 8 cm FOV, 14.4–15.21/3.3–3.9 ms TR/TE and scan time of 10 min).[46] The image acquisition resulted in an image resolution of 156 µm × 156 µm × 500 µm. Hyun et al. designed a semiautomatic segmentation algorithm to measure cortical thickness.[44]

Clinical Applications

The technological developments over the past few years have made quantitative MRI of bone structure more clinically practical. There has been a substantial improvement in fracture discrimination by including structural information in addition to BMD. Wehrli et al. showed that topological bone parameters investigated in 79 women (29 with vertebral fracture) could much better discriminate the fracture group from the nonfracture group than BMD.[47] Many researchers have concluded that MRI based in vivo assessment of trabecular bone has great promise as a tool for monitoring osteoporosis treatment. However, till now no current recommendations are there from ISCD to use it in diagnosis of osteoporosis, prediction of fracture risk or monitoring of treatment.

In the future, bone MR imaging may be proposed for patients who are undergoing treatment but have diskrepant findings with clinical, biochemical, and "conventional" imaging markers, and may replace biopsy when this would be advocated.

High-resolution Peripheral Quantitative Computed Tomography (HR-pQCT)

A dedicated extremity imaging system has been designed for trabecular-scale imaging. This device has the advantage of significantly higher SNR and spatial resolution compared to MDCT and MRI. The radiation dose is several orders of magnitude lower compared to whole body CT, and primarily does not involve critical, radiosensitive organs. However, a disadvantage is that it is limited to peripheral skeletal sites and presently only a limited number of devices are installed.

Image acquisition scan set-up: A standard, manufacturer recommended scan protocol has been used in the majority of the published literature to date.[48] There are several different protocol modifications that have been employed for developmental studies in children and adolescents to account for patient size and designed to avoid radiation exposure to the epiphyseal growth plate. The typically used 6 cm field of view (FOV) is reconstructed across a 1536×1536 matrix using a modified Feldkamp algorithm, yielding 82 µm isotropic voxels.[49] The total scan time is 2.8 minutes and results in an effective dose to the subject of approximately 4.2 µSv—several orders of magnitude smaller than clinical CT and comparable to DXA and other planar radiographic modalities.

Image analysis and postprocessing: The reconstructed images are analyzed using a standard protocol provided by the manufacturer which include segmentation and approximate contour delineation. The cortical bone compartment is segmented using a 3D Gaussian smoothing filter and then trabecular compartment is identified by digital subtraction of the cortical bone from the region enclosed by the periosteal contours. The linear attenuation values of the tomographic images are converted to hydroxyapatite (HA) mineral densities using a beam-hardening correction and phantom calibration procedure.

Morphometric analysis: Unlike MRI and MDCT, which have a large slice thickness relative to the in-plane resolution, the high isotropic resolution of HRpQCT (82 μm) permits direct, 3D assessment of important measurements like inter-trabecular distances, trabecular number, average trabecular thickness and bone volume fraction (BV/TV).

According to ISCD pQCT of the forearm at the ultradistal radius predicts hip, but not spine, fragility fractures in postmenopausal women. There is lack of sufficient evidence to support this position for men. Pharmacologic treatment can be initiated if the fracture probability, as assessed by pQCT of the radius in conjunction with clinical risk factors, is sufficiently high.

Multidetector Computed Tomography (MDCT)

Spiral CT generates densitometric data, which is used to assess mass lesions. Efforts are being made to use this data to assess BMD in the lumbar spine. A recent study calculated bone mineral density from spiral CT data by using equation BMD = 0.77 × mean BMD MDCT where mean BMD on MDCT was average of densities of L1–L3 vertebrae as calculated on spiral CT and 0.77 is conversion factor. They found significant correlation between BMD data obtained from spiral CT and QCT.[50] Ito et al. demonstrated that MDCT depicted trabecular microarchitecture of the thoracic spine (T12) which better separated patients with, and without, vertebral fractures than did BMD of the spine, obtained by DXA.[51]

In addition, advent of MDCT enables analysis of the hip, a clinically important site of fracture, which was not possible with 2D single slices due to their poor precision. However, high radiation dose remains a matter of concern.

MANAGEMENT OF OSTEOPOROTIC COMPRESSION FRACTURES: PERCUTANEOUS VERTEBROPLASTY

Treatment of acute osteoporotic fractures has been largely conservative, with therapy emphasizing pain control using narcotic or anti-inflammatory medications and immobilization.[52] Vertebroplasty aims to alleviate pain and improve mobility, with secondary goal of stabilizing the vertebral body. A study by Klazen CA et al. have shown that vertebroplasty resulted in significant greater pain relief than did conservative treatment.[53] A large study including vertebroplasty for 500 vertebral fractures concluded that percutaneous vertebroplasty was effective in relieving the pain associated with osteoporosis-induced vertebral compression fractures (VCFs), and the analgesic effect was long lasting when no new VCF occurred.[54] The age of fracture has minimal impact on outcome following single-level vertebroplasty, with good outcomes noted among acute, subacute and chronic fractures.[55]

Indications

For percutaneous vertebroplasty for osteoporotic vertebral compression fractures (VCF) are as follows:

- Painful VCF refractory to medical therapy.
- Painful VCF associated with osteonecrosis (Kümmell's disease).
- Unstable VCF that demonstrates movement at the wedge deformity.
- Conditions in which reinforcement of the vertebral body or pedicle is desired, before a posterior surgical stabilization procedure or inter body fusion, in patients with osteoporosis.
- Although routine prophylactic treatment is not advocated, unaffected vertebra in patients with multiple compressions in whom further collapse would lead to pulmonary compromise as a result of kyphosis, may rarely be considered for vertebroplasty.

Patients who are improving on conservative medical therapy are not considered to be the candidates. Some physicians advocate not treating patients with greater than 20–30% spinal canal compromise from retropulsed fracture fragments.[56]

Procedure

The procedure is done under conscious sedation under fluoroscopy/CT/CT-fluoroscopy guidance. Patient is placed prone on the fluoroscopic/CT table. Vertebroplasty needle (11/13G needle with biopsy set) is introduced under fluoroscopic guidance through the pedicle into the involved vertebral body up to the junction of anterior third and posterior two-thirds and bone cement, an acrylic polymer—PMMA (polymethylmethacrylate) is injected with the aim of almost completely filling the osteoporotic collapsed vertebral body, care been taken not to have any spillage beyond the posterior margin of the vertebral body **(Figs. 8A and B)**.

Postprocedure Care

Nowadays the procedure is routinely being done on outpatient basis, with a 2 hours observation period after vertebroplasty. Focal pain at the puncture sites may last 2 for days which usually responds to analgesics.

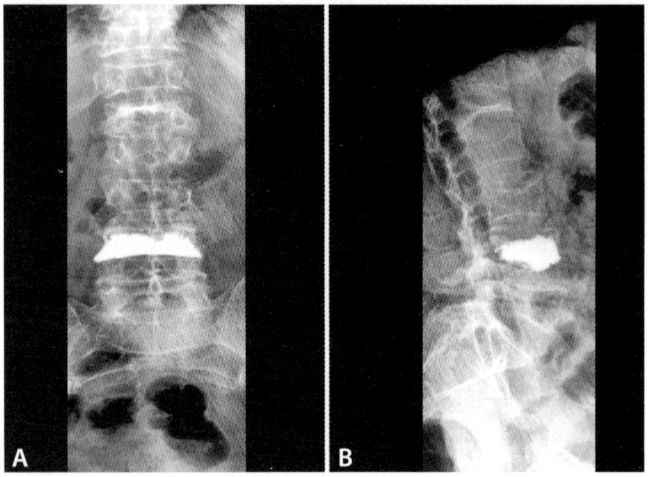

Figs. 8A and B: Vertebroplasty AP (A) and lateral (B) view shows filling of PMMA on both sides of L4 vertebral body in a patient with osteoporotic collapse.

Complications

Complication rate of vertebroplasty procedure ranges from 1% to 10% with higher rates being reported in the treatment of neoplastic collapse than the osteoporotic collapse.

- Leakage of PMMA into adjacent structures because of vertebral cortical destruction/fracture, causing nerve root/spinal cord compression.
- Injection into vertebral venous plexus leading to pulmonary embolism.
- Fracture of rib, transverse process or pedicle.
- Paravertebral hematoma, epidural abscess.
- Seizure or respiratory arrest from over sedation.
- Swallowing difficulties from esophageal compression in a cervical vertebroplasty.
- Death from massive PMMA pulmonary embolization.

There have been concerns that vertebroplasty may increase the risk of fracture at an adjacent level. Jensen et al. found no statistically significant difference in the rates of adjacent level fractures between a group of patients previously treated with vertebroplasty who returned with new fractures and a control group of patients who presented with multiple painful fractures.[57] They postulated that these new fractures were more likely the result of the natural history of osteoporosis rather than the presence of a vertebroplasty.

REFERENCES

1. Prevention and management of osteoporosis. World Health Organ Tech Rep Ser; 2003. p. 921.
2. Lane JM, Riley EH, Wirganowicz PZ. Osteoporosis: Diagnosis and treatment. JBJS. 1996;78-A:618-31.
3. Fitzpatrick LA. Secondary causes of osteoporosis. Mayo Clin Proc. 2002;77:453-68.
4. Jergas M, Gluer CC. Assessment of fracture risk by bone density measurements. Seminars in Nuclear Medicine. 1997;27(3):261-75.
5. WHO. Assessment of fracture risk and its application to screening for postmenopausal osteoporosis: technical report series 843. WHO, Geneva; 1994.
6. Sartoris DJ, Resuik D. Current and innovative methods for noninvasive bone densitometry. RCNA. 1990;28(2):257-78.
7. Guglielmi G, Muscarella S, Leone A, et al. Imaging of metabolic bone diseases. Radiol Clin North Am. 2008;46(4):735-54.
8. Kanis JA, on behalf of the World Health Organization Scientific Group. Assessment of osteoporosis at the primary healthcare level: technical report. World Health Organization Collaborating Centre for Metabolic Bone Diseases, University of Sheffield, UK; 2008.
9. Kanis JA. An update on the diagnosis of osteoporosis. Curr Rheumatol Rep. 2000;2(1):62-6.
10. International Society of Clinical Densitometry (ISCD). Official positions of the (International Society for Clinical Densitometry: updated 2005).
11. Blake GM, Fogelman I. The clinical role of dual energy X-ray absorptiometry. European Journal of Radiology. 2009;71:406-14.
12. World Health Organization. FRAX WHO fracture risk assessment tool. Available at: *http://www.shef.ac.uk/FRAX/*.
13. Marwaha RK, Tandon N, Kaur P, et al. Establishment of age-specified bone mineral density reference range for Indian females using dual-energy X-ray absorptiometry. J Clin Densitom. 2011 (Epub ahead of print).
14. Cann CE. Quantitative CT for determination of bone mineral density—a review. Radiology. 1988;166:509-22.
15. Ryan PJ. Overview of role of BMD measurements in managing osteoporosis. Seminars in Nuclear Medicine 1997;27(3):197-209.
16. Sartoris DJ. Clinical value of bone densitometry. AJR. 1994; 163:133-5.
17. Guglielmi G, Muscarella S. Axial CT in the diagnosis of osteoporosis. Clin Cases Miner Bone Metabol. 2005;2(2):110-2.
18. Engelke K, Adams JE, Armbrecht G, et al. Clinical use of quantitative computed tomography and peripheral quantitative computed tomography in the management of osteoporosis in adults: the 2007 ISCD Official Positions. J Clin Densitom. 2008;11(1):123-62.
19. Ito M, Hayashi K, Ishida Y, et al. Discrimination of spinal fracture with various bone mineral measurements. Calcif Tissue Int. 1997;60(1):11-5.
20. Grampp S, Jergas M, Lang P, et al. Quantitative CT assessment of the lumbar spine and radius in patients with osteoporosis. AJR. 1996;167:133-40.
21. Agarwal MM, Mandal AK, Khandelwal N, et al. Need for measurement of bone mineral density in patients of prostate cancer before and after orchidectomy: role of quantitative computer tomography. J Assoc Physicians India. 2007;55:486-90.
22. Bansal SC, Khandelwal N, Sen R, et al. Correlation between biochemical bone markers and bone mineral density in the evaluation of osteoporosis. J Pharm Res. 2011;4(8):2853-5.

23. Bansal SC, Khandelwal N, Rai DV, et al. Comparison between the QCT and the DEXA scanners in the evaluation of BMD in the lumbar spine. J Clin Diagn Res. 2011;5(4):694-9.
24. Miller P. Controversies in bone mineral density diagnostic classification. Calcif Tiss Int. 2000;66:317-9.
25. Faulkner R, von Stetten E, Miller P. Diskordance in patient classification using T-scores. J Clin Densitom. 1999;2:343-50.
26. Felsenberg D, Gowin W. Bone densitometry by dual energy methods. Radiology. 1999;39(3):186-93.
27. Zemel B, Bass S, Binkley T, et al. Peripheral quantitative computed tomography in children and adolescents: the 2007 ISCD Pediatric Official Positions. J Clin Densitom. 2008;11(1):59-74.
28. Brennan BM, Mughal Z, Roberts SA, et al. Bone mineral density in childhood survivors of acute lymphoblastic leukemia treated without cranial irradiation. J Clin Endocrinol Metab. 2005;90:689-94.
29. Ekman A, Michaëlsson K, Petrén-Mallmin M, et al. Dual X-ray absorptiometry of hip, heel ultrasound, and densitometry of fingers can discriminate male patients with hip fracture from control subjects: a comparison of four different methods. J Clin Densitom. 2002;5(1):79-85.
30. Langton CM, Langton DK. Comparison of bone mineral density and quantitative ultrasound of the calcaneus: site matched correlation and discrimination of axial BMD status. BJR. 2000;73:31-5.
31. Cepollaro C, Gonnelli S, Pondrelli C, et al. The combined use of ultrasound and densitometry on the prediction of vertebral fractures. BJR. 1997;70:691-6.
32. Mark AM. Presenting male osteoporosis; prevalence risks, diagnosis and imaging tests. Urol Clin N Am. 2004;31:321-30.
33. Huda W, Morin RL. Patients doses in bone mineral densitometry. BJR. 1996;69:422-5.
34. Khaw KT, Reeve J, Luben R, et al. Prediction of total and hip fracture risk in men and women by quantitative ultrasound of the calcaneus: EPIC-Norfolk prospective population study. Lancet. 2004;363(9404):197-202.
35. Li CQ, Magland JF, Rajapakse CS, et al. Implications of resolution and noise for in vivo micro-MRI of trabecular bone. Med Phys. 2008;35:5584.
36. Krug R, Banerjee S, Han ET, et al. Feasibility of in vivo structural analysis of high-resolution magnetic resonance images of the proximal femur. Osteoporos Int. 2005;16:1307.
37. Krug R, Han ET, Banerjee S, et al. Fully balanced steady-state 3D-spin-echo (bSSSE) imaging at 3 Tesla. Magn Reson Med. 2006;56:1033.
38. Krug R, Carballido-Gamio J, Burghardt AJ, et al. Assessment of trabecular bone structure comparing magnetic resonance imaging at 3 Tesla with high-resolution peripheral quantitative computed tomography ex vivo and in vivo. Osteoporos Int. 2008;19:653.
39. Krug R, Stehling C, Kelley DA, et al. Imaging of the musculoskeletal system in vivo using ultra-high field magnetic resonance at 7 T. Invest Radiol. 2009;44:613.
40. Kazakia GJ, Hyun B, Burghardt AJ, et al. In vivo determination of bone structure in postmenopausal women: a comparison of HR-pQCT and high-field MR imaging. J Bone Miner Res. 2008;23:463.
41. Wehrli FW, Song HK, Saha PK, et al. Quantitative MRI for the assessment of bone structure and function. NMR Biomed. 2006;19:731.
42. Wehrli FW. Structural and functional assessment of trabecular and cortical bone by micro magnetic resonance imaging. J Magn Reson Imaging. 2007;25:390.
43. Carballido-Gamio J, Krug R, Huber MB, et al. Geodesic topological analysis of trabecular bone microarchitecture from high-spatial resolution magnetic resonance images. Magn Reson Med. 2009;61:448.
44. Hyun B, Newitt DC, Majumdar S. Assessment of Cortical Bone Structure Using High-Resolution Magnetic Resonance Imaging. Proceedings 13th Scientific Meeting, International Society for Magnetic Resonance in Medicine; Miami.
45. Techawiboonwong A, Song HK, Leonard MB, et al. Cortical bone water: *in vivo* quantification with ultrashort echo-time MR imaging. Radiology. 2008;248:824.
46. Goldenstein J, Kazakia G, Majumdar S. In vivo evaluation of the presence of bone marrow in cortical porosity in postmenopausal osteopenic women. Ann Biomed Eng; 2009.
47. Wehrli FW, Gomberg BR, Saha PK, et al. Digital topological analysis of in vivo magnetic resonance microimages of trabecular bone reveals structural implications of osteoporosis. J Bone Miner Res. 2001;16:1520.
48. Laib A, Hauselmann HJ, Ruegsegger P. In vivo high resolution 3D-QCT of the human forearm. Technol Health Care. 1998;6:329.
49. Feldkamp LA, Davis LC, Kress JW. Practical cone-beam algorithm. J Opt Soc Am A. 1984;1:6
50. Thomas ML, Boris BK, Thomas L, et al. In vitro and in vivo spiral CT to determine bone mineral density: initial experience in patients at risk for osteoporosis. Radiology. 2004;231:805-11.
51. Ito M, Ikeda K, Nishiguchi M, Shindo H, et al. Multidetector row CT imaging of vertebral microstructure for evaluation of fracture risk. J Bone Miner Res. 2005;20(10):1828-36.
52. Jenson ME, Dion JE. Percutaneous vertebroplasty in the treatment of osteoporotic compression fractures. Neuroimaging Clinics of North America. 2000;10(3):547-68.
53. Klazen CA, Lohle PN, de Vries J, et al. Vertebroplasty versus conservative treatment in acute osteoporotic vertebral compression fractures (Vertos II): an open-label randomised trial. Lancet. 2010;376(9746):1085-92.
54. Tanigawa N, Kariya S, Komemushi A, et al. Percutaneous vertebroplasty for osteoporotic compression fractures: long-term evaluation of the technical and clinical outcomes. AJR. 2011;196:1415-8.
55. Rad AE, Kallmes DF. Correlation between preoperative pain duration and percutaneous vertebroplasty outcome. Am J Neuroradiol. 2011;32:1842-5.
56. Jensen ME, Dion JE. Percutaneous vertebroplasty in the treatment of osteoporotic compression fractures. Neuroimaging Clin N Am. 2000;10:547-68.
57. Jensen ME, Kallmes DF, Short JG, et al. Percutaneous vertebroplasty does not increase the risk of adjacent vertebral fracture—a retrospective study. Proceedings of the ASNR; Atlanta 2000 April 3-8.

CHAPTER 198

Benign Bone Tumors and Tumor-like Conditions

Mahesh Prakash, Niranjan Khandelwal

INTRODUCTION

Bone tumors may be defined as a new growth arising in a bone or derived from cells which are components of skeletal tissue.[1] The majority of benign true tumor of bone are detected in children and young adults. Benign bone tumors can be classified according to their matrix production and/or predominant cell type into cartilage forming, bone-forming, fibrous, vascular and other connective tissue lesions.[2,3] The term "tumor-like lesions of bone" denotes various conditions of non-neoplastic nature originating from or affecting the bone and presenting as solitary or multiple bone lesions. A broad classification of benign bone tumor and tumor like lesions is depicted in **Table 1**. For diagnosis of bone tumors and tumor-like lesion, there is need for close cooperation of radiologist, orthopedician and pathologists; however, the role of radiologist is most important. The primary aim of imaging should be to make specific diagnosis (if possible) or narrowing of the differential diagnosis which can be a guide for further intervention and management.

Table 1: Benign bone tumors and tumor like lesions.[4]

Benign bone tumors	*Tumor-like lesions*
Bone-forming tumors • Enostosis • Osteoma • Osteoid osteoma • Osteoblastoma	**Fibro-osseous lesions** • Nonossifying fibroma • Fibrous dysplasia • Osteofibrous dysplasia • Periosteal desmoid
Cartilage-forming tumors • Enchondroma • Osteochondroma • Periosteal chondroma • Chondroblastoma • Chondromyxoid fibroma	**Cystic lesions** • Simple bone cyst • Aneurysmal bone cyst • Intraosseous ganglion • Epidermoid cyst • Subchondral cyst
Connective tissue tumors • Desmoplastic fibroma • Benign fibrous histiocytoma • Ossifying fibroma • Myxoma • Lipoma	**Giant cell-containing lesions** • Giant cell reparative granuloma • Brown tumor • Pigmented villondoular synovitis
Vascular tumors • Hemangioma • Lymphangioma • Glomous tumor	**Others** • Eosinophilic granuloma • Pseudotumors
Others/semimalignant • Giant cell tumor • Ameloblastoma	

IMAGING MODALITIES

Before radiological evaluation, consideration of patient's data (age, gender) and clinical information of concerned patient are very useful for diagnosis as many lesions of bone show predilection for particular age group and gender.[2,3]

Radiography

Despite availability of a host of imaging modalities, plain radiographs continue to play a major role in the diagnostic evaluation of bone neoplasms. Plain radiographs demonstrate location of the tumor in the body, segment involved—whether epiphysis, metaphysis or diaphysis, growth characters of the lesion, such as margin-well defined/ill-defined, presence or absence of periosteal reaction and the appearance of tumor matrix—whether calcified or not, which are all important parameters to arrive at a proper diagnosis.

The pointers to the benign nature of a bone tumor include the following:

1. *Area of geographic bone destruction:* It is well circumscribed and is characterized by a sharp transition between the destroyed area and the normal bone (i.e. narrow zone of transition—less than 1 cm).
2. *Sclerotic margin:* It indicates slow growth and is generally seen in benign lesions located at the metaphysis. Certain tumors stimulate surrounding sclerosis which may obscure the central lytic area, such as osteoid osteoma.
3. *Periosteal reaction:* In general, periosteal reaction is not a feature of benign bone tumors unless a fracture has occurred except in a very few lesions, such as osteoblastoma, osteoid osteoma and chondromyxoid fibroma. Periosteal reaction is radiographically described as solid or interrupted. Solid periosteal reaction is defined as a single layer of new bone greater than 1 mm in thickness which is usually of uniform density. When seen, solid periosteal reaction indicates benign pathology.[1,3] It is seen in osteoid osteoma and osteoblastoma.
4. *Tumor matrix:* Presence of calcification in the form of rings, flocculant patches or stippled flecks point to the cartilaginous origin of the tumor. A ground glass haze indicates fibrous lesions. Osteoid matrix is seen in bone forming tumors.

Computed Tomography

Computed tomography (CT) can be used for radiographic information where conventional radiography has limited information like in the region of complex anatomy and superimposition of bony elements (pelvis, spine and scapula). Computed tomography is superior to radiography in determination of the epicenter of a bone lesion, whether it is in cortex, medulla or periosteal in location.[3,5,6]

Other advantages of CT over radiography to detect cortical alteration (breech, scalloping, expansion) and detection of periosteal reaction. Computed tomography is most valuable imaging modality in detection of subtle matrix calcifications and therefore it is very useful for diagnosis of a bone- or cartilage-forming benign bone tumor.[3-6]

Magnetic Resonance Imaging

Magnetic resonance imaging (MRI) is the most accurate method for demonstrating extent of tumors, especially intramedullary component.[7] Magnetic resonance imaging (MRI) has also demonstrated significant potential for tumor characterization. On T1-weighted images, most bone tumors show decrease in signal intensity because of marked contrast with hyper-intense fat of the marrow. On T2-weighted images most of the tumors are of high intensity making it difficult to separate tumor from fat but easy to differentiate tumor from surrounding muscles. Presence of atypical signal patterns help in predicting a dominant tissue component, e.g. high signal intensity on T1W images may be due to fat, as seen in lipoma, hemangioma, medullary bone infarct or hemorrhage as seen in aneurysmal bone cyst.[8]

MR is the best technique for demarcating the soft tissue component of bone tumors and its relationship to adjacent joint and neurovascular structures.[7,8]

Generally only few bone tumors have a classical radiological picture. Similarly, biopsy of the lesion is not always the ultimate answer. On the other hand, some tumors difficult to diagnose histologically but have a typical radiographic appearance, e.g. osteoid osteoma. Others with unusual radiographic features exhibit a characteristic histological appearance, e.g. aneurysmal bone cysts. Thus, close correlation of clinical history, histology and radiology are always essential to achieve highest diagnostic accuracy.

BONE-FORMING TUMORS

Enostosis

These lesions are commonly known as 'bony islands' are usually asymptomatic. Histologically, bone Island consist of dense intramedullary lamellar bone with normal haversian canals. Enostosis are commonly found in spine, ribs and pelvis.[9] It is usually seen as oval, densely sclerotic intramedullary lesions. Usually a bone island is aligned in the long axis of trabeculae **(Figs. 1A and B)**. Its only significance lies in the fact that it may be confused with osteoblastic metastases. Scintigraphy and MRI are helpful in the differentiation, as bony islands usually do not exhibit an increase tracer uptake on bone scans. On MRI, enostosis shows hypointense signal on both T1W and T2W sequences **(Figs. 2A and B)** while sclerotic metastasis shows halo of surrounding marrow edema on fluid sensitive sequences.[10]

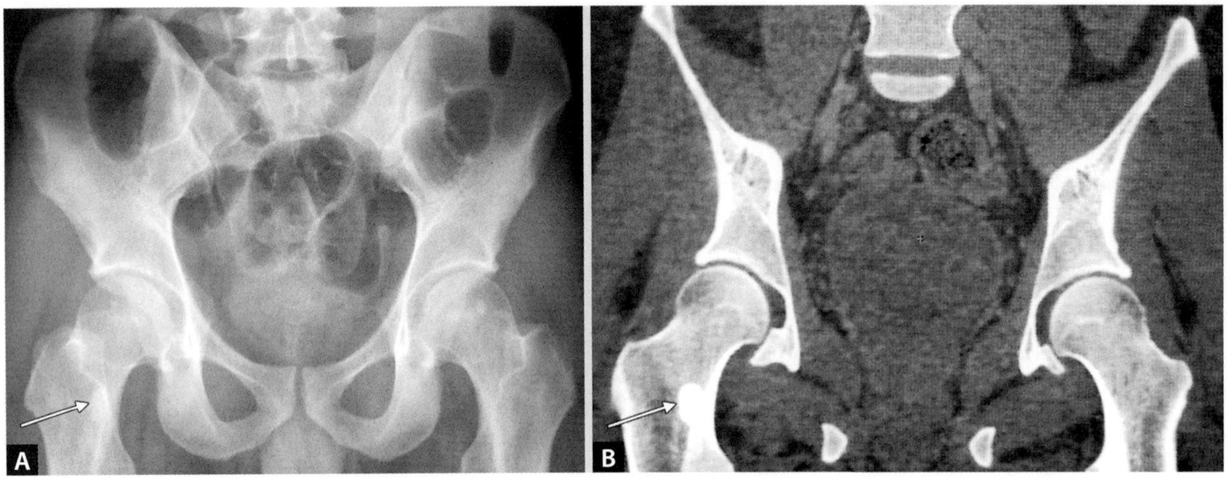

Figs. 1A and B: Enostosis: Radiograph (A) and CT coronal reconstruction (B) of pelvis shows well-defined oval sclerotic lesion (arrow) in intertrochanteric region of right femur.

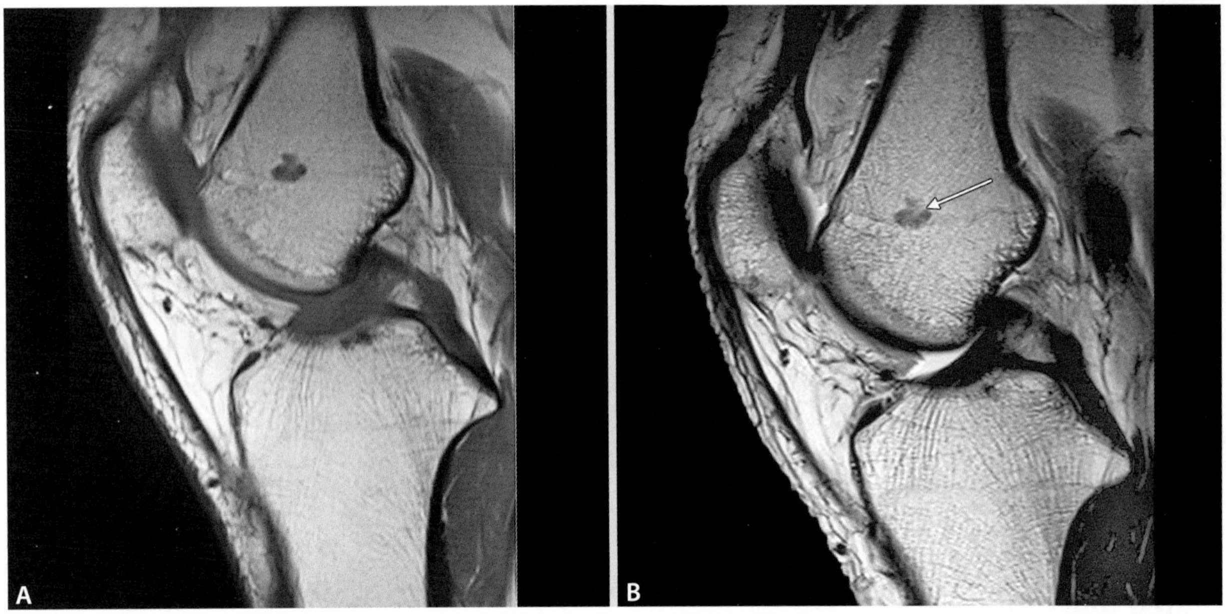

Figs. 2A and B: Enostosis—T1W (A) and T2W (B) sagittal MR images show well-defined lobulated lesion in lower end of femur which shows hypointense signal on both sequences (arrow).

Osteoma

Histologically, an osteoma is composed of both dense and woven bone and arises from the cortex. Common sites include outer table of skull, paranasal sinuses (frontal/ethmoid) and mandible. They are generally asymptomatic, but may cause sinus obstruction, proptosis, etc. Radiologically, osteoma is seen as a well circumscribed lesion arises from the cortex, which protrudes from the surface of the affected bone. It demonstrates same density as cortex on X-ray and CT scan **(Fig. 3)**. On MRI, osteoma shows hypointense signal on both T1- and T2W images.[11] Multiple osteomas occur as a part of Gardner's syndrome.

Osteoid Osteoma

Osteoid osteoma is a fairly common tumor, accounting for approximately 10–12% of all benign tumors.[12] These tumors usually affects patients between 5 and 25 years of age. Clinically most patients presents with pain that is especially severe at night and relieved by aspirin or other nonsteroidal anti-inflammatory agents.

More than half of tumors are located in proximal femur and tibia. They occur less frequently in the upper extremities than in the lower extremities. Osteoid osteoma also frequently affect the tubular bones of the hands and feet. They are, however, less common in the spine, where they affect the posterior arches of the vertebrae. Histologically, the lesion consists of a nidus which is usually less than 1 cm in diameter and surrounded by variable degree of sclerotic bone depending upon location. The nidus contains interlacing trabeculae at various stages of ossification within a stroma of loose, vascular connective tissue. Osteoid osteoma can be cortical (the most common type), cancellous or medullary, and subperiosteal.[11] The latter two types produce less sclerotic bone than those in the cortex do, making radiologic diagnosis difficult.

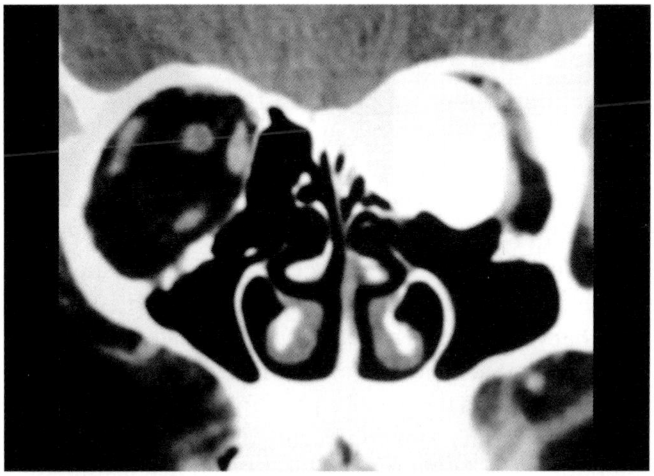

Fig. 3: Large osteoma: Computed tomography (coronal section) of paranasal sinus shows large well-defined bony lesion arising from ethmoid sinus causing compression of left orbital structures.

Radiographically, the lesion appears as well defined lytic lesion, surrounded by reactive sclerosis **(Figs. 4A and B)**. Nidus may be purely radiolucent or contain a dense center. Intra-articular osteoid osteomas may be either cancellous or periosteal and have little reactive bone or periosteal new bone formation.[11]

Computed tomography is very useful in showing the nidus, which can vary in its degree of ossification. Computed tomography appears to display the nidus better than MRI. Intense bone marrow edema adjacent to nidus is very useful to detect and localized the lesion on MRI **(Fig. 5)**, however, nidus may not readily visible if it is very small.[13] The tumor nidus typically shows hypo to intermediate signal on T1W images and low to high signal on T2W images. The nidus shows enhancement with gadolinium. Intra-articular osteoid osteomas produce joint effusions and synovial proliferation. Radionuclide bone scans have been used for many years to help diagnosis of osteoid osteomas. Bone scintigraphy, which is a highly sensitive method of detecting osteoid osteoma typically shows increased flow to the lesion on immediate images and a focus of increased activity on skeletal equilibrium images with double density sign.[14] Many times, osteomyelitis can mimick osteoid osteoma clinically as well radiographically; however, presence of soft tissue extension favors the diagnosis of osteomyelitis.

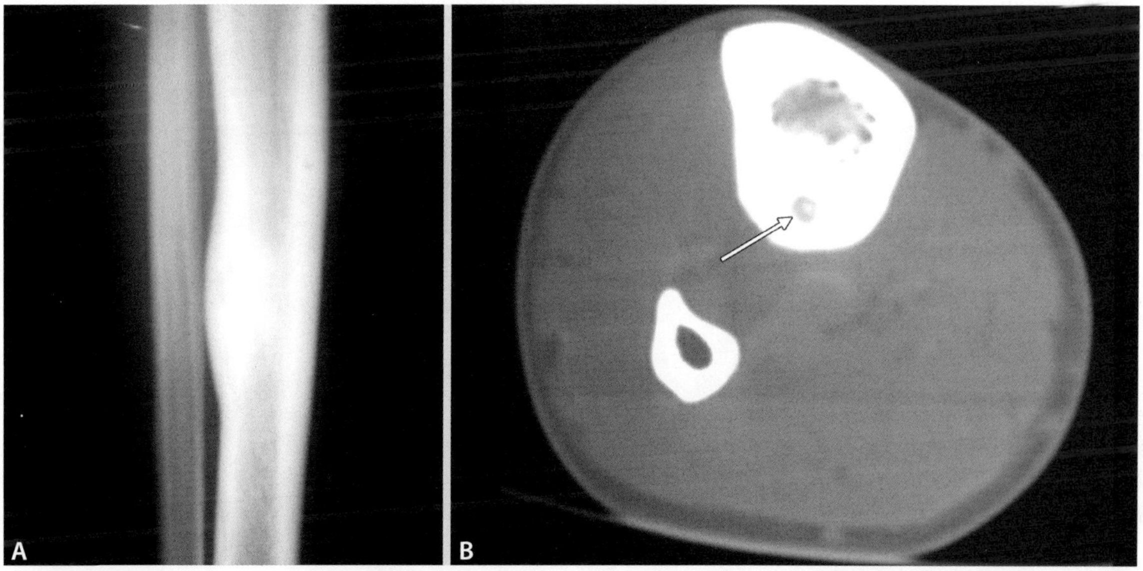

Figs. 4A and B: Osteoid osteoma: (A) Radiograph of leg shows dense sclerosis and solid periosteal reaction in the diaphysis of tibia; (B) CT scan axial section reveals well-defined lytic lesion with calcified nidus (arrow) associated with gross adjacent sclerosis.

Osteoblastoma

Osteoblastoma is rare bone forming tumors and most commonly occurs in patients in the second and third decade of life. This tumor is more common in males than in females. Histologically the osteoblastoma is closely related to osteoid osteomas except that bony trabeculae are broader and longer with absence of surrounding sclerotic halo. Size is an important consideration in distinguishing between these two types of tumors. If the size of lesion is less than 2 cm in diameter than it is likely of be osteoid osteomas, whereas tumors larger than 2 cm are usually osteoblastoma.[15]

The most common location of osteoblastoma is spine where it classically affects posterior elements **(Figs. 6A and B)**. The other common locations are proximal femur and talus. On plain X-ray, spinal osteoblastoma is osteolytic lesion with destruction of overlying cortex and may extend to in the spinal canal. In the long bones osteoblastoma appear radiologically as round or oval lucent tumors in the medulla. Periosteal reaction is common. Computed tomography demonstrate extent of lesion in complex bony structures like spine and pelvis better than radiography. Magnetic resonance imaging features may be nonspecific but helps to determine extension of vertebral lesion into spinal canal and spinal foramina.[16]

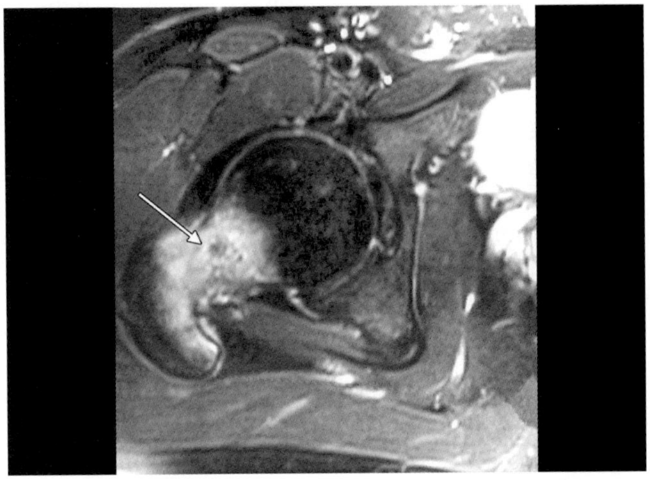

Fig. 5: Osteoid osteoma: T2W fat suppressed MRI (axial section) shows small nidus in neck of femur associated with extensive surrounding edema.

CARTILAGE-FORMING TUMORS

Osteochondroma

Osteochondromas are common lesions of the growing skeleton. It is the most common benign neoplasm and constitutes 20–50% of all benign tumors.[17] They arise from bony metaphysis with cartilage cap covering. These tumors are either pedunculated or sessile **(Fig. 7)**. Multiple osteochondroma occur as a manifestation of diaphyseal aclasis, an inherited disorder with autosomal dominance **(Fig. 8)**. The long axis of the osteochondroma pedicle or stalk is almost always directed away from the adjacent joint. The direct communication between the osteochondroma and the cortex and marrow cavity of the bone from which it arises is a distinctive feature, that is particularly well demonstrated on computed tomography and magnetic resonance imaging. T2/PD-weighted MR image is useful to demonstrate an cartilaginous cap **(Figs. 9A and B)**. The cap can be quite thick in early childhood like the normal physis, becomes thinner with age. After epiphyseal closure, growth of the osteochondroma

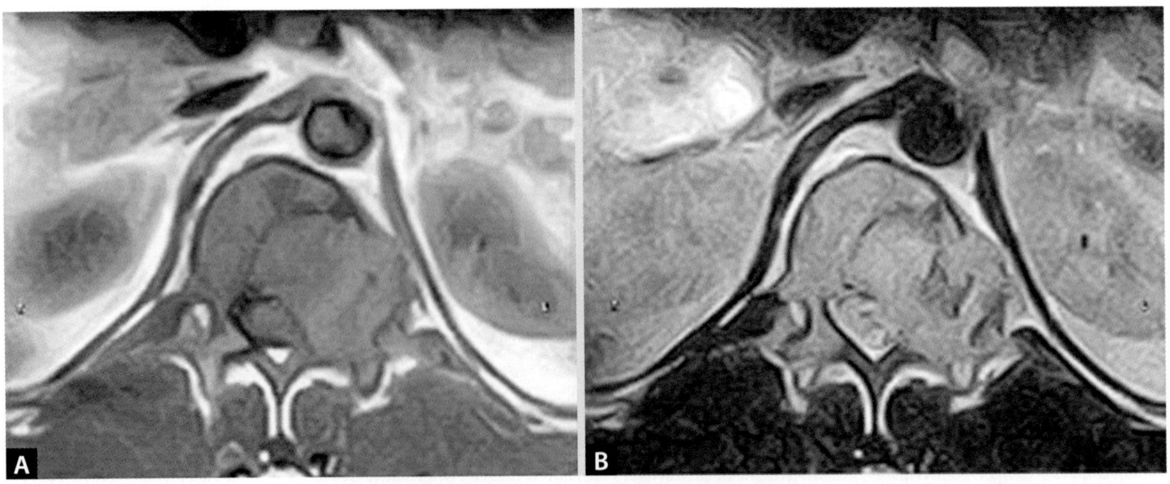

Figs. 6A and B: Osteoblastoma: MRI axial section, T1 and T2WI images reveal heterogeneous signal mass lesion, predominantly involving posterior elements of vertebra extending into spinal canal.

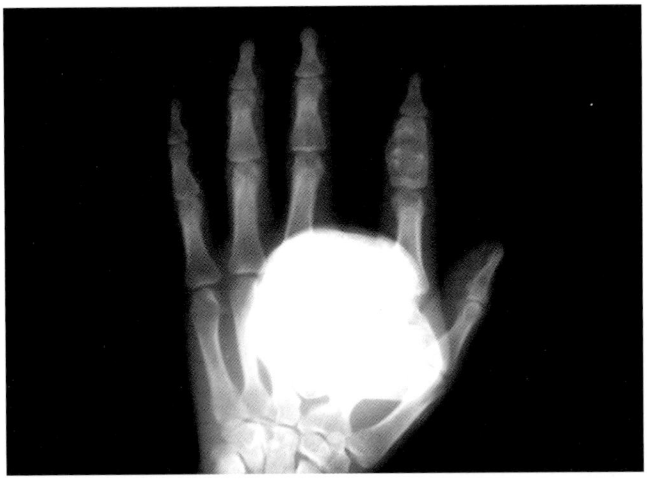

Fig. 7: Sessile osteochondroma: Radiograph of the left hand shows a large well-defined calcified lesion having a broad-based attachment to second metacarpal. An enchondroma showing typical central spotty calcification is also present in the middle phalanx of the index finger.

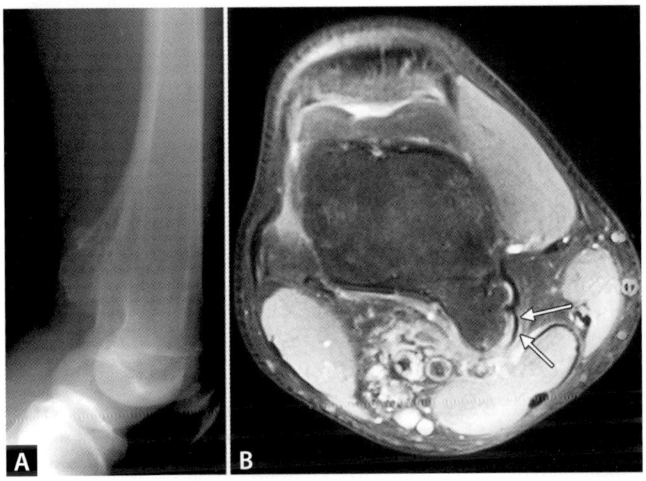

Figs. 9A and B: Pedunculated osteochondroma: (A) Radiograph of lower end of femur (Lateral view) shows large well-defined bony outgrowth, with broad based attachment to femur; (B) MRI (PD fat sat), axial section of the same patient shows clear demonstration of continuity of marrow and cortex of host bone into osteochondroma with covering cartilage cap (arrows).

ceases. Because most osteochondromas are asymptomatic, they are usually discovered incidentally. However, mechanical irritation of adjacent soft tissues or nerves, vascular injuries, fracture of the stalk, or malignant transformation can produce symptoms.

Malignant transformation into low-grade chondrosarcoma occurs in 1% of osteochondromas; however, the risk is 10–30% in cases of multiple osteochondromatosis.[17] Malignant transformation should be considered when

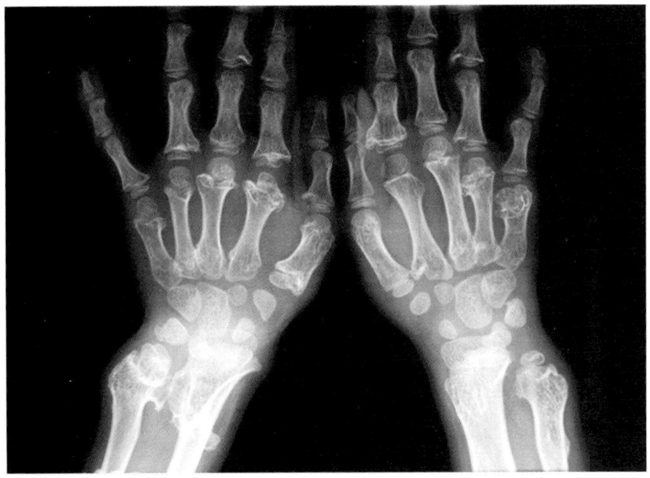

Fig. 8: Diaphyseal aclasis: Radiograph of bilateral hands (PA view) show multiple osteochondromas and deformities involving multiple bones of hands and forearm.

the osteochondroma grows after epiphyseal closure. Malignancy occurs in the cartilaginous cap, which becomes thickened. After skeletal maturity, the cartilage cap should not be thicker than 2 cm. Pain and cartilage cap growth are the sign of malignant transformation.[18]

Enchondroma

Enchondromas accounts for 12% of benign bone tumors.[18] These are most frequently located in the large and small tubular bones of the hands and feet **(Fig. 10)**. Like other cartilaginous tumors, enchondromas exhibit a lobulated growth pattern that results in asymmetric expansion of the medullary cavity and endosteal scalloping. Tumor matrix may be radiolucent or show calcification. Characteristic cartilaginous ring and arc pattern of calcifications are seen on radiographs and CT images. On MR imaging, the tumor is isointense to muscle on T1-weighted and exhibits a heterogeneous, predominantly high T2-weighted signal.[19] Contrast enhanced MRI may demonstrate a pattern of thin arcs and rings.

Ollier's disease is a nonheritable disorder of cartilage proliferation in which enchondromas involve multiple bones, especially those of the hands and may result in skeletal deformity **(Fig. 11)**. Enchondromatosis accompanied by multiple hemangiomas is known as Maffucci's syndrome. Calcified phleboliths may be demonstrated radiographically in the hemangiomatous soft tissue masses. Lesions associated with both Ollier's disease and Maffucci's syndrome carry a significant risk of malignant degeneration.[20]

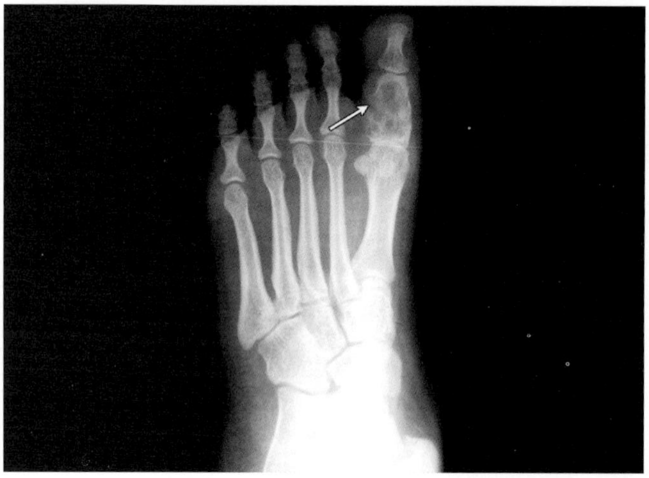

Fig. 10: Enchondroma: Radiograph of foot shows sharply demarcated expansile lesion in proximal phalynx of great toe having endosteal scalloping and cortical breech (arrow).

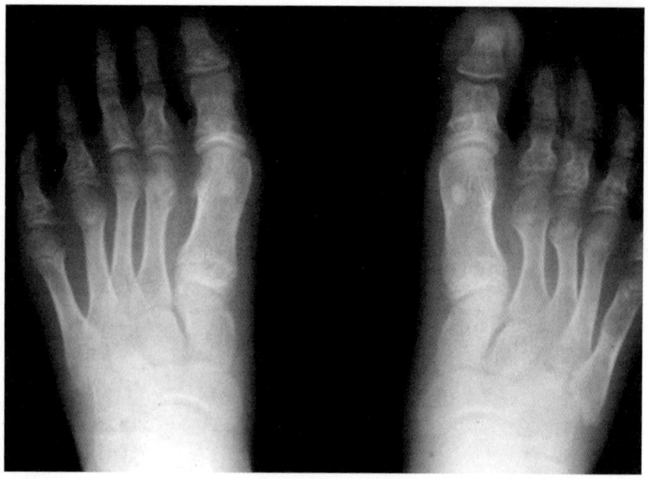

Fig. 11: Ollier's disease: Radiograph of feet shows relatively well-defined expansile lytic lesions involving most of the phalanges, with varying amounts of calcification within them.

Chondroblastoma

It is less common than enchondroma. Chondroblastoma is composed of primitive cartilage cells, usually occurs in the age group of 10–25 years. It is typically located in epiphysis and apophysis of bone, most often the proximal humerus, distal femur and proximal tibia.[17] On plain X-ray, chondroblastoma is an eccentric, lucent, well-defined lesion with sclerotic borders. Periosteal reaction, far from the lesion is another common feature suggesting an accompanying inflammatory process. Approximately one-third of chondroblastoma have a calcified matrix which can be better seen on CT scan **(Fig. 12)**.

The tumor shows signal intensity similar to that of muscle on MR imaging; however, the rim of the tumor has lower signal intensity. On T2-weighted images, the signal intensity of the tumor is low to intermediate. This tumor also shows extensive surrounding inflammation which may be confused with more aggressive lesion. Malignant transformation of chondroblastoma is extremely uncommon.[21] The differential diagnosis of epiphyseal lesions includes giant cell tumor, osteomyelitis, subchondral cyst and Langerhans cell histiocytosis.

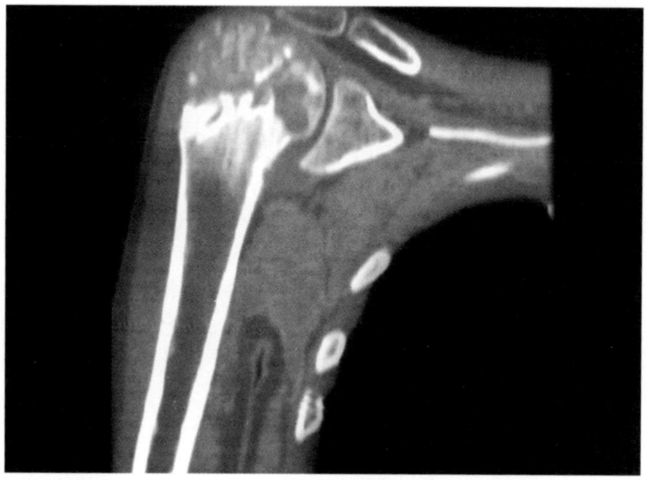

Fig. 12: Chondroblastoma: CT (coronal reformation) shows expansile lytic lesion in epiphysis (characteristic location) of upper humerus with matrix calcification.

Chondromyxoid Fibroma

Chondromyxoid fibroma is rare and commonly affects males and patients younger than 35 years.[18] Histologically, it is composed of chondroid, myxoid and fibrous tissue in varying amounts. The common locations of tumor are ilium, tibia and bones of foot. These tumors are located characteristically in metadiaphyseal location unlike chondroblastoma and do not cross an open growth plate. On plain radiograph, it appears as a well marginated central or eccentric lucent lesion, with sclerotic margins and cortical thinning **(Fig. 13)**. Half of the lesions may show parallel orientation to the long axis of the involved bone. Matrix calcification and periosteal new bone formation usually do not occur.

FIBROUS TUMORS/LESIONS

Fibrous Cortical Defects and Nonossifying Fibroma

Fibrous cortical defect and nonossifying fibroma are basically similar benign fibrous lesions located

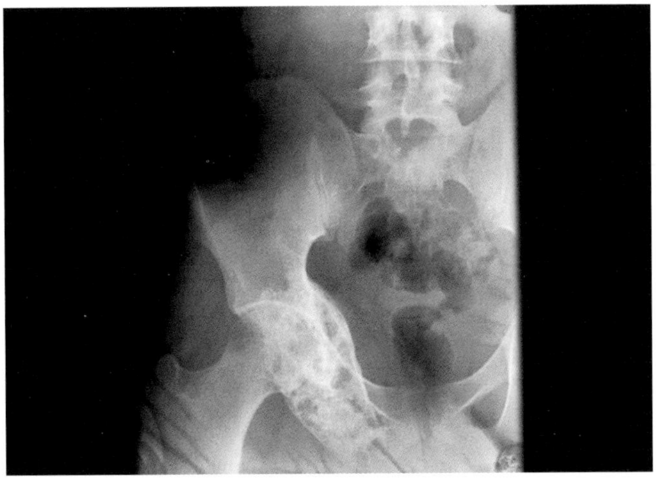

Fig. 13: Chondromyxoid fibroma: Radiograph of right hip shows large expansile lesion with sclerotic border and trabeculations involving right acetabulum.

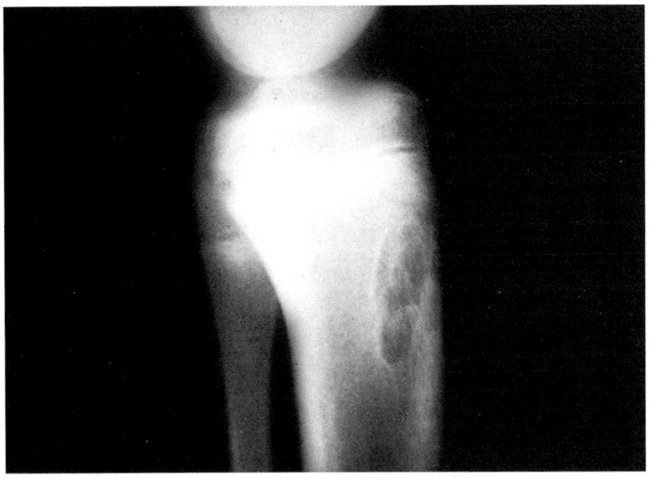

Fig. 14: Nonossifying fibroma: Lateral radiograph of leg shows an eccentric geographic lytic lesion in the medulla of proximal tibial metaphysis.

slightly differently, nonossifying fibroma being located eccentrically in the medullary cavity **(Fig. 14)** and fibrous cortical defect seen superficially affecting the cortex **(Fig. 15)**. Pathologically, these lesions are composed of fibrous tissue, xanthoma cells and giant cells. The common location of lesion are in the bones around the knee joints. These lesions are usually asymptomatic and do not require specific treatment. On plain radiography, the lesion appears as well-marginated eccentric lytic lesion with scalloped margin. Its inner border is often sclerotic and may appear multilocular due to corrugations. Differential diagnosis includes unicameral bone cyst, aneurysmal bone cyst, fibrous dysplasia, and chondromyxoid fibroma. The signal intensity of nonossifying fibroma is equal to or less than muscle on T1-weighted MR images and hypointense on T2-weighted images.[22] Postcontrast images usually show heterogeneous enhancement.

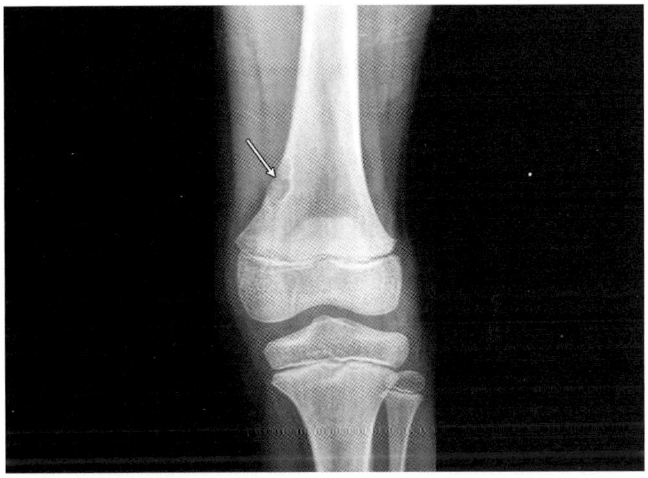

Fig. 15: Fibrous cortical defect: Radiograph of knee (AP view) show eccentric well-defined lytic lesion in lower end of femur which is limited to cortex (arrow).

Fibrous Dysplasia

Fibrous dysplasia is disorders where bone is replaced by abnormal fibrous tissue. Fibrous dysplasia can be monostotic, polyostotic, monomelic, or polymelic. It is more common in young females. It is occasionally seen in the first decade of life. In a small percentage of cases (2–3%), fibrous dysplasia is associated with endocrine disorders, especially precocious puberty in girls (McCune–Albright syndrome).[23,24] Although it is not a true neoplasm, fibrous dysplasia involving a long bone may mimic a bone tumor or cyst. This type of fibrous dysplasia causes expansion of the medullary cavity of tubular bones, endosteal scalloping and trabeculation. The margin is sclerotic **(Fig. 16)**. The lesion may appear as ground glass or radiolucent, and this depends upon amount of fibrous tissue within the lesion. Bowing of the affected long bone may occur; when the affected bone is femur, the resulting deformity is called a "shepherd's crook" **(Fig. 17)**. Thinning and destruction of the bony cortex may be seen on CT or MR images. Soft tissue extension of the lesion is unusual. On T1-weighted MR images, the signal intensity of fibrous dysplasia is similar to that of skeletal muscle. Although the signal of pure fibrous tissue is hypointense on T2-weighted images, the signal of fibrous dysplasia is variable.

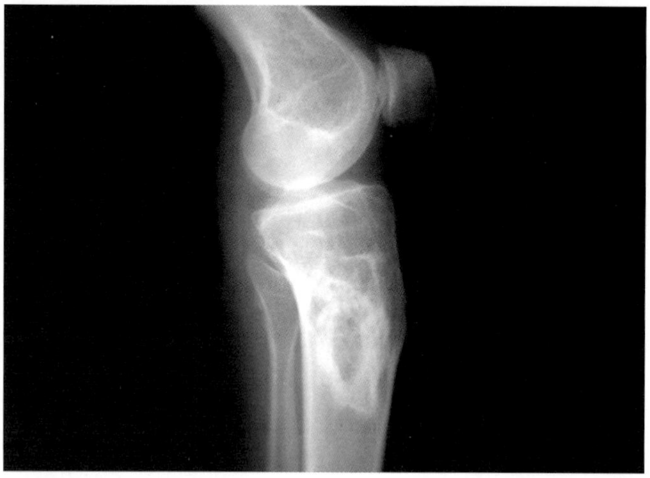

Fig. 16: Fibrous dysplasia: Lateral radiograph of knee joint shows a well-defined lytic lesion in proximal tibial metaphysis with surrounding sclerotic rind which is characteristic of fibrous dysplasia.

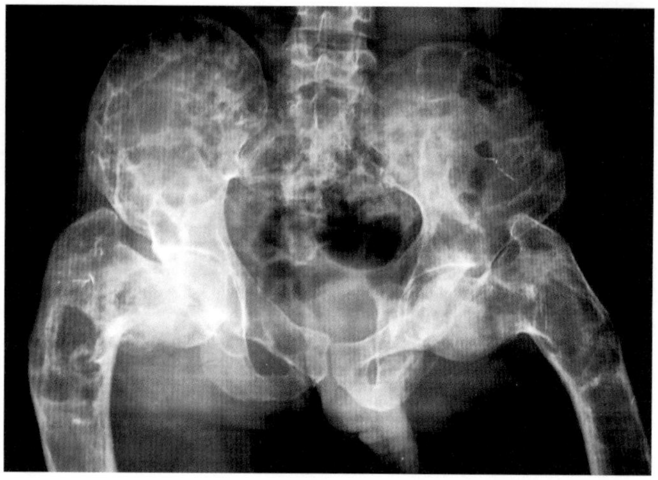

Fig. 17: Polystotic fibrous dysplasia: Radiograph of pelvis shows multiple lytic lesions involving pelvic bones and bilateral femora with characteristic Shepherd's crook deformity.

Osteofibrous Dysplasia

It is a rare lesion that is usually confined to the tibia but can also involve the fibula. Most cases occur during the first decade of life. On plain X-ray, the lesion appears as an eccentric, lucent, solitary or multiloculated, lesion involving the anterior aspect of tibia. CT is very helpful in determining its intracortical location, an important feature in distinguishing osteofibrous dysplasia from fibrous dysplasia.[25]

Desmoplastic Fibroma

Desmoplastic fibroma is rare accounting for only 0.1% of benign bone tumors. This lesion usually seen in the second and third decades of life. Histologically, there is infiltration of abnormal fibrous tissue in the bone and at times it is confused with low grade fibrosarcoma of bone. They are mostly located in the metadiaphysis of long bones but may invade the epiphysis. Femur, tibia and humerus are most commonly affected.[26] On radiography, the lesion has aggressive appearance and present as lytic expansile lesion with internal trabeculation and sclerotic margin. Computed tomography may demonstrate cortical breech and adjacent soft tissue if any. Magnetic resonance imaging typically shows intermediate to low signal on fluid sensitive sequences.[27]

VASCULAR AND CONNECTIVE TISSUE TUMORS

Hemangioma

Hemangioma is slowly growing lesions of bone composed of newly formed vascular spaces. About 50% of hemangiomas of bone occur in vertebrae and are most commonly located in lower thoracic and upper lumbar regions.[28] Twenty percent of hemangiomas occur in skull. Small bones of the hand and feet may also be affected.

Hemangioma of the vertebra has a typical radiographic picture in the form of coarse vertical striations on the plain radiographs and Polka dot appearance on CT[29] **(Figs. 18A and B)**. It shows high intensity on both T1W and T2W images. In the skull, hemangioma generally affects the calvarium and is seen as an expansile lytic lesion, which has a sunburst appearance with striations radiating from the center. In the short and long bones, the lesion lacks characteristic features and may be difficult to differentiate from other expansile central lesions such as aneurysmal bone cyst, chondromyxoid fibroma or enchondroma.

Lipoma

Intraosseous lipoma is a rare benign neoplasm occurs between 5 and 70 years of age. The proximal femur, tibia and calcaneum are the most common sites of involvement. On plain radiographs lipoma appears as a well-defined osteolytic lesion with a thin sclerotic rim. Bone expansion and trabeculations may be seen within the lesion. Cortical erosion and periosteal reaction are characteristically absent. In the calcaneum, the lesion usually occurs along the plantar margin where a "triangle" is formed by major trabecular groups and there may be a calcified nidus. CT scan shows typical "Fat" density (–60 to –120 HU) and lack of contrast enhancement. On MR, lipoma typically shows high signal intensity on T1 weighted image and iso to hyperintense signal on T2 weighted image.[30]

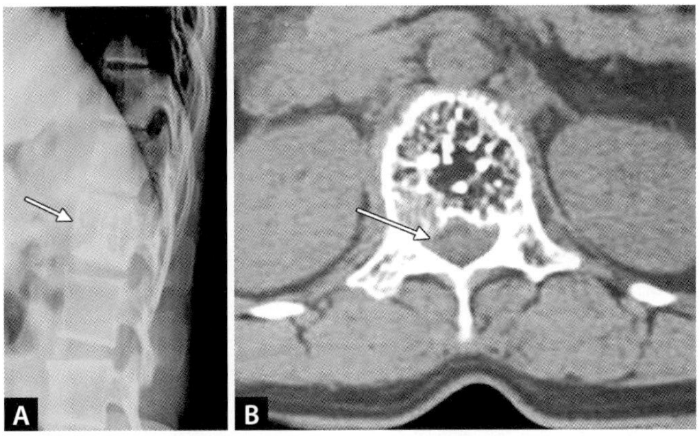

Figs. 18A and B: Hemangioma of vertebra: (A) Lateral radiograph of dorsolumbar spine shows mild expansion of L1 vertebral body with coarse vertical striations (arrow); (B) Axial CT scan of the same patient shows 'Polka dot' appearance due to vertical trabeculae cut in cross section. In addition there is focal disruption of the posterior cortex of vertebral body (arrow).

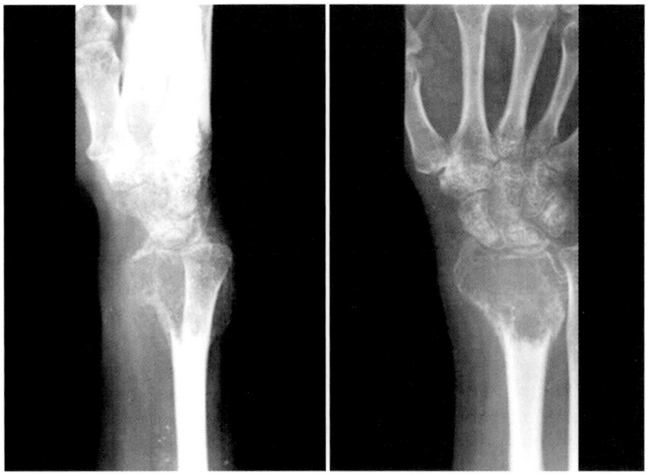

Fig. 19: Giant cell tumor: Radiograph of the left wrist shows an expansile subarticular lytic lesion in the distal end of radius. Cortex appears intact.

OTHER TUMORS

Giant Cell Tumor

Giant cell tumor (GCT) constitutes about 5% of all bone tumors and slightly less than 20% of all benign tumors.[31] The tumor originates from undifferentiated cells of the supporting tissues of bone marrow. As opposed to other benign tumors, GCT has a female predilection and mostly occurs after the closure of epiphysis, with a peak in the third decade.

Giant cell tumors arise eccentrically in the metaphysis with tendency to approach the adjacent subarticular cortex as they enlarge **(Fig. 19)**. Forty to fifty percent of lesions occur around the knee.[31] Involvement of distal radius is seen in 10–12% which otherwise is an uncommon site for bone tumors. Other sites are sacrum, short tubular bones and vertebral bodies. Classical radiographic picture is that of a well defined eccentric lytic lesion which expands the bone and is usually not surrounded by a sclerotic rim **(Fig. 20)**. Cortical penetration with or without an associated soft tissue mass is seen in 33–50% of cases. The solid portion of a giant cell tumor is usually low to intermediate signal intensity at T1- and T2-weighted images. This has been attributed to its high collagen content, high cellularity or presence of hemosiderin.[32] Giant cell tumor is the most common lesion associated with secondary ABC. Following contrast administration, there is diffuse enhancement of the solid component and peripheral or septal enhancement of cystic areas **(Figs. 21A and B)**. Giant cell tumors are aggressive benign neoplasms with a high rate of recurrence.

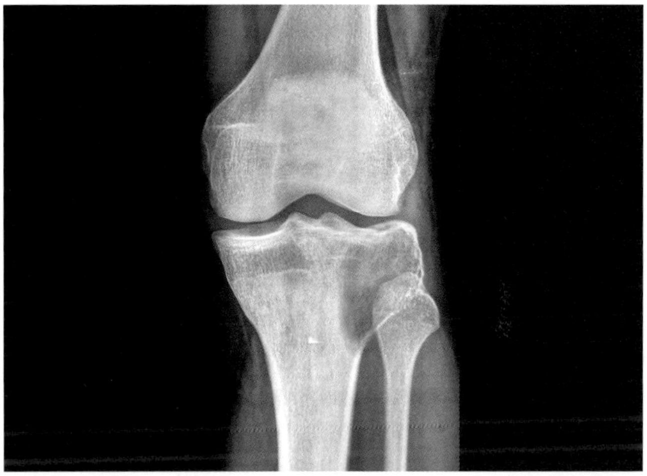

Fig. 20: Giant cell tumor: Radiograph of the knee shows an eccentric expansile subarticular lytic lesion in proximal end of tibia without sclerotic margin.

TUMOR-LIKE LESIONS

Simple Bone Cyst

A bone cyst is a fluid filled lesion with fibrous lining. It occurs in metaphysis of long bones and adjacent to physis in children and young adults. Common locations are proximal humerus and femur.[28] Calcaneum and ileum are less common sites. On plain radiograph, the lesion appears as moderately expansile, well marginated with or without sclerosis **(Fig. 22)**. The cortex may be thinned out and may lead to pathological fracture. "Fallen fragment" sign has been described as pathognomonic features of bone cyst when fragment of bone settles at the base of

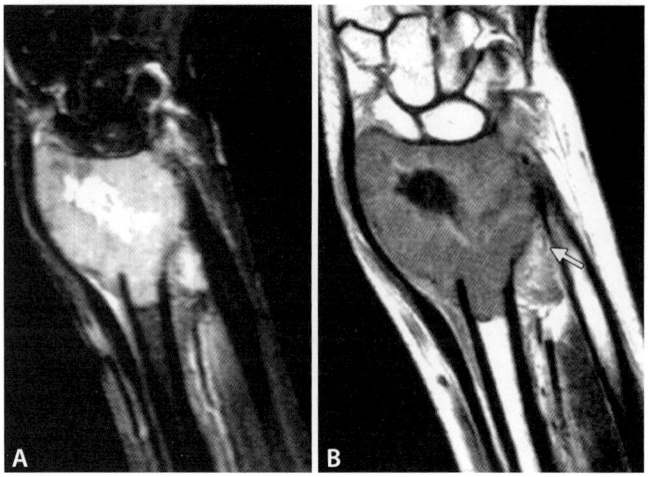

Figs. 21A and B: Giant cell tumor: (A) Coronal MR images of left forearm of the previous patient (Fig. 19) showing expansile subarticular epiphyseal lesion of radius which is hyperintense on T2W image with central cystic area; (B) Postcontrast image shows homogeneous enhancement of solid component and no enhancement of cystic area. The cortical line on the lateral side is intact but shows disruption with extension of the tumor into the soft tissues on the medial aspect (arrow).

lesion due to simple nature of fluid. "Rising bubbles" sign is also based on similar principles.[33] CT and MRI can confirm the cystic nature of the lesion. The fluid contents are usually of low intensity on T1-weighted images and hypertense on T2- weighted images.[34] However, hemorrhage into the cyst can alter the signal characteristics of the lesion.

Aneurysmal Bone Cyst

Aneurysmal bone cyst is solitary, expansile radiolucent lesion and generally located in metaphysis of long bones. Other sites are dorsolumbar spine, small bones of hand, feet and pelvis. Pathologically, the lesion contains multiples cystic spaces containing various stages of blood. Radiologically, the lesion appears as expansile, lytic sharply circumscribed with thin cortex. The characteristic features are its ballooned out appearance and trabeculated appearance **(Fig. 23)**. CT may demonstrate fluid-fluid level and thin rim of bone overlying the lesion. MRI shows the various stages of blood products which appear as layers of different signal intensity on both T1- and T2W images[28] **(Figs. 24A and B)**. The differential diagnosis includes giant cell tumor, osteoblastoma, chondroblastoma, osteosarcoma and simple bone cyst.

Eosinophilic Granuloma

Eosinophilic granuloma is the most benign form of histiocytosis X, which is a disease of unknown etiology characterized by proliferation of histiocytes. Eosinophilic granuloma constitutes 60–80% of Langerhans cell histiocytosis. Bone lesion may be solitary (85%) or multiple (20%) with peak incidence between 5 and 10 years.[35] The preferred sites being skull, mandible, spine and long bones.

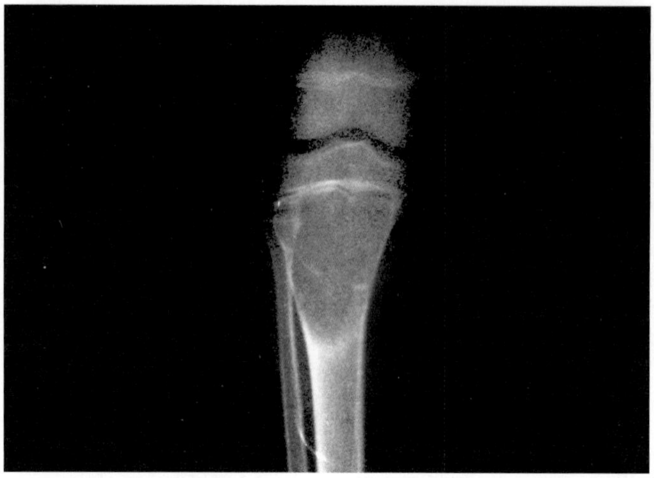

Fig. 22: Bone cyst: Radiograph of knee joint show mildly expansile lytic lesion in metaphysis of tibia with thinning of cortex and septation.

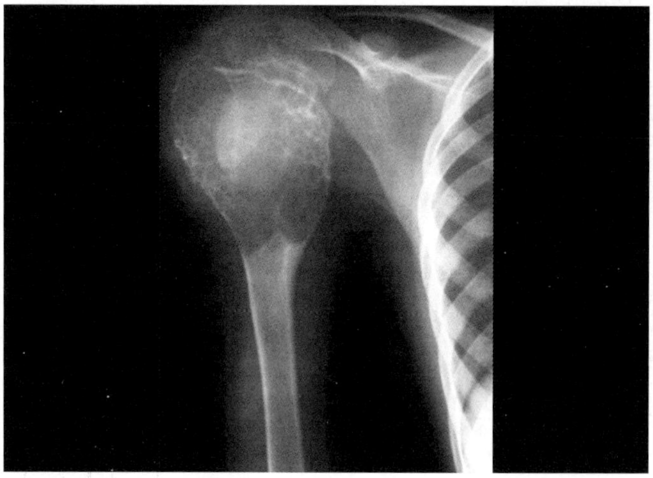

Fig. 23: Aneurysmal bone cyst: Radiograph of shoulder joint shows multiloculated very expansile lytic lesion, involving upper end of humerus.

The skull lesion on radiographs is seen as a punched out lytic lesion having a bevelled appearance due to unequal involvement of outer and inner table with a variably sclerotic margin **(Fig. 25)**. The center of the lesion has a sclerotic focus which is often termed as a button sequestrum. In the mandible, lytic lesion may cause floating teeth. In the spine, typically the vertebral body is affected, and there may be complete lysis resulting in

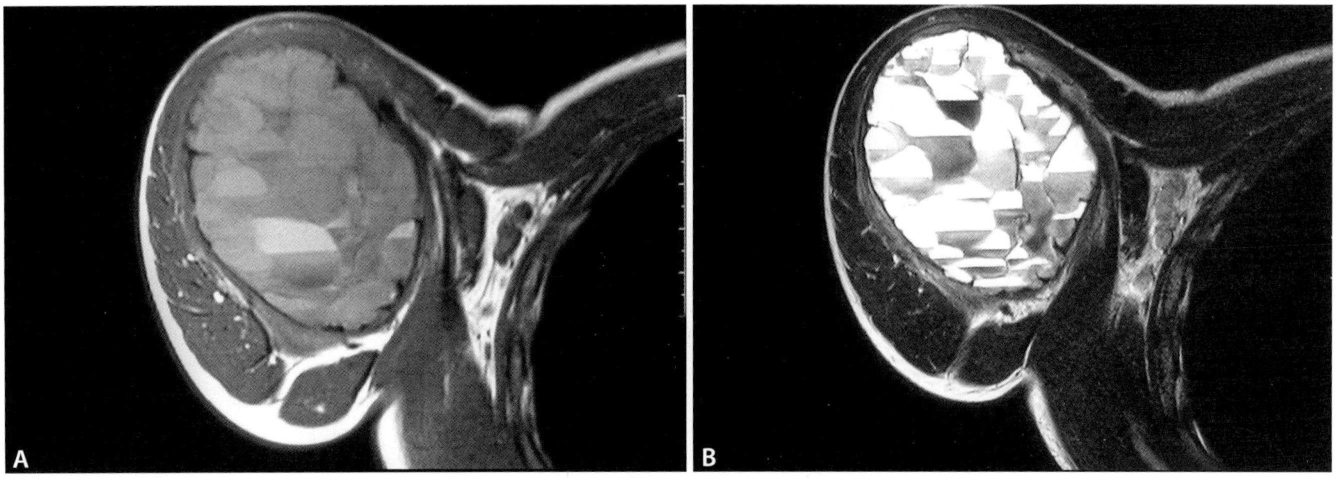

Figs. 24A and B: Aneurysmal bone cyst: (A and B) MRI of the same patient, axial T1- and T2W images shows well-defined multiloculated expansile lesion with extensive fluid-fluid/hemorrhage levels.

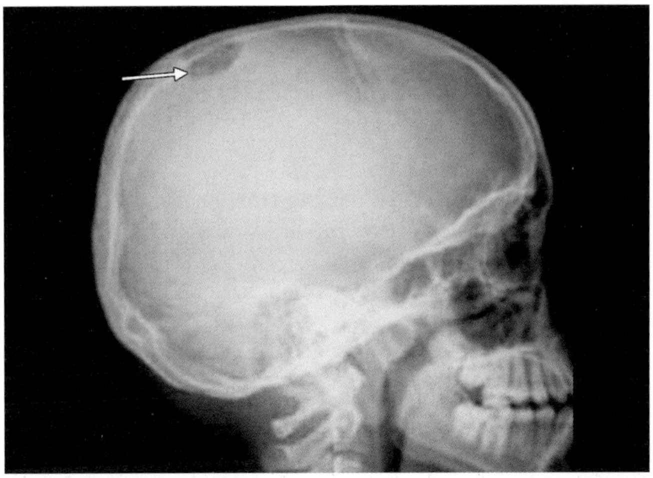

Fig. 25: Eosinophilic granuloma: Lateral radiograph of skull shows a well-defined lytic lesion with bevelled edges in the parietal bone (arrow).

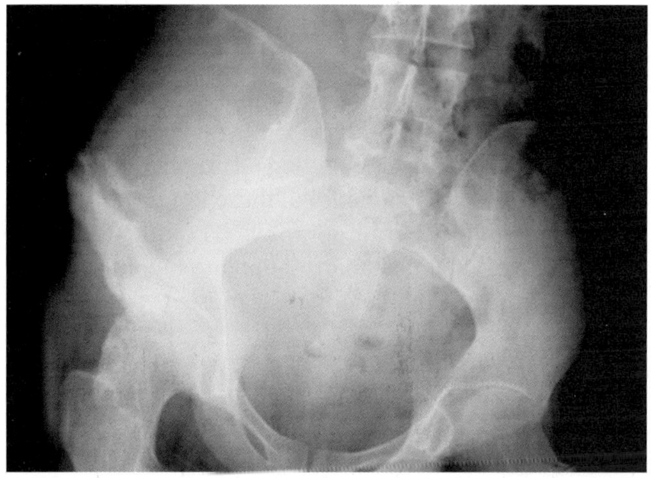

Fig. 26: Hemophilic pseudotumor: AP radiograph of pelvis reveals a large well-defined lytic lesion in the right iliac bone with an associated soft tissue mass.

a solitary collapsed vertebra with a preserved disk space. In the long bones, the lesions are generally diaphyseal or metaphyseal in location and cause endosteal scalloping. Benign type of periosteal reaction is considered typical.

Pseudotumor of Hemophilia

Hemophilia is a bleeding disorder that occurs in males. Repetitive hemorrhage within the bone may result expansile geographic lesion which can simulate neoplasm **(Fig. 26)**. The common locations are femur, pelvis, tibia and hand. Computed tomography scan better demonstrate the bony erosion/destruction with adjacent hematoma **(Fig. 27)**. Magnetic resonance imaging shows variable heterogeneous signals, in form of various stages of blood products.[36]

Brown Tumor of Hyperparathyroidism

Brown tumors represent focal, bone replacing lesions, encountered both in primary or secondary hyperparathyroidism. They represents hemorrhage and breakdown product of hemoglobin. The lesions most often occur in metaphyses and diaphyses and the common bones involved are mandible, pelvis, ribs and femur.[37]

On plain radiographs, the lesions are seen as slightly trabeculated, solitary or multiple expansile lytic lesions with well defined margins **(Fig. 28)**. Differentiation from a simple bone cyst is difficult when the lesion is solitary. Associated skeletal osteoporosis and biochemical changes, sclerotic appearance of brown tumor after removal of parathyroid adenoma and the marked activity with scintigraphy are helpful in the diagnosis.[37,38]

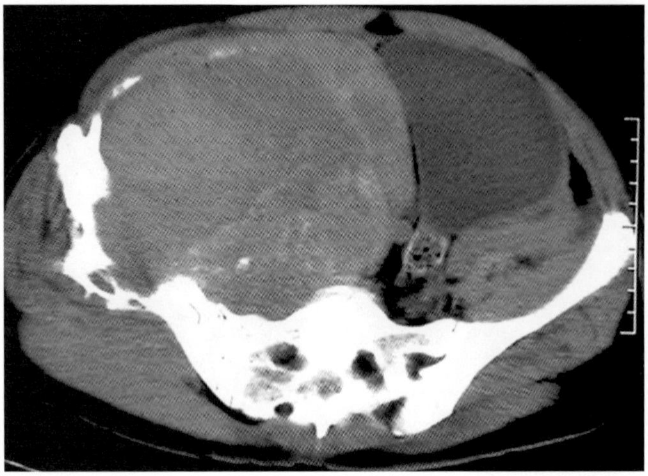

Fig. 27: Axial NCCT scan of the same patient shows erosion of the right ilium with a large soft tissue mass that has a variegated appearance with hyperdense areas within it suggestive of hemorrhage.

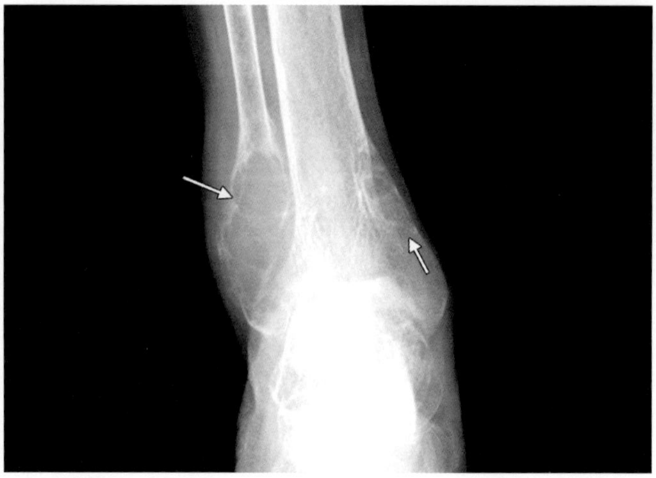

Fig. 28: Brown tumors: Radiograph of left ankle of young man with hyperparathyroidism shows multiple well-defined expansile multiloculated lytic lesions in lower end of tibia and fibula.

CONCLUSION

Some of the bony tumor and tumor-like lesions have characteristic imaging features; however, many others may have overlap imaging findings. Thorough knowledge of radiographic characteristics of these lesions on various imaging modalities (radiography, CT and MRI) with patient data and clinical information are helpful to make diagnosis or to reach differential diagnosis.

REFERENCES

1. Greenfield BG. The solitary lesion. Radiology of Bone Disease 5th edn. Philadelphia: JB Lippincott; 1990. pp. 580-732.
2. Forest M, Coindre JM, Diebold J. Pathology of tumors. In: Forest M, Tomeno B, Vanel D (Eds). Orthopedic surgical pathology: diagnosis of tumors and pseudotumoral lesions of bone and joints. Churchill livingstone, Epindburgh; 1997. pp. 71-516.
3. Resnick D. Tumors and tumor like lesions of bone: radiolographic principles. In: Resnick D (Ed). Diagnosis of bone and joint disorders. Saunders, Philadelphia; 1995. pp. 3613-27.
4. Woertler K. Benign bone tumor and tumor-like lesions: value of cross sectional imaging. Eur Radiol. 2003;13:1820-35.
5. Resnick D, Kyriakos M, Greenway GD. Tumors and tumor like lesions of bone: Imaging and pathology of specific of bone lesions. In: Resnick D (Ed). Diagnosis of bone and joint disorders. Saunders, Philadelphia; 1995. pp. 3628-938.
6. Magid D. Two dimensional and three dimensional computed tomographic imaging in musculoskeletal tumors. Radiol Clin North Am. 1993;31:425-47.
7. Berquist TH. Magnetic resonance imaging of primary skeletal neoplasms. Radiol Clin North Am. 1993;31: 411-24.
8. Moulton JS, Bvaley SE, Biedel JS. Bone and soft tissue tumors. In Clinical Magnetic Resonance Imaging, 2nd edn; 1996. pp. 2042-77.
9. Greenspan A. Bone island (enostotsis): current concept: a review. Skeletal Radiol. 1995;24:111-5.
10. Schweitzer ME, Levine C, Mitchell DG, et al. Bull's eyes and halos: useful discriminators of osseous metastases. Radiology. 1993;188:249-52.
11. Cerase A, Priolo F. Skeletal benign bone forming lesions. Eur J Radiol. 1998;27:91-7.
12. Bloem JL, Kroon HM. Osseous lesions. Radiol Clin of North America. 1993;31:261-5.
13. Davies M, Cassar-Pullicino VN, Davies MA, et al. The diagnostic accuracy of MR imaging in osteoid osteoma. Skeletal Radiol. 2002;31:559-69.
14. Brown LM. Bone scintigraphy in benign and malignant tumors. Radiol Clin of North Am. 1993;31:731-8.
15. Motamedi K, Seeger LL. Benign bone tumors. Radiol Clin N Am. 2011;49:1115-34.
16. Motamedi K, Ilaslan H, Seeger LL. Imaging of lumbar spine neoplasms. Semin Ultrasound CT MR. 2004;25:474-89.
17. Giudici MA, Moser RP, Kransdorf MJ. Cartilaginous bone tumors. Radiol Clin of North Am. 1993;31:237-59.
18. Robbin MR, Murphey MD. Benign chondroid neoplasms of the bone. Semin Musculoskeletal Radiol. 2000;4: 45-58.
19. Steven S, Srinivas K, Javicr B. MR imaging of tumors and tumor like lesions of the upper extremity. Magn Reson Imaging Clin of N Am. 2004;12:349-59.
20. Holtz P, Sundaram M. Enchondroma. Orthopaedics. 1995;18:509-10.
21. Mermelstein LE, Friedlaender GE, Katz LD. Chondroblastoma. Orthopaedics. 1997;20:67-71.
22. Jee Wh, Choe BY, Kang HS, et al. Non ossifying fibroma: characteristics at MR imaging with pathologic correlation. Radiology. 1998;209:197-202.

23. Hudson TM, Stiles RG, Monson DK. Fibrous lesions of bone. Radiol Clin of North Am. 1993;31:279-97.
24. Lucas E, Sundaram M, Boccini T. Polyostotic fibrous dysplasia. Orthopaedics. 1995;18:311-3.
25. Zeanah WR, Hudson TM, Springfield DS. Computed tomography of ossifying fibroma of the tibia. J Comput Assist Tomogr. 1983;7:688-91.
26. Robbin MR, Murphey MD, Temple HD, et al. Imaging of musculoskeletal fibromatosis. Radiographics. 2001;21: 585-600.
27. Frick MA, Sundaram M, Unni KK, et al. Imaging findings in desmoplastic fibroma of bone: distinctitive T2 characterstics. AJR. 2005;184:1762-7.
28. Conway WF, Hayes CW. Miscellaneous lesions of bone. Radiol Clin of North Am. 1993;31(2):339-58.
29. Persaud T. The polka dot sign. Radiology. 2008;246:980-1.
30. Propeck T, Bullard MA, Linj, et al. Radiologic pathologic correlation of intraosseous lipomas. Am J Roentgenology. 2000;175:673-8.
31. Manaster BJ, Doyle AJ. Giant cell tumors of bone. Radiol Clin of North Am. 1993;31(2):299-323.
32. Nomikos George, Murphey M, Kransdof MJ. Primary bone tumors of the lower extremities. Radiol Clin of North America. 2002;40:971-90.
33. Jordanov MI. The "rising bubble" sign: a new aid in the diagnosis of unicarmeral bone cyst. Skeletal Radiol. 2009;38:597-600.
34. Parman LM, Murphey MD. Alphabet soup: cystic lesions of bone. Semin Musculoskelet Radiol. 2000;4:89-101.
35. Marin C, Warrier RP. Langerhan's cell histiocytosis. Orthop Clin of North Am. 1996;27(3):615-23.
36. Wilson DA, Prince JR. MR imaging of hemophilic pseudotumors. AJR. 1988;150:349.
37. Richardson ML, Pozz-mucelli RS, Kanter AS. Bone mineral changes in primary hyperparathyroidism. Skeletal Radiology. 1986;15:85-95.
38. Hayes CW, Conway WF. Hyperparathyroidism. Radiol Clin North Am. 1991;29:85-96.

CHAPTER 199

Malignant Bone Tumors

Anju Garg

INTRODUCTION

Primary malignant bone tumors are relatively rare and are responsible only for about 1% of all deaths from neoplasia.[1]

The determination of the nature and extent of the tumor is crucial for appropriate decision-making regarding the utility of limb salvage procedures, chemotherapy, radiation therapy or combined therapy in managing skeletal neoplasms. The correct diagnosis and an accurate staging, therefore, becomes more than just an academic exercise, as it determines the appropriate therapy and prognosis. Conventional radiography along with cross-sectional imaging modalities, particularly magnetic resonance imaging play a very important role in the detection, establishing the nature, assessing extent and in follow-up in all suspected cases of bone tumors.

CLASSIFICATION OF PRIMARY MALIGNANT BONE TUMORS

Primary bone tumors are generally classified according to their cell of origin or histogenesis. However, the exact cell of origin of a tumor is not always certain, therefore, such a classification often depends on the cells which predominate in the fully developed lesion. **Table 1** gives a modified version of the WHO classification.[2]

Table 1: Histological typing of primary malignant bone tumors (Modified from WHO classification)[2].

I. Bone forming tumors	• Osteosarcoma • Parosteal osteosarcoma • Periosteal osteosarcoma • Telangiectatic osteosarcoma and other types
II. Cartilage forming tumors	• Chondrosarcoma • Mesenchymal chondrosarcoma • Clear cell chondrosarcoma
III. Giant cell tumor	Malignant giant cell tumor
IV. Marrow tumors	• Ewing's sarcoma • Primary lymphoma of bone (Lymphosarcoma of bone) • Multiple myeloma
V. Vascular tumors	Angiosarcoma
VI. Other connective tissue tumors	• Fibrosarcoma • Malignant fibrous histiocytoma • Liposarcoma
VII. Other miscellaneous tumors	• Chordoma • Adamantinoma • Neurosarcoma
VIII. Unclassified tumors	Undifferentiated sarcoma

General Principles of Diagnosis

A reasonable differential diagnosis can be achieved for most bone tumors using the patient's age, location of the lesion and its radiographic appearance. However, the final diagnosis is histological, often requiring an imaging guided biopsy.

The *age* of the patient plays an important role in establishing the diagnosis and may lead to the correct histological diagnosis even when the tumor is radiographically atypical. The preferential time of origin of the various tumors is summarized in **Table 2**. In very young patients, malignant bone tumors are likely to be metastases from neuroblastoma or leukemia. In the first decade, the most likely primary bone tumors are Ewing's sarcoma and later, osteosarcoma. In adolescence and adult life various primary tumors are probable. In older age groups, most bone tumors are metastatic carcinomas. Multiple myeloma also occurs in this age group.

The *site of origin or location* of a lesion is also of diagnostic significance with respect to which bone is involved and which portion of the bone, i.e. epiphysis, metaphysis or diaphysis **(Table 3)**. Many primary osseous neoplasms develop in areas of rapid bone growth, especially the distal femur and the proximal tibia and humerus. As the tumors of a given cell type typically arise in a location where the homologous normal cells are most active, the predilection of many bone tumors for the metaphysis and physeal regions of an enlarging tubular bone is not unexpected.[3] Furthermore, the vascular anatomy peculiar to this region, consisting of looped vessels and sinusoidal channels, promote sluggish blood flow and, with it, metastatic seeding of tumor (and infection).

Certain tumors, because of their derivation, predominate in one or more particular areas of the skeleton, e.g. chordomas, developing from the remnant of the primitive notochord, are typically seen at the cranial and caudal limits of the vertebral column whereas, a variety of neoplasms related to dentition are virtually confined to the mandible or maxilla.

The *morphological features* of the bone tumors generally reflect their tissue of origin. The pattern of bone destruction, the growth rate of the lesion, the presence and nature of the visible tumor matrix, internal trabeculation, cortical erosion, penetration, expansion and the periosteal response are some of the features which need to be analyzed.

Determining the *histological type* of the tumor, by fine needle aspiration cytology or biopsy, should be the last step in the patient's pretreatment evaluation as the reaction of tissue to the biopsy alters the imaging appearance of tumor obscuring its true anatomic extent and local aggressiveness. Also, if the biopsy is done at the final stage of evaluation, the definitive surgical procedure can be done at the same operation with the diagnosis made on the frozen section. Imaging studies can be of value in identifying the specific area of a tumor that should be biopsied and in planning how to get there without undue tissue contamination.

Staging of Bone Tumors

The universal TNM staging system used for most carcinomas is not commonly used for bone sarcomas because of the rarity with which these sarcomas metastasize to lymph nodes. A special staging system adopted by the musculoskeletal society first described by Enneking and co-authors[4] has gained acceptance in which malignant bone tumors are staged by assessment of the histological grade(G), the local extent (T) and the presence or absence of regional or distant metastases **(Table 4)**.

Grade: The grade of a tumor is a measure of its potential to metastasize. It is based primarily on histological features and therefore requires a preoperative biopsy. A sarcoma is classified as either low-grade or high-grade. In general, a low-grade lesion is biologically less active and requires a relatively conservative surgical procedure. Conversely, a high grade lesion usually necessitates a more radical procedure, because of its more aggressive nature.

Local extent: The anatomic extent is either intracompartmental (A) or extracompartmental (B). A "compartment" is defined as an anatomic structure or space bounded by natural barriers to tumor extension. Tumors confined

Table 2: Age and malignant tumors.

Age (years)	*Tumors*
<1	Neuroblastoma
1–10	Ewing's—tubular bones
10–30	Osteosarcoma, Ewing's—flat bones
30–40	• Fibrosarcoma, malignant fibrous histiocytoma, parosteal sarcoma, malignant giant cell tumor, lymphomas • Metastatic carcinoma, multiple myeloma, chondrosarcoma
>40	Metastatic carcinoma, multiple myeloma, chondrosarcoma

Table 3: Preferential site of origin of various malignant tumors of bone.

Epiphysis	Giant cell tumor (after fusion of growth plate)
Metaphysis	• Osteosarcoma • Parosteal sarcoma • Chondrosarcoma • Fibrosarcoma • Giant cell tumor (before fusion of growth plate)
Diaphysis	• Ewing's tumor • Myeloma • Reticulum cell sarcoma • Adamantinoma • Malignant fibrous histiocytoma

Table 4: Enneking surgical staging of musculoskeletal sarcoma.[5]

Stage (M)	*Grade*	*Site (T)*	*Metastasis (M)*
IA	Low (G1)	Intracompartmental (T1)	No (MO)
IB	Low (G1)	Extracompartmental (T2)	No (MO)
IIA	High (G2)	Intracompartmental (T1)	No (MO)
IIB	High (G2)	Extracompartmental (T2)	No (MO)
III	Any (G)	Any (T)	Yes (MI) Regional/Distant

to the compartment of origin usually are less aggressive and require less radical surgery than those extending into the adjacent compartment. Small nodules of tumor may be found separate from the main body of the tumor, but usually remain within the same anatomic compartment. Extracompartmental spread may occur via direct tumor invasion of an adjacent compartment or by contamination resulting from fracture, hemorrhage, or an operative procedure, such as an unplanned resection or poorly planned biopsy.

Metastases: The third component of the staging system is the presence or absence of nodal or distant metastases. Regional lymph node involvement is much less common with musculoskeletal sarcomas than are pulmonary metastases, but both are equally poor prognostic factors.

IMAGING MODALITIES

Conventional radiographic techniques still remain the mainstay in initial diagnosis and work-up of a patient suspected to have any bony pathology. Cross-sectional studies are required following conventional radiography, in cases of suspected malignant bone tumors for (a) staging of tumor, (b) determining the site and route of biopsy, (c) providing measurements needed for an anticipated surgical procedure, and (d) evaluation of residual and/or recurrent disease after therapy.

Conventional Radiography

Plain radiographs can demonstrate the location of the lesion, the pattern of bone destruction, size and shape of the lesion, presence and nature of the visible tumor matrix, trabeculation, periosteal response and the presence and characteristics of the adjacent soft tissue mass. This information combined with the site of the lesion and the age of the patient allows formulation of a reasonable diagnosis in most cases. Malignant lesions are generally poorly defined lesions with a wide zone of transition, a moth-eaten or permeative pattern of bone destruction, an interrupted periosteal reaction of the sunburst or onion-skin type and an adjacent soft tissue mass. However, some aggressive benign lesions may also show the same pattern on plain radiographs.

Chest radiographs should be obtained in all cases of malignant skeletal tumors to evaluate for pulmonary metastases, particularly in patients with osteosarcoma.

Magnetic Resonance Imaging

Due to its excellent contrast resolution and multiplanar capabilities, MRI has now virtually replaced CT as the imaging modality for assessing the local extent, local staging and follow-up of malignant bone tumors. Magnetic resonance imaging (MRI) is the best imaging modality in assessing (1) intra- and extracompartmental extent of bone tumors, (2) neurovascular and juxta-articular involvement and (3) in detection of skip lesions, leading to a more accurate staging.[5] Intra-articular extension still remains a difficult problem. When the lesion is far from the joint or obviously within the joint, the diagnosis is easy, but when the tumor abuts the joint, involvement of the joint is often over evaluated. Involvement is suggested when the hyaline cartilage is penetrated or more commonly when the tumor extends through the capsule. Joint effusion does not necessarily mean involvement.[6]

The MR imaging protocol for bone tumor evaluation should include an initial large field of view T1 or inversion recovery sequence to detect any skip lesions and for planning subsequent sequences. T1 and T2 or inversion recovery sequences of the involved area should then be acquired in axial, coronal and/or sagittal planes, using the surface coil, to show the complete extent of the tumor in all three dimensions, along with its relation to the adjacent joint and neurovascular bundle.

Magnetic resonance imaging features are usually nonspecific in differentiating benign from malignant tumors. Both benign and malignant tumors are generally seen as low signal on T1- and high signal on T2-weighted images. Thus, intraosseus extent and skip lesions are well evaluated on T1W images due to the contrast between the high signal marrow and the low signal tumor, whereas the extraosseus extent is better assessed on T2W images due to the contrast provided by the low signal muscles to the high signal tumor. Fat suppression techniques can suppress the adjacent bright fat to further increase the contrast on T2W images **(Figs. 1A to C)**. Contrast enhancement delineates the exact extent of the tumor, defines viable tumor and necrotic areas and helps in differentiating edema from tumor tissue and identifying residual/recurrent tumor from scar or fibrotic tissue in treated cases.

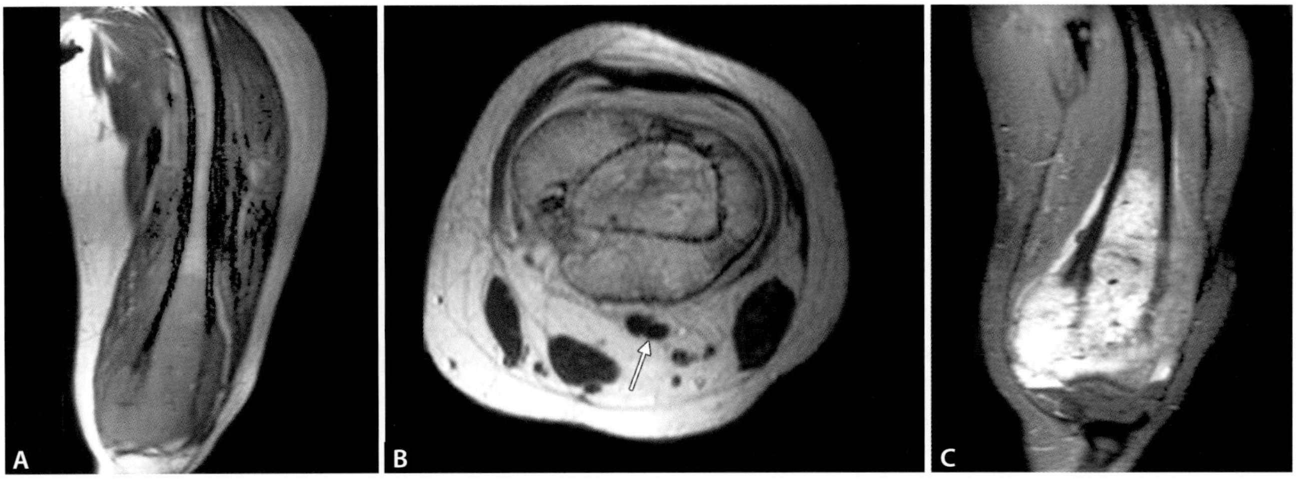

Figs. 1A to C: MRI showing local staging of distal femoral osteosarcoma: (A) Coronal T1-weighted sequence demonstrates the intraosseous extent; (B) Axial T2-weighted sequence demonstrates the extraosseous extent. The periosteum is intact and the neurovascular bundle (arrow) is well-separated from the tumor; (C) Coronal STIR image shows the soft tissue extension well, however, the intramedullary extension is not well-appreciated.

Dynamic contrast enhanced MR imaging has been used to determine response to chemotherapy. In patients who respond to chemotherapy, MR images show a reduction in enhancement, whereas patients who do not respond show little or no reduction. Dynamic contrast-enhanced MR images should be acquired in short time intervals, since reactive changes may show contrast enhancement indistinguishable from that of tumor in the later phases of enhancement. Subtraction MR imaging has been used to increase the detection of early arterial enhancement of residual tumor.[6]

Magnetic resonance spectroscopy provides a means of molecular characterization of the tumors and is a promising modality in the evaluation of malignant bone and soft tissue tumors. Preliminary studies have shown that choline levels are elevated in many malignant musculoskeletal tumors. However, similar findings may be seen in some benign tumors like giant cell tumor of bone.[7]

Diffusion weighted MRI has been found useful in assessing tumor response to therapy. Effective therapy in bone tumors leads to breakdown of tumor cell membranes resulting in increased diffusion of water in the tumor on diffusion weighted images. Even though the tumor bulk may not reduce significantly, increase in the apparent diffusion coefficient (ADC) value indicates a response to treatment.[8]

Computed Tomography

With the easier availability of MRI, the role of computed tomography (CT) in the evaluation of malignant bone tumors has reduced considerably. However, CT still remains superior to MRI in detection and characterization of matrix mineralization (osteoid or chondroid), in assessment of cortical involvement, bone trabeculation and periosteal reaction. CT can be used to demonstrate the morphological features of the tumor in areas which are not well evaluated by plain radiography, e.g. pelvis, shoulder, vertebrae, etc. and where MRI is contraindicated. Computed tomography is also the investigation of choice for detecting pulmonary metastases.

Nuclear Medicine

Radionuclide scanning using both traditional technetium labeled phosphonate compounds and newer positron emitters is an important adjunctive modality.

^{99m}Technetium methylene diphosphonate (^{99m}Tc MDP) bone scan has traditionally been used as the first additional investigation in most instances to detect whether the lesion is monostotic or accompanied by other skeletal lesions. The major limitation of bone scanning is its lack of specificity as a number of bone disorders may have similar scintigraphic appearances. These lesions need to be characterized further by other imaging modalities. The role of ^{99m}Tc MDP bone scan for monitoring response to treatment is limited because it is not always possible to distinguish active disease from healing.

FDG-PET is assuming an increasingly important role in evaluation of skeletal metastatic disease. FDG accumulation in skeletal lesions reflect direct uptake by tumor, in contrast to ^{99m}Tc MDP activity on conventional bone scans, which reflects increased new bone formation in response to destruction of bone by tumor. The role of FDG-PET in the imaging algorithm of primary musculoskeletal tumors is not well defined. Its role in the initial diagnosis is limited. It cannot replace biopsy because it cannot consistently differentiate benign from malignant bone tumors. In the patient with a documented bone tumor it can—(a) guide a biopsy to the most active tissue, (b) predict overall survival, (c) distinguish recurrent tumor from post-therapeutic changes, (d) monitor response to neoadjuvant chemotherapy and also may identify poorly responding patients earlier in therapy.[9]

Recently, another positron emitter fluorine-18 sodium fluoride (NaF) has been used as a PET bone imaging agent. The bone uptake of this agent is two-fold higher and blood clearance much faster than ^{99m}Tc MDP which makes it much more sensitive and selective than conventional bone scan for diagnosis and detection of bone metastases.[10]

The use of low-dose CT or MRI in conjunction with PET improves the sensitivity and specificity of the PET imaging techniques.

Angiography

Angiography has limited specificity in differentiating between benign and malignant tumors as there are no characteristic angiographic features of malignancy. However, two signs, i.e. encasement of normal vessels and presence of tumor vessels occur with greater frequency in malignant tumors.

Currently conventional angiography has been largely replaced by noninvasive CT and MR angiography techniques. Conventional angiography still remains useful for pretherapy planning in selected cases and in therapeutic interventions. In planning limb salvage procedures, it can be used to map the vascular supply of a potential vacularized bone graft. Preoperative selective arterial embolization can substantially lower the risk of hemorrhage from hypervascular bone tumors, such as giant cell tumor and metastatic renal cancer. Conventional angiography also has been used to deliver intra-arterial infusion chemotherapy to some malignant bone tumors.[1]

Ultrasonography

With the advent of CT and MRI, ultrasonography (US) has been relegated to the role of an adjunct imaging modality in the evaluation of musculoskeletal tumors. Ultrasonography plays no useful role in diagnosis or staging but has proven to be of value in guiding needle biopsy of those lesions with a large extraosseous component.[9] Color Doppler flow imaging with duplex analysis has a role in monitoring tumor response to chemotherapy in patients with high grade sarcomas, provided there is a soft tissue component. Response is predicted on the basis of changes in intratumoral blood flow and changes in resistive indices in the limb arteries. Post-surgery ultrasonography can be of value in detecting sarcoma recurrence, particularly when orthopedic hardware is present.[11]

OSTEOSARCOMA

Osteosarcoma is the commonest primary malignant bone tumor in the young. It is characterized by the production of osteoid or bone by the tumor cells. The malignant cells also retain the potential to form fibrous tissue or cartilage. Thus, the constituents of the tumor matrix are highly variable and can include osteoid tissue, calcification, fibrous tissue, cartilaginous tissue or a combination of these tissues. They can be classified according to their main tissue component and their site of origin **(Table 5)**.

Intraosseous Osteosarcoma

Conventional or central osteosarcomas account for approximately 75–85% of all osteosarcomas.

Clinical Presentation

Age: About 80% of patients are under the age of 30 years.[12] Age range is 2–92 years. The median age of patients with osteosarcoma arising in tubular bones is 17 years. Flat bones are affected at median age of 25 years.

Sex: The male:female ratio is 2:1.

Clinical picture: Most patients present with pain and a palpable mass. Symptoms are usually present for several months, the swelling having been attributed to trauma or infection in the first place. Systemic symptoms and pathological fractures are common. Serum alkaline phosphatase may be elevated with larger tumors.

Table 5: Classification of osteosarcoma.

a. *Intraosseous osteosarcoma*: • Conventional (osteoblastic, fibroblastic, chondroblastic) • Telangiectatic • Small cell • Low-grade • Cortical
b. *Surface osteosarcoma*: • Periosteal (chondroblastic) • High-grade periosteal • Juxtacortical (parosteal)
c. Extraosseous osteosarcoma
d. Multicentric osteosarcoma
e. Secondary osteosarcoma

Site: The typical lesion affects the metaphyseal region of the growing end of a long bone. About 50–75% are found in the distal femur or the proximal tibia. Other common sites include proximal humerus and femur. Rarer sites include the ilium, ribs, vertebrae and jaw bones. Extension of the tumor into the diaphysis and/or epiphysis is common. About 10% of the tumors arise in the diaphysis. Distant spread is mainly via the blood stream with early metastases to the lungs.

Imaging Features

On plain radiographs, the tumor may be predominantly osteosclerotic (25%) or osteolytic (25%), but more frequently it is of the mixed osteosclerotic/osteolytic type (50%). The classical appearance is that of a focal lesion in the metaphyseal end of a long bone showing a moth-eaten or permeative pattern of destruction with a wide zone of transition. The tumor breaks through the cortex early in the course of the disease leading to a soft tissue mass. This mass is first unmineralized but later shows ill-defined tumor bone within it. Mineralization of the tumor osteoid leads to a cloud-like density in the region known as the *cumulus cloud* appearance. The medullary lesion is predominantly lytic but mineralization leads to a characteristic associated medullary sclerosis. A Codman's triangle may form at the margin of the lesion due to subperiosteal extension of the tumor lifting the periosteum **(Figs. 2A and B)**. Bone spicules can be seen perpendicularly or radially in a "sunburst"or "sunray" pattern following the line of extended Sharpey's fibers **(Figs. 3A and B)**. A lamellated (onion skin) pattern of periosteal reaction resembling that of Ewing's sarcoma may sometimes be seen. In contrast to cortical bone, the articular cartilage is more resistant to tumor invasion and is not violated until late in the course of disease.[13,14]

Magnetic resonance imaging is the investigation of choice following conventional radiographs. An obvious heterogeneous tumor can be seen within the bone, often associated with a soft tissue mass, with low signal intensity on T1-weighted images and high signal intensity on STIR or T2-weighted images **(Figs. 4A to D)**. Areas with increased sclerosis may show lower signal intensity on both T1 and T2-weighted images. Peritumoral edema in the marrow tends to be of an intermediate signal intensity on STIR and T1-weighted images and does not disrupt the normal architecture.[15] Both intramedullary and extraosseous extensions are accurately demonstrated as is involvement of the neurovascular bundle and extension into the adjacent joint **(Figs. 5A to D)**. Intramedullary 'skip' lesions may also be identified.

The classical osteosarcoma has been described above, but a variety of appearances may be observed. The tumor bone may be entirely sclerotic **(Figs. 6A and B)** or the tumor may be entirely lytic when it is difficult to differentiate from Ewing's sarcoma. A chondroblastic variety of osteosarcoma may occur when a large part of the tumor is composed of cartilage.

The rare *telangiectatic osteosarcoma*[16] is characterized by the formation of large septated blood filled cavities and presents usually as a lytic lesion resembling an aggressive

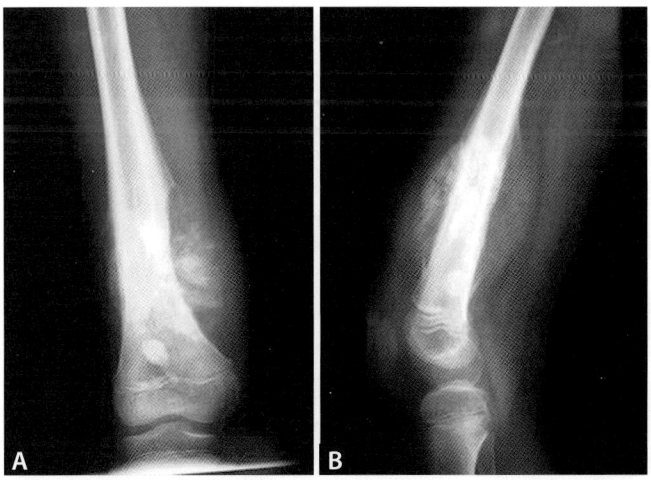

Figs. 2A and B: Conventional central osteosarcoma: AP and lateral radiographs of the distal femur in a 14-year-old boy showing a classical osteosarcoma with mixed lytic and sclerotic areas, extraosseous mass with tumor bone formation and Codman's triangles at the upper and lower margins of the lesion.

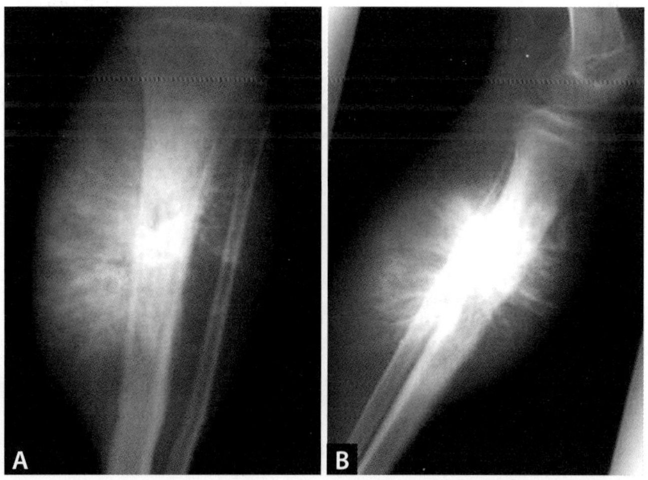

Figs. 3A and B: Osteosarcoma of the metadiaphyseal region of tibia shows a mixed lesion with a large soft tissue component and the characteristic "sunburst" or spiculated periosteal reaction.

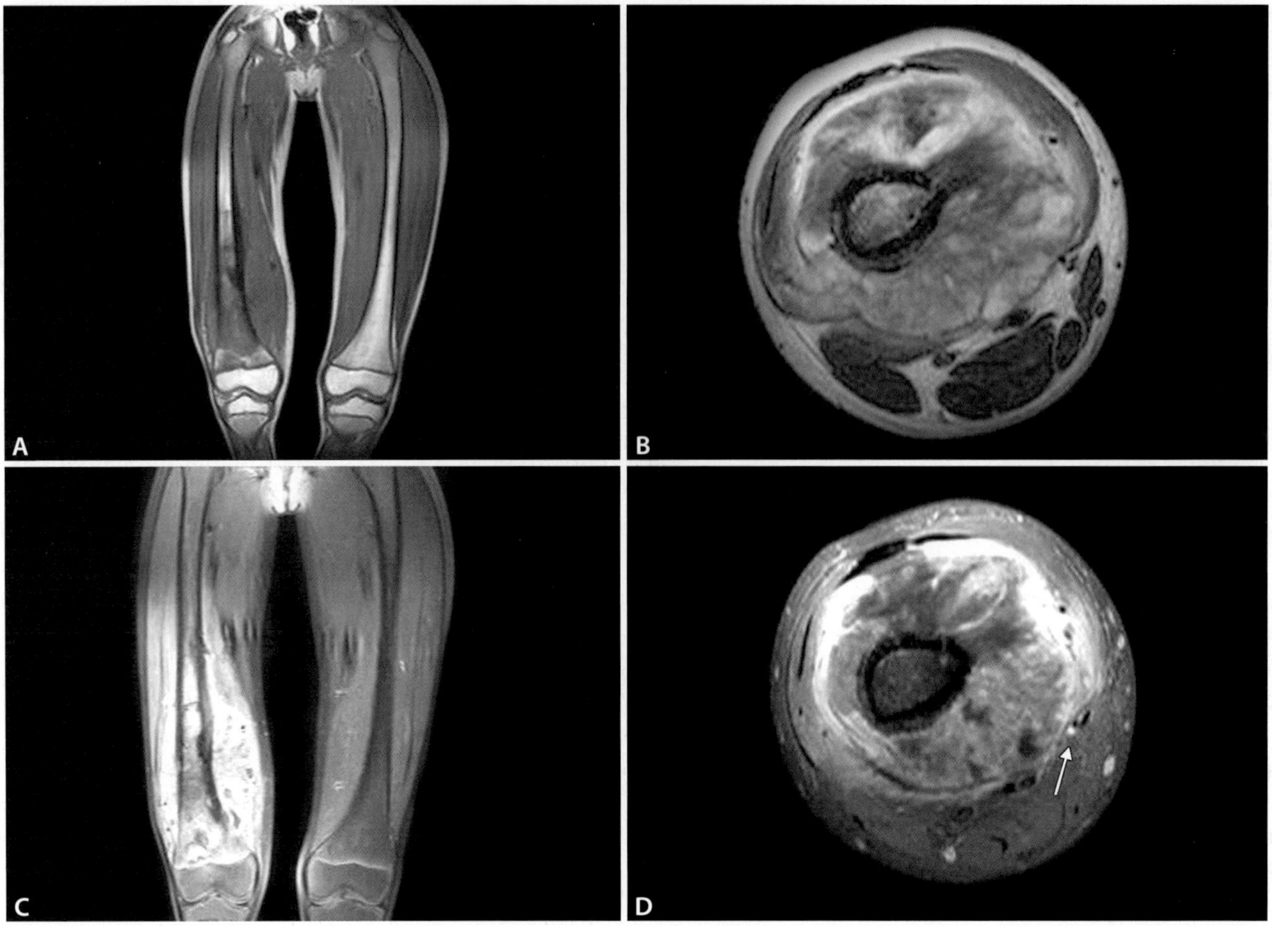

Figs. 4A to D: MRI osteosarcoma (same case as in Figure 2): (A) A coronal T1W MR image shows the large tumor as a predominantly hypointense mass with evidence of cortical destruction; (B) Axial T2W image shows the cortical disruption with soft tissue extension of the tumor mass with loss of fat planes with the neurovascular bundle. Contrast-enhanced coronal (C) and axial (D) MR images show heterogeneous enhancement of the tumor mass (arrow).

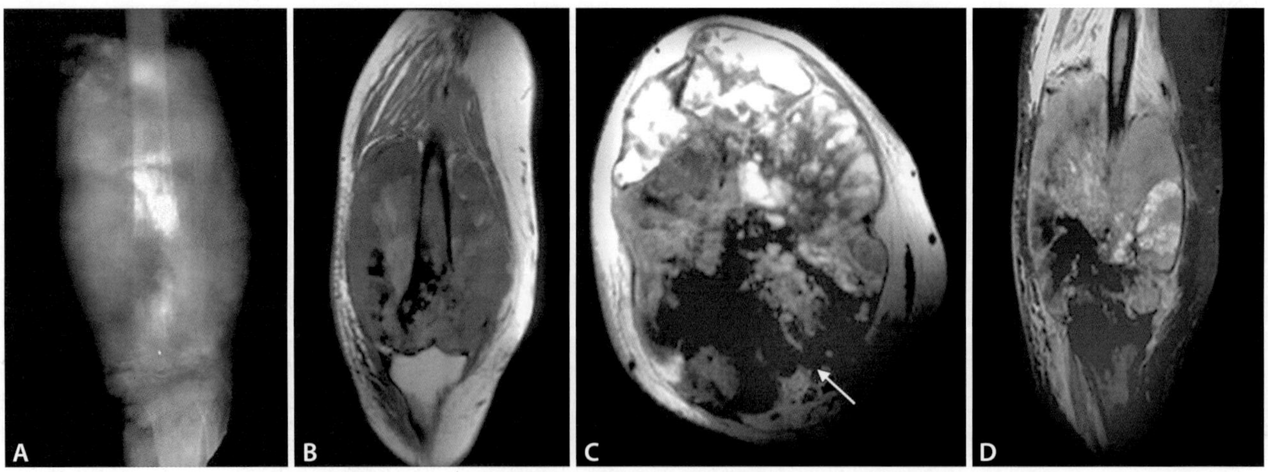

Figs. 5A to D: Osteosarcoma of distal femur: (A) AP radiograph showing a destructive lesion in the distal femur with extensive cloud like mineralization in the intra- and extraosseous component; (B) A coronal T1W MR image shows the large tumor as a predominantly hypointense mass with evidence of cortical destruction; (C) An axial T2W image shows a heterogeneous mass which is completely encasing the neurovascular bundle (arrow); (D) T2W (fat-suppressed) coronal image shows the intra-articular extension of the tumor into the knee joint.

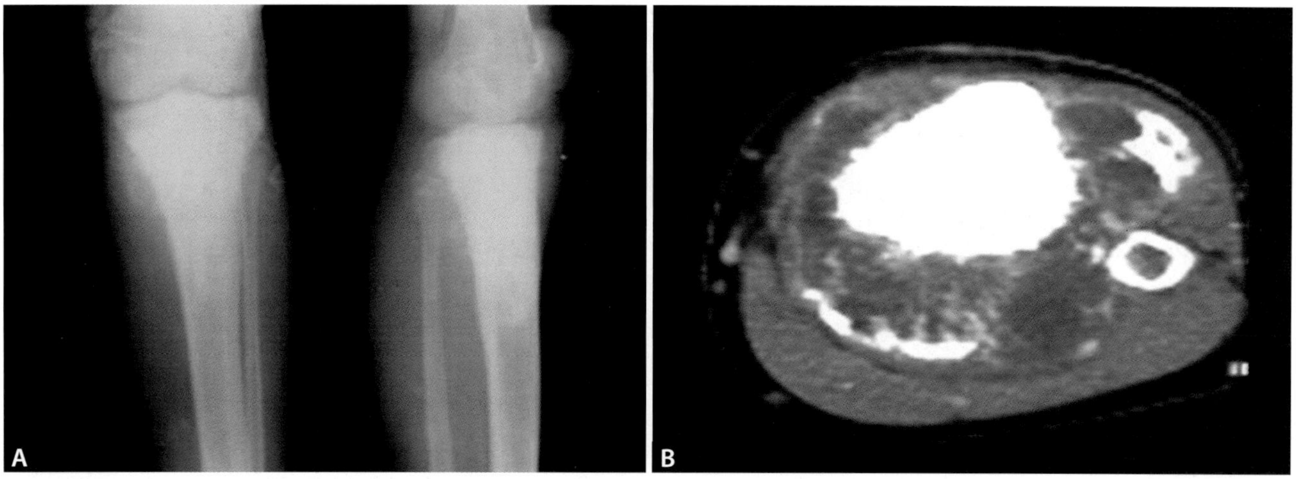

Figs. 6A and B: Osteosarcoma—osteoblastic variety: (A) AP and lateral radiographs show a purely osteosclerotic lesion of the proximal metaphysis of the tibia; (B) CT shows mineralization of tumor matrix within the soft tissue component and a spiculated periosteal reaction.

aneurysmal bone cyst (ABC). The femur, tibia and humerus are most commonly involved. It arises frequently in the diaphysis and extends into the metaphysis. It lacks visible bone production. A predominant lytic lesion is seen on plain radiographs **(Fig. 7A)**. Subtle matrix mineralization may be demonstrated by CT. Extensive hemorrhage and blood-fluid levels can be seen on both CT and MRI **(Fig. 7B)**, mimicking ABC. However, the presence of thick peripheral, septal and nodular enhancement of solid viable tissue on post contrast studies **(Fig. 7C)** helps distinguish telangiectatic osteosarcoma from ABC. Although the prognosis for this type of osteosarcoma is poor as compared to conventional osteosarcoma, effective chemotherapy has improved survival.

Small cell osteosarcoma[17] (approximately 1%) is similar to conventional osteosarcomas in its clinical presentation and radiographic appearance. Histologically, it contains solid areas of small round cells or spindle-shaped cells resembling those seen in Ewing's sarcoma. The significance of this entity is its extremely poor prognosis.

Low-grade osteosarcoma[18] also referred to as intraosseous well-differentiated osteosarcoma, is a rare type of osteosarcoma which presents in an older age group (median age 30 years) with a long-standing history. The radiographic features vary from predominantly osteolytic or ground glass to predominantly sclerotic. The tumor may show geographic destruction and is frequently expansile with regular cortical destruction and solid periosteal reaction. It has a good prognosis. Due to its relatively benign appearance, the tumor may be mistaken for fibrous dysplasia, osteoblastoma or a low-grade chondroid tumor. However, CT and MRI will show extraosseous extension which should aid in the diagnosis.

Intracortical osteosarcomas are the rarest form of osteosarcoma, accounting for less than 1% of cases. All reported cases had arisen in the cortex of femur or tibia. The tumor appears as a small lytic lesion surrounded by thickened cortex, resembling an osteoid osteoma or osteoblastoma. These tumors have a better prognosis than the conventional intramedullary osteosarcoma.

The main *differential diagnoses* of osteosarcoma in its early stages are osteomyelitis and trauma. A long history may indicate that infection is unlikely. Once the plain radiograph reveals a medullary lesion, the diagnosis usually lies between osteosarcomas and other malignancies, including metastasis. Of the benign lesions, osteoblastoma, giant cell tumor, osteoid osteoma and osteomyelitis, particularly the sclerosing variety of Garré has to be considered.

Osteosarcoma spreads via the bloodstream leading to pulmonary metastases. These contain osteoid, take up bone-seeking isotopes and ultimately ossify. The metastases are often subpleural in location and commonly associated with a pneumothorax. It is essential to exclude the presence of lung metastases with CT for purposes of staging before starting therapy **(Figs. 8A to C)**.

The prognosis of osteosarcoma has improved greatly with the use of chemotherapy and limb-preserving surgery. Presently the treatment requires multiple cycles of chemotherapy before surgical resection. Dynamic contrast enhanced MRI has been used with considerable success in some centers to predict the degree of chemotherapy response and to identify active tumor remnants in recurrences.[19]

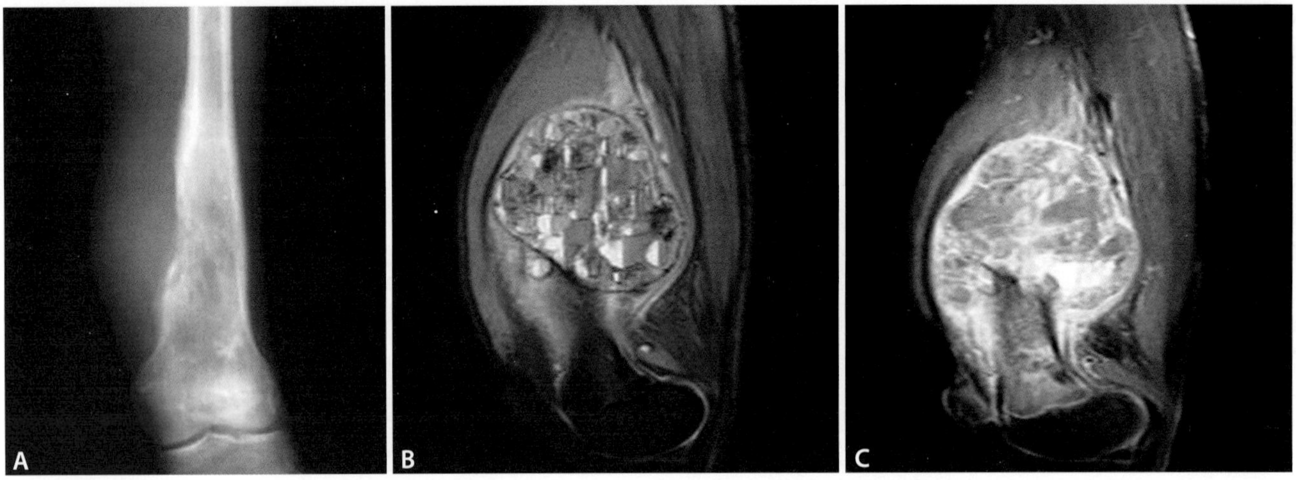

Figs. 7A to C: Telangiectatic osteosarcoma: (A) AP radiograph of the distal femur shows a predominantly lytic lesion in the distal femur with irregular cortical destruction and a large soft tissue component; (B) Sagittal T2W fat-suppressed MR image shows the characteristic blood-fluid levels within the tumor; (C) On contrast enhancement, marked peripheral and septal enhancement is seen.

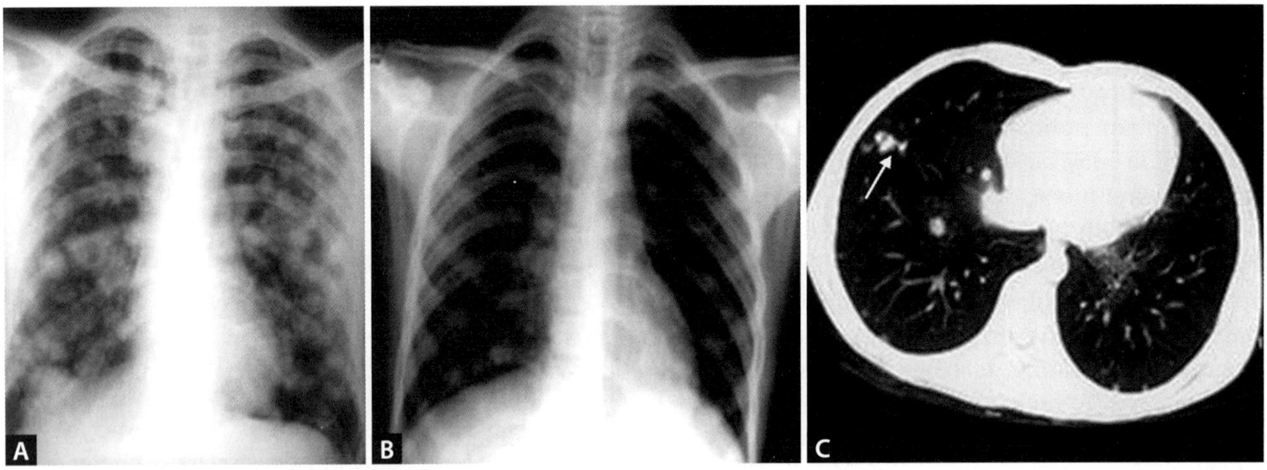

Figs. 8A to C: Pulmonary metastases from osteosarcoma: (A) Multiple dense rounded opacities are seen scattered through both the lung fields suggestive of osteoblastic metastases; (B) In another case, plain radiograph of the chest shows a few ill-defined opacities suspicious of metastases; (C) Axial CT scan shows multiple nodular metastatic lesions scattered in both lung fields. Ossification can be seen in some (arrow).

Surface Osteosarcomas

Surface osteosarcomas arise from the surface of the bone and account for 4–10% of osteosarcomas. They include the periosteal, paraosteal and high-grade surface osteosarcomas.

Periosteal Osteosarcoma[20]

Periosteal osteosarcoma is an intermediate grade chondroblastic osteosarcoma accounting for 1–2% of all osteosarcomas. The age distribution, gender and presenting features are similar to conventional osteosarcomas. This entity is characteristically diaphyseal in location and the center of the tumor is located on the surface of the bone with a saucer-like shallow area of adjacent cortical bone destruction. The crater contains striated, radiating mineralization. Tumor mineralization is best shown by CT. Absence of marrow involvement is easily seen on CT/MR imaging. Magnetic resonance imaging classically shows hyperintensity on T2W images due to the chondroblastic nature of the lesion.

Juxtacortical/Parosteal Osteosarcoma

This uncommon tumor is attached to the surface of the affected bone and has a tendency to encircle it. It generally occurs in the 20–40 years age group and affects both sexes equally. This tumor is almost exclusively found in long bones, with 70% occurring around the knee specially the posterior aspect of femur.[21]

The characteristic feature is of a dense bony mass abutting or enveloping the distal femoral metaphysis **(Fig. 9A)**.[21] In its early growth, a well-defined radiolucent line separates the tumor from the normal cortex. Medullary involvement needs to be evaluated on CT or MRI **(Figs. 9B to D)**. Magnetic resonance imaging shows a low signal equivalent to normal cortex in the poorly cellular ossified element with a variable increase in signal intensity from the peripheral more active element of the tumor.[22] Eventually both cortex and medulla become involved by the tumor. The differential diagnosis includes a heavily mineralized osteochondroma and juxtacortical myositis ossificans, which is differentiated by its peripheral mineralization pattern.

High-grade Surface Osteosarcoma

This is a very rare lesion arising from the surface of the bone but having the same histological features as conventional central osteosarcomas. It, therefore, has a very much poorer prognosis than other osteosarcomas. The radiological features are similar to those of periosteal osteosarcoma but more aggressive in that the tumor is usually larger and there is a greater degree of cortical erosion.[23]

Extraosseous Osteosarcoma

Occasionally, osteosarcomas may arise in an extraosseous site. The most common site is the soft tissues of the thigh, but they can also be found in the pleura, dura of brain, heart valves, retroperitoneum, axilla, breast, etc. These rare tumors present the same histological pattern as other osteosarcomas. They usually present as large soft tissue masses which may not be close to bone. The radiological appearance is nonspecific. Mineralization of the matrix can suggest the diagnosis but differentiation from other soft tissue sarcomas which calcify (e.g. chondrosarcoma, fibrosarcoma, synovial sarcoma) is difficult.[12]

Primary Multifocal Osteosarcoma[24]

Children between the age of 5 and 10 years are predominantly affected, adolescents and adults can rarely be affected. A characteristic radiological appearance is seen with densely osteoblastic lesions, all about the same size and maturity involving the metaphyses of long bones **(Fig. 10)**. Spinal involvement may occur, presenting as an irregular, nodular radiopaque mass or ivory vertebra. Initially, they are confined to bone, but later spread into the soft tissues. The similar size of all the lesions with absence of lung metastases differentiates this disease from metastatic osteosarcoma. However, lung metastases do appear later in the course of the disease and the disease is invariably fatal.

Secondary Osteosarcoma

Secondary osteosarcomas occur following malignant degeneration of benign disorders most commonly seen after radiotherapy and in Paget's disease. Rarely osteosarcoma develops in association with osteonecrosis, fibrous dysplasia, osteogenesis imperfecta, metal prosthesis and chronic osteomyelitis.[12]

Radiation therapy may lead to development of osteosarcoma. The criteria for diagnosing a *postradiation*

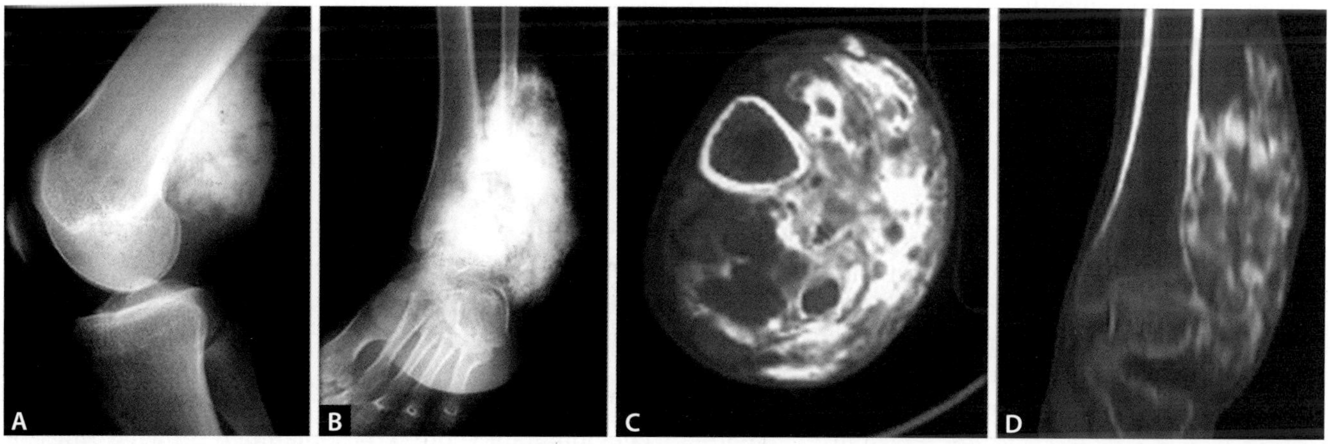

Figs. 9A to D: (A) Paraosteal osteosarcoma: Lateral radiograph of the knee shows a dense, lobulated mass arising from the posterior distal femur. This is the classical location for parosteal osteocarcoma; (B) Paraosteal Osteosarcoma: In another case, AP radiograph of the ankle shows a dense homogeneous mass of bone overlying the distal fibula and tibia; (C and D) Axial and coronal reformatted CT sections show the cleavage plane separating the lesion from the underlying bone.

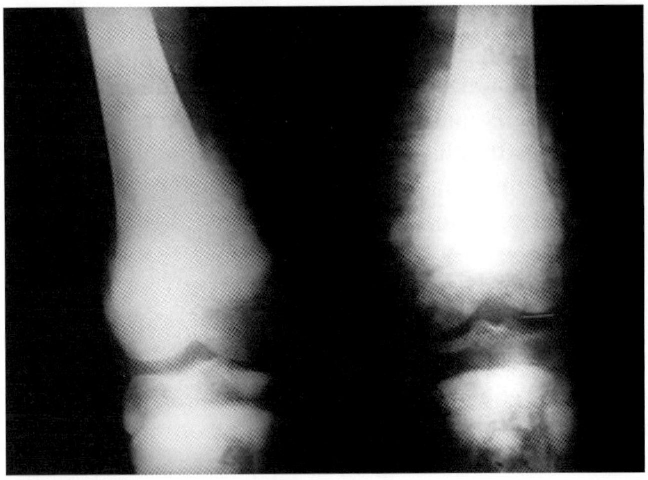

Fig. 10: Multifocal osteosarcoma: AP radiograph of bilateral knees of a 16-year-old boy shows dense osteoblastic lesions involving the metaphyses of both femora and tibia.

sarcoma (PRS) include following: (i) a history of radiation therapy, (ii) development of a neoplasm in the radiation field, (iii) a latent period of several years and (iv) histological proof of a sarcoma, which differs significantly from that initially treated.

Precise threshold dosage is unknown, but it is considered that a minimal dose of 30 Gy is required to induce a PRS and it is also suggested that concurrent chemotherapy increases the risk of sarcoma development. The treated tumors which most commonly result in development of PRS are breast carcinoma, lymphoma, head and neck cancers and gynecological malignancies. The most common sites are pelvic and shoulder girdle and the most common PRS is an osteosarcoma followed by malignant fibrous histiocytoma. Radiologically, there is evidence of bone destruction, soft tissue mass, matrix mineralization and periosteal reaction. There may also be associated features of radiation changes in the underlying bone in the form of radiation osteitis and marrow infarction. The prognosis is usually poor.[25]

Malignant change has also been reported to occur in about 1% patients with Paget's disease.[26] In at least 50% this is an osteosarcoma, in 25% a fibrosarcoma or malignant fibrous histiocytoma and in the rest other cell types are seen. Radiologically, the most common sites for Paget's disease, the pelvis and the femur, are common locations for malignant change. CT and MRI show an area of bone destruction with a wide zone of transition and a large soft tissue mass.[12]

CHONDROSARCOMA

Chondrosarcoma is a malignant tumor of chondrogenic origin that remains essentially cartilaginous throughout its evolution. It arises from chondroblasts and collagenoblasts, thus producing only cartilage and collagen. It is the third most common primary malignant tumor of bone after multiple myeloma and osteosarcoma, accounting for about 10% of all primary bone tumors. It usually develops later in life than osteosarcoma and carries a much better prognosis because metastases often occur late. A high-grade chondrosarcoma. However, behaves in a fashion very similar to an osteosarcoma.

Chondrosarcoma can be divided into two broad categories which are: primary and secondary. A primary chondrosarcoma is believed to be malignant from the outset while a secondary chondrosarcoma arises in a pre-existing bony lesion, usually an enchondroma or an osteochondroma and rarely in chondromyxoid fibroma or chondroblastoma. A chondrosarcoma may also be classified according to its histological grade as low grade (grade 1: 45–50% of cases), myxoid (grade 2: 30–40% of cases), high grade (grade 3: 8–25% of cases) or dedifferentiated, which refers to the development of an adjacent high grade nonchondroid neoplasm, typically osteosarcoma or malignant fibrous histiocytoma. Other distinct varieties include mesenchymal and clear cell chondrosarcoma.[27]

Clinical Presentation

Age: About half the patients are above 40 years of age with a mean peak incidence at about 50 years. It is rare in children and should be differentiated from the chondroblastic variety of osteosarcoma.

Sex: Male:female incidence is 1.5–2:1.

Site: The common sites are the pelvis, ribs and proximal ends of femur and humerus. It is relatively rare distal to the knee and elbow joints. According to its epicentre, chondrosarcoma can be classified into 2 types which are: central, when it is intramedullary and peripheral, when it arises from the surface of the bone. Rarely, chondrosarcomas may arise in an extraosseous site.

Imaging Features[27,28]

Radiologically the *central tumors* are seen as large, osteolytic, expansile, round or oval lesions which are well marginated with endosteal thickening or thinning **(Figs. 11A and B)**. There is evidence of cartilaginous matrix mineralization which may be stippled, nodular or conglomerate (popcorn) sometimes showing rings or arcs. Computed tomography may show calcification of the matrix when it is not visible on plain radiographs **(Figs. 12A and B)**. As chondrosarcomas are slow growing tumors, reactive changes occur in the normal bone, so that as endosteal resorbtion takes place, periosteal new bone is laid down and bone expansion occurs. Deep endosteal cortical scalloping (greater than two-thirds) is suggestive of chondrosarcoma as opposed to chondroma. Periosteal reaction is common and is seen in almost 50% of cases.

As the tumor grows, tumor margination may be lost and the tumor tissue may invade the overlying cortex to extend into the adjacent soft tissues. A soft tissue mass out of proportion to the size of the intraosseous lesion may be present **(Fig. 13A)**. In the pelvic tumors, this mass is not easily demonstrated on conventional radiography. CT and MRI can demonstrate the soft tissue extension with much greater accuracy. On MRI, cartilage shows characteristic increased signal intensity on T2-weighted images and a multilobulated, septated appearance. The lesion is slightly hypointense to muscle on T1-weighted images and may show focal areas of hyperintensity due to trapped marrow **(Figs. 11B, 13B and C)**.

Most chondrosarcomas are poorly vascularized and therefore show minimal enhancement after intravenous contrast on CT and MRI, typically showing a peripheral or septal enhancement pattern **(Fig. 13D)**. The presence of clearcut enhancement, especially if it is only in a part of the tumor, is a feature which favors dedifferentiation into a more malignant tumor, usually a malignant fibrous histiocytoma, with a more adverse prognosis.

Most of the *peripheral chondrosarcomas* probably arise from benign osteochondromas. The distinction between active osteochondroma and low-grade

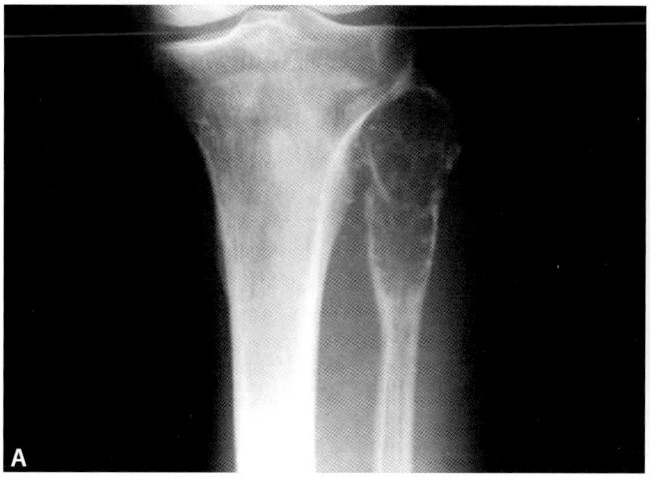

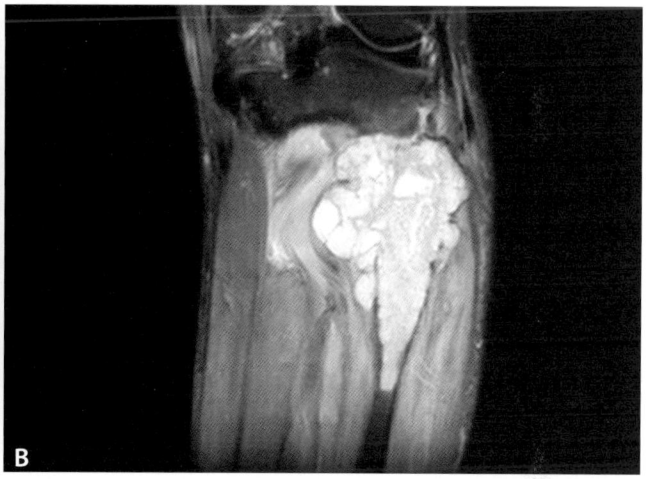

Figs. 11A and B: Conventional chondrosarcoma: (A) Plain radiograph shows an osteolytic, expansile lesion in the upper end of the fibula with faint calcification seen within; (B) Coronal T2W fat-suppressed MR image shows the characteristic hyperintense, lobulated lesion with internal septations.

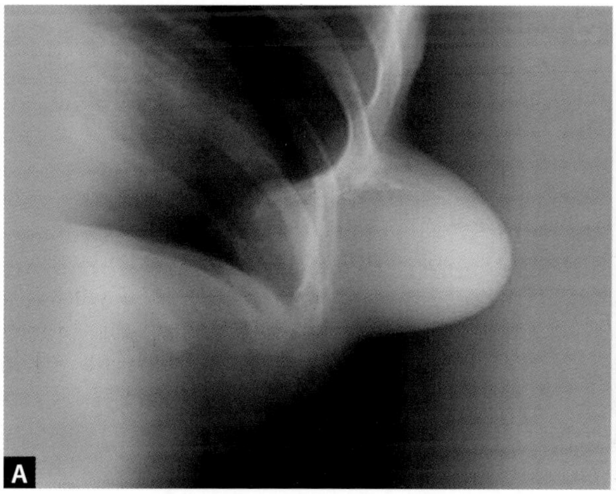

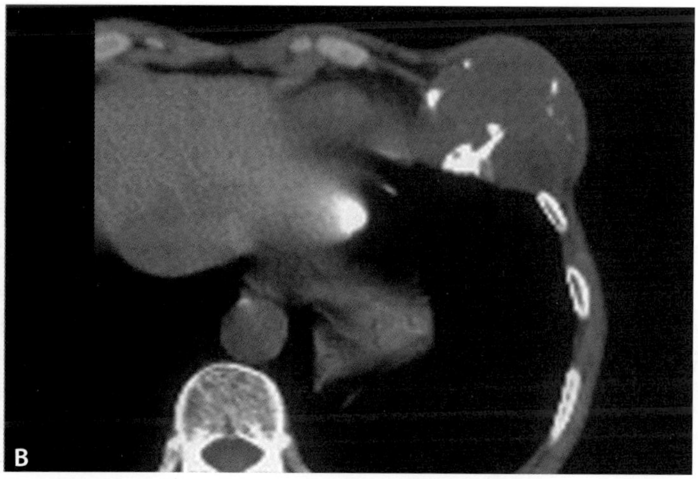

Figs. 12A and B: Chondrosarcoma: (A) A large expansile lesion in the anterior end of the left 7th rib; (B) CT shows specks of calcification within the lesion.

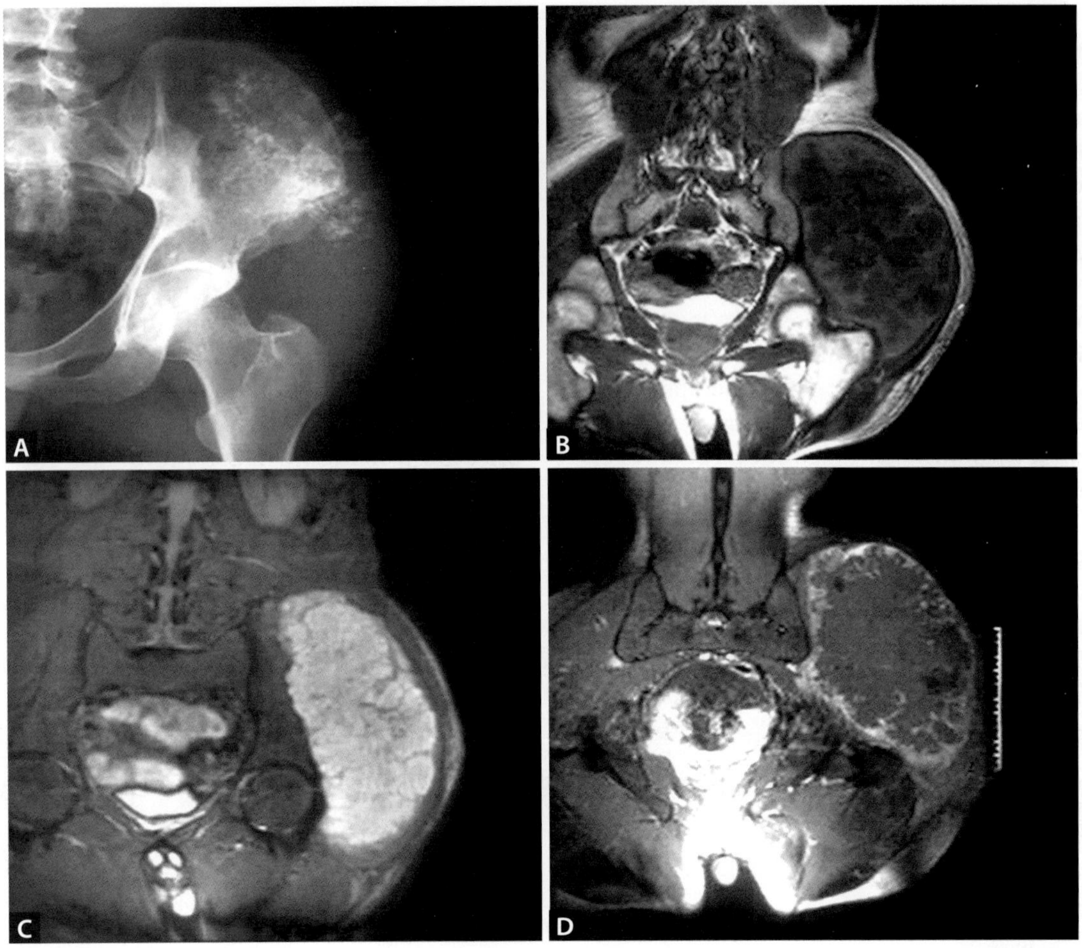

Figs. 13A to D: Conventional chondrosarcoma: (A) Radiograph of the hemipelvis shows a mass extending from the left iliac blade with the characteristic 'popcorn' calcification of a cartilaginous matrix; (B) T1W MR image shows the large soft tissue component of the chondrosarcoma as a low signal intensity lobulated mass; (C) On a coronal T2W MR image, the tumor is seen as lobulated mass of high signal intensity with septations of low signal intensity; (D) After intravenous administration of gadolinium, a coronal T1W MR image shows irregular peripheral and septal enhancement.

chondrosarcoma can be extremely difficult. Clinical features such as recent onset of pain or presence of an enlarging mass may suggest a malignant transformation. Radiologically, there may be destruction of part of a well-formed calcified cap or ossified stem of such a structure. The thickness of the cartilage cap cannot be assessed radiographically unless it abuts some other structure, e.g. a vessel or viscus filled with contrast medium. It can be readily identified by USG, CT or MRI and the thicker the cap, the more likely it is that malignant degeneration has supervened. Most osteochondromas have cartilage caps less than 5 mm thick and a cap in excess of 20 mm is likely to be malignant. Unfortunately the wide separation between these figures makes this observation of limited value.[29]

The prognosis of chondrosarcoma is good when complete resection is achieved before metastatic spread. When metastatic spread occurs, it is generally owing to invasion by the tumor of regional venous channels. Parenchymal metastases to the lungs are therefore, not uncommon. Metastases elsewhere, particularly to the skeleton, are rare; similarly regional lymph nodes are also only rarely involved.

The prognosis is better for peripheral tumors in the limbs than with central tumors, e.g. in the pelvis. Failure to remove the complete tumor leads to local recurrence and often breakdown of the overlying skin. The tumor shows a poor response to radiotherapy and cytotoxic drugs.

Other Varieties of Chondrosarcoma

Mesenchymal chondrosarcoma[30] is an uncommon entity. It occurs typically in the spine or the nonpelvic flat bones and at a younger age as compared to the conventional chondrosarcomas. Histologically, it has a much more cellular malignant matrix than the conventional chondrosarcoma. Radiologically, it is indistinguishable from a central chondroid calcification. Local recurrence and disseminated metastases occur earlier and more frequently.

Clear cell chondrosarcomas[31] are low-grade chondrosarcomas with a long history. They almost always involve the ends of long bones (femur or humerus) after closure of the epiphyseal plate. Radiographically, they are usually lytic and may show a loculated or a "soap-bubble" appearance. They may be indistinguishable from chondroblastoma or even chondromyxoid fibroma. The presence of a painful lesion and a soft tissue mass suggests the provisional diagnosis of chondrosarcoma and makes a biopsy obligatory.

FIBROSARCOMA

Fibrosarcomas of bone are rare malignant tumors that contain spindle-shaped cells that produce no osteoid in either the primary lesion or in any metastatic deposits. They may be primary or can occur secondarily in Paget's disease, chondrosarcoma, bone infarction, following irradiation and even in sinus tracts of osteomyelitis.

Clinical Presentation

Age: Most of the tumors occur between 20 and 50 years.

Sex: Equal in both sexes.

Clinical picture: Pain, swelling and pathological fractures are the common presenting features.

Site: The tubular bones are more frequently involved in younger patients , the flat bones in older patients. Almost 50% of these tumors arise in the lower limbs, particularly around the knee. The femur, tibia and humerus account for approximately two thirds of the tumors and the classical location within these bones are the condyles of the femur and the epicondyles of the humerus. Other frequent sites include the innominate bones, skull and facial bones. The majority develop primarily in bone and may either be medullary or periosteal in location, while a few arise primarily in soft tissue and cause secondary bone changes. Metastases occur to the lungs, central skeleton and viscera in a large percentage of cases.

Imaging Features[32]

The tumor is essentially osteolytic, provokes little new bone formation and usually lacks calcification or ossification **(Figs. 14A and B)**. The medullary variety is characterized by an irregular area of radiolucency. The zone of transition

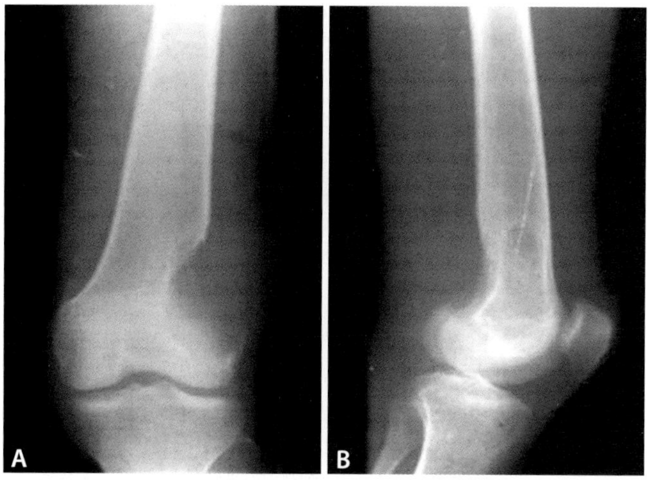

Figs. 14A and B: Fibrosarcoma: (A) AP; (B) Lateral radiographs of the knee show an osteolytic lesion with a short zone of transition in the distal femur. Note the absence of a periosteal reaction and tumor matrix mineralization.

may vary from narrow to diffusely permeative in highly aggressive tumors. With very low-grade tumors a minimal degree of sclerosis may surround the radiolucency. Slowly growing tumors may thin and expand the cortex, but with a diffuse infiltrative pattern it is more usual for cortical destruction to occur. The subsequent soft-tissue extensions are without calcification or ossification and periosteal new bone formation is unremarkable. This feature may differentiate it from osteosarcoma or chondrosarcoma.

Periosteal tumors, however, frequently exhibit shaggy ill-defined periosteal new bone formation. Destruction of the outer side of the cortex frequently takes place, but the erosion is usually clearly defined, almost as though a piece of bone has been removed surgically. In this respect considerable variance is shown from the poor definition of the edge of most malignant tumors. Secondary involvement of bone may result also from a fibrosarcoma arising in soft tissue.

The major differential diagnoses are lytic osteosarcoma, dedifferentiated chondrosarcoma and metastases. The more aggressive ill-defined varieties may be indistinguishable from malignant round cell tumors.

MALIGNANT FIBROUS HISTIOCYTOMA[12]

Malignant tumors that contain both histiocytic and fibroblastic cells are called malignant fibrous histiocytomas (MFH). Although arising much more commonly in soft tissue, these neoplasms are being diagnosed with increasing frequency and are now the main primary malignant tumor of fibrous origin affecting bone. It is believed that many tumors diagnosed in the past as fibrosarcomas were in fact MFH. They can be primary or secondary to radiation or pre-existing bone infarcts.

Clinical Presentation

Age: Can occur in all age groups with a predilection for the fourth decade, but are rare in children.

Sex: Males are affected twice as often as females.

Clinical picture: The patient presents with localized pain and swelling of insidious onset. Pathological fracture is common.

Site: The ends of long bones, particularly around the knee are commonly involved. Other bones involved are the humerus, ribs, craniofacial bones and the spine.

Imaging Features[32]

The radiological features of MFH are similar to fibrosarcoma. It is seen as a lytic lesion with geographic, moth-eaten or permeative destruction. Most tumors penetrate the cortex, produce extraosseous masses and often stimulate some periosteal reaction. Occasionally punctate, soft tissue calcification is present. Most cases present with multiple skeletal lesions and the initial impression is of skeletal metastases rather than of a primary or multifocal bone tumor. The main differential diagnosis is malignant round cell tumor.

MALIGNANT ROUND CELL TUMORS (MRCT)

This is a group of highly malignant tumors involving the bones, characterized histologically by numerous small round cells. It includes Ewing's sarcoma, peripheral primary neuroectodermal tumor (PNET), primary lymphoma of bone (formerly reticulum cell sarcoma), metastatic neuroblastoma and small cell osteosarcoma.

EWING'S SARCOMA[33]

Ewing first identified this tumor in the early 1920s. It is composed of tumor cells derived from the connective tissue framework of the bone marrow. It is a highly malignant tumor and the second most frequent bone tumor in children and adolescents. Although its etiology is still unknown, cytogenetic analysis shows a specific constant reciprocal translocation between chromosomes 11 and 22 which is shared with extraskeletal Ewing's sarcoma, PNET and Askin tumors.

Clinical Presentation

Age: Seventy-five percent of patients are under the age of 20 years, most are between 5 and 15 years.

Sex: Males are affected twice as often as females.

Clinical picture: Characteristically, the presentation is of a sick child with localized pain and swelling for few weeks or months. Pain is persistent and often severe. Fever with raised ESR may occur.

Site: Any bone in the body may be affected. Long bones, especially of the lower extremity are most commonly involved. Of the flat bones the most commonly involved are the ilium and the ribs. The scapula, ischium, pubis and bones of distal appendicular skeleton may also be affected. Most cases show extensive involvement of the diaphysis or the metadiaphyseal region.

Usually a single bone is involved, but multiple lesions occur at presentation in 10% of cases and more commonly later in the disease as Ewing's sarcoma spreads by direct infiltration and hematogenous route to other bones and the lungs. About 60% have bone metastases at autopsy.

Imaging Features[34]

The classical appearance is of a central, diaphyseal, permeative lesion with a wide zone of transition **(Figs. 15A and B)**. Larger lytic foci of moth-eaten or geographic destruction may also occur. Lesions are usually lytic but may be mixed with areas of sclerosis especially when the metaphyseal region or flat bones are involved. Saucerization is an early and characteristic sign. This irregular defect effaces the outside of the bone, showing as a marginal scalloping effect. It occurs when the tumor grows through the haversian

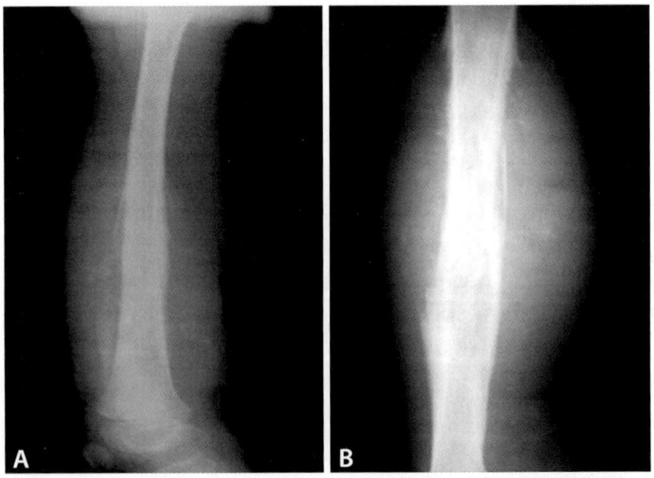

Figs. 15A and B: (A) Ewing's sarcoma of the femur shows an ill-marginated, lytic-sclerotic lesion with cortical irregularity, laminar periosteal reaction, with a large soft tissue mass in the metadiaphyseal region; (B) In another case involving the femoral diaphysis "saucerization" is well seen, with peripheral Codman's triangles and a large soft tissue mass.

system and presents subperiosteally. Subsequent spread usually leads to a very large well-defined soft tissue mass. The classic multilaminar (onion peel) periosteal reaction is uncommon, but confirms the periodic activity of the lesion. An incomplete laminar periosteal reaction is more common with marginal Codman's triangles. The "hair-on-end" periosteal reaction may also be seen **(Figs. 16A and B)** which has been found to be thinner and more hair-like than in osteosarcoma.

Ewing's sarcoma of flat bones is characterized by a larger soft tissue component relative to the osseous involvement than is seen in the long bone. Approximately one third of the cases affecting flat bones show diffuse sclerosis which is due to reactive bone formation, rather than actual tumor bone **(Figs. 17A and B)**. CT, and particularly MRI **(Figs. 18A to C)** show the large extraosseous component, the complete intraosseous extent and 'skip' metastases.

Ewing's sarcoma is one of the more aggressive tumors with a tendency towards recurrence and metastases. It is the most common primary malignant tumor to metastasize to bone **(Figs. 19A to C)**. Skip lesions are common.

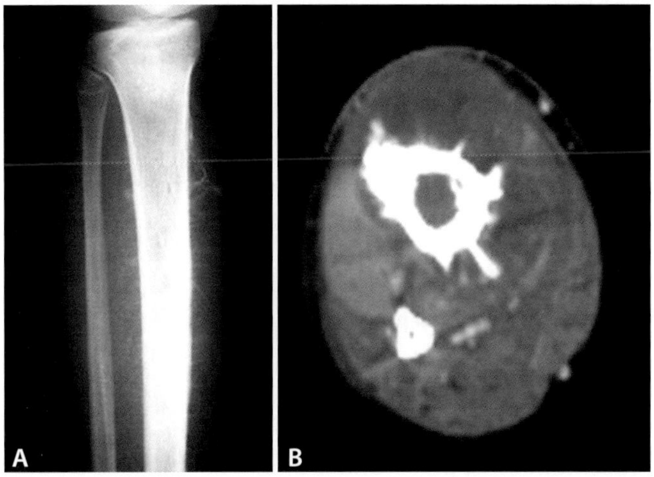

Figs. 16A and B: Ewing's sarcoma: (A) Conventional radiograph shows a permeative lesion in the tibial diaphysis with a soft tissue component with spiculated periosteal reaction better appreciated on the axial CT scan (B).

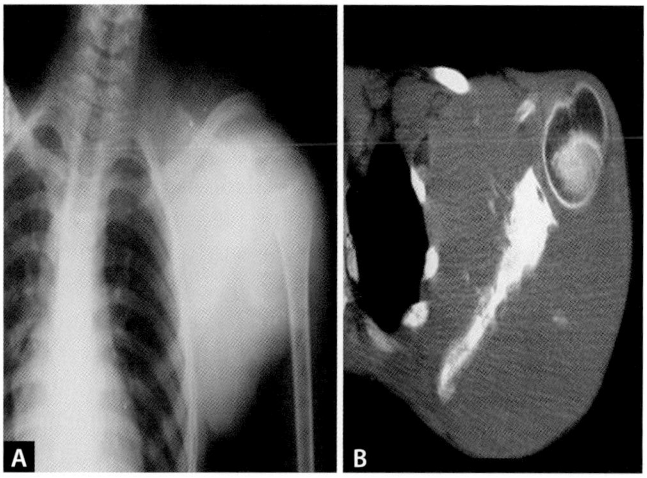

Figs. 17A and B: Ewing's sarcoma: (A) Plain radiograph; (B) Axial CT section of left shoulder shows a dense sclerotic involvement of the scapula with a large soft tissue mass.

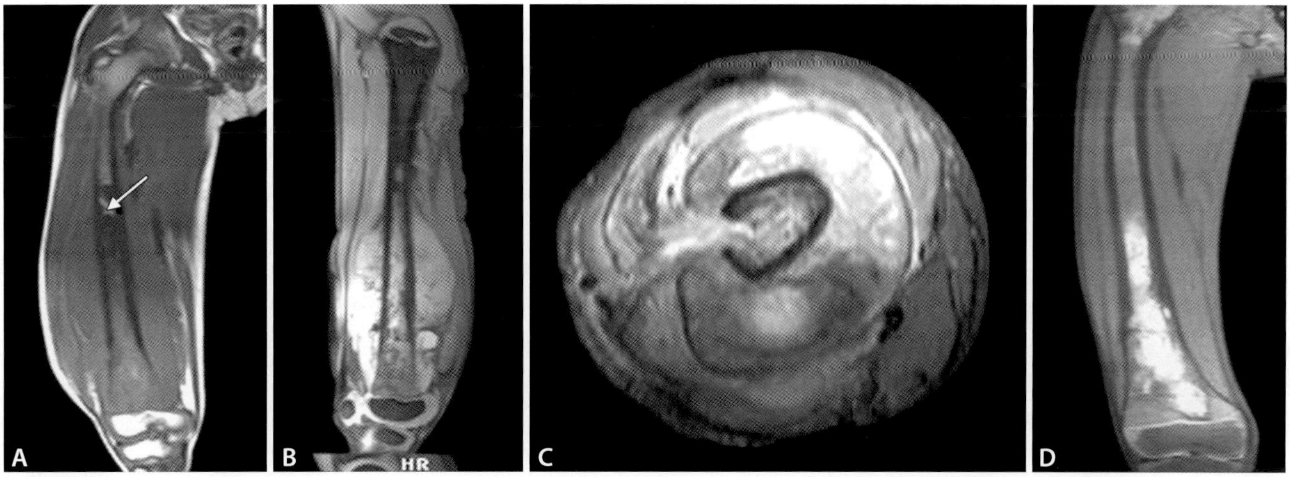

Figs. 18A to D: Ewing's sarcoma: (A) A T1W coronal scan shows the intramedullary extent of the tumor as low signal intensity of the marrow with a small "skip" lesion proximally (arrow); (B) The extraosseous component is better appreciated on the STIR coronal image; (C) The axial T2W image shows the tumor within the femur as high signal intensity with cortical discontinuity. Soft tissue component can be seen surrounding the femoral diaphysis, displacing the neurovascular bundle posteromedially; (D) After radiotherapy, there is marked reduction in the soft tissue mass with well-defined high signal intensity mass within the bone suggesting necrotic change.

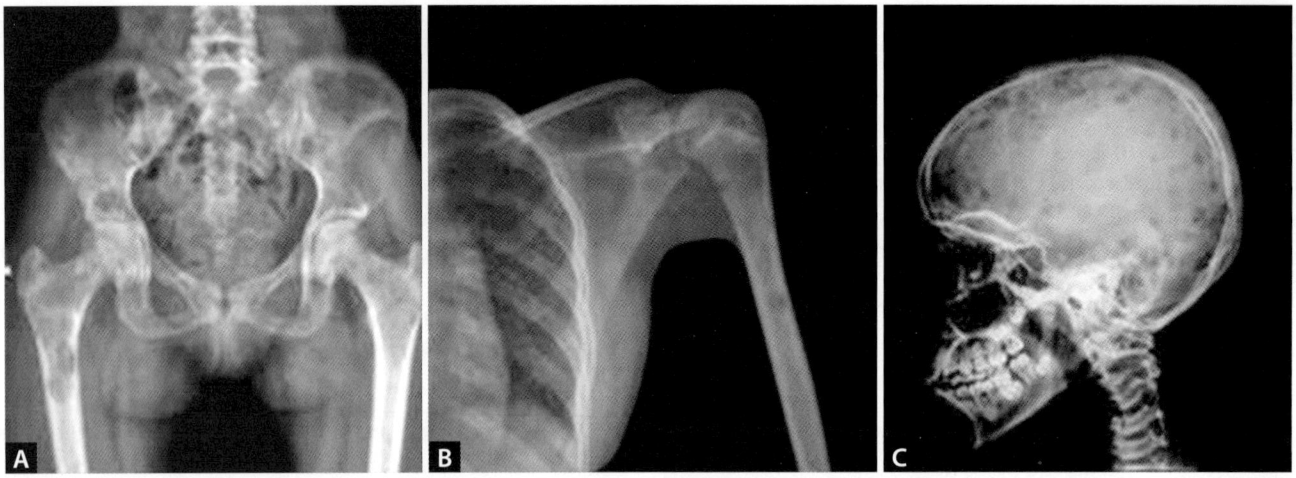

Figs. 19A to C: Ewing's sarcoma with skeletal metastses: (A) Pelvic radiograph shows the primary tumor as a large predominantly lytic lesion in the left iliac bone with multiple lytic bony metastases in the right iliac blade and both the femora; (B) Humeral shaft; (C) Skull.

Secondary spread to the lungs also occurs frequently involving the lung parenchyma and pleura.

Differential diagnosis in the early stages is with osteomyelitis or occasionally trauma. Each of these may produce a periosteal reaction with little bone destruction. In Ewing's sarcoma, a well defined soft tissue mass is seen while in infection the soft tissue component is ill-defined. In later stages Ewing's sarcoma may be indistinguishable from a lytic osteosarcoma. Primary lymphoma is a differential in patients over the age of 30 years. Langerhan's cell histiocytosis may occasionally mimic Ewing's sarcoma, specially when presenting at an early destructive stage and involving the pelvis.[12]

Ewing's sarcoma is usually treated with multiple cycles of multidrug chemotherapy for local and metastatic disease and radiation therapy or limb salvage for local control of tumor. Resectable lesions in the extremities have a better prognosis than those found in the pelvis or other bones of the axial skeleton.[35] Pretreatment dynamic enhanced MRI has a potential role for determining outcome and may be used in the decision to intensify treatment.[36] With treatment, the soft tissue mass decreases in size and the intraosseous portion becomes necrotic with a higher signal on T2W imaging **(Fig. 18D)**. MRI is also more accurate than standard radiography, CT or scintigraphy in the diagnosis of recurrent Ewing's sarcoma.

Rarely, extraskeletal Ewing's sarcoma (EES) may develop in the soft tissues at any location. The most common sites of occurrence of EES are the trunk, extremities and retroperitoneum. Although it is a soft tissue primary tumor, it can cause changes in the cortex of adjacent bone. Extraskeletal Ewing's sarcoma is more common in adults and is associated with a high incidence of local recurrence and distant metastases.[37]

Primitive Neuroectodermal Tumor of Bone (PNET)[12]

These rare tumors of bone resemble Ewing's tumors clinically except that they are commoner in the female sex. They arise in the metaphyses and diaphyses of the lower limbs, humerus, pelvis and scapula. Radiologically, they resemble Ewing's sarcoma in being destructive ill-defined neoplasms which readily spread into the soft tissues. *Askin tumor* is a rare PNET of the thoracopulmonary region occurring in children and young adults. Radiologically, in 70% of patients, it presents as a pleural disorder. A soft-tissue mass involving the chest wall is seen in about half the patients and a subpleural pulmonary mass with pleural involvement in about one quarter.

Non-Hodgkin's Lymphoma of Bone[38] (Lymphosarcoma, Reticulum Cell Sarcoma)

Primary lymphoma of bone is a rare extranodal lymphoma, histologically identical with others arising in lymphoid or soft tissue but presenting initially as a localized solitary bone lesion. It constitutes only 3–4% of all primary malignant bone tumors. The skeletal system may be secondarily involved in about 30% of malignant lymphomas.

Clinical Presentation

Age: The majority of patients are between 20 and 50 years of age.

Sex: Male:female ratio is 2:1.

Clinical picture: Patients usually present with localized dull aching pain, often of long duration. A palpable mass may be present.

Site: The common sites are the diaphysis of long bones, particularly femur, tibia and humerus. Flat bones can also be involved.

Imaging Features

The osseous destruction in this tumor is usually markedly permeative or moth-eaten in type with an associated soft tissue mass. Relative absence of cortical destruction is a characteristic feature. Nearly half the cases show some reactive sclerosis, however, a purely sclerotic appearance is very rare **(Figs. 20A and B)**. Pathological fracture is common and may be the initial complaint. It occurs more frequently in this disease than with any other primary malignant bone tumor as the symptoms are mild and of long duration. Proximal spread within the bone, sometimes with "skip" areas, may be seen. MRI typically shows extensive involvement of the medullary canal with little cortical destruction but a large soft tissue mass.[12]

The main differential diagnosis is Ewing's sarcoma which can present an identical picture. An older age group and the lack of systemic symptoms aid in differentiating the two. Like Ewing's sarcoma, this tumor shows good response to local radiotherapy and adjuvant chemotherapy.

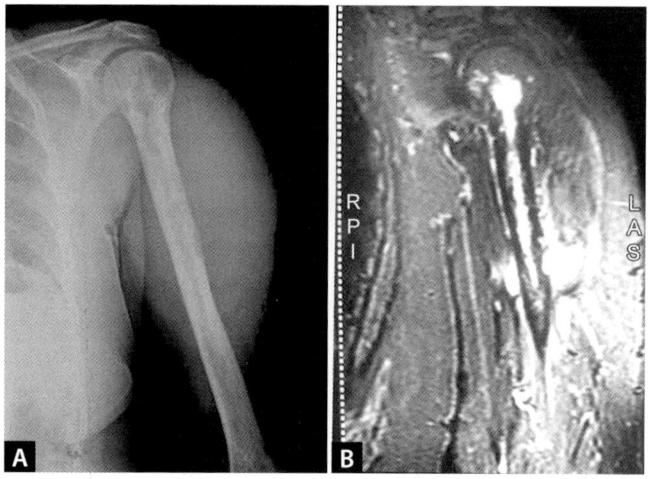

Figs. 20A and B: Non-Hodgkin's lymphoma: (A) AP radiograph of the humerus shows a mixed lytic and sclerotic lesion involving proximal half of the shaft with little cortical destruction and a large soft tissue component; (B) Sagittal T2W fat-suppressed MR image through the shaft shows the extent of medullary involvement.

Hodgkin's Lymphoma of Bone

Hodgkin's lymphoma of the bone occurs more commonly as a secondary manifestation of systemic Hodgkin's disease and rarely as a primary bone involvement. Between 10 and 20% of patients with Hodgkin's disease develop skeletal disease. Pain is the most common initial symptom. The main site is the vertebral body of the lower thoracic and upper lumbar spine. Other bones to be involved are the ilium, scapula, sternum, ribs and femur.

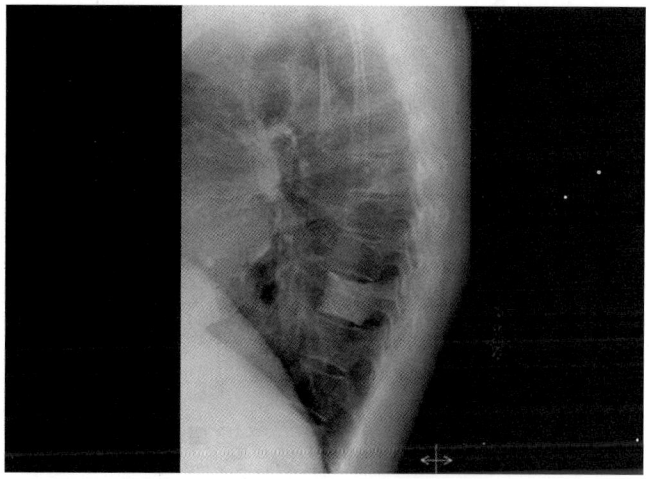

Fig. 21: Ivory vertebra seen as a homogeneous increased density of a solitary thoracic vertebra.

Imaging Features

Radiographically, most lesions are osteolytic (75%). Sclerotic lesions may also occur (15%),and a mixed destruction with periosteal reaction can be seen in a few cases. Occasionally, a marked sclerotic reaction can be seen as an ivory vertebra **(Fig. 21)**. In the lumbar vertebrae, lytic destruction is more common with exuberant periosteal reaction.[38]

CHORDOMA

Chordoma[39] is a neoplasm which arises from ectopic cellular remnants of the notochord which have persisted within the nucleus pulposus of the intervertebral disk or from aberrant cell rests of notochord tissue within the vertebral bodies. This tumor has a predilection for the sacrococcygeal and spheno-occipital regions.

Clinical Presentation

Age: The peak incidence is between 50 and 70 years. Range between 30 and 70 years.

Sex: Incidence is equal below 40 years, but over 40, male : female ratio is 2:1.

Clinical picture: Patients present with pain. Other symptoms relate to pressure on local structures-rectal/

vesical dysfunction in the sacral region, cranial nerve palsies in the spheno-occipital region.

Site: About 90% of cases occur in the sacrococcygeal (50%) and basisphenoid (40%) regions with rare involvement of other vertebrae. Distant metastases are rare, mainly involving lymph nodes, liver and lungs.

Imaging Features

Sacral lesions usually show a large area of bone destruction with well-defined, scalloped margins and a large soft tissue mass. Amorphous calcification may occur within the mass. Calcification may be seen in approximately 50% of cases on plain films and in 85% cases on CT **(Figs. 22A and B)**. In the spheno-occipital region, the dorsal aspect of the sella and clivus may be destroyed, with a soft tissue mass indenting the nasopharyngeal air-space. Here, the differential diagnosis is from chondrosarcoma whereas in the sacrum the possibility of plasmacytoma or giant cell tumor should also be considered. CT or MRI are invaluable for demonstrating the extent of bone destruction and soft tissue mass **(Figs. 23A to C)**.

If the tumor primarily involves the spine, the radiographic picture is nonspecific. C2 vertebral body is the most commonly involved vertebra. Bone destruction is present with or without involvement of the intervertebral disc and two or more vertebrae may be involved. Chordoma is the only primary malignant bone tumor that crosses the joint space. The presence of bone destruction of two contiguous vertebrae with a large soft tissue component may simulate spinal tuberculosis. An ivory vertebra can also occur.[38]

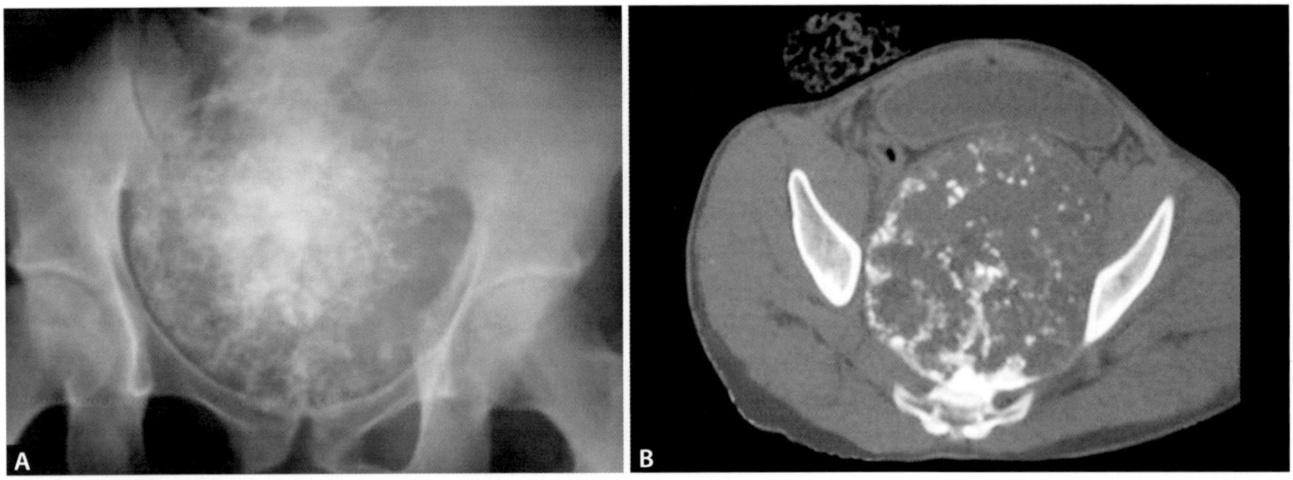

Figs. 22A and B: Chordoma of the sacrum: Plain radiograph (A) and CT (B) showing a large pelvic mass with calcification.

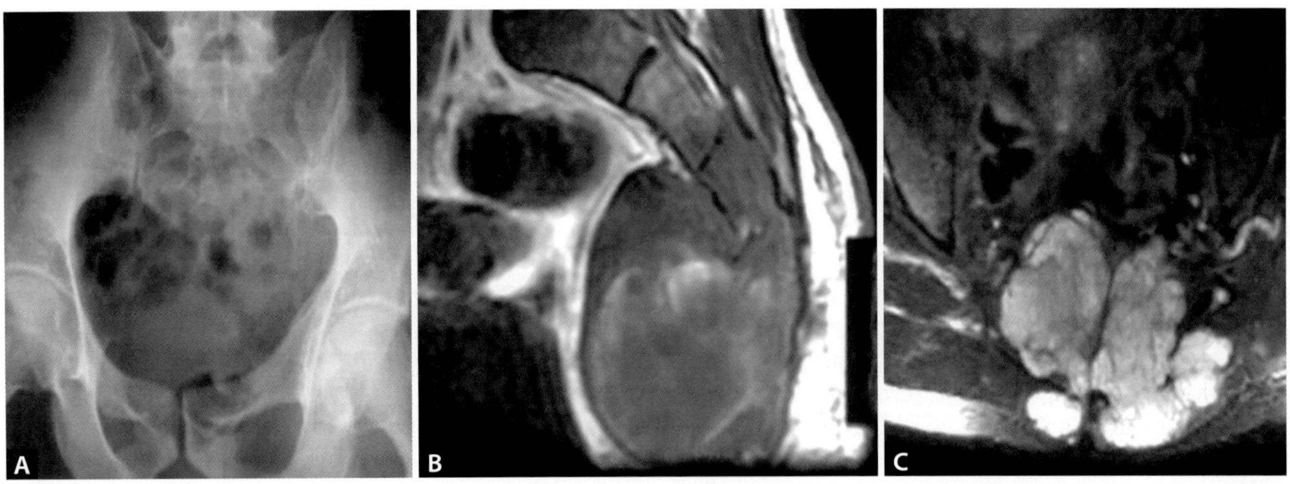

Figs. 23A to C: Chordoma of the sacrum: (A) Plain radiograph shows a lytic lesion destroying the distal half of the sacrum; (B and C) T1W sagittal and T2W axial MR images show the large tumor with inhomogeneous signal intensity arising from the distal sacrum.

Treatment is limited by the region involved. Ideally, resection (often partial) is combined with radiotherapy. The recurrence rate is high, but the tumor metastasizes late.

LIPOSARCOMA

Intraosseous liposarcoma is extremely rare despite the extensive fatty content of the bone marrow. It is four times as common in males as in females and the mean age of presentation is the fourth decade (range: 15–55 years).

Most tumors affect the long bones of the lower limbs. Radiologically, appearance varies from local geographic bone destruction to a permeative pattern. CT and MRI provide characteristic diagnostic information due to the nonhomogeneous fatty content of the tumor.

VASCULAR TUMORS OF THE BONE

Angiosarcoma

Angiosarcoma[40] is a rare vascular tumor of bone, affecting all ages. Male : female ratio is 2:1. Any bone can be affected, but the vertebrae and femur are most commonly involved. Multiple lesions occur in one-third cases.

Radiologically, a multilocular or "soap bubble" appearance may be seen. The lesion often involves a considerable length of bone. Reactive sclerosis may be seen at the margins of some tumors. In less well differentiated sarcomas marginal demarcation is poor. CT and MRI appearances are nonspecific. This is a highly malignant tumor usually treated by surgery and radiotherapy with a 5 years survival rate of under 10%.

Hemangioendothelioma

Hemangioendothelioma[12] is a rare low-grade endothelial tumor which affects a wide age group of patients and presents as a multifocal lesion in 25% of cases. The radiological features of individual lesions are nonspecific but the presence of multifocal disease, either within the same bone or in different bones, is a clue to the diagnosis. Each lesion is typically lytic although mixed lytic/sclerotic tumors can be seen. Periosteal reaction, cortical destruction and extraosseus extension are uncommon.

MALIGNANT GIANT CELL TUMOR

True malignant giant cell tumors are rare, accounting for less than 5% of the giant cell tumors in most series. Most of them are secondary malignancies arising in previously irradiated conventional giant cell tumor of bone. A few are either malignant from the outset, or are termed evolutionary malignant giant cell tumors, arising at a site of recurrent giant cell tumor previously treated by surgery but without radiation therapy. The radiologist alone often cannot predict with any accuracy whether the tumor is benign or malignant as some of the most benign appearing tumors may show metastases.[38]

ADAMANTINOMA OF LONG BONES[41]

This is a rare tumor typically involving the midshaft of the tibia. Its pathogenesis is unknown. It was originally thought to be of epithelial origin comparable to the histologically similar ameloblastoma of the jaw, but is now known to be unrelated.

Clinical Presentation

Age: Most cases occur between 10 and 50 years with an average age of 35 years.

Sex: Male:female ratio is 5:4, but a higher female incidence is found at the younger end of the age range.

Clinical picture: Local pain and tenderness of several months to several years duration is the most common presenting complaint.

Site: More than 90% occur in the tibia, mostly in the mid shaft. Other bones involved include fibula, ulna, femur and occasionally even the short bones. Tumors with multiple foci in the same long bone may sometimes occur.

Imaging Features

Adamantinomas can be situated in the cortex or the medullary space. Plain radiographs thus, show an eccentric or central osteolytic lesion in the shaft of the bone with a well defined margin, causing mild expansion of the bone. A multiloculated appearance and satellite lesions are useful diagnostic features. Periosteal reaction is uncommon. Magnetic resonance imaging is invaluable in local staging of adamantinoma for features like extension into the marrow cavity, extraosseus extension and multifocal lesions. A lobulated growth pattern is typical, but there are no specific signal characteristics. Intense, uniform enhancement is seen following contrast enhanced studies.[42]

Differential diagnosis includes metastatic carcinoma, plasmacytoma, aneurysmal bone cyst and active fibrous dysplasia. Adamantinomas grow at a slow rate but are characterized by local recurrences and eventual metastases to the lung. Extensive local resection is the usual form of treatment.

MULTIPLE MYELOMA

Multiple myeloma[43] is the most common primary malignant neoplasm of bone. It is a predominant plasma cell dyscrasia. There is production of an abnormal paraprotein leading to a wide M-band on plasma electrophoresis. Production of light chain immunoglobulins results in Bence Jones proteinuria in over half the patients. Hypercalcemia, hypercalciuria and amyloidosis can occur, but serum alkaline phosphatase and serum phosphorus are normal.

Clinical Presentation

Age: This is a disease of the elderly. Seventy-five percent of those affected are over the age of 50 with a peak over 80 years.

Sex: A male predominance of up to 2:1 is seen.

Clinical picture: Persistent bone pain is the most common symptom which is worse during the day, is relieved by rest and aggravated by weight bearing. Pathological fracture is a common complication. Associated weight loss, anemia and cachexia occur. Bacterial infections occur in 10% of cases, most of which are respiratory in nature.

Laboratory findings reveal a normochromic, normocytic anemia, thrombocytopenia, hypercalcemia, hyperglobulinemia with a reversed A:G ratio, hyperuricemia and Bence Jones' proteinuria. ESR is often raised over 100 mm/h. Bone marrow biopsy confirms the plasma cell dyscrasia.

Site: The spine, pelvis, skull, ribs and scapula are the most frequently involved bones.

Imaging Features

The preferred initial imaging examination for the diagnosis and staging of myeloma (according to the 2009 International Myeloma Working Group consensus statement) remains the skeletal survey. Patients suspected of having multiple myeloma based on bone marrow aspirate results or hypergammaglobulinemia should undergo a radiographic skeletal survey.[44]

The classical appearance of multiple myeloma on plain radiographs consists of well-defined, osteolytic "punched-out" lesions throughout the skeleton, most characteristic in the skull **(Figs. 24A and B)**. These lesions can also be seen in the pelvic bones, clavicles, ribs, and long bones. These lesions may be differentiated from lytic metastatic lesions by the more uniform size of the lesions in multiple myeloma. Generalized osteopenia is another important form of presentation **(Figs. 25A and B)**. A pathological fracture affects about half of the patients at some time or the other. Examples of purely sclerotic myeloma have been occasionally reported. They may take the form of diffuse osteosclerosis, patchy sclerotic areas throughout the skeleton and very rarely, small numbers of focal sclerotic lesions.

Involvement of the spine is usually in the lower thoracic and upper lumbar regions and is seen as diffuse osteopenia. Pathological vertebral collapse involving a single or multiple vertebrae is a common occurrence. Pedicular involvement, although rare can occur in multiple myeloma patients and so the usefulness of this feature to differentiate multiple myeloma from metastatic disease appears doubtful.[38]

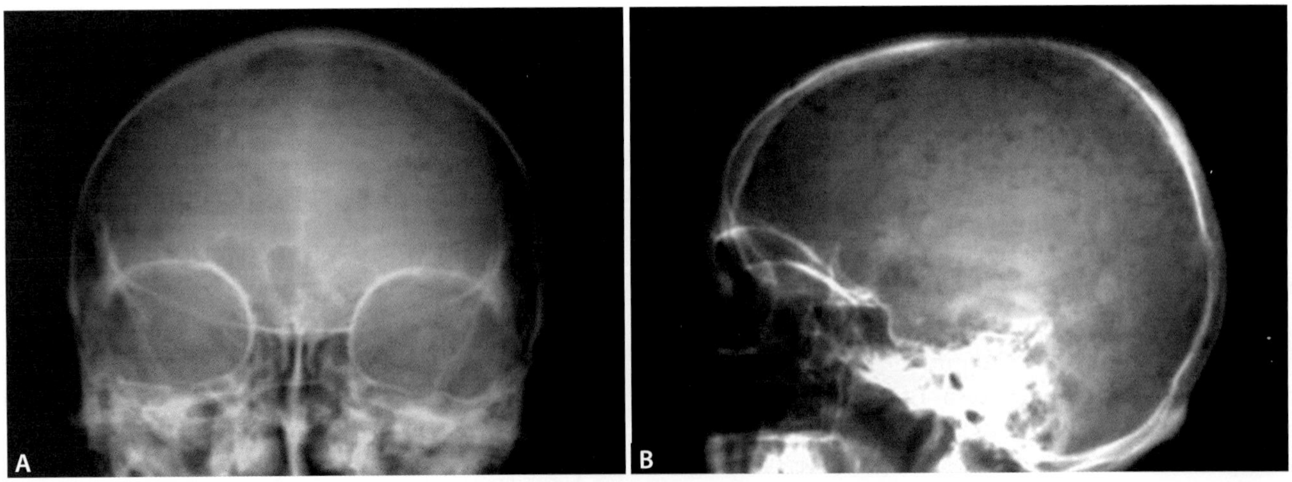

Figs. 24A and B: Multiple myeloma: (A) AP and (B) lateral skull radiographs showing small, well-defined, 'punched out' lesions in the calvarium.

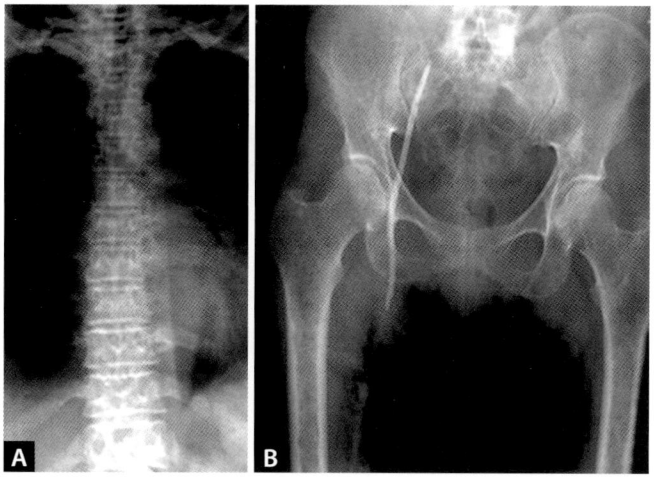

Figs. 25A and B: Multiple myeloma: Radiographs of the dorsal spine (A) and pelvis (B) of the same patient as in Figure 24 show osteoporosis with small discrete lesions in the femora.

Scintigraphy using standard technetium-99m (^{99m}Tc) may underestimate myelomatous lesions, as many lesions are cold probably because of their nonreactive pathology. Uptake of radionuclide depends on the osteoblastic activity which is deficient in patients with non fractured melanoma deposits. Symptomatic lesions are more likely to be detected by a combination of radiography and scintigraphy. A study by Erten et al. appeared to demonstrate that whole body scintigraphy with technetium-99m 2-methoxy-isobutyl-isonitrile (^{99m}Tc-MIBI) may be a useful adjunct for the diagnostic imaging of multiple myeloma.[45] The authors reported that in 24 patients, ^{99m}Tc-MIBI demonstrated the extent and intensity of bone marrow infiltration equally as well as MRI, and they suggested that ^{99m}Tc-MIBI may serve as an alternative to MRI in cases in which MRI is not readily available or when its use is limited.

PET/CT scanning can be helpful in the staging and post-therapeutic monitoring of multiple myeloma by providing functional detection of high metabolic lesions.[46] However, a preliminary report by Nanni et al.[47] in a small population of patients indicates that carbon-11 (^{11}C)-choline PET/CT scanning may be more sensitive than FDG-PET/CT scanning for detecting myeloma lesions.

Magnetic resonance imaging is highly sensitive to marrow infiltration from myeloma. Several MR imaging patterns of multiple myeloma infiltration have been described. These include normal marrow, a micronodular pattern (also termed variegated or salt-and-pepper), a focal pattern and a diffuse pattern. Focal lesions also may be seen in the setting of a micronodular or diffuse pattern of disease. On T1W images, the affected areas are low in signal intensity. With T2-weighting a heterogeneous increase in signal intensity is seen.[48] MRI, although sensitive to the presence of disease, is not disease specific. Additional tests must be employed to diagnose myeloma, such as measurement of gamma-globulin levels and direct aspiration of bone marrow to assess for plasmacytosis. Because of this, MRI may understage or overstage patients with myeloma.

Vertebral body compression fractures occur frequently in patients with multiple myeloma. The differentiation between osteoporotic vertebral collapse and that due to myeloma may be difficult even on MRI **(Figs. 26A and B)**. Diffusion-weighted imaging and opposed-phase (in-phase–out-of-phase) imaging have been advocated to help differentiate insufficiency fractures from pathologic compression fractures.

Staging: Morbidity and mortality, in myeloma patients, are directly related to the stage of disease at initial diagnosis. In 1975, Durie and Salmon[49] proposed the initial clinical staging system for multiple myeloma. The system was revised in 2003[50] and is now referred to as the Durie/Salmon PLUS system, since additional information from advanced imaging modalities has been added:

- Stage IA: normal skeletal survey or single lesion
- Stage IB: 5 focal lesions or mild diffuse spine disease
- Stage IIA/B: 5 to 20 focal lesions or moderately diffuse spine disease
- Stage IIIA/B: >20 focal lesions or severe diffuse spine disease
- Subclasses A and B (A = normal renal function, B = abnormal renal function).

Mild, moderate and diffuse spine disease is established by MR imaging. Moderate diffuse disease is defined as vertebral body signal intensity brighter than adjacent disk on a T1-weighted sequence. Severe diffuse disease is defined as vertebral body signal intensity less than or equal to the adjacent disk on a T1-weighted sequence. Mild disease has not been precisely defined.

The most important differential diagnosis in this age group is metastases. Features which help in distinguishing the two, are summarized in **Table 6**. Taken together, these features may give an indication of the correct diagnosis.

The overall prognosis of multiple myeloma is poor. Over 90% patients die within 3 years. The treatment is usually palliative with the aim of minimizing suffering, with radiotherapy and chemotherapy.

PLASMACYTOMA (SOLITARY MYELOMA)

A plasmacytoma represents a localized form of plasma cell proliferation, which is apparently solitary at presentation

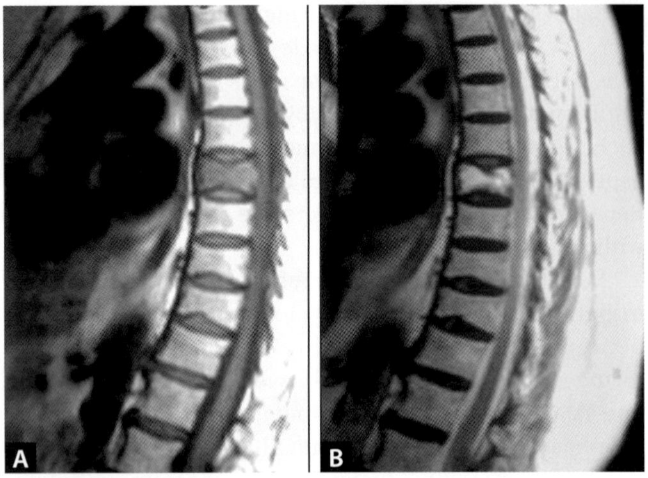

Figs. 26A and B: Multiple myeloma: T1W (A) and T2W (B) sagittal MR images of the dorsal spine show complete alteration of the marrow signal in the seventh thoracic vertebra, hypointense on T1W and hyperintense on T2W images, with evidence of collapse. A posterior convexity of the involved vertebra suggests a malignant etiology.

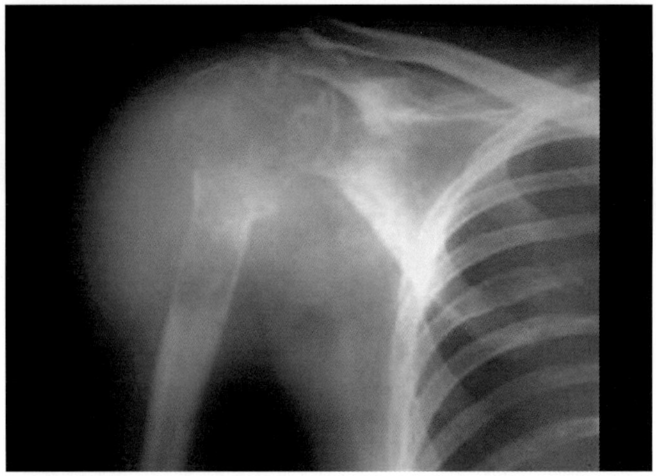

Fig. 27: Plasmacytoma: An expansile, lytic lesion with sparse, thin trabeculations is seen in the upper end of humerus.

Table 6: Distinguishing features between multiple myeloma and metastases.

	Multiple myeloma	***Metastases***
1.	Vertebral pedicles and posterior elements less commonly involved Destruction of intervertebral disk may occur	Destruction of vertebral pedicles
2.	Soft tissue mass associated with a bony lesion	Soft tissue extension is relatively uncommon
3.	Mandible involved commonly	Mandible involved rarely
4.	Radionuclide studies may give false negative results	Radionuclide studies are very sensitive
5.	Serum alkaline phosphatase may be normal	Serum alkaline phosphatase is always raised in disseminated disease

and may remain localized for many years, but is potentially capable of transition to generalized myelomatosis.

Clinical Presentation

Age: Although few cases present below the age of 40 years, the overall age of presentation tends to the earlier and the age range wider, than in generalized myelomatosis.

Clinical picture: Presentation may be with local pain as a result of fracture, but uncomplicated plasmacytoma may cause no symptoms.

Site: The lesion predominantly affects sites containing persistent red marrow. The mandible, ilium, vertebrae, ribs and proximal femur are the commonly involved bones. Peripheral lesions are rare.

Imaging Features

A plasmacytoma arises in the medulla and the bone changes usually resemble a benign lesion. The characteristic appearance is that of a geographic, radiolucent lesion which is highly expansile with apparent trabeculation or a "soap bubble" appearance **(Fig. 27)**.

Involvement of the vertebral body is common, sometimes leading to early collapse. Sometimes a whole vertebral body is lost, with geographical destruction of the margins of the adjoining vertebral bodies, usually posteriorly. Coarse trabecular strands of increased density may give a network appearance in the area of destruction. Exceptionally, the lesion may be entirely sclerotic. Scintigraphy and CT/MRI do not give any specific information, however, the finding of apparently solitary plasmacytoma in the spine should be investigated with whole spine MRI to identify further radiographically occult lesions.[51]

The most important differential diagnosis is an osteolytic metastasis. In the vertebrae such metastases are likely to involve the pedicles most commonly. Chordoma, brown tumors of hyperparathyroidism, hemophilic pseudotumor, hydatid cyst, fibrous dysplasia and giant cell tumor can also be considered in the differential diagnosis.

Seventy percent of patients who have what seems to be a solitary plasmacytoma, develop diffuse multiple myeloma and die within 3 years. Progression to multiple myeloma has been documented in cases up to 23 years after the initial presentation and thus long-term follow-up of these patients is essential.[52]

POEMS Syndrome

An uncommon condition with the acronym POEMS is characterized by a chronic, progressive polyneuropathy, organomegaly (hepatosplenomegaly), endocrinopathy (commonly diabetes mellitus), M-proteins (plasma cell dyscrasia) and skin changes (hirsutism, pigmentation, edema).[53] It is usually seen in young men and radiologically presents with multiple sclerotic lesions, most commonly in the spine and pelvis. The lesions may be uniformly sclerotic or appear target-like, with a peripheral margin of bone sclerosis. Ivory vertebrae and areas resembling bone islands may be seen. Bone proliferation is seen at sites of tendon and ligament attachments. Irregular bony excrescences involving the posterior elements of the spine are characteristically seen. Digital clubbing and periostitis in tubular bones simulate the findings of hypertrophic osteoarthropathy.[54]

METASTATIC BONE DISEASE

Metastases are the most common malignant tumors of the skeletal system. Approximately 70% of all malignant tumors are metastatic in origin, with only 30% being primary in nature.[38] Postmortem studies show that their incidence is much higher than may be detected *in vivo*. Bony metastases are present in approximately 25% of all deaths from malignant disease.[55] Most of the osseous metastases are from a primary extraskeletal focus, the majority are epithelial in origin. The most common primary sites are in the breast, lung, prostate, kidney, thyroid and bowel. With the exception of tumors of the central nervous system and basal cell carcinoma of the skin, almost every malignant tumor can metastasize to bone.

Bone involvement in metastases occurs by means of 3 main mechanisms: (1) direct extension, (2) retrograde venous flow and (3) seeding with tumor emboli via the blood circulation which is the most common route of spread. Venous tumor emboli get arrested at a distant capillary bed. As the tumor emboli have to pass through the pulmonary bed, metastatic cancer to bone is a relatively late occurrence and generally occurs after pulmonary metastases have appeared.[56] Retrograde venous embolism is probably the major mechanism when spread from intra-abdominal cancer involves the vertebrae. Increased intra-abdominal pressure causes blood to be diverted from the systemic caval system to the valveless vertebral venous plexus of Batson; this diversion allows the caudal and cranial flow of blood.

Clinical Presentation

Age: Most patients are older than 40 years. In children <5 years, skeletal metastases usually occur from neuroblastoma, between 10 and 25 years, Ewing's sarcoma and osteosarcoma and between 20 and 35 years Hodgkin's lymphoma is the most common source.

Sex: In females, carcinoma breast is responsible for majority of all bone metastases followed by carcinomas of thyroid, kidney and uterus. In males, carcinoma prostate is the most common primary focus, followed by carcinoma lung.

Site: They are most often found in the axial skeleton and other sites of residual red marrow. Thus, the common sites for metastases are vertebrae, pelvis, proximal femora and humerii, skull and ribs. Metastases to bones of hand and feet are rare and almost 50% of these are due to carcinoma of the lung.

Clinical picture: The lesions may be entirely asymptomatic or present with vague bone pains. Occasionally a pathological fracture through the metastatic lesion may bring it to notice. Weight loss, cachexia, anemia and even fever may be seen in the later stages.

Imaging Features

Plain radiographs: As a metastatic lesion grows in the medullary cavity, the surrounding bone is remodeled by means of either osteoclastic or osteoblastic processes. The relative degree of resultant bone resorption or deposition is highly variable and depends on the type and location of the tumor. The relationship between the osteoclastic and osteoblastic remodeling processes determines whether a predominant lytic, sclerotic, or mixed pattern is seen on radiographs. The majority (75%) of metastases are *osteolytic*. Lesions usually appear in the medullary cavity, spread to destroy the medullary bone and then involve the cortex, usually without the development of much periosteal reaction. Soft tissue extension is relatively uncommon. At least 30% bone destruction is necessary before the lytic lesions can be detected on plain radiographs.

Some metastases (15%) are predominantly *osteoblastic*, e.g. from prostate, stomach and carcinoid. The increased density of the blastic metastases is due to the laying down of new bone, which is non-neoplastic in nature, but is a reactive response of the local osteoid tissue to the presence of tumor. *Mixed osteolytic and osteosclerotic* metastasis (10%) occur from carcinoma breast and occasionally, lung.

Breast in females and prostate in males, are the most common primary tumors metastasizing to bone.

Breast metastases are commonly lytic **(Figs. 28A and B)**, but 10% may be osteoblastic and in another 10% can be mixed. Diffuse infiltration of the whole marrow may occur and may only become evident radiologically when sclerosis occurs after therapy. Skeletal metastases from *prostate* are predominantly blastic or mixed **(Figs. 29A and B)**. Purely lytic lesions are rare. Individual lesions may sometimes show a florid "sunburst' appearance, simulating osteosarcoma **(Fig. 30)**. Metastases from the *lung* occur most commonly to the axial skeleton, however, metastases to hand and foot are most commonly from bronchogenic carcinoma **(Fig. 31)**. The squamous cell and oat cell carcinomas of lung produce lytic metastases, while adenocarcinomas and bronchial carcinoid which metastasize to bone in about 10% of cases, produce focal or diffuse densely blastic lesions.

Hypernephroma and *thyroid* carcinoma generally show lytic, expansile metastases also called "blow-out metastases" **(Fig. 32)**. The incidence of skeletal metastases from the *gastrointestinal tract* is under 7%, but as these malignancies are more common than kidney and thyroid, they are encountered commonly. They are usually lytic, but sclerotic metastases may occur. Calcification is also a feature. *Cervical carcinoma* usually involves bone by contiguous spread to the bony pelvis. Blood borne metastases are uncommon and usually lytic, but may rarely be osteoblastic or mixed. Carcinoma of the *uterine body* is an adenocarcinoma and like that of the *ovary*, may produce osteoblastic metastases, particularly of the vertebrae.

Nuclear medicine: The value of establishing the presence of multiple skeletal lesions cannot be over-emphasized,

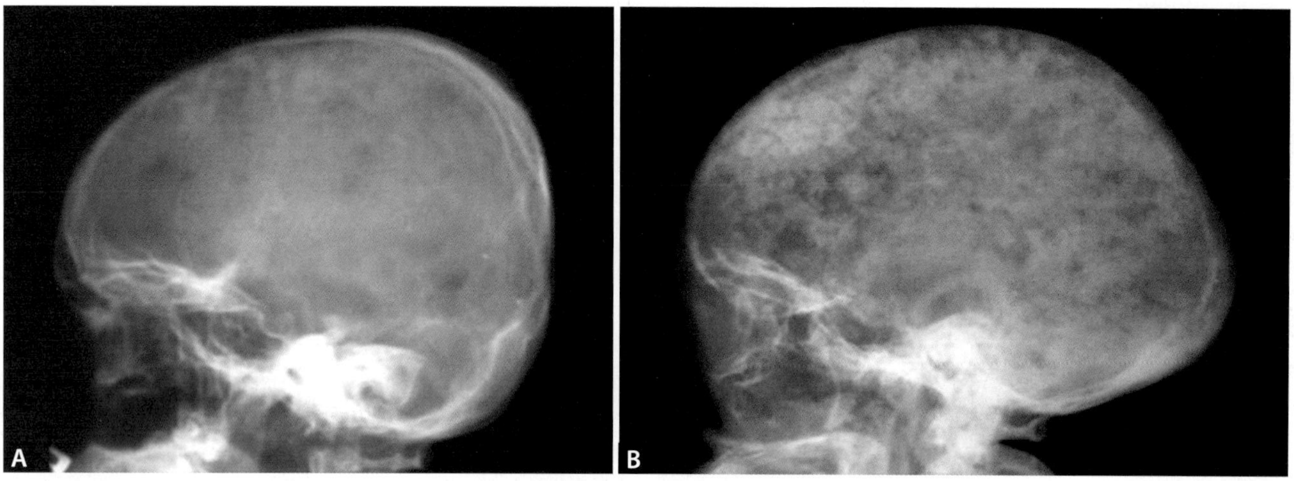

Figs. 28A and B: Skeletal metastases: Lateral radiographs of the skull of two different patients show multiple ill-defined lytic lesions of varying sizes in the calvarium.

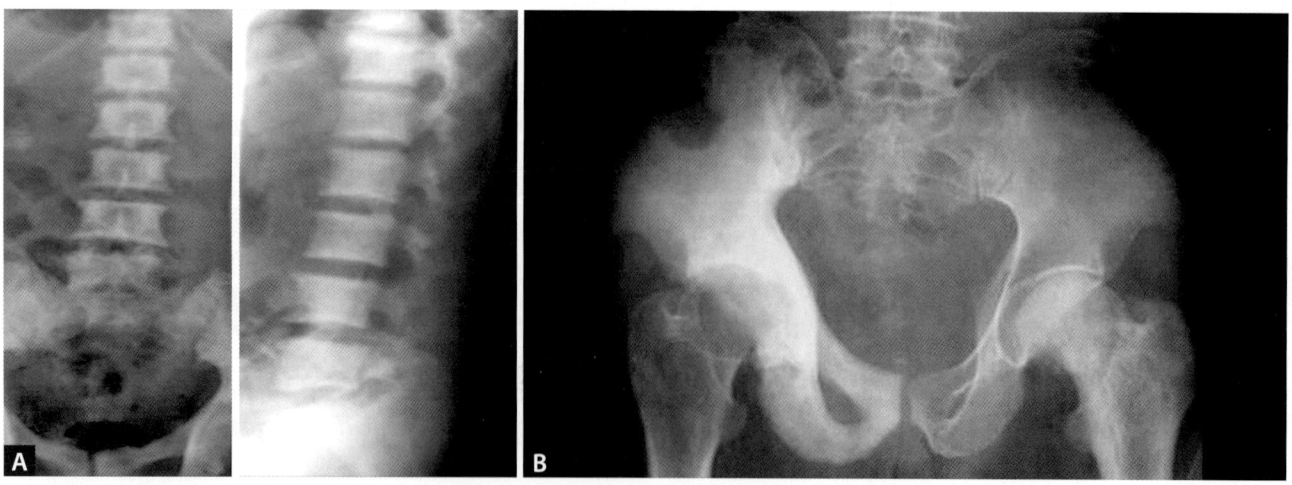

Figs. 29A and B: Metastases from carcinoma prostate: (A) AP and lateral radiographs of the lumbar spine show characteristic osteoblastic metastases; (B) Radiograph of pelvis shows diffuse sclerosis in the right iliac bone and left femoral head.

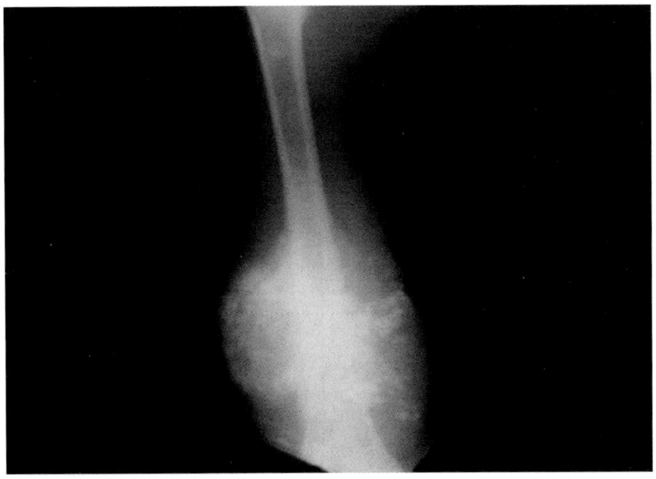

Fig. 30: Metastasis from carcinoma prostate: AP radiograph of the femur shows osteoblastic metastasis with extensive 'sunburst' periosteal reaction resembling osteosarcoma.

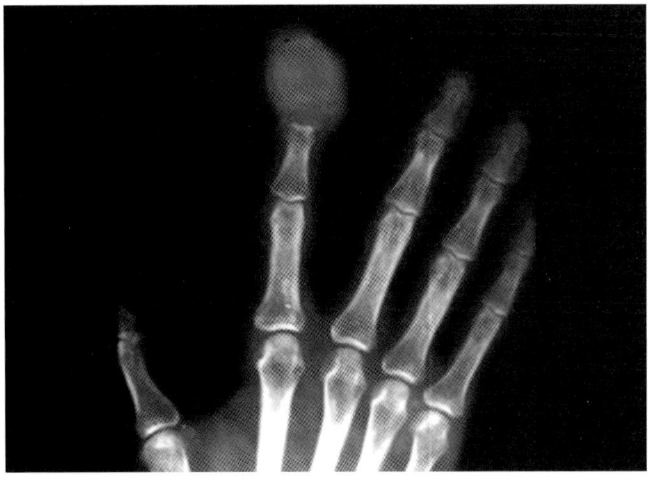

Fig. 31: Metastasis from carcinoma lung: A lytic lesion involves the terminal phalanx of the index finger.

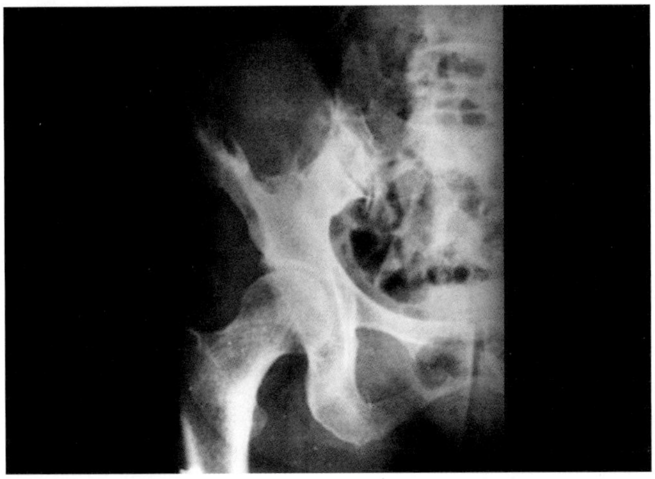

Fig. 32: Metastasis from a hypernephroma. A large lytic lesion is seen in the left iliac blade.

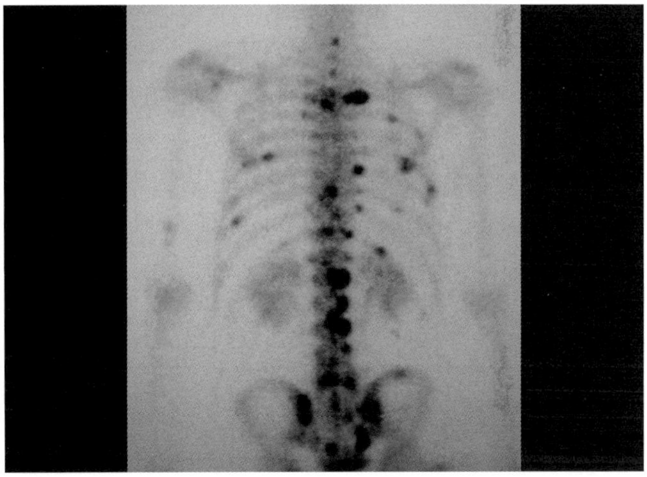

Fig. 33: Skeletal scintigraphy in metastatic disease of the skeleton shows multiple randomly distributed focal lesions scattered throughout the skeleton, particularly the spine, ribs and pelvis.

as individual metastatic lesions may mimic primary malignant tumors of bone. For this purpose, *bone scintigraphy* remains the most cost-effective method.[57] Several patterns of scintigraphic abnormality may be seen. The most common is one of multiple sites of increased skeletal activity typically in the axial skeleton **(Fig. 33)**. The abnormal uptake on scintigraphy depends upon intact local blood flow and increased osteoblastic activity. Lesions which outgrow their blood supply or stimulate no osteoblastic response may appear as photopenic or "cold spots". Occasionally a combination of both 'hot' and 'cold' lesions may be seen. A super scan appearance, i.e. generalized increase in skeletal activity with reduced or absent renal activity is typically seen in diffuse osteoblastic metastatic disease from breast or prostate **(Fig. 34)**.

FDG-PET is more sensitive and specific than bone scan for detecting bone metastases. It detects all types of bone metastases, however, it is more sensitive for detecting lytic metastases than sclerotic metastases. The increased avidity of lytic lesions for FDG is because of the high glycolytic rate and relative hypoxemia that are characteristic of these lesions in contrast to sclerotic lesions, which are relatively acellular, less aggressive and not prone to hypoxia.[9] FDG-PET has the additional advantage of detecting extraskeletal metastatic disease as well.

Sodium Fluoride PET is very sensitive for detecting both osteolytic and osteoblastic lesions and is superior to bone scintigraphy for diagnosing skeletal metastases. Evan Sapir and colleagues compared bone scintigraphy, NaF PET and NaF PET/CT in patients with high risk prostate

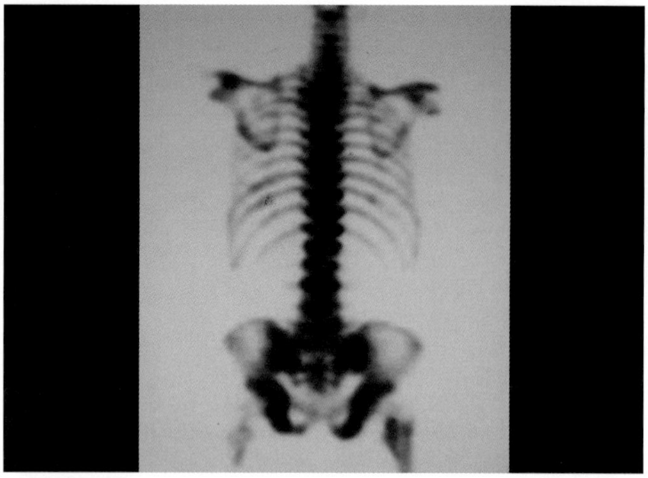

Fig. 34: Technetium-99m bone scintiscan in a case of prostatic carcinoma. This image shows diffuse and intense uptake in most of the bones. Patchy rib lesions are also seen, but renal uptake is absent.

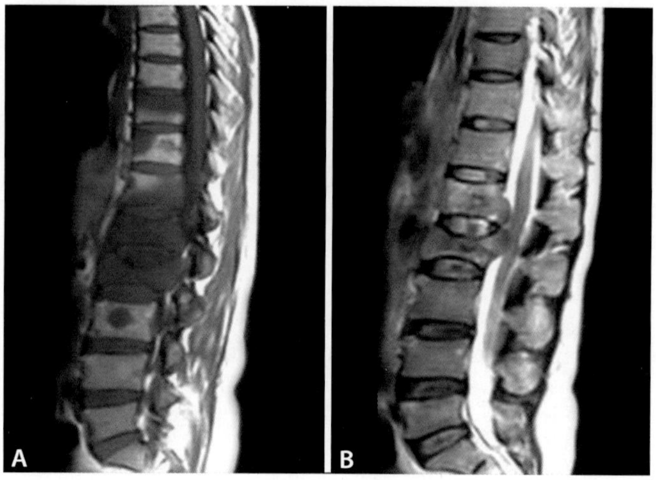

Figs. 35A and B: Skeletal metastases: (A) T1W and (B) T2W sagittal MR images of the lumbar spine in a patient with hypernephroma, show multiple lesions in the vertebrae appearing hypointense on T1W and hyperintense on T2W sequences. The disk spaces are spared even when there is a contiguous involvement of vertebra.

cancer and found that NaF PET/CT was the most accurate modality for detecting bone metastases.[58]

MRI depicts early hematogenous dissemination of the tumor to the bone marrow before reactions in adjacent bone are detectable on ^{99m}Tc scintiscans. Metastatic seeding in the bone marrow is characterized by long T1 relaxation times, whereas T2 relaxation times are variable, depending on tumor morphology. Lesions are seen as focal or diffuse areas of hypointensity on T1-weighted images and as areas of intermediate or high signal intensity on T2-weighted images **(Figs. 35A and B)**. Tumor deposits typically appear hyperintense against a dark background of suppressed signal intensity within fat on STIR images. Osteoblastic metastases may appear hypointense on all pulse sequences. The identification of a 'halo' of high signal intensity around a lesion is a highly specific feature of metastasis on T2W sequences.[59] In vertebrae, additional criteria for malignancy include bulging of the posterior margin of the vertebral body, signal intensity changes that extend into the pedicle and paraosseous tumor spread.

Diffusion weighted MRI is highly sensitive to cellularity and the mobility of free water molecules, which are responsible for the differences between benign and malignant fractures. Using a single-shot echo-planar DWI pulse sequence with a high *b* factor, Chan et al. showed that apparent diffusion coefficient values are useful in differentiating benign osteoporotic fractures from malignant vertebral body compression fractures.[60]

Differential Diagnosis

A solitary metastasis may resemble a primary malignant bone tumor, a primary benign tumor of aggressive nature, e.g. a giant cell tumor, infection and miscellaneous disorders such as Paget's disease. The most important factor in the differential diagnosis is the patient's age. The second important factor is the presence of multiple bone deposits. Other features are the diaphyseal location, involvement of vertebral bodies and then pedicles, the lack of bone expansion, absence of florid periosteal reaction, tumor bone or soft tissue mass. No one investigation, apart from biopsy, can provide a specific diagnosis of a metastasis or its site of origin.

CONCLUSION

Conventional radiographic techniques remain of fundamental importance in the analysis of bone tumors and tumor-like lesions. Radiographic information combined with data concerning the clinical presentation, site of the lesion, and the age of the patient allows formulation of a reasonable diagnosis in most cases. Though CT scan may be preferred to MR imaging in analyzing the internal features and morphology of a lesion, MR imaging has virtually replaced CT in its ability to detect the presence of a lesion and demonstrate its extent with respect to compartmental anatomy, i.e. in the staging of the tumor.

REFERENCES

1. Cobby M, Watt I. Tumours and tumour-like conditions of bone (1). In: Sutton D (Ed). Textbook of Radiology and Medical Imaging, 7th edition. Churchill Livingstone; 2003;2:1247-86.
2. Schajowicz F. Tumours and tumour-like lesions of bones and joints. New York, Springer-Verlag; 1981.
3. Johnson LC. A general theory of bone tumors. Bull NY Acad Med. 1953;29:164-71.
4. Enneking WF. Staging of musculoskeletal neoplasms. Skeletal Radiol. 1985;13:183-94.
5. Nomikos GC, Murphey MD, Kransdorf MD, et al. Primary bone tumors of lower extremities. RCNA. 2002;40:971-90.
6. Stoller DW. Bone and soft tissue tumors in Magnetic Resonance Imaging in Orthopaedics and Sports Medicine, 3rd edn. Lippincott Williams and Wilkins; 2007.
7. Chien-Kuo Wang, Chun-Wei Li, Tsyh-Jyi Hsieh, et al. Characterization of bone and soft-tissue tumors with *in vivo* 1H MR spectroscopy: Initial results. Radiology. 2004;232:599-605.
8. Hayashida Y, Yakushiji T, Awai K, et al. Monitoring therapeutic response of primary bone tumors by diffusion-weighted image: initial results. Eur Radiol. 2006;16:2637-43.
9. Hwang S, Panicek DN. The evolution of musculoskeletal tumour imaging. RCNA. 2009;47(3):435-53.
10. Evan-Sapir E. PET/CT in Malignant bone disease. Sem Musculoskeletal Radiol. 2007;11:312-21.
11. Van der Woude HJ, Van der Shueren G. Ultrasound in musculoskeletal tumours with emphasis on its role in tumour follow up. RCNA. 1999;37(4):753-66.
12. Stoker DJ, Saifuddin A. Bone Tumours (2): Malignant lesions in Grainger and Allison's Diagnostic Radiology. Churchill Livingstone. 2007;3:1059-81.
13. Ellis JH, Siegel CL, Martel W, et al. Radiologic features of well-differentiated osteosarcoma. AJR. 1988;151: 739-42.
14. Kumar N, Daoid R, Madewell JE, et al. Radiographic spectrum of osteogenic sarcoma. AJR. 1991;157:1243-8.
15. Miller SL, Hoffer FA. Malignant and Benign bone tumours. RCNA. 2001;39(4):673-99.
16. Murphey MD, wan Jaovisidha S, Temple HT, et al. Telangiectatic Osteosarcoma: Radiologic-Pathologic Comparison. Radiology. 2003;229:545-53.
17. Edeiken J, Raymond AK, Ayala AG, et al. Small Cell osteosarcoma. Skeletal Radiol. 1987;16:621-8.
18. Choong PF, Pritchard DJ, Rock MG, et al. Low grade central osteogenic sarcoma. A long-term follow-up of 20 patients. Chir Orthop. 1996;322:198-206.
19. Van der Woude HJ, Bloom JL, Hogendoorn PC. Preoperative evaluation and monitoring chemotherapy in patients with high grade osteogenic and Ewing's sarcomas: A review of current imaging modalities. Skeletal Radiology. 1998;27:57-71.
20. Murphey MD, Jelinek JS, Temple HT, et al. Imaging of Periosteal Osteosarcoma: Radiologic-Pathologic Correlation. Radiology. 2004;233:129-38.
21. Okada K, Frassica FJ, Sim FH, et al. Parosteal sarcoma: A clinicopathological study. J Bone Joint Surg. 1994;76A: 366-78.
22. Jelinek JS, Murphey MD, Kransdorf MJ, et al. Parosteal sarcoma: Value of MR imaging and CT in the prediction of histologic grade. Radiology. 1996;201:837-42.
23. Okada K, Kubota H, Ebina T, et al. High grade surface osteosarcoma of the humerus. Skeletal Radiol. 1995;24: 531-4.
24. Parham DM, Pratt CB, Parvey LS, et al. Childhood multifocal osteosarcoma: Clinicopathological and radiologic correlates. Cancer. 1985;55:2653-8.
25. Sheppard DG, Libshitz H. Post radiation sarcomas: a review of the clinical and imaging features in 63 cases. Clin Radio. 2001;56:22-9.
26. Moore TE, King AA, Kathol MH, et al. Sarcoma in Paget disease of bone: Clinical, radiologic, and pathologic features in 22 cases. AJR. 1991;156:1199-203.
27. Murphey MD, Walker EA, Wilson AJ, et al. From the Archives of the AFIP: Imaging of primary chondrosarcoma-radiologic-pathologic correlation. Radiographics. 2003;23:1245-78.
28. Brien EW, Mirra JM, Luck JV Jr. Benign and malignant cartilage tumors of bone and joint: Their anatomic and theoretical basis with an emphasis on radiology, pathology and clinical biology. II. Juxta cortical cartilage tumors. Skeletal Radiol. 1999;28:1-20.
29. Lee YK, Yao L Wirth CR. MR imaging of solitary osteochondromas: Report of eight cases. AJR. 1987;149: 557-60.
30. Nakashuma Y, Unni KK, Shives TC, et al. Mesenchymal chondrosarcoma of bone and soft tissue. A review of 111 cases. Cancer. 1986;57:2444-53.
31. Collins NS, Koyama T, Swee RG, et al. Clear cell chondrosarcoma: Radiographic, computed tomographic and magnetic resonance findings in 34 patients with pathologic correlation. Skeletal Radiol. 2003;32:687-94.
32. Taconis WK, Mulder JD. Fibrosarcoma and malignant fibrous histiocytoma of long bone: Radiographic features and grading. Skeletal Radiol. 1984;11:237-45.
33. Eggli KD, Quiogue T, Moser RP. Ewing's sarcoma. RCNA. 1993;31:325-37.
34. Zelanzny A, Reinus WR, Wilson AJ. Quantitative analysis of the plain radiographic appearance of Ewing's sarcoma of bone. Invest Radiol. 1997;32:59-65.
35. Sailer SL, Harmon DC, Nakin HJ, et al. Ewing's sarcoma: surgical resection as a prognostic factor. Int J Radiat Oncol Biol Phys. 1988;15:43-52.
36. Hoffer FF, Reddick WE, Gronemeyer SA, et al. Dynamic enhanced MR imaging of Ewing's sarcoma. Paediatric Radiol. 2000;30:86.
37. Weshi AS, Allam A, Ajarim D, et al. Extraskeletal Ewing's sarcoma family of tumors in adults: Analysis of 57 patients from a single institution. Clin Oncol. 2010;22:374-81.
38. Yochum TR, Rowe LJ. Tumors and tumor-like processes. In: Yochum TR, Rowe LJ (Eds). Essentials of Skeletal Radiology,

3rd edition. Philadelphia: Lippincott Williams and Wilkins. 2005.pp.1137-72.
39. Papagelopoulos PJ, Mavrogenis AF, Galanis EC, et al. Chordoma of the spine: Clinicopathological features, diagnosis and treatment. Orthopaedics. 2004;27:1256-63.
40. Lomasney LM, Martinez S, Demos TC, Harrelson JM. Multifocal vascular lesions of bone: Imaging characteristics. Skeletal Radiol. 1996;25:255-61.
41. Keenay GL, Unni KK, Beabout JW, et al. Adamantinoma of long bones. A clinicopathological study of 85 cases. Cancer. 1989;64:730-7.
42. Van der Woude HJ, Hazelbag HM, Bloem JL, et al. MRI of adamantinoma of long bones in correlation with histopathology. AJR. 2004;183:1737-44.
43. Singer CRJ. Multiple myeloma. Br Med J. 1997;314:960-3.
44. Dimopoulos M, Terpos E, Comenzo RL, Tosi P, Beksac M, Sezer O, et al. International myeloma working group consensus statement and guidelines regarding the current role of imaging techniques in the diagnosis and monitoring of multiple Myeloma. Leukemia. 2009;23(9):1545-56.
45. Erten N, Saka B, Berberoglu K, et al. Technetium-99m 2-methoxy-isobutyl-isonitrile uptake scintigraphy in detection of the bone marrow infiltration in multiple myeloma: correlation with MRI and other prognostic factors. Ann Hematol. 2007;86(11):805-13.
46. Wiesenthal AA, Nguyen BD. ^{18}F-FDG PET/CT staging of multiple myeloma with diffuse osseous and extra-medullary lesions. Clin Nucl Med. 2007;32(10):797-801.
47. Nanni C, Zamagni E, Cavo M, et al. ^{11}C-choline vs. ^{18}F-FDG PET/CT in assessing bone involvement in patients with multiple myeloma. World J Surg Oncol. 2007;5:68.
48. Walker R, Barlogie B, Haessler J, Tricot G, Anaissie E, Shaughnessy JD Jr. Magnetic resonance imaging in multiple myeloma: Diagnostic and clinical implications. J Clin Oncol. 2007;25(9):1121-8.
49. Durie BG, Salmon SE. A clinical staging system for multiple myeloma. Correlation of measured myeloma cell mass with presenting clinical features, response to treatment, and survival. Cancer. 1975;36(3):842-54.
50. Durie BG, Kyle RA, Belch A, Bensinger W, Blade J, Boccadoro M. Myeloma management guidelines: a consensus report from the Scientific Advisors of the International Myeloma Foundation. Hematol J. 2003;4(6):379-98.
51. Moulopoulos LA, Dimopdulous MA, Weber D, et al. MRI in the imaging of solitary plasmacytoma of bone. J Clin Oncol. 1993;11:1311-5.
52. Tanaka M, Shibui S, Nomura K. Solitary plasmacytoma of the skull: A case report. Jpn J Clin Oncol. 1998;28(10):626.
53. Brandon C, Martel W, Weatherbee L, et al. Case report 572. Osteosclerotic myeloma (POEMS) syndrome. Skeletal Radiol. 1989;18:542.
54. Martinez-Lavin M, Vargas As, Cabre J, et al. Features of hypertrophic osteoarthropathy in patients with POEMS syndrome—A meta-analysis. J Rheumatol. 1997;24:2267.
55. Abrams HL, Sprio R, Goldstein N. Metastasis in carcinoma. Analysis of 1000 autopsied cases. Cancer. 1950;3:74-85.
56. Galasko CSB. The anatomy and pathways of skeletal metastases. In: Weiss L, Gilbert HA (Eds). Bone Metastassis. GK Hall, Boston. 1981.pp.49-63.
57. Rosenthal DI. Radiological diagnosis of bone metastases. Cancer. 1997;80:1595-607.
58. Evan-Sapir E, Mester U, Mishani G, et al. The detection of bone metastases inpatients with high risk prostate cancer: ^{99m}Tc-MDP planar bone scintigraphy, single and multi-field-of-view SPECT, ^{18}Fluoride PET, and ^{18}Fluoride PET/CT. J Nucl Med. 2006;47:287-97.
59. Schweitzer ME, Levine C, Mitchell DG, et al. Bull's eyes and halos: Useful MR discriminators of osseus metastases. Radiology. 1993;188:249-52
60. Chan JH, Peh WC, Tsui EY, Chau LF, Cheung KK, Chan KB, et al. Acute vertebral body compression fractures: discrimination between benign and malignant causes using apparent diffusion coefficients. Br J Radiol. 2002;75(891):207-14.

CHAPTER 200

Magnetic Resonance Imaging of the Knee

Sapna Singh

INTRODUCTION

The knee is one of the important weight-bearing joints capable of performing complex and extensive movements. It is therefore most frequently affected by traumatic and degenerative condition.

Since, its inception magnetic resonance imaging (MRI) has been found to be a very informative imaging method widely accepted by the orthopedic community for evaluating the knee joint. Magnetic resonance imaging should reduce the number of diagnostic arthroscopies and select the patients for therapy oriented arthroscopy.[1,2]

Soft tissue discrimination with MR imaging is excellent and differentiation can be made among cortex, marrow, ligaments, tendons, muscles, synovium, vascular and cartilage elements.[3] This differentiation is not possible with conventional radiographic techniques. Additional advantages of MR imaging are multiplanar and thin section capabilities and the ability to evaluate subchondral bone and marrow. Magnetic resonance is the recommended imaging modality than CT for the evaluation of bone contusions and occult knee fractures, including tibial plateau fractures of the knee. Magnetic resonance has supplanted nuclear scintigraphy in the characterization of osteonecrosis and can be used to assess the integrity of overlying articular cartilage surfaces. Kinematic and dynamic MR techniques provide an improved perspective for assessing the biomechanics of the patellofemoral joint and the normal functions of the ligamentous structures of the knee.

The rapid development of 3T MR imaging has revolutionized musculoskeletal imaging. The gain in the signal-to-noise ratio (SNR) improves image quality with increased signal and higher spatial resolution, there is potential for improved diagnostic accuracy.

The ligamentous and cartilaginous structures are elucidated in better detail on a 3T MR scanner. The smaller structures, such as the posterolateral corner are also assessed better.

IMAGING PROTOCOLS/TECHNICAL FACTORS

An ideal MR technique should yield images with good contrast and spatial resolution of the osseous and soft tissue structures of the knee in a reasonable time to maximize patient acceptability. The use of a dedicated knee coil is mandatory for a quality study because it improves the signal to noise ratio. Using a small field of view (FOV) in the range of 10–14 cm greatly improves the spatial resolution and facilitates optimal assessment of the small anatomical structures of the knee. A matrix of 256 × 256 is usually standard.

Patient Positioning

The patient is placed supine, feet first with the leg in full extension. The knee is placed in 10–15° of external rotation to realign the anterior cruciate ligament parallel with the sagittal imaging plane. This is typically the position of the knee in the relaxed state and no effort at externally rotating the knee needs to be made in the majority of patients. The knee is placed in a dedicated knee coil to produce a uniform signal intensity across the image and foam pads are used to immobilize the knee within the center of the coil. Only one knee can be imaged at a time.

Slice Thickness

Four millimeter sections are used for axial, coronal and sagittal images of the knee.[4] When needed, submillimeter resolution can be obtained with three-dimensional Fourier transformation (3DFT) volume protocols. In the children, 3 mm slices allow optimal medial to lateral joint coverage in the sagittal plane and anterior to posterior coverage in the coronal plane.

Imaging Planes and Pulse Sequences

Acquisition of images in three orthogonal planes is helpful in defining and characterizing abnormalities.[4,5] An axial acquisition through the patellofemoral joint is used as the initial localizer for subsequent sagittal and coronal plane images. Menisci and cruciate ligaments are best evaluated on sagittal images with coronal views for secondary visualization and confirmation of pathology. The medial and lateral collateral ligaments are best displayed on coronal images. The articular cartilage surfaces of medial and lateral compartments are assessed in both coronal and sagittal planes. The patellofemoral joint including patellar facet and trochlear groove is best seen on axial images.

Short echo time (TE) conventional spin-echo (CSE) images generally provide the best contrast for anatomical evaluation. The more rapidly acquired, fast spin-echo (FSE) pulse sequences with short echo train length have no significant disadvantages compared to conventional spin echo techniques in the evaluation of the knee. Three-dimensional Fourier transformation (3DFT) imaging provides the highest spatial resolution with an acceptable signal to noise ratio while allowing image reconstruction in any plane. STIR and fat-saturated FSE pulse sequences are best for the evaluation of bone contusions and other marrow abnormalities. A knee protocol that works well includes fast spin-echo PD and T2W in the sagittal plane, a STIR sequence in the coronal plane, T1W coronal images, T2W axial images and a sequence for articular cartilage.

Intravenous gadolinium is useful in assessment of inflammatory arthritides as it causes enhancement of the pannus. The biomechanics of patellar tracking can be assessed with kinematic technique with a cine loop display of acquired images.

An MR imaging of the knee includes evaluation of the menisci, the anterior and posterior cruciate ligaments, the medial and lateral collateral ligaments, the extensor mechanism of the knee, the articular cartilage and the evaluation of bone marrow.

MENISCI

Magnetic resonance imaging (MRI) is the modality of choice for evaluating a patient with suspected meniscal pathology. By displaying the morphology of meniscal tear MR provides valuable information for determining the need for operative intervention and predicting the feasibility of meniscal repair.

Normal Anatomy

The menisci are C-shaped fibrocartilaginous structures situated within the knee joint between the femoral condyles and the tibial plateau. Functions of the menisci include—transmission of axial and torsional forces across the joint,[6] cushioning of mechanical loading, limitation of comprehensive displacement, distribution of synovial fluid, increasing of the surface area for femoral condylar motion and prevention of synovial impingement.[7]

The periphery of the menisci are thick and convex and attach to the inside of the joint capsule. Facing the intercondylar notch, the meniscus tapers to a thin free edge. Tibial attachments to the meniscus are made through meniscofemoral, meniscotibial and coronary ligaments of the joint capsule.

Microanatomy of the Menisci

The menisci are predominantly made up of type I collagen arranged into bundles. Most of the bundles course circumferentially parallel to the long axis of the meniscus. A smaller number of fibers are oriented in a radial fashion functioning as stabilizing tie fibers. With axial loading of the joint, the circumferential orientation of most of the collagen bundles allows for meniscal deformation, the development of "hoop stresses" and a relatively even distribution of the load across the joint surfaces. Up to one-third of the peripheral meniscus is vascularized and innervated (the "red zone") whereas the remaining inner two-thirds or more is strictly fibrocatilagnious (the "white zone").[6]

Macroanatomy and MRI Appearance

The menisci are C-shaped structures that are conventionally described as having three segments **(Figs. 1A to C)**:

1. Anterior horn
2. Body
3. Posterior horn.

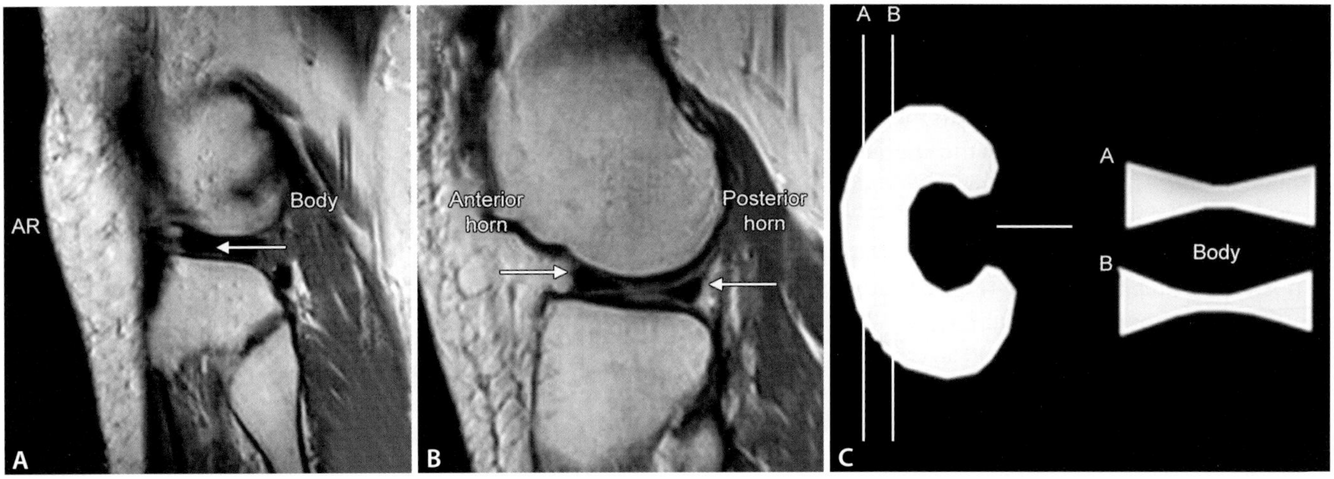

Figs. 1A to C: Sagittal T2W MR images of the knee showing a bow-tie configuration of the body of the lateral meniscus (A) and the symmetric equal size anterior and posterior horns (B); Schematic diagram of the body of the meniscus seen as a bow-tie (C). Normal diffuse low signal intensity of the meniscus is seen throughout—Normal lateral meniscus.

Each meniscus measures approximately 5 mm in height along its periphery and tapers to a thin inner edge and hence shows a triangular shape when cut in cross section **(Fig. 2)**. The upper margin is called the superior articular surface whereas the lower margin is called the inferior articular surface. The superior articular surface is completely visible to the arthroscopist, the inferior to some extent, while the outer nonarticular capsular surface is not seen.

The menisci demonstrate diffusely low signal on all MRI pulse sequences because of their fibrocartilaginous nature. Meniscal pathology is best demonstrated on sequences that use a short echo time TE (<20 millisecond), i.e. T1-weighted, proton density and gradient echo images. If a fast spin echo technique is used, the echo train length should be kept below four to five and the interecho space minimized to reduce the blurring effect inherent to this technique that can obscure a meniscal tear.[8,9] The menisci can also be evaluated by 3D volumetric acquisitions and radial imaging. Radial imaging in which multiple planes are rotated from the center of each meniscus or center of tibia can section portions of both the medial and lateral meniscus in views similar to conventional arthrogram.

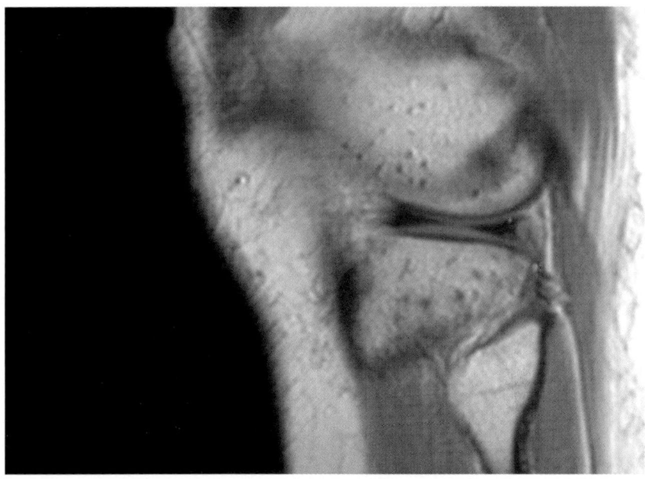

Fig. 2: Sagittal proton density MR image through the lateral meniscus showing the normal triangular shape of the meniscus thick peripherally and tapering to a thin inner edge. The normal meniscus measures 3–5 mm in height along its periphery.

Medial Meniscus

The semicircular medial meniscus has a wide posterior horn, narrows anteriorly and has a more open C-shaped configuration than the more circular lateral meniscus. The anterior horn is roughly 1/3–1/2 as large as the posterior horn on sagittal images. The body of the meniscus is seen as a bow-tie shaped structures on the two most peripheral sagittal slices through the meniscus when 3 or 4 mm thick slices are obtained.[10]

The medial meniscus is attached to the joint capsule along its entire peripheral circumference. It is attached to medial femoral condyle and tibial plateau by the coronary ligament (deep fibers of medial collateral ligament). The less mobile medial meniscus attachment to the deep layer of the MCL and the capsule makes the medial meniscus more susceptible to injury.

Lateral Meniscus

The lateral meniscus forms a tight C-shape (more circular than the medial meniscus) and is symmetric in width from anterior to posterior. The lateral meniscus is relatively mobile, it is more loosely attached to the joint capsule especially along its posterolateral aspect where the popliteus tendon courses through its intra-articular tunnel. There is no direct attachment of the lateral meniscus to the fibular collateral ligament or lateral collateral ligament.

The meniscofemoral ligaments course from the posterior horn of the lateral meniscus, along either side of posterior cruciate ligament (PCL), to attach to the inner margin of the medial femoral condyle. The ligament of Humphrey courses anterior to PCL, whereas the ligament of Wrisberg passes posterior to it. One of these two limbs is present in approximately 70% of the knees and both are present in only 6%.[6]

Anatomic Variants

Discoid Meniscus

A discoid meniscus is a dysplastic meniscus in which the meniscus is disc shaped rather than C-shaped. The lateral meniscus is most commonly affected with a reported incidence of around 3%. Often a discoid meniscus is enlarged and affects the anterior or posterior horns of the meniscus asymmetrically. On sagittal images using 4–5 mm slice thickness, a discoid meniscus exhibits a continuous or bow-tie appearance on three or more consecutive images **(Figs. 3A to C)**. Central tapering seen in normal menisci is lost in discoid fibrocartilage. Coronal images show the extension of the discoid meniscus apex towards or into the intercondylar notch. Although often encountered incidentally, discoid menisci are more prone to undergo cystic degeneration with subsequent tears and multiple tears within the same meniscus are not uncommon.[11]

Meniscus Flounce (Buckled Meniscus)

Occasionally, the medial meniscus demonstrates an undulating or buckled appearance on sagittal MR images. This redundancy is a normal variant that is related, at least in part to knee position. Close inspection of the meniscus is needed, however because a meniscal tear may occasionally result in a similar appearance.[12]

Meniscal Ossicle

This is an embryologic variant or sequelae of prior trauma. It is a small focus of ossification within the meniscus and usually involves the posterior horn of the medial meniscus.[13] Although mostly asymptomatic, a meniscal ossicle may cause mechanical symptoms or pain and can be mistaken for a loose body on radiographs or MRI.

ABNORMAL MENISCUS

Meniscal Degenerations and Tears

The rotation of femur against a fixed tibia during flexion and extension places the menisci at risk for injury. Degeneration and tears of the meniscus demonstrate increased signal attributed to the imbibed synovial fluid.

MR Grading of Meniscal Tears

The MRI diagnosis of a meniscal tear is based on the alteration of intrameniscal signal characteristic. A MRI grading system divides increased intrameniscal signal into three grades according to their configuration and relation to articular surface.[14]

Grade 1: In Grade 1 a nonarticular focal or globular intra-substance increased signal is seen **(Fig. 4)**. Histologically,

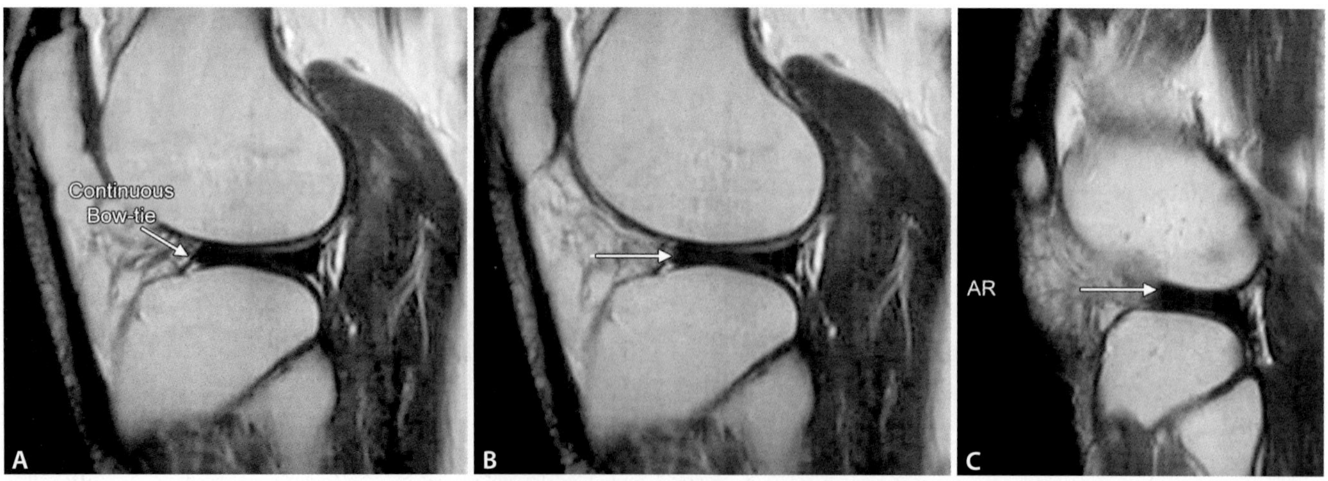

Figs. 3A to C: Consecutive 4 mm T2W sagittal MR images through the lateral meniscus showing a continuous bow-tie appearance on three sections—Discoid meniscus.

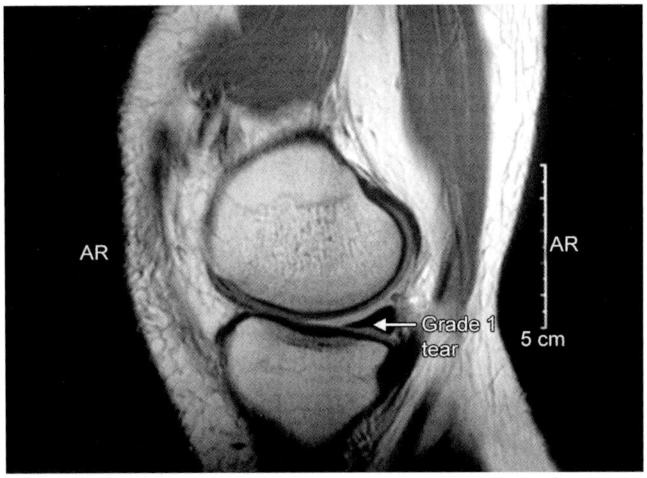

Fig. 4: Proton density sagittal MR image showing intrasubstance focal/globular increased signal within the posterior horn of the medial meniscus—Grade 1 meniscal signal.

grade 1 signal intensity correlates with foci of early mucinous degeneration and chondrocyte deficient or hypocellular regions. Grade 1 signal intensity may be observed in asymptomatic athletes and normal volunteers and is not clinically significant.[15]

Grade 2: In Grade 2 a horizontal, linear intrasubstance increased signal extends from the capsular periphery of the meniscus but does not involve an articular meniscal surface **(Figs. 5A and B)**. Areas and bands of mucinous degeneration are more extensive in Grade 2 than in Grade 1.

Grade 3: A meniscus is considered Grade 3 when the area of increased signal intensity communicates or extends to at least one articular surface **(Figs. 6A and B)**.

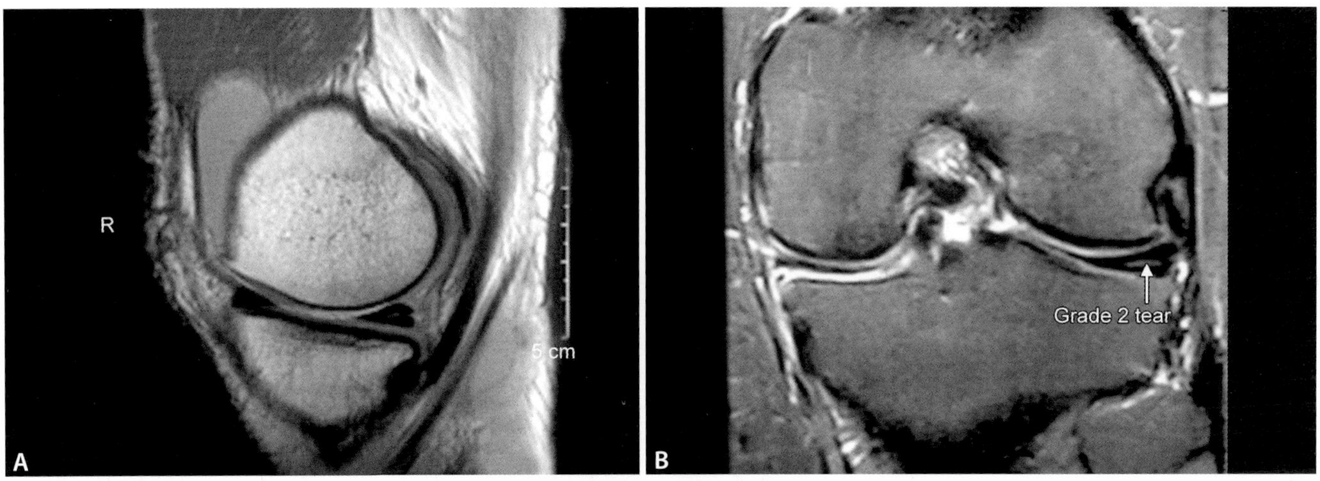

Figs. 5A and B: T2W sagittal MR image (A) and STIR coronal image (B) showing a horizontal, linear intrasubstance increased signal extending from the capsular periphery of the meniscus but not involving an articular meniscal surface—Grade 2 meniscal signal.

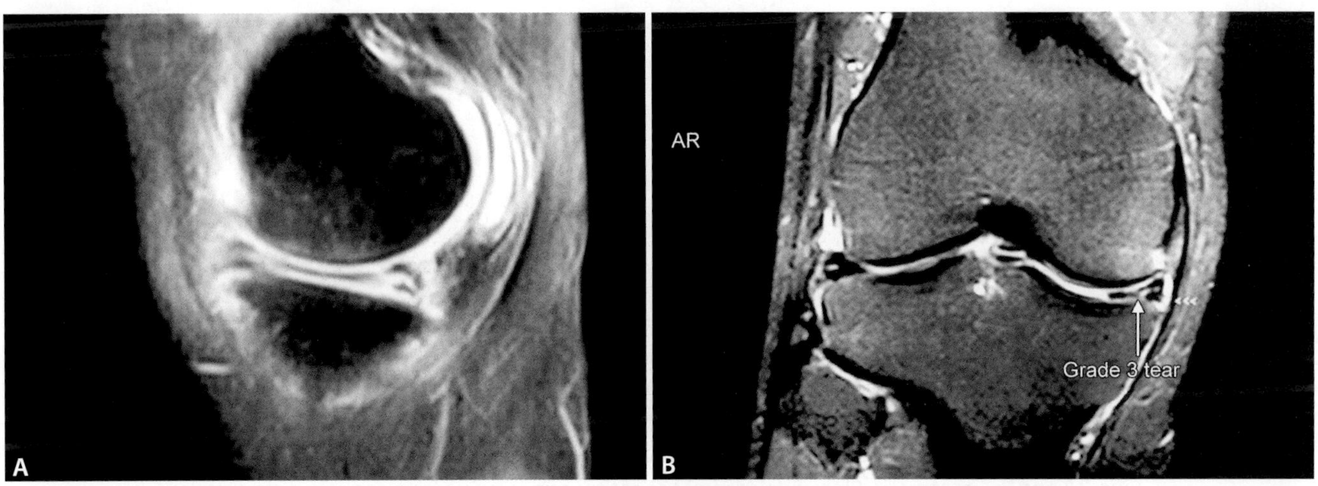

Figs. 6A and B: T2W fat-suppressed sagittal (A) and STIR coronal (B) MR images showing increased signal intensity within the meniscus communicating or extending to the inferior articular surface—Grade 3 meniscal signal.

Abnormal Morphology

In addition to abnormal signal intensity the morphology, i.e. size and shape of the meniscus should be assessed when evaluating meniscal lesions. The normal meniscus measures 3–5 mm in height. The medial meniscus varies in width from 6 mm at the anterior horn to 12 mm at the posterior horn. The lateral meniscus is approximately 10 mm in width throughout its length. Irregularity of the meniscal margin, a focal defect in one of its articular surfaces or an abnormally small meniscal segment may be indicative of a tear **(Figs. 7A and B)**. Focal step like contour deformities and wedge defects in the contour of the articular surface "Notch sign" may be the only sign present in some tears.[16] If a smaller than normal meniscal segment is observed, a thorough search should be performed to identify a displaced fragment.

CLASSIFICATION OF MENISCAL TEARS

Meniscal tears are divided into two basic types: vertical and horizontal. Vertical tears are often of a traumatic origin whereas horizontal tears are usually secondary to meniscal degeneration. Vertical tears are further subdivided into radial (perpendicular to the long axis of the meniscus) and longitudinal (parallel to the long axis) varieties **(Fig. 8)**.

Horizontal Tears

A horizontal or oblique tear extends through the meniscus along a plane parallel to the tibial plateau, separating the meniscus into superior and inferior fragments **(Fig. 9)**. Also called a horizontal cleavage tear this is the most common type of tear to be associated with a meniscal cyst.[17] The cyst occurs as a result of fluid extending through the tear by a ball valve effect and collecting either within the meniscus (intrameniscal cyst) **(Figs. 10A and B)** or at the meniscocapsular junction (parameniscal cyst) **(Figs. 11A and B)**. If a cyst is seen along the meniscocapsular junction an underlying meniscal tear should be excluded because the cysts tend to recur after resection if the underlying tear is not repaired. There are three criteria for the diagnosis of a meniscal cyst:

1. Horizontal tear
2. Fluid accumulation bright on T2
3. Flat lining against the outside margin of the meniscus.

The connection with the joint space is often lost, so they do not fill with contrast on MR arthrography. The synovial fluid is absorbed and is replaced by a gelatinous substance.

Radial/Free Edge Tears

Radial tears extend perpendicular to the long axis of the meniscus. These range from a small injury along its free edge to a large tear extending through its entire circumference. Magnetic resonance images obtained perpendicular to the orientation of a radial tear demonstrate the tear as a small gap or cleft in the meniscus *(cleft sign)* which can sometimes be observed to move across the meniscus on successive images *(marching cleft sign)*.[18] If the orientation of the imaging plane is in the same direction as a full thickness radial tear, a section through the same plane of the tear will demonstrate an absent meniscus or high signal intensity resulting in the so called *ghost sign*. A partial thickness radial tear will demonstrate blunting or abrupt truncation of the apex of the meniscus *(truncated triangle sign)*. A full thickness

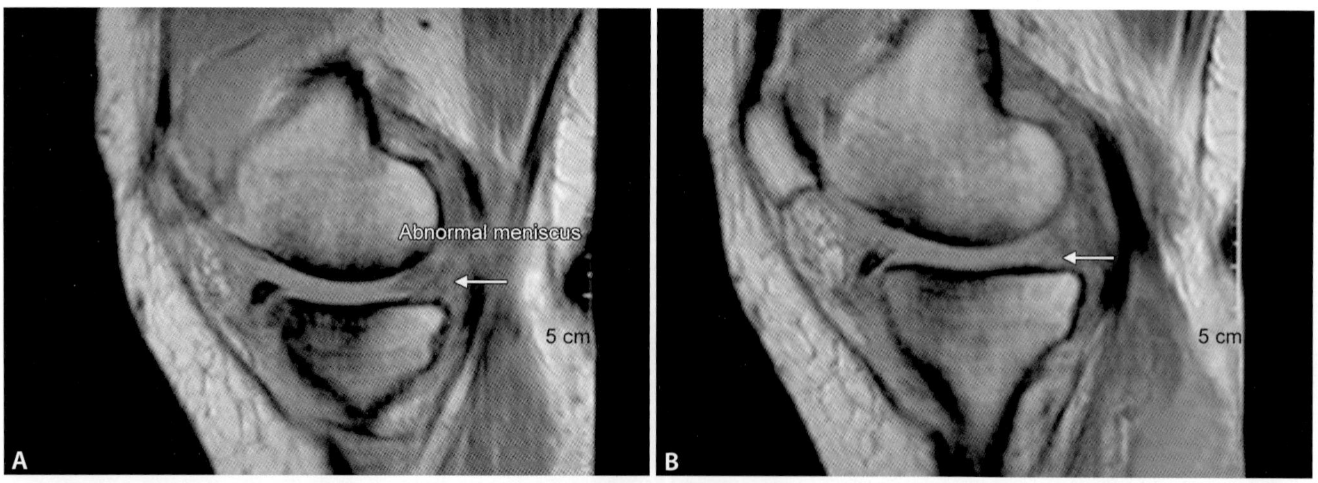

Figs. 7A and B: Consecutive PD sagittal MR images of the knee showing irregularity and abnormally small posterior horn of the medial meniscus suggestive of a tear.

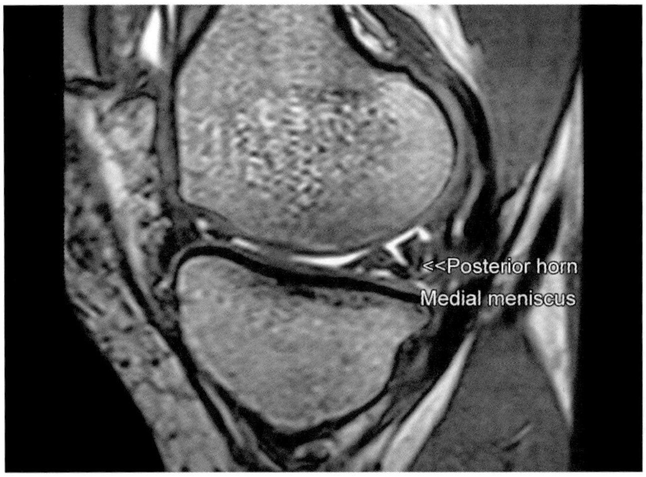

Fig. 8: Double echo steady state (DESS) sequence sagittal MR image showing a vertical longitudinal tear of the posterior horn of the medial meniscus seen as a vertically oriented linear focus of abnormal signal intensity within the substance of the meniscus along its long axis.

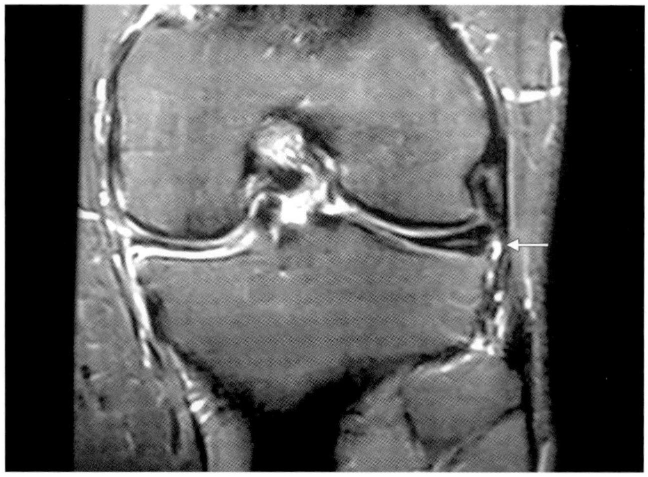

Fig. 9: STIR coronal MR image showing a horizontal tear in the body of the lateral meniscus.

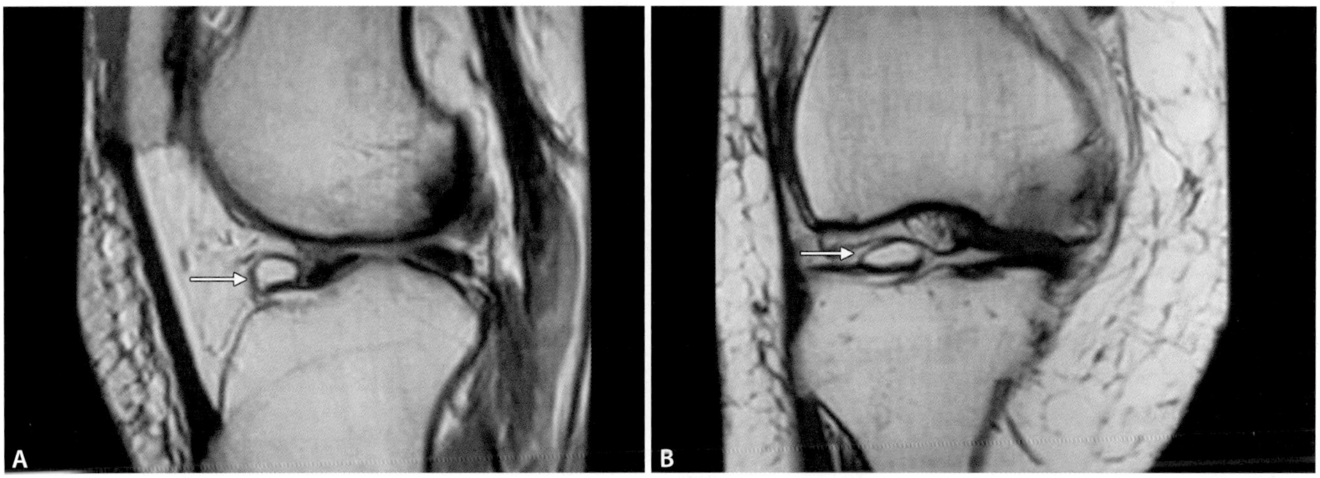

Figs. 10A and B: Sagittal and coronal MR images showing a meniscal cyst giving a slightly swollen appearance to the meniscus.

radial tear severely compromises meniscal function by disrupting the critical circumferential collagen bundles such that the meniscus can no longer develop the "hoop stresses" necessary to disperse an axial load.[19] The middle third of the lateral meniscus is a common location for radial tears, probably because of its more circular shape and decreased radius of curvature, its increased mobility and excessive loading during valgus stress.

Root tears: Root tears are full thickness radial tears at the central tibial attachments of the menisci. Radial tears should be suspected in cases of peripheral subluxation of the involved meniscus.[20] On posterior coronal MR images abrupt loss or blunting of the normal meniscotibial attachment and foreshortening of the meniscus towards the posterior aspect of the intercondylar notch are seen.

Longitudinal Tears

Vertical longitudinal tears make up the common bucket handle tear that occurs in about 10% of meniscal tears. The normal meniscus has a body width of about 9 mm, which is seen on sagittal images as a single slab of meniscal tissue that has a shape similar to a bow-tie. When the inner edge of the meniscus displaces, a bucket handle tear is easily diagnosed by noting only one instead of the normal two body segments present on the outermost sagittal images through the meniscus. This is called the *"absent bow-tie*

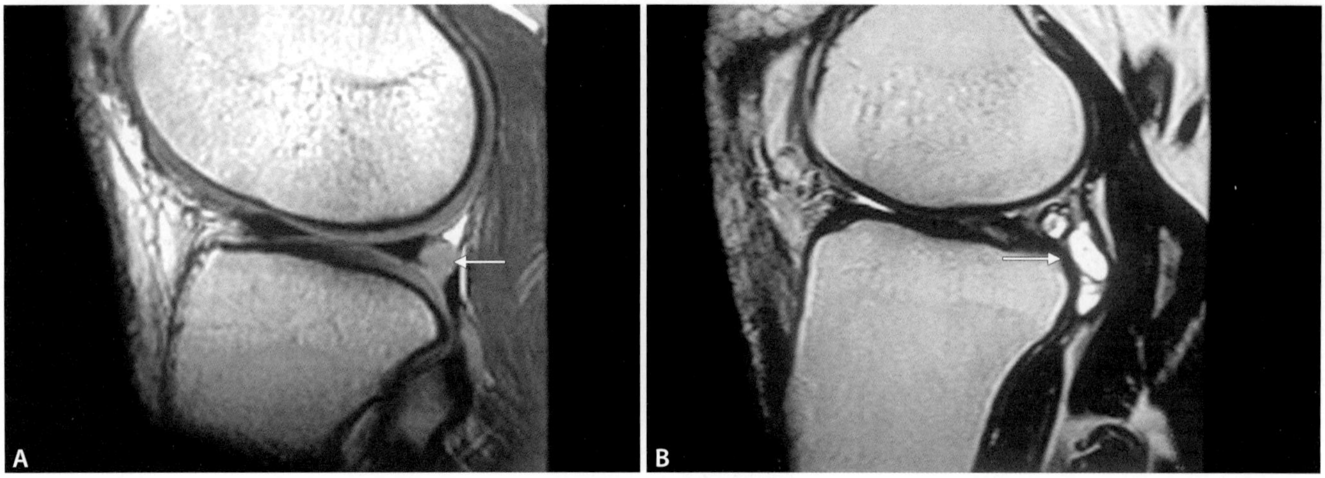

Figs. 11A and B: Sagittal PD (A) and T2W (B) MR images showing a fluid signal intensity structure at the meniscocapsular junction—Parameniscal cyst.

sign"[10] and may be the only indication of a bucket handle tear. Normally, there are only two structures in the intercondylar fossa, the anterior and the posterior cruciate ligament. Any other structure in the intercondylar fossa is abnormal and a displaced meniscal fragment is the most likely possibility. A displaced meniscal fragment, usually, but not always, can be found, especially in the intercondylar notch and a careful inspection for a fragment should always be made when only one body segment is seen on the sagittal images **(Fig. 12)**.[21,22] The displaced meniscal fragment can lie in front of the posterior cruciate ligament (PCL) which is called a "double PCL sign" **(Figs. 13A to C)**. The displaced fragment may also flip over the anterior horn of the affected meniscus which is called an *"anterior flipped meniscus sign"*. On coronal images a truncated appearance of the meniscus may be seen **(Figs. 14A to C)**. A new sign has been described recently for the diagnosis of bucket handle tears called the *"V sign"*. The V sign is seen on the axial images and is seen at the junction of the displaced fragment and the meniscus, which is in place. The acute angle created accounts for the appearance as an inverted V. The V sign, when seen on axial images, is highly suggestive of a bucket handle tear.[23]

Peripheral Tears

If a tear is confined to the outer one-third of the meniscus, it is described as a peripheral tear because this changes the therapeutic plan for the patient. Except for the peripheral 10–25% of the meniscus which is supplied by the perimeniscal capillary plexus the meniscus in adults is relatively avascular. Because of the rich vascularity in peripheral portion of the meniscus (red zone), this type of tear is more likely to heal with conservative therapy or operative repair, whereas tears confined to the inner white zone of the meniscus (avascular) have to be debrided or resected.[24]

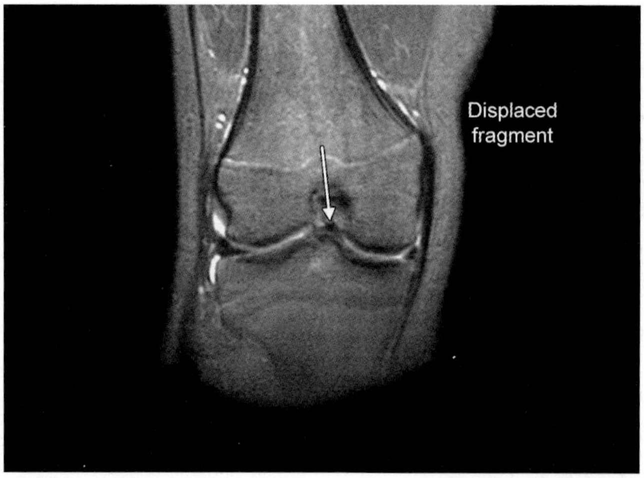

Fig. 12: STIR coronal MR image showing the displaced fragment lying within the intercondylar notch—Bucket handle tear of the medial meniscus.

Meniscocapsular Separation

A meniscocapsular separation refers to an injury in which the meniscus separates from the adjacent capsule. This can lead to meniscal instability if unrecognized and is most commonly seen along the medial meniscus, which is more tightly adherent to the joint capsule. It can also occur along the posterolateral corner of the joint where the lateral meniscus is attached by the popliteal meniscal fascicles. This injury is diagnosed when true fluid signal intensity is seen interposed between the meniscus and

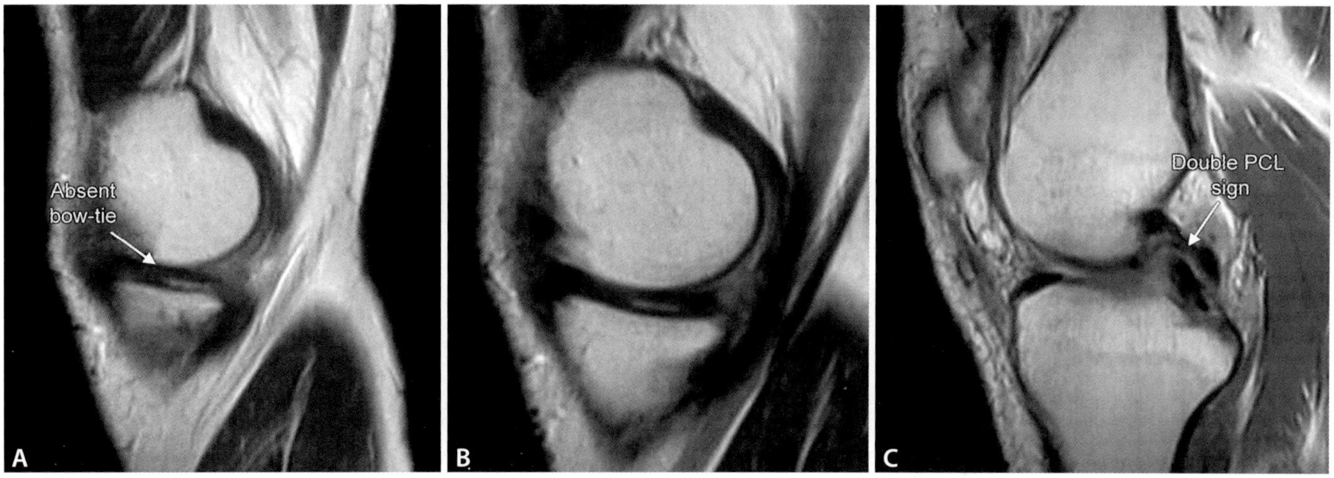

Figs. 13A to C: T2W sagittal MR images showing *Absent bow-tie* sign (A and B) and a displaced meniscal fragment beneath the posterior cruciate ligament designated as a *double PCL* sign (C); Bucket handle tear of the medial meniscus.

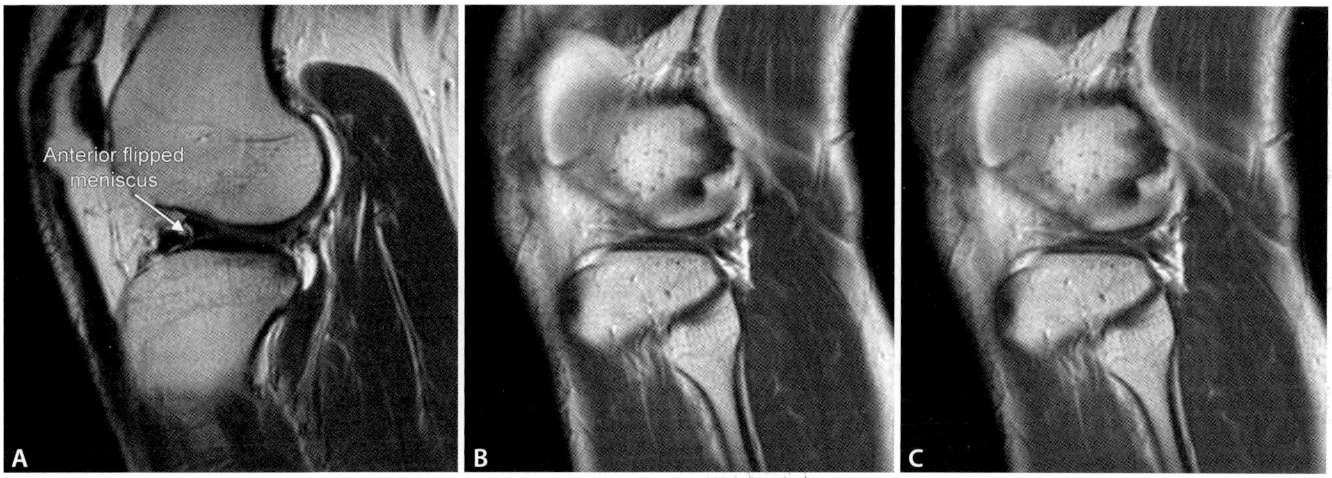

Figs. 14A to C: T2W sagittal MR images showing the displaced fragment flip over the anterior horn of the lateral meniscus (A) with an absent bow-tie sign (B and C); Bucket handle tear of the lateral meniscus.

adjacent capsule or when the popliteal meniscal fascicles are disrupted.

IMAGING CHALLENGES

Although MRI is extremely accurate in diagnosing meniscal pathology, there are numerous imaging pitfalls and artifacts that may simulate a tear and lead to an erroneous diagnosis. These are especially common in the posterior horn of the lateral meniscus.

Potential Pitfalls

Transverse Intrameniscal Ligament

On sagittal scans, the attachment of the transverse ligament to the anterior horn of the medial or lateral meniscus may be mistaken for a tear. This pitfall is avoided by following the meniscal fragment on successive sagittal scans, recognizing that it is contiguous with the normal ligament coursing across the infrapatellar fat.

Meniscofemoral Ligaments

Similarly, the attachment of the meniscofemoral ligaments of Humphrey or Wrisberg to the posterior horn of the lateral meniscus may be mistaken for a tear on sagittal scans. Again, examination of sequential sagittal or appropriate coronal scans should allow for accurate diagnosis.[25]

Popliteus Tendon

There is usually at least a small amount of fluid within the popliteus tendon sheath that can be mistaken for a tear at the junction of the posterior horn and body of the lateral meniscus on sagittal or coronal scans.[26]

Magic Angle Effect

The posterior horn of the lateral meniscus courses slightly upwards as it extends into the posterior intercondylar notch. As a result, artifactually increased signal may be seen within the meniscus on short TE sequences because of the magic angle artifact. This is due to the magic angle phenomenon caused by 55 degree orientation of this meniscus with respect to the static magnetic field. The signal, however, is often of a rather diffuse nature and disappears on long TE images (>40 milliseconds).[27]

Pulsation Artifact from the Popliteal Artery

Phase artifacts propagating from the popliteal artery may mimic a tear in the posterior horn of the lateral meniscus on sagittal scans. Misdiagnosis can be avoided by recognizing the alternating lines of increased and decreased signal propagating across the entire image at that level.

Surgical Considerations in Meniscal Tear

When faced with a meniscal tear, the surgeon has three options: (i) leave the tear alone, (ii) attempt a primary meniscal repair, (iii) perform a partial or complete meniscectomy. The paramount goal is to preserve as much meniscal tissue as possible to lessen the probability of developing osteoarthritis.[28] Several features have been shown to be correlated with a higher probability of a successful meniscal repair and these features should be included in the MRI report by the radiologist.

Tear Location

The most important factor in predicting the success of a meniscal repair is where the tear is located in the meniscus, e.g. a tear in the periphery of the meniscus (within 3 mm of its capsular surface) has the highest probability for healing because of the excellent vascularity in that region.[24]

Blind spots for the arthroscopist include the anterior horn of each meniscus, the extreme inner portion of the posterior horn of the medial meniscus, and the undersurface of both menisci. It is also important to describe any meniscal tissue that has become displaced into a para-articular "gutter" so that the arthroscopist is able to probe for and resect the fragment, which might otherwise be missed.

Tear Morphology and Length

Vertical longitudinal tears have the best prognosis for healing because they do not disrupt the circumferential collagen bundles that are important for maintaining normal meniscal function.

Small partial tears (involving less than half the height of the meniscus) and radial tears measuring less than 5 mm in length also have a higher rate of healing than do larger tears.[24,29] A radial tear extending through the meniscus to the capsule is essentially unrepairable because of the complete disruption of the circumferential collagen bundles. Most horizontal tears are also not amenable to repair and the surgeon typically resects either the superior or inferior flap, leaving the other *in situ*.

Accuracy of MR in the Diagnosis of Meniscal Tears

The accuracy of MR imaging of meniscal tears is greater than 90% in most series and the negative predictive value approaches 100%.[30,31] An additional advantage of MR imaging is the ability to evaluate extra-articular cause of knee pain masquerading as meniscal disease.

LIGAMENTS AND TENDONS OF THE KNEE

Excellent spatial resolution and unparalleled contrast resolution have allowed MRI to emerge as the dominant imaging modality for diagnosis of ligament and tendon pathology of the knee joint. There are several mechanisms of injury associated with ligament and tendon disruptions, a knowledge of which enables the radiologist to analyze systematically the structures of the knee affected and maximize the detection of pathology.

CENTRAL STRUCTURES OF THE KNEE

Anatomy of Anterior Cruciate Ligament

The anterior cruciate ligament (ACL) provides central support of the knee joint, contributing the most significant stabilizing mechanism against excessive anterior translation of the tibia. The ACL is a fan-shaped structure, with a tightly bound femoral attachment that expands broadly at the tibial attachment. The ACL is 11 mm wide and 31–38 mm long. The individual fascicles of the ACL are divided into two longitudinal fiber bundles, the longer and stronger anteromedial bundle (AMB) and the shorter posterolateral bundle (PLB).[32]

MR Appearance of ACL

T2W sagittal 3–4 mm thickness images are recommended for evaluating the ACL. It is also well-visualized on the axial and coronal images. The normal ACL has straight, taut fibers that run parallel to the roof of the intercondylar notch **(Figs. 15A and B)**. It typically has a striated

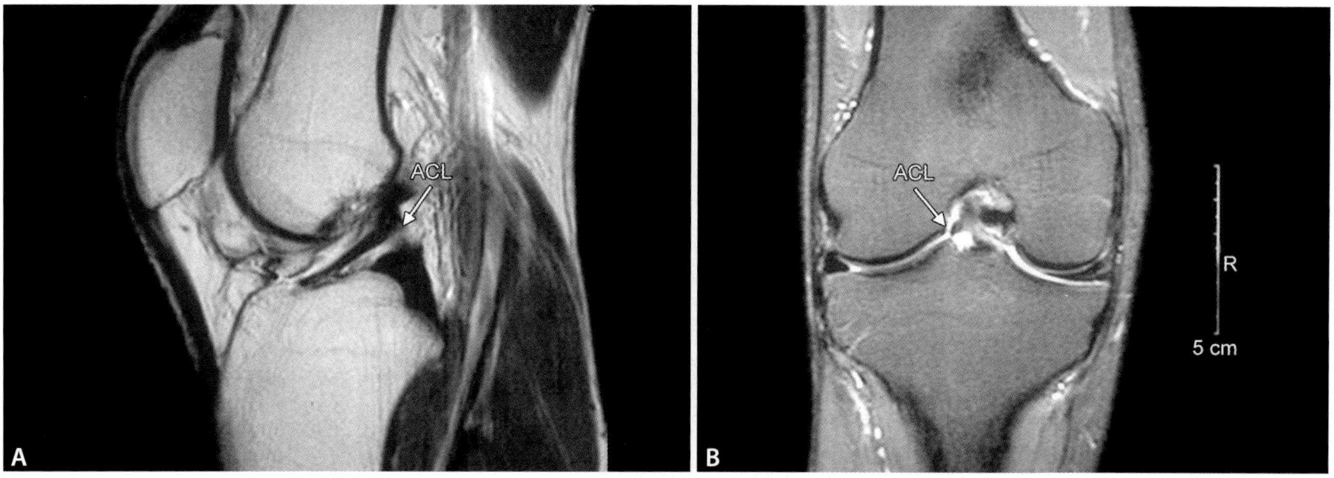

Figs. 15A and B: T2W sagittal MR image (A) of the knee depicting the normal ACL with straight, taut fibers that run parallel to the roof of the intercondylar notch. STIR coronal MR image (B) showing the ACL as a triangular structure within the notch.

appearance with some high signal within it especially at its insertion on the tibia.

ACL Tears

The most common mechanism of ACL tear is external rotation of femur on a fixed tibia combined with valgus force (i.e. twisting injury).

On MRI, an ACL tear is diagnosed by alterations in signal intensity, morphology and the course of the ligament. An increased signal intensity within the ACL on proton density and T2W images indicates an acute or subacute injury. A cloud like or amorphous mass of increased signal intensity may be evident within the ligament reflecting edema or hemorrhage **(Figs. 16A and B)**.

A complete ACL tear can be diagnosed when the ligament is either absent (*"empty notch sign"* in coronal images) **(Figs. 17A and B)** or discontinuous. An irregular or wavy contour and disruption of fibers also suggests a complete tear.[33]

Indirect Signs of ACL Tear

- Buckling (abnormal high arc) of the posterior cruciate ligament giving rise to a "question mark" configuration **(Fig. 18)**
- Undulation and redundancy of the patellar tendon
- *Uncovered lateral meniscus sign:* This sign is positive if a vertical line drawn tangentially to the most posterior margin of the lateral tibial plateau intersects any part of the posterior horn of the lateral meniscus. A positive uncovered lateral meniscus sign indicates that the lateral meniscus does not subluxate anteriorly with the tibia in an ACL injury
- Anterior tibial subluxation larger than 5 mm with respect to femur is a very sensitive and specific sign of complete ACL tear. If the distance between two parallel lines drawn tangential to the posterior lateral femoral condyle and posterior lateral tibial plateau is more than 5 mm, it is a sensitive ancillary sign of complete ACL tear **(Figs. 19A and B)**. This sign offers improved discrimination of complete from partial tears which is clinically important since the presence of partial tear is not considered an indication for surgical reconstruction.[34]
- Lateral notch sign in which the deep lateral femoral notch exceeds 2 mm in depth.
- Bone bruises/contusions in the midportion of the lateral femoral condyle and posterior portion of the lateral tibial plateau.[35,36] These so called kissing contusions are representative of edema and hemorrhage caused by impaction trabecular microfractures that occur when the ACL ruptures **(Figs. 20A to C)**.
- Avulsion fracture of the lateral tibial rim (Segond fracture) is also suggestive of ACL tear.
- Joint effusion/hemarthrosis is a common finding associated with ACL injuries[37] **(Fig. 20C)**.
- A tibial spine avulsion is an uncommon but specific finding for ACL injury. Chronic tears of ACL may present with slumping of the distal fragment over the tibial indicating increased laxity of the ligament which may also be attenuated. In chronic tears, edema and synovitis are usually not present. MR also has an important role in defining partial tears of the ACL because these injuries are difficult to differentiate from complete ACL tears clinically. The detection of a discrete area or focus of increased signal intensity

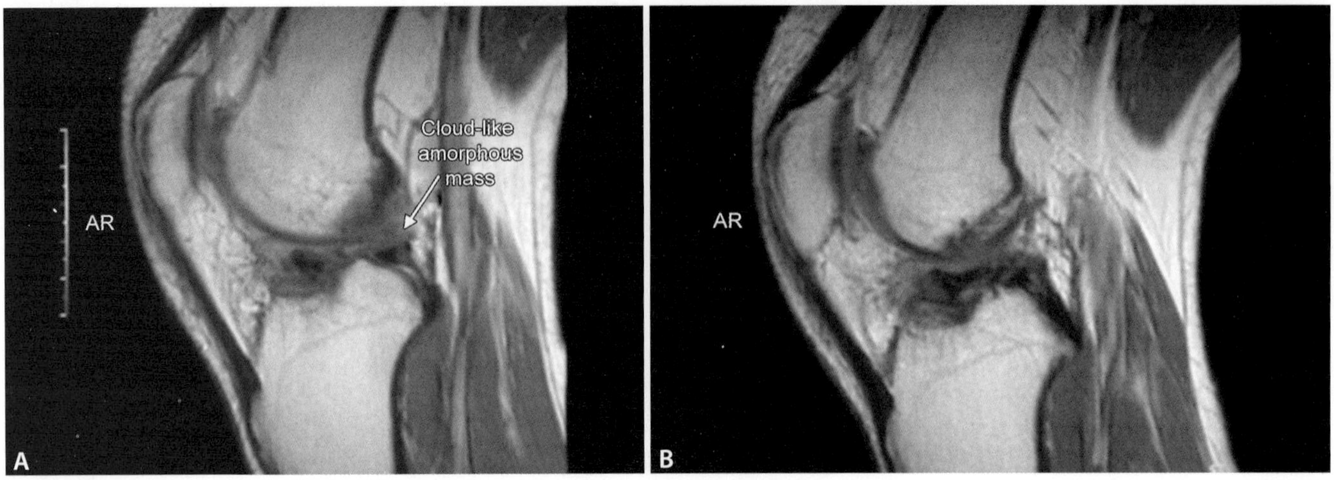

Figs. 16A and B: T2W sagittal MR images of the knee showing complete disruption of ACL fibers with a cloud-like amorphous mass of increased signal intensity in the region of ACL reflecting edema and hemorrhage—Complete ACL tear

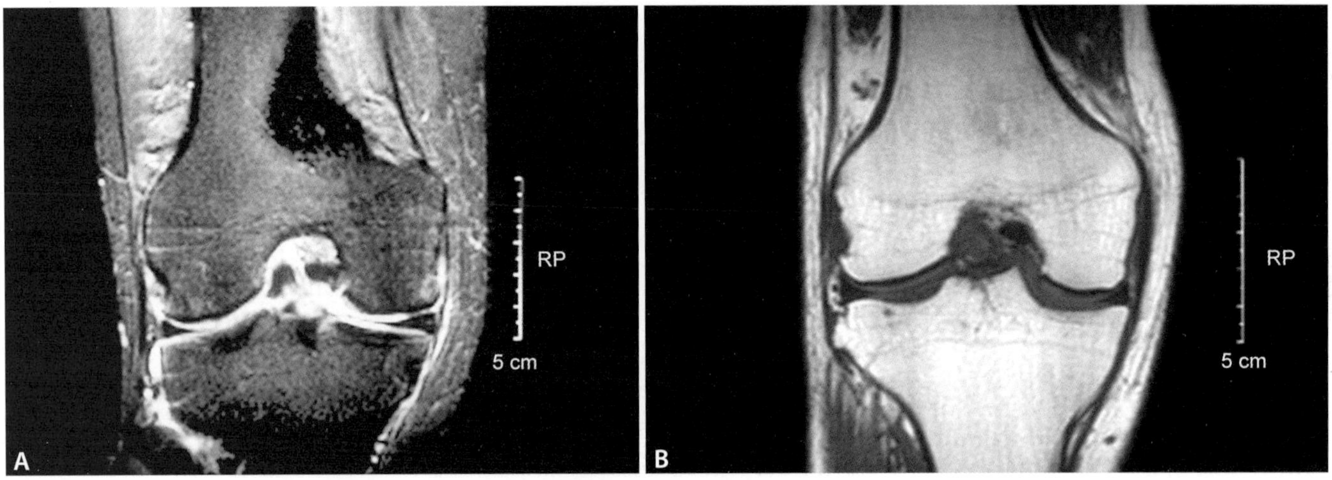

Figs. 17A and B: STIR coronal image (A) of the knee showing normal ACL and PCL in the intercondylar notch. T1W coronal image (B) shows the anterior cruciate ligament to be absent ("empty notch" sign) in a case of ACL tear.

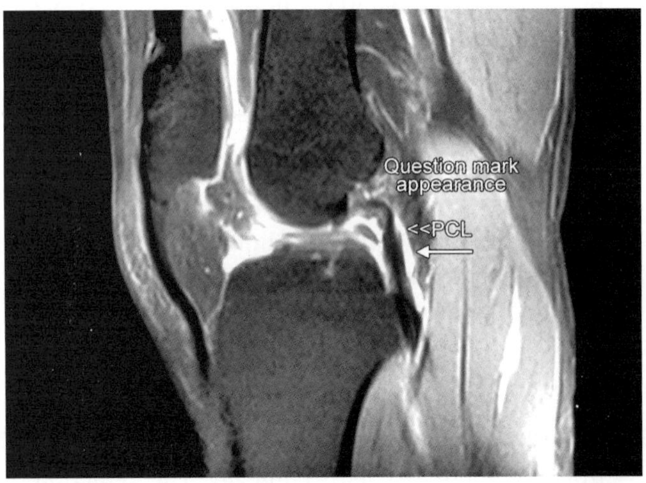

Fig. 18: T2W fat-suppressed sagittal image of knee showing abnormal high arc (buckling) of the posterior cruciate ligament giving rise to a "question mark" configuration (arrow)—Indirect sign of ACL tear.

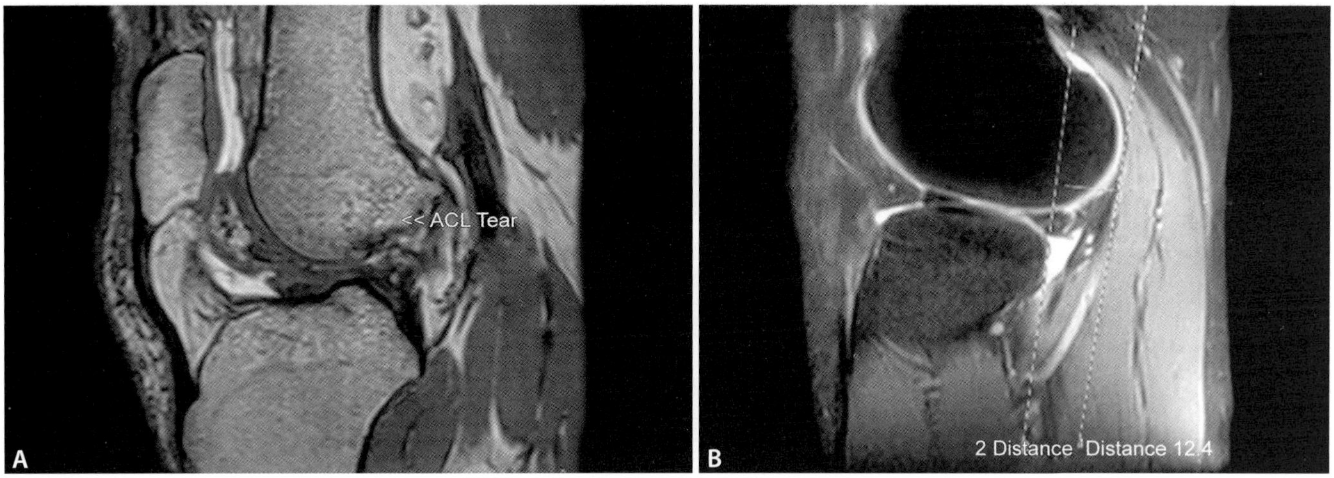

Figs. 19A and B: DESS sagittal (A) and T2W fat-suppressed sagittal (B) MR images of the knee showing cloud-like amorphous mass of increased signal in the region of ACL with anterior tibial translation larger than 5 mm with respect to femur—Indirect sign of complete ACL tear.

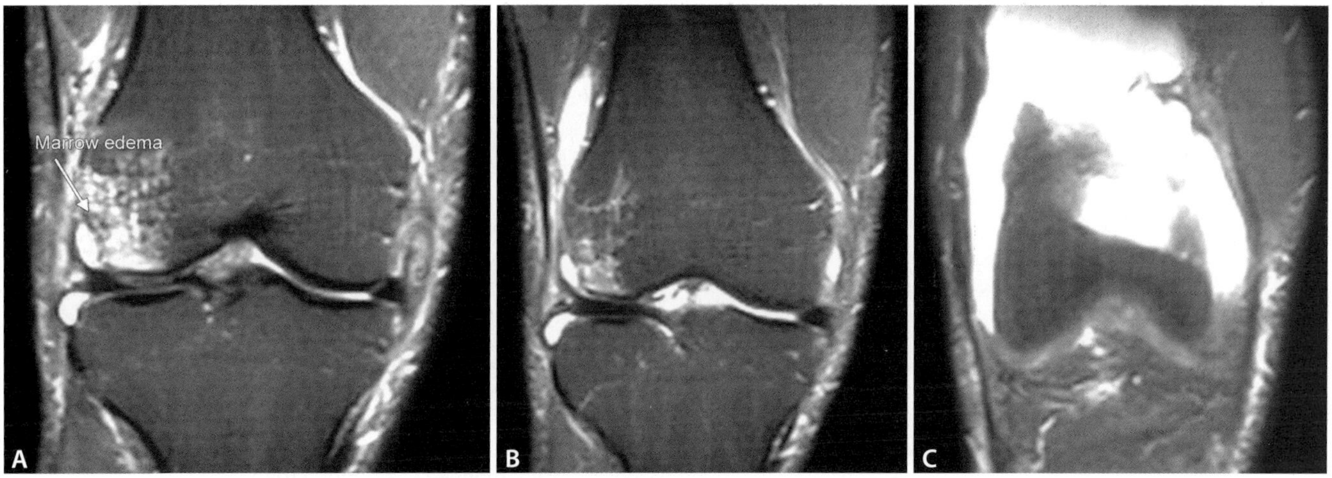

Figs. 20A to C: STIR coronal MR images of the knee showing marrow edema in the lateral femoral condyle and suprapatellar joint effusion—Indirect signs of ACL tear.

within the substance of the ACL is consistent with a diagnosis of partial tear **(Figs. 21A and B)**. In partial tear, although the bulk of the ligament appears to be intact with a relatively normal axis, there may be localized angulation of the ligament at the site of fiber disruption. False-negative diagnosis may result from the formation of scar tissue with adherence of anterior cruciate ligament to the post cruciate ligament simulating a normal course and signal of the anterior cruciate ligament. Foci of myxoid degeneration within the anterior cruciate ligament, partial volume averaging with the lateral femoral condyle and periligamentous or intraligamentous fat should be differentiated from partial ACL tears to avoid false-positive diagnosis.

O'Donoghue triad: A triad of ACL injury associated with medial collateral ligament disruption and medial meniscus tear is known as O'Donoghue triad **(Figs. 22A to C)**.

Accuracy of MR in ACL Tears

Accuracy of MRI for the ACL is extremely high approaching 95–100% in almost all reported series.[4]

Posterior Cruciate Ligament

Anatomy of the PCL

The posterior cruciate ligament (PCL) originates in the lateral aspect of the medial femoral condyle, crosses the

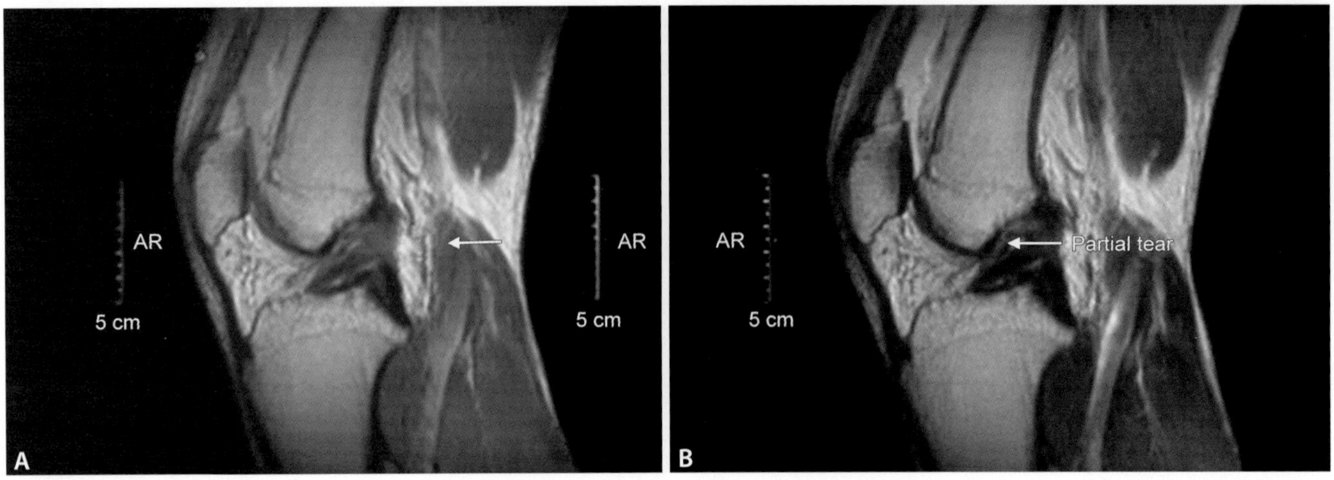

Figs. 21A and B: Proton density (A) and T2W (B) sagittal MR images showing a discrete area of increased signal intensity within the substance of the ACL, the ligament appearing intact—Partial tear of ACL.

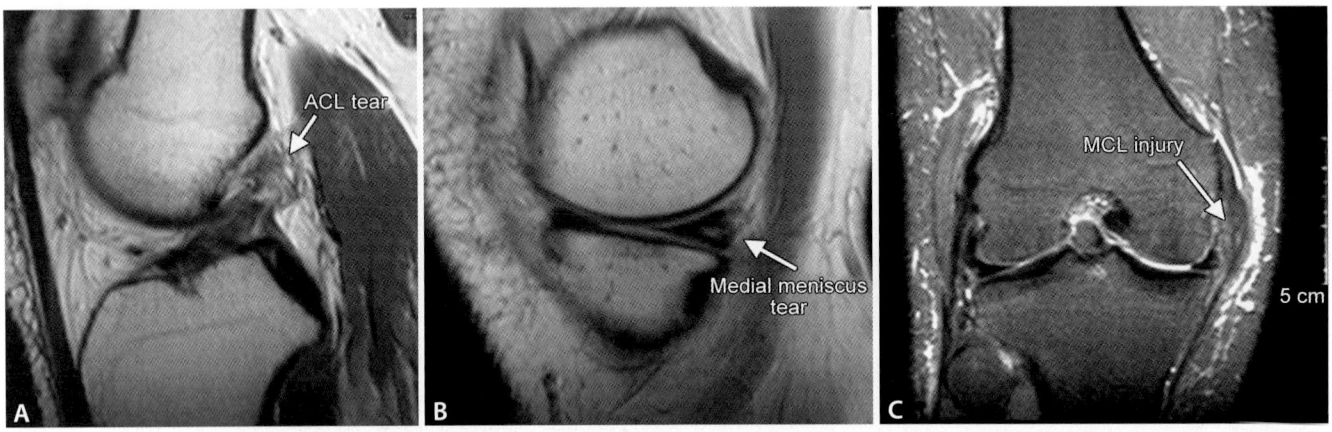

Figs. 22A to C: T2W sagittal (A and B) and STIR coronal (C) MR images showing ACL tear, medial meniscus tear and injury of the medial collateral ligament—O'Donoghue triad.

ACL and attaches to the posterior intercondylar fossa of tibia.[38] It averages 38 mm in length and 13 mm in width at its midportion. The PCL provides central support of the knee joint and protects against excessive posterior translation of tibia, stabilizes the joint against excessive varus and valgus stress and restricts external rotation of tibia.

MR Appearance of PCL

On MRI, the PCL is normally depicted as a band-like structure of low signal intensity. In sagittal images it has an arcuate shape with the knee in neutral position **(Figs. 23A and B)**.

PCL injury MR findings of PCL injury are anatomic disruption, increased signal intensity in the ligament and redundancy of an avulsed ligament.

Injuries to the PCL are classified as follows **(Figs. 24A to C)**:

- *Grade 1* is consistent with intraligamentous edema and hemorrhage and appears as foci of increased signal in a ligament with otherwise intact borders.
- *Grade 2* injuries represent partial tears.
- *Grade 3* abnormalities represent complete tears.

Aggressive surgical treatment of PCL tears is recently becoming more common since chronic knee instability with early degenerative arthritis has become better appreciated with chronic injuries of the PCL.

MEDIAL STRUCTURES OF THE KNEE

Anatomy

Medially, the supporting structures of the knee are arranged in three layers. The invested deep fascia of the sartorius

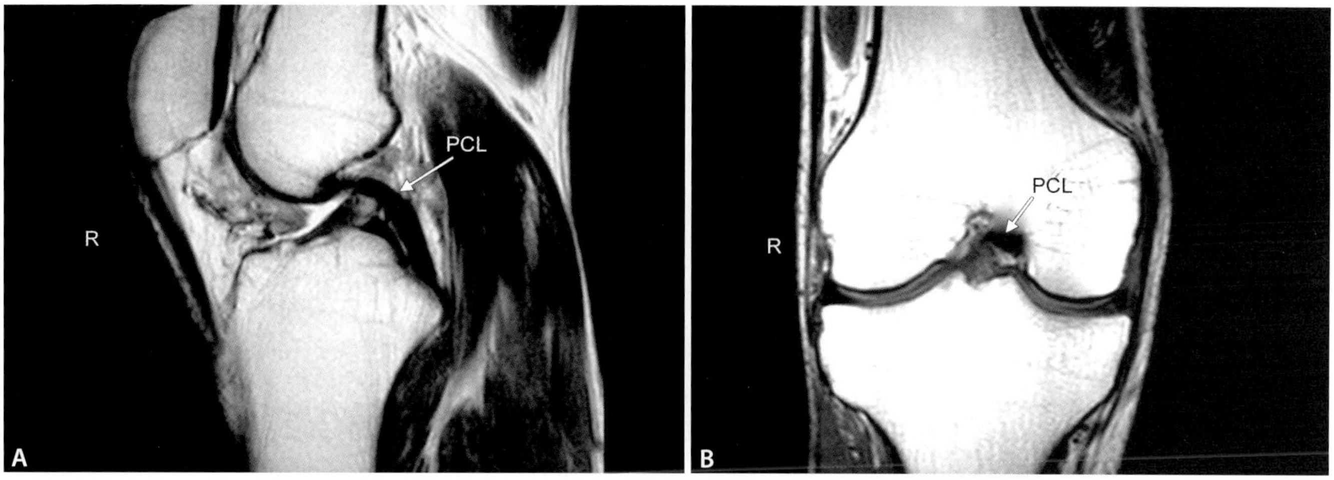

Figs. 23A and B: T2W sagittal (A) MR image of knee showing normal PCL (arrow) as a band-like structure of low signal intensity having an arcuate shape. T1W coronal MR image (B) showing the normal PCL (arrow) as a triangular structure within the intercondylar notch.

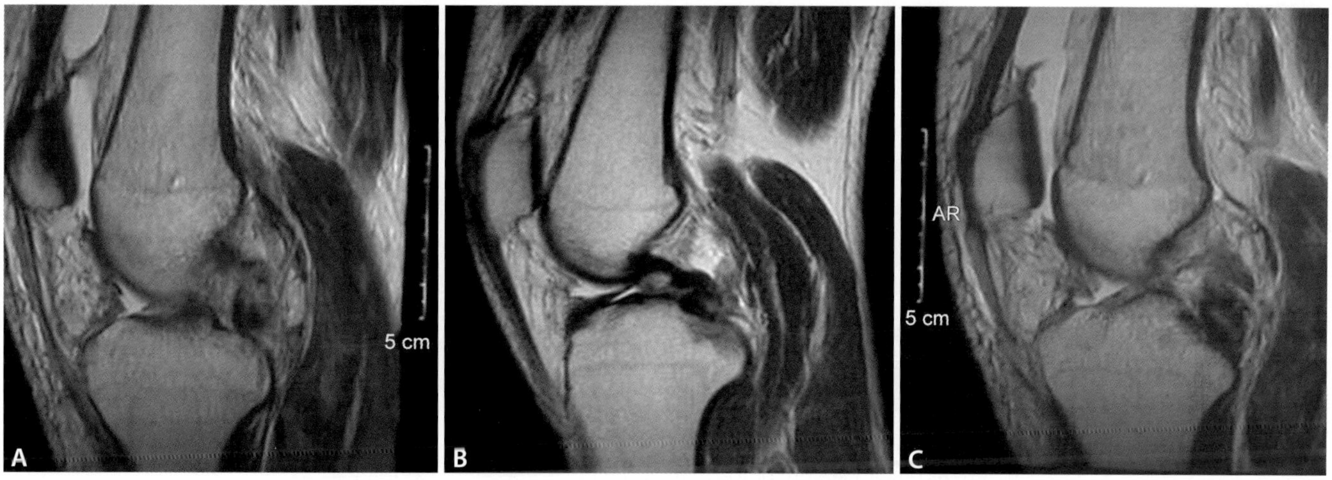

Figs. 24A to C: T2W sagittal MR images showing Grade 1 tear of the PCL seen as intraligamentous edema and hemorrhage (A) Grade 2 tear seen as partial tear of the tibial attachment (B) and Grade 3 tear seen as a complete disruption of the ligament (C).

muscle, which overlies the gastrocnemius muscle, forms the most superficial layer.[39] The tibial collateral ligament, the superficial component of the medial collateral ligament (MCL), forms the middle layer. The deepest layer is comprised of the meniscofemoral and meniscotibial ligaments, which constitute the deep components of the MCL. The MCL stabilizes the knee against excessive valgus force and hyperextension. The tibial collateral ligament, the primary support structure, extends from the medial epicondylar region of the femur to the medial surface of the proximal tibia and spans about 8–9 cm in length.[40]

Magnetic Resonance Imaging

On MRI, the MCL is best displayed on coronal images and appears as a smooth structure of low signal intensity that extends from the medial femoral epicondyle to the proximal tibial metaphysis **(Fig. 25)**. At the level of the joint line the superficial and deep portions of the ligament are separated by a bursa and surrounding fat which should not be mistaken for a localized meniscocapsular separation.

MCL Injury

Twisting injuries cause a large number of MCL injuries.

In Grade 1 injury a slight contour irregularity or thickening of the ligament may be seen but there is no discontinuity of its fibers. Edema and hemorrhage are identified in the soft tissue and subcutaneous fat paralleling the MCL **(Figs. 26A and B)**.

In Grade 2 discontinuity of some fibers may be evident.

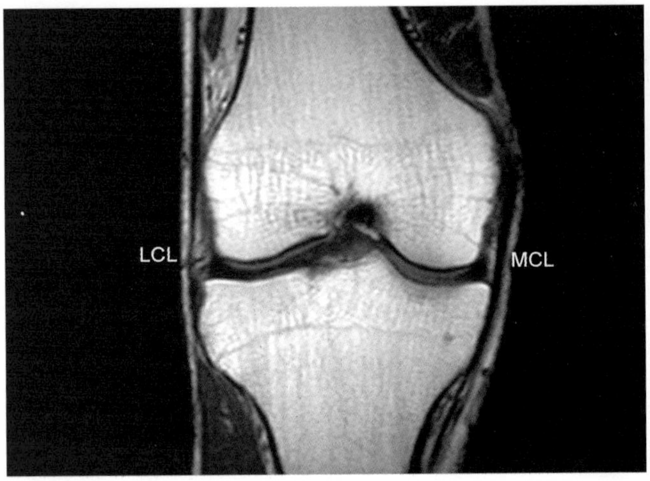

Fig. 25: T1W coronal MR image of the knee showing the normal medial collateral ligament (MCL) as a low signal intensity structure that extends from the medial femoral epicondyle to the proximal tibial metaphysis.

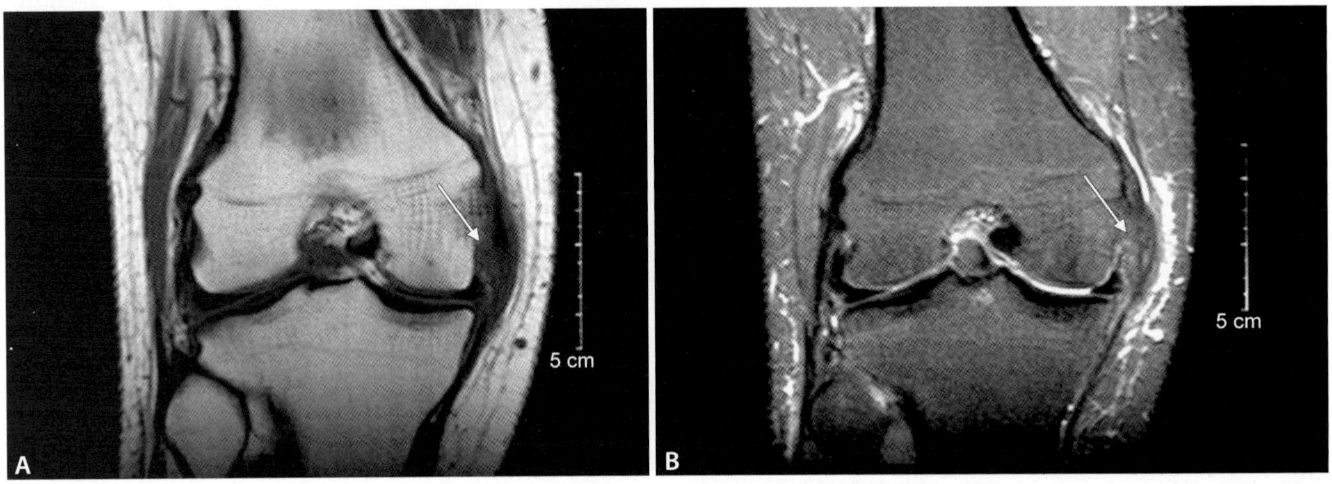

Figs. 26A and B: T1W coronal MR image (A) and STIR coronal image (B) showing Grade 1 MCL injury as edema and hemorrhage in the soft tissue and subcutaneous fat paralleling the MCL with slight contour irregularity of the ligament (arrows).

In Grade 3 frank discontinuity of all its fibers is seen **(Figs. 27A and B)**. Two findings that may be encountered on conventional radiography are predictive of underlying MCL injury. Pellegrini–Stieda disease or calcification around the medial femoral condyle represents chronic partial or complete tears of the MCL.[41] The reverse Segond fracture is an avulsion fracture of medial tibial plateau at the attachment of the deep fibers of the MCL. This finding is associated with PCL disruption and peripheral medial meniscal tear.

POSTEROMEDIAL STRUCTURES OF THE KNEE

Anatomy

The tendon of the semimembranosus muscle and the posterior oblique ligament are the main support structures in the posteromedial aspect of the knee.[42] The posterior oblique ligament is formed by the union of the posterior fibers of the MCL and the medial capsular ligament. The semimembranosus muscle originates from the posterolateral portion of the ischial tuberosity, and inserts on the posteromedial surface of the medial tibial condyle.

Magnetic Resonance Imaging

Posteromedial corner injuries usually result from a valgus stress combined with rotational forces. The semimembranosus tendon is the largest tendon in the popliteal fossa. It has a fusiform configuration and appears uniformly hypointense on all imaging sequences. A strain of the semimembranosus tendon is manifested by loss of continuity at the insertion and high signal on T2-weighted and STIR sequences owing to edema and hemorrhage.

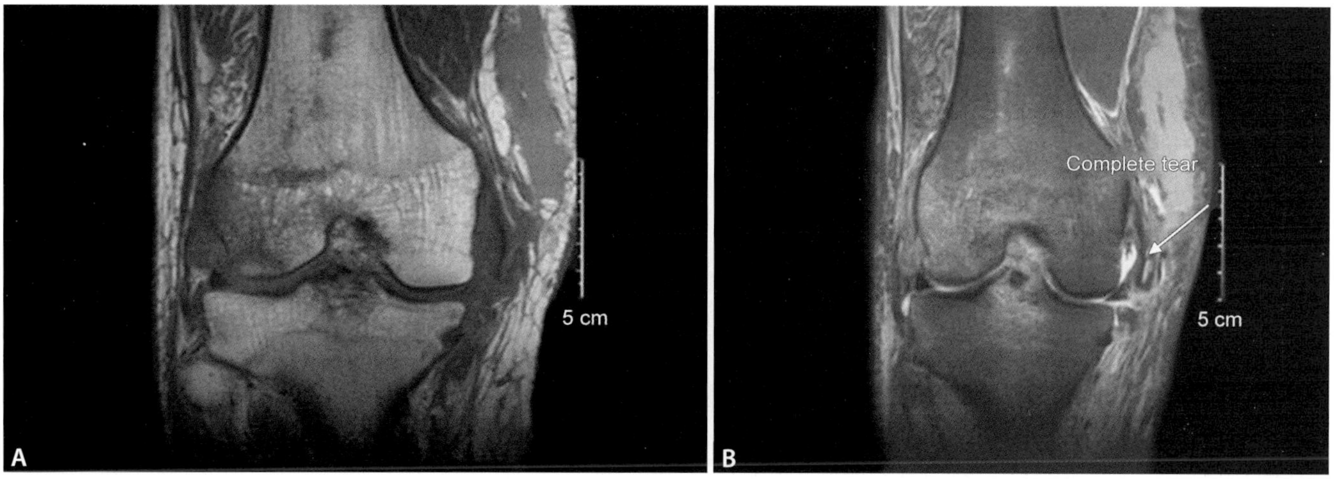

Figs. 27A and B: TIW (A) and STIR (B) coronal MR images showing a complete distruption of the MCL with extensive edema and hemorrhage in the adjacent soft tissues and subcutaneous fat. Extensive bone marrow contusions are also noted—Complete MCL tear.

Accompanying fluid within the tendon sheath is a common finding. A focus of marrow edema may be present when the posterior oblique ligament avulses.

POSTEROLATERAL CORNER OF THE KNEE

Anatomy

The posterolateral corner of the knee is composed of ligaments, muscles and tendons that are static restraints to posterior translation, varus angulations and external rotation of the knee. Also called the arcuate ligament complex, they include the fibular ligament or LCL, popliteus muscle and tendon, popliteofibular ligament, biceps femoris tendon, fabellofibular ligament, arcurate ligament and the lateral head of gastrocnemius. The fibular collateral ligament or lateral collateral ligament (LCL) is 5–7 cm long, arising from a tubercle on the lateral femoral condyle directly above the groove of the popliteus tendon origin. It inserts on the lateral surface of the head of the fibula, joining the biceps femoris tendon to form the conjoined tendon **(Figs. 28A and B)**. The main function of the LCL is to stabilize the knee against varus forces.[43]

The fabellofibular ligament courses from the fibular styloid process to the fabella, a normal sesamoid bone within the lateral gastrocnemius tendon. The arcuate ligament is as Y-shaped structure that represents thickening of the posterolateral joint capsule.

Magnetic Resonance Imaging

The LCL and iliotibial tract are most vulnerable when a varus force is applied to the knee when it is in flexion or internal rotation. The iliotibial tract and LCL are best visualized in entirety in the coronal planes. These are seen as low signal intensity structures on all pulse sequences and nearly uniform in thickness.

Soft tissue edema characterizes the MRI findings associated with acute iliotibial tract and LCL injuries. Contour changes, such as thickening and irregularity, are more typical of subacute or old injuries. Complete tears with discontinuity and retraction of the fibers may produce a ribbon-like deformity of the LCL **(Figs. 29A to C)**. Most complete ruptures involve the conjoined tendon and may produce a small avulsion of the styloid process of the fibular head. When this occurs, marrow edema in the proximal fibula is usually evident on T2-weighted and STIR images.

A direct varus force to the knee produces injuries to the posterolateral corner when the knee is locked in hyperextension **(Figs. 30A to F)**. Most injuries involving the posterolateral structures are optimally depicted using a coronal oblique plane that is oriented parallel to the popliteus tendon.[44] Acute injuries of the popliteus muscle most commonly involve the myotendinous junction, whereas avulsion injuries of fibular insertion are less common. When the popliteal tendon tears, hemorrhage and edema in the muscle and tendon produce focal and high signal on T2-weighted sequences. Edema of the adjacent soft tissue structures can also be observed. Complete tears of the popliteal tendon cause enlargement of the muscle belly and the retracted tendon terminates abruptly. Isolated popliteal injuries are rare, because most are associated with concomitant injuries of the arcuate ligament complex.

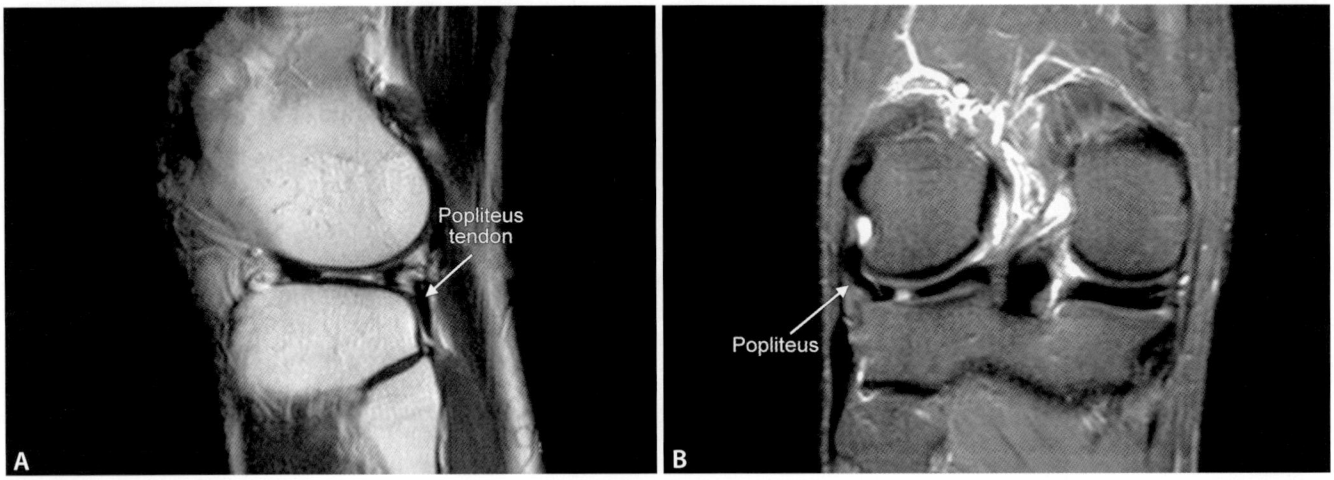

Figs. 28A and B: PD sagittal MR image (A) and STIR coronal (B) MR images of the knee showing the popliteal muscle that arises as a tendon from the lateral femoral condyle just anterior and inferior to the LCL, courses in a posteromedial direction to insert at the medial aspect of tibia, attaches to the lateral meniscus forming the popliteomeniscal ligament and has a third attachment site on the styloid process of the fibula.

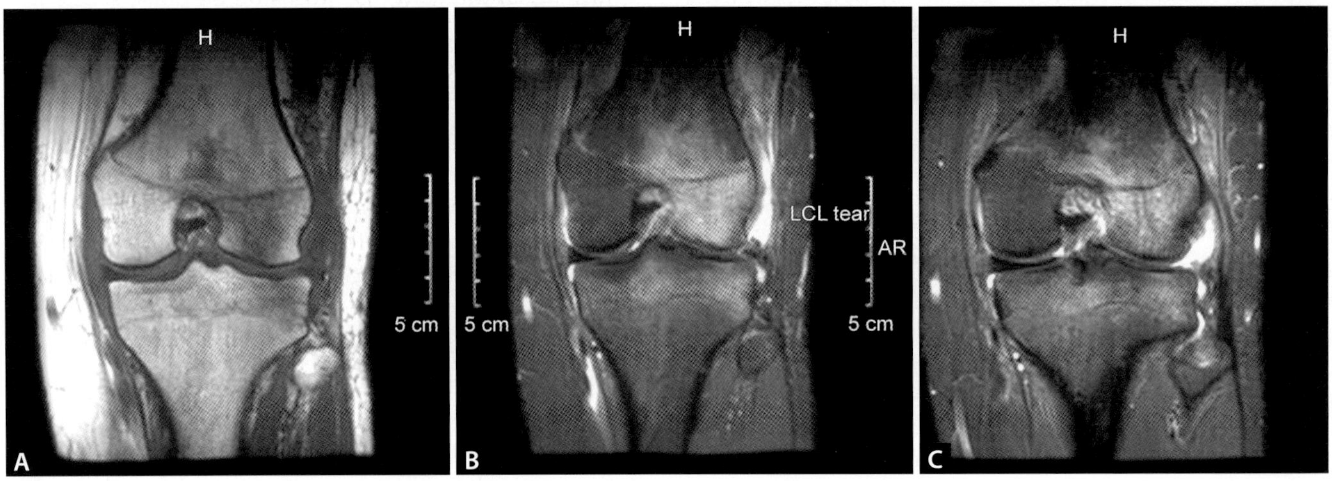

Figs. 29A to C: T1W (A) and STIR coronal (B and C) MR images showing complete discontinuity and retraction of the fibers of the LCL producing a ribbon-like deformity. Extensive contusions are seen in the lateral femoral condyle and lateral aspect of the tibial plateau—Complete tear of LCL.

POSTERIOR STRUCTURES OF THE KNEE

Anatomy

The gastrocnemius, soleus, and plantaris muscles form the superficial muscles of the calf. The gastrocnemius muscle arises as two heads from the posterior surface of the medial and lateral femoral condyles. The tendons of the gastrocnemius muscles along with the soleus tendon form the Achilles tendon, which inserts on the posterior tubercle of the calcaneus. The primary action of the gastrocnemius muscle is plantar flexion of the foot but also serves as a passive supportive structure of the posterior joint capsule.

Magnetic Resonance Imaging

Gastrocnemius injuries most commonly are caused by hyperextension of the knee or when the tibia posteriorly dislocates during knee flexion.[45] Acute injuries of the proximal gastrocnemius include interstitial edema of the myotendinous junction and surrounding soft tissues.[46] Occasionally, an intramuscular hematoma forms a space-occupying mass in the muscle. Magnetic resonance imaging can assess the chronicity of the hematoma by the general appearance of the products of hemoglobin degradation. A complete rupture of the gastrocnemius head is associated with retraction of the muscle belly.

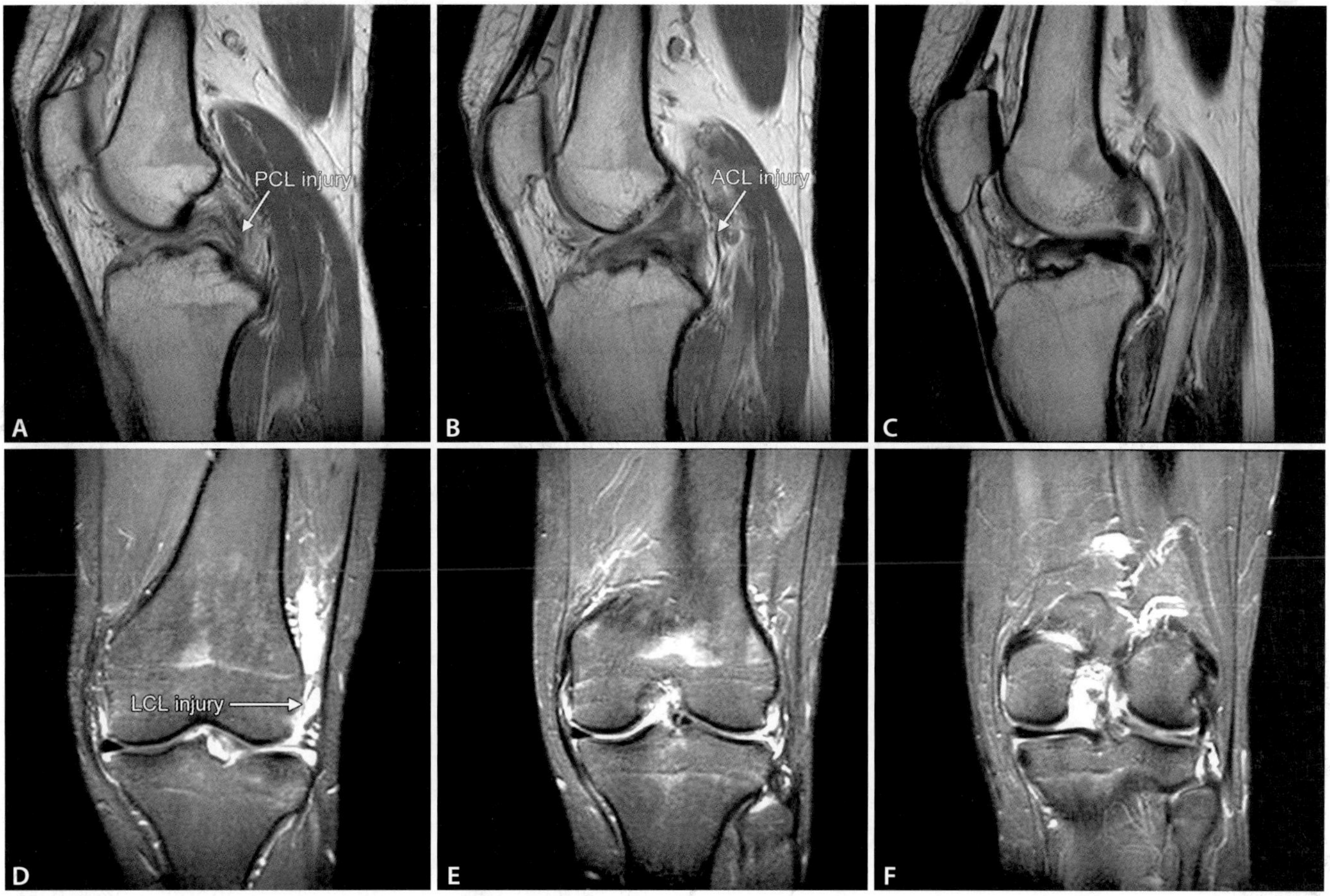

Figs. 30A to F: T2W sagittal (A to C) and STIR coronal (D to F) MR images showing a tear of the PCL, ACL and the lateral collateral ligament—Multiligament injury of the knee.

KNEE DISLOCATIONS

A dislocation of the knee is a severe injury that is caused by high-energy trauma, such as motor vehicle and motorcycle accidents, falls, and industrial accidents. Knee dislocations are important because they produce extensive disruption of the ligaments that stabilize the knee and the surrounding soft tissue structures, including the popliteal artery.[47]

Magnetic Resonance Imaging

A knee dislocation is classified according to the position of the tibia relative to the femur. There are five different types of dislocations: (i) anterior, (ii) posterior, (iii) lateral, (iv) medial, and (v) posterolateral. Posterior and posterolateral dislocations have a high association with complete tears of the popliteus and conjoined tendons, manifested by retraction, hemorrhage, and muscle edema. In general, both cruciate ligaments are likely to be torn. Complete disruption of one or both of the collateral ligaments is expected with this severe injury. Concomitant meniscal injury is also common. Frequently, the pattern of bone contusions allows definition of the type of knee dislocation. This is an important observation because posterior and posterolateral dislocations have a high association with peroneal nerve injury.[47]

ANTEROLATERAL CORNER OF THE KNEE

Normal Anatomy

Anterolateral corner of the knee include the iliotibial band (ITB), the anterior oblique band (AOB) of the LCL, and the capsular ligament. Together, these structures contribute to anterior and posterolateral stability. The ITB is an extension of the tensor fasciae latae with distal attachments to the lateral femoral condyle, the lateral patella, and the tubercle of Gerdy at the anterolateral aspect of the tibia.

Iliotibial Band Injury

Iliotibial band (ITB) injury is the most common injury to the anterolateral corner. Tearing most often involves the posterior fibers that interdigitate with the anterior oblique band (AOB). These are usually well demonstrated on coronal MR images.

Segond Fracture

The Segond fracture, or avulsion of the anterolateral aspect of the lateral tibial plateau, is a radiographic entity that signifies underlying trauma to the anterolateral corner structures of the knee. These lesions, like all anterolateral corner injuries, are highly suggestive of the presence of an underlying ACL tear (75–100%), meniscal tear (66–75%) or posterolateral corner injury.

Iliotibial Band Friction Syndrome

Iliotibial band friction syndrome (ITBFS) refers to lateral knee pain arising from the friction that occurs as the iliotibial band passes over the lateral femoral epicondyle during repetitive flexion and extension of the knee. This injury is seen most often in individuals who participate in long-distance running and cycling. On MR images, ill-defined signal abnormality signifying soft tissue edema is present within the fat deep to the iliotibial band.

ANTERIOR STRUCTURES OF THE KNEE OR THE EXTENSOR MECHANISM OF THE KNEE

Anatomy

The main soft tissue structures in the anterior aspect of the knee are the components of the extensor mechanism and include the quadriceps tendon, patellar tendon, the medial and lateral patellar retinacula.[48] The four muscle groups that form the quadriceps tendon include the rectus femoris, vastus lateralis, vastus medialis and the vastus intermedius. The quadriceps tendon inserts on the superior pole of the patella and causes extension of the knee joint **(Fig. 31A)**. The medial and lateral patellar retinacula are extensions of the vastus medialis and lateralis respectively and contribute to passive stabilization of the patella **(Fig. 31B)**.

The layers of the quadriceps tendon can be visualized best in sagittal plane on MRI as uniform low signal intensity bands with intervening higher signal intensity fat separating each layer. The layered configuration of the quadriceps tendon enables discrimination between partial and full tears. Discontinuity of any of the tendinous layers is consistent with partial tears often involving the rectus femoris component. Transection of all the layers is diagnostic of a complete rupture and may be associated with a mass of edematous tissue and hemorrhage seen as high signal on T2W images.[49] A patella baja (low riding patella) and undulating appearance of the patellar tendon is associated.

The patellar tendon also has homogeneous low signal intensity appearance except for small occasional triangular areas of intermediate signal intensity directly below the patella and adjacent to the tibial tuberosity. The normal thickness of the tendon does not exceed 7 mm in its proximal part. A large collection of adipose tissue, the infrapatellar fat pad of Hoffa, rests just posterior to the patellar tendon. The patellar tendon ruptures less frequently than the quadriceps tendon.

Patellar Tendinosis (Jumper's Knee)

Most patellar ligament injuries are the result of repetitive forced extension of the knee as seen in the context of basketball, volleyball, soccer, tennis and track

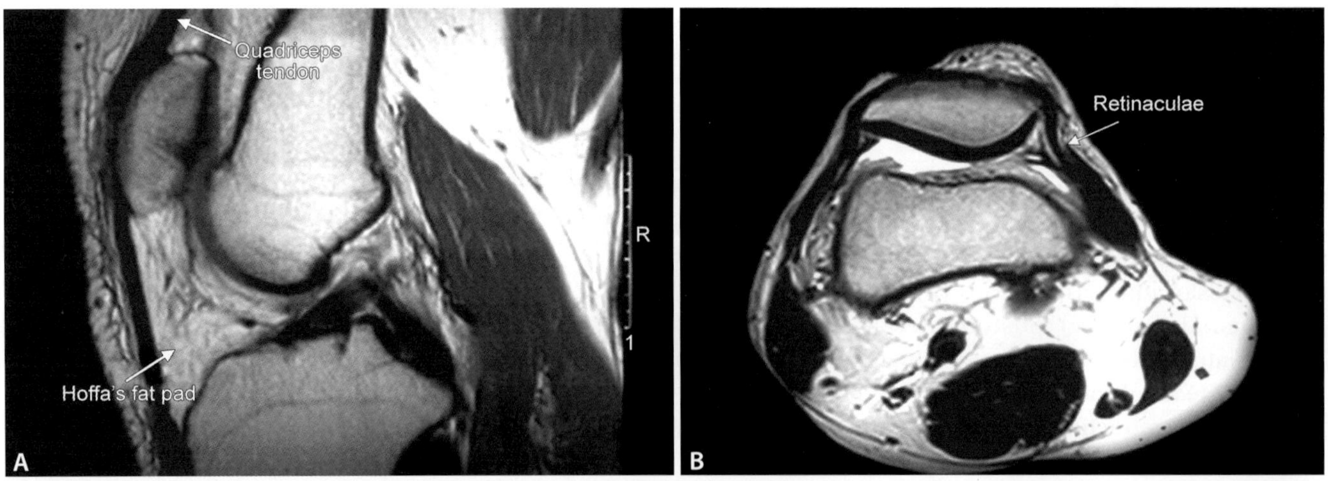

Figs. 31A and B: T2W sagittal MR image (A) showing the normal quadriceps tendon inserting on the superior pole of the patella, the patellar tendon and the infrapatellar Hoffa's fat pad. T2W axial (B) MR image showing the medial and lateral patellar retinaculae.

events—hence the name jumper's knee. This form of injury manifests as thickening and partial tearing of the proximal patellar tendon and is well seen on sagittal MR images as increased tendon thickness greater than 7 mm or as intrasubstance high signal intensity. Similar changes can be seen in both symptomatic and asymptomatic individuals. In symptomatic patients, the findings may be accompanied by patellar tracking disorders in as many as 45% of patients.

Acute Patellar Tendon Disruption

A minority of patellar ligament injuries are complete tendon disruption resulting from acute macrotrauma in the setting of sports-related activity. This most commonly occurs near the patellar attachment and is best seen on sagittal MR images as discontinuity of the patellar ligament with buckling of the tendon, retraction of the patella, and fluid signal in the intervening gap.

Patellar Tendon–Lateral Femoral Condyle Friction Syndrome

Patellar tendon–lateral femoral condyle friction syndrome refers to the constellation of MRI findings that corresponds to the clinical entity known as fat-pad impingement syndrome. Affected patients are both athletes and nonathletes who experience chronic anterior knee pain that localizes to the inferior patellar pole on physical examination. The etiology is unknown, but it is likely related to friction onto the fat interposed between the patellar ligament and the lateral femoral condyle due to abnormal patellar tracking or alignment. MRI findings include abnormal obliteration of the fat planes, abnormal signal, and enhancement within the lateral soft tissues of the inferior patellofemoral joint. Most patient demonstrate patellar alignment abnormality, such as patella alta or lateral subluxation. Patients typically respond well to conservative treatment, which usually entails taping the superior pole of the patella.

Retinacular tears are characterized by areas of high signal on T2 and STIR sequences secondary to edema and hemorrhage.[50] The medial retinaculum is thinner than the lateral and frequently tears. The avulsed free end of the retinaculum is often frayed and thickened and fluid may dissect around a muscular slip of the vastus medialis muscle.

PATELLOFEMORAL JOINT

Patellofemoral Joint Anatomy

The shape of the patella and femoral trochlear groove are important for the function of the patellofemoral joint.

Patellar shape: Wiberg has proposed a three part classification to encompass the majority of patellar facet configurations. In type I configuration, both facets are gently concave, symmetrical and nearly equal in size. In type II which is the most common the medial facet is smaller than the lateral. In type III configuration the medial facet is distinctly markedly smaller with marked lateral predominance.[51] Dysplastic patellar shapes have a variety of unusual configurations and are commonly observed with chondromalacia, recurrent dislocation and patellofemoral instability.

Femoral Trochlear Groove

The femoral trochlear groove provides a mechanical restraint that helps stabilize and serve as a guide for the patella as it articulates with the groove during joint function. In the axial plane the posterior apex of a normal patella is centered directly above the intercondylar femoral sulcus. The sulcus angle is formed by the highest points of the medial and lateral femoral condyles and the lowest point of the intercondylar sulcus and measures 138° ± 6° **(Fig. 32A)**. Shallow sulcus angles (larger sulcus angle measurements) predispose to patellar instability.

Patella Alta and Patella Baja

In the sagittal plane the patella is in normal position when in semiflexion of the knee the greatest diagonal length of the patella approximately equals the distance between the inferior pole of the patella and the tibial tuberosity (patellar tendon length) **(Fig. 32B)**. A truly high riding patella (patella alta) most commonly results from a patellar tendon tear but is also associated with lateral patellar subluxations, recurrent dislocations and spastic neuromuscular disorders **(Figs. 33A to C)**. A low riding patella (patella baja or profunda) occurs in quadriceps tendon rupture but is also found with paralytic neuromuscular disorders, achondroplasia and juvenile rheumatoid arthritis.

KINEMATIC MR IMAGING

Kinematics is a term to describe movement of a body without reference to force or mass. Kinematic MR imaging was first used for the evaluation of the patellofemoral joint in 1988. Although conventional computed tomography (CT) and cine CT have also been used to perform kinematic studies of the patellofemoral joint, kinematic MR imaging has the advantage of showing the various soft tissue components (i.e. medial and lateral retinacula, patellar tendon, quadriceps muscles) that are involved in the stability and function of the joint.

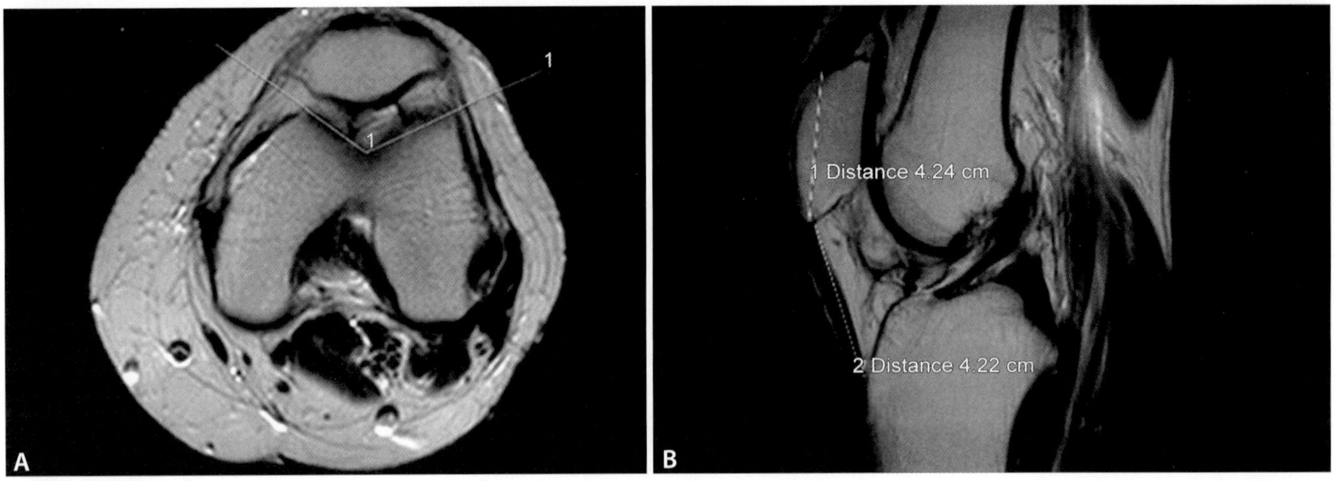

Figs. 32A and B: T1W axial (A) image showing the normal sulcus angle formed by the highest points of the medial and lateral femoral condyles and the lowest point of the intercondylar sulcus. T2W sagittal (B) MR image showing the normal position of the patella (the greatest diagonal length of the patella equals the patellar tendon length).

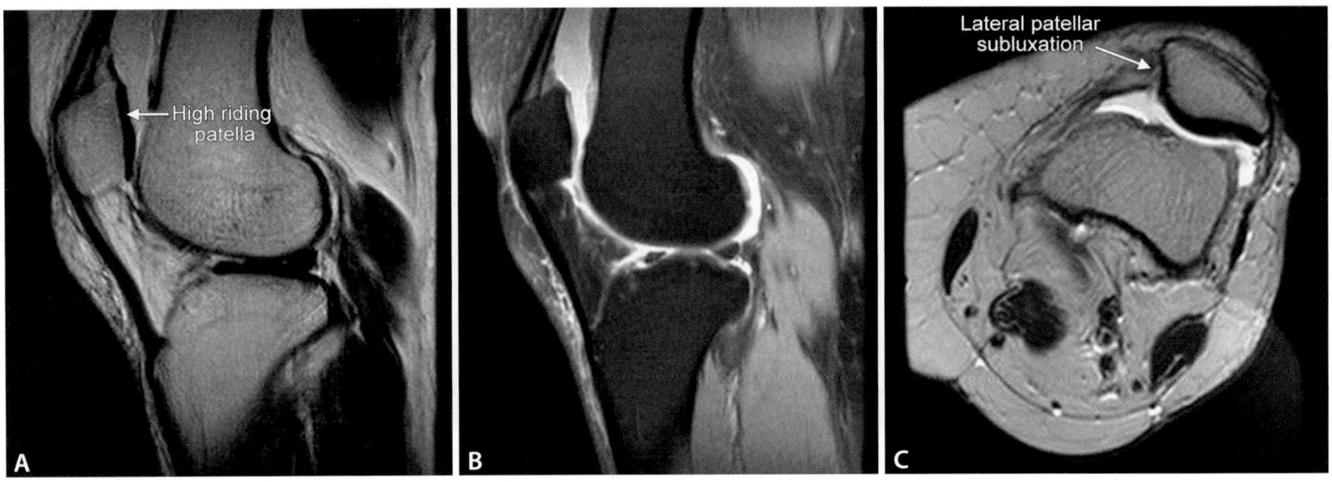

Figs. 33A to C: Proton density (A) and T2W fat-suppressed sagittal (B) MR images showing a high riding patella with axial T2W MR image (C) revealing a lateral patellar subluxation—Patella alta.

Techniques

Incremental, Passive Positioning Technique

The technique involves obtaining multiple axial images at different section locations and both the patellofemoral joints are passively flexed into incremental positions using a nonferromagnetic positioning device. The use of a special positioning device is crucial because direct anterior or lateral pressure may occur with the patient placed in prone position that is sufficient to displace the patella and give an erroneous appearance of patellar subluxation.

The MR images are obtained using a T1-weighted spin echo, or spoiled gradient echo pulse sequences at several different slice locations while the joint is progressively flexed at 5° increments from 5° to 30°. This procedure should be repeated at three different section locations so that the entire excursion of the patella can be evaluated as it articulates with the femoral trochlear groove.[51]

Active Movement or Dynamic Technique

Faster MR imaging techniques (e.g. ultrafast spoiled gradient recalled acquisition in the steady state (GRASS), turbo fast low angle shot (FLASH) have been developed recently that provide significant improvements in temporal resolution and allow images to be obtained during active or dynamic movement of the patellofemoral joint. MR images typically are obtained at a temporal resolution of one image per second or faster using these fast scan techniques. The primary advantage of using active movement kinematic MR imaging technique is that the patellofemoral joint may be examined in terms of influence of the activated muscles and other related soft tissue structures on patellar alignment and tracking. Compared with the incremental, passive positioning technique, a more physiological examination is obtained and in certain instances abnormal patellar tracking is more apparent during active movement.

Motion Triggered Cine Technique

In this technique, a special nonferromagnetic device incorporates a trigger system that senses the motion of the patella. The patient is placed supine on the positioning device and a single patellofemoral joint is flexed and extended repeatedly while gradient echo images are obtained using a circular surface coil.

Active Movement, Loaded Technique

In this, active movement against an externally applied load or resistance is applied.[52] With the patient in prone position the movement against this resistance primarily requires activation of the extensor mechanism of the knee. This method enables identification of abnormalities that may not be observed during unloaded examination.

Abnormalities that may be seen on kinematic MR include lateral or medial subluxation of patella and lateral patellar tilt or excessive lateral pressure syndrome.

Kinematic MR study can be combined with routine MR study of the knee since both the procedures can be completed within an acceptable time and can provide a more thorough examination of the knee specially in cases of suspected patellofemoral incongruency.

MR IMAGING OF THE ARTICULAR CARTILAGE

The articular surfaces of the knee are covered by hyaline cartilage. By deforming under pressure the articular cartilage greatly increases the effective contact area between femoral condyles and tibial plateaus, significantly decreasing the pressure transmitted across these joints. The menisci are also helpful in distributing forces across the knee joint. The cartilaginous matrix of articular cartilage allows the knee to withstand large local pressures, up to 5 times normal pressures.

Articular Cartilage Structure and Damage

Articular cartilage is composed of an extracellular matrix maintained by a relatively small population of chondrocytes.[53] The framework of the matrix is composed primarily of collagen, which is a highly ordered structure with organization of fibers in a pattern of arcades with densely packed fibers parallel to the surface forming a covering layer. Proteoglycan molecules are the other major solid constituent of the extracellular matrix of cartilage and are located within the collagen framework and covering, where they attract water into cartilage because of their hydrophilic nature. Articular cartilage function is lost with damage to chondrocytes, collagen or proteoglycans. In early damage there is loss of the collagen organization resulting in swelling of the cartilage with increased water content and loss of proteoglycans. With more severe injury cracks, fissures, and focal defects form in the cartilage. When defects form in the cartilage repair response generally results in fibrocartilage, which incompletely fills the defect and which does not reproduce the biomechanical properties of the highly structured normal articular cartilage. This fibrocartilage generally degenerates within a year.

MRI of Articular Cartilage

Initial evaluation of the articular cartilage used primarily T1-weighted images. Because of its hydropic composition normal hyaline cartilage demonstrates intermediate signal intensity on T1-weighted images compared with the low signal intensity of the cortex and fibrocartilaginous menisci. On conventional T2-weighted images also hyaline cartilage displays an intermediate signal intensity. In the presence of joint effusion T2-weighted images create an arthrogram like effect with hyperintense synovial fluid improving the delineation of thinner cartilage surfaces (e.g. medial and lateral compartments). There is poor contrast; however, between articular cartilage and subchondral bone on conventional T2-weighted images and in the absence of joint effusion, surface or contour irregularities may not be resolved. The demand for improved preoperative detection and characterization of articular cartilage damage has resulted in recent improvements in the accuracy of MRI of articular cartilage with use of sequences optimized for articular cartilage evaluation.

STIR and gradient echo images may also depict morphological changes of the articular cartilage. With STIR image contrast it is possible to differentiate the brighter signal intensity of fluid from intermediate to high signal intensity of articular cartilage. This sequence is also useful in demonstrating early changes of subchondral bone in areas of overlying articular cartilage damage. Areas of fluid within articular cartilage fissures and fragmentation can also be visualized on STIR images. Gradient echo imaging is useful with respect to imaging geometry, speed and contrast. Three-dimensional imaging significantly improves signal to noise ratios at high spatial resolution. With gradient echo techniques articular cartilage demonstrates high signal intensity. However, articular cartilage and articular fluid show similar high signal intensity, and significant cartilaginous injuries may be missed using gradient echo techniques if joint fluid and articular cartilage are isointense. Fat-suppressed T2-weighted fast spin echo techniques are useful in separating the cartilage-fluid interface and identifying early changes of articular cartilage degeneration **(Fig. 34A)**.[54] A fat-suppressed three-dimensional spoiled gradient echo technique (3D SPGR)[55-57] is also used.

Another recent development includes dual echo steady state (DESS) imaging which combines the principles of heavily T2-weighted steady state sequence and gradient echo imaging **(Fig. 34B)**. All three imaging planes are useful; however, the sagittal plane is the best single plane for evaluation of articular cartilage because it provides near orthogonal images of most of the articular cartilage surfaces in the knee. Intra-articular contrast or MR arthrography is useful for detection of loose bodies or for evaluation of osteochondral defects for assessment of integrity of overlying articular cartilage.

MRI Assessment of Articular Cartilage Injury

Arthroscopic grading system for correlation with MR findings is as follows:

- Minimal articular cartilage change with localized softening and minimal or no break in the articular surface.
- Areas of fibrillation or fissuring with an irregular roughened surface.
- Definite fibrillation with fissuring extending to the subchondral region and a classic "crab meat" appearance.
- Absence of articular cartilage with possibly eburnated subchondral bone.

Despite high accuracy for detection of most articular cartilage defects, certain defects are poorly visualized with MRI because of limited resolution. Cartilage softening and loss of proteoglycan from cartilage are often not seen with routine MRI. The use of high field strength 3.0T MR imaging system is becoming widespread in clinical practice and has the potential to improve clinical cartilage imaging. These 3.0 T systems can produce images of articular cartilage with higher spatial resolution and thinner section thickness than a 1.5 T system without sacrificing signal to noise ratio (SNR) or prolonging acquisition time.[58, 59]

MR also has a role in the follow-up of cartilaginous injuries. Arthroscopy is too invasive for follow-up of these lesions.[51]

QUANTITATIVE CARTILAGE MR IMAGING

Using high field MR imaging at 3.0T visulization of cartilage and related pathology has been improved. Volumetric quantitative cartilage MR imaging has been developed as a tool to monitor the progression of osteoarthritis and evaluate new pharmacological cartilage protective therapies. Cartilage consists of approximately 70% water and the remainder predominantly of type II collagen fibers and glycosaminoglycans (GAG). The GAG macromolecules contain negative charge and attract

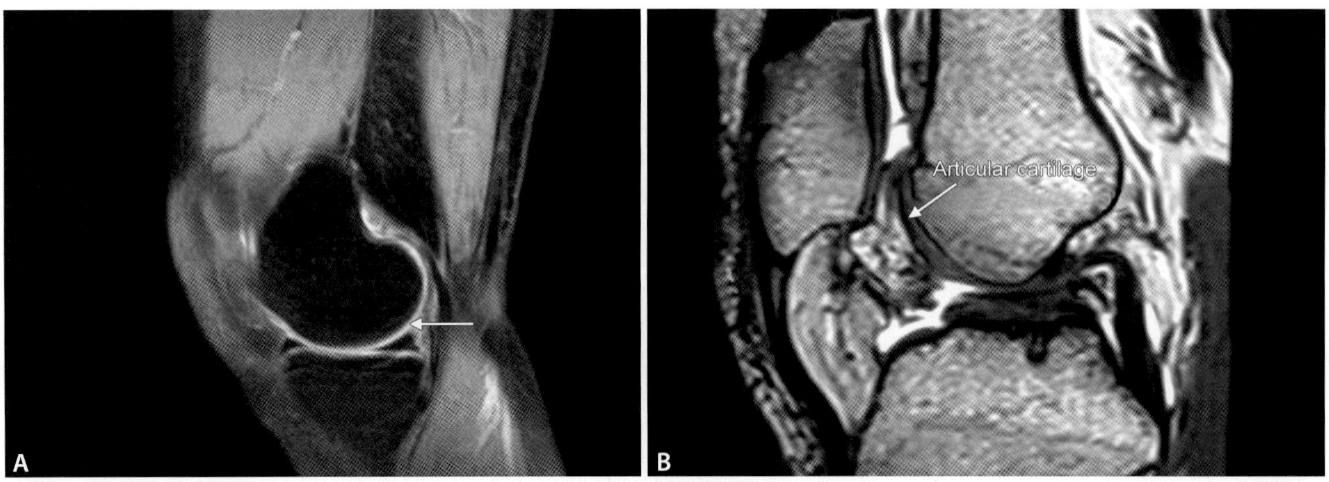

Figs. 34A and B: Sagittal fat-suppressed T2W (A) MR image showing the articular cartilage as high signal intensity. Double echo steady-state (DESS) sequence (B) for articular cartilage showing the intermediate gray signal articular cartilage. The thickness of the cartilage varies with the thickest cartilage seen at the patella and thinnest seen at the tibial plateau.

sodium ions (Na^+). The most common MR contrast agent, gadopentetate dimeglumine (Gd-DTPA) has a negatives charge and will therefore show a lower concentration in cartilage areas of high GAG concentrations following penetration by diffusion. Gadopentetate dimeglumine concentrations in cartilage can be quantified and this technique has been defined as dGEMRIC or delayed gadolinium enhanced MR imaging of cartilage. The quantitative findings have a particularly important role in evaluating early osteoarthritis at a stage when the changes are potentially still reversible.[60]

Chondromalacia Patellae

The term chondromalacia patellae meaning softening of the patellar cartilage is widely used to designate a clinical syndrome of retropatellar pain, patellofemoral crepitus and quadriceps wasting which is associated with softening or fibrillation of the articular cartilage of patella.[61] The clinical observations that symptoms are self-limiting, may settle spontaneously and that chondromalacia patellae does not progress to fully developed osteoarthritis in later life, suggest that the two diseases are different entities. Patients with chondromalacia patellae have cartilaginous thinning, focal signal or focal contour defects in the patellar cartilage on T2-weighted MR images.

Osteoarthritis

Osteoarthritis (OA) affects the knee more frequently than any other joint. The MR findings in degenerative arthrosis/osteoarthritis vary from osteophytic spurring to compartment collapse, denuded articular cartilage, torn and degenerative meniscal fibrocartilage and diminished marrow signal intensity in areas of subchondral sclerosis **(Figs. 35A to C)**. The various alterations in the subchondral bone microstructure associated with the different stages of OA include the following:[62]

- **Bone marrow edema-like lesions:** Bone marrow edema-like lesions (BMELs) are defined on MR imaging as monocystic subchondral areas of ill-defined hyperintensity on STIR and T2W sequences and areas of hypointensity on T1W sequences. BMELs may increase or decrease over time and larger BMELs are seen more frequently in subjects who have pain.[63]
- **Subchondral cyst-like lesions:** These lesions have a characteristic appearance on MR imaging and are seen as well-defined round areas of fluid like signal intensity on non-enhanced imaging. They are a consequence of traumatic bone necrosis following impact of two opposing articular surfaces.
- **Synovitis:** It occurs not only as a secondary phenomenon related to cartilage degeneration but also plays a role in the progression of cartilage loss. Synovial inflammation is believed to contribute to pain in patients who have knee OA.
- **Joint effusion:** It is commonly detected in patients who have moderate to advanced OA and reflects synovial activation secondary to ligament injury, loose bodies, hyaline cartilage deterioration and meniscal damage. Only contrast-enhanced images can differentiate between synovium and joint effusion.
- **Subchondral bone attrition:** Subchondral bone attrition is defined as a depression or flattening of the subchondral bony surface unrelated to gross fracture. It is considered to be a predictor of knee pain in cases of OA.
- **Periarticular cysts and bursae:** A wide spectrum of periarticular cystic lesions may be encountered in knee OA. Popliteal (Baker's cysts) of the gastrocnemius

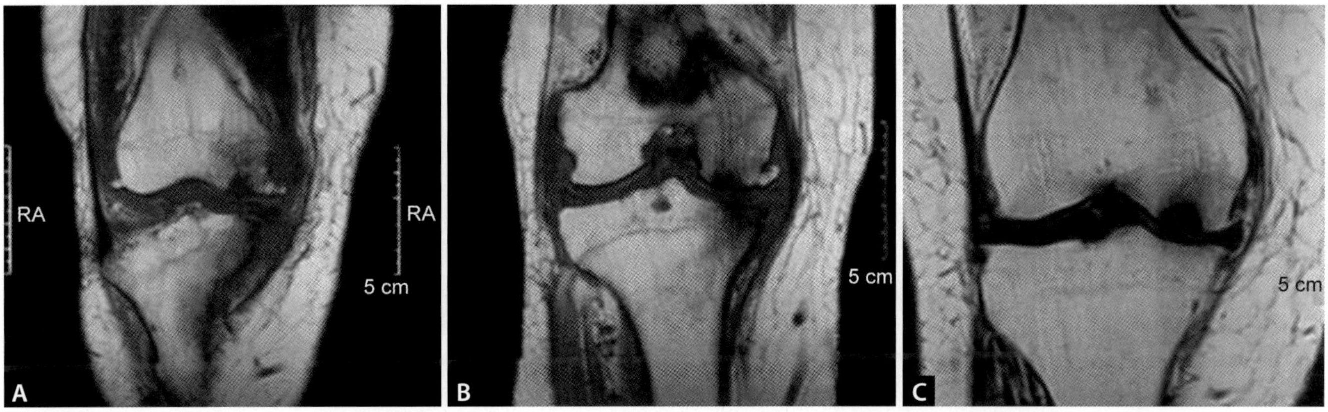

Figs. 35A to C: T1W coronal MR images of the knee showing osteophytic spurring, denuded articular cartilage, mild medial compartment collapse and subchondral sclerosis—Osteoarthritis.

semimembranosus bursae arise between medial head of the gastrocnemius muscle and the more medial semimembranosus tendon. A narrow neck connecting the cyst to the joint may be seen on axial images **(Figs. 36A and B)**. Popliteal cysts may arise from any condition that causes an increase in synovial fluid within the joint and are frequently seen in association with tears of the posterior horn of the medial meniscus.[4,51] Atypical locations for other cysts include the tibiofibular joint and the bursa between the lateral head of the gastrocnemius and biceps femoris. With MR evaluation a cyst can be differentiated from a popliteal artery aneurysm or venous malformation which may have a similar clinical appearance. In contrast to popliteal cysts, ganglion cysts are viscous synovium filled masses with mucopolysaccharide rich contents. Septations are common within ganglia. There is usually a connection or stalk traceable to the joint. Other bursites like prepatellar bursites and pes anserine bursites may also be seen. Parameniscal cysts are also a common finding in knee OA.

- **Loose bodies:** Chondral fragments (intermediate signal intensity) and loose bodies (high signal intensity of marrow fat) may be associated with more advanced degenerative disease. A T1-weighted image in at least one plane should be included in the study to improve the identification of loose bodies that contain marrow fat. The exclusive use of fat-suppressed sequences may lead to the loose bodies being missed. In addition to the patellofemoral, medial and lateral compartments of the knee, changes in the tibiofibular joint which may also be affected by degenerative arthrosis are well seen by MRI **(Figs. 37A to D)**.

The ability of MRI to accurately assess hyaline cartilage surfaces may give MR an advantage over plain film radiography in preoperative planning for joint replacement procedures, especially in unicondylar arthroplasties for osteoarthritis.[64] Tailored MR imaging producing high spatial and contrast resolution images is proving to be an important tool in the early detection and surveillance of progression of osteoarthritis.[65] Therapeutic techniques, such as chondrocyte transplantation requires high resolution and volumetric MR imaging studies for accurate identification of focal articular cartilage defects and generalized cartilage loss. Creation of cartilage models by three dimensional MR image rendering may be helpful for preoperative planning of orthopedic surgical procedures in advanced cases of osteoarthritis.

EVALUATION OF THE SYNOVIUM

Synovial reaction and proliferation are characterized on MR images by changes in the contour of synovial reflections. Although the synovium cannot be imaged directly, a corrugated surface along Hoffa's infrapatellar fat pad is evident in the early stages of synovial irritation. This irregular infrapatellar fat pad sign is seen in patients with rheumatoid arthritis, pigmented villonodular synovitis (PVNS), hemophilia and hemorrhagic effusions with reactive synovium.

Gd-DTPA contrast enhanced T1-weighted MR images are useful in the accurate identification of pannus tissue. Pannus tissue is seen as an area of increased signal intensity on these contrast enhanced images adjacent to the low signal intensity joint fluid.[66]

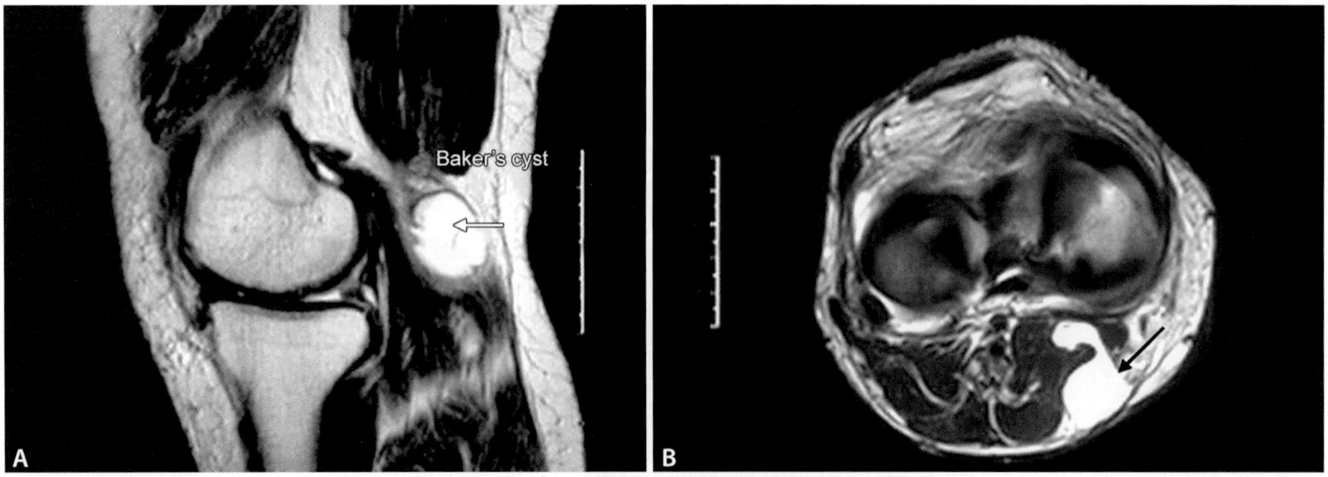

Figs. 36A and B: T2W sagittal (A) and T2W axial (B) MR images of the knee showing fluid intensity cystic structure between the medial head of gastrocnemius and the more medial semimembranosus tendon—Popliteal/Baker's cyst.

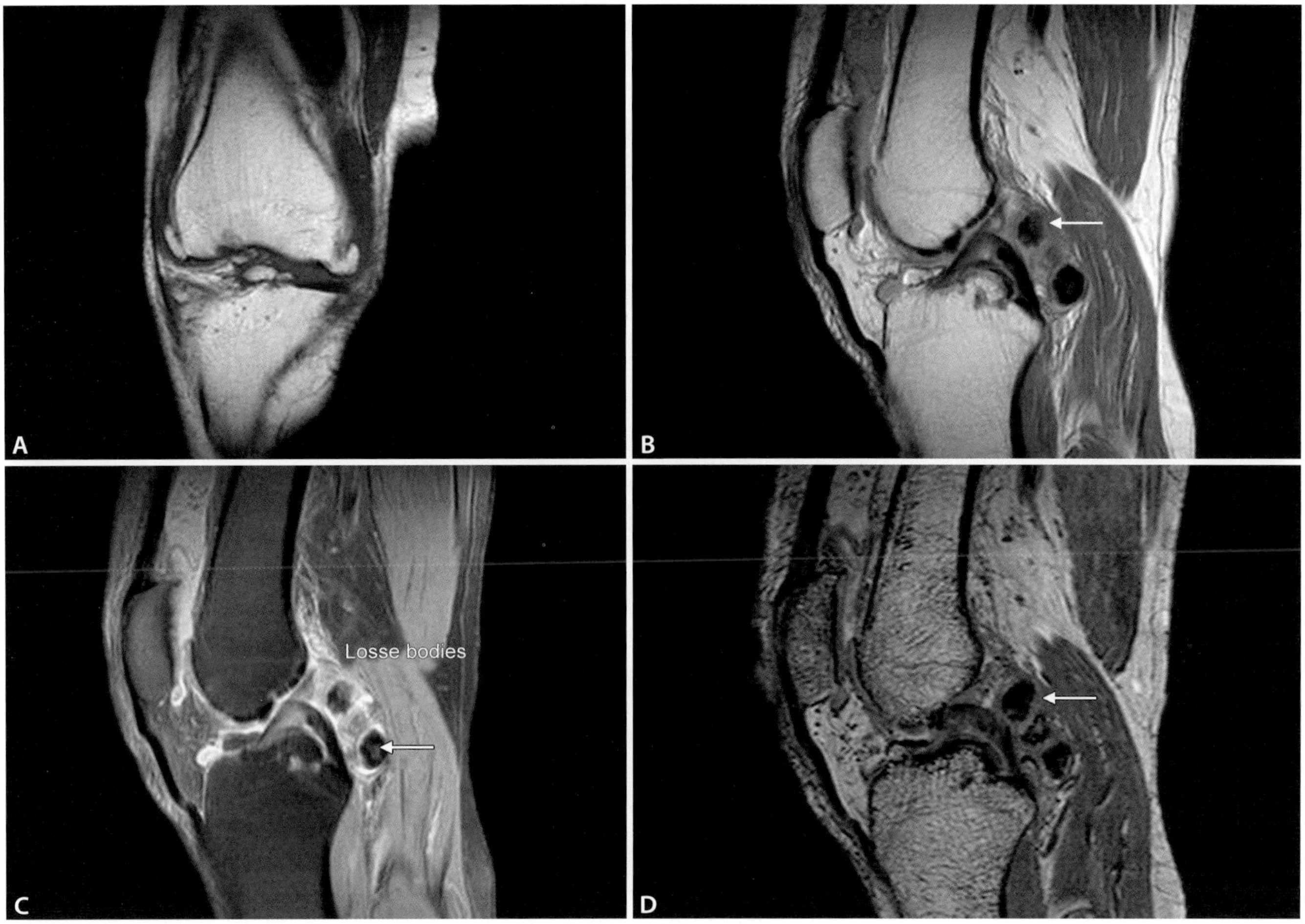

Figs. 37A to D: T1W coronal (A) T2W sagittal (B) fat-suppressed T2W sagittal (C) and DESS sequence (D) showing osteophytic spurring at femur, patella and multiple loose bodies. The loose bodies show high signal marrow fat on T1W images (A) with signal suppression on fat-suppressed images (B).

Rheumatoid Arthritis

Rheumatoid arthritis (RA) typically presents with joint effusions and bony and cartilaginous erosions. Marginal and subchondral erosions with diffuse loss of hyaline articular cartilage are evident on both medial and lateral femoral articular surfaces. An irregular fat pad may be seen in the more active stages of the disease. Hypertrophied synovial masses remain relatively low in signal intensity on T1 and T2W images. The gadolinium DTPA contrast enhanced images are useful in identifying the pannus or granulation tissue that grows on the surfaces of articular cartilage in rheumatoid arthritis **(Figs. 38A to D)**.[66]

The ability to map out pannus is useful in examining patients with inflammatory arthritis when synovectomy is considered. MRI determined synovial membrane and effusion volumes are sensitive markers and predictors of disease activity and treatment outcome in RA. Osteonecrosis and infarcts in rheumatoid arthritis can also be identified on MR scans before radiographic changes are evident.

Tuberculosis of the Knee

Magnetic resonance imaging is excellent for detecting early changes of tuberculosis. Synovial proliferalation seen in TB is typically hypointense on T2-weighted images. On administration of IV contrast the hypertrophied synovium is intensely enhancing. Marrow edema, osteomyelitis, cortical erosions, myositis, cellulitis, abscesses and skin ulceration/sinus formation can be seen in the bone and adjacent soft tissues **(Figs. 39A to C)**.

Juvenile Rheumatoid Arthritis

In juvenile rheumatoid arthritis (JRA) or Still's disease MRI studies demonstrate synovitis with irregularity of Hoffa's

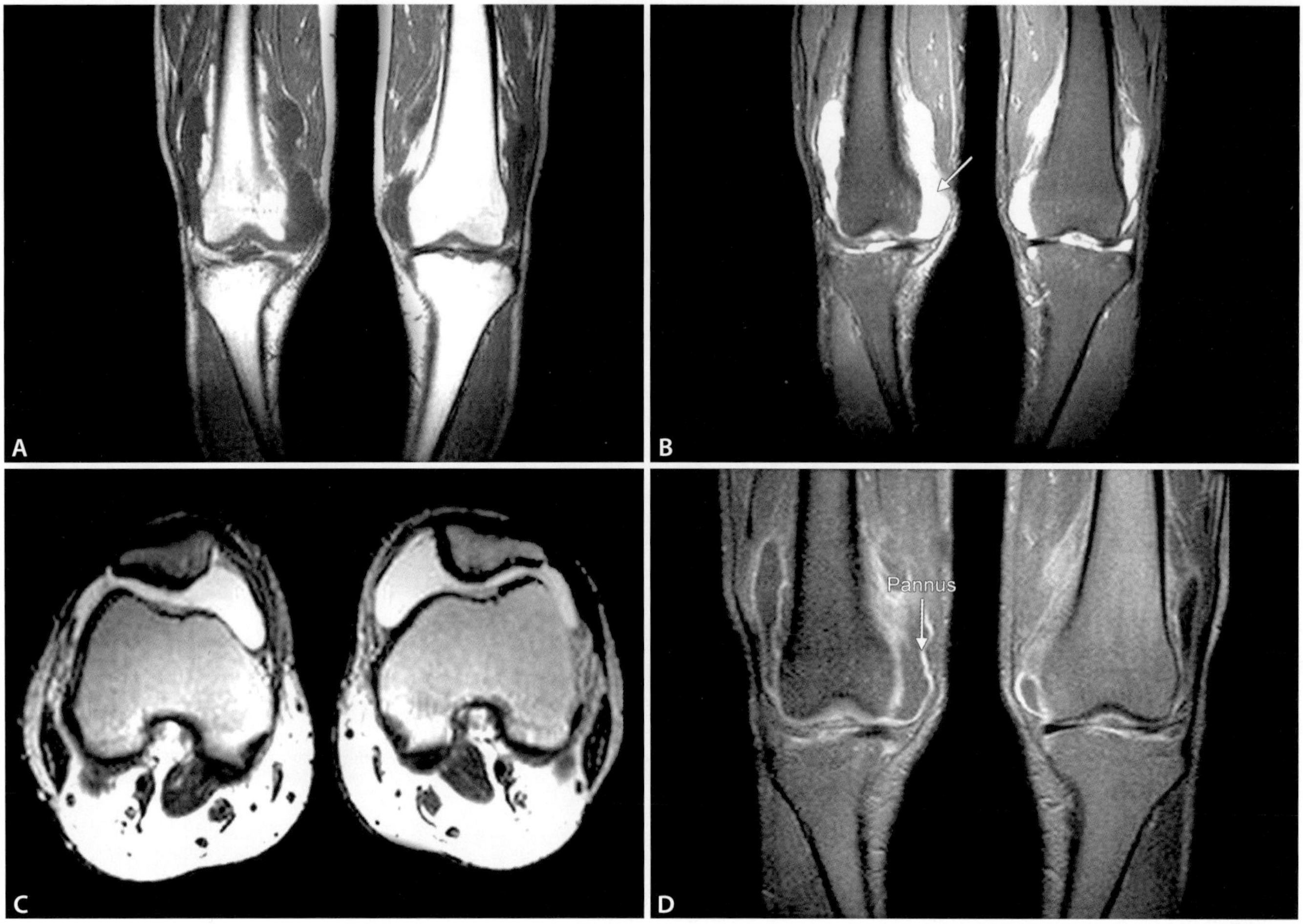

Figs. 38A to D: T1W coronal: (A) STIR coronal (B) axial T2W (C) and postcontrast T1W coronal (D) showing joint effusion with enhancing pannus growing on the surface of the articular cartilage in both the knees—Rheumatoid arthritis.

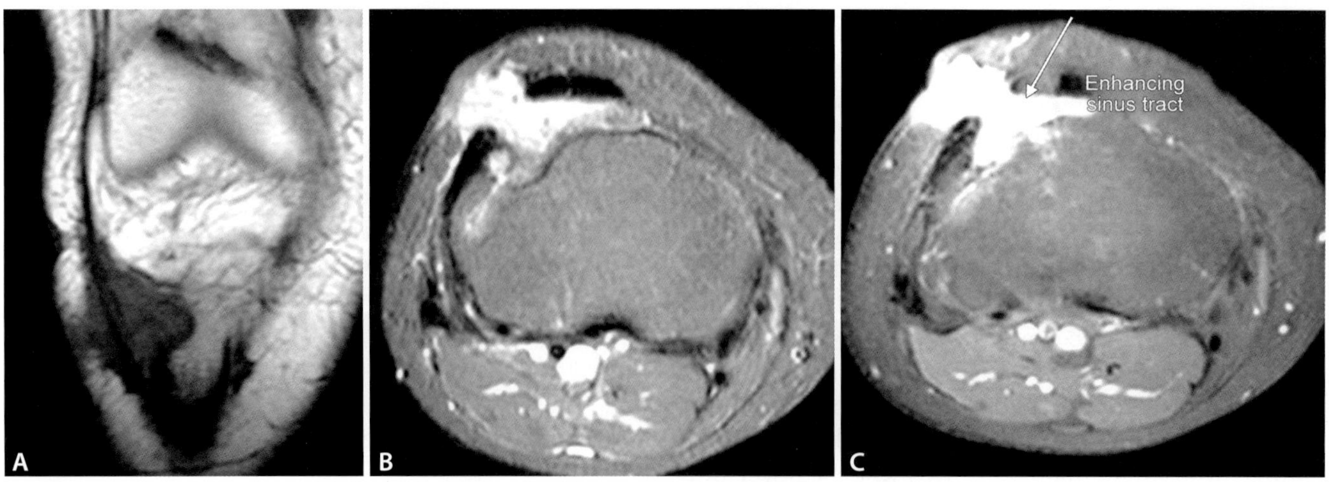

Figs. 39A to C: T1W coronal: (A) postcontrast T1W axial (B and C) MR images showing irregularity of the lateral tibial plateau with enhancing synovium and an enhancing sinus tract from the bone to the skin surface—Tuberculosis.

infrapatellar fat pad in the early stage. Articular cartilage erosions and synovial hypertrophy can also be identified. Hypoplastic menisci, with small anterior and posterior horns and body have also been described in patients with JRA on MR studies. An enlarged epiphysis, widening of the intercondylar notch and squaring of the inferior margin of the patella are radiographic findings also detected on MR. MR evaluation of signs of disease progression, such as pannus tissue changes may be a cost-effective way of monitoring the effectiveness of therapy. MR studies may also be used for serial follow-up of functional status in patients with JRA.[5]

Pigmented Villonodular Synovitis

Pigmented villonodular synovitis (PVNS) may also affect the knee. PVNS may present as a focal mass but more frequently is monoarticular. Histologically, the lesions present with fibrous synovial proliferation, infiltration by histiocytes, multinucleated giant cells and hemosiderin laden macrophages and hemosiderin staining of the synovium presumably from recurrent hemorrhage. These lesions present on MRI as characteristic proliferative synovial focal masses containing hypointense signal on all pulse sequences **(Figs. 40A to D)**. The signal loss results from proton dephasing from local magnetic field inhomogeneity caused by magnetic susceptibility effects of the iron containing byproducts of hemoglobin. Bony erosions are better visualized on MR than on plain films.[5,51]

Hemophilia

Subchondral and intraosseous cysts or hemorrhage can be identified on coronal and sagittal MR images. Hemosiderin

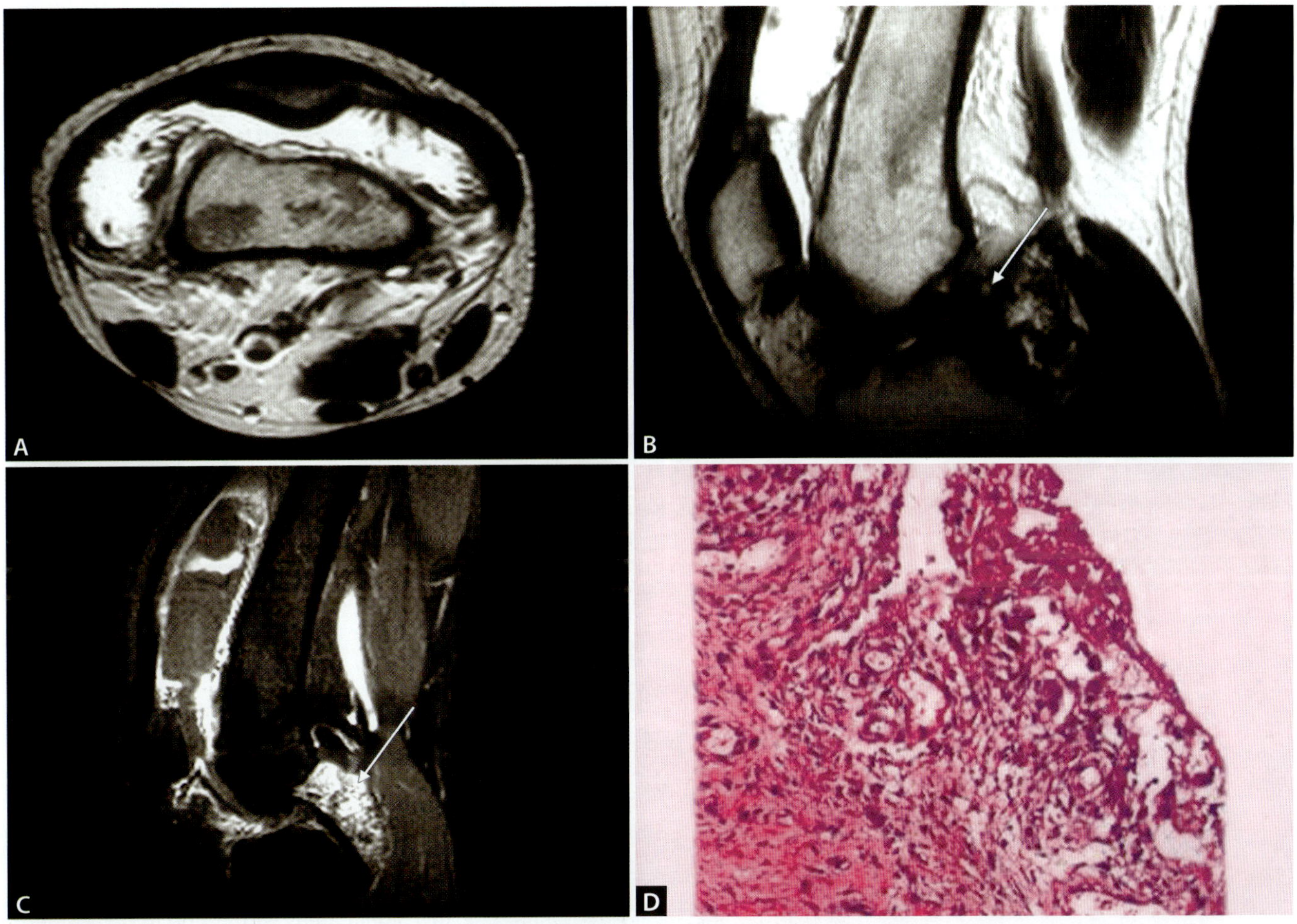

Figs. 40A to D: Axial T2W (A) and sagittal (B) images showing synovial thickening and associated effusion with scattered low signal areas of hemosiderin within (arrow). Low signal mass seen posterior to PCL. Postcontrast image (C) showing enhancement of the thickened synovium and the focal mass posterior to PCL (arrow). Biopsy (D) showing histiocytes with hemosiderin pigment—Pigmented villonodular synovitis (PVNS).

and fibrous tissue formed from repeated episodes of joint hemorrhage demonstrate low signal intensity on T1 and T2-weighted images **(Figs. 41A to C)**. Signal loss in these conditions is usually more uniform in its involvement of the joint synovium and focal masses characteristic of PVNS are not usually seen in chronic hemorrhagic conditions.

Synovial Chondromatosis of the Knee

It is a process associated with metaplastic changes within the synovium that produce multiple cartilaginous islands in the synovium. These cartilaginous islands may become dislodged producing both calcified and noncalcified loose bodies. Lesions contain enough calcium to be detected on plain films. They are low in signal intensity on all MR pulse sequences.

Deferiprone-induced Arthropathy

Deferiprone (DFP) is widely used as an iron chelator in thalassemia patients. The arthropathy consists of musculoskeletal stiffness, joint pain and joint effusion. Arthroscopy reveals excess iron in the synovium and cartilage. MRI in these cases reveals irregular thickening of the cartilage with subchondral erosions and cartilage intrusions in the subchondral defects. Synovial thickening and enhancement, synovial bands and effusions have been described. The symptoms decrease with dose reduction or temporary discontinuation of drug **(Figs. 42A to C)**.

MR IMAGING OF BONE MARROW ABNORMALITIES OF THE KNEE

Entities that affect the bone marrow are varied and include trauma, osteonecrosis, infection, tumors and metabolic disorders. Bone marrow typically demonstrates a similar response regardless of the insult, i.e. increased fluid content in the form of edema, hemorrhage pus or tumor. A systematic approach of analyzing the pattern of the marrow pathology and associated abnormalities helps in arriving at a specific diagnosis.

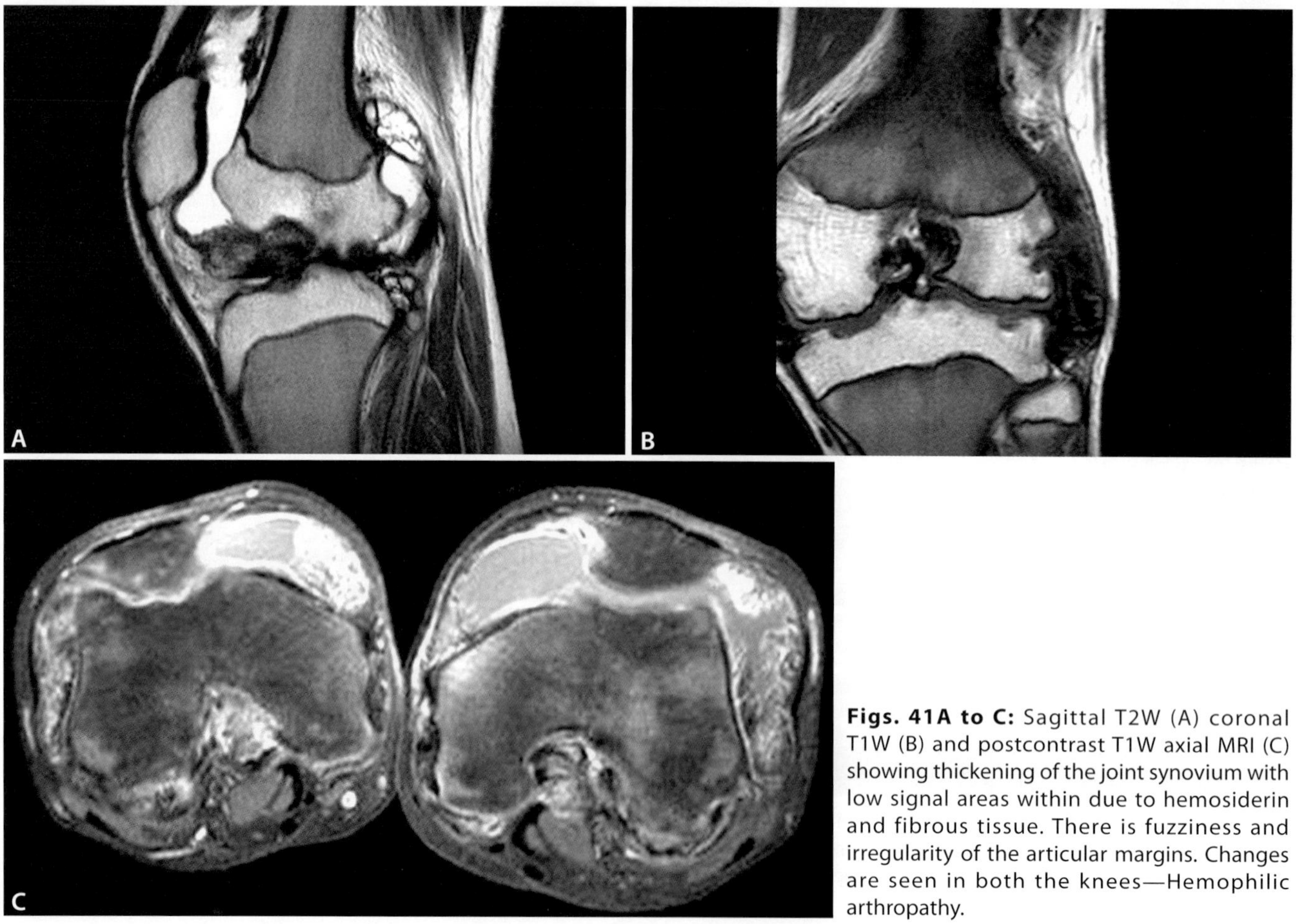

Figs. 41A to C: Sagittal T2W (A) coronal T1W (B) and postcontrast T1W axial MRI (C) showing thickening of the joint synovium with low signal areas within due to hemosiderin and fibrous tissue. There is fuzziness and irregularity of the articular margins. Changes are seen in both the knees—Hemophilic arthropathy.

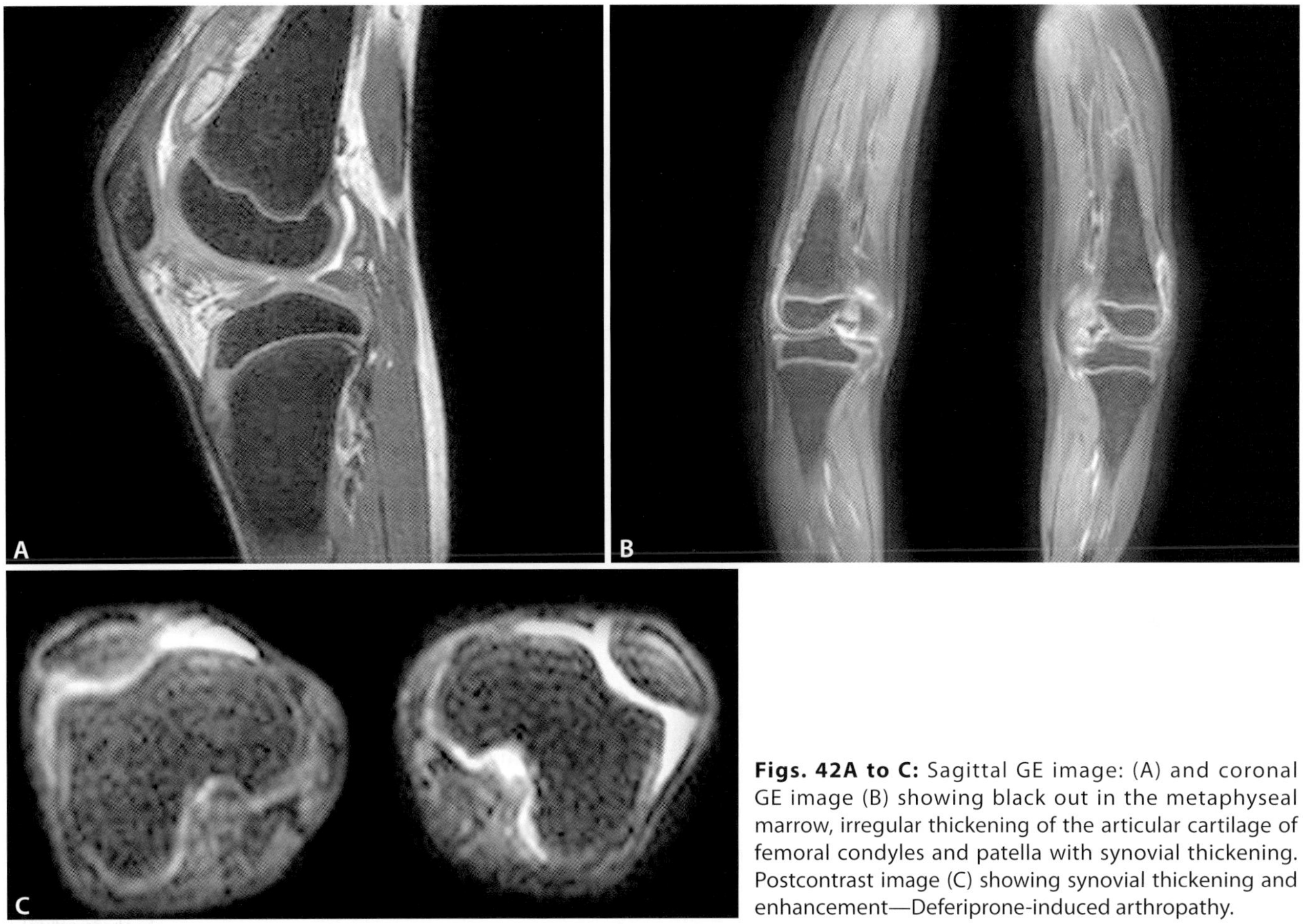

Figs. 42A to C: Sagittal GE image: (A) and coronal GE image (B) showing black out in the metaphyseal marrow, irregular thickening of the articular cartilage of femoral condyles and patella with synovial thickening. Postcontrast image (C) showing synovial thickening and enhancement—Deferiprone-induced arthropathy.

Trauma

The ability of MRI to detect clinically significant bony injuries that are undetected on radiographic studies has probably been MRI's most important attribute in clinical practice. MRI may be very helpful in evaluating patients with acute knee pain. Occult bony injuries are an important component of the cause of symptoms. Lynch has classified bony injuries as:[51]

Lynch type I: An acute impaction force on a bone results in marrow hemorrhage and edema, disruption of trabeculae and interstitial fluid leakage within the marrow space. On MRI these type I bony injuries known as bone bruises/contusions are identified by the vague, geographic, edema-like pattern hypointense on T1 and hyperintense on T2 and STIR images **(Fig. 43)**. Majority of the bone bruises show signal resolution at 3 months. A minority <5% fail to resolve by 3 months probably secondary to repetitively

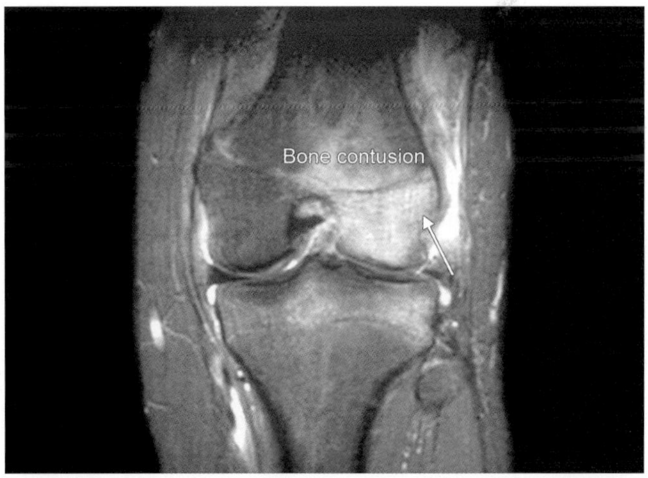

Fig. 43: STIR coronal MR images in a case of trauma showing areas of geographic bone marrow edema seen as hyperintense signal in the lateral femoral condyle and the posterolateral tibial plateau—Type I bony injury.

applied trauma. A method of grading severity of marrow edema particularly trauma induced marrow edema is based on diffusion imaging. Diffusion imaging represents a precise method of evaluating water movement. Trabecular disruption leads to increased multidirectional movement of water; hence, a recorded change in marrow diffusion is an objective marker of the severity of marrow injury. A high recorded diffusion coefficient can be used as on early indicator of severe marrow injury and can be optimally managed by a nonweight-bearing regimen. Five classic contusion patterns have been described in the knee.[67, 68]

1. The *pivot shift injury* occurs in skiers and American football players as a result of rapid deceleration with simultaneous change in direction. The tibia undergoes external rotation with the knee in flexion. On MRI, bone bruises are seen in the posterolateral tibial plateau and midportion of the lateral femoral condyle. This pattern is highly suggestive of an ACL injury.
2. The *dashboard injury* occurs in passengers in automobiles who undergo traumatic impact of the anterior proximal tibia with the dashboard while their knee is in flexion. An identical injury pattern can result from a fall onto bent knee. This injury will manifest on MRI as a bone contusion at the site of impact. A significant association has been demonstrated with injury to the PCL.
3. *Hyperextension injury* of the knee occurs with a direct blow to the anterior tibia on to the planted foot, results in "kissing contusions" of the anterior aspect of the proximal tibia and the distal femur. This finding on MRI is suggestive of additional trauma to the PCL, ACL, or menisci.
4. The *clip injury* result from pure valgus stress onto the partially flexed knee joint. Classically, this injury is seen in American football players who experience a blow to the lateral knee with the foot planted. It may also occur in a pedestrian struck by a car. The direct impact to the lateral knee will result in bone contusion at the lateral femoral condyle and lateral tibial plateau. The distractive forces at the medial joint compartment may result in coexisting MCL and medial meniscal tears (O'Donoghue triad). A smaller contusion in the medial femoral condyle at the MCL attachment may also be present as a result of the avulsive stress. Small contusion at the posterior lip of the medial tibial plateau has been described and attributed to contrecoup impaction as the knee relocates following the ACL tear.
5. *Lateral patellar dislocation* occurs in the setting of internal rotation of the femur with the knee in flexion. The resultant contraction of the quadriceps tendon in this configuration causes the patella to dislocate laterally. Bone contusions occur at the inferomedial patella and the anterior aspect of the lateral femoral condyle from the contact that occurs on relocation.

Lynch type II: These lesions reveal an interruption in the cortical bone on T1-weighted scans **(Fig. 44A)**. These are seen as regions of increased signal intensity on T2-weighted images and those lesions usually represent acute traumatic injuries with medullary hemorrhage and edema.

Lynch type III: Lesions present as regions of profound signal loss immediately adjacent to the cortical bone on T1 both and T2-weighted scan. Type III lesions most likely represent degenerative type subchondral sclerosis.[64]

Acute and Chronic Avulsive Injuries

Distraction injuries result in a small avulsion fracture related to a tendinous, ligamentous or capsular attachment on the bone. The associated marrow edema is much less extensive than the marrow edema seen with an impaction injury because cortical rather than medullary bone is involved.[69] The avulsed fragment is difficult to detect on MRI as the disproportionate edema and hemorrhage in the adjacent soft tissues masks the small osseous fragment. An example is Segond fracture. A Segond fracture represents an avulsion of the lateral tibial rim at the attachment site of the lateral capsular ligament **(Fig. 44B)**. Although the fracture fragment is typically small, cortical and obscured by soft tissue edema, this injury is important to identify, because it indicates substantial meniscoligamentous injury and anterolateral instability of the knee which may cause long-term disability if not recognized.

Thigh and shin splints cause traction periostitis.[70] In addition to the expected periosteal edema or fluid MRI reveals marrow edema and even cortical signal abnormalities that indicate osseous stress injuries of varying degrees.

Fatigue and Insufficiency Fractures

Fatigue fractures occur when abnormal stress is applied to normally mineralized bone whereas insufficiency fractures result from normal activities applied to the weakened bone. MRI reveals a spectrum of findings from periosteal edema alone to progressively severe marrow edema **(Figs. 45A and B)** to a hypointense fracture line in cancellous or cortical bone. MR has been advocated as a problem solving modality in suspected stress fracture in

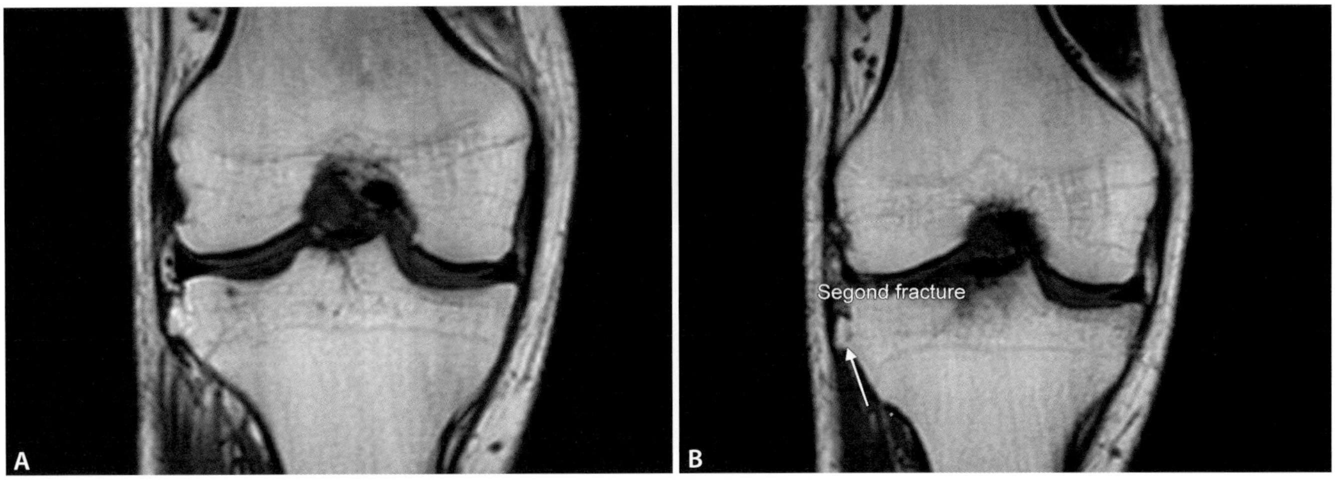

Figs. 44A and B: T1W coronal image showing an interruption in the cortical bone seen as linear low signal in the tibial spine—Grade 2 bony injury. Also seen is avulsion of the lateral tibial rim slightly below the level of the joint—Segond fracture.

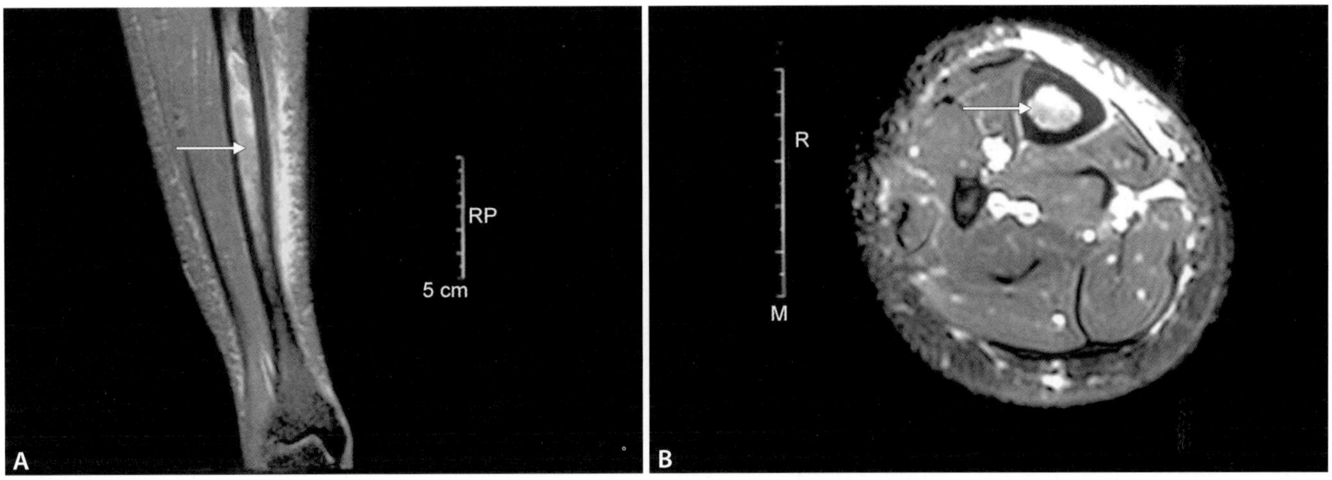

Figs. 45A and B: STIR coronal (A) and STIR axial (B) images showing edema in the subcutaneous tissues, extensive bone marrow edema seen as hyperintense signal with no evidence of cortical irregularity or periosteal reaction—Stress fracture in tibia.

a patient[71] with negative plain radiographs and equivocal bone scan. MR may secure the diagnosis if the fracture line is identified.

Stress Fractures

Stress fractures can result from either normal stress placed on deficient bone, as would occur in the osteoporotic elderly individual or, excessive stress placed on normal bone, as would occur in the running, jumping, or hurdling athlete.

Radiogrpahy is unreliable for detecting these lesions, particularly in the early stages. MRI, with a reported sensitivity and specificity as high as 88 and 100%, respectively, is the modality of choice. On MRI, stress fractures appear as as linear low-signal-intensity bands, away from the joint on T1-weighted and T2-weighted images. Increased signal intensity may be seen aroud the impacted fracture site on T2-weighted images, reflecting the associated edema.

Spontaneous Osteonecrosis

As its name implies, spontaneous osteonecrosis of the knee (SPONK) is a condition that affects the knee and results in an area of subchondral necrosis. Although long thought to represent a form of primary osteonecrosis, recent studies have concluded that this lesion is actually a subchondral insufficiency fracture that results in a devitalized segment of bone between the fracture line and overlying articular cartilage.[72] Osteonecrosis may cause osteoarthritis particularly when the necrotic defect is large.

This entity needs to be differentiated from osteochondritis dissecans. Spontaneous osteonecrosis is a distinct clinicopathological entity characterized by an older age of onset (most commonly an elderly woman), an abrupt onset of symptoms, acute onset of pain, a predilection for the weight bearing surface of medial femoral condyle and a unique MRI appearance. The patients who develop osteonecrosis are elderly and osteoporotic. The osteoporotic bone is susceptible to microfracture leading to accumulation of fluid within the subchondral bone seen as extensive edema on the MR images. The fluid leads to increased intraosseous pressure compromising blood flow and ultimately resulting in osteonecrosis. However, osteonecrosis is not an inevitable outcome. Patients may recover completely and in these patients the MR signal may return to normal. Current studies suggest that spontaneous osteonecrosis of the knee actually represents a subchondral insufficiency fracture.[68] The lesion in osteochondritis dissecans is typically in a different location on the lateral aspect of medial femoral condyle. Histologically, the osteochondritic lesion is composed of hyaline articular cartilage covering a metabolically active ossific nucleus. The lesion in osteonecrosis consists of dead bone. Loose bodies are a frequent result of osteochondritis—in fact, they may be the presenting symptom in osteochondritis dissecans but they are unusual in osteonecrosis.

Initial radiographs are often normal in spontaneous osteonecrosis even though the pain is severe, and the patient is unable to ambulate. On MRI, extensive edema-like signal is seen in the medial femoral condyle along with a linear subchondral focus of low signal intensity that represents the insufficiency fracture **(Figs. 46A and B)**.[73] Medial meniscal tears have also been reported in association with spontaneous osteonecrosis.

Medullary Infarction

Several factors, e.g. steroids, trauma, vasculitis are known to predispose to the development of focal areas of medullary infarction. Medullary infarcts result in geographic areas of ischemic and devitalized marrow that produce a characteristic MRI appearance; a geographic focus of typically heterogeneous signal within the marrow that is surrounded by characteristic low signal intensity, serpentine border on T1-weighted images. This border often demonstrates a classic double-line sign on T2-weighted images.[70] This is one of the few medullary lesions that usually contain some central fat. The presence of central fat is characteristic of this lesion.

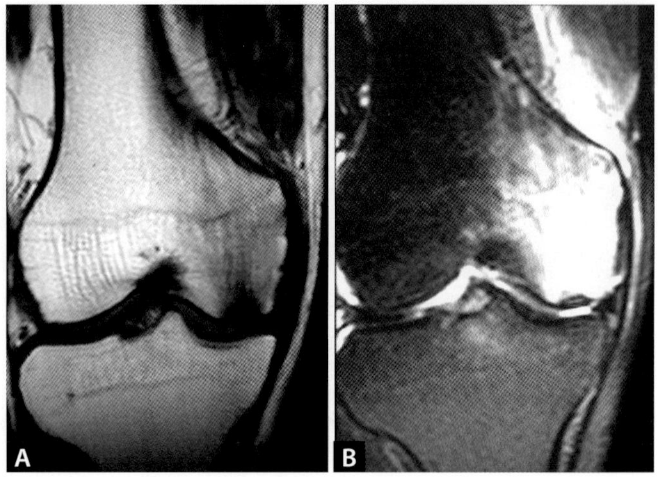

Figs. 46A and B: T1W coronal (A) and STIR coronal (B) MR images showing extensive marrow edema in the medial femoral condyle along with a crescentic subchondral focus of low signal intensity—Spontaneous osteonecrosis of the knee.

Osteochondritis Dissecans

A special form of subchondral osteonecrosis is termed osteochondritis dissecans. This entity is most frequently seen in adolescents and young adults and refers to fragmentation, and often separation, of a portion of subchondral bone, typically along the lateral aspect of the medial femoral condyle.[74] The cause of this lesion is uncertain, but it is suggested by some to result from repetitive trauma that produces shear forces across the cartilage. The alternative theory, more popular recently is that osteochondritis dissecans is an avascular lesion attributed to an insufficient end arterial blood supply to the subarticular trabeculae and poor anastomoses with the neighboring systems resulting in the infarctions of small wedge-shaped pieces of bone immediately beneath the articular cartilage. Though there is disagreement about the etiology of osteochondritis dissecans there is agreement on the pathological changes. A fragment of avascular bone with overlying articular cartilage is separated from the underlying normal bone by a layer of fibrous tissue that forms a barrier to revascularization. The fragment may separate completely to form a loose body or it may remain in its crater in the femoral condyle. Radiographic findings include a geographic, subchondral lucency along the non-weight-bearing surface of the medial femoral condyle.

Magnetic resonance imaging plays an important role in detecting the lesion if plain films are normal. A crescentic or ovoid focus of subchondral signal abnormality is evident. The primary concern when evaluating a focus of osteochondritis dissecans is whether the fragment of subchondral bone is unstable (i.e. at risk of evolving into a displaced loose body in the joint), in which case it likely requires operative intervention. Several MRI features have been shown to be suggestive of an unstable fragment. These include fluid tracking between the fragment and host bone, i.e. high signal interface, focal cystic areas beneath the fragment or a 5 mm or larger defect in the overlying cartilage **(Figs. 47A to C)**.[75]

Transient Bone Marrow Edema Syndrome (Transient Osteoporosis)

Transient bone marrow edema syndrome (also known as transient osteoporosis) was first described in the hip.

In the knee, the lateral femoral condyle is usually involved, although involvement of the medial femoral condyle and tibial plateau has also been described. Affected patients present with an acute onset of pain usually not associated with trauma. Resolution of pain and edema usually takes place within 6–12 months. Long-term sequelae do not occur. MRI findings include diffuse edema (low signal on T1-weighted images and high signal on T2-weighted or STIR sequences) without a focal area of signal abnormality typical of osteonecrosis.[76]

There is a considerable difference in clinical prognosis and treatment of transient osteoporosis as compared to spontaneous osteonecrosis. Hence, it is important to differentiate between these two entities. The differentiating features include as follows:

- Absence of low signal intensity in subchondral areas on T2W MR images is indicative of complete reversibility.
- When present a length of 14 mm and a thickness of 4 mm for these subchondral low signal intensity areas is indicative of evolution to collapsed osteonecrosis. Deeply located low signal lines with respect to subchondral bone also indicate irreversible osteonecrosis.
- Absence of focal deformity of the epiphyseal contour is indicative of complete reversibility.
- Spontaneous osteonecrosis of the knee typically involves medial femoral condyle while transient osteoporosis is more commonly seen in the lateral femoral condyle.

Reflex Sympathetic Dystrophy

The exact cause of reflex sympathetic dystrophy (RSD) is unclear, but it is believed to represent sequelae from hyperactivity of the sympathetic nervous system. In many cases it occurs after a recent episode of trauma. It results in circulatory changes and may progress to muscle atrophy, contractures, pale skin, and loss of hair on the extremity. MRI reveals diffuse, patchy bone marrow edema, which does not progress to the subchondral collapse seen in osteonecrosis. MRI findings which suggest the diagnosis of RSD include skin thickening, contrast enhancement, muscular atrophy, soft tissue edema and joint effusions.[77]

Infection

Capsular distension and joint effusions can be seen in MR scans of infected joints but are nonspecific findings.[78] A septic joint may be further characterized by intra-articular debris and synovitis from hematogenous seeding. In cases of osteomyelitis, the metaphysis, an active site of bone formation in children may show signal abnormalities (low signal on T1 bright signal on T2 or STIR images) restricted to this region. Marrow infiltration and soft tissue extension of osteomyelitis can be demonstrated using STIR and fat-suppressed T2W image **(Figs. 48A to D)**. Supportive

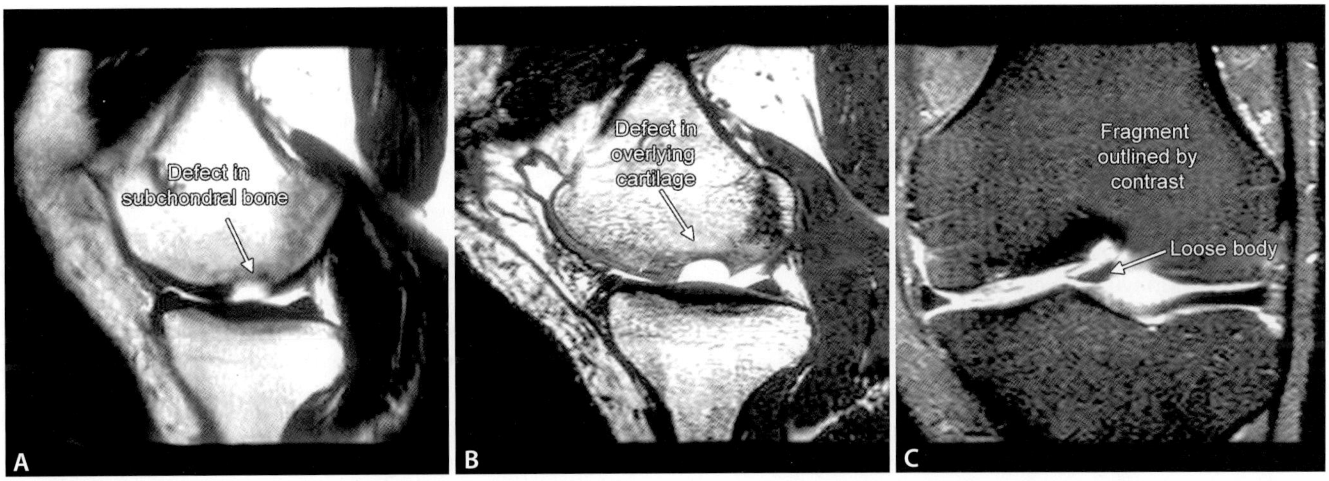

Figs. 47A to C: Sagittal T2W (A) DESS sagittal plane (B) images showing a defect in the subchondral bone and overlying cartilage. Indirect MR arthrography image (C) showing the displaced fragment outlined by contrast—Osteochondritis dessicans.

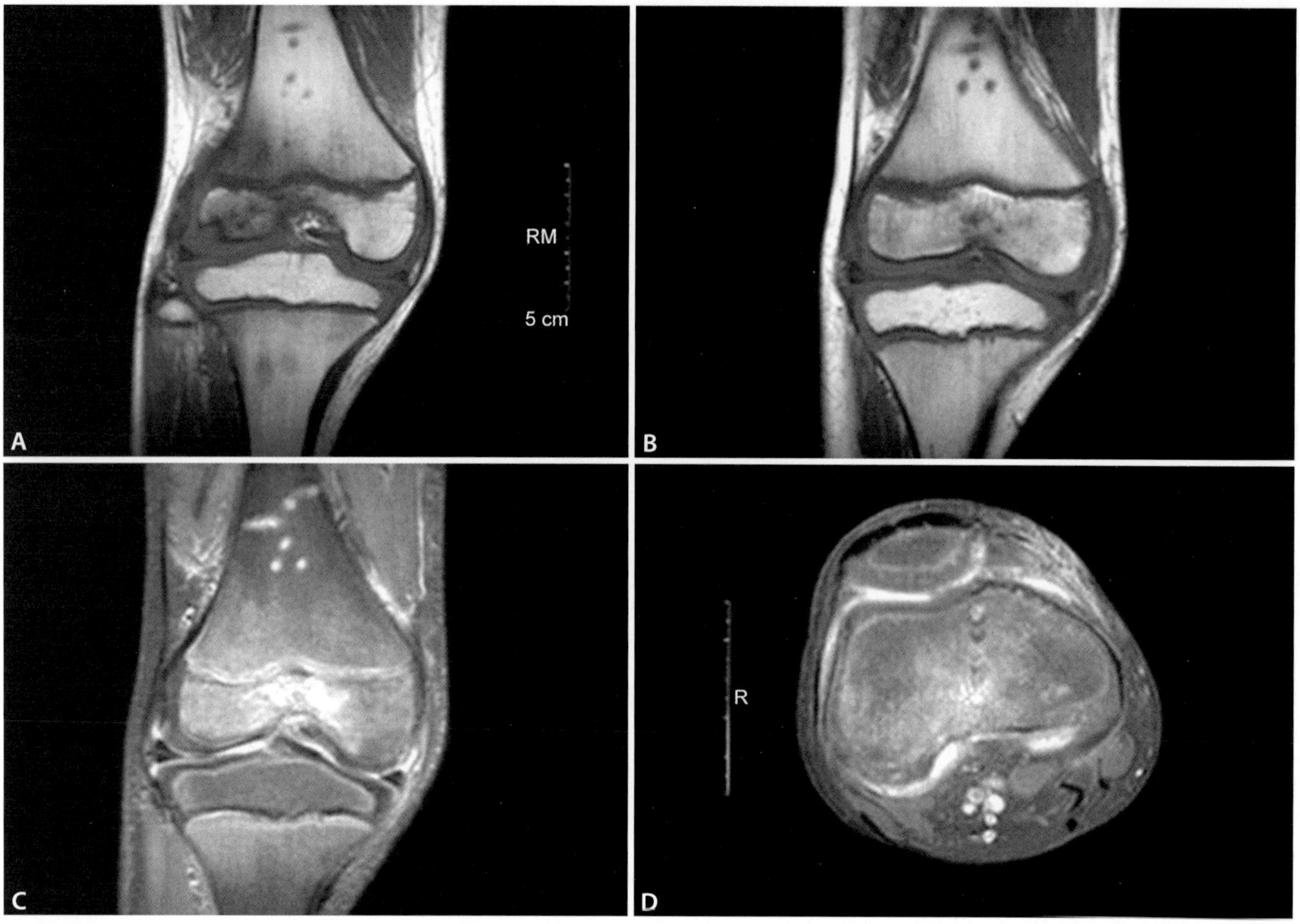

Figs. 48A to D: T1 coronal (A) and (B) postgadolinium coronal (C) postgadolinium T1 axial (D) images showing erosion of the articular margin of femur, fuzziness of the articular margins, marrow signal alteration, joint effusion and thick-enhancing synovium—Septic arthritis.

findings include overlying cortical destruction and an abscess or fistula extending to bone. A low signal intensity rim sign has been described in chronic infection resulting from trauma. This rim of fibrous tissue or reactive bone displays low signal on all pulse sequences and surrounds the area of active bone disease.

MR is also used to evaluate subacute osteomyelitis including Brodie's abscess. In Brodie's abscess the focus of involvement of osteomyelitis is hyperintense on STIR and fat-suppressed T2W images. The sclerotic margin displays low signal on all pulse sequences and there may be fluid in communication with the central infected focus.[5]

Bone Neoplasms

Magnetic resonance imaging has become an important component in the evaluation of primary bone neoplasms because of its ability to detect and accurately determine the local extent of disease. MRI and MR spectroscopy may also be helpful in following a patient's response to therapy. **Osteogenic sarcoma is one of the most common primary bone tumors emanating from the distal femur.** The extent of intramedullary disease is best defined with T1-weighted spin echo or STIR images while T2-weighted images may provide information about full extent disease and edema into the soft tissues. Encasement of major vessels and nerves as well as involvement of multiple muscular compartment may all be evaluated by MR and may decrease the efficacy of limb salvage surgery **(Figs. 49A to D)**.[79]

Infiltrative neoplasms, such as leukemia and lymphoma may present with knee pain indistinguishable from that caused by internal derangements of knee. These lesions need to be distinguished from signal inhomogeneity of normal marrow bone in metaphyses caused by variations in extent of hematopoietic marrow. Most types of marrow pathology result in signal intensity that is lower than that of skeletal muscle or intervertebral disc on T1-weighted images whereas hematopoietic

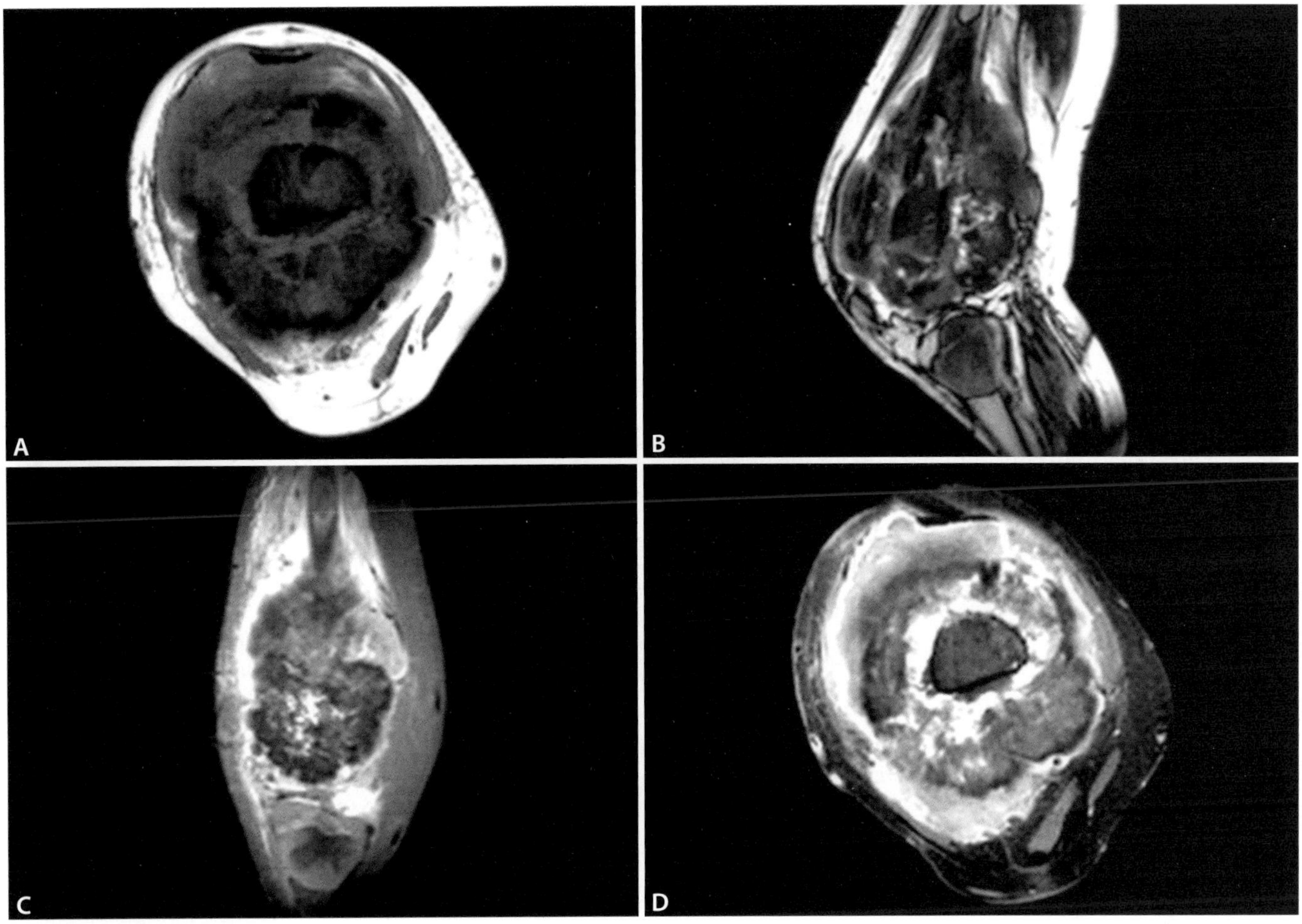

Figs. 49A to D: T1 axial (A) T2 sagittal (B) and T1 postcontrast coronal (C) and axial (D) MR images showing an irregular circumferential heterogeneous mass arising from the lower metadiaphyseal region of femur with cortical destruction, spiculated periosteal reaction, new bone formation, infiltration of medulla and multicompartment muscle involvement. Skip/metastatic focus also seen in upper tibia—Osteogenic sarcoma lower end femur.

marrow demonstrates signal intensity that is slightly higher than that of skeletal muscle or disc on T1-weighted images (owing to the relatively high amount of fat present even in red marrow). Other features of red marrow include signal intensity that parallels the signal intensity of other areas of known hematopoietic marrow, bilateral symmetry, scattered foci of fatty signal within the region of concern and an abrupt margination at the level of a closed physis. Also in contrast to the normal hematopoietic marrow, infiltrative disorders usually present a homogeneous low signal intensity mass on T1-weighted images and show well-defined margin.

Magnetic resonance imaging is also helpful in evaluating benign bony neoplasm. MRI characterizes the components of an osteochondroma better than other imaging techniques such as CT. The cartilaginous cap is well visualized by MRI and should be less than 1 cm in the non-neoplastic disease.[51]

MR ARTHROGRAPHY

Intra-articular contrast material enhances the diagnostic capabilities of MR imaging especially in the depiction of small structure and subtle disease.

Technique

The direct MR arthrographic technique does not differ from conventional arthrography. The knee is placed in a slightly bent, recumbent position for the usually used anterolateral access. The patella is pulled laterally and the puncture is made mid-patella or above with the needle entering the joint beneath the surface of the patella. To be able to fill the knee joint with a small volume of dissolved contrast medium, compression is applied to the soft tissues 15–20 cm above the joint cavity with an elastic bandage to prevent entry of the contrast medium into the suprapatellar recess. The injection is carried out under sterile conditions.

The total amount of the dilute contrast mixture (Gd-DTPA) injected should be 30–40 mL. After the injection, active and passive movements of the knee joint are carried out several times to achieve uniform distribution in the joint. An arthrographic effect or indirect MR arthrography can also be achieved with joint fluid enhancement following intravenous injection of Gd-DTPA. This method is referred to as indirect MR arthrography since no articular injection is required. The role of MR arthrography is in the following lesions:

Meniscal Lesions

Magnetic resonance arthrography has been shown to have a greater accuracy than conventional MRI for the detection of meniscal retears.[80] Because gadolinium-based contrast material has a lower viscosity than synovial fluid, it is more likely to be imbibed into a small cleft and, thereby, highlight the presence of a tear.

Cartilage Lesions

Administration of intra-articular contrast agent allows excellent delineation of the cartilage surface and provides good discrimination of cartilaginous lesions which have been graded from I to IV.[81] Magnetic resonance arthrography allows detection of grade 2 to IV lesions however grade 1 lesions still remain difficult to detect by arthrography since grade 1 lesions have no surface abnormality that is detected by intra-articular Gd-DTPA solution. On delayed sequences, however, an enhancement effect in cartilaginous areas with altered intrachondral structures can be observed. This is caused by diffusion of contrast material into the hyaline cartilage, although the thickness and surface of the cartilage may still appear normal in grade 1 lesions.

Osteochondritis Dissecans

Osteochondritis dissecans (OCD) is a lesion that characteristically affects the articular cartilage and subchondral bone with the potential of fragmentation and separation. Early detection of osteochondral lesion is desirable because the onset of degenerative arthritis in patients with OCD is estimated to occur 10 years earlier than in normal individuals. Management and prognosis of these osteochondral lesions depend on the stability of the fragment within its bony crater and the status of the overlying articular cartilage. Magnetic resonance arthrography is more accurate than MR in staging these osteochondral lesions of the knee.[82]

Intra-articular Bodies

The knee is affected most commonly by intra-articular bodies. These may consist of bone, cartilage or both bone and cartilage. Imaging is necessary to confirm the clinical diagnosis and to localize these bodies before surgery, because intra-articular bodies may be missed during arthroscopy. Radiography and conventional tomography are useful only when radiopaque intra-articular bodies are present. MR arthrography has the greatest sensitivity (86%) which is significantly more sensitive than conventional MRI.[83]

Plica Synovialis

The three plicae of the knee (suprapatellar plica, medial patellar plica and infrapatellar plica) are remnants of the embryologic synovium that separate the joint into different compartments during gestation. Partial plical remnants are often identified at arthroscopy but are incidental findings without clinical significance. Some plicae may persist into adult life and cause anterior knee pain, clicking, catching or locking of the knee when these plicae become inflamed and thickened by trauma or overuse.

The mediopatellar plica which extends from underneath the quadriceps and slides over the medial femoral condyle with knee movement is of great pathologic importance. The plica is usually attached closely to the femoral condyle and is not visualized when there is insufficient synovial fluid to outline. Differentiation between knee injuries and mediopatellar plica is important to avoid unnecessary arthroscopy. MR arthrography enables assessment of thickened plicae and should be considered as an alternative to diagnostic arthroscopy in patients with mediopatellar plica.[84]

POSTOPERATIVE EVALUATION OF THE KNEE

New developments and improvements in the ligamentous and meniscal surgery and cartilage repair procedures have led to an increased incidence of these procedures being performed. Subsequently there is an increase in the postoperative imaging studies and it is imperative for the radiologist to know the normal imaging appearance and complication of these procedures.

Imaging of the ACL Graft

The most commonly injured ligament in the knee is the ACL. ACL deficient knees can result in changes in mechanics causing secondary meniscal and cartilage injury. Hence, reconstruction of ACLs is being undertaken more commonly.

Fast spin echo is preferred over conventional spin echo because of the decreased metallic artifact seen with fast spin echo.[85] An addition, an oblique sagittal scan is often performed in the plane of the graft to allow better visualization of the ACL graft on one slice. Use of thinner 3 mm sections reduces volume averaging artifacts and provides better delineation of the neoalignment. An ACL neoalignment is considered intact if a smooth well-defined low signal intensity band is seen along its entire course on both T1- and T2-weighted images. The MR criteria used to assess disruption are contour irregularity, increased signal intensity within the ligament on T2-weighted images and discontinuity of the ligament.

Graft Rupture

Spontaneous graft rupture is rare and is frequently secondary to trauma. The same criteria used to diagnose a torn native ACL are used to diagnose a ruptured ACL graft and include discontinuity of normal fibers **(Figs. 50A and B)** and abnormal signal intensity within the substance of the graft which is usually fluid signal intensity interrupting the graft.

Graft Impingement

Graft impingement occurs when the graft abnormally contacts either the wall or the roof of the intercondylar notch. Impingement can lead to stretching, erosion, remodeling and tearing of the graft.

In impingement MRI shows the tibial tunnel to project anterior to a line drawn along the intercondylar roof and extended to the tibial plateau (Blumensaat's line). The distal two-thirds of the graft show increased signal intensity on T2W images;[86] however, this is never fluid signal intensity unlike in graft rupture.

Arthrofibrosis

Following ACL reconstruction loss of terminal extension (extension lag) is one of the major causes of morbidity. One of the major etiologies causing extension lag is localized anterior arthrofibrosis. In this condition, a focal fibrous nodule develops anterior to the distal portion of the ACL within the intercondylar notch. The nodule physically impairs terminal extension of the knee. The bluish discoloration of this rounded lesion resembles an eyeball on arthroscopy and has been named the cyclops lesion.[87] Cyclops lesion can be identified on MRI. On T1 and proton density weighted images, nodular intermediate signal intensity mass is seen at the anterior distal aspect of the graft in the intercondylar notch. On T2-weighted images the nodule has a heterogeneous but predominantly low signal intensity.

Postoperative Meniscus

The criteria for diagnosing meniscal tears in the virgin meniscus do not apply to the postmeniscectomy knee because there can be residual abnormal signal intensity and morphology. This is especially important when greater than 25% of the meniscus is removed in which the remaining meniscus can appear foreshortened with an irregular margin. In addition, abnormal signal can also be seen in stable meniscal remnants. The specificity of these findings for meniscal retear is lower than that for tears in non-

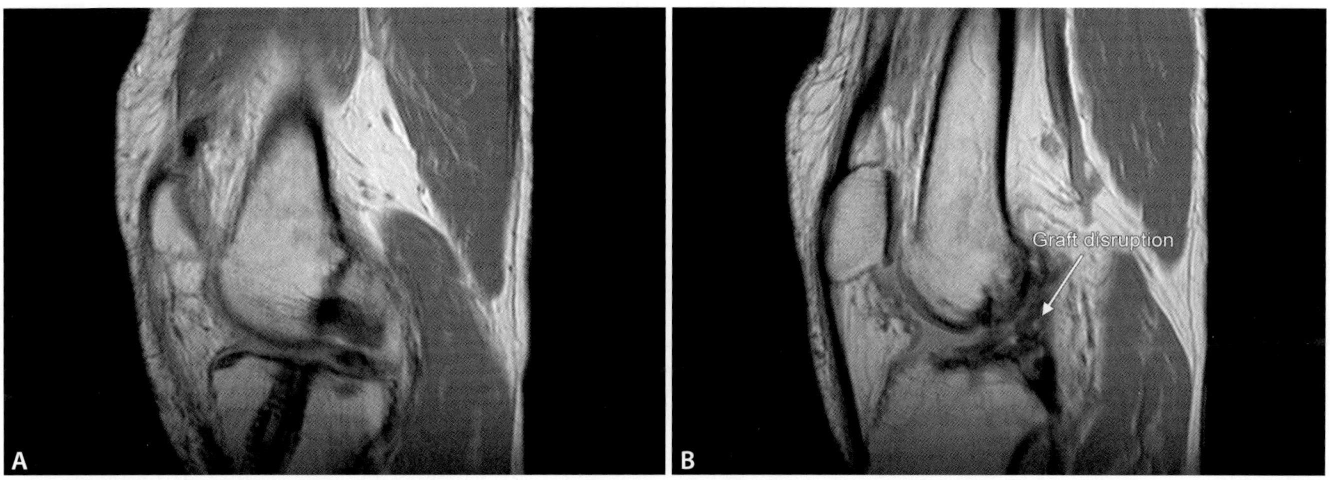

Figs. 50A and B: T2W sagittal MR images in a postoperative knee with ACL graft showing discontinuity of the graft fibers with high-signal intensity within—Graft disruption.

operative menisci. Several studies have reported an accuracy of 66–80% in the postoperative meniscus.[80]

Signal changes within the meniscus at a site distant from the original tear, fluid signal intensity in the meniscus remnant and a displaced fragment are specific signs of a meniscal retear but are not very sensitive. Direct MR arthrography increases the accuracy of diagnosing retears of the postoperative meniscus.

Postoperative Articular Cartilage

The development of new cartilage repair procedures that transplant or potentially reform hyaline like articular cartilage has led to an accurate noninvasive evaluation of the cartilage lesions following repair procedures.

Magnetic resonance imaging has been used to assess incorporation of grafts, assess vascularity of grafts evaluate the congruency between the graft and the native cartilage and bone and assess the donor site. One complication associated with this procedure is incongruence of the graft. Other complications include loose bodies, avascular necrosis of the donor site and condylar fracture which are all detected by MRI.

Autologous chondrocyte implantation involves harvesting chondrocytes from the relative nonweight bearing surfaces such as intercondylar notch. The chondrocytes are grown ex vivo and replaced into the periosteal covered site of the cartilage defect. Chondrocytes progress through several stages. Initially in the proliferative stage there is formation of a jelly-like substance. The second stage (7–12 weeks) known as the transition stage involves formation of a type II collagen framework. From 13 weeks to 3 years the maturation stage involves remodeling of the collagen framework resulting in firm hyaline tissue. MRI can assess the rate of and characteristics of growth cartilage and its incorporation within the native cartilage.[88] The state of the underlying subchondral bone can also be assessed by MRI.

Magnetic resonance and arthroscopy are complementary examinations for follow-up of autologous chondrocyte implants in knee. Asthroscopy is better used for assessing the cartilage surface and MR is better used for assessing lesions deep within the cartilage and underlying bone.[89,90]

CONCLUSION

Magnetic resonance imaging is clearly the imaging modality of choice for detecting and exploring joint, osseous and soft tissue injuries in the knee. MRI plays a pivotol role in making a precise diagnosis and then guiding treatment decisions. It is also extremely helpful in imaging the postoperative knee and in determining the response to therapy. It should be the goal of any radiologist who interprets MRI examinations of the knee to be able not only to recognize the normal anatomy and accurately diagnose pathology but also to develop a better grasp of the surgical implications of the imaging findings. By thinking like an arthroscopist, one can provide a more clinically relevant report and by doing so add value to the work-up of a patient with any knee pathology.

REFERENCES

1. Reicher MA, Bassett LW, Gold RH. High resolution MRI of the knee joint. Pathologic correlations. AJR. 1985;145:903-9.
2. Reicher MA, Hartzman S, Duckwiler GR, et al. Meniscal injuries. Detection using MR imaging. Radiology. 1986;159:753-7.
3. Hartzman S, Reicher MA, Bassett LW, et al. MR imaging of the knee. Chronic disorder. Radiology. 1987;162:553-7.
4. Kaplan PA. Knee. In: Kaplan PA, Helms CA, Dussault R, Anderson MW, Major NM (Eds). Musculoskeletal MRI. WB Saunders; 2001.
5. Stoller DW, Cannon WD, Anderson LJ. The knee. In: Stoller DW (Ed). Magnetic Resonance Imaging in Orthopaedics and Sports Medicine, 2nd edition. Lippincott Raven; 1997.
6. Bassett GC. The meniscus. Orthopaedics. 1992;15:35-42.
7. Koski JA, Ibarra C, Rodeo SA, Warren RF. Meniscal injury and repair: Clinical status. Orthop Clin North Am. 2000;31:419-35.
8. Escobedo EM, Hunter JC, et al. Usefulness of turbo spin-echo MR imaging in the evaluation of meniscal tears. Comparison with a conventional spin echo sequence. AJR. 1996;167:1223-7.
9. Kowalchuk RM, Kneeland JB, Dalinka MK, et al. MRI of the knee. Value of short echo time fast spin echo using high performance gradients versus conventional spin echo imaging for the detection of meniscal tears. Skeletal Radiol. 2000;29:520-4.
10. Helms CA, Laorr A, Cannon WD. The absent bow-tie sign in Bucket handle tears of the menisci in knee. AJR. 1998;170:57-61.
11. Ryu KN, Kim IS, Kim EJ, et al. MR imaging of tears of discoid lateral menisci. AJR. 1998;171:963-7.
12. Yu JS, Cosgarea AJ, Kaeding CC, Wilson D. Meniscal flounce MR imaging. Radiology. 1997;203:513-5.
13. Schnarkowski P, Tirman PF, Fuchigami KD, et al. Meniscal ossicle: Radiographic and MR imaging findings. Radiology. 1995;196:47-50.
14. Hajek PC, Gylys Morin VM, Baker LL, et al. The high signal intensity meniscus of the knee magnetic resonance evaluation and in vivo correlation. Investigative Radiology. 1987;22:883-90.
15. Kaplan PA, Nelson NL, Garvin KL, et al. MR of the knee. The significance of high signal in the meniscus that does not clearly extend to the surface. AJR. 1991;156:333-6.
16. Davis SJ, Teresi LM, et al. The "Notch" sign: Meniscal contour deformities as indicators of tear in MR imaging of the knee. J Comput Assist Tomography. 1990;14:975-80.

17. Campbell SE, Sanders TG, Morrison WB. MR imaging of meniscal cysts: Incidence, location and clinical significance. AJR. 2001;177:409-13.
18. Harper KW, Helms CA, Lambert HS III, Higgins LD. Radial Meniscal tears : Significance incidence and MR appearance. Am J Roentgenol. 2005;185:1429-34.
19. Tuckman GA, Miller WJ, Remo JW, et al. Radial tears of the menisci: MR findings. AJR. 1994;163:395-400.
20. Ozkor G, Circi E Gone U, et al. Radial tears in the root of the posterior horn of the medial meniscus. Knee Surg Sports Traumatol Arthrosc. 2008;16:849-54.
21. Wright DH, De Smet AA, Norris M. Bucket handle tears of the medial and lateral menisci of the knee: Value of MR imaging in detecting displaced fragments. AJR. 1995;165:621-5.
22. Singson R, Feldman F, Staron R, Kiernan H. MR imaging of displaced meniscal bucket handle tear of the medial meniscus. AJR. 1991;156:121-4.
23. Rao N, Patel Y, Opsha O, et al. Use of the V-sign in the diagnosis of bucket handle meniscal tear of the knee. Skeletal Radiol. 2012;41(3):293-7. Epub 2011 Jun 10.
24. Belzer JP, Cannon WD. Meniscus tears: Treatment in the stable and unstable knee. J Am Acad Orthop Surg. 1993;1:41-7.
25. Vahey TN, Bennett HT, Arrington LE, et al. MR imaging of the knee: Pseudotear of the lateral meniscus caused by the meniscofemoral ligament. AJR. 1990;154:1237-9.
26. Watanabe AT, Carter BC, et al. Normal variations in MR imaging of the knee: Appearance and frequency. AJR. 1989;153:341-4.
27. Peterfy CG, Janzen DL, Tirman PF, et al. Magic-angle phenomenon: A cause of increased signal in the normal lateral meniscus on short TE MR images of the knee. AJR. 1994;163:149-54.
28. Henning CE, Lynch MA. Current concepts of meniscal function and pathology. Clin Sports Med. 1985;4:259-64.
29. Matava MJ, Eck K, Totty W. Magnetic resonance imaging as a tool to predict meniscal reparability. Am J Sports Med. 1999;27:436-43.
30. Reicher MA, Hartzman S, Bassett LW, et al. MR imaging of the knee traumatic disorders. Radiology. 1987;162:547-51.
31. Crues JV, Mink J, Levy TL, et al. Meniscal tears of the knee: Accuracy of MR imaging. Radiology. 1987;164:445-8.
32. Bencardino JT, Rosenber ZS, Brown RR, et al. Traumatic musculotendinous injuries of the knee: Diagnosis with MR imaging. Radiographics. 2000;20:103-20.
33. Lee JK, Yao L, Phelps CT, et al. Anterior cruciate ligament tears. MR imaging compared with arthroscopy and clinical tests. Radiology. 1988;166:861-4.
34. Chan WP, Peterfy C, Fritz RC, Genant HK. MR diagnosis of complete tears of the anterior cruciate ligament of the knee: Importance of anterior subluxation of tibia. AJR. 1994;162: 355-60.
35. Kaplan PA, Gehl RH, Dussault RG, Anderson MW, Diduch DR. Bone contusions of the posterior lip of the medial tibial plateau (countercoup injury) and associated internal derangements of the knee at MR imaging. Radiology. 1999;211:747-53.
36. Graf BK, Cook DA, De Smat AA, Keene JS. Bone bruises on magnetic resonance imaging evaluation of anterior cruciate ligament injuries. Am J Sports Med. 1993;21:220-3.
37. Tung GA, Davis LM, Wiggins ME, Fadale PD. Tears of the anterior cruciate ligament: Primary and secondary signs at MR imaging. Radiology. 1993;188:661-7.
38. Covey DC, Sapega AA. Anatomy and function of the posterior cruciate ligament. Clin Sports Med. 1994;13:509-18.
39. D Maesaneer M, Von Roy F, Lenchik L, et al. Three layers of the medial capsular and supporting structures of the knee: MR imaging-anatomic correlation. Radiographics. 2000;20:83-9.
40. Schweitzer MS, Tran D, Deely DM, Hume EL. Medial collateral ligament injuries: Evaluation of multiple signs, prevalence and location of associated bone bruises and assessment with MR imaging. Radiology. 1995;194:825-9.
41. Mendes LF, Preeterklieber ML, Cho JH, et al. Pellegrini Stieda disease: A heterogeneous disorder not synonymous with ossification/calcification of the tibial collateral ligament–anatomic and imaging investigation. Skeletal Radiol. 2006;35: 916-22.
42. Loredo R, Hodler J, Pedowitz R, et al. Posteromedial corner of the knee: MR imaging with gross anatomic correlation. Skeletal Radiol. 1999;28:305-11.
43. Recondo JA, Salvador E, Villanua JA, et al. Lateral stabilising structures of the knee: Functional anatomy and injuries assessed with MR imaging. Radiographics. 2000;20:91-102.
44. Yu JS, Salonen DC, Hodler J. Posterolateral aspect of the knee: Improved MR imaging with a coronal oblique technique. Radiology. 1996;198:199-204.
45. Hayes CW, Brigido MK, Jamadar DA, Propeck T. Mechanism based pattern approach to classification of complex injuries of the knee depicted at MR imaging. Radiographics. 2000;20:121-34.
46. Menz MJ, Lucas GL. Magnetic resonance imaging of a rupture of the medial head of the gastrocnemius muscle. J Bone Joint Surg Am. 1991;73:1260-1.
47. Yu JS, Goodiwn D, Salonen D, et al. Complete dislocation of the knee: Spectrum of associated soft tissue injuries depicted by MR imaging. AJR. 1995;164:135-9.
48. Yu JS, Petersilge C, Sartoris DJ, et al. MR imaging of injuries of the extensor mechanism of the knee. Radiographics. 1994;14:541-51.
49. Nance EP, Kaye JJ. Injuries of the quadriceps mechanism. Radiology. 1982;142:301-7.
50. Quinn SF, Brown TR, Demlow TA. MR imaging of patellar retinacular ligament injuries. J Magn Reson Imaging. 1993;3: 843-7.
51. Crues JV, Manji SA, Shellock FG. Knee. In: Stark D, Bradley WG (Eds): Magnetic Resonance Imaging, 3rd edition. Mosby; 1999.
52. Shellock FG, Mink JH, Deutsch AL, et al. Patellofe-moral joint: Identification of abnormalities with active movement 'unloaded' versus 'loaded' kinematic MR imaging techniques. RSNA. 1993;188:575-8.
53. Buckwalter JA, Mankin HG. Articular cartilage tissue design and chondrocyte matrix interactions. J Bone Joint Surg Am. 1997;79:600-11.

54. Bradella MA, Tirman PFJ, Peterfy CG, et al. Accuracy of T2 weighted fast spin-echo MR imaging with fat saturation in detecting cartilage defects in the knee: Comparison with arthroscopy in 130 patients. AJR. 1999;172:1073-80.
55. Hardy PA, Recht MP, Piraino DW. Fat-suppressed MRI of articular cartilage with spatial-spectral excitation pulse. J Magn Reson Imaging. 1998;8:1279-87.
56. Disler DG, McCauley TR, Kelman CG, et al. Fat suppressed three-dimensional spoiled gradient-echo MR imaging of hyaline cartilage defects in the knee: Comparison with standard MR imaging and arthroscopy. AJR. 1996;167:127-32.
57. Erickson SJ, Waldochmidt JG, Czervionke LF, et al. Hyaline cartilage truncation artifact as a cause of trilaminar appearance with fat suppressed three-dimensional spoiled gradient recalled sequences. Radiology. 1996;201:260-4.
58. Kijowski R, Blankenpaker DG, Davis KW, et al. Comparison of 1.5 and 3.0 T MR Imaging for Evaluating the Articular Cartilage of the Knee Joint. Radiology. 2009;250:839-48.
59. Wong S, Steinbach L, Zhao J, et al. Comparative study of imaging at 3.0 T versus 1.5 T of the knee. Skeletal Radiol. 2009;38:761-9.
60. Link TM, Stahl R, Woertler K, et al. Cartilage imaging, motivation, techniques, current and future significance. Eur Radiol. 2007;17:1135-46.
61. McCauley TR, Kier R, Lynch KJ, et al. Chondromalacia patellae: Diagnosis with MR imaging. AJR. 1992;158:101-5.
62. Crema MD, Roemer FW, Marra MD, et al. MR Imaging of Intra and periarticular Soft tissues and subchondral bone in knee osteoarthritis. Radiol Cl N Am. 2009;47:687-701.
63. Kijowski R, Stanton P, Fine J, Smet AD. Subchondral bone marrow edema in patients with degeneration of the articular cartilage of the knee joint. Radiology. 2006;238:943-9.
64. Waldochmidt JG, Braunstein EM, Buckwalter KA. Magnetic resonance imaging of osteoarthritis. Rheum Dis Clin North Am. 1999;25:451-65.
65. Buckwalter JA, Mankin HJ. Articular cartilage repair and transplantation. Arthritis Rheum. 1998;41:1331-42.
66. McGonagle D, Gibbon W, O'Connor P, et al. Characteristics magnetic resonance imaging entheseal changes of knee synovitis in spondyloarthropathy. Arthritis Rheum. 1998;41:694-700.
67. Sanders TG, Medynski MA, Feller JF. Bone contusion patterns of the knee at MR imaging: Footprint of the mechanism of injury. Radiographics. 2000;20:135-51.
68. Baltazar R, Ma C, Shankman S, Beltran J. Knee. In: Haaga JR, Dogra VS, Forsting M, Gilkeson RC, Kwon HA H, Sundaram M (Eds): CT and MRI of the whole Body, 5th edition. Mosby; 2009.
69. Palmer WE, Levine SM, Dupuy DE. Knee and shoulder fractures: Association of fracture detection and marrow oedema on MR images with mechanism of injury. Radiology. 1997;204:395-401.
70. Anderson MW, Ugalde U, Batt M, et al. Shin splints: MR appearance in a preliminary study. Radiology. 1997;204:177-80.
71. Anderson MW, Greenspan A. Stress fractures. Radiology. 1996;199:1-12.
72. Yamamoto T, Bullough PG. Subchondral insufficiency fracture of the femoral head and medial femoral condyle. Skeletal Radiol. 2000;29:40-4.
73. Frosberg PK, Braunstein EM, Buckwalter KA. Osteonecrosis, transient osteoporosis and transient bone marrow edema. Radiol Clin North Am. 1996;34:273-91.
74. Hughston JC, Hergenroeder PT, et al. Osteochondritis dissecans of the femoral condyles. J Bone Joint Surg. 1984;66:1340-8.
75. DeSmet A, Fisher DR, Graf BK, et al. Osteochondritis dissecans of the knee: Value of MR imaging in determining lesion stability and the presence of articular cartilage defects. AJR. 1990;155:549-53.
76. Wambeek N, Munk PL, Lee MJ, Meek RN. Intra-articular regional migratory osteoporosis of the knee. Skeletal Radiol. 2000;29:97-100.
77. Schweitzer ME, Mandel S, Schwartzman RJ, et al. Reflex sympathetic dystrophy revisted: MR imaging findings before and after infusion of contrast material. Radiology. 1995;195:211-4.
78. Graif M, Schweitzer ME, Deery D, et al. The septic versus nonspecific inflamed joint: MRI characteristics. Skeletal Radiol. 1999;28:616-20.
79. Sundaram M, McGuire MH, Herbold DR, et al. Magnetic resonance imaging in planning limb salvage surgery for primary malignant tumours of bone. J Bone Joint Surg. 1986;68:809-19.
80. Applegate GR, Flannigan BD, Tolin BS, et al. MR diagnosis of recurrent tears in the knee: Value of intra-articular contrast material. AJR. 1993;161:821-5.
81. Kramer J, Recht MP, Imhof H, et al. Postcontrast MR arthrography in assessment of cartilage lesions. J Comput Assist Tomography. 1994;18:218.
82. Kramer J, Stiglbauer R, Engel A, et al. MR contrast arthrography in osteochondrosis dissecans. J Comput Assist Tomography. 1992;18:254-60.
83. Brossmann J, Priedler KW, Daenen B. Imaging of osseous and cartilaginous intra-articular bodies in the knee: Comparison of MR imaging and MR arthrography with CT and CT arthrography in cadavers. Radiology. 1996;200:509-17.
84. Kobayashi Y, Murkami R, Tajima H. Direct MR arthrography of plica synovialis mediopatellaris. Acta Radiol. 2001;42:286-90.
85. Schatz JA, Potter HG, Rodeo SA, et al. MR imaging of anterior cruciate ligament reconstruction. AJR. 1997;169:223-8.
86. Howell SM, Berns GS, Farley TE. Unimpinged and impinged anterior cruciate ligament grafts: MR signal intensity measurements. Radiology. 1991;179:639-43.
87. Recht MP, Piraino DW, Cohen MAH, et al. Localised anterior arthrofibrosis (cyclopos lesion) after reconstruction of the anterior cruciate ligament: MR imaging findings. AJR. 1995;165:383-5.
88. Alparslan L, Winalski CS, Boutin RD, et al. Postoperative magnetic resonance imaging of articular cartilage repair. Seminars in Musculoskeletal. Radiology. 2001;5:345.
89. Ho YY, Wang SC. Postoperative evaluation of the knee after autologous chondrocyte implantation: What Radiologists Need to Know. Radiographics. 2007;27:207-20.
90. Gnannt R, Chhabra A, Theodoropoubs JS, et al. MR imaging of postoperative knee. Journal of Magnetic Resonance Imaging. 2011;5:1007-21.

CHAPTER 201

Magnetic Resonance Imaging of Hip and Pelvis

Anjali Prakash

INTRODUCTION

The primary weight-bearing joint is the hip joint. The pelvis is responsible for transferring the weight of the whole body to both the feet and at the same time, it allows for extensive hip movement. Hip disorders are a potential source of disability in patients of all age groups. Diagnostic imaging has a significant role in the diagnosis and staging of disease. Early diagnosis is potent of delaying the onset of arthritis and the requirement of total hip replacement. Magnetic resonance imaging (MRI) is the most preferred choice for the diagnosis of most hip disorders, where plain radiographs are nondiagnostic.

NORMAL ANATOMY

The pelvis is a very complex structure which is composed of an osseous ring formed by the innominate bones and the sacrum with numerous muscles attached for support and ambulation. The sacroiliac joint does not allow much movement and the weight is transmitted by articulating surfaces. The hip is a ball and socket joint which gains stability by the anterolateral orientation of the acetabulum and the anterior position of the femoral head with regard to the femoral shaft. Medially, the osseous acetabulum is deficient in its inferior extent, with osseous discontinuity in the region of the acetabular notch. A soft tissue structure, the transverse ligament, spans this region, thus completing the socket morphology of the acetabulum.

There is absence of cartilage in the center of the acetabulum, but its peripheral margin is covered with articular cartilage which leads to an inverted horseshoe configuration of the acetabular articular surface. The acetabulum is centrally filled with fatty tissue termed as pulvinar. The femoral articulating surface also has a region without articular cartilage which is called the fovea capitus. It corresponds to the proximal attachment site of the ligamentum teres. This structure courses along the medial joint space to a distal attachment site at the transverse ligament. The fovea capitus should not be mistaken for an osteochondral lesion.

Four distinct facets have been described in the hip, of which three have corresponding tendon attachment sites. The anterior facet of the hip is located on the anterolateral surface of the trochanter. It has an oval shape and shares a medial border with the intertrochanteric line. The second of four facets, the lateral facet, has an inverted triangular shape, with the most caudal portion comprising the clearly visible part of the trochanter at physical examination. The posterior superior border of the lateral facet is in contact with the superoposterior facet, the third facet of the greater trochanter. The most cranial part of the greater trochanter is the facet which has an oblique transverse orientation. The posterior facet accounts for the fourth and final facet and is comprised of the most posterior aspect of the trochanter. It borders the lateral and superoposterior facets and has a curved shape in a mediolateral direction.

These facets with their corresponding tendon attachments march around the greater trochanter from its anterior to posterior extent. The muscular attachments to these facets facilitate the wide range of motion elicited at this articulation. The facets of the greater trochanter have bursae that are intimately associated with them. These include the subgluteus minimus and medius bursae. These bursae are located under the gluteus minimus and medius tendon osseous attachment sites, respectively. In addition, there is a subgluteus maximus bursa, the largest of the three that covers the posterior facet and a portion of the lateral facet.[1]

Similarly, the attachment sites of the proximal hamstring tendons correspond to changes in osseous contour. The proximal hamstring attachment complex is composed of the semimembranosis, semitendinosis, and biceps femoris tendons. Except for the short head of the biceps femoris, these three arise from the posterolateral ischial tuberosity, lateral and inferomedial facets. The semimembranosus tendon originates from the superolateral facet while the semitendinosis and long head of the biceps femoris form a conjoint tendon that attaches to the inferomedial facet. In rare cases, the conjoint tendon is not present and the two tendons arise separately. The coronal plane on MR imaging is superior in visualization of the proximal hamstring attachment to these facets. In the transverse plane, the semimembranosis tendon can be found anterolaterally to the conjoint tendon. More distally, the tendon runs more medial and anterior to the other two hamstring tendons.

The acetabular labrum comprises of fibrocartilaginous tissue that is attached to the acetabular rim. It is primarily an avascular structure that is triangular in its cross-section and appears to be thickest at its osterosuperior extent. Inferiorly, the acetabular labrum coalesces with the transverse ligament in the region of the acetabular notch. On MR imaging, the normal labrum demonstrate variations in both its morphology and signal intensity. The three types of morphology are: triangular, circular, flat, and absent. Triangular is the most common shape; the labrum usually demonstrates homogeneously low signal intensity. However, an age-related pattern of increased intralabral signal on both T1- and T2-weighted sequences has been documented in asymptomatic patient populations.

The appearance of the hip on MRI varies depending on the type of sequence and the skeletal maturity of the patient. Cortical bone produces a thin sharply defined black line. Thicker cortex is noted in the femoral diaphysis. Higher signal is always present within the medullary cavity of both the femoral head and acetabulum. In the adult, the epiphysis is filled completely with fatty marrow that is high in signal on all sequences, except STIR and fat saturation techniques, in which the epiphysis becomes dark **(Figs. 1A and B)**. The nonossified epiphyseal cartilage of the child is homogeneous and moderately high in signal **(Figs. 2A and B)**. Maturation replaces the cartilage with larger amounts of fatty marrow within the bony epiphysis.

The immature metaphysis contains hematopoietic marrow and is intermediate in signal on all sequences. The adult metaphysis contains a mix of fatty and hematopoietic marrow that is lower in signal than the epiphysis and is often heterogeneous. Hematopoietic marrow dominates in younger patients and fatty marrow in older patients. This may be due to decreased blood supply of the marrow with age and a change from the sinusoidal blood flow of

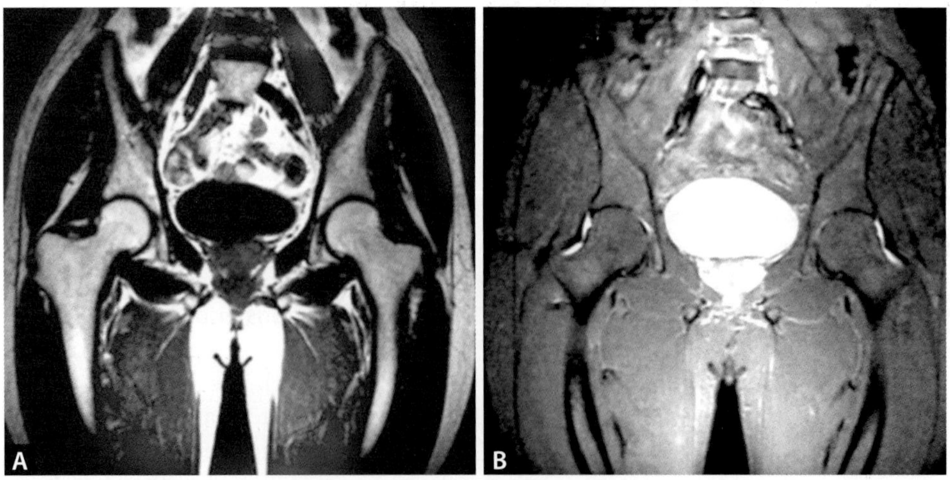

Figs. 1A and B: (A) T1W coronal image of bilateral hips and pelvis; (B) STIR coronal image showing fatty marrow of the femoral head, which is suppressed on STIR. Cortical outline is sharply defined and black on both sequences—Normal appearance.

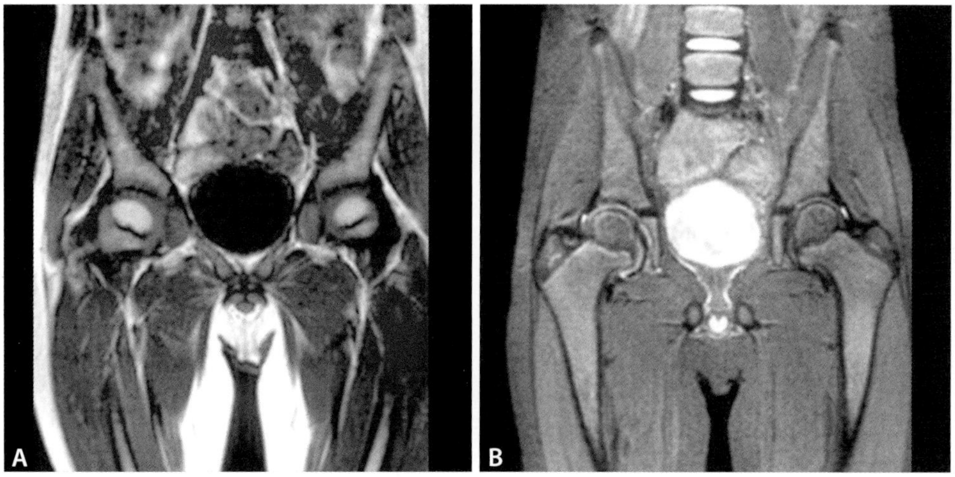

Figs. 2A and B: (A) T1W coronal image and (B) STIR coronal image shows moderately high signal in the epiphyseal cartilage with ossifying femoral head exhibiting fatty marrow in a child.

hematopoietic marrow to the more sparse capillary flow in fatty marrow.

The physeal scar separating the epiphysis from the metaphysis is seen on all MR examinations of the hip. The inability to identify some part of the physeal scar indicates an examination of inadequate quality. The physeal scar, best seen on T1W images is seen as a thin black line on all sequences **(Fig. 3)**.

The trabecular pattern within the femoral head and neck is reinforced by two regions of increased trabeculation corresponding to areas of relative increase in stress. The largest of these areas runs from the apex of the femoral head inferolaterally crossing the physeal plate to the medial femoral neck. This region is referred to as primary weight-bearing trabecula. Primary weight-bearing trabeculae produce a fan shaped area of lower signal within the femoral head and neck, produced by increased concentration of calcium relative to fat **(Fig. 4)**. A second area of trabecular prominence runs from the inferomedial femoral head laterally and across the neck towards the greater trochanter.

The articular cartilage of the femoral head and acetabulum produces a thin, smooth uniform intermediate signal, the signal being higher on STIR, gradient and fat saturation technique **(Fig. 5)**.

TECHNIQUE

The technique used for performing MRI of the hip is designed to image both hips and the entire pelvis. Hip MRI is best performed on a 1.5/3 tesla magnet. There is no true hip coil and hip imaging is best performed with a shoulder coil, a small field of view wrap coil.[2] In addition to high resolution surface coil images, larger field of view body coil images are also used to detect occult sacral or pubic fractures, pelvic masses which may simulate hip pain.

Magnetic resonance examination of the hip begins with a triplane localization which is a low resolution gradient recalled echo imaging technique. This facilitates accurate positioning. The hip MR is performed using a surface coil to optimize the ratio of signal-to-noise. Standard hip MR protocol consists of T1-weighted (TR-600 msec/ TE-14 msec) and STIR coronal sequences. In the axial plane, T1-weighted (TR-600 msec/TE-14 msec) and T2-weighted fat-saturation (TR-3000 msec/TE-90 msec) sequences are obtained. The latter is performed to gather a true fluid-sensitive sequence. Additionly, T1-weighted (TR-600 msec/TE-14 msec) sagittal, proton-density fat-saturation (TR-3000 msec/TE-30 msec) coronal sequences are acquired. A new proton-density (TR-3000 msec/TE-30 msec) axial oblique sequence to look for abnormal femoral head-neck offset is also done.[2] The coronal localizer is used to obtain an axial oblique plane by angling the slices parallel to the femoral neck **(Figs. 6A and B)**. Additional technical parameters for standard hip MR include a slice thickness of 5 mm, and field of view (FOV)-36 cm, 34 cm, and 24 cm for the coronal, axial, and sagittal sequences respectively. The axial oblique images can be obtained at a slice thickness of 24 cm.

Routine MR imaging of the hip is appropriate for identifying occult fracture, marrow abnormality, avascular necrosis (AVN) and musculotendinous pathology.

Magnetic resonance arthrography (MRA) of the hip is specifically indicated at the detection of labral pathology, osteochondral lesions, intra-articular bodies, and

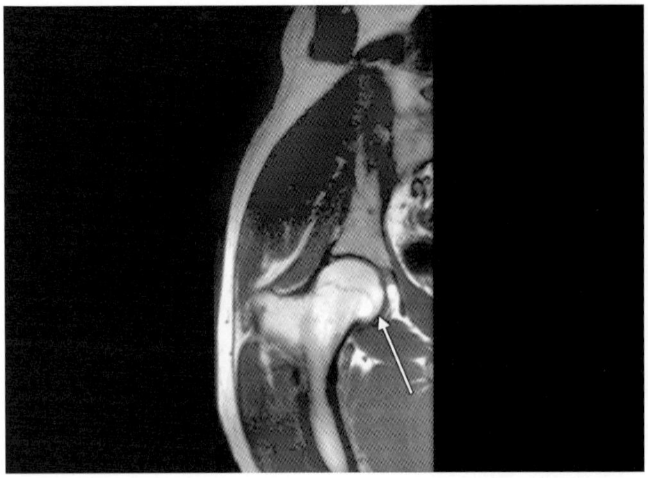

Fig. 3: T1W coronal image of the right hip showing normal physeal scar seen as a thin hypointense line separating epiphysis from metaphysis.

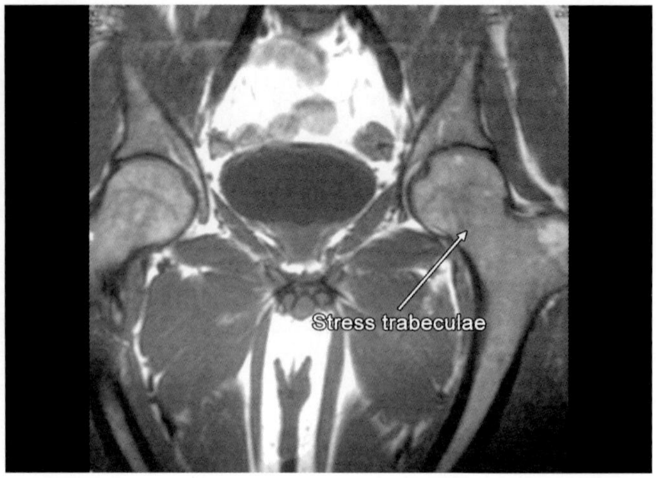

Fig. 4: T1W coronal image of both hips—Stress trabeculae seen as fan-shaped region of hypointensity in the femoral neck.

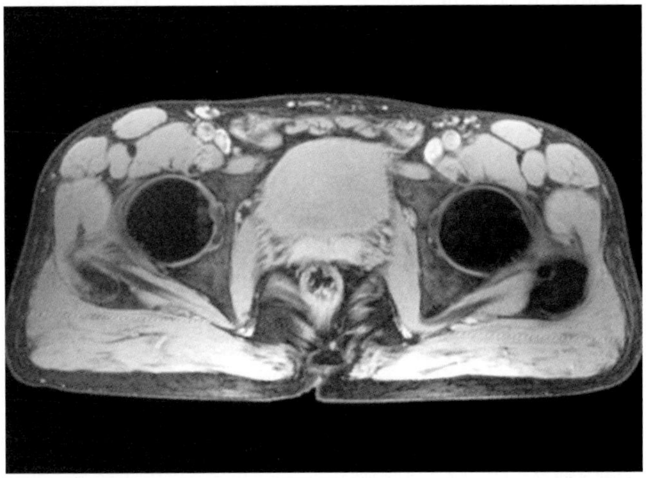

Fig. 5: T2W multiple echo data image combination (MEDIC) axial scan depicts normal intermediate signal articular cartilage.

preoperative assessment of developmental dysplasia of the hip.

MR arthrography of the hip involves two steps. Initially, the joint injection is performed in the fluoroscopic suite. The patient is placed on the fluoroscopic table with the knees slightly bent by keeping a pillow under the knees. The patient's feet are taped together at the toes to allow around 15° of internal rotation of the hip. The hip joint is accessed through an anterolateral approach by using a 20 gauge spinal needle. This is performed by inserting a needle in the skin at the mid intertrochanteric line. The angle of the needle is kept parallel to the femoral neck at a 45° angle with the target site near the midfemoral neck. An alternative lateral approach involves perpendicular skin entry of the needle with the target site at the lateral cortex of the midfemoral neck. After instillation of iodinated

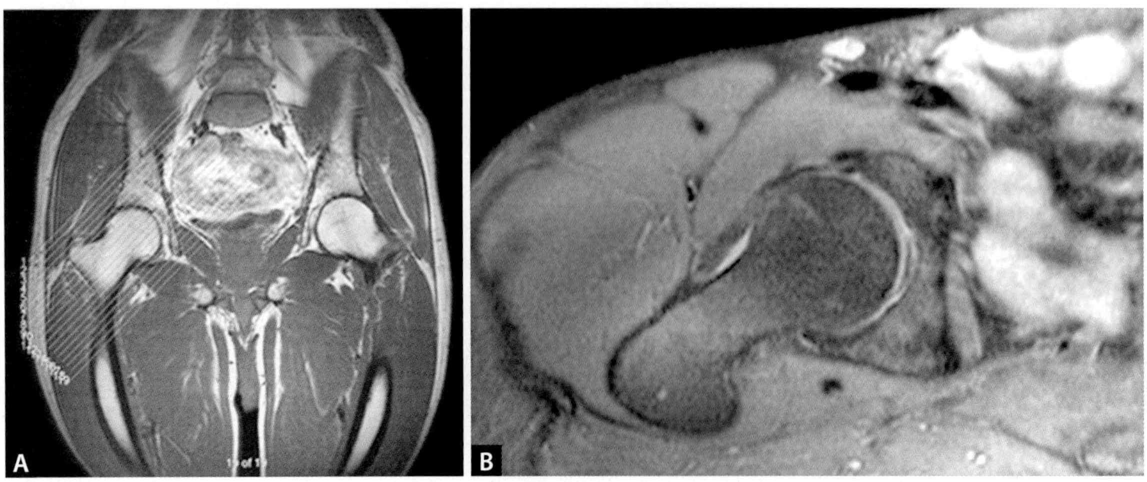

Figs. 6A and B: (A) T1W coronal; (B) Used as localizer to obtain axial oblique PDWI.

contrast material to document the intra-articular position of the needle, a 1:200 dilution of gadolinium contrast is injected as the joint capacity of the hip ranges from 8 to 20 mL[1,2] 10 mL as the appropriate volume. The second step is the actual MR imaging in the MR suite. T1-weighted fat-saturation (TR = 600 msec/TE = 14 msec) sequences in all three planes is acquired. An additional set of fluid-sensitive T2-weighted fat-saturated (TR = 3000 msec/TE = 90 msec) images are acquired in the coronal plane hip MRA protocol also includes the proton density (TR = 3000 msec/TE =30 msec) axial oblique images. Slice thickness-5 mm, FOV-24 for all sequences, and image matrix size 320 × 224 except for the sagittal plane, which is 256 × 224.[1]

Evaluation of the acetabular labrum and cartilage will be improved upon due to increased signal to noise and contrast to noise ratios on a 3 T magnet.

HIP AND PELVIS: EVALUATION OF STRUCTURES

Coronal (Figs. 7A and B)

Osseous Structures

Acetabulum, femoral head and neck, greater and lesser trochanter, sacrum, ilium and sacroiliac joints.

Nonosseous Structures

Suprafoveal articular cartilage over the femoral head, lateral dome and superior labrum, hip abductors, short external rotator tendons attachments, iliopsoas, iliofemoral ligament gluteal muscles, adductors/abductors, hamstrings, quadriceps.

Axial (Figs. 8A to C)

Osseous Structures

Acetabulum, femoral neck, greater and lesser trochanter, sacrum, ilium, sacroiliac joint.

Nonosseous Structures

Muscles: Gluteus maximus, medius, minimus, sartorius, rectus femoris, gracilis, pectineus, adductor longus, brevis, and magnus, tensor fascia lata, piriformis, obturator internus and externus, gemelli superior and inferior, quadratus femoris.

Sciatic nerve: Cartilage over anterior and posterior wall, bare area of acetabulum.

Sagittal

Anterior labrum.

AVASCULAR NECROSIS

Osteonecrosis refers to bone death secondary to interruption of the blood supply. The term avascular necrosis (AVN) describes the occurrence of osteonecrosis in the epiphysis.

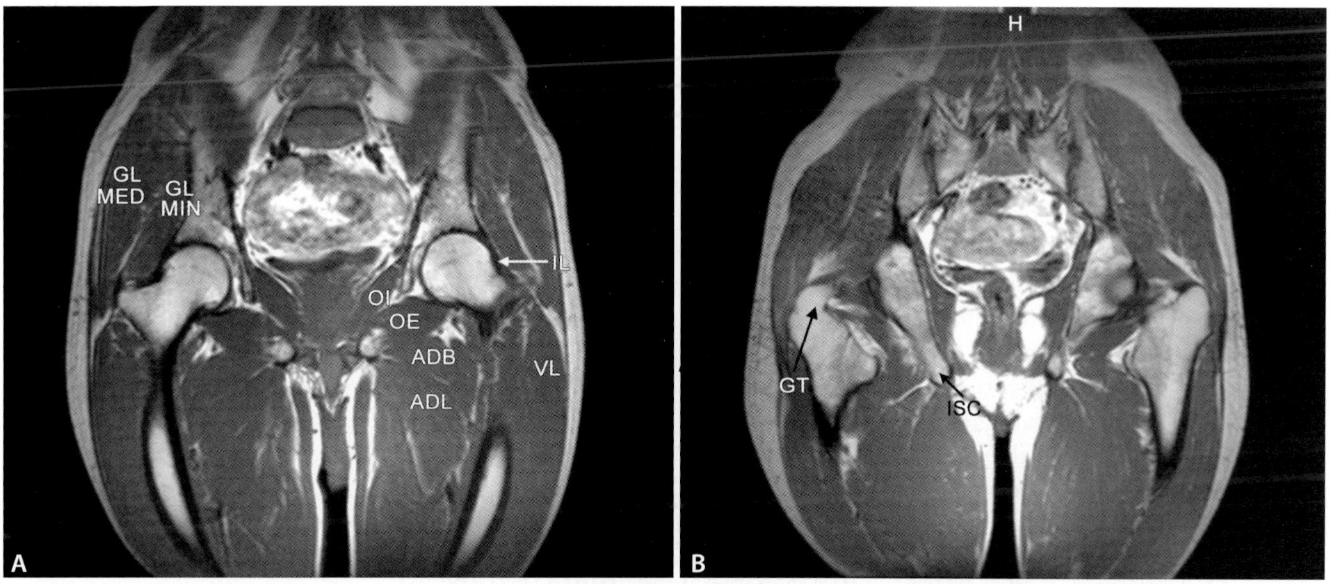

Figs. 7A and B: T1W coronal images of both hips anterior (A) to posterior (B) depicting normal anatomy.
Abbreviations: GL MED: Gluteus medius; GL MIN: Gluteus minimus; OI: Obturator internus; OE: Obturator externus; ADB: Abductor brevis; ADL: Abductor longus; VL: Vastus lateralis; IL: Iliofemoral ligament; GT: Greater trochanter; ISC: Ischium.

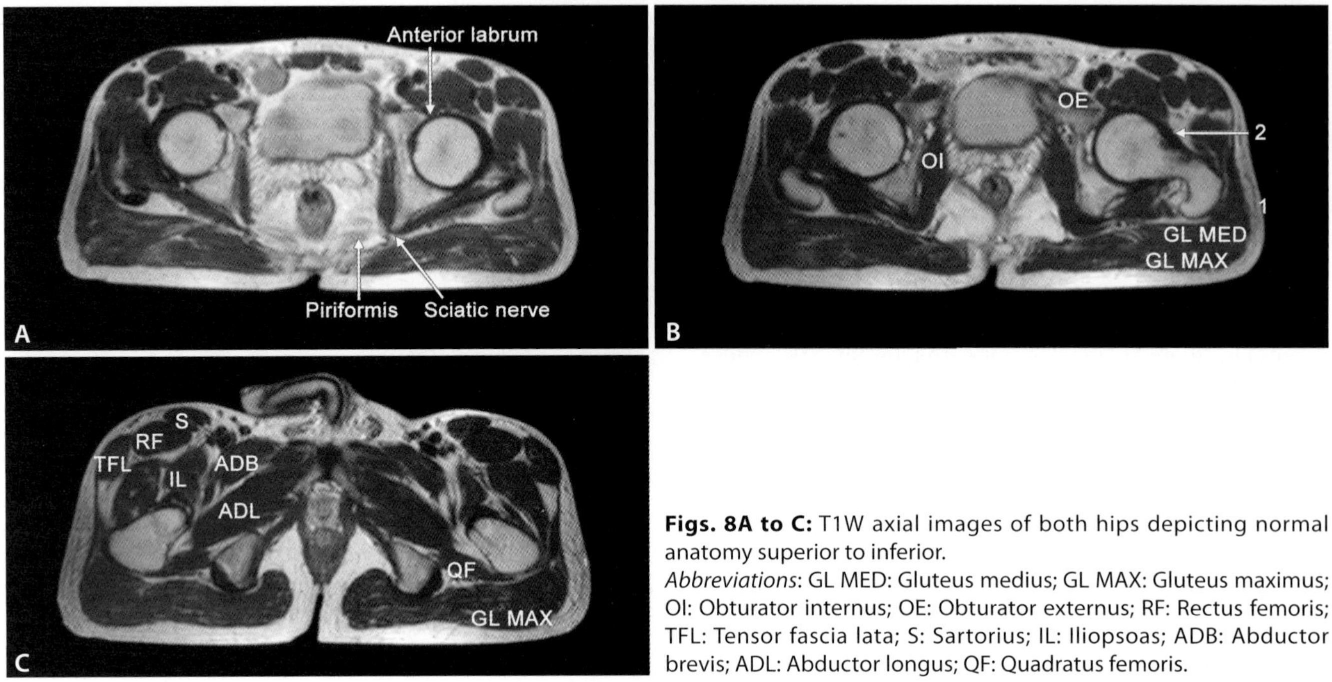

Figs. 8A to C: T1W axial images of both hips depicting normal anatomy superior to inferior.
Abbreviations: GL MED: Gluteus medius; GL MAX: Gluteus maximus; OI: Obturator internus; OE: Obturator externus; RF: Rectus femoris; TFL: Tensor fascia lata; S: Sartorius; IL: Iliopsoas; ADB: Abductor brevis; ADL: Abductor longus; QF: Quadratus femoris.

Cause and Pathogenesis

The most common cause of AVN is trauma.[3] In the hip, AVN occurs as a complication of displaced femoral neck fracture or hip dislocation. The risk of AVN is related to the degree of fracture displacement and a delay in reduction.

Blood supply to the femoral head is derived primarily from the medial circumflex artery. This is a branch of the profunda femoris artery. The medial and lateral circumflex artery sends branches with the capsular reflections (retinacula) of the hip joint to the femoral head. These branches are oriented along the long axis of the femoral head. Consequently, a subcapital fracture or a fracture of the femoral neck traverses these branches, which renders the head susceptible to ischemic necrosis. In some individuals blood supply to the femoral head reaches via the foveal artery which runs in the ligamentum teres. This artery may also be disrupted in the setting of trauma.

In the newborn and infants the purulent joint effusion of septic arthritis can also cause AVN of the femoral head.

A myriad of conditions are also associated with the development of nontraumatic AVN, common among these are corticosteroid use and alcoholism. Other predisposing conditions include hemoglobinopathies, coagulopathies, collagen vascular disease, Caisson disease, marrow storage disease, pancreatitis, chemotherapy, radiation, and pregnancy. Approximately 5% of cases of AVN are labeled idiopathic.[4] Various pathophysiological mechanisms have been proposed and include some form of arterial or venous insufficiency or extravascular compression in the context of a rigid bony compartment. There is resultant marrow edema, which forms the basis of therapeutic core decompression in an effort to lower intermedullary pressure.

The first phase is interruption of blood supply. The second pathological phase of AVN is characterized by a rim of hyperemia surrounding the infarcted marrow. Centripetal neovascularization of the necrotic zone characterizes the third pathological phase. Dead bone is resorbed and trabecular structure gets weakened. During this time, the weakened bone may collapse. Without fracture, the bone slowly heals. With fracture there is progressive deformity, joint narrowing and degenerative arthritis.

Presentation

Patients who have AVN typically present with intermittent groin pain of gradual onset that is present at rest, exacerbated by weight bearing and it may radiate to the knee or buttocks. Movement of hip is associated with pain; particularly on internal rotation. Avascular necrosis is not always painful. Hips with stage I, II disease may be completely asymptomatic.

MRI OF AVN

Bone marrow is composed of three separate cell types—hematopoietic cells, osteocytes, and marrow fat cells.

When these cells are exposed to an ischemic insult, they die at a different rate. Hematopoietic cells tend to die within 6–12 hours after insult, whereas osteocytes live up to 12–48 hours after blood flow is interrupted while fat cells live up to 5 days after the ischemic insult. MR imaging depiction depends on a change in the normally high signal intensity of marrow on T1W images and intermediate signal intensity on T2W images. Although the histological definition of osteonecrosis means death of osteocytes, the MR imaging changes in osteonecrosis reflect the death and replacement of normal fat cells.

A basic MR imaging protocol for suspected AVN includes coronal T1W spin echo (SE) and coronal short tau inversion recovery (STIR) or fat-suppressed fast turbo spin echo (TSE). In case of marrow abnormalities, a small field of view fat suppressed PD/T2 and cartilage specific sequence should be used. IV contrast is given to differentiate between viable and necrotic tissue. Similar differentiation can be done without contrast as a viable tissue appears hypointense on T1 and intermediate/high on T2/STIR sequences. Contrast-enhancement increases SNR is, important for providing images with special resolution in the preoperative evaluation of head contour and to monitor the vascularized graft.

The most common MR appearance of AVN is that of a circumscribed geographic circumscribed subchondral lesion in the anterosuperior portion of the femoral head[5] **(Figs. 9A and B)**. This site represents the most peripheral site in the intraosseous circulation of the proximal femur. The lesion is bounded by a low signal on T1W images. This correlates histologically with the reactive interface between viable and nonviable bone.

Another sign, seen on T2W images, in patients who have AVN is the *double line sign.* This consists of an outer low intensity rim and an inner high intensity band on T2W images **(Fig. 10)** and has been described in up to 80% of cases.[6-8] The high intensity component of this sign is believed to represent a zone of hyperemia and granulation tissue at the reactive interface between viable and nonviable bone. This sign was introduced by Mitchell and was considered as pathognomonic for AVN. It has been noted that transposition of the frequency and phase encoding axis results in the reversal of the positions of the bright and dark rims, suggesting the possibility of a chemical shift artifact as the etiology behind this sign. The newer TSE sequences that are used have an inherent artifact, the "bright fat" due to JJ coupling effect. Therefore, this sequence is applied with spectral fat saturation and thus the double line sign is not seen and is instead manifested as the "bright band" sign. This bright line/band corresponds to the vascular and repair tissue at the periphery of the necrosis. It is seen in fat suppressed turbo (fast) spin echo T2 and contrast-enhanced T1W images.[9] The artifactual nature of the double line sign does not reduce its diagnostic value for the diagnosis of AVN when conventional T2W SE or nonfat-suppressed turbo spin echo sequences are applied.

Mitchell proposed a classification system based on the appearance of the center region signal, bounded by a low signal rim on T1 and T2W images.

Class A lesions have fat like signal characteristics—high signal intensity on T1 and intermediate signal intensity on T2W images **(Figs. 11A and B)**. Class A lesions represent early stage disease. These changes are found in

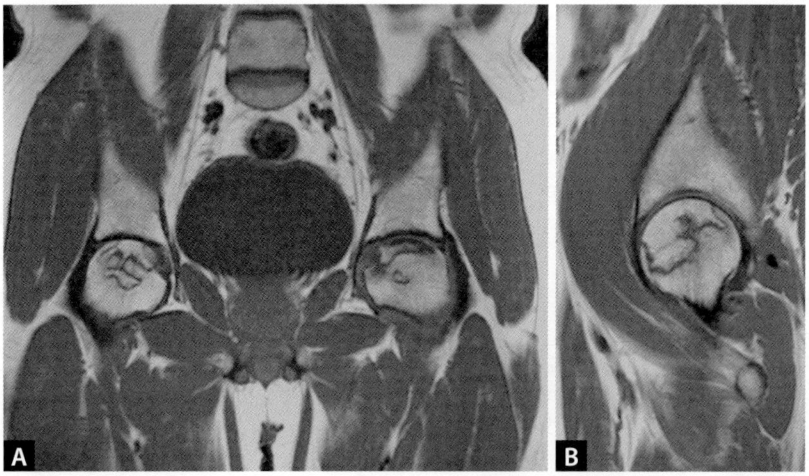

Figs. 9A and B: T1W axial image of both hips (A) and T1W sagittal image of right hip (B) showing characteristic serpiginous area of altered signal intensity of the anterosuperior part of the femoral head—AVN.

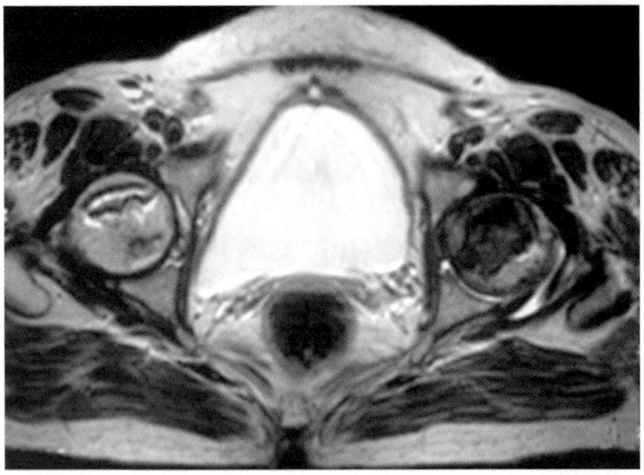

Fig. 10: T2W axial image of both hips showing the 'double line' sign—Outer hypointense and inner hyperintense rim—AVN.

the asymptomatic individuals who have radiographically and scintigraphically normal hips.

Class B lesions demonstrate signal characteristics that are similar to subacute blood-high signal on T1W and T2W images.

Class C lesions demonstrate signal characteristics that have fluid like features—low signal intensity on T1W and high signal intensity on T2W images **(Figs. 12A and B)**.

Class D demonstrates low signal intensity on T1W and T2W images. Class D lesions are believed to represent a late stage—the fibrous tissue like signal result from fibrosis, scarring, and osteonecrosis.

Cases with larger areas of abnormality most commonly have mixed characteristics with an incomplete surrounding

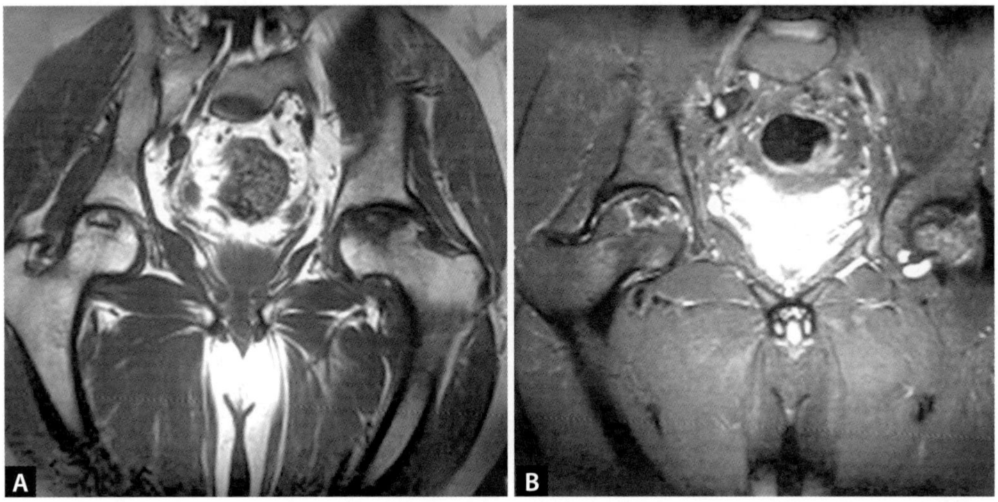

Figs. 11A and B: Mitchell class A and D AVN: T1W coronal (A), STIR coronal image of both hips (B) shows area of altered signal in both femoral heads with fat-intensity signal on T1W and STIR on the right side-class A and hypointense signal on the left side-class D.

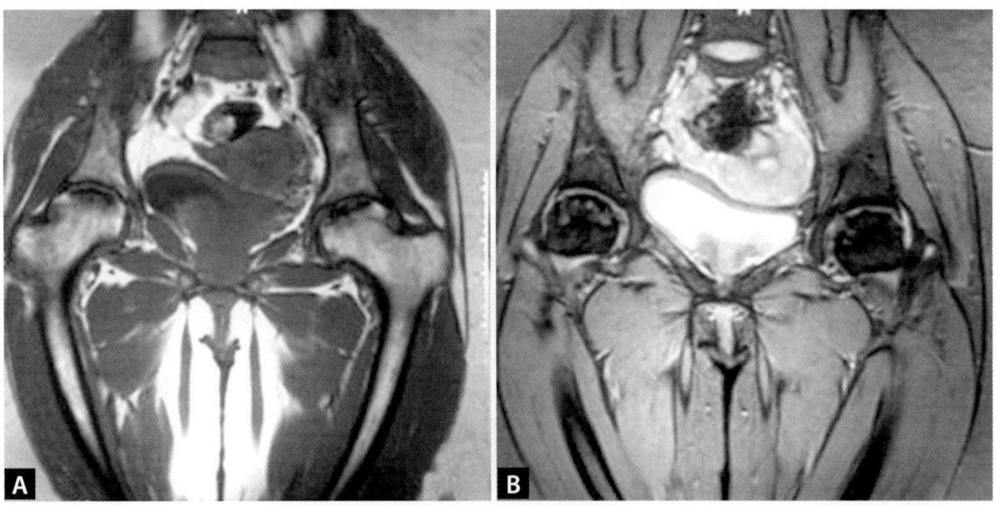

Figs. 12A and B: Mitchell class C and D AVN: T1W coronal image (A), T2W fat-suppressed coronal image of both hips (B) show bilateral areas of altered signal in femoral head showing hypointensity on T1W and mixed hypo- and hyperintensity on T2WI.

rim and heterogeneous central signal. This classification is not widely used as it does not correlate with radiographic staging and prognosis.[10]

Subchondral fractures in AVN may occur. These are seen as low SI lines on T1-weighted MR images and can be differentiated from subchondral insufficiency fractures in osteoporotic women on the basis of the shape of the lesion. In AVN, the low signal band is smooth, concave to the articular surface and circumscribes the entire necrotic segment, whereas in insufficiency fractures, the low signal intensity band is irregular, discontinuous and convex to the articular surface[11] **(Figs. 13A and B)**.

Secondary findings: These give supportive evidence of osteonecrosis. One such finding is the premature conversion of hematopoietic marrow into fatty marrow in the intertro-chanteric region[8] **(Figs. 14A and B)**.

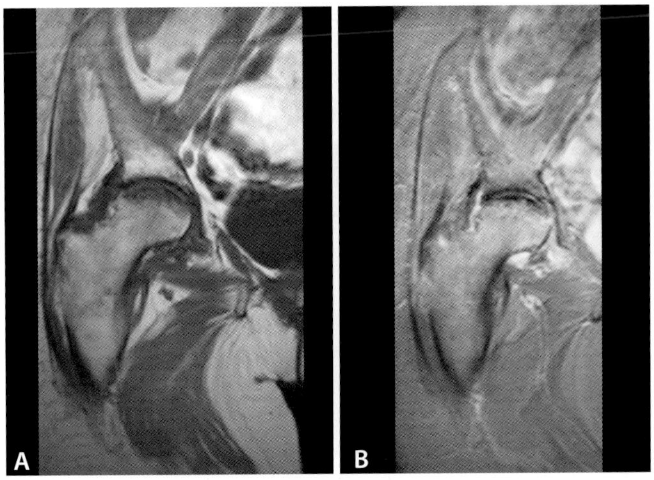

Figs. 13A and B: T1W coronal (A) and STIR coronal (B) depict insufficiency fracture of osteoporosis as irregular, discontinuous low signal intensity lines

An increased amount of synovial fluid is an important but nonspecific evidence of AVN **(Fig. 15)**. A small amount of synovial fluid is seen in up to 84% of normal hips, grade 3 effusions that distend the joint capsule are seen in approximately 50% of patients with femoral head collapse. Joint effusion is due to associated synovitis and is correlated with pain, being found with bone marrow edema (BME). Bone marrow edema may be visible in up to 30–59% of patients with AVN.[12] It is located within the femoral head, neck and intertrochanteric region, as a reaction to subchondral fracture and blockage of venous drainage. Subchondral abnormalities, presence of doubleline/ band, bilateral involvement point to AVN related bone marrow edema. There is diffuse enhancement in transient osteoporosis, whereas no enhancement is seen in necrotic part in AVN. Bone marrow edema is never found in the early stages of avascular necrosis as earlier thought. It develops after the onset of pain, typically in advanced disease and is correlated with necrotic volume and articular collapse. Bone marrow edema is also associated with failure of core decompression, failure of vascularized bone grafting and is a poor prognostic indicator.

Conventional MR imaging detects morphological changes in the femoral head after repair process has begun.[13,14] Use of gadolinium-enhanced imaging has demonstrated both enhancing and nonenhancing components of the AVN lesion. Areas that enhance correspond to viable areas within the AVN lesion, whereas nonenhancing areas correspond to necrotic marrow **(Figs. 16A and B)**. Decreased enhancement of the femoral

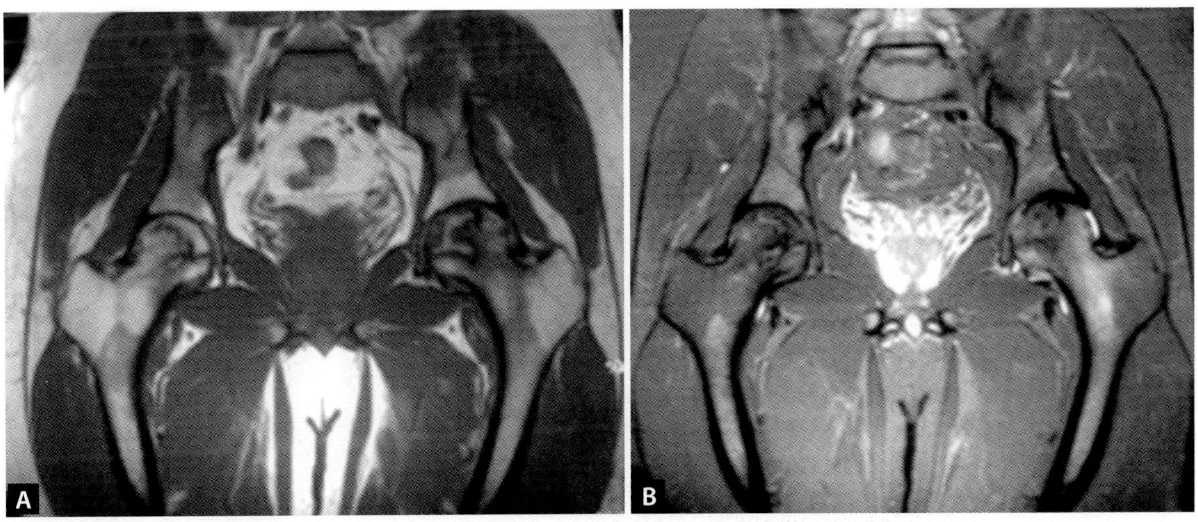

Figs. 14A and B: T1W coronal (A) and STIR coronal (B) images of both hip showing increase in intertrochanteric fatty marrow on the right side with marrow edema on the left side with bilateral AVN.

head is analogous to the scintigraphic cold spot. Perfusion MR[15] (dynamic contrast-enhanced MR-DCE-MRI) is now being used to assess early femoral head ischemia. Delayed peak enhancement is noted in hips where MRI shows no changes. The delayed time to peak may be due to reactive hyperemia with vasodilatation. This may be a method to detect occult osteonecrosis of the femoral head. There is increased peak enhancement in the proximal femur and decreased perfusion (stasis) in the intertrochanteric area in advanced osteonecrosis. Diffusion MR[16] was also investigated as a method to stage osteonecrosis. The ADC values in hip AVN are significantly higher than normal marrow but diffusion weighted MRI fails to distinguish between different stages of avascular necrosis. Preliminary studies have shown that proton MR spectroscopy can detect changes in the lipid/water spectra of patients with AVN before any evidence of morphological changes appears.[17]

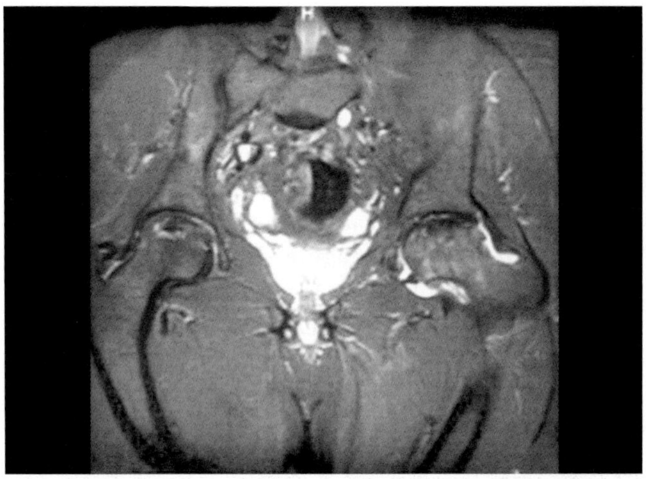

Fig. 15: STIR coronal image of both hips showing joint effusion on the left side with bilateral AVN.

Magnetic Resonance Imaging and Prognostic Indicators

A normal MR image is a good predictor of disease absence and is rare in case of biopsy proven disease.[9,10] When AVN is present, the percentage of weight bearing surface that is involved by the AVN lesion, is the most reliable factor in predicting outcome.

The size of the necrosis is crucial in prediction of the occurrence of a fracture or a further joint destruction. Methods of quantification vary from the simple to the sophisticated, requiring advanced software. The extent of femoral head involvement has been estimated with MR imaging as percentage of the weight bearing area, index of necrotic extent and absolute necrotic volume.

Shimizu et al.[18] assessed the extent and location of the necrotic fragment using coronal MR images. The femoral head is viewed as a circle. If the necrotic fragment involves less than 25% of the diameter of the circle, there is less likelihood of lesion progressing to collapse. Determining the location of the lesion also helps in identifying future deterioration. The weight bearing surface of the femoral head is defined as a segment extending from the medial aspect of the acetabulum to the lateral aspect of the acetabular roof. If more than 2/3rds of the weight bearing surface is involved, there is a 74% chance of collapse of the femoral head. Sagittal MR imaging can also be used to assess the extent and location of the necrotic fragment. If the reactive interface does cross the zenith (12 o'clock position), there is an 82% chance of collapse **(Figs. 17A and B)**.

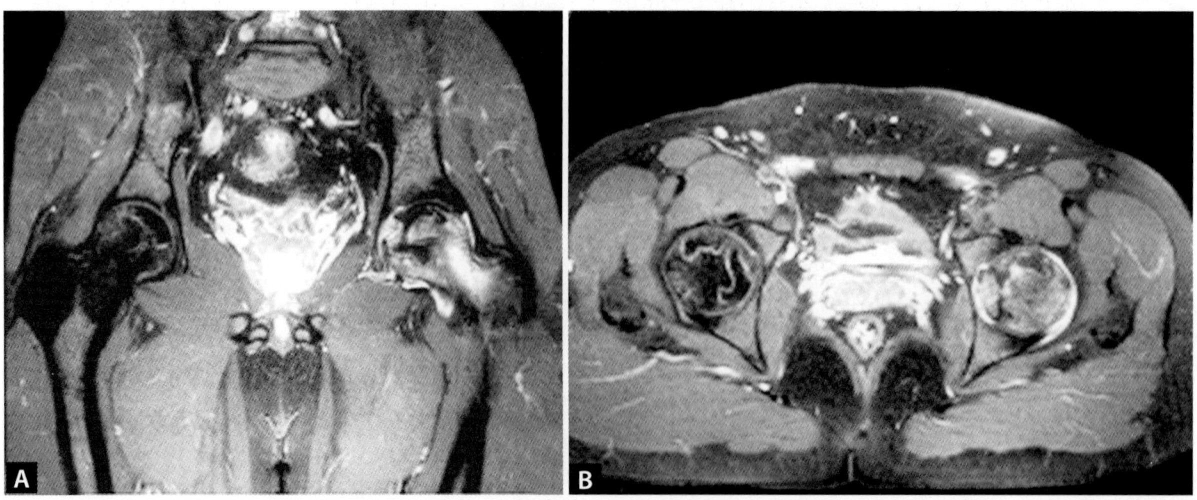

Figs. 16A and B: Bilateral AVN: T1W coronal (A) and T1W axial (B) fat-suppressed, postgadolinium image of both hips showing necrotic nonenhancing areas with enhancing viable interface and viable fragments.

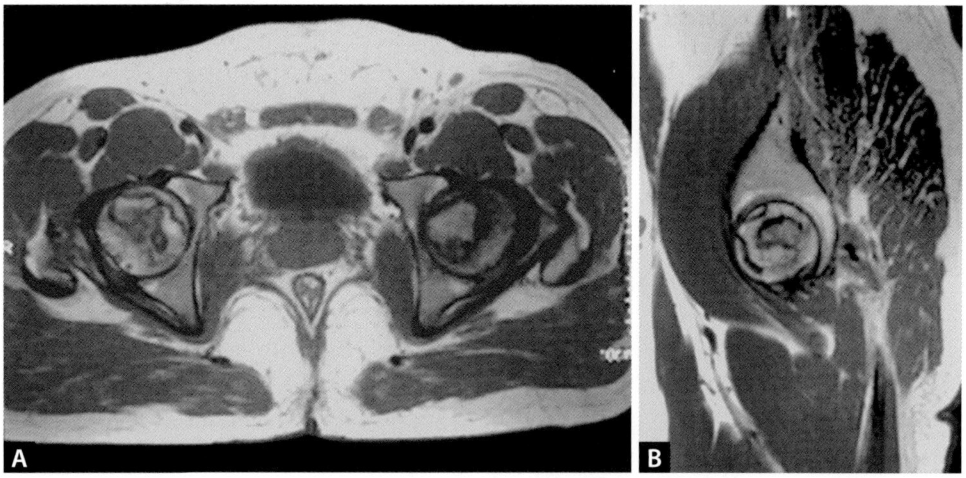

Figs. 17A and B: T1W axial image of bilateral hips (A) and T1W sagittal image of right hip (B) show bilateral AVN with >30% involvement of femoral head. The lesion is seen to cross the 12 o'clock position with an increased likelihood of collapse on the right side.

Two high-risk markers of disease may be observed in patients who have clinically suspected AVN.[19] These are an early conversion from hematopoietic to fatty marrow and a dense intact physeal scar. The presence of either of these findings and the absence of definite disease warrants a follow-up in patients with risk factors for AVN and hip pain.

Pitfalls in Diagnosis[20]

- Occasionally normal red marrow can be present in the femoral head, leading to a misinterpretation.
- Synovial herniation pit, which represents a tiny defect in the bone that allows joint fluid to fill this space, can be erroneously identified as an area of AVN **(Fig. 18)**.
- Subchondral bone cysts resulting from degenerative joint disease of the hip may appear similar to AVN, but the low signal margins of the cyst are smooth and regular, rather than serpiginous as with AVN **(Figs. 19A and B)**.
- Fovea central is, a normal anatomic finding, can be diagnosed as a site of AVN **(Fig. 20)**.

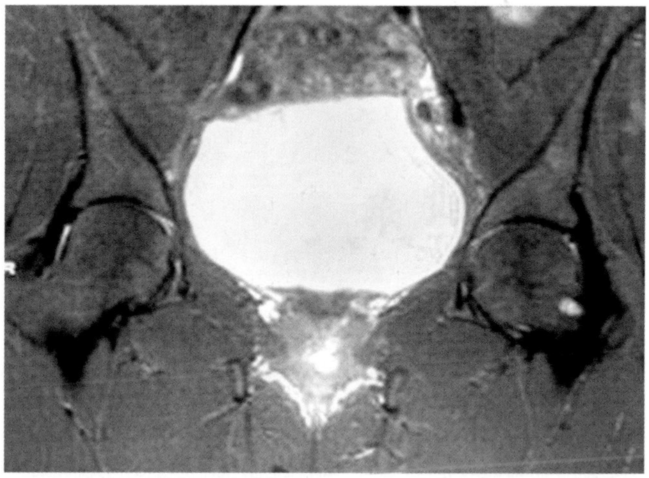

Fig. 18: T2W fat-suppressed coronal image of both hips shows herniation pit in the characteristic location.

Staging

Arlet and Ficat[21] devised a widely used staging system for hip AVN, based on clinical and plain radiographic findings:

- *Stage 0*: Represents biopsy proven AVN in asymptomatic patients with normal radiographs and bone scan
- *Stage 1*: Patients may have normal radiographs, abnormal bone scans and is associated with hip pain and decreased range of motion
- *Stage 2*: Femoral head osteoporosis with areas of cystic lucency and sclerosis
- *Stage 3*: There is subchondral collapse (crescent sign) of the femoral head with preservation of joint space
- *Stage 4*: There is frank cortical collapse of the femoral head
- Stage 5: Superimposed degenerative joint disease.

Magnetic resonance is an integral part of several staging systems. The most critical part in all systems is the loss of spherical contour of the femoral head; MRI is to be used in precollapse stages of AVN.

The Toulouse, France-based Association *Internationale de Recherche sur la Circulation Osseuse (the association research circulation osseous)*[22] have proposed a more comprehensive staging system (ARCO classification, **Table 1**).

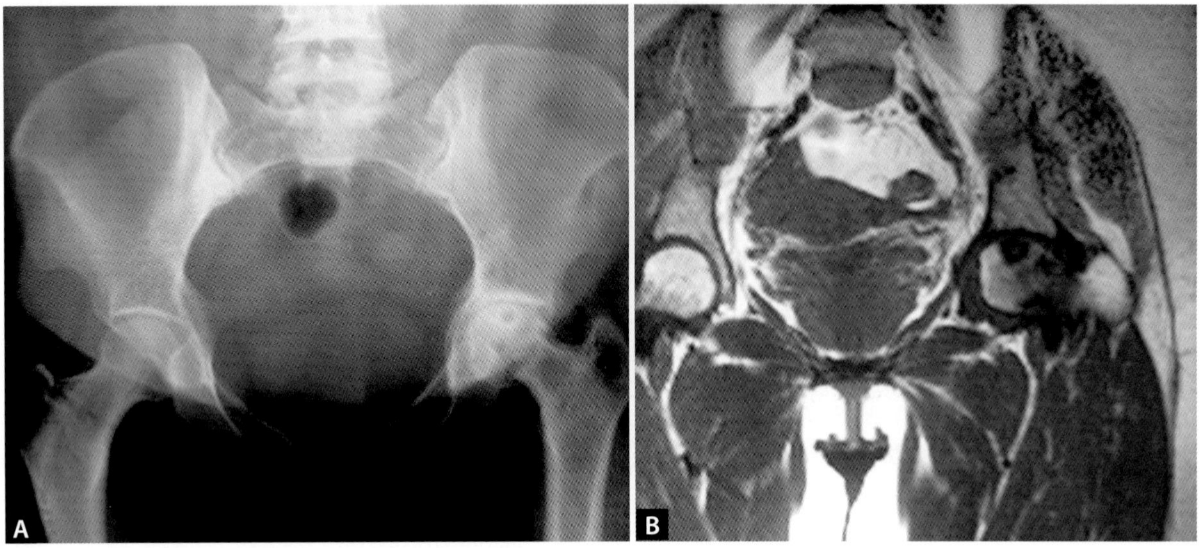

Figs. 19A and B: X-ray pelvis and both hips (A) AP view shows decreased joint space on the left with subchondral cystic changes and osteophytes; (B) T1W coronal image of both hips depicting subchondral cyst with osteophytes—Degenerative changes.

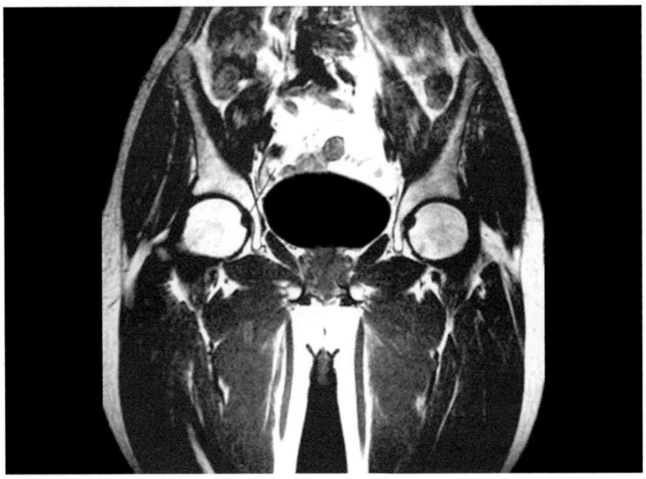

Fig. 20: T1W coronal image of both hips: Normal fovea central is seen on both sides.

Table 1: International classification: AVN of femoral head.

Stage	*Findings*
0	Bone biopsy AVN. All other tests normal
I	Scintigraphic or MRI positive lesions, subdivided based on locations (medial, central or lateral) and percentage of femoral head involved
IA	<15%
IB	15–30%
IC	>30% involvement
II	• *Radiographs*: Osteosclerosis, cystic osteopenia or mottled femoral head without collapse or acetabular involvement • Scintigraphy or MRI positive lesions subdivided based on location (medial, central, or lateral), and percentage of involvement
IIA	<15%
IIB	15–30%
IIC	>30%
III	*Radiographs*: Crescent sign lesions subdivided based on location (medial, central and lateral) and percentage of involvement.
IIIIA	<15% involvement or <2 mm depression of femoral head
IIIB	15–30% involvement or 2–4 mm depression of femoral head
IIIC	>30% involvement or >4 mm depression of femoral head
IV	*Radiographs*: Flattened articular surface, joint space narrowing, acetabular changes and osteophytosis

Study Choice and Work-up

Radiographs are used in the initial work-up of clinically suspected AVN; an anteroposterior (AP) and frog leg lateral projection should be obtained (this increases the likelihood of detecting a subchondral fracture. If the radiographs are positive for advanced disease, further imaging is unnecessary except in the determination of clinically occult contralateral disease in patients, at risk for AVN. A negative radiographic examination requires additional imaging.

Radionuclide imaging for AVN is performed with a bone-seeking agent ^{99m}Tc MDP or marrow-seeking agent, such as ^{99m}Tc sulfur colloid. Early in the course of disease a cold photopenic zone may be observed in the anterosuperior part of the femoral head, which is virtually pathognomic for AVN. Later the reactive hyperemia and reparative response may result in a doughnut sign. Between the two phases is a window where bone scan may be normal.[23]

The principal role of MRI is in establishing the diagnosis of AVN in patients with normal or equivocal radiographs. It is also used for screening high-risk populations or for evaluating the opposite side with known unilateral disease. Its sensitivity reaches 100% in symptomatic patients and is 10–20% greater than scintigraphy. Magnetic resonance imaging is 90% specific and 95% sensitive in distinguishing patients with AVN from normal patients or those with other disorders. MR can be used to evaluate the volume of osteonecrotic involvement of the femoral head relative to the cross-sectional area. This may assist in the decision to perform a core decompression or a rotational osteotomy. Clinically, occult AVN may be present for an average of 5.5 years[24] before the onset of disease symptoms. A limited protocol for rapid screening has shown good correlation with full MR examination in determining presence and for characterizing the extent of AVN.

Prognosis

The natural history of AVN is typically of progression, though the rate of progression is unpredictable. The most important prognostic indicators are the size and location of the lesion. The lesions themselves do not increase in size and small lesions remain stable. The larger the area involved, the more likely it is to collapse. As the lateral weight-bearing portion gets involved, the likelihood of collapse increases. In case of CRF, MRI positive asymptomatic, radiographically occult lesions have been seen to disappear without therapy.[25]

Patients, whose disease is discovered prior to articular collapse, are candidates for a host of operative interventions, aimed at preserving the femoral head. These include core decompression, rotational osteotomy, etc. Hip arthroplasty is performed in cases of femoral head collapse and intractable pain. The results of hip replacement in patients with AVN are poorer than those of age related controls.

Computed tomography plays an adjunctive role in evaluation of AVN and may be useful in defining the disease in patients who have a contraindication to MR imaging. Computed tomography is also the technique of choice for detecting subchondral fractures.

MONITORING OF TREATMENT

The MR features indicating normal incorporation of the graft includes enhancement surrounding the graft, revascularization of the previously necrotic area, reduction in bone marrow edema and an increase in signal of the necrotic bone. Dynamic CEMRI shows vascular ingrowth at 1–7 months postsurgery.

MINIMAL AVN

This entity is seen as a small and eccentrically located focal lesion at the femoral head, believed to be as a result of single episode of infarction rather than recurrent ischemia.[26] This does not lead to articular collapse. Differential diagnosis includes bone tumors, synovial herniation pits.

BONE MARROW EDEMA SYNDROME

The "bone marrow edema (BME) syndrome" of the femoral head is a generic term which refers to a lesion pattern seen on MR imaging and is characterized by alteration in the intensity of marrow signal within the femoral head suggestive of medullary infiltration by interstitial edema. There are four morphologic criteria on T1-weighted SE images that indicate the presence of the bone marrow edema syndrome of the femoral head.[27] First, the lesion must involve the femoral head. Generally, it involves the upper pole and reaches the subchondral bone. It may extend further into the femoral neck and in rare cases, subtle marrow changes may also involve the acetabulum. The lesion does not have any definite margins and the transition zone between the lesion and the adjacent marrow is large. The lesion signal is homogeneous, without obvious focal round or lobulated changes and without residual intra-lesional fatty areas. Finally, the lesion signal intensity reduces moderately on T1-weighted SE images. All these features must be seen on T1-weighted images. The lesion's signal intensity is intermediate to high on T2-weighted SE images and high on STIR and fat-saturated intermediate- or T2-weighted images. After intravenous contrast injection, homogeneous and moderate-to-marked signal intensity enhancement shows on T1-weighted SE, subtle focal changes may also be noticed in the subchondral area. These additional changes may represent clues to a more specific diagnosis. A moderate joint effusion is usually present. The adjacent soft tissues generally remain normal.

The pathophysiology of the bone marrow edema syndrome remains unknown. Links with ischemia, fractures and reflex sympathetic dystrophy syndrome have been suggested. The bone marrow edema syndrome is nonspecific and could probably be a result of various causes. Subsequently, the bone marrow edema syndrome of the femoral head shows a variable time course, depending on the underlying causes that include transient osteoporosis of the hip, idiopathic bone marrow edema of the hip, traumatic or stress fracture of the femoral head, hip osteoarthritis and femoral head osteonecrosis. It is crucial to make distinction between these conditions because of their different outcomes.

Transient osteoporosis of the hip[28] is a rare clinical entity which is characterized by the spontaneous appearance and resolution over time of pain in hip as well as the associated delayed appearance of marked osteoporosis of the femoral head.[28] This was first described by Curtiss and Kincaid[29] in pregnant women during third trimester, since then most cases have been observed in middle aged men. Generally only one hip is patients' typical time course of clinical and radiographic changes. The beginning of unilateral hip pain is spontaneous, it may be gradual or rapid in onset and is aggravated by weight-bearing. After a plateau phase, pain progressively decreases until complete regression by 6–12 months after the onset, without residual sequelae.

Initial radiographs are normal, but marked osteoporosis of the femoral head with preserved joint space is seen on radiographs obtained several weeks after the onset of symptoms. The bone resorption can be so intense that the conventional radiographs may fail to distinguish the subchondral bone plate. Follow-up radiographs demonstrate a return to a normal appearance. Radionuclide studies with bone-seeking agents show presence of abnormal accumulation. On MR imaging, the bone marrow edema syndrome is observed **(Figs. 21A to C)**. The severity of osteopenia does not correlate with the extent of marrow edema. Vande Berg et al.[30] described small subchondral areas of low signal intensity in 30% of patients with BME syndrome. Lesions that were <4 mm thick or 12.5 mm long returned to normal as opposed to those that were larger and continued on to collapse representing progression to AVN. In transient osteoporosis diffuse homogeneous enhancement is seen in contra-distinction to AVN, where enhancement is heterogeneous with avascular foci of low signal.

An intra-articular osteoid osteoma may also cause marrow edema in a similar distribution to transient osteoporosis. A cortically based, small round lesion must be searched for, though these disease processes affect different age groups. In some or the majority of cases of transient osteoporosis of the femoral head the diagnosis of transient osteoporosis of the femoral head remains presumptive, until demonstration of complete resolution of clinical and radiological changes. Transient osteoporosis does not recur in the same joint but may involve another lower limb epiphysis, a situation called migratory transient osteoporosis.

Transient osteoporosis requires no treatment, other than protected weight-bearing and mild analgesics.

Insufficiency or Stress Fractures of the Femoral Head

Insufficiency fractures of the femoral head are one of the causes of the bone marrow edema syndrome of the femoral head. In addition to bone marrow edema, two morphological changes are diagnostic clues for insufficiency fractures, although they can also be observed in transient osteoporosis. In insufficiency fractures, marked and focal osteopenia is generally lacking on radiographs. First, impaction fractures of the trabecular bone appear as thin low signal intensity bands or lines or more globular speckled areas of low signal intensity on the T2- or enhanced T1-weighted SE images. They should not be confused with the reactive interface or rim that surrounds marrow infarcts. The plane of impaction fractures runs parallel to the subchondral bone plate at a small distance from the articular surface and does not delineate a large marrow area. It is surrounded by marrow edema on both sides (with no residual fat in the subchondral area) and it does not show the double-line sign on T2-weighted spin echo images. These lines are more prominent on

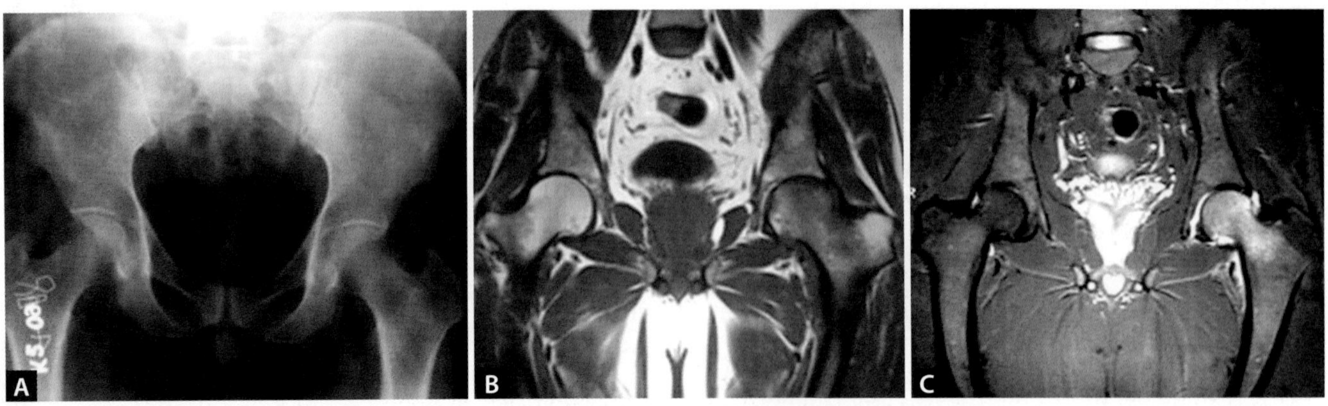

Figs. 21A to C: X-ray pelvis and both hips (A) of a patient with hip pain shows no abnormality; T1W coronal image (B) and STIR coronal image (C) of the same patient show homogeneous area of altered signal intensity seen as hypointense on T1W and bright on STIR images involving the left femoral head, extending to intertrochanteric region—Bone marrow edema.

T2-weighted than on T1-weighted sequences. Second, subtle focal deformity of the subchondral bone plate is occasionally visible in the anterosuperior or lateral aspects of the femoral head, just below the acetabular roof margin. This probably represents diskrete impaction of the bone plate separating the articular cartilage from the underlying bony trabeculae. These depressions of the subchondral bone plate remain limited and are not as abrupt or as marked as the overt fractures that occur in epiphyseal osteonecrosis.

Femoral Head Osteonecrosis and BMEs

Avascular necrosis of the hip can result in extensive marrow edema which can be observed in femoral head osteonecrosis. Femoral head osteonecrosis can develop as an isolated predominant finding, mainly in elderly patients, in a manner reminiscent to on T1-weighted SE images. There is no residual fat within the necrotic lesion and there is no interface at its periphery. In this case of the bone marrow edema syndrome, careful analysis of the subchondral area on T2- or fat-saturated intermediate-weighted images usually shows additional features suggestive of epiphyseal osteonecrosis. A crescent-shaped low signal intensity area is seen in the subchondral area, delineated at its lower aspect by edema. Femoral head deformity can be observed and indicates epiphyseal collapse compatible with femoral head osteonecrosis. It is important to differentiate this from insufficiency fracture. A low signal intensity subchondral area with a thickness equal or superior to 4 mm (thicker than the articular space) on T2-weighted images suggests an irreversible lesion. Marked femoral head contour deformity also indicates osteonecrosis, in systemic osteonecrosis (the condition observed in patients with multiple marrow infarcts associated with inflammatory diseases, alcohol abuse or steroid treatment) and in post-traumatic osteonecrosis, extensive head and neck edema can occur. In this condition, a focal ischemic lesion involves the upper pole of the femoral head, and marrow edema occurs more distally, in the femoral head and neck and spares the proximal lesion. Therefore, this lesion pattern does not correspond to a true bone marrow edema syndrome. The T1-weighted SE image better displays the ischemic femoral head lesion, because this lesion contains residual marrowfat and is surrounded by a low signal intensity rim.

In Osteoarthritis, bone marrow edema may be seen. This is recognized in rapidly progressing osteoarthritis. The presence of cartilage abrasion is seen as a diagnostic clue.

A careful and systematic analysis of the MR images is recommended if bone marrow edema syndrome of the femoral head is noted given the variable outcomes observed in the numerous conditions showing this syndrome.[27] Analysis of the T1-weighted SE images is mandatory to differentiate a true "bone marrow edema syndrome" from other lesions in which marrow edema can also be a predominant feature like tumors, infection, cysts and systemic osteonecrosis. Second, after confirmation of the bone marrow edema syndrome on T1-weighted SE images, high-resolution T2-weighted SE sequences are useful to assess (a) the articular cartilage, (b) the subchondral bone plate and (c) the subchondral marrow. If the articular cartilage is abnormal, the lesion is clinically irreversible (osteoarthritis or osteonecrosis); if the subchondral bone plate is interrupted and the epiphysis lacks sphericity, the lesion is irreversible; if a fluid-like signal intensity plane is visible underneath the epiphyseal contour (cleft fracture), the lesion is irreversible. After exclusion of a cartilage lesion and obvious fracture of the subchondral bone plate, detection and quantitative assessment of possible focal subchondral changes (low signal intensity subchondral area on T2- or enhanced T1-weighted SE images), is done. The lack of any additional focal changes in the subchondral edematous marrow area indicates a favorable prognosis, i.e. spontaneous resolution of the lesions and symptoms. The presence of a crescent-shaped low signal intensity area in the subchondral region with a thickness equal or superior to 4 mm on T2-weighted images is suggestive of an irreversible lesion. In some situations, the prognosis remains uncertain and follow-up MR studies obtained 3 months later represent a valid alternative to further evaluate the femoral head lesion.

FEMOROACETABULAR IMPINGEMENT

Femoroacetabular impingement is a recently recognized cause of hip pain in all age groups and a proposed mechanism in the development of early osteoarthritis.[31,32]

Femoroacetabular impingement refers to abnormal relationship between the femur, typically the junction between the anterior/ superior femoral head and neck, and the acetabular rim. Repetitive contacts between the two may instigate chondral lesions and labral tears leading to early degenerative disease. A number of predisposing conditions have been described with deformities of the femur and/or the acetabulum which result in abnormal contact between these two structures, such as Legg–Calvé–Perthes, slipped capital femoral epiphysis, coxa magna, hip dysplasia, and fractures of the femoral neck are known to predispose to femoroacetabular impingement.

However, a subset of patients who have no history of developmental or acquired disease of the hip joint may also be predisposed to femoroacetabular impingement. Clinically femoroacetabular impingement is characterized by anterior inguinal pain and decreased range of motion with flexion, adduction and internal rotation.

Classically, there are two types of femoroacetabular impingement. The first has been labeled cam impingement and is most often found in young athletic males. The second has been labeled pincer impingement and is more common in middle aged and older females.

Cam Impingement

In cam type impingement of the hip, the predominant abnormality is in the contour of the anterior/superior femoral head–neck junction with a normal morphology of the acetabulum. Normally, the anterior/superior femoral head–neck junction has a concave configuration. However, this junction is either flattened or convex in cam type impingement. In addition, the femoral head may become somewhat aspherical due to this morphologic abnormality. During forceful motion, especially flexion, the nonspherical portion of the femoral head is squeezed under the acetabular rim. This abnormal contact results in damage predominately to the acetabular cartilage in a rather constant location along the anterosuperior acetabular rim. Chondral abrasion or avulsion in turn leads to a tear or detachment of the acetabular labrum **(Figs. 22A to D)**. Repetitive osseous impingement can then result in osteophyte formation on the anterior femoral neck; worsening the problem further. The decreased head-neck offset may be due to a subclinical slipped capital femoral epiphysis.[33]

Radiographs of patients with cam impingement may appear normal initially because these abnormalities are too subtle to be observed easily. On an AP view of the hip, the normal concavity along the lateral aspect of the femoral head–neck junction becomes flattened or slightly convex, this has been referred to as the pistol-grip deformity and more recently as an abnormal epiphyseal extension. This is found in 40% of patients who develop osteoarthritis of the hip. This same abnormality can be seen on the frog lateral view, loss of the normal concavity along the anterior femoral head-neck junction can also be appreciated on a true lateral view.

The MR imaging shows the same morphologic abnormalities. Epiphyseal extension is best seen on coronal sequences as they most closely approximate the AP view of the hip. The abnormal femoral head-neck offset on the anterior/superior head–neck junction often shows

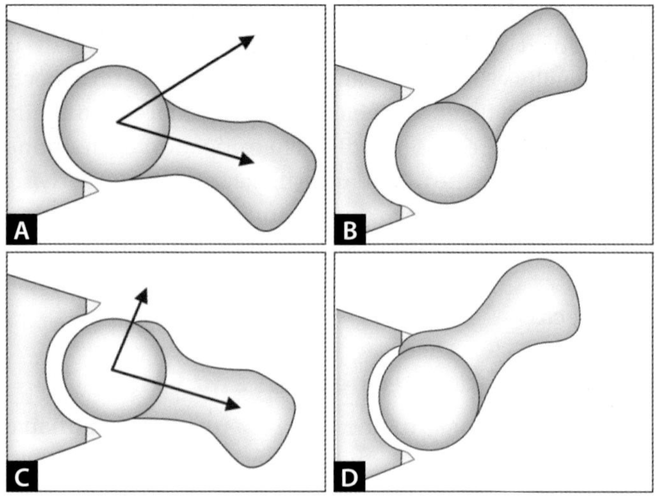

Figs. 22A to D: Schematic diagram through the femoral neck in the axial oblique plane alpha angle is measured, the normal angle = 42° (A); A normal femoral head/neck junction allows clearance of the acetabular labrum during flexion of the hip (B); Abnormal head/neck offset with an alpha angle greater than 55° (C); This creates an abnormal contact on the acetabular labrum during hip flexion (D)—Cam impingement.

best on oblique (oblique axial or oblique sagittal) images that parallel the femoral neck to measure the sphericity of the femoral head as well as the abnormal offset at the femoral head–neck junction.[34,35]

Quantitative measurement is done by measuring the alpha angle. The alpha angle is measured on an oblique image through the center of the femoral neck. A line is drawn along the long axis of the femoral neck bisecting a circle which outlines the femoral head. A second line is then drawn from the center of the circle to the point at which the femoral head or neck protrudes beyond the confines of the circle anteriorly. The angle formed by these two lines comprises the alpha. An alpha angle greater than 50° is abnormal although using a threshold of 55° may be more specific to impingement. The alpha angle will be greater in many causes of impingement due to an abnormality of the shape of the femoral head–neck junction, such as a wide femoral neck, osteophytes or posterior displacement of the femoral head[33] **(Figs. 23A to C)**.

Magnetic resonance arthrography helps in visualizing the cartilage and labral lesions that are often associated with femoroacetabular impingement. The labrum is present in approximately three fourths of the circumference of the acetabulum and absent along its inferior aspect. When degeneration is present, the labrum shows globular foci of increased signal intensity on the T2 and proton density weighted images frequently associated with a volume increase of the labrum. A labral tear is established when

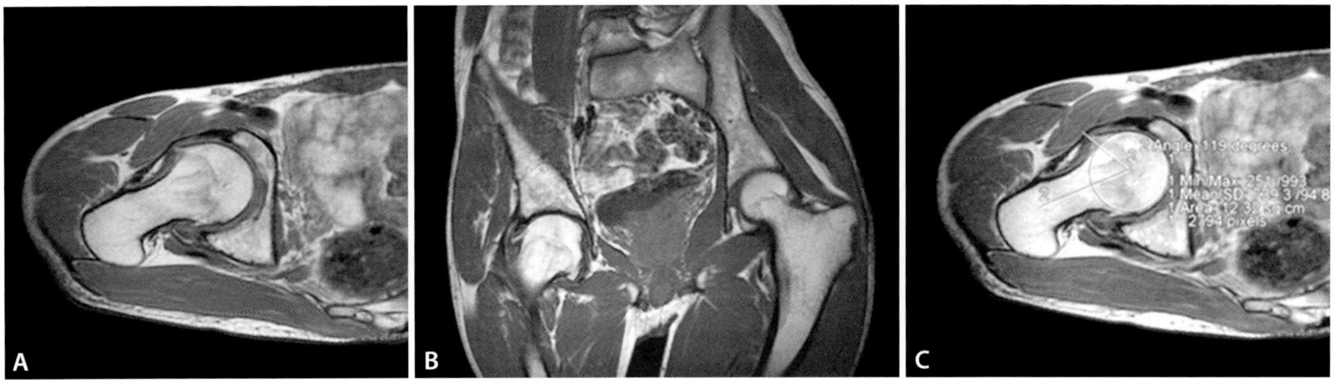

Figs. 23A to C: Abnormal head/neck offset in the right hip of a young adult, appreciated on the axial oblique image (A) with degenerative changes seen on T1W coronal image (B) alpha angle measures 119° (C).

contrast material can be seen traversing or undercutting the labrum. Displacement of the labrum or the presence of a paralabral cyst can increase diagnostic confidence. Since most labral tears occur in the anterior/superior labrum, it appears that oblique and sagittal planes are the most useful in detecting these tears. With age, the shape of the acetabular labrum tends to become rounded and irregular. However, an absent labral segment at MR arthrography should always be considered abnormal in patients with symptoms suggesting a pathologic labral condition. A normal cleft along the anteroinferior and posteroinferior labrum near its junction with the transverse ligament which spans the inferior aspect of the acetabulum along the acetabular notch is seen. The presence of gadolinium in this cleft should not be misinterpreted as a labral tear. In addition, there is a normal recess superficial to the superior labrum and as gadolinium enters this recess, the appearance can mimic a labral tear. A triad of MR arthrographic findings has been described in patients with cam type femoroacetabular impingement. The triad consists of an abnormally increased alpha angle, an anterior/superior acetabular cartilage lesion, and an anterior/superior acetabular labral tear.[36]

Pincer Impingement

In pincer type impingement, the predominant abnormality is with the morphology of the acetabulum with a relatively normal contour of the proximal femur. Some of the abnormalities in acetabular morphology are acetabular retroversion, anterior and/or lateral over-coverage, and protrusio acetabulae. All these conditions increase either the relative depth of the acetabulum or the circumferential over-coverage of the femoral head. Continued impact of the relatively normal femoral neck against the acetabular rim leads to pincer abutment and lesions in the acetabular rim. The first lesion to appear is degeneration of the labrum

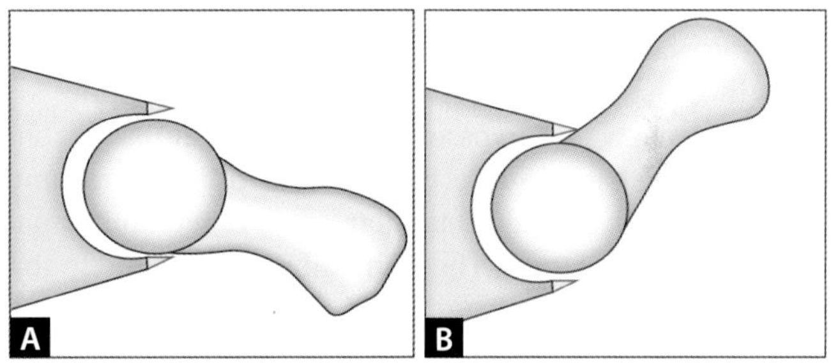

Figs. 24A and B: Schematic diagram through the femoral neck in the axial oblique plane. Redundant acetabulum with over coverage of the femoral head (A) which causes abnormal linear contact with the labrum during flexion (B)—Pincer impingement.

with formation of an intrasubstance cyst or ossification of the rim responsible for additional deepening of the acetabulum and worsening of the over-coverage. The repetitive abutments occur more often anteriorly and can result in chondral injury in the conter-coup region of the posteroinferior acetabulum. Acetabular cartilage lesions are typically limited to a small region on the acetabular rim. In contrast cam impingement is characterized by deeper cartilage lesions (some of which are very large flaps) and more extensive labral tears **(Figs. 24A and B)**.

On a properly positioned anteroposterior (AP) view of the pelvis, the anterior rim of the acetabulum should always project medial to the posterior rim of the acetabulum. A retroverted acetabulum is present when the anterior rim of the acetabulum projects lateral to the posterior rim on a true AP view of the pelvis. This typically involves the superior half of the anterior acetabular rim. The edge of the anterior and posterior rims of the acetabulum will crossover on the AP view of the pelvis, the crossover sign. Care must be taken as slight craniocaudal or transverse angulation can either mimic or obscure true retroversion of the acetabulum. On cross-sectional imaging (CT or MR), retroversion can be identified if the anterior rim of the acetabulum is lateral to the posterior rim on the first axial image that includes the femoral head. Retroversion results in a prominent anterolateral acetabular rim creating an obstacle for flexion and internal rotation movements and thus predisposing to femoroacetabular impingement. Acetabular over-coverage can also be seen on an AP view of the pelvis. It can be identified as abnormal lateral extension of sloping of its most lateral portion. A center edge angle of greater than 40° has been proposed as evidence of acetabular over-coverage.

The association between femoroacetabular impingement and so-called synovial herniation pits of the femoral neck is not entirely clear. There is a high prevalence of these cysts in patients with femoroacetabular impingement, it is possible that these cysts are more common in patients with dysplastic hips and/or pincer type impingement than in those with purely cam type impingement. An association between an os acetabuli and hip impingement is also suggested. Some believe that this heterotopic bone formation on the acetabular rim is due to abnormal contact with the femur. The mineralization may be in the soft tissues or in the labrum.

Although femoroacetabular impingement has been classified as cam type and pincer type, many patients have components of both although one component predominates.[37] Treatment of femoroacetabular impingement focuses on potential abnormalities of both the femur and the acetabulum.

HERNIATION PITS

Conversion defects (herniation pits) result from an abrasive effect of the anterior hip capsule in an area of the anterosuperior subcapital region of the femoral neck. This phenomenon is common affecting 4–5%[38] of adults and occurs in an area where there are normal cortical defects. The medullary canal is exposed to erosion from the overlying soft tissue and synovium, which create a subcortical pit. Previously considered an incidental finding, these are now considered as potential imaging indicators for femoroacetabular impingement.

On MR images herniation pits show marrow replacement in the subcapital region with a rim of low signal on all pulse sequences corresponding to an area of sclerosis. Internally the lesions are composed primarily of fibrocartilaginous tissue and fluid components. Lesions show a low to intermediate signal intensity on T1 and are of variable signal intensity on T2WI, those with fibrous component being low and those with fluid being hyperintense on T2WI[39] **(Figs. 25A and B)**.

Symptomatic herniation pit are generally larger than 1 cm, and it is postulated that movement of iliopsoas may cause progressive invagination of soft tissue leading to symptoms.

The differential diagnosis includes osteoid osteoma, avascular necrosis, abscess and ganglion. The location and imaging characteristics allow distinction.

FRACTURE

Fractures of the pelvis, hip and proximal femur are usually identified at radiography. Computed tomography adds substantially in further evaluation of complex pelvic fractures. MR imaging adds another dimension to the study of hip trauma as immediate changes in the appearance of marrow, are identified on MR. Thus, it is

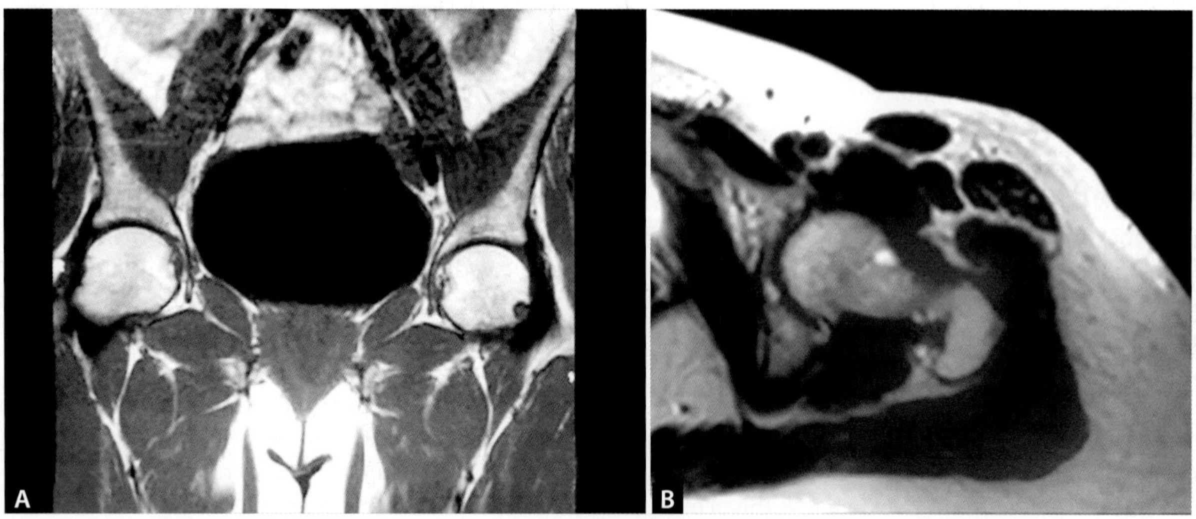

Figs. 25A and B: Herniation pit seen as a smooth well-marginated lesion in anterosuperior aspect of right femoral head with fluid characteristics on T1W coronal image (A) and T2W axial image of both hips (B).

useful in nondisplaced fractures, stress fractures, occult fractures, insufficiency fractures and fractures in axial plane that cannot be identified on CT.

Magnetic Resonance Imaging

The fracture disrupts the trabecular pattern and produces bleeding within the marrow. Trabeculae may be impacted, producing a black line on T1W images, and a higher signal may be seen on T2W images, because of associated hemorrhage **(Figs. 26A and B)**.

Screening MRI, with only coronal T1W studies are advocated as an inexpensive method for rapid evaluation of patients. This is of value in the elderly and the osteopenic, when a delay in diagnosis and therapy equates with higher morbidity.

Contrast-enhanced MR perfusion of the femoral head may be useful to assess femoral head perfusion after femoral neck fracture to aid the clinician in deciding between joint preserving surgery and hip arthroplasty.[40]

STRESS FRACTURES

Magnetic resonance imaging can contribute to the diagnosis of stress fractures. Stress fractures can be further divided into fatigue and insufficiency fractures.

Fatigue fractures occur commonly in pelvis and hips. Fatigue fractures result from increased or abnormal stress applied to normal bone. Magnetic resonance imaging is sensitive and specific because it shows the fracture line as a linear low signal band/line on both T1W and T2W images with surrounding marrow edema. Increased signal may be seen within the fracture site on fluid sensitive sequences because of hemorrhage within the fracture site. The signal alterations related with stress injury resolve by 6–12 weeks. Stress reactions occur along the medial aspect of the femoral neck (compressive surface) or superior surface (tensile surface). Additional locations include pubic rami and sacrum.

In the pelvis fatigue fractures are seen in the sacrum. These are frequently bilateral in the supra-acetabular region of ilium **(Figs. 27A to C)**.

Insufficiency fractures occur from normal strain on a bone weakened by osteoporosis, osteomalacia, steroids, rheumatoid arthritis, etc. In a clinical setting of osteoporosis and a painful hip, even in absence of trauma an occult fracture may be present. A limited MRI examination consisting of coronal and axial images of the entire pelvis using T1 and fat-suppressed T2W sequences can be used. Magnetic resonance demonstrates low signal fracture line surrounded by marrow edema. Multiple fractures coexist. The most common location for insufficiency fractures of hip and pelvis are subcapital, intertrochanteric, sacral, supra-acetabular, pubic bones, and pubic rami.

OSTEOCHONDRAL INJURY[41,42]

It can occur due to impaction injuries that result in laceration of the articular cartilage and microfracture of the underlying subchondral trabeculae. In the hip joints osteochondral lesions occur following hip dislocation. In anterior dislocation of the hip impaction is typically located along the posterolateral aspect of the femoral head whereas following posterior dislocations the anterior margin is involved.

These have been classified by MR imaging into 4 grades depending on the integrity of the articular cartilage, the degree of attachment and displacement of the subchondral

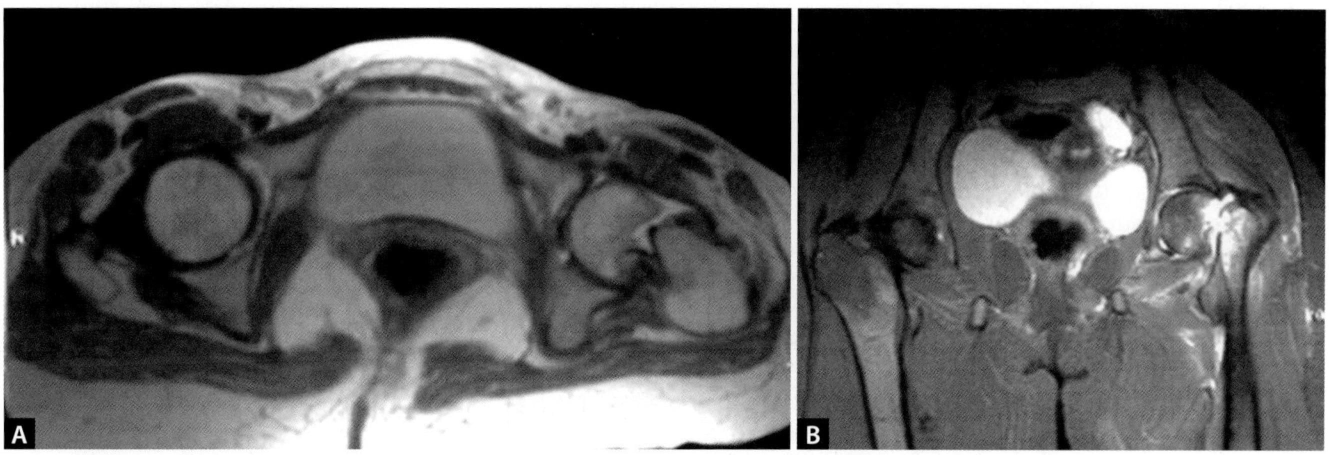

Figs. 26A and B: Fracture neck left femur: T2W axial (A) and STIR coronal (B) images of both hips show marrow edema and fluid at the fracture site.

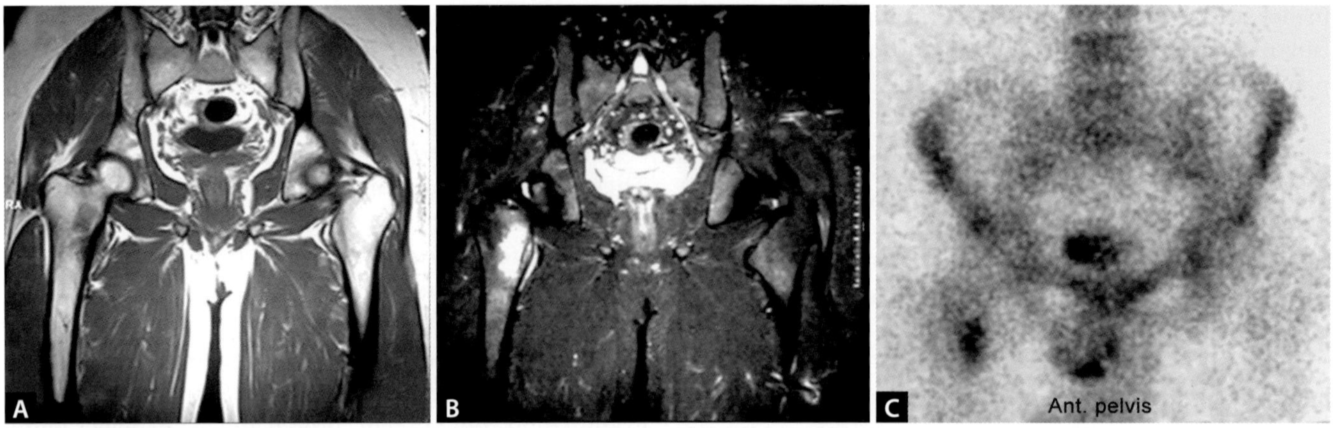

Figs. 27A to C: T1W coronal image of both hips (A) and STIR coronal image of both hips (B) showing an area of edema on the compressive medial surface of the right femur (hypo on T1WI and hyper on STIR) with associated soft tissue swelling and corresponding hot spot on the bone scan (C)—Stress reaction.

fragment. Grade 1 lesions present as intact articular cartilage with signal changes in the subchondral bone. Grade 2 lesions show partial detachment of the cartilage and subchondral fragment. Grade 3 lesions contain a completely detached nondisplaced fragment. Grade 4 is a detached and displaced osteochondral fragment located away from the parent bone.

Magnetic resonance imaging can help determine the exact location and size of the lesion, the integrity of the overlying lesion, the degree of attachment/ displacement of the cartilage and viability of the osteochondral fragment. Fragment stability can be assessed on T2W sequence. A low signal intensity line in the interface between normal bone and osteochondral fragment has been related to healing and stability as opposed to a high signal intensity interface, which indicates fluid underneath the nonattached part of the fragment and the donor site.

Loose bodies are an important cause of chronic debilitating symptoms, including joint pain and locking. The identification of cartilaginous loose bodies remains difficult on both conventional and arthrographic MR imaging scans. T2W images may improve the detection of loose bodies. On T1W images, these fragments increase in signal intensity as they imbibe gadolinium and become isointense with surrounding solution and may therefore escape detection. On MR arthrography cartilage fragments are visualized because they appear hypointense as compared to bright contrast solution.

TRAUMATIC MUSCULOTENDINOUS INJURIES[43,44]

Musculotendinous injuries are among the most common form of sport-related injury to the pelvis and hip. The pelvic ring and proximal femur are the sites of origin or insertion for several major muscle groups, including the abdominal, gluteal, adductors, hamstrings and iliopsoas muscles. The injuries occur as a result of blunt direct trauma or secondary to indirect trauma from excessive tension or forceful contraction. The injuries can be categorized on the basis of the mechanism of trauma and the site of involvement. These include tendinous avulsion injury, muscle contusion and myotendinous strain.

Avulsion Injury

Acute avulsion injury at the tendinous insertion site results from forceful eccentric muscle contraction or passive lengthening. It is manifested on MR as a hematoma and periosteal stripping at the tendinous attachment site. Waviness and retraction of the torn end of the tendon along with a fragment of bone or cartilage may be present. Avulsion injuries about the hip joint occur primarily at six sites:

1. Ischial tuberosity
2. Anterosuperior iliac spine
3. Anteroinferior iliac spine
4. Lesser trochanter
5. Greater trochanter
6. Pubic bone.

Muscle Contusions

These are secondary to direct trauma usually by a blunt object. They often occur deep in the muscle belly and tend to be less symptomatic than strains because the latter are commonly localized in the superficial muscle layers. Common sites of muscle contusion about the hip joint include the gluteal region and proximal thigh. Muscle contusions are seen in MR examinations of clinically suspected hip fractures and negative radiographs.

The MR imaging appearance varies according to the severity of the lesion. Diffuse edematous changes of the muscle are manifested by a feathery MR imaging appearance on STIR and T2W images along with an increased muscle girth. Intramuscular hemorrhages may develop with more severe trauma.

Muscle Strain—Myotendinous Strain

Strain injuries affect the myotendinous junction, the weakest point of the musculotendinous unit. The most common strained muscles about the hip joint are the rectus femoris and the hamstrings. In the first-degree strains implying minor degrees of fiber disruption, there is interstitial edema and hemorrhage at the myotendinous junction extending into the fascicles producing a feathery pattern. Partial tears without retraction characterize the second-degree tears. Hematoma and perifascial fluid collections may also be seen. Third-degree tears refer to complete rupture of the myotendinous unit. Magnetic resonance imaging is used for preoperative assessment of the extent of retraction.

Gluteus Medius Tendon Tear—Greater Trochanteric Pain Syndrome

The rotator cuff lesions of the hip involve tears of the abductor musculature, namely the gluteus medius and minimus. Proposed causes include friction of the iliotibial band with the underlying tendons, abnormal gait leading to altered biomechanics, repitative stress in runners and trauma. It more commonly affects middle-aged to elderly women who complain of chronic pain around hip or groin region, mimicking intra-articular hip pathology. It is also seen in recreational runners and participants of step aerobics. The most common symptom is lateral hip pain which has a broad differential diagnosis including entities likebursitis,tendonitis,muscleinsufficiencyfractures,nerve entrapment, muscle strain and bursitis **(Figs. 28A and B)**. Small focal tears are more common than diffuse avulsions. Various MR findings, such as increased T2 signal superior to the greater trochanter and atrophy of the gluteal muscles may be seen. This increased signal is considered to be the most specific and accurate for a tear. The increased signal lateral to the greater trochanter most likely represents sub gluteus maximus bursitis.[44]

LABRUM

The acetabular labrum is a rim of fibrocartilaginous tissue around the margin of the acetabulum that deepens the acetabular fossa and provides additional coverage for the femoral head. Nerves that play a role in pain and proprioception innervate the labrum. The labrum does not form a complete circle and is continued inferolaterally as the transverse ligament across the acetabular notch. The normal labrum is a triangular structure on axial and coronal imaging that is attached to the rim of the acetabulum. The normal labrum is low in signal on all imaging sequences.

Labral tear is now being recognized as a initial point for the beginning of degenerative joint disease. The torn labral fragment gets separated from the acetabular rim and loses its capacity for cushioning and protecting the adjacent articular cartilage. Loading forces across the joint

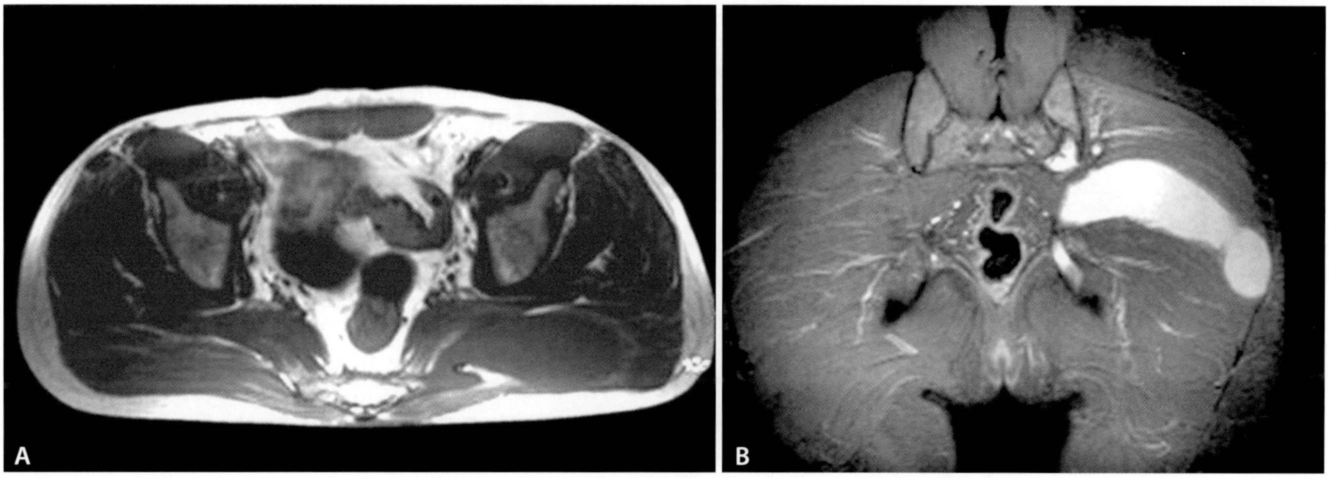

Figs. 28A and B: T1W axial image (A) and STIR coronal image (B) of the pelvis show well-marginated area of altered signal in the gluteus maximus suggestive of a tear.

are no longer distributed evenly over the entire cartilage surface. Repetitive impaction by the femoral head on the acetabulum results in the development of chondral defects and progressive arthritis.

Acetabular labral tears are seen in the setting of osteoarthritis and congenital hip dysplasia, chronic stress from athletic events or a traumatic event may lead to presence of tear. Patients present with persistent pain, clicking, and decreased range of motion. The morphology of the normal labrum is triangular, without any sulcus and of homogeneously low signal intensity **(Fig. 29)**. Tears of the labrum are diagnosed whenever contrast material extends into the labral substance or undermines its base at the interface between fibrocartilage and articular cartilage. An abnormal labrum shows linear or diffuse high signal. There may also be deformity in the contour of the labrum (loss of normal triangular shape). A labral tear may lead to the formation of a paralabral cyst when the tear passes through the capsule allowing the joint fluid to leak. Paralabral cysts are more medial in location to the iliopsoas bursae and contiguous with the acetabular rim. Identification of a paralabral cyst is an indirect sign of a labral tear. Acetabular labral tears may occur at any location. In setting of osteoarthritis and congenital hip dysplasia, the superior acetabular labrum is most frequently degenerated and torn, whereas in posterior dislocation complex labral tears may be seen.

One pitfall in imaging is the extension of acetabular cartilage along the medial aspect of the labrum, which should not be confused with a labral tear/detachment.

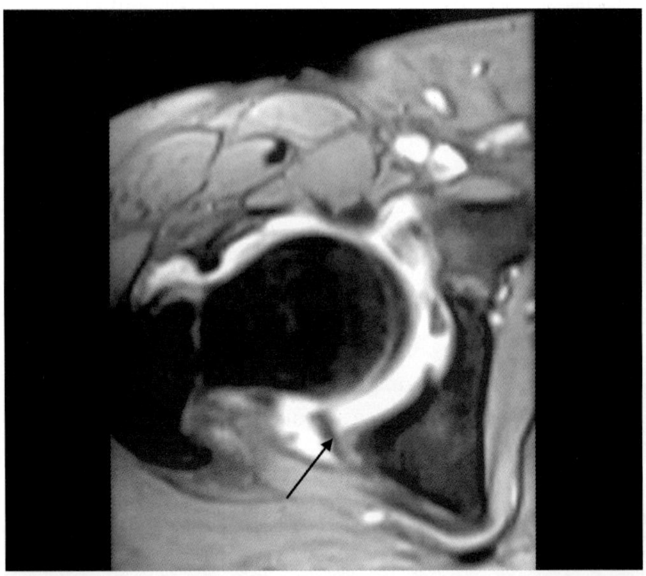

Fig. 29: T2W medic axial image of the right hip shows hyperintense articular cartilage, with the labrum (arrow) appearing hypointense—Normal.

The iliopsoas tendon crosses anterior to the labrum. This relationship is important to understand as the normal high signal between the two low signal intensity structures could mimic a labral tear.

The treatment of acetabular labral tears is conservative in the initial 4–6 weeks with limited weight bearing and in some cases by steroid injection.

BURSAE

There are several bursae in the hip region, which can get inflamed. *The iliopsoas bursa* is the largest bursa in the body and communicates with the hip joint in 15% of population. The iliopsoas bursa is located anterior to the hip joint and adjacent to femoral vessels. It lies between the psoas muscle and the anteromedial surface of the hip joint. The bursa measures 3–7 cm in length and is 2–4 cm in width. It gets distended in inflammatory, infective or degenerative disease. Patient may have groin pain and a palpable mass. It is not seen unless distended with fluid. Postcontrast scanning delineates the bursa better as the lining of the bursa enhances and the fluid does not. Asymptomatic bursal fluid may occur in the presence of joint effusion due to communication with the joint.

Greater trochanteric bursitis is another cause of hip pain, with patient localizing the pain to lateral aspect of the hip; this results from repetitive hip flexion. The findings on MR consist of no perceptible abnormality on T1W images. On T2 images, there is increased signal paralleling the greater trochanter.[20] A focus of interdigitating high signal may be seen around the tendons of the greater trochanter. Clinically, it may not be possible to differentiate bursitis from gluteus medius/minimus tears.

PIRIFORMIS SYNDROME

The sciatic nerve exits the pelvis at the greater sciatic notch and is located immediately anterior to the piriformis muscle. The sciatic nerve can split through piriformis, and a portion of the nerve can be superficial to the piriformis muscle. Due to this variation in location of the sciatic nerve, compression, hypertrophy or injury to the piriformis muscle can cause irritation to the sciatic nerve, mimicking radicular symptoms of disk disease.

Magnetic resonance imaging may show asymmetry in size of one piriformis compared to opposite side. In case of trauma, high signal may be noted.

MAGNETIC RESONANCE IN POSTARTHROPLASTY

Initially MRI had a limited role in postoperative assessment of hip arthroplasty due to severe susceptibility artifact.

With modification of imaging parameters, MRI can be used in patients with newer implants. The artifacts can be reduced by use of higher bandwidth, fast spin echo, instead of spin echo STIR instead of fat sat T2, avoiding gradient echo sequences, lowering echo time, orienting the frequency encoding direction along the longitudinal axis of the implant use of a large frequency encoding matrix.[45]

Magnetic resonance imaging plays a significant role in the assessment of soft tissues adjacent to the prosthesis. Trochanteric bursitis, avulsion of the gluteus tendons and short external rotators can be identified on MRI.

ARTHRITIS

Arthropathies commonly affect the following joints of the pelvis: The sacroiliac joint, the hips and to a lesser extent the symphysis pubis. The hips are target for many arthritides. Primary and secondary arthritis are common. Rheumatoid arthritis can affect the hip, often bilaterally symmetrically with axial joint space narrowing. Infection, calcium pyrophosphate dihydrate deposition (CPPD) disease and occasionally gout also involve the hip. The hip is a preferred site for several unusual articular disease, including pigmented villonodular synovitis (PVNS) and primary synovial chondromatosis.

Radiography remains the primary modality by which arthropathy of the hip is evaluated. Magnetic resonance imaging provides information regarding the extent of disease and visualization of surrounding soft tissue. Magnetic resonance imaging can demonstrate extent of synovial hypertrophy (pannus) that is common to all inflammatory arthritis but not evident on radiographs.

Pannus shows low signal on T1 and high signal intensity on T2 images.[36] It may be difficult to differentiate from synovial fluid. Pannus shows slightly higher signal intensity on short TR images and has more heterogeneous and mildly lower signal intensity on long TR images. Pannus and synovitis enhances more dramatically and diffusely compared to synovial fluid which enhances only peripherally. Fibrotic component of pannus may be of low SI on T2W images. These are often more prominent in seronegative spondyloarthropathy and reflect inactive disease or therapeutic effect.

Magnetic resonance imaging of inflammatory arthritis allows determination of the extent of pannus, degree of bone erosion and cartilage thinning. Magnetic resonance imaging can be used to monitor therapy by quantitating the volume of pannus.

Pigmented Villonodular Synovitis (PVNS)

It is an uncommon disorder characterized by synovial proliferation with hemosiderin deposition in the involved synovial tissue. Pressure erosions of bone by the synovial masses may occur. Pigmented villonodular synovitis occurs most commonly in 2nd and 5th decades and is usually monoarticular. The knee is the most often involved joint but it can also occur in the hip.

Magnetic Resonance Imaging

Hemosiderin deposition is pathognomic of the condition and is seen as large globular areas of low signal intensity on all imaging sequences with blooming on gradient echo imaging. Pigmented villonodular synovitis is characterized by low signal intensity on T1W and T2W images distinguishing it from almost all tumors and inflammatory conditions, which have high signal on T2W images.[46]

Primary Synovial Chondromatosis

This results from metaplastic proliferation of synovium with formation of multiple cartilaginous or osseous loose bodies. It is not associated with degenerative change, until later in the course of disease. On conventional radiography, it is not possible to differentiate it from PVNS.

Magnetic Resonance Imaging

Magnetic resonance imaging makes the differentiation possible as synovial chondromatosis follows the signal characteristics of cartilage. Cartilaginous loose bodies are low in signal on T1 and higher in signal on T2 images. Ossified loose bodies may be diffusely dense and sclerotic (low signal on all pulse sequences) or may have low signal cortical margin with a fatty center (chewy nougat).[47]

Amyloid Arthropathy

It is a rare entity and typically presents in patients of renal failure with clinical features similar to rheumatoid arthritis. There may be erosions within acetabulum and femoral head and neck that show low signal on T1 and low to intermediate signal on T2 images. History and absence of hemosiderin, allows it to be differentiated from PVNS.

INFECTION

The MRI protocol for diagnosis of soft tissue infections and osteomyelitis differs from the routine protocol. Additional imaging sequences using fat suppressed T1 FSE sequences pre- and post-IV gadolinium are performed to enable the diagnosis of sinus tracts and abscesses. The presence of bone marrow edema and enhancement on MR images is very sensitive for osteomyelitis and the absence of these findings excludes the presence of acute osteomyelitis. The distinction between para-articular cellulitis and osteomyelitis can be made with MR imaging, which is also useful in defining the extent of osteomyelitis before surgery.

Soft tissue infection about the hips can involve the joint or surrounding muscles. Hip joint infection is common in infancy and childhood. Magnetic resonance imaging shows early cartilage destruction. Any case of monoarticular arthritis should be considered infectious unless proved otherwise.

Tubercular arthritis: Articular manifestations of musculoskeletal TB are second to spinal disease in frequency of presentation. The most commonly involved are the hip and knee followed by the sacroiliac joint, shoulder, elbow and ankle. Magnetic resonance demonstrates synovitis and joint effusion. Indolent infections like tuberculosis result in prominent synovitis and MRI can then simulate a noninfectious inflammatory arthritis. Magnetic resonance imaging may demonstrate intraosseous involvement earlier than with other modalities; tuberculous marrow infiltration demonstrates signal characterization similar to that of osteomyelitis **(Figs. 30A and B)**.

Sacroiliitis is a nonspecific term suggesting an inflammatory process involving the sacroiliac joints. A variety of disease process affect this joint including HLA-B27 spondyloarthropathies such as ankylosing spondylitis, psoriasis and Reiter's syndrome. Other common conditions that affect these joints include osteoarthritis, gout, rheumatoid arthritis, and infection, including tuberculosis. The asymmetry of appearance aids the differential diagnosis, as ankylosing spondylitis is generally bilateral and symmetric.

In contrast to the hip, conventional radiography of the sacroiliac joints is often difficult even with specialized projections. The complex shape of the sacrum and iliac bones, curved nature of SI joints and the overlapping bowel gases make the assessment suboptimal with early changes being difficult to interpret.

Magnetic Resonance Imaging

The normal sacroiliac joint is well-depicted with MR imaging.[48] It clearly distinguishes the synovial and ligamentous compartments of the sacroiliac joint. The ligamentous part of the joint is posterior and obliquely oriented and contains adipose tissue with focal areas of low signal intensity representing loose connective tissue and the interosseous sacroiliac ligaments. The synovial compart-ment of the sacroiliac joint is anterior and more vertically oriented corresponding to the inferior one-half to two-thirds on plain radiographs MR imaging allows identification of the hyaline cartilage in the synovial compartment as a thin zone of intermediate signal, the maximum thickness of the cartilage is 5 mm. The iliac and sacral cortices are seen as areas of low signal intensity on either side of the cartilage **(Fig. 31)**.

The most characteristic finding of sacroiliitis at MR imaging is loss of the normal thin band of intermediate signal intensity representing cartilage on T1W images. Altered signal intensity in the sacral and iliac cortices with adjacent marginal irregularity and deeper defects in the juxtaposed marrow are seen on T1W images. Erosions are more prominent anteroinferiorly and on the iliac side of the synovial compartment where cartilage is thinned and subchondral bone is not well protected. Area of increased signal is seen on T2 images in the synovial compartment.

Magnetic resonance imaging is an accurate method for assessing early sacroiliac joint disease. It is more sensitive than CT in detecting cartilage loss, edema, and small

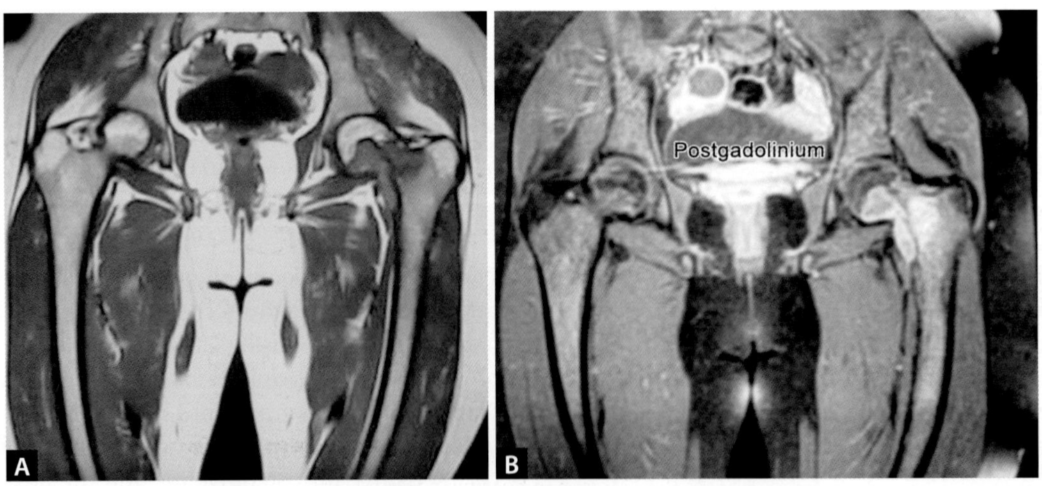

Figs. 30A and B: T1W coronal image of the pelvis (A) and T1W coronal postgadolinium image (B) show an area of cortical erosion in the femoral neck with associated marrow edema—Tubercular arthritis.

erosions. The use of dynamic gadolinium enhanced MR imaging has shown to be more sensitive than conventional MR imaging. Rapid (>90% increase in signal intensity curve) articular and periarticular enhancement represents active sacroiliitis.[49] Intra-articular enhancement is noted in patients with active sacroiliitis. The fluid within the joint space does not enhance whereas the inflammatory reaction (phlegmon) may enhance **(Figs. 32 and 33)**.

The cause of sacroiliitis cannot be distinguished with MR imaging. Unilateral disease with prominent edema in the soft tissue and marrow adjacent to the joint suggests infection. The advantages of MR evaluation are direct visualization of cartilage, imaging in the oblique coronal plane for evaluation of synovial compartment and lack of ionizing radiation as most patients of sacroiliitis are young and of reproductive age group.

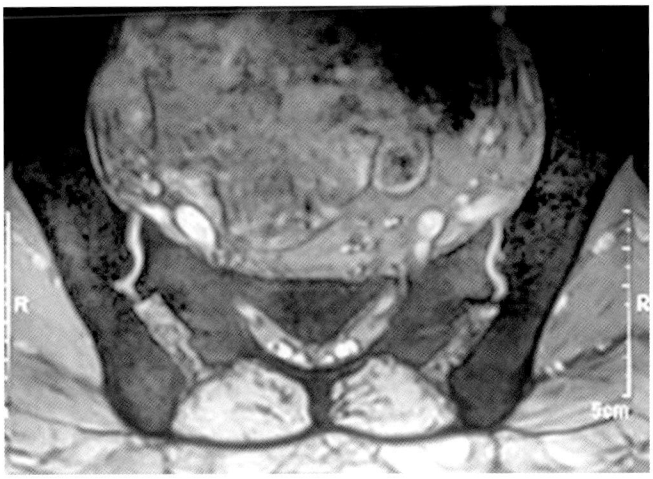

Fig. 31: Gradient T2W axial image shows vertical anterior synovial part of the joint and posterior obliquely oriented ligamentous part—Normal sacroiliac joint.

NERVES

The largest nerve adjacent to the hip joint is the sciatic nerve. It is located immediately posterior to the posterior column of the acetabulum and lateral to the L4–S3 nerve roots. The nerve exits the infrapiriformis portion of the greater sciatic foramen and courses between the ischial tuberosity and greater trochanter surrounded by fat. It is located between quadratus femoris muscle anteriorly and gluteus maximus posteriorly. On MRI, the sciatic nerve is identified as intermediate signal intensity stippled structure surrounded by fat just lateral to the ischial tuberosity on axial images.

The sciatic nerve can be compressed by a nearby mass or may be traumatized by a direct blow resulting in swelling of the nerve with an increased signal on T2W images.

Magnetic resonance imaging of acetabular fractures can be used to detect subclinical injury to the sciatic nerve. The injured nerve shows perineural or intraneural enhancement.[50] The common sites of nerve enhancement include the greater sciatic foramen adjacent to the piriformis muscle and at the hip external rotator muscles, adjacent to the posterior wall of acetabulum. Preoperative detection of such abnormalities warrants intraoperative monitoring as these patients would be at risk for further (iatrogenic) nerve injury. Compared with neurological examinations and SEP (somatosensory evoked potential) monitoring, MR may be a more sensitive indicator of sciatic nerve trauma.

Fibrolipomatous hematoma may be seen in relation to sciatic nerve in which fascicles of the nerve are surrounded by fat.

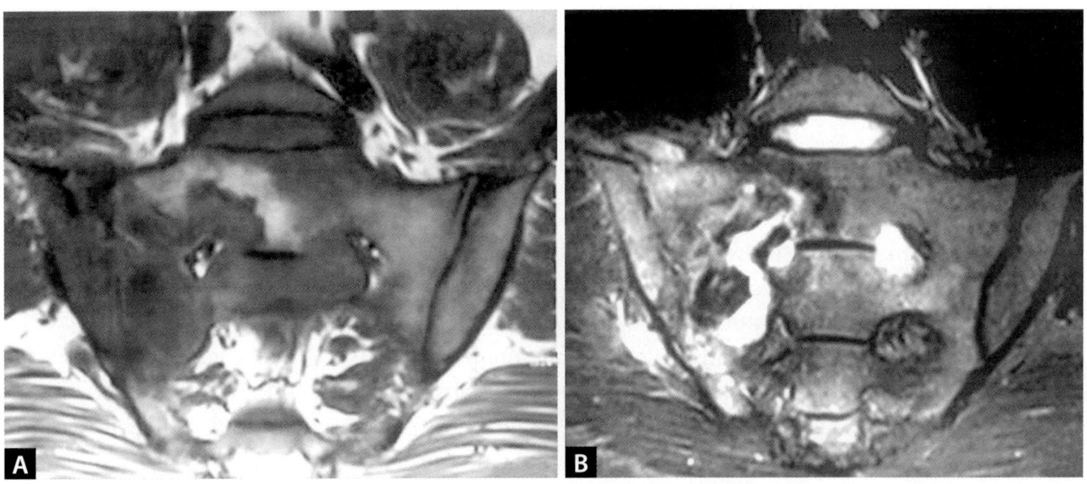

Figs. 32A and B: T1W coronal image of both sacroiliac joints (A) and T2W coronal image (B) show altered signal in the right sacral ala and iliac blade, with articular erosion and decreased joint space—Right sacroiliitis.

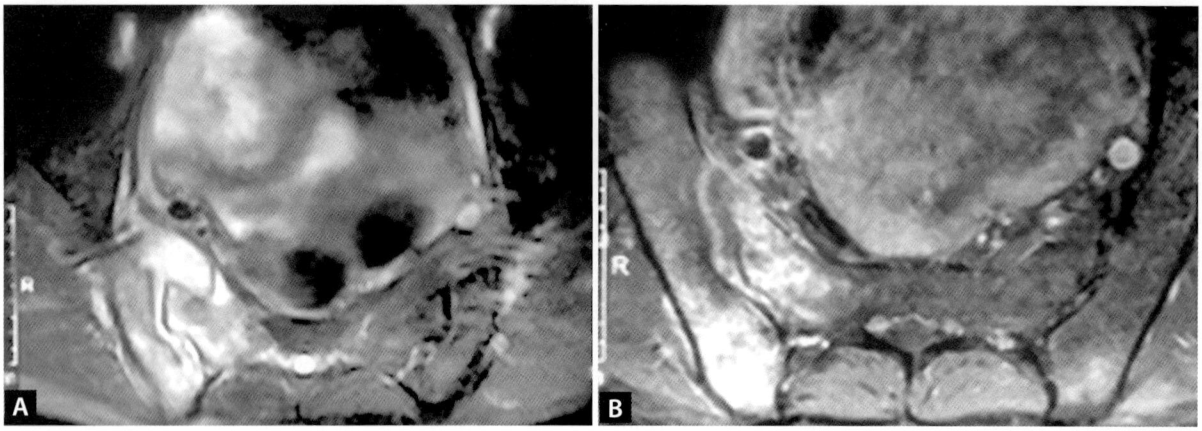

Figs. 33A and B: T2W axial (A) and STIR axial (B) images of both sacroiliac joints showing altered signal in right sacroiliac joint with widened joint space and periarticular collection—Tubercular sacroiliitis.

MARROW REPLACEMENT PROCESSES

The bone marrow of the pelvis and hips shows higher signal than muscle on T1W images because of large amount of red marrow that persists in this region throughout life. The epiphysis and apophysis (trochanters) have high signal fatty marrow on T1W images. Occasionally, a small rim of red marrow may parallel the subchondral bone of the femoral epiphysis—a normal variant. Thick stress trabeculae and linear physeal scars at the femoral head/neck junction can be seen as low signal lines on MRI.

Replacement of the marrow fat by cellular tumor or a cellular marrow packing process decreases signal intensity on T1W images. On Fat Sat T2W images and STIR sequence, the marrow abnormality generally increases in signal intensity with the exception of marrow fibrosis, Gaucher's disease and osteoblastic metastasis. Separation of metastasis from foci of hematopoietic marrow may be difficult. Uniform or peripherally located ring like high signal suggests metastasis, while centrally located high signal suggests focal red marrow[51]—benign etiology.

TUMORS

The hip and pelvis is not a site unique to any particular bone tumor. Neoplastic involvement about the hip, both benign and malignant can involve either the osseous structures or soft tissues. Magnetic resonance imaging can provide localization and characterization information which are essential in staging and preoperative planning. Advantages of MRI include multiplanar imaging, superior contrast resolution and lack of ionizing radiation.

The multiplanar capability of MRI is important in assessing osseous neoplasms about the hip for surgical planning. Detection of hip joint invasion is important because resection of structures on both sides of the joint is then required. Involvement is best seen on coronal and sagittal images with soft tissue mass within the articulation and with associated effusion. Absence of joint effusion in cases of osseous malignancy about the hip excludes joint involvement.

Numerous primary osseous neoplasms occur about the hip. The following are commonly encountered.

Osteoid Osteoma

Osteoid osteoma is common, accounting for 10-12% primary benign lesions. These lesions are seldom larger than 1.5-2 cm in diameter and are classified by their location.

Cortical-75%— tibia and femur.

Cancellous-25%—are most common about the hip with the proximal femur involved more frequently than the acetabulum.

Magnetic Resonance Imaging

Magnetic resonance imaging is usually not necessary to detect these lesions and variable appearance has been reported. The nidus may show low to intermediate signal intensity on T2W images if it is mineralized or may be similar to fat if it is nonmineralized. On long TR images extensive marrow edema surrounding the nidus may obscure it. An associated joint effusion may be seen with contrast enhancement of the nidus. A reactive soft tissue mass may be seen with osteoid osteoma on MR a manifestation of associated inflammatory lesion.

Chondroblastoma

A benign chondroid neoplasm that involves primarily the epiphysis of young patients between 10 and 20 years of age. One of the most common sites—proximal femur is involved in 16% of the cases. Less frequently involved is the iliac bone in area of triradiate cartilage.

Magnetic Resonance Imaging

On T1W images MRI shows marrow replacement. Most chondroblastomas retain low to intermediate signal intensity on long TR images. This is probably related to high cellularity, fibrosis or areas of chondroid mineralization. Magnetic resonance imaging may also show extensive surrounding edema and hip effusion.

Chondrosarcoma

It occur predominantly in males between the age of 30 and 60 years. The tumor arises *de novo* in the medullary cavity or as a secondary complication of a pre-existing enchondroma. The preferred location are metadiaphysis of long bones (femur and humerus), the flat bones especially pelvis and vertebrae.

Magnetic Resonance Imaging

On MRI, they are seen as slightly expansible, multilobulated, inhomogeneous lesions with low to intermediate signal intensity on T1WI and high signal intensity on T2WI. Areas of decreased signal intensity on T2WI may represent calcified cartilaginous foci. Hemorrhages of different ages may be seen within the tumor. Contrast-enhancement occurs in a focal or diffuse fashion and the degree of enhancement may correspond to the degree of malignancy. Cortical break-through and soft tissue mass indicate malignancy **(Fig. 34)**.

Chordomas

Chordomas originate from sacrum and coccyx (60%), clivus (30%) and spine especially C2 (10%). Sacrococcygeal chordomas occur in 40–60 years old patients with male predominance. Occipital chordomas are usually diagnosed in 20–40 years old patients without gender predilection.

Magnetic Resonance Imaging

Chordomas are destructive lesions with osseous expansion and large soft tissue mass with mixed signal intensity low to intermediate on T1WI, intermediate to high on T2WI. Internal septation may be seen. Hyperintense foci on T1WI represent subacute hemorrhage (methemoglobin) or possibly proteinaceous material and hypointense foci on T2WI are caused by hemosiderosis, calcifications or bone fragments. Contrast enhancement is heterogeneous and moderate to marked. In the sacrum the tumor grows anteriorly and may contain cystic areas **(Figs. 35A and B)**.

Among soft tissue tumors and tumor like lesions—lipomas, hemangiomas, arteriovenous malformations, benign neural tumors, ganglions, and PVNS can be diagnosed with high accuracy with MR.

CONCLUSION

Magnetic resonance imaging is the diagnostic modality of choice for most disorders of the hip and pelvis in evaluating cases with radiographic findings that are inconclusive or do not explain the patient's complaints. In the evaluation of hip and pelvis, MRI is often the problem solving technique bypassing bone scintigraphy and CT. With MRI one can stage the pathology of the hip and pelvis to prognosticate and influence therapeutic decisions.

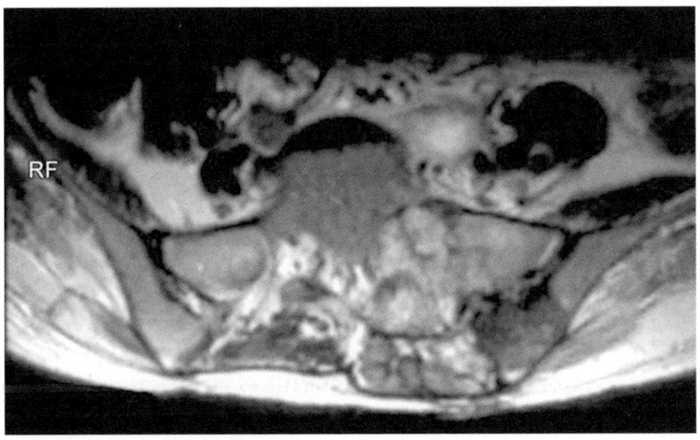

Fig. 34: T2W axial image of the pelvis shows destruction of the left sacral ala with lobulated soft tissue mass—Chondrosarcoma.

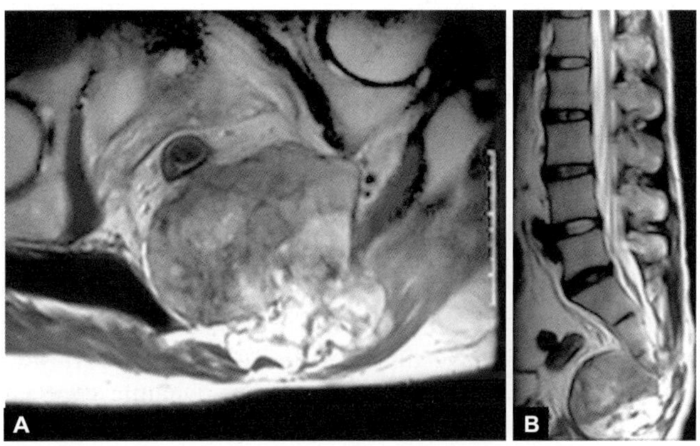

Figs. 35A and B: T2W axial image (A) and T2W sagittal image of the pelvis (B) show a lobulated mixed signal intensity mass arising from sacrum and projecting into presacral space anteriorly—Chordoma.

REFERENCES

1. Hong RJ, Hughes TH, Gentili A, et al. Magnetic resonance of the hip. J Magn Reson Imaging. 2008;27:435-45.
2. Potter HG, Schachar J. High resolution non contrast MRI of the hip. J Magn Reson Imaging. 2010;31:268-78.
3. Solomon L. Mechanism of ischemic necrosis. Orthop Clin North Am. 1985;16:655.
4. Hungerford DS, Zizic TM. Pathogenesis of ischemic necrosis of the femoral head. In: Hungerfod DS (Ed) The Hip. Philadelphia: Mosby. 1983;62:249.
5. Coleman BG, Kressel HY, Dalinka MK, et al. Radiographically negative avascular necrosis detection with MR imaging. Radiology. 1988;168:525-8.
6. Mitchell DG, Rao VM, Dalinka MK, et al. Femoral head avascular necrosis: Correlation of MR imaging, radiographic staging, radionuclide imaging and clinical findings. Radiology. 1987;162(3):709-15.
7. Mitchell DG, Steinberg ME, Dalinko MK, et al. Magnetic resonance imaging of the ischemic hip. Alterations within the osteonecrotic, viable and reactive zones. Clin Orthop. 1989;244:60-72.
8. Mitchell DG, Rao UM, Dalinka MK, et al. Hematopoietic and fatty bone marrow distribution in the normal and ischemic hip: New observations with 1.5T MR imaging. Radiology. 1986;161(1):199-202.
9. Malizos KN, Karantanas AH, Varitimidis SE, et al. Osteonecrosis of the femoral head: etiology, imaging and treatment. Eur J Radiol. 2009;63:16-28.
10. Karantanas AH, Drakonaki EE. The role of MR imaging in vascular necrosis of the femoral head. Semin Musculoskelet Radiol. 2011;15:281-300.
11. Ikemura S, Yamamota T, Motomura G, et al. MRI evaluation of collapsed femoral head in patients 60 years old or older: differentiation of subchondral insufficiency fracture from osteonecrosis of the femoral head. Am J Roentgenol. 2010;195(1):W63-8.
12. Huang GH, Chan WP, Chang YC. MR imaging of bone marrow edema and joint effusion in patients with osteonecrosis of the femoral head: relationship to pain. AJR. 2003;181:545-9.
13. Nadel DN, Debatin JT, Richardson LW. Detection of acute avascular necrosis of the femoral head in dogs: Dynamic contrast enhanced MR imaging vs spin echo and STIR sequences. Am J Roentgenol. 1992;159:1255.
14. Van de Berg B, Malghem J, Labaisse MA, et al. Avascular necrosis of the hip. Comparison of contrast enhanced and nonenhanced MR imaging with histological correlation. Radiology. 1992;182:445.
15. Chan WP, Liu YJ, Huang GS, et al. Relationship of the idiopathic osteonecrosis of the femoral head to perfusion changes in the proximal femur by dynamic contrast enhanced MRI. AJR. 2011;196:637-43.
16. Oner AY, Aggunlu L, Akpek S, et al. Staging of hip avascular necrosis: Is there need for DWI? Acta Radiol. 2001;52:111-7.
17. Hou CH, Shih TT, Liu CY, et al. Proton MR spectroscopy of the femoral head-evaluation of patients at risk for vascular necrosis. J Magn Reson Imaging. 2006;(2):409-17.
18. Shimizu K, Moriya H, Akita T, et al. Prediction of collapse with magnetic resonance imaging of avascular necrosis of the femoral head. J Bone Joint Surg. 1994;76A:215-21.
19. Jiang CC, Shih TT. Epiphyseal scar of the femoral head: Risk factor of osteonecrosis. Radiology. 1994;191(2):409-12.
20. Kaplan, Helms, Dussault, Anderson, Major: Hip and pelvis. Musculoskeletal MRI (1st edn) Philadelphia: WB Saunders; 2001.pp.333-62.
21. Arlet J, Ficat RP. Diagnostic de l' osteonecroses femoraoccipitale primitive an stade 1 (stade preradiologic) (in French). RPV Chir Orthop. 1968;54:637-48.
22. Association for Research on Osseous Circulation. Committee on Terminology and Classification. ARCO News. 1992;4:41.
23. Beltran J, Herman LJ, Burk JM, et al. Femoral head avascular necrosis: MR imaging with clinical pathological and radionuclide correlation. Radiology. 1988;166:215.
24. Bradway JK, Morrey BF. The natural history of the silent hip in bilateral atraumatic osteonecrosis. J Arthroplasty. 1993;8(4):383-7.
25. Kopecky KK, Braunstein EM, Brandt KD, et al. Apparent avascular necrosis of the hip: Appearance and spontaneous resolution of MR findings in renal allograft recipient. Radiology. 1991;179:523-7.
26. Saito S, Ohzono K, Ono K. Minimal osteonecrosis as a segmental infarct within the femoral head. Clin Orthop Relat Res. 1998;(231):35-50.
27. Van de Berg BC, Lecovet FE, Koutaissoff S. Bone marrow edema of the femoral head and transient osteoporosis of the hip. Eur J Radiol. 2008;67:68-77.
28. Kaplan SS, Stegman CJ. Transient osteoporosis of the hip. J Bone Joint Surg Am. 1985;67A:490-2.
29. Curtiss PH, Kincaid WE. Transitory demineralisation of the hip in pregnancy. J Bone Surg Am. 41A:1237-1333.
30. Vande Berg BE, Malghemm JJ, Labaisse MA, et al. MR imaging of avascular necrosis and transient marrow edema of the femoral head. Radiographics. 1993;13(3):501-20.
31. Kassarjian A, Brisson M, Palmer WE. Femoroacetabular impingement. Eur J Radiol. 2007;63:29-35.
32. Ganz R, Parvizi J, Beck M, Leuing M, Notzli H, et al. Femoroactabular impingement: a cause of osteoarthritis of the hip.Clin Orthop Relat Res. 2003;417:112-20.
33. Siebenrock KA, Wahab KH, Werlen S, Kalhor M, et al. Abnormal extension of the femoral head epiphysis as a cause of cam impingement Clin Orthop Relat Res. 2004;418:54-60.
34. Notzli HP, Wyss TF, Stoecklin CH, Schmid MR, et al. The contour of the femoral head-neck junction as a predictor for the risk of anterior impingement. J Bone Joint Surg Br. 2002;84:556-60.
35. Ito K, Minka A, Leunig M, Werlen S, Ganz R. Femoroacetabular impingement and the cam effect: an

MRI based quantitative anatomical study of the femoral head-neck offset. J Bone Joint Surg Br. 2001;83:171-6.
36. Kassarjian A, Yoon LS, Belzile E, et al. Triad of arthrographic findings in patients with cam type femoroacetabular impingement. Radiology. 2005;236:588-92.
37. Anderson SE, Siebenrock KA, Tannast M. Femoroacetabular impingement: evidence of an established hip abnormality. Radiology. 2010;257:8-13.
38. Haaga JR, Lanzieri CF, Gilkeson RC. The hip: In: Murphy MD, Peterrilge CA (Eds). CT and MR Imaging of the Whole Body (4th edn) 1909-38. Mosby.
39. Nokis SR, Vogler JB, Spritzer CE, et al. Herniation pits of the femoral neck: Appearance at MR imaging. Radiology. 1989;172:231-4.
40. Lang P, Mauz M, Schirner W, et al. Acute fracture of the femoral neck: Assessment of femoral head perfusion with gadopentetate Dimeglumine—Enhanced MR imaging. AJR. 1993;160:335-41.
41. Bencardino JT, Palmer WE. Imaging of hip disorders in athletes. Radiol Clin North Am. 2002;40(2):(vi-vii):267-87.
42. Boutin RD, Newman JS. MR imaging of sports related hip disorders. Magn Reson Imaging Clin N Am. 2003;11(2):255-81.
43. Sadro C. Current concepts in magnetic resonance imaging of the adult hip and pelvis. Semin Roentgenol Vol XXXV. 2000.pp.231-48.
44. Kingzett Taylor, Tirman PFJ, Feller J, et al. Tendinosis and tears of gluteus medius and maximus muscles as a cause of hip pain: MR imaging findings. AJR. 1999;173:1123-6.
45. Sheikh A, Schweitzer M. Imaging in pre and postoperative assessment in joint preserving and replacing surgery. Radiol Clin North Am. 2009;47:761-75.
46. Flandry F, Hughston J, McCann S, et al. Diagnostic features of diffuse pigmented villonodular synovitis of the knee. Clin Orthop. 1994;298:212-20.
47. Heimano G, Abdelwahab IF, Kelin M, et al. Synovial chondromatosis. Skeletal Radiol. 1995;24:298-300.
48. Murphey MD, Wetzel LH, Bramble JM, et al. Sacroiliitis: MR imaging findings. Radiology. 1991;180:239-44.
49. Bollow M, Broun J, Hamm B, et al. Early sacroiliitis in patients with spondyloarthropathy: Evaluation with dynamic gadolinium enhanced MR imaging. Radiology. 1995;194:529-36.
50. Potter HG, Montgomery KD, Heise CW, et al. MR imaging of Acetabular fractures: Value in detecting femoral head injury, intra-articular fragments and sciatic nerve injury. AJR. 1993;163:881-6.
51. Schweitzer ME, Levine C, Mitchell DG, et al. Bull's eyes and halos: useful MR discriminators of osseous metastasis. Radiology. 1993;188:249-52.

CHAPTER 202

Magnetic Resonance Imaging of Shoulder and Temporomandibular Joints

Mahesh Prakash, Paramjeet Singh

SHOULDER JOINT

Various imaging modalities have been used to assess the shoulder joint like, radiography, computed tomography (CT), ultrasonography (USG) and magnetic resonance imaging (MRI). Although each modality has its own advantages and disadvantages, MR imaging provides the comprehensive and accurate assessment of shoulder.[1] Clinical examination is important and usually help in providing the proper choice of subsequent investigative modality. Radiographs and computed tomography are useful to demonstrate osseous structures of shoulder girdle however they provide poor or limited evaluation of soft tissue anatomy. Ultrasonography has also been used to visualize pathology of rotator cuff and bursae of the joint with variable success.[2-4] This technique is however operator dependent and needs high end equipment.[5] The MRI, because of its excellent soft tissue contrast, imaging capability in any desired plane and nonionizing noninvasive nature, is an ideal modality for evaluation of shoulder joint.[6]

MR IMAGING PROTOCOLS

Improved coil designs have helped to improve the signal to noise ratio and provide adequate spatial resolution in MR imaging of shoulder. Proper immobilization and comfort of the patient, off axis small FOV imaging capability, high matrix size and elimination of phase wrap are desirable requisites for imaging the shoulder.

During MR imaging of shoulder, patient is placed in supine position with their arm on the side of body in partial external rotation. After localizer images, joint should be imaged in axial, coronal-oblique and sagittal-oblique planes.[7] Coronal-oblique plane is selected parallel to the course of supraspinatus tendon. The sagittal-oblique images are done parallel to glenoid surface. The imaging sequences may vary in different institutions depending on available hardware and other factors and have been being changed over the years. Previously we had used proton/T2 turbo spin-echo (TSE) and gradient-echo sequences in axial planes, T1 spin-echo and proton/T2 TSE sections oblique coronal planes and oblique sagittal sections using T1 SE and T2 TSE sequences. An STIR, turbo inversion recovery or fat suppressed T2 TSE sequence were additionally used in one of the planes. The basic sequences presently done in our institution on 3 Tesla MR machine are listed in **Table 1**.

MR ARTHROGRAPHY

MR arthrography with intra-articular contrast is performed by injecting 12–15 cc mixture of gadolinium dimeglumine (2 mmol/L), normal saline, lidocaine and iodinated contrast media into joint cavity with a 20G spinal needle through either anterior or posterior approach under fluoroscopic guidance.[8,9] The gadolinium concentration of 2 mmol/L is achieved by mixing 0.5 mL of contrast in 50 mL of saline. T1 fat suppressed sections are taken in axial,

Table 1: Standard pulse sequences for MRI examination of the shoulder at 3 tesla.

Pulse sequence	*FOV (cm)*	*Slice thickness (mm)*	*Matrix*	*TR/TE*
Axial PD with fat saturation	14	3	256 × 256	3000/43
Sagittal oblique PD with fat saturation	14	3	256 × 256	3000/43
Coronal oblique T1	14	3	256 × 256	650/24
Coronal oblique T2 with fat saturation	14	3	256 × 256	3000/89
Sagittal oblique T1	14	3	256 × 256	650/24
Axial T2	14	3	256 × 256	3000/89

Abbreviations: FOV: Field of view; TR: Repetition time; TE: Echo time.

oblique coronal and sagittal planes. Additional imaging in an abducted externally rotated (ABER) arm may also be done to assess capsule-labral pathology.

NORMAL ANATOMY

Shoulder joint is a ball and socket joint formed by articulation between head of humerus and glenoid of scapula. Structurally it is a weak joint because of disparity of articulating surface area between small and shallow glenoid cavity in comparison to the humeral head. However, this arrangement provides the glenohumeral joint with the greatest range of motion of any articulation in human body. Stability to this unstable joint is provided by following structures:

- Coracoacromial arch (CCA) consisting of acromian, coracoacromial ligament (CAL), coracoid process and the acromioclavicular joint (AC joint).
- Musculotendinous cuff of shoulder.
- Glenoid labrum along with capsule and glenohumeral ligaments.
- The muscles attaching the humerus to pectoral girdle, i.e. long head of biceps and triceps, coracobrachialis, teres major, etc.

OSSEOUS STRUCTURES

The osseous structures of shoulder joint include proximal humerus, scapula and clavicle. The proximal humerus consists of head, neck, greater and lesser tuberosities. The humeral head is typically round with slight flattening of posteroinferior surface. This flattening should not be confused with Hill-Sachs lesion which is seen at or above the level of coracoid process.[10] The anatomic neck forms the oblique circumference and separates head from tuberosities. The acromian and glenoid of scapula makes articulation with humeral head and clavicle to become components of shoulder joint. The acromian is posterior landmark and articulates with clavicle. The coracoid process is anterior landmark of shoulder with variable morphology.[11] The glenoid is important structure which articulates with humeral head to form shoulder joint. The glenoid is pear or oval shaped in coronal plane.[12] The lateral end of clavicle articulates with acromian to form acromioclavicular (AC) joint.

LIGAMENTS

The joint capsule is loose and permits free movements. It is least supported inferiorly where dislocations are common. Medially the capsule is attached to the scapula beyond the supraglenoid tubercle and margins of the labrum and laterally to the anatomical neck of humerus. The capsule is reinforced anteriorly and inferiorly by several thickenings namely the anterior and posterior bands of inferior glenohumeral ligament (IGHL) with an inferior axillary recess, the more variable middle GHL (MGHL) and the smallest superior GHL (SGHL). They all extend to the anatomical neck of humerus and stabilize the joint variably. The coracohumeral ligament (CHL) extends from lateral aspect of coracoid process to the neck of humerus and is a key structure in impingement and instability syndromes. Transverse humeral ligament bridges the bicipital groove and holds tendon of long head of biceps brachii. The glenoid labrum is a fibrocartilaginous ovoid rim attached to the margins of the glenoid cavity. It is often deficient anterosuperiorly. It functions to deepen the glenoid cup and is a site of capsuloligamentous attachment. It is more mobile superiorly and functions with biceps tendon as a mobile 'biceps labral complex' that slides over the superior glenoid.

MUSCULOTENDINOUS ANATOMY

From anterior to posterior, subscapularis muscle (SCM), biceps, supraspinatus muscle (SSM), infraspinatus muscle (ISM) and teres minor (TM) muscles together with their tendons form the rotator cuff. All originates from the scapula and insert on the humerus. Of these tendons, the supraspinatus tendon (SST), infraspinatus tendon (IST) and teres minor insert on their respective notches on the greater tuberosity while subscapularis tendon (SCT) attaches to the lesser tuberosity. The SST and IST fibers may partially fuse posteriorly to form a conjoint tendon (an area sometimes referred to as posterior rotator interval). The gap between SCT and SST, named anterior rotator cuff interval (RCI) is filled with fibrofatty tissue. The CHL, SGHL and biceps tendon (BT) lie beneath it in that order. The long head of BT originates from the supraglenoid tubercle, crosses the joint obliquely through RCI, attaches to superior labrum and exits the joint into bicipital groove. The bicipital groove is hooded by transverse humeral ligament.

BURSAE

Numerous bursae are related to shoulder joint, which can be communicating or noncommunicating with the joint. The subscapularis, subcoracoid, infraspinatus and peri bicipital bursae are communicating bursae. Bursa superior to AC joint and those related to coracobrachialis, teres major, long head of triceps and lattisimus dorsi do not communicate with the joint. The SASDB, the largest bursa in the body is lined with areolar tissue and synovium, which allow free sliding motion of adjacent structures. They are fused and considered as one and do not communicate with the joint.

NORMAL MR APPEARANCE

Axial Sections (Figs. 1 and 4)

These show the cuff muscles as intermediate signal intensity structures. Highest sections show SSM, followed posteriorly by ISM and TM and their tendons. The tendons appear darker than muscles and can be traced to greater tuberosity. Biceps tendon is seen anterosuperiorly and SCT anterior to the scapula at midsuperior head level. Bicipital groove is best seen on these sections lateral to lesser tuberosity. Anterior and posterior labra are particularly well seen on axial sections. The GHL are low intensity structures and better seen in presence of fluid in the joint or on MR arthrograms. The SGHL lies superiorly and follows the concavity of coracoid on its lateral aspect. The MGHL closely follows posterior margin of SCT and IGHL lies at lower head level. The articular cartilage appears bright on T2 and gradient images and best evaluated in axial sections.

Coronal Sections (Figs. 2 and 4)

The rotator cuff tendon structures are best evaluated on oblique coronal sections. The mid to anterior sections show the SST (along with AC joint). The sections posterior to this show conjoint tendons of SST and IST and TM. The tendons can be traced to greater tuberosity. The SASDB appears as a thin bright line beneath the deltoid muscle on T1/T2WI. The anterior sections also show SST and biceps tendon passing beneath it as well as coracohumeral, coracoacromial and coracoclavicular ligaments. The superior labrum is best evaluated for injury in the coronal plane. Axillary pouch is seen medial and inferior to humeral head.

Sagittal Sections (Figs. 3 and 4)

These provide a cross-sectional view of all the muscles of shoulder. Mid and lateral sagittal images show the SST/IST

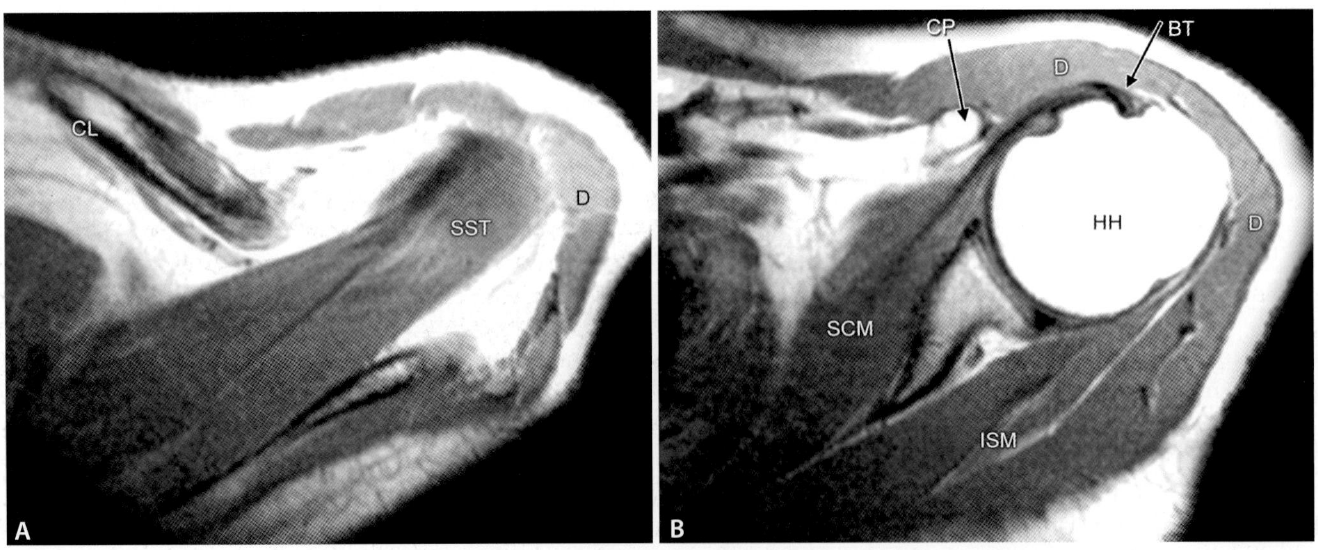

Figs. 1A and B: Axial T1-weighted sections of shoulder (normal anatomy).
Abbreviations: BT, biceps tendon; CL, clavicle; CP, coracoid process; D, deltoid muscle; HH, humeral head; ISM, infraspinatus muscle; SCM, subscapularis muscle; SST, supraspinatus tendon.

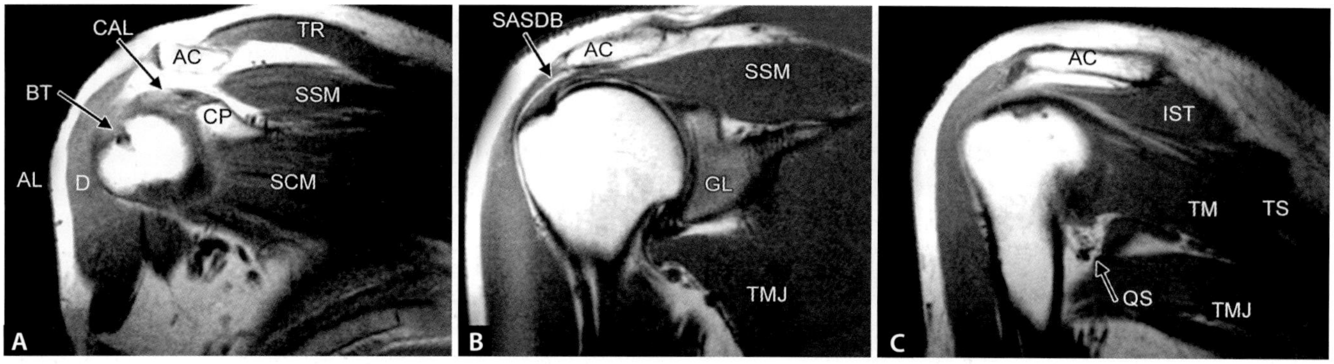

Figs. 2A to C: (A to C—anterior to posterior) Oblique coronal T1-weighted sections (normal anatomy).
Abbreviations: AC: Acromian process; BT: Biceps tendon; CAL: Coracoacromial ligament; CP: Coracoid process; D: Deltoid muscle; GL: Glenoid; IST: Infraspinatus tendon; QS: Quadrilateral space; SASDB: Subacrominal subdeltoid bursa; SCM: Subscapularis muscle; SSM: Supraspinatus muscle; TM: Teres minor; TMJ: Teres major; TR: Trapezius; TS: Triangular space.

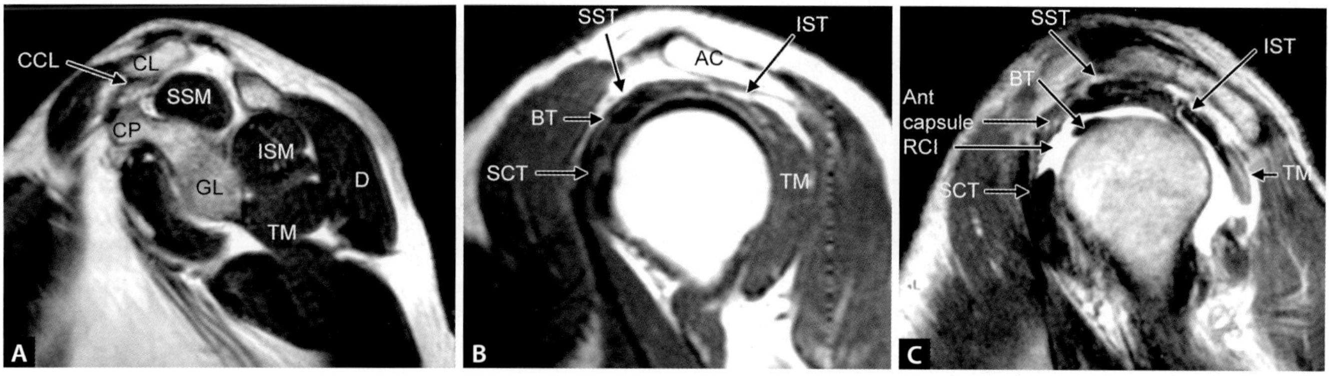

Figs. 3A to C: Oblique sagittal T1 (A and B—medial to lateral) and T2-weighted sections (C) (normal anatomy)
The intra-articular course of biceps tendon can be seen coursing through the rotator cuff interval.
Abbreviations: AC: Acromian process; BT: Biceps tendon; CCL: Coracoclavicular ligament; CL: Clavicle; CP: Coracoid process; D: Deltoid muscle; GL: Glenoid; ISM: Infraspinatus muscle; IST: Infraspinatus tendon; RCI: Rotator cuff interval; SCT: Subscapularis tendon; SSM: Supraspinatus muscle; SST: Supraspinatus tendon; TM: Teres minor.

conjoint tendon as a low signal structure between humeral head and acromion. The morphological abnormalities of acromion (i.e. anterior sloping) are best shown on these images. The long head of biceps can be seen passing anteroinferiorly between SST and SCT through the rotator cuff interval. More medially coracoacromial ligament can be seen arching over the rotator cuff interval along with AC joint in profile. The SGHL can be seen lying beneath the long head of biceps, the MGHL anterior to medial humeral head and IGHL along with a thick inferior labrum along the inferior aspect of the glenoid cavity **(Figs. 4A to F)**.

SHOULDER IMPINGEMENT SYNDROME

Impingement syndrome is a clinical diagnosis in which pain is felt in shoulder due to encroachment of the rotator cuff and associated soft tissues between the humeral head and overlying coracoacromial arch. The CCL is a triangular strong structure limiting the space available to rotator cuff during abduction. Abnormalities involving one or more of the components of CCA results in narrowing of the acromiohumeral distance.

Rotator cuff impingement can be classified as follows:
- Primary extrinsic impingement
- Secondary extrinsic impingement
- Intrinsic impingement.

Primary Extrinsic Impingement

This is due to the abnormalities of the CCA and can be subacromial or subcoracoid types.

Possible etiologies of subacromial impingement are as follows:
- Subacromial spur
- Hypertrophic changes in AC joint
- Unstable os acromial (failure to fuse by 25 years)
- Subacromial subdeltoid bursitis

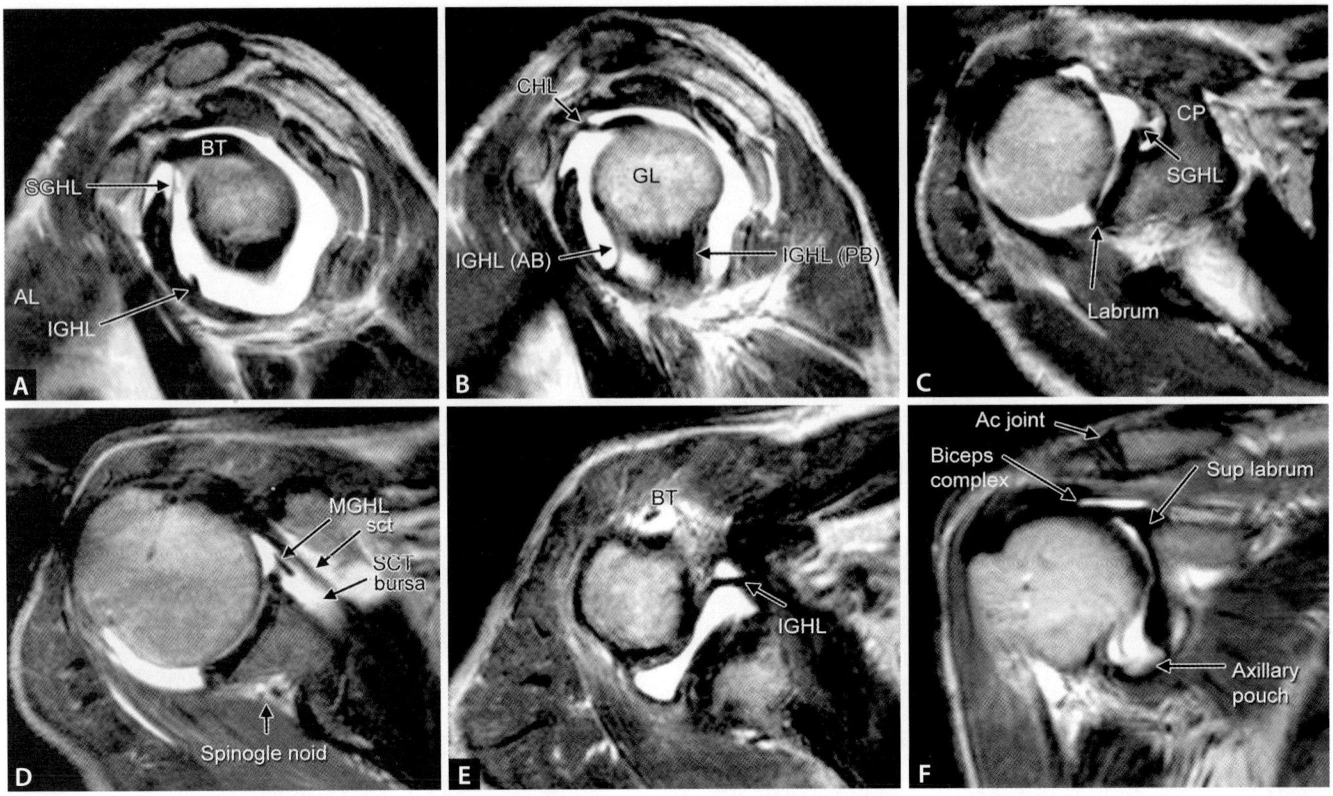

Figs. 4A to F: Sagittal (A and B), axial (C, D and E) and coronal (F) T2 TSE sections of a joint distended with effusion shows ligamentous anatomy. The SGHL is seen coursing down from its coracoid attachment (A and C). IGHL is seen with thick anterior and posterior bands outlining a distended axillary recess (B). The MGHL is seen as a thin hypointense band beneath SCT (D). The bicep-labral complex is firmly attached to the glenoid rim (Type I) (F). Biceps tendon is seen in bicipital groove (E).
Abbreviations: AC: Acromian process; BT: Biceps tendon; CHL: Coracohumeral ligament; CP: Coracoid process; GL: Glenoid; IGHL: Inferior glenohumeral ligament; AB: Anterior band; PB: Posterior band; MGHL: Middle glenohumeral ligament; SCT: Subscapularis tendon; SGHL: Superior glenohumeral ligament.

- Thickening of the coracoacromial ligament
- Laterally downsloping acromian process (Type III).

As seen on oblique sagittal plane (outlet view on plain radiographs) the anterior acromion is straight in Type I, curved in Type II and anteriorly hooked in Type III morphology **(Figs. 5A to C)**.[13] Type II configuration is most common and Type III is most commonly associated with rotator cuff pathology. Anterior part of SST is most commonly affected in subacromial type impingement alone or along with other tendons in 95% cases. The cuff along with subacromial bursa is entrapped along the undersurface of CCA.

The subcoracoid impingement can be due to reduced distance between coracoid process and the medial aspect of humeral head leading to compression of SCT and biceps long head.

Secondary Extrinsic Impingement

Here the abnormality lies in the stability of the glenohumeral joint in the setting of a normal CCA. It usually occurs in young athletes involved in sports demanding overhead arm movements. Possible underlying defect of static stabilizers (glenohumeral ligaments) leads to overload on secondary stabilizers (cuff structures) and a reduced acromiohumeral gap.

Internal Impingement

It is due to contact between undersurface of rotator cuff and glenoid rim due to throwing with arm in abduction and maximal external rotation. Supraspinatus hypertrophy or an abnormality of the greater tuberosity may also be contributory factors.

ROTATOR CUFF TENDINOPATHY AND TEARS

Rotator cuff disease is one of the most common causes of shoulder pain and indication for MRI evaluation of shoulder. Multiple etiologies have been implicated in the development of degenerative changes (tendinopathy) in the rotator cuff tendons near greater tuberosity.

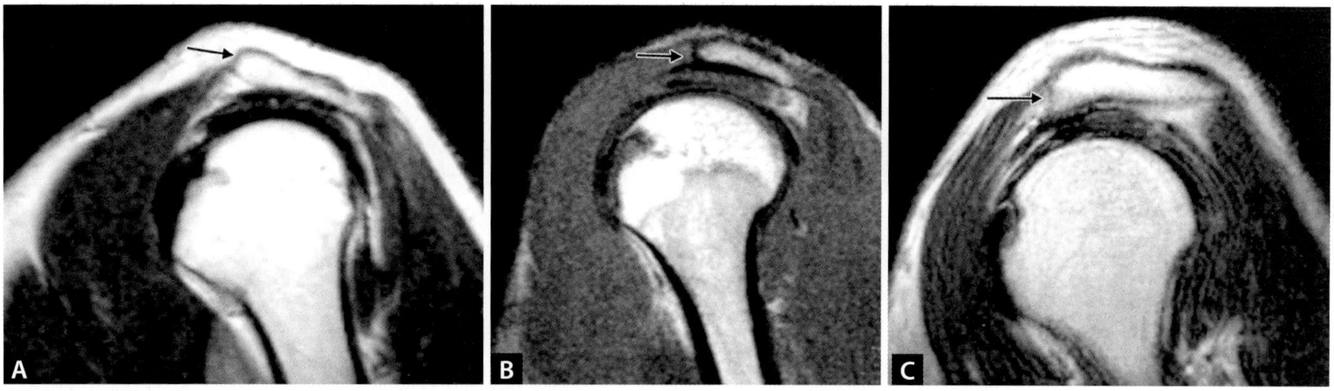

Figs. 5A to C: Type I (A), Type II (B) and Type III (C) acromian morphologies.

Aforementioned rotator cuff impingement between CCA and humeral head is most often implicated. Acute and chronic trauma, sports, overuse, aging, collagen, vascular and metabolic diseases are also associated with rotator cuff tendinopathy and tears. Vascular insufficiency leading to degeneration in critical zone may also play a role in rotator cuff tears (RCT). Critical zone, approximately 1 cm from the insertion of the supraspinatus tendon at the greater tuberosity, is the most susceptible area for tears.

Neer described three clinicopathologic stages of impingement.[14]

Stage I: There is reversible edema and hemorrhage within the distal supraspinatus tendon usually in young patient (<25 years) and is managed conservatively.

Stage II: There is tendinitis and thickening with fibrosis. Bursal pathology aggravates the condition by compromising subacromial space. Patient are usually between 25 and 40 years of age. No radiographic changes are seen in stage I and II.

Stage III: These are characterized by partial or a full thickness tears of rotator cuff or biceps tendon usually seen in patients older than 40 years of age. Osseous changes in the form of degenerative changes at greater tuberosity and acromial osteophyte formation are seen on radiographs.

Impingement is a process of progressive wear and tear. MR interpretation in early stages is often equivocal. The injured tendon may appear thickened due to mucoid degeneration; however histology of tendons of asymptomatic people also show similar changes. The term 'tendinosis or tendinopathy' is preferred over tendinitis as no inflammatory changes are seen within these tendons. In contrast to these intrasubstance changes of tendinosis, 'tendon surface degeneration' is seen as irregularity of surface and may be indistinguishable from or coexist with 'partial tears'. There may also be associated features of bursal and peribursal inflammation.

MR Appearance

Seeger[15] has classified impingement on coronal MR images into three types:

Type 1: Normal low-signal intensity on T1 and T2WI and normal morphology of the SST. Areas of increased signal intensity are noted on proton and GRE images.

Type 2: High-signal intensity of supraspinatus tendon on T1WI. If T2WI also reveal high signal intensity, which is not involving the entire thickness, it may represent partial tear (bursal or articular surface or intrasubstance).

Type 3: High-signal intensity is found on T1 and T2WI traversing full thickness suggestive of complete rotator cuff tear, with or without tendon retraction.

Carrino et al.[16] described more extensive MR grading for rotator cuff tears.

Grade 0 (Normal): Uniform low-signal intensity of the tendons.

Grade I: Increased signal intensity in tendon, more obvious on T1WI and proton images but not seen or less obvious on T2WI **(Figs. 6A and B)**.

Grade II (Tendinosis/Tendinitis): Increased signal intensity on T2WI that does not involve articular or superior surface. The tendon may be thin, thick or irregular, similar to Neer stage II **(Figs. 7A and B)**.

Grade III (Degeneration): Increased signal intensity on T2WI in one or multiple areas but signal changes do not meet criteria for partial or complete tear.

Grade IV (Partial tear): Increased signal intensity on T2WI that involve the inferior (articular) or superior (bursal) surface of the tendons **(Fig. 8)**.

Grade V: Full thickness tear with few spared fibers **(Figs. 9A and B)**.

Grade VI: Full thickness tear without tendon retraction **(Fig. 10)**.

Grade VII: Full thickness tear with tendon retraction.

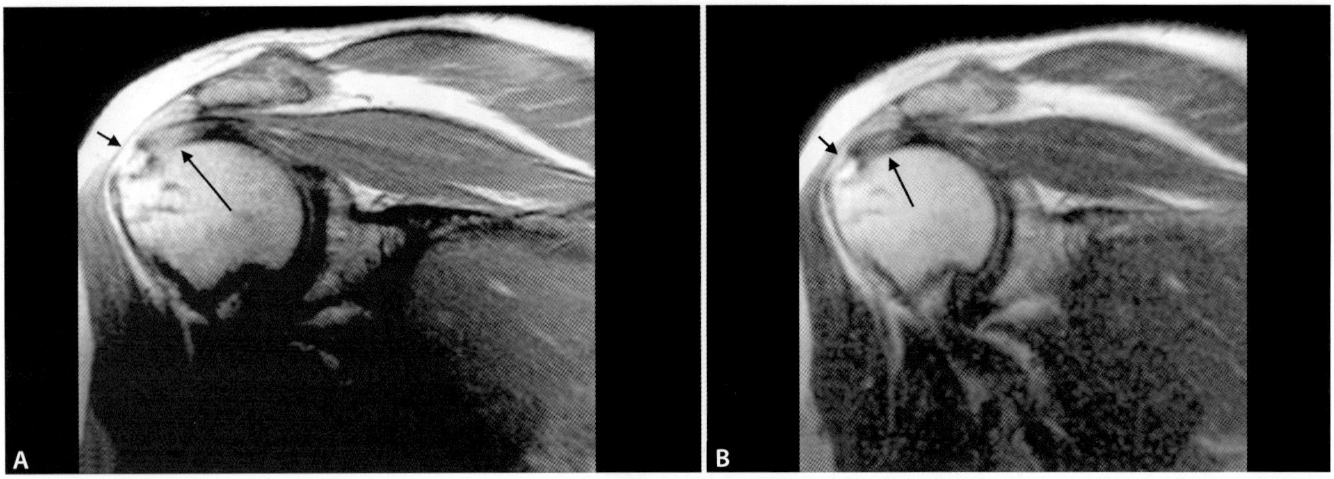

Figs. 6A and B: Proton (A) and T2 TSE (B) coronal sections show increased signal within the SST (A, long arrow), however T2WI (B) shows less pronounced signal changes in the tendon suggesting tendinopathy. Partial retraction at the insertion site with cyst formation is also noted (short arrow).

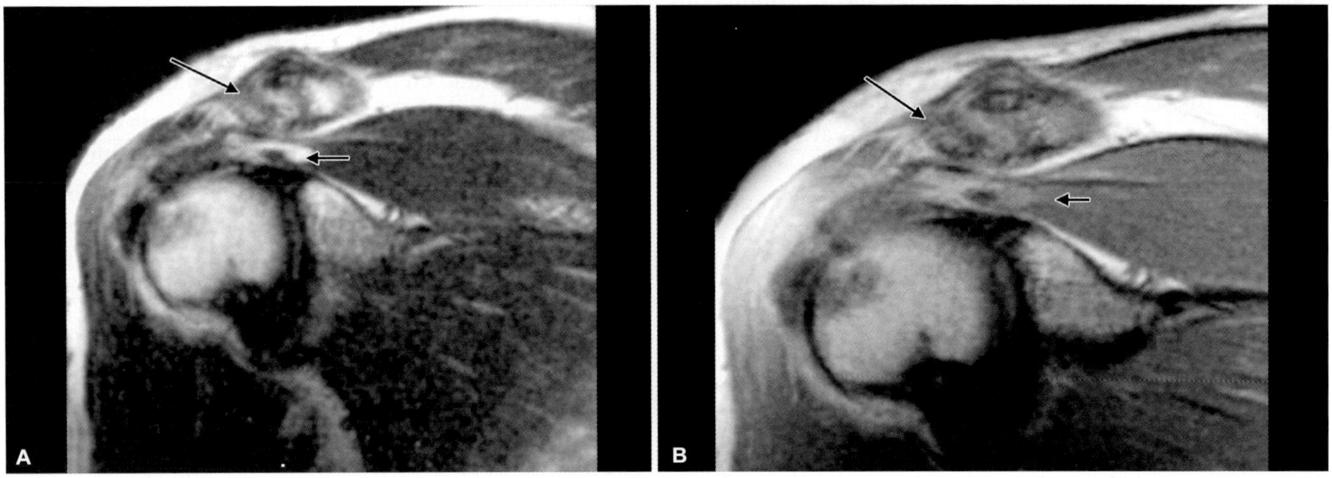

Figs 7A and B: Proton (A) and T2 TSE (B) coronal sections show impingement of the SST at the undersurface of AC joint which shows gross arthropathic hypertrophy (long arrow) leading to intrasubstance increased signal (tear) at the musculotendinous junction on both the images (short arrow).

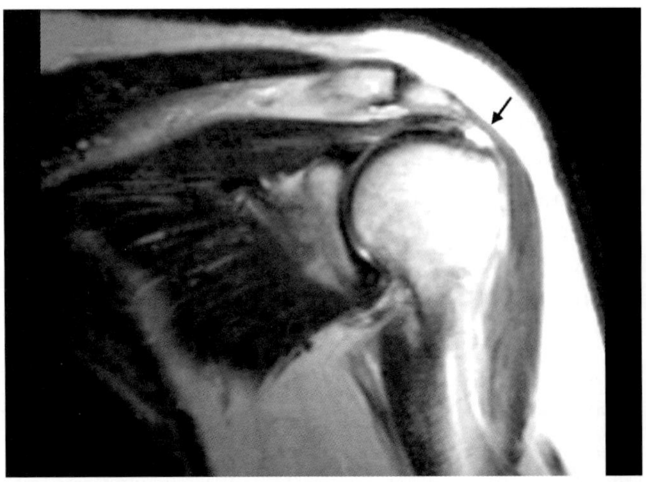

Fig. 8: T2 TSE coronal section shows a small articular surface tear as a focus of bright signal area along the undersurface of the SST (arrow).

An increase in T2 signal intensity along with abnormality in tendon morphology increases the confidence level of diagnosing a tear. Partial tears are better shown on T2WI (with fat suppression), particularly in presence of joint effusion as a discontinuity or fraying of the tendon **(Figs 9A and B)**. Partial tears are classified as Grade I, II or III depending on involvement of less than 25%, 25–30% or more than 50% of the tendon thickness.

Complete rotator cuff tears occur at sites of previous tendinopathy and can be diagnosed with greater confidence on MRI than the debatable early tendon pathology and partial tears. Full thickness tears can be classified as small (less than 1 cm or involvement of one tendon only) **(Fig. 11)**, medium (1–3 cm or involvement of two tendons) and massive (more than 3–5 cm or involvement of three or more tendons). Massive tears of the

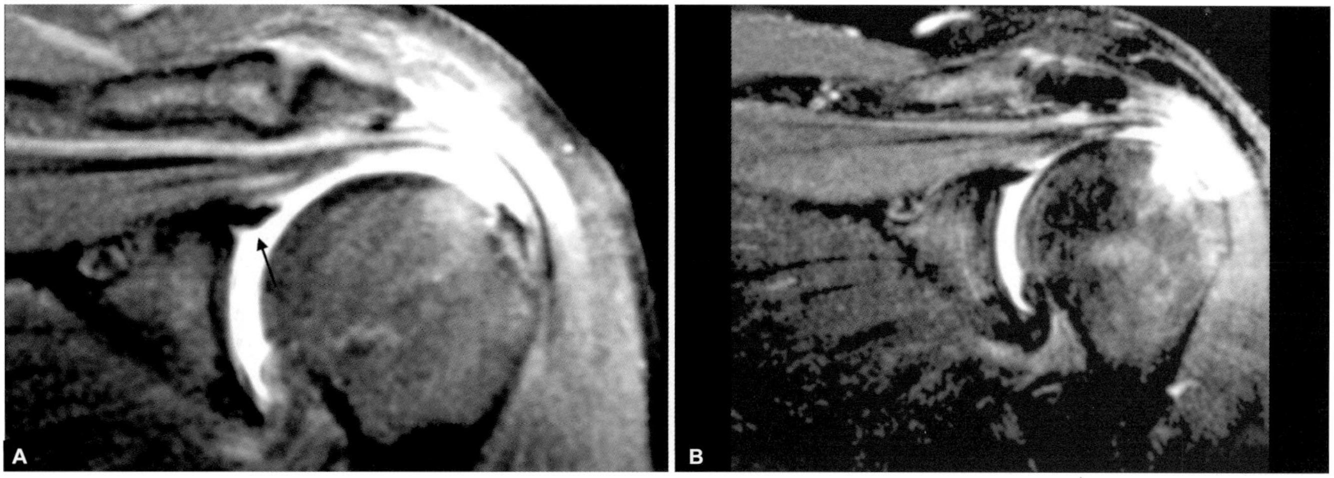

Figs. 9A and B: MR arthrogram (A) and fat-saturated T2 TSE coronal sections (B) show a near full thickness tear at the critical zone of SST on the articular surface with a few intact fibers. There is no retraction of the tendon. Fat-saturated images show the defect and edema at the greater tuberosity better. A sublabral recess (arrow) can be noted beneath the undersurface of the superior labrum.

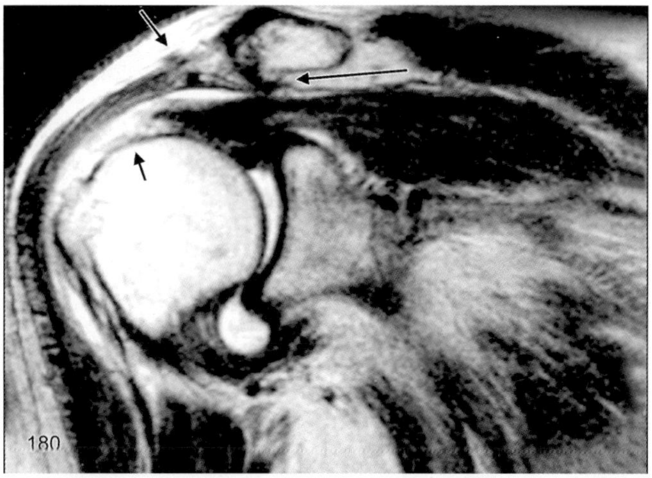

Fig. 10: T2 TSE coronal section: Full thickness tear of SST without tendon retraction (short arrows). There is fluid in the SASDB and axillary recess. AC joint osteophyte is noted (long arrow).

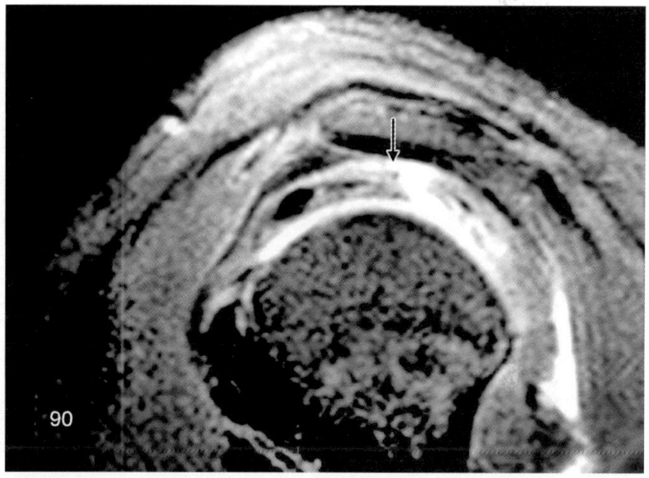

Fig. 11: Sagittal fat-suppressed T1 MR arthrographic image showing tear of posterior SST and possibly IST (conjoint tendon) with a full thickness defect outlined by the contrast in posterior rotator interval (arrow).

rotator cuff may also involve the subscapularis and biceps with or without dislocation **(Fig. 12)**. Both anteroposterior and mediolateral measurements of tears as well as quality of torn margins should be noted as these are important information from surgical point of view. Undersurface tears of posterior SST and IST, humeral head chondromalacia and fraying of posterosuperior labrum are hallmarks of internal impingement syndrome seen in overhead throwers **(Fig. 11)**.

Sometimes tears may not show T2 hyperintensity due to granulation or fibrosis and appear to be normal. Although less specific, knowledge of secondary signs of rotator cuff tear is useful in such difficult cases. MR may show fatty atrophy of muscle belly in complete tears as T1 hyperintensity and loss of volume **(Fig. 13)**. Humeral head may be apposed to the acromion in such chronic cases. Tendons may be completely nonvisualized due to musculotendinous retraction in complete tears. Tendon retraction, loss of peribursal/subdeltoid fat plane and fluid in the subdeltoid subacromial bursa can be seen in 92% patients with complete rotator cuff tear **(Figs. 14A and B)**.[17] However, bursal fluid can also be found in impingement (43%), labral abnormality (29%), bursitis (19%), tendinitis (14%) and even in normal people **(Fig. 15)**.[18] Joint effusion can be seen in both partial and complete tears. Marrow signal changes and cyst formation in the greater tuberosity

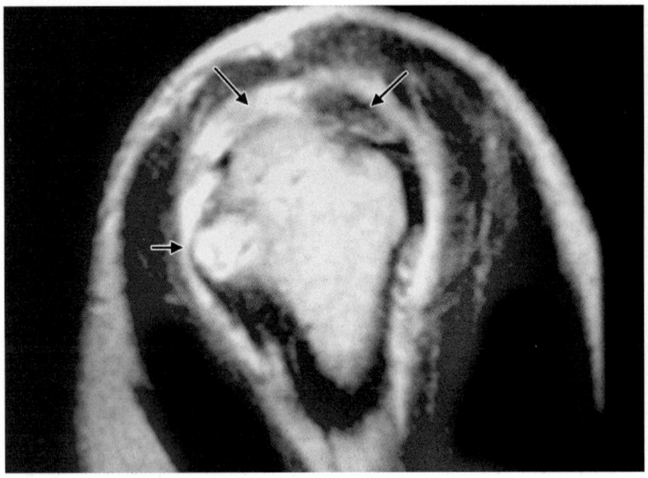

Fig. 12: Oblique sagittal T2 TSE section through the rotator cuff shows a massive tear involving SCT, SST as well as the IST (from anterior to posterior—arrows) seen as increased T2 signal replacing normal low signal of the tendons.

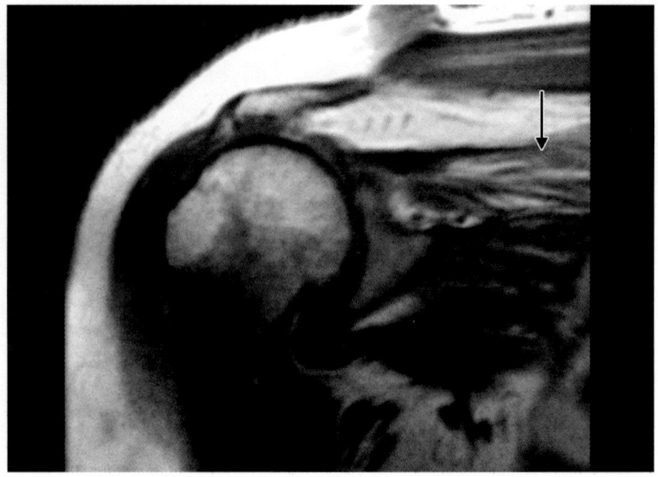

Fig. 13: T1 SE coronal section: Chronic rotator cuff tear with SST retraction, atrophy of the muscle and fatty changes seen as T1 hyperintensity (arrow).

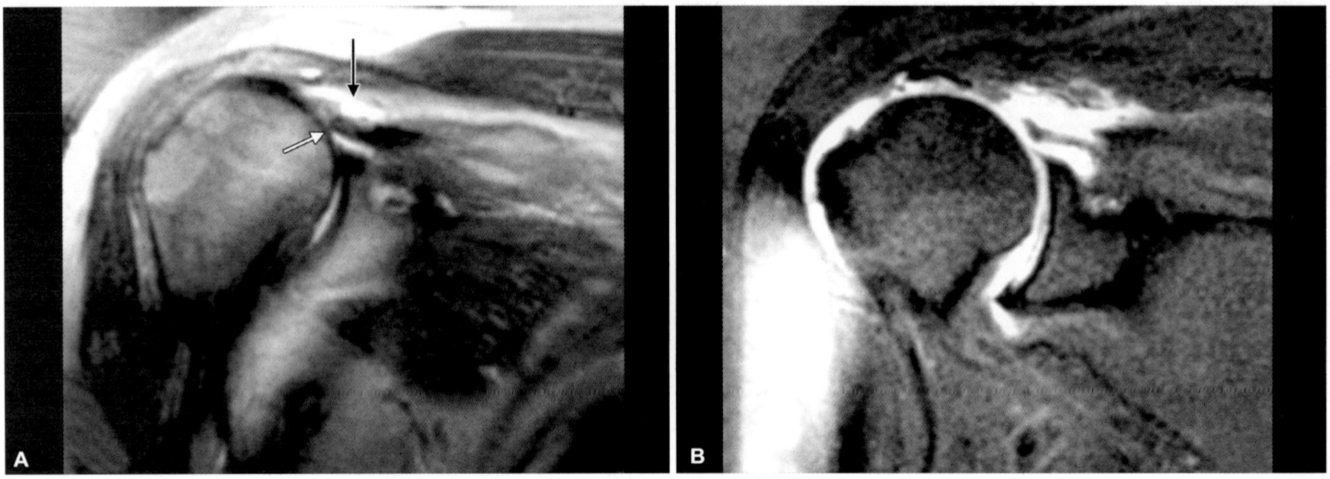

Figs. 14A and B: T2 TSE and arthrographic coronal sections show complete tear of SST (white arrow) with tendon retraction and fluid in the SASDB (black arrow) (A). There is free spillage of intra-articular contrast into the SASD bursa (B).

on fat suppressed T2 WI and osseous changes like AC joint osteophytosis and subacromial spurs are secondary signs of cuff tendinopathy and indicate advanced disease (***see* Figs. 9 and 10**). Artifactually increased signal may be noted within the tendons on proton images due to 'magic angle effect' in areas where the tendon courses at 55° angle in relation to the magnetic field. Normal signal on T2WI differentiates this from actual tendinopathy.

According to Zlatkin and colleagues[19] sensitivity and specificity of MR for imaging partial and full thickness tears are 91% and 88% respectively with 89% accuracy. MR arthrography though not used routinely, is useful in difficult cases and is gaining in popularity (***see* Figs. 9 and 14B**).[20] It is superior to conventional T2WI for evaluating partial tears particularly on the articular side and differentiating small complete tears (with fibrosis) from partial tears. It is also helpful for diagnosing associated instability and capsulolabral disorders.

INSTABILITY

Shoulder joint is one of the most mobile joints in the body. But this mobility comes at the expense of stability as the joint architecture which allows maximum mobility also predis-poses it to dislocation.

Glenohumeral joint is relatively shallow with a large humeral head in comparison to glenoid fossa. The structures responsible for maintaining joint stability are dynamic stabilizers (rotator cuff) and static stabilizers

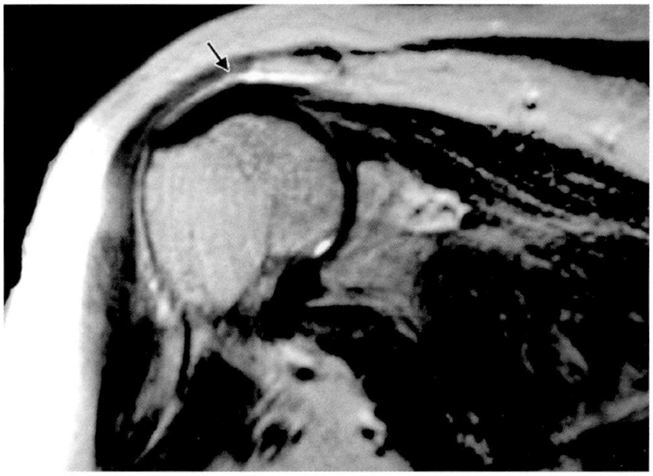

Fig. 15: T2 TSE coronal section: The SASDB shows fluid (arrow) in absence of any visible rotator cuff tear.

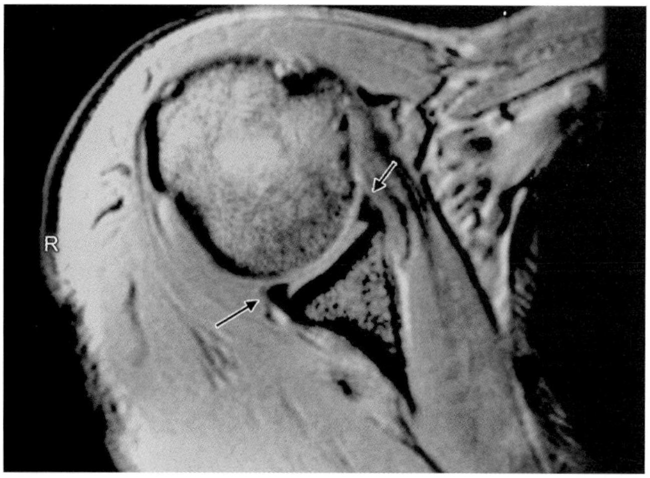

Fig.16: Gradient-echo axial section shows normal anterior and posterior triangular labra undercut by a bright appearing articular cartilage (arrows).

(glenoid labrum, joint capsule, GHL and periarticular soft tissue) **(Figs. 4A and B)**. Pathology of any of these structures can predispose to instability.

Anterior and posterior bands are thickenings of anterior and posterior margins of IGHL, which prevent anterior and posterior dislocation respectively. Most important static stabilizer of shoulder is anterior band of inferior GHL, which prevents anterior dislocation.[21]

For practical purpose, shoulder instability can be broadly classified into two types: unidirectional traumatic instability and multidirectional nontraumatic instability, former being more common.[22] As the name implies unidirectional traumatic instability follows trauma, is unidirectional, usually anterior and is unilateral. Anterior instability is often associated with anteroinferior labral tear with or without glenoid rim fracture (Bankart lesion). This condition usually requires surgery and has been given a name traumatic, unidirectional, Bankart, surgery (TUBS).[22] MR imaging aids in planning surgical management in these patients as it can show associated capsulolabral-ligamentous defects, rotator cuff injury as well as osseous lesions.

Multidirectional nontraumatic instability is seen in young without history of trauma. It is often bilateral and invariably has an inferior component. These patients can voluntarily dislocate their shoulders. Basic pathology here seems to be capsular laxity which is difficult to assess by MRI. Treatment is usually conservative. These lesions are also named AMBRI (atraumatic, multidirectional, bilateral, rehabilitation, inferior capsular shift).[22] As MR plays little role in evaluation of multidirectional instability subsequent discussion will mainly focus on unidirectional instability (labral tears).

Imaging Techniques for Labral Tears

The shape of labrum varies from individual to individual (triangular, rounded, blunted, crescent shaped, etc). Most commonly, it is triangular anteriorly and rounded or triangu-lar posteriorly **(Fig. 16)**. Few horizontal notches and vertical clefts along anterior aspect of labrum are considered normal. When seen posteriorly, these are considered tears.

Labral tear is seen as either complete absence of a portion of labrum, displacement of labrum from glenoid rim or linear area of increased signal intensity within the labrum on T2WI. Abnormal labral appearance in MRI is classified into 4 types as follows:

Type I—Increased signal within the labrum not extending to the surface consistent with degeneration.

Type II—Frayed appearance of labrum with normal signal.

Type III—Increased signal within labrum extending to the surface consistent with tear and

Type IV—Combined features of Type II and Type III **(Fig. 17)**. Type II–IV labra are considered pathological. MR arthrography is the technique of choice for diagnosing labral pathology. Injected contrast distends the joint cavity and better delineates morphology of labrum and GHL. Contrast entering the labrum or tracking beneath the labrum to the external surface of joint also suggests tear **(Fig. 18)**. Positioning the arm is abduction and external rotation (ABER) has been shown to increase the sensitivity of MR arthrography.[23] This position puts tension on and improves evaluation of anterior band of IGHL and anterior inferior labrum.

MR arthrography has sensitivity of 91% and specificity of 93% for labral tears.[24] Conventional MRI, CT arthrography

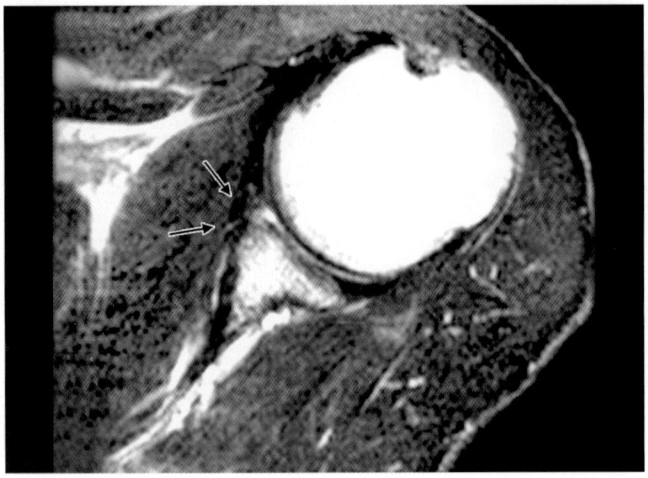

Fig. 17: T2 TSE axial section at the inferior head level: Bankart lesion is seen as a fragmented anterior inferior labrum with a defect at its base reaching the articular surface (arrows). The glenoid rim shows edema as increased signal.

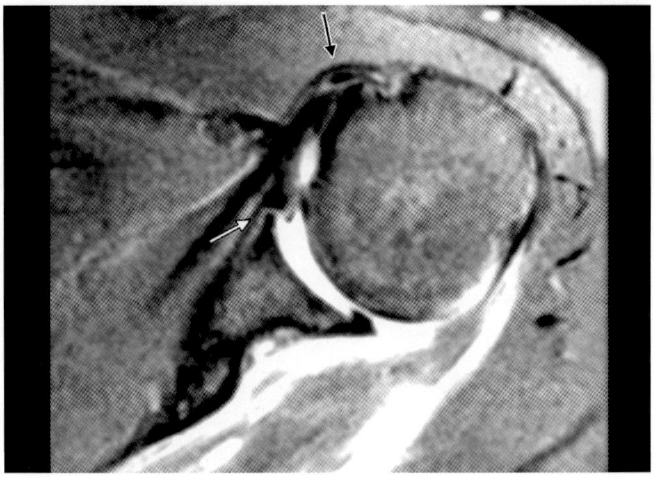

Fig. 18: MR arthrogram shows a detached labrum with contrast outlining its base (white arrow). Partially sectioned MGHL may at times mimic a labral fragment. Also note the medially dislocated biceps tendon from its groove and lying anterior to the SCT (black arrow).

and radiographic arthrography are alternative techniques for evaluation of labrum. Conventional MRI has shown variable accuracy with sensitivity ranging from 78% to 93% and specificity from 68% to 87%.[25,26] Relatively few studies have compared the accuracy of various techniques. However, one study by Chandnani et al.[27] compared CT arthrography, MR and MR arthrography and showed MR arthrography to be the most sensitive modality among these (96%).

MR Findings in Patients with Instability

Findings in anterior instability typically include anteroinferior labral tear with rupture of scapular periosteum (Bankart lesion), Bankart fracture (bony Bankart) and Hill Sach's lesion **(Figs. 17 and 19)**. When humeral head dislocates anteriorly it can cause fracture of anterior glenoid rim (Bankart fracture) and can produce impaction fracture in superior posterolateral aspect of humeral head (Hill Sach's lesion). On axial images, this is identified as a compression defect in the normally round posterolateral humeral head superior to the coracoid process (as opposed to normal defect of head below it) **(Figs. 19 and 20)**.[28] There may be associated marrow edema in recent injuries. Identification of these lesions is important as they predispose to recurrent dislocation with minimal trauma and may affect surgical planning.[29]

Some terms are used to describe Bankart variants. Glenolabral articular disruption (GLAD) lesions are described as tears of anteroinferior glenoid labrum with injury to glenoid articular cartilage. Scapular periosteum remains intact and holds labrum in place in GLAD. Loose bodies can occur in joint from detached avulsed articular cartilage fragment.[30] In anterior labroligamentous periosteal sleeve avulsion (ALPSA) lesion, there is tear of anterior labrum with periosteal stripping and displacement of labrum medially. Healing occurs typically with synovial fibrosis.[31] Humeral avulsion of GHL (HAGL) lesions include detachment of capsule and IGHL from their anterior humeral attachment site. These lesions are uncommon cause of instability.[32] Perthe's lesion is described as an anterior labral tear having a scapular attachment with an intact periosteal sleeve **(Fig. 21)**.[31]

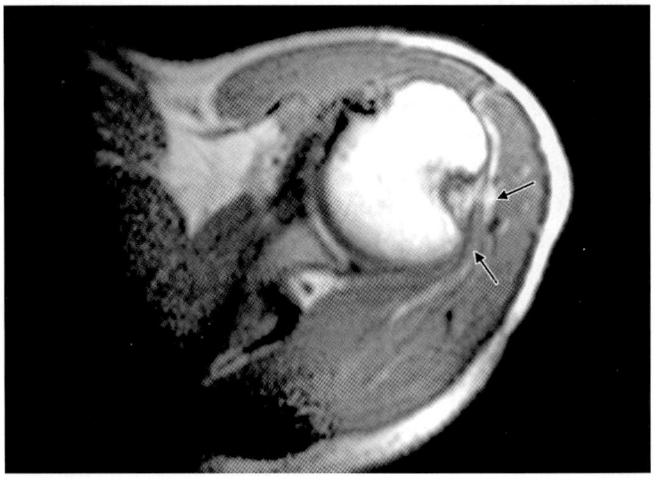

Fig. 19: T1 SE axial section: There is a wedge-shaped defect at the posterosuperior aspect of the humeral head representing Hill Sach's lesion (arrows) due to anterior dislocation of shoulder.

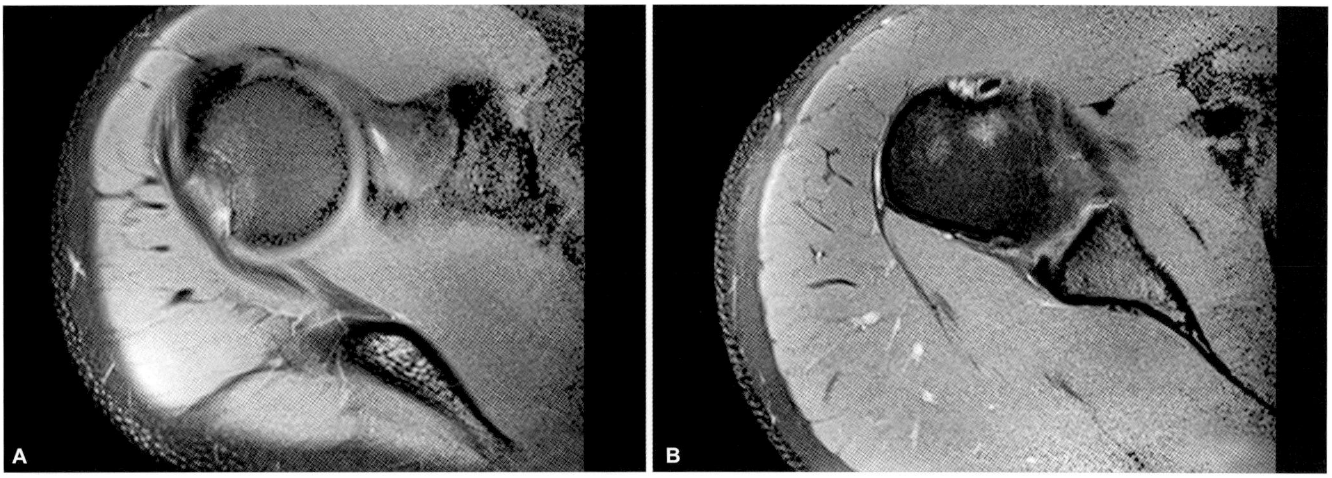

Figs. 20A and B: PD fat sat axial sections (A and B) in another patient show typical Hill Sach's defect in humeral head with anteroinferior glenoid injury.

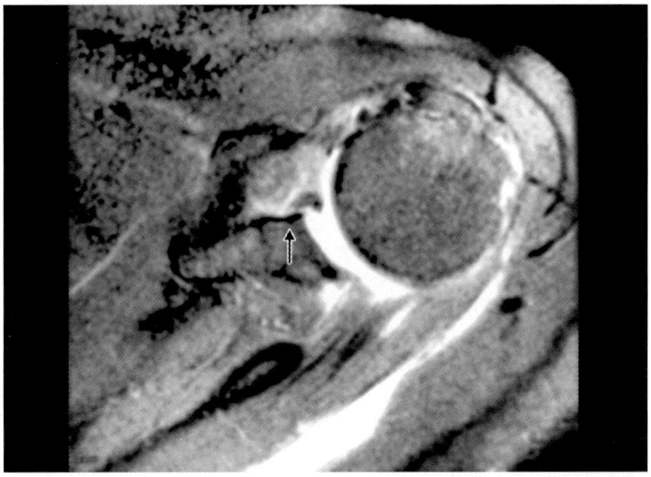

Fig. 21: MR arthrogram axial section showing avulsed labrum with a sleeve attached to the periosteum of the scapular neck consistent with Perthe's variation of Bankart lesion (arrow).

Three variations in anterior capsule insertion have been described.[33] Type I capsule inserts near the labrum, in Type II, it inserts just medial to the labrum and in Type III, capsule is attached greater than 1 cm from the labral margin. Whether Type III capsule predisposes to or is the result of anterior instability is not clear and debatable. However, a large capacious anterior pouch/subscapularis bursa is a frequent secondary finding in patients with recurrent anterior subluxation.

A close scrutiny of rotator cuff interval should also be done in all patients of clinical instability with rotator cuff tear as capsule is weak in this area. The tear of the capsule may be isolated or associated with SST/SCT tears as well as biceps tendon dislocation.[34]

Superior labrum anterior to posterior (SLAP) lesions are important cause of traumatic instability. These lesions are typically seen in young people involved in sports activity requiring overhead movement of humeral head like bowlers. They are believed to be caused by repetitive contact of humeral head with posterosuperior labrum. Consequently labrum becomes weak and tears away. Gradually tear progresses from posterior to anterior direction. The SLAP lesions were originally classified into four types by Snyder,[35] depending on the nature of labral injury and whether there is associated biceps tendon damage.

Type I: Fraying of glenoid labrum, but biceps tendon and labrum are not torn from glenoid (managed conservatively).

Type II: Stripping of labrum along with biceps tendon from glenoid (repaired surgically).

Type III: Bucket handle tear of labrum leaving biceps attachment to glenoid intact.

Type IV: Extension of bucket handle tear into biceps tendon.

This original classification was later expanded on basis of arthroscopic findings; however, their clinical implication is questionable.

Type V: Bankart tear extending posterosuperiorly to biceps labral complex.

Type VI: Unstable flap or radial tear with separation of biceps from its anchor.

Type VII: Superior labral tear extending anteriorly beneath the middle GHL.

Type VIII: Superior labral tear with posterior extension, similar but more extensive tham type II.

Type X: Rotator interval extension.

Type IX: Circumferential labral tear.

The SLAP lesions are associated with anterior instability and cuff tears. They are difficult to diagnose but important to identify as they respond well to arthroscopic repair.

Labral tears can be associated with labral cysts or ganglia which can cause compression neuropathy. These form because of one way valve mechanism leading to accumulation of joint fluid within them.

Anterior instability may also result from subscapularis injury. Subscapularis tears are seen after anterior dislocation over 40 years of age and after posterior dislocation at any age. Plain films and MRI may show lesser tuberosity fracture **(Fig. 22)**. Pfirrman et al.[36] graded subscapularis injury into four grades. Grade 0 tear is normal morphology. Grade I tear involves less than one fourth and grade II tears involve greater than one fourth of subscapularis width. Grade III is complete detachment.

Posterior instability is much less common than anterior (2–4%). It is usually a result of anterior direct blow on shoulder or seizures. Imaging findings in addition to subscapularis tears include teres minor injury, posterior labral and capsular tear and anteromedially located reverse Hill Sach's lesion **(Figs. 23A and B)**.[37]

Pitfalls

Some anatomic variants that can mimic labral tear should be kept in mind while interpreting shoulder MR. The most significant normal variation is a deficient attachment of labrum in the anterosuperior quadrant of glenoid (sublabral foramen or recess). At superior portion of the labrum three types of attachments are seen.

Type I: Labrum firmly attached to glenoid rim **(*see* Fig. 4)**.

Type II: A small recess is present between labrum and the cartilage **(*see* Fig. 9)**.

Type III: A large sublabral recess is present.

Sublabral recess is seen in 30% of patients[38] and should be differentiated from a SLAP tear on MR arthrography by observing location and configuration of contrast. The SLAP tears are usually seen at or posterior to biceps tendon attachment while the recess is seen anterior to

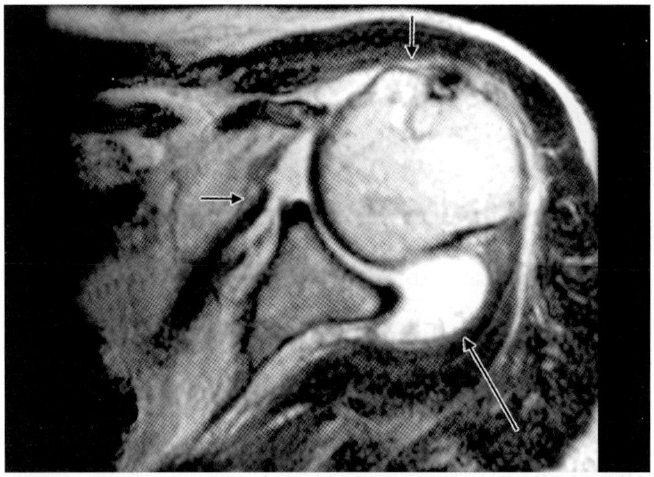

Fig. 22: T2 TSE axial section shows a SCT tendon tear in a case of massive RCT. The retracted tendon fibers (black arrow) and marrow edema at the lesser tuberosity (arrowhead) can be seen. A redundant posterior capsule indicates shoulder instability (long arrow).

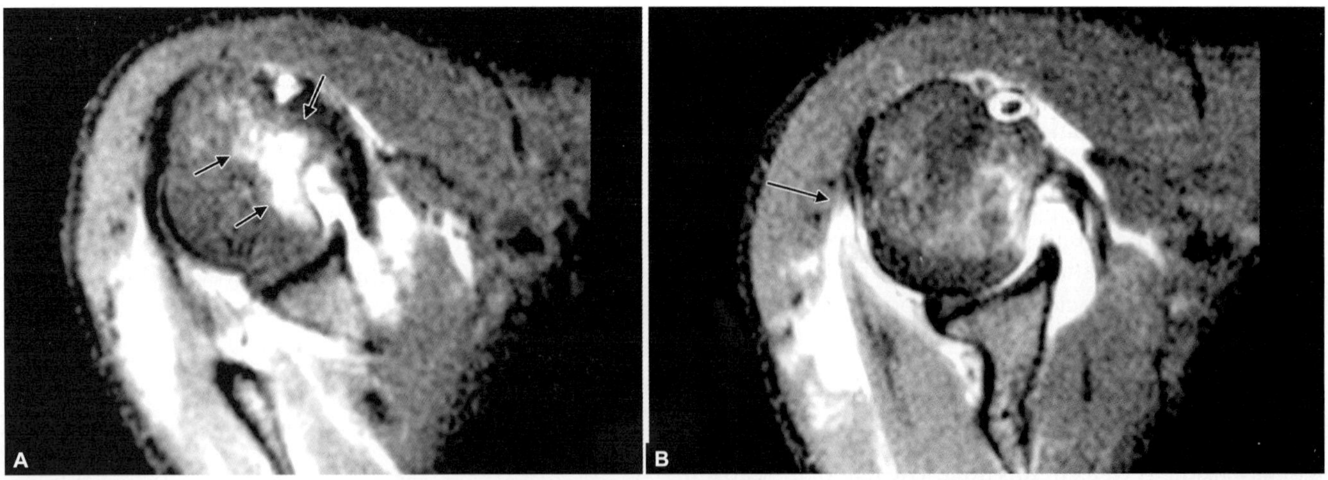

Figs. 23A and B: Turbo inversion recovery axial sections show classical anteromedial bony defect of reverse Hill Sach's lesion due to posterior dislocation (arrows in A) and associated teres minor tendon tear (arrows in B). The posterior labrum is infolded and heterogeneous in signal.

it. Contrast in sublabral recess is seen as a thin line with smooth margins that runs along the glenoid. Contrast in a tear has irregular margins, globular shape and is seen to enter into labral substance.[39] Occasionally contrast may be seen filling both sublabral recess and tear. This has been likened to a double chocolate or cream filled cookie (Oreo sign).

A sublabral hole seen in 17% normal people and is present at 2 o'clock position in pear-shaped glenoid cavities. Association of thick MGHL and a absent anterosuperior labrum has been termed 'Buford complex' and is also a normal variant.

The bright signal of hyaline cartilage between glenoid rim and labrum and the gap between MGHL and anterior glenoid can mimic tears of labrum. Following GHL on consecutive images can solve this problem.

ABNORMALITIES OF BICEPS TENDON

Bicipital Tendinopathy/Rupture

This usually occurs in middle aged or older patients with rotator cuff disease due to impingement of biceps tendon during flexion at shoulder joint beneath coracoacrominal ligament and anterior acromian.

This impingement may cause tendinopathy (or tenosynovitis) with flattening and thinning of tendon that may lead to complete rupture of the tendon **(Figs. 24A and B)**. Bicipital tendinopathy may also occur in patients with glenohumeral instability and attrition at the groove. Early bicipital tendinopathy often goes undetected on MR studies. MRI reveals increased signal intensity within the abnormal tendon.[40] 'Magic angle effect' can also lead to fallacious increased signal intensity within the tendon.

Morphologic abnormalities such as fraying, flattening and absence of tendon may sometime be identified. Disproportionate amount of fluid in bicipital tendon sheath as compared to the joint fluid may suggest bicipital abnormality, i.e. tenosynovitis.

Bicipital Tendon Dislocations

Bicipital tendon dislocation usually occurs with the chronic rotator cuff tears that have extended to involve the subscapularis tendons. The symptoms are usually masked by those of rotator cuff tears.

Some fibers of subscapularis along with deep fibers of coracohumeral and the superior GHL complex forms the pulley for biceps tendon and the bicipital groove is hooded by transverse humeral ligament. When all the three structures are disrupted, tendons of long head of biceps dislocates medially posterior to subscapularis tendon into the joint, where it may be mistaken for a detached anterior labrum. Rarely when subscapularis tendon remains intact, with the disruption of other two ligaments, biceps tendon displaces extra-articularly, anterior to subscapularis muscle.[41] On axial MR images, bicipital groove is empty with medially dislocated tendon in cases of biceps dislocations **(Fig. 25)**.

NERVE ENTRAPMENT SYNDROMES

The following two nerve entrapment syndromes are uncommon but important causes of shoulder pain.

Quadrilateral Space Compression Syndrome

Quadrilateral space is bounded by teres minor superiorly, teres major inferiorly, shaft of humerus laterally and long

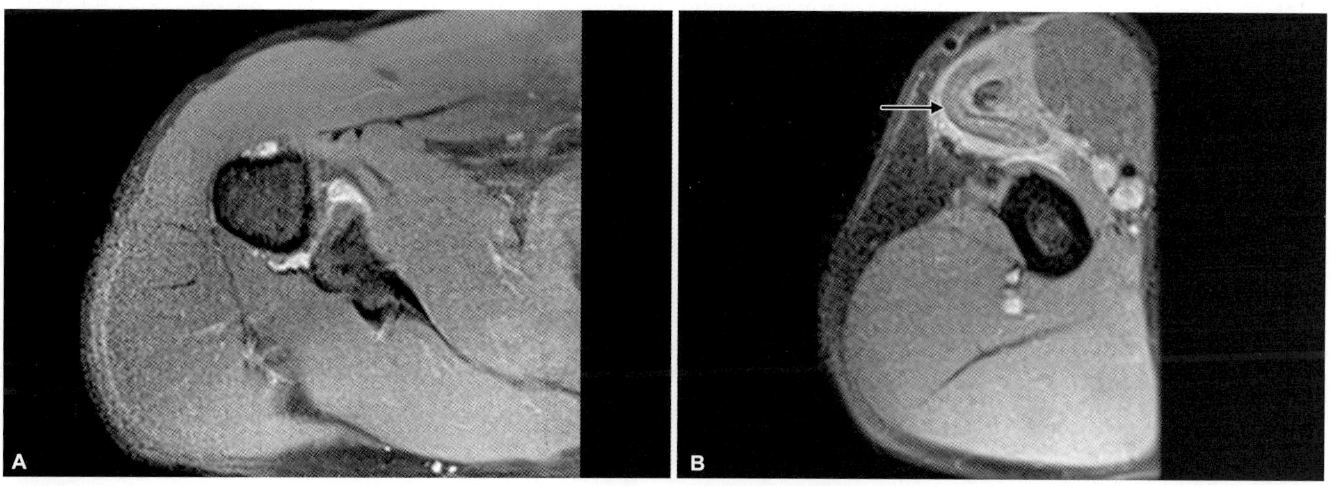

Figs. 24A and B: PD fat-saturated axial section at the level of glenoid (A) shows empty bicipital groove suggestive of complete rupture of biceps tendon. Retracted biceps tendon (arrow) seen in upper arm (B).

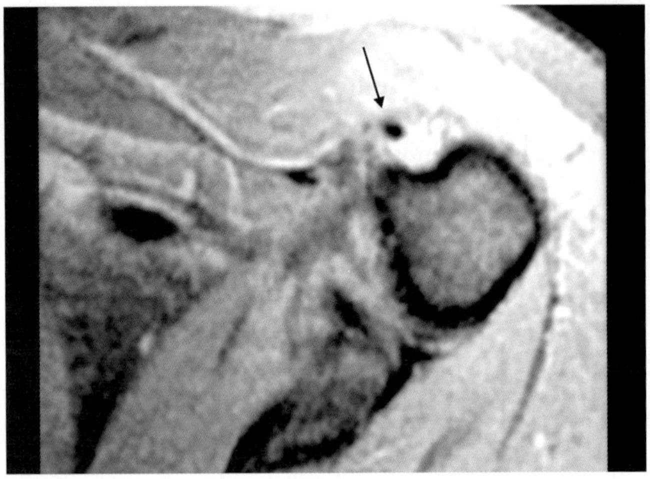

Fig. 25: Fat-suppressed T2 TSE axial section: Biceps tendon is seen dislocated medially (arrow) with an empty bicipital groove.

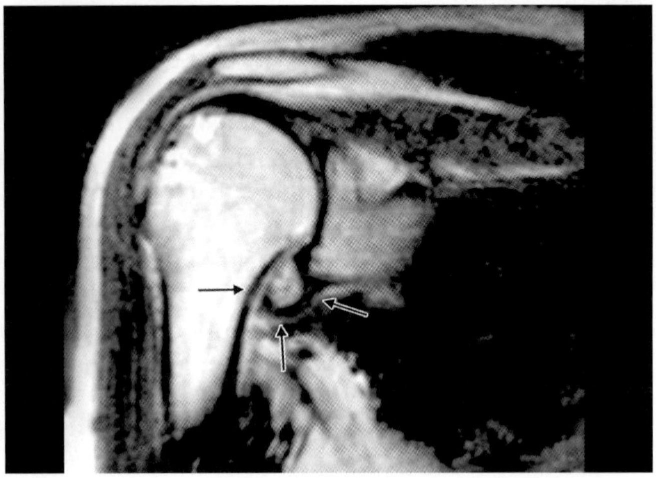

Fig. 26: T2 TSE coronal section: The axillary pouch (arrows) shows an abnormally thick wall (more than 4 mm) indicative of adhesive capsulitis in a patient with frozen shoulder after trauma.

head of biceps medially. Axillary nerve and posterior humeral circumflex artery and vein pass through it. Patients present with pain and paresthesia in axillary nerve distribution and muscle atrophy of teres minor and major muscles. MR imaging does not show actual entrapment but excludes other causes of shoulder pain and only shows atrophy of teres minor with major muscle.[42] MR angiography or DSA may be helpful by showing occlusion of posterior circumflex humeral artery.

Suprascapular Nerve Entrapment

Suprascapular nerve passes through supraspinatus notch to enter supraspinatus fossa beneath supraspinatus muscles. Further posteriorly it passes through spinoglenoid notch to enter into the intraspinatus fossa. It supplies both supraspinatus as well as infraspinatus muscle. Compression of nerve at the level of suprascapular notch results in atrophy of both muscles and compression at the level of spinoglenoid notch results in atrophy of infraspinatus muscle only. Compression may be because of neoplasm, hematoma or most commonly ganglion cyst. MR shows fatty replacement of involved muscle and soft tissue lesion responsible for compression.[43]

Ganglion cysts are either associated with labral tears or typically arise from a posterior capsular defect and present at spinoglenoid notch. They appear isointense to muscle on T1WI and hyperintense on T2WI. They are often septate and may show rim enhancement on gadolinium administration.

ADHESIVE CAPSULITIS

Adhesive capsulitis (frozen shoulder) is a clinical syndrome of pain and restricted joint movement secondary to thickening and contraction of the synovial sheath and joint capsule. It is most commonly seen in 40–60 years old females. It may be associated with trauma, osteoarthritis or rheumatic disorders.

On MRI, abnormal soft tissue may be seen in the rotator cuff interval encasing SGHL or coracohumeral ligament and may extend to undersurface of the biceps anchor.

Joint capsule and synovial thickening of more than 4 mm at the level of axillary recess is a useful MR criterion to diagnose this condition **(Fig. 26)**.[44] Postgadolinium enhancement of the rotator cuff interval or axillary recess may be present, increasing the diagnostic accuracy.

MR arthrography, though not preferred for diagnosis, reveals decreased joint volume (less than 10 cc) decreased fluid volume in biceps tendon sheath and axillary recess, corrugations of capsule with thickening and rotator interval abnormality.

CALCIFIC TENDINITIS

Formation of calcific deposits in the tendon is a degenerative process. Calcification of rotator cuff most commonly occurs in supraspinatous tendon but can occur in other tendons.[45] The size of deposition may vary from few millimeter to several centimeter. MR examination shows linear or globular area of decreased signal in all pulse sequences however T2* GRE has more sensitivity and specificity to demonstrate hypointensity in the tendon **(Figs. 27A and B)**.

ARTHRITIS

The shoulder joint is frequently involved in osteoarthritis and other infective/inflammatory arthropathies. MR

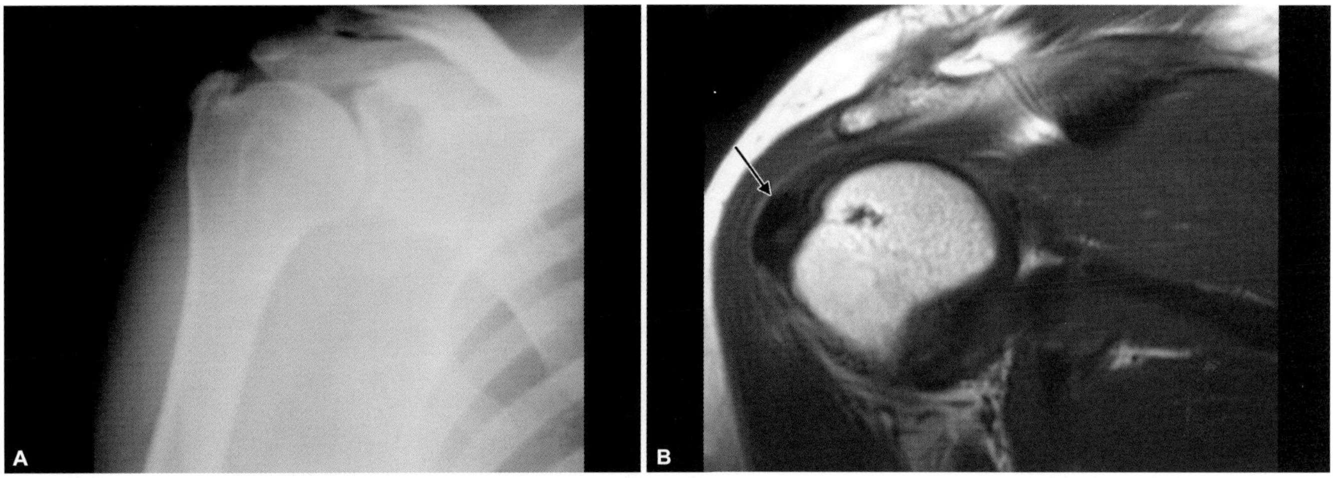

Figs. 27A and B: Radiographs of shoulder: (A) shows globular calcification near greater tuberosity. T1W coronal section (B) shows globular area of hypointense signal (arrow) in the supraspinatus tendon suggestive of calcific tendinitis.

imaging can demonstrate early inflammatory soft tissue and osseous changes and can be used as a sensitive monitoring tool.

OSTEOARTHRITIS

Osteoarthritis of shoulder is characterized by chondral erosions, osteophyte formation, subchondral cyst, sclerosis and synovitis.[46] Humeral head sclerosis and cartilage loss are usually central or superior in location. MRI is very good to identify cartilage thinning and loss. Subchondral cysts are seen in both humeral head and glenoid. Inferior capsule may be enlarged with contration of anterior capsule. Loose bodies occur in glenohumeral joint and subacromial bursa which appear isointense to bone or hypointense on T2W images.

INFECTIVE ARTHRITIS

Septic arthritis is a clinical diagnosis relying on physical and laboratory parameters and microbiologic assessment of joint aspirate. Usually, it affects older age group (average 65 years). The source of infection is either hematogenous or local. Immunocompromised status and pre-existing degenerative joint disease increases risk of septic arthritis.

However, typical systemic and local symptoms may be absent in indolent infections like tuberculosis. Conventional radiographs, may show associated osteoarthritis, osteomyelitis or serve as a baseline study to monitor disease progression or response to treatment, but are insensitive to pick up early marrow or soft tissue changes. MR demonstrates these well along with bone changes, however its specificity is low.[47]

Inflammation of synovial lining and joint effusion, the earliest pathologic changes and associated bone marrow edema are seen well on fat-saturated T2WI and post contrast T1WI **(Figs. 28A and B)**. Further progression of disease leads to cartilage destruction manifesting as joint space narrowing and marginal erosion of bare area. Subchondral bone changes in form of edema, subchondral cyst formation and bone destruction follow when disease becomes subacute. Osteomyelitis, bone destruction and joint ankylosis are features of chronic septic arthritis. Rotator cuff tears can also be seen in subacute and chronic disease. MR cannot distinguish septic from nonseptic arthritis. Combination of bone erosions with marrow edema favors infectious etiology.

Tuberculosis of shoulder joint is infrequent and has indolent clinical presentation. Patients usually presents with pain and restriction of movement for long duration. MRI is very useful to demonstrate synovial thickening, erosions, bone edema and periarticular collections **(Figs. 29A and B)**.

RHEUMATOID ARTHRITIS

Rheumatoid arthritis (RA) is a chronic inflammatory joint disease, which involves synovial lining of joints. With disease progression there is involvement of articular cartilage, bone at joint margins and periarticular soft tissue. Shoulder joint becomes involved later in the disease process**.** Proliferative synovitis involves glenohumeral joint, AC joint and bursae around shoulder. Rotator cuff also becomes involved as disease progresses.

Magnetic resonance imaging is useful for detecting early changes of RA including synovitis, joint effusion and

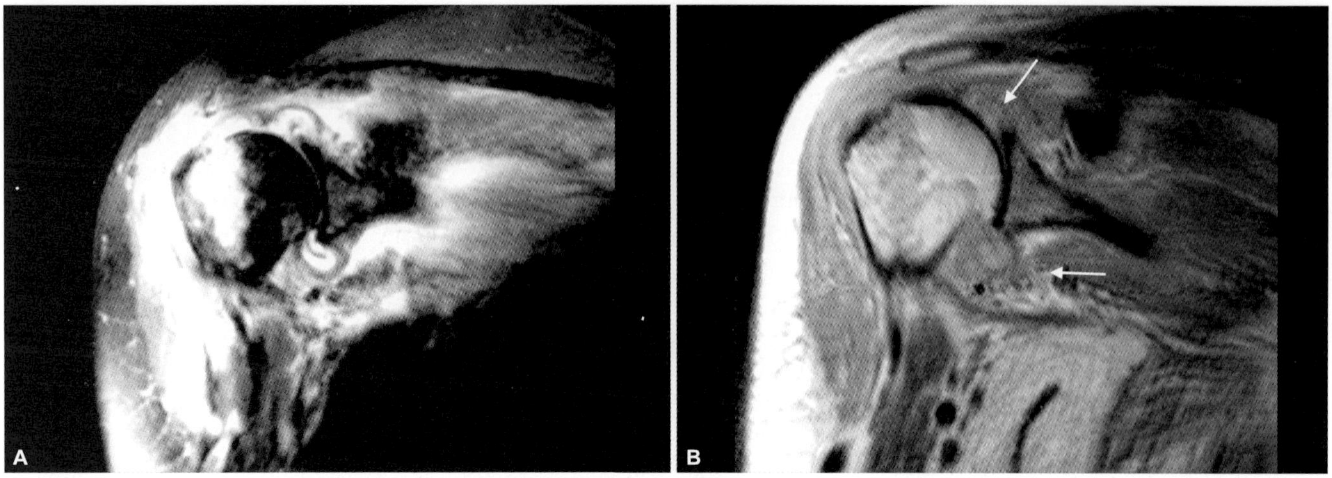

Figs. 28A and B: T2 TSE fat-suppressed coronal section (A) reveals marked bone marrow and periarticular soft tissue edema and synovial thickening in a case of septic arthritis. T1 SE postcontrast (B) shows enhancement of the synovium and the periarticular tissue (arrows).

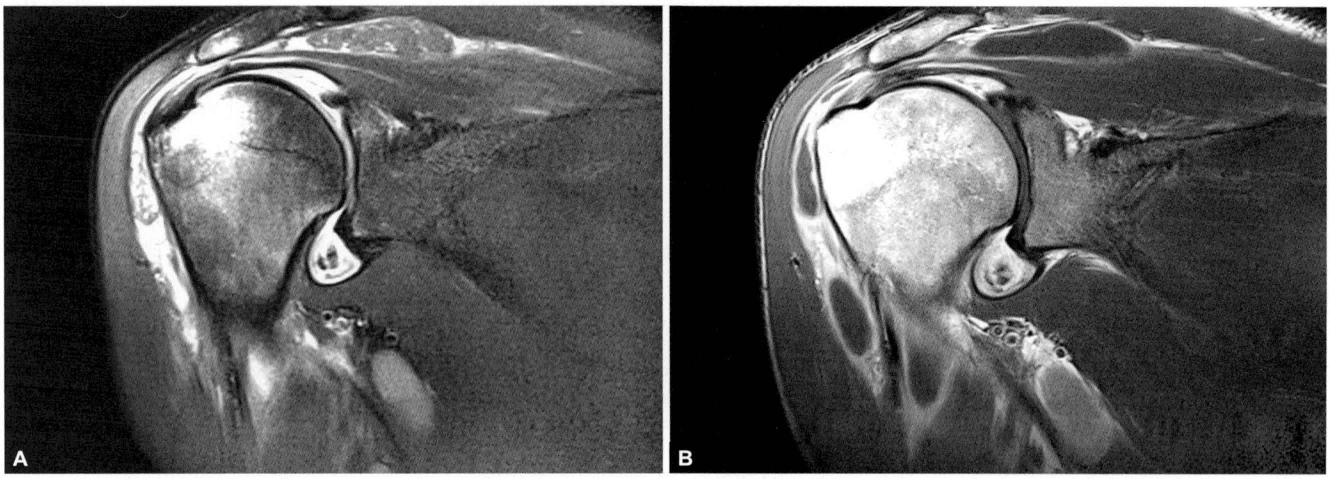

Figs. 29A and B: Tubercular arthritis: T2W fat-saturated (A) and T1 fat-saturated postcontrast coronal section (B) show joint effusion, synovial thickening, erosions and periarticular collections.

marginal erosions. Marginal erosions are seen as low-signal areas on T1WI and variable signal intensity on T2WI. MRI may be superior to ultrasound, CT or conventional radiographs for detecting marginal erosions.[48]

Cartilage destruction is difficult to evaluate with routine shoulder protocol including MR arthrography, as it is very thin. Rotator cuff tears are commonly seen in RA due to destructive synovitis near greater tuberosity.

Presence, size and extent of synovial cysts, clinically evident soft tissue swellings of subacromial and subdeltoid bursitis and simultaneous arthritic involvement of AC joint, all well-known manifestations of RA can be well shown by MR.

AVASCULAR NECROSIS

It is associated with trauma, steroid use, sickle cell anemia and alcoholism. It can be differentiated from osteoarthritis by signal abnormality confined to the humeral head and sparing of glenoid. The Neer classification for shoulder AVN is similar to Ficat classification for hip osteonecrosis.[49] MR may show focal subarticular dark signal, a dark line encircling normal marrow or a double line sign early on and fragmentation and collapse of head later. Metadiaphyseal lesions may show classical serpiginous low intensity line surrounding high intensity center (in chronic infarcts) and high-intensity rim in more acute infarcts.

NEOPLASMS

Magnetic resonance imaging is the imaging modality of choice for characterizing and staging both primary and secondary musculoskeletal neoplasms and tumor like lesions. MR shows joint involvement, soft tissue and osseous components, involvement of neurovascular structures as well as helps in tissue characterization. T1WI (for marrow involvement), T2WI (for soft tissue extension), STIR and postgadolinium fat suppressed T1WI diagnose and stage tumors well. Metastatic disease is by far the commonest malignant tumor around shoulder followed by myeloma, osteosarcoma, chondrosarcoma and Ewing's sarcoma **(Figs. 30A and B)**. Frequent benign lesions comprise osteo-chondroma, chondroma, chondroblastoma and giant cell tumor. Common soft tissue lesions around the shoulder are hemangioma **(Figs. 31A and B)**, lipoma **(Figs. 32A and B)** and extra-abdominal desmoid.[50]

TEMPOROMANDIBULAR JOINT

Temporomandibular dysfunction (TMJ) is common condition that may affect up to 28% of the population.[51] The most common cause of TMJ dysfunction is internal derangement, which is defined as an abdominal relationship of the disc to the condyle. The TMJ dysfunction is best evaluated with magnetic resonance imaging due to excellent demonstration of disc morphologic changes, disc displacement and various other abnormalities of TM joint.[52]

MR Imaging Technique

Magnetic resonance imaging of TMJ is performed by using the body coil as transmitter and dual surface coils as receiver (simultaneous examination of both sides is preferred as TMJ disorders often involve both sides). Axial plane is used for localization of condyle and planning of sagittal and coronal images. Sagittal images are obtained

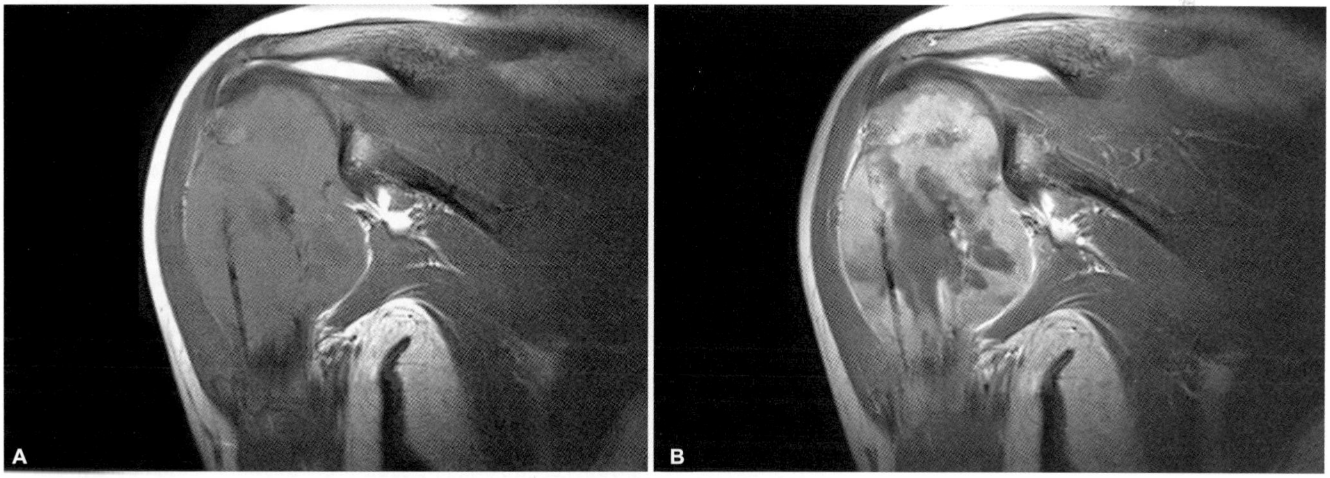

Figs. 30A and B: Ewing's sarcoma: T1W coronal (A) and postcontrast T1W, coronal section (B) show malignant mass arising from metadiaphysis of right humerus associated with cortical destruction and adjacent soft tissue.

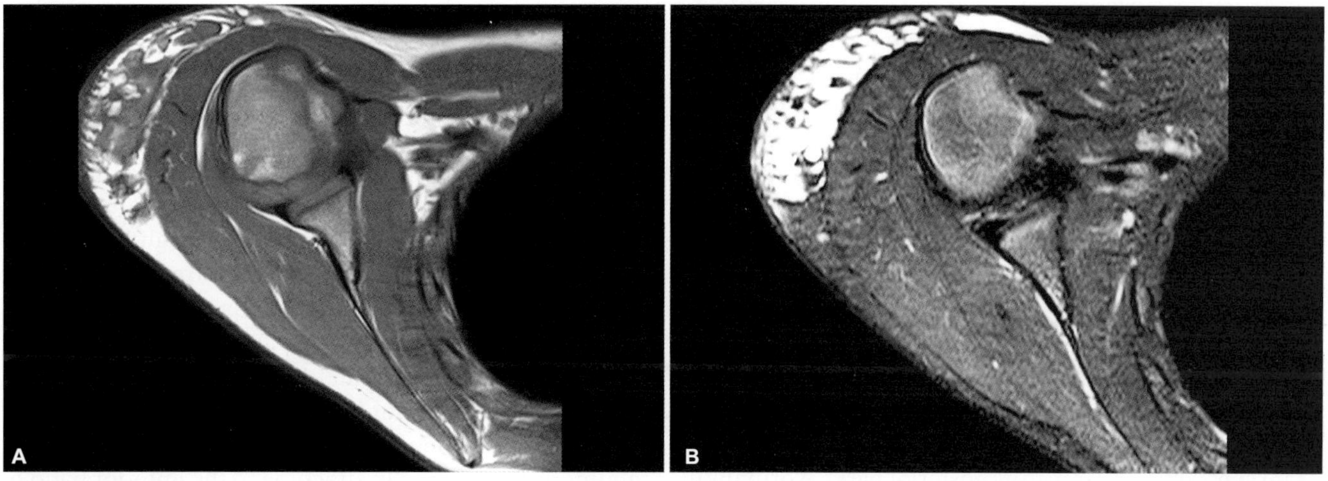

Figs. 31A and B: Soft tissue hemangioma: T1W axial (A) and T2W fat-saturated axial section (B) of shoulder show altered signal soft tissue lesion superficial to deltoid muscle limited to subcutaneous tissue.

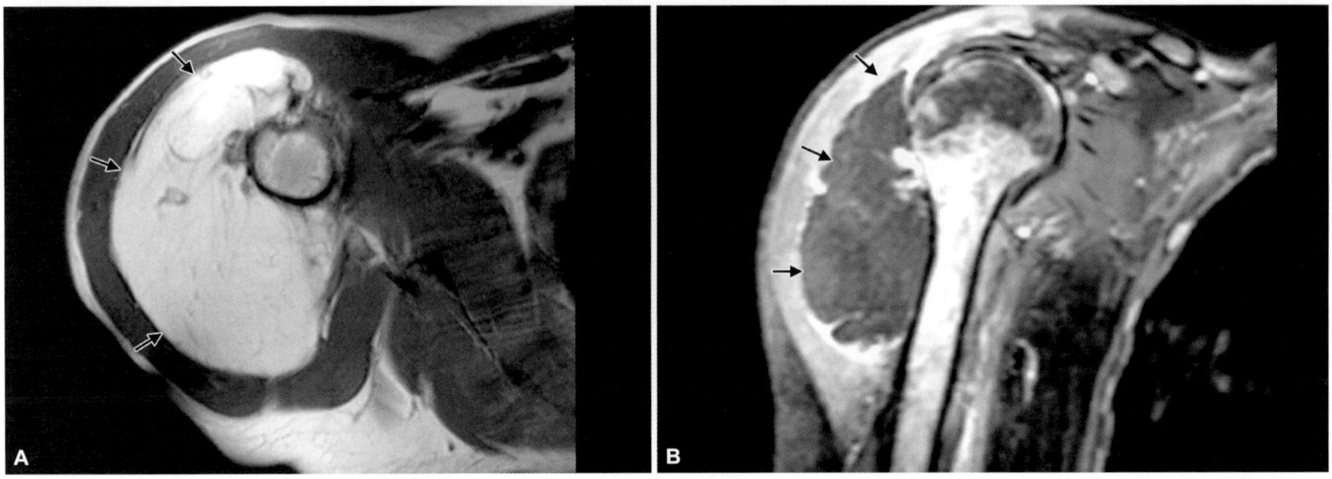

Figs. 32A and B: T1 axial section: A lipoma (arrows) in relation to the SASDB showing high-signal of fat (A). The inversion recovery image shows dark signal due to fat saturation (B).

in both closed and open mouth positions, in a plane perpendicular to the horizontal long axes of mandibular condyles **(Fig. 33)**. Coronal images are acquired along the horizontal long axes of condyles in closed mouth position. Out of these sagittal plane is standard plane of imaging. The preferred sequences are T1 spin echo (shows fat as bright), T2 turbo spin echo (fluid sensitive) and proton density images. Functional joint dynamics at incremental mouth opening can be shown with small flip angle gradient echo imaging.

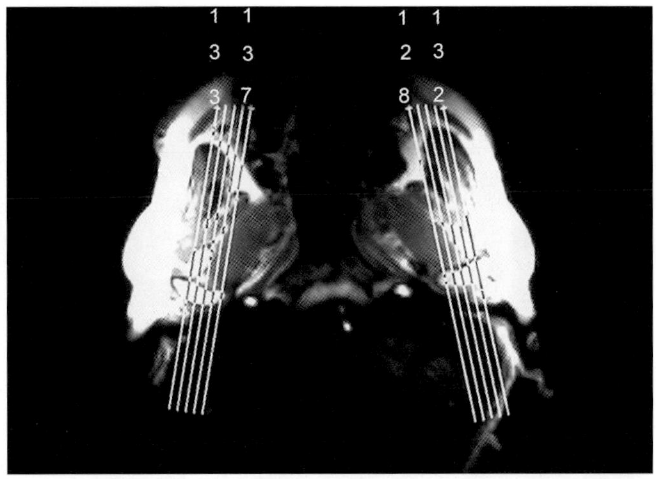

Fig. 33: For TMJ imaging sagittal images are planned perpendicular to the horizontal axes of mandibular condyles on axial scout images as shown. The coronal images are planned perpendicular to the above prescribed sagittal plane.

NORMAL ANATOMY AND MR APPEARANCE (FIGS. 34 TO 37)

TM joint is a diarthrodial synovial joint. Its articular surfaces are formed by articular eminence and anterior part of mandibular (glenoid) fossa superiorly and head of mandibular condyle inferiorly **(Figs. 34A and B)**. Articular surfaces are covered by a fibrocartilage. Mandibular condyles are elliptical in shape with their long axes converging posteriorly at around 15° **(Figs. 35A to C)**.[53] An intra-articular disc divides the joint into upper and lower compartments **(Figs. 34 and 35)**. The disc is composed of avascular fibrous connective tissue which merges with peripheral capsule. It is oval in shape, measuring approximately 18 mm in anteroposterior dimension and 20 mm in mediolateral extension. It is biconcave in sagittal plane and crescent shaped in coronal plane. Two localized thickenings are present in the disc, called anterior and posterior bands. Posterior band is thicker than the anterior band. Consequently the disc is 2 mm thick in its anterior part, 1 mm centrally and 3 mm in its posterior part.[54] Normally in a closed mouth position, posterior band is located directly above the condyle, central thin zone between articular eminence and condyle and anterior band below articular eminence. Disc is attached posteriorly to temporal bone and posterior subcondylar area through a fibrofatty vascular connective tissue called posterior attachment, retrodiskal tissue or bilaminar zone through its superior and inferior lamina. This structure restrains its anterior movement. Joint is covered by a loose connective tissue capsule, attached superiorly to articular eminence and circumference of mandibular fossa and inferiorly to neck of condyle. The superior head of lateral pterygoid inserts on anterior capsule and adjacent condylar neck with its tendinous fibers directly attaching to the anterior band of the disc and helps in mouth opening. Medial pterygoid and

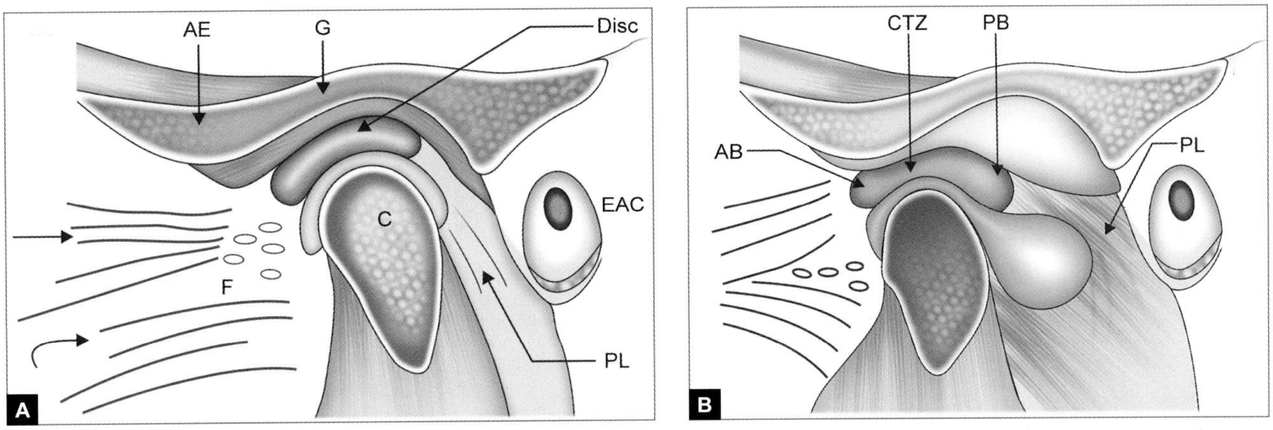

Figs. 34A and B: Diagrammatic representation of TMJ anatomy: (A) Close mouth position—Oval disc lies between the condyle (C) and glenoid fossa (G). More anteriorly the articular eminence is seen (AE). The retrodiscal tissue (PL) acts as the posterior attachment. Bright lateral pterygoid fat plane (F), external auditory canal (EAC), superior (straight arrow) and inferior (curved arrow) bellies of lateral pterygoid muscles are also labeled. (B) Open mouth position—the condyle and the disc move anteriorly together to a position below the articular eminence with central thin zone interposed between the two.
Abbreviations: AB: Anterior band; PB: Posterior band; CTZ: Central thin zone.

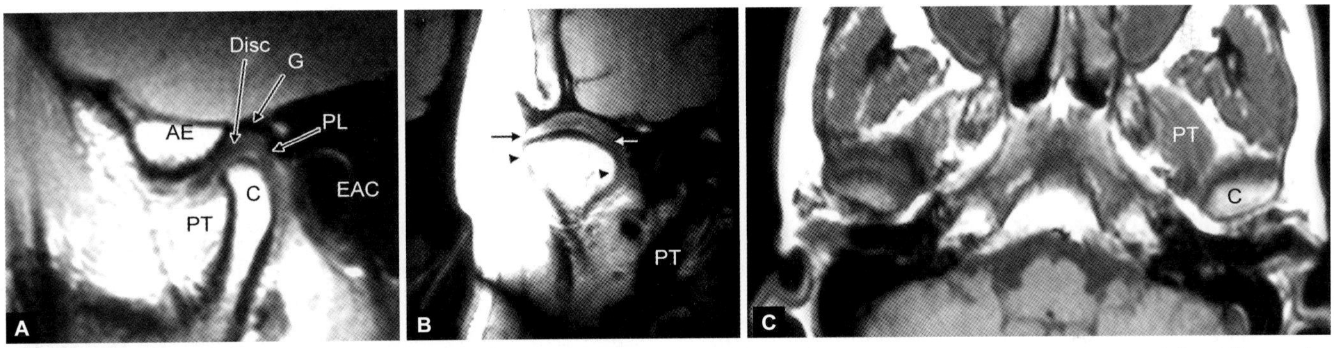

Figs. 35A to C: (A) Sagittal proton WI showing normal anatomy (Compare with figure 2): The marrow in the condyle and articular eminence appear bright in signal. The articular margins of temporal bone are dark and well-defined. The disc shows intermediate signal; (B) Coronal proton WI : The crescent-shaped disc (white arrow) and lateral attachment of disc (black arrow) are seen. The lateral and medial poles of the condyle (arrowheads) can be seen with disc attaching just beneath them; (C) Axial anatomy T1WI: Elliptical condyles with posteriorly converging horizontal axes in relation to skull base.
*Abbreviations***:** C: Condyle; PT: Inferior belly of lateral pterygoid muscle.

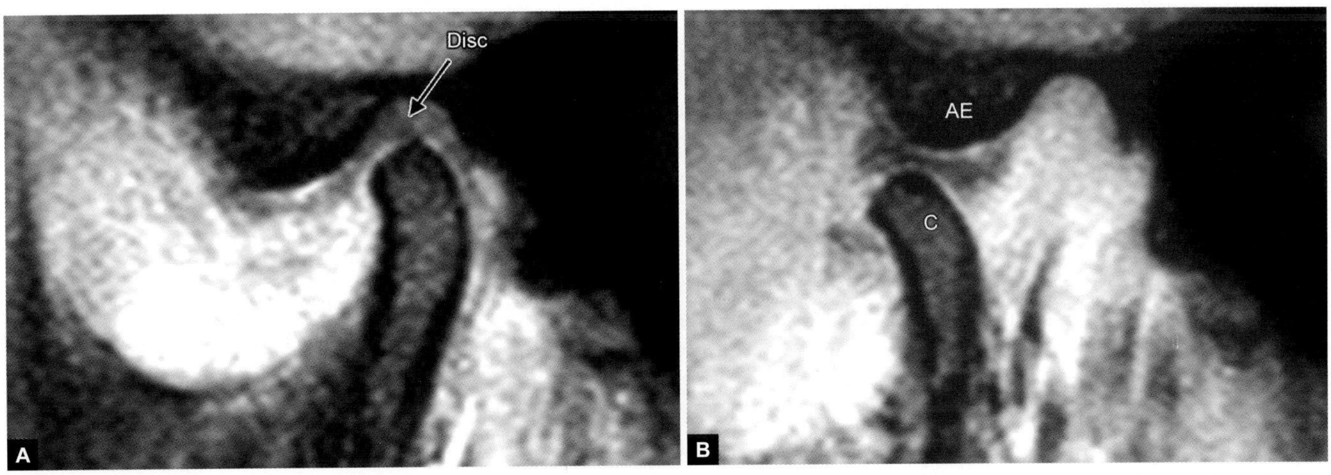

Figs. 36A and B: (A) Close mouth and (B) open mouth positions showing location of disc (arrow) in relation to the condyle (C). The posterior band lies just superior to condyle in (A) and the condyle lies opposite the articular eminence (AE) with interposed thin zone between them in open mouth position (B).

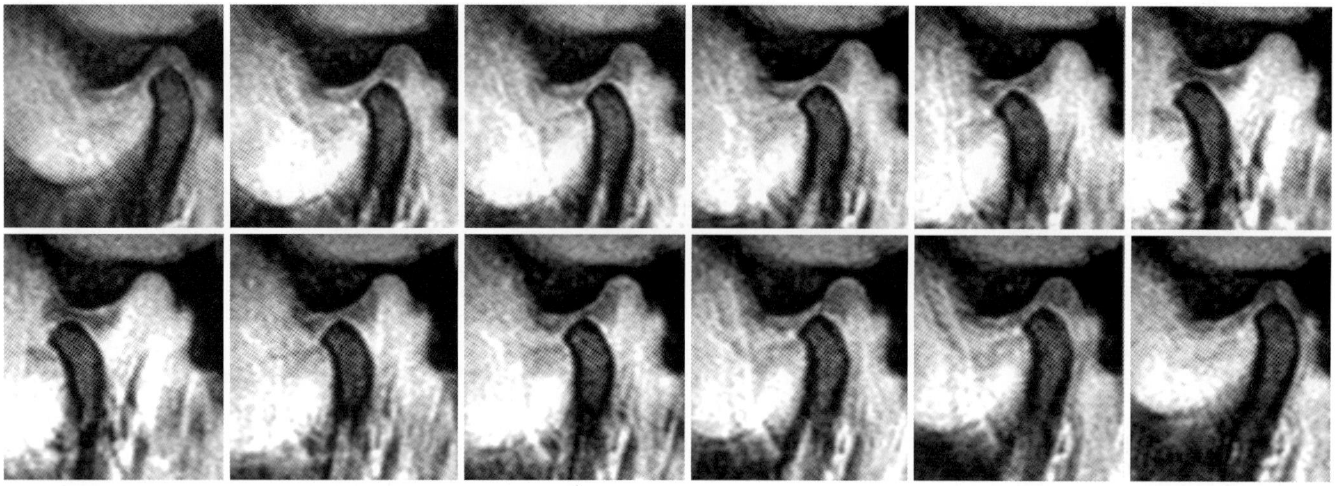

Fig. 37: Fast gradient-echo serial sagittal sections showing condylar translation in the glenoid fossa and its constant relationship with the disc (upper row—mouth opening and lower row—mouth closing). The posterior band at 12 o'clock position in the closed mouth position (first frame upper row). The head opposed to articular eminence with thin zone of disc interposed between the two (last frame upper row). Note the expansion of the posterior soft tissues as mouth opens.

temporalis muscles with their mandibular insertions also assist mandibular movements. Temporomandibular and sphenomandibular/stylomandibular ligaments reinforce the lateral and medioposterior capsule respectively.

Normal MR Appearance

The cortices of condyle and temporal component of the TMJ have smooth outline and low-signal intensity **(Fig. 35A)**. The articular covering and synovium shows high-signal. Intra-articular disc shows low-signal intensity as it is composed of fibrous tissue, however the posterior disc attachment has relatively high-signal intensity because of fatty tissue. The attachment of superior belly of lateral pterygoid to anteromedial disc and adjacent condyle can also be demonstrated as low intensity structure. The medial pterygoid muscle lies inferiorly. The low-signal maxillary vessels can be seen between pterygoid muscles and mandibular condyle. The low-signal temporomandibular ligament can be seen as laterally supporting structures on coronal images **(Fig. 35B)**.

Movements

The TM joint movements take place at both compartments. Translation occurs predominantly in the upper compartment and both rotation and translation in the lower compartment. During jaw opening, initially the condyles rotate in lower compartment followed by translatory movement in upper and subsequently in the lower joint compartment. During translation there is sliding movement of intra-articular disc along with condyle in relation to mandibular fossa. During all movements the central disc remains located between the condyle and the articular tubercle with anterior and posterior bands acting as functional guides. In contrast to the 12 o'clock location of posterior band in closed mouth position; in open mouth position the apex of the condyle lies opposite the articular eminence with interposed central thin zone between the two and there is marked expansion of the tissue in the region of posterior attachment **(Figs. 34 to 36)**. The disc does not move in the mediolateral direction unless these attachments are torn.

DISEASES OF TEMPOROMANDIBULAR JOINT

Temporomandibular joint (TMJ) disorders are more prevalent in young and middle age females. Patients with TMJ disorders present with complaints of myofacial pain syndrome (pain and muscle tenderness around the joint) and biomechanical dysfunction (clicking, crepitus and limitation of jaw movements).

INTERNAL DERANGEMENT

Internal derangement is defined as altered morphological and functional relationship between articular surface of the temporal bone, disc and mandibular condyle.

DISC DISPLACEMENTS

This is the most common TMJ disorder.[55] Normally the posterior band is at 12 o'clock position in relation to mandibular condyle. Displacement is said to have occurred when this relationship is altered. Disc can displace in anterior, posterior, anteromedial, anterolateral and sometimes purely in lateral and medial directions.[56] Anterior and posterior displacements are seen best in sagittal images. Lateral and medial displacements are best seen in coronal images.

Disc displacement is further categorized into 'displacement without reduction' and 'displacement with reduction'. When an anteriorly displaced disc fails to return to normal position on jaw opening it is called displacement without reduction **(Figs. 38A and B)**. These patients can not open their mouths fully (closed lock jaw).[57] In displacement with reduction, displaced disc returns to normal position relative to condyle during jaw opening leading to reciprocal clicking **(Figs. 39A and B)**.[58]

Most common disc displacement is anterior however, often it also has an anteromedial or anterolateral component **(Figs. 40A and B)**. Such displacements are also called rotational displacements. Further the disc displacement may be complete or partial when only the medial or lateral part of the disc is displaced. In pure medial and lateral disc displacements sagittal images will show no disc between condyle and mandibular fossa. Instead pulled up lateral or medial capsular tissue respectively will be seen, giving it an empty appearance (empty fossa sign).

DISC DEFORMITY AND OSTEOARTHRITIS

Internal derangements of TMJ are progressive disorders. The reducing disc leads to nonreducing disc in due course of time and a chronically displaced disc slowly gets

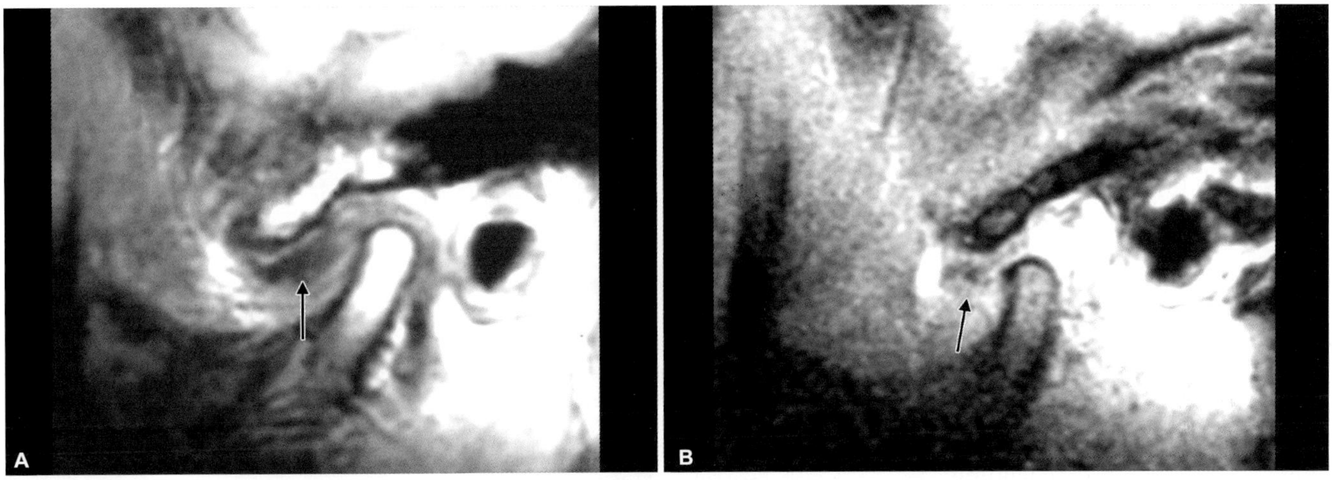

Figs. 38A and B: Nonreducing disc: Sagittal section (A) closed mouth and (B) open mouth. The nonreducing anteriorly displaced disc is shown (arrows).

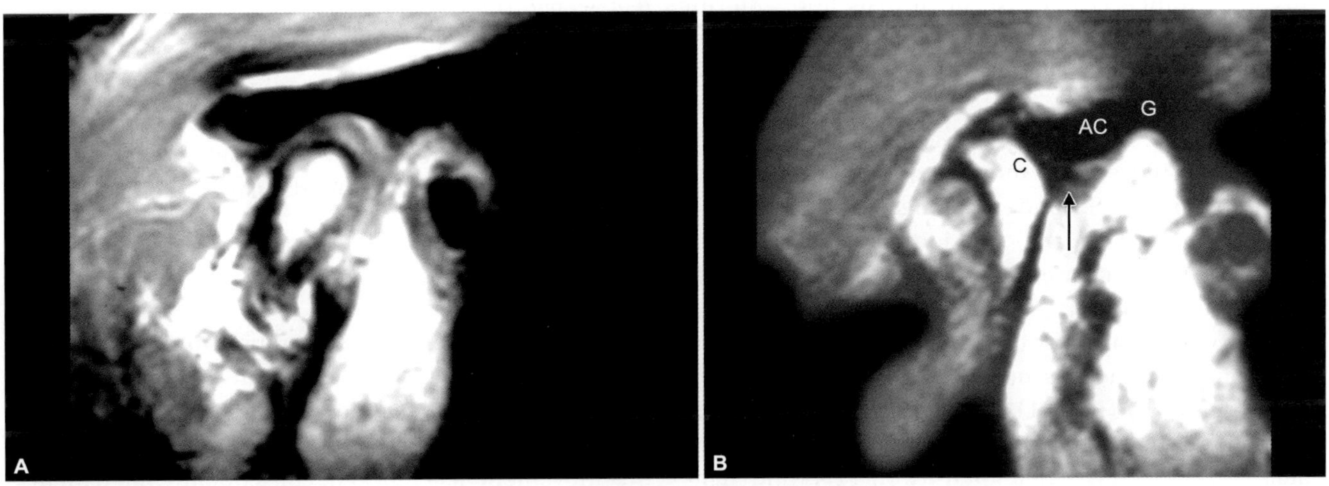

Figs. 39A and B: Reducing disc: Sagittal section (A) closed mouth and (B) open mouth. (A) There is mild anterior displacement of the disc; (B) Dislocation of condyle into infratemporal fossa anterior to the articular eminence. The eminence and the reduced disc (arrow) prevents condyle from returning to the glenoid fossa.

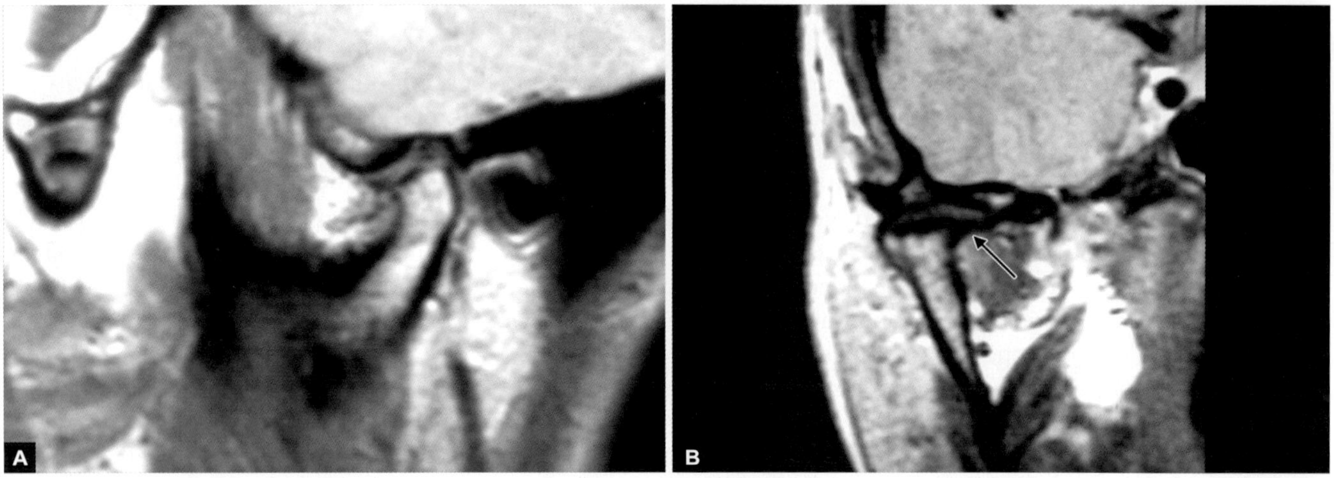

Figs. 40A and B: (A) Proton-weighted sagittal section: The disc is not well seen in the glenoid fossa; (B) Coronal section: The disc is anteromedially displaced (arrow).

deformed and later leads to osteoarthritis of the joint.[59] The above stages of displaced disc are also graded as acute (reducing disc with normal morphology), subacute (non-reducing disc with deformity) and chronic (adhesions, fibrosis, perforation and degenerative joint disease).[60] Disc deformity is important to identify as it is treated with diskectomy while disc repositioning is done for disc displacements.

Earliest MR findings of disc deformity is thickening of posterior band. As the disease progresses disc assumes rounded, biconvex or sigmoid shape instead of normal biconcave configuration. It may also show fissuring and surface irregularity. In some of the cases, the disc may show severely diminished volume.

Another tissue alteration seen in association with chronic disc displacement is formation of 'pseudodisc'. This appearance is because of fibrosis and anterior displacement of posterior attachment which comes to occupy the normal position of disc between condyle and mandibular fossa and simulates disc because of its low-signal intensity. Perforations are seen in 5–15% patients with disc displacement, more frequently at posterior disc attachment.[61] Secondary changes because of disc deformity include synovitis and joint effusion. It is best seen on T2 WI as increased signal intensity in upper, lower or both compartments.

Marrow abnormality in form of marrow edema, osteonecrosis or sclerosis in the condyle can be secondary to disc deformity **(Fig. 41)**. Normal marrow in condyle shows high signal intensity on both T1 and T2 WI. Marrow edema is seen as low-signal intensity on T1WI and high-signal intensity on T2WI. Osteonecrosis and sclerosis show low-signal intensity on T1WI and variable signal intensity on T2WI. Long standing disc displacement without reduction can lead to osteoarthritis in TM joints. It is characterized by osteophyte formation with flattening and irregularity of articular surfaces **(Figs. 42A and B)**.

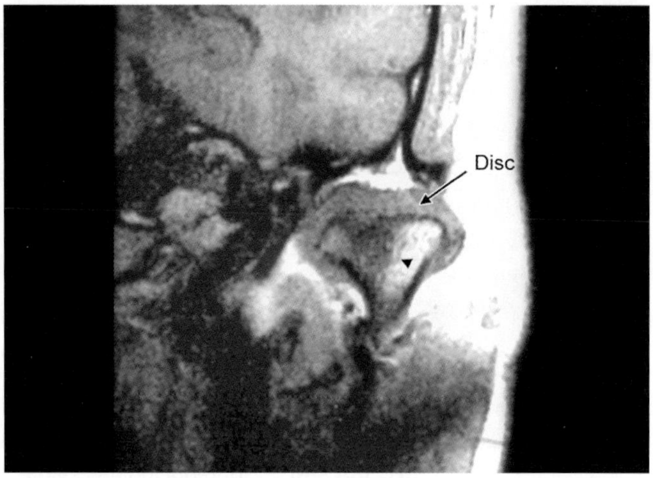

Fig. 41: Coronal T1WI: Low intensity area in the medial part of the condyle (arrowhead) in case of displaced disc (arrow) likely representing a focus of avascular necrosis.

STUCK DISC

Upper compartment permits translational movements only, in which the disc slides or translates relative to the mandibular fossa. This movement is important in later part of jaw opening. In pathology of upper compartment, this movement gets blocked, consequently the patient is not able to open his mouth fully. This can cause pain and discomfort.

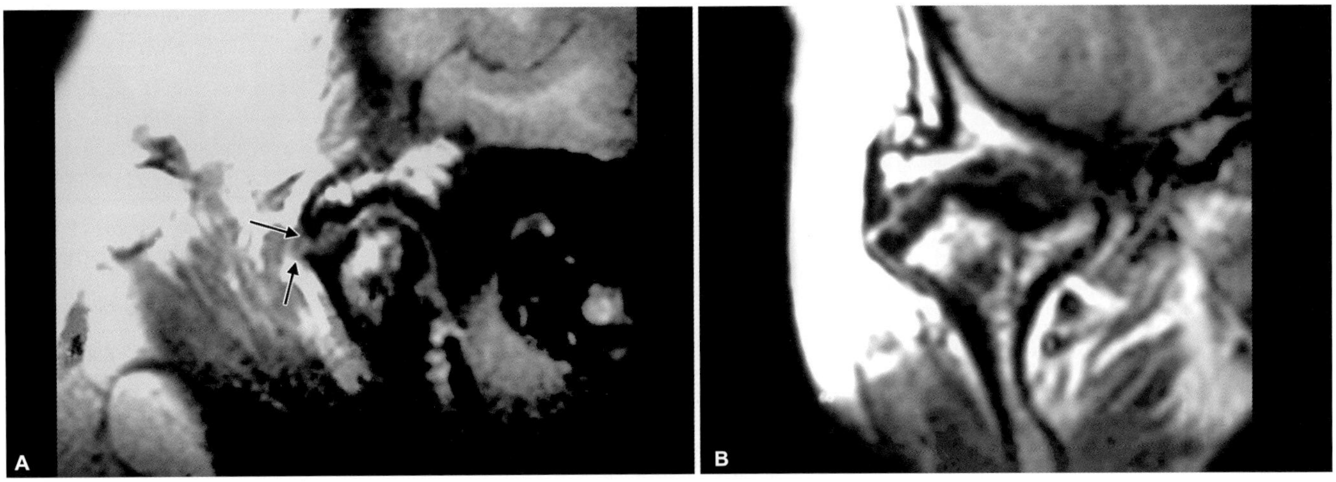

Figs. 42A and B: Sagittal (A) and coronal (B) T1-weighted sections: Articular surface irregularity, subchondral sclerosis and osteophytes (arrows) along anterior glenoid rim and condyle in a case with osteoarthritis of TMJ.

OPEN LOCK JAW

In contrast to 'closed lock state' described above, in 'open lock jaw', after wide opening of the mouth patient is not able to close mouth temporarily or permanently due to the dislocation of condyles in infratemporal fossa anterior to articular eminence. The latter prevents the condyle from returning back into glenoid fossa. On the other hand, a reducing disc may do the same **(Figs. 39A and B)**.

Further indications of imaging of TM joint are demonstration of loose bodies, postoperative evaluation, mandibular asymmetry, trauma, infective/noninfective arthritis and neoplasia.

OSTEONECROSIS AND OSTEOCHONDRITIS DISSECANS

Low-signal areas on T1WI within the marrow of mandibular condyle may represent above two conditions. Increased signal on T2 WI may indicate presence of edema and may be a precursor of osteonecrosis. The probable precipitating factors are local trauma and disc displacement **(Fig. 41)**.[62] Loose bodies may be seen within the joint in osteochondritis dissecans as hypointense structures.

POSTOPERATIVE IMAGING

MR is valuable in demonstrating joint mobility and postoperative adhesions/fibrosis after disc repositioning surgery and diskectomy and also for evaluation of alloplastic implants. Contrast administration may be useful in postoperative evaluations of the joint.

EVALUATION OF MANDIBULAR ASYMMETRY

This is multifactorial and could be due to trauma or internal derangement. Unilateral condylar hyperplasia on long side may be seen in these patients.[63] In children with facial asymmetry, decreased condylar growth or degenerative joint changes on short side may be demonstrated in response to displaced disc **(Figs. 43A to C)**.[64]

INFECTIONS AND ARTHRITIDES

Infections of TM joint are rare and seen postoperatively or through spread from adjacent structures, i.e. ear cavity.[65] Fluid sensitive sequences (T2 TSE) and postcontrast imaging provide valuable information in infections. TM joint is involved in 50% of patients with rheumatoid arthritis, ankylosing spondylitis, psoriatic arthritis and pseudogout. MR imaging shows soft tissue involvement, erosions and synovial proliferation.[66]

TUMORS AND TUMOR-LIKE CONDITIONS

Synovial chondromatosis is reported in TMJ[67] and MR may show joint expansion with low intensity foci within it. Pigmented villonodular synovitis is also reported in TMJ. Osteochondroma is also a common tumor of the mandibular condyle and needs to be differentiated from osteoma and hypertrophic condylar changes **(Figs. 44A and B)**. Metastatic disease from a remote site (mostly adenocarcinoma from breast) can present around the TMJ in less than 1% cases. Synovial cysts, simple bone cyst,

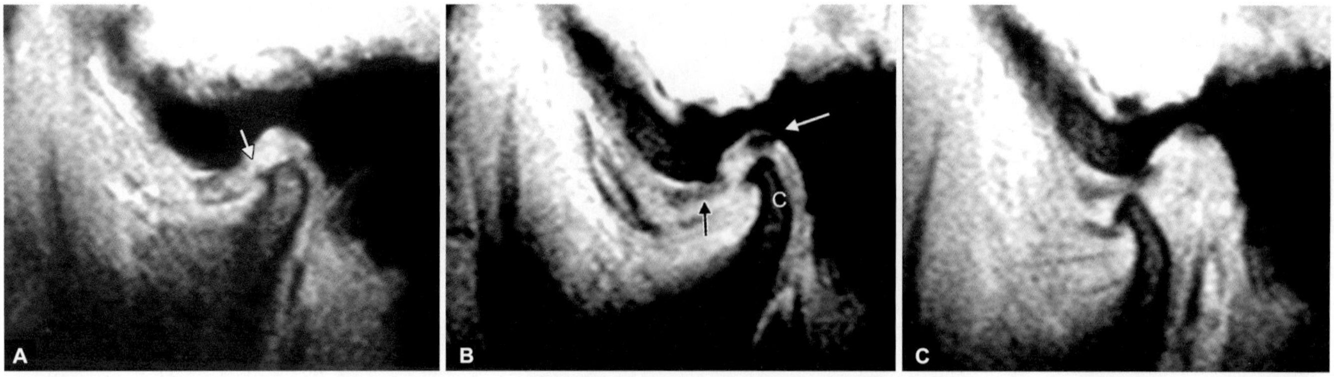

Figs 43A to C: Mandibular asymmetry due to disc dislocation (A) right side—closed mouth (B) left side—closed mouth (C) left side—open mouth. The left condyle is hypoplastic (B). There is anterior dislocation of the disc on this side (black arrow) with fibrosis of posterior attachment (white arrow). The disc is nonreducing (C). The right sided disc also shows features of degeneration (arrow in A).

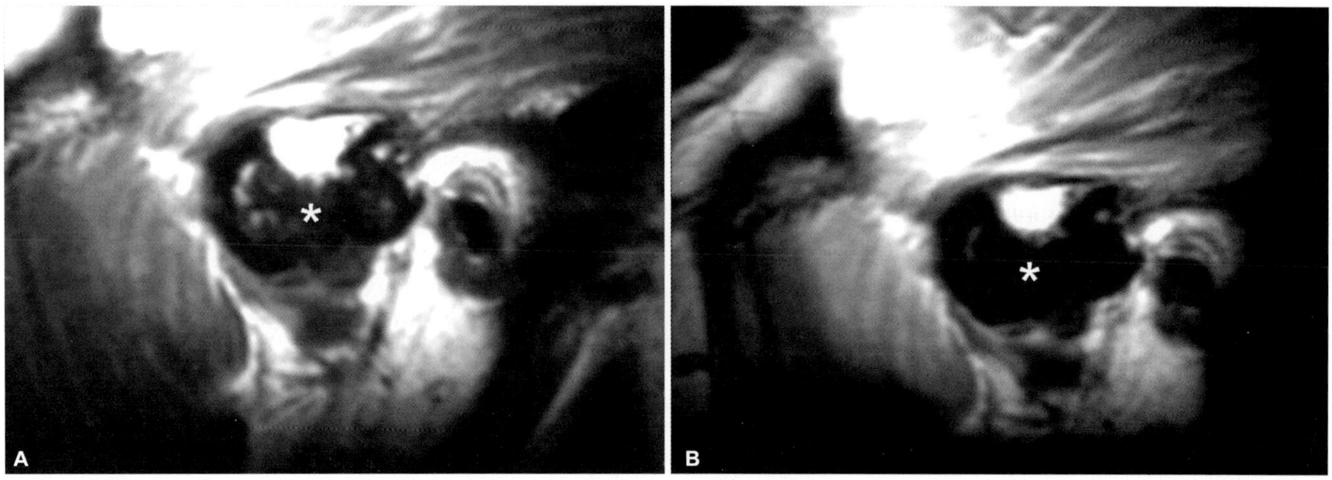

Figs. 44A and B: T1WI (A) and T2WI (B) show a densely sclerotic lesion in the articular eminence (asterisks) suggestive of osteoma.

eosinophilic granuloma, chondrosarcoma, lymphoma and synovial sarcoma are all reported in TMJ or mandibular condyle.

REFERENCES

1. Stoller DW, Wolf EM, LI AE, et al. The shoulder, Chapter 8. In: Magnetic Resonance Imaging in Orthopaedics and Sports Medicine, 3rd edition. Philadelphia: Lippincott, Williams and Wilkins; 2007. p. 1131.
2. Mack LA, Matsen FA III, Kilcoyne RF, et al. US evaluation of rotator cuff. Radiology. 1985;157:205-9.
3. Middleton WD, Edelstein G, Reinus WR, et al. Sonographic detection of rotator cuff tears. Am J Roentgenol. 1985;144:349-53.
4. Van Holsbeeck M, Strouse PJ. Sonography of the shoulder: evaluation of the subacromial subdeltoid bursa. Am J Roentgenol. 1993;160:561-4.
5. Martinoli C, Bianchi S, Prato N, et al. US of the shoulder: nonrotator cuff disorders. Radiographics. 2003;23:381-401.
6. Berquist TH. MRI of the Musculoskeletal System, 3rd edition. New York: Raven Press; 1990. pp. 517-607.
7. Cook TS, Stein JM, Simonson S, Kim W. Normal and variant anatomy of the shoulder on MRI. Magn Reson Imaging Clin N Am. 2011;19:595-608.
8. Chung CB, Dwek JR, Feng S, et al. MR arthrography of the glenohumeral joint: A tailored approach. Am J Roentgenol. 2001;177:217-19.
9. Chung CB, Corrente L, Resnick D. MR arthrography of the shoulder joint. MRI Clinics of North Am. 2004;12:217-9.
10. Rudez J, Zanetti M. Normal anatomy, variants and pitfalls on shoulder MRI. Eur J Radiol. 2008;68:25-35.
11. Gumina S, Postacchini F, Orsina L, et al. The morphometry of the coracoid process: its aetiologic role in subcoracoid impingement syndrome. Int Orthop. 1999;23:198-201.
12. Prescher A, Klompen T. The glenoid notch and its relation to the shape of glenoid cavity of the scapula. J Anat. 1997;190:457-60.
13. Bigliani LU, et al. Morphology of acromion and its relationship to rotator cuff tears. Orthop Trans. 1986;10:216.

14. Neer CS. Anterior acromioplasty for the chronic impingement syndrome: A preliminary report. J Bone Joint Surg (Am). 1972;54:41-50.
15. Seeger LL, Gold RH, Bassett LW, et al. Shoulder impingement syndrome: MR findings in 53 shoulders. AJR. 1988;150:343-7.
16. Carrino JA, McCauley TR, Katz LD, et al. Rotator cuff: Evaluation with fast spin echo versus conventional spin echo imaging. Radiology. 1997;202:533-9.
17. Zlatkin MB, Reicher MA, Kellerhouse ME, et al. The painful shoulder: MR imaging of the glenohumeral joint. J Comput Assist Tomogr. 1988;12:995-1001.
18. Mirowitz SA. Normal rotator cuff: MR imaging with conventional and fat suppression techniques. Radiology. 1991;180:735-40.
19. Zlatkin MB, Iannotti JP, Roberts MC, et al. Rotator cuff tears: Diagnostic performance of MR imaging: comparison with arthrography and correlation with surgery. Radiology. 1989;172:223-9.
20. Hoddler J, Kursunoglu-Brahme S, Syndler SJ, et al. Rotator cuff disease: Assessment with MR arthrography versus standard MR imaging in 36 patients with arthroscopic confirmation. Radiology. 1992;182:431-3.
21. Turkel SJ, Panio MW, Marshal JL, et al. Stabilising mechanisms preventing anterior dislocation of the glenohumeral joint. J Bone Joint Surg (Am). 1981;63:1208-17.
22. Cleeman E, Flatow EL. Shoulder dislocations in the young patient. Orthop Clin North Am. 2000;3:217-29.
23. Kwak SM, Brown RR, Trudell D, et al. Gleno-humeral joint: Comparison of shoulder positions at MR arthrography. Radiology. 1998;208:375-80.
24. Palmer WE, Caslowitz PL. Anterior shoulder instability: Diagnostic criteria determined from prospective analysis of 121 MR arthrograms. Radiology. 1995;197:819-25.
25. Garneau RA, Renfrew DL, Moore TE, et al. Glenoid labrum: Evaluation with MR imaging. Radiology. 1991;179.519-22.
26. Legan JM, Burkhard TK, Goff WB II, et al. Tears of the glenoid labrum: MR imaging of 88 arthroscopically confirmed cases. Radiology. 1991;179:241-6.
27. Chandnani VP, Yeager TD, De Berardino T, et al. Glenoid labral tears: Prospective evaluation with MR imaging, MR arthrography and CT arthrography. Am J Roentgenol. 1993;161:1229-53.
28. Richards RD, Sartoris DJ, Pathria MN, et al. Hill Sach's lesion and normal humeral groove: MR imaging features allowing their differentiation. Radiology. 1994;190:665-8.
29. Sugaya H, Moriishi J, Dohi M, et al. Glenoid rim morphology in recurrent anterior glenohumeral instability. J Bone Joint Surg Am. 2003;85:878-84.
30. Sanders TG, Tirman PF, Linares R, et al. The glenolabral articular disruption lesion: MR arthrography with arthroscopic correlation. Am J Roentgenol. 1999;172:171-5.
31. Levine WN, Flatow EL. The pathophysiology of shoulder instability. Am J Sports Med. 2000;28:910-7.
32. Bui-Mansfield LT, Taylor DC, Uhorchak JM, et al. Humeral avulsions of the glenohumeral ligament: Imaging features and a review of the literature. Am J Roentgenol. 2002;179:649-55.
33. Mosley HF, Overgaard B. The anterior capsular mechanism in recurrent anterior dislocation of the shoulder morphological and clinical studies with special reference to glenoid labrum and the glenohumeral ligaments. J Bone Joint Surg. 1962;44:913-27.
34. Bigoni JB, Christine B, Chung MD. MR imaging of the rotator cuff interval. Magn Reson Imaging Clin North Am. 2004;12:61-73.
35. Snyder SJ, Karzel RP, Del Pizzo, et al. SLAP lesions of the shoulder. Arthroscopy. 1990;6:274-9.
36. Pfirrman CWA, Zannette M, Weishaupt D, et al. Subscapularis tendon tears: Detection and grading at MR arthrography. Radiology. 1999;213:709-14.
37. Tung GA, Hou DD. MR arthrography of the posterior labrocapsular complex: Relationship with glenohumeral joint alignment and clinical posterior instability. Am J Roentgenol. 2003;180:369-75.
38. Stoller W. MR arthrography of the glenohumeral joint. Radiolol Clin North Am. 1997;35:97-116.
39. Jee WH, McCauley TR, Kalz LD, et al. Superior labral anterior posterior (SLAP) lesions of the glenoid labrum: Reliability and accuracy of MR arthrography for diagnosis. Radiology. 2001;218:127-32.
40. Erickson SJ, Fitzgerald SW, Quinn SF, et al. Long bicipital tendon of the shoulder: Normal anatomy and pathologic findings on MR imaging. Am J Roentgenol. 1992;158:1091-6.
41. Bennet WF. Visualisation of the anatomy of the rotator interval and bicipital sheath. Arthroscopy. 2001;17:107-11.
42. Linker CS, Helms CA, Fritz RC. Quadrilateral space syndrome: Findings at MR imaging. Radiology. 1993;188:675-6.
43. Fritz RC, Helms CA, Steinback LS, et al. Suprascapular nerve entrapment: evaluation with MR imaging. Radiology. 1992;183:437.
44. Emig EW, Schweitzer ME, Karasick D, et al. Adhesive capsulitis of the shoulder: MR diagnosis. Am J Roentgenol. 1995;164:1457-9.
45. Rockwood C, Uhthoff HK, Dervin G, et al. Calcifying tendinitis, chapter 8. In: Rockwood C, Matsen III F, Wirth M, Lippt S (Eds). The Shoulder, 3rd edition. Philadelphia: Saunders; 2004. p. 1033.
46. Lee E, Flatow E. The shoulder and arm, Chapter 12. In: Weinstein S, Buckwalter J (Eds). Turek' Orthopedics, 6th edition. Philadelphia: Lippinkot Williams and Wilkins; 2005. p. 345.
47. Learch TJ, Farooki S. Magnetic resonance imaging of septic arthritis. Clinical Imaging. 2000;24:336-42.
48. Alasaarela E, Suramo I, Tervonen O, et al. Evaluation of humeral head erosions in rheumatoid arthritis: A comparison of ultrasonography, magnetic resonance

imaging, computed tomography and plain radiography. Br J Rheumatol. 1998;37:1152-6.
49. Neer CS. Shoulder Reconstruction. Philadelphia: WB Saunders; 1990. p. 194.
50. Enzinger FM, Weiss SW. Soft Tissue Tumors. St. Louis, MO: CV Mosby; 1983.
51. Guralnick W, Kaban LB, Merrill RG. Temporomandibular joints afflictions. N Engl J Med. 1978;299:123-9.
52. Tomas X, Pomes J, Berenguer J, et al. MR Imaging of temporomandibular joint dysfunction: A pictorial review. Radiographics. 2006;26:765-81.
53. Yale SH. Radiographic evaluation of the temporomandibular joint. J Am Dent Assoc. 1969;79:102-7.
54. Hansson T, Oberg T, Carlsson GE, et al. Thickness of soft tissue layers and articular disc in the temporomandibular joint. Acta Odontol Scand. 1977;35:77-83.
55. Paesani D, Westesson PL, Hatala M, et al. Prevalence of internal derangement in patients with craniomandibular disorders. Am J Orthod Dentofacial Orthop. 1992; 101:41-7.
56. Katzberg RW, Westesson PL, Tallents RH, et al. Temporomandibular joint: MR assessment of rotational and sideways disc displacements. Radiology. 1988;169:741-8.
57. Wikes CH. Arthrography of the temporomandibular joint in patients with temporomandibular joint pain dysfunction syndrome. Minn Med. 1978;39:319-23.
58. Farrar WB. Characteristics of the condylar path in internal derangement of the TMJ. J Prosthet Dent. 1978;39:319-23.
59. Wikes CH. Internal derangement of the temporomandibular joint: Pathological variations. Arch Otolaryng Head Neck Surg. 1989;115:469-77.
60. Hasso AN, Christiansen EL, Alder ME. The temporomandibular joint. Radiol Clin North Am. 1989;27:301.
61. Westesson PL, Bronstein SL, Leidberg JL. Internal derangement of the temporomandibular joint: Morphological description with correlation to joint function. Oral Surg Oral Med Oral Path. 1985;59:323-31.
62. Schellhas KP, Wikes CH, Fritts HM, et al. MR of osteochondritis dissecans and avascular necrosis of the mandibular condyle. AJNR. 1989;10:3-12.
63. Jonck LM. Facial asymmetry and condylar hyperplasia. Oral Surg Oral Med Oral Pathol. 1975;40:567-73.
64. Katzberg RW, Tallents RH, Hayakawa K, et al. Internal derangements of the temporomandibular joint: Findings in paediatric age group. Radiology. 1985;154:125-7.
65. Thomson HG. Septic arthritis of the temporomandibular joint complicating otitis externa. J Otolaryngol Otol. 1989;103:319-21.
66. Smith HJ, Larheim TA, Aspestrand F. Rheumatic and non-rheumatic disease in the temporomandibular joint: Gadolinium enhanced MR imaging. Radiology. 1992;185: 229-34.
67. Heffez LB. Imaging of internal derangements and synovial chondromatosis of the temporomandibular joint. Radiol Clin North Am. 1993;31:149-62.

CHAPTER 203

Magnetic Resonance Imaging in Bone Marrow Disorders

Veena Chowdhury

INTRODUCTION

Normal bone marrow lies within the skeleton, and it provides red blood cells, platelets and white blood cells to meet the requirements for oxygenation, coagulation and immunity. Traditionally, bone marrow evaluation has been established with biopsy or aspiration. Techniques, such as scintigraphy or computed tomography are nonspecific and insensitive.

Magnetic resonance imaging (MRI) with its excellent spatial and contrast resolution is the only imaging technique that allows direct visualization of the bone marrow. Magnetic resonance imaging can depict hematopoietic and fatty marrow separately and is therefore a useful technique for noninvasive evaluation of pathologic bone marrow conditions.[1,2] Magnetic resonance imaging provides information at the level of cellular and chemical composition in addition to gross morphologic data. The signal intensity, morphology and location of pathological findings on MRI can be used to provide more accurate diagnosis, to guide treatment and to follow therapy related changes. Various MRI techniques are utilized to accentuate chemical and cellular composition of normal marrow and marrow diseases. Magnetic resonance imaging is more sensitive than specific in marrow disorders but an integration of clinical and radiologic data helps in suggesting an accurate diagnosis.

Normal bone marrow has three primary components:

1. The osseous component consisting of primary and secondary trabeculae of cancellous bone which provide the structural framework for myeloid and fat cells.
2. The red marrow which is composed of leukocytes and platelet precursors is hematopoietically active.
3. The yellow marrow contains fat which is hematopoietically inactive. The chemical composition and vascular supply of these types of marrow are different and the hematopoietic marrow composition changes with age as the bone marrow is a dynamic organ.[2-4]

DISTRIBUTION OF NORMAL BONE MARROW AND NORMAL CONVERSION

Almost all marrows are hematopoietic in a newborn. Conversion of red to yellow marrow commences in the immediate postnatal period beginning in the terminal phalanges of hand and feet. Conversion is continuous from peripheral to central with respect to the skeleton and from diaphysis to metaphysis in long bones. This conversion is not entirely symmetric. Red marrow is predominantly localized to the axial skeleton.

In less than 10 years of age, yellow marrow is seen in most of the diaphysis of long bones of arms, legs and cranium **(Fig. 1)**.[1-3]

At 10–20 years, yellow marrow is seen predominantly in the limbs with residual red marrow in the femoral and humeral metaphysis.

By 25 years, conversion is usually complete, and red marrow is situated in the axial skeleton, sternum, ribs, proximal humerii and femur, calcaneum and calvaria while yellow predominates the remainder of long bones **(Figs. 2A to C)**. Regional differences between the two sexes have been demonstrated.

In a young adult, the red marrow has approximately 40% water, 40% fat and 20% protein. At 60 years of age, the percentage of fat in hematopoietically active marrow can be as high as 70% **(Figs. 3A and B)**. Yellow marrow contains 80% fat, 15% water and 5% proteins. These changes vary and are dependent on factors, such as disease, athletic activities and therapies.[4-7]

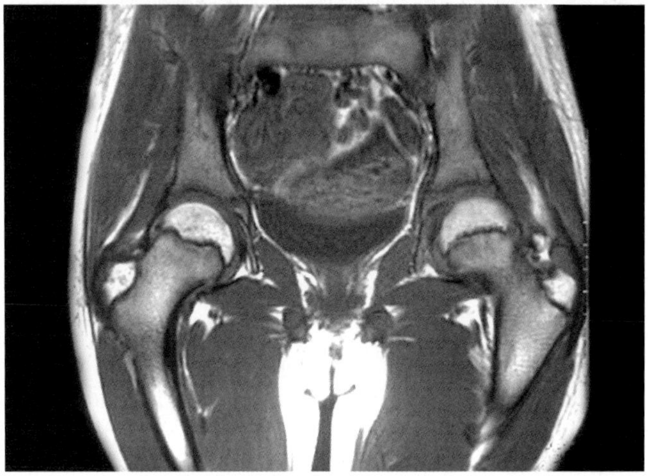

Fig. 1: T1W coronal image of the pelvis showing high-signal yellow marrow (signal identical to subcutaneous fat) in the femoral epiphysis, apophysis and the femoral diaphysis. Red marrow has intermediate signal intensity (higher than adjacent muscle) is seen present in the proximal femoral metaphysis and in the pelvic bones. Marked symmetry of distribution seen bilaterally: Normal marrow pattern in childhood (1–10 years).

MR IMAGING TECHNIQUES FOR EVALUATION OF NORMAL BONE MARROW

The MR signal intensities in the bone marrow are determined by the proportion of its constituents, i.e. water, fat and protein as well as artifacts induced by bone trabeculae, diffusion and uptake of contrast media. Although the contribution of each constituent is not entirely understood, the relaxation of water depends on its environment. Different signal characteristics can be identified from bound water, complex bound water, free water and structured water. However, the exact state of water in specific tissue is not known.

Fat also occurs in various states and the signal intensity depends on the protons in the methyl groups and unsaturated fatty acids. Further, fat cells in marrow differ from those elsewhere in the body as these cells decrease during periods of increased hematopoietic activity. In the case of marrow a critical determinant of its signal character is its fat content and the fat content varies according to the age and anatomic locations.[1-7]

Appearances of bone marrow on MRI sequences depend on the distribution of red hematopoietically active marrow, and yellow hematopoietically inactive marrow, density of the trabeculae which varies with age, gender and anatomical region.[6-8] Hence, the appearance of bone marrow varies with the pulse sequence and the relative fractions of fatty and red marrow. Therefore, sequences displaying differences between fat and water signal are useful. An optimal protocol for the detection and characterization of marrow abnormalities uses a T1-weighted sequence and either a T2-weighted/fast T2-weighted spin echo sequence (SE) with fat suppression or a short inversion time, inversion recovery

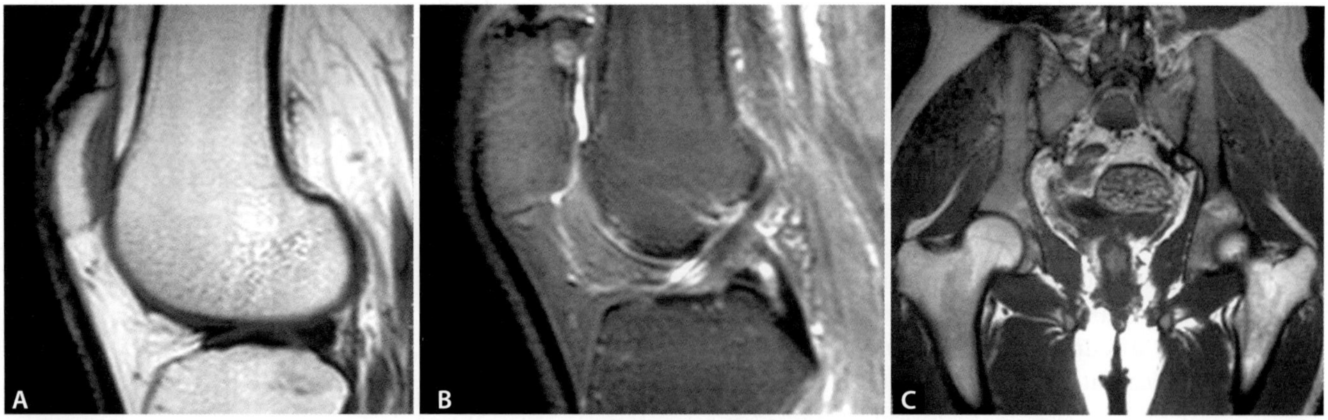

Figs. 2A to C: T1W sagittal (A) and STIR sagittal (B) images of the knee showing normal yellow marrow in the diaphysis and the distal metaphysis of the femur. T1W coronal image of the pelvis (C) showing intermediate signal intensity red marrow in the proximal femoral metaphysis and pelvic bones: Normal marrow pattern in an adult >25 years of age.

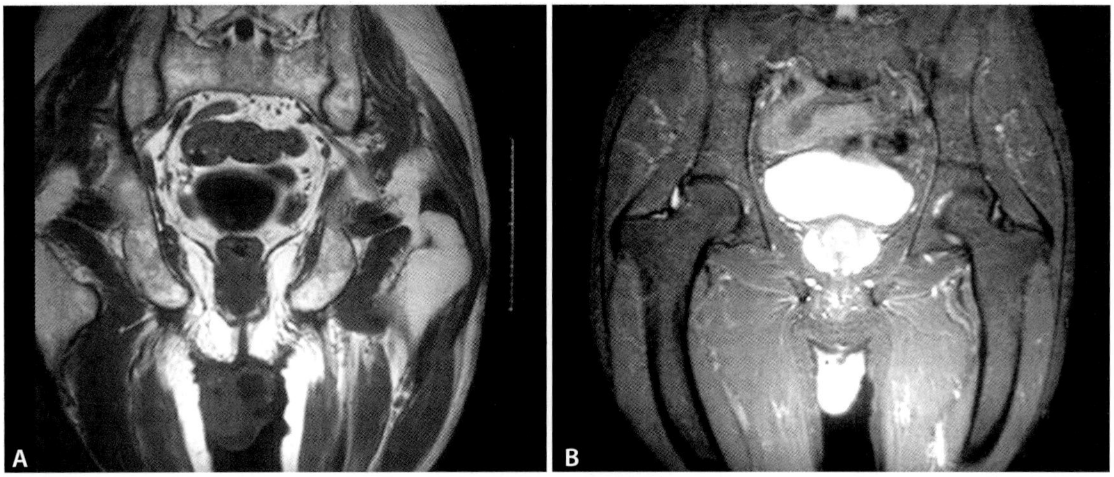

Figs. 3A and B: T1W coronal image of the pelvis (A) in a 70-year-old showing high-signal yellow marrow in the proximal femoral metaphyses and foci of yellow marrow in the pelvic bones; STIR coronal image of the pelvis (B) shows complete suppression of the signal indicating fatty marrow: Normal marrow pattern for > 60 years of age.

(STIR) sequence. The addition of other sequences will be influenced by the disease process and the anatomic region being evaluated.

SE and fast SE sequences: The T1W SE sequence remains a fundamental tool in MR imaging of the bone marrow as yellow marrow contains 80% fat and 15% water. The signal of fat is the highest and shorter than the signal of water. The short T1 of normal fatty marrow produces excellent contrast on these sequences and pathologic lesions which have a low-signal are easy to detect. The signal intensity of normal non-hematopoietic (yellow) marrow is isointense to subcutaneous fat on T1W and less than subcutaneous fat on T2W images **(Fig. 1)**. Hematopoietic marrow contains 40% fat and 40% water. Hence, the signal intensity of red marrow is less than fat but hyperintense to muscles **(Figs. 1 and 2C)**. There is little contrast between hematopoietic marrow and pathologic lesions as both have a low-signal intensity.[3,4,9] The differentiating feature is that the signal intensity of pathological lesions is usually less than that of the intervertebral disks in the spine and less than that of the muscle in the extremities.

On the basis of T1W signal characteristics, the various pathologies have been characterized by Hanrahan and Shah in a recently published article in December 2011.[10] The differential diagnosis is based on conditions causing a focal or of diffuse increase in T1 signal intensity of the marrow in various locations of the spine. Causes of focal T1 signal in crease in any marrow may be a normal variant, solitary hemangioma, metastasis, lipoma, bone marrow hemorrhage or degenerative disk disease.

Focal T1 signal decrease at the end plate may occur in degenerative changes, osteomyelitis and amyloid while T1 signal changes in the body are seen in atypical hemangioma, fracture, malignancy, metastasis, myeloma, lymphoma and fibrous dysplasia. Primary bone tumor and fracture involve the posterior elements.

Diffuse or multifocal increase in T1 signal is seen in osteoporosis, chronic malnutrition, multiple hemangiomas and prior radiation therapy. Diffuse or mulifocal decrease in T1 signal is seen in hematopoietic hyperplasia, renal osteodystrophy, spondyloarthropathy, myelofibrosis, hemosiderosis, sarcoidosis and neoplasms.

The T2-weighted SE sequences are rarely more informative than T1-weighted sequence in contrast to most other body regions because the poor contrast between fatty marrow and hematopoietic marrow. Also, there is little difference between pathologic and fatty marrow both of which show a high-signal intensity on T2W images. This problem is most pronounced on turbo-spin-echo (TSE) sequences, but the use of fat suppression solves this problem. Fat-suppressed sequences are useful to increase the contrast between normal and pathologic marrows and also between red and yellow marrows. The two widely used fat suppression techniques are the STIR sequence and the fat-saturated SE sequence.[3,11]

STIR sequence: This sequence has an excellent contrast between marrow and pathological lesions due to the additive values of T1 and T2-weighted sequences along with the suppression of fat signal, as nulling of fat signal and addition of signal from other tissues increases the contrast sensitivity. This sequence can be obtained when a 180° inversion pulse is used and the inversion time is chosen to cancel the signal of fat. Hence, fatty marrow has a low-signal on STIR **(Fig. 3B)** and hematopoietic marrow has an indeterminate signal equal to muscle.[4,11]

The STIR sequence is of great value for pathological lesions associated with increased water and prolonged T1 and T2 values. The main advantages of STIR are due to (i) additive T1 and T2 contrast, (ii) marked fat suppression, (iii) a two-field increase in the magnetization range of spin echo sequences. As a result, STIR images demonstrate an extraordinary high contrast, conspicuousness and sensitivity for the detection of bone marrow pathology. Pathological lesions have a high-signal intensity due to increased cells, fluid and edema. The STIR sequence has a high sensitivity but a low specificity. Normal marrow is seen as signal void, hematopoietic marrow as low-signal intensity and pathological lesions are seen as high-signal intensity.

The main drawback of the STIR sequence is that it cancels every signal identical to fat, e.g. blood in hematoma or contrast-enhanced tissue. Further, a very homogeneous magnetic field is required; therefore, this sequence is not efficient on every MR unit. The other disadvantage includes a relatively long imaging time and a low signal to noise ratio. The combination of T1W SE sequence with a STIR or fat suppressed fast SE T2W sequence forms the basis of most bone marrow imaging protocols.[11]

Gradient-recalled echo (GRE) imaging is most useful for assessing the amount of trabecular bone and paramagnetic elements, e.g. iron or calcification. Gradient-recalled echo sequence permits faster scanning times, but the images are more susceptible to magnetic field inhomogeneities, chemical shift effects and magnetic susceptibility. The effect of magnetic field inhomogeneities can be exploited when bone marrow is imaged.

Normal trabecular bone pattern results in intrinsic magnetic field inhomogeneities and reduction in T2 relaxation time with a decrease in the signal intensity on T2-weighted images. Trabecular bone and paramagnetic substances cause artifactual signal loss resulting in hypointense marrow regardless of the type of marrow.[3,4,12]

Opposed phase GRE sequences are highly sensitive for the detection of red marrow that is visualized as low-signal intensity or sometimes a signal void. This is due to:

- The imaging parameters with the phases of the fat and water protons opposed
- The susceptibility effects of iron containing compounds in the bone marrow
- The susceptibility effects from bony trabeculae in the bone marrow. These effects are more intense with increasing echo time. If a pathology replaces normal marrow, fat will be obliterated and no marrow subtraction will occur. The difference between the signal produced by normal marrow which always contains fat and water is emphasised on opposed phase sequences.[3,4,12]

Chemical shift imaging is similar to the opposed phase GRE technique based on the chemical shift between the protons of fat and water. The difference in resonance frequency between water and fat protons can be used. At 1.5 tesla (T), the difference is 220 Hz. Initially both fat and water acquire transverse magnetization vectors that are in plane. The read-out gradient is normally centered on the echo which appears symmetrically on the 90° pulse with respect to the 180° pulse. Hence, the signal is proportional to the sum of water and fat protons (in phase imaging). By shifting the read-out window, it is possible to obtain images, the contrast of which is related to the difference between the quantities of water and fat protons (opposed phase imaging) **(Figs. 4A and B)**. This is as a result of the frequency difference after a given time when the vectors are exactly out of phase. After a further period of time the spins will be in phase again. At 1.5T fat and water are in phase every 4.5 msec. This means that out of phase images are acquired with an echo time of 2.25 msec. This phenomenon is known as the 'Dixon effect' also termed as chemical shift. Chemical shift imaging improves the sensitivity of MRI to bone marrow infiltration by systemic disease as seen in Hodgkin's disease, non-Hodgkin's lymphoma or leukemia. The therapy of systemic disease, such as leukemia can be monitored as there is quantitative assessment of the relative water fraction. A further refinement of this technique is the development of quantitative chemical shift imaging where the quantitative assessment of fat fraction can be calculated.[3,13,14]

It has been suggested that a decrease in signal intensity greater than 20% on out-of-the-phase images compared within phase images should be used as a cutoff threshold for normalcy to allow distinction between benign and malignant causes of vertebral marrow abnormalities **(Figs. 5A and B)**. It has been concluded that any lesion that is not composed of fat on T1-weighted images and that decreases less than 20% of its signal intensity on out-of-phase images compared to in phase images should be considered suspicious for malignancy.[15]

Diffusion imaging using echoplanar imaging (EPI) is difficult to apply outside the brain. Single shot SE

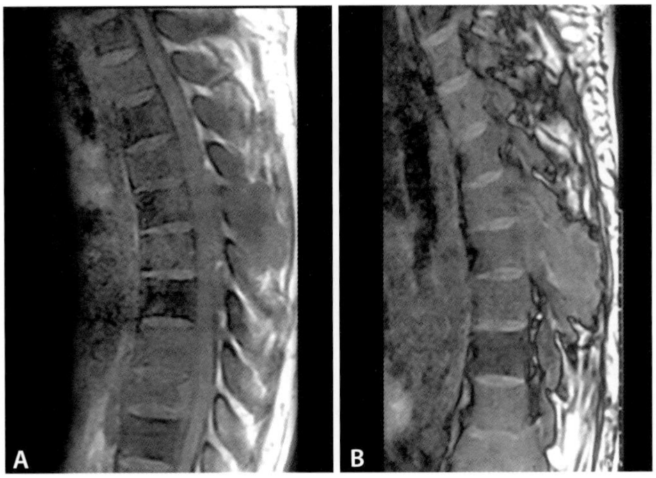

Figs. 4A and B: MR images of the dorsolumbar spine in phase (A) and opposed phase (B) showing neoplastic (metastatic) lesions as high-signal on the opposed phase images as compared to the in phase images due to replacement of fat in these lesions.

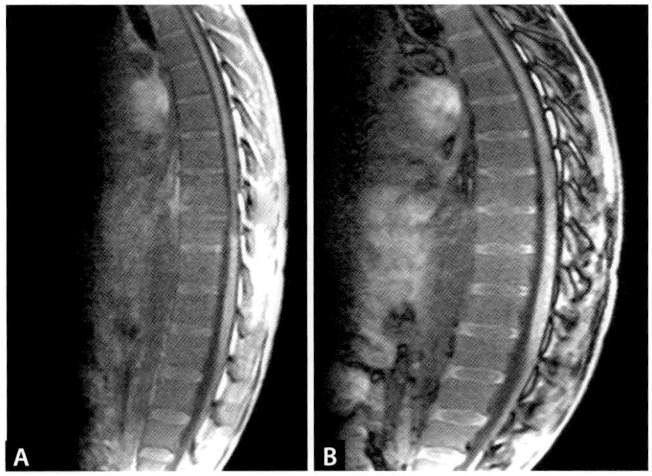

Figs. 5A and B: MR images of the spine revealing a decrease of signal less than 20% on the opposed phase images (B) as compared to the in phase images (A) suggesting a malignant etiology.

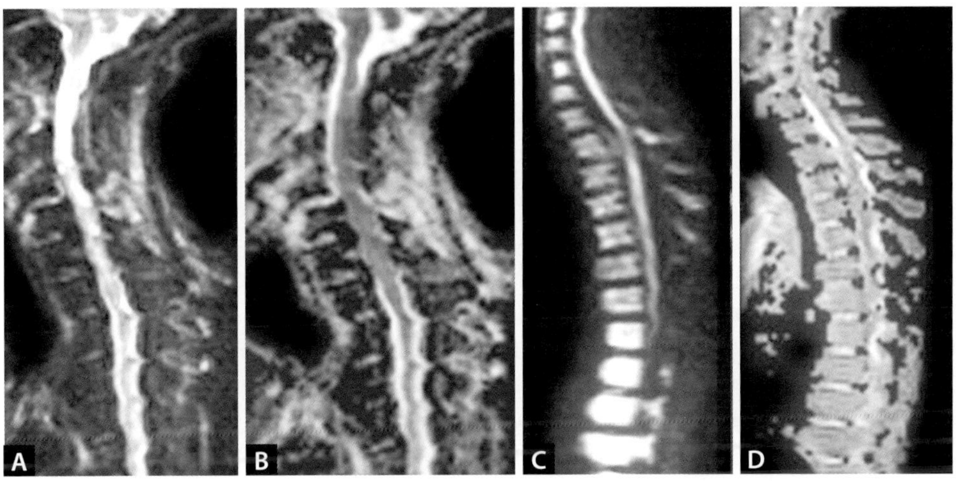

Figs. 6A to D: Diffusion-weighted MR imaging of the spine (A) showing the normal vertebral bodies as hypointense with the normal ADC map (B); Diffusion-weighted imaging (C) in a case of acute leukemia showing a restricted diffusion in the vertebral bodies which show a corresponding low signal on ADC map (D).

sequences are applied to the spine to differentiate benign and malignant vertebral fractures. The rapidity of the EPI pulse sequence enables data acquisition with increasing 'b' values thus enabling accurate calculation of apparent diffusion coefficient (ADC). On all DW images fat marrow signals are nulled **(Figs. 6A to D)**. Normal vertebral bodies are hypointense on both DW images and STIR images because the fat marrow signal is suppressed, and there is negligible amount of free water content in the interstitial space. Thus, there are minimal amount of mobile protons available for generating a MR signal. Diffusion weighted MR imaging is useful for differentiating benign fracture edema and tumor infiltration of the vertebral body.[3,13,14] DWI is also useful in distinguishing progressive changes in bone marrow among treatment sequelae, fracture or tumor which can be difficult on conventional MRI. DWI may show decreased signal intensity of metastatic disease of the vertebral marrow with successful treatment. In a study, decreased DWI signal of the spine was seen after 2 months of therapy in patients with clinical improvement whereas persistent abnormal hyperintense signal was found when there was no clinical improvement.[16] In addition to the tumor evaluation, DWI may be useful for differentiation of degenerative and infectious end-plate abnormalities. DWI showed hyperintensity in patients with infection and no hyperintensity in degenerative end plates with ADC values of infectious end plates significantly higher than normal and degenerative end plates.

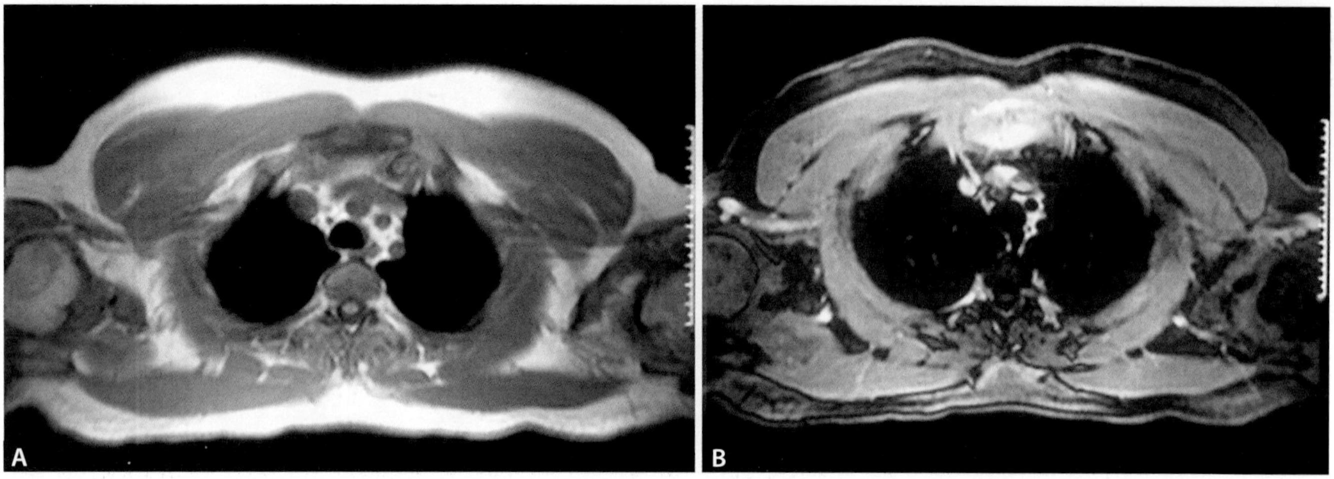

Figs. 7A and B: MR images of the sternum showing signal alteration seen as hypointense signal on T1W image (A) which shows intense enhancement on postcontrast image (B)—Tuberculosis of the sternum.

Contrast-enhanced marrow imaging: Normal marrow signal does not show a visible change after the injection of gadolinium chelates. Certain pathological lesions exhibit a strong signal increase with contrast. Therefore, the absence of uptake practically rules out involvement of the marrow. A pre-injection T1 sequence is mandatory because enhanced signal of the lesion may make it equal to the signal intensity of fatty marrow masking the lesion. The uptake is best seen on T1W fat presaturated sequences.[3,4,17] It has been stated that in case of normal STIR images no relevant additional information is found with contrast enhanced T1-weighted images while in the case of abnormal STIR images significant additional information is obtained on administration of gadopentetate dimeglumine. Thus, the administration of contrast is strongly recommended with cases with abnormal STIR images[18] **(Figs. 7A and B)**.

RECENT ADVANCES IN MR IMAGING OF BONE MARROW

Dynamic Contrast-enhanced MR Imaging and Bone Marrow Perfusion

Dynamic contrast-enhanced MR studies with gadolinium chelates have been applied by investigators in order to generate estimates of the volume of normal or pathological marrow before and after treatment. Dynamic Gd-DTPA enhanced MR scans reveal increased blood volume (increased enhancement) of the neoplastic infiltration compared to normal marrow. The enhancement is significantly higher in marked marrow infiltration as compared to mild or no infiltration and the enhancement is significantly higher in lesions with higher vessel density than in lesions with low vessel density. A potential role for dynamic contrast enhanced MRI is being explored in the assessment of the percentage of necrosis present within a bone tumor after treatment. It has been seen that the percentage of necrosis following chemotherapy plays a role in the patient prognosis. Dynamic MRI has a potential valuable role for noninvasively assessing the treatment response during neoadjuvant therapy. Bone marrow perfusion measured with dynamic contrast-enhanced MR imaging (DCE) in acute myeloid leukemia (AML) patients in complete remission is associated with outcome and survival.[19] Bone marrow perfusion assessed by dynamic contrast enhanced MR has also been studied in patients with osteoporosis. Studies have shown that a decreasing marrow perfusion and increasing marrow fat content accompany a reduction in bone density.[20]

CONTRAST-ENHANCED MR IMAGING OF THE BONE MARROW USING IRON OXIDE PARTICLES

A new class of contrast agents with respect to bone marrow imaging is the group of ultrasmall superparamagnetic iron oxide particles (USPIO). These particulate iron oxide contrast agents are phagocytosed by macrophages in the normal bone marrow, where they induce a T2 shortening effect. The principle is similar to MR imaging of the liver with super paramagnetic iron oxide particles (SPIO). However, SPIO, used for liver imaging have a diameter of >50 mm, whereas USPIO used for bone marrow imaging have a diameter of < 50 mm. Ultra small superparamagnetic iron oxide particle (USPIO) particles are not taken up in neoplastic infiltrates which do not contain macrophages.[21] Thus, USPIO may be used to differentiate hypercellular normal and neoplastic marrow. After infusion of USPIO at a dose of 2.6 mg/kg body weight, the normal marrow shows a USPIO induced signal loss as opposed to focal neoplastic infiltrates. The neoplastic infiltrates do not show any signal loss with USPIO thus enabling differentiation from normal bone marrow, the neoplastic infiltrates stand out as bright lesions.[22] Metz et al. found a significantly increased number of detected focal bone marrow lesions (<1 cm) in patients of non-Hodgkin's-lymphoma after administration of USPIO (FERUMOXTRAN-10) compared to non-enhanced scans.[23]

MR SPECTROSCOPY

In additional to DWI, proton MR spectroscopy is used to assess bone marrow changes with varying bone minerals densities. Magnetic resonance spectroscopy (MRS) allows the noninvasive quantitative assessment at the molecular level. In this technique, the global MR signal from bone is divided into the two major segments of water and lipid separated by 3.1 ppm. The spectra of proton MRS have a water peak, originating mostly from red marrow, and a lipid peak, arising from yellow marrow. The lipid signal is composed of at least eight fractions, the largest of which is from the methylene group at 1.6 ppm. Signal peaks can vary among subjects and are influenced not only by the water–lipid proton quantity and the tissue environment but also by the surface coil and the distance between the voxel and surface coil. Because of these variables, instead of measuring the absolute signal peak for signal quantification, a lipid–water ratio is often measured. The fat fraction value determined from MRS has been adopted as a predictor of bone marrow fat content in most studies. MRS has been used to illustrate the increase in fat content with age. It has been shown that a decrease in cancellous bone is accompanied by a corresponding increase in fat cells and decrease in arterial capillaries and sinuses in bone marrow. Not only has it been shown that vertebral marrow fat increases as bone marrow density decreases, but also inferences of osseous quality may be made. It has also been found that using MRS, the percentage fat fraction was higher in lumbar vertebral bodies of subjects with weakened bone compared with the control group, suggesting it could serve as a measure of bone quality. Increased bone density will cause greater magnetic field inhomogeneity and wider spectral peaks as opposed to narrow peaks due to decreased bone mineral density.[24]

WHOLE BODY MRI

Recent advances in MR technology have made whole body MRI (WBMRI) possible in a single session. Whole body turbo STIR, the introduction of rolling table platform with integrated surface coils and sequences, such as breath hold gradient echo have substantially reduced scan time. The scan time has been reduced to less than 15 minutes without compromising the spatial resolution. Whole body MRI provides excellent soft tissue contrast and has high sensitivity in the detection of marrow lesions and hence is under investigation as a screening and staging modality in oncology patients.[25]

Although MRI has not replaced bone marrow biopsy for the diagnosis of bone marrow disease, WBMRI is useful in evaluating the number and location of bone marrow lesions. In particular, WBMRI has proved useful for detecting multifocal bone marrow involvement throughout the skeleton. In almost all cases of bone marrow involvement, WBMRI is also useful in targeting marrow biopsy due to the favorable contrast between tumors and normal tissue on the STIR sequences in cases of multiple myeloma. WBMRI is also more sensitive and specific than radiographic skeletal survey in assessing the extent of multiple myeloma which is critical in determining the appropriate therapy.[26]

Magnetic resonance imaging is safe and convenient and costs less than scintigraphy. Furthermore, compared to PET, WBMRI does not require special equipment as a cyclotron and it provides good spatial resolution. Whole body MRI can detect more abnormal lesions in diabetes mellitus patients than ^{18}F-FDG PET. Therefore WBMRI can be used as a feasibility study in patients who cannot undergo pretreatment PET CT.

Whole body MRI also detects extramedullary lesions, such as the lymph nodes in non-Hodgkin's lymphoma. Although FDG-PET has been reported to be able to detect involvement of lymph nodes better than other modalities in the initial stage, WBMRI is an effective method for evaluation of both bone marrow and extramedullary lesions of the patients with non-Hodgkin's lymphoma.[27]

3T MRI

Higher magnetic field strength MRI has the advantage of increased signal to noise ratio which can be used to improve contrast and spatial resolution. Another advantage is that more rapid scanning time is associated with reduced patient motion artifacts.

COMBINED PET AND MR IMAGING

An additional development taking place is combining PET and MR imaging, either by retrospective spatial registration of data from PET and MR imaging obtained on separate PET and MR machines or sequential data acquisition on combined PET-MR scanners. PET-MR imaging is superior to PET-CT, because of the improved intrinsic soft tissue contrast and direct bone marrow depiction using MRI.

NORMAL MR APPEARANCES OF BONE MARROW

Hematopoietically active red marrow is mildly hypointense to muscle on T1-weighted images and the signal intensity is slightly increased on T2-weighted images. With increasing age there is fatty replacement and the signal intensity of hematopoietic marrow shows a progressive increase on T1W images that clearly exceeds that of muscle.

Hematopoietically inactive yellow marrow has high-signal intensities on T1W images due to its high fat content and a slight decrease in signal intensity on T2W images, i.e. it follows the signal pattern of subcutaneous fat.

Four patterns of bone marrow distribution have been described in the *appendicular skeleton* and these patterns reflect the conversion pattern of red to yellow marrow.

1. Low-signal intensity red marrow in all parts of long bones at birth.
2. High-signal intensity yellow marrow in the diaphysis with low-signal intensity red marrow in the metaphysis at 3–12 months.
3. High-signal intensity yellow marrow in the diaphysis with foci of yellow marrow in the distal metaphysis at 1–5 years and proximal metaphysis at 6–10 years.
4. Homogeneous yellow diaphyseal and distal metaphyseal marrow at 25 years of age.[1,2,28]

The *vertebral marrow* is hematopoietic and demonstrates a low-signal intensity in the first two decades of life. The intensity is homogeneous with areas of high-signal intensity along the basivertebral vein centrally. The hematopoietic marrow is replaced by fatty marrow with increase in age, the replacement may be diffuse or focal.

In children less than 10 years the signal intensity of vertebral marrow is lower than the adjacent intervertebral disk on T1W images.

After 10 years the signal intensity is greater than the adjacent disk **(Fig. 8)** and a lower signal intensity suggests replacement by tumor infection or hyperplastic marrow.[7,28]

The *pelvis* shows hematopoietic marrow in the first two decades of life. Red to yellow conversion starts in the acetabulum and anterior ilium.[8,28] The signal intensity is heterogeneous and greater than that of muscle but less than that of fat on T1W images **(*see* Fig. 1)**. High-signal intensity fatty marrow is seen by the third decade of life **(Figs. 3A and B)**.

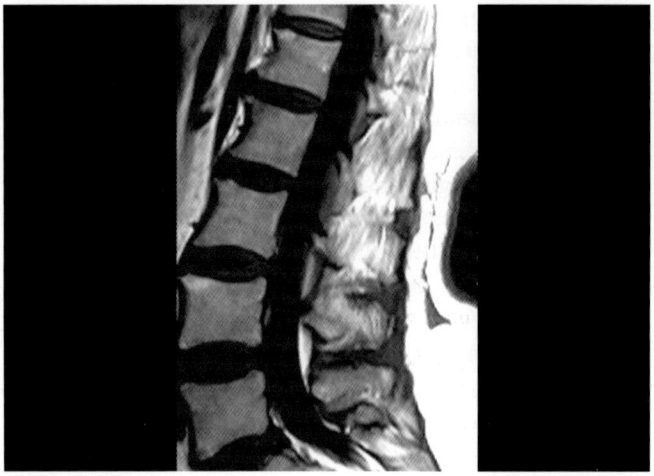

Fig. 8: T1W sagittal image of the lumbosacral spine showing normal signal intensity of the vertebrae which is greater than the adjacent intervertebral disks.

IMAGING OF BONE MARROW DISORDERS

Non-neoplastic hematologic conditions and neoplastic conditions affecting the bone marrow are disease processes that affect the marrow and can be broadly categorized as follows, based on the MRI pattern.

- Reconversion of fatty marrow to hematopoietic marrow due to hyperplasia
- Marrow infiltration or replacement with regular or malignant cells
- Depletion of hematopoietic marrow
- Depletion of myeloid elements with fibrosis
- Deposition of metabolic products
- Sequelae of bone marrow transplant.

Reconversion of Fatty Marrow to Hematopoietic Marrow

Reconversion of fatty marrow to hematopoietic marrow takes place when the demand of the body exceeds the capacity of existing red marrow store. This occurs in hematologic disorders such as severe chronic anemia, thalassemia, sickle cell disease and hereditary spherocytosis. It also occurs in chronic infection, chronic cardiac decompensation, hyperparathyroidism, endurance athletes and heavy smokers.[2,29]

The pattern of reconversion is opposite of that of physiological marrow conversion. Reconversion begins in the axial skeleton in the vertebrae and flat bones of the pelvis and progresses peripherally to the long bones of the extremities, the proximal bones before the distal long bones. Epiphyses are usually spared and reconversion occurs only in the severely affected.[1,2,30]

In sickle cell disease, thalassemia, hemolytic anemia and myeloid hyperplasia, there is reconversion of yellow marrow to hematopoietic marrow. This is because the erythrocytes produced in the bone marrow are either less efficient at transporting oxygen or have a shorter life than normal or there is a combination of both factors.[1,2,31]

Magnetic resonance imaging: Hyperplastic hematopoietic cells lead to a reduction in signal intensity on T1W images although the signal intensity is still equal to or greater than that of muscle. On T2W images the signal intensity may be equal or hypointense to that of fatty marrow. The reconversion tends to be symmetrical.

In sickle cell disease and thalassemia, there is marked expansion of the hematopoietic bone marrow seen as decreased signal intensity on T1W images throughout the femur and axial skeleton **(Figs. 9A to F)**.

Complications of hemolytic anemias due to repeated transfusion leads to excessive iron deposition in the liver, spleen and marrow. The marrow appears hypointense on T2W and GRE images. In severe hemosiderosis the signal also decreases on T1W images. The complete signal loss in the marrow results in a "black marrow".[1,2,31,32]

Medullary infarction is another complication of sickle cell disease. Acute infarct is seen as decreased signal intensity on T1W and increased signal intensity on T2W images. Chronic infarct is seen as fatty marrow centrally with a hypointense rim due to reactive or sclerotic bone.

Grading of reconversion has been done in order to quantify the extent.[32]

Grade I and II indicate a low level of hematopoietic marrow and may be encountered without any apparent cause and sometimes in young obese women. Grades III and IV can be generally attributed to an underlying cause. It is however difficult to differentiate foci of reconverted bone marrow in an atypical location, e.g. diaphysis of long bones from a malignant process and metastases.

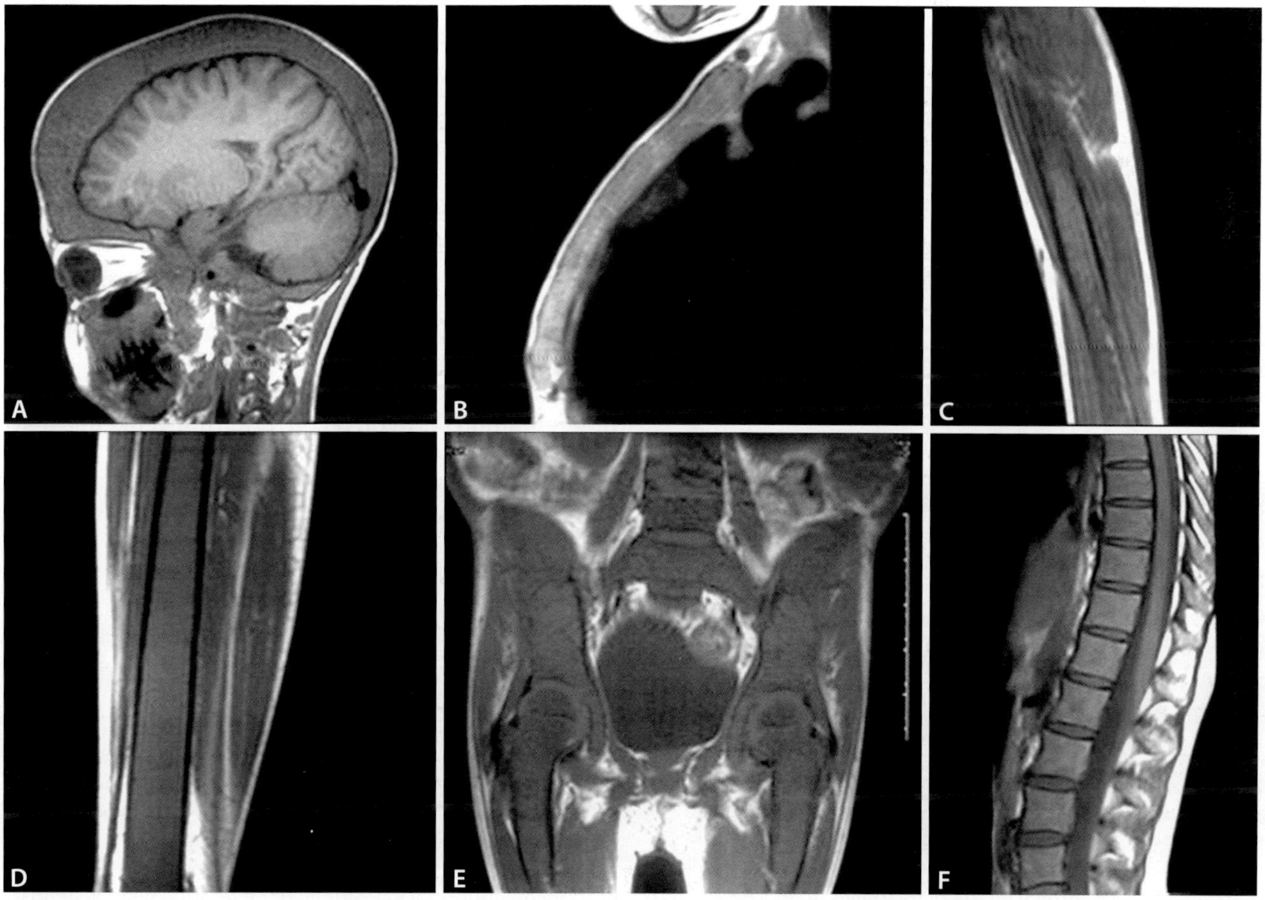

Figs. 9A to F: T1W images of skull (A), sternum (B), humerus (C), femur (D), pelvis (E) and dorsolumbar spine (F) showing medullary expansion and red marrow reconversion. The hematopoietic marrow is seen as decreased signal intensity on these T1W images throughout the axial and appendicular skeleton—Thalassemia.

On SE sequences appearances of reconverted hematopoietic marrow are nonspecific and neoplastic process may appear similar. Differentiating criteria narrowing the differential diagnosis are tabulated in **Table 1**.[1,2,31,32]

Marrow Replacement or Infiltration

Marrow replacement or infiltration may be due to neoplastic diseases, such as leukemia, lymphoma, metastasis and inflammation. The understanding of the location of infiltrative and metastatic lesion is important. Distally occurring metastases in the sites of yellow marrow suggest extensive red marrow involvement or replacement in proximal sites. The location of tumors primary to the red marrow is dependent on the age of the patient.[1,33]

Leukemias

Leukemias are neoplasms of the hematopoietic stem cells and are characterized by diffuse replacement of the bone marrow by neoplastic cells. Leukemia comprises one-third of all malignancies in childhood and acute lymphatic leukemia is the most common.

Table 1: Differentiating features of reconverted and malignant marrows.

Reconversion marrow	*Malignancy*
Follows the normal pattern of marrow distribution and is bilaterally symmetrical	Asymmetric and geographic
Signal intensity equal to than muscle on STIR and fat-saturated T2W images	Signal intensity more muscle
No cortical break or soft tissue mass	Cortical break with mass
No contrast-enhancement present	Contrast-enhancement present

All leukemias involve accumulation of abnormal cells from the myelocytic or lymphocytic groups in the bone marrow. The red marrow is preferentially infiltrated by leukemic cells. The calvaria, spine, flat bones, proximal end of the long bones and subsequently the appendicular skeleton is involved **(Figs. 10A to C)**.

Magnetic resonance imaging: In acute lymphatic leukemias, the immature blast cells accumulate rapidly leading to a diffuse decrease in signal intensity on T1W images **(Fig. 11A)**. On T2W images the signal intensity remains unchanged **(Fig. 11B)** or increases, because of the high water content of leukemic cells **(Figs. 12A and B)**. The tumor deposits are best visualized when the surrounding marrow contains a large number of fat cells.[1,2,33,34]

Bone marrow necrosis (BMN) is an unusual entity that has been reported to occur in close association with malignancy, particularly acute lymphocytic leukemia. Bone marrow necrosis is characterized by a loss of myeloid tissue and marrow fat without trabecular destruction which is unlike a vascular necrosis. About 91% of patients have malignancy, with acute lymphocytic leukemia representing 18% of cases.[35] MR findings of BMN are similar to those of avascular necrosis but are more diffuse and involve the axial skeleton without vertebral collapse. AVN involves the periarticular locations and may progress to vertebral fracture.

Chronic Leukemias

In chronic leukemias there is massive overproduction of cells with limited capacity for differentiation and function.

Magnetic resonance imaging: The changes are most profound in chronic myeloid leukemia. The general pattern of involvement is diffuse but may be multifocal when differentiation between reconverted and leukemic marrow

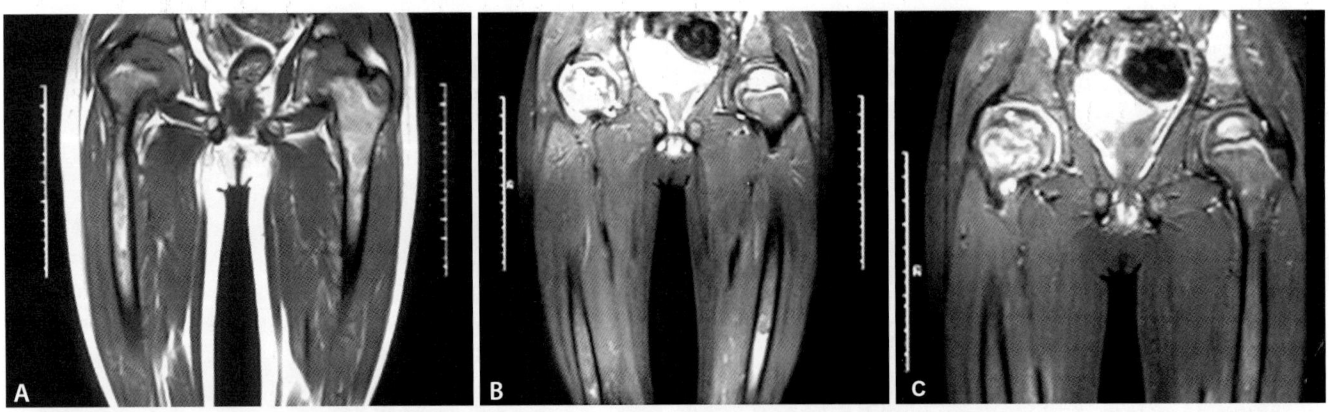

Figs. 10A to C: T1W coronal image of the pelvis (A) in a 5-year-old child showing abnormal low-signal in the femoral head instead of the high-signal fat normally seen at this age. Few foci of abnormal signal are also seen in the femoral diaphysis and iliac blades. STIR coronal images of the pelvis (B and C) show these foci in the femoral head, diaphysis and iliac blades to be high-signal (higher than muscle) which is abnormal—Leukemic infiltration of marrow.

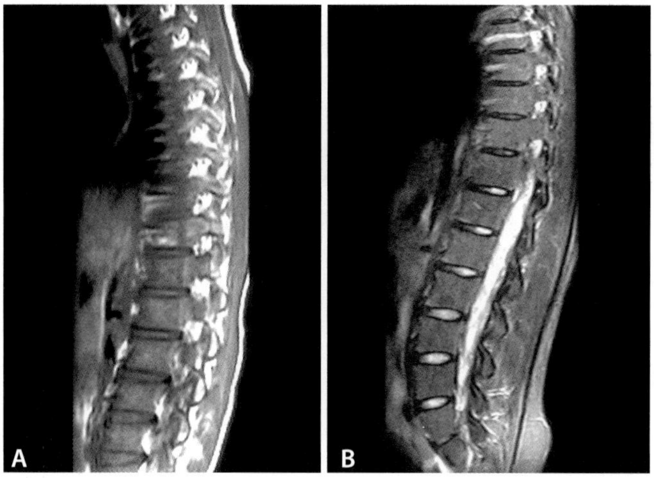

Figs. 11A and B: T1W sagittal image of the dorsolumbar spine (A) showing diffuse abnormal signal in the vertebrae, the signal being lower than the adjacent intervertebral disks; T2W sagittal image (B) showing no increase in signal—This is the typical appearance of most leukemias on T2W sequence.

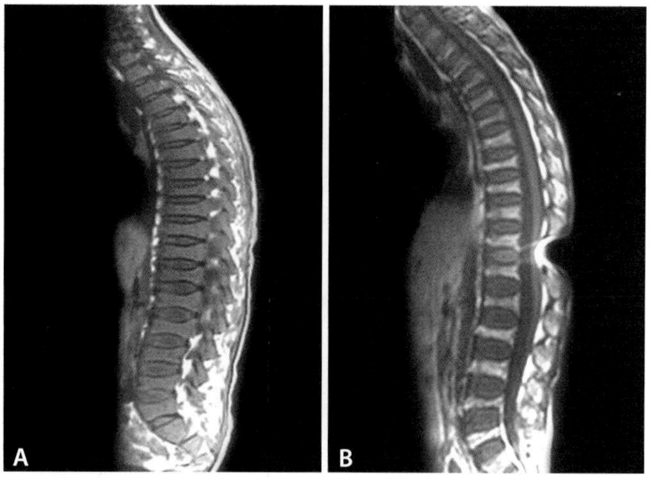

Figs. 12A and B: T1W images of the spine in a case of ALL showing a diffuse low signal of the vertebral bodies in the active stage. The vertebrae also show reduced height (A). In the stage of remission (B) the vertebral bodies show a replacement of the marrow with fat.

may not be possible even with the use of differences in T1 relaxation times. Gradient echo and STIR sequences have a higher rate of detection as lesions appear hyperintense relative to normal marrow **(Figs. 13A to D)**.[36]

Lymphomas

Lymphomas are a heterogeneous group of tumors of the lymphoid tissue which can arise anywhere in the body. Marrow involvement is more common in non-Hodgkin's lymphoma (NHL) while Hodgkin's disease primarily involves the lymph nodes. Infiltration of bone marrow is found in 5–15% of patients with Hodgkin's and 20 to 40% of patients with non Hodgkin's disease. Extranodal involvement of the bone marrow indicates a poor prognosis.

In Hodgkin's lymphoma marrow involvement is detected more often with MR than with marrow biopsy. In low-grade NHL the involvement is diffuse and biopsy is superior **(Figs. 14A to C)**. In high-grade lymphomas the involvement is more focal and MRI is more efficient.

Magnetic resonance imaging: In both types of lymphoma the marrow deposits are nodular in contrast to leukemias. These appear as focal areas of decreased signal intensity of T1W images and increased signal intensity on GRE and STIR images. These findings are not specific and may be seen with metastasis as well as in inflammatory conditions. The nodular nature of lymphomatous marrow deposits allows MR mapping to select the site of biopsy because blind bone marrow biopsy may give false-negative results.[37,38] A soft tissue mass around an apparent intact cortical bone raises concern for lymphoma, though it may be found in small cell malignancies also **(Figs. 15A to E)**.

Metastasis

Metastatic infiltration of the marrow occurs by haematogenous spread. The hematopoietic marrow is predominantly affected because of its rich vascular supply. The most common metastasis in children are from neuroblastoma, rhabdomyosarcoma and Ewing's sarcoma while in adults they are from the prostate, breast, lung and kidney.

Site: In young children proximal and distal metaphysis of the long bones, flat bones and spine are the areas of vessel rich cellular marrow.

In adolescent and adults the spine, flat bones, proximal humeral and femoral metaphysis are common sites. Remainder of the appendicular skeleton can be involved at any age when there is extensive disease.[3,39]

Magnetic resonance imaging: MR can detect intramedullary lesions not visible on plain films and before any osteoblastic reaction is detected on the bone scan. With newer coils and sequences the whole skeleton can be studied. Whole body MRI is very sensitive in detecting metastases and has a superior sensitivity compared to bone and bone marrow scintigraphy. T1W SE sequences display fat and water and metastasis usually have a lower signal as compared to water on this sequence **(Figs. 16A to C)**. They are easily visualized in yellow marrow but barely seen in red marrow. A homogeneous, fat signal rules out metastases and this sequence may be sufficient.

On T2W fat saturation and STIR images, metastasis are relatively hyperintense to normal marrow which indicates increased water content due to hypercellularity. The STIR

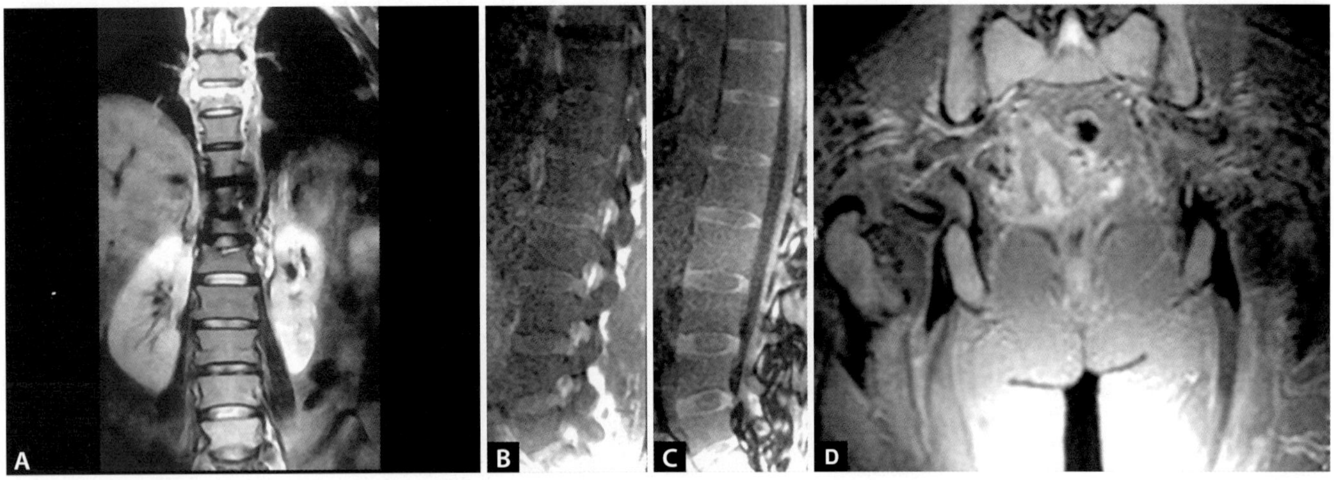

Figs. 13A to D: STIR coronal image of the spine (A) showing diffuse marrow infiltration seen as high-signal intensity in the vertebrae (higher signal than adjacent muscle). In phase (B) and opposed phase (C) images showing a brighter signal of the vertebral marrow on opposed phase images as compared to the in phase images s/o diffuse marrow infiltration. STIR coronal image (D) showing diffuse high-signal in the pelvic bones and the femori—Proven case of chronic myeloid leukemia (CML).

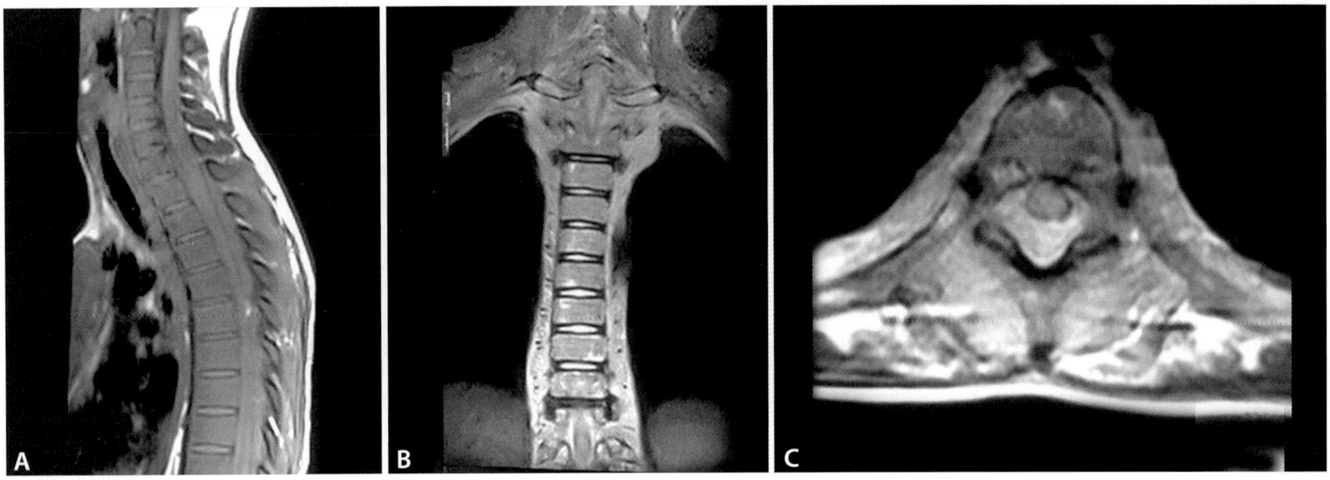

Figs. 14A to C: T1W sagittal image (A), STIR coronal (B) and T2W axial (C) images of the spine showing diffuse marrow signal alteration in the vertebrae seen as low-signal on T1, high-signal on STIR with associated soft tissue masses in B/L paravertebral, paraspinal and dorsal epidural regions—Proven non-Hodgkin's lymphoma.

sequence is used for screening **(Fig. 17)**. Osteoblastic/sclerotic metastasis remain hypointense on all sequences **(Figs. 18A and B)**.

Magnetic resonance has proved helpful in cases of *pathologic fractures* in distinguishing benign and malignant causes.[3,39] The key features that help differentiate between benign and malignant causes of vertebral collapse are tabulated in **Table 2**.

A sign called the "fluid sign" has been described by Baur et al. in cases of osteoporotic vertebral compression fracture. The fluid sign is defined as a focal or triangular area of strong hyperintensity in the vertebral body because of acute collapse. They stated that the "fluid sign" can be used as an additional sign of osteoporotic vertebral compression fractures although tumor cannot be excluded.[40]

Diffusion images provide excellent distinction as the signal of metastasis is higher and that of osteoporotic collapse is lower than normal marrow. In malignant acute vertebral fracture, there is replacement of the fat marrow cells in the vertebral bodies by an accumulation of tumor cells. Signal enhancement in tumor masses on T2W images reflects mainly intracellular water. The diffusion of water molecules inside the tumor cells is restricted resulting in signal hyperintensity on DW images. The apparent diffusion coefficient (ADC) of malignant vertebral body

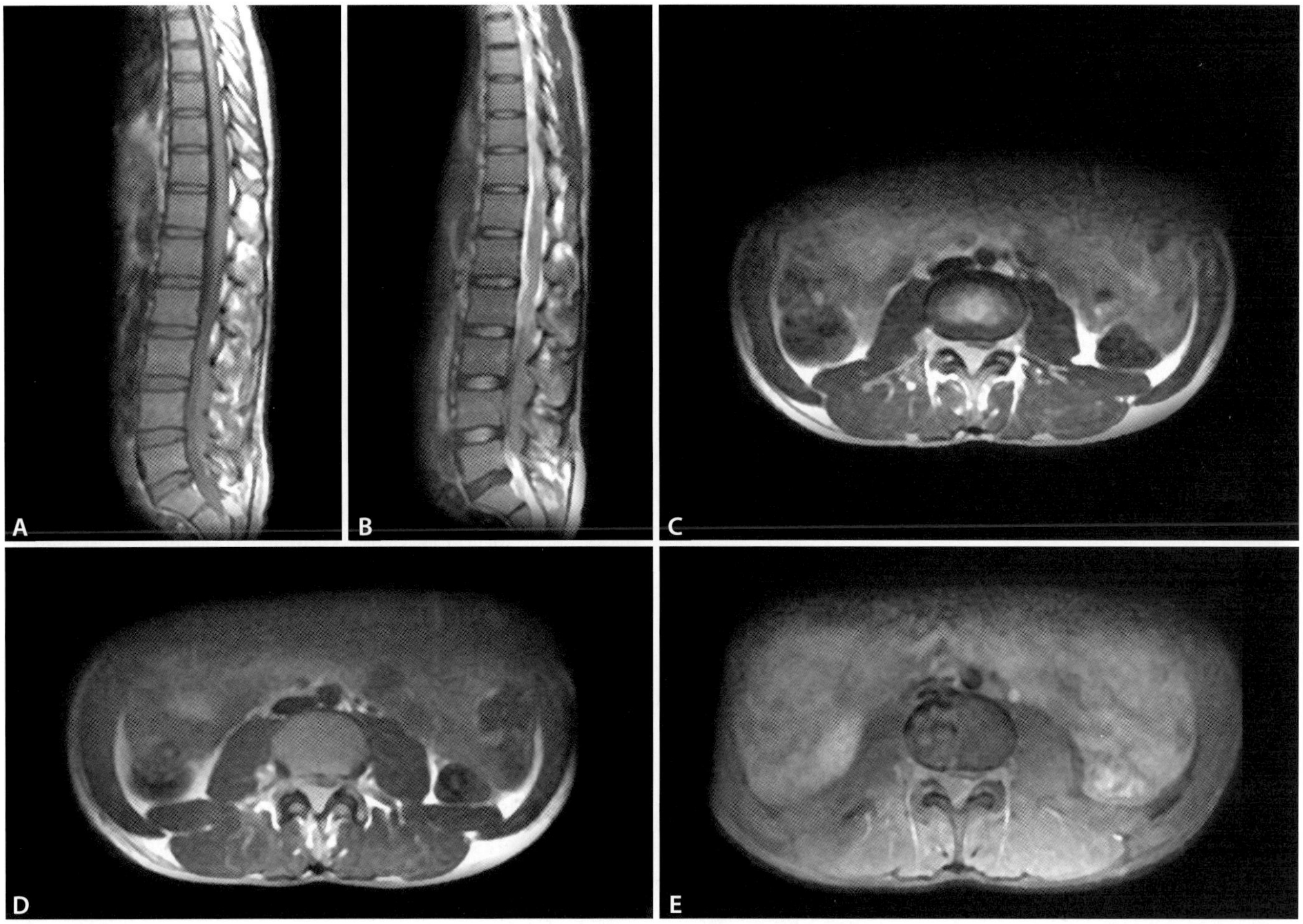

Figs. 15A to E: T1W sagittal (A), T2W sagittal (B) and T2W axial (C and D) MR images of the lumbosacral spine showing an epidural soft tissue mass hypointense on T1W and isointense to the cord on T2W images encasing the cauda equina nerve roots with extension into the neural foramina and consequent widening of the same. Postcontrast axial T1W image (E) shows minimal enhancement. No evidence of cortical destruction of the bone seen—Non-Hodgkin's lymphoma.

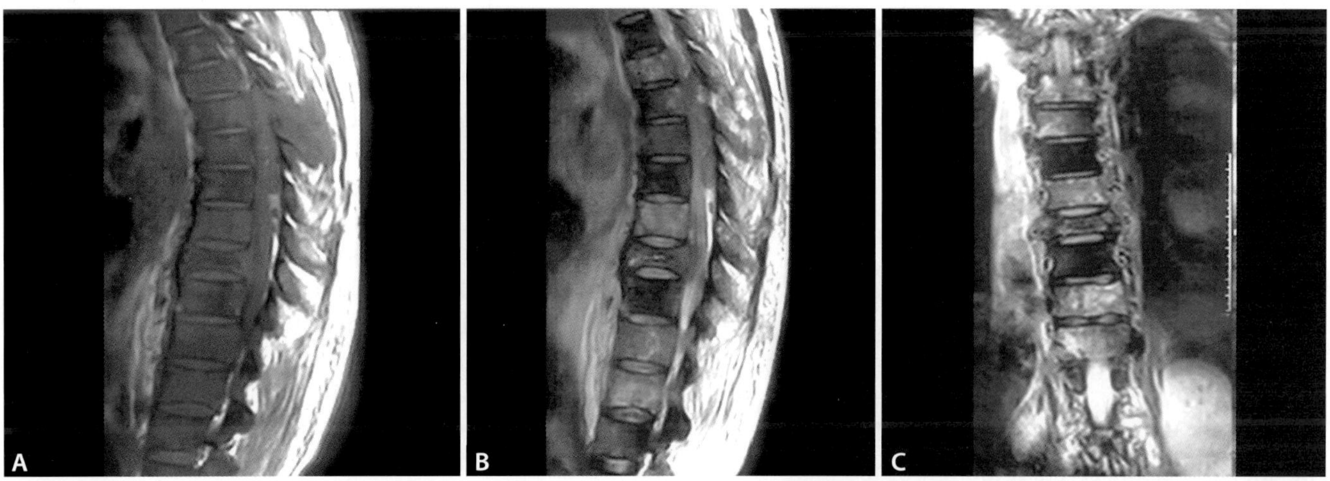

Figs. 16A to C: Sagittal T1W (A), sagittal T2W (B) and STIR coronal (C) images of the spine showing multiple areas of signal alteration involving the vertebrae and posterior elements with associated soft tissue mass and collapse of D9 vertebra—Metastases in a case of CA breast.

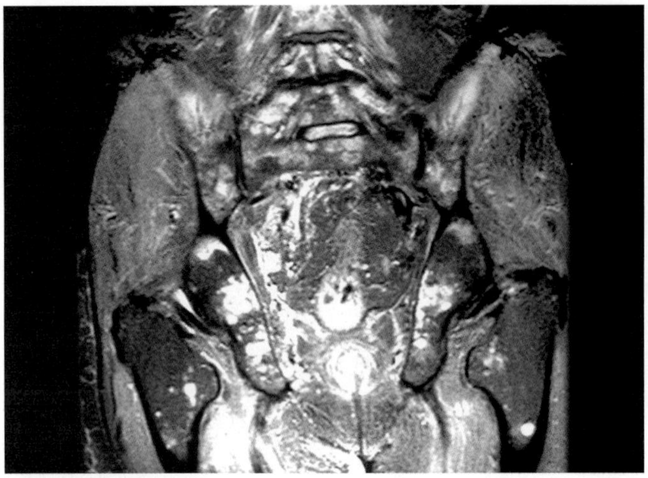

Fig. 17: STIR coronal image of the pelvis showing multiple round to oval hyperintense foci studded in the spine, the pelvic bones, B/L femori—Metastases.

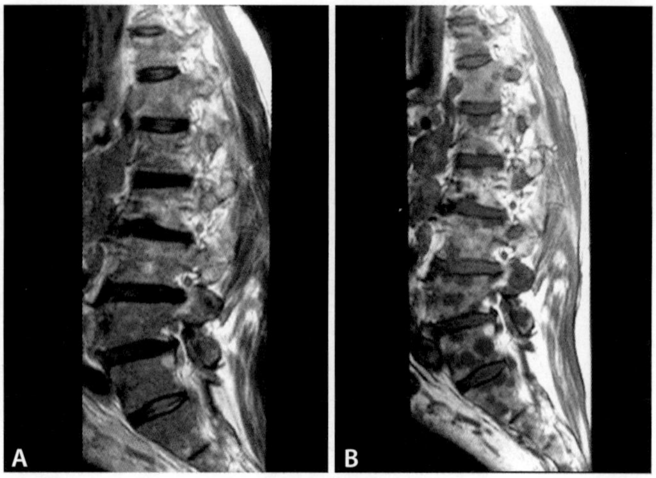

Figs. 18A and B: T1W sagittal (A) and T2W sagittal (B) MR images in a patient with carcinoma prostate showing multiple round hypointense foci on T1W which remain hypointense to isointense on T2W images—Sclerotic metastases.

Table 2: Differentiating features of benign and malignant vertebral collapse.

Benign vertebral collapse (Figs. 19A and B)	*Malignant vertebral collapse (Figs. 20A and B)*
Normal signal intensity in non-fractured vertebrae	Abnormal signal intensity in other non-fractured vertebrae
Abnormal signal intensity parallels fracture	Abnormal signal intensity of entire fractured vertebra
Flat posterior border of fractured vertebra	Convex posterior border of fractured vertebra
Other vertebral deformities with normal signal intensity	No vertebral deformities with normal signal intensity
Rare paravertebral mass	Occasional paravertebral mass
Abnormal signal intensity stabilizes with time	Progresses to destruction

fractures is more than the normal vertebral bodies. Benign acute fractures have an increased amount of water in the interstitial space thus increasing water mobility.[13,14,41] In the presence of diffusion sensitizing gradients these characteristics result in lower signal attenuation compared with stronger dephasing of more mobile extracellular water with signal attenuation. Therefore, more restricted diffusion is present in malignant compression fractures with packed tumor cells than in benign compression fractures with more mobile water in the extracellular volume fraction. Simple qualitative analysis of data from different diffusion weighted images may raise the question whether T2 shine through effect contributes to the appearance observed. A too low or too high "b"value in diffusion weighted imaging can fail to differentiate between benign and malignant etiologies. It has been concluded in several studies that using a "b" value of 300 s/mm^2 with a single shot echoplanar imaging sequence may be useful in differentiating metastatic tumor infiltration from benign fracture edema of the spine.[42,43] Quantification of diffusion in abnormal vertebra using ADC value is helpful in differentiating malignant and benign collapse. Apparent diffusion coefficients (ADC) are significantly lower in metastatic disease than in benign bone marrow edema. Bone marrow cellularity can also be assessed by the ADC measurements. The mean ADC for the normal disks and normal bone marrow has been found to be 1.5 $\times 10^{-3}$ and 0.3 $\times 10^{-3}$ mm^2/s respectively. In contrast to the spinal cord, bone marrow has an isotopic diffusion and shows no signs of anisotropy. In several studies normal bone marrow has been found to have an ADC value of <0.5 $\times 10^{-3}$ mm^2/s.[44-46] Higher ADC values were found in benign edema of osteoporotic fractures (1.61 $\times 10^{-3}$) vs neoplastic fractures (0.71 $\times 10^{-3}$) and metastases (0.69 $\times 10^{-3}$).[47]

Metastasis are better demonstrated on opposed phase imaging **(*see* Figs. 4A and B)** chemical shift imaging and on contrast enhanced images.

On gradient-echo sequences the trabecular destruction in metastatic infiltration results in a higher signal intensity than is seen with normal bone. Normal marrow on this sequence produces low-signal intensity because of the combined effects of fat water nulling and magnetic field heterogeneity due to normal trabeculae.[12,41]

Multiple Myeloma and Plasmacytoma

Multiple myeloma and plasmacytoma result in deposits of neoplastic plasma cells throughout the bone marrow which may be secretory monoclonal immunoglobulins or

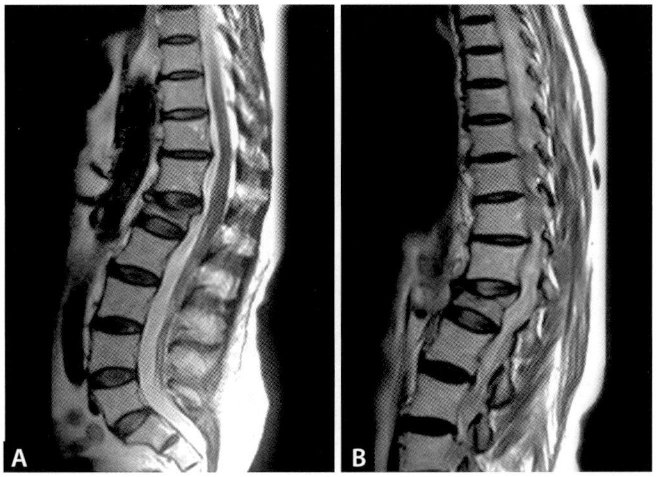

Figs. 19A and B: T1W sagittal (A) and T2W sagittal (B) MR images of the dorsolumbar spine showing collapse of L1 vertebra which is showing high signal along the fracture with flat posterior border of the collapsed vertebra and normal signal in other vertebrae with no paravertebral mass seen—Benign osteoporotic vertebral collapse.

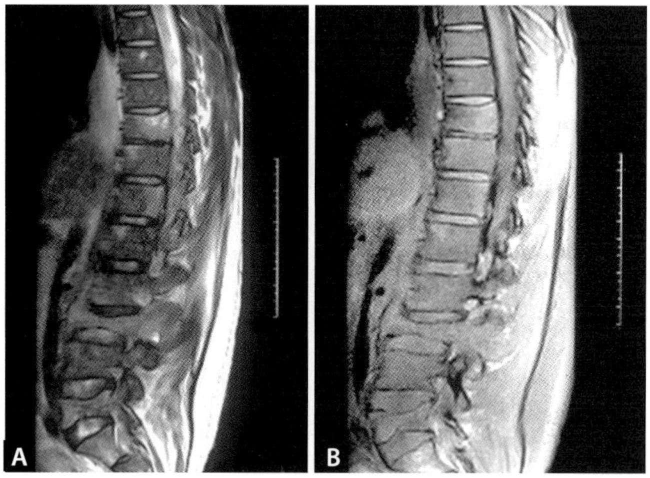

Figs. 20A and B: T2W sagittal (A) and fat-suppressed T2W sagittal (B) images of the dorsolumbar spine showing collapse of L3 vertebra which shows convex posterior border with associated paravertebral mass with signal alteration in several other vertebrae—Malignant vertebral collapse from lymphoma.

they may be nonsecretory. Due to the lack of associated osteoblastic activity nuclear bone scans and radiographs are often normal in multiple myeloma, making MRI the most sensitive imaging method for lesion detection.[48] More marrow lesions are detected with MRI than by a bone scan or plain radiographs. In radiographically diagnosed solitary plasmacytoma MR reveals a more diffuse involvement in one-third patients. This is important as MR involvement of the spinal bone marrow is correlated with prognosis.

Magnetic resonance imaging: The pattern may be focal, multifocal or diffuse. These are seen as multiple foci of low-signal intensity on T1W images and increased signal intensity on T2W and STIR images. The diffuse pattern is due to increased cellularity and decreased signal intensity on T1W images. MR imaging correlates with the clinical severity. Stabler et al have found five infiltration patterns of multiple myehoma on MR imaging. These are: (i) normal appearing marrow with low-grade interstitial infiltration, (ii) focal pattern, (iii) diffuse (iv) mixed focal and diffuse, and (v) salt and pepper appearance. The infiltration patterns correlated with the clinical staging in their study. They concluded that MR is of prognostic value and like laboratory parameters, biopsies and radiographs MR imaging can be a supporting pillar in the staging and planning treatment of patients with multiple myeloma.[49] A greater than 40% increase in signal intensity compared with the baseline after contrast administration correlates with diffuse tumor infiltration of marrow.[48] MR may help confirm the response to therapy. Reconstituted fatty tissue is seen as diffuse or multifocal increase in signal intensity on T1W images **(Figs. 21A to C)** with less contrast enhancement which is regarded as evidence of successful therapy.[3,50]

Waldenstrom Macroglobulinemia

Waldenstrom macroglobulinemia is a dyscrasia marked by diffuse infiltration of the hematopoietic marrow by plasma cells resulting in increased cellularity in the presence of decreased fatty tissue. The cellularity of the lesion determines its MR signal and MRI shows marrow involvement in 90% of cases with clinical evidence of gammopathy.

Magnetic resonance imaging: Normal hematological marrow has a signal intensity equal or increased relative to adjacent muscles and the intervertebral disk appears as a structure of decreased signal intensity. The disease is initially seen as a focal decrease in intensity which becomes diffuse with progression of the disease. The change of bone marrow is associated with increased contrast enhancement which correlates with the cellularity indices and possibly reflects the number of intramedullary plasma cells.

After successful therapy the MR signal intensity of the bone marrow returns to normal. This suggests that MRI may be a noninvasive method of assessing response to therapy.[3,51]

Infections

Osteomyelitis is an infection of medullary bone caused by bacteria and the most common infecting organisms are

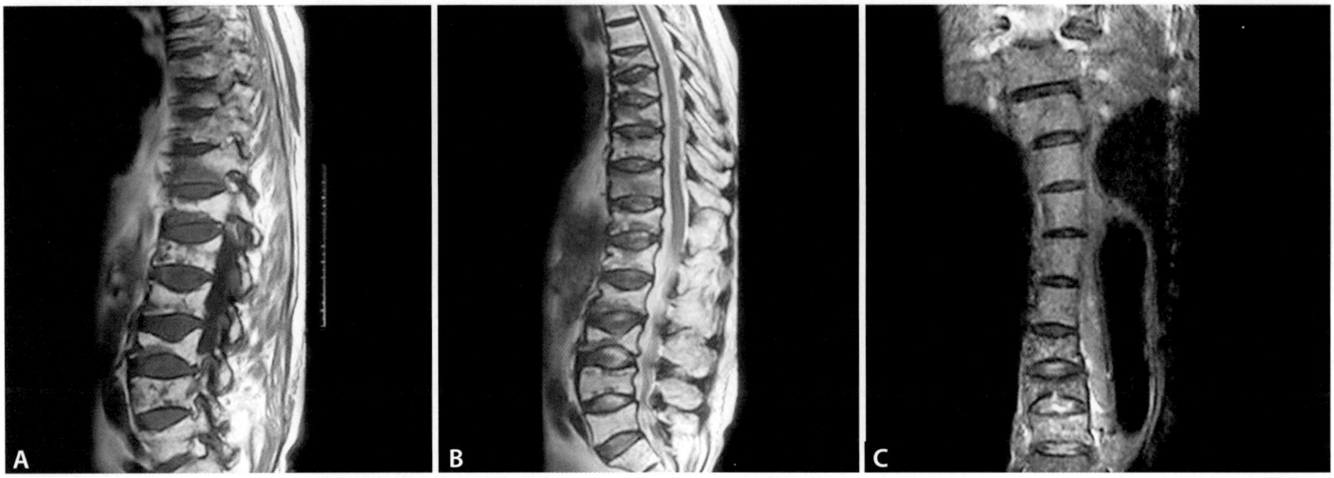

Figs. 21A to C: T1W sagittal (A), T2W sagittal (B) and STIR coronal (C) MR images showing collapse of multiple vertebrae with heterogeneous marrow signal of vertebral bodies predominantly hyperintense on both T1W and T2W images s/o fatty marrow replacement. Areas of active marrow infiltration/edema are noted involving D11 and few other lower dorsal and lumbar vertebrae seen as hypointense on T1W, hyperintense on T2W and STIR images with associated (L) paravertebral mass—Proven case of multiple myeloma on treatment showing fatty marrow replacement with residual active marrow infiltration in few vertebrae.

Staphylococcus aureus, *Streptococcus* and *Pneumococcus*. Less common organisms are *H. influenzae*, *E. coli* and *Pseudomonas*. Occasionally fungi, viruses and parasites are the causative agents.[2,3]

There are three major causes of pathogenesis:

1. Hematogenous, beginning in the metaphysis of long bones, juxtachondral portion of flat bones or spiral end plates. This is commonly seen in infancy and childhood.
2. Direct inoculation due to trauma/surgery. In neonates the intact vascular communication between metaphysis and epiphysis leads to epiphyseal involvement in up to 70%. Between 1 year and skeletal maturity the cartilage provides a barrier to joint involvement except in the hip where the femoral head is intra-articular.
3. In adults the location of infection depends on the mechanism and the presence of medical conditions, such as diabetes, spinal cord injury, etc.[1-3]

Imaging: Routine radiographs are fairly specific in the late stages. Three phase bone scan is very sensitive but specificity is poor in complications.

Magnetic resonance imaging: Osteomyelitis causes marrow infiltration by replacement with inflammatory cells resulting in increased extracellular water or fluid which causes a decreased signal intensity on T1W images and increased signal intensity on T2W fat-saturated images as well as contrast enhanced and STIR images.

Fat-suppressed images increase the specificity and conspicuity of bony changes **(Figs. 22A to D)**. Edema on STIR images and enhancement on contrast administration are the two most common findings in osteomyelitis.

Acute osteomyelitis causes marrow replacement due to infiltration by inflammatory cells, hemorrhage, fibrin, debris and edema. The margins are typically ill-defined against the surrounding marrow.

The sensitivity of the STIR sequence leads to overestimation of infection when there is associated neuropathic disease or septic arthritis. In such cases the contrast enhanced fat-saturated T1W images are important.

Contrast enhancement of the infected bone is intense with a surrounding rim of enhancement while in septic arthritis there may be a small amount of subarticular marrow enhancement. Hence, the location and volume of marrow abnormality allows differentiation of osteomyelitis from sympathetic marrow changes.

Secondary signs of infection, such as cellulitis, cortical disruption, sinus tracts, soft tissue abscesses and periosteal reaction help distinguish osteomyelitis.[2,3,52]

Healed osteomyelitis appears as localized fat replacement within hematopoietic marrow.

Chronic osteomyelitis exhibits the same signal pattern as acute osteomyelitis but the foci are surrounded by a sclerotic rim seen as a signal void which clearly delineates the extent of the lesion. Sequestrated bone appears as a signal void while infarct is seen as "double line" with associated muscle infarction.

Intraosseous abscess may be seen in chronic infections following surgery or trauma. In the acute stage there is an increased signal intensity on STIR and T2W

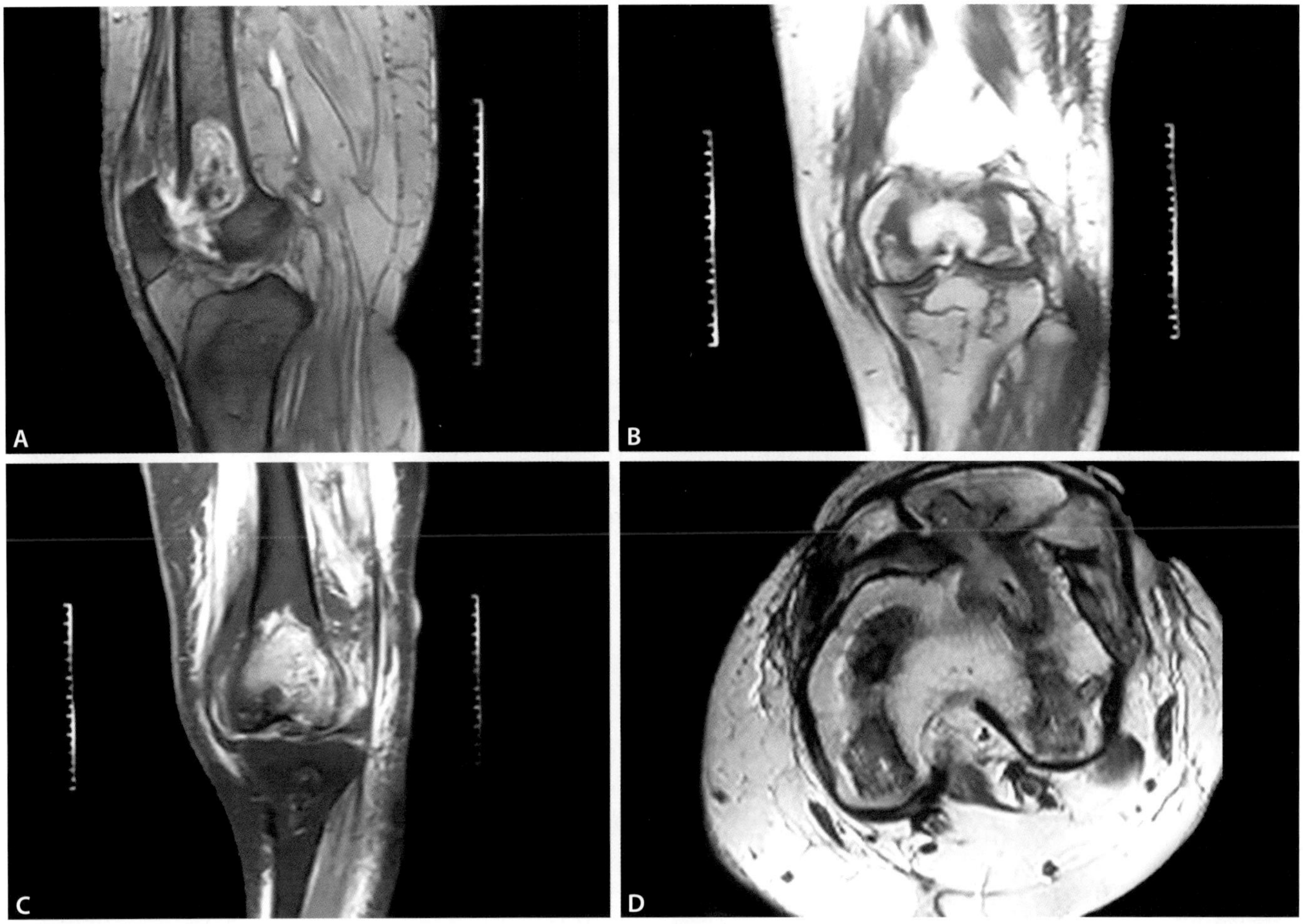

Figs. 22A to D: Fat-suppressed sagittal (A), T1W coronal (B), STIR coronal (C) and T2W axial (D) MR images of the knee showing an area of marrow signal alteration in the metadiaphyseal region of lower femur. Signal alteration is also seen in patella and upper end tibia. Cortical destruction with cloacae formation seen in anterior aspect of femur, posterior aspect of patella, joint effusion with edema seen in muscles—Chronic osteomyelitis of femur with intramedullary abscess and associated infective arthritis.

images. A low-signal intensity rim is seen on all sequences secondary to fibrosis or reactive bone formation.[52,53]

Myeloid Depletion

Myeloid depletion refers to the loss of hematopoietic tissue. This is also known as *aplastic anemia*. Aplastic anemia is a panmyelopathy thought to result from suppression of the multipotent myeloid cells with decrease in the erythroid, myeloid and megaloid precursors. The myeloid depletion manifests as cytopenia of the erythrocytes, leukocytes and thrombocytes. There is a resultant decrease in the cellularity due to decrease in the hematopoietic marrow which is replaced by fatty marrow.

Causes have not been identified but provoking factors are viral infections, drugs, toxic substances, hepatitis and unknown causes.[3,54]

Magnetic resonance imaging: There is a homogeneous increase in signal intensity in the hematopoietic marrow on T1W and T2W images approaching the signal intensity of fat **(Figs. 23A and B)**. Chemical shift imaging may help in differentiation of changes in vertebral marrow due to replacement of hematopoietic marrow from vertebral marrow changes associated with physiologic conversion to fatty marrow with associated degenerative changes **(Figs. 24A to C)**.

After treatment, recovering marrow is seen as areas of decreased signal intensity within the background of fatty marrow. The hematopoietically active cell nests return mainly in the marrow space of the vertebral body.[3,54]

Depletion of Myeloid Elements with Fibrosis

Myelofibrosis is characterized by replacement of normal marrow cells by fibrotic tissue. Primary myelofibrosis is rare in children and is generally seen post-chemotherapy or radiation therapy for leukemia, lymphoma or metastasis.

In adults myeloproliferative disorders, metastasis, leukemia, lymphoma, tuberculosis and toxins are the varied causes.[3,55]

In myelofibrosis polyclonal activation of fibroblasts occurs which secrete collagen, causing fibrosis. This results in extramedullary hematopoiesis in liver and spleen and immature blood cells in the peripheral blood. In myelofibrosis the predominant radiographic feature is osteosclerosis that may be found in 30–70% of the patients and it is most evident in the bones of the axial skeleton in particular spine and pelvis.

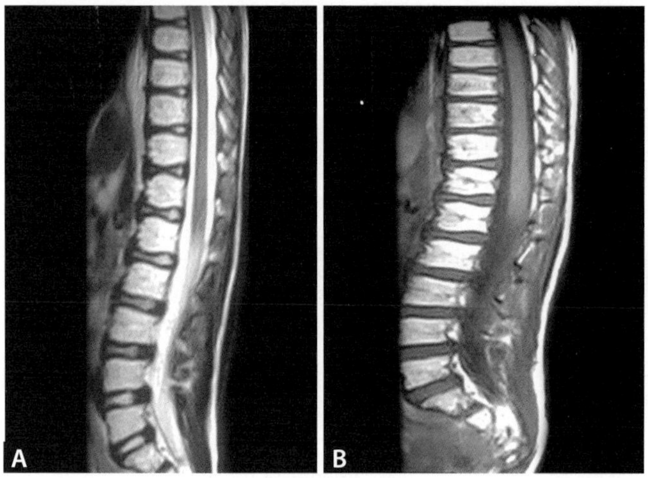

Figs. 23A and B: Sagittal T1W (A) and sagittal T2W (B) MR images of the dorsolumbar spine showing high-signal of the vertebral marrow on both T1W and T2W images s/o fatty marrow—Aplastic anemia.

Magnetic resonance imaging: MRI is very sensitive in assessing the extent of the disease and shows low-signal intensity changes both in T1 and T2 weighted images due to replacement of marrow fat by collagen and reticulin fibers **(Figs. 25A to C)**. On STIR images the signal intensity is greater than muscle.

Differential Diagnosis of Gaucher's Disease and Hemosiderosis

In Gaucher's disease, associated bone infarcts may be present while in hemosiderosis, excessive iron deposition can cause almost a complete signal loss resulting in a "black marrow".[54,55]

Deposition of Metabolic Products

Gaucher's disease is the most common lysosomal storage disorder which is caused by a genetic deficiency of glucosylceramide in macrophages leading to an increase in glucocerebrosidase with deposition in the brain, spleen, liver and bone marrow. Eighty percent of patients have skeletal abnormalities.

Magnetic resonance imaging can be used in the early diagnosis of Gaucher's disease and for demonstrating improvement after enzyme therapy. The severity of the change depends on the extent to which medullary cavity is infiltrated by Gaucher cells. Accumulation of these cells leads to osteoporosis, localized destruction and ischemic necrosis.

Infiltration of the marrow with Gaucher cells increases the T1 relaxation time and shortens the T2 relaxation time causing a low-signal intensity of the affected marrow on

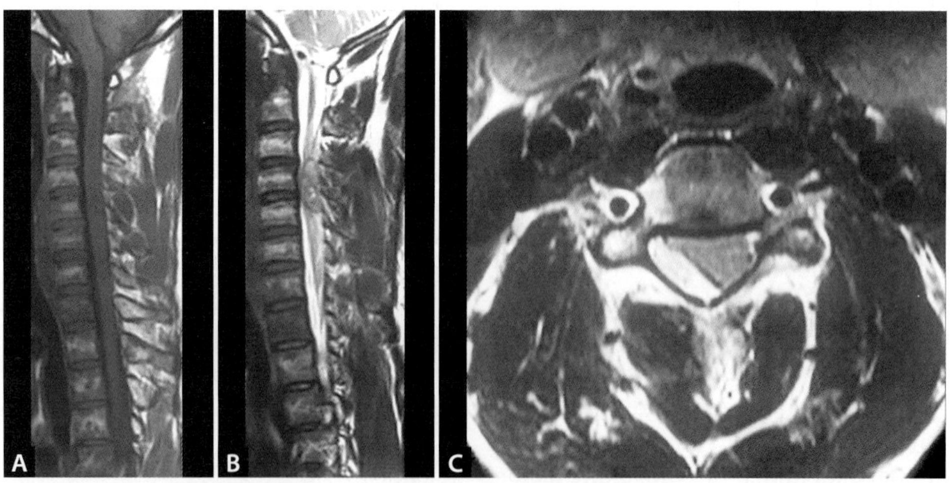

Figs. 24A to C: T1W sagittal (A) and T2W sagittal (B) MR images of the cervicodorsal spine showing replacement of the normal marrow with the high signal foci of fatty marrow. T2W axial (C) shows an epidural hematoma causing compression and displacement of the spinal cord at C3–C4 vertebral level—Aplastic anemia.

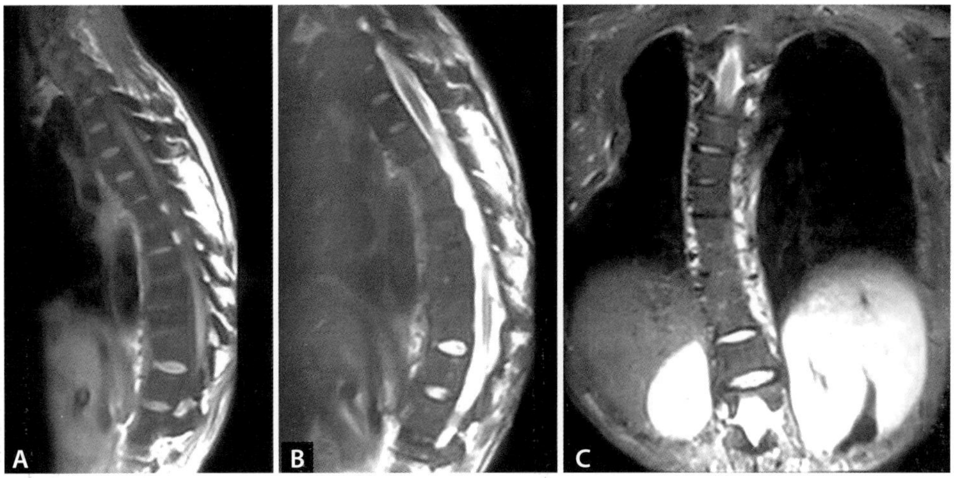

Figs. 25A to C: T1W sagittal (A), T2W sagittal (B) and STIR coronal (C) images showing a diffuse low-signal in all the vertebral bodies—Myelofibrosis.

both T1W and T2W images. These appearances are similar to those in other infiltrative processes but the low-signal intensity on T2W images allows differentiation from tumor processes. This low-signal intensity is due to fibrosis.[1,2,56] Bone marrow infiltration starts proximal and increasingly affects more peripheral areas of the appendicular skeleton. Bone marrow infarction is also a typical finding related to Gaucher's disease and is characterized by a serpinginous pattern with a bright signal in fat-saturated T2W or STIR sequences.

Iron overload (Hemosiderosis): This disorder can be primary or secondary following multiple transfusions and hemolytic anemias.

Magnetic resonance imaging: The iron deposition can be patchy or uniform in distribution involving the pelvis, spine and metaphysis or diaphysis of long bones. Excessive iron deposition can cause nearly a complete signal loss resulting in a "black marrow".[31,32,37]

MR IMAGING OF THERAPY-INDUCED CHANGES OF BONE MARROW

Post-therapy alteration can be observed as early as 2 weeks after treatment especially on STIR imaging. The early findings are marrow edema and necrosis seen as increased signal intensity.

Between 3 and 6 weeks, the signal becomes heterogeneous due to fat predominance best seen on T1W SE images. Late changes occur after 6 weeks to 14 months. These may be of two types:

1. Homogeneous high-signal pattern on T1W images due to fatty replacement.
2. Band like pattern of peripheral intermediate signal intensity due to red marrow around a central zone of high-signal intensity due to fatty marrow.

Postradiation changes are dose related and preferentially affect the hematopoietic marrow. Initial changes are edema and necrosis followed by compensatory proliferation and hypertrophy of the fat cells **(Fig. 26)**.

Doses <2 Gy induce no visible changes on T1W images. Doses between 8 and 15 Gy produce characteristic vertebral changes. A distinct horizontal demarcation between normal and damaged marrow is often seen and the visualization of changes depends on the magnetic field strength.[33,34,57]

Radiation treatment-induced complications in marrow include osteonecrosis, AVN, fractures, and radiation-induced neoplasm, and depend on factors, such as radiation dose, patient age, size of the radiation field, and beam energy. Cell death and devascularization of bone occur after doses exceeding 5000 cGy.[58] These events impair hematopoietic regeneration and normal bone formation. Osteonecrosis/AVN is localized within the radiation portal and usually is diagnosed years after RT. Typical locations include the mandible, clavicle, humeral head, rib and femur. On MRI, the presence of high-signal intensity inside a low-intensity peripheral rim on T2-weighted images (the "double line" sign) is specific for diagnosis of AVN. Fractures of irradiated bones, such as sacral insufficiency fractures or collapsed vertebrae, can occur within a few months of RT and may present diagnostic challenges by mimicking osseous metastases. Correct diagnosis is imperative to avoid unnecessary biopsies and to guide proper clinical management.

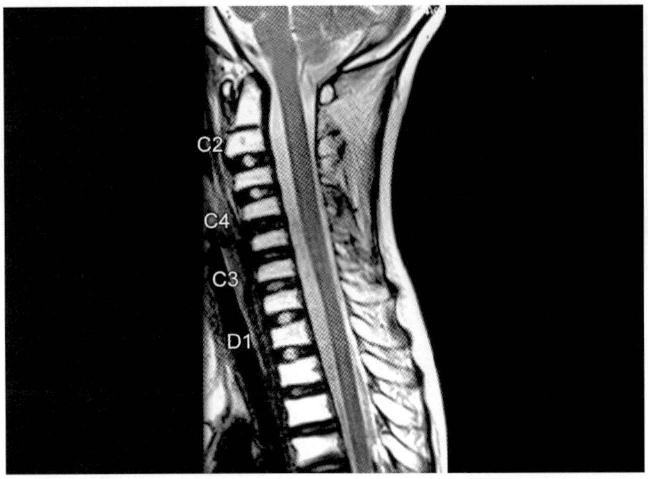

Fig. 26: T2W sagittal MR images of the cervical spine in a case of carcinoma breast (postradiation) revealing increased signal in the vertebral marrow s/o fatty replacement.

In patients with osteoporosis (such as postmenopausal women), fracture risk after RT is substantially increased. Multiple fractures may develop within 24 months. The incidence of RT-induced sacral fractures seen on MRI is 20–80%. The fracture lines usually parallel to the sacroiliac joints and show ill-defined margins in all sequences. Magnetic resonance imaging may demonstrate the fractures earlier than CT by revealing surrounding edema, before fracture lines become visible on CT.

CHANGES IN MARROW SIGNAL DUE TO CHEMOTHERAPY

Upon initiation of chemotherapy, marrow signal becomes hypointense on T1-weighted images and hyperintense in fat-suppressed T2-weighted and STIR images, reflecting marrow congestion. About 3–4 weeks into chemotherapy, reconversion from fatty marrow to hematopoietic marrow can occur, and is readily recognized as it usually occurs in the reverse sequence of marrow conversion, both bilaterally and symmetrically. After chemotherapy, depletion of hematopoietic marrow may result in predominantly fatty marrow.

Several drugs used in oncology patients can cause various side effects in immature and mature skeletons, some of which can be misdiagnosed as tumors on MRI. Osteopenia, fractures, osteonecrosis, and AVN are well-known complications of prolonged administration of steroids in patients of all ages. In children, methotrexate can cause osteopenia, severe bone pain and metaphyseal insufficiency fracture (described as methotrexate osteopathy). In breast cancer treatment, both hormonal therapy with aromatase inhibitors in postmenopausal women and chemotherapy-induced ovarian failure in premenopausal women can cause significant loss of bone mass, increasing the risk of fractures.

Bisphosphonates (BP) are osteoclast inhibitors that can be used for the treatment of bone loss and bone pain in metastatic disease and multiple myeloma. Cases of osteonecrosis of the jaw in patients treated with bisphosphonates have been recently and increasingly reported.[58] Oversuppression of bone turnover and antiangiogenic effects of bisphosphonates are considered to be contributing factors.

The effects of granulocyte-colony stimulating factor (G-CSF) in bone marrow are often encountered in MRI, as G-CSF is increasingly used in conjunction with chemotherapy. G-CSF is an agent used to promote hematopoietic activity (specifically, stimulation of granulocyte cell line) in order to decrease the incidence of chemotherapy-induced neutropenia. Multiple areas of red marrow develop in conjunction with increasing neutrophil counts. However, there is no apparent relationship between the number of treatment courses of G-CSF and the extent of red marrow reconversion. The signal characteristics of the changes in marrow are similar to those of red marrow in both pediatric and adult patients. Although, this drug-induced red marrow can simulate marrow disease on MRI, combined knowledge of the effects of G-CSF on marrow and the clinical status of individual patients can help avoid misdiagnosing this treatment-related effect as an interval development of metastases.[58]

NEW THERAPY REGIMENS

Angiogenesis-inhibiting drugs, such as thalidomide to be useful for treating hematologic malignancy depend on neovascularization, and these agents were recently added to some treatment regimens for patients with advanced myeloma. The antiangiogenesis is intended to stop cancer progression by suppressing tumor recruitment of new blood supply. As such, antiangiogenic drugs are generally tumorostatic, not cytotoxic. Thus, a successful therapeutic inhibition of angiogenesis can be expected to slow or stop tumor growth, but not to cause tumor regression or disappearance. Accordingly, MR imaging may show a persistent high bone marrow cellularity under antiangiogenic treatment. Signs of a response to this treatment are rather a delayed, less steep and smaller bone marrow enhancement after intravenous administration of small molecular Gd-chelates compared to pretreatment studies.

Treatment effects of various chemotherapeutic regimen on the bone marrow in patients with leukemia and lymphoma can be detected with ^{31}P MR spectroscopy. The treatment induced change in tumor pH with an alkaline shift is related temporally to increases in the phosphodiester/beta-adenosine triphosphate ratio and occurs before alterations in tumor size are documented. The changes in the ^{31}P MR spectral profile cannot only be detected by direct investigations of the bone marrow itself, but also by MR spectroscopy of the serum of the patients. The ^{31}P MR spectral profile of the serum changes in responding patients resemble that of normal serum with typical higher peak intensities as compared to nontreated and nonresponding patients.[58]

BONE MARROW TRANSPLANTATION

After bone marrow transplantation, the evolution of distinct MR signal patterns of the bone marrow has been described. During the first post-transplantation days, the bone marrow shows a decline in signal intensity on T1-weighted images and an increased signal intensity on T2-weighted images, probably due to a treatment-induced edema. Within 3 months from bone marrow transplantation, a characteristic band pattern appears on T1-weighted MR images of the spine. This band consists of a peripheral T1-hypointense zone and a central T1-hyperintense zone. At histologic examination, the peripheral zone corresponded to repopulating hematopoietic marrow and the central zone to marrow fat. This pattern may be seen for several months. Subsequently, the band pattern gradually evolves into homogeneous appearance of the marrow after successful bone marrow transplantation. On late post-transplantation studies, years after bone marrow transplantation, MR shows that the signal intensity of the post-transplant bone marrow is higher as compared to the normal matched controls.[59]

In some patients, residual marrow abnormalities are observed on MR images after bone marrow transplantation and the administration of high dose myeloablative chemotherapy, in the same way that they may occur after conventional chemotherapy and conditioning chemotherapy regimens. For example, sharply defined focal low-signal intensity areas of marrow on T1-weighted images have been reported in patients who are in complete remission after transplantation. Patients with these abnormalities do not have poorer outcome than those with normal post-transplantation MR imaging findings. Spectroscopy, perfusion studies or markers of tumor cell proliferation help to differentiate these residual marrow abnormalities.[58]

FOCAL DISORDERS OF THE BONE MARROW

Marrow Edema

This develops as a result of various stimuli causing increased vascular permeability or hyperperfusion leading to an abnormal expansion of interstitial fluid.

Bone diseases causing edema include trauma, tumor, infection and ischemia.

Imaging features: Radiographic changes, such as osteoporosis, bony destruction or new bone formation are well seen but accompanying marrow edema can only be visualized with MRI. Marrow edema is the first and often the only manifestation of a osseous disease process.

Magnetic resonance imaging: The interstitial fluid accumulation of edema causes an increase in the T1 and T2 relaxation times on SE sequences. T1W images have an excellent negative contrast, i.e. edema is dark, fat is bright and T2W images have an excellent positive contrast, i.e. edema dark, lesions are bright. STIR images have a high-signal intensity for edema with low-signal intensity for normal fat.[2,60]

Ischemia

The causes of avascular necrosis are multifactorial but the radiologic appearances are similar. Vascular obstruction occurs in the venous system in the epiphysis of long bones and in small carpal or tarsal bones.

Scintigraphy and MR imaging have been used to demonstrate hyperemia and edema within the marrow. Ischemia may lead to bone infarct or osteonecrosis depending on its severity, size and location.[61]

Osteonecrosis

The fatty marrow in the subchondral region with sparse vascularity is most often affected. Hematopoietic cells die within the first 6 hours of anoxia while osteocytes, osteoblasts and osteoclasts survive up to 48 hours. Fat cells become vulnerable 2–5 days following the insult. An adequate circulation allows repair to begin with a fibrous demarcation of necrotic area. This is usually asymptomatic.

Magnetic resonance imaging: In the early stages when the radiograph is normal, focal subchondral lines of altered signal intensity, low-signal intensity on T1W and high on T2W images due to free water are seen. A "double line" sign consisting of two parallel stripes of low and high-signal indicate irreversibility.[2,62,63]

Bone Infarction

The metadiaphyseal regions of tubular bones regardless of the dominating marrow type is the favored site for infarction. This is due to the vascular anatomy and blood supply of tubular bones. Predisposing conditions are sickle cell disease, hyperglobulinemia and Gaucher's disease. In 20% cases of sickle cell disease the infarcts may be multiple.

Magnetic resonance imaging: In the early stage there is decreased signal intensity on T1W and increased signal intensity on T2W images due to accompanying edema. These changes are linear or geographical. When scalloped in outline they are painful.

Infarcts in the late stages are generally calcified seen as decreased signal intensity on all sequences. Due to the partial blood supply to the peripheral marrow cavity, the infarct exhibits a peripheral line due to a subcortical double contour giving the "bone in bone" appearance. Infarcts may become infected and cause osteomyelitis.[62,63]

Transient Osteoporosis

Transient osteoporosis or transient marrow edema syndrome most often involves the hip joint. This is probably an ischemic process that induces marrow edema in the proximal femur with extension into the acetabulum.

Magnetic resonance imaging: MR changes of subchondral effusion and edema are accompanied by a positive bone scan.

Trauma

Direct or indirect trauma can involve the bone marrow and mild marrow changes have been termed as bone bruises **(Fig. 27)**. These may be due to edema, blood and hyperemia.

Magnetic resonance imaging: Conventional radiographs are generally normal. On MR these are seen as geographic areas of decreased signal intensity on T1W and increased signal intensity on T2W images. Bone bruises are most often seen in the juxta-articular and subchondral areas of the distal femur and proximal tibia in association with ligamentous and meniscal injuries. Bone bruises resolve within 6–9 weeks.[60,61,63]

Occult Fractures

These are trabecular bone microfractures which may be diagnosed on MR in the absence of conventional radiographic signs.

Magnetic resonance imaging: The use of STIR or a fat suppressed T2W sequence is helpful for screening for an occult fracture. These subchondral occult fractures are well seen as a linear signal void on all sequences surrounded by an ill-defined band of decreased signal intensity on T1W and increased signal intensity on T2W images[64] **(Figs. 28A and B)**.

Avulsion Fracture

Avulsion fracture in the juxta-articular region is a special type of occult fracture which may be missed on conventional radiography but is well visualized on MR imaging.

Stress Fracture

Stress fractures are caused by an imbalance between the strength of the bone and the stress applied. These may be seen after marching, jogging, chronic cough, etc.[65]

Imaging: Conventional radiographs show a juxtacortical transverse or oblique sclerotic band with a thin radiolucent line within this band.

Magnetic resonance imaging can visualize the pathophysiologic changes accompanying a stress fracture. This consists of a band like signal void surrounded by marrow edema. The signal void band represents trabecular microfractures and intratrabecular callus formation.

Differentiation of stress fractures from occult intraosseous fractures is difficult. Stress fractures are almost always metaphyseal or diaphyseal while occult fractures are typically subchondral or epiphyseal and have a precipitating cause.

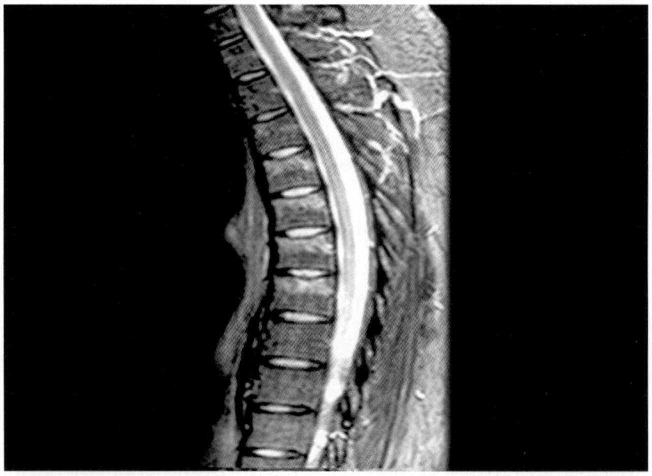

Fig. 27: T2W sagittal MR image of the spine in a case of trauma showing bone marrow edema/contusions in multiple dorsal vertebrae.

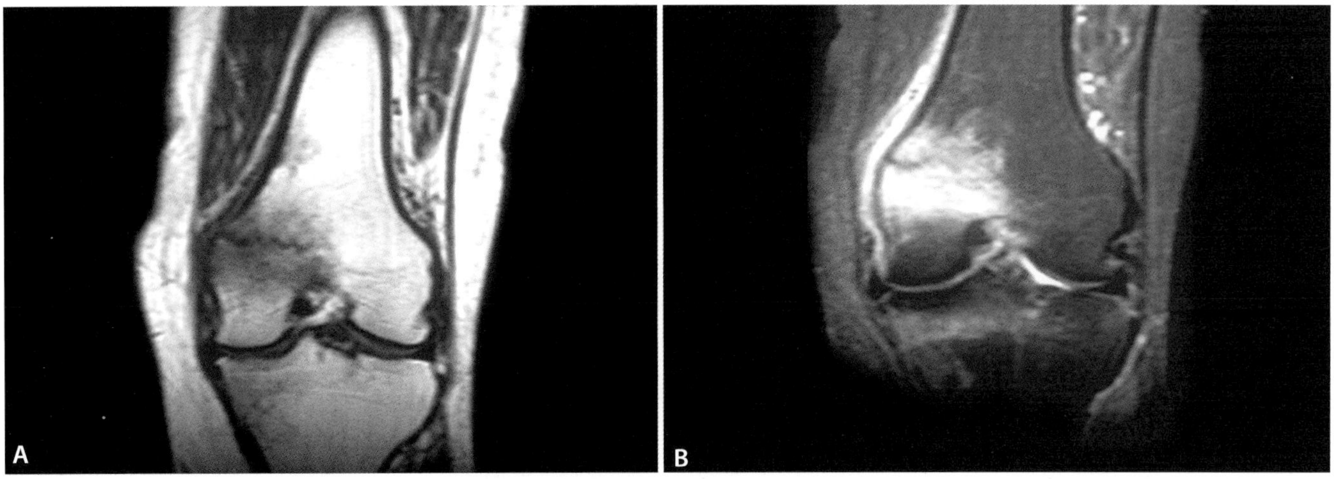

Figs. 28A and B: T1W coronal (A) and STIR coronal (B) MR images of the knee showing a linear fracture line in the medial femoral condyle with surrounding bone marrow edema in a case where X-ray knee was normal—Occult fracture knee.

CONCLUSION

Imaging characteristics of normal bone marrow changes through life and familiarity with these changes is important to correctly approach bone marrow pathology. Neoplastic disease of the bone marrow is a frequent pathology and has different morphologic patterns. A number of bone marrow pathologies are characterized by a depletion of normal hematopoietic bone marrow cells. Storage diseases and hemoglobinopathies have typical bone marrow patterns, which are well visualized with MRI. A number of pathologies go along with increased or decreased vascularity of bone marrow. For standard imaging of bone marrow T1W and STIR sequences are the fundamental sequences. The addition of newer imaging techniques and advances in MR imaging has enabled a better characterization of the various pathologies and helped in narrowing the differential diagnosis.

REFERENCES

1. Moore SG, Bisset GS III, Siegal MJ, et al. Pediatric musculoskeletal MR imaging. Radiology. 1991;179:345-60.
2. Siegel MJ, Luker GD. Bone marrow imaging in children. Magnetic Resonance Imaging Clinics North America. 1996;4:771-96.
3. Vogler JB III, Murphy WA. Bone marrow imaging. Radiology. 1988;168:679-93.
4. Waitches SG, Zanvin JK, Poznanski AK. Sequences and rate of bone marrow conversion in the femora of children as seen on MR imaging: Are accepted standards accurate? AJR. 1994;162:1399-406.
5. Moore DG, Dawson KL. Red and yellow marrow in the femur: Age-related changes in the appearance at MR imaging. Radiology. 1990;175:219-23.
6. Dooms GC, Fischer MR, Hricak H, et al. Bone marrow imaging: Magnetic resonance studies related to age and sex. Radiology. 1985;155:429-32.
7. Taccone A, Oddone M, Dell Acqua AD, et al. MRI "road map' of normal age-related bone marrow: Thorax, pelvis and extremities. Pediatric Radiology. 1995;25:596-606.
8. Dawson KL, Moore SG, Rowland JM. Age-related marrow changes in the pelvis. MR and anatomic findings. Radiology. 1992;183:47-51.
9. Babyn PS, Ranson M, McConville ME. Normal bone marrow: Signal characteristics and fatty conversion. Magnetic Resonance Imaging Clinics North America. 1998;6:473-95.
10. Hanharan CJ, Shah LM. MRI of Spinal Bone Marrow: Part 2, T1-weighted imaging-based differential diagnosis. AJR. 2011;197:1309-21.
11. Jones KM, Unger EC, Granstrom P, et al. Bone marrow imaging using STIR at 0.5 and 1-5T Magnetic Resonance Imaging. 1992;10:169-76.
12. Sebag GH, Moore SG. Effects of trabecular bone on the appearance of marrow in gradient-echo imaging of the appendicular skeleton. Radiology. 1990;174:855-9.
13. Rosen BR, Fleming DM, Kushner DC. Hematologic bone marrow disorders: Quantitative chemical shift MR imaging. Radiology. 1988;169:799-804.
14. Glover GH. Multipoint Dixon technique for water and fat proton and susceptibility imaging. JMRI. 1991;1:521-30.
15. Zajick DC, Morrison WB, Schweitzer ME, et al. Benign and malignant processes: Normal values and differentiation with chemical shift MR imaging in vertebral marrow. Radiology. 2005;237:590-6.
16. Byun WM, Shin SO, Chany Y, et al. Diffusion weighted MR imaging of metastatic disease of the spine: assessment of response to therapy. AJNR. 2002;23:906-12.
17. Enlemann R, Vassollo B, Bongartz G. Musculoskeletal neoplasms with fast low angle shot MR imaging with and without Gd-DTPA. Radiology. 1990;176:489-95.

18. Mahnken AH, Wildberger JE, Adam G, et al. Is there a need for contrast enhanced T1 weighted MRI of the spine after inconspicuous short T inversion recovery imaging? Eur Radiol. 2005;15:1387-92.
19. Chen BB, Hsu CY, Yu CW, et al. Dynamic contrast enhanced MR imaging measurement of vertebral bone marrow perfusion may be indicator of outcome of acute myeloid leukemia patients in remission. Radiology. 2011;258:821-31.
20. Griffith JF, Yeung DKW, Antonio GE, et al. Vertebral bone mineral density, marrow perfusion and fat content in healthy men and men with osteoporosis: dynamic contrast enhanced MR imaging and MR spectroscopy. Radiology. 2005;236(3):945-51.
21. Simon GH, Raatchen HJ, Wendland MF, et al. Ultra small super-paramagnetic iron oxide enhanced MR imaging of normal bone marrow in rodents original research original research. Acad Radiol. 2005;12:1190-7.
22. Paldrup Link HE, Rummeny EJ, Ihssen B, et al. Iron-oxide-enhanced MR imaging of bone marrow in patients with Non-Hodgkin lymphoma: differentiation between tumour infiltration and hypercellular bone marrow. Eur Radiol. 2002;12:1557-66.
23. Metz S, Lohr S, Settles M, et al. Ferumoxtran-10-enhanced MR imaging of the bone marrow before and after conditioning therapy in patients with non-Hodgkin lymphomas. Eur Radiol. 2006;16:598-607.
24. Schellinger D, Lin CS, Hatipaglu HG, et al. Potential value of vertebral proton MR spectroscopy in determining bone weakness. AJNR. 2001;22:1620-7.
25. Ghanem N, Altehoefer C, Kelly T, et al. Whole body MRI in comparison to skeletal scintigraphy in detection of skeletal metastases in patients with solid tumours. *In Vivo.* 2006;20:173-82.
26. Ghanom N, Lohrmann C, Engelhardt M, et al. Whole body MRI in the detection of bone marrow infiltration in patients with plasma cell neoplasm in comparison to radiological skeletal survey. Eur Radiol. 2006;16:1205-14.
27. Mikami MI, Nagai K, Yoshida K, et al. Detection of bone marrow and extramedullary involvement in patients with non-Hodgkin's lymphoma by whole-body MRI: comparison with bone and ^{67}Ga scintigraphies. Eur Radiol. 2004;14:1074-81.
28. Ricci C, Cova M, Kang YS, et al. Normal age-related patterns of cellular and fatty bone marrow distribution in the axial skeleton. MR imaging study. Radiology. 1989;172:805-10.
29. Shellock FG, Morris E, Deutsch AL, et al. Hematopoietic bone marrow hyperplasia, high prevalence on MR images of the knee in asymptomatic marathon runners. AJR. 1992;158: 335-8.
30. Emery JL, Follet GF. Regression of bone marrow haematopoiesis from the terminal digits in the foetus and infants. Br J Hematology. 1964;10:485-99.
31. Levin TL, Sheth SS, Ruzal-Shapiro C, et al. MRI marrow observations in thalassemia: The effects of primary disease, transfusional therapy and chelation. Pediatric Radiology. 1995;25:605-13.
32. Levin TL, Sheth SS, Hurlet A. MR marrow signs of iron overload in transfusion dependent patients with sickle cell disease. Pediatric Radiology. 1995;25:614-9.
33. McKinstry CS, Steiner RE, Young AT, et al. Bone marrow in leukemia and aplastic anaemia. MR imaging before, during and after treatment. Radiology. 1987;162:701-7.
34. Jensen KE, Thomsen C, Henriksen O, et al. Changes in T1 relaxation processes in the bone marrow following treatment in children with acute lymphoblastic leukemia. Pediatric Radiology. 1990;20:464-8.
35. Janssens AM, Offner FC, Van Hove WZ. Bone marrow necrosis. Lancer. 2000;88:1769-80.
36. Jensen KE, Sorensen PG, Thomsen C, et al. Pro-longed T1 relaxation of haemopoietic bone marrow in patients with chronic leukemia. Acta Radiol. 1990;31:445-9.
37. Shields AF, Porter BA, Chunchley S, et al. The detection of bone marrow involvement by lymphoma using magnetic resonance imaging. J Clin Onco. 1987;5:225-30.
38. White LM, Scheweitzer ME, Khalili K, et al. MR imaging of primary lymphoma of bone: Variability of T2-weighted signal intensity. AJR. 1998;170:1243-7.
39. Vanel D, Bittoun J, Tardivan A. MRI of bone metastasis. European Radiology. 1998;8:1345-51.
40. Baur A, Stabler A, Arbogast S, et al. Acute osteoporotic and neoplastic vertebral compression fractures: fluid sign at MR imaging. Radiology. 2002;225:730-5.
41. Baur A, Stabler A, Bruning R. Diffusion weighted MR imaging of bone marrow—differentiation of benign versus pathologic fractures. Radiology. 1998;207:349-56.
42. Oztekin O, Ozan E, Adibelli ZH, et al. SSH – EPI diffusion weighted MR imaging of the spine with low b values: is it useful in differentiating malignant metastatic infiltration from benign fracture edema? Skeletal Radiol. 2009;38:651-8.
43. Tang G, Liu Y, Li W, et al. Optimization of b value in diffusion weighted MRI for the differential diagnosis of benign and malignant vertebral fractures. Skeletal Radiol. 2007;36:1035-41.
44. Dietrich O, Herlihy A, Dannels WR, et al. Diffusion-weighted imaging of the spine using radial k-space trajectories, MAGMA. 2001;12:23-31.
45. Feydy A, Drape JL, Argaud C, et al. Diffusion-weighted MRI and ADC measurement of tumoral bone marrow. In: Proc Intl Soc Mag Reson Med. 2001;9:2117.
46. Chan JH, Peh WC, Tsui EY, et al. Acute vertebral body compression fractures: discrimination between benign and malignant causes using apparent diffusion coefficients. Bj J Radiol. 2002;75:207-14.
47. Herneth AM, Philipp MO, Naude J, et al. Vertebral metastases: assessment with apparent diffusion coefficient. Radiology. 2002;225:889-94.

48. Hwang S, Panicek DM. Magnetic resonance imaging of bone marrow in oncology part 2. Skeletal Radiology. 2007;36:1017-27.
49. Stabler A, Baur A, Bartt, et al. Contrast Enhancement and Quantitative Signal Analysis in MR Imaging of Multiple Myeloma: Assessment of focal and diffuse growth patterns in marrow correlated with biopsies and survival rates. AJR. 1996;167:1029-36.
50. Rahmouni A, Divine M, Mathieu D. MR appearance of multiple myeloma of the spine before and after treatment. AJR. 1993;160:1053-7.
51. Moulopoulos LA. Waldenstrom macroglobulinemia. MR imaging of the spine and CT of the abdomen and pelvis. Radiology. 1993;188:669-73.
52. Cohen MD, Cary DA, Kleiman M, et al. Magnetic resonance differentiation of acute and chronic osteomyelitis in children. Clinical Radiology. 1990;41:53-6.
53. Erdman WA, Tamburno F, Jayson HT, et al. Osteomyelitis: Characteristics and pitfalls of diagnosis with MR imaging. Radiology. 1991;180:533-9.
54. Kaplan PA, Asleson RJ, Klanen LW, et al. Bone marrow patterns in aplastic anaemia: Observations with 1.5T MR imaging. Radiology. 1987;164:441-4.
55. Kaplan KR, Mitchell DG, Steiner RM. Polycythemia vera and myelofibrosis; Correlation of MR imaging, clinical and lab findings. Radioloogy. 1992;183:329-34.
56. Rosenthal DI, Scott JA, Barianger J. Evaluation of Gaucher's disease using magnetic resonance imaging. Journal Bone and Joint Surgery (Am). 1986;68:802-8.
57. Cosamassina F, Ruggiero D, Caramella C, et al. Haematopoietic bone marrow recovering after radiation therapy: MR evaluation. Blood. 1989;73:1677-81.
58. Daldrup-link HE, Henning T, Link TM, et al. MR imaging of therapy-induced changes of bone marrow. Eur Radiol. 2007;17:743-61.
59. Boothnoyd AE, Sebag G, Brunelle F. MR appearances of bone marrow in children following bone marrow transplant. Pediatric Radiology. 1991;21:291-2.
60. Wilson AJ, Murphy WA, Hardy DC, et al. Transient osteoporosis—transient bone marrow oedema. Radiology. 1988;167:757-60.
61. Pory NT, Singer WS, Bartel E. Hip pain in three children accompanied by transient abnormal findings on MR images. Radiology. 1989;171:147-9.
62. Imhof H, Breitenseher M, Trattnig S. Imaging of avascular necrosis of bone. European Radiology. 1997;7:180-6.
63. Bloem JL. Transient osteoporosis of the hip: MR imaging. Radiology. 1988;167:753-5.
64. Lee JK, Yao L. Stress fractures: MR imaging. Radiology. 1988;169:217-20.
65. Staffard S, Rosenthal ADI, Gerbaardt MC, et al. MRI in stress fractures. AJR 1986;147:553-6.

CHAPTER 204

Radiological Evaluation of Appendicular Trauma

Atin Kumar, Arun Kumar Gupta

INTRODUCTION

Skeletal trauma is one of the most common forms of injuries suffered by people in everyday life. The extremities are the most often affected. The emergency radiologist plays a key role in the work-up of such patients as the initial evaluation requires radiographic examination. The radiograph has to be well-performed and accurately interpreted. It provides diagnostic evidence of the presence of fracture or dislocation along with the severity and extent of the trauma. The radiographs are also essential to check for accuracy of fracture reduction and to monitor bone healing.

CLINICAL EVALUATION

The features pointing towards underlying fracture include deformity, swelling, ecchymosis, marked local tenderness, abnormal mobility and crepitus on palpation and impairment of function. It is important to assess the state of the circulation and neural integrity in the limb distal to the fracture, both at the time of initial presentation and after any intervention.

The radiologist should also be aware of the mechanism of the injury as well as the time interval from the injury to the radiographic examination. This helps the radiologist to know what and where to look for in the radiograph. The radiologist can also look for specific injuries that are known to be associated with the mechanism of the injury.

RADIOLOGICAL EVALUATION

Definitions and Classification

A *fracture* is a disruption in the continuity of the bone. A *dislocation* is a complete disruption of a joint with loss of congruity between the articular surfaces. *Subluxation* is a minor disruption of the joint where some part of the articular surfaces remain in contact.

The fractures are clinically classified into open or closed fractures. The open fractures are those which penetrate the overlying skin and the fracture site is exposed to the external environment whereas closed fractures are those with intact overlying skin and hence no exposure to the environment. This makes the open fractures amenable to the risk of infection because of contamination by microorganisms.

The radiographic evaluation of fracture should work on the basic principle of obtaining at least two views of the involved bone, ideally perpendicular to each other, with each view including two joints adjacent to the involved bone. This helps the radiologist eliminate the risk of missing an associated dislocation or subluxation at a site remote from the apparent primary injury. Additional views should be obtained if there is any doubt or in specific situations like an oblique view for scaphoid fracture. It is estimated that about 5% of fractures are seen only on one view and about 5% of fractures require additional views to be detected **(Figs. 1A and B)**. In children, especially if

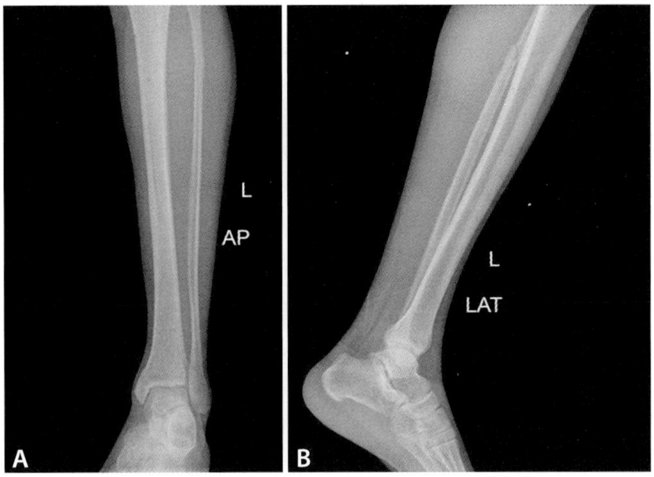

Figs. 1A and B: Anteroposterior (AP) and lateral radiographs of the leg show a fracture of the upper shaft of fibula which is visualized only on the lateral view and is almost not seen on the AP view.

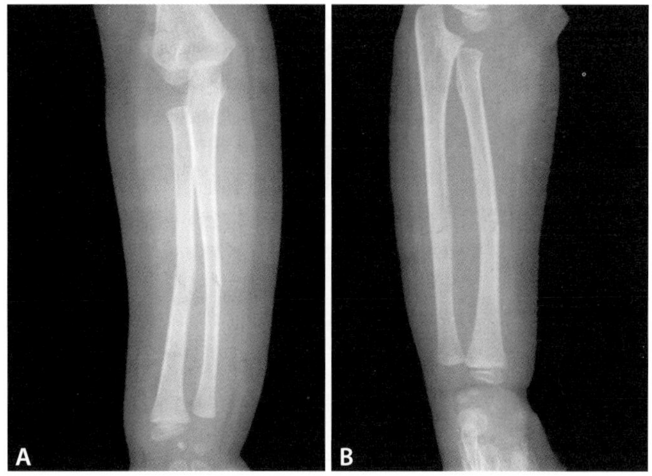

Figs. 2A and B: Anteroposterior and lateral radiographs of the forearm show greenstick fractures of the shaft of radius and ulna.

there is involvement of the ossification centers which are not fused, it may be necessary to obtain a radiograph of the normal, unaffected side for comparison.

The complete radiographic evaluation of a trauma patient should consist of the following:

1. Osseous evaluation.
2. Soft-tissue evaluation.

Osseous Evaluation

Presence or Absence of Bony Injury

A careful examination of all the bones included in the radiograph must be done for detection or ruling out a fracture. A fracture can appear as any of the following—an obvious disruption in continuity of bone, abnormal line of radiolucency, cortical irregularity or increase in bone density (due to impacted or compression fractures). Sometimes the fracture may be 'occult' which are clinically suspected but are not visualized on the initial radiograph. They may be detected subsequently on a follow-up radiography or scintigraphy. Scaphoid fractures are an example.

Anatomic Location and Extent of the Fracture

When describing a fracture it is important to specify the location within the long bone. In case of a fracture involving shaft of a long bone it should be described whether it is located in proximal, middle or distal thirds of bone or at junction of any two parts. It can also be described in terms of involvement of anatomic point of reference, e.g. supracondylar fracture of humerus. For fractures located near bone ends, mention should be made of any intra-articular extension as this will alter the subsequent management of the patient.

Types of Fracture

Complete or incomplete: The fracture is classified as complete, if it involves the entire width of the bone to involve both the cortices and incomplete if only some of the bony trabeculae are completely severed while others are bent or remain intact.[1] Incomplete fractures are more likely to be seen in children. Angular deformities are common without any displacement in incomplete fractures.

The complete fractures are further classified as:

a. *Simple*: One fracture line separating the bone into two fragments.
b. *Comminuted*: Two or more fracture lines with 3 or more fragments. A 'butterfly' fragment can be seen, if a small triangular fragment gets isolated on the concave side of the injury.

The incomplete fractures can be of following types:

a. *Greenstick (Hickory stick) fractures* **(Figs. 2A and B)**: Fractures occurring due to angulation forces primarily in infants and young children below 10 years of age because of the relatively greater component of pliable woven bone. The fracture affects the tension or the convex side of the bone. The bone bends with the convex side showing a horizontal break in the continuity of the cortex whereas the other concave side remains intact.[1] The greenstick fractures heal without any complications in most instances.

b. *Torus (buckling) fractures*: Fractures occurring due to longitudinal compressive forces over a soft bone of young child. The fracture affects the compressive (concave) side of the bone. The cortex bulges outward due to compressive forces at the site of injury. They occur mostly in the metaphysis and are very painful.[1]

c. *Plastic bowing fractures* ***(Figs. 3A and B)***: No true fracture is seen. It occurs when the force on the bone is not sufficient enough to cause a cortical disruption but instead leads to bowing of the bone.

Direction of Fracture Line

This is described with respect to the longitudinal axis of the bone.[2] Based on this, the fractures can be classified into:

a. *Transverse fracture* ***(Figs. 4A and B)***: The fracture line is perpendicular to the long axis of the bone. In long bones it occurs as a result of angulation force. This type of fracture is usually stable and unlikely to be displaced after reduction.

b. *Oblique fracture*: The fracture line runs oblique to the long axis of the bone and the angle is <90°.

c. *Spiral fracture* ***(Fig. 5)***: The fracture line turns and twists around the shaft and encircles it atleast once. It occurs as a result of twisting force to the limb. This type of fracture is prone to be displaced after reduction.[2]

Spatial Relationship of the Fragments

This is described in terms of apposition/displacement, alignment/angulation, rotation and distraction/overriding.

a. *Apposition*: It refers to the state of bony contact at the fracture site and the resultant shift of the fragments relative to each other. This classifies fractures into undisplaced and displaced. The displacement is described with reference to the direction of shift of the distal fragment. An undisplaced fracture with a fine fracture line is termed as 'hairline' fracture.

b. *Alignment*: It refers to the position of the distal fragment with respect to the proximal fragment. It can be lateral/medial displacement or tilt/angulation. The angulation of the distal fragment medially is termed 'varus' and laterally is termed 'valgus'.

c. *Rotation*: It refers to the rotation of the distal fragment over the longitudinal axis. It can be internal or external rotation. To comment on rotation, the proximal and distal joints must be included in the radiograph.

d. *Overriding/distraction*: A longitudinal separation of the bony fragments in the long axis of the bone with resultant increased distance between the two fragments is termed distraction. If the bony fragments overlap on each other it is termed overriding and leads to foreshortening of the limb **(Figs. 4A and B)**.

Presence of Special Features

The special features that need to be commented upon in a radiograph include:

a. *Impaction*: When the two fragments are driven into each other. This occurs due to compressive forces. The classical radiolucent fracture line is not seen but instead a subtle radiopaque line is seen at the site which may be the only marker of the fracture. It is

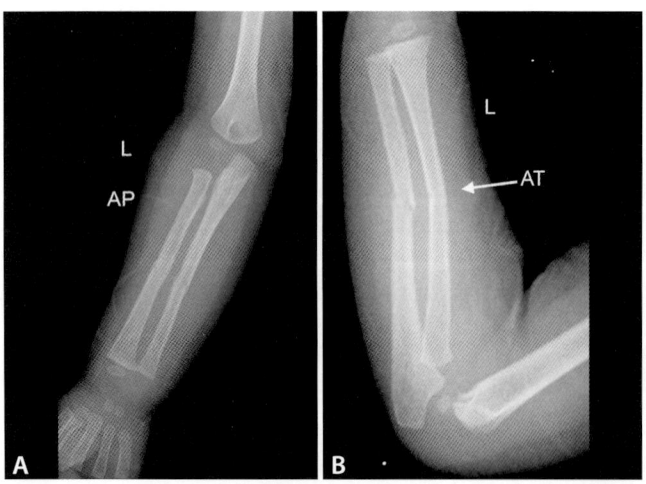

Figs. 3A and B: Anteroposterior and lateral radiographs of the forearm show plastic bowing fracture without an obvious cortical break in the midshaft of radius (arrow). A complete fracture of the adjacent ulna is associated.

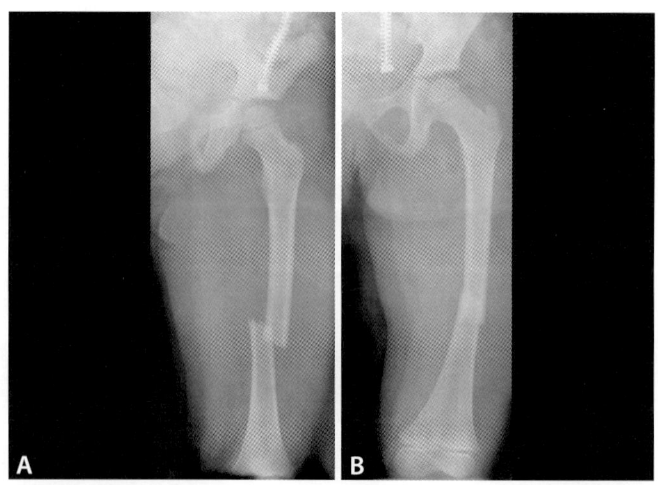

Figs. 4A and B: Anteroposterior and oblique radiographs of the left thigh show a transverse fracture of the shaft of ulna with overriding of the bone fragments.

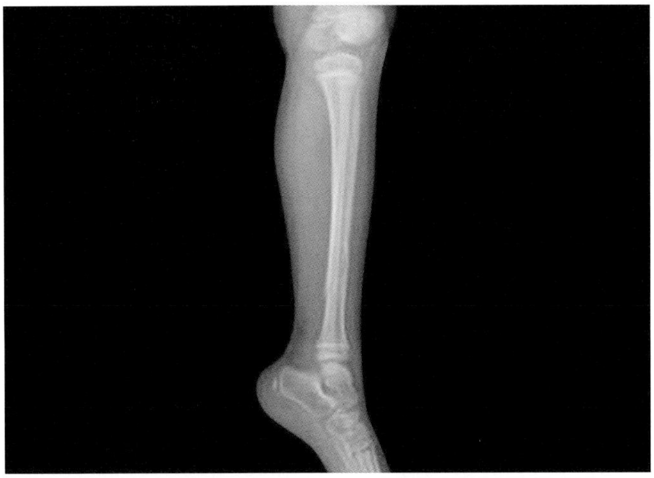

Fig. 5: Lateral radiograph of leg showing a spiral fracture through the lower shaft of tibia.

important to obtain additional views in this situation in case of a doubt.

b. *Depression*: It represents an inward bulging of the outer bony surface. It is a type of impaction fracture. This gives rise to a 'double cortical line'. It is seen most commonly at tibial plateau and radial head in extremities and in frontal bone in the skull.
c. *Compression*: It represents an impaction fracture involving the spinal vertebral body due to hyperflexion forces.
d. *Avulsion*: It involves tearing away of a portion of the bone usually at insertion of a muscle or ligament due to forceful pulling. The frequent sites are tuberosities of tubular bones, elbow, lateral metatarsal and lower cervical spinous processes. A small cortical avulsion is termed a 'flake' fracture. 'Chip' or 'corner' fracture represents avulsion of a small fragment of bone from the corner of a phalanx or other short or long tubular bone. Corner chip fractures at metaphyseal ends in children should raise the suspicion of battered baby syndrome.

Presence of Associated Abnormalities of the Adjacent Joints

It may be commonly associated with certain types of mechanisms of injuries and some specific fractures. Examples include a femoral shaft fracture associated with hip joint dislocation, a lower end tibial fracture associated with upper end fibula fracture, etc. The joints may be dislocated or subluxated. When dislocation is associated with a fracture, it is termed as fracture dislocation. A fracture through a joint surface may involve the cartilage only (chondral fracture) or cartilage and underlying bone (osteochondral fracture).

Presence of Special Types of Fractures

The fractures may be due to excessive stress or due to underlying bone weakening disorder. A normal classical fracture occurs due to excessive trauma to a normal bone without underlying abnormality. The ends of the fracture are sharply marginated and the adjacent bone appears healthy in acute settings. However, if the underlying bone is weakened by a localized (tumor) or systemic disease process (osteopenia due to any cause, metastases, multiple myeloma), then even a normal trauma (which is otherwise insufficient to cause fracture) can lead to a fracture. Such fractures are termed *pathological fractures*. These fractures are usually transverse with smooth margins. A *stress (fatigue)* fracture is caused by repetitive stress on normal bone. The stress itself is insufficient to cause fracture but over a period of time it leads to the development of fracture. These are commonly seen in runners, dancers and gymnasts. The metatarsals, tibia and fibula are commonly affected bones. These fractures become radiologically evident about 2–4 weeks after trauma as a faint transverse radiolucent line often surrounded by a callus **(Figs. 6A and B)**. *Insufficiency fractures* are special type of fractures which occur as a result of chronic repetitive normal stress on a pathological (often osteoporotic) bone. They can occur even with normal walking in a person with underlying osteopenia. They occur commonly in patients of osteomalacia, Paget's disease and rickets. Radiographically they are seen as linear lucencies on the convex surface of the bone that are oriented perpendicular to the long axis of the bone. They are often multiple and bilateral.

Involvement of Growth Plate/Physis: Seen in Children

These fractures result in growth arrest and deformity. The *Salter-Harris* classification is used most commonly for such fractures.[3] This classifies the physeal injuries into the following five types:

Type 1: Fracture through the growth plate. The radiograph appears normal.

Type 2: Fracture through the displaced growth plate with involvement of the metaphysis. The metaphyseal fragment is called as the 'Thurston-Holland sign'. This type is the most commonly seen in about 75% of cases.

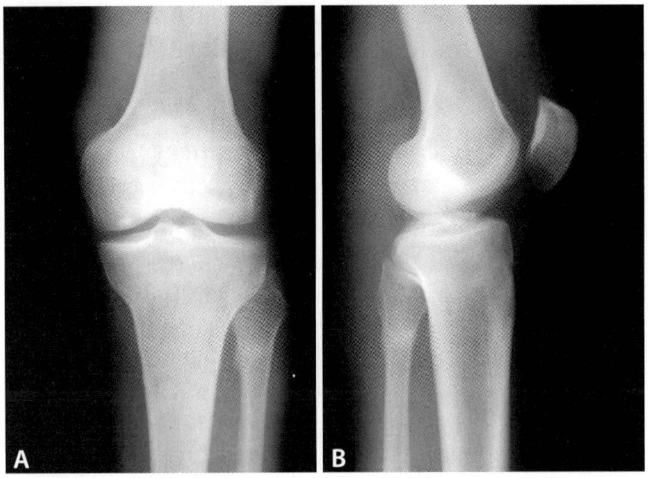

Figs. 6A and B: Anteroposterior and lateral radiographs of the knee joint show a stress fracture of the proximal shaft of fibula.

Type 3: Fracture through the growth plate with involvement of the epiphysis. The resultant intra-articular fracture often requires open reduction treatment.

Type 4: Obliquely oriented vertical fracture passing though the metaphysis, growth plate and epiphysis.

Type 5: Crush fracture leading to compressive deformity of the growth plate. The initial radiographs are normal. Subsequently due to growth arrest there occurs progressive angulation deformity. Hence, it is advisable to follow-up these children for atleast 2 years following injury.

Radiographs may not detect the epiphyseal injuries or their displacement especially if only one side alone is radiographed. Hence, it is important to radiograph the opposite limb for comparative evaluation.

Soft-tissue Evaluation

a. *Soft-tissue swelling*: Almost always present adjacent to the site of acute fracture.
b. *Obliteration or displacement of fat stripes*: Also gives a clue to underlying soft tissue swelling associated with a fracture. Commonly seen in fractures around the wrist joint.
c. *Joint capsular swelling*: May be seen due to joint effusion/hemarthrosis secondary to an intra-articular fracture. The capsular distension is also evident by bulging of fat planes around it. It is a good sign to detect fractures near elbow joint. If there is leak of bone marrow fat from within the medullary cavity into the joint along with blood (lipo-hemarthrosis), then a fat-fluid level may be visualized. It is better evident on CT or MRI.

FRACTURE HEALING

The pathological process of healing of fractures occurs in following phases which last for about 10 days each.[4]

- Circulatory or inflammatory phase—it comprises of:
  - Stage of hematoma
  - Stage of subperiosteal and endosteal cellular proliferation
  - Stage of callus formation
- Consolidation or reparative phase
- Remodeling or mechanical phase.

Radiologically the fracture line shows increase in its width in the first few days due to resorption of its margins. In the next 2–4 weeks the healing occurs by formation of callus. In cases of simple undisplaced fractures the healing occurs by primary union wherein the predominant callus formation is endosteal (internal) which obliterates the fracture line. In cases of complex displaced fractures the healing occurs by secondary union wherein the predominant callus formation is periosteal (external). The callus is initially radiolucent when it contains fibrous tissue and cartilage. At this stage the fracture may be clinically united. Gradually the callus gets remodeled and also gets ossified to give the radiodense white line appearance consistent with radiographic union. In a young adult the total process takes around 4–6 weeks while it may take up to 12 weeks in elderly.[5]

COMPLICATIONS OF FRACTURE

The various complications occur at multiple time intervals post injury. They are divided into immediate, intermediate and delayed complications.

Immediate Complications

a. *Vascular injury*: Most commonly with penetrating trauma, sharp bony fragments in open or communited fractures or even due to operative manipulation. The popliteal artery, distal superficial femoral artery and the brachial artery are involved most frequently.
b. *Nerve and soft tisssue injury*: The adjacent nerves, muscles, ligaments and tendons may show varying severity of injury.
c. *Compartment syndrome*: Results from increased pressure within a muscular compartment secondary to hemorrhage and edema. It leads to muscle necrosis and may be limb or life threatening. Anterior compartment of leg and anterior compartment of forearm are common sites.
d. *Fat embolism*: Associated with fracture of a major bone most commonly femur. Usually, it is not of any

clinical significance as it occurs in minor degree. It leads to emboli of fat globules from the bone marrow into the vessels and get lodged in small vessels of lung and brain. There is a classical symptom free period of about 2 days between the injury and symptoms of fat embolism. It is clinically evident by cerebral disturbance, drowsiness, coma, tachypnea, dyspnea and petechial rash over the body.[6,7] Chest radiograph may reveal bilateral diffuse air space consolidation in peripheral distribution with normal sized heart. Brain changes are best evident on MRI in the form of bilateral small T2 hyperintense lesions in deep white matter and corpus callosum which may show restricted diffusion.[8]

e. *Gas gangrene*: Occurs in open wounds which get infected by *Clostridium perfringens*.

Intermediate Complications

a. *Infection*: Occurs in the form of osteomyelitis and is seen in open fractures and those which have undergone operative intervention. Most commonly by *Staphylococcus aureus*. Tibia and femur are the frequently involved bones.

b. *Post-traumatic ossification* **(*Fig. 7*)**: Also known as myositis ossificans which is a misnomer as there is no infective lesion of the muscle. It is heterotropic bone formation occurring deep to the muscles. The common sites are elbow and thigh. The new bone formation occurs in the hematoma beneath the stripped periosteum and the joint capsule. The children are more prone as the periosteum is loosely attached and gets stripped following trauma. On radiograph the classical hallmark is the clearly recognizable pattern of its evolution over a period of 2 months. At the end of 2 months when the lesion is fully formed, the characteristic zonal appearance may be seen. The central part is radiolucent representing immature bone formation. It is surrounded by a dense peripheral zone of ossification. The outermost part of this ossification zone shows definite well-organized cortical bone. A thin lucent zone may separate this cortical layer from the ossific mass. If the ossification reaches up to the bone surface it mimics parosteal osteosarcoma. Computed tomography and MRI may help to confirm the diagnosis. Biopsy is conformatory.[9]

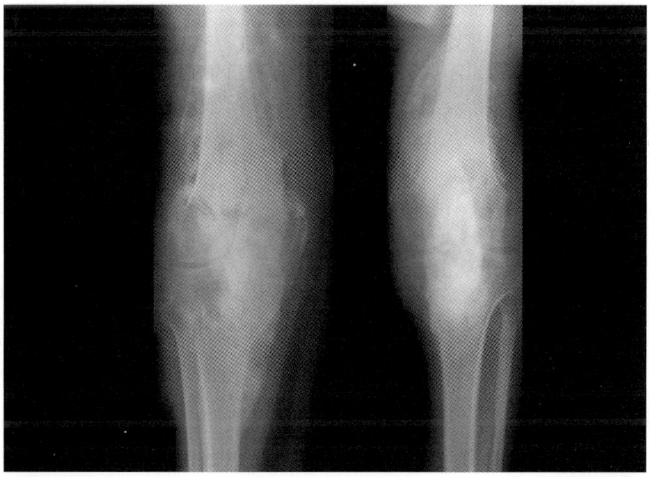

Fig. 7: Anteroposterior radiograph bilateral knee joints show extensive soft tissue ossification around bilateral knee joints suggestive of myositis ossificans.

c. *Sudeck's post-traumatic osteodystrophy*: Also known as reflex sympathetic dystrophy syndrome or post-traumatic painful osteoporosis. The hand or foot are commonly involved. The patient presents about 2 months after injury with extremely painful and tender swollen extremity which is hyperemic and glossy with marked stiffness of the small joints. Colles' fracture is the most common cause in upper limb. The radiograph shows diffuse soft-tissue swelling with gradually progressive patchy osteoporosis which is more than that expected by disuse osteoporosis. The bone scan may show diffuse area of increased uptake.

d. *Post-traumatic osteolysis*: It refers to dissolution of bone following trauma. Most commonly involves distal end of clavicle and pubic bones.

e. *Synostosis*: May occur between bones which are closely opposed like radius-ulna and tibia-fibula.

Delayed Complications

a. *Abnormal healing process*: These occur secondary to multiple factors including inadequate blood supply, distraction, inadequate immobilization, interposition of soft tissues, infection and pathological weakness of bone. The term delayed union is used to describe a fracture which does not unite within a reasonable period of time (16–18 weeks) depending on patient's age and the fracture site. Nonunion is diagnosed if the fracture fails to unite. The most common sites are midclavicle, ulna and tibia. The radiograph shows characteristic features after few months which include rounding of fracture edges, smoothening of margins with sclerosis, gap between the two fragments, demonstration of mobility (on serial stress radiographs or on fluoroscopy), lack of callus formation and pseudoarthrosis **(Figs. 8A and B)**. Pseudoarthrosis refers to formation of false joint-like cavity with synovial-like capsule between the ends of the two fragments. If formed, a pseudoarthrosis requires refracture and

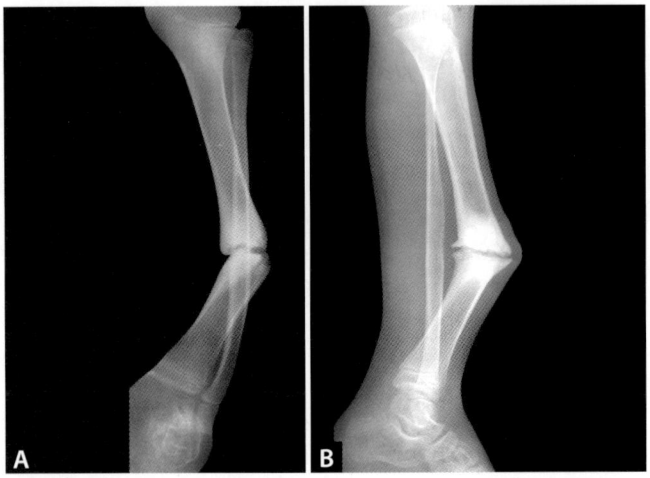

Figs. 8A and B: Anteroposterior and lateral radiographs of the leg. Six months after trauma shows an old nonunited fracture of the shaft of tibia with rounding of fracture edges, marginal sclerosis, gap between the fracture ends and formation of pseudoarthrosis.

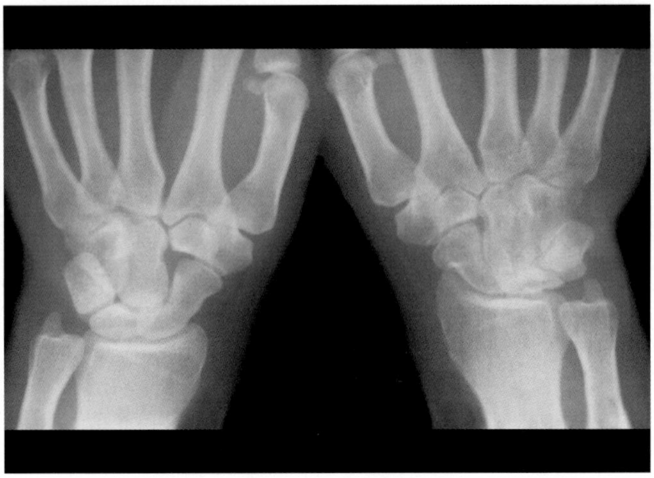

Fig. 9: Anteroposterior radiograph—bilateral wrist joints. The left lunate is showing an old fracture with marked sclerosis of the bone consistent with avascular necrosis (Kienbock's disease).

removal for the process of healing. Malunion refers to a union of fracture fragments in an imperfect anatomical position which results in unacceptable deformity. It usually requires surgical correction.

b. *Avascular necrosis* **(*Fig. 9*)**: Also known as osteonecrosis. It occurs due to loss of blood supply secondary to fracture. The process may take months to years. The most commonly affected bones are femoral head, scaphoid, humeral head and talus. On radiograph it appears as a sharply defined dense bone in contrast to the surrounding disuse osteoporosis. This progresses to loss of height of the involved part with shrunken, crumpled appearance. Bone scan with ^{99m}Technetium may be helpful. Magnetic resonance imaging shows the features earliest.
c. *Disuse osteoporosis*: Mild to moderate degree osteoporosis secondary to pain and immobilization.
d. *Post-traumatic arthritis*: Degenerative changes in the joint. The predisposing factors include intra-articular fracture, malaligned fracture and avascular necrosis. Seen most commonly in weight bearing joints such as knee, hip and ankle.

Imaging Modalities

Plain radiograph: It is the first line investigation for any skeletal trauma of the extremities. A minimum of two radiographic projections ideally perpendicular to each other should be acquired to conclusively rule out fracture. Additional views are taken if necessary. The detailed radiographic evaluation has been discussed above.

Ultrasonography: It has been shown to have an increasing role in the detection of fractures in the acute setting of trauma as well as monitoring of fracture healing. It is also helpful in joint pathologies for detection of effusion (hemarthrosis), ligaments and tendinous injuries.

Radioisotope scanning: With 99m Technetium diphosphonate is useful in detection of occult fractures. The scan may become positive after 24 hours in acute setting. It is also helpful in detection of stress fractures.

Computed tomography: It is markedly superior to radiograph for detection of bony injuries. It is reserved for areas of complex bony anatomy or where the radiographs are equivocal. Multiplanar reformats in all three planes gives a complete overview of the presence and extent of the bony injury alongwith its relation to surrounding structures. In addition, the soft tissues can also be well evaluated which gives it an added advantage over radiographs. It is commonly used to assess fractures of tibial plateau, ankle and epiphyseal injuries. In addition it can assess complications like vascular injury by CT angiography.

Magnetic resonance imaging: It has become the investigation of choice for detailed evaluation of injuries of joints and soft tissues. It has advantages of excellent depiction of soft tissue injuries including those of ligaments, tendons, menisci and cartilage besides detection of bony injuries by marrow edema. It can detect subtle bone injuries like occult fractures and bone contusions which may sometimes not be evident on both radiographs and

CT. It is also the best modality to detect complications like avascular necrosis. Use of contrast MR arthrography also enables better depiction of articular and periarticular injuries like those of labrum, cartilage and menisci.

UPPER LIMB TRAUMA

Dislocation of the Shoulder

Glenohumeral joint is the most common joint of the body to dislocate. It is seen usually in adults and elderly. It is classified into subtypes depending upon the direction of displacement of the humeral head into anterior, posterior, superior and inferior direction.

Anterior dislocation: It is the most frequent (95% cases). The humeral head can dislocate anteriorly to lie in subglenoid, subcoracoid, or subclavicular position. The subglenoid dislocation is accompanied by fracture of greater tuberosity whereas subcoracoid dislocation can occur without bony injury and is prone to recurrence **(Fig. 10)**. The Hill-Sach's defect (impaction of the humeral head) and avulsion of the inferior glenoid rim (Bankart's lesion) are often seen especially with recurrent dislocations. Magnetic resonance imaging with MR arthrography is more sensitive in detecting these lesions.[10]

Posterior dislocation: Occur as a result of violent muscle contraction as in epileptic convulsion or following electric shock.

Inferior dislocation: Also known as *Luxatio Erecta*. It occurs secondary to severe hyperabduction trauma with humeral head locked in abduction under the subgleniod position.

Superior dislocation: It is rare. It occurs secondary to considerable force and most commonly occurs secondary to rotator cuff tear.

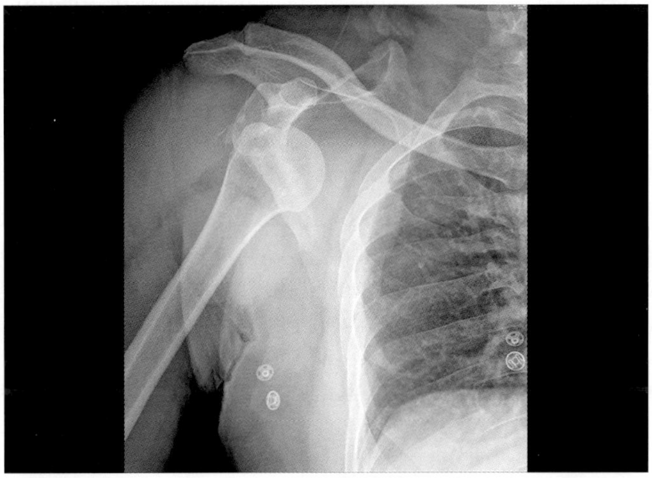

Fig. 10: Anteroposterior radiograph of the right shoulder shows anteroinferior dislocation of the right humerus.

The radiological evaluation of shoulder dislocation should consist of a true anteroposterior and a trans-scapular view since it may be missed in the anteroposterior views with internal and external rotation which are routinely done for any shoulder pathology.[11] The AP view can diagnose a shoulder dislocation but the anterior and posterior varieties cannot be differentiated on it. Fracture of the glenoid rim or the greater tuberosity may be seen in this view. Recurrent anterior dislocations would show the Hill-Sach's deformity. In posterior dislocations, on AP radiograph the normal parallelism between the humeral head and the anterior rim of glenoid is absent. The 'light bulb' or the 'tennis racquet' appearance on the AP view along with widening of the joint space more than 6 mm are clue to diagnosis of posterior dislocation of shoulder. Since the head is fixed in internal rotation, there occurs no change in the appearance of the head on external rotation view.[12]

Fracture of Neck of Humerus

The frontal AP views of the shoulder with humerus in internal and external rotation are usually sufficient to detect majority of humeral fractures. The fractures of the neck are described by Neer classification[13] which includes four different areas of involvement—the anatomic neck, surgical neck, greater tuberosity and lesser tuberosity. The total number of fractures and their angulations are taken into account to classify the fractures into four parts—1, 2, 3 and 4. The fragments are considered displaced if there is atleast 1 cm of separation or 45° angulation. Most common (80%) are one part fractures. The surgical neck which lies immediately distal to the tuberosities is the most commonly fractured region **(Fig. 11)**. The axillary nerve may be involved by these fractures. It is important to note that an impacted fracture can be easily overlooked in this region.

Fracture of Shaft of Humerus

These can involve the proximal, middle or distal shaft of the humerus. The fracture orientation can be transverse, oblique or spiral. There can be marked angulation, overlap or displacement of the fragments. Transverse fracture of the middle shaft is the most common fracture in this region. A fracture in the proximal shaft should be carefully evaluated to look for underlying pathology as metastatic deposits are common in this part of the bone.

Fracture of Distal Humerus

The fractures of this region are classified according to their relationship with humeral condyles and the shape of the fracture line.

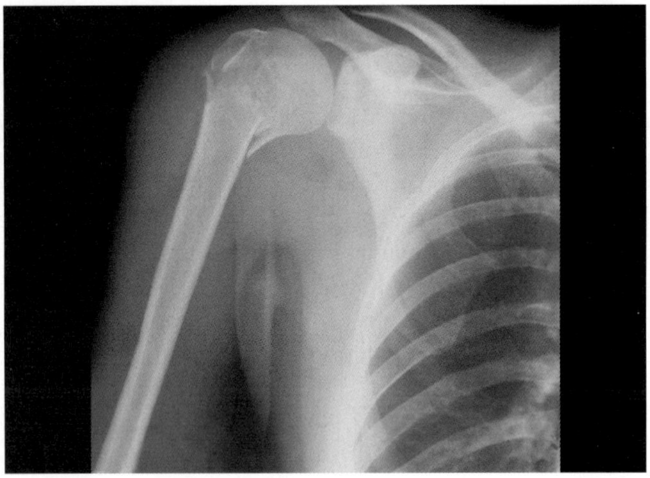

Fig. 11: Anteroposterior radiograph of the left arm shows fracture at the surgical neck of the humerus.

a. *Supracondylar fractures*: The fracture line runs superior to the level of condyles. This is seen most commonly in children after fall on outstretched hand. The distal fragment is displaced and angulated posteriorly. The lateral view shows the displacement and the fracture best. Elevation of anterior and posterior fat pads are also indirect signs of underlying fracture. The fracture may be associated with development of Volkman's ischemic contracture. The brachial artery may also be injured.
b. *Intercondylar fractures*: The fracture line runs between the medial and lateral condyles and extends into the supracondylar region to form a 'T' or a 'Y' configuration. This is more commonly seen in adults. If the fracture involves both condyles it is termed transcondylar fracture.
c. *Condylar fractures*: Fracture running through either of the lateral or medial humeral condyle. Fracture of the lateral condyle is the second most common fracture of this region in children and can often result in nonunion. The ulnar nerve may be injured in lateral condyle fractures. If a small fragment gets detached it can lead to loose body within the joint.
d. *Epicondylar fractures*: They are avulsion injuries of the epicondyles due to strong pull of the flexor or extensor tendons. The medial epicondyle fractures are seen in sportspersons with throwing action. In children, due to the apophysis being unossified, the fracture may not be radiologically evident.

Dislocation of the Elbow

It is the most common joint to be dislocated in children and third most common in adults (after shoulder and interphalangeal joints).[14] The most common type is posterior or posterolateral dislocation which describes the position of the radius and ulna relative to the humerus **(Figs. 12A and B)**. It is often associated with fractures of the radial head, coronoid process, capitulum or the medial epicondyle. Post-traumatic ossification can also be seen following posterior dislocations.

The other form of dislocation of the elbow is 'pulled elbow'. It occurs in young children less than 5 years of age due to traction to the elbow as in lifting the child from the floor by holding the hand. It leads to slippage of the humeral head out of the annular ligament. It leads to immediate crying of the child with forearm held in midpronation. It is not evident radiographically. The treatment involves just simple supination of the forearm.

Fracture of the Head and Neck of Radius

It is the most common injury of the elbow region in young adults and occurs due to fall on outstretched hand. It usually is a hairline fracture oriented vertically involving the articular surface. Since the fracture is often nondisplaced, it is sometimes difficult to visualize on routine AP and lateral views of the elbow. Displacement of anterior and posterior fat pads on the lateral view may aid in the diagnosis. The presence of posterior fat pad is a more reliable and consistent indicator of underlying fracture of the radial head. The radial neck fracture is usually an impacted fracture at its junction with the head.

Fracture of Upper End of Ulna

Olecranon fractures are the second most common fractures of this region in adults. They occur after fall on the point of elbow. The fracture line is best visualized on lateral view. The coronoid process may rarely be fractured in association with posterior dislocation of the elbow or by avulsion by brachialis muscle.

Fractures of the Shaft of the Radius and Ulna

The radius and ulna can be fractured in isolation but are both fractured in association in a large number of patients when it is called both bones ('B-B') fracture. The fractures of this region are prone to displacement with angulation and rotation and hence often require surgical correction. There are increased chances of compartment syndrome after fractures of this region.

A fracture of the proximal ulnar shaft with dislocation of the radial head is known as *Monteggia fracture dislocation* **(Figs. 13A and B)**.

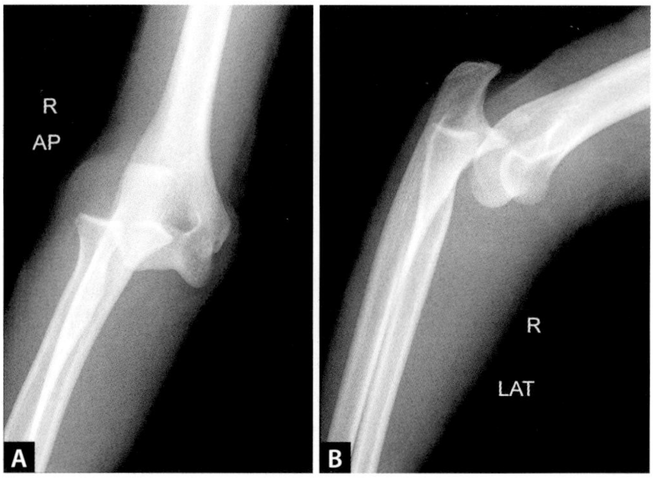

Figs. 12A and B: Anteroposterior and lateral radiographs of the elbow show posterolateral dislocation of the elbow.

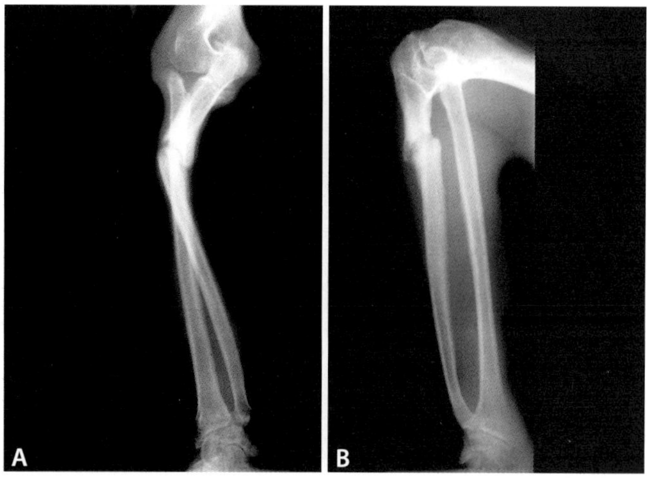

Figs. 13A and B: Anteroposterior and lateral radiographs of the forearm show an old nonunited fracture of the upper shaft of ulna with dislocation of the radial head consistent with *Monteggia's fracture dislocation*.

An isolated fracture of distal ulnar shaft is termed as *Nightstick* or *Parry fracture*.

A fracture of the distal shaft of radius at the junction of middle and distal third with dislocation of the distal radio-ulnar joint is termed as *Galeazzi* or *Reversed Monteggia fracture*.

Fractures of Distal End of Radius

Fractures of the distal part of radius are common injuries of adulthood especially in females.[15]

A fracture of the distal end of radius with posterior angulation of the distal fragment is termed as *Colles' fracture* **(Figs. 14A and B)**. The fracture line is seen around 2–3 cm proximal to the articular surface of the radius. The distal fragment is tilted dorsally so that on lateral view it gives rise to classical 'dinner-fork' deformity. A fracture of ulnar styloid process is associated in 60% of cases. Complications include malunion and Sudeck's post-traumatic osteodystrophy.

A fracture of the distal radius with anterior angulation of the distal fragment is termed as *Smith's fracture* or *Reversed Colles' fracture*.

A fracture of the posterior rim of the distal radial articular surface with associated proximal dislocation of the carpus is termed *Barton's fracture*. The involvement of volar radial rim is termed *Reverse Barton's fracture*.

Fracture of the radial styloid process is termed *Chauffeur's fracture*.

A fracture through the distal radial epiphysis is common in children. The epiphysis gets slipped posteriorly and is usually associated with a small metaphyseal fracture

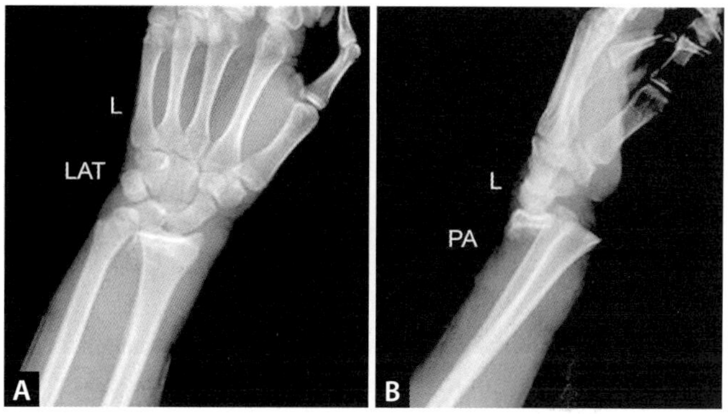

Figs. 14A and B: Anteroposterior and oblique radiographs of the hand show *Colles' fracture* of the radius.

making it a Type 2 Salter Harris injury. This is equivalent of a *Colles' fracture* of adult.

Fractures of the Carpal Bones

Scaphoid is the most common carpal bone to be fractured. It is usually seen in adults with fall on outstretched hand. Clinically there is tenderness in the anatomical snuffbox. The standard views to detect a scaphoid fracture include PA, lateral, external oblique and a PA view with ulnar deviation.[16] About 70% of fractures involve the waist of scaphoid followed by proximal and distal poles **(Figs. 15A and B)**. Nondisplaced fractures are difficult to identify. If there is high clinical suspicion but no fracture line is visible on initial radiograph, then precautionary immobilization is done and the radiograph is repeated after 2 weeks. The fracture line may be better evident by this time. A bone scan may detect the fracture earlier. Fractures

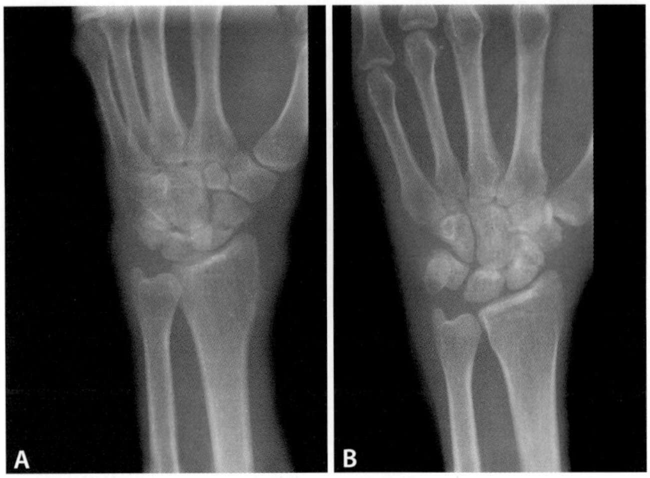

Figs. 15A and B: Anteroposterior and oblique radiographs of the wrist joint show a fracture through the waist of scaphoid bone.

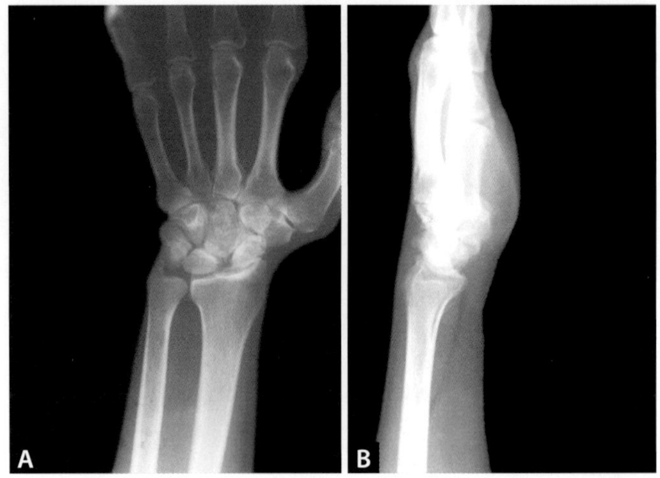

Figs. 16A and B: Anteroposterior and lateral radiographs of the wrist show scapho-lunate dislocation with increased distance between the scaphoid and lunate (*Terry Thomas sign*) and signet ring appearance of the scaphoid.

through the waist or proximal to it make the proximal part of scaphoid prone to avascular necrosis as the nutrient artery enters the bone through the distal part of the waist. The chances of avascular necrosis increases with more proximal fracture line. The avascular part is seen as more dense compared to the rest of the bone and the other surrounding bones. The scaphoid fractures are also more prone to nonunion.

Triquetrum is the second most common carpal bone to be fractured. An avulsion fracture at the site of attachment of the radiocarpal ligament is termed *Fischer's fracture*. It is identified on lateral radiograph of the wrist.

Lunate fractures are uncommon. *Kienbock's disease* is avascular necrosis of the lunate which may be secondary to a fracture **(Fig. 9)**.

Dislocation of the Wrist

Dislocations affecting the wrist are mainly of 2 types: (a) single carpal dislocations and (b) multiple carpal dislocations.[17]

Single Carpal Dislocations

Lunate dislocation is the most common of all carpal bones. The lunate displaces anteriorly with forward tilt so that the concave lower articular surface faces anteriorly. This is best seen on the lateral view.

The scaphoid is the second most common bone to subluxate. It usually undergoes rotatory subluxation so that it rotates anteriorly and moves laterally to cause scapho-lunate dissociation. The distance between the scaphoid and lunate on AP view is increased to more than 4 mm (known as *Terry Thomas sign)*. In addition the scaphoid appears small and circular in shape (*signet ring sign)* **(Figs. 16A and B)**.

Multiple Carpal Dislocations

The most common in perilunate dislocation where the lunate bone maintains its spatial relationship with the radius but rest of all the carpal bones get dislocated dorsally. It is best visualized on lateral view. This type of dislocation may be associated with fracture of the scaphoid.

Fractures and Dislocations of the Hand

Anteroposterior, lateral and oblique projections are the most commonly used views to image injuries of this region. Collimated views may be required if a single digit is to be evaluated.

Among the metacarpals, the first metacarpal base is most commonly injured. An oblique intra-articular fracture through the base of first metacarpal with dorsal and radial displacement of the shaft is known as *Bennet's fracture*. A comminuted *Bennet's fracture* is termed *Ronaldo's fracture*.

A transverse fracture of the neck of the fifth metacarpal with volar angulation of the distal fragment is termed *Boxer's fracture*.

Fractures of the phalanges are more common than metacarpal fractures. An avulsion chip fracture at the base of distal phalanx at the insertion of extensor tendon leads to *Mallet finger* with the finger fixed in moderate flexion and cannot be extended.

LOWER LIMB TRAUMA

Dislocations of the Hip

The dislocations of the hip are classified as anterior or posterior.[18]

Posterior Dislocation

It is the most common type accounting for approximately 80% of hip dislocations. It occurs when there is a blow to the knee with hip in flexed position. The femoral head displaces posteriorly to lie outside the acetabulum on its lateral and superior aspect. This often produces a fracture of the posterior acetabular rim with rarely a small fracture of the anterior femoral head. These fractures are best seen on CT scan. The sciatic nerve may also be injured. Clinically there is medial rotation of the leg with limb shortening.

Anterior Dislocation

It accounts for about 15% of hip dislocations and is caused by forced abduction and extension of the femur. Clinically the limb is seen to lie in abduction. The head may be dislocated anteriorly and superiorly (subspinous or iliac type) with the femur extended and abducted or the head may get dislocated anteriorly and inferiorly (obturator type) with the femur abducted and externally rotated. The acetabulum usually does not show any fracture.[19]

Fractures of the Proximal Femur

Fracture of the neck of femur is a common injury seen in elderly especially in females with underlying osteoporosis.[20] Complications include avascular necrosis, osteoarthritis and nonunion. AP view of pelvis, coned AP view of ipsilateral hip and horizontal beam lateral view are the usual radiographs for detection. The fractures of this region are classified into intracapsular and extracapsular types depending upon the relationship of the fracture line to the joint capsule.

Intracapsular Fractures

The intracapsular fractures include all fractures above the level of trochanters. They account for about 60% of all proximal femoral fractures. The intracapsular fractures are more prone to undergo nonunion and avascular necrosis.

Subcapital fracture occurs at the junction of head with neck and is the most common type of intracapsular fracture. These fractures may be impacted without displacement or may show variable degrees of displacement.

Midcervical fracture at the middle part of the neck and basicervical fractures just above the level of trochanters are the other types of intracapsular fractures. These regions may be more commonly fractured with underlying pathological lesion.

Extracapsular Fractures

These include all fractures at or below the level of the trochanters.

The intertrochanteric fractures constitute of a fracture line running obliquely to involve both the trochanters **(Fig. 17)**. These fractures are generally comminuted. These fractures unite easily without significant complications.

The trochanteric fractures involve avulsion injuries of the greater or the lesser trochanter.

Subtrochanteric fractures occur below the level of the trochanters or may be seen as an extension of intertrochanteric fractures. It is usually seen in younger patients with significant trauma or superimposed over pathological bone in elderly.

Fractures of the Shaft of Femur

These occur at all ages and are a result of severe violence. The fracture orientation may be spiral, oblique or transverse. The fractures may be associated with significant soft tissue hemorrhage. The femoral artery may commonly get injured most commonly at the level of the adductor canal. Radiograph should always include both the proximal hip and the distal knee joint because of high incidence of ipsilateral associated injuries.

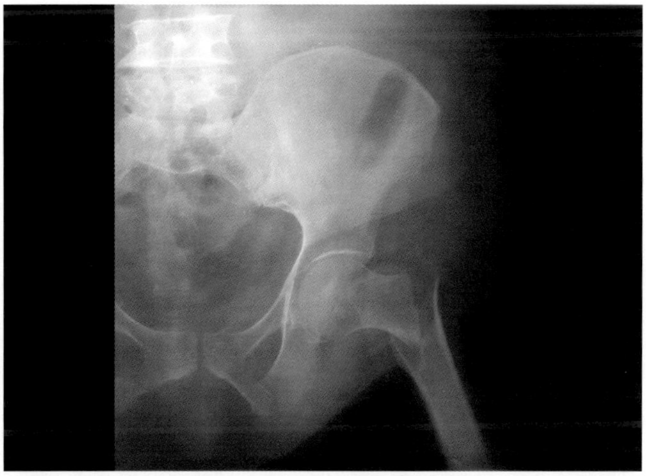

Fig. 17: Anteroposterior radiograph of the left hip joint shows an intertrochanteric fracture of the left femur.

The supracondylar fracture of the femur produces posterior angulation and displacement of the distal fragment due to the pull of the gastrocnemius muscle.

The condylar fractures often involve the articular surface and need to be corrected to prevent delayed osteoarthritis. The condyles may be injured in isolation or there may be extension of a supracondylar fracture into the intercondylar area with a 'T' or 'Y' configuration. Injury of the popliteal artery must be looked for with these fractures.

Fractures of the Patella

The patella gets fractured either by direct trauma or by indirect mechanism of strong quadriceps contraction. Direct trauma often leads to a comminuted fracture while the quadriceps mechanism usually results in a transverse or oblique fracture **(Figs. 18A and B)**. The transverse fracture line is at the mid part. These fractures at best visualized on AP and lateral view except a rare vertical fracture which may be seen only on the sunrise or the skyline view. A superolateral accessory ossification center in a bipartite patella may simulate an acute fracture but can be differentiated by its typical location, well defined sclerotic margins and being bilateral.

Dislocation of the Patella

The patella most commonly dislocates laterally. It may occur secondary to a sudden change in direction while dancing or running or may occur following direct trauma. The dislocation is usually transient and gets reduced easily. The patella may rarely get dislocated in vertical direction with locking in the intercondylar notch or in horizontal direction with inversion and locking of superior pole of patella in the knee joint.

The dislocations may be associated with an osteochondral fragment on the medial facet of the patella or the lateral femoral condyle. Computer tomography scan may be required for the diagnosis as the fragment needs to be removed to prevent future occurrence of osteoarthritis.

Fractures of the Proximal Tibia

Fracture of the lateral tibial plateau is much more common than that of the medial tibial plateau **(Figs. 19A and B)**. It is also known as bumper fracture as is commonly seen in car accidents but this mechanism constitutes only 25% of etiology.[21] It may be more commonly seen in various other injury mechanisms including vertical compression and twisting. The common classification followed is the Hohl classification:[22] Type 1 is a vertical split of the joint margin, Type 2 is a compression of lateral plateau by impaction of lateral femoral condyle, Type 3 is a split peripheral vertical fracture with compression of the medial articular surface of the lateral tibial plateau, Type 4 is fracture of medial tibial plateau and Type 5 is bicondylar fracture with 'Y' or 'T' configuration.

These fractures may be associated with ligament injuries. Hence on radiograph it is important to look for avulsion fractures at the site of ligamentous attachments. Lipohemarthrosis may be seen in tibial plateau fractures and is identified on horizontal beam lateral radiograph. CT scan and MRI are often indicated to look for the exact extent of the fracture and the associated ligamentous injuries.

An avulsion fracture of the lateral tibial plateau at the site of attachment of the iliotibial tract is termed as

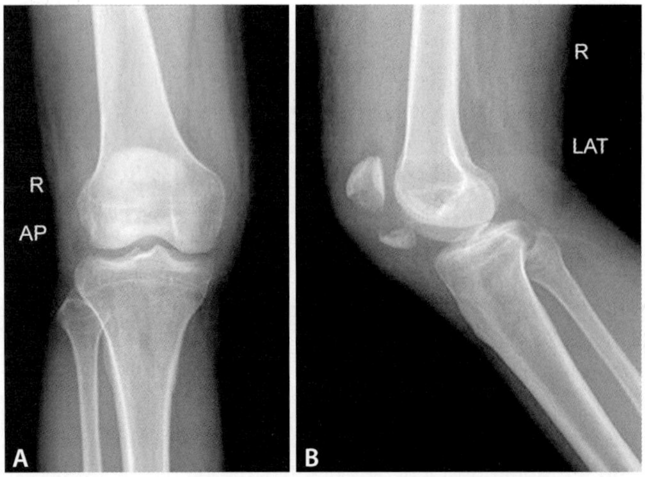

Figs. 18A and B: Anteroposterior and lateral radiographs of the knee joint show a fracture through the midpart of patella with separation of the fracture fragments due to associated muscle pull.

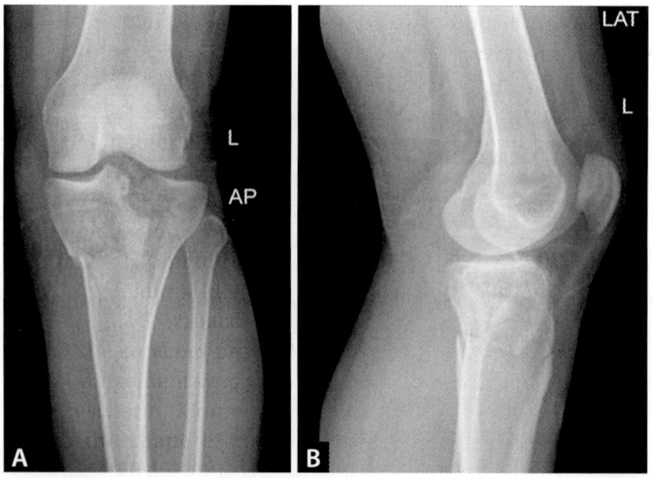

Figs. 19A and B: Anteroposterior and lateral radiographs of the knee joint show fracture of the lateral tibial plateau extending into the proximal metaphysis.

segond's fracture. It is commonly associated with injuries of the anterior cruciate ligament and meniscal injuries.

Fractures of the anterior and posterior tibial spine (intercondylar eminence) usually result from avulsion injuries at the origin of anterior and posterior cruciate ligaments.

Fractures of Shaft of Tibia and Fibula

Fractures of shaft of tibia are often associated with fractures of fibula **(Figs. 20A and B)**. The fibular fracture is commonly at upper and middle third region whereas the tibial fractures are usually at middle and lower third region. Hence, it is important to image the complete length of both bones in the radiograph so as to avoid missing associated fracture. The fractures of this region are prone to development of compartment syndrome.

An undisplaced spiral fracture in a child around 2 years of age is called as toddler's fracture.

Midshaft of the tibia alongwith proximal tibial metaphysis, fibular shaft and femoral neck are the common sites for stress fractures. They are seen in athletic individuals or those involved in strenuous running. Clinically it presents with pain during activity with relief on rest.

Fractures of the Distal Tibia and Fibula

Fractures of the medial and lateral malleoli occur due to adduction and abduction injuries. The medial malleolus fractures are generally transverse or oblique **(Fig. 21)** whereas those of the lateral malleolus are usually spiral. There may also be avulsion injuries at the malleoli. The distal tibio-fibular joint may also show diastasis associated with the malleolar fractures.

Fractures of the Talus

Fractures of the talus are second only to the calcaneus as a site of injury in the ankle region. Most common injuries are the avulsion fractures. It occurs at the anterosuperior part of the talar neck at the site of attachment of the joint capsule. The other common type of fracture is the vertical fracture of the talar neck occurring in an automobile accident. Such fractures are often complicated by avascular necrosis of the proximal part of talus. The likelihood of developing avascular necrosis increases with more anterior neck fracture. The talar dome is also a common site for development of osteochondral fractures.[23] These occur in typical location of middle third of lateral margin or posterior third of the medial margin of talar dome. If there is doubt in detection of osteochondral fractures on plain radiograph, CT scan can be done which clearly shows the fracture line.

Fractures of the Calcaneum

The calcaneus is the most frequent tarsal bone to get injured. About 75% of the fractures are intra-articular with involvement of the subtalar joint and the rest 25% are extra-articular.[24,25] The intra-articular fractures are most commonly caused by fall from height and are compression fractures. They are often bilateral (10%) and/or associated with fractures of the thoracolumbar spine. These fractures usually have associated depression of the posterior facet of the subtalar joint. The subtle compression fractures of the calcaneum can be best detected on lateral radiograph of ankle by measuring the Beohler's angle. It is the angle between a line joining the superior most part of anterior process of calcaneum to

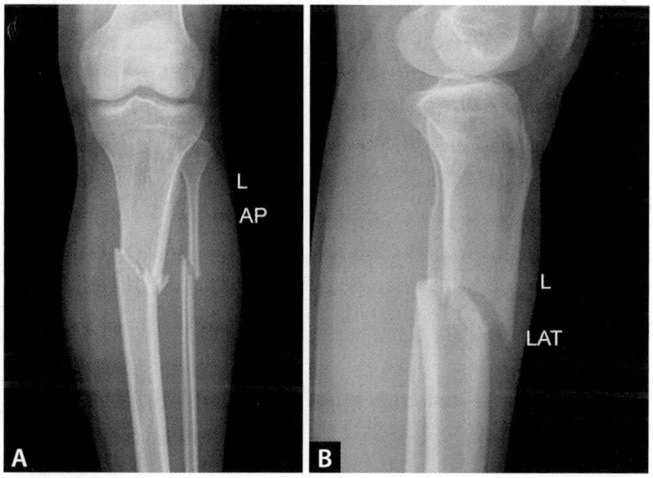

Figs. 20A and B: Anteroposterior and lateral radiograph of the proximal leg show fractures of upper shafts of both tibia and fibula.

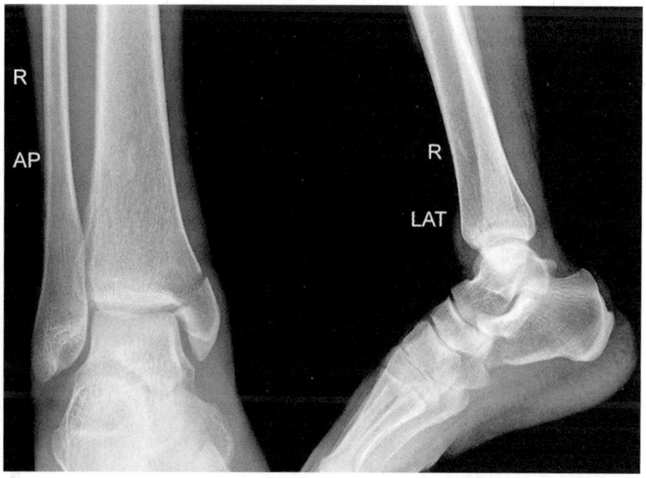

Fig. 21: Anteroposterior and lateral radiograph of the ankle joint show a transverse fracture of the medial malleolus.

the superior point of posterior facet and a line joining the superior point of posterior facet to posterosuperior margin of calcaneum tuberosity. Normally the angle between these two lines ranges from 28° to 40°. A Boehler's angle of less than 28° represents a depression of the calcaneus and hence a fracture. The extra-articular fractures are mainly avulsion injuries and may involve the anterior process (most common), superior aspect of tuberosity, plantar aspect of tuberosity or the sustentaculum tali.

Dislocations of the Foot

The talus is the most common foot bone to dislocate. The dislocation may involve the talotibial, talocalcaneal (subtalar) and the talonavicular joints.

Lisfranc's dislocation is a dislocation at tarsometatarsal junction. The second, third and the fourth metatarsals dislocate laterally, with or without associated fractures. Fracture of the base of second metatarsal is characteristic. The first metatarsal may dislocate laterally with other metatarsals (homolateral type) or may deviate medially (divergent type).

Chopart's dislocation is medial dislocation of the talonavicular and calcaneocuboid joints of the foot.

CONCLUSION

For an accurate interpretation of a radiograph of skeletal trauma, it is important for the radiologist to be aware of the clinical details including the time interval from injury and mechanism of injury. The traumatized region should always be imaged in atleast two different planes with inclusion of both the proximal and distal joints to the injured bone. A knowledge of the common injuries, their radiographic manifestations, the special radiographic views for that region if any, the pitfalls in diagnosis and the associated injuries is paramount for the radiologist. It is important not to miss an injury not only because of the treatment implications but also because many of these are medicolegal cases in which the radiograph forms part of concrete irrefutable radiological evidence. Comparative evaluation with the contralateral normal limb may be required especially in children. The use of other imaging modalities including ultrasound, CT, MRI and scintigraphy may be indicated in specific situations as and when indicated. The radiologist also has a role in the detection of post-traumatic early and delayed complications during the follow-up of the patient.

REFERENCES

1. Felson B. Roentgenology of fractures and dislocations. New York: Grune and Straton; 1978.
2. Rogers LF. Radiology of skeletal trauma, Vols 1 and 2, 2nd edition. New York: Churchill Livingstone; 1992.
3. Salter RB, Harris WR. Injuries involving the epiphyseal plate. J Bone Joint Surg. 1963;45:587.
4. Cruess RL, Dumont J. Current concepts, fracture healing. Can J Surg. 1975;18:403.
5. Hulth A. Current concepts in fracture healing. Clinical Orthopaedics. 1989;249:265.
6. Bulger EM, Smith DG, Maier RV, Jurkovich GJ. Fat embolism syndrome: A 10-year review. Arch Surg. 1997;132:435-9.
7. Shaikh N, Parchani A, Bhat V, Kattren MA. Fat embolism syndrome: Clinical and imaging considerations: Case report and review of literature. Indian J Crit Care Med. 2008;12:32-6.
8. Gupta B, Kaur M, D'souza N, Dey CK, Shende S, Kumar A, Gamangatti S. Cerebral fat embolism: A diagnostic challenge. Saudi J Anaesth. 2011;5(3):348-52.
9. Nuovo MA, Norman A, Chumas J, Ackerman LV. Myositis ossificans with atypical clinical, radiographic, or pathologic findings: a review of 23 cases. Skeletal Radiol. 1992;21:87-101.
10. Workman TL, Burkhard TK, Resnick D, et al. Hill Sach lesion: comparison of detection with MR imaging, radiography and arthroscopy. Radiology. 1992;185:847.
11. Pavlov H, Freiberger RH. Fractures and dislocations about the shoulder. Semin Roentgenol. 1978;13:85-91.
12. Kerr R. Diagnostic imaging of upper extremity trauma. Radiol Clin North Am. 1989;27(5):891-908.
13. Neer CS II. Displaced proximal humeral fractures. Part 1-classification and evaluation. Journal Bone Joint Surg (Am). 1970;52:1077.
14. Linscheid RL, Wheeler DK. Elbow dislocations. JAMA. 1965;194:1171.
15. Goldfarb CA, Yin Y, Gilula LA, Fisher AJ, Boyer MI. Wrist fractres: what the clinican wants to know. Radiology. 2001;219:11-28.
16. Munk PL, Lee MJ, Logan PM, et al. Scaphoid bone waist fractures, acute and chronic: imaging with different techniques. Am J Roentgenol. 1997;168:779-86.
17. Fisher MR, Rogers LF, Hendrix RW. A systematic approach to the diagnosis of carpometacarpal dislocations. Radiographics. 1982;2:612-27.
18. Epstein HC. Traumatic dislocations of the hip. Clin Orthop. 1973;92:116.
19. Erb RE, Steele JR, Nance EP Jr, Edwards JR. Traumatic anterior dislocation of the hip: spectrum of plain film and CT findings. Am J Roentgenol. 1995;165:1215-9.
20. Sutton David. Textbook of Radiology and Imaging, 7th edition. Churchill Livingstone; 2003;2:1371-416.
21. Newberg AH, Greenstein R. Radiographic evaluation of tibial plateau fracture. Radiology. 1978;126:319.
22. Hohl M. Tibial condylar fractures. J Bone Joint Surg (Am). 1967;49:1455.
23. Canale ST, Belding RH. Osteochondral lesions of the talus. J Bone Joint Surg [Am]. 1980;62A:97-102.
24. Greenspan A. Imaging of the foot and ankle. Curr Opin Orthop. 1996;7:61-8.
25. Karasick D. Fractures and dislocations of the foot. Semin Roentgen. 1994;24:152.

CHAPTER 205

Imaging of Soft Tissue Lesions

Ashu Seith Bhalla, Sanjay Thulkar

INTRODUCTION

Soft tissue pathologies encompass a wide spectrum of entities. Patients often present with nonspecific clinical findings, such as an ill-defined soft tissue swelling or a discrete palpable mass, with or without accompanying tenderness or pain. With equivocal clinical findings, imaging can confirm the presence of a soft tissue lesion or identify a suspected 'mass' as normal tissue.

The objectives of initial imaging evaluation are detecting the suspected lesion, establishing a diagnosis or formulating a differential diagnosis and radiological staging (if the lesion is neoplastic).[1,2] The evaluation of soft tissue pathology has undergone dramatic evolution with advances in magnetic resonance imaging (MRI).

IMAGING MODALITIES

- Plain radiography
- Ultrasonography (USG)
- Magnetic resonance imaging (MRI)
- Computed tomography (CT)
- Positron emission tomography-computed tomography (PET-CT).

Plain Radiography

On conventional radiography, the appreciation of difference in radiodensity is made difficult by the fact that most organs are composed of chemicals whose atomic numbers are relatively low and closely related. For practical purposes, soft tissue organs may be regarded as having the same radiographic density as that of water (or urine or blood). Only fat and gas will give a discernible radiodensity less than that of muscle. Distinction between structures is hence usually possible only by the presence of surrounding fat. Fat is readily distinguished from other soft tissues provided a primary X-ray beam of lower energy is used, i.e. about 15 kV less than for bone radiography for the same region. Density differences can also be maximized using postprocessing in digital radiography.

Increased radiodensity may be seen in soft tissues with mineralization (calcification or ossification), hemosiderin deposition and certain foreign bodies. Soft tissue calcifications can be suggestive and at times characteristic of a specific diagnosis. Radiographs may also be diagnostic of a palpable lesion caused by an underlying skeletal deformity (e.g. bony exostosis) masquerading as a soft tissue mass.

Decreased radiodensity is observed with fat or air-containing lesions.

In addition, radiographs are the best initial methods of assessing *coexistent osseous involvement*, such as osseous remodeling, periosteal reaction, osseous destruction or new bone formation. In most cases, two views at right angles are mandatory to delineate soft tissue planes and the adjacent cortical bone.[1,3]

Unlike intraosseous tumors the biologic activity of a soft tissue mass cannot be reliably assessed by its growth rate. A slow growing soft tissue mass that may remodel adjacent bone may still be malignant on histologic examination.

Ultrasonography

Ultrasonography (USG) is a readily available, noninvasive and relatively inexpensive method of detecting and determining the size and consistency of a soft tissue mass. It should be the initial screening modality used in soft tissue pathology, and may suffice in several cases. Ultrasonography is of value in distinguishing cystic from solid masses. It is invaluable in the evaluation of arteriovenous malformations and hemangiomas. More accurate staging and characterization of a soft tissue mass, however, requires MRI. Doppler is a useful adjunct in assessing tumor vascularity.[4] USG is also useful for image guided interventions.

Elastography is an adjunct tool to high resolution USG in the evaluation of soft tissue lesions. Assessment of stiffness of masses using elastography helps in their characterization.[5]

Magnetic Resonance Imaging

Magnetic resonance imaging has emerged as the preferred modality for imaging soft tissue lesions. MRI is superior to CT in delineating the extent of a soft tissue mass and in defining its relationship to adjacent neurovascular structures. Superior soft tissue contrast resolution and discrimination of tissues on MRI is based on multiple tissue parameters including T1 and T2 relaxation times, proton density, etc. which are significantly different for different soft tissues.

Technique: Positioning of patient and the choice of proper surface coils for the study of soft tissue lesions is essential to minimize motion artifacts and to obtain optimal signal to noise ratio. Evaluation of trunk and thighs is most efficacious using the body coil with the patient supine. If a gluteal soft tissue lesion is suspected, prone position may be helpful to avoid distortion of the posterior soft tissues. The body coil also allows comparison of both lower extremities and can provide complete evaluation of the entire osseous or soft tissue region of interest.

Numerous pulse sequences can be used to evaluate soft tissue masses, including spin echo sequences, short tau inversion recovery (STIR) sequence and gradient echo sequences. New sequences have been developed to decrease the examination time or improve the specificity. Fast spin echo T2-weighted sequences give a strong T2-weighted image and save time. Their main drawback is high-signal intensity of fat similar to that of water, which is not convenient for evaluation of musculoskeletal tumors. To be used adequately, a fat presaturation method must be employed with this sequence.

Short tau inversion recovery (STIR) sequences are very useful in detecting subtle abnormalities and are frequently added to the spin echo sequences. Although STIR imaging increases lesion conspicuity, it has lower signal-to-noise ratio than spin echo imaging and is also more susceptible to degradation by motion. STIR imaging can thus be an adjunct. Gradient echo imaging is a useful supplement in demonstrating hemosiderin because of its greater magnetic susceptibility. Gradient echo images may also be better in some instances to demonstrate the lesion fat interface and to detect small surrounding vessels.

Contrast enhancement following intravenous gadolinium injection will show up soft tissue lesions due to their vascularization and perfusion but contrast enhancement is rarely necessary and hence should not be used routinely. Fat suppressed T2-weighted or STIR sequences generally suffice without the additional cost of contrast medium. In equivocal cases contrast enhancement may be useful in distinguishing cystic from solid lesions, and thus identifying the most appropriate site for biopsy.[6,7]

Dynamic contrast-enhanced MR: Different dynamic contrast-enhanced MR imaging techniques have been developed, e.g. region of interest technique, first pass technique and gadolinium-enhanced MR imaging subtraction technique, etc. Rapid contrast uptake is an indicator of malignancy in a soft tissue tumor.[8] With the increasing use of adjuvant chemotherapy in the management of soft tissue sarcomas, these techniques can be expected to be used more often to assess angiogenesis and response.[6,7]

Dynamic susceptibility-weighted contrast-enhanced MR imaging also has been used wherein a threshold dynamic susceptibility contrast ratio (percentage) of 30.7% is reported to have an accuracy of 84.6% for differentiating malignant from benign tumors.[9]

Lesion characterization: Despite the superiority of MRI in identifying, delineating and staging soft tissue tumors, it remains limited in precisely characterizing soft tissue masses, with most lesions demonstrating prolonged T1 and T2 relaxation times. A majority of soft tissue masses have a nonspecific low to intermediate signal on T1 and high signal on T2-weighted images. A correct histologic diagnosis based on imaging studies alone is achieved in perhaps only 25–30% of cases. Investigators, however, feel that this percentage is increasing and ultimately will approach the range of 75–90%.[10] It is useful to use muscle as a reference tissue when assessing T1-weighted scans, with cysts showing lower signal and solid tumors slightly increased signal intensity. Simple cystic lesions (ganglion, meniscal cyst, bursa, fat necrosis, lymphocele) have a characteristic homogeneous, very low and very high signal on T1 and T2-weighted images, respectively. Conversely, some soft tissue masses (scar/fibrous tissue), chronic hematoma, aggressive fibromata, pigmented villonodular synovitis, aneurysm and vascular malformation show a low signal or signal void on both sequences. There are instances, however, in which a specific diagnosis may be made or strongly suspected, e.g. fat containing lesions. Some soft tissue masses (lipoma, subacute hematoma, hemangioma, intralesional hemorrhage and well-differentiated liposarcoma) demonstrate a characteristic high-signal on T1 and T2-weighted images. Lipoma, aggressive fibromatosis (desmoids), nerve sheath tumors, myxomas and soft tissue secondaries tend to be multiple. Hence, some lesions can be accurately diagnosed on MRI, e.g. lipoma/liposarcoma, benign vascular lesions such as hemangioma, arteriovenous malformation, pseudoaneurysm, hemosiderin-laden lesions, such as pigmented villonodular synovitis (PVNS), fibromatosis and some neurogenic tumors.[2]

Magnetic resonance imaging may also give potentially useful histological information in that the T2 signal may correlate with tumor cellularity and presence of myxoid matrix.[11]

An important limitation of MRI is its relative inability to detect soft tissue calcification; consequently, a diagnosis that may be readily apparent on radiographs frequently remains nonspecific on MR images. It must be emphasized that it is essential to interpret MR images in conjunction with appropriate corresponding plain radiographs and other imaging studies, if available.[2,12]

Traumatic lesions, such as soft tissue hematoma and myositis ossificans can mimic a malignant tumor in view of the varying signal intensities of the altered blood. In these cases, it is helpful to have a clinical history of trauma, use intravenous gadolinium chelate and perform a plain radiograph to assess the presence of calcification. Myositis ossificans can produce an intense diffuse enhancement, but hematoma does not enhance. Careful follow-up and histological review are required for indeterminate lesions. Infection can also mimic a malignant soft tissue tumor and clinical history is important in this regard.

Benign vs malignant differentiation: It was earlier thought that MRI would correctly differentiate benign from malignant masses on the basis of signal intensity appearances on T1- and T2-weighted images. Subsequent work has shown that signal intensity patterns are not a good discriminator between benign and malignant tumors. Definite characterization of tumor types into benign and malignant is difficult, but it is useful to assess various criteria **(Table 1)**, which can help make the distinction.[13,14] MRI is also useful in the postoperative setting in distinguishing seromas (fluid collections) from recurrent or residual tumor.[15,16]

MR imaging depicts characteristics of a malignant soft tissue tumor as an ill-defined heterogeneous mass that encases neurovascular structures and invades bone **(Figs. 1A and B)**. Edema in adjacent muscles is another MRI feature that has been strongly associated with malignant soft tissue neoplasms. In contrast, the well-defined homogeneous lesion that does not invade adjacent bone and neurovascular structures and maintains soft tissue planes is suggestive of a benign process. However, there is considerable overlap. A significant proportion of malignant soft tissue tumors may have well-defined margins with a so called pseudocapsule and relatively homogeneous signal intensity. It is important that the full extent of any soft tissue mass together with its relationship to the adjacent joint and surrounding anatomical structures be clearly demonstrated. Intravenous contrast is useful if a lesion is not pure blood, pure water or pure fat. If the lesion enhances, a tumor should be suspected and biopsy of the enhancing area be obtained.

MR Spectroscopy

Investigators have reported that proton spectroscopy can help differentiate malignant from benign tumors by demonstrating the presence of water-soluble choline metabolites in malignant lesions.[17]

Diffusion-weighted imaging: Diffusion weighted imaging may also be useful in differentiation of benign and malignant tumors, with benign lesions demonstrating higher ADC values and malignant lesions showing lower values. Though there is a substantial overlap in the ADC values of benign and malignant tumors; however, the presence of

Table 1: Criteria for differentiating benign and malignant soft tissue tumors.

- Location
- Signal intensity
- Signal homogeneity
- Size (growth rate)
- Tumor margin
- Compartment spread
- Neurovascular invasion
- Adjacent soft tissues
- Bone infiltration/destruction

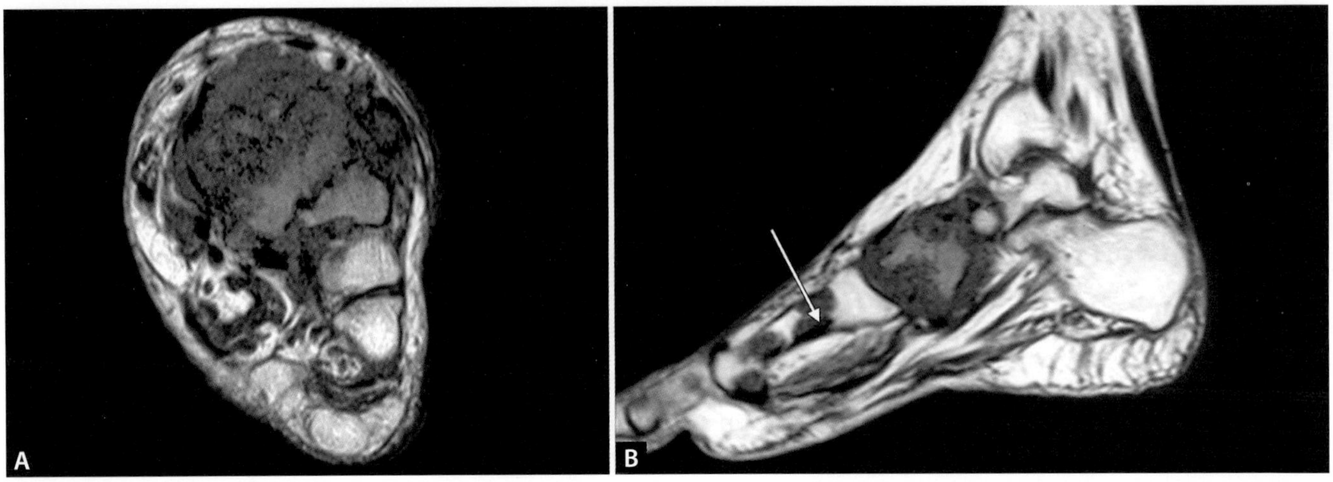

Figs. 1A and B: Malignant mass: Axial (A) and sagittal (B) T1W images showing a heterogeneous soft tissue mass which is invading the adjoining tarsal bones with encasement of the neurovascular bundle. Also metastatic lesions are seen in the metatarsals on the sagittal image (arrow).

extremely low ADC values (relative to adjoining muscles) in soft tissue tumors suggests malignancy.[18,19] ADC also correlates with tumor cellularity in soft tissue sarcomas with lower values seen in malignant nonmyxoid tumors compared to benign tumors. In one study in malignant nonmyxoid tumors had a mead ADC of 0.94 × 10^{-3} mm^2/sec compared with 1.31 94 × 10^{-3} mm^2/sec for benign nonmyxoid tumors.[20]

Staging

The staging system most commonly used for soft tissue tumor is the one proposed by American Joint Committee (AJC).[21] The staging of the tumor requires the use of multiple imaging planes with a variety of pulse sequences. Coronal T1-weighted images show extent of tumor, with transverse sections using pathology sensitive sequences (T2-weighted, STIR, fat-suppressed T2-weighted) more clearly depict compartmental spread and neurovascular invasion. The staging of soft tissue sarcomas is determined by the size of the tumor, the histologic grade, and lymph nodal spread or distant metastases. The American Joint Committee on Cancer (AJCC) has detailed staging using the four criteria of tumor size, nodal status, grade, and metastasis (TNGM). The T stage is detailed below. N0/N1 refers to regional lymph nodes, while M0/M1 represent distant metastasis. Histological grade of the tumor varies from G1 to G3. The tumor is then further stage into four stages (I–IV). Presently the 7th edition of the system is in use. CT scan of the chest is recommended for tumors more than 5 cm (T2) or for those with moderate to poor differentiation (grades 2–4). Nodal involvement is rare.

T Stage:

- Tx : Primary tumor cannot be assessed.
- T0 : No evidence of primary tumor.
- T1 : Tumor ≤5 cm in greatest dimension. T1a—Superficial tumor, T1b—Deep tumor.
- T2 : Tumor >5 cm in greatest dimension. T2a—Superficial tumor. T2b—Deep tumor.

Location

The location of the lesion also aids in narrowing the differential diagnosis, and MRI can accurately localize the lesions. The locations include intramuscular, intermuscular, subcutaneous, and intra-articular/periarticular. An extensive lesion may be multicompartmental and the differential diagnosis of such lesions is angiomatous lesions, neurofibromatosis, fibromatosis, lipomatosis, myxoma (Mazabraud syndrome), metastases, or lymphoma. An intracompartmental lesion refers to one that has not crossed any natural anatomic boundaries. These boundaries may be cortical bone, articular cartilage, joint capsule, major fascial plane, tendon, or ligament. Aggressive lesions may invade surrounding tissues and cross anatomic boundaries. It is important to identify and report these invasions on MR. The spread may be along vascular channels or even poorly planned biopsy paths.[10]

Tumor recurrence vs post-therapy changes: MRI plays a major role in the detection of tumor recurrence. MR imaging is also useful in follow-up for evaluating the treatment response, especially in infiltrative tumors involving major neurovascular structures that receive adjuvant radiation or chemotherapy.[11]

T2-weighted/STIR images can be used to demonstrate tumor recurrence which is shown as a high signal intensity mass. There is, however, difficulty in separating the changes related to recent treatment, particularly radiotherapy. Radiotherapy may result in soft tissue trabeculation, increase in fatty marrow as well as focal marrow abnormalities. Rarely, patients may develop radiation-induced malignancies in the irradiated field. Chemotherapy also alters the imaging appearance of a tumor. Chemotherapy-induced hemorrhage may result in an increase in the size of the mass. Familiarity with post-surgical appearances is also important. Myocutaneous flaps demonstrate time-dependent changes in size, signal intensity, and enhancement which help distinguish them from recurrent tumors on MR. Recurrent tumor appears as a discrete nodule or mass with signal characteristics that characteristically mirror those of the original tumor. Use of unenhanced T1-weighted fat-suppressed and gradient-echo sequences helps differentiate post-treatment hemorrhage from tumor recurrence.[22] The use of contrast enhancement is helpful in distinguishing recurrent tumor from radiation-induced inflammation and necrosis, tumor takes contrast medium early, whereas inflammatory reaction enhances later.[13,14] MR spectroscopy and diffusion-weighted images are useful adjuncts in this setting.

Computed Tomography

In general, computed tomography (CT) has been replaced by MRI in the evaluation of patients with soft tissue masses. Although adipose tissue within a mass may be identified equally well with either CT or MRI, further characterization of fat containing masses (other than simple lipoma) is better seen with MRI. CT is unequivocally superior in detecting subtle calcification or ossification in the soft tissues not detectable on radiographs and may be complementary to MRI. The zonal pattern of mineralization essential to the radiologic diagnosis of early myositis ossificans may be seen on CT, whereas radiographs remain nonspecific. CT also details involvement of the adjacent bone. CT remains the examination of choice for the evaluation of chest to rule out pulmonary metastases.

PET-CT

PET-CT is covered in detail in the chapter on nuclear medicine.

SOFT TISSUE LESIONS

Soft tissue lesions will be discussed under the following heads:

- Artifacts
- Calcification and ossification in soft tissues

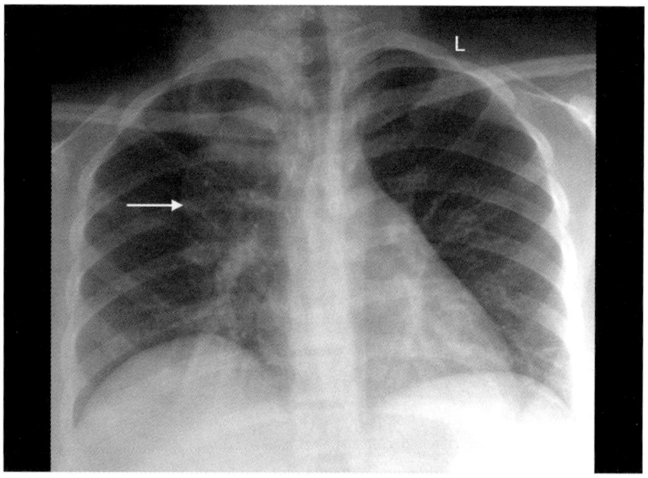

Fig. 2: Artifact: Frontal chest radiograph of a young girl with artifact caused by overlying hair braid (arrow).

- Air in the soft tissues
- Fat in soft tissues
- *Soft tissue masses*:
  - Cystic soft tissue lesions
  - Inflammatory lesions
  - Soft tissue tumors.

ARTIFACTS

The radiologist must be aware of various misleading appearances which can be produced due to normal structures casting soft tissue shadows, e.g. in the skull, shadow of the pinna, plaited hair **(Fig. 2)** or wrinkled scalp of a newborn may cause added densities. Substances on the skin, such as lead ointment or pigments used in tattoos, may cause confusing opacities. Another possible source of error is the appearance of a thin dark line where two soft tissue shadows overlap—the so-called 'Mach effect'. This may simulate a fracture.

CALCIFICATION AND OSSIFICATION IN SOFT TISSUES

Calcification of the soft tissues is seen in many diseases and trauma. Abnormal tissue calcification can be subdivided into three major categories **(Table 2)**.[3]

1. Metastatic in previously undamaged tissues, with elevated serum of calcium and phosphate levels.
2. Dystrophic calcification in injured tissue with normal serum levels.
3. Idiopathic calcification or calcinosis in previously normal tissues with normal serum levels.

Metastatic calcification is commonly widespread, fairly symmetrical and bilateral in distribution. Dystrophic

Table 2: Conditions showing soft tissue calcification and/or ossification.[3]

1. *Metastatic calcification* (Normal tissue, elevated Ca × P ion product) A. *Hypercalcemia*: • Hyperparathyroidism (primary) • Vitamin D intoxication • Milk–alkali syndrome • Metastases to bone • Malignancies diseases, e.g. multiple myeloma, leukemia B. *Hyperphosphatemia*: • Hyperparathyroidism (secondary) • Idiopathic hyperphosphatemia • Hypoparathyroidism, etc.
2. *Dystrophic calcification* (Altered or necrotic tissue with normal Ca × P ion product) A. *Metabolic diseases*: • Pseudohypoparathyroidism, pseudopseudohypoparathyroidism • Crystal deposition disease—calcium pyrophosphate deposition disease, hydroxyapatite deposition disease, hemochromatosis B. *Collagen vascular diseases*: • Scleroderma • Crest syndrome (calcinosis, Raynaud's phenomenon, esophageal ectasia, sclerodactyly, telangiectasia) • Dermatomyositis C. *Parasitic infestations and infections*: • Tuberculosis • Leprosy • Cysticercosis • Dracunculosis D. *Vascular calcification*: • Arterial, e.g. atherosclerosis, venous E. Injection site F. *Miscellaneous*: • Blunt trauma • Thermal injury • Fat necrosis • Tumor calcification
3. *Idiopathic calcification:* • Calcific peritendinitis • Calcific bursitis • Calcinosis circumscripta • Idiopathic calcinosis universalis • Tumoral calcinosis
4. *Soft tissue tumors*

calcification is usually limited to the site of injury and tends to be more focal and asymmetrically distributed.

Calcification/ossification may also be seen within soft tissue tumors.

Metastatic Calcification

Prolonged elevation of product of serum calcium and phosphate due to any cause may lead to calcium deposition in soft tissues. Arterial and cartilaginous calcifications are well recognized in hyperparathyroidism. Arterial calcification is frequently seen in patients on renal dialysis and in this group one may also find quite gross periarticular calcification similar to the appearance of tumoral calcinosis. This may occur with relatively normal values of serum calcium and appears to be related to the rising levels of serum phosphate.[3]

Dystrophic Calcification

Metabolic Diseases

Soft tissue calcification may also be observed in patients with pseudohypoparathyroidism and pseudopseudohypoparathyroidism. In the latter condition the diagnostic areas are hands and feet, where soft tissue calcification is associated with characteristic shortening of the first, fourth and fifth metacarpals and metatarsals.

Collagen Vascular Diseases

Scleroderma, Raynaud's Phenomenon

Calcification in the fingers is an important and striking feature of soft tissue necrosis associated with Raynaud's phenomenon. It is, therefore, common in patients with diffuse systemic sclerosis (scleroderma). The calcium deposits are often very dense and sharply localized near the fingertips with associated soft tissue loss.

Dermatomyositis

Dermatomyositis is more common in women in their third to fifth decade. It is frequently associated with widespread calcification, both in the skin itself and in subcutaneous connective tissue. Fibrosis and calcification in muscles may lead to flexion contractures. Raised muscle enzymes occur during the active stage of the disease. The patients may suffer from proximal muscle weakness and vasculitis. A severe form of the disease affecting children under 10 years of age causes extensive muscle damage and fibrosis with particularly widespread calcification. Radiographically, soft tissue calcification is indistinguishable from idiopathic calcinosis universalis.[1,3]

Parasitic Infestations

Of the parasitic infestations, cysticercosis cellulosae is the most common cause of soft tissue calcification, seen in Asian subcontinent. They appear to have a predilection for skeletal muscle, subcutaneous tissue and brain. On radiographs, calcified cysts are seen as elongated ovoids with their long axis roughly aligned with the direction of muscle fibers **(Fig. 3)**. Typically guinea worm *(Dracunculus medinensis)* is seen as a coiled worm **(Fig. 4)** which in course of time may disintegrate to a more

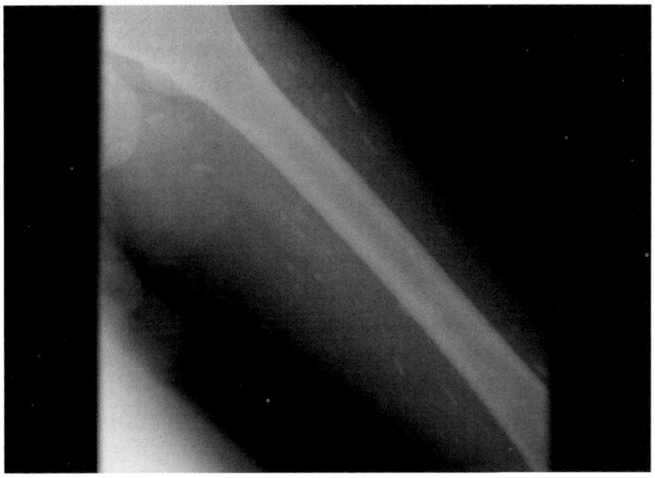

Fig. 3: Calcified cysticerci seen as elongated ovoid structures roughly aligned with the direction of muscles in the thigh on plain radiograph.

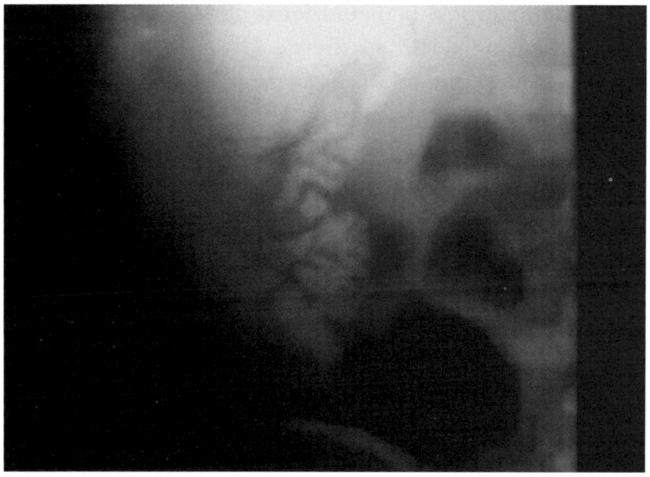

Fig. 4: Calcified guinea worm: A coiled calcified guinea worm is seen in the soft tissues in the right lumbar region on plain X-ray of the abdomen.

amorphous appearance. Calcification may occur as part of healing process of any infective lesion but is particularly associated with tuberculosis where calcified lymph nodes are commonly seen.[1,3]

Vascular Calcification

Atheromatous calcification is an inevitable consequence of aging and may range from localized irregular plaques to extensive tram-like calcification involving most of the aorta and pelvic vessels and extending into lower limbs. The finer "pipe stem calcification" of Monckeberg's medial sclerosis shows a similar tendency to favor the lower limbs, a feature well recognized in diabetes. Mural calcification in a vein is rarely seen, but calcified phleboliths are extremely common especially in the pelvis. Phleboliths may also be seen in hemangiomas.

Idiopathic Calcification

Idiopathic Calcinosis Universalis

Idiopathic calcinosis universalis is a rare disorder of unknown cause affecting infants and children. The calcifiation laid down in longitudinal bands **(Fig. 5)**, initially occurs in the subcutaneous fat of the extremities and subsequently appears in muscles, ligaments and tendons. The calcific deposits coalesce, enlarge and can break through the skin surface. Serum biochemistry is normal in these patients.[1,3]

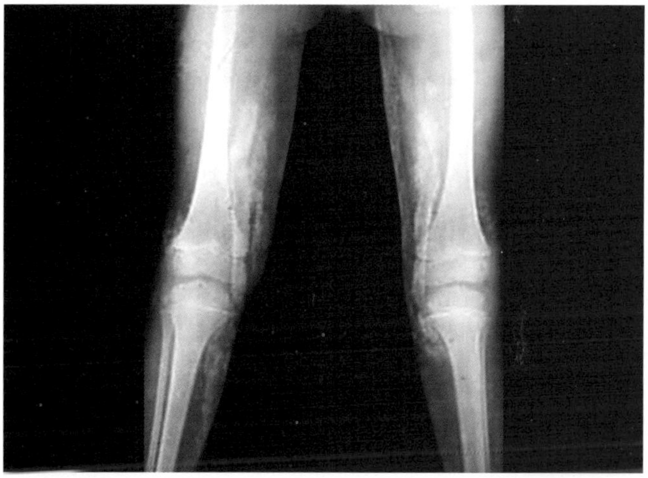

Fig. 5: Idiopathic calcinosis universalis: Calcification laid down in longitudinal bands seen in the soft tissues of both lower extremities on the plain radiograph.

Calcinosis Circumscripta

Deposits of calcium in subcutaneous tissues in a circumscribed form occur in a variety of diseases most frequently in and around joints, e.g. acrosclerosis, scleroderma, dermatomyositis, renal osteodystrophy with secondary hyperparathyroidism.

Tumoral Calcinosis

The condition consists of large painless juxta-articular calcified masses, frequently in soft tissues of hips, shoulders, elbows or smaller joints. There is a familial tendency. The etiology is unknown, but a metabolic defect and trauma are considered as some of the factors. The condition becomes manifest in second to third decade with the majority of individuals having an inborn error of phosphate metabolism. Similar appearances can occur in renal osteodystrophy.

On radiographs, loculated dense homogeneous masses of calcification occur in the periarticular soft tissues. Radiolucent septa separate aggregates of calcification giving a multiloculated appearance. Large periarticular calcifications may have fluid levels. The bones are normal. The masses grow progressively and recur after incomplete excision. Radionuclide scan will show intense increase in uptake over all the areas of involvement.[3] On MRI, there is a variable high and low signal intensity on T2-weighted (T2W) images from these calcific masses, often with large areas of signal void.[23]

OSSIFICATION

Many calcifying lesions may proceed to ossification and radiological distinction is neither always easy nor necessarily important. Heterotopic ossification occurs secondary to trauma, surgery, burn or paralysis. Soft tissue uptake on isotope bone scanning can occur before the ossification is evident radiographically. The basic defect is the inappropriate differentiation of fibroblasts into osteoblasts following an inflammatory lesion in the soft tissues.

Myositis Ossificans

Myositis ossificans is a benign, self-limiting response to soft tissue injury. The reactive lesions are composed mainly of hypercellular fibrous tissue which evolves into mature bone. Bone formation usually becomes evident within 6–8 weeks after the onset of symptoms. The condition is most common in the 2nd and 3rd decades of life.[18] Myositis ossificans is heterotopic bone (sometimes cartilage) forming in muscles, tendons and fascia following trauma **(Figs. 6 and 7)**. After muscle damage, what initially may appear to be a hematoma can subsequently show the fine, lacy calcification. During the first 2 weeks following trauma, a warm and painful soft tissue mass develops. In the subsequent 2 weeks, amorphous densities develop in the mass possibly with periosteal reaction. During this initial period of 4 weeks, the process histologically resembles a parosteal osteosarcoma, and the MRI features are nonspecific. There is usually, however, a thin line of separation between the ossification and adjacent bone which helps in differentiation. Subsequently, the post-traumatic myositis ossificans matures (ossifies) in a peripheral to central pattern and is associated with a reduction in the size of the mass, factors which also help

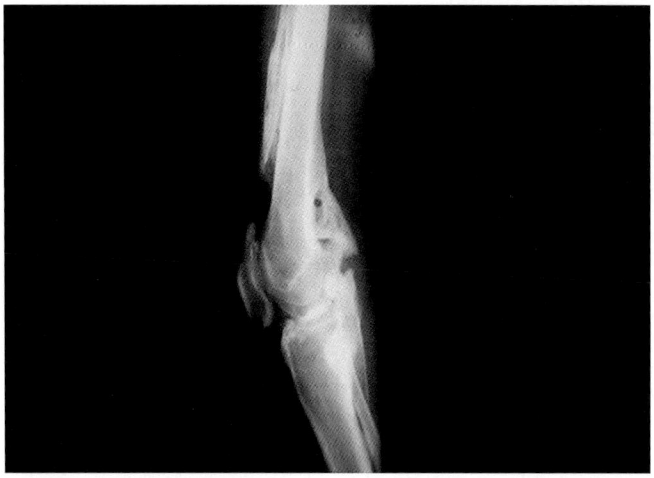

Fig. 6: Post-traumatic myositis ossificans seen involving the soft tissues adjacent to the lower end of femur and upper end of tibia on the plain radiograph.

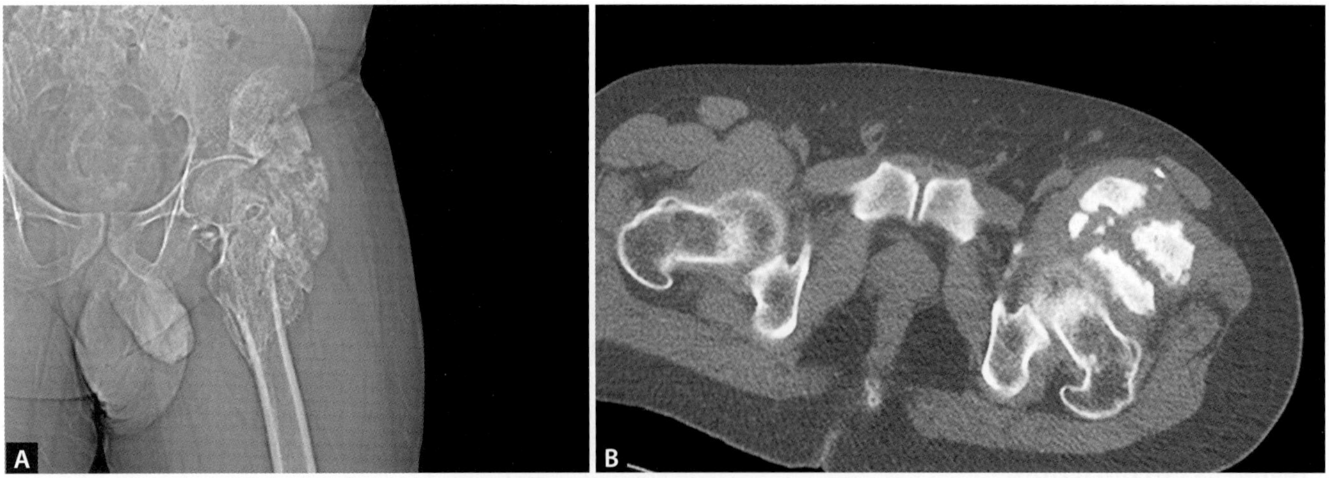

Figs. 7A and B: Myositis ossificans: CT scout (A) and axial image (B) reveal inhomogeneous, dense ossification involving the muscles of anterior compartment of the thigh and inguinal region. The "bone mass" is separate from the underlying bone.

to distinguish it from a malignant process. About 30% of cases resolve entirely.[18]

Magnetic resonance imaging appearance of myositis ossificans depends on the age of the lesion. Early lesions appear isointense to muscle on T1-weighted images and on T2WI signal intensity is greater than that of fat, with diffuse surrounding soft tissue edema. Intermediate lesions are similar but typically demonstrate a rim of curvilinear decreased intensity at the periphery corresponding to ossification. Mature (late) lesions are well-defined inhomogeneous masses with a signal intensity approximating that of fat on T2 and T1-weighted images. A rim of decreased signal intensity is seen around the lesion with similar areas of ossification within, with no evidence of associated edema.[2,24]

Once mature, CT can also delineate the extent of the lesion.

Surgical resection is best left until after maturation is complete which can be assessed on MRI or isotope bone scanning, otherwise, a high recurrence rate results. The soft tissues around the elbow and thigh are common sites for developing this complication.

Repeated minor trauma may result in bone formation, particularly in tendinous or ligamentous insertions. Heterotopic bone is known as "rider's bone" when it arises in the adductor longus muscle, "Pellegrini-Stieda lesion" adjacent to adductor tubercle of distal femur, "fencer's bone" in brachialis muscle and "dancer's bone" in the soleus.[3]

Extensive ossification, particularly round the pelvic girdle is sometimes found in patients with paraplegia. The bone, which is usually attached to the underlying skeleton, is frequently extensive, tending to invest neighboring joints in coarse amorphous bands.

Myositis Ossificans Progressiva (Fibrodysplasia Ossificans Progressiva)

Myositis ossificans progressiva: It is an inherited disorder with autosomal dominant inheritance. It is characterized by congenital malformations of the great toes and progressive heterotopic ossification, which appears in specific anatomic patterns. The disorder usually manifests between birth and 10 years with abnormal ossification first commencing in the neck, then on the shoulders, arms, chest and eventually on the feet. Dorsal involvement precedes ventral involvement **(Figs. 8A to C)**. The patients are usually bed-ridden by the age of 30 years.[25]

Soft Tissue Masses with Calcification/Ossification

The presence of calcified matrix within a lesion suggests a differential diagnosis of chondro-osseus type tumors. Linear, spiculated and amorphous central calcification are seen in osteosarcomas. On the other hand, stippled and curvilinear calcifications are typical of cartilaginous tumors, such as soft tissue chondroma and chondrosarcoma. As detailed peripheral calcification may be seen in myositis ossificans, and also in ossifying fibromyxoid tumors. Other tumors that may show calcification are lipoma, liposarcoma, malignant fibrous histiocytoma, synovial sarcoma, and rhabdomyosarcoma.[18]

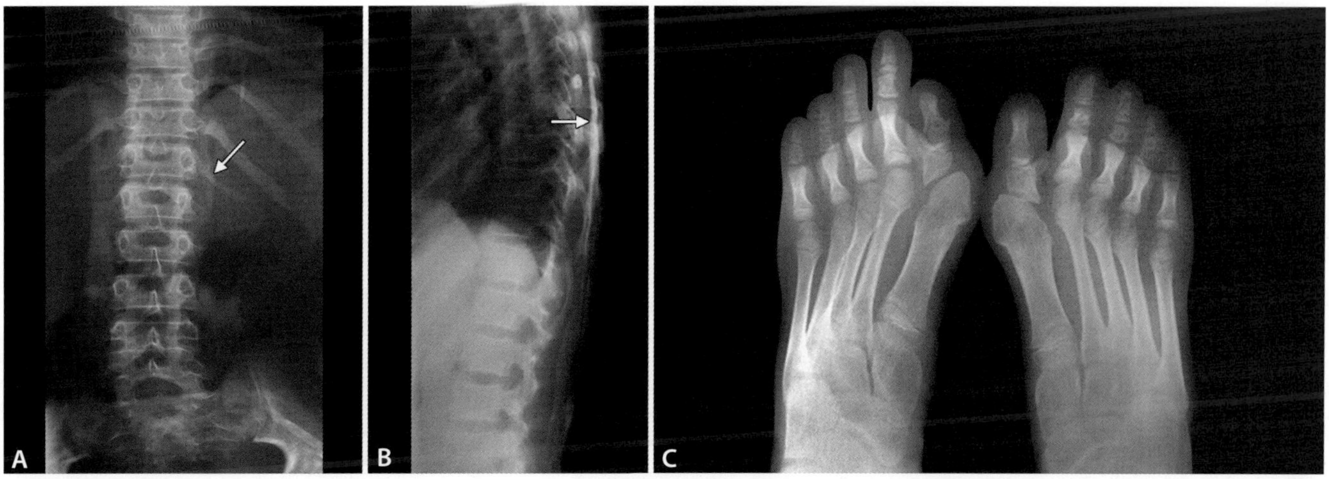

Figs. 8A to C: Myositis ossificans progressiva: Plain radiographs of dorsolumbar spine frontal (A) and lateral (B) views of a 20-year-old male reveal dense ossification in the paraspinal region, involving the dorsal soft tissues. Bilateral great toes are deformed (C) with short broad proximal phalanges and metatarsals.

AREAS OF DECREASED DENSITY

Air in the Soft Tissues

Air Leaks (Surgical Emphysema)

Air may be driven into the tissues by positive pressure from respiratory tract following fracture of the paranasal sinuses, rupture of trachea, bronchi or puncture of the lung by a fractured rib. Similar appearances are seen following chest surgery. The skin and muscle bundles are separated from each other and from the ribs by coalescing areas of radiolucent air **(Fig. 9)**.

Air Formed within the Soft Tissues

Air within the skeletal soft tissues usually arises as a result of infection, e.g. coliform infection especially in diabetes. Soft tissue injury, especially if associated with extensive muscle damage and foreign body penetration as in shrapnel wounds may be complicated by infection with anaerobic organisms, particularly clostridia. This may take the form of cellulitis which tends to be confined to the superficial tissues where pockets of gas may be visible radiographically. Much more serious is true gas gangrene (clostridial myositis), where necrotic muscle is rapidly colonized by anaerobic organisms **(Fig. 10)**. Radiological feature of gas gangrene which distinguishes it from anaerobic cellulitis, is the pectinate appearance of gas infiltrating individual groups of muscle fibers.

Air Introduced from Outside

Air may be introduced as a result of penetrating wounds or compound fractures. Manipulation of such injuries may cause air to be sucked into the wound, particularly if there are torn or retracted muscles.[1,3]

FAT IN THE SOFT TISSUES

Fat normally produces translucencies in certain well defined areas—in front of lower end of humerus, infrapatellar region, and in front of the Achilles tendon. Obliteration of these translucencies indicates edema or hemorrhage into the fat. Displacement or obliteration of the translucency in front of the elbow suggests presence of a fracture, and is a useful sign in diagnosing occult fractures.[26]

Fracture may also lead to release of fat from the marrow cavity besides hemorrhage. The fat then floats on the blood and a horizontal ray film of the injured area may show fat blood interface. This condition is referred to as lipohemarthrosis. Fat containing masses (lipomas/ liposarcomas) may also be recognized as translucent areas within muscles. These will be discussed subsequently.

SOFT TISSUE MASSES

Cystic Soft Tissue Lesions

Bursae

Bursae lined with synovial cells are usually found over bony prominences. Bursae superficial to the patella and olecranon are so well known that the symptoms related to these have been given such terms as "house maid's knee" and "student's elbow", respectively. Septic bursitis usually results from invasion of bacteria through a skin abrasion. US findings include a fluid-filled collection surrounded by

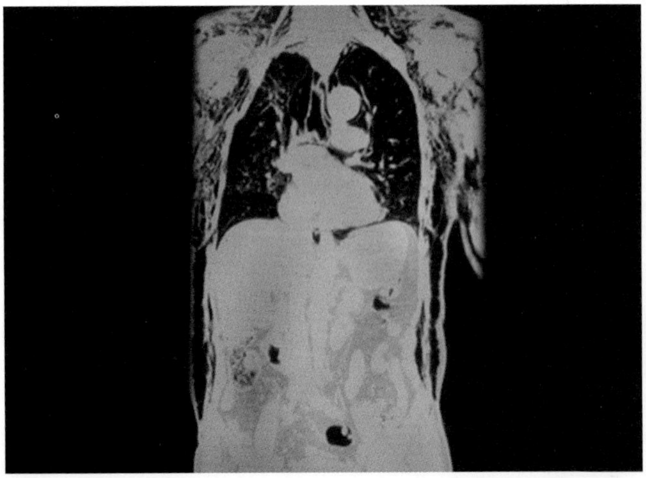

Fig. 9: Surgical emphysema: Coronal MPR of CT chest-abdomen of a 70-year-old man obtained following trauma reveals air tracking through the subcutaneous tissues, intra- and intermuscular planes of the thorax and abdomen.

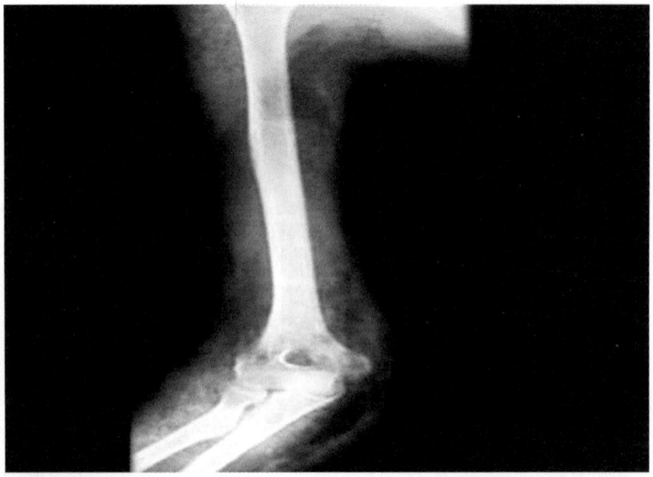

Fig. 10: Gas gangrene: Plain radiograph of the arm showing extensive air in the soft tissues and the muscles of arm and forearm.

a thickened bursal wall. The specific anatomic location is the clue to the diagnosis, however, only needle aspiration of the distended bursa can confirm the sepsis.[3]

Cystic Masses around the Knee

Cystic masses around the knee include synovial cysts, meniscal cyst or ganglion cyst. Ultrasonography demonstrates exact location of the cyst, relationship with adjacent structures and nature of the cyst fluid or septations within the cyst. A differential diagnosis between cyst, abscess and hematoma cannot always be established on USG, but clinical setting will help to make a final diagnosis in most cases. MRI is ideally suited for diagnosis of either of these conditions, and can differentiate amongst popliteal, meniscal and ganglion cysts by delineating their site and relationship to the joint.[2]

Inflammatory Lesions

Cellulitis or abscesses may present as soft tissue masses. Though the clinical presentation of acute lesions is characteristic, these may simulate a malignancy in a subacute or chronic clinical scenario. This is especially true in case of tubercular ("cold abscesses"). Ultrasonography and MRI can help differentiate between the two, i.e. demonstrate extent of liquefaction and hence further surgical/percutaneous drainage. Cellulitis appears as thickened subcutaneous tissues which demonstrate low-signal intensity stranding on T1-weighted images and, high- signal intensity stranding on T2-weighted images with moderate to contrast enhancement **(Figs. 11A to C)**.

An abscess, on the other hand, appears as a well-defined focal fluid collection that is hypointense on T1W and hyperintense on T2W with rim enhancement. The signal intensity of the contents can, however, be variable in the presence of blood or proteinaceous material within the abscess cavity **(Figs. 12A and B)**. Abscesses can, however, simulate necrotic tumors on imaging.[27]

Soft Tissue Tumors

Soft tissue tumors are a heterogeneous group of lesions which arise from different nonepithelial, extraskeletal elements, which include adipose tissue, smooth and skeletal muscle, tendon, cartilage, fibrous tissue, blood vessels, and lymphatic structures. They are relatively uncommon lesions that occur in the trunk, extremities or head and neck. The new WHO classification of soft

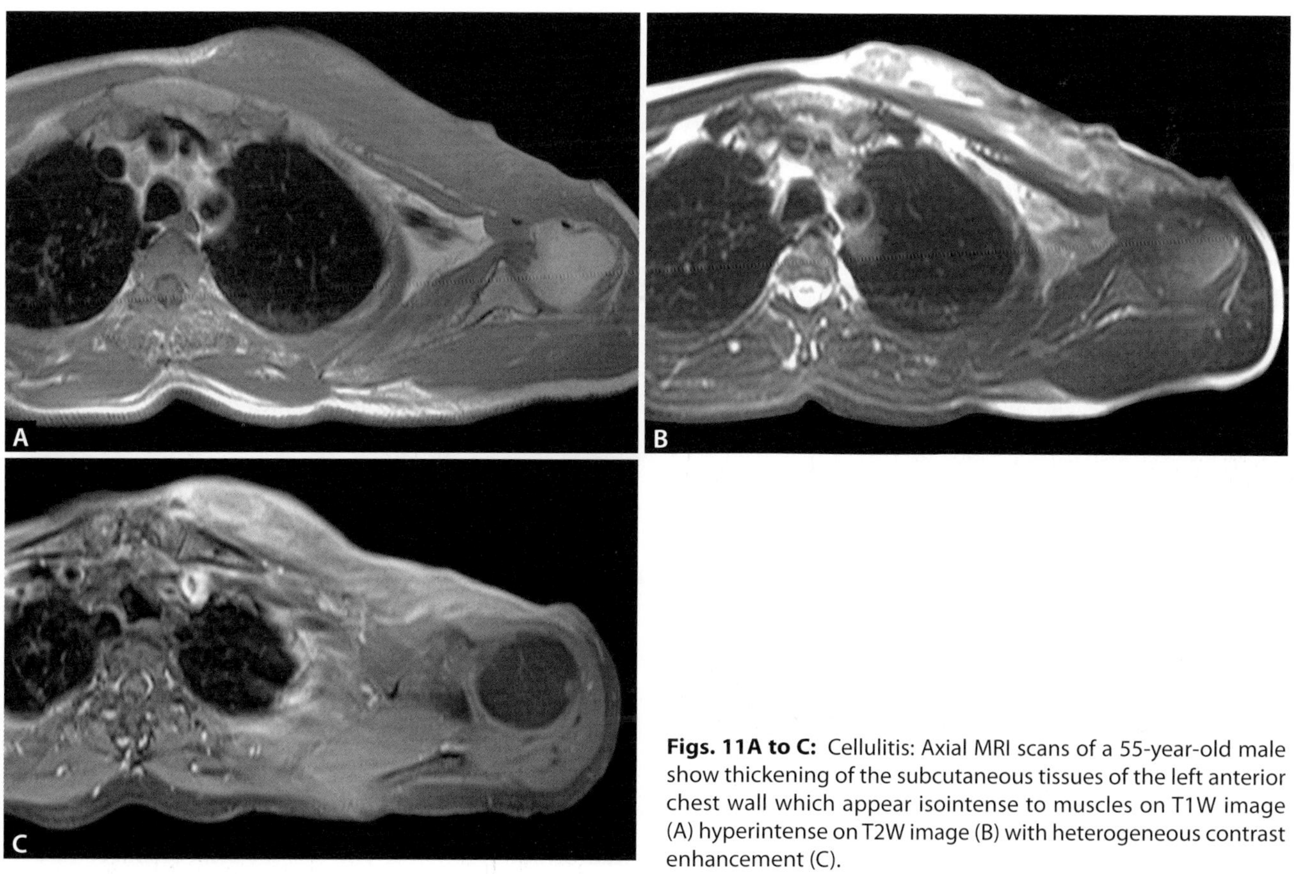

Figs. 11A to C: Cellulitis: Axial MRI scans of a 55-year-old male show thickening of the subcutaneous tissues of the left anterior chest wall which appear isointense to muscles on T1W image (A) hyperintense on T2W image (B) with heterogeneous contrast enhancement (C).

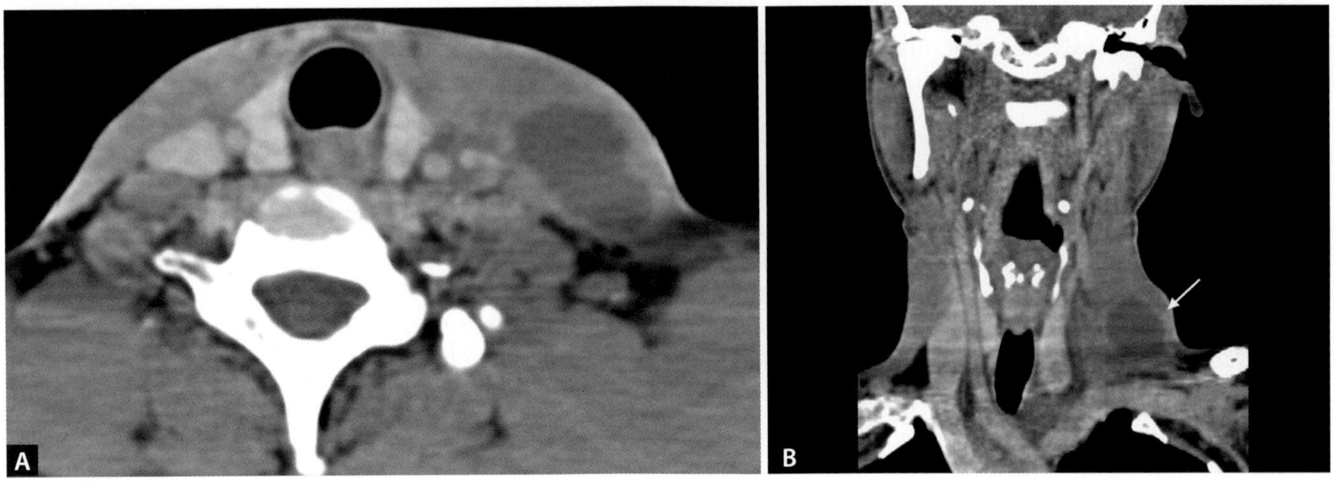

Figs. 12A and B: Tubercular abscess: Axial CECT (A) and coronal MPR (B) images of a 30-year-old man reveal an enlarged, heterogeneous left sternocleidomastoid muscle with a large necrotic area within (arrow). The aspirate was AFB positive.

tissue tumors was introduced in late 2002. The nine major groups of tumors under this pathological classification system include adipocytic tumors, vascular tumors, fibroblastic/myofibroblastic tumors, fibrohistiocytic tumors, smooth muscle tumors, skeletal muscle tumors, pericytic (perivascular) tumors, chondro-osseous tumors and tumors of uncertain differentiation.[28] Each of the histologic subtypes can be further subdivided depending on their biological behavior into benign, intermediate (have malignant potential) or malignant. Benign tumors far more common than the malignant forms. Peripheral nerve sheath tumors are not included in the classification but are discussed here as these show relatively characteristic imaging features.

Adipocytic Tumors

Lipoma is the most common benign soft tissue tumor. It is usually a solitary lesion (although multiple lesions may be present occasionally) and is composed of mature adipose tissue. Soft tissue lipomas are categorized by anatomic location as either superficial (subcutaneous) or deep. Depending on the size and location of the lesion, the radiograph may be unremarkable or demonstrate a mass of fat density **(Fig. 13)**.

On CT, the tumor is well-defined and homogeneous **(Fig. 14)** with a low tissue attenuation (approx. -65 to -120 HU) and without enhancement following administration of intravenous contrast. On MR imaging the signal intensity of lesion parallels that of subcutaneous fat on all pulse sequences **(Figs. 15A and B)** being hyperintense on both T1 and T2-weighted images. When a lipoma is encapsulated, a surrounding fibrous capsule of low-signal intensity on MR and attenuation similar to that of muscle on CT may be delineated. The lesion may contain thin septae.[29]

Cartilage and bone formation considered as metaplastic may be occasionally seen in a lipoma, particularly if it is long standing. There are numerous lipoma variants, *viz.* lipoblastoma, hibernoma and lipomatosis. Amongst these, *lipoblastoma* is a tumor of immature fat which occurs in young children. A mixture of fat and nonadipose tissue is seen on imaging of these lesions.[29] Besides soft tissues, benign lipomatous lesions may also affect bone, joints or tendon sheaths. Diffuse *lipomatosis* is characterized by diffuse overgrowth of mature adipose tissue infiltrating through the soft tissue of the affected extremity or the abdomen **(Figs. 16A and B)**.

Liposarcoma: The WHO classification recognizes several subtypes of liposarcoma: well-differentiated, dedifferentiated, myxoid, pleomorphic and mixed. Amongst these, the well-differentiated form is the most common (50%), and it does not metastasize. CT and MRI appearance of liposarcoma reflects its degree of differentiation **(Figs. 17A and B)**.[2,15] MR imaging features that suggest a diagnosis of well-differentiated liposarcoma vs lipoma include prominent internal septae more than 2 mm in thickness and nodular nonadipose areas. The gadolinium enhancement of nonadipose regions is variable ranging from mild to marked.[29,30]

Vascular Lesions

Benign vascular lesions can broadly be divided into two distinct groups: hemangiomas and vascular malformations. While the former are considered as true

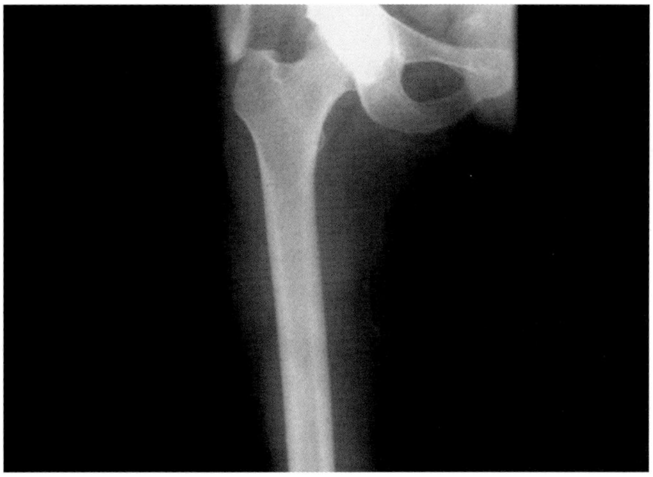

Fig. 13: Lipoma: A fat density mass seen in medial part of right thigh suggestive of lipoma on plain radiograph.

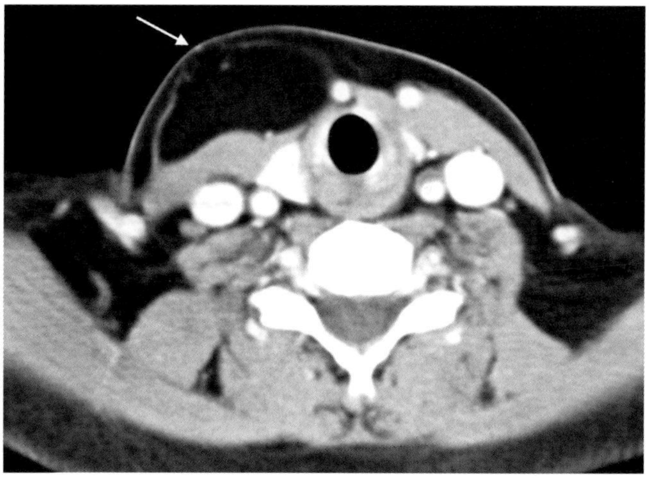

Fig. 14: Lipoma: Axial CECT image showing well-defined, homogeneous, fat-attenuation lesion in the subcutaneous plane of left side of the neck (arrow).

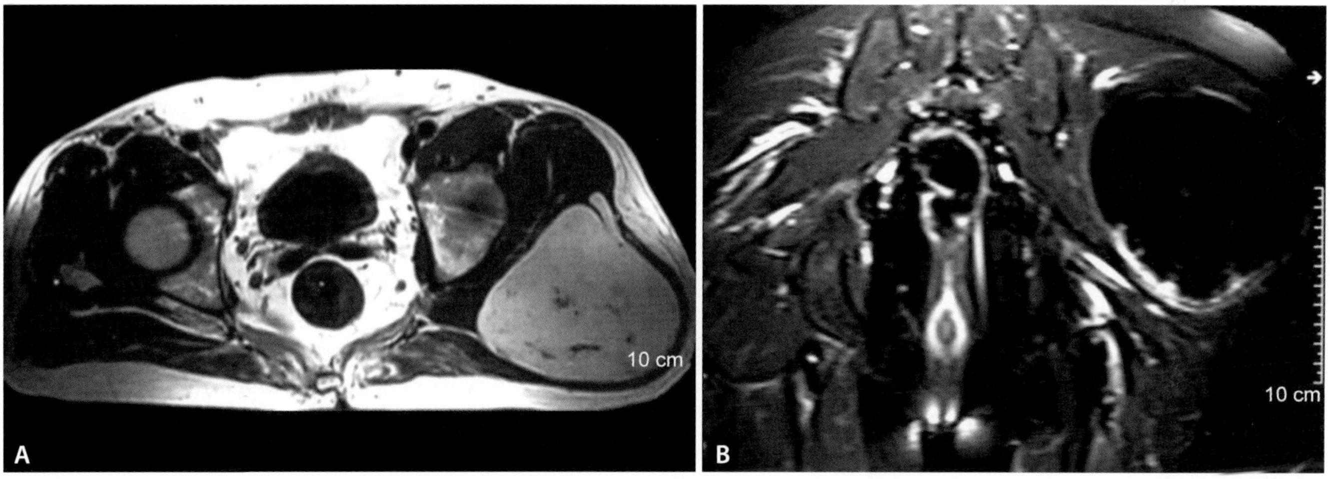

Figs. 15A and B: Lipoma: Axial T1WI (A) and coronal fat-saturated T2WI (B) showing a well defined, homogeneous mass lesion in left gluteal region with signal intensity similar to subcutaneous fat on both sequences. Fine strands are seen within.

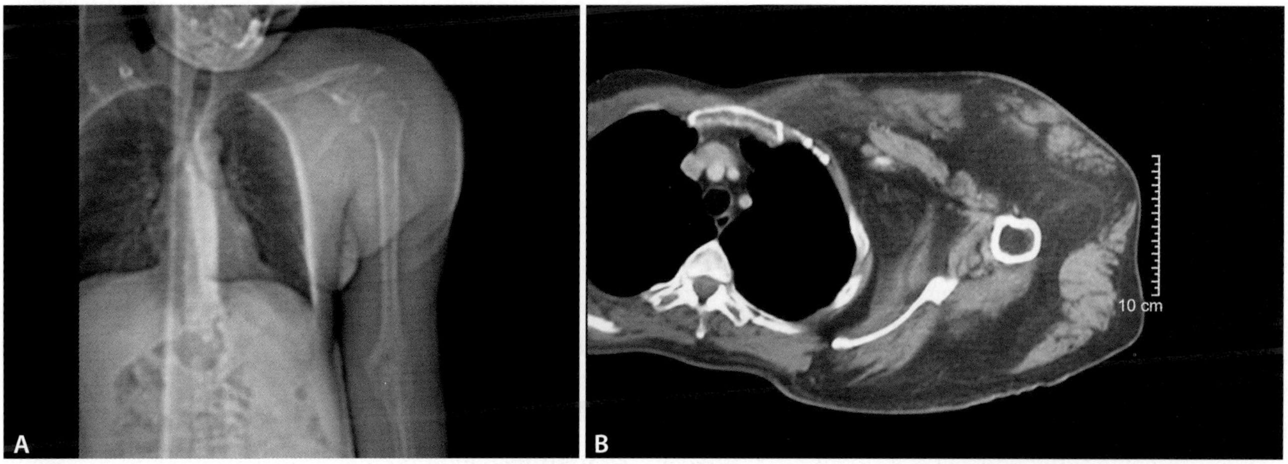

Figs. 16A and B: Lipomatosis: CT scout film (A) of a middle-aged man reveals marked increase in soft tissues around the left shoulder and upper arm, with mass effect on the left hemithorax. Axial CECT (B) reveals this to be fat diffusely distributed in the subcutaneous and intermuscular planes.

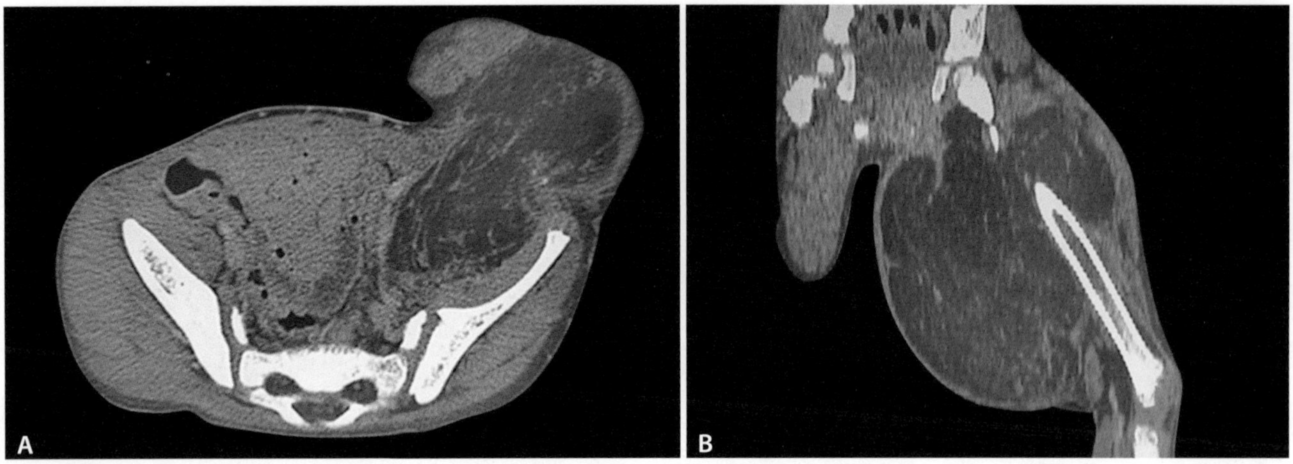

Figs. 17A and B: Liposarcoma (well-differentiated): Axial CECT (A) and coronal MPR (B) showing a well-defined fat-attenuation lesion with prominent internal septae located in the pelvis, inguinal region and upper thigh.

neoplastic lesions, vascular malformations are disorders of vascular morphogenesis.[31] Differentiation between the two groups has significant therapeutic and prognostic implications. Vascular lesions are the most common soft tissue lesions in children and young adults.

Hemangioma

Hemangioma is among the most frequent tumors to involve the soft tissues. Soft tissue hemangiomas represent a broad-spectrum of benign endothelial neoplasms that histologically resemble normal blood vessels. Hemangioma may be divided into common hemangiomas of infancy, congenital hemangiomas, and kaposiform hemangioendothelioma.

Common hemangiomas of infancy, also known as infantile or juvenile hemangiomas. These are present at birth and are usually evident by 3 months of age. These lesions undergo two phases: proliferative phase and involuting phase. The proliferative phase is during the first few months of life and is characterized by rapid endothelial growth. The lesion size tends to stabilize by about 9 to 10 months of age, after which the involuting phase continues slowly for the next several years up to 7–10 years of age. The hemangioma is replaced by fibrofatty tissue during this phase.[27] *Congenital hemangioma* demonstrate a different clinical course—these are either rapidly involuting, i.e. the lesion does not go through a proliferative phase and involutes by about 14 months of age; or noninvoluting wherein the lesion continues to grow for several years. *Noninvoluting hemangiomas* grow proportionally with the child without undergoing involution and may present in adulthood.

Common sites of hemangiomas include face and neck (60%), trunk (25%) and extremities (15%).[27] Diagnosis is evident clinically in most cases, with a characteristic strawberry-like appearance in cutaneous lesions. Deeper lesions however, in which the overlying skin may be normal or have only slight bluish discoloration. Ultrasonography is often sufficient for diagnosis, MR may be required to demonstrate extent for presurgical planning or for treatment response evaluation.

Radiographs are often normal or reveal a nonspecific soft tissue mass. Phleboliths may be seen in some cases **(Fig. 18A)**. Ultrasonography typically reveals a complex mass with anechoic channels with phleboliths and acoustic shadowing **(Fig. 18B)**. Noncontrast CT generally shows a poorly defined lesion with attenuation similar to that of skeletal muscle with significant enhancement on the contrast administration **(Figs. 19A and B)**. Phleboliths are easily detected on CT. MRI often shows characteristic imaging appearance, allowing distinction from other soft tissue masses[2,32] **(Figs. 20A and B)**. On T1W image, hemangioma shows a poorly marginated mass of low to intermediate signal intensity. Areas of high-signal intensity representing fat or slow flowing blood may be seen as fine delicate lace-like strands to thick coarse bands. On T2-weighted images, soft tissue hemangiomas reveal a well-marginated mass with very high-signal intensity in areas of vascular components, whereas regions of adipose tissue are of intermediate intensity or isointense to subcutaneous fat. The areas of high-signal intensity are caused by vessels with slow flow and are seen as circular and/or linear or serpentine vessels.

Kaposiform hemangioendothelioma: It is a vascular neoplasm of infancy that may display an infiltrative growth pattern. These lesions have a borderline malignant potential

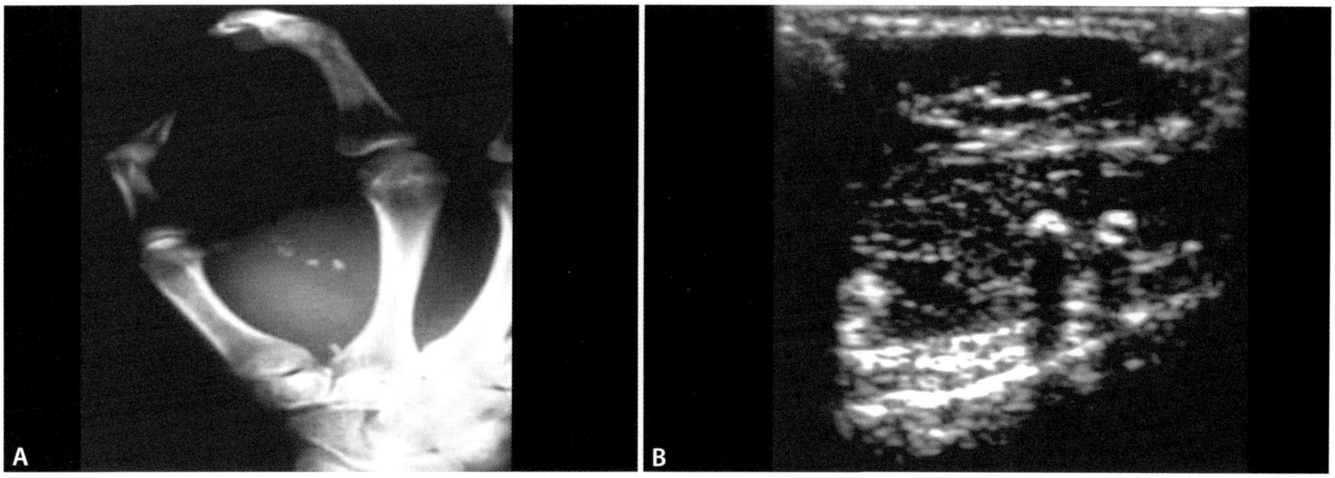

Figs. 18A and B: Hemangioma: (A) Plain radiograph showing soft tissue mass with phleboliths between first and second metacarpals; (B) Ultrasonography of the mass shows an isoechoic solid lesion with acoustic shadowing from phleboliths.

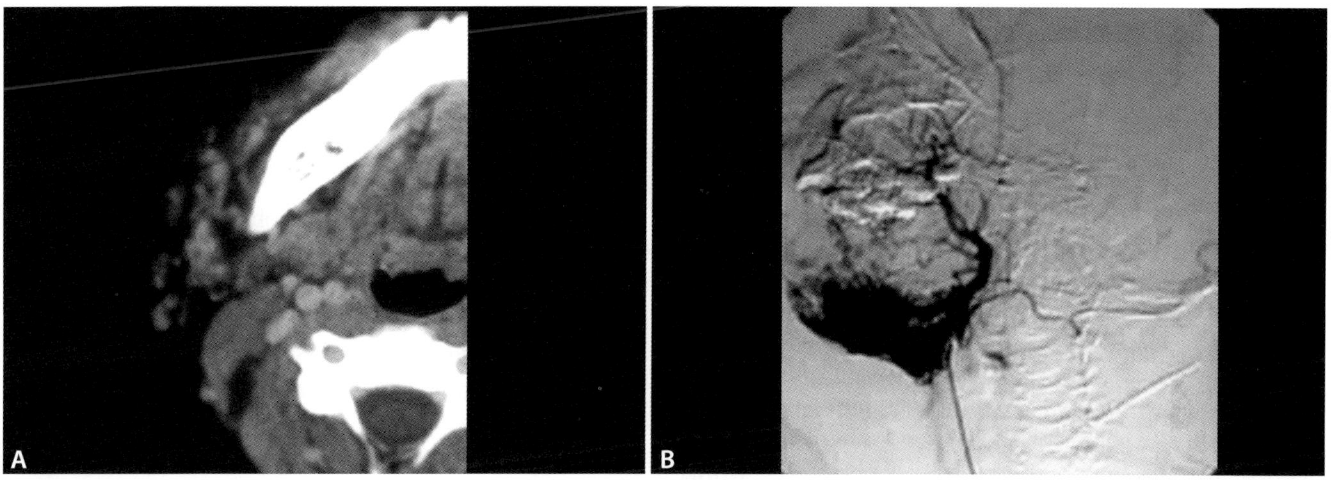

Figs. 19A and B: (A) CT scan showing hemangioma involving the soft tissues superficial to the body and ramus of the mandible on right side. The mass shows multiple serpiginous channels; (B) Selective right common carotid, digital subtraction angiography shows features suggestive of hemangioma with vascular supply from right lingual artery.

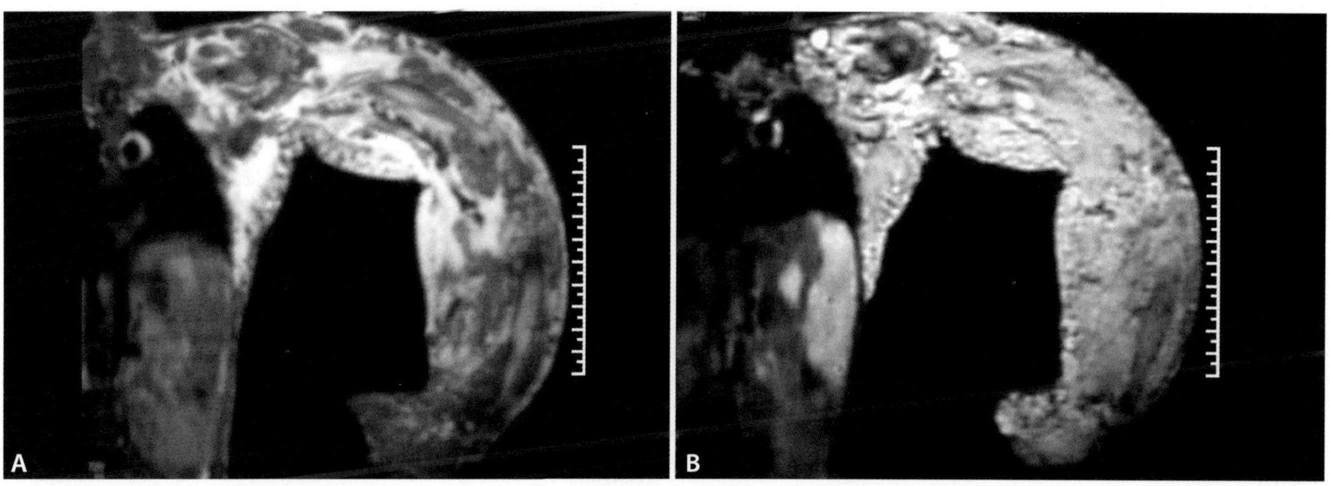

Figs. 20A and B: SE T1W (A) and T2W (B) coronal scans demonstrating diffuse hemangioma involving left upper limb, axilla, shoulder and left chest wall. There are multiple oblong, linear and serpiginous regions which are hypointense on T1W and hyperintense on T2W images. Evidence of fat overgrowth in soft tissues seen. The bones of upper limb are also seen to be involved.

as they can occasionally metastasize to regional lymph nodes, though distant metastases have not been reported. Kaposiform hemangioendothelioma often presents in the first year of life, being present at birth in about 50% patients with most common site being the extremities followed by head and neck. Kaposiform hemangioendothelioma is different from spindle cell hemangioendothelioma, which is seen in older patients being a reactive vascular proliferation that develops within a pre-existing vascular malformation. About half the patients may be associated with Kasabach–Merritt phenomenon (a coagulopathy with profound thrombocytopenia). On MR imaging, these lesions ill-defined margins, involvement of multiple tissue planes, cutaneous thickening and stranding of the subcutaneous fat, and destructive changes or remodeling of adjacent bones.[27]

Soft Tissue Angiosarcoma

Angiosarcoma is a malignant vascular tumor occurring at any age, with peak in the 7th decade. It has high incidence of local recurrence and distant metastasis. Predisposing risk factors for this malignancy include chronic lymph edema, previous radiotherapy, foreign bodies, immune suppression and familial syndromes such as type 1 neurofibromatosis, Klippel–Trénaunay–Weber syndrome, and Maffucci syndrome.

On MR, the tumors show intermediate signal intensity on T1W images and high signal on T2W images, with contrast enhancement. There is often aggressive infiltration of adjacent tissues. Areas of hemorrhage or necrosis may be seen within. Vascular structures within the tumor appear as flow voids if high flow, and high signal intensity areas on T2W images, if low flow.

Vascular Malformations

Soft tissue vascular malformations can be categorized with combined MRI and MR angiography, as either high-flow (arteriovenous malformations, arteriovenous fistula) or low-flow (venous, lymphatic, capillary, and combined). These are present at birth, though they may not be evident and subsequently grow with the growth of the child. These may show rapid growth during puberty, pregnancy or following trauma (including iatrogenic trauma). Unlike hemangiomas, vascular malformations do not involute or regress.

High-flow Vascular Malformations

Arteriovenous malformations (AVMs): These malformations are comprised of an abnormal network of tortuous and dysplastic vascular channels, referred to as nidus which is interposed between enlarged feeding arteries and draining veins. The clinical presentation is of a pulsatile mass with palpable thrill and localized warmth. The complications of these lesions include: hemorrhage, ischemia from arterial steal, asymmetric overgrowth or even high-output cardiac failure.[27]

Magnetic resonance imaging shows imaging enlarged feeding arteries and draining veins, which appear as tortuous channels and flow on spin-echo images and high-signal intensity channels on gradient-echo images, without a well-defined mass. Sometimes, they assume a mass like appearance. CT/MR angiography can be used to demonstrate the vascular supply which aids in planning subsequent interventions **(Figs. 21A and B)**.[27]

Arteriovenous fistula (AVF): The fistula comprises of usually a single large vascular channel between an artery

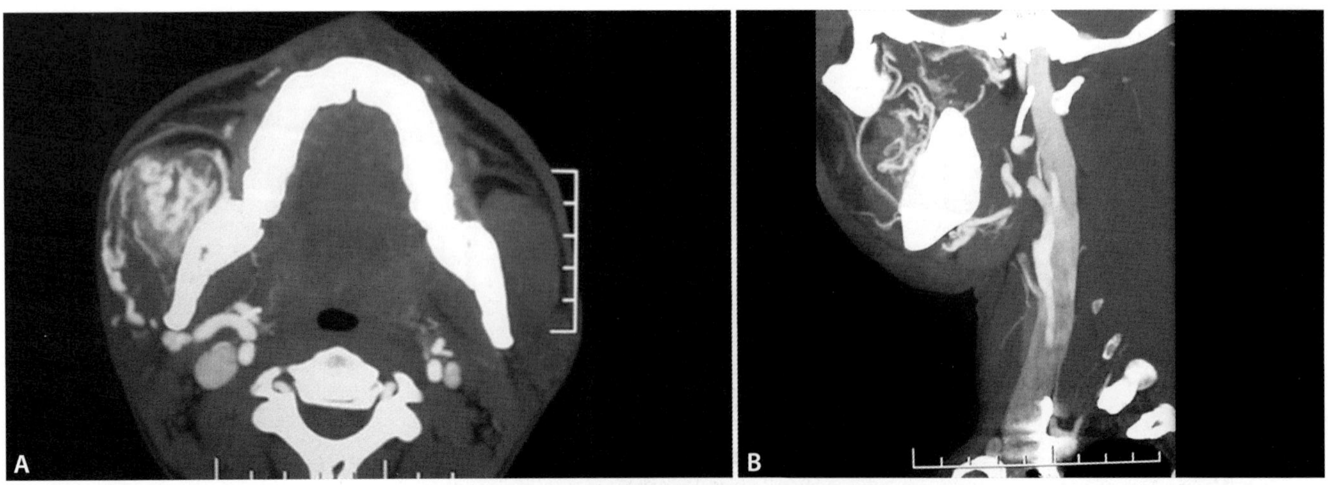

Figs. 21A and B: High flow AVM: CT angiography of a 22-year-old male presenting with gum bleed showing a large nidus involving the right masseter and infratemporal fossa with rapid venous filling.

and a vein, with no intervening nidus. It may be congenital, or develop following a penetrating trauma.[27]

Low-flow Vascular Malformations

Venous malformations: These are the most common form of all vascular malformations, often misnamed as cavernous hemangiomas. They often present at birth as soft, fluctuant masses with overlying skin discoloration. These lesions increase in size with gravity (dependent position) and Valsalva maneuver. Superficial varices may also be evident.

On USG and MR imaging, venous malformations appear either as dilated veins or more often lobulated multilocular masses. These locules represent venous lakes separated from each other by interstitial septa. Phleboliths may be seen within, with Doppler evaluation revealing venous flow pattern.[27,31]

Lymphatic malformations: The common term used for these lesions is lymphangioma or cystic hygroma. They are slow flow, cystic malformations. The size of the cysts varies from few millimeters (microcystic) to larger variable sized (in centimeters) cystic spaces (macrocystic variant or cystic hygroma). Cystic lymphangiomas (hygromas) are the most common type and are usually located in the neck or axilla. These are composed of unilocular or multilocular spaces containing serous or chylous proteinaceous material. Sonography of cystic hygroma shows a multiloculated cystic mass with septae of variable thickness. Cystic lesions complicated by hemorrhage or infection may appear solid.

Ultrasonography and CT shows a lymphangioma as a unilocular or multilocular cystic mass **(Figs. 22A and B)**. On MRI typical appearance is heterogeneous with a low-signal intensity, similar to or slightly less than that of muscle on T1-weighted images and high-signal intensity greater than that of fat on T2-weighted images, reflecting the preponderance of fluid-filled cystic spaces. Focal heterogeneities within the lesions represent fibrous septa which are seen as low intensity linear structures. On contrast administration, the septae may show enhancement.[27,31]

Fibroblastic/Myofibroblastic Tumors

Fibroblastic and myofibroblastic tumors comprise a large group of mesenchymal tumors with varied biologic behavior and diverse anatomic locations. About 76% of these tumors are benign, 13% of intermediate category, and 11% malignant.[18] They form about 12% of soft tissue tumors in children and adolescents, with 50% of cases presenting within the 1st year of life, and further 71% in the 1st decade.[33,34] Also, they are one of the most common soft tissue tumors in adults. There are four broad categories of fibrous proliferations referred to as benign fibrous proliferations, fibromatoses, fibrosarcomas, and fibrous proliferations of infancy and childhood.[11] The benign lesions include nodular fasciitis, fibromatosis colli, myofibroma, giant cell angiofibroma, etc. *Myositis ossificans* is also now classified under benign fibrous proliferations.

Fibromatosis refers to a family of soft tissue lesions characterized by intermediate malignant potential, i.e. they are locally infiltrative and tend to recur but do not metastasize. The fibromatosis are classified on the basis of their anatomic location as either superficial or deep. The superficial group includes palmar, plantar and penile fibromatosis. The deep or musculoaponeurotic

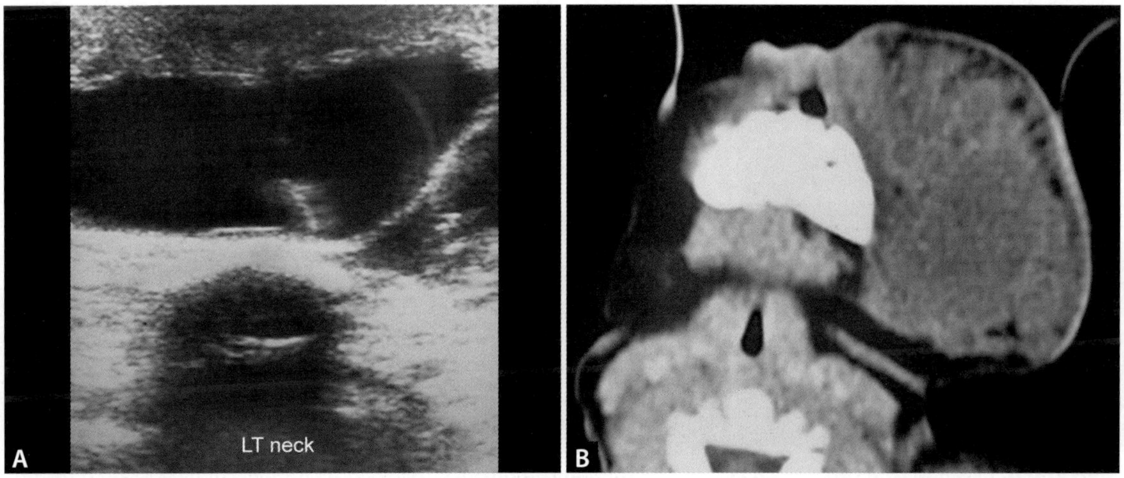

Figs. 22A and B: Lymphangioma USG (A) and CECT (B) of a 2-month-old infant showing a large cystic mass with few septae on left side of neck.

fibromatosis include extra-abdominal, abdominal, intra-abdominal and extremity fibromatosis. The descriptive term desmoid tumor was coined to emphasize the band-like or tendon-like character of the lesion ("Desmos" meaning band or tendon). These masses of fibromatoses are usually solitary although synchronous multicentric lesions may occur.

Radiographs are usually nonspecific but may reveal a mass. Bone involvement may be seen in the form of a pressure erosion, scalloping without invasion or destruction, or stimulation of periosteum producing a "frond-like" periosteal reaction. Bone reaction is more common in patients with multiple recurrences. On CT, the lesion is seen as a nonspecific soft tissue mass **(Fig. 23)**. On MRI, the deep fibromatoses was initially described as demonstrating decreased signal intensity on all pulse sequences, reflecting the fibrous nature of the tumor, subsequently, great variability of MRI characteristics of these lesions have been observed. Typically, the lesion has a heterogeneous signal intensity approximately similar to fat on T2-weighted and muscle on T1-weighted images **(Figs. 24A and B)**. The heterogeneous signal reflects varying proportions of collagen, spindle cells and mucopolysaccharide within the tumor. Those fibrous tumors that are hypocellular tumors with dense collagenous components have lower T2 signal intensity while those with higher cellularity or larger amounts of extracellular myxoid matrix have higher signal intensity.[11] Fibromatosis typically demonstrates moderate to marked enhancement following the administration of intravenous Gd-DTPA.

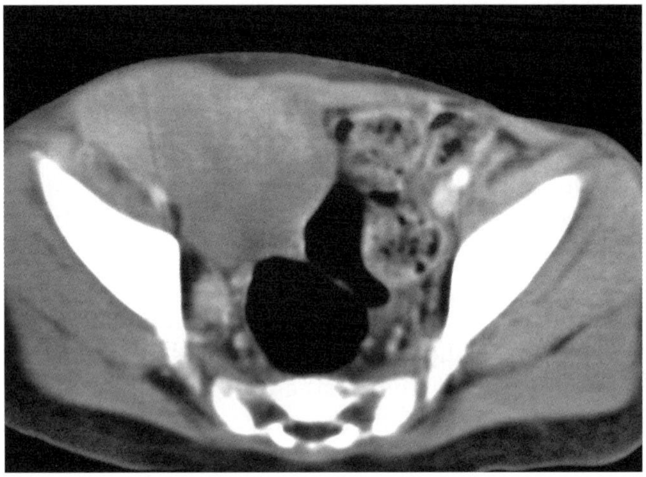

Fig. 23: Fibromatosis: CECT of a 24-year-old female showing a large, heterogeneous left pelvic mass.

Solitary fibrous tumor, hemangiopericytoma and inflammatory pseudotumor are also classified as intermediate lesions, while fibrosarcoma is the malignant tumor. *Inflammatory myofibroblastic tumor*, commonly known as referred to as inflammatory pseudotumor commonly occurs in the orbit but also at other sites, such as lung, trachea, skull base and thyroid. These tumors may be associated with fibrosing mediastinitis and retroperitoneal fibrosis. Histologically the tumors show myofibroblastic spindle cells and an inflammatory infiltrate comprising of plasma cells, lymphocytes, and eosinophils.[18] It could represent a reparative response to infection. Extraorbital pseudotumors are less responsive to steroid therapy than orbital pseudotumors and may show perineural spread.[35] On imaging, these lesions appear as well-circumscribed or poorly defined masses with extensive surrounding inflammatory changes. They are commonly T1 hypo-/ isointense with variable intensity on T2W images. Some tumors may be hypointense on T2W images.

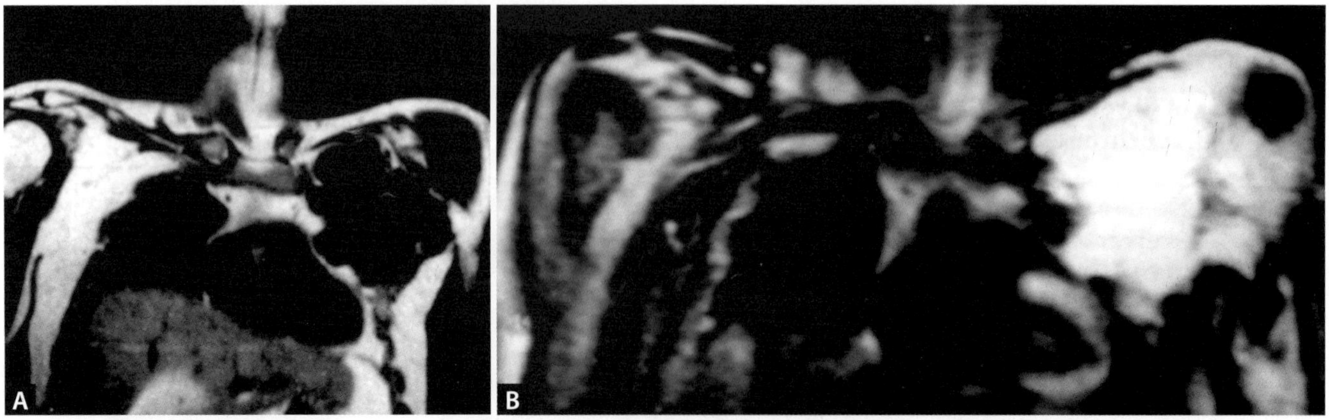

Figs. 24A and B: T1W and STIR coronal scans of a patient of fibromatosis showing large lobulated mass located over the left infraclavicular region. The mass is isointense on T1W (A) and hyperintense on STIR (B) sequences.

Fibrohistiocytic Tumors

The classification of this group is of tumors is controversial and is currently under revision. The benign forms include pigmented villonodular synovitis (PVNS) and giant cell tumor of the tendon sheath (GCTTS) while the intermediate forms include dermatofibrosarcoma protuberans. Malignant forms include *malignant fibrous* histiocytoma.[36]

Dermatofibrosarcoma Protuberans

Dermatofibrosarcoma protuberans is a rare tumor seen in middle-age adults but also reported in children, commonly found on the trunk or proximal extremities. The site of origin of the tumor is dermis, but it spreads locally into the deeper tissues. Clinical presentation is of slow-growing subcutaneous plaque or nodule with overlying skin discoloration simulating a vascular lesion. MR imaging is indicated only in atypical cases or in large tumors to look for deep infiltration. MR reveals a well-defined mass which is The mass is usually iso- to hypointense to muscle on T1W images, hyperintense on T2W images with uniform or patchy enhancement.[36]

Malignant Fibrous Histiocytoma

Malignant fibrous histiocytoma is a highly controversial entity. Once considered the most common soft tissue tumor in adults, it is now considered a diagnosis of exclusion. The term is now refers to a small group of pleomorphic sarcomas (about 5%) that do not show a definite line of differentiation.[36] The extremities, especially thigh, are the most common location of this often large mass. This lesion may also occur as second malignancy at sites of previous surgery/radiotherapy. MR imaging is nonspecific, revealing a soft tissue mass often located adjacent to a long bone and involving the underlying cortex. The lesion is usually of intermediate T1 signal intensity, heterogeneously high T2 signal intensity with enhancement of the solid components with a gadolinium contrast agent.[36]

Smooth Muscle Tumors

The tumors in this group include leiomyoma, angio-leiomyoma and leiomyosarcoma.

Leiomyoma

There are two groups within leiomyoma, one being the pelvic tumor seen in females and the other being tumors occurring in deep soft tissues of either sex. Nonuterine deep soft tissues leiomyoma is rare. The MR description of the second group is thus confined to few cases in literature. These are reported as well-defined masses which are slightly hyperintense to muscle on T1W images and with heterogeneous high signal intensity on T2W images. The tumors may show calcification within.

Leiomyosarcoma

It accounts for about 6% cases of deep soft tissue sarcomas and shows a more heterogeneous MR appearance. These are large, bulky masses and seldom show calcification.[18,36]

Skeletal Muscle Tumors

This group includes rhabdomyoma and rhabdomyosarcoma. Rhabdomyoma is commonly found in the heart, while extracardiac rhabdomyoma is extremely rare and hence is not being discussed in detail.

Rhabdomyosarcoma

Rhabdomyosarcoma accounts for more than half of soft-tissue sarcomas seen in children. This tumor is thought to arise from primitive mesenchymal cells that are committed to develop into striated muscle. It can be found anywhere within the body, i.e. even in sites that lack striated muscle. The histological variants of the tumor include embryonal, alveolar, and pleomorphic variants. Embryonal type is the most common variant seen in children. The alveolar form occurs in older children and young adults. The pleomorphic type is primarily an adult tumor found in the extremities. The lesion may have an association with syndromes such as Beckwith-Wiedemann syndrome and neurofibromatosis. Common sites include pelvis **(Fig. 25)**, head and neck, genitourinary tract and less often extremities.

MR features are nonspecific. Rhabdomyosarcomas appear to be well or poorly defined masses with low signal intensity on T1W images, high signal intensity on T2W images and variable contrast enhancement **(Figs. 26A and B)**. Presence of internal necrosis is a poor prognostic sign in neonates.[36]

Pericytic Tumors

Pericytic tumors are neoplasms that have a characteristic tendency to grow in a circumferential perivascular pattern and comprise of contractile cells. These include glomus tumors and myopericytoma. Soft tissue glomus tumors are rare and are distinct from, and hence should not be mistaken for, the common head and neck paraganglionomas (glomus vagale, etc.) which are neuroendocrine tumors. Hemangiopericytoma was earlier included in this category but is now considered to be more closely related to solitary fibrous tumors. These rare tumors occur in the extremities as cutaneous nodules and occasionally in the sinonasal cavity. Being rare entities their imaging is not being discussed here.[18,28]

Chondro-osseous Tumors

The benign tumor in this category is soft tissue chondroma while the malignant lesions include mesenchymal chondrosarcoma and extraskeletal osteosarcoma.

Mesenchymal Chondrosarcoma

These are rare tumors occurring in 2nd or 3rd decades of life. The common site is the craniofacial region. On MR images, these lesions show heterogeneous high signal intensity on T2W images with heterogeneous contrast enhancement **(Figs. 27A to C)**. Plain radiographs and CT reveal the characteristic chondroid matrix calcifications.[18]

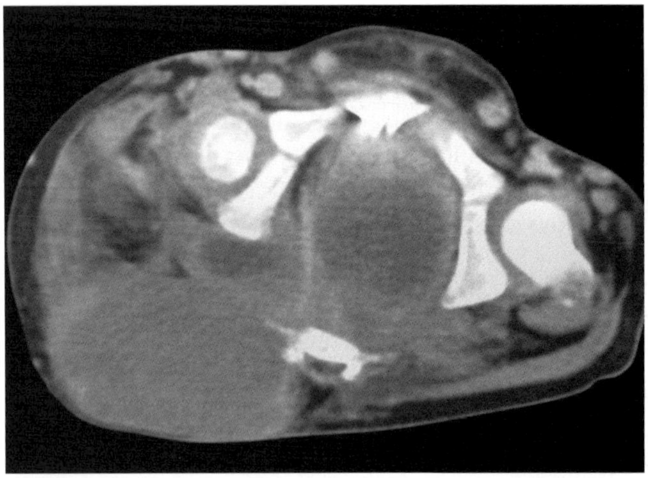

Fig. 25: Rhabdomyosarcoma: Axial CECT of a 5-year-old male patient showing an ill-defined presacral mass with extension into bilateral gluteal regions (right > left).

Extraskeletal Osteosarcoma

Extraskeletal osteosarcomas occur in older patients compared to their osseous counterparts. These are high-grade malignancies and have no attachment to the bone or periosteum. The predisposing factors include previous irradiation and even previous trauma. These tumors are often large at presentation Plain radiographs and CT demonstrate the amorphous ossification seen in these tumors, which is typically most prominent in the centre (unlike myositis ossificans). MR features are nonspecific with tumors often showing necrosis and hemorrhage.[18,33]

Tumors of Uncertain Origin

This category includes tumors that show an uncertain/ no definite line of differentiation. These are uncommon tumors and include myxoma and synovial sarcoma.

Synovial Sarcoma

Synovial sarcoma is the fourth most common soft tissue tumor and affects the extremities, particularly around the knee joint (popliteal fossa) in majority of the cases. Despite its name the lesion does not arise from the synovium, it is extra-articular in location, being near the knee joint. Adolescents and young adults are most often affected. Although the radiographic appearance is not characteristic, the finding of a soft tissue mass near a joint of a young patient is highly suggestive **(Figs. 28A to C)**. About 30% masses show calcification.[37]

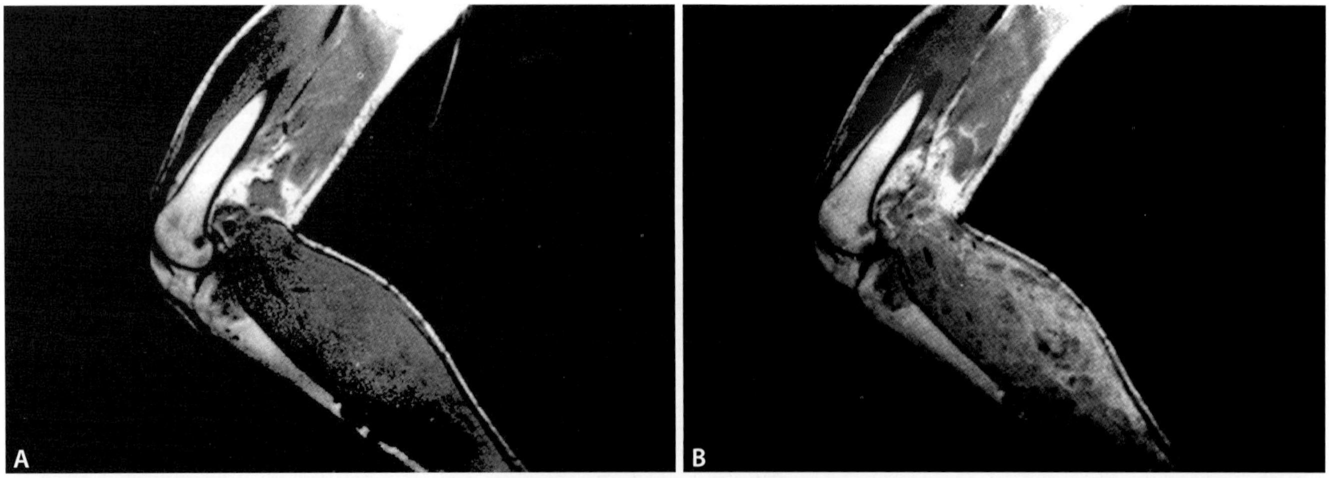

Figs. 26A and B: Rhabdomyosarcoma: SE T1W (A) and postcontrast sagittal (B) scans showing the tumor involving all muscle compartments of left leg and inner part of left thigh with secondary involvement of left tibia and lower end of femur.

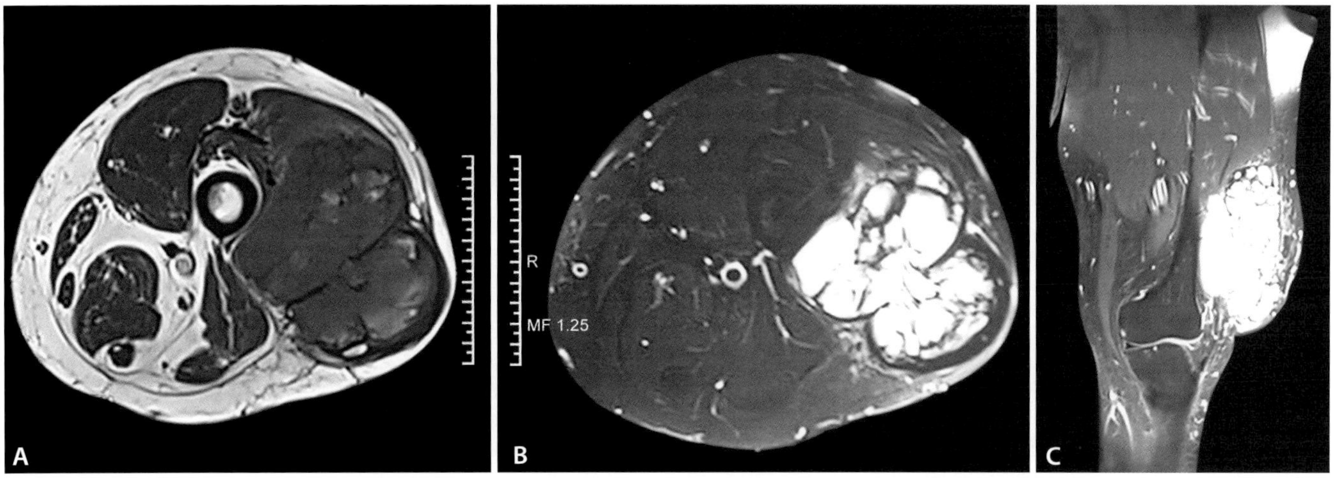

Figs. 27A to C: Chondrosarcoma: MRI of 44-year-old male showing heterogeneous mass lesion in the medial compartment of thigh, which is hypointense on T1W image (A) with hyperintense areas within. On T2W fat-suppressed images (B and C) the lesion show high signal intensity.

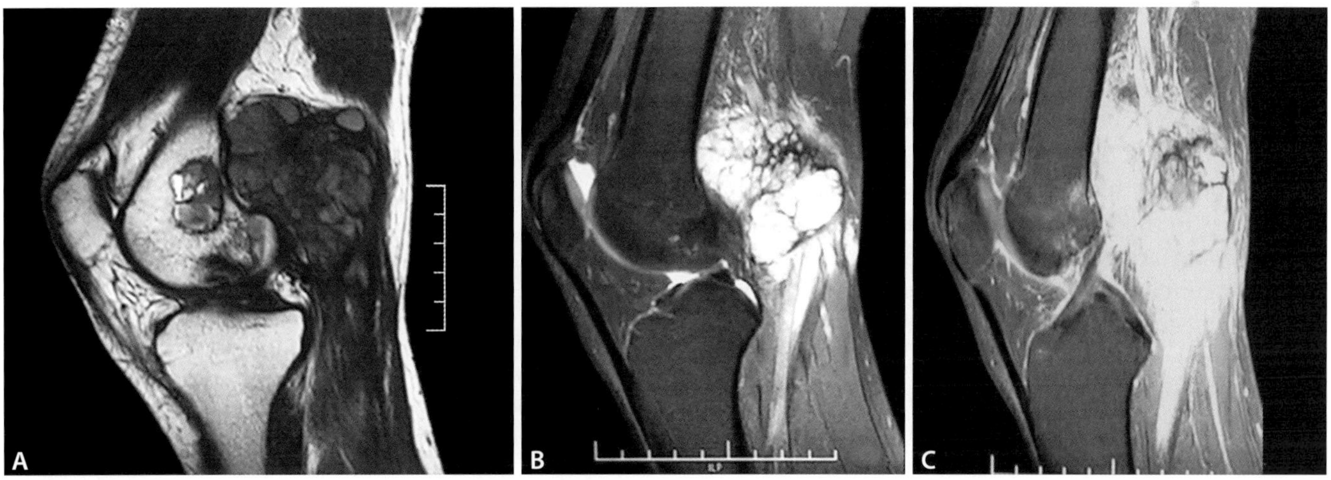

Figs. 28A to C: Synovial sarcoma: T1W (A), T2W (B) and postcontrast (C) MR images of a 21-year-old male showing a heterogeneous, solid, lobulated extra-articular mass located just behind the knee joint. Intraosseous extension is seen into the adjoining femur.

Miscellaneous

Neurogenic Tumors

Neurogenic tumors are not listed in the WHO classification of soft tissue tumors, but are being discussed as these may present as soft tissue masses. These lesions include schwannoma, neurofibroma, and malignant peripheral nerve sheath tumor.[38]

CT and MRI remain the primary modalities for the evaluation of neurogenic neoplasms, of which, MRI is superior. Imaging usually shows a fusiform shaped mass and the nerve can often be seen entering and exiting the mass as a tubular structure, a sign that is virtually pathognomonic. This sign is seen in lesions involving large nerve trunks and not in lesions of small nerves. Plexiform neurofibroma shows diffuse nerve thickening, often including nerve branches, producing a serpentine appearance on imaging and reflecting the irregular, convoluted gross appearance. Diffuse neurofibromas infiltrate the subcutaneous tissues and appear as fine linear branching lesions. Distinction between neurofibroma and schwannoma may be possible, particularly with MRI. Classically, the nerve is eccentric to the mass (although within the capsule) in schwannoma, rather than being central or obliterated by the mass as in neurofibroma. Neurogenic neoplasms show a signal intensity similar to or slightly higher than that of skeletal muscle on T1-weighted imaging. Typically T2-weighted images demonstrate a high-signal intensity with a variable degree of heterogeneity **(Figs. 29A and B)**.[2,38]

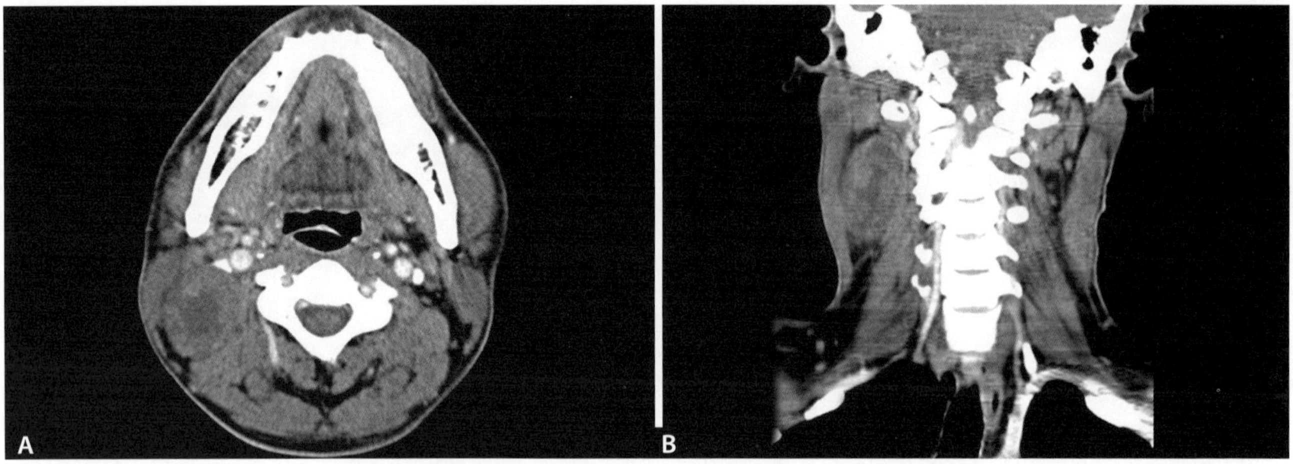

Figs. 29A and B: Neurogenic tumor: CECT of a 31-year-old male showing an ovoid, right carotid space heterogeneous mass lesion displacing the vessels anteriorly.

EXTRASKELETAL EWING'S SARCOMA AND PRIMITIVE NEUROECTODERMAL TUMOR

Both of these lesions are malignant soft tissue sarcomas which are likely neuroectodermal in origin. Their peak age of occurrence is the 2nd/3rd decade. They are aggressive neoplasms with high recurrence rates with frequent metastases to the lungs. MR appearance is nonspecific. On CT, Ewing's sarcomas may show low attenuation areas within or contain areas with lower attenuation than that in the adjacent muscle—features that correspond with cellular necrosis seen at microscopy **(Fig. 30)**. Intratumoral hemorrhage, adjoining bone destruction and lymphadenopathy may also be seen.

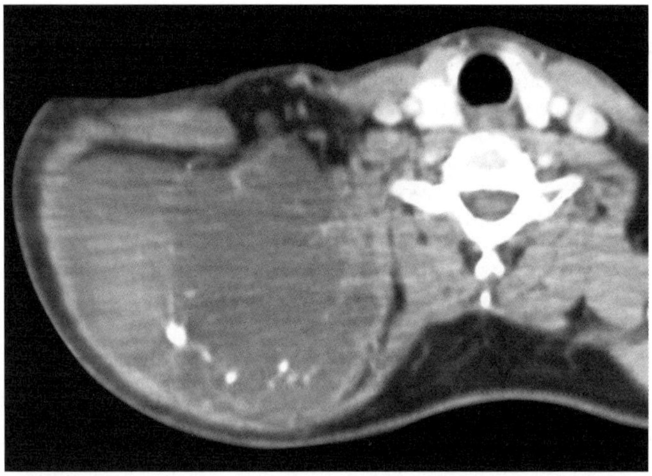

Fig. 30: Primitive neuroectodermal tumor: CECT of a 18-year-old girl showing a large heterogeneous, necrotic mass lesion in the right scapular region.

SUMMARY

Ultrasound and MRI would suffice for evaluation of most soft tissue lesions, while plain radiographs and CT are useful adjuncts to demonstrate associated osseous changes or matrix mineralization/ossification. MRI is the method of choice for their assessment and staging but MRI does not provide histologic diagnosis. Soft tissue involvement is often underestimated by CT. Indeterminate lesions will require biopsy and careful follow-up. Once histology has confirmed that a lesion is malignant, CT scanning of thorax is required to determine the presence or absence of intrapulmonary metastases.

ACKNOWLEDGMENT

We acknowledge the valuable contribution of Professor Sushma Vashisht, Former Head, Department of Radiodiagnosis, AIIMS, New Delhi, India to the chapter.

REFERENCES

1. Davies AM. Imaging of soft tissues. In: Grainger RG, Alison DJ (Eds). Diagnostic Radiology: A Textbook of Medical Imaging. New York: Churchill Livingstone; 2001. pp.2075-96.
2. Krausdorj MS, Berquist TH. Musculoskeletal Neoplasms in MRI of the Musculoskeletal System, 4th edition. Lippincott William and Wilkins, Philadelphia; 2001.pp.842-955.
3. Eddiken's De. Calcinosis Calcifications and Myositis Ossificans. In: Edeiken J, Dalinka M, Karasick D (Eds). Roentgen diagnosis of disease of bone. William and Willkins; 1990.pp.1369-400.
4. Newman JS, Adler RS, Bude RO, et al. Detection of soft tissue hyperemia—value of power Doppler sonography. AJR. 1994;163:385-9.

5. Potolicchio PM, Luna A, Mateo PC, Barrientos EA, Manzi E, Rivera MR. Assessment of Muscular Lesions with Sonoelastography. Presented at RSNA 2011 LL-MKE2209.
6. Shah GV, Fischbein NJ, Gandhi D, Mukherji SK. Dynamic contrast-enhanced MR imaging. Top Magn Reson Imaging. 2004;15:71-7.
7. Verstraete KL, Vanzieleghem B, De Deeney, et al. Static, dynamic and first pass, MR imaging of musculoskeletal lesions using Gadodiamide injection. Acta Radiol. 1995;36:27-36.
8. van Rijswijk CS, Geirnaerdt MJ, Hogendoorn PC, et al. Soft-tissue tumors: value of static and dynamic gadopentetate dimeglumine-enhanced MR imaging in prediction of malignancy. Radiology. 2004;233(2):493-502.
9. Razek AA, Elsorogy LG, Soliman NY, Nada N. Dynamic susceptibility contrast perfusion MR imaging in distinguishing malignant from benign head and neck tumors: a pilot study. Eur J Radiol. 2011;77(1):73-9.
10. Walker EA, Salesky JS, Fenton ME, Murphey MD. Magnetic Resonance Imaging of malignant soft tissue neoplasms in the adult. Radiologic Clinics of North America. 2011;49(6):1219-34.
11. Dinauer PA, Brixey CJ, Moncur JT, Smith JCF, Murphey MD. Pathologic and MR imaging features of benign fibrous soft-tissue tumors in adults. Radiographics. 2007;27:173-87.
12. Chang AE, Matory YL, Dwyer AJ, et al. Magnetic resonance imaging versus computed tomography in the evaluation of soft tissue tumours of the extremities. Ann Surg. 1987;205:340-8.
13. Garcia-Gomez JM, Vidal C, Marti-Bonmati L, et al. Benign/malignant classifier of soft tissue tumours using MR imaging. MAGMA. 2004;16:194-201.
14. Pang KK, Hughes T. MR imaging of the musculoskeletal soft tissue mass: is heterogeneity a sign of malignancy? J Chin Med Assoc. 2004;66:655-61.
15. Davies AM, Hall AD, Strouhal PD, et al. The MR imaging appearances and natural history of seromas following excision of soft tissue tumours. Eur Radiol. 2004;14(7):1196-202.
16. Davies AM, Mehr A, Parsonage S, et al. MR imaging in the assessment of residual tumour following inadequate primary excision of soft tissue sarcomas. Eur Radiol. 2004;14(3):506-13.
17. Wang CK, Li CW, Hsieh TJ, Chien SH, Liu GC, Tsai KB. Characterization of bone and soft-tissue tumors with *in vivo* 1H MR spectroscopy: initial results. Radiology. 2004;232:599-605.
18. Razek AA, Huang BY. Soft tissue tumors of the head and neck: imaging-based review of the WHO classification. Radiographics. 2011;31:1923-54.
19. Nagata S, Nishimura H, Uchida M, et al. Diffusion-weighted imaging of soft tissue tumors: usefulness of the apparent diffusion coefficient for differential diagnosis. Radiat Med. 2008;26(5):287-95.
20. Schnapauff D, Zeile M, Niederhagen MB, et al. Diffusion-weighted echo-planar magnetic resonance imaging for the assessment of tumor cellularity in patients with soft-tissue sarcomas. J Magn Reson Imaging. 2009;29(6):1355-9.
21. Soft tissue sarcoma. In: Edge SB, Byrd DR, Compton CC, et al. (Eds). AJCC Cancer Staging Manual, 7th edition. New York, NY: Springer; 2010.pp.291-6.
22. Garner HW, Kransdorf MJ, Bancroft LW, Peterson JJ, Berquist TH, Murphey MD. Benign and malignant soft-tissue tumors: Posttreatment MR imaging. Radiographics. 2009;29:119-34.
23. Hug I, Guncaga J. Tumoral calcinosis with sedimentation sign. Br J Radiol. 1974;47:734-6.
24. Shirkhoda A, Armin AR, Bis KG, et al. MR imaging of myositis ossificans, variable patterns at different stages. J MRI. 1995;5:287-92.
25. Sakhalkar VS. Dalvi RB, Pradhan MR, Colaco MP, Merchant RH. Myositis Ossificans Progressiva. 1994;31:1413-5.
26. O'Dwyer H, O'Hullivan P, Fitzgerald D, et al. The fat pad sign following elbow trauma in adults: Its usefulness and reliability in suspecting occult fracture. J Comput Assist Tomogr. 2004;28:562-5.
27. Navarro OM, Laffan EE, Ngan BY. Pediatric soft-tissue tumors and pseudotumors: MR imaging features with pathologic correlation part 1. Imaging approach, pseudotumors, vascular lesions, and adipocytic tumors. Radiographics. 2009;29:887-906.
28. Fletcher CDM, Unni KK, Mertens F (Eds). World Health Organisation classification of tumours. Pathology and genetics of tumours of soft tissue and bone. Lyon: IARC Press, 2002.
29. Murphey MD, Carroll JF, Flemming DJ, Pope TL, Gannon FH, Kransdorf MJ. Benign Musculoskeletal Lipomatous Lesions Radiographics. 2004;24:1433-66.
30. Drevelegas A, Pilavaki M, Chourmouzi D. Lipomatous tumours of soft tissue: MR appearance with histological correlation. Eur J Radiol. 2004;50:257-67.
31. Mulliken JB, Glowacki J. Hemangiomas and vascular malformations in infants and children: a classification based on endothelial characteristics. Plast Reconstr Surg. 1982;69:412-22.
32. Vilanova JC, Barcelo J, Smirniotopoulos JG, et al. Hemangioma from head to toe: MR imaging with pathologic correlation. Radiographics. 2004;24:367-85.
33. Vilanova JC, Woertler K, Narváez JA, et al. Soft-tissue tumors update: MR imaging features according to the WHO classification. Eur Radiol. 2007;17(1):125-38.
34. Wu JS, Hochman MG. Soft-tissue tumors and tumor like lesions: a systematic imaging approach. Radiology. 2009; 253(2):297-316.
35. Park SB, Lee JH, Weon YC. Imaging findings of head and neck inflammatory pseudotumor. Am J Roentgenol. 2009;193(4):1180-6.
36. Laffan EE, Ngan BY, Navarro OM. Pediatric soft-tissue tumors and pseudotumors: MR imaging features with pathologic correlation. Part 2. tumors of fibroblastic/myofibroblastic, so-called fibrohistiocytic, muscular, lymphomatous, neurogenic, hair matrix, and uncertain origin. Radiographics. 2009;e36. Published online 10.1148/rg.e36.
37. Murphey MD, Gibson MS, Jennings BT, Crespo-Rodríguez AM, Fanburg-Smith J, Gajewski DA. Imaging of synovial sarcoma with padiologic-pathologic correlation. Radiographics. 2006;26:1543-65.
38. Nam SJ, Kim S, Lim BJ, et al. Imaging of primary chest wall tumors with radiologic-pathologic correlation. Radiographics. 2011;31:749-70.

CHAPTER 206

A Systematic Approach to Imaging of Breast Lesions

Smriti Hari, Sanjay Thulkar, Arun Kumar Gupta

INTRODUCTION

Imaging is essential for accurate diagnosis of breast disease and early detection of breast cancer. Mammography and ultrasound (US) are the first-line investigations for imaging the breasts. Magnetic resonance imaging (MRI) is a valuable adjunctive diagnostic tool because of its high sensitivity for breast pathology. Mammography is the only screening modality, which has been proven to reduce mortality from breast cancer through early detection.[1] Sensitivity of mammography in detection of breast cancers in the screening set-up ranges from 83 to 95%.[2] However, it decreases to as low as 30–48% in patients with radiographically dense and glandular breasts.[3]

IMAGING TECHNIQUES

Mammography (Basic Physics, Equipment and Technique)

Effective mammography requires consistent high-quality images with optimal contrast, high resolution and low radiation dose. The mammography equipment and technique used have to take into account the wide variation in breast size, variation in the relative amounts of fat, glandular and stromal tissue present, and the low inherent contrast between normal and abnormal breast tissue. Dedicated mammography X-ray equipment **(Fig. 1)** with following features is necessary for producing high-quality images:

- Tube current should be as high as possible in order to keep exposure time short. Movement unsharpness may occur when exposure time exceeds 1 sec.

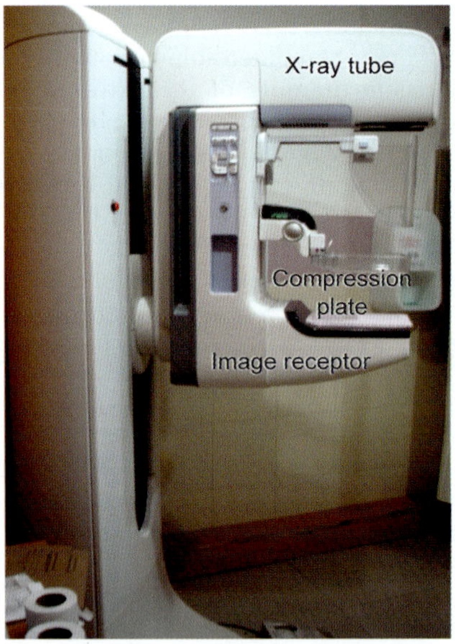

Fig. 1: Mammography equipment. Modern mammography machines automatically select target/filter combination, kVp and tube current according to breast density and the thickness of the compressed breast.

- Special X-ray tubes with molybdenum or rhodium anodes are required to produce the low energy X-rays necessary to achieve high tissue contrast. The spectrum is refined further by adding filters at the source of the X-ray beam to remove the very low energy photons which are likely to be absorbed in the breast and not contribute in the image formation. The most commonly used target-filter combination of molybdenum target with 0.03 mm molybdenum filter is well suited for the average sized breasts. The peak kilovoltage is in the range 26–30 kV.

- High spatial resolution is required to identify microcalcifications measuring in the order of 100 μm. Small focal spot of the X-ray tube (0.3 mm for routine mammography and 0.1 mm for magnification mammography) and high resolution film-screen combinations improve the spatial resolution of the mammography, which may be up to 15–20 lp/mm.
- Grids are used for all mammographic studies to reduce scattered radiation and to increase contrast, especially in the dense or thick breast.
- Modern mammography machines automatically select target/filter combination, kVp and tube current according to breast density and the thickness of the compressed breast. This allows for the selection of a higher energy X-ray spectrum for large breasts to provide sufficient penetration and prevent excessive radiation. In addition, automatic exposure control devices control the exposure duration so that the optimum optical density of the mammograms is maintained over a wide range of breast sizes and densities. The automatic exposure control device, either a phototimer or ionization chamber, is normally positioned 3 cm posterior to the nipple, where the most dense glandular tissue is likely to be present.
- Good breast compression with radiolucent compression paddle is mandatory for mammography. Breast compression results in uniform thickness and hence uniform exposure and density in most parts of the breast. The overlapping tissues are separated and spread evenly which improves their visualization. Firm compression of the breast closer to film or image receptor reduces the geometric blur and magnification. Compression also stabilizes the breast and reduces the movement blur. Mammography cannot be performed if breast compression is not possible. Such situations may include uncooperative women, presence of wound, recent surgery or tender breasts.
- Single side emulsion film is used with a single intensifying screen in order to ensure optimum resolution. Especially designed cassettes ensure good film-screen contact.
- Optimum film density and contrast are achieved by an extended processing time of up to 3.5 minutes together with a lower developer temperature (34°C) than for general radiography.

For accurate detection and characterization of the breast abnormalities on mammography, good quality control is essential. It is required at several steps; acceptance and periodic maintenance of the equipment, positioning and exposure, film processing, viewing conditions and the interpretation. The quality control requirements of mammography are probably more stringent than any other imaging modality.

RADIATION DOSE

Modern mammographic examinations are safe and the mean glandular radiation dose to the breast is approximately 2 mGy (0.2 rad) per exposure. With present mammographic equipment, there is little or no radiation related risk to the women over 40 years of age.[4]

Mammography Projections

The standard mammographic examination consists of a mediolateral-oblique (MLO) and craniocaudal (CC) view of each breast. These provide two orthogonal images for basic imaging evaluation of the breast. The MLO view is obtained with the tube angled at 45° to the horizontal, with compression applied obliquely across the chest wall, perpendicular to the long axis of the pectoralis major muscle **(Fig. 2A)**. Entire breast cannot be included in any single mammographic view. More breast tissue is demonstrated on the MLO projection than on any other view.

The standard CC view is obtained with a vertical X-ray beam. Positioning is achieved by pulling the breast up and forward, away from the chest wall, with compression applied from above **(Fig. 2B)**. The CC projection demonstrates the subareolar, medial and lateral portions of the breast, however, tissue in the posterolateral aspect of the breast may not be demonstrated completely. The criteria for well-positioned MLO and CC views are given in **Table 1**.

Table 1: Criteria for well-positioned mediolateral-oblique and craniocaudal views

Criteria for a well-positioned MLO view ***(Fig. 3A):***
• The nipple should be seen in profile.
• The pectoralis muscle should extend inferior to the posterior nipple line (PNL) an imaginary line drawn from the nipple to the pectoralis muscle or film edge and perpendicular to the pectoralis muscle
• An open inframammary fold should be visible
• There should be no skin folds superimposed on the breast
Criteria for a well-positioned CC view ***(Fig. 3B):***
• The nipple should be demonstrated in profile
• The PNL on the CC view is drawn from the nipple to the pectoralis muscle or film edge. The length of the PNL on the CC view should be within 1 cm of its length on the MLO projection.

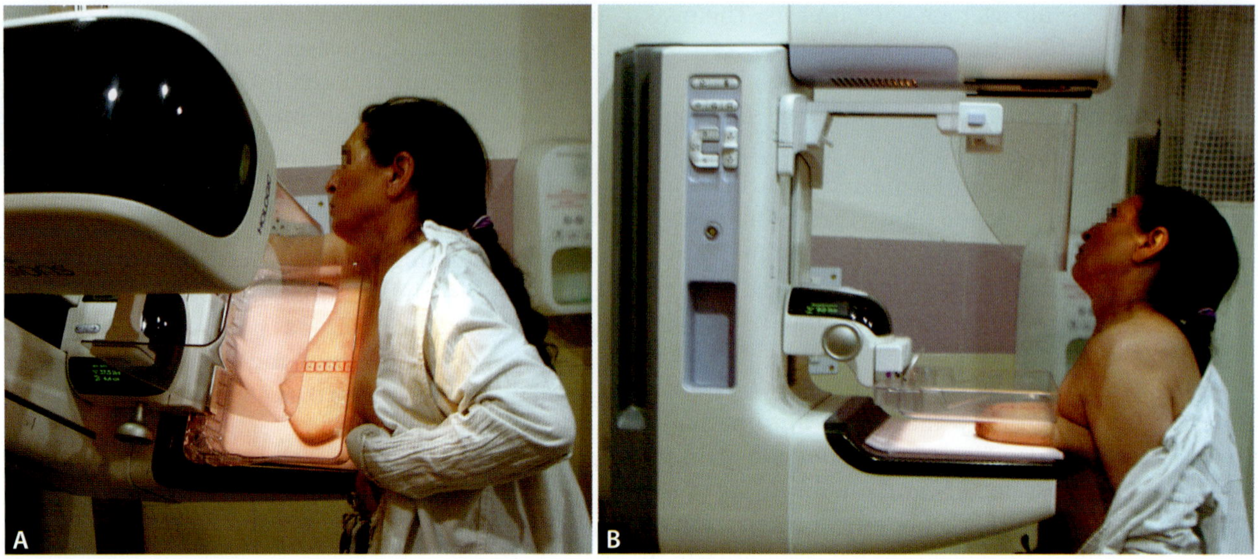

Figs. 2A and B: Positioning for MLO and CC views: (A) *MLO view*: The MLO view is obtained with the tube angled at 45° to the horizontal, with compression applied obliquely across the chest wall, perpendicular to the long axis of the pectoralis major muscle; (B) *CC view*: Positioning is achieved by pulling the breast up and forward, away from the chest wall, with compression applied from above.

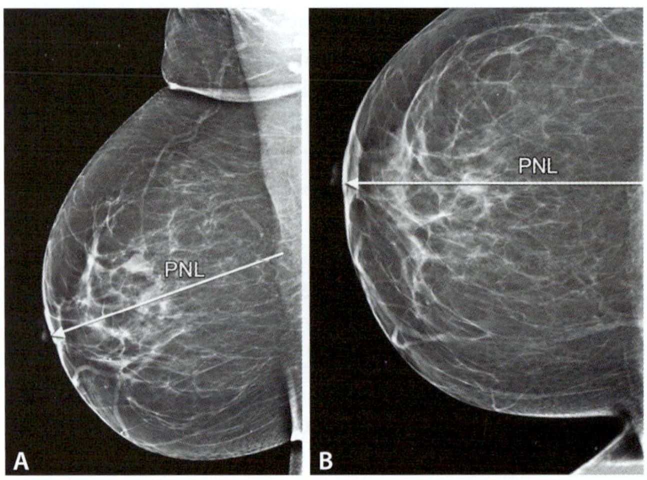

Figs. 3A and B: Well-positioned MLO and CC views: (A) A well-positioned MLO view should include breast tissue from high in the axilla to just below the inframammary fold. The pectoralis muscle should extend inferior to the posterior nipple line (PNL) an imaginary line drawn from the nipple to the pectoralis muscle or film edge and perpendicular to the pectoralis muscle; (B) An adequately positioned CC view should demonstrate the subareolar, medial and lateral portions of the breast. The PNL on the CC view is drawn from the nipple to the pectoralis muscle or film edge. The length of the PNL on the CC view should be within 1 cm of its length on the MLO projection.

Supplementary Views

Supplementary views may be taken to solve specific diagnostic problems.

Rolled views may separate normal fibroglandular elements into their individual components. These views are performed by "rolling" the breast tissue and compressing the breast in the same projection in which the finding was first discovered. On the rolled view, a summation shadow would be separated into its normal fibroglandular components, whereas true masses will retain their shape and persist.

Magnification view is obtained by increasing the object-film distance, producing an 'air gap' and using a fine focal spot to increase resolution. This is particularly helpful for detailed analysis of microcalcifications and the margins of small mass lesions.

Spot compression view is obtained by using a small compression paddle with or without magnification. By compression, the breast tissue overlying a small lesion is displaced, allowing for better demonstration of its morphologic features. This technique is also very helpful in analyzing asymmetrical soft tissue shadows, either by confirming that the shadow represents normal glandular tissue or by demonstrating that an underlying lesion is present.

An extended CC view can be performed by rotating the patient's body to display the lateral or medial breast tissue better than possible with a standard CC view. For demonstration of tissue in the most posterolateral part of the breast, the patient is rotated medially to bring the lateral part of the breast and axillary tail over the film, while excluding the medial portion of the breast. For medial breast lesions, the patient is rotated laterally to bring the medial part of the breast over the film, while excluding the outer breast tissue.

NORMAL MAMMOGRAPHIC ANATOMY

The breast contains 15–20 lobes, each drained by a lactiferous duct with an opening in the nipple. The main duct branches repeatedly within the breast and the most distal branches of the duct system are called the terminal ducts **(Fig. 4)**. The terminal duct consists of intralobular and extralobular portions. The intralobular portion, together with the acini, forms a lobule. The extralobular terminal duct and the lobule form a terminal ductal lobular unit. Terminal ductal lobular unit is the site of origin of most malignant and benign disease of the breast.

The mammographic appearance of the breast depends on the relative amounts of fat and glandular tissue that are present. The young woman's breast contains a large amount of glandular tissue which appears as soft tissue density on the mammogram; in older women, when involution of the glandular tissue has occurred most of the breast tissue appears of fatty density.

Normal lymph nodes are often seen in the axilla and within the breast (intramammary lymph nodes), in the upper outer quadrant. A normal lymph node is an oval or lobulated dense mass with a radiolucent fatty hilum.

The nipple is usually everted and it should be seen in profile on at least one mammographic view so that the retroareolar region can be visualized without its superimposition. The nipple can be inverted since birth as a normal variant; however, recent nipple inversion is of concern for a retroareolar mass.

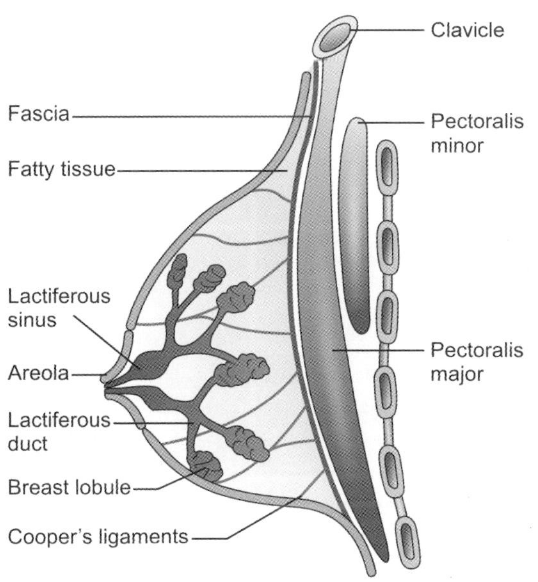

Fig. 4: Schematic representation of the breast anatomy.

Interpretation and Reporting of Mammograms

Mammograms should be viewed in optimum lighting conditions, light from around the films and extraneous light in the viewing room should be excluded as far as possible. The films should be checked for correct identification labeling and for radiographic quality. The standard MLO and CC views are studied with the right and left breast films 'back to back' so that symmetry of the breast tissue can be examined.

American College of Radiology (ACR) has devised the Breast Imaging Reporting and Data System (BI-RADS), a standardized method for describing the morphology of breast lesions and categorizing the findings in an unambiguous report. A lexicon of descriptive terms is an integral part of BI-RADS and is intended to provide a common language for lesion description and assessment. The first step in mammographic interpretation should be the assessment of parenchymal density as the diagnostic accuracy of mammogram decreases with increased density of breast. The ACR BI-RADS divides breast parenchyma into four major categories based on the mammographic density **(Table 2)**.

The abnormal mammographic finding is then categorized as a mass, calcification, architectural distortion or asymmetry.

Mass

The ACR BI-RADS lexicon defines a breast mass as a three-dimensional space-occupying lesion which is seen in two mammographic views. Masses are assessed for their size, shape, margins and density **(Table 3)**. Evaluation of a mass is most optimal in a spot compression magnification view in which the mass is superimposed over the surrounding fat. The shape of a mass may be round, oval, lobulated or irregular **(Figs. 6A to D)** and as the shape becomes more irregular, the probability of malignancy increases. Margins are generally described as circumscribed (sharply defined), indistinct, spiculated **(Figs. 7A to D)** or microlobulated.

Table 2: ACR BI-RADS categories of breast density.

*CACR BI-RADS categories of breast density **(Figs. 5A to D)***
1. Breast tissue almost entirely fatty (dense glandular tissue occupying <25% of the breast parenchyma)
2. Scattered fibroglandular tissue (dense glandular tissue occupying 25–50% of the breast parenchyma)
3. Heterogeneously dense parenchyma (dense glandular tissue occupying 50–75% of the breast parenchyma)
4. Extremely dense breast (dense glandular tissue occupying >75% of the breast parenchyma)

Table 3: ACR BI-RADS mass descriptors in mammography

Characteristic	*Term*	*Description*
Shape	Round	Spherical
	Oval	Elliptical
	Lobular	2–3 gentle lobulations
	Irregular	Neither round nor oval
Margin	Circumscribed	Margins from a sharp, abrupt transition with the surrounding tissue
	Microlobulated	Short undulations at the surface of the lesion
	Obscured	Normal surrounding tissue hides the true edge of the lesion
	Indistinct	Demarcation between the mass and surrounding tissue is not clearly defined
	Spiculated	Sharp lines radiating from the margins of the mass
Density	High	More dense relative to glandular parenchyma
	Equal	Similar density relative to glandular parenchyma
	Low	Less dense relative to glandular parenchyma
	Fat containing	Internal lucent area suggestive of fat

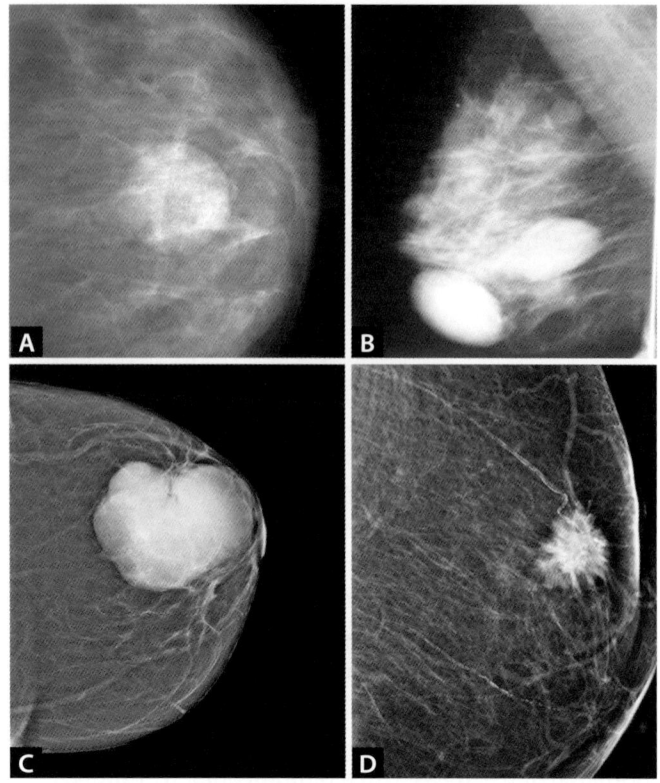

Figs. 6A to D: ACR BI-RADS descriptors for mass shape on mammography: (A) Round; (B) Oval; (C) Lobulated; (D) Irregular.

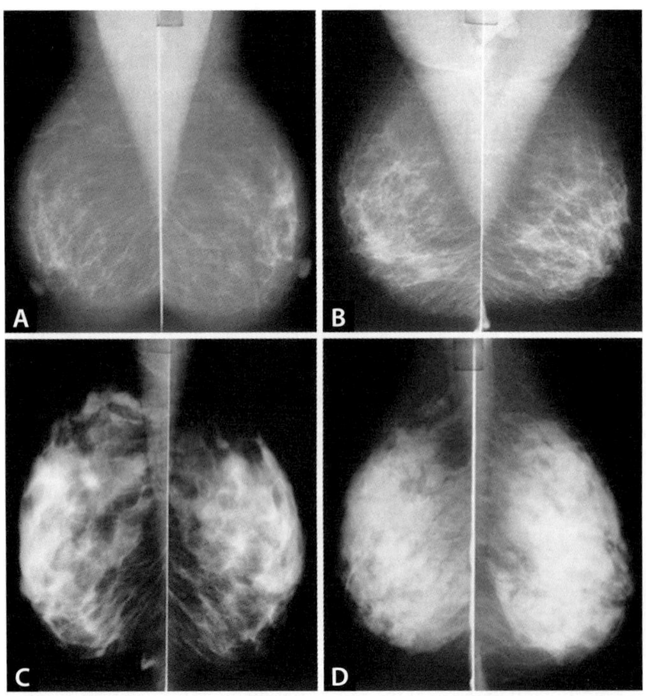

Figs. 5A to D: ACR categories of breast parenchymal density. (A) *Category 1*: Breast tissue almost entirely fatty; (B) *Category 2*; Scattered fibroglandular tissue; (C) *Category 3*: Heterogeneously dense parenchyma; (D) *Category 4*: Extremely dense breast.

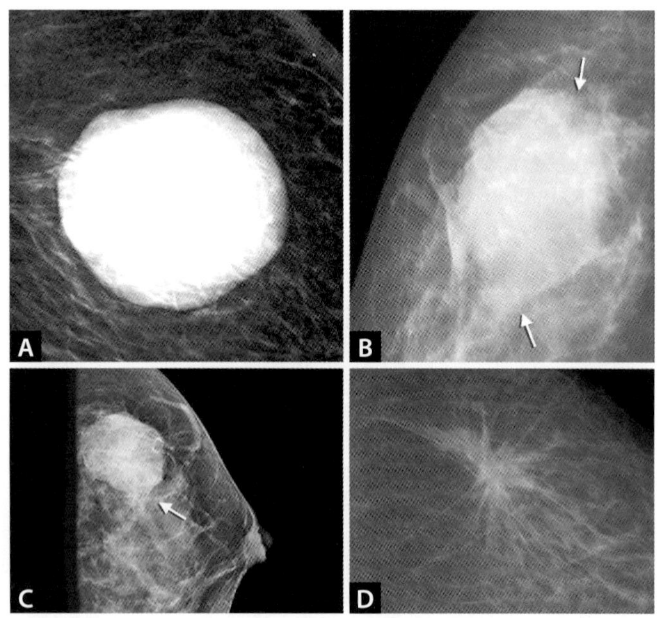

Figs. 7A to D: ACR BI-RADS descriptors for mass margins on mammography. (A) Circumscribed (sharply defined); (B) Obscured; (C) Indistinct; (D) Spiculated.

Benign masses do not invade tissue margins and therefore tend to have well circumscribed borders. Because breast cancers invade the basement membrane and extend into the surrounding glandular tissue, they produce irregularly shaped masses with indistinct or spiculated margins. Microlobulated masses have small undulations and are more worrisome for malignancy than are smooth masses. When all or part of the margin is abutting the normal glandular parenchyma and not amenable to precise evaluation, the term obscured margin is used. Spiculated margin is characterized by thin lines radiating from the central portion of the mass and is significant for malignancy. Spiculations are produced either by the intense fibrotic reaction to the cancer or by growth of the tumor into the surrounding glandular tissue. The density is described as high, equal or low relative to glandular breast parenchyma **(Figs. 8A to C)**. Density of the mass is not helpful for characterization of the masses. Exception is fat containing masses which are always benign and are described as such.

Calcification

Calcifications are commonly encountered on mammograms but majority of these are the result of benign processes. All calcifications are evaluated for their number, size, shapes, distribution and any characteristic morphology **(Table 4)**. Calcifications are broadly classified into typically benign calcifications, those with intermediate concern and those having high probability of malignancy. Most benign calcifications are larger than 0.5 mm. Typically benign calcifications include lucent-centered calcifications (skin calcifications or fat necrosis), vascular calcifications, popcorn calcifications of involuted fibroadenoma, eggshell or rim calcifications, long rod like ductal calcifications and coarse dystrophic calcifications **(Figs. 9A to E)**.

Calcifications with intermediate concern include amorphous and coarse heterogeneous calcifications **(Figs. 10A and B)**. The BI-RADS term "amorphous" describes intermediate calcifications that are tiny, roundish" flake-like" particles too small and vague to characterize further. "Coarse heterogeneous" calcifications are a new addition to the fourth edition of BI-RADS. These calcifications are irregular, conspicuous and larger than 0.5 mm. They are associated most often with benign conditions, such as fibrosis or fibroadenomas, but can occasionally be seen within malignant lesions.

Calcifications with high probability of malignancy are irregular, smaller than 0.5 mm (microcalcifications) and are pleomorphic (varying in size and shape and density) **(Fig. 11A)**. On screening mammography, pleomorphic calcifications often herald the presence of DCIS, which is the diagnosis in 25–48% of all cancers found at screening. DCIS develops in breast duct epithelium, remains within the duct basement membrane and grows along the duct. Individual calcifications form within the DCIS tumor as a result of cell death and necrosis in the comedo form of DCIS. The ACR BI-RADS term for these calcifications is "fine linear or fine linear branching (casting) calcifications" because the calcifications form an irregular cast of the duct. The calcifications may look like little broken needles with pointy ends or may have a "dot-dash" appearance with both round and linear shapes. They are much smaller, less dense and less well-defined than the linear calcifications in benign secretory disease, which can be mistaken for DCIS. Another suspicious calcification form described is "fine heterogeneous calcifications";

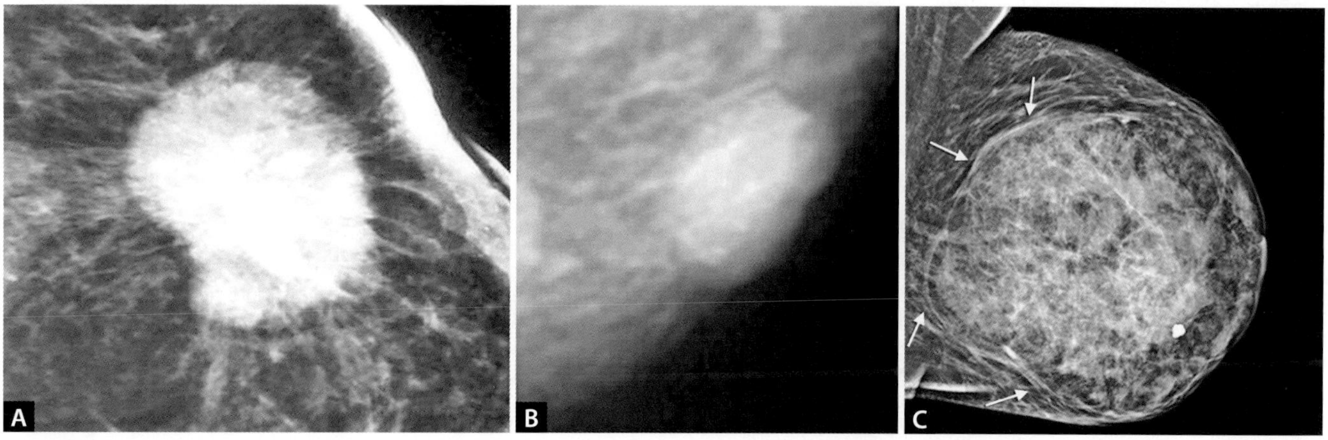

Figs. 8A to C: ACR BI-RADS descriptors for mass density (as compared to the fibroglandular parenchyma) on mammography. (A) High density mass; (B) Isodense mass; (C) Low density mass. MLO view showing a large heterogeneous mass in the breast (arrows) containing areas of fat density within, consistent with the diagnosis of hamartoma.

Table 4: Specific ACR BI-RADS terms for description of calcifications.

Characteristic	***Term***	***Description***
Distribution	Grouped or clustered	Five or more calcifications in a cubic centimeter of tissue constitutes a cluster
	Ductal	Fine linear branching pattern produced by calcification of necrotic cancer cells within a duct
	Segmental	Calcifications within a single duct network of a lobe
	Regional	Randomly distributed calcifications not conforming to a duct and usually occupying a quadrant or more
	Diffusely scattered	Randomly distributed calcifications throughout the entire breast
Number	<5	Unlikely to represent cancer
	5–10	Indeterminate
	>10	More likely to be associated with cancer
Morphology (Typically benign)	Skin Vascular	Sharply defined with lucent center Parallel tram-track calcification
	Coarse or "popcorn like"	Characteristic of involuting fibroadenoma
	Large rod like	Secretory calcifications—Calcified debris in the duct lumen (solid rods)
		Calcified inflammatory reaction around a duct (lucent-centered rods)
	Round spherical	Concretions formed in the acini of microcystically dilated lobules
	Rim or eggshell	Very thin, benign calcifications that appear as calcium deposited on the surface of a sphere
	Suture	Typically linear or tubular in appearance and knots are frequently visible
	Dystrophic	Large (>0.5 mm), irregular (post-trauma or radiotherapy)
	Punctate	Round or oval and very small (<0.5 mm) but very sharply defined, pinpoint deposits
Morphology (Intermediate)	Amorphous or indistinct Coarse heterogeneous	Round or flake-shaped deposits those are too small or hazy to characterize Irregular, dense calcifications >0.5 mm in size
Morphology (Higher probability of malignancy)	Pleomorphic Fine heterogeneous Fine branching	Irregular, vary in size and shape and are <0.5 mm Rounded but very tiny, irregularly shaped calcifications Thin, discontinuous, irregular particles that form in a linear pattern and are <1 mm in width/calcifications of necrotic tumor in the lumen of a duct that is irregularly involved by breast cancer

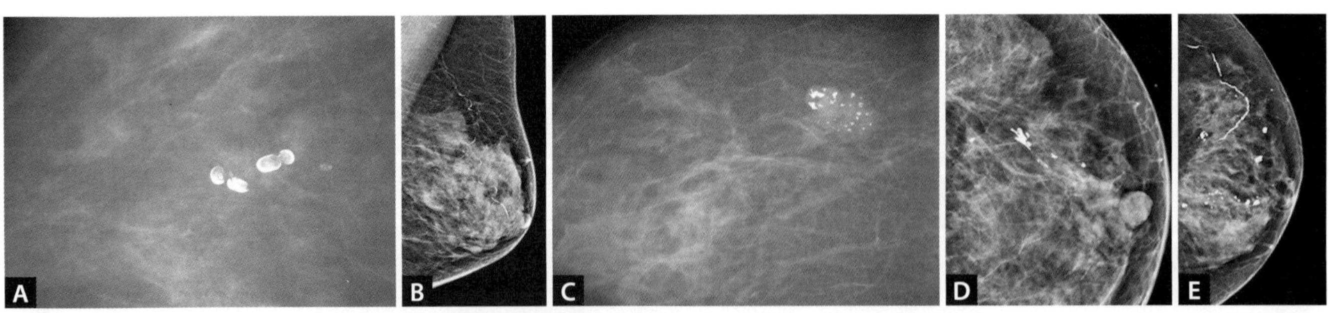

Figs. 9A to E: Typically benign calcifications. (A) Lucent-centered calcifications consistent with skin calcifications; (B) Vascular calcification; (C) Popcorn calcifications within involuted fibroadenoma; (D) Rod-like ductal calcifications; (E) Coarse dystrophic calcifications seen in a postoperative, irradiated breast.

this term reflects more rounded but very tiny, irregularly shaped calcifications that form in small rounded pockets of necrotic tumors such as DCIS or in fibrocystic disease or sclerosing adenosis **(Fig. 11B)**.

Amorphous, pleomorphic and coarse heterogeneous types of calcification may, at times, be difficult to separate but can have different prognostic implications. Pleomorphic calcifications, together with fine, linear

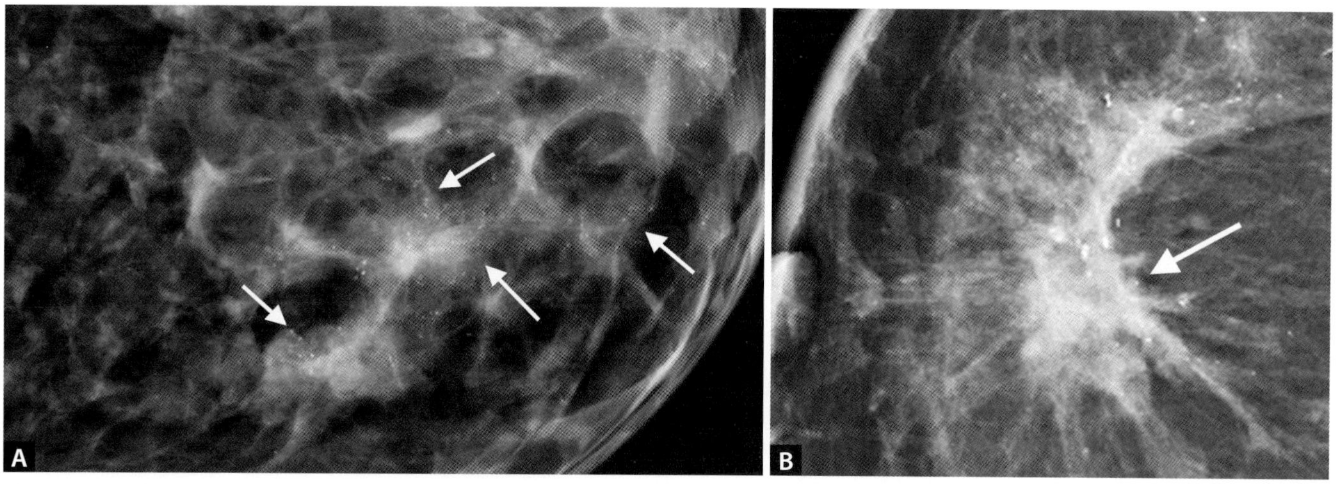

Figs. 10A and B: Calcifications of intermediate concern. (A) Amorphous calcifications (arrows) are tiny, flake-like particles too small and vague to characterize further; (B) Coarse heterogeneous calcifications are a new addition to the fourth edition of BI-RADS. These calcifications are irregular, conspicuous and larger than 0.5 mm.

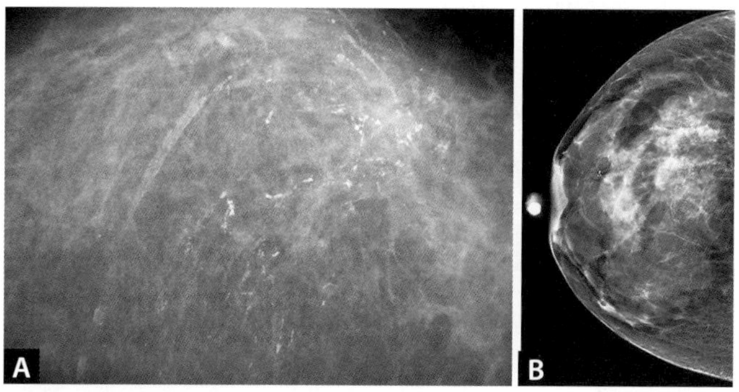

Figs. 11A and B: Calcifications having high probability of malignancy. (A) Pleomorphic calcifications are irregular, smaller than 0.5 mm (microcalcifications) and vary in size, shape and density; (B) Fine heterogeneous calcifications are more rounded but very tiny and irregularly shaped

branching calcifications, have the highest probability for malignancy. Amorphous calcifications differ from pleomorphic calcifications in their conspicuity or density. Their edges are not defined as sharply as are those in the pleomorphic category. They may present with only a slightly higher density than surrounding glandular tissue, accounting for their difficult detection. Of the three types of calcifications described, pleomorphic are the most suspicious, coarse heterogeneous are the least suspicious and amorphous are between the former and the latter. Approximately 20% of lesions associated with amorphous calcifications are malignant and of these, 90% represent DCIS.[5] As a rule, it is unusual to have calcifications that are exclusively of one shape. Most are mixtures of different forms; however, it is the most worrisome of these forms that should direct subsequent management.

The number of calcifications is also important; fewer than five calcifications in a cluster rarely represent cancer. The distribution of calcifications **(Figs. 12A to D)** within the breast often may allow separation into benign and malignant status with increased accuracy. The terminal duct lobular unit is the anatomic site of origin of most intraductal carcinomas. When this concept is kept in mind, calcifications oriented in a "linear" or multiple linear (segmental) orientation assume greater importance, even if the individual calcification shape is of intermediate concern. For example, linear or segmental arrangements of coarse heterogeneous calcifications are more worrisome than a regional distribution of the same calcifications. Grouped or clustered microcalcifications occupy less than 1 cm^3 of tissue and are composed of at least five elements. A cluster of coarse heterogeneous calcifications is less worrisome than a linear or segmental distribution; however, calcifications in the category of higher probability of malignancy (pleomorphic and fine linear) almost always require tissue diagnosis, regardless of distribution. As the distribution becomes less focal, as in "regional" (>2 cm^3 of breast tissue not conforming to a duct and usually occupying a quadrant or more), or distributed randomly throughout the breast (diffuse/scattered), the suspicion for malignancy diminishes.

ARCHITECTURAL DISTORTION

The term architectural distortion is used to describe focal distortion or tethering of the trabeculae, focal spiculations and retraction of the parenchyma. The hallmark of this feature is a series of thin, straight lines or spiculations

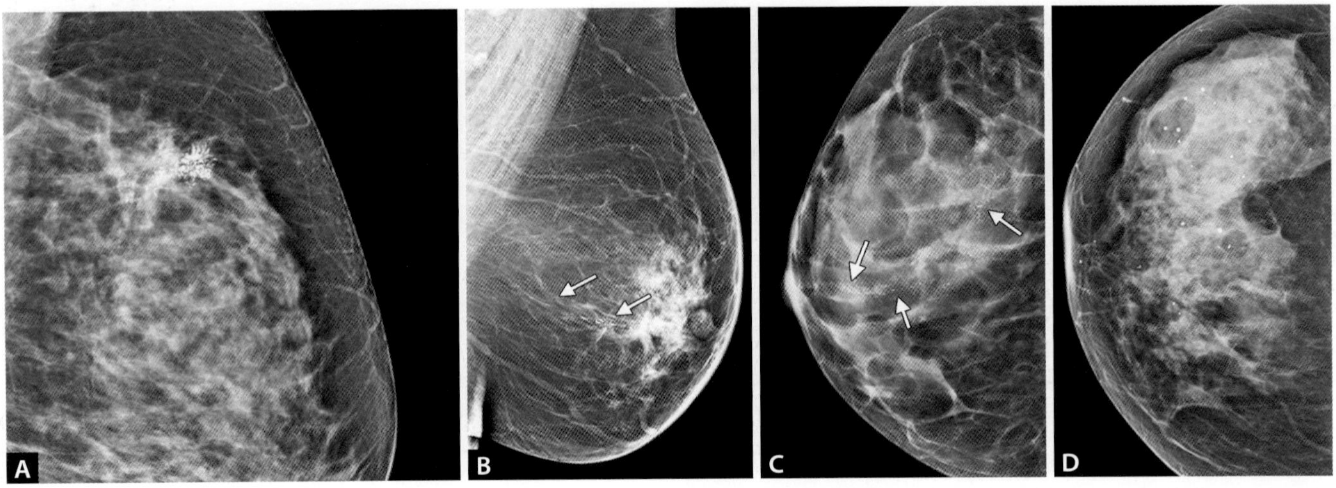

Figs. 12A to D: ACR BI-RADS descriptors for distribution of calcifications: (A) Clustered; (B) Ductal; (C) Segmental; (D) Scattered/Diffuse

radiating from an area that does not have features of a mass or focal asymmetry **(Fig. 13)**; however, these radiating spicules also may be identified from the edge of a mass or focal asymmetry. In this situation, they become part of the margin description (spiculated) for the mass or asymmetry. There are situations in which it becomes difficult or impossible to determine whether one is dealing with a spiculated mass or architectural distortion; however, the presence of these radially oriented lines, whether originating from a mass, focal asymmetry, or a point, strongly suggest the presence of malignancy. Differential diagnosis of architectural distortion includes complex sclerosing lesion/radial scar, carcinoma and postoperative scarring. Once surgical scar is excluded from appropriate clinical history and physical examination, localized areas of architectural distortion require histological diagnosis.

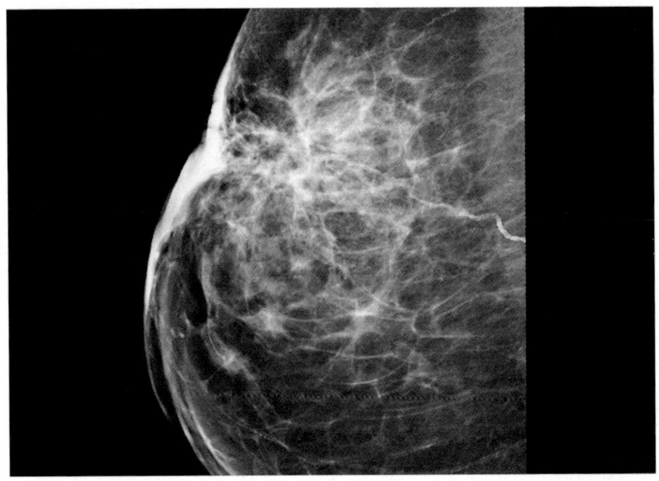

Fig. 13: Architectural distortion. Mammogram showing multiple thin, straight lines radiating from a central area that does not have features of a mass. There is associated focal skin thickening and retraction.

FOCAL ASYMMETRY

It is important to differentiate an asymmetry versus a focal asymmetry versus a mass. A soft tissue finding identified only on one view, without matching tissue in a similar location in the contralateral breast, represents an asymmetry. This is in contradistinction to focal asymmetry and mass, both of which are soft tissue findings seen on two views, lying at a comparable depth when one view is compared with another and showing similar density and shape on those views. Focal asymmetry lacks convex outward borders on both views **(Figs. 14A and B)**, whereas mass displays consistent convex margins. Focal asymmetry is confined to a small area of the breast (within a quadrant) and may represent a subtle, but important, sign of malignancy (often an infiltrating lobular carcinoma), especially if it is associated with palpable abnormality or it is a new or evolving finding on serial mammograms.[6] Conversely, global asymmetry occupies a large portion of the breast (more than one quadrant). This asymmetry is usually on the basis of normal variation or secondary to the effects of hormone replacement therapy. The term "density" has been removed from the discussion of asymmetries because it is more accurately used as a descriptor of X-ray attenuation.

BREAST EDEMA

Breast edema is recognized on mammograms as diffusely increased density and coarse trabecular pattern in an enlarged breast with thickened skin. The causes of an edematous breast are as follows:

- *Primary breast cancer*: Lymphatic spread from an advanced primary tumor or inflammatory carcinoma can lead to breast edema

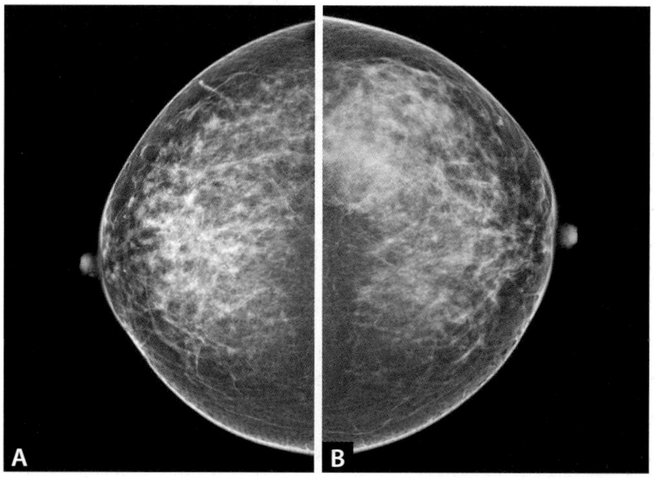

Figs. 14A and B: Focal asymmetry. Bilateral CC views showing focal asymmetry in the left breast outer quadrant which was also seen on the MLO view. Ultrasound showed a suspicious mass. Invasive ductal carcinoma on histopathology.

- Axillary lymph node metastasis
- Breast abscess
- *Radiotherapy*: Breast edema develops progressively following radiotherapy treatment, reaches a maximum at 6 months and resolves approximately 18 months after treatment
- Cardiac or renal failure may cause unilateral or bilateral breast edema.

Abnormal Axillary Lymph Nodes

Normal lymph nodes are commonly seen on mammograms and are well-defined, having a peripheral area of soft tissue density and a central radiolucent area. Intramammary lymph nodes most commonly occur in the upper outer quadrant and show the same features. Pathological lymph nodes are enlarged and show loss of central fatty lucency. Enlarged lymph nodes may be due to benign conditions such as infection, sarcoidosis or malignant conditions like lymphoma, leukemia or metastasis. Metastatic lymph nodes from breast cancer may contain microcalcifications. Coarse calcification is seen in tubercular nodes.

AMERICAN COLLEGE OF RADIOLOGY BI-RADS ASSESSMENT CATEGORIES

The mammographic findings are categorized from BI-RADS 0 to BI-RADS 6, which are primarily aimed for communication of significance of the mammographic findings to the referring physician and to recommend the most appropriate management **(Table 5)**.

Mammographic Assessment is Incomplete

Category 0

Incomplete evaluation: Repeat mammography, additional views or investigations like US or MRI (but not biopsy) are recommended.

Mammographic Assessment is Complete: Final Categories

Category 1

Negative: There is nothing to comment on. The breasts are symmetric and no masses, architectural distortion or suspicious calcifications are present.

Category 2

Benign Finding: Like category 1, this is a "normal" assessment, but here, the film reader chooses to describe a benign finding in the mammography report. Involuting, calcified fibroadenomas, multiple secretory calcifications, fat-containing lesions such as oil cysts, lipomas, galactoceles and mixed-density hamartomas all have characteristically benign appearances. The reader may also choose to describe intramammary lymph nodes, vascular calcifications, implants or architectural distortion clearly related to prior surgery while still concluding that there is no mammographic evidence of malignancy.

Category 3

Probably benign finding—initial short-interval follow-up suggested: A finding placed in this category should have less than a 2% risk of malignancy. Lesions appropriately placed in this category include a nonpalpable, circumscribed mass on a baseline mammogram (unless it can be shown to be a cyst, an intramammary lymph node, or another benign finding), a focal asymmetry and a cluster of punctate calcifications.

Management of Probably Benign Lesions

Probability of malignancy in such lesions is very small, usually less than 2% and hence, routine biopsy of all such lesions is not necessary. Instead, a short-term (normally 6 months later) follow-up mammography of the same breast is performed to determine the stability of the lesion. The follow-up is aimed to prove the benign diagnosis short of biopsy and not to determine whether the lesion is benign or malignant. If the lesion is stable, the follow-up is continued usually for two years.[7]

Table 5: ACR BI-RADS mammographic assessment categories.

Category	Description	Likelihood of malignancy	Examples	Next step in evaluation
0	Incomplete; need additional imaging evaluation, or comparison with previous examinations	Unknown	Asymmetry, mass, calcifications on screening mammography	Special mammographic views, US, MRI; obtain previous examinations
1	Negative	No mammographic evidence of malignancy	Normal mammography	Routine screening
2	Benign finding	No mammographic evidence of malignancy	Intramammary lymph node, oil cyst, vascular calcifications, calcifying fibroadenoma	Routine screening
3	Probably benign finding	Less than 2%	Benign-appearing solid mass or clustered calcifications	Follow-up imaging (mammography or US) at six and 12 months
4	Suspicious abnormality	5–95%	Complex or solid mass, indeterminate clustered calcifications	Biopsy
5	Highly suggestive of malignancy	Greater than 95%	Spiculated mass	Biopsy
6	Known malignancy	100%	Biopsy-proven	Definitive treatment

Any change in morphology on follow-up mammogram warrants immediate biopsy. Such a lesion, even if proved malignant subsequently, does not significantly affect the stage and prognosis in majority.

Category 4

Suspicious abnormality—biopsy should be considered: This category is reserved for findings that do not have the classic appearance of malignancy and the probability of malignancy is greater than category 3. Probability of malignancy in the BI-RADS 4 category is very large, from 5 to 95%. By subdividing category 4 into 4A, 4B and 4C, it is encouraged that relevant probabilities for malignancy be indicated within this category so the patient and her physician can make an informed decision on the ultimate course of action.

BI-RADS 4A category is used if the lesion is sampled, but with a very low probability for malignancy. A malignant pathology report is not expected and a 6-month follow-up after a benign biopsy is appropriate. Examples of findings placed in this category may be a palpable, partially circumscribed solid mass with US features suggestive of a fibroadenoma, a palpable complicated cyst or a breast abscess.

BI-RADS 4B includes lesions with an intermediate probability of malignancy. Biopsy is recommended and close radio-pathological correlation is warranted. Follow-up in case of a benign result depends on the concordance between imaging and pathological features: a partially circumscribed mass with ill-defined margins with a fibroadenoma result is acceptable, but in case of a diagnosis of papillary lesion, surgery should be proposed.

BI-RADS 4C includes findings of moderate concern, but not classic (as in category 5) for malignancy. Examples of findings placed in this category are, solid, irregular masses with ill-defined margins or recent cluster of fine pleomorphic calcifications. A malignant result is expected in this category. In case of a benign biopsy result, 6-month follow-up is mandatory to rule out a false-negative report.

Category 5

Highly suggestive of malignancy—appropriate action should be taken: (Almost certainly malignant): This category 5 is used for findings that are classic breast cancers, with a ≥95% likelihood of malignancy. A spiculated, irregular high-density mass, a segmental or linear arrangement of fine linear calcifications or an irregular spiculated mass with associated pleomorphic calcifications are examples of lesions that should be placed in this category.

Category 6

Known biopsy-proven malignancy—appropriate action should be taken: This category is reserved for lesions identified on the imaging study with biopsy proof of malignancy prior to definitive therapy.

Indications for Mammography

Mammography is not performed in pregnant or lactating women and is generally avoided in women below 30 years

Table 6: Indications for mammography.

• Screening asymptomatic women aged 50 years and over • Screening asymptomatic women aged 35 years and over who have a high-risk of developing breast cancer – Women who have one or more first degree relatives diagnosed with premenopausal breast cancer – Women with histologic risk factors found at previous surgery, e.g. atypical ductal hyperplasia • Symptomatic women aged 35 years and over with breast lump or other clinical evidence of breast cancer • Search of the occult primary tumor in patients presenting with metastases • Surveillance of the breast following local excision of breast cancer • Breast lump in a male

of age. Major indications for mammography are listed in **Table 6**.

DIGITAL MAMMOGRAPHY

Because of the stringent technical requirements of the mammography, it was the last imaging technique to go digital. Full field digital mammography is now gradually replacing screen-film (conventional) mammography.

FULL FIELD DIGITAL IMAGING

Digital systems may be direct radiography (DR) units, which have a built-in digital detector, thus completely replacing screen film mammography or computed radiography (CR) units, which consist of add-on digital conversion detectors that only replace the screen film cassette system in a screen film unit.

Computed radiography systems use photostimulable phosphor imaging plates that can be loaded into a conventional bucky assembly. The CR image can be presented on film or displayed on a high resolution monitor. Image acquisition in CR is a two-stage process requiring transfer of the CR plate to the readout device.

Most important component of the digital mammography system is digital detector. It converts the X-rays into digital signals and replaces the film. The detectors can be broadly divided into two types. The indirect digital detectors convert X-rays into light and then into a digital signal. These detectors use amorphous silicon, charge-couple devices (CCD) or photostimulable phosphors. The direct digital detectors, often called flat panel detectors, do not have this light conversion step; instead the substrate used is a photoconductive material that is able to directly convert the X-ray photons into a digital image. Amorphous selenium detectors and crystal silicon detectors are direct digital detectors.[8] The overall design of the mammography unit (including X-ray tube, gantry, compression paddles), technique of performing the mammography and amount of radiation involved remains similar to those of the film-screen mammography.

Advantages and Applications of the Digital Mammography

Digital mammography images are available for viewing immediately and dark-room, which is frequently a major source of image degradation and artifacts, is eliminated. The advantages of digital mammography over screen-film mammography are as follows:

- Better contrast characteristics and dynamic range.
- Post processing such as manipulations of the contrast, brightness, edge enhancement, zoom-pan, etc.
- Better archival, storage and communication, i.e. PACS and tele-mammography.

When compared with the screen-film mammography, major limitations of digital mammography are the cost and lower spatial resolution. The full field digital mammography units are several times more expensive than conventional mammography units. The spatial resolution of the current digital mammography systems is about 6–8 lp/mm, i.e. about half of what is possible with screen-film mammography. However, better dynamic range and post processing abilities compensate for this so that the lesion detection and characterization on digital mammography is not affected adversely.

Newer applications of the digital mammography are exciting. These include computer-aided detection (CAD) and diagnosis, digital breast tomosynthesis (DBT) and dual energy contrast enhanced mammography.

Computer-aided Detection

Computer-aided detection is a computer software system that is designed to aid the film reader by highlighting the areas of concern (calcifications and masses). These areas are then carefully assessed by the radiologist. The CAD thus decreases the chances of overlooking these abnormalities. It may help inexperienced radiologists and also acts as a second opinion to the experienced radiologists. Use of CAD in screening set-ups improves the cancer detection rates.[9] The CAD software correctly prompts around 90% of all cancers, with 86–88% of all masses and 98% of microcalcifications correctly marked. Specificity however, is a problem with CAD and high rate of false-positive prompts is common.

Digital Breast Tomosynthesis

The dense glandular tissue in conventional mammography is frequently a source of both false positives and false

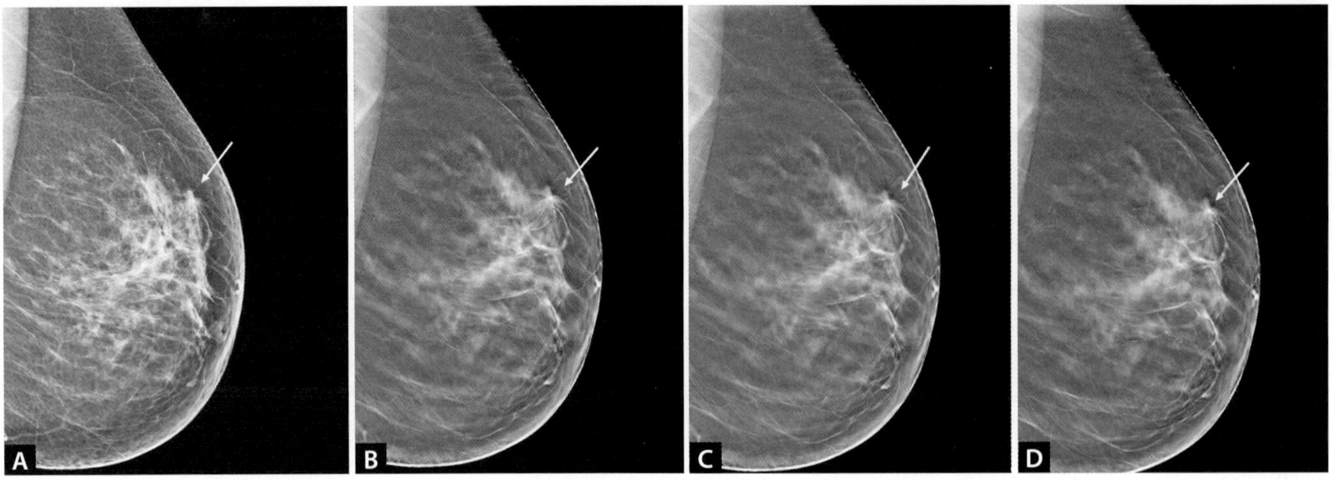

Figs. 15A to D: Digital breast tomosynthesis: Conventional MLO view (A) shows a subtle area of architectural distortion (arrow) in the upper part of right breast. 1 mm thin contiguous tomographic slices (B to D) convincingly show the irregular spiculations radiating from this area (arrows), thus increasing the diagnostic confidence.

negatives. The overlapping glandular tissue may hide the mass and in others, it may simulate a mass when none exists. Digital breast tomosynthesis is an emerging digital imaging technique that provides sectional images which help to distinguish the glandular breast tissue from true lesions, especially in dense breasts. Multiple projections are acquired at different depths by a digital detector from a mammographic X-ray source that moves gradually in a small arc over the compressed breast. The total dose is similar to single-view breast examination. These projection image datasets are reconstructed using specific algorithms in the form of sections similar to the CT. Each individual slice presents a planar mammogram in either the CC or MLO view. As each reconstructed slice may be as thin as 0.5 mm, masses and mass margins that may otherwise be superimposed with out-of-plane structures are more visible in the reconstructed slice **(Figs. 15A to D)**. It is more useful in characterization of the masses and asymmetries than in the evaluation of calcifications.[10]

The potential benefits of DBT include improvement in screening sensitivity, improvement in lesion size at detection, improvement in characterization and decrease in recall rates.[11] The DBT may be useful in both screening and diagnostic evaluation of the breast. Neither has been proved in randomized controlled trials. The primary benefit of DBT would be expected to be for noncalcified mammographic findings such as masses, asymmetries and distortion.

CONTRAST-ENHANCED DIGITAL MAMMOGRAPHY

Combining high-resolution digital mammography with the functional information obtained with contrast enhancement offers another potential derivative application for digital mammography. The advantage of contrast-enhanced digital mammography would be to obtain functional contrast information attributed to malignant neovascularity directly linked to high-quality anatomic information.

There are two main methods described for contrast-enhanced digital mammography: serial examinations over time and dual energy imaging.[12] Both use iodinated contrast material and modified digital mammography units for imaging. The patient's breast is placed in compression in a single view such as the MLO. Before contrast injection, a noncontrast image is obtained. Next, following contrast administration, a series of images are obtained. There is insufficient visible enhancement to allow primary interpretation and for this reason the enhanced images are subtracted from the baseline image leaving areas of enhancement visible. Using this methodology, enhancement curves can be obtained. Weaknesses of this type of study include the ability to only image the breast in a single projection at a time. For this reason, dual energy methods have been developed to allow imaging of both breasts with a single contrast administration. Dual energy mammography requires a modified mammographic machine that is capable of producing both normal mammographic images and images obtained at higher energy (45–50 kV).[13] The patient is injected with contrast and placed in compression. Two paired exposures are obtained, one at low kilovolts and the other at high kilovolts. A subtraction image is produced that highlights areas of iodine concentration or enhancement. The mammographic image at low energy can be used as a routine grayscale mammographic interpretation.

This technique does not allow for kinetic assessment of enhancement curves.

Early work has shown technical and clinical feasibility of contrast-enhanced digital mammography. The actual number of patients studied to date has been limited so the application of this technique for future potential clinical use is uncertain.

BREAST ULTRASOUND

Ultrasound is the most valuable and readily used adjunct to mammography for the diagnosis of breast diseases.

Technique

Breast US should be performed with broadband linear electronically focused high frequency transducers. The center frequency should be 10 MHz, with frequency ranging as high as 17 MHz in the near field and as low as 5 MHz deeper in the image field, thus enabling greater penetration of the posterior breast tissue and pectoralis muscle. The patient is examined in the supine oblique position. The side being examined is raised and the arm is placed above the head to ensure that the breast is evenly distributed over the chest wall. If the US is being done as a targeted examination, proper area to scan must be determined from the mammogram or clinical examination. The direction of scanning is in the transverse and longitudinal directions. Scanning in the radial (parallel to the ducts) and anti-radial (perpendicular to ducts) planes is of value in demonstrating ductal abnormalities. If lesion is identified, its presence is confirmed with 90° rotation of the transducer. The morphology of the lesion should be carefully assessed. For the purpose of accurate follow-up, it is crucial to consistently and completely document the lesion size and location. The specific location, including laterality (right or left breast), the clock-face location and the distance from the nipple, should be accurately annotated on the images and documented in the reports. The length of the transducer face (footprint), usually between 3.5 and 5 cm, can be used to estimate the distance from the nipple. Extended field of view imaging is a helpful tool to image large lesions that extend beyond the width of the transducer footprint or to better depict relationships among multiple lesions. It is often helpful to place the transducer slightly off center to the nipple and then use angulation to image the retroareolar tissues.

Investigations into the use of Doppler US of breast lesions have produced mixed results. Because Doppler technique relies on increased vascularity (which can be seen in both benign and malignant lesions), significant overlap of positive findings is not unexpected. As color Doppler equipment has become more and more sensitive, vascular signals can be found in normal, benign and malignant tissue. Penetrating vessels are more likely to be present in malignant tumors.[14] There are several potential causes of false-positive Doppler results (inflammatory lesions, recent fine needle aspiration and some vascular fibroadenomas) and false-negative results (poorly vascularized tumors, insensitive Doppler parameters and incidental cancers) on color Doppler US.

Normal Anatomy

The skin, which is normally 1–3 mm thick, appears as two parallel echogenic lines. The subcutaneous fat layer is demonstrated superficially as hypoechoic tissue compared to the glandular tissue from which it is separated by a well-defined scalloped margin. Normal ducts are often visible in the subareolar region, as anechoic tubular structures. The US appearance of the glandular tissue depends on how much involution of the glandular tissue has taken place. The young glandular breast contains a well-defined layer of glandular tissue, within which round or oval well-defined, hypoechoic fat lobules may be present. As involution takes place, more of the breast is composed of fat. In the completely involuted breast, US shows hypoechoic fat lobules separated by fine curvilinear septa of increased echogenicity. Fat lobules can be distinguished by their unique spindle shape, which merges with the rest of the parenchyma at different angles and planes of imaging. By contrast, masses remain discrete with distinctive borders in all planes of imaging. Deep to the glandular tissue, a retromammary fat layer is seen and behind this pectoral muscle can be seen sharply demarcated by its echogenic fascia. Costochondral cartilages appear as hypoechoic oval masses deep to the muscle and calcified ribs show prominent shadowing. Beneath the thoracic wall, a linear echogenic interface can be seen that includes chest wall, pleura and lung border. Anatomic structures that can be seen in axilla include blood vessels, lymph nodes and the proximal portions of the pectoral muscles.

Indications for Breast Ultrasound

No longer used only to differentiate masses as cystic versus solid, US today contributes significantly to the characterization of solid masses through feature analysis. As the density of breast is higher and the tissues are more sensitive to radiation in women less than 30 years of age, US is the imaging technique of choice in these women and in lactating and pregnant women. Breast US is valuable in the assessment of the mammographically 'dense' breast. It is also successfully used as a 'second-look' procedure when an abnormality has been detected using MRI or scintimammography. The main indications for breast US have been summarized in **Table 7**.

Table 7: Indications for breast ultrasound.

- Symptomatic breast lumps in women aged less than 30 years
- Breast lump developing during pregnancy or lactation
- Assessment of mammographic abnormality
- Assessment of MRI or scintimammography detected lesions
- Clinical breast mass with negative mammogram
- Breast inflammation
- The augmented breast
- Breast lump in a male
- Guidance of needle biopsy or localization

In the absence of a suspicious clinical lesion, a negative US and mammography has a very high negative predictive value for malignant disease. Main disadvantage of US is that its performance is operator dependent and it can be time consuming. Ultrasound does not always detect cancers that are visualized mammographically.

ACR BI-RADS Ultrasound Lexicon Descriptors

Acknowledging the expanded role of breast US, the BI-RADS lexicon has been developed for reporting breast US findings[15] **(Table 8)**.

On US, a mass is evaluated by its shape, orientation, margin, lesion boundary, echo pattern and posterior acoustic features. A mass can be oval, round, lobulated or

Table 8: ACR BI-RADS ultrasound lexicon descriptors for breast lesions.

Characteristic	***Term***	***Description***
Shape	Oval	Elliptical (may include 2–3 undulations)
	Round	Spherical
	Irregular	Neither round nor oval in shape
Orientation	Parallel	Wider than tall
	Not parallel	Taller than wide
Margin	Circumscribed	Well-defined or sharp margin with an abrupt transition between the lesion and the surrounding tissue
	Angular	Some or all of the margin has sharp corners, often forming acute angles
	Indistinct	No clear demarcation between a mass and its surrounding tissue
	Microlobulated	Short cycle undulations impart a scalloped appearance to the margin of the mass
	Spiculated	Margin characterized by sharp lines projecting from the mass
Echo pattern	Anechoic	Without internal echoes
	Hyperechoic	Increased echogenicity relative to fat
	Complex	Mass contains both anechoic and echogenic components
	Isoechoic	Same echogenicity as fat
	Hypoechoic	Decreased echogenicity relative to fat
Lesion boundary	Abrupt interface	Sharp demarcation between the lesion and surrounding tissue; imperceptible or a thin well-defined echogenic capsule
	Echogenic halo	No sharp demarcation between the lesion and surrounding tissue, which is bridged by an echogenic transition zone
Posterior acoustic features	No posterior acoustic features	No posterior shadowing or enhancement
	Enhancement	Increased posterior echoes
	Shadowing	Decreased posterior echoes; edge shadows are excluded
	Duct changes	Abnormal caliber
Surrounding tissue	Cooper's ligaments edema	Thickening Increased echogenicity of surrounding tissue
	Architectural distortion	Disruption of normal anatomic planes
	Skin thickening	Normal skin is 2 mm or less in thickness except in the periareolar area and lower breast
Special cases	Clustered microcysts	A cluster of tiny anechoic foci 2–3 mm in diameter with thin intervening septations and no discrete solid components
	Complicated cysts	Cysts having homogeneous, low-level echoes. May also have fluid-fluid, or fluid-debris levels
	Mass in or on skin	These masses are clinically apparent and may include sebaceous or epidermal inclusion cysts, keloids, moles and neurofibromas
	Lymph nodes	Bean-shaped, well-defined with an echogenic hilum

irregular **(Figs. 16A to C)**. By definition, orientation refers to the relationship the mass has to the skin **(Figs. 17A and B)**. In general, benign solid masses are parallel to the skin. When a mass is taller than it is wide, it is a suspicious sonographic finding. When describing mass margins, the most important distinction is between circumscribed and noncircumscribed margins **(Figs. 18A to E)**. Circumscribed margins are well defined or sharp, with an abrupt transition between the lesion and the surrounding tissue. Noncircumscribed margins encompass the remaining margin descriptors, including microlobulated, indistinct, angular and spiculated. Microlobulated margins demonstrate a scalloped appearance. Indistinct margins are not clearly demarcated from the surrounding tissue. Angular margins demonstrate sharp corners, often with acute angles, in distinction from spiculated margins, which appear more as lines projecting from a mass. The interface of the mass and its surrounding breast parenchyma is called the "lesion boundary" in the ACR BI-RADS atlas. Lesion boundary should be described as an abrupt interface, which is seen as a sharp demarcation between the lesion and the surrounding tissue, or an echogenic halo, a surrounding echogenic transition zone. An echogenic halo is a suspicious US finding. The BI-RADS US descriptors shown to have a high predictive value for benignity include a circumscribed margin (90%), parallel orientation (78%) and an oval shape (78%).[16] The features most predictive of malignancy are an irregular shape (62%), spiculated margins (86%) and nonparallel orientation (69%).

The internal echogenicity of the mass may be anechoic, hyperechoic, complex, hypoechoic or isoechoic. The patient's fat should serve as the internal control to which the echogenicity of all lesions should be compared. Generally,

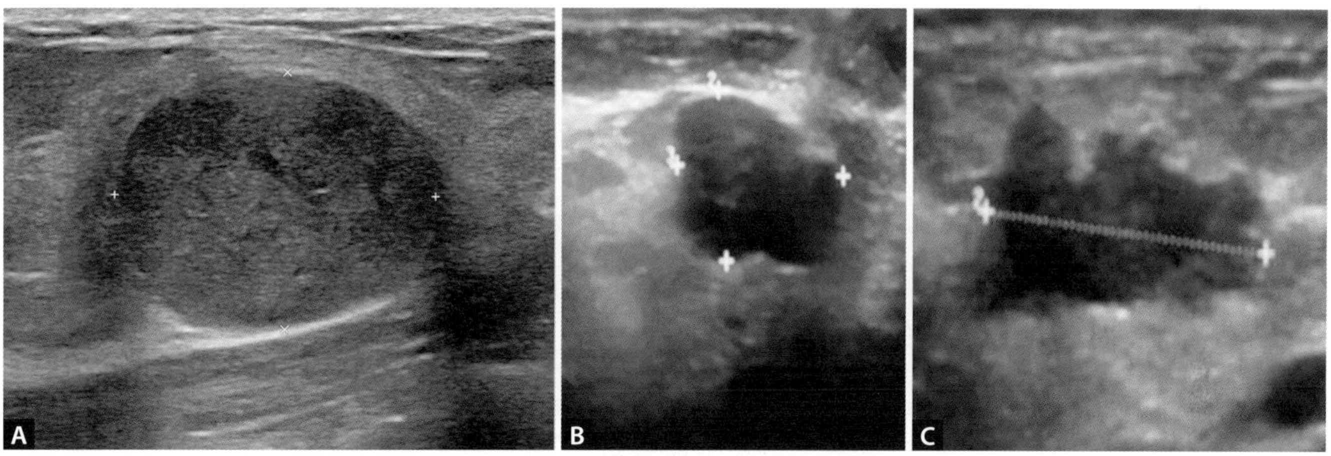

Figs. 16A to C: ACR BI-RADS descriptors for mass shape on ultrasound. (A) Oval; (B) Lobulated; (C) Irregular.

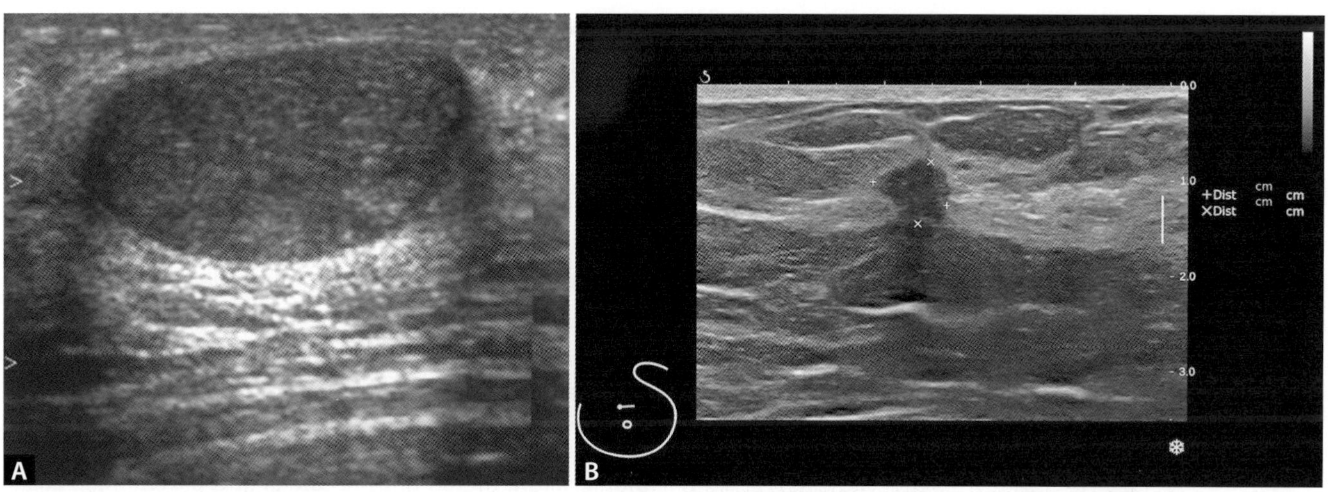

Figs. 17A and B: Orientation of a mass to skin on ultrasound. (A) Parallel orientation (wider than taller); (B) Antiparallel orientation (taller than wider).

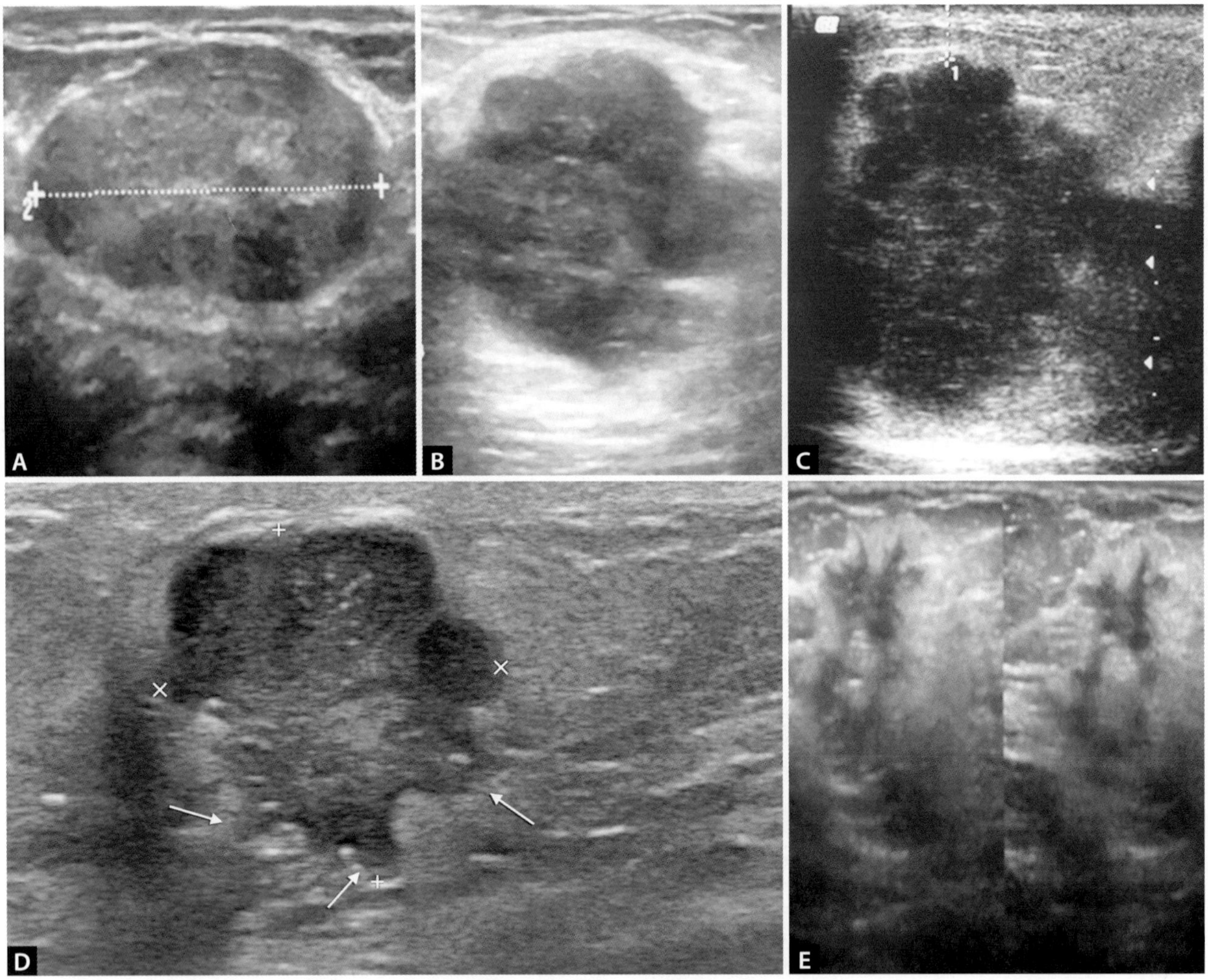

Figs. 18A to E: ACR BI-RADS descriptors for mass margins on ultrasound. (A) Circumscribed; (B) Indistinct; (C) Microlobulated; (D) Angular (arrows); (E) Spiculated.

lesions that are hyperechoic to the subcutaneous fat are benign. Because a majority of both malignant and benign solid breast masses are hypoechoic, other features, such as margin characteristics, establish the level of suspicion.

Posterior acoustic features **(Figs. 19A and B)** may or may not be seen when imaging solid masses. Posterior acoustic shadowing is a suspicious finding and may be seen in cases of invasive carcinoma, postoperative scar, complex sclerosing lesion, or macrocalcifications. Posterior acoustic enhancement is an indeterminate US finding that can be associated with a variety of entities, including simple cysts, complicated cysts, fibroadenoma, papilloma, complex cystic mass, invasive ductal carcinoma and lymphoma.

After complete US evaluation the appropriate ACR BI-RADS category should be assigned to guide further management **(Table 9)**.

Challenges in Assigning Final Assessment Categories and the Influence of Clinical Factors

For a lesion with benign characteristics, although data support follow-up of probably benign lesions, an important clinical factor that influences BI-RADS final assessment categorization is the age of the patient. For an older patient, the threshold for biopsy should be lowered and biopsy may be warranted even in the setting of probably benign imaging features.

Despite benign imaging features at US or mammography, palpable solid lesions are frequently subjected to biopsy, which leads to a large number of benign results of biopsies and incurs both financial and psychologic costs. Recent data support the fact that a solid mass need not be subjected to biopsy simply because it is palpable.[17] For

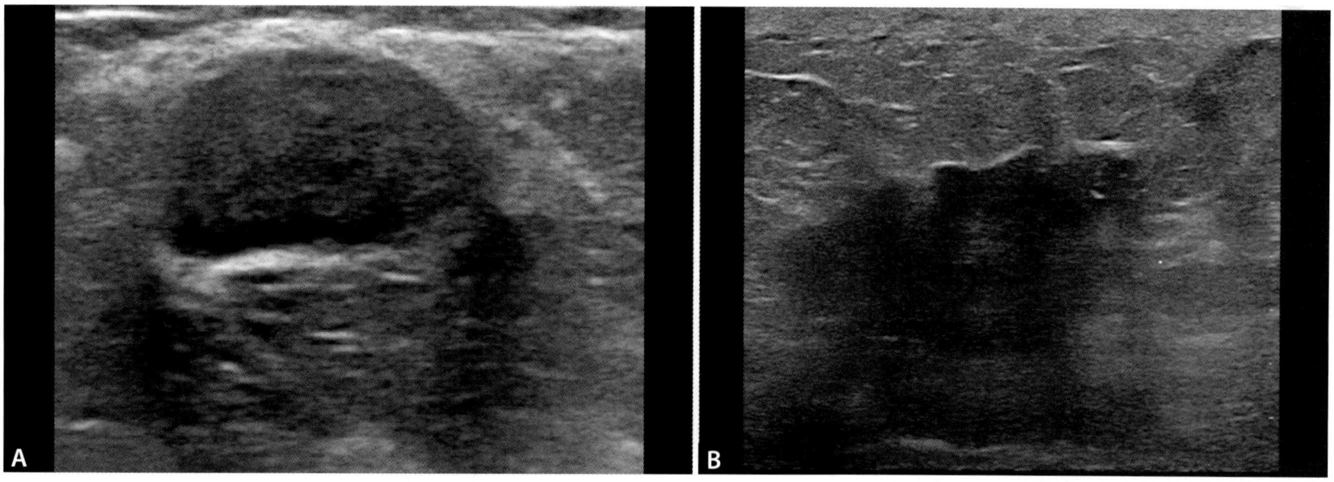

Figs. 19A and B: Posterior acoustic features of a mass on ultrasound. (A) Posterior acoustic enhancement; (B) Posterior acoustic shadowing.

Table 9: ACR BI-RADS ultrasound assessment categories.

Category	*Description*	*Likelihood of malignancy*	*Examples*	
0	Incomplete; need additional imaging evaluation, or comparison with previous examinations	Unknown	Postoperative scar/ recurrence	MRI; obtain previous examinations
1	Negative	No US evidence of malignancy	Normal US	Negative findings at US do not exclude breast cancer in the setting of a suspicious mammographic finding. If the patient is being evaluated for a palpable abnormality and the findings with both US and mammography are negative, the report should stress the importance of clinical assessment and further management should be based on the clinical level of concern
2	Benign finding	No US evidence of malignancy	Simple cysts, breast implants, stable postsurgical changes, and probable fibroadenomas noted to be unchanged at successive US studies	
3	Probably benign finding	<2%	A solid mass with circumscribed margins, an oval-shaped and parallel orientation	Follow-up imaging (mammography or US) at 6 and 12 months
4	Suspicious abnormality	3–95%	Solid masses with benign features (e.g. fibroadenomas), if the lesion is clinically palpable. Complicated cysts and some complex cystic and solid masses (e.g. clinically apparent abscesses)	Fine-needle aspiration, percutaneous or surgical biopsy
5	Highly suggestive of malignancy	>95%	Spiculated mass	Percutaneous or surgical biopsy
6	Known malignancy	100%	Biopsy-proven	Definitive treatment

palpable masses with benign imaging characteristics, the range of reported negative predictive values is 97–100%.[18] Therefore such lesions should be managed with short-interval follow-up rather than with biopsy.

There are situations in which clinical factors are more important than the imaging appearance of a lesion. An abscess often demonstrates a complex internal echo pattern and can be indistinguishable from an invasive carcinoma. However, in the correct clinical setting (a young lactating patient with clinical signs of infection and a mass that is tender to palpation), the likelihood of malignancy is low and it should be categorized as a BI-RADS 3 lesion with recommendation of follow-up.

Contrast-enhanced Ultrasound

During the last few years, US contrast agents have been developed that increase blood echogenicity and improve US image quality by detection of slow and low-volume blood flow in small tumor vessels (<5 mm) within the focal lesions in the breast. Commonly used US contrast agents include Sonovue (sulfur hexafluoride microbubbles coated with phospholipids) and Levovist (galactose microparticles coated with palmitic acid). Various studies involving contrast-enhanced ultrasound (CEUS) in breast masses have shown differences in the vascularity pattern in benign and malignant lesions. Malignant lesions tend to have greater number of vessels, irregular vessels running to the center of the mass and greater enhancement[19] **(Figs. 20A and B)**. Several studies have proven the potential of CEUS of the breast in differentiating malignant from benign breast lesions, with varying sensitivities (67–95%) and specificities (58–82%) depending on the patient population being studied, the type of equipment and the criteria used for interpretation of the CEUS images.[20] The CEUS may also be helpful to assess the extent of infiltrative breast carcinoma or to evaluate the tumor response after chemotherapy. Another interesting potential clinical application is the differentiation between postoperative change and recurrence.

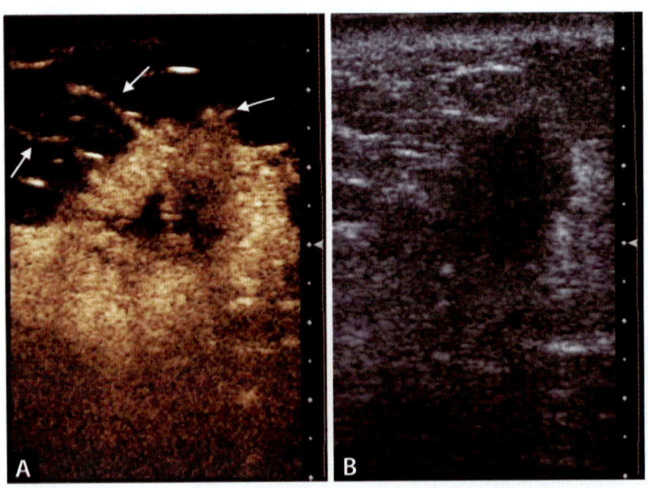

Figs. 20A and B: Contrast enhanced ultrasound in a 43-year-old lady with invasive ductal carcinoma. Ultrasound image obtained 30 seconds after contrast injection shows intense early enhancement of the irregular mass lesion with ductal extension (arrows).

Ultrasound Elastography

Ultrasound elastography explores the simple principle of tissue response to a given amount of external pressure; a harder tissue (breast malignancies tend to be schirrhous and therefore harder) shows less distortion to externally applied pressure than softer tissue (normal breast tissue and benign breast masses tend to be softer). Static US elastography provides a color coded map of elasticity that is superimposed on the real-time grayscale image.[21] Invasive breast cancers have been shown to be stiffer than benign or normal tissues. Invasive cancers often produce areas of stiffness which are appreciably larger than the grayscale abnormality. The US static elastography has been hampered by significant interobserver variability and lack of quantification. Shear wave elastography (SWE) is a new quantitative technique of obtaining elastography images where an acoustic radiation force impulse (ARFI) is induced in the tissues by a focused US beam and an ultrafast imaging sequence captures in real time the propagation of the resulting shear waves.[22] The production of ARFI impulse by the probe rather than the operator (as in static US elastography) means shear wave elastography is more reproducible than static elastography. Within a given region of interest (ROI), defined by an electronic cursor, values for the max stiffness, mean stiffness and standard deviation are produced **(Fig. 21)**. Areas of stiffness can thus be clearly mapped. Preliminary studies have demonstrated good separation of elasticity values measured in kilopascals between fat (3 kPa), dense parenchyma (45 kPa), benign lesions (<80 kPa) and malignant lesions (>100 kPa). It is envisaged that shear wave elastography will provide a useful adjunct to routine US in differentiation of benign and malignant lesions, though its role is not yet established in larger studies.

DYNAMIC CONTRAST-ENHANCED BREAST MRI

Neoangiogenesis by the malignant tumor serves as the basis for breast cancer detection by MR imaging. The neovasculature of cancers does not resemble blood vessels

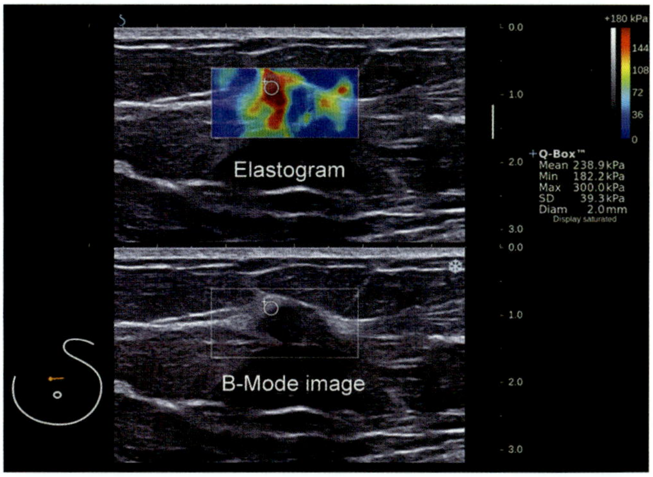

Fig. 21: Shear wave elastography: B-mode ultrasound image shows a subtle, 7 mm size, irregular solid mass. The real-time elastography image shows peritumoral stiffness (red areas) with high mean elasticity value of 238.9 kPa in the operator marked region of interest (ROI). Ultrasound-guided core biopsy confirmed invasive ductal carcinoma.

found in normal tissue or benign lesions. These new blood vessels have increased permeability (i.e. "leakiness") resulting in early tumor uptake of contrast on MR imaging. In many, but not all cancers, this leaky vasculature also results in rapid washout of contrast, producing a dynamic enhancement pattern that helps to differentiate malignant from benign enhancing breast lesions.

Basic MR Technique for Breast Cancer Imaging

Since the early development of breast MRI, numerous technical developments, variations and innovations have been described. This section describes the basic features of a breast MR imaging protocol common to nearly all imaging facilities.

Coils and Patient Positioning

For breast MR imaging, the patient is placed in the prone position with the breasts in the 'cups' of the coil, with judicious padding to minimize patient motion and transmitted vibration. Immobilization should be achieved by gently fixating the breast in the section-encoding direction (craniocaudal direction for transverse protocols).

Prone patient positioning minimizes the effects of respiratory motion on images and helps to move the breasts away from the chest wall and the resulting artifacts from cardiac and respiratory movement. Patient comfort is vital, as the breast MR examination can last 30 minutes or longer and any patient discomfort is likely to manifest as movement during or between scans.

MR Field Strength

The current recommendations require that breast MR imaging be performed at 1.5 T or higher. The higher field strength enables the acquisition of high-resolution imaging with adequate signal to noise ratio (SNR) and enables the use of fat suppression. Imaging at 3.0 T provides an opportunity for even greater improvement in SNR, increased image resolution and faster imaging.[23]

Imaging Protocols

Gadolinium-enhanced T1-weighted imaging: Common to all breast MRI protocols for cancer evaluation is the use of gadolinium-based contrast agents to depict enhancing lesions on T1-weighted gradient echo (GE) sequences, e.g. fast field echo, fast low angle shot (FLASH), fast imaging with steady precession (FISP) and gradient recalled acquisition in a steady state (GRASS). Imaging should be done with adequate resolution so that the morphologic features of the enhancing lesions are clearly demonstrated. Higher imaging matrices allow for improved in-plane resolution. Both 2D and 3D sequences are useful and the choice normally depends on local practice. 3D GE sequences provide better resolution and thinner slices (3 mm or less) without interslice gaps however; they may be susceptible to field inhomogeneity.

Implementation of the dynamic enhanced imaging requires careful monitoring by the radiologist. Precontrast T1W imaging should be checked carefully to ensure adequate breast coverage and lack of severe artifacts. A 0.1 mmol/kg Gd-DTPA should be injected via an intravenous catheter placed in an antecubital vein before the patient is positioned in the coil. The patient must not be moved in and out of the magnet for the injection, to prevent motion and unnecessary time loss in the early postcontrast phase. The contrast agent is injected with a power injector at a rate of 3 mL/sec, followed by a 20 mL saline flush. The first postcontrast acquisition is started after the volume of contrast material has been injected (i.e. during the application of the saline flush). Hand injections can also be used. T1 weighted scans are obtained at every 1 minutes for at least 5–7 minutes after contrast injection. It is important to use the same T1 sequence and scan technique which was used for precontrast scan.

Bilateral imaging helps to avoid diagnostic errors (e.g. in patients with nonmass like enhancement or enhancing foci). To categorize these areas or foci, it is very helpful to be able to assess symmetry by comparing with the contralateral breast.

Plane of Imaging

Sagittal or axial planes of acquisition are preferred, as these planes allow for better depiction of the ductal organization of the breast glandular tissue than does the coronal plane. Sagittal imaging provides the opportunity for much higher in-plane resolution because of the small imaging field of view (FOV) obtainable. However, simultaneous bilateral sagittal imaging requires longer imaging time and can lead to inadvertent exclusion of breast tissue in the axillary region. Axial imaging is therefore often used for bilateral breast MR imaging.

Fat Suppression

The ACR guidelines encourage the use of fat suppression techniques because, after contrast injection, enhancing lesions may become isointense to adjacent fatty tissue. Active fat suppression means that the signal from fatty tissue is specifically eliminated by additional radiofrequency pulses or by choosing selective water excitation. Both types add to the acquisition time and require a very homogeneous magnetic field across the entire FOV, which is difficult to achieve with bilateral imaging.

Subtraction does not require extra-acquisition time and is not influenced by magnetic field inhomogeneities, which is why it is the preferred type of fat suppression for dynamic bilateral imaging. The main disadvantage of subtraction is that it may suffer from patient motion: Subtraction errors occur if the precontrast mask and the postcontrast image are not entirely congruent due to even subtle patient motion.

Nongadolinium-enhanced Sequences

In addition to the standard dynamic gadolinium-enhanced T1W imaging, the breast MR imaging examination is generally supplemented with a T2-weighted (T2W) sequence. T2W imaging can depict nonenhancing structures that correlate to mammographic or palpable findings, including simple or complex cysts and dilated retroareolar ducts. T2W imaging can also help characterize certain benign lesions such as simple cysts, myxoid fibroadenoma or lymph nodes as these have very high signal intensity on T2W scans, whereas most cancers are dark.[24]

Kinetic Analysis

Kinetic data can be evaluated by visually assessing the lesion enhancement pattern, by placing a region of interest (ROI) to obtain kinetic curves and by using a CAD system. The ROIs should be placed with wide window settings into the area that exhibits strongest enhancement on the first postcontrast image. Softwares which demonstrate color coded areas of high enhancement with respect to predetermined threshold have now been developed and should be used if available, to place the ROI accurately. The ROI should include not more than 3–4 pixels and care should be taken to ensure that the ROI is within the lesion throughout the entire dynamic series. If there is unrecognized patient movement during dynamic scans, the lesion moves out of the prescribed ROI after the first postcontrast image leading to false washout pattern. To quantify enhancement, the increase in signal intensity relative to baseline precontrast signal intensity is measured and is plotted over time.

Normal MRI Appearances

Normal glandular tissue has intermediate signal intensity on T1- and T2-weighted sequences, whereas fat is of high signal. The fibrous trabeculae are seen as fine low signal intensity structures traversing the subcutaneous fat. Low axillary and intramammary lymph nodes can be recognized through their characteristic bean shape and central fatty hilum. The skin is of intermediate signal and uniformly thin except in the areolar region where it may be few millimeters in thickness. After intravenous gadolinium, the nipple, blood vessels and lymph nodes normally enhance. Normal glandular parenchyma can also enhance gradually, especially in the second half of the menstrual cycle, reflecting hormonal-induced glandular proliferation. This enhancement, referred to as background enhancement is often diffuse, patchy and progressive. Rarely, it may be intense or focal and difficult to interpret. Hence, if possible, breast MRI should be performed after menstruation in second week of the cycle.[25]

Interpretation of Breast MRI

For differential diagnosis of enhancing lesions in breast MR imaging, morphologic information (type of enhancement, mass shape and margins, distribution of nonmass like enhancement, internal architecture), kinetic information (initial enhancement increase and delayed phase enhancement) and information related to lesion signal intensity on T2W and T1W precontrast non-fat-suppressed images is analyzed systematically.

When interpreting breast MR imaging studies, the first step is to categorize any abnormal enhancement according to the ACR BI-RADS-MRI lexicon, published as a part of the American College of Radiology's Breast Imaging Reporting and Data System Atlas: a mass, an area of nonmass like enhancement or a focus.

Mass

A mass is a 3D space occupying lesion within the breast. Usually, it has a visible correlate on precontrast T1- or T2-weighted images. Masses are described in terms of shape, margin and internal enhancement characteristics **(Table 10)**.

- Shape—A mass can be round, oval, lobulated, or irregular **(Figs. 22A to D)**. Lobulated masses have an undulating contour. Irregular masses have an uneven shape that cannot be characterized as round, oval, or lobulated.
- Margin—Margins can be described as smooth or spiculated **(Figs. 23A and B)**. Spiculated margins frequently are a feature of malignant breast lesions and radial scars.
- Internal enhancement characteristics—Enhancement patterns of masses have been divided into the following six types:
  - Homogeneous enhancement is uniform and confluent enhancement throughout the mass **(Fig. 23A)**.
  - Heterogeneous enhancement is nonuniform enhancement that shows variations within the mass **(Fig. 23B)**.
  - Rim enhancement is enhancement mainly concentrated at the periphery of the mass **(Fig. 23C)**. This type of enhancement is most frequently a feature of high-grade invasive ductal cancer,[26] fat necrosis and cysts with inflammation.
  - Dark internal nonenhancing septations within an enhanced lesion are typical of fibroadenomas, especially when the lesion has smooth or lobulated borders.
  - Enhanced internal septations are usually a feature of malignant lesions.
  - Central enhancement is enhancement of a nidus within a mass that is usually more pronounced than the rest of the enhanced mass. Central enhancement has been associated with high-grade ductal cancer and vascular breast tumors.

Table 10: IACR BI-RADS mass descriptors in MRI

Characteristic	***Term***	***Description***
Shape	Round	Spherical
	Oval	Elliptical
	Lobular	Undulating contour
	Irregular	Uneven shape
	Smooth	
Margin	Irregular	
	Spiculated	Sharp lines projecting from the mass
	Homogeneous	Uniform enhancement
	Heterogeneous	Nonuniform enhancement
Internal enhancement	Rim enhancing	Enhancement concentrated at the periphery
	Internal nonenhancing septations	Dark septations within an enhanced lesion
	Enhancing septae	Enhanced internal septations
	Central enhancement	Enhancement of central nidus more than rest of the mass

Nonmass-like Enhancement

Nonmass-like enhancement means that enhancement occurs in an area of the fibroglandular tissue that otherwise appears normal on precontrast images. There is no space-occupying effect **(Fig. 24)**. The enhancing area usually has no correlate on fat-suppressed or non-fat-suppressed T2-weighted images. The distinction between mass and nonmass-like enhancement is important for further differential diagnosis. In a mass, the differential diagnostic consideration is either invasive breast cancer or a benign solid tumor (e.g. fibroadenoma). In nonmass-like enhancement, the main differential diagnosis is between intraductal or diffuse (e.g. lobular) cancer and mastopathic changes (focal adenosis), hormonal stimulation, or inflammatory changes. Features of nonmass-like enhancement such as internal enhancement pattern, symmetry and the distribution are assessed **(Table 11)**, with major emphasis on whether it is oriented

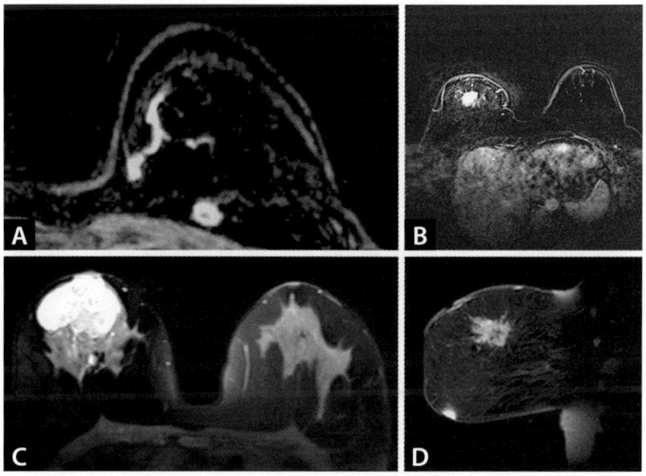

Figs. 22A to D: ACR BI-RADS descriptors for mass shape on MRI: (A) Round; (B) Oval; (C) Irregular; (D) Spiculated.

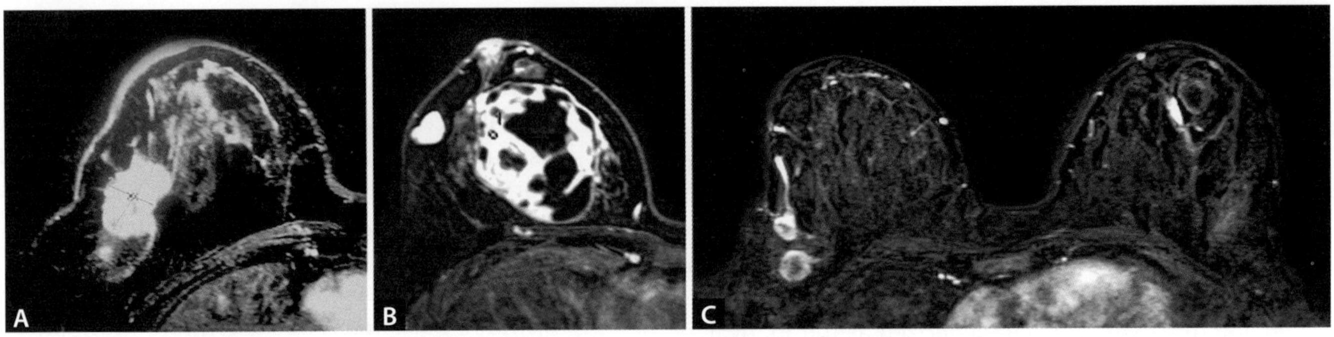

Figs. 23A to C: ACR BI-RADS descriptors for internal enhancement characteristics of a mass on MRI: (A) Homogeneous; (B) Heterogeneous; (C) Rim enhancement.

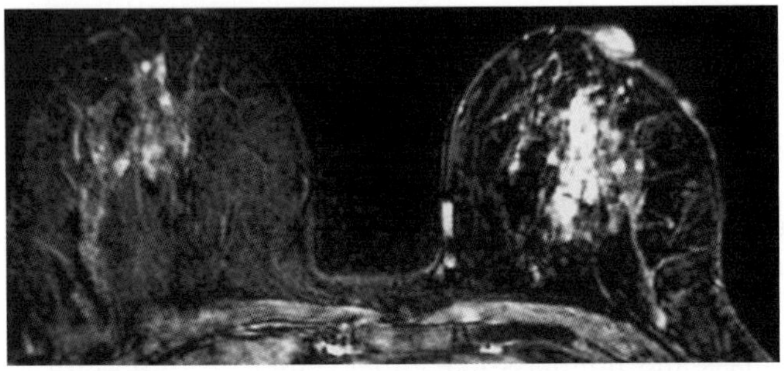

Fig. 24: Nonmass-like enhancement: Enhancement occurs in an area of the fibroglandular tissue that otherwise appears normal on precontrast images and there is no space-occupying effect.

along the distribution of the ducts (ductal or segmental enhancement) or not (linear, focal, regional or diffuse).

Distribution

- A focal area is enhancement occupying less than 25% of the volume of a breast quadrant that has fat or normal glandular tissue between abnormally enhanced components. This type of enhancement usually manifests as clumped, irregular contrast enhancement.
- Linear enhancement is a sheet of enhancement that does not conform to the shape of a ductal system.
- Ductal enhancement conforms to the shape of a ductal system, pointing towards the nipple.
- Segmental enhancement is conical and probably represents one or more ductal systems. Ductal and segmental distribution of enhancement may be associated with *in situ* ductal cancer or invasive ductal cancer, atypical ductal hyperplasia, papillary neoplasms, or sclerosing adenosis.[27]
- Regional enhancement is geographic enhancement involving one or more segments of the breast. A specific ductal or segmental configuration cannot be discerned.
- Multiple regions of enhancement are distributed in several areas of the breast.
- Diffuse enhancement is uniform enhancement of the entire parenchyma of the breast, usually associated with benign processes or normal fibroglandular tissue.

Internal Enhancement Pattern

The internal enhancement patterns are homogeneous, heterogeneous, clumped, stippled or punctate and reticular or dendritic. In the reticular or dendritic pattern, the normal fat-glandular tissue interface is lost. This finding is usually associated with inflammatory breast cancer or lymphatic involvement.

Symmetry is helpful in further characterization of nonmass like enhancement. Bilateral symmetric nonmass like enhancement in any distribution is more often caused by benign changes than by malignant lesions.

FOCUS

Focus is defined as an enhancing area of less than 5 mm that is too small to be further characterized. Foci are frequently stable on follow-up images and may result from hormonal changes. A focus may correspond to a very small invasive breast cancer, DCIS, a papilloma, a small fibroadenoma, an intramammary lymph node and so forth. Further management of a focus depends on other findings in the same or the opposite breast (symmetry is always reassuring), on corresponding findings from mammography or US and on the personal risk status of the patient.

ASSOCIATED FINDINGS

Associated findings with or without enhancement should be noted. These findings include nipple retraction or inversion, skin retraction, skin thickening, skin invasion, pectoralis muscle or chest wall invasion, high signal

Table 11: ACR BI-RADS descriptors of nonmass-like enhancement in MRI.

Characteristic	*Descriptor*	*Illustration*
Distribution	Linear	Enhancement in a line that may not conform to a duct
	Ductal	Enhancement in a line that may branch, conforming to a duct
	Segmental	Triangular area of enhancement, apex pointing to nipple, suggesting a duct and its branches
	Regional	Enhancement in a large volume of tissue not conforming to a ductal distribution
	Multiple	Enhancement in at least two large volumes of tissues not conforming to a ductal distribution, multiple geographic areas, patchy areas of enhancement
	Diffuse	Enhancement distributed uniformly throughout the breast
Internal enhancement pattern	Homogeneous	Confluent uniform enhancement
	Heterogeneous	Nonuniform enhancement in a random pattern
	Clumped	Punctuate dot-like, enhancing foci
	Stippled or punctate	Cobblestone-like enhancement, with occasional confluent areas
	Reticular or dendritic	Enhancement with finger-like projections extending toward nipple
Symmetry	Bilaterally symmetrical	Mirror-image enhancement
	Bilaterally asymmetrical	More in one breast than in the other

intensity in ducts on unenhanced images, abnormal signal void, hematoma, edema, lymphadenopathy and cysts.

Kinetic Curve Assessment

The analysis of enhancement kinetics is achieved by measuring the signal intensity in a small area of a lesion and tracking its course over the dynamic series to yield the kinetic curve (also referred to as time-signal intensity curve).

The most suspicious curve pattern derived from the fastest-enhancing part of a lesion is chosen to describe the enhancement curve. Early phase enhancement, i.e. enhancement within the first 2 minutes after contrast injection or until the curve starts to change, indicates the velocity and degree with which enhancement occurs and may be slow, medium, or rapid.

Delayed phase enhancement refers to signal intensity changes that occur immediately after the early signal intensity increase, as early as 3 minutes after injection. Immediately after the early initial increase, the signal intensity may (a) decline again, yielding a so-called washout curve (type 3) **(Fig. 25A)**; (b) exhibit a sharp bend and plateau (type 2) **(Fig. 25B)**; or (c) continue to rise after the early phase, yielding persistent enhancement until the delayed postcontrast phase (type 1) **(Fig. 25C)**. The main difference is that in types 2 (plateau) and 3 (washout) curves, peak enhancement is reached early, usually within the first 2 minutes. This is the time course observed in most invasive breast cancers. Lesions with rapid early enhancement followed by a delayed phase plateau or washout have a positive predictive value of 77% for malignancy.[28] In persistent kinetics, the enhancement continues until the delayed postcontrast phase. This is the time course observed in most benign changes.

While enhancement kinetics is useful for the differential diagnosis of morphologically equivocal masses, it may be misleading and should, therefore, not be used for classification of nonmass-like enhancement. The reason is that in nonmass-like enhancement, the differential diagnosis includes DCIS and lobular cancers—two disease states known to exhibit inconsistent angiogenic activity.

Sensitivity and Specificity of MRI

Detection of invasive breast carcinoma is extremely reliable on MR imaging as the sensitivity approaches 100%.[29] The sensitivity of breast MR imaging is not impaired by the density of the fibroglandular tissue or by scar tissue (e.g. after lumpectomy), radiation therapy, or prosthetic breast implants. It can therefore, detect cancers which are occult on mammography and US. Normal breast MRI excludes the presence of gross focus of invasive cancer with high reliability. However, breast MRI has lower specificity and this is one of its biggest limitations. The detection of cancer relies on contrast enhancement but this can also be seen in many benign conditions like fibroadenoma, papilloma, fibrocystic disease and lymph nodes **(Table 12)**. This results in significant false positive examinations and hence unnecessary biopsies. False negative breast MRI examinations can also occur but these are rare. Nonenhancing invasive breast cancers are exceedingly rare. More often, the reason for failure

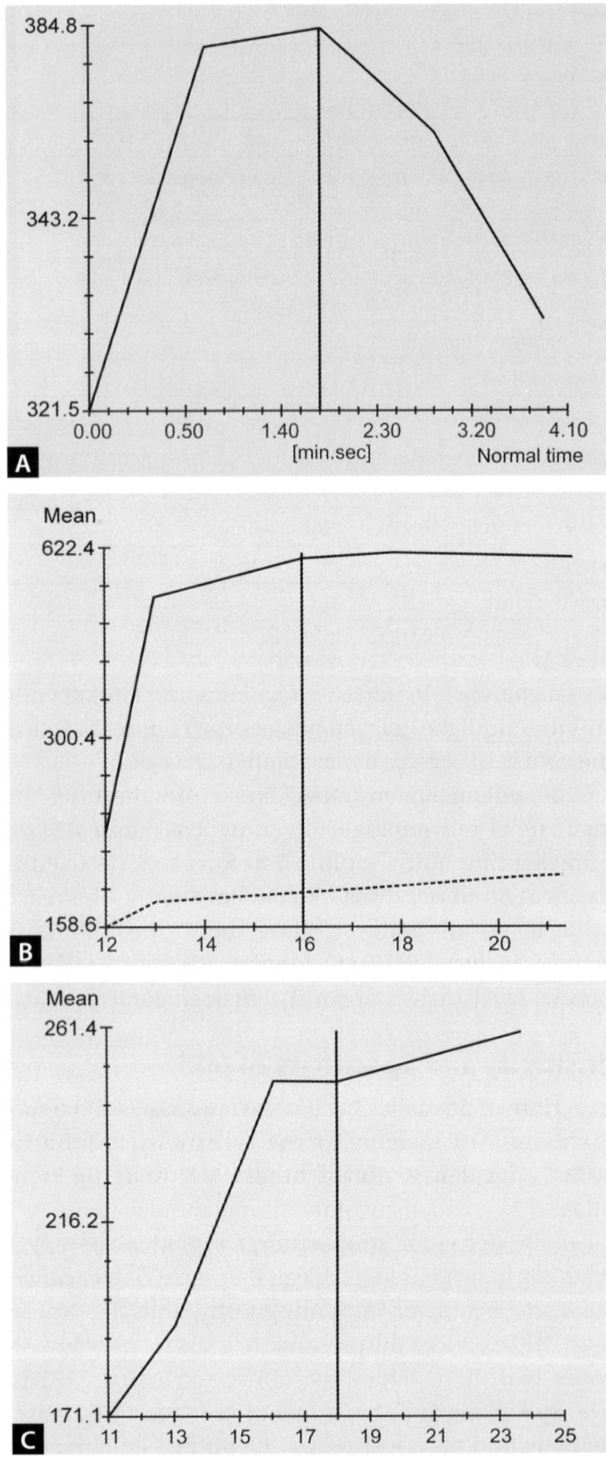

Figs. 25A to C: Kinetic analysis of enhancing mass lesions on DCEMRI: (A) *Type 3 curve*: Immediately after the early initial increase, the signal intensity declines rapidly yielding a type 3 or washout curve; (B) *Type 2 curve*: After the initial rise in signal intensity there is a plateau with sustained contrast enhancement; (C) *Type 1 curve*: Signal intensity continues to rise after the early phase, yielding persistent enhancement until the delayed postcontrast phase.

Table 12: Challenges in MR interpretation.

False-positive:
• Fibrocystic change
• Hormone-related enhancement
• Focal fibrosis, scar, fat necrosis
• Intraductal papilloma
• Fibroadenomas
• Intramammary lymph node
False-negative:
• Strong background enhancement
• Nonenhancing DCIS
• Nonenhancing invasive lobular carcinoma
• Recent radiotherapy

to diagnose invasive cancer with breast MR imaging is early and strong enhancement in the surrounding normal fibroglandular tissue that may mask the enhancing cancer. Invasive lobular carcinoma, well differentiated invasive ductal carcinoma and few DCIS may be missed on breast MRI. A recent meta-analysis of 44 studies has estimated the sensitivity and specificity of MRI for the diagnosis of breast cancer as 90% and 72% respectively.[30]

Because of the potential issue of a false-negative examination, a negative MRI examination should not deter biopsy of a suspicious lesion (BIRADS 4 or 5) on mammography or US. Breast MRI is best used as an adjunct to conventional imaging, complementing but never replacing basic mammography and US.

Indications for MRI

As breast MRI is expensive and time consuming, it is used in selected situations. Some of the indications of breast MRI are well defined while others are controversial. These are discussed below. Major indications for DCEMRI are listed in **Table 13**.

Newer advances in breast MRI include diffusion weighted imaging (DWI) and proton MR spectroscopy (1H MRS).

PROTON MR SPECTROSCOPY

1H MRS is a technique that is used to suppress water and lipid signals to enhance the weaker signals from hydrogen atoms of metabolites with small molecular weights. The hallmark of breast MR spectroscopic examination is the detection of choline and its derivatives (collectively referred to as "total choline," or tCho), at 3.2 ppm. Elevated tCho has been shown more frequently in malignant than in benign enhancing breast lesions **(Figs. 26A and B)**. A region of interest is outlined after the dynamic gadolinium acquisition and MRS examination is performed within that voxel. Depending on the voxel size, signal averaging for 4–6 minutes is required to produce a single MR spectrum, representing the metabolite profile of that volume of tissue. 1H MRS is highly sensitive for all breast cancers, regardless of histology. Although 1H MRS shows promising results in the differentiation of benign and malignant breast lesions, a review of published results so far shows that the technique has a false-negative rate of approximately 4–18% and a false-positive rate of 14–18%. The use of 1H MRS as an adjunctive examination to contrast enhanced MRI may provide added specificity in characterizing malignant breast lesions.[31] In addition to being used for breast cancer diagnosis, 1H MRS has also been assessed in monitoring breast cancer response to chemotherapy. The choline levels in tumor may decrease much before the decrease in tumor size in good responders.[32]

Table 13: Indications for DCEMRI.

- *Screening*:
  - Women at a high-risk of breast cancer
  - Obscured breast tissue (Silicon implant)
- *Diagnosis*:
  - Suspicious lesion on mammography, negative US
  - Bloody nipple discharge
  - Indeterminate palpable findings with negative mammogram and US
  - Occult breast primary in patients with axillary metastases
- *Staging*:
  - Chest wall invasion
  - Extent of cancer in patients with limited mammographic evaluation
  - Dense breasts
  - Implants
  - Infiltrating lobular cancer
  - DCIS without microcalcifications
- *Goals of breast staging with MRI*:
  - Preoperative mapping before BCT to reduce the rate of positive margins
  - Detection of multifocal or multicentric cancer
  - Detection of occult contralateral cancer
  - Detection of residual disease when initial lumpectomy is incomplete
- *Treatment*:
  - Early assessment of response to neoadjuvant chemotherapy
  - Residual disease after completion of neoadjuvant chemotherapy
  - Differentiation of recurrence/postoperative scar

DIFFUSION-WEIGHTED IMAGING

Invasive breast cancers demonstrate restricted diffusion (lower apparent diffusion coefficient) relative to normal breast tissue or benign breast lesions.[33] This restricted diffusion of water in invasive cancers, renders these lesions bright on diffusion-weighted images **(Fig. 27)** and can potentially help identify malignant lesions when dynamic contrast-enhanced imaging is equivocal. Benign lesions with high intrinsic T2 signal intensity can also appear bright on diffusion-weighted imaging (DWI) because of the phenomenon of "T2 shine through". An ADC pixel map should be generated from the component diffusion-weighted images produced from 2 or more DWI sets as hypointensity on these images confirms the restriction of diffusion. Thus, use of ADC quantification rather than DWI inspection alone is recommended for breast lesion characterization. The use of optimized ADC cut off improves breast lesion characterization without decreasing sensitivity,[34] with a potential reduction in the number of negative biopsies.

NUCLEAR MEDICINE IN BREAST IMAGING

Nuclear medicine techniques require intravenous administration of a radiotracer (technetium 99m methoxyisobutyl isonitrile [MIBI]) and a camera that detects radiotracer activity. ^{99m}Tc-sestamibi preferentially accumulates in malignant tissue and this differential uptake is imaged. Its uptake and retention in the lesion

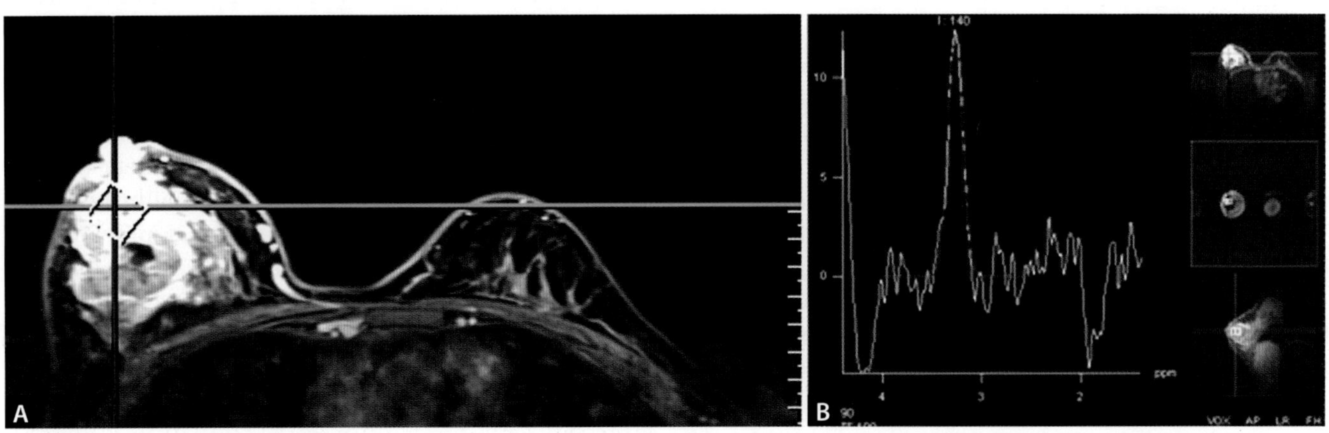

Figs. 26A and B: MR spectroscopy in a malignant lesion. Single voxel MR spectroscopy showing markedly elevated choline peak.

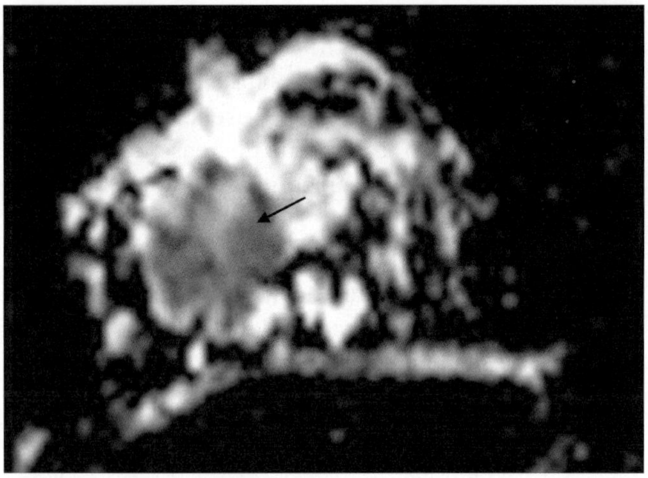

Fig. 27: Diffusion weighted MR imaging. ADC pixel map in a malignant lesion showing hypointensity (arrow) confirming the marked restriction of diffusion.

depends on the regional blood flow, angiogenesis and metabolic activity. The use of traditional gamma camera and radiotracer to image the breast is termed scintimammography, where patients lie prone with breast dependent and imaging is performed in the lateral and anteroposterior positions. Malignant lesions are seen as focal increased uptake. A recent meta-analysis has reported the sensitivity and specificity values to be 85.2% and 86.6% respectively.[35] The sensitivity however drops to 48% in lesions smaller than 1 cm due to the poor spatial resolution of these cameras.[36] This spurred the development of high resolution, small field of view, breast specific gamma cameras which could reliably image subcentimeter cancers and could image in positions comparable to mammography. The imaging of breast with these high resolution cameras and radiotracers is referred to as breast-specific gamma imaging.

Breast-specific Gamma Imaging

Breast-specific gamma imaging (BSGI) addresses the limited tumor visibility (minimum size, 15–20 mm) of large field-of-view sestamibi imaging. It provides optimal spatial resolution and sensitivity and is targeted at 95% detection rate of lesions 5 mm in diameter. For BSGI, the breast is positioned and compressed in a manner similar to a mammogram examination after intravenous injection of 20 mCi of technetium sestamibi. Routine CC and MLO views are obtained, with additional images as necessary resulting in an approximate 45-minute total examination time. If a focal area of uptake is seen, especially if there was no concern on mammogram, a directed US can be performed to determine if there is a suspicious finding that warrants biopsy.

The BSGI has shown improved sensitivity of 90% and specificity of 82% for lesions less than 1 cm.[37] As its diagnostic accuracy is not affected by density of the breast, BSGI is a useful adjunct to clinical examination and mammography in evaluation of women with dense breasts. It has been used to screen high-risk women for occult cancer. Sestamibi scan is particularly useful in patients with BI-RADS 3 lesions on mammography that are normally advised short-term follow-up. Scintimammography has high negative predictive value and hence it can be used in these patients to rule out malignancy, particularly if the follow-up is not possible. Sestamibi scintimammography has a role in prediction of treatment response to neoadjuvant chemotherapy in patients with locally advanced breast cancer.

Positron Emission Tomography

The ^{18}F-FDG positron emission tomography (PET) has emerged as another imaging tool for many malignancies, including breast cancer. Rapidly dividing neoplastic cells have higher glucose metabolism compared with nonmalignant cells and hence, show preferential uptake of ^{18}F-FDG. The ^{18}F-FDG PET however, has poor anatomic resolution like other nuclear medicine techniques. Introduction of the hybrid FDG PET/CT scanner, in which the FDG-PET scanner is equipped with a high-resolution multidetector CT for simultaneous acquisition of the FDG-PET and CT data, has greatly enhanced the spatial resolution of this technique. The FDG PET/CT has proved to be useful in the following:

- Detection of breast cancers in mammographically dense breast, those with implants and those presenting with occult primary when other imaging modalities are indeterminate. A positive FDG-PET scan of the breast is highly suspicious for cancer with a high positive predictive value of 96%.
- Locoregional staging of breast cancer: Whole body FDG PET can correctly estimate the true local and distant extent of the disease. PET can detect metastases to axillary lymph nodes as well as nodes at unsuspected areas such as internal mammary or supraclavicular lymph nodes owing to its large field of view.
- Detection of unsuspected distant metastases: ^{99m}Tc-MDP bone scan has better sensitivity for sclerotic bone metastases and PET is more sensitive for lytic bone metastases. PET is unsatisfactory for detection of brain and small pulmonary metastases.

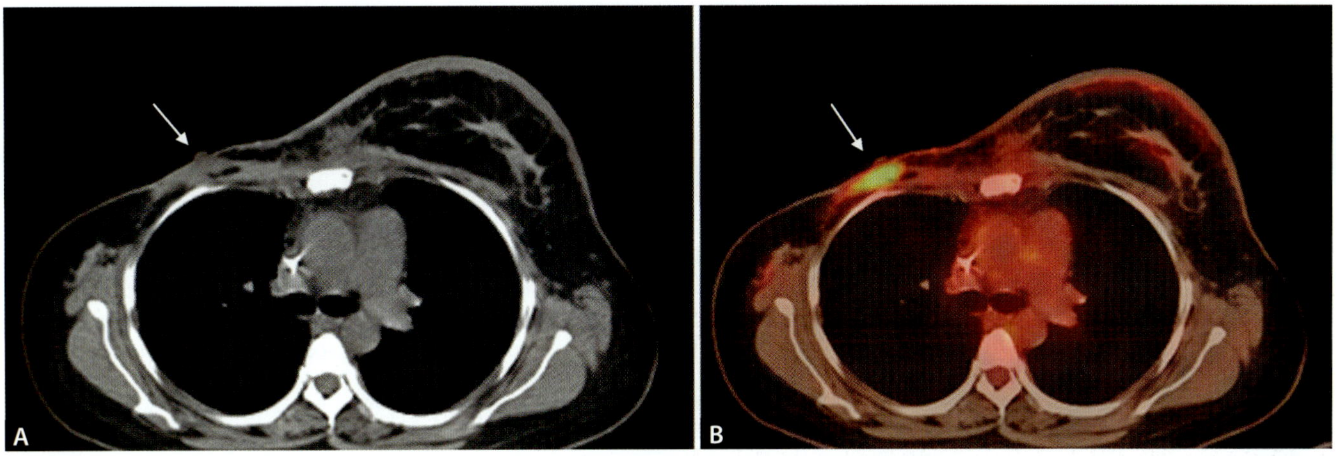

Figs. 28A and B: FDG PET-CT images showing recurrence in the pectoral muscles (arrows) in an operated patient of breast cancer.

- Detection of recurrences in soft issues **(Figs. 28A and B)**.
- Early prediction of tumor response in patients with locally advanced breast cancer undergoing neoadjuvant chemotherapy. Decreased uptake with chemotherapy suggests that pathologic remission may be achieved. Persistent high uptake with treatment predicts poor response.[38]
- Differentiation of scar tissue from cancer recurrence.

Limitations

Diagnostic accuracy of FDG-PET is dependent on tumor size and histology. The sensitivity of FDG-PET is 92% for lesions larger than 2 cm, but is only 53% for primary lesions smaller than 5 mm.[39] PET also has poor sensitivity for detection of ductal carcinoma in situ and slow growing cancers such as invasive lobular carcinoma. PET is not suitable for screening even for high-risk patients, as negative study has limited value.

Positron Emission Mammography

Positron emission mammography (PEM) is a high spatial resolution (2 mm), dedicated breast positron emission tomography device that can provide anatomical and functional information. Dual moving head detectors are mounted opposite each other on compression paddles attached to a portable compact scanner to obtain tomographic images of the breast in the CC and MLO positions. A recent multicenter study compared the performance of PEM with MRI in evaluating the disease extent in breast cancer and in evaluating the impact on surgical management. PEM and MRI had comparable sensitivity, although MRI more accurately depicted the need for mastectomy. PEM had greater specificity. Integration of PEM and MRI increased cancer detection to 74% versus 60% identified with MRI alone.[40]

REFERENCES

1. Tabár L, Vitak B, Chen TH, et al. Swedish two-county trial: impact of mammographic screening on breast cancer mortality during 3 decades. Radiology. 2011;260(3):658-63.
2. Mushlin AI, Kouides RW, Shapiro DE. Estimating the accuracy of screening mammography: a meta-analysis. Am J Prev Med. 1998;14:143-53.
3. Boyd NF, Guo H, Martin LJ, et al. Mammographic density and the risk and detection of breast cancer. N Engl J Med. 2007;356:227-36.
4. Mettler FA, Upton AC, Kelsey CA, et al. Benefits versus risks from mammography: a critical assessment. Cancer. 1996;77:903-9.
5. Berg WA, Arnoldus CL, Teferra E, et al. Biopsy of amorphous breast calcifications: pathologic outcome and yield at stereotactic biopsy. Radiology. 2001;221:495-503.
6. Leung JWT, Sicles EA. Developing asymmetry identified on mammography: correlation with imaging outcome and pathologic findings. Am J Roentgenol. 2007;188:667-75.
7. Sickles E. Periodic mammographic follow-up of probably benign lesions: results in 3184 consecutive cases. Radiology. 1991;179:463-8.
8. D'Orsi CJ, Newell MS. Digital mammography: clinical implementation and clinical trials. Semin Roentgenol. 2007;42(4):236-42.
9. Noble M, Bruening W, Uhl S, et al. Computer-aided detection mammography for breast cancer screening: systematic review and meta-analysis. Arch Gynecol Obstet. 2009;279(6):881-90.
10. Poplack SA, Tosteson TD, Kogel CA, et al. Digital breast tomosynthesis: initial experience in 98 women with abnormal digital screening mammography. Am J Roentgenol. 2007; 189:616-23.

11. Gur D, Abrams GS, Chough DM, et al. Digital breast tomosynthesis: observer performance study. Am J Roentgenol. 2009;193:586-91.
12. Dromain C, Balleyguier C, Adler G, et al. Contrast-enhanced digital mammography. Eur J Radiol. 2009;69:34-42.
13. Lewin IM, Isaacs PK, Vance V, et al. Dual energy contrast enhanced digital subtraction mammography: feasibility. Radiology. 2003;229:261-8.
14. Raza S, Baum JK. Solid breast lesions: Evaluation with power Doppler US. Radiology. 1997;203:164-8.
15. Mendelson EB, Baum JK, Berg WA, et al. Breast imaging reporting and data system, BI-RADS: ultrasound, 1. Reston, VA: American College of Radiology; 2003.
16. Stavros AT, Thickman D, Rapp CL, et al. Solid breast nodules: use of sonography to distinguish between benign and malignant lesions. Radiology. 1995;196(1):123-34.
17. Graf O, Helbich TH, Fuchsjaeger MH, et al. Follow-up of palpable circumscribed noncalcified solid breast masses at mammography and US: can biopsy be averted? Radiology. 2004;233(3):850-6.
18. Raza S, Goldkamp AL, Chikarmane SA, Birdwell RL. US of breast masses categorized as BI-RADS 3, 4, and 5: pictorial review of factors influencing clinical management. Radiographics. 2010;30(5):1199-213.
19. Ozdemir A, Kilic K, Ozdemir H, et al. Contrast-enhanced power Doppler sonography in breast lesions: Effect on differential diagnosis after mammography and grey scale sonography. J Ultrasound Med. 2004;23:183-95.
20. Kook SH, Kwag HJ. Value of contrast-enhanced power Doppler sonography using a microbubble echo-enhancing agent in evaluation of small breast lesions. J Clin Ultrasound. 2003;31:227-38.
21. Burnside ES, Hall TJ, Sommer AM, et al. Differentiating benign from malignant solid breast masses with US strain imaging. Radiology. 2007;245(2):401-10.
22. Athanasiou A, Tardivon A, Tanter M, et al. Breast lesions: quantitative elastography with supersonic shear imaging-preliminary results. Radiology. 2010;256(1):297-303.
23. Pinker K, Grabner G, Bogner W, et al. A combined high temporal and high spatial resolution 3 Tesla MR imaging protocol for the assessment of breast lesions: initial results. Invest Radiol. 2009;44(9):553-8.
24. Ballesio L, Savelli S, Angeletti M, et al. Breast MRI: Are T2 IR sequences useful in the evaluation of breast lesions? Eur J Radiol. 2009;71(1):96-101.
25. Morris EA. Diagnostic breast MR imaging: current status and future directions. Radiol Clin N Am. 2007;45:863-80.
26. Matsubayashi R, Matsuo Y, Edakuni G, et al. Breast masses with peripheral rim enhancement on dynamic contrast-enhanced MR images: correlation of MR findings with histologic features and expression of growth factors. Radiology. 2000;217:841-8.
27. Liberman L, Morris EA, Dershaw DD, et al. Ductal enhancement on MR imaging of the breast. AJR. 2003;181:519-25.
28. Kuhl CK, Mielcareck P, Klaschik S, et al. Dynamic breast MR imaging: are signal intensity time course data useful for differential diagnosis of enhancing lesions? Radiology. 1999;211:101-10.
29. Saslow D, Boetes C, Burke W, et al. American Cancer Society guidelines for breast screening with MRI as an adjunct to mammography. CA Cancer J Clin. 2007;57(2):75-89.
30. Peters NH, Borel Rinks IH, Zuithoff NP, et al. Meta-analysis of MR imaging in the diagnosis of breast lesions. Radiology. 2008;246:116-24.
31. Bartella L, Morris EA, Dershaw DD, et al. Proton MR spectroscopy with choline peak as malignancy marker improves positive predictive value for breast cancer diagnosis: Preliminary study. Radiology. 2006;239(3):686-92.
32. Meisamy S, Bolan PJ, Baker EH, et al. Neoadjuvant chemotherapy of locally advanced breast cancer: predicting response with in vivo (1) H MR spectroscopy—a pilot study at 4T. Radiology. 2004;233:424-31.
33. Kuroki Y, Nasu K, Kuroki S, et al. Diffusion-weighted imaging of breast cancer with the sensitivity encoding technique: analysis of the apparent diffusion coefficient value. Magn Reson Med Sci. 2004;32:79-85.
34. Partridge SC, DeMartini WB, Kurland BF, et al. Quantitative diffusion-weighted imaging as an adjunct to conventional breast MRI for improved positive predictive value. Am J Roentgenol. 2009;193(6):1716-22.
35. Liberman M, Sampalis F, Mulder DS, Sampalis JS. Breast cancer diagnosis by scintimammography: a meta-analysis and review of the literature. Breast Cancer Res Treat. 2003;80(1):115-26.
36. Khalkhali I, Villanueva-Meyer J, Edell SL, et al. Diagnostic accuracy of ^{99m}Tc-sestamibi breast imaging: multicenter trial results. J Nucl Med. 2000;41(12):1973-9.
37. Brem RF, Floerke AC, Rapelyea JA, Teal C, Kelly T, Mathur V. Breast-specific gamma imaging as an adjunct imaging modality for the diagnosis of breast cancer. Radiology. 2008;247(3):651-7.
38. Smith IC, Welch AE, Hutcheon AW, et al. PET using 18-FDG to predict the pathologic response of breast cancer to primary chemotherapy. J Clin Oncol. 2000;18:1676-88.
39. Kumar R, Das CJ. Hybrid PET-dynamic CECT in the management of breast cancer. Eur J Nucl Med Mol Imaging. 2009;36(3):413-5.
40. Berg WA, Madsen KS, Schilling K, et al. Comparative effectiveness of positron emission mammography and MRI in the contralateral breast of women with newly diagnosed breast cancer. Am J Roentgenol. 2012;198(1):219-32.

CHAPTER 207

Benign and Malignant Lesions of the Breast

Smriti Hari, Ashu Seith Bhalla, Sanjay Thulkar

INTRODUCTION

The primary role of breast imaging is to detect and characterize abnormalities that could represent malignancy. A large number of benign conditions of the breast are diagnosed and managed clinically. Imaging of benign conditions is required to detect underlying suspicious abnormalities, if any, and to evaluate patients of symptomatic breast diseases with equivocal clinical findings. Mammography is the primary breast imaging modality; ultrasound and MRI have an important complementary role. Imaging findings are generally suggestive but not specific for most breast lesions.

PROLIFERATIVE BENIGN LESIONS OF THE BREAST

Benign proliferative breast disease is a pathological term used to describe breast conditions wherein there is more glandular and/or fibrotic tissue than expected for the patient's age and parity. It involves the lobules or ducts or both. The tissue is also morphologically abnormal. These conditions include fibrocystic disease, adenosis, fibroadenoma, cyst, ductal hyperplasia, and papilloma. These may coexist.

Fibrocystic Disease

This is the most common benign diagnosis in symptomatic women. It is a nonspecific term which includes variations in the breast that histologically range from normal physiological changes to premalignant proliferative conditions. The breast is an end organ for cyclic hormonal changes during normal menstruation. The breast parenchyma is hyperemic and edematous in luteal phase of the menstruation. The response of the breast parenchyma to these hormonal changes varies considerably; from minimal to severe, time to time and woman to woman. This heterogeneous response of breast leads to variable symptoms, such as cyclical pain and lumpiness with clinical findings of nonspecific nodularity and tenderness. In addition, there is a long-term age related actual involution resulting in replacement of glandular tissue with fat. The range of breast changes is often included under the broad heading of aberrations in normal development and involution (ANDI) of the breast.

Imaging findings are also variable. These include increased mammographic density or heterogeneous echotexture of the breast. Diffuse imaging findings do not correlate with histological changes and there is overlap in the normal and pathological conditions. Hence, imaging diagnosis of fibrocystic disease is discouraged.[1] Indication of imaging in symptomatic patient is to detect the underlying focal lesion, if any. If detected, further characterization and management such as biopsy or follow-up should be recommended.

Adenosis

Adenosis represents enlargement of the lobule secondary to a benign proliferation of the blunt ending intralobular ductules (acini). This proliferation is primarily an elongation and multiplication of the acini accompanied by overgrowth of epithelial and connective tissue elements in the lobule. If connective tissue proliferation is a predominant finding, then the term 'sclerosing adenosis' is used. Adenosis is a relatively common benign condition of the breast, which is included under benign proliferative conditions.

Mammographically, adenosis rarely forms a visible mass. On occasion, it may be the cause of isolated cluster of uniform microcalcifications. These are extremely small deposits that precipitate in the acini of the lobule and their cystic dilated ends. These calcifications may be diffuse and scattered bilaterally. Adenosis may also cause nonspecific patchy or homogeneous areas of increased density. Adenosis is not visible by ultrasound.

Fibroadenoma

Fibroadenoma is the most common benign tumor of the breast in women of childbearing age. Fibroadenoma develops from overgrowth of the stromal connective tissue within the lobule. This idiopathic proliferation of collagen expands the lobule while simultaneously surrounding and compressing the acini and terminal ducts. Histologically, the proportion of stromal elements found in a fibroadenoma may vary, producing very cellular adenomas or preponderantly fibrotic lesions.

Clinical breast examination reveals a firm, mobile, non-tender mass. Fibroadenoma may be single or multiple, unilateral or bilateral, vary in size from few millimeters to a very large size, though most are less than 3 cm in diameter. Fibroadenomas in women older than 35 years or those which are rapidly growing are excised. Fibroadenomas are hormone-dependent lesions. They regress with age and necrosis within the tumor results in coarse calcification. Fibroadenomas are not premalignant lesions. As there is epithelium within fibroadenoma, cancer can develop just as it can in normal ductal epithelium. Hence, ill-defined margins, microcalcifications and increase in size on follow- up should arouse concern.

On mammography, fibroadenoma is seen as a well-defined, round or oval mass with smooth margins **(Fig. 1A)**. Fibroadenomas may have somewhat flattened contours which if present help to distinguish them from cysts. Because, fibroadenomas follow the structure of the lobule, their margins are often lobulated. Occasionally, they have microlobulated margins. In the presence of microlobulation, however, cancer should be suspected. Fibroadenoma may be partly or completely surrounded by a radiolucent halo. Many fibroadenomas calcify as they undergo myxoid degeneration with age. There may be heavy, central, amorphous calcification or coarse, sharp, intermittent popcorn calcification. In postmenopausal age, there may be complete resolution of the soft tissue component of the fibroadenoma resulting in no residual soft tissue density on mammogram, but calcification remains unchanged.

On ultrasound, fibroadenomas are typically solid, round or oval, well-circumscribed, homogeneously hypoechoic masses that are wider than taller **(Fig. 1B)**. Like any round or oval masses, fibroadenomas may exhibit lateral wall refractive shadowing; the sidelobe artifact. Posterior acoustic enhancement is frequently seen. Fibroadenomas can, however, produce varying sonographic appearances, including ill-defined margins and posterior acoustic shadowing in more fibrotic adenomas.[2]

Magnetic resonance imaging (MRI) is not recommended for a mammographically well-defined mass

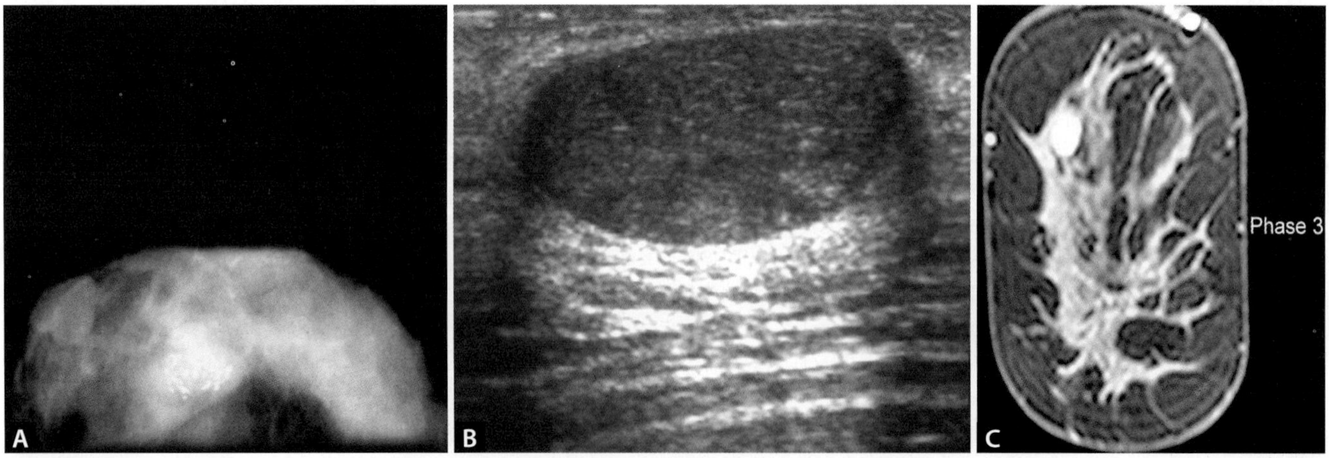

Figs. 1A to C: Fibroadenoma: (A) Mammogram shows a well-defined lobulated superficial mass. Another similar mass shows coarse benign calcifications within it; (B) Ultrasound shows a well-defined oval hypoechoic mass with distal acoustic enhancement; (C) Fibroadenoma is seen as a well-defined, round, homogeneously enhancing mass on contrast-enhanced T1-weighted MRI scan of another woman.

that is suspected to be a fibroadenoma. If MRI is performed, predominantly fibrous fibroadenomas are hypointense on all sequences and show no enhancement. Fibroadenomas, which are cellular and contain adenomatous or myxoid tissue, show an intermediate to high-signal intensity on T2-weighted images and most have well-circumscribed margins with low intensity internal septae. The enhancement is significant and homogeneous; usually delayed (type 1) **(Fig. 1C)**. Visualization of nonenhancing septae is diagnostic of fibroadenoma.[3]

A fibroadenoma with a diameter of more than 6 cm is defined as a giant fibroadenoma. It may fill a large part of the breast. It is a benign lesion and most commonly seen in adolescent females. Phyllode tumor is a close differential diagnosis however; it is generally seen in later decades of life. Lactating fibroadenoma occurs in young females, and is associated with pregnancy or lactation. The lactating fibroadenoma may attain enormous size. Juvenile fibroadenoma is another variant which may be seen in teenage females. It often grows rapidly and becomes very large.

Cysts

Breast cysts develop when lumina of ducts or acini become dilated and lined by atrophic epithelium. Simple cysts are common lesions and vary in size from microscopic to large palpable masses. These are frequently bilateral and multiple but all may not be identified clinically or by imaging. Cysts are common in perimenopausal age but may be seen in women of all ages. Cysts are benign lesions. Cysts may remain stable for many years or spontaneously resolve.

On mammography, a cyst is typically seen as well-defined, round or oval mass **(Fig. 2A)**. The cyst may be of variable size, solitary or may occur in clumps. A tense cyst is round, but a lax cyst may vary in shape depending upon the degree of compression applied. Calcification is infrequent and it may be seen as a thin peripheral rim or flecks of calcium near the periphery. Rarely, microcysts may contain milk of calcium fluid which on erect lateral mammography layers on the cyst floor forming so-called 'tea-cup' calcification. Cysts cannot be accurately diagnosed by mammography, because they cannot be distinguished from other well-circumscribed masses, unless they display characteristic pattern of calcification. However, bilateral multiple benign morphology masses on mammography most commonly represent cysts.[1]

Ultrasound has an important role in the diagnosis of breast cysts. Typical simple breast cyst is sharply marginated, anechoic with posterior acoustic enhancement **(Fig. 2B)**. It may have angular margin, few thin septations or echogenic debris in the dependent part. These features do not necessarily make it suspicious for malignancy and can be ignored.[4] Posterior enhancement may not be seen if the cyst is small or close to the chest wall. Sometimes, multiple cysts may be seen forming a cluster **(Fig. 2C)**. Ultrasound diagnosis of simple breast cyst is important as it obviates the need of any FNAC, treatment or follow-up. Cysts with debris, wall thickening and septations are referred to as complicated cysts. Chances of malignancy in a complicated cyst are less than 0.5% and hence, most complicated cysts are appropriately assigned BIRADS 3 category.[5] Intracystic tumors are rare. If present, these are commonly intracystic papillomas; intracystic cancer is extremely rare. Indications for aspiration of complicated cysts include suspicion of cyst being an abscess, significant enlargement on follow-up, solid mass in the cyst or suspicious mammographic

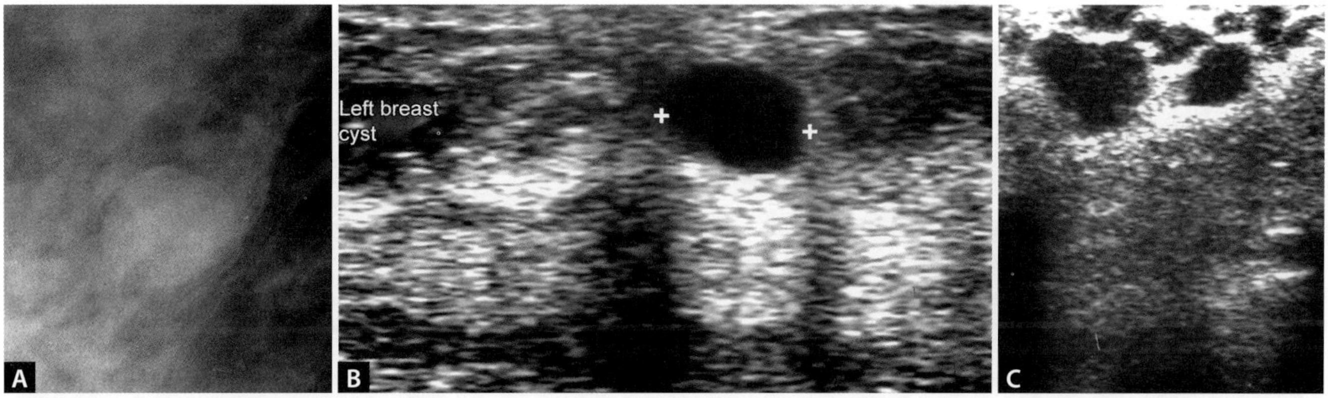

Figs. 2A to C: Breast cyst: (A) Mammogram shows a small, round, sharply circumscribed, low density mass; (B) Ultrasound shows sharply defined, anechoic cyst with distal acoustic enhancement; (C) Ultrasound shows multiple small clustered cysts in another woman.

findings. Symptomatic cysts may also require ultrasound guided aspiration; however, half of these recur over two years.

On MRI, most cysts are hypointense on T1-weighted images and brightly hyperintense on T2-weighted images. The presence of proteinaceous contents or blood products can modify the signal intensity pattern.

Intraductal Papilloma

Papilloma results from proliferation of the ductal epithelium. They project into the lumen of the duct and connected by a fibrovascular stalk to the epithelial lining. The duct around them can dilate forming a cystic structure giving the appearance of an intracystic papilloma. Benign papilloma is the most common cause of unilateral nipple discharge.[6] Most are located within few centimeters from the nipple in the major subareolar ducts and are usually single.

On mammography, most papillomas are not seen. Larger papillomas are seen as round or oval mass with benign morphology **(Fig. 3A)**. Sometimes, they grow over a long length of the duct filling, but not enlarging it. Occasionally, mulberry-like calcification may be seen in the subareolar region. Ultrasound is the preferred modality for the evaluation of nipple discharge. On ultrasound, a typical finding of papilloma is a dilated duct with solid round or oval intraluminal mass **(Fig. 3B)**. Ductography shows dilated duct with intraluminal filling defect or complete obstruction of a duct with a meniscus **(Fig. 3C)**. On MRI, large papillomas behave similar to fibroadenomas.[7] Multiple papillomas arise more distally and are associated with increased risk of cancer.[8]

Duct Ectasia

Duct ectasia primarily affects the major ducts in the subareolar region. There is nonspecific dilatation of one or more ducts. It is generally associated with periductal inflammation. The distended ducts are filled with secretions and cellular debris.

On mammography, dilated ducts may or may not be appreciated. Ectatic ducts with thickened walls or periductal fibrosis are more visible. Intraluminal debris may calcify and produce calcifications called secretory deposits, resembling broken sticks. Ultrasound shows one or more dilated ducts without intraluminal mass. Depending on the composition of the contents, the duct may be anechoic, show debris or may be hyperechoic. Ductography is usually unnecessary, and it shows a dilated duct with attenuated peripheral branches.

Ductal Epithelial Hyperplasia

Ducts are lined with a single layer of epithelial cells. In ductal hyperplasia, there is the benign multilayered cellular proliferation of the epithelium. If atypical cells are found in these, it is called atypical ductal hyperplasia (ADH). It is a high-risk condition as some of these progresses into ductal carcinoma in situ (DCIS). Ductal hyperplasia is incidentally diagnosed on biopsy and does not have specific clinical or imaging features. Sometimes, suspicious masses or calcifications may be seen on mammography.

MISCELLANEOUS BENIGN BREAST CONDITIONS

Lipoma

As fat is frequently the preponderant tissue in the breast, it is difficult to differentiate a true lipoma from normal fat. Most lipomas are superficial and form a palpable mass. These are freely movable and generally soft. On mammography, they are lucent, have thin capsule and mass effect with displacement of surrounding structures **(Fig. 4)**. They are hypoechoic on ultrasound, just like the normal breast fat.

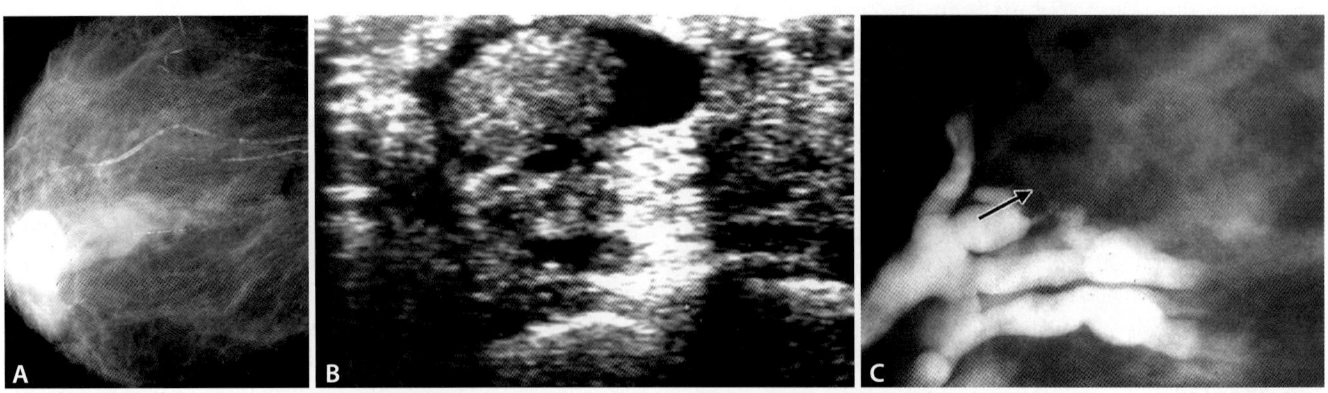

Figs. 3A to C: Duct papilloma: (A) Mammogram shows a small well-defined mass in subareolar location along with dilated duct; (B) Ultrasound shows a papilloma within a dilated duct; (C) Ductogram shows an abrupt cut-off of a duct with meniscus formation (arrow).

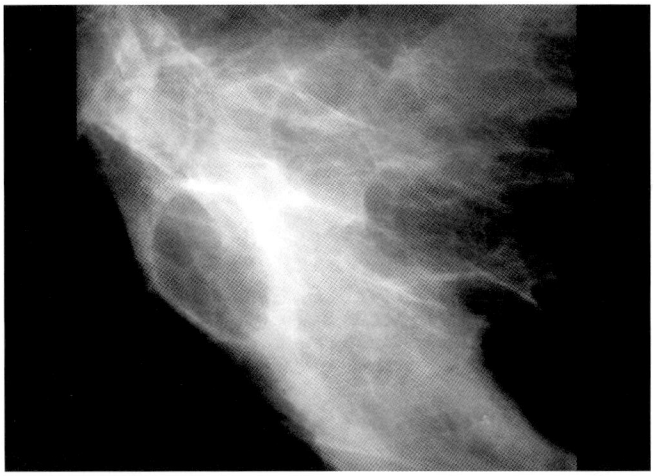

Fig. 4: Lipoma: Mammogram shows a well-defined fat density mass with a capsule.

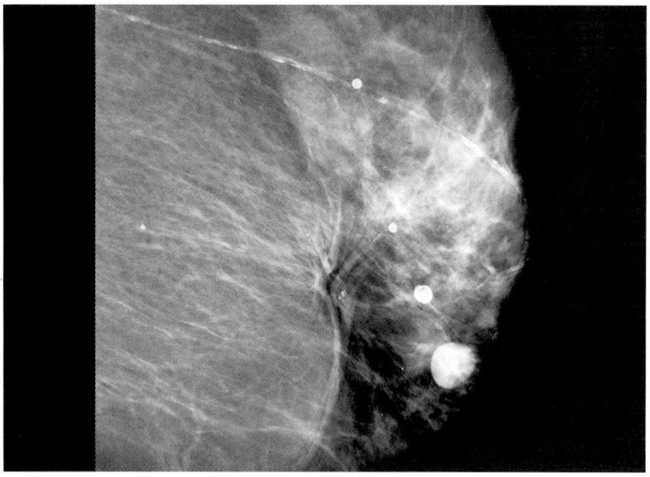

Fig. 5: Fat necrosis: Mammogram shows multiple round calcified nodules suggestive of oil cyst formation at the operative site.

Fat Necrosis

Fat necrosis is an inflammatory process of breast related to prior trauma or surgery. Patients are mostly asymptomatic and history of definite trauma is not always present. Some patients have a palpable painful mass with skin thickening or retraction. Occasionally, necrosed fat may form a gelatinous oil cyst with fibrous wall. Fat necrosis is an important lesion because it comes in the differential diagnosis of carcinoma and abscess on mammography.

Mammographically, there is a wide spectrum of appearances. Most lesions are superficial in location. Surgical bed is also a common site. Fat necrosis may appear as a spiculated or irregular mass. Calcification is common in fat necrosis and may produce several patterns. Oil cyst shows a round smooth lucent mass, sometimes with calcified thin rim with eggshell appearance **(Fig. 5)**. Cluster of microcalcifications or coarse calcification may also be seen. Post-traumatic oil cysts show varying echogenicity on ultrasound. MRI features of fat necrosis are variable and cannot be distinguished from malignancy. If a fat density is demonstrated within the center of the lesion on nonfat suppressed unenhanced T1-weighted images, fat necrosis can be confirmed.

Galactocele

Galactocele is a cyst filled with inspissated milk. It occurs during pregnancy or lactation and may persist long after cessation of lactation. It may be unilateral or bilateral or may present with multiple palpable masses.

Mammographic features vary with the fat content of the cyst. It may be a well-defined dense lesion like a cyst or a radiolucent mass surrounded by dense lactating breast parenchyma. The usual site is the retroareolar central breast area. Ultrasound shows features of a simple or complicated cyst or a solid mass with posterior enhancement **(Fig. 6)**.

Radial Scar

Radial scar, also known as sclerosing duct hyperplasia, is a lesion of unknown etiology, possibly related to chronic inflammatory process or obliterative changes in blood vessels. There is no palpable mass and no history of trauma. Most are found incidentally on histopathology and some are detected on mammography. Radial scars cannot be accurately diagnosed on core biopsy and require an excisional biopsy. Radial scar is not a premalignant condition, but it may rarely contain ADH and DCIS.

Mammographically, it is a spiculated lesion that cannot be differentiated from a cancer **(Fig. 7)**. Central dense mass may or may not be seen. If central mass is absent, it appears like a spiculated architectural distortion only, which is well seen in one view but difficult to appreciate in the other.[9] Microcalcifications are rare. Ultrasound appearance is also similar to cancer and it shows an irregular, ill-defined, hypoechoic mass. On MRI, an irregular mass with variable contrast enhancement is seen.

Hamartoma

Hamartoma or fibroadenolipoma is an uncommon lesion which results from fibrous and adenomatous proliferation. The mammographic appearance is characteristic and is seen as sharply defined mass containing admixture of both fatty and soft tissue density. Ultrasound appearance is also similar and shows hypoechoic and hyperechoic areas within a well-defined mass.

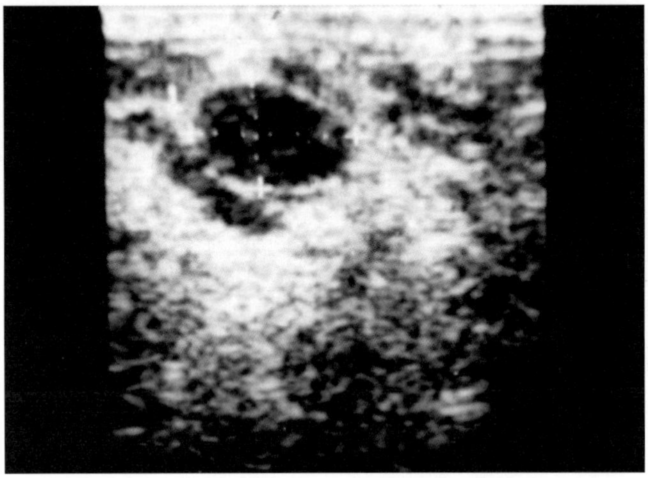

Fig. 6: Galactocele: Ultrasound shows a cyst with debris in vicinity of a prominent duct.

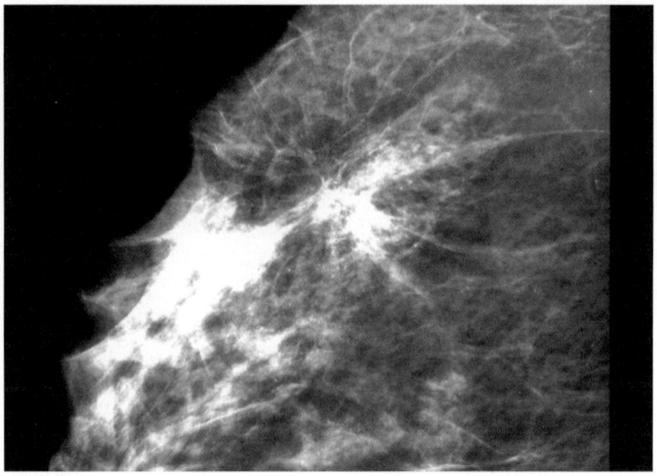

Fig. 7: Radial scar: Mammogram shows spiculated architectural distortion. The spicules are long and there is no central high density mass.

Pseudoangiomatous Stromal Hyperplasia

Pseudoangiomatous stromal hyperplasia (PASH) is a rare benign tumor that is seen in young women. It results from fibrous, glandular and vascular proliferation of the stroma. On mammography and ultrasound, these appear similar to fibroadenomas.[10]

Desmoid Tumor

Desmoid tumor, also known as fibromatosis, is a locally invasive, benign spindle cell tumor. It usually occurs in abdominal wall but may rarely be seen in the breast. It tends to develop deep in the breast, along the pectoralis fascia. Most patients have history of trauma or surgery. On mammography, it is seen as round or irregular mass with ill-defined or spiculated margins.[3]

Diabetic Mastopathy

It is a rare fibrous tumor that is found in young women with type 1 diabetes. It probably represents an autoimmune inflammatory process. They present with a hard palpable breast mass. Usual mammographic appearance is that of an asymmetric density. Ultrasound shows an ill-defined hypoechoic mass with posterior shadowing.[11]

Superficial Thrombophlebitis (Mondor's Disease)

It is a thrombophlebitis of superficial veins of the breast. It is clinically diagnosed and characterized by thickened and painful cord like veins. History of trauma, surgery or breast biopsy may be present in some patients. It is a self-limiting process. It is difficult to demonstrate on mammography. The thrombosed vein may be seen as an elongated and beaded cord like opacity on mammography **(Fig. 8A)**. A thrombosed subcutaneous vein can also be demonstrated on ultrasound **(Fig. 8B)**.

Breast Infections

Breast infections may be in the form of acute mastitis associated with lactation or a breast abscess. Acute mastitis may progress to form an abscess. Patient presents with painful, localized or diffuse enlargement of the breast, with erythematous and edematous overlying skin. Breast infections are usually diagnosed and managed clinically.

Mammography is not required in acute mastitis. Breast abscess is painful and mammography is also difficult to perform. If performed, abscess formation is easily missed through the dense, edematous breast. In others, it is usually seen as a well or ill-defined mass. Overlying skin thickening is often present. Ultrasound is preferred in evaluation of painful and tender breast as it does not require breast compression. It is useful to localize the abscess, to exclude underlying inflammatory breast cancer and for diagnostic or therapeutic aspiration.[12] On ultrasound, an abscess is seen as a complex irregular mass with solid/cystic components **(Fig. 9)**. Gross subcutaneous edema is usually associated which is seen as multiple thin, fluid filled clefts beneath the skin. MRI is not required for evaluation of breast infections. If performed, it shows intense enhancement and secondary changes, such as skin thickening, retraction or architectural distortion. The enhancement tends to be delayed and diffuse but it cannot be differentiated from inflammatory carcinoma.

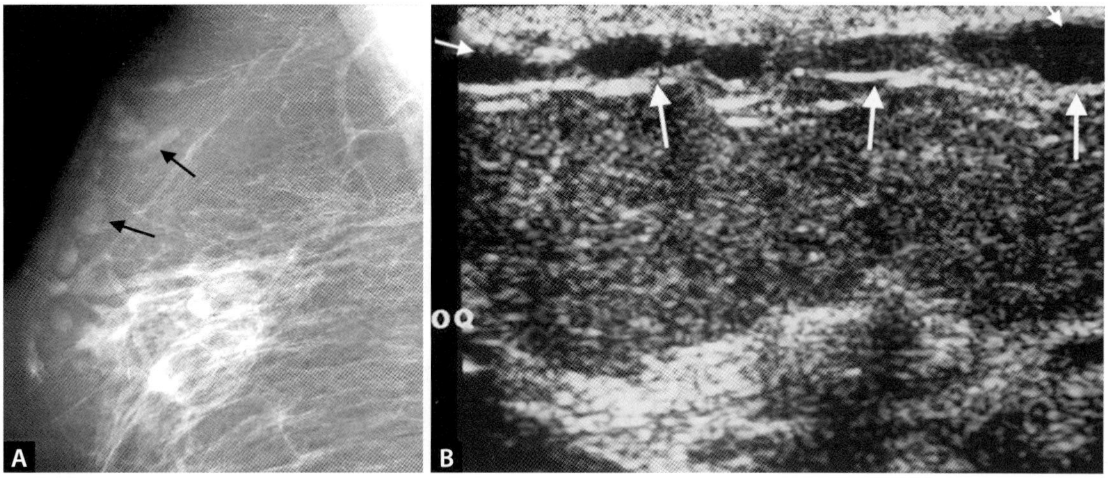

Figs. 8A and B: Mondor's disease: (A) Mammogram shows superficial tortuous linear opacities (arrows) representing a thrombosed vein; (B) Thrombosed subcutaneous vein (arrows) can be seen on ultrasound also.

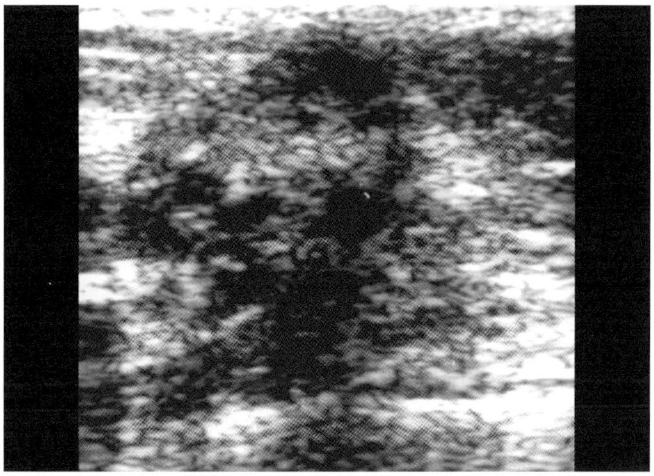

Fig. 9: Breast abscess: Ultrasound shows an irregular complex solid cystic mass.

Breast Tuberculosis

Tuberculosis of the breast is uncommon. It has variable mammographic appearances. There are three types of lesions seen on mammography.[13] Nodular form is seen as a dense mass with irregular or spiculated margin, with or without calcification **(Fig. 10A)**. It is the most common mammographic feature of breast tuberculosis and may mimic carcinoma.[14] Diffuse involvement produces multiple caseating confluent foci of tuberculosis. These also result in skin thickening, ulceration and sinus formation. Mammography shows dense breast, or skin thickening with or without lymphadenopathy. These findings may mimic inflammatory carcinoma. Sclerosing form of breast tuberculosis is a slow growing process with excessive fibrosis rather than caseation. Entire breast is hard with nipple retraction. Mammography is not contributory as it shows uniformly increased density of one breast. Ultrasound features of breast tuberculosis are nonspecific and these include a hypoechoic mass or abscess **(Fig. 10B)**, skin thickening, sinuses and duct ectasia.[15] CT is useful in demonstrating the underlying chest wall involvement.

Granulomatous mastitis is an idiopathic chronic inflammatory condition. Patients usually present with vague lumps. Clinical evaluation may mimic cancer. Mammography shows nonspecific features, such as asymmetric increased density or an ill-defined mass. Ultrasound shows an irregular mass, multiple tubular hypoechoic foci or nonspecific focal hypoechoic areas in the breast.[16] Diagnosis is established on biopsy only.

Breast Implants

Implants are used for cosmetic augmentation of the breast or for breast reconstruction after mastectomy. These are silicone rubber bags filled with silicone gel or saline. These are usually placed behind the breast tissue and anterior to pectoralis muscle. A fibrous capsule normally forms around the implant because of foreign body reaction. Implants appear semiovoid and opaque on mammography and these are anechoic on ultrasound **(Figs. 11A and B)**. During mammography, only the breast tissue anterior to implant can be pulled forward and compressed. Hence, complete visualization of breast parenchyma is not possible on mammography and this interferes with cancer detection. Ultrasound and MRI are useful for evaluation of implants. Magnetic resonance imaging is the modality of

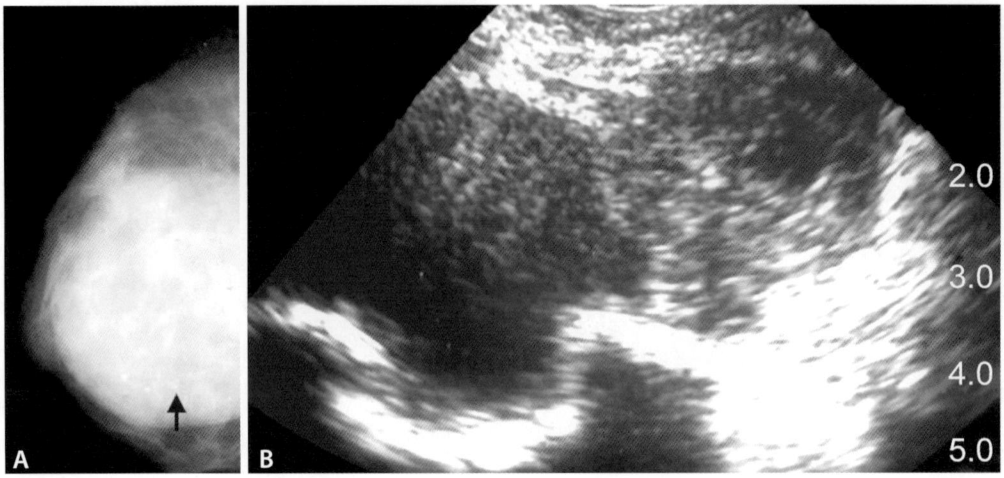

Figs. 10A and B: Breast tuberculosis: (A) Mammogram shows a large mass with nonspecific morphology; (B) Ultrasound shows a complex solid cystic mass with chest wall involvement.

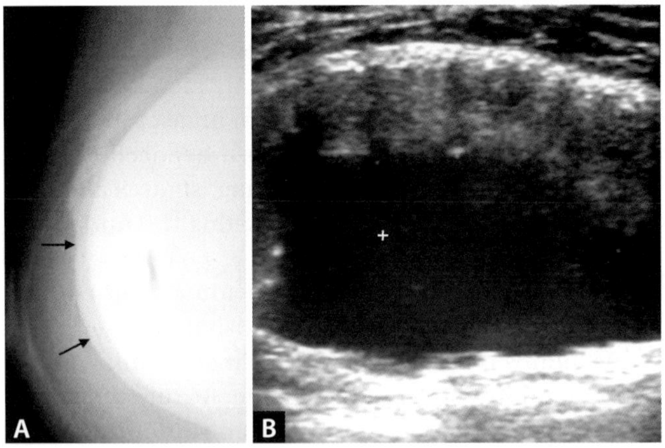

Figs. 11A and B: Breast implant: (A) Mammogram shows the implant as a large, semiovoid well-defined opacity. Surrounding fibrous capsule formation is also seen (arrows); (B) Implant shows anechoic fluid content on ultrasound.

choice. Plain MRI is sufficient. Water and fat suppressed (silicone only) T2-weighted MR sequences are particularly useful. Silicone is hypointense on T1-weighted images and hyperintense on T2-weighted images.

Common complications of implants are capsular contractions causing pain and deformity of the breast and implant rupture. Rupture may occur spontaneously due to capsular contracture or during the closed capsulotomy, a procedure in which a surgeon manually compress the capsule to break it and relieve the pain. Rupture can be intracapsular in which the extravasated gel remain inside fibrous capsule or it may be extracapsular leading to spread of the gel in breast parenchyma. The sequelae of noncontained silicone include granuloma formation, fibrosis, and migration. Migration of silicone into the axilla can involve the brachial plexus, resulting in neuropathy.

On ultrasound, intracapsular rupture is seen as folded membranes representing collapsed envelope in stepladder pattern within the anechoic gel. On MRI, collapsed envelope is seen as low intensity membranes floating in hyperintense gel on T2-weighted sequences.[17] With extracapsular rupture, ultrasound shows multiple hyperechoic foci in the breast. Extravasated gel in the parenchyma is very echogenic and produces shadowing.[18] On MRI, the extravasated gel appears as foci of low-signal intensity on T1-weighted sequences and high-signal intensity on T2-weighted sequences.[19]

MALIGNANT LESIONS OF THE BREAST

Breast cancer is the most common cancer in women in the developed world, where the incidence ranges from 60 to 90 cases per 100,000 women per year. The incidence is low in Asia and Africa however; it is rising in the developed and urbanized countries in these regions. In India, breast cancer is most common cancer in women in urban areas where the age averaged incidence ranges from 1 to 29.2 cases per 100,000 women per year. In rural India, the incidence is 7.6 to 9.7 per 100,000 women per year.[20]

Risk Factors for Breast Cancer

Female gender and increasing age are the most important risk factors for development of breast cancer. Other risk factors include early menarche, late menopause, nulliparity or late first pregnancy and decreased breastfeeding. All of these factors increase the overall duration of endogenous estrogen exposure; a hormone known to play a major role in the development of breast cancer. Exogenous estrogen exposure in hormonal replacement therapy (HRT) also increases the risk of breast cancer. Family history of breast cancer in a first degree relative is also a risk factor, especially if they had breast cancer at an early age. The familial inheritance of the risk may be associated with or without genetic mutations. Women with Li-Fraumeni-Cowden syndromes have a high-risk. History of benign breast disease, especially atypical hyperplasia also increases the risk of breast cancer. Mammographic breast density has also been identified as a risk factor. Women with more than 75% glandular density on mammogram are at four fold greater risk for breast cancer development.[21]

BRCA1 and *BRCA2* genes mutations are major risk factors and these account for 5–10% of all breast cancers. The chances of breast cancer in the carriers of these mutations are variable in different races and range from 45–85%.[22] They also have increase a risk for ovarian cancer, especially with BRCA1 mutation. Breast cancer arising in these women is frequently aggressive and triple negative; negative for estrogen receptor (ER), progesterone receptor (PR) and human epidermal growth factor receptor (HER2). Management options in BRCA mutation carriers include close surveillance, chemoprevention and prophylactic bilateral mastectomy.

Diagnosis of the Breast Cancer

Breast cancer may be detected in preclinical stage on screening mammography. Others are detected by self breast examination (SBE) or clinical breast examination (CBE). Symptomatic breast cancers present with a palpable mass, focal tenderness, nipple discharge, skin retraction or ulceration, or sometimes as a metastatic disease with occult primary site. Mammography is the primary modality for detection of breast cancer; ultrasound and MRI complement mammography in detection of breast cancer. Approach to the breast imaging and role of various imaging modalities in detection of breast cancer has been covered in the preceding chapter. However, there are no characteristic features of breast cancer on imaging. It is interesting to note that mammographic interpretation has a category of definitely benign lesions (BIRADS 2), but there is no category of definitely malignant lesions. Mammography only detects lesions which are either suspicious (BIRADS 4) or highly suspicious (BIRADS 5) for malignancy. Hence, all such lesions need to be subjected to biopsy for the definitive diagnosis of breast cancer. Image guided breast biopsy is an important tool for the diagnosis of breast cancer, and it is described in detail in the following chapter. Pathological analysis routinely consists of assessment of invasion, histopathological characterization and immunohistochemical analysis for ER, PR and HER2 receptor status. Uncommonly, classification of breast cancer into luminal and basal type, based on genetic expressions and molecular biology may be performed.[23] It is expensive, however, with growing trends for targeted treatment protocols; such analysis is likely to increase in future.

BREAST CANCER SCREENING

Cancer screening is aimed at detection of a cancer when it is small, asymptomatic, and early stage. Chances of cure are highest with such cancers. Primary purpose of any screening program that targets healthy population, is to reduce deaths from the disease and not just its early diagnosis. Mammography screening achieves this goal.

Mammography Screening

Mammography screening is the most widely used cancer screening modality in the world. It has been studied extensively and no other imaging modality has been subjected to as large scale and extensive research as mammography. There is level 1 evidence to suggest that mammography screening reduces the breast cancer mortality significantly in the screened population and it is cost effective. This evidence has primarily come from eight large randomized screening trials (RCTs) started in 1970s and early 80s in which half of women were invited to screening and the other half were not. These trials along with early benefits from these are given in **Table 1**.[24] Many of these trials are continuously analyzed. Health Insurance Plan (HIP) of New York was the first trial and it also included CBE along with mammography. Twin county trial consisted of two simultaneous trials conducted at Swedish counties of Ostergotland and Kopparberg. It is the largest screening trial for which longest follow-up is available. National Breast Screening Studies (NBSS) of Canada performed two separate screenings for women of age groups 40–49 and 50–75 years, respectively. These were similar to HIP. The data and long-term follow-up of these trials have been analyzed and debated several times to determine the exact quantum of benefits from mammography screening. Overall, mammography screening effectively reduces the overall breast cancer mortality by 28–45%.[25] Most recent meta-analysis for US preventive services task force (USPSTF) also confirmed that mammography screening significantly reduces breast cancer mortality in women aged 39–69 years.[26] A three decade follow-up of the twin county trial has shown that cost effectiveness and number

Table 1: Randomized controlled trials of mammography screening.

RCT	*Years of start*	*Number of women*	*Age group*	*Mammography Interval (Months)*	*Early mortality reduction*
HIP, New York, USA	1963	62,000	40–64	12	29%
Two county, Sweden	1978	162,981	40–74	24	37%
Malmo, Sweden	1976	42,000	45–69	18	18%
Stockholm, Sweden	1981	59,176	40–64	24	20%
Gothenburg, Sweden	1982	52,000	39–59	18	14%
Edinburg, UK	1978	45,130	45–64	12	16%
NBSS 1, Canada	1980	50,430	40–49	12	Nil
NBSS 2, Canada	1980	39,476	50–59	12	30%

of deaths prevented by screening improve over time.[27] Analysis of community screening programs, outside the RCTs, in developed countries of Europe, America and Australia have also shown that the implementation of screening mammography reduces breast cancer deaths by as high as 35–50%.[28-30] Reviews and data analysis from the RCTs have been performed several times and using variable methods. Some concluded that there is no benefit with screening mammography.[31] However, such reviews are few and their analysis is considered flawed by most experts.[32] Early detection is beneficial for diagnosis and treatment of any cancer and breast cancer is certainly not an exception to this logic.

There are some variations in the recommendations for mammography screening. American College of Radiology and American Cancer Society recommend mammography every year from 40 to 74 years of age. However, USPSTF recommends two yearly mammography in the 50–75 years age group.[33] In some European countries, mammography is offered every two years from 50 to 70 or 74 years. After the age of 75 years, mammography is not cost effective in term of number of lives saved as there are other competing causes of death.

Mammography screening must be organized and optimized for it to be successful. Mammography is the most regulated and legislated imaging modality in Europe and America. Licensing and accreditation of the facilities, regular QA programs, tests and training programs of radiographers and radiologists, reporting standards are regularly monitored and audit of the outcome performed.

Screening mammography is a high cost venture. At least 414 women must be screened for seven years to prevent one breast cancer death.[27] It has several other drawbacks as well, which frequently generates controversies. Most important among these are false positive mammograms and overdiagnosis. After a regular screening round, some women are recalled at the facility for additional imaging and/or biopsy. Although majority of them will not have a cancer, it causes anxiety in all of them and also increases the cost of screening. About half of women screened for 10 years have at least one recall and may be a biopsy.[34] Screening mammography has also led to manifold increase in the DCIS detection rates.[35] This leads to biopsy and surgery, including mastectomies, in women with mammographic lesions. This may be unnecessary in some women since all DCIS do not grow into invasive carcinoma and cancer would have never been diagnosed in their lifetime, had screening not been done. Overdiagnosis and overtreatment of such indolent breast cancers is considered a major disadvantage of mammographic screening and often criticized. However, since there is no way to predict which DCIS will progress into IDC, this limitation of mammographic screening should be accepted for overall benefits. Screening mammography also does not detect all breast cancers. Some aggressive cancers may get diagnosed in between two sequential rounds of the screening. These are called interval cancers and their incidence may range from 10–43% in different age groups.[36]

True benefits from screening mammography have also been debated. In recent years, improved breast cancer treatment with better chemo/hormonal therapy and targeted therapy have improved the survival and it is difficult to determine the absolute contribution of screening mammography in reducing overall breast cancer mortality.[37] It is estimated that mammography has contributed by two-third and adjuvant treatment by one-third in present day breast cancer mortality reduction in developed countries.[30]

MRI Screening

Familial breast cancers account for 10–15% of all breast cancers and about half of these patients are BRCA1 and BRCA2 mutations carriers. Cancer occurs in these women at younger age and hence, screening must be started much earlier. Mammographic breast density is high in young women and as expected, the performance of mammography is poor in detection of breast cancer in these women. Magnetic resonance imaging does not depend on breast density and it is the most sensitive tool for breast cancer detection in these women.[38,39] Breast MRI is recommended for screening of high risk women, if risk quantification is more than 25%.[39,40] Generally, annual breast MRI and mammograms are performed with six months gap between these two tests, resulting in imaging surveillance at every sixth months. Screening should be started at younger age of 25–30 years. Higher sensitivity of breast MRI comes with high false positive rates. This leads to higher number of benign breast biopsies, when compared with mammographic screening.

Ultrasound Screening

Ultrasound, as a sole modality, has never been used for breast cancer screening. However, it is routinely used to evaluate mammographically dense breasts. It can show mammographically occult breast cancers in asymptomatic women with negative mammograms. However, the detection rate is less than 1%.[41,42] A blinded screening trial (ACRIN 6666) comparing ultrasound and mammography for cancer detection in high-risk women found mammographic detection rate of 7.6 cancers per 1000 women screened. It increased to 11.8 cancers with combined mammography and ultrasound use.[43] Additional cancers detected on ultrasound were invasive and node negative and hence, these women actually benefited from ultrasound screening. However, ultrasound is not likely to be used for population screening because of its inability to visualize microcalcifications, operator dependency, time consuming nature, and high false-positive rates mostly from complicated cysts.[5]

Breast Cancer Screening in Developing Countries

Population-based screening mammography is expensive and resource intensive. Hence, it is not an immediate option in countries with limited resources. SBE and CBE are widely encouraged for early diagnosis, or more precisely, to decrease the proportion of advanced breast cancers at presentation. However, the only randomized controlled trial on SBE for breast cancer screening has shown no benefits.[44] Breast Health Global Initiative (BHGI), a nonprofit organization working in this area, has recommended the use of traditional 'triple test' assessment comprising CBE, imaging (diagnostic mammography or ultrasound) and FNAC or biopsy for early diagnosis of breast cancer in low resource countries.[45]

IMAGING FEATURES OF BREAST CANCER

Breast cancer is a group of malignant breast lesions. All breast cancers are believed to arise from the terminal duct lobular unit (TDLU). It is the distal most part of the ductal branching system which opens into the lobule of the gland and is the site of most active cellular proliferation. Breast cancers are classified into various pathological subtypes according to the WHO system. These cannot be determined on imaging. There are no imaging features which are specific to any pathological subtype of the breast cancer. Actually, imaging features are not even specific for cancer. However, some imaging characteristics are somewhat more commonly associated with particular type of cancer than others.

Preinvasive Breast Lesions

Preinvasive breast lesions include ductal carcinoma in situ (DCIS) and lobular carcinoma *in situ* (LCIS). Ductal carcinoma *in situ* is the precursor of invasive breast cancer. On the other hand, most LCIS do not become invasive and this entity is hence, regarded as a high-risk condition rather than a true cancer.

Ductal Carcinoma *in Situ*

Ductal carcinoma *in situ* lies along a spectrum of preinvasive lesions of the breast tissue, with histologic progression from ADH to DCIS and then to the invasive ductal carcinoma (IDC). The pathological classification of DCIS is based on the nuclear grade of the tumor cells (low, intermediate, or high), the architectural pattern of tumor growth (solid, papillary, micropapillary, or cribriform), and the presence or absence of comedonecrosis.

Ductal carcinoma *in situ* are usually small but can grow to large size and become symptomatic. Presentations of DCIS include mammographically detected mass or calcification, palpable mass, Paget's disease, or an incidental finding on breast biopsy. DCIS is a precursor of invasive ductal carcinoma however, only some of DCIS develop into invasive cancer, while other remains indolent forever. True incidence of IDC in patients with DCIS is unknown. On mammography, DCIS is characterized by microcalcifications, usually of linear branching type **(Fig. 12)**. Less commonly, DCIS can produce a mass

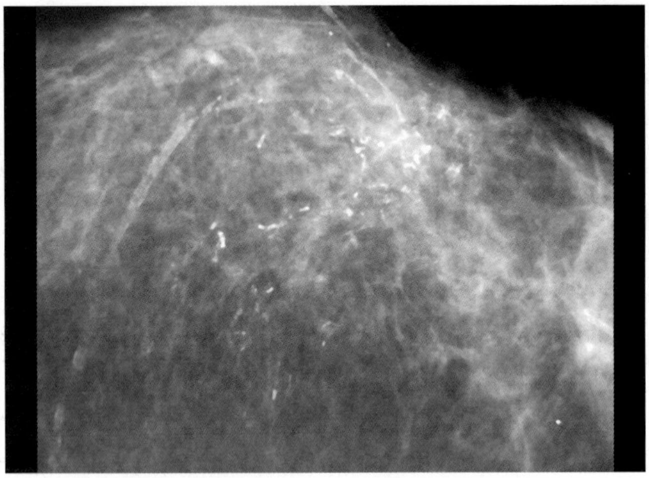

Fig. 12: DCIS: Mammogram shows pleomorphic, linear branching microcalcifications in the ductal orientation.

with ill-defined or lobulated borders, with or without calcification. Ultrasound is unsuitable to detect microcalcifications. Associated soft tissue component and architectural distortion may be appreciated as a hypoechoic mass on ultrasound. Calcifications are not seen on MRI; however, overall sensitivity of MRI is higher than mammography in detection of DCIS.[46] Both can detect DCIS not detected by the other modality. On MRI, about half of DCIS are seen as enhancing masses. Others show nonmass-like enhancement or no enhancement.[47] All three patterns of enhancement curves can be seen with DCIS. DCIS is treated with mastectomy or breast conservation treatment (lumpectomy followed by radiotherapy). Since, it is not an invasive cancer, axillary dissection is not required.

Lobular Carcinoma *in Situ*

Atypical lobular hyperplasia (ALH) and lobular carcinoma *in situ* (LCIS) are not true cancers but are high-risk or premalignant conditions. These are asymptomatic and incidentally detected on breast biopsy. Pathologically, these represent spectrum of atypical proliferation of loosely cohesive cells in the TDLU. LCIS is often multifocal and bilateral. It does not cause any clinical or imaging abnormalities. About one-third of the women with LCIS ultimately develop invasive lobular carcinoma (ILC) in the same or contra lateral breast.[1] Management options include close surveillance or prophylactic mastectomy.

Invasive Breast Cancer

Invasive or infiltrating ductal carcinoma (IDC) is the most common histologic subtype of breast cancer. It is designated not otherwise specified (NOS) as it is not categorized into specific types, such as medullary, lobular, mucinous, etc. In SEER data of National Cancer Institute, IDC (NOS) constituted 83.9% of all invasive breast cancers.[48] Others include invasive lobular (7.4%), medullary (3.1%), mucinous (2.3%) and Paget's disease (1%). Other subtypes accounted for less than 1% each. Depending on the nuclear pleomorphism and mitotic activity, all breast cancers are also graded histologically into grade 1 (well differentiated), grade 2 (moderately differentiated) and grade 3 (poorly differentiated). This tumor grading has prognostic significance.

Invasive Ductal Carcinoma

Invasive ductal carcinoma (NOS) is undifferentiated and has no specific histologic pattern. Desmoplastic reaction is common in IDC which accounts for its most common presentation of hard mass on palpation and spiculated mass on mammography **(Fig. 13A)**. It may also be seen as malignant calcifications, architectural distortion or any combination of these. Ultrasound and MRI show a mass having one or more malignant features described in previous chapter **(Figs. 13B and C)**. Irregular mass with rim enhancement or heterogeneous internal enhancement is the most common MR appearance of IDC.

Invasive Lobular Carcinoma

Invasive lobular carcinoma (ILC) is the second most common invasive breast cancer and a large number of these are multicentric or bilateral. Histologically, these show diffuse tumor foci invading the stroma. They spread in the form of a single file (line) of noncohesive malignant cells through intervening normal parenchyma, instead of a well formed mass. They do not evoke desmoplastic response. Because of these features, ILC are difficult to detect on clinical examination, mammography and even on MRI. Clinical presentation may be of an ill-defined mass, nonspecific induration or tenderness. Other patients may present with symptoms from distant metastases. Mammographically, asymmetric breast density is the most common finding. Other mammographic findings include spiculated or ill-defined mass, or a normal mammogram.[1] Calcifications are distinctly rare. Ultrasound is useful to detect underlying mass in an asymmetric density seen on mammography. MRI does not detect all ILC; however, it is more accurate than mammography for detection of ILC.[49] On MRI, ILC are most commonly seen as enhancing mass with variable contrast enhancement patterns. Others may be seen as diffuse area of enhancement that is difficult to differentiate from normal parenchyma.[50] MRI detects

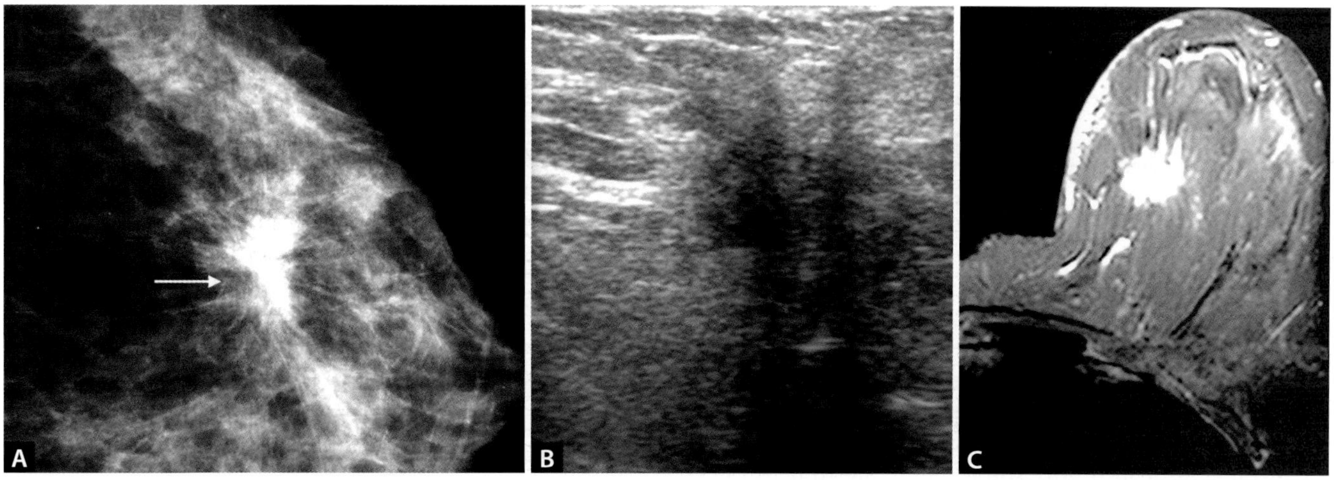

Figs. 13A to C: IDC: (A) Mammogram shows a high density, irregular, spiculated mass (arrow); (B) Ultrasound shows a hypoechoic, irregular, spiculated mass with distal acoustic shadowing; (C) Contrast-enhanced T1-weighted MRI scan of another woman shows a spiculated, intensely enhancing mass.

additional foci of cancer in more than 50% of patients diagnosed with ILC.[51]

Medullary Carcinoma

Medullary carcinoma is usually seen in younger age. It is a rapidly growing tumor and often large in size when detected.[1] Histologically, they are high grade tumors with abundant infiltration by inflammatory cells. Desmoplastic process is uncommon. The prognosis is poor as most have early lymphovascular invasion, lymph node and distant metastases. On mammography, a well defined or ill-defined mass, without spiculations or calcification is seen **(Fig. 14)**. On ultrasound, they are hypoechoic, well-circumscribed or lobulated. Distal acoustic enhancement may be seen. These ultrasound features often simulate benign masses.

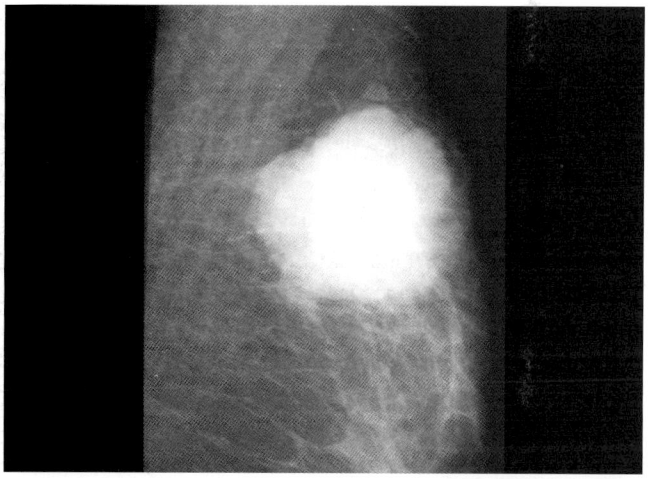

Fig. 14: Medullary carcinoma: Mammogram shows a round mass with lobulated, partially indistinct margin.

Mucinous Carcinoma

Mucinous (or colloid) carcinoma is a well-differentiated, slow growing tumor. It is generally seen in older women and has a better prognosis. It is characterized by abundant mucin production. Usual mammographic finding is of a low density mass with ill-defined or microlobulated margins **(Fig. 15)**. Calcification or desmoplastic reaction is uncommon. Ultrasound shows a well-defined, hypoechoic mass with microlobulated margins and posterior acoustic enhancement in some.[52] Rarely, it is seen as a complex cystic-solid mass on ultrasound. MR features are similar to mammography; however, the contrast enhancement pattern is frequently of benign type. Unlike most other breast cancers, mucinous cancer can demonstrate high signal intensity on T2-weighted images.

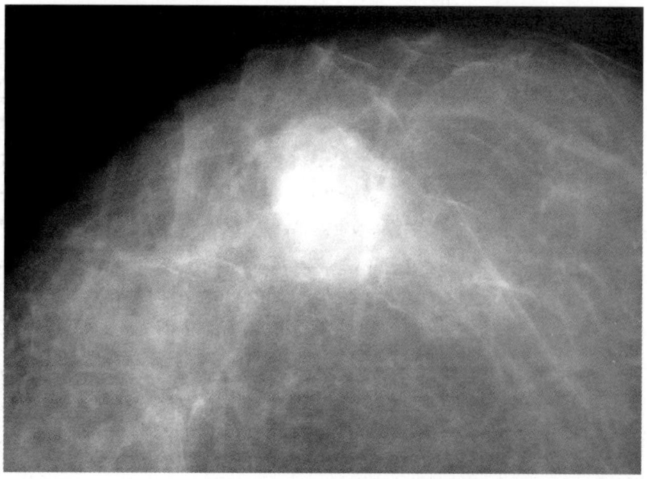

Fig. 15: Mucinous carcinoma: Mammogram shows an ill-defined, low density round mass.

Tubular Carcinoma

Tubular carcinoma is a rare well-differentiated invasive carcinoma which demonstrates poorly formed ductal structures. About one-third of these are multicentric and bilateral. They are slow growing and have better prognosis. On mammography, a small spiculated or ill-defined mass is usually seen.[1] Uncommonly, calcifications may be seen. There are no specific MR features.

Papillary Carcinoma

Papillary carcinoma is seen with advanced age. There is villous epithelial proliferation that eventually fills the ductal lumen. Papillary carcinoma can develop as an intracystic lesion, although it is likely that the cyst represents a secondarily dilated duct.[1] These are slow growing and do not have desmoplastic reaction. On mammography, papillary carcinomas are seen as well circumscribed masses because of their cystic nature. This is the only breast cancer which is commonly cystic on ultrasound; usual sonographic appearance is a complex solid-cystic mass or intracystic tumor with multiple fronds projecting into the lumen of the cyst **(Figs. 16A and B)**.

Triple Negative Breast Cancer

Triple negative breast cancer (TNBC) is the term used for invasive breast cancers of any histologic type which are negative for ER, PR and HER2 receptors on immunohistochemistry. These are now separately classified because of their distinct clinical, radiological and prognostic features. TNBC are characterized by occurrence at younger age, aggressive behavior, early metastases and are refractory to treatment. Triple negative breast cancer are also difficult to diagnose on mammography. These are usually seen as well-defined or ill-defined masses. Spiculations and calcifications are rare. Hence, these may be difficult to differentiate from benign masses.[53] On ultrasound also, these have benign features of circumscribed masses with frequent posterior acoustic enhancement. MRI is most useful their diagnosis. These are seen as mass or nonmass for like lesions with intense type 3 enhancement curve. These are frequently multicentric and are well demonstrated on MRI.[54]

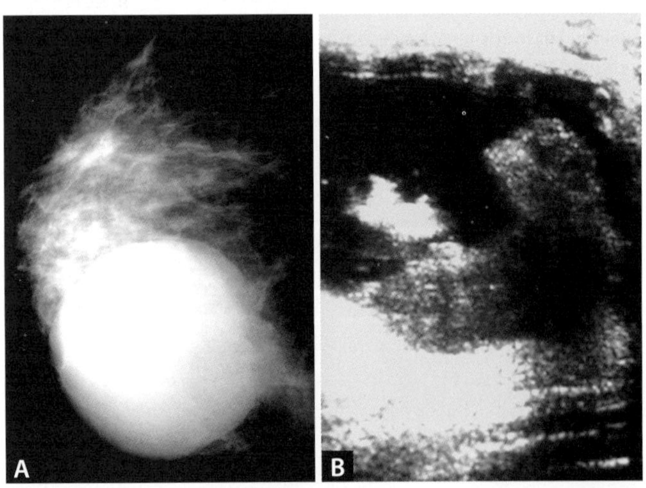

Figs. 16A and B: Intracystic papillary carcinoma: (A) Mammogram shows a large well-defined mass with some distortion of the posterior margin; (B) Ultrasound shows a complex cyst with irregular solid component projecting intraluminally from the posterior wall.

STAGING AND TREATMENT OF BREAST CANCER

Breast cancer is staged according to the TNM staging system of AJCC. An overview of the staging system is given in **Table 2**. After the diagnosis of breast cancer, clinical staging is performed based on both clinical as well as imaging findings. The clinical stage is denoted as cTNM. For metastatic work-up, chest X-ray, ultrasound of the abdomen and bone scan is sufficient in stage I and II tumors. Computed tomography or PET is recommended for stage III cancers. Surgery is the primary treatment of breast cancer in resectable patients and this includes breast conservation therapy or mastectomy. After surgery, a final or pathological stage is assigned and it is denoted as pTNM. Final stage of the disease and other risk factors are considered to decide for adjuvant (postoperative) treatment with radiotherapy, chemotherapy and hormone therapy.[55]

Preoperative Breast Imaging

Surgery, either mastectomy or breast conservation surgery (BCS), is the mainstay of breast cancer treatment. Preoperative mammography, sometimes complemented with MRI, is important in patient selection for breast conservation. If mastectomy is planned, the role of mammography is limited to evaluation of the contralateral breast.

Main purpose of mammographic evaluation prior to BCS is to assess the extent and size of the tumor and to exclude multiple cancers. Breast cancers that are larger than 5 cm are generally not treated with BCT. Mammography detects additional cancer in about 10% patients **(Fig. 17)**. Multifocal (located in same quadrant or within 4 cm) tumor can be considered for BCT. However, the extent of surgical resection will be wide and may not achieve the

Table 2: Overview of staging of breast cancer.

Tis	*Carcinoma in situ*		*T-stage*		
T1	< 2 cm		T1a: Up to 5 mm T1b: Up to 1 cm T1c: Up to 2 cm		
T2	2–5 cm				
T3	>5 cm				
T4	Chest wall/skin involvement		T4a: Chest wall invasion T4b: Skin invasion T4c: Both chest wall and skin invasion T4d: Inflammatory breast cancer		
N-stage					
N0 N1 N2 N3	No LN pathy Mobile level I,II axillary LN Fixed level I,II axillary LN or internal mammary LN Level III axillary, internal mammary, supraclavicular LN		N2a: Fixed or matted level I/II axillary LN N2b: Internal mammary LN without axillary LN N3a: Level III axillary LN N3b: Both axillary and internal mammary LN N3c: Supraclavicular LN		
M-stage					
M0 M2	No distant metastases Distant metastases				
Stage Groups					
	N0	N1	N2	N3	M1
T1	IA	IIA	IIIA	IIIC	IV
T2	IIA	IIB	IIIA	IIIC	IV
T3	IIB	IIIA	IIIA	IIIC	IV
T4	IIIB	IIIB	IIIB	IIIC	IV

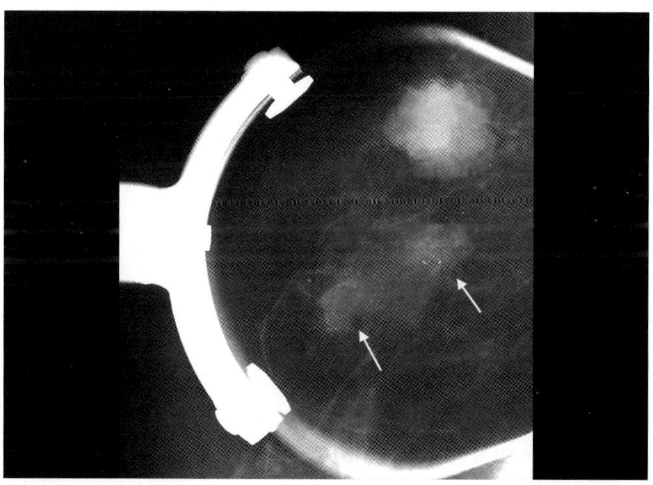

Fig. 17: Multifocal breast cancer: Spot compression mammogram shows two small ill-defined masses with microcalcifications (arrows) adjacent to an already diagnosed microlobulated index tumor.

desired cosmesis. Also, women with multiple cancers have propensity to develop more cancers after the surgery resulting in treatment failure.[56] Multicentric (located in different quadrant) cancer is an absolute contraindication for BCT. Presence of suspicious calcification in and around the tumor should be carefully assessed. Clustered calcifications away from the tumor may indicate skip tumor areas. Invasive carcinoma frequently has associated component of DCIS which might extend along the ducts over a large area away from the tumor. This is known as extensive intraductal component (EIC). It is a frequent cause of positive margins in the surgically resected specimen.[57] Presence of linear branching calcifications extending from the primary tumor is a strong indicator of presence of EIC. Indeed, tumor may be more extensive than suspected on mammography. Many DCIS, especially the noncomedo type, are not always calcified and hence, not appreciated on mammography.[58,59] Contralateral breast must also be carefully evaluated on mammography to detect additional cancer, if any.

Preoperative mammographic evaluation is unsatisfactory in women with dense glandular breasts. Breast MRI is superior to mammography for preoperative evaluation of both breasts.[60] Routine preoperative MRI in women already diagnosed with breast cancer detects mammographically occult ipsilateral multicentric cancer in 20% women and contralateral synchronous cancer in 3–5% women[61,62] **(Fig. 18)**. Extent of surgical resection may

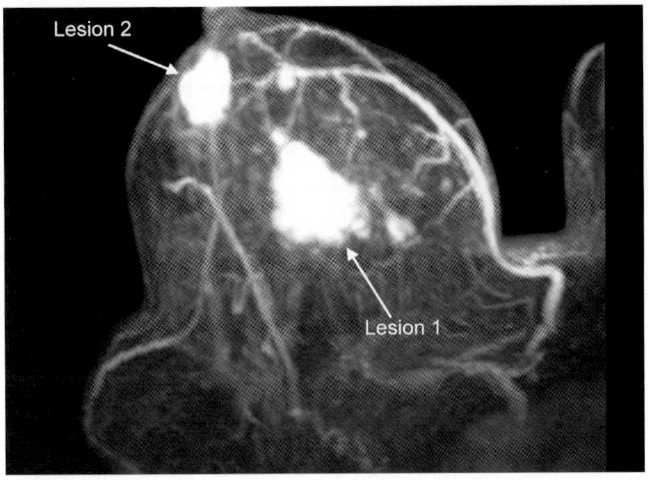

Fig. 18: Mutlicentric breast cancer: MIP image of a contrast-enhanced MRI shows a subareolar cancer in addition to an already diagnosed index tumor.

be increased if multifocal cancer is detected. Similarly, BCS is converted into mastectomy if multicentric cancer is detected on MRI. Women in whom contralateral breast cancer is detected by MRI are also benefited as both cancers can be treated at the same time. Overall, preoperative breast MRI changes surgical management in 13% women; however, it may be due to false-positive MRI finding in half of these.[62] False-positive MRI, which results in unnecessarily more extensive breast surgery or mastectomy, is an important area of concern.[55] MRI is also useful for assessment of pectoralis muscle in patients with deep seated tumors, as this cannot be evaluated on mammography.[63] Abnormal enhancement of the muscle is a specific indicator of muscle invasion, loss of fat plane is unreliable to diagnose muscle invasion. Breast MRI is the most preferred modality for preoperative breast evaluation, but not yet considered mandatory. Mammography remains the basic requirement of preoperative evaluation of the breasts before BCT.

Breast Conservation Therapy

Breast conservation therapy (BCT) consists of wide local excision of the tumor with negative margins (breast conservation surgery or BCS), followed by radiotherapy of the breast. It retains the affected breast and hence, has a cosmetic and psychological advantage over mastectomy. BCT has low recurrence rates and its overall survival rates are comparable with those of mastectomy.[64,65] BCT is the preferred treatment modality for breast cancer in carefully selected patients. It is generally offered for the tumors up to 5 cm in size (T2). Ratio of tumor size and breast size is also considered. Patients with small breasts and large tumor size may be unsuitable, although some use neoadjuvant chemotherapy (NACT) for reduction of tumor size and to make it suitable for BCT. Large or multicentric tumors, pregnancy and collagen vascular diseases are contraindications for BCT. Finally, patient's preference is also taken into account while selecting BCT or mastectomy.

Mastectomy

Mastectomy is the traditional surgery for breast cancer. It is performed in patients with contraindications for BCS or in those who opt for it. Total mastectomy removes skin, nipple-areola and fascia anterior to pectoralis major along with the entire breast parenchyma. When combined with simultaneous axillary dissection, it is termed as modified radical mastectomy (MRM). Reconstruction of the breast for cosmetic purpose is also possible after skin sparing mastectomy. It is done in same sitting using myocutaneous flaps with intact vascular pedicle, such as transverse rectus abdominis muscle (TRAM) flap or latissimus dorsi (LD) flap to create a breast mound. Silicone or saline implants are also used for breast reconstruction.

Management of Axilla

Axillary lymph node involvement is the most important prognostic indicator for breast cancer survival. Axillary lymph node dissection is a standard part of surgery, whether BCS or mastectomy, in patients with invasive breast cancer. It is performed in same sitting. It is both therapeutic as well as a staging procedure used to determine pathological N-stage. Axillary lymph nodes are divided into three groups: level I, II and III which are located lateral, posterior and medial to pectoralis minor muscle respectively. Level III axillary nodes are also called as infraclavicular nodes. Axillary lymph node dissection however, is a morbid procedure. It causes disruption of major lymphatic channels and fibrosis, which may be further complicated by axillary irradiation. This leads to various problems like lymphedema of the arm, sensory loss and restricted shoulder movements. This may be reported by up to one-third of the patients after axillary dissection and it is difficult to treat.

Sentinel lymph node mapping and biopsy is a technique which helps to avoid axillary dissection in some of the patients who do not have axillary lymph nodes on clinical examination. In this, a radiotracer (^{99m}Tc labeled sulphur colloid) along with a blue dye is injected in or around the tumor. The lymphatics draining the tumor take up this dye with the radiotracer and course towards axilla. Intraoperatively, the first lymph node (sentinel node) draining the tumor is identified using a hand held gamma camera sensor. This lymph node is removed and analyzed with frozen sections. If it is free of tumor, it is presumed that axillary nodes are also uninvolved and axillary dissection is avoided. If the sentinel node is involved, axillary dissection is performed to pathologically stage the axilla. False negative rates of sentinel lymph node biopsy are low and its ability to correctly stage the axilla is comparable with direct axillary dissection.[66]

However, sentinel lymph node biopsy is a time consuming and expensive procedure. The sentinel lymph node may not be localized in some patients and axillary dissection has to be performed. Allergic reactions to dye may also occur. Preoperative ultrasound evaluation of the axilla in patients selected for sentinel lymph node biopsy is fast gaining acceptance. It helps to avoid sentinel lymph node biopsy in some patients. A detailed description of ultrasound and ultrasound guided FNAC of axillary lymph nodes is given in next chapter.

Perioperative Breast Imaging

If the tumor is nonpalpable, preoperative mammography or ultrasound guided hookwire localization is required before the BCS. These procedures are described in detail in next chapter. Although uncommonly utilized, intraoperative ultrasound is useful to assess gross tumor margins more accurately. Use of intraoperative ultrasound results in better margins of resection and lowers the chances of residual tumor.[67] Immediate postoperative mammograms may sometimes be requested but these are difficult to perform and interpret. The breast is tender and adequate compression cannot be given to the recently operated breast. The postoperative hematoma and edema also makes the mammographic interpretation difficult and residual mass, if any, cannot be reliably excluded on mammogram. Diagnosis of residual breast cancer after surgery and the decision to re-excise is primarily based on detection of positive tumor margins on postoperative histopathology and not on imaging. However, postoperative MRI after positive margins is desirable, if it was not performed preoperatively. It can identify gross residual tumor or unsuspected multifocal cancer and aid in planning of the extent of re-excision or to consider mastectomy.[68]

Adjuvant Treatment

Adjuvant (postoperative) treatment is given to treat microscopic disease. Radiotherapy (RT) is used for local adjuvant treatment and is aimed at eradicating microscopic residual disease if any, so that chances of local recurrence are reduced. Systemic adjuvant treatment consists of chemotherapy or hormonal therapy, or more commonly, both. It is aimed at eradicating circulating micrometastases, if any, so that chances of distant metastatic recurrence are reduced.

Radiotherapy is given to all patients after BCS. Generally, a total of 45–50 Gy of whole breast RT is given, which may be followed by 10–16 Gy of boost RT to the tumor bed. After mastectomy, radiotherapy is given to patients with adverse factors only, such as those with large tumors, close margins, lymphovascular invasion and axillary lymph node involvement.[55]

Chemotherapy and hormonal therapy is the mainstay of systemic adjuvant treatment of breast cancer. All tumors of >1 cm require adjuvant chemotherapy. Standard anthracycline based chemotherapy includes combination of 5 FU and cyclophosphamide along with doxorubicin or epirubicin (FAC). Newer regimes also incorporate taxanes.[55] Hormonal therapy with tamoxifen, an estrogen analogue, is given for five years to all patients with ER positive breast cancers. It significantly improves the disease free survival and overall survival in these patients.[69] HER2 overexpression by the breast cancer is associated with high risk of early recurrence and resistance to standard chemotherapy and hormonal therapy. Trastuzumab (Herceptin) is a monoclonal antibody against HER2 protein. It improves survival in HER2 positive patients when given for one year alongwith or after adjuvant chemotherapy.[55]

ADVANCED BREAST CANCER

Locally Advanced Breast Cancer

This term is used for breast cancers which are inoperable at presentation but without distant metastases **(Fig. 19)**. It includes all T4 tumors (invasion of chest wall, skin or both), those with fixed axillary lymph nodes and inflammatory breast cancer. Some breast surgeons also include large (>5 cm) but operable tumors in LABC. The pretreatment work up includes core biopsy for the diagnosis and receptors status, as well as metastatic work-up to exclude distant metastases. These patients are treated with neoadjuvant chemotherapy with the intention of down staging the tumor and making it operable.

Inflammatory Breast Cancer

Inflammatory breast cancer (IBC) is an aggressive form of invasive duct carcinoma and accounts for 2.5% of all breast cancers.[70] Histopathologically, there is diffuse infiltration and obstruction of dermal lymphatics. It is characterized

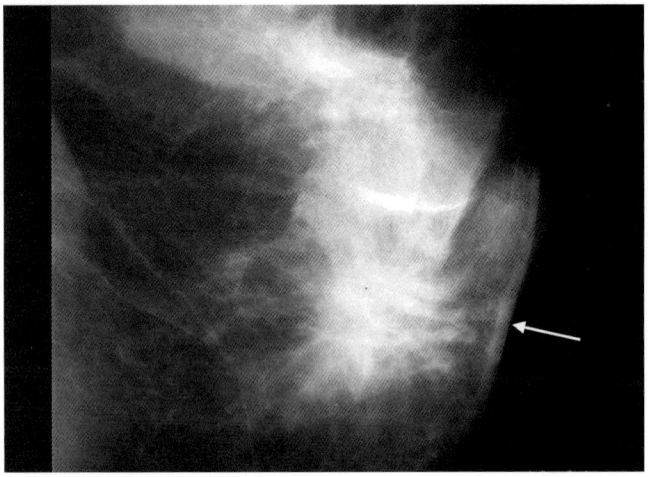

Fig. 19: Locally advanced breast cancer: Mammogram shows a large, infiltrating, spiculated mass with thickening and retraction of overlying skin (arrow).

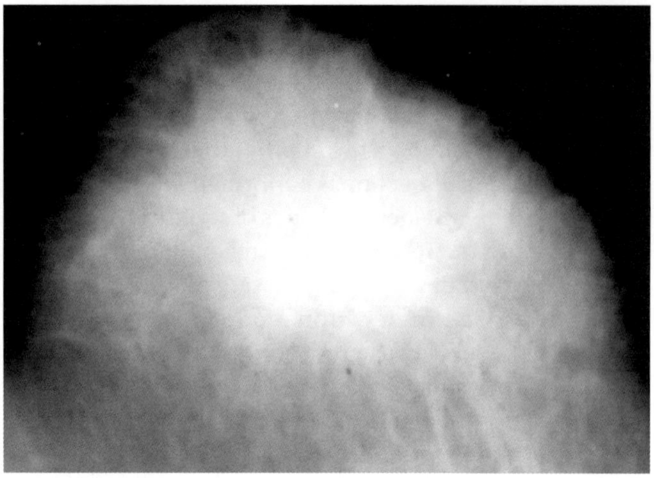

Fig. 20: Inflammatory breast cancer: Mammogram shows diffuse increase in breast density along with thickening of trabeculi and skin. No definite mass is seen.

by younger age, rapid progression, early metastases and high mortality. Patients present with enlarged painful breast with diffuse erythema, edema, sloughing and ulceration of the skin over the breast. Clinical presentation mimics acute mastitis and the tumor, though sizable, is difficult to palpate.

The diagnosis is usually clinical. Mammography is difficult to perform in a painful breast. Usual mammographic finding is of a dense edematous breast with skin and trabecular thickening **(Fig. 20)**. Hence, primary tumor is uncommonly identified on mammography. Ultrasound is useful and it locates the primary tumor in more than half of patients.[71] It is seen as irregular or lobulated mass on ultrasound, usually large in size. Multicentric and diffusely infiltrating IBC is not localized on ultrasound. MRI and PET-CT are most accurate for evaluation of primary tumor as well as distant metastases.[70] MRI detects primary tumor in nearly all patients with IBC. The primary tumor is most often seen as single or multiple confluent masses with type three enhancement curve and skin involvement in majority of lesions.[72]

Neoadjuvant Chemotherapy

Locally advanced breast cancer (LABC) is the most common indication for neoadjuvant chemotherapy (NACT). Patients with large but operable tumors who desire for BCT instead of mastectomy are also offered NACT. Traditional anthracycline based chemotherapy is used. Majority of tumors respond well to chemotherapy and become operable. Mastectomy or BCT is offered after successful NACT, depending on the residual tumor size. About 15–25% patients achieve pathological complete response with NACT.[55]

Response to NACT is assessed with clinical examination and imaging. Mammography, ultrasound, MRI and PET have been used for response assessment. Prediction of response after initial one or two cycles is important. Good responders can be continued with NACT while it can be stopped in nonresponders. For this purpose, combination of mammography and ultrasound is more useful than clinical assessment alone.[73] PET-CT is also useful but MRI is most accurate.[74] Response to NACT is depicted by decrease in size and degree of contrast enhancement on MRI and decrease in SUV on PET.[75,76] Diffusion weighted MRI evaluation is also useful to predict the response to NACT. Low pretreatment ADC values and high post one cycle ADC values predict good response.[77,78] After completion of NACT, residual tumor size is an important consideration for surgical planning. Both MRI and PET are highly sensitive to identify patients with pathological complete response, however, with moderate specificity.[79] Hence, all patients need to be operated, even if complete resolution of tumor is seen on post NACT scans.

It is prudent to insert a metallic marker clip in these tumors before starting NACT. If the tumor disappears on mammography, the marker clip is used to perform preoperative hook wire localization and surgery.[80]

Metastatic Breast Cancer

Metastatic breast cancer (MBC) is stage IV breast cancer that has spread beyond the breast, regional lymph nodes and chest wall. Common sites of breast cancer metastases are liver, bone, lung, distant lymph nodes and brain, however, any organ in the body can be involved. ER/PR positive cancers tend to spread to bones while receptor negative cancers are more likely to involve the liver.

Lobular carcinoma has propensity for serosal deposits involving pleura and peritoneum. Most women with MBC have already diagnosed breast cancer but small proportion of women present with symptoms of metastatic disease and breast cancer is subsequently diagnosed during work up for the occult primary cancer. Symptoms of MBC are nonspecific and include cough or dyspnea, bone pain, lymphadenopathy or fatigue. Radionuclide bone scan, ultrasound, CT scan and PET-CT are usually employed for diagnosis and response assessment of breast cancer metastases.

Bone is the most common site of distant metastases from breast cancer.[81] These preferentially involve spine and pelvis but any bone can be involved. Radionuclide bone scan is the primary imaging modality for detection of bone metastases.[82] It is sensitive, however, specificity is moderate. False positive bone scan results are mainly from degenerative and inflammatory lesions. X-ray or CT-evaluation is required if metastases cannot be differentiated reliably from these on bone scan. On radiographs, bone metastases of breast cancer may be osteolytic, sclerotic or mixed **(Fig. 21)**. PET is equally sensitive as bone scan but more specific. MRI is the most accurate modality for diagnosis of bone metastases from breast cancer.[83] However, it is not used as a routine investigation. PET-CT and MRI are also useful to monitor treatment response of the bone metastases. Liver metastases are hypovascular and hence, are identified on venous phase of the CT **(Fig. 22)**. Some liver metastases may be small and diffuse giving rise to the appearance of pseudo-cirrhosis.[84] Ascites and shrinkage of liver outline may also be present with these. Focal fatty infiltration is common in patients on chemo- or hormonal therapy. This may also be misinterpreted as metastases on CT. Lack of mass effect and preserved liver architecture is helpful to differentiate these from metastases. MRI is required in equivocal cases. Lung metastases from breast cancer are usually seen as single or multiple nodules. Breast cancer is a common cause of unusual manifestation of lung metastases, such as lymphangitis carcinomatosis, airspace consolidation and endobronchial metastases.[85] Breast cancer is the most common cause of ovarian metastases and its clinicoradiological features are usually similar to that of primary ovarian cancer. Breast cancer metastases to small bowel produce long segment strictures and those to stomach may produce antral narrowing similar to linitis plastica.

Clinical and imaging diagnosis of metastases is usually unequivocal in majority. In others, biopsy may be required. If not already known, ER, PR and HER2 status must be determined on biopsy; either from the breast lesion or the metastatic site.

Treatment of MBC is aimed at palliation and prolonging survival. Patients with less extensive metastases, fewer symptoms and late development of metastases perform better. Chemotherapy is the mainstay of treatment in all MBC. Patients with ER/PR positive MBC are initially treated with hormonal therapy. HER2 positive patients benefit from trastuzumab. Other treatment options include bisphosponates (pamidronate ro zolidronic acid) to patients with bone metastases and radiotherapy to brain metastases and painful bone metastases.[55]

Occult Primary Breast Cancer

Mammography is standard part of work-up in women presenting with metastatic adenocarcinoma anywhere

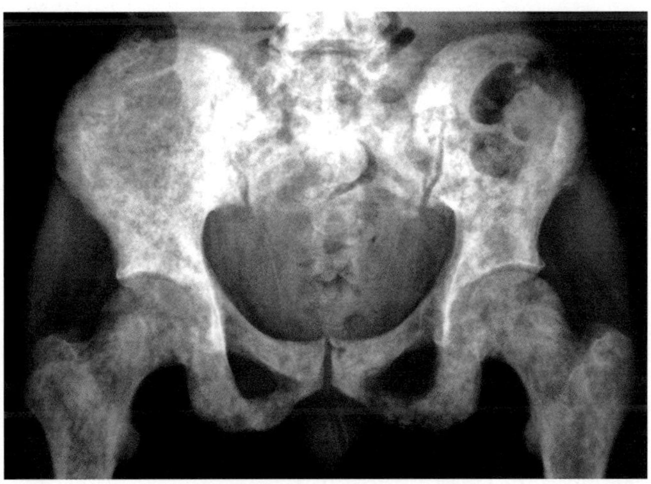

Fig. 21: Bone metastases: Pelvic radiograph shows multiple diffuse lytic and sclerotic metastases in all pelvic bones and both proximal femoral bones.

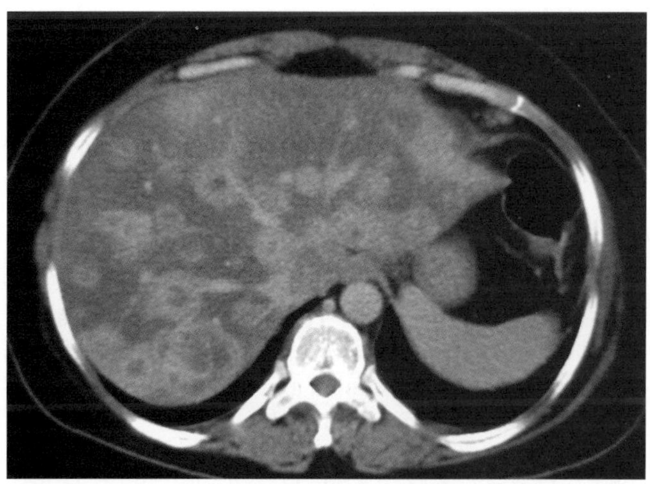

Fig. 22: Liver metastases: Multiple liver metastases are seen. In spite of being hypovascular, they appear hyperdense in the background of fatty infiltration of the liver.

from an occult primary site. Women presenting with axillary lymphadenopathy only are also evaluated with mammography. If clinical examination and mammography are negative but axillary lymph node biopsy is suspicious of primary breast carcinoma, MRI is recommended. MRI identifies mammographically occult breast cancer in majority of these patients.[86] If primary is not identified, the patients are treated with mastectomy or radiotherapy.

POST-TREATMENT BREAST IMAGING AND FOLLOW-UP

Patients treated with BCT need regular bilateral mammographic follow-up. It is primarily required to detect recurrence of cancer in treated or contralateral breast. A baseline mammogram of the treated breast should be obtained at three to six months after completion of the radiotherapy. This mammogram is compared with future serial mammograms. Patients treated with mastectomy are also followed with annual screening mammograms of the contralateral breast, as they are at high-risk for development of second breast cancer. Breast cancer survivors have three-fold increased risk of developing contralateral breast cancer. They are also at some risk for endometrial cancer, lung cancer, angiosarcoma and acute leukemia.[55]

Several postsurgery and radiotherapy changes are apparent on follow-up mammogram after the BCT. A fibrous scar develops at the operative site which is seen as an ill-defined density with adjacent architectural distortion **(Fig. 23)**. Metallic surgical clips, intended to mark the tumor bed for boost radiation, may also be seen at the operative site. Sometimes, the fibrous scar has spiculated appearance and appears suspicious **(Fig. 24)**. However, it does not have high central density as in the case of a true mass. Exact site of the lumpectomy site must be known and review of preoperative mammograms is useful to determine this. Careful evaluation of scar in both CC and MLO views is also helpful. Unlike solid mass, the scar is a two dimensional structure formed by approximation and fibrosis of the lumpectomy cavity. Hence, size and density of the scar varies considerably in two views. Seroma is a fluid collection that is frequently seen at the operative site. It is usually seen as a round or oval mass which may persist for up to two years[87] **(Figs. 25A and B)**. It can be reliably characterized on ultrasound. Debris or septations are commonly seen in seroma and this should not lead to ultrasound guided aspiration.

Radiation changes are seen in the form of diffuse thickening of trabeculi and skin; alongwith an overall increase in breast density **(Fig. 23)**. The changes are similar to breast edema due to any other cause. The severity of these changes varies in different patients, however; these remain stable or decrease on follow-up mammograms. Some distortion of the breast outline is also apparent after BCT and the degree of this depends on the extent of the excision. In addition to above changes, there may be development of benign calcifications in post-treatment mammograms. The causes include fat necrosis, sutural calcifications and radiation induced dystrophic calcifications **(Figs. 23 and 25)**.

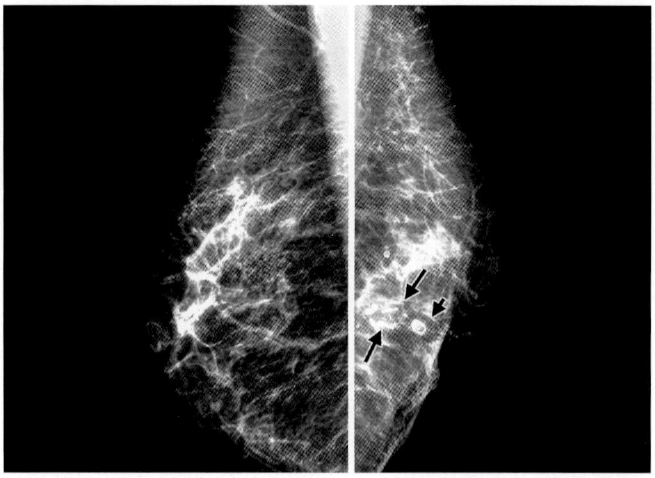

Fig. 23: Post-treatment bilateral mammogram: Left breast shows fibrous scar at the operative site (arrows) with metallic clips placed intraoperatively to mark the tumor bed. Foci of dystrophic calcifications and fat necrosis (arrowhead) are seen. There is diffuse trabecular thickening and increased density of the left breast, secondary to radiotherapy, as compared to the right breast.

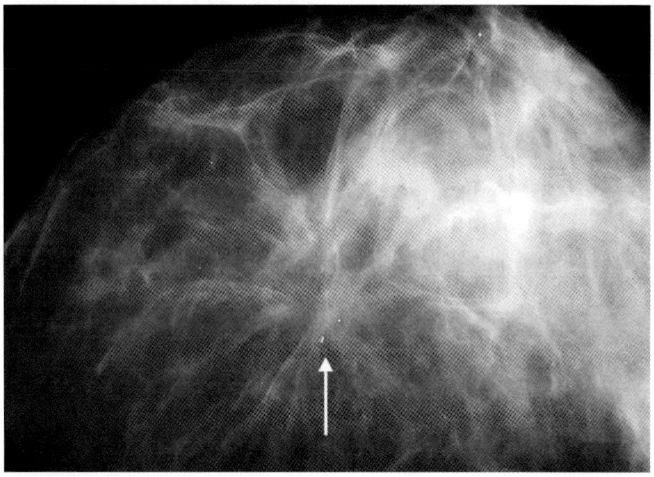

Fig. 24: Postoperative scar: Mammogram shows a spiculated scar (arrow) at the operative site. This is an expected finding and does not suggest recurrence.

Local recurrence at operative site occurs rarely and is seen in 2–7% of women followed for 10 years.[55]

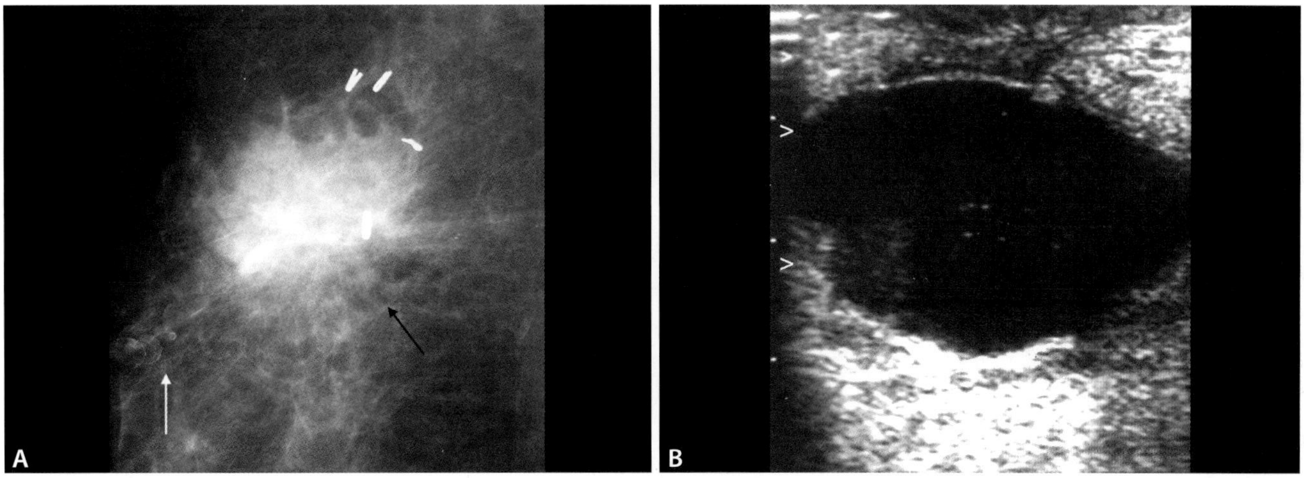

Figs. 25A and B: Seroma: (A) Mammogram shows an irregular mass at operative site (black arrow). Adjacent sutural calcification is also seen (white arrow); (B) Ultrasound shows it as a cyst with internal debris.

Younger age at diagnosis, high grade and ER/PR negative breast tumors are more prone for local recurrence. Mammography is the primary modality of follow-up and detection of recurrences. However, its accuracy is lowered because of distortion of breast parenchyma by the post-treatment changes. Majority of local recurrences are detected by mammography or by patients themselves on breast self-examination, while few are diagnosed on clinical breast examination.[88] The recurrences are most often seen as increased density and/or size of the scar, new mass or suspicious calcifications on mammography. Their morphology is usually similar to that of the primary breast cancers in these patients and hence, review of the preoperative mammogram is useful for the detection of a recurrence.[89] MRI and percutaneous biopsy should be promptly obtained in case of suspicion of recurrence on mammogram.[90]

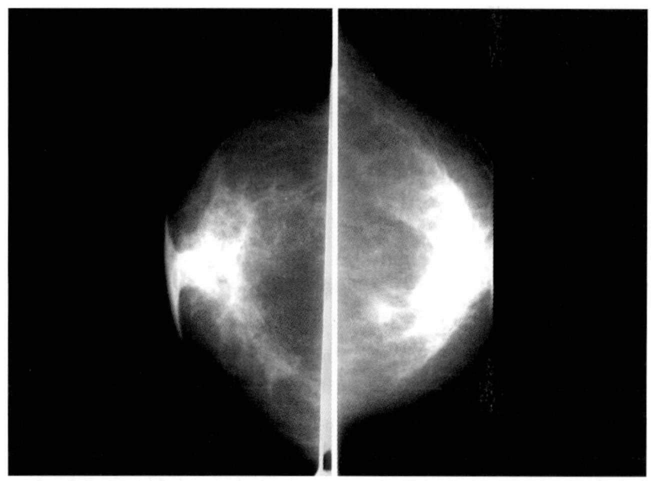

Fig. 26: Paget's disease: Mammography shows nipple and areolar thickening in right breast with a subareolar mass.

MISCELLANEOUS MALIGNANT LESIONS OF THE BREAST

Paget's Disease

In this condition, a centrally located ductal carcinoma grows along the ducts into the nipple with eczematous changes at the summit of the nipple (pagetoid changes). Nipple changes range from mild itching to extensive scaling, erosions and ulceration in the nipple. Erosion extends to the areola and may cover a larger area of the skin. Fifty percent patients have a palpable mass. This disease is usually unilateral.

On mammography and ultrasound, underlying malignant mass or calcification is seen in most patients **(Fig. 26)**. Nipple and areolar thickening is also present.[91] Malignant type of calcifications may be seen extending from deeper carcinoma to the nipple. MRI is recommended if mammogram is equivocal or normal.

Phyllodes Tumor

Phyllodes tumor (or phylloid tumor) is a stromal tumor composed of the epithelial elements of connective tissue stroma, similar to fibroadenoma. Its malignant potential is variable from completely benign lesion to fully malignant sarcoma. Most are benign. Clinically, they present as round multinodular palpable tumors like fibroadenomas. On mammography and ultrasound, they are well-defined and indistinguishable from fibroadenomas **(Figs. 27A and B)**. Occasionally, cystic component may be seen on ultrasound.[2] Phyllodes tumors are treated with wide local

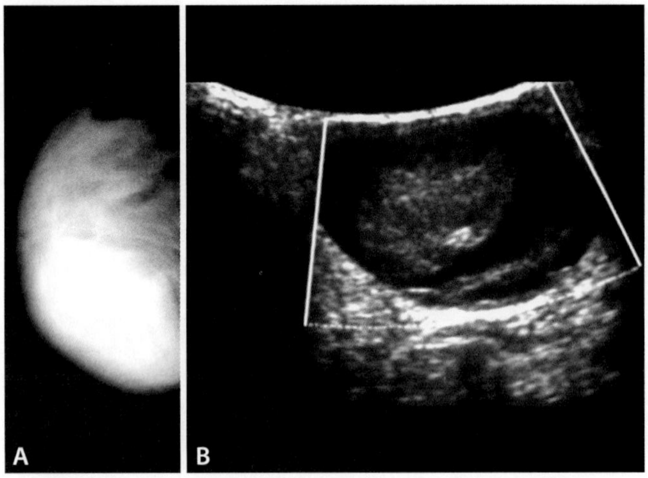

Figs. 27A and B: Phyllodes tumor: (A) Mammogram shows a dense breast with an ill-defined large mass in the inferior aspect of the breast; (B) Ultrasound shows a large hypoechoic mass with fluid clefts.

excision. Approximately 20% of these recur, if margins of excision are inadequate.[55] As malignant phyllodes tumor is a sarcoma, axillary lymphadenopathy is less common and lung metastases are more common.

Sarcoma

Sarcomas are rare tumors of breast. These include phyllodes tumor, angiosarcoma, fibrosarcoma, liposarcoma, malignant fibrous histiocytoma and osterosarcoma. Their imaging features are nonspecific. Angiosarcoma is an aggressive, rapidly growing vascular tumor of young age. Presentation is similar to IBC. Magnetic resonance imaging shows a strongly enhancing, ill-defined, infiltrative mass with skin invasion. It metastasizes early and is rapidly fatal.

Metastases to Breast

Metastases to breast from other sites are rare. Usual primary sites of cancer are melanoma, lung, stomach, cervix and ovary. Clinically, there are multiple palpable masses. In one-third of these patients, this maybe the first manifestation of an occult primary cancer.[55] Another form of metastasis to breast is cross lymphatic spread from the contralateral advanced breast cancer causing localized thickening of the skin.

On mammography, metastases to breast are usually multiple and bilateral **(Fig. 28)**. These are seen as well-defined or ill-defined masses. Spiculations and calcifications are not commonly seen.

Although rare, lymphoma can secondarily involve the breasts. Large axillary lymph nodes are usually associated.

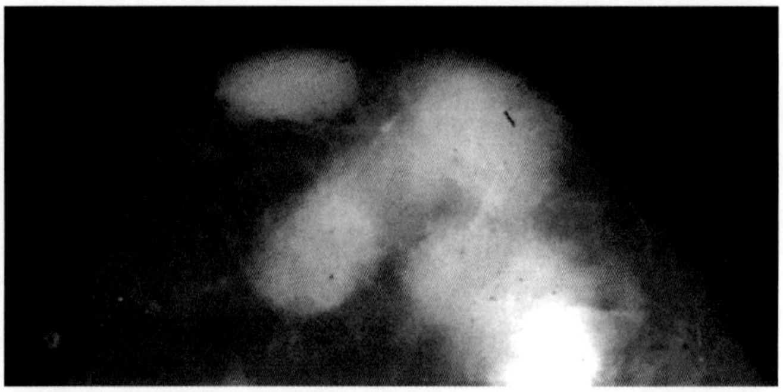

Fig. 28: Metastases: Mammogram shows multiple variable sized metastatic masses in the breast from primary carcinoma of the nasopharynx.

Mammographically, single or multiple ill-defined masses are seen. Spiculations and calcification are not seen. Lymphomatous lesion may also be seen as increased asymmetric density in the breast. Ultrasound shows single or multiple nonspecific solid masses.[92]

Male Breast Cancer

Male breast cancer accounts for about 1% of all breast cancers. Breast cancer in male patients occurs at an older age group than in female patients. Risk factors include Klinefelter syndrome, BRCA mutation carriers, undescended testis, chronic liver disease and alcoholism.[55] Gynecomastia is not a risk factor. Clinically, there is a painless hard mass. Nipple discharge or ulceration is seen in 25% cases. Mammographic features of male breast cancer are similar to those in females.[93] Pathology and treatment of male breast cancer is also same. Due to small size of the breast, BCT is not performed.

REFERENCES

1. Kopans DB. Histologic, pathologic and imaging correlation. In: Kopans DB (Ed). Breast Imaging. Lippincott, Williams and Wilkins. Philadelphia, 3rd edn; 2007. pp. 783-888.
2. Goel NB, Knight TE, Pandey S, et al. Fibrous lesions of the breast: imaging-pathologic correlation. Radiographics. 2005;25:1547-59.
3. Liberman L, Morris E, Lee MJY, et al. Breast lesions detected on MR imaging: features positive predictive value. AJR. 2002;179:171-8.
4. Venta LA, Kim JP, Pelloski CE, et al. Management of complex breast cysts. AJR. 1999;173:1331-6.
5. Berg WA, Sechtin AG, Marques H, Zhang Z. Cystic breast masses and ACRIN 6666 experience. Radiol Clin N Am. 2010;48:931-87.
6. Lau S, Kuchenmeister I, Stachs A, et al. Pathologic nipple discharge: surgery is imperative in post menopausal women. Ann Surg Oncol. 2005;12:546-51.

7. Orel SG, Dougherty CS, Reynolds C, et al. MR imaging in patients with nipple discharge: initial experience. Radiology. 2000;216:248-54.
8. Neal L, Tortorelli CL, Nasser A. Clinicians guide to imaging and pathologic findings in benign breast disease. Mayo Clin Proc. 2010;85:274-9.
9. Ciatto S, Morrone D, Catarazi S, et al. Radial scars of the breast. Review of 38 consecutive mammography diagnoses. Radiology. 1993;187:757-60.
10. Hargaden GC, Yeh ED, Georgian-Smith D, et al. Analysis of mammographic and sonographic features of pseudoangiomatous stromal hyperplasia. AJR. 2008;191:359-63.
11. Wong KT, Tse GM, Yang WT. Ultrasound and MR imaging of diabetic mastopathy. Clin Radiol. 2002;57:730-5.
12. Hook GW, Ikeda DM. Treatment of breast abscess with US guided percutaneous needle drainage without indwelling catheter placement. Radiology. 1999;213:579-82.
13. Sabate JM, Clotet M, Gomez A, et al. Radiologic evaluation of uncommon and reactive breast disorders. Radiographics. 2005;24:411-24.
14. Sakr AA, Fawzy RK, Fadaly G, Baky MA, et al. Mammographic and sonographic features of tuberculous mastitis. Eur J Radiol. 2004;51:54-60.
15. Oh K, Kim JH, Kook SH. Imaging of tuberculous disease involving breast. Eur Radiol. 1998;8:1475-80.
16. Memis A, Bilgen I, Ustun EE, et al. Granulomatous mastitis: imaging features with histopathological correlation. Clin Radiol 2001;57:1001-6.
17. Herborn CU, Marincek B, Erfmann D, et al. Breast augmentation and reconstructive surgery: MR imaging of implant rupture and malignancy. Eur Radiol. 2002;12:2198-206.
18. Debruhl ND, Gorczyca DP, Ahn CY, et al. Silicone breast implants: US evaluation. Radiology. 1993;189:95-8.
19. Caskey CI, Berg WA, Hamper UM, et al. Imaging spectrum of extracapsular silicone: Correlation of US, MR imaging, mammographic and histopathologic findings. Radiographics. 1999;19:S39-51.
20. Indian Council of Medical Research: National Cancer Registry Programme. Consolidated report of population based cancer registries 2001-2004. Available at www.icmr.nic.in/ncrp.
21. Boyd NF, Guo H, Martin LJ, et al. Mammographic density and the risk and detection of breast cancer. N Engl J Med. 2007;356:227.
22. Brose MS, Rebbeck TR, Catzone KA, et al. Cancer risk estimates for BRCA1 mutation carriers identified in a risk evaluation program. J Natl Cancer Inst. 2002;94:1365.
23. Perou CM, Sorlie T, Eisen MB, et al. Molecular portraits of human breast tumours. Nature. 2000;406:747-52.
24. Kopans DB. Screening mammography. In: Kopans DB (Ed). Breast Imaging. Lippincott, Wiliams and Wilkins. Philadelphia, 3rd edn; 2007. pp. 121-90.
25. Tabar I, Vitak B, Chen HH, et al. Beyond randomized controlled trials: organized mammographic screening substantially reduces breast cancer mortality. Cancer. 2001;91:1724-31.
26. Nelson HD, Tyne K, Naik A, et al. Screening for breast cancer: an update for the US Preventive Services Task Force. Ann Intern Med. 2009;151:727-42.
27. Tabar L, Vitak B, Chen THH, et al. Swedish two county trial: impact of mammographic screening on breast cancer mortality during 3 decades. Radiology. 2010;260: 658-63.
28. Paci E, Duffy SW, Giorgi D, et al. Quantification of the effect of mammographic screening on fatal breast cancers: the Florence programme 1990-96. Br J Cancer. 2002;87:65-9.
29. Elmore JG, Armstrong K, Lehman CD, Fletcher SW. Screening for breast cancer. JAMA. 2005;293:1245-56.
30. Schopper D, de Wolf C. How effective are breast cancer screening programmes by mammography? Review of current evidence. Eur J Cancer. 2009;45:1916-23.
31. Gotzsche PC, Olsen O. Is screening for breast cancer with mammography justifiable? Lancet. 2000;355:129-34.
32. Bock K, Borisch B, Cawson J, et al. Effect of population based screening on breast cancer mortality. Lancet. 2011; 378:1775-6.
33. Cologne N, Petitti DB, DeWitt TG, et al. Screening for breast cancer: US preventive services task force recommendation statement. Ann Intern Med. 2009;151:716-26.
34. Elmore JG, Barton MB, Moceri VM, et al. Ten year risk of false positive screening mammograms and clinical breast examinations. N Engl J Med. 1998;338:1089.
35. Ernster VL, Ballard BR, Barlow WE, et al. Detection of ductal carcinoma in situ in women undergoing screening mammography. J Natl Cancer Inst. 2002;94:1546-54.
36. Bordas P, Jonsson H, Nystom L, Lenner P. Interval cancer incidence and episode sensitivity in Norrbotten mammography screening programme. Sweden. J Med Screen. 2009;16:39.
37. Kalager M, Zelen M, Langmark F, et al. Effect of screening mammography on breast cancer mortality in Norway. N Engl J Med. 2010;163:1203-10.
38. Warner E, Plewes DB, Hill KA, et al. Surveillance of BRCA1 and BRCA2 mutation carriers with magnetic resonance imaging, ultrasound, mammography and clinical breast examination. JAMA. 2004;292:1317-25.
39. Gilbert FJ, Warren RM, Kwan-Lin G, et al. Cancers in BRCA1 and BRCA2 carriers and in women with high risk for breast cancer: MR imaging and mammographic features. Radiology. 2009;254:358-68.
40. Saslow D, Boetes C, Burke W, et al. American Cancer Society guidelines for breast screening with MRI as an adjunct to mammography. CA Cancer J Clin. 2007; 57:75-89.
41. Corsetti V, Houssami N, Ferrari A, et al. Breast screening with ultrasound in women with mammography negative dense breasts: evidence on incremental cancer detection, false positives and associated cost. Eur J Cancer. 2004;4: 539-44.
42. Nothaker M, Duda V, Hahn M, et al. Early detection of breast cancer: benefits and risks of supplemental breast ultrasound in asymptomatic women with mammographically dense breasts. A systematic review. BMC Cancer. 2009;9:335.

43. Berg WA, Blume JD, Cormac JB, et al. Combined screening with ultrasound and mammography vs mammography only in women at elevated risk of breast cancer. JAMA. 2008;299:2151-63.
44. Thomas DB, Gao DL, Ray RM, et al. Randomized trial of breast self-examination in Shanghai: final results. J Natl Cancer Inst. 2002:94:1445-57.
45. Anderson BO, Shyyan R, Eniu A, et al. Breast cancer in limited resources countries: an overview of the Breast Health Global Initiative 2005 guidelines. Breast J. 2006;12:S3-15.
46. Kuhl CK, Shrading S, Bieling HB, et al. MRI for diagnosis of pure ductal carcinoma in situ: a prospective observational study. Lancet. 2007;370:485-92.
47. Morris EA: Breast cancer imaging with MRI. RCNA. 2002; 40:443-86.
48. Stalsberg H, Thomas DB. Age distribution of histologic types of breast cancer. Int J Cancer. 1993;54:1-7.
49. Weinstein SP, Orel SG, Heller R, et al. MR imaging of the breast in patients with invasive lobular carcinoma. AJR. 2001;176:399-406.
50. Yeh ED, Slanetz PJ, Edmister WB, et al. Invasive lobular carcinoma: spectrum of enhancement and morphology on magnetic resonance imaging. Breast J. 2003;9:13-8.
51. Liberman L, Morris EA, Dershaw DD, et al. MR imaging of ipsilateral breast in women with percutaneously proved breast cancer. AJR. 2003;180:901-10.
52. Lam WW, Chu WC, Tse GM, et al. Sonographic appearance of mucinous carcinoma of the breast. AJR. 2004;182:1069-74.
53. Yang WT, Dryden M, Broglio K, et al. Mammographic features of triple negative primary breast cancers in young premenopausal women. Breast Cancer Res Treat. 2008; 111:405-10.
54. Dogan BE, Gonzalez-Angulo AM, Gilcreae M, et al. Multimodality imaging of triple negative breast tumours with mammography, ultrasound and MRI. AJR. 2010;194: 1160-6.
55. Burstein HJ, Harris JR, Morrow M. Malignant tumours of the breast. In: DeVita VT, Lawrence TS, Rosenberg SA (Eds) Cancer: Principles and Practice of Oncology. 9th edn. Wolter Kluwer, Lippincott, Williams and Wilkins. Philadelphia; 2011. pp. 1401-46.
56. Kutz JM, Jacquemier J, Amalric R, et al. Breast conserving therapy for macroscopically multiple cancers. Ann Surg. 1991;212:38-44.
57. Kurniawan ED, Wong MH, Windle I, et al. Predictors of surgical margin status in breast conserving surgery within a breast screening program. Ann Surg Oncol. 2008; 15(9):2542-9.
58. Holland R, Hendricks J, Verbee K, et al. Extent, distribution and mammographic/histologic correlations of breast ductal carcinoma in situ. Lancet. 1990;335:519.
59. Umetsu T, Yuen S, Kasami M, et al. Comparison of magnetic resonance imaging, multidetector row computed tomography, ultrasonography and mammography for tumour extension of breast cancer. Breast Cancer Res Treat. 2008;112:461-74.
60. Berg WA, Gutlerrez L, NessAlver MS, et al. Diagnostic accuracy of mammography, clinical examination, US, and MR imaging in preoperative assessment of breast cancer. Radiology. 2004;233:830-49.
61. Lehman CD, Gatsonis C, Kuhl CK, et al. MRI evaluation of contralateral breast in women with recently diagnosed breast cancer. N Engl J Med. 2007;356:1295-303.
62. Plana MN, Carreira C, Muriel A, et al. Magnetic resonance imaging in preoperative assessment of patients with primary breast cancer: systematic review of diagnostic accuracy and meta-analysis. Eur Radiol. 2012;22:26-38.
63. Morris EA, Schwartz LH, Drotman MB, et al. Evaluation of pectoralis major muscle in patients with posterior breast tumours on breast MR images: early experience. Radiology. 2000;214:67-72.
64. Veronesi U, Cascinelli N, Mariani L, et al. Twenty year follow up of a randomized study comparing breast conserving surgery with radical mastectomy for early breast cancer. N Engl J Med. 2002;347:1227-32.
65. Fisher B, Anderson S, Bryant J, et al. Twenty year follow up of a randomized trial comparing total mastectomy, lumpectomy, and lumpectomy plus irradiation for the treatment of invasive breast cancer. N Engl J Med. 2002; 347:1233-7.
66. Mansel RE, Fellowfield L, Kissin M, et al. Randomized multicenter trial of sentinel node biopsy versus standard axillary treatment in operable breast cancer: the ALMANC trial. J Natl Cancer Inst. 2006;98:599.
67. Moore MM, Whitney LA, Cerilli I, et al. Intraoperative ultrasound is associated with clear lumpectomy margins for palpable infiltrating ductal breast cancer. Ann Surg. 2001;233:761-8.
68. Lee JM, Orel SG, Czerniecki BJ, Solin LJ, Schnall MD. MRI before re-excision surgery in patients with breast cancer. AJR. 2004;182:473-80.
69. Early breast cancer trialist group. Effects of chemotherapy and hormonal therapy for early breast cancer on recurrence and 15-year survival: an overview of the randomized trials. Lancet. 2005;365:1687.
70. Robertson FM, Bondy M, Yang W, et al. Inflammatory breast cancer: the disease, the biology, the treatment. CA Cancer J Clin. 2010;60:351-75.
71. Le-Petraus H, Uppendahl L, Stafford J. Sonographic features of inflammatory breast cancer. Semin Roentgenol. 2011;46:275-9.
72. Le-Petross H, Cristofanilli M, Carkaci S, et al. MRI features of inflammatory breast cancer. AJR. 2011;197:W769-6.
73. Peintinger F, Kuerer HM, Anderson K, et al. Combination of mammography and sonography is useful in predicting tumor response in breast cancer patients after neoadjuvant chemotherapy. Ann Surg Oncol. 2006;13:1443-9.
74. Choi JH, Lim HI, Lee SK, et al. The role of PET CT to evaluate the response to neoadjuvant chemotherapy in advanced breast cancer: comparison with ultrasonography and magnetic resonance imaging. J Surg Oncol. 2009;4:1-6.

75. Yeh E, Slanetz P, Kopans DB, et al. Prospective comparison of mammography, sonography and MRI in patients undergoing neoadjuvant chemotherapy for palpable breast cancer. AJR. 2006;184:868-77.
76. Wang Y, Zhang C, Liu J, Huang G. Is ^{18}F-FDG PET accurate to predict neoadjuvant therapy response in breast cancer? a meta-analysis. Breast Cancer Res Treat. 2012;131:357-69.
77. Park SH, Moon WK, Cho N, et al. Diffusion weighted MRI imaging: pretreatment prediction of response to neoadjuvant chemotherapy in patients with breast cancer. Radiology. 2010;257:56-63.
78. Fangberget A, Nilsen LB, Hole KH, et al. Neoadjuvant chemotherapy in breast cancer response evaluation and prediction of response to treatment using dynamic contrast enhanced and diffusion weighted MRI imaging. Eur Radiol. 2011;21:1188-99.
79. Park SH, Moon WK, Cho N, et al. Comparison of diffusion weighted MR imaging and FDG PET/CT to predict pathological complete response to neoadjuvant chemotherapy in patients with breast cancer. Eur Radiol. 2012;22:18-25.
80. Nadeem R, Chagla LS, Harris O, et al. Tumour localization with a metal coil before administration of neoadjuvant chemotherapy. Breast. 2005;14:403-7.
81. Hamaoka T, Madewell JE, Podoloff DA, et al. Bone imaging in metastatic breast cancer. J Clin Oncol. 2004; 22:2942-53.
82. Costelloe CM, Rohren EM, Madewell JE, et al. Imaging bone metastases in breast cancer: techniques and recommendations for diagnosis. Lancet Oncol. 2009; 10:606-14.
83. Liu T, Cheng T, Xu W, et al. A meta-analysis of ^{18}FDG-PET, MRI and bone scintigraphy for diagnosis of bone metastases in patients with breast cancer. Skeletal Radiol. 2011;40:523-32.
84. Brookes M, MacVicar D, Husband J. Metastatic carcinoma of the breast: the appearances of metastatic spread to abdomen and pelvis as demonstrated by CT. Br J Radiol. 2007;80:284-92.
85. Jung JM, Kim HH, Park SH, et al. Thoracic manifestations of breast cancer and its therapy. Radiographics. 2004; 24:1269-85.
86. Olson JA Jr, Morris EA, Van Zee KA, et al. Magnetic resonance imaging facilitates breast conservation for occult breast cancer. Ann Surg Oncol. 2000;7:411-5.
87. Brenner RJ, Pfaff JM. Mammographic features after conservation therapy for malignant breast disease: serial findings standardized by regression analysis. AJR. 1996; 167:171-8.
88. Montgomery DA, Krupa K, Cooke TG. Follow-up in breast cancer: Does routine clinical examination improve outcome? A systematic review of literature. Br J Cancer. 2007;97: 1632-41.
89. Gunhan-Bilgen I, Oktay A. Mammographic features of local recurrence after conserving surgery and radiation therapy: comparison with that of the primary tumour. Acta Radiologica. 2007;48:390-7.
90. Dao TH, Rahmount A, Campana F, et al. Tumour recurrence versus fibrosis in the irradiated breast: differentiation with dynamic gadolinium contrast enhanced MR imaging. Radiology. 1993;187:751-5.
91. Gunhan-Bilgen I, Oktay A. Paget's disease of breast. Clinical, mammographic, sonographic and pathologic findings in 52 cases. Eur J Radiol. 2006;60:256-63.
92. Yang WT, Lane DL, Le-Petross HT, et al. Breast lymphoma: imaging findings in 32 tumours. Radiology. 2007;245:692-702.
93. Dershaw DD, Borgen PI, Deutch BM, et al. Mammographic findings in men with breast cancer. AJR. 1993;160:267-70.

CHAPTER 208

Breast Interventions

Smriti Hari, Sanjay Thulkar

INTRODUCTION

Breast interventions primarily comprise of biopsy of the suspicious breast lesions so as to obtain accurate pathological diagnosis. Breast biopsy is the mainstay of definitive and timely diagnosis of breast cancer and its treatment. Preoperative wire localization has both diagnostic and therapeutic applications. Ablative procedures for breast cancer treatment are still considered investigational.

BREAST BIOPSY

Mammography and other breast imaging modalities can detect nonpalpable breast abnormalities which may represent breast cancer and hence, image-guided procedure for their sampling is mandatory for timely diagnosis of the breast cancer. The techniques and instrumentation of these procedures have evolved over years with improvement in accuracy of the diagnosis. Although image-guided breast biopsy is performed primarily for imaging detected nonpalpable breast lesions and palpable lesions are subjected to manually guided percutaneous biopsy. However, even in palpable lesions, image-guided biopsy should be done as it improves the accuracy of diagnosis.[1] Special skills beyond those acquired in general radiology are required for radiologist who performs these procedures. As several of these techniques involve special equipment, assistance of an experienced technologist is desirable. The radiologist must have the basic knowledge of diagnostic breast imaging, limitations of imaging, cancer risks and treatment options for breast cancer so as to select appropriate lesion and the biopsy technique. This knowledge is also required for meaningful discussion with the patient, referring clinician and the pathologist. After the biopsy, follow-up of patient to diagnose and treat any complications is mandatory. Pathology results of the biopsy must also be correlated with baseline imaging findings to ensure that these are concordant with imaging.

BREAST BIOPSY TECHNIQUES

Surgical Biopsy

Surgical excision biopsy is the most accurate technique for the diagnosis of breast cancer as it completely removes the abnormality and hence, there is no chance of sampling error. For nonpalpable lesions, this is performed after preoperative hookwire localization, so as to guide the surgeon to the exact location of the lesion. Surgical excision biopsy is the gold standard of breast cancer diagnosis and it is still routinely performed at few centers. However, the procedure is invasive and disfiguring. This disadvantage is especially important considering the fact that majority of breast biopsy results are benign and resultant scar and disfigurement of breast may be unacceptable to these patients. Even in patients with malignant diagnosis, this leads to two surgical procedure, one diagnostic and then another for treatment, leading to increased patient anxiety and cost of the treatment.

Percutaneous needle biopsy expedites the breast cancer diagnosis and is cost-effective. With modern biopsy techniques and instrumentations, the diagnostic accuracy is also nearly comparable to that of surgical excision biopsy. Percutaneous biopsy can be a fine needle aspiration cytology or core biopsy.

Fine Needle Aspiration Cytology

Fine needle aspiration cytology (FNAC) is a simple, less expensive and less traumatic technique. Generally, a 20–22 G needle is used to make multiple excursions in the lesion and fluid containing dislodged cells is aspirated to make smears for cytological diagnosis. Results of FNAC are immediately available. However, FNAC has several limitations. It requires the availability of an experienced breast cytologist who can establish the adequacy of aspirated sample on site and also interpret it accurately. It has high insufficiency and false-negative rates. A negative FNAC cannot reliably exclude the presence of breast cancer. FNAC is especially unsuitable for nonpalpable breast lesions as up to 34% of FNAC samples may be insufficient for diagnosis.[2] Insufficiency rate is much higher for calcifications than for masses. FNAC gives cytological diagnosis only, i.e. it cannot differentiate *in situ* from invasive cancer. Modern treatment protocols often require immunohistochemical analysis for hormonal receptor status and this is difficult to obtain on FNAC. Benign FNAC results are often nonspecific and definitive diagnosis of a benign condition is rarely made. This affects the radiologic–pathologic correlation and may be a limitation in deciding further management. Diagnosis of papillary lesions is inaccurate on FNAC and it cannot differentiate fibroadenoma from phyllodes tumor.[3] FNAC results are frequently interpreted as atypical or suspicious only, which leads to a second more invasive biopsy. This leads to increased cost and delay in the diagnosis of breast cancer.[4] Although extremely rare, false-positive results on FNAC leading to an unnecessary surgery are also known. Because of these disadvantages, breast FNAC is less commonly employed at present and most breast care centers do not rely on breast FNAC to make the management decisions.

Core Needle Biopsy

Several of the disadvantages of FNAC have been addressed by percutaneous core needle biopsy (CNB) of the breast, and this has become the standard of care for biopsy of breast lesions; whether palpable or not. Accuracy of CNB is better than FNAC and it allows cellular and architectural evaluation. With this, specific diagnosis of benign and malignant conditions can be made. The cores are also suitable for immunohistochemical and genetic analysis. However, CNB of breast is more traumatic, more expensive and requires higher skills to perform when compared with FNAC. Results of CNB are not immediately available and take few days at least.

Breast CNB is commonly performed using spring loaded automated core biopsy needles, commonly known as biopsy guns. Earlier smaller gauge (16 or 18 G) biopsy needles were used, but these suffered from lower sample sufficiency rates. Introduction of 14 G core needles significantly improved the accuracy of breast CNB[5] **(Figs. 1A and B)**. False-negative rates of 14 G CNB range from 0 to 9%.[6] Long throw (2 cm), 14 G caliber is the standard size of biopsy guns used for breast CNB and smaller gauge biopsy guns which are routinely used in other body parts are not recommended for breast CNB. Typically, a minimum of 4–5 cores are obtained during a breast CNB.

Vacuum-assisted Biopsy

Directional vacuum-assisted biopsy (VAB) of breast is a modified and improved technique of large core breast biopsy. It was introduced in late 1990s.[7] It can be used under ultrasound, stereotactic or MR guidance. The VAB device consists of a main unit housing the vacuum generator and the operating console and disposable biopsy probe (needle) attached to it **(Fig. 2)**. The probe consists of an outer cannula with a sample notch and an inner cutting cannula. When activated, a vacuum is applied which sucks and holds the tissue at the sample notch. Next, the inner cannula advances with high speed rotation to cut and enclose the tissue core within. Without removing the

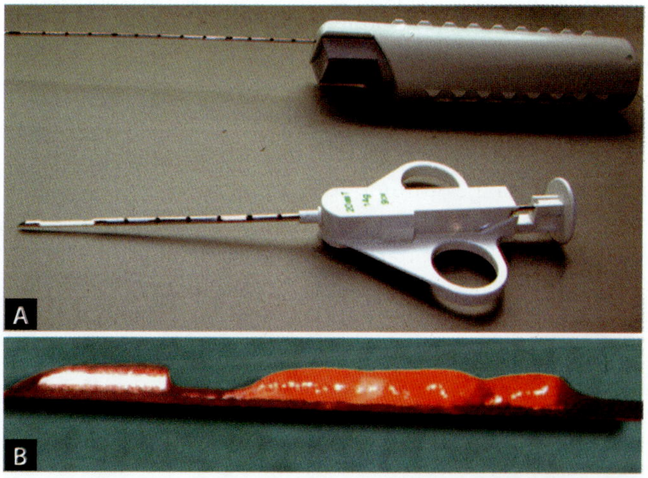

Figs. 1A and B: Core needle biopsy of breast: (A) 14 G biopsy guns; (B) Open sample notch of the biopsy gun showing harvested tissue specimen.

probe from the breast, the cut sample is then transported outside to the sample chamber using activation of another vacuum. Vacuum is also used to aspirate the oozed blood preventing hematoma formation. Saline irrigation or instillation of local anesthetic at the biopsy site through the probe is also possible during the procedure. All the steps of VAB are automated and contiguous multiple cores of tissue can be harvested without removing the probe from the breast. Some of the currently available VAB devices include Mammotome® (previously Johnson and Johnson; now Devicor, Cincinnati, USA), Eviva® and Atec® (previously Suros; now Hologic, Beford, USA) and Encore® (previously Senorx; now Bard, Tempe, USA). Thick calibre (11–7 G) probes are typically used in VAB.

Advantages of VAB

Major advantage of the VAB is that it allows fast acquisition of multiple, large and contiguous tissue cores with single needle insertion into the breast. When compared with CNB using biopsy guns, a 10-fold greater tissue volume is obtained per core.[8] The probe can be rotated 360 degrees within the lesion facilitating removal of tissue around the probe. Small lesions can be completely removed thereby eliminating the chances of sampling errors. Unlike biopsy guns, very accurate needle placement is not mandatory for VAB. The sample notch can be directed to the lesion and it can pull the lesion into the notch. This feature is particularly valuable when a small cluster of calcification is targeted. In VAB, the probe is placed close to or within the lesion before actually taking the biopsy and hence chance of cutting needle sliding by the side of the lesion, rather than penetrating it, is also eliminated. After the first few cores obtained during CNB, subsequent cores tend to contain tissue as well as clots. This does not happen in VAB as the oozing blood is continuously removed and all the harvested cores are of good quality.

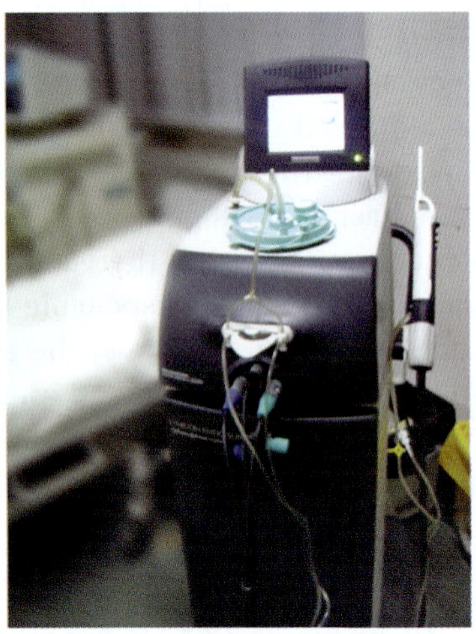

Fig. 2: VAB device: Mammotome® unit with attached biopsy probe.

Larger tissue removal with VAB increases the accuracy of breast biopsy. False-negative rates of VAB range from 0.6 to 5.2%.[6] The results of VAB are almost as good as surgical biopsy and negative predictive value as high as 99.9% can be achieved with VAB.[9,10] Vacuum-assisted biopsy is also more accurate than CNB in terms of frequency of histological underestimation, false-negatives and need for rebiopsy.[11,12]

Marker Clip Placement with VAB

Vacuum-assisted biopsy probes also allow placement of radiopaque marker clips at the biopsy site before the removal of the probe from the breast **(Figs. 3A and B)**. If the small lesion is completely removed during the biopsy and histopathology result is positive for cancer, this clip can be used to direct preoperative hookwire placement to

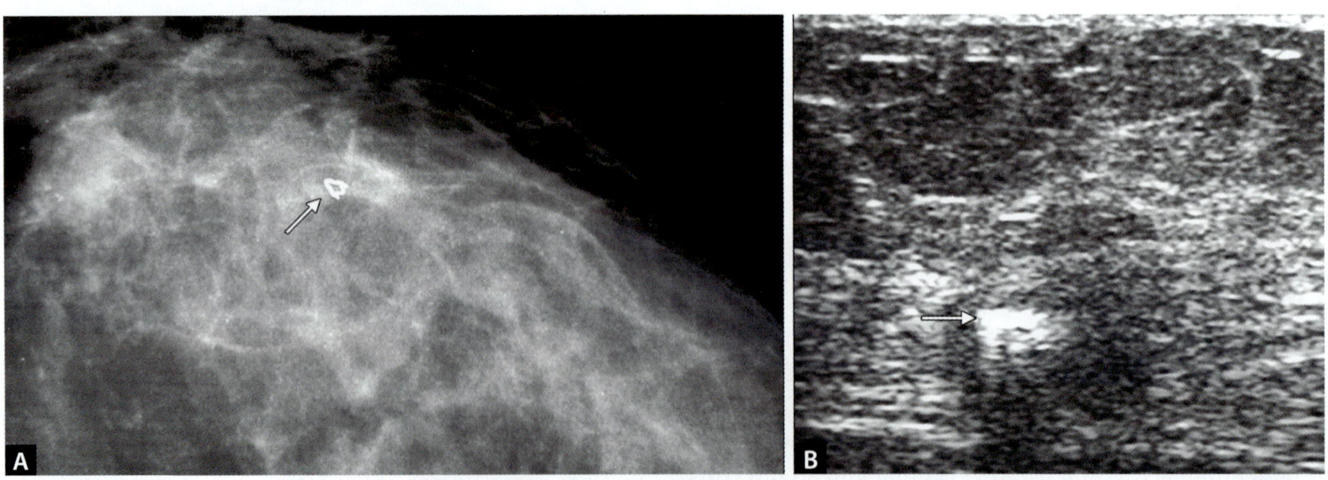

Figs. 3A and B: Marker clips: (A) Metallic marker clip Mammomark® deployed at the biopsy site (arrow) after VAB is seen on postbiopsy mammogram; (B) Gel-coated marker clip (arrow) can also be visualized on ultrasound.

guide breast conservation surgery. If the result is benign, the small marker clip is left as such in the breast. Some marker clips have both metal and a gel which expands into the tissue. This type of clip can be visualized both on mammography and ultrasound for hookwire localization. Placement of marker clip is also important for breast mass of any size that is being considered for neoadjuvant chemotherapy.[13,14] After chemotherapy, some breast cancers may completely disappear on imaging and in this situation, tumor site can be identified with marker clip only and the surgery can be performed after performing hookwire localization of the marker clip.

Disadvantages of VAB

Vacuum-assisted biopsy is more expensive than CNB using biopsy guns. The main unit with operating console as well as disposable biopsy probes are expensive. VAB probes are up to 10 times more expensive than the biopsy guns. One of the approaches towards better cost-effectiveness is that it could be selectively used as an alternative to open surgical biopsy for patients with nondiagnostic initial biopsy.[15] This approach is currently followed at author's institute. VAB also lacks the convenience of CNB. The probe is heavier and an experienced assistant is required during the procedure. However, advantages of VAB far outweigh the disadvantages and it has become the standard of breast biopsy in most breast care centers.

Complete Lesion Removal with VAB

It is important to note that VAB instrument is intended for tissue sampling only and not for therapeutic removal of the lesion. Even if complete imaging evidence of the malignant lesion is removed with VAB, cancer is still found on surgery in majority of the patients.[16,17] Surgery for breast cancer requires en bloc removal of the tumor with adequate margins of normal parenchyma around it and not just the gross tumor removal. However, this is not an issue with the benign lesions. Although uncommonly performed, VAB has been used as a minimally invasive technique to remove small benign breast masses with high patient satisfaction rates.[18,19] VAB leaves a very small, 3–4 mm, scar on the breast and results in excellent cosmesis when compared with surgical removal of a benign mass.

Lesion Selection for Breast Biopsy

Breast biopsy is indicated in all lesions classified as BIRADS 4 (suspicious) or BIRADS 5 (highly suspicious). BIRADS 3 lesions have less than 2% chance of malignancy and these are best managed with imaging follow-up without significant delay in diagnosis or treatment of breast cancer. However, sometimes biopsy needs to be performed in BIRADS 3 lesions as well. Such situations include inability to follow-up, anxious patient who refuse for follow-up, planned pregnancy and presence of another breast lesion which is already diagnosed as breast cancer.

Selection of Guiding Modality

Image-guided breast biopsy can be performed under ultrasound, mammographic (stereotactic) or MR guidance. Ultrasound is the most commonly used modality, if the breast lesion is unequivocally demonstrated on ultrasound. No special ultrasound equipment is required and the modality as well as expertise is widely available. The procedure is real time and fast. The lying position is also comfortable to the patient. Ultrasound guided procedures also allow greater flexibility of the approach and the puncture site. The needle can be inserted oblique or near parallel to the chest wall. Lesions located close to the chest wall, in the axillary tail or in the subareolar location may be difficult to position under stereotactic biopsy but these can be readily targeted with ultrasound guidance.

Microcalcifications only or masses which are seen on mammography only are indications for stereotactic breast biopsy. Personal preference and experience with biopsy techniques also govern the selection of guiding modality. At some centers, stereotactic biopsy is the preferred modality for all types of lesions, including masses that can be seen on ultrasound. MR-guided biopsy is cumbersome, expensive and time consuming. However, with increasing use of breast MRI and its higher sensitivity, MR guided biopsy is required for lesions which are visible on MRI only. It is worthwhile to perform a careful 'second look' targeted breast ultrasound in an attempt to localize the MRI detected lesion. Many of the MR positive breast lesions can be demonstrated like this and ultrasound-guided biopsy can be performed.[20,21]

Suspicious areas of focal asymmetry or architectural distortion are generally not subjected to percutaneous biopsy. Excision biopsy is preferred in these situations. A suspicious dilated duct is also excised surgically unless there is an associated mass or calcification which can be used as a target for image-guided percutaneous biopsy.

Prebiopsy Assessment

Imaging on basis of which the breast biopsy has been recommended must be carefully evaluated. It should be ensured that a clearly visible abnormality is present which can be targeted accurately. Appropriate biopsy technique and guiding modality is then selected. If the imaging is inadequate or presence of the lesion is doubtful, additional imaging must be done before scheduling the biopsy. A brief history should be obtained from the patient and at the same time biopsy procedure, its risks and post-biopsy instructions may also be conveyed to the patient. History of allergy to betadine or lignocaine, if any, should also be asked. No claims about outcome of the biopsy or future management should be made. The patient should be aware that a rebiopsy or excision may be required if the biopsy specimen is considered inadequate for definite pathological opinion. Informed consent must be obtained before the biopsy. Preprocedural coagulation profile is not required, unless patient has a bleeding tendency or is taking anticoagulants. Patients on aspirin or NSAID should stop it 3–5 days before the biopsy. Prophylactic antibiotics are not routinely required, however, these can be considered based on individual clinical judgment in patients with diabetes, rheumatic heart disease, artificial heart valves or joint replacement.

Ultrasound-guided Breast Biopsy

Wide availability, low cost, and ease of convenience to both the radiologist and the patient makes ultrasound the preferred modality for breast biopsy. Linear, 7.5 MHz (or more) transducer should be used. CNB must be performed with 14 G long through (2 cm or more) biopsy guns, even for a small subcentimeter lesion. Preprocedure test fire of the biopsy gun should be avoided. Correct patient positioning is important for ultrasound-guided breast biopsy. Ipsilateral arm of the patient should be raised above the head. Supine patient position is good for medial quadrant lesions. For lateral quadrant lesions, ipsilateral anterior supine oblique position is should be made, preferably with a pillow under the patient's shoulder. This helps to spread and thin out the breast parenchyma over the lesion. Ultrasound unit should be aligned in such a way that a right-handed radiologist can conveniently scan with left hand and hold the needle in right hand, without twisting his or her body to see the image on the monitor.

Technique

After preliminary scanning, skin puncture site should be carefully chosen. Free hand technique with needle visualization in longitudinal plane of the scan field is used for ultrasound-guided breast biopsy. Instead of choosing shortest skin to lesion distance, puncture site should be at least 1 cm or more away from the edge of the transducer. This increases the distance which the needle has to travel in the breast, but it makes the needle path parallel to chest wall, thereby reducing the chances of injury or penetration of the chest wall. The needle remains parallel to the transducer improving the needle visibility **(Fig. 4)**.

The skin should be cleaned with betadine and the draped with sterile sheets. Transducer surface is also cleaned or covered with sterile cover, as per the local practice. Local anesthesia should be given using 5–10 cc of 1% lignocaine and 22 or 23 G needle. Local anesthetic should be injected under ultrasound guidance, first close to the lesion, then along the needle tract and finally, in the subcutaneous tissue at the puncture site. Raising a skin wheal with local anesthetic at the puncture site greatly reduces the pain during biopsy. A small skin incision is given at the puncture site using number 11 scalpel blade. Needle is then carefully inserted and turned horizontally. Some resistance may be felt initially as the needle penetrates through the fascia and ligaments attached to the skin, the needle advancement should be carefully controlled so as to avoid sudden give-in and deep penetration. In hard breast, counter pressure from opposite direction may be required to facilitate needle penetration. The needle should always be kept parallel to the chest wall and in the plane of the long axis of the transducer, i.e. the scan plane. Otherwise, the needle tip may not be seen. To achieve this transducer-needle alignment, sometimes, the transducer needs to be rotated or repositioned during advancement of the needle. The needle tip should just pierce the lesion, if it is large enough, and has been stabilized with the transducer pressure **(Fig. 5A)**. Patient should be warned that a 'thud' sound will be heard and she should not get scared or make sudden jerky moves. If an assistant is helping in taking the samples, phrases like 'fire now' should be avoided as it may upset or scare the patient. The gun is then fired under realtime guidance. Before removing the needle, scanning in longitudinal and transverse planes should be done so as to ensure that the sample notch part of the gun is truly

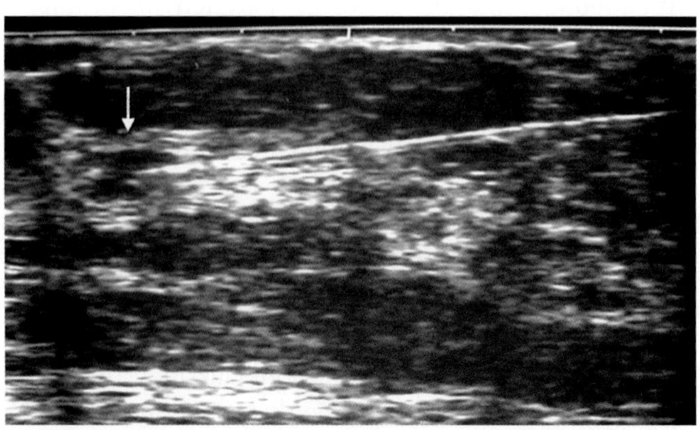

Fig. 4: Ultrasound-guided CNB: Horizontal needle approach improves the needle visualization, especially for targeting of small mass (arrow).

within the lesion **(Figs. 5B and C)**. It does not matter if the needle tip has crossed beyond the lesion. The needle is withdrawn; sample is retrieved and transferred to the sample bottle containing 10% formalin. The needle should not be dipped in formalin; instead, a scalpel blade should be used to remove the tissue from the sample notch. In this way multiple, at least 4–5 samples are collected and sample bottle is labeled. After the biopsy, light compression is applied at the biopsy site for about 10 minutes.

Technique of ultrasound-guided VAB is similar to that of ultrasound-guided CNB using biopsy gun **(Fig. 6A)**. The skin incision should be little wider so as to accommodate the large caliber VAB probes. The probe (needle) of VAB is not fired inside the lesion. Instead of hitting the lesion from the side, the probe tip is positioned below the lesion, in such a way that the sample notch remains just beneath the lesion **(Fig. 6B)**. This helps obtain contiguous core of the lesion, beginning from the deeper part of the lesion and then probe gradually moves superficially through the lesion for each subsequent core. The probe of the VAB is thick and not removed from the breast until the end of the biopsy procedure. If it is placed in the superficial part, most part of the lesion will be obscured beneath the acoustic shadowing of the probe after obtaining initial cores. If a small lesion is completely removed during VAB, a marker clip must be deployed at the biopsy site through the probe before taking it out from the breast.

Stereotactic Breast Biopsy

The principle of stereotactic biopsy is based on the trigonometric determination of depth of the target lesion in the breast. The breast is positioned and compressed in the stereotactic unit and pair of mammographic spot exposures (stereo images) is obtained with +15 degree and –15 degree tube angulations. Relative position of the target will change in both views because of the parallax shift due to different tube angulations. Lesion situated close to the detector moves less and lesion situated away from the detector moves more in these two images. This movement is compared with the movements of a marker with known depth (reference marker at the base) to determine the depth (z-coordinate) of the target lesion in the breast. Actual process involves complex trigonometric calculations, which are fortunately performed by the system computer. The x- and y-coordinates are same in both views.

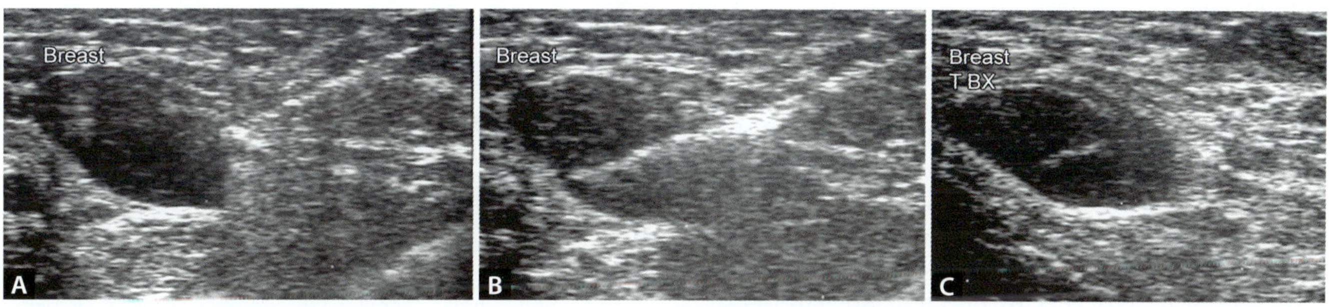

Figs. 5A to C: Ultrasound-guided CNB: (A) The tip of the biopsy needle is positioned at the periphery of the mass; (B) The mass and the needle are stabilized and the needle is fired. Area of sample notch is seen within the center of the mass indicating accurate positioning and sampling; (C) After withdrawal of the needle, small echogenic area of hemorrhage is seen within the mass at the site of biopsy.

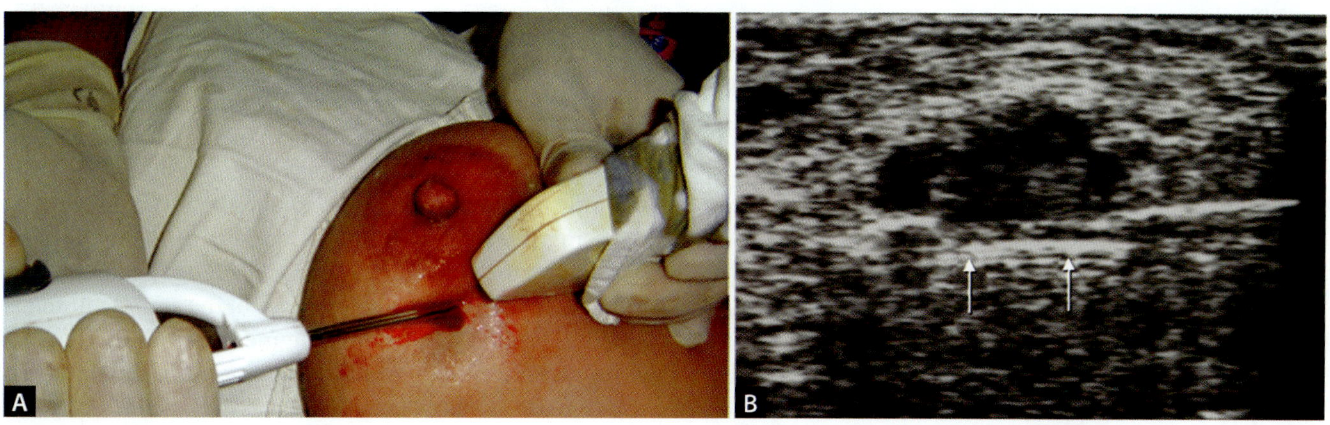

Figs. 6A and B: Ultrasound-guided VAB: (A) Biopsy procedure is being performed with Mammotome® probe and transducer aligned in the same plane; (B) The open sample notch (arrows) is positioned just beneath the mass.

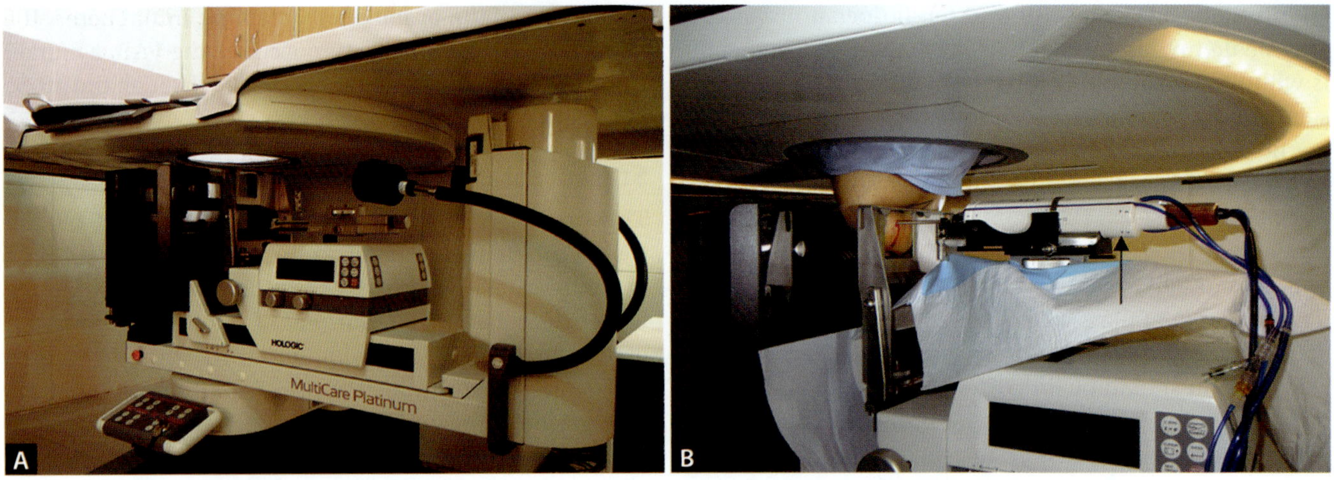

Figs. 7A and B: Dedicated prone table stereotactic biopsy: (A) Equipment (Multicare®, Hologic); (B) Stereotactic biopsy being performed using Atec® VAB device.

Equipment

Stereotactic biopsy equipment are of two types: dedicated prone table and add-on erect stereotactic device. Both of these were film based in past but now digital systems are used as they make the procedure simpler and faster. In dedicated prone table unit, the patient lies prone on the table and the breast hangs down through an opening in the table **(Figs. 7A and B)**. The patient is comfortable and breast remains stable during the procedure which is performed below the table. As the patient does not see the procedure, her anxiety is reduced. There is also more working space for the radiologist. The lesion can be approached from any side (360°) around the breast. Dedicated prone table stereotactic biopsy units are more expensive, require large space and cannot be used for diagnostic mammography. Hence, these are cost effective only if stereotactic biopsy is being routinely performed in the department. As thickness of the table will always remain between the chest wall and the breast, lesions situated too close to the chest wall may be difficult to access.

Add-on stereotactic biopsy device is actually an accessory device which can be attached to a standard diagnostic mammography unit to perform stereotactic biopsy **(Figs. 8A and B)**. It is cheaper and cost-effective. However, the biopsy can be performed in erect (sitting) patient position only. It is inconvenient to both the patient and the radiologist as working space is limited. The needle must be inserted from cranial aspect only, even if the lesion is located in caudal part of the breast. The chances of breast movement resulting in unnoticed shifting of the target lesion during biopsy are more likely. The patient closely watches the approach and insertion of the biopsy needle in her breast and hence, there are high chances of fainting and vasovagal reactions.

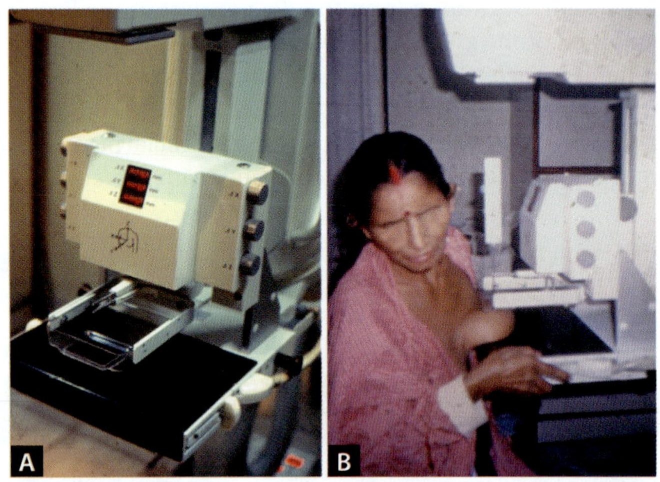

Figs. 8A and B: Add on erect stereotactic biopsy equipment: (A) Biopsy unit (Opdima®, Siemens); (B) Stereotactic biopsy is being performed with biopsy gun in a sitting position.

Technique

The technique of stereotactic biopsy is same for both types of units. The breast is positioned and compressed with a compression plate having an open window. An initial spot image is obtained without tube angulation to ensure that the lesion is seen in the center of the window. Once this is confirmed, a pair of stereo images is obtained without releasing the breast compression **(Fig. 9A)**. At the user interface of the computer, total needle length and distance from tip of the needle to the center of the sample notch is entered. Needle length must be measured in fired status of the needle. Single or multiple targets are then marked with mouse clicks in both images and transmitted to the device. Care must be taken to mark same part of the lesion in both images. The x-, y- and z-coordinates are calculated and displayed by the unit. The needle holder position is then moved and adjusted to appropriate position.

Presence of adequate breast tissues (thickness), both proximal and deep to the lesion, in compressed position of the breast is essential in stereotactic breast biopsy. The core biopsy sample is obtained from the sample notch and not from the tip of the needle. If the lesion is too close to the skin, the gun will have to be fired while the sample notch is partially outside the breast. This is not recommended. Similarly, if the lesion is too close to the table (bucky), the needle tip will puncture the skin and hit the table. These situations are called insufficient stroke margins and biopsy cannot be done. Some stereotactic units detect these errors automatically and warn the operator, while in others, safety of the stroke margin has to be calculated and determined by the radiologist. Changing breast position or rolling the breast before compression is sometimes is useful in such situations. Prone table biopsy units are better in these situations as they allow greater flexibility in choosing the direction of needle entry.

Site preparation and biopsy procedure is same as that for ultrasound-guided breast biopsy. Needle is inserted through the needle holder in its selected final position. A pre-fire pair of stereo images is obtained with needle fully inserted **(Fig. 9B)**. In both of these images, the needle tip should be seen just before and at the same distance from the target. After that, the gun is fired and another set of post-fire stereo images is obtained **(Fig. 9C)**. The needle tip should have symmetrically crossed the lesion in both of these images. The biopsy gun is them removed and sample retrieved. Subsequently, each target is selected, transmitted and fresh needle insertions are made to obtain multiple cores. It is not necessary to obtain pre- and post-fire images for each subsequent core if these images are satisfactory during first sample. However, if the lesion has moved or if there is asymmetry of needle tip—lesion relationship in pre- or post-fire images, a fresh pair of stereo images without needle should be obtained and biopsy continued with fresh target setting. When biopsy is being performed with vacuum assisted probe, the probe is rotated in the same position to obtain multiple cores from all directions around the probe. At the end, the needle is withdrawn from the breast and compression is released.

Specimen Radiography

If the target lesion has calcifications, specimen radiography of the harvested cores is essential to document retrieval of calcifications in the specimen **(Fig. 9D)**. This is recommended both after ultrasound-guided and stereotactic core biopsy. The cores may be placed on a wet slide or film so that they do not stick to it and specimen radiography is performed on standard mammography unit using lowest exposure factors. Demonstration of calcifications in cores eliminates the risk of sampling error

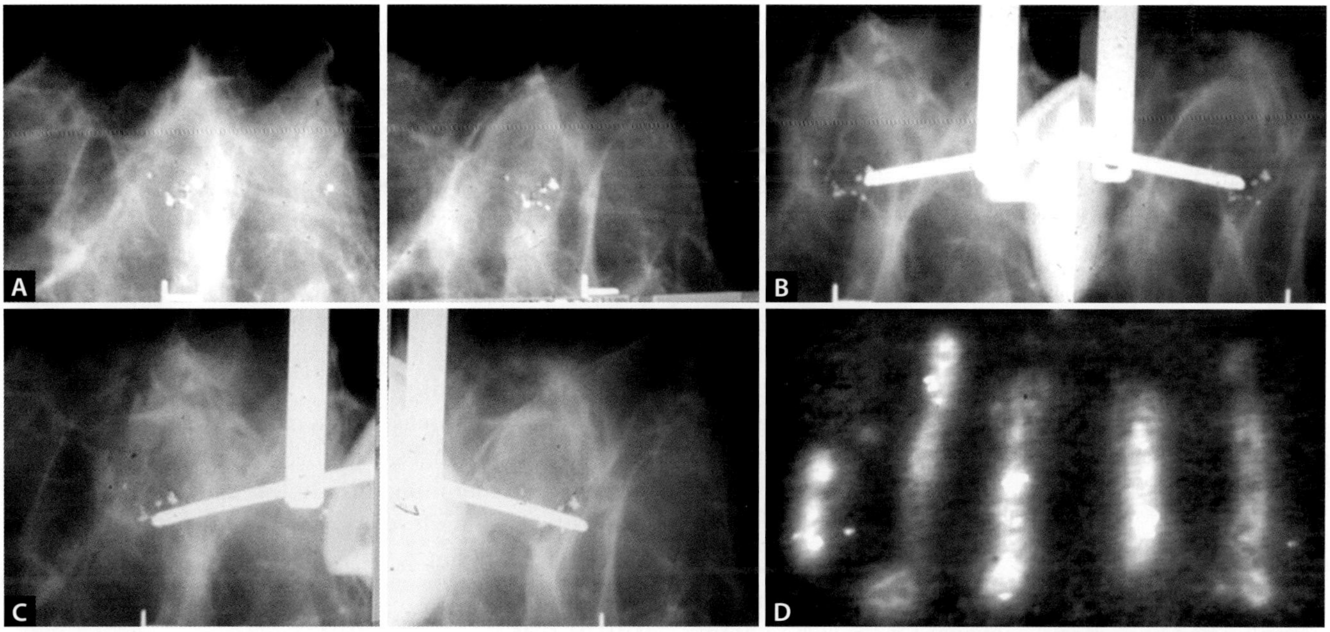

Figs. 9A to D: Stereotactic biopsy: (A) Pair of stereo images obtained at +10 and –10 degrees. Targets are marked in both images on the lesion, i.e. cluster of calcifications in this case; (B) Prefire pair of images show needle tip close to the lesion in both images; (C) Postfire images show that needle has traversed the lesion; (D) Specimen radiography of the samples shows presence of calcifications in multiple cores, confirming accurate targeting and sampling.

and improves the chances of specific diagnosis. If the calcifications are not demonstrated, pathological diagnosis can still be made however, the accuracy of the diagnosis is lower than when calcifications are demonstrated.[22,23] Specimen mammography of cores is not required when the target is a mass lesion without calcification.

Postbiopsy Care

After ultrasound-guided or stereotactic core biopsy of the breast, a continuous light pressure is maintained over the biopsy site (and not at the skin puncture site) at least for 10 minutes to achieve good hemostasis. Sometimes, a longer compression is needed. After that the skin is cleaned with alcohol and the incision is closed using sterile adhesive tape. Procedure and instructions must be written in postbiopsy notes and explained to the patient. The patient should be advised to keep the biopsy site dry and watch for obvious bleeding or sudden breast enlargement; the latter would indicate internal bleed and hematoma formation. Although this is rare, the patient can apply light pressure herself and contact the radiologist immediately should this happen. A telephone number of the radiologist should be provided to her for this purpose. Patient should be asked to avoid strenuous ipsilateral arm movements, such as lifting heavy weights, pushing something exercise or cooking activities. The tape on the wound can be removed after 48 hours.

Mild pain and some heaviness of the breast may be experienced by the patient immediately after the biopsy. Ice fomentation using ice cubes in a plastic bag is useful to relieve post-biopsy pain and also to reduce chances of bleeding. Routine analgesics are not required and should be avoided as for as possible. Patients should also be told that small bruising or discoloration of the skin due to ecchymosed blood can occur and this clears subsequently. Local skin inflammation or small serous ooze from incision site may rarely be seen which is also self-limiting. The wound should be kept clean and dry and no ointment, etc. should be applied. Prolonged bloody or purulent discharge from the wound however, should be evaluated clinically as well radiologically to determine if any treatment is required.

COMPLICATIONS OF BREAST BIOPSY

Percutaneous core biopsy breast is a safe procedure and complications are rare. Vasovagal reaction, hematoma formation and infection are main complications. Excessive bleeding or pain during biopsy necessitating termination of the procedure is extremely rare. Minor complication rate is 1.4%.[9] Significant hematoma formation or infection, defined as those requiring medical or surgical treatment, occur only in 0.1% cases. Small hematoma formation at the biopsy site is an expected finding and it can be seen on ultrasound for a week in majority of patients.[24] Complication rates of biopsy with biopsy gun and VAB are similar.[25]

Vasovagal reaction is a potential but unpredictable risk of breast biopsy. It is caused by anxiety, fear and pain. It is characterized by complaints of lightheadedness or fainting and signs of sweating, skin flushing and bradycardia. Distracting light conversation with patient during the biopsy procedure is helpful to avoid it. The patient should not be left alone during the biopsy. If vasovagal reaction occurs, she should be immediately placed in a supine position with feet raised and pulse and blood pressure monitored. This is usually adequate and active treatment with atropine is not generally required. Strict aseptic precautions during the biopsy are essential to minimize the chances of infection. A good compression after the biopsy and patient compliance of the post-biopsy instructions are important to reduce the chances of major hematoma formation.

Although complications of breast biopsy are uncommon, psychological impact of breast biopsy is important. The patient is worried and disturbed ever since she is told that there is a suspicious lesion in her breast that could be a cancer. Anxiety about the biopsy procedure itself is an additional cause of fear. These factors must also be considered while interacting with the patient.

Percutaneous breast biopsy does not cause seeding of tumor cells along the biopsy tract so as to cause spread or recurrence of the tumor in the breast or skin.[26] Although displaced tumor cells can be rarely found along the needle tract on histological examination of excised specimen, these cells probably do not sustain long enough to produce tumor seeding.[27,28] Needle tract cell displacement is more common with automated gun biopsies than with VAB, as unlike with biopsy guns, only single-time needle insertion is required with VAB.

Percutaneous breast biopsy generally does not produce any long-term changes, scarring or architectural distortion on follow-up mammograms. In less than 2% cases, a tiny round opacity may develop, which is seen in only one view of the mammogram.[29]

MRI-guided Breast Biopsy

Magnetic resonance imaging of breast is generally used as a problem solving modality. It is also being used for high-risk screening and preoperative staging of breast cancer.

Contrast-enhanced breast MRI is the most sensitive modality for breast cancer detection, which means that some breast lesions are seen only on MRI and not on conventional imaging. These are the lesions which require biopsy using MR guidance.

MRI-guided breast biopsy is performed with special breast coils and needle guide known as aiming device. It allows access on lateral aspect of breast only and hence, medially located lesions require deep needle insertion. Two types of localization devices are available. Most commonly used is a grid type device, a plate with multiple holes. The patient is positioned prone with breast in the coil. Mild compression is given with grid plate itself and contrast enhanced MRI is performed. A fiducial (marker), usually a vitamin E capsule, is also placed in one of the holes. The lesion is localized in axial and sagittal planes. Its location and distance with respect to fiducial is determined. The needle holder is fixed in the grid hole which is in line with the lesion. Depth is determined by counting the sagittal slices between needle holder and the lesion. A co-axial needle is first introduced up to the lesion, through which biopsy is taken using MR compatible biopsy gun or VAB probe.[30] The other type of aiming device has a bar and column, which can be moved in horizontal and vertical directions respectively, instead of a grid. The lesion and fiducial are localized and bar and columns moved to align the needle holder with the lesion for performance of biopsy.

MRI-guided breast biopsy is difficult, time-consuming and expensive. It requires special hardware in the form of a special imaging coil with window for biopsy and localization device and MR compatible needles, usually made of titanium of nickel alloys. The biopsy must be done with contrast enhanced MRI, which means that the procedure must be completed within 30–40 minutes when the lesion is enhancing and hence visible. The patient needs to be moved in and out of the gantry several times during the biopsy, making it cumbersome and time consuming. As the lesion is seen only because of contrast enhancement *in vivo*, specimen imaging cannot be done.

Histopathological Correlation

Core biopsy is a reliable method of diagnosis of breast abnormalities. When malignancy is found, definitive surgery is undertaken. However, some cancers can be missed on core biopsy. False-negative rates of core breast biopsy can be as high as 9% for gun biopsy and 5% for VAB.[6] Core biopsy is a sampling procedure and sampling error cannot be eliminated altogether. However, steps should be taken to achieve best possible accuracy of the procedure. Accurate target setting and relationship of the needle with the lesion should be verified on imaging during breast biopsy. Whenever applicable, specimen radiography must be done to verify presence of calcifications in the harvested samples. After biopsy, the results of the biopsy should always be correlated with imaging findings. A rebiopsy is essential if the sample is considered inadequate for definitive pathological diagnosis. Rebiopsy, preferably a surgical excision biopsy, should also be performed when there is imaging-histologic discordance or if a high-risk lesions like atpyical ductal hyperplasia (ADH) is reported on core biopsy.

Imaging-histologic discordance is a situation when imaging findings are not consistent with the pathology report. Benign core biopsy diagnosis for a spiculated mass lesion or pleomorphic microcalcifications is not expected. Imaging histologic-discordance occurs in 3–7% of core biopsies and malignancy is found in about one-fourth of these cases on surgical excision.[31,32] Even if benign diagnosis of core biopsy is acceptable, such as for BIRADS 4 lesions, it should be closely followed up with six monthly mammograms to rule out any sampling error.[33,34] Any suspicious development on follow-up mammogram is an indication for rebiopsy.

Histological underestimation is another limitation of core biopsy. When core biopsy result are correlated with final histopathology of the surgical specimen, a lesion diagnosed ADH a on core biopsy may turn out to be ductal carcinoma-*in situ* (DCIS) or DCIS on core biopsy may turn out to be an invasive cancer. Histological underestimation occurs when core biopsy samples do not represent the pathologically most aggressive part of the lesion and this can occur in up to 40% of gun biopsies and 16% of VABs.[35] Hence, high-risk lesions like ADH should be subjected to rebiopsy with excision.

Close audit of the biopsy results at an individual center should be regularly performed to maintain the standard and accuracy of breast biopsy. Overall, malignant results are expected in 20–40% of all breast biopsies performed. This is known as positivity rate or positive predictive value (PPV) of the breast biopsy. If higher PPV is encountered, it indicates low index of suspicion on breast imaging. This means that some lesions which could have been cancers, are not being recommended for biopsy and therefore, missed. On the other hand, if the PPV is low, the index of suspicion is very high and some lesions best suited for follow-up only are being referred for unnecessary biopsies.

PREOPERATIVE HOOKWIRE LOCALIZATION

Needle hookwire localization followed by surgical excision was the standard procedure for obtaining pathological diagnosis of nonpalpable but suspicious breast lesions seen on the mammograms. With development of accurate percutaneous core biopsy techniques, hookwire localization is now rarely performed for initial diagnosis. At present, it is mainly used as a preoperative localization procedure for therapeutic excision (breast conservation surgery) of already diagnosed but nonpalpable breast cancer. Hookwire localization prior to breast conservation surgery helps to precisely resect the cancer with clear margins. Indications of hookwire localization for diagnostic surgical excision biopsy include nonavailability of stereotactic biopsy facility or re-biopsy after inconclusive or discordant percutaneous core breast biopsy. It is also recommended for biopsy of vaguely defined breast abnormalities lesions; such as suspicious focal asymmetry or architectural distortion without associated mass. Needle localization for excision biopsy helps to achieve accurate lesion retrieval with minimal removal of breast parenchyma.

Early preoperative localization procedures were performed using various types of dyes, such as methylene blue or evans blue, mixed with iodinated contrast. The dye was injected in the lesion through a needle introduced under mammographic guidance. The dye could be seen on post-localization films and also intraoperatively. However, spread of the dye and amount of tissue stained was unpredictable, leading to missed lesions or excision of much larger breast tissue than actually required. Charcoal powder was also used instead of aqueous dyes, so as to restrict the spread over large area, but this was also not very accurate.

Accuracy and reliability of preoperative needle localization greatly improved after the development of various needle–hookwire combinations. Kopan's needle-hookwire assembly is most widely used. It consists of a 20 G needle and a thin flexible wire which can be introduced through it. The distal end of the wire is folded back forming a sharp angle and overbent so that it has a spring action **(Fig. 10)**. The needle is introduced under mammographic guidance. After correct needle placement, the hookwire is introduced and needle withdrawn over it. This exposes the hook of the wire which then anchors itself in the lesion. Then it can only be removed surgically. A modification of this hook-wire has a thick stiffened segment just proximal to the hook. This rigid segment of wire is useful to the surgeon as it allows manual palpation of the target lesion intraoperatively. Some versions of hookwire have double folded hook forming a barb, which prevent their displacement with in or out of the breast. Another type of needle hookwire assembly has a retractable curved J-tip instead of the angled hook. In this design, after positioning of the needle, the wire is advanced. The end of the wire which comes out of the needle forms a J shaped curve and gets anchored. If final hookwire position is unsatisfactory, the curved part of the wire can be retracted back into the needle and repositioning can be performed. The needle stays in the breast after deployment and it provides a stiff guide to the surgeon.

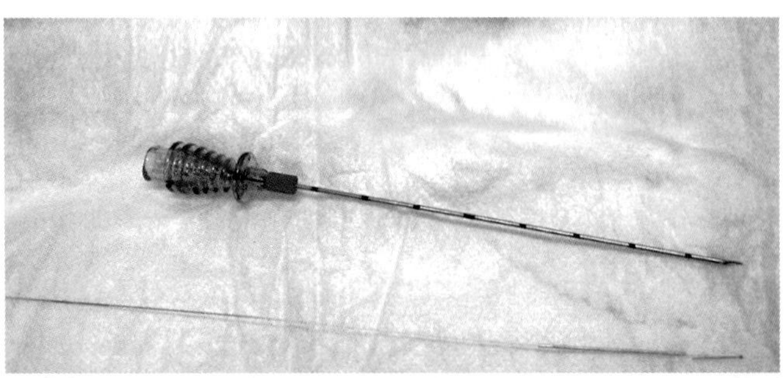

Fig. 10: Kopan's needle-hookwire assembly: It consists of a 20G needle and a hookwire.

Equipment

Needle localization is usually performed under mammographic guidance. However, it may also be performed under ultrasound guidance if the lesion is clearly defined on ultrasound. Magnetic resonance compatible needle hookwire assemblies are also available to localize the lesions seen only on MRI. Needle localization can be performed on all standard mammography machines. Only requirement is a special compression plate for needle localization. There are two types of compression plates. Alpha-numeric plate is the most widely used. It has a rectangular open window under which the lesion is positioned. There are radiopaque alpha-numeric centimeter markers on the margins of the window. The fenestrated compression plate has rows of multiple small round holes, like a sieve, instead of a single open window. These are also marked. The needle is introduced through the hole overlying the lesion. This type of compression is not preferred by many, as lesion frequently gets positioned under the solid part of the plate, rather than under the hole. Both digital and film based mammography machines are suitable for needle localization. However, digital systems are preferred as images at each step are immediately available and procedure is therefore much faster.

Technique

Films on the basis of which needle localization has been recommended are reviewed and appropriate guiding modality and approach is selected. The procedure is scheduled just before the surgery. Informed consent inclusive of needle localization and excision is usually obtained by the surgeon. Mammographic needle localization is performed with the patient in a sitting position. An approximate area of lesion, based on the baseline films, is marked on the skin and breast is positioned in the craniocaudal view. The breast is compressed with the alpha-numeric window compression plate, with skin mark in the center. A scout image is obtained **(Fig. 11A)** but breast compression is not released. If the lesion is seen well within the window, its x- and y-axis location is determined using the alpha-numeric markers in the image. The point is marked on the skin at the crossing of same coordinates, as visible on the compression plate. Availability of movable cross-hair shadow marker in the light beam of mammography unit is greatly useful to mark the exact point on the skin.

After the skin entry point is marked, skin is prepared and local anesthetic is injected. If the target lesion is a mass or architectural distortion, care should be taken not to inject too much local anesthetic as it can obscure lesion. The localization needle without hookwire is then inserted vertically into the breast. Too improve the accuracy of needle hitting the target, the light beam of the mammography unit is turned on during insertion. It should be ensured that the shadow of the needle hub on the breast surrounds the needle entry point **(Fig. 11B)**. This maintains the needle in the direction of the X-ray beam and the needle remains perfectly perpendicular to the lesion. The needle is inserted to maximum depth and another image is obtained. With perfect positioning, the needle is seen enface in the form of a dot superimposed on the lesion **(Fig. 11C)**. Needle positioning is inaccurate if some length of the shaft is seen or if the needle is more than 5 mm away from the target. If this occurs, the needle should be withdrawn and re-inserted. After satisfactory positioning, the compression released gradually. While the compression is being released, the breast bounces back and this may cause needle tip to come out from the lesion. To prevent this, the needle should be firmly supported and mild pressure is maintained to keep the needle tip deep in the breast during compression release. If the needle is not held, the needle hub may get entangled at the border of the compression plate window and come out with it. The breast is then repositioned in orthogonal (mediolateral) view using same compression plate. Then the exposure is made and the image obtained **(Fig. 11D)**. The needle should be seen crossing the lesion with tip about 1 cm beyond the lesion in this image. If this is not the case, then needle should be withdrawn accordingly while the breast is still compressed. Exact length to be withdrawn can be determined with the help of centimeter markings seen in the image. Presence of centimeter marks on the needle is useful in this depth adjustment.

After needle tip adjustment, the hookwire is inserted into the needle with the hook closed. The wire is inserted till a black mark on the wire reaches the hub. The tip of the hook is just at the needle tip at this position. A slight resistance to further advancement of wire is also be felt. The outside wire is then firmly held in position and needle withdrawn over it, releasing the hook in the breast. Wire should not be pushed during the withdrawal of the needle, as the hook may move further beyond the lesion, especially in fatty breasts.

After hookwire deployment, a mediolateral film is obtained for the surgeon **(Fig. 11E)**, CC view is not necessary. Procedure is considered successful if the hookwire is in the lesion or within 1 cm of it. If the wire is further away, procedure should be repeated with additional hookwire placement. The wire entry site is lightly covered with a gauze piece taking care that the wire is free to move in and out of the breast with changes in breast shape in supine and erect position of the patient. The wire should not be plastered to the breast at the skin entry site; otherwise the hook end of the wire inside the breast may get dislodged as the patient moves. The patient is then sent to the operation theater along with post-localization film, with lesion marked on it, and a written note about the procedure and final hookwire-lesion relationship.

Specimen Radiography

The surgeon dissects the breast using hookwire *in situ*. The approach is usually along the wire. Rarely, a separate incision is made guided by the palpation of the thickened part of the wire and lesion approached. The breast tissue around the hook and the thickened wire segment is resected and sent to the mammography room for specimen radiography. The specimen radiography is done on mammography unit with minimal exposure factors **(Fig. 11F)**. Mild compression may be required, if the specimen is large. The specimen mammogram should confirm that the target lesion, along with good margins, has been removed within the resected specimen. The specimen mammogram must be correlated carefully with baseline mammogram for this purpose. This is especially important if the lesion has calcifications; all foci of suspicious calcifications should be within the specimen. Successful lesion removal should be communicated to the surgeon, who is waiting in the OT, so that the breast can be closed and sutured. If the lesion is incompletely seen

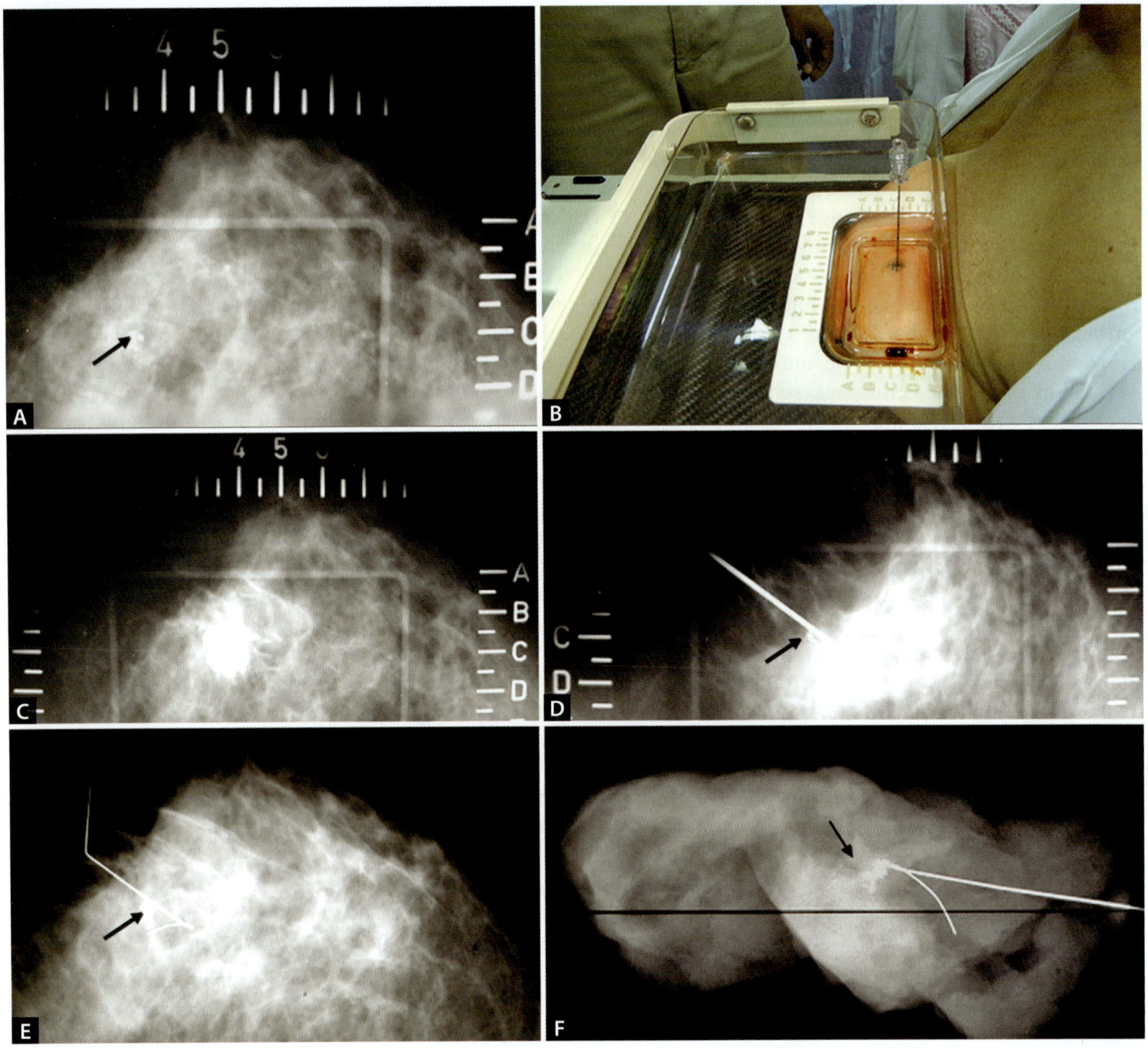

Figs. 11A to F: Preoperative hookwire localization: (A) Craniocaudal scout view shows cluster of calcification (arrow) in the center of the window of the compression plate. Its coordinates are determined in this film and skin entry point is marked; (B) Needle is inserted vertically. Note that the needle entry point is in the center of the shadow of the hub; thereby ensuring correct needle alignment in the direction of X-ray beam; (C) Another film is obtained. Needle is seen end on with its hub overlapping the lesion in this view; (D) Mediolateral view obtained thereafter shows that the needle tip has just crossed the lesion (arrow). Then the hookwire is inserted and the needle is withdrawn; (E) Post-hookwire localization mammogram shows hookwire anchored correctly within the lesion (arrow); (F) Specimen radiograph of the excised tissue confirms accurate removal of the lesion (arrow).

or seen extending up to the margins, this should also be communicated in details, so that additional resection at the appropriate site is attempted.[36]

Complications

Preoperative hookwire localization is a well-established safe procedure. Complications are rare. These mainly include vasovagal reaction, bleeding and pain. Unusual complications include hooking of pectoralis muscle and pneumothorax due to entry of the needle into the chest.

Migration of the hookwire after successful placement is an uncommon but serious problem. Risk factors for this include entirely fatty breast, excessive arm movements after the wire placement and delay in surgery. Hookwire migration can also occur intraoperatively. Surgeon may hold and pull the wire during dissection and wire may come out. The wire may also get cut during dissection. The deeper segment of the wire then gets retracted and lost in the breast. If the surgeon is not familiar with this procedure, he should be cautioned about these complications.

Special Techniques of Localization

Placement of two or more hookwires in the same breast may be required for multiple lesions or to mark the extent of a large lesion (Hookwire Bracketing) before breast conservation surgery.[37] Stereotactic guidance is generally not preferred for needle localization procedures but this may be required for lesions seen in one view only. Needle localization can be accurately and quickly performed under ultrasound guidance and this modality should be preferred if the lesion is visible on ultrasound. Another advantage of ultrasound-guided needle localization is that it can be performed with anterior approach. Most surgeons prefer anterior approach for dissection. As with mammographic needle localization, post-localization mammogram and specimen radiography should also be performed after ultrasound-guided localization. Magnetic resonance imaging guided hookwire localization is also possible with MR compatible needle-hookwire devices. It is required for the lesions seen on MRI only.

Hematoma-guided localization has also been found useful for breast conservation surgery of nonpalpable breast cancers.[38,39] After a core biopsy, a small hematoma is always formed at the biopsy site. If the biopsy result is malignant and surgery is planned within 4–5 weeks, the small hematoma can be identified with intraoperative ultrasound. This can be used as a guide for dissection, without the need for any preoperative localization procedure. Radioguided occult lesion localization (ROLL) is another technique in which a radioisotope containing colloid (also used for sentinel lymph node mapping) is injected into the tumor. Tumor is then localized intraoperatively using handheld gamma probe.[40]

MISCELLANEOUS BREAST INTERVENTIONS

Ductography

Ductography (or galactography) was a commonly performed procedure for evaluation of patients with nipple discharge, as ductal anatomy is not well seen on mammogram. With the advent of high resolution ultrasound and contrast enhanced MRI of the breast, ductal evaluation is now possible with reasonable accuracy with these modalities, and hence, ductography is rarely performed at present.

Indications of ductography include spontaneous solitary duct discharge that is serosanguineous, or bloody. Causes of such duct discharge are papilloma, fibrocystic disease, duct ectasia and carcinoma.[41] Bilateral nipple discharge or discharge elicited by squeezing only is physiological not requiring ductography.

Ductography should be performed during active discharge. A 27 or 30 G ductography cannula is used which is connected to a syringe containing 3–5 mL of nonionic contrast. All air form the cannula, tube and syringe must be removed. The duct is identified with a gentle squeeze and cannulated with gentle probing. The contrast is slowly injected till the patient feels some fullness. Usually, less than 1 cc of contrast is required. The cannula is then securely taped on the breast and mediolateral and craniocaudal mammographic views are obtained. Additional contrast can be injected if ductal opacification is incomplete.

Ductography demonstrates ductal anatomy of the drainage territory of the cannulated duct **(Fig. 12A)**. The size of the ductal territory is highly variable; this may be a small segment of the breast or it may cover a large area of the breast. Normal ducts show uniform and orderly branching of the ducts with smooth tapering from nipple to periphery. Single or multiple filling defects in the duct are most commonly produced by papillomas **(Fig. 12B)**, sometime by fibrocystic disease, blood clots, air bubbles or rarely by carcinoma. Abrupt cut-off may be produced by papilloma or a carcinoma. Ductal dilatation with abrupt tapering of distal ducts is a characteristic feature of duct ectasia **(Fig. 12C)**. Beaded appearance of the duct with multiple opacified cysts is seen in fibrocystic disease.[42]

Cyst Aspiration

Percutaneous cyst aspiration may be required for analysis of the contents of complex breast cysts. These usually represent inflammatory pathology, and extremely rarely, malignancy. Breast cyst aspiration may also be performed for symptomatic relief of large simple breast cysts. Breast cyst aspiration is best performed under ultrasound guidance using 18G needle **(Fig. 13)**. Complete evacuation of the cyst should be attempted. If the fluid is clear or serous, cytological evaluation is not required.[43] If the fluid is bloody or purulent, it should be sent for cytological examination. Residual solid lesion after cyst aspiration is an indication for biopsy.

Ultrasound-guided Axillary Lymph Node FNAC

All patients with breast cancer require axillary lymph node dissection for sampling and pathological staging

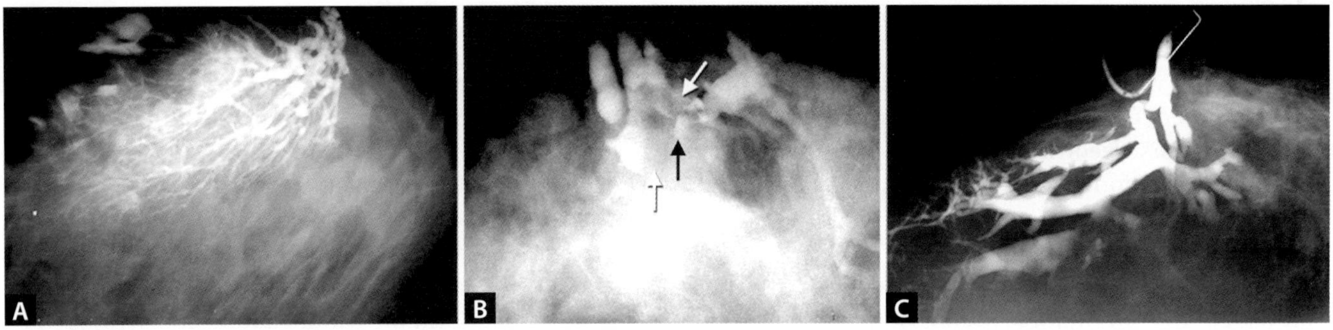

Figs. 12A to C: Ductogram: (A) Normal ductogram shows uniform branching pattern of the nondilated ducts opacified in segment of the breast; (B) Subareolar papilloma is seen as a filling defect (arrows) within a mildly dilated duct; (C) Duct ectasia is seen as moderately dilated ducts with pruning of side branches.

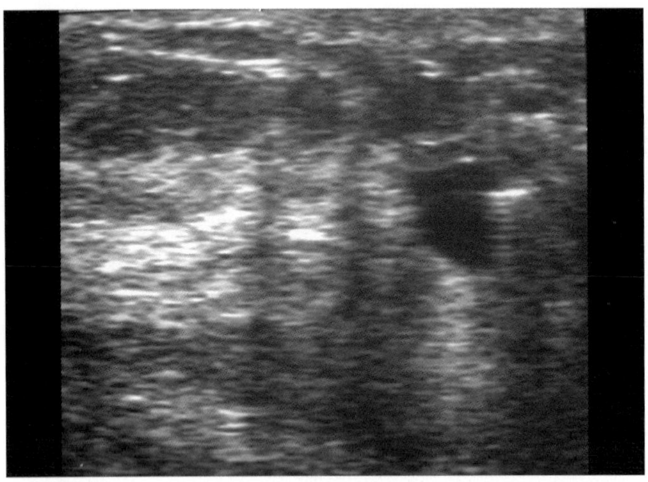

Fig. 13: Ultrasound-guided cyst aspiration: Needle tip is seen within the cyst with accompanied reverberations characteristically seen during cyst aspiration.

of the nodes, irrespective of their clinical nodal status. However, this procedure is morbid and many of the patients develop shoulder stiffness and lymphedema of the arm subsequently. Sentinel lymph node staging helps avoid axillary lymph dissection in some of the patients who do not have axillary lymphadenopathy on clinical examination. In this procedure, a dye and radionuclide (^{99m}Tc labeled sulfur colloid) is injected around the tumor. The first node draining the tumor area is localized with scintigraphy probe and excised. If this node is not pathologically involved, distal axillary lymph nodes are considered to be disease free and axillary dissection is avoided. However, the technique of sentinel lymph node staging is cumbersome, time consuming and expensive.

Ultrasound of axilla in clinically node negative patients, with ultrasound-guided FNAC of abnormal lymph nodes so detected, is fast gaining acceptance. Patients with confirmed axillary lymph node involvement can then be spared of sentinel lymph node staging and directly taken for axillary lymph node dissection. On ultrasound, size criteria or Doppler evaluation are not useful for identification of abnormal axillary lymph nodes. Lymph nodes of any size with focal or diffuse cortical thickening (more than 3 mm) or presence of hypoechoic deposits are considered suspicious[44] **(Figs. 14A and B)**. Absence of fatty hilum is also a reliable feature.[45] Abnormal lymph nodes are subjected to ultrasound-guided FNAC. Core biopsy is also done at some centers but FNAC is generally sufficient, as aim is to confirm the presence of malignancy and histological analysis is not essential. Overall, ultrasound-guided FNAC of axillary lymph nodes has high sensitivity and specificity of 80 and 98% respectively for axillary lymph node staging.[46]

ABLATIVE PROCEDURES FOR BREAST CANCER

Radiofrequency ablation (RFA) of small breast cancer is feasible and complete ablation of tumor and adjacent margin of breast parenchyma can be achieved **(Figs. 15A and B)**. Several feasibility studies have reported good pathological tumor ablation in most patients.[47,48] Major advantage of RFA of breast cancer, is minimally invasive treatment of breast cancer with best cosmetic outcome. High intensity focused ultrasound (HIFU) is also useful for thermal ablation of small breast cancers. RFA and HIFU for breast cancers are still considered investigational as it is difficult to reliably confirm and document complete tumor ablation and long-term results are not known. However, these procedures have reasonable potential to become an option for minimally invasive treatment of breast cancer in future, if large studies and long-term results are available.

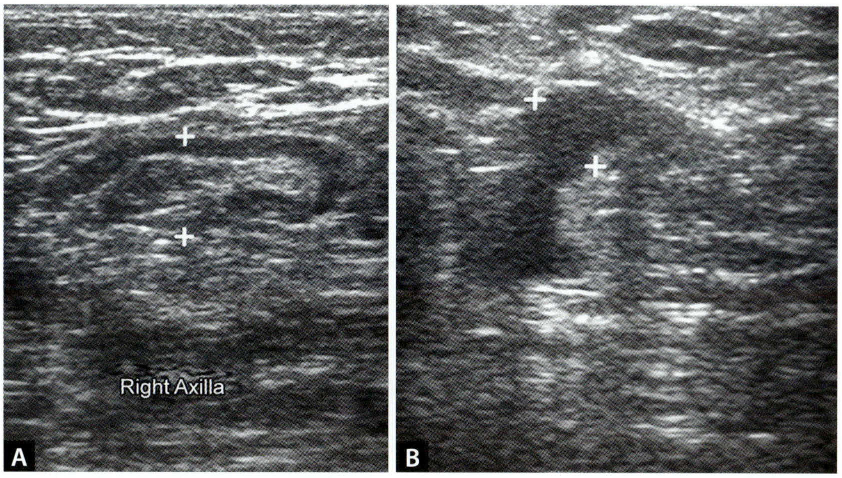

Figs. 14A and B: Ultrasound of axillary lymph nodes: (A) Central echogenic fatty hilum constitutes the most prominent part of a normal axillary lymph node. Peripheral cortex is seen as a thin hypoechoic rim of uniform thickness around the hilum; (B) A metastatic axillary lymph node showing irregular cortical thickening with normal fatty hilum.

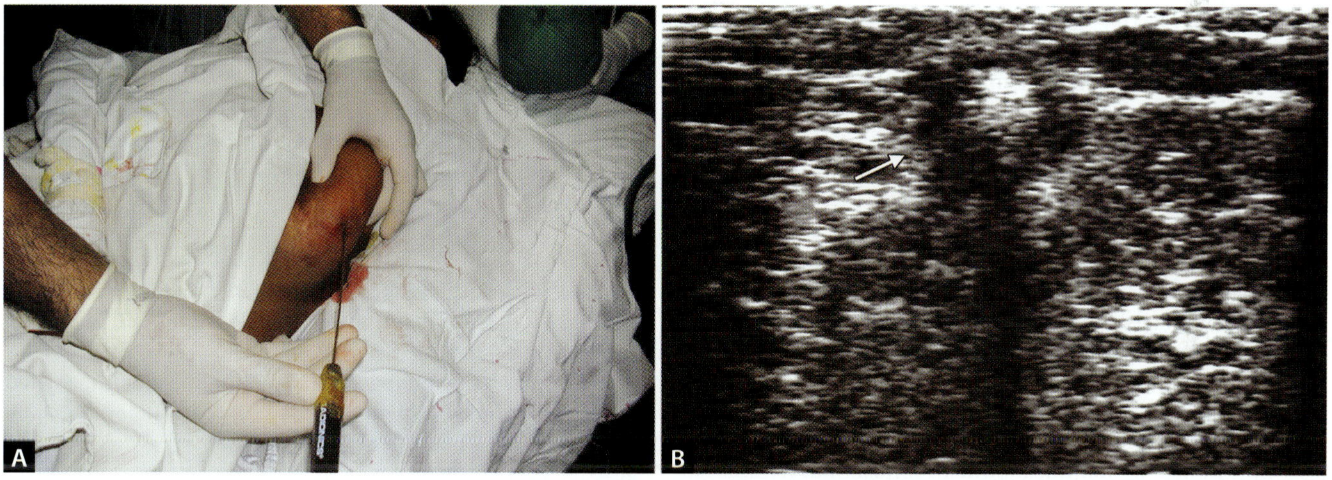

Figs. 15A and B: Breast cancer RFA: (A) RFA probe is percutaneously inserted into the breast mass using same technique as that for biopsy; (B) An echogenic area forms within the tumor (arrow) as energy is deposited during RFA procedure.

REFERENCES

1. Liberman L, Ernberg LA, Heerdt A, et al. Palpable breast masses: is there a role of percutaneous imaging-guided core biopsy? AJR. 2000;175:774-87.
2. Pisano ED, Fajardo LL, Tsimikas J, et al. Rate of insufficient samples from fine needle aspiration for non-palpable breast lesions in an multicenter clinical trial: the Radiologic Diagnostic Oncology Group 5 study. Cancer. 1998;82:678-88.
3. Tse MG, Tan PH. Diagnosing breast lesions by fine needle aspiration cytology or core biopsy: which is better? Breast Cancer Res Treat. 2010;123:1-8.
4. Hukinen K, Kiwisaari L, Heikkelis PS, Von Simitten K, Leidenius M. Unsuccessful preoperative fine needle aspiration cytology or core biopsy, led to increased cost of the diagnostic work-up in breast cancer. Acta Oncol. 2008;47:1037-45.
5. Parker SH, Jobe WE, Dennis MA, et al. US guided automated large core breast biopsy. Radiology. 1993;187:507-11.
6. O'Flyn EAM, Wilson ARM, Michel MJ. Image-guided breast biopsy: state-of-the-art. Clin Radiol. 2010;65:259-70.
7. Burbank F, Parker SH, Fogarty TJ. Stereotactic breast biopsy: improved tissue harvesting with mammotome. Am Surg. 1996;62:738-44.
8. Berg WA, Krebs TL, Campassi C, Magder LS, Sun CC. Evaluation of 14 and 11 gauge directional vacuum assisted biopsy probes and 14 gauge biopsy guns in a breast parenchymal model. Radiology. 1997;205:203-8.
9. Kettritz U, Rotter K, Schrer I, et al. Stereotactic vacuum-assisted breast biopsy in 2874 patients: a multicenter study. Cancer. 2004;100:245-51.
10. Jackman RJ, Marzoni FA Jr, Rosenberg J. False negative diagnosis at stereotactic vacuum-assisted needle breast

biopsy: long-term follow-up of 1280 lesions and review of literature. AJR. 2009;192:341-51.

11. Shah VJ Raju U, Chitale D, et al. False negative core needle biopsies of the breast: an analysis of clinical, radiologic and pathologic findings in 27 consecutive cases of missed breast cancer. Cancer. 2003;1519:1824-31.
12. Cho N, Moon WK, Cha JH, et al. Sonographically guided core biopsy of the breast: comparison of 14 gauge automated gun and 11 gauge directional vacuum assisted biopsy methods. Korean J Radiol. 2005;6:102-9.
13. Nadeem R, Chagla LS, Harris O, et al. Tumour localization with a metal coil before administration of neoadjuvant chemotherapy. Breast. 2005;14:403-7.
14. Oh JL, Nguyen G, Whitman GJ, et al. Placement of radiopaque clips for tumour localization in patients undergoing neoadjuvant chemotherapy and breast conservation therapy. Cancer. 2007;110:2420-7.
15. Carpentier E, Maruani A, Michenet P, et al. Can US guided vacuum assisted biopsies be an alternative to diagnostic surgery in cases of non-diagnostic core needle biopsy? J Radiol. 2005;86:475-80.
16. Liberman L, Dershaw DD, Rosen PP, et al. Percutaneous removal of malignant mammographic lesions at stereotactic vacuum assisted biopsy. Radiology. 1998;206: 711-5.
17. March DE, Coughlin BF, Barham RB, et al. Breast masses: removal of all US evidence during biopsy by using a hand held vacuum assisted device—initial experience. Radiology. 2003;227:549-55.
18. Fine RE, Whitworth PW, Kim JA, et al. Low risk palpable breast masses removal using a vacuum assisted hand held device. Am J Surg. 2003;186:362-7.
19. Thurley P, Evans A, Hamilton L, James J, Wilson R. Patient satisfaction and efficacy of vacuum-assisted excision biopsy of fibroadenomas. Clin Radiol. 2009;64:381-5.
20. LaTrenta LR, Menel JH, Morris EA, et al. Breast lesions detected with MR imaging: utility and histopathologic importance of identification with ultrasound. Radiology. 2003;227:85-61.
21. Meissnitzer M, Dershaw DD, Lee CH, Morris EA. Targeted ultrasound of the breast in women with abnormal MRI findings for whom biopsy has been recommended. AJR. 2009;193:1025-9.
22. Liberman L, Smolkin JH, Dershaw D, et al. Calcification retrieval at stereotactic 11 gauge directional vacuum assisted breast biopsy. Radiology. 1998;208:251-60.
23. Margolin FR, Kaufman L, Jacobs RP, Denny SR, Schrumpf JD. Stereotactic core biopsy of malignant calcifications: diagnostic yield of cores with and without micro-calcifications on specimen radiographs. Radiology. 2004;233:251-4.
24. Huber S, Wagner M, Medl M, Czembirek H. Benign breast lesions minimally invasive vacuum-assisted biopsy with 11-gauge needles: patient acceptance and effect on follow-up imaging. Radiology. 2003;226:783-90.
25. Philpotts LE, Hooley RJ, Lee CH. Comparison of automated versus vacuum assisted biopsy methods for sonographically guided core biopsy of the breast. AJR. 2003;180: 347-51.
26. Parker SH, Burbank, F Jackman RJ, et al. Percutaneous large core breast biopsy: a multi-institutional study. Radiology. 1994;193:359-64.
27. Diaz LK, Wiley EL, Venta LA. Are malignant cells displaced by large core biopsy of the breast? AJR. 1999;173:1303-13.
28. Hoorntie LE, Schipper ME, Kaya A, et al. Tumour cell displacement after 14 G breast biopsy. Eur J Surg Oncol. 2004;30:520-5.
29. Lamm RL, Jackman RJ. Mammographic abnormalities caused by percutaneous stereotactic biopsy of histologically benign lesions evident on follow-up mammograms. AJR. 2000;174:753-6.
30. Albiter M, Boyer B, Britton P, et al. Interdisciplinary consensus on the uses and technique of MR-guided vacuum assisted breast biopsy (VAB): results of a European consensus meeting. Eur J Radiol. 2009;72:289-94.
31. Liberman L, Drotman M, Morris EA, et al. Imaging-histologic discordance at percutaneous breast biopsy. Cancer. 2000;89:2538-46.
32. Ciatto S, Houssami N, Ambrogetti D, et al. Accuracy and underestimation of malignancy of breast core needle biopsy: the Florence experience of over 4000 consecutive biopsies. Breast Cancer Res Treat. 2007;101:291-7.
33. Jackman RJ, Nowels KW, Roderiguez-Soto J, et al. Stereotactic, automated, large-core needle biopsy of nonpalpable breast lesions: false negative and histologic underestimation rates after long-term follow-up. Radiology. 1999;210:799-805.
34. Youk JH, Kim EK, Kim MJ, Oh KK. Sonographically guided 14-gauge core needle biopsy of breast masses: a review of 2420 cases with long-term follow-up. AJR. 2008;190: 202-7.
35. Hoorntie LE, Peeters PH, Mati WP, et al. Vacuum assisted breast biopsy: a critical review. Eur J Cancer. 2003;39: 1676-3.
36. Schaefer FK, Eden I, Schaefer PJ, et al. Factors associated with one step surgery in case of nonpalpable breast cancer. Eur J Radiol. 2007;64(3):426-32.
37. Kirstien LJ, Rafferty E, Spencht MC, et al. Outcome of multiple wire localization for larger breast cancers: when can mastectomy be avoided? J Am Coll Surg. 2008;207: 342-6.
38. Thompson M, Tillman RH, Margulies A, et al. Hematoma-directed ultrasound guided (HUG) breast lumpectomy. Ann Surg Oncol. 2007;14:148-56.
39. Arentz C, Baxter K, Boneti C, et al. Ten years experience with hematoma directed ultrasound guided breast lumpectomy. Ann Surg Oncol. 2010;17:378-83.
40. Nadeem R, Chagla LS, Harris O, et al. Occult breast lesions: a comparison between radioguided occult lesion localization (ROLL) vs wire guided lumpectomy (WGL). Breast. 2005;14:283-9.
41. Tabar L, Dean PB, Pentek Z. Galactography: the diagnostic procedure of choice for nipple discharge. Radiology. 1983;149:31-8.

42. Bassett LW, Kim CH. Ductography. In: Dershaw DD (Ed) Imaging-guided interventional breast techniques. Springer, New York; 2003. pp. 1-30.
43. Ciatto S, Cariaggi P, Bularisis P. The value of routine cytologic examination of breast cyst fluid. Acta Cytol. 1987;31:301-4.
44. Choi YJ, Ko EY, Han B, et al. High resolution ultrasonographic features of axillary lymph node metastases in patients with breast cancer. Breast. 2009;18:119-22.
45. Cho N, Moon WK, Han W, et al. Preoperative sonographic classification of axillary lymph nodes in patients with breast cancer: node-to-node correlation with surgical histology and sentinel node biopsy results. AJR. 2009;193:1731-7.
46. Houssami N, Ciatto S, Turner RM, Cody HS 3rd, Macaskill P. Preoperative ultrasound guided needle biopsy of axillary nodes in invasive breast cancer: meta-analysis of its accuracy and utility in staging the axilla. Ann Surg. 2011;254:243-51.
47. Manenti G, Bolacchi F, Perretta T, et al. Small breast cancers: in vivo percutaneous US-guided radiofrequency ablation with dedicated cool-tip radiofrequency system. Radiology. 2009;251:339-46.
48. Zhao Z, Wu F. Minimally invasive thermal ablation of early-stage breast cancer: a systematic review. Eur J Surg Oncol. 2010;36:1149-55.

CHAPTER 209

PET-CT in Management of Breast Cancer

Rakesh Kumar, Punit Sharma, Arun Malhotra

INTRODUCTION

Breast cancer is the most commonly diagnosed cancer and the leading cause of cancer death in females, accounting for 23% (1.38 million) of the total new cancer cases and 14% (458,400) of the total cancer deaths worldwide in 2008. Around half of the breast cancer cases and 60% of the deaths are estimated to occur in economically developing countries.[1] Increased risk of breast cancer is associated with reproductive factors, including a long menstrual history, nulliparity, recent use of postmenopausal hormone therapy or oral contraceptives and late age at first birth.[2] Alcohol consumption also increases the risk of breast cancer.[3] In many Asian countries, including India, incidence and mortality rates have been rising,[4] with changes in reproductive patterns, physical inactivity and obesity being the main risk factors.[5,6] Increase in breast cancer awareness and screening may be partially responsible for the rising incidence in these populations.

Breast cancers arise from the epithelial cells in the breast cancer ducts. The most important histologic feature in the primary tumor is the absence or presence of tumor invasion beyond the ductal architecture (ductal carcinoma *in situ* and invasive carcinoma respectively). Major histological architectural patterns are ductal, lobular, or mixed carcinomas.[7] In addition to morphologic analysis, biopsy material is routinely assayed for phenotypic features that include the expression of hormone receptors (estrogen receptor [ER] and progesterone receptor [PR]) and HER2/neu (also known as cerbB2), typically by immunohistochemistry or fluorescent *in situ* hybridization. These markers predict tumor aggressiveness and behavior and are also targets for specific therapy.[8]

Imaging plays an important role in early detection of breast cancer and in directing therapy. Mammography, breast ultrasound and magnetic resonance imaging (MR imaging) are the primary diagnostic modalities to evaluate breast pathology. ^{18}F-Fluorodeoxyglucose (FDG) positron emission tomography-computed tomography (PET-CT) has now emerged as another imaging tool for many malignant neoplasms, including breast cancer. Malignant cells generally have enhanced glucose metabolism compared with non-malignant cells and therefore exhibit increased glycolytic activity. This feature of malignant cells forms the basis for imaging with FDG PET-CT. A brief overview of utility of PET-CT in patients with breast cancer is presented below.

PRIMARY MALIGNANCY

Most studies have suggested that the degree of FDG uptake is somewhat correlated with breast cancer phenotype such as histologic type (higher uptake in ductal vs lobular cancers), tumor histologic grade and indices of cellular proliferation (higher uptake with higher levels of proliferation). Low uptake is seen in ductal carcinoma *in situ* and well-differentiated forms such as grade I lobular breast cancer.[9,10] Overall, the sensitivity of ^{18}F-FDG PET in detecting primary breast cancer is 64–96%, specificity is 73–100%, positive predictive value is 81–100% and negative predictive value is 52–89%.[11] Because primary breast cancer detection requires the ability to depict occult, non-palpable, small (<1 cm) invasive and *in situ* malignant lesions, whole-body FDG-PET is not used in primary breast cancer detection. It is not currently indicated for breast cancer detection, mainly due to its poor spatial resolution.[12,13] In fact, the sensitivity of PET to detect breast lesions is in the range of 60% for lesions smaller than 1 cm and in the range of 90% in case of larger tumors (>2 cm). The absence of FDG uptake in breast lesions smaller than 2 cm does not exclude the presence of malignant disease. Conversely, the detection of high and focal FDG uptake in the breast has a strong positive value for cancer.[14] Moreover, FDG uptake may vary according to breast cancer histological type, with less sensitivity to detect lobular carcinoma than invasive ductal carcinoma. To overcome these problems, new dedicated high-resolution PET scans, such as positron emission mammography (PEM), have been recently implemented, but their role in clinical practice is still to be established.[15]

Dual time point imaging has been demonstrated to be advantageous in head and neck, lung, pancreatic, and cervical malignancies. Similarly, it has been proposed that dual time point FDG-PET may improve the sensitivity and accuracy of FDG-PET in assessing patients with primary breast cancer. It has been shown that sensitivities of the dual time imaging method in detecting invasive breast cancer measuring larger than 10 mm, 4–10 mm and noninvasive breast cancer were 90.1%, 82.7% and 76.9%, respectively.[16] In addition, invasive ductal cancer showed a significantly higher standardized uptake value (SUV) than those of invasive lobular and mixed types, which are relatively well-differentiated invasive cancers. Therefore, dual point imaging can result in higher SUV values, helping to differentiate between benign and malignant processes.

Some of the limitations of PET alone can be overcome with PET-CT. PET-CT combination is particularly useful for specific types of patients, such as those with dense breasts or with implants. Although younger, premenopausal patients or the patients with dense breasts have higher SUVs, the accuracy of ^{18}F-FDG PET studies in diagnosing malignant breast tumors may not be significantly affected because of the high contrast between the tumor and the surrounding uptake of this radiotracer.[17] It has been shown that FDG PET-CT may improve breast cancer detection after mammaplasty.[18] Furthermore, PET-CT has advantages with respect to the assessment of local tumor recurrence and the detection of metastases in the lymph node and distant areas. These advantages mean that this combined method is also useful for imaging patients who underwent reconstruction with breast implants after mammary carcinoma resection.[19-21] PET-CT also has a potential advantage over PET for evaluating small lesions in which the uptake may be artifactually lowered due to the partial volume effect of PET.[22] FDG-PET being a whole body imaging modality, the contralateral breast is invariably screened when the ipsilateral breast with the known cancer is being evaluated. This may lead to detection of unknown primary in contralateral breast. In one series FDG PET-CT detected tumor in the contralateral breast in 2.1% (5 of 234) of patients and accounted for 41.6% (5 of 12) of the bilateral breast tumors in this series.[23]

POSITRON EMISSION MAMMOGRAPHY

Positron emission mammography (PEM) uses a dedicated instrument for breast cancer detection that is equipped with two parallel photon detectors in a configuration similar to mammography compressors. As an organ-specific instrument, it can provide high spatial resolution compressed-breast images.[15] The advantages of PEM, compared with whole-body PET, include higher spatial resolution, shorter imaging time and reduced attenuation. In initial studies, the sensitivity of PEM was reported to be about 90%.[24] A recent prospective study compared the imaging sensitivity of PEM with that of PET-CT in relation to tumor size. The results showed that PEM had significantly higher sensitivity in small-sized tumors <2 cm than PET-CT. PEM may be used for diagnosis and characterization of small lesions as a supplementary imaging modality for PET-CT.[25] However, the clinical data regarding dedicated positron breast-imaging devices are still limited.

LOCOREGIONAL STAGING

FDG-PET-CT for Axillary Disease

Axillary lymph node involvement is the most important prognostic factor in patients with breast cancer. Many early studies of FDG-PET for breast cancer were focused on detecting axillary metastases. These studies showed sensitivities of largely 85–90% and higher,[26,27] suggesting the feasibility of FDG-PET as a noninvasive method for axillary staging and potential substitute for axillary nodal dissection. However, the population of patients in these earlier studies was heavily weighted toward more advanced breast cancer than found in typical screened populations. More recent studies with a larger fraction of T1 primary cancers demonstrated lower sensitivities for axillary nodal metastases, as low as 20–30%.[12] These studies also indicated that the sensitivity of FDG-PET for axillary nodal metastases depended on both axillary tumor burden and FDG uptake in the primary tumor. A recently published systematic review on the use of FDG-PET for assessment of axillary lymph node status in early breast cancer, including 26 studies and 2591 patients, indicated a sensitivity of 63% and a specificity of 94%. As a consequence, the authors conclude that replacing sentinel node evaluation with PET, while avoiding local adverse effects, may lead to false-negative results with high risk of relapse and to false-positive results, with patients undergoing unnecessary axillary dissection.[28] These results indicate the limitation of FDG-PET in detecting micrometastases and small tumor-infiltrated axillary lymph nodes. Further studies comparing FDG-PET with sentinal lymph node (SLN) biopsy support the latter for early-stage disease and confirm the limited sensitivity of FDG-PET for axillary nodal metastases in this clinical setting (20–40%), particularly in small (1–15 mm) and isolated lesions.[12,29] Thus, FDG-PET is not sufficiently accurate to replace SLN biopsy in patients with early-stage breast cancer. In locally advanced disease, sensitivity and specificity are increasing, yielding clinically relevant results. In this stage of disease, a positive PET scan is highly specific for the presence of lymph node invasion in the axilla and can be used as a staging procedure before preoperative therapy.[30] Hence, FDG-PET may have a clinical role for patients with a high likelihood of axillary metastases, such as those patients with locally advanced disease and for patients with advanced axillary disease, plexopathy, or symptomatic metastases.[31] Although SLN biopsy is highly sensitive for axillary metastases in early breast cancer and well tolerated by patients, it requires a prolonged surgical session, lymphoscintigraphy, a considerable pathologic work-up and additional cost. If some of the patients with axillary metastases could be identified before the SLN biopsy, axillary lymph node dissection may be performed directly without SLN biopsy. To identify the patients with axillary metastases, some have suggested the use of FDG-PET directed ultrasound with ultrasound-guided biopsy, or a combination of both. For FDG-PET, most of the studies demonstrate specificities in the range of 93–100%.[12,27] The high specificity of FDG-PET could direct the subgroup of patients with axillary disease determined by FDG-PET to targeted sampling (e.g. by ultrasound) or to axillary lymph node dissection and avoid the need for SLN biopsy.

For the immediate future, it appears unlikely that any noninvasive imaging method will provide the same sensitivity as that of SLN biopsy. Thus, SLN biopsy will likely remain the procedure of choice for the staging of axillae, ultrasound the procedure of choice for the sampling of palpable nodes or screening of high-risk axillae and FDG-PET an adjunct tool for high-risk patients and for advanced or recurrent axillary disease, possibly in conjunction with MRI.

FDG-PET-CT for Other Regional Lymph Nodes

Breast cancer can often spread to other regions besides the ipsilateral axilla, including the internal mammary nodes, the supraclavicular nodes and the mediastinal nodes. Evidence has indicated the ability of PET to reveal the involvement of internal mammary lymph nodes and/or distant disease in patients diagnosed with early breast cancer **(Figs. 1A to C)**. In a retrospective study on 73 early breast cancer patients, FDG uptake was detected in mediastinal and/or internal mammary nodes in 40% of them, while CT scan was positive only in 23%. In this study, sensitivity and specificity of PET and CT were, respectively, 85% vs 54% and 90% vs 85%.[32] Moreover, some reports have suggested that internal mammary FDG uptake predicts treatment failure patterns of disease consistent with internal mammary nodal involvement and progression.[33] The likelihood of an extra-axillary lymph node finding on FDG-PET is affected by the position of the tumor (medial vs lateral). The presence of extra-axillary nodal uptake on FDG-PET, combined with medial tumor location, indicated a high-risk of subsequent disease progression.[34]

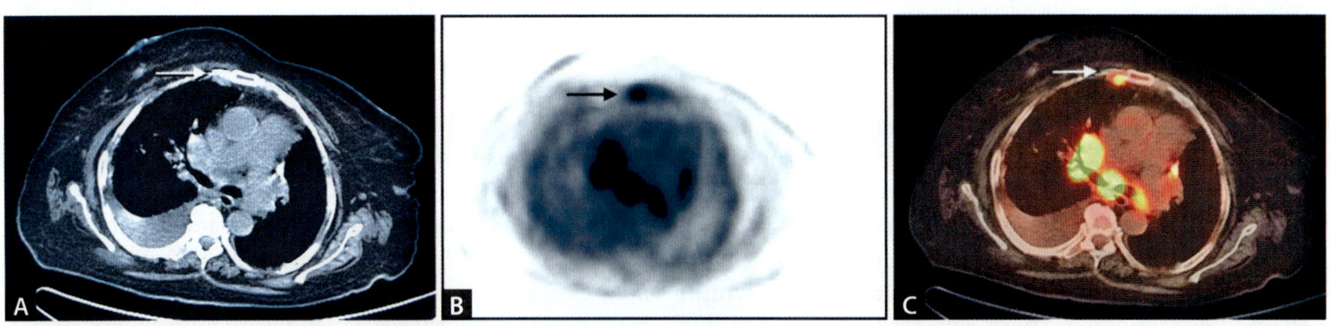

Figs. 1A to C: A 70-year-old lady with invasive ductal carcinoma of left breast. CT (A) image of chest was essentially normal. PET (B) and PET-CT (C) images showed increased FDG uptake in right internal mammary lymph node (arrows), suggesting metastasis. Also noted were multiple FDG-avid mediastinal nodes. Findings were confirmed at postoperative histopathology.

SYSTEMIC STAGING

Distant Metastasis

The presence of distant metastases, outside the breast and regional nodes, is an important factor predicting prognosis and directing the intensity of care, because metastatic (stage IV) breast cancer has a low likelihood of cure. Because of the low yield, cost and distress associated with investigating detected abnormalities that are for the most part false positives, baseline systemic staging is neither performed nor recommended[35] before surgery and axillary staging in patients with early-stage breast cancer.[36-38] In the patients with more advanced disease (such as LABC or inflammatory breast cancer), however, some evidence supports the use of systemic imaging staging at the diagnosis to rule out stage IV disease, which would significantly alter treatment options because of the high likelihood of distant metastases.[39,40] Baseline systemic imaging staging needs to survey the chest, abdomen, pelvis and bones and includes chest radiography or CT, abdominal ultrasound or CT and bone scintigraphy. According to current National Comprehensive Cancer Network (NCCN) Practice Guidelines,[41] FDG-PET or PET-CT is recommended as a staging option for patients with either locally advanced breast cancer or inflammatory breast carcinoma (T3/T4d) especially when standard staging findings are equivocal **(Figs. 2A to C)**. FDG-PET-CT is helpful in identifying unsuspected regional lymph node and distant metastasis in such scenarios.

Bone Metastasis

Bone is the most common site for breast cancer metastasis, and bone metastases will develop in 30–85% of patients with metastatic breast cancer during the course of disease.[42,43] Bone also represents the first site of metastasis for 26–50% of patients with metastatic breast carcinoma.[43,44] Bone metastases in breast cancer can be osteoblastic (bone formation), osteolytic (bone resorption), or mixed lesions. Up to half of all bone metastases from breast cancer tend to show osteolytic changes. Breast cancer preferentially metastasizes to the spine and pelvis, followed by ribs, skull and femur.[44] Bone scintigraphy (BS) is the most widely used tool to identify bone metastases. However, this technique is less sensitive than high-resolution CT and MRI and needs adequate correlation with radiological investigation in case of doubtful bone uptake. In particular, lytic lesions are frequently underestimated by BS and additional investigations are needed.[45] Recently, hybrid SPECT-CT in patients with breast cancer has been shown to be superior to planar scintigraphy for characterizing equivocal BS lesions.[46]

A recent retrospective study, performed at Memorial Sloan-Kettering Cancer Center supports the use of PET in detecting bone metastases for metastatic breast cancer, but due to its retrospective nature, this study was not able to assess whether FDG-PET may replace BS in this setting.[47] FDG PET-CT is a sensitive tool for bone metastases, with

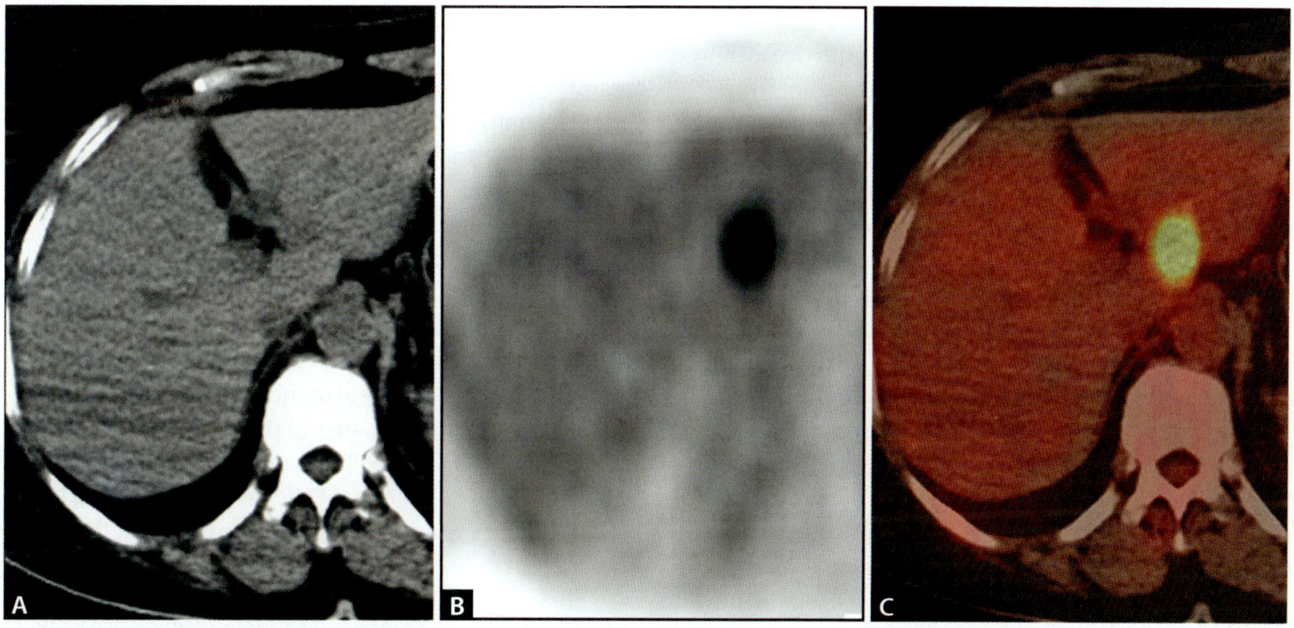

Figs. 2A to C: A 65-year-old lady with inflammatory breast cancer underwent baseline FDG-PET-CT. Noncontrast CT (A) image of liver was normal. PET (B) and PET-CT (C) images showed solitary FDG avid metastasis in liver. This changed the management from curative to palliative.

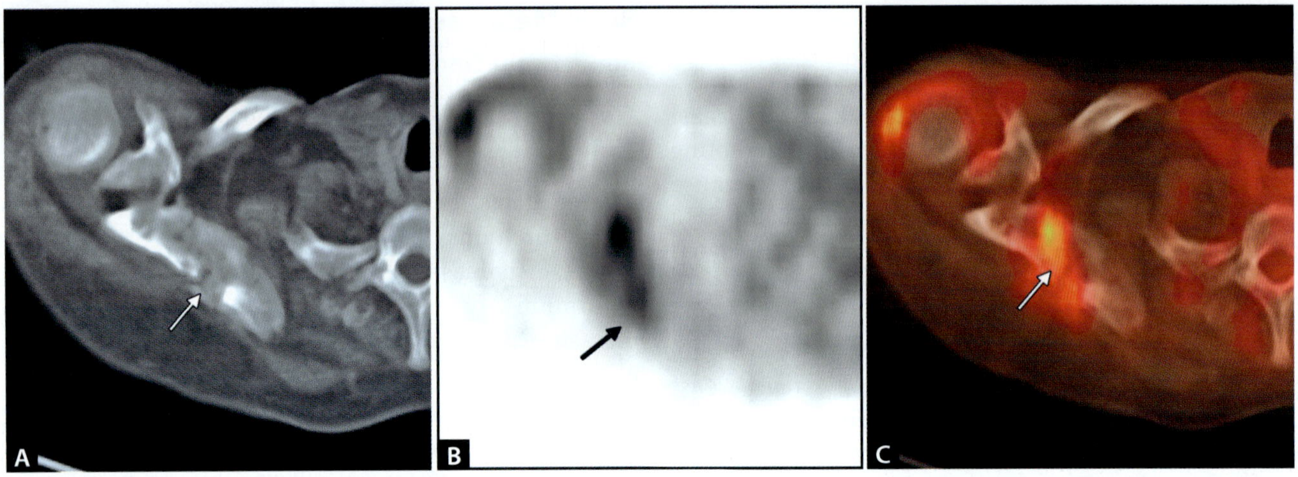

Figs. 3A to C: A 47-year-old previously treated breast cancer patient. CT (A) images showed mixed lytic sclerotic lesion in right scapula which showed FDG uptake in PET (B) and PET-CT (C) images (arrows). This was suspicious for bone metastasis. The lesion was not much FDG-avid (SUVmax-2.1).

an acknowledged high accuracy for lytic lesions at risk of complications such as pain and fracture, whereas a low FDG uptake has been detected in sclerotic metastases **(Figs. 3A to C)**. This observation could be related to the notion that FDG-negative sclerotic bone lesions may no longer be metabolically active or even that they may not contain malignant cells.[48] However, this may not be entirely true.

^{18}F-Fluoride PET-CT for Bone Metastasis

Another interesting application of PET in the evaluation of bone metastases is the use of ^{18}F-Fluoride, a bone imaging agent for PET. The combination of the better spatial resolution of PET-CT and the improved image quality achieved by the favorable pharmacokinetic characteristics of ^{18}F-Fluoride, has led to its use in the evaluation of skeletal metastases. However, increased ^{18}F-Fluoride uptake is not specific for tumoral bone involvement and the high sensitivity of ^{18}F-Fluoride PET may also be associated with a higher detection rate of benign bone lesions. As in the case of BS, lesions detected on ^{18}F-Fluoride PET often require correlation with CT or MRI for further validation. ^{18}F-Fluoride PET has been shown to be more accurate than bone scan in detecting both sclerotic and lytic lesions in breast cancer and to be a valid alternative to BS in patients at high-risk of metastatic bone disease.[49] The high detection rate of metastases by ^{18}F-Fluoride PET-CT could be used as a staging procedure in high-risk breast cancer patients who have a high probability of bone involvement. Moreover, the early identification of bone metastases may enable adequate treatment to prevent bone complications such as fractures and pain. Considering the low sensitivity of FDG-PET-CT for small osteoblastic bone lesions, the integrated use of ^{18}F-Fluoride PET-CT in doubtful cases could be of interest.

RESPONSE TO CHEMOTHERAPY

An interesting potential application of PET is the early identification of treatment effectiveness through a comparison of the levels of radiotracer uptake before and after 1 or 2 cycles of systemic therapy. In fact, while morphological changes due to effective therapy are not detectable until late in the course of treatment, metabolic changes generally occur earlier.[50,51] At least two sequential FDG-PET scans are warranted for the early prediction of treatment response; the first scan is usually performed at baseline, before therapy is administered and the second one is obtained after the first or second cycle. Evaluation of tumor response with FDG-PET has several advantages over anatomically based criteria. Some therapeutic agents, such as biological drugs, are cytostatic rather than cytotoxic and do not change the tumor size despite their effectiveness.[52] PET response criteria in solid tumors (PERCIST Criteria) have been developed recently. The PERCIST criteria for treatment response are based on SUV measurement. SUL, one of the many variants of SUV, defined as SUV corrected for lean body mass, was selected for use by PERCIST because SUL has been shown to be less susceptible to variations in patient body weight than other SUV metrics.[53] According to PERCIST, response to therapy is evaluated as a continuous variable and expressed as percentage change in SUL peak between the pre-treatment and post-treatment scans.

Neoadjuvant Chemotherapy

Neoadjuvant chemotherapy has gained acceptance in treating locally advanced breast cancer. The advantages of neoadjuvant treatment over conventional adjuvant chemotherapy include improved rates of complete resection and the ability to convert mastectomy candidates to breast conservation candidates. If neoadjuvant chemotherapy is selected, monitoring tumor response to treatment by assessing the residual tumor size is essential to determine the best course of surgical action. The modalities that exist at this time to assess a tumor's response to neoadjuvant treatment include physical exam (PE), MR imaging and mammography (MG). These three modalities (PE, MG and MR imaging) have been found to carry both significant false positive and false negative rates.[54,55] In addition, chemotherapy itself may induce significant biologic changes of the tumor, affecting imaging findings differently. PET-CT might overcome some of these limitations. In a recent study, the PET definition of NR (nonresponder) as less than 50% reduction in tumor SUV was more predictive of pNR (pathologic nonresponder) compared with MR imaging or clinical breast examination (CBE).[56] PET-CT response for neoadjuvant chemotherapy also correlates well with histopathological response **(Figs. 4A to D)**.[57]

Lymph node assessment in patients receiving neoadjuvant chemotherapy can also provide information regarding prognosis as well as treatment planning. A recent prospective study compared PE, MG, MR imaging and PET-CT in tumor and lymph node assessment in patients with T3/T4 tumors receiving neoadjuvant chemotherapy.[58] The results showed PE and PET scan after neoadjuvant chemotherapy to be highly specific for nodal disease, but with poor sensitivity and accuracy. In addition, baseline PET and PE were shown to be more accurate and sensitive in predicting the final nodal status

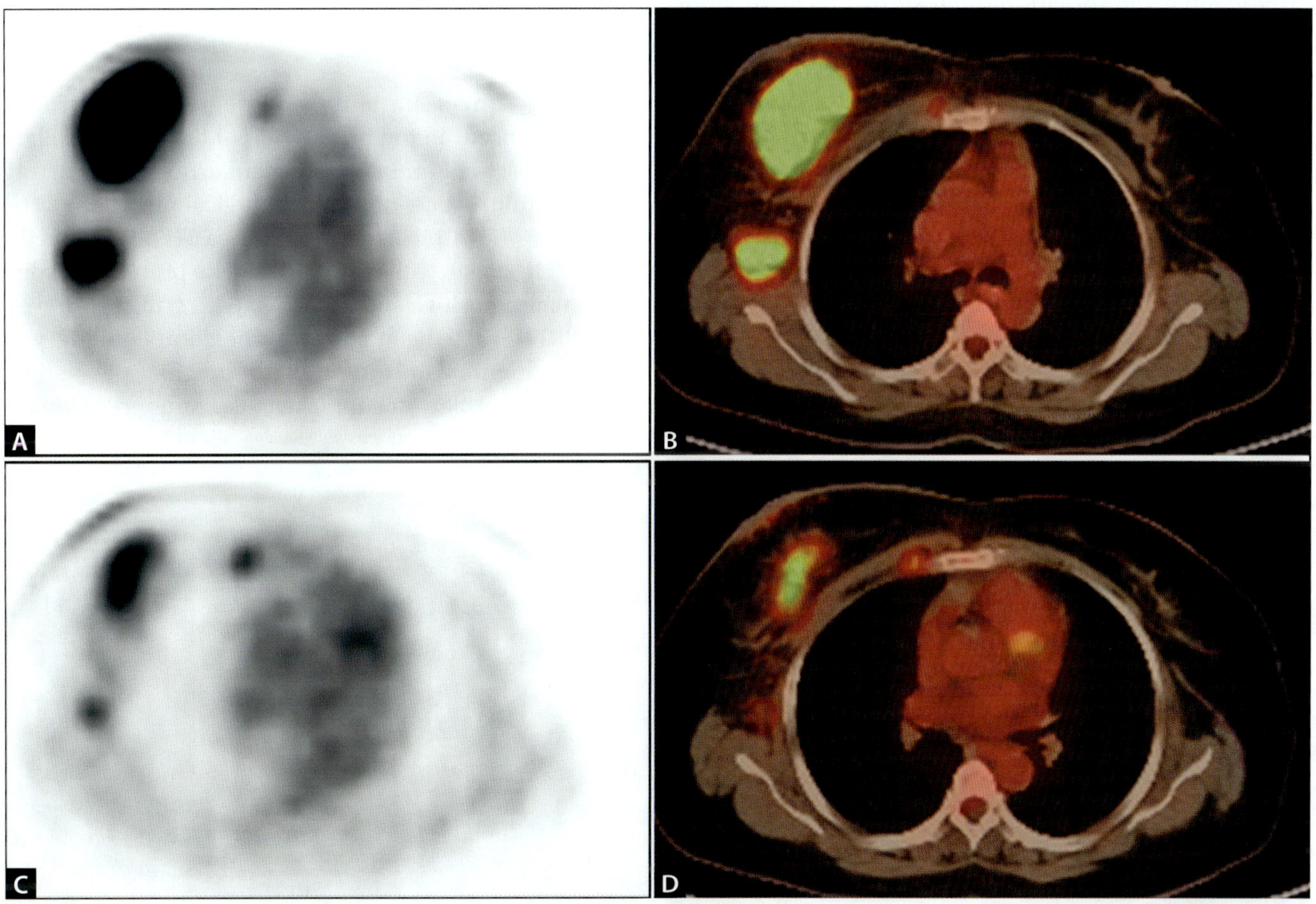

Figs. 4A to D: A 43-year-old lady with ductal carcinoma of right breast with ipsilateral axillary lymph node metastasis. Baseline PET (A) and PET-CT (B) images show FDG avid primary breast mass with FDG avid metastatic axillary nodes. PET-CT was repeated after 3 cycles of neoadjuvant chemotherapy to response. Postchemotherapy images (C and D) showed significant reduction in size as well as FDG uptake of both the primary tumors as well as lymph nodes. The PET-CT impression was responder which was confirmed on histopathology.

than the post neoadjuvant evaluation by either PE or PET, but none was sufficient to replace pathologic staging. FDG-PET has the potential to provide valuable staging information and possibly predict tumor response, but its role in the evaluation of lymph node involvement after neoadjuvant chemotherapy is yet to be clearly defined.

Adjuvant Chemotherapy in Metastatic Disease

The clinical utility of sequential FDG-PET in patients with metastatic disease undergoing chemotherapy has been evaluated in small case series studies. Some studies suggested that imaging as early as after 1 cycle of chemotherapy could predict response. In most of them, a significant decrease in tumor FDG uptake was observed after the first course of therapy, whereas no substantial decrease was detected in non-responding patients. These preliminary observations were confirmed in a more recent study, which confirmed the predictive ability of FDG-PET in the identification of early response to treatment, superior to conventional imaging procedures performed after three chemotherapy cycles. Most studies showed, similar to neoadjuvant therapy, that response is accompanied by substantial drops in FDG uptake, typically 40–250% or more from the pretherapy baselines.[59] There is a relative paucity of studies that had evaluated the role of metastatic disease other than bone and axillary lymph nodes.

A particularly vexing clinical problem for breast cancer clinicians is the evaluation of response of bone metastases. Bone metastases are not considered evaluable for response by RECIST criteria. ^{18}F-Fluoride PET, because it images bone metastases through a mechanism similar to bone scintigraphy, may yield comparable results to that of former. In fact a fluoride PET flare response has been reported similar to BS.[60] In contrast, FDG-PET might image hypermetabolism in the tumor itself and therefore provide useful information. A recent study showed that both metabolic and structural changes on FDG PET-CT predicted bone metastasis time to progression.[61] In interpreting FDG-PET studies to evaluate bone metastasis response, it is important to recognize that although an absence of uptake after therapy indicates a good response to treatment and favorable prediction for time to progression, it does not indicate an absence of disease. Although FDG-PET has been a highly successful modality in monitoring response to treatment, tumor recurrence, and restaging, one must keep in mind the phenomenon of "metabolic flare," which is a transient increase in FDG activity very early in the course of therapy. Such an increase occurs 7–10 days after initiating hormonal therapy because of partial estrogen-like agonist effects of tamoxifen and should not be construed as disease progression.

RESTAGING

In breast cancer patients, locoregional recurrence commonly occur in the breast, skin of the breast, axillary nodes, chest wall and supraclavicular nodes; occurring mostly within 5 years of primary surgical resection.[62] The evaluation of local recurrence in the breast **(Figs. 5A and B)**, skin, or chest wall with FDG-PET can be problematic due to both false positive and false negative results. However, FDG-PET-CT has been shown to be complementary to MRI in patients with symptoms of brachial plexopathy suspected of axillary or supraclavicular tumor recurrence,

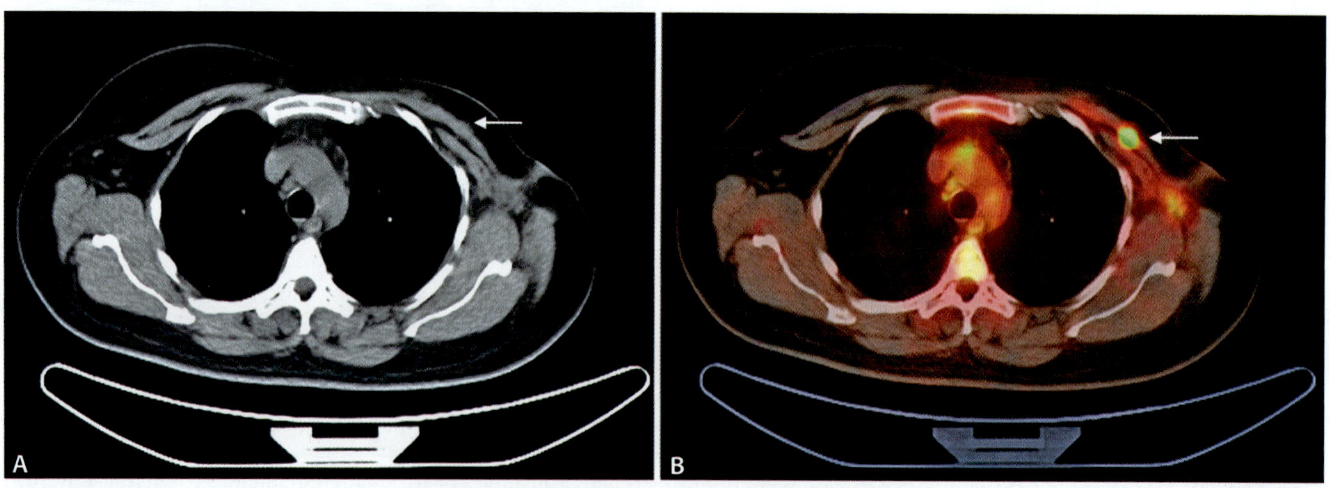

Figs. 5A and B: A 38-year-old lady with left breast cancer, postmastectomy and axillary dissection. PET-CT was done for restaging. CT (A) images failed to show any definite abnormality. PET-CT (B) images show focal FDG uptake in the left chest wall (arrows) suggestive of local recurrence. Findings were confirmed with FNAC.

because either tumor recurrence or treatment-induced scarring can be responsible for the symptoms.[63,64]

Neoplastic involvement of internal mammary nodes may go undetected at initial diagnosis and, if not adequately treated, may give rise to intrathoracic recurrence in the follow-up period. A number of studies have pointed towards the value of PET-CT in new or recurrent locally advanced breast cancer (LABC). Experience with imaging patients with LABC shows that the prevalence of internal mammary FDG uptake can be as high as 25% and that the presence of internal mammary FDG uptake predicts treatment failure patterns of disease consistent with internal mammary nodal involvement and progression.[33,65]

FDG-PET-CT can be helpful in the evaluation for distant metastases in patients who have been previously treated for their primary disease, particularly in those with advanced stages of disease, equivocal CT findings and in asymptomatic patients with elevated tumor markers. In a meta-analysis of FDG-PET for the evaluation of breast recurrence and metastases, a median sensitivity and specificity of 93% and 82%, respectively, was reported in a patient-based analysis.[66] It has been shown that FDG-PET detects a significantly greater number (about twofold) of extra-axillary lymph node metastases. Neoplastic spread to mediastinal nodes is common in patients with advanced disease. FDG PET has been shown to have higher sensitivity and specificity than CT for this site.[67] Bone is the most frequent site of recurrence after treatment for primary breast cancer; nearly 70% of patients with advanced disease have skeletal metastases. It has been shown that FDG-PET is superior to bone scintigraphy in the detection of osteolytic metastases and bone scintigraphy detects significantly more osteoblastic metastases.[48] FDG uptake is a more direct reflection of metabolically active tumor cells in bone, whereas bone scintigraphy reflects a reparative process occurring in bone tissues adjacent to tumor cells. Although FDG-PET cannot replace BS, it can help to clarify staging in the case of difficult or equivocal conventional staging. Use of PET-CT is very useful in such circumstances. In a study for detection of systemic metastases, PET-CT added incremental diagnostic confidence in 60% of patients who had positive FDG uptake compared with FDG-PET alone.[68] The boost in confidence was caused by better anatomic localization of FDG foci in over half of the cases and fewer equivocal readings. For the evaluation of pulmonary metastases, there was a tendency for the readers of PET-CT or CT alone to overestimate disease, probably because any pulmonary nodule seen on CT in this patient group is considered suspicious and to underestimate disease with PET alone because of the small size of these lesions. Slightly fewer hepatic metastases were detected at CT alone compared with PET-CT or PET alone indicating that FDG-PET enhances slightly the sensitivity for detecting metastatic disease in the liver.[69,70] Keeping in mind these advantages of PET-CT, some investigators have recommended the use of PET-CT for the detection of local and distant recurrences in patients previously treated for primary breast cancer because the combination of CT and PET overcomes the limitations of each modality when used separately. This needs to be confirmed in larger prospective trials using FDG-PET-CT based algorithms.

Prognostication

Predicting tumor behavior and in particular the likelihood of cancer relapse or progression, is an increasingly important part of directing breast cancer therapy and is traditionally done by *in vitro* assay of tumor biopsy material. Early data suggest that parameters from radiotracer imaging may also carry prognostic information for breast cancer. A study showed that the level of FDG uptake in the primary tumor was predictive of disease-free survival.[71] Other studies showed that the patterns of perfusion, measured by PET or MRI and kinetics of FDG uptake are prognostically significant.[72,73] Although it is unlikely that one would perform MRI or PET solely to gather prognostic information, such information may be readily available from scans obtained for staging or response evaluation and therefore, merits further investigation.

RECEPTOR IMAGING

Although molecular imaging of breast cancer is still not commonly used in daily clinical practice, its application portfolio is expanding rapidly. Increasingly more breast cancer–specific targets are imaged such as the estrogen receptor (ER), growth factors and growth factor receptors. The presence of ERs and PRs is predictive of a successful response to hormone therapy. Whereas ER expression alone is associated with a favorable response to hormone therapy, PR expression has been shown to have additional value to predict a successful response to tamoxifen.[74] The presence of both receptors is more predictive than either receptor alone. Imaging of the ER with the PET tracer 16-alpha-[(18)F]fluoro-17-beta-estradiol (FES) has shown a good correlation between FES tumor uptake and ER density.[75] FES uptake is readily visualized and quantified in primary and metastatic breast cancer and can identify heterogeneous ER expression, for example, loss of ER expression in metastases arising from ER-expressing primary tumors.[76] The level of FES uptake has been shown to be predictive of response to endocrine therapy,[77] including heavily pretreated patients. Serial FES PET can also measure the pharmacodynamic effect of drugs on estradiol binding to the ER, yielding insights into determinants of drug efficacy.[78]

HER2 (ErbB2) expression in breast cancer has become an important indicator of prognosis and an increasingly important target for therapy. Wide arrays of labelled tracers are being clinically evaluated for this purpose. Recently, a study used ^{111}Indium-trastuzumab SPECT to image the human epidermal growth factor receptor 2 (HER2) and showed that in most patients with metastatic HER2- positive disease more lesions were detected than with conventional staging procedures.[79] Various PET-CT tracers are being evaluated for this purpose. This includes ^{18}F-labeled Affibody molecules, ^{68}Ga-DOTA-Affibody molecule and ^{89}Zr-Trastuzumab.[80,81] Few clinical studies with these tracers are underway and may define its role in clinical imaging.

FUTURE DIRECTIONS

Several methods have addressed tumor biosynthesis as an indicator of tumor growth, with approaches targeted to protein synthesis and membrane synthesis. The uptake of labeled amino acids, such as ^{11}C-methionine, has been shown to correlate with tumor growth and changes in uptake provide an early indication of breast cancer response to therapy.[82] Aberrant cellular proliferation is a fundamental property of cancer, including breast cancer. Assay of breast tissue for cellular proliferation, typically by assay of MIB-1 (Ki-67), is routinely performed in many centers. ^{18}F-Fluorothymidine (^{18}F-FLT) is an imaging marker for DNA synthesis and correlates well with Ki-67. FLT PET-CT appears especially promising for measuring the early effects of therapy on breast cancer growth, as suggested by recent studies[83] that showed ability of serial FLT PET-CTs to identify early responders, and importantly, nonresponders. This is an exciting area of imaging research and likely to be of clinical importance in the future.

Tumor vascularity has been recognized as being important in cancer growth and metastasis and in the systemic delivery of therapeutic agents.[84] Antiangiogenic agents such as bevacizumab are now used as part of US. Food and Drug Administration–approved breast cancer treatments.[85] For these reasons, the ability to image and quantify tumor perfusion and neovasculature is a clinically important need. Tumor perfusion is one of the earliest physiologic properties to be measured and advances in methodology have led to increasingly quantitative approaches. The most physiologically robust and quantitative measures of tumor blood flow use freely diffusible imaging probes. One example is the use of $^{150}H_2O$ to measure tumor blood flow by PET, which yields measures of tumor blood flow in mL/min/g. $^{150}H_2O$ PET has been shown to yield reliable estimates of tumor blood flow for breast cancer.[86] Recent studies have shown that serial measures of breast cancer perfusion by $^{150}H_2O$ PET in the neoadjuvant setting are highly predictive of response and survival.[87] Simplifying things further, studies have suggested that dynamic FDG-PET and kinetic analysis may yield estimates of tumor perfusion, inferred from the FDG delivery (K1) kinetic parameter, comparable to $^{150}H_2O$ PET. Studies have shown that this parameter is predictive of response[88] and recent studies have suggested that changes in FDG K1 with therapy in the neoadjuvant setting are comparable to changes in perfusion from $^{150}H_2O$ in ability to predict response and survival.[73] Thus, it may be possible to obtain information from dynamic FDG-PET on both tumor perfusion and metabolism that is clinically predictive. This approach, therefore, merits further investigation.

Although tumor perfusion imaging measures the physiologic consequences of angiogenesis, perfusion is not specific to tumor neovessels and is influenced by physiologic parameters not necessarily related to tumor angiogenesis.[84] Targeted imaging probes can noninvasively and specifically assess tumor neovasculature. PET probes based on labeled peptides that bind specifically to integrins expressed in neovessels have been studied in animals and tested in humans.[89] Such agents may be especially helpful for therapies directed at tumor neovasculature, such as bevacizumab.

Cell death, or apoptosis, is a fundamental part of normal cellular physiology and an early indicator of therapeutic response. Methods for imaging cell death based on extension of annexin V staining *in vitro*, which indicates apoptotic cells through binding to phosphatidylserines. The earlier study used ^{99m}Tc-annexin and SPECT to measure apoptosis in animal models and patients.[90] Methods for annexin-based apoptosis imaging have been developed for PET and are currently under investigation.

Another exciting development is the availability of clinical PET-MRI systems. These systems will combine the excellent resolution of MRI with functional information rendered by PET, but with a lesser radiation dose. As breast cancer treatment becomes increasingly targeted and individualized, demands on breast cancer diagnostic modalities have increased. We hope that in future with combination of multiple PET radiopharmaceuticals we will be able to provide specific information as desired by the treating oncologist.

CONCLUSION

PET-CT is a powerful metabolic imaging method for breast cancer. Currently, it has limited role in primary tumor detection and axillary nodal staging. The major utility of PET-CT lies in detection on extra-axillary nodal metastasis and distant metastasis. It also appears to be very useful for monitoring treatment response and detection of recurrent disease. The availability of newer tracers, hybrid PET-MRI and positron emission mammography might redefine its role in management of breast cancer.

REFERENCES

1. Jemal A, Bray F, Center MM, Ferlay J, Ward E, Forman D. Global cancer statistics. CA: A Cancer Journal for Clinicians. 2011;61:69-90.
2. Hulka BS, Moorman PG. Breast cancer: hormones and other risk factors. Maturitas. 2001;38:103-13.
3. Baan R, Straif K, Grosse Y, et al. Carcinogenicity of alcoholic beverages. Lancet Oncol. 2007;8:292-3.
4. Parkin DM, Whelan S, Ferlay J, Storm H, et al. Cancer Incidence in Five Continents. Vol I to VIII. Cancer Base No. 7. Lyon: IARC Press; 2005.
5. Colditz GA, Sellers TA, Trapido E. Epidemiology-identifying the causes and preventability of cancer? Nat Rev. 2006;6:75-83.
6. Ito Y, Ioka A, Tanaka M, Nakayama T, Tsukuma H. Trends in cancer incidence and mortality in Osaka, Japan: evaluation of cancer control activities. Cancer Sci. 2009;100:2390-5.
7. Schnitt SJ. Traditional and newer pathologic factors. J Natl Cancer Inst Monogr. 2001;2001:22-6.
8. Walker RA. Immunohistochemical markers as predictive tools for breast cancer. J Clin Pathol. 2008;61:689-96.
9. Avril N, Menzel M, Dose J, et al. Glucose metabolism of breast cancer assessed by ^{18}F-FDG PET: histologic and immunohistochemical tissue analysis. J Nucl Med. 2001;42:9-16.
10. Bos R, van Der Hoeven JJ, van Der Wall E, et al. Biologic correlates of ^{18}fluorodeoxyglucose uptake in human breast cancer measured by positron emission tomography. J Clin Oncol. 2002;20:379-87.
11. Scheidhauer K, Walter C, Seemann MD. FDG PET and other imaging modalities in the primary diagnosis of suspicious breast lesions. Eur J Nucl Med Mol Imaging. 2004;31 (suppl 1):S70-9.
12. Rosen EL, Eubank WB, Mankoff DA. FDG PET, PET/CT and breast cancer imaging. Radiographics. 2007;27:S215-29.
13. Lim HS, Yoon WY, Chung TW, et al. FDG PET/CT for the detection and evaluation of breast diseases: usefulness and limitations. Radiographics. 2007;27:S197-213.
14. Kang BJ, Lee JH, Yoo IeR, et al. Clinical significance of incidental finding of focal activity in the breast at ^{18}F-FDG PET/CT. Am J Roentgenol. 2011;197:341-7.
15. MacDonald L, Edwards L, Lewellen T, et al. Clinical Imaging Characteristics of the Positron Emission Mammography Camera: PEM Flex Solo II. J Nucl Med. 2009;50:1666-75.
16. Mavi A, Urhan M, Yu JQ, et al. Dual time point ^{18}F-FDG PET imaging detects breast cancer with high sensitivity and correlates well with histologic subtypes. J Nucl Med. 2006;47:1440-6.
17. Mavi A, Cermik TF, Urhan M, Puskulcu H, Basu S, Cucchiara AJ, Yu JQ, Alavi A. The Effect of Age, Menopausal State, and Breast Density on ^{18}F-FDG Uptake in Normal Glandular Breast Tissue. J Nucl Med. 2010;51:347-52.
18. Kobe K, Chin T, Aoki R, Hyakusoku H. A False-Positive Fluorodeoxyglucose Positron Emission Tomography (FDG-PET) Imaging Result for a Patient After Augmentation Mammaplasty. Aesthetic Plastic Surgery. 2009;33:611-5.
19. Juweid ME, Cheson BD. Positron-emission tomography and assessment of cancer therapy. N Engl J Med. 2006;354: 496-507.
20. Muzaffar AR, Rohrich RJ. The silicone gel-filled breast implant controversy: an update. Plast Reconstr Surg. 2002;109:742-7.
21. Spear SL, Spittler CJ. Breast reconstruction with implants and expanders. Plast Reconstr Surg. 2001;107:177-87.
22. Noh DY, Yun IJ, Kang HS, Kim YC, Kim JS, Chung JK. Detection of cancer in augmented breasts by positron emission tomography. Eur J Surg. 1999;165:847-51.
23. Nadig MR, Kumar R, Patel CD, et al. Detection of contralateral breast cancer in patients with known breast cancer undergoing PET-CT scan for restaging. J Nucl Med. 2007;48(Suppl):367 P (1572).
24. Berg WA, Weinberg IN, Narayanan D, Lobrano ME, Ross E, Amodei L, et al. High resolution fluorodeoxyglucose positron emission tomography with compression ("positron emission mammography") is highly accurate in depicting primary breast cancer. Breast J. 2006;12:309-23.
25. Eo JS, et al. Imaging sensitivity of dedicated positron emission mammography in relation to tumor size. The Breast. 2011;doi:10.1016/j.breast.2011.08.002.
26. Crippa F, Gerali A, Alessi A, Agresti R, Bombardieri E. FDG-PET for axillary lymph node staging in primary breast cancer. Eur J Nucl Med Mol Imaging. 2004;31 (suppl 1):S97-102.
27. Eubank W, Mankoff D. Current and future uses of positron emission tomography in breast cancer imaging. Semin Nucl Med. 2004;34:224-40.
28. Cooper K, Harnan S, Meng Y, et al. Positron emission tomography (PET) for assessment of axillary lymph node status in early breast cancer: a systematic review and meta-analysis. Eur J Surg Oncol. 2011;37:187-98.
29. Powles T, Murray I, Brock C, Oliver T, Avril N. Molecular positron emission tomography and PET/CT imaging in urological malignancies. Eur Urol. 2007;51:1511-20.

30. Van der Hoeven JJM, Krak NC, Hoekstra OS, et al. ^{18}F-2-Fluoro-2-Deoxy-D-Glucose positron emission tomography in staging of locally advanced breast cancer. J Clin Oncol. 2004;22:1253-9.
31. Eubank WB, Mankoff DA. Evolving role of positron emission tomography in breast cancer imaging. Semin Nucl Med. 2005;35:84-99.
32. Eubanks WB, Markoff D, Bhattacharya M, et al. Impact of FDG-PET on defining the extent of disease and on the treatment of patients with recurrent or metastatic breast cancer. Am J Roentgenol. 2004;183:479-86.
33. Bellon JR, Livingston RB, Eubank WB, et al. Evaluation of the internal mammary lymph nodes by FDG-PET in locally advanced breast cancer (LABC). Am J Clin Oncol. 2004;27:407-10.
34. Tran A, Pio BS, Khatibi B, Czernin J, Phelps ME, Silverman DH. ^{18}F-FDG PET for staging breast cancer in patients with inner-quadrant versus outer quadrant tumors: comparison with long-term clinical outcome. J Nucl Med. 2005;46:1455-9.
35. Carlson RW, Anderson BO, Burstein HJ, et al. Invasive breast cancer. J Natl Compr Canc Netw. 2007;5:246-312.
36. Puglisi F, Follador A, Minisini AM, et al. Baseline staging tests after a new diagnosis of breast cancer: further evidence of their limited indications. Ann Oncol. 2005;16:263-6.
37. Ravaioli A, Pasini G, Polselli A, et al. Staging of breast cancer: new recommended standard procedure. Breast Cancer Res Treat. 2002;72:53-60.
38. Hodgson NC, Gulenchyn KY. Is there a role for positron emission tomography in breast cancer staging? J Clin Oncol. 2008;26:712-20.
39. Shenkier T, Weir L, Levine M, Olivotto I, Whelan T, Reyno L. Clinical practice guidelines for the care and treatment of breast cancer: Treatment for women with stage III or locally advanced breast cancer. CMAJ. 2004;170:983-94.
40. Chia S, Swain SM, Byrd DR, Mankoff DA. Locally advanced and inflammatory breast cancer. J Clin Oncol. 2008;26:786-90.
41. Carlson RW, Allred DC, Anderson BO, et al. NCCN Clinical Practice Guidelines in Oncology TM. Breast Cancer. Version 2.2011.
42. Hortobagyi GN. Bone metastases in breast cancer patients. Semin Oncol. 1991;18:11-5.
43. Hamaoka T, Madewell JE, Podoloff DA, Hortobagyi GN, Ueno NT. Bone imaging in metastatic breast cancer. J Clin Oncol. 2004;22:2942-53.
44. Pivot X, Asmar L, Hortobagyi GN, Theriault R, Pastorini F, Buzdar A. A retrospective study of first indicators of breast cancer recurrence. Oncology. 2000;58:185-90.
45. Haubold-Reuter BG, Duwell S, Schilcher BR, et al. The value of bone scintigraphy, bone marrow scintigraphy and fast spin magnetic resonance imaging in staging of patients with malignant solid tumors: A prospective study. Eur J Nucl Med. 1993;20:1063-9.
46. Sharma P, Singh H, Kumar R, Bal CS, Thulkar S, Seenu V, Malhotra A. Bone scintigraphy in breast cancer: added value of hybrid SPECT-CT and its impact on patient management. Nucl Med Commun. 2012;33:139-47.
47. Morris PG, Lynch C, Feeney JN, et al. Integrated Positron Emission Tomography/Computed Tomography may render bone scintigraphy unnecessary to investigate suspected metastatic breast cancer. J Clin Oncol. 2010;28:3154-9.
48. Cook GJ, Houston S, Rubens R, et al. Detection of bone metastases in breast cancer by ^{18}FDG PET: differing metabolic activity in osteoblastic and osteolytic lesions. J Clin Oncol. 1998;16:3375-9.
49. Schirrmeister H, Guhlmann A, Elsner K, et al. Sensitivity in detecting osseous lesions depends on anatomic localization: planar bone scintigraphy versus ^{18}F PET. J Nucl Med. 1999;40:1623-9.
50. Wahl RL, Zasadny K, Helvie M, et al. Metabolic monitoring of breast cancer chemohormonotherapy using positron emission tomography: initial evaluation. J Clin Oncol. 1993;11:2101-11.
51. Jansson T, Westlin JE, Ahlstrom H, et al. Positron emission tomography studies in patients with locally advanced and/or metastatic breast cancer: a method for early therapy evaluation? J Clin Oncol. 1995;13:1470-7.
52. Michaelis LC, Ratain MJ. Measuring response in a post-RECIST world: from black and white to shades of grey. Nat Rev Cancer. 2006;6:409-14.
53. Wahl RL, Jacene H, Kasamon Y, et al. From RECIST to PERCIST: Evolving Considerations for PET response criteria in solid tumors. J Nucl Med. 2009;50:122S-50S.
54. Homer MJ. Mammographic interpretation: a practical approach. New York: McGraw-Hill; 1991.pp.4-5.
55. Orel SG, Schnall MD, LiVolsi VA, et al. Suspicious breast lesions: MR imaging with radiologic-pathologic correlation. Radiology. 1994;190:485-93.
56. Chen X, Moore MO, Lehman CD, et al. Combined use of MRI and PET to monitor response and assess residual disease for locally advanced breast cancer treated with neoadjuvant chemotherapy. Acad Radiol. 2004;11:1115-24.
57. Kumar A, Kumar R, Seenu V, Gupta SD, Chawla M, Malhotra A, Mehta SN. The role of ^{18}F-FDG PET/CT in evaluation of early response to neoadjuvant chemotherapy in patients with locally advanced breast cancer. Eur Radiol. 2009;19:1347-57.
58. Prati R, Minami CA, Gornbein JA, et al. Accuracy of clinical evaluation of locally advanced breast cancer in patients receiving neoadjuvant chemotherapy. Cancer. 2009;115:1194-202.
59. Couturier O, Jerusalem G, N'Guyen JM, Hustinx R. Sequential positron emission tomography using [^{18}F]fluorodeoxyglucose for monitoring response to chemotherapy in metastatic breast cancer. Clin Cancer Res. 2006;12:6437-43.
60. Wade AA, Scott JA, Kuter I, Fischman AJ. Flare response in ^{18}F-fluoride ion PET bone scanning. AJR. 2006;186:1783-6.
61. Tateishi U, Gamez C, Dawood S, Yeung HW, Cristofanilli M, Macapinlac HA. Bone metastases in patients with metastatic breast cancer: morphologic and metabolic monitoring of response to systemic therapy with integrated PET/CT. Radiology. 2008;247:189-96.

62. Katz A, Strom EA, Buchholz TA, et al. Locoregional recurrence patterns after mastectomy and doxorubicin-based chemotherapy: implications for postoperative irradiation. J Clin Oncol. 2000;18:2817-27.
63. Hathaway PB, Mankoff DA, Maravilla KR, et al. The value of combined FDG-PET and magnetic resonance imaging in the evaluation of suspected recurrent local-regional breast cancer: preliminary experience. Radiology. 1999;210:807-14.
64. Ahmad A, Barrington S, Maisey M, et al. Use of positron emission tomography in evaluation of brachial plexopathy in breast cancer patients. Br J Cancer. 1999;79:478-82.
65. Danforth DN Jr, Aloj L, Carrasquillo JA, et al. The role of [F-18]-FDG-PET in the local/regional evaluation of women with breast cancer. Breast Cancer Res Treat. 2002;75:135-46.
66. Isasi CR, Moadel RM, Blaufox MD. A meta-analysis of FDG-PET for the evaluation of breast cancer recurrence and metastases. Breast Cancer Res Treat. 2005;90:105-12.
67. Eubank WB, Mankoff DA, Takasugi J, et al. [F-18]-fluorodeoxyglucose positron emission tomography to detect mediastinal or internal mammary metastases in breast cancer. J Clin Oncol. 2001;19:3516-23.
68. Tatsumi MCC, Mortzikos KA, Fishman EK, et al. Initial experience with FDG-PET/CT in the evaluation of breast cancer. Eur J Nucl Med Mol Imaging. 2006;33:254-62.
69. Haug AR, Schmidt GP, Klingenstein A, et al. [F-18]- fluoro-2-deoxyglucose positron emission tomography/computed tomography in the follow-up of breast cancer with elevated levels of tumor markers. J Comput Assist Tomogr. 2007;31:629-34.
70. Radan L, Ben-Haim S, Bar-Shalom R, et al. The role of FDG-PET/CT in suspected recurrence of breast cancer. Cancer. 2006;107:2545-51.
71. Oshida M, Uno K, Suzuki M, et al. Predicting the prognoses of breast carcinoma patients with positron emission tomography using 2-deoxy-2-fluoro[18F]-D-glucose. Cancer. 1998;82:2227-34.
72. Semple SI, Gilbert FJ, Redpath TW, et al. The relationship between vascular and metabolic characteristics of primary breast tumours. Eur Radiol. 2004;14:2038-45.
73. Dunnwald LK, Gralow JR, Ellis GK, et al. Tumor metabolism and blood flow changes by positron emission tomography: relation to survival in patients treated with neoadjuvant chemotherapy for locally advanced breast cancer. J Clin Oncol. 2008;26:4449-57.
74. Bardou VJ, Arpino G, Elledge RM, et al. Progesterone receptor status significantly improves outcome prediction over estrogen receptor status alone for adjuvant endocrine therapy in two large breast cancer databases. J Clin Oncol. 2003;21:1973.
75. MacGuire AH, Dehdashti F, Siegel BA, et al. Positron tomographic assessment of 16 alpha-[18F] fluoro-17 beta-estradiol uptake in metastatic breast carcinoma. J Nucl Med. 1991;8:1526-31.
76. Dehdashti F, Mortimer JE, Siegel BA, et al. Positron tomographic assessment of estrogen receptors in breast cancer: comparison with FDG-PET and *in vitro* receptor assays. J Nucl Med. 1995;36:1766-74.
77. Linden HM, Stekhova SA, Link JM, et al. Quantitative fluoroestradiol positron emission tomography imaging predicts response to endocrine treatment in breast cancer. J Clin Oncol. 2006;24:2793-9.
78. Mankoff DA, Link JM, Linden HM, Sundararajan L, Krohn KA. Tumor receptor imaging. J Nucl Med. 2008;49:49S-163S.
79. Chopra A. ^{89}Zr-Labeled trastuzumab, a humanized monoclonal antibody against epidermal growth factor receptor 2; Molecular Imaging and Contrast Agent Database (MICAD) [Internet]. Bethesda (MD): National Center for Biotechnology Information (US) 2004-2010, 2010.
80. Dijkers EC, Oude Munnink TH, Kosterink JG, Browers AH, Jager PL, de Jong JR, et al. Biodistribution of ^{89}Zrtrastuzumab and PET imaging of HER2-positive lesions in patients with metastatic breast cancer. Clin Pharmacol Ther. 2010;87:586-92.
81. Miao Z, Ren G, Jiang L, Liu H, Webster JM, Zhang R, et al. A novel 18F-labeled two-helix scaffold protein for PET imaging of HER2-positive tumor. Eur J Nucl Med Mol Imaging. 2011. *doi:10.1007/s00259-011-1879-9.*
82. Jansson T, Westlin JE, Ahlstrom H, Lilja A, Langstrom B, Bergh J. Positron emission tomography studies in patients with locally advanced and/or metastatic breast cancer: a method for early therapy evaluation? J Clin Oncol. 1995;13:1470-7.
83. Kenny L, Coombes RC, Vigushin DM, Al-Nahhas A, Shousha S, Aboagye EO. Imaging early changes in proliferation at 1 week post chemotherapy: a pilot study in breast cancer patients with 39-deoxy-39-[^{18}F]fluorothymidine positron emission tomography. Eur J Nucl Med Mol Imaging. 2007;34:1339-47.
84. Jain RK. Antiangiogenic therapy for cancer: current and emerging concepts. Oncology (Williston Park). 2005;19:7-16.
85. Hayes DF, Miller K, Sledge G. Angiogenesis as targeted breast cancer therapy. Breast. 2007;16:S17-9.
86. Wilson CBJH, Lammertsma AA, McKenzie CG, Sikora K, Jones T. Measurements of blood flow and exchanging water space in breast tumors using positron emission tomography: a rapid and non-invasive dynamic method. Cancer Res. 1992;52:1592-7.
87. Mankoff DA, Dunnwald LK, Gralow JR, et al. Changes in blood flow and metabolism in locally advanced breast cancer treated with neoadjuvant chemotherapy. J Nucl Med. 2003;44:1806-14.
88. Tseng J, Dunnwald LK, Schubert EK, et al. ^{18}F-FDG kinetics in locally advanced breast cancer: correlation with tumor blood flow and changes in response to neoadjuvant chemotherapy. J Nucl Med. 2004;45:1829-37.
89. Beer AJ, Haubner R, Sarbia M, et al. Positron emission tomography using [^{18}F]galacto-RGD identifies the level of integrin avb3 expression in man. Clin Cancer Res. 2006;12:3942-9.
90. Blankenberg F, Ohtsuki K, Strauss HW. Dying a thousand deaths: radionuclide imaging of apoptosis. QJ Nucl Med. 1999;43:170-6.

Index

Page numbers followed by *b* refer to box, *f* refer to figure, *fc* refer to flow chart, and *t* refer to table.

A

B

C

D

E

F

G

H

I

J

K

L

M

N

O

P

Q

R

T

U

V

W

X

Y

Z